DORLAND'S ILLUSTRATED MEDICAL DICTIONARY

32nd EDITION

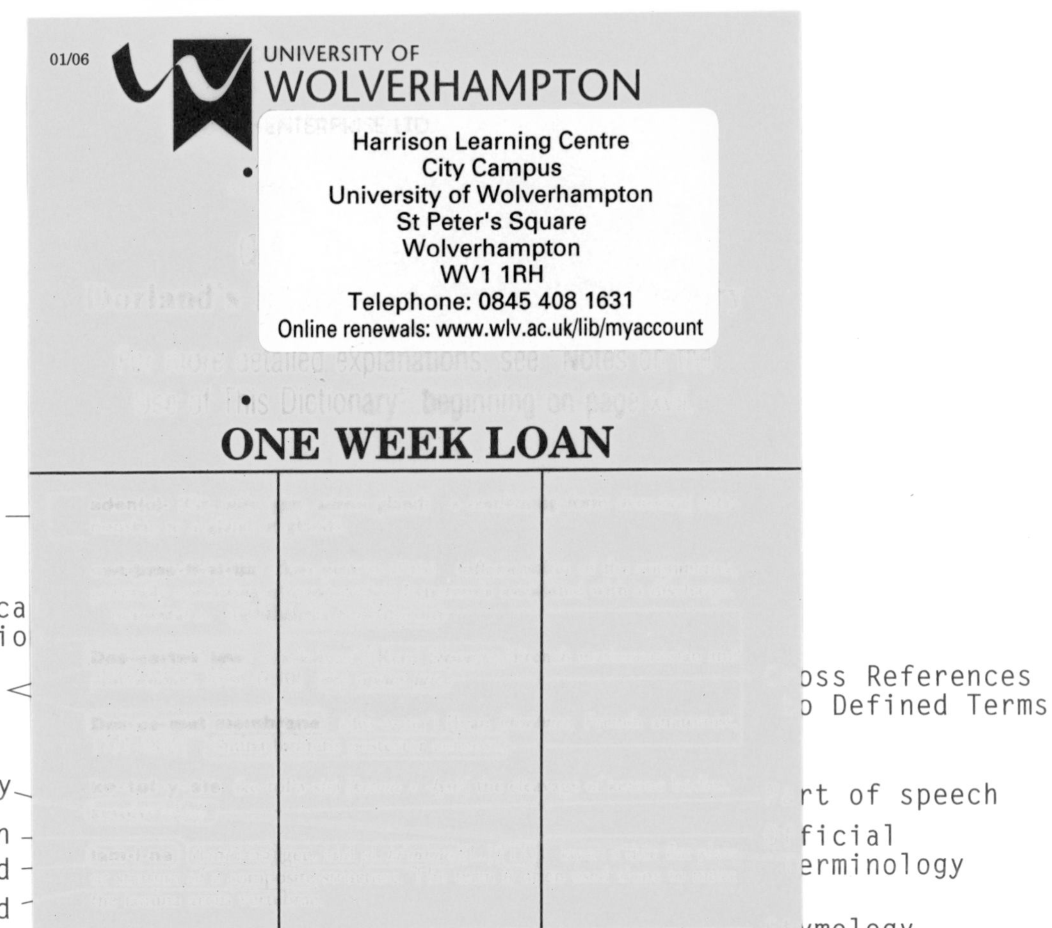

Combining Form

Biographica
Informatio

Eponyms

Run-on Entry

Pronunciation

Headword

Genitive and Plural

oss References
o Defined Terms

rt of speech

ficial
erminology

ymology

nonym

Abbreviations

SA sinoatrial

Main Entry — Plural

seg·men·tum (seg-menʹtəm) pl. *segmenʹta* [L.] [TA] segment: a part of an organ or other structure set off by natural or arbitrarily established boundaries.

Subentry — Definition

segmenʹta medulʹlae spinaʹlis [TA] segments of spinal cord: small sections of the spinal cord, to each of which is attached anterior and posterior roots of one of the 31 pairs of spinal nerves; there are 8 cervical, 12 thoracic, 5 lumbar, 5 sacral, and one or more coccygeal segments.

Subsubentry

segmenʹta cervicaʹlia [**1–8**] the eight cervical segments; in official terminology the term is considered an alternative to *pars cervicalis medullae spinalis* (q.v.).

Multiple Definitions

state (stāt) [L. *status*] 1. condition or situation; see also *status.* 2. the crisis, or the turning point of an attack of disease.

Cross Reference to Defined Terms

dreamy s. a state of altered consciousness lasting for a few minutes and accompanied by hallucinations; associated with temporal lobe lesions. See also *temporal lobe epilepsy*, under *epilepsy*, and *petit mal status*, under *status.*

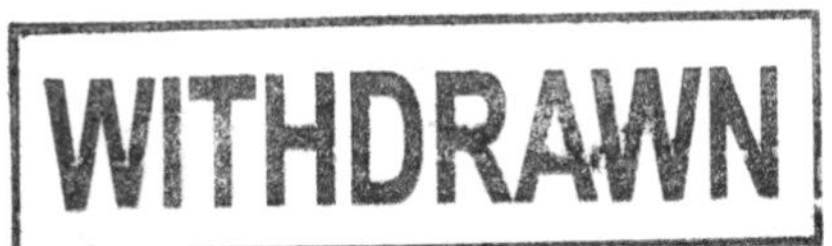

DORLAND'S ILLUSTRATED MEDICAL DICTIONARY

32nd EDITION

ELSEVIER
SAUNDERS

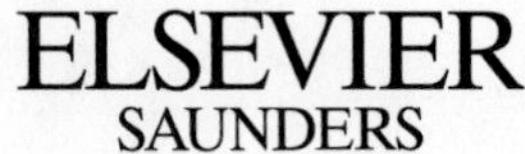

1600 John F. Kennedy Blvd.
Ste 1800
Philadelphia, PA 19103-2899

DORLAND'S ILLUSTRATED MEDICAL DICTIONARY
32nd edition

ISBN: 978-1-4160-6257-8 (Standard)
978-1-4160-6256-1 (Deluxe)
978-0-8089-2418-0 (International)

Notices

Knowledge and best practice in this field are constantly changing. As new research and experience broaden our understanding, changes in research methods, professional practices, or medical treatment may become necessary.
Practitioners and researchers must always rely on their own experience and knowledge in evaluating and using any information, methods, compounds, or experiments described herein. In using such information or methods they should be mindful of their own safety and the safety of others, including parties for whom they have a professional responsibility.
With respect to any drug or pharmaceutical products identified, readers are advised to check the most current information provided (i) on procedures featured or (ii) by the manufacturer of each product to be administered, to verify the recommended dose or formula, the method and duration of administration, and contraindications. It is the responsibility of practitioners, relying on their own experience and knowledge of their patients, to make diagnoses, to determine dosages and the best treatment for each individual patient, and to take all appropriate safety precautions.
To the fullest extent of the law, neither the Publisher nor the authors, contributors, or editors, assume any liability for any injury and/or damage to persons or property as a matter of products liability, negligence or otherwise, or from any use or operation of any methods, products, instructions, or ideas contained in the material herein.

Library of Congress Cataloging-in-Publication Data

ISBN: 978-1-4160-6257-8 (Standard)
978-1-4160-6256-1 (Deluxe)
978-0-8089-2418-0 (International)

Listed here are the latest translated editions of this book together with the languages for the translations and the publishers:

Chinese (*28th Edition*)—Xi'an World Publishing Corp., Xi'an, China
Indonesian (*26th Edition*)—E.G.C. Medical Publishers, Jakarta, Indonesia
Italian (*28th Edition*)—Edizioni Scientifiche Internazionali (ESI), Milan, Italy
Japanese (*28th Edition*)—Hirokawa Publishing Company, Tokyo, Japan
Portuguese (*28th Edition*)—Editiora Manole Ltda., São Paulo, Brazil
Spanish (*30th Edition*)—Elsevier España, S.A., Madrid, Spain

Chief Lexicographer: Douglas M. Anderson, MA
Senior Lexicographer: Patricia D. Novak, PhD
Lexicographer: Jefferson Keith, MA
Assistant Lexicographer: Michelle A. Elliott, MA
Publishing Services Manager: Patricia Tannian
Senior Project Manager: Linda Van Pelt
Design Direction: Steve Stave

Printed in the United States of America

Last digit is the print number: 9 8 7 6 5 4 3 2 1

CONSULTANTS

Daniel Albert, MD, MS
Retina Research Foundation
Emmett A. Humble Distinguished Director of the University of Wisconsin, Eye Research Institute
F.A. Davis Professor
Department of Ophthalmology and Visual Sciences
University of Wisconsin Medical School and Public Health
Madison, Wisconsin

Anne Marie Block, PhD, FACMG
Associate Professor of Oncology
Director, Clinical Cytogenetics Laboratory
Deparment of Pathology and Laboratory Medicine
Roswell Park Cancer Institute
Buffalo, New York

Beau Benjamin Bruce, MD
Fellow, Neuro-ophthalmology
Associate, Department of Ophthalmology
Emory University School of Medicine
Atlanta, Georgia

Duane E. Haines, PhD
Professor Emeritus of Surgery
Professor of Neurology
Professor of Neurosurgery
The University of Mississippi Medical Center
Jackson, Mississippi

Laura J. McCloskey, PhD
Assistant Professor of Pathology Anatomy, and Cell Biology
Jefferson Medical College of Thomas Jefferson University
Associate Director
Clinical Laboratories
Director, JHN, IC, Immunology, Specimen Processing, and Referral Testing
Jefferson University Hospital
Philadelphia, Pennsylvania

Richard N. Mitchell, MD
Lawrence J. Henderson Associate Professor of Pathology and Health Sciences and Technology
Harvard Medical School
Staff Pathologist, Department of Pathology
Brigham and Women's Hospital
Boston, Massachusetts

Keith Moore, PhD, FIAC, FRSM
Professor Emeritus, Division of Anatomy
Department of Surgery
Faculty of Medicine
Former Chair of Anatomy and Associate Dean for Basic Medical Sciences
Faculty of Medicine
University of Toronto
Toronto, Ontario, Canada

William Petri
Wade Hampton Frost Professor of Epidemiology
Professor of Medicine, Microbiology, and Pathology
Chief of the Division of Infectious Diseases and International Health
University of Virginia Health System
Charlottesville, Virginia

Alvin G. Telser, PhD
Associate Professor Emeritus
Department of Cell and Molecular Biology
Northwestern University
Feinberg School of Medicine
Chicago, Illinois

PREFACE

This new edition of *Dorland's Illustrated Medical Dictionary* carries on a tradition of excellence that stretches back for more than a century. Its nearly 124,000 entries are by far the largest number to be found in a single-volume medical dictionary. The entries are enhanced by 1525 illustrations, nearly all in full color, each chosen for its ability to clarify the description given in the definition. About 500 of our illustrations are new in this edition, keeping the dictionary fresh and up to date. We are confident that the 32nd edition will continue to provide its users with the same authoritativeness, comprehensiveness, and currency that they have come to expect from *Dorland's*.

In the creation of any dictionary, the demands of providing the fullest coverage possible must be balanced against the need to keep the size of the volume within reasonable limits. In this edition, we have adopted a space-saving feature familiar from standard English dictionaries, the use of run-on entries to give related parts of speech without definitions. These are confined to fairly colorless terms, such as adjectives meaning "pertaining to. . . ." This change has allowed us to decrease the size of the book somewhat while maintaining the coverage that *Dorland's* users have long been used to.

Dorland's also continues to include the familiar electronic resources. The accompanying CD-ROM contains supplementary appendices comprising a tabular listing of selected terms in anatomy and a listing of surgical equipment not covered in the main section of the dictionary, as well as audio phonetics for over 35,000 medical terms. The content of the A to Z section of the dictionary is also available at www.dorlands.com; access can be obtained using the PIN included inside the front cover of this book.

As in previous editions, we have relied on a number of works containing official and standard nomenclatures for guidance. For anatomy, we have used the *Terminologia Anatomica*, as approved by the Federative International Committee on Anatomical Terminology. In enzyme nomenclature, we have relied heavily on the Recommendations of the Nomenclature Committee of the International Union of Biochemistry and Molecular Biology on the Nomenclature and Classification of Enzymes. For prokaryotes, we have used the "Taxonomic Outline of the Archaea and Bacteria," by GM Garrity and JG Holt, in Volume 1 of *Bergey's Manual of Systemic Bacteriology*, 2nd edition, together with the descriptions that have been published to date. For viruses, we have relied on the Universal Virus Database of the International Committee on Taxonomy of Viruses (ICTVdB). Psychiatric terminology is based on the *Diagnostic and Statistical Manual of Mental Disorders*, 4th edition (DSM-IV), published by the American Psychiatric Association. Drugs are identified as being included in the *United States Pharmacopeia* or the *National Formulary*. Abbreviations included in this volume, both in the vocabulary and the "Selected Abbreviations" appendix, that appear in the "Do not use" lists of the Joint Commission (JHACO), both the official list and the potential inclusions, carry the notation "*(on the JCAHO 'Do Not Use' List)*." We gratefully acknowledge our indebtedness to the compilers, editors, and publishers of these works and we emphasize that any inaccuracies that may have arisen from our transcription or interpretation of this material are our sole responsibility.

As always, we are indebted to our consultants for their work in reviewing the vocabulary and for their invaluable expert guidance in selecting new material, deleting obsolete terms, and revising existing entries. We are also grateful to the many users who, over the years, have provided opinions, information, corrections, criticism, and innumerable suggestions, as well as their praise and support. To them we owe a debt of gratitude; their ongoing interest has helped to maintain *Dorland's* position as the most comprehensive and authoritative medical dictionary available.

DOUGLAS M. ANDERSON

Chief Lexicographer
Elsevier

CONTENTS

INDEX TO TABLES

INDEX TO PLATES

INDEX TO APPENDICES

NOTES ON THE USE OF THIS DICTIONARY

Main Entries and Subentries

Main entries appear in boldface type, with bullets indicating syllabication. Terms consisting of two or more words are ordinarily given as subentries under the noun, as is traditional in medical dictionaries; subentries are also set in boldface type, and each is set on a new line. Although this arrangement may be confusing at first to those accustomed to general dictionaries, it has the advantage of allowing related terms to be grouped together (for example, all the *lymphocyte* entries appear under the main entry *lymphocyte*).

According to this scheme, *Howell-Jolly bodies*, *ketone bodies*, and *pineal body* are all to be found under the main entry *body*, and *carotid pulse*, *dicrotic pulse*, and *paradoxical pulse* are to be found under the main entry *pulse*. It is important for the user to bear in mind that it is impossible to provide entries for every variation of every term, so that a phrase that is not found under one main entry should be sought under a synonymous main entry. For example, the same entity may be described as a disease or a syndrome (as *Fabry disease—Fabry syndrome*, which is to be found under *disease*). In such cases, the main entry should be consulted for references to synonymous terms under which the desired phrase may be found.

Example:

treatment... the management and care of a patient for the purpose of combating disease or disorder. See also under *care*, *maneuver*, *method*, *technique*, *test*, and *therapy*.

In subentries, the main entry word is represented only by the initial letter, e.g., *cogwheel r.* under *respiration*, unless it occurs in the plural form. Regular English plurals are represented by the initial letter followed by *'s*, as *b's* for *bones* under *bone*. Irregular plurals, such as *teeth* under *tooth*, and Latin plurals, such as *foramina* under *foramen*, are spelled out in full.

Chemical Compounds

Exceptions to the use of subentries are made for specific acids and for enzymes and enzyme deficiencies. Names of specific acids will be found as main entries under the first word of the name, for examples, *sulfuric acid* under *S*, as will enzyme names, for example, *acetyl-CoA carboxylase* under *A*. Enzyme deficiencies, when they occur as separate entries, will be found as main entries immediately following the entry for the enzyme in question, for examples, *carbamoyl phosphate synthetase deficiency* after *carbamoyl phosphate synthetase*.

Chemical compounds having a binary name will be found under the first word, so that *aluminum acetate*, *aluminum hydroxide*, and *aluminum sulfate* are all located under *aluminum*, and *ferric citrate* is found under *ferric*.

Drug Names

Drugs are to be found under the active moiety, if that is a main entry. For example, *prednisolone acetate*, *prednisolone hemisuccinate*, and *prednisolone sodium phosphate* all appear under *prednisolone*. If the active moiety is not itself a main entry then the entire drug name appears as a main entry, for example, *methadone hydrochloride* under *M*.

Syllabication

Acceptable word divisions are indicated for main entries by the use of bullets within the entry word; syllabication is based on pronunciation. Not all syllable breaks are given; for example, the separation of a single vowel from the beginning or end of a word is not allowed and is not shown. Likewise, single letters should not be separated from the word elements to which they belong in compound words. In many cases a word may be broken at places other than the ones indicated; for example, different pronunciations imply different sets of breaks, so that *melanocyte* could be divided *mel•a•no•cyte* or *me•lano•cyte*, depending on which syllable, the first or second, is stressed. In any case, breaks that could confuse a reader as to the meaning of a word are to be avoided.

Sequence of Entries

Main Entries

Main entries will be found alphabetized on the sequence of letters, regardless of spaces or hyphens that may occur between them. (Special rules govern terms that begin with proper names, which are mainly eponyms; see below.) Thus the following sequences will be found:

formboard	**heart**
form-class	**heartbeat**
forme	**heart block**
form-family	**heartburn**

Subentries

Subentries, like main entries, are alphabetized letter by letter. The main entry word, whether it is represented by the initial letter, the initial plus *'s*, or a spelled-out plural, is ignored in alphabetizing subentries, as are prepositions, conjunctions, and articles. Inflected forms, such as genitives and plurals of Latin words, are treated as if they were nominative singular. (For what is meant by "inflected forms," see "Presentation of Plurals and Other Inflections," p. xix.) The following forms, all from *os craniale* "cranial bone," are considered equivalent for purposes of alphabetization: *os craniale*, *ossis cranialis*, *ossa cranialia*, and *ossium cranialium*.

In accordance with the above rules, the following sequences of subentries are found under *ganglion* and *prolapse*:

ganglion	**prolapse**
Andersch ganglia	anal p.
ganglia aorticorenalia	p. of anus
auditory g.	p. of cord
Auerbach g.	frank p.
g. autonomicum	p. of iris

A special case is that of what may be called inverted subentries, in which the initial word or words are moved to the end of the entry, set off by a comma. This is done in order to allow related terms to fall together in the subentry list; such inversions are especially common in the anatomical vocabulary for anterior/posterior structures and the like. These terms are alphabetized as usual up to the comma marking the inversion; words following the comma, however, are not counted except within the group of repeated entries:

lobe
inferior l., left
inferior l., right
inferior l. of left lung
inferior l. of right lung

Proper Names

A number of main entries are included for terms beginning with a proper name, usually eponymic terms; these give information about the term's origin (most often a bit of biographical information) and cross-references to entries where definitions may be found. These cross-references can be helpful in giving an indication of where to look for an entry that may go by more than one name (such as disease or syndrome). Entries of this sort are alphabetized as entries for the proper name only, following this set of rules:

(1) The *'s*, if one occurs, is never counted for alphabetization. *Jackson's law*, *Jackson membrane*, *Jackson safety triangle*, *jacksonian* appear in that order.
(2) Words following the name are not counted for alphabetical order unless the names are the same. Thus, *Addison disease* precedes *Addison planes*.
(3) Only the first name in a term containing more than one proper name is counted for alphabetization unless the entries are the same in all other respects. *Babinski reflex*, *Babinski-Frohlich syndrome*, *Babinski-Nageotte syndrome*, *Babinski-Vaquez syndrome* appear in that order.
(4) Umlauts (*ö*, *ü*) are ignored for purposes of alphabetization. *Löwe ring*, *Lowe syndrome*, *Lowe-Terry-MacLachlan syndrome*, *Löwenberg canal*, *Löwenthal tract*, *Lower rings* appear in that order.
(5) Names beginning *Mac* or *Mc* are alphabetized as if spelled *Mac*.

Subentries that begin with a proper name also follow the above rules for sequencing.

Proper nouns (or capitalized entries) appear before common nouns (or lower case entries). Thus *Bacillus* precedes *bacillus*.

Chemical Terms

In the alphabetization of chemical names, italic prefixes (e.g., *o*-, *p*-, *m*-, *trans*-, *cis*-) are ignored, as are numbers, Greek letters, and the prefixes D-, L-, *d*-, *l*-, (+)-, and (−)-. When a prefix is spelled out, however, the term is to be found under the fully spelled out form, for example, *levodopa* under *L*, *orthocresol* under *O*, and *beta-naphtholsulfonic acid* under *B*.

Indication of Pronunciation

A phonetic spelling of a term appears in parentheses after the boldface entry word. The pronunciation is given for all main entries; it is generally not given for subentries but does appear in some subentries that are foreign phrases. As a rule, the most common pronunciation is given, with no effort to list the variants, although exceptions to this do occur. The phonetic spelling is kept as simple as possible, with few diacritical marks; the only special character used is ə, the schwa, used to represent the unstressed vowel sound heard at the end of *sofa*. The schwa is also used in combination with *r* in unstressed syllables to represent the sound heard in the second syllable of *sulfur* or *other*.

There are four basic rules:

(1) An unmarked vowel ending a syllable (an "open" syllable) is long. Thus *ma* represents the pronunciation of *may*.
(2) An unmarked vowel in a syllable ending in a consonant (a "closed" syllable) is short. Thus *not* represents the pronunciation of *knot*.
(3) A long vowel in a closed syllable is indicated by a macron. Thus *māt* represents the pronunciation of *mate*.
(4) A short vowel that ends or itself constitutes a syllable is indicated by a breve. Thus *ĭ-mūn'* represents the pronunciation of *immune*.

Primary (') and secondary (") stresses are shown in polysyllabic words, with unstressed syllables followed by hyphens, as in *rep"lĭ-kā'shən*. Monosyllables have no stress mark unless they are part of a compound term, in which case each word is given a stress mark for clarity. Thus, *broun* is used to represent *brown*, but *den'is broun'* is used for *Denis Browne splint*. Primary stresses are also given as part of the boldface subentries for foreign phrases. However, even in compound terms, stresses are omitted from prepositions, conjunctions, and other similar small words.

It is impossible with *Dorland's* simplified phonetics to represent the native pronunciations of many foreign words and proper names. These are shown as closely as possible in English phonetics.

Pronunciation Guide

Vowels

(For the use of breves and macrons, see the four rules above.)

ə	sof*a*	ŏ	g*o*t
ā	m*a*te	ū	f*u*el
ă	b*a*t	ŭ	b*u*t
ē	b*ea*m	aw	*a*ll
ĕ	m*e*t	oi	b*oi*l
ī	b*i*te	o͞o	b*oo*m
ĭ	b*i*t	o͝o	b*oo*k
ō	h*o*me	ou	f*ow*l

Consonants

b	*b*ook	s	*s*igh
d	*d*og	t	*t*in
f	*f*og	w	*w*ood
g	*g*et	z	size, pha*s*e
h	*h*eat	ch	*ch*in
j	*j*ewel, *g*em	ks	si*x*
k	*c*art, pi*ck*	kw	*qu*ote
l	*l*ook	ng	si*ng*
m	*m*ouse	sh	*sh*ould
n	*n*ew	th	*th*in, *th*an
p	*p*ark	zh	mea*s*ure
r	*r*at		

Presentation of Plurals and Other Inflections

In main entries for foreign (nearly always Greek or Latin) nouns, the original and anglicized plurals are given after the phonetic spelling; irregular plurals of English nouns are also given.

Example:

sto·ma (sto′mə) pl. *stomas, sto′mata*...
tooth (tooth) pl. *teeth*...

The original foreign plural is often given a separate boldface listing in its proper alphabetical place in the vocabulary.

Example:

sto·ma·ta (sto′mə-tə) [Gr.] plural of *stoma*.

Latin is used, especially in anatomy, to form phrases of the type "the X of Y," for example, *arcus aortae*, "the arch of the aorta." The prepositional phrase introduced by "of" corresponds to the Latin genitive case (*aortae* "of the aorta," from *aorta*). For this reason, the genitive case (= English "of") for Latin nouns is also frequently given, introduced by the abbreviation *gen*.

Examples:

pa·pil·la...gen. and pl. *papil′lae*...
os[1]...gen. *o′ris*, pl. *o′ra*...
os[2]...gen. *os′sis*, pl. *os′sa*...

Latin and Greek (and a number of other languages, such as German and Russian, for that matter) are said to be inflected, that is, words change form to show how they are related to other words in a sentence. An example of this is the "aortae" phrase given above, where the change in the ending of the word corresponds to the use of the English preposition "of." Other Latin inflected forms are found in subentries; these forms will be the objects in a prepositional phrase. For example, under the main entry *fissura*, there is the subentry *f. in ano*; *ano* is the object of the preposition *in* and is one of the half-dozen or so different inflected forms of *anus*, which is a main entry in the Dictionary and has listed with it the genitive and plural form *ani*. As in all subentries, differences in singular and plural forms do not count for alphabetizing, nor do prepositions or conjunctions (e.g., *et* "and," *in* "in"); thus under the main entry *fissura*, the subentry *f. in ano* precedes *f. ansoparamedianis cerebelli*.

Etymology

Information on the origin of a word appears in brackets after the phonetic spelling or a plural form of the entry when that is given. The information is necessarily brief, and the reader must often reason from the etymon, the original word from which other words are derived, to the meaning. For example, for the main entry *dualism* the etymological section reads [L. *duo* two]. L. stands for Latin (languages are either abbreviated or spelled out; see "Abbreviations Used in This Dictionary," p. xxi). The word *duo* is the etymon, and "two" is the English translation of the etymon, not of the entry. The reader proceeds from *duo* to *dual* to *dualism*. Furthermore, space limitations preclude the listing of all the stages in the passage from the etymon to the modern derivative (i.e., the entry). For example, the etymological part of the entry for *vein* is simply [L. *vena*]; in full, it would be [Middle English *veine*, from Old Fr., from L. *vena*].

For those foreign words or phrases taken into English entire, only the language is given, with a translation given within quotation marks.

Example:

déjà vu [Fr. "already seen"]...

If the meaning of the foreign word or phrase is the same as that of the entry word, no translation is given.

There are three further additions:

(1) Many technical terms of Greek or Latin derivation are listed twice as main entries (and both times with meaning and cross-references), first as an independent word (with an etymology), then as a combining form (without an etymology), e.g., *ectomy* and *-ectomy*.

(2) There is an essay, "Fundamentals of Medical Etymology" (see p. xxiii), which explains the basic rules for the derivation and composition of Greek, Latin, and Greco-Latin terms in medicine. Appendix 1 is an analytical word list of Greek and Latin roots, prefixes, and combining forms; the list is an aid for the analysis of existing medical terms and the creation of new ones.

(3) The prefixes (e.g., *hyper-*, *hypo-*), suffixes (e.g., *-ia*, *-oid*), and combining forms (e.g., *action-*, *-emia*) from the analytical word list are also listed as main entries in the vocabulary.

Official Publications

Certain terms listed in official publications are identified by an abbreviation in brackets. In main entries, these abbreviations usually appear after the etymology (or after the phonetic spelling if no etymology is given). In subentries, they appear immediately after the boldface subentry word. When a term has more than one meaning, the abbreviation is placed at the beginning of the definition to which it applies. The following abbreviations are used:

[DSM-IV]	*Diagnostic and Statistical Manual of Mental Disorders* of the American Psychiatric Association, 4th Edition, 1994
[EC]	Enzyme Commission number (e.g., citrate (*si*)-synthase...[EC 2.3.3.1]) from the Recommendations of the Nomenclature Committee of the International Union of Biochemistry and Molecular Biology on the Nomenclature and Classification of Enzymes published in *Enzyme Nomenclature* (1992), with updates published electronically at http://www.chem.qmul.ac.uk/iubmb/enzyme/
[TA]	*Terminologia Anatomica* (1998)
[NF]	*The National Formulary*, 24th edition (2006)
[USP]	*The United States Pharmacopeia*, 29th edition (2006)

Placement of Definitions and Cross-References

With few exceptions, a definition is given in only one place for two or more synonymous terms. Entries for the synonyms provide cross-references to the term where the definition is to be found. Such cross-references are in place of a definition and are set in roman type:

mas·to·plas·ty (mas′to-plas″te) mammaplasty.

The definition will be found at *mammaplasty*. In many cases, a list of synonyms is given at the end of the entry where the definition appears. This list is introduced by the phrase "called also" and the synonyms are set in italic type.

Cross-references from one subentry to another subentry under the same main heading use the abbreviated form of the main entry:

syndrome
  hypersomnia-bulimia s. Kleine-Levin s.

Cross-referencing has also been used for earlier terms that have been supplanted and for variant spellings of a term. In such instances, the definition is attached to the term that is currently the preferred term. A word of warning is, however, warranted here. In some instances, preference for one term over another may be slight or even nonexistent, while in others, different spellings or terms may be preferred by different authorities, by different specialties, or in different regions. In such cases, the practice of defining words only at one place has been adhered to as a means of keeping down the size of the Dictionary by avoiding duplication of definitions, and the user should remember that the appearance of a cross-reference or definition does not always indicate a preference for one form or synonym over another.

Related Entries

Cross-references to related entries or to entries where additional information may be found are also given. They are identified by "see also," "cf.," and "q.v." (or "qq. v."). (For the abbreviations, see "Abbreviations Used in This Dictionary," p. xxi.) Cross-references introduced by "see also" or "cf." are set in italic type.

Run-On Entries

As a space-saving device, one or more undefined forms (usually adjectives) related to the main entry may occur at the end of the main entry definition. Their meaning is basically the same as that of the main entry, but they have different grammatical functions. They are set in bold type and given a stress mark, and they are followed by a part-of-speech label. Alternative forms with the same part of speech are separated by commas, with a single part-of-speech label following.

Example:

adac·ty·ly...a developmental anomaly characterized by the absence of digits on the hand or foot. **adac′tylous** *adj*

Official Terminology

In general, when a term is included in one of the official publications listed in the preceding section ("Official Publications"), its definition appears at the official term. Thus the definition for "pelvic bone" is found at *os coxae*; a cross-reference to the official term is found at the subentry under *bone*. Exceptions have been made in a few cases where the nonofficial term is so common or important that it makes the most sense to put the definition on the unofficial term (for example, *heart* is defined, not *cor*).

Entries Containing a Proper Name

Entries containing a proper name are generally entered twice. The definition for the entity is given in a subentry under the appropriate main entry, as *Down syndrome* under *syndrome*. Biographical, geographical, or other information attached to the proper name is given in a main entry (see "Proper Names" in the section "Sequence of Entries," p. xviii.) A cross-reference is given from the main entry for the proper name to the subentry where the term is defined. For example:

Down syndrome (disease) (doun) [John Langdon Haydon *Down*, English physician, 1828–1896] see under *syndrome*.

Form of Eponyms

The tendency in recent years has been to drop the *'s* from medical eponyms and to use the nonpossessive form of the personal name. Although this tendency is far from universal and the possessive is still commonly found, it was decided after much debate that for the sake of consistency the *'s* would be omitted from eponymic entries for the 31st edition of *Dorland's*. Exceptions were made for a very few categories (such as the entries for *law*) where there is a large amount of nonmedical terminology and the possessive is still the rule in general use. This decision should by no means, however, be taken as a proscription of the possessive eponym, and whether or not to use the possessive is very much a matter of individual preference. The user should be aware that some terms, such as *Apgar score*, have never had an *'s* and that for some terms, such as *Christmas disease* and *Down syndrome*, the nonpossessive form is always preferred. On the other hand, use of the eponym by itself to stand for the entity, as in the common phrase "living with Alzheimer's," requires the possessive form; "living with Alzheimer" has an entirely different meaning.

Symbols and Abbreviations

Symbols, abbreviations, and acronyms are included as main entries; definitions consist of the term for which the symbol or the abbreviation stands, with a translation if the term is in a foreign language. These terms will usually be found at the appropriate places in the vocabulary; some terms, however, are self-explanatory and have no entry, such as the names of organizations and phrases like the following:

q.h. [L.] *qua'que ho'ra* (every hour).

In a few cases, the definition is placed at the abbreviation or acronym instead of at the term for which it stands, for example, *ELISA*; in such cases, the abbreviation, not the term, is what is actually in use.

Abbreviations appear both with and without periods. This should not be taken to denote proper usage, since abbreviations may appear either way; at the present the trend is away from the use of the period for most abbreviations.

A list of selected abbreviations also appears in Appendix 2.

Abbreviations Used in This Dictionary

a.	artery (L. *arteria*); agar
aa.	arteries (L. *arteriae*)
ant.	anterior
Ar.	Arabic
A.S.	Anglo-Saxon
c.	about (L. *circa*)
cf.	compare (L. *confer*)
def.	definition
dim.	diminutive
EC	Enzyme Commission
e.g.	for example (L. *exempli gratia*)
Fr.	French
gen.	genitive
Ger.	German
Gr.	Greek
i.e.	that is (L. *id est*)
inf.	inferior
It.	Italian
L.	Latin
l.	ligament (L. *ligamentum*)
lat.	lateral
ligg.	ligaments (L. *ligamenta*)
m.	muscle (L. *musculus*)
med.	medial; median
mm.	muscles (L. *musculi*)
n.	nerve (L. *nervus*)
neg.	negative
NF	National Formulary
nn.	nerves (L. *nervi*)
obs.	obsolete
pl.	plural
Port.	Portuguese
post.	posterior
qq. v.	which (things) see (L. *quae vide*)
q.v.	which see (L. *quod vide*)
sing.	singular
Sp.	Spanish
sup.	superior
TA	Terminologia Anatomica
USAN	United States Adopted Names
USP	United States Pharmacopeia
v.	vein (L. *vena*)
vv.	veins (L. *venae*)

FUNDAMENTALS OF MEDICAL ETYMOLOGY

By Joseph M. Patwell, PhD

Twenty-six hundred years ago the Asiatic Greeks of Ionia and the Italian Greeks in Magna Graecia began the speculative and investigational sciences, pushing the then Greek to its limits, pushing beyond those limits, riveting new meanings onto old words, smithing new words for new ideas and discoveries—*philosophia*, "the love of wisdom," was supposedly first used by Pythagoras.

The sciences still go their robust way, iconoclastic but also indebted to and respectful of their ancient tradition. In anatomy, surgery, clinical medicine, and laboratory medicine, Greek, Latin, and Greco-Latin have always formed well over ninety per cent of the technical terms. Knowing the fundamentals of Greek and Latin word formation is immensely helpful in learning the vocabulary of modern medicine or of any modern science and is absolutely necessary for anyone coining a word for a new hypothesis, theory, process, or entity. The purpose of this introduction is to present those fundamentals in as practical and concise a form as possible; any statements contrary to historical and comparative linguistic fact that are made in the following pages are deliberate in keeping with this purpose.

Alphabet and Pronunciation

The Latin alphabet is a modification of one of the many Greek alphabets. The order and shape of the Latin letters are the same as in ours except that the Classical Latin alphabet has no *j*, *u*, or *w*, which are improvements dating from the Middle Ages.

The consonants of the Latin alphabet have about the same values as the English except that *c*, *ch*, *g*, *s*, *t*, and *v* are pronounced as in *c*old, *ch*rome, *g*et, *s*o, *t*in, and *w*ine, and not as in *c*ent, *ch*ill, *g*em, ro*s*e, men*t*ion, and *v*ine. *Ph* and *th* may be pronounced as in *ph*ilosophy and *th*eology.

Latin vowels may be long or short. The short vowels are pronounced very much like the American w*a*nder, b*e*d, *i*t, h*o*pe, and p*u*t; short *y* sounds like the *ü* in German *dünn*. The long vowels are pronounced as in f*a*ther, h*e*y, mar*i*ne, st*o*ve, and r*u*de; long *y* is pronounced like the *ü* in the German *über*.

Words are stressed on the next-to-last syllable, called the penult, if that syllable contains a long vowel or diphthong or is followed by two or more consonants, otherwise on the syllable before the penult.

The Greek alphabet used today is based on that used in Athens by the end of the fifth century BCE. The accompanying table shows one modern English pronunciation of each ancient Greek character in terms of English.

Capital	Small Letter	Sound	Name	Transcription
Α	α	f*a*ther	alpha	a
Β	β	*b*arbarism	beta	b
Γ	γ	*g*rammar	gamma	g
Δ	δ	*d*iet	delta	d
Ε	ε	*e*lephant	epsilon	e
Ζ	ζ	*z*oology	zeta	z
Η	η	r*a*bies	eta	ē
Θ	θ, ϑ	*th*eory	theta	th
Ι	ι	mach*i*ne	iota	i
Κ	κ	s*k*eleton	kappa	k or c (Latin)
Λ	λ	*l*ithograph	lambda	l
Μ	μ	*m*usic	mu	m
Ν	ν	*n*eolithic	nu	n
Ξ	ξ	e*x*egesis	xi	x
Ο	ο	*o*belisk	omicron	o
Π	π	s*p*asm	pi	p
Ρ	ρ	a*r*achnid	rho	r
Σ	σ, ς	*s*ymbol	sigma	s
Τ	τ	s*t*adium	tau	t
Υ	υ	*ü*, *ü*ber (German)	upsilon	y
Φ	φ	*ph*oto	phi	ph
Χ	χ	Ba*ch* (German)	chi	ch
Ψ	ψ	di*ps*omania	psi	ps
Ω	ω	*o*cher, Sh*aw*	omega	ō

The vowels are α, ε, η, ι, ο, υ, ω, most of which may be followed by ι or υ to form diphthongs, the most common of which are shown below.

Diphthong	Sound	Transcription
αι	*ai*sle	ae, e, or ai
αυ	*ou*t	au
ει	*ei*ght	i or ei
ευ	*eu*phony	eu
οι	po*i*son	oe, e, or oi
ου	gh*ou*l	ou or u
υι	s*ui*te	ui

Transliteration

The Romans transliterated kappa with *c*, not *k*, and chi with *ch*, not *kh*; thus *ch*ara*c*ter, not *kh*ara*k*ter. This Dictionary transliterates kappa with *k* in its etymologies in order to make immediately clear the nature of the underlying Greek sound: Spelling *cystis* for *kystis*, cyst, could cause doubt whether the sound was "kystis" or "systis." Similar difficulties with chi are less likely, and therefore *Dorland's* retains the traditional *ch*; hence our etymological spelling is *charakter*.

Classical Greek ει was pronounced as in *skein*, but by the end of the fourth century BCE it was pronounced as in *seize;* thus the city that Alexander the Great founded in Egypt, *Alexandreia*, became Alexandria in Latin. English generally prefers the Latin transliteration, but the use of *ei* for ει is growing. This Dictionary transliterates ει with *ei* in its etymologies.

The Romans transliterated Greek αι and οι with their own *ae* and *oe*, which had nearly the same pronunciation. By late antiquity the Greek and Latin diphthongs had become simple vowels, having gone through the regular progression *ai*sle to *ai*r to *ai*m, and the spelling wavered between the old diphthongs and the new pronunciation. This vacillation persists in English: the British prefer the diphthongs (*oe*dema, h*ae*morrhage); the Americans, the simple vowel (*e*dema, h*e*morrhage). In the etymologies of this Dictionary Greek αι and οι are transliterated by *ai* and *oi*, and Latin *ae* and *oe* retained, for clarity's sake.

The Greeks especially but also the Romans had the same troubles with aitch (*h*) that Cockneys do, dropping it where it belonged and adding it where it did not. In Greek, initial *h-* ordinarily remained in simple words (*haima*, blood) but would either assimilate with or disappear before a prefix. For assimilation, *hypo* and *haima* make *hyphaimos*, suffused with blood (first appearing in Hippocrates); for disappearance, *a-*, *an-*, and *haima* make *anaimia*, anemia (first appearing in Aristotle), not *ahaimia* and *ahemia*.

Latin usually preserved initial *h-* even after prefixes *(Homo habilis, habilitas, inhabilitas; honor, honestus, inhonestus)*, but very much of our Latin has come through French with inconsistent (to say the least) spellings and pronunciations: *able*, *ability*, and *inability*, not *hable*, *hability*, and *inhability*; *honor* and *honest*, not *onor* and *onest*.

Speakers of American English generally have no difficulty with *h-* and treat it as a full consonant when adding prefixes; thus we have *inharmonious*, not *anarmonious*; *ahaptoglobinemia*, not *anaptoglobinemia*; and *anhydride*, not *anydride* or *ahydride*.

Greek words are written with several accents (´ ` ˆ) that now indicate the stressed syllable. Words beginning with a vowel, diphthong, or rho (ρ) are written with a so-called breathing mark over the initial vowel or rho or over the second element of the diphthong (ἑτεροδοξία, *heterodoxia;* αἰσθητικός, *aisthētikos*; ῥυθμός, *rhythmos*). The *rough* breathing mark (ʽ) indicates that the syllable begins with an aspiration (aitch) as in *heterodoxia*, above, and words beginning with the rough breathing are usually transcribed into English with an initial *h*. Words beginning with a rho or an upsilon always have a rough breathing (ὑπέρ, *hyper;* ῥεῦμα, *rheuma)*. The smooth breathing (ʼ) shows the absence of aspiration and so has no effect on pronunciation (ἀρωματικός, *arōmatikos;* αὐτογράφος, *autographos*).

The other conventions for transliterations from Greek are as follows: Gamma (γ), which before gamma (γ), kappa (κ), chi (χ), or xi (ξ) has the sound of *n* as in *finger*, is transcribed as *n.** Initial rho and its rough breathing (ῥ) are transcribed as *rh*, not *hr*, as *rheuma*, above; double rho (ρρ) is transcribed as *rrh* (διάρροια, *diarrhoea*, *diarrhea*). Upsilon (υ) is transcribed as *y* (ῥυθμός, *rhythmos*) except in diphthongs, where it is reproduced by *u* (ῥεῦμα, *rheuma*).

A few Greek words have come into English unchanged (σκελετόν, skeleton; αυτόματον, automaton); most Greek words have passed into English through Latin, undergoing slight change (Greek στέρνον, *sternon*; Latin *sternum*); and some Greek words have passed through a secondary intermediary language, such as French, with still further change (Greek χειρουργία, *cheirourgia*; Latin *chirurgia*; French *cirurgerie*; English *surgery*). Other changes are accounted for by our tendency to drop Greek and Latin inflectional endings (ἀξίωμα, *axioma*, becomes axiom; *dorsalis* becomes dorsal) or replace them with a final mute *e* as if the words have come into English through French (γονοφόρος, *gonophoros*, becomes gonophore; *spina* becomes spine).

Word Formation

The most frequent, the most important, and the seemingly most capricious changes in Greek or Latin words (or in English words, for that matter) arise not when the words pass from Greek or Latin into English, but when these words are first formed in the original language.

Many words in English and nearly all words in the Classical languages are combinations of roots and affixes. The root of a word contains the basic, lexical meaning, and the affixes give the root its shape as a word. (Affixes for the most part are prefixes and suffixes, including the inflections, added before or after the root, respectively.)

For example, in the English *love, loves, lover, lovers, loving, loved, lovingly, unloved*, and *unlovable*, the root is *love*, and the various prefixes (*un-*) and suffixes (*-s*, *-r*, *-r-s*, *-ing*, *-ingly*, etc.) form the root into a word and modify that word for use in an utterance.

In English a root may very often function as an independent word, as *love, hate, smile, frown, milk;* these "root words" are extremely rare in the Classical languages. Nearly always in Latin and Greek, and usually in English, a word is a complex consisting of a form of a root and one or more affixes, which are not independent words themselves but may be used only to modify the root in some way (as *un-*, *-er*, *-ed*); such words are called "derived words."

When the root remains unchanged from derived word to derived word (a "regular" or "weak" root) and the affixes remain unaffected in their surroundings, the entire system of derived words has a transparent, instantly comprehended simplicity, as in *love* and its forms. So in Latin and Greek: there is a systematic clarity to derivations of the Latin root *laud-* (praise)—the nouns *laudis* and *laudatory* (praise, praiser); the principal parts of the regular verb, *laudo* (I praise), *laudare* (to praise); and the adjectives *laudabilis* and *laudatorius* (laudable, laudatory). There is also a regular system in the Greek root *pau-* (stop): the nouns

*During World War II, *Ancistrodon* (from ἄγκιστρον, fishhook, and ὀδοντ-, tooth) was reformed to *Agkistrodon*, which is the official spelling. *Ancistrodon* and *Ankistrodon* are both correct, but not *Agkistrodon*: Greek ἄγγελος (messenger) becomes *angelus* in Latin and *angel* in English, not *aggelus* and *aggel*.

pausis (pause) and *paustēr* (reliever, calmer); the regular principal parts of the verb *pauō* (I stop), *pausō* (I shall stop); and the adjectives *pausteōn* (to be ended) and *paustērios* (relieving, calming).

Difficulties arise in English, Latin, and Greek with roots that change from word to word ("irregular" or "strong" roots) as in the English *sing, sang, sung, song;* and one says *singer,* not *songer; unsung,* not *unsing;* and *unsingable,* not *unsungable*. One example will suffice. The root *ten-* (stretch) appears in Latin and Greek (and also in English in *thin*). In Latin the root is as regular as the English *talk,* and the derivations are obvious: *tendo* (tendon), *ten*sio (tension), *ten*ius (tenuous, thin), ex*ten*uatus (stretched out, thinned out, weakened). In Greek, however, the same root appears as *ten-, tein-, ton-, ta-, tan-*, and *tain-*. Indeed, the rules for ancient Greek word formation would make a heavy book, and therefore, for efficiency's sake, the list of prefixes, suffixes, and combining forms (Appendix 1, p. 2101) gives examples of which affixes are attached to which forms of the root, for both the methodical Latin and the exuberant Greek.

In the Latin system there is an inconsistency affecting many common Latin and therefore English words: Latin roots with short vowels will have the normal, strong vowel in simple, unprefixed words but a reduced, weakened vowel in prefixed words.

Consider the Latin root *făc-* (do, make). The normal *ă* remains in unprefixed words; hence the principal parts of the verb are:

făcio	I make
făcere	to make
făctus	made

Other unprefixed derivatives are:

facies	thing made or formed, face, "facies"
factor	factor
factura	as in manu*facture*
faction-	faction
factiosus	factious
facil-	doable, feasible, easy

From *facil-* are derived in turn:

facultat-	faculty
facilitat-	facility

Now let us add the prefix *ex* to the root *fac-*. *Ex* assimilates to *ef-* before *f* and changes the meaning of *fac-* to "complete." This or any prefix will cause a short *ă* to become a short *ĭ* before one consonant and a short *ĕ* before two consonants. Note the changes in the principal parts of the prefixed verb:

efficio	from	*exfacio*
efficere	from	*exfacere*
effectus	from	*exfactus*

It is from words like *efficio* that one can most clearly understand the derivations of Latin words. One forms the present participle by dropping the final *-re* from the present active infinitive, which is the form used in the etymologies of *Dorland's*, and adding *-nt* (verbs like *efficio* drop the final *-ere* and add *-ient*). The present participle of *efficio, efficere* is *efficient-* (efficient). And from the present participle is derived the noun *efficientia* (efficiency).

From the last principal part, *effectus*, one forms derivatives by dropping the *-us* and adding other suffixes. Thus from *effect-* one derives

effectum	effect
effector	effector
effectivus	effective

Occasionally the Romans would recompose a prefixed form according to the unprefixed norm. The most common example, and perfect for medical use, is *calefacio*, I warm, not *caleficio*, and therefore *calefacient-*, not *caleficient-*.

Alas, there are exceptions. *Tenant* comes to English not directly from the Latin *tenēre*, to hold, which would give us *tenent*, but through the French *tenir*, and in French all verbs form their present participles in *-ant*, therefore *tenant*; a *locum tenens* is a *lieu tenant*.

Assimilation may affect the consonants between roots and affixes. In English the *v* in dri*v*e and thri*v*e becomes voiceless and changes to *f* before the voiceless suffix *-t* that forms the nouns *drift* and *thrift*. In Latin, assimilation is usually minimal and obvious: *scribo* ("I write") and *scriba* ("writer, scribe") alternate with *scripsi* ("I wrote") and *scriptura* ("writing, scripture"). Occasionally the assimilation between Latin roots, prefixes, and suffixes may cause enough distortion to result in confusion. Below are listed some common Latin prefixes (most of them are also used as prepositions) showing the assimilation of the prefix to the following element. Note that the prefix *in-* has two sources and hence two uses: as a spatial prefix meaning *in*, *on*, or *into* (*in*scribe, *im*bibe, *il*luminate, *ir*radiate) and the antonymous prefix (*in*sensitive, *im*mature, *il*legible, *ir*reverent).

Consonant Changes		English
ad-	before *c* becomes *ac-*	*ac*celerate
ad-	before *f* becomes *af-*	*af*finity
ad-	before *g* becomes *ag-*	*ag*glutinant
ad-	before *p* becomes *ap-*	*ap*pendix
ad-	before *s* becomes *as-*	*as*similate
ad-	before *t* becomes *at-*	*at*trition
ex-	before *f* becomes *ef-*	*ef*fusion
in-	before *l* becomes *il-*	*il*linition
in-	before *m* becomes *im-*	*im*mersion
in-	before *r* becomes *ir-*	*ir*radiation
ob-	before *c* becomes *oc-*	*oc*clusion
sub-	before *f* becomes *suf-*	*suf*focate
sub-	before *p* becomes *sup-*	*sup*pository
trans-	before *s* becomes *tran-*	*tran*spiration

In Greek, assimilation may cause drastic changes to a word, and the phonetic laws governing these assimilations are far beyond the limits of this Dictionary. Fortunately, however, Greek prefixes are fairly regular. Like Latin prefixes, they may also function as prepositions of motion or location. Most Greek prefixes end in a vowel, which is maintained when the following element begins with a consonant and is lost (elided) when that element begins with a vowel: for example, the iota in *epi* ("on, upon") is unchanged in *epi*demic and is elided before *o* in *ep*onychium ("cuticle"). When a Greek prefix ends in a consonant and the following element begins with a consonant, assimilation takes place with results as in Latin: the nu (*n*) of *syn* ("with") changes in *symphatheia* and *syllogismos* (sympathy and syllogism). Note that the prevocalic prefix *an-* has two sources and therefore two uses: it is the spatial preposition *ana* ("up, back"), as in *ana*bolism and *an*ode; and it is the antonymous prefix *a-*, *an-*, as in *a*theist and *an*odyne, coming from the same source as Latin and English antonymous prefixes *in-* and *un-*.

Below are listed some common Greek prefixes with examples of elision and assimilation.

Preposition	Combining Forms	English
amphi	amphi-	*amphi*crania
	amph-	*amph*eclexis
ana	ana-	*ana*bolism
	an-	*an*ode
anti	anti-	*anti*gen
	ant-	*ant*helminthic
apo	apo-	*apo*physis
	ap-	*ap*andria
dia	dia-	*dia*thermy
	di-	*di*uretic
ek	ek-	*ec*topia
ex	ex-	*ex*osmosis
en	en-	*en*ostosis
	em-	*em*bolus
epi	epi-	*epi*nephrine
	ep-	*ep*arterial
hyper	hyper-	*hyper*trophy
hypo	hypo-	*hypo*dermic
	hyp-	*hyp*axial
kata	kata-	*cata*lepsy
	kat-	*cat*ion
meta	meta-	*meta*morphosis
	met-	*met*encephalon
para	para-	*para*mastoid
	par-	*par*otid
peri	peri-	*peri*toneum
pro	pro-	*pro*gnosis
syn	syn-	*syn*thesis
	sym-	*sym*physis
	syl-	*syl*lepsis
	sy-	*sy*stole

Many Latin suffixes have been naturalized in English for centuries, and little comment is needed on their morphology and use. Some common suffixes of particular use in medicine are listed below with their English derivatives. Note that the suffixes *-abilis* and *-alis/-aris* are attached to verb stems of the first conjugation (the infinitives end in *-āre*, as in *laudāre* to praise); and *-ibilis* and *-ilis* are used with the other conjugations (*vidēre*, *visibilis*; *legĕre*, *legibilis*; *audīre*, *audibilis*).

Latin components	English
avis + -arium	avi*ary*
dormio (dormitus) + -orium	dormit*ory*
nutrio (nutritus) + -io	nutrit*ion*
moveo (motus) + -or	mot*or*
porosus + -tas	poros*ity*
frio + -abilis	fri*able*
edo + -ibilis	ed*ible*
corpus (corporis) + -alis	corpor*al*
febris + -ilis	febr*ile*
oculus + -aris	ocul*ar*
cilium + -arius	cili*ary*
sensus + -orius	sens*ory*
reticulum + -atus	reticul*ate*
morbus + -idus	morb*id*
aborior (abortus) + -ivus	abort*ive*
squama + -osus	squam*ous*
adeps (adipis) + -osus	adip*ose*
prae + caveo (cautus) + -io + -arius	precaut*ionary*

Greek suffixes in general have not been naturalized in English as the Latin have, with spectacular exception of the family of suffixes represented by verbs in *-izō* (-ize), agent nouns in *-istēs* (-ist), and verbal nouns in *-ismos* (-ism).

So far we have examined the various forms of roots, root words, and derived words; only compound words remain. A compound word is one formed from two (or more) independent words, the first word modifying, dependent upon, or being object of the next. In English, *housewife*, *kidney transplant*, *salesman*, *schoolboy*, *store-bought*, *backbreaking*, and *anteater* are compound words. In English the individual elements undergo little if any change from their basic, lexical forms but remain isolated, as it were, and receive their new meaning solely from juxtaposition (an example is the difference between *house guest* and *guest house*).

The conditions are vastly different in Latin and Greek; in the Classical languages one must use so-called combining forms of substantives (i.e., nouns and adjectives including past participles) that are often considerably different from the lexical forms.

In Latin all native compound words ordinarily will consist of the stem of the first word; then the connecting vowel, usually -i-, sometimes -u-; then the stem of the second word; then the inflection: magn-i-ficient-ia, *magnificientia*, magnificence. In science there are many compounds like *dorsoradial* and *frenosecretory* with Latin words and Greek connecting vowels (see the next paragraph); the true Latin forms for such compounds would be *dorsiradialis* and *frenisecretorius*.

In Greek the rules for forming compound words are much more complicated. If the first substantive of a Greek compound ends in *-a* (but not *-ma*) or *-ē*, one nearly always changes that vowel to *-o-*:

glōssa, tongue + *ptōsis*, fall = glossoptosis
phōnē, voice, sound + *logos*, word, reason, study = *phōnologia*, phonology

Substantives ending in *-on*, *-os*, or *-ys* usually drop the final consonant and leave the vowel unchanged:

osteon, bone + *arthritis*, gout (first appears in Hippocrates) = osteoarthritis
myelos, marrow + *poiēsis*, production = myelopoiesis
pachys, thick + *derma*, skin = pachydermia (first appears in Hippocrates)

If the second element begins with a vowel, one merely drops the final *-a* or *-ē* from the first element without adding *-o-*:

archē, beginning, chief, rule + *enteron*, intestine = archenteron
bradys, slow, dull + *akusis*, hearing = bradyacousia

There are exceptions:

idea, idea + *logos* = ide*o*logy is regular,
but
genea, family, lineage + *logos* = *genealogia*, gene*a*logy is irregular, as are
architektōn not *archotektōn*, arch*i*tect
archetypos not *archotypos*, arch*e*type

Indeed the regular *archo-* is extremely rare compared with *arche-* and *archi-* and is therefore "irregular."

Forming compounds from other substantives is complicated by the fact that one cannot generally predict the combining form of a substantive from the lexical entry, and in fact one usually predicts the lexical entry from the combining form, not vice versa.

In Greek, substantives ending in *-ma* have a stem or combining form in *-mat-*; so *haima* (blood), *haimat-* and *poiēsis* (making, "poesy") make *haimatopoiēsis*, hematopoiesis. But Hippocrates himself uses *haimorrhagia*, hemorrhage, not *haimatorrhagia*. And no one could predict from the nominative *gynē* (woman), which looks like a regular noun, a combining form *gynaik-*, whence gynecology; or from *gala* (milk), *galakt-*, whence galactophorous.

Latin is not so irregular, but even so the combining stem of *lac* (milk) is *lact-* (lactacidemia); of *cor* (heart), *cord-* (cordial); of *miles* (soldier), *milit-* (military); of *rex* (king), *reg-* (regicide); and of *nomen* (name), *nomin-* (nominate). The combining form of *homo* (human being, man) is *homin-* (hominoid ape), but Cicero himself uses *homicida* (murderer, homicide), not *hominicida*.

Prefixes, Suffixes, and Combining Forms Used in Medical Etymology

For a list of Greek and Latin elements used in medical terminology, see Appendix 1 on page 2101.

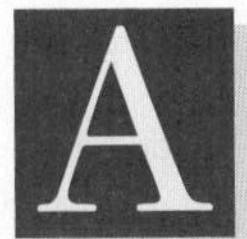

A accommodation; adenine or adenosine; alanine; ampere; anode; anterior; (as a subscript) alveolar gas.

A. [L.] an′num (year).

A absorbance; activity (def. 3); admittance; area; mass number.

A_2 aortic second sound.

Å angstrom.

AI primary auditory cortex; see *auditory cortex*, under *cortex.*

AII secondary auditory cortex; see *auditory cortex*, under *cortex.*

a accommodation; atto-; (as a subscript) arterial blood.

a. [L.] an′num (year); a′qua (water); arte′ria (artery).

a-[1] [Gr.] an inseparable prefix denoting want or absence; appears as *an-* before stems beginning with a vowel or with *h*.

a-[2] [L.] a prefix denoting separation, or away from.

a acceleration (def. 2); activity (def. 2); specific absorptivity.

ā [L.] an′te (before).

α alpha, the first letter of the Greek alphabet; symbol for *Bunsen coefficient*, the heavy chain of IgA (see *immunoglobulin*), the α chain of hemoglobin, and the probability of *Type I error.*

α- a prefix designating (1) the carbon atom adjacent to the principal functional group, e.g., α-amino acids, succeeding letters, β, γ, δ, etc., being used to designate succeeding carbon atoms in the chain; (2) the specific rotation of an optically active substance, e.g., α-D-glucose; (3) the orientation of an exocyclic atom or group, e.g., 3α-hydroxy-5α-androstan-17-one (androsterone); (4) a plasma protein migrating with the α band (subdivided into α_1 and α_2 bands) in protein electrophoresis, e.g., α-fetoprotein; (5) one in a series of related chemical compounds, particularly a series of stereoisomeric, isomeric, polymeric or allotropic forms, e.g., α-carotene; and (6) one in a group of related entities, e.g., α-ray. For compounds prefixed with the symbol α-, see the unprefixed form.

AA achievement age; Alcoholics Anonymous; amino acid.

$\overline{\text{AA}}$ [Gr. *ana* of each] $\overline{\text{aa}}$.

aa. [L.] arteriae (arteries).

$\overline{\text{aa}}$ an abbreviation used in prescription writing, following the names of two or more ingredients and signifying "of each"; also written $\overline{\text{AA}}$ and *ana.*

AAA American Association of Anatomists.

AAAS American Association for the Advancement of Science.

AABB American Association of Blood Banks.

AACP American Academy of Child Psychiatry.

AAD American Academy of Dermatology.

AADP American Academy of Denture Prosthetics.

AADS American Association of Dental Schools.

AAE American Association of Endodontists.

AAFP American Academy of Family Physicians.

Aa•ge•naes syndrome (ah′gĕ-nēz) [Oyestein *Aagenaes*, Norwegian pediatrician, 20th century] see under *syndrome.*

AAI American Association of Immunologists.

AAID American Academy of Implant Dentistry.

AAIN American Association of Industrial Nurses.

AAMA American Association of Medical Assistants.

AAMC Association of American Medical Colleges.

AAMR American Association on Mental Retardation.

AAMT American Association for Medical Transcription.

AAN American Academy of Neurology.

AANP American Association of Naturopathic Physicians.

AAO American Association of Orthodontists; American Academy of Ophthalmology; American Academy of Otolaryngology; American Academy of Osteopathy; amino acid oxidase.

AAOMR American Academy of Oral and Maxillofacial Radiology.

AAOP American Academy of Oral Pathology.

AAOS American Academy of Orthopaedic Surgeons.

AAP American Academy of Pediatrics; American Academy of Pedodontics; American Academy of Periodontology; American Association of Pathologists; Association of Academic Physiatrists.

AAPA American Academy of Physician Assistants; American Association of Pathologists' Assistants.

AAPB American Association of Pathologists and Bacteriologists.

AAPMR American Academy of Physical Medicine and Rehabilitation.

AARC American Association for Respiratory Care.

Aar•on sign (ar′ən) [Charles Dettie *Aaron*, American physician, 1866–1951] see under *sign.*

Aar•skog syndrome (ahr′skog) [Dagfinn Charles *Aarskog*, Norwegian pediatrician, born 1928] see under *syndrome.*

Aar•skog-Scott syndrome (ahrs′kog skot′) [D.C. *Aarskog*, Charles I. *Scott*, Jr., American pediatrician, 20th century] Aarskog syndrome; see under *syndrome.*

AAS anabolic-androgenic steroid.

Aase syndrome (ahz) [Jon Morton *Aase*, American pediatrician, born 1936] see under *syndrome.*

AATA American Art Therapy Association.

AAV adeno-associated virus; see *Dependovirus.*

AB [L.] Ar′tium Baccalau′reus (Bachelor of Arts).

Ab antibody.

ab Latin preposition meaning *from.*

ab- [L. *ab* from] prefix meaning *away from, from.*

abac•a•vir sul•fate (ə-bak′ə-vir) a nucleoside analogue reverse transcriptase inhibitor used as an antiretroviral in the treatment of human immunodeficiency virus infection; administered orally.

abac•te•ri•al (a″bak-tēr′e-əl) free from bacteria.

Aba•die sign (ah-bah-de′) [Joseph Louis Irenée *Abadie*, French neurologist, 1873–1946] see under *sign.*

abap•tis•ton (a″bap-tis′tən) pl. *abaptis′ta* [*a-*[1] + Gr. *baptein* to dip] a trephine so shaped that it will not penetrate the brain.

abar•og•no•sis (a″bar-əg-no′sis) [*a-*[1] + *baro-* + Gr. *gnosis* knowledge] baragnosis.

ab•ar•thro•sis (ab″ahr-thro′sis) [*ab-* + L. *arthrosis*] diarthrosis.

ab•ar•tic•u•lar (ab″ahr-tik′u-lər) 1. not affecting a joint. 2. remote from a joint.

ab•ar•tic•u•la•tion (ab″ahr-tik″u-la′shən) [*ab-* + L. *articulatio* joint] 1. a dislocation of a joint. 2. junctura synovialis.

aba•sia (ə-ba′zhə) [*a-*[1] + Gr. *basis* step + *-ia*] inability to walk. **aba′sic, abat′ic** *adj*

a.-asta′sia astasia-abasia.

a. atac′tica abasia characterized by uncertainty of movement, due to a defect of coordination.

choreic a. inability to walk due to chorea of the lower limbs.

paralytic a. inability to walk due to paralysis of the muscles of the lower limbs.

paroxysmal trepidant a. astasia-abasia caused by spastic stiffening of the lower limbs on attempting to stand; called also *spastic a.*

spastic a. paroxysmal trepidant a.

trembling a., a. tre′pidans inability to walk due to trembling of the lower limbs.

ab•a•ta•cept (ab″ə-ta′sept) a synthetic fusion protein produced by recombinant technology, comprising the extracellular domain of human cytotoxic T lymphocyte–associated antigen 4 (CTLA-4) linked to a portion of human immunoglobulin G1 (IgG1), which acts as an inhibitor of T-cell activation; used in the treatment of moderate to severe rheumatoid arthritis unresponsive to other medications, administered intravenously.

abate (ə-bāt′) to lessen or decrease.

abate•ment (ə-bāt′mənt) a decrease in the severity of a pain or a symptom.

ab•bau (ahp′bou) [Ger. "decomposition," "breakdown"] 1. exergonic breakdown of chemical substances. 2. decomposition of chemical substances. 3. catabolic products.

Ab•be condenser (ah′bə) [Ernst Karl *Abbe*, German physicist, 1840–1905] see under *condenser.*

Ab•be flap, operation (ab′e) [Robert *Abbe*, American surgeon, 1851–1928] see under *flap* and *operation.*

Ab•be-Zeiss counting chamber (apparatus) (ah′bə tsīs′) [E.K. *Abbe;* Carl *Zeiss*, German optician, 1816–1888] Thoma-Zeiss counting chamber.

Ab•bo•ki•nase (ab″o-ki′nās) trademark for a preparation of urokinase.

Ab•bott method (ab′ət) [Edville Gerhardt *Abbott*, American surgeon, 1870–1938] see under *Table of Methods.*

Ab•bott-Mil•ler tube (ab′ət mil′ər) [William Osler *Abbott*, American physician, 1902–1943; T. Grier *Miller*, American physician, 1886–1981] see *Miller-Abbott tube*, under *tube.*

Ab•bott-Raw•son tube (ab′ət raw′sən) [W.O. *Abbott;* Arthur J. *Rawson*, American medical physicist, 1896–1963] see under *tube.*

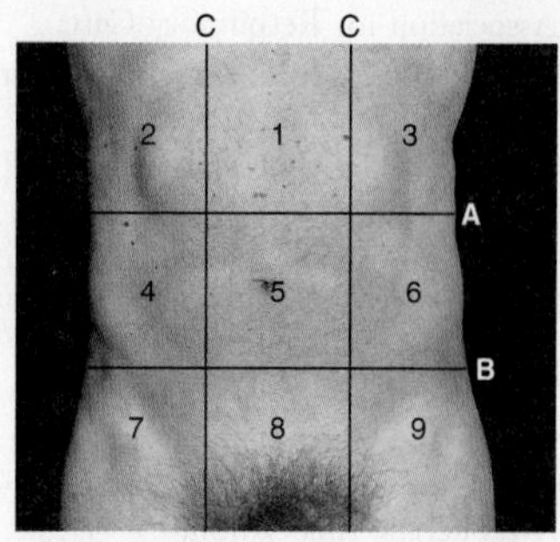

■ Regions of abdomen: *1*, epigastric region; *2*, right hypochondrium; *3*, left hypochondrium; *4*, right flank; *5*, umbilicus; *6*, left flank; *7*, right groin; *8*, pubic region; *9*, left flank. *A*, transpyloric plane; *B*, transtubercular plane; *C*, midclavicular line.

ABC argon beam coagulator; aspiration biopsy cytology; avidin-biotin complex.

ABCD a cancer chemotherapy regimen consisting of Adriamycin (doxorubicin), bleomycin, CCNU (lomustine), and dacarbazine.

ab·cix·i·mab (ab-sik′sĭ-mab) a human-murine monoclonal antibody Fab fragment that inhibits the aggregation of platelets, used as an antithrombotic in percutaneous transluminal coronary angioplasty; administered by intravenous infusion.

ab·do·men (ab′də-mən, ab-do′mən) [L., possibly from *abdere* to hide] [TA] that portion of the body which lies between the thorax and the pelvis; it contains a cavity *(abdominal cavity)* separated by the diaphragm from the thoracic cavity above and by the plane of the pelvic inlet from the pelvic cavity below and lined with a serous membrane, the peritoneum. This cavity contains the abdominal viscera (see Plate 50) and is enclosed by a wall *(abdominal wall)* formed by the abdominal muscles, the vertebral column, and the ilia. Called also *belly* and *venter.* It is divided into nine regions by four imaginary lines projected onto the anterior wall (see illustration); two of the lines pass horizontally around the body (the upper at the level of the cartilages of the ninth ribs, the lower at the tops of the crests of the ilia), and two extend vertically on each side of the body from the cartilage of the eighth rib to the center of the inguinal ligament. The regions are: three upper—right hypochondrium, epigastric region, left hypochondrium; three middle—right flank (right lateral region), umbilicus, left flank (left lateral region); and three lower—right groin (right inguinal region), pubic region, left flank (left inguinal region).

acute a. any abdominal condition of abrupt onset, usually with pain, due to inflammation, perforation, obstruction, infarction, or rupture of intra-abdominal organs; emergency surgical intervention is usually required. Called also *surgical a.*

boat-shaped a., carinate a. scaphoid a.

gridiron a. an abdomen criss-crossed with scars from multiple surgical procedures, such as may occur in severe forms of Munchausen syndrome.

navicular a. scaphoid a.

a. obsti′pum congenital shortness of the rectus abdominis muscle.

pendulous a. a relaxed condition of the abdominal wall, so that the anterior abdominal wall hangs over the pubis.

scaphoid a. an abdomen whose anterior wall is hollowed out, seen in children with cerebral disease. Called also *boat-shaped, carinate,* or *navicular a.*

surgical a. acute a.

ab·dom·i·nal (ab-dom′ĭ-nəl) [L. *abdominalis*] pertaining to the abdomen. Called also *celiac.*

abdomin(o)- [L. *abdomen,* q.v.] a combining form denoting relationship to the abdomen.

ab·dom·i·no·cen·te·sis (ab-dom″ĭ-no-sen-te′sis) [*abdomino-* + *-centesis*] abdominal paracentesis.

ab·dom·i·no·cys·tic (ab-dom″ĭ-no-sis′tik) abdominovesical.

ab·dom·i·no·gen·i·tal (ab-dom″ĭ-no-jen′ĭ-təl) pertaining to the abdomen and the reproductive organs.

ab·dom·i·no·hys·ter·ec·to·my (ab-dom″ĭ-no-his″tər-ek′tə-me) abdominal hysterectomy.

ab·dom·i·no·hys·ter·ot·o·my (ab-dom″ĭ-no-his″tər-ot′ə-me) abdominal hysterotomy.

ab·dom·i·no·plas·ty (ab-dom′ĭ-no-plas″te) plastic surgery of the surface of the abdomen. **abdominoplas′tic** *adj*

ab·dom·i·nos·co·py (ab-dom″ĭ-nos′kə-pe) laparoscopy.

ab·dom·i·no·scro·tal (ab-dom″ĭ-no-skro′təl) pertaining to the abdomen and scrotum.

ab·dom·i·no·tho·rac·ic (ab-dom″ĭ-no-thə-ras′ik) pertaining to the abdomen and thorax; thoracoabdominal.

ab·dom·i·no·uter·ot·o·my (ab-dom″ĭ-no-u-tər-ot′ə-me) abdominal hysterotomy.

ab·dom·i·no·vag·i·nal (ab-dom″ĭ-no-vaj′ĭ-nəl) pertaining to the abdomen and the vagina.

ab·dom·i·no·ves·i·cal (ab-dom″ĭ-no-ves′ĭ-kəl) 1. abdominocystic. 2. pertaining to or connecting the abdominal cavity and urinary bladder. Called also *abdominocystic* and *vesicoabdominal.*

ab·du·cens (ab-doo′sənz) [L. "drawing away"] serving to abduct a part, used in names of structures (e.g., nervus abducens).

ab·du·cent (ab-doo′sənt) [L. *abducens*] abducting, or effecting a separation, as an abducent nerve.

ab·duct (ab-dukt′) [*ab-* + *duct*] to draw away from the median plane or (in the digits) from the axial line of a limb.

ab·duc·tio (ab-duk′she-o) [L.] [TA] abduction.

ab·duc·tion (ab-duk′shən) the act of abducting or state of being abducted.

ab·duc·tor (ab-duk′tor) [L.] that which abducts; see under *musculus.*

ABE acute bacterial endocarditis; see *infective endocarditis,* under *endocarditis.*

Abel·cet (a′bəl-set) trademark for a preparation of amphotericin B lipid complex.

ab·em·bry·on·ic (ab″em-bre-on′ik) [*ab-* + *embryonic*] away from the embryo.

ab·e·quose (ab′ə-kwōs) an unusual sugar found to be a polysaccharide somatic antigen of *Salmonella* species.

Ab·er·ne·thy fascia (ab′ər-ne″the) [John *Abernethy,* British surgeon and anatomist, 1764–1831] see *fascia iliaca.*

ab·er·ran·cy (ab-er′ən-se) aberration (def. 3).

acceleration-dependent a. aberrancy resulting from the occurrence of impaired intraventricular conduction as the heart attains a specific critical rate.

bradycardia-dependent a. deceleration-dependent a.

deceleration-dependent a. aberrancy resulting from the occurrence of impaired intraventricular conduction after long pauses or slowing of the heart to a critical rate.

tachycardia-dependent a. acceleration-dependent a.

ab·er·rant (ă-ber′ənt, ab′ər-ənt) wandering or deviating from the usual or normal course.

ab·er·ra·tio (ab″ər-a′she-o) [L., from *aberrare* to wander away from] aberration (def. 1).

a. tes′tis situation of the testis in a part distant from the path which it takes in normal descent.

ab·er·ra·tion (ab″ər-a′shən) [L. *aberratio,* q.v.] 1. deviation from the usual course or condition. 2. unequal refraction or focalization of light rays by a lens, resulting in degradation of the image they produce. 3. in cardiology, aberrant electrical impulse conduction.

chromatic a. unequal deviation of light rays of different wavelengths passing through a refractive medium, resulting in fringes of color around the image produced; called also *newtonian a.*

chromatic a., lateral difference in magnification due to differences in position of the principal points for light of different wavelengths; also a difference of focal length.

chromatic a., longitudinal difference in position along the axis for the focal points of light, produced by unequal deviation of light rays of different wavelengths by a lens.

chromosome a. an irregularity in the number or structure of chromosomes that may alter the course of development of the embryo, usually in the form of a gain (duplication), loss (deletion), exchange (translocation), or alteration in sequence (inversion) of genetic material. See illustration and see *genetic disease,* under *disease.*

dioptric a. spherical a.

distantial a. a blurring of vision for distant objects.

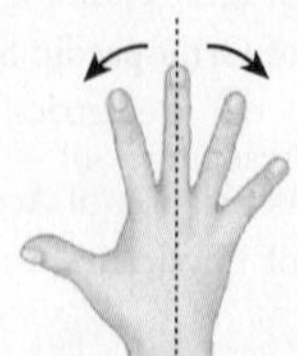

■ Abduction of the fingers.

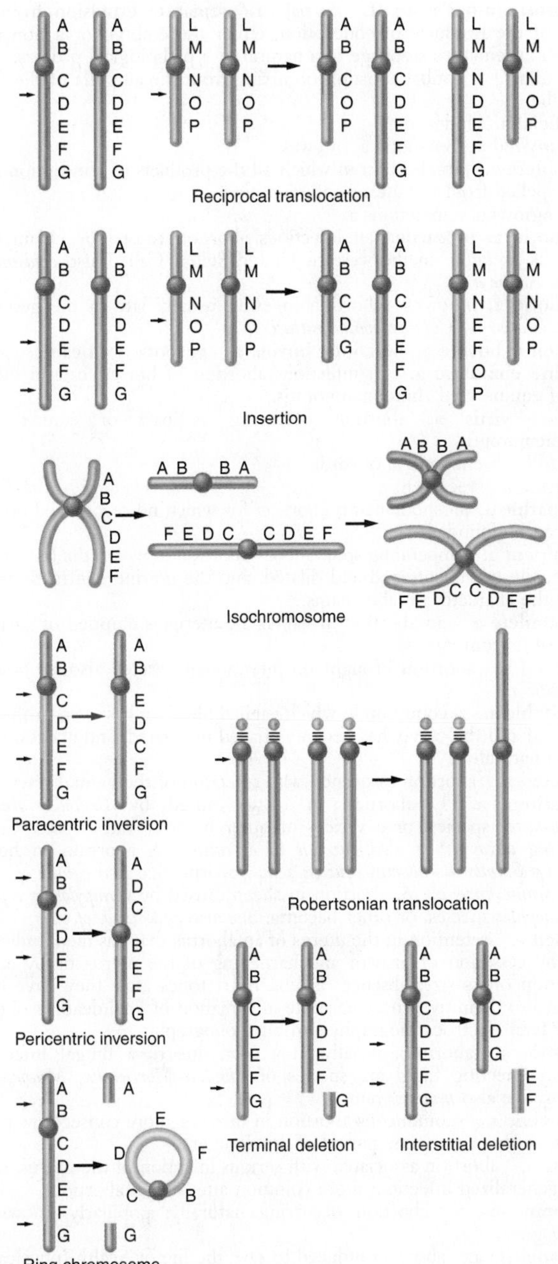

■ Different types of chromosome aberrations. Genes are indicated by letters; breaks are indicated by small arrows.

intraventricular a. aberrant conduction within the ventricles of an impulse generated in the supraventricular region; it is characterized by a bizarre, usually wide QRS complex. Abnormalities due to fixed organic defects in conduction are excluded.

lateral a. deviation of a ray from the focal point, measured on a line perpendicular to the axis at the focal point.

longitudinal a. deviation of a ray from the focal point, measured along the optic axis.

mental a. any pathological deviation from normal mental activity, usually limited to a circumscribed deviation in an otherwise adapted individual.

meridional a. unequal refraction of light rays as a result of variation of refractive power in different portions of the same meridian of a lens.

negative spherical a. unequal refraction of light rays by a lens, the peripheral rays being focused farther from the lens than the paraxial rays.

newtonian a. chromatic a.

penta-X chromosomal a. the occurrence of five X chromosomes in a female.

positive spherical a. unequal refraction of light rays by a lens, the peripheral rays being focused closer to the lens than the paraxial rays.

spherical a. zonal aberration in relation to an axial point; see *negative spherical a.* and *positive spherical a.* Called also *dioptric a.*

tetra-X chromosomal a. the occurrence of four X chromosomes in a female or tetra-XY in the male.

triple-X chromosomal a. the occurrence of three X chromosomes in a female or triple-XY in the male.

zonal a. unequal refraction of light rays by a lens, the rays passing through different zones being focused at different distances from the lens.

abeta•lipo•pro•tein•emia (a-ba″tə-lip″o-pro″te-ne′me-ə) an autosomal recessive disorder of lipoprotein metabolism (gene locus: 4q22-q24) in which lipoproteins containing apolipoprotein B (chylomicrons, very-low-density lipoproteins, and low-density lipoproteins) are not synthesized; it is characterized by acanthocytes in plasma, hypocholesterolemia, progressive ataxic neuropathy, pigmentary retinal degeneration, defective intestinal lipid absorption, and deficiency of fat-soluble vitamins.

normotriglyceridemic a. a variant of abetalipoproteinemia in which apolipoprotein (apo) B-48 is present, but apo B-100 is absent; chylomicrons are formed but low-density lipoproteins are not, and some fat absorption may occur.

ab•frac•tion (ab-frak′shən) pathological loss of tooth structure owing to biomechanical forces (flexion, compression, or tension) or chemical degradation; it is most visible as V-shaped notches in the cervical area of a tooth.

ABG arterial blood gases.

ABI ankle-brachial index.

ab•i•a•tro•phy (a-bi-ă′trə-fe) premature and endogenous loss of vitality or tissue substance. See also *abiotrophy.*

ab•i•ent (ab′e-ənt) avoiding the source of stimulation; said of a response to a stimulus. Cf. *adient.*

Abi•es (a′be-ēz) the firs, a genus of evergreens of the family Pinaceae, mainly found in North America. *A. balsa′mea* (L.) Mill. is the balsam fir, which yields Canada balsam.

abi•et•ic ac•id (ab″e-et′ik) an acid resin that is the major active component of rosin (q.v.); it is used in the manufacture of soaps, and its esters are used in the manufacture of lacquers and varnishes.

Abil•i•fy (ə-bil′ĭ-fi) trademark for preparations of aripiprazole.

abi•on•er•gy (a″bi-on′ər-je) [*a-*^{1} + Gr. *bio-* life + *ergon* work] abiotrophy.

abi•os•is (a″bi-o′sis) [*a-*^{1} + *bio-* + *-osis*] absence of life.

abi•ot•ic (a″bi-ot′ik) pertaining to or characterized by absence of life; incapable of living; antagonistic to life.

Abio•tro•phia (a-bi-o-tro′fe-ə) a genus of gram-positive bacteria of the family Aerococcaceae, found growing in satellite colonies around other bacteria, especially *Staphylococcus aureus;* many are penicillin-resistant. They are found as normal flora in the upper respiratory, urogenital, and gastrointestinal tracts, and have been implicated in some cases of bacterial endocarditis. The type species is *A. defectiva.*

A. adia′cens former name for *Granulicatella adiacens.*

A. defecti′va a species found in cases of infective endocarditis; formerly called *Streptococcus defectivus.*

abi•ot•ro•phy (a″bi-ot′rə-fe) [*a-*^{1} + *bio-* + *-trophy*] progressive loss of vitality of certain tissues or organs, leading to disorders or loss of function; applied especially to degenerative hereditary diseases of late onset, e.g., Huntington disease. **abiotro′phic** *adj*

retinal a. any of a group of age-dependent, genetically determined diseases of the retina, such as retinitis pigmentosa and neuronal ceroid-lipofuscinosis.

ab•ir•ri•ta•tion (ab-ir-ĭ-ta′shən) 1. diminished responsiveness to stimulation. 2. atony.

abi•u•ret (a-bi′u-ret) [*a-*^{1} + *biuret*] not giving a positive reaction to the biuret test.

abi•u•ret•ic (ə-bi″u-rĕ′tik) not responsive to the biuret test.

ab•lac•ta•tion (ab″lak-ta′shən) [*ab-* + *lactation*] the weaning of a child or the cessation of milk secretion.

ablas•tem•ic (a″blas-tem′ik) [*a-*^{1} + *blastemic*] not concerned with germination.

ablas•tin (a″blas′tin) an antibody, produced by rats infected with trypanosomes, that inhibits reproduction of trypanosomes; it has no other known function and is neither a lysin nor an opsonin.

ab•late (ab-lāt′) [L. *ablatus* removed] to remove, especially by cutting; to extirpate.

ab•la•tio (ab-la′she-o) [L.] ablation.

a. placen′tae abruptio placentae.

ab•la•tion (ab-la′shən) [L. *ablatus* carried away] 1. separation or detachment; extirpation; eradication. 2. removal or destruction of a part, especially by cutting.

alcohol a. see *chemical a.*

androgen a. see under *deprivation.*

catheter a. delivery of destructive electrical energy, usually high energy or radiofrequency alternating current, via electrodes on a catheter.
chemical a. destruction of tissue by injection of small amounts of alcohol or phenol; used in the treatment of tachyarrhythmias and hypertrophic cardiomyopathy and for the destruction of tumor cells in the treatment of cancer.
electrical a. fulguration; the term is used particularly to describe destruction of areas of myocardial tissue in the treatment of tachyarrhythmias.
endometrial a. removal of the endometrium; methods used include radiofrequency, electrical energy, lasers, and hot and cold liquids.
immune a. immunoablation.
photochemical a. laser ablation of tissue in which light absorbed by the tissue dissociates molecular bonds.
photomechanical a. laser ablation of tissue in which the absorption of light energy causes stress in excess of the tissue's strength.
photothermal a. laser ablation of tissue in which light is absorbed by the tissue and converted to heat, resulting in coagulation, necrosis, and vaporization.
radiofrequency a., radiofrequency catheter a. the destruction of precisely controlled areas of tissue by heat induced by low-frequency electromagnetic waves, used for a variety of purposes, including the treatment of arrhythmias and the reduction of tumors.
rotational a. rotablation.
transurethral needle a. (TUNA) a form of radiofrequency ablation using interstitial needles inserted via the urethra into the lateral lobes of the prostate, the heat producing localized necrotic lesions of prostatic tissue; used in the treatment of benign prostatic hyperplasia.

ABLB alternate binaural loudness balance; see under *test.*

able·pha·ria (a″blĕ-far′e-ə) cryptophthalmos. **ableph′arous** *adj*

ableph·a·ron (a″blef′ə-ron) cryptophthalmos.

ab·lu·ent (ab′loo-ənt) 1. detergent. 2. a cleansing agent.

ab·lu·mi·nal (ab-loo′mĭ-nəl) directed away from the lumen of a tubular structure.

ab·lu·tion (ab-loo′shən) [L. *ablutio* a washing] the act of washing or cleansing; the application of water by the hand, which may be covered with a bath mitt or towel.

ab·lu·to·ma·nia (ab-loo″to-ma′ne-ə) [L. *ablutio* a washing + *-mania*] obsessional preoccupation with cleanliness, washing, or bathing, often accompanied by compulsive rituals, a common symptom in obsessive-compulsive states.

ABMT autologous bone marrow transplantation; see *bone marrow transplantation*, under *transplantation.*

ab·nor·mal (ab-nor′məl) [*ab-* + *normal*] not normal; contrary to the usual structure, position, condition, behavior, or rule.

ab·nor·mal·i·ty (ab″nor-mal′ĭ-te) 1. the quality or fact of being abnormal. 2. a malformation, deformity, or anomaly.
congenital a. birth defect.
potential a. of glucose tolerance (pot AGT) a statistical classification containing individuals who have a significantly higher than average risk of developing diabetes mellitus, such as identical twins of type 2 diabetics.
previous a. of glucose tolerance (prev AGT) a statistical classification containing individuals once having had diabetes mellitus, gestational diabetes, or impaired glucose tolerance, but who now have normal glucose tolerance.

ab·oma·si·tis (ab″o-mə-si′tis) inflammation of the abomasum.

ab·o·ma·so·pexy (ab″o-ma′so-pek″se) surgical fixation of the abomasum to correct right or left displacement of the abomasum (see under *displacement*).

ab·o·ma·sot·omy (ab″o-ma-sot′ə-me) surgical cutting into the abomasum, usually to remove a bezoar or impaction.

ab·oma·sum (ab″o-ma′sum) [*ab-* + L. *omasum*] the fourth stomach of a ruminant, comparable in structure and function to the stomach of a nonruminant; it contains gastric glands that secrete gastric juice. **aboma′sal** *adj*

ab·orad (ab-or′ad) directed away from the mouth.

ab·oral (ab-or′əl) opposite to, away from, or remote from the mouth.

ab·orig·i·nal (ab-ə-rij′ĭ-nəl) native to the place inhabited.

abort (ə-bort′) [L. *aboriri* to miscarry] 1. to check the usual course of a disease. 2. to cause, undergo, or experience termination of a pregnancy before the fetus is viable. 3. to become checked in development.

abor·tient (ə-bor′shənt) abortifacient.

abor·ti·fa·cient (ə-bor″tĭ-fa′shənt) [L. *abortio* abortion + *-facient*] 1. causing abortion. 2. an agent that causes abortion; called also *abortient.*

abor·tion (ə-bor′shən) [L. *abortio*] 1. premature expulsion from the uterus of the products of conception, either the embryo or a nonviable fetus. 2. premature stoppage of a natural or a pathological process.
ampullar a. a tubal abortion occurring from the ampulla of the fallopian tube.
artificial a. induced a.
chlamydial a. enzootic a. of ewes.
complete a. an abortion in which all the products of conception have been expelled from the uterus and identified.
contagious a. infectious a.
enzootic a. of cattle an infectious abortion caused by chlamydiae; known as *foothill a.* in the western United States. Called also *epidemic* or *epizootic bovine a.*
enzootic a. of ewes abortion in ewes, usually late in the gestation period, caused by *Chlamydophila psittaci.*
epidemic bovine a., epizootic bovine a. enzootic a. of cattle.
equine epizootic a. an infectious abortion of horses, caused by the virus of equine viral rhinopneumonitis.
equine virus a. abortion occurring as part of equine viral rhinopneumonitis.
foothill a. enzootic a. of cattle.
habitual a. recurrent a.
idiopathic a. a spontaneous abortion for which no recognized organic cause can be found.
imminent a. impending spontaneous abortion in which the bleeding is profuse, the cervix softened and dilated, and the uterine contractions approach the character of labor pains.
incomplete a. an abortion in which the uterus is emptied of part but not all of its contents.
induced a. abortion brought on intentionally; called also *artificial* or *therapeutic a.*
inevitable a. a condition in which vaginal bleeding has been profuse or prolonged and the cervix has become effaced or dilated, and abortion will proceed naturally.
infected a. abortion associated with infection of the genital tract.
infectious a. 1. abortion in cattle caused by *Brucella abortus, Campylobacter* species, or a variety of other bacteria and viruses. Called also *Bang disease.* See also *enzootic a. of cattle.* 2. abortion in horses caused by *Salmonella abortus equi* or a herpesvirus. See also *equine epizootic a.* and *equine virus a.* 3. abortion in sheep caused by *Campylobacter fetus, Chlamydophila* species, or other bacteria. See also *enzootic a. of ewes.*
missed a. retention in the uterus of an abortus that has died, indicated either by cessation of growth and hardening of the uterus or by actual diminution of its size; absence of fetal heart tones after they have been heard is also definitive; more accurate information of fetal death is obtainable by fetal electrocardiography and ultrasonography.
mycotic a. abortion, usually in a cow, due to a fungal infection; common infecting fungi are species of *Absidia, Mortierella, Mucor,* and *Rhizopus.* See also *mucormycosis.*
recurrent a. spontaneous abortion in three or more consecutive pregnancies, at about the same period of development.
septic a. abortion associated with serious infection of the uterus, leading to generalized infection; more common after illegal abortions.
spontaneous a. abortion occurring naturally; popularly known as *miscarriage.*
therapeutic a. abortion induced to save the life or health (physical or mental) of a pregnant woman; sometimes performed after rape or incest.
threatened a. a condition in which there is bloody discharge from the uterus but the loss of blood is usually less than in inevitable abortion and there is no dilation of the cervix; it may proceed to actual abortion or the symptoms may subside and the pregnancy go to full term.
tubal a. extrusion of the conceptus through the open end of the uterine tube into the abdominal cavity, occurring in tubal pregnancy.
vibrio a. an infectious abortion of cattle, sheep, and goats, caused by *Campylobacter fetus.*

abor·tive (ə-bor′tiv) [L. *abortivus*] 1. incompletely developed. 2. abortifacient (def. 1). 3. cutting short the course of a disease.

abor·tus (ə-bor′təs) [L.] a fetus weighing less than 500 g (17 oz) or being of less than 20 completed weeks' gestational age at the time of expulsion from the uterus, having no chance of survival.

abouche·ment (ah-bo͞osh-maw′) [Fr.] the termination of a vessel in a larger one.

abou·lia (ə-boo′le-ə) abulia.

ABP arterial blood pressure.

ABR auditory brainstem response.

abra·chia (ə-bra′ke-ə) [*a-*[1] + L. *brachia*] congenital absence of the upper limbs.

abra·chi·a·tism (ah-bra′ke-ah-tiz″əm) abrachia.

abra·chio·ce·pha·lia (ə-bră″ke-o-sĕ-fa′le-ə) acephalobrachia.

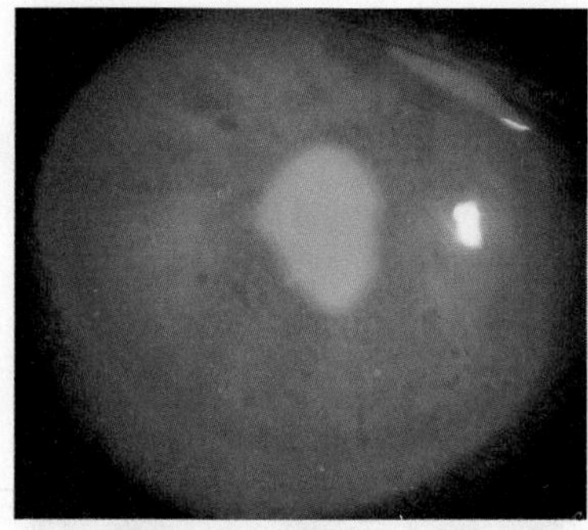

■ Corneal abrasion, with epithelial defect demonstrated by fluorescein staining.

abra•chio•ceph•a•lus (ə-brā″ke-o-sef′ə-lus) acephalobrachius.

abra•chi•us (ə-bra′ke-əs) an individual exhibiting abrachia.

abrad•ant (ə-bra′dənt) abrasive.

abrade (ə-brād′) to rub away the external covering or layer of a part; see also *planing*.

abrad•er (ə-bra′dər) an instrument used for abrading; called also *abrasor*.

Abrams heart reflex (a′brəmz) [Albert *Abrams*, American physician, 1863–1924] see under *reflex*.

abra•sio (ə-bra′se-o) [L.] abrasion.

a. cor′neae corneal abrasion.

abra•sion (ə-bra′zhən) [L. *abrasio*] 1. the wearing away of a substance or structure (such as the skin or the teeth) through some unusual or abnormal mechanical process. 2. an area of body surface denuded of skin or mucous membrane by such a process.

air a. a type of microabrasion in which a jet of air blows tiny particles against the tooth or cavity surface.

corneal a. a rubbing off of the superficial layers of the cornea.

abra•sive (ə-bra′siv) 1. causing abrasion. 2. a substance used for abrading, grinding, or polishing.

abra•sor (ə-bra′zər) abrader.

Ab•rax•ane (ə-brak′sān) trademark for a preparation of paclitaxel.

ab•re•ac•tion (ab″re-ak′shən) [*ab-* + *reaction*] the reliving of an experience in such a way that previously repressed emotions associated with it are released, usually also resulting in insight.

motor a. an abreaction achieved through motor or muscular expression.

Abri•ko•sov (Abri•kos•soff) tumor (ah″bre-kos′of) [Aleksei Ivanovich *Abrikosov* (or *Abrikossoff*), Russian pathologist, 1875–1955] see *granular cell tumor*, under *tumor*.

abrin (a′brin) a powerful phytotoxin or toxalbumin, present in the seeds of *Abrus precatorius* (jequirity bean) and used in the synthesis of immunotoxins; formerly used topically in certain chronic eye disorders.

abrism (a′brizm) poisoning by the jequirity bean; see *abrin*.

ab•rup•tio (ab-rup′she-o) [L., from *abrumpere* to break off from] a rending asunder.

a. placen′tae premature detachment of a placenta, often attended by maternal systemic reactions in the form of shock, oliguria, and coagulation abnormalities.

Abrus (a′brəs) a genus of trees of the family Leguminosae, found in warm regions. *A. precato′rius* L. is found in tropical and subtropical Asia and the Americas; its seed (called *jequirity bean, rosary pea*, or *crab's eye*) is used for rosary beads and jewelry but contains the toxalbumin abrin (q.v.).

abs- [L. *abs*, variant of *ab*] a prefix meaning *away from, from*.

ab•scess (ab′ses) [L. *abscessus*, from *ab* away + *cedere* to go] a localized collection of pus within tissues, organs, or confined spaces. See also *empyema*.

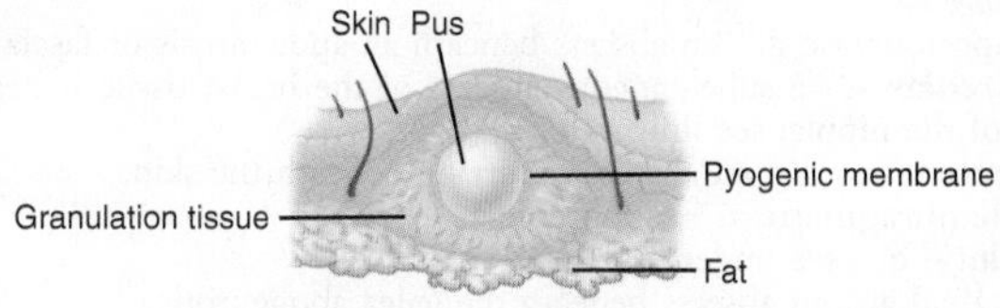

■ Cross section of abscess.

acute a. an abscess that runs a relatively short course, producing fever and painful local inflammation.

alveolar a. apical a. (def. 2).

amebic a. an abscess seen in amebiasis, usually in the liver but sometimes in the lungs, spleen, or brain.

amebic liver a. the abscess formed in hepatic amebiasis, resulting from liquefaction necrosis due to entrance of *Entamoeba histolytica* into the portal circulation.

anorectal a. an abscess arising in the anorectum.

apical a. 1. an abscess at the apex of an organ. 2. inflammation of tissues around the apex of a tooth, with pus formation, owing to infection that has spread from pulp infection through a carious lesion or because of an injury causing pulp necrosis. Called also *alveolar a., dentoalveolar a.*, and *periapical a.*

apical a., acute an apical abscess of a tooth characterized by rapid onset, acute pain, tenderness of the tooth to touch, pus formation, and swelling of tissues in a later stage.

apical a., chronic an apical abscess of a tooth characterized by an intermittent discharge of pus through a sinus tract, with gradual onset, little or no swelling of the affected tissue, and only slight discomfort.

appendiceal a., appendicular a. an intra-abdominal abscess near the vermiform appendix in perforating appendicitis; called also *periappendiceal a.*

Bartholin a., bartholinian a. abscess of the excretory duct of the Bartholin gland.

Bezold a. an abscess in the neck resulting from acute mastoiditis *(Bezold mastoiditis)* in which pus tracts have formed deep to the superior portion of the sternocleidomastoid muscle and along the posterior belly of the digastric muscle.

bicameral a. an abscess having two chambers or pockets; see *collar-button a.*

bile duct a. cholangitic a.

biliary a. abscess of the gallbladder or some part of the biliary tract.

bone a. an abscess seen in osteomyelitis.

brain a. an abscess affecting the brain as a result of extension of an infection (e.g., otitis media) from an adjacent area or through bloodborne infection. Called also *pyencephalus* and *pyocephalus*.

broad ligament a. an abscess between the folds of the broad ligament of the uterus; called also *parametric* or *parametrial a.*

Brodie a. a roughly spherical region of bone destruction, filled with pus or connective tissue, usually found in the metaphyseal region of long bones and caused by *Staphylococcus aureus*.

canalicular a. a mammary abscess that communicates with a lactiferous duct.

caseous a. an abscess that contains cheeselike material, as in pulmonary tuberculosis. Called also *cheesy a.*

central mammary a. a mammary abscess in the deep parenchyma of the breast; it may be unicentric or multicentric. See illustration.

cervical a. streptococcal lymphadenitis of swine.

cheesy a. caseous a.

cholangitic a. an abscess in the liver complicating cholangitis; called also *bile duct a.*

chronic a. cold a. (def. 1).

circumtonsillar a. peritonsillar a.

cold a. 1. an abscess of comparatively slow development, with relatively minimal symptoms of inflammation. Called also *chronic a.* 2. tuberculous a.

collar button a. a superficial abscess connected with a deeper one by a fistulous tract.

dental a. an abscess in or around a tooth.

dentoalveolar a. apical a. (def. 2).

diffuse a. an uncircumscribed abscess whose pus is diffused in the surrounding tissues.

Douglas a. an abscess in the rectouterine pouch.

Dubois a. abscess of the thymus in congenital syphilis; called also *Dubois disease* and *thymic a.*

epidural a. a collection of pus located between the dura mater and surrounding bone; see *intracranial epidural a.* and *spinal epidural a.* Called also *extradural a.*

epiploic a. an abscess in the omentum; called also *omental a.*

extradural a. epidural a.

fecal a. an abscess containing pus and fecal matter, usually pericolic or perirectal, resulting from lower bowel perforation; extension to the skin or mucosa leads to a fecal fistula.

frontal a. a brain abscess in the frontal lobe.

gas a. a localized collection of seropurulent material containing gas produced by gas-forming bacteria. Called also *tympanitic* or *Welch a.*

gingival a. a localized, painful, inflammatory lesion of the gingivae, usually limited to the marginal gingiva or interdental papilla. See also *periodontal a.*

gravitation a., gravity a. an abscess in which the pus migrates or gravitates to a lower or deeper portion of the body.

heel a. abscess of the heel of a sheep with lameness and suppuration at the skin-horn junction, usually as an extension of the infection of interdigital dermatitis. Called also *infectious bulbar necrosis.*

helminthic a. worm a.

hot a. an acute abscess with symptoms of local inflammation.

hypostatic a. wandering a.

interlobular a., interlobular mammary a. a mammary abscess found within the lactiferous ducts of the breast; called also *periductal* or *periductal mammary a.* See illustration.

intersphincteric a. an anorectal abscess deep to the internal anal sphincter.

intra-abdominal a. an abscess in the absominal cavity outside the intestine, usually following perforation of the appendix or some other part of the intestine.

intracranial epidural a. an epidural abscess of the brain, located between the dura mater and the skull, which may cause dangerously increased intracranial pressure.

intradural a. a brain abscess within the layers of the dura mater.

intramastoid a. mastoid a.

ischiorectal a. an anorectal abscess in the ischiorectal fossa.

jowl a. streptococcal lymphadenitis of swine.

kidney a. renal a.

lacrimal a. an abscess in or around the lacrimal sac.

lateral a., lateral alveolar a. periodontal a.

mammary a. an abscess of the breast, often due to *Staphylococcus aureus* or streptococcal bacteria, usually seen in lactating women. Types include subcutaneous, subareolar, interlobular, central mammary, and retromammary. See illustration.

mastoid a. an abscess within the mastoid process and the air cells, as a complication of mastoiditis. Called also *intramastoid a.* and *mastoid empyema.*

metastatic a. a secondary abscess, usually of embolic origin, in which organisms are carried by the circulation to a point distant from the primary lesion.

metastatic tuberculous a. tuberculous gumma.

migrating a. wandering a.

miliary a. any of a group of small multiple abscesses.

Munro a. see under *microabscess.*

omental a. epiploic a.

palatal a. an apical abscess of a maxillary tooth which erupts or extends toward the palate.

pancreatic a. a circumscribed collection of pus adjacent to the pancreas after an episode of acute pancreatitis or trauma to the pancreas.

parafrenal a. abscess of a preputial gland.

parametrial a., parametric a. broad ligament a.

paranephric a. an abscess in the vicinity of the kidney, extending outside the renal fascia. Cf. *perinephric a.*

parietal a. periodontal a.

Pautrier a. see under *microabscess.*

pelvic a. abscess of the pelvic peritoneum, usually of the rectouterine pouch.

pelvirectal a. an abscess lying immediately above the levator ani muscle, in close relation to the wall of the rectum.

perianal a. a superficial anorectal abscess occurring beneath the perianal skin.

periapical a. apical a. (def. 2).

periappendiceal a., periappendicular a. appendiceal a.

pericolic a. an intra-abdominal abscess near the colon as a result of perforation complicating diverticulitis; called also *peridiverticular a.*

pericoronal a. an abscess around the crown of a partially erupted tooth.

peridental a. periodontal a.

peridiverticular a. pericolic a.

periductal a., periductal mammary a. interlobular a.

perinephric a. an abscess outside the parenchyma of the kidney but within the renal capsule. Cf. *paranephric a.* and *perinephritis.*

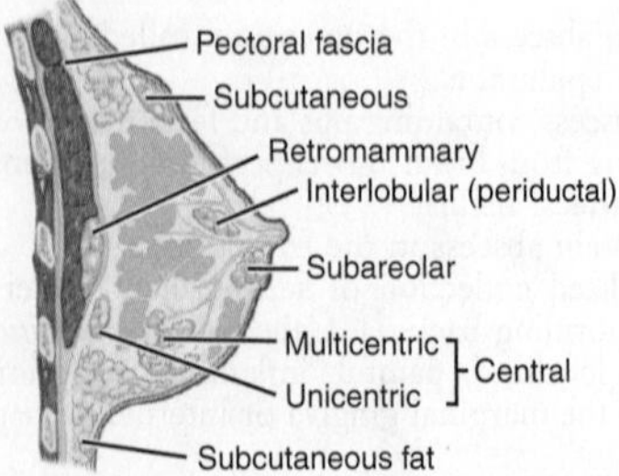

■ Abscesses of breast.

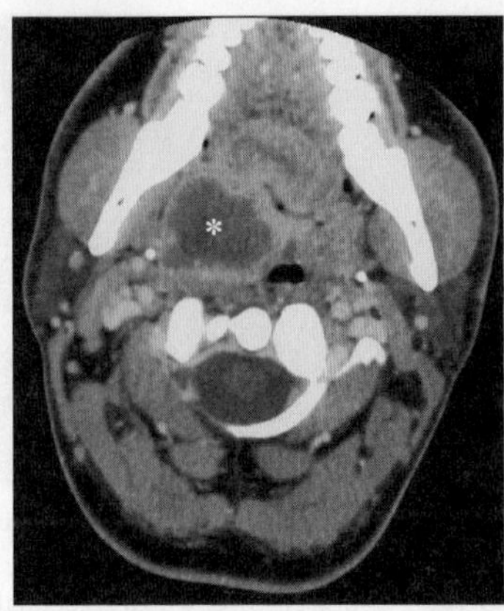

■ Peritonsillar abscess. Enhanced CT cross section of neck shows the abscess as a low-density mass *(asterisk)* with a thick rim, in the expected location of the tonsillar pillar. The oropharynx and tongue are displaced.

periodontal a. an abscess in the periodontal tissue; it may involve the supporting periodontal tissue or the soft tissue wall of a periodontal pocket. Called also *lateral a., lateral alveolar a., parietal a.,* and *peridental a.* See also *gingival a.*

peritoneal a. peritonitis complicated by abscess.

peritonsillar a. an abscess in the peritonsillar tissue extending into the tonsil capsule, resulting from suppuration of the tonsil; called also *quinsy.*

periureteral a. an abscess around the ureter.

phlegmonous a. an abscess associated with acute inflammation of the subcutaneous connective tissues.

phoenix a. an abscess with symptoms identical to those of an acute apical abscess, developing from a chronic apical granuloma and suddenly becoming symptomatic.

Pott a. an abscess associated with tuberculosis of the spine.

premammary a. an abscess located in the skin and subcutaneous tissues of the breast.

psoas a. an abscess that arises from disease of the lumbar or nearby vertebrae, with pus descending in the sheath of the psoas muscle.

pulp a., pulpal a. 1. an inflammation of the dental pulp, associated with a circumscribed collection of necrotic tissue and pus arising from breakdown of leukocytes and bacteria, sometimes walled off with connective tissue. 2. whitlow.

renal a. an abscess within the parenchyma of the kidney, caused by bacterial infection.

residual a. an abscess occurring at the site of a previous, incompletely resolved abscess.

retromammary a. a mammary abscess in the soft tissue behind the breast parenchyma; see illustration.

retroperitoneal a. subperitoneal a.

retropharyngeal a. a suppurative inflammation of the lymph nodes in the posterior and lateral walls of the pharynx.

retrotonsillar a. an abscess behind a tonsil caused by any of the common pyogenic bacteria, usually occurring with or closely following acute tonsillitis or pharyngitis.

ring a. a ring-shaped abscess at the periphery of the cornea.

root a. a chronic or acute abscess in supporting structures of the root of a tooth; when it is of endodontic origin, called *apical a.;* when periodontal in origin, called *periodontal a.*

satellite a. a secondary abscess arising from, and situated near, a primary abscess.

septicemic a. an abscess due to septicemia.

spinal epidural a. an epidural abscess between the dura mater and the surrounding vertebrae; the most common sites are the lumbar and cervical regions. Initial symptoms are pain, weakness, and sensory deficits, and if untreated it may progress to cause paralysis.

stercoraceous a., stercoral a. fecal a.

sterile a. an abscess from which microorganisms cannot be isolated.

stitch a. an abscess that develops adjacent to a stitch or suture; called also *suture a.*

subaponeurotic a. an abscess beneath an aponeurosis or fascia.

subareolar a. a subcutaneous abscess of the breast tissue beneath the areola of the nipple; see illustration.

subcutaneous a. an abscess occurring beneath the skin.

subdiaphragmatic a. subphrenic a.

subdural a. see under *empyema.*

subgaleal a. an abscess beneath the galea aponeurotica.

subhepatic a. an abscess situated beneath the liver.

submammary a. an abscess beneath the mammary gland.

subpectoral a. an abscess beneath the pectoral muscles.

subperiosteal a. a bone abscess situated just below the periosteum.

subperitoneal a. an abscess between the parietal peritoneum and the abdominal wall.

subphrenic a. an abscess beneath the diaphragm; called also *subdiaphragmatic a.*

subscapular a. an abscess between the serratus anterior and the posterior thoracic wall.

sudoriparous a. sweat gland a.

superficial a. an abscess occurring near the surface.

suprahepatic a. an abscess occurring in the suspensory ligament between the liver and the diaphragm.

supralevator a. an anorectal abscess occurring above the levator ani muscle and below the pelvic peritoneum.

suture a. stitch a.

sweat gland a. an abscess in a sweat gland, such as occurs in hidradenitis suppurativa; called also *sudoriparous a.*

syphilitic a. an abscess found in the bones during tertiary syphilis.

thecal a. an abscess in an enveloping sheath, such as a tendon sheath.

Thornwaldt a. Tornwaldt a.

thymic a. Dubois a.

toe a. abscess of the toe of a sheep with lameness and suppuration at the coronet, usually involving one digit of a front foot.

Tornwaldt (Thornwaldt) a. an abscess occurring in the adenoids, usually associated with adenoidism.

tuberculous a. an abscess due to infection with tubercle bacilli (*Mycobacterium tuberculosis).*

tubo-ovarian a. abscess of the uterine tube and ovary.

tympanitic a. gas a.

tympanocervical a. an abscess arising in the tympanum and extending to the neck. See also *Bezold a.*

tympanomastoid a. an abscess of the tympanum and mastoid.

urinary a. an abscess caused by extravasation of infection-containing urine.

verminous a. worm a.

vitreous a. abscess of the vitreous body due to infection, trauma, or foreign body.

von Bezold a. Bezold a.

wandering a. an abscess that burrows in the tissues and finally points at a distance from the site of origin; called also *hypostatic a.* and *migrating a.*

Welch a. gas a.

worm a. an abscess caused by or containing worms. Called also *helminthic* or *verminous a.*

ab•scis•sa (ab-sis′ə) [L. (*linea*) *abscissa* cut-off line, from *abscindere* to cut off] the horizontal coordinate in a two-dimensional coordinate system; the horizontal distance of a point from *y*- (or vertical) axis. Denoted by *x*. Cf. *ordinate.*

ab•scis•sion (ab-sĭ′zhən) [L. *abscindere* to cut off] removal by cutting.

ab•scon•sio (ab-skon′se-o) pl. *absconsio′nes* [L.] the cavity of a bone receiving and concealing the head of another bone.

ab•scop•al (ab-sko′pəl) pertaining to the effect on nonirradiated tissue resulting from irradiation of other tissue of the organism.

ab•sence (ab′sens) 1. absence epilepsy. 2. absence seizure.

abs. feb. [L.] absen′te feb′re (while fever is absent).

Ab•sid•ia (ab-sid′e-ə) a genus of fungi of the family Mucoraceae. *A. corymbi′fera* (called also *A. ramo′sa, Mucor corymbifer*, and *M. ramosus*) grows on bread and decaying vegetation and sometimes causes mucormycosis and otomycosis.

ab•sinthe (ab′sinth) 1. absinthium (def. 1). 2. a liqueur made from an extract of *Artemisia absinthium* and other bitter herbs; its use has been banned because it contains neurotoxins and prolonged ingestion can cause trismus, amblyopia, optic neuritis, and convulsions.

ab•sin•thi•um (ab-sin′the-um) 1. a plant of the species *Artemisia absinthium* (common wormwood). 2. the dead leaves and flowering tops of *A. absinthium*, formerly used as a bitter tonic. 3. an oil extracted from *A. absinthium* and used in absinthe.

ab•so•lute (ab′sə-lo͞ot) [L. *absolutus*, from *absolvere* to set loose] free from limitations; unlimited; uncombined.

ab•sorb (ab-sorb′) [L. *absorbēre*] 1. to take in or assimilate, as to take up substances into or across tissues, e.g., the skin, intestine, or renal tubules. 2. to react with radiation energy so as to attenuate it. 3. to retain specific wavelengths of radiation incident upon a substance, either increasing its temperature or changing the energy state of its molecules.

ab•sorb•able (ab-sorb′ə-bəl) capable of being absorbed.

ab•sor•bance (ab-sor′bəns) 1. in analytical chemistry, the negative logarithm of the transmittance, $-\log_{10}(I/I_0)$, where I is the light intensity transmitted by the solution under analysis and I_0 is the intensity transmitted by the pure solvent or other reference solution. Symbol *A*. Formerly referred to as *absorbancy* or *optical density.* 2. in radiation physics, the negative logarithm of the transmittance, defined as the ratio of the radiant energy transmitted by an object (I) to the incident radiant energy (I_0).

ab•sor•ban•cy (ab-sor′bən-se) absorbance.

ab•sor•be•fa•cient (ab-sor″bə-fa′shənt) [L. *absorbere* to absorb + *facient*] 1. causing or promoting absorption. 2. absorbent (def. 3).

ab•sor•bent (ab-sor′bənt) [*ab-* + *sorbent*] 1. able to take in, or suck up and incorporate. 2. a tissue structure involved in absorption. 3. a substance that absorbs or promotes absorption.

ab•sorp•ti•om•e•ter (ab-sorp″she-om′ə-tər) [*absorption* + *-meter*] 1. an instrument for measuring the solubility of gas in a liquid. 2. a device for measuring the layer of liquid absorbed between two glass plates; used as a hematoscope.

ab•sorp•ti•om•e•try (ab-sorp″she-om′ə-tre) in radiology, the measurement of the degree to which the radiation emitted by a radioisotope is completely dissipated within a tissue.

dual energy x-ray a. (DEXA) an imaging technique that uses two low-dose x-ray beams with different levels of energy to produce a detailed image of body components; used primarily to measure bone mineral density.

dual photon a. measurement of the bone mineral content in the axial skeleton, particularly the lumbar spine, by comparing transmission of the two separate photoelectric energy peaks emitted by gadolinium 153 through both soft and bone tissues.

ab•sorp•tion (ab-sorp′shən) [L. *absorptio*] 1. the uptake of substances into or across tissues such as the skin, intestine, or renal tubules. 2. in psychology, devotion of thought to one object or activity, with inattention to others. 3. radiation a. 4. in chemistry, the penetration of a substance within the inner structure of another. Cf. *adsorption.*

agglutinin a. the removal of antibody from an immune serum by treatment with particulate antigen (usually bacteria) homologous to that antibody, followed by separation of the antigen-antibody complex.

chemical a. absorption (def. 4).

digestive a. the passage of the end products of digestion from the gastrointestinal tract into the blood and lymphatic vessels and the cells of tissues; this can take place by either diffusion or active transport.

enteral a. intestinal a.

external a. the absorption of foods, poisons, or other agents through the skin or mucous membrane.

internal a. digestive absorption.

interstitial a. removal of waste matter by the absorbent system.

intestinal a. the uptake from the intestinal lumen of fluids, solutes, proteins, fats, and other nutrients into the intestinal epithelial cells, blood, lymph, or interstitial fluids of the intestine.

net a. the difference between uptake and efflux from a tissue or cell.

parenteral a. absorption otherwise than through the digestive tract.

radiation a. the taking up of energy by matter with which the radiation interacts. Cf. *attenuation* (def. 3).

ab•sorp•tive (ab-sorp′tiv) capable of absorbing; absorbent; pertaining to absorption.

ab•sorp•tiv•i•ty (ab″sorp-tiv′ĭ-te) a measure of the amount of light absorbed by a solution, defined as the absorbance per unit concentration per unit length of light path. By Beer's law (q.v.) absorptivity is proportional to the concentration of the absorbing solute. Called also *absorbancy index, absorption constant, absorption coefficient,* and *extinction coefficient.*

molar a. (ε) absorptivity defined in terms of concentrations expressed in moles per liter.

specific a. (a) absorptivity defined in terms of concentrations expressed in grams per liter.

abst abstract.

ab•sti•nence (ab′sti-nəns) a refraining from the use of or indulgence in food, stimulants, or sexual activity.

periodic a. rhythm method.

abstr abstract.

ab•stract (ab′strakt) [L. *abstractum*, from *abstrahere* to draw off] a summary or epitome of a book, paper, or case history.

ab•strac•tion (ab-strak′shən) [L. *abstractus*, past part. of *abstrahere* to draw away] 1. the withdrawal of any ingredient from a compound. 2. a condition in which the teeth or other maxillary and mandibular structures are lower than the normal position, away from the occlusal plane, thereby lengthening the face. Cf. *attraction* (def. 2).

ab•ter•min•al (ab-tur′mĭ-nəl) [*ab-* + L. *terminus* end] moving from the end toward the center; said of electric currents in muscle.

ab•tor•sion (ab-tor′shən) extorsion.

abu•lia (ə-boo′le-ə) [*a-*[1] + Gr. *boulē* will + *-ia*] 1. lack of will or willpower; inability to make decisions. 2. akinetic mutism that is less than total. Called also *aboulia.* **abu′lic** *adj*

abuse (ə-būs′) misuse or wrong use, particularly excessive use of anything.

child a. physical, emotional, or sexual abuse of children, usually by parents, relatives, or caretakers. See also *battered-child syndrome,* under *syndrome.*

drug a. substance a.

physical a. any act resulting in a nonaccidental physical injury, including not only intentional assault but also the result of unreasonable punishment.

psychoactive substance a. substance a.

sexual a. any act of a sexual nature performed in a criminal manner, as with a child or with a nonconsenting adult, including rape, incest, sodomy, oral copulation, and penetration of genital or anal opening with a foreign object; also included are lewd and lascivious acts with a child or any sexual act which could be expected to irritate, trouble or offend a child performed by one motivated by an abnormal sexual interest in children, as well as acts related to sexual exploitation of children, including activities related to pornography or prostitution involving minors and coercion of minors to perform obscene acts.

substance a. [DSM-IV] a substance use disorder characterized by the use of a mood- or behavior-altering substance in a maladaptive pattern resulting in significant impairment or distress, such as failure to fulfill social or occupational obligations or recurrent use in situations in which it is physically dangerous to do so or which end in legal problems, but without fulfilling the criteria for substance dependence (q.v.). Specific disorders are named for their etiology, e.g., alcohol abuse, anabolic steroid abuse. DSM-IV includes specific abuse disorders for alcohol, amphetamines or similar substances, cannabis, cocaine, hallucinogens, inhalants, opioids, PCP or similar substances, and sedatives, hypnotics, or anxiolytics.

abut (ə-but′) to touch, adjoin, or border upon.

abut•ment (ə-but′mənt) 1. that on which or at which abutting occurs. 2. a part of a structure that sustains thrust or pressure. 3. a tooth or root used as an anchorage for either a fixed or a removable dental prosthesis, or any other device serving the same purpose. See also under *tooth.*

auxiliary a. secondary a.

implant a. the part of a subperiosteal, intraperiosteal, or intraosseous implant that protrudes into the oral cavity and serves as an abutment for retaining and stabilizing a denture.

intermediate a. a natural tooth or root, without other natural teeth in proximal contact, that is used as an abutment, in addition to two terminal abutments. Called also *pier.*

isolated a. an intermediate abutment, particularly one used to support a removable partial denture.

multiple a. an abutment resulting from the fixed splinting of two or more adjacent natural teeth to serve as a unit in the support and retention of a fixed or removable partial denture.

primary a. a tooth used for direct support of a denture.

secondary a. a natural tooth used in addition to the primary abutments to provide support or indirect retention for a removable partial denture; called also *auxiliary a.*

terminal a. a natural tooth located at an extremity of a fixed partial denture and used for the support and retention of the prosthesis.

ABVD a cancer chemotherapy regimen consisting of Adriamycin (doxorubicin), bleomycin, vinblastine, and dacarbazine, used for treatment of Hodgkin disease.

AC 1. acromioclavicular; air conduction; alternating current; axiocervical. 2. a cancer chemotherapy regimen consisting of Adriamycin (doxorubicin) and cyclophosphamide.

Ac actinium.

a.c. [L.] an′te ci′bum (before meals).

ACA American College of Angiology; American College of Apothecaries.

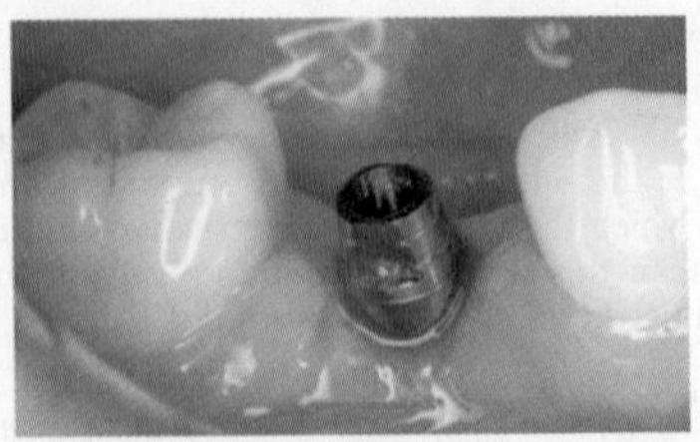

■ Implant abutment.

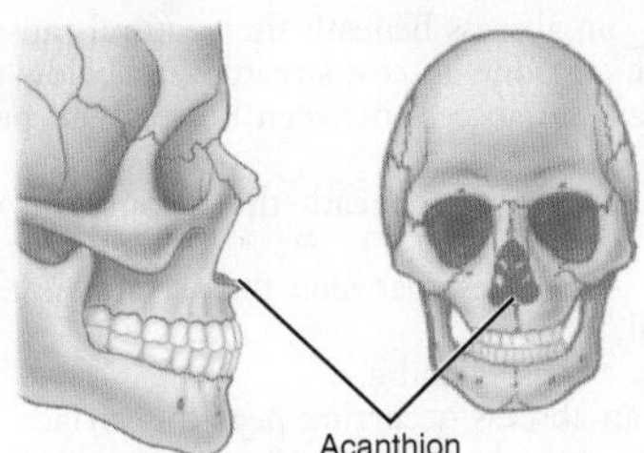

Aca•cia (ə-ka′shə) [L., from Gr. *akakia*] a genus of shrubs and trees of the family Leguminosae. *A. ca′na* is a selenium accumulator that can cause selenium poisoning in livestock. *A. ca′techu* Willd. is a small tree native to India and Burma that yields catechu. *A. georgi′nae* F. M. Bail. is an Australian tree whose leaves can cause fatal fluoroacetate poisoning in livestock. *A. se′negal* is an African tree that yields acacia (gum arabic).

aca•cia (ə-ka′shə) 1. a plant of the genus *Acacia.* 2. [NF] the dried, gummy exudate from the stems and branches of *Acacia senegal,* occurring as spheroids, flakes, powder, granules, or spray-dried acacia and prepared as a mucilage or syrup; used as a suspending agent, emollient, and demulcent in pharmaceutical preparations. Called also *gum arabic.*

acal•cu•lia (a″kal-ku′le-ə) [*a-*[1] + L. *calculare* to reckon + *-ia*] inability to do simple arithmetical calculations. Cf. *dyscalculia.*

ACAM2000 (ak′am) trademark for a preparation of smallpox vaccine.

acam•pro•sate cal•ci•um (ə-kam′pro-sāt) a synthetic compound used for the maintenance of abstinence from alcohol in the treatment of alcoholism, administered orally. Although its mechanism of action is uncertain, it is believed to interact with biochemical systems altered in alcoholism to restore the normal balance between neuronal excitation and inhibition.

acamp•sia (ə-kamp′se-ə) [*a-*[1] + Gr. *kamptein* to bend + *-ia*] rigidity or inflexibility of a part or of a joint.

acan•tha (ə-kan′thə) [Gr. *akantha* thorn] 1. spina (def. 1). 2. processus spinosus vertebrae.

acan•tha•ceous (ak″an-tha′shəs) bearing prickles or spines.

acan•tha•me•bi•a•sis (ə-kan″thə-me-bi′ə-sis) infection with a species of *Acanthamoeba;* the most common manifestations are granulomatous amebic encephalitis and *Acanthamoeba* keratitis.

Acan•tha•moe•ba (ə-kan″thə-me′bə) [*acanth-* + *amoeba*] a genus of free-living ameboid protozoa of the order Centramoebida found usually in fresh water or moist soil. Certain species, such as *A. astronyxis, A. castellanii, A. culbertsoni, A. hatchetti, A. polyphaga,* and *A. rhysodes,* may occur as human pathogens. See also *acanthamebiasis.*

Acan•thas•ter (a″kan-thas′tər) a genus of starfish. *A. plan′ci* is the crown-of-thorns starfish, a venomous species.

acan•thes•the•sia (ə-kan″thes-the′zhə) [*acanth-* + *esthesia*] perverted sensibility with a feeling as of pressure of a sharp point.

Acan•thia lec•tu•la•ria (ə-kan′the-ə lek″too-lar′e-ə) *Cimex lectularius.*

acan•thi•on (ə-kan′the-on) [Gr. *akanthion* little thorn] a point at the tip of the anterior nasal spine.

acanth(o)- [Gr. *akantha,* thorn] a combining form meaning thorny or spiny, or denoting a relationship to a sharp spine or thorn.

Acan•tho•bdel•lid•ea (ə-kan″tho-dĕ-lid′e-ə) an order of leeches of the class Hirudinea, which have spines on the surface of the body.

Acan•tho•ceph•a•la (ə-kan″tho-sef′ə-lə) [*acantho-* + Gr. *kephalē* head] the thorny-headed worms, a phylum of parasites often infesting animals, so called because of the proboscis projecting anteriorly that is covered with thornlike spines for attachment to the digestive tract of the host. In some systems of classification, they are considered to be a class of the phylum Nemathelminthes.

acan•tho•ceph•a•lan (ə-kan″tho-sef′ə-lən) any individual of the phylum Acanthocephala; called also *thorny-headed worm.*

acan•tho•ceph•a•li•a•sis (ə-kan″tho-sef″ə-li′ə-sis) infestation of the intestine of a vertebrate with any species of the phylum Acanthocephala.

acan•tho•ceph•a•lous (ə-kan″tho-sef′ə-ləs) pertaining to or caused by worms of the phylum Acanthocephala.

Acan•tho•ceph•a•lus (ə-kan″tho-sef′ə-ləs) a genus of worms of the phylum Acanthocephala; some species are parasitic in fish.

Acan•tho•chei•lo•ne•ma (ə-kan″tho-ki″lo-ne′mə) a genus of filarial nematodes, of unclear status, closely related to *Mansonella.* The species

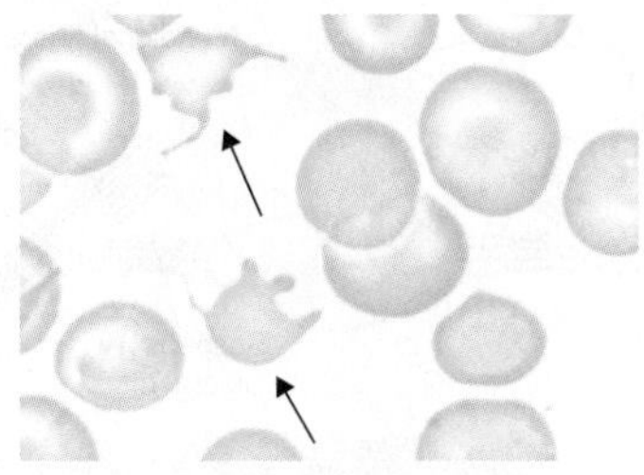

■ Acanthocytes *(arrows).*

A. per'stans and *A. streptocer'ca* have both been reclassified as species of *Mansonella.*

acan•tho•chei•lo•ne•mi•a•sis (ə-kan″tho-ki″lo-ne-mi′ə-sis) infection with a species of *Acanthocheilonema*, having symptoms similar to those of mansonellosis.

acan•tho•cyte (ə-kan′tho-sīt) [*acantho-* + *-cyte*] a spiculed erythrocyte with five to ten spiny protoplasmic projections of varying lengths distributed irregularly over its surface; seen in abetalipoproteinemia, malnutrition, liver diseases, and a few other conditions. Called also *acanthrocyte* and *spur cell.*

acan•tho•cy•to•sis (ə-kan″tho-si-to′sis) [*acanthocyte* + *-osis*] 1. the presence of acanthocytes in the blood. 2. abetalipoproteinemia.

acan•thoid (ə-kan′thoid) [*acanth-* + *-oid*] resembling a spine; spinous.

acan•thol•y•sis (ak″an-thol′ĭ-sis) [*acantho-* + *-lysis*] disruption of the intercellular connections between keratinocytes of the epidermis. A primary type is caused by lysis of intercellular cement substance, and secondary types occur with conditions such as types of pemphigus or dyskeratosis. There is often secondary disruption of desmosomes, as well as a defined sequence of cellular degenerative events. **acantholyt′ic** *adj*

ac•an•tho•ma (ak″an-tho′mə) pl. *acanthomas, acantho′mata* [*acanth-* + *-oma*] a tumor composed of epidermal or squamous cells.
  a. adenoi′des cys′ticum multiple trichoepithelioma.
  clear cell a., Degos a. an erythematous, dome-shaped plaque or papule, with some crusting or scaling, usually found on the lower leg in older adults; it is characterized by acanthotic epithelium containing large, pale, glycogen-rich squamous cells.
  a. fissura′tum a benign, firm, skin-colored or erythematous nodule, grossly resembling basal cell epithelioma, occurring on the bridge of the nose or behind the ear, resulting from constant minor mechanical trauma caused by poorly fitting glasses. Called also *granuloma fissuratum.*
  pilar sheath a. a benign tumor of the hair follicle, usually occurring as an asymptomatic lesion on the upper lip of middle-aged adults; it is characterized by a central keratin-filled cavity lined by stratified squamous epithelium that projects into the connective stroma.

Acan•tho•pa•ryph•i•um (ə-kan″tho-pə-rif′e-əm) [*acantho-* + Gr. *paryphē* border] a genus of trematodes of the family Echinostomatidae.
  A. tyrosenen′se a species originally seen as an intestinal parasite of birds; it causes human intestinal infections in Korea, with salt water mollusks as the vector.

acan•tho•pel•vis (ə-kan″tho-pel′vis) [*acantho-* + *pelvis*] a pelvis with a sharp, prominent pubic crest.

Acan•tho•phis (ə-kan′tho-fis) a genus of snakes of the family Elapidae. *A. antarc′ticus* is the death adder of Australia and New Guinea. See table at *snake.*

Acan•tho•po•di•na (ə-kan″tho-po-di′nə) [*acantho-* + Gr. *pous* foot] a suborder of ramicristate amebae that have finely tipped, filiform, or furcate hyaline subpseudopodia produced from a broad hyaline lobe.

acan•tho•po•di•um (ə-kan″tho-po′de-əm) *pl.* acanthopo′dia. A thornlike or spikelike pseudopodium occurring on trophozoites of the genus *Acanthamoeba.*

ac•an•tho•sis (ak″an-tho′sis) [*acanth-* + *-osis*] diffuse hyperplasia of the spinous layer of the skin. Called also *hyperacanthosis.*
  a. ni′gricans diffuse velvety acanthosis with dark pigmentation, found in areas of body folds such as the axillae or groin. One type in adults accompanies internal carcinomas and is called *malignant acanthosis nigricans.* There is also a benign, nevoid form in adults that is more or less generalized and may accompany endocrine disturbances. A benign form seen in children is called *pseudoacanthosis nigricans.*

ac•an•thot•ic (ak″an-thot′ik) marked by acanthosis.

acan•thro•cyte (ə-kan′thro-sīt) acanthocyte.

acan•thro•cy•to•sis (ə-kan″thro-si-to′sis) acanthocytosis.

a ca•pi•te ad cal•cem (a cap′ĭ-te ad kal′sem) [L.] from head to heel, the classic order for describing symptoms.

Aca•ra•pis (a-kar′ə-pis) a genus of mites. *A. woo′di* is a tracheal mite of the honeybee, the cause of Isle of Wight disease.

acar•bose (a′kahr-bōs) an α-glucosidase inhibitor produced by fermentation by *Actinoplanes utahensis,* used as an antihyperglycemic agent in treatment of type 2 diabetes mellitus; administered orally.

acar•dia (a-kahr′de-ə) [*a-*[1] + Gr. *kardia* heart] congenital absence of the heart.

acar•di•ac (a-kahr′de-ak) having no heart.

acar•di•a•cus (a″kahr-di′ə-kus) acardius.

acar•di•us (a-kahr′de-əs) [*a-*[1] + *cardia*] an imperfectly formed free twin fetus, lacking a heart and invariably lacking other body parts as well; called also *fetus acardiacus.*
  a. ace′phalus holoacardius acephalus.
  a. acor′mus holoacardius acormus.
  a. amor′phus holoacardius amorphus.
  a. an′ceps hemiacardius.

aca•ri (ak′ə-ri) [L.] plural of *acarus.*

acar•i•an (ə-kar′e-ən) pertaining to the acarids or mites.

ac•a•ri•a•sis (ak″ə-ri′ə-sis) [*acar-* + *-iasis*] infestation with acarids (ticks or mites); see also *mange.* Called also *acaridiasis* and *acarinosis.*
  chorioptic a. see under *mange.*
  demodectic a. see under *mange.*
  nasal a. infestation of the nasal cavity or sinuses of a dog by the nasal mite *Pneumonyssus caninum,* which causes mild rhinitis.

acar•i•cide (ə-kar′ĭ-sīd) [*acari* + *-cide*] 1. destructive to mites. 2. an agent that destroys mites.

ac•a•rid (ak′ə-rid) 1. a mite or tick of the order Acarina. 2. a mite of the family Acaridae.

Acar•i•dae (ə-kar′ĭ-de) a family of small mites. Genera of medical interest include *Acarus* and *Tyrophagus.* Several species cause skin rashes, such as grocers' itch, copra itch, and vanillism.

acar•i•dan (ə-kar′ĭ-dən) acarid.

acar•i•di•a•sis (ə-kar″ĭ-di′ə-sis) acariasis.

Ac•a•ri•na (ak″ə-ri′nə) an order of arthropods of the class Arachnida, including the ticks and mites.

ac•a•rine (ak′ə-rīn) acarid (def.1).

acar•i•no•sis (ə-kar″ĭ-no′sis) acariasis.

acar•i•o•sis (ə-kar″e-o′sis) acariasis.

acar(o)- [L. *Acarus* a genus of mites, from Gr. *akari*] a combining form denoting relationship to mites.

ac•a•ro•der•ma•ti•tis (ak″ə-ro-dur″mə-ti′tis) any skin inflammation caused by mites.
  a. urticarioi′des grain itch.

ac•a•roid (ak′ə-roid) [Gr. *akari* a mite + *eidos* form] resembling a mite.

ac•a•rol•o•gist (ak″ə-rol′ə-jist) a specialist in acarology.

ac•a•rol•o•gy (ak″ə-rol′ə-je) [*acaro-* + *-logy*] the scientific study of mites and ticks.

ac•a•ro•pho•bia (ak″ə-ro-fo′be-ə) [*acaro-* + *-phobia*] irrational fear of mites or of other minute animate (insects, worms) or inanimate (pins, needles) objects, sometimes accompanied by fear of parasites crawling beneath the skin.

Acar•to•myia (ə-kar″to-mi′yə) a genus of culicine mosquitoes.

Ac•a•rus (ak′ə-rəs) [L., from Gr. *akari* a mite] a genus of small mites of the family Acaridae. They are often ectoparasitic, causing itch, mange, and other skin diseases.
  A. folliculo′rum *Demodex folliculorum.*
  A. galli′nae *Dermanyssus gallinae.*
  A. hor′dei the barley bug, a mite that burrows under the skin.
  A. rhyzoglyp′ticus hyacin′thi the onion mite, which is found on decaying onions and produces onion mite dermatitis in persons who handle them.
  A. si′ro a mite that causes vanillism in vanilla pod handlers; called also *Tyrophagus siro* and *Tyroglyphus siro.*

ac•a•rus (ak′ə-rəs) pl. *a′cari* [L.] mite.

ACAT acyl CoA:cholesterol acyltransferase; see *sterol* O*-acyltransferase.*

acat•a•la•se•mia (a″kat-ə-la-se′me-ə) acatalasia.

acat•a•la•sia (a″kat-ə-la′zhə) a rare autosomal recessive disorder (gene locus: 11p13) due to virtual absence of catalase activity, observed mainly in Japan and Switzerland. It is usually asymptomatic, but in approximately 50 per cent of the Japanese cases it is characterized by a syndrome of oral ulcerations and gangrene and is called also *Takahara disease.* See also *hypocatalasia.*

ac·a·thex·is (ak″ə-thek′sis) [*a-*[1] + Gr. *kathexis* a retention] a lack of the emotional charge (cathexis) with which an object or idea would normally be invested; detachment of feelings from thoughts and ideas.

ac·a·this·ia (ak″ə-thĭ′zhə) akathisia.

acau·dal (a-kaw′dəl) acaudate.

acau·date (a-kaw′dāt) [*a-*[1] + *caudate*] lacking a tail.

ACC American College of Cardiology.

Acc accommodation.

ac·cel·er·ant (ak-sel′ər-ənt) a catalyst.

ac·cel·er·a·tion (ak-sel″ər-a′shən) [L. *acceleratio,* from *ad-* intensification + *celerare* to quicken] 1. a quickening, as of the pulse rate or respiration. 2. in physics, the time rate of change of velocity; symbol *a.*

a. of gravity standard gravity.

negative a. a slowing.

psychomotor a. generalized physical and emotional overactivity in response to internal and external stimuli, such as that seen in the manic phase of bipolar disorder.

ac·cel·er·a·tor (ak-sel′ər-a″tər) [L. "hastener"] 1. an agent or apparatus that is used to increase the rate at which an object proceeds or a substance acts or at which some reaction occurs. 2. any nerve or muscle which hastens the performance of a function. 3. any of a group of chemicals used in the vulcanization of rubber or other polymerization reactions; they frequently cause dermatitis in workers.

linear a. an accelerator that propels high-energy particles in a linear beam, using energy from an electromagnetic field; its medical use is in radiotherapy to penetrate tissue and minimize the radiation dose at the surface of the body.

particle a. an apparatus that accelerates charged particles to such high speeds that when they bombard a target they cause nuclear reactions.

serum prothrombin conversion a. (SPCA) factor VII; see under *coagulation factors,* at *factor.*

a. uri′nae musculus bulbospongiosus.

ac·cel·er·in (ak-sel′ər-in) factor VI, formerly considered to be one of the coagulation factors (q.v.).

ac·cel·er·om·e·ter (ak-sel″ər-om′ĕ-tər) an instrument for measuring the acceleration (rate of change of velocity) of an object.

ac·cen·tu·a·tion (ak-sen″choo-a′shən) [L. *accentus* accent] increased loudness or distinctness; intensification.

ac·cep·tor (ak-sep′tər) a substance which unites with another substance; specifically a substance which unites with hydrogen or oxygen in an oxidoreduction reaction and so enables the reaction to proceed. Cf. *donor.*

hydrogen a. in oxidation and reduction occurring anaerobically in body tissue, the substance that is reduced.

ac·cess (ak′ses) [L. *accessus,* past part. of *accedere* to approach] a means of approaching something.

arteriovenous a. a tube that begins at an artery and ends at a vein, the usual means of vascular access for hemodialysis apparatus to blood vessels; see also *arteriovenous fistula* and *arteriovenous shunt.*

hemodialysis a., hemodialysis vascular a., vascular a. a tube connecting two parts of the circulatory system to provide access for hemodialysis; the usual method is arteriovenous access, although in some cases venovenous access is used.

venovenous a. a tube that begins at a vein and ends at a vein, used as vascular access in hemodialysis and continuous venovenous hemofiltration.

ac·ces·si·flex·or (ak-ses′ə-flek″sər) any accessory flexor muscle.

ac·ces·sion·al (ak-sesh′ən-əl) [L. *accessus,* past part. of *accedere* to approach] pertaining to that which has been added or acquired.

ac·ces·so·ri·us (ak″ses-o′re-əs) [L. "supplementary"] accessory; used in naming certain structures thought to serve a supplementary function.

ac·ces·so·ry (ak-ses′ə-re) [L. *accessorius*] supplementary or affording aid to another similar and generally more important thing; complementary; concomitant.

ac·ci·dent (ak′sĭ-dənt) an unforeseen occurrence, especially one of an injurious character; an unexpected complicating occurrence in the regular course of a disease.

cerebrovascular a. stroke syndrome.

ac·ci·den·tal (ak″sĭ-den′təl) 1. occurring by chance, unexpectedly, or unintentionally. 2. nonessential; not innate or intrinsic.

ac·ci·dent prone (ak′sĭ-dənt prōn) specially susceptible to accidents owing to psychological factors.

ac·cli·ma·ta·tion (ə-kli″mə-ta′shən) acclimation.

ac·cli·ma·tion (ak″lĭ-ma′shən) physiological or psychological adjustment to a new environment. Called also *acclimatation* and *acclimatization.*

ac·cli·ma·ti·za·tion (ə-kli″mə-tĭ-za′shən) acclimation.

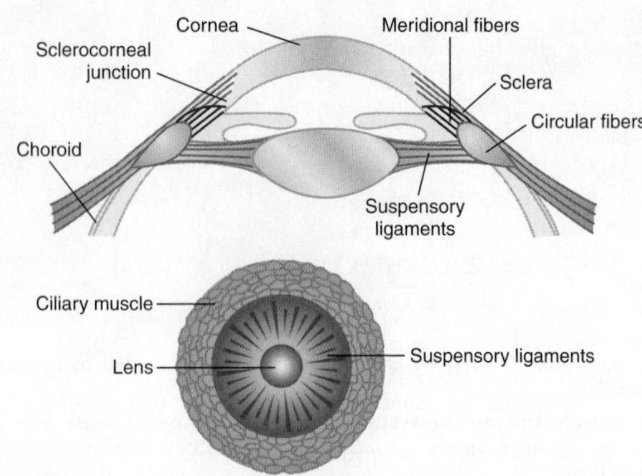

■ Structures involved in accommodation of the lens; tension on the suspensory ligaments works to keep the lens relatively flat whereas the meridional and circular fibers of the ciliary muscle counteract the pull of the ligaments and when contracted allow the lens to assume a more spherical shape.

Ac·co·late (ak′ə-lāt) trademark for a preparation of zafirlukast.

ac·colé (ah-ko-la′) see *appliqué form,* under *form.*

ac·com·mo·da·tion (ə-kom″ə-da′shən) [L. *accommodare* to adjust to] 1. adjustment, especially that of the position and shape of the lens of the eye for focusing at various distances (see illustration). Symbol A or a. 2. nerve a.

absolute a. the accommodation of either eye separately.

binocular a. accommodation in both eyes in coordination with convergence.

excessive a. accommodation of the eye that is continually above the normal.

histologic a. a group of changes in the morphology and function of cells following changed conditions.

negative a. adjustment of the eye for focusing at long distances by relaxation of the ciliary muscle.

nerve a. the rise in the threshold during the passage of a constant, direct electric current because of which only the make and break of the current stimulates the nerve.

positive a. adjustment of the eye for focusing at short distances by contraction of the ciliary muscle.

relative a. the change in accommodation that is possible with a fixed amount of convergence.

subnormal a. insufficient power of accommodation of the eye.

ac·com·mo·da·tive (ə-kom′ə-da″tiv) pertaining to, of the nature of, or affecting accommodation.

ac·com·mo·dom·e·ter (ə-kom″ə-dom′ĕ-tər) [*accommodation* + *-meter*] a device for measuring the accommodative capacity of the eye.

ac·com·plice (ah-kom-plēs′) [Fr.] a bacterium which accompanies the chief infecting agent in a mixed infection and which influences the virulence of the chief organism.

ac·couche·ment (ah-ko͞osh-maw′) [Fr.] 1. childbirth. 2. delivery.

a. forcé (for-sa′) ["forced delivery"] rapid forcible delivery from below by any one of several methods; originally applied to rapid dilation of the cervix with the hands, followed immediately by version and extraction of the fetus.

ac·cou·cheur (ah-koo-shur′) [Fr.] obstetrician.

ac·cou·cheuse (ah-koo-shooz′) [Fr.] midwife.

ACCP American College of Chest Physicians.

ac·cre·men·ti·tion (ak″rə-men-tish′ən) [L. *ad-* to + *crementum* increase] growth or increase by the addition of similar tissue.

ac·cre·tio (ə-kre′she-o) [L.] abnormal adhesion of parts normally separate.

a. cor′dis, a. pericar′dii a form of adhesive pericarditis in which adhesions extend from the pericardium to the pleurae, diaphragm, and chest wall.

ac·cre·tion (ə-kre′shən) [L. *ad-* to + *crescere* to grow] 1. growth by addition of material. 2. accumulation. 3. adherence of parts normally separated.

ac·cum·bens (ă-kum′bens) [L., pres. part. of *accumbere* to recline] nucleus accumbens.

Ac·cu·Neb (ak′u-neb) trademark for preparations of albuterol sulfate.

Ac·cu·pril (ak′u-pril″) trademark for a preparation of quinapril hydrochloride.

ac·cu·ra·cy (ak′u-rə-se) the closeness of the expected value to the true value of the measured or estimated quantity; a measure that depends on both precision and bias. Cf. *precision* (def. 1).

Ac·cu·ret·ic (ak″u-ret′ik) trademark for a combination preparation of quinapril hydrochloride and hydrochlorothiazide.

Ac·cu·tane (ak′u-tān″) trademark for a preparation of isotretinoin.

Ac·cu·zyme (ak′u-zīm) trademark for a combination preparation of papain and urea.

ACD acid citrate dextrose; see *anticoagulant citrate dextrose solution*, under *solution*.

ACE American College of Endocrinology; angiotensin-converting enzyme; see *peptidyl-dipeptidase A*.

ac·e·bu·to·lol (as″ə-bu′tə-lol) a cardioselective β_1-adrenergic blocking agent with intrinsic sympathomimetic activity; its uses are similar to those of propranolol.

a. **hydrochloride** [USP] the hydrochloride salt of acebutolol, used for the treatment of hypertension, angina pectoris, and arrhythmias; administered orally.

acec·li·dine (ə-sek′lĭ-dēn) a synthetic cholinergic agonist similar to the natural alkaloids arecoline and pilocarpine; used to reduce intraocular pressure in glaucoma.

ace·clo·fen·ac (ə-se′klo-fen″ak) a nonsteroidal antiinflammatory drug chemically related to diclofenac, used in treatment of osteoarthritis, rheumatoid arthritis, and ankylosing spondylitis.

acel·lu·lar (a-sel′u-lər) not made up of or containing cells.

ace·lo·mate (a-se′lə-māt) not having a coelom or body cavity.

ace·lous (a-se′ləs) [*a-*[1] + *cel-*[2] + *-ous*] not concave on either surface; said of the vertebral centra of certain animals.

ace·nes·the·sia (a-sēn″es-the′zhə) [*a-*[1] + *cenesthesia*] absence of the normal sense of physical existence and well-being and of the regular functioning of the bodily organs.

ace·no·cou·ma·rol (ə-se″no-koo′mə-rol) a coumarin derivative used as an oral anticoagulant; it acts by inhibiting the hepatic synthesis of vitamin K–dependent coagulation factors (prothrombin and factors VII, IX, and X) and proteins C and S.

acen·tric (a-sen′trik) [Gr. *akentrikos* not centric] 1. not central; not located in the center. 2. a chromosome lacking a centromere, so that the chromosome will not survive subsequent cell divisions.

Ace·on (a′se-on) trademark for a preparation of perindopril erbumine.

ACEP American College of Emergency Physicians.

ace·pha·lia (a″sĕ-fa′le-ə) [*a-*[1] + *cephal-* + *-ia*] congenital absence of the head.

aceph·a·lo·bra·chia (a-sef″ə-lo-bra′ke-ə) [*a-*[1] + *cephalo-* + *brachia*] congenital absence of the head and upper limbs.

aceph·a·lo·bra·chi·us (a-sef″ə-lo-bra′ke-us) a fetus exhibiting acephalobrachia.

aceph·a·lo·car·dia (a-sef″ə-lo-kahr′de-ə) [*a-*[1] + *cephalo-* + *cardia*] congenital absence of the head and heart.

aceph·a·lo·car·di·us (a-sef″ə-lo-kahr′de-us) a fetus exhibiting acephalocardia.

aceph·a·lo·chi·ria (a-sef″ə-lo-ki′re-ə) [*a-*[1] + *cephalo* + *chir-* + *-ia*] congenital absence of the head and hands.

aceph·a·lo·chi·rus (a-sef″ə-lo-ki′rəs) a fetus exhibiting acephalochiria.

aceph·a·lo·cyst (a-sef′ə-lo-sist″) [*a-*[1] + *cephalo-* + *cyst*] a true hydatid cyst that fails to produce brood capsules; called also *sterile cyst*.

aceph·a·lo·gas·ter (a-sef″ə-lo-gas′tər) [*a-*[1] + *cephalo-* + *gaster*] a fetus exhibiting acephalogastria.

aceph·a·lo·gas·tria (a-sef″ə-lo-gas′tre-ə) congenital absence of the head, thorax, and upper part of the abdomen.

aceph·a·lo·po·dia (a-sef″ə-lo-po′de-ə) [*a-*[1] + *cephalo-* + *pod-* + *-ia*] congenital absence of the head and feet.

aceph·a·lo·po·di·us (a-sef″ə-lo-po′de-us) a fetus exhibiting acephalopodia.

aceph·a·lo·rha·chia (a-sef″ə-lo-ra′ke-ə) [*a-*[1] + *cephalo-* + *rhachi-* + *-ia*] congenital absence of the head and vertebral column.

aceph·a·lo·sto·mia (a-sef″ə-lo-sto′me-ə) [*a-*[1] + *cephalo-* + *stom-* + *-ia*] congenital absence of the head, but having a mouthlike structure on the superior aspect of the fetus.

aceph·a·los·to·mus (a-sef″ə-los′tə-məs) a fetus exhibiting acephalostomia.

aceph·a·lo·tho·ra·cia (a-sef″ə-lo-tho-ra′se-ə) [*a-*[1] + *cephalo-* + *thorac-* + *-ia*] congenital absence of the head and thorax.

aceph·a·lo·tho·rus (a-sef″ə-lo-tho′rəs) a fetus exhibiting acephalothoracia.

aceph·a·lous (a-sef′ə-ləs) headless.

aceph·a·lus (a-sef′ə-ləs) pl. *aceph′ali* [*a-*[1] + *-cephalus*] a headless fetus.

a. **dibra′chius** an acephalus with both upper limbs more or less undeveloped.

a. **di′pus** an acephalus with both lower limbs more or less undeveloped.

a. **monobra′chius** an acephalus with only one upper limb.

a. **mo′nopus** an acephalus with only one foot or lower limb.

a. **parace′phalus** a fetus with a partially formed cranium but no brain.

a. **sym′pus** an acephalus with the two lower limbs fused into one.

aceph·a·ly (a-sef′ə-le) acephalia.

ac·e·pro·ma·zine maleate (as″ə-pro′mə-zēn) [USP] a tranquilizer used in veterinary medicine to immobilize large animals.

Acer (a′sər) the maples, a genus of flowering trees and shrubs of the family Aceraceae. *A. ru′brum* is the red or swamp maple, whose wilted or dry leaves can cause hemolytic anemia in livestock.

Ace·ra·ria (as″ə-rar′e-ə) a genus of nematodes. *A. spira′lis* parasitizes the esophagus of fowls.

ace·ro·la (ă-sə-ro′lə) 1. any of various species of trees of the genus *Malpighia*, especially *M. glabra*, *M. punicifolia*, or *M. urens*. 2. the fruit of these trees, one of the richest natural sources of vitamin C (about 1690 mg per 100 g of pitted fruit); it can be used in the diet of individuals allergic to citrus fruits. Called also *Barbados cherry*.

acer·vu·line (ə-sur′vu-līn) [L. *acervulus* little heap] aggregated; said of certain glands.

acer·vu·lus (ə-sur′vu-ləs) pl. *acer′vuli* [L., dim. of *acervus* a heap] in Fungi Imperfecti, a conidioma with a saucer-shaped surface where conidia form underneath a dome of tissue that ruptures at maturity to release the conidia.

ac·e·tab·u·la (as″ə-tab′u-lə) plural of *acetabulum*.

Ace·ta·bu·la·ria (as″ə-tab″u-lar′e-ə) a genus of large unicellular green algae having a giant single nucleus. Inter- and intraspecies grafting and other genetic experiments have been used to study the morphogenetic influences of nuclear and cytoplasmic information, and their interplay.

ac·e·tab·u·lec·to·my (as″ə-tab″u-lek′tə-me) [*acetabulum* + *-ectomy*] excision of the acetabulum.

ac·e·tab·u·lo·plas·ty (as″ə-tab′u-lo-plas″te) [*acetabulum* + *-plasty*] plastic reconstruction of the acetabulum. **acetabuloplas′tic** *adj*

ac·e·tab·u·lum (as″ə-tab′u-ləm) pl. *acetab′ula* [L. "vinegar-cruet," from *acetum* vinegar] [TA] the large cup-shaped cavity on the lateral surface of the os coxae in which the head of the femur articulates; called also *acetabular bone*, *cotyloid cavity*, and *os acetabuli*. **acetab′ular** *adj*

sunken a. Otto pelvis.

Ace·ta·dote (ə-se′tə-dōt) trademark for a preparation of acetylcysteine.

ac·e·tal (as′ə-təl) 1. any of a class of organic compounds of the formula $RCH(OR')_2$, where R and R′ are organic radicals, formed by combination of an aldehyde molecule with two alcohol molecules. 2. $CH_3CH(OC_2H_5)_2$, a colorless volatile liquid used as a solvent and in cosmetics.

ac·et·al·de·hyde (as″ət-al′də-hīd″) a colorless flammable liquid with a pungent odor, used in the manufacture of acetic acid, perfumes, and flavors. It is also an intermediate in the metabolism of alcohol. If ingested, it may cause irritation of mucous membranes, lacrimation, photophobia, conjunctivitis, corneal injury, rhinitis, anosmia, bronchitis, pneumonia, pleurisy,

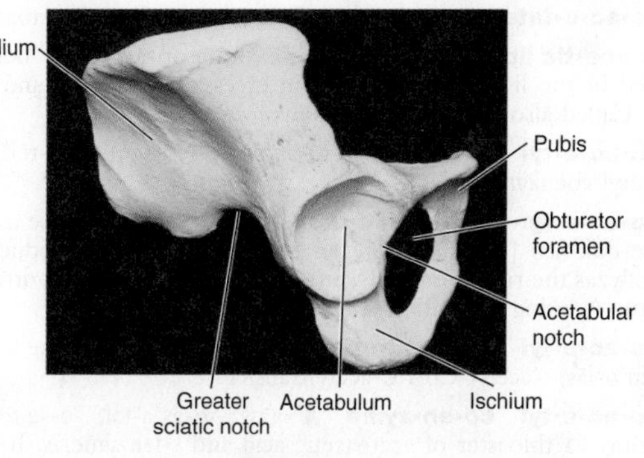

■ Acetabulum.

headache, and unconsciousness. Called also *acetic aldehyde, ethanal,* and *ethylaldehyde.*

ac•et•al•de•hyde de•hy•dro•gen•ase (as″ət-al′də-hīd de-hi′dro-jen-ās) aldehyde dehydrogenase (NAD^+).

acet•a•mide (ə-set′ə-mīd) colorless crystals used in organic synthesis and as a general solvent when melted.

ac•et•am•i•dine (as″ət-am′ĭ-dēn) the imine of acetamide, used in the synthesis of imidazoles and pyrimidines; it is irritating to the skin and mucous membranes.

ace•ta•min•o•phen (ə-se″tə-min′ə-fen) [USP] the amide of acetic acid and *p*-aminophenol, having analgesic and antipyretic effects similar to aspirin's but only weak antiinflammatory effects. Administered orally and rectally. Called also *paracetamol.*

***p*-acet•ani•si•dine** (ə-sēt″ə-ni′sĭ-dēn) methacetin.

ac•et•ar•sol (as″ət-ahr′sol) a pentavalent arsenical used as an anthelmintic in veterinary medicine.

ac•et•ar•sone (as″ət-ahr′sōn) acetarsol.

ace•tas (ə-se′təs) [L.] acetate.

ac•e•tate (as′ə-tāt) a salt or ester or the conjugate base of acetic acid.

ac•e•tate–CoA li•gase (as′ĕ-tāt ko-a′ li′gās) [EC 6.2.1.1] an enzyme of the ligase class that catalyzes the formation of acetyl coenzyme A from acetate and coenzyme A, as well as analogous reactions linking propionic or acrylic acid to coenzyme A. The enzyme occurs in the mitochondrial membrane and cytosol. Called also *acetyl CoA synthetase.*

ac•et•a•zol•a•mide (as″et-ə-zol′ə-mīd) [USP] a carbonic anhydrase inhibitor with a wide variety of uses, including adjunctive treatment of glaucoma and epilepsy, treatment of familial periodic paralysis, prophylaxis and treatment of acute mountain sickness, and as a urinary alkalizer in the prophylaxis and treatment of uric acid renal calculi; administered orally, intravenously, and intramuscularly.

Ace•test (as′ə-test) trademark for a reagent tablet containing sodium nitroprusside, aminoacetic acid, dibasic sodium phosphate, and lactose, turning purple in the presence of ketone bodies in urine, blood, plasma, or serum; the intensity of the color reaction indicates the acetoacetate or acetone concentration, ranging from a pale lavender through a dark purple as the concentration increases.

ace•tic (ə-se′tik, ə-set′ik) pertaining to vinegar or its acid; sour.

ace•tic ac•id (ə-se′tik) 1. the two-carbon carboxylic acid, CH_3COOH, which is the characteristic component of vinegar, and, mostly in the form of acetyl coenzyme A, an important biochemical intermediate. 2. [NF] a preparation used as a solvent and menstruum and as a pharmaceutic necessity in the preparation of aluminum subacetate topical solution. Systematic name: *ethanoic acid.*

glacial a. a. [USP] anhydrous acetic acid, used as a solvent, as a caustic and vesicant, and as a pharmaceutic necessity.

acet•i•fy (ə-sēt′ĭ-fi, ə-set′ĭ-fi) to turn into acetic acid or vinegar.

ac•e•tim•e•ter (as″ə-tim′ə-tər) [*acet-* + *-meter*] an apparatus for determining the amount of acetic acid present in a solution.

ac•e•tin (as′ə-tin) a glyceryl acetate, usually containing one acetyl group but sometimes two or three; used in tanning and as a food additive and a solvent for dyes.

Ace•ti•vib•rio (ə-se″tĭ-vib′re-ə) [*aceto-* + *vibrio*] a genus of anaerobic, gram-positive, straight or slightly curved rod-shaped bacteria of the family Clostridiaceae, made up of cells that are motile with flagella and produce acetic acid as the principal acid from carbohydrates. The organisms are found in the intestines of pigs. The type species is *A. celluloly′ticus.*

acet(o)- a prefix denoting the presence of the acetyl radical or of acetic acid molecules.

ac•e•to•ac•e•tate (ə-se″to-as′ə-tāt) a salt or anion of acetoacetic acid.

ace•to•ace•tic ac•id (ə-se″to-ə-se′tik) one of the ketone bodies (q.v.) produced in the liver and occurring in excess in the urine and blood in ketosis. Called also *diacetic* or *β-ketobutyric acid.*

ac•e•to•ac•e•tyl CoA (as″ə-to-as′ə-təl, ə-se′to-as-ə-tēl″ ko-a′) acetoacetyl coenzyme A.

ac•e•to•ac•e•tyl-CoA re•duc•tase (as″ə-to-as′ə-təl, ə-se′to-as-ə-tēl″ ko-a′ re-duk-tās) [EC 1.1.1.36] an enzyme of the oxidoreductase class that catalyzes the reduction of 3-ketoacyl coenzyme A to 3-hydroxybutyryl coenzyme A, using NADPH as an electron donor.

ac•e•to•ac•e•tyl CoA thi•o•lase (as″ə-to-as′ə-təl, ə-se′to-as-ə-tēl″ ko-a′ thi′o-lās) acetyl-CoA *C*-acetyltransferase.

ac•e•to•ac•e•tyl co•en•zyme A (as″ə-to-as′ə-təl, ə-se′to-as-ə-tēl″ ko-en′zīm) a thioester of acetoacetic acid and coenzyme A. It is an important metabolic intermediate in the oxidation of fatty acids, as a fuel for the citric acid cycle in brain and nervous tissue, and as a precursor of cholesterol. Written also *acetoacetyl CoA.*

Ace•to•bac•te•ra•ceae (ə-se″to-bak″tər-a′se-e) [L. *acetum* vinegar + *-bacter*] a family of aerobic, gram-negative, acetic acid–producing bacteria of the order Rhodospirillales; organisms of medical interest are contained in the genus *Roseomonas.*

ace•to•form (ə-se′to-form) methenamine.

ac•e•to•hex•a•mide (as″ə-to-hek′sə-mīd) [USP] a sulfonylurea compound used as a hypoglycemic in the treatment of type 2 diabetes mellitus; administered orally.

ac•e•to•hy•drox•am•ic ac•id (AHA) (as″ə-to-hi″droks-am′ik) [USP] an inhibitor of bacterial urease used in the prophylaxis and treatment of struvite renal calculi whose formation is favored by urease-producing bacteria and as an adjunct in the treatment of urinary tract infections caused by urease-producing bacteria; administered orally.

acet•o•in (ə-set′o-in) a ketone product formed in the fermentation of glucose by certain bacteria, especially species of Enterobacteriaceae, and detected by the Voges-Proskauer test.

ac•e•tol•y•sis (as″ə-tol′ĭ-sis) the decomposition of an organic compound using acetic acid or acetic anhydride.

ac•e•tom•e•ter (as″ə-tom′ə-tər) acetimeter.

ac•e•to•mor•phine (as″ə-to-mor′fēn) diacetylmorphine.

ac•e•to•na•tion (as″ə-to-na′shən) combination with acetone.

ac•e•tone (as′ə-tōn) 1. dimethylketone, a flammable colorless, volatile liquid with a pleasant ethereal odor; it is a commonly used solvent and is one of the ketone bodies (q.v.) produced in ketoacidosis. 2. [NF] a preparation of acetone used as a solvent and as an antiseptic.

ac•e•ton•emia (as″ə-to-ne′me-ə) excessive acetone or ketone bodies in the blood; see *ketonemia.*

ac•e•to•ni•trile (as″ə-to-ni′trīl) a colorless liquid with an ethereal odor used as an extractant, solvent, and chemical intermediate; when it is ingested or inhaled one of its metabolic products is inorganic cyanide.

ac•e•to•nu•mer•a•tor (as″ə-to-noo′mər-a″tər) an instrument for estimating the amount of acetone in the urine.

ac•e•ton•uria (as″ə-to-nu′re-ə) ketonuria.

ac•e•to•or•ce•in (as″ə-to-or′sēn) orcein dissolved in acetic acid, used in making squash preparations of polytene chromosomes.

ac•e•to•sol•uble (as″ə-to-sol′u-bəl) soluble in acetic acid.

ace•tous (as′ə-təs) pertaining to, producing, or resembling acetic acid.

ace•to•white (ə-se′to-hwīt) [*aceto-* + *white*] having a white coloration due to acetowhitening.

ace•to•whit•en•ing (ə-se″to-hwi′tən-ing) the process by which certain subclinical lesions of the skin or mucous membranes, especially warts caused by human papillomavirus, become temporarily colorless when acetic acid is applied topically.

acet•phe•nar•sine (as″ət-fen-ahr′sēn) acetarsone.

ac•e•tract (as′ə-trakt) [*acetic acid* + *extract*] an extract of a medicinal herb prepared using acetic acid as the menstruum.

ac•e•tri•zo•ate (as″ə-tri-zo′āt) a water-soluble, iodinated radiographic contrast medium, used as *sodium acetrizoate* in hysterosalpingography.

ace•tum (ə-se′təm) pl. *ace′ta* [L.] vinegar.

ac•e•tu•rate (ə-set′u-rāt) USAN contraction for *N*-acetylglycinate.

ac•e•tyl (as′ə-təl, as′ə-tēl″, ə-se′təl) [*acet-* + *-yl*] the monovalent radical, CH_3CO—.

a. chloride a colorless, corrosive, toxic, flammable liquid used as a reagent for forming acetate esters of alcohols.

a. peroxide a highly irritating, flammable, explosive compound used as an initiator and catalyst for resins.

ac•e•tyl•an•drom•e•dol (as″ə-təl-, as″ə-tēl-an-drom′ə-dol) andromedotoxin.

acet•y•lase (ə-set′ə-lās) an enzyme that catalyzes the addition or removal of an acetyl group; the most common are acetyltransferases.

acet•y•la•tion (ə-set″ə-la′shən) the introduction of an acetyl group into the molecule of an organic compound.

acet•y•la•tor (ə-set″ə-la′tər) an organism capable of metabolic acetylation; in humans, acetylator status (fast or slow) is determined by the rate of acetylation of sulfamethazine.

ac•e•tyl•cho•line (ACh) (as″ə-təl- , as″ə-tēl-ko′lēn) a reversible acetic acid ester of choline; it is a cholinergic agonist and serves as a neurotransmitter at the myoneural junctions of striated muscles, at autonomic effector cells innervated by parasympathetic nerves, at the preganglionic synapses of the sympathetic and parasympathetic nervous systems, and at various sites in the central nervous system. ACh has few therapeutic applications owing to its diffuse action and rapid hydrolysis by acetylcholinesterase (AChE); synthetic derivatives are used for more specific, prolonged action. ACh is used as a vasodilator in pharmacoangiography, administered by intraarterial infusion.

a. chloride [USP] a miotic administered by instillation into the anterior chamber of the eye during intraocular surgical procedures.

ac•e•tyl•cho•lin•er•gic (as″ə-təl- , as″ə-tēl-ko″lin-ur′jik) cholinergic.

ac•e•tyl•cho•lin•es•ter•ase (AChE) (as″ə-təl-, as″ə-tēl-ko″lĭ-nes′tə-rās) [EC 3.1.1.7] an enzyme of the hydrolase class that catalyzes the cleavage of acetylcholine to choline and acetate; it is found in the central nervous system, particularly in gray matter of nerve tissue, in red blood cells, and in motor endplates of skeletal muscle. Called also *choline esterase I* and *true cholinesterase.* Cf. *cholinesterase.*

ac•e•tyl CoA (as′ə-təl, as″ə-tēl′ ko-a′) acetyl coenzyme A.

ac•e•tyl-CoA C-ac•e•tyl•trans•fer•ase (as′ə-təl-ko-a′ as″ə-təl-trans′fər-ās, as″ə-tēl′ko-a′ as″ə-tēl-trans′fər-ās) [EC 2.3.1.9] an enzyme of the transferase class that catalyzes the synthesis of acetoacetyl coenzyme A from two molecules of acetyl coenzyme A; it can also act as a thiolase, catalyzing the reverse reaction and generating two-carbon units from the four-carbon product of fatty acid oxidation. A mitochondrial form is involved in ketone body synthesis, and a cytoplasmic form is involved in the synthesis of cholesterol and other isoprenoids.

ac•e•tyl-CoA C-acyl•trans•fer•ase (as′ə-təl-ko-a′ a″səl-trans′fər-ās, as″ə-tēl′ko-a′ a″səl-trans′fər-ās) [EC 2.3.1.16] any of several enzymes of the transferase class that catalyze the conversion of a 3-ketoacyl CoA to acetyl coenzyme A and an acyl coenzyme A with its chain length shortened by two carbons; the reaction converts fatty acid chains to two-carbon units via beta oxidation. See also individual enzymes, e.g., *α-methylacetoacetyl CoA thiolase.* Called also *β-ketothiolase.*

ac•e•tyl-CoA car•box•yl•ase (as′ə-təl-, as″ə-tēl′ko-a′ kahr-bok′sə-lās) [EC 6.4.1.2] a biotin-containing enzyme of the ligase class that catalyzes the carboxylation of acetyl coenzyme A to form malonyl coenzyme A. The reaction is the key rate-controlling step in the synthesis of fatty acids from acetyl groups, and the enzyme requires citrate or isocitrate for activity.

ac•e•tyl-CoA:α-glu•cos•am•i•nide N-ac•e•tyl•trans•fer•ase (as′ə-təl-ko-a′ gloo″kōs-am′ĭ-nīd as″ə-təl-trans′fər-ās, as″ə-tēl′ko-a′ gloo″kōs-am′ĭ-nīd as″ə-tēl-trans′fər-ās) heparan-α-glucosaminide *N*-acetyltransferase.

ac•e•tyl-CoA syn•the•tase (as′ə-təl-, as″ə-tēl′ko-a′ sin′thə-tās) acetate–CoA ligase.

ac•e•tyl co•en•zyme A (as′ə-təl, as″ə-tēl′ ko-en′zīm) acetyl CoA, a thioester of coenzyme A and acetic acid, the acetyl groups being derived from carbohydrates, fatty acids, and amino acids. Acetyl CoA can enter the tricarboxylic acid cycle, can be used to acetylate numerous compounds, and can be a precursor of steroids and other isoprenoid compounds. Excess acetyl coenzyme A may be converted to fats for storage or may appear as ketone bodies.

ac•e•tyl•cys•te•ine (as″ə-təl-, as″ə-tēl-sis′te-ēn) [USP] the *N*-acetyl derivative of L-cysteine used as a mucolytic agent for adjunct therapy in bronchopulmonary disorders to reduce the viscosity of mucus and facilitate its removal, administered by instillation or nebulization; and as an antidote for acetaminophen poisoning, administered orally or intravenously.

ac•e•tyl•di•hy•dro•lipo•am•ide (as″ə-təl-, as″ə-tēl″di-hi″dro-lĭ-po-am′īd) acetyl bound to lipoamide, an intermediate in the reaction catalyzed by the pyruvate dehydrogenase complex (q.v.).

acet•y•lene (ə-set′ə-lēn) a colorless, volatile, explosive gas; it is the simplest of a class of unsaturated (triple-bonded) hydrocarbons, the alkynes.

ac•et•yl•eu•ge•nol (as″ə-təl-u′jə-nol) an essential oil that is a minor constituent of oil of cloves.

***N*-ac•e•tyl•ga•lac•to•sa•mine (GalNAc)** (as″ə-təl-, as″ə-tēl-gal″ak-tōs′ə-mēn) the acetyl derivative of galactosamine; it is a component of structural glycosaminoglycans, of glycolipids, and of membrane glycoproteins.

***N*-ac•e•tyl•ga•lac•to•sa•mine-4-sul•fa•tase** (as″ə-təl-, as″ə-tēl″gal-ak-tōs′ə-mēn sul′fə-tās) [EC 3.1.6.12] a lysosomal enzyme of the hydrolase class that catalyzes the cleavage of sulfate groups from the 4 position of *N*-acetylgalactosamine residues. The reaction is important in the degradation of dermatan sulfate; deficiency of the enzyme, an autosomal recessive trait, results in Maroteaux-Lamy syndrome (mucopolysaccharidosis VI). Called also *arylsulfatase B.*

***N*-ac•e•tyl•ga•lac•to•sa•mine-6-sul•fa•tase** (as″ə-təl-, as″ə-tēl-gal″ak-tōs′ə-mēn sul′fə-tās) [EC 3.1.6.4] a lysosomal enzyme of the hydrolase class that catalyzes the cleavage of the sulfate group from the 6 position of sulfated galactose residues in keratan sulfate or of sulfated *N*-acetylgalactosamine residues in chondroitin 6-sulfate as a step in the degradation of these glycosaminoglycans. Deficiency of the enzyme, an autosomal recessive trait, results in Morquio syndrome, type A.

α-*N*-ac•e•tyl•gal•ac•to•sa•min•i•dase (as″ə-təl-, as″ə-tēl-gal″ak-tōs″ə-min′ĭ-dās) [EC 3.2.1.49] a lysosomal hexosaminidase specifically catalyzing the cleavage of terminal, α-linked, nonreducing *N*-acetylgalactosamine residues from glycoconjugates. Deficiency of the enzyme, an autosomal recessive trait, is a cause of infantile neuroaxonal dystrophy. Called also *α-galactosidase B.*

β-*N*-ac•e•tyl•gal•ac•to•sa•min•i•dase (as″ə-təl-, as″ə-tēl-gal″ak-tōs″ə-min′ĭ-dās) [EC 3.2.1.53] a lysosomal hexosaminidase specifically catalyzing the cleavage of terminal, β-linked, nonreducing *N*-acetylgalactosamine residues from gangliosides or other glycosides.

***N*-ac•e•tyl•glu•co•sa•mine (GlcNAc)** (as″ə-təl-, as″ə-tēl″gloo-kōs′ə-mēn) the acetyl derivative of glucosamine; it is a component of structural glycosaminoglycans, of glycolipids, and of membrane glycoproteins.

***N*-ac•e•tyl•glu•co•sa•mine-6-sul•fa•tase** (as″ə-təl-, as″ə-tēl″gloo-kōs′ə-mēn sul′fə-tās) [EC 3.1.6.14] a lysosomal enzyme that catalyzes the cleavage of sulfate groups from the 6 position of *N*-acetylglucosamine residues in heparan sulfate and keratan sulfate, a step in the degradation of these glycosaminoglycans. Deficiency of the enzyme, an autosomal recessive trait, results in Sanfilippo syndrome, type D.

α-*N*-ac•e•tyl•glu•co•sa•min•i•dase (as″ə-təl-, as″ə-tēl″gloo-kōs″ə-min′ĭ-dās) [EC 3.2.1.50] a lysosomal hexosaminidase specifically catalyzing the cleavage of terminal, α-linked, nonreducing *N*-acetylglucosamine residues from glycosides; the reaction is necessary for the degradation of heparan sulfate. Deficiency of the enzyme, an autosomal recessive trait, results in Sanfilippo syndrome, type B.

β-D-ac•e•tyl•glu•co•sa•min•i•dase (as′ə-təl-, as′ə-tēl″gloo-kōs″ə-min′ĭ-dās) a lysosomal hexosaminidase now recognized as the same enzyme as β-*N*-acetylhexosaminidase (q.v.).

N^4-(β-*N*-ac•e•tyl•glu•co•sa•min•yl)-L-as•par•a•gin•ase (as″ə-təl-, as″ə-tēl″gloo-kōs″ə-min′əl as-par′ə-jin″ās) [EC 3.5.1.26] official nomenclature for *aspartylglucosaminidase.*

β-*N*-ac•e•tyl•glu•cos•amin•yl•gly•co•pep•tide β-1,4-ga•lac•to••syl•trans•fer•ase (as″ə-təl-, as″ə-tēl″gloo-kōs″ə-min′əl-gli″ko-pep′tīd gal″ak-tōs″əl-trans′fər-ās) [EC 2.4.1.38] EC nomenclature for *glycoprotein 4-β-galactosyltransferase.*

***N*-ac•e•tyl•glu•cos•am•i•nyl•phos•pho•trans•fer•ase** (as″ə-təl-, as″ə-tēl″gloo-kos″ə-min″əl-fos″fo-trans′fər-ās) UDP-*N*-acetylglucosamine–lysosomal-enzyme *N*-acetylglucosaminephosphotransferase.

***N*-ac•e•tyl•glu•ta•mate** (as″ə-təl-, as″ə-tēl-gloo′tə-māt) *N*-acetylglutamic acid in dissociated form.

***N*-ac•e•tyl•glu•ta•mate syn•the•tase** (as″ə-təl-, as″ə-tēl-gloo′tə-māt sin′thə-tās) amino-acid *N*-acetyltransferase.

***N*-ac•e•tyl•glu•tam•ic ac•id** (as″ə-təl-, as″ə-tēl″gloo-tam′ik) glutamic acid acetylated at its N-terminus, a necessary cofactor in the synthesis of carbamoyl phosphate catalyzed by carbamoyl-phosphate synthase (ammonia). The molecule is an allosteric activator of this enzyme and hence a positive regulator of ureagenesis.

***N*-ac•e•tyl•hex•os•amine** (as″ə-təl-, as″ə-tēl″hek-sōs′ə-mēn) a hexosamine acetylated at its amino group, such as *N*-acetylglucosamine or *N*-acetylgalactosamine.

β-*N*-ac•e•tyl•hex•os•amin•i•dase (as″ə-təl-, as″ə-tēl″hek-sōs″ə-min′ĭ-dās) [EC 3.2.1.52] a lysosomal enzyme of the hydrolase class that catalyzes the cleavage of *N*-acetylhexosamine residues from gangliosides or other glycosides; it is necessary for the degradation of keratan sulfate and also ganglioside GM_2 and related compounds. The enzyme comprises two polypeptide chains, α and β, which are arranged into three isozymes: A (αβ), B (ββ), and S (αα). Lack of isozyme A activity, due to a defect in the α chain, causes Tay-Sachs disease; lack of isozymes A and B, due to a defect in the β chain, causes Sandhoff disease. The enzyme is usually called *hexosaminidase.*

acet•y•li•za•tion (ə-set″əl-ĭ-za′shən) acetylation.

***N*-ac•e•tyl•man•no•sa•mine** (as″ə-təl-, as″ə-tēl″mə-nōs′ə-mēn) mannosamine acetylated at its amino group, an intermediate in the biosynthesis and degradation of sialic acids and sialoglycoconjugates.

***N*-ac•e•tyl•mu•ram•ate** (as″ə-təl-, as″ə-tēl-mūr′ə-māt) a salt, ester, or anionic form of *N*-acetylmuramic acid.

***N*-ac•e•tyl•mu•ram•ic ac•id** (as″ə-təl-, as″ə-tēl″mu-ram′ik) a polysaccharide constituent of bacterial cell walls; it is composed of *N*-acetylglucosamine coupled to lactic acid.

***N*-ac•e•tyl•neu•ra•min•ate** (as″ə-təl-, as″ə-tēl″noo͝-ram′ĭ-nāt) a salt, ester, or anionic form of *N*-acetylneuraminic acid.

***N*-ac•e•tyl•neu•ram•i•nate ly•ase** (as″ə-təl-, as″ə-tēl″noo͝-ram′ĭ-nāt li′ās) [EC 4.1.3.3] a cytoplasmic enzyme of the lyase class that catalyzes the cleavage of a pyruvate residue from *N*-acetylneuraminate to form *N*-acetylmannosamine as a step in the degradation of sialic acids and sialoglycoconjugates.

***N*-ac·e·tyl·neu·ra·min·ic ac·id** (as″ə-təl-, as″ə-tēl-noor″ə-min′ik) the acetyl derivative of the amino sugar neuraminic acid; it occurs in many glycoproteins, glycolipids, and polysaccharides.

ac·e·tyl·sal·i·cyl·ic ac·id (ASA) (ə-se′təl-sal″ə-sil′ik) chemical name for *aspirin.*

ac·e·tyl·stro·phan·thi·din (as″ə-təl-, as″ə-tēl″stro-fan′thə-din) a synthetic fast-acting digitalis-like preparation.

ac·e·tyl·sul·fa·di·a·zine (as″ə-təl-, as″ə-tēl″sul″fə-di′ə-zēn) the form in which sulfadiazine is excreted in the urine, often occurring in dark green crystalline spheres.

ac·e·tyl·sul·fa·guan·i·dine (as″ə-təl-, as″ə-tēl″sul″fə-gwan′ĭ-dēn) the form in which sulfaguanidine is excreted in the urine, often occurring in thin oblong crystalline plates.

ac·e·tyl·sul·fa·thi·a·zole (as″ə-təl-, as″ə-tēl-sul″fə-thi′ə-zōl) the form in which sulfathiazole is excreted in the urine, often occurring in the form of sheaves-of-wheat crystals.

ac·e·tyl·trans·fer·ase (as″ə-təl-, as″ə-tēl-trans′fər-ās) an acyltransferase specifically catalyzing the transfer of an acetyl group, often acetyl coenzyme A, to another compound. Those forming esters or amides are also called *acetylases.*

ac·e·tyl·tri·bu·tyl cit·rate (as″ə-təl-, as″ə-tēl″tri-bu′təl) [NF] a compound derived by the esterification and acetylation of citric acid, used as a plasticizer in pharmaceutical preparations.

ac·e·tyl·tri·eth·yl cit·rate (as″ə-təl-, as″ə-tēl″tri-eth′əl) [NF] a compound derived by the esterification and acetylation of citric acid, used as a plasticizer in pharmaceutical preparations.

ACG American College of Gastroenterology; angiocardiography; apexcardiogram.

AcG accelerator globulin (factor V; see *coagulation factors*, under *factor*).

ACh acetylcholine.

ACHA American College of Hospital Administrators.

ach·a·la·sia (ak″ə-la′zhə) [*a-*[1] + *chalasia*] failure of the smooth muscle fibers of the gastrointestinal tract to relax at a point of junction of one part with another; usually used to denote esophageal achalasia.

a. of cardia, cardial a. esophageal a.

cricopharyngeal a. achalasia of the cricopharyngeal muscle; see *Asherson syndrome*, under *syndrome.*

esophageal a. failure of the lower esophageal sphincter to relax with swallowing due to degeneration of ganglion cells in the wall of the organ. The thoracic esophagus also loses its normal peristaltic activity and becomes dilated (megaesophagus).

pelvirectal a. congenital megacolon.

sphincteral a. failure of a sphincter to relax in response to a normal physiological stimulus, usually seen in the gastrointestinal tract.

Achard syndrome (ah-shahr′) [Émile Charles *Achard*, French physician, 1860–1944] see under *syndrome.*

Achard-Thiers syndrome (ah-shahr′ tērz′) [É.C. *Achard;* Joseph *Thiers*, 20th-century French physician] see under *syndrome.*

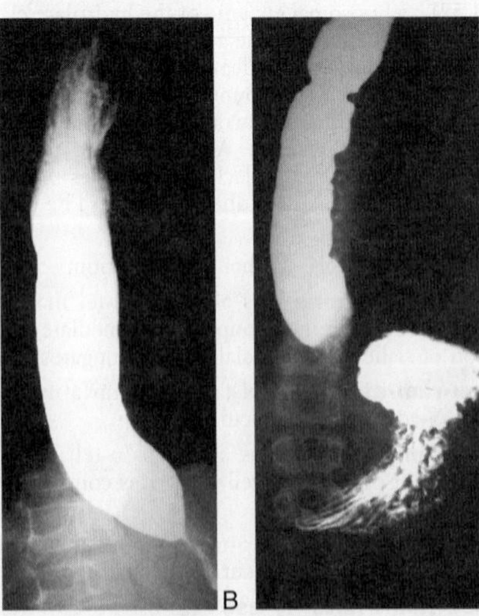

■ Barium meal demonstrating esophageal achalasia in a 9-year-old patient. *(A)*, The enlarged esophagus shows very slow emptying and a typical "carrot" or "bird beak" appearance; *(B)* some feeble esophageal contractions are seen but the esophageal walls remain widely separated and so peristalsis is absent.

Ach·a·ti·na (ak″ə-ti′nə) a genus of large land snails of the family Achatinidae, order Stylommatophora, originally native to Africa. *A. fuli′ca* serves as an intermediate host of the rat lungworm *Angiostrongylus cantonensis.*

Acha·tin·i·dae (ak″ə-tin′ĭ-de) a family of African land snails of the suborder Stylommatophora, order Pulmonata; it includes the genus *Achatina.*

AChE acetylcholinesterase.

ache (āk) 1. a continuous, fixed pain, as distinguished from twinges. 2. to suffer such pain.

achei·lia (ə-ki′le-ə) [*a-*[1] + *cheil-* + *-ia*] congenital absence of one or both lips.

achei·lous (ə-ki′lus) lacking lips; exhibiting acheilia.

achei·ria (ə-ki′re-ə) [*a-*[1] + *cheir-* + *-ia*] 1. congenital absence of one or both hands. 2. lack of feeling of the hands or a feeling of their absence, sometimes occurring in conversion disorder.

achei·ro·po·dia (ə-ki″ro-po′de-ə) [*a-*[1] + *cheir-* + *pod-* + *-ia*] congenital absence of hands and feet.

achei·rus (ə-ki′rəs) [L.] an individual exhibiting acheiria.

Achil·lea (ak″ə-le′ə, ə-kil′e-ə) [Gr. *achilleios* pertaining to the hero Achilles, who is supposed to have used a plant of the genus medicinally] a large genus of herbs occurring in the northern hemisphere, including *A. millefo′lium*, one of the species known as yarrow, which is used medicinally.

Achil·les bur·sa, jerk (reflex), tendon (ə-kil′ēz) [Gr. *Achilleus* Greek hero, whose mother held him by the heel to dip him in the Styx] see *bursa tendinis calcanei, triceps surae jerk*, under *jerk*, and *tendo calcaneus.*

achil·lo·bur·si·tis (ə-kil″o-bər-si′tis) retrocalcaneal bursitis.

achil·lo·dy·nia (ə-kil″o-din′e-ə) [*Achilles* (tendon) + *-odynia*] 1. pain in the Achilles tendon. 2. retrocalcaneal bursitis.

ach·il·lor·rha·phy (ak″ĭ-lor′ə-fe) [*Achilles* (tendon) + *rhaphy*] suture of the Achilles tendon.

achil·lo·te·not·o·my (ə-kil″o-tə-not′ə-me) [*Achilles* + Gr. *tenōn* tendon + *tomē* cut] surgical division of the Achilles tendon.

plastic a. elongation of the Achilles tendon by plastic operation.

achil·lot·o·my (ak″ĭ-lot′ə-me) achillotenotomy.

achi·ria (ə-ki′re-ə) 1. acheiria. 2. inability to tell which side of the body has been touched; cf. *dyschiria.*

achi·rus (ə-ki′rəs) acheirus.

achlor·hy·dria (a″klor-hi′dre-ə) [*a-*[1] + *chlorhydria*] absence of hydrochloric acid from maximally stimulated gastric secretions; a result of gastric mucosal atrophy. Called also *gastric anacidity.*

achlor·hy·dric (a″klor-hi′drik) characterized by achlorhydria.

Ach·lya (ak′le-ə) a genus of funguslike chromists of the order Saprolegniales, which form molds on certain fish and insects.

Acho·le·plas·ma (a″ko-le-plaz′mə) [*a-*[1] + *chole-* + *plasma*] a genus of bacteria of the family Acholeplasmataceae, made up of spherical cells bounded by a triple-layered membrane but lacking a cell wall, and not requiring serum or cholesterol for growth. The type species is *A. laidlaw′ii.*

A. granula′rum a species found in the nasal cavities of swine and reported to have been isolated from the synovial fluid of arthritic pigs. Called also *Mycoplasma granularum.*

A. laidlaw′ii a species isolated from human clinical specimens, from the body cavities of cattle, swine, and birds, and from soils. Called also *Mycoplasma laidlawii.*

Acho·le·plas·ma·ta·ceae (a-ko″le-plaz″mə-ta′se-e) a family of bacteria of the order Acholeplasmatales, made up of organisms that do not require sterol for growth. It contains the genus *Acholeplasma.*

Acho·le·plas·ma·ta·les (a-ko″le-plaz″mə-ta′lēz) an order of bacteria of the class Mollicutes, containing the single family Acholeplamataceae.

acho·lia (a-ko′le-ə) [*a-*[1] + *chol-* + *-ia*] absence of bile, such as from ductal atresia or failure of secretion. **acho′lic** *adj*

acho·lu·ric (a″ko-lu′rik) not characterized by choluria; said of jaundice.

achon·dro·gen·e·sis (a-kon″dro-jen′ə-sis) the severest of the chondrodysplasias, a hereditary disorder characterized by hypoplasia of bone, micromelia, enlarged head, shortened trunk, and deficient or absent ossification of the lower spine and pubis. It is divided into type I (further subdivided into Ia and Ib) and type II, which differ in site of mutation and mode of inheritance; all are lethal before or shortly after birth.

achon·dro·pla·sia (a-kon″dro-pla′zhə) [*a-*[1] + *chondroplasia*] an autosomal dominant disorder caused by mutation in the fibroblast growth factor receptor 3 (*FGFR3*) gene (locus: 4p16.3), which encodes a transmembrane receptor protein-tyrosine kinase that binds fibroblast growth factor and

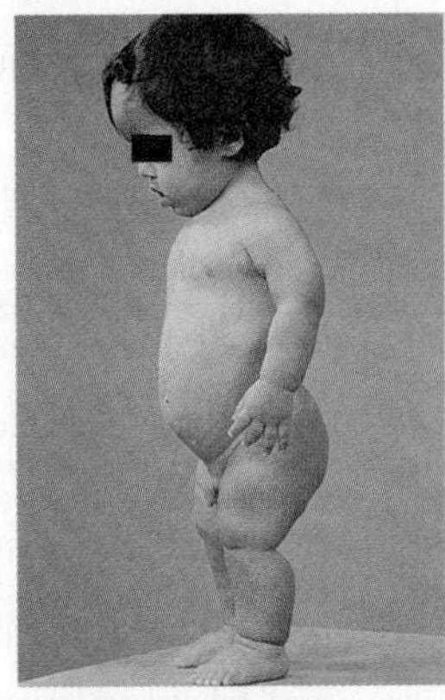

■ Child with achondroplasia showing short stature, short limbs and fingers, normal length of the trunk, a relatively large head, prominent forehead, and depressed nasal bridge.

inhibits proliferation of chondrocytes within the growth plate, causing ligand-independent activation of the gene. It is characterized by disturbance of epiphyseal chondroblastic growth and maturation, causing inadequate enchondral bone formation and resulting in dwarfism with short limbs, normal trunk, small face, normal vault, lordosis, and trident hand. See also *achondroplastic dwarf,* under *dwarf.* **achondroplas′tic** *adj*

achon•dro•plas•ty (a-kon′dro-plas″te) achondroplasia.

achor•dal (a-kor′dəl) achordate.

achor•date (a-kor′dāt) without a notochord; used with reference to animals which are not chordates.

achres•tic (ə-kres′tik) not using some normal tool or process, as the inability of those with achrestic anemia (q.v.) to utilize vitamin B_{12}.

achro•ma•sia (ak″ro-ma′zhə) 1. hypopigmentation. 2. achromatosis (def. 2).

achro•mat (ak′ro-mat) [*a-*[1] + *chromat*] 1. an achromatic objective. 2. monochromat.

achro•mate (ə-kro′māt) monochromat.

achro•mat•ic (ak″ro-mat′ik) [*a-*[1] + *chromatic*] 1. staining with difficulty. 2. refracting light without decomposing it into its component colors. 3. colorless. 4. monochromatic (def. 2).

achro•ma•tism (ə-kro′mə-tiz-əm) 1. the quality or condition of being achromatic. 2. monochromatic vision.

achro•ma•tize (ə-kro′mə-tīz) to render achromatic.

achro•ma•to•phil (ak″ro-mat′o-fil) [*a-*[1] + *chromato-* + *-phil*] 1. having no affinity for stains. 2. an organism or tissue element that does not stain easily.

achro•ma•to•phil•ia (ə-kro″mə-to-fil′e-ə) the property of resisting the coloring action of stains.

achro•ma•top•sia (ə-kro″mə-top′se-ə) monochromatic vision.

achro•ma•to•sis (ə-kro″mə-to′sis) [*a-*[1] + *chromat-* + *-osis*] 1. hypopigmentation. 2. lack of staining power in a cell or tissue.

achro•ma•tous (ə-kro′mə-tus) colorless.

achro•ma•tu•ria (ə-kro″mə-tu′re-ə) [*a-*[1] + *chromaturia*] the excretion of colorless urine, such as from hyperhydration.

achro•mia (ə-kro′me-ə) hypopigmentation.
cortical a. a condition in which an area of the cerebral cortex shows disappearance of ganglion cells.

achro•mic (ə-kro′mik) colorless.

Achro•mo•bac•ter (ə-kro″mo-bak′tər) [*a-*[1] + *chromo-* + *-bacter*] a genus of gram-negative, nonfermentative, peritrichously flagellated, rod-shaped bacteria of the family Alcaligenaceae, found in water and the human intestinal tract and sometimes associated with significant infections.

achro•mo•cyte (ə-kro′mo-sīt) a crescent-shaped red cell artifact that stains more faintly than intact red cells; cf. *ghost cell.* Called also *demilune body* and *achromic erythrocyte.*

achro•mo•phil (ə-kro′mo-fil) [*a-*[1] + *chromo-* + *-phil*] achromatophil.

achro•moph•i•lous (a″kro-mof′ĭ-ləs) having no affinity for stains.

achro•mo•trich•ia (a-kro″mo-trik′e-ə) loss of pigment in the hair, as in canities, leukotrichia, or poliosis. Called also *hypochromotrichia.*

Achro•my•cin (ak″ro-mi′sin) trademark for preparations of tetracycline hydrochloride.

ach•roo•am•y•loid (a-kro″o-am′ə-loid) [*a-*[1] + Gr. *chroa* color + *amyloid*] amyloid in its early nonstainable stage.

ach•roo•dex•trin (ə-kro″o-dek′strin) [*a-*[1] + Gr. *chroa* color + *dextrin*] any of the lower-molecular-weight dextrins not colored by iodine.

achy•lia (ə-ki′le-ə) [Gr. *achylos* juiceless + *-ia*] absence of hydrochloric acid and pepsinogen (pepsin) in the gastric juice; called also *a. gas′trica.*

achy•mia (ə-ki′me-ə) imperfect, insufficient, or absence of formation of chyme.

acic•u•lar (ə-sik′u-lər) [L. *acicularis*] shaped like a needle or needle point.

acic•u•lum (ə-sik′u-lum) a bent, finger-like spine or bristle found in certain flagellates.

ac•id (as′id) [L. *acidum* from *acidus* sharp, sour] any of a large class of chemical substances defined by three chemical concepts of increasing generality. An *Arrhenius acid* is a substance that lowers the pH (increases the hydrogen ion concentration) when added to an aqueous solution; such substances have a sour taste, turn litmus red, and react with alkalis to form salts. A *Bronsted-Lowry acid* is a species that acts as a proton donor in solution; e.g., the ammonium ion (NH_4^+) can donate a proton, leaving ammonia (NH_3); such species are termed conjugate acid-base pairs. A *Lewis acid* is a species that can accept a pair of electrons to form a covalent bond; e.g., BF_3 in the reaction $BF_3 + NH_3 \rightarrow BF_3NH_3$. Aqueous solutions of certain compounds that dissociate in solution, e.g., hydrogen chloride, are designated acids by names beginning with *hydro-*, e.g., hydrochloric acid. Most other common inorganic acids are *oxo acids* (q.v.); common organic acids include carboxylic acids, sulfonic acids, and phenols. The name of the anion formed by the removal of hydrogen from an acid (its conjugate base) and the names of salts and esters of acids are formed by removing the suffix *-ic* and the word *acid* and adding the suffix *-ate*, except for oxo acids ending in *-ous*, when the suffix is *-ite*. For particular acids, see the specific name.
amino a. see at *amino.*
bile a. see under *B.*
binary a. an acid which contains only two elements, e.g., HCl; called also *hydracid.*
carboxylic a. any acid containing the carboxyl (—COOH) group, including amino acids and fatty acids.
a. citrate dextrose (ACD) anticoagulant citrate dextrose solution.
conjugate a. a chemical species that is formed from its conjugate base by addition of a proton, e.g., ammonium (NH_4^+) is the conjugate acid of ammonia (NH_3).
dicarboxylic a. any of various organic acids that contain two carboxyl groups, such as azelaic acid, glutaric acid, iminodiacetic acid, or oxalic acid. See also *dicarboxylicaciduria.*
fatty a. see under *F.*
haloid a. an acid which contains no oxygen in the molecule but is composed of hydrogen and a halogen element.
hydroxy a. an organic acid that contains an additional hydroxyl group.
inorganic a. an acid containing no carbon atoms.
monobasic a. an acid having but one replaceable hydrogen atom and therefore yielding only one series of salts, e.g., HCl.
nucleic a. see under *N.*
organic a. an acid containing one or more carbon atoms, often specifically a carboxylic acid.
oxo a. 1. oxyacid. 2. keto acid; see under *K.*
oxygen a. an acid that contains oxygen; an oxyacid.
polybasic a. an acid which contains two or more hydrogen atoms which may be neutralized by alkalis and replaced by organic radicals.
sulfo-a. an acid in which oxygen or carbon is replaced by sulfur.
ternary a. an acid which contains three distinct radicals.
thio a. an acid formed by replacement of an oxygen atom in an oxo acid or carboxylic acid by a sulfur atom, e.g., thiophosphoric acid (H_3PSO_3) or thioacetic acid (CH_3COSH).
tribasic a. an acid that has three replaceable hydrogen atoms.

ac•id•al•bu•min (as″id-al′bu-min) a protein that dissolves in acids and shows an acid reaction.

ac•id al•pha-glu•co•si•dase (as′id al′fə gloo-ko′sĭ-dās) glucan 1,4-α-glucosidase.

ac•id al•pha-glu•co•si•dase de•fi•cien•cy (as′id al′fə gloo-ko′sĭ-dās) glycogen storage disease, type II.

Ac•id•ami•no•coc•ca•ceae (as″id-ə-me″no-kok-a′se-e) a family of anaerobic, gram-negative bacteria of the order Clostridiales; organisms of medical interest are contained in the genera *Acidaminococcus, Dialister, Selenomonas,* and *Veillonella.*

Ac•id•ami•no•coc•cus (as″id-ə-me″no-kok′əs) [*acid* + *amino* + *coccus*] a genus of bacteria of the family Acidaminococcaceae, found in the intestinal tract of normal humans and pigs, made up of gram-negative anaerobic cocci. The type species is *A. fermen′tans.*

ac•id–CoA li•gase (GDP-forming) (as′id ko-a′ li′gās form′ing) [EC 6.2.1.10] an enzyme of the ligase class that catalyzes the formation of acyl coenzyme A from long chain fatty acids (12 or more carbons) and coenzyme A, using the energy derived from GTP hydrolysis. The enzyme occurs in the mitochondrial matrix and thus can activate any free fatty acids appearing there. Called also *acyl CoA synthetase (GDP-forming).*

ac•i•de•mia (as″ĭ-de′me-ə) a decreased pH (increased hydrogen ion concentration) of the blood. For acidemias characterized by increased concentration of a specific acid, see at the acid (e.g., *isovalericacidemia).*

organic a. increased concentration of one or more organic acids in the blood.

acid-fast (as′id-fast) not readily decolorized by acid after staining, a characteristic of certain bacteria, particularly *Mycobacterium tuberculosis, Mycobacterium leprae,* and some species of *Nocardia.* See under *stain.*

ac•id α-glu•co•si•dase (as′id gloo-ko′sĭ-dās) glucan 1,4-α-glucosidase.

ac•id α-glu•co•si•dase de•fi•cien•cy (as′id gloo-ko′sĭ-dās) glycogen storage disease, type II.

acid•ic (ə-sid′ik) of or pertaining to an acid; acid-forming.

acid•i•fi•a•ble (ə-sid′ə-fi″ə-bəl) susceptible of being made acid.

acid•i•fi•er (ə-sid″ĭ-fi′ər) 1. an agent that causes acidity. 2. an agent used to increase gastric acidity.

acid•i•fy (ə-sid′ĭ-fi) 1. to render acid, as by addition of a strong acid. 2. to become acid.

ac•i•dim•e•ter (as″ĭ-dim′ə-tər) [L. *acidum* acid + *-meter*] an instrument used in performing acidimetry.

ac•i•dim•et•ry (as″ĭ-dim′ə-tre) the determination of the amount of free acid in a solution.

ac•id•ism (as′ĭ-diz-əm) a condition due to introduction into the body of acids from outside.

acid•i•ty (ə-sid′ĭ-te) [L. *aciditas*] the quality of being acid or sour; containing acid (hydrogen ions).

ac•id li•pase (as″id li′pās) 1. sterol esterase. 2. a lipase with an acid pH optimum.

ac•id li•pase de•fi•cien•cy (as″id li′pās) 1. Wolman disease. 2. cholesteryl ester storage disease.

ac•id mal•tase (as′id mawl′tās) glucan 1,4-α-glucosidase.

ac•id mal•tase de•fi•cien•cy (as′id mawl′tās) glycogen storage disease, type II.

ac•i•do•gen•ic (as″ĭ-do-jen′ik) producing acid or acidity, especially acidity of the urine.

acid•o•phil (ə-sid′o-fil″) [L. *acidum* acid + Gr. *-phil*] 1. a structure, cell, or other histologic element staining readily with acid dyes. 2. one of the hormone-producing acidophilic cells of the adenohypophysis; types include corticotrophs, lactotrophs, lipotrophs, and somatotrophs. Called also *alpha cell* and *A cell.* 3. an organism that grows well in highly acid media. 4. acidophilic.

alpha a. somatotroph.

epsilon a. lactotroph.

acid•o•phile (ə-sid′o-fīl″) 1. acidophil. 2. acidophilic.

ac•i•do•phil•ic (as″ĭ-do-fil′ik) 1. readily stained with acid dyes. 2. growing in highly acid media; said of microorganisms. Called also *acidophil, acidophile,* and *oxyphilic.*

ac•i•do•sis (as″ĭ-do′sis) 1. the accumulation of acid and hydrogen ions or depletion of the alkaline reserve (bicarbonate content) in the blood and body tissues, resulting in a decrease in pH. 2. the pathologic condition resulting from this process; see also *acidemia.* Cf. *alkalosis.* **acido′sic, acidot′ic** *adj*

compensated a. a condition in which the compensatory mechanisms have returned the pH toward normal; see *compensated metabolic a.* and *compensated respiratory a.*

compensated metabolic a. a state of metabolic acidosis in which the pH of the blood has been returned toward normal by respiratory compensatory mechanisms.

compensated respiratory a. respiratory acidosis in which the pH of the blood has been returned toward normal by renal compensatory mechanisms.

diabetic a. see under *ketoacidosis.*

distal renal tubular a. renal tubular acidosis without the usual lowering of the pH of urine in the distal tubules. A nonhereditary type seen in infant boys is called *Lightwood syndrome,* and an autosomal dominant type seen later in life is called *Butler-Albright syndrome.* See also *generalized distal renal tubular a.* Called also *type 1 renal tubular a.*

generalized distal renal tubular a. distal renal tubular acidosis associated with hyporeninemic hypoaldosteronism, usually associated with diabetes mellitus. Called also *type 4 renal tubular a.*

hypercapnic a. respiratory a.

hyperchloremic a. metabolic acidosis accompanied by elevated plasma chloride.

lactic a. a metabolic acidosis occurring as a result of excess lactic acid in the blood, due to conditions causing impaired cellular respiration. It occurs most commonly in disorders in which O_2 is inadequately delivered to tissues, e.g., shock, septicemia, or extreme hypoxemia, but it can also result from exogenous or endogenous metabolic defects. Initially manifesting as hyperventilation, it progresses to mental confusion and coma.

metabolic a. any of the various kinds of acidosis in which the acid-base status of the body shifts toward the acid side because of loss of base or retention of acids other than carbonic acid (fixed or nonvolatile acids), in contrast to respiratory acidosis. Called also *nonrespiratory a.*

nonrespiratory a. metabolic a.

proximal renal tubular a. renal tubular acidosis caused by malfunction of the proximal tubules. Mild forms are often accompanied by bicarbonaturia; severe forms such as Fanconi syndrome may be free of bicarbonaturia but show increased excretion of other solutes. Called also *type 2 renal tubular a.*

renal hyperchloremia a. renal tubular a.

renal tubular a. (RTA) a variety of metabolic acidosis resulting from impairment of renal function; it is usually accompanied by hyperchloremic acidosis, high urinary pH, bicarbonaturia, and lowered excretion of ammonium and titratable acids. Two types are distinguished according to whether the primary dysfunction is in distal or proximal tubules; see *distal renal tubular a.* and *proximal renal tubular a.*

respiratory a. acidosis due to excess retention of carbon dioxide in the body, as opposed to metabolic acidosis; it is seen in chronic obstructive pulmonary disease and other conditions that interfere with normal ventilation. Called also *hypercapnic a.*

starvation a. a type of metabolic acidosis produced by accumulation of ketone bodies which may accompany a caloric deficit. Called also *starvation ketoacidosis.*

type 1 renal tubular a. distal renal tubular a.

type 2 renal tubular a. proximal renal tubular a.

type 4 renal tubular a. generalized distal renal tubular a.

uremic a. a type of metabolic acidosis seen in chronic renal disease in which the ability to excrete acid is decreased.

ac•i•dos•teo•phyte (as″ĭ-dos′te-o-fīt″) [Gr. *akis* point + *osteo-* + *-phyte*] a sharp-pointed osteophyte.

ac•id phos•pha•tase (as′id fos′fə-tās) [EC 3.1.3.2] an enzyme of the hydrolase class that catalyzes the cleavage of orthophosphate from orthophosphoric monoesters under acid conditions. The enzyme is found in mammalian liver, spleen, bone marrow, plasma and formed blood elements, and prostate gland. The determination of serum acid phosphatase activity is an important diagnostic test. Called also *phosphomonoesterase.*

acid•u•lat•ed (ə-sid′u-lāt″ed) rendered acid in reaction.

acid•u•lous (ə-sid′u-ləs) somewhat acid.

ac•id•u•ria (as″ĭ-du′re-ə) excess of acid in the urine; types are usually named for the acid in question, such as aminoaciduria, dicarboxylicaciduria, glutaricaciduria, and so on.

organic a. excessive excretion of one or more organic acids in the urine.

ac•id•uric (as″ĭ-doo′rik) [L. *acidum* acid + *durare* to endure] acid-tolerant; said of bacteria which are able to withstand a degree of acidity usually fatal to nonsporulating bacteria.

ac•i•dyl (as′ĭ-dəl) any acid radical.

acid•y•la•tion (ə-sid″ə-la′shən) acylation.

Aci-jel (a′sĭ-jel) trademark for a bland, nonirritating, water-dispersible, buffered acid jelly for intravaginal use.

ac•i•nar (as′ĭ-nər) pertaining to or affecting one or more acini.

ac•i•ne•sia (as″ĭ-ne′zhə) akinesia.

ac•i•net•ic (as″ĭ-net′ik) akinetic (def. 1).

Ac•i•net•o•bac•ter (as″ĭ-net″o-bak′tər) [*a-*[1] + *cineto-* + *-bacter*] a genus of bacteria of the family Moraxellaceae, consisting of gram-negative, paired coccobacilli that are aerobic, catalase-positive, and oxidase-negative. The organisms are widely distributed in nature and are part of the normal mammalian flora, but can cause severe primary infections in compromised hosts. The type species is *A. calcoace′ticus.*

ac•i•ni (as′ĭ-ni) [L.] genitive and plural of *acinus.*

acin•ic (ə-sin′ik) acinar.

acin•i•form (ə-sin′ĭ-form) [*acini* + *form*] shaped like an acinus, or grape.

acin•i•tis (as″ĭ-ni′tis) inflammation of the acini of a gland.

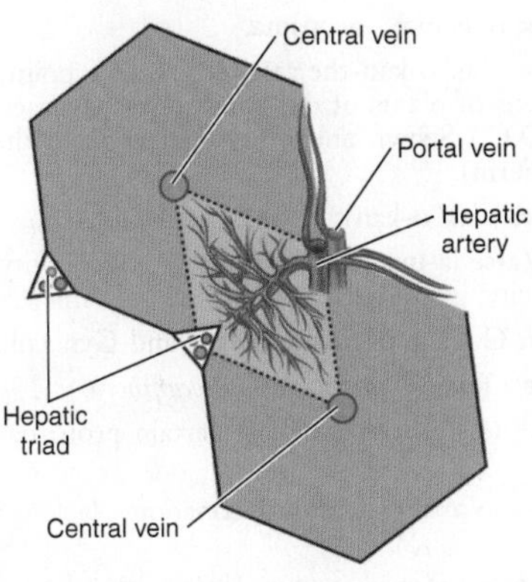

■ Liver acinus: hepatic lobules are represented by hexagons *(solid lines)*; liver acinus is represented by rhombus *(dotted line)*.

ac•i•nose (as'ĭ-nōs) [L. *acinosus* grapelike] 1. made up of acini. 2. acinar.

ac•i•no•tu•bu•lar (as″ĭ-no-too'bu-lər) composed of tubular acini or of tubules ending in acini.

ac•i•nous (as'ĭ-nəs) acinar.

ac•i•nus (as'ĭ-nəs) pl. *a'cini* [L. "grape"] a small saclike dilation, particularly in the lung or a gland. See also *alveolus.*

hepatic a., liver a., a. of liver a functional unit of the liver, smaller than a portal lobule, being a diamond-shaped mass of liver parenchyma surrounding a portal tract.

pancreatic a. one of the secretory units of the exocrine pancreas, where pancreatic juice is produced.

pulmonary a. terminal respiratory unit.

thyroid acini thyroid follicles.

ac•i•pen•ser•in (as″ĭ-pen'sər-in) a toxic substance from the gonads of the sturgeon *Acipenser.*

Ac•i•pHex (as'ĭ-feks″) trademark for a preparation of rabeprazole sodium.

ac•i•tret•in (as″e-tret'in) a substance related to tretinoin, used in treatment of severe psoriasis; administered orally.

ackee (ă'ke) akee.

aclad•i•o•sis (ə-klad″e-o'sis) an ulcerative type of dermatomycosis that was seen in southern Asia and the Balkans and was caused by a species of *Acladium.*

Acla•di•um (ə-kla'de-um) a former genus of Fungi Imperfecti, now reclassified.

acla•sia (ə-kla'zhə) aclasis.

acla•sis (ak'lə-sis) [*a-*[1] + Gr. *klasis* a breaking] pathologic continuity of structure, as in multiple exostoses.

diaphyseal a. multiple exostoses.

tarsoepiphyseal a. dysplasia epiphysealis hemimelica.

aclas•tic (a-klas'tik) 1. pertaining to or characterized by aclasis. 2. not refracting.

Aclo•vate (a'klo-vāt″) trademark for a preparation of alclometasone dipropionate.

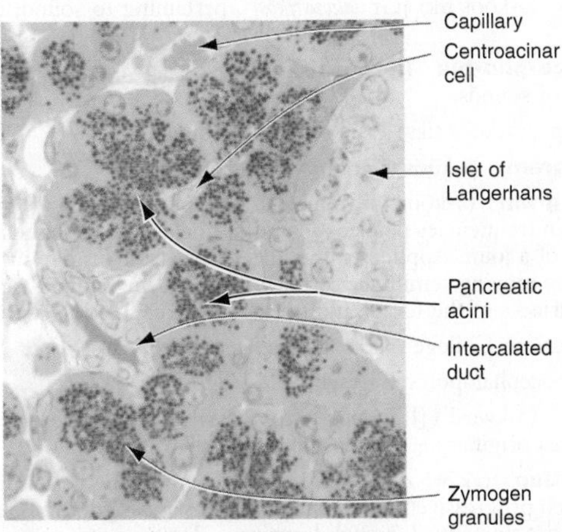

■ Acini of pancreas.

aclu•sion (ə-kloo'zhən) [*a-*[1] + *occlusion*] absence of occlusion of the opposing tooth surfaces.

ac•me (ak'me) [Gr. *akmē* highest point] the crisis or critical stage of a disease.

ac•ne (ak'ne) [possibly a corruption of Greek *akmē* a point or of *achnē* chaff] 1. any of numerous inflammatory diseases of the pilosebaceous unit of the skin. 2. a. vulgaris.

a. agmina'ta lupus miliaris disseminatus faciei.

a. artificia'lis contact a.

atrophic a., a. atro'phica acne vulgaris in which, after the disappearance of small papular lesions, a stippling of tiny atrophic pits and scars remains.

bromide a. acne caused by ingestion of bromide compounds, one of the most common manifestations of bromism; it does not include comedo formation.

a. cachectico'rum acneiform eruptions on the skin of persons suffering from anemia or other debilitating conditions.

chlorine a. chloracne.

comedonal a., comedone a. acne vulgaris in which most of the lesions are comedones, usually on the forehead or chin.

common a. a. vulgaris.

a. congloba'ta, conglobate a. a severe, chronic form of acne seen primarily in males, beginning during late puberty and often continuing in later life, characterized by comedones (often double or triple), large abscesses with interconnecting sinuses, and cysts containing clear or seropurulent material; pronounced and disfiguring scarring remains after healing.

contact a. acne produced by contact with any of numerous chemicals, including those used in cosmetic or grooming agents (see *cosmetic a.* and *pomade a.*) or in industry (see *occupational a.*). Called also *a. artificialis* and *a. venenata.*

contagious a. of horses, contagious pustular a. a contagious disease of the skin in horses caused by infection with *Corynebacterium pseudotuberculosis,* characterized by groups of pustules, especially in areas in contact with the harness; when ruptured, the pustules release greenish pus that dries and forms a crust.

cosmetic a., a. cosme'tica a type of contact acne, usually of a low grade, seen on the chin and cheeks of persons habitually using facial cosmetics. The usual lesions are closed comedones or papular pustules.

cystic a., a. cys'tica acne with formation of cysts that enclose a mixture of keratin and sebum in varying proportions.

a. deter'gicans a type of mechanical acne caused by too frequent washing of acne lesions with comedogenic soaps, rough cloths, or abrasive pads.

drug-induced a. a. medicamentosa.

a. estiva'lis acne characterized by keratotic papules, seen in the summer or after a vacation in the sun; called also *Mallorca a.*

excoriated a., a. excoriée des filles, a. excoriée des jeunes filles a superficial type seen most often in girls and young women, caused by the compulsive neurotic habit of picking and squeezing minute, trivial, or nonexistent facial lesions; this produces secondary lesions that can leave scars.

a. fronta'lis a. varioliformis.

a. ful'minans a rare form of severe cystic acne occurring primarily in teenage boys, characterized by highly inflammatory nodules and plaques that undergo suppurative degeneration, leaving ulcerations; this is accompanied by fever, weight loss, anemia, leukocytosis, elevated erythrocyte sedimentation rate, and polyarthritis.

halogen a. acne due to ingestion of salts of bromine, chlorine, or iodine, such as in cold remedies, expectorants, sedatives, analgesics, and vitamins. See *bromide a., chlorine a.,* and *iodide a.*

hypertrophic a. acne vulgaris that heals and leaves hypertrophic scars.

a. indura'ta a progression of papular acne, with deep-seated and destructive lesions that may produce severe scarring.

infantile a. acne vulgaris in infants after three months of age; this type usually has comedones that are more prominent than those of neonatal acne, and may result in scarring.

a. inver'sa hidradenitis suppurativa.

iodide a., iodine a. acne caused by ingestion of iodide compounds.

a. keloid, keloid a., keloidal a., a. keloida'lis development of persistent, hard, follicular plaques along the posterior hairline of the scalp that fuse to form a thick, sclerotic, hypertrophic, pseudokeloidal band extending across the occiput; usually occurring in males of black African descent. Called also *dermatitis papillaris capillitii, keloidal folliculitis,* and *folliculitis keloidalis.*

a. keloida'lis nu'chae acne keloidalis specifically on the neck.

Mallorca a. a. estivalis.

a. mecha'nica, mechanical a. aggravation of existing acne lesions by mechanical factors that deform the skin, such as friction, rubbing, stretching, pressure, pinching, or pulling. The irritation may be provoked by such factors as chin straps, articles of clothing, orthopedic casts, backpacks, chairs, or car or bus seats.

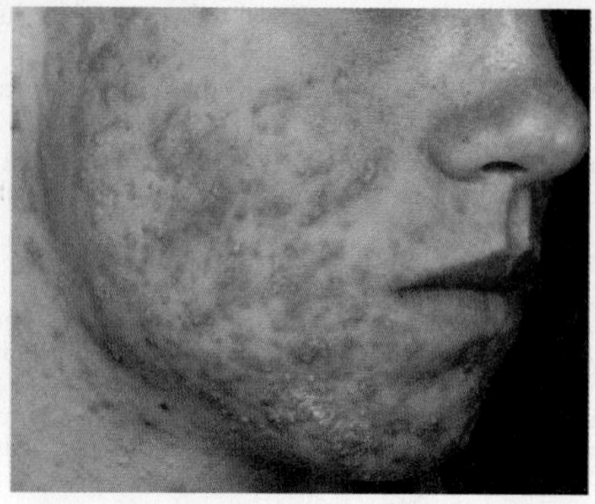

■ Nodulocystic acne.

a. medicamento′sa any type of acne resulting from reaction to medication, such as to a steroid or the salt of a halogen (see *halogen a.*). Called also *drug-induced a.*

a. necro′tica milia′ris a rare, chronic form of folliculitis of the scalp, occurring principally in adults, with formation of tiny superficial pustules that can be destroyed by scratching. See also *a. varioliformis.*

neonatal a., a. neonato′rum a type of acne vulgaris commonly seen in newborn infants, chiefly characterized by papules, pustules, and facial comedones; it usually resolves spontaneously within a few weeks.

nodulocystic a., a. nodulocys′tica a type of severe cystic acne, usually seen in young men, with subcutaneous nodules that may become inflamed and leave scars.

occupational a. contact acne caused by exposure to industrial chemicals, such as oils, tars, waxes, or chlorinated hydrocarbons (see *chloracne*).

oil a. a type of contact acne consisting of follicular acneiform eruptions on the backs of the hands, back of the neck, forearms, face, and thighs, caused by contact with water-insoluble cutting oils.

papular a. a type of acne vulgaris characterized by numerous inflammatory papules; this type often progresses to acne indurata.

papulopustular a., a. papulopustulo′sa a type of acne vulgaris with both papules and inflamed pustules; see *papular a.* and *pustular a.*

pomade a. a type of contact acne seen primarily in persons of African descent who groom their scalps and facial hair with greasy lubricants; characteristics are closed comedones and a few papular pustules around the face.

premenstrual a. acne of a cyclic nature, appearing shortly before menses (or occasionally after).

pustular a., a. pustulo′sa acne vulgaris in which the lesions show central suppuration.

a. rosa′cea rosacea.

a. scrofuloso′rum papulonecrotic tuberculid.

a. sim′plex a. vulgaris.

tropical a., a. tropica′lis a type of severe acne vulgaris seen in hot and moist environments such as tropical climates; characteristics include large painful cysts, nodules, and pustules with formation of conglobate abscesses and frequent scarring, usually on the back, nape of the neck, buttocks, thighs, and upper arms.

a. urtica′ta a skin eruption characterized by edematous papular wheals resembling acne papules, usually on the trunk, upper arms, or neck, but sometimes on the scalp or face; it affects middle-aged women most often, and the cause is unknown. It is not a true form of acne.

a. variolifor′mis a rare condition, with persistent brown papular pustules, usually on the brow and scalp; probably a deep variant of acne necrotica miliaris. Called also *a. frontalis* and *folliculitis varioliformis.*

a. venena′ta contact a.

a. vulga′ris the usual form of acne, a chronic inflammatory disease of the pilosebaceous units; lesions usually occur on the face, chest, and back. The inflamed glands may form small papules (which may surround comedones to give them black centers), or they may form pustules or cysts. The exact cause of acne is unknown, but many factors have been implicated, including hormones, hereditary factors, drugs, stress, and bacteria such as *Propionibacterium acnes* and *Malassezia furfur*. Called also *common a.* and *a. simplex.*

ac·ne·form (ak′ne-form) acneiform.

ac·ne·gen (ak′nə-jen) a substance that causes acne.

ac·ne·gen·ic (ak″ne-jen′ik) [*acne* + *-genic*] causing or capable of producing acne.

ac·ne·iform (ak-ne′ĭ-form″) resembling acne.

ac·ne·mia (ak-ne′me-ə) [*a-*[1] + Gr. *knēmē* leg] atrophy of the calves of the legs.

ACNM American College of Nurse-Midwives.

ac·o·as·ma (ak″o-as′mə) acousma.

Ac·o·can·the·ra (ak″o-kan-the′rə) [Gr. *akōkē* a point, edge + *anthēros* blooming] a genus of plants of the family Apocynaceae, native to Africa. *A. schim′peri* (A.D.C.) Schwf. and other species yield the toxic glycoside ouabain (acocantherin).

ac·o·can·ther·in (ak″o-kan′thər-in) ouabain.

acoe·lom·ate (a-se′lə-māt) 1. lacking a body cavity. 2. an animal lacking a body cavity, as the platyhelminths.

ACOG American College of Obstetricians and Gynecologists.

Ac·o·kan·the·ra (ak″o-kan-the′rə) *Acocanthera.*

acol·u·mel·late (a″kol-u-mel′āt) of certain protozoa and fungi, lacking columellae.

acon·a·tive (ə-kon′ə-tiv) without conation; lacking any desire or impulse to act.

acon·i·tase (ə-kon′ĭ-tās) aconitate hydratase.

***cis*-acon·i·tate** (ə-kon′ĭ-tāt) an intermediate in the interconversion of citrate and isocitrate in the tricarboxylic acid cycle, formed by dehydration of either compound.

acon·i·tate hy·dra·tase (ə-kon′ĭ-tāt hi′drə-tās) [EC 4.2.1.3] an enzyme of the lyase class that catalyzes the interconversion of citrate and isocitrate, a reaction of the tricarboxylic acid cycle (q.v.). The enzyme, a nonheme iron protein, is named for the *cis*-aconitate formed as an intermediate in the dehydration and rehydration reaction. Called also *aconitase.*

ac·o·nite (ak′ə-nīt) [L *aconitum;* Gr. *akoniton*] a poisonous substance from the dried tuberous root of *Aconitum napellus,* which contains aconitine and other related alkaloids; it causes potentially fatal ventricular fibrillation and respiratory paralysis. It was formerly given internally as a febrifuge and gastric anesthetic and is used in Chinese herbal medicine and homeopathy as an analgesic, antiinflammatory, and cardiac tonic. Called also *monkshood* and *wolfsbane.*

acon·i·tine (ə-kon′ĭ-tin) [L. *aconitina, aconitia*] a poisonous alkaloid, the active principle of aconite.

Ac·o·ni·tum (ak″ə-ni′təm) [L.] a genus of poisonous herbs of the family Ranunculaceae. *A. napel′lus* is wolf's bane (or wolfsbane), the source of aconite.

aco·rea (ə-kor′e-ə) [*a-*[1] + Gr. *korē* pupil] absence of the pupil of the eye.

aco·ria (ə-kor′e-ə) [*a-*[1] + Gr. *koros* satiety + *-ia*] a form of polyphagia due to loss of the sensation of satiety, a condition in which patients never feel that they have eaten enough.

acorn (a′korn) the fruit of an oak tree (see *Quercus*). Many types are ground up for food; because they contain gallic acid and tannic acid, they are poisonous if eaten in large amounts.

ACOS American College of Osteopathic Surgeons.

Acos·ta disease (ah-ko′stah) [José de *Acosta,* 1539–1600, Spanish Jesuit missionary who first described it after his travels in Peru in 1590] acute mountain sickness.

acou- [Gr. *akouein* to hear] a combining form denoting relationship to hearing.

acous·ma (ə-kōōz′mə) pl. *acous′mata* [Gr. *akousma* a thing heard] a simple auditory hallucination, e.g., buzzing or ringing sounds.

acous·mat·am·ne·sia (ə-kōōz″mat-am-ne′zhə) [*acousma* hearing + *amnesia*] inability to recall sounds.

acous·tic (ə-kōōs′tik) [Gr. *akoustikos*] pertaining to sound; called also *phonic.*

acous·ti·co·pho·bia (ə-kōōs″tĭ-ko-fo′be-ə) [*acoustic* + *-phobia*] irrational fear of sounds.

acous·tics (ə-kōōs′tiks) the science of sounds.

acous·ti·gram (ə-kōōs′tĭ-gram) acoustogram.

acous·to·gram (ə-kōōs′to-gram) the graphic tracing of the curves, delineated in frequencies per second and decibel levels, of sounds produced by motion of a joint. Applied to the knee joint, an acoustogram shows the sound of the moving semilunar cartilages, the moving contact between the articular surfaces of the femur and tibia, and the circulation of the synovia.

ACP American College of Physicians; acid phosphatase.

ACPS acrocephalopolysyndactyly.

ac·quired (ə-kwīrd′) [L. *acquirere* to obtain] not genetic, but produced by influences originating outside the organism.

ac·qui·si·tion (ak″wĭ-zĭ′shən) 1. in psychology, the period in learning during which progressive increments in response strength can be measured. Also the process involved in such learning. 2. term used in magnetic resonance imaging for the capture of data.

ac·qui·si·tus (ə-kwis′ĭ-təs) [L.] acquired.

ACR American College of Radiology.

ac·ral (ak′rəl) [*acr-* + *-al*[1]] pertaining to an extremity or apex; affecting the limbs (extremities).

acra·nia (ə-kra′ne-ə) [*a-*[1] + *crani-* + *-ia*] a developmental anomaly characterized by partial or complete absence of the cranium.

acra·ni·al (ə-kra′ne-əl) having no cranium.

Acra·ni·a·ta (ə-kra″ne-a′tə) a subphylum of Chordata comprising species without a true skull.

acra·ni·us (ə-kra′ne-əs) a fetus exhibiting acrania.

Ac·rel gan·gli·on (ahk′rel) [Olof (or Olaf) *Acrel*, Swedish surgeon, 1717–1806] see under *ganglion.*

Ac·re·mo·ni·el·la (ak″rə-mo-ne-el′ə) a genus of Fungi Imperfecti of the form-class Hyphomycetes, form-family Dematiaceae; it resembles *Acremonium* and has reportedly been isolated from lung lesions.

ac·re·mo·ni·o·sis (ak″rə-mo-ne-o′sis) infection with the fungus *Acremonium*, producing fever and gummalike swellings.

Ac·re·mo·ni·um (ak″rə-mo′ne-əm) a genus of Fungi Imperfecti of the form-class Hyphomycetes, form-family Moniliaceae; formerly called *Cephalosporium*. Some species produce cephalosporin antibiotics.

A. coenophi′alum a species endophytic in the grass *Festuca arundinacea*, causing the disease fescue foot in cattle and sheep.

A. falcifor′me a species that causes eumycotic mycetoma.

A. kilien′se a species that causes eumycotic mycetoma.

A. lo′liae an endophytic species that infests the grass *Lolium perenne* and causes ryegrass staggers in grazing animals.

A. reci′fei a species that causes eumycotic mycetoma.

ac·rid (ak′rid) [L. *acer, acris* sharp] pungent; producing an irritation.

ac·ri·dine (ak′rĭ-dēn) a tricyclic compound comprising two benzene rings linked by one of pyridine; a dye used in the synthesis of dyes and drugs.

a. orange see under *orange.*

acrit·i·cal (a-krit′ĭ-kəl) [*a-*[1] + *critical*] having no crisis, said especially of febrile diseases ending by lysis.

acrit·o·chro·ma·cy (ə-krit″o-kro′mə-se) monochromatic vision.

ac·ri·vas·tine (ak″rĭ-vas′tēn) an antihistamine (H_1 receptor antagonist) used in treatment of seasonal allergic rhinitis; administered orally.

ACRM American Congress of Rehabilitation Medicine.

acr(o)- [Gr. *akron* extremity, from *akros* extreme] a combining form denoting relation to an extremity, top, or summit, or to an extreme.

ac·ro·ag·no·sis (ak″ro-ag-no′sis) [*acro-* + *a-*[1] + Gr. *gnōsis* knowledge] lack of sensory recognition of a limb; lack of acrognosis.

ac·ro·an·es·the·sia (ak″ro-an″es-the′zhə) [*acro-* + *anesthesia*] loss of sensation in the extremities.

ac·ro·ar·thri·tis (ak″ro-ahr-thri′tis) [*acro-* + *arthritis*] arthritis affecting the extremities.

ac·ro·blast (ak′ro-blast) [*acro-* + *-blast*] Golgi material in the spermatid from which the acrosome develops.

ac·ro·brachy·ceph·a·ly (ak″ro-brak″ĭ-sef′ə-le) [*acro-* + *brachycephaly*] a condition resulting from fusion of the coronal suture, causing abnormal shortening of the anteroposterior diameter of the skull.

ac·ro·cen·tric (ak″ro-sen′trik) [*acro-* + *centric*] having the centromere near one end of the replicating chromosome, so that one arm is much longer than the other; see also under *chromosome*. Cf. *metacentric* and *submetacentric.*

ac·ro·ce·pha·lia (ak″ro-sə-fa′le-ə) [*acro-* + *cephal-* + *-ia*] oxycephaly.

ac·ro·ce·phal·ic (ak″ro-sə-fal′ik) oxycephalic.

ac·ro·ceph·a·lo·poly·syn·dac·ty·ly (ACPS) (ak″ro-sef″ə-lo-pol″e-sin-dak′tə-le) [*acrocephaly* + *polysyndactyly*] any of a group of inherited disorders characterized by acrocephaly and syndactyly, with polydactyly as an additional feature.

a., type I Pfeiffer syndrome.

a., type II Carpenter syndrome.

a., type III Sakati-Nyhan syndrome.

a., type IV Goodman syndrome.

ac·ro·ceph·a·lo·syn·dac·tyl·ia (ak″ro-sef″ə-lo-sin″dak-til′e-ə) acrocephalosyndactyly.

ac·ro·ceph·a·lo·syn·dac·ty·lism (ak″ro-sef″ə-lo-sin-dak′tə-liz-əm) acrocephalosyndactyly.

ac·ro·ceph·a·lo·syn·dac·ty·ly (ak″ro-sef″ə-lo-sin-dak′tə-le) [*acrocephaly* + *syndactyly*] any of a group of autosomal dominant disorders in which craniostenosis is associated with acrocephaly and syndactyly, sometimes with additional anomalies. The term is occasionally used to denote Apert syndrome (acrocephalosyndactyly, type I).

a., type I Apert syndrome.

a., type III Chotzen syndrome.

a., type V Pfeiffer syndrome.

ac·ro·ceph·a·lous (ak″ro-sef′ə-ləs) oxycephalic.

ac·ro·ceph·a·ly (ak″ro-sef′ə-le) oxycephaly.

a.-syndactyly the characteristic shape of the head seen in acrocephalosyndactyly.

ac·ro·chor·don (ak″ro-kor′dən) [*acro-* + *chordo-*] a type of papillomatous skin lesion, sometimes slightly discolored, usually seen on the neck, upper chest, or axilla of middle-aged women. The epidermis is hyperplastic and encloses a dermal connective tissue stalk composed of loose, edematous collagen fibers; larger lesions may be pedunculated and are called *soft fibromas*. Called also *skin tag, cutaneous tag* or *papilloma*, and *fibroepithelial polyp.*

ac·ro·ci·ne·sis (ak″ro-si-ne′sis) [*acro-* + Gr. *kinēsis* motion] excessive motility; abnormal freedom of movement. Called also *acrokinesia.*

ac·ro·ci·net·ic (ak″ro-si-net′ik) affected with acrocinesis.

ac·ro·con·trac·ture (ak″ro-kən-trak′chər) [*acro-* + *contracture*] contracture of an extremity; contracture of muscles of the hand or foot.

ac·ro·cy·a·no·sis (ak″ro-si″ə-no′sis) [*acro-* + *cyanosis*] symmetrical cyanosis of the extremities, with persistent, uneven blue or red discoloration of the skin of the digits, wrists, and ankles accompanied by profuse sweating and coldness of the digits. Called also *Raynaud sign.*

ac·ro·der·ma·ti·tis (ak″ro-dur″mə-ti′tis) [*acro-* + *dermatitis*] inflammation involving the skin of the extremities, especially the hands and feet.

chronic atrophic a., a. chro′nica atro′phicans a chronic, diffuse type seen in later stages of Lyme disease, usually confined to the limbs, seen most often in Europe and in women; characteristics include an erythematous, edematous, pruritic phase followed by sclerosis and atrophy.

a. conti′nua a variant of localized pustular psoriasis characterized by a chronic inflammatory eruption of the digits, palms, and soles; it sometimes becomes more generalized, with a thin annular vesiculopustular border that gradually extends and recurs, leaving inflamed, mildly exfoliating skin. Called also *a. perstans, Hallopeau a.*, and *dermatitis repens.*

a. enteropa′thica a severe gastrointestinal and cutaneous disease of neonates and infants, due to an autosomal recessive disorder of zinc uptake (gene locus: 8q24.3); babies suffer from failure to thrive and alopecia. The skin lesion is a vesiculopustular dermatitis, preferentially located around body orifices and on the head, hands, and feet. Gastrointestinal symptoms include diarrhea and steatorrhea.

Hallopeau a. a. continua.

infantile a., papular a. of childhood, a. papulo′sa infan′tum Gianotti-Crosti syndrome.

a. per′stans a. continua.

ac·ro·der·ma·to·sis (ak″ro-dur″mə-to′sis) pl. *acrodermato′ses* [*acro-* + *dermatosis*] any disease involving the skin of the extremities.

ac·ro·dol·i·cho·me·lia (ak″ro-dol″ĭ-ko-me′le-ə) [*acro-* + *dolicho-* + *-melia*] abnormal or disproportionate length of hands and feet.

ac·ro·dyn·ia (ak″ro-din′e-ə) [*acr-* + *-odynia*] a disease of early childhood characterized by pink, swollen, painful fingers and toes; listlessness, irritability, failure to thrive, and photophobia; rashes, profuse perspiration, loss of teeth, and sometimes redness of the cheeks and tip of the nose. Most cases are toxic neuropathies caused by mercury poisoning; individual sensitivity may also be a factor. Called also *erythredema polyneuropathy* and *Bilderbeck, Selter, Swift, Swift-Feer*, or *pink disease.*

ac·ro·dys·pla·sia (ak″ro-dis-pla′zhə) acrocephalosyndactyly.

ac·ro·es·the·sia (ak″ro-es-the′zhə) [*acro-* + *esthesia*] 1. increased sensitiveness. 2. pain in the extremities.

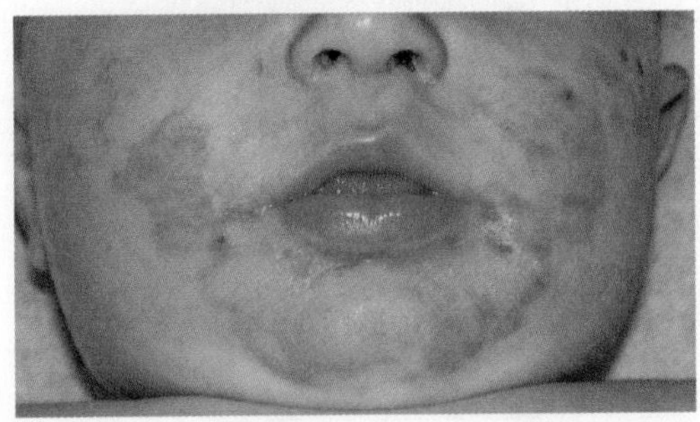

■ Acrodermatitis enteropathica with typical U-shaped distribution.

acrog·e·nous (ə-kroj′ə-nəs) produced at the apex of a conidiophore; said of conidia.

ac·ro·ger·ia (ak″ro-je′re-ə) a rare condition consisting of partial progeria, primarily of the skin, which is thin and parchmentlike, especially on the hands and feet; in some cases it is inherited in autosomal recessive fashion. Called also *metageria.*

ac·rog·no·sis (ak″rog-no′sis) [*acro-* + Gr. *gnōsis* knowledge] sensory recognition of the limbs and of the different portions of each limb in relation to each other.

ac·ro·hy·po·ther·my (ak″ro-hi′po-thur″me) [*acro-* + *hypothermy*] abnormal coldness of the hands and feet.

ac·ro·ker·a·to·elas·toi·do·sis (ak″ro-ker″ə-to-e-las″toi-do′sis) [*acro-* + *kerato-* + *elastoidosis*] a rare skin disorder consisting of elastosis with small keratotic papules or plaques on the hands and feet; it is usually inherited in autosomal dominant fashion and becomes evident after puberty. Cf. *focal acral hyperkeratosis.*

ac·ro·ker·a·to·sis (ak″ro-ker″ə-to′sis) a condition involving keratosis (horny growths) on the skin of the upper and lower limbs.

paraneoplastic a. Bazex syndrome.

a. verrucifor′mis an autosomal dominant geroderma allelic with Darier disease, caused by mutation in the *ATP2A2* gene (locus: 12q23-q24.1), which encodes a calcium-transporting ATPase of the sarcoplasmic reticulum. It is characterized by closely grouped warty papules on the backs of the hands, elbows, knees, and feet. It is sometimes associated with diffuse hyperkeratosis of the palms and soles.

ac·ro·ki·ne·sia (ak″ro-kĭ-ne′zhə) acrocinesis.

acro·le·in (ak-ro′le-in) a volatile, acrid, highly toxic liquid from the decomposition of glycerin; it is one of the degradation products of cyclophosphamide and is thought to be the cause of hemorrhagic cystitis and neoplasms of the bladder in patients treated with oral cyclophosphamide.

ac·ro·mac·ria (ak″ro-mak′re-ə) arachnodactyly.

ac·ro·me·ga·lia (ak″ro-mə-ga′le-ə) acromegaly.

ac·ro·meg·a·lo·gi·gan·tism (ak″ro-meg″ə-lo-ji′gan-tiz-əm) gigantism and acromegaly due to hypersecretion of growth hormone beginning before puberty and continuing into maturity.

ac·ro·meg·a·loid·ism (ak″ro-meg′ə-loid-iz-əm) a bodily condition resembling acromegaly but not due to pituitary disorder.

ac·ro·meg·a·ly (ak″ro-meg′ə-le) [*acro-* + *-megaly*] a chronic disease of adults caused by hypersecretion of growth hormone, characterized by enlargement of many parts of the skeleton, especially distal portions such as the nose, ears, jaws, fingers, and toes. Joint pain resulting from osteoarthrosis occurs, and the joint spaces are increased because of cartilage proliferation. Complications resulting from increased growth hormone secretion include insulin resistance and glucose intolerance, airway obstruction, hypertension, cardiomyopathy, and abnormalities of calcium and bone metabolism. **acromegal′ic** *adj*

ac·ro·mel·al·gia (ak″ro-məl-al′jə) erythromelalgia.

ac·ro·mel·ic (ak″ro-me′lik) [*acro-* + *mel-* + *-ic*] pertaining to or affecting the end of a limb.

ac·ro·meta·gen·e·sis (ak″ro-met″ə-jen′ə-sis) [*acro-* + *meta-* + *-genesis*] undue growth of the extremities.

ac·ro·mic·ria (ak″ro-mik′re-ə) [*acro-* + *micr-* + *-ia*] hypoplasia of the extremities of the skeleton, including the nose, jaws, fingers, and toes; the converse of acromegaly.

acromi(o)- [L. *acromion,* q.v.] a combining form denoting relationship to the acromion.

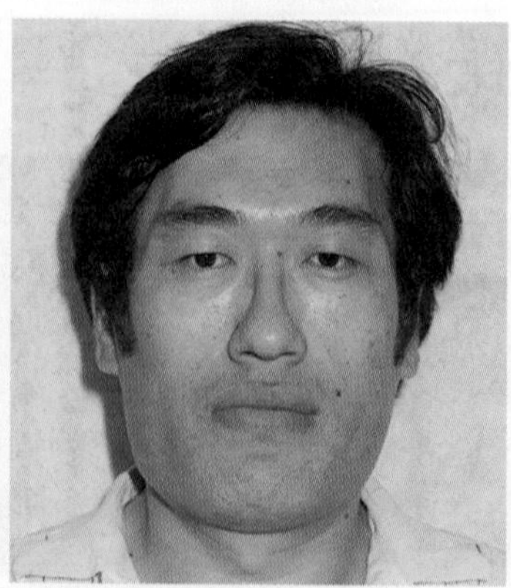

■ Acromegaly, showing characteristic skeletal enlargement.

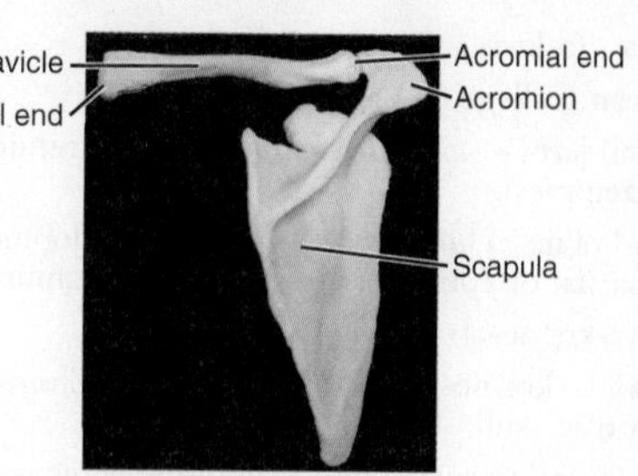

■ Posterior (dorsal) surface of the scapula, showing the acromion.

acro·mio·cla·vic·u·lar (ə-kro″me-o-klə-vik′u-lər) pertaining to the acromion and clavicle, especially to the articulation between the acromion and clavicle. See also *articulatio acromioclavicularis.*

acro·mio·cor·a·coid (ə-kro″me-o-kor′ə-koid) pertaining to the acromion and the coracoid process; called also *coracoacromial.*

acro·mio·hu·mer·al (ə-kro″me-o-hu′mər-əl) pertaining to the acromion and humerus.

acro·mi·on (ə-kro′me-ən) [*acro-* + Gr. *ōmos* shoulder] [TA] the lateral extension of the spine of the scapula, projecting over the shoulder joint and forming the highest point of the shoulder; called also *acromial process* and *acromion scapulae.* **acro′mial** *adj*

acro·mio·nec·to·my (ə-kro″me-o-nek′tə-me) resection of the distal end of the acromion, done in the treatment of acromioclavicular arthritis.

acro·mio·plas·ty (ə-kro′me-o-plas″te) surgical removal of an anterior spur of the acromion to relieve mechanical compression of the rotator cuff during movement of the glenohumeral joint; called also *anterior acromioplasty.* **acromioplas′tic** *adj*

acro·mio·scap·u·lar (ə-kro″me-o-skap′u-lər) pertaining to the acromion and scapula.

acro·mio·tho·rac·ic (ə-kro″me-o-tho-ras′ik) pertaining to the acromion and thorax.

acrom·pha·lus (ə-krom′fə-ləs) [*acr-* + *omphalus*] 1. undue prominence of the navel; sometimes a sign of umbilical hernia. 2. the center of the navel.

ac·ro·myo·to·nia (ak″ro-mi″o-to′ne-ə) [*acro-* + *myotonia*] contracture of the hand or foot resulting in spastic deformity.

ac·ro·my·ot·o·nus (ak″ro-mi-ot′o-nəs) acromyotonia.

ac·ro·nar·cot·ic (ak″ro-nahr-kot′ik) both acrid and narcotic.

ac·ro·neu·ro·sis (ak″ro-noo̅-ro′sis) [*acro-* + *neurosis*] any neuropathy of the extremities.

ac·ro·nym (ak′ro-nim) [*acro-* + Gr. *onoma* name] a word formed by the initial letters of the principal components of a compound term, as laser or maser.

ac·ro·os·te·ol·y·sis (ak″ro-os″te-ol′ĭ-sis) osteolysis involving the distal phalanges of the fingers and toes.

ac·ro·pach·ia (ak″ro-pak′e-ə) [*acro-* + *pachy-* + *-ia*] 1. clubbing. 2. hypertrophic osteopathy.

ac·ro·pachy (ak′ro-pak″e) clubbing.

thyroid a. clubbing of digits accompanying severe autoimmune thyroid disease.

ac·ro·pachy·der·ma (ak″ro-pak″ĭ-dur′mə) [*acro-* + *pachy-* + *derma*] thickening of the skin of the limbs, as seen in acromegaly and pachydermoperiostitis.

a. with pachyperiostitis pachydermoperiostosis.

ac·ro·pa·ral·y·sis (ak″ro-pə-ral′ĭ-sis) [*acro-* + *paralysis*] paralysis of the extremities.

ac·ro·par·es·the·sia (ak″ro-par″es-the′zhə) [*acro-* + *paresthesia*] 1. paresthesia of limbs and tips of other extremities due to nerve compression at any of several levels, or polyneuritis. 2. a disease marked by attacks of tingling, numbness, and stiffness in the limbs, chiefly the fingers, hands, and forearms, sometimes with pain, pallor of the skin, or slight cyanosis.

ac·ro·pa·thol·o·gy (ak″ro-pə-thol′ə-je) [*acro-* + *pathology*] the pathology of diseases affecting the extremities.

acrop·a·thy (ă-krop′ə-the) [*acro-* + *-pathy*] any disease of the extremities.

ac·ro·pep·tide (ak″ro-pep′tīd) a protein fraction obtained by heating protein to above 140°C in nonaqueous solvents.

acrop·e·tal (ə-krop′ə-təl) [*acro-* + *-petal*] developing from the base toward the summit; pertaining to the production of conidia in fungi.

ac•ro•pho•bia (ak″ro-fo′be-ə) [*acro-* + *-phobia*] irrational fear of heights.

ac•ro•pig•men•ta•tion (ak″ro-pig″mən-ta′shən) hyperpigmentation of the skin of the extremities.

reticulate a. of Dohi dyschromatosis symmetrica hereditaria.

reticulate a. of Kitamura an autosomal dominant pigmentary genodermatosis caused by mutations in the *KRT5* gene (locus:12q13), which encodes keratin 5, characterized by slightly depressed, hyperpigmented macules arranged in a reticulate pattern on the dorsal extremities, appearing in early childhood. It most commonly occurs in Asian ethnic groups. Some authorities consider it to be the same disorder as Dowling-Degos disease.

ac•ro•pleu•rog•e•nous (ak″ro-ploo-roj′ə-nəs) produced at the apex and on the sides of a conidiophore; said of conidia.

ac•ro•pus•tu•lo•sis (ak″ro-pus″tu-lo′sis) pustulosis of the extremities.

infantile a. a congenital condition characterized by small pruritic pustules of the hands and feet; episodes last one to two weeks, followed by a remission of a few weeks and another episode. It is usually seen in infants of African descent and resolves completely by age 2 or 3 years.

ac•ro•scle•ro•der•ma (ak″ro-skler″o-dur′mə) acrosclerosis.

ac•ro•scle•ro•sis (ak″ro-sklə-ro′sis) [*acro-* + *sclerosis*] a type of systemic scleroderma of the hands and feet, especially the digits (sclerodactyly), as well as the face and neck, in combination with Raynaud phenomenon. Called also *acroscleroderma.*

ac•ro•sin (ak′ro-sin) [EC 3.4.21.10] a type of serine endopeptidase stored in the acrosomes of mammalian spermatozoa, as the inactive precursor proacrosin; after activation it is believed to aid penetration of the zona pellucida of the oocyte.

ac•ro•some (ak′ro-sōm) [*acro-* + *-some*] the caplike, membrane-bound structure derived from Golgi elements found at the anterior portion of the head of a spermatozoon; it contains lysosomal enzymes and a proteolytic enzyme, which are believed to facilitate entry of spermatozoa into oocytes. Called also *acrosomal cap.* See also *acrosome reaction,* under *reaction.*

ac•ro•sphe•no•syn•dac•tyl•ia (ak″ro-sfe″no-sin″dak-til′e-ə) acrocephalosyndactyly.

ac•ro•spi•ro•ma (ak″ro-spi-ro′mə) [*acro-* + *spiroma*] 1. an adnexal tumor of the distal portion of a sweat gland, such as a hidradenoma or poroma. 2. sometimes used as a synonym for *poroma.*

eccrine a. clear cell hidradenoma.

ac•ros•te•al•gia (ak″ros-te-al′jə) [*acr-* + *ostealgia*] a painful apophysitis of the bones of the extremities.

ac•ro•syn•dac•ty•ly (ak″ro-sin-dak′tə-le) [*acro-* + *syndactyly*] fusion of the terminal portion of two or more digits, with clefts or sinuses present between their proximal phalanges.

ac•ro•ter•ic (ak″ro-ter′ik) pertaining to the tips or outermost parts.

acrot•ic (ă-krot′ik) [*a-*[1] + Gr. *krotos* beat] pertaining to absence or weakness of the pulse.

ac•ro•tism (ak′ro-tiz-əm) [*a-*[1] + Gr. *krotos* beat + *-ism*] absence or imperceptibility of the pulse.

ac•ro•tropho•dyn•ia (ak″ro-trof″o-din′e-ə) [*acro-* + *troph-* + *-odynia*] a trophic disorder with neuritis and paresthesia from exposure of extremities to cold and moisture.

acryl•a•mide (ə-kril′ə-mīd) a vinyl monomer used in the production of polymers with many industrial uses. The polymers are nontoxic but exposure to acrylamide can cause peripheral neuropathy, polyneuritis, and central nervous system lesions.

acry•late (ə-kril′āt) a salt, ester, or conjugate base of acrylic acid.

acryl•ic (ə-kril′ik) pertaining to or containing polymers of acrylic acid, methacrylic acid, or acrylonitrile; as acrylic resins (q.v.), used in various medical and dental applications.

acryl•ic ac•id (ə-kril′ik) a readily polymerizing liquid used as a monomer for acrylic polymers; see also *acrylic.*

ac•ry•lo•ni•trile (ak″rə-lo-ni′trīl) a colorless halogenated hydrocarbon used in the making of plastics and as a pesticide; its vapors are irritant to the respiratory tract and eyes, can cause systemic poisoning, and are carcinogenic. Called also *2-propenenitrile* and *vinyl cyanide.*

ACS American Cancer Society; American Chemical Society; American College of Surgeons.

ACSM American College of Sports Medicine.

act (akt) something done; a performance involving motor activity.

reflex a. a relatively fixed action or pattern of response performed as a result of the triggering of a reflex arc and usually without involvement of the higher centers.

Ac•taea (ak-te′ə) [L., from Gr. *aktē* elder tree] a genus of plants of the family Ranunculaceae. *A. odora′ta* (bitter weed) and *A. richardso′ni* (rubber weed) are poisonous to sheep and goats.

ac•ta•pla•nin (ak″tə-pla′nin) any of various glycopeptide antibiotics used as veterinary growth stimulants, derived from species of *Actinoplanes,* containing a chlorophenyl group, glucose, mannose, rhamnose, and other amino acids.

ACTH adrenocorticotropic hormone; see *corticotropin.*

Ac•thar (ak′thahr) trademark for preparations of corticotropin.

Act-HIB (akt′hib) trademark for a preparation of *Haemophilus* b conjugate vaccine.

ACTH•oma (ak-to′mə) a type of pancreatic endocrine tumor that arises from islet cells, secretes corticotropin, and causes Cushing syndrome; these are often malignant.

Ac•threl (ak′threl) trademark for a preparation of corticorelin ovine triflutate.

Ac•ti•cin (ak′tĭ-sin) trademark for a preparation of permethrin.

Ac•ti-Di•one (ak″tĭ-di′ōn) trademark for a preparation of cycloheximide.

Ac•ti•gall (ak′tĭ-gawl″) trademark for a preparation of ursodiol.

ac•ti•graph (ak′tĭ-graph) a device worn on the wrist for measuring body movements over time and studying circadian rhythms; it can be used when the patient is asleep to estimate sleep quantity and quality.

ac•tig•ra•phy (ak-tig′rə-fe) the use of an actigraph to measure periods of rest and activity; used in the evaluation of patients with insomnia or suspected wake/sleep cycle abnormalities.

Ac•tim•mune (ak′tĭ-mūn) trademark for a preparation of interferon gamma-1b.

ac•tin (ak′tin) a structural protein present in all eukaryotic cells, important both as a component of the cytoskeleton and for its role in cell motility. In the absence of salt, it exists as a 42-kD globular monomer *(G-actin);* in the presence of potassium chloride and adenosine triphosphate it polymerizes, forming long fibers *(F-actin).* It binds over 60 families of cytoplasmic proteins, and genetic defects in the actin system cause a wide variety of diseases, including muscular dystrophy, hemolytic anemia, and cardiomyopathies. In combination with myosin it is responsible for muscular contraction and for the pinching off of daughter cells in cytokinesis. See Plate 32 and see also *actomyosin.*

act•ing out (ak′ting out) the expression of unconscious feelings and fantasies in behavior; reacting to present situations as if they were the original situation that gave rise to the feelings and fantasies, i.e., acting out of a transference. Often applied imprecisely to any sort of disapproved impulsive behavior.

ac•tin•ic (ak-tin′ik) [*aktin-* + *-ic*] pertaining to those rays of light beyond the violet end of the spectrum that produce chemical effects.

ac•ti•nic•i•ty (ak″tĭ-nis′ĭ-te) actinism.

ac•tin•i•form (ak-tin′ĭ-form) [*aktin-* + *form*] formed like a ray; radiate.

α-ac•tin•in (ak′tə-nin) a 100-kD protein occurring as a dimer and found in muscle, fibroblasts, and epithelial cells; it binds actin filaments to one another and to cell membranes and in the Z band holds the actin fibers in a lattice array. See also *vinculin.*

ac•ti•nism (ak′tĭ-niz-əm) [*aktin-* + *-ism*] the property of radiant energy that produces chemical changes, as in photography or heliotherapy; called also *actinicity.*

ac•tin•i•um (Ac) (ak-tin′e-əm) [Gr. *aktis* ray] a rare metallic chemical element occurring in the ores of uranium and having radioactive properties; atomic number 89, atomic weight 227.

actin(o)- [Gr. *aktis,* gen. *aktinos* a ray] a combining form denoting relation to a ray or to radiation, or shaped like a ray.

ac•ti•no•bac•il•lo•sis (ak″tĭ-no-bas″ĭ-lo′sis) a disease of domestic animals and occasionally humans, resembling actinomycosis but caused by species of *Actinobacillus.* In cattle and sheep the species is *A. lignieresii;* characteristics in cattle include granulomatous lesions in the throat and mouth *(wooden tongue)* and in sheep, suppurative lesions of the skin and lungs. In horses and pigs the species is *A. equuli* and the disease is more commonly known as *equulosis* (q.v.).

Ac•ti•no•ba•cil•lus (ak″tĭ-no-bə-sil′us) [*actino-* + *bacillus*] a genus of gram-negative, fermentative, nonmotile, coccoid or rod-shaped bacteria of the family Pasteurellaceae, part of the normal mammalian microflora. They are potentially pathogenic for humans and for cattle, sheep, horses, and pigs, causing granulomatous lesions.

A. actinomycetemco′mitans a species that is found in association with species of *Actinomyces* in actinomycotic lesions and septicemias; the etiologic role is unclear. It has also been isolated from the human gingival crevice.

A. equu′li a species that is found normally on mucous membranes but can also cause equulosis in horses and pigs.

A. ho′minis a rare species that is commensal in the human upper respiratory tract and can cause respiratory infections.

A. ligniere′sii a species that is primarily a commensal and pathogen of domestic animals, causing actinobacillosis; occasionally it infects humans.

A. su′is a species isolated from horses, pigs, and cattle. It produces pneumonia and septicemia in pigs. The organisms have also been isolated from human clinical blood and respiratory and wound specimens.

A. ure′ae a species that has occasionally been isolated from the nasal passages and can cause ozena and other respiratory infections. Formerly called *Pasteurella ureae.*

Ac•ti•no•bac•te•ria (ak″tĭ-no-bak-tēr′e-ə) [*actino-* + *bacteria*] 1. a morphologically and physiologically diverse phylum of bacteria grouped together on the basis of 16S rRNA sequence analysis, containing a large number of medically important organisms. 2. the sole class of bacteria of this phylum, divided into several phylogenetically distinct subclasses; medically important organisms are included in the subclasses Actinobacteridae and Coriobacteridae.

Ac•ti•no•bac•te•ri•dae (ak″tĭ-no-bak-tēr′ĭ-de) a large, diverse subclass of bacteria of the class Actinobacteria; it contains two orders, Actinomycetales and Bifidobacteriales.

Ac•ti•no•ba•cu•lum (ak″tĭ-no-bak′u-ləm) [*actino-* + L. *baculum* staff] a genus of gram-positive, anaerobic or facultatively anaerobic bacteria of the family Actinomycetaceae, consisting of nonmotile, nonsporulating, non–acid-fast, straight to slightly curved rods, which may exhibit branching. *A. schaa′lii, A. massi′liae,* and *A. urina′le* cause urinary tract infections in humans and *A. sui′s* is an important cause of urinary tract infections and abortion in sows. The type species is *A. suis.*

ac•ti•no•chem•is•try (ak″tĭ-no-kem′is-tre) [*actino-* + *chemistry*] photochemistry.

ac•ti•no•con•ges•tin (ak″tĭ-no-kən-jes′tin) congestin.

ac•ti•no•der•ma•ti•tis (ak″tĭ-no-dur″mə-ti′tis) actinic dermatitis.

ac•tin•o•lyte (ak-tin′ə-līt) [*actino-* + Gr. *lytos* soluble, from *lyein* to loosen] any substance that is markedly changed by light.

Ac•ti•no•ma•du•ra (ak″tĭ-no-mə-dōōr′ə) [*actino-* + *Madura* (now *Madurai*), a city in India] a genus of bacteria of the family Thermomonosporaceae, consisting of non–acid-fast organisms that form nonfragmenting branched filaments.

A. madu′rae a species distributed worldwide in soil, and a common cause of actinomycotic mycetoma.

A. pelletie′ri a species found in Africa, India, and North and South America, and a common cause of actinomycotic mycetoma.

ac•ti•nom•e•ter (ak″tĭ-nom′ə-ter) [*actino-* + *-meter*] an instrument for measuring radiation intensity, particularly that from the sun or other sources capable of causing photochemical reactions.

ac•ti•nom•e•try (ak″tĭ-nom′ə-tre) the measurement of the photochemical power of light.

ac•ti•no•my•ce•li•al (ak″tĭ-no-mi-se′le-əl) 1. pertaining to the mycelium of an actinomyces. 2. actinomycetic.

Ac•ti•no•my•ces (ak″tĭ-no-mi′sēz) [*actino-* + Gr. *mykēs* fungus] a genus of bacteria of the family Actinomycetaceae, consisting of gram-positive, irregularly staining, straight or slightly curved rods that form branched filaments; organisms are asporogenous, non–acid-fast, nonmotile, and chemo-organotrophic. The type species is *A. bo′vis.*

A. asteroi′des *Nocardia asteroides.*

A. bo′vis a non–acid-fast, facultatively anaerobic species of serologic group B, a normal inhabitant of animal mucous membranes, and the etiologic agent of actinomycosis in cattle.

A. brasilien′sis *Nocardia brasiliensis.*

A. dentocario′sus *Rothia dentocariosa.*

A. eppinge′ri *Nocardia asteroides.*

A. europae′us an anaerobic species isolated from skin abscesses.

A. israe′lii a non–acid-fast anaerobic species of serologic group D, parasitic in the mouth and proliferating in necrotic tissue. It is the etiologic agent of human actinomycosis and sometimes actinomycotic mycetoma, and it occasionally causes infection in cattle.

A. mey′eri a species that is a normal inhabitant of the human oral cavity and is sometimes found in abscesses and other infections.

A. mu′ris, A. mu′ris-rat′ti *Streptobacillus moniliformis.*

A. naeslun′dii an aerobic species of serologic group A. It is a normal inhabitant of the oral cavity and an etiologic agent of human actinomycosis and periodontal disease.

A. odontoly′ticus a facultatively anaerobic species of serologic group E. It is a natural inhabitant of the human oral cavity and has been found in dental caries.

A. radin′gae an anaerobic species isolated from soft tissue infections of the chest, breast, and back.

A. turicen′sis an anaerobic species isolated from infections of the genitourinary tract.

A. visco′sus a facultative anaerobic species of serologic group F. It is found in the oral cavity of humans, hamsters, and rats, and is a cause of dental caries in laboratory animals; pathogenicity for humans has not been established.

ac•ti•no•my•ces (ak″tĭ-no-mi′sēz) pl. *actinomyce′tes.* A bacterium of the genus *Actinomyces.*

Ac•ti•no•my•ce•ta•ceae (ak″tĭ-no-mi″sə-ta′se-e) a family of bacteria of the suborder Actinomycineae, order Actinomycetales, consisting of gram-positive, nonsporulating, irregularly shaped rods that tend to form branched filaments. It contains the genera *Actinobaculum, Actinomyces, Arcanobacterium,* and *Mobiluncus.*

Ac•ti•no•my•ce•ta•les (ak″tĭ-no-mi″sə-ta′lēz) an order of bacteria of the subclass Actinobacteridae (class Actinobacteria), made up of elongated cells that tend to form branching filaments; medically important organisms are included in the suborders Actinomycineae, Corynebacterineae, Micrococcineae, Micromonosporineae, Propionibacterineae, Pseudonocardineae, Streptomycineae, and Streptosporangineae.

ac•ti•no•my•cete (ak″tĭ-no-mi′sēt) any bacterium of the order Actinomycetales.

nocardioform a′s a morphological group of actinomycetes characterized by a fugacious mycelium that breaks up into bacillary or coccal forms; all genera in this group are gram-positive and aerobic.

ac•ti•no•my•ce•tes (ak″tĭ-no-mi-se′tēz) plural of *actinomyces* and *actinomycete.*

ac•ti•no•my•cet•ic (ak″tĭ-no-mi-set′ik) of or caused by actinomyces; of or pertaining to bacteria of the order Actinomycetales or diseases caused by such organisms.

ac•ti•no•my•ce•tin (ak″tĭ-no-mi-se′tin) a substance derived from cultures of the actinomycete *Streptomyces albus;* it lyses dead bacteria.

ac•ti•no•my•ce•to•ma (ak″tĭ-no-mi″sə-to′mə) [*actino-* + *mycetoma*] actinomycotic mycetoma.

ac•ti•no•my•cin (ak″tĭ-no-mi′sin) a large, complex family of antibiotics obtained from cultures of various species of *Streptomyces,* which have antibacterial, antifungal, and cytotoxic properties. Actinomycin D (see *dactinomycin*) is an antineoplastic agent.

Ac•ti•no•my•ci•neae (ak″tĭ-no-mi-sin′e-e) a suborder of bacteria of the order Actinomycetales, containing the single family Actinomycetaceae.

ac•ti•no•my•co•ma (ak-tĭ-no-mi-ko′mə) [*actinomyces* + *-oma*] a tumorlike swelling seen in actinomycosis.

ac•ti•no•my•co•sis (ak″tĭ-no-mi-ko′sis) [*actino-* + *mycosis*] an infectious disease caused predominantly by *Actinomyces israelii* in humans and by *A. bovis* in cattle. The most common sites are the submandibular region, thorax, and abdomen. Characteristics include fever, weight loss, and intraperitoneal and pelvic abscesses, including in the liver and sometimes the lung (resulting from aspiration). In cattle there is cervical lymphadenitis, called lumpy jaw. Pus from a suppurative lesion may contain yellow clusters called sulfur granules.

ac•ti•no•my•cot•ic (ak″tĭ-no-mi-kot′ik) pertaining to or affected with actinomycosis.

ac•ti•no•phage (ak-tin′o-fāj) a virus that causes the lysis of actinomycetes.

Ac•ti•no•pla•nes (ak″tĭ-no-pla′nēz) [*actino-* + Gr. *planēs* one who wanders] a genus of bacteria of the family Micromonosporaceae, consisting of saprophytic forms found on a wide variety of plant material and in soil. The type species is *A. philippinen′sis.*

A. teichomyce′ticus a species that is the source of teicoplanin.

A. utahen′sis a species that produces acarbose.

ac•ti•no•ther•a•py (ak″tĭ-no-ther′ə-pe) phototherapy.

ac•tion (ak′shən) [L. *actio*] any performance of function or movement either of any part or organ or of the whole body.

ball-valve a. the intermittent obstruction caused by a free or partially attached foreign body in a tubular or cavitary structure, as by a foreign body in a bronchus, a stone in a bile duct, or a tumor in the cardiac atrium.

buffer a. an action that tends to stabilize an inanimate system or a body function or state, such as pH, blood pressure, [Ca^{2+}], etc.; most commonly used to denote the stabilization of pH by acid-base buffers (tampon a.).

capillary a. the transport of a fluid in a tube, caused by adhesion of the fluid to the tube wall.

contact a. contact catalysis.

cumulative a. action of increased intensity, as may be evidenced after administration of several doses of a drug due to the accumulation of the drug in the body so that the biological effect is greater than after the first dose. Called also *cumulative effect.*

reflex a. a response, often involuntary, resulting from the passage of excitation potential from a receptor to a muscle or gland, over a reflex arc.

specific a. the action of a drug which is exerted on a certain definite pathogenic organism.

tampon a. buffer a.

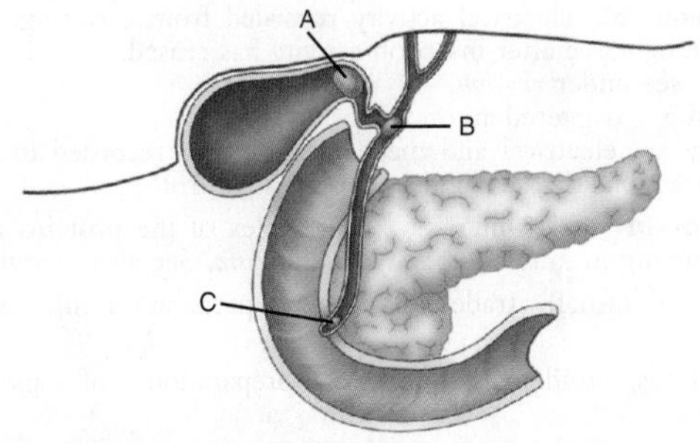

■ Ball-valve action. Calculi obstructing the cystic duct *(A)*, common hepatic duct *(B)*, and common bile duct *(C)*.

trigger a. an action that releases energy whose character has no relation to the process which released it.

Ac•tiq (ak′tik) trademark for a preparation of fentanyl citrate.

Ac•ti•site (ak′tĭ-sīt″) trademark for fibers impregnated with tetracycline hydrochloride, for use in the treatment of periodontal disease.

Ac•ti•vase (ak′tĭ-vās) trademark for a preparation of alteplase.

ac•ti•vate (ak′tĭ-vāt) to render active.

ac•ti•va•tion (ak″tĭ-va′shən) 1. the act or process of rendering active. 2. the transformation of a proenzyme into an active enzyme by the action of a kinase or another proenzyme. 3. the process by which the central nervous system is stimulated into activity through the mediation of the reticular activating system. 4. the deliberate induction of a pattern of electrical activity in the brain in electroencephalography.

allosteric a. increase in enzyme activity by binding of an effector at an allosteric site that causes at the catalytic site either increased binding affinity of the enzyme for the substrate or increased rate of catalytic turnover.

contact a. initiation of the intrinsic pathway of coagulation through interaction of factor XII with various electronegative surfaces, such as collagen fibers, skin, or sebum in vivo, or particulate silicates in vitro.

lymphocyte a. stimulation of lymphocytes by specific antigen or nonspecific mitogens resulting in macromolecular synthesis (RNA, protein, and DNA) and production of lymphokines; it is followed by proliferation and differentiation of the progeny into various effector and memory cells.

ac•ti•va•tor (ak′tĭ-va″tər) 1. a substance that combines with an enzyme to increase its catalytic activity. 2. a substance that stimulates the development of a particular structure in the embryo. Cf. *inductor* and *organizer.* 3. functional a. 4. a chemical or other form of energy that causes another substance to become reactive or that induces a chemical reaction.

bow a. a functional activator whose two halves are connected by a wire bow or safety-pin loop; between the halves of the anterior area, a layer of rubber is attached as a shock absorber and to open the bite in front. Called also *Schwarz a.*

functional a. a myofunctional removable orthodontic appliance that acts as a passive transmitter of the force produced by the function of the activated muscle, and applied to the teeth and alveolar processes to effect tooth movement. Called also *Andresen appliance*, *monoblock a.*, and *monoblock appliance.*

monoblock a. a removable orthodontic appliance utilizing muscle forces to achieve therapeutic correction; called also *Andresen appliance* and *functional a.*

plasminogen a. any of a group of substances that have the ability to cleave plasminogen and convert it into plasmin, its active form; see *t-plasminogen a.* and *u-plasminogen a.*

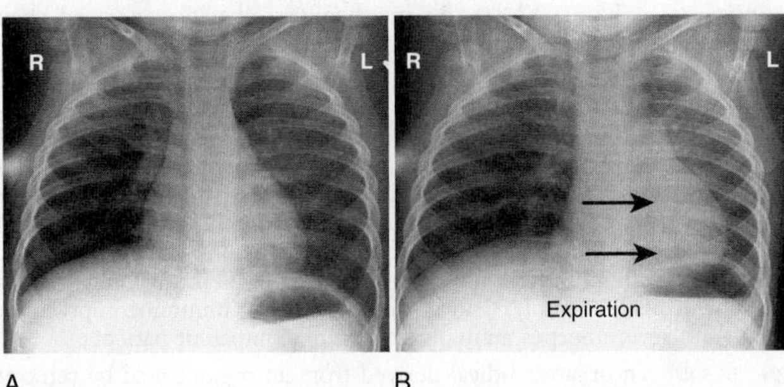

■ Ball-valve action caused by foreign body in the right main stem bronchus. *(A)*, Inspiration appears normal. *(B)* On expiration, the right lung remains hyperinflated due to trapping of air from the ball-valve effect of the foreign body. The left lung shows normal decrease in volume and the heart has shifted to the left *(arrows)*.

polyclonal a. a mitogen that activates lymphocytes of many antigenic specificities, in contrast to an antigen, which only activates cells specific for the antigen. Some polyclonal activators activate T cells; others activate B cells.

prothrombin a. any of the substances in the intrinsic or extrinsic pathways of coagulation including factors III, VII, X, and XII.

Schwarz a. bow a.

single-chain urokinase-type plasminogen a. (scu-PA) prourokinase.

tissue plasminogen a. (TPA, t-PA), t-plasminogen a. [EC 3.4.21.68] a serine endopeptidase synthesized by endothelial cells, the major physiologic activator of plasminogen; when bound to fibrin clots it catalyzes the conversion of plasminogen to plasmin by hydrolysis of a specific arginine-valine bond. It can be produced by recombinant technology for use in therapeutic thrombolysis.

u-plasminogen a. [EC 3.4.21.73], **urinary plasminogen a.** a serine endopeptidase that acts as a plasminogen activator by catalyzing the preferential cleavage of plasminogen at the same arginine-valine bond where t-plasminogen activator (t-PA) cleaves. It is produced in the kidney and excreted in the urine and is used (usually called urokinase, q.v.) to induce therapeutic thrombolysis; unlike t-PA or prourokinase (single chain urokinase-type plasminogen activator) it does not require fibrin for activity. Called also *urokinase*, particularly when used as a pharmaceutical.

ac•tive (ak′tiv) characterized by action; not passive; not expectant.

optically a. capable of rotating the plane of polarization of a light wave.

Ac•ti•vel•la (ak″tĭ-vel′ə) trademark for a combination preparation of estradiol and norethindrone acetate.

ac•ti•vin (ak′tĭ-vin) any of several polypeptide growth and differentiation factors, members of the transforming growth factor-β superfamily of proteins, that are synthesized in the pituitary gland and gonads and stimulate the secretion of follicle-stimulating hormone; they also play roles in neuroendocrine regulation, modulate production of other hormones, and affect gonadal functions such as steroid production. They are signaling proteins that act through a heteromeric complex of receptor serine/threonine kinases, signaling particular transcriptional responses. Their actions oppose those of inhibins (q.v.), with which they share subunits, the activins comprising dimers of either or both of the inhibin beta subunits.

ac•tiv•i•ty (ak-tiv′ĭ-te) [L. *agere* to do, drive] 1. the state of being active; the ability to produce some effect; the extent of some function or action. 2. a thermodynamic quantity that represents the effective concentration of a solute in a nonideal solution; if concentrations are replaced by activities, the equations for equilibrium constants, electrode potentials, osmotic pressure, boiling point elevation, freezing point depression, and vapor pressures of volatile solutes are converted from approximations that hold only for dilute solutions to exact equations that hold for all concentrations. The activity is equal to the product of the concentration and the activity coefficient, a dimensionless number measuring deviation from nonideality. Symbol *a.* 3. for radioactivity, the number of disintegrations per unit time of a radioactive material, measured in curies or becquerels. Symbol *A.* 4. in electroencephalography and electromyography, the presence of recordable electrical energy in a muscle or nerve. Called also *electrical a.* 5. optical a.

alpha a. see under *rhythm.*

background a. in measurements of physical or physiological processes, the ongoing generalized, sometimes artifactual, activity from which the more specific activity in question must be distinguished.

bactericidal a. the rate of killing of bacteria in a given inoculum by a particular antibiotic or disinfectant; for effective treatment it should be at least 99.9 percent. See also *serum bactericidal a.*

beta a. see under *rhythm.*

continuous muscle a., continuous muscle fiber a. Isaacs syndrome.

a's of daily living (ADL) basic tasks, such as bathing and eating, routinely performed daily by the average person in a given society; rehabilitation following illness or injury often aims to help patients achieve independence in performing them. See also *instrumental a's of daily living.*

delta a. see under *rhythm.*

discrete a. pathologically reduced electrical activity on a recording from a muscle during maximal voluntary contractions, so that the normal interference pattern (q.v.) is lacking and several discrete motor unit action potentials can be identified.

electrical a. activity (def. 4).

end-plate a. spontaneous activity recorded close to motor end plates in normal muscle. There are two types: *monophasic* (or *end-plate noise*) consists of dense, steady, entirely negative potentials with low amplitude and high frequency, similar to the miniature end-plate potentials of experimental animals; *biphasic* (or *end-plate spikes*) consists of irregular, alternately negative and positive spike potentials that come in short bursts with high frequencies.

enzyme a. the catalytic effect exerted by an enzyme, expressed as units per milligram of enzyme (specific activity) or as molecules of substrate

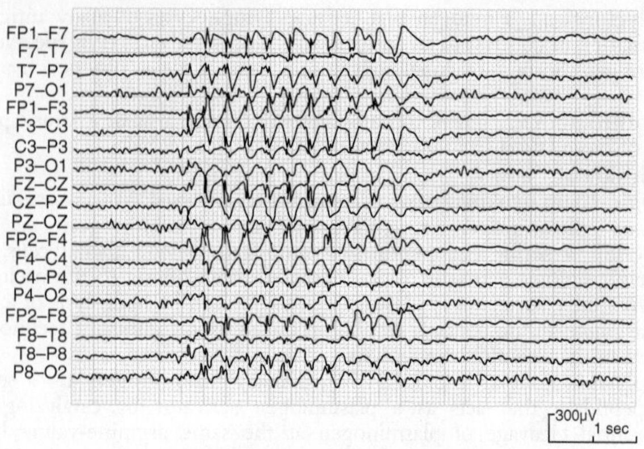

■ Epileptiform activity during an absence seizure, characterized by high-amplitude, 3-Hertz spike and wave discharge emerging from a normal electroencephalographic (EEG) background, rarely lasting longer than 2 to 10 seconds, and abruptly stopping with resumption of normal activity. The discharge is strictly regular, bilateral, and most prominent in frontal leads (Fp1–F7, Fp1–F3, FZ–CZ, Fp2–F4, Fp2–F8).

transformed per minute per molecule of enzyme (molecular activity). The conventional unit of enzyme activity is the International Unit (IU), equal to one micromole of substrate transformed per minute. A proposed coherent Système Internationale (SI) unit is the katal (kat), equal to one mole of substrate transformed per second.

epileptiform a. interictal activity on an electroencephalogram, characterized by paroxysmal spike, polyspike, or sharp wave discharges; it may occur in patients who have never had a seizure, and it does not occur in all epileptics. Called also *epileptiform discharges.*

insertion a., insertional a. the electrical activity caused by insertion or movement of a needle electrode; it is prolonged in neuropathies and myopathies and is diminished in some metabolic disorders.

instrumental a's of daily living (IADL) tasks more complex than activities of daily living, such as shopping and preparing meals, that are often performed in the course of a normal day by a person living independently in a community setting.

intermittent rhythmic delta a. slow, paroxysmal, relatively constant delta activity seen on the electroencephalogram, associated frequently with metabolic disorders or diffuse encephalopathies and sometimes with subfrontal, deep midline, or posterior fossa lesions; it may be stronger occipitally in children and frontally in adults.

intrinsic sympathomimetic a. (ISA) the ability of a β-blocker to stimulate β-adrenergic receptors weakly during beta-blockade. Called also *partial agonist a.*

involuntary a. electrical activity consisting of motor unit action potentials that are involuntary; cf. *spontaneous a.*

leukemia-associated inhibitory a. (LIA) the inhibition of normal marrow cells of donors from forming colonies of granulocytes and macrophages, induced in vitro by the presence of cell extracts, or of culture media conditioned by cells, from the bone marrow, spleen, or blood of patients with acute leukemia.

nonsuppressible insulinlike a. (NSILA) insulin-like growth factors.

optical a. the ability of a chemical compound to rotate the plane of polarization of plane-polarized light.

partial agonist a. intrinsic sympathomimetic a.

plasma renin a. a measurement of the enzymatic activity of renin in vitro; angiotensinogen is added to a sample containing renin and the amount of angiotensin I generated is measured.

polymorphic delta a. continuous irregular slow activity that is variable in duration and amplitude and may change little with sleep or other physiological alterations; it may be related to deafferentation of an area of the cortex, to metabolic factors, or to the presence of subcortical cerebral lesions and tumors.

pulseless electrical a. (PEA) continued electrical rhythmicity of the heart in the absence of effective mechanical function; it may be due to uncoupling of ventricular muscle contraction from electrical activity or may be secondary to cardiac damage with respiratory failure and cessation of cardiac venous return. Called also *electromechanical dissociation.*

serum bactericidal a. the bactericidal activity of an antibiotic or disinfectant in the serum of a specific patient. See also *serum bactericidal activity test*, under *test.*

slow a. electrical activity with frequencies below 8 per second.

specific a. 1. activity per unit weight of a radioactive material, or the activity of a radioisotope per unit weight of the element (including stable isotopes) present. 2. the catalytic effect of an enzyme expressed as units per milligram of enzyme.

spontaneous a. electrical activity recorded from a resting, unstimulated muscle or nerve after insertion activity has ceased.

theta a. see under *rhythm.*

triggered a. triggered automaticity.

voluntary a. electrical and mechanical activity recorded in a muscle during contractions that are under conscious control.

ac•to•my•o•sin (ak″to-mi′o-sin) a complex of the proteins actin and myosin occurring in muscle. Cf. *actin* and *myosin.* See also *myosin ATPase.*

Ac•to•nel (ak′tə-nəl) trademark for a preparation of risedronate sodium.

Ac•tos (ak′tōs) trademark for a preparation of pioglitazone hydrochloride.

acu- [L. *acus* needle] a combining form denoting relationship to a needle.

Ac•u•a•ria (ak″u-a′re-ə) a genus of nematodes that infest birds. *A. spira′lis* is found in the proventriculus and esophagus of fowls, causing lesions that may be fatal.

acu•i•ty (ə-ku′ĭ-te) [L. *acuitas* sharpness] clarity or clearness, especially of the vision.

Vernier a. displacement threshold.

visual a. (V, VA) the ability to discriminate visually between forms, measured by Snellen test type or, sometimes, by Landolt rings.

Acu•lar (ak′u-lar) trademark for preparations of ketorolac tromethamine.

acu•le•ate (ə-ku′le-āt) [L. *aculeatus* thorny] covered with sharp points; pointed.

acu•mi•nate (ə-ku′mĭ-nāt) [L. *acuminatus*] sharp-pointed.

acu•point (ak′u-point) any of the specific sites for needle insertion in acupuncture; stimulation of acupoints also forms the basis of other therapies, including acupressure and moxibustion. There are 361 basic, named acupoints along the 12 principal and two of the collateral meridians, and a large number of other points derived from clinical experience; most acupoints are areas of high electrical conductance on the body surface. Called also acupuncture point.

acu•pres•sure (ak′u-presh″ər) [*acu-* + *pressure*] the use of pressure applied, usually with the hands, at acupoints in order to release muscular tension for therapeutic purposes. According to traditional theory, the release of tension allows qi to flow through the meridians and restore balance to the body's systems; biologically, acupressure may relieve pain by sensory gating or by the release of endorphins.

acu•punc•ture (ak′u-punk″chər) [*acu-* + *puncture*] a practice originally developed in traditional Chinese medicine (see under *medicine*) in which fine needles are inserted into specific exterior body locations (acupoints) and manipulated for relief of pain, induction of surgical anesthesia, and therapy for a variety of conditions. According to traditional theory, the goal of acupuncture is the prevention and treatment of disease by correcting disturbances in the flow of qi (q.v.); biologically, the effects of acupuncture may result from the release of neurotransmitters such as endorphins and serotonin. Other means of stimulating the acupoints, including lasers, ultrasound, and electricity, may also be used. See also *acupressure* and *moxibustion.*

auricular a. acupuncture performed using points on the ear that have been mapped to specific anatomic areas of the body.

Korean hand a. a system of acupuncture in which the hand is considered to be a representation of the entire body, and stimulation of specific points on the hand is used to obtain effects in distant areas of the body.

acus (a′kəs) [L.] a needle or needlelike process.

acute (ə-kūt′) [L. *acutus* sharp] having a short and relatively severe course.

acy•a•not•ic (a-si″ə-not′ik) characterized by absence of cyanosis.

acy•clic (a-sik′lik, a-si′klik) 1. in chemistry, having an open-chain structure; aliphatic. 2. occurring independently of a cycle, such as the menstrual cycle. 3. aliphatic.

acy•clo•vir (a-si′klo-vēr) [USP] a synthetic acyclic purine nucleoside with selective antiviral activity against herpes simplex virus (types 1 and 2, human herpesvirus 3, Epstein-Barr virus, and cytomegalovirus). It is used in the treatment of genital and mucocutaneous herpesvirus infections in certain patients, both immunocompromised and nonimmunocompromised; administered orally or topically.

a. sodium the monosodium salt of acyclovir, used intravenously in the treatment of herpes simplex and herpes genitalis in immunocompromised patients and severe herpes genitalis in immunocompetent patients.

acyl (a′səl) an organic radical derived from an organic acid by removal of the hydroxyl group from the carboxyl group.

ac•yl•ase (a′sə-lās) amidase (def. 1).

ac•yl•a•tion (a″sə-la′shən) the introduction of an acyl radical into the molecule of a chemical compound.

ac•yl CoA (a′səl ko-a′) acyl coenzyme A.

ac•yl CoA:cho•les•ter•ol ac•yl•trans•fer•ase (a′səl ko-a′ kə-les′tər-ol a″səl-trans′fər-ās) sterol *O*-acyltransferase.

ac•yl-CoA de•hy•dro•gen•ase (a′səl ko-a′ de-hi′dro-jən-ās) [EC 1.3.99.3] any of several enzymes of the oxidoreductase class that catalyze the oxidation of acyl coenzyme A thioesters to the enoyl coenzyme A form, using a flavin electron acceptor. The reaction is a step in the degradation of fatty acids and the *trans* isomer of enoyl coenzyme A is formed exclusively. Individual enzymes are specific for certain ranges of acyl chain lengths. See also *electron transfer flavoprotein*, under *flavoprotein*.

long-chain a.-CoA d. (LCAD) deficiency a defect in mitochondrial beta oxidation due to a mutation in the gene (locus: 2q34-q35) encoding the acyl-CoA dehydrogenase that acts on long chain length fatty acids. It is clinically similar to MCAD deficiency, but urinary excretion is of long-chain dicarboxylic acids and skeletal muscle weakness and cardiac enlargement may also be present.

medium-chain a.-CoA d. (MCAD) deficiency a defect in mitochondrial beta oxidation due to a mutation in the gene (locus: 1p31) encoding acyl-CoA dehydrogenase that acts on medium chain length fatty acids. It is characterized by recurring episodes of hypoglycemia, vomiting, and lethargy, with urinary excretion of medium-chain dicarboxylic acids, minimal ketogenesis, and low plasma and tissue levels of carnitine.

short-chain a.-CoA d. (SCAD) deficiency a defect in mitochondrial beta oxidation due to a mutation in the gene (locus: 12q22-qter) encoding the acyl-CoA dehydrogenase that acts on short chain length fatty acids. Clinical presentation is variable, but myopathy and abnormalities of carnitine accumulation and excretion are often present.

acyl-CoA de•sat•ur•ase (a′səl-ko-a′ de-sach′ə-rās) stearoyl-CoA 9-desaturase.

ac•yl CoA syn•the•tase (a′səl-ko-a′ sin′thə-tās) 1. any enzyme of the ligase class that catalyzes the formation of an activated acyl coenzyme A thioester; individual enzymes are specific for a range of fatty acid chain lengths. See also individual enzymes: *acetate–CoA ligase*, *butyrate–CoA ligase*, and *long-chain-fatty-acid–CoA ligase*. 2. long-chain-fatty-acid–CoA ligase.

ac•yl CoA syn•the•tase (GDP-forming) (a′səl ko-a′ sin′thə-tās form′ing) acid–CoA ligase (GDP-forming).

ac•yl co•en•zyme A (a′səl ko-en′zīm) a thiol ester of a carboxylic acid, particularly a long-chain fatty acid, and coenzyme A. Its formation is the first step in fatty acid oxidation, leading to the sequential production of two-carbon groups and progressively shorter acyl coenzyme A compounds until the entire chain is degraded. Also written *acyl CoA*.

ac•yl•glyc•er•ol (a″səl-glis′ər-ol) glyceride.

2-ac•yl•glyc•er•ol *O*-ac•yl•trans•fer•ase (a″səl-glis′ər-ol a″səl-trans′fər-ās) [EC 2.3.1.22] an enzyme of the transferase class that catalyzes the transfer of the acyl group from palmitoyl coenzyme A or other long-chain acyl coenzyme A to a monoglyceride to form a diglyceride. The reaction occurs in the intestinal mucosa, synthesizing triglycerides from monoglycerides produced during digestion. Called also *acylglycerol palmitoyltransferase* and *monoglyceride acyltransferase*.

ac•yl•glyc•er•ol li•pase (a″səl-glis′ər-ol li′pās) [EC 3.1.1.23] an enzyme of the hydrolase class that catalyzes the cleavage of the last long-chain fatty acyl group from monoglycerides formed during the digestion of lipids. It occurs in the small intestine.

ac•yl•glyc•er•ol pal•mi•to•yl•trans•fer•ase (a″səl-glis′ər-ol pal″mĭ-to″əl-trans′fər-ās) 2-acylglycerol *O*-acyltransferase.

***N*-ac•yl•neu•ra•min•ate cy•ti•dyl•yl•trans•fer•ase** (a″səl-noo-ram′ĭ-nāt si″tĭ-dil-əl-trans′fər-ās) [EC 2.7.7.43] an enzyme of the transferase class that catalyzes the transfer of a cytidylyl group from CTP to a sialic acid to form the corresponding CMP-sialic acid, a nucleotide sugar compound that donates sialic acid residues in the biosynthesis of gangliosides.

***N*-ac•yl•neu•ra•min•ic ac•id** (a″səl-noor″ə-min′ik) sialic acid.

***N*-ac•yl•sphin•go•sine** (a″səl-sfing′go-sēn) ceramide.

acyl•sphin•go•sine de•acyl•ase (a″səl-sfing′go-sēn de-a′səl-ās) ceramidase.

ac•yl•trans•fer•ase (a″səl-trans′fər-ās) 1. [EC 2.3] one of a subclass of enzymes of the transferase class that catalyze the transfer of an acyl group from a donor (often the corresponding acyl coenzyme A derivative) to an acceptor compound. Many form esters or amides. 2. a further division of this subclass, a sub-subclass [EC 2.3.1], to distinguish it from the other sub-subclass, aminoacyltransferases. Called also *transacylase*.

acys•tia (a-sis′te-ə) [*a-*[1] + *cyst-* + *-ia*] congenital absence of the bladder.

AD[1] [L.] au′ris dex′tra (right ear).

AD[2] alcohol dehydrogenase.

ad [L. *ad* to] used in writing prescriptions to indicate that a substance (usually a diluent) be added up to a certain amount.

ad- [L. *ad* to] a prefix meaning to or toward, addition to, nearness, or intensification.

-ad[1] [L. *ad* to] an adverbial suffix meaning toward, as in caudad, cephalad.

-ad[2] [Gr. *-as*, gen. *-ados*] a suffix denoting a group, or derivation from or connection with.

ADA adenosine deaminase; American Dental Association; American Diabetes Association; American Dietetic Association; Americans with Disabilities Act; Australian Dental Association.

Ad•a•cel (ad′ə-sel) trademark for a preparation of tetanus toxoid, reduced diphtheria toxoid, and acellular pertussis vaccine, adsorbed (Tdap).

adac•tyl•ia (a″dak-til′e-ə) adactyly.

adac•ty•ly (a-dak′tə-le) [*a-*[1] + Gr. *daktylos* finger] a developmental anomaly characterized by the absence of digits on the hand or foot. **adac′tylous** *adj*

Ada•gen (ad′ə-jen) trademark for a preparation of pegademase.

Ad•a•lat (ad′ə-lat) trademark for preparations of nifedipine.

ada•lim•u•mab (a″də-lim′u-mab) a recombinant human IgG1 monoclonal antibody that binds to and blocks the action of tumor-necrosis factor α, used to alleviate the signs and symptoms of and inhibit the progression of structural damage in rheumatoid arthritis; administered subcutaneously.

ad•a•man•tane (ad″ə-man′tān) 1. a saturated hydrocarbon consisting of four fused cyclohexanes, having a camphorlike smell and subliming at room temperature. 2. *(pl.)* a group of antiviral drugs related to this compound, used in prophylaxis and treatment of influenza A.

ad•a•man•tine (ad″ə-man′tin) pertaining to the enamel of the teeth.

ad•a•man•ti•no•ma (ad″ə-man″tĭ-no′mə) ameloblastoma.

a. of long bones a rare tumor usually occurring in the tibia and probably of epithelial origin; it resembles an ameloblastoma of the jaw microscopically but is believed to be unrelated to it.

pituitary a. craniopharyngioma.

ad•a•man•to•blast (ad″ə-man′to-blast) [Gr. *adamas* a hard substance + *-blast*] ameloblast.

ad•a•man•to•blas•to•ma (ad″ə-man″to-blas-to′mə) ameloblastoma.

ad•a•man•to•ma (ad″ə-man-to′mə) ameloblastoma.

ADAMHA Alcohol, Drug Abuse, and Mental Health Administration, an agency of the United States Public Health Service.

Adam•kie•wicz arteries (ah-dahm-kyĕ′vich) [Albert *Adamkiewicz*, Polish pathologist, 1850–1921] see *rami spinales arteriae vertebralis*, under *ramus*.

Ad•ams operation (ad′əmz) [William *Adams*, English surgeon, 1810–1900] see under *operation*.

Ad•ams-Stokes attack, syndrome (syncope) (ad′əmz stōks′) [Robert *Adams*, Irish physician, 1791–1875; William *Stokes*, Irish physician, 1804–1878] see under *attack* and *syndrome*.

ad•ams•ite (ad′əmz-īt) phenarsazine chloride.

Ad•an•so•nia (ad″an-so′ne-ə) [Michel *Adanson*, French naturalist, 1727–1806] a genus of trees of the family Bombacaceae. *A. digita′ta* is the baobab, a huge tree of Africa and India. In Africa, the young leaves and seeds are eaten as food and the pulp is used as a diaphoretic.

ad•an•so•ni•an (ad″an-so′ne-ən) named for Michel *Adanson;* see *numerical taxonomy*, under *taxonomy*.

a•dap•a•lene (ə-dap′ə-lēn) a synthetic retinoic acid analogue applied topically in the treatment of acne vulgaris; it acts similarly to retinoic acid but binds selectively to certain nuclear retinoic acid receptors.

ad•ap•ta•tion (ad″ap-ta′shən) [L. *adaptare* to fit] 1. the adjustment of an organism to its environment, or the process by which it enhances such fitness. 2. the normal adjustment of the eye to variations in intensity of light. 3. the decline in the frequency of firing of a neuron, particularly of a receptor, under conditions of constant stimulation. 4. in dentistry, *(a)* the proper fitting of a denture, *(b)* the degree of proximity and interlocking of restorative material to a tooth preparation, *(c)* the exact adjustment of bands to teeth. 5. in microbiology, the adjustment of bacterial physiology to a new environment; see *genetic a.* and *phenotypic a.*

auditory a. abnormal decrease in auditory sensitivity as a result of auditory stimulation.

color a. 1. fading of hue and dulling of brightness of visual perceptions with prolonged stimulation. 2. adjustment of vision to degree of brightness or color tone of illumination indoors or out; includes *dark a.*

dark a. the adaptation of the eye to vision in the dark or in reduced illumination (night vision), with build-up of rhodopsin in the retinal rods; called also *scotopic a.*

genetic a. the natural selection of the progeny of a mutant better suited to a new environment, as in the development of bacterial strains resistant to certain antibiotics.

light a. adaptation of the eye to vision in the sunlight or in bright illumination (photopia), with reduction in the concentration of the photosensitive pigments of the eye; called also *photopic a.*

phenotypic a. a change in the structural and physiological properties of an organism in response to a genetic mutation or to a change in environment.

photopic a. light a.

retinal a. the adjustment of the photoreceptor cell of the eye to the surrounding illumination.

scotopic a. dark a.

social a. adjustment and adaptation of a person to other individuals and community groups working together for a common purpose.

adap·tin (ə-dap′tin) any of a family of polypeptides that mediate the binding of clathrin to the membrane of coated vesicles and select the specific proteins to be transported.

ad·ap·tom·e·ter (ad″ap-tom′ə-tər) [*adaptation* + *-meter*] an instrument for measuring the time required for retinal adaptation: i.e., for regeneration of the visual purple. It is used to help detect night blindness, vitamin A deficiency, and retinitis pigmentosa.

color a. an instrument using colored and neutral filters and control of illuminant to demonstrate adaptation of the eye to color or light.

ad·ax·i·al (ad-ak′se-əl) located alongside of, or directed toward, the axis.

ADCC antibody-dependent cell-mediated cytotoxicity.

add. [L.] ad′de (add); adda′tur (let there be added).

ad·der (ad′ər) 1. *Vipera berus.* 2. any of numerous venomous snakes of the families Elapidae and Viperidae; see table at *snake.*

death a. *Acanthophis antarcticus*, an extremely venomous elapid snake of Australia and New Guinea that has a short, stout body and a tail with a spine at the tip.

puff a. *Bitis arrietans*, an extremely venomous, brightly colored, viperine snake found in Africa and Arabia; when annoyed it inflates its stubby body and hisses loudly.

Ad·der·all (ad′ər-ahl″) trademark for a combination preparation of amphetamine and dextroamphetamine, used in the treatment of attention-deficit/hyperactivity disorder and narcolepsy.

ad·dict (ad′ikt) a person who cannot resist a habit, especially the use of drugs or alcohol, for physiological or psychological reasons.

ad·dic·tion (ə-dik′shən) 1. the state of being given up to some habit or compulsion. 2. strong physiological and psychological dependence on a drug or other psychoactive substance; see *drug a.*

alcohol a. alcoholism, particularly that in which physiological dependence is present.

drug a. a state of heavy dependence on a drug; sometimes defined as physical dependence but usually also including emotional dependence, i.e., compulsive or pathological drug use. It is often used synonymously with substance dependence.

Ad·dis count, test (ad′is) [Thomas *Addis*, American physician, 1881–1949] see under *count* and *test.*

Ad·di·son disease (ad′ĭ-sən) [Thomas *Addison*, English physician, 1793–1860] see under *disease.*

Ad·di·son planes, point (ad′ĭ-sən) [Christopher *Addison*, English anatomist, 1869–1951] see under *plane* and *point.*

ad·di·so·ni·an (ad″ĭ-so′ne-ən) named for Thomas *Addison*, as *addisonian crisis* and *addisonian syndrome.*

ad·di·son·ism (ad′ĭ-sən-iz″əm) addisonian syndrome.

Ad·di·son-Schil·der disease (ad′ĭ-sən shil′dər) [T. *Addison;* Paul Ferdinand *Schilder*, Austrian-born neurologist in the United States, 1886–1940] adrenoleukodystrophy.

ad·di·tive (ad′ĭ-tiv) 1. characterized by addition; see also under *effect.* 2. a substance, such as a flavoring agent, preservative, or vitamin, added to another substance (such as a food or drug) that is to be ingested.

feed a. a chemical, such as a drug or nutritional supplement, that is added to animal feed.

ad·dress·in (ə-dres′in) a molecule on the surface of vascular endothelial cells that mediates the attachment of specific leukocytes, particularly lymphocytes, to the endothelium, binding with their homing receptors.

ad·du·cent (ə-du′sənt) performing adduction.

ad·du·cin (ə-doo′sin) a protein that binds to both actin and spectrin and is thought to play a role in the spectrin-actin complex of the erythrocyte membrane.

ad·duct[1] (ə-dukt′) [L. *adducere* to draw toward] to draw toward the median plane or (in the digits) toward the axial line of a limb.

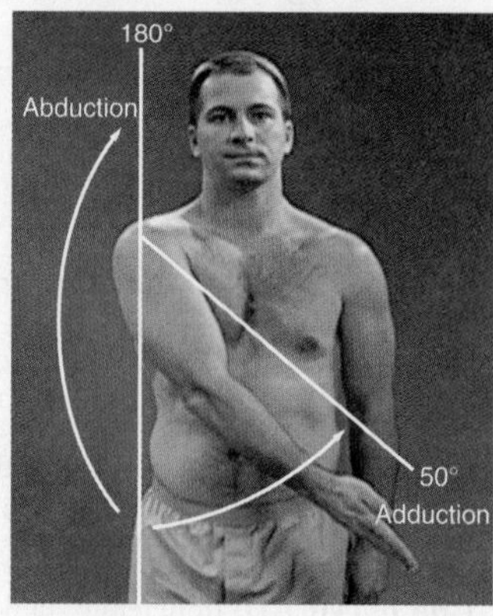

■ Adduction and abduction of the shoulder.

ad·duct[2] (ă′dukt) inclusion complex.

ad·duc·tio (ad-duk′she-o) [L.] [TA] adduction.

ad·duc·tion (ə-duk′shən) the act of adducting or the state of being adducted.

ad·duc·tor (ə-duk′tər) [L.] that which adducts; see under *musculus.*

adef·o·vir dip·i·vox·il (ə-def′o-vir dip″e-vok′sil) a nucleoside reverse transcriptase inhibitor administered orally in treatment of hepatitis B.

Ad·e·le·i·na (ad″ə-le-i′nə) a suborder of homoxenous or heteroxenous protozoa (order Eucoccidiida, subclass Coccidia) parasitic in the intestinal epithelium and associated glands of invertebrates, characterized by syzygy during development that usually involves a macrogamete and microgamont, with the latter producing one to four sporozoites enclosed in an envelope. Representative genera include *Haemogregarina*, *Hepatozoon*, and *Klossiella.*

-adelphus [Gr. *adelphos* brother] a word termination denoting a symmetrical pair of twins conjoined at the site indicated by the stem to which it is affixed; cf. *-pagus.*

ad·e·nal·gia (ad″ə-nal′jə) [*aden-* + *-algia*] pain in a gland; called also *adenodynia.*

aden·dric (a-den′drik) adendritic.

aden·drit·ic (a″den-drit′ik) [*a-*[1] + *dendritic*] lacking dendrites.

ad·e·nec·to·my (ad″ə-nek′tə-me) [*aden-* + *-ectomy*] surgical removal of a gland.

ad·en·ec·to·pia (ad″ə-nek-to′pe-ə) [*aden-* + *ectopia*] malposition or displacement of a gland.

ade·nia (ə-de′ne-ə) chronic great enlargement of the lymphatic glands, as in lymphoma.

aden·ic (ə-den′ik) 1. glandular (def. 1). 2. adenoid (def. 2).

aden·i·form (ə-den′ĭ-form) [*aden-* + *form*] adenoid (def. 2).

ad·e·nine (ad′ə-nēn) 1. a major purine base (see illustration at *base*). In animal and plant cells it usually occurs condensed with ribose or deoxyribose to form the nucleosides adenosine and deoxyadenosine. As such, it is a component of nucleic acids, of certain nucleotides, and of many coenzymes. Symbol A. 2. [USP] a preparation of adenine used to improve the preservation of whole blood.

a. arabinoside vidarabine.

a. nucleotide adenylic acid.

ad·e·nine phos·pho·ri·bo·syl·trans·fer·ase (ad′ə-nēn fos″fo-ri′bo-səl-trans′fer-ās) [EC 2.4.2.7] an enzyme of the transferase class that catalyzes the transfer of ribose 5-phosphate from phosphoribosylpyrophosphate to adenine to form AMP. The enzyme salvages adenine within the cell.

ad·e·nine phos·pho·ri·bo·syl·trans·fer·ase de·fi·cien·cy (ad′ə-nēn fos″fo-ri′bo-səl-trans′fer-ās) an autosomal recessive disorder of purine salvage (gene locus:16q24.3), resulting in accumulation of the insoluble purine 2,8-dihydroxyadenine; clinical signs range from none to nephrolithiasis (causing colic, hematuria, urinary tract infection, and dysuria) to acute renal failure and permanent kidney damage, with greater severity generally correlated with lower residual enzyme activity.

ad·e·ni·tis (ad″ə-ni′tis) inflammation of a gland; see also *lymphadenitis.*

Bartholin a. inflammation of the greater vestibular gland (Bartholin gland) resulting from acute infection of the gland.

cervical a. see under *lymphadenopathy.*

mesenteric a. see under *lymphadenitis.*

phlegmonous a. inflammation of a gland and the surrounding connective tissue; called also *adenophlegmon.*

tuberculous cervical a. see under *lymphadenitis.*

vestibular a. chronic inflammation of the lesser vestibular glands, which produces small, extremely painful ulcerations of the vestibular mucosa.

Ade•ni•um (ə-de′ne-um) a genus of African plants of the family Apocynaceae; they contain cardioactive glycosides such as somalin that are close in structure and action to the digitalis glycosides.

aden(o)- [Gr. *adēn,* gen. *adenos* gland] a combining form denoting relationship to a gland or glands.

ad•e•no•ac•an•tho•ma (ad″ə-no-ak″an-tho′mə) [*adeno-* + *acanth-* + *-oma*] an adenocarcinoma in which some or the majority of the cells exhibit squamous differentiation; called also *adenosquamous* or *adenoid squamous cell carcinoma.*

ad•e•no•am•e•lo•blas•to•ma (ad″ə-no-ə-mel″o-blas-to′mə) adenomatoid odontogenic tumor.

ad•e•no•blast (ad′ə-no-blast″) [*adeno-* + *-blast*] an embryonic cell that gives rise to glandular tissue.

ad•e•no•car•ci•no•ma (ad″ə-no-kahr″sĭ-no′mə) carcinoma derived from glandular tissue or in which the tumor cells form recognizable glandular structures; adenocarcinomas may be classified according to the predominant pattern of cell arrangement, as papillary, alveolar, etc., or according to a particular product of the cells, as mucinous adenocarcinoma.

acinar a. 1. see under *carcinoma.* 2. the most common neoplasm of the prostate, usually arising in the peripheral acini. Histological abnormalities of the acini may include size distortions ranging from giant to tiny, irregular architectural arrangements, and abnormal epithelium that is sometimes cribriform.

acinic cell a., acinous a. see under *carcinoma.*

alveolar a. bronchioloalveolar carcinoma.

ampullary a. adenocarcinoma near the ampulla of Vater, seen most often in persons over 60 years old; common symptoms are obstructive jaundice, weight loss, and abdominal pain.

bronchioalveolar a., bronchiolar a. bronchioloalveolar carcinoma.

bronchioloalveolar a., bronchoalveolar a. bronchioloalveolar carcinoma.

bronchogenic a. the usual type of adenocarcinoma of the lung, as distinguished from the subtype *bronchioloalveolar carcinoma.*

clear cell a. a rare malignant tumor of the female genital tract, resembling a renal cell carcinoma and containing tubules or small cysts with some cells that are hobnail-shaped and others whose cytoplasm is clear, containing abundant glycogen and inconspicuous stroma. It may occur in the ovary, uterus, cervix, or vagina. One form has been linked to in utero exposure to diethylstilbestrol. Called also *clear cell carcinoma* and *mesonephroma.*

digital papillary a. a type of adnexal carcinoma found as a solitary lesion on a hand or foot, representing a digital papillary adenoma that has undergone malignant transformation. Called also *eccrine papillary a.*

ductal a. of the prostate adenocarcinoma of columnar epithelium in the peripheral prostatic ducts; it may project into the urethra, causing obstruction and hematuria.

eccrine a. hidradenocarcinoma.

eccrine papillary a. digital papillary a.

endometrioid a. the most common form of endometrioid carcinoma, containing tumor cells differentiated into glandular tissue with little or no stroma.

follicular a. follicular carcinoma of thyroid gland.

gastric a. any of a group of common stomach cancers, usually located in the antrum; it may present as a bulky mass with central ulceration invading the wall, a mass that narrows the antral lumen, a polypoid lesion, or a tumor that spreads superficially over the mucosal surface. It is common in Japan, China, Eastern Europe, South America, and certain other places, but the incidence is decreasing in North America and Western Europe. There may be links to certain dietary substances such as nitrosamines and benzo[a]pyrene. Called also *gastric carcinoma* and *a. of the stomach.*

a. of infantile testis yolk sac tumor.

a. of kidney renal cell carcinoma.

a. of lung a type of bronchogenic carcinoma made up of cuboidal or columnar cells in a discrete mass, usually at the periphery of the lungs. Most such tumors form glandular structures containing mucin, although a minority are solid and without mucin. Growth is slow, but there may be early invasion of blood and lymph vessels, giving rise to metastases while the primary lesion is still asymptomatic. Two types are distinguished, *bronchogenic a.* and *bronchioloalveolar carcinoma.*

mucinous a. mucinous carcinoma.

papillary a., polypoid a. an adenocarcinoma whose tumor elements are arranged as fingerlike processes or as a solid spherical nodule projecting from an epithelial surface. See also *papillary carcinoma.*

polymorphous low-grade a. terminal duct carcinoma.

a. of the prostate acinar a. (def. 2).

renal a. renal cell carcinoma.

sebaceous a. see under *carcinoma.*

a. of the stomach gastric a.

sweat gland a. hidradenocarcinoma.

terminal duct a. see under *carcinoma.*

urachal a. adenocarcinoma in the urachal region of the dome of the urinary bladder, sometimes extending outwards into the abdomen; the tumor usually has a thick mucous coating, leading to excretion of mucus in the urine.

Aden•o•card (ə-den′o-kahrd) trademark for a preparation of adenosine.

ad•e•no•cele (ad′ə-no-sēl″) [*adeno-* + *-cele*[1]] cystadenoma.

ad•e•no•cel•lu•li•tis (ad″ə-no-sel″u-li′tis) inflammation of a gland and the tissue around it.

ad•e•no•cys•tic (ad″ə-no-sis′tik) having both glandular (adenoid) and cystic elements.

ad•e•no•cys•to•ma (ad″ə-no-sis-to′mə) cystadenoma.

papillary a. lymphomatosum adenolymphoma.

ad•e•no•cyte (ad′ə-no-sīt″) [*adeno-* + *-cyte*] a mature secretory cell of a gland.

ad•e•no•dyn•ia (ad″ə-no-din′e-ə) [*aden-* + *-odynia*] adenalgia.

ad•e•no•fi•bro•ma (ad″ə-no-fi-bro′mə) a tumor composed of connective tissue containing glandular structures.

a. edemato′des a tumor composed of glandular and connective tissue elements in which there is marked edema of the stroma, as in nasal polyp.

ad•e•no•fi•bro•sis (ad″ə-no-fi-bro′sis) fibroid change in a gland.

ad•e•nog•e•nous (ad″ə-noj′ə-nəs) [*adeno-* + *-genous*] originating from glandular tissue.

ad•e•nog•ra•phy (ad″ə-nog′rə-fe) [*adeno-* + *-graphy*] radiography of a gland or glands. **adenograph′ic** *adj*

ad•e•no•hy•po•phys•e•al (ad″ə-no-hi-po-fiz′e-əl) adenohypophysial.

ad•e•no•hy•poph•y•sec•to•my (ad″ə-no-hi-pof″ĭ-sek′tə-me) excision or ablation of the adenohypophysis.

ad•e•no•hy•po•phys•i•al (ad″ə-no-hi-po-fiz′e-əl) pertaining to the adenohypophysis; spelled also *adenohypophyseal.*

ad•e•no•hy•poph•y•sis (ad″ə-no-hi-pof′ĭ-sis) [*adeno-* + *hypophysis*] [TA] the anterior lobe of the hypophysis (pituitary gland), which originates in the buccal epithelium of the embryo; it secretes hormones that regulate the functioning of the thyroid gland, gonads, adrenal cortex, and other endocrine organs. The adenohypophysis comprises the pars tuberalis; the pars distalis, which is its main body; and the pars intermedia, which secretes β-endorphin, melanotropins, and other regulators but is sometimes considered to be part of the neurohypophysis (q.v.). Called also *anterior pituitary, anterior lobe of hypophysis,* and *lobus anterior hypophyseos* [TA alternative]. See illustration at *hypophysis.*

ad•e•noid (ad′ə-noid) [*aden-* + *-oid*] 1. tonsilla pharyngealis. 2. pertaining to a tonsilla pharyngealis. 3. resembling a gland.

ad•e•noid•ec•to•my (ad″ə-noid-ek′tə-me) [*adenoid* + *-ectomy*] excision of the adenoids.

ad•e•noid•ism (ad′ə-noid″iz-əm) a syndrome resulting from great enlargement of the adenoids.

ad•e•noid•i•tis (ad″ə-noid-i′tis) inflammation of the adenoid tissue of the nasopharynx.

ad•e•noids (ad′ə-noidz) popular name for the pharyngeal tonsils; used particularly when they are hypertrophied, which occurs primarily in preadolescents and adolescents. See also *adenoidism.*

ad•e•no•li•po•ma (ad″ə-no-lĭ-po′mə) a tumor composed of both glandular and fatty tissue elements. Cf. *lipoadenoma.*

ad•e•no•log•a•di•tis (ad″ə-no-log″ə-di′tis) [*adeno-* + Gr. *logades* whites of the eyes + *-itis*] 1. ophthalmia neonatorum. 2. inflammation of the glands of the conjunctiva.

ad•e•no•lym•phan•gi•tis (ad″ə-no-lim″fan-ji′tis) lymphadenitis and lymphangitis occurring together as the result of obstructive lymphedema.

acute a., episodic a. periodic occurrence of lymphangitis and lymphadenitis in filarial lymphedema, characterized by tenderness and swelling of the affected limb, with red streaks running along its length, and lymph node enlargement. It is accompanied by fever, chills, and malaise.

ad•e•no•lym•phi•tis (ad″ə-no-lim-fi′tis) lymphadenitis.

ad•e•no•lym•pho•cele (ad″ə-no-lim′fo-sēl) [*adeno-* + *lymphocele*] lymphadenocele.

ad•e•no•lym•pho•ma (ad″ə-no-lim-fo′mə) [*adeno-* + *lymphoma*] a benign tumor of the parotid gland characterized by cystic spaces lined by tall, columnar, eosinophilic epithelial cells, overlying a lymphoid tissue–containing stroma. Called also *Warthin tumor* and *papillary cystadenoma lymphomatosum.*

ad•e•no•ma (ad″ə-no′mə) [*adeno-* + *-oma*] a benign epithelial tumor in which the cells form recognizable glandular structures or in which the cells are clearly derived from glandular epithelium.

Adenoma

acidophilic a. in a classification system formerly used for pituitary adenomas, an adenoma whose cells stain with acid dyes; most adenomas that secreted excessive amounts of growth hormone were in this group. See *growth hormone–secreting a.*
acidophil stem-cell a. a rapidly growing plurihormonal adenoma; usually a null-cell adenoma, seen in young patients; its single cell type secretes both prolactin and growth hormone and is presumed to be a stem cell for both lactotrophs and somatotrophs.
ACTH-secreting a. corticotroph a.
adnexal a. an adenoma of the skin appendages (adnexa).
a. of the adrenal cortex, adrenocortical a. a benign tumor of the adrenal cortex, usually small and unilateral; most types cause endocrine symptoms. See *cortisol-producing a.*, *aldosterone-producing a.*, *feminizing tumor*, and *virilizing tumor.*
adrenocorticotropic hormone–secreting a. corticotroph a.
aggressive digital papillary a. digital papillary a.
aldosterone-producing a., aldosterone-secreting a. a benign aldosteronoma, usually small and unilateral.
alpha subunit a. a variant of glycoprotein adenoma that secretes only one subunit of the glycoprotein hormones; most are endocrine-inactive, although a few are endocrine-active.
a. alveola′re an adenoma whose cells are arranged like those of an alveolar gland.
apocrine a. any of numerous adnexal adenomas having differentiation toward apocrine gland tissue.
basal cell a. a benign, encapsulated, slow-growing, painless salivary gland tumor of intercalated duct or reserve cell origin, usually seen in males in the parotid gland or upper lip. Solid, canalicular, trabecular-tubular, and membranous types have been distinguished histologically, but all show little myoepithelial cell participation, stromal differentiation, or metaplasia.
basophil a., basophilic a. in a classification system formerly used for pituitary adenomas, an adenoma whose cells stain with basic dyes; most adenomas that secreted excessive amounts of adrenocorticotrophic hormone were in this group.
bile duct a. a small firm white nodule with multiple bile ducts embedded in a fibrous stroma.
bronchial a's adenomas situated in the submucosal tissues of large bronchi, thought to be derived from neuroendocrine cells. Sometimes composed of well-differentiated cells and usually circumscribed, they are almost always carcinoid in histologic form. Although termed *adenomas,* these tumors are now recognized as being of low-grade malignancy.
canalicular a. the canalicular type of basal cell adenoma.
carcinoma ex pleomorphic a. see under *carcinoma.*
chief cell a. adenoma of the parathyroid gland composed of solid masses of small chief cells similar to those seen in the normal gland.
chromophobe a., chromophobic a. a pituitary adenoma composed of cells that lack acidophilic or basophilic granules; this is the same entity as the more precisely named *null-cell a.*
colloid a. macrofollicular a.
cortical a's minute tumors in the renal cortex, arising from the renal tubules; some authorities consider these to be simply small renal cell carcinomas.
corticotrope a., corticotrope cell a. corticotroph a.
corticotroph a., corticotroph cell a. a pituitary adenoma made up predominantly of corticotrophs; excessive corticotropin secretion may cause Cushing disease or Nelson syndrome. Called also *ACTH-secreting* or *adrenocorticotropic hormone–secreting a.* and *corticotropinoma.*
cortisol-producing a. the most common adenoma of the adrenal cortex; it secretes cortisol and causes Cushing syndrome.
digital papillary a. a type of solitary, nodular adnexal adenoma on a hand or foot in an adult, thought to originate in eccrine glands; it may extend deeply and even impinge on bone and will recur unless thoroughly excised. These lesions often have malignant transformation and are then called *digital papillary adenocarcinoma.* Called also *aggressive digital papillary a.*
eccrine a. any of numerous adnexal adenomas having differentiation toward eccrine gland tissue.
eccrine papillary a. digital papillary a.
embryonal a. trabecular a.
endocrine-active a. functioning a.
endocrine-inactive a. nonfunctioning a.
eosinophil a., eosinophilic a. growth hormone–secreting a.
fetal a. microfollicular a.
a. fibro′sum fibroadenoma.
follicular a. adenoma of the thyroid in which the cells are arranged in the form of follicles. It is sometimes subclassified as either *macrofollicular a.*, *microfollicular a.*, *trabecular a.*, or *Hürthle cell a.*; however, many adenomas are mixtures of types, and all types have similar clinical characteristics.
functional a., functioning a. a pituitary adenoma that secretes excessive amounts of a hormone; see *prolactinoma*, *corticotroph a.*, *gonadotroph a.*, *growth hormone–secreting a.*, and *thyrotroph a.* Called also *hyperfunctional* or *hyperfunctioning a.* and *endocrine-active a.*
gastric a. adenomatous polyp of stomach.
glycoprotein a., glycoprotein hormone a. a pituitary adenoma that causes excessive secretion of one of the three glycoprotein hormones (follicle-stimulating hormone, luteinizing hormone, and thyrotropin); see *gonadotroph a.* and *thyrotroph a.*
gonadotrope a., gonadotroph a., gonadotroph cell a. a rare type of pituitary adenoma made up of gonadotroph-like cells that secrete excessive amounts of follicle-stimulating hormone or luteinizing hormone, or both; it may cause precocious puberty, visual disturbances, or hypogonadism.
growth hormone cell a. growth hormone–secreting a.
growth hormone–secreting a. a pituitary adenoma made up of somatotroph-like cells that secrete excessive amounts of growth hormone; it may cause gigantism in children or acromegaly in adults. Called also *somatotrope a.*, *somatotroph a.*, and *eosinophilic a.*
hepatocellular a. a benign circumscribed tumor of the liver, usually in the right lobe; growth is in a sheetlike fashion and it may be highly vascular with a tendency to hemorrhage and with areas of necrosis. Women are affected more often than men and use of oral contraceptives has been implicated in some cases. Called also *liver cell a.*
Hürthle cell a. a benign Hürthle cell tumor, usually considered a subtype of the follicular adenomas. Called also *oncocytic a.*, *oxyphilic a.*, and *oncocytoma.*
hyperfunctional a., hyperfunctioning a. functioning a.
islet cell a. a benign islet cell tumor.
a's of kidney cortical a's.
lactotrope a., lactotroph a. prolactinoma.
langerhansian a. islet cell a.
liver cell a. hepatocellular a.
macrofollicular a. a follicular adenoma composed of large follicles filled with colloid and lined with flat epithelium. Called also *colloid a.*
malignant pleomorphic a. any of several malignant epithelial neoplasms arising in a pre-existing pleomorphic adenoma, usually in the salivary glands of an older adult; it occurs in several types, usually divided into *carcinoma ex pleomorphic a.* and *malignant mixed tumor.*
mammosomatotroph a. a plurihormonal adenoma composed of mammosomatotrophs, a single cell type secreting both growth hormone and prolactin; cf. *mixed somatotroph-lactotroph a.*
membranous a. the membranous type of basal cell adenoma.
microfollicular a. a follicular adenoma with small closely packed follicles lined with epithelium; called also *fetal a.*
mixed-cell a. a pituitary adenoma containing more than one cell type, usually making it plurihormonal; see *plurihormonal a.*
mixed somatotroph-lactotroph a. the most common type of mixed-cell adenoma, containing two cell types that produce respectively growth hormone and prolactin. Cf. *mammosomatotroph a.*
monomorphic a. any of a group of benign salivary gland tumors that lack connective tissue changes and are each predominantly composed of a single cell type; included are basal cell adenomas, adenolymphomas, and oxyphilic adenomas. Cf. *pleomorphic a.*
mucinous a. an epithelial tumor whose cells produce mucin.
nephrogenic a. nephrogenic metaplasia.
nipple a. a benign lesion of the breast, clinically resembling Paget disease of the breast, consisting of ductal and stromal proliferation beneath the nipple, which presents as a mass, ulceration, or erosion, with a

Adenoma *Continued*

serous or bloody discharge. Called also *papillary a., erosive adenomatosis of nipple, florid papillomatosis of nipple,* and *subareolar duct papillomatosis.*
nonfunctional a., nonfunctioning a. a pituitary adenoma that does not secrete excessive amounts of any hormone; many null-cell adenomas are of this type. Called also *nonsecreting* or *nonsecretory a.* and *endocrine-inactive a.*
nonsecreting a., nonsecretory a. nonfunctioning a.
null-cell a. a pituitary adenoma whose cells give negative results on tests for staining and hormone secretion; although classically they were considered to be composed of sparsely granulated or degranulated (nonfunctioning) cells, some contain functioning cells and may be associated with a hyperpituitary state such as acromegaly or Cushing syndrome. These tumors are often discovered clinically only when they have grown large and are pressing on surrounding structures. Called also *chromophobic a.*
oncocytic a. 1. oncocytoma. 2. Hürthle cell a.
a. ova'rii testicula're androblastoma (def. 2).
oxyphilic a., oxyphilic granular cell a. 1. oncocytoma. 2. Hürthle cell a.
papillary a. 1. nipple a. 2. see *digital papillary a.*
papillary cystic a. papillary cystadenoma.
papillary eccrine a. digital papillary a.
Pick testicular a., Pick tubular a. androblastoma (def. 1).
pituitary a. a benign neoplasm of the anterior pituitary gland; some contain hormone-secreting cells *(functioning adenomas)* but some are not secretory *(nonfunctioning adenomas).*
pleomorphic a. a benign, slow-growing tumor of the salivary gland, occurring as a small, painless, firm nodule, usually of the parotid gland, but also found in any major or accessory salivary gland anywhere in the oral cavity. It is most often seen in women in the fifth decade. Histologically, the tumor presents a variety of cells: cuboidal, columnar, and squamous cells, showing all forms of epithelial growth. See also *malignant pleomorphic a.*

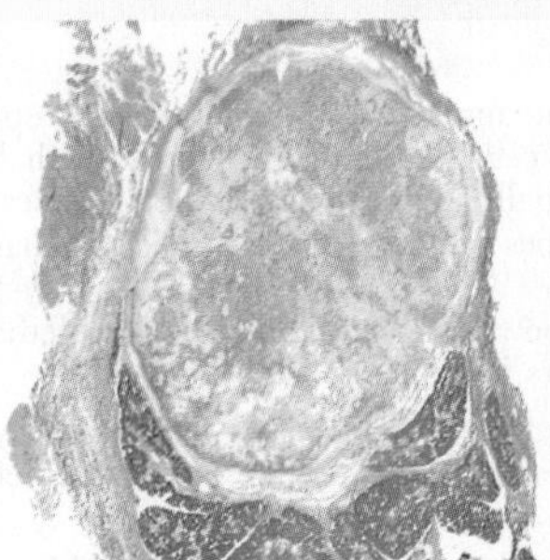

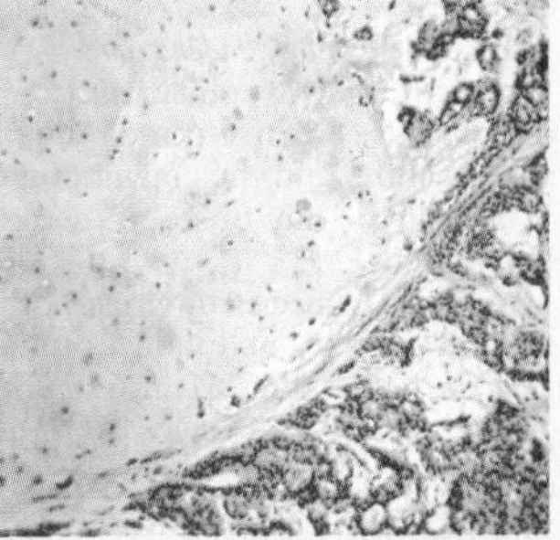

■ Pleomorphic adenoma. *(A)*, Low-power view showing well-demarcated tumor with adjacent normal salivary gland parenchyma; *(B)*, high-power view showing the mixture of epithelial and myoepithelial cells in a chondroid matrix material.

plurihormonal a. an endocrine-active adenoma that secretes two or more hormones, usually growth hormone and one or more of the glycoprotein types, so that its effects are similar to those of a combination of other adenomas such as the growth hormone–secreting adenoma and the glycoprotein hormone adenoma; it may be mixed-cell or a single cell type. Varieties include *acidophil stem-cell a., mammosomatotroph a.,* and some types of *alpha subunit a.*
prolactin cell a., prolactin-secreting a. prolactinoma.
sebaceous a., a. seba'ceum 1. see under *hyperplasia.* 2. *Pringle type adenoma sebaceum:* misnomer for a type of hamartoma of the face seen in tuberous sclerosis complex; it does not involve the sebaceous glands. 3. *Balzer type adenoma sebaceum:* nevoid hyperplasia of the sebaceous glands, seen as multiple pale papules or nodules of the face.
serrated a. a dysplastic condition of the colon characterized by polyps having a serrated or sawtooth appearance and malignant potential, often developing into adenocarcinoma.
somatotrope a., somatotroph a. growth hormone–secreting a.
sweat gland a. hidradenoma.
thyroid stimulating hormone–secreting a. thyrotroph a.
thyrotrope a., thyrotroph a., thyrotroph cell a. a rare type of pituitary adenoma made up of thyrotroph-like cells that secrete excess thyrotropin and cause hyperthyroidism; called also *TSH-secreting a.* and *thyroid stimulating hormone–secreting a.*
toxic a., toxic thyroid a. toxic multinodular goiter.
trabecular a. a follicular adenoma whose cells are closely packed to form cords or trabeculae, with only a few small follicles; called also *embryonal a.*
trabecular-tubular a. the trabecular-tubular type of basal cell adenoma.
TSH-secreting a. thyrotroph a.
tubular a. 1. an adenoma whose cells are arranged in tubules, as occurs with adenomatous polyps of the colon, some fibroadenomas of the breast, and androblastoma. 2. androblastoma (def. 1). 3. the most common type of adenomatous polyp of the colon, usually seen in middle-aged to elderly people; its tubules are highly variable in size and often occur singly, although small and large groups of tubules are also seen. Its potential for malignant transformation is uncertain.
a. tubula're testicula're ova'rii androblastoma (def. 2).
villous a. an uncommon type of adenomatous polyp of the colon that is large, soft, and papillary and often premalignant.

ad•e•no•ma•la•cia (ad″ə-no-mə-la′shə) [*adeno-* + *malacia*] abnormal softening of a gland.

ad•e•no•ma•toid (ad″ə-no′mə-toid) resembling adenoma.

ad•e•no•ma•to•sis (ad″ə-no-mə-to′sis) a condition characterized by development of numerous adenomatous growths.
erosive a. of nipple nipple adenoma.
multiple endocrine a. multiple endocrine neoplasia.
a. o′ris enlargement of the mucous glands of the lip without secretion or inflammation.
pluriglandular a., polyendocrine a. multiple endocrine neoplasia.
porcine intestinal a. porcine proliferative enteritis.
pulmonary a. 1. bronchioloalveolar carcinoma. 2. a chronic contagious neoplastic lung disease of adult sheep and goats, caused by a retrovirus with adenomatous proliferation in the alveoli and small bronchioles. Called also *jaagsiekte* and *jagziekte.*

ad•e•nom•a•tous (ad″ə-nom′ə-təs) 1. pertaining to an adenoma. 2. pertaining to nodular hyperplasia of a gland.

ad•e•no•mec•to•my (ad″ə-no-mek′tə-me) [*adenoma* + *-ectomy*] surgical removal of an adenoma.

ad•e•no•meg•a•ly (ad″ə-no-meg′ə-le) enlargement of a gland.

ad•e•no•mere (ad′ə-no-mēr″) [*adeno-* + *-mere*] the blind terminal portion of a developing gland, becoming the functional portion of the organ.

ad•e•no•myo•fi•bro•ma (ad″ə-no-mi″o-fi-bro′mə) a fibroma containing adenomatous and myomatous tissue.

ad•e•no•my•o•ma (ad″ə-no-mi-o′mə) [*adeno-* + *myoma*] 1. a benign tumor consisting of smooth muscle and glandular elements. 2. see *adenomyosis.*

ad•e•no•my•o•ma•to•sis (ad″ə-no-mi″o-mə-to′sis) the formation of multiple adenomyomatous nodules in the parauterine tissues or in the uterus.

ad•e•no•my•o•ma•tous (ad″ə-no-mi-o′mə-tus) pertaining to or resembling adenomyoma.

ad•e•no•myo•sar•co•ma (ad″ə-no-mi″o-sahr-ko′mə) a mixed mesodermal tumor in which striated muscle cells are one component.
embryonal a. Wilms tumor.

ad•e•no•my•o•sis (ad″ə-no-mi-o′sis) a benign condition characterized by endometrial glands and stroma within the myometrium, accompanied by hypertrophy of the myometrium. If the lesion forms a circumscribed tumor-like nodule, it is called *adenomyoma.* Called also *endometriosis interna* or *uterina.*
a. exter′na endometriosis.
stromal a. stromatosis.
a. tu′bae the growth of the endometrium into the lumen of the uterine tube from the uterus, replacing the endosalpinx.
a. u′teri adenomyosis.

ad•e•non•cus (ad″ə-nong′kəs) adenomegaly.

ad•e•no•neu•ral (ad″ə-no-noor′əl) pertaining to a gland and a nerve.

ad•e•nop•a•thy (ad″ə-nop′ə-the) [*adeno-* + *-pathy*] lymphadenopathy.

ad•e•no•phar•yn•gi•tis (ad″ə-no-far″in-ji′tis) [*adeno-* + *pharyngitis*] inflammation of the adenoids and pharynx, usually involving the tonsils.

ad•e•no•phleg•mon (ad″ə-no-fleg′mon) [*adeno-* + *phlegmon*] phlegmonous adenitis.

ad•e•noph•thal•mia (ad″ə-nof-thal′me-ə) [*aden-* + *ophthalmia*] inflammation of the meibomian glands.

ad•e•no•pit•u•i•cyte (ad″ə-no-pĭ-tu′ĭ-sīt) see *pituicyte.*

ad•e•no•sar•co•ma (ad″ə-no-sahr-ko′mə) a mixed tumor composed of sarcomatous and glandular elements, such as a Wilms tumor.

embryonal a. Wilms tumor.

Aden•o•scan (ə-den′o-skan) trademark for a preparation of adenosine.

ad•e•no•scle•ro•sis (ad″ə-no-sklĕ-ro′sis) [*adeno-* + *sclerosis*] the hardening of a gland.

aden•o•sine (ə-den′o-sēn) 1. a purine nucleoside, adenine linked by its N9 nitrogen to the C1 carbon of ribose. It is a component of ribonucleic acid (RNA) and its nucleotides play major roles in the reactions and regulation of metabolism. Symbol A. 2. [USP] a preparation of adenosine, which acts as a cardiac depressant of automaticity in the sinus node and conduction in the atrioventricular node and also as a vasodilator; used as an antiarrhythmic in the treatment of paroxysmal supraventricular tachycardia and as a diagnostic adjunct, in conjunction with myocardial perfusion imaging, to induce coronary artery vasodilation in patients unable to exercise adequately to undergo an exercise stress test; administered intravenously.

cyclic a. monophosphate (3′,5′-AMP, cAMP, cyclic AMP) a cyclic nucleotide, adenosine 3′,5′-cyclic monophosphate, that serves as an intracellular and, in some cases, extracellular "second messenger" mediating the action of many peptide or amine hormones. The nucleotide binds to cAMP-dependent kinases and releases free (catalytically active) subunits.

a. diphosphate (ADP) a nucleotide, the 5′-pyrophosphate of adenosine, involved in energy metabolism; it is produced by hydrolysis of ATP and converted back to ATP by the processes of oxidative phosphorylation and substrate-level phosphorylation.

a. monophosphate (AMP) a nucleotide, the 5′-phosphate of adenosine, involved in energy metabolism; it is produced by hydrolysis of ATP and converted to ADP by adenylate kinase. Called also *adenylic acid.*

a. phosphate any of the three interconvertible compounds in which adenosine is attached through its ribose group to one *(a. monophosphate)*, two *(a. diphosphate)*, or three *(a. triphosphate)* phosphoric acid molecules.

a. triphosphate (ATP) a nucleotide, the 5′-triphosphate of adenosine, involved in energy metabolism and required for RNA synthesis; it occurs in all cells and is used to store energy in the form of high-energy phosphate bonds. The free energy derived from hydrolysis of ATP is used to drive metabolic reactions including the synthesis of nucleic acids and proteins, to move molecules against concentration gradients (active transport), and to produce mechanical motion (contraction of microfibrils and microtubules).

aden•o•sine de•am•i•nase (ADA) (ə-den′o-sēn de-am′ĭ-nās) [EC 3.5.4.4] an enzyme of the hydrolase class that catalyzes the deamination of adenosine to form inosine, a reaction of purine metabolism. Absence of enzyme activity, an autosomal recessive trait, has been found in many individuals with severe combined immunodeficiency disease.

aden•o•sine ki•nase (ə-den′o-sēn ki′nās) [EC 2.7.1.20] an enzyme of the transferase class that catalyzes the phosphorylation of adenosine by ATP to form ADP. The reaction is part of the purine salvage mechanism.

aden•o•sine•tri•phos•pha•tase (ə-den″o-sēn-tri-fos′fə-tās) [EC 3.6.1.3] an enzyme of the hydrolase class that catalyzes the hydrolysis of ATP to ADP. The reaction is a result of the concerted action of proteins using ATP to drive processes such as muscle contraction, maintenance of concentration gradients, membrane transport, and regulation of ion concentrations. Called also *ATPase.* See also *myosin ATPase*, *Na^+,K^+-ATPase*, *Ca^{2+}-ATPase*, *dynein ATPase*, and *H^+,K^+-ATPase.*

ad•e•no•sis (ad″ə-no′sis) 1. any disease of the glands. 2. the abnormal development or formation of glandular tissue.

blunt duct a. a form of mammary dysplasia characterized by dominance of the proliferation of the epithelial parenchyma; it is often accompanied by fibrosis and cystic disease of the breast.

mammary sclerosing a., sclerosing a. of breast a form of disease of the breast characterized by multiple firm tender nodules, fibrous tissue, mastodynia, and sometimes small cysts; histologically, it may resemble carcinoma.

a. vagi′nae the presence in the vagina of multiple ectopic areas of glandular (columnar) epithelium.

ad•e•no•squa•mous (ad″ə-no-skwa′məs) having both glandular (adenoid) and squamous elements.

aden•o•syl (ə-den′o-sil″) the radical formed from adenosine on loss of an H or OH group, particularly from the 5′ position.

aden•o•syl•co•ba•la•min (AdoCbl) (ə-den″o-səl-ko-bal′ə-min) a cobalamin derivative in which the substituent is deoxyadenosyl. It is one of two metabolically active forms synthesized upon ingestion of vitamin B_{12} and is the predominant form in the liver; it acts as a coenzyme in the reaction catalyzed by methylmalonyl-CoA mutase.

S-aden•o•syl•ho•mo•cys•te•ine (ə-den″o-səl-ho″mo-sis′tēn) the compound remaining after the methyl group of *S*-adenosylmethionine has been transferred to an acceptor; it is a potent inhibitor of transmethylation reactions and is rapidly hydrolyzed.

S-aden•o•syl•me•thi•o•nine (ə-den″o-səl-mə-thi′o-nēn) a reaction product of ATP and methionine in which the sulfur atom of methionine is bound to the ribose of adenosine; it serves as a methyl donor in transmethylation reactions.

ad•e•no•tome (ad′ə-no-tōm″) [*adeno-* + *-tome*] an instrument for excision of the adenoids.

ad•e•no•ton•sil•lar (ad″ə-no-ton′sĭ-lər) pertaining to the pharyngeal (adenoid) tonsils.

ad•e•no•ton•sil•lec•to•my (ad″ə-no-ton″sil-ek′tə-me) removal of the adenoids and tonsils.

ad•e•nous (ad′ə-nəs) glandular (def. 1).

Ad•e•no•vi•ri•dae (ad″ə-no-vir′ĭ-de) the adenoviruses: a family of DNA viruses having a nonenveloped icosahedral virion 80–110 nm in diameter with 252 capsomers. The genome consists of a single linear molecule of double-stranded DNA (MW 20–30 × 10^6, size 36–38 kbp). Viruses contain at least ten structural proteins and are ether-resistant and acid-stable; some are heat-sensitive. Replication occurs in the nucleus and structural proteins are synthesized in the cytoplasm; assembly occurs in the nucleus and virions are released by cell destruction. Host range is generally narrow and transmission may be direct or indirect. Genera include *Mastadenovirus* and *Aviadenovirus.*

ad•e•no•vi•rus (ad′ə-no-vi″rəs) any virus belonging to the family Adenoviridae. For naming of adenovirus species, see *Aviadenovirus* and *Mastadenovirus.* **adenovi′ral** *adj*

a's of birds *Aviadenovirus.*

conditionally replicative a. mutant adenoviruses that can replicate only inside certain types of tumor cells, infecting those cells with lethal abnormalities and thus being potentially useful in gene therapy for cancer.

enteric a. any of several serotypes of adenoviruses that cause diarrhea in children.

fowl a. a species of viruses of the genus *Aviadenovirus* that is lethal for chicken embryos and induces tumors in newborn hamsters.

mammalian a's *Mastadenovirus.*

ad•e•nyl (ad′ə-nəl) 1. the radical of adenine. 2. a term sometimes (incorrectly) used for *adenylyl.*

aden•yl•ate (ə-den′ə-lāt) the dissociated form of adenylic acid.

aden•yl•ate cy•clase (ə-den′ə-lāt si′klās) [EC 4.6.1.1] an enzyme of the lyase class that catalyzes the formation of 3′,5′-cyclic adenosine monophosphate (cAMP) from ATP. The enzyme occurs in plasma cell membranes and is activated by certain hormones (epinephrine, vasopressin, glucagon, and corticotropin). The resultant cyclic AMP serves as an important metabolic regulator. Called also *adenyl cyclase* and *adenylyl cyclase.*

aden•yl•ate de•am•i•nase (ə-den′ə-lāt de-am′ĭ-nās) AMP deaminase.

aden•yl•ate ki•nase (ə-den′ə-lāt ki′nās) [EC 2.7.4.3] any of a family of structurally and functionally related enzymes of the transferase class that catalyze the reaction 2ADP = ATP + AMP. The enzymes occur predominantly in muscle and provide a means of using both high-energy phosphate bonds from ATP for muscle contraction. The reaction makes AMP concentration a sensitive indicator of depletion of the high-energy phosphate pool and also maintains balance in the nucleotide pool. Called also *AMP kinase.*

ad•e•nyl cy•clase (ad′ə-nəl si′klās) adenylate cyclase.

ad•e•nyl•ic ac•id (ad″ə-nil′ik) phosphorylated adenosine, usually referring to adenosine monophosphate (q.v.).

ad•e•nylo•suc•ci•nase (ad″ə-nəl-o-suk′sĭ-nās) adenylosuccinate lyase.

ad•e•nylo•suc•ci•nate (ad″ə-nəl-o-suk′sĭ-nāt) adenylate with succinate substituted for the C6 amino group, an intermediate in the biosynthesis of adenylate.

ad•e•nylo•suc•ci•nate ly•ase (ad″ə-nəl-o-suk′sĭ-nāt li′ās) [EC 4.3.2.2] an enzyme of the lyase class that catalyzes the cleavage of adenylosuccinate to form fumarate and AMP. The enzyme occurs in the liver, where it catalyzes several steps in purine nucleotide biosynthesis; in muscle it is involved in the utilization of energy. Called also *adenylosuccinase.*

ad•e•nylo•suc•ci•nate syn•thase (ad″ə-nəl-o-suk′si-nāt sin′thās) [EC 6.3.4.4] an enzyme of the ligase class that catalyzes the substitution of succinate for the carbonyl oxygen of inosine monophosphate, a step in the biosynthesis of adenosine monophosphate.

ad•e•nyl•yl (ad′ə-nəl-əl) the radical formed by removal of OH from the phosphate group of adenosine monophosphate.

ad•e•nyl•yl cy•clase (ad′ə-nəl-əl si′klās) adenylate cyclase.

ad•e•nyl•yl•trans•fer•ase (ad″ə-nəl-əl-trans′fər-ās) one of the nucleotidyltransferases [EC 2.7.7] that catalyzes the transfer of an adenylyl residue from one compound to another.

ad•e•qua•cy (ad′ə-kwə-se) the state of being sufficient for a specific purpose.

velopharyngeal a. sufficient velopharyngeal closure so that air and hence sound cannot enter the nasopharyngeal and nasal cavities. Cf. *velopharyngeal insufficiency.*

ader•mia (ə-dur′me-ə) dermal aplasia.

ader•mine (ə-dur′mēn) pyridoxine; vitamin B_6.

ADH alcohol dehydrogenase; antidiuretic hormone (see *vasopressin*).

Ad•hat•o•da (ad-hat′o-də) a genus of plants of the family Acanthaceae. *A. va′sica* is the Malabar nut tree, used in India for its antispasmodic and expectorant properties.

ad•her•ence (ad-hēr′əns) the act or condition of sticking to something.

immune a. the adherence of antigen-antibody complexes or cells coated with antibody or complement to cells bearing complement receptors or Fc receptors. The agglutination reaction between antigen-antibody complexes or antibody coated cells and indicator cells, usually human erythrocytes, bearing complement receptors is used as a detector system in complement fixation tests (immune adherence hemagglutination assay).

ad•he•sin (ad-he′zin) any of a group of molecular components of the exterior cell wall of bacteria, involved in adhesion processes. See *adhesion* (def. 1).

ad•he•sio (ad-he′ze-o) pl. *adhesio′nes* [L. "clinging together"] adhesion.

a. interthala′mica [TA] interthalamic adhesion: a mass of gray matter connecting the thalami across the midline of the third ventricle; it develops as a secondary adhesion and may be absent in 20 to 25 per cent of human brains.

ad•he•si•ol•y•sis (ad-he″se-ol′ĭ-sis) adhesiotomy.

ad•he•sion (ad-he′zhən) [L. *adhaesio*, from *adhaerere* to stick to] 1. the property of remaining in close proximity, as that resulting from the physical attraction of molecules to a substance, or the molecular attraction existing between the surfaces of contacting bodies. 2. the stable joining of parts to each other, as in wound healing or some pathological process; sometimes done artificially such as in bonding materials to a tooth. 3. a fibrous band or structure by which parts abnormally adhere.

amniotic a's fibrous adhesions from the amnion to the fetus; see *amniotic band*, under *band.*

focal a. a specialized area of the plasma membrane, characterized by clusters of integrins that transduce transmembrane signals and link actin filaments of the cytoskeleton to the extracellular matrix. Called also *focal contact.*

interthalamic a. adhesio interthalamica.

primary a. healing by first intention.

secondary a. healing by second intention.

sublabial a. abnormal union of the sublabial mucosa of the upper lip to the alveolar process, as seen in cleft lip.

traumatic uterine a's adhesions of the uterus, most often in the cervical canal, frequently in the uterine cavity, and sometimes in both; they are usually caused by trauma or infection and may cause amenorrhea. See also *Asherman syndrome*, under *syndrome.*

ad•he•si•ot•o•my (ad-he″ze-ot′ə-me) the cutting or division of adhesions; called also *adhesiolysis.*

ad•he•sive (ad-he′siv) 1. sticky; tenacious. 2. a substance that causes close adherence of adjoining surfaces.

cyanoacrylate a. any of a group of adhesives and cements containing cyanoacrylate, widely used in surgery and dentistry.

dental a. a chemical capable of forming a mechanical or chemical bond to tooth structures or restorative materials.

denture a. a substance composed of various types of gum, used to help stabilize a denture base on the underlying mucosa.

ad•he•sive•ness (ad-he′siv-nis) the property of remaining adherent.

platelet a. the physical property of platelets by which they stick to a variety of materials in vivo and in vitro, particularly as it occurs in the initial formation of a clot and in the maintenance of hemostasis.

Adhib. [L.] adhiben′dus (to be administered).

ADHR autosomal dominant hypophosphatemic rickets.

adi•a•do•cho•ci•ne•sia (a-di″ə-do″ko-sĭ-ne′zhə) adiadochokinesia.

adi•a•do•cho•ci•ne•sis (a-di″ə-do″ko-sĭ-ne′sis) adiadochokinesia.

adi•a•do•cho•ki•ne•sia (ə-di″ə-do″ko-kĭ-ne′zhə) [*a-*[1] + *diadochokinesia*] a dyskinesia consisting of inability to perform the rapid alternating movements of diadochokinesia. Called also *adiadochocinesia, adiadochokinesis,* and *adiadokokinesia.*

adi•a•do•cho•ki•ne•sis (a-di″ə-do″ko-kĭ-ne′sis) adiadochokinesia.

adi•a•do•ko•ki•ne•sia (a-di″ə-do″ko-kĭ-ne′zhə) adiadochokinesia.

adi•a•do•ko•ki•ne•sis (a-di″ə-do″ko-kĭ-ne′sis) adiadochokinesia.

Ad•i•an•tum (ad″e-an′təm) [*a-*[1] + Gr. *dianein* to moisten] the maidenhair ferns, a genus of the family Polypodiaceae. *A. peda′tum* is a species found in North America and eastern Asia that has been used as an expectorant and demulcent.

adi•a•pho•ria (a″di-ə-for′e-ə) [Gr. "indifference"] nonresponse to stimuli as a result of previous exposure to similar stimuli; see also *refractory period*, under *period.*

adi•a•spi•ro•my•co•sis (ad″e-ə-spi″ro-mi-ko′sis) a pulmonary disease of many species of rodents and occasionally of humans, caused by the inhalation of spores of the fungus *Emmonsia parva* and *E. crescens.* It is marked by huge spherules in the lungs (adiaspores) without endospores, with symptoms ranging from the subclinical to a bilateral pneumonia. The condition is often confused with the tissue phase of *Coccidioides immitis* infection.

adi•a•spore (ad′e-ə-spor″) a spore produced by the soil fungi *Emmonsia parva* and *E. crescens*, which, after inhalation into the lungs, enlarges to form a huge spherule without endospores.

adi•a•ther•man•cy (a-di″ə-thur′mən-se) [*a-*[1] + *dia-* + *thermansis* heating] the condition of being impervious to heat waves.

Ad•ie pupil, syndrome (a′de) [William John *Adie*, English neurologist, 1886–1935] see *tonic pupil*, under *pupil*, and see under *syndrome.*

ad•i•ent (ad′e-ənt) tending toward the source of stimulation; positive. Cf. *abient.*

ad•i•pec•to•my (ad″ĭ-pek′tə-me) [*adip-* + *-ectomy*] lipectomy.

Ad•i•pex-P (ad′ĭ-peks-pe) trademark for a preparation of phentermine hydrochloride.

adip•ic (ə-dip′ik) [L. *adeps* fat] fatty.

adip(o)- [L. *adeps*, gen. *adipis* lard, fat] a combining form denoting relationship to fat.

ad•i•po•cele (ad′ĭ-po-sēl″) [*adipo-* + *-cele*[1]] fat hernia.

ad•i•po•cel•lu•lar (ad″ĭ-po-sel′u-lər) composed of connective tissue and fat.

ad•i•po•cer•a•tous (ad″ĭ-po-ser′ə-təs) pertaining to or resembling adipocere.

ad•i•po•cere (ad′ĭ-po-sēr″) [*adipo-* + *cera*] a peculiar waxy substance formed during the decomposition of animal bodies, and seen especially in human bodies buried in moist places; it consists principally of insoluble salts of fatty acids.

ad•i•po•cyte (ad′ĭ-po-sīt) fat cell.

ad•i•po•cy•to•kine (ad″ĭ-po-si′to-kīn) a general term for any of a number of bioactive factors, synthesized and secreted by adipose tissue, that modulate the physiological function of other tissues. Called also *adipokine.*

ad•i•po•gen•e•sis (ad″ĭ-po-jen′ə-sis) [*adipo-* + *-genesis*] lipogenesis.

ad•i•po•gen•ic (ad″ĭ-po-jen′ik) lipogenic.

ad•i•pog•e•nous (ad″ĭ-poj′ə-nəs) lipogenic.

ad•i•po•he•pat•ic (ad″ĭ-po-hə-pat′ik) pertaining to or marked by fatty degeneration of the liver.

ad•i•poid (ad′ĭ-poid) lipoid.

ad•i•po•kine (ad′ĭ-po-kīn) adipocytokine.

ad•i•po•ki•ne•sis (ad″ĭ-po-kĭ-ne′sis) the mobilization of fat in the body, often with the liberation of free fatty acids into the blood plasma; see also *lipolytic hormones*, under *hormone.*

ad•i•po•kin•et•ic (ad″ĭ-po-kĭ-net′ik) pertaining to, characterized by, or promoting adipokinesis.

ad•i•po•ki•nin (ad″ĭ-po-ki′nin) former name for β-lipotropin.

ad•i•pol•y•sis (ad″ĭ-pol′ĭ-sis) [*adipo-* + *-lysis*] lipolysis.

ad•i•po•lyt•ic (ad″ĭ-po-lit′ik) lipolytic.

ad•i•pom•e•ter (ad″ĭ-pom′ə-tər) an instrument for measuring the thickness of the skin fold to determine obesity.

ad•i•po•ne•cro•sis (ad″ĭ-po-nə-kro′sis) necrosis of adipose tissue; see *panniculitis.*

a. subcuta′nea neonato′rum subcutaneous fat necrosis of newborn.

ad•i•po•nec•tin (ad-ĭ-po-nek′tin) an adipocytokine important in insulin resistance and energy homeostasis. Plasma and adipose tissue levels are reduced in diabetic and obese persons; adiponectin has also been found in the synovial fluid of patients with inflammatory joint disease.

ad•i•po•pec•tic (ad″ĭ-po-pek′tik) pertaining to, characterized by, or promoting adipopexis.

ad•i•po•pex•ia (ad″ĭ-po-pek′se-ə) adipopexis.

ad•i•po•pex•ic (ad″ĭ-po-pek′sik) adipopectic.

ad•i•po•pex•is (ad″ĭ-po-pek′sis) [*adipo-* + *pexis*] the fixation or storing of fats.

ad•i•pos•al•gia (ad″ĭ-pōs-al′jə) [*adipo-* + *-algia*] adiposis dolorosa.

ad•i•pose (ad′ĭ-pōs) [L. *adiposus* fatty] 1. fatty. 2. the fat present in the cells of adipose tissue.

ad•i•po•sis (ad″ĭ-po′sis) [*adip-* + *-osis*] 1. obesity. 2. fatty change of an organ or tissue; see under *change.*

a. cerebra′lis cerebral adiposity.

a. doloro′sa nodular circumscribed lipomatosis in which the adipose deposits are tender or painful because of pressing against adjacent nerves. It is usually seen in women, and sometimes there are accompanying pulmonary complications that can be fatal. Called also *Anders disease, Dercum disease,* and *lipomatosis dolorosa.*

a. hepa′tica fatty change of the liver.

a. tubero′sa sim′plex a disorder resembling adiposis dolorosa, marked by development in the subcutaneous tissue of fatty masses that may be painful to pressure.

a. universa′lis a deposit of fat generally throughout the body, including the internal organs.

ad•i•pos•i•tas (ad″ĭ-pos′ĭ-təs) [L.] obesity.

ad•i•po•si•tis (ad″ĭ-po-si′tis) panniculitis.

ad•i•pos•i•ty (ad″ĭ-pos′ĭ-te) obesity.

cerebral a. obesity due to a lesion in the brain, especially the hypothalamus, as in adiposogenital dystrophy. Called also *adiposis cerebralis.*

pituitary a. obesity formerly believed to be due to pituitary insufficiency but actually due to a lesion of the diencephalon such as a tumor that impinges on the pituitary gland.

ad•i•po•stat•ic (ad″ĭ-po-stat′ik) acting to slow or halt formation of adipose tissue.

ad•i•po•su•ria (ad″ĭ-po-su′re-ə) [*adipo-* + *-uria*] lipiduria.

adip•sia (ə-dip′se-ə) [*a-*[1] + *dipsia*] absence of thirst, or abnormal avoidance of drinking.

ad•i•tus (ad′ĭ-təs) pl. *ad′itus* [L. "approach"] the entrance or approach to an organ or part.

a. ad an′trum mastoi′deum [TA] an opening between the epitympanum and the mastoid antrum.

a. laryn′gis [TA] laryngeal inlet; the aperture by which the pharynx communicates with the larynx; called also *laryngeal aperture.*

a. orbita′lis [TA] orbital opening: the opening to the orbit in the cranium; called also *anterior opening of orbital cavity.*

ad•junct (ad′junkt) an accessory or auxiliary agent or measure.

ad•just•ment (ə-just′mənt) 1. the act or process of modification of physical parts made in response to changing conditions. 2. in psychology, the relative degree of harmony between an individual's needs and the requirements of the environment. 3. a modification made in a denture after its completion and insertion in the mouth. 4. the mechanism for raising and lowering the tube of a microscope to bring the object being examined into focus. 5. in chiropractic, any of a number of manual and mechanical interventions, most often applied to the spine, in which controlled and directed forces are applied to a joint in order to correct structural dysfunction and restore normal nerve function. Called also *manipulation* and *spinal manipulation.*

occlusal a. selective grinding of occlusal surfaces of the teeth to eliminate premature contacts and occlusal interferences. Called also *occlusal equilibration.* See also *milling-in.*

ad•ju•vant (aj′ə-vənt, ă-joo′vənt) [L. *adjuvans* aiding] 1. assisting or aiding. 2. a substance that aids another, such as an auxiliary remedy. 3. in immunology, a nonspecific stimulator of the immune response, such as BCG vaccine.

A. 65 trademark for a water-in-oil emulsion containing antigen in peanut oil with Arlacel A and aluminum monostearate as the emulsifying agent.

aluminum a. an aluminum-containing compound, such as aluminum hydroxide or alum, that by combining with soluble antigen forms a precipitate; slow release of the antigen from the precipitate on injection causes prolonged, strong antibody response.

Freund a. a water-in-oil emulsion incorporating antigen, in the aqueous phase, into lightweight paraffin oil with the aid of an emulsifying agent. On injection, this mixture *(Freund incomplete a.)* induces strong persistent antibody formation. The addition of killed, dried mycobacteria, e.g., *Mycobacterium butyricum,* to the oil phase *(Freund complete a.)* elicits cell-mediated immunity (delayed hypersensitivity), as well as humoral antibody formation.

mycobacterial a. Freund complete a.; see *Freund a.*

ad•ju•van•tic•i•ty (aj″ə-vən-tis′ĭ-te, ă-joo″vən-tis′ĭ-te) the ability to nonspecifically stimulate the immune response.

ADL activities of daily living.

Ad•ler (ahd′lər) Alfred, 1870–1937. Austrian psychiatrist. A student of Freud who developed his own psychoanalytic theory stating that the need for superiority and power is a more driving force than Freud's postulated unconscious sexual libido. Adler concentrated on overt personality manifestations and was the first to use such terms as inferiority complex and compensation.

ad lib. [L.] ad lib′itum (at pleasure).

ad•me•di•al (ad-me′de-əl) situated near the median plane.

ad•me•di•an (ad-me′de-ən) toward the median plane, or midline of the body.

ad•mi•nic•u•la (ad″mĭ-nik′u-lə) [L.] plural of *adminiculum.*

ad•mi•nic•u•lum (ad″mĭ-nik′u-ləm) pl. *adminic′ula* [L.] a prop or support.

a. lin′eae al′bae [TA] posterior attachment of linea alba: the expansion of fibers extending from the superior pubic ligament to the posterior surface of the linea alba.

ad•mit•tance (*A*) (ad-mit′əns) the measure of how readily an alternating current flows in a circuit; it is the ratio of peak current to peak voltage, the reciprocal of impedance. The unit of admittance is the siemens.

acoustic a. the ease of energy flow through the middle ear. See also *acoustic immittance.*

admov. [L.] ad′move (add); admovea′tur (let there be added).

ad nau•se•am (ad naw′se-əm) [L.] to the extent of producing nausea.

ad•ner•val (ad-nur′vəl) 1. situated near a nerve. 2. toward a nerve, said of an electric current which passes through muscle toward the entrance point of a nerve.

ad•neu•ral (ad-noor′əl) [*ad-* + *neural*] adnerval.

ad•nexa (ad-nek′sə) [L., pl.] appendages. **adnex′al** *adj*

cutaneous a. skin appendages.

a. of eye ocular adnexa.

a. mastoi′dea the structures in the mastoid (posterior) wall of the middle ear, including the mastoid antrum and its aditus and the mastoid air cells.

ocular a., a. o′culi the eyelids, lacrimal apparatus, and other accessory structures adjacent to the eye; called also *eye* or *ocular appendages, structurae oculi accessoriae* [TA], *accessory structures of eye,* and *accessory visual structures.*

skin a. skin appendages.

a. u′teri uterine appendages.

ad•nex•ec•to•my (ad″nek-sek′tə-me) [*adnexa* + *-ectomy*] excision or removal of adnexa, especially the adnexa uteri.

ad•nex•i•tis (ad″nek-si′tis) inflammation of the adnexa uteri.

AdoCbl adenosylcobalamin.

ad•o•les•cence (ad″o-les′əns) [L. *adolescentia*] the period of life beginning with the appearance of secondary sex characters and terminating with the cessation of somatic growth, roughly from 11 to 19 years of age; cf. *puberty.*

ad•o•les•cent (ad″o-les′ənt) 1. pertaining to adolescence. 2. an individual during the period of adolescence.

ad•or•al (ad-or′əl) [*ad-* + *oral*] toward or near the mouth.

ADP adenosine diphosphate.

ADPKD autosomal dominant polycystic kidney disease.

Ad pond. om. [L.] ad pon′dus om′nium (to the weight of the whole).

ad•re•nal (ə-dre′nəl) [*ad-* + *renal*] 1. pertaining to either of two glands located just above the kidneys; see *glandula suprarenalis.* Called also *suprarenal.* 2. glandula suprarenalis.

ad•re•nal•ec•to•mize (ə-dre′nəl-ek′to-mīz) to excise one or both adrenal glands.

ad•re•nal•ec•to•my (ə-dre″nəl-ek′tə-me) [*adrenal* + *-ectomy*] excision of one *(unilateral adrenalectomy)* or both *(bilateral adrenalectomy)* adrenal glands; called also *suprarenalectomy.*

Adren•a•lin (ə-dren′ə-lin) trademark for preparations of epinephrine.

adren•a•line (ə-dren′ə-lin) epinephrine.

a. acid tartrate epinephrine bitartrate.

adren•a•lin•emia (ə-dren″ə-lin-e′me-ə) the presence of epinephrine in the blood.

adren•a•lin•uria (ə-dren″ə-lin-u′re-ə) the presence of epinephrine in the urine.

adren•al•ism (ə-dren′əl-iz-əm) any disorder of adrenal function, whether decreased (adrenal or adrenocortical insufficiency) or increased (hyperadrenalism or hyperadrenocorticism).

adre•na•li•tis (ə-dre″nəl-i′tis) inflammation of the adrenal glands; called also *adrenitis.*

autoimmune a. Addison disease caused by autoantibodies to cells of the adrenal cortex, the most common type of the disease in Europe and North America.

adre•nal•op•a•thy (ə-dre″nəl-op′ə-the) [*adrenal* + *-pathy*] any disease of the adrenal glands. Called also *adrenopathy.*

adren•a•lo•tro•pic (ə-dren″ə-lo-tro′pik) [*adrenal* + *-tropic*] 1. adrenotropic. 2. pertaining to the developmental stage preceding puberty, during which adrenal androgen secretion increases.

ad•ren•ar•che (ad″rən-ahr′ke) [*adren-* + *arche*] augmentation of adrenal cortical secretion, involving especially androgens, a physiologic change that occurs at approximately the age of eight years in both sexes.

ad•ren•er•gic (ad″ren-ur′jik) 1. activated by, characteristic of, or secreting epinephrine or related substances, particularly referring to the sympathetic nerve fibers that liberate norepinephrine at a synapse when a nerve impulse passes. See also under *receptor.* Cf. *cholinergic* and *sympathomimetic.* 2. an agent that produces such an effect.

adre•nic (ə-dren′ik) adrenal (def. 1).

ad•re•ni•tis (ad″rə-ni′tis) adrenalitis.

adren(o)- [*ad-* near + *ren* kidney] a combining form denoting relationship to the adrenal gland.

adre•no•cep•tive (ə-dre″no-sep′tiv) pertaining to the sites on effector organs that are acted upon by adrenergic transmitters.

adre•no•cep•tor (ə-dre″no-sep′tər) adrenergic receptor.

adre•no•cor•ti•cal (ə-dre″no-kor′tĭ-kəl) pertaining to or arising from the adrenal cortex.

adre•no•cor•ti•co•hy•per•pla•sia (ə-dre″no-kor″tĭ-ko-hi″pər-pla′zhə) adrenal cortical hyperplasia.

adre•no•cor•ti•coid (ə-dre″no-kor′tĭ-koid″) corticosteroid.

adre•no•cor•ti•co•mi•met•ic (ə-dre″no-kor″tĭ-ko-mi-met′ik) producing effects similar to those of the adrenocortical hormones (corticosteroids).

adre•no•cor•ti•co•tro•phic (ə-dre″no-kor″tĭ-ko-tro′fik) adrenocorticotropic.

adre•no•cor•ti•co•troph•in (ə-dre″no-kor′tĭ-ko-tro″fin) corticotropin.

adre•no•cor•ti•co•tro•pic (ə-dre″no-kor″tĭ-ko-tro′pik) having a stimulating effect on the adrenal cortex; called also *adrenocorticotrophic* and *corticotropic.*

adre•no•cor•ti•co•trop•in (ə-dre″no-kor″tĭ-ko-tro′pin) corticotropin.

adre•no•dox•in (ə-dre″no-dok′sin) an iron-sulfur protein occurring in the mitochondria of the adrenal cortex and serving as an electron carrier in the series of redox reactions by which adrenal steroid hormones are biosynthesized from cholesterol.

ad•re•no•gen•ic (ə-dre″no-jen′ik) adrenogenous.

ad•re•nog•e•nous (ad″ren-oj′ə-nəs) [*adreno-* + *-genous*] produced or arising in an adrenal gland.

ad•re•no•gram (ə-dre′no-gram) a radiograph of the adrenal glands.

ad•re•no•ki•net•ic (ə-dre″no-kĭ-net′ik) adrenotropic.

adre•no•leu•ko•dys•tro•phy (ə-dre″no-loo″ko-dis′trə-fe) an X-linked recessive disease of childhood (gene locus: Xq28), in which deficient peroxisomal fatty acid degradation results in the accumulation of very long chain fatty acids in the tissues. It is marked by progressive adrenal dysfunction and diffuse abnormality of the cerebral white matter, with neurologic degeneration leading to severe dementia and deterioration of speech, vision, hearing, and gait. Death occurs within a few years of onset. Called also *Addison-Schilder disease.*

adre•no•lyt•ic (ə-dre″no-lit′ik) [*adreno-* + *-lytic*] inhibiting the action of adrenergic nerves; inhibiting the response to epinephrine. Cf. *adrenergic blocking agent,* under *agent.*

adre•no•med•ul•lary (ə-dre″no-med′u-lar″e) pertaining to or originating in the adrenal medulla. Called also *medulloadrenal.*

adre•no•me•dul•lin (ə-dre″no-med′u-lin) a peptide originally isolated from human pheochromocytoma, having vasodilator, diuretic, and natriuretic activity.

adre•no•med•ul•lo•tro•pic (ə-dre″no-med″u-lo-tro′pik) having a stimulatory influence on the adrenal medulla.

adre•no•meg•a•ly (ə-dre″no-meg′ə-le) [*adreno-* + *-megaly*] enlargement of one or both of the adrenal glands.

adre•no•mi•met•ic (ə-dre″no-mi-met′ik) sympathomimetic.

adre•no•my•elo•neu•rop•a•thy (ə-dre″no-mi″ə-lo-nŏŏ-rop′ə-the) a phenotypic variant of adrenoleukodystrophy manifested primarily by spinal cord degeneration and peripheral neuropathy; it affects mainly adults.

ad•ren•op•a•thy (ad″rən-op′ə-the) adrenalopathy.

adre•no•pause (ad-re′no-pawz) a decrease with age in the secretion of certain adrenal hormones; it is most noticeable with dehydroepiandrosterone and its sulfate.

adre•no•pri•val (ad-re′no-pri″vəl) pertaining to or characterized by adrenocortical insufficiency.

adre•no•re•cep•tor (ə-dre″no-re-sep′tər) adrenergic receptor.

adre•no•stat•ic (ə-dre″no-stat′ik) 1. inhibiting the activity of the adrenal glands. 2. an agent that inhibits the activity of the adrenal glands.

adre•nos•te•rone (ă″drĕ-nos′tər-ōn) an androgenic steroid isolated from the adrenal cortex.

adre•no•tox•in (ə-dre′no-tok″sin) any substance that is toxic to the adrenals.

adre•no•tro•phic (ə-dre″no-tro′fik) [*adreno-* + *-trophic*] adrenotropic.

adre•no•tro•phin (ə-dre′no-tro″fin) corticotropin.

adre•no•tro•pic (ə-dre″no-tro′pik) [*adreno-* + *-tropic*] having specific affinity for or growth-promoting or hormonal secretory influence on the adrenal glands; see also *adrenocorticotropic* and *adrenomedullotropic.*

adre•no•tro•pin (ədre′no-tro″pin) corticotropin.

Adri•a•my•cin (a″dre-ə-mi′sin) trademark for preparations of doxorubicin hydrochloride.

adro•mia (ə-dro′me-ə) [*a-*[1] + *dromo-* + *-ia*] absence of conduction in nerve of muscle.

Adru•cil (a′droo-sil) trademark for a preparation of fluorouracil.

ad•rue (ad-roo′a) *Cyperus articulatus,* a grasslike plant of the West Indies whose root is aromatic tonic, antiemetic, and anthelmintic.

Ad•son forceps, test (maneuver) (ad′sən) [Alfred Washington *Adson,* American neurosurgeon, 1887–1951] see under *forceps* and *test.*

Ad•son-Brown forceps (ad′sən broun′) [A.W. *Adson;* James Barrett *Brown,* American plastic surgeon, 1899–1971] see under *forceps.*

ad•sorb (ad-sorb′) to attract and retain other material on the surface; to conduct the process of adsorption.

ad•sor•bate (ad-sor′bāt) a substance taken up on a surface by adsorption.

ad•sor•bent (ad-sor′bənt) 1. pertaining to or characterized by adsorption. 2. an agent that attracts other materials or particles to its surface by adsorption.

ad•sorp•tion (ad-sorp′shən) [L. *ad-* to + *sorption*] the attachment of one substance to the surface of another; the concentration of a gas or a substance in solution in a liquid on a surface in contact with the gas or liquid, resulting in a relatively high concentration of the gas or solution at the surface. Cf. *absorption.*

agglutinin a. the taking up by bacteria suspended in diluted antiserum of those agglutinins specific for that microorganism.

immune a. the use of antigen as a specific adsorbent for antibody or the use of antibody or antiserum as a specific adsorbent for antigen; the antigen-antibody complex is removed by filtration or centrifugation.

ad•ster•nal (ad-stur′nəl) toward or near the sternum.

adst. feb. [L.] adstan′te feb′re (while fever is present).

ADTA American Dance Therapy Association.

ad•ter•mi•nal (ad-tur′mĭ-nəl) [*ad-* + *terminal*] moving from the center toward the end of a muscle; said of an electric current.

ad•tor•sion (ad-tor′shən) intorsion.

adult (ə-dult′) [L. *adultus* grown up] 1. having attained full growth or maturity. 2. a living organism that has attained full growth or maturity.

adul•ter•ant (ə-dul′tər-ənt) a substance used as an addition to another substance for adulteration.

adul•te•ra•tion (ə-dul″tər-a′shən) addition of an impure, cheap, or unnecessary ingredient to cheat, cheapen, or falsify a preparation; in legal terminology, incorrect labeling, including dosage not in accordance with the label.

ad•um•bra•tion (ad″əm-bra′shən) 1. an inherent property of the focal spot which causes the production of double images. 2. in radiology, the giving forth of a shadow.

Adv. [L.] adver′sum (against).

Ad•vair (ad′vār) trademark for a combination preparation of fluticasone propionate and salmeterol xinafoate.

ad•vance (ad-vans′) [Fr. *avancer*] to perform the operation of advancement.

ad•vance•ment (ad-vans′mənt) 1. surgical detachment, as of a muscle or tendon, followed by reattachment at a point farther forward than the original position. 2. orthognathic surgery in which the mandible is moved forward.

capsular a. the artificial attachment of Tenon capsule in such a way as to draw forward the insertion of an ocular muscle.

ad•ven•ti•tia (ad″ven-tish′e-ə) [L. *adventicius* foreign, from without] 1. adventitial. 2. tunica adventitia.

ad•ven•ti•tial (ad″ven-tish′əl) pertaining to the tunica adventitia; called also *adventitious.*

ad•ven•ti•tious (ad″ven-tish′əs) [*ad-* + *venire* to come] 1. accidental or acquired; not natural or hereditary. 2. found somewhere other than in the normal or usual place. 3. adventitial.

ad•ver•sive (ad-vur′siv) opposite; as the turning to one side in an adversive seizure.

Ad 2 vic. [L.] ad du′as vi′ces (at two times, for two doses).

Ad•vil (ad′vil) trademark for preparations of ibuprofen.

ady•nam•ic (a-di-nam′ik) asthenic.

adys•pla•sia (a″dis-pla′zhə) severe dysplasia in which an organ or part is shrunken and sometimes ectopic, and initially appears to be absent.

hereditary renal a. an autosomal dominant condition in which a kidney is severely dysplastic, nonfunctional, and often ectopic; if bilateral, as in the oligohydramnios sequence, the infant usually dies soon after birth.

A-E, AE above-elbow; see under *amputation.*

ae- for words beginning thus, see also those beginning *e-*.

Ae•by muscle, plane (a′be) [Christopher Theodore *Aeby*, Swiss anatomist, 1835–1885] see *musculus depressor labii inferioris*, and see under *plane.*

aec- for words beginning thus, see also words beginning *ec-*.

aeci•um (e′se-əm) pl. *ae′cia* [Gr. *aikia* injury] a cup-shaped fruiting body of a rust fungus; see *rust* (def. 3).

AED automatic external defibrillator.

Ae•des (a-e′dēz) [Gr. *aēdēs* unpleasant] a genus of mosquitoes of the tribe Aedini, subfamily Culicinae, having broad appressed scales on the head and scutellum. The palpi in the female are short and sparsely tufted and have three segments of equal length; in the male, the palpi are long and tufted. In addition to the vectors listed below, the following species are annoying because of their bites: *A. al′drichi*, *A. commu′nis*, *A. excru′cians*, *A. punc′tor*, *A. sti′mulans*, and *A. vex′ans.* Also written *Aëdes.*

A. aegyp′ti the yellow fever mosquito, which breeds near houses and transmits urban yellow fever, dengue, and sometimes filariasis and encephalitis.

A. africa′nus an arboreal mosquito that attacks monkeys and is a vector of the yellow fever virus and the Zika virus over much of Central Africa.

A. albopic′tus the Asian tiger or forest day mosquito, a species that transmits yellow fever, equine encephalomyelitis, and dengue.

A. atlan′ticus a North American species that is a vector of eastern equine encephalitis and of *Dirofilaria immitis.*

A. canaden′sis a North American species that is a vector of eastern equine encephalitis and La Crosse virus.

A. cine′reus a North American species that is a vector for equine encephalomyelitis.

A. flaves′cens a species found on certain islands in the Pacific, a transmitter of filariasis.

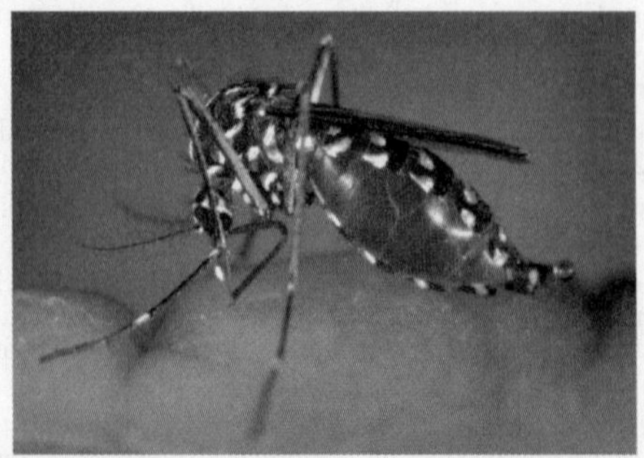

■ *Aedes albopictus* female partially engorged during feeding.

A. ingra′mi a species found in the pool from which Uganda S virus was isolated in 1947.

A. leucocelae′nus a South American species that transmits jungle yellow fever.

A. mela′nimon a species that is a vector of California encephalitis.

A. polynesien′sis a species found on certain islands in the South Pacific, a vector of filaria and dengue.

A. pseudoscutella′ris a species found on certain islands in the Pacific, a transmitter of filariasis.

A. scapula′ris a vector of the Cache Valley virus in Trinidad.

A. serra′tus a South American species that is a vector of Oropouche virus.

A. simp′soni a vector of jungle yellow fever in Africa.

A. sollic′itans the common salt-marsh mosquito of the Atlantic and Gulf coasts of the United States, a vector of equine encephalomyelitis.

A. spen′cerii a species found on the prairies of western Canada.

A. taeniorhyn′chus a New World species that is the vector of a number of diseases, including equine encephalitis, dengue in Florida, and wuchereriasis.

A. to′goi a Japanese species that serves as a vector of *Brugia malayi*, which causes filariasis malayi.

A. triseria′tus a species that transmits La Crosse encephalitis.

A. varipal′pus a species found along the Pacific coast of North America.

Ae•di•ni (a-e-di′ni) a tribe of mosquitoes of the subfamily Culicinae, including the genera *Aedes*, *Armigeres*, *Haemagogus*, and *Psorophora.*

aed•oeo•ceph•a•lus (ēd″e-o-sef′ə-lus) [Gr. *aidoia* genitals + *-cephalus*] a fetus with no mouth, a nose like a penis, and only one orbit.

Aeg. [L.] ae′ger, ae′gra (the patient).

Ae•gyp•ti•a•nel•la (e-jip″she-ə-nel′ə) [*Egypt*, where the organism was first described] a bacterial genus incertae sedis within the family Anaplasmataceae, parasitic in erythrocytes of wild and domestic birds and transmitted by ticks of the genus *Argas.* Organisms form inclusions that on Romanowsky staining appear as purple intracytoplasmic bodies. The type species is *A. pullo′rum.*

aelu•ro•pho•bia (e-loo″ro-fo′be-ə) [Gr. *ailouros* cat + *-phobia*] ailurophobia.

Aelu•ro•stron•gy•lus (e-loo″ro-stron′jə-lus) a genus of nematodes of the family Angiostrongylidae. *A. abstru′sus* is a lungworm that causes verminous bronchitis or pneumonia in cats.

-aemia see *-emia.*

AEP auditory evoked potential.

aequa•tor (e-kwa′tər) [L. "equalizer"] equator.

aequor•in (e-kwor′in) a protein isolated from the jellyfish *Aequora aequora*, bioluminescent in proportion to the amount of calcium ions present and injected into cells to measure calcium concentration; now largely replaced by fluorescent dyes.

aer•at•ed (ār′āt-əd) [L. *aeratus*] 1. charged with air. 2. charged with carbon dioxide. 3. oxygenated.

aer•a•tion (ār-a′shən) 1. the exchange of carbon dioxide for oxygen by the blood in the lungs. 2. the charging of a liquid with air or gas.

aer•emia (ār-e′me-ə) [*aer-* + *-emia*] air embolism.

aer(o)- [Gr. *aēr* air] a combining form denoting relationship to air or gas.

aero•al•ler•gen (ār″o-al′ər-jən) an airborne particle capable of producing an allergic reaction in sensitized individuals.

aer•obe (ār′ōb) [*aero-* + Gr. *bios* life] a microorganism that can live and grow in the presence of free oxygen.

facultative a. a microorganism that can live under either aerobic or anaerobic conditions.

obligate a. a microorganism that requires molecular oxygen for growth.

aer•o•bic (ār-o′bik) 1. having molecular oxygen present. 2. growing, living, or occurring in the presence of molecular oxygen. 3. requiring oxygen for respiration. 4. designed to increase oxygen consumption by the body; see *aerobic exercise*, under *exercise.*

Aero•Bid (ār′o-bid″) trademark for preparations of flunisolide.

aero•bi•ol•o•gy (ār″o-bi-ol′ə-je) [*aero-* + *biology*] the branch of biology that deals with the distribution of living organisms by the air, either the exterior or outdoor air *(extramural a.)* or the indoor air *(intramural a.).*

aero•bi•o•sis (ār″o-bi-o′sis) [*aero-* + *biosis*] life in the presence of molecular oxygen. **aerobiot′ic** *adj*

aero•cele (ār′o-sēl″) [*aero-* + *-cele*[1]] pneumatocele (def. 1).

epidural a. a collection of air between the dura mater and the wall of the vertebral column.

intracranial a. pneumocephalus resulting from trauma.

Aero·coc·ca·ceae (ār″o-kŏ-ka′se-e) a family of gram-positive, nonmotile, non–spore-forming, facultatively aerobic to microaerophilic cocci of the order Lactobacillales, occurring singly or in pairs, tetrads, or short chains; medically important organisms are contained in the genus *Aerococcus.*

Aero·coc·cus (ār″o-kok′əs) [*Aero-* + *coccus*] a genus of aerobic, gram-positive cocci of the family Aerococcaceae. The type species is *A. vi′ridans.*

A. uri′nae a species that is a rare cause of urinary tract infections, soft tissue infection, septicemia, and endocarditis.

A. vi′ridans a widely occurring species that is a part of the normal skin flora; it is an opportunistic pathogen that causes a variety of illnesses, including endocarditis, septic arthritis, and urinary tract infections.

aero·der·mec·ta·sia (ār″o-dur″mek-ta′zhə) subcutaneous emphysema.

aer·o·di·ges·tive (ār″o-dĭ-jes′tiv) [*aero* + digestive] pertaining to the respiratory and digestive tracts, or parts of them, considered together.

aer·odon·tal·gia (ār″o-don-tal′jə) [*aero-* + *odontalgia*] barodontalgia.

aer·odon·tics (ār″o-don′tiks) a branch of dentistry concerned with effects on the teeth of high altitude flying.

aero·em·bo·lism (ār″o-em′bo-liz-əm) air embolism.

aero·gas·tria (ār-o-gas′tre-ə) the presence of gas in the stomach; stomach bubble. See also *magenblase.*

blocked a. retention of air in the stomach due to spasm of the esophagus.

aero·gel (ār′o-jel″) a porous solid formed by replacing the liquid of a gel with a gas, such as rigid plastic foam.

aero·gen (ār′o-jen″) an aerogenic, or gas-producing, bacterium.

aero·gen·e·sis (ār″o-jen′ə-sis) [*aero-* + *-genesis*] gas production.

aero·gen·ic (ār-o-jen′ik) producing gas; said of bacteria that liberate free gaseous products.

aer·og·e·nous (ār-oj′ə-nəs) aerogenic.

Aero·late (ār′o-lāt) trademark for preparations of theophylline.

aer·ol·y·sin (ār-ol′ĭ-sin) a cytolysin produced by *Aeromonas hydrophila.*

aero·med·i·cine (ār″o-med′ə-sin) aviation medicine.

Aero·mo·na·da·ceae (ār″o-mo″nə-da′se-e) a family of gram-negative, primarily aquatic, bacteria of the order Aeromonadales, consisting of straight, rigid, non–spore-forming, usually motile rods; organisms are facultatively anaerobic, chemo-organotrophic, and oxidase- and catalase-positive. Most are aquatic and some are pathogenic. Medically important organisms are contained in the genus *Aeromonas.*

Aero·mo·na·da·les (ār″o-mo″nə-da′lēz) an order of gram-negative, facultatively anaerobic, oxidase-positive, and generally catalase-negative, rod-shaped bacteria of the class Gammaproteobacteria, phylum Proteobacteria; members are mainly aquatic. It contains the family Aeromonadaceae; the family Succinivibrionaceae has also tentatively been placed in this order.

Aero·mo·nas (ār″o-mo′nəs) [*aero-* + Gr. *monas* unit] a genus of gram-negative bacteria of the family Aeromonadaceae, consisting of small, straight, rigid, non–spore-forming rods with polar flagella, occurring singly or in pairs or short chains; organisms are facultatively anaerobic, chemo-organotrophic, and catalase-positive. They are primarily aquatic, found in salt and fresh water, sewage, and soil, and cause various different diseases.

A. ca′viae a species found in fresh water and sewage and on domestic and wild mammals, birds, and fish; it causes gastroenteritis and wound infections in humans.

A. hydro′phila a species that causes red leg in frogs. In humans it is a cause of cellulitis, wound infections, acute diarrheal disease, septicemia, and urinary tract infections.

A. so′bria a species found in fresh water, sewage, and fish.

aer·op·a·thy (ār-op′ə-the) [*aero-* + *-pathy*] any disease due to change in atmospheric pressure, such as decompression sickness or air sickness.

aero·peri·to·ne·um (ār″o-per″ĭ-to-ne′um) pneumoperitoneum.

aero·pha·gia (ār″o-fa′jə) [*aero-* + *-phagia*] excessive swallowing of air, usually an unconscious process associated with anxiety, resulting in abdominal distention or belching, often interpreted by the patient as signs of a physical disorder.

aer·oph·a·gy (ār-of′ə-je) aerophagia.

aero·phil (ār′o-fil″) [*aero-* + *-phil*] an aerophilic organism.

aero·phil·ic (ār″o-fil′ik) requiring air for proper growth; aerobic.

aer·oph·i·lous (ār-of′ĭ-lus) aerophilic.

aero·pho·bia (ār-o-fo′be-ə) [*aero-* + *-phobia*] irrational fear of drafts or fresh air, often connected with the idea of harmful airborne influences.

aero·plank·ton (ār″o-plank′ton) the organisms (bacteria, pollen, etc.) present in the air.

Aero·seb-Dex (ār′o-seb-deks′) trademark for preparations of dexamethasone.

Aero·seb-HC (ār′o-seb″) trademark for a preparation of hydrocortisone.

aero·si·a·loph·a·gy (ār″o-si″ə-lof′ə-je) sialoaerophagy.

aero·si·nus·itis (ār″o-si″nəs-i′tis) barosinusitis.

aer·o·sis (ār-o′sis) the production of gas in the tissues or organs of the body.

aer·o·sol (ār′o-sol) 1. a colloid system, a type of sol, in which the continuous phase (dispersion medium) is a gas, e.g., fog. 2. a liquid stored under pressure along with a propellant so that it can be dispensed as a fine mist, e.g., a bactericidal solution that can be finely atomized for the purpose of sterilizing the air of a room. 3. a solution of a drug that can be atomized into a fine mist for inhalation therapy.

aero·sol·i·za·tion (ār″o-sol″ĭ-za′shən) conversion into an aerosol. See also *nebulization.*

Aero·spo·rin (ār″o-spor′in) trademark for a preparation of polymyxin B sulfate.

aero·tax·is (ār″o-tak′sis) [*aero-* + *-taxis*] a movement of an organism in response to the presence of molecular oxygen.

aer·oti·tis (ār″o-ti′tis) barotitis.

a. me′dia barotitis media.

aero·tol·er·ant (ār″o-tol′ər-ənt) able to survive or to grow slowly in an aerobic environment; said of certain anaerobic microorganisms.

aero·to·nom·e·ter (ār″o-tə-nom′ə-tər) [*aero-* + *tonometer*] an instrument for measuring the partial pressure of the gases in the blood.

aer·ot·ro·pism (ār-ot′ro-piz″əm) [*aero-* + *tropism*] movement of an organism toward *(positive a.)* or away from *(negative a.)* a supply of air.

aes- for words beginning thus, see also those beginning *es-*, *et-*.

aes·cu·la·pi·an (es″ku-la′pe-ən) pertaining to Aesculapius, or to the art of medicine.

Aescu·la·pi·us (es″ku-la′pe-əs) [L., from Gr. *Asklēpios*, son of Apollo and Coronis, tutelary god of medicine] the Greek god or deified hero of medicine and healing. See also under *staff.*

aes·cu·lin (es′ku-lin) esculin.

Aes·cu·lus (es′ku-ləs) [L.] a genus of trees of the family Hippocastanaceae; most species contain the coumarin glycoside esculin, which makes them toxic to livestock. *A. hippocasta′num* L. is the horse chestnut, which is used medicinally. *A. glab′ra* is the buckeye.

aesthesi(o)- for words beginning thus, see those beginning *esthesi(o)-*.

aes·thet·ic (es-thet′ik) esthetic.

aes·thet·ics (es-thet′iks) esthetics.

aestiv(o)- for words beginning thus, see those beginning *estiv(o)-*.

aet. [L.] ae′tas (age).

aetio- for words beginning thus, see those beginning *etio-*.

AF atrial fibrillation.

AFCR American Federation for Clinical Research.

afe·brile (a-feb′ril) without fever; called also *apyretic* and *apyrexial.*

afe·tal (a-fe′təl) without a fetus.

af·fect (af′ekt) the external expression of emotion attached to ideas or mental representations of objects; cf. *mood.* **affec′tive** *adj*

blunted a. severe reduction in the intensity of affect; seen in schizophrenic disorders, frontotemporal dementia, and certain other conditions.

constricted a. restricted a.

flat a. lack of signs expressing affect.

inappropriate a. affect that is incongruent with the situation or with the content of a patient's ideas or speech.

labile a. an affect in which a person has rapid changes in emotion not necessarily related to external events or stimuli.

pseudobulbar a. episodes of uncontrollable laughing and crying seen in patients with neurologic conditions; called also *emotional incontinence.*

restricted a. reduction in the intensity of affect, to a somewhat lesser degree than is characteristic of blunted affect.

af·fec·tion (ə-fek′shən) a state of emotion or feeling.

af·fec·tiv·i·ty (af″ek-tiv′ĭ-te) the capacity to feel emotions; the degree of responsiveness or susceptibility to emotional stimuli.

af·fec·to·mo·tor (ə-fek″to-mo′tər) [*affect* + *motor*] characterized by mental excitement and muscular hyperactivity, as in the manic phase of bipolar disorder.

af·fer·ent (af′ər-ənt) [L. *ad-* to + *ferre* to carry] 1. conveying toward a center; called also *centripetal.* 2. something that so conducts; see under *fiber* and *nerve.* Cf. *corticipetal.*

af·fil·i·a·tion (ə-fil″e-a′shən) a social drive to be associated with others in interdependent relationships, involving using others for help or support without making them responsible for problems.

af·fin·i·ty (ə-fin′ĭ-te) [L. *affinitas* relationship] 1. a special attraction for a specific element, organ, or structure. 2. chemical a. 3. in immunology, a thermodynamic expression of the strength of interaction between a single antigen-binding site and a single antigenic determinant (and thus of the stereochemical compatibility between them), most accurately applied to interactions among simple, uniform antigenic determinants such as haptens. Expressed as the association constant (K liters $mole^{-1}$), which, owing to the heterogeneity of affinities in a population of antibody molecules of a given specificity, actually represents an average value (mean intrinsic association constant). Cf. *avidity.*

chemical a. the tendency of an atom or compound to combine by chemical reaction with atoms or compounds of unlike composition.

electron a. the energy released when a single electron is combined with an isolated atom; its value is determined by the effective charge on the nucleus and the size and electronic configuration of the atom.

af·flux (af′luks) [L. *affluxus, affluxio*] the rush of blood or liquid to a part.

af·flux·ion (ə-fluk′shən) afflux.

af·fri·cate (af′rĭ-kət) a consonantal speech sound made up of a plosive followed by a fricative, such as *ch* or *j.* Called also *affricative.*

af·fric·a·tive (ə-frik′ə-tiv) affricate.

AFib atrial fibrillation.

afi·brin·o·gen·emia (a″fi-brin″o-jə-ne′me-ə) lack of fibrinogen (coagulation factor I) in the blood; cf. *hypofibrinogenemia.*

congenital a. a rare autosomal recessive hemorrhagic coagulation disorder caused by mutations in any of the three genes (locus: 4q28) encoding fibrinogen subunits, characterized by complete incoagulability of the blood; hemorrhagic manifestations vary from mild to serious.

Afip·ia (ə-fip′e-ə) [Armed Forces Institute of Pathology] a genus of bacteria of the family Bradyrhizobiaceae, consisting of gram-negative rods.

A. fe′lis a species that has been found in lymph nodes and skin lesions of humans, but has not been proven to cause disease.

AFl atrial flutter.

af·la·tox·i·co·sis (af″lə-tok″sĭ-ko′sis) an often fatal type of mycotoxicosis affecting turkeys and other farm animals fed on peanut meal or seedlings of peanut plants *(Arachis hypogaea)* contaminated with the molds *Aspergillus flavus* and related species, which produce aflatoxin. Symptoms include liver necrosis, bile duct proliferation, and cirrhosis, and, with prolonged feeding, hepatocellular carcinoma and cholangiocarcinoma. Called also *x disease.*

af·la·tox·in (af′lə-tok″sin) a toxic factor produced by *Aspergillus flavus* and *A. parasiticus,* molds contaminating seedlings of peanut plants *(Arachis hypogaea).* Domestic fowl and other animals fed with infected peanut meal may die of aflatoxicosis, hepatocellular carcinoma, or cholangiocarcinoma. It has also been implicated as a cause of human hepatic carcinoma.

Aflu·ria (a-floo′re-ə) trademark for a preparation of influenza virus vaccine.

AFO ankle-foot orthosis.

AFP alpha fetoprotein.

AFS American Fertility Society.

af·ter·birth (af′tər-bərth) the placenta and membranes, delivered from the uterus after the birth of the child. Called also *secundina, secundinae,* and *secundines.*

af·ter·care (af′tər-kār) 1. the care and treatment of a convalescent patient, especially one who has undergone surgery; called also *aftertreatment.* 2. the continuing outpatient treatment and rehabilitation services provided within the community to psychiatric patients following discharge from the hospital.

af·ter·cat·a·ract (af″tər-kat′ə-rakt) see under *cataract.*

af·ter·cur·rent (af′tər-kur″ənt) a current produced in a muscle and nerve after cessation of an electric current that has been flowing through it.

af·ter·de·po·lar·iza·tion (af″tər-de-po″lər-ĭ-za′shən) a depolarizing afterpotential, sometimes occurring in tissues not normally excitable. It is frequently one of a series, failing to reach threshold and self-perpetuating; triggered automaticity may result.

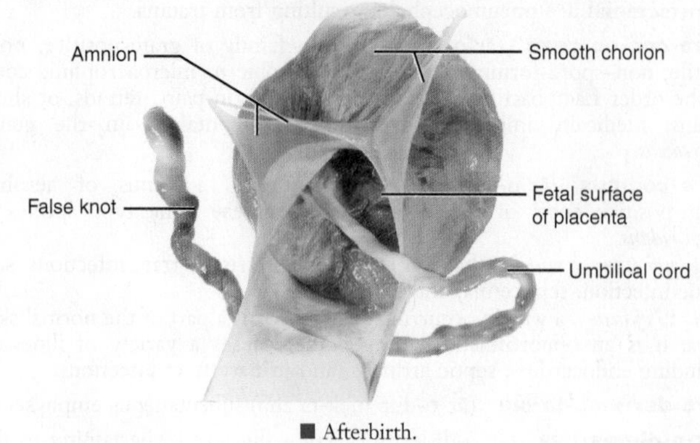

■ Afterbirth.

delayed a. (DAD) an afterdepolarization occurring after full repolarization, and generally during a period of hyperpolarization, of the cells initially depolarized in the main (spike) potential.

early a. (EAD) an afterdepolarization occurring before full repolarization of the cells initially depolarized in the main (spike) potential, thus arising from a low membrane potential.

late a. delayed a.

af·ter·dis·charge (af″tər-dis′chahrj) the portion of the response to stimulation in a nerve which persists after the stimulus has ceased.

af·ter·gil·ding (af″tər-gild′ing) the histologic application of gold salts to nerve tissue after fixation and hardening.

af·ter·im·age (af′tər-im″əj) a visual impression persisting briefly after cessation of the stimuli causing the original image; called also *accidental* or *negative image* and *aftervision.*

negative a. an afterimage in which the brights and darks are reversed from, and the colors are complementary to, the original image.

positive a. an afterimage in which the bright, dark, and colored areas are the same as in the original image.

af·ter·im·pres·sion (af″tər-im-presh′ən) aftersensation.

af·ter·load (af′tər-lōd″) in cardiac physiology, the force against which cardiac muscle shortens. In isolated muscle it is the force resisting shortening after the muscle is stimulated to contract; in the intact heart it is the pressure against which the ventricle ejects blood, as measured by the stress acting on the ventricular wall following the onset of contraction, determined largely by the peripheral vascular resistance and by the physical characteristics of and blood volume in the arterial system. It is often estimated by determining systolic arterial pressure, from which can be determined the systolic wall stress; see also *Laplace's law,* under *law.*

af·ter·math (af′tər-math) mowed second-growth grass, which sometimes causes *fog fever (aftermath disease)* when eaten by ruminants. Called also *fog.*

af·ter·move·ment (af″tər-mo͞ov′mənt) spontaneous elevation of the upper limb by idiomuscular contraction after benumbing it by powerful pressure against a rigid object; called also *Kohnstamm phenomenon.*

af·ter·pains (af′tər-pānz) the cramplike pains felt after the birth of the child, due to the contractions of the uterus.

af·ter·per·cep·tion (af″tər-pər-sep′shən) the perception of a sensation after the stimulus producing it has ceased.

af·ter·po·ten·tial (af″tər-po-ten′shəl) the small action potential generated following termination of the spike or main potential; it has a negative and a positive phase.

negative a. the period following termination of the spike potential during which there is a lag in the return of the potential of an excitable cell membrane to resting potential.

positive a. the period following termination of the negative afterpotential, during which the potential of an excitable cell membrane is more negative than the resting potential. It is paradoxically called *positive* because it was first detected outside the cell, where the polarity is reversed.

af·ter·sen·sa·tion (af″tər-sen-sa′shən) a sensation lasting after the stimulus that produced it has been removed; called also *afterimpression.*

af·ter·taste (af′tər-tāst) a taste continuing after the substance producing it has been removed.

af·ter·treat·ment (af″tər-trēt′mənt) aftercare (def. 1).

af·ter·vi·sion (af″tər-vizh′ən) afterimage.

afunc·tion (a-funk′shən) loss of function.

AFX atypical fibroxanthoma.

AG atrial gallop.

Ag antigen; silver (L. *argen'tum*).

AGA American Gastroenterological Association.

aga•lac•tia (a″gə-lak'she-ə) [*a-*[1] + *galacto-* + *-ia*] absence or failure of the secretion of milk; called also *agalactosis.*

contagious a. a contagious disease of goats and sheep in southern Europe and North Africa, usually caused by *Mycoplasma agalactiae;* symptoms include arthritis and eye lesions, with mastitis in females.

mastitis-metritis-a. lactation failure in swine; see under *failure.*

agal•ac•to•sis (a-gal″ak-to'sis) agalactia.

aga•lac•tous (a″gə-lak'təs) 1. suppressing the secretion of milk. 2. not nursed; artificially fed.

agal•or•rhea (a-gal″o-re'ə) [*a-*[1] + Gr. *gala* milk + *rhoia* flow] absence or arrest of the flow of milk.

agam•ete (ag'ə-mēt) [*a-*[1] + *gamete*] the product of multiple fission in protozoa.

agam•ma•glob•u•lin•emia (a-gam″ə-glob″u-lĭ-ne'me-ə) [*a-*[1] + *gamma globulin* + *-emia*] absence of all classes of immunoglobulins in the blood; the term was used before assays sensitive enough to detect very low levels of globulins were developed, and most such disorders are really hypogammaglobulinemias (q.v.); see also *dysgammaglobulinemia* and *immunodeficiency.*

acquired a. common variable immunodeficiency.

Bruton a. X-linked a.

common variable a. see under *immunodeficiency.*

lymphopenic a. severe combined immunodeficiency.

X-linked a., X-linked infantile a. a primary X-linked immunodeficiency disorder (gene locus: Xq21.3-q22) caused by mutation of the gene encoding Bruton tyrosine kinase. It is characterized by absence of circulating B lymphocytes, absence of plasma cells and germinal centers in lymphoid tissues, and very low levels of circulating immunoglobulins. The pathogenic defect appears to be a failure of pre-B cells to differentiate into mature B cells, express surface immunoglobulins, and produce antibody. Patients are unusually prone to bacterial infection and many have symptoms resembling those of rheumatoid arthritis. Called also *Bruton a.* or *disease* and *X-linked hypogammaglobulinemia.*

agam(o)- [Gr. *agamos* unmarried] a combining form meaning asexual.

Aga•mo•fi•la•ria (ə-gam″o-fĭ-lar'e-ə) a name given to filarial worms which are known only in immature stages and which cannot be assigned to any known genus or species.

aga•mo•gen•e•sis (ag″ə-mo-jen'ə-sis) asexual reproduction.

aga•mo•ge•net•ic (ag″ə-mo-jə-net'ik) reproducing asexually.

aga•mog•o•ny (ag″ə-mog'ə-ne) asexual reproduction.

aga•mont (ag'ə-mont) schizont.

aga•mous (ag'ə-məs) 1. asexual. 2. having no recognizable sexual organs.

agan•gli•on•ic (a-gang″gle-on'ik) pertaining to or characterized by the absence of ganglion cells.

agan•gli•on•o•sis (a-gang″gle-on-o'sis) [*a-*[1] + *ganglion* + *-osis*] congenital absence of parasympathetic ganglion cells, as in congenital megacolon.

agar (ag'ahr) [Malay *agar-agar*] [NF] a mucilaginous complex sulfated polymer of galactose units, extracted from *Gelidium cartilagineum, Gracilaria confervoides,* and related red algae. It melts at 100°C and solidifies into a gel at 40°C, is not digested by most bacteria, and as a gel is used in the preparation of solid culture media for microorganisms, as a bulk laxative, in making emulsions, as a supporting medium in procedures such as immunodiffusion and electrophoresis, and as the principal component in reversible hydrocolloid dental impression material. See under *culture medium* for specific agars.

agar•ic (ə-gar'ik, ag'ə-rik) [Gr. *agarikon* a sort of tree fungus] 1. any of various mushrooms, especially any species of *Agaricus.* 2. a preparation of rotten wood mixed with fungi or dried mushrooms.

fly a. *Amanita muscaria.*

Agar•i•ca•ceae (ə-gar″ĭ-ka'se-e) a family of mushrooms (order Agaricales); it includes the genera *Agaricus, Chlorophyllum, Clitocybe, Lepiota,* and *Paxillus.*

Agar•i•ca•les (ə-gar″ĭ-ka'lēz) the mushrooms, a large order of perfect fungi of the subphylum Basidiomycotina, class Holobasidiomycetes; some are edible, some poisonous, and some hallucinogenic. Families of medical importance include Agaricaceae, Amanitaceae, Coprinaceae, and Strophariaceae.

Agar•i•cus (ə-gar'ĭ-kəs) [Gr. *agarikon* a sort of tree fungus] a genus of mushrooms of the family Agaricaceae. *A. campes'tris* is a common edible variety found in fields. *A. musca'rius* has been renamed *Amanita muscaria.* See also *agaric.*

agas•tria (a-gas'tre-ə) absence of the stomach, either as a congenital condition or after gastrectomy. **agas'tric** *adj*

Aga•ve (ə-ga've) [Gr. *agauē* noble] a genus of plants of the family Amaryllidaceae; many species have spiny-margined leaves and tall candelabra-shaped inflorescences. Some species serve as a source of a Mexican alcoholic beverage, and others contain saponins.

A. america'na the century plant, a species whose juice is cathartic and diuretic and has been used as an abortifacient.

A. lecheguil'la lechuguilla, a species that grows in the southwestern United States and Mexico; it contains sapotoxins that cause diarrhea, as well as a photodynamic substance that causes lechuguilla fever in sheep and goats.

AGE advanced glycation end product.

age (āj) 1. the duration of individual existence measured in units of time. 2. the measure of some individual attribute in terms of the chronological age of an average normal individual showing the same degree of proficiency, e.g., achievement age.

achievement a. a measure of achievement expressed in terms of the chronological age of an average child showing the same degree of attainment.

anatomical a. age expressed in terms of the chronological age of the average individual showing the same body development.

Binet a. mental age as determined by Binet test.

bone a. osseous development shown radiographically, stated in terms of the chronologic age at which the development is ordinarily attained.

chronologic a. the age of a person expressed in terms of the period elapsed from the time of birth.

coital a. the age of a conceptus defined by the time elapsed since the coitus that led to fertilization.

conceptual a. the age of a conceptus defined by the time elapsed since fertilization. Called also *fertilization a.*

developmental a. age estimated from the degree of anatomical development. In psychology, the age of an individual as determined by the degree of emotional, mental, anatomical, and physiologic maturation.

emotional a. the age of an individual expressed in terms of the chronological age of an average normal individual showing the same degree of emotional maturity.

fertilization a. conceptual a.

functional a. the combined expression of the chronological, emotional, mental, and physiological ages of an individual.

gestational a. the age of a conceptus or pregnancy. In human clinical practice, pregnancy is timed from onset of the last normal menstrual period (menstrual age), which is about two weeks longer than the fertilization age. Elsewhere the onset may be timed from estrus, coitus, artificial insemination, vaginal plug formation, fertilization, or implantation.

height a. the age on a height growth chart at which a child's actual height is the same as the 50th percentile height.

menstrual a. conceptus age defined by the time elapsed since the onset of the mother's last normal menstrual period (LNMP).

mental a. the score achieved by a person in an intelligence test, expressed in terms of the chronological age of an average normal individual showing the same degree of attainment.

physical a., physiological a. the age of an individual expressed in terms of the chronological age of a normal individual showing the same degree of anatomical and physiological development.

postovulatory a. conceptus age defined by the time elapsed since release of the secondary oocyte from the ovary.

Age•le•ni•dae (ag″ə-len'ĭ-de) a large family of common spiders that build sheetlike or funnel-shaped webs in grass or under rocks or boards; it includes the genus *Tegenaria,* to which the hobo spider (*T. agrestis,* q.v.) belongs.

Agen•er•ase (a-jen'ə-rās) trademark for a preparation of amprenavir.

agen•e•sia (a″jə-ne'zhə) agenesis.

agen•e•sis (a-jen'ə-sis) [*a-*[1] + *-genesis*] absence of an organ, usually referring to such absence resulting from failure of appearance of its primordium in embryonic development. Cf. *aplasia.*

adrenal a. failure of development of adrenal glands, a usually lethal condition; cf. *congenital adrenal hypoplasia.*

callosal a. defect of the callosal structures of the brain.

gonadal a. complete failure of gonadal development, as in Turner syndrome.

nuclear a. Möbius syndrome.

ovarian a. failure of development of the ovaries, as in Turner syndrome.

renal a. failure of development of the kidneys; see also *hereditary renal adysplasia,* under *adysplasia.*

sacral a. caudal regression syndrome.

agen·i·tal·ism (a-jen′ĭ-təl-iz″əm) 1. absence of the genitalia. 2. a condition caused by failure to secrete gonadal hormones. See also *agonadism*.

ageno·so·mia (a-jen″o-so′me-ə) congenital absence or rudimentary development of the genitals and eventration of the lower part of the abdomen.

ageno·so·mus (a-jen″o-so′məs) [*a-*[1] + *geno-* + *sōma* body] a fetus exhibiting agenosomia.

agent (a′jənt) [L. *agens* acting] any power, principle, or substance capable of producing an effect, whether physical, chemical, or biological.

adrenergic blocking a. a compound that selectively inhibits response to sympathetic impulses and to catecholamines and other adrenergic amines. See *alpha-adrenergic blocking a.*, *beta-adrenergic blocking a.*, and *adrenergic neuron blocking a.*

adrenergic neuron blocking a. a substance that inhibits the release of norepinephrine from postganglionic adrenergic nerve endings.

alkylating a. a highly reactive compound that can substitute alkyl groups for the hydrogen atoms of certain organic compounds. Such agents are cytotoxic, producing their effects by the scission and cross-linking of DNA chains, and are not cell cycle–specific, but cell killing occurs primarily in rapidly proliferating tissues in which there is not time between mitoses for DNA repair systems to reverse the effects of the agent. Classes of antineoplastic alkylating agents include nitrogen mustards, ethylenimine derivatives, alkyl sulfonates, nitrosoureas, triazenes, and platinum compounds. Hematopoietic, reproductive, and epithelial tissues are particularly sensitive to alkylating agents, and their use may cause depressed blood cell counts, amenorrhea or impaired spermatogenesis, damage to intestinal mucosa, alopecia, and increased risk of malignancy.

alpha-adrenergic blocking a. an agent that induces adrenergic blockade at α-adrenergic receptors.

antianxiety a. a drug that reduces anxiety; the group includes the benzodiazepines (diazepam and congeners) as well as some nonbenzodiazepines such as buspirone, meprobamate, and hydroxyzine. Called also *minor tranquilizer*.

beta-adrenergic blocking a. an agent that induces adrenergic blockade at either β_1- or β_2-adrenergic receptors or at both.

blocking a. an agent that inhibits a biological action, such as movement of an ion across the cell membrane, passage of a neural impulse, or interaction with a specific receptor.

calcium channel blocking a. any of a group of drugs that inhibit the entry of calcium into cells or inhibit the mobilization of calcium from intracellular stores, resulting in slowing of atrioventricular and sinoatrial conduction and relaxation of arterial smooth and cardiac muscle; used in the treatment of angina, cardiac arrhythmias, and hypertension.

chelating a. 1. a compound that combines with metal ions by means of two or more coordinating positions to form stable ring structures, e.g., heme. 2. a substance used to reduce the concentration of free metal ion in solution by complexing it. Called also *metal complexing a.* and *chelator*.

cholinergic blocking a. a substance that blocks or inactivates acetylcholine.

clearing a. an agent used in staining technique for fixed cells, which has the same refractive index as that of protein particles.

complexing a. ligand.

contrast a. see under *medium*.

coupling a. a substance used to coat filler particles in a resin matrix composite so that the particles bind to the resin matrix.

depolarizing neuromuscular blocking a. a nicotinic agonist that blocks neural transmission at the myoneural junction by binding to the nicotinic receptors of the motor end plate to produce prolonged depolarization of the postsynaptic membrane.

doping a. dopant.

Eaton a. *Mycoplasma pneumoniae*.

emulsifying a. emulsifier.

fixing a's agents, such as formalin, alcohol, acids, salts of heavy metals, or mixtures of these, that precipitate the proteins of cells or tissues and render them insoluble.

fluorescent whitening a. optical whitening a.

ganglionic blocking a. a drug that blocks nerve impulses at autonomic ganglionic synapses; used for initial control of blood pressure in patients with acute dissecting aortic aneurysm, production of controlled hypotension during surgery, and treatment of autonomic hyperreflexia.

hypomethylating a's a group of drugs that inhibit the methylation of DNA and are used as antineoplastics.

inotropic a. any of a class of agents affecting the force of muscle contraction, particularly a drug affecting the force of cardiac contraction; positive inotropic agents, such as digitalis glycosides or catecholamines, increase and negative inotropic agents, such as calcium antagonists, decrease the force of cardiac muscle contractions. All such drugs currently used act indirectly, as by affecting sodium pump, calcium transport, or cyclic AMP production, rather than by directly affecting myofibrils or troponin complexes.

levigating a. a material used for moistening a solid before reducing it to a powder.

luting a. lute (def. 1).

metal complexing a. chelating a.

molecularly targeted a's a group of antineoplastic drugs that target cancer cell–specific pathways on the molecular level, interfering with processes such as growth regulation, cell cycle control, apoptosis, or other mechanisms.

neuromuscular blocking a. a compound that causes paralysis of skeletal muscle by blocking neural transmission at the neuromuscular junction.

nondepolarizing neuromuscular blocking a. a compound that blocks neural transmission at the myoneural junction by inhibiting the action of acetylcholine by competitive binding to the nicotinic receptors of the motor end plate without depolarizing the postsynaptic membrane.

nonsteroidal antiinflammatory a. see under *drug*.

optical whitening a. a substance added to something else to produce brightness by absorbing invisible ultraviolet light and reflecting it as visible blue light; these are added to detergents, paper, and textiles to give them a white color. Called also *fluorescent whitening a.* See also *blankophore*.

A. Orange a herbicide and defoliant containing 2,4-D and 2,4,5-T and the contaminant dioxin; it is suspected of being teratogenic and possibly carcinogenic.

oxidizing a. a substance capable of accepting electrons from another substance, thereby oxidizing the second substance and itself becoming reduced.

phase-specific a. a cytotoxic agent that has its maximum effect at a given phase of the cell growth cycle.

Pittsburgh pneumonia a. *Legionella micdadei*.

potassium channel blocking a. any of a class of antiarrhythmic agents that inhibit the movement of potassium ions through the potassium channels, thus prolonging repolarization of the cell membrane.

progestational a. any of a group of hormones secreted by the corpus luteum and placenta and in small amounts by the adrenal cortex, including progesterone; they induce the formation of a secretory endometrium. Many are now also produced synthetically, and their uses include contraception, hormone replacement therapy, and treatment of menstrual disorders, of endometriosis, of infertility, of hormonally responsive carcinomas, and of anorexia and significant weight loss associated with AIDS or cancer. Called also *gestagen*, *progestagen*, *progestin*, *progestogen*, and *progestational hormone*.

psychoactive a., psychotropic a. see under *substance*.

reducing a. a substance capable of donating electrons to another substance, thereby reducing the second substance and itself becoming oxidized.

sclerosing a. a chemical irritant injected into a vein in sclerotherapy. Called also *sclerosant*.

sodium channel blocking a. any of a class of antiarrhythmic agents that prevent ectopic beats by acting on partially inactivated sodium channels to inhibit abnormal depolarizations.

surface-active a. a substance that exerts a change on the surface properties of a liquid, especially one that reduces its surface tension, such as a detergent. Called also *surfactant*.

transforming a. a substance that produces transformation in a cell, e.g., a DNA fragment from a bacterial (donor) cell that, when introduced into another bacterial (recipient) cell, is incorporated into the chromosome and produces a permanent, inherited change.

wetting a. a substance that lowers the surface tension of water to promote wetting.

AGEP acute generalized exanthematous pustulosis.

AGEPC acetyl glyceryl ether phosphoryl choline; see *platelet-activating factor*, under *factor*.

ager·a·sia (ă-jər-a′zhə) [*a-*[1] + Gr. *gēras* old age] an unusually youthful appearance in a person of advanced years.

ageu·sia (ə-goo′zhə) [*a-*[1] + Gr. *geusis* taste] absence of the sense of taste; called also *ageustia* and *gustatory anesthesia*. ageu′sic *adj*

ageus·tia (ə-gōōs′te-ə) ageusia.

ag·ger (aj′er) pl. *ag′geres* [L. "mound"] an eminence or projection.

a. na′si [TA] ridge of nose: a ridgelike elevation midway between the anterior extremity of the middle nasal concha and the inner surface of the dorsum of the nose; called also *nasoturbinal concha*.

ag·ger·es (aj′ər-ēz) [L.] plural of *agger*.

ag·glom·er·at·ed (ə-glom′ər-āt″əd) [L. *agglomeratus*, from *ad* together + *glomus* mass] crowded into a mass.

ag·glu·ti·na·ble (ə-gloo′tĭ-nə-bəl) capable of agglutination.

ag·glu·ti·nant (ə-gloo′tĭ-nənt) [L. *agglutinans* gluing] 1. promoting union by adhesion. 2. a tenacious or gluey substance that holds parts together during the process of healing.

ag·glu·ti·na·tion (ə-gloo″tĭ-na′shən) [L. *agglutinatio*] 1. the action of an agglutinant substance. 2. the process of union in the healing of a wound. 3. the clumping together in suspension of antigen-bearing cells,

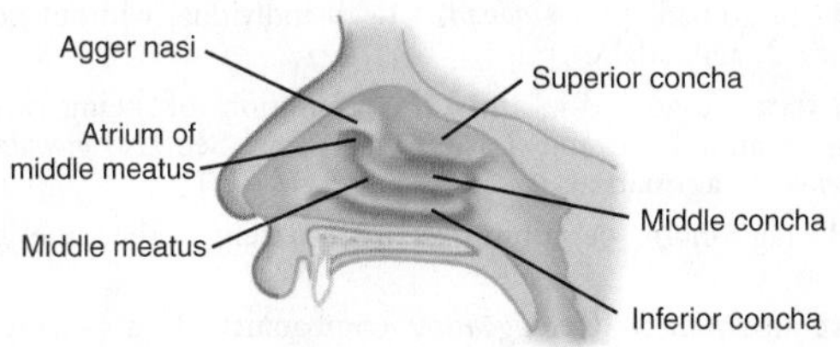

■ Agger nasi, an elevation anterior to the middle concha on the lateral nasal wall, above the atrium of the middle meatus.

microorganisms, or particles in the presence of specific antibodies (agglutinins). Called also *clumping*.

acid a. the nonspecific agglutination of microorganisms at relatively low hydrogen ion concentration; it occurs without participation of antibody.

bacteriogenic a. clumping of cells due to bacterial action. See *T agglutinin*, under *agglutinin*.

cold a. agglutination with cold agglutinins (q.v.), occurring more efficiently below 37°C than at 37°C.

cross a. the agglutination of particulate antigen by antibody raised against a different but related antigen; see also *group a.*

group a. agglutination, usually to a lower titer, of various members of a group of biologically related organisms or corpuscles by an agglutinin specific for one of that group. For instance, the specific agglutinin of typhoid bacilli may agglutinate other members of the colon-typhoid group, such as *Escherichia coli.*

H a. the agglutination of motile bacteria in the presence of antibody to the heat-labile flagellar antigens.

intravascular a. clumping of particulate elements (usually referring to red blood cells) within the blood vessels, such as after an injury. Called also *sludging of blood.*

O a. the agglutination of bacteria in the presence of antibody to the heat-stable somatic antigen.

passive a. agglutination in antiserum of particles owing to adsorbed specific soluble antigen.

platelet a. the clumping together of platelets under the influence of platelet agglutinins.

salt a. agglutination that occurs in salt solutions of certain concentrations.

spontaneous a. the agglutination of bacteria or other cells in physiologic salt solution due to the lack of sufficient surface polar groups to give stable suspensions in the presence of electrolytes.

Vi a. agglutination of bacteria containing Vi antigen on their surface, in the presence of specific agglutinin.

ag·glu·ti·na·tive (ə-gloo′tĭ-na″tiv) promoting adhesion or agglutination.

ag·glu·ti·na·tor (ə-gloo′tĭ-na″tər) something which agglutinates; an agglutinin.

ag·glu·ti·nin (ə-gloo′tĭ-nin) 1. antibody that aggregates a particulate antigen, e.g., bacteria, following combination with the homologous antigen in vivo or in vitro. 2. any substance other than antibody, e.g., lectin, that is capable of agglutinating particles.

anti-Rh a. an agglutinin not normally present in human plasma but which may be produced in an Rh^- mother carrying an Rh^+ fetus or after transfusion of Rh^+ blood into an Rh^- patient. See *blood group.*

chief a. major a.

cold a. (CA) antibody that agglutinates erythrocytes or bacteria more efficiently at temperatures below 37°C than at 37°C. See *cold agglutinin syndrome*, under *syndrome*, and *paroxysmal cold hemoglobinuria*, under *hemoglobinuria.*

complete a. see *antibody.*

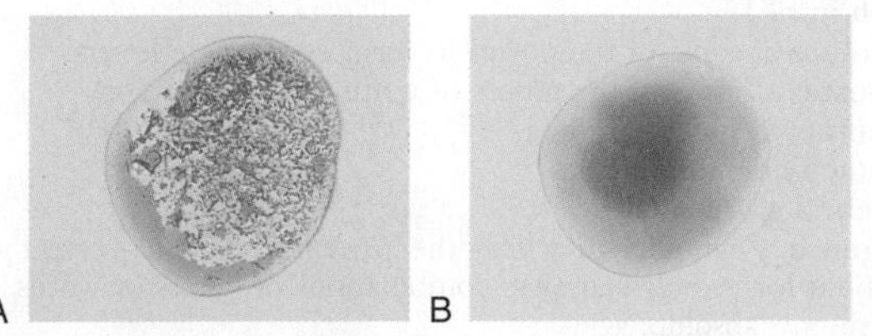

■ Agglutination occurring on addition of anti-human immunoglobulin to erythrocytes carrying antibody *(A)* and not occurring when it is added to erythrocytes lacking antibody *(B).*

cross a., cross-reacting a. an agglutinin which, although formed in response to one particulate antigen, also has specific action on a different but related antigen.

flagellar a. an agglutinin specific for the flagella of a microorganism.

group a. an agglutinin that has a specific action on certain organisms or cells but will also agglutinate other closely related species.

H a. see under *antigen.*

immune a. any agglutinating antibody.

incomplete a. see under *antibody.*

leukocyte a. an antibody capable of agglutinating leukocytes; leukocyte autoagglutinins and isoagglutinins are associated with a variety of disorders, both with and without frank leukopenia. Called also *leukoagglutinin.*

major a. the specific agglutinin present at highest titer in an antiserum. Called also *chief a.*

minor a. a specific or cross-reacting agglutinin present in an antiserum at lower titer than the major agglutinin. Called also *partial a.*

O a. see under *antigen.*

partial a. minor a.

platelet a. an antibody capable of agglutinating platelets; platelet autoagglutinins and isoagglutinins are associated with a variety of disorders, both with and without frank thrombocytopenia. Called also *thromboagglutinin.*

saline a. complete antibody.

somatic a. an agglutinin specific for the body of a microorganism.

T a. a natural antibody present in normal human sera that causes agglutination of erythrocytes treated with neuraminidase or incubated with neuraminidase-producing bacteria causing exposure of the T antigen.

warm a. an agglutinin more reactive at 37° C than at lower temperatures.

ag·glu·tin·o·gen (ag″loo-tin′o-jen) 1. any substance which, acting as an antigen, stimulates the production of agglutinin. 2. the particulate antigen used in conducting agglutination tests.

ag·glu·ti·no·gen·ic (ə-gloo″tĭ-no-jen′ik) pertaining to the production of agglutinin; producing agglutinin.

ag·glu·ti·no·phil·ic (ə-gloo″tĭ-no-fil′ik) agglutinating readily.

ag·glu·to·gen·ic (ə-gloo″to-jen′ik) agglutinogenic.

Ag·gra·stat (ag′grə-stat) trademark for a preparation of tirofiban hydrochloride.

ag·gre·can (ag′rə-kan) the major structural proteoglycan of cartilage, consisting of a 210-kD core protein to which are linked about 100 chondroitin sulfate and a number of keratan sulfate and oligosaccharide chains; it binds to a link protein and to hyaluronan, creating large aggregates.

aggred. feb. [L.] aggredien′te feb′re (while the fever is coming on).

Ag·gre·ga·ta (ag″rə-ga′tə) [L. *aggregare* to add to] a genus of coccidian protozoa (suborder Eimeriina, order Eucoccidiida), the life cycle of which involves schizogony in a crustacean and sporogony and gametogony in a cephalopod.

ag·gre·gate[1] (ag′rə-gāt) [L. *aggregatus*, from *ad* to + *grex* flock] to crowd or cluster together.

ag·gre·gate[2] (ag′rə-gət) 1. crowded or clustered together. 2. a mass or assemblage.

ag·gre·ga·tion (ag″rə-ga′shən) 1. massing of materials together as in clumping. 2. a clumped mass of material.

familial a. a concentration of cases of a disease in families; the occurrence of more cases of a given disorder in close relatives of a person with the disorder than in control families.

platelet a. a clumping together of platelets, part of a sequential mechanism leading to the initiation and formation of a thrombus or hemostatic plug. It can be induced in vitro, and probably in vivo, by agents such as ADP, thrombin, and collagen.

ag·gre·gom·e·ter (ag″rə-gom′ə-tər) an instrument that measures platelet aggregation by detecting changes in optical density of plasma or solution caused by clustering of platelets.

ag·gre·gom·e·try (ag″rə-gom′ə-tre) the measurement of platelet aggregation by means of an aggregometer.

Ag·gre·nox (ag′rə-noks) trademark for a combination preparation of aspirin and extended-release dipyridamole.

ag·gres·sin (ə-gres′in) any of a postulated group of nontoxic substances produced by pathogenic bacteria that inhibit the mechanisms of host resistance.

ag·gres·sion (ə-gresh′ən) [L. *aggressus*, from *ad* to + *gradi* to step] a form of behavior which leads to self-assertion; it may arise from innate drives and/or a response to frustration; it may be manifested by destructive and attacking behavior, by covert attitudes of hostility and obstructionism, or by a healthy self-expressive drive to mastery.

ag•ing (āj′ing) the gradual changes in the structure of any organism that occur with the passage of time, that do not result from disease or other gross accidents, and that eventually lead to the increased probability of death as the individual grows older. Cf. *senescence.*

ag•i•ta•tion (aj″ĭ-ta′shən) excessive, purposeless cognitive and motor activity or restlessness, usually associated with a state of tension or anxiety. Called also *psychomotor a.*

ag•i•to•graph•ia (aj″ĭ-to-graf′e-ə) [L. *agitare* to hurry + *graph-* + *-ia*] a dysgraphia with excessively rapid writing and unconscious omission or distortion of words or parts of words; it is usually associated with logorrhea.

ag•i•to•la•lia (aj″ĭ-to-la′le-ə) logorrhea.

ag•i•to•pha•sia (aj″ĭ-to-fa′zhə) logorrhea.

Agit. vas. [L.] agita′to va′se (the vial being shaken).

Ag•kis•tro•don (ag-kis′trə-don) [Gr. *ankistron* fishhook + Gr. *odous* tooth] a genus of venomous snakes of the family Crotalidae. *A. contor′trix* is the copperhead of North America and *A. pisci′vorus* is the water moccasin or cottonmouth of North America. The Southeast Asian species *A. rhodosto′ma* has been renamed *Calloselasma rhodostoma.* Called also *Ancistrodon.* See table at *snake.*

aglo•mer•u•lar (a″glo-mer′u-lər) having no glomeruli; said of a kidney in which the glomeruli have been absorbed or in which they have never formed (as in some fishes).

aglos•sia (a-glos′e-ə) [*a-*[1] + *gloss-* + *-ia*] congenital absence of the tongue.

aglos•so•sto•mia (a″glos-o-sto′me-ə) [*a-*[1] + *glosso-* + *stom-* + *-ia*] a congenital anomaly characterized by a malformed mouth and absence of the tongue.

aglu•con (a-gloo′kon) 1. the nonsugar portion of a glucoside. 2. aglycon.

aglu•cone (a-gloo′kōn) aglucon.

aglu•ti•tion (a-gloo-tish′ən) aphagia.

agly•ce•mia (a″gli-se′me-ə) [*a-*[1] + *glyc-* + *-emia*] virtually total absence of sugar from the blood; see also *hypoglycemia.*

agly•con (a-gli′kon) the noncarbohydrate group of a glycoside molecule; called also *genin.*

agly•cone (a-gli′kōn) aglycon.

agly•cos•uric (a-gli″ko-sur′ik) free from glycosuria.

ag•mi•nate (ag′mĭ-nāt) aggregate[2] (def. 1).

ag•na•thia (ag-na′the-ə) [*a-*[1] + *gnath-* + *-ia*] a congenital anomaly characterized by absence of the lower jaw. **agnath′ic, agnath′ous** *adj*

ag•na•thus (ag-na′thəs) a fetus exhibiting agnathia.

ag•nea (ag-ne′ə) agnosia.

ag•ni (ug-ne′) [Sanskrit] according to ayurveda, the digestive and metabolic energy created by the doshas that transforms nourishment into forms (ojas) that are used by the body and mind.

ag•no•gen•ic (ag″no-jen′ik) [Gr. *agnōs* unknown, obscure + *-genesis*] idiopathic.

ag•no•sia (ag-no′zhə) [*a-*[1] + *gnosia*] loss of the power to recognize the import of sensory stimuli; the varieties correspond with the several senses and are distinguished as *auditory, visual, olfactory, gustatory,* and *tactile.*

acoustic a. auditory a.

apperceptive a. lack of the ability to analyze and orient using visual representations and their spatial relationships. Called also *visual-spatial* or *visuospatial a.*

auditory a. inability to recognize the significance of sounds; called also *acoustic a.*

body-image a. autotopagnosia.

environmental a. inability to orient oneself to a familiar environment, although one may be able to locate it on a map or picture, owing to a lesion in the right temporal or occipital lobe. Cf. *topographagnosia.*

face a., facial a. prosopagnosia.

finger a. inability to recognize, indicate on command, name, or choose the individual fingers of one's own hand or the hands of others. Also written *fingeragnosia.*

ideational a. loss of the special associations which make up the idea of an object from its component ideas.

tactile a. inability to recognize familiar objects by touch. Cf. *astereognosis* and *stereoanesthesia.*

time a. loss of comprehension of the succession and duration of events.

visual a. inability to recognize familiar objects by sight, usually due to a lesion in one of the visual association areas. Called also *psychic blindness.*

visual-spatial a., visuospatial a. apperceptive a.

-agogue [Gr. *agōgos* leading, inducing] a word termination denoting an agent that leads or induces.

ago•nad (a-go′nad) [*a-*[1] + *gonad*] 1. an individual without gonads; see *agonadism.* 2. agonadal.

ago•nad•ism (a-go′nad-iz″əm) the condition of being without sex glands, as in anorchism and Turner syndrome. See also *gonadal agenesis,* under *agenesis.* **agonad′al** *adj*

ag•o•nal (ag′ə-nəl) pertaining to or occurring at the time just before death.

ag•o•nist (ag′ə-nist) [Gr. *agōnistēs* combatant] 1. a person or thing involved in a struggle or competition. 2. agonistic muscle. 3. in pharmacology, a drug that has affinity for and stimulates physiologic activity at cell receptors normally stimulated by naturally occurring substances.

ag•o•nis•tic (ag″ə-nis′tik) pertaining to a struggle or competition; as an agonistic muscle, counteracted by an antgonistic muscle.

ag•o•ny (ag′ə-ne) [Gr. *agōnia*] severe pain or extreme suffering.

ag•o•ra•pho•bia (ag″ə-rə-fo′be-ə) [Gr. *agora* marketplace + *-phobia*] [DSM-IV] intense, irrational fear of open spaces, characterized by marked fear of venturing out alone or of being in public places where escape would be difficult or help might be unavailable. It may be associated with panic attacks (see *panic disorder,* under *disorder*) or may occur independently (called *a. without history of panic disorder* in DSM-IV).

a. without history of panic disorder [DSM-IV] agoraphobia with fear of having an attack of one or only a few incapacitating or embarrassing symptoms, which the person may or may not have had in the past, rather than a full panic attack.

agou•ti (ə-goo′te) [Fr., from Guarani *acuti*] 1. a rodent of the genus *Dasyprocta,* about the size of a rabbit and with brown and gray fur, found in tropical America; it is a reservoir for the protozoan *Trypanosoma cruzi* and the tapeworm *Echinococcus vogeli.* 2. the pattern of alternating bands of color on the individual hairs of the fur of certain mammals. 3. pertaining to or characterized by such a pattern.

-agra [Gr. *agra* a catching, seizure] a word termination denoting a seizure of acute pain.

agraffe (ah-grahf′) [Fr.] a clamplike instrument for maintaining the edges of a wound in apposition.

ag•ram•ma•ti•ca (ag″rə-mat′ĭ-kə) agrammatism.

agram•ma•tism (a-gram′ə-tiz-əm) [Gr. *agrammatos* unlettered] inability to speak grammatically because of brain injury or disease, usually with simplified sentence structure (telegraphic speech) and errors in tense, number, and gender. See also *jargon aphasia* and *syntactical aphasia.* Called also *agrammatologia* and *dysgrammatism.*

agram•ma•to•lo•gia (a-gram″ə-to-lo′jə) agrammatism.

agran•u•lar (a-gran′u-lər) lacking granules.

agran•u•lo•cyte (a-gran′u-lo-sīt″) nongranular leukocyte.

agran•u•lo•cy•to•sis (a-gran″u-lo-si-to′sis) 1. any condition involving greatly decreased numbers of granulocytes; see also *leukopenia, neutropenia,* and *granulocytopenia.* 2. more specifically, a symptom complex characterized by marked decrease in the number of circulating granulocytes; severe neutropenia results in lesions of the throat, other mucous membranes, gastrointestinal tract, and skin; in most cases it is caused by sensitization to drugs, chemicals, or radiation affecting the bone marrow and depressing granulopoiesis. Called also *malignant* or *pernicious leukopenia* and *Schultz syndrome.*

feline a. panleukopenia.

infantile genetic a. Kostmann syndrome.

infectious feline a. panleukopenia.

agran•u•lo•plas•tic (a-gran″u-lo-plas′tik) [*a-*[1] + *granule* + *plastic*] forming nongranular cells only; not forming granular cells.

agraph•es•the•sia (ə-graf″es-the′zhə) inability to recognize characters drawn on the skin, a form of tactile agnosia; called also *graphanesthesia.*

agraph•ia (ə-graf′e-ə) [*a-*[1] + *-graph* + *-ia*] impairment or loss of the ability to write; it takes two forms, one involving poor morphology of written letter forms and the other a reflection of the aphasia also observed in spoken language. See also *dysgraphia.* Called also *graphomotor aphasia.* **agraph′ic** *adj*

absolute a. loss of the power to form even single letters.

acoustic a. loss of the power of writing from dictation.

a. amnemo′nica jargon a.

a. atac′tica absolute a.

cerebral a. mental a.

jargon a. agraphia in which the patient can write correctly formed letters but forms only senseless combinations of letters or words.

literal a. absolute a.

mental a. agraphia due to inability to put thoughts into phrases.

motor a. inability to write because of lack of motor coordination.

musical a. loss of the power to write musical symbols.

optic a. inability to copy written or printed words, but with ability to write from dictation.

verbal a. ability to write single letters, with loss of ability to combine them into words or sentences.

Ag•ri•mo•nia (ag″rĭ-mo′ne-ə) a genus of flowering herbs of the family Rosaceae. *A. eupatoria* is the usual cause of meadow grass dermatitis.

Ag•rio•li•max (ag″re-o-li′maks) a genus of slugs. *A. lae′vis* is a species that serves as an intermediate host for the rat lungworm *Angiostrongylus cantonensis.*

Ag•ro•bac•te•ri•um (ag″ro-bak-te′re-əm) [Gr. *agros* field + *bacterium*] a former genus of bacteria of the family Rhizobiaceae, members of which are now included in the genus *Rhizobium.*

Ag•ro•stem•ma (ag″ro-stem′ə) a genus of herbs of the family Caryophyllaceae. *A. githa′go* (called also *Lychnis githago*) is the corn cockle, a flowering plant whose seeds may contaminate human or animal food and cause githagism.

Agros•tis (ə-gros′tis) a genus of grasses (family Gramineae). *A. al′ba* is Johnson grass, whose pollen causes hay fever.

Ag•ry•lin (ag′rə-lin) trademark for a preparation of anagrelide hydrochloride.

agryp•not•ic (ă″grip-not′ik) [Gr. *agrypnos* sleepless] 1. promoting wakefulness. 2. an agent that promotes wakefulness.

AGS American Geriatrics Society.

AGT antiglobulin test.

agy•ria (a-ji′re-ə) [*a-*[1] + *gyr-* + *-ia*] a malformation in which the convolutions of the cerebral cortex are not fully formed, so that the brain surface is smooth; called also *lissencephaly.*

agy•ric (a-ji′rik) 1. pertaining to or characterized by agyria. 2. having no gyri.

ah hyperopic astigmatism.

AHA acetohydroxamic acid; American Heart Association; American Hospital Association.

ahap•to•glo•bin•emia (a-hap″to-glo″bĭ-ne′me-ə) the presence of little or no haptoglobin in the blood serum; indicative of recent hemolysis.

AHCPR Agency for Health Care Policy and Research, an agency of the United States Public Health Service.

AHDI Association for Healthcare Documentation Integrity.

AHF antihemophilic factor (factor VIII; see *coagulation factors,* under *factor*).

AHG 1. antihemophilic globulin (factor VIII; see *coagulation factors,* under *factor*). 2. antihuman globulin; see under *test.*

Ahu•ma•da-del Cas•ti•llo syndrome (ah-oo-mah′thah dāl kahs-te′yo) [Juan Carlos *Ahumada* Sotomayor, Argentine gynecologist, 1890–1976; Enrique Benjamin *del Castillo,* Argentine endocrinologist, 1897–1969] see under *syndrome.*

A-hy•dro•Cort (a-hi′dro-kort″) trademark for a preparation of hydrocortisone sodium succinate.

AI anaphylatoxin inactivator; aortic incompetence; aortic insufficiency; apical impulse; aromatase inhibitor; artificial insemination.

Ai•car•di syndrome (ĕ-kahr-de′) [J. *Aicardi,* French neurologist, 20th century] see under *syndrome.*

AICC anti-inhibitor coagulant complex.

AICD activation-induced cell death; automatic implantable cardioverter-defibrillator.

aich•mo•pho•bia (īk″mo-fo′be-ə) [Gr. *aichmē* spearpoint + phobia] irrational fear of sharp-pointed objects, often connected with the fear that one might use the object to stab someone.

AID artificial insemination by donor; see *donor insemination,* under *insemination.*

aid (ād) help or assistance; by extension, applied to any device by which a function can be improved or augmented, as a hearing aid.

bone-anchored hearing a. a hearing aid that allows direct bone conduction of sound to the cochlea by means of a sound-processing device attached to an osseointegrated titanium fixture implanted posterior to the ear.

first a. the initial emergency care and treatment of an injured or ill person before definitive medical and surgical management can be secured.

hearing a. a device that amplifies sound to help deaf persons hear, often referring specifically to devices worn on the body. See also *assistive listening devices,* under *device.*

pharmaceutic a., pharmaceutical a. see under *necessity.*

prosthetic speech a. speech-aid prosthesis.

speech a. 1. an appliance that improves speech. 2. see under *therapy.*

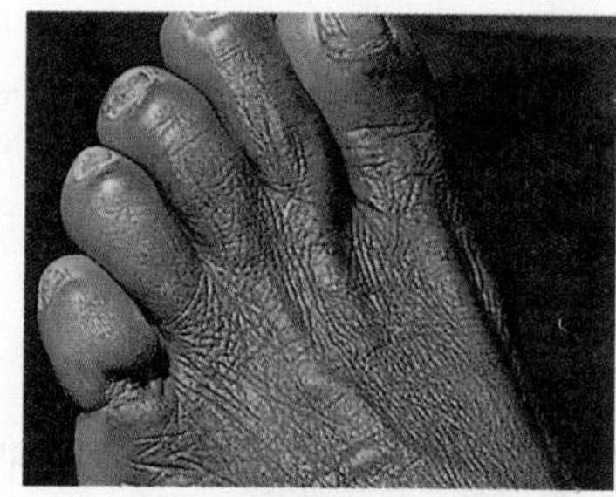

■ Ainhum.

AIDS acquired immunodeficiency syndrome.

AIH American Institute of Homeopathy; artificial insemination by husband.

AIHA American Industrial Hygiene Association; autoimmune hemolytic anemia.

AIIC Association des Infirmières et Infirmiers du Canada.

AILD angioimmunoblastic lymphadenopathy with dysproteinemia.

ail•ment (āl′mənt) any disease or affection of the body, usually referring to slight or mild disorder.

ai•lu•ro•pho•bia (i-loor″o-fo′be-ə) [Gr. *ailouros* cat + *-phobia*] irrational fear of cats.

ain•hum (i′num, ān′hum, Port. īn′yoom) [Port., from Yoruba *eyun* to saw] a disease affecting the toes, especially the fifth toe, and sometimes the fingers, seen chiefly in black adult males in Africa, in which a linear constriction around the affected digit leads to spontaneous amputation of the distal part of the digit. Called also *dactylolysis spontanea.*

AIP acute intermittent porphyria.

air (ār) [L. *aer,* from Gr. *aēr*] the gaseous mixture that makes up the earth's atmosphere; it is an odorless, colorless gas, consisting of about 1 part by volume of oxygen to 4 parts of nitrogen, the proportion varying somewhat according to conditions. It also contains small amounts of carbon dioxide, ammonia, argon, and other gases and organic matter.

alveolar a. see under *gas.*

liquid a. air liquefied by great pressure; on evaporation it produces intense cold. Liquid air has been used to produce local anesthesia, to treat neuralgia and herpes zoster, and as a source of oxygen for medical use.

residual a. see under *volume.*

tidal a. see under *volume.*

air•borne (ār′born) suspended in, transported by, or spread by air, as an infectious disease or a pathogen.

Air•bra•sive (ār′bra-siv) trademark for *(a)* an instrument for preparing a cavity in a tooth or removing deposits from teeth by application of silicon carbide or aluminum oxide by air blast; *(b)* the abrasive cutting powder used with the instrument.

air•flow (ār′flo) 1. any flowing of air. 2. the flow rate of air through the airways; see *flow* (def. 2).

air•sac•cu•li•tis (ār″sak-u-li′tis) inflammation of the air sacs in birds.

air•sick•ness (ār′sik-nis) sickness due to change in air pressure and to the movements experienced in an airplane, marked by nausea, salivation, and cold sweats. Written also *air sickness.*

air•way (ār′wa) 1. the route for passage of air into and out of the lungs; see also *respiratory system,* under *system.* 2. a device for securing unobstructed passage of air into and out of the lungs during general anesthesia or when the patient is not ventilating properly.

Brain a. laryngeal mask a.

conducting a. the lower and upper airways together, from the nares to the terminal bronchioles.

endotracheal a. an endotracheal tube that serves as an airway.

esophageal obturator a. a hollow tube inserted into the esophagus to maintain upper airway patency in unconscious persons and to permit positive-pressure ventilation through the face mask connected to the tube.

laryngeal mask a. a device for maintaining a patent airway without tracheal intubation, consisting of a tube connected to an oval inflatable cuff that seals the larynx. Called also *Brain a.*

lower a. the airway from the inferior end of the larynx to the ends of the terminal bronchioles.

nasopharyngeal a. a hollow tube inserted into a nostril and directed along the floor of the nose to the nasopharynx to prevent the tongue from blocking off passage of air in unconscious persons.

oropharyngeal a. a hollow tube inserted into the mouth and back of the throat to prevent the tongue from blocking off passage of air in unconscious persons.

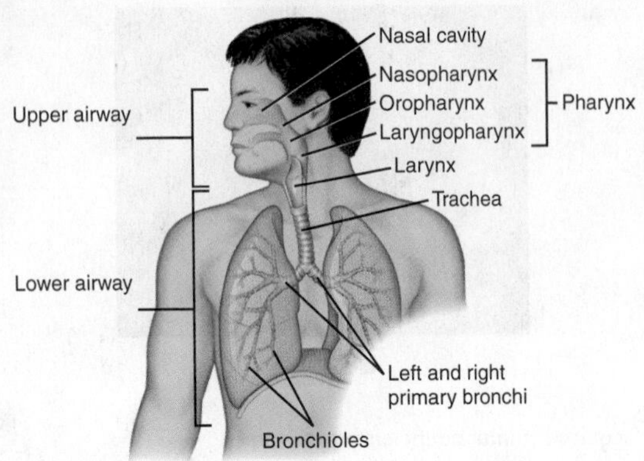

■ The larynx marks the division between upper and lower airways.

upper a. the airway from the nares and lips to the larynx.

AIS androgen insensitivity syndrome.

AIUM American Institute of Ultrasound in Medicine.

AJCC American Joint Committee on Cancer.

Ajel·lo·my·ces (a″jə-lo-mi′sēz) a genus of fungi of the family Gymnoascaceae. *A. capsula′tus*, the perfect stage of *Histoplasma capsulatum*, is the etiologic agent of classic histoplasmosis. *A. dermati′tidis*, the perfect stage of *Blastomyces dermatitidis*, is the etiologic agent of North American blastomycosis.

A-K, AK above-knee; see *transfemoral amputation*, under *amputation*.

ak- for words beginning thus, see also words beginning *ac-*.

akaryo·mas·ti·gont (a-kar″e-o-mas′tĭ-gont) [*a-*[1] + *karyo-* + *mastigont*] a condition characteristic of certain flagellate protozoa in which the mastigont system is not associated with a nucleus. Cf. *karyomastigont*.

ak·a·this·ia (ak″ə-thĭ′zhə) [*a-*[1] + Gr. *kathisis* a sitting down + *-ia*] a condition of motor restlessness in which there is a feeling of muscular quivering, an urge to move about constantly, and an inability to sit still, a common extrapyramidal side effect of neuroleptic drugs.

tardive a. a variant of tardive dyskinesia in which a person cannot remain still.

AK-Dex (ak′deks) trademark for preparations of dexamethasone sodium phosphate.

Ak-Di·late (ak-di′lāt) trademark for preparations of phenylephrine hydrochloride.

akee (ăk′ee) 1. *Blighia sapida.* 2. the fruit of *B. sapida;* its whitish, ripe aril is cooked and consumed as a delicacy in the West Indies. The uncooked fruit and aril contain the toxic amino acids hypoglycin A and B, and ingestion without cooking causes Jamaican vomiting sickness. Called also *ackee.*

Åker·lund deformity (ek′ər-loond) [Åke Olof *Åkerlund*, Swedish radiologist, 1885–1958] see under *deformity*.

aki·ne·sia (a″kĭ-ne′zhə) [*a-*[1] + *kinesi-* + *-ia*] 1. absence, poverty, or lack of control of voluntary muscle movements. 2. the temporary paralysis of a muscle by the injection of procaine. **akinet′ic** *adj*

a. al′gera a condition characterized by generalized pain associated with movement of any kind.

O'Brien a. paralysis of the orbicularis oculi muscle produced by injection of an anesthetic solution directly over the orbital branch of the seventh nerve as it emerges from behind the ear and extends toward the orbital region along the ramus of the jaw, permitting better exposure of the bulb of the eye.

aki·ne·sis (a″kĭ-ne′sis) akinesia.

akin·es·the·sia (ə-kin″es-the′zhə) absence or loss of movement sense or kinesthesia.

Akin·e·ton (a-kin′ə-ton) trademark for preparations of biperiden.

aki·ya·mi (ah″ke-yah′me) nanukayami.

ak·lo·mide (ak′lo-mīd) a coccidiostatic agent used in poultry.

Ak·ne-My·cin (ak′ne-mi″sin) trademark for a preparation of erythromycin.

Ak·o·kan·the·ra (ak″o-kan-the′rə) *Acocanthera.*

ako·ria (ə-kor′e-ə) acoria.

AK-Pred (ak′pred) trademark for preparations of prednisolone sodium phosphate.

AKPro (ak′pro) trademark for a preparation of dipivefrin hydrochloride.

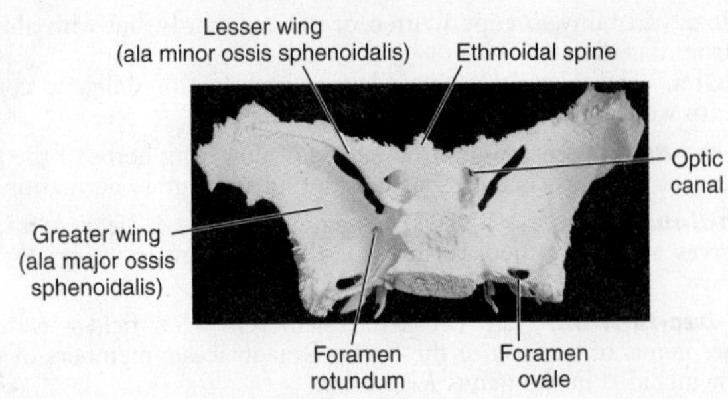

■ Superior view of ala major ossis sphenoidalis (greater wing of sphenoid bone) and ala minor ossis sphenoidalis (lesser wing of sphenoid bone).

AK-Tate (ak′tāt) trademark for a preparation of prednisolone acetate.

Aku·rey·ri disease (ah-ku′ra-re) [*Akureyri*, town in Iceland where more than 1000 cases occurred in 1948] epidemic neuromyasthenia.

Akur·za (a-kur′zə) trademark for a preparation of salicylic acid.

Al aluminum.

-al[1] [L. *-alis* adjective-forming suffix] an adjective-forming suffix meaning pertaining to or characterized by, as *arterial, diarrheal.*

-al[2] [L. *-alia*, neuter plural of *-alis*] a noun-forming suffix denoting an act or process, as *denial.*

-al[3] [from *aldehyde*] a suffix used in forming the names of chemical compounds, indicating presence of the aldehyde group, —CHO, as chloral.

ALA aminolevulinic acid.

Ala alanine.

ala (a′lə) pl. *a′lae* [L. "wing"] wing; a winglike structure or process.

a. cris′tae gal′li [TA] a small winglike process on the anterior part of the crista galli of the ethmoid bone.

a. of ilium a. ossis ilii.

a. lo′buli centra′lis [TA] wing of central lobule (HII and HIII): the lateral hemispheric extension of the central lobule of the vermis in the anterior lobe of the cerebellum; it is subdivided into inferior (HII) and superior (HIII) parts.

a. ma′jor os′sis sphenoida′lis [TA] greater wing of sphenoid bone: a large wing-shaped process arising from either side of the body of the sphenoid bone; its cerebral surface forms the anterior part of the floor of the middle cranial fossa, and its orbital surface forms the chief part of the lateral wall of the orbit. Called also *major* or *temporal wing of sphenoid bone.*

a. mi′nor os′sis sphenoida′lis [TA] lesser wing of sphenoid bone: the thin triangular plate of bone that extends horizontally and laterally from either side of the anterior part of the body of the sphenoid bone; it articulates with the frontal bone and helps form the roof of the orbit and the floor of the anterior cranial fossa. Called also *minor* or *small wing of sphenoid bone.*

a. na′si [TA] wing of nose: the flaring cartilaginous expansion forming the outer side of each naris. See also *cartilago alaris major nasi.*

a. os′sis i′lii [TA] wing of ilium: the expanded superior portion of the ilium which forms the lateral boundary of the greater pelvis.

a. os′sis sa′cri [TA], a. of sacrum the upper surface of the lateral part of the sacrum.

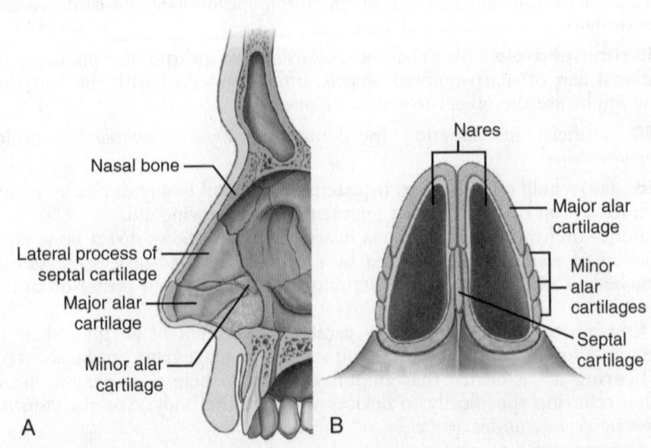

■ The major and minor alar cartilages of the ala nasi in a view of the lateral wall of the nasal cavity *(A)* and an inferior view of the nares *(B)*.

a. of vomer, a. vo′meris [TA] wing of vomer: one of the two lateral expansions on the superior border of the vomer, coming into contact with the sphenoidal process of the palatine bone and the vaginal process of the medial pterygoid plate.

alac·ri·ma (a-lak′rĭ-mə) [*a-*[1] + *lacrima*] deficiency of secretion of tears. The hereditary form is autosomal dominant and is characterized by deficient lacrimation from infancy, punctate corneal epithelial erosions, hypoplasia of the lacrimal gland, and anosmia. Alacrima also occurs in association with dysautonomia, anhidrotic ectodermal dysplasia, and adnexal abnormalities, or as an isolated congenital defect.

alac·ta·sia (a″lak-ta′zhə) malabsorption of lactose due to deficiency of lactase; see *lactase deficiency.*

alae (a′le) [L.] plural of *ala.*

Ala·gille syndrome (ah-lah-zhēl′) [Daniel *Alagille,* French pediatrician, born 1925] see under *syndrome.*

Ala·jou·a·nine syndrome (ah′lah-zhoo-ah-nēn′) [Théophile *Alajouanine,* French neurologist, 1890–1980] see under *syndrome.*

Al·a·mast (al′ə-mast″) trademark for a preparation of pemirolast potassium.

Åland eye disease (ah′lahnt) [Åland Islands, Finnish islands in the Baltic Sea, where it was first observed in the 1960′s] Forsius-Eriksson syndrome.

al·a·nine (Ala, A) (al′ə-nēn) 1. a nonessential amino acid, 2-aminopropanoic acid, occurring in proteins; high levels also occur free in plasma. It is synthesized from pyruvate. See also table at *amino acid.* 2. [USP] a preparation of alanine used as a dietary supplement.

β-a. an ω-amino acid, β-aminopropionic acid; it is not found in proteins but occurs both free and in several peptides, is a precursor of acetyl coenzyme A and several related compounds, and is an intermediate in the catabolism of uracil and cytosine.

al·a·nine ami·no·trans·fer·ase (al′ə-nēn ə-me″no-trans′fər-ās) alanine transaminase.

al·a·nine–gly·ox·y·late ami·no·trans·fer·ase (al′ə-nēn gli-ok′sə-lāt ə-me″no-trans′fər-ās) alanine–glyoxylate transaminase.

al·a·nine–gly·ox·y·late trans·am·i·nase (al′ə-nēn gli-ok′sə-lāt trans-am′ĭ-nās) [EC 2.6.1.44] an enzyme of the transferase class that catalyzes the transamination of glyoxylate to form glycine, using alanine as an amino group donor. Deficiency of the hepatic peroxisomal enzyme, an autosomal recessive trait, causes primary hyperoxaluria, type I.

β-al·a·nin·emia (al″ə-nēn-e′me-ə) hyper-β-alaninemia.

β-al·a·nine–α-ke·to·glu·ta·rate trans·am·i·nase (al′ə-nēn ke″to-gloo′tə-rāt trans-am′ĭ-nās) an enzyme activity that transfers the amino group from β-alanine to α-ketoglutarate, forming glutamate and malonate semialdehyde as a step in the metabolism of β-alanine. The enzyme can also act on γ-aminobutyrate and *S*-β-aminoisobutyrate; it has been listed as a secondary activity of the enzyme 4-aminobutyrate transaminase but may be a separate enzyme. Deficiency of this enzyme activity causes hyper-β-alaninemia.

β-al·a·nine–py·ru·vate ami·no·trans·fer·ase (al′ə-nēn pi′roo-vāt ə-me″no-trans′fər-ās) β-alanine–pyruvate transaminase.

β-al·a·nine-py·ru·vate trans·am·i·nase (al′ə-nēn pi′roo-vāt trans-am′ĭ-nās) [EC 2.6.1.18] a mitochondrial enzyme of the transferase class that catalyzes the transfer of the amino group from β-alanine to pyruvate, forming alanine and malonate semialdehyde. The enzyme can also act on *R*-β-aminoisobutyrate.

al·a·nine trans·am·i·nase (ALT) (al′ə-nēn trans-am′ĭ-nās) [EC 2.6.1.2] an enzyme of the transferase class that catalyzes the reversible transfer of an amino group from alanine to α-ketoglutarate to form glutamate and pyruvate, with pyridoxal phosphate as a cofactor. The reaction transfers nitrogen for excretion or for incorporation into other compounds. The enzyme is found in serum and body tissues, especially in the liver. Serum enzyme activity (SGPT) is greatly increased in liver disease and also elevated in infectious mononucleosis. Called also *alanine aminotransferase* and *glutamic-pyruvic transaminase (GPT).*

β-al·a·nine trans·am·i·nase (al′ə-nēn trans-am′ĭ-nās) 1. β-alanine–α-ketoglutarate transaminase. 2. β-alanine–pyruvate transaminase.

Al·an·son amputation (al′ən-sən) [Edward *Alanson,* English surgeon, 1747–1823] see under *amputation.*

al·a·nyl (al′ə-nəl) the acyl radical of alanine.

alar (a′lər) [L. *alaris*] pertaining to an ala, or wing.

ALARA as low as reasonably achievable (exposure dose of radiation).

Ala·ria (ə-la′re-ə) a genus of trematodes that are intestinal parasites of birds and mammals, which become infected after they eat uncooked or undercooked frogs. Infection is usually subclinical, but a fatal human case has been reported.

ala·ri·a·sis (al″ə-ri′ə-sis) infection of the intestines with the trematode *Alaria.*

ALAS 5-aminolevulinate synthase.

ALAT alanine aminotransferase.

alate (a′lāt) [L. *alatus* winged] having wings; winged.

alat·ro·flox·a·cin mes·y·late (ə-lat″ro-flok′sə-sin) a fluoronaphthyridone antibacterial related to the fluoroquinolones, effective against a broad spectrum of gram-positive and gram-negative organisms, used in the treatment of infections due to susceptible organisms. Alatrofloxacin is the prodrug of trovafloxacin; following intravenous infusion, it is rapidly converted to the active drug.

al·ba (al′bə) gen. and pl. *al′bae* [L., feminine of *albus*] white; used as an adjective in names of certain anatomical tissues or structures, such as substantia alba, and of certain diseases, such as pityriasis alba.

Al·ba·lon (al′bə-lon) trademark for preparations of naphazoline hydrochloride.

Al·ba·my·cin (al″bə-mi′sin) trademark for preparations of novobiocin.

Al·bar·rán gland (ahl-bah-rahn′) [Joaquín *Albarrán* y Domínguez, Cuban surgeon in Paris, 1860–1912] see under *gland.*

al·be·do (al-be′do) [L.] whiteness.

a. re′tinae edema of the retina.

Al·bee operation (al′be) [Fred Houdlett *Albee,* U.S. Army surgeon, 1876–1945] see under *operation.*

al·ben·da·zole (al-ben′də-zōl) [USP] a broad-spectrum benzimidazole anthelmintic used against many helminths and in the treatment of hydatid disease and neurocysticercosis and to treat ruminant infestations by either roundworms or flatworms.

Al·ben·za (al-ben′zə) trademark for a preparation of albendazole.

Al·bers-Schön·berg disease (ahl′berz-shurn′bərg) [Heinrich Ernst *Albers-Schönberg,* German radiologist, 1865–1921] osteopetrosis.

Al·bert diphtheria stain (al′bərt) [Henry *Albert,* American physician, 1878–1930] see *Stains and Staining Methods,* under *stain.*

Al·bert disease, operation, suture (ahl′bert) [Eduard *Albert,* Austrian surgeon, 1841–1900] see under *disease, operation,* and *suture.*

al·bi·cans (al′bĭ-kanz) gen. *albican′tis* pl. *albican′tia* [L., from *albus* white] white; see *corpus albicans.*

al·bi·du·ria (al″bĭ-du′re-ə) [L. *albidus* whitish + *uria*] the discharge of white or pale urine; cf. *chyluria.* Called also *albinuria.*

al·bi·dus (al′bĭ-dəs) [L., from *albus* white] whitish.

Al·bi·ni nodules (ahl-be′ne) [Giuseppe *Albini,* Italian physiologist, 1827–1911] see under *nodule.*

al·bi·nism (al′bĭ-niz-əm) [Port. *albino,* from L. *albus* white + *-ism*] a group of genetic abnormalities of melanin synthesis causing hypomelanosis or amelanosis of the eyes and skin. It may affect the eyes only *(ocular albinism)* or eyes, hair, and skin *(oculocutaneous albinism).* **albinot′ic** *adj*

autosomal recessive ocular a. a type of albinism formerly believed to be an autosomal recessive form of ocular albinism but now considered to belong within the phenotypes of oculocutaneous albinism types 1 and 2.

brown a., brown oculocutaneous a. a phenotypic variant of oculocutaneous albinism type 2 seen in persons from normally dark-skinned groups; pigmentation is deficient but not absent and photophobia is less severe than in other tyrosinase-positive types. The red reflex and nystagmus are present and visual acuity is moderately reduced.

Nettleship-Falls ocular a., Nettleship-Falls type ocular a. ocular a. type 1.

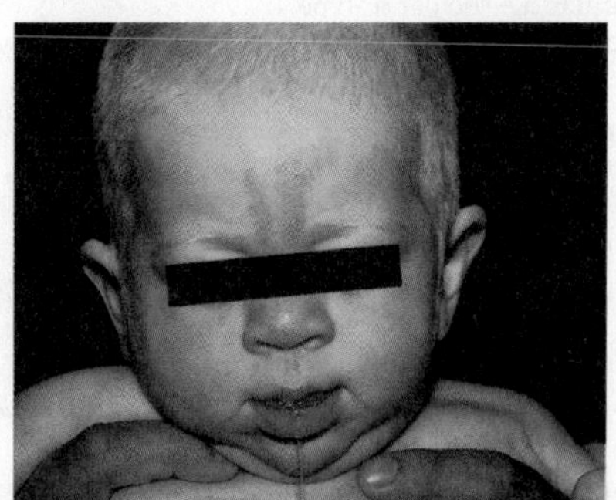

■ Albinism; the fingers are those of a normally pigmented adult.

ocular a. (OA) X-linked albinism that affects primarily the eyes, with pigment of the hair and skin being normal or only slightly diluted. It is characterized by reduced visual acuity, retinal hypopigmentation, the presence of macromelanosomes in the eyes, nystagmus, photophobia, and hypoplasia of the fovea.

type 1 (OA1) the classic type of ocular albinism, caused by mutations in the *GPR143* (or *OA1*) gene (locus: Xp22.3), which encodes a G protein–coupled receptor expressed exclusively by melanocytes and retinal pigment epithelium. It is characterized by reduced pigmentation of the irides, nystagmus, head nodding and tilting, photophobia, decreased visual acuity, and strabismus. The pupillary reflex is present, the fundi of the eyes are depigmented, and the choroidal vessels stand out. Heterozygous females show translucent irides and a mosaic of pigmentation in the fundus due to lyonization and may also show nystagmus and photophobia. Called also *Nettleship-Falls ocular a.* and *X-linked ocular a.*

type 2 (OA2) Forsius-Eriksson syndrome, formerly thought to be a form of ocular albinism.

oculocutaneous a. (OCA) albinism characterized by partial or total absence of melanin from the melanocytes of the skin, hair, and eyes, with additional ocular defects including hypoplastic fovea, photophobia, nystagmus, and decreased visual acuity. There are a number of types, varying in incidence and in genetic, biochemical, and clinical characteristics. Inheritance is autosomal recessive, except for a few families which appear to exhibit an autosomal dominant pattern, which may be due to incomplete penetrance or quasidominance.

type 1a (OCA1A) a type caused by mutations in the *TYR* (tyrosinase) gene (locus: 11q14–q21) that result in a complete absence of tyrosinase activity and consequent inability of cells to synthesize melanin. It is characterized by absence of pigment in hair, skin, and eyes. Signs include white hair throughout life, skin that is pink and highly susceptible to neoplasias, absence of pigmented nevi or freckles, gray to blue eyes with prominent red reflexes from the fundi. Called also *tyrosinase-negative a.*

type 1b (OCA1B) a type caused by mutations in the *TYR* (tyrosinase) gene (locus: 11q14–q21) that lead to reduced tyrosinase activity, characterized by yellow hair, fair skin, and severe ocular abnormalities. The hair and skin are white at birth but become pigmented in infancy. The eyes are blue at birth and darken with age; from the age of 3 years, transillumination of the iris reveals a cartwheel effect. Pigmentation of the fundus is slight or absent and the macular reflex is absent or minimal. Called also *yellow mutant a.*

type 2 (OCA2) the most common type of oculocutaneous albinism, caused by a mutation in the *P* (or *OCA2*) gene (locus: 15q11.2–q12) which encodes a membrane protein involved in regulating melanosomal pH. It is characterized by reduced, but usually visible, pigmentation of hair, skin, and eyes; the phenotype is highly variable, ranging from nearly normal pigmentation to almost none; pigmentation increases with age, and pigmented nevi may occur. The eyes usually develop some pigment, and visual acuity improves from infancy through adolescence. Newborns usually have pigmented hair but occasionally it is white, so that affected infants resemble those with OCA1A. Called also *tyrosine-positive a.*

type 3 (OCA3) a type caused by a mutation in the *TYRP1* gene (locus: 9p23), which encodes a protein involved in melanin synthesis. It occurs in persons of black African descent and is characterized by red to reddish brown coloration of the skin, hair, and iris; photophobia and nystagmus are mild and visual acuity is normal or nearly normal. Called also *red* or *rufous a.* and *xanthism.*

type 4 (OCA4) a type caused by mutations in the *MATP* gene (locus: 5p13.3), which encodes a transporter that mediates melanin synthesis; it is rare worldwide but is one of the most common forms of albinism in Japan. The phenotype is highly variable and resembles that of OCA2.

red a., rufous a. oculocutaneous a. type 3.

temperature-sensitive oculocutaneous a. a phenotypic variant of oculocutaneous albinism type 1b in which activity of the abnormal tyrosinase ceases above 35°C, so that the hair on warmer areas of the body is light and becomes progressively darker on the cooler areas (the extremities).

tyrosinase-negative oculocutaneous a. (ATN) oculocutaneous a. type 1a.

tyrosinase-positive oculocutaneous a. oculocutaneous a. type 2.

X-linked ocular a. ocular a. type 1.

yellow mutant oculocutaneous a. oculocutaneous a. type 1b.

al·bi·no (al-bi′no) an individual with albinism.

al·bi·noid·ism (al-bĭ-noid′iz-əm) [*albinism* + *-oid* + *-ism*] hypopigmentation of structures derived from the neural crest (iris, skin, and hair), but without the ocular defects seen in albinism.

al·bin·uria (al″bĭ-nu′re-ə) albiduria.

Al·bi·nus muscle (ahl-bi′noos) [Bernard Siegfried *Albinus*, German anatomist and surgeon in the Netherlands, 1697–1770] see *musculus risorius* and *musculus scalenus medius.*

al·bo·pap·u·loid (al″bo-pap′u-loid) [L. *albus* white + *papuloid*] white and papuloid.

Al·brecht bone (ahl′brekt) [Karl Martin Paul *Albrecht*, German anatomist, 1851–1894] basiotic bone.

Al·bright hereditary osteodystrophy, syndrome (awl′brīt) [Fuller *Albright*, American physician and endocrinologist, 1900–1969] see *pseudohypoparathyroidism* and see under *syndrome.*

al·bu·gin·ea (al″bu-jin′e-ə) [L., from *albus* white] tunica albuginea, particularly the tunica albuginea testis; see entries under *tunica.*

al·bu·gin·e·ot·o·my (al″bu-jin″e-ot′ə-me) [*albuginea* + *-tomy*] incision of the tunica albuginea testis.

al·bu·gin·e·ous (al″bu-jin′e-əs) [L. *albugineus*] pertaining to or resembling a tough whitish layer of fibrous tissue (tunica albuginea testis).

al·bu·gi·ni·tis (al″bu-jĭ-ni′tis) inflammation of any one of the albugineous tissues or tunics.

al·bu·men (al-bu′mən) [L., from *albus* white] 1. egg white. 2. albumin.

al·bu·mim·e·ter (al″bu-mim′ə-tər) albuminimeter.

al·bu·min (al-bu′min) [*albumen* + *-in*] 1. any protein that is soluble in water and moderately concentrated salt solutions and is coagulable by heat. 2. the major plasma protein, approximately 60 per cent of the total, which is responsible for much of the plasma colloidal osmotic pressure and serves as a transport protein for large organic anions such as fatty acids, bilirubin, and many drugs; it also carries hormones such as cortisol and thyroxine when their specific binding globulins are saturated. It is synthesized in the liver. Decreased serum albumin *(hypoalbuminemia)* occurs in protein malnutrition, active inflammation, and serious hepatic and renal disease. Called also *serum a.* and *seralbumin.*

a. A the normal type of human serum albumin, as opposed to electrophoretic variants.

acid a. albumin altered by the action of an acid.

aggregated a. heat-denatured albumin human; labeled radioactively (technetium 99m), its uses include lung imaging, radionuclide venography, and assessment of peritoneovenous shunt patency. Called also *macroaggregated a. (MAA).* See table at *technetium.*

alkali a. any albumin which has been treated with an alkali.

blood a. albumin (def. 2).

derived a. any albumin denatured by chemical action, as albuminate.

egg a. a glycoprotein that constitutes 20 per cent of the white of hens' eggs; called also *ovalbumin.*

a. human [USP] a preparation of serum albumin fractionated from human whole blood, serum, plasma, or placentas; used as a plasma volume expander in the treatment of various conditions including hypovolemia, hypoproteinemia, severe burns, adult respiratory distress syndrome, acute nephrotic syndrome, and acute liver failure, and to increase the binding capacity for bilirubin in the treatment of hyperbilirubinemia. Administered intravenously.

iodinated I 125 a. [USP] a solution containing normal human albumin adjusted to provide no more than 37 MBq (1 mCi) of radioactivity (from ^{125}I) per milliliter, used as a diagnostic aid in determining blood or plasma volume and cardiac output.

iodinated I 131 a. [USP] a solution containing normal human albumin adjusted to provide no more than 37 MBq (1 mCi) of radioactivity (from ^{131}I) per milliliter, used as a diagnostic aid in determining blood or plasma volume and cardiac output.

macroaggregated a. (MAA) aggregated a.

a. microspheres sonicated microbubbles, mean size 2–4.5 µm, created by heat treatment and sonication of diluted albumin human in the presence of octafluoropropane gas; injected intravenously as a diagnostic adjunct in echocardiography.

native a. an albumin in its natural state, i.e., not denatured.

serum a. albumin (def. 2).

vegetable a. any albumin of vegetable origin.

Al·bu·mi·nar (al-bu′mĭ-nahr) trademark for preparations of albumin human.

al·bu·mi·nate (al-bu′mĭ-nāt″) albumin denatured by a base or an acid, characterized by solubility in dilute acids or alkalis and by being insoluble in dilute salt solutions, water, or alcohol; called also *derived albumin* and *derived protein.*

al·bu·min·a·tu·ria (al-bu″mĭ-nă-tu′re-ə) proteinuria in which there is an excess of albuminates in the urine.

al·bu·min·emia (al-bu″mĭ-ne′me-ə) the presence of albumin in the blood plasma or serum; proteinemia.

al·bu·mi·nim·e·ter (al-bu″mĭ-nim′ə-tər) [*albumin* + *-meter*] an instrument used in determining the proportion of albumin present, as in the urine.

al·bu·mi·nim·e·try (al-bu″mĭ-nim′ə-tre) the determination of the proportion of albumin present.

al·bu·mi·no·cho·lia (al-bu″mĭ-no-ko′le-ə) [*albumin* + *chol-* + *-ia*] the presence of albumin in the bile.

al•bu•mi•no•cy•to•log•i•cal (al-bu″mĭ-no-si″to-loj′ĭ-kəl) pertaining to the level of protein as albumin in relation to number of cells present in cerebrospinal fluid.

al•bu•mi•noid (al-bu′mĭ-noid″) [*albumin* + *-oid*] 1. resembling albumin. 2. fibrous protein. 3. a scleroprotein.

al•bu•mi•nol•y•sis (al-bu″mĭ-nol′ĭ-sis) the splitting up of albumins.

al•bu•mi•nom•e•ter (al-bu″mĭ-nom′ə-tər) albuminimeter.

al•bu•mi•nop•ty•sis (al-bu″mĭ-nop′tĭ-sis) [*albumin* + Gr. *ptyein* to spit] presence of albumin in the sputum.

al•bu•mi•no•re•ac•tion (al-bu″mĭ-no-re-ak′shən) the reaction of the sputum to tests for albumin; the presence of albumin (positive reaction) is indicative of pulmonary inflammation.

al•bu•mi•nor•rhea (al-bu″mĭ-no-re′ə) [*albumin* + *-rrhea*] excessive excretion of albumins.

al•bu•mi•nous (al-bu′mĭ-nəs) containing, charged with, or of the nature of an albumin.

al•bu•min•uria (al″bu-mĭ-nu′re-ə) 1. the most common kind of proteinuria, characterized by presence of albumin in the urine. 2. sometimes used as a synonym for *proteinuria* in general.

Al•bu•nex (al-bu′neks) trademark for a contrast agent used in echocardiography.

Al•bu•tein (al′bu-tēn) trademark for preparations of albumin human.

al•bu•ter•ol (al-bu′tər-ol) [USP] a β-adrenergic agonist, specific for β_2-adrenergic receptors; administered by inhalation as a bronchodilator for the treatment and prophylaxis of bronchospasm associated with bronchitis, pulmonary emphysema, or other chronic obstructive airway disease, the treatment of asthma-associated bronchospasm, and the prophylaxis of exercise-induced bronchospasm. Called also *salbutamol.*

a. **sulfate** [USP] the sulfate salt of albuterol, having the same actions as the base; administered orally or parenterally in the symptomatic treatment of bronchial asthma and the treatment of bronchospasm associated with bronchitis, pulmonary emphysema, or other chronic obstructive airway disease.

Al•caine (al′kān) trademark for a preparation of proparacaine hydrochloride.

Al•ca•li•ge•na•ceae (al″kə-lij″ə-na′se-e) a family of bacteria of the order Burkholderiales, consisting of gram-negative, aerobic, chemoorganotrophic, motile or nonmotile rods or coccobacilli occurring singly, in pairs, or rarely in chains; it includes soil and water bacteria, as well as avian and mammalian pathogens. Medically important genera include *Alcaligenes, Achromobacter, Bordetella, Oligella,* and *Taylorella.*

Al•ca•li•ge•nes (al″kə-lij′ə-nēz) [Ar. *al-qily* potash + Gr. *gennan* to produce] a widespread genus of gram-negative, aerobic, rod-shaped, alkaline-producing bacteria of the family Alcaligenaceae, found in the intestines of vertebrates and as part of normal skin flora; it is occasionally the cause of opportunistic infections.

A. denitri′ficans a species isolated from a variety of clinical specimens.

A. faeca′lis a species isolated from hospital environments and from blood, sputum, and urine specimens. It is a cause of nosocomial septicemia in immunocompromised patients, generally arising from contaminated hemodialysis or intravenous fluids.

A. xylosox′idans a species that has been found in the respiratory tracts of patients with cystic fibrosis, as well as in cases of bacteremia.

al•cap•ton•uria (al-kap″to-nu′re-ə) alkaptonuria.

al•cap•ton•uric (al-kap″to-nu′rik) alkaptonuric.

al•clo•met•a•sone di•pro•pi•o•nate (al-klo-met′ə-sōn″) [USP] a synthetic corticosteroid used topically for the relief of inflammation and pruritus in corticosteroid-responsive dermatoses.

Al•cock canal (al′kok) [Benjamin *Alcock,* Irish professor of anatomy; born 1801, date of death unknown] canalis pudendalis.

al•co•gel (al′ko-jel) a gel that has alcohol as its dispersion medium.

al•co•hol (al′kə-hol) [Ar. *al kuhl* fine powder of antimony or other distilled substance] 1. any of a class of organic compounds formed from the hydrocarbons by substitution of one or more hydroxyl groups for an equal number of hydrogen atoms; the term is extended to various substitution products that are neutral in reaction and that contain one or more of the alcohol groups. 2. ethanol. 3. [USP] an official preparation of ethanol, used in pharmacy as a disinfectant, solvent, and preservative; applied topically as a rubefacient, disinfectant, astringent, hemostatic, and coolant; and used internally in sclerotherapy and in the treatment of pain, of spasticity, and of poisoning by methyl alcohol or ethylene glycol.

absolute a. dehydrated a.

***tert*-amyl a.** amylene hydrate.

aromatic a. an aromatic compound in which the side chain on the benzene ring contains a hydroxyl group; e.g., phenol.

azeotropic isopropyl a. [USP] a preparation containing 91–93 per cent isopropyl alcohol by volume and water.

benzyl a. [NF] a clear colorless oily liquid used as a bacteriostatic in solutions for injection and topically as a local anesthetic. Called also *benzenemethanol, phenylcarbinol,* and *phenylmethanol.*

butyl a. [NF] a clear, colorless, mobile liquid, C_4H_9OH, with a characteristic odor, occurring in four isomeric forms; used as a solvent.

cetostearyl a. [NF] a mixture of stearyl alcohol and cetyl alcohol, used as an emulsifier; the official preparation consists of at least 40 per cent stearyl alcohol and at least 90 per cent of stearyl and cetyl alcohols combined.

cetyl a. [NF] a solid fatty alcohol prepared by hydrogenation of palmitic acid or by saponification of spermaceti, used as an emulsifying and stiffening agent.

dehydrated a. [USP] an extremely hygroscopic, transparent, colorless, volatile liquid with characteristic odor and burning taste, containing at least 99.5 per cent ethanol by volume; used as a solvent and administered by injection into nerves and ganglia for relief of pain. Called also *absolute a.*

denatured a. ethanol which has been rendered unfit for internal use by addition of an adulterant such as methanol or acetone, but which may still be used for other purposes including industrial processes, as a solvent, on the skin as a cooling agent, and as a skin disinfectant.

dihydric a. an alcohol containing two hydroxyl groups.

diluted a. [NF] a mixture of alcohol and water, used as a solvent; the official preparation contains 41 to 42 per cent ethanol by weight, or 48.4 to 49.5 per cent by volume, at 15.56° C.

ethyl a. ethanol.

fatty a. any of a group of high molecular weight primary alcohols, usually straight chain; they may be synthetic or derived from natural oils and are used in pharmacy and as solvents, detergents, and emulsifiers.

glyceryl a., glycyl a. glycerin.

grain a. ethanol.

isoamyl a. one of the isomeric forms of amyl alcohol; used as a solvent and in pharmacy.

isopropyl a. [USP] an isomer of propyl alcohol and a homologue of ethyl alcohol, having disinfectant properties similar to those of ethyl alcohol; used as a solvent and disinfectant and applied topically as an antiseptic. Called also *dimethyl carbinol* and *isopropanol.*

isopropyl rubbing a. [USP] a preparation containing 68–72 per cent isopropyl alcohol in water, used as a rubefacient.

lanolin a′s [NF] a mixture of aliphatic alcohols, triterpenoid alcohols, and sterols, obtained by hydrolysis of lanolin; used as an emulsifying agent in the preparation of water-in-oil emulsions. Called also *wool a′s.*

methyl a. [NF] a clear, colorless, flammable liquid, CH_3OH, with characteristic odor, miscible with alcohol, ether, and water; it has many industrial and household uses, including in solvents and antifreeze. Called also *methanol.* See also *methanol poisoning,* under *poisoning.*

monohydric a. an alcohol containing only one hydroxyl group.

nicotinic a., nicotinyl a. a vasodilator with properties similar to those of nicotinic acid, used in peripheral vascular disorders.

palmityl a. cetyl a.

pantothenyl a. 1. panthenol. 2. dexpanthenol.

phenethyl a., phenylethyl a. [USP] a colorless liquid with a roselike odor and a sharp, burning taste, occurring in a number of natural essential oils; used as an antimicrobial agent in pharmaceutical preparations. Called also *benzyl carbinol.*

polyhydric a. polyol.

polyvinyl a. [USP] a water-soluble synthetic resin, represented by the formula $(C_2H_4O)_n$, in which n varies between 500 and 5000; used as a viscosity-increasing agent in pharmaceutical preparations and as a lubricant and protectant in ophthalmic preparations.

primary a. an alcohol in which the carbon atom attached to the hydroxyl group carries a single alkyl group and two hydrogen groups. See illustration.

***n*-propyl a.** a clear colorless liquid with an alcohol-like odor, miscible with water and most organic solvents; used as a solvent for resins.

rubbing a. [USP] a preparation of acetone, methyl isobutyl ketone, and 68.5 to 71.5 per cent ethanol; used as a rubefacient.

secondary a. an alcohol in which the carbon atom attached to the hydroxyl group carries two alkyl groups and one hydrogen group. See illustration.

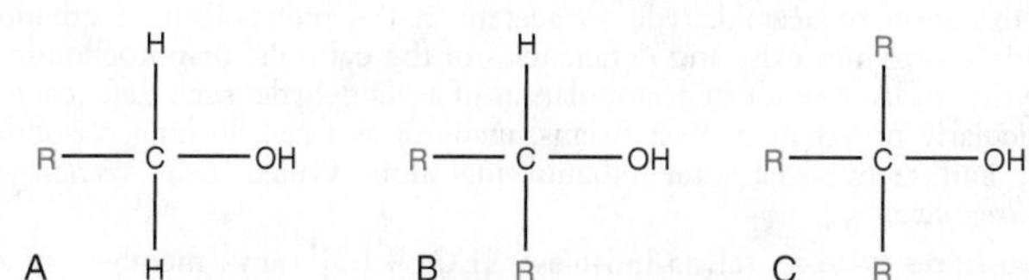

■ Chemical structure of primary *(A)*, secondary *(B)*, and tertiary *(C)* alcohols.

stearyl a. 1. a solid alcohol prepared from stearic acid by catalytic hydrogenation; used as an emollient and emulsifying agent. 2. [NF] an official preparation, containing at least 90 per cent stearyl alcohol, the remainder consisting mainly of cetyl alcohol.

sugar a. a polyhydric alcohol having no more than one hydroxy group attached to each carbon atom, formed by the reduction of the carbonyl group of a sugar to a hydroxyl group.

tertiary a. an alcohol in which the carbon atom attached to the hydroxyl group carries three alkyl groups. See illustration.

tertiary amyl a. amylene hydrate.

trihydric a. an alcohol containing three hydroxyl groups.

unsaturated a. alcohol that is derived from unsaturated hydrocarbons (alkenes, or olefins).

wood a. methyl a.

wool a's lanolin a's.

al•co•hol de•hy•dro•gen•ase (al′kə-hol de-hi′dro-jən-ās) [EC 1.1.1.1] an enzyme of the oxidoreductase class that catalyzes the reversible oxidation of primary or secondary alcohols to aldehydes using NAD^+ as an electron acceptor. The reaction is the first step in the metabolism of alcohols by the liver. Abbreviated AD and ADH.

al•co•hol de•hy•dro•gen•ase (NADP⁺) (al′kə-hol de-hi′dro-jən-ās) [EC 1.1.1.2] an enzyme of the oxidoreductase class that catalyzes the reversible oxidation of primary (or secondary) alcohols to aldehydes (or ketones), using $NADP^+$ as an electron acceptor.

al•co•hol de•hy•dro•gen•ase (NAD(P)⁺) (al′kə-hol de-hi′dro-jən-ās) [EC 1.1.1.71] an enzyme of the oxidoreductase class that catalyzes the reversible oxidation of primary or secondary alcohols to aldehydes or ketones respectively, using NAD^+ or $NADP^+$ as an electron acceptor. The enzyme also interconverts retinol and retinal.

al•co•hol•emia (al″kə-hol-e′me-ə) the presence of alcohol in the blood.

al•co•hol•ic (al″kə-hol′ik) 1. pertaining to or containing alcohol. 2. a person suffering from alcoholism (q.v.).

al•co•hol•ism (al′kə-hol-iz-əm) a disorder characterized by a pathological pattern of alcohol use that causes a serious impairment in social or occupational functioning. In DSM-IV it is covered by alcohol abuse and alcohol dependence.

al•co•hol•i•za•tion (al″kə-hol″i-za′shən) treatment by application or injection of alcohol.

al•co•hol•ize (al′kə-hol-īz″) 1. to treat with alcohol. 2. to transform into alcohol.

al•co•hol•om•e•ter (al″kə-hol-om′ə-tər) [*alcohol* + *-meter*] an instrument used in determining the percentage of alcohol in a solution.

al•co•hol•y•sis (al″kə-hol′ĭ-sis) [*alcohol* + *-lysis*] a process analogous to hydrolysis, but in which alcohol takes the place of water.

al•co•sol (al′kə-sol) a sol in which the dispersion medium is alcohol.

al•cu•ro•ni•um chlo•ride (al-ku-ro′ne-əm) a nondepolarizing skeletal muscle relaxant used in general anesthesia for surgical procedures.

Al•dac•ta•zide (al-dak′tə-zīd) trademark for a preparation of spironolactone with hydrochlorothiazide.

Al•dac•tone (al-dak′tōn) trademark for a preparation of spironolactone.

Al•dara (al-dar′ə) trademark for a preparation of imiquimod.

al•dar•ic ac•id (al-dar′ik) any of various dicarboxylic acids resulting from oxidation of both terminal groups of an aldose to carboxyl groups, such as glutaric acid.

al•de•hyde (al′də-hīd) [*al*cohol + L. *de* away from + *hyd*rogen] 1. any one of a large class of organic compounds containing the group —CHO, that is, with the carbonyl group, C═O, occurring at the end of the carbon chain. 2. a suffix used to denote a compound occurring in aldehyde conformation. 3. acetaldehyde.

acetic a. acetaldehyde.

formic a. formaldehyde.

glyceric a. glyceraldehyde.

al•de•hyde de•hy•dro•gen•ase (NAD⁺) (al′də-hīd de-hi′dro-jən-ās) [EC 1.2.1.3] an enzyme of the oxidoreductase class that catalyzes the oxidation of various aldehydes, using NAD^+ as an electron acceptor, including the oxidation of acetaldehyde to acetate in the metabolism of ethanol. Multiple isozymes exist and deficiencies of the cytosolic or mitochondrial isozymes of liver result in accumulation of acetaldehyde; such deficiencies, particularly prevalent in East Asians, manifest as facial flushing, vasodilation, and tachycardia after ethanol ingestion. Called also *acetaldehyde dehydrogenase*.

al•de•hyde-ly•ase (al″də-hīd-li′ās) [EC 4.1.2] any member of a sub-subclass of enzymes of the lyase class that catalyze cleavage of a C—C bond in a molecule containing a hydroxyl group and a carbonyl group to form two smaller molecules, each being an aldehyde or a ketone; chemically, it is the reverse of an aldol condensation. Called also *aldolase*.

al•de•hyde ox•i•dase (al′də-hīd ok′sĭ-dās) [EC 1.2.3.1] an enzyme of the oxidoreductase class that catalyzes the oxidation of aldehydes to the corresponding acids, generating a superoxide anion. It is a molybdoflavoprotein found in liver tissue, catalyzing the oxidation of a wide variety of heterocyclic compounds and xenobiotics. Activity of this enzyme is believed to be deficient in molybdenum cofactor deficiency.

al•de•hyde re•duc•tase (al′də-hīd re-duk′tās) [EC 1.1.1.21] an enzyme of the oxidoreductase class that catalyzes the reduction of aldoses to form alditols, using NADPH as an electron donor. In galactosemia due to galactokinase deficiency, catalysis of the reduction of galactose to galactitol by aldehyde reductase in the lens of the eye results in cataract formation. Called also *aldose reductase*.

Al•der anomaly (ahl′dər) [Albert von *Alder*, German physician, 1888–1951] see under *anomaly*.

Al•der-Reil•ly anomaly, bodies (ahl′dər ri′le) [A. von *Alder;* William Anthony *Reilly*, 20th-century American pediatrician] see under *anomaly* and *body*.

al•des•leu•kin (al″dəs-loo′kin) a recombinant interleukin-2 product used as an antineoplastic and biological response modifier in the treatment of metastatic renal cell carcinoma and malignant melanoma; administered by intravenous infusion.

al•di•carb (al′dĭ-kahrb) a carbamate pesticide used as an insecticide; in some countries, also used as a rodenticide.

Al•din•a•mide (al-din′ə-mīd) trademark for preparations of pyrazinamide.

al•di•tol (al′dĭ-tol) the polyhydroxy alcohol produced by reduction of the aldehyde group of an aldose.

al•do•bi•on•ic ac•id (al″do-bi-on′ik) 1. an oxidized disaccharide derivative containing an aldose linked to an aldonic acid. 2. more frequently, an incorrectly used term denoting an aldobiuronic acid.

Al•do•clor (al′do-klor) trademark for a combination preparation of methyldopa and chlorothiazide.

al•do•hex•ose (al″do-hek′sōs) any aldose containing six carbon atoms, such as glucose or mannose. Cf. *ketohexose*.

al•do•lase (al′do-lās) 1. aldehyde-lyase. 2. fructose bisphosphate aldolase.

Al•do•met (al′do-met) trademark for preparations of methyldopa.

al•don•ic ac•id (al-don′ik) a carboxylic acid resulting from oxidation of the aldehyde group of an aldose to a carboxyl group, e.g., gluconic acid.

al•do•pen•tose (al″do-pen′tōs) any ketose containing five carbon atoms, such as arabinose.

Al•do•ril (al′do-ril″) trademark for combination preparations of methyldopa and hydrochlorothiazide.

al•dose (al′dōs) one of two subgroups of monosaccharides, being those having a terminal carbonyl (aldehyde) group; it is further subdivided on the basis of the number of carbon atoms in the sugar; see *aldotetrose, aldopentose, aldohexose*, etc. Examples are glucose, galactose, and mannose.

al•dose 1-epim•er•ase (al′dōs ə-pim′ər-ās) [EC 5.1.3.3] an enzyme of the isomerase class that catalyzes interconversion of the α- and β-forms of D-glucose, L-arabinose, D-xylose, D-galactose, lactose, and maltose. Commonly called *mutarotase*.

al•dose re•duc•tase (al′dōs re-duk′tās) aldehyde reductase.

al•do•side (al′do-sīd) a glycoside formed from an aldose; e.g., a glucoside.

al•dos•ter•one (al-dos′tər-ōn) the major mineralocorticoid secreted by the adrenal cortex; it promotes retention of sodium and bicarbonate, excretion of potassium and hydrogen ions, and secondary retention of water. Large excesses can invoke plasma volume expansion, edema, and hypertension. The secretion of aldosterone is stimulated by low plasma potassium concentration and angiotensin II.

al•dos•ter•one syn•thase (al-dos′tər-ōn sin′thās) an isozyme of steroid 11β-monooxygenase that catalyzes the last three steps (11-hydroxylation, 18-hydroxylation, and 18-oxidation) in the synthesis of aldosterone from deoxycorticosterone. It includes the activities of steroid 11β-monooxygenase [EC 1.14.15.4] and corticosterone 18-monooxygenase [EC 1.14.15.5].

al•dos•ter•one syn•thase de•fi•cien•cy (al-dos′tər-ōn sin′thās) a disorder of steroidogenesis caused by mutations in the *CYP11B2* gene (locus: 8q21) that result in a deficiency of aldosterone synthase activity, impairing the biosynthesis of aldosterone and causing salt wasting. It occurs as two types: *type I*, in which decreased hydroxylation of corticosterone results in corticosterone and deoxycorticosterone accumulation, and *type II,* in which decreased oxidation of the 18-hydroxy intermediate results in elevated levels of this compound and corticosterone. Called also *corticosterone methyl oxidase deficiency.*

al·dos·ter·on·ism (al-dos′tə-ro-niz″əm) an abnormality of electrolyte metabolism caused by excessive secretion of aldosterone; called also *hyperaldosteronism.*

primary a. aldosteronism arising from oversecretion of aldosterone by an adrenal cortical adenoma, characterized typically by hypokalemia, alkalosis, muscular weakness, polyuria, polydipsia, and hypertension. Called also *Conn syndrome.*

pseudoprimary a. signs and symptoms identical to those of primary aldosteronism but caused by factors other than excessive aldosterone secretion.

secondary a. aldosteronism due to extra-adrenal stimulation of aldosterone secretion; it is commonly associated with edematous states, such as those accompanying nephrotic syndrome, hepatic cirrhosis, heart failure, or malignant hypertension.

al·dos·ter·ono·gen·e·sis (al-dos″tər-o″no-jen′ə-sis) the production of aldosterone by the adrenal cortex.

al·dos·ter·o·no·ma (al″do-ster″o-no′mə) a tumor of the adrenal cortex that secretes aldosterone, causing primary aldosteronism; the majority are adenomas, but few are carcinomas. Called also *aldosterone-secreting tumor.*

al·dos·ter·ono·pe·nia (al-dos″tər-o″no-pe′ne-ə) hypoaldosteronism.

al·dos·ter·on·uria (al-dos″tər-o-nu′re-ə) hyperaldosteronuria.

al·do·tet·rose (al″do-tet′rōs) any aldose containing four carbon atoms, such as erythrose.

al·do·tri·ose (al″do-tri′ōs) an aldose containing three carbon atoms; see *glyceraldehyde.*

al·dox·ime (al-dok′sīm) the —CH═NOH radical formed by the union of an aldehyde with hydroxylamine.

Al·drich syndrome (awl′drich) [Robert Anderson *Aldrich,* American pediatrician, 1917–1999] Wiskott-Aldrich syndrome; see under *syndrome.*

Al·drich-Mees lines (awl′drich mās′) [C.J. *Aldrich,* American physician, early 20th century; *R.A. Mees,* Dutch scientist, 20th century] Mees′ lines.

al·drin (al′drin) a chlorinated hydrocarbon insecticide, closely related to dieldrin; if ingested or absorbed through the skin by a human or other animal, it causes neurotoxic reactions that can be fatal, including tremors, ataxia, and convulsions.

alec·i·thal (a-les′ĭ-thəl) [*a-*[1] + *lecith-* + *-al*[1]] without yolk; applied to eggs with very little yolk, as those of mammals and many of the invertebrates.

alef·a·sept (ə-lef′ə-sept) a dimeric fusion protein with immunosuppressive qualities, used in treatment of plaque psoriasis; administered by intramuscular injection.

al·em·tuz·u·mab (al″əm-tuz′u-mab″) a recombinant, DNA-derived, humanized monoclonal antibody directed against the CD antigen CD52, which is present on B and T lymphocytes, many monocytes, macrophages, and NK cells, and certain granulocytes; administered intravenously as an antineoplastic in the treatment of B-cell chronic lymphocytic leukemia.

alen·dro·nate sodium (ə-len′dro-nāt) a bisphosphonate calcium-regulating agent used to inhibit the resorption of bone in the treatment of osteitis deformans and of hypercalcemia related to malignancy, and in the treatment and prophylaxis of osteoporosis; administered orally.

Alesse (ə-les′) trademark for a combination preparation of levonorgestrel and ethinyl estradiol.

aleu·ke·mia (a″loo-ke′me-ə) 1. leukopenia. 2. aleukemic leukemia.

aleu·ke·mic (a″loo-ke′mik) leukopenic.

aleu·kia (a-loo′ke-ə) leukopenia.

alimentary toxic a. (ATA) a rare form of mycotoxicosis associated with the ingestion of grain that has overwintered in the field and become contaminated with fungi that contain trichothecenes; characteristics include skin inflammation, vomiting, diarrhea, and hemorrhages that can be fatal. Causative fungi include members of the genera *Alternaria, Fusarium, Myrothecium, Piptocephalis, Thamnidium, Trichoderma, Trichothecium, Verticillium,* and others.

aleu·ko·cyt·ic (a-loo″ko-sit′ik) leukopenic.

aleu·ko·cy·to·sis (a-loo″ko-si-to′sis) [*a-*[1] + *leukocyte* + *-osis*] leukopenia.

aleu·rio·co·nid·i·um (ə-lo͝o″re-o-kə-nid′e-əm) [Gr. *aleuron* flour + *conidium*] a terminal or lateral conidium that is released by dissolution of its attachment to the mycelium. Called also *aleuriospore.*

aleu·rio·spore (ə-lo͝o′re-o-spor) aleurioconidium.

al·eu·rone (ə-lo͞or′ōn, al′yə-rōn″) granules of protein occurring in the endosperm of ripe seeds, particularly those concentrated in the outer layer of the endosperm of cereal grains.

al·eu·ro·noid (ə-lu′ro-noid″) resembling flour.

Al·ex·an·der deafness (hearing loss) (al″eg-zan′dər) [Gustav *Alexander,* Austrian otologist, 1873–1932] see under *deafness.*

Al·ex·an·der disease (al″eg-zan′dər) [W. Stewart *Alexander,* English pathologist, 20th century] see under *disease.*

Al·ex·an·der operation (al″eg-zan′dər) [William *Alexander,* English surgeon, 1844–1919] see under *operation.*

Al·ex·an·der technique (al″eg-zan′dər) [Frederick Matthias *Alexander,* Australian actor, 1869–1955] see under *technique.*

Al·ex·an·der-Ad·ams operation (al″eg-zan′dər ad′əmz) [William *Alexander;* James Alexander *Adams,* Scottish gynecologist, 1857–1930] see *Alexander operation,* under *operation.*

alex·ia (ə-lek′se-ə) [*a-*[1] + Gr. *lexis* word + *-ia*] a form of receptive aphasia in which there is loss of the ability to understand written language as a result of a cerebral lesion; cf. *dyslexia.* Called also *optical alexia, visual aphasia,* and *word blindness.* alex′ic *adj*

cortical a. a form of sensory aphasia due to lesions of the left parietal lobe, especially the gyrus angularis.

motor a. alexia in which the patient understands written or printed material but cannot read it aloud.

musical a. loss of the ability to read music; called also *music blindness.*

optical a. alexia.

subcortical a. alexia due to interruption of the connection between the optic center and the parietal lobe, including the gyrus angularis of the dominant hemisphere.

alex·i·phar·mac (ə-lek″sĭ-fahr′mək) antidote.

alex·i·thy·mia (ə-lek″sĭ-thi′me-ə) [*a-*[1] + Gr. *lexis* word + *-thymia*] inability to recognize or describe one's emotions.

aley·dig·ism (a-li′dig-iz″əm) absence of androgen secretion by Leydig cells, as occurs in hypogonadotropic hypogonadism.

Al·ez·zan·dri·ni syndrome (ahl″ĕ-tsahn-dre′ne) [Arturo Alberto *Alezzandrini,* Argentine ophthalmologist, born 1932] see under *syndrome.*

al·fa·cal·ci·dol (al″fə-kal′sĭ-dol) a synthetic analogue of calcitriol, to which it is converted in the liver; used in the treatment of hypocalcemia, hypophosphatemia, rickets, and osteodystrophy associated with various medical conditions including chronic renal failure and hypoparathyroidism, administered orally or intravenously.

al·fal·fa (al-fal′fə) [Sp., from Ar. *al fasfasah*] *Medicago sativa.*

Al·fen·ta (al-fen′tə) trademark for a preparation of alfentanil hydrochloride.

al·fen·ta·nil hy·dro·chlo·ride (al-fen′tə-nil) [USP] an opioid analgesic of rapid onset and short duration derived from fentanyl, used as a primary agent for the induction of general anesthesia, as an adjunct in the maintenance of general anesthesia, and as a supplement to regional or local anesthesia; administered intravenously.

Al·fer·on N (al′fēr-on) trademark for a preparation of interferon alfa-n3.

Al·flo·rone (al′flo-rōn) trademark for preparations of fludrocortisone.

al·fu·zo·sin hy·dro·chlo·ride (al-fu′zo-sin) an alpha-adrenergic blocking agent that is selective for the $alpha_1$-adrenergic receptors of the lower urinary tract, causing relaxation of smooth muscles of the bladder neck and prostate; used to improve urine flow in men with benign prostatic hyperplasia, administered orally.

ALG antilymphocyte globulin.

al·ga (al′gə) any individual organism of the algae.

al·gae (al′je) [L., pl., "seaweeds"] a large group included in the kingdom Protista, now classified into several different phyla. They are cryptogamous plantlike organisms in which the body is unicellular or consists of a thallus. Algae include the seaweeds and many unicellular fresh-water plants, most of which contain chlorophyll, and they account for about 90 per cent of the earth's photosynthetic activity. al′gal *adj*

blue-green a. *Cyanobacteria.*

brown a. Phaeophyta.

al·ga·ro·ba (al″gə-ro′bə) algarroba.

al·gar·ro·ba (al″gə-ro′bə) [Ar. *al kharrubah*] 1. carob (defs. 1, 2). 2. mesquite.

alge- [Gr. *algēsis* sense of pain, from *algos* pain] a combining form denoting relationship to pain.

al·ge·don·ic (al″jə-don′ik) [*alge-* + *hedonic*] characterized by or relating to both pleasure and pain.

al·ge·fa·cient (al″jə-fa′shənt) [L. *algere* to be cold + *-facient*] cooling; refrigerant.

al·ge·sia (al-je′ze-ə) 1. nociception. 2. excessive sensitivity to pain, a type of hyperesthesia. **alge′sic, alget′ic** *adj*

al·ge·si·chro·nom·e·ter (al-je″zĭ-kro-nom′ə-tər) [*algesi-* + *chrono-* + *-meter*] an instrument for recording the time required to produce a painful impression.

al·ge·sim·e·ter (al″jə-sim′ə-tər) [*algesi-* + *-meter*] an instrument used in measuring the sensitiveness to pain, such as by pricking with a sharp object or by applying measurable amounts of heat or pressure. Called also *algesiometer* and *algometer*. Cf. *dolorimeter*.

Björnström a. an apparatus for determining the sensitiveness of the skin.

Boas a. an instrument for determining the sensitiveness over the epigastrium.

al·ge·sim·e·try (al″jə-sim′ə-tre) the measurement of sensitiveness to pain.

algesi(o)- [Gr. *algēsis* sense of pain, from *algos* pain] a combining form denoting relationship to pain.

al·ge·sio·gen·ic (al-je″ze-o-jen′ik) [*algesio-* + *-genic*] dolorific.

al·ge·si·om·e·ter (al-je″ze-om′ə-tər) algesimeter.

al·ges·the·sia (al″jes-the′zhə) [*alge-* + *esthesia*] 1. nociception. 2. any painful sensation.

al·ges·the·sis (al″jes-the′sis) algesthesia.

al·ges·tone ace·to·phen·ide (al-jes′tōn) a progestin with actions similar to those of progesterone.

-algia [Gr., from *algos* pain + *-ia*] a word termination denoting a painful condition.

al·gi·cide (al′jĭ-sīd) [*algae* + *-cide*] a substance which is destructive to algae.

al·gid (al′jid) [L. *algidus*] chilly or cold.

al·gin (al′jin) sodium alginate, a purified carbohydrate (sodium mannuronate) extracted from brown algae species and used as a stabilizing colloid in numerous pharmaceuticals, cosmetics, and foods.

al·gi·nate (al′jĭ-nāt) any salt of alginic acid. Soluble alginates, such as sodium, potassium, and magnesium alginates, form a viscous sol that can be changed into a gel by a chemical reaction with compounds such as calcium sulfate, a property which makes them useful as materials for taking dental impressions. See also *magnesium alginate*, under *magnesium*.

al·gin·ic ac·id (al-jin′ik) [NF] a hydrophilic colloidal carbohydrate extracted with dilute alkali from species of brown seaweed of the class Phaeophyceae; used as a tablet binder and emulsifying agent.

algi(o)- [Gr. *algos* pain] a combining form denoting relationship to pain.

al·gio·mo·tor (al″je-o-mo′tər) producing painful movements, such as spasm or dysperistalsis.

al·gio·mus·cu·lar (al″je-o-mus′ku-lər) algiomotor.

al·gio·vas·cu·lar (al″je-o-vas′ku-lər) pertaining to vascular action resulting from painful stimulation. Called also *algovascular*.

al·glu·cer·ase (al-gloo′sər-ās″) a modified form of β-glucocerebrosidase, prepared from pooled human placental tissue, used to replace glucocerebrosidase (glucosylceramidase) in the treatment of type 1 Gaucher's disease; administered by intravenous infusion.

al·glu·co·si·dase al·fa (al-gloo-ko′sĭ-dās al′fə) a recombinant form of the enzyme α-1,4-glucosidase, used in treatment of glycogen storage disease, type II; administered by intravenous infusion.

alg(o)- [Gr. *algos* pain] a combining form denoting relationship to pain.

al·go·dys·tro·phy (al″go-dis′trə-fe) [*algo-* + *dystrophy*] complex regional pain syndrome type 1.

al·go·gen·e·sia (al″go-jə-ne′zhə) [*algo-* + Gr. *gennan* to produce] the production of pain.

al·go·gen·e·sis (al″go-jen′ə-sis) algogenesia.

al·go·gen·ic (al-go-jen′ik) dolorific.

al·go·lag·nia (al″go-lag′ne-ə) [*algo-* + Gr. *lagneia* lust] any psychosexual disorder associated with the derivation of pleasure from experiencing or inflicting physical or psychological pain.

active a. sadism.

passive a. masochism.

al·gom·e·ter (al-gom′ə-tər) [*algo-* + *-meter*] algesimeter.

pressure a. an instrument for measuring sensitivity to pressure.

al·gom·e·try (al-gom′ə-tre) algesimetry.

al·go·pho·bia (al″go-fo′be-ə) [*algo-* + *phobia*] exaggerated, irrational fear of pain.

al·go·rithm (al′gə-rith-əm) 1. a step-by-step method of solving a problem or making decisions, as in making a diagnosis. 2. an established mechanical procedure for solving certain mathematical problems.

al·go·spasm (al′go-spaz″əm) [*algo-* + *spasm*] painful spasm or cramp.

al·go·vas·cu·lar (al″go-vas′ku-lər) algiovascular.

ali·as·ing (a′le-əs-ing) 1. introduction of an artifact or error in sampling of a periodic signal when the sampling frequency is too low to properly capture the signal. 2. in pulsed Doppler ultrasonography, an artifact occurring when the velocity of the sampled object exceeds the pulse repetition frequency of the sampling system; the system cannot sample rapidly enough for Doppler frequency determination. 3. an artifact appearing in magnetic resonance imaging when a part being examined is larger than the field of view; an image of the area outside the field of view appears as an artifact inside the field of view. Called also *aliasing artifact* and *wraparound artifact*.

al·i·cy·clic (al″ĭ-sik′lik, -si′klik) having the properties of both aliphatic and cyclic substances.

Al·i·dase (al′ĭ-dās) trademark for a preparation of hyaluronidase for injection.

alien·a·tion (āl″e-ən-a′shən) [L. *alienatio*, from *alienus* strange, foreign] 1. estrangement from society; feelings of being an outsider, foreigner, or outcast. 2. estrangement from one's self; feelings of unreality or depersonalization. 3. alienation of affect; isolation of ideas from feelings, avoidance of emotional situations, and other efforts to estrange one's self from one's feelings.

ali·enia (a-li-e′ne-ə) [*a-*[1] + *lien-* + *-ia*] asplenia.

al·i·flu·rane (al″ĭ-floo′rān) an inhalation anesthetic.

ali·form (al′ĭ-form) [*ala* + *form*] shaped like a wing.

align·ment (ə-līn′mənt) [Fr. *aligner* to put in a straight line] in dentistry, bringing natural or artificial teeth into line, so that they form the two regular parabolic curves of the dental arches and reestablish a harmonious relationship with the supporting structures and with the opposite dentition.

al·i·ment (al′ə-ment) [L. *alimentum*] food or nutritive material.

al·i·men·ta·ry (al″ə-men′tər-e) pertaining to food or nutritive material, or to the organs of digestion.

al·i·men·ta·tion (al″ə-men-ta′shən) the act of giving or receiving nutriment.

artificial a. the giving of food or nourishment to persons who cannot take it in the usual way.

forced a. 1. the feeding of a person against his or her will. 2. the giving of more food to a person than his or her appetite calls for.

parenteral a. see under *nutrition*.

rectal a. the administration of concentrated nourishment by instillation into the rectum.

total parenteral a. see under *nutrition*.

Alim·ta (a-lim′tə) trademark for a preparation of pemetrexed disodium.

ali·na·sal (al″ĭ-na′səl) pertaining to the ala nasi.

al·i·phat·ic (al″ĭ-fat′ik) [Gr. *aleiphar*, *aleiphatos* oil] pertaining to any member of one of the two major groups of organic compounds; those having a straight or branched chain structure. Cf. *cyclic*.

alipo·gen·ic (a-lip″o-jen′ik) not lipogenic; not forming fat.

alipo·tro·pic (a-lip″o-tro′pik) having no influence on the metabolism of fat.

al·i·quot (al′ĭ-kwot) [L. "some, several"] the part of a number which will divide it without a remainder; e.g., 2 is an aliquot of 6. By extension, any portion that bears a known quantitative relationship to a whole or to other portions of the same whole, as an aliquot portion of a solution or specimen, e.g., plasma or serum; a sample of a whole taken to determine the quantitative composition of the whole.

alis·ki·ren (a-lis-ki′ren) an inhibitor of plasma renin activity, interfering with the renin-angiotensin-aldosterone system; administered orally in treatment of hypertension.

ali·sphe·noid (al-ĭ-sfe′noid) [*ala* + *sphenoid*] 1. pertaining to the greater wing of the sphenoid. 2. a cartilage of the fetal chondrocranium on either side of the basisphenoid bone; later in development it forms most of the greater wing of the sphenoid bone. See also *postsphenoidal part of sphenoid bone*, under *part*.

al·i·tret·i·noin (al″ĭ-tret′ĭ-noin″) 9-*cis*-retinoic acid; an endogenous retinoid used as a topical antineoplastic in the treatment of AIDS-related cutaneous Kaposi sarcoma.

aliz·a·rin (ə-liz′ə-rin) [Ar. *ala sara* extract] a red crystalline dye, prepared synthetically or obtained from madder; its compounds are used as indicators.

a. No. 6 purpurin (def. 1).

a. red S sodium alizarinsulfonate.

a. yellow, a. yellow g see under *yellow.*

al•i•zar•i•no•pur•pu•rin (al″ĭ-zar″ĭ-no-pur′pu-rin) purpurin (def. 1).

al•ka•le•mia (al″kə-le′me-ə) [*alkali* + *-emia*] increased pH or decreased hydrogen ion concentration of the blood.

al•ka•les•cence (al″kə-les′əns) slight or incipient alkalinity.

al•ka•les•cent (al″kə-les′ənt) having a tendency to alkalinity.

al•ka•li (al′kə-li) [Ar. *al-qily* potash] any of a class of compounds which form soluble soaps with fatty acids, turn red litmus blue, have pH values greater than 7.0, and form soluble carbonates. Essentially the hydroxides of cesium, lithium, potassium, rubidium, and sodium, they include also the carbonates of these metals and of ammonia.

al•ka•lig•e•nous (al″kə-lij′ə-nəs) yielding an alkali.

al•ka•lim•e•ter (al″kə-lim′ə-tər) [*alkali* + *-meter*] an instrument for measuring the alkali contained in any mixture.

al•ka•lim•e•try (al″kə-lim′ə-tre) the measurement of the alkalis present in any substance.

al•ka•line (al′kə-līn, -lin) 1. having the reactions of an alkali. 2. having a pH greater than 7.0.

al•ka•line phos•pha•tase (ALP) (al′kə-līn, -lin fos′fə-tās) [EC 3.1.3.1] an enzyme of the hydrolase class that catalyzes the cleavage of orthophosphate from orthophosphoric monoesters under alkaline conditions. Differing forms of the enzyme occur in normal and malignant tissues. The activity in serum is useful in the clinical diagnosis of many illnesses. Deficient bone enzyme activity, an autosomal recessive trait, causes hypophosphatasia. Called also *phosphomonoesterase.*

leukocyte a. p. (LAP) the isozyme of alkaline phosphatase occurring in the leukocytes, specifically in the neutrophils; LAP activity is used in the differential diagnosis of neutrophilia, being lowered in chronic myelogenous leukemia but elevated in a variety of other disorders.

al•ka•lin•i•ty (al″kə-lin′ĭ-te) the fact, quality, or degree of being alkaline.

al•ka•lin•i•za•tion (al″kə-lin″ĭ-za′shən) alkalization.

al•ka•lin•ize (al′kə-lin-iz″) alkalize.

al•ka•lin•uria (al″kə-lĭ-nu′re-ə) [*alkaline* + *-uria*] an alkaline condition of the urine.

al•ka•li•za•tion (al″kə-li-za′shən) the act of making alkaline.

al•ka•lize (al′kə-līz) to make alkaline; called also *alkalinize.*

al•ka•liz•er (al′kə-li″zər) an agent that neutralizes acids or causes alkalinization.

al•ka•lo•gen•ic (al″kə-lo-jen′ik) alkaligenous.

al•ka•loid (al′kə-loid″) [*alkali* + *-oid*] one of a large group of nitrogenous basic substances found in plants. They are usually very bitter and many are pharmacologically active. Examples are atropine, caffeine, coniine, morphine, nicotine, quinine, and strychnine. The term is also applied to synthetic substances *(artificial a's)* which have structures similar to plant alkaloids, such as procaine.

belladonna a's a group of anticholinergic alkaloids occurring in belladonna *(Atropa belladonna)*; see *belladonna.*

ergot a's a group of chemically related alkaloids either derived from ergot or synthesized; some cause ergotism while others are medicinal. Included are ergocornine, ergocristine, ergocryptine, ergonovine, ergotamine, and lysergic acid diethylamide.

vinca a's alkaloids produced by the Madagascar periwinkle, *Vinca rosea;* they are cytotoxic and cell cycle–specific for the M phase of cell division, acting by binding to tubulin, leading to arrest of cells in metaphase.

al•ka•lom•e•try (al″kə-lom′ə-tre) [*alkaloid* + *-metry*] the dosimetric administration of alkaloids.

al•ka•lo•sis (al″kə-lo′sis) a pathologic condition resulting from accumulation of base, or from loss of acid without comparable loss of base in the body fluids, and characterized by decrease in hydrogen ion concentration (increase in pH). Cf. *acidosis.* **alkalot′ic** *adj*

altitude a. increased alkalinity in blood and tissues occurring in mountain sickness.

compensated a. alkalosis in which compensatory mechanisms have returned the pH toward normal; see *compensated metabolic a.*, and *compensated respiratory a.*

compensated metabolic a. a state of alkalosis in which the pH of the blood has been returned toward normal by respiratory compensation.

compensated respiratory a. a respiratory alkalosis in which the pH of the blood has been returned toward normal through retention of acid or excretion of base by renal mechanisms.

hypochloremic a. metabolic alkalosis marked by hypochloremia together with hyponatremia and hypokalemia, resulting from the loss of sodium chloride and hydrochloric acid due to prolonged vomiting.

hypokalemic a. a type of metabolic alkalosis associated with a low serum potassium level; retention of alkali or loss of acid occurs in the extracellular (but not intracellular) fluid compartment, although the pH of the intracellular fluid may be below normal. It may be caused by hypertrophy and hypoplasia of the juxtaglomerular cells, as in Bartter syndrome.

metabolic a. a disturbance in which the acid-base status of the body shifts toward the alkaline side because of retention of base or loss of noncarbonic, or fixed (nonvolatile), acids.

respiratory a. a state due to excess loss of carbon dioxide from the body, usually as a result of hyperventilation; hyperventilation may be either psychogenic or physical in nature, with the most common physical problems being disordered regulation in the central nervous system and pulmonary conditions.

al•kal•uria (al″kə-lu′re-ə) 1. the presence of an alkali in the urine. 2. alkalinuria.

al•ka•mine (al′kə-mēn) an alcohol that contains an amine group.

al•kane (al′kān) any of a class of saturated hydrocarbons with straight or branched chain structures, with general formula C_nH_{2n+2}.

al•kan•nin (al′kə-nin) a red powder, the coloring ingredient of alkanet; used as a colorant and, in the form of alkannin paper, as an indicator: alkalis turn the paper blue, acids red.

al•kap•ton•uria (al-kap″to-nu′re-ə) an autosomal recessive aminoacidopathy caused by mutations in the *HGD* gene (locus: 3q21-q23), which encodes homogentisate 1,2-dioxygenase; enzyme deficiency results in accumulation of homogentisic acid. Manifestations include elevated concentrations of homogentisic acid in urine, which darkens on standing or undergoing alkalinization; ochronosis; and arthritis.

al•kap•ton•uric (al-kap″to-nu′rik) 1. pertaining to, characterized by, or causing alkaptonuria. 2. an individual with alkaptonuria.

al•ka•tri•ene (al″kə-tri′ēn) an unsaturated aliphatic hydrocarbon containing three double bonds.

al•kene (al′kēn) an unsaturated aliphatic hydrocarbon containing one double bond.

Al•ker•an (al-ker′ən) trademark for preparations of melphalan.

al•kyl (al′kəl) the radical which results when an aliphatic hydrocarbon loses one hydrogen atom.

a. (C12–15) benzoate [NF] the esters of a mixture of C12 to C15 alcohols and benzoic acid, used as an oleaginous vehicle and emollient in pharmaceutical preparations.

a. sulfonate a member of a class of alkylating agents comprising a series of symmetrical *bis*-substituted straight chain esters of methanesulfonic acid with a bridge of methylene groups that varies in length; compounds having a methylene bridge of intermediate length (4 or 5 methylene groups) have the highest therapeutic index. Written also *alkylsulfonate.*

al•kyl•amine (al′kəl-ə-mēn″) an amine containing an alkyl radical.

al•kyl•ate (al′kə-lāt) to cause alkylation; see also *alkylating agent*, under *agent.*

al•kyl•a•tion (al″kə-la′shən) the substitution of an alkyl group for an active hydrogen atom in an organic compound.

al•kyne (al′kīn) an unsaturated hydrocarbon containing a triple bond between two carbon atoms; the alkynes are members of the acetylene series.

ALL acute lymphoblastic leukemia.

al•la•ches•the•sia (al″ə-kes-the′zhə) allesthesia.

optical a. visual allesthesia.

Al•lan-Hern•don-Dud•ley syndrome (al′ən hurn′dən dud′le) [William *Allan*, American physician and geneticist, 1881–1943; Claude Nash *Herndon*, American geneticist, 20th century; Florence C. *Dudley*, American geneticist, 20th century] see under *syndrome.*

al•lan•ti•a•sis (al″an-ti′ə-sis) [*allanto-* + *-iasis*] a type of sausage poisoning from sausages containing the toxins of *Clostridium botulinum.* See *botulism.*

allant(o)- [Gr. *allas*, gen. *allantos* sausage] a combining form denoting relationship to a sausage or to the allantois.

al•lan•to•cho•ri•on (ə-lan″to-kor′e-on) a compound membrane formed by fusion of the allantois and chorion.

al•lan•to•gen•e•sis (al″an-to-jen′ə-sis) the formation and development of the allantois.

al•lan•toid (ə-lan′toid) [*allanto-* + Gr. *-oid*] 1. resembling the allantois. 2. sausage-shaped.

al•lan•toi•de•an (al″ən-toi′de-ən) 1. pertaining to the allantois. 2. any animal with an allantois during its embryonic development; in the plural, *amniotes* is the more usual term.

al•lan•toi•do•an•gi•op•a•gous (al″ən-toi″do-an″je-op′ə-gəs) joined by the vessels of the umbilical cord; see under *twin.*

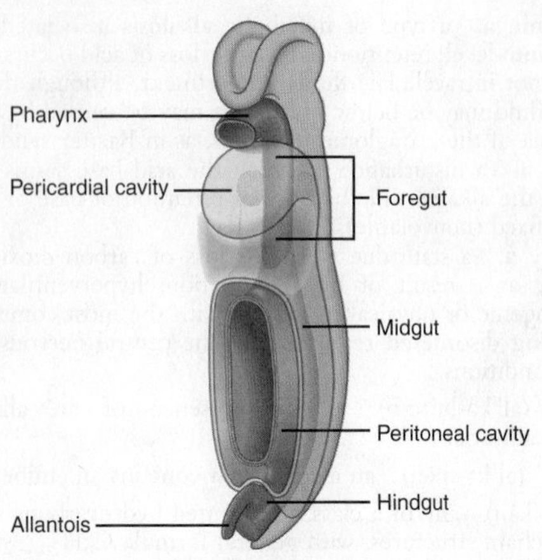

■ The small allantois of an early human embryo, shown in relation to the developing foregut, midgut, and hindgut.

al·lan·toi·do·an·gi·op·a·gus (al″ən-toi″do-an″je-op′ə-gəs) [*allantoid* + *angio-* + *-pagus*] twin fetuses joined by the vessels of the umbilical cord; allantoidoangiopagous twins. Called also *omphaloangiopagus.*

al·lan·to·in (ə-lan′to-in) the diureide of glyoxylic acid, found in human allantoic fluid and fetal urine; it is also found in many plants, and as a urinary excretion product of purine metabolism in most mammals but not in humans or related primates. It is produced synthetically by the oxidation of uric acid for use as an astringent and keratolytic, often as a component of multi-ingredient dermatological preparations.

al·lan·to·in·uria (ə-lan″to-in-u′re-ə) the presence of allantoin in the urine; this is normal in most mammals but abnormal in humans and related primates.

al·lan·to·is (ə-lan′to-is) [*allanto-* + *eidos* form] an initially tubular ventral diverticulum of the hindgut of embryos of reptiles, birds, and mammals. In reptiles and birds, it expands to a large sac for storing urine and, after fusing with the chorion which lines the shell, provides for gas exchange. The allantois is prominent in some mammals (carnivores, ungulates); in others such as humans, it is vestigial except that it becomes the urachus and its blood vessels give rise to those of the umbilical cord. **allanto′ic** *adj*

Al·leg·ra (ə-leg′rə) trademark for preparations containing fexofenadine hydrochloride.

al·lele (ə-lēl′) [Gr. *allēlōn* of one another, from *allos* other] one of the two or more alternative forms of a gene that can occur at a particular chromosomal locus and that determine alternative characters in inheritance. In diploid species, there are two alleles, identical or differing, for each specific locus of an autosomal chromosome, one on each chromosome of a homologous pair. **allel′ic** *adj*

codominant a. one of two or more alleles at a locus that are each fully expressed in a heterozygote and thus each contribute to the phenotype.

dominant a. an allele that is phenotypically expressed when present either in the homozygous or heterozygous state. Cf. *recessive a.*

hypomorphic a. a mutant allele whose effect is subnormal expression of a normal phenotype.

multiple a's alleles of which there are more than two alternative forms possible at any one locus.

null a. silent a.

recessive a. an allele that is phenotypically expressed only in the homozygous (or hemizygous, for X-linked traits) state. Cf. *dominant a.*

silent a. an allele that codes for a nonfunctional or undetectable product.

al·le·lism (ə-le′liz-əm) the existence of alleles, or their relationship to one another.

multiple a. the existence in a population of more than two alleles at a locus.

allel(o)- [Gr. *allēlōn* of one another, from *allos* other] a combining form denoting relationship to another.

al·le·lo·chem·ics (ə-le″lo-kem′iks) chemical interactions between species, involving release of active chemical substances, such as scents, pheromones, and toxins.

al·le·lo·tax·is (ə-le″lo-tak′sis) [*allelo-* + Gr. *-taxis*] the development of an organ from several embryonic structures.

al·le·lo·taxy (ə-le′lo-tak″se) allelotaxis.

Al·le·mann syndrome (ah′lə-mahn) [Richard *Allemann*, Swiss physician, 1893–1958] see under *syndrome.*

Al·len's law (al′ənz) [Frederick Madison *Allen*, American physician, 1879–1964] see under *law.*

Al·len test (al′ən) [Edgar Van Nuys *Allen*, American physician, 1900–1961] see under *test.*

Al·len-Doi·sy test, unit (al′ən doi′se) [Edgar V. *Allen*, American anatomist, 1892–1943; Edward Adelbert *Doisy*, American biochemist, 1893–1986] see under *test* and *unit.*

al·ler·gen (al′ər-jən) [*allergy* + *-gen*] an antigenic substance capable of producing immediate-type hypersensitivity (allergy).

pollen a. any protein antigen of weed, tree, or grass pollens capable of causing allergic asthma or rhinitis; pollen allergen extracts are used in skin testing for pollen sensitivity and in immunotherapy (desensitization) for pollen allergy.

al·ler·gen·ic (al″ər-jen′ik) acting as an allergen; inducing allergy.

al·ler·gist (al′ər-jist) a physician who specializes in the diagnosis and treatment of allergic conditions.

al·ler·gi·za·tion (al″ər-jĭ-za′shən) active sensitization or the introduction of allergens into the body.

al·ler·gize (al′ər-jīz) to subject to sensitization; to make allergic.

al·ler·goid (al′ər-goid) an allergen rendered less allergenic but not less antigenic (formation of IgE but not of IgG blocking antibody is decreased) by formalin or glutaraldehyde treatment.

al·ler·gol·o·gist (al-ər-gol′ə-jist) a specialist in allergology.

al·ler·gol·o·gy (al″ər-gol′ə-je) the branch of medicine devoted to the study of allergy, its etiology, diagnosis, and treatment. **allergolog′ical** *adj*

al·ler·go·sis (al″ər-go′sis) any allergic disease.

al·ler·gy (al′ər-je) [*all-* + *ergon* work] 1. a state of hypersensitivity induced by exposure to a particular antigen (allergen) resulting in harmful immune responses on subsequent exposures; the term is usually used to refer to hypersensitivity to an environmental antigen (atopic allergy or contact dermatitis) or to drug allergy. 2. The medical specialty dealing with diagnosis and treatment of allergic disorders. **aller′gic** *adj*

atopic a. atopy.

bacterial a. hypersensitivity to a bacterial antigen, e.g., delayed-type hypersensitivity to *Mycobacterium tuberculosis.*

bronchial a. allergy affecting the bronchi; see *allergic asthma.*

buckwheat a. an allergic reaction to buckwheat, *Fagopyrum esculentum*, characterized primarily by photosensitivity; seen in susceptible persons who eat the grain and ruminants that eat excessive numbers of buckwheat plants. Called also *fagopyrism.*

cold a. any condition in which signs and symptoms of allergy are produced by exposure to cold, e.g., cold urticaria.

contact a. the allergic condition seen with allergic contact dermatitis.

delayed a. see under *hypersensitivity.*

drug a. an allergic reaction occurring as the result of unusual sensitivity to a drug.

food a., gastrointestinal a. an adverse immune-mediated reaction to food, having a variety of manifestations involving the skin and the gastrointestinal and respiratory tracts.

fragrance a. an allergic reaction to chemicals in certain types of colognes, perfumes, and other fragrances, sometimes manifested as a type of allergic contact dermatitis.

hereditary a. atopy.

immediate a. see under *hypersensitivity.*

latent a. allergy that is not manifested by symptoms but may be detected by tests.

latex a. allergy to natural rubber latex, a type IV hypersensitivity reaction; see also *latex* (def. 1).

physical a. any condition in which signs and symptoms of allergy are produced by exposure to cold (cold urticaria or angioedema), heat (cholinergic urticaria), or light (photosensitivity).

pollen a. hay fever.

polyvalent a. a simultaneous allergic response to several allergens.

spontaneous a. atopy.

sun a. popular term for *idiopathic photodermatosis.*

Al·les·che·ria (al″əs-kēr′e-ə) a former genus of fungi. *A. boy′dii* is now called *Pseudallescheria boydii.*

al·les·che·ri·a·sis (al″əs-kə-ri′ə-sis) former name for *pseudallescheriasis.*

al·les·the·sia (al″es-the′zhə) [*all-* + *esthesia*] a dysesthesia in which a sensation, as of pain or touch, is experienced at a point remote from that at which the stimulus is applied or occurs, as in allochiria. Called also *allachesthesia* and *alloesthesia.*

visual a. a condition in which visual images are transposed from one half of the visual field to the other, either vertically or horizontally; called also *optical allachesthesia.*

al·le·thrin (al'ə-thrin) a synthetic analogue of the natural insecticides cinerin, jasmolin, and pyrethrin, used as an insecticide.

All·fen (awl'fen) trademark for preparations of guaifenesin.

All·grove syndrome (awl'grōv) [Jeremy *Allgrove*, British pediatric endocrinologist, born 1948] see under *syndrome.*

al·li·ance (ə-li'əns) a union formed for the furtherance of interests of the members; an agreement to cooperate for specific purposes.

National A. for the Mentally Ill (NAMI) a self-help and national advocacy group composed of persons with mental illnesses and their family members.

therapeutic a. a conscious contractual relationship between therapist and patient in which each agrees to work together to work toward a resolution of the patient's problems.

working a. therapeutic a.

al·li·cin (al'ĭ-sin) an oily substance, extracted from garlic, which has antibacterial activity. See also *Allium.*

al·li·ga·tion (al"ĭ-ga'shən) the process of finding the cost of a mixture of known quantities of ingredients, each of known value, or of determining the quantities of solutions of various strengths to be used to form a mixture of a particular strength.

Al·lis sign (al'is) [Oscar Huntington *Allis*, American surgeon, 1836–1921] see under *sign.*

al·lit·er·a·tion (ə-lit"ər-a'shən) [*ad-* + *litera* letter] a speech disorder in which the patient uses words containing the same consonant sounds.

Al·li·um (al'e-əm) [L. "garlic"] a genus of flowering plants with bulbous stem bases, of the family Liliaceae. *A. ce'pa* is the onion and *A. sati'vum* is the garlic (q.v.).

all(o)- [Gr. *allos* other] a combining form denoting a condition differing from the normal or a reversal, or referring to another.

al·lo·al·bu·min (al"o-al-bu'min) any genetic variant of albumin.

al·lo·an·ti·body (al"o-an'tĭ-bod"e) isoantibody.

al·lo·an·ti·gen (al"o-an'tĭ-jən) an antigen present in allelic forms encoded at the same gene locus in different individuals of the same species.

al·lo·an·ti·se·rum (al"o-an"tĭ-sēr'əm) an antiserum raised in an individual of a species and directed against antigens of genetically nonidentical members of the same species.

al·lo·bar (al'o-bahr) [*allo-* + Gr. *baros* weight] a form of a chemical element having an atomic weight different from that of the naturally occurring form.

al·lo·bi·o·sis (al"o-bi-o'sis) [*allo-* + *biosis*] the condition of altered reactivity which an organism manifests under changed environmental or physiologic conditions.

al·lo·cen·tric (al"o-sen'trik) focused on the thoughts and feelings of others; not egocentric.

al·lo·chei·ria (al"o-ki're-ə) allochiria.

al·lo·ches·the·sia (al"o-kes-the'zhə) allesthesia.

al·lo·chi·ria (al"o-ki're-ə) [*allo-* + *chir-* + *-ia*] dyschiria in which, if one extremity is stimulated, the sensation is referred to the opposite side; called also *allocheiria.* allochi'ral *adj*

al·lo·chro·ism (al"o-kro'iz-əm) [*allo-* + Gr. *chroa* color + *-ism*] change or variation in color, as in certain minerals. allochro'ic *adj*

al·lo·chro·ma·cy (al"o-kro'mə-se) the formation of other coloring agents from a dye that is unstable in solution.

al·lo·cor·tex (al"o-kor'teks) [*allo-* + *cortex*] [TA] the older, original part of the cerebral cortex, comprising the archicortex and the paleocortex. It does not have the six-layered histologic structure of the larger, phylogenetically newer isocortex. Called also *heterotypical cortex.*

Al·lo·der·ma·nys·sus (al"o-dur"mə-nis'əs) former name for *Liponyssoides.*

al·lo·dyn·ia (al"o-din'e-ə) [*all-* + *-odynia*] pain resulting from a non-noxious stimulus to normal skin.

al·lo·erot·i·cism (al"o-ə-rot'ĭ-siz-əm) [*allo-* + *eroticism*] 1. sexual feeling directed to another person. 2. the final stage in the development of object relationships, a state of maturity, characterized both by direction of erotic energies to another and also by the ability to form a love relationship with that other. Cf. *autoeroticism, heteroeroticism.* alloerot'ic *adj*

al·lo·es·the·sia (al"o-es-the'ze-ah) allesthesia.

al·log·a·my (al-og'ə-me) cross fertilization.

al·lo·ge·ne·ic (al"o-jə-ne'ik) 1. having cell types that are antigenically distinct. 2. in transplantation biology, denoting individuals (or tissues) that are of the same species but antigenically distinct, as opposed to *syngeneic* and *xenogeneic.* Called also *homologous.* See also *allograft* and *allogeneic transplantation.*

al·lo·gen·ic (al"o-jen'ik) allogeneic.

al·lo·graft (al'o-graft) a graft of tissue between individuals of the same species but of disparate genotype; types of donors are cadaveric, living related, and living unrelated (see under *donor*). Called also *allogeneic graft* and *homograft.*

al·lo·group (al'o-groop) an allotype linkage group, especially of allotypes for the four IgG subclasses, which are closely linked and inherited as a unit.

al·lo·im·mune (al"o-ĭ-mūn') specifically immune to an allogeneic antigen.

al·lo·im·mu·ni·za·tion (al"o-im"u-nĭ-za'shən) an immune response generated in an individual or strain of one species by an alloantigen from a different individual or strain of the same species, such as that occurring after transplantation of an organ.

al·lo·isom·er·ism (al"o-i-som'ər-iz-əm) isomerism which does not appear in the structural formula.

al·lo·ker·a·to·plas·ty (al"o-ker'ə-to-plas"te) [*allo-* + *keratoplasty*] repair of the cornea by the use of foreign material.

al·lo·ki·ne·sis (al"o-ki-ne'sis) [*allo-* + *-kinesis*] movement that is not performed voluntarily but is produced passively or occurs by reflex. allokinet'ic *adj*

al·lo·lac·tose (al"o-lak'tōs) a derivative of lactose formed in cells of *Escherichia coli;* it is the physiological inducer of β-galactosidase in these cells.

al·lom·er·ism (ə-lom'ər-iz-əm) [*allo-* + *merism*] change of chemical constitution without change in the crystalline form. Cf. *allomorphism.*

al·lo·met·ric (al"o-met'rik) [*allo-* + *metric*] denoting the change of proportion between organs or parts during the growth of an organism; pertaining to allometry.

al·lo·met·ron (al"o-met'ron) [*allo-* + Gr. *metron* measure] an evolutionary change in bodily form or proportion as expressed in measurements and indices.

al·lom·e·try (al-om'ə-tre) the measurement of changing shape of an organism with increase in size, i.e., the determination of the relationship of two varying dimensions, usually linear.

al·lo·mor·phism (al"o-mor'fiz-əm) [*allo-* + *morph-* + *-ism*] change of crystalline form without change in chemical constitution. Cf. *allomerism.*

al·lon·o·mous (al"on'ə-məs) [*allo-* + *nom-* + *-ous*] regulated by stimuli from the outside.

al·lo·path (al'o-path) a term sometimes applied to a practitioner of allopathy.

al·lop·a·thist (al-op'ə-thist) allopath.

al·lop·a·thy (al-op'ə-the) [*allo-* + *-pathy*] a term applied to that system of therapeutics in which diseases are treated by producing a condition incompatible with or antagonistic to the condition to be cured or alleviated. Called also *heteropathy.* Cf. *homeopathy.* allopath'ic *adj*

al·lo·phan·am·ide (al"o-fan-am'īd) biuret.

al·lo·phan·ate (al"o-fan'āt) a salt of allophanic acid.

al·lo·phan·ic ac·id (al"o-fan'ik) urea carbonic acid which does not occur as the free acid but only in salts or compounds; its amide (allophanamide) is biuret.

al·lo·phe·nic (al"o-fe'nik) [*allo-* + *phen-* + *-ic*] 1. of or relating to single individuals originating from more than one conceptus. 2. having orderly coexistence of cells with different phenotypes ascribable to known allelic genotypic differences; mosaic.

al·loph·thal·mia (al"of-thal'me-ə) heterophthalmia.

al·lo·pla·sia (al"o-pla'zhə) [*allo-* + *-plasia*] heteroplasia.

al·lo·plast (al'o-plast) [*allo-* + *-plast*] an inert foreign body used for implantation into tissue.

al·lo·plas·tic (al"o-plas'tik) 1. pertaining to an alloplast. 2. pertaining to or characterized by alloplasty.

al·lo·plas·ty (al'o-plas"te) [*allo-* + *-plasty*] in psychoanalytic theory, adaptation by alteration of the external environment (alloplastic change). Cf. *autoplasty* (def. 2).

al·lo·preg·nane·di·ol (al"o-preg"nān-di'ol) an isomer of pregnanediol occurring in female urine.

al·lo·psy·chic (al"o-si'kik) [*allo-* + *psychic*] pertaining to the mind in its relation to the external world.

al·lo·pur·i·nol (al"o-pūr'ĭ-nol) [USP] an isomer of hypoxanthine; used in the treatment of hyperuricemia of gout and the prophylaxis and treatment of that secondary to blood dyscrasias or cancer chemotherapy, for prophylaxis of recurrent formation of uric acid and oxalate renal calculi, and for prophylaxis and treatment of uric acid nephropathy. Both allopurinol and its primary metabolite, oxypurinol, are potent inhibitors of xanthine oxidase and reduce serum levels and urinary excretion of uric acid.

al•lo•re•ac•tive (al″o-re-ak′tiv) [*allo-* + *reactive*] pertaining to the immune response in reaction to a transplanted allograft.

al•lo•rec•og•ni•tion (al″o-rek″og-nĭ′shən) recognition of antigen after allogeneic transplantation; see *recognition* (def. 3).

al•lo•rhyth•mia (al″o-rith′me-ə) [*allo-* + *rhythm* + *-ia*] irregularity in the rhythm of the heart beat or pulse that recurs in a regular fashion.

al•lo•rhyth•mic (al″o-rith′mik) affected with or of the nature of allorhythmia.

all or none (awl or nun) 1. the principle that the heart muscle, under whatever stimulus, will contract to the fullest extent or not at all; stimulation of any single atrial or ventricular muscle fiber causes the action potential to travel over the entire atrial or ventricular mass, or not to travel at all. 2. in muscles other than cardiac muscle, and in nerves, stimulation of an individual fiber causes an action potential to travel over the entire fiber or not to travel at all. Called also *all-or-none law*.

al•lose (al′ōs) an aldohexose epimeric with glucose at carbon 3.

al•lo•sen•si•ti•za•tion (al″o-sen″sĭ-ti-za′shən) sensitization to alloantigens (isoantigens), as to Rh antigens during pregnancy (see *Rh isoimmunization*). Called also *isosensitization*.

al•lo•sta•sis (al″o-sta′sis, ə-los′tə-sis) maintenance by an organism of internal physical or psychological stability by making changes during situations of challenge; see *allostatic load*, under *load*. **allostat′ic** *adj*

al•lo•ster•ism (al′o-ster″iz-əm) allostery.

al•lo•ste•ry (al′o-ster″e) the condition in which the binding of a substrate, product, or other effector to a subunit of a multi-subunit enzyme or other protein at a site (allosteric site) other than the functional site alters its conformation and functional properties, such as by affecting binding of other ligands at the functional site (cooperativity). **alloster′ic** *adj*

al•lo•therm (al′o-thərm″) [*allo-* + *therm*] 1. poikilotherm. 2. heterotherm.

al•lo•tope (al′o-tōp) a site on the constant or nonvarying portion of an antibody molecule that can be recognized by a combining site of other antibodies. Cf. *idiotope*.

al•lo•to•pia (al″o-to′pe-ə) malposition.

al•lo•top•ic (al″o-top′ik) dystopic.

al•lo•tox•in (al′o-tok″sin) [*allo-* + *toxin*] any substance formed by tissue change within the body which serves as a defense against toxins by neutralizing their poisonous properties.

al•lo•trans•plan•ta•tion (al″o-trans-plan-ta′shən) [*allo-* + *transplantation*] allogeneic transplantation.

allotri(o)- [Gr. *allotrios* strange] a combining form meaning strange or foreign.

al•lot•ri•odon•tia (ə-lot″re-o-don′shə) [*allotrio-* + *odont-* + *-ia*] 1. the transplantation of teeth from one individual into the mouth of another. 2. the existence of teeth in abnormal places, as in dermoid cysts.

al•lot•rio•geu•stia (ə-lot″re-o-goo′ste-ə) [*allotrio-* + Gr. *geusis* taste + *-ia*] abnormal sense of taste or appetite.

al•lo•tri•os•mia (al″o-tri-os′me-ə) heterosmia.

al•lo•trope (al′o-trōp) an allotropic form.

al•lo•tro•phic (al″o-tro′fik) rendered non-nutritious by the process of digestion.

al•lo•tro•pic (al″o-tro′pik) 1. exhibiting allotropism. 2. preoccupied with the ideas, actions, and feelings of others; said of a personality that is inclined to be preoccupied by others rather than oneself; not self-centered.

al•lot•ro•pism (ə-lot′rə-piz″əm) [*allo-* + *tropism*] the existence of a substance in two or more distinct forms (allotropic forms) with distinct physical properties, e.g., graphite and diamond, allotropic forms of carbon.

al•lot•ro•py (ə-lot′rə-pe) 1. allotropism. 2. direction of one's interest more toward others than toward oneself.

al•lo•type (al′o-tīp) [*allo-* + *type*] any of several allelic variants of a protein that are characterized by antigenic differences (allotypic markers), especially allelic variants of immunoglobulin heavy and light chains. Cf. *isotype* and *idiotype*.

Am a's [alpha chain marker] allotypes of human α2 chains (IgA2 heavy chains); two markers designated A2m(1) and A2m(2) have been identified.

Gm a's [gamma chain marker] allotypes of human γ chains (IgG heavy chains); 25 markers designated Gm(1) through Gm(25) have been identified. Each marker occurs only in certain specific IgG subclasses. A specific allotype (allelic γ chain) may have more than one marker.

Inv a's Km a's.

Km a's [kappa chain marker] allotypes of human κ light chains; three markers designated Km(1), Km(2), and Km(3) have been identified. Km(2) always occurs with Km(1), thus the possible serotypes are Km(1), Km(1,2), and Km(3). Called also *Inv a's*.

Oz a. an allotypic antigenic marker on the λ chain of human immunoglobulins, equivalent to the Km allotypes on κ light chains.

al•lo•typ•ic (al″o-tip′ik) characterized by allotypes.

al•lo•ty•py (al″o-ti′pe) the condition of being an allotype; used particularly in describing immunoglobulins and other serum proteins.

al•low•ance (ə-lou′əns) something permitted or allowed.

recommended daily a. popularly used synonym for *recommended dietary a.*

recommended dietary a. (RDA) the amount of nutrient and calorie intake per day considered necessary for maintenance of good health, calculated for males and females of various ages and recommended by the Food and Nutrition Board of the National Research Council. Popularly called *recommended daily a.*

al•lox•an (ə-lok′san) an oxidized product of uric acid that, when administered to experimental animals, tends to destroy the islet cells of the pancreas, producing alloxan diabetes. Called also *uroxin*.

al•lox•an•tin (al″ok-san′tin) a diabetogenic compound derived from alloxan by reduction.

al•lox•a•zine (ə-lok′sə-zēn) a heterocyclic compound that is isomeric with isoalloxazine, which is the parent structure of riboflavin.

al•loy (al′oi) [Fr. *aloyer* to mix metals] a mixture of two or more metals or of one or more metals with certain metalloids that are mutually soluble in the molten condition; distinguished as binary, ternary, quaternary, etc., depending on the number of metals in the mixture. An alloy may also be classified on the basis of its behavior when solidified.

amalgam a. an alloy, composed chiefly of silver, tin, and copper, that is mixed with mercury to form dental amalgam; it is prepared by melting its components and casting it in an ingot that is afterward cut into small particles (filings), or it may be produced in the form of spheres.

solid solution a. an alloy whose molecules are in a solid solution; commonly used in dentistry.

al•loy•age (ə-loi′əj) the combining of metals into alloys.

al•lyl (al′əl) [*allium* + *-yl*] a univalent organic group, $—CH_2═CHCH_2$.

a. chloride a compound derived by the chlorination of propylene, used in the preparation of other allyl compounds, of thermosetting resins, and of pharmaceuticals and insecticides; it is toxic by ingestion, inhalation, and skin absorption and affects the lungs, kidneys, and liver.

a. isothiocyanate [USP] a volatile oil derived from sinigrin, which is found in the seeds of black mustard and horseradish; used as a counterirritant in ointments and plasters, in the preparation of flavors, and in the manufacture of war gas. It can cause fatal gastroenteritis in animals consuming the plants.

al•lyl•am•ine (al″əl-am′in) a caustic liquid with an ammoniacal odor, used in the manufacture of pharmaceuticals.

al•lyl•gua•ia•col (ă″ləl-gwi′ə-kol) eugenol.

al•ly•sine (ă-li′sēn) a product of the oxidative deamination of lysine, formed by the action of lysyl oxidase. It is an intermediate in the formation of cross-linkages in collagens.

ALM acral-lentiginous melanoma.

Al•mei•da disease (ahl-ma′də) [Floriano Paulo de *Almeida*, Brazilian physician, 1898–1977] paracoccidioidomycosis.

al•mond (ah′mənd) [Fr. *amande*, from L. *amygdala* almond] 1. *Prunus dulcis*. 2. the fruit or seed of *Prunus dulcis*, source of almond oil and bitter almond oil (see under *oil*). Called also *amygdala*.

bitter a. 1. *Prunus dulcis* var. *amara*. 2. the fruit or seed of *P. dulcis* var. *amara*, which contains the toxin amygdalin; it is a source of bitter almond oil and almond oil (see under *oil*).

sweet a. 1. *Prunus dulcis* var. *dulcis*. 2. the fruit or seed of *P. dulcis* var. *dulcis*; a source of almond oil (see under *oil*).

al•mo•ner (al′mə-nər) a person who dispenses alms.

hospital a. *Brit.*, a person trained in dispensing the social service funds of a hospital, and in administering social service work.

al•mo•trip•tan ma•late (al″mo-trip′tan) a selective serotonin receptor agonist used in the acute treatment of migraine; administered orally.

alo•chia (ə-lo′ke-ə) [*a-*[1] + *lochia*] absence of the lochia.

Alo•cin•ma (a″lo-sin′mə) a genus of fresh water snails of the family Helicidae. *A. longicor′nis* is a species found in China that can serve as an intermediate host of the liver fluke *Clonorchis sinensis*.

Alo•cril (al′o-kril) trademark for a preparation of nedocromil sodium.

Al•oe (al′ə-we) [L. *alöe*, from Gr. *aloē*] a large genus of succulent plants of the family Liliaceae, found in southern Africa and elsewhere. Several

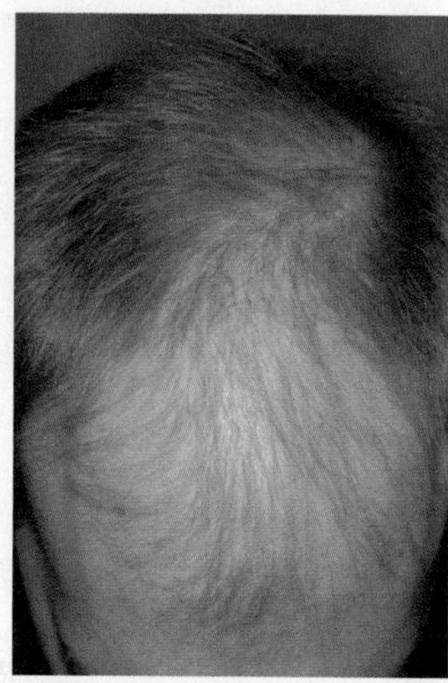

■ Androgenetic alopecia showing frontal and vertex thinning typical for men.

species, such as *A. barbaden'sis* (called also *A. ve'ra*), *A. fe'rox*, and *A. per'ryi*, have juice that contains the cathartic barbaloin. See also *aloe*.

al·oe (al'o) 1. any plant of the genus *Aloe*. 2. [USP] the dried juice of the leaves of various plants of the genus *Aloe*, which has cathartic properties and is also used as an ingredient of *compound benzoin tincture* and other dermatologic and cosmetic preparations. **aloet'ic** *adj*

al·o·in (al'o-in) a mixture of active principles, chiefly barbaloin, extracted from aloes; it has been used as a cathartic.

Al·o·mide (al'o-mīd") trademark for a preparation of lodoxamide tromethamine.

al·o·pe·cia (al"o-pe'shə) [Gr. *alōpekia* a disease in which the hair falls out] lack or loss of hair from skin areas where it normally is present. Called also *atrichia*, *baldness*, and *calvities*.

a. adna'ta congenital a.

androgenetic a., a. androgene'tica, androgenic a. progressive, diffuse, symmetric loss of scalp hair. In men it may begin in the twenties or early thirties, with hair loss from the vertex and the frontoparietal regions; in some men it progresses to finally leave only a sparse peripheral rim of scalp hair. This is also called *male pattern a.* or *baldness*. In women it may begin later, with less severe hair loss in the front area of the scalp. This is also called *female pattern a.* or *baldness*. In affected areas, hair follicles produce finer and lighter terminal hairs until terminal hair production ceases; the phase called anagen becomes longer, while telogen becomes shorter. The etiology is unknown but may be a combination of genetic factors and increased response of hair follicles to androgens.

a. area'ta patchy, nonscarring, asymmetric hair loss, sometimes reversible, occurring in sharply defined areas of the scalp or beard. The etiology is unknown; in some patients there may be an autoimmune component, and in others genetic factors may play a role. See also *ophiasis*. Called also *a. circumscripta* and *pelade*.

a. ca'pitis tota'lis a. totalis.

chemical a. traumatic alopecia caused by a chemical applied to the hair or scalp, such as a hair relaxer product, usually with scarring of the scalp.

cicatricial a., a. cicatrisa'ta hair loss associated with scarring, usually irreversible and found on the scalp. It may be secondary to a process such as cancer, a burn, infection, or sarcoidosis or due to a primary disease process such as Graham Little syndrome, lichen planus follicularis, or pseudopelade.

a. circumscrip'ta a. areata.

congenital a., a. congenita'lis congenital absence of the scalp hair, which may occur alone or be part of a more widespread disorder.

diffuse a. gradual loss of hair across the entire scalp without itching or other signs, usually seen in females; it may occur following childbirth, high fever, or emotional stress, or may be a sign of iron deficiency or reaction to a medication.

drug a., drug-induced a. transient hair loss caused by administration of certain drugs, such as heparin or antimitotics such as cyclophosphamide, methotrexate, and colchicine.

female androgenetic a., female androgenic a., female pattern a., female pattern androgenetic a. see *androgenetic a.*

a. follicula'ris folliculitis decalvans.

hot comb a. see *follicular degeneration syndrome*, under *syndrome*.

involutional a. a. senilis.

lipedematous a. a rare type of alopecia in which the scalp is edematous and has additional subcutaneous fat, seen most often in dark-skinned females; the etiology is unknown.

male androgenetic a., male androgenic a., male pattern a., male pattern androgenetic a. see *androgenetic a.*

marginal a., a. margina'lis traumatic marginal a.

a. medicamento'sa drug-induced a.

moth-eaten a. syphilitic a.

a. mucino'sa follicular mucinosis.

occipital a., postoperative a. a type of pressure alopecia in the occipital region after the patient has had a prolonged surgical procedure.

postpartum a. telogen effluvium occurring shortly after childbirth.

premature a. androgenetic alopecia at a young age, usually in young men from teenage years to the early twenties.

pressure a. traumatic alopecia due to persistent pressure on the scalp, such as in babies lying on their backs, adults having prolonged surgical procedures, or ill persons having prolonged bed rest.

psychogenic a. hair loss owing to severe emotional stress; it is often of the alopecia areata type. Called also *stress a.*

radiation a., radiation-induced a. transient alopecia following exposure to ionizing radiation.

scarring a. cicatricial a.

seborrheic a., a. seborrhe'ica alopecia associated with excessive oiliness of the scalp, dandruff, and other signs of seborrheic dermatitis.

senescent a., senile a., a. seni'lis thinning of the hair in old age, owing to slowing down of metabolism and fewer nutrients being able to reach the hair follicles; it occurs about equally in men and women and is not related to androgenetic alopecia.

stress a. psychogenic a.

syphilitic a., a. syphili'tica alopecia involving the eyebrows, beard, and scalp in secondary syphilis; it occurs in small, irregular scattered patches, resulting in a moth-eaten appearance. Called also *moth-eaten a.*

total a., a. tota'lis complete loss of hair from the entire scalp, resulting from progression of alopecia areata.

traction a. traumatic alopecia due to continuous or prolonged traction on the hair, such as in certain hairstyles or in the habit of compulsively twisting one's own hair.

traumatic a. a type of telogen effluvium caused by injury to the hair follicles, such as by rubbing, traction, or a chemical agent, and confined to the areas thus traumatized.

traumatic marginal a. traction alopecia occurring along the scalp margin.

triangular a., a. triangula'ris bilateral rounded triangular areas of alopecia in the anterior temporal area, seen most often as a component of male pattern androgenetic alopecia.

universal a., a. universa'lis loss of hair over the entire body, resulting from progression of alopecia areata.

al·o·pe·cic (al"o-pe'sik) 1. pertaining to alopecia. 2. bald.

Alo·prim (al'o-prim) trademark for a preparation of allopurinol.

Alor (ə-lor') trademark for a combination preparation of aspirin and hydrocodone bitartrate.

Alora (ə-lor'ə) trademark for a preparation of estradiol.

alo·se·tron hy·dro·chlo·ride (ə-lo'sə-tron) a selective antagonist of specific serotonin receptors, used in the treatment of severe chronic irritable bowel syndrome in women; administered orally.

Alox·i (a-lok'se) trademark for a preparation of palonosetron hydrochloride.

ALP alkaline phosphatase.

Al·pers syndrome (al'pərz) [Bernard Jacob *Alpers*, American neurologist, 1900–1981] see under *syndrome*.

al·pha (al'fə) [A, α] the first letter of the Greek alphabet. See also α-.

al·pha$_2$-an·ti·plas·min (al'fə an"tĭ-plaz'min) see under *antiplasmin*.

al·pha$_1$-an·ti·tryp·sin (al'fə an"tĭ-trip'sin) 1. a plasma protein of the serpin group, an α_1-globulin with M_r of 53,000, produced primarily in the liver; it is an acute phase reactant and inhibits the activity of elastase, cathepsin G, trypsin, and other proteolytic enzymes. Deficiency of this protein is associated with development of emphysema. Also written *α_1-antitrypsin*. Called also *alpha$_1$-protease* or *proteinase inhibitor*. 2. alpha$_1$-proteinase inhibitor (human).

Al·pha Chy·mar (al'fə ki'mər) trademark for a preparation of chymotrypsin.

al·pha fe·to·pro·tein (al'fə fe"to-pro'tēn) a plasma protein produced by the fetal liver, yolk sac, and gastrointestinal tract; serum levels decline markedly by the age of one year but are again elevated in many hepatocellular carcinomas and teratocarcinomas and embryonal cell carcinomas; elevated levels may also be seen in benign liver disease, such as cirrhosis and viral hepatitis. Used in monitoring the response of hepatomas and germ cell neoplasms to treatment and in antenatal diagnosis of neural tube defects (indicated by elevated amniotic fluid alpha-fetoprotein levels).

Al•pha•gan (al′fə-gan) trademark for a preparation of brimonidine tartrate.

al•pha glob•u•lin (al′fə glob′u-lin) see *α-globulins*, under *globulin.*

al•pha-1,4-glu•co•si•dase de•fi•cien•cy (al′fə gloo-ko′sĭ-dās) glycogen storage disease, type II.

Al•pha•her•pes•vi•ri•nae (al″fə-hur″pēz-vir-i′ne) the herpes simplex virus and related viruses, a subfamily of Herpesviridae. Genera of medical and veterinary importance include *Iltovirus, Mardivirus, Simplexvirus,* and *Varicellovirus.*

al•pha-lo•be•line (al′fə lo′bə-lēn) lobeline.

al•pha•lyt•ic (al″fə-lit′ik) 1. blocking α-adrenergic receptors. 2. alpha-adrenergic blocking agent.

al•pha$_2$-mac•ro•glob•u•lin (al′fə mak′ro-glob″u-lin) α_2-macroglobulin.

al•pha•mi•met•ic (al″fə-mi-met′ik) 1. stimulating or mimicking stimulation of α-adrenergic receptors. 2. an alpha-adrenergic agent.

Al•pha•nate (al′fə-nāt″) trademark for a preparation of antihemophilic factor (human).

Al•pha•Nine SD (al′phə-nīn″) trademark for a preparation of coagulation factor IX (human).

Al•pha•pap•il•lo•ma•vi•rus (al″fə-pap″ĭ-lo′mə-vi″rəs) a genus of viruses of the family Papillomaviridae that contains several of the human papillomaviruses.

Al•pha•pro•teo•bac•te•ria (al″fə-pro″te-o-bak-tēr′e-ə) [*alpha* the first letter of the Greek alphabet + *Proteobacteria*] a class of bacteria of the Proteobacteria, grouped together on the basis of 16S rRNA sequence analysis; organisms of medical interest are included in the orders Caulobacterales, Rhizobiales, Rickettsiales, and Sphingomonadales.

Al•pha•ret•ro•vi•rus (al″fə-ret′ro-vi″rəs) a genus of the family Retroviridae, characterized by a dense, spherical, symmetrically located inner core. These are not found in humans but can cause serious diseases in other animals. Species include avian leukosis virus and Rous sarcoma virus. alpharetrovi′ral *adj*

al•pha-to•coph•er•ol (al′fə to-kof′ər-ol) vitamin E.

Al•pha•trex (al″fə-treks′) trademark for preparations of betamethasone dipropionate.

Al•pha•vi•rus (al′fə-vi″rəs) [*alpha* the first letter of the Greek alphabet + *virus*] a genus of viruses of the family Togaviridae that cause encephalitis or febrile illness with rash or arthralgia, including eastern, western, and Venezuelan equine encephalitis viruses, chikungunya virus, Everglades virus, igbo-ora virus, Mayaro virus, o'nyong-nyong virus, Ross River virus, Semliki Forest virus, and Sindbis virus. Formerly called *group A arboviruses.* alphavi′ral *adj*

al•pha•vi•rus (al′fə-vi″rəs) any virus belonging to the genus *Alphavirus.*

Al•port syndrome (al′port) [Arthur Cecil *Alport*, South African–born English physician, 1880–1959] see under *syndrome.*

al•pra•zo•lam (al-pra′zo-lam) [USP] a short-acting benzodiazepine used as an antianxiety agent in the treatment of anxiety disorders and panic disorders and for short-term relief of anxiety symptoms, administered orally.

al•pros•ta•dil (al-pros′tə-dil) [USP] name for prostaglandin E_1 when used pharmaceutically as a vasodilator and platelet aggregation inhibitor; used for the temporary maintenance of patent ductus arteriosus until corrective or palliative surgery can be performed in neonates with congenital heart defects; administered intravenously or intra-arterially. It is also administered by intracavernosal injection, intraurethral suppository, or the rectal route to facilitate erection in men with impotence; an intracavernosal injection is used as an aid in diagnosis of erectile dysfunction and in imaging of penile vasculature.

ALPS autoimmune lymphoproliferative syndrome.

Al•rex (al′reks) trademark for a preparation of loteprednol.

ALS amyotrophic lateral sclerosis; antilymphocyte serum.

al•ser•ox•y•lon (al″sər-ok′sə-lon) a purified extract of *Rauwolfia serpentina*, containing reserpine and other amorphous alkaloids; used orally as an antihypertensive.

Al•stroe•me•ria (al-strə-me′re-ə) [Baron Klos von *Alstroemer*, Swedish botanist, 19th century] A genus of flowering South American plants of the family Amaryllidaceae. Several species are popular ornamental plants and are sources of allergic contact dermatitis.

Al•ström syndrome (ahl′strəm) [Carl-Henry *Alström*, Swedish geneticist, 1907–1993] see under *syndrome.*

ALT alanine transaminase.

Al•tace (al′tās) trademark for a preparation of ramipril.

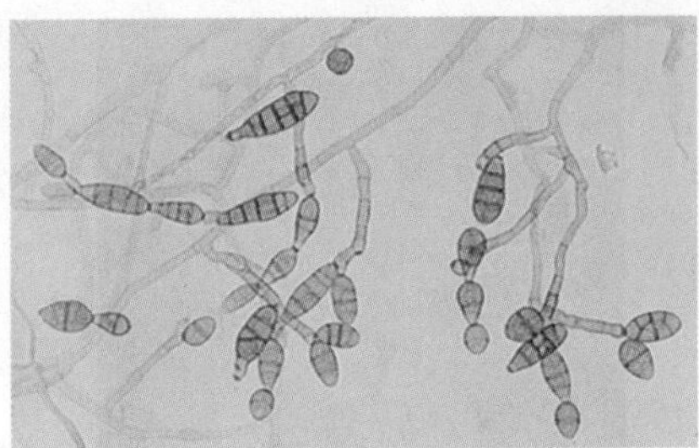

■ *Alternaria*, with dematiaceous conidia borne in chains on short conidiophores. Multicelled conidia have angular cross-walls and taper distally.

Alt. dieb. [L.] alter′nis die′bus (every other day).

Al•te•mei•er procedure (awl-tə-mi′ər) [William A. *Altemeier*, American surgeon, 1910–1983] see under *procedure.*

al•te•plase (al′tə-plās) [USP] a tissue plasminogen activator (see under *activator*) produced by recombinant DNA technology; used in fibrinolytic therapy for acute myocardial infarction and as a thrombolytic in the treatment of acute ischemic stroke and acute pulmonary embolism, administered intravenously.

al•ter (awl′tər) to castrate, as housepets or livestock.

al•ter•ego•ism (awl″tər-e′go-iz-əm) interest and sympathy for persons who are in the same situation as or are otherwise similar to one's self.

al•ter•nans (awl-tur′nanz) [L., pres. part. of *alternare* to do by turns] 1. alternating; see *pulsus alternans*, under *pulsus.* 2. alternation.

cardiac a. alternation of the heart.

electrical a. alternating variations in the amplitude of specific electrocardiographic waves over successive cardiac cycles.

mechanical a. alternation of the heart, used particularly in contrast with electrical alternans.

pul′sus a. see under *pulsus.*

total a. pulsus alternans in which alternate beats are so weak that they are not detected, causing apparent halving of the pulse rate.

Al•ter•na•ria (awl″tər-nar′e-ə) a genus of Fungi Imperfecti of the form-class Hyphomycetes, form-family Dematiaceae; it has dark-colored conidia and somewhat resembles *Trichophyton.* It causes several diseases of plants and is a common allergen in human bronchial asthma; it occasionally causes alternariosis of the skin or lung.

al•ter•nar•ia•tox•i•co•sis (awl″tər-nar″e-ə-tok-sĭ-ko′sis) a form of mycotoxicosis in animals caused by members of the genus *Alternaria.*

al•ter•nar•i•o•sis (awl″tər-nar-e-o′sis) infection by species of *Alternaria*, usually seen as a cutaneous or lung infection in weak or immunocompromised patients.

al•ter•nate (awl′tər-nət) 1. following in turns. 2. pertaining to every other one in a series. 3. occurring in place of another; acting as a substitute.

al•ter•nat•ing (awl′tər-nāt″ing) 1. occurring in regular succession. 2. alternately direct and reversed.

al•ter•na•tion (awl″tər-na′shən) [L. *alternare* to do by turns] the succession of two opposing or different events in turn.

a. of generations the regular alternation of two or more different forms or of different modes of reproduction in the life cycle; it may be used specifically for the alternating formation of diploid and haploid generations.

a. of the heart alternating variation in the intensity of the heartbeat or pulse over successive cardiac cycles of regular rhythm. Called also *mechanical alternans.* Cf. *electrical alternans.*

Al•te•ro•mo•na•da•ceae (awl″tər-o-mo″nə-da′se-e) the sole family of the order Alteromonadales; medically important organisms are contained in the genus *Shewanella.*

Al•te•ro•mo•na•da•les (awl″tər-o-mo″nə-da′lēz) [L. *alter* another + Gr. *monas* unit, from *monos* single] an order of chiefly marine bacteria of the class Gammaproteobacteria, phylum Proteobacteria, consisting of gram-negative, straight or curved rods that are motile by a single polar flagellum. Organisms are non–spore-forming, facultatively anaerobic or strictly aerobic, and chemo-organotrophic; most are nonpathogenic. It contains the single family Alteromonadaceae.

Al•thaea (al-the′ə) a genus of Old World herbs having terminal clusters of showy flowers; *A. officina′lis*, the marshmallow, is used medicinally.

Alt. hor. [L.] alter′nis ho′ris (every other hour).

Al•tin•ac (al′tin-ak) trademark for preparations of tretinoin.

Alt•mann fluid (ahlt′mahn) [Richard *Altmann*, German histologist, 1852–1900] see under *fluid.*

Alt•mann-Gersh method (ahlt′mahn gersh′) [R. *Altmann;* Isidore *Gersh*, American anatomist,1907–1998] see under *method*.

Al•to•prev (al′to-prev) trademark for a preparation of lovastatin.

Al•tra•cin (al-tra′sin) trademark for a preparation of bacitracin.

al•tret•amine (al-tret′ə-mēn) [USP] an antineoplastic agent used in the palliative treatment of ovarian carcinoma; administered orally. Although structurally related to certain alkylating agents, it does not appear to act similarly; its activity is related to the degree to which it is demethylated by the hepatic microsomal enzyme system, but the exact mechanism is unknown. Called also *hexamethylmelamine*.

al•trose (al′trōs) an aldohexose isomeric with glucose at carbons 2 and 3.

al•tru•ism (al′troo-iz-əm) unselfish concern for the needs or interests of others, providing gratification vicariously or from their responses.

Alu-Cap (al′u-kap) trademark for a preparation of dried aluminum hydroxide gel.

Alu•drox (al-u′droks) trademark for a preparation of aluminum hydroxide gel, magnesium hydroxide, and simethicone.

al•um (al′əm) [L. *alumen*] 1. an odorless, colorless crystalline substance, with local astringent and styptic properties and a sweet taste, prepared from bauxite and sulfuric acid, with the addition of ammonium *(ammonium a.)* or potassium *(potassium a.)*. It is also used as an adjuvant in adsorbed vaccines and toxoids. 2. any of a group of double sulfates formed on the type of this compound.

ammonium a. [USP] alum prepared with the addition of ammonium; used topically as an astringent.

burnt a., dried a., exsiccated a. ammonium or potassium alum heated to drive off the water of crystallization; used as an astringent.

potassium a. [USP] alum prepared with the addition of potassium; used topically as an astringent.

alu•mi•na (ə-loo′mĭ-nə) 1. aluminum oxide. 2. *(in pharmaceuticals)* aluminum hydroxide.

hydrated a. aluminum hydroxide.

alu•mi•nat•ed (ə-loo′mĭ-nāt″əd) charged with alum.

al•u•min•i•um (al″u-min′e-əm) aluminum.

alu•mi•no•sis (ə-loo″mĭ-no′sis) a form of pneumoconiosis caused by the presence of aluminum-bearing dust in the lungs; cf. *bauxite pneumoconiosis*.

alu•mi•num (Al) (ə-loo′mĭ-nəm) an extremely light, whitish, lustrous, metallic element, obtainable from bauxite or clay: specific gravity, 2.699; atomic weight, 26.982; atomic number, 13. It is very malleable and ductile and has many industrial uses. In dentistry it is used for the manufacture of instruments for the fabrication of dentures, obturators, and other prosthetic devices and as a base for artificial dentures. The aluminum of the pharmacopeia is a fine, free-flowing, silvery powder, free from gritty or discolored particles. Aluminum compounds are used chiefly for their antacid and astringent properties. Excessive amounts in the body have a variety of toxic effects; see *aluminum poisoning*, under *poisoning*.

a. acetate a salt, $C_6H_9AlO_6$, prepared by the reaction of aluminum hydroxide and acetic acid; used in solution as an astringent.

a. aminoacetate dihydroxyaluminum aminoacetate.

a. ammonium sulfate ammonium alum.

basic a. carbonate an aluminum hydroxide–aluminum carbonate complex, available only in the form of *basic aluminum carbonate gel* (see under *gel*).

a. chloride [USP] aluminum chloride hexahydrate, $AlCl_3{\bullet}6H_2O$, used topically as an astringent and anhidrotic.

a. chlorohydrate [USP] the hydrate of aluminum chloride hydroxide, $Al_2Cl(OH)_5$, having astringent and anhidrotic properties; used as an antiperspirant and as an anhidrotic in the treatment of hyperhidrosis. Called also *a. hydroxychloride*.

colloidal a. hydroxide aluminum hydroxide gel.

a. glycinate dihydroxyaluminum aminoacetate.

a. hydrate a. hydroxide.

a. hydroxide $Al(OH)_3$, used as an antacid and as a phosphate binder in treatment of urolithiasis and hyperphosphatemia; the usual form is *aluminum hydroxide gel* or *dried aluminum hydroxide gel* (see under *gel*). It is also used as an adjuvant in adsorbed vaccines and toxoids.

a. hydroxychloride a. chlorohydrate.

a. monostearate [NF] a combination of aluminum with variable proportions of stearic acid and palmitic acid; used in preparation of a suspension of penicillin G procaine.

a. oxide a compound, occurring naturally as corundum and in hydrated form as bauxite, that is the raw material in aluminum production; impure crystalline forms include emery, ruby, and sapphire. Very fine grains are used in the production of abrasives, refractories, ceramics, catalysts, laboratory wares, and fluxes, to strengthen dental ceramics, and in chromatography.

a. phosphate $AlPO_4$, used as an adjuvant in adsorbed toxoids and vaccines, as a component (with calcium sulfate and sodium silicate) in dental cements, and, in the form of aluminum phosphate gel, as an antacid.

a. potassium sulfate potassium alum.

a. silicate Al_2SiO_5, the silicate salt of aluminum. It occurs in several different hydrated forms in nature that have pharmaceutical or dental uses; see *attapulgite*, *bentonite*, *fuller's earth*, *kaolin*, and *zeolite*. See also *silicatosis*.

a. subacetate a basic aluminum acetate, used topically in solution as an astringent.

a. sulfate [USP] a powerful astringent, $Al_2(SO_4)_3{\bullet}xH_2O$, used topically as a local antiperspirant; also used as a pharmaceutical necessity in the preparation of aluminum subacetate topical solution.

alun•dum (ə-lun′dəm) electrically fused aluminum oxide used in making laboratory appliances that must withstand intense heat.

Al•u•pent (al′u-pent) trademark for preparations of metaproterenol sulfate.

Al•ur•ate (al′ūr-āt) trademark for a preparation of aprobarbital.

Alus•tra (a-lus′trə) trademark for a preparation of hydroquinone.

Alu-Tab (al′u-tab) trademark for a preparation of dried aluminum hydroxide gel.

al•vei (al′ve-i) [L.] genitive and plural of *alveus*.

al•veo•bron•chi•ol•i•tis (al″ve-o-brong″ke-o-li′tis) inflammation of the bronchioles and alveoli of the lungs.

al•veo•lal•gia (al″ve-o-lal′jə) [*alveolo-* + *-algia*] pain in a dental alveolus, such as after tooth extraction. See also *dry socket*, under *socket*.

al•ve•o•la•ri•za•tion (al-ve-o″lə-rĭ-za′shən) the formation of new pulmonary alveoli; most occurs in the fetus or infant, but some occurs throughout life.

al•ve•o•late (al-ve′ə-lāt) marked by honeycomb-like pits; called also *faveolate*.

al•ve•o•lec•to•my (al″ve-o-lek′tə-me) [*alveol-* + *-ectomy*] subtotal or complete excision of the alveolar process of the maxilla or mandible.

al•ve•o•li (al-ve′o-li) genitive and plural of *alveolus*.

al•ve•o•li•tis (al″ve-o-li′tis) 1. inflammation of a pulmonary alveolus. 2. inflammation of a dental alveolus; called also *odontobothritis*.

allergic a. hypersensitivity pneumonitis.

cryptogenic fibrosing a. idiopathic pulmonary fibrosis.

extrinsic allergic a. hypersensitivity pneumonitis.

fibrosing a. idiopathic pulmonary fibrosis.

lymphocytic a. alveolitis with inflammatory CD4 or CD8 cells in the alveoli. A type with CD4 cells is seen in early stages of sarcoidosis, and a type with CD8 cells is seen in hypersensitivity pneumonitis.

a. sic′ca doloro′sa dry socket.

alveol(o)- [L. *alveolus, q.v.*] a combining form denoting relationship to an alveolus, especially a dental alveolus.

al•ve•o•lo•cap•il•lary (al-ve″ə-lo-kap′ĭ-lar″e) pertaining to the pulmonary alveoli and capillaries.

al•ve•o•lo•cla•sia (al-ve″ə-lo-kla′zhə) [*alveolo-* + Gr. *klasis* breaking] destruction of the dental alveolus; see *marginal periodontitis*, under *periodontitis*.

al•ve•o•lo•den•tal (al-ve″ə-lo-den′təl) pertaining to a tooth and its alveolus.

al•ve•o•lo•gen•e•sis (al-ve″ə-lo-jen′ə-sis) the formation and development of pulmonary alveoli.

al•ve•o•lo•la•bi•al (al-ve″ə-lo-la′be-əl) pertaining to the alveolar processes and the lips.

al•ve•o•lo•lin•gual (al-ve″ə-lo-ling′gwəl) pertaining to the alveolar processes and the tongue.

al•ve•o•lo•me•rot•o•my (al-ve″ə-lo″mə-rot′ə-me) [*alveolo-* + *mero-*[1] + *-tomy*] excision of part of the alveolar process.

al•ve•o•lo•na•sal (al-ve″ə-lo-na′səl) pertaining to the alveolar point and the nasion.

al•ve•o•lo•pal•a•tal (al-ve″ə-lo-pal′ə-təl) pertaining to the alveolar process and palate.

al•ve•o•lo•plas•ty (al-ve′ə-lo-plas″te) [*alveolo-* + *-plasty*] conservative contouring of the alveolar process, in preparation for immediate or future denture construction. **alveoloplas′tic** *adj*

interradicular a., intraseptal a. the surgical removal of the interradicular bone and collapsing of the cortical plates on each other to achieve an acceptable or more desirable contour.

al•ve•o•lot•o•my (al″ve-ə-lot′ə-me) [*alveolo-* + *-tomy*] incision into a dental alveolus; see also *alveolectomy*.

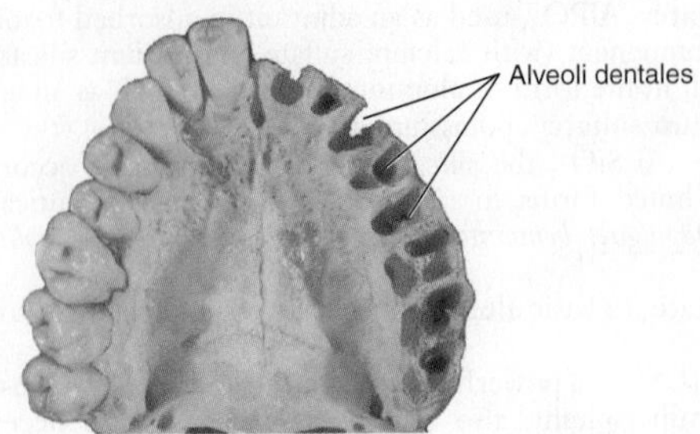

■ Alveoli dentales maxillae (dental alveoli of the maxilla).

al·ve·o·lus (al-ve′ə-ləs) gen. and pl. *alve′oli* [L., dim. of *alveus* hollow] a small saclike structure, especially in the jaws or lungs. Cf. *acinus*. **alve′olar** *adj*

dental a., a. denta′lis [TA] one of the cavities or sockets in the alveolar process of the mandible or maxilla, in which the roots of the teeth are held by fibers of the periodontal ligament. Called also *alveolar cavity* and *tooth socket*. See also *alveoli dentales mandibulae* and *alveoli dentales maxillae*.

alve′oli denta′les mandi′bulae [TA] the dental alveoli of the mandible.

alve′oli denta′les maxil′lae [TA] the dental alveoli of the maxilla.

primitive alveoli, primordial alveoli terminal sacs.

pulmonary alveoli, alve′oli pulmo′nis alveoli of lung: small polyhedral outpouchings along the walls of the alveolar sacs and alveolar ducts; through these walls gas exchange takes place between alveolar gas and pulmonary capillary blood.

al·ve·rine citrate (al′vĕ-rēn) an anticholinergic used as a smooth muscle relaxant in disorders of the gastrointestinal and genitourinary tracts.

Al·ves·co (al-ves′ko) trademark for a preparation of ciclesonide.

al·ve·us (al′ve-əs) gen. and pl. *al′vei* [L.] a trough or a canal.

a. hippocam′pi [TA], **a. of hippocampus** the thin layer of white matter that covers the ventricular surface of the hippocampus.

al·vim·o·pan (al-vim′o-pan) a peripherally-acting antagonist to μ-opioid receptors, used to accelerate the time needed for recovery of the intestinal tract after resection of part of the small or large intestine.

alym·phia (a-lim′fe-ə) [*a-*[1] + *lymph-* + *-ia*] deficiency or absence of the lymph.

alym·pho·cy·to·sis (a-lim″fo-si-to′sis) lymphocytopenia.

alym·pho·pla·sia (a-lim-fo-pla′zhə) failure of development of lymphoid tissue.

Alz·hei·mer disease (dementia), etc. (awltz′hi-mər) [Alois *Alzheimer*, German neurologist, 1864–1915] see *primary degenerative dementia*, under *dementia*, and see under *cell* and *disease*, and at *Stains and Staining Methods*, under *stain*.

AM [L.] Ar′tium Magis′ter (Master of Arts).

Am 1. americium. 2. see under *allotype*.

am ametropia; meter angle; myopic astigmatism.

AMA Aerospace Medical Association; American Medical Association; Australian Medical Association.

ama (ah′mə) [Sanskrit] according to ayurveda, physical and mental toxins that are produced by poor digestion and living habits and accumulate and clog the channels of the body.

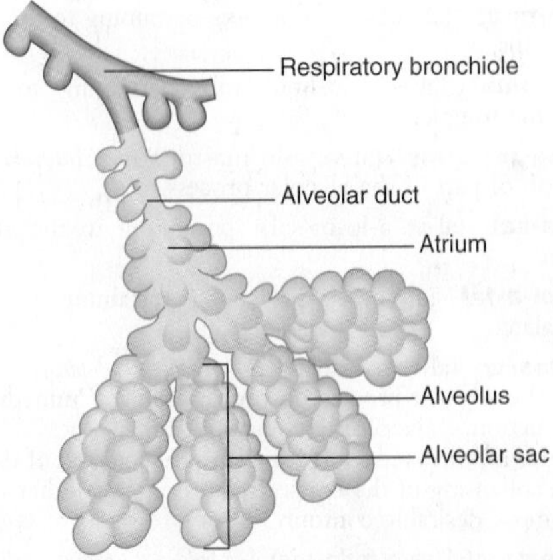

■ Alveoli pulmonis (pulmonary alveoli) and associated structures.

am·a·cri·nal (am″ə-kri′nəl) amacrine.

am·a·crine (am′ə-krēn) [*a-*[1] + *macro-* + *inos*] 1. having no long processes. 2. amacrine cell; see under *cell*.

Am·a·dori product (ah″mah-dor′e) [Mario *Amadori*, Italian chemist, 1886–1941] see under *product*.

amal·gam (ə-mal′gəm) [Gr. *malagma* poultice or soft mass] an alloy in which mercury is one of the components.

dental a. an amalgam containing mercury, silver, tin, copper, and sometimes zinc, which is prepared by mixing mercury with amalgam alloy to form a silvery, soft paste for condensation into the prepared cavity where it hardens to form a dental restoration.

retrograde a. see under *filling*.

amal·ga·mate (ə-mal′gə-māt″) to unite a metal in an alloy with mercury; to form an amalgam. Cf. *triturate*.

amal·ga·ma·tion (ə-mal′gə-ma′shən) trituration (def. 3).

amal·ga·ma·tor (ə-mal′gə-māt″ər) triturator.

AMAN acute motor axonal neuropathy.

Am·a·ni·ta (am″ə-ni′tə) [Gr. *amanitai* a sort of fungus] a genus of mushrooms of the family Amanitaceae, order Agaricales, several of which are poisonous.

A. musca′ria fly agaric, a species that produces muscarine and ibotenic acid; ingestion causes intoxication resembling drunkenness, followed by loss of consciousness.

A. pantheri′na a species that produces muscarine; ingestion causes intoxication followed by loss of consciousness.

A. phalloi′des the destroying angel or death cup, a species that produces a hemolysin and a mixture of amatoxins such as phalloidin, which are protoplasmic poisons; ingestion causes potentially fatal mushroom poisoning (see under *poisoning*).

A. ver′na the death angel, a highly poisonous species that contains peptide toxins similar to those of *A. phalloides*.

A. viro′sa the destroying angel, a highly poisonous species that contains peptide toxins similar to those of *A. phalloides*.

Am·a·ni·ta·ceae (am″ə-ni-ta′se-e) a family of mushrooms (order Agaricales), which includes the genus *Amanita*.

ama·ni·tine (ə-mă-nĭ′tin) a poisonous glycoside found in the deadly species of *Amanita*.

aman·i·to·tox·in (ə-man′ĭ-to-tok″sin) amatoxin.

aman·ta·dine hy·dro·chlo·ride (ə-man′tə-dēn) [USP] 1-aminoadamantane, an antiviral of the adamantane group, used for prophylaxis and treatment of influenza A. Because it augments the release of dopamine, it is also used as an antidyskinetic in treatment of parkinsonism and drug-induced extrapyramidal reactions; administered orally.

am·a·ranth (am′ə-ranth) 1. any plant of the genus *Amaranthus*. 2. a red dye, formerly made from amaranth plants but now made synthetically as an azo dye; formerly used in food, drugs, and cosmetics (FD&C Red No. 2) but now banned by the FDA for any of those uses.

Am·a·ran·thus (am″ə-ran′thəs) [L., from Gr. *amarantos* unfading] a genus of herbs of the family Amarantaceae, a source of the dye amaranth. Several species have medical and food uses, and some in the western United States cause hay fever. Some are high in nitrates and oxalates and can cause nitrite or oxalate poisoning in ruminants.

A. retroflex′us pigweed or prince's feather, a species found in pastures that contains oxalates and nitrates and can cause neurologic or kidney disorders in cattle and pigs. See also *oxalate poisoning*, under *poisoning*.

am·a·rine (am′ə-rēn) [L. *amarus* bitter] a poisonous crystalline base from oil of bitter almonds; also prepared artificially.

am·a·roid (am′ə-roid) any of a group of bitter principles of vegetable origin that stimulate the secretion of saliva and gastric juice.

am·a·roi·dal (am″ə-roi′dəl) somewhat bitter; also resembling a bitter in properties.

Am·a·ryl (am′ə-rəl) trademark for a preparation of glimepiride.

am·a·se·sis (am″ə-se′sis) [*a-*[1] + Gr. *masēsis* chewing] inability to chew food.

amas·tia (ə-mas′te-ə) [*a-*[1] + *mast-* + *-ia*] congenital absence of the mammae; sometimes applied to masculine breast characteristics in an adult female. Called also *amazia*.

amas·ti·gote (ə-mas′tĭ-gōt) [*a-*[1] + Gr. *mastix* whip] a morphologic stage in the life cycle of some kinetoplastid protozoa; the oval or round cell has a nucleus, kinetoplast, and basal body but has neither an undulating membrane nor an external flagellum. Called also *Leishman-Donovan body*. Cf. *choanomastigote*, *epimastigote*, *opisthomastigote*, *promastigote*, and *trypomastigote*.

amatho·pho·bia (ə-math″o-fo′be-ə) [Gr. *amathos* sand + *-phobia*] irrational dread of dust.

am·a·tol (am′ə-tol) a war explosive, being a mixture of trinitrotoluene and ammonium nitrate; moderately toxic by ingestion, inhalation, and absorption through the skin; highly irritating.

am·a·tox·in (am′ə-tok″sin) any in a class of cyclic hepatotoxins found in *Amanita phalloides* and other mushrooms of the genera *Amanita,* as well as species of *Chlorophyllum* and *Galerina;* ingestion causes potentially fatal mushroom poisoning (see under *poisoning*). Called also *Amanita toxin.*

am·au·ro·sis (am″aw-ro′sis) [L., from Gr. *amaurōsis* darkening] 1. blindness. 2. in a more limited sense, loss of vision in which there is no apparent lesion of the eye, such as from disease of the optic nerve, spine, or brain. Cf. *amblyopia.* **amaurot′ic** *adj*

central a., a. centra′lis, cerebral a. amaurosis due to disease of the central nervous system.

a. congenita of Leber Leber congenital a.

diabetic a. loss of vision due to diabetes mellitus, such as diabetic retinopathy or diabetic cataracts.

a. fu′gax a transient episode of blindness or partial blindness affecting one eye, caused by ischemia of the eye and lasting ten minutes or less. Sometimes used synonymously with *transient monocular blindness* (q.v.).

intoxication a. toxic amblyopia.

Leber congenital a. a genetically heterogeneous, autosomal recessive disorder of the retina, characterized by severe or complete loss of vision that becomes apparent early in infancy, with absent or attenuated electroretinogram responses, inattention to visual stimuli, sluggish pupillary responses, nystagmus, roving eye movements, hyperopia, and photophobia. Called also *a. congenita of Leber* and *congenital retinal blindness.*

a. partia′lis fu′gax sudden transitory partial blindness.

reflex a. blindness caused by the reflex action of a remote irritation.

saburral a. blindness that occurs in an attack of acute gastritis.

toxic a. toxic amblyopia.

uremic a. loss of vision due to uremia.

ama·zia (ə-ma′zə) [*a-*[1] + *maz-* + *-ia*] amastia.

am·be·no·ni·um chlo·ride (am″bə-no′ne-əm) a cholinesterase inhibitor used in the treatment of myasthenia gravis to treat the symptoms of muscular weakness and fatigue; administered orally.

amb(i)- [L.] an inseparable prefix meaning on all sides.

am·bi·dex·ter·i·ty (am″bĭ-dek-ster′ĭ-te) the ability to perform acts requiring manual skill with either hand, some ordinarily being performed with one and some with the other.

am·bi·dex·trism (am″bĭ-dek′striz-əm) ambidexterity.

am·bi·dex·trous (am″bĭ-dek′strəs) pertaining to or characterized by ambidexterity.

Am·bi·en (am′be-ən) trademark for a preparation of zolpidem tartrate.

am·bi·ent (am′be-ənt) [L. *ambire* to surround] surrounding; encompassing; prevailing.

am·bi·lat·er·al (am″bĭ-lat′ər-əl) [*ambi-* + *lateral*] pertaining to or affecting both the right and the left side. Cf. *bilateral.*

am·bi·le·vos·i·ty (am″bĭ-lə-vos′ĭ-te) the inability to perform acts requiring manual skill with either hand.

am·bi·le·vous (am″bĭ-le′vəs) [*ambi-* + *levo-* + *-ous*] pertaining to or characterized by ambilevosity.

Am·bil·har (am′bil-hahr) trademark for preparations of niridazole.

am·bi·o·pia (am″be-o′pe-ə) [L.] diplopia.

am·bi·sex·u·al (am″bĭ-sek′shoo-əl) [*ambi-* + *sexual*] 1. bisexual. 2. hermaphroditic. 3. denoting sexual characteristics common to both sexes, e.g., pubic hair.

am·bi·sin·is·ter (am″bĭ-sin′is-tər) [*ambi-* + *sinister*] ambilevous.

am·bi·si·nis·trous (am″bĭ-sĭ-nis′trəs) ambilevous.

Am·Bi·some (am′bĭ-sōm) trademark for a preparation of amphotericin B liposomal complex.

am·biv·a·lence (am-biv′ə-ləns) [*ambi-* + L. *valentia* strength, power] the simultaneous existence of conflicting attitudes, emotions, ideas, or wishes toward the same object. **ambiv′alent** *adj*

am·bi·ver·sion (am″bĭ-vur′zhən) a balance of introversion and extroversion.

am·bi·vert (am′bĭ-vərt) a person who is intermediate between an extrovert and an introvert.

ambly- [Gr. *amblys* dull] a combining form denoting dullness.

am·bly·a·phia (am-ble-a′fe-ə) [*ambly-* + Gr. *haphē* touch + *-ia*] tactile hypoesthesia.

am·bly·chro·ma·sia (am″ble-kro-ma′zhə) the condition of staining faintly or of having little chromatin.

am·bly·chro·mat·ic (am″ble-kro-mat′ik) [*ambly-* + *chromatic*] feebly staining.

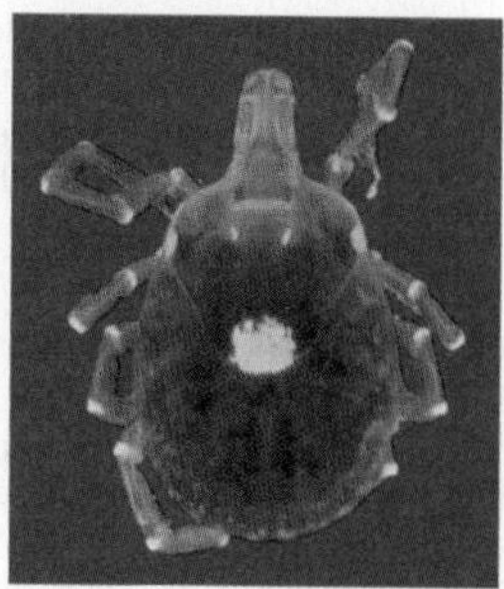

■ *Amblyomma americanum* adult female.

am·bly·geu·stia (am″ble-goo′ste-ə) hypogeusia.

Am·bly·om·ma (am″ble-om′ə) [*ambly-* + Gr. *omma* eye] a genus of ticks of the family Ixodidae, some of which transmit diseases.

A. america′num the Lone Star tick of the southern United States, a vector of Rocky Mountain spotted fever in humans and tick paralysis in humans and dogs.

A. cajennen′se the Cayenne tick, a species of Central and South America that has a vicious bite and attacks many different mammals and birds; it transmits Rocky Mountain spotted fever to humans.

A. coo′peri a South American species that feeds on rodents in Brazil and is a vector for Rocky Mountain spotted fever.

A. hebrae′um the bont tick, an African species that transmits heartwater to sheep, goats, and cattle and boutonneuse fever and African tick-bite fever to humans.

A. macula′tum the Gulf Coast tick, a species found along the coast of the Gulf of Mexico; immature forms feed on rodents and birds, and adult ticks feed on larger mammals, sometimes spreading heartwater and tick paralysis.

A. ova′le a tropical tick of dogs and tapirs that can transmit tick paralysis.

A. variega′tum an African species that feeds on domestic animals and transmits the virus causing Nairobi sheep disease and the rickettsiae causing heartwater in domestic animals and African tick-bite fever in humans.

am·bly·ope (am′ble-ōp) a person with amblyopia.

am·bly·o·pia (am″ble-o′pe-ə) [*ambly-* + *-opia*] impairment of vision due to abnormal development, without detectable organic lesion of the eye. Cf. *amaurosis.* **amblyop′ic** *adj*

alcoholic a. see *nutritional a.* and *toxic a.*

ametropic a. amblyopia with a high refractive error in both eyes.

anisometropic a. amblyopia that exists in both eyes but to different degrees.

a. ex anop′sia amblyopia resulting from disuse.

arsenic a. amblyopia due to arsenic poisoning.

color a. impairment of color vision, caused by toxic or other influences.

deficiency a. nutritional a.

deprivation a. amblyopia due to a media opacity in the visual axis.

nocturnal a. abnormal dimness of vision at night.

nutritional a. central or cecocentral scotomata due to poor nutrition; seen in alcoholics and patients with severe nutritional deprivation or vitamin B_{12} deficiency, as in pernicious anemia. Complete recovery is possible with good diet and B vitamins; prolonged deficiency results in permanent loss of central vision.

quinine a. amblyopia following large doses of quinine; thought to be due to anemia of the retina.

reflex a. amblyopia resulting from peripheral irritation.

strabismic a. amblyopia resulting from suppression of vision in one eye to avoid diplopia.

tobacco a. nutritional or toxic amblyopia caused by ingestion of tobacco.

toxic a. amblyopia due to poisoning, as from tobacco or alcohol.

traumatic a. amblyopia due to injury.

uremic a. amblyopia due to uremia.

am·blyo·scope (am′ble-o-skōp″) [*amblyopia* + *-scope*] a hand-held reflecting stereoscope that can measure convergence and divergence, measure or train binocular vision, or stimulate vision in an amblyopic eye.

major a. a large, table-mounted amblyoscope that has greater freedom for adjustment than a simple amblyoscope.

Am·blys·to·ma (am-blis′to-mə) Ambystoma.

am·bo (am′bo) ambon.

ambo- [L. *ambo* both] a combining form signifying both, on both sides.

am·bo·cep·tor (am′bo-sep″tər) [*ambo-* + L. *capere* to take] Ehrlich's term for complement-fixing antibody, which he thought had two receptors, one for antigen, one for complement; now used colloquially to denote the anti–sheep red blood cell antibody used in complement fixation tests.

am•bon (am′bon) the ring of fibrocartilage forming the edge of the sockets in which the heads of long bones are lodged.

am•bo•sex•u•al (am″bo-seks′u-əl) ambisexual.

am•bri•sen•tan (am-brĭ-sen′tan) an antagonist to endothelin receptors, having potent vasodilator action; administered orally in treatment of pulmonary artial hypertension.

Am•bro•sia (am-bro′zhə) [L., from Gr. *ambrotos* immortal] a genus of annual plants of the family Compositae, which produce quantities of windborne pollen and are important causes of hay fever. *A. artemisiaefo′lia* is the common or small ragweed; *A. tri′fida* is the giant ragweed.

am•bros•te•rol (am-bros′tə-rol) a phytosterol with a melting point of 147° to 149°C; found in the pollen of ragweed *(Ambrosia)*.

am•bu•lance (am′bu-ləns) [Fr.] a vehicle for conveying the sick or injured and equipped with apparatus for rendering emergency treatment.

am•bu•lant (am′bu-lənt) ambulatory.

am•bu•la•tion (am″bu-la′shən) walking.

am•bu•la•to•ry (am′bu-lə-tor″e) [L. *ambulare* to walk] 1. walking or able to walk; not confined to bed. 2. denoting a condition that can be treated without admission to a hospital. 3. pertaining to a procedure perfomed on an outpatient basis, whether in a hospital or a freestanding facility.

Am•bys•to•ma (am-bis′to-mə) a genus of salamanders used for experimental purposes; see *axolotl*. Called also *Amblystoma*.

am•cin•o•nide (am-sin′ə-nīd″) [USP] a synthetic corticosteroid used topically for the relief of inflammation and pruritus in corticosteroid-responsive dermatoses.

am•di•no•cil•lin (am-de′no-sil″in) a semisynthetic penicillin effective against many gram-negative bacteria and used in the treatment of urinary tract infections; administered intravenously or intramuscularly. Called also *mecillinam*.

a. pivoxil an ester of amdinocillin, administered orally in the treatment of urinary tract infections; the form used can be the ester or the hydrochloride salt of the ester.

AME apparent mineralocorticoid excess.

ame•ba (ə-me′bə) pl. *ame′bae* or *amebas* [L., from Gr. *amoibē* change] 1. a type of sarcodine protozoa of the superclass Rhizopoda that move their bodies by cytoplasmic extrusions called *pseudopodia*. Some are parasitic; see *amebiasis* and *amebic dysentery*. Also spelled *amoeba*. 2. any of various other cells or organisms resembling these protozoa. ame′bic *adj*

ramicristate amebae one of two subgroups of ameboid protozoa (class Lobosa), characterized by mitochondria with branching, tubular cristae; they are typically "naked" i.e., without a test. In this group are the orders Centramoebida, Euamoebida, and Leptomyxida. Called also *gymnamoebae*. The group is sometimes referred to as the subclass Gymnamoebia.

shelled amebae, testate amebae one of two subgroups of ameboid protozoa (class Lobosa), characterized by a body enclosed in a test, tectum, or other complex membrane external to the plasma membrane and glycocalyx. The order Arcellinida is in this group. The group is sometimes referred to as the subclass Testacealobosia.

amebi- a combining form denoting a relationship to an ameba.

ame•bi•a•sis (am″e-bi′ə-sis) [*ameb-* + *-iasis*] infestation with amebae, especially *Entamoeba histolytica*. Although other protozoa such as *Acanthamoeba*, *Balamuthia*, *Hartmannella*, and *Naegleria* can infect humans, this term usually refers specifically to infections with *E. histolytica*.

a. cu′tis cutaneous manifestations of amebiasis, usually in the form of painful ulcers or verrucous plaques. It is primarily seen in patients with active intestinal or hepatic disease, including from direct extension of intestinal amebiasis after surgery or extension of a hepatic abscess spontaneously or after surgery, although sometimes there is direct implantation of trophozoites on the skin with or without preexisting skin lesions.

hepatic a. 1. amebic hepatitis. 2. invasion of liver parenchyma by trophozoites of *Entamoeba histolytica*, leading to an amebic liver abscess. Called also *amebic hepatitis*.

intestinal a. amebic dysentery.

pleuropulmonary a., pulmonary a. amebic infection in the thoracic space, secondary to intestinal amebiasis and usually associated with amebic liver abscesses; it may affect the pleura, diaphragm, lung, or bronchi.

ame•bi•ci•dal (ə-me″bĭ-si′dəl) lethal to amebae; cf. *antiamebic*.

ame•bi•cide (ə-me′bĭ-sīd) [*amebi-* + *-cide*] an agent that kills amebae; cf. *antiamebic*. amebici′dal *adj*

ame•bi•form (ə-me′bĭ-form) shaped like or resembling an ameba.

ame•bi•o•sis (am″e-bi-o′sis) amebiasis.

ameb(o)- [L., from Gr. *amoibē* change] a combining form denoting a relationship to an ameba.

ame•bo•cyte (ə-me′bo-sīt″) [*amebo-* + *-cyte*] ameboid cell.

ame•bo•flag•el•late (ə-me″bo-flag′ə-lāt) [*amebo-* + *flagellate*] a microorganism having both an ameboid and a flagellate stage in its life cycle; said of certain protozoa.

ame•boid (ə-me′boid) [*amebo-* + *-oid*] resembling an ameba in form or in movements.

ame•boid•ism (ə-me′boid-iz-əm) a type of motility characteristic of amebae and certain other cells, occurring as a result of protrusion of pseudopods.

am•e•bo•ma (am″e-bo′mə) a tumorlike mass in the intestine, produced by localized inflammation due to amebiasis.

ame•bu•la (ə-me′bu-lə) [dim. of *ameba*] 1. the small ameboid daughter cell occurring following reproduction in certain rhizopod amebae. 2. the motile ameboid stage of a spore prior to aggregation in certain protozoa or on germination of the spore in others. Also written *amoebula*.

amel•a•no•sis (ə-mel″ə-no′sis) [*a-*[1] + *melanosis*] complete lack of melanin in the tissues. See also *hypomelanosis*.

ame•lia (ə-me′le-ə) [*a-*[1] + *-melia*] congenital absence of a limb or limbs; cf. *meromelia* and *phocomelia*.

amel•i•fi•ca•tion (ə-mel″ĭ-fĭ-ka′shən) [*amel-* + L. *facere* to make] the development of enamel cells into enamel.

amel•io•ra•tion (ə-mēl″yə-ra′shən) [L. *ad* to + *melior* better] improvement, as of the condition of a patient.

amel(o)- [Middle English *amel* enamel, from Old Fr. *esmal*] a combining form denoting enamel.

am•e•lo•blast (am′ə-lo-blast″) [*amelo-* + *-blast*[1]] a cylindrical epithelial cell in the innermost layer of the enamel organ which takes part in the elaboration of the enamel prism. The ameloblasts cover the dental papilla. Called also *adamantoblast*, *ganoblast*, and *enameloblast*.

am•e•lo•blas•to•ma (am″ə-lo-blas-to′mə) [*ameloblast* + *-oma*] a type of odontogenic tumor of tissue characteristic of the enamel organ but not differentiated to the point of enamel formation; it usually originates in the mandibular molar-ramus area and is usually benign but locally invasive. Ameloblastomas are often classified on the basis of histologic appearance, the most common subtypes being *follicular*, *cystic*, *acanthomatous*, *plexiform*, *basal cell*, and *granular cell;* they are also sometimes classified as *multicystic* versus *unicystic*. Called also *adamantinoma*.

acanthomatous a. ameloblastoma in which the cells occupying the position of the stellate reticulum have undergone squamous metaplasia.

basal cell a. a rare form of ameloblastoma microscopically resembling a basal cell carcinoma of the skin.

cystic a. ameloblastoma in which the follicular islands have undergone central cystic degeneration.

extraosseous a. a benign nonaggressive ameloblastoma occurring in the gingiva surrounding the alveolar bone; it resembles the intraosseous form histologically and is believed to originate in surface epithelium or odontogenic remnants.

follicular a. ameloblastoma composed of numerous discrete islands of tumor cells that mimic the normal dental follicle.

granular cell a. ameloblastoma in which the cytoplasm of the central neoplastic cells takes on a coarsely granular eosinophilic appearance.

malignant a. ameloblastoma exhibiting metastases that histologically resemble the primary lesion; cf. *ameloblastic carcinoma*.

melanotic a. melanotic neuroectodermal tumor.

multicystic a. ameloblastoma containing multiple cystic spaces; it may exhibit any or all of the histologic patterns described as subtypes of the lesion and is more aggressive and recurs more frequently than does unicystic ameloblastoma. Cf. *unicystic a.*

peripheral a. extraosseous a.

pigmented a. melanotic neuroectodermal tumor.

pituitary a. craniopharyngioma.

plexiform a. ameloblastoma, often cystic, in which the neoplastic cells have formed an interconnected network of strands.

plexiform unicystic a. a variant of unicystic ameloblastoma in which there is ameloblastic proliferation in an epithelial network on the cyst wall; it occurs in young adults, usually in the mandibular molar area.

solid a. multicystic a.

spindle cell a. malignant ameloblastoma in which the central portions of the tumor cell islands have become elongated.

unicystic a. ameloblastoma containing a single cystic space, characterized by intraluminal or mural growth; it may be a unilocular ameloblastoma or ameloblastic transformation of the epithelial lining of an odontogenic cyst. Cf. *multicystic a.*

am•e•lo•den•ti•nal (am″ə-lo-den′tĭ-nəl) pertaining to the enamel and dentin of a tooth.

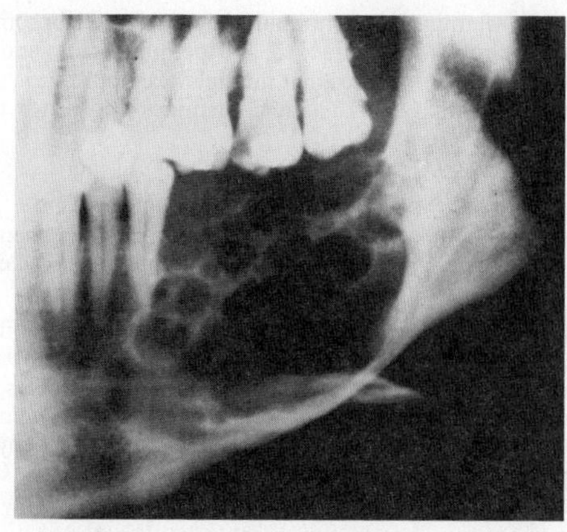

■ Multicystic ameloblastoma of the left body of the mandible.

am•e•lo•gen•e•sis (am″ə-lo-jen′ə-sis) [*amelo-* + *genesis*] the elaboration of dental enamel by ameloblasts.

a. **imperfec′ta** an autosomal dominant or X-linked disorder in which there is faulty development of the dental enamel owing to agenesis, hypoplasia, or hypocalcification of the enamel. It is marked by enamel that is very thin and friable and frequently stained in various shades of brown. Called also *hereditary brown enamel.*

am•e•lo•gen•ic (am″ə-lo-jen′ik) forming enamel; pertaining to amelogenesis.

am•e•lo•gen•in (am″ə-lo-jen′in) any of several proteins secreted by ameloblasts and forming the organic matrix of tooth enamel.

am•e•lus (am′ə-ləs) an individual exhibiting amelia.

Amen (a′men) trademark for a preparation of medroxyprogesterone acetate.

ame•nia (ə-me′ne-ə) [*a-*[1] + *men-* + *-ia*] amenorrhea.

amen•or•rhea (ə-men″o-re′ə) [*a-*[1] + *menorrhea*] absence or abnormal stoppage of the menses; called also *amenia.* **amenorrhe′al** *adj*

dietary a. amenorrhea accompanying loss of weight due to dietary restriction that is less extreme than that seen in anorexia nervosa and is not associated with psychological problems. Called also *nutritional a.*

dysponderal a. amenorrhea associated with disorder of weight, such as obesity or extreme underweight.

hypogonadotropic a. amenorrhea caused by failure to maintain a critical body fat-to-lean ratio, resulting in hypothalamic suppression; seen most often in women who engage in strenuous exercise, such as athletes, dancers, and those who are excessively weight conscious.

hypothalamic a. amenorrhea associated with disorders of the hypothalamus.

lactation a. absence of the menses associated with lactation.

nutritional a. dietary a.

ovarian a. amenorrhea resulting from deficiency of ovarian hormones.

physiologic a. absence of menses not due to organic disorder, such as that occurring in pregnancy.

pituitary a. absence of the menses owing to pituitary deficiency.

premenopausal a. physiologic decrease of menstruation during establishment of the climacterium.

primary a. failure of menstruation to occur at puberty.

relative a. menstrual flow which is less than normal for the individual; called also *oligomenorrhea.*

secondary a. cessation of menstruation after it has once been established at puberty.

traumatic a. amenorrhea due to adhesions, frequently a result of curettage, as in Asherman's syndrome.

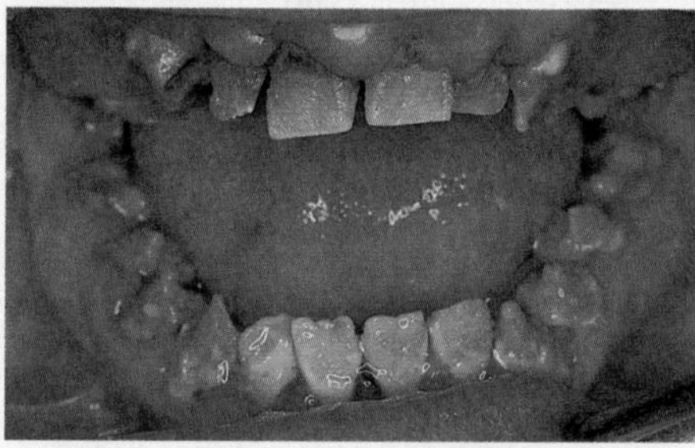

■ Amelogenesis imperfecta, hypocalcified type.

amen•sal•ism (a-men′səl-iz-əm) symbiosis in which one population (or individual) is adversely affected and the other is unaffected.

Amerge (ə-merj′) trademark for a preparation of naratriptan hydrochloride.

Amer•i•caine (ə-mer′ə-kān″) trademark for preparations of benzocaine.

Amer•i•can Type Cul•ture Col•lec•tion (ATCC) an organization established in Rockville, MD, as a depository for reference cultures. It maintains and distributes authentic reference strains of algae, bacteria, fungi, and protozoa; bacteriophages and viruses; and cell lines of animal tissues.

am•er•ic•i•um (Am) (am″ər-is′e-əm) the chemical element of atomic number 95, atomic weight 243, obtained by cyclotron bombardment of uranium and plutonium.

am•er•ism (am′ər-iz-əm) [*a-*[1] + *merism*] the quality of not splitting into segments or fragments.

am•er•is•tic (am″ər-is′tik) [*a-*[1] + *meristic*] not split into segments.

Ames test (āmz) [Bruce Nathan *Ames*, American biochemist, born 1928] see under *test.*

ame•tab•o•lon (am-ə-tab′o-lon) an animal that develops without undergoing metamorphosis.

ame•tab•o•lous (a″mə-tab′ə-ləs) not undergoing metamorphosis.

ameta•chro•mo•phil (ə-met″ə-kro′mo-fil) orthochromophil.

ameta•neu•tro•phil (ə-met″ə-noo′tro-fil) orthochromophil.

ameth•o•caine (ə-meth′o-kān) BAN for *tetracaine.*

ameth•op•ter•in (am″əth-op′tə-rin) methotrexate.

ame•tria (a-me′tre-ə) [*a-*[1] + *metr-* + *-ia*] congenital absence of the uterus.

am•e•trom•e•ter (am″ə-trom′ə-tər) [*ametropia* + *-meter*] an instrument for measuring the degree of ametropia.

am•e•tro•pia (am″ə-tro′pe-ə) [Gr. *ametros* disproportionate + *-opia*] discrepancy between the size and refractive powers of the eye, such that images are not brought to a proper focus on the retina; consequently hyperopia, myopia, or astigmatism are produced. See illustration at *refraction.* **ametrop′ic** *adj*

axial a. ametropia due to lengthening of the eyeball along the optic axis.

curvature a. ametropia due to variations in the curvature of the surface of the eye.

index a. ametropia due to alterations in the refractive index media of the eye.

position a. ametropia due to faulty position of the crystalline lens.

refractive a. ametropia due to fault in the dioptric system of the eye.

Ame•vive (am′ə-vēv) trademark for a preparation of alefacept.

Amh mixed astigmatism with myopia predominating over hyperopia.

AMI acute myocardial infarction.

am•i•an•thoid (am″e-an′thoid) [Gr. *amianthos* asbestos + *-oid*] having the appearance of asbestos.

-amic chemical suffix denoting a compound in which one carboxyl group of a dicarboxylic acid is replaced by a carboxamide group.

Am•i•car (am′ĭ-kar) trademark for preparations of aminocaproic acid.

am•i•clor•al (am″ĭ-klor′əl) a compound closely related to glucopyranose, administered as a veterinary feed additive.

ami•cro•scop•ic (a-mi″kro-skop′ik) submicroscopic.

amic•u•la (ə-mik′u-lə) [L.] plural of *amiculum.*

amic•u•lum (ə-mik′u-ləm) pl. *amic′ula* [L.] 1. a coat or covering. 2. a. olivare.

a. oliva′re [TA], a. of olive a capsule of myelinated fibers that surrounds the inferior olivary nucleus; called also *amiculum* and *siliqua olivae.*

ami•dap•sone (ă-mĭ-dap′sōn) a member of the dapsone group used as an antiviral in poultry.

am•i•dase (am′ĭ-dās) 1. [EC 3.5.1.4] an enzyme of the hydrolase class that catalyzes the formation of a monocarboxylic acid and ammonia by cleavage of the C—N bond of a monocarboxylic acid amide. 2. more generally, a term used in the recommended and trivial names of some amidohydrolases, particularly those acting on linear amides [EC 3.5.1].

Ami•date (am′ĭ-dāt) trademark for a preparation of etomidate.

am•ide (am′īd) [*am*monia + *-ide*] an organic compound derived from ammonia by substituting an acyl radical for hydrogen, or from an acid by replacing the —OH group by —NH_2.

niacin a., nicotinic acid a. niacinamide.

am•i•dine (am′ĭ-dēn″) any compound containing the amidino group.

am·i·dine-ly·ase (am'ĭ-dēn li'ās) [EC 4.3.2] a sub-subclass of enzymes of the lyase class that catalyze the cleavage of a carbon-nitrogen bond to eliminate the amidino group from an amidine such as adenylosuccinate or argininosuccinate.

am·i·dino (am-ĭ-dēn'o) the chemical group —C(=NH)—NH_2. As a prefix (amidino-), it indicates the presence in a compound of this group.

am·i·dino·hy·dro·lase (am-ĭ-dēn″o-hi'dro-lās) [EC 3.5.3] systematic name for enzymes of the hydrolase class that catalyze the hydrolysis of C—N bonds in linear amidines.

am·i·dino·trans·fer·ase (am-ĭ-dēn″o-trans'fər-ās) [EC 2.1.4] a sub-subclass of enzymes of the transferase class that catalyze the transfer of an amidino group from one compound to another. Called also *transamidinase*.

amido- a prefix indicating the presence of the radical NH_2 along with the radical CO.

am·i·do·ben·zene (ə-me″do-, am″ĭ-do-ben'zēn) aniline.

am·i·do·gen (ə-me'do-jen″) the hypothetic radical NH_2, found in amido compounds.

am·i·do·hy·dro·lase (ə-me″do-, am″ĭ-do-hi'dro-lās) systematic name for enzymes of the hydrolase class that catalyze the cleavage of carbon-nitrogen bonds in linear [EC 3.5.1] or cyclic [EC 3.5.2] amide compounds. Called also *deamidase*.

am·i·do-li·gase (ə-me″do-, am″ĭ-do-li'gās) [EC 6.3.5] systematic name for enzymes of the ligase class that catalyze the transfer of the amide nitrogen from glutamine to an acceptor molecule, driven by the concomitant hydrolysis of ATP to ADP or AMP and forming an amide or amidine group on the acceptor.

am·i·dol·y·sis (am″id-ol'is-is) the cleaving of small proteins by removal of amides. **amidolyt'ic** *adj*

am·i·do·phos·pho·ri·bo·syl·trans·fer·ase (ə-me″do-, am″ĭ-do-fos″fo-ri″bo-səl-trans'fər-ās) [EC 2.4.2.14] an enzyme of the transferase class that catalyzes the first committed step in purine nucleotide biosynthesis, the transfer of an amino group to phosphoribosylpyrophosphate from glutamine, forming phosphoribosylamine as well as glutamate and pyrophosphate. The reaction is inhibited by purine nucleotides.

Am·i·dos·to·mum (am″ĭ-dos'to-məm) a genus of nematodes of the superfamily Strongyloides. *A. an'seris* is parasitic in the mucous membrane of the intestinal tract of ducks and geese and may kill young birds by its excessive consumption of their blood.

am·i·dox·ime (am-ĭ-dok'sīm) any of a class of compounds formed from the amidines by substituting hydroxyl for a hydrogen atom of the amide group.

am·i·fos·tine (am″ĭ-fos'tēn) [USP] a chemoprotectant used to prevent renal toxicity in cisplatin chemotherapy; administered by intravenous infusion.

am·i·ka·cin (am″ĭ-ka'sin) [USP] a semisynthetic aminoglycoside antibiotic derived from kanamycin A, effective against a wide range of aerobic gram-negative bacilli and some gram-positive bacteria.

a. sulfate [USP] the sulfate salt of amikacin, used in the treatment of a wide variety of serious infections caused by susceptible gram-negative organisms; administered intramuscularly and intravenously.

Am·i·kin (am'ĭ-kin) trademark for a preparation of amikacin sulfate.

amil·o·ride hy·dro·chlo·ride (ə-mil'ə-rīd) [USP] a potassium-sparing diuretic that inhibits the reabsorption of sodium in the distal and proximal convoluted tubules and the collecting tubule; used in conjunction with a loop or thiazide diuretic for the treatment of edema and hypertension and for the prophylaxis and treatment of hypokalemia; administered orally.

am·il·ox·ate (am″il-ok'sāt) [USP] a cinnamate compound that absorbs ultraviolet B radiation; used topically as a sunscreen. Called also *isoamyl methoxycinnamate*.

amim·ia (a-mim'e-ə) [*a*-[1] + Gr. *mimos* actor, mime + *-ia*] loss of the power of expression by the use of signs or gestures.

am·i·na·tion (am″ĭ-na'shən) the creation of an amine, either by addition of an amino group to an organic acceptor compound or by reduction of a nitro compound.

amine (ə-mēn', am'in) an organic compound containing nitrogen; any member of a group of chemical compounds formed from ammonia by replacement of one or more of the hydrogen atoms by organic (hydrocarbon) radicals. The amines are distinguished as *primary*, *secondary*, and *tertiary*, according to whether one, two, or three hydrogen atoms are replaced. The amines include allylamine, arylamine, ethylamine, methylamine, phenylamine, propylamine, and many other compounds.

biogenic a. a type of amine synthesized by both plants and animals and frequently involved in signaling; prominent examples are neurotransmitters such as acetylcholine, catecholamines, and serotonin. Others are hormones or components of vitamins, phospholipids, bacteria, and ribosomes and include cadaverine, choline, histamine, muscarine, putrescine, and spermine.

sympathomimetic a's amines that mimic the actions of the sympathetic nervous system, comprising the catecholamines and drugs that mimic their actions.

vasoactive a's amines that cause vasodilation and increase small vessel permeability, e.g., histamine and serotonin.

amine-ly·ase (ə-mēn', am'in li'ās) [EC 4.3.3] any member of a sub-subclass of enzymes of the lyase class that catalyze the cleavage of a carbon-nitrogen bond within an amine.

amine ox·i·dase (cop·per-con·tain·ing) (ə-mēn', am'in ok'sĭ-dās kop'ər kən-tān'ing) [EC 1.4.3.6] a group of enzymes of the oxidoreductase class that catalyze the oxidative deamination of diamines, including histamine, to form aminoaldehydes, ammonia, and hydrogen peroxide. The enzymes can also convert primary monoamines to aldehydes. They are copper proteins and may contain pyridoxal phosphate. Called also *diamine oxidase*.

amine ox·i·dase (fla·vin-con·tain·ing) (ə-mēn', am'in ok'sĭ-dās fla'vin kon-tān'ing) [EC 1.4.3.4] a flavoprotein (FAD) enzyme of the oxidoreductase class that catalyzes the oxidative deamination of primary amines to form aldehydes and hydrogen peroxide. Substrates include serotonin, norepinephrine, epinephrine, dopamine, and also some secondary and tertiary amines. It occurs in several isozymes. Called also *monoamine oxidase (MAO)*. See also *monoamine oxidase inhibitor*, under *inhibitor*.

am·in·er·gic (am″ĭ-nur'jik) activated by, characteristic of, or secreting one of the biogenic amines.

ami·no (ə-me'no, am'ĭ-no″) the monovalent chemical group —NH_2. As a prefix (amino-) it indicates the presence in a compound of the group —NH_2.

ami·no·ace·tic ac·id (ə-me″no-ə-se'tik) glycine.

ami·no ac·id (AA) (ə-me'no) any organic compound containing an amino (—NH_2) and a carboxyl (—COOH) group. The 20 α-amino acids listed in the accompanying table are the amino acids from which proteins are synthesized by formation of peptide bonds during ribosomal translation of messenger RNA. Other amino acids occurring in proteins, such as hydroxyproline in collagen, are formed by posttranslational enzymatic modification of amino acid residues in polypeptide chains. There are also several important amino acids, such as the neurotransmitter γ-aminobutyric acid, that have no relation to proteins.

α-a. a. an amino acid whose amino and carboxyl groups are both attached to the same carbon atom.

branched-chain a. a's leucine, isoleucine, and valine; they are incorporated into proteins or catabolized for energy.

essential a. a's the nine α-amino acids required for protein synthesis that cannot be synthesized by humans and must be obtained in the diet: histidine, isoleucine, leucine, lysine, methionine, phenylalanine, threonine, tryptophan, and valine.

excitatory a. a's a group of nonessential amino acids that act as excitatory neurotransmitters in the central nervous system, including glutamic acid or L-glutamate, aspartic acid or L-aspartate, and the excitotoxins.

nonessential a. a's the eleven α-amino acids required for protein synthesis that are synthesized by humans and are not specifically required in the diet: alanine, arginine, asparagine, aspartic acid, cysteine, glutamic acid, glutamine, glycine, proline, serine, and tyrosine.

ω-a. a. an amino acid whose amino and carboxyl groups are attached to opposite ends of a carbon chain.

sulfur a. a's amino acids that contain sulfur, such as methionine, cysteine, and homocysteine.

ami·no-ac·id *N*-ac·e·tyl·trans·fer·ase (ə-me'no as'id as″ə-tēl-trans'fər-ās) [EC 2.3.1.1] an enzyme of the transferase class that catalyzes the transfer of an acetyl group from acetyl coenzyme A to the N-terminus of glutamate to form *N*-acetylglutamate. It can also act on aspartate and, slowly, on some other amino acids. Deficiency of the enzyme causes an aminoacidopathy with hyperammonemia but no oroticaciduria, similar to that seen in carbamoyl phosphate synthetase deficiency. Called also *N-acetylglutamate synthetase*.

ami·no·ac·id·emia (ə-me″no-as″ĭ-de'me-ə) an excess of amino acids in the blood; called also *hyperaminoacidemia*.

ami·no·ac·i·dop·a·thy (ə-me″no-as″ĭ-dop'ə-the) any of a group of inborn errors of metabolism caused by defects in enzymatic steps in the metabolic pathway of one or more amino acids or in a protein mediator necessary for transport of certain amino acids into or out of cells.

D-ami·no-ac·id ox·i·dase (ə-me'no as'id ok'sĭ-dās) [EC 1.4.3.3] an enzyme of the oxidoreductase class that catalyzes the oxidative deamination of D-amino acids to form 2-keto acids, producing hydrogen peroxide as

Name (Symbols)	Structural Formula	Name (Symbols)	Structural Formula
Alanine (Ala, A)	HOOC — CH(NH$_2$) — CH$_3$	Leucine (Leu, L)	HOOC — CH(NH$_2$) — CH$_2$ — CH(CH$_3$) — CH$_2$
Arginine (Arg, R)	HOOC — CH(NH$_2$) — CH$_2$ — CH$_2$ — CH$_2$ — NH — C(=NH) — NH$_2$	Lysine (Lys, K)	HOOC — CH(NH$_2$) — CH$_2$ — CH$_2$ — CH$_2$ — CH$_2$ — NH$_2$
Asparagine (Asn, N)	HOOC — CH(NH$_2$) — CH$_2$ — C(=O) — NH$_2$	Methionine (Met, M)	HOOC — CH(NH$_2$) — CH$_2$ — CH$_2$ — S — CH$_3$
Aspartic Acid (Asp, D)	HOOC — CH(NH$_2$) — CH$_2$ — COOH	Phenylalanine (Phe, F)	HOOC — CH(NH$_2$) — CH$_2$ —
Cysteine (Cys, C)	HOOC — CH(NH$_2$) — CH$_2$ — SH	Proline (Pro, P)	HOOC, H, N
Glutamic Acid (Glu, E)	HOOC — CH(NH$_2$) — CH$_2$ — CH$_2$ — COOH	Serine (Ser, S)	HOOC — CH(NH$_2$) — CH$_2$ — OH
Glutamine (Gln, Q)	HOOC — CH(NH$_2$) — CH$_2$ — CH$_2$ — C(=O) — NH$_2$	Threonine (Thr, T)	HOOC — CH(NH$_2$) — CH(OH) — CH$_3$
Glycine (Gly, G)	HOOC — CH(NH$_2$) — H	Tryptophan (Trp, W)	HOOC — CH(NH$_2$) — CH$_2$ — (H, N)
Histidine (His, H)	HOOC — CH(NH$_2$) — CH$_2$ — (H, N, N)	Tyrosine (Tyr, Y)	HOOC — CH(NH$_2$) — CH$_2$ — — OH
Isoleucine (Ile, I)	HOOC — CH(NH$_2$) — CH(CH$_3$) — CH$_2$ — CH$_3$	Valine (Val, V)	HOOC — CH(NH$_2$) — CH(CH$_3$) — CH$_3$

■ The 20 α-amino acids specified by the genetic code. The three-letter and single-letter symbols are used in presenting the sequence of a polypeptide or protein (e.g., Gly-Phe-Tyr); by convention, the N-terminal residue is shown at the left; the C-terminal residue at the right.

a byproduct. The enzyme is a flavoprotein found in the cytoplasm of kidney, brain, and liver; its metabolic role is unclear.

L-ami•no-ac•id ox•i•dase (ə-me′no as′id ok′sĭ-dās) [EC 1.4.3.2] an enzyme of the oxidoreductase class that catalyzes the oxidative deamination of L-amino acids to form 2-keto acids, producing hydrogen peroxide as a byproduct. The enzyme is a flavoprotein, present in liver and kidney and found in snake venom. It acts on all naturally occurring monocarboxylic L-amino acids except serine and threonine. The mammalian enzymes also attack 2-hydroxy acids; their function is unclear.

ami•no•ac•id•u•ria (ə-me″no-as″ĭ-du′re-ə) an excess of amino acids in the urine; many types are called by the name of the amino acid plus the suffix *-uria*, such as cystinuria, lysinuria, and tryptophanuria. Called also *hyperaminoaciduria.*

overflow a. aminoaciduria caused by excessive levels of a given amino acid in the blood.

renal a. aminoaciduria caused by defective transport mechanisms for amino acids in the renal tubules.

ami•no•acyl (ə-me″no-a′səl) an acyl radical of an amino acid, e.g., alanyl, glycyl, etc.

a. adenylate an amino acid residue linked via an acid anhydride bond to the 5′ phosphate of adenosine monophosphate; it is a high energy intermediate in the synthesis of aminoacyl-tRNA.

a.-tRNA an amino acid residue joined by an ester linkage to the 2′ or 3′ hydroxyl group of the terminal adenosine residue of a transfer RNA (see also *translation*).

ami•no•acy•lase (ə-me″no-a′sə-lās) [EC 3.5.1.14] an enzyme of the hydrolase class that catalyzes the cleavage of the acyl group from acylated L-amino acids. It occurs in the kidney and acts on a variety of substrates, including hippuric acid and benzamide.

ami•no•acyl-his•ti•dine di•pep•ti•dase (ə-me″no-a′səl his′tĭ-dēn di-pep′tĭ-dās) X-His dipeptidase.

ami•no•acyl•trans•fer•ase (ə-me″no-a″səl-trans′fər-ās) [EC 2.3.2] a sub-subclass of enzymes of the transferase class that catalyze the transfer of an aminoacyl group from one molecule to another with formation of an ester or an amide linkage.

ami•no•acyl-tRNA syn•the•tase (ə-me″no-a′səl sin′thə-tās) any of the group of ligases that catalyze the ATP-driven formation of a bond between an amino acid and a tRNA, activating the amino acids as a step in protein synthesis. Individual enzymes are highly specific for one amino acid and for any tRNA corresponding to that amino acid; they are known by the name of the amino acid acted on, e.g., alanyl-tRNA synthetase (formally called alanine–tRNA ligase, EC 6.1.1.7).

α-ami•no•adip•ate (ə-me″no-ə-dip′āt) the anionic form of α-aminoadipic acid.

2-ami•no•ad•i•pate trans•am•i•nase (ə-me″no-ə-dip′āt trans-am′ĭ-nās) [EC 2.6.1.39] an enzyme of the transferase class that catalyzes the oxidative deamination of α-ketoglutarate to form glutamate. The reaction is a step in the degradation of lysine and hydroxylysine. Called also *2-aminoadipate aminotransferase.*

α-ami•no•adip•ic ac•id (ə-me″no-ə-dip′ik) a dicarboxylic amino acid occurring as an intermediate in the degradation of lysine and hydroxylysine. Written also *2-aminoadipic acid.*

α-ami•no•adip•ic•ac•id•uria (ə-me″no-ə-dip″ik-as″ĭ-du′re-ə) excretion of α-aminoadipic acid in the urine.

α-ami•no•adip•ic semi•al•de•hyde syn•thase (ə-me″no-ə-dip′ik sem″e-al′də-hīd sin′thās) a bifunctional enzyme comprising the two enzyme activities lysine-ketoglutarate reductase (q.v.) and saccharopine dehydrogenase (q.v.) and catalyzing the first two steps in the major pathway of lysine degradation. Deficiency of the enzyme, an autosomal recessive trait, causes hyperlysinemia or its variant saccharopinuria.

***p*-ami•no•azo•ben•zene** (ə-me″no-a″zo-ben′zēn) a yellow azo dye; it is carcinogenic.

o-ami·no·azo·tol·u·ene (ə-me″no-az″o-tol′u-ēn) a red crystalline azo dye that is actively carcinogenic.

ami·no·ben·zene (ə-me″no-ben′zēn) aniline.

ami·no·ben·zo·ate (ə-me″no-ben′zo-āt) *p*-aminobenzoate, any salt or ester of *p*-aminobenzoic acid.

a. potassium [USP] the potassium salt of *p*-aminobenzoic acid, administered orally as an antifibrotic in the treatment of dermatologic disorders marked by fibrosis or nonsuppurative inflammation.

a. sodium the monosodium salt of *p*-aminobenzoic acid, which has been used in combination with sodium salicylate as an analgesic.

p-ami·no·ben·zo·ic ac·id (PAB, PABA) (ə-me″no-ben-zo′ik) a substance required for the synthesis of folic acid by many organisms. PABA is included in the B vitamin complex, although it is not an essential nutrient for humans. It also absorbs ultraviolet light, specifically ultraviolet B, and is used as *aminobenzoic acid* [USP] as a topical sunscreen.

p-ami·no·bi·phen·yl (ə-me″no-bi-fen′əl) a nitrogen-substituted arylamine formerly used in dyemaking and certain other industrial processes; because of its toxicity and carcinogenicity, it is now used mainly to induce cancer in laboratory animals. Written also *4-aminobiphenyl.* Called also *p-aminodiphenyl*, *p-biphenylamine*, and *xenylamine.*

γ-ami·no·bu·ty·rate (ə-me″no-bu′tə-rāt) the conjugate base of γ-aminobutyric acid.

4-ami·no·bu·ty·rate trans·am·i·nase (ə-me″no-bu′tə-rāt trans-am′ĭ-nās) [EC 2.6.1.19] an enzyme of the transferase class that catalyzes the transfer of an amino group from γ-aminobutyrate (GABA) to α-ketoglutarate, forming glutamate and succinate semialdehyde. The reaction occurs predominantly in the liver and in the neurons of the brain. The enzyme can also act on β-alanine and β-aminoisobutyrate. Deficiency of the enzyme, an autosomal recessive trait, causes psychomotor retardation, hypotonia, hyperreflexia, and accelerated linear growth, with high levels of GABA, homocarnosine, and β-alanine in the cerebrospinal fluid. See also *β-alanine–α-ketoglutarate transaminase.* Called also *GABA transaminase* and *aminobutyrate aminotransferase.*

γ-ami·no·bu·tyr·ic ac·id (GABA) (ə-me″no-bu-tēr′ik) an ω-amino acid formed in the metabolism of L-glutamic acid; it is the principal inhibitory neurotransmitter in the brain but is also found in several extraneural tissues, including kidney and pancreatic beta cells. In the brain, it is released from presynaptic cells upon depolarization, and via receptor binding it modulates membrane chloride permeability and inhibits postsynaptic cell firing. Called also *4-aminobutyric acid.*

ami·no·ca·pro·ic ac·id (ə-me″no-kə-pro′ik) [USP] a preparation of ε-aminocaproic acid, used orally and intravenously for treatment of acute bleeding syndromes due to excessive fibrinolysis and for the prevention and treatment of postsurgical hemorrhage.

ε-ami·no·ca·pro·ic ac·id (ə-me″no-kə-pro′ik) an ω-amino acid that inhibits plasminogen activators and, to a lesser degree, plasmin.

7-ami·no·ceph·a·lo·spo·ran·ic ac·id (ə-me″no-sef″ə-lo-spor-an′-ik) the active nucleus of the semisynthetic cephalosporins, structurally related to the penicillin nucleus (6-aminopenicillanic acid) and obtained by hydrolysis of cephalosporin C; modification of positions 3 and 7 of this nucleus results in antibiotics with a variety of antibacterial and pharmacologic characteristics.

Amino-Cerv (ə-me′no-surv″) trademark for a combination preparation of sodium propionate, methionine, cystine, inositol, and urea.

ami·no·cyc·li·tol (ə-me″no-sik′lĭ-tol) aminoglycoside.

ami·no·di·ni·tro·phe·nol (ə-me″no-di-ni″tro-fe′nol) dinitroaminophenol.

p-ami·no·di·phen·yl (ə-me″no-di-fen′əl) *p*-aminobiphenyl.

ami·no·glu·teth·i·mide (ə-me″no-gloo-teth′ĭ-mīd) [USP] an inhibitor of the enzymatic conversion of cholesterol to pregnenolone, thereby reducing corticosteroid synthesis and an aromatase inhibitor that inhibits conversion of androstenedione to estrone in peripheral tissues; used in the treatment of Cushing syndrome and as an investigational drug in the treatment of breast carcinoma; administered orally. It was formerly used as an anticonvulsant, but this use has been discontinued because of the adrenal suppressant effect.

ami·no·gly·co·side (ə-me″no-gli′ko-sīd) any of a group of antibiotics (e.g., amikacin, gentamicin, streptomycin) derived from various bacterial species, especially those of genus *Streptomyces*, or produced synthetically. Aminoglycosides inhibit bacterial protein synthesis by binding with the 30S ribosomal subunit and are bactericidal.

p-ami·no·hip·pu·rate (ə-me″no-hip′u-rāt) a salt, conjugate base, or ester of *p*-aminohippuric acid. See also *p-aminohippurate clearance*, under *clearance.*

p-a. sodium [USP] the sodium salt of *p*-aminohippuric acid; administered by intravenous injection to measure effective renal plasma flow and to determine the functional capacity of the tubular excretory mechanism.

p-ami·no·hip·pu·ric ac·id (PAH, PAHA) (ə-me″no-hĭ-pūr′ik) the glycine amide of *p*-aminobenzoic acid, which is filtered by the renal glomeruli and secreted into the urine by the proximal tubules. See also *p-aminohippurate sodium* and see *p-aminohippurate clearance*, under *clearance.*

ami·no·hy·dro·lase (ə-me″no-hi′dro-lās) systematic name for some enzymes of the hydrolase class that catalyze the hydrolysis of an amino group from a cyclic amidine [EC 3.5.4] or a nitrile [EC 3.5.5]. Cf. *deaminase.*

ami·no·hy·droxy·ben·zo·ic ac·id (ə-me″no-hi-drok″se-ben-zo′ik) a group of chemotherapeutic agents used in the treatment of infections with acid-fast bacilli.

ami·no·iso·bu·ty·rate (ə-me″no-i″so-bu′tər-āt) an anionic form of aminoisobutyric acid.

β-ami·no·iso·bu·ty·rate–py·ru·vate trans·am·i·nase (ə-me″no-i″so-bu′tər-āt pi′roo-vāt trans-am′ĭ-nās) an enzyme of the transferase class that catalyzes the oxidative deamination of *R*-β-aminoisobutyrate, transferring the amino group to pyruvate; the reaction is a step in the catabolism of thymine. Deficiency of the enzyme, an autosomal recessive trait, causes β-aminoisobutyricaciduria. In EC nomenclature, called (R)-*3-amino-2-methylpropionate–pyruvate transaminase.* Called also *β-aminoisobutyrate–pyruvate aminotransferase.*

ami·no·iso·bu·tyr·ic ac·id (ə-me″no-i″so-bu-tir′ik) an amino acid not occurring in proteins; the *R*-β- isomer is produced in the degradation of thymine and excreted in excess in β-aminoisobutyricaciduria; the *S*-β-isomer is a metabolite of valine; and the α- form, which does not occur naturally, is used in studies of transport and cytokinin effects.

β-ami·no·iso·bu·tyr·ic·ac·id·uria (ə-me″no-i″so-bu-tir″ik-as-ĭ-du′re-ə) excessive excretion of *R*-β-aminoisobutyric acid in the urine, occurring as a benign metabolic variant due to deficiency of β-aminoisobutyrate–pyruvate transaminase; it also occurs in certain illnesses in which rapid tissue destruction and deoxyribonucleic acid catabolism occur. Called also *hyper-β-aminoisobutyricaciduria.*

ami·no·lev·u·lin·ate (ə-me″no-lev″u-lin′āt) the conjugate base of aminolevulinic acid.

ami·no·lev·u·lin·ate de·hy·dra·tase (ə-me″no-lev″u-lin′āt de-hi′drə-tās) porphobilinogen synthase.

5-ami·no·lev·u·lin·ate syn·thase (ə-me″no-lev″u-lin′āt sin′thās) [EC 2.3.1.37] an enzyme of the transferase class that catalyzes the condensation of the succinyl group from succinyl coenzyme A with glycine to form δ-aminolevulinate. It is a pyridoxal phosphate protein and the reaction occurs in mitochondria as the first step of the heme biosynthetic pathway. The enzyme is a key regulatory enzyme in heme biosynthesis and, in liver at least, is feedback inhibited by heme. Abbreviated ALAS. Written also *δ-aminolevulinate synthase.*

ami·no·lev·u·lin·ic ac·id (ALA) (ə-me″no-lev″u-lin′ik) δ-aminolevulinic acid; an intermediate in the synthesis of heme, produced from succinyl-CoA and glycine. Two molecules of ALA are condensed to form porphobilinogen. Blood and urinary ALA levels are increased in lead poisoning, and urinary levels are increased in a variety of porphyrias.

a. a. hydrochloride the hydrochloride salt of aminolevulinic acid, applied topically in the treatment of nonhyperkeratotic actinic keratoses of the face and scalp. It is metabolized to protoporphyrin IX, a photosensitizer, which accumulates in the skin at the sites of application; upon exposure of the sites to light of appropriate energy and wavelength together with oxygen, a photodynamic reaction occurs with cytotoxic effects.

am·i·nol·y·sis (am″ə-nol′ə-sis) [*amine* + *-lysis*] reaction with an amine, resulting in the addition of (or substitution by) an imino group, —NH—.

ami·no·meth·ane (ə-me″no-meth′ān) methylamine.

ami·no·meth·yl (ə-me″no-meth′əl) a methylated amino group, the acyl radical of methylamine (aminomethane).

***(R)*-3-ami·no-2-meth·yl·pro·pi·o·nate–py·ru·vate trans·am·i·nase** (ə-me″no-meth″əl-pro′pe-ən-āt pi′roo-vāt trans-am′ĭ-nās) [EC 2.6.1.40] EC nomenclature for *β-aminoisobutyrate–pyruvate transaminase.*

ami·no·ni·tro·thi·a·zole (ə-me″no-ni″tro-thi′ə-zōl) a green or orange-colored powder used in the treatment and prevention of blackhead in turkeys.

6-ami·no·pen·i·cil·lan·ic ac·id (ə-me″no-pen″ĭ-səl-an′ik) the active nucleus common to all penicillins; it may be obtained from cultures of *Penicillium* to which no side-chain precursors have been added. Substitution at the 6-amino position results in semisynthetic penicillins with a variety of antibacterial and pharmacologic characteristics.

ami·no·pen·i·cil·lin (ə-me″no-pen″ĭ-sil′in) any in a group of penicillin derivatives that have an amino group substitution; they have a broad spectrum of activity but are destroyed by β-lactamase.

ami·no·pen·ta·mide sul·fate (ə-me″no-pen′tə-mīd) [USP] an anticholinergic with atropine-like action; used as an antiemetic and antidiarrheal in veterinary practice.

ami·no·pep·ti·dase (ə-me″no-pep′tĭ-dās) any member of a sub-subclass of enzymes of the hydrolase class that catalyze the hydrolytic cleavage of the N-terminal amino acid or dipeptide from a peptide chain; they are exopeptidases and occur in plasma and many tissues.

***p*-ami·no·phe·nol** (ə-me″no-fe′nol) a dye intermediate and photographic developer and the parent compound of acetaminophen; it is a potent allergen that causes dermatitis as well as asthma and methemoglobinemia on inhalation.

am·i·noph·yl·line (am″ĭ-nof′ə-lin) [USP] a salt of theophylline prepared from theophylline and aqueous ethylenediamine, used as a bronchodilator for the prevention and treatment of symptoms of asthma and of reversible bronchospasm associated with chronic bronchitis, emphysema, or other chronic obstructive pulmonary disease; administered orally, rectally, or intravenously. It is also administered intravenously as an antidote to dipyridamole toxicity.

ami·no·pu·rine (ə-me″no-pu′rēn) a purine that is a component of nucleic acid and the nucleotides; the aminopurines include adenine and guanine.

ami·no·py·rine (ə-me″no-pi′rēn) a compound chemically related to antipyrine, used in liver function tests. See *aminopyrine breath test*, under *test.*

ami·no·quin·o·line (ə-me″no-kwin′o-lēn) a heterocyclic compound derived from quinoline by the addition of an amino group.

4-a's a group of antimalarial compounds effective against the erythrocytic stage of *Plasmodium;* it includes amodiaquine, chloroquine, and hydroxychloroquine.

8-a's a group of antimalarial compounds effective against the exoerythrocytic stage of *Plasmodium;* of this group, only primaquine is widely used.

amin·o·rex (ə-min′o-reks) an amphetamine lying midway between dextroamphetamine and methamphetamine in central nervous system–stimulating effect and having anorectic actions; it has been a drug of abuse.

ami·no·sa·lic·y·late (ə-me″no-sə-lis′ə-lāt) any salt of *p*-aminosalicylic acid; aminosalicylates are antibacterials effective against mycobacteria and have been used as tuberculostatics.

a. sodium [USP] the dihydrated sodium salt of *p*-aminosalicylic acid, an antibacterial effective against mycobacteria; administered orally as a tuberculostatic.

ami·no·sal·i·cyl·ic ac·id (ə-me″no-sal-ĭ-sil′ik) [USP] pharmaceutical name for *p-aminosalicylic acid;* administered orally as a tuberculostatic.

5-ami·no·sal·i·cyl·ic ac·id (5-ASA) (ə-me″no-sal-ĭ-sil′ik) mesalamine.

***p*-ami·no·sal·i·cyl·ic ac·id (PAS, PASA)** (ə-me″no-sal-ĭ-sil′ik) an analogue of *p*-aminobenzoic acid (PABA) that inhibits folic acid synthesis in *Mycobacterium tuberculosis* and is bacteriostatic, inhibiting growth and multiplication of the tubercle bacillus; available as *aminosalicylic acid* [USP].

ami·no·si·dine sul·fate (ə-me″no-si′din) paromomycin sulfate.

am·i·no·sis (am″ĭ-no′sis) the pathologic production of amino acids in the body.

Ami·no·sol (ə-me′no-sol) trademark for an amino acid preparation for intravenous injection.

ami·nos·uria (ə-me″no-su′re-ə) aminuria.

Ami·no·syn (ə-me′no-sin) trademark for a crystalline amino acid solution for intravenous administration; it contains a mixture of essential and nonessential amino acids but no peptides.

ami·no·tol·u·ene (ə-me″no-tol′u-ēn) toluidine.

ami·no·trans·fer·ase (ə-me″no-trans′fər-ās) transaminase.

3-ami·no·tri·az·ole (ə-me″no-tri′ə-zōl) amitrole.

am·in·uria (am″ĭ-nu′re-ə) an excess of amines in the urine.

ami·o·da·rone hy·dro·chlo·ride (ə-me′o-də-rōn″) a potassium channel blocking agent that prolongs the action potential duration and refractory period of all cardiac fibers; administered orally or by intravenous infusion in the treatment and prophylaxis of ventricular arrhythmias.

Am·i·paque (am′ĭ-pāk) trademark for metrizamide.

ami·sul·pride (am″ĭ-sul′prīd) a substituted benzamide that is a dopamine antagonist and is used as an antipsychotic; administered orally.

Am·i·ti·za (am″ĭ-ti′zə) trademark for a preparation of lubiprostone.

ami·to·sis (am″ĭ-to′sis) [*a*-[1] + *mitosis*] division of the nucleus by constriction without the formation of a spindle, condensation of chromosomes, or disruption of the nuclear membrane.

ami·tot·ic (am″ĭ-tot′ik) of the nature of amitosis; not occurring by mitosis.

am·i·traz (am′ĭ-traz) [USP] a topical acaricide used on cattle, sheep, pigs, and dogs.

am·i·trip·ty·line hy·dro·chlo·ride (am″ĭ-trip′tə-lēn) [USP] a tricyclic antidepressant of the dibenzocycloheptadiene group, also having sedative effects; it is also used in the treatment of enuresis, chronic pain, peptic ulcer, and bulimia nervosa. Administered orally and intramuscularly.

am·i·trole (am′ĭ-trol) an herbicide used on non-food crops; its use is restricted because it is an epigenetic carcinogen. Called also *3-aminotriazole.*

AML acute myelogenous leukemia.

am·lex·a·nox (am-lek′sə-noks″) a topical antiulcerative used in the treatment of recurrent aphthous stomatitis.

am·lo·di·pine bes·yl·ate (am-lo′dĭ-pēn″) a calcium channel blocking agent used in the treatment of hypertension and chronic stable and vasospastic angina; administered orally.

am·me·ter (am′me-tər) [*am*pere + *-meter*] an instrument calibrated to read in amperes or subdivisions of amperes the amount of electric current flowing in a circuit.

Am·mi (am′e) a genus of plants of the family Umbelliferae, native to Mediterranean countries. *A. ma′jus* and *A. visna′ga* contain psoralens and in large amounts are toxic to animals.

Am·mon fissure, operation (ah′mən) [Friedrich August von *Ammon,* German ophthalmologist and pathologist, 1799–1861] see under *fissure* and *operation.*

Am·mon's horn (am′ənz) [*Ammon,* a ram-headed god of the Egyptians] hippocampus proprius.

am·mo·ne·mia (ă-mo-ne′me-ə) hyperammonemia.

am·mo·nia (ə-mōn′yə) [Zeus *Ammon,* near whose temple in Libya it was formerly obtained] a colorless alkaline gas, NH_3, having a penetrating odor; it is soluble in water. Excessive levels in the blood are toxic (see *hyperammonemia*). It forms compounds in the form of ammonium (q.v.).

a. hemate a compound of ammonia and hematein, used as a violet-black stain for microscopic specimens.

a. N 13 [USP] ammonia in which a portion of the molecules are labeled with ^{13}N; administered intravenously for use in positron emission tomography of the cardiovascular system, brain, and liver.

am·mo·ni·a·cal (am″o-ni′ə-kəl) containing ammonia or treated with excess ammonia.

am·mo·nia-ly·ase (ə-mōn′yə-li′ās) [EC 4.3.1] a sub-subclass of enzymes of the lyase class that catalyze the formation of a C═C bond in a molecule by liberation of ammonia, e.g., histidine ammonia-lyase.

am·mo·ni·ate (ə-mo′ne-āt) 1. to treat or to combine with ammonia. 2. the product of combination with ammonia.

am·mo·ni·emia (ə-mo″ne-e′me-ə) hyperammonemia.

am·mo·ni·fi·ca·tion (ə-mo″nĭ-fĭ-ka′shən) the formation of ammonia by the action of bacteria on proteins.

am·mo·ni·o·mag·ne·si·um phos·phate (ə-mo″ne-o-mag-ne′ze-əm) ammonium magnesium phosphate.

am·mo·ni·um (ə-mo′ne-əm) the hypothetical radical, NH_4; it forms salts analogous to those of the alkaline metals.

a. alum see under *alum.*

a. bicarbonate NH_4HCO_3, having a slight ammoniacal odor and used in pharmacy to produce ammonium carbonate and as an expectorant.

a. carbamate $NH_2CO_2NH_4$, having an ammoniacal odor and used in pharmacy to produce ammonium carbonate.

a. carbonate [NF] a mixture of ammonium bicarbonate and ammonium carbamate in varying proportions, used as an ingredient of aromatic ammonia spirit and as a source of ammonia in smelling salts. It has also been used as an expectorant. Called also *hartshorn* and *sal volatile.*

a. chloride [USP] a systemic and urinary acidifying agent and diuretic administered orally or by intravenous infusion. It is also administered orally as an expectorant. Called also *a. muriate* and *sal ammoniac.*

a. lactate lactic acid neutralized with ammonium hydroxide, applied topically as a humectant in ichthyosis vulgaris and xerosis.

a. magnesium phosphate struvite.

a. molybdate [USP] the hexaammonium salt of molybdic acid, used as a supplement in parenteral feeding solutions and as a reagent.

a. muriate a. chloride.

a. nitrate NH_4NO_3; a chemical used in fertilizers, in matches, and in the manufacture of nitrous oxide gas and freezing compounds; it may accumulate in plants and lead to nitrite poisoning in livestock.

a. oxalate $NH_4OOCCOONH_4$; used as a test solution.

a. phosphate [NF] the diammonium salt of phosphoric acid, $(NH_4)_2HPO_4$, used as a buffering agent in pharmaceutical preparations. See also *struvite.*

a. tartrate a white crystalline compound soluble in water and alcohol; used in Cohn solution.

am•mo•ni•uria (ə-mo″ne-u′re-ə) hyperammonuria.

am•mo•nol•y•sis (am″o-nol′ĭ-sis) a process analogous to hydrolysis, but in which ammonia takes the place of water, resulting in attachment of (or replacement by) an amino group, NH_2.

am•mo•no•tel•ic (ə-mo″no-tel′ik) [*ammonia* + Gr. *telikos* belonging to the completion, or end] having ammonia as the chief excretory product of nitrogen metabolism, as in fresh-water fishes.

Am•mo•sper•moph•i•lus (am″o-spər-mof′ĭ-ləs) the antelope squirrels, a genus found in the deserts of western North America. *A. leucu′rus* is a natural host of a plague-transmitting flea.

am•ne•sia (am-ne′zhə) [Gr. *amnēsia* forgetfulness] lack or loss of memory; inability to remember past experiences.

anterograde a. impairment of memory for events occurring after the onset of amnesia; inability to form new memories. Cf. *retrograde a.*

circumscribed a. loss of memory for all events during a discrete, specific period of time. Called also *localized a.*

concussion a., concussive a. posttraumatic a.

continuous a. loss of memory for all events after a certain time, continuing up to and including the present.

dissociative a. [DSM-IV] a dissociative disorder characterized by a sudden loss of memory for important personal information, usually circumscribed or selective amnesia, rarely generalized or continuous amnesia, and which is not due to the direct effects of a psychogenic substance or a general medical condition; the amnesia may follow severe psychological stress or may be an unconscious response to internal conflicts or an intolerable life situation; complete recovery of memory almost always occurs.

episodic a. amnesia for a particular episode or a small area of experience.

generalized a. loss of memory encompassing the individual's entire life.

infantile a. the usual inability to recall the events of infancy and early childhood.

lacunar a. partial loss of memory; amnesia for certain isolated experiences.

localized a. 1. circumscribed a. 2. lacunar a.

neurological a. loss of memory caused by disease of or injury to the nervous system.

postconcussion a., postconcussional a. posttraumatic a.

posthypnotic a. a directed forgetfulness of the subject for experiences undergone while in the hypnotic state.

posttraumatic a. amnesia resulting from concussion or other head trauma. Called also *concussion, concussive, postconcussion,* or *traumatic a.* See also *amnestic syndrome,* under *syndrome.*

psychogenic a. dissociative a.

retrograde a. inability to recall events that occurred before the actual onset of amnesia; loss of memories of past events. Cf. *anterograde a.*

selective a. loss of memory for a group of related events but not for other events occurring during the same period of time.

tactile a. astereognosis.

transient global a. an episode of short-term memory loss, usually nonrecurrent, and lasting a few hours, without other signs or symptoms of neurological impairment; the cause is usually unknown but is occasionally an ischemic or epileptic attack.

traumatic a. posttraumatic a.

visual a. alexia.

am•ne•si•ac (am-ne′se-ak) a person affected with amnesia.

am•ne•sic (am-ne′sik) affected with or characterized by amnesia.

am•nes•tic (am-nes′tik) 1. amnesic. 2. causing amnesia.

amni(o)- [*amnion,* q.v.] a combining form denoting relationship to the amnion.

am•nio•cele (am′ne-o-sēl) omphalocele.

am•nio•cen•te•sis (am″ne-o-sen-te′sis) percutaneous transabdominal puncture of the uterus to obtain amniotic fluid.

am•nio•cho•ri•al (am″ne-o-kor′e-əl) pertaining to the amnion and chorion.

am•nio•cyte (am′ne-o-sīt) a cell of fetal origin in an amniotic fluid specimen, obtained during amniocentesis.

am•nio•gen•e•sis (am″ne-o-jen′ə-sis) [*amnio-* + *-genesis*] the development of the amnion.

am•ni•og•ra•phy (am″ne-og′rə-fe) [*amnio-* + *-graphy*] radiography of the gravid uterus after injection of opaque media into the amniotic fluid, outlining the amniotic cavity and fetus.

am•nio•in•fu•sion (am″ne-o-in-fu′zhən) introduction of solutions into the amnion, as to induce abortion, to counteract the late decelerations caused by cord compression, or to dilute thick meconium.

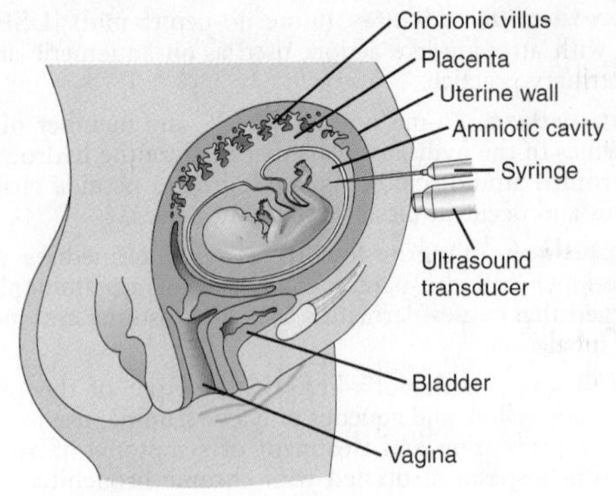

■ Amniocentesis.

am•ni•on (am′ne-on) [Gr. "bowl"; "membrane enveloping the fetus"] the thin but tough extraembryonic membrane of reptiles, birds, and mammals that lines the chorion and contains the embryo and later the fetus, with the amniotic fluid around it; in mammals it is derived from trophoblast by folding or splitting. See also *amniotic sac,* under *sac.*

a. nodo′sum a nodular condition of the fetal surface of the amnion, usually appearing near the insertion of the cord; it may be associated with multiple congenital abnormalities, especially hypoplastic kidneys and oligohydramnios.

am•ni•on•ic (am″ne-on′ik) amniotic.

am•ni•o•ni•tis (am″ne-o-ni′tis) inflammation of the amnion.

Am•ni•o•plas•tin (am-ne-o-plas′tin) trademark for the dried and sterilized amnionic membrane applied to prevent adhesions after craniotomy.

am•ni•or•rhea (am″ne-o-re′ə) [*amnio-* + *-rrhea*] the escape of amniotic fluid.

am•ni•or•rhex•is (am″ne-o-rek′sis) [*amnio-* + *-rrhexis*] rupture of the amnion.

am•nio•scope (am′ne-o-skōp″) an endoscope used in amnioscopy.

am•ni•os•co•py (am″ne-os′kə-pe) direct observation of the fetus and the color and amount of the amniotic fluid by means of a specially designed endoscope inserted through the uterine cervix.

Am•ni•o•ta (am-ne-o′tə) a major group of vertebrates comprising those which develop an amnion, including reptiles, birds, and mammals; opposed to Anamniota.

am•ni•ote (am′ne-ōt) any animal or group belonging to the Amniota.

am•ni•ot•ic (am″ne-ot′ik) pertaining to or developing an amnion.

am•ni•o•tome (am′ne-ə-tōm″) [*amnio-* + *-tome*] an instrument for cutting the fetal membranes.

am•ni•ot•o•my (am″ne-ot′ə-me) [*amnio-* + *-tomy*] deliberate rupture of the fetal membranes to induce labor.

amo•bar•bi•tal (am″o-bahr′bĭ-təl) an intermediate-acting barbiturate used orally as a sedative and hypnotic, particularly for preoperative sedation; called also *amylobarbitone.*

a. sodium [USP] the monosodium salt of amobarbital, administered orally, intravenously, and intramuscularly as a hypnotic and sedative, particularly for preoperative sedation, and intravenously in the emergency treatment of convulsions.

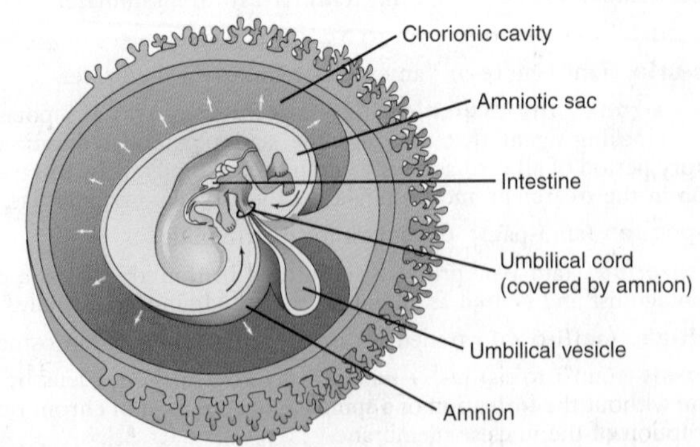

■ Amnion and other extraembryonic membranes surrounding a human embryo at 10 weeks; the amnion has enveloped the umbilical cord.

am·o·di·a·quine (am″o-di′ə-kwin) [USP] a 4-aminoquinoline compound with antiinflammatory and antiprotozoal properties.
 a. **hydrochloride** [USP] the dihydrated dihydrochloride salt of amodiaquine, having the same actions as the base; administered orally in the treatment of malaria.

amoeb- for words beginning thus, see also words beginning *ameb(i)(o)-*.

Amoe·ba (ə-me′bə) [L., from Gr. *amoibē* change] a genus of ramicristate amebae, protozoa now classified in the order Euamoebida; species have a vesicular nucleus, usually one contractile vacuole, and lobopodia, and are usually free living. Numerous species once included in this genus have been assigned to other genera.
 A. pro′teus a species found in fresh water and widely studied in the laboratory.

amoe·ba (ə-me′bə) ameba.

Amoe·bi·da (ə-me′bid-ə) in older systems of classification, an order of ramicristate amebae, protozoa of the class Lobosa, mostly living in fresh water; they are typically uninucleate and have mitochondria but no flagellate stage. A newer classification has assigned most families formerly in this order to other orders, including Centramoebida, Euamoebida, and Leptomyxida.

Amoe·bo·tae·nia (ə-me″bo-te′ne-ə) a genus of tapeworms of the family Dipylidiidae. *A. cunea′ta* is found in the intestines of fowls and causes hemorrhagic enteritis.

amoe·bu·la (ə-me′bu-lə) [dim. of *amoeba*] amebula.

amok (ə-mok′) [Malay "furious attack"] a culture-specific syndrome first reported in the Malay people, almost always male, consisting of a sudden outburst of indiscriminate aggressive or homicidal fury provoked by a perceived slight or insult or possibly unprovoked (running amok). Spelled also *amuck.*

amo·rol·fine hy·dro·chlo·ride (ə-mo′rol-fēn) a heterocyclic compound used as an antifungal agent, applied topically to the skin or nails.

amorph (a′morf) silent allele.

amor·phia (ə-mor′fe-ə) [*a-*[1] + *morph-* + *-ia*] the fact or quality of being amorphous.

amor·phism (ə-mor′fiz-əm) amorphia.

amor·pho·syn·the·sis (a-mor″fo-sin′thə-sis) [*a-*[1] + *morpho-* + *synthesis*] defective perception of somatic sensations from one side of the body, such as astereognosis or lack of position sense on one side. It may be accompanied by a generalized faulty awareness of spatial relationships and is often a sign of a parietal lobe lesion. Cf. *asomatognosia.*

amor·phous (ə-mor′fəs) [*a-*[1] + *morph-* + *-ous*] 1. having no definite form; shapeless. 2. having no specific orientation of atoms. 3. in pharmacy, not crystallized.

amor·phus (ə-mor′fəs) [*a-*[1] + Gr. *morphē* form] a shapeless malformed fetus. See also *holoacardius amorphus.*

am·o·site (a′mə-sīt″) a mineral in the amphibole class of asbestos, used industrially but now restricted because it causes asbestosis and certain forms of cancer such as mesotheliomas. Called also *brown asbestos.*

Amoss sign (a′məs) [Harold Lindsay *Amoss*, American physician, 1886–1956] see under *sign.*

amo·tio (ə-mo′she-o) gen. *amotio′nis* pl. *amotio′nes* [L., from *amovēre* to move away from] removal or detachment.
 a. re′tinae retinal detachment.

amox·a·pine (ə-mok′sə-pēn) [USP] a tricyclic antidepressant of the dibenzoxazepine class used for the treatment of symptoms of depression in neurotic and psychotic depressive disorders and endogenous and reactive depression; administered orally.

amox·i·cil·lin (ə-mok″sĭ-sil′in) [USP] a semisynthetic derivative of ampicillin effective against a broad spectrum of gram-positive and gram-negative bacteria; used especially in the treatment of infections due to susceptible strains of *Haemophilus influenzae, Escherichia coli, Proteus mirabilis, Neisseria gonorrhoeae,* streptococci (including *Streptococcus faecalis* and *S. pneumoniae*), and nonpenicillinase-producing staphylococci. It is administered orally.

Amox·il (ə-mok′sil) trademark for preparations of amoxicillin.

AMP adenosine monophosphate.
 3′,5′-AMP, cyclic AMP cyclic adenosine monophosphate.

amp former abbreviation for *ampere.*

AMP de·am·i·nase (de-am′ĭ-nās) [EC 3.5.4.6] an enzyme of the hydrolase class that catalyzes the deamination of AMP to form inosine monophosphate. Isoenzyme A (myoadenylate deaminase) is present in large amounts in muscle tissue and is a major source of ammonium ions during muscle contraction. Deficiency of this isoenzyme, an autosomal recessive trait, is characterized by muscle fatigue following exercise. Two additional isoenzymes have been identified: isoenzyme B, found in liver, kidney, and testes, and isoenzyme C, found in heart muscle. Called also *adenylate deaminase.*

am·per·age (am′pər-əj) the amount of electric current expressed in amperes or milliamperes.

am·pere (A) (am′pēr) [André M. *Ampère*, 1775–1836] the base SI unit of electric current, defined as the constant current that if maintained in two parallel straight conductors (of infinite length and negligible circular cross section) separated by a distance of 1 meter in a vacuum, produces a force between the conductors of 2×10^{-7} newton per meter of length; it is equivalent to one coulomb per second. Formerly abbreviated amp.

am·phet·a·mine (am-fet′ə-mēn″) 1. racemic amphetamine, (±)-α-methylphenethylamine, a sympathomimetic amine that has a stimulating effect on both the central and peripheral nervous systems. It relaxes bronchial muscle, increases heart rate and blood pressure, contracts the sphincter of the urinary bladder, and depresses the appetite. Abuse of this drug and its salts may lead to strong psychic dependence, to marked tolerance, and to mild physical dependence associated with tachycardia, increased blood pressure, restlessness, irritability, insomnia, personality changes, and, in the severe form of chronic intoxication, psychosis similar to schizophrenia. Abrupt withdrawal can cause severe fatigue, mental depression, and abnormalities in the electroencephalogram. 2. any of a group of closely related compounds having similar actions, including amphetamine and its salts, dextroamphetamine, and methamphetamine.
 a. **aspartate** the aspartate salt of amphetamine, having the same actions and uses as the sulfate salt; administered orally.
 a. **sulfate** [USP] the sulfate salt of amphetamine, having the same actions as the base, used orally in the treatment of narcolepsy and attention-deficit/hyperactivity disorder; it was formerly used as an anorectic in the treatment of obesity.

amphi- [Gr. *amphi* on both sides] a prefix meaning on both sides; around or about; double.

am·phi·ar·thro·sis (am″fe-ahr-thro′sis) [*amphi-* + *arthrosis*] junctura cartilaginea. **amphiarthro′dial** *adj*

Am·phib·ia (am-fib′e-ə) [*amphi-* + Gr. *bios* life] a class of vertebrate animals that breathe by means of gills in the larval state, but after metamorphosis generally breathe by means of lungs; orders include Anura (frogs and toads) and Caudata (salamanders).

am·phib·i·ous (am-fib′e-əs) capable of living both on land and in water.

am·phi·blas·tic (am″fe-blas′tik) [*amphi-* + *blast-* + *-ic*] denoting the complete but unequal cleavage of a telolecithal egg.

am·phi·blas·tu·la (am″fĭ-blas′tu-lə) [*amphi-* + *blastula*] a blastula with unequal blastomeres.

am·phi·bol·ic (am″fĭ-bol′ik) uncertain, vacillating, or having the potential to go in more than one of various directions.

am·phi·ce·lous (am″fe-se′lus) [*amphi-* + Gr. *koilos* hollow] concave on both sides; said of the vertebral centra of certain cold-blooded vertebrates. Called also *dicelous.*

am·phi·cen·tric (am″fĭ-sen′trik) [*amphi-* + *centric*] beginning and ending in the same vessel, as a branch of a rete mirabile.

am·phi·chro·ic (am″fĭ-kro′ik) [*amphi-* + Gr. *chrōma* color] exhibiting two colors; affecting both red and blue litmus.

am·phi·chro·mat·ic (am″fĭ-kro-mat′ik) amphichroic.

am·phi·cyte (am′fĭ-sīt) [*amphi-* + *-cyte*] a satellite cell (def. 1).

am·phi·cyt·u·la (am″fĭ-sit′u-lə) [*amphi-* + *cytula*] a fertilized telolecithal egg.

am·phi·di·ar·thro·sis (am″fĭ-di″ahr-thro′sis) [*amphi-* + *diarthrosis*] a joint having the nature of both a ginglymus and articulatio plana (arthrodia), as the articulation of the mandible.

am·phi·gas·tru·la (am″fĭ-gas′troo-lə) [*amphi-* + *gastrula*] a gastrula composed of cells unequal in size in its upper and lower hemispheres.

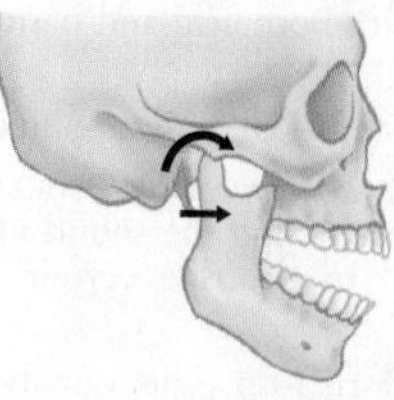

■ Amphidiarthrosis, exemplified by the temporomandibular joint. Arrows show the gliding component (arthrodia or articulatio plana) and hinge component (ginglymus) of movement.

am·phi·ge·net·ic (am″fĭ-jə-net′ik) produced by means of both sexes; said of reproduction.

am·phi·gon·a·dism (am″fĭ-go′nə-diz-əm) 1. possession of both ovarian and testicular tissue by the same animal. 2. true hermaphroditism.

am·phig·o·ny (am-fig′o-ne) sexual reproduction.

am·phi·leu·ke·mic (am″fĭ-loo-ke′mik) [*amphi-* + *leukemic*] showing leukemic changes which vary in degree with the changes in the organ.

Am·phim·er·us (am-fim′ər-əs) a genus of trematodes. *A. nover′ca* is a biliary-duct parasite of dogs and foxes and occasionally of hogs and humans. *A. pseudofeli′neus* infects cats and coyotes in the central United States.

am·phi·mor·u·la (am″fĭ-mor′u-lə) [*amphi-* + *morula*] the morula resulting from unequal cleavage, the cells of the two hemispheres being of unequal size.

am·phi·nu·cle·us (am″fĭ-noo′kle-əs) [*amphi-* + *nucleus*] a nucleus that consists of a single body made of spindle fibers and centrosome, around which the chromatin is massed; it is the ordinary form of protozoan nucleus. Called also *centronucleus.*

am·phi·path (am′fĭ-path) a molecule showing amphipathic properties.

am·phi·path·ic (am″fĭ-path′ik) of or relating to molecules containing groups with characteristically different properties, e.g., both hydrophilic and hydrophobic properties.

am·phi·reg·u·lin (am″fe-reg′u-lin) a 78–amino acid glycoprotein, originally identified in cultures from human breast carcinoma cells; it is 38 per cent identical with epidermal growth factor and can inhibit the growth of several carcinoma cell lines while stimulating the proliferation of normal cells.

Am·phis·to·ma (am-fis′tə-mə) [*amphi-* + *stoma*] a genus of parasitic trematodes, many species of which have been reassigned to other genera.

A. co′nicum *Paramphistomum cervi.*
A. ho′minis *Gastrodiscoides hominis.*
A. watso′ni *Watsonius watsoni.*

am·phis·tome (am-fis′tōm) paramphistome.

am·phi·sto·mi·a·sis (am″fĭ-sto-mi′ə-sis) paramphistomiasis.

am·phi·the·a·ter (am″fĭ-the′ə-tər) an operating room or lecture room with seats arranged in tiers for students or spectators.

am·phit·ri·chous (am-fit′rĭ-kəs) [*amphi-* + *trich-* + *-ous*] having a single flagellum, or a single tuft of flagella, at each end; said of a bacterial cell. See *flagellum.*

am·phit·y·py (am-fit′ĭ-pe) the condition of showing both types.

ampho- [Gr. *amphō* both] a combining form signifying both, on both sides.

am·pho·chro·ma·to·phil (am″fo-kro-mə′tə-fil) 1. amphophilic cell. 2. amphophilic.

am·pho·chro·mo·phil (am″fo-kro′mə-fil) [*ampho-* + *chromophil*] 1. amphophilic cell. 2. amphophilic.

Am·pho·cin (am′fo-sin) trademark for a preparation of amphotericin B.

am·pho·cyte (am′fo-sīt) amphophilic cell.

am·pho·gen·ic (am″fo-jen′ik) [*ampho-* + *-genic*] producing offspring of both sexes.

Am·pho·jel (am′fo-jəl) trademark for preparations of aluminum hydroxide gel.

am·pho·lyte (am′fo-līt) [*ampho-* + *electrolyte*] amphoteric electrolyte.

am·pho·phil (am′fo-fil) 1. amphophilic cell. 2. amphophilic.

am·pho·phile (am′fo-fīl″) 1. amphophil. 2. amphophilic cell.

am·pho·phil·ic (am-fo-fil′ik) [*ampho-* + *-philic*] stainable with either acid or basic dyes; see also *amphophilic cell,* under *cell.* Called also *amphophil, amphophile,* and *amphophilous.*

a.-basophil staining with both acid and basic stains, but having a greater affinity for basic ones.

gram-a. tending to stain both positive and negative with Gram stain.

a.-oxyphil staining with both acid and basic dyes but having a greater affinity for the acid ones.

am·phoph·i·lous (am-fof′ĭ-ləs) amphophilic.

am·phor·ic (am-for′ik) [L. *amphoricus,* from Gr. *amphora* jar] 1. pertaining to a bottle. 2. resembling the sound made by blowing across the mouth of a bottle, used to describe certain high-pitched auscultatory sounds.

am·pho·ric·i·ty (am″fə-ris′ĭ-te) the quality of being amphoric; see *cavernous voice,* under *voice.*

am·pho·ril·o·quy (am″fə-ril′o-kwe) [L. *amphora* jar + *loqui* to speak] cavernous voice.

am·pho·roph·o·ny (am″fə-rof′ə-ne) [Gr. *amphoreus* jar + *phonē* voice] cavernous voice.

Am·pho·tec (am′fo-tek) trademark for a preparation of amphotericin B cholesteryl complex.

am·pho·ter·ic (am-fə-ter′ik) [Gr. *amphoteros* pertaining to both] having opposite characters; capable of acting either as an acid or as a base; combining with both acids and bases; affecting both red and blue litmus.

am·pho·ter·i·cin B (am″fə-ter′ĭ-sin) [USP] one of two polyene antifungal antibiotics (the other, amphotericin A, is not used clinically), derived from a strain of *Streptomyces nodosus* and effective against a wide range of fungi and against some species of *Leishmania.* It is used intravenously or by intracavitary instillation in the treatment of progressive, potentially fatal fungal infections and as a secondary drug in the treatment of mucocutaneous leishmaniasis and topically in the treatment of superficial candidiasis.

a. B cholesteryl complex amphotericin B complexed with cholesteryl sulfate in a 1:1 ratio; administered by intravenous infusion in the treatment of disseminated aspergillosis in patients refractory to or intolerant of conventional amphotericin B therapy.

a. B lipid complex amphotericin B complexed with two phospholipids in a 1:1 drug-to-lipid ratio; administered by intravenous infusion in the treatment of invasive fungal infections in patients who are refractory to or intolerant of conventional amphotericin B therapy.

a. B liposomal complex amphotericin B intercalated into a single bilayer liposome; administered by intravenous infusion in the treatment of severe systemic fungal infections and visceral leishmaniasis in patients refractory to or intolerant of conventional amphotericin B therapy.

am·pho·ter·ic·i·ty (am″fə-tər-is′ĭ-te) amphoterism.

am·pho·ter·ism (am-fo′tər-iz-əm) the condition or quality of possessing both basic and acid properties.

am·phot·er·ous (am-fot′ər-əs) amphoteric.

am·phot·o·ny (am-fot′ə-ne) [*ampho-* + Gr. *tonos* tension] a condition in which both sympathicotonia and vagotony are said to exist; hypertonia of the entire sympathetic nervous system.

am·pi·cil·lin (am″pĭ-sil′in) [USP] a semisynthetic, acid-resistant, penicillinase-sensitive penicillin of the aminopenicillin group, effective against a broad spectrum of gram-positive and gram-negative bacteria, used in the treatment of infections caused by susceptible organisms; administered orally.

a. sodium [USP] the monosodium salt of ampicillin, having the same actions and uses as the base; administered intramuscularly or intravenously.

AMP ki·nase (ki′nās) adenylate kinase.

am·plex·a·tion (am″plek-sa′shən) [L. *amplexus* embrace] treatment of fractured clavicle by an apparatus which fixes the shoulder and embraces the chest and neck.

am·plex·us (am-plek′səs) [L.] an embrace, as in the sexual clasping of the female by the male frog; see *pseudocopulation.*

am·pli·fi·ca·tion (am″plĭ-fĭ-ka′shən) [L. *amplificatio*] the act or result of increasing in number, size, power, or other variable, such as the increase of an auditory or visual stimulus as a means of improving its perception.

DNA a. 1. an in vitro technique used to increase the number of copies of a specific segment of DNA to aid in its detection; see *nucleic acid amplification technique,* under *technique.* 2. a term sometimes used to denote in vivo gene amplification, particularly that associated with malignancy.

gene a. 1. selective replication of a specific gene or genes disproportionate to their representation in the parent molecule, such as that occurring in specific cells in response to signals of cell development or to stress from the environment. A common place where this occurs is in malignant cells. 2. a term sometimes used to denote in vitro nucleic acid amplification (q.v.), even though the sequence amplified may not correspond precisely to a gene.

nucleic acid a. increase in the number of copies of a specific nucleic acid sequence, either DNA or RNA; usually used to denote an in vitro nucleic acid amplification technique (q.v.).

RNA a. an in vitro technique used to increase the number of copies of a specific segment of RNA to aid in its detection; see *nucleic acid amplification technique,* under *technique.*

am·pli·fi·er (am′plĭ-fī″ər) 1. an electronic device that increases the strength of an input signal. 2. an apparatus for increasing the magnification of a microscope.

am·pli·tude (am′plə-tōōd) [L. *amplus* full] 1. largeness or fullness; wideness or breadth of range or extent. 2. in a phenomenon that occurs in waves, the maximal deviation of a wave from the baseline, measured as either *peak a.* or *peak-to-peak a.*

a. of accommodation range of accommodation; see under *range.*

a. of convergence the difference in the power required to turn the eyes from their far point to their near point of convergence.

peak a. the maximal deviation of a wave in just one direction from the baseline.

peak-to-peak a. the sum of the peak amplitude in a positive direction and that in a negative direction from the baseline.

am·poule (am′pūl) ampule.

am·pren·a·vir (am-pren′ə-vir) an HIV protease inhibitor that causes formation of immature, noninfectious viral particles; used in treatment of human immunodeficiency virus infection; administered orally.

Am·prol (am′prol) trademark for a preparation of amprolium.

am·pro·li·um (am-pro′le-əm) [USP] a thiamine analogue used in veterinary medicine for the prevention and treatment of coccidiosis.

Am·pro·vine (am′pro-vēn) trademark for a preparation of amprolium.

am·pul (am′pūl) ampule.

am·pule (am′pūl) [Fr. *ampoule*] a small glass or plastic container capable of being sealed so as to preserve its contents in a sterile condition; used principally for containing sterile parenteral solutions.

am·pul·la (am-pul′ə) gen. and pl. *ampul′lae* [L. "a jug"] a flasklike dilation of a tubular structure.

biliaropancreatic a. ampulla hepatopancreatica.

a. biliaropancrea′tica TA alternative for *ampulla hepatopancreatica*.

bony a., anterior a. ossea anterior.

bony a., lateral a. ossea lateralis.

bony a., posterior a. ossea posterior.

a. canali′culi lacrima′lis [TA] ampulla of lacrimal canaliculus: a dilation of a lacrimal canaliculus just before it opens into the lacrimal sac.

a. duc′tus deferen′tis [TA] ampulla of ductus deferens: the enlarged and tortuous distal end of the ductus deferens; called also *Henle a.* and *a. of vas deferens.*

duodenal a., a. duode′ni [TA] the superior part of the duodenum, often seen only radiographically after a barium meal; called also *bulbus duodeni* [TA alternative] and *duodenal bulb* or *cap.* A true duodenal ampulla is seen in some other mammalian species.

Henle a. a. ductus deferentis.

hepatopancreatic a., a. hepatopancrea′tica [TA] the dilatation formed by junction of the common bile duct and pancreatic duct just before they open together into the lumen of the duodenum; called also *biliaropancreatic a., ampulla biliaropancreatica* [TA alternative], and *a. of Vater.*

a. of lacrimal canaliculus a. canaliculi lacrimalis.

a. membrana′cea ante′rior [TA] anterior membranous ampulla: the dilation at the end of the anterior membranous semicircular duct.

a. membrana′cea latera′lis [TA] lateral membranous ampulla: the dilation at the end of the lateral membranous semicircular duct.

a. membrana′cea poste′rior [TA] posterior membranous ampulla: the dilation at the end of the posterior membranous semicircular duct.

membranous a., anterior a. membranacea anterior.

membranous a., lateral a. membranacea lateralis.

membranous a., posterior a. membranacea posterior.

a. os′sea ante′rior [TA] anterior bony ampulla: the dilatation at one end of the anterior semicircular canal, lodging the anterior membranous ampulla (ampulla membranacea anterior).

a. os′sea latera′lis [TA] lateral bony ampulla: the dilatation at one end of the lateral semicircular canal, lodging the lateral membranous ampulla (ampulla membranacea lateralis).

a. os′sea poste′rior [TA] posterior bony ampulla: the dilatation at one end of the posterior semicircular canal, lodging the posterior membranous ampulla (ampulla membranacea posterior).

phrenic a. a dilation sometimes seen at the lower end of the esophagus.

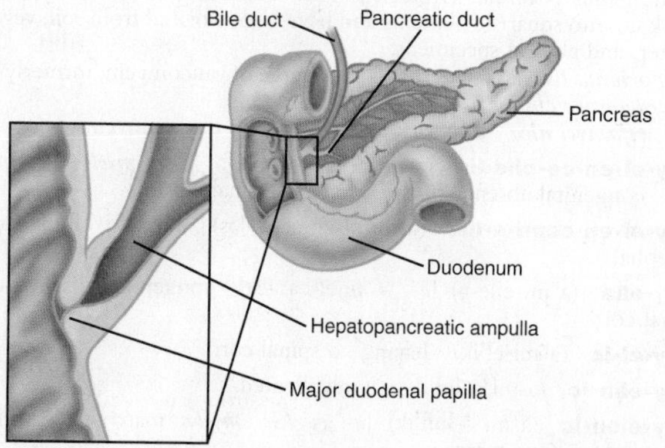

■ Ampulla hepatopancreatica (hepatopancreatic ampulla), receiving the common bile and pancreatic ducts and entering the duodenum at the major duodenal papilla.

rectal a., a. rec′ti [TA] the dilated portion of the rectum just proximal to the anal canal.

a. of Thoma one of the small terminal expansions of an interlobar artery in the pulp of the spleen.

a. tu′bae uteri′nae [TA] ampulla of uterine tube: the thin-walled, almost muscle-free, midregion of the uterine tube; its mucosa is greatly plicated.

a. of vas deferens a. ductus deferentis.

a. of Vater a. hepatopancreatica.

am·pul·lae (am-pul′e) [L.] genitive and plural of *ampulla.*

am·pul·lar (am-pul′ər) pertaining to an ampulla, especially to the ampulla hepatopancreatica.

am·pul·lary (am′pu-la″re) ampullar.

am·pul·late (am-pul′āt) flask-shaped.

am·pul·lec·to·my (am″pul-ek′tə-me) surgical removal of an ampulla, especially the hepatopancreatic ampulla.

am·pul·li·tis (am″pul-li′tis) inflammation of an ampulla, especially of the ampulla ductus deferentis.

am·pul·lu·la (am-pul′oo-lə) [L.] any minute ampulla, like many of those of the lymphatic and lacteal vessels.

am·pu·ta·tion (am″pu-ta′shən) [L. *amputare* to cut off, or to prune] the removal of a limb or other appendage or outgrowth of the body.

above-elbow (A-E) a. amputation of the upper limb between the elbow and the shoulder.

above-knee (A-K) a. transfemoral a.

Alanson a. circular amputation in which the stump is shaped like a hollow cone.

Alouette a. amputation at the hip, with a semicircular outer flap to the greater trochanter and a large internal flap from within outward; called also *Alouette operation.*

aperiosteal a. amputation with complete removal of the periosteum from the end of the stump of the bone; called also *Bunge a.*

Béclard a. hip disarticulation with cutting of the posterior flap first.

below-elbow (B-E) a. amputation of the upper limb between the wrist and the elbow.

below-knee (B-K) a. transtibial a.

Bier a. osteoplastic amputation of the lower limb with a bone flap cut out of the tibia and fibula above the stump; called also *Bier operation.*

Boyd a. amputation at the ankle with removal of the talus and fusion of the tibia and calcaneus.

Bunge a. aperiosteal a.

Callander a. a tenoplastic knee disarticulation with long anterior and posterior flaps, the patella being removed to leave a fossa for the end of the divided femur.

Carden a. a single flap transfemoral amputation done just above the knee.

central a. an amputation in which the scar is at or near the center of the stump.

chop a. guillotine a.

Chopart a. amputation of the foot, with the calcaneus, talus, and other parts of the tarsus being retained; called also *Chopart operation* and *mediotarsal a.*

cinematic a., cineplastic a. kineplasty.

circular a. an amputation performed by means of a single flap and by a circular cut in a direction vertical to the long axis of a limb.

closed a. amputation in which flaps are made from the skin and subcutaneous tissue and sutured over the end of the bone; called also *flap a.*

coat-sleeve a. a circular amputation with a single skin flap made very long for closing of the end.

congenital a. absence of a limb at birth, usually because of constriction of the part by an encircling amniotic band; see *amniotic band syndrome,* under *syndrome.*

a. in contiguity an amputation at a joint.

a. in continuity an amputation elsewhere than at a joint.

cutaneous a. amputation in which the flaps are composed entirely of skin.

double-flap a. closed amputation in which two flaps are formed.

Dupuytren a. shoulder disarticulation.

eccentric a. an amputation in which the scar is not at the center of the stump.

Ertl a. see under *procedure.*

Farabeuf a. amputation of the lower limb with a large external flap.

flap a. closed a.

flapless a. guillotine a.

forequarter a. interscapulothoracic a.

Gritti a. knee disarticulation in which the patella is fused to the distal end of the femur. Called also *Gritti operation.*

Gritti-Stokes a. a modification of Gritti amputation using an oval anterior flap; called also *Stokes a.* or *operation.*

guillotine a. rapid amputation of a limb by a circular sweep of the knife and a cut of the saw, the entire cross-section being left open for dressing; done when primary closure of the stump is contraindicated, owing to the possibility of recurrent or developing infection. Called also *chop a.*, *flapless a.*, and *open a.*

Guyon a. transtibial amputation just above the malleoli.

Hancock a. a modification of Pirogoff amputation in which a part of the astragalus (talus) is retained in the flap, the lower surface being sawed off, and the cut surface of the calcaneus being brought into contact with it; called also *Hancock operation.*

Hey a. disarticulation of the tarsus from the metatarsus with removal of a part of the medial cuneiform bone. Called also *Hey operation.* Cf. *Lisfranc a.*

hindquarter a. hemipelvectomy.

interilioabdominal a., interinnominoabdominal a., interpelviabdominal a. hemipelvectomy.

interscapulothoracic a. amputation of the upper limb with removal of the scapula and the clavicle; called also *forequarter a.*

Jaboulay a. hemipelvectomy.

kineplastic a. kineplasty.

Kirk a. a tenoplastic transfemoral amputation done just above the femoral condyles, with the tendon of the quadriceps femoris muscle sutured over the end of the divided femur.

Langenbeck a. amputation in which the flaps are cut from without inward.

Larrey a. shoulder disarticulation with an incision extending from the acromion about three inches down the arm, splitting the deltoid muscle, and from this point going around the arm to the center of the axilla; called also *Larrey operation.*

Le Fort a. a modification of Pirogoff amputation in which the calcaneus is sawed through horizontally instead of vertically.

linear a. amputation by a simple straight division of all the tissues.

Lisfranc a. 1. amputation of the foot between the tarsus and the metatarsus. 2. shoulder disarticulation.

long above-knee (A-K) a. transfemoral amputation in which the femur is divided in the supracondylar region

long below-knee (B-K) a. transtibial amputation in which the division is in the distal third of the tibia.

Mackenzie a. an amputation similar to Syme amputation except that the flap is taken from the inner side of the ankle.

Maisonneuve a. amputation by breaking the bone, followed by cutting of the soft parts.

major a. amputation of the lower limb above the ankle or of the upper limb above the wrist.

Malgaigne a. subastragalar a.

mediotarsal a. Chopart a.

minor a. amputation of a hand or foot, or of a part thereof.

mixed a. amputation performed by a combination of the circular and flap methods.

musculocutaneous a. an amputation in which the flap consists of muscle and skin.

oblique a. oval a.

open a. guillotine a.

osteoplastic a. an amputation in which the cut surface of one bone is brought into contact with the cut surface of another so as to unite, thus providing a better stump.

oval a. an amputation in which the incision consists of two reversed spirals; called also *oblique a.* and *loxotomy.*

periosteoplastic a. subperiosteal a.

phalangophalangeal a. amputation of a digit at a phalangeal joint.

Pirogoff a. amputation of the foot at the ankle, part of the calcaneus being left in the lower end of the stump.

pulp a. pulpotomy.

racket a. an amputation in which there is a single longitudinal incision continuous below with a spiral incision on each side of the limb.

ray a. amputation of a metacarpal or metatarsal and all the phalangeal segments distal to it.

rectangular a. an amputation with a long and a short rectangular skin flap, such as Teale amputation.

Ricard a. amputation of the foot with disarticulation of the tibia from the calcaneus, astragalectomy, and the placing of the calcaneus in the mortise between the tibia and fibula.

root a. excision of the root of a tooth; amputation of the root of a single-rooted tooth is called *apicoectomy,* and that of one root of a two-rooted mandibular tooth is *hemisectomy.* Called also *radiectomy* and *radisectomy.*

short below-knee (B-K) a. transtibial amputation in which the division is in the proximal third of the tibia.

spontaneous a. loss of a part without surgical intervention, as in leprosy, diabetes mellitus, or Buerger disease.

Stokes a. Gritti-Stokes a.

subastragalar a. amputation of the foot, leaving the astragalus (talus) in the lower end of the stump; called also *Malgaigne a.*

subperiosteal a. an amputation in which the cut end of the bone is covered with a flap of periosteum; called also *periosteoplastic a.*

Syme a. ankle disarticulation with removal of both malleoli; called also *Syme operation.*

Teale a. amputation with preservation of a long rectangular flap of muscle and integument on one side of the limb and a short rectangular flap on the other.

transfemoral a. amputation of the lower limb between the knee and the hip; called also *above-knee (A-K) a.*

a. by transfixion amputation performed by thrusting a long knife through the limb and cutting the flaps from within outward.

transmetatarsal a. amputation of the anterior part of the foot across the metatarsal bones.

transtibial a. amputation of the lower limb between the ankle and the knee. Called also *below-knee (B-K) a.*

traumatic a. amputation of a part by accidental injury.

Tripier a. an amputation similar to a Chopart amputation except that a part of the tarsus is removed.

Vladimiroff-Mikulicz a. a type of osteoplastic amputation of the foot with incision of the calcaneus and talus.

am•pu•tee (am″pu-te′) a person who has had one or more limbs amputated.

am•ri•none (am′rĭ-nōn) inamrinone.

Am•rix (am′riks) trademark for a preparation of cyclobenzaprine hydrochloride.

AMRL Aerospace Medical Research Laboratories.

AMS American Meteorological Society.

ams. amount of a substance.

AMSA American Medical Student Association.

am•sa•crine (am′sə-krēn) an antineoplastic agent that inhibits DNA synthesis, used to treat some forms of leukemia; administered intravenously.

Am•sler charts, grid (ahm′zlər) [Marc *Amsler,* Swiss ophthalmologist, 1891–1968] see under *chart* and *grid.*

AMTA American Music Therapy Association.

amu atomic mass unit.

amuck (ə-muk′) [Malay *amok*] 1. amok. 2. *(colloq.)* wild, frenzied, or uncontrollable.

amu•sia (ə-mu′ze-ə) [Gr. *amousia* want of harmony] a form of auditory agnosia in which a person has lost the ability to recognize or produce music; cf. *paramusia.*

instrumental a. amusia in which the patient has lost the power of playing a musical instrument.

sensory a. loss of the ability to comprehend musical sounds; called also *tone deafness.*

vocal motor a. amusia in which the patient cannot sing in tune.

Am•visc (am′visk) trademark for a preparation of hyaluronan.

AMWA American Medical Women's Association; American Medical Writers Association.

amy•cho•pho•bia (ə-mi″ko-fo′be-ə) [Gr. *amychē* a scratch + *-phobia*] irrational fear of being scratched, as by the claws of a cat.

Am•y•co•la•top•sis (am″ĭ-ko″lə-top′sis) a genus of nonmotile, gram-positive, non–acid fast, aerobic, chemo-organotrophic bacteria of the family Pseudonocardiaceae, comprising organisms formerly included in the genus *Nocardia.* Organisms form branching substrate hyphae that break up into squarish elements and have been isolated from soil, vegetable matter, and clinical specimens.

A. orienta′lis a species that is the source of vancomycin; formerly called *Nocardia orientalis.*

A. rifamyci′nica a species that synthesizes the rifamycins.

amy•el•en•ce•pha•lia (ə-mi″əl-en-sə-fa′le-ə) [*a-*[1] + *myelo-* + *encephal-* + *-ia*] congenital absence of the brain and spinal cord.

amy•el•en•ceph•a•lus (ə-mi″əl-en-sef′ə-ləs) a fetus exhibiting amyelencephalia.

amy•elia (a″mi-e′le-ə) [*a-*[1] + *myel-* + *-ia*] congenital absence of the spinal cord.

amy•el•ic (a″mi-el′ik) having no spinal cord.

amy•elin•ic (a-mi″ə-lin′ik) unmyelinated.

amy•elon•ic (a-mi″ə-lon′ik) [*a-*[1] + Gr. *myelos* marrow] 1. amyelic. 2. having no bone marrow.

amy•elus (a-mi′ə-ləs) [*a-*[1] + Gr. *myelos* marrow] a fetus exhibiting amyelia.

amyg•da•la (ə-mig′də-lə) [Gr. *amygdalē* almond] 1. almond. 2. in anatomical nomenclature, an almond-shaped structure. 3. corpus amygdaloideum.

amyg•da•lin (ə-mig′də-lin) a cyanogenetic glycoside (*l*-mandelonitrile-β-gentiobioside) found in seeds and other plant parts of the bitter almond and other members of the family Rosaceae, often the cause of cyanide poisoning in animals eating them in large amounts. It is split by enzymatic hydrolysis into glucose, benzaldehyde, and hydrocyanic acid. See also *Laetrile* and *laetrile.*

amyg•da•line (ə-mig′də-lēn″) [L. *amygdalinus*] 1. like an almond. 2. tonsillar.

amygdal(o)- [Gr. *amygdalē* almond] a combining form denoting relationship to an almond-shaped structure or to the tonsil.

amyg•da•lof•u•gal (ə-mig″də-lof′ə-gəl) carrying impulses away from the amygdaloid body; see *ventral amygdalofugal tract,* under *tract.*

amyg•da•lo•hip•po•cam•pec•to•my (ə-mig″də-lo-hip″o-cam-pek′tə-me) [*amygdalo-* + *hippocampus* + *-ectomy*] surgical removal of all or part of the amygdala, hippocampus, and parahippocampal gyrus; done for the treatment of temporal lobe epilepsy resistant to medical treatment.

amyg•da•loid (ə-mig′də-loid) [*amygdalo-* + *-oid*] resembling an almond or tonsil.

am•yl (am′əl) [Gr. *amylon* starch] the univalent radical, —C_5H_{11}. amyl′ic *adj*

a. acetate a colorless limpid liquid, the acetic acid ester of amyl alcohol, CH_3•CO•OC_5H_{11}; it has the odor of bananas and is also called *banana oil.*

a. nitrite [USP] a mixture of the nitrite esters of 3-methyl-1-butanol and 2-methyl-1-butanol, a flammable clear liquid with an ethereal odor, volatile at low temperatures and administered by inhalation. It is a vasodilator and is used as a diagnostic aid in tests of reserve cardiac function and diagnosis of certain heart murmurs; it has also been used in the treatment of acute angina pectoris, although it has largely been replaced by other agents. It is also used in treatment of cyanide poisoning to promote formation of methemoglobin, which combines with the cyanide ion to form nontoxic cyanmethemoglobin. It is abused to produce euphoria and as a sexual stimulant and may cause methemoglobinemia, hemolytic anemia, and immunologic disorders.

am•y•la•ceous (am″ə-la′shəs) [L. *amylaceus*] starchy; containing starch; of the nature of starch.

am•y•lase (am′ə-lās) an enzyme of the hydrolase class that catalyzes the hydrolysis of α-1,4-glucosidic linkages in polysaccharides.

α-a. [EC 3.2.1.1] an endoamylase catalyzing the hydrolysis of internal α-1,4-glucosidic linkages in polysaccharides that contain three or more glucose residues, yielding a mixture of linear and branched oligosaccharides. The enzyme is secreted by the salivary glands and pancreas of mammals.

β-a. [EC 3.2.1.2] an exoamylase occurring in plants and bacteria; it cleaves alternate glucosidic bonds to remove maltose units from the polysaccharide chains.

am•y•las•uria (am″ə-lās-u′re-ə) an excess of amylase in the urine, a sign of pancreatitis. Called also *diastasuria.*

am•y•le•mia (am″ə-le′me-ə) [*amyl-* + *-emia*] an excess of starch in the blood.

am•y•lene (am′ə-lēn) a flammable liquid hydrocarbon of five isomeric forms.

a. hydrate [NF] a clear, colorless liquid with a camphoraceous odor, miscible with alcohol, chloroform, ether, and glycerin; used as a solvent in pharmaceutical preparations. See also *amylism.*

am•yl•in (am′ə-lin) a 37–amino acid polypeptide with over 40 per cent homology with calcitonin gene–related peptide, occurring packaged with insulin in the beta cell secretory granules in normal pancreatic islets; it is also a major component of islet amyloid in patients with type 2 diabetes. Amylin inhibits insulin-stimulated glycogen synthesis in isolated skeletal muscle and inhibits insulin-induced glucose utilization in vivo. Called also *islet amyloid polypeptide.*

am•y•lism (am′ə-liz-əm) poisoning by amylene hydrate.

amyl(o)- [Gr. *amylon* starch] a combining form denoting relationship to starch.

am•y•lo•bar•bi•tone (am″ə-lo-bahr′bĭ-tōn) amobarbital.

am•y•lo•dex•trin (am″ə-lo-dek′strin) any of the class of water-soluble dextrins staining blue with iodine and formed in the early stages of hydrolysis of starch.

am•y•lo•dys•pep•sia (am″ə-lo-dis-pep′se-ə) [*amylo-* + *dyspepsia*] inability to digest starch-containing foods.

am•y•lo•gen•e•sis (am″ə-lo-jen′ə-sis) [*amylo-* + *-genesis*] the biosynthesis of starch.

am•y•lo•gen•ic (am″ə-lo-jen′ik) 1. producing starch. 2. of or pertaining to amylogenesis.

am•y•lo-1,6-glu•co•si•dase (am″ə-lo-gloo-ko′sĭ-dās) [EC 3.2.1.33] an enzyme of the hydrolase class that catalyzes the cleavage of terminal α-1,6-glucoside linkages, releasing free glucose residues. In mammals, the enzyme also has a transferase activity on the same polypeptide chain (see *oligo-1,4-1,4-glucantransferase*) and can hydrolyze such linkages occurring at points of branching in glycogen molecules by first transferring to nearby chains those triglucosides adjacent to branch points, thereby exposing the α-1,6-linked branch points to the glucosidase activity. In concert with glycogen phosphorylase, the enzyme can thus degrade glycogen to free glucose and glucose 1-phosphate. Both liver and muscle isoforms exist; deficiency of one or both isoforms results in glycogen storage disease, type III. Called also *debranching enzyme (of glycogen).*

am•y•loid (am′ə-loid) [*amylo-* + *-oid*] 1. resembling starch; characterized by starchlike staining properties. 2. a substance produced by the action of sulfuric acid on cellulose, which gives a blue color when treated with iodine. 3. the pathologic extracellular proteinaceous substance deposited in amyloidosis; it is a waxy eosinophilic material that exhibits a green birefringence under polarized light when stained with Congo red. Amyloid deposits are composed primarily of straight, nonbranching fibrils 7.5–10 nm in diameter and of indefinite length, arranged either in bundles or in a feltlike meshwork; each fibril is composed of identical polypeptide chains arranged in stacked antiparallel β-pleated sheets. Although different forms have similar appearance, the protein in each is different.

a. A, AA a. a pathological fibrillar low-molecular-weight protein formed by cleavage of serum amyloid A (SAA) protein. It is deposited in the tissues secondary to chronic inflammatory conditions; see *AA amyloidosis,* under *amyloidosis.*

Aβ a. an abnormal, neurotoxic peptide, either 40 or 42 amino acids in length, found in aggregates in the cerebrovascular walls and the cores of the plaques in Alzheimer disease. It is derived from a large transmembrane glycoprotein, amyloid precursor protein. Called also *amyloid-β* or *β-amyloid peptide.*

AL a., a. L a pathological fibrillar low-molecular-weight protein derived from circulating monoclonal immunoglobulin light chains, usually λ chains; it may be composed of whole chains, fragments, or both. It is deposited in the tissues in AL amyloidosis (q.v.).

am•y•loi•do•gen•e•sis (am″ĭ-loi-do-jen′ə-sis) the formation of amyloid.

am•y•loi•do•gen•ic (am″ĭ-loi-do-jen′ik) causing formation of amyloid.

am•y•loi•do•ma (am″ə-loi-do′mə) a tumor that contains amyloid; some occur in conjunction with amyloidosis and others are idiopathic.

am•y•loi•do•sis (am″ə-loi-do′sis) [*amyloid-* + *-osis*] a group of conditions of diverse etiologies characterized by the accumulation of insoluble amyloid in various organs and tissues of the body, which compromises vital function. The associated disease states may be inflammatory, hereditary, or neoplastic, and the deposition can be local or generalized (systemic). The most widely used classification is based on the chemistry of the amyloid fibrils.

AA a. amyloidosis in which the deposited fibrillar material is AA amyloid, occurring secondary to a chronic inflammatory condition, either infectious (e.g., tuberculosis, osteomyelitis) or noninfectious (e.g., rheumatoid arthritis, Crohn disease). It usually affects the kidneys, spleen, and liver. Called also *reactive* or *secondary a.*

a. of aging senile a.

AL a. 1. systemic amyloidosis in which the deposited fibrillar material is AL amyloid; it may be due to either aberrant synthesis or processing of immunoglobulin light chains. It is associated with tumors or dyscrasias of immunoglobulin-producing plasma cells and involves some combination of the skin and subcutaneous tissue, nerve tissue, liver, spleen, heart, kidney, intestine, and tongue. Treatment usually includes chemotherapy or stem cell transplantation. Called also *immunoglobulin light chain a., light chain–related a.,* and *primary a.* 2. rarely, a localized form of amyloidosis with deposition of AL amyloid.

ATTR a. the most common form of hereditary amyloidosis, in which any of numerous mutations of the *TTR* gene (locus: 18q11.2-q12.1), which encodes transthyretin, cause systemic autosomal dominant disorders characterized by polyneuropathies, cardiomyopathies, and variable organ involvement. See also *familial amyloid polyneuropathy,* under *polyneuropathy.* Called also *transthyretin* and *TTR a.*

$β_2$-microglobulin a. a condition sometimes seen in end-stage kidney disease, characterized by excessive plasma $β_2$-microglobulin, some of which is catabolized to form amyloid deposits.

dialysis a. hemodialysis-associated a.

familial a. hereditary a.

familial visceral a. a group of rare, autosomal dominant systemic amyloidoses, not associated with transthyretin, caused by mutations in any of a large number of genes and characterized by deposition of amyloid in the viscera without neuropathy. It is manifested by nephropathy, arterial hypertension, hepatosplenomegaly, albuminuria, hematuria, and pitting edema.

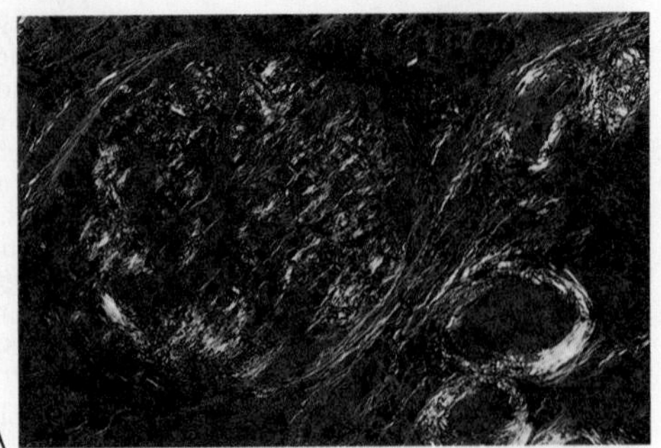

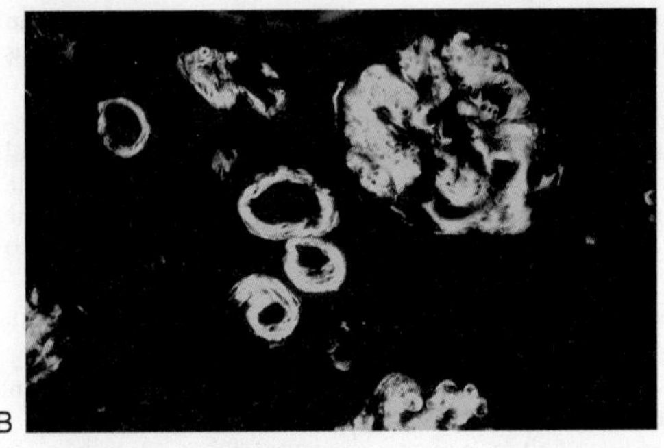

■ Amyloidosis. *(A)*, Apple-green birefringence of deposits under polarized light (Congo red). *(B)*, Fluorescence of deposits under ultraviolet light (thioflavine T).

Affected patients usually die within ten years of onset of clinical manifestations. Called also *Ostertag* or *Ostertag type a.*

hemodialysis-associated a. amyloidosis occurring in patients on long-term hemodialysis, caused by the deposition of beta$_2$-microglobulin, which cannot be removed from the blood by hemodialysis, in the joints, synovial membranes, and tendon sheaths. Manifestations include carpal tunnel syndrome and arthritis. Called also *dialysis a.*

hereditary a. any inherited form of amyloidosis. The term is usually used to denote various systemic autosomal dominant disorders of amyloid deposition involving the nervous system (polyneuropathies). The most common form is ATTR amyloidosis, which is associated with various point mutations of the *TTR* gene; rare mutations of other proteins can also be a cause. The term is less commonly used to describe AA amyloidosis in which the fibril deposition is associated with an inherited disease (e.g., familial Mediterranean fever). Subclassifications are based on clinical presentation and the biochemical composition of the fibrils deposited; originally the subclasses were distinguished on the basis of kinship. Called also *familial* or *heredofamilial a.;* see also *familial amyloid polyneuropathy*, under *polyneuropathy.*

heredofamilial a. hereditary a.

immunoglobulin light chain a. AL a.

lichen a. the most common form of amyloidosis affecting the skin, characterized by symmetrical distribution on the shins and thighs, and occasionally elsewhere, of translucent, yellow to brown, discrete, pruritic papules. Called also *papular a.* and *lichen amyloidosus.*

light chain–related a. AL a.

macular a. a type of amyloidosis affecting the skin, more common among dark-skinned individuals, characterized by ill-defined, sometimes pruritic gray to brown macules, usually on the upper back and sometimes on the breasts, buttocks, arms, ankles, and thighs.

nodular a. localized amyloidosis consisting of single or multiple, amyloid-containing nodular masses beneath the mucous membranes or skin; the most common mucous membrane sites are in the lung, urinary bladder, larynx, tongue, and conjunctiva, and the most common skin sites are on the limbs, trunk, genitals, and face.

Ostertag a., Ostertag type a. familial visceral a.

papular a. lichen a.

primary a. AL a.

reactive a. AA a.

renal a. amyloid deposits in the kidneys; in the *primary type* the fibrils are mainly of AL amyloid, and in *secondary types* they are of AA amyloid. Secondary types may accompany inflammatory disorders such as rheumatoid arthritis or paraplegias, chronic infectious diseases such as tuberculosis or leprosy, and neoplastic diseases such as multiple myeloma. Called also *amyloid nephropathy* or *nephrosis.*

secondary a. AA a.

senile a. amyloidosis seen in the elderly, usually involving the heart, brain, pancreas, or spleen, typically due to the deposition of normal or mutant transthyretin. Called also *a. of aging.*

transthyretin a., TTR a. ATTR a.

am·y·lol·y·sis (am″ə-lol′ə-sis) [*amylo-* + *-lysis*] the degradation of starch to water-soluble dextrins and sugars, particularly that catalyzed by enzymes. **amylolyt′ic** *adj*

am·y·lo·pec·tin (am″ə-lo-pek′tin) a highly branched, water-insoluble glucan, the more prevalent of the two constituents of starch (see also *amylose*); it consists of a chain of glucose residues in α-(1,4) linkage to which branches are formed by α-(1,6) linkages. It stains violet to red-violet with iodine.

am·y·lo·pec·ti·no·sis (am″ə-lo-pek″tĭ-no′sis) glycogen storage disease, type IV.

am·y·lo·pha·gia (am″ə-lo-fa′jə) [*amylo-* + *-phagia*] the habit of eating starch, such as laundry starch, a form of pica.

am·y·lo·plas·tic (am″ə-lo-plas′tik) [*amylo-* + *-plastic*] forming starch.

am·y·lor·rhea (am″ə-lo-re′ə) [*amylo-* + *rrhea*] the presence of an abnormal amount of starch in the stools.

am·y·lose (am′ə-lōs) a linear, water-soluble glucan, a lesser constituent of starch (see also *amylopectin*); it consists of a chain of glucose residues in α-(1,4) linkage and it stains blue with iodine.

am·y·lo-1:4,1:6-trans·glu·co·si·dase (am″ə-lo-trans″gloo-ko′sĭ-dās) 1,4-α-glucan branching enzyme.

am·y·lu·ria (am″əl-u′re-ə) [*amylo-* + *uria*] an excess of starch in the urine.

amyo·es·the·sia (a″mi-o-es-the′zhə) [*a-*[1] + *myo-* + *esthesia*] muscular anesthesia.

amyo·pla·sia (a-mi″o-pla′zhə) [*a-*[1] + *myo-* + *-plasia*] lack of muscle formation.

a. conge′nita a generalized lack of muscular development and growth, with contracture and deformity at most of the joints; called *congenital multiple arthrogryposis* and *arthrogryposis multiplex congenita.*

amyo·sta·sia (a-mi″o-sta′zhə) [*a-*[1] + *myo-* + *stasis*] a tremor of the muscles, seen especially in locomotor ataxia.

amyo·stat·ic (a-mi″o-stat′ik) marked by amyostasia or muscular tremors.

amyo·to·nia (a″mi-o-to′ne-ə) [*a-*[1] + *myotonia*] atonic condition of the musculature of the body; called also *myatonia* and *myatony.*

amyo·tro·phia (a-mi″o-tro′fe-ə) [*a-*[1] + *myotrophia*] amyotrophy.

neuralgic a. neuralgic amyotrophy.

a. spina′lis progressi′va progressive muscular atrophy.

amyo·tro·phic (a-mi″o-tro′fik) pertaining to or characterized by amyotrophy.

amy·ot·ro·phy (a″mi-ot′rə-fe) atrophy of muscle tissue.

diabetic a. lumbosacral radiculoplexus neuropathy associated with uncontrolled diabetes; called also *Bruns-Garland syndrome.*

neuralgic a. pain across the shoulder and upper arm, with atrophy and paralysis of the muscles of the shoulder girdle.

am·y·ous (am′e-əs) [*a-*[1] + *myo-* + *-ous*] deficient in muscular tissue.

Am·y·tal (am′ĭ-təl) trademark for preparations of amobarbital.

amyx·ia (ə-mik′se-ə) [*a-*[1] + *myx-* + *-ia*] absence of mucus.

An anodal; anode.

an-[1] the form of *a-* neg. used before a vowel or *h;* see *a-*[1].

an-[2] the form of the prefix *ana-* used before a vowel or *h;* see *ana-*.

ANA American Neurological Association; American Nurses Association; antinuclear antibodies.

ana (an′ah) [Gr.] so much of each; usually written āā (q.v.).

ana- [Gr. *ana* up, back, again] a prefix meaning upward, excessive, or again.

Ana·bae·na (an″ə-be′nə) a genus of cyanobacteria that sometimes contaminates water, giving it an offensive odor and danger of cyanobacteria poisoning.

anab·a·sine (ə-nab′ə-sēn) an alkaloid, from the plant *Anabasis aphylla*, which closely resembles nicotine; it is used as an insecticide.

ana·bi·o·sis (an″ə-bi-o′sis) [Gr. *anabiōsis* a reviving] restoration of vital processes after their apparent cessation.

ana·bi·ot·ic (an″ə-bi-ot′ik) apparently lifeless, but still capable of living.

ana·bol·ic (an″ə-bol′ik) pertaining to or serving to promote anabolism.

anab·o·lism (ə-nab′ə-liz″əm) [Gr. *anabolē* a throwing up] any constructive metabolic process by which organisms convert substances into other components of the organism's chemical architecture. Called also *assimilation* and *integration.*

anab•o•lite (ə-nab′ə-līt″) any product of anabolism or of a constructive metabolic process.

Ana•car•di•a•ce•ae (an″ə-kahr″de-a′se-e) a family of leafy plants found in many parts of the world. Many species have urushiols in their bark, leaves, and other parts and cause urushiol dermatitis. Among the more common genera are *Anacardium, Mangifera, Rhus, Schinus,* and *Semecarpus.*

Ana•car•di•um (an″ə-kahr′de-əm) a genus of tropical flowering trees of the family Anacardiaceae. *A. occidenta′le,* native to the Americas, is the cashew nut tree; its bark, leaves, and nut shells cause severe urushiol dermatitis.

ana•cata•did•y•mus (an″ə-kat″ə-did′ə-məs) anakatadidymus.

ana•cat•es•the•sia (an″ə-kat″es-the′zhə) [*ana-* + *cata-* + *esthesia*] a hovering feeling or perception.

an•acid•i•ty (an″ə-sid′ĭ-te) [*an-*[1] + *acidity*] lack of normal acidity.
gastric a. achlorhydria.

anac•la•sis (ə-nak′lə-sis) [Gr. *anaklasis* reflection] reflection or refraction of light.

ana•cli•sis (an″ə-kli′sis) [*ana-* + Gr. *klinein* to lean] physical and emotional dependence on another for protection and gratification; used to refer to the normal dependence of an infant on its mother or to excessive leaning on others for emotional support in an older individual.

ana•clit•ic (an″ə-klit′ik) 1. pertaining to anaclisis. 2. exhibiting excessive emotional dependency.

ana•co•bra (an″ə-ko′brə) cobra venom treated with formaldehyde and heat.

an•acou•sia (an″ə-koo′zhə) anakusis.

ana•crot•ic (an″ə-krot′ik) 1. pertaining to the ascending limb of a pulse tracing. 2. characterized by a notch, i.e., two waveforms in the ascending limb of the pulse tracing. Called also *anadicrotic.*

anac•ro•tism (ə-nak′rə-tiz-əm) [*ana-* + Gr. *krotos* beat + *-ism*] the presence of an anacrotic pulse.

an•acu•sis (an″ə-koo′sis) anakusis.

Ana•cys•tis (an″ə-sis′tis) *Microcystis.*

ana•di•crot•ic (an″ə-di-krot′ik) anacrotic (def. 2).

ana•did•y•mus (an″ə-did′ĭ-məs) [*ana-* + *didymus*] conjoined twins that are divided below but united toward the cephalic pole; called also *duplicitas inferior* and *duplicitas posterior.*

ana•dip•sia (an″ə-dip′se-ə) [*ana-* + *dipsia*] extreme thirst; see *hyperdipsia* and *polydipsia.*

an•adre•nal•ism (an″ə-dre′nəl-iz-əm) absence or failure of adrenal function.

an•adre•nia (an″ə-dre′ne-ə) anadrenalism.

Ana•drol (an′ə-drol) trademark for a preparation of oxymetholone.

an•aer•obe (an′ə-rōb) [*an-*[1] + *aerobe*] a microorganism that lives and grows in the complete, or almost complete, absence of molecular oxygen.
aerotolerant a. a microorganism that is normally anaerobic but can grow slowly under aerobic conditions.
facultative a. a microorganism that can grow under either anaerobic or aerobic conditions.
obligate a. a microorganism that can grow only in the complete absence of molecular oxygen; some are killed by oxygen.

an•aer•o•bic (an″ə-ro′bik) 1. lacking molecular oxygen. 2. growing, living, or occurring in the absence of molecular oxygen; pertaining to an anaerobe.

an•aer•o•bi•o•sis (an″ə-ro″bi-o′sis) [*an-*[1] + *aero-* + *biosis*] metabolic processes occurring in the absence of molecular oxygen.

An•aero•bi•o•spi•ril•lum (an-ār″o-bi-o-spi-ril′əm) a genus of gram-negative bacteria of the family Succinivibrionaceae, consisting of helical rods.
A. succiniciprodu′cens a species that sometimes causes septicemia and diarrhea.

An•aero•coc•cus (an-ār″o-kok′əs) a genus of anaerobic, gram-positive bacteria of the family Peptostreptococcaceae.
A. hydrogena′lis a species isolated from various types of infections.
A. lactoly′ticus a species isolated from urinary tract infections, diabetic ulcers, and other infections.
A. prevo′tii a species isolated from various types of infections.

an•aero•gen•ic (an″ə-ro-jen′ik) [*an-*[1] + *aero-* + *-genic*] 1. producing little or no gas. 2. suppressing the formation of gas by the gas-producing bacteria.

Anaf•ra•nil (ə-naf′rə-nil) trademark for a preparation of clomipramine hydrochloride.

an•a•gen (an′ə-jen) the long first phase of the hair cycle, during which synthesis and growth take place.

ana•go•ge (an″ə-go′je) anagogy.

ana•gog•ic (an″ə-goj′ik) [*ana-* + Gr. *agogē* leading] pertaining to the moral, uplifting, progressive strivings of the unconscious.

ana•go•gy (an″ə-gŏ′je) psychic material that has an idealistic quality.

anag•o•tox•ic (ə-nag′o-tok″sik) acting antagonistically to toxin; counteracting toxic action.

an•ag•re•lide hy•dro•chlo•ride (an-ag′rə-līd) an agent used to reduce elevated platelet counts and the risk of thrombosis in the treatment of hemorrhagic thrombocythemia; administered orally.

ana•kata•did•y•mus (an″ə-kat″ə-did′ĭ-məs) [*ana-* + *cata-* + *didymus*] conjoined twins that are separate above and below, but united in the middle.

ana•khré (ah-nah-kra′) [Fr., from native West African name] goundou.

an•a•kin•ra (an″ə-kin′rə) a recombinant, nonglycosylated form of the human interleukin-1 receptor antagonist, used as an antiinflammatory in the treatment of rheumatoid arthritis; administered subcutaneously.

an•ak•me•sis (an-ak′me-sis) [*an-*[1] + Gr. *akmēnos* full grown] arrest of maturation; specifically, increase of granulocyte precursors in the marrow with lack of further maturation, as seen in agranulocytosis.

an•aku•sis (an″ə-koo′sis) [*an-*[1] + Gr. *akouein* to hear] total deafness. Called also *anacusis* and *anacousia.*

an•al•bu•min•emia (an″al-bu″mĭ-ne′me-ə) 1. absence of albumin in the blood serum. 2. hypoalbuminemia.

ana•lep•tic (an″ə-lep′tik) [Gr. *analepsis* a repairing] 1. stimulating, invigorating, or restorative. 2. a drug that acts as a central nervous system stimulant, such as caffeine.

an•al•ge•sia (an″əl-je′ze-ə) [*an-*[1] + *algesia*] 1. absence of sensibility to pain; absence of pain on noxious stimulation. 2. the relief of pain without loss of consciousness.
audio a. audioanalgesia.
breakthrough a. analgesia administered for the relief of breakthrough pain.
continuous epidural a. a method of pain relief consisting of continuous bathing of lumbar or thoracic nerve roots within the epidural space with an injected anesthetic solution; used during labor and childbirth, in general surgery for blockage of pain pathways below the umbilicus, and postoperatively. Called also *continuous epidural anesthesia.*
epidural a. see under *block.*
infiltration a. see under *anesthesia.*
paretic a. loss of the sense of pain accompanied by partial paralysis.
patient controlled a. a technique for pain control using an infusion pump so that small doses of an opioid can be administered intravenously by the patient; it includes safeguards against overdose.
patient controlled epidural a. patient controlled analgesia in which an opioid or local anesthetic is administered into the epidural space via a catheter.
relative a. in dental anesthesia, a maintained level of conscious sedation, short of general anesthesia, in which the pain threshold is elevated, usually induced in inhalation of nitrous oxide and oxygen.
rescue a. breakthrough a.
spinal a. analgesia produced by injection of an opioid into the subarachnoid space around the spinal cord; cf. *spinal anesthesia.*

an•al•ge•sic (an″əl-je′zik) 1. relieving pain. 2. not sensitive to pain. 3. an agent that alleviates pain without causing loss of consciousness.
narcotic a. opioid a.
nonsteroidal antiinflammatory a. (NSAIA) see under *drug.*
opiate a., opioid a. any of a class of compounds that bind with a number of closely related specific receptors (opioid receptors) in the central nervous system to block the perception of pain or affect the emotional response to pain; such compounds include opium and its derivatives, as well as a number of synthetic compounds, and are used for moderate to severe pain. Chronic administration or abuse may lead to dependence.

an•al•get•ic (an″əl-jet′ik) analgesic.

an•al•gia (an-al′jə) analgesia (def. 1).

an•al•gic (an-al′jik) analgesic (def. 2).

anal•i•ty (a-nal′ĭ-te) the psychic organization of all the sensations, impulses, and personality traits derived from the anal stage (q.v.) of psychosexual development.

an•al•ler•gic (an″ə-lur′jik) not allergic; not causing anaphylaxis or hypersensitivity.

ana•log (an′ə-log) [shortening of *analogue*] 1. pertaining to electronic equipment in which data are represented by electrical signals or physical magnitudes having continuously varying values. Cf. *digital* (def. 3). 2. analogue.

anal·o·gous (ə-nal′ə-gəs) [Gr. *analogos* according to a due ratio, conformable, proportionate] resembling or similar in some respects, as in function or appearance, but not in origin or development; cf. *homologous* (def. 1).

ana·logue (an′ə-log) 1. a part or organ having the same function as another, but of a different evolutionary origin; cf. *homologue* (def. 1). 2. a chemical compound with a structure similar to that of another but differing from it in respect to a certain component; it may have a similar or opposite action metabolically. Cf. *homologue* (def. 2).

folic acid a. a structural analogue of folic acid; see *folic acid antagonist*, under *antagonist*.

homologous a. a part that is similar to another in both function and structure.

insulin a. a compound prepared from insulin that has been altered by recombinant technology so that it still has the chemical activity of insulin but has different pharmacokinetics.

metabolic a. a closely similar compound which tends to replace an essential metabolite.

nucleoside a. a structural analogue of a nucleoside, including both purine analogues and pyrimidine analogues.

purine a. a structural analogue of one of the purine bases (e.g., adenine, guanine), able to inhibit the biosynthesis of purine bases or to mimic them such that the analogues interfere with the synthesis or function of nucleic acids. Their clinical uses include antineoplastic, immunosuppressive, and antiviral agents.

pyrimidine a. a structural analogue of one of the pyrimidine bases (e.g., cytosine, thymine, uracil), able to inhibit the biosynthesis of pyrimidine bases or to mimic them such that the analogues interfere with the synthesis or function of nucleic acids. Their clinical uses include antineoplastic, antipsoriatic, antiviral, and antifungal agents.

substrate a. a substance with a structure similar to the natural substrate of an enzyme and which, because of this similarity, in some cases inhibits the action of the enzyme, as in competitive inhibition.

anal·o·gy (ə-nal′ə-je) [Gr. *analogia* equality of ratios, proportion] the quality of being analogous; resemblance or similarity in function or appearance, but not in origin or development.

an·al·pha·li·po·pro·tein·emia (an-al″fə-lip″o-pro″te-ne′me-ə) 1. absence of high-density lipoproteins (alpha lipoproteins) in the blood. 2. Tangier disease.

An·al·pram-HC (an′al-pram) trademark for preparations of hydrocortisone acetate.

anal·y·sand (ə-nal′ĭ-sand) one who is being psychoanalyzed.

anal·y·sis (ə-nal′ĭ-sis) pl. *anal′yses* [*ana-* + *-lysis*] 1. separation into component parts or elements; the act of determining the component parts of a substance. 2. psychoanalysis. **analyt′ic** *adj*

Analysis

activation a. a quantitative or qualitative determination of trace levels of atoms possessing certain types of nuclei in a sample by bombarding it with radioactivity and analyzing the emanating radiation.

affected sib-pair a. sib-pair a.

behavior a. Skinner model for examination and prediction of the behavior of individuals in the environment based on theories of operant and respondent conditioning and social learning and depending on observation.

bioimpedance a. a method for analyzing the water content of the body through variations in bioimpedance between different types of tissue.

bite a. occlusal a.

bivariate a. any of various statistical methods for analysis of the association between one independent and one dependent variable.

blood gas a. the laboratory determination of the pH and the partial pressures and concentrations of oxygen and carbon dioxide in the blood.

bootstrap a. see *bootstrap*.

bradykinetic a. cineradiographic study of motor activity.

cephalometric a. measurement of the head, using the vector quantities distance and direction, based on the tracing of the radiograph of the living head, usually in the lateral view.

character a. psychoanalysis of the personality traits and character defenses particular to an individual.

chromatographic a. chromatography.

chromosome a. karyotyping.

cluster a. in epidemiology, statistical techniques used to analyze observations that are clustered in subgroups.

colorimetric a. analysis based on the principle that in certain instances the color intensity of a solution is proportional to the concentration of a specific substance in that solution.

computer-aided semen a. (CASA), **computer-assisted semen a.** any of various methods of automated, objective, standardized evaluation of sperm concentration and movement in a semen sample, assessing the individual's potential fertility or infertility. Most techniques use video recordings showing movements of multiple spermatozoa.

a. of covariance (ANCOVA) a statistical procedure used with one dependent variable and multiple independent variables of both categorical (ordinal, dichotomous, or nominal) and continuous types; it is a variation of analysis of variance that adjusts for confounding by continuous variables; see also *a. of variance*.

decision a. a statistical method used for delineating the probabilities of various outcomes by determining the probabilities of each option available at each point where a decision can be made; often graphed as a decision tree to display the array of choices and outcomes as nodes and branches.

densimetric a. analysis by ascertaining the specific gravity of a solution and estimating the amount of matter dissolved.

discriminant function a. a form of multivariate analysis useful when the dependent variable is nominal or dichotomous and the independent variables are continuous; used to find the combination of variables that maximizes the separation between categories for the dependent variable. In recent years it has largely been replaced by logistic regression.

dot blot a. see *dot blot*, under *blot*.

Downs a. radiographic cephalometric criteria developed by Downs as an aid in orthodontic diagnosis.

ego a. in a psychoanalytic treatment, the analysis of the strengths and weaknesses of the ego, especially its defense mechanisms against unacceptable unconscious impulses.

end-group a. evaluation of the degree of linearity and branching of polysaccharide by determination of the number of end groups; determination of the amino- and carboxyl-terminal amino acids of a protein permitting an evaluation of the number of peptide chains per molecule as well as the state of purity of the protein.

gasometric a. the measurement of the different components of a gaseous mixture.

gravimetric a. a form of quantitative analysis in which the sample is purified by precipitation or combustion before being dried, weighed, and analyzed.

group a. group therapy in which interpretation is given to the patients and insight is evoked on the basis of the communication and interactions occurring within the group.

linkage a. a statistical method for determining linkage (q.v.) of loci by studying genotypes and phenotypes of parents and offspring.

log-linear a. a form of multivariate analysis useful for examining the effects of multiple independent variables, at least some of which are categorical, on a nominal dependent variable; it is used to construct models for the evaluation of relationships between categorical variables.

multipoint linkage a. linkage analysis that examines the segregation of a particular locus in relation to that of three or more linked marker loci, using recombination frequencies to determine likelihoods for various chromosomal locations.

multivariate a. any of various statistical methods for analyzing more than two variables simultaneously.

nearest neighbor sequence a. a technique for determining the nearest neighbor frequency (q.v.) for a nucleic acid; one nucleotide at a time, radioactive labeling of a nucleotide is followed by enzymatic digestion that transfers the label to the 3′-adjacent nucleotide, and the labeled products are then analyzed.

Northern blot a. see *Northern blot*, under *blot*.

occlusal a. an analysis of the contact of the teeth in centric relation and during excursions of the mandible to determine if occlusal dysfunction is present. Called also *bite a.*

organic a. the analysis of animal and vegetable tissues.

Analysis *Continued*

power a. a statistical procedure used to determine the number of subjects in a study required to show a significant difference at a predetermined level of significance and size of effect; it is also used to determine the power of a test from the sample size, size of effect, and level of significance in order to determine the risk of Type II error when the null hypothesis is accepted.
proximate a. quantitative analysis separating and identifying categories of compounds in a mixture.
pulse-chase a. a method for examining a cellular process occurring over time: organisms, cells, or organelles are briefly exposed to a radioactive compound (pulse) and washed; then they are exposed to the same compound, but in a nonradioactive form, for varying lengths of time (chase), and their characteristics over time are observed.
qualitative a., qualitive a. the determination of the nature of the constituents of a compound or a mixture of compounds.
quantitative a., quantitive a. the determination of the proportionate quantities of the constituents of a compound.
radiochemical a. direct or indirect identification or determination of the content of specific elements in a substance through measurement of the disintegration rates of radionuclides.
regression a. interpretation of a finite population of data by exploring the relationship between several variables using the principle of regression; see *regression* (def. 5).
segregation a. a statistical method for determination of the mode of inheritance of a disorder or trait by examination of its transmission within families.
sequential a. a statistical technique in which the sample size is not fixed in advance; rather, sampling is stopped as soon as significant results are observed. The criteria for stopping the trials at each sample size are set so that the overall probability (for all sample sizes) of falsely rejecting the null hypothesis at any step is held to a preset level. Cf. *hypothesis test.*
sib-pair a. a form of linkage analysis that examines pairs of siblings who are both affected by a particular genetic disorder, analyzing the genome for other loci at which the sibs share alleles more often than the 50 per cent that would be expected by chance.
Southern blot a. see *Southern blot*, under *blot.*
Southwestern blot a. see *Southwestern blot*, under *blot.*
spectroscopic a., spectrum a. analysis by means of determining the wavelength(s) at which electromagnetic energy is absorbed by a sample.
survival a. statistical analysis that evaluates the timing of events, particularly survival but also by extension other nonrecurrent events occurring in a cohort over time, such as relapse, death, or marriage. It involves following the cohort, plotting the occurrence of events, and calculating their probabilities for each time interval. See also *Kaplan-Meier survival curve*, under *curve.*
transactional a. a type of psychotherapy based on an understanding of the interactions (transactions) between patient and therapist and between patient and others in the environment. It focuses primarily on ego states, principally the Parent, Adult, and Child.
ultimate a. the determination of the proportions of elements in a chemical compound.
a. of variance (ANOVA) a statistical method for analyzing the effects of each of one or more categorical (nominal, ordinal, or dichotomous) independent variables on a continuous dependent variable as well as on each other, examining more than two groups simultaneously; if the null hypothesis that the variables' effects do not differ and all outcomes are drawn from the same population is true, then the means of all outcome groups approximate each other. To test the hypothesis, the variability between group means is compared to that within groups using the *F*-test; if their ratio approximates 1.0 then the null hypothesis cannot be rejected. When a single independent variable is tested the method is sometimes called *one-way ANOVA;* when multiple independent variables are tested, N-*way ANOVA.*
vector a. analysis of a directed quantity to determine both its magnitude and its direction, e.g., analysis of the scalar electrocardiogram to determine the magnitude and direction of the electromotive force for one complete cycle of the heart.
volumetric a. quantitative analysis of solutions of known volume but unknown strength: reagents of known concentration are added by volume to the solution until a reaction endpoint is reached; the most common method is by titration.
Western blot a. see *Western blot*, under *blot.*

ana•lyst (an′ə-list) 1. one who performs analysis. 2. psychoanalyst.

ana•lyte (an′ə-līt) a substance undergoing analysis.

ana•ly•zer (an′ə-li″zer) 1. a device used in the analysis of the physical or chemical characteristics of a sample or system. 2. a device, such as a Nicol prism, that transmits only plane polarized light, as in the eyepiece of a polariscope. 3. a nervous receptor together with its central connections, by means of which sensitivity to stimulations is differentiated.
amino acid a. an analytical instrument that separates, identifies, and measures quantities of amino acids and related compounds.
blood gas a. an instrument for measuring partial pressures of oxygen, carbon dioxide, carbon monoxide, and nitrogen in blood.
breath a. an instrument for determining the volume and composition of respired gases; some types are specifically designed for detecting alcohol in the breath.
image a. an instrument that counts, measures, and classifies cells and images viewed on microscopes, photographs, transparencies, etc.
oxygen gas a. an instrument for measuring the oxygen content of a gaseous mixture, or dissolved oxygen in a liquid, or saturation of blood hemoglobin with O_2 or partial pressure of O_2 in blood.
pulse height a. an electronic circuit designed to respond to voltage pulses only within a certain range, or window, of amplitudes.
voice a. an electronic instrument that prints out waveforms corresponding to vocal characteristics; used for analysis of voice and speech problems or identification of a particular speaker.

An•a•me (an′ə-me) a genus of spiders of the family Theraphosidae, including the venomous bird spiders.

Ana•mir•ta (an″ə-mir′tə) a genus of East Indian flowering vines of the family Menispermaceae. *A. coc′culus* L. Wight & Arn is cocculus indicus, a poisonous variety whose seeds yield picrotoxin.

an•am•ne•sis (an″am-ne′sis) [Gr. *anamnēsis* a recalling] 1. recollection. 2. a medical or psychiatric patient case history, particularly using the patient's recollections; cf. *catamnesis.* 3. immunologic memory.

an•am•nes•tic (an″am-nes′tik) 1. pertaining to anamnesis. 2. aiding the memory.

An•am•ni•o•ta (an″am-ne-o′tə) [*an-*[1] + Gr. *amnion*] a major group of vertebrates comprising those which develop no amnion, including fishes and amphibians; opposed to Amniota.

an•am•ni•ote (an-am′ne-ōt″) any animal or group belonging to the Anamniota.

an•am•ni•ot•ic (an″am-ne-ot′ik) [*an-*[1] + *amnion*] having no amnion.

ana•morph (an′ə-morf″) [*ana-* + *-morph*] the stage of a fungus where reproduction results from mitosis of a parent cell by means of conidia only (asexual spores), as opposed to a teleomorph. See also *imperfect fungus*, under *fungus.* Called also *asexual stage* or *state* and *imperfect stage* or *state.*

ana•mor•pho•sis (an″ə-mor-fo′sis) [*ana-* + *morphosis*] an ascending progression or change of form in the evolution of a group of animals or plants.

an•an•cas•tic (an″an-kas′tik) obsessive-compulsive.

an•an•da•mide (an-an′də-mīd) an endocannabinoid produced in the brain.

ana•phase (an′ə-fāz) [*ana-* + *phase*] the stage of cell division following metaphase, in which the kinetochores separate and the chromatids lined up on the spindle move to the poles (anaphase A), followed by lengthening of the spindle microtubules with consequent elongation of the cell and further separation of the poles (anaphase B). In mitosis, all pairs of chromatids are separated, resulting in a diploid number of chromosomes. In meiosis I, the chiasmata release and one of each pair of homologous chromosomes (each consisting of a pair of chromatids) moves to each pole, resulting in a haploid number of chromosomes; in meiosis II, the sister chromatids separate and move to opposite poles.

ana•phia (ə-na′fe-ə) [*an-* + Gr. *haphē* touch + *-ia*] tactile anesthesia.

ana•pho•re•sis (an-ə-fə-re′sis) the passage of charged particles toward the positive pole (anode) in electrophoresis.

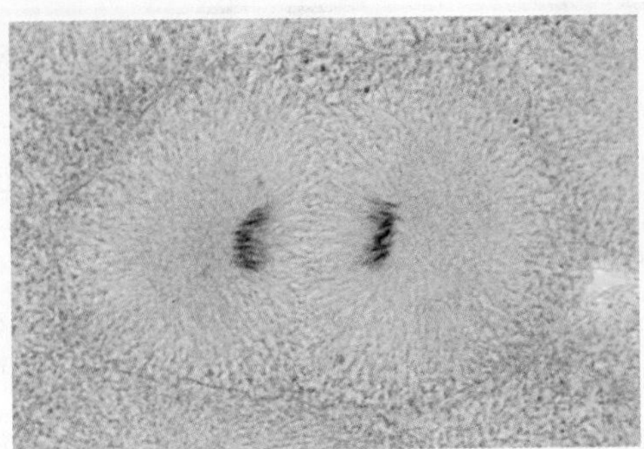

■ Anaphase stage of mitosis.

ana•pho•ria (an″ə-for′e-ə) [*ana-* + Gr. *phoros* carrying + *-ia*] a tendency for the visual axes of both eyes to divert above the horizontal plane.

an•aph•ro•dis•iac (an″af-ro-diz′e-ak) 1. repressing sexual desire. 2. a drug or medicine that allays sexual desire.

ana•phy•lac•to•gen (an″ə-fə-lak′to-jen) an antigen capable of inducing anaphylaxis.

ana•phy•lac•to•gen•e•sis (an″ə-fə-lak″to-jen′ə-sis) the production of anaphylaxis.

ana•phy•lac•to•gen•ic (an″ə-fə-lak″to-jen′ik) producing anaphylaxis.

ana•phy•lac•toid (an″ə-fə-lak′toid) resembling anaphylaxis.

ana•phyl•a•tox•in (an″ə-fil′ə-tok″sin) a substance produced by complement activation that causes the release of histamine and other mediators of immediate hypersensitivity from basophils and mast cells, thereby producing signs and symptoms of immediate hypersensitivity (anaphylaxis) without involvement of IgE. The anaphylatoxins are low-molecular-weight complement cleavage products, C3a, C4a, and C5a, which bind to specific receptors on mast cells and basophils; C4a has comparatively weak anaphylatoxin activity; C5a is also a chemotactic factor for granulocytes and macrophages.

ana•phy•lax•is (an″ə-fə-lak′sis) [*ana-* + *phylaxis*] 1. systemic or generalized anaphylaxis; a type I hypersensitivity reaction (see under *hypersenstivity reaction*) in which exposure of a sensitized individual to a specific antigen or hapten results in urticaria, pruritus, and angioedema, followed by vascular collapse and shock and often accompanied by life-threatening respiratory distress. Common agents causing anaphylaxis include Hymenoptera venom, pollen extracts, certain foods, horse and rabbit sera, heterologous enzymes and hormones, and certain drugs, such as penicillin and lidocaine. 2. a general term originally applied to the situation in which exposure to a toxin resulted not in development of immunity (prophylaxis) but in hypersensitivity. The term was extended to include all cases of systemic anaphylaxis in response to foreign antigens, as well as a variety of experimental models, such as e.g., passive cutaneous anaphylaxis. Anaphylaxis has now been subsumed under the more general concept of type I (immediate) hypersensitivity. **anaphylac′tic** *adj*

active a. the anaphylactic state produced in an individual by the injection of a foreign immunogen; distinguished from *passive anaphylaxis*.

aggregate a. an anaphylactic reaction initiated by the formation of large amounts of antigen-antibody complexes upon injection of the antigen. The complexes activate complement, producing anaphylatoxins (C3a and C5a) that trigger the release of mediators of immediate hypersensitivity from basophils and mast cells.

antiserum a. passive a.

generalized a. anaphylaxis (def. 1).

inverse a. 1. anaphylaxis in which the shocking agent is antibody rather than antigen. 2. anaphylactic shock produced by a single intravenous injection into guinea pigs of Forssman antibody, which interacts with Forssman antigen in their tissues. Called also *reverse a.*

local a. anaphylaxis confined to a limited area, e.g., passive cutaneous anaphylaxis.

passive a. anaphylaxis occurring in a normal individual as a result of the injection of the serum of a previously sensitized individual; called also *antiserum a.*

passive cutaneous a. (PCA) a passively transferred local anaphylactic reaction used in the study of reaginic antibodies; the skin of an animal is sensitized by intradermal injection of serum from a sensitized animal, and after a 24- to 72-hour latent period the antigen and Evans blue dye are injected intravenously. Reaction of the antigen with skin-fixed antibody causes the release of histamine, which increases vascular permeability, permits leakage of the albumin-bound dye, and produces a blue spot at the site of the intradermal injection.

reverse a. anaphylaxis following the injection of antigen succeeded by the injection of antiserum; also local reactions from the union of circulating antibodies with antigen fixed by tissue cells.

systemic a. anaphylaxis (def. 1).

ana•phy•lo•tox•in (an″ə-fil′o-tok″sin) anaphylatoxin.

ana•pla•sia (an″ə-pla′zhə) [*ana-* + *-plasia*] a loss of differentiation of cells and of their orientation to one another and to their axial framework and blood vessels, a characteristic of tumor tissue; called also *dedifferentiation* and *undifferentiation.*

Ana•plas•ma (an″ə-plaz′mə) [Gr. *anaplasma* something without form] a genus of tick-borne bacteria of the family Anaplasmataceae, consisting of small, gram-negative, often pleomorphic, coccoid to ellipsoidal cells that are nonmotile and non–spore-forming. Organisms are parasitic in cells of the hematopoietic system and associated tissues, occurring in cytoplasmic vacuoles and often forming inclusion bodies (morulae); they cause disease in canids, ruminants, and humans. The type species is *A. margina′le*.

A. margina′le a species that causes disease in ruminants.

A. o′vis a species that causes anaplasmosis in sheep and goats.

A. phagocyto′philum a species containing organisms formerly classified in the genus Ehrlichia; it causes human granulocytic anaplasmosis, tick-borne fever in ruminants, and canine and equine granulocytic anaplasmosis. Formerly called *Ehrlichia phagocytophila.*

A. pla′tys a species that causes infectious cyclic thrombocytopenia in dogs. Formerly called *Ehrlichia platys.*

Ana•plas•ma•ta•ce•ae (an″ə-plaz″mə-ta′se-e) a family of bacteria of the order Rickettsiales, consisting of small, gram-negative, often pleomorphic, coccoid to ellipsoidal organisms parasitic in cells of the blood and hematopoietic system in some mammals and birds and transmitted by arthropods and helminths. Organisms grow in a cytoplasmic vacuole, and in blood smears stained with Romanowsky stain they appear as dense, bluish-purple inclusions known as morulae. There are two morphological forms: dense-core and reticulate cells. They cause disease in mammals and birds. The family includes the genera *Aegyptianella, Anaplasma, Ehrlichia, Neorickettsia* and *Wolbachia.*

ana•plas•mo•da•stat (an″ə-plaz-mo′də-stat″) any of a group of chemical agents for control of anaplasmosis in animals.

ana•plas•mo•sis (an″ə-plaz-mo′sis) 1. infection with organisms of the genus *Anaplasma.* 2. a disease of cattle and related ruminants marked by fever, anemia, and icterus; caused by *Anaplasma marginale* or *A. ovis,* which is transmitted by ticks and other blood-sucking arthropods. Called also *gallsickness* or *gall sickness.*

canine granulocytic a. an infection of dogs with *Anaplasma phagocytophilum*, characterized by fever, lethargy, and anorexia with lymphopenia and thrombocytopenia.

equine granulocytic a. a usually nonfatal infection of horses with *Anaplasma phagocytophilaum*, seen in California and eastward into the midwestern United States; characteristics include fever, limb edema, and anemia. Formerly called *equine ehrlichiosis.*

human granulocytic a. (HGA) infection with *Anaplasma phagocytophilum*, transmitted by ticks of the genus *Ixodes.* It affects primarily neutrophils, is characterized by flulike symptoms with leukopenia and thrombocytopenia, and ranges in severity from asymptomatic to severe or occasionally fatal. Formerly called *human granulocytic ehrlichiosis.*

ana•plas•tic (an″ə-plas′tik) [*ana-* + *plastic*] characterized by anaplasia or reversed development; said of cells. Called also *undifferentiated.*

ana•ple•ro•sis (an″ə-plĕ-ro′sis) [Gr. "filling up, restoration"] anaplerotic reaction.

ana•ple•rot•ic (an″ə-plĕ-rot′ik) [*anaplerosis*] pertaining to a filling up or restoration; see under *reaction.*

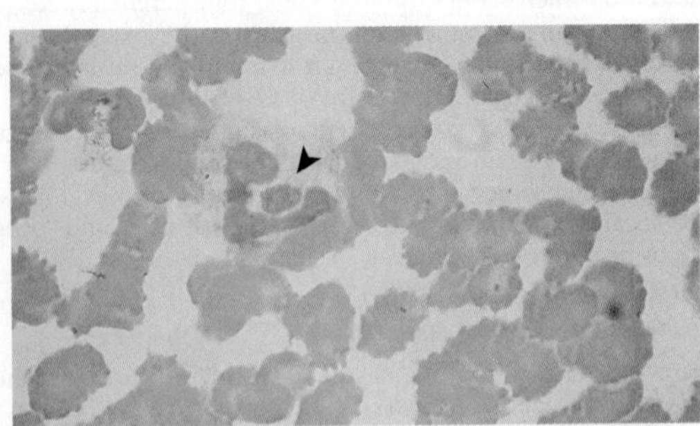

■ Human granulocytic anaplasmosis; a peripheral blood smear shows a morula *(arrowhead)* containing *Anaplasma phagocytophilum* in a neutrophil (Wright stain).

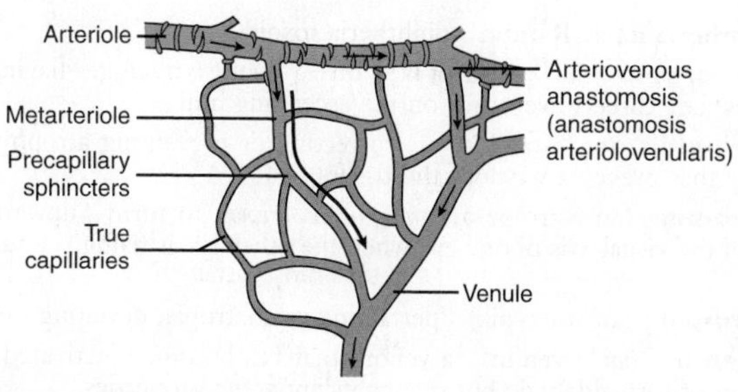

■ Dermal vasculature showing arteriovenous anastomoses.

Ana•plex DM (an′ə-pleks″) trademark for a combination preparation of dextromethorphan hydrobromide, brompheniramine maleate, and pseudoephedrine hydrochloride.

Ana•plex HD (an′ə-pleks″) trademark for a combination preparation of hydrocodone bitartrate, brompheniramine maleate, and pseudoephedrine hydrochloride.

Ana•po•lon (an″ə-po′lon) trademark for a preparation of oxymetholone.

an•apoph•y•sis (an″ə-pof′ĭ-sis) [*ana-* + *apophysis*] an accessory vertebral process, especially an accessory process of a thoracic or lumbar vertebra.

Ana•prox (an′ə-proks) trademark for a preparation of naproxen sodium.

anap•tic (ə-nap′tik) marked by anaphia (tactile anesthesia).

an•a•rith•mia (an″ə-rith′me-ə) [*an-* + Gr. *arithmos* number] acalculia.

an•ar•rhex•is (an″ə-rek′sis) [*ana-* + *-rrhexis*] the operation of refracturing a bone.

an•ar•thria (an-ahr′thre-ə) [*an-* + *arthr-*[2] + *-ia*] severe dysarthria (q.v.) resulting in speechlessness.

ana•sar•ca (an″ə-sahr′kə) [*ana-* + *sarco*] generalized massive edema.

ana•sar•cous (an″ə-sahr′kəs) affected with or of the nature of anasarca.

an•a•scit•ic (an″ə-sit′ik) without ascites.

an•a•stig•mat•ic (an″ə-stig-mat′ik) not astigmatic; corrected for astigmatism.

anas•to•mose (ə-nas′tə-mōs) 1. to connect with one another by anastomosis, as arteries and veins. 2. to create a connection between two formerly separate structures.

anas•to•mo•sis (ə-nas″tə-mo′sis) pl. *anastomo′ses* [Gr. *anastomōsis* opening, outlet] 1. a connection between two vessels. See also *rete.* 2. an opening created by surgical, traumatic, or pathological means between two normally separate spaces or organs. Cf. *shunt.* **anastomot′ic** *adj*

antiperistaltic a. enterostomy in which the intestinal segments are so joined that the directions of the peristaltic waves in the two conjoined portions are opposed.

a. arteriolovenula′ris [TA] arteriolovenular anastomosis: a vessel that directly interconnects the arterial and venous systems and that acts as a shunt to bypass the capillary bed. Called also *a. arteriovenosa* [TA alternative] and *arteriovenous a.*

a. arterioveno′sa TA alternative for *a. arteriolovenularis.*

arteriovenous a. 1. a. arteriolovenularis. 2. arteriovenous shunt (def. 2).

biliary-enteric a., bilioenteric a. surgical anastomosis of one end of the biliary duct to the small intestine.

Braun a. formation of an anastomosis between the afferent and efferent intestinal loops just distal to a gastroenteric stoma to prevent unwanted mixing of gastric and duodenal contents.

Clado a. the anastomosis between the appendicular and ovarian arteries in the appendiculo-ovarian ligament.

crucial a., cruciate a. an arterial anastomosis in the proximal part of the thigh, formed by the anastomotic branch of the sciatic, the internal circumflex, the first perforating, and the transverse portion of the external circumflex.

end-to-end a. 1. an anastomosis connecting the end of an artery and that of some other vessel, either directly or with a synthetic graft. 2. anastomosis of two sections of colon, such as with partial colectomy or when an ileostomy is closed.

end-to-side a. 1. an anastomosis connecting the end of one vessel with the side of a larger one. 2. anastomosis between two sections of colon with the smaller segment terminating at a stoma in the side of the larger one.

Galen a. ramus communicans nervi laryngei superioris cum nervo laryngeo inferiore.

Glenn a. see under *operation.*

heterocladic a. an anastomosis between branches of different arteries.

homocladic a. an anastomosis between two branches of the same artery.

Hyrtl a. see under *loop.*

ileoanal a. anastomosis of the terminal ileum and anus following colectomy, often in conjunction with creation of a reservoir from the terminal ileum; performed in the management of ulcerative colitis.

ileoanal pull-through a. anastomosis of an ileoanal reservoir to the anal canal by means of a short conduit of ileum pulled through the rectal cuff and sutured to the anus; done to allow continent elimination of feces following colectomy in the management of ulcerative colitis. See also *Duhamel operation*, *Soave operation*, and *Swenson operation*, under *operation.* Called also *ileoanal pull-through procedure.*

ileorectal a. surgical anastomosis of the ileum and rectum after total colectomy, done in treatment of ulcerative colitis.

intestinal a. the establishment of a communication between two portions of the intestinal tract.

isoperistaltic a. enterostomy in which the intestinal segments are so joined that the peristaltic waves in the two conjoined portions progress in the same direction.

microvascular a. anastomosis of microvessels, such as with a free flap.

portal-systemic a., portosystemic a. 1. a naturally occurring anastomosis between the portal and systemic venous circulations. 2. see under *shunt.*

postcostal a. a longitudinal linkage of the seven highest intersegmental arteries in the embryo that gives rise to the vertebral artery.

Potts a. see under *operation.*

precapillary a. anastomosis between small arteries just before they become capillaries.

precostal a. a longitudinal anastomosis of intersegmental arteries in the embryo that gives rise to the thyrocervical and costocervical trunks.

pyeloileocutaneous a. a rare type of ileal conduit that connects the renal pelvis to the abdominal wall.

a. of Riolan the part of the marginal artery of the colon that is an anastomosis of the superior and inferior mesenteric arteries.

Roux-en-Y a. any Y-shaped anastomosis in which the small intestine is included; after division of the small intestine segment, the distal end is implanted into another organ, such as the stomach or esophagus, and the proximal end into the small intestine below the anastomosis to provide drainage without reflux.

stirrup a. an arterial branch sometimes seen connecting the dorsalis pedis and external plantar arteries.

Sucquet-Hoyer a. segmentum arteriale anastomosis arteriovenosae glomeriformis.

terminoterminal a. surgical anastomosis between the distal end of an artery and the proximal end of the corresponding vein and between the proximal end of the artery and the distal end of the vein.

transureteroureteral a. transureteroureterostomy.

ureterocolonic a. anastomosis of a ureter to part of the colon, either a detached segment like an ileal conduit or an in situ segment so that urine empties into the colon, sometimes as a continent urinary diversion. Called also *ureterocolostomy.*

ureteroileal a., ureteroileocutaneous a. ileal conduit.

ureterointestinal a. surgical attachment of a ureter to part of the intestine, as either an ileal conduit, a neobladder, or a continent urinary diversion. Called also *ureteroenterostomy.*

ureterosigmoid a. surgical implantation of the ureter into the sigmoid colon; this was one of the earliest types of continent urinary diversion. Called also *ureterosigmoidostomy.*

ureteroureteral a. ureteroureterostomy.

Waterston a. see under *operation.*

an•as•tral (an-as′trəl) [*an-*[1] + *astral*] lacking, or pertaining to the lack of, an aster; used in reference to a mitotic spindle.

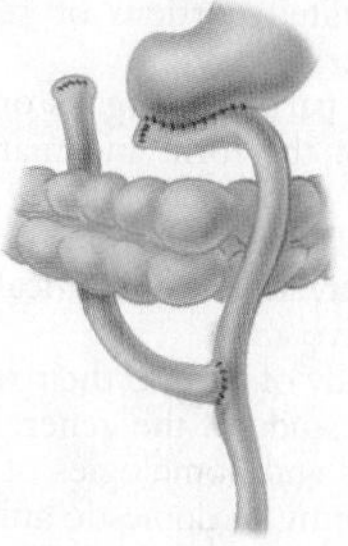
■ Roux-en-Y anastomosis

anas·tro·zole (ə-nas′trə-zōl) a nonsteroidal aromatase inhibitor that lowers levels of serum estradiol by interfering with its production in peripheral tissues and is used in chemotherapy for advanced carcinoma of the breast in postmenopausal women; administered orally.

anat. anatomical; anatomy.

ana·tom·ic (an″ə-tom′ik) anatomical.

ana·tom·i·cal (an″ə-tom′ĭ-kəl) pertaining to anatomy, or to the structure of an organism.

ana·tom·i·co·med·i·cal (an-ə-tom″ĭ-ko-med′ĭ-kəl) pertaining to anatomy and medicine or to medical anatomy.

ana·tom·i·co·path·o·log·i·cal (an″ə-tom″ĭ-ko-path″o-loj′ĭ-kəl) pertaining to anatomic pathology.

ana·tom·i·co·phys·i·o·log·i·cal (an-ə-tom″ĭ-ko-fiz″e-o-loj′ĭ-kəl) pertaining to anatomy and physiology.

ana·tom·i·co·sur·gi·cal (an-ə-tom″ĭ-ko-sur′jĭ-kəl) pertaining to anatomy and surgery.

anat·o·mist (ə-nat′ə-mist) a person skilled or learned in anatomy; a specialist in the science of anatomy.

anat·o·my (ə-nat′ə-me) [*ana-* + *-tomy*] 1. the science of the structure of the body and the relation of its parts; it is largely based on dissection, from which it obtains its name. 2. dissection of an organized body.

applied a. anatomy as applied to diagnosis and treatment.

artificial a. the study of anatomical structure by use of models or other artificial means.

artistic a. the study of anatomy as applied to drawing, painting, and sculpture.

clastic a. anatomy studied by the aid of models in which various layers can be removed to show the position of organs and parts underneath.

clinical a. anatomy as applied to clinical practice.

comparative a. a comparison of the structure of different animals and plants, one with another.

corrosion a. anatomy studied by means of corrosive agents that remove the tissues not intended to be observed.

dental a. the study of the structure of the teeth and their correlated parts.

descriptive a. the study or description of individual parts of the body; called also *systematic a.*

developmental a. the field of study concerned with the changes that cells, tissues, organs, and the body as a whole undergo from fertilization of a secondary oocyte to the resulting offspring; it includes both prenatal (embryology and fetology) and postnatal development.

general a. the study of the structure and composition of the body, and its tissues and fluids in general.

gross a. anatomy that deals with structures that can be distinguished with the unaided eye; called also *macroscopic a.*

histologic a. histology.

homologic a. the study of the correlated parts of the body in different animals.

macroscopic a. gross a.

medical a. anatomy concerned with the study of points connected with the physical examination and localization of internal abnormalities.

microscopic a., minute a. histology.

morbid a., pathological a. anatomic pathology.

physiognomonic a. the study of the external expression of the body surface, especially of the face.

physiological a. the study of the organs with respect to their normal functions.

plastic a. the study of anatomy by the aid of models and manikins, especially those that can be taken apart.

practical a. anatomy studied by means of demonstration and dissection.

radiological a. the study of the anatomy of organs and tissues using radiological techniques.

regional a. descriptive anatomy arranged according to the regions of the body; the study of limited portions or regions of the body and the relationships of their parts.

special a. the study of particular organs or parts.

surface a. the study of the form and markings of the surface of the body, especially in relation to deeper parts.

surgical a. the study of limited portions or regions of the body, with a view to the diagnosis and treatment of surgical conditions.

systematic a. descriptive a.

topographic a. the study of parts in their relation to surrounding parts.

transcendental a. the study of the general design and morphology of the body and the analogies and homologies of its parts.

veterinary a. the anatomy of domestic animals.

x-ray a. radiological a.

ana·tox·in (an′ə-tok″sin) [*ana-* + *toxin*] toxoid. **anatox′ic** *adj*

diphtheria a., a.-Ramon diphtheria toxoid.

ana·tri·crot·ic (an″ə-tri-krot′ik) on a pulse tracing, having two notches, i.e., three waveforms, on the ascending limb.

ana·tro·phic (an″ə-tro′fik) 1. correcting or preventing atrophy. 2. a remedy that prevents waste of the tissues.

ana·tro·pia (an″ə-tro′pe-ə) [*ana-* + Gr. *trepein* to turn] upward deviation of the visual axis of one eye when the other eye is fixing. **anatrop′ic** *adj*

ana·tro·pic (an″ə-tro′pik) pertaining to anatropia; deviating upward.

ana·ven·in (an″ə-ven′in) a venom that has become inactivated by the addition of formaldehyde but retains its antigenic properties.

ANCA antineutrophil cytoplasmic autoantibody (or antibody).

An·cef (an′sef) trademark for a preparation of cefazolin sodium.

an·chor (ang′kər) a means by which something is held securely.

endosteal implant a. a metal implant in the shape of a ship's anchor, usually made of a chromium-cobalt alloy, which is placed deep into the bone to provide retention for an implant denture.

an·chor·age (ang′kər-əj) 1. surgical fixation of a displaced viscus. 2. in operative dentistry, the fixation of fillings or of artificial crowns or bridges. 3. in orthodontics, the nature and degree of resistance to displacement offered by an anatomical unit when force is applied to cause movement during a procedure. 4. in tissue cell culture, the attachment of proliferating cells to a solid surface.

cervical a. an orthodontic anchorage in which the back of the neck is used for resistance through a strap fitted around the neck.

compound a. an orthodontic anchorage in which the resistance is obtained from two or more teeth.

extramaxillary a. extraoral a.

extraoral a. an orthodontic anchorage in which the resistance unit is outside of the oral cavity, the force being transmitted to the teeth by means of headgear attached to the teeth. Called also *extramaxillary a.*

intermaxillary a. an orthodontic anchorage in which the resistance units situated in one jaw are used to effect tooth movement in the other jaw. Called also *maxillomandibular a.*

intraoral a. an orthodontic anchorage in which the resistance units are all located within the oral cavity.

maxillomandibular a. intermaxillary a.

multiple a. an orthodontic anchorage in which more than one type of resistance unit is used. Called also *reinforced a.*

occipital a. an orthodontic anchorage in which the resistance is borne by the top and back of the head, and the force is transmitted to the teeth by means of the headgear and heavy elastics connected with attachment on the teeth.

precision a. see under *attachment.*

reciprocal a. anchorage in which the movement of one or more dental units is balanced against the movement of one or more opposing dental units. Cf. *reciprocal force.*

reinforced a. multiple a.

simple a. an orthodontic anchorage in which larger teeth or groups of teeth and their location are used to move teeth of lesser size; the resistance to the movement comes solely from resistance to tipping movement of the anchored unit.

stationary a. an orthodontic anchorage in which the resistance to the movement of one or more dental units comes from the resistance to bodily movement of the anchorage unit; a questionable concept of anchorage implying that selected teeth remain stable.

an·cil·la·ry (an′sĭ-lar″e) [L. *ancillaris* relating to a maid servant] assisting in the performance of a service or the achievement of a result.

an·cip·i·tal (an-sip′ĭ-təl) [L. *anceps* two headed] having two heads or two edges.

An·cis·tro·don (an-sis′tro-don) *Agkistrodon.*

an·cis·troid (an-sis′troid) [Gr. *ankistron* fishhook + *-oid*] uncinate.

An·co·bon (an′ko-bon) trademark for a preparation of flucytosine.

an·co·ne·al (ang-ko′ne-əl) cubital.

an·co·ni·tis (ang″ko-ni′tis) inflammation of the elbow joint.

ANCOVA analysis of covariance.

an·crod (an′krod) a proteinase obtained from the venom of the Malayan pit viper *Agkistrodon rhodostoma*; it reduces the blood concentration of fibrinogen and is used as an anticoagulant in the treatment of deep vein thrombosis and the prevention of postoperative thrombosis.

ancyl(o)- for words beginning thus, see also words beginning *ankyl(o)-*.

An·cy·los·to·ma (ang″kĭ-los′tə-mə, an″sĭ-los′tə-mə) [*ancylo-* + *stoma*] a genus of hookworms, nematode parasites of the family Ancylostomatidae.

A. america′num *Necator americanus.*

A. brazilien′se a hookworm found in cats and dogs in tropical and subtropical regions of the Americas, from Brazil to the southeastern

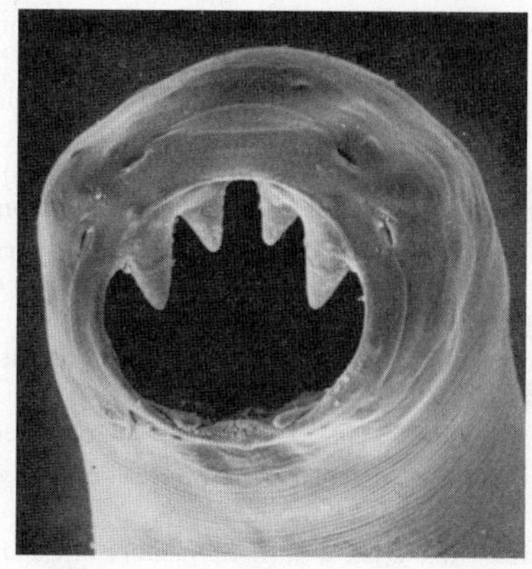

■ Scanning electron micrograph of mouth of *Ancylostoma duodenale* showing the two pairs of teeth.

United States. Its larvae may cause cutaneous larva migrans in humans (see under *larva*).

A. cani′num the most common hookworm of dogs; it also infects cats, and its larvae may cause cutaneous larva migrans in humans (see under *larva*).

A. ceylo′nicum *A. braziliense.*

A. duodena′le the common European or Old World hookworm, which inhabits the small intestine and causes ancylostomiasis. Males are 10 to 12 mm long and females are somewhat larger.

A. tubaefor′mis a common hookworm of cats.

an•cy•lo•sto•mat•ic (an″kĭ-lo-stə-mat′ik, an″sĭ-lo-stə-mat′ik) caused by *Ancylostoma.*

An•cy•lo•sto•ma•ti•dae (ang″kĭ-lo-, an″sĭ-lo-sto-mat′ĭ-de) the hookworms, a family of often parasitic phasmid nematodes that includes the genera *Ancylostoma, Bunostomum, Gaigeria, Necator,* and *Uncinaria.* See also *hookworm disease*, under *disease*.

an•cylo•stome (an-kil′ə-stōm, an-sil′ə-stōm) 1. an individual of the genus *Ancylostoma.* 2. an individual of the family Ancylostomidae; a hookworm.

an•cy•los•to•mi•a•sis (an″sĭ-los″to-mi′ə-sis) 1. a type of hookworm disease in carnivores, caused by members of the genus *Ancylostoma.* 2. cutaneous larva migrans (def. 1).

An•cy•lo•sto•mi•dae (ang″kĭ-lo-, an″sĭ-lo-sto′mĭ-de) Ancylostomatidae.

An•cy•los•to•mum (an″kĭ-los-to′məm, an″sĭ-los-to′məm) *Ancylostoma.*

an•cy•roid (an′sə-roid) [Gr. *ankyra* anchor + *oid*] shaped like an anchor or hook.

An•der•nach ossicles (ahn′der-nahk) [Johann Winther von *Andernach*, German physician, 1487–1574] one of the ossa suturalia; see *os suturale.*

An•ders disease (an′dərs) [James Meschter *Anders*, American physician, 1854–1936] adiposis dolorosa.

An•dersch ganglion, nerve (ahn′dərsh) [Carolus Samuel *Andersch*, German anatomist, 1732–1777] see *ganglion inferius nervi glossopharyngei* and *nervus tympanicus.*

An•der•sen disease, syndrome (an′dər-sən) [Dorothy Hansine *Andersen*, American pathologist, 1901–1963] see under *disease* and *syndrome.*

An•der•sen syndrome (an′dər-sen) [Ellen D. *Andersen*, Norwegian geneticist, late 20th century] Andersen-Tawil syndrome.

An•der•sen-Ta•wil syndrome (an′dər-sen tah′wil) [E.D. *Andersen;* Al-Rabi N. *Tawil*, American neurologist, born 1958] see under *syndrome.*

An•der•son splint (an′dər-son) [Roger *Anderson*, American orthopedic surgeon, 1891–1971] see under *splint.*

An•der•son-Hynes pyeloplasty (an′dər-sən hīnz) [J.C. *Anderson*, British surgeon, 20th century; W. *Hynes*, British surgeon, 20th century] dismembered pyeloplasty; see under *pyeloplasty.*

An•des disease (an′dēz) [*Andes* Mountains in Peru, where it was first observed] chronic mountain sickness.

An•dre•sen appliance (ahn′drə-sən) [Viggo *Andresen*, Norwegian orthodontist, 1870–1950] see *functional activator*, under *activator.*

andr(o)- [Gr. *anēr, andros* man] a combining form denoting relationship to the male.

an•dro•blas•to•ma (an″dro-blas-to′mə) 1. a rare, benign tumor of the testis that histologically resembles the fetal testis; there are three varieties: diffuse stromal, mixed (stromal and epithelial), and tubular (epithelial). Sertoli cells in the epithelial elements may produce estrogen and cause feminization. Called also *gonadal stromal tumor, Pick testicular* or *tubular adenoma, tubular adenoma,* and *Sertoli cell tumor.* 2. a rare tumor of the ovary, usually occurring in young women; both Sertoli cells (sex cord origin) and Leydig cells (stromal origin) are present. The tumor may cause masculinization and hirsutism, although occasionally estrogenic activity results. Called also *Sertoli-Leydig cell tumor* and *arrhenoblastoma.*

An•droc•to•nus (an-drok′tə-nəs) the fat-tailed scorpions, a genus of the family Buthidae found in North Africa and parts of Asia. *A. austra′lis* is a yellow species with a deadly sting.

an•dro•de•do•tox•in (an″dro-de′do-tok″sin) a poisonous principle from the leaves of rhododendrons.

An•dro•derm (an′dro-durm″) trademark for a preparation of testosterone.

an•droe•ci•um (an-dre′she-əm) stamen.

an•dro•ga•lac•to•ze•mia (an″dro-gə-lak″to-ze′me-ə) [*andro-* + *galacto-* + Gr. *zēmia* loss] lactation from the male breast.

An•dro•gel (an′dro-jel) trademark for a preparation of testosterone.

an•dro•gen (an′dro-jən) [*andro-* + *-gen*] any substance that promotes masculinization; see *adrenal a′s* and *testosterone.*

adrenal a′s the 19-carbon steroids synthesized by the adrenal cortex that function as weak steroids or steroid precursors, including dehydroepiandrosterone, dehydroepiandrosterone sulfate, and androstenedione.

an•dro•gen•e•sis (an″dro-jen′ə-sis) [*andro-* + *-genesis*] development of a zygote that contains only paternal chromosomes, as after fertilization of an oocyte whose chromosomes are absent or inactivated.

an•dro•ge•net•ic (an″dro-jə-net′ik) 1. pertaining to androgenesis. 2. caused by androgens.

an•dro•gen•ic (an″dro-jen′ik) 1. producing masculine characteristics. 2. pertaining to an androgen.

an•dro•ge•nic•i•ty (an″dro-jə-nis′ĭ-te) the quality of exerting a masculinizing effect.

an•dro•gen•i•za•tion (an″dro-jen-ĭ-za′shən) masculinization.

an•drog•e•nized (an-droj′ə-nīzd) showing the effects of a response to androgens.

an•drog•e•nous (an-droj′ə-nəs) [*andro-* + *-genous*] pertaining or tending to the production of male rather than female offspring.

an•dro•gyne (an′dro-jīn) 1. a person characterized by androgyny; see also *pseudohermaphrodite.* 2. female pseudohermaphrodite.

an•drog•y•nism (an-droj′ĭ-niz″əm) 1. androgyny. 2. pseudohermaphroditism.

an•drog•y•noid (an-droj′ĭ-noid) 1. pseudohermaphrodite. 2. androgynous.

an•drog•y•nous (an-droj′ĭ-nəs) pertaining to or characterized by androgyny; see also *pseudohermaphrodite.* Called also *androgynoid, bisexual,* and *intersexual.*

an•drog•y•ny (an-droj′ĭ-ne) 1. sexual ambiguity, either physical or psychological; called also *androgynism* and *bisexuality.* 2. female pseudohermaphroditism.

An•droid (an′droid) trademark for a preparation of methyltestosterone.

an•droid (an′droid) [*andr-* + *-oid*] resembling a man; see *male.* Called also *androidal* and *andromorphous.*

an•droi•dal (an-droi′dəl) android.

an•dro•log•ic (an″drə-loj′ik) pertaining to andrology or to health conditions specific to males.

an•dro•log•i•cal (an″drə-loj′ĭ-kəl) andrologic.

an•drol•o•gist (an-drol′ə-jist) a specialist in andrology.

an•drol•o•gy (an-drol′ə-je) [*andro-* + *-logy*] scientific study of the male body and diseases and conditions specific to males, such as diseases of the male reproductive organs.

An•drom•e•da (an-drom′ə-də) [L.] a genus of shrubs and trees of the family Ericaceae; some species contain andromedotoxin.

an•drom•e•do•tox•in (an-drom′ə-do-tok″sin) [*Andromeda* + *toxin*] a poisonous crystalline principle found in plants such as species of *Andromeda, Azalea, Kalmia,* and *Rhododendron.* In sheep and other livestock that graze on the plants, it causes salivation, nasal discharge, emesis, and central nervous system symptoms that may include paralysis, coma, and death. Called also *acetylandromedol* and *grayanotoxin.*

an•dro•mi•met•ic (an″dro-mĭ-met′ik) [*andro-* + *mimetic*] exerting influences of the sort promoted by testosterone and other androgens. See also *masculinization.*

an•dro•mor•phous (an″dro-mor′fəs) [*andro-* + *morph-* + *-ous*] android.

an•drop•a•thy (an-drop′ə-the) [*andro-* + *-pathy*] any disease peculiar to males.

an•dro•pause (an′dro-pawz) [*andro-* + *pause*] a variable complex of symptoms, including a reduction in Leydig cell numbers and a decline in androgen production, occurring in men after middle age, purported to be analogous to menopause in women.

an•droph•i•lous (an-drof′ĭ-ləs) anthropophilic.

an•dro•stane (an′dro-stān) the 19-carbon tetracyclic hydrocarbon nucleus, $C_{19}H_{32}$, that is the parent structure of the androgens; used in steroid nomenclature.

an•dro•stane•di•ol (an″dro-stān-di′ol, -stān′de-ol) an androgen, $C_{19}H_{32}O_2$, implicated as a regulator of gonadotropin secretion.

a. **glucuronide** a metabolite of dihydrotestosterone formed in the peripheral tissues; plasma and urinary concentrations are used to estimate peripheral androgen activity.

an•dro•stene (an′dro-stēn) a cyclic hydrocarbon nucleus, $C_{19}H_{30}$, with one double bond; used in androgen nomenclature.

an•dro•stene•di•ol (an″dro-stēn-di′ol, -stēn′de-ol) a testosterone metabolite, $C_{19}H_{30}O_2$, occurring in two isomeric forms, 3-*trans*,17-dihydroxy Δ^5-androstene and 3-*cis*,17-dihydroxy Δ^5-androstene, that may contribute to gonadotropin secretion.

an•dro•stene•di•one (an″dro-stēn-di′ōn, -stēn′de-ōn) an anabolic-androgenic steroid produced by the testis, adrenal cortex, and ovary, occurring as two types, Δ^4-androstenedione and Δ^5-androstenedione. Androstenediones can be converted metabolically to testosterone and other androgens.

an•dros•ter•one (an-dros′tər-ōn) an androgen degradation product, 3α-hydroxy-5α-androstan-17-one, $C_{19}H_{30}O_2$; in some species it exerts weak androgenlike effects.

AN-DTPA trademark for a kit for the preparation of technetium Tc 99m pentetate.

-ane a word termination denoting a saturated open-chain hydrocarbon, C_nH_{2n+2}.

an•ec•do•tal (an″ek-do′təl) [Gr. *anekdotos* not published] based on descriptions of unmatched individual cases rather than on controlled studies.

an•ec•dy•sis (an-ek′dĭ-sis) [*an-*[1] + *ecdysis*] a long period during the molting cycle of arthropods when there are no signs of either recovery from a molt or preparations for the next molt.

an•echo•ic (an-ə-ko′ik) [*an-*[1] + *echo* + *-ic*] 1. without echoes, as an anechoic chamber. 2. sonolucent.

an•ec•ta•sis (an-ek′tə-sis) [*an-*[1] + *ectasis*] primary atelectasis.

An•ec•tine (an-ek′tin) trademark for preparations of succinylcholine chloride.

an•e•jac•u•la•tion (an″e-jak″u-la′shən) failure of ejaculation of semen from the urinary meatus in sexual intercourse.

An•el probe, syringe (ah-nel′) [Dominique *Anel*, French surgeon, 1679–1730] see under *probe* and *syringe*.

an•elec•trot•o•nus (an″ə-lek-trot′ə-nəs) [*ana-* + *electrotonus*] lessened irritability of a nerve in the region of the positive pole or anode during the passage of an electric current. **anelectroton′ic** *adj*

Anel•lo•vi•rus (ə-nel′o-vi″rəs) a genus of nonenveloped DNA viruses that has not been assigned to a family; it includes the pathogenic species Torque teno virus.

ane•mia (ə-ne′me-ə) [*an-*[1] + *-emia*] a reduction below normal in the concentration of erythrocytes or hemoglobin in the blood, measured per mm^3 or by volume of packed red cells per 100 mL of blood; it occurs when the equilibrium is disturbed between blood loss (through bleeding or destruction) and blood production. **ane′mic** *adj*

Anemia

achrestic a. any of various types of megaloblastic anemia that resemble pernicious anemia but are unresponsive to therapy with vitamin B_{12}.
achylic a. iron deficiency a.
acquired sideroachrestic a., acquired sideroblastic a. refractory sideroblastic a.
acute posthemorrhagic a. hemorrhagic a.
anhematopoietic a. aplastic a.
aplastic a. any of a diverse group of anemias characterized by bone marrow failure with reduction of hematopoietic cells and their replacement by fat, resulting in pancytopenia, often accompanied by granulocytopenia and thrombocytopenia. It may be hereditary; it may be secondary to causes such as toxic, radiant, or immunologic injury to bone marrow stem cells or their microenvironment; it may be associated with various diseases; or it may be idiopathic.
Arctic a. polar a.
aregenerative a. an anemia characterized by bone marrow failure, so that functional marrow cells are regenerated slowly or not at all; the term has been used to denote specific disorders with this characteristic, including aplastic anemia and pure red cell anemia.
autoimmune hemolytic a. (AIHA) any of a large group of anemias involving autoantibodies against red cell antigens. Those due to warm-reactive antibodies, usually IgG but occasionally IgM or IgA, may be idiopathic or secondary to autoimmune diseases, hematologic neoplasms, viral infections, or immunodeficiency diseases, and usually involve sequestration of sensitized erythrocytes by the spleen. Those due to cold-reactive antibodies, usually IgM but occasionally IgG, include cold agglutinin syndrome and paroxysmal cold hemoglobinuria and usually involve complement-dependent intravascular hemolysis or sequestration of erythrocytes by the liver.
***Bartonella* a.** Oroya fever.
Blackfan-Diamond a. congenital hypoplastic a. (def. 1).
a. of chronic disease, a. of chronic disorders mild to moderate anemia secondary to any of numerous chronic diseases lasting more than two months, such as infections, inflammatory conditions, or malignancies, characterized by hypoferremia in combination with siderosis of the reticuloendothelial system.
congenital aregenerative a. congenital hypoplastic a. (def. 1).
congenital dyserythropoietic a. any of several rare hereditary anemias, mostly types of macrocytic anemia, characterized by nuclear anomalies of the erythrocytes, such as multinuclearity, karyorrhexis, or macrocytosis. The most common type (called also *HEMPAS*) is an autosomal recessive condition characterized by multinuclear erythrocytes and a positive acidified serum test.
congenital hemolytic a. 1. hemolytic anemia that is present from birth and in which the lifespan of red blood cells is diminished, such as occurs in hereditary spherocytosis. 2. hereditary spherocytosis.
congenital hypoplastic a. 1. a genetically diverse anemia, often associated with other congenital anomalies, encountered in the first year of life and characterized by deficiency of red cell precursors in an otherwise normally cellular bone marrow; it is unresponsive to hematinics and often requires multiple blood transfusions. Called also *Blackfan-Diamond a.* or *syndrome*, *Diamond-Blackfan a.* or *syndrome*, *congenital pure red cell a.* or *aplasia*, *congenital aregenerative a.*, and *erythrogenesis imperfecta*. 2. Fanconi syndrome (def. 1).
congenital a. of newborn erythroblastosis fetalis.
congenital nonspherocytic hemolytic a. any of a heterogeneous group of inherited anemias characterized by shortened red blood cell survival, lack of spherocytosis, and normal osmotic fragility associated with erythrocyte membrane defects, multiple intracellular enzyme deficiencies or other defects, or unstable hemoglobins. The most common enzyme defects are in glucose-6-phosphate dehydrogenase or pyruvate kinase.
congenital pernicious a. a rare disorder seen in children, clinically similar to the pernicious anemia of adults but differing in that gastric acid secretion is normal, the gastric mucosa is not atrophied, and development is delayed.
congenital sideroachrestic a. hereditary sideroblastic a.
Cooley a. thalassemia major.
cow's milk a. milk anemia in infants fed exclusively on cow's milk.
deficiency a. anemia caused by lack of a specific substance required for normal hemoglobin synthesis and erythrocytic maturation and arising by several means, such as malabsorption or poor dietary intake. See *folic acid deficiency a.*, *iron deficiency a.*, and *scorbutic a.* Called also *nutritional a.*
Diamond-Blackfan a. congenital hypoplastic a. (def. 1).
dilution a. hydremia.
dimorphic a. anemia with erythrocytes of two different sizes, such as with combined deficiencies of vitamin B_{12} and iron or after a blood transfusion.

Anemia *Continued*

drug-induced hemolytic a., drug-induced immune hemolytic a. immune hemolytic anemia induced by drugs, classified by mechanism as *penicillin type*, in which the drug, acting as a hapten bound to the red cell membrane, induces the formation of specific antibodies; *methyldopa type*, in which the drug, possibly by inhibition of suppressor T cells, induces the formation of anti-Rh antibodies; or *stibophen* or "*innocent bystander*" *type*, in which circulating drug-antibody immune complexes bind nonspecifically to red cells. The first two types usually involve warm-reactive antibodies and accelerated sequestration of red cells by the reticuloendothelial system; the third usually involves cold-reactive antibodies and complement-dependent intravascular hemolysis.
elliptocytic a. hereditary elliptocytosis.
equine infectious a. a disease of equines caused by a lentivirus and spread through the blood by inoculation, especially by blood-sucking insects; characteristics include abrupt fevers and recurring attacks of malaise. Called also *infectious a. of horses* and *swamp fever*.
Fanconi a. Fanconi syndrome (def. 1).
feline infectious a. a cyclic type of hemolytic anemia in domestic cats caused by infection of red blood cells with the rickettsia *Haemobartonella felis*, which may be spread from cat to cat during fights; acute cases are characterized by fever, jaundice, anorexia, and splenomegaly and can be fatal. Called also *haemobartonellosis*.
folic acid deficiency a. macrocytic anemia due to deficiency of folic acid. Called also *nutritional macrocytic a.*
goat's milk a. milk anemia in infants fed exclusively on goat's milk.
ground itch a. hookworm a.
Heinz body a's a group of hemolytic anemias of diverse etiology with the common morphologic characteristic of having Heinz bodies within affected erythrocytes.
hemolytic a. any of a group of acute or chronic anemias characterized by excessive hemolysis (shortened survival of mature erythrocytes) and inability of bone marrow to compensate with new erythrocytes. There are two major groups: the *inherited anemias* are generally due to intrinsic cell defects such as in the erythrocyte membrane, glycolytic pathway, glutathione metabolism, or hemoglobin molecule; these include *congenital hemolytic* and *congenital nonspherocytic hemolytic a.* The *acquired anemias* are due to the actions of extrinsic agents such as infectious agents, poisons, physical trauma, or antibodies; these include *autoimmune, immune, infectious,* and *toxic hemolytic a.*
hemolytic a. of newborn erythroblastosis fetalis.
hemorrhagic a. anemia caused by the sudden and acute loss of blood; called also *acute posthemorrhagic a.*
hereditary iron-loading a. hereditary sideroblastic a.
hereditary sideroachrestic a., hereditary sideroblastic a. an X-linked anemia, usually detected in childhood or early adulthood, characterized by an abundance of ringed sideroblasts, hypochromic, microcytic erythrocytes, poikilocytosis, weakness, and iron overload in later years. Called also *Rundles-Falls syndrome.*
hookworm a. hypochromic microcytic anemia that occurs as part of hookworm disease (q.v.). Called also *ground itch a.*
hypochromic a. anemia characterized by a disproportionate reduction of red cell hemoglobin and an increased area of central pallor in the red cells. It may be hereditary (e.g., hereditary sideroblastic anemia, thalassemia minor) or acquired (e.g., iron deficiency anemia). Called also *Faber syndrome.*
hypochromic microcytic a. any anemia with microcytes that are hypochromic (reduced in size and in hemoglobin content); the most common type is iron deficiency anemia.
a. hypochro′mica sideroachres′tica heredita′ria hereditary sideroblastic a.
hypoplastic a. any of various anemias caused by some degree of erythrocytic hypoplasia without leukopenia or thrombocytopenia, which may develop into aplastic anemia.
immune hemolytic a., immunohemolytic a. an acquired hemolytic anemia in which hemolysis takes place in response to isoantibodies or autoantibodies produced on exposure to drugs, toxins, or other antigens. See also *autoimmune hemolytic a., drug-induced immune hemolytic a.,* and *erythroblastosis fetalis.*
infectious hemolytic a. hemolytic anemia due to an incompletely compensated decrease in red blood cell survival secondary to infection.
infectious a. of horses equine infectious a.
iron deficiency a. a type of hypochromic microcytic anemia caused by low or absent iron stores and serum iron concentration; there is elevated free erythrocyte porphyrin, low transferrin saturation, elevated transferrin, low serum ferritin, and low hemoglobin concentration. Symptoms may include pallor, angular stomatitis and other oral lesions, gastrointestinal complaints, retinal hemorrhages and exudates, and thinning and brittleness of the nails, occasionally leading to spoon nails (koilonychia).

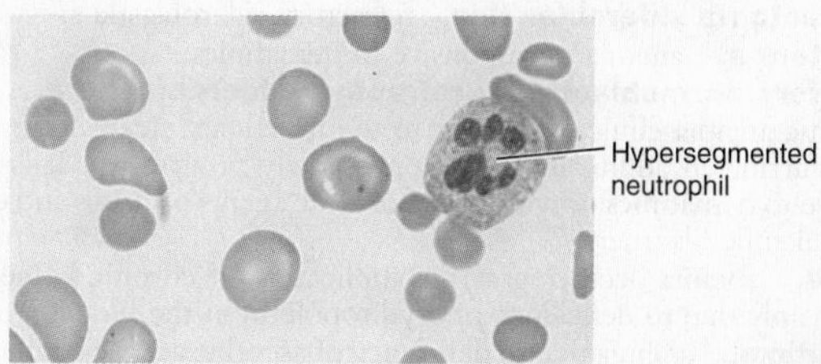

■ Megaloblastic anemia, showing a characteristic hypersegmented neutrophil.

juvenile pernicious a. congenital pernicious a.
leukoerythroblastic a. leukoerythroblastosis.
macrocytic a. any of various anemias of diverse etiology that are characterized by erythrocytes that are larger than normal and lack the usual central area of pallor; mean corpuscular volume and mean corpuscular hemoglobin are also elevated. See *folic acid deficiency a.* and *tropical macrocytic a.*
Mediterranean a. thalassemia major.
megaloblastic a. any anemia characterized by megaloblasts in the bone marrow, such as pernicious anemia.
megalocytic a. macrocytic a.
microangiopathic a., microangiopathic hemolytic a. thrombotic thrombocytopenic purpura.
microcytic a. any anemia characterized by microcytes (erythrocytes smaller than normal), such as iron deficiency anemia or β-thalassemia. See also *hypochromic microcytic a.*
milk a. iron deficiency anemia in infants fed a diet of only milk; see *cow's milk a.* and *goat's milk a.*
mountain a. a misnomer for *mountain sickness.*
myelopathic a., myelophthisic a. leukoerythroblastosis.
nonspherocytic hemolytic a. see *congenital nonspherocytic hemolytic a.*
normochromic a. anemia in which the hemoglobin content of the red cells as measured by the MCHC is in the normal range.
normocytic a. anemia with erythrocytes of normal size but a proportionate decrease in hemoglobin content, packed red cell volume, and number of erythrocytes per cubic millimeter of blood.
nutritional a. deficiency a.
nutritional macrocytic a. folic acid deficiency a.
osteosclerotic a. anemia due to bone marrow failure associated with osteosclerosis, as a result of the effect on bone marrow of changes in the bones.
pernicious a. a type of megaloblastic anemia usually seen in older adults, caused by impaired intestinal absorption of vitamin B_{12} due to lack of availability of intrinsic factor; it is often characterized by pallor, achlorhydria, glossitis, gastric mucosal atrophy, weakness, antibodies against gastric parietal cells or intrinsic factor, and neurologic manifestations.
physiologic a. the normocytic, normochromic anemia that occurs in infants at the age of two or three months, owing to normal depression of erythropoiesis and hemoglobin synthesis, probably resulting as an adjustment to the changeover from placental to pulmonary oxygenation.
polar a. an anemic condition that occurs during exposure to low temperature; it is initially microcytic but later becomes normocytic. Called also *Arctic a.*
posthemorrhagic a. of newborn anemia of the newborn due to hemorrhage, such as into the placenta or from umbilical vessels; it may range from mild to severe.
primary acquired sideroblastic a. refractory sideroblastic a.
pure red cell a. anemia characterized by absence of red cell precursors in the bone marrow. It may be acquired or congenital; the latter is called *congenital hypoplastic a.*
pyridoxine-responsive a. a form of sideroblastic anemia in which there is a therapeutic response to pyridoxine; it affects predominately young or middle-aged males.

Anemia *Continued*

a. refracto′ria sideroblas′tica refractory sideroblastic a.
refractory a. anemia unresponsive to hematinics.
refractory normoblastic a., refractory sideroblastic a. a sideroblastic anemia clinically similar to the hereditary sideroblastic form but occurring in adults and often only slowly progressive. It is unresponsive to hematinics or withdrawal of toxic agents or drugs and can be a preleukemic disorder.
renal a. anemia occurring as a complication of chronic kidney disease, mainly due to deficiency of erythropoietin in the blood.
scorbutic a. anemia due to deficiency of ascorbic acid (vitamin C); in naturally occurring human scurvy the anemia is generally normocytic, although in experimentally induced vitamin C deficiency the anemia is of the megaloblastic type.
sickle cell a. a hereditary hemolytic anemia, seen primarily in West Africa and in people of West African descent, and less often in the Mediterranean basin and a few other areas. It is an autosomal recessive disorder in which mutation of the *HBB* gene (locus: 11p15.5), which encodes the β-globin chain, results in hemoglobin S, which has decreased solubility in the deoxygenated state and results in abnormal sickle-shaped erythrocytes *(sickle cells).* Homozygous individuals have 85 to 95 percent sickle cells and have the full-blown syndrome with accelerated hemolysis, increased blood viscosity and vaso-occlusion, arthralgias, acute attacks of abdominal pain, ulcerations of the lower extremities, and periodic attacks of any of the conditions called *sickle cell crises.* The heterozygous condition is called *sickle cell trait* and is usually asymptomatic. See also *sickle cell disease,* under *disease.* Called also *sicklemia.*
sideroachrestic a., sideroblastic a. any of a heterogeneous group of acquired and hereditary anemias with diverse clinical manifestations; commonly characterized by large numbers of ringed sideroblasts in the bone marrow, ineffective erythropoiesis, variable proportions of hypochromic erythrocytes in the peripheral blood, and usually increased levels of tissue iron. The two most common kinds are hereditary sideroblastic anemia and refractory sideroblastic anemia.
sideropenic a. any of a group of anemias characterized by low levels of iron in the plasma; it includes iron deficiency anemia and the anemias of chronic disorders.
slaty a. a term applied to a gray discoloration of the face in poisoning by silver.
spherocytic a. hereditary spherocytosis.
splenic a. congestive splenomegaly.
spur cell a. anemia in which the red blood cells have a bizarre spiculated shape and are destroyed prematurely, primarily in the spleen; it is an acquired form occurring in severe liver disease and represents an abnormality in the cholesterol content of the cell membrane.
toxic hemolytic a. anemia due to a toxic agent such as a drug, bacterial lysin, or snake venom.
tropical macrocytic a. a type of nutritional macrocytic anemia seen in impoverished tropical regions, resembling pernicious anemia but without achlorhydria and only erratically responsive to vitamin B_{12}. The etiology is often related to folate deficiency, and administration of folic acid usually produces marked improvement.
X-linked sideroblastic a. hereditary sideroblastic a.

an•e•mom•e•try (an″ə-mom′ə-tre) velocimetry.

Anem•o•ne (ə-nem′o-ne) a large genus of plants of the family Ranunculaceae with divided leaves and conspicuous flowers of sepals. Most species contain ranunculin, which converts enzymatically to protoanemonin, an irritant toxin that can cause the poisoning called anemonism. *A. pulsatil′la* and certain other species contain anemonin rather than its precursors, and have been used medicinally.

anem•o•ne (ə-nem′o-ne) 1. a flower of the genus *Anemone.* 2. something that resembles these flowers.
sea a. any of various marine invertebrates of the class Anthozoa; some have painful stings.

anem•o•nism (ə-nem′o-niz-əm) poisoning by plants of the genus *Anemone.*

anem•o•nol (ə-nem′o-nol) a highly toxic volatile oil from various species of *Anemone* and from other ranunculaceous plants.

Anem•o•nop•sis (ə-nem″ə-nop′sis) a genus of herbs. *A. califor′nica* Hook and Arn., a species found in the southwestern United States and northern Mexico, is the source of mansa.

an•e•mo•pho•bia (an″ə-mo-fo′be-ə) [Gr. *anemos* wind + *-phobia*] irrational fear of wind or of drafts.

an•en•ce•pha•lia (an″ən-sə-fa′le-ə) anencephaly.

an•en•ce•phal•ic (an″ən-sə-fal′ik) exhibiting anencephaly; having no brain.

an•en•ceph•a•lous (an″ən-sef′ə-ləs) anencephalic.

an•en•ceph•a•lus (an″ən-sef′ə-ləs) an infant exhibiting anencephaly.

an•en•ceph•a•ly (an″ən-sef′ə-le) [*an-*[1] + Gr. *enkephalos* brain] congenital absence of the calvaria, with cerebral hemispheres missing or reduced to small masses attached to the base of the cranium; complete absence of the brain is rare. Cf. *meroanencephaly.*

an•en•ter•ous (an-en′tər-əs) [*an-*[1] + *entero-* + *-ous*] lacking intestines.

aneph•ric (a-nef′rik) without kidneys.

aneph•ro•gen•e•sis (a″nef-ro-jen′ə-sis) [*a-*[1] + *nephrogenesis*] congenital absence of kidney tissue.

an•ep•i•plo•ic (an-ep″ĭ-plo′ik) devoid of omentum.

an•er•gia (an-ur′je-ə) anergy.

an•er•gic (an-ur′jik) [*an-*[1] + Gr. *ergon* work] 1. characterized by abnormal inactivity; inactive. 2. marked by lack of energy. 3. pertaining to anergy.

an•er•gy (an′ər-je) 1. lack of energy, extreme passivity. 2. diminished reactivity to all antigens; it may take the form of diminished immediate hypersensitivity, diminished delayed hypersensitivity, or both. Cf. *immunologic tolerance.*
negative a. transient reduction in reactivity to allergens in a sensitized individual, occurring as a result of intervening events, such as cachexia.
positive a. reduction in reactivity to allergens in a sensitized individual, owing to alterations in the immune response in the course of disease, as in tuberculosis.
T-cell a. anergy (def. 2).

an•er•oid (an′ər-oid) [*a-*[1] + Gr. *nēros* liquid + *-oid*] not containing liquid.

an•eryth•ro•pla•sia (an″ə-rith″ro-pla′zhə) [*an-*[1] + *erythro-* + *-plasia*] anerythropoiesis.

an•eryth•ro•plas•tic (an″ə-rith″ro-plas′tik) pertaining to or characterized by anerythropoiesis.

an•eryth•ro•poi•e•sis (an″ə-rith″ro-poi-e′sis) [*an-*[1] + *erythropoiesis*] deficient or absent erythropoiesis; see also *erythropenia.* Called also *anerythroplasia.*

an•eryth•ro•re•gen•er•a•tive (an″ə-rith″ro-re-jen′ər-a″tiv) characterized by lack of regeneration of erythrocytes; see also *aregenerative.*

Anes•ta•con (ə-nes′tə-kon) trademark for a preparation of lidocaine hydrochloride.

anes•the•ci•ne•sia (an-es″the-sĭ-ne′zhə) [*an-*[1] + *esthesi-* + *cinesi-* + *-ia*] loss of sensibility and motor power.

anes•the•ki•ne•sia (an-es″the-kĭ-ne′zhə) anesthecinesia.

an•es•the•sia (an″es-the′zhə) [*an-*[1] + *esthesia*] 1. loss of sensation, usually by damage to a nerve or receptor; called also *numbness.* 2. loss of the ability to feel pain, caused by administration of a drug or by other medical interventions; cf. *anesthetic* (def. 2).
acupuncture a. regional anesthesia using the principles of acupuncture.
ambulatory a. anesthesia performed on an outpatient basis for ambulatory surgery.
angiospastic a. loss of sensibility dependent on spasm of the blood vessels.
balanced a. anesthesia that uses a combination of drugs, each in an amount sufficient to produce its major or desired effect to the optimum degree and keep its undesirable or unnecessary effects to a minimum.
basal a. anesthesia that acts as a basis for further and deeper anesthesia; a state of narcosis produced by preliminary medication so profound that the added inhalation anesthetic necessary to produce surgical anesthesia is greatly reduced.
Bier local a. Bier block.
block a. regional a.
brachial plexus a. see under *block.*

bulbar a. lack of sensation caused by a lesion of the pons.
caudal a. see under *block.*
closed circuit a. inhalation anesthesia maintained by the continuous rebreathing of a relatively small amount of anesthetic gas and a basal amount of oxygen, normally used with an absorption apparatus for the removal of carbon dioxide.
compression a. loss of sensation resulting from pressure on a nerve.
conduction a. regional a.
continuous epidural a. see under *analgesia.*
crossed a. hemianesthesia cruciata.
dissociated a., dissociation a. loss of sensitivity to pain, heat, and cold without loss of other tactile senses; seen in syringomyelia.
a. doloro'sa spontaneous pain in a denervated part; pain in an area or region that is anesthetic; called also *anesthesia dolorosa.*
electric a. anesthesia induced by passage of an electric current.
endotracheal a. anesthesia produced by introduction of a gaseous mixture through a wide-bore tube inserted into the trachea through either the mouth or the nose.
epidural a. see under *block.*
facial a. loss of sensation caused by a lesion of the facial nerve.
gauntlet a. loss of sensation in the hand and wrist; called also *glove a.*
general a. a reversible state of unconsciousness, produced by anesthetic agents, with absence of pain sensation over the entire body and a greater or lesser degree of muscular relaxation; the drugs producing this state can be administered by inhalation, intravenously, intramuscularly, or rectally.
girdle a. loss of sensation in a zone encircling the hips.
glove a. gauntlet a.
gustatory a. ageusia.
high pressure a. anesthesia produced by controlled application of pressure to a nerve trunk or its branches.
hypnosis a. production of insensibility to pain during surgical procedures by means of hypnotism.
hypotensive a. anesthesia accompanied by deliberate lowering of blood pressure to reduce blood loss and improve usability of the surgical field.
hypothermic a. anesthesia accompanied by the deliberate lowering of the body temperature. See also *cryoanesthesia.*
hysterical a. loss of tactile sensation occurring as a symptom of a conversion disorder, often recognizable by its lack of correspondence with nerve distributions.
infiltration a. the production of local anesthesia by deposition of anesthetic solution into a superficial area.
inhalation a. anesthesia produced by the inhalation of vapors of a volatile liquid or gaseous anesthetic agent.
insufflation a. anesthesia produced by blowing a mixture of gases or vapors through a tube introduced into the respiratory tract.
intercostal a. see under *block.*
intrapulpal a. a local anesthetic effect produced by the administration of an anesthetic agent directly into the dental pulp.
intraspinal a. spinal a. (def. 1).
intravenous a. 1. anesthesia produced by introduction of an anesthetic agent into a vein, usually in a limb to which a pneumatic tourniquet has been applied. 2. Bier block.
intravenous regional a. Bier block.
local a. anesthesia confined to one area of the body; see also *regional a.*
lumbar epidural a. anesthesia produced by injection of the anesthetic agent into the epidural space at the second or third lumbar interspace.
muscular a. loss or lack of muscle sense.
nausea a. loss of the sensation of nausea that is normally stimulated by noxious and disgusting substances.
olfactory a. anosmia.
open a. general inhalation anesthesia utilizing a cone or ether mask; there is no significant rebreathing of expired gases.
paraneural a. perineural block.
paravertebral a. see under *block.*
peridural a. epidural a.
perineural a. see under *block.*
peripheral a. loss of sensation which is due to changes in the peripheral nerves.
plexus a. anesthesia produced by the injection of a local anesthetic around a nerve plexus.
pressure a. anesthesia caused by pressure on a nerve.
rectal a. anesthesia induced by introduction of an anesthetic agent into the rectum.
regional a. the production of insensibility of a part by interrupting the sensory nerve conductivity from that region of the body; it may be produced by either *field block* or *nerve block* (see under *block*). Called also *block, blockade, block a.*, and *conduction a.*
sacral a. see under *block.*
saddle block a. see under *block.*
segmental a. loss of sensation caused by lesions of nerve roots.
semiclosed a. general inhalation anesthesia in which there is partial rebreathing of the exhaled gases, with a carbon dioxide absorber in the circuit.
semiopen a. general inhalation anesthesia administered by use of a partially open circuit; there is partial rebreathing of the exhaled gases without a carbon dioxide absorber in the circuit.
spinal a. 1. regional anesthesia produced by injection of a local anesthetic into the subarachnoid space around the spinal cord; cf. *epidural a.* Called also *intraspinal a.* or *block* and *subarachnoid a.* or *block.* 2. see under *anesthesia.* 3. loss of sensation due to a spinal lesion.
subarachnoid a. spinal a. (def. 1).
surgical a. the degree of anesthesia at which surgery may safely be performed; ordinarily used to designate such depth of general anesthesia.
tactile a. loss or impairment of the sense of touch; called also *anaphia.* Cf. *paraphia.*
thalamic hyperesthetic a. thalamic syndrome; see under *syndrome.*
thermal a. thermoanesthesia.
topical a. anesthesia produced by application of a local anesthetic directly to the area involved, as to the oral mucosa or the cornea.
transsacral a. sacral block.
traumatic a. loss of sensation caused by injury to a nerve.
unilateral a. hemianesthesia.
visceral a. loss or lack of the visceral sense.

an•es•the•si•ol•o•gist (an″əs-the″ze-ol′ə-jist) a physician or dentist specializing in anesthesiology. Cf. *anesthetist.*

an•es•the•si•ol•o•gy (an″əs-the″ze-ol′ə-je) [*anesthesia* + *-logy*] the branch of medicine that studies anesthesia and anesthetics.

an•es•the•si•o•phore (an″əs-the′ze-o-for″) [*anesthesia* + *-phore*] the portion of the molecule of a chemical compound which is responsible for its anesthetic action.

an•es•thet•ic (an″əs-thet′ik) 1. characterized by anesthesia (def. 1); called also *numb.* 2. producing anesthesia (defs. 1, 2). 3. a drug or agent that is used to abolish the sensation of pain.
general a. an agent that produces general anesthesia.
local a. an agent whose anesthetic action is limited to an area of the body determined by the site of its application; it produces its effect by blocking nerve conduction.
topical a. a local anesthetic applied directly to the area to be anesthetized, usually the mucous membranes or the skin.

anes•the•tist (ə-nes′thə-tist) a nurse or technician trained to administer anesthetics. Cf. *anesthesiologist.*

anes•the•ti•za•tion (ə-nes″thə-tĭ-za′shən) the production of insensibility to pain.

anes•the•tize (ə-nes′thə-tīz) to put under the influence of anesthetics.

an•es•trum (an-es′trəm) anestrus.

an•es•trus (an-es′trəs) 1. abnormal lack of ovarian activity in a female mammal; the term is sometimes extended to include any prolonged lack of sexual responsiveness. 2. a period of the estrous cycle during which there is no ovarian activity; in cats, horses, sheep, goats, and certain other species this occurs annually for periods of weeks to months. Called also *diestrus.*

an•e•thole (an′ə-thōl) [NF] a flavoring agent for drugs, obtained from anise and fennel oils and other sources, or prepared synthetically.

Ane•thum (ə-ne′thəm) [L., from Gr. *anēthon*] a genus of plants of the family Umbelliferae, originally native to Asia. *A. graveo′lens* is dill, whose fruit is carminative and stimulant.

an•e•to•der•ma (an″ə-to-dur′mə) [Gr. *anetos* slack + *derma*] a rare type of localized elastolysis producing circumscribed areas of soft, thin, wrinkled skin that may protrude as small outpouchings. It may be primary and accompanied by inflammatory lesions, or secondary to syphilis, leprosy, or tuberculosis. See also *atrophoderma.* Called also *atrophia cutis, atrophia maculosa*, and *macular atrophy.*
Jadassohn a., Jadassohn-Pellizari a. primary anetoderma after an inflammatory or urticarial eruption; the lesions are round or oval erythematous macules that become atrophic, wrinkled, and pale protrusions. It is usually seen in females between age 10 and 40. Cf. *Schweninger-Buzzi a.*
Schweninger-Buzzi a. a progressive primary type of anetoderma without any preceding inflammatory condition, characterized by the abrupt appearance of many blue to white macules, some of which protrude; usually seen in women. Cf. *Jadassohn a.*

an•eu•ga•my (an-u′gə-me) [*an-*[1] + *eugamy*] union of gametes in one or both of which the chromosomes have not been reduced to the normal haploid number, resulting in an abnormal number of chromosomes (aneuploidy) in the zygote.

an•eu•ploid (an′u-ploid) [*an-*[1] + *euploid*] 1. a chromosome number that is not an exact multiple of the normal diploid number. 2. an individual or cell having an aneuploid number of chromosomes.

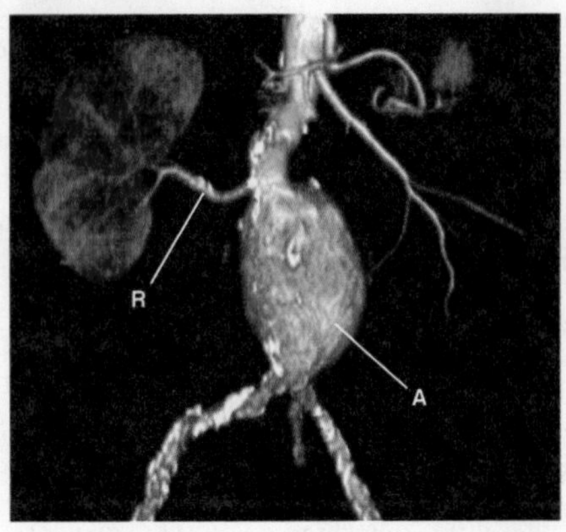

■ Abdominal aortic aneurysm. Three-dimensional shaded-surface display of axial contrast-enhanced CT scan, which shows the juxtarenal aneurysm *(A)* and its relation to other surrounding structures, including the right renal arteries *(R)* proximally and the aortic bifurcation distally.

an•eu•ploi•dy (an′u-ploi″de) [*an-*[1] + *euploidy*] any deviation from an exact multiple of the haploid number of chromosomes, whether fewer (hypoploidy, as in Turner syndrome) or more (hyperploidy, as in Down syndrome).

aneu•rine (an-u′rin) [*a-*[1] + Gr. *neuron* nerve] thiamine.

aneu•ro•gen•ic (a″noo-ro-jen′ik) pertaining to or characterized by absence of formation of nerve fibers.

an•eu•rysm (an′u-riz″əm) [Gr. *aneurysma* a widening] a sac formed by the dilatation of the wall of an artery, a vein, or the heart; it is filled with fluid or clotted blood, often forming a pulsating tumor.

abdominal a., abdominal aortic a. a common type of aneurysm, found in the abdominal aorta, usually in an area of severe atherosclerosis.

ampullary a. saccular a.

aortic a. aneurysm of the aorta.

aortic sinusal a. aneurysm arising in the aortic sinuses; it is a rare, usually congenital lesion that begins as fingerlike projections in the right or noncoronary sinuses and can progress to rupture, usually into the right ventricle or atrium, causing volume overload and congestive heart failure.

arterial a. aneurysm in the wall of an artery; the chief signs are formation of a pulsating tumor, often a bruit *(aneurysmal bruit)* heard over the swelling, and sometimes symptoms from pressure on contiguous parts.

arteriosclerotic a. an aneurysm arising in a large artery, most commonly the abdominal aorta, as a result of weakening of the wall in severe atherosclerosis; called also *atherosclerotic a.*

arteriovenous a. a communication, either congenital or traumatic, between an artery and a vein; arterial blood may flow directly into the vein *(aneurysmal varix)* or be carried into it by a connecting sac *(varicose aneurysm)*.

arteriovenous pulmonary a. pulmonary arteriovenous fistula.

atherosclerotic a. arteriosclerotic a.

atrial septal a. a rare malformation of the interatrial septum in which the sac protrudes into one of the atria; it may cause cerebral embolism.

axillary a. aneurysm of the axillary artery.

berry a. a saccular aneurysm of a cerebral artery, usually at the junction of vessels in the circle of Willis; its narrow neck of origin and larger dome resemble those of a berry. Called also *cerebral a.*

brain a. berry a.

cardiac a. ventricular a.

cerebral a. berry a.

Charcot-Bouchard a. a type of miliary aneurysm found in the small vessels affected by hypertension; not thought to be a cause of bleeding.

cirsoid a. racemose a.

compound a. an aneurysm in which some layers of the vessel wall are ruptured and others are only dilated; called also *mixed a.*

congenital cerebral a. berry a.

cylindroid a. the uniform dilatation of a considerable part of an artery; called also *tubular a.*

dissecting a. longitudinal splitting of the arterial wall resulting from hemorrhage, producing a tear in the intima and establishing communication with the lumen; it usually affects the aorta *(aortic dissection)* but may also affect other large arteries.

ectatic a. an aneurysm formed by distention of a section of an artery without rupture of any of its coats.

embolomycotic a. mycotic a.

false a. 1. an aneurysm in which the entire wall is injured and the blood is contained by the surrounding tissues, with eventual formation of a sac communicating with the artery (or heart); called also *aneurysmal hematoma.* 2. pseudoaneurysm.

fusiform a. a spindle-shaped arterial aneurysm in which the stretching process affects the entire circumference of the artery, as opposed to a *saccular aneurysm.* Called also *Richet a.*

hernial a. an aneurysm whose sac is formed by an inner coat projecting through the outer.

infected a. an aneurysm produced by growth of bacteria or fungi in the vessel wall, or infection arising within a preexisting arteriosclerotic aneurysm.

innominate a. aneurysm of the innominate artery (brachiocephalic trunk).

intracranial a. any aneurysm found within the cranium.

lateral a. an aneurysm that projects from one side of an artery.

luetic a. syphilitic a.

miliary a. aneurysm of a tiny artery, usually in the retina or inside the skull.

mixed a. compound a.

mycotic a. 1. an infected aneurysm resulting from infective endocarditis, either by hematogenous seeding of bacteria to atherosclerotic arteries or by lodging of septic emboli in the vasa vasorum. 2. occasionally, any aneurysm resulting from an infectious cause other than syphilitic aortitis.

Park a. an arteriovenous aneurysm at the elbow, establishing communication between the brachial artery and the brachial and median basilic veins.

Pott a. aneurysmal varix (def. 2).

racemose a. a condition in which the blood vessels become dilated, lengthened, and tortuous; called also *cirsoid a., cirsoid varix,* and *diffuse arterial ectasia.*

Rasmussen a. dilatation of an artery in a tuberculous cavity, sometimes rupturing to produce hemorrhage.

renal a. an aneurysm within the kidney.

Richet a. fusiform a.

saccular a., sacculated a. an eccentric, localized distended sac affecting only a part of the circumference of the arterial wall, as opposed to a *fusiform aneurysm.* Called also *ampullary a.*

serpentine a. an elongated and varicose senile condition of certain arteries, such as the splenic, iliac, and temporal.

spurious a. 1. false a. (def. 1). 2. pseudoaneurysm.

suprasellar a. aneurysm of the internal carotid artery above the sella turcica.

syphilitic a. an aortic aneurysm, usually of the ascending aorta, occurring in cases of cardiovascular syphilis; called also *luetic a.*

traumatic a. an aneurysm caused by injury.

true a. an aneurysm whose sac is formed by the arterial walls, at least one of which is unbroken.

tubular a. cylindroid a.

varicose a. an aneurysm in which the artery communicates with contiguous veins by means of an intervening sac.

venous a. aneurysm of a vein; called also *phlebangioma.*

ventricular a. an aneurysmal dilatation of a portion of the wall of a ventricle, usually the left, or, rarely, a saccular protrusion through it (*false a.* of the heart). It is usually consequent to myocardial infarction but other causes, such as bacterial endocarditis or trauma, have been described.

verminous a., worm a. an aneurysm of equines caused by the nematode *Strongylus vulgaris,* usually in the anterior mesenteric artery. Called also *verminous mesenteric arteritis.*

an•eu•rys•mal (an″u-riz′məl) pertaining to or resembling an aneurysm.

an•eu•rys•mat•ic (an″u-riz-mat′ik) aneurysmal.

an•eu•rys•mec•to•my (an″u-riz-mek′tə-me) [*aneurysm* + *-ectomy*] extirpation of an aneurysm by removal of the sac.

an•eu•rys•mo•plas•ty (an″u-riz′mo-plas″te) [*aneurysm* + *-plasty*] plastic reconstruction of an aneurysmal artery.

an•eu•rys•mor•rha•phy (an″u-riz-mor′ə-fe) [*aneurysm* + *-rrhaphy*] the operation of suturing an aneurysm.

an•eu•rys•mot•o•my (an″u-riz-mot′ə-me) [*aneurysm* + *-tomy*] the operation of incising the sac of an aneurysm.

an•eu•so•my (an′u-so″me) the condition of being made up of cells that contain different numbers of chromosomes. It occurs widely in flowering plants. In animals, it generally denotes a diploid organism with subpopulations of aneuploid somatic cells.

segmental a. in human cytogenetics, a term used incorrectly to describe a genetic imbalance within a pair of chromosomes, caused by deletion or duplication of a segment of one homologue of the pair.

ANF antinuclear factor; see *antinuclear antibodies,* under *antibody.*

angei- for words beginning thus, see those beginning *angi-*.

An·gel·i·ca (an-jel′ĭ-kə) [L., from Gr. *angelikos* angelic] a genus of plants of the family Umbelliferae. Two species have medicinal properties: *A. archange′lica*, the garden angelica, found along the coasts of the Baltic and North Seas, and *A. sinen′sis*, Chinese angelica or dong quai, which is native to China.

an·gel·i·ca (an-jel′ĭ-kə) 1. any plant of the genus *Angelica*. 2. a medicinal preparation *A. archangelica*, which has carminative, cholagogic, and spasmolytic properties and stimulates the secretion of gastric juice. All parts of the plant are medicinal: the fruit is used for fevers and colds, urinary tract infections, dyspepsia, and loss of appetite; the root is used for dyspepsia and loss of appetite; and the leaves have been used as a diuretic and diaphoretic.

Chinese a. dong quai.

An·gel·man syndrome (ān′jəl-mən) [Harry *Angelman*, British physician, 1915–1996] see under *syndrome.*

An·ge·luc·ci syndrome (ahn″jə-loo′che) [Arnaldo *Angelucci*, Italian ophthalmologist, 1854–1934] see under *syndrome.*

An·ger camera (ang′gər) [Hal Oscar *Anger*, American electrical engineer, born 1920] see under *camera.*

An·ghe·les·cu sign (ahn-jə-les′koo) [Constantin *Anghelescu*, Romanian surgeon, 1869–1948] see under *sign.*

an·gi·al·gia (an″je-al′jə) [*angi-* + Gr. *algos* pain + *-ia*] pain in a blood vessel; called also *angiodynia.*

an·gi·as·the·nia (an″je-əs-the′ne-ə) [*angi-* + *asthenia*] instability or loss of tone in the vascular system.

an·gi·ec·ta·sia (an″je-ek-ta′zhə) angiectasis.

an·gi·ec·ta·sis (an″je-ek′tə-sis) [*angi-* + *ectasis*] abnormal, usually gross dilatation and often lengthening of a blood or lymphatic vessel; see also *lymphangiectasis* and *vasodilation.* Called also *hemangiectasia.*

an·gi·ec·tat·ic (an″je-ek-tat′ik) pertaining to or characterized by angiectasis.

an·gi·ec·to·my (an″je-ek′tə-me) [*angi-* + *-ectomy*] excision or resection of a vessel.

an·gi·ec·to·pia (an″je-ek-to′pe-ə) [*angi-* + *ectopia*] abnormal position or course of a vessel.

an·gi·i·tis (an″je-i′tis) pl. *angii′tides* [*angi-* + *-itis*] vasculitis.

allergic granulomatous a. Churg-Strauss syndrome.

cutaneous leukocytoclastic a. see under *vasculitis.*

granulomatous central nervous system a. 1. hypersensitivity vasculitis. 2. primary central nervous system a.

hypersensitivity a. see under *vasculitis.*

isolated central nervous system a., isolated a. of central nervous system primary central nervous system a.

leukocytoclastic a. hypersensitivity vasculitis.

necrotizing a. systemic necrotizing vasculitis.

primary central nervous system a., primary a. of central nervous system an idiopathic vasculitis affecting small and medium-sized intracranial vessels, marked by headache, progressive intellectual deterioration, and recurrent cerebral infarcts. Called also *granulomatous* or *isolated central nervous system a.* and *granulomatous, isolated,* or *primary central nervous system vasculitis.*

an·gi·na (an-ji′nə, an′jĭ-nə) [L.] 1. a. pectoris. 2. any spasmodic, choking, or suffocative pain.

abdominal a., a. abdomina′lis, a. abdo′minis intestinal a.

a. cor′dis a. pectoris.

a. cru′ris intermittent claudication.

a. decu′bitus cardiac pain occurring in a recumbent position.

a. of effort, effort-associated a. stable a. pectoris.

herpes a., a. herpe′tica herpangina.

intestinal a. cramping postprandial abdominal pain caused by ischemia of the smooth muscle of the intestine in patients with intestinal vascular insufficiency conditions such as nonocclusive mesenteric ischemia. Called also *abdominal a.*

a. inver′sa Prinzmetal a.

Ludwig a. a severe form of cellulitis of the submaxillary space and secondary involvement of the sublingual and submental spaces, usually resulting from an infection in the mandibular molar area or a penetrating injury of the floor of the mouth. Elevation of the tongue, difficulty in eating and swallowing, edema of the glottis, fever, rapid breathing, and moderate leukocytosis are the most common symptoms.

microvascular a. angina pectoris resulting from ischemia caused by microvascular dysfunction.

a. pec′toris a paroxysmal thoracic pain, often radiating to the arms, particularly the left, sometimes accompanied by a feeling of suffocation and impending death; it is most often due to ischemia of the myocardium and precipitated by effort or excitement. It is subdivided into *stable* and *unstable a. pectoris.* Called also *a. cordis, angor pectoris, Heberden disease,* and *Rougnon-Heberden disease.*

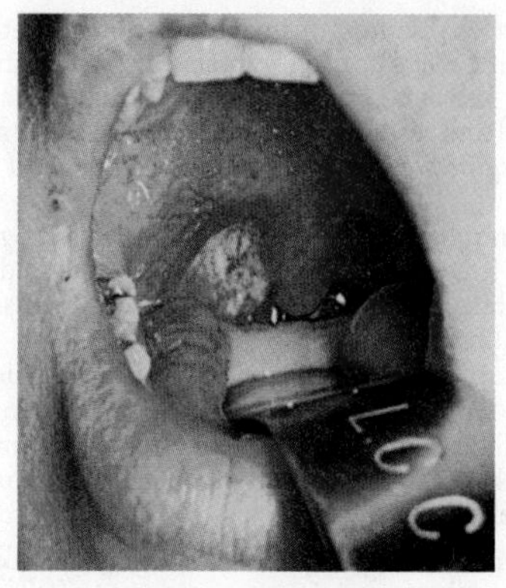

■ Vincent angina.

a. pec′toris elec′trica pain and tightness in the chest on effort, without specific electrocardiographic changes, persisting for several weeks following electrical injury.

preinfarction a. 1. angina pectoris preceding a myocardial infarction. 2. unstable a. pectoris.

Prinzmetal a. a variant of angina pectoris, often considered a form of unstable angina, in which the attacks occur during rest, exercise capacity is often well preserved, and attacks are associated electrocardiographically with elevation of the ST segment. Focal spasm of an epicardial coronary artery causes transient abrupt reduction of arterial diameter, resulting in myocardial ischemia. Called also *variant a. pectoris* and *vasospastic a.*

pseudomembranous a. necrotizing ulcerative gingivostomatitis.

silent a. an episode of coronary insufficiency in which no pain is experienced.

stable a., stable a. pectoris, typical a. angina pectoris occurring in attacks of predictable frequency and duration after provocation by circumstances that increase myocardial oxygen demands, such as exercise, emotional stress, or excitement, the precipitating circumstances tending to remain constant across episodes. Called also *a. of effort* and *effort-associated a.* Cf. *unstable a.*

unstable a., unstable a. pectoris angina pectoris that occurs unpredictably or suddenly increases in severity or frequency; attacks may occur without provocation, such as during sleep or rest, may not respond to nitroglycerin, and may be of unusually long duration. Prinzmetal angina is often included in this category. Cf. *stable a. pectoris.*

variant a., variant a. pectoris, vasospastic a. Prinzmetal a.

Vincent a. a type of membranous pharyngitis consisting of painful ulceration with edema and hyperemic patches; it represents spread of necrotizing ulcerative gingivitis to the oropharynx.

an·gi·nal (an-ji′nəl, an′jə-nəl) pertaining to or characteristic of angina.

an·gin·i·form (an-jin′ĭ-form) resembling angina.

an·gi·noid (an′jĭ-noid) anginiform.

an·gino·pho·bia (an″jin-o-fo′be-ə) [*angina* + *-phobia*] irrational dread of choking.

an·gi·nous (an′jĭ-nəs) anginal.

angi(o)- [Gr. *angeion* vessel] a combining form denoting relationship to a vessel, usually a blood vessel.

an·gio·ac·cess (an″je-o-ak′ses) vascular access.

an·gio·atax·ia (an″je-o-ə-tak′se-ə) [*angio-* + *ataxia*] irregular tension of the blood vessels.

an·gio·blast (an′je-o-blast″) [*angio-* + *-blast*[1]] 1. the mesenchymal tissue of the embryo from which the blood cells and blood vessels differentiate; called also *angioderm.* 2. an individual vessel-forming cell; called also *vasoformative cell.* **angioblas′tic** *adj*

an·gio·blas·to·ma (an″je-o-blas-to′mə) 1. hemangioblastoma. 2. angioblastic meningioma.

an·gio·car·dio·gram (an″je-o-kahr′de-o-gram) the film produced by angiocardiography.

an·gio·car·di·og·ra·phy (an″je-o-kahr″de-og′rə-fe) [*angio-* + *cardiography*] angiography of the heart and great vessels; contrast material may be injected into a blood vessel or one of the cardiac chambers. Images obtained can be analyzed to determine parameters of ventricular function, including ventricular ejection fractions, cardiac output, ejection rates, stroke volume, end-diastolic volume, and end-systolic volume, as well as to test the effects of exercise. Called also *cardioangiography.*

equilibrium radionuclide a. radionuclide angiocardiography in which images are taken at specific phases of the cardiac cycle over a series of several hundred cycles. Timing of image recording is set, or gated, by the occurrence of specific electrocardiographic waveforms, and the data can be used to determine average activity during specific cardiac cycle phases or can be accumulated and displayed in rapid sequence, as a movie. Called also *multiple gated acquisition* or *MUGA scanning* and *gated cardiac blood pool imaging.*

first pass radionuclide a. radionuclide angiocardiography in which a rapid sequence of images is taken immediately after administration of a bolus of radionuclide, recording only the initial transit of the isotope through the central circulation.

gated equilibrium radionuclide a. equilibrium radionuclide a.

radionuclide a. angiocardiography in which the contrast material is a radionuclide, usually a compound of technetium Tc 99m such as Tc 99m pyrophosphate or Tc 99m–labeled red blood cells, and images are obtained using a gamma camera.

an•gio•car•dio•ki•net•ic (an″je-o-kahr″de-o-kĭ-net′ik) [*angio-* + *cardiokinetic*] 1. affecting the motions or movements of the heart and blood vessels. 2. any agent that affects the movements of the heart and vessels.

an•gio•car•di•tis (an″je-o-kahr-di′tis) [*angio-* + *carditis*] inflammation of the heart and great blood vessels.

an•gio•cen•tric (an″je-o-sen′trik) angiogenic (def. 1).

an•gio•chei•lo•scope (an″je-o-ki′lo-skōp″) [*angio-* + *cheilo-* + *-scope*] an instrument for observing blood circulation of the lips under magnification.

An•gio-Con•ray (an″je-o-kon′ra) trademark for a preparation of iothalamate sodium.

an•gio•crine (an′je-o-krīn) [*angio-* + *endocrine*] denoting vasomotor disorders of endocrine origin.

an•gio•cri•no•sis (an″je-o-krĭ-no′sis) a vasomotor disorder of endocrine origin.

an•gio•cyst (an′je-o-sist″) [*angio-* + *cyst*] angioblastic cyst.

an•gio•derm (an′je-o-dərm) angioblast (def. 1).

an•gio•der•ma•ti•tis (an″je-o-dur″mə-ti′tis) [*angio-* + *dermatitis*] inflammation of the vessels of the skin; when this occurs in association with an arteriovenous fistula, it is known as *pseudo–Kaposi sarcoma.*

an•gio•di•as•co•py (an″je-o-di-as′kə-pe) [*angio-* + *diascopy*] direct visual inspection of blood vessels of the extremities, a light being held behind the part.

an•gi•odyn•ia (an″je-o-din′e-ə) [*angi-* + *-odynia*] angialgia.

an•gio•dys•pla•sia (an″je-o-dis-pla′zhə) small abnormalities of blood or lymphatic vessels.

papular a. small superficial papular lesions around the face, considered by some to be a variant of angiolymphoid hyperplasia with eosinophilia but lacking the lymphocytic response and eosinophils.

an•gio•dys•tro•phia (an″je-o-dis-tro′fe-ah) [*angio-* + *dystrophy*] any disorder of blood vessels caused by a defective supply of nutrients.

an•gio•dys•tro•phy (an″je-o-dis′trə-fe) angiodystrophia.

an•gio•ec•tat•ic (an″je-o-ek-tat′ik) angiectatic.

an•gio•ec•ta•sia (an″je-o-ek-ta′zhə) angiectasis.

an•gio•ede•ma (an″je-o-ə-de′mə) [*angio-* + *edema*] a vascular reaction involving the deep dermis or subcutaneous or submucosal tissues, representing localized edema caused by dilatation and increased permeability of capillaries, with development of giant wheals. Urticaria is the same reaction occurring in superficial portions of the dermis. *Type 3* is caused by a mutation in the *F12* gene (locus: 5q33-qter), which encodes factor XII, and affects only women; it is precipitated or exacerbated by high estrogen levels. Called also *angioneurotic edema* and *Quincke disease* or *edema.*

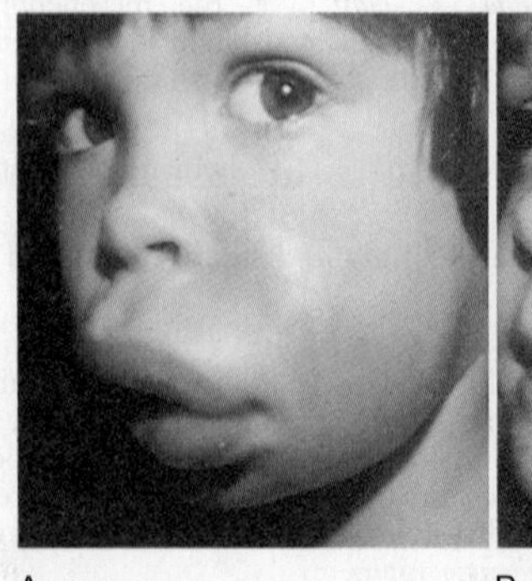
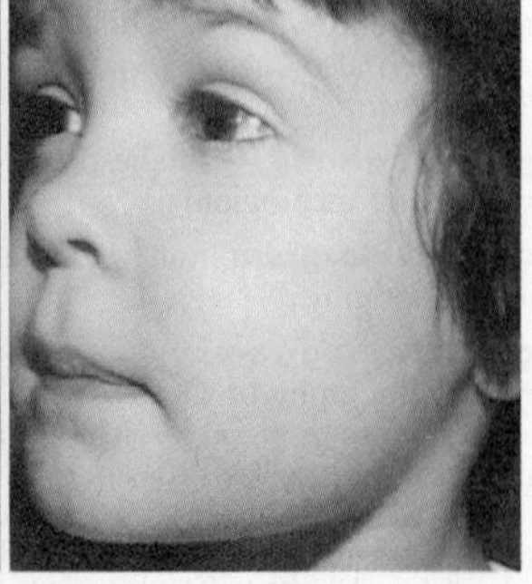

A B

■ *(A),* Angioedema of sudden onset; *(B),* complete resolution within 24 hours.

hereditary a. an autosomal dominant disorder manifested as recurrent episodes of edema of the skin, upper respiratory tract, and gastrointestinal tract with increased levels of several vasoactive mediators of anaphylaxis; it may result in life-threatening laryngeal edema. Although precipitating events are often unidentifiable, factors such as minor trauma, sudden changes in environmental temperature, and sudden emotional stress can initiate attacks. There are three types: two are clinically indistinguishable and are caused by mutations in the *C1NH* gene (locus: 11q11-q13.1), while the third is caused by mutation in the *F12* gene (locus: 5q33-qter), which encodes factor XII.

type 1 a type caused by mutations in *C1NH* that result in abnormally low levels of C1 inhibitor.

type 2 a type in which mutations in *C1NH* cause expression of dysfunctional C1 inhibitor, so that activity is markedly decreased although the level of C1 inhibitor is normal or elevated.

type 3 a type caused by mutations in *F12*, occurring only in women and precipitated or exacerbated by elevated levels of estrogen; C1 inhibitor level and activity are normal.

vibratory a. angioedema due to vibratory stimuli to the skin. One type is an autosomal dominant disorder and is accompanied by cholinergic urticaria; another type is seen with prolonged occupational exposure to vibration.

an•gio•ede•ma•tous (an″je-o″ə-de′mə-təs) pertaining to or characterized by angioedema.

an•gio•en•do•the•li•o•ma (an″je-o-en″do-the″le-o′mə) hemangioendothelioma.

endovascular papillary a., papillary intralymphatic a. a rare, low-grade type of angiosarcoma, seen mainly in children, characterized by anastomosing blood vessels and outpouchings in the skin or subcutaneous tissue. Called also *Dabska tumor.*

an•gio•en•do•the•lio•ma•to•sis (an″je-o-en″do-the″le-o-mə-to′sis) [*angio-* + *endotheliomatosis*] intravascular proliferation of tumors derived from endothelial cells; there are both benign and malignant varieties.

reactive a. a rare, benign variant in which there is proliferation of cells with endothelial cell markers within small capillaries in the skin; it is considered to be a reactive process, although many cases are idiopathic.

systemic proliferating a. cutaneous and visceral intravascular proliferation of tumor cells believed to be of endothelial origin, with obstruction of vascular lumina and thromboses; it occurs in a benign, self-limited form in which involvement is limited to the cutaneous vasculature and in a malignant, systemic, usually fatal form in which various organs as well as cutaneous and central nervous system vessels may be involved, with variable clinical manifestations. The malignant form has been noted to frequently follow or precede lymphoma.

an•gio•fi•bro•ma (an″je-o-fi-bro′mə) [*angioma* + *fibroma*] a lesion characterized by fibrous tissue and vascular proliferation; it often occurs as one or more small, flesh-colored papules, particularly on the face.

juvenile nasopharyngeal a., nasopharyngeal a. a benign tumor of the nasopharynx composed of fibrous connective tissue with abundant endothelium-lined vascular spaces, usually occurring during puberty in boys. Nasal obstruction may become total, with hyponasality, discomfort in swallowing, auditory tube obstruction, and massive epistaxis.

an•gio•fol•lic•u•lar (an″je-o-fŏ-lik′u-lər) pertaining to a lymphoid follicle (lymphoid nodule) and its blood vessels.

an•gio•gen•e•sis (an″je-o-jen′ə-sis) [*angio-* + *genesis*] 1. development of blood vessels in the embryo. 2. any formation of new blood vessels; see also *neovascularization* (def. 2) and *revascularization.* Called also *angiopoiesis* and *vasculogenesis.*

tumor a. the induction of the growth of blood vessels from surrounding tissue into a tumor by a diffusible protein factor released by the tumor cells.

an•gio•gen•ic (an″je-o-jen′ik) 1. pertaining to angiogenesis; called also *angiopoietic* and *vasculogenic.* 2. arising in the circulatory system.

an•gio•gram (an′je-o-gram″) a radiograph of blood vessels taken during angiography.

an•gio•gran•u•lo•ma (an″je-o-gran″u-lo′mə) [*angio-* + *granuloma*] an angioma of the skin or oral mucous membranes that contains granulation tissue, representing a vasoproliferative inflammatory response; after it develops, ulcerates, and suppurates, it is referred to as a *pyogenic granuloma.*

an•gio•graph (an′je-o-graf″) angiogram.

an•gi•og•ra•phy (an″je-og′rə-fe) [*angio-* + *-graphy*] the radiographic visualization of blood vessels following introduction of contrast material; used as a diagnostic aid in such conditions as stroke syndrome and myocardial infarction. See also *arteriography* and *phlebography.* Called also *vasography.*

cerebral a. angiography of the vascular system of the brain.

computed tomography a. (CTA) a minimally invasive form of angiography in which contrast material is injected intravenously through a small

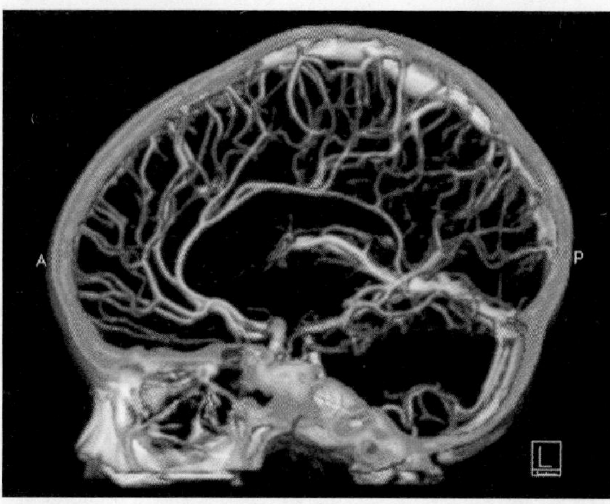

■ Computed tomography angiography used for selective imaging of the cerebral blood vessels.

needle or cannula and precise, detailed images of the vascular system are produced by computed tomography. It has numerous applications including screening, diagnosis, and planning for surgery.

coronary a. angiography of the coronary arteries.

digital subtraction a. an angiographic technique that produces images by subtracting background structures and enhancing the contrast of those areas that change in density between a preliminary "mask" image and subsequent images.

fluorescein a., fluorescence a. examination of the vasculature of the fundus of the eye with rapid serial photography after intravenous injection of fluorescein to act as a contrast agent.

ICG a., indocyanine green a. a technique similar to fluorescein angiography, for examining the fundus of the eye after intravenous injection of the dye indocyanine green.

intra-arterial digital subtraction a. a type of arteriography that uses electronic circuitry to subtract the background of bone and soft tissue to provide a useful image of the arteries injected with contrast medium.

intravenous digital subtraction a. a type of phlebography that uses electronic circuitry to subtract the background of bone and soft tissue to provide a useful image of the veins injected with contrast medium.

magnetic resonance a. (MRA) a form of magnetic resonance imaging used to study blood vessels and blood flow, used for detection of abnormalities in the vessels of the head and neck, for evaluation of the peripheral vasculature of the lower extremities, and for the detection of coronary artery disease.

pulmonary a. angiography of the pulmonary vessels, used to detect pulmonary embolism or less frequently to delineate pulmonary arteriovenous malformations, pulmonary varices, or pulmonary vessel anatomy.

retinal a. examination of the vasculature of the eye after injection of a contrast medium, such as fluorescein sodium or indocyanine green.

an•gio•he•mo•phil•ia (an″je-o-he′mo-fil′e-ə) von Willebrand disease.

an•gio•hy•a•li•no•sis (an″je-o-hi″ə-lĭ-no′sis) [*angio-* + *hyalinosis*] hyaline degeneration of the walls of blood vessels.

an•gi•oid (an′je-oid) [*angi-* + *-oid*] resembling a blood vessel.

an•gio•im•mu•no•blas•tic (an″je-o-im″u-no-blas′tik) characterized by the presence of immunoblasts (lymphoblasts) and an inflammatory infiltrate in small blood vessels infiltrating lymph nodes.

an•gio•in•va•sive (an″je-o-in-va′siv) tending to invade the walls of blood vessels.

an•gio•ker•a•to•ma (an″je-o-ker″ə-to′mə) [*angio-* + *keratoma*] a discrete, skin colored or reddish telangiectasia having a tendency to undergo secondary epithelial changes such as acanthosis or hyperkeratosis. An underlying vascular abnormality is present in many cases. Called also *angiokeratosis* and *telangiectatic wart.*

a. circumscrip′tum a rare type of angiokeratoma, seen mainly in girl infants or young children, characterized by usually unilateral papules and small nodules that may coalesce to form plaques.

a. cor′poris diffu′sum, diffuse a. 1. telangiectasias in the "bathing suit" area of the trunk, as seen in Fabry disease. 2. occasionally, a synonym for Fabry disease.

a. of Fordyce small vascular papules that become keratotic, found along the superficial veins of the scrotum and occasionally over the penis, inguinal area, or upper thigh; seen in older men, usually those with a history of venous obstruction. Similar lesions may occur on the vulva in women. Called also *a. of scrotum.*

a. of Mibelli symmetrical discrete, aggregated or confluent, soft, slightly darkened vascular papules on the backs of the fingers, toes, elbows, and knees; they may later become hyperkeratotic. Most cases are seen in children or young adults, often those with a history of chilblains, cold sensitivity, or frostbite.

a. of scrotum a. of Fordyce.

solitary a. angiokeratoma that takes the form of a small, bluish black, usually solitary warty papule, generally on the lower limb and appearing in childhood or adolescence.

an•gio•ker•a•to•sis (an″je-o-ker″ə-to′sis) angiokeratoma.

an•gio•ki•ne•sis (an″je-o-kĭ-ne′sis) vasomotion.

an•gio•ki•net•ic (an″je-o-kĭ-net′ik) vasomotor.

an•gio•leio•my•o•ma (an″je-o-li″o-mi-o′mə) [*angio-* + *leiomyoma*] a leiomyoma arising from vascular smooth muscle, usually occurring as a solitary nodular, sometimes painful, subcutaneous tumor on the lower extremity, more deeply situated than ordinary leiomyoma; usually seen in middle-aged women. Called also *angiomyoma* and *vascular leiomyoma.*

an•gio•lipo•leio•my•o•ma (an″je-o-lip″o-li-o-mi-o′mə) [*angio-* + *lipo-* + *leiomyoma*] a benign tumor composed of blood vessel, adipose tissue, and smooth muscle elements, such as occurs in the kidney in association with tuberous sclerosis, where it is usually called *angiomyolipoma.*

an•gio•li•po•ma (an″je-o-lĭ-po′mə) [*angio-* + *lipoma*] a frequently painful type of lipoma that contains clusters of thin-walled proliferating blood vessels.

an•gi•ol•o•gy (an″je-ol′ə-je) [*angio-* + *-logy*] 1. the study of the blood and lymph vessels of the body. 2. the sum of knowledge about the blood and lymph vessels.

an•gio•lu•poid (an″je-o-loo′poid) [*angio-* + *lupoid*] a rare cutaneous manifestation of sarcoidosis, found on the cheek, on the bridge of the nose, or near the eyes; it consists of discolored nodular lesions that coalesce to form plaques.

an•gio•lym•phan•gi•o•ma (an″je-o-lim-fan″je-o′mə) a mixed angioma in which lymph vessels and blood vessels are involved.

an•gio•lym•phi•tis (an″je-o-lim-fi′tis) lymphangitis.

an•gi•ol•y•sis (an″je-ol′ĭ-sis) [*angio-* + *-lysis*] retrogression or obliteration of blood vessels, such as occurs during embryonic development.

an•gi•o•ma (an″je-o′mə) [*angio-* + *-oma*] a tumor whose cells tend to form blood vessels *(hemangioma)* or lymph vessels *(lymphangioma);* a tumor made up of blood vessels or lymph vessels. Called also *endothelioma angiomatosum* and *vascular tumor.*

a. arteria′le racemo′sum a dilatation and complex intertwining of many new-formed and altered vessels of small caliber with subsequent involvement of normal vessels.

arteriovenous a. of brain cerebral arteriovenous malformation.

capillary a. cherry a.

cavernous a. see under *hemangioma.*

cherry a. a bright red to purple, smooth, dome-shaped lesion representing a telangiectatic vascular disturbance, usually found on the trunk or proximal end of a limb; these are common in elderly persons, but the onset may be earlier in adult life. Called also *capillary a., De Morgan spot,* and *senile a.*

a. cu′tis vascular nevus.

fissural a. a hemangioma occurring in embryonal fissures (clefts) of the face, neck, or lips.

hypertrophic a. angioma with proliferation of endothelial tissue.

a. lympha′ticum lymphangioma.

senile a. cherry a.

a. serpigino′sum a rare type of generalized essential telangiectasia characterized by groups of orange to red dots on the skin that enlarge and form new dots at the periphery with central clearing, which produces annular or serpiginous patterns. The eruption usually occurs on the lower limbs in girls and young women. Called also *Hutchinson disease.*

spider a. a telangiectasis with a red central portion and branching lines like a silhouette of a spider with its legs; it is caused by dilatation and ramification of superficial cutaneous arteries, and may occur singly or in groups. Spider angiomas may be congenital (nevoid) or acquired, such as in

■ Cherry angiomas.

association with pregnancy or liver disease. See also *vascular nevus*, under *nevus*. Called also *arterial* or *vascular spider*, *nevus araneus*, *spider nevus*, and *spider telangiectasia*.

tufted a. a rare, benign, slow-growing vascular tumor of the skin and subcutaneous tissue, characterized by erythematous macules or papules that may spread to form plaques over a wide area; the condition is usually seen in children.

a. veno′sum racemo′sum the swellings caused by severe varicosity of superficial veins.

venous a. of brain congenital angioma of the brain, composed of abnormal branches of veins, usually with a common center, found most often near the ventricular wall; it is often asymptomatic.

an•gi•o•ma•toid (an″je-o′mə-toid) 1. resembling an angioma. 2. a mass of dilated, twisted vessels that resembles an angioma.

an•gi•o•ma•to•sis (an″je-o-mə-to′sis) a diseased state of the vessels with the formation of multiple angiomas.

bacillary a. a disorder of neovascular proliferation, caused by *Bartonella henselae* and *B. quintana;* its manifestations range from subcutaneous or dermal nodules and papules to more widespread disease involving the lymph nodes, liver, spleen, bone marrow, brain, lungs, bowel, and uterine cervix.

cerebroretinal a. von Hippel-Lindau disease.

encephalofacial a., encephalotrigeminal a. Sturge-Weber syndrome.

hepatic a. peliosis hepatis.

a. of retina von Hippel disease.

retinocerebral a. von Hippel-Lindau disease.

an•gi•om•a•tous (an″je-om′ə-təs) of the nature of angioma.

An•gio•max (an′je-o-maks) trademark for a preparation of bivalirudin.

an•gio•meg•a•ly (an″je-o-meg′ə-le) [*angio-* + *-megaly*] enlargement of blood vessels, causing swelling, such as of the eyelids.

an•gio•myo•li•po•ma (an″je-o-mi″o-lĭ-po′mə) [*angio-* + *myo-* + *lipoma*] a benign tumor containing vascular, adipose, and muscle elements; it occurs most often as a renal tumor with smooth muscle elements (more correctly called *angiolipoleiomyoma*) usually in association with tuberous sclerosis, and is considered to be a hamartoma.

an•gio•my•o•ma (an″je-o-mi-o′mə) [*angio-* + *myoma*] angioleiomyoma.

an•gio•myo•sar•co•ma (an″je-o-mi″o-sahr-ko′mə) a tumor made up of elements of angioma, myoma, and sarcoma.

an•gio•myx•o•ma (an″je-o-mik-so′mə) a chorioangioma containing capillary-like blood vessels; it may extend into the umbilical cord and often contains myxomatous tissue resembling that in the normal cord.

an•gio•ne•cro•sis (an″je-o-nə-kro′sis) [*angio-* + *necrosis*] necrosis of the walls of blood vessels.

an•gio•neu•ral•gia (an″je-o-noo͝-ral′jə) [*angio-* + *neuralgia*] burning pain in an extremity with edema and redness.

an•gio•neu•rec•to•my (an″je-o-noo͝-rek′tə-me) [*angio-* + *neurectomy*] excision of vessels and nerves.

an•gio•neu•rop•a•thy (an″je-o-noo͝-rop′ə-the) [*angio-* + *neuropathy*] 1. angiopathic neuropathy. 2. any neuropathy affecting primarily the blood vessels; a disorder of the vasomotor system, as angiospasm, angioparalysis, or vasomotor paralysis. **angioneuropath′ic** *adj*

an•gio•neu•rot•ic (an″je-o-noo͝-rot′ik) angioneuropathic.

an•gio•neu•rot•o•my (an″je-o-noo͝-rot′ə-me) [*angio-* + *neurotomy*] the cutting of vessels and nerves.

an•gio•no•ma (an″je-o-no′mə) [*angio-* + *noma*] ulceration of a blood vessel.

an•gio•pa•ral•y•sis (an″je-o-pə-ral′ə-sis) [*angio-* + *paralysis*] vasomotor paralysis.

an•gio•pa•re•sis (an″je-o-pə-re′sis) vasoparesis.

an•gio•path•ol•o•gy (an″je-o-pə-thol′ə-je) the pathology of, or the changes seen in, diseases of the blood vessels.

an•gi•op•a•thy (an-je-op′ə-the) [*angio-* + *-pathy*] any disease of the blood vessels or lymphatics.

cerebral amyloid a., congophilic a. vascular amyloidosis affecting small and medium-sized arteries of the leptomeninges and cerebral cortex, resulting in microinfarcts or in hemorrhage; it may be asymptomatic or may result in hemorrhagic stroke or dementia. Most cases are sporadic and occur most often in the elderly. A hereditary form with autosomal dominant inheritance also exists.

an•gio•phak•o•ma•to•sis (an″je-o-fak″o-mə-to′sis) [*angio-* + *phakomatosis*] von Hippel-Lindau disease.

an•gio•plas•ty (an′je-o-plas″te) [*angio-* + *-plasty*] an angiographic procedure for elimination of areas of narrowing in blood vessels. **angioplas′tic** *adj*

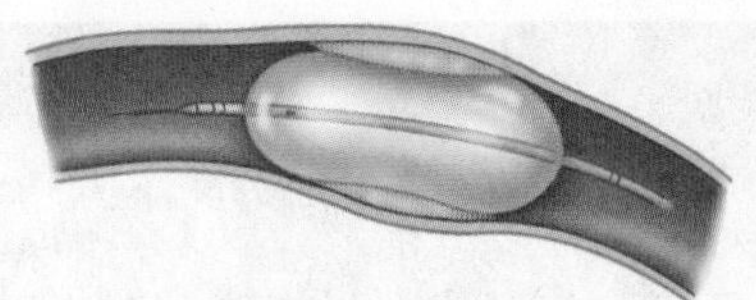

■ Balloon angioplasty, the expanded balloon pressing against a stenotic site in an artery.

balloon a. angioplasty using a balloon catheter that is inflated inside an artery, stretching the intima and leaving a ragged interior surface after deflation, which triggers a healing response and breaking up of plaque. See also *percutaneous transluminal a.*

laser a. angioplasty using a laser, usually an excimer laser, inserted through a tube for vaporization of plaque; sometimes used prior to balloon angioplasty.

percutaneous transluminal a. a type of balloon angioplasty in which the catheter is inserted through the skin and through the lumen of the vessel to the site of narrowing.

percutaneous transluminal coronary a. (PTCA) percutaneous transluminal angioplasty to enlarge the lumen of a sclerotic coronary artery, an alternative to bypass cardiac surgery for selected patients with ischemic heart disease.

percutaneous transluminal renal a. (PTRA) percutaneous transluminal angioplasty to enlarge the lumen of a sclerotic renal artery, preserve renal function, and treat renovascular hypertension.

an•gio•poi•e•sis (an″je-o-poi-e′sis) [*angio-* + *-poiesis*] angiogenesis.

an•gio•poi•et•ic (an″je-o-poi-et′ik) angiogenic (def. 1).

an•gio•pres•sure (an′je-o-presh″ər) the application of pressure to a blood vessel to control hemorrhage.

an•gio•re•tic•u•lo•en•do•the•li•o•ma (an″je-o-rĕ-tik″u-lo-en″do-the-le-o′mə) Kaposi sarcoma.

an•gio•re•tic•u•lo•ma (an″je-o-re-tik″u-lo′mə) hemangioblastoma.

an•gi•or•rha•phy (an″je-or′ə-fe) [*angio-* + *rrhaphy*] the suturing of a vessel or vessels, particularly of blood vessels.

arteriovenous a. the suturing of an artery to a vein, so as to divert the arterial current into the vein.

an•gio•sar•co•ma (an″je-o-sahr-ko′mə) [*angio-* + *sarcoma*] a malignant neoplasm arising from vascular endothelial cells; the term may be used generally or may denote a specific histologic subtype, usually hemangiosarcoma but sometimes lymphangiosarcoma or hemangiopericytoma.

cutaneous a. angiosarcoma of the skin, usually of the scalp or face, characterized by violaceous patches and nodules, sometimes with ulceration and bleeding.

hepatic a. a malignant tumor of the liver characterized by dilated sinusoids with hypertrophied or necrotic hepatocytes that leave vascular channels lined by malignant cells. It usually affects older men and has been linked to exposure to toxins such as vinyl chloride gas, inorganic arsenic compounds, and thorium dioxide. Called also *Kupffer cell sarcoma*.

an•gio•scin•tig•ra•phy (an″je-o-sin-tig′rə-fe) scintigraphy of the vascular system.

an•gio•scle•ro•sis (an″je-o-sklĕ-ro′sis) [*angio-* + *sclerosis*] hardening of walls of blood vessels; see *arteriosclerosis* and *phlebosclerosis*.

an•gio•scope (an′je-o-skōp″) [*angio-* + *-scope*] 1. a fiberoptic catheter for viewing the inside of a blood vessel. 2. a microscope for observing capillary blood vessels.

an•gi•os•co•py (an″ge-os′kə-pe) 1. use of a fiberoptic angioscope to visualize the lumen of a blood vessel. 2. visualization of capillary blood vessels with a special microscope (angioscope).

an•gio•sco•to•ma (an″je-o-sko-to′mə) [*angio-* + *scotoma*] a cecocentral scotoma caused by shadows of the retinal blood vessels.

an•gio•sco•tom•e•try (an″je-o-sko-tom′ə-tre) [*angio-* + *scotoma* + *-metry*] the plotting or mapping of the scotoma caused by the shadow of retinal blood vessels; used particularly in the diagnosis of glaucoma.

an•gio•spasm (an′je-o-spaz″əm) [*angio-* + *spasm*] vasospasm.

an•gio•spas•tic (an″je-o-spas′tik) vasospastic.

an•gio•sperm (an′je-o-spərm″) [*angio-* + *sperm*] a true flowering plant; a plant having its seeds in an enclosed ovary.

an•gio•stat•in (an″je-o-stat′in) 1. an angiogenesis inhibitor. 2. a 38-kD fragment of plasminogen that inhibits the growth of new blood vessels; it is produced by proteolytic cleavage of plasminogen and by certain types of tumor cells.

an•gio•ste•no•sis (an″je-o-stə-no′sis) [*angio-* + *stenosis*] narrowing of the caliber of a vessel.

an·gi·os·te·o·sis (an″je-os″te-o′sis) [*angi-* + *osteosis*] ossification or calcification of a vessel.

an·gi·os·to·my (an″je-os′tə-me) [*angio-* + *-stomy*] 1. the creation of an opening into a blood vessel. 2. the opening so made.

an·gio·stron·gy·li·a·sis (an″je-o-stron″jĭ-li′ə-sis) infection by a nematode of the genus *Angiostrongylus.* In humans the usual species is the rat lungworm, *A. cantonensis,* and infection comes after eating contaminated raw snails, slugs, or paratenic hosts such as prawns or crabs. The larval worms migrate to the central nervous system and cause eosinophilic meningitis. In dogs the most common infecting species is *A. vasorum* and the worms are found in the pulmonary arteries.

An·gio·stron·gy·li·dae (an″je-o-stron-jil′ĭ-de) a family of nematodes that includes the genera *Aelurostrongylus* and *Angiostrongylus.* Several species are lungworms in mammals.

an·gio·stron·gy·lo·sis (an″je-o-stron″jĭ-lo′sis) angiostrongyliasis.

An·gio·stron·gy·lus (an″je-o-stron′jĭ-ləs) [*angio-* + Gr. *strongylos* round] a genus of parasitic nematodes of the family Angiostrongylidae.

A. cantonen′sis the rat lungworm, a species that parasitizes the domestic rat primarily in Australia and many Pacific islands. Larval development occurs in snails, slugs, and planarians; in rats, the adult worms are found in the bronchioles. Human infection is caused by ingestion of larvae in raw seafood; see *angiostrongyliasis.*

A. costaricen′sis a species that normally inhabits the mesenteric arteries of rodents but has been found in the mesenteric and nearby arteries of humans in Central America and Brazil.

A. vaso′rum a species parasitic in dogs; see *angiostrongyliasis.*

an·gio·te·lec·ta·sis (an″je-o-tə-lek′tə-sis) pl. *angiotelec′tases* [*angio-* + *tel-* + *ectasis*] dilatation of the minute arteries and veins.

an·gio·ten·sin (an″je-o-ten′sin) any of a family of polypeptide vasopressor hormones formed by the catalytic action of renin on angiotensinogen. Called also *angiotonin.*

a. I a decapeptide cleaved from angiotensinogen by renin; it has some biological activity but serves mainly as a precursor to a. II.

a. II an octapeptide hormone formed by the action of angiotensin-converting enzyme (peptidyl-dipeptidase A) on angiotensin I, chiefly in the lungs but also at other sites, including the blood vessel walls, uterus, and brain. It is a powerful vasopressor and stimulator of aldosterone and vasopressin secretion, and it also functions as a neurotransmitter. Its vasopressor action raises blood pressure and diminishes fluid loss in the kidney by restricting blood flow.

a. III a heptapeptide degradation product of a. II, having less vasopressor activity than the parent compound.

a. amide an amide derivative of angiotensin and a powerful vasoconstrictor and vasopressor, used in the treatment of certain hypotensive states; usually administered by slow intravenous infusion.

an·gio·ten·sin·ase (an″je-o-ten′sin-ās) any of a group of plasma or tissue peptidases that cleave and inactivate angiotensin.

an·gio·ten·sin-con·vert·ing en·zyme (an″je-o-ten′sin kən-vurt′ing en′zīm) peptidyl-dipeptidase A.

an·gio·ten·sin·o·gen (an″je-o-ten-sin′o-jen) a serum α_2-globulin secreted in the liver and produced in many organs, which is cleaved by renin to give rise to angiotensin I. Called also *renin substrate.*

an·gio·tome (an′je-o-tōm″) [*angio-* + *-tome*] any one of the segments of the vascular system of the embryo.

an·gi·ot·o·my (an″je-ot′ə-me) [*angio-* + *-tomy*] the cutting or severing of a blood or lymphatic vessel.

an·gio·to·nia (an″je-o-to′ne-ə) vasotonia.

an·gio·ton·ic (an″je-o-ton′ik) [*angio-* + *tonic*] vasotonic.

an·gio·to·nin (an″je-o-to′nin) angiotensin.

an·gio·tro·phic (an″je-o-tro′fik) [*angio-* + *-trophic*] vasotrophic.

an·gi·tis (an-ji′tis) angiitis.

An·gle classification, splint (ang′gəl) [Edward Hartley *Angle,* American orthodontist, 1855–1930] see under *classification* and *splint;* see also *malocclusion.*

an·gle (ang′gəl) [L. *angulus*] 1. the area or point of junction of two intersecting borders or surfaces. 2. the degree of divergence of two intersecting lines or planes. Symbol θ.

Angle

For specific anatomic structures not found here, see under *angulus.*

a. of aberration a. of deviation.
acetabular a. the angle between the acetabular line and Hilgenreiner line, normally between 27° and 30° in the neonatal hip; used in the radiographic assessment of developmental dysplasia of the hip. Called also *acetabular index.*
acromial a. angulus acromii.
acromial a. of scapula angulus lateralis scapulae.
alpha a. the angle formed by the intersection of the visual axis with the optic axis at the nodal point. It is *positive* when the visual axis crosses the cornea on the nasal side of the optic axis, as in most individuals; *negative* when the visual axis crosses the cornea on the temporal side of the optic axis; and *nil* when the visual axis and the optic axis coincide.
Alsberg a. see under *triangle.*

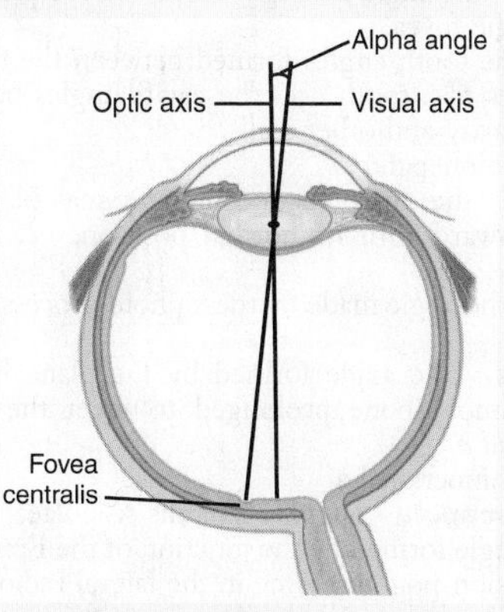

■ Positive alpha angle.

alveolar a. the angle between a line running through a point beneath the nasal spine and the most prominent point of the lower border of the alveolar process of the superior maxilla and the cephalic horizontal (glabella to opisthocranion).
anorectal a. the angle formed by the anorectal flexure; it flexes to maintain continence and straightens during defecation.
a. of anterior chamber of eye the angle formed at the border of the anterior chamber of the eye by the trabecular reticulum, the ciliary body, and the part of the iris attached to the ciliary body.
a. of aperture the angle between two lines from the focus of a lens to the ends of its diameter.
auriculo-occipital a. the angle between lines from the auricular point to the lambda and opisthion.
axial a. an angle whose formation is partially dependent on the axial wall of a tooth cavity preparation, such as the axiodistal angle or the buccoaxial angle. See table of *cavity angles* and illustration of *tooth angles.*
axial line a. any line angle that is parallel with the long axis of a tooth. For names of various angles see table of *cavity angles* and illustration of *tooth angles.*
Baumann a. on an anteroposterior radiograph of the distal humerus, the angle formed by a line perpendicular to the long axis of the humerus and a line tangential to the straight epiphyseal border of the distal lateral metaphysis, normally 70°–75°; a larger angle indicates cubitus varus and a smaller, cubitus valgus.
Bennett a. the angle formed by the sagittal plane and the path of the advancing condyle during lateral movement of the mandible, as viewed in the horizontal plane. See also *Bennett movement,* under *movement.*
beta a. the angle between the radius fixus and a line joining the bregma and the hormion.
biorbital a. the angle formed by intersection of a posterior extension of the axes of the two orbits.
Broca a. ophryospinal a.

Angle *Continued*

buccal a's the angles formed between the buccal surface and the other surfaces of a posterior tooth, or between the buccal wall of a tooth cavity and other walls, named according to the surfaces which participate in their formation. See table of *cavity angles* and illustration of *tooth angles.*
cardiodiaphragmatic a. the angle formed by the junction of the shadows of the heart and diaphragm in posteroanterior radiographs of the chest; called also *cardiophrenic a.*
cardiohepatic a. the angle formed by the horizontal limit of hepatic dullness with the upright line of cardiac dullness in the fifth right intercostal space, close to the sternal border; called also *Ebstein a.*
cardiophrenic a. cardiodiaphragmatic a.
carrying a. the accustomed angle of a person's elbow; the angle formed laterally by the axes of the arm and forearm when the forearm is extended in the anatomical position.
cavity a's the angles formed by the junction of two or more walls of a tooth cavity, named according to the walls participating in their formation. See accompanying table.
cavosurface a. the angle formed by the junction of a wall of a tooth cavity preparation and a surface of the crown of the tooth.
center-edge a. of Wiberg the angle formed by a line drawn perpendicular to a baseline that passes through the center of the femoral heads and a line connecting the center of the femoral head and the superior border of the acetabulum, used in radiographic evaluation of the hip joint; it is less than 20° in developmental dysplasia of the hip.
cephalic a's various angles of the skull or face.
cephalometric a. measurement of intersecting anthropometric lines on tracings made of oriented head films in radiologic orthodontic diagnosis.
cerebellopontine a. the angle between the cerebellum and the pons.
chi a. the angle between two lines from the hormion to the staphylion and to the basion, respectively.
Cobb a. an angle measuring scoliosis as seen on a radiograph: for a given group of vertebrae, lines are drawn across the vertebral column on the upper surface of the upper vertebra and the lower surface of the lower vertebra. The angle measured may be either that between these two lines or that between lines drawn perpendicular to them.
collodiaphyseal a. the angle formed by the intersection of the long axes of the neck and shaft of the femur.

Cavity Angles

Line Angles (Formed by the Junction of Two Walls)

Axiodistal	Gingivoaxial
Axiogingival	Labiogingival
Axioincisal	Linguoaxial
Axiolabial	Linguodistal
Axiolingual	Linguogingival
Axiomesial	Linguomesial
Axio-occlusal	Linguopulpal
Axiopulpal	Mesiobuccal
Buccoaxial	Mesiogingival
Buccodistal	Mesiolabial
Buccogingival	Mesiolingual
Buccomesial	Mesio-occlusal
Buccopulpal	Mesiopulpal
Distobuccal	Pulpoaxial
Distogingival	Pulpodistal
Distolabial	Pulpolabial
Distolingual	Pulpolingual
Disto-occlusal	Pulpomesial
Distopulpal	

Point Angles (Formed by the Junction of Three Walls)

Axiodistogingival	Distopulpolingual
Axiodisto-occlusal	Gingivobuccoaxial
Axiolabiogingival	Gingivolinguoaxial
Axiolinguogingival	Mesiobuccopulpal
Axiomesiogingival	Mesiolinguopulpal
Axiomesio-occlusal	Mesiopulpolabial
Distobuccopulpal	Mesiopulpolingual
Distolinguopulpal	Pulpobuccoaxial
Distopulpolabial	Pulpolinguoaxial

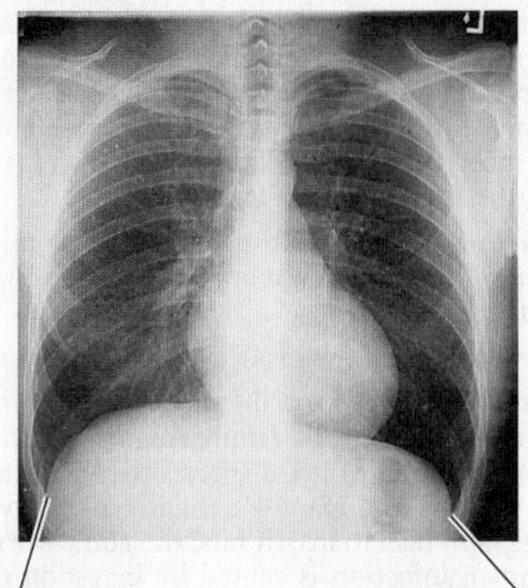

■ Costophrenic angles on a posteroanterior (PA) projection chest radiograph.

condylar a. the angle between the planes of the basilar clivus and the foramen magnum.
a. of convergence the angle between the visual axis and the median line when an object is looked at.
a. of convexity a radiographic cephalometric measurement formed by connecting the nasion, point A, and pogonion (NAP), which reflects the convexity or concavity of the facial profile.
coronary a. angulus frontalis ossis parietalis.
costal a. angulus costae.
costophrenic a. the angle formed at the junction of the costal and diaphragmatic pleurae. See also *recessus costodiaphragmaticus pleuralis.*
costovertebral a. the angle formed on either side of the vertebral column, between the last rib and the lumbar vertebrae.
craniofacial a. the angle between the basifacial and basicranial axes at the middle of the ethmoidosphenoid suture.
critical a. the angle of incidence at which a ray of light passing from one medium to another of different density changes from refraction to total reflection; called also *limiting a.*
cusp a. 1. the angle made by the slopes of a cusp of a tooth with the plane that passes through the tip of the cusp and that is perpendicular to a line bisecting the cusp, measured mesiodistally or buccolingually. 2. the angle made by the slopes of a cusp with a perpendicular line bisecting the cusp, measured mesiodistally or buccolingually. 3. one half of the included angle between the buccal and lingual or mesial and distal cusp inclines.
cusp plane a. the incline of the cusp plane in relation to the plane of occlusion.
Daubenton a. an angle formed by junction of the opisthiobasial and opisthionasial lines; called also *occipital a.*
a. of declination Mikulicz a.
a. of deviation the angle between a refracted ray and the incident ray prolonged; called also *a. of aberration.*
a. of direction the angle through which the eye must move to bring the image onto the fovea.
distal a's 1. the tooth angles formed between the distal surface and the other surfaces of a tooth. 2. the cavity angles between the distal wall of a tooth cavity and other walls.
Ebstein a. cardiohepatic a.
elevation a. 1. the angle made by the visual plane when moved upward or downward with its normal position. 2. Alsberg triangle; see under *triangle.*
epigastric a. the angle made by the xiphoid process with the body of the sternum.
ethmocranial a. the angle formed by the plane of the cribriform plate of the ethmoid bone prolonged to meet the basicranial axis; called also *ethmoid a.*
ethmoid a. ethmocranial a.
external a. of scapula angulus lateralis scapulae.
facial a. the angle formed by the junction of the Frankfort horizontal plane and the nasion-pogonion line in the lateral radiographic cephalometric tracing. Used to express the degree of retrusion or protrusion of the chin. See also *prognathism* and *retrognathism.*

filtration a. angulus iridocornealis.
frontal a. of parietal bone angulus frontalis ossis parietalis.
gamma a. the angle formed by junction of the line of fixation and the optic axis at the center of rotation of the eye.
gonial a. the angle formed by the intersection of the body of the mandible and the ascending mandibular ramus; an important consideration in prognathic procedures. Called also *angulus mandibulae* [TA].
horizontal a. in dental radiology, an angle measured within a horizontal plane, at which the central ray of the useful beam is projected relative to a vertical plane of reference.
a. of incidence the angle made with the perpendicular by a ray of light which strikes a denser or a rarer medium; see *refraction.*
incisal a. one of the angles formed by the junction of the incisal and the mesial or distal surfaces of an anterior tooth; called the *mesial* and the *distal incisal angle,* respectively.
incisal guide a. the angle formed with the horizontal plane by drawing a line in the sagittal plane between incisal edges of the maxillary and mandibular central incisors when the teeth are in centric occlusion.
incisal mandibular plane a. one of the three angles composing the Tweed triangle, designating the axial inclination of the lower incisor to the mandibular plane in the lateral cephalometric radiograph.
a. of inclination inclinatio pelvis.
inferior a. of duodenum flexura duodeni inferior.
inferior a. of parietal bone, anterior angulus sphenoidalis ossis parietalis.
inferior a. of parietal bone, posterior angulus mastoideus ossis parietalis.
inferior a. of scapula angulus inferior scapulae.
infrasternal a. of thorax angulus infrasternalis.
inner a. of humerus margo medialis humeri.
iridial a., iridocorneal a., a. of iris angulus iridocornealis.
Jacquart a. ophryospinal a.
a. of jaw angulus mandibulae.
kappa a. the angle between the pupillary axes.
kyphotic a. the superior angle formed by intersection of two lines drawn on the lateral chest radiogram, tangential to the anterior borders of the second and eleventh intervertebral spaces; an index of the degree of deformity in thoracic kyphosis.
labial a's the angles formed between the labial surface and other surfaces of an anterior tooth, or between the labial wall of a tooth cavity and other walls; named according to the surfaces participating in their formation. See table of *cavity angles* and illustration of *tooth angles.*
lambda a. the angle between the pupillary axis and the line of sight.
lateral a. of eye angulus oculi lateralis.
lateral a. of scapula angulus lateralis scapulae.
limiting a. critical a.
line a. an angle formed by the junction of two planes; used to designate the junction of two surfaces of a tooth, or of two walls of a tooth cavity preparation. Line angles of the posterior teeth include the mesio-occlusal, linguo-occlusal, mesiolingual, distolingual, mesiobuccal, distobuccal, bucco-occlusal, and disto-occlusal angles. Those of the anterior teeth include the labioincisal, linguoincisal, mesiolabial, distolabial, mesiolingual, and distolingual angles. See table of *cavity angles* and illustration of *tooth angles.*
lingual a's the angles formed between the lingual and other surfaces of a tooth, or between the lingual wall of a tooth cavity preparation and other walls; named according to the surfaces which participate in their formation, e.g., the linguopulpal angle is formed at the junction of the lingual and pulpal walls of a cavity preparation. See table of *cavity angles* and illustration of *tooth angles.*
Louis a., Ludwig a. angulus sterni.
lumbosacral a. sacrovertebral a.
a. of mandible, mandibular a. angulus mandibulae.
mastoid a. of parietal bone angulus mastoideus ossis parietalis.
maxillary a. the angle between two lines extending from the point of contact of the upper and lower central incisors to the ophryon and the most prominent point of the lower jaw (pogonion).
medial a. of eye angulus oculi medialis.
medial a. of scapula angulus superior scapulae.
mesial a's the angles formed between the mesial surface and other surfaces of a tooth, or between the mesial wall of a tooth cavity and other walls, named according to the surfaces participating with the mesial in their formation. See table of *cavity angles* and illustration of *tooth angles.*
metafacial a. the angle between the base of the skull and the pterygoid process; called also *Serres a.*
meter a. a unit of convergence of the eye: that amount of convergence required for binocular fixation of an object at 1 meter and using 1 diopter of accommodation.
Mikulicz a. an angle formed by two planes, one passing through the long axis of the epiphysis of the femur and the other through the long axis of the diaphysis; it is normally 130 degrees. Called also *a. of declination.*
minimum separabile a., minimum separable a. 1. the smallest angle of separation at which the eye recognizes two points, lines, or objects as being separate. 2. minimum visible a.
minimum visible a., minimum visual a. the angle which the minimum separabile subtends at the eye; 60 seconds of arc is usually taken as standard for a normal eye.
a. of mouth angulus oris.
a. of Mulder the angle formed by the intersection of the facial line of Camper and a line from the root of the nose to the spheno-occipital suture.
nu a. the angle between the radius fixus and a line joining the hormion and nasion.
occipital a. Daubenton a.
occipital a. of parietal bone angulus occipitalis ossis parietalis.
olfactive a., olfactory a. the angle formed by the line of the olfactory fossa and the os planum of the sphenoid bone.
ophryospinal a. the angle at the anterior nasal spine between lines from the auricular point and the glabella; called also *Broca a., Jacquart a.,* and *Topinard a.*
optic a. visual a.
orofacial a. one of the facial angles formed by the junction of the Frankfort horizontal plane with the nasion-pogonion plane.
parietal a. the angle formed by junction of lines passing through the extremities of the transverse bizygomatic diameter and the maximum transverse frontal diameter; called also *Quatrefages a.*
a. of pelvis inclinatio pelvis.
pelvivertebral a. inclinatio pelvis.
phrenopericardial a. the space or angle between the pericardium and the diaphragm.
Pirogoff a. venous a.
point a. any angle formed by the junction of three surfaces of a tooth crown, or three walls of a tooth cavity preparation, named according to the tooth surfaces or the cavity walls participating in its formation. Point angles on the posterior teeth include the mesiolinguo-occlusal, mesiobucco-occlusal, distolinguo-occlusal, and distobucco-occlusal angles. Point angles on the anterior teeth include the mesiolabioincisal, mesiolinguoincisal, distolabioincisal, and distolinguoincisal angles. See table of *cavity angles* and illustration of *tooth angles.*
a. of polarization the angle at which light reflected from a surface is most completely polarized.
principal a. refracting a.
a. of pubis angulus subpubicus.
Q a. the angle formed by the intersection of a line connecting the center of the patella and the anterior iliac spine (representing the line of pull of the quadriceps tendon) and a line connecting the center of the patella and the center of the tibial tuberosity; in a normal knee it is 15 degrees.
Quatrefages a. parietal a.
Ranke a. the angle between the horizontal plane of the skull and a line through the center of the maxillary alveolar margin and the center of the nasofrontal suture.
a. of reflection the angle that a reflected ray makes with a line perpendicular to the reflecting surface.
refracting a. the angle between the two refracting faces of a prism; called also *principal a.*
a. of refraction the angle between a refracted ray and a line perpendicular to the refracting surface; see *refraction.*
a. of rib angulus costae.
rolandic a., a. of Rolando the angle formed by junction of the median plane and the central sulcus (fissure of Rolando).
sacrovertebral a. the angle formed at the junction of the sacrum with the lowest lumbar vertebra; called also *lumbosacral a.*
Serres a. metafacial a.

sigma a. the angle between the radius fixus and a line from the staphylion to the hormion.
somatosplanchnic a. the angle formed by junction of the somatic and splanchnic layers of the mesoblast in the embryo.
sphenoid a., sphenoidal a. 1. an angle at the top of the sella turcica between lines from the nasal point and from the tip of the rostrum of the sphenoid. 2. angulus sphenoidalis ossis parietalis.
sphenoidal a. of parietal bone angulus sphenoidalis ossis parietalis.
squint a. the angle by which the visual line of the squinting eye deviates from a line drawn to the object which should be fixed; called also *squint deviation.*
sternal a. angulus sterni.
sternoclavicular a. the angle formed by junction of the sternum and clavicle.
a. of sternum angulus sterni.
subcostal a. angulus infrasternalis.
subpubic a. angulus subpubicus.
subscapular a. a transverse depression on the costal or ventral surface of the scapula, where the bone appears bent on itself perpendicular to and passing through the glenoid cavity.
substernal a. angulus infrasternalis.
superior a. of duodenum flexura duodeni superior.
superior a. of parietal bone, anterior angulus frontalis ossis parietalis.
superior a. of parietal bone, posterior angulus occipitalis ossis parietalis.
superior a. of scapula angulus superior scapulae.
a. of Sylvius the angle formed by junction of the lateral sulcus (fissure of Sylvius) and a line perpendicular to the horizontal plane tangential to the highest point of the hemisphere.
tentorial a. the angle between the basicranial axis and the plane of the tentorium.
tooth a's the angles formed by the junction of two or more surfaces of a tooth, named according to the surfaces participating in their formation (see illustration).
Topinard a. ophryospinal a.
torsion a., a. of torsion the angle between the axes of any two different portions of long bones, such as between the head and neck of the femur and its long axis.
tuber a. the angle formed by junction of two lines, one parallel with the superior surface of the tuber calcanei and the other joining the anterior and posterior articular facets; normally about 30 degrees.
urethrovesical a. an angle formed by junction of the bladder wall and the urethra; analysis of such angles was formerly considered to be a way of gauging the risk for stress incontinence. Called also *vesicourethral a.*
venous a. the angle formed by junction of the internal jugular and subclavian veins; called also *Pirogoff a.*
vertical a. in dental radiology, the angle measured within a vertical plane, at which the central ray of the useful beam is projected relative to a horizontal plane of reference.
vesicourethral a. urethrovesical a.
a. of Virchow the angle between the nasobasilar line and the nasosubnasal line.
visual a. the angle formed between two lines extending from the nodal point of the eye to the extremities of the object seen; called also *optic a.*
Vogt a. the angle between the nasobasilar and alveolonasal lines.
Weisbach a. the angle at the alveolar point between lines passing from the basion and from the middle of the frontonasal suture.
Welcker a. angulus sphenoidalis ossis parietalis.
xiphoid a's the angles formed by the borders of the xiphoid notch.
Y a. the angle between the radius fixus and a line joining the lambda and the inion.

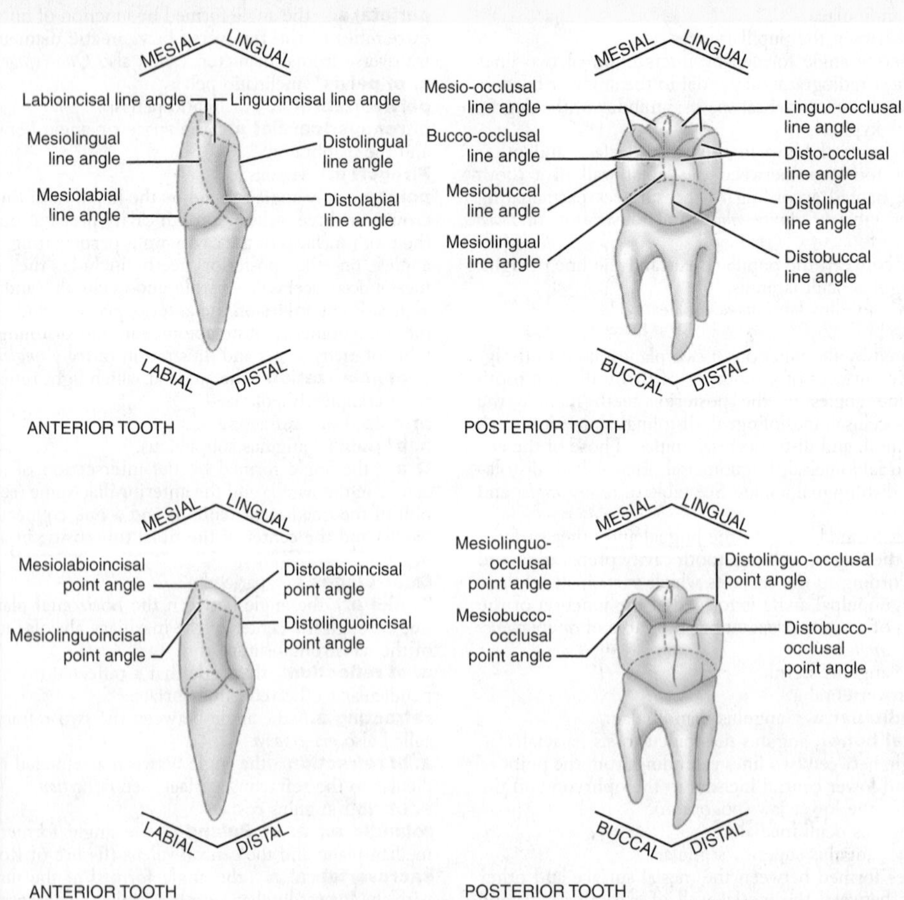

■ Tooth angles: *Top,* line angles; *Bottom,* point angles.

an•gor (ang′gor) [L. "a strangling"] angina.

a. a′nimi a feeling of life slipping away and impending death.

a. ocula′ris a condition marked by fear of imminent blindness and by sudden attacks of mist before the eyes, possibly due to angiospasm of ocular vessels.

a. pec′toris angina pectoris.

Ång•ström's law, unit (ang′strəmz) [Anders Jonas *Ångström*, Swedish physicist, 1814–1874] see under *law*, and see *angstrom*.

ang•strom (Å) (ang′strəm) a unit of length used for atomic dimensions and light wavelengths; it is defined in terms of the wavelength of the red line of cadmium but is nominally equivalent to 10^{-10} meter. Called also *Angström unit*.

An•guil•lu•la (ang-gwil′u-lə) [L. "little eel"] a genus of nematode parasites, many species of which have been reassigned to other genera.

A. ace′ti *Turbatrix aceti*.

A. intestina′lis, **A. stercora′lis** *Strongyloides stercoralis*.

An•guil•lu•li•na pu•tre•fa•ci•ens (ang-gwil″u-li′nə pu″trə-fa′she-ənz) *Ditylenchus dipsaci*.

an•gu•lar (ang′gu-lər) [L. *angularis*] sharply bent; having corners or angles.

an•gu•la•tion (ang″gu-la′shən) [L. *angulatus* bent] 1. formation of a sharp obstructive angle, as in the intestine, the ureter, or similar tubes. 2. deviation from a straight line, as in a poorly set bone.

an•gu•li (ang′gu-li) [L.] genitive and plural of *angulus*.

an•gu•lus (ang′gu-ləs) gen. and pl. *an′guli* [L.] angle; used for a triangular area or the angle of a particular structure or part of the body.

a. acro′mii [TA] acromial angle: the easily palpable subcutaneous bony point where the lateral border of the acromion becomes continuous with the spine of the scapula.

a. cos′tae [TA] costal angle: a prominent line on the external surface of a rib, slightly anterior to the tubercle, where the rib is bent in two directions and at the same time twisted on its long axis; called also *angle of rib*.

a. fronta′lis os′sis parieta′lis [TA] frontal angle of parietal bone: the anterosuperior angle of the parietal bone, which is membranous at birth and forms part of the anterior fontanelle; called also *anterior superior angle of parietal bone* and *coronary angle*.

a. infe′rior sca′pulae [TA] inferior angle of scapula: the angle formed by the junction of the medial and lateral borders of the scapula.

a. infrasterna′lis [TA] infrasternal angle of thorax: the angle on the anteroinferior surface of the thorax, the apex of which is the sternoxiphoid junction, and the sides of which are the seventh, eighth, and ninth costal cartilages; it partially delimits two sides of the triangular epigastric region on the ventral body surface; called also *subcostal* or *substernal angle*.

a. i′ridis, a. iridocornea′lis [TA] iridocorneal angle: a narrow recess between the sclerocorneal junction and the attached margin of the iris, marking the periphery of the anterior chamber of the eye; it is the principal exit site for the aqueous humor. Called also *filtration angle*, *iridial angle*, and *angle of iris*.

a. latera′lis sca′pulae [TA] lateral angle of scapula: the head of the scapula, which bears the glenoid cavity and articulates with the head of the humerus; called also *acromial* or *external angle of scapula* and *condyle of scapula*.

a. mandi′bulae [TA] angle of mandible: the angle created at the junction of the posterior edge of the ramus and the lower edge of the mandible; called also *angle of jaw*, *gonial angle*, and *mandibular angle*.

a. mastoi′deus os′sis parieta′lis [TA] mastoid angle of parietal bone: the posteroinferior angle of the parietal bone, which articulates with the posterior part of the temporal bone and the occipital bone; called also *posterior inferior angle of parietal bone*.

a. occipita′lis os′sis parieta′lis [TA] occipital angle of parietal bone: the posterosuperior angle of the parietal bone, which during fetal life participates in the formation of the posterior fontanelle; called also *posterior superior angle of parietal bone*.

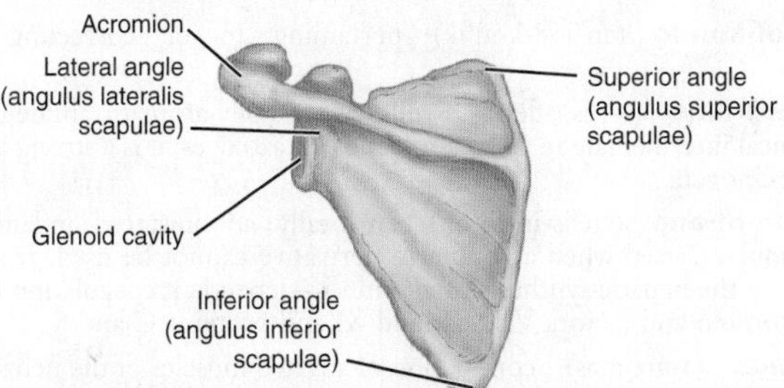

■ Scapula, showing the lateral, superior, and inferior angles.

a. o′culi latera′lis [TA] lateral angle of eye: the angle formed by the lateral junction of the superior and inferior eyelids.

a. o′culi media′lis [TA] medial angle of eye: the angle formed by the medial junction of the superior and inferior eyelids.

a. o′ris [TA] angle of mouth: the angle formed at either side of the mouth by the junction of the upper and the lower lip.

a. sphenoida′lis os′sis parieta′lis [TA] sphenoid angle of parietal bone: the anteroinferior angle of the parietal bone, which articulates with the greater wing of the sphenoid bone and the frontal bone; called also *anterior inferior angle of parietal bone* and *Welcker angle*.

a. ster′ni [TA] sternal angle: the angle formed on the anterior surface of the sternum at the junction of its body and manubrium; called also *Louis* or *Ludwig angle*.

a. subpu′bicus [TA] subpubic angle: the apex of the pubic arch; the angle formed at the point of meeting of the conjoined rami of the ischial and pubic bones of the two sides of the body. Called also *subpubic arch* and *arch of pelvis*.

a. supe′rior sca′pulae [TA] superior angle of scapula: the angle made by the superior and medial borders of the scapula.

an•hal•o•nine (an″hə-lo′nēn) a crystalline alkaloid from *Lophophora williamsii*, with the pharmacologic properties of mescaline.

An•ha•lo•ni•um le•win•ii (an-″hə-lo′ne-əm loo-win′e-e) *Lophophora williamsii*.

an•ha•phia (an-ha′fe-ə) anaphia.

an•he•do•nia (an″he-do′ne-ə) [*an*[1] + Gr. *hēdonē* pleasure + *-ia*] total loss of feeling of pleasure in acts that normally give pleasure.

an•hi•dro•sis (an″hĭ-dro′sis, an″hi-dro′sis) [*an-*[1] + *hidr-* + *-osis*] 1. absence or severe deficiency of sweating, usually due to absence or paralysis of the sweat glands or to obstruction of the sweat ducts. See also *hypohidrosis*. 2. a condition in horses where they cannot sweat; in hot climates they may develop severe dyspnea and inability to work. Called also *dry coat* and *puff disease*. Defs. 1 and 2 called also *anidrosis* and *hidroschesis*.

thermogenic a. tropical anhidrotic asthenia.

an•hi•drot•ic (an″hĭ-drot′ik) 1. pertaining to or characterized by anhidrosis. 2. antiperspirant.

an•hy•drase (an-hi′drās) an older, common term used in naming some enzymes of the hydro-lyase (q.v.) sub-subclass.

an•hy•dre•mia (an″hi-dre′me-ə) [*an-*[1] + *hydremia*] deficiency of water in the blood. See also *dehydration* and *hypovolemia*.

an•hy•dride (an-hi′drīd) [*an-*[1] + *hydride*] a chemical compound derived from a substance, especially an acid, by the abstraction of a molecule of water. The anhydrides of bases are oxides; those of alcohols are ethers.

acetic a. a colorless mobile liquid of a pungent acetic odor, the anhydride of acetic acid.

acid a. an anhydride formed by dehydration of an acid or one that forms an acid upon hydration; if bimolecular, it can be composed of two molecules of the same acid (e.g., acetic anhydride or pyrophosphate), or it can be a mixed anhydride.

arsenous a. arsenic trioxide.

chromic a. chromic acid.

mixed a. an acid anhydride composed of two different acids, e.g., adenosine triphosphate or an aminoacyl adenylate.

perosmic a. osmium tetroxide.

phthalic a. a reactive, low-molecular-weight compound with a wide variety of industrial uses, including the manufacture of dyes, pharmaceuticals, and insecticides, and as a hardener for resins. It is an allergen that causes skin irritation, and if its fumes are inhaled it can cause *epoxy resin lung*, a form of hypersensitivity pneumonitis.

silicic a. silica.

sorbitol a. sorbitan.

sulfurous a. sulfur dioxide.

trimellitic a. (TMA) a low-molecular-weight reactive chemical used in the manufacture of plastics, epoxy resin, coatings, and paints; inhalation of its dust or fumes produces a variety of respiratory symptoms. See under *flu* and *pneumonitis*.

anhydr(o)- [Gr. *anydros* waterless, from *an-*[1] + *hydōr* water] deprived of water; anhydrous.

an•hy•dro•chlo•ric (an″hi-dro-klor′ik) achlorhydric.

an•hy•dro•sug•ar (an-hi″dro-shoog′ər) a sugar from which one or more molecules of water have been removed, resulting in the formation of an internal acetal structure.

an•hy•drous (an-hi′drəs) [Gr. *anydros* waterless, from *an-*[1] + *hydōr* water] 1. deprived of water. 2. of an inorganic compound, not containing water, either in the form of water of crystallization or as water adsorbed to the surface.

ani•a•cin•am•i•do•sis (ə-ni-ə-sin-am″ĭ-do′sis) any disorder due to niacinamide deficiency; see *pellagra*.

ani•a•ci•no•sis (ə-ni″ə-sĭ-no′sis) pellagra.

Anich•kov (Anitsch•kow) cell (myocyte) (ah-nich′kof) [Nikolai Nikolaevich *Anichkov* (or *Anitschkow*), Russian pathologist, 1885–1964] see under *cell.*

an•ic•ter•ic (an″ik-ter′ik) not associated with jaundice.

anid•e•us (ə-nid′e-əs) [*an-*[1] + *idea*] holoacardius amorphus. **anid′ean** *adj*
embryonic a. a blastoderm in which no embryonic axis develops.

an•idro•sis (an″ĭ-dro′sis) anhidrosis.

an•idrot•ic (an″ĭ-drot′ik) 1. anhidrotic (def. 1). 2. antiperspirant.

a•nid•u•la•fun•gin (ə-nid″u-lə-fun′jin) an antifungal antibiotic of the echinofungin class, used primarily in treatment of *Candida* infections; administered by intravenous injection.

an•ile (a′nīl) [L. *anus* old woman] 1. like an old woman. 2. senile; in one's dotage.

an•i•ler•i•dine (an″ĭ-ler′ĭ-dēn) [USP] a synthetic opioid analgesic used for the relief of moderate to severe pain, as premedication for general anesthesia, as a postoperative sedative, and as an obstetric analgesic; administered intramuscularly, subcutaneously, or intravenously. Abuse of this drug may lead to dependence.
a. hydrochloride [USP] the hydrochloride salt of anileridine; administered orally in the treatment of moderate to severe pain.

an•i•lid (an′ĭ-lid) anilide.

an•i•lide (an′ĭ-līd) any compound formed from aromatic amines by substitution of an acyl group for the hydrogen of NH_2.

an•i•line (an′ĭ-lin) [Ar. *an-nil* indigo plant] a colorless oily liquid arylamine derived from coal tar or indigo, made commercially by reducing nitrobenzene. It is slightly soluble in water and freely so in ether and alcohol. Combined with other substances, especially chlorine and the chlorates, it forms the aniline colors or dyes. It is an important cause of serious industrial poisoning *(anilinism)*, and high doses or long exposure may be carcinogenic. Called also *amidobenzene* and *aminobenzene*.

ani•lin•gus (a″nĭ-ling′gəs) [L. *anus*, q.v. + *lingere* to lick] sexual stimulation of the anus with the lips or tongue.

an•i•lin•ism (an′ĭ-lin-iz-əm) a condition produced by exposure to aniline, and marked by methemoglobinemia and aplastic anemia, vertigo, muscular weakness, cyanosis, and digestive derangement.

an•i•lism (an′ĭ-liz-əm) anilinism.

anil•i•ty (ə-nil′ĭ-te) [L. *anus* old woman] 1. the state of existing as or like an old woman. 2. senility; dotage.

an•i•ma (an′ĭ-mə) [L., the animating spirit present in any animal] 1. the soul. 2. in jungian psychology, the soul or inner being of a person, as opposed to the *persona*, the social role or facade presented to the world; because the inner and outer facades are often opposing, Jung also used the term to refer to the feminine aspect of a man's soul, the analogous masculine aspect of a woman's soul being termed the *animus*.

an•i•mal (an′ĭ-məl) [L. *animalis*, from *anima* life, breath] 1. a living organism having sensation and the power of voluntary movement and requiring for its existence oxygen and organic food; animals constitute one of the five kingdoms of living organisms. 2. pertaining to such an organism. 3. any animal organism other than a human being.
control a. see *control* (def. 2).
conventional a. an experimental animal that has not been reared under gnotobiotic conditions.
decerebrate a. an experimental animal that has been subjected to decerebration; such an animal exhibits rigid extension of the lower limbs, with strong tonic contraction of the extensor muscles and to some extent the flexor muscles. See also *decerebrate*, and see *decerebrate rigidity*, under *rigidity*.
experimental a. an animal which is used as a subject of experimental procedures in the laboratory.
Houssay a. an experimental animal deprived of both pituitary gland and pancreas; see *Houssay phenomenon*, under *phenomenon*.
hyperphagic a. an experimental animal in which the cells of the ventromedial nucleus of the hypothalamus have been destroyed, abolishing its awareness of the point at which it should stop eating; excessive eating and savageness characterize such an animal.
Long-Lukens a. an experimental animal deprived of the pancreas and adrenal glands.
spinal a. an animal whose spinal cord has been severed, thus cutting off communication with the brain.
thalamic a. an animal in which the brainstem has been transected just above the thalamus.

an•i•ma•tion (an″ĭ-ma′shən) 1. the state of being alive. 2. liveliness of spirits.
suspended a. a temporary state of apparent death.

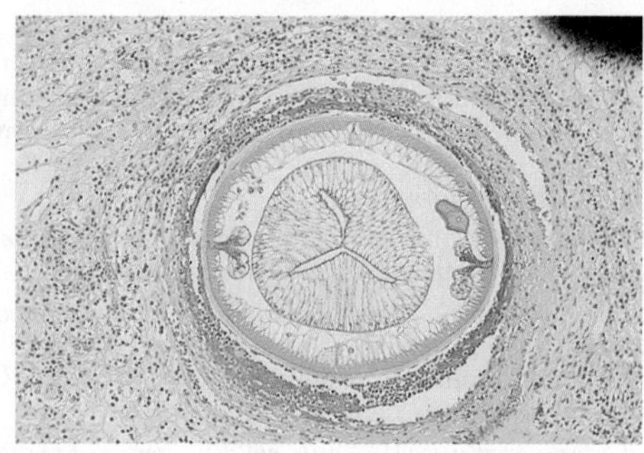

■ Cross-section of *Anisakis* larva found in small bowel following surgery for acute obstruction (H & E stain).

an•i•mism (an′ĭ-miz-əm) [L. *anima* soul] the belief that nonliving objects and phenomena (such as clouds) are inhabited and motivated by a nonphysical agent; it is a characteristic of the thinking of early childhood.

an•i•mus (an′ĭ-məs) [L., the rational part of the mind; intellect or motivations] 1. disposition. 2. ill will or hostility; animosity. 3. in jungian psychology, the masculine aspect of a woman's soul or inner being; see *anima*.

an•ion (an′i-on) [*ana-* + *ion*] an ion carrying a negative charge owing to a surplus of electrons; in an electrolytic cell anions migrate toward the anode, the positively charged electrode.

an•ion•ic (an″i-on′ik) pertaining to or containing an anion.

an•ion•ot•ro•py (an″e-on-ot′rə-pe) [*anion* + Gr. *tropos* a turning] a type of tautomerism in which the migrating group is a negative ion rather than the more usual hydrogen ion. Cf. *prototropy*.

an•irid•ia (an″ĭ-rid′e-ə) [*an-*[1] + *irid-* + *-ia*] absence of the iris; a usually bilateral, hereditary anomaly that is rarely complete, a rudimentary stump usually being visible on gonioscopy.

an•i•sa•ki•a•sis (an″ĭ-sə-ki′ə-sis) infection with a nematode of the family Anisakidae. Human infection is usually caused by third-stage larvae of the genera *Anisakis* and *Pseudoterranova*, which are eaten in undercooked infected marine fish (e.g., herring); the larvae then burrow into the stomach wall, producing an eosinophilic granulomatous mass. Called also *eosinophilic granuloma*.

An•i•sa•ki•dae (an″ĭ-sak′ĭ-de) a family of nematodes, many of which cause anisakiasis when raw fish are eaten. Genera include *Anisakis* and *Pseudoterranova*.

an•i•sa•ki•do•sis (an″ĭ-sak″ĭ-do′sis) anisakiasis.

An•i•sa•kis (an″ĭ-sa′kis) [Gr. *an-* + *is-* + *akis* point] a genus of nematodes of the family Anisakidae; the usual infecting species is *A. mari′na.* It parasitizes the stomachs of marine mammals and birds, where it reaches the adult stage. Infective third-stage larvae occur in various marine fishes, and humans who eat raw fish may get anisakiasis.

an•ise (an′is) [L. *anisum*] 1. *Pimpinella anisum.* 2. the fruit of *P. anisum;* a source of anise oil. It is also used for dyspepsia and as an expectorant and in homeopathy for the treatment of shoulder pain and lumbago. 3. any of several other similar fruits.
Chinese a. star a.
Japanese star a. 1. *Illicium religiosum.* 2. the poisonous fruit of *I. religiosum.*
star a. 1. *Illicium verum.* 2. the dried ripe fruit of *I. verum;* a source of anise oil. It is also used for loss of appetite and for cough and bronchitis; in ayurveda, it is used to treat a wide variety of conditions.

an•is•ei•ko•nia (an″is-i-ko′ne-ə) [*anis-* + Gr. *eikōn* image + *-ia*] a condition in which the ocular image of an object as seen by one eye differs in size and shape from that seen by the other.

an•is•ei•kon•ic (an″is-i-kon′ik) pertaining to or correcting aniseikonia.

o-an•is•i•dine (ə-nis′ĭ-dēn) a yellow to red oily aromatic amine used as a chemical intermediate in the manufacture of azo dyes; it is a strong irritant and carcinogen.

an•is•in•di•one (an″is-in-di′ōn) an orally administered indanedione anticoagulant, used when a coumarin derivative cannot be used. It acts by inhibiting the hepatic synthesis of vitamin K–dependent coagulation factors (prothrombin and factors VII, IX, and X) and proteins C and S.

anis•mus (ə-niz′məs) contraction of striated muscles of the pelvic floor instead of the normal relaxation when a person strains to defecate; the result is constipation. Called also *pelvic floor dyssynergia*.

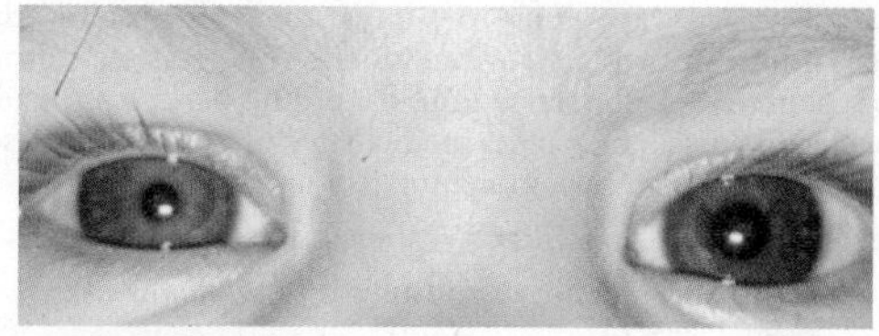
■ Anisocoria; iris heterochromia is also present.

anis(o)- [Gr. *anisos* unequal, uneven] a combining form meaning unequal or dissimilar.

an•iso•ac•com•mo•da•tion (an-i″so-ə-kom″ə-da′shən) a difference in the accommodative capacity of the two eyes.

an•iso•chro•ma•sia (an-ī″so-kro-ma′zhə) [*aniso-* + Gr. *chrōma* color] a condition in which only the peripheral zone of an erythrocyte is colored; seen in some forms of anemia. Called also *anisochromia.*

an•iso•chro•mat•ic (an-i″so-kro-mat′ik) [*aniso-* + *chromatic* color] 1. not of the same color throughout. 2. pertaining to solutions used for testing color blindness, containing two pigments which are distinguished by both the normal and the color blind eye. Cf. *pseudoisochromatic.*

an•iso•chro•mia (an″i-so-kro′me-ə) [*aniso-* + *chrom-* + *-ia*] anisochromasia.

an•iso•co•ria (an-i″so-kor′e-ə) [*aniso-* + *cor-* + *-ia*] inequality in diameter of the pupils.

an•iso•cy•to•sis (an-i″so-si-to′sis) [*aniso-* + *cyt-* + *-osis*] presence in the blood of erythrocytes with excessive variation in size; see also *macrocythemia* and *microcythemia.* Called also *anisopoikilocytosis.*

an•iso•dac•ty•lous (an-i″so-dak′tə-ləs) [*aniso-* + *dactylo-* + *-ous*] having corresponding digits of unequal length.

an•iso•dac•ty•ly (an-i″so-dak′tə-le) a condition characterized by having corresponding digits of unequal length.

an•iso•di•a•met•ric (an-i″so-di″ə-met′rik) characterized by different dimensions in different diameters.

an•iso•dont (an-i′so-dont) [*anis-* + Gr. *odous* tooth] 1. one who has unequal, asymmetric teeth. 2. an animal having irregular, asymmetric teeth, as in certain reptiles.

an•iso•gam•ete (an-i″so-gam′ēt) a gamete of different size and structure from the one with which it unites. See *macrogamete* and *microgamete.*

an•iso•ga•met•ic (an-i″so-gə-met′ik) characterized by the production of gametes of different size and structure.

an•isog•a•mous (an″i-sog′ə-məs) having conjugating elements (gametes) that differ in size or structure.

an•isog•a•my (an″i-sog′ə-me) [*aniso-* + Gr. *gamos* marriage] in the most restrictive sense, fertilization of a large motile female gamete by a small motile male gamete; the term is often used more generally to mean the sexual union of two dissimilar gametes (heterogamy), particularly in lower organisms.

an•iso•ico•nia (an-i″so-i-ko′ne-ə) aniseikonia.

an•iso•kary•o•sis (an-i″so-kar″e-o′sis) [*aniso-* + *kary-* + *-osis*] inequality in the size of the nuclei of cells.

An•iso•lo•bis (an-i″so-lo′bis) a genus of beetles, the earwigs. Nymphs and adults of *A. euborel′lia* (Lucas) are intermediate hosts of helminth parasites.

an•iso•mas•tia (an-i″so-mas′te-ə) [*aniso-* + *mast-* + *-ia*] inequality in the size of the breasts.

an•iso•me•lia (an-i″so-me′le-ə) [*aniso-* + *-melia*] inequality between paired limbs.

an•iso•mer•ic (an-i″so-mer′ik) not isomeric.

an•iso•met•rope (an-i″so-met′rōp) a person with anisometropia.

an•iso•me•tro•pia (an-i″so-mə-tro′pe-ə) [*an-* + Gr. *isometros* of equal measure + *-opia*] an error of refraction in which a person's two eyes have different refractive powers. **anisometrop′ic** *adj*

an•iso•me•tro•pic (an-i″so-mĕ-tro′pik) pertaining to or characterized by anisometropia.

An•iso•mor•pha (an-i″so-mor′fə) a genus of insects.

*A. bupr**estoi′des*** the walking stick; a species of orthopterous insects capable of discharging an irritating fluid.

an•iso•pho•ria (an″i-so-for′e-ə) [*aniso-* + *phoria*] a condition in which the balance of the vertical muscles of one eye differs from that of the other eye, so that the visual lines do not lie in the same horizontal plane.

an•iso•pia (an″i-so′pe-ə) [*aniso-* + *-opia*] inequality of vision in the two eyes.

an•iso•pi•esis (an-i″so-pi-e′sis) [*aniso-* + *-piesis*] variation or inequality in the blood pressure as registered in different parts of the body.

an•iso•poi•ki•lo•cy•to•sis (an-i″so-poi″kĭ-lo-si-to′sis) presence in the blood of erythrocytes of abnormal sizes and shapes; anisocytosis with poikilocytosis.

an•i•sos•mot•ic (an″i-soz-mot′ik) not having the same osmotic pressure or not containing the same effective concentration of osmotically active components.

an•iso•spore (an-i′so-spor″) [*aniso-* + *spore*] 1. a sexual spore, the male and female differing in size or shape. 2. an asexual spore produced by a heterosporous organism. See *isospore.*

an•isos•po•rous (an″ĭ-sos′pə-rəs) having anisospores.

an•isos•then•ic (an-i″sos-then′ik) [*aniso-* + *sthenic*] not having equal strength; said of paired muscles.

an•iso•ton•ic (an-i″so-ton′ik) 1. showing a variation in tonicity or tension. 2. having an osmotic pressure differing from that of a solution with which it is compared.

an•isot•ro•pal (an″i-sot′ro-pəl) anisotropic.

an•iso•tro•pic (an-i″so-tro′pik) [*aniso-* + *tropic*] 1. having unlike properties in different directions, as in any unit lacking spherical symmetry. 2. doubly refracting or having a double polarizing power.

an•i•so•tro•pine meth•yl•bro•mide (an-i″so-tro′pēn) an orally administered anticholinergic that produces relaxation of visceral smooth muscle and has been used as an adjunct in the treatment of peptic ulcer.

an•isot•ro•py (an″i-sot′rə-pe) the quality or condition of being anisotropic.

an•is•trep•lase (an-is-trep′lās) a thrombolytic agent, primarily used to clear coronary vessel occlusions associated with myocardial infarction; administered intravenously.

an•i•su•ria (an″i-su′re-ə) [*anis-* + *-uria*] a condition marked by alternating oliguria and polyuria.

ani•tis (a-ni′tis) anusitis.

ani•trog•e•nous (a″ni-troj′ə-nəs) not nitrogenous.

Anitsch•kow see *Anichkov.*

an•kle (ang′kəl) [A.S. *anclēow*] 1. tarsus (def. 1). 2. by extension, the joint between the leg and foot (articulatio talocruralis), or the region of the leg and foot including and immediately adjacent to this joint. 3. hock.

tailor's a. an abnormal bursa over the lower end of the fibula in tailors, from pressure caused by sitting on the floor with the legs crossed in front.

ankyl(o)- [Gr. *ankylos* bent or crooked] a combining form meaning bent, or denoting fusion or adhesion.

an•ky•lo•bleph•a•ron (ang″kə-lo-blef′ə-ron) [*ankylo-* + Gr. *blepharon* eyelid] the adhesion of the ciliary edges of the eyelid to each other.

a. filifor′me adna′tum congenital adhesion of the margins of the upper and lower lids by filamentous bands.

an•ky•lo•chei•lia (ang″kə-lo-ki′le-ə) [*ankylo-* + *cheilo-* + *-ia*] adhesion of the lips to each other.

an•ky•lo•col•pos (ang-kə-lo-kol′pos) [*ankylo-* + Gr. *kolpos* vagina] atresia or imperforation of the vagina.

an•ky•lo•dac•ty•ly (ang″kə-lo-dak′tə-le) [*ankylo-* + Gr. *daktylos* finger] fusion or adhesion of fingers or toes to one another. Cf. *syndactyly.*

an•ky•lo•glos•sia (ang″kə-lo-glos′e-ə) [*ankylo-* + *glossa* + *-ia*] restricted movement of the tongue, resulting in speech difficulty. Called also *adherent tongue, lingua frenata,* and *tongue-tie.* See also *complete a.* and *partial a.*

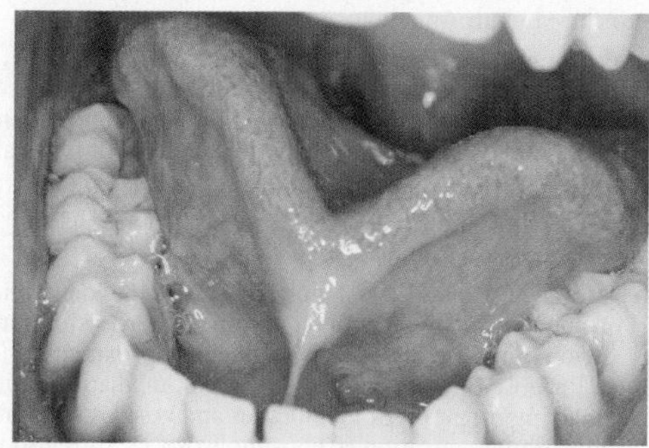
■ Ankyloglossia.

complete a. ankyloglossia resulting from fusion between the tongue and the floor of the mouth.

partial a. ankyloglossia resulting from a short lingual frenum or one which is attached too near the tip of the tongue.

a. supe′rior an unusual association of an extensive adhesion of the tongue to the palate, sometimes with deformities of the extremities.

an•ky•lo•poi•et•ic (ang″kə-lo-poi-et′ik) [*ankylo-* + Gr. *poiein* to make] producing or characterized by ankylosis.

An•ky•lo•pro•glypha (ang″kə-lo-pro-glif′ə) Proteroglypha.

an•ky•losed (ang′kə-lōzd) fused or obliterated, as a joint.

an•ky•lo•ses (ang″kə-lo′sēz) plural of *ankylosis.*

an•ky•lo•sis (ang″kə-lo′sis) pl. *ankylo′ses* [Gr. *ankylōsis*] immobility and consolidation of a joint due to disease, injury, or surgical procedure.

artificial a. arthrodesis.

bony a. the union of the bones of a joint by proliferation of bone cells, resulting in complete immobility; called also *true a.*

cricoarytenoid joint a. fixation of the cricoarytenoid joint due to inflammation; characterized by hoarseness, cough, and difficulty in expectoration.

extracapsular a. ankylosis due to rigidity of structures exterior to the joint capsule.

false a. fibrous a.

fibrous a. reduced mobility of a joint due to proliferation of fibrous tissue; called also *false a.* and *spurious a.*

intracapsular a. obliteration of joint motion due to disease, injury, or surgical procedure within the joint capsule.

spurious a. fibrous a.

stapedial a. fixation of the footplate of the stapes in otosclerosis, causing a conductive hearing loss.

true a. bony a.

An•ky•los•to•ma (ang″kə-los′to-mə) *Ancylostoma.*

an•ky•lo•sto•mi•a•sis (ang″kə-lo-sto-mi′ə-sis) ancylostomiasis.

an•ky•lot•ic (ang″kə-lot′ik) pertaining to or marked by ankylosis.

an•ky•lot•o•my (ang″kə-lot′ə-me) [*ankylo-* + *-tomy*] frenotomy for relieving ankyloglossia.

an•ky•rin (ang′kə-rin) a membrane protein of erythrocytes and brain that anchors spectrin to the plasma membrane at the sites of anion channels. Defects of ankyrin lead to elliptocytosis, spherocytosis, and pyropoikilocytosis.

an•ky•roid (ang′kĭ-roid) ancyroid.

an•lage (ahn-lah′gə, an′lāj) pl. *anla′gen* [Ger. "a laying on"] primordium.

AN-MAA trademark for a kit for the preparation of technetium Tc 99m albumin aggregated.

AN-MDP trademark for a kit for the preparation of technetium Tc 99m medronate.

ANNA-1 type 1 antineuronal antibody; see *anti-Hu antibody,* under *antibody.*

ANNA-2 type 2 antineuronal antibody; see *anti-Ri antibody,* under *antibody.*

an•neal (ə-nēl′) 1. to heat a material, such as glass or metal, followed by controlled cooling to remove internal stresses and induce a desired degree of toughness, temper, or softness of the material. 2. to homogenize an amalgam alloy ingot by heating it in an oven. 3. to degas; see *degassing* (def. 2). 4. in molecular biology, to cause the association or reassociation of single-stranded nucleic acids so that double-stranded molecules are formed, often by heating followed by cooling.

an•nec•tent (ə-nek′tənt) [L. *annectens*] connecting or joining; spelled also *annectant.*

an•ne•lid (an′ə-lid) 1. any member of the phylum Annelida. 2. of or pertaining to the phylum Annelida.

An•ne•li•da (ə-nel′ĭ-də) [Fr. *anneler* to arrange in rings, from L. *anellus* a little ring] a phylum of metazoan invertebrates comprising the segmented worms, and including marine annelids, freshwater annelids and earthworms, and leeches (class Hirudinea); only the latter are of medical interest.

an•nel•lide (an′ə-līd) a type of conidiogenous cell formed in blastic conidiogenesis, having multiple ringlike scars around its tip resulting from release of successive conidia.

an•nex•in (ə-nek′sin) any of a family of Ca^{2+}-dependent phospholipid-binding proteins, which share a common primary structure in the C-terminal region, four or eight repeats of an approximately 70 amino acid sequence. Proposed functions include roles in mediation of intracellular calcium signals, aggregation of membranes and vesicles, and ion channel formation. Some inhibit activation of phospholipase A_2, thus also inhibiting synthesis of prostaglandins and other arachidonic acid derivatives.

An•no•na (ə-no′nə) a genus of trees and shrubs of the family Annonaceae, found in tropical regions of the Americas. *A. murica′ta* L. is the soursop, source of a popular edible fruit. The bark, fruit, and leaves of various species are used in native medicine, and the seeds of some have emetic properties and are poisonous for fish and insects.

an•nu•lar (an′u-lər) [L. *annularis*] shaped like a ring. See also *circular.*

an•nu•li (an′u-li) [L.] genitive and plural of *annulus.*

an•nu•lo•aor•tic (an″u-lo-a-or′tĭk) [*annulus* + *aortic*] pertaining to the aorta and the fibrous ring of the heart at the aortic orifice.

an•nu•lo•plas•ty (an′u-lo-plas″te) [*annulus* + *-plasty*] plastic repair of a cardiac valve by shortening the circumference of its annulus. **annulo-plas′tic** *adj*

DeVega a. a method for repair of an incompetent tricuspid valve by placing a series of purse-string sutures around the valve annulus to reduce it to the size of the obturator.

Kay a. a method for repairing a tricuspid valve with a dilated annulus but little prolapse: by placing several sutures at the commissures, the posterior leaflet is drawn forward toward the anterior cusp and their surface area of approximation is increased.

an•nu•lor•rha•phy (an″u-lor′ə-fe) [*annulus* + *-rrhaphy*] closure of a hernial ring or defect by sutures.

an•nu•lus (an′u-ləs) gen. and pl. *an′nuli* [L., from *anus* ring] a ring or ringlike structure; in official anatomical terminology, spelled *anulus* [TA], q.v. for terms not found here.

a. cilia′ris orbiculus ciliaris.

a. ova′lis limbus fossae ovalis.

an′nuli tra′cheae cartilagines tracheales.

Vieussens a. 1. limbus fossae ovalis. 2. ansa subclavia.

Ano•cen•tor (a″no-sen′tər) a genus of ticks of the family Ixodidae.

A. ni′tens a yellow-brown species usually found on horses in the West Indies and the southern United States; it transmits *Babesia caballi,* an etiologic agent of equine babesiosis. Called also *Dermacentor nitens.*

ano•chro•ma•sia (an″o-kro-ma′zhə) 1. absence of the usual staining reaction from a tissue or cell. 2. a condition in which the erythrocytes show a piling up of hemoglobin at the periphery so that the center is pale.

ano•ci•as•so•ci•a•tion (ə-no″se-ə-so″se-a′shən) [*a-*[1] + L. *nocere* to injure + *association*] the blunting of harmful association impulses; a method of anesthesia designed to minimize the effect of surgical shock.

ano•ci•ated (ə-no′se-āt″əd) in a condition of anociassociation.

ano•ci•a•tion (ə-no″se-a′shən) anociassociation.

ano•coc•cy•ge•al (a″no-kok-sij′e-əl) pertaining to the anus and coccyx.

an•ode (an′ōd) [Gr. *ana-* up + *hodos* way] 1. in an electrochemical cell, the electrode at which oxidation occurs, i.e., the positive electrode in an electrolytic cell or a storage battery. It is the negative electrode in a voltaic cell that is delivering current. 2. the positive electrode of devices such as electron tubes, x-ray tubes, and electrophoresis cells. Symbol A. Cf. *cathode.* **ano′dal** *adj*

hooded a. in radiology, an anode incorporating a copper shield to overcome problems of secondary ray emission.

rotating a. in radiology, an anode in the form of a disk with the target material annealed to its rim; the anode is continuously rotated so that the electron stream strikes only a small part of the target at one time, thus allowing heat dissipation.

ano•derm (a′no-dərm) the epithelial lining of the anal canal.

an•od•mia (an-od′me-ə) [*an-*[1] + Gr. *odmē* smell + *-ia*] anosmia.

an•odon•tia (an″o-don′shə) [*an-*[1] + *odont-* + *-ia*] congenital absence of the teeth; it may involve all *(total a.)* or only some of the teeth *(partial a., hypodontia),* and both the deciduous and the permanent dentition, or only teeth of the permanent dentition. See also *Kennedy classification* and *Skinner classification,* under *classification.* Called also *anodontism* and *edentia.*

partial a. hypodontia.

total a. a rare condition characterized by congenital absence of all teeth, both deciduous and permanent.

true a., a. ve′ra total or partial (hypodontia) congenital absence of the teeth.

an•odon•tism (an″o-don′tiz-əm) anodontia.

an•o•dyne (an′o-dīn) [*an-*[1] + Gr. *odynē* pain] 1. relieving pain. 2. a medicine that relieves pain; the anodynes include opium, morphine, codeine, aspirin, and others.

Ano•geis•sus (a″no-ji′səs) a genus of trees of the family Combretaceae, found in southern Asia. *A. latifo′lia* is the source of ghatti gum.

an•oi•kis (an-oi′kis) [Gr. *anoikos* homeless] apoptosis triggered by separation from the extracellular matrix.

p-anol (a′nol) an intermediate in the production of estrogens; it is readily polymerized to form active carcinogenic and estrogenic substances.

Ano•lor (an′o-lor) trademark for a combination preparation of butalbital, acetaminophen, and caffeine.

anom•a•lad (ə-nom′ə-lad) sequence (def. 2).

 amniotic band a. see under *syndrome.*

anomal(o)- [Gr. *anōmalos* irregular] a combining form meaning irregular or uneven.

anom•a•lo•scope (ə-nom′ə-lo-skōp″) [*anomalo-* + *-scope*] an instrument used in testing for anomalies of color vision by having the subject match mixed spectral lines.

anom•al•ot•ro•phy (ə-nom″əl-ot′ro-fe) [*anomalo-* + *-trophy*] abnormality of nutrition.

anom•a•lous (ə-nom′ə-ləs) [Gr. *anōmalos*] irregular; marked by deviation from the natural order. Applied particularly to congenital and hereditary defects.

anom•a•ly (ə-nom′ə-le) [Gr. *anōmalia*] marked deviation from the normal standard, especially as a result of congenital defects.

 acquired Pelger-Huët a. pseudo–Pelger-Huët a.

 Alder a., Alder constitutional granulation a., Alder-Reilly a. an autosomal dominant condition in which leukocytes of the myelocytic series, and sometimes all leukocytes, contain coarse azurophil granules called *Alder-Reilly bodies;* it is usually clinically unimportant but is sometimes associated with Hurler syndrome or other pathological conditions.

 Aristotle a. if the first and second fingers are crossed and a pencil is placed between them, the person feels two pencils.

 Axenfeld a. a developmental anomaly consisting of posterior embryotoxon and iris processes to the Schwalbe ring. Called also *arcus juvenilis* and *posterior embryotoxon.* See also *anterior chamber cleavage syndrome,* under *syndrome.*

 body stalk a. limb–body wall complex.

 Chédiak-Higashi a., Chédiak-Steinbrinck-Higashi a. see under *syndrome.*

 chromosomal a., chromosome a. see under *aberration.*

 collie eye a. an autosomal recessive ocular defect seen in collies and a few other breeds of dog, characterized by an area of choroidal hyperplasia lateral to the optic disk, sometimes with colobomas, retinal detachment, and intraocular hemorrhaging.

 congenital a. a developmental anomaly present at birth; it may be a malformation, disruption, deformation, or dysplasia.

 developmental a. 1. a structural abnormality of any type. 2. a defect resulting from imperfect development of the embryo.

 Ebstein a. a malformation of the tricuspid valve, the septal and posterior leaflets being adherent to the wall of the right ventricle to a varying degree, producing tricuspid deficiency, and the anterior leaflet being normally attached to the annulus fibrosus; usually associated with an atrial septal defect. Called also *Ebstein disease.*

 Freund a. stenosis of the upper thoracic aperture from shortening of the first rib, resulting in deficient expansion of the apex of the lung.

 Jordans a. presence of lipid vacuoles in the cytoplasm of granulocytes, monocytes, and occasionally plasma cells and lymphocytes; some affected persons develop muscular dystrophy while others develop ichthyosis.

 May-Hegglin a. an autosomal dominant disorder of blood cell morphology, caused by mutations in the *MYH9* gene (locus: 22q11.2), which encodes a component of nonmuscle myosin. It is characterized by blue, RNA-containing cytoplasmic inclusions similar to Döhle bodies in most of the granulocytes, accompanied by abnormally large, poorly granulated platelets and sometimes thrombocytopenia, usually without other distinguishing features.

 Pelger-Huët a. a benign autosomal dominant defect of neutrophils and eosinophils caused by mutations in the *LBR* gene (locus: 1q42.1), which encodes the lamin B receptor, in which their nuclei are bilobed or dumbbell-shaped and have a coarse and lumpy structure.

 Peters a. a developmental defect in structures around the anterior chamber of the eye, characterized by corneal clouding and sometimes adhesions of the iris, lens, and cornea; it is often accompanied by other defects such as dwarfism and mental retardation.

 Poland a. see under *syndrome.*

 pseudo–Pelger-Huët a. an acquired condition clinically similar to Pelger-Huët anomaly, occurring in myelodysplastic syndrome and some leukemias; it is also seen occasionally as a reversible effect of drug toxicity.

 Rieger a. a developmental anomaly consisting of posterior embryotoxon, hypoplasia of iris stroma, and usually glaucoma. See also *anterior chamber cleavage syndrome,* under *syndrome.*

 Uhl a. congenital hypoplasia of the myocardium of the right ventricle, resulting in decreased output of the right side of the heart.

 Undritz a. hereditary hypersegmentation of neutrophils; see under *hypersegmentation.*

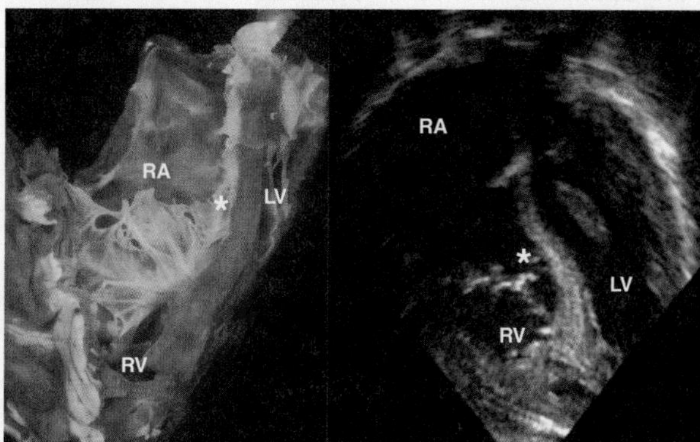

■ Ebstein anomaly, in a clinical specimen *(left)* and apical four-chamber view *(right).* There is significant displacement of the septal leaflet of the tricuspid valve *(asterisk),* with associated valve dysplasia. *LV,* left ventricle; *RA,* right atrium; *RV,* right ventricle.

an•o•mer (an′o-mər) [*ana-* + *-mere*] either of a pair of cyclic diastereoisomers of a sugar or glycoside, differing only in the configuration at the reducing carbon atom and resulting from the new point of symmetry created by ring formation; they are designated α- and β- to denote position of the hydroxyl group below and above the plane of the ring, respectively.

an•o•mer•ic (an″o-mer′ik) pertaining to an anomer; denoting the reducing carbon atom in an anomer.

ano•mia (ə-no′me-ə) anomic aphasia.

an•onych•ia (an″o-nik′e-ə) [*an-*[1] + *onych-* + *-ia*] absence of a nail or nails.

anon•y•mous (ə-non′ĭ-məs) nameless; innominate.

ano•per•i•ne•al (a″no-per-ĭ-ne′əl) pertaining to the anus and perineum.

Anoph•e•les (ə-nof′ə-lēz) [Gr. *anōphelēs* hurtful] 1. a large genus of mosquitoes of the tribe Anophelini, subfamily Anophelinae, characterized by long slender palpi, nearly as long as the proboscis, and by holding the body at an angle with the surface on which it rests while the head and proboscis are in line with the body. Many species are vectors of malaria, and some are vectors of *Wuchereria bancrofti.* It has been subdivided into several subgenera, including *Cellia, Kerteszia, Nyssorhynchus,* and one called *Anopheles.* 2. a subgenus of genus *Anopheles.*

Malaria-Carrying *Anopheles* Species

Subgenus *Anopheles*
- *A.* (*A.*) *anthropophagus*
- *A.* (*A.*) *atroparvus*
- *A.* (*A.*) *aztecus*
- *A.* (*A.*) *bancroftii*
- *A.* (*A.*) *campestris*
- *A.* (*A.*) *claviger*
- *A.* (*A.*) *donaldi*
- *A.* (*A.*) *freeborni*
- *A.* (*A.*) *labranchiae*
- *A.* (*A.*) *letifer*
- *A.* (*A.*) *messeae*
- *A.* (*A.*) *nigerrimus*
- *A.* (*A.*) *pseudopunctipennis*
- *A.* (*A.*) *punctimacula*
- *A.* (*A.*) *quadrimaculatus*
- *A.* (*A.*) *sacharovi*
- *A.* (*A.*) *sinensis*
- *A.* (*A.*) *whartoni*

Subgenus *Cellia*
- *A.* (*C.*) *aconitus*
- *A.* (*C.*) *annularis*
- *A.* (*C.*) *arabiensis*
- *A.* (*C.*) *balabacensis*
- *A.* (*C.*) *culicifacies*
- *A.* (*C.*) *dirus*
- *A.* (*C.*) *farauti*
- *A.* (*C.*) *flavirostris*
- *A.* (*C.*) *fluviatilis*
- *A.* (*C.*) *funestus*
- *A.* (*C.*) *gambiae*
- *A.* (*C.*) *hilli*
- *A.* (*C.*) *karwari*
- *A.* (*C.*) *koliensis*
- *A.* (*C.*) *leucosphyrus*
- *A.* (*C.*) *ludlowae*
- *A.* (*C.*) *maculatus*
- *A.* (*C.*) *melas*
- *A.* (*C.*) *merus*
- *A.* (*C.*) *minimus*
- *A.* (*C.*) *moucheti*
- *A.* (*C.*) *multicolor*
- *A.* (*C.*) *nili*
- *A.* (*C.*) *pattoni*
- *A.* (*C.*) *pharoensis*
- *A.* (*C.*) *philippinensis*
- *A.* (*C.*) *pulcherrimus*
- *A.* (*C.*) *punctulatus*
- *A.* (*C.*) *sergentii*
- *A.* (*C.*) *stephensi*
- *A.* (*C.*) *subpictus*
- *A.* (*C.*) *sundaicus*
- *A.* (*C.*) *superpictus*
- *A.* (*C.*) *tessellatus*

Subgenus *Nyssorhynchus*
- *A.* (*N.*) *albimanus*
- *A.* (*N.*) *albitarsis*
- *A.* (*N.*) *aquasalis*
- *A.* (*N.*) *argyritarsis*
- *A.* (*N.*) *darlingi*
- *A.* (*N.*) *nuneztovari*
- *A.* (*N.*) *triannulatus*

Subgenus *Kerteszia*
- *A.* (*K.*) *bellator*
- *A.* (*K.*) *cruzii*

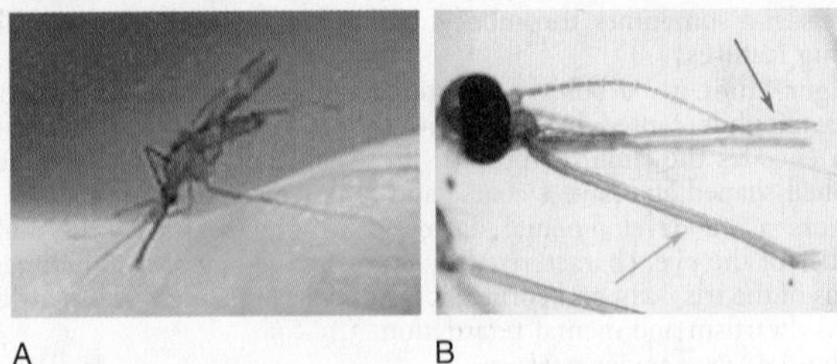

■ *Anopheles* adult. *(A)*, Female feeding, showing the characteristic head and body posture; *(B)*, close-up of head showing the length of the palpi *(red arrow)* in relation to that of the proboscis *(blue arrow)*.

Anoph•e•li•nae (ə-nof″ə-li′ne) a subfamily of mosquitoes of the family Culicidae. It includes one tribe, Anophelini, which contains the genera *Anopheles* and *Chagasia*.

anoph•e•line (ə-nof′ə-lēn) pertaining to or caused by mosquitoes of the tribe Anophelini.

Anoph•e•li•ni (ə-nof″ə-li′ni) a tribe of mosquitoes of the subfamily Anophelinae; genera of medical interest include *Anopheles* and *Chagasia*.

anoph•e•lism (ə-nof′ə-liz-əm) infestation of a district with anopheline mosquitoes.

an•o•pho•ria (an-o-for′e-ə) [Gr. *anō* upward + Gr. *pherein* to bear] hyperphoria.

an•oph•thal•mia (an″of-thal′me-ə) [*an-*[1] + *ophthalm-* + *-ia*] a developmental defect characterized by complete absence of the eyes (rare) or by the presence of vestigial eyes.

an•oph•thal•mos (an″of-thal′mos) anophthalmia.

ano•plas•ty (a′no-plas″te) [*anus* + *-plasty*] a plastic or restorative operation on the anus. **anoplas′tic** *adj*

An•op•lo•ceph•a•la (an″op-lo-sef′ə-lə) [Gr. *anoplos* unarmed + Gr. *kephalē* head] a genus of tapeworms of the family Anoplocephalidae, found in horses.

An•op•lo•ce•phal•i•dae (an″op-lo-sə-fal′ĭ-de) a family of medium-sized or large tapeworms of the order Cyclophyllidea, found as parasites in various species of mammals. Genera of medical or veterinary importance include *Anoplocephala*, *Bertiella*, *Moniezia*, *Paranoplocephala*, and *Thysanosoma*.

An•o•plu•ra (an″o-ploo′rə) [Gr. *anoplos* unarmed + *oura* tail] an order of insects, the sucking lice, characterized by claws and sucking mouth parts; genera of medical or veterinary interest include *Haematopinus*, *Linognathus*, *Pediculus*, *Phthirus*, *Polyplax*, and *Solenopotes*.

an•or•chia (an-or′ke-ə) congenital absence of the testis in a male; it may be either unilateral or bilateral. See also *hypogonadism* and *vanishing testes syndrome*. Called also *anorchidism* and *anorchism*.

an•or•chic (an-or′kik) anorchid (def. 1).

an•or•chid (an-or′kid) [*an-*[1] + *orchis*] 1. lacking testes or not having testes in the scrotum; called also *anorchic* and *anorchidic*. 2. a male who lacks testes or whose testes are not in the scrotum.

an•or•chid•ic (an″or-kid′ik) anorchid (def. 1).

an•or•chi•dism (an-or′kĭ-diz″əm) anorchia.

an•or•chism (an-or′kiz-əm) anorchia.

ano•rec•tal (a″no-rek′təl) pertaining to the anus and rectum or to the junction region between the two.

ano•rec•tic (an″o-rek′tik) [Gr. *anorektos* without appetite for] 1. pertaining to anorexia; having no appetite. 2. a substance that diminishes the appetite. Called also *appetite suppressant*, *anorexic*, and *anorexigenic*.

ano•rec•ti•tis (a″no-rek-ti′tĭs) inflammation of the anorectum.

ano•rec•to•plas•ty (a″no-rek′to-plas″te) [*ano-* + *rectoplasty*] plastic surgery of the anus and rectum. **anorectoplas′tic** *adj*

posterior sagittal a. plastic surgery to create a functional anus and rectum in children with imperforate anus or other anorectal malformations. Called also *Peña procedure*.

ano•rec•tum (a″no-rek′təm) [*anus* + *rectum*] the anus and rectum considered together as a single unit.

ano•ret•ic (an″o-ret′ik) anorectic.

an•orex•ia (an″o-rek′se-ə) [Gr. "want of appetite"] lack or loss of the appetite for food.

a.-cachexia anorexia-cachexia syndrome.

a. nervo′sa [DSM-IV] an eating disorder primarily affecting females, usually with onset in adolescence, characterized by refusal to maintain a normal minimal body weight, intense fear of gaining weight or becoming obese, and a disturbance of body image resulting in a feeling of being fat or having fat in certain areas even when extremely emaciated, undue reliance on body weight or shape for self-evaluation, and amenorrhea. Associated features often include denial of the illness and resistance to psychotherapy, depressive symptoms, markedly decreased libido, and obsessions or peculiar behavior regarding food, such as hoarding. The disorder is divided into two subtypes, a *restricting* type, in which weight loss is achieved primarily through diet or exercise, and a *binge-eating/purging* type, in which binge eating or purging behavior also occurs regularly; the latter type resembles *bulimia nervosa*, which is not diagnosed in the presence of anorexia nervosa.

ano•rex•i•ant (an″o-rek′se-ənt) anorectic (def. 2).

ano•rex•ic (an″o-rek′sik) anorectic.

ano•rex•i•gen (an″o-rek′sĭ-jen) [*anorexia* + *-gen*] anorectic (def. 2).

ano•rex•i•gen•ic (an″o-rek″sĭ-jen′ik) [*anorexia* + *-genic*] 1. producing anorexia, or diminishing the appetite. 2. anorectic (def. 2).

an•or•gan•ic (an″or-gan′ik) denoting tissue (e.g., bone) from which the organic material has been removed.

an•or•gas•mia (an″or-gaz′me-ə) inability or failure to experience orgasm.

an•or•gas•my (an-or-gaz′me) [*an-*[1] + *orgasm*] anorgasmia.

an•or•thog•ra•phy (an″or-thog′rə-fe) [*an-*[1] + *ortho-* + *-graphy*] agraphia.

an•or•tho•pia (an″or-tho′pe-ə) [*an-*[1] + *ortho-* + *-opia*] 1. distorted vision in which straight lines appear as curves or angles, and symmetry is incorrectly perceived. 2. strabismus.

an•or•tho•scope (an-or′thə-skōp″) [*an-*[1] + *ortho* + *-scope*] an instrument for combining two disconnected pictures in one perfect visual image.

ano•scope (a′nə-skōp) [*anus* + *-scope*] a speculum for examining the anus and lower rectum.

anos•co•py (a-nos′kə-pe) examination of the anus and lower rectum by means of an anoscope.

ano•sig•moi•dos•co•py (a″no-sig″moi-dos′kə-pe) [*anus* + *sigmoid* + *-scopy*] endoscopic examination of the anus, rectum, and sigmoid colon. **anosigmoidoscop′ic** *adj*

an•os•mia (an-oz′me-ə) [*an-*[1] + *osm-*[1] + *-ia*] absence of the sense of smell; called also *anosphresia* and *olfactory anesthesia*. **anosmat′ic, anos′mic** *adj*

a. gustato′ria the loss of the power to smell foods.

preferential a. lack of ability to sense certain odors only.

a. respirato′ria loss of smell due to nasal obstruction.

ano•sog•no•sia (an-o″sog-no′zhə) [*a-*[1] + *noso-* + *gnosia*] unawareness or denial of a neurological deficit such as hemiplegia; see also *Anton syndrome*, under *syndrome*, and *asomatognosia*.

an•os•phre•sia (an″os-fre′zhə) [*an-*[1] + *osphresi-* + *-ia*] anosmia.

ano•spi•nal (a″no-spi′nəl) pertaining to the anus and the spinal cord.

an•os•teo•pla•sia (an-os″te-o-pla′zhə) [*an-*[1] + *osteo-* + *-plasia*] defective bone formation.

an•os•to•sis (an″os-to′sis) [*an-*[1] + *osteo-* + *-osis*] defective development of bone.

an•otia (an-o′shə) [*an-*[1] + *ot-* + *-ia*] congenital absence of one or both external ears.

ano•tro•pia (an″o-tro′pe-ə) [*ano-* + Gr. *trepein* to turn] a condition in which the visual axes tend to rise above the object looked at.

an•otus (an-o′təs) [*an-*[1] + *ot-* + *-ous*] a fetus lacking the external ears.

ano•ure•thral (a″no-u-re′thrəl) pertaining to or connecting the anus and urethra. Called also *urethroanal*.

ANOVA analysis of variance.

ano•vag•i•nal (a″no-vaj′ĭ-nəl) pertaining to or connecting the anus and vagina.

an•ova•ria (an″o-var′e-ə) anovarism.

an•ovar•i•an•ism (an″o-var′e-ən-iz-əm) anovarism.

an•ovar•ism (an-o′vər-iz-əm) [*an-*[1] + *ovary*] absence of the ovaries; see also *hypogonadism* and *Turner syndrome*. Called also *anovarianism*.

ano•ves•i•cal (a″no-ves′ĭ-kəl) pertaining to or connecting the anus and urinary bladder.

an•ov•u•lar (an-ov′u-lər) anovulatory.

an•ov•u•la•tion (an″ov-u-la′shən) absence of ovulation.

hypothalamic a. anovulation caused by failure of the hypothalamus to secrete enough luteinizing hormone–releasing hormone. The most common causes are functional, such as excessive exercise, weight loss, or emotional distress. In a minority of women there is a primary cause such as aberration of neuromodulators within the brain.

an·ov·u·la·to·ry (an-ov′u-lə-tor″e) not accompanied by discharge of an oocyte.

anox·ia (ə-nok′se-ə) a total lack of oxygen; often used interchangeably with *hypoxia* to mean a reduced supply of oxygen to the tissues. **anox′ic** *adj*

altitude a. see under *sickness*.

anemic a. anoxia resulting from a decrease in amount of hemoglobin or number of erythrocytes in the blood. Cf. *anemic hypoxia*.

anoxic a. anoxia resulting from interference with the source of oxygen. Cf. *hypoxic hypoxia*.

histotoxic a. particularly severe histotoxic hypoxia.

myocardial a. failure of coronary blood flow to keep up with myocardial needs.

a. neonato′rum anoxia of the newborn.

stagnant a. particularly severe stagnant hypoxia.

anox·i·ate (ə-nok′se-āt) to put into a state of anoxia.

ANP atrial natriuretic peptide.

ANS anterior nasal spine; autonomic nervous system.

an·sa (an′sə) gen. and pl. *an′sae* [L. "handle"] a loop or looplike structure.

a. cervica′lis [TA] a nerve loop in the neck that supplies the infrahyoid muscles and that presents an anterior (superior) root, which connects with the hypoglossal nerve (and actually consists of fibers of the second or first cervical nerve), and an inferior root (nervus descendens cervicalis), which connects with the second and third cervical nerves. Called also *loop of hypoglossal nerve*.

a. lenticula′ris [TA] a small fiber tract arising in the globus pallidus of the lenticular nucleus and extending around the medial border of the internal capsule to join and mingle with the fibers of the fasciculus lenticularis, some of which synapse with cells in the subthalamic nucleus, nucleus of the prerubral field (field H of Forel), and the zona incerta, and others of which continue to the ventral nuclei of the thalamus.

a. nephro′ni a long, U-shaped part of the renal tubule, extending through the medulla from the end of the proximal convoluted tubule to the beginning of the distal convoluted tubule. It begins with a *descending limb* having a thick-walled segment called the *proximal straight tubule*, followed by a thin-walled segment called the *thin* or *attenuated tubule;* this is followed by the *ascending limb*, which sometimes includes the distal end of the attenuated tubule and always ends with a long thick-walled segment called the *distal straight tubule*. The loops vary in the lengths of their segments according to their locations in the kidney. Called also *loop of Henle*.

a. peduncula′ris [TA] peduncular loop: a complex grouping of fibers connecting the amygdaloid nucleus, the piriform area, and the anterior part of the hypothalamus, and various thalamic nuclei. The fiber bundles pass below the internal capsule, a principal bundle being the inferior peduncle of the thalamus.

a. subcla′via [TA] subclavian loop: nerve filaments that pass anterior and posterior to the subclavian artery to form a loop interconnecting the middle and inferior cervical ganglia; called also *a. of Vieussens* and *Vieussens annulus*.

a. of Vieussens a. subclavia.

a. vitelli′na an embryonic vein that connects the yolk sac with the umbilical vein.

an·sae (an′se) [L.] genitive and plural of *ansa*.

An·said (an′sād) trademark for a preparation of flurbiprofen.

an·sate (an′sāt) [L. *ansatus*, from *ansa* handle] having a handle; loop-shaped.

Ans·bach·er unit (ahns′bahk-ər) [Stefan *Ansbacher*, German-born biologist in the United States, 1905–1995] see under *unit*.

an·ser·ine[1] (an′sər-īn) [L. *anser* goose] pertaining to or like a goose.

an·ser·ine[2] (an′sər-ēn) [L. *anser* goose] a dipeptide related to carnosine, composed of β-alanine and methylated histidine; it was first identified in goose muscle and occurs in the skeletal muscle of birds and some mammals, but not humans.

an·se·ri·nus (an″sə-ri′nəs) [L.] anserine[1].

an·si·form (an′sĭ-form) loop-shaped.

An·so·ly·sen (an″so-li′sən) trademark for preparations of pentolinium tartrate.

AN-Sul·fur Col·loid (sul′fur kol′oid) trademark for a kit for the preparation of technetium Tc 99m sulfur colloid.

ant. anterior.

ant- see *anti-*.

ant (ant) any of several crawling insects of the family Formicoidae. See *Formica* and *Solenopsis*.

fire a. 1. any ant of the genus *Solenopsis*. 2. any ant with a fierce sting.

An·ta·buse (an′tə-būs″) trademark for a preparation of disulfiram.

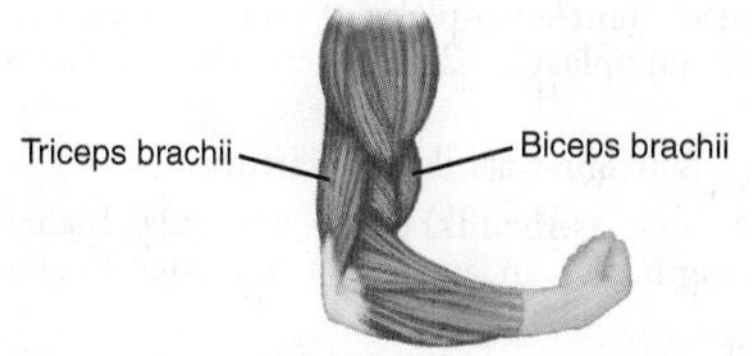

■ Antagonist. The triceps brachii extends the forearm at the elbow while the biceps brachii, its antagonist, flexes the elbow.

ant·ac·id (ant-as′id) [*ant-* + *acid*] 1. counteracting acidity. 2. a substance that counteracts or neutralizes acidity, usually of the stomach.

An·ta·gon (an′tə-gon) trademark for a preparation of ganirelix acetate.

an·tag·o·nism (an-tag′ə-niz″əm) [Gr. *antagōnisma* struggle] opposition or contrariety between similar things, as between muscles, medicines, or organisms; cf. *antibiosis*.

bacterial a. the antagonistic (inhibiting) effect of one bacterial organism on another by reason of its production of an antibiotic (antibiosis) or by its superior competitive ability to absorb nutrients.

metabolic a. interference with the metabolism or function of a given chemical compound by another bearing a close structural resemblance, the similarity in structure being the basis of the interference. For the various forms of such interference, see under *inhibition*.

an·tag·o·nist (an-tag′ə-nist) [Gr. *antagōnistēs* an opponent] 1. a substance that tends to nullify the action of another, as a drug that binds to a cell receptor without eliciting a biological response, blocking binding of substances that could elicit such responses. 2. antagonistic muscle. 3. a tooth in one jaw that articulates with a tooth in the other jaw.

α-adrenergic a. alpha-adrenergic blocking agent.

β-adrenergic a. beta-adrenergic blocking agent.

aldosterone a. any of a group of compounds that block the action of aldosterone and function as potassium-sparing diuretics; they compete with aldosterone for receptor sites, thus blocking the aldosterone-dependent exchange of sodium and potassium in the distal renal tubules.

angiotensin receptor a., angiotensin II receptor a. any of a class of antihypertensive agents that block the vasoconstrictor and aldosterone-secreting effects of angiotensin II by competitive binding with angiotensin receptors. Called also *angiotensin receptor* or *angiotensin II receptor blocker*.

competitive a. a substance that competes with a substrate or with an enzyme which ordinarily attacks the substrate, thus interfering with usual metabolic activity. The antagonist is usually a substrate analogue. See *antimetabolite*.

enzyme a. an antimetabolite that interferes with the normal action of an enzyme. See *enzyme inhibition*, under *inhibition*.

folic acid a. an antimetabolite of folic acid; those used as chemotherapeutic agents are competitive inhibitors of dihydrofolate reductase: trimethoprim is used as an antibacterial, pyrimethamine as an antimalarial, and methotrexate as an antineoplastic. Called also *antifol* and *antifolate*.

H_1 receptor a. any of a large number of agents that block the action of histamine by competitive binding to the H_1 receptor. Such agents also have sedative, anticholinergic, and antiemetic effects, the exact effect varying from drug to drug, and are used for the relief of allergic symptoms and as antiemetics, antivertigo agents, sedatives, and antidyskinetics in parkinsonism. This group is traditionally called the *antihistamines*.

H_2 receptor a. an agent that blocks the action of histamine by competitive binding to the H_2 receptor; used to inhibit gastric secretion in the treatment of peptic ulcer.

insulin a's hormones, antibodies, and other factors that block the action of insulin, such as epinephrine, somatotropin, glucocorticoids, and glucagon.

leukotriene receptor a. any of a class of antiasthmatic drugs that bind competitively to leukotriene receptors in the airways, thus inhibiting bronchoconstriction caused by leukotriene-mediated inflammatory response.

metabolic a. an antimetabolite that interferes with the utilization of a substance essential in metabolism.

narcotic a., opioid a. an agent that opposes the action of narcotics on the nervous system.

ant·a·lar·min (ant-ə-lahr′min) a peptide that acts as an antagonist to corticotropin-releasing hormone and thus damps the alarm reaction.

ant·al·gic (ant-al′jik) 1. counteracting or avoiding pain, as a posture or gait assumed so as to lessen pain. 2. analgesic.

ant·al·ka·line (ant-al′kə-līn″, -lin″) [*ant-* + *alkali*] 1. neutralizing alkalinity. 2. an agent that neutralizes alkalis.

ant·aph·ro·di·si·ac (ant″af-ro-diz′e-ak) 1. abrogating the sexual instinct. 2. an agent that allays sexual impulses; called also *anterotic*.

ant·ap·o·plec·tic (ant″ap-o-plek′tik) [*ant-* + *apoplectic*] 1. relieving or preventing stroke (apoplexy). 2. an agent that alleviates stroke. Spelled also *antiapoplectic.*

ant·arth·rit·ic (ant″ahr-thrit′ik) antiarthritic.

ant·as·then·ic (ant″as-then′ik) [*ant-* + *asthenic*] 1. alleviating weakness, or restoring strength. 2. an agent that alleviates weakness and restores strength.

ant·asth·mat·ic (ant″az-mat′ik) antiasthmatic.

ant·atro·phic (ant″ə-tro′fik) correcting or opposing the progress of atrophy.

an·taz·o·line (an-taz′o-lēn) an ethylenediamine derivative used as an antihistaminic.

a. hydrochloride the hydrochloride salt of antazoline, used topically to treat minor skin irritations.

a. phosphate [USP] the phosphate salt of antazoline, applied topically to the eyes in the treatment of allergic conjunctivitis.

ante- [L. *ante* before] a prefix meaning prior to or in front of.

an·te·bra·chi·um (an″te-bra′ke-əm) [*ante-* + L. *brachium* arm] [TA] the part of the upper limb of the body between the elbow and the wrist; called also *forearm.*

an·te·car·di·um (an″te-kahr′de-əm) [*ante-* + Gr. *kardia* heart] epigastrium.

an·te·ce·dent (an″tə-se′dənt) [L. *antecedere* to go before, precede] a precursor.

plasma thromboplastin a. (PTA) factor XI; see under *coagulation factors,* at *factor.*

an·te ci·bum (an′te si′bəm) [L.] before meals, usually abbreviated *a.c.* in prescriptions, etc.

an·te·cu·bi·tal (an″te-ku′bĭ-təl) situated anterior to the cubitus, or elbow.

an·te·flect (an′te-flekt) to bend anteriorly.

an·te·flexed (an′te-flekst) in a condition of anteflexion.

an·te·flex·ion (an-te-flek′shən) [*ante-* + *flexion*] forward curvature of an organ or part, so that its top is turned anteriorly, such as the normal forward curvature of the uterus.

an·te·grade (an′tĭ-grād) anterograde.

an·te·lo·ca·tion (an″te-lo-ka′shən) [*ante-* + L. *locatio* placement] the forward displacement of an organ.

an·te mor·tem (an′te mor′təm) [L.] before death.

an·te·mor·tem (an″te-mor′təm) [L.] occurring before death.

an·te·na·tal (an″te-na′təl) [*ante-* + *natal*] prenatal.

an·ten·na (an-ten′ə) pl. *anten′nae.* A feeler of an arthropod; one of the two lateral appendages on the anterior segment of the head of arthropods.

An·te·par (an′te-pahr) trademark for a preparation of piperazine citrate and piperazine phosphate.

an·te·par·tal (an″te-pahr′təl) antepartum.

an·te·par·tum (an″te-pahr′təm) [L.] occurring before parturition, or childbirth, with reference to the mother. Cf. *prenatal.* Spelled also *ante partum.* Called also *antepartal* and *prepartal.*

ant·ephi·al·tic (ant″ef-e-al′tik) [*ant-* + Gr. *ephialtēs* nightmare] alleviating or preventing nightmare.

an·te·po·si·tion (an″te-pə-zish′ən) forward displacement, as of the uterus.

an·te·pros·tate (an″te-pros′tāt) [*ante-* + *prostate*] glandula bulbourethralis.

an·te·py·ret·ic (an″te-pi-ret′ik) [*ante-* + *pyretic*] occurring before the stage of fever.

an·te·ri·ad (an-tēr′e-ad) toward the anterior surface of the body.

an·te·ri·or (an-tēr′e-ər) [L. "before"] 1. situated in front of or in the forward part of an organ. 2. [TA] in humans and other bipeds, toward the belly surface of the body; called also *ventral.* 3. in quadruped anatomy, a term sometimes used as a synonym for *cranial.*

antero- [L. *anterior* before] a prefix signifying before.

an·tero·clu·sion (an″tər-o-kloo′zhən) mesioclusion.

an·tero·col·lis (an″tər-o-kol′is) spasmodic torticollis in which the head is drawn forward.

an·tero·ex·ter·nal (an″tər-o-ek-stur′nəl) anterolateral.

an·tero·grade (an′tər-o-grād″) [*antero-* + L. *gredi* to go] moving or extending anteriorly; called also *antegrade.*

an·tero·in·fe·ri·or (an″tər-o-in-fēr′e-ər) situated anteriorly and inferiorly.

an·tero·in·ter·nal (an″tər-o-in-tur′nəl) anteromedial.

an·tero·lat·er·al (an″tər-o-lat′ər-əl) situated anteriorly and to one side; preferred to *anteroexternal.*

an·tero·lis·the·sis (an″tər-o-lis′thə-sis) [*antero-* + Gr. *olisthanein* to slip] spondylolisthesis; cf. *retrospondylolisthesis.*

an·tero·me·di·al (an″tər-o-me′de-əl) situated anteriorly and to the medial side; preferred to *anterointernal.*

an·tero·me·di·an (an″tər-o-me′de-ən) situated anteriorly and toward the median plane.

an·tero·pos·te·ri·or (an″tər-o-pos-tēr′e-ər) from front to back of the body, such as the direction of a radiographic projection.

an·tero·sep·tal (an″tər-o-sep′təl) situated in front of a septum, particularly the atrioventricular septum.

an·tero·su·pe·ri·or (an″tər-o-soo-pēr′e-ər) situated anteriorly and superiorly.

ant·erot·ic (ant″ə-rot′ik) antaphrodisiac.

an·tero·ven·tral (an″tər-o-ven′trəl) situated anteriorly and toward the ventral surface.

an·te·tor·sion (an″te-tor′shən) an increase in the torsion angle of the femur, causing internal deviation of the thigh.

an·te·ver·sion (an″te-vur′zhən) [*ante-* + *version*] the forward tipping or tilting of an organ or part, with the entire organ or part being tipped forward but not bent at an angle, as opposed to *anteflexion;* for example, the normal tipping forward of the entire uterus relative to the pelvic axis.

femoral a. inward twisting of the femur so that the knees and feet turn inward, usually seen in children or in persons with osteoarthritis of the hip.

ant·he·lix (ant′he-liks) [*ant-* + Gr. *helix* coil] antihelix.

ant·hel·min·thic (ant″həl-min′thik) anthelmintic.

ant·hel·min·tic (ant″həl-min′tik) [*ant-* + Gr. *helmins* worm] 1. destroying parasitic worms; called also *anthelminthic, vermicidal,* and *vermifugal.* 2. an agent that destroys parasitic worms; called also *vermicide* and *vermifuge.*

an·the·lot·ic (ant″he-lot′ik) [*ant-* + Gr. *hēlos* nail] 1. effective against corns. 2. a remedy for corns.

An·the·mis (an′thə-mis) [L., from Gr. *anthemis*] a genus of composite-flowered plants (family Compositae). *A. cotu′la,* or mayweed, is a contact allergen that has been associated with severe allergic contact dermatitis with bullous lesions; it also contains cyanogenetic compounds that can cause cyanide poisoning in livestock.

A. no′bilis *Chamaemelum nobile* (Roman chamomile); see *Chamaemelum.*

ant·hem·or·rhag·ic (ant″hem-ə-raj′ik) antihemorrhagic.

an·ther (an′thər) [Gr. *anthēros* blooming] the portion of the stamen of flowering plants containing the microsporangia (pollen sacs) in which haploid microspores (pollen grains) are formed.

an·ther·id·i·um (an″thər-id′e-um) pl. *antherid′ia* [*anther-* + Gr. *idion* a diminutive ending] male organ of a cryptogamic plant or fungus in which microgametes are produced. Cf. *archegonium.*

an·thero·zoid (an′thər-o-zoid″) the motile fertilizing cell of certain fungi.

ant·her·pet·ic (ant″hər-pet′ik) antiherpetic.

An·tho·my·ia (an″tho-mi′yə) a genus of small black houseflies. Two species of medical importance were formerly assigned to this genus; see *Fannia canicularis* and *F. scalaris.*

An·tho·my·ii·dae (an″tho-mi′ə-de) [Gr. *anthos* flower + *myia* fly] in some systems of classification, a family of the order Diptera; the only genus of medical importance is *Fannia.*

An·tho·xan·thum (an″tho-zan′thəm) a genus of grasses (family Gramineae). *A. odora′tum* is sweet vernal grass, whose pollen causes hay fever.

An·thox·i·um (an-thok′se-um) a genus of grasses. *A. odora′tum* is sweet vernal grass, a species used as fodder for horses and cattle in the British Isles; since it contains dicumarol, animals consuming excessive amounts of it can suffer fatal hemorrhaging. It causes hay fever in susceptible humans.

An·tho·zoa (an″tho-zo′ə) [Gr. *anthos* flower + *zoia* animal] a class of invertebrates of the phylum Cnidaria, including animals with large polyps and no medusa stage; it includes corals and sea anemones. Some species are toxic, especially if a person in swimming bumps against them and has a skin abrasion.

an·thra·cene (an′thrə-sēn) a colorless crystalline hydrocarbon derived from coal tar and used in the manufacture of anthracene dyes.

an·thra·cene·di·one (an″thrə-sēn-di′ōn) any of a class of derivatives of anthraquinone; some have antineoplastic properties. Cf. *mitoxantrone hydrochloride.*

■ Anthracycline. For daunorubicin, R_1 = —CH_3; for doxorubicin, R_1 = —CHOH.

anthrac(o)- [Gr. *anthrax* charcoal, carbuncle] a combining form denoting relationship to coal or carbon, or to a carbuncle.

an·thra·coid (an′thrə-koid) [*anthrac-* + *-oid*] resembling anthrax or a carbuncle.

an·thra·com·e·ter (an″thrə-kom′ə-tər) [*anthraco-* + *-meter*] an instrument for measuring the carbon dioxide of the air.

an·thra·co·ne·cro·sis (an″thrə-ko-nə-kro′sis) [*anthraco-* + *necrosis*] necrotic transformation of a tissue into a black dry mass.

an·thra·co·sil·i·co·sis (an″thrə-ko-sil″ĭ-ko′sis) [*anthraco-* + *silicon*] a type of mixed dust pneumoconiosis consisting of both anthracosis and silicosis, caused by coal with a high silica content. Called also *silicoanthracosis.*

an·thra·co·sis (an-thrə-ko′sis) [*anthraco-* + *-osis*] blackening of lung tissue caused by deposition of inhaled carbon in the lungs, seen in many individuals, particularly smokers and those who live in industrial or urban environments. Fibrosis is minimal or absent and the presence of carbon particles is of little or no functional or pathologic significance. Accumulation of large amounts of carbon in the lungs, seen primarily in coal miners, may result in coal workers' pneumoconiosis. **anthracot′ic** *adj*
 a. lin′guae black hairy tongue.

an·thra·co·ther·a·py (an″thrə-ko-ther′ə-pe) [*anthraco-* + *therapy*] treatment with charcoal.

an·thra·cy·cline (an″thrə-si′klēn) any of a class of antineoplastic antibiotics, including daunorubicin and doxorubicin, produced by *Streptomyces peucetius* or *S. coeruleorubidus* and having a four-ring system to which a daunosamine molecule is attached by glycoside linkage (see illustration). Although the precise mechanism of action is unknown, anthracyclines can damage DNA by intercalation, metal ion chelation, and the generation of free radicals and can inhibit enzyme activity critical to DNA function. The use of these drugs is limited by dose-related cardiotoxicity.

An·thra-Derm (an′thrə-dərm) trademark for a preparation of anthralin.

an·thra·lin (an′thrə-lin) [USP] an anthraquinone derivative that reduces DNA synthesis and mitotic activity in hyperplastic epidermis, restoring the normal rate of epidermal cell proliferation and keratinization; used topically in the treatment of psoriasis. Called also *dithranol.*

an·thra·nil·ate (an″thrə-nil′āt) 1. a salt, anion, or ester of anthranilic acid. 2. a chemical compound containing this structure.

an·thra·nil·ic ac·id (an″thrə-nil′ik) a cyclic aromatic compound, the *ortho* form of aminobenzoic acid; it is a product of tryptophan catabolism.

an·thra·quin·one (an″thrə-kwin′ōn) 1. the 9, 10 quinone derivative of anthracene, used in dye manufacture. 2. more commonly, any of the usually highly colored derivatives, yellow, orange, red, red-brown, or violet, of this compound, some of which are used as dyes. Anthraquinones occur in aloe, cascara sagrada, senna, and rhubarb, and have cathartic properties. The antineoplastic mitoxantrone is a synthetic derivative.

an·thrax (an′thraks) [Gr. "coal," "carbuncle"] an infectious disease caused by infection with *Bacillus anthracis.* In herbivores it is acquired through ingestion of the bacillus or its spores from infected pastures. In carnivores it is acquired indirectly when they eat carcasses of infected animals. Humans can become infected by contact with infected animals, their bodily discharges, or contaminated animal products. Types named for primary routes of inoculation include *cutaneous, gastrointestinal,* and *inhalational.* **anthrac′ic** *adj*
 agricultural a. anthrax in a human contracted by contact with infected animals or their bodily discharges.
 cutaneous a. the most common type of anthrax in humans, due to inoculation of *Bacillus anthracis* into superficial wounds or abrasions. It begins with a small, painless, pruritic papular lesion that may have satellite lesions and enlarges, ulcerates, and becomes crusted with a black eschar; this is surrounded by spreading edema *(malignant edema)* and induration. The eschar may either heal or progress to a systemic condition, sometimes involving the meninges, accompanied by high fever and severe toxemia.
 gastrointestinal a. anthrax due to ingestion of poorly cooked meat contaminated with *Bacillus anthracis.* Spores become deposited in the submucosa of the intestinal tract, where they germinate, multiply, and produce toxin, resulting in massive edema that may obstruct the intestine, with hemorrhage and necrosis. Called also *intestinal a.*
 industrial a. anthrax contracted by a person working with contaminated meat or meat products.
 inhalational a. a highly fatal form of anthrax due to inhalation of dust containing anthrax spores, which are transported by the alveolar pneumocytes to regional lymph nodes where they germinate, multiply, and produce toxin. Characteristics include hemorrhagic edematous mediastinitis, pleural effusions, dyspnea, cyanosis, stridor, and shock. It is usually an occupational disease, most often affecting those who handle and sort contaminated wools and fleeces. Called also *pulmonary a.* and *ragpicker's* or *woolsorter's disease.*
 intestinal a. gastrointestinal a.
 malignant a. anthrax.
 meningeal a. anthrax meningitis.
 oropharyngeal a. a rare variant of gastrointestinal anthrax having its focus in the mouth or oropharynx, with throat pain and ulceration of mucous membranes.
 pulmonary a. inhalational a.
 symptomatic a. blackleg.

anthrop(o)- [Gr. *anthrōpos* man, human being] a combining form denoting a relationship to human beings.

an·thro·po·bi·ol·o·gy (an″thrə-po-bi-ol′ə-je) the biological study of human beings and the anthropoid apes.

an·thro·po·cen·tric (an″thrə-po-sen′trik) [*anthropo-* + *centric*] with a human bias; considering human beings the center of the universe.

an·thro·pog·e·ny (an″thrə-poj′ə-ne) [*anthropo-* + *-geny*] the evolution and development of human beings.

an·thro·pog·ra·phy (an″thrə-pog′rə-fe) [*anthropo-* + *-graphy*] the branch of anthropology that deals with the distribution of the varieties of humans, as distinguished by factors such as physical character, institutions, or customs. Cf. *ethnography.*

an·thro·poid (an′thrə-poid) [*anthropo-* + *-oid*] resembling a human being, as an anthropoid ape.

An·thro·poi·dea (an″thrə-poi′de-ə) a suborder of primates characterized by well-developed brains and upright walking stance; it includes human beings (family Hominidae) and the anthropoid apes (family Pongidae). Cf. *Hominoidea.*

an·thro·po·ki·net·ics (an″thrə-po-kĭ-net′iks) [*anthropo-* + *kinetics*] the study of the total human being in action, with integrated applications from the special fields of the biological and physical sciences, psychology, and sociology.

an·thro·pol·o·gy (an″thrə-pol′ə-je) [*anthropo-* + *-ology*] the scientific study of human beings, their origins, historical and cultural development, and ethnicity.
 criminal a. a branch of anthropology that deals with criminals and crimes.
 cultural a. a branch of anthropology that deals with human beings in relation to their fellows and to their environment.
 physical a. a branch of anthropology that deals with the physical characteristics of human beings.

an·thro·pom·e·ter (an″thrə-pom′ə-tər) an instrument especially designed for measuring dimensions of the human body.

an·thro·pom·e·trist (an″thrə-pom′ə-trist) a person skilled in anthropometry.

an·thro·pom·e·try (an″thrə-pom′ə-tre) [*anthropo-* + *-metry*] the science that deals with the measurement of the size, weight, and proportions of the human body. **anthropomet′ric** *adj*

an·thro·po·mor·phism (an″thrə-po-mor′fiz-əm) [*anthropo-* + *morph-* + *-ism*] the attribution of human form or character to nonhuman objects.

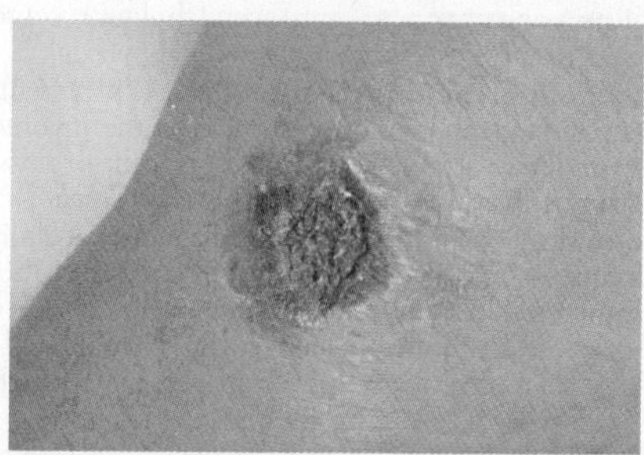

■ Cutaneous anthrax lesion.

an·thro·pon·o·my (an″thrə-pon′ə-me) [*anthropo-* + Gr. *nomos* law] the science that deals with the laws of human development in relation to environment and to other organisms.

an·thro·po·no·sis (an″thrə-pə-no′sis) [*anthropo-* + Gr. *nosos* disease] a disease that is spread from humans to humans; said of diseases with some varieties that spread from animals to humans *(zoonoses)* and others that spread from humans to humans, particularly in reference to parasitic disease such as dry cutaneous leishmaniasis in which the disease can be spread from one human to another by an appropriate vector. **anthroponot′ic** *adj*

an·thro·pop·a·thy (an″thrə-pop′ə-the) [*anthropo-* + *-pathy*] the ascription of human emotions to nonhuman subjects.

an·thro·po·phil·ic (an″thrə-po-fil′ik) [*anthropo-* + *-philic*] preferring human beings to other animals, such as a mosquito or a dermatophyte. Cf. *anthropozoophilic* and *zoophilic.*

an·thro·po·pho·bia (an″thrə-po-fo′be-ə) [*anthropo-* + *-phobia*] irrational dread of human society.

an·thro·pos·co·py (an″thrə-pos′kə-pe) [*anthropo-* + *-scopy*] the judging of the type of body build by inspection rather than by anthropometry.

an·thro·po·zoo·phil·ic (an″thrə-po-zo″o-fil′ik) [*anthropo-* + *zoophilic*] attracted to both human beings and animals, such as certain mosquitoes and fungi. Cf. *anthropophilic* and *zoophilic.*

anti- [Gr. *anti* against] a prefix signifying counteracting, effective against, opposing, or opposite; sometimes shortened to *ant-*.

an·ti·abor·ti·fa·cient (an″te-ə-bor″tĭ-fa′shənt) an agent that prevents abortion or promotes successful pregnancy.

an·ti·ad·re·ner·gic (an″te-ad″rə-nur′jik) 1. opposing the effects of impulses conveyed by adrenergic postganglionic fibers of the sympathetic nervous system. 2. an agent that opposes the effects of impulses conveyed by adrenergic postganglionic fibers. Called also *sympatholytic.* Cf. *anticholinergic.*

an·ti·ag·glu·ti·nin (an″te-ə-gloo′tĭ-nin) a substance that opposes the action of an agglutinin.

an·ti·al·bu·min (an″te-al-bu′min) a precipitin for albumin.

an·ti·ame·bic (an″te-ə-me′bik) 1. destroying or suppressing the growth of amebas. 2. an antiprotozoal agent that particularly attacks amebas.

an·ti·ana·phy·lax·is (an″te-an-ə-fə-lak′sis) a condition in which the anaphylaxis reaction is not obtained because of the presence of free antibodies in the blood; the state of desensitization to antigens.

an·ti·an·dro·gen (an″te-an′drə-jən) any substance capable of inhibiting the biological effects of androgens.

an·ti·ane·mic (an″te-ə-ne′mik) 1. counteracting or preventing anemia. 2. an agent that counteracts or prevents anemia.

an·ti·an·gi·nal (an″te-an-ji′nəl) 1. preventing or alleviating angina. 2. an agent that prevents or alleviates angina.

an·ti·an·gi·o·gen·ic (an″te-an″je-o-jen′ik) inhibiting or preventing neovascularization of tumors; see *angiogenesis inhibitor*, under *inhibitor.*

an·ti·anoph·e·line (an″te-ə-nof′ə-lēn) directed against anopheline mosquitoes or their larvae.

an·ti·an·ti·body (an″te-an′tĭ-bod″e) an antibody directed against antigenic determinants on other antibody (immunoglobulin) molecules.

an·ti·an·ti·tox·in (an″te-an′tĭ-tok″sin) an antibody, formed in immunization with an antitoxin, which counteracts the effect of the latter.

an·ti·an·xi·e·ty (an″te-ang-zi′ə-te) reducing anxiety. Called also *anxiolytic.* See also under *agent.*

an·ti·ap·o·plec·tic (an″te-ap″o-plek′tik) antapoplectic.

an·ti·ap·op·tot·ic (an″te-ap″op-tot′ic, an″te-ap″o-tot′ic) inhibiting apoptosis.

an·ti·a·rin (an-te′ə-rin) a poisonous principle from the upas tree, *Antiaris toxicaria;* formerly used as a heart depressant.

An·ti·a·ris (an″te-ă′rĭs) [Javanese *antiar*] a genus of plants of the family Moraceae, having fleshy fruit and milky juice. *A. toxica′ria* is the Bohun upas or upas tree, an Indonesian species that yields a latex used as an arrow poison. The major toxic principle is a digitalis-like cardioactive glycoside, α-antiarin.

an·ti·ar·rhyth·mic (an″te-ə-rith′mik) 1. preventing or alleviating cardiac arrhythmia. 2. an agent that prevents or alleviates cardiac arrhythmia.

an·ti·ar·thrit·ic (an″te-ahr-thrit′ik) [*anti-* + *arthritic*] 1. alleviating arthritis. 2. an agent that alleviates arthritis.

an·ti·asth·mat·ic (an″te-az-mat′ik) [*anti-* + *asthmatic*] 1. affording relief in asthma. 2. an agent that prevents or treats the symptoms of asthma.

an·ti·ath·ero·gen·ic (an″te-ath″ər-o-jen′ik) combating the formation of atheromatous lesions in arterial walls.

an·ti·au·tol·y·sin (an″te-aw-tol′ĭ-sin) a substance which opposes the action of autolysin.

an·ti·bac·te·ri·al (an″te-, an″ti-bak-tēr′e-əl) 1. destroying or suppressing the growth or reproduction of bacteria. Cf. *bactericidal* and *bacteriostatic.* 2. a substance that destroys or suppresses the growth or reproduction of bacteria.

an·ti·bech·ic (an″te-, an″ti-bek′ik) antitussive.

an·ti·bi·o·gram (an″te-, an″ti-bi′o-gram) the susceptibility profile of a given microorganism when exposed to a battery of antimicrobial agents.

an·ti·bi·o·sis (an″te-, an″ti-bi-o′sis) [*anti-* + *biosis*] 1. an association between two organisms that is detrimental to one of them. 2. a relationship between one organism and an antibiotic produced by another.

an·ti·bi·ot·ic (an″te-, an″ti-bi-ot′ik) [*anti-* + *biotic*] 1. destructive of life. 2. a chemical substance having the capacity, in dilute solution, to kill or inhibit growth of microorganisms. Antibiotics that are sufficiently nontoxic to the host are used as chemotherapeutic agents to treat infectious diseases. The term was originally restricted to substances produced by microorganisms, but has been extended to include synthetic and semisynthetic compounds of similar chemical activity.

antineoplastic a., antitumor a. any of a class of antineoplastic agents that act by binding DNA and preventing RNA, and therefore protein, synthesis; they are thus cell cycle nonspecific.

broad-spectrum a. an antibiotic that is effective against a wide range of bacteria, both gram-positive and gram-negative.

β-lactam a. any of a group of antibiotics, including the cephalosporins and the penicillins, whose chemical structure contains a β-lactam ring; their mechanism of action is inhibition of the synthesis of the bacterial peptidoglycan wall.

an·ti·body (an′tĭ-bod″e) an immunoglobulin molecule that has a specific amino acid sequence by virtue of which it interacts only with the antigen that induced its synthesis in cells of the lymphoid series (especially plasma cells), or with antigen closely related to it. Antibodies are classified in groups named according to their mode of action, such as agglutinins, bacteriolysins, hemolysins, opsonins, precipitins, and others. See *immunoglobulin.*

Antibody

acetylcholine receptor a's anti–acetylcholine receptor a's.

anaphylactic a. IgE antibody causing anaphylaxis.

anti–acetylcholine receptor (anti-AChR) a's circulating autoantibodies against the acetylcholine receptors of the myoneural junction. High titers are demonstrable in about 85 per cent of myasthenia gravis patients; false positives are rare. Called also *acetylcholine receptor a's.*

anticardiolipin a. an antibody directed against cardiolipin, seen with increased frequency in systemic lupus erythematosus; its presence correlates with increased risk for thrombotic events.

anti-CCP a. an antibody against cyclic citrullinated peptide (see under *peptide*), seen almost exclusively in persons with rheumatoid arthritis and indicating a severe prognosis.

anti-D a. antibody directed against the "Rh_0" or "D" antigen of the Rh blood group.

anti-DNA a. see *antinuclear a's.*

anti-dsDNA a. a type of antinuclear antibody specific for double-stranded DNA, found in the serum of patients with systemic lupus erythematosus.

anti-GBM a's antibodies against the glomerular basement membrane; see *anti-GBM antibody nephritis*, under *nephritis.*

antigliadin a's circulating IgA and IgG antibodies to gliadin, found in the serum of patients with celiac disease; measurement of these antibodies is used in diagnosis of celiac disease.

anti–glomerular basement membrane a's anti-GBM a's.

Antibody *Continued*

anti-Ha a. anti–SS-B a.
anti-HCV a. antibody directed against the hepatitis C virus.
anti-Hu a. any of the polyclonal IgG autoantibodies directed against the proteins of the Hu antigen family; they are associated with paraneoplastic sensory neuronopathy and encephalomyelitis in small cell lung carcinoma and, more rarely, sarcoma and neuroblastoma. Called also *type 1 antineuronal antibody (ANNA-1).*
anti-idiotype a. antibody that binds selectively to a specific idiotope.
anti-La a. anti–SS-B a.
antimicrosomal a's organ-specific autoantibodies directed against a thyroid microsomal antigen, demonstrable in almost all patients with Hashimoto thyroiditis.
antimitochondrial a's circulating antibodies directed against inner mitochondrial membrane antigens; they are seen in almost all patients with primary biliary cirrhosis, and occasionally in other liver diseases. Called also *mitochondrial a's.*
antineuronal a., type 1 (ANNA-1) anti-Hu a.
antineuronal a., type 2 (ANNA-2) anti-Ri a.
antineutrophil cytoplasmic a. see under *autoantibody.*
antinuclear a's (ANA) antibodies directed against nuclear antigens; ones against a variety of different antigens are almost invariably found in systemic lupus erythematosus and are frequently found in rheumatoid arthritis, scleroderma (systemic sclerosis), Sjögren syndrome, and mixed connective tissue disease. Antinuclear antibodies may be detected by immunofluorescent staining. Serologic tests are also used to determine antibody titers against specific antigens.
antiphospholipid a's a group of antibodies against phosphorylated polysaccharide esters of fatty acids, thought to be markers of a hypercoagulable state of the blood; included are anticardiolipin antibodies and lupus anticoagulant.
anti–Purkinje cell a. (APCA) anti-Yo a.
antireceptor a's autoantibodies against cell-surface receptors, e.g., those directed against acetylcholine receptors in myasthenia gravis, against TSH receptors in Graves disease, against insulin receptors in type B insulin resistance with acanthosis nigricans, and against β_2-adrenergic receptors in some patients with allergic disorders.
anti-Ri a. an autoantibody having neuronal binding characteristics similar to those of anti-Hu antibody but directed against a different RNA-binding site; it is associated with paraneoplastic opsoclonus-myoclonus in small cell lung carcinoma and cancer of the breast and fallopian tube. Called also *type 2 antineuronal antibody (ANNA-2).*
anti-Ro a. anti–SS-A a.
antisperm a. (ASA) any of various surface-bound antibodies found on sperm after infection, trauma to the testes, or vasectomy; they interfere with the fertilization process or result in nonviable zygotes.
anti-SS-A a. an antinuclear antibody that occurs in Sjögren syndrome and systemic lupus erythematosus. Called also *anti-Ro a.*
anti-SS-B a. an antinuclear antibody that occurs in Sjögren syndrome and systemic lupus erythematosus. Called also *anti-La a.*
antithyroglobulin a's autoantibodies directed against thyroglobulin, demonstrable in about 50 to 75 per cent of patients with Hashimoto thyroiditis and in about one-third of patients with other types of thyroiditis, Graves disease, and thyroid carcinoma.
antithyroid a's see *antimicrosomal a's* and *antithyroglobulin a's.*
anti-Yo a. polyclonal IgG autoantibody directed against Purkinje cells and associated with paraneoplastic cerebellar degeneration in small cell lung carcinoma and cancer of the breast or ovary. Called also *anti–Purkinje cell antibody (APCA).*
auto-anti-idiotypic a's autologous anti-idiotype antibodies that suppress the immune response in many experimental situations; auto-anti-idiotypic antibodies occur in certain autoimmune disorders.
autologous a. self-derived antibody; autoantibody.
bispecific a. antibody in which each of two antigen-binding sites is specific for separate antigenic determinants. It is an artificial antibody produced in the laboratory, formed by reassociating half molecules of two different antibody specificities to form a hybrid or bispecific antibody with antigen-binding sites of separate specificities. Called also *hybrid a.*
blocking a. any antibody that by combining with an antigen blocks another immunologic reaction with the antigen. In most patients, immunotherapy (hyposensitization or desensitization) for allergic disorders induces IgG blocking antibodies that can bind the allergen and prevent it from binding to cell-fixed IgE, triggering immediate hypersensitivity; it can thus induce partial immunologic tolerance. Blocking antibodies directed against tumor-specific antigens have been suggested as one mechanism allowing tumors to escape immune surveillance. Blocking antibodies can prevent agglutination in serologic tests (see *incomplete a.*).
cell-bound a., cell-fixed a. any antibody bound to a cell surface either by its antigen-combining sites to cell-surface antigenic determinants or by other sites to specific cell-surface receptors (Fc receptors, IgE receptors).
cold a., cold-reactive a. antibody, usually IgM but occasionally IgG, that reacts less efficiently with antigen at 37°C than at lower temperatures.
complement-fixing a. antibody that activates complement when reacted with antigen; IgM and IgG (the usual complement-fixing antibodies) fix complement by the classical pathway, whereas IgA fixes complement by the alternative pathway. See also *complement fixation,* under *fixation.*
complete a. antibody capable of agglutinating cells in physiologic saline solution. Called also *saline agglutinin.* Cf. *incomplete a.*
cross-reacting a. an antibody that combines with an antigen other than the one that induced its production.
cytophilic a. cytotropic a.
cytotoxic a. any specific antibody directed against cellular antigens, which when bound to the antigen, activates the complement pathway or activates killer cells, resulting in cell lysis.
cytotropic a. antibody that binds to mast cells and basophils at specific receptors; subsequent binding of antigen to the cell-fixed antibody triggers release of mediators of immediate hypersensitivity. Such antibodies produced by the animal itself in response to antigenic challenge or transferred from another animal of the same species *(homocytotropic* or *reaginic antibodies* or *reagin)* are always of the IgE class. In some cases IgG, IgA, or IgM from one species (heterocytotropic antibodies) can sensitize tissues of another species; e.g., rabbit IgG can sensitize guinea pig skin for passive cutaneous anaphylaxis.
depleting a. a type of monoclonal antibody that binds to elements on the cell membranes of leukocytes and depletes the population of circulating leukocytes, thus causing immunosuppression.
Donath-Landsteiner a. an IgG antibody directed against the P blood group antigen; it binds to red cells at low temperatures and induces complement-mediated lysis on warming, and is responsible for hemolysis in paroxysmal cold hemoglobinuria.
duck virus hepatitis yolk a. yolk antibody derived from chicken eggs, used for treatment of duck virus hepatitis.
7E3 a. a monoclonal antibody that blocks glycoprotein IIb/IIIa receptors, used experimentally as an anticoagulant.
Forssman a. heterophile antibody directed against the Forssman antigen.
Goodpasture a. a type of circulating antibody against basement membrane antigens, present in Goodpasture syndrome.
heteroclitic a. antibody produced in response to immunization with one antigen but having a higher affinity for a second antigen that was not present during immunization.
heterocytotropic a. see *cytotropic a.*
heterogenetic a., heterophil a., heterophile a. antibody directed against heterophile antigens. Heterophile sheep erythrocyte agglutinins appear in the serum of patients with infectious mononucleosis (see *Paul-Bunnell test* under *test*).
homocytotropic a. see *cytotropic a.*
hybrid a. bispecific a.
immune a. antibody induced by immunization or by transfusion incompatibility, in contrast to the natural antibodies.
incomplete a. 1. antibody that binds to erythrocytes or bacteria but does not produce agglutination; the nonagglutinating antibody is detectable with the antiglobulin (Coombs) test. For example, IgG anti-Rh antibodies do not agglutinate erythrocytes in physiologic saline whereas IgM antibodies do (the large IgM molecule can cross-link the erythrocytes at a wider separation so that there is less electrostatic repulsion due to the zeta potential). 2. a univalent antibody fragment, e.g., Fab fragment.
indium-111 antimyosin a. a monoclonal antibody against myosin, labeled with indium 111; it binds selectively to irreversibly damaged myocytes and is used in infarct avid scintigraphy.
isophil a. antibody against red blood cell antigens produced in members of the species from which the red cells originated.
mitochondrial a's antimitochondrial a's.

Antibody *Continued*

monoclonal a's chemically and immunologically homogeneous antibodies produced by hybridomas, used as laboratory reagents in radioimmunoassays, ELISA, and immunofluorescence assays; also used experimentally in cancer immunotherapy.

natural a's antibodies present in the serum of normal individuals in the apparent absence of any contact with the specific antigen, probably induced by exposure to cross-reacting antigens. They may result from unknown exposure to naturally occurring antigens, e.g., food or bacterial flora.

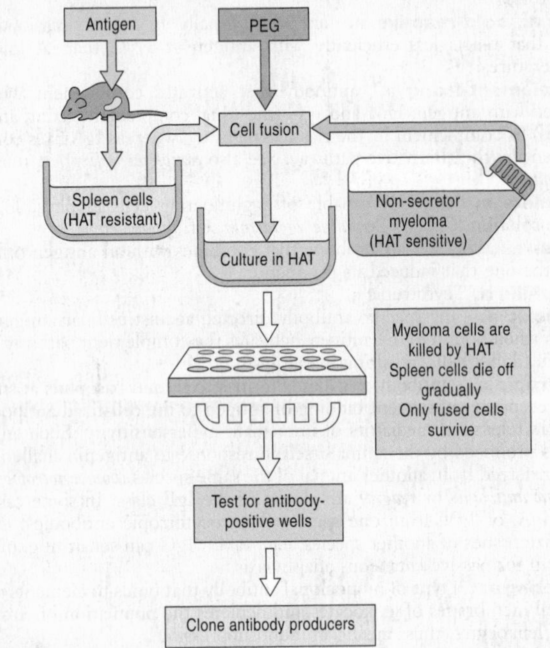

■ Monoclonal antibody production. *HAT*, HAT medium; *PEG*, polyethylene glycol.

neutralizing a. see *viral neutralization*, under *neutralization*.

OKT3 monoclonal a. a mouse monoclonal antibody directed against T3 lymphocytes and used to prevent or treat rejection after organ transplantation.

opsonizing a. see *opsonin*.

panel-reactive a. (PRA) 1. the pre-existing anti-HLA antibody in the serum of a potential allograft recipient that reacts with specific antigen in a panel of leukocytes (see *antibody screening*, under *screening*). A higher percentage of PRA indicates a higher risk of a positive crossmatch. 2. the percentage of such antibody in the recipient's serum.

P-K a's Prausnitz-Küstner a's.

polyclonal a. antibody produced by more than one clone of antibody-synthesizing plasma cells (B lymphocytes); antibody that is not monoclonal, e.g., that produced by immunizing an animal.

Prausnitz-Küstner a's cytotropic IgE antibodies responsible for cutaneous anaphylaxis; see *Prausnitz-Küstner reaction*, under *reaction*.

protective a. antibody responsible for immunity to an infectious agent observed in passive immunity.

reaginic a. reagin.

Rh a's antibodies directed against Rh antigen(s) of human erythrocytes. Not normally present, but may be produced when Rh-negative persons receive Rh-positive blood by transfusion or when an Rh-negative person is pregnant with an Rh-positive fetus.

saline a. complete a.

sensitizing a. a loosely used term, applied to antibodies that are attached to body cells and that "sensitize" the cells or render them susceptible to destruction by body defenses.

thyroid colloidal a's antibodies to antigens in the thyroid colloid such as thyroglobulin or CA_2, seen in Hashimoto disease.

TSH-displacing a. (TDA) TSH-binding inhibitory immunoglobulins.

warm a., warm-reactive a. antibody, usually IgG but occasionally IgM or IgA, that reacts more efficiently with antigen at 37°C than at lower temperatures.

---

an·ti·bra·chi·um incorrect spelling of *antebrachium*.

an·ti·bro·mic (an″te-bro′mik) [*anti-* + Gr. *brōmos* smell] deodorant.

an·ti·ca·chec·tic (an″te-, an″ti-kə-kek′tik) 1. preventing or relieving cachexia. 2. an agent that prevents or relieves cachexia.

an·ti·cal·cu·lous (an″te-, an″ti-kal′ku-ləs) antilithic (def. 1).

an·ti·car·cin·o·gen (an″te-, an″ti-kahr-sin′ə-jen) an agent that counteracts the effect of a carcinogen.

an·ti·car·ci·no·gen·ic (an″te-, an″ti-kahr″sin-o-jen′ik) inhibiting or preventing the development of carcinoma.

an·ti·car·io·gen·ic (an″te-, an″ti-kar″e-o-jen′ik) suppressing the development of caries; anticarious.

an·ti·car·i·ous (an″te-, an″ti-kar′e-əs) anticariogenic.

an·ti·cat·a·lyst (an″te-, an″ti-kat′ə-list) a substance that retards the action of a catalyzer by acting on the catalyzer itself.

an·ti·cat·a·lyz·er (an″te-, an″ti-kat′ə-līz″ər) anticatalyst.

an·ti·ca·thex·is (an″te-, an″ti-kə-thek′sis) [*anti-* + *cathexis*] in psychoanalytic theory, the energy required for the ego to maintain repression of unacceptable ideas and impulses.

an·ti·ceph·a·lal·gic (an″te-sef-ə-lal′jik) curing or preventing headache.

an·ti·cho·le·litho·gen·ic (an″te-, an″ti-ko″lə-lith″o-jen′ik) 1. serving to prevent the formation of gallstones. 2. an agent that opposes formation of gallstones.

an·ti·cho·les·ter·emic (an″te-, an″ti-kə-les″tər-e′mik) 1. promoting a reduction of cholesterol levels in the blood. 2. an agent that reduces cholesterol levels in the blood. Called also *anticholesterolemic*.

an·ti·cho·les·te·rol·emic (an″te-kə-les″tər-ol-e′mik) anticholesteremic.

an·ti·cho·lin·er·gic (an″te-, an″ti-ko″lin-ur′jik) [*anti-* + *cholinergic*] 1. blocking the passage of impulses through the parasympathetic nerves. 2. an agent that blocks the passage of impulses through the parasympathetic nerves. Called also *parasympatholytic*. Cf. *antiadrenergic*.

an·ti·cho·lin·es·ter·ase (an″te-, an″ti-ko″lin-es′tər-ās) cholinesterase inhibitor.

an·ti·chy·mo·sin (an″te-ki′mo-sin) an antibody that prevents the action of rennin on milk.

an·ti·ci·pate (an-tis′ĭ-pāt) [*ante-* + L. *capere* to take] to occur or recur before the regular time; said of a disease or of symptoms. See *anticipation*.

an·ti·ci·pa·tion (an-tis″ĭ-pa′shən) 1. the manifestation of a hereditary disease at a progressively earlier age in successive generations; it can be caused by expansion of triplet repeats in some genetic disorders, but can also be an artifact arising from the greater likelihood of detecting a mildly affected parent having a severely affected child, rather than the reverse, or from other ascertainment bias. 2. looking forward to future events, experiences, or emotions, preexperiencing them; it can be used as a defense mechanism.

an·ti·clin·al (an″te-, an″ti-kli′nəl) [*anti-* + Gr. *klinein* to slope] sloping in opposite directions, as opposite sides of triangular structures.

an·tic·ne·mi·on (an″tik-ne′me-on) [*anti-* + Gr. *knēmē* leg] the shin.

an·ti·co·ag·u·lant (an″te-, an″ti-ko-ag′u-lənt) 1. preventing blood clotting. 2. an agent that prevents blood clotting; see *anticoagulant therapy*, under *therapy*.

circulating a. a substance present in the blood that inhibits normal clotting and thus may cause a hemorrhagic syndrome; it may be directed against a specific coagulation factor and may accompany various hematologic and nonhematologic diseases.

lupus a. a circulating anticoagulant that inhibits the conversion of prothrombin to thrombin, found in 5–10 per cent of patients with systemic lupus erythematosus, but also seen in other disorders. Although associated with a prolonged partial thromboplastin time, it rarely causes abnormal bleeding and, paradoxically, increases the risk of thromboembolism. Called also *lupus inhibitor*.

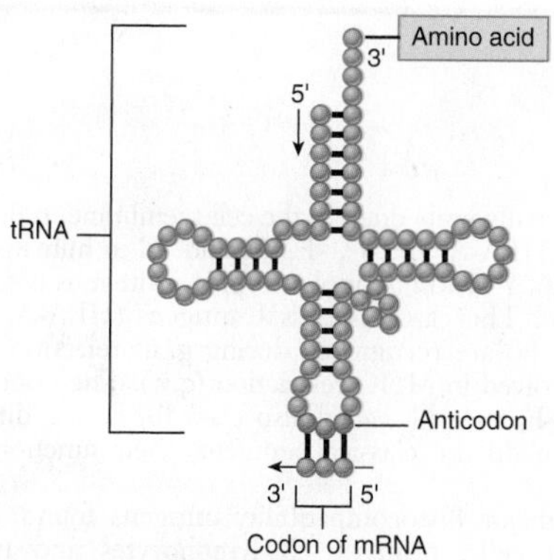

■ Anticodon. The three nucleotides *(pink)* on a transfer RNA bind to a complementary messenger RNA codon.

an·ti·co·ag·u·la·tion (an″te-, an″ti-ko-ag″u-la′shən) 1. the prevention of coagulation. 2. anticoagulant therapy.

an·ti·co·ag·u·la·tive (an″te-ko-ag′u-lə-tiv) anticoagulant (def. 1).

an·ti·coc·cid·i·al (an″te-kok-sid′e-əl) coccidiostatic.

an·ti·co·don (an″te-, an″ti-ko′don) a triplet of nucleotides in transfer RNA that is complementary to the codon in messenger RNA that specifies the amino acid.

an·ti·com·ple·ment (an″te-, an″ti-kom′plə-mənt) a substance that opposes or counteracts the action of a complement.

an·ti·com·ple·men·ta·ry (an″te-, an″ti-kom″plə-men′tə-re) capable of reducing or destroying the power of a complement.

an·ti·con·cep·tive (an″te-, an″ti-kən-sep′tiv) contraceptive.

an·ti·con·vul·sant (an″te-, an″ti-kən-vul′sənt) 1. preventing or relieving convulsions. 2. an agent that prevents or relieves convulsions.

an·ti·con·vul·sive (an″te-, an″ti-kən-vul′siv) anticonvulsant.

an·ti·cro·tin (an″te-kro′tin) the antitoxin of crotin.

an·ti·cu·ra·re (an″te-, an″ti-koo-rah′re) an agent that counteracts the action of curare on skeletal muscle.

an·ti·cus (an-ti′kəs) [L.] anterior.

an·ti·cy·tol·y·sin (an″te-, an″ti-si-tol′ĭ-sin) a substance opposing the action of cytolysin.

an·ti·cy·to·tox·in (an″te-, an″ti-si′to-tok″sin) a substance that opposes the action of a cytotoxin.

an·ti-D antibody against the "D" or "Rh_0" antigen, one of the Rh factors; see *Rh_0(D) immune globulin* under *globulin.*

an·ti·de·pres·sant (an″te-, an″ti-de-pres′ənt) 1. preventing or relieving depression; stimulating the mood of a depressed patient. 2. an agent that prevents or relieves depression.

atypical a. any of a number of antidepressant drugs with varying structures and pharmaceutical properties that do not belong to the tricyclic or tetracyclic antidepressants or monoamine oxidase inhibitors.

tetracyclic a. an antidepressant drug that includes four fused rings in its chemical structure.

tricyclic a. any of a group of antidepressant drugs that contain three fused rings in their chemical structure and that potentiate the action of catecholamines; the tricyclic antidepressants include a number of compounds, which may be grouped into four classes on the basis of chemical structure: dibenzazepines, dibenzocycloheptadienes, dibenzoxazepines, and dibenzoxepines.

an·ti·di·a·bet·ic (an″te-, an″ti-di″ə-bet′ik) 1. preventing or alleviating diabetes. 2. an agent that prevents or alleviates diabetes mellitus.

an·ti·di·a·be·to·gen·ic (an″te-, an″ti-di″ə-bet″o-jen′ik) 1. preventing the development of diabetes. 2. an agent that prevents development of diabetes mellitus.

an·ti·di·ar·rhe·al (an″te-, an″ti-di″ə-re′əl) 1. counteracting diarrhea. 2. an agent that counteracts diarrhea.

an·ti·di·ar·rhe·ic (an″te-, an″ti-di″ə-re′ik) antidiarrheal.

an·ti·di·u·re·sis (an″te-, an″ti-di″u-re′sis) suppression of urinary excretion.

an·ti·di·uret·ic (an″te-, an″ti-di″u-ret′ik) 1. suppressing the rate of urine formation. 2. an agent that slows the rate of urine formation.

an·ti·do·tal (an″tĭ-do′təl) serving as an antidote.

an·ti·dote (an′tĭ-dōt) [L. *antidotum,* from Gr. *anti* against + *didonai* to give] a remedy for counteracting a poison.

chemical a. an antidote that reacts chemically with a poison to form a harmless compound.

mechanical a. an antidote that prevents the absorption of a poison.

physiologic a. an antidote that counteracts the effects of a poison by producing opposing physiologic effects.

"universal" a. a mixture of 2 parts activated charcoal, 1 part magnesium oxide, and 1 part tannic acid; given when the exact poison is not known. There is no true "universal" antidote and this mixture is no longer recommended by most authorities; activated charcoal alone is preferred.

an·ti·dot·ic (an″tĭ-dot′ik) antidotal.

an·ti·drom·ic (an″te-drom′ik) [Gr. *antidromein* to run in a contrary direction] conducting impulses in a direction opposite to the normal; see under *conduction.* Cf. *orthodromic.*

an·ti·dys·en·ter·ic (an″te-, an″ti-dis″ən-ter′ik) 1. preventing, alleviating, or curing dysentery. 2. an agent that prevents, alleviates, or cures dysentery.

an·ti·dys·ki·net·ic (an″te-, an″ti-dis″kĭ-net′ik) 1. relieving or preventing dyskinesia. 2. an agent that relieves or prevents dyskinesia.

an·ti·ec·ze·mat·ic (an″te-ek″zə-mat′ik) 1. alleviating eczema. 2. an agent that alleviates eczema.

an·ti·edem·a·tous (an″te-e-dem′ə-təs) antiedemic (def. 1).

an·ti·edem·ic (an″te-ə-dem′ik) 1. preventing or alleviating edema. 2. an agent that prevents or alleviates edema.

an·ti·emet·ic (an″te-ə-met′ik) 1. preventing or alleviating nausea and vomiting. 2. an agent that prevents or alleviates nausea and vomiting; see also *antinauseant.*

an·ti·en·zyme (an″te-en′zīm) [*anti-* + *enzyme*] an agent that prevents or retards the action of an enzyme, such as a protease inhibitor or an antibody.

an·ti·ep·i·lep·tic (an″te-ep″ĭ-lep′tik) 1. combating epilepsy. 2. an agent that combats epilepsy.

an·ti·ep·i·the·li·al (an″te-ep″ĭ-the′le-əl) destructive to epithelial cells.

an·ti·es·tro·gen (an″te-es′trə-jen) a substance capable of inhibiting the biological effects of estrogens.

an·ti·es·tro·gen·ic (an″te-es-trə-jen′ik) counteracting or suppressing estrogenic activity.

an·ti·feb·rile (an″te-, an″ti-feb′ril) antipyretic (def. 1).

an·ti·fib·ril·la·to·ry (an″te-, an″ti-fib′rĭ-lə-tor″e) 1. preventing or stopping fibrillation of the heart. 2. an agent that prevents or stops fibrillation of the heart.

an·ti·fi·bri·nol·y·sin (an″te-, an″ti-fi″brĭ-nol′ĭ-sin) antiplasmin.

an·ti·fi·bri·no·lyt·ic (an″te-, an″ti-fi″brĭ-no-lit′ik) 1. inhibiting fibrinolysis. 2. an agent that inhibits fibrinolysis.

an·ti·fi·brot·ic (an″te-, an″ti-fi-brot′ik) 1. causing regression of fibrosis. 2. an agent that causes regression of fibrosis.

an·ti·fi·lar·i·al (an″te-, an″ti-fĭ-lar′e-əl) 1. suppressing or killing filaria. 2. an agent that suppresses or kills filaria.

an·ti·flat·u·lent (an″te-, an″ti-flat′u-lənt) 1. relieving or preventing flatulence. 2. an agent that relieves or prevents flatulence.

an·ti·flux (an′tĭ-fluks) a substance that prevents the attachment of solder.

an·ti·fol (an′tĭ-fōl) folic acid antagonist.

an·ti·fo·late (an″tĭ-fo′lāt) folic acid antagonist.

an·ti·fun·gal (an″te-, an″ti-fung′gəl) 1. destroying fungi, or suppressing their reproduction or growth; effective against fungal infections. 2. an agent that destroys fungi or inhibits their growth; called also *antimycotic.*

azole a. any of a group of antifungals characterized by the presence of an azole ring structure, which includes the triazoles and the imidazoles (qq.v.). They are usually fungistatic but can be fungicidal at higher concentrations, and act by interfering with the enzyme activity of cytochrome P-450, decreasing the production of ergosterol and so damaging the cell membrane by altering its permeability and functions.

an·ti·ga·lac·tic (an″te-, an″ti-gə-lak′tik) [*anti-* + *galactic*] 1. diminishing or stopping lactation. 2. an agent that has this effect. Called also *lactifuge.*

an·ti·gen (an′tĭ-jən) [*antibody* + *-gen*] any substance capable, under appropriate conditions, of inducing a specific immune response and of reacting with the products of that response, that is, with specific antibody or specifically sensitized T lymphocytes, or both. Antigens may be soluble substances, such as toxins and foreign proteins, or particulate, such as bacteria and tissue cells; however, only the portion of the protein or polysaccharide molecule known as the antigenic determinant (q.v.) combines with antibody or a specific receptor on a lymphocyte. Abbreviated Ag.

Antigen

allogeneic a. 1. an antigen that occurs in some but not all individuals of the same species, e.g., histocompatibility antigens. 2. isoantigen.
Am a's see under *allotype.*
Au a., Australia a. former name for *hepatitis B surface a.*
blood group a's the antigens responsible for specificities of blood groups; those of the ABO and Lewis blood groups were the first to be characterized. They are formed by sequential addition of monosaccharide moieties to any of several different types of precursor substances; addition of one moiety produces the Lewis antigen, addition of a second produces the H antigen, and addition of a third produces either the A or the B antigen. Secreted blood group antigens (in individuals with the secretor phenotype) are glycoproteins, and red cell antigens are glycosphingolipids; the oligosaccharide chains determining blood group specificity are the same in both.
cancer a. 125 (CA 125) a surface glycoprotein associated with müllerian epithelial tissue; elevated serum levels are often associated with epithelial ovarian carcinomas, particularly with nonmucinous tumors, but are also seen in some other malignant and various benign pelvic disorders. See also *cancer antigen 125 (CA 125) assay,* under *assay.*
capsular a. K a.
carcinoembryonic a. (CEA) a glycoprotein secreted into the glycocalyx coating the luminal surface of gastrointestinal epithelia. Originally thought to be a specific antigen of the fetal digestive tract and adenocarcinoma of the colon, CEA is now known to occur normally in feces and pancreaticobiliary secretions and to appear in the plasma in a diverse group of neoplastic and non-neoplastic conditions, including cancers of the colon, pancreas, stomach, lung, and breast, alcoholic cirrhosis and pancreatitis, inflammatory bowel disease, rectal polyps, and cigarette smoking. The primary use of CEA is in monitoring response to treatment of colorectal cancer.
CD a. any of a number of cell surface markers expressed by leukocytes and used to distinguish cell lineages, developmental stages, and functional subsets; such markers can be identified by specific monoclonal antibodies and are numbered CD1, CD2, CD3, etc. Markers used to identify T lymphocyte subsets were formerly called *T antigens.* See also *CD system,* under *system.*
class I a's major histocompatibility antigens found on virtually every cell except for human erythrocytes; they are found on molecules consisting of two noncovalently bound chains. One, a 44-kD polymorphic glycoprotein partially embedded in the cell membrane, is determined by an MHC gene (HLA-A, -B, -C, -E, -F, and -G in humans); the other, β_2-microglobulin, a 12-kD nonpolymorphic protein, is determined by a non-MHC gene. The classical class I antigens (HLA-A, -B, and -C, called also class Ia) are recognized during graft rejection and are also the antigens involved in MHC restriction (q.v.). The nonclassical antigens (HLA-E, -F, and -G, called also class Ib) have a different tissue distribution than do the classical antigens; their functions are under investigation.

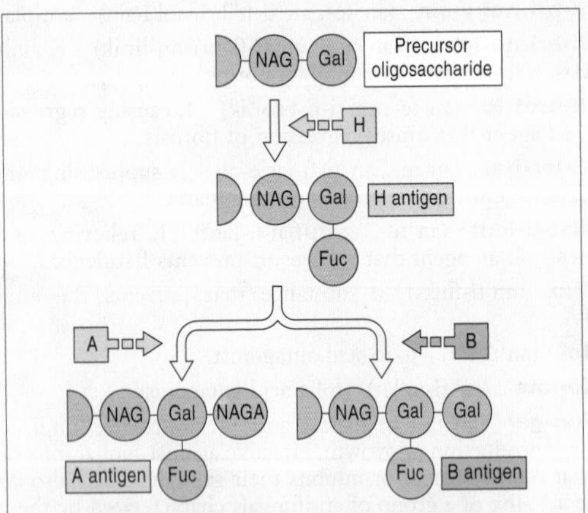

Blood group (phenotype)	Genotypes	Antigens	Antibodies to ABO in serum
A	AA, AO	A	anti-B
B	BB, BO	B	anti-A
AB	AB	A and B	none
O	OO	H	anti-A and anti-B

■ Blood group antigens. *(Diagram),* Synthesis of ABO groups. The enzyme produced by the H gene attaches a fucose residue *(Fuc)* to the terminal galactose *(Gal)* of the precursor oligosaccharide. Individuals possessing an A gene then attach *N*-acetylgalactosamine *(NAGA)* to this galactose; those with a B gene attach another galactose, producing A and B antigens, respectively. NAG=*N*-acetylglucosamine. *(Table),* Genotypes and antigens of the ABO system.

class II a's major histocompatibility antigens found only on immunocompetent cells, primarily B lymphocytes and macrophages; they are found on molecules consisting of two noncovalently bound chains, the 34,000-dalton α chain and 29,000-dalton β chain, both glycoproteins partially embedded in the cell membrane and both determined by MHC genes. The human HLA-D, -DR, -DP, and -DQ loci are all associated with antigenic determinants on class II antigen molecules.
class III a's a term used to refer to nonhistocompatibility antigens mapping in the major histocompatibility complex, e.g., the complement components C2, C4, factor B.
common a. an antigenic determinant group (epitope) that is present in two or more different antigen molecules and frequently leads to cross-reactions among them.
common acute lymphoblastic leukemia a. (CALLA) a tumor-associated antigen, CD10, occurring on lymphoblasts in about 80 per cent of patients with acute lymphoblastic leukemia (ALL) and also in 40–50 per cent of patients with blastic phase chronic myelogenous leukemia (CML). It does not occur on normal lymphoid cells except during fetal development.
common leukocyte a's leukocyte common a's.
complete a. an antigen that both stimulates the immune response and reacts with the products (e.g., antibody) of that response.
conjugated a. antigen produced by coupling a hapten to a protein carrier molecule through covalent bonds; when it induces immunization, the resultant immune response is directed against both the hapten and the carrier.
cross-reacting a. 1. an antigen that combines with antibody produced in response to a different but related antigen, owing to similarity of antigenic determinants. 2. identical antigens in two bacterial strains, so that antibody produced against one strain will react with the other.
D a. one of the Rh factors, an antigen of the Rh blood group, important in the development of isoimmunization in Rh-negative persons exposed to the blood of Rh-positive persons.
delta a. a 32- to 37-nm RNA particle coated with hepatitis B surface antigen.
E a. one of the Rh factors, an antigen of the Rh blood group system.
epithelial membrane a. a protein specific to the epithelial membrane; used as an immunohistochemical marker for epithelium.
extractable nuclear a's ENA; protein antigens, not containing DNA, that are extractable from cell nuclei in phosphate-buffered saline; anti-ENA antibodies are a component of the antinuclear antibodies occurring in systemic lupus erythematosus and other connective tissue diseases.
febrile a's a standard panel of serologic antigens *(Salmonella, Proteus, Francisella tularensis,* and *Brucella)* used in screening patients with unexplained fever.
flagellar a. H a. (def. 1).
Forssman a. a heterophile antigen that induces production of anti-sheep hemolysin, found in a variety of different animals, mainly in organs and not in erythrocytes (guinea pig, horse); sometimes it is found only in erythrocytes (sheep), and occasionally in both organs and erythrocytes (chicken). In the original and strict sense, the antigen is typified by that found in the guinea pig kidney, characterized by heat stability and solubility in alcohol; the antigenic determinant is polysaccharide in nature. Its antibody is absorbed by tissues containing the antigen and contains no lysin for bovine cells and little or no agglutinin for sheep cells. The term has been broadened to refer loosely to any antigen producing sheep hemolysin, although antibodies to them may not be identical, as they are in the case of the true Forssman antigen.
Gm a's see under *allotype.*
Goodpasture a. a type of autoantibody seen in Goodpasture syndrome.
H a. [*Hauch,* q.v.] 1. the precursor of the A and B blood group antigens. Normal type O individuals lack enzymes to convert H antigen to

A or B antigens. Those individuals having the rare *Bombay phenotype* lack the ability to make H antigen and thus are phenotypically type O whether or not they possess A or B genes. Called also *H substance.* 2. one of the bacterial flagellar antigens important in the serological classification of enteric bacilli, especially *Salmonella.* Cf. *O a.*
H-2 a's the major histocompatibility antigens in mice.
hepatitis a., hepatitis-associated a. (HAA) former name for *hepatitis B surface a.*
hepatitis B core a. (HBcAg) a core protein antigen of the hepatitis B virus present inside complete virions (Dane particles) and in the nuclei of infected hepatocytes, indicating the presence of replicating hepatitis B virus; the antigen is not present in the blood of infected individuals, but anti-HBc antibodies appear during the acute infection; they do not protect against reinfection.
hepatitis B e a. (HBeAg) an antigen of hepatitis B virus sometimes present in the blood during acute infection, usually disappearing afterward but sometimes persisting in chronic disease. Anti-HBe antibodies appear transiently during convalescence and do not protect against reinfection.
hepatitis B surface a. (HBsAg) a coat protein antigen of the hepatitis B virus present on complete virions (Dane particles) and smaller spherical and filamentous particles circulating in the blood of individuals with active or chronic infections, being first detectable several weeks prior to clinical disease and peaking with the appearance of symptoms. Anti-HBs antibodies appear in the blood in late convalescence and are protective against reinfection. See also *hepatitis B vaccine (recombinant),* under *vaccine.*
heterogeneic a. xenogeneic a.
heterogenetic a. heterophile a.
heterologous a. an antigen that reacts with an antibody that is not the one (the homologous antigen) that induced its formation.
heterophil a., heterophile a. any of a group of cross-reacting antigens occurring in several species and having a species distribution that does not correspond to phylogenetic relationships, such as the Forssman antigen. Called also *heterogenetic a.*
high frequency a's, high incidence a's public a's (def. 1).
histocompatibility a's systems of allelic alloantigens that can stimulate an immune response that leads to transplant rejection when the donor and recipient are mismatched. Called also *transplantation a's.* See *human leukocyte a's.*
histocompatibility a's, major the antigens in the major histocompatibility complex; HLA antigens in humans and H-2 antigens in mice.
histocompatibility a's, minor systems of allelic alloantigens that can cause transplant rejection, but with a long delay (up to 100 days); about 15–30 such systems have been found in mice.
HLA a's human leukocyte antigens.
homologous a. 1. the antigen that induces the formation of an antibody. 2. isoantigen.
Hu a. a family of four RNA-binding proteins (HuD, HuC/ple21, Hel-N1, and Hel-N2) that are expressed in neurons and are believed to play an important role in the development and maintenance of the nervous system; they are also expressed in the cells of small cell lung carcinoma, sarcoma, and neuroblastoma, and antibodies to them are associated with neurologic paraneoplastic syndromes.
human leukocyte a's (HLA) histocompatibility antigens governed by genes of the HLA complex (the human major histocompatibility complex), a region on the short arm of chromosome 6 containing several genetic loci, each having multiple alleles. Loci are designated by letters; the classical loci are HLA-A, -B, -C, -E, -F, -G, -DP, -DQ, and -DR (there are at least three subloci in the D region). Alleles at each locus are designated by numbers, e.g., HLA-A1, provisional designations being indicated by "w" (for "workshop"), e.g., HLA-DRw10. The A, B, C, and DR antigens are defined and typed by serologic reactions. The D antigens are defined and typed by one-way mixed lymphocyte culture (MLC) using panels of HLA-D-homozygous typing cells. The SB (for "secondary B cell") antigens are defined and typed by primed lymphocyte typing. See *class I, class II,* and *class III a's.*
H-Y a. a minor histocompatibility antigen present in all tissues of normal males and coded for by a structural gene on the short arm of the Y chromosome; it is thought to promote the differentiation of indifferent gonads into testes, thus determining male sex.
I a. see *cold agglutinin syndrome,* under *syndrome.*
i a. see *cold agglutinin syndrome,* under *syndrome.*
Ia a's [*I* region–*a*ssociated] class II histocompatibility antigens found on the surface of mouse B cells, macrophages, and accessory cells. They are also found on granulocyte precursors but disappear during maturation. Ia antigens are governed by the Ia genes of the H-2 complex (q.v.).
Inv group a's see *Km allotypes,* under *allotype.*
isogeneic a. isoantigen.
isophile a. isoantigen.
K a. [Ger. *Kapsel* capsule] a surface antigen found on the capsule of bacteria, external to the cell wall, such as the *Salmonella* Vi antigen or some found on pneumococci. Called also *capsular a.*
Km a's see under *allotype.*
Kveim a. a saline suspension of human sarcoid tissue prepared from the spleen or lymph nodes of a patient with active sarcoidosis.
La a. SS-B a.
LD a's lymphocyte-defined a's.
leukocyte common a's (LCA) a group of glycoproteins, antigenically similar but of different molecular weights, found on B cells, T cells, thymocytes, and leukopoietic cells. Called also *common leukocyte a's.*
leukocyte function–associated a. 1 (LFA-1) a β_2 integrin expressed on most lymphocytes, granulocytes, and monocytes that mediates leukocyte adhesion; it also plays a role in antibody-dependent cellular cytotoxicity.
leukocyte function–associated a. 2 (LFA-2) a cell membrane glycoprotein, perhaps related to the immunoglobulins, expressed on thymocytes and NK cells that mediates leukocyte adhesion.
leukocyte function–associated a. 3 (LFA-3) a cell surface glycoprotein expressed on a wide variety of cells that serves as a ligand for LFA-2.
leu-M1 a. an antigen present on granulocytes and Reed-Sternberg cells in Hodgkin disease, except in the lymphocyte-predominant diffuse subtype.
low frequency a's, low incidence a's private a's (def. 1).
Ly a's cell-surface markers differentiating subpopulations of murine T lymphocytes: Ly 1, Ly 2, and Ly 3. Most thymocytes and undifferentiated peripheral T cells are Ly $1^+2^+3^+$; helper cells are Ly $1^+2^-3^-$; cytotoxic T cells and suppressor cells are Ly $1^-2^+3^+$.
Lyb a's cell-surface markers on murine B lymphocytes: Lyb 1,2,3,4, and 5. Lyb 1,2, and 4 are found on all B cells, Lyb 3 and 5 on a subset of mature B cells.
lymphocyte-defined (LD) a's major histocompatibility antigens defined and typed by the mixed lymphocyte reaction (MLR), e.g., HLA-D antigens.
Lyt a's Ly a's.
M a. M protein (def. 2).
Mitsuda a. lepromin.
mumps skin test a. [USP] preparation of killed mumps virus, used in the mumps skin test (q.v.).
nuclear a's the components of cell nuclei with which antinuclear antibodies (q.v.) react.
O a. [*ohne Hauch,* q.v.] the lipopolysaccharide-protein somatic antigens of gram-negative bacteria, important in the serological classification of enteric bacilli. See *lipopolysaccharide.* Cf. *H a.*
oncofetal a. an antigenic gene product that is expressed during fetal development, partially or completely repressed in adult tissues, and derepressed in some tissues that have undergone neoplastic transformation; oncofetal antigens, e.g., alpha-fetoprotein, carcinoembryonic antigen, and pancreatic oncofetal antigen, are thus useful tumor markers.
organ-specific a. any antigen that occurs exclusively in a particular organ and serves to distinguish it from other organs. Two types of organ specificity have been proposed: (1) first-order or tissue specificity is attributed to the presence of an antigen characteristic of a particular organ in a single species; (2) second-order organ specificity is attributed to an antigen characteristic of the same organ in many, even unrelated species. Called also *tissue-specific a.*
Oz a. an antigenic marker on the lambda chain of human immunoglobulins, equivalent to Km allotypes on kappa light chains. Together with Kern markers, they delineate three types of human lambda chain.
pancreatic oncofetal a. (POA) a glycoprotein, mol. wt. 800,000, found in fetal and neoplastic pancreatic tissue but not in that of normal adults; it also occurs at lower levels in the serum of patients with cancer at other sites and some normal adults.
pan–T-cell a. an antigen present on several different types of T cells.

Antigen *Continued*

partial a. hapten.
Pl(A1) a. the most commonly expressed antigen of platelets; patients not expressing this isoantigen are at risk for transfusion-induced hematologic disorders of platelets, such as thrombocytopenic purpura.
platelet a. any of several isoantigens expressed by platelets.
pollen a. see under *allergen.*
Pr a. see *cold agglutinin syndrome,* under *syndrome.*
private a's 1. blood group antigens that occur in only a few kindreds *(low frequency blood groups).* Called also *low frequency a's.* 2. HLA antigens found only on the gene product of a single allele. 3. a tumor antigen expressed only on a particular type of chemically induced tumor. Cf. *public a's.*
proliferating cell nuclear a. (PCNA) a 36-kD trimeric nuclear acidic protein that acts as an auxiliary factor in DNA replication and repair; its levels in the body correlate with the rates of DNA synthesis and it is commonly used as a marker for proliferating cells.
prostate-specific a. (PSA) a serine endopeptidase secreted by the epithelial cells of the prostate gland; serum levels are elevated in benign prostatic hyperplasia and prostate cancer. Measurement of PSA serum levels is used as a screening test for prostate cancer.
prostate-specific membrane a. (PSMA) a substance often expressed by the most aggressive clones of prostate cancer cells; monoclonal antibody tests for PSMA appear to be more sensitive than those using prostate-specific antigen alone in finding circulating prostate cancer cells and may be useful in identifying patients with a high risk of advanced disease.
public a's 1. blood group antigens that occur in the general population at high frequencies; see *high frequency blood group,* under *blood group.* Called also *high frequency a's.* 2. HLA antigens occurring on the products of several allelic genes. Cf. *private a's.*
recall a. an antigen to which an individual has previously been sensitized and which is subsequently administered as a challenging dose to elicit a hypersensitivity reaction.
Rh a. see under *factor.*
RNP a. [*ribo*nucleo*p*rotein] one of the extractable nuclear antigens.
Ro a. SS-A a.
SD a's serologically defined a's.
self-a. autoantigen.
sequestered a's the cellular constituents of tissue (e.g., lens of the eye) sequestered anatomically from the lymphoreticular system during embryonic development and thus thought not to be recognized as "self." Should such tissue be exposed to the lymphoreticular system during adult life, an autoimmune response would be elicited.
sero-defined (SD) a's, serologically defined (SD) a's major histocompatibility antigens defined by serologic reactions, e.g., HLA-A, HLA-B, and HLA-C antigens.
shock a. an antigen capable of eliciting anaphylactic shock in a sensitized animal.
skin test a. the antigen used in a skin test (see under *test*).
Sm a. [after a patient, *Smith*] an uncharacterized nuclear antigen that is a nonhistone acidic protein not complexed with DNA or RNA; anti-Sm antibodies make up a part of the antinuclear antibodies in about one-third of patients with systemic lupus erythematosus, but do not occur in other connective tissue diseases, except mixed connective tissue disease.
somatic a's antigens, usually cell surface antigens, of the body of a bacterial cell, in contrast to flagellar or capsular antigens. See *O a.*
species-specific a's antigens restricted to a single species and found in all members of the species.
SS-A a. a ribonucleoprotein extractable nuclear antigen; see also *anti-SS-A antibody,* under *antibody.*
SS-B a. a ribonucleoprotein extractable nuclear antigen; see also *anti-SS-B antibody,* under *antibody.*
T a. 1. any of several antigens, coded for by the viral genome, associated with transformation of infected cells by certain DNA tumor viruses, such as SV 40. Called also *tumor a.* 2. an antigen present on human erythrocytes that is exposed by treatment with neuraminidase or contact with certain bacteria. See *T agglutinin* under *agglutinin.* 3. see *CD a.*
θ a. Thy 1 a.
Tac a. the receptor for interleukin 2.
T-dependent a. an antigen that requires the presence of helper T cells to stimulate antibody production by B cells; most antigens are T-dependent.
theta a., Thy 1 a. a cell-surface marker occurring on all murine T lymphocytes.
T-independent a. an antigen that can trigger B cells to produce antibodies without the participation of T cells; most are polymers with a simple repeating pattern and are B cell mitogens; only IgM is produced and few memory cells are formed.
tissue-specific a. organ-specific a.
TL a. [*t*hymus *l*eukemia] a differentiation antigen, first discovered on thymic leukemia cells, that occurs on thymocytes but not peripheral T cells in some strains of mice.
transplantation a's histocompatibility a's.
tumor a. 1. T a. (def. 1). 2. tumor-specific a. 3. tumor-associated a.
tumor-associated a. (TAA) an antigen that is associated with tumor cells; it may also be found under other conditions, as on normal cells during fetal life (oncofetal antigen) or on normal adult cells specific to certain organs (organ-specific antigen), or may occur normally on many cells but at a lower level.
tumor rejection a. (TRA) tumor-specific transplantation a.
tumor-specific a. (TSA) any cell-surface antigen of a tumor that does not occur on normal cells of the same origin.
tumor-specific transplantation a. (TSTA) any of the cell surface histocompatibility antigens of a given tumor that evoke a specific immune response on transplantation to a syngeneic host.
VDRL a. an alcohol solution containing 0.03 per cent cardiolipin, 0.99 per cent cholesterol, and enough lecithin to produce standard reactivity. See *VDRL test,* under *test.*
very late activation (VLA) a. β_1 integrin.
Vi a. a K antigen of the bacteria causing typhoid fever (*Salmonella enterica* subsp. *enterica* serovar Typhi), originally thought to be responsible for virulence.
a. X UDP-*N*-acetylglucosamine pyrophosphorylase.
xenogeneic a. an antigen common to members of one species but not to members of other species; called also *heterogeneic a.*

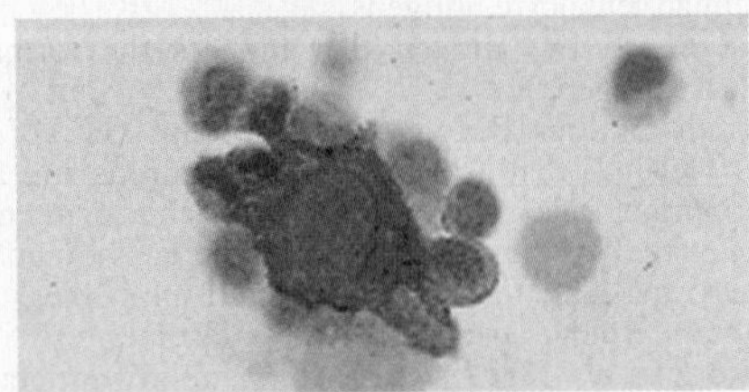

■ Tumor-associated antigen used to detect micrometastases. Cytokeratins are expressed as tumor-associated antigens in some malignancies; cells from a lymph node draining a tumor site were stained by immunoalkaline phosphatase using a monoclonal antibody against a cytokeratin; the positive result, staining pink, indicates a carcinoma cell expressing cytokeratin.

an·ti·gen·emia (an″tĭ-jə-ne′me-ə) [*antigen* + *-emia*] the presence of antigen in the blood.

an·ti·gen·emic (an″tĭ-jen-e′mik) exhibiting antigenemia.

an·ti·gen·ic (an-tĭ-jen′ik) having the properties of an antigen.

an·ti·ge·nic·i·ty (an″tĭ-jə-nis′ĭ-te) the property of being able to induce a specific immune response or the degree to which a substance is able to stimulate an immune response. Called also *immunogenicity.*

an·ti·glau·co·ma (an″te-, an″ti-glaw-ko′mə, an″te-, an″ti-glou-ko′mə) preventing or alleviating glaucoma.

an·ti·glob·u·lin (an′tĭ-glob″u-lin) an antibody directed against gamma globulin; see also under *test.*

an·ti·goit·ro·gen·ic (an″te-, an″ti-goi″tro-jen′ik) preventing or inhibiting the development of goiter.

an·ti·go·nado·tro·pic (an″te-go″nə-do-tro′pik) inhibiting the secretion or actions of the gonadotropins.

an·ti·grav·i·ty (an″te-, an″ti-grav′ĭ-te) counteracting the pull of gravity.

an·ti·hal·lu·cin·a·to·ry (an″te-, an″ti-hə-loo′sĭ-nə-tor″e) counteracting hallucinogenesis; suppressing hallucinations.

an·ti-HBc antibody to hepatitis B core antigen (HB_cAg).

an·ti-HBs antibody to hepatitis B surface antigen (HB_sAg).

an·ti·he·lix (an″te-he′liks) [TA] the prominent semicircular ridge seen on the lateral aspect of the auricle of the external ear, anteroinferior to the helix; called also *anthelix.*

an·ti·hel·min·tic (an″te-, an″ti-hel-min′tik) anthelmintic.

an·ti·he·mag·glu·ti·nin (an″te-, an″ti-he″mə-gloo′tĭ-nin) a substance whose action is antagonistic to hemagglutinin.

an·ti·he·mol·y·sin (an″te-, an″ti-he-mol′ə-sin) any agent that opposes the action of a hemolysin.

an·ti·he·mo·lyt·ic (an″te-, an″ti-he″mo-lit′ik) preventing hemolysis.

an·ti·he·mo·phil·ic (an″te-, an″ti-he″mo-fil′ik) 1. counteracting hemophilia. 2. an agent that counteracts hemophilia.

an·ti·hem·or·rhag·ic (an″te-, an″ti-hem″o-raj′ik) 1. preventing or stopping hemorrhage. 2. an agent that prevents or stops hemorrhage.

an·ti·her·pes (an″te-, an″ti-hur′pēz) antiherpetic.

an·ti·her·pet·ic (an″te-, an″ti-hər-pet′ik) 1. acting against herpes. 2. an agent that acts against herpes.

an·ti·het·er·ol·y·sin (an″te-, an″ti-het″ər-ol′ĭ-sin) a substance that counteracts heterolysin.

an·ti·his·ta·mine (an″te-, an″ti-his′tə-mēn) an agent that counteracts the action of histamine. While the term can broadly include any agent that blocks any histamine receptor, in practice it is usually used to denote those blocking H_1 receptors (H_1 receptor antagonists), which are the drugs conventionally used to treat allergic reactions and are also components of many cough and cold preparations. Agents blocking H_2 receptors are usually called histamine H_2 receptor antagonists, and include the agents used to inhibit gastric secretion in peptic ulcer. See also *histamine.*

an·ti·his·ta·min·ic (an″te-, an″ti-his-tə-min′ik) 1. counteracting the effect of histamine. 2. antihistamine.

an·ti·hor·mone (an″te-, an″ti-hor′mōn) any substance that opposes the action of a hormone.

an·ti·hy·per·cho·les·ter·ol·emic (an″te-, an″ti-hi″pər-kə-les″tər-ol-e′mik) 1. effective in decreasing or preventing an excessively high level of cholesterol in the blood. 2. an agent that decreases or prevents high levels of cholesterol in the blood.

an·ti·hy·per·gly·ce·mic (an″te-, an″ti-hi″pər-gli-se′mik) 1. counteracting high levels of glucose in the blood. 2. an agent that counteracts high levels of glucose in the blood.

an·ti·hy·per·ka·le·mic (an″te-, an″ti-hi″pər-kə-le′mik) 1. effective in decreasing or preventing an excessively high level of potassium in the blood. 2. an agent that decreases or prevents high levels of potassium in the blood.

an·ti·hy·per·lip·i·de·mic (an″te-, an″ti-hi″pər-lip″ĭ-de′mik) 1. promoting a reduction of lipid levels in the blood. 2. an agent that reduces lipid levels in the blood.

an·ti·hy·per·lipo·pro·tein·emic (an″te-, an″ti-hi″pər-lip″o-pro″tēn-e′mik) 1. promoting a reduction of lipoprotein levels in the blood. 2. an agent that reduces levels of lipoproteins in the blood.

an·ti·hy·per·ten·sive (an″te-, an″ti-hi″pər-ten′siv) 1. counteracting high blood pressure. 2. an agent that counteracts high blood pressure.

an·ti·hyp·not·ic (an″te-, an″ti-hip-not′ik) 1. preventing or hindering sleep. 2. an agent that prevents or hinders sleep.

an·ti·hy·po·gly·ce·mic (an″te-, an″ti-hi″po-gli-se′mik) 1. counteracting hypoglycemia. 2. an agent that counteracts hypoglycemia.

an·ti·hy·po·ten·sive (an″te-, an″ti-hi″po-ten′siv) 1. counteracting low blood pressure. 2. an agent that counteracts low blood pressure.

an·ti·ic·ter·ic (an″te-ik-ter′ik) 1. relieving jaundice. 2. an agent that has this effect.

an·ti·id·io·type (an″te-id′e-o-tīp) an antibody directed against an idiotypic determinant of another antibody. See *idiotype–anti-idiotype network,* under *network.*

an·ti·in·fec·tive (an″te-in-fek′tiv) 1. capable of killing or suppressing activity of infectious agents; cf. *antimicrobial.* 2. an agent that suppresses or kills infectious agents.

an·ti·in·flam·ma·to·ry (an″te-in-flam′ə-tor″e) 1. counteracting or suppressing inflammation. 2. an agent that counteracts or suppresses inflammation.

an·ti·in·su·lin (an″te-in′su-lin) a substance that counteracts the action of insulin; see also *insulin antagonists,* under *antagonist.*

an·ti·is·che·mic (an″te-is-kem′ik) 1. relieving or preventing ischemia. 2. an agent that relieves or prevents ischemia.

an·ti·isol·y·sin (an″te-i-sol′ĭ-sin) a substance that counteracts an isolysin.

an·ti·ke·to·gen·e·sis (an″te-, an″ti-ke″to-jen′ə-sis) inhibition of the formation of ketone bodies.

an·ti·ke·to·gen·ic (an″te-, an″ti-ke″to-jen′ik) preventing or inhibiting the formation of ketone bodies.

an·ti·leish·ma·ni·al (an″te-, an″ti-lēsh-ma′ne-əl) 1. effective against protozoa of the genus *Leishmania.* 2. an agent having this effect.

an·ti·lep·rot·ic (an″te-, an″ti-lep-rot′ik) 1. therapeutically effective against leprosy. 2. an agent with this effect.

an·ti·leu·ko·ci·din (an″te-, an″ti-loo-ko′sĭ-din) a substance that counteracts leukocidin; called also *antileukotoxin.*

an·ti·leu·ko·cyt·ic (an″te-, an″ti-loo″ko-sit′ik) leukocytolytic.

an·ti·leu·ko·tox·in (an″ti-loo′ko-tok″sin) antileukocidin.

an·ti·leu·ko·tri·ene (an″te-, an″ti-loo″ko-tri′ēn) an agent that interferes with leukotriene synthesis or binding; used in the treatment of asthma.

an·ti·lew·is·ite (an″tĭ-loo′ĭ-sīt) dimercaprol; called also *British anti-lewisite,* or *BAL.*

an·ti·li·pe·mic (an″te-, an″ti-lĭ-pe′mik) antihyperlipidemic.

an·ti·lip·i·de·mic (an″tĭ-lip″ĭ-de′mik) antihyperlipidemic.

an·ti·lipo·tro·pic (an″te-, an″ti-lip″o-tro′pik) interfering with the mobilization of fat in the liver.

an·ti·lip·ot·rop·ism (an″te-, an″ti-lip-ot′rə-piz-əm) interference with the mobilization of fat in the liver.

An·ti·lir·i·um (an″tĭ-lir′e-əm) trademark for a preparation of physostigmine salicylate.

an·ti·lith·ic (an″te-, an″ti-lith′ik) [*anti-* + *lithic*] 1. preventing formation of calculi. 2. an agent that prevents formation of calculi.

an·ti·ly·sin (an″te-, an″ti-li′sin) [*anti-* + *lysin*] a substance that opposes the action of a lysin.

an·ti·ly·sis (an″te-, an″ti-li′sis) the inhibition or suppression of lysis.

an·ti·lyt·ic (an″te-, an″ti-lit′ik) pertaining to antilysis; inhibiting or suppressing lysis.

an·ti·ma·lar·i·al (an″te-, an″ti-mə-lar′e-əl) 1. therapeutically effective against malaria. 2. an agent having this quality.

an·ti·me·phit·ic (an″te-, an″ti-mə-fit′ik) preventing or neutralizing mephitic substances.

an·ti·mere (an′tĭ-mēr) [*anti-* + *-mere*] one of the opposite corresponding parts of an organism which are symmetrical with respect to the longitudinal axis of its body; cf. *metamere.*

an·ti·mes·en·ter·ic (an″te-, an″ti-mez′ən-ter″ik) designating the part of the intestine that is opposite to the site of attachment of the mesentery.

an·ti·me·tab·o·lite (an″te-, an″ti-mə-tab′o-līt) a substance bearing a close structural resemblance to one required for normal physiological functioning, and exerting its effect by interfering with the utilization of the essential metabolite. For various ways in which antimetabolites inhibit metabolic processes, see under *inhibition.*

an·ti·meta·stat·ic (an″te-met″ə-stat′ik) inhibiting metastasis.

an·ti·met·he·mo·glo·bin·emic (an″te-, an″ti-met-he″mo-glo″bĭ-ne′-mik) 1. effective in reducing the production of methemoglobin; effective in the treatment of methemoglobinemia. 2. an agent that produces such effects.

an·ti·me·tro·pia (an″te-, an″ti-mə-tro′pe-ə) [Gr. *antimetrein* to measure out in turn + *-opia*] difference in refractive error between the two eyes, e.g., hyperopia in one eye with myopia in the other.

an·ti·mi·cro·bi·al (an″te-, an″ti-mi-kro′be-əl) 1. killing microorganisms, or suppressing their multiplication or growth. 2. an agent that kills microbes or inhibits their growth. Cf. *antibiotic.*

an·ti·min·er·alo·cor·ti·coid (an″te-, an″ti-min″ər-əl-o-kor′tĭ-koid) a substance that suppresses the secretion or opposes the action of mineralocorticoids.

An·ti·minth (an′tĭ-minth) trademark for a preparation of pyrantel pamoate.

an·ti·mi·tot·ic (an″te-, an″ti-mi-tot′ik) 1. inhibiting or preventing mitosis. 2. an agent that inhibits or prevents mitosis.

an·ti·mon·ic (an″tĭ-mon′ik) containing antimony in its pentad valency.

an·ti·mo·nid (an″tĭ-mo′nid) any binary compound of antimony.

an·ti·mo·ni·ous (an″tĭ-mo′ne-əs) containing antimony in its triad valency.

an·ti·mo·ni·um (an″tĭ-mo′ne-əm) gen. *antimo′nii* [L.] antimony.

an·ti·mo·ny (Sb) (an′tĭ-mo″ne) a crystalline metallic element with a bluish luster, atomic number 51, atomic weight 121.75, forming various medicinal and poisonous salts. See also *antimony poisoning* and *antimony pneumoconiosis*. antimo′nial *adj*

a. potassium tartrate [USP] a trivalent antimony compound used as an antischistosomal, especially for treatment of *Schistosoma japonicum* infections, administered intravenously; now rarely used because of its toxicity.

a. sodium dimercaptosuccinate sodium stibocaptate.

a. sodium tartrate [USP] a trivalent antimony compound having the same actions and uses as the potassium tartrate but more water-soluble and less irritant when injected; now rarely used because of its toxicity.

an·ti·mo·nyl (an-tim′o-nil″) the univalent radical SbO—.

an·ti·mül·le·ri·an (an″te-, an″ti-mu-ler′e-ən) inhibiting the development of müllerian ducts, such as an antimüllerian hormone.

an·ti·mus·ca·rin·ic (an″te-, an″ti-mus′kə-rin′ik) 1. acting against the toxic effects of muscarine. 2. blocking the muscarinic receptors. 3. an agent that does these things.

an·ti·mu·ta·gen (an″te-, an″ti-mu′tə-jen) a substance that antagonizes the mutagenic effects of other substances.

an·ti·my·as·then·ic (an″te-, an″ti-mi″əs-then′ik) 1. counteracting or relieving muscular weakness in myasthenia gravis. 2. an agent that counteracts or relieves myasthenia gravis.

an·ti·my·co·bac·te·ri·al (an″te-, an″ti-mi″ko-bak-te′re-əl) 1. effective against mycobacteria. 2. an agent having this effect.

an·ti·my·cot·ic (an″ti-mi-kot′ik) antifungal.

an·ti·myd·ri·at·ic (an″ti-mid″re-at′ik) 1. reversing dilation of the pupil. 2. an agent that reverses dilation of the pupil.

an·ti·nar·cot·ic (an″ti-nahr-kot′ik) counteracting narcotic depression.

an·ti·na·tri·ure·sis (an″te-, an″ti-na″tre-u-re′sis) opposition to normal natriuresis.

an·ti·nau·se·ant (an″te-, an″ti-naw′ze-ənt) 1. preventing or relieving nausea. 2. an agent that prevents or relieves nausea; see also *antiemetic*.

an·ti·neo·plas·tic (an″te-, an″ti-ne″o-plas′tik) 1. inhibiting or preventing the development of neoplasms; checking the maturation and proliferation of malignant cells. 2. an agent having such properties.

an·ti·neo·plas·tons (an″te-ne″o-plas′tonz) a group of antineoplastic peptides and amino acid derivatives, originally isolated from blood and urine, that inhibit the growth of tumor cells; used investigationally in the treatment of cancer.

an·ti·ne·phrit·ic (an″te-, an″ti-nə-frit′ik) counteracting inflammation of the kidneys.

an·ti·neu·ral·gic (an″te-, an″ti-noo͝-ral′jik) counteracting neuralgia.

an·ti·neu·rit·ic (an″te-, an″ti-noo͝-rit′ik) counteracting neuritis.

an·ti·neu·ro·tox·in (an″ti-noor′o-tok″sin) a substance that counteracts a neurotoxin.

an·ti·neu·tri·no (an″te-, an″ti-noo-tre′no) the antiparticle of the neutrino.

an·ti·neu·tron (an″te-, an″ti-noo′tron) an elementary particle without a charge and with a mass and spin equal to that of a neutron, but with magnetic moment opposite to that of a neutron; the antiparticle of a neutron.

an·tin·i·ad (an-tin′e-ad) toward the antinion.

an·tin·ion (an-tin′e-on) [*anti-* + *inion*] the frontal pole of the head; the median frontal point farthest from the inion. anti′nial *adj*

an·ti·no·ci·cep·tive (an″te-, an″ti-no″sĭ-sep′tiv) blocking or reducing sensitivity to painful stimuli; cf. *analgesic*.

an·ti·nu·cle·ar (an″te-, an″ti-noo′kle-ər) destructive to or reactive with components of the cell nucleus, as antinuclear antibody.

an·ti·odon·tal·gic (an″te-o″don-tal′jik) relieving toothache.

an·ti·on·co·gene (an″te-ong′ko-jēn″) tumor suppressor gene.

an·ti·op·so·nin (an″te-op′so-nin) a substance that has an inhibitory influence on opsonins; called also *antitropin*.

an·ti·ov·u·la·to·ry (an″te-ov′u-lə-tor″e) suppressing ovulation.

an·ti·ox·i·dant (an″te-ok′sĭ-dənt) 1. preventing or delaying oxidation. 2. a substance that prevents or delays oxidation, such as any of numerous synthetic or natural substances added to something to prevent or delay its deterioration by action of oxygen in the air. Rubber, paints, vegetable oils, and prepared foods commonly contain antioxidants.

an·ti·ox·i·da·tion (an″te-ok-sĭ-da′shən) the prevention of oxidation.

an·ti·oxy·gen (an″te-ok′sĭ-jen) antioxidant.

an·ti·par·al·lel (an″te-, an″ti-par′ə-lel) denoting molecules that are arranged side by side, but in opposite directions. For example, the strands of deoxyribonucleic acid are antiparallel, with their 5′ to 3′ linkages running in opposite directions.

an·ti·par·a·lyt·ic (an″te-, an″ti-par″ə-lit′ik) relieving paralysis.

an·ti·par·a·sit·ic (an″te-, an″ti-par″ə-sit′ik) 1. destroying parasites. 2. an agent that destroys parasites.

an·ti·para·sym·patho·mi·met·ic (an″te-, an″ti-par″ə-sim″pə-tho-mĭ-met′ik) opposing or blocking a parasympathomimetic agent or effect.

an·ti·par·kin·so·ni·an (an″te-, an″ti-pahr″kin-so′ne-ən) 1. effective against parkinsonism. 2. an agent having this effect.

an·ti·par·ti·cle (an′tĭ-pahr″tĭ-kəl) either of a pair of particles, as an electron and a positron, that are identical in mass and spin but opposite in charge and magnetic moment; the collision of two antiparticles results in annihilation.

an·ti·pe·ri·od·ic (an″te-, an″ti-pēr″e-od′ik) preventing periodic recurrence of symptoms, as in malaria.

an·ti·per·i·stal·sis (an″te-, an″ti-per″ĭ-stawl′sis) peristalsis that impels intestinal contents in the reverse direction from normal; called also *retrograde* or *reversed peristalsis*.

an·ti·per·i·stal·tic (an″te-, an″ti-per′ĭ-stawl′tik) 1. pertaining to or causing antiperistalsis. 2. diminishing peristaltic action. 3. an agent that diminishes peristaltic action.

an·ti·per·spir·ant (an″te-, an″ti-pur′spər-ant) 1. inhibiting or preventing sweating. 2. an agent that inhibits or prevents sweating.

an·ti·phago·cyt·ic (an″te-, an″ti-fa-go-sit′ik) counteracting or opposing phagocytosis.

an·ti·phlo·gis·tic (an″te-, an″ti-flo-jis′tik) 1. counteracting inflammation and fever. 2. an agent that counteracts inflammation and fever.

an·ti·plas·min (an″te-, an″ti-plaz′min) a substance in the blood that inhibits plasmin.

α_2-a. the most important inhibitor of fibrinolysis, an α_2-globulin, M_r 53,000, found in large quantities in normal blood; it is synthesized predominantly in the liver and functions by forming stable complexes with free plasmin. It is also cross-linked to fibrin by the action of coagulation factor XIII and inhibits the binding of plasminogen to fibrin. Deficiency of this protein, an autosomal recessive trait, is associated with severe bleeding, including hemarthrosis.

an·ti·plas·mo·di·al (an″tĭ-plaz-mo′de-əl) antimalarial.

an·ti·plas·tic (an″te-, an″ti-plas′tik) [*anti-* + *plastic*] 1. unfavorable to the healing process. 2. suppressing cell formation. 3. myelosuppressive.

an·ti·plate·let (an″te-, an″ti-plāt′lət) directed against or destructive to blood platelets; called also *antithrombocytic*. See also *platelet inhibitor*, under *inhibitor*.

an·ti·pneu·mo·coc·cal (an″te-, an″ti-noo″mo-kok′əl) destroying or inhibiting the growth of *Streptococcus pneumoniae*.

an·ti·pneu·mo·coc·cic (an″te-, an″ti-noo″mo-kok′sik) antipneumococcal.

an·ti·po·dag·ric (an″te-, an″ti-pə-dag′rik) effective against gout.

an·tip·o·dal (an-tip′ə-dəl) occupying opposite positions, as of a cell or body; diametrically opposed.

an·ti·pode (an′tĭ-pōd) something occupying a directly opposed position. In chemistry, a molecule whose atoms are arranged in a directly opposite manner.

an·ti·poly·cy·the·mic (an″te-, an″ti-pol″e-si-the′mik) 1. effective against polycythemia. 2. an agent with this effect.

an·ti·port (an′tĭ-port) a cotransport mechanism that couples the transport of two compounds across a membrane in opposite directions. Cf. *symport*.

an·ti·port·er (an′te-port″ər) a membrane transport protein that mediates the cotransport of substances in opposite directions.

an·ti·po·sia (an″tĭ-po′zhə) antipathy to drinking.

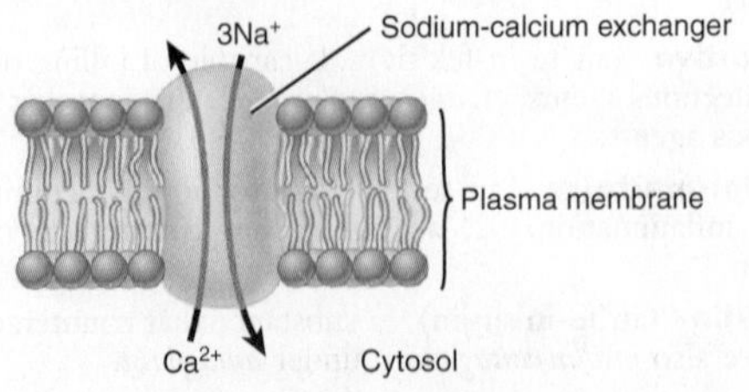

■ Antiport: sodium-calcium exchanger. The electrochemical gradient of Na^+ is used to pump Ca^{2+} out of the cell and thereby regulate the cytosolic Ca^{2+} level.

an•ti•pre•ci•pi•tin (an″te-, an″ti-pre-sip′ĭ-tin) a substance antagonistic in its action to precipitin.

an•ti•pro•ges•tin (an″te-, an″ti-pro-jes′tin) a substance that inhibits the formation, transport, or action of progestational agents, e.g., mifepristone.

an•ti•pro•lif•er•a•tive (an″te-, an″ti-pro-lif′ər-ə-tiv) 1. blocking proliferation, especially of cancer cells. 2. an agent that blocks the proliferation of cancer cells.

an•ti•pro•throm•bin (an″te-, an″ti-pro-throm′bin) 1. directed against prothrombin. 2. any of a diverse group of anticoagulants that retard the conversion of prothrombin to thrombin by any means.

an•ti•pro•to•zo•al (an″te-, an″ti-pro-tə-zo′əl) 1. destroying protozoa, or checking their growth or reproduction. 2. an agent that destroys parasites or checks their growth or reproduction.

an•ti•pro•to•zo•an (an″te-, an″ti-pro-tə-zo′ən) antiprotozoal.

an•ti•pru•rit•ic (an″te-, an″ti-proo-rit′ik) 1. relieving or preventing itching. 2. an agent that relieves or prevents itching.

an•ti•pso•ri•at•ic (an″te-, an″ti-sor″e-at′ik) 1. effective against psoriasis. 2. an agent with that effect.

an•ti•psy•cho•mo•tor (an″te-, an″ti-si′ko-mo′tər) suppressing or inhibiting hyperactivity or hyperkinesis.

an•ti•psy•chot•ic (an″te-, an″ti-si-kot′ik) 1. effective in treatment of psychosis. 2. an agent for treating psychosis. Antipsychotics are a chemically diverse group (including phenothiazines, thioxanthenes, butyrophenones, dibenzoxazepines, dibenzodiazepines, dihydroindolones, and diphenylbutylpiperidines), although they are pharmacologically similar; used to treat schizophrenic, paranoid, schizoaffective, and other psychotic disorders; acute delirium and dementia and manic episodes; to control the movement disorders associated with Huntington chorea, Gilles de la Tourette syndrome, and ballismus; and to treat intractable hiccups and severe nausea and vomiting. Antipsychotic agents bind to dopamine, histamine, muscarinic cholinergic, α-adrenergic, and serotonin receptors. Blockade of dopaminergic transmission in various areas is thought to be responsible for their major effects: antipsychotic action by blockade in the mesolimbic and mesocortical areas; extrapyramidal side effects (dystonia, akathisia, parkinsonism, and tardive dyskinesia) by blockade in the basal ganglia; and antiemetic effects by blockade in the chemoreceptor trigger zone of the medulla. Sedation and autonomic side effects (orthostatic hypotension, blurred vision, dry mouth, nasal congestion, and constipation) are caused by blockade of histamine, cholinergic, and adrenergic receptors. Called also *neuroleptic.*

an•ti•pu•tre•fac•tive (an″te-, an″ti-pu″trə-fak′tiv) counteracting putrefaction.

an•ti•pyo•gen•ic (an″te-, an″ti-pi″o-jen′ik) [*anti-* + *pyogenic*] pyostatic.

an•ti•py•re•sis (an″te-, an″ti-pi-re′sis) [*anti-* + Gr. *pyressein* to have a fever] the therapeutic use of antipyretics.

an•ti•py•ret•ic (an″te-, an″ti-pi-ret′ik) [*anti-* + *pyretic*] 1. relieving or reducing fever; called also *antifebrile.* 2. an agent that relieves fever; called also *febrifuge.*

an•ti•py•rine (an″te-pi′rēn) [USP] a pyrazolone analgesic and antipyretic. Because it can cause agranulocytosis, it has been replaced by safer and more effective agents. Now used as a component of antipyrine and benzocaine otic solution; as a component of antipyrine, benzocaine, and phenylephrine otic solution; and complexed with chloral hydrate in dichloralphenazone. Called also *phenazone.*

an•ti•py•rot•ic (an″te-, an″ti-pi-rot′ik) [*anti-* + *pyrotic*] 1. therapeutically effective against burns. 2. an agent with this effect.

an•ti•ra•chit•ic (an″te-, an″ti-rə-kit′ik) therapeutically effective against rickets.

an•ti•ra•di•a•tion (an″te-, an″ti-ra″de-a′shən) capable of counteracting the effects of radiation; effective against radiation injury.

an•ti•re•flux (an″te-, an″tĭ-re′fluks) counteracting gastroesophageal reflux.

an•ti•re•sorp•tive (an″te-, an″ti-re-sorp′tiv) opposing resorption, such as that occurring in osteoporosis; said of drugs or other therapeutic measures.

an•ti•ret•ro•vi•ral (an″te-, an″ti-ret′ro-vi″rəl) 1. effective against retroviruses. 2. an agent having this effect.

an•ti•rheu•mat•ic (an″te-, an″ti-roo-mat′ik) [*anti-* + *rheumatic*] 1. relieving or preventing rheumatism or other rheumatoid conditions. 2. an agent for relieving or preventing rheumatoid conditions.

an•ti•ri•cin (an″te-ri′sin) a substance such as an antitoxin that opposes the action of ricin.

an•ti•rick•ett•si•al (an″te-, an″ti-rĭ-ket′se-əl) 1. effective against rickettsiae. 2. an agent having this quality.

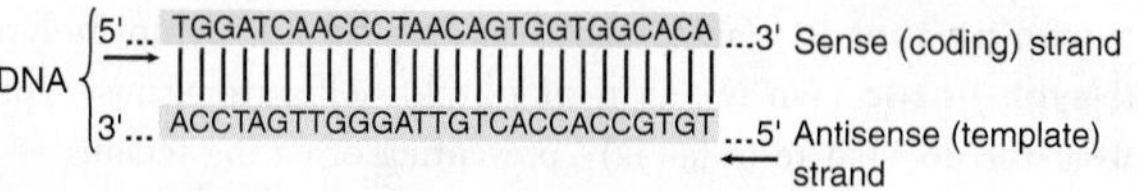

■ Antisense strand of DNA, complementary to the sense (coding) strand and serving as a template for RNA synthesis.

an•ti•ro•bin (an″tĭ-ro′bin) the antitoxin of robin, a poison of the locust tree.

an•ti•schis•to•so•mal (an″te-, an″ti-shis″to-so′məl) 1. suppressing or killing schistosomes. 2. an agent that suppresses or kills schistosomes.

an•ti•scor•bu•tic (an″te-, an″ti-skor-bu′tik) [*anti-* + *scorbutus*] effective in the prevention or relief of scurvy.

an•ti•seb•or•rhe•ic (an″te-, an″ti-seb″o-re′ik) 1. effective in the prevention or relief of seborrheic dermatitis or of the excessive secretion of sebum. 2. an agent that prevents or relieves seborrheic dermatitis or excessive secretion of sebum.

an•ti•se•cre•to•ry (an″te-, an″ti-sə-kre′to-re) 1. inhibiting or diminishing secretions, such as in the stomach; called also *secretoinhibitory.* 2. an agent that inhibits or prevents secretions.

an•ti•sense (an″te-, an′ti-sens) pertaining to the strand of a double-stranded molecule that does not directly encode the product but is complementary to it; see under *strand* and *RNA.*

an•ti•sep•sis (an″tĭ-sep′sis) [*anti-* + *sepsis*] 1. the prevention of sepsis by antiseptic means. 2. any procedure that reduces to a significant degree the microbial flora of skin or mucous membranes. Cf. *disinfection.*

an•ti•sep•tic (an″tĭ-sep′tik) 1. pertaining to antisepsis. 2. preventing decay or putrefaction. 3. a substance that inhibits the growth and development of microorganisms without necessarily killing them. Cf. *disinfectant.*

an•ti•se•rum (an″tĭ-se′rəm) a serum that contains antibody or antibodies; it may be obtained from an animal that has been immunized either by injection of antigen into the body or by infection with microorganisms containing the antigen. Antisera may be monovalent (specific for one antigen) or polyvalent (specific for more than one antigen).

Erysipelothrix rhusiopathiae a. an antiserum prepared by hyperimmunization of horses with *Erysipelothrix rhusiopathiae,* used for prevention and treatment of swine erysipelas.

an•ti•si•al•a•gogue (an″te-, an″ti-si-al′ə-gog) 1. counteracting the formation of saliva. 2. an agent that prevents secretion of saliva.

an•ti•si•al•ic (an″te-, an″ti-si-al′ik) 1. checking the secretion of saliva. 2. an agent that checks the secretion of saliva.

an•ti•sid•er•ic (an″te-, an″ti-sĭ-der′ik) [*anti-* + *sider-* + *-ic*] incompatible with iron.

an•ti•so•cial (an″te-, an″ti-so′shəl) 1. denoting behavior that violates the rights of others, societal mores, or the law. 2. denoting the specific personality traits seen in antisocial personality disorder.

an•ti•spas•mod•ic (an″te-, an″ti-spaz-mod′ik) 1. relieving spasms, usually of smooth muscles and sometimes of voluntary muscles. Cf. *antispastic.* 2. an agent that relieves spasms. Called also *spasmolytic.*

biliary a. an agent that relieves spasm of the biliary duct and sphincter.

bronchial a. an agent that relieves bronchial spasm.

an•ti•spas•tic (an″te-, an″ti-spas′tik) antispasmodic with specific reference to skeletal muscle.

an•ti•staph•y•lo•coc•cal (an″te-, an″ti-staf″ə-lo-kok′əl) 1. killing or suppressing staphylococci. 2. an agent that kills or suppresses staphylococci.

an•ti•staph•y•lo•he•mol•y•sin (an″te-, an″ti-staf″ə-lo-he-mol′ĭ-sin) antistaphylolysin.

an•ti•staph•y•lol•y•sin (an″te-, an″ti-staf-ə-lol′ĭ-sin) an antibody that opposes the action of staphylolysin.

an•ti•ste•ril•i•ty (an″te-, an″ti-stə-ril′ĭ-te) combating sterility or promoting fertility.

an•ti•strep•to•coc•cal (an″te-, an″ti-strep″to-kok′əl) 1. effective against streptococci. 2. an agent having this effect.

an•ti•strep•to•ki•nase (an″te-, an″ti-strep″to-ki′nās) an antibody that inhibits streptokinase.

an•ti•strep•tol•y•sin (an″te-, an″ti-strep-tol′ĭ-sin) an antibody that inhibits streptolysin.

an•ti•su•do•rif•ic (an″te-, an″ti-soo″də-rif′ik) antiperspirant.

an·ti·sym·pa·thet·ic (an″te-, an″ti-sim″pə-thet′ik) sympatholytic.

an·ti·syph·i·lit·ic (an″te-, an″ti-sif″ĭ-lit′ik) effective against syphilis.

an·ti·te·tan·ic (an″te-tə-tan′ik) preventing or curing tetanus.

an·ti·the·nar (an″te-the′nar) [*anti-* + *thenar*] situated opposite to the palm or the sole.

an·ti·ther·mic (an″te-thur′mik) [*anti-* + *thermic*] antipyretic (def. 1).

an·ti·throm·bin (an″te-throm′bin) [*anti-* + *thrombin*] any naturally occurring or therapeutically administered substance that neutralizes the action of thrombin and thus limits or restricts blood coagulation. Six naturally occurring antithrombins have been designated by Roman numerals I to VI; antithrombins I and III are the most common and significant ones. Heparin is also considered an antithrombin.

a. I fibrin; referring to the capacity of fibrin to adsorb large amounts of thrombin and thus neutralize (but not inactivate) it.

a. III an α_2-globulin of the serpin family synthesized in the liver and found in plasma and various extravascular sites, which inactivates thrombin in a time-dependent irreversible reaction. It also inhibits certain other proteinases with serine active sites, including coagulation factors Xa, XIIa, XIa, and IXa, and kallikrein. Inherited deficiency of the protein, a rare autosomal dominant disorder, is associated with recurrent deep vein thrombosis and pulmonary emboli; the complications are prevented and, in conjunction with heparin, treated with a preparation of antithrombin III from pooled human plasma, administered intravenously.

an·ti·throm·bo·cyt·ic (an″te-, an″ti-throm″bo-sit′ik) antiplatelet.

an·ti·throm·bo·plas·tin (an″te-, an″ti-throm″bo-plas′tin) any agent or substance that prevents or interferes with the interaction of the blood coagulation factors as they generate prothrombinase.

an·ti·throm·bot·ic (an″te-, an″ti-throm-bot′ik) 1. preventing or interfering with the formation of thrombi. 2. an agent that prevents or slows the formation of thrombi; see also *anticoagulant* and *thrombolytic.*

an·ti·thy·roid (an″te-thi′roid) counteracting the functioning of the thyroid, especially in its synthesis of thyroid hormones.

an·ti·thy·ro·tox·ic (an″te-thi″ro-tok′sik) counteracting the toxic effects of excessive amounts of thyroid hormones.

an·ti·thy·ro·tro·pic (an″te-thi″ro-tro′pik) inhibiting the secretion or actions of thyrotropin.

an·ti·ton·ic (an″te-ton′ik) reducing tone or tonicity of muscle or other tissue.

an·ti·tox·ic (an″te-, an″ti-tok′sik) 1. effective against a poison. 2. pertaining to antitoxin.

an·ti·tox·i·gen (an″te-tok′sĭ-jən) antitoxinogen.

an·ti·tox·in (an″tĭ-tok′sin) 1. antibody against a toxin. 2. a purified antiserum from animals (usually horses) immunized by injections of a toxin or toxoid, administered as a passive immunizing agent to neutralize a specific bacterial toxin, e.g., botulinus, tetanus, or diphtheria.

botulinal a., botulinum a., botulinus a. botulism a.

botulism a. [USP] an equine antitoxin against the toxins produced by the type A and type B and/or type E strains of *Clostridium botulinum;* administered intravenously in the postexposure prophylaxis and treatment of botulism, other than infant botulism.

bovine a. antitoxin containing antibodies derived from the cow instead of from the horse, for use on persons who are hypersensitive to horse serum.

***Clostridium perfringens* types C and D a.** an antitoxin prepared from serum of animals hyperimmunized with toxins of *C. perfringens* types C and D, administered immediately after birth for prevention of enterotoxemia in calves, lambs, and suckling pigs.

diphtheria a. [USP] equine antitoxin from horses immunized against diphtheria toxin or the toxoid; administered intramuscularly or intravenously in the treatment of suspected cases of diphtheria.

equine a. an antitoxin derived from the blood of healthy horses that have been immunized against a specific bacterial toxin.

tetanus a. [USP] equine antitoxin from horses that have been immunized against tetanus toxin or toxoid; used for the passive prevention and treatment of tetanus. It is rarely used, tetanus immune globulin being preferred.

an·ti·tox·in·o·gen (an″te-, an″ti-tok-sin′o-jen) [*antitoxin* + *-gen*] an antigen that stimulates the production of antitoxin, i.e., a toxin or toxoid.

an·ti·trag·i·cus (an″tĭ-traj′ĭ-kəs) see under *musculus.*

an·ti·tra·gus (an″te-tra′gəs) [*anti-* + *tragus*] [TA] a projection opposite the tragus, bounding the cavitas conchae posteroinferiorly and continuous above with the antihelix.

an·ti·trep·o·ne·mal (an″te-, an″ti-trep″o-ne′məl) effective against *Treponema;* cf. *antisyphilitic.*

an·ti·trich·o·mo·nal (an″te-, an″ti-trik″o-mo′nəl) 1. killing or suppressing *Trichomonas.* 2. an antiprotozoal agent that kills or suppresses *Trichomonas.*

an·ti·tris·mus (an″te-triz′məs) a spasm that prevents the closure of the mouth.

an·ti·trope (an′tĭ-trōp) [*anti-* + Gr. *trepein* to turn] any organ that forms a symmetrical pair with another.

an·ti·tro·pic (an″tĭ-tro′pik) corresponding, but oppositely oriented, as a right and a left glove.

an·ti·tro·pin (an″tĭ-tro′pin) antiopsonin.

an·ti·try·pan·o·so·mal (an″te-, an″ti-trĭ-pan″ə-so′məl) 1. killing or suppressing trypanosomes. 2. an agent that kills or suppresses trypanosomes.

α_1-an·ti·tryp·sin (an″tĭ-trip′sin) alpha$_1$-antitrypsin.

an·ti·tu·ber·cu·lar (an″te-, an″ti-too-bur′ku-lər) 1. therapeutically effective against tuberculosis; called also *antituberculous.* 2. an agent with this characteristic.

an·ti·tu·ber·cu·lin (an″te-too-bur′ku-lin) an antibody developed following the injection of tuberculin.

an·ti·tu·ber·cu·lot·ic (an″te-too-bur″ku-lot′ik) antitubercular.

an·ti·tu·ber·cu·lous (an″te-too-bur′ku-ləs) antitubercular (def. 1).

an·ti·tu·bu·lin (an″te-too′bu-lin) 1. an agent that prevents the polymerization of tubulin, and thus the formation of microtubules in a cell. 2. directed against tubulin, as antitubulin antibodies.

an·ti·tu·mor·i·gen·ic (an″tĭ-too″mər-ĭ-jen′ik) counteracting tumor formation.

an·ti·tus·sive (an″te-, an″ti-tus′iv) 1. relieving or preventing cough. 2. an agent that relieves or prevents cough.

an·ti·ty·phoid (an″te-ti′foid) counteracting or preventing typhoid fever.

an·ti·ul·cer·a·tive (an″te-ul′sə-ra″tiv, an″te-ul′sər-ə-tiv) 1. preventing ulcers or promoting their healing. 2. an agent that prevents or treats ulcers.

an·ti·uro·lith·ic (an″te-u″ro-lith′ik) 1. preventing the formation of urinary calculi. 2. an agent that prevents formation of urinary calculi.

an·ti·vac·ci·na·tion·ist (an″te-vak″sĭ-na′shən-ist) a person who is opposed to vaccination.

an·ti·ven·ene (an″te-, an″ti-vĕ-nēn′) antivenin.

an·ti·ven·in (an″te-, an″ti-ven′in) [*anti-* + L. *venenum* poison] an antitoxin used in treatment of poisoning by animal venom.

black widow spider a. a. *(Latrodectus mactans).*

crotalid a. an antivenin against the venom of crotalid snakes (pit vipers, including rattlesnakes); see *a. (Crotalidae) polyvalent* and see *Crotalidae polyvalent immune Fab,* under *Fab.*

a. (Crotalidae) polyvalent [USP] a lyophilized preparation containing specific venom-neutralizing globulins obtained from the serum of horses immunized with the venoms of *Crotalus atrox* (western diamondback rattlesnake), *C. adamanteus* (eastern diamondback rattlesnake), *C. durissus terrificus* (tropical rattlesnake), and *Bothrops atrox;* used to neutralize the effects of envenomation by pit vipers native to North, Central, and South America.

Fab a. see *Crotalidae polyvalent immune Fab,* under *Fab.*

a. *(Latrodectus mactans)* [USP] a lyophilized preparation containing specific venom-neutralizing globulins obtained from the serum of horses immunized with the venom of *Latrodectus mactans* (the black widow spider); occasionally used to treat the symptoms of black widow spider bites. Called also *black widow spider a.*

a. *(Micrurus fulvius)* [USP], **North American coral snake a.** a lyophilized preparation containing specific venom-neutralizing globulins obtained from the serum of horses immunized with the venom of *Micrurus fulvius* (the eastern coral snake); used to neutralize the effects of envenomation by the eastern coral snake *(M. fulvius fulvius)* and the Texas coral snake *(M. fulvius tenere).*

polyvalent crotaline a. a. (Crotalidae) polyvalent.

an·ti·ven·om (an″te-, an″ti-ven′om) antivenin.

an·ti·ven·om·ous (an″te-, an′ti-ven′ə-məs) antitoxic (def. 1).

An·ti·vert (an′tĭ-vert″) trademark for preparations of meclizine hydrochloride.

an·ti·vi·ral (an″te-, an″ti-vi′rəl) 1. destroying viruses or suppressing their replication. 2. an agent that destroys viruses or suppresses their replication.

an·ti·vi·rot·ic (an″te-, an″ti-vi-rot′ik) antiviral.

an·ti·vi·ta·min (an″te-, an″ti-vi′tə-min) a substance that interferes with the synthesis or metabolism of a vitamin.

an•ti•vivi•sec•tion (an″te-, an″ti-viv″ĭ-sek′shən) opposition to vivisection.

an•ti•vivi•sec•tion•ist (an″te-, an″ti-viv″ĭ-sek′shən-ist) an individual opposed to vivisection.

an•ti•xen•ic (an″te-, an″ti-ze′nik) [*anti-* + *xen-* + *-ic*] pertaining to the reaction of living tissue to any foreign substance.

an•ti•xe•roph•thal•mic (an″te-, an″ti-zēr″of-thal′mik) counteracting xerophthalmia.

An•ti•zol (an′tĭ-zol) trademark for a preparation of fomepizole.

ant•odon•tal•gic (ant″o-don-tal′jik) antiodontalgic.

An•ton syndrome (ahn′ton) [Gabriel *Anton*, German neuropsychiatrist, 1858–1933] see under *syndrome.*

An•ton-Ba•bin•ski syndrome (ahn′ton bə-bin′ske) [G. *Anton;* Joseph François Félix *Babinski*, French physician, 1857–1932] Anton syndrome.

ant•oph•thal•mic (ant″of-thal′mik) relieving ophthalmia.

an•tra (an′trə) [L.] plural of *antrum.*

an•trec•to•my (an-trek′tə-me) [*antr-* + *-ectomy*] surgical excision of an antrum, such as the pyloric antrum of the stomach.

an•tri•tis (an-tri′tis) 1. inflammation of an antrum, usually referring to the pyloric antrum. 2. maxillary sinusitis.

antr(o)- [L. *antrum*, q.v.] a combining form denoting relationship to an antrum, or sinus; often used with specific reference to the maxillary antrum, or sinus.

an•tro•at•ti•cot•o•my (an″tro-at″ĭ-kot′ə-me) atticoantrotomy.

an•tro•buc•cal (an″tro-buk′əl) pertaining to or communicating between the maxillary antrum (maxillary sinus) and the oral cavity.

an•tro•cele (an′tro-sēl) [*antro-* + *-cele*[1]] a cystic accumulation of fluid in the maxillary antrum (sinus).

an•tro•du•o•de•nal (an″tro-doo″o-de′nəl) [*antro-* + *duodenal*] pertaining to the pyloric antrum and the duodenum.

an•tro•du•o•de•nec•to•my (an″tro-doo″o-de-nek′tə-me) surgical removal of the pyloric antrum and adjacent portion of the duodenum, formerly done in the treatment of duodenal ulcer.

an•tro•dyn•ia (an″tro-din′e-ə) [*antro-* + *-odynia*] pain in an antrum.

an•tro•na•sal (an″tro-na′zəl) pertaining to the maxillary antrum and the nose.

an•tro•phose (an′tro-fōz) [*antro-* + *phose*] a phose originating in the central ocular mechanism.

an•tro•py•lo•ric (an″tro-pi-lor′ik) pertaining to or affecting the pyloric part of the stomach, including its antrum.

an•tro•scope (an′trə-skōp″) [*antro-* + *-scope*] an instrument for illuminating and examining the maxillary antrum.

an•tros•co•py (an-tros′kə-pe) inspection of an antrum using an antroscope.

an•tros•to•my (an-tros′tə-me) [*antro-* + *-stomy*] the operation of making an opening into an antrum for purposes of drainage.

an•trot•o•my (an-trot′ə-me) [*antro-* + *-tomy*] antrostomy.

an•tro•tym•pan•ic (an″tro-tim-pan′ik) pertaining to the mastoid antrum and the tympanic cavity.

an•trum (an′trəm) pl. *an′tra, antrums* [L., from Gr. *antron* cave] a cavity or chamber, such as one within a bone or organ. an′tral *adj*

a. au′ris meatus acusticus externus.

cardiac a. the short conical portion of the esophagus below the diaphragm, its base being continuous with the cardiac orifice of the stomach.

ethmoid a. bulla ethmoidalis.

follicular a. a cavity filled with follicular fluid on one side of a vesicular ovarian follicle in its later stages of growth just prior to ovulation.

frontal a. sinus frontalis.

gastric a. a. pyloricum.

a. of Highmore sinus maxillaris.

mastoid a., a. mastoi′deum [TA] an air space in the mastoid portion of the temporal bone, communicating with the tympanic cavity and the mastoid cells; called also *tympanic a.* and *mastoid cavity.*

maxillary a. sinus maxillaris.

pyloric a., a. pylo′ricum [TA] the dilated portion of the pyloric part of the stomach, distal to the body of the stomach and proximal to the pyloric canal. Called also *gastric a.* and *a. of stomach.*

retained gastric a. gastric antrum retained after a partial gastrectomy; see under *syndrome.*

a. of stomach a. pyloricum.

tympanic a. a. mastoideum.

An•try•pol (an′trə-pol) trademark for a preparation of suramin hexasodium.

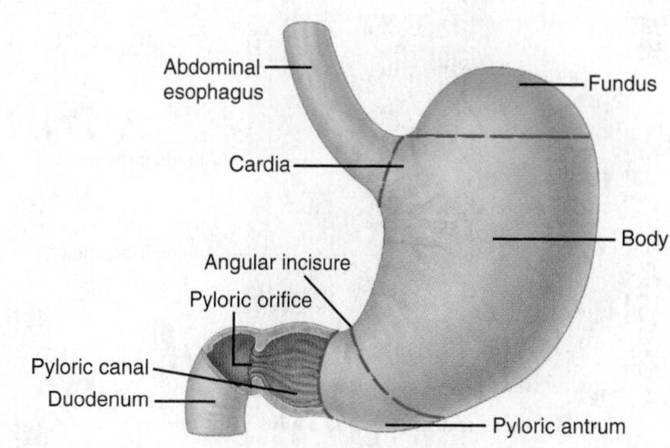

■ Antrum pyloricum (pyloric antrum) in relation to other parts of the stomach.

ANTU alphanaphthyl thiourea, a compound used as a rodenticide; it produces massive pulmonary edema and pleural effusion in rats and many other mammals.

An•tu•rane (an′choo-rān) trademark for a preparation of sulfinpyrazone.

Anu•sol (an′u-sol) trademark for preparations of hydrocortisone acetate.

a•nu•cle•ar (a-noo′kle-ər) anucleate.

anu•cle•ate (a-noo′kle-it) having no nucleus; used especially of cells that have lost their nuclei during maturation (such as erythrocytes) or through a pathologic process. Called also *anuclear* and *anucleated.*

a•nu•cle•at•ed (a-noo′kle-āt″əd) anucleate.

ANUG acute necrotizing ulcerative gingivitis.

anu•lo•plas•ty (an′u-lo-plas″te) annuloplasty.

anu•lus (an′u-ləs) gen. and pl. *a′nuli* [L., from *anus* ring] ring: preferred spelling in official terminology (TA) for a circular or ringlike structure; spelled also *annulus.* See also *circle* and *circulus.*

atrioventricular anuli, atrioventricular valve anuli see *a. fibrosus dexter/sinister cordis.*

a. conjunc′tivae [TA] conjunctival ring: a ring at the junction of the conjunctiva and cornea.

a. femora′lis [TA] femoral ring: the abdominal opening of the femoral canal, normally closed by the crural septum and peritoneum.

a. fibrocartilagi′neus membra′nae tym′pani [TA] fibrocartilaginous ring of tympanic membrane: the margin of the pars tensa of the tympanic membrane, which attaches to the sulcus tympanicus.

a. fibro′sus dex′ter/sinis′ter cor′dis [TA] right/left fibrous ring of heart: one of the dense fibrous rings that surround the right and left atrioventricular orifices. To these rings, either directly or indirectly, are attached the atrial and ventricular muscle fibers. The rings form part of the cardiac skeleton. Called also *Lower rings.*

a. fibro′sus dis′ci intervertebra′lis [TA] anulus fibrosus of intervertebral disk: the circumferential ringlike portion of an intervertebral disk, composed of fibrocartilage and fibrous tissue.

a. inguina′lis profun′dus [TA] deep inguinal ring: an aperture in the fascia transversalis for the spermatic cord or for the round ligament; called also *abdominal ring* and *internal inguinal ring.*

a. inguina′lis superficia′lis [TA] superficial inguinal ring: an opening in the aponeurosis of the external oblique muscle for the spermatic cord or for the round ligament; called also *external inguinal ring.*

a. i′ridis ma′jor [TA] greater ring of iris: the less coarsely striated outer concentric circle on the anterior surface of the iris; called also *greater circle of iris.*

a. i′ridis mi′nor [TA] lesser ring of iris: the more coarsely striated inner concentric circle on the anterior surface of the iris; called also *lesser circle of iris.*

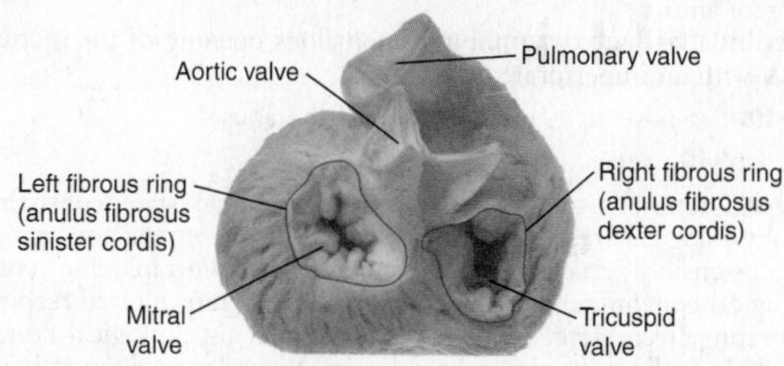

■ Anuli fibrosi cordis (fibrous rings of heart), one surrounding each of the two atrioventricular valves.

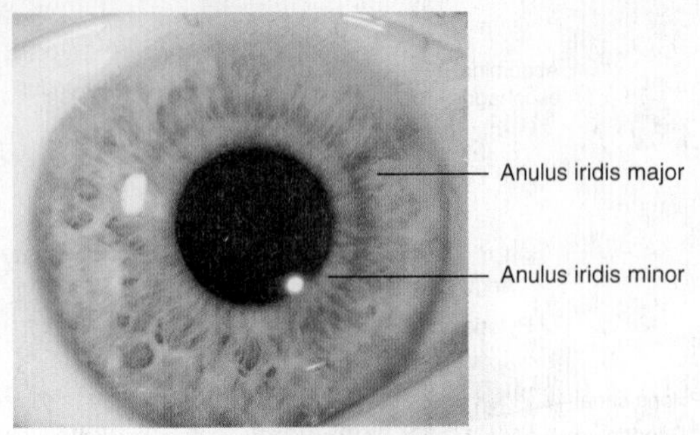

■ Anulus iridis major and anulus iridis minor.

a. lympha′ticus car′diae [TA] cardiac lymphatic ring: a chain of lymph nodes (paracardial lymph nodes) around the cardiac opening of the stomach.

mitral a., mitral valve a. see *a. fibrosus dexter/sinister cordis.*

a. of spermatozoon a dark ringlike structure at the posterior end of the middle piece of a spermatozoon. Called also *ring centriole.*

a. tendi′neus commu′nis [TA] common tendinous ring: the annular ligament of origin common to the recti muscles of the eye, attached to the edge of the optic canal and the inner part of the superior orbital fissure; called also *anulus of Zinn, Zinn ligament* or *ring,* and *common annular tendon.*

tricuspid a., tricuspid valve a. see *a. fibrosus dexter/sinister cordis.*

a. tympa′nicus [TA] tympanic anulus or ring: the bony ring forming part of the temporal bone at the time of birth and developing into the pars tympanica of the bone.

a. umbilica′lis [TA] umbilical ring: the aperture in the abdominal wall through which the umbilical cord communicates with the fetus. After birth it is felt for some time as a distinct fibrous ring surrounding the umbilicus; these fibers later shrink progressively. Called also *umbilical canal.*

a. urethra′lis musculus sphincter urethrae internus.

a. of Zinn a. tendineus communis.

Anu•ra (ə-nu′rə) an order of amphibians, including the frogs and toads.

anu•ran (ə-nu′rən) any member of Anura.

an•ure•sis (an″u-re′sis) 1. urinary retention. 2. anuria.

an•uret•ic (an-u-ret′ik) 1. pertaining to or characterized by urinary retention. 2. anuric.

an•uria (an-u′re-ə) [*an-*[1] + *-uria*] suppression of urine formation and excretion; called also *anuresis.* **anu′ric** *adj*

obstructive a., postrenal a. anuria resulting from obstruction of the ureters or urethra.

prerenal a. anuria resulting from fall of blood pressure below the level necessary to maintain adequate filtration pressure in the glomeruli.

renal a. anuria due to disease within the kidney itself, in spite of adequate glomerular filtration pressure and patency of the ureters.

an•u•rous (an-u′rəs) [*an-*[1] + Gr. *oura* tail] acaudate.

anus (a′nəs) gen. and pl. *a′ni* [L. "ring, circle"] [TA] the distal or terminal orifice of the digestive tract, located in the gluteal cleft. **a′nal** *adj*

artificial a. an opening from the colon formed by the creation of a colostomy.

ectopic a. an anus that opens in an abnormal location; see *a. vesicalis* and *a. vestibularis.*

imperforate a. persistence of the anal epithelial plug, so that the anus is closed. The defect is not always complete; sometimes a narrow opening permits passage of contents of the colon. When the anus is completely imperforate, there is simply a dimple in the skin of the perineum; this condition is often associated with atresia of the lower rectum. Called also *anal atresia, atresia ani,* and *proctatresia.*

a. of Rusconi blastopore.

a. vesica′lis anomalous opening of the rectum into the bladder with an imperforate anus.

a. vestibula′ris, vulvovaginal a. anomalous opening of the rectum on the vulva with an imperforate anus.

anus•i•tis (a-nəs-i′tis) inflammation of the anus.

an•vil (an′vil) incus.

an•xi•e•ty (ang-zi′ə-te) the unpleasant emotional state consisting of psychophysiological responses to anticipation of unreal or imagined danger, ostensibly resulting from unrecognized intrapsychic conflict. Physiological concomitants include increased heart rate, altered respiration rate, sweating, trembling, weakness, and fatigue; psychological concomitants include feelings of impending danger, powerlessness, apprehension, and tension. Cf. *fear.*

castration a. see under *complex.*

free-floating a. severe, generalized anxiety having no apparent connection to any specific object, situation, or idea.

performance a. a social phobia characterized by extreme anxiety and episodes of panic when performance, particularly public performance, is required.

separation a. apprehension due to removal of significant persons or familiar surroundings, common in infants 12 to 24 months old; see also under *disorder.*

situational a. anxiety occurring specifically in relation to a situation or object.

anx•io•lyt•ic (ang″ze-o-lit′ik) 1. antianxiety. 2. antianxiety agent.

An•ze•met (an′zə-met″) trademark for preparations of dolasetron mesylate.

AO ankle orthosis; atrioventricular opening.

AOA American Optometric Association; American Orthopsychiatric Association; American Osteopathic Association.

AOMA American Occupational Medical Association.

aor•ta (a-or′tə) pl. *aortas, aor′tae* [L., from Gr. *aortē*] [TA] the main trunk from which the systemic arterial system proceeds. It arises from the left ventricle of the heart; passes upward (*pars ascendens aortae* or *ascending aorta*), bends over (*arcus aortae* or *aortic arch*), and then proceeds downward (*pars descendens aortae* or *descending aorta*); the latter is divided into an upper, thoracic part (*pars thoracica aortae*) and a lower, abdominal part (*pars abdominalis aortae*). At about the level of the fourth lumbar vertebra it divides into the two common iliac arteries. **aor′tal, aor′tic** *adj*

abdominal a. pars abdominalis aortae.

a. abdomina′lis TA alternative for *pars abdominalis aortae.*

a. ascen′dens TA alternative for *pars ascendens aortae.*

ascending a. pars ascendens aortae.

a. descen′dens TA alternative for *pars descendens aortae.*

descending a. pars descendens aortae.

dextropositioned a. overriding a.

overriding a. a congenital anomaly occurring in tetralogy of Fallot, in which the aorta is displaced to the right so that it appears to arise from both ventricles and straddles the ventricular septal defect.

palpable a. an aorta that is easily palpable, on account of a thin retracted abdominal wall.

paravisceral a. thoracoabdominal a.

primordial a. either of two main vascular trunks before fusion into a single aorta in the early embryo.

thoracic a. pars thoracica aortae.

a. thora′cica TA alternative for *pars thoracica aortae.*

thoracoabdominal a. the lower part of the thoracic aorta and the upper part of the abdominal aorta, where the visceral branches originate.

ventral a. a single short vascular segment that, in fishes, in some amphibians, and in the embryo of higher vertebrates, connects the heart with the arteries in the pharyngeal arches. In mammalian development, it becomes continuous with the aortic arch.

aor•tae (a-or′te) [L.] genitive and plural of *aorta.*

aor•tal (a-or′təl) aortic.

aor•tal•gia (a″or-tal′jə) [*aorta* + *-algia*] pain in the region of the aorta.

aor•tec•to•my (a″or-tek′tə-me) [*aorta* + *-ectomy*] excision of part of the aorta.

aor•ti•co•me•di•as•ti•nal (a-or″tĭ-ko-me″de-ə-sti′nəl) pertaining to the aorta and mediastinum.

aor•ti•co•pul•mo•nary (a-or″tĭ-ko-pool′mo-nar″e) pertaining to or lying between the aorta and pulmonary artery. Called also *aortopulmonary* and *pulmoaortic.*

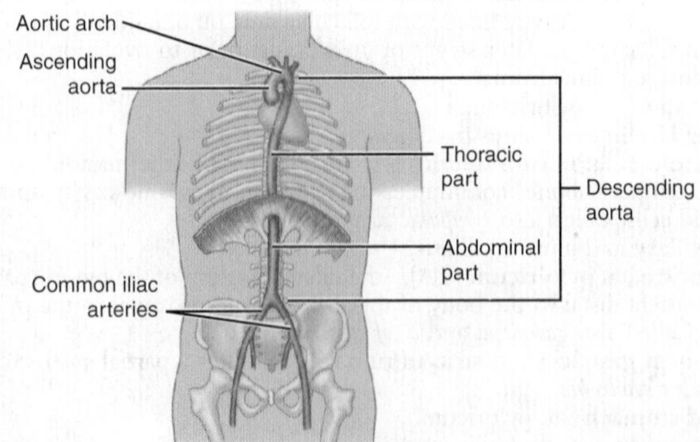

■ Aorta, arising from the left ventricle, ascending, arching, then descending through the thorax to the abdomen, where it divides into the common iliac arteries.

aor·ti·co·re·nal (a-or″tĭ-ko-re′nəl) pertaining to the aorta and the kidneys.

aor·ti·tis (a″or-ti′tis) [*aorta* +*-itis*] inflammation of the aorta.
Döhle-Heller a. syphilitic a.
nummular a. aortitis with white circular patches on the inner coat of the vessel.
rheumatic a. inflammation of the aorta due to rheumatism, which may progress to patchy fibrosis.
syphilitic a. aortitis caused by syphilis; its complications include insufficiency of the aortic valve, stenosis or occlusion of the coronary orifices, and aortic aneurysm. Called also *Döhle-Heller a.*

aor·to·bi·fem·o·ral (a-or″to-bi-fem′ə-rəl) pertaining to the aorta and both femoral arteries.

aor·to·bron·chi·al (a-or″to-brong′ke-əl) pertaining to or connecting the aorta and a bronchus.

aor·to·ca·val (a-or″to-ka′vəl) pertaining to or connecting the aorta and vena cava.

aor·to·cor·o·nary (a-or″to-kor′ə-nar-e) pertaining to or communicating with the aorta and coronary arteries.

aor·to·du·o·de·nal (a-or″to-doo″o-de′nəl) pertaining to or connecting the aorta and duodenum.

aor·to·en·ter·ic (a-or″to-en-ter′ik) pertaining to or connecting the aorta and gastrointestinal tract.

aor·to·esoph·a·ge·al (a-or″to-e-sof″ə-je′əl) pertaining to or connecting the aorta and esophagus.

aor·to·fem·o·ral (a-or″to-fem′ə-rəl) pertaining to the aorta and the femoral artery.

aor·to·gas·tric (a-or″to-gas′trik) pertaining to or connecting the aorta and stomach.

aor·to·gram (a-or′to-gram) the radiographic record resulting from aortography.

aor·tog·ra·phy (a″or-tog′rə-fe) [*aorta* + *-graphy*] radiography of the aorta after the intravascular injection of radiopaque medium.
digital subtraction a. digital subtraction angiography of the aorta.
retrograde a. radiography of the aorta after passage of a catheter through a peripheral artery to the aorta and the rapid injection of a radiopaque medium.
translumbar a. radiography of the aorta after injection of a radiopaque medium into it through a needle inserted into the lumbar area at about the level of the 12th thoracic vertebra.

aor·to·il·i·ac (a-or″to-il′e-ak) pertaining to the aorta and the iliac artery.

aor·to-os·ti·al (a-or″to-os′te-əl) pertaining to the aortic sinus and the coronary ostia.

aor·top·a·thy (a″or-top′ə-the) [*aorta* + *-pathy*] any disease of the aorta.

aor·to·pexy (a-or′to-pek″se) [*aorta* + *-pexy*] suturing of the anterior walls of the aortic arch and right subclavian artery to the sternum in order to pull the attached trachea to an open position; performed for relief of airway obstruction caused by compression of the trachea in tracheomalacia.

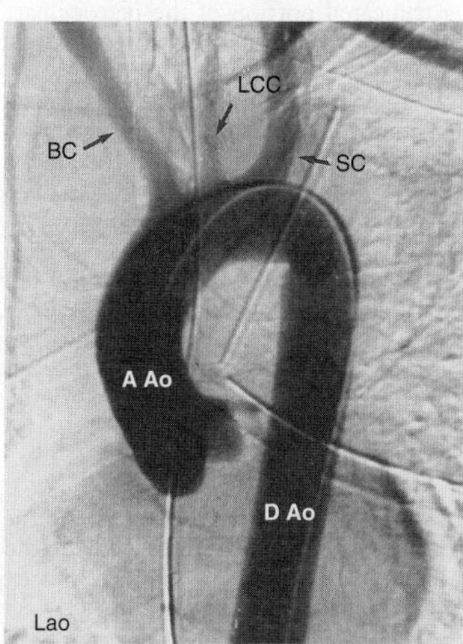

■ Digital subtraction aortography of a normal aortic arch, in a left anterior oblique *(Lao)* projection. *A Ao*, ascending aorta; *D Ao*, descending aorta; *BC*, brachiocephalic artery; *LCC*, left common carotid artery; *SC*, left subclavian artery.

aor·to·plas·ty (a-or′to-plas″te) [*aorta* + *-plasty*] surgical repair of the aorta; see also *aortic reconstruction.* **aortoplas′tic** *adj*

aor·to·pul·mo·nary (a-or″to-pool′mə-nar″e) aorticopulmonary.

aor·to·re·nal (a-or″to-re′nəl) pertaining to or connecting the aorta and a renal artery.

aor·tor·rha·phy (a″or-tor′ə-fe) [*aorta* + *-rrhaphy*] suture of the aorta.

aor·to·scle·ro·sis (a-or″to-sklə-ro′sis) arteriosclerosis in the aorta.

aor·tot·o·my (a″or-tot′ə-me) [*aorta* + *-tomy*] incision of the aorta.

AOTA American Occupational Therapy Association.

AP action potential; angina pectoris; anterior pituitary (gland); anteroposterior; arterial pressure.

ap- see *apo-*.

APA American Pharmaceutical Association; American Podiatric Association; American Psychiatric Association; American Psychological Association.

ap·a·con·i·tine (ap″ə-kon′ĭ-tēn) [*ap-* + *aconitine*] a poisonous base derived from aconitine.

Apaf-1 apoptotic protease activating factor 1.

apal·les·the·sia (ə-pal″es-the′zhə) pallanesthesia.

apan·cre·at·ic (a-pan″kre-at′ik) lacking a pancreas or due to absence of the pancreas.

Apan·sporo·blas·ti·na (a″pan-spor″o-blas-ti′nə) [*a-*[1] + *pansporoblast*] a suborder of parasitic protozoa (order Microsporida, class Microsporea) in which a pansporoblastic membrane is usually absent, being vestigial when present, and never persisting as a sporophorous vesicle; the sporoblast is most often dinucleate. Representative genera include *Encephalitozoon*, *Glugea*, and *Nosema*.

apar·a·lyt·ic (a-par″ə-lit′ik) without paralysis.

apar·a·thy·roid·ism (a-par″ə-thi′roid-iz-əm) aparathyrosis.

apar·a·thy·ro·sis (a-par″ə-thi-ro′sis) absence or deficiency of the parathyroid glands; see also *hypoparathyroidism*. Called also *aparathyroidism*.

apa·reu·nia (a″pə-roo′ne-ə) impossibility of sexual intercourse.

ap·ar·thro·sis (ap″ahr-thro′sis) [Gr. *aparthrōsis*] junctura synovialis.

ap·a·thet·ic (ap″ə-thet′ik) indifferent; undemonstrative.

ap·a·thy (ap′ə-the) [Gr. *apatheia*] lack of feeling or emotion; indifference.

ap·a·tite (ap′ə-tīt) [Gr. *apatan* to deceive] any of a group of minerals with the general formula $10Ca^{2+}$: $6PO_4^{3-}$: X^- where X is a monovalent anion such as a chloride, carbonate, fluoride, or hydroxyl ion; when it contains a hydroxyl ion the compound is hydroxyapatite (q.v.), an important inorganic constituent of teeth and bones.

ap·a·zone (ap′ə-zōn) a pyrazolone derivative having antiinflammatory, analgesic, antipyretic, and uricosuric effects; used for treatment of rheumatoid arthritis, osteoarthritis, and gout. Called also *azapropazone*.

APB atrial premature beat; see *atrial premature complex*, under *complex*.

APC atrial premature complex; activated protein C (see under *protein*).

APCA anti–Purkinje cell antibody; see *anti-Yo a.*, under *antibody*.

APCC anti-inhibitor coagulant complex.

APD atrial premature depolarization (see *atrial premature complex*, under *complex*); pamidronate (aminohydroxypropylidene diphosphonate).

ape (āp) an imprecise term used to refer to most of the larger Old World monkeys.
anthropoid a. any member of the family Pongidae; some are used in laboratory experiments because of their relationship to human beings.

APECED autoimmune polyendocrinopathy-candidiasis–ectodermal dysplasia; autoimmune polyendocrinopathy-candidiasis–ectodermal dystrophy.

ap·ei·do·sis (ap″i-do′sis) [*ap-* + Gr. *eidos* form] progressive disappearance of characteristic form in either the histologic or clinical aspect of a disease.

apel·lous (a-pel′əs) [*a-*[1] + L. *pellis* skin] 1. skinless; not covered with skin; not cicatrized; said of a wound. 2. having no prepuce.

ape·ri·ent (ə-pēr′e-ənt) [L. *aperiens* opening] laxative.

ape·ri·od·ic (a″pēr-e-od′ik) having no definite period; said of membranes that have no definite periods of vibration of their own, but are free to take up any vibrations imparted to them.

aper·i·stal·sis (a-per″ĭ-stawl′sis) [*a-*[1] + *peristalsis*] absence of usual peristalsis.

aper·i·tive (ə-per′ĭ-tiv) 1. stimulating the appetite. 2. laxative.

Apert syndrome (ah-pār′) [Eugène *Apert*, French pediatrician, 1868–1940] see under *syndrome*.

ap·er·tog·na·thia (ə-pur″tog-na′the-ə) open bite.

ap·er·tom·e·ter (ap″ər-tom′ə-tər) an apparatus for measuring the angle of aperture of microscopical objectives.

ap·er·tu·ra (ap″ər-too′rə) gen. and pl. *apertu′rae* [L., from *aperire* to open] aperture: an opening or orifice in the body.

a. canali′culi coch′leae [TA] opening of cochlear canaliculus: the external opening of the cochlear canaliculus on the margin of the jugular foramen in the temporal bone.

a. canali′culi vesti′buli [TA] opening of vestibular canaliculus: the external opening for the vestibular canaliculus, located on the posterior surface of the petrous part of the temporal bone, lateral to the opening for the internal acoustic meatus.

a. duc′tus nasolacrima′lis [TA] opening of nasolacrimal duct: the opening in the inferior nasal meatus through which tears flow out of the nasolacrimal duct.

a. exter′na cana′lis caro′tici [TA] external opening of carotid canal: a large, circular opening on the inferior surface of the petrous part of the temporal bone, through which the internal carotid artery enters the carotid canal.

a. inter′na canali′culi co′chleae [TA] internal opening of cochlear canaliculus: the opening of the cochlear canaliculus into the subarachnoid space.

a. inter′na canali′culi vesti′buli [TA] internal opening of vestibular canaliculus: the opening in the elliptical recess of the bony labyrinth through which the endolymphatic duct enters the petrous part of the temporal bone.

a. inter′na cana′lis caro′tici [TA] internal opening of carotid canal: the opening in the apex of the petrous part of the temporal bone, through which the internal carotid artery exits the carotid canal and enters the cranial cavity.

a. latera′lis ventri′culi quar′ti [TA] lateral aperture of fourth ventricle: an opening at the end of each lateral recess of the fourth ventricle by which the ventricular cavity communicates with the subarachnoid space; called also *foramen of Luschka* and *foramen of Key and Retzius.*

a. media′na ventri′culi quar′ti [TA] median aperture of fourth ventricle: a deficiency in the lower portion of the roof of the fourth ventricle through which the ventricular cavity communicates with the subarachnoid space; called also *foramen of Magendie.*

a. nasa′lis poste′rior TA alternative for *choana* (def. 2).

a. pel′vis infe′rior [TA] pelvic outlet: the inferior, very irregular aperture of the minor pelvis, bounded by the coccyx, the sacrotuberous ligaments, part of the ischium, the sides of the pubic arch, and the pubic symphysis.

a. pel′vis supe′rior [TA] pelvic inlet: the superior aperture of the minor pelvis, bounded by the crest and pecten of the pubic bones, the arcuate lines of the ilia, and the anterior margin of the base of the sacrum; called also *pelvic brim.*

a. pirifor′mis [TA] piriform aperture: the anterior end of the bony nasal opening, connecting the external nose with the skull; called also *anterior nasal aperture* and *base of nose.*

a. si′nus fronta′lis [TA] opening of frontal sinus: the external opening of the frontal sinus into the nasal cavity; its structure is variable, but it usually drains into the middle meatus. Called also *frontal ostium*, *frontal sinus ostium*, and *ostium of frontal sinus.*

a. si′nus sphenoida′lis [TA] opening of sphenoid sinus: a round opening just above the superior nasal concha, connecting the sphenoid sinus and the nasal cavity. Called also *sphenoid ostium*, *sphenoid sinus ostium*, and *ostium of sphenoid sinus.*

a. thora′cis infe′rior [TA] inferior thoracic aperture: the irregular opening at the inferior part of the thorax bounded by the twelfth thoracic vertebra, the twelfth ribs, and the curving edge of the costal cartilages as they meet the sternum; called also *thoracic outlet.*

a. thora′cis supe′rior [TA] superior thoracic aperture: the elliptical opening at the superior end of the thorax, bounded by the first thoracic vertebra, the first ribs and cartilage, and the upper margin of the manubrium sterni. Called also *thoracic inlet.* NOTE: In clinical usage, the term "thoracic outlet syndrome" refers to this structure, not to the apertura thoracis inferior.

a. tympa′nica canali′culi chor′dae tym′pani [TA] tympanic aperture of canaliculus for chorda tympani: the opening in the posterior part of the middle ear through which the chorda tympani nerve enters the tympanic cavity.

ap·er·tu·rae (ap″ər-too′re) [L.] genitive and plural of *apertura.*

ap·er·ture (ap′ər-chər) [L. *apertura*, q.v.] 1. an opening, or orifice; see also *apertura.* 2. the diameter of a microscope objective lens or the (adjustable) diameter of the iris diaphragm of a camera lens.

angle of a., angular a. the angle formed at a luminous point between the most divergent rays that are capable of passing through the objective of a microscope; called also *a. of lens.*

cloacal a. the posterior opening on the body surface of the cloaca in vertebrates such as birds, reptiles, fish, and amphibians. Called also *vent.*

laryngeal a. aditus laryngis.

lateral a. of fourth ventricle apertura lateralis ventriculi quarti.

a. of lens angle of a.

median a. of fourth ventricle apertura mediana ventriculi quarti.

nasal a., anterior apertura piriformis.

nasal a., posterior choana (def. 2).

numerical a. a measure of the efficiency of a microscope objective, being the product of the sine of one-half the angle of the aperture times the lowest refractive index of any medium between the objective and the specimen; usually abbreviated NA.

orbital a. aditus orbitalis.

piriform a. apertura piriformis.

thoracic a., inferior apertura thoracis inferior.

thoracic a., superior apertura thoracis superior.

tympanic a. of canaliculus for chorda tympani apertura tympanica canaliculi chordae tympani.

apex (a′peks) pl. *apexes, a′pices* [L.] 1. the superior aspect of a body, organ, or part, or the pointed extremity of a conical structure such as the heart or lung; called also *tip.* 2. the point of greatest activity, or the point of greatest response to any type of stimulation, such as electrical stimulation of a muscle. **ap′ical** *adj*

a. of arytenoid cartilage a. cartilaginis arytenoideae.

a. auri′culae [TA] a point sometimes present on the posterior superior part of the helix of the ear. Cf. *tuberculum auriculare.*

a. of bladder a. vesicae urinariae.

a. ca′pitis fi′bulae [TA] apex of head of fibula: a process pointing upward on the posterior surface of the head of the fibula, giving attachment to the arcuate popliteal ligament of the knee joint and part of the biceps tendon.

cardiac a. a. cordis.

a. cartila′ginis arytenoi′deae [TA] apex of arytenoid cartilage: the upper part of the arytenoid cartilage, which bends posteriorly and medially and connects with the corniculate cartilage.

a. cor′dis [TA] apex of heart: the blunt rounded extremity of the heart formed by the left ventricle; it is directed ventrally, inferiorly, and to the left.

a. cor′nus posterio′ris medul′lae spina′lis [TA] apex of posterior horn of spinal cord: the extremity of the posterior horn of the spinal cord, which is capped by the posteromarginal nucleus (Rexed lamina I) and the substantia gelatinosa (Rexed lamina II). Called also *a. of dorsal horn of spinal cord.*

a. cus′pidis den′tis [TA] the apex of the cusp of a tooth.

a. den′tis [TA] apex of dens: the tip of the dens of the axis.

a. of dorsal horn of spinal cord a. cornus posterioris medullae spinalis.

a. of head of fibula a. capitis fibulae.

a. of heart a. cordis.

a. lin′guae [TA] tip of tongue: the most distal portion of the tongue.

a. of lung a. pulmonis.

a. na′si [TA] tip of nose: the most distal portion of the nose.

a. os′sis sacra′lis TA alternative for *a. ossis sacri.*

a. os′sis sa′cri [TA] apex of the sacrum: the caudal end of the body of the fifth sacral vertebra, which articulates with the coccyx.

a. par′tis petro′sae os′sis tempora′lis [TA] apex of petrous part of temporal bone: the truncated portion of the petrous part of the temporal bone that is directed anteriorly and medially and ends at the medial opening of the carotid canal.

a. patel′lae [TA] apex of patella: the inferiorly directed blunt point of the patella, to which the patellar ligament is attached.

a. of petrous part of temporal bone a. partis petrosae ossis temporalis.

a. of posterior horn of spinal cord a. cornus posterioris medullae spinalis.

a. pro′statae [TA], **a. of prostate gland** the lower portion of the prostate, located just superior to the pubococcygeal muscle.

a. pulmo′nis [TA] apex of the lung: the rounded upper extremity of either lung, extending upward as high as the first thoracic vertebra.

a. ra′dicis den′tis [TA], **root a.** apex of root of tooth: the terminal end of the root of a tooth.

a. of sacrum a. ossis sacri.

a. of tongue a. linguae.

a. of urinary bladder, a. vesi′cae urina′riae [TA] the superior area of the urinary bladder, opposite to the fundus; it is at the junction of the superior and inferolateral surfaces of the bladder, and from it the middle umbilical ligament (urachus) extends to the umbilicus. Called also *summit of bladder* and *summit of urinary bladder.*

apex·car·dio·gram (a″peks-kahr′de-o-gram) a graphic record, in the form of a simple displacement curve, of the thrust of the apex of the heart as manifested on the surface of the body. Abbreviated ACG.

apex·car·di·og·ra·phy (a″peks-kahr″de-og′rə-fe) a method of graphically recording the pulsations of the anterior chest wall over the apex of the heart.

apex·i·fi·ca·tion (a-pek″sĭ-fĭ-ka′shən) treatment of an immature tooth whose pulp has died by creating an environment that encourages a calcified barrier to form over the open apex; done by cleaning the tooth and applying a paste.

apex·o·gen·e·sis (a″peks-o-jen′ĕ-sis) normal development of the root apex of a tooth.

APF acidulated phosphate fluoride; see *sodium fluoride and phosphoric acid gel*, under *gel*, and *sodium fluoride and acidulated phosphate topical solution*, under *solution*.

Ap·gar score (scale) (ap′gahr) [Virginia *Apgar*, American anesthesiologist, 1909–1974] see under *score*.

APHA American Public Health Association.

APhA American Pharmacists Association.

apha·cia (ə-fa′shə) aphakia.

apha·gia (ə-fa′jə) [*a-*[1] + *-phagia*] 1. inability to swallow; see also *dysphagia*. 2. refusal to swallow.

apha·kia (ə-fa′ke-ə) [*a-*[1] + *phak-* + *-ia*] absence of the lens of the eye; it may occur congenitally or from trauma, but is most commonly caused by extraction of a cataract. **apha′cic, apha′kic** *adj*

apha·lan·gia (a-fə-lan′jə) [*a-*[1] + *phalang-* + *-ia*] a developmental anomaly characterized by absence of a digit or of one or more phalanges of a finger or toe.

Aphan·i·zo·men·on (ə-fan″ĭ-zo-men′on) a genus of cyanobacteria that sometimes contaminate water and can cause cyanobacteria poisoning.

Aphan·o·as·cus (ə-fan″o-as′kəs) a genus of fungi of the family Gymnoascaceae. *A. fulves′cens* and *A. steroca′ria* are keratinophilic soil fungi that occasionally cause hyalohyphomycosis.

apha·sia (ə-fa′zhə) [*a-*[1] + Gr. *phasis* speech] any of a large group of language disorders involving defect or loss of the power of expression by speech, writing, or signs, or of comprehending spoken or written language, due to injury or disease of the brain or to psychogenic causes. Less severe forms are known as *dysphasia*. See also *agrammatism, dysphasia*, and *paraphasia*.

acoustic a. auditory a.

acquired epileptic a. Landau-Kleffner syndrome.

amnesic a., amnestic a. anomic a.

anomic a. defective recall of words, such as names of objects, with intact abilities of comprehension and repetition. Called also *amnesic a., amnestic a., nominal a.*, and *anomia*.

associative a. conduction a.

auditory a. a form of receptive aphasia in which sounds are heard but convey no meaning to the person affected, due to disease of the subcortical pathways leading to the main auditory center of the brain, or disease of the center itself; called also *acoustic a.* and *word deafness*.

Broca a. motor a.

central a. a term that has been used as a synonym for various aphasias that involve disturbance in word selection, grammar, and sentence structure apart from elementary auditory or visual comprehension and the ability to write legible characters and speak aloud. Many are presumed to be due to lesions of brain centers *(motor speech areas)*. See *global a., motor a.*, and *receptive a.*

combined a. aphasia of two or more forms occurring concomitantly in the same person.

commissural a. conduction a.

complete a. global a.

conduction a. a type of aphasia characterized by normal comprehension but inability to repeat words correctly; said to be caused by lesions in the pathways connecting the Broca motor speech and Wernicke areas. Called also *associative a.* and *commissural a.*

expressive a. motor a.

expressive-receptive a. global a.

fluent a. a type of receptive aphasia in which speech is well articulated with satisfactory melodic intonation, syllable stress, and phrasing but has gross errors in grammatical structure and is lacking in content.

frontocortical a. motor a.

functional a. aphasia associated with a psychogenic disorder.

gibberish a. jargon a.

global a. aphasia involving all the functions of spoken or written language and comprehension; called also *central a., complete a., expressive-receptive a.*, and *total a.*

graphomotor a. agraphia.

impressive a. receptive a.

intellectual a. true a.

jargon a. utterance of meaningless phrases, either neologisms or incoherently arranged known words (see *agrammatism*); it is sometimes a symptom of certain types of schizophrenia. Written also *jargonaphasia*.

mixed a. global a.

motor a. aphasia in which there is impairment of the ability to speak and write, owing to a lesion in the insula and surrounding operculum, including the Broca motor speech area. The patient understands many written and spoken words but has difficulty uttering the words. Cf. *receptive a.* Called also *Broca a., expressive a., frontocortical a., nonfluent a.*, and *logaphasia*.

nominal a. anomic a.

nonfluent a. motor a.

primary progressive a. deterioration of speech and language ability over a period of years without significant loss of memory or of ability to understand language, seen in certain degenerative brain diseases.

receptive a. inability to understand written, spoken, or tactile speech symbols, due to disease of the auditory and visual word centers. Cf. *motor a.* Called also *impressive a., sensory a.*, and *Wernicke a.*

semantic a. aphasia characterized by a lack of recognition of the full significance of words and phrases, or faulty use of words, phrases, or sentences; words heard, seen, spoken, or written are misunderstood or used incorrectly in place of other words in the same class.

sensory a. receptive a.

syntactical a. a type of agrammatism in which some necessary elements for coherent sentences are lacking.

tactile a. anomic aphasia characterized by inability to name objects that are touched. Cf. *tactile agnosia*.

total a. global a.

transcortical a. a type of conduction aphasia believed to be caused by a lesion of a pathway between the speech center and other cortical centers, but often reflecting large lesions in brain areas other than the perisylvian region of the hemisphere dominant for speech and language. The patient may repeat words *(echolalia)* but cannot speak independently.

true a. aphasia due to a lesion of any one of the speech centers; called also *intellectual a.*

visual a. alexia.

Wernicke a. receptive a.

apha·si·ac (ə-fa′ze-ak) aphasic (def. 2).

apha·sic (ə-fa′zik) 1. pertaining to or affected with aphasia. 2. a person affected with aphasia.

apha·si·ol·o·gist (ə-fa″ze-ol′ə-jist) a specialist in aphasiology.

apha·si·ol·o·gy (ə-fa″ze-ol′ə-je) the scientific study of aphasia and the specific neurologic lesions producing it.

aphas·mid (a-faz′mid) [*a-*[1] + *phasmid*] a nematode belonging to the subclass Aphasmidia. Cf. *phasmid*.

Aphas·mid·ia (a-faz-mid′e-ə) a subclass of Nematoda comprising those organisms which do not possess phasmids, and including the superfamilies Trichuroidea, Mermithoidea, and Dioctophymoidea.

ap·he·li·ot·ro·pism (ap″he-le-ot′rə-piz-əm) negative heliotropism.

aphe·mia (ə-fe′me-ə) [*a-*[1] + *-phemia*] 1. apraxia of speech. 2. formerly common name for a type of motor aphasia.

aphe·pho·bia (af″ə-fo′be-ə) haphephobia.

aph·e·re·sis (af-ə-re′sis) [Gr. *aphairesis* removal] any procedure in which blood is withdrawn from a donor, a fluid or solid portion (plasma, leukocytes, platelets, etc.) is separated and retained, and the remainder is retransfused into the donor. Types include erythrocytapheresis, leukapheresis, lymphocytapheresis, plasmapheresis, and plateletpheresis. Called also *hemapheresis* and *pheresis*.

apho·nia (a-fo′ne-ə) [*a-*[1] + *phon-* + *-ia*] 1. loss of voice. Cf. *dysphonia*. 2. mutism.

hysteric a. loss of speech due to emotional conflicts in conversion disorder.

spastic a. see under *dysphonia*.

aphon·ic (a-fon′ik) 1. pertaining to or affected with aphonia. 2. without audible voice.

apho·no·ge·lia (a″fo-no-je′le-ə) [*a-*[1] + *phono-* + *gelōs* laughter] inability to laugh aloud.

aphose (a′fōz) [*a-*[1] + *phose*] any phose or subjective visual sensation due to absence or interruption of light.

aphos·pha·gen·ic (a-fos″fə-jen′ik) due to deficiency of phosphorus.

aphos·pho·ro·sis (a-fos″fə-ro′sis) a deficiency of dietary phosphorus in animals, particularly grazing cattle, characterized by inappetence, lameness, osteomalacia, bone fragility, decline in milk production, and lowered fertility.

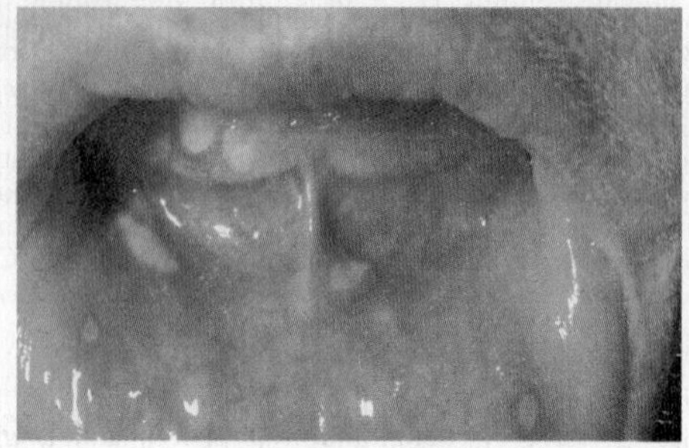
■ Multiple aphthae in aphthous stomatitis.

aphot·es·the·sia (a″fōt-es-the′zhə) [*a-*[1] + *phot-* + *esthesia*] reduced sensitivity of the retina to light resulting from excessive exposure to rays of the sun.

aphot·ic (a-fot′ik) without light; totally dark.

aphra·sia (ə-fra′zhə) [*a-*[1] + Gr. *phrasis* utterance] inability to speak or to understand phrases. See also *aphasia* and *mute*.

aph·ro·dis·ia (af″ro-diz′e-ə) [Gr. *aphrodisia* sexual pleasures] sexual excitement.

aph·ro·dis·iac (af″ro-diz′e-ak) 1. exciting the libido. 2. any drug that arouses the sexual instinct.

Aph·ro·dyne (af″ro-dīn′) trademark for a preparation of yohimbine hydrochloride.

aph·tha (af′thə) pl. *aph′thae* [L., from Gr. "thrush"] a small ulcer, such as the round lesion with a grayish exudate surrounded by a red halo characteristic of recurrent aphthous stomatitis.

Bednar aphthae symmetric excoriation of the hard palate over the pterygoid plates in infants; thought to be due to pressure of the nipple against the palate during nursing, or to sucking of the tongue or foreign objects.

epizootic aphthae foot-and-mouth disease in cattle.

Mikulicz aphthae periadenitis mucosa necrotica recurrens.

recurring scarring aphthae periadenitis mucosa necrotica recurrens.

aph·thae (af′the) [L.] 1. plural of *aphtha*. 2. recurrent aphthous stomatitis.

Aph·tha·sol (af′thə-sol) trademark for a preparation of amlexanox.

aph·thoid (af′thoid) [*aphtha* + *-oid*] 1. resembling thrush; thrushlike. 2. an exanthema resembling that of thrush.

aph·thon·gia (af-thon′jə) [*a-*[1] + Gr. *phthongos* sound] aphasia due to spasm of the speech muscles.

aph·tho·sis (af-tho′sis) any condition marked by aphthae.

aph·thous (af′thəs) pertaining to, characterized by, or affected with aphthae.

Aph·tho·vi·rus (af′tho-vi″rəs) [*aphtha* + *virus*] a genus of viruses of the family Picornaviridae; the one medically important species is foot-and-mouth disease virus.

ap·i·ca·lis (ap″ĭ-ka′lis) [L., from *apex*, gen. *apicis*, top] 1. apical. 2. [TA] a general term denoting relationship to or location at an apex.

api·cec·to·my (a″pĭ-sek′tə-me) [*apic-* + *-ectomy*] excision of the apex of the petrous portion of the temporal bone.

ap·i·ces (ap′ĭ-sēz) [L.] plural of *apex*.

api·ci·tis (a″pĭ-si′tis) [*apic-* + *-itis*] inflammation of an apex, as the apex of a tooth, of the lung, or of the petrous portion of the temporal bone (petrositis).

apic(o)- [L. *apex* top, summit] a prefix denoting a relationship to the top, as of an organ or other structure.

api·co·ec·to·my (a″pĭ-ko-ek′tə-me) [*apico-* + *-ectomy*] excision of the apical portion of a tooth through an opening made in the overlying labial, buccal, or palatal alveolar bone; see also *root amputation*. Called also *root resection*.

Ap·i·com·plexa (ap″ĭ-kəm-plek′sə) [*apico-* + *complex*] a phylum of uninucleate, parasitic tissue-dwelling protozoa characterized by an apical complex, with one or more microspores usually present at some stage of development. Flagella and cilia are absent in the adult stage, and many mature apicomplexans glide by means of ultrastructural ridges and fibers on the body surface. They typically reproduce either asexually by means of multiple fission (forming merozoites or schizozoites) or by endodyogeny; or sexually by syngamy. The phylum comprises two classes: Perkinsea and Sporozoea. Called also *Sporozoa*.

ap·i·com·plex·an (ap″ĭ-kəm-plek′sən) 1. any protozoan of the subphylum Apicomplexa. 2. pertaining or relating to protozoa of the subphylum Apicomplexa.

apicoplast (a′pĭ-ko-plast) an organelle found in protozoa of the subphylum Apicomplexa, having its own genome; it is a nonphotosynthetic chloroplastlike structure.

api·cos·to·my (a″pĭ-kos′tə-me) dental trephination.

api·cot·o·my (a″pĭ-kot′ə-me) puncture of the apex of the petrous portion of the temporal bone.

apic·u·late (ə-pik′u-lāt) having an apiculus.

apic·u·lus (ə-pik′u-ləs) a short pointed projection at or near the end of a conidium or spore.

Api·dae (ap′ĭ-de) the bees, a family of flying insects with relatively large bodies, of the order Hymenoptera; many species can sting. Genera include *Apis* and *Bombus*.

Api·dra (a′pĭ-drə) trademark for a preparation of insulin glulisine.

APIM [Fr.] Association Professionnelle Internationale des Médecins (International Professional Association of Physicians).

apio·ther·a·py (a″pe-o-ther′ə-pe) treatment with bee venom.

api·pho·bia (a″pĭ-fo′be-ə) [L. *apis* bee + *-phobia*] irrational fear of bees.

Apis (a′pis) a genus of bees of the family Apidae, smaller than the bumblebees (genus *Bombus*). *A. melli′fera* is the most common type of honeybee, which can sting if bothered.

apis·i·na·tion (a″pis-ĭ-na′shən) [L. *apis* bee] poisoning by a bee sting.

api·tox·in (a′pĭ-tok″sin) the toxic protein constituent of bee venom.

api·tu·i·tar·ism (a″pĭ-too′ĭ-tər-iz″əm) 1. lack of pituitary tissue; it may be congenital, as with anencephaly, or acquired, as by hypophysectomy. 2. hypopituitarism.

A.P.L. trademark for a preparation of chorionic gonadotropin.

apla·cen·tal (a-plə-sen′təl) [*a-*[1] + *placenta*] having no placenta.

aplan·a·tism (ə-plan′ə-tiz-əm) freedom from spherical aberration and coma; said of a lens. **aplanat′ic** *adj*

apla·sia (ə-pla′zhə) [*a-*[1] + *-plasia*] lack of development of an organ or tissue. Cf. *agenesis* and *hypoplasia*.

a. axia′lis extracortica′lis conge′nita Pelizaeus-Merzbacher disease.

a. cu′tis conge′nita a usually lethal congenital condition consisting of localized failure of development of skin, usually of the scalp but sometimes of the trunk or limbs. The defects are usually covered by a thin translucent membrane or scar tissue, or may be raw, ulcerated, or covered by granulation tissue.

dermal a. lack of skin development in a circumscribed area; see *focal dermal hypoplasia*, under *hypoplasia*.

germinal a., germinal cell a. Sertoli-cell–only syndrome.

Michel a. lack of development of the internal ear, which causes Michel deafness.

nuclear a. Möbius syndrome.

pure red cell a. severe normochromic, normocytic anemia, reticulocytosis, and erythroblastopenia in bone marrow that produces the other cellular elements in a normal way. It occurs as a primary chronic form *(congenital hypoplastic anemia)*, in chronic forms secondary to immune disorders, or in an acute form that is self-limited and associated with drugs or infection.

retinal a. retinal dysplasia, defs. 1 and 2.

Scheibe a. partial aplasia of the saccule and cochlear duct, which causes Scheibe deafness.

thymic a. absence of the thymus gland, as in DiGeorge syndrome.

thymic-parathyroid a. DiGeorge syndrome.

aplas·tic (a-plas′tik) [*a-*[1] + *plastic*] pertaining to or characterized by aplasia; anatomically undeveloped from the primordium or from a stem cell.

Aplec·ta·na (ə-plek′tə-nə) a genus of nematodes parasitic in the intestinal tract of amphibians and reptiles.

apleu·ria (a-ploor′e-ə) [*a-*[1] + *pleur-* + *-ia*] absence of ribs.

Ap·li·graf (ap′lĭ-graf) trademark for a preparation of graftskin.

Ap·li·sol (ap′lĭ-sol) trademark for a preparation of purified protein derivative tuberculin.

APN advanced practice nurse.

ap·nea (ap′ne-ə) [*a-*[1] + *-pnea*] cessation of breathing. **apne′ic** *adj*

central a., central sleep a. sleep apnea resulting from failure of stimulation by the respiratory centers in the medulla; both hereditary varieties and varieties accompanying other brainstem disorders have been observed.

deglutition a. a temporary arrest of the activity of the respiratory nerve center during an act of swallowing.

initial a. a condition in which an infant fails to establish sustained respiration within two minutes of delivery.

late a. cessation of respiration in an infant for more than 45 seconds after spontaneous breathing has been established and sustained.

mixed a. sleep apnea with aspects of both central and obstructive types.

a. neonato′rum initial a.

obstructive a., obstructive sleep a. sleep apnea resulting from collapse or obstruction of the airway with the inhibition of muscle tone that occurs during REM sleep. In adults it is seen primarily in middle-aged obese individuals, with a male predominance; in children it is often seen accompanying conditions such as adenotonsillar hypertrophy, Down syndrome, or morbid obesity.

primary a. cessation of breathing resulting when a fetus or newborn infant is deprived of oxygen; exposure to oxygen and stimulation usually restore respiration.

secondary a. a period of time following primary apnea during which continued asphyxia of the fetus or newborn, with a fall in blood pressure and heart rate, necessitates artificial ventilation for resuscitation and reestablishment of ventilation.

sleep a. transient periods of cessation of breathing during sleep. It may result in hypoxemia and vasoconstriction of pulmonary arterioles, producing pulmonary arterial hypertension. The two primary types are *central sleep a.* and *obstructive sleep a.*

traumatic a. cessation of pulmonary ventilation following physical injury. See also under *asphyxia.*

ap•neu•mia (ap-noo′me-ə) [*a-*[1] + *pneum-* + *-ia*] congenital absence of the lungs.

ap•neu•sis (ap-noo′sis) [*a-*[1] + *pneusis*] a condition marked by maintained inhalational activity unrelieved by exhaling, each inhalation being long and cramplike; it follows excision of the pneumotaxic center in the upper part of the pons. **apneu′stic** *adj*

ap(o)- [Gr. *apo* from] a prefix denoting separation or derivation from. Also, *ap-*.

ap•o•cam•no•sis (ap″o-kam-no′sis) apokamnosis.

apo•chro•mat (ap″o-kro′mat) [*apo-* + *chromatic aberration*] an apochromatic objective; see under *objective.*

apo•chro•mat•ic (ap″o-kro-mat′ik) free from chromatic and spherical aberration; see under *objective.*

apo•crine (ap′o-krin) [Gr. *apokrinesthai* to be secreted] denoting that type of glandular secretion in which the free end or apical portion of the secreting cell is cast off along with the secretory products that have accumulated therein.

apo•crin•i•tis (ap″o-krin-i′tis) [*apo-* + Gr. *krinein* to separate] hidradenitis suppurativa.

ap•o•crus•tic (ap″o-krus′tik) 1. astringent and repellent. 2. an astringent and repellent agent.

apoc•y•nin (ə-pos′ĭ-nin) a cardiotonic found in species of *Apocynum,* formerly used like digitalis but now considered poisonous; animals consuming the plants may develop an increased pulse rate with fever that can be fatal.

Apoc•y•num (ə-pos′ĭ-nəm) the dogbanes, a genus of poisonous North American plants of the family Apocynaceae, noted for their digitalis-like cardioactive principles. *A. cannabi′num* L. (Canadian or Indian hemp) and *A. androsaemifo′lium* L. contain apocynin.

apo•dal (ə-po′dəl) having no feet; see also *symmelia.*

Ap•o•de•mus (ap″o-de′məs) a genus of Old World field mice of the family Muridae, containing some species that are reservoirs of infectious diseases. Species include *A. sylva′ticus,* the wood mouse, *A. agra′rius,* the Manchurian striped field mouse, and *A. flavicol′lis,* the yellow-necked field mouse.

apo•dia (a-po′de-ə) [*a-*[1] + *pod-* + *-ia*] 1. a congenital anomaly characterized by absence of one or both feet. 2. apodal symmelia.

apo•en•zyme (ap″o-en′zīm) the protein component of an enzyme that is separable from the prosthetic group (cofactor or coenzyme) but that requires the presence of the prosthetic group to form the functioning compound (holoenzyme).

ap•o•fer•ri•tin (ap″o-fer′ĭ-tin) a colorless protein closely related to transferrin, of molecular weight 460,000, produced in the mucosal cells of the small intestine; it binds iron and forms ferritin.

apo•gam•ia (ap″o-gam′e-ə) apogamy.

apog•a•my (ə-pog′ə-me) [*apo-* + Gr. *gamein* to wed] 1. reproduction without conjugation of gametes and usually without meiosis, as in certain seed plants. 2. parthenogenesis.

apo•kam•no•sis (ap″o-kam-no′sis) abnormal liability to fatigue in myasthenia; a feeling of tiredness, numbness, and heaviness in a limb motion.

apo•lar (a-po′lər) [*a-*[1] + *polar*] not having poles or processes.

apo•lipo•pro•tein (ap″o-lip″o-pro′tēn) any of the protein constituents of lipoproteins; grouped by function in four classes A, B, C, and E (the former apo D is now apo A-III).

a. A a class of apolipoproteins, apo A-I, -II, -III, and -IV, that occur primarily in high-density lipoproteins (HDL) and in lesser amounts in chylomicrons; apo A-I is the activator of lecithin-cholesterol acyltransferase (LCAT), which forms cholesteryl esters in HDL.

a. B a class of apolipoproteins recognized by specific cell-surface receptors that mediate endocytosis of lipoprotein particles; apo B-100 on very-low-density, intermediate-density, and low-density lipoproteins is recognized by LDL receptors on liver and extrahepatic cells; apo B-48 on chylomicrons is recognized by chylomicron remnant receptors on liver cells.

a. C a class of apolipoproteins, apo C-I, -II, and -III, that occur in very-low-density and high-density lipoproteins and chylomicrons; apo C-II activates lipoprotein lipase, which hydrolyzes triglycerides for transfer from VLDL and chylomicrons to tissues.

a. D a. A-III.

a. E an apolipoprotein, apo E, that occurs in all classes of lipoproteins; it may be involved in the conversion of very-low-density to intermediate-density lipoprotein and its clearance from the circulation.

ap•o•mix•ia (ap″o-mik′se-ə) apomixis.

ap•o•mix•is (ap″o-mik′sis) [*apo-* + Gr. *mixis* a mingling] 1. asexual reproduction in a species normally reproducing sexually, as in certain seed plants. 2. apogamy.

apo•mor•phine hy•dro•chlo•ride (ap″o-mor′fēn) [USP] a derivative of morphine with structural similarities to dopamine and acting as a dopamine D_2-receptor agonist; administered subcutaneously in the diagnosis of parkinsonism.

ap•o•neu•rec•to•my (ap″o-noo͝-rek′tə-me) [*aponeurosis* + *-ectomy*] excision of the aponeurosis of a muscle.

ap•o•neu•rol•o•gy (ap″o-noo͝-rol′ə-je) [*aponeurosis* + *-logy*] the sum of knowledge regarding aponeuroses and fasciae.

ap•o•neu•ro•gen•ic (ap″o-noor″o-jen′ik) arising from an aponeurosis; used specifically of the aponeurosis of the levator superioris palpebrae muscle. See *aponeurogenic ptosis,* under *ptosis.*

ap•o•neu•ror•rha•phy (ap″o-noo͝-ror′ə-fe) [*aponeurosis* + *-rrhaphy*] suture of an aponeurosis; fasciorrhaphy.

ap•o•neu•ro•ses (ap″o-noo͝-ro′sēz) plural of *aponeurosis.*

ap•o•neu•ro•sis (ap″o-noo͝-ro′sis) pl. *aponeuro′ses* [Gr. *aponeurōsis*] 1. [TA] a white, flattened or ribbonlike tendinous expansion, usually serving to connect a muscle with the parts that it moves. 2. a term formerly applied to certain fasciae. **aponeurot′ic** *adj*

abdominal a. the conjoined tendons of the oblique and transverse muscles on the abdomen.

a. of biceps muscle of arm, bicipital a. a. musculi bicipitis brachii.

a. bicipita′lis TA alternative for *a. musculi bicipitis brachii.*

epicranial a. galea aponeurotica.

a. epicrania′lis TA alternative for *galea aponeurotica.*

extensor a. see under *expansion.*

falciform a. of rectus abdominis muscle falx inguinalis.

femoral a. fascia lata.

a. glutea′lis [TA] gluteal aponeurosis: a dense sheet of fascia lying between the iliac crest and the superior border of the gluteus maximus; from it arises a part of the gluteus medius muscle.

a. of insertion the connection of a muscle with the part or parts that it moves.

a. lin′guae [TA], **lingual a.** the connective tissue framework of the tongue, supporting and giving attachment to the intrinsic and extrinsic muscles; composed of the connective tissue layer of the tunica mucosa, the lingual septum, and the posterior transverse expansion of the septum which attaches to the hyoid bone.

a. mus′culi bici′pitis bra′chii [TA] aponeurosis of biceps muscle of arm: an expansion of the tendon of the biceps brachii muscle by which it is attached to the fascia of the forearm and to the ulna; called also *bicipital a., a. bicipitalis* [TA alternative], *lacertus fibrosus musculi bicipitis brachii* [TA alternative], *bicipital fascia, semilunar fascia,* and *fibrous fasciculus of biceps muscle.*

a. of occipitofrontal muscle galea aponeurotica.

a. palati′na [TA] palatine aponeurosis: a fibrous sheet in the anterior part of the soft palate, derived mainly from the tendons of the two tensor muscles, giving attachment to the musculus uvulae and to the palatopharyngeus and levator veli palatini muscles.

a. palma′ris [TA] palmar aponeurosis: bundles of fibrous tissue radiating toward the bases of the fingers from the tendon of the palmaris longus muscle; called also *Dupuytren* or *volar fascia.*

pharyngeal a. fascia pharyngobasilaris.

a. planta′ris [TA] plantar aponeurosis: bands of fibrous tissue radiating toward the bases of the toes from the medial process of the tuber calcanei; called also *plantar fascia.*

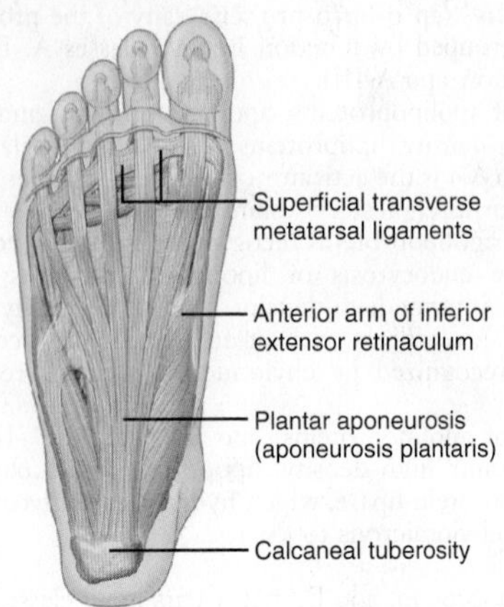

■ Aponeurosis plantaris (plantar aponeurosis).

supraspinous a. a dense fascia that partly envelops the supraspinous muscle.

temporal a. fascia temporalis.

a. of Zinn see *fibrae zonulares.*

ap·o·neu·ro·si·tis (ap″o-nŏŏ-ro-si′tis) [*aponeurosis* + *-itis*] inflammation of an aponeurosis.

ap·o·neu·ro·tome (ap″o-noor′o-tōm) a knife for cutting aponeuroses.

ap·o·neu·rot·o·my (ap″o-nŏŏ-rot′ə-me) [*aponeurosis* + *-tomy*] surgical cutting of an aponeurosis.

Ap·o·nom·ma (ap″o-nom′ə) a genus of ticks of the family Ixodidae that infest reptiles.

A. hydrosau′ri a species that is the primary vector for *Rickettsia honei* in Australia, causing Flinders Island spotted fever.

apoph·y·sa·ry (ə-pof′ə-ză-re) apophyseal.

apoph·y·ses (ə-pof′ə-sēz) plural of *apophysis.*

apoph·y·si·al (ə-pof′ə-se″əl, ap″o-fiz′e-əl) apophyseal.

ap·o·phys·i·ary (ap″o-fiz′e-ar″e) apophyseal.

apoph·y·sis (ə-pof′ə-sis) pl. *apoph′yses* [Gr. "an offshoot"] 1. [TA] any outgrowth or swelling, especially a bony outgrowth that has never been entirely separated from the bone of which it forms a part, such as a process, tubercle, or tuberosity. 2. in fungi, a V-shaped swelling of the sporangiophore just below the columella. See illustration at *mold.* **apophys′eal** *adj*

annular a. epiphysis anularis.

basilar a. pars basilaris ossis occipitalis.

cerebral a. glandula pinealis.

odontoid a. dens axis.

pterygoid a. processus pterygoideus ossis sphenoidalis.

ring a. epiphysis anularis.

apoph·y·si·tis (ə-pof″ə-si′tis) inflammation of an apophysis, especially a disorder of the foot caused by disease of the epiphysis of the calcaneus.

a. tibia′lis adolescen′tium Osgood-Schlatter disease.

Apo·phy·so·my·ces (ap″o-fiz″o-mi′sēz) [*apophysis* (def. 2) + Gr. *mykēs* fungus] a genus of fungi of the family Mucoraceae. *A. e′legans* is a soil saprobe that occasionally causes mucormycosis.

apo·plas·mat·ic (ap″o-plaz-mat′ik) pertaining to substances that are produced by cells and form a constituent part of the tissues of an organism, such as fibers of connective tissue or the matrix of bone and cartilage.

ap·o·plec·ti·form (ap″o-plek′tĭ-form) resembling apoplexy.

ap·o·plec·toid (ap″o-plek′toid) resembling apoplexy.

ap·o·plex·ia (ap″o-plek′se-ə) [Gr. *apoplēxia*] apoplexy.

ap·o·plexy (ap′o-plek″se) [Gr. *apoplēxia*] 1. stroke syndrome. 2. hemorrhage into an organ. **apoplec′tic** *adj*

abdominal a. spontaneous intraperitoneal hemorrhage due to rupture of an intra-abdominal blood vessel, independent of any trauma to the abdomen.

adrenal a. massive hemorrhage into the adrenal glands, as seen in Waterhouse-Friderichsen syndrome.

bulbar a. stroke syndrome affecting the substance of the pons.

pituitary a. sudden massive degeneration with hemorrhagic necrosis of the pituitary gland, associated with a pituitary tumor; it is signaled by abrupt headache followed by loss of sight, diplopia, drowsiness, confusion or other mentally deranged states, and coma.

spinal a. hematomyelia.

apo·pro·tein (ap″o-pro′tēn) the protein moiety of a conjugated protein or protein complex. See also *apolipoprotein.*

ap·op·to·sis (ap″op-to′sis, ap″o-to′sis) [Gr. "a falling off"] a morphologic pattern of cell death affecting single cells, marked by shrinkage of the cell, condensation of chromatin, formation of cytoplasmic blebs, and fragmentation of the cell into membrane-bound apoptotic bodies that are eliminated by phagocytosis. It is a mechanism for cell deletion in the regulation of cell populations, as of B and T lymphocytes following cytokine depletion. Often used synonymously with *programmed cell death* (q.v.). **apoptot′ic** *adj*

chondrocyte a. apoptosis of chondrocytes, which may occur normally but is increased in various degenerative conditions, with weakening or destruction of cartilage.

apop·to·some (ə-pop′tə-sōm) [*apoptosis* + *-some*] a complex of apoptotic protease activating factor 1 (Apaf-1), caspase 9, cytochrome *c*, and other proteins; it is formed when deoxyadenosine triphosphate (dATP) and cytochrome c (released from mitochondria) bind to the C-terminal of and activate Apaf-1, which in turn binds and activates caspase 9. Caspase 9 activates caspase 3 and initiates a cascade that results in apoptosis.

apo·re·pres·sor (ap″o-re-pres′ər) an inactive form of a repressor (q.v.), requiring binding of a corepressor to become a functional repressor.

apos·ta·sis (ə-pos′tə-sis) [Gr.] the end or crisis of an attack of disease.

apos·thia (ə-pos′the-ə) [*a-*[1] + *posth-* + *-ia*] congenital absence of the prepuce.

apoth·e·cary (ə-poth′ə-kar″e) [Gr. *apothēke* storehouse] pharmacist.

ap·o·the·ci·um (ap″o-the′se-əm) an open or expanded fruiting body seen in lichens and actinomycetous fungi (see *ascocarp*), having asci contained on its exposed surface.

APP amyloid precursor protein.

ap·pa·ra·tus (ap″ə-ră′təs) pl. *apparatus* or *apparatuses* [L., from *ad-* to + *parare* to make ready] an arrangement of a number of parts acting together in the performance of some special function; used in anatomical nomenclature to designate a number of structures or organs which act together in serving some particular function.

Abbe-Zeiss a. Thoma-Zeiss counting chamber.

biliary a. the parts concerned in the formation, conduction, and storage of bile, including the secreting cells of the liver, bile ducts, and gallbladder.

branchial a. pharyngeal a.

Brown-Roberts-Wells a. the equipment used in the Brown-Roberts-Wells technique of stereotactic surgery; see under *technique.*

Charnley a. see under *prosthesis.*

ciliary a. corpus ciliare.

cytopharyngeal a. a cytopharynx with walls supported by nematodesmata; see *rhabdos.*

Desault a. see under *bandage.*

Golgi a. see under *complex.*

Jaquet a. a recording apparatus for venous and cardiac impulses.

juxtaglomerular a. a complex in the kidney comprising the juxtaglomerular cells, macula densa, and lacis cells of the polkissen; it is the site of tubuloglomerular feedback for autoregulation of the glomerular filtration rate. Called also *juxtaglomerular complex.*

Kirschner a. see under *wire.*

a. lacrima′lis [TA] lacrimal apparatus: the system concerned with the secretion and circulation of the tears and the normal fluid of the conjunctival sac; it consists of the lacrimal gland and ducts, and associated structures. See Plate 15.

Leksell a. the equipment used in the Leksell technique of stereotactic surgery; see under *technique.*

masticatory a. the organs and structures involved in mastication, including the teeth and jaws and their supporting structures, temporomandibular joints, mandibular muscles, accessory facial muscles, tongue, lips, cheeks, and oral mucosa together with their innervation. Called also *organs of mastication* and *masticatory system.*

mucociliary a. on the inner surface of the respiratory tract, a layer of columnar epithelial cells covered by a thin mucous layer and many projecting cilia that beat in a rhythmic manner to bring about mucociliary clearance (see under *clearance*).

parabasal a. in protozoa of the phylum Parabasalia, the structure comprising the parabasal body and the fibril or thread that connects it to the basal body.

a. of Perroncito a mass of fibrils in the form of spirals and networks with newly formed axons which develop in the cut stump of a nerve during regeneration; called also *Perroncito spirals.*

pharyngeal a. the pharyngeal arches, pouches, membranes, and grooves considered as a unit; called also *branchial a.*

pilosebaceous a. see under *unit.*

respiratory a. see under *system.*

Riechert-Mundinger a. the equipment used in the Riechert-Mundinger technique of stereotactic surgery; see under *technique.*

Sayre a. an apparatus for suspending a patient during the application of a plaster-of-Paris jacket.

Soxhlet a. an apparatus by which fatty or lipid constituents can be extracted from solid matter by repeated treatment with distilled solvent.

spindle a. see *spindle* (def. 2).

subneural a. see under *cleft.*

sucker a. pericapillary end foot.

Taylor a. see under *brace.*

Tiselius a. an apparatus for the electrophoretic separation of the proteins of blood serum, plasma, and other body fluids.

Todd-Wells a. the equipment used in the Todd-Wells technique of stereotactic surgery; see under *technique.*

vasomotor a. the neuromuscular mechanism controlling the constriction and dilation of blood vessels and thus the amount of blood supplied to a part.

vestibular a. the structures in the internal ear concerned with reception and transduction of stimuli of equilibrium; they include the semicircular canals, the utricle, and the saccule.

ap•pear•ance (ə-pēr′əns) a coming into view; outward aspect.

batwing a. 1. seen in pulmonary edema. 2. a characteristic appearance of the fourth ventricle, resembling the wings of a bat, seen in Joubert syndrome.

urea nitrogen a. the amount of urea in grams produced by a person's body over a specific period of time, closely related to the amount of nitrogen that has not been absorbed by the body. It is calculated as the sum of the urea excreted in the urine plus that found in the blood by calculating blood urea nitrogen. A low figure indicates efficient use of dietary protein. The person's intake of protein must also be known, because a low urea nitrogen appearance is also seen with a low protein diet or malnutrition.

ap•pen•dage (ə-pen′dəj) a thing or part appended; see also *adnexa* and *appendix.*

atrial a., auricular a. auricula atrii.

cutaneous a's skin a's.

endolymphatic a. an outgrowth of the otic vesicle that forms the endolymphatic duct and sac during embryonic development; called also *endolymphatic diverticulum.*

epidermal a's skin a's.

a. of epididymis appendix epididymidis.

epiploic a's appendices omentales.

eye a's, a's of eye ocular adnexa.

a's of the fetus the trophoblast derivatives and extraembryonic or fetal membranes, including the umbilical cord, amnion, yolk sac, and chorion (fetal part of placenta).

fibrous a. of liver appendix fibrosa hepatis.

ocular a's ocular adnexa.

omental a's appendices omentales.

skin a's, a's of the skin the hair, nails, sebaceous glands, sweat glands, and mammary glands; called also *cutaneous* or *skin adnexa.*

testicular a., a. of the testis appendix testis.

uterine a's the ovaries, uterine tubes, and uterine ligaments; called also *adnexa uteri.*

a. of ventricle of larynx sacculus laryngis.

vesicular a's of epoöphoron appendices vesiculosae epoophori.

ap•pen•da•gi•tis (ə-pen″də-ji′tis) inflammation of an appendage, particularly of the epiploic appendages.

epiploic a. inflammation of one or more of the epiploic appendages of the colon, with pain and tenderness over the affected area.

ap•pen•dec•to•my (ap″en-dek′tə-me) surgical removal of the vermiform appendix.

delayed a. a method of treating appendicitis complicated by an inflammatory mass or abscess; nonsurgical treatment is given initially and appendectomy is performed during the same hospital admission.

interval a. a method of treating appendicitis complicated by an inflammatory mass or abscess; nonsurgical treatment is given and the patient's condition is monitored for several weeks and appendectomy is performed during a second hospital admission.

ap•pen•di•cal (ə-pen′dĭ-kəl) appendicular (defs. 1 and 2).

ap•pen•dic•e•al (ap″en-dis′e-əl) appendicular (defs. 1 and 2).

ap•pen•di•cec•to•my (ə-pen″dĭ-sek′tə-me) [*appendix* + *-ectomy*] appendectomy.

ap•pen•di•ces (ə-pen′dĭ-sēz) [L.] plural of *appendix.*

ap•pen•di•ci•tis (ə-pen″dĭ-si′tis) inflammation of the vermiform appendix.

actinomycotic a. appendicitis caused by *Actinomyces israelii.*

acute a. appendicitis of acute onset requiring surgical intervention; symptoms usually include pain in the right lower abdominal quadrant with local and referred rebound tenderness, overlying muscle spasm, and cutaneous hyperesthesia; fever with presence of polymorphonuclear leukocytes results from the localized infection. Periumbilical colicky pain may be present, due to blockage of the appendix by a fecalith; other symptoms and signs may vary according to the location of the appendix or presence of adhesive bands or kinking.

amebic a. appendicitis caused by infection with *Entamoeba histolytica.*

chronic a. 1. appendicitis characterized by fibrotic thickening of the wall of the organ due to previous acute inflammation. 2. a term formerly applied to chronic or recurrent pain in the appendiceal area in the absence of evidence of acute inflammation.

foreign-body a. acute appendicitis, usually obstructive, due to a foreign body in the lumen.

fulminating a. acute appendicitis marked by sudden onset and often early death.

gangrenous a. acute appendicitis complicated by gangrene of the organ, owing to interference with the blood supply.

left-sided a. appendicitis on the left side of the abdomen, owing to situs inversus.

lumbar a. a type of appendicitis in which the appendix is posterior, lying against the peritoneum behind or below the cecum.

obstructive a. a common type of acute appendicitis caused by obstruction of the lumen of the appendix, such as by a fecalith.

perforating a., perforative a. acute appendicitis with perforation of the organ.

purulent a. suppurative a.

recurrent a., relapsing a. repeated episodes of acute appendicitis.

segmental a. inflammation confined to a segment of the appendix; it may be proximal, central, or distal.

stercoral a. appendicitis in which a fecal concretion is the assumed cause.

subperitoneal a. appendicitis in which the appendix is buried under the peritoneum instead of being free in the peritoneal cavity.

suppurative a. purulent infiltration of the walls of the appendix; called also *purulent a.*

traumatic a. acute appendicitis caused by trauma, such as something external or a medical procedure.

verminous a. appendicitis due to the presence of a worm in the appendix, usually causing obstruction.

appendic(o)- [L. *appendix,* q.v., gen. *appendicis*] a combining form denoting relation to an appendix, especially to the vermiform appendix.

ap•pen•di•co•ce•cos•to•my (ə-pen″dĭ-ko-se-kos′tə-me) 1. surgical creation of a new opening between the appendix and cecum, often including connection to a stoma on the skin surface for administration of an antegrade continence enema. 2. the opening so established.

ap•pen•di•co•cele (ə-pen′dĭ-ko-sēl) hernia containing the vermiform appendix.

ap•pen•di•co•lith (ə-pen′dĭ-ko-lith) a calculus in the vermiform appendix.

ap•pen•di•co•li•thi•a•sis (ə-pen″dĭ-ko″lĭ-thi′ə-sis) [*appendix* + *lithiasis*] obstruction of the lumen of the vermiform appendix with calculi. Called also *appendicular lithiasis.*

ap•pen•di•col•y•sis (ə-pen″dĭ-kol′ĭ-sis) [*appendix* + *-lysis*] the surgical division of adhesions about the appendix.

ap•pen•di•cop•a•thy (ə-pen″dĭ-kop′ə-the) [*appendix* + *-pathy*] any diseased condition of the vermiform appendix.

ap•pen•di•cos•to•my (ə-pen″dĭ-kos′tə-me) [*appendix* + *-stomy*] surgical creation of an opening from the surface of the abdominal wall into the vermiform appendix for the purpose of irrigating or draining the large intestine.

ap•pen•di•co•ves•i•cal (ə-pen″dĭ-ko-ves′ĭ-kəl) pertaining to or connecting the vermiform appendix and the urinary bladder.

ap•pen•di•co•ves•i•cos•to•my (ə-pen″dĭ-ko-ves″ĭ-kos′tə-me) surgical transference of the isolated appendix so that it can be used as a conduit for urinary diversion from the bladder to the skin in children with cloacal exstrophy or neurogenic bladder, making a route for insertion of a catheter. Called also *Mitrofanoff procedure.*

ap•pen•dic•u•lar (ap″en-dik′u-lər) 1. pertaining to the vermiform appendix. 2. pertaining to any appendix. Defs. 1 and 2 called also *appendiceal.* 3. pertaining to an appendage.

ap•pen•dix (ə-pen′diks) pl. *appendixes, appen′dices* [L., from *appendere* to hang upon] a supplementary, accessory, or dependent part attached to a main structure; called also *appendage.* Frequently used alone to denote the vermiform appendix (see *a. vermiformis*).

appen′dices adipo′sae co′li TA alternative for *appendices omentales.*

auricular a. auricula atrii.

cecal a. a. vermiformis.

a. epididy′midis [TA] appendix of epididymis: a remnant of the mesonephros sometimes found on the head of the epididymis; called also *appendage of epididymis.*

epiploic appendices appendices omentales.

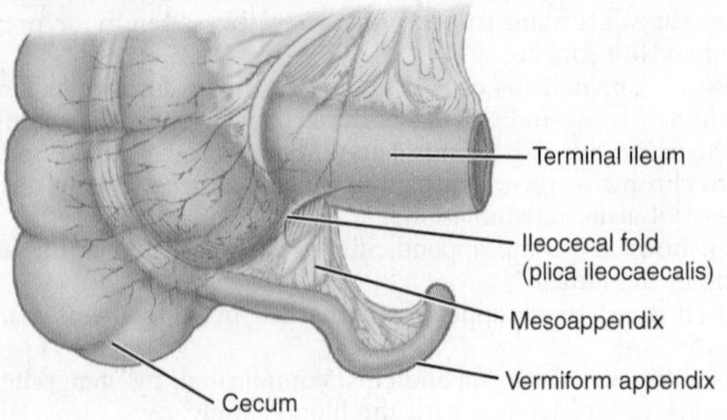

■ Vermiform appendix and adjacent structures.

appen′dices epiplo′icae TA alternative for *appendices omentales.*
fatty appendices of colon appendices omentales.
a. fibro′sa he′patis [TA], **fibrous a. of liver** a fibrous band at the left extremity of the liver, being the atrophied remnant of formerly more extensive liver tissue.
Morgagni a. 1. a. testis. 2. *(in the pl.)* appendices vesiculosae epoöphori.
omental appendices, appen′dices omenta′les [TA] peritoneum-covered tabs of fat, 2 to 10 cm long, attached in rows along the taeniae of the colon; called also *appendices epiploicae, appendices adiposae coli* [TA alternatives], *epiploic appendices,* and *fatty appendices of colon.*
a. tes′tis [TA] the remnant of part of the müllerian duct (paramesonephric duct) on the upper end of the testis; called also *hydatid of Morgagni, morgagnian cyst, sessile hydatid,* and *testicular appendage.*
a. of ventricle of larynx sacculus laryngis.
a. vermicula′ris a. vermiformis.
vermiform a., a. vermifor′mis [TA] a wormlike diverticulum of the cecum, varying in length from 7 to 15 cm, and measuring about 1 cm in diameter. Called also *appendix* and *cecal a.*
appen′dices vesiculo′sae epoo′phori [TA] vesicular appendages of epoophoron: small pedunculated structures attached to the uterine tubes near their fimbriated end, being remnants of the mesonephric ducts; called also *hydatids of Morgagni, Morgagni appendices,* and *morgagnian cyst.*
xiphoid a. processus xiphoideus.

ap·per·cep·tion (ap″ər-sep′shən) [L. *ad* to + *percipere* to perceive] conscious perception and appreciation; the power of receiving, appreciating, and interpreting sensory impressions. **appercep′tive** *adj*

ap·per·son·a·tion (ə-pur″so-na′shən) appersonification.

ap·per·son·i·fi·ca·tion (ap″ər-son″ĭ-fĭ-ka′shən) unconscious identification with another person or delusional belief that one is another person; it may be associated with various mental disorders, particularly schizophrenia.

ap·pe·stat (ap′ə-stat) [*appetite* + *stat*] the brain center (probably in the hypothalamus) concerned with controlling the amount of food intake.

ap·pe·tite (ap′ə-tīt) [L. *appetere* to desire] a natural longing or desire, especially the natural and recurring desire for food.

ap·pe·ti·tion (ap″ə-tish′ən) [L. *ad* toward + *petere* to seek] the directing of desire toward a definite purpose or object.

ap·pet·i·tive (ə-pet′ĭ-tiv″) characterized by approach, or exciting approach behavior; said of stimuli or behavior. Cf. *aversive.*

ap·pla·na·tion (ap″lə-na′shən) [L. *applanatio*] undue flatness, as of the cornea.

ap·pla·nom·e·ter (ap″lə-nom′ĕ-tər) applanation tonometer.

ap·ple (ap′əl) 1. *Malus sylvestris.* L. 2. the edible fruit of *M. sylvestris.* In dried and powdered form it is used as an antidiarrheal; its seeds are cyanogenetic, and ingestion of large quantities can cause cyanide poisoning. 3. something that resembles this fruit.
Adam's a. prominentia laryngea.
bitter a. colocynth.
Indian a., May a. podophyllum.
thorn a. 1. *Datura stramonium.* 2. stramonium (def. 2).

ap·pli·ance (ə-pli′əns) in dentistry, a general term referring to various devices used to provide a function or therapeutic effect, e.g., dental prostheses, obturators, or orthodontic appliances.
Andresen a. functional activator.
Begg a. an orthodontic appliance consisting of a light wire and brackets permitting the tipping of tooth crowns, horizontal buccal tubes on the anchor molars to prevent their tipping, and elastics. See also *Begg technique,* under *technique.*
Bimler a. a removable orthodontic appliance believed to stimulate reflex muscle activity, which in turn produces the desired tooth movement. Called also *Bimler stimulator.*
craniofacial a. a device used to immobilize and/or reduce mandibular or midfacial fractures.
Crozat a. a removable orthodontic appliance, usually made of a precious metal, used to align teeth during orthodontic therapy. Called also *crozat* and *Walker a.*
Denholz a. an orthodontic appliance consisting of a wire assembly containing a vestibular acrylic screen and open coil spring segments that fit over the wire arch.
edgewise a. a fixed, multiunit orthodontic appliance using a rectangular labial arch wire ligated to brackets cemented to individual teeth or to bands encircling the teeth. So called because the bracket is machined so that the rectangular arch wire is inserted with its long cross section horizontal instead of vertical as in the ribbon arch bracket. Called also *edgewise attachment.*
expansion plate a. any orthodontic appliance equipped with an expansion plate. Called also *split plate a.*
extraoral a. an orthodontic appliance using a resistance unit outside of the oral cavity; see under *anchorage.*
fixed a. an appliance that is cemented to the teeth or attached by means of an adhesive material. Called also *permanent a.*
Fränkel a. function corrector.
habit-breaking a. an orthodontic appliance designed to correct faulty habits, such as finger-sucking, tongue-thrusting, infantile swallowing.
Hawley a. see under *retainer.*
Jackson a. a removable orthodontic appliance retained in position by crib-shaped wires, bent to follow the outline of the buccal and lingual contours of the bicuspid and molar teeth, and united by cross wires lying in the occlusal embrasures. Called also *Jackson crib.*
Johnston twin wire a. twin wire a.
jumping-the-bite a. Kingsley a.
Kesling a. an occlusal splint made of soft acrylic resin or latex rubber that fits over the occlusal and incisal surfaces of the teeth; it is designed to hold the mandible in a certain relationship to the maxilla to treat bruxism.
Kingsley a. an active plate appliance having a bite plate with an inclined anterior plane to move the mandible forward by jumping the bite. Called also *jumping-the-bite a., jumping-the-bite plate,* and *Kingsley plate.*
labiolingual a. an orthodontic appliance for intermaxillary therapy, consisting of a maxillary labial arch introduced into horizontal buccal tubes attached to the anchor bands and lingual arches of the same diameter fitted into vertical or horizontal tubes fastened to the lingual side of the anchor bands.
monoblock a. functional activator.
orthodontic a. a device, either fixed to the teeth or removable, that applies force to the teeth and their supporting structures to produce changes in their relationship to each other and to control their growth and development. Used in orthodontic therapy to move the teeth into esthetically or physiologically better positions, such as better alignment within the dental arch or with the opposing dentition. Called also *braces.*
permanent a. fixed a.
prosthetic a. a device affixed to or implanted in the body, designed to take the place, or perform the function, of a missing body part, such as an artificial limb or a complete or partial denture.
removable a. any orthodontic appliance that the patient is able to insert and remove from the mouth.
ribbon arch a. an orthodontic appliance consisting of a flattened wire inserted into a special bracket against the labial and buccal surfaces of the teeth; usually done to move the teeth laterally. Called also *ribbon arch.*
Schwarz a. a removable orthodontic appliance with a tissue-borne anchorage and appurtenances of wire for tooth movement.
split plate a. expansion plate a.
twin wire a. an orthodontic appliance using fixed lingual arches and a labial arch consisting of a pair of round wires attached to brackets on the anterior teeth. Called also *Johnston twin wire a.* and *twin wire.*
universal a. an orthodontic appliance that combines the edgewise and ribbon arch techniques, affording precise control of individual teeth in all

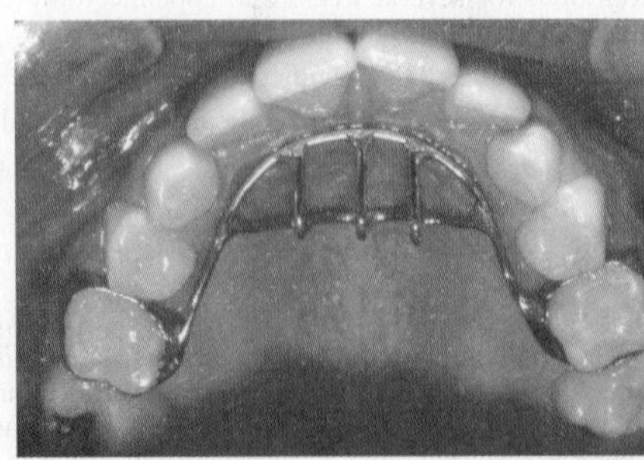

■ Habit-breaking appliance cemented to the molars and used as a reminder to interrupt a finger-sucking habit.

planes of space; it consists of bands or brackets or both for all the teeth in both arches.

Walker a. Crozat a.

ap·pli·ca·tor (ap′lĭ-ka″tər) an instrument for putting something (such as a remedy) onto a surface.

sonic a. an electromechanical transducer used in the local application of sound for therapeutic purposes, as in the treatment of muscular ailments.

ap·pli·qué (ap″lĭ-ka′) see under *form.*

ap·po·si·tion (ap″ə-zish′ən) [L. *appositio*] the placing of things next to each other; specifically, the deposition of successive layers upon those already present, as in cell walls. Called also *juxtaposition.*

ap·pre·hen·sion (ap″re-hen′shən) 1. perception and understanding. 2. anticipatory fear or anxiety.

ap·proach (ə-prōch′) 1. the method used to reach some goal. 2. the specific anatomic dissection by which an organ or part is exposed in surgery.

Risdon a. a surgical method of exposing the ascending ramus of the mandible by means of an incision made below and behind the angle of the mandible, for treatment of fractures, e.g., condylar fractures, or for reconstructive surgery.

Trager A. service mark for a bodywork technique whose purpose is to train patients to develop awareness of movement patterns that relieve pain and promote relaxation. It consists of two components: tablework, in which the practitioner, in a meditative state, uses touch and gentle passive movement to assist the person in experiencing new movement patterns, and Mentastics, in which the patient is taught a series of movements designed to relieve tension.

ap·prox·i·mal (ə-prok′sĭ-məl) situated close together.

ap·prox·i·mate (ə-prok′sĭ-māt″) 1. to bring close together, or into apposition. 2. approximal.

ap·prox·i·ma·tion (ə-prok″sĭ-ma′shən) the act or process of bringing closer together or into apposition.

successive a. shaping.

ap·ra·clon·i·dine hy·dro·chlo·ride (ap″rə-klon′ĭ-dēn) [USP] an α_2-adrenergic receptor agonist used to reduce intraocular pressure in the treatment of open-angle glaucoma and the treatment and prevention of ocular hypertension; administered topically.

aprac·tag·no·sia (ə-prak″tag-no′zhə) [*apractic* + *agnosia*] a type of agnosia marked by inability to use objects or perform skilled motor activities, due to lesions in the lower occipital or parietal lobes; subtypes include *ideomotor apraxia* and *sensory apraxia.*

ap·ra·my·cin (ap″rə-mi′sin) an aminoglycoside antibiotic, part of the nebramycin complex, effective against a wide variety of aerobic gram-negative bacilli; used as the sulfate salt in the treatment of enteric colibacillosis in swine.

aprax·ia (ə-prak′se-ə) [Gr. "a not acting," "want of success"] loss of ability to carry out familiar, purposeful movements in the absence of paralysis or other motor or sensory impairment. Cf. *dyspraxia.* **aprac′tic, aprax′ic** *adj*

akinetic a. loss of ability to carry out spontaneous movement.

amnestic a. loss of ability to carry out a movement on command as a result of inability to remember the command, although ability to perform the movement is present.

Bruns a. gait a.

buccofacial a. facial a.

classic a. ideokinetic a.

Cogan oculomotor a., congenital oculomotor a. an absence or defect of horizontal eye movements, so that when the patient tries to look at an object off to one side, the head must turn to bring the eyes into line with the object and the eyes exhibit nystagmus; the cause is probably a brain lesion. Called also *Cogan syndrome.*

constructional a. a type of deficit in motor skills characterized by lack of ability to copy simple drawings or to reproduce patterns created with building blocks or matchsticks.

dressing a. inability to dress oneself properly, often on just one side, as a result of a lesion in the parietal lobe, usually on the nondominant side. See also *unilateral neglect,* under *neglect.*

facial a. apraxia of the facial muscles with inability to carry out movements for expression, articulation, and other functions; caused by a lesion in either the supramarginal gyrus or the motor association area on the dominant side. It may be associated with ideokinetic apraxia. Called also *buccofacial a.*

gait a., a. of gait a disorder of gait and equilibrium caused by a lesion in the frontal lobe, commonly seen in elderly persons and those with Alzheimer disease; the person walks with a broad-based gait, taking short steps and placing the feet flat on the ground. Called also *Bruns a.* and *frontal ataxia.*

ideational a. sensory a.

ideokinetic a., ideomotor a. inability to carry out movements that are part of normal activities when requested, in imitation of a demonstration, or even when the person spontaneously wishes to do them. The name is derived from the older concept that ideas were not linked to movements. Called also *transcortical a.*

Liepmann a. apraxia.

motor a. impairment of skilled movements that is greater than or different in form from that caused by weakness of the affected parts; the patient appears clumsy rather than weak.

ocular a. gaze paralysis.

ocular motor a., oculomotor a. defective or absent voluntary eye movements, often owing to a brain lesion. It may be congenital (see Cogan oculomotor a.) or acquired as a result of a brain lesion or ataxia-telangiectasia.

sensory a. loss of ability to make proper use of an object, due to lack of perception of its proper nature and purpose or to gross disorganization of a plan of usage. Called also *ideational a.*

a. of speech a speech disorder similar to motor aphasia, due to apraxia of mouth and neck muscles because of a lesion interfering with coordination of impulses from Broca's motor speech area. Called also *aphemia.*

transcortical a. ideokinetic a.

aprep·i·tant (ə-prep′ĭ-tənt) an antagonist of substance P, used as an antiemetic; administered orally.

Apres·a·zide (ə-pres′ə-zīd) trademark for combination preparations of hydralazine hydrochloride and hydrochlorothiazide.

Apres·o·line (ə-pres′o-lēn) trademark for preparations of hydralazine hydrochloride.

APRI AST to platelet ratio index.

Apri·so (ə-pre′zo) trademark for a preparation of mesalamine.

APRN advanced practice registered nurse.

ap·ro·bar·bi·tal (ap″ro-bahr′bĭ-təl) an intermediate-acting barbiturate, used as a sedative and hypnotic; administered orally. Abuse of this drug may lead to dependence.

aproc·tia (ə-prok′she-ə) imperforate anus.

apro·so·dia (a″pro-so′de-ə) aprosody.

motor a. inability to modulate speech and gestures to convey emotional content, usually owing to a lesion in a frontal lobe.

sensory a. inability to comprehend the emotional content of the speech and gestures of others, usually owing to damage in part of a temporal lobe.

apros·o·dy (a-pros′ə-de) severe dysprosody.

apro·so·pia (ap″ro-so′pe-ə) [*a-*[1] + *prosopo-* + *-ia*] partial or complete congenital absence of structures of the face.

apro·so·pus (ə-pro′sə-pəs) a fetus exhibiting aprosopia.

apro·tic (a-pro′tik) denoting a substance that neither accepts nor donates protons.

apro·ti·nin (ap″ro-ti′nin) [USP] a single-chain polypeptide of the serpin group that inhibits multiple mediators, resulting in attenuation of inflammatory responses, of fibrinolysis, and of thrombin generation; used as an antihemorrhagic to reduce perioperative blood loss in patients undergoing cardiopulmonary bypass during coronary artery bypass graft; administered intravenously.

APS American Physiological Society; antiphospholipid (antibody) syndrome.

APTA American Physical Therapy Association.

ap·ter·ous (ap′tər-əs) [*a-*[1] + Gr. *pteron* wing] wingless.

ap·ti·tude (ap′tĭ-tōōd) natural ability and skill in certain lines of endeavor.

Ap·ti·vus (ap′tĭ-vəs) trademark for a preparation of tipranavir.

APTT, aPTT activated partial thromboplastin time.

ap·ty·a·lia (ap″ti-a′le-ə, a″ti-a′le-ə) aptyalism.

ap·ty·a·lism (ap-ti′ə-liz-əm, a-ti′ə-liz-əm) deficiency or absence of the saliva.

APUD [*a*mine *p*recursor *u*ptake (and) *d*ecarboxylation] see under *cell.*

apud·o·ma (a″pəd-o′mə) any tumor composed of cells with APUD properties.

apul·mo·nism (a-pool′mo-niz-əm) [*a-*[1] + *pulmon-* + *-ism*] apneumia.

apus (a′pəs) [*a-*[1] + Gr. *pous* foot] sirenomelus.

apy·e·tous (a-pi′ə-təs) [*a-*[1] + Gr. *pyon* pus] showing no pus; nonpurulent.

apyk·no·mor·phous (ə-pik″no-mor′fəs) [*a-*[1] + *pyknomorphous*] not pyknomorphous; not having the stainable cell elements compactly placed; said of certain nerve cells.

apy·ous (a-pi′əs) [*a-*[1] + Gr. *pyon* pus] having no pus; nonpurulent.

apy·rene (a′pi-rēn) [*a-*[1] + Gr. *pyrēn* fruit stone, nucleus] having no nucleus or nuclear material; said of certain spermatozoa.

apy·ret·ic (a″pi-ret′ik) [*a-*[1] + *pyretic*] afebrile.

apy·rex·ia (a″pi-rek′se-ə) [*a-*[1] + *pyrexia*] 1. absence of fever. 2. the intermission of fever.

apy·rex·i·al (a″pi-rek′se-əl) afebrile.

apy·ro·gen·ic (a-pi″ro-jen′ik) [*a-*[1] + *pyrogenic*] not producing fever.

AQ achievement quotient.

Aq. [L.] a′qua (water).
 Aq. dest. a′qua destilla′ta (distilled water).
 Aq. pur. a′qua pu′ra (pure water).
 Aq. tep. a′qua tep′ida (tepid water).

aq·ua (ah′kwə, ak′wə) pl. *a′quae* [L.] water.
 a. o′culi aqueous humor.
 a. re′gia a mixture of one part concentrated nitric acid to three or four parts concentrated hydrochloric acid; it is able to dissolve gold and platinum.

Aqua·bir·na·vi·rus (ah″kwə-bur′nə-vi″rəs) [L. *aqua* water + *bi*segmented *RNA* + *virus*] a genus of viruses of the family Birnaviridae that infect fish, mollusks, and crustaceans; it includes a single species, infectious pancreatic necrosis virus, which is the cause of infectious pancreatic necrosis of fish.

Aq·ua·chlo·ral (ah-kwə-klor′əl) trademark for a preparation of chloral hydrate.

aq·uae (ah′kwe, ak′we) [L.] plural of *aqua.*

aq·uae·duc·tus (ak″we-duk′təs) [L.] aqueductus.

aq·ua·gen·ic (ak″wə-jen′ik) caused by water or by contact with water.

Aq·ua·MEPH·Y·TON (ak″wə-mef′ĭ-tən) trademark for a preparation of phytonadione.

aq·ua·pho·bia (ak″wə-fo′be-ə) [*aqua-* + *-phobia*] irrational fear of water, i.e., of swimming or of being near water where one might fall in and drown.

aqua·po·rin (ak″wə-po′rin) any of a family of proteins, composed of four identical 28-kD subunits surrounding a central, water-permeable pore and found in the plasma membranes of plant and animal cells, that permit passage of water and very small solutes. Called also *water channel.*

aq·ua·punc·ture (ak′wə-pungk″chər) [*aqua* + *puncture*] the subcutaneous injection of water.

Aq·ua·reo·vi·rus (ak″wə-re′o-vi″rəs) [L. *aqua* water + *reovirus*] a genus of viruses of the family Reoviridae that infect fresh- and salt-water fish and invertebrates; some species cause economically important diseases of fish.

aq·ua·re·sis (ak″wə-re′sis) the excretion of water that is free of electrolytes.

aq·ua·ret·ic (ak″wə-ret′ik) 1. pertaining to or causing aquaresis. 2. a substance that causes aquaresis.

Aq·ua·ten·sen (ak″wə-ten′sən) trademark for a preparation of methyclothiazide.

aquat·ic (ə-kwaht′ik) inhabiting or frequenting water.

aq·ue·duct (ak′wə-dukt″) a passage or channel in a body structure or organ; see also *aqueductus.*
 cerebral a. aqueductus mesencephali.
 cochlear a. aqueductus cochleae.
 a. of Cotunnius 1. aqueductus vestibuli. 2. canaliculus cochleae.
 fallopian a., a. of Fallopius canalis nervi facialis.
 a. of mesencephalon, a. of midbrain aqueductus mesencephali.
 a. of Sylvius aqueductus mesencephali.
 ventricular a. aqueductus mesencephali.
 vestibular a. aqueductus vestibuli.

aq·ue·duc·tus (ak″wə-duk′təs) gen. and pl. *aqueduc′tus* [L., from *aqua* water + *ductus* canal] a passage or channel in a body structure or organ, especially a channel for the conduction of fluid; called also *aqueduct* and *aquaeductus.*
 a. ce′rebri TA alternative for *a. mesencephali.*
 a. coch′leae [TA] cochlear aqueduct: a small channel that connects the scala tympani with the subarachnoid space; called also *perilymphatic duct.*
 a. mesence′phali [TA] aqueduct of mesencephalon: the narrow channel in the mesencephalon that connects the third and fourth ventricles; called also *aqueduct of Sylvius, a. cerebri* [TA alternative], and *cerebral aqueduct.*
 a. vesti′buli [TA] aqueduct of vestibule: a small canal extending from the vestibule of the internal ear to open onto the posterior surface of the petrous part of the temporal bone. It lodges the endolymphatic duct and an arteriole and a venule. Called also *vestibular aqueduct* and *aqueduct of Cotunnius.*

aque·ous (a′kwe-əs) 1. watery; prepared with water. 2. aqueous humor.

aq·uip·a·rous (ak-wip′ə-rəs) [*aqua* + *-parous*] producing water or a watery secretion.

AR alarm reaction; aortic regurgitation; artificial respiration.

Ar argon.

ara-A adenine arabinoside; see *vidarabine.*

ar·a·ban (ar-ə-ban) any of a group of pentosans composed of L-arabinose residues; they are major constituents of gums and pectins.

ar·a·bic ac·id (ar′ə-bik) arabin.

ar·a·bin (ar′ə-bin) an amorphous carbohydrate gum composed of residues of arabinose, rhamnose, galactose, and an aldobionic acid composed of glucuronic acid and galactose; its salts with calcium, potassium, and magnesium are the main constituents of gum arabic (acacia). Called also *arabic acid.*

arab·i·nose (ə-rab′ĭ-nōs) an aldopentose epimeric with ribose at the 2 carbon, occurring naturally in both D- and L-forms, widely distributed in plants in the form of complex polysaccharides, glycosides, and mucilages and also occurring in some bacteria.

ar·a·bin·o·side (ar″ə-bin′o-sīd) a glycoside of arabinose.

arab·in·o·sis (ə-rab″ĭ-no′sis) poisoning by arabinose, which may produce nephrosis.

arab·i·no·su·ria (ə-rab″ĭ-nōs-u′re-ə) the presence of arabinose in the urine.

arab·i·no·syl·cy·to·sine (ə-rab″ĭ-no-səl-si′to-sēn) cytarabine.

arab·i·tol (ə-rab′ĭ-tol) a sugar alcohol formed by the reduction of the carbonyl group of arabinose.

arab(o)- related to, or having the same stereochemical arrangement as, arabinose.

ara-C arabinosylcytosine; see *cytarabine.*

arach·ic ac·id (ə-rak′ik) arachidic acid.

arach·i·date (ə-rak′ĭ-dāt) a salt (soap), ester, or anionic form of arachidic acid.

ar·a·chid·ic (ar″ə-kid′ik) [L. *arachis* peanut] pertaining to or caused by peanuts or other members of the genus *Arachis.*

ar·a·chid·ic ac·id (ar″ə-kid′ik) a saturated 20-carbon fatty acid found in vegetable oils such as peanut oil and in fish oils. Called also *eicosanoic acid.* See table accompanying *fatty acid.*

arach·i·don·ate (ə-rak″ĭ-don′āt) a salt, ester, or anion of arachidonic acid.

arach·i·don·ate 5-lip·oxy·gen·ase (ə-rak″ĭ-don′āt lĭ-pok′sə-jən-ās) [EC 1.13.11.34] an enzyme of the oxidoreductase class that catalyzes the oxidation of arachidonate at the 5 position to form 5-hydroperoxyeicosatetraenoic acid (5-HPETE). The reaction occurs in leukocytes, particularly neutrophils, as the first step of the lipoxygenase pathway for conversion of arachidonic acid to leukotrienes.

arach·i·don·ate 12-lip·oxy·gen·ase (ə-rak′ĭ-don″āt lĭ-pok′sə-jən-ās) [EC 1.13.11.31] an enzyme of the oxidoreductase class that catalyzes the oxidation of arachidonate at the 12 position to form 12-hydroperoxyeicosatetraenoic acid (12-HPETE). The reaction occurs primarily in platelets and is the first step of the lipoxygenase pathway for conversion of arachidonic acid to the leukotriene 12-hydroxyeicosatetraenoic acid (12-HETE).

arach·i·don·ate 15-lip·oxy·ge·nase (ə-rak′ĭ-don′āt lĭ-pok′sə-jən-ās) [EC 1.13.11.33] an enzyme of the oxidoreductase class that catalyzes the oxidation of arachidonate at the 15 position to form 15-hydroperoxyeicosatetraenoic acid (15-HPETE). The reaction occurs primarily in vascular endothelium and is the first step in the conversion of arachidonic acid to 15-hydroxyeicosatetraenoic acid (15-HETE) and to lipoxins.

arach·i·don·ic ac·id (ə-rak″ĭ-don′ik) a polyunsaturated 20-carbon essential fatty acid (see table at *fatty acid*) occurring in animal fats and also formed by biosynthesis from dietary linoleic acid. It is a precursor in the biosynthesis of leukotrienes, prostaglandins, and thromboxanes.

Ara·chis (ar′ə-kis) a genus of herbs of the family Leguminosae, having yellow flowers, originally native to southern Brazil. *A. hypogae′a* is the peanut, source of peanut oil. See also *aflatoxin.*

arach·ne·pho·bia (ə-rak″nə-fo′be-ə) arachnophobia.

arach·nid (ə-rak′nid) any member of the class Arachnida.

Arach·ni·da (ə-rak′nĭ-də) [Gr. *arachnē* spider] a class of the Arthropoda; orders include Araneae (the spiders), Acarina (the ticks and mites), and Scorpionida (the scorpions).

arach•nid•ism (ə-rak'nĭ-diz-əm) the condition produced by the bite of a venomous spider; envenomation by a spider. Called also *araneism* and *arachnoidism.*
 necrotic a. spider envenomation marked by necrosis at the site of the bite, resulting in slow-healing, ulcerating lesions.

arach•ni•tis (ar"ak-ni'tis) [*arachno-* + *-itis*] arachnoiditis.

arachn(o)- [Gr. *arachnē* spider] a combining form denoting relationship to the arachnoid membrane or to a spider.

arach•no•dac•tyl•ia (ə-rak"no-dak-til'e-ə) arachnodactyly.

arach•no•dac•ty•ly (ə-rak"no-dak'tə-le) [*arachno-* + Gr. *daktylos* finger] a condition characterized by abnormal length and slenderness of the fingers and toes; called also *acromacria, dolichostenomelia,* and *spider finger.* Sometimes used in the past as a synonym for *Marfan syndrome.*
 congenital contractural a. (CCA) an autosomal dominant syndrome caused by mutations in the *FBN2* gene (locus: 5q23-q31), which encodes fibrillin 2. It is characterized by long, thin extremities; multiple joint contractures; kyphoscoliosis; and malformed auricles of the ears. Called also *distal arthrogryposis type 9* and *Beals syndrome.*

arach•no•gas•tria (ə-rak"no-gas'tre-ə) [*arachno-* + *gastr-* + *-ia*] the prominent network of veins on the protuberant abdomen caused by ascites, especially in cirrhosis.

arach•noid (ə-rak'noid) 1. resembling a spider's web. 2. arachnoidea mater.
 a. of brain, cranial a. arachnoidea mater cranialis.
 spinal a., a. of spinal cord arachnoidea mater spinalis.

arach•noi•dal (ar"ak-noi'dəl) pertaining to the arachnoidea mater.

arach•noi•dea (ar"ak-noi'de-ə) pl. *arachnoi'deae* [Gr. *arachnoidēs* like a cobweb] arachnoidea mater.

arach•noi•dea ma•ter (ar"ak-noi'de-ə ma'tər, mah'ter) [TA] a delicate membrane interposed between the dura mater and the pia mater, separated from the pia mater by the subarachnoid space.
 a. m. crania'lis [TA] the arachnoidea covering the brain; called also *arachnoid of brain, cranial arachnoid,* and *a. m. encephali* [TA alternative].
 a. m. ence'phali TA alternative for *a. m. cranialis.*
 a. m. et pi'a ma'ter TA alternative for *leptomeninx.*
 a. m. spina'lis [TA] spinal arachnoid: the arachnoidea covering the spinal cord; called also *arachnoid of spinal cord.*

arach•noid•ism (ə-rak'noid-iz"əm) arachnidism.

arach•noid•i•tis (ə-rak"noid-i'tis) [*arachnoid* + *-itis*] inflammation of the arachnoidea mater; called also *arachnitis.*
 chronic adhesive a. thickening and adhesions of the leptomeninges in the brain or spinal cord, resulting from previous meningitis, other disease processes, or trauma; it is sometimes secondary to therapeutic or diagnostic injection of substances into the subarachnoid space. The signs and symptoms vary with extent and location. See also *spinal a.*
 spinal a., spinal adhesive a. chronic adhesive arachnoiditis in the spinal arachnoid, with root and spinal cord symptoms similar to those caused by pressure from a tumor.

arach•noid ma•ter (ə-rak'noid ma'tər, mah'ter) arachnoidea mater.
 cranial a. m. arachnoidea mater cranialis.
 spinal a. m. arachnoidea mater spinalis.

arach•nol•y•sin (ar"ak-nol'ə-sin) [*arachno-* + *lysin*] the active hemolytic principle of spider venom.

arach•no•me•lia (ə-rak"no-me'le-ə) [*arachno-* + *-melia*] an autosomal recessive skeletal defect in calves and lambs in which the limbs are long, thin, and fragile, resembling the legs of a spider.

arach•no•pho•bia (ə-rak"no-fo'be-ə) [*arachno-* + *-phobia*] irrational fear of spiders.

Ar•a•len (ăr'ə-len) trademark for preparations of chloroquine.

aral•kyl (ə-ral'kəl) an organic group in which an aryl group has replaced an alkyl hydrogen.

Ar•a•mine (ar'ə-min) trademark for a preparation of metaraminol.

Ar•an's law (ah-rahnz') [François Amilcar *Aran,* French physician, 1817–1861] see under *law.*

Ar•an-Du•chenne muscular atrophy (disease) (ah-rahn' du-shen') [F.A. *Aran;* Guillaume Benjamin Amand *Duchenne,* French neurologist, 1806–1875] spinal muscular atrophy; see under *atrophy.*

Aran•e•ae (ə-rān'e-e) an order of the Arachnida comprising the spiders; it is divided into the suborders Labidognatha and Orthognatha.

Ar•a•ne•i•da (ar"ə-ne'ĭ-də) Araneae.

ara•ne•ism (ə-ra'ne-iz-əm) arachnidism.

Ar•a•nesp (ar'ə-nesp) trademark for a preparation of darbepoetin alfa.

Aran•ti•us bodies (nodules), etc. (ə-ran'shəs) [Julius Caesar *Arantius (Aranzi),* Italian anatomist and physician, 1530–1589] see *ductus venosus* and *ligamentum venosum;* see *noduli valvularum semilunarium valvae aortae,* under *nodulus;* and see under *ventricle.*

Aran•zi (ah-rahn'tse) Arantius.

ara•phia (ə-ra'fe-ə) dysraphism.

Ar•a•va (ar'ə-və) trademark for a preparation of leflunomide.

ar•bor (ahr'bər) pl. *ar'bores* [L.] a treelike structure or part; a structure or system resembling a tree with its branches.
 a. bronchia'lis [TA] bronchial tree: the bronchi and their branching structures.
 dendritic a. see under *tree.*
 a. vi'tae 1. *Thuja occidentalis.* 2. a. vitae cerebelli.
 a. vi'tae cerebel'li [TA] the treelike outline of white substance seen in a median section of the cerebellum; called also *medullary body of vermis.*
 a. vi'tae u'teri plicae palmatae.

ar•bo•re•al (ahr-bo're-əl) 1. pertaining to trees or to a treelike part; see *arbor.* 2. inhabiting or attached to trees.

ar•bo•res (ahr-bor'ēz) [L.] plural of *arbor.*

ar•bo•res•cent (ahr"bə-res'ənt) [L. *arborescens*] branching like a tree; called also *dendriform* and *dendroid.*

ar•bo•ri•za•tion (ahr"bə-rĭ-za'shən) 1. the branching termination of certain nerve cell processes. 2. a form of the termination of a nerve fiber when in contact with a muscle fiber. 3. the treelike appearance of capillary vessels in inflamed conditions.

ar•bo•vi•rus (ahr'bo-vi"rəs) [from *ar*thropod-*bo*rne + virus] any member of an epidemiologic class of viruses (the arboviruses) that replicate in blood-feeding arthropods and are transmitted by bite to the host. Arboviruses can be grouped serologically; the original groups were designated A, B, and C, but new groups are named from the first member of the group to be discovered. Arboviruses are contained in the families Arenaviridae, Bunyaviridae, Flaviviridae, Reoviridae, Rhabdoviridae, and Togaviridae; a few are unclassified. "Arbovirus" has no relationship to viral chemistry, morphology, or replication and so has no standing as a legitimate taxonomic term. **arbovi'ral** *adj*
 group A a's *Alphavirus.*
 group B a's *Flavivirus.*

ar•but•amine hy•dro•chlo•ride (ahr-bu'tə-mēn") a synthetic catecholamine used as a diagnostic aid in cardiac stress testing in patients unable to exercise sufficiently for the test; administered intravenously through a device that determines and delivers the dose as a function of the heart rate through the procedure.

ARC AIDS-related complex; American Red Cross; anomalous retinal correspondence.

arc (ahrk) [*arcus*] 1. a structure or projected path having a curved or bowlike outline. 2. a visible electrical discharge generally taking the outline of an arc. 3. in neurophysiology, the pathway of neural reactions.
 auricular a., binauricular a. a measurement from the center of one auditory meatus to that of the other.
 bregmatolambdoid a. the arc extending along the course of the sagittal suture from the bregma to the lambda.
 carbon a. an electrical discharge between carbon electrodes that gives off an intense white light.
 mercury a. an electric discharge between electrodes in mercury vapor in a vacuum tube; it gives off light rich in ultraviolet rays.
 nasobregmatic a. the arc extending from the nasion to the bregma.
 naso-occipital a. the arc extending from the nasion to the most inferior part of the external occipital protuberance.
 neural a. a series of two or more neurons connecting certain receptors and effectors, and constituting the pathway for neural reactions and reflexes; called also *sensorimotor a.*
 nuclear a. vortex lentis.
 reflex a. the neural arc used in a reflex action; an impulse travels to a nerve center over afferent fibers and the response travels outward from the center to an effector organ or part over efferent fibers. See illustration.
 sensorimotor a. neural a.

ar•cade (ahr-kād') an anatomical structure composed of a series of arches.
 arterial a's a series of anastomosing arterial arches as in the intestinal branches of the superior mesenteric artery.
 Flint a. a series of arteriovenous arches at the base of the renal pyramids.
 a. of Fröhse a fibrous arch formed by the superficial layer of the supinator muscle next to the biceps brachii tendon, forming part of the radial tunnel.
 lower dental a., mandibular dental a. arcus dentalis mandibularis.
 marginal a. arteria marginalis coli.
 maxillary dental a., upper dental a. arcus dentalis maxillaris.

Ar•ca•no•bac•te•ri•um (ahr-ka"no-bak-tēr'e-əm) [L. *arcanus* secret + *bacterium*] a genus of irregular, rod-shaped, non–spore-forming,

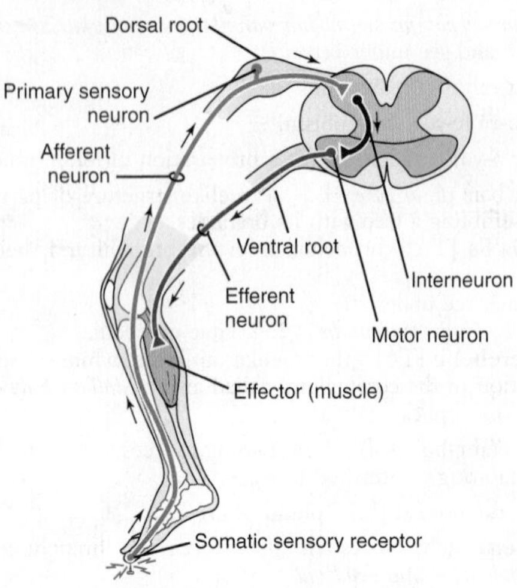

■ Simple reflex arc by which sensory input leads to a muscular movement. A receptor transduces a painful stimulus into an action potential, which is conveyed by the afferent neuron to the central nervous system (CNS) and then passed on to the target organ by an efferent neuron, where the electrical signals are converted to muscle motion.

gram-positive bacteria of the family Actinomycetaceae; organisms are nonmotile, facultatively anaerobic, and catalase-negative. The type species is *A. haemoly'ticum.*

A. bernar'diae a species that causes actinomycosis and sometimes other infections.

A. haemoly'ticum a species that causes human and animal infection. In adolescents, infection is manifested by pharyngitis and a scarlatiniform rash similar to those seen in streptococcal infection.

A. pyo'genes a toxicogenic species that causes acute pyogenic lesions in cattle, sheep, and pigs, interdigital dermatitis in sheep, and foot rot in pigs, and has been isolated from human pharyngitis and skin lesions. Formerly called *Corynebacterium pyogenes.*

ar·cate (ahr'kāt) arcuate.

Ar·cel·la (ahr-sel'ə) [L., dim. of *arca* box, chest] a genus of testate amebae, protozoa of the order Arcellinida, characterized by a few slender lobopodia and a transparent test to which the body of the organism is attached by numerous strands of ectoplasm.

Ar·cel·lin·i·da (ahr″sə-lin'ĭ-də) an order of testate amebae, free-living protozoa of the class Lobosa, phylum Sarcomastigophora; all species are enclosed in a test, tectum, or other external membrane that is composed of either organic or inorganic material or both and has a definite aperture through which pseudopodia (lobopodia or filopodia) can be extruded. A representative genus is *Arcella.* Called also *Testacea.*

arch (ahrch) [L. *arcus* bow] a structure with a curved or bowlike outline. arc'ual *adj*

Arch

For specific anatomic structures not listed here, see under *arcus.*

abdominothoracic a. the lower boundary of the anterior aspect of the thorax.

alveolar a. an arch formed by the ridge of the alveolar process of the mandible or maxilla; see *arcus alveolaris mandibulae* and *arcus alveolaris maxillae.*

anterior a. of atlas arcus anterior atlantis.

anterior carpal a. palmar carpal a.

anterior palatine a. arcus palatoglossus.

a. of aorta arcus aortae.

aortic a. 1. arcus aortae. 2. any of a group of paired vessels arching from the ventral to the dorsal aorta through the branchial arches of fishes and the pharyngeal arches of amniote embryos. In mammalian development, arches 1 and 2 disappear; arch 3 joins the common to the internal carotid; the left arch 4 remains as the arch of the definitive aorta while the right arch 4 joins the aorta to the subclavian artery; arch 5 is absent or disappears; and the ventral halves of arch 6 form the pulmonary arteries while the connections to the dorsal aorta are lost, although the left half, or ductus arteriosus, serves as an arterial shunt until birth.

axillary a. a muscular slip occasionally arising from the cranial border of the latissimus dorsi muscle, crossing the axilla anterior to the axillary vessels and nerves, and joining the under surface of the tendon of the pectoralis major, the coracobrachialis, or the fascia of the biceps brachii muscle.

a. of azygos vein arcus venae azygou.

basal a. apical base.

branchial a's paired arched columns that bear the gills in lower aquatic vertebrates and that, in the embryos of higher vertebrates, appear in comparable form before subsequent modification into structures of the head and neck. Each one contains a cartilaginous bar, consisting of right and left halves. In humans these are called *pharyngeal arches* because gills do not develop.

cervical aortic a. a rare, usually asymptomatic, congenital anomaly in which the aortic arch has an abnormally superior location, occasionally extending to the thoracic inlet or into the neck.

a's of Corti a series of arches in the organ of Corti formed by inner and outer pillar cells.

costal a. arcus costalis.

a. of cricoid cartilage arcus cartilaginis cricoideae.

crural a. ligamentum inguinale.

deep crural a. tractus iliopubicus.

deep palmar a. arcus palmaris profundus.

deep palmar venous a. arcus venosus palmaris profundus.

deep plantar a. arcus plantaris profundus.

dental a. the curving structure formed by a line described by the buccal surfaces or through the central grooves of the molars and bicuspids of the teeth in their normal position, viewed from the incisal and occlusal aspects. See also *arcus dentalis mandibularis* and *arcus dentalis maxillaris.*

distal transverse a. of foot arcus pedis transversus distalis.

dorsal carpal a. rete carpale dorsale.

dorsal venous a. of foot arcus venosus dorsalis pedis.

double aortic a. a congenital anomaly in which the aorta divides into two branches which embrace the trachea and esophagus and reunite to form the descending aorta.

epiphyseal a. the embryonic structure in the roof of the third ventricle from which the pineal gland develops.

fibrous a. of soleus muscle arcus tendineus musculi solei.

first pharyngeal a. the first of the pharyngeal arches in the human embryo, later differentiating into the sphenomandibular and anterior malleolar ligaments, malleus, and incus; it also gives rise to two prominences (the *maxillary* and *mandibular prominences*), from which the maxilla and mandible develop. Called also mandibular a.

fixed lingual a. a space-retaining appliance consisting of an arch wire designed to fit the lingual surface of the teeth, and soldered to metal crowns or orthodontic bands. Called also *stationary lingual a.*

a's of foot the longitudinal and transverse arches of the foot considered together.

glossopalatine a. arcus palatoglossus.

Haller a's see *ligamentum arcuatum laterale* and *ligamentum arcuatum mediale.*

hemal a. one of the cartilaginous structures surrounding the caudal vein in the tail of the vertebrate embryo, formed by the ventrad growth of the ventrolateral arcualia. In fish, the arches are also present in the thoracic region. Cf. *neural a.*

hyoid a. second pharyngeal a.

iliopectineal a. arcus iliopectineus.

inferior dental a. arcus dentalis mandibularis.

inferior palpebral a. arcus palpebralis inferior.

inguinal a. ligamentum inguinale.

ischiopubic a. angulus subpubicus.

jugular venous a. arcus venosus jugularis.

Langer axillary a. axillary a.

lateral Haller a. ligamentum arcuatum laterale.

lateral longitudinal a. of foot pars lateralis arcus pedis longitudinalis.

lateral lumbocostal a. ligamentum arcuatum laterale.

lingual a. a wire appliance made to conform to the lingual aspect of the dental arch; used to promote or to prevent movement of the teeth in orthodontic therapy.

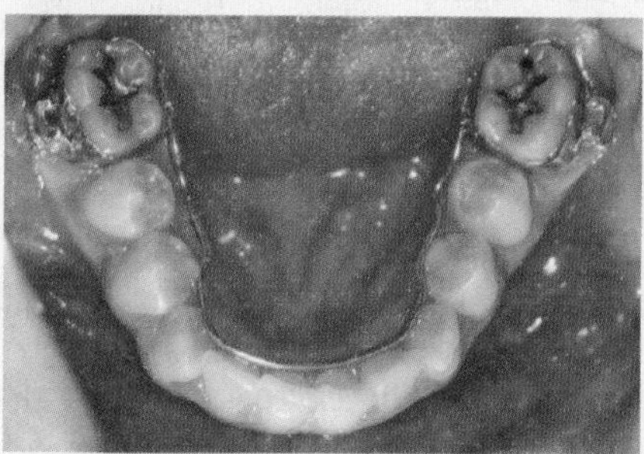

■ Lingual arch used to maintain space for premolars after premature loss of the primary molars.

longitudinal a. of foot arcus pedis longitudinalis.
malar a. arcus zygomaticus.
mandibular a. 1. first pharyngeal a. 2. arcus dentalis mandibularis.
maxillary a. 1. palatal a. 2. arcus dentalis maxillaris.
medial Haller a. ligamentum arcuatum mediale.
medial longitudinal a. of foot pars medialis arcus pedis longitudinalis.
medial lumbocostal a. ligamentum arcuatum mediale.
metatarsal a. transverse a. of foot.
nasal a. the arch formed in the embryo by the nasal bones and by the nasal processes of the maxilla.
neural a. one of the cartilaginous structures surrounding the embryonic spinal cord, formed by the dorsad growth of the dorsolateral arcualia; it is the primordium of the vertebral arch. Cf. *hemal a.*
open pubic a. a congenital anomaly in which the pubic arch is not fused, the bodies of the pubic bones being spread apart.
oral a. palatal a.
palatal a. the arch formed by the roof of the mouth from the teeth on one side of the maxilla to the teeth on the other or, if the teeth are missing, from the residual dental arch on one side to that on the other. Called also *maxillary a.*, *palatomaxillary a.*, and *oral a.*
palatoglossal a. arcus palatoglossus.
palatomaxillary a. palatal a.
palatopharyngeal a. arcus palatopharyngeus.
palmar carpal a. an arch formed by anastomosis of the palmar carpal branches of the radial and ulnar arteries. Called also *anterior carpal a.*
paraphysial a. the embryonic structure in the roof of the third ventricle of vertebrates from which the paraphysis develops.
passive lingual a. an orthodontic appliance for maintaining space and preserving arch length when bilateral primary molars are prematurely lost.
a. of pelvis angulus subpubicus.
pharyngeal a's term used to denote the branchial arches (q.v.) in human embryos. The *first* and *second pharyngeal arches* (qq.v.) contribute to the formation of the upper and lower jaws and the hyoid bone. The third pharyngeal arch develops into the greater horn of the hyoid bone and the caudal part of its body; the fourth and sixth arches develop into the laryngeal cartilages. In the human embryo, the sixth arch is actually the fifth in number but is so named for reasons of comparative anatomy and evolution; it does not appear on the surface.
pharyngopalatine a. arcus palatopharyngeus.
plantar a. 1. arcus plantaris profundus. 2. arcus venosus plantaris. 3. the hollow on the sole of the foot; see *arcus pedis longitudinalis* and *transverse a. of foot.*
plantar venous a. arcus venosus plantaris.
popliteal a. ligamentum popliteum arcuatum.
postaural a's branchial a's.
posterior a. of atlas arcus posterior atlantis.
posterior carpal a. rete carpale dorsale.
posterior palatine a. arcus palatopharyngeus.
primordial costal a's arches formed in the embryo from costal processes of the vertebrae, later developing into ribs.
proximal transverse a. of foot arcus pedis transversus proximalis.
pubic a. arcus pubicus.
pulmonary a's the most caudal of the aortic arches; they become the pulmonary arteries.
residual a., residual dental a. the curved contour of the ridge remaining after tooth removal.
ribbon a. see under *appliance.*
a. of ribs arcus costalis.
right aortic a. a congenital anomaly in which the aorta is displaced to the right and passes behind the esophagus, thus forming a vascular ring that may cause compression of the trachea and esophagus.
Riolan a. the arch formed by the mesentery of the transverse colon.
second pharyngeal a. in the human embryo, the pharyngeal arch just caudal to the first pharyngeal arch; it later differentiates into the stapes, styloid process of temporal bone, stylohyoid ligament, lesser horn of the hyoid bone, and cranial part of the hyoid bone. Called also *hyoid a.*
Shenton a. see under *line.*
stationary lingual a. fixed lingual a.
subpubic a. angulus subpubicus.
superciliary a. arcus superciliaris.
superficial femoral a. ligamentum inguinale.
superficial palmar a. arcus palmaris superficialis.
superficial palmar venous a. arcus venosus palmaris superficialis.
superficial plantar a. arcus plantaris superficialis.
superior dental a. arcus dentalis maxillaris.
superior palpebral a. arcus palpebralis superior.
tendinous a. arcus tendineus.
tendinous a. of levator ani muscle arcus tendineus musculi levatoris ani.
tendinous a. of lumbodorsal fascia ligamentum lumbocostale.
tendinous a. of pelvic fascia arcus tendineus fasciae pelvis.
tendinous a. of soleus muscle arcus tendineus musculi solei.
a. of thoracic duct arcus ductus thoracici; see *ductus thoracicus.*
thyrohyoid a. the third pharyngeal (branchial) arch, which becomes represented by the greater horn of the hyoid bone.
transverse a. of foot an arch on the plantar surface of the foot, formed by the navicular, cuneiform, cuboid, and five metatarsal bones. Called also *metatarsal a.*
Treitz a. an arch sometimes found in the paraduodenal fold, composed of the left superior colic artery and the inferior mesenteric vein.
venous a's of kidney venae arcuatae renis.
vertebral a. arcus vertebrae.
visceral a's branchial a's.
V-shaped a. a dental arch which narrows and comes to a point at the lingual junction of the maxillary central incisors.
Zimmermann a. an inconstant, rudimentary arch of the embryo, supposed to explain the origin of certain occasionally occurring vessels between the fourth aortic and the pulmonary arch.
zygomatic a. arcus zygomaticus.

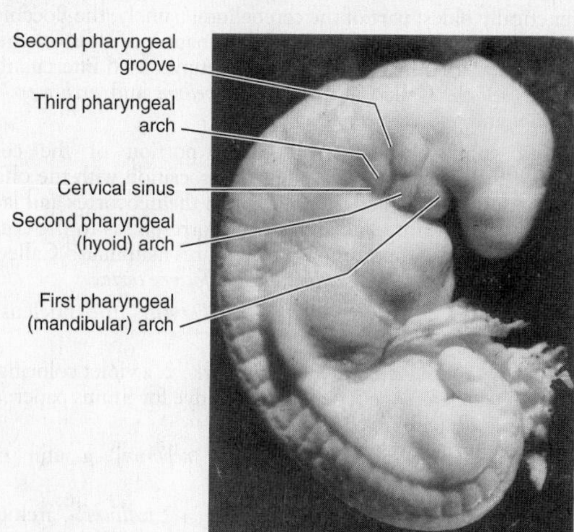

■ Pharyngeal arches in a stage 13, 4.5-week-old embryo.

arch- See *archi-*.

Ar·chaea (ahr-ke′ə) [Gr. *archaios* ancient, from *archē* beginning, from *archein* to begin] in the three-domain system of classfication, one of the two large divisions into which prokaryotes are grouped, genetically distinct from bacteria and sharing some molecular features with the eukaryotes. Organisms are diverse in shape and size, may or may not have a cell wall, and occur both as unicellular forms and as filaments or aggregations. They are subclassfied into methanogenic, sulfate-reducing, halophilic, and thermophilic groups. Members are predominantly terrestrial or aquatic organisms, living mainly in extreme environments, such as submarine hydrothermal vents and subterranean salt deposits; some occur as symbionts in the digestive tracts of animals. None are human pathogens. Cf. *Bacteria*.

archae(o)- for words beginning thus, see also those beginning *arche(o)-*.

ar·chaeo·cer·e·bel·lum (ahr″ke-o-ser″ə-bel′əm) archicerebellum.

ar·chaeo·cor·tex (ahr″ke-o-kor′teks) archicortex.

ar·cha·ic (ahr-ka′ik) [Gr. *archaios* ancient] very ancient; pertaining to early evolutionary stages.

ar·che·go·nium (ahr″kə-go′ne-əm) [*arche-* + Gr. *gonos* offspring] the female organ of a cryptogamic plant taking part in the formation of sexually produced spores; cf. *antheridium*.

arch·en·ceph·a·lon (ahrk″ən-sef′ə-lon) [*arche-* + *encephalon*] the primordial brain, anterior to the end of the notochord, from which the midbrain and the forebrain are developed.

arch·en·ter·on (ahrk-en′tər-on) [*arche-* + *enteron*] the primordial digestive cavity of those embryonic forms whose blastula becomes a gastrula by invagination; called also *gastrocoele* and *primordial gut*.

arche(o)- [Gr. *archaios* ancient, from *archē* beginning, from *archein* to begin] a combining form meaning first, beginning, original, primitive. Written also *archae(o)-*.

ar·cheo·cer·e·bel·lum (ahr″ke-o-ser″ə-bel′əm) archicerebellum.

ar·cheo·cor·tex (ahr″ke-o-kor′teks) archicortex.

ar·che·spore (ahr′kə-spor) [*arche-* + *-spore*] the mass of cells that give rise to spore mother cells; called also *archesporium* and *archispore*.

ar·che·spo·ri·um (ahr″kə-spo′re-əm) archespore.

ar·che·type (ahr′kə-tīp) [*arche-* + *type*] an ideal, original, or standard type or form.

archi- [Gr., from *archein* to begin, to rule] a prefix meaning (1) chief or principal, (2) beginning, original, or primitive. Written *arch-* before a vowel.

ar·chi·blast (ahr′kĭ-blast) [*archi-* + *-blast*] 1. the components of an oocyte that actively form the embryo, as distinguished from the yolk. 2. His′ term for the fundamental part of the blastodermic layers as distinguished from the parablast or peripheral portion of the mesoderm.

ar·chi·blas·tic (ahr″kĭ-blas′tik) derived from or pertaining to the archiblast.

ar·chi·carp (ahr′kĭ-kahrp) 1. the group of cells, including the ascogonium, that give rise to the fruiting body of ascomycetous fungi. Cf. *ascocarp*. 2. archegonium.

ar·chi·cer·e·bel·lum (ahr″kĭ-ser″ə-bel′əm) [*archi-* + *cerebellum*] [TA] the phylogenetically oldest part of the cerebellum; namely, the flocculonodular lobe. Because this lobe is the site of termination of most of the projections of vestibular afferents, the term is sometimes used interchangeably with *vestibulocerebellum*. Called also *archaeocerebellum* and *archeocerebellum*. Cf. *neocerebellum* and *paleocerebellum*.

ar·chi·cor·tex (ahr″kĭ-kor′teks) [TA] the portion of the cerebral cortex that, with the paleocortex, develops in association with the olfactory system, and which is phylogenetically older than the neocortex and lacks its layered structure. The embryonic archicortex corresponds to the cortex of the dentate gyrus and hippocampus in mature mammals. Called also *archaeocortex* or *archeocortex*, *archipallium*, and *olfactory cortex*.

ar·chi·kary·on (ahr-kĭ-kar′e-on) [*archi-* + *karyon*] the nucleus of a zygote.

ar·chil (ahr′kil) 1. the lichen *Roccella tinctoria*. 2. a violet coloring from this and other lichens, employed as an indicator dye for litmus paper: alkalis give a blue color, and acids a red color.

ar·chi·neph·ron (ahr″kĭ-nef′ron) [*archi-* + *nephron*] a unit of the pronephros.

ar·chi·pal·li·um (ahr″kĭ-pal′e-əm) [*archi-* + *pallium*] archicortex. **archipal′lial** *adj*

ar·chi·spore (ahr′kĭ-spor) archespore.

ar·chi·stome (ahr′kĭ-stōm) [*archi-* + *-stome*] blastopore.

ar·chi·stri·a·tum (ahr″kĭ-stri-a′təm) [*archi-* + *striatum*] the primordial corpus striatum, which becomes the amygdaloid body.

ar·chi·tec·ton·ic (ahr″kĭ-tek-ton′ik) pertaining to architectural pattern.

ar·ci·form (ahr′sĭ-form) [L. *arcus* bow + *form*] bow-shaped; arcuate.

Ar·co·bac·ter (ahr′ko-bak″tər) [L. *arcus* bow + *-bacter*] a genus of bacteria of the family Campylobacteraceae, consisting of gram-negative, slender, curved rods. Organisms are non–spore-forming, microaerobic to aerobic, and chemo-organotrophic; grow at 15°C; and have a single polar flagellum at one or both ends of the cell. Pathogenicity is unknown, but several species have been isolated from clinical specimens. The type species is *A. nitrofi′gilis*.

A. butz′leri a species that is associated with enteritis, bacteremia, and appendicitis in humans and enteritis and abortion in other animals.

A. skir′rowi a species found in the feces of ruminants and pigs with diarrhea.

arc-quad·rant (ahrk-kwod′rənt) an arc guidance system that has a 90° arc.

arc·ta·tion (ahrk-ta′shən) [L. *arctare* to draw together] stenosis.

Arc·to·mys (ahrk′tə-mis) *Marmota*.

Arc·to·staph·y·los (ahrk″to-staf′ə-lōs) a genus of North American evergreen plants of the family Ericaceae. *A. uva-ur′si* is the bearberry or uva ursi, a shrub whose leaves are used medicinally (see *uva ursi*). *A. manzani′ta* Parry is manzanita, a small shrub or tree of the western United States whose leaves are used as a medicinal tea, astringent, tonic, and diuretic.

ar·cu·al·ia (ahr″ku-a′le-ə) nodules of cartilage in the continuous mesenchymal sheath in close apposition to the external surface of the notochord in vertebrate embryos, typically occurring in double pairs, one pair dorsolateral and one pair ventrolateral to the notochord; the dorsolateral pairs give rise to the neural arches, while the ventrolateral pairs give rise to the rudiments of the ribs and the hemal arches.

ar·cu·ate (ahr′ku-āt) [L. *arcuatus* bow shaped] shaped like an arc; arranged in arches.

ar·cu·a·tion (ahr-ku-a′shən) [L. *arcuatio*] curvature; especially an abnormal curvature.

ar·cus (ahr′kəs) pl. *ar′cus* [L. "a bow"] arch: a structure having a curved or bowlike outline.

a. **alveola′ris mandi′bulae** [TA] alveolar arch of mandible: the superior free border of the alveolar process of the mandible. Called also *alveolar border* or *alveolar limbus of mandible*, and *limbus alveolaris mandibulae*.

a. **alveola′ris maxil′lae** [TA] alveolar arch of maxilla: the inferior free border of the alveolar process of the maxilla; called also *alveolar border* or *alveolar limbus of maxilla*, and *limbus alveolaris maxillae*.

a. **ante′rior atlan′tis** [TA] anterior arch of atlas: the more slender portion joining the lateral masses of the atlas ventrally, constituting about one-fifth of the entire circumference of the atlas.

a. **aor′tae** [TA] arch of aorta: the continuation of the ascending aorta, giving rise to the brachiocephalic trunk, and the left common carotid and left subclavian arteries; it continues as the thoracic aorta. Called also *aortic arch*.

a. **cartila′ginis cricoi′deae** [TA] arch of cricoid cartilage: the slender anterior portion of the cricoid cartilage.

a. **cor′neae** a white or gray opaque ring in the corneal margin, present at birth, or appearing later in life, and becoming quite frequent

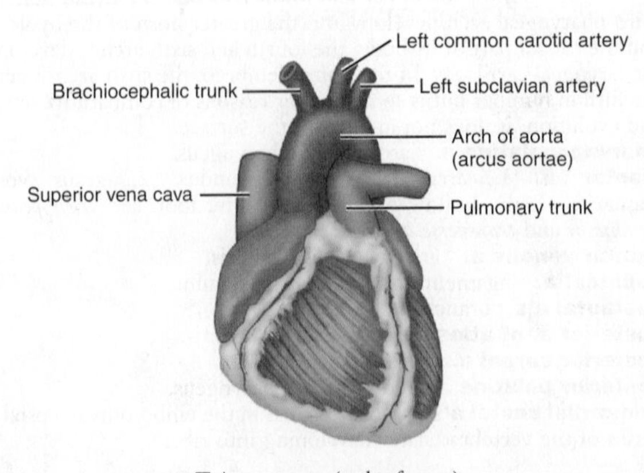

■ Arcus aortae (arch of aorta).

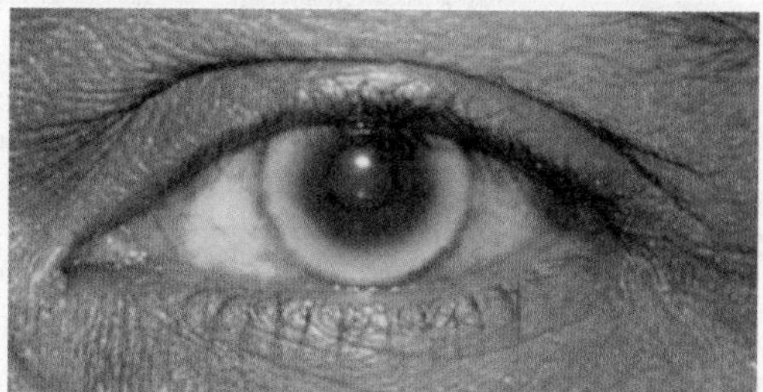

■ Arcus corneae.

in those over 50; it results from cholesterol deposits in or hyalinosis of the corneal stroma and may be associated with ocular defects or with familial hyperlipidemia. Called also *a. juvenilis*, *a. lipoides corneae*, and *a. senilis*.

a. **costa'lis** [TA] costal arch: the anterior portion of the apertura thoracis inferior, consisting of the costal cartilages of ribs 7 to 10, inclusive; called also *costal margin* and *arch of ribs*.

a. **denta'lis infe'rior** TA alternative for *a. dentalis mandibularis*.

a. **denta'lis mandibula'ris** [TA] mandibular dental arcade: the portion of the dental arch formed by the teeth of the mandible. Called also *arcus dentalis inferior* [TA alternative], *inferior dental arch*, *mandibular arch*, and *lower dental arcade*.

a. **denta'lis maxilla'ris** [TA] maxillary dental arcade: the portion of the dental arch formed by the teeth of the maxilla. Called also *arcus dentalis superior* [TA alternative], *superior dental arch*, *maxillary arch*, and *upper dental arcade*.

a. **denta'lis supe'rior** TA alternative for *a. dentalis maxillaris*.

a. **duc'tus thora'cici** [TA] the arch of the thoracic duct; see *ductus thoracicus*.

a. **iliopecti'neus** [TA] iliopectineal arch: the fascial partition that separates the lacuna musculorum and the lacuna vasorum; called also *iliopectineal fascia*.

a. **inguina'lis** TA alternative for *ligamentum inguinale*.

a. **juveni'lis** 1. a. corneae. 2. Axenfeld anomaly.

a. **lipoi'des cor'neae** a. corneae.

a. **margina'lis co'li** TA alternative for *arteria marginalis coli*.

a. **palatoglos'sus** [TA] palatoglossal arch: the anterior of the two folds of mucous membrane on either side of the oropharynx, connected with the soft palate and enclosing the palatoglossal muscle; called also *glossopalatine arch*, *anterior palatine arch*, and *anterior column* or *pillar of fauces*.

a. **palatopharyn'geus** [TA] palatopharyngeal arch: the posterior of the two folds of mucous membrane on each side of the oropharynx, connected with the soft palate and enclosing the palatopharyngeal muscle; called also *pharyngopalatine arch*, *posterior palatine arch*, and *posterior column* or *pillar of fauces*.

a. **palma'ris profun'dus** [TA] deep palmar arch: an arterial arch formed by the terminal part of the radial artery and its anastomosis with the deep branch of the ulnar, and extending from the base of the metacarpal bone of the little finger to the proximal end of the first interosseous space; it gives off palmar metacarpal arteries and perforating branches.

a. **palma'ris superficia'lis** [TA] superficial palmar arch: an arterial arch formed by the terminal part of the ulnar artery and its anastomosis with the superficial palmar branch of the radial, giving rise to the palmar digital arteries and supplying blood to the palmar aspect of the hands and fingers.

a. **palpebra'lis infe'rior** [TA] inferior palpebral arch: an arch derived from the inferior medial palpebral artery, supplying the lower lid of the eye.

a. **palpebra'lis supe'rior** [TA] superior palpebral arch: an arch derived from the superior medial palpebral artery, supplying the upper lid of the eye.

a. **parietooccipita'lis** the curved convolution formed by the backward continuation into the occipital lobe of the superior postcentral sulcus.

a. **pe'dis longitudina'lis** [TA] longitudinal arch of foot: the arch running longitudinally along the sole of the foot, consisting of lateral and medial parts (see *pars lateralis arcus pedis longitudinalis* and *pars medialis arcus pedis longitudinalis*).

a. **pe'dis transver'sus dista'lis** [TA] distal transverse arch of foot: a shallow arch that forms the distal part of the transverse arch of the foot, formed by the proximal heads of the metatarsal bones.

a. **pe'dis transver'sus proxima'lis** [TA] proximal transverse arch of foot: the deeper proximal part of the transverse arch of the foot, formed by the cuneiform bones and the cuboid bone.

a. **planta'ris profun'dus** [TA] deep plantar arch: the deep arterial arch in the foot, formed by the anastomosis of the lateral plantar artery with the deep plantar branch of the dorsal artery of the foot, and giving off the plantar metatarsal arteries. Called also *plantar arch*.

a. **planta'ris superficia'lis** [TA] superficial plantar arch: a rarely occurring superficial arterial arch, formed by anatosmosis between the medial and lateral plantar arteries.

a. **poste'rior atlan'tis** [TA] posterior arch of atlas: the slender portion joining the lateral masses of the atlas dorsally, constituting about two-fifths of the entire circumference of the atlas.

a. **pu'bicus** [TA], **a. pu'bis** pubic arch: the arch formed by the conjoined rami of the ischial and pubic bones of the two sides of the body.

a. **seni'lis** a. corneae.

a. **supercilia'ris** [TA] superciliary arch: a smooth elevation arching superolaterally from the glabella, slightly superior to the margin of the orbit.

a. **tendi'neus** [TA] tendinous arch: a linear thickening of fascia over some part of a muscle, such as that over the soleus or the obturator internus.

a. **tendi'neus fas'ciae pel'vis** [TA] tendinous arch of pelvic fascia: a thickening of the superior fascia, extending from the ischial spine to the posterior part of the body of the pubis.

a. **tendi'neus mus'culi levato'ris a'ni** [TA] tendinous arch of levator ani muscle: a linear thickening of the fascia covering the obturator internus muscle, from which the levator ani takes origin.

a. **tendi'neus mus'culi so'lei** [TA] tendinous arch of soleus muscle: an aponeurotic band in the front part of the soleus muscle, extending from a tubercle on the neck of the fibula to the soleal line of the tibia.

a. **ve'nae azy'gou** [TA] arch of azygos vein: an arch formed by the azygos vein above the root of the right lung.

a. **veno'sus dorsa'lis pe'dis** [TA] dorsal venous arch of foot: a transverse venous arch across the dorsum of the foot near the bases of the metatarsal bones.

a. **veno'sus jugula'ris** [TA] jugular venous arch: a transverse connecting trunk between the anterior jugular veins of either side.

a. **veno'sus palma'ris profun'dus** [TA] deep palmar venous arch: a venous arch accompanying the deep palmar arterial arch.

a. **veno'sus palma'ris superficia'lis** [TA] superficial palmar venous arch: a venous arch accompanying the superficial palmar arterial arch.

a. **veno'sus planta'ris** [TA] plantar venous arch: the deep venous arch that accompanies the plantar arterial arch.

a. **ver'tebrae** [TA] vertebral arch: the bony arch on the dorsal aspect of a vertebra, composed of the laminae and pedicles.

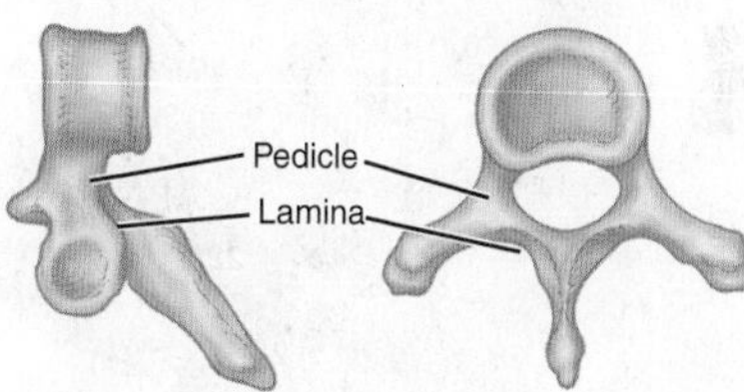

■ Arcus vertebrae (vertebral arch). The vertebral arch consists anteriorly of a pair of pedicles and posteriorly of a pair of laminae.

a. **zygoma'ticus** [TA] zygomatic arch: the arch formed by the articulation of the broad temporal process of the zygomatic bone and the slender zygomatic process of the temporal bone, giving attachment to the masseter muscle and serving as a line of demarcation between the temporal and infratemporal fossae; called also *malar arch*.

ARD acute respiratory disease (of any undefined form); acute respiratory distress (see under *syndrome*).

ar•de•par•in so•di•um (ahr-de-par'in) a low molecular weight heparin used as an anticoagulant and antithrombotic in the prophylaxis of deep vein thrombosis and pulmonary thromboembolism after knee replacement surgery; administered subcutaneously.

ar•dor (ahr'dor) [L.] intense heat.

a. **uri'nae** a scalding sensation during the passage of urine.

ARDS acute respiratory distress syndrome; adult respiratory distress syndrome.

Ar•du•an (ahr'du-an) trademark for a preparation of pipecuronium bromide.

ar•ea (ār'e-ə) pl. *a'reae* or *areas* [L.] 1. a limited space. 2. in anatomy, a specific surface or a region with a given function.

Area

See also entries under *region.*

acoustic a's auditory cortex.
a. amygdaloi'dea ante'rior [TA], **anterior amygdaloid a.** a poorly differentiated transition zone in the corticomedial part of the amygdaloid body, through which the nuclei are continuous with adjacent areas.
aortic a. the area on the thorax over the medial end of the right second costal cartilage.
association a's areas of the cerebral cortex (excluding the primary areas) that are connected with each other and with the neothalamus by numerous fibers passing through the corpus callosum and the white matter of the hemispheres; these areas are responsible for the higher mental and emotional processes, such as memory, learning, speech, and the interpretation of sensations.
auditory a's auditory cortex.
auditory association a. a sensory association area for auditory stimuli.
auditory receiving a's auditory cortex.
Bamberger a. an area of cardiac dullness in the left intercostal region, suggestive of pericardial effusion.
bare a. of liver a. nuda hepatis.
basal seat a. denture-bearing a.
B-dependent a. thymus-independent a.
Betz cell a. primary somatomotor a.
brain a. cortical a.
Broca motor speech a. an area comprising parts of the opercular portion of the inferior frontal gyrus; injury to this area may result in a minor form of motor aphasia.
Broca parolfactory a. a. subcallosa.
Brodmann a's areas of the cerebral cortex distinguished by hypothesized differences in the arrangement of their six cellular layers and identified by numbers; although the histologic basis is in dispute, the topographic numbering is widely used as a descriptor for mapping cortical locations that control different functions of the nervous system and the body.

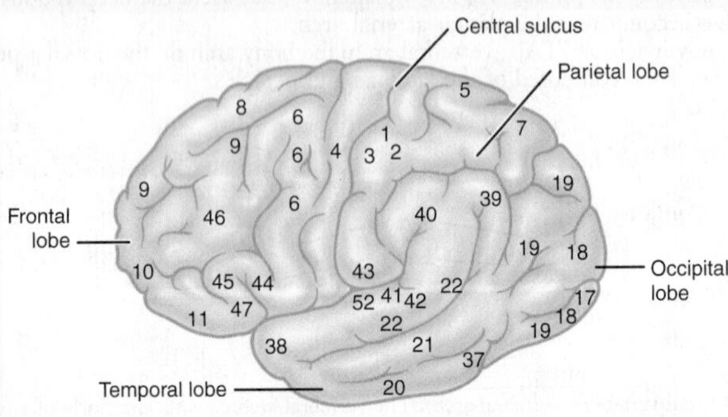

■ Lateral view of the cerebral hemisphere, showing some of the Brodmann areas.

catchment a. the geographical area that a specialized health care facility is responsible for serving.
a. centra'lis macula lutea.
a. cerebrovasculo'sa a membrane-covered, reddish, spongy mass, consisting of thin-walled blood vessels and variable amounts of ependyma, choroid plexus, and glial tissue, that replaces the forebrain in anencephaly.
cingulate a. the area comprising the cingulate gyrus and isthmus, an important component of the limbic system.
a. coch'leae TA alternative for *a. cochlearis.*
cochlear a., a. cochlea'ris [TA] the anterior part of the inferior portion of the fundus of the internal acoustic meatus, near the base of the cochlea; called also *a. cochleae* [TA alternative].
Cohnheim a's dark, polygonal areas of myofibrils seen on cross-section of a poorly fixed muscle fiber.
contact a. of tooth a. contingens dentis.
a. contin'gens den'tis [TA] contact area of tooth: the area of the mesial or distal surface of a tooth that touches the adjoining tooth.
cortical a. any portion of the cerebral cortex that can be differentiated functionally from its neighbors; see names of specific areas and see also *cortex, field,* and *zone.*
cribriform a. of renal papilla, a. cribro'sa papil'lae rena'lis [TA] the tip of a renal pyramid, which is perforated by 10–25 openings for the papillary ducts.
a. of critical definition that part of an optic image within which the detail is clear.
denture-bearing a., denture foundation a., denture-supporting a. the surface of the oral tissues (residual alveolar ridge) that supports a denture. Called also *basal seat a.* and *stress-bearing a.*
dermatomic a. dermatome.
eloquent a's eloquent brain.
embryonic a. see under *disc.*
entorhinal a. Brodmann area 28, the inferior and posterior parts of the piriform area, including the caudal part of the parahippocampal gyrus.
eye a. see *frontal eye field* and *occipital eye field.*
a. of facial nerve a. nervi facialis.
a's of Forel see under *field.*
fusion a. Panum a.
gastric a's, a'reae gas'tricae [TA] small patches of gastric mucosa, 1 to 5 mm in diameter, separated by the plicae villosae and containing the foveolae gastricae (gastric pits).
germinal a. embryonic disc.
gustatory receiving a. the primary receiving area for taste sensations; thought to be in or near the opercular part of the postcentral gyrus.
hypoglossal a., a. hypoglos'si the portion of the mouth beneath the tongue.
hypophysiotropic a. the part of the hypothalamus that contains neurons that secrete hormones that regulate adenohypophysial cells.
hypothalamic a., anterior a. hypothalamica rostralis.
hypothalamic a., dorsal a. hypothalamica dorsalis.
hypothalamic a., intermediate a. hypothalamica intermedia.
hypothalamic a., lateral a. hypothalamica lateralis.
hypothalamic a., posterior a. hypothalamica posterior.
a. hypothala'mica dorsa'lis [TA] dorsal hypothalamic area: the most dorsal part of the hypothalamus, comprising the entopeduncular nucleus and the nucleus of the ansa lenticularis. Called also *dorsal hypothalamic region.*
a. hypothala'mica interme'dia [TA] intermediate hypothalamic area: the part of the hypothalamus comprising the lateral hypothalamic region and the following nuclei: arcuate, tuberal, ventromedial hypothalamic, dorsomedial hypothalamic, dorsal hypothalamic, posterior periventricular, and infundibular. Called also *intermediate hypothalamic region* and *tuberal region.*
a. hypothala'mica latera'lis [TA] lateral hypothalamic area: a part of the intermediate hypothalamic area lateral to the fornix and the mammillothalamic fasciculus; called also *lateral hypothalamic region.*
a. hypothala'mica poste'rior [TA] posterior hypothalamic area: the most posterior part of the hypothalamus, consisting of the lateral and medial nuclei of the mammillary body and the posterior hypothalamic nucleus. Called also *posterior hypothalamic region* and *mammillary region.*
a. hypothala'mica rostra'lis [TA] anterior hypothalamic area: the most anterior part of the hypothalamus, lying adjacent to the lamina terminalis and superior to the optic chiasm, and comprising the lateral and medial preoptic nuclei, the supraoptic and paraventricular nuclei, and the anterior hypothalamic nucleus; called also *preoptic a.* or *region, anterior hypothalamic region,* and *chiasmatic region.*
impression a. the surface of the oral structures recorded in an impression.
insular a. the cortex of the insula.
a. intercondyla'ris ante'rior ti'biae [TA] anterior intercondylar area of tibia: the broad area between the superior articular surfaces of the tibia; called also *anterior intercondylar fossa of tibia.*
a. intercondyla'ris poste'rior ti'biae [TA] posterior intercondylar area of tibia: a deep notch separating the condyles on the posterior surface of the tibia; called also *posterior intercondylar fossa of tibia.*

Kiesselbach a. an area on the anterior part of the nasal septum above the intermaxillary bone, which is richly supplied with blood vessels and is a common site of nosebleed; called also *Little a.*
Laimer-Haeckerman a. a triangular area of sparse musculature just below the pharyngoesophageal junction, where Zenker diverticulum most frequently develops.
language a. any nerve center of the cerebral cortex, usually in the dominant hemisphere, controlling the understanding or use of language.
Little a. Kiesselbach a.
a. of Martegiani a slightly enlarged, funnel-shaped space anterior to the optic disk, marking the posterior opening of the hyaloid canal.
a. medullovasculo´sa a median elongated area of vascular granulation-like tissue in rachischisis.
mesobranchial a. the pharyngeal floor of the embryo, between the pharyngeal arches and pouches of each side.
midarm muscle a. a value used to estimate lean body mass, calculated by the formula

$$\frac{[\text{midarm circumference (in cm)} - (\pi \times \text{triceps skinfold (in cm)})]^2}{4\pi} - n$$

where n is 10 for males and 6.5 for females.
mirror a. the reflecting surface of the cornea and lens when illuminated through the slit lamp.
motor a. any area of the cerebral cortex primarily involved in stimulating muscle contractions; often used alone to refer to the primary somatomotor area. See also *premotor a.*, *sensorimotor a.*, and *Broca motor speech a.*
motor speech a. see *Broca motor speech a.* and *Wernicke second motor speech a.*
a. ner´vi facia´lis [TA] area of facial nerve: the part of the fundus of the internal acoustic meatus where the facial nerve enters the facial canal.
a. nu´da he´patis [TA] bare area of liver: a large part of the diaphragmatic surface of the liver that lacks a peritoneal covering; its boundaries are formed by the coronary ligament of the liver and the triangular ligaments.
olfactory a. 1. an area of the cerebral cortex, including the olfactory bulb, tract, and trigone, the anterior portion of the gyrus cinguli, and the uncus. 2. substantia perforata rostralis.
Panum a. the area on the retina of one eye over which a point-sized image can range and still provide a stereoscopic image with a specific point of stimulus on the retina of the other eye. Called also *fusion a.*
parastriate a. Brodmann area 18, an area of the occipital cortex partly surrounding the striate cortex and having some of the functions of an association area for visual sensations.
a. pellu´cida the central clear part of the embryonic disc, as seen in the bird egg.
periamygdaloid a. the intermediate part of the piriform area, between the piriform area and the entorhinal area; it covers the amygdaloid body.
peristriate a. Brodmann area 19, an area of the occipital cortex partly surrounding the striate cortex and having some functions of an association area for visual sensations.
piriform a. an area in the rhinencephalon, pear-shaped in some species but not in humans; it includes the lateral olfactory process or gyrus, the limen insulae, the uncus, and part of the parahippocampal gyrus; subdivided into the prepiriform area, the periamygdaloid area, and the entorhinal area. Called also *piriform lobe.*
postcentral a. the sensory area just posterior to the central sulcus of the cerebral hemisphere, the primary receiving area for general sensations; called also *postrolandic a.* and *somesthetic cortex.*
post dam a. posterior palatal seal a.
posterior palatal seal a. the soft tissues along the junction of the hard and soft palates on which pressure can be applied by a denture to aid in its retention; called also *post dam a.*
a. postre´ma a small tongue-shaped area on the lateral wall of the fourth ventricle, between the funiculus separans and the tuberculum gracile, in which the blood-brain barrier may be modified. See also *circumventricular organs,* under *organ.*
postrolandic a. postcentral a.
precentral a. primary somatomotor a.
prefrontal a. the cortex of the frontal lobe immediately in front of the premotor cortex, concerned chiefly with associative functions.
premotor a. the motor cortex of the frontal lobe immediately in front of the precentral gyrus.
preoptic a. 1. a. preoptica. 2. a. hypothalamica rostralis.
a. preop´tica [TA] preoptic area: several groups of cells in the median plane immediately below the rostral commissure of the telencephalon that are functionally related to the hypothalamus; called also *preoptic region.*
prepiriform a. the anterior part of the piriform area, consisting primarily of the lateral olfactory gyrus.
pressure a. an area subjected to excessive pressure with consequent displacement of tissue or fluid.
pretectal a., a. pretecta´lis [TA] an area at the junction of the mesencephalon and diencephalon, extending from a position dorsolateral to the commissure of the epithalamus toward the cranial colliculus, within which is situated the pretectal nucleus; called also *pretectal region.*
primary a's areas of the cerebral cortex comprising the motor and sensory (primary receiving) areas. Cf. *association a's.*
primary receiving a's, primary receptive a's the areas of the cerebral cortex that receive the thalamic projections of the primary sensory modalities. Called also *sensory a's* or *centers.*
primary somatomotor a. an area in the posterior part of the frontal lobe just anterior to the central sulcus, corresponding to Brodmann area 4; different regions control motor activity of specific parts of the body. Called also *Betz cell a., motor a., precentral a., rolandic a.,* and *Rolando zone.*
projection a's those areas of the cerebral cortex that receive the most direct projection of the sensory systems of the body.
pyriform a. piriform a.
receiving a's, receptive a's primary receiving a's.
relief a. the portion of the surface of the mouth upon which pressures or forces are reduced or eliminated in prosthodontic therapy. See also *relief* (def. 3).
rest a. the prepared surface of a tooth or fixed restoration into which the rest fits, giving support to a removable partial denture. Called also *rest seat.*
a. retrooliva´ris [TA], **retroolivary a.** the most caudal part of the lateral region of the medulla oblongata, towards the posterolateral sulcus.
rolandic a. primary somatomotor a.
rugae a. the portion of the mouth in which rugae are found; called also *rugae zone.*
SI a. first somatosensory a.
SII a. second somatosensory a.
saddle a. the edentulous portion of the dental arch upon which a fixed or removable prosthesis rests.
sensorimotor a. the cortex of the pre- and postcentral gyri—the motor area and the primary receiving area for general sensations, respectively.
sensory a's primary receiving a's.
sensory association a. an association area around the borders of a primary receiving area, where sensory stimuli are interpreted.
septal a. the area on either cerebral hemisphere comprising the area subcallosa and the corresponding half of the septum pellucidum; the area has olfactory, hypothalamic, and hippocampal connections.
silent a. 1. an area of the brain in which pathologic conditions may occur without producing symptoms obvious to the clinician. 2. association a.
somatic sensory a., somatosensory a. either of the two cortical regions where conscious perception of somatic sensations occurs, called the *first* or *primary somatosensory area* and the *second* or *secondary somatosensory area.*
somatosensory a., first, somatosensory a., primary the cortical projection area in the postcentral gyrus for receiving into consciousness somatosensory information initiated by stimulation of receptors in the skin, joints, muscles, and viscera. Called also *SI a.*
somatosensory a., second, somatosensory a., secondary a cortical projection area lateral and posterior to the primary somatosensory area; it receives somatic sensations mainly from the skin, particularly sensations of pain and of movement across the skin. Called also *SII a.*
somesthetic a. somatosensory a.
a. spina´lis X [TA] the innermost region of the layers of the spinal cord as described by Rexed; see *Rexed laminae,* under *lamina.* Called also *lamina spinalis X* [TA alternative].

Area *Continued*

stress-bearing a. 1. the portion of the mouth capable of providing support for a denture. 2. surfaces of oral structures which resist forces, strains, or pressures brought upon them during function. 3. denture-bearing a.
striate a. see under *cortex.*
strip a. a strip of cerebral cortex between the motor and premotor areas, thought to be suppressor in function.
a. subcallo′sa [TA], **subcallosal a.** a small area of cortex on the medial surface of each cerebral hemisphere, between the anterior and posterior parolfactory sulci.
a. of superficial cardiac dullness a triangular area of dullness observed on percussion of the chest, corresponding to that area of the heart not covered by lung tissue.
supplementary a's small motor and sensory areas of the cerebral cortex in addition to the primary areas.
supplementary motor a. an area in the gyrus frontalis medius just above the cingulate gyrus and anterior to the part of the first somatomotor area that mediates movements of the lower extremity.
supporting a. 1. the surface of the mouth available for support of a denture. 2. those areas of the maxillary and mandibular edentulous ridges which are considered best suited to carry the forces of mastication when the dentures are in function.
suppressor a's areas of the cerebral cortex whose activation is thought to suppress or prevent movement; see also *strip a.*
taste receiving a. gustatory receiving a.
T-dependent a. thymus-dependent a.
thymus-dependent a. any of the areas of the peripheral lymphoid organs populated by T lymphocytes, e.g., the periarteriolar lymphatic sheath in the spleen, the paracortex in lymph nodes, and the parafollicular areas of gut-associated lymphoid tissue. Called also *paracortex, T-dependent a.,* and *tertiary cortex.*
thymus-independent a. any of the areas of the peripheral lymphoid organs populated by B lymphocytes, e.g., the lymph nodules (lymphoid follicles) of the spleen, lymph nodes, and gut-associated lymphoid tissue. Called also *B-dependent a.* and *T-independent a.*
T-independent a. thymus-independent a.
trigger a. see under *zone.*
a. under the curve (AUC) the area enclosed between a probability curve with nonnegative values and the axis of the quality being measured; of the total area under a curve, the proportion that falls between two given points on the curve defines a probability density function (see under *function*).
vagus a. trigonum nervi vagi.
ventral tegmental a. the part of the mesencephalon lying medial to the substantia nigra and containing large numbers of dopaminergic neurons; it sends projections to various limbic structures and the cerebral cortex.
vestibular a. a rounded triangular elevation lateral to foveae of the fourth ventricle over which pass the striae medullares; it extends into the lateral recess, where it forms the *auditory,* or *acoustic, tubercle.*
vestibular a. of internal acoustic meatus, inferior a. vestibularis inferior meatus acustici interni.
vestibular a. of internal acoustic meatus, superior a. vestibularis superior meatus acustici interni.
a. vestibula′ris infe′rior mea′tus acus′tici inter′ni [TA] inferior vestibular area of internal acoustic meatus: the lower portion of the fundus of the internal acoustic meatus, transmitting fibers of the saccular nerve.
a. vestibula′ris supe′rior mea′tus acus′tici inter′ni [TA] superior vestibular area of internal acoustic meatus: the upper portion of the fundus of the internal acoustic meatus, transmitting fibers of the utricular and superior ampullary nerves.
visual a. see under *cortex.*
visual a., first striate cortex.
visual a., second parastriate a.
visual a., third peristriate a.
visual association a's the peristriate and parastriate areas considered together.
visual receiving a. visual cortex.
visuopsychic a's visual association a's.
visuosensory a. striate cortex.
vocal a. rima glottidis.
watershed a. any of several areas over the convexities of the cerebral or cerebellar hemispheres, distant from the circle of Willis, where the vascular beds of two cerebral arteries meet and form anastomoses. At times of prolonged systemic hypotension, these are particularly susceptible to infarction, with those fed by the largest arterial branches being the first affected. See also *watershed infarction,* under *infarction.*
Wernicke a., Wernicke second motor speech a. originally a term denoting a language center thought to be confined to the posterior part of the superior temporal gyrus adjacent to the transverse temporal gyri; the term now includes a wider zone that encompasses the supramarginal and angular gyri as well; called also *Wernicke field* or *zone.*

ar•e•a•ta (ar″e-a′tə) [L., fem. of *areatus* dried up] occurring in patches.

Ar•e•ca (ar′ə-kə) [from Malayalam *atekka*] a genus of palm trees (family Palmae), native to southern Asia and nearby islands. *A. ca′techu* L. is the betel palm, an East Indian species that is the source of areca (betel).

ar•e•ca (ar′ə-kə) 1. any palm tree of the genus *Areca.* 2. the dried ripe seed of *Areca catechu,* a common masticatory in India and elsewhere in Asia. It contains the alkaloid arecoline and astringent tannins and has parasympathomimetic and anthelmintic properties. Called also *areca nut* and *betel nut.* See also *betel.*

arec•o•line (ə-rek′o-lēn) a cholinomimetic alkaloid obtained from areca (betel nut) having both muscarinic and nicotinic effects, used as an ingredient of the veterinary anthelmintic *drocarbil.*

Are•dia (ə-re′de-ə) trademark for a preparation of pamidronate disodium.

are•flex•ia (a″re-flek′se-ə) [*a-*^{1} + *reflex* + *-ia*] absence of reflexes.
  detrusor a. failure of the detrusor urinae muscle to respond to stimuli, usually owing to a lesion of a lower motoneuron, resulting in failure to empty the bladder completely on urination.

are•gen•er•a•tive (a″re-jen′ər-ə-tiv) characterized by absence of regeneration; applied especially to blood cells in aplastic anemia.

ar•e•na•ceous (ar″ə-na′shəs) sandy; gritty.

Are•na•vi•ri•dae (ə-re″nə-vir′ĭ-de) the arenaviruses: a family of RNA viruses having a pleomorphic virion 50–300 nm in diameter consisting of a lipid bilayer envelope, with large peplomers, surrounding a coiled nucleocapsid with two members and a variable number of ribosomes. The genome consists of two circular molecules of ambisense single-stranded RNA, designated L (MW 1.1×10^6) and S (MW $2.2–2.8\times10^6$) (size of total genome 10–14 kb). Viruses contain three major polypeptides, including a transcriptase, and are ultraviolet- and gamma radiation–sensitive. Replication and assembly occur in the cytoplasm; virions are released by budding through the plasma membrane. Host ranges are narrow. There is a single genus, *Arenavirus.*

Are•na•vi•rus (ə-re′nə-vi″rəs) [L. *arena* sand + *virus* (from the granules that give the virions a sandy appearance)] arenaviruses; a genus of viruses of the family Arenaviridae, some of which cause hemorrhagic fevers. It includes lymphocytic choriomeningitis virus, Lassa virus, and the viruses of the Tacaribe complex (Amapari, Flexal, Guanarito, Junin, Machupo, Parana, Pichinde, Sabia, Tacaribe, and Tamiami viruses). Rodents are common hosts.

are•na•vi•rus (ə-re′nə-vi″rəs) any virus belonging to the family Arenaviridae. **arenavi′ral** *adj*
  New World a's Tacaribe complex.
  Old World a's former name for the LCMV-LASV complex.

ar•e•noid (ar′ə-noid) [L. *arena* sand + *-oid*] resembling sand.

are•o•la (ə-re′o-lə) pl. *are′olae* [L., dim. of *area* space] 1. any minute space or interstice in a tissue; see *areolar tissue,* under *tissue.* 2. a circular area of a different color, surrounding a central point, such as around a pustule or vesicle, the pupil of the eye, or the nipple of the breast. **are′olar** *adj*
  a. mam′mae [TA], **a. of mammary gland, a. of nipple** the darkened ring surrounding the nipple of a breast.
  second a. a ring that surrounds the areola mammae during pregnancy.

are•o•lae (ə-re′o-le) [L.] genitive and plural of *areola.*

are•o•li•tis (ar″e-o-li′tis) inflammation of the areola of the breast.

Ar•ey rule (ār′e) [Leslie Brainerd *Arey,* American anatomist, 1891–1988] see under *rule.*

ARF acute renal failure.

Ar•fon•ad (ahr′fon-ad) trademark for a preparation of trimethaphan camsylate.

Arg arginine.

Ar•gand burner (ahr-gah′) [Aimé *Argand,* Swiss physicist, 1755–1803] see under *burner.*

Ar•gas (ahr′gəs) a genus of ticks of the family Argasidae, some of which transmit diseases.

A. america′nus *A. persicus.*

A. brump′ti a species found in Africa whose bite causes local inflammation.

A. minia′tus *A. persicus.*

A. per′sicus the tampan tick, one of the most important blood-sucking parasites of poultry, which produces a weakened condition of flocks, with great economic losses. In numerous tropical and subtropical countries it acts as the carrier of fowl spirochetosis. Called also *A. americanus* or *A. miniatus, tampan, miana bug,* and *Mianeh bug.*

A. reflex′us an ectoparasite of pigeons and other roosting birds, which can also attack humans and cause skin inflammation.

ar•ga•sid (ahr′gə-sid) 1. pertaining to ticks of the family Argasidae. 2. a tick of the family Argasidae; called also *argasid* or *soft tick.* 3. pertaining to ticks of the genus *Argas.*

Ar•gas•i•dae (ahr-gas′ĭ-de) the soft ticks, a family of the superfamily Ixodoidea, distinguished from the hard ticks (Ixodidae) by absence of the scutum. Genera of medical or veterinary interest include *Argas, Ornithodoros,* and *Otobius.*

ar•gat•ro•ban (ahr-gat′ro-ban″) a type of direct thrombin inhibitor derived from L-arginine, used as an anticoagulant in the prophylaxis and treatment of heparin-induced thrombocytopenia, administered intravenously.

ar•ge•ma (ahr′jə-mə) a white ulcer of the cornea.

Ar•gem•o•ne (ahr-jem′ə-ne) a genus of herbs of the family Papaveraceae, originally native to the Americas, having prickly leaves and yellow or white flowers. *A. mexica′na* is the prickly poppy, which contains argemone oil and can cause epidemic dropsy.

ar•gen•taf•fin (ahr-jen′tə-fin) [L. *argentum* silver + *affinis* having affinity for] having an affinity for silver and chromium salts; said of tissues. See also under *cell.*

ar•gen•taf•fi•no•ma (ahr″jən-taf″ĭ-no′mə) carcinoid tumor

ar•gen•ta•tion (ahr″jen-ta′shən) [L. *argentum* silver] staining with a silver salt.

ar•gen•tic (ahr-jen′tik) [L. *argentum* silver] containing silver.

ar•gi•nase (ahr′jĭ-nās) [EC 3.5.3.1] an enzyme of the hydrolase class that catalyzes the hydrolysis of arginine to form ornithine and urea, which is the last step of the urea cycle. In mammals there are two isoforms, *arginase 1,* expressed mainly in the liver and in macrophages, and *arginase 2,* expressed mainly in extrahepatic tissues.

ar•gi•nase de•fi•cien•cy (ahr′jĭ-nās) an autosomal recessive aminoacidopathy caused by mutations in the *ARG1* gene (locus: 6q23), which encodes arginine 1. Arginine is elevated in blood and urine and may cause secondary cystinuria; oroticaciduria is common, but hyperammonemia is rare. Clinical signs include psychomotor retardation, hepatomegaly, and scalp discoloration. Called also *argininemia* and *hyperargininemia.*

ar•gi•nine (ahr′jĭ-nēn) 1. a nonessential amino acid, 2-amino-5-guanidinovaleric acid, produced by the hydrolysis or digestion of proteins. It is one of the hexone bases and supplies the amidine group for the synthesis of creatine. Arginine is also formed by the transfer of a nitrogen atom from aspartate to citrulline in the urea cycle. It then gives off urea, to form ornithine. Symbols Arg and R. See table at *amino acid.* 2. [USP] a preparation of L-arginine used in the treatment of hyperammonemia and as a diagnostic aid in the assessment of pituitary function (see *arginine stimulation test,* under *test*).

a. **glutamate** a salt composed of L-arginine and L-glutamic acid, used as an adjunct in the treatment of hyperammonemia; administered intravenously.

a. **hydrochloride** [USP] the monohydrochloride salt of L-arginine, used as an adjunct in the treatment of hyperammonemia and as a stimulant of growth hormone release by the pituitary in arginine stimulation tests (see under *test*); administered intravenously.

ar•gi•nine car•boxy•pep•ti•dase (ahr′jĭ-nēn kahr-bok″se-pep′tĭ-dās) lysine carboxypeptidase.

ar•gi•ni•ne•mia (ahr′jĭ-nĭ-ne′me-ə) arginase deficiency.

ar•gi•ni•no•suc•cin•ase (ahr″jĭ-ne″no-suk′sĭ-nās) argininosuccinate lyase.

ar•gi•ni•no•suc•cin•ase de•fi•cien•cy (ahr″jĭ-ne″no-suk′sĭ-nās) argininosuccinicaciduria.

ar•gi•ni•no•suc•cin•ate (ahr″jĭ-ne″no-suk′sĭ-nāt) the anionic form of argininosuccinic acid.

ar•gi•ni•no•suc•cin•ate ly•ase (ahr″jĭ-ne″no-suk′sĭ-nāt li′ās) [EC 4.3.2.1] an enzyme of the lyase class that catalyzes the cleavage of argininosuccinate to form fumarate and arginine. The reaction is part of the urea cycle in the liver (see illustration at *urea cycle,* under *cycle*). Deficiency of the enzyme, an autosomal recessive trait, results in argininosuccinicaciduria. Called also *argininosuccinase.*

ar•gi•ni•no•suc•cin•ate syn•thase (ahr″jĭ-ne″no-suk′sĭ-nāt sin′thās) [EC 6.3.4.5] an enzyme of the ligase class that catalyzes the condensation of citrulline and aspartate to form argininosuccinate. The reaction is a part of the urea cycle in the liver (see illustration at *urea cycle,* under *cycle*). Deficiency of enzyme activity causes citrullinemia. Written also *argininosuccinate synthetase.*

ar•gi•ni•no•suc•ci•nate syn•thase de•fi•cien•cy (ahr″jĭ-ne″no-suk′sĭ-nāt sin′thās) citrullinemia.

ar•gi•ni•no•suc•cin•ic ac•id (ahr″jĭ-ne″no-suk-sin′ik) a compound formed by the condensation of aspartic acid and citrulline as a step in the urea cycle (q.v.).

ar•gi•ni•no•suc•cin•ic•ac•i•de•mia (ahr″jĭ-ne″no-sək-sin″ik-as″ĭ-de′me-ə) the presence in the blood of argininosuccinic acid.

ar•gi•ni•no•suc•cin•ic•ac•id•uria (ahr″jĭ-ne″no-suk-sin″ik-as″ĭ-du′re-ə) 1. an autosomal recessive aminoacidopathy caused by mutations in the *ASL* gene (locus: 7cen-q11.2), which encodes argininosuccinate lyase, characterized by urinary excretion of argininosuccinic acid with hyperammonemia, argininosuccinicacidemia, and hypercitrullinemia. Neonatal and late onset forms exist, and clinical findings, which vary widely in severity, include mental retardation, seizures, ataxia, hepatomegaly, and friable hair. Called also *argininosuccinase* or *argininosuccinate lyase deficiency.* 2. excretion of argininosuccinic acid in the urine.

ar•gi•nyl (ahr′jĭ-nəl) the acyl radical of arginine.

ar•gi•pres•sin (ahr″jĭ-pres′in) arginine vasopressin.

ar•gon (Ar) (ahr′gon) [Gr. *argos* inert] a chemical element, atomic number 18, discovered in the atmosphere in 1895. One of the inert gases, atomic weight 39.948.

Ar•gyll Rob•ert•son pupil (pupil sign) (ahr-gil′ rob′ərt-sən) [Douglas Moray Cooper Lamb *Argyll Robertson,* Scottish physician, 1837–1909] see under *pupil.*

ar•gyr•emia (ahr″jə-re′me-ə) [Gr. *argyros* silver + *-emia*] the presence of silver or silver salts in the blood.

ar•gyr•ia (ahr-jir′e-ə) a permanent ash gray discoloration of the skin, conjunctiva, and internal organs that results from long-continued use of silver salts. Called also *argyrosis.*

a. **nasa′lis** argyric discoloration of the nasal mucosa.

ar•gyr•i•a•sis (ahr″jə-ri′ə-sis) argyria.

ar•gyr•ic (ahr-jir′ik) 1. pertaining to or caused by silver. 2. pertaining to argyria.

ar•gyr•ism (ahr′jə-riz-əm) argyria.

Ar•gyr•ol (ahr′jə-rol) trademark for mild silver protein; see under *silver.*

ar•gy•ro•phil (ahr′jə-ro-fil, ahr-ji′ro-fil) [Gr. *argyros* silver + *-phil*] capable of binding silver salts, which may subsequently be reduced by light or by a reducing agent to give a black deposit of silver; said of tissues and tissue elements.

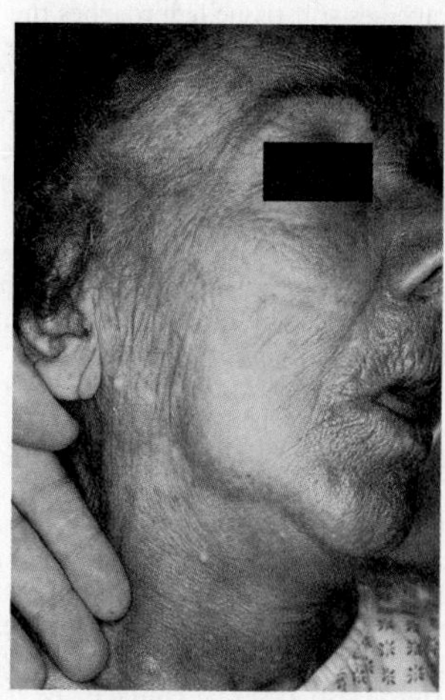

■ Argyria.

ar·gy·ro·phil·ic (ahr″jə-ro-fil′ik) argyrophil.

ar·gy·ro·sis (ahr″jə-ro′sis) [Gr. *argyros* silver] argyria.

arhin·en·ce·pha·lia (a″rin-en″sə-fa′le-ə) arrhinencephalia.

arhin·ia (ə-rin′e-ə) arrhinia.

Arias-Ste·lla reaction (ahr′yahs-sta′yə) [Javier *Arias-Stella*, Peruvian pathologist, born 1924] see under *reaction*.

ari·bo·fla·vin·o·sis (a-ri″bo-fla″vĭ-no′sis) [*a-*[1] + *riboflavin* + *-osis*] deficiency of riboflavin in the diet. It produces a syndrome chiefly marked by cheilosis or cheilitis, angular stomatitis, glossitis associated with a purplish red or magenta-colored tongue that may show fissures, corneal vascularization, dyssebacia, and anemia.

Ar·i·cept (ar′ĭ-sept) trademark for a preparation of donepezil hydrochloride.

ar·il (ar′il) [L. *arillus* dried grape] an accessory covering or appendage of seeds.

ar·il·lode (ar′ĭ-lōd) an appendage of certain seeds attached to the micropyle or raphe.

Arim·i·dex (ə-rim′ĭ-deks) trademark for a preparation of anastrozole.

ar·i·pip·ra·zole (ar″ĭ-pip′rə-zōl) an antipsychotic with partial agonist activity at dopamine D_2 and serotonin 5-HT_{1A} receptors and anatagonist activity at serotonin 5-HT_{2A} receptors; administered orally in the treatment of schizophrenia and of acute manic and mixed episodes of bipolar disorder.

Aris·to·cort (ə-ris′to-cort) trademark for preparations of triamcinolone.

Aris·to·lo·chia (ə-ris″to-lo′ke-ə) [L., from Gr. *aristos* best + *lochia*] a large genus of shrubs and herbs of the family Aristolochiaceae; many species contain aristolochic acid. High doses may be toxic, causing kidney damage or diarrhea.

aris·to·lo·chic ac·id (ə-ris″to-lo′kik) a phenanthrene-carboxylic acid derivative, the major bitter aromatic principle of herbs of the genus *Aristolochia* and related species; high doses can be toxic, causing kidney damage, diarhea, and other symptoms.

Aris·to·span (ə-ris′to-span) trademark for preparations of triamcinolone hexacetonide.

Ar·is·tot·le anomaly (ar′is-tot″əl) [*Aristotle*, Greek philosopher, 384–322 B.C.] see under *anomaly*.

arith·mo·ma·nia (ə-rith″mo-ma′ne-ə) [Gr. *arithmos* number + *mania*] compulsive counting, as paces when walking, steps in a staircase, etc., a common symptom in obsessive-compulsive disorder.

Arix·tra (ə-riks′trə) trademark for a preparation of fondaparinux sodium.

Ar·i·zo·na (ar″ĭ-zo′nə) see *Salmonella enterica* subsp. *arizonae*.

Arlt recess, sinus, trachoma (ahrlt) [Carl Ferdinand Ritter von *Arlt*, Austrian ophthalmologist, 1812–1887] see under *trachoma* and see *sinus of Maier*.

arm (ahrm) [A.S. *earm*] 1. brachium (def. 1). 2. in common usage, the entire upper limb (*membrum superius* [TA]). 3. a slender part or extension, usually having mobility and independent function, that projects from a main structure. 4. an extension or projection by which a removable partial denture is retained in position in the mouth.

bar clasp a. a clasp arm that serves as an extracoronal retainer, originating from the denture base, a major or minor connector, or the framework of a denture, traverses soft tissue, approaches the tooth undercut area from a gingival direction, and terminates in a retentive undercut lying gingival to the height of contour.

bird a. a wasted condition of the forearm due to atrophy of the muscles.

chromosome a. either of the two segments of the chromosome separated by the centromere; the symbol p indicates the short arm and q the long arm.

circumferential clasp a. a clasp arm that originates above the height of contour, traverses part of the suprabulge portion of the tooth, approaches the tooth undercut from an occlusal direction, and terminates in a retentive undercut lying gingival to the height of contour.

clasp a. an extension or projection of the clasp of a partial denture, helping to stabilize and retain it in the mouth.

glass a. a painful condition of the upper arm due to an injury to the long tendon of the biceps muscle or to the tendon of the supraspinatus muscle, at times resulting in subdeltoid bursitis.

reciprocal a. a clasp arm located in such a manner as to reciprocate any force arising from an opposing clasp arm on the same tooth.

retention a., retentive a. a rigid clasp that engages the infrabulge area at the terminal end of the arm.

stabilizing a. a rigid clasp arm that contacts the tooth at or occlusal to the surveyed height of contour.

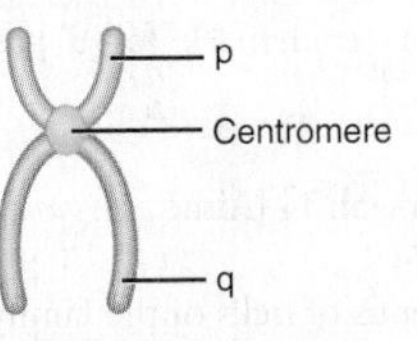

■ Chromosome arms.

ar·ma·dil·lo (ahr″mə-dil′o) [Sp. "little armored thing"] one of a group of burrowing mammals of the order Edentata, family Dasypodidae, that have horny shields on the dorsal surface of the body; one species in South America is a reservoir for *Trypanosoma cruzi*.

ar·ma·men·tar·i·um (ahr″mə-men-tar′e-əm) [L.] the equipment of a practitioner or institution, including books, instruments, medicines, and surgical appliances.

Ar·man·ni-Eb·stein cells, kidney, lesion (degeneration) (ahr-mah′ne eb′shtīn) [Luciano *Armanni*, Italian pathologist, 1839–1903; Wilhelm *Ebstein*, German internist, 1836–1912] see under *cell*, *kidney*, and *lesion*.

ar·ma·ture (ahr′mə-choor) [L. *armatura* a defensive apparatus] 1. the iron bar or keeper across the open end of a horseshoe magnet. 2. a protective organ or structure.

ARMD age-related macular degeneration.

Ar·mig·er·es (ahr-mij′ər-ēz) a genus of mosquitoes of the tribe Aedini, subfamily Culicinae. *A. obtur′bans* transmits dengue in Japan.

Ar·mil·li·fer (ahr-mil′ĭ-fər) a genus of pentastomes, wormlike endoparasites of the phylum Pentastomida.

A. armilla′tus a species whose adults are found in the lungs and trachea of the python and whose larvae are found in the internal organs of monkeys, lions, and occasionally humans in Africa. Formerly called *Porocephalus armillatus*.

A. monilifor′mis a species whose larvae are parasitic in humans in China, the Philippines, and other nearby islands.

Ar·mo·ra·cia (ahr″mo-ra′shə) a genus of flowering herbs of the family Cruciferae. *A. lapathifo′lia* is the horseradish plant, whose root yields the condiment horseradish; it can cause fatal gastroenteritis in livestock. Formerly called *Cochlearia armoracia*.

Ar·mour (ahr′mər) trademark for a preparation of porcine thyroid, which contains levothyroxine and liothyronine.

arm·pit (ahrm′pit) the domed space inferior to the floor of the axilla and between the arm and thoracic wall.

Arndt's law (ahrnts) [Rudolf *Arndt*, German psychiatrist, 1835–1900] see under *law*.

ARN acute retinal necrosis.

Arndt-Schulz law (ahrnt′ shoolts′) [R. *Arndt*; Hugo *Schulz*, German pharmacologist, 1853–1932] Arndt's law.

Ar·neth classification, count, formula, index (ahr-net′) [Joseph *Arneth*, German physician, 1873–1955] see under *classification*, *count*, *formula*, and *index*.

Ar·ni·ca (ahr′nĭ-kə) [L.] a genus of composite-flowered plants (family Compositae), known also as *leopard's bane*, *wolfsbane*, and *mountain tobacco*. The dried flowerheads of *A. monta′na* are called *arnica* and are used medicinally.

ar·ni·ca (ahr′nĭ-kə) 1. any plant of the genus *Arnica*. 2. the dried flower heads of *Arnica montana;* they contain arnicin, arnisterol, anthoxanthins, tannin, and resins and are used topically in tincture form for contusions, sprains, and superficial wounds, and as a counterirritant. Called also *wolfsbane* and *leopard's bane*.

Ar·nold canal, etc. (ahr′nəld) [Philipp Friedrich *Arnold*, German anatomist, 1803–1890] see under *canal*, *ligament*, *nerve*, and *syndrome*.

Ar·nold-Chi·a·ri malformation (deformity, syndrome) (ahr′nəld ke-ah′re) [Julius *Arnold*, German pathologist, 1835–1915; Hans *Chiari*, Austrian pathologist, 1851–1916] see under *malformation*.

aro·ma (ə-ro′mə) [Gr. *arōma* spice] fragrance or odor, especially that of a spice or medicine or of articles of food or drink.

Aro·ma·sin (ə-ro′mə-sin) trademark for a preparation of exemestane.

aro·ma·tase (ə-ro′mə-tās) an enzyme activity occurring in the endoplasmic reticulum and catalyzing the conversion of testosterone to the aromatic compound estradiol, proceeding via three successive hydroxylations, loss of a carbon atom, and rearrangement.

aro·ma·ther·a·py (ə-ro′mə-ther″ə-pe) the therapeutic use of essential oils extracted from plants by steam distillation or expression; they may be used by inhalation, introduced internally (orally, rectally, or intravaginally), or applied topically by means of compresses, baths, or massage.

ar•o•mat•ic (ar″o-mat′ik) [L. *aromaticus;* Gr. *arōmatikos*] 1. having a spicy odor. 2. in organic chemistry, denoting a compound containing a ring system stabilized by a closed circle of conjugated double bonds or nonbonding electron pairs, such as benzene, naphthalene, or the arylamines.

ar•o•mat•ic-L-ami•no-ac•id de•car•box•y•lase (ar″o-mat′ik ə-me′no as′id de″kahr-bok′sə-lās) [EC 4.1.1.28] an enzyme of the lyase class that catalyzes the decarboxylation of aromatic amino acids, notably converting dopa to dopamine, tryptophan to tryptamine, and hydroxytryptophan to serotonin. The enzyme is bound to a pyridoxal phosphate cofactor and occurs particularly in liver, kidney, brain, and vas deferens; the reaction is important in the biosynthesis of catecholamines and of melanin.

aro•ma•ti•za•tion (ə-ro″mə-tĭ-za′shən) chemical conversion to an aromatic form.

arous•al (ə-rou′zəl) 1. a state of responsiveness to sensory stimulation or excitability. 2. the act or state of waking from or as if from sleep. 3. the act of stimulating to readiness or to action.

sexual a. physical and psychological responses to mental or physical erotic stimulation, including altered respiration, muscular tension, pulse, and blood flow to the genitals as well as increased interest in sexual activity.

ar•pri•no•cid (ahr-pri′no-sid) a coccidiostat used in poultry.

ARPKD autosomal recessive polycystic kidney disease.

ar•range•ment (ə-rānj′mənt) the disposal or positioning of parts.

anterior tooth a. the arrangement of anterior teeth for esthetic or phonetic effects.

tooth a. 1. the positioning of teeth on a denture for specific purposes. 2. the setting of teeth on temporary bases.

Ar•ra•non (ăr′ə-non) trademark for a preparation of nelarabine.

ar•rec•tor (ə-rek′tər) pl. *arrecto′res* [L., from *arrigere,* to set up or raise] raising, or that which raises. Cf. *erector.*

a. pi′li pl. *arrecto′res pilo′rum* [L. "raiser of the hair"] musculus arrector pili.

ar•rec•to•res (ar″ek-to′res) [L.] plural of *arrector.*

ar•rest (ə-rest′) stoppage; the act of stopping.

cardiac a. sudden cessation of the pumping function of the heart, with disappearance of arterial blood pressure, connoting either ventricular fibrillation or ventricular standstill; it usually leads to death unless corrected but may be temporary or paroxysmal.

deep transverse a. the condition during delivery in which the occiput of the fetus turns and stops in the transverse diameter of the pelvis.

developmental a. a temporary or permanent cessation of the process of development.

epiphyseal a. interruption of growth at the epiphysis of a bone by diaphyseal-epiphyseal fusion.

heart a. cardiac a.

maturation a. interruption of the process of development before it is complete; applied especially to failure of maturation of granulocytes, with myeloblasts and promyelocytes predominating, as seen in certain forms of leukemia.

sinus a. a halt, usually transient, in the normal cardiac (sinus) rhythm due to a slowing or cessation of impulse initiation by the sinus node, lasting for an interval that is not an exact multiple of the normal cardiac cycle; either ectopic pacemakers assume control of the rhythm or periods of ventricular asystole occur. See also *sinus pause,* under *pause.*

ar•rest•ed (ə-rest′əd) detained; stopped. In obstetrics, the head of the fetus is said to be arrested when it is *detained,* but not *impacted,* in the pelvic cavity.

ar•res•tin (ə-res′tin) any of a family of inhibitory proteins that bind to phosphorylated G protein–coupled receptors and so block their interaction with G proteins. In the retina, arrestin binds activated phosphorylated rhodopsin and prevents it from binding transducin, thus deactivating rhodopsin as part of the visual cycle.

ar•rha•phia (ə-ra′fe-ə) [*a-*[1] + *-rrhaphy*] status dysraphicus.

Ar•rhe•ni•us equation, formula, theory (doctrine) (ə-re′ne-əs) [Svante August *Arrhenius,* Swedish chemist, 1859–1927] see under *equation, formula,* and *theory.*

ar•rhe•no•blas•to•ma (ə-re″no-blas-to′mə) androblastoma (def. 2).

ar•rhin•en•ce•pha•lia (ə-rin″ən-sə-fa′le-ə) [*a-*[1] + *rhinencephalon*] congenital absence of the rhinencephalon.

ar•rhin•ia (ə-rin′e-ə) [*a-*[1] + *rhin-* + *-ia*] congenital absence of the nose.

ar•rhyth•mia (ə-rith′me-ə) [*a-*[1] + *rhythm* + *-ia*] 1. a disturbance in or loss of regular rhythm. 2. especially, any variation from the normal rhythm of the heartbeat; it may be an abnormality of either the rate, regularity, or site of impulse origin or the sequence of activation. The term encompasses abnormal regular and irregular rhythms as well as loss of rhythm. Cf. *dysrhythmia* and see also entries under *rhythm.*

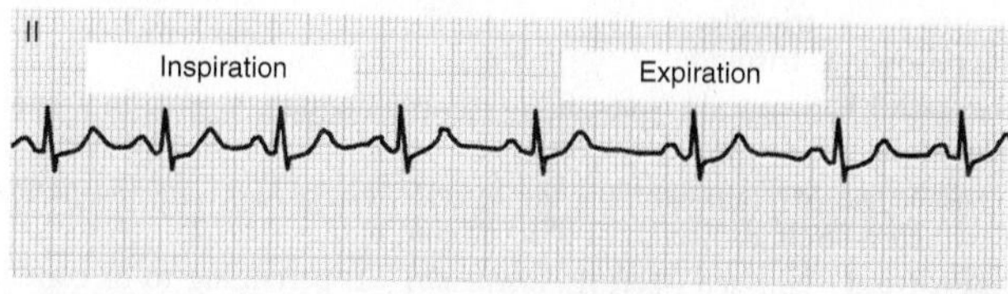

■ Phasic arrhythmia; the rhythm strip shows the heart rate increasing with inspiration and decreasing with expiration.

chronic a. continuous a.

compound a. an arrhythmia with multiple disturbances in rhythm.

continuous a. irregularity in the force, quality, and sequence of the pulse beat, continuing as a permanent phenomenon; called also *chronic* or *perpetual a.*

juvenile a. sinus arrhythmia occurring in children.

nodal a. arrhythmia occurring when the atrioventricular node or surrounding junctional tissue is acting as pacemaker.

nonphasic a. a form of sinus arrhythmia in which the irregularity is not linked to the phases of respiration. Cf. *phasic a.*

perpetual a. continuous a.

phasic a. a form of sinus arrhythmia linked to the phases of respiration, the heart rate increasing with inhalation and decreasing with exhalation. Cf. *nonphasic a.*

sinus a. the physiologic cyclic variation in heart rate related to vagal impulses to the sinoatrial node, which can be linked to or independent of the phases of respiration (see *phasic a.* and *nonphasic a.*). It is common, particularly in children, and is not considered abnormal.

sinus a., nonrespiratory nonphasic a.

sinus a., respiratory phasic a.

supraventricular a. an arrhythmia originating in the atria, including the atrioventricular node; it may be either a bradyarrhythmia or a tachyarrhythmia.

ventricular a. an arrhythmia originating in the ventricles.

ar•rhyth•mic (ə-rith′mik) [*a-*[1] + Gr. *rhythmos* rhythm] 1. characterized by absence of rhythm. 2. pertaining to or characterized by arrhythmia.

ar•rhyth•mo•gen•esis (ə-rith″mo-jen′ə-sis) [*arrhythmia* + *genesis*] the development of an arrhythmia.

ar•rhyth•mo•gen•ic (ə-rith″mo-jen′ik) [*arrhythmia* + *-genic*] producing or promoting arrhythmia.

ar•rhyth•mo•ki•ne•sis (ə-rith″mo-kĭ-ne′sis) [*arrhythmia* + *kinesis*] a dyskinesia consisting of defective ability to perform voluntary successive movements of a definite rhythm. Cf. *adiadochokinesia.*

Ar•ro•yo sign (ah-ro′yo) [Carlos F. *Arroyo,* American physician, 1892–1928] asthenocoria.

ARRS American Roentgen Ray Society.

ar•sa•nil•ic ac•id (ahr″sə-nil′ik) [USP] an arsenical antibacterial used in veterinary practice for the prevention and treatment of swine dysentery.

ar•se•ni•a•sis (ahr″sə-ni′ə-sis) chronic arsenic poisoning.

ar•se•nic[1] **(As)** (ahr′sə-nik) [L. *arsenicum, arsenium,* or *arsenum;* from Gr. *arsēn* strong] a nonmetallic element, occurring as a brittle, lustrous, grayish solid, with a garlicky odor. Atomic number, 33; atomic weight, 74.922; specific gravity, 5.73; it is toxic by inhalation and ingestion and is carcinogenic. Although arsenic and its compounds have been widely employed in medicine, it is now rarely used and is important only in the treatment of certain tropical parasitic diseases. See also *arsenic poisoning,* under *poisoning.*

a. chloride a. trichloride.

a. disulfide, red a. sulfide a poisonous compound, used as a pigment, in fireworks, in shot manufacture, and in the leather industry; called also *realgar.*

a. trichloride a very poisonous fuming liquid, $AsCl_3$, which readily liberates highly irritant hydrochloric acid; it is used in war gas and as an intermediate for organic chemicals.

a. trioxide an oxidized form of arsenic, with a sweetish taste and erythropoietic effect; used in weed killers, sheep dips, and rodenticides. It is also administered intravenously as an antineoplastic in the treatment of acute promyelocytic leukemia. Called also *white a., arsenous acid,* and *arsenous anhydride.*

a. trisulfide a poisonous substance, occurring in nature as the mineral orpiment; used as a pigment and sometimes as a medicine. Called also *a. yellow* and *auripigment.*

white a. a. trioxide.
a. yellow a. trisulfide.

ar•sen•ic[2] (ahr-sen′ik) pertaining to or containing arsenic in a pentavalent state.

ar•sen•ic ac•id (ahr-sen′ik) the hydrate, H_3AsO_4, of arsenic pentoxide, which is itself also referred to as arsenic acid.

ar•sen•i•cal (ahr-sen′ĭ-kəl) [L. *arsenicalis*] 1. pertaining to or containing arsenic. 2. a drug or other compound (such as a pesticide) containing arsenic; all arsenicals are toxic and some are carcinogenic.

ar•sen•i•cal•ism (ahr-sen′ĭ-kəl-iz″əm) chronic arsenic poisoning.

ar•sen•i•cism (ahr-sen′ĭ-siz″əm) chronic arsenic poisoning.

ar•sen•i•co•sis (ahr-sen″ĭ-ko′sis) chronic arsenic poisoning.

ar•se•nide (ahr′sə-nīd) any compound of arsenic with another element, in which arsenic is the negative element.

ar•sen•i•ous (ahr-sen′e-əs) arsenous.

ar•se•nism (ahr′sə-niz″əm) chronic arsenic poisoning.

ar•se•nite (ahr′sə-nīt) any salt of arsenous acid.

arseno- a prefix indicating the chemical group —As:As—.

ar•se•no•ther•a•py (ahr″sə-no-ther′ə-pe) [*arsenic* + *therapy*] treatment of disease by the use of arsenic and arsenical preparations.

ar•se•nous (ahr′sə-nəs) containing arsenic in its lower or triad valency.
a. oxide arsenic trioxide.

ar•se•nous ac•id (ahr′sə-nəs) the hydrate, H_3AsO_3, of arsenic trioxide, which is itself also referred to as arsenous acid.

ar•sine (ahr′sēn) any member of a peculiar group of volatile arsenical bases, formed when arsenous acid is brought in contact with albuminous substances. The typical arsine is AsH_3, arsenous hydride or arseniuretted hydrogen, a very poisonous gas, and some of its compounds have been used in warfare. A major industrial use is in the production of microelectronic components. It is carcinogenic and also causes hemolysis, jaundice, gastroenteritis, and nephritis.

ar•sin•ic ac•id (ahr-sin′ik) an organic compound containing the —AsO_2H functional group.

ar•son•ic ac•id (ahr-son′ik) an organic compound containing the —$AsO(OH)_2$ functional group.

ar•so•ni•um (ahr-so′ne-əm) the univalent radical or ion, AsH_4, which acts in combination like the ammonium ion, NH_4.

ars•phen•a•mine (ahrs-fen′ə-mēn) the first medicine specific for the treatment of syphilis, yaws, and other spirillum infections, later replaced by oxophenarsine and then by penicillin. Called also *salvarsan*.

ART Accredited Record Technician; assisted reproductive technology; automated reagin test.

Ar•tane (ahr′tān) trademark for preparations of trihexyphenidyl.

ar•te•fact (ahr′tə-fakt) artifact.

ar•tem•e•ther (ahr-tem′ə-thər) a derivative of artemisinin, used in combination with lumefantrine in the treatment of malaria; administered intramuscularly.

Ar•te•mi•sia (ahr″tə-mis′e-ə) [L., from Gr. *artemisia* from *Artemis* Diana] a genus of aromatic composite-flowered plants (family Compositae) widely distributed in dry areas in the temperate and cool regions of the world; some species are used medicinally.
A. absin′thium common wormwood (q.v.) or absinthium (def.1).
A. an′nua sweet wormwood; a Eurasian species used in Chinese medicine to control fever and as an antimalarial; it is the source of artemisinin.
A. vulga′ris mugwort; the source of moxa and also used orally.

ar•te•mis•i•nin (ahr″tə-mis′ĭ-nin) 1. an antimalarial lactone derived from *Artemisia annua*, effective against schizonts of *Plasmodium vivax* and *Plasmodium falciparum*. Artemisinin and its derivatives are rapid-acting but are subject to recrudescence and are used in combination with other, longer-acting antimalarials. 2. any of the antimalarial drugs derived from this compound.

ar•te•ral•gia (ahr″tər-al′jə) pain emanating from an artery, such as headache from an inflamed temporal artery.

ar•ter•ec•to•my (ahr″tər-ek′tə-me) arteriectomy.

ar•te•ria (ahr-tēr′e-ə) pl. *arte′riae* [L. *arteria;* from Gr. *artēria*, possibly from *aēr* air + *tērein* to keep, because the arteries were thought to contain air, or from *aeirein* to lift or attach] [TA] artery.

Arteria

a. alveola′ris infe′rior [TA] inferior alveolar artery: *origin*, maxillary artery; *branches*, dental, peridental, mental, and mylohyoid rami; *distribution*, lower jaw, lower lip, and chin. Called also *inferior dental artery* and *mandibular artery*.

arte′riae alveola′res superio′res anterio′res [TA] anterior superior alveolar arteries: *origin*, infraorbital artery; *branches*, dental and peridental rami; *distribution*, incisor and canine regions of upper jaw, maxillary sinus. Called also *anterior dental arteries*.

a. alveola′ris supe′rior poste′rior [TA] posterior superior alveolar artery: *origin*, maxillary artery; *branches*, dental and peridental rami; *distribution*, molar and premolar regions of upper jaw, maxillary sinus. Called also *posterior dental artery*.

a. angula′ris [TA] angular artery: *origin*, facial artery; *branches*, none; *distribution*, lacrimal sac, lower eyelid, nose.

a. appendicula′ris [TA] appendicular artery: *origin*, ileocolic artery; *branches*, none; *distribution*, vermiform appendix. Called also *vermiform artery*.

a. arcua′ta pe′dis [TA] arcuate artery of foot: *origin*, dorsalis pedis artery; *branches*, deep plantar branch and dorsal metatarsal arteries; *distribution*, foot, toes.

arte′riae arcua′tae re′nis [TA] arcuate arteries of kidney: *origin*, interlobar artery; *branches*, interlobular artery and arteriolae rectae; *distribution*, parenchyma of kidney.

a. ascen′dens [TA] ascending artery: an inconstant branch of the inferior mesenteric artery that anastomoses with the middle colic artery.

a. auricula′ris poste′rior [TA] posterior auricular artery: *origin*, external carotid artery; *branches*, auricular and occipital branches, stylomastoid artery; *distribution*, middle ear, mastoid cells, auricle, parotid gland, digastric and other muscles.

a. auricula′ris profun′da [TA] deep auricular artery: *origin*, maxillary artery; *branches*, none; *distribution*, skin of auditory canal, tympanic membrane, temporomandibular joint.

a. axilla′ris [TA] axillary artery: *origin*, continuation of subclavian artery; *branches*, subscapular rami, and superior thoracic, thoracoacromial, lateral thoracic, subscapular, and anterior and posterior circumflex humeral arteries; *distribution*, upper limb, axilla, chest, shoulder.

arte′riae azy′goi vagi′nae [TA] rami vaginales arteriae uterinae.

a. basila′ris [TA] basilar artery: *origin*, from junction of right and left vertebral arteries; *branches*, pontine, anterior inferior cerebellar, mesencephalic, superior cerebellar, and posterior cerebral arteries; *distribution*, brainstem, internal ear, cerebellum, posterior cerebrum.

a. brachia′lis [TA] brachial artery: *origin*, continuation of axillary artery; *branches*, profunda brachii, nutrient of humerus, superior ulnar collateral, inferior ulnar collateral, radial, and ulnar arteries; *distribution*, shoulder, arm, forearm, hand.

a. brachia′lis superficia′lis [TA] superficial brachial artery: an occasional vessel that arises from high bifurcation of the brachial artery and assumes a more superficial course than usual.

a. bucca′lis [TA] buccal artery: *origin*, maxillary artery; *branches*, none; *distribution*, buccinator muscle, mucous membrane of mouth. Called also *buccinator artery*.

a. bul′bi pe′nis [TA] artery of bulb of penis: *origin*, internal pudendal artery; *branches*, none; *distribution*, bulbourethral gland, bulb of penis. Called also *bulbourethral artery*.

a. bul′bi vesti′buli [TA] artery of bulb of vestibule: *origin*, internal pudendal artery; *branches*, none; *distribution*, bulb of vestibule of vagina, greater vestibular glands.

a. caeca′lis ante′rior [TA] anterior cecal artery: *origin*, ileocolic; *branches*, none; *distribution*, cecum. Spelled also *a. cecalis anterior*.

a. caeca′lis poste′rior [TA] posterior cecal artery: *origin*, ileocolic; *branches*, none; *distribution*, cecum. Spelled also *a. cecalis posterior*.

a. callo′sa media′na [TA] median callosal artery: *origin*, anterior communicating artery; *distribution*, runs above the lamina terminalis to supply anterior hypothalamic and subcallosal areas and corpus callosum.

a. callosomargina′lis [TA] callosomarginal artery: *origin*, postcommunicating part of anterior cerebral artery; *branches*, anteromedial frontal, intermediomedial frontal, posteromedial frontal, cingular, and paracentral branches; *distribution*, medial and superolateral surfaces of cerebral hemisphere.

a. cana′lis pterygoi′dei artery of pterygoid canal: 1. [TA] *origin*, maxillary artery; *branches*, pterygoid; *distribution*, roof of pharynx, auditory tube. Called also *vidian artery*. 2. *origin*, internal carotid artery; *branches*, none; *distribution*, pterygoid canal, anastomosing with the artery of the pterygoid canal that branches from the maxillary artery.

arte′riae caroticotympa′nicae [TA] caroticotympanic arteries: branches of the petrous part of the internal carotid artery that supply the tympanic cavity.

a. caro′tis commu′nis [TA] common carotid artery: *origin*, brachiocephalic trunk (right), aortic arch (left); *branches*, external and internal carotid arteries; *distribution*, see *a. carotis externa* and *a. carotis interna*. See illustration.

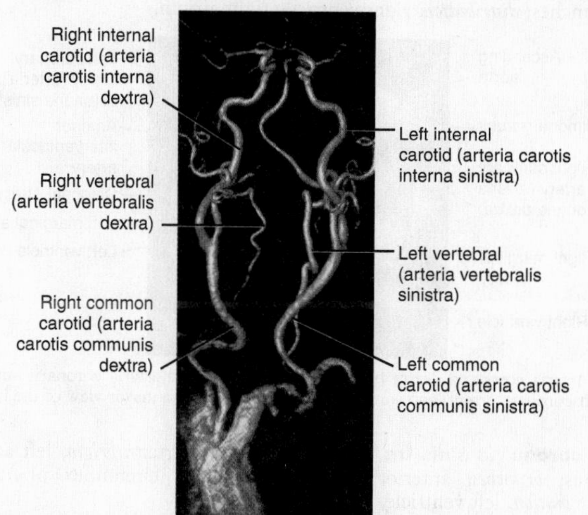

■ Enhanced CT scan of carotid vessels.

a. caro′tis exter′na [TA] external carotid artery: *origin*, common carotid; *branches*, superior thyroid, ascending pharyngeal, lingual, facial, sternocleidomastoid, occipital, posterior auricular, superficial temporal, maxillary; *distribution*, neck, face, skull.

a. caro′tis inter′na [TA] internal carotid artery: divided into four parts: cervical *(pars cervicalis)*, petrous *(pars petrosa)*, cavernous *(pars cavernosa)*, and cerebral *(pars cerebralis)*; *origin*, common carotid; *branches*, numerous, including (petrous part) caroticotympanic arteries; (cavernous part) tentorial basal, tentorial marginal, meningeal, and cavernous branches, and inferior hypophysial artery; (cerebral part) ophthalmic, superior hypophysial, posterior communicating, anterior choroidal, anterior cerebral, and middle cerebral arteries; *distribution*, middle ear, brain, pituitary gland, orbit, choroid plexus. See illustration.

a. cau′dae pancre′atis [TA] artery to tail of pancreas: *origin*, splenic artery; *branches and distribution*, supplies branches to tail of pancreas, and accessory spleen (if present).

a. ceca′lis ante′rior a. caecalis anterior.

a. ceca′lis poste′rior a. caecalis posterior.

arte′riae centra′les anterolatera′les [TA] anterolateral central arteries: *origin*, sphenoid part (M1 segment) of middle cerebral artery; *branches;* two sets of branches, proximal lateral and distal lateral; *distribution*, anterior lenticular and caudate nuclei and internal capsule of brain. Called also *anterolateral thalamostriate arteries*, *lenticulostriate arteries*, and *lateral striate arteries*.

arte′riae centra′les anteromedia′les [TA] anteromedial central arteries: *origin*, anterior communicating artery and precommunicating part (A1 segment) of anterior cerebral artery; *branches*, none; *distribution*, anterior and medial corpus striatum. Called also *anteromedial thalamostriate arteries*.

arte′riae centra′les posterolatera′les [TA] posterolateral central arteries: *origin*, postcommunicating part of posterior cerebral artery; *branches*, none; *distribution*, cerebral peduncle, posterior thalamus, colliculi, medial geniculate and pineal bodies. The group includes the thalamogeniculate artery and the peduncular and posterior medial and lateral choroidal branches.

arte′riae centra′les posteromedia′les arte′riae ce′rebri posterio′ris [TA] posteromedial central arteries of posterior cerebral artery: *origin*, precommunicating part (P1 segment) of posterior cerebral artery; *branches*, none; *distribution*, anterior thalamus, lateral wall of third ventricle, and globus pallidus of lentiform nucleus. Called also *paramedian arteries*.

arte′riae centra′les posteromedia′les arte′riae communican′tis posterio′ris [TA] posteromedial central arteries of posterior communicating artery: *origin*, posterior communicating artery; *branches*, anterior and posterior branches; *distribution*, medial thalamic surface and walls of third ventricle.

a. centra′lis re′tinae [TA] central retinal artery: *origin*, ophthalmic artery; *branches*, superior and inferior nasal, and superior and inferior temporal; *distribution*, courses within dural sheath and then pierces and runs within optic nerve (extraocular part) to retina (intraocular part). Called also *central artery of retina* and *artery of Zinn*.

a. ce′rebri ante′rior [TA] anterior cerebral artery: divided into two parts, the *precommunicating part (pars precommunicalis)*, and the *postcommunicating part (pars postcommunicalis); origin*, internal carotid artery; *branches*, (precommunicating part) anteromedial central arteries; (postcommunicating part) distal medial striate, medial frontobasal, polar frontal, callosomarginal (and its branches), and pericallosal (and its branches) arteries; *distribution*, orbital, frontal, and parietal cortex, corpus callosum, diencephalon, corpus striatum, internal capsule, and choroid plexus of lateral ventricle. The artery is often described as comprising a number of segments; see *segments of anterior cerebral artery*, under *segment*.

a. ce′rebri me′dia [TA] middle cerebral artery: the larger terminal branch of the internal carotid artery. It begins as single vessel *(sphenoid part* or *pars sphenoidalis)* and branches at the limen insulae, turning posterosuperiorly, usually into inferior terminal branches (rami terminales inferiores) that distribute below the sylvian fissure, and superior terminal branches (rami terminales superiores) that distribute above the sylvian fissure. The superior and inferior branches run first in the sylvian fissure *(insular part* or *pars insularis)*, through the inner aspects of the opercula *(opercular part)*, and finally end along the lateral surface of the cerebral hemisphere. *Branches*, anterolateral central, polar temporal, anterior temporal, and insular arteries, anterior temporal, middle temporal, posterior temporal, and temporooccipital branches, branch to angular gyrus, lateral frontobasal, prefrontal, anterior parietal, and posterior parietal arteries, and arteries of precentral, central, and postcentral sulci; *distribution*, orbital, frontal, parietal, and temporal cortex, corpus striatum, internal capsule. Called also *sylvian artery*. See also specific parts and see *segments of middle cerebral artery*, under *segment*.

a. ce′rebri poste′rior [TA] posterior cerebral artery: divided into four segments: the *precommunicating part (pars precommunicalis)*, the *postcommunicating part (pars postcommunicalis)*, the *lateral occipital artery*, and the *medial occipital artery; origin*, terminal bifurcation of basilar artery; *branches*, (precommunicating part) posteromedial central, short circumferential, thalamoperforating, and collicular arteries; (postcommunicating part) posterolateral central and thalamogeniculate arteries, and medial and lateral posterior choroidal, and peduncular branches; (lateral occipital artery) anterior, intermediate, and posterior temporal branches; (medial occipital artery) parietal, parietooccipital, calcarine, and occipitotemporal branches, and dorsal branch to corpus callosum; *distribution*, occipital and temporal cortex, diencephalon, midbrain, choroid plexus of lateral and third ventricles, and visual area of cerebral cortex and other structures associated with the visual pathway. See also *segments of posterior cerebral artery* under *segment*.

a. cervica′lis ascen′dens [TA] ascending cervical artery: *origin*, inferior thyroid artery or directly from thyrocervical trunk; *branches*, spinal branches; *distribution*, muscles of neck, vertebrae, vertebral canal.

a. cervica′lis profun′da [TA] deep cervical artery: *origin*, costocervical trunk; *branches*, none; *distribution*, deep neck muscles.

a. choroi′dea ante′rior [TA] anterior choroidal artery: *origin*, cervical part of internal carotid or sometimes middle cerebral artery; *branches*, many small branches; *distribution*, interior of brain, including choroid plexus of lateral ventricle and adjacent parts.

arte′riae cilia′res anterio′res [TA] anterior ciliary arteries: *origin*, muscular arteries; *branches*, episcleral and anterior conjunctival arteries; *distribution*, iris, conjunctiva.

arte′riae cilia′res posterio′res bre′ves [TA] short posterior ciliary arteries: *origin*, ophthalmic artery; *branches*, none; *distribution*, choroid coat of eye. Called also *short ciliary arteries*.

arte′riae cilia′res posterio′res lon′gae [TA] long posterior ciliary arteries: *origin*, ophthalmic artery; *branches*, none; *distribution*, iris, ciliary processes. Called also *long ciliary arteries*.
arte′riae circumferentia′les bre′ves [TA] short circumferential arteries: *origin*, basilar artery and precommunicating part of posterior cerebral artery; *branches*, none; *distribution*, part of the ventrolateral surface of the pons.
a. circumflex′a fe′moris latera′lis [TA] lateral circumflex femoral artery: *origin*, deep femoral artery; *branches*, ascending, descending, and transverse branches; *distribution*, hip joint, thigh muscles.
a. circumflex′a fe′moris media′lis [TA] medial circumflex femoral artery: *origin*, deep femoral artery; *branches*, deep, superficial, ascending, transverse, and acetabular branches; *distribution*, hip joint, thigh muscles.
a. circumflex′a hu′meri ante′rior [TA] anterior circumflex humeral artery: *origin*, axillary artery; *branches*, none; *distribution*, shoulder joint and head of humerus, long tendon of biceps, tendon of pectoralis major muscle.
a. circumflex′a hu′meri poste′rior [TA] posterior circumflex humeral artery: *origin*, axillary artery; *branches;* none; *distribution*, deltoideus, shoulder joint, teres minor and triceps muscles.
a. circumflex′a i′lium profun′da [TA] deep circumflex iliac artery: *origin*, external iliac artery; *branches*, ascending branches; *distribution*, iliac region, abdominal wall, groin.
a. circumflex′a i′lium superficia′lis [TA] superficial circumflex iliac artery: *origin*, femoral artery; *branches*, none; *distribution*, groin, abdominal wall.
a. circumflex′a sca′pulae [TA] circumflex artery of scapula: *origin*, subscapular artery; *branches*, none; *distribution*, inferolateral muscles of the scapula.
a. cochlea′ris commu′nis [TA] common cochlear artery: *origin*, labyrinthine artery; *branches*, vestibulocochlear, proper cochlear, and spiral modiolar arteries; *distribution*, cochlea and vestibule.
a. cochlea′ris pro′pria [TA] proper cochlear artery: *origin*, common cochlear artery; *branches*, none; *distribution*, cochlea. Called also *cochlear artery*.
a. co′lica dex′tra [TA] right colic artery: *origin*, superior mesenteric artery; *branches*, none; *distribution*, ascending colon. See illustration at *arteria mesenterica superior*.
a. co′lica me′dia [TA] middle colic artery: *origin*, superior mesenteric artery; *branches*, none; *distribution*, transverse colon. Called also *accessory superior colic artery*.
a. co′lica sinis′tra [TA] left colic artery: *origin*, inferior mesenteric; *branches*, none; *distribution*, descending colon.
a. collatera′lis me′dia [TA] middle collateral artery: *origin*, profunda brachii artery; *branches*, none; *distribution*, triceps muscle, elbow joint.
a. collatera′lis radia′lis [TA] radial collateral artery: *origin*, profunda brachii artery; *branches*, none; *distribution*, brachioradialis and brachialis muscles.
a. collatera′lis ulna′ris infe′rior [TA] inferior ulnar collateral artery: *origin*, brachial artery; *branches*, none; *distribution*, arm muscles at back of elbow.
a. collatera′lis ulna′ris supe′rior [TA] superior ulnar collateral artery: *origin*, brachial artery; *branches*, none; *distribution*, elbow joint, triceps muscle.
a. collicula′ris [TA] collicular artery: *origin*, precommunicating part of posterior cerebral artery; *branches*, none; *distribution*, corpora quadrigemina (superior and inferior colliculi) of the tectum of the mesencephalon. Called also *a. quadrigeminalis* [TA alternative] and *quadrigeminal artery*.
a. co′mitans ner′vi ischia′dici [TA] accompanying artery of sciatic nerve: *origin*, inferior gluteal artery; *branches*, none; *distribution*, accompanies sciatic nerve. Called also *artery to sciatic nerve* and *sciatic artery*.
a. co′mitans ner′vi media′ni [TA] accompanying artery of median nerve: *origin*, anterior interosseous artery; *branches*, none; *distribution*, median nerve, muscles of front of forearm. Called also *median artery*.
a. commissura′lis media′na [TA] median commissural artery: *origin*, anterior communicating artery; *branches*, none; *distribution*, supraoptic commissures and optic chiasm.
a. commu′nicans ante′rior [TA] anterior communicating artery: *origin*, precommunicating part of anterior cerebral artery; *branches*, anteromedial central arteries; *distribution*, establishes connection between the right and left anterior cerebral arteries.
a. commu′nicans poste′rior [TA] posterior communicating artery: establishes connection between internal carotid and posterior cerebral arteries; *branches*, posteromedial central, thalamotuberal, and mammillary arteries, artery of tuber cinereum, and branches to the optic chiasm, oculomotor nerve, and hypothalamus.
arte′riae conjunctiva′les anterio′res [TA] anterior conjunctival arteries: *origin*, anterior ciliary arteries; *branches*, none; *distribution*, conjunctiva.
arte′riae conjunctiva′les posterio′res [TA] posterior conjunctival arteries: *origin*, medial palpebral arteries; *branches*, none; *distribution*, caruncula lacrimalis, conjunctiva.
a. corona′ria dex′tra [TA] right coronary artery: *origin*, right aortic sinus; *branches*, conus artery and atrial, atrioventricular node, intermediate atrial, posterior interventricular, right marginal, and sinoatrial node branches; *distribution*, right ventricle, right atrium.

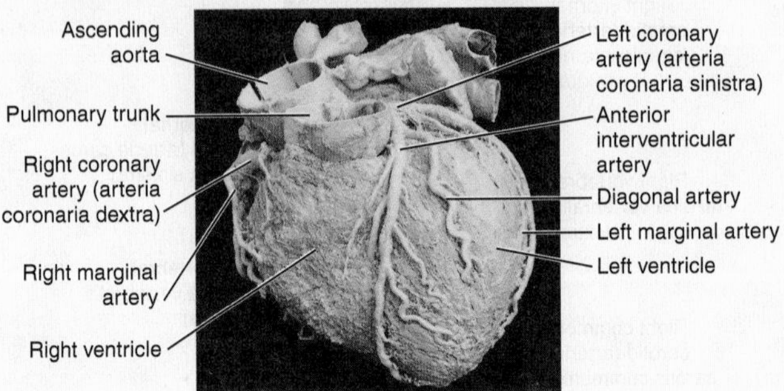

■ Arteria coronaria dextra (right coronary artery) and arteria coronaria sinistra (left coronary artery) and some of their branches in an anterior view of the heart.

a. corona′ria sinis′tra [TA] left coronary artery: *origin*, left aortic sinus; *branches*, anterior interventricular and circumflex branches; *distribution*, left ventricle, left atrium.
arte′riae cortica′les radia′tae [TA] cortical radiate arteries: arteries originating from the arcuate arteries of the kidney and distributed to the renal glomeruli. Called also *interlobular arteries of kidney* and *arteriae interlobulares renis* [TA alternative].
a. cremaste′rica [TA] cremasteric artery: *origin*, inferior epigastric artery; *branches*, none; *distribution*, cremaster muscle, coverings of spermatic cord. Called also *external spermatic artery*.
a. cys′tica [TA] cystic artery: *origin*, right branch of hepatic artery proper; *branches*, none; *distribution*, gallbladder.
a. descen′dens ge′nus [TA] descending genicular artery: *origin*, femoral artery; *branches*, saphenous, articular; *distribution*, knee joint, upper and medial leg.
arte′riae digita′les dorsa′les ma′nus [TA] dorsal digital arteries of hand: *origin*, dorsal metacarpal arteries; *branches*, none; *distribution*, dorsum of fingers.
arte′riae digita′les dorsa′les pe′dis [TA] dorsal digital arteries of foot: *origin*, dorsal metatarsal arteries; *branches*, none; *distribution*, dorsum of toes.
arte′riae digita′les palma′res commu′nes [TA] common palmar digital arteries: *origin*, superficial palmar arch; *branches*, proper palmar digital arteries; *distribution*, fingers. Called also *common volar digital arteries* and *ulnar metacarpal arteries*.
arte′riae digita′les palma′res pro′priae [TA] proper palmar digital arteries: *origin*, common palmar digital arteries; *branches*, none; *distribution*, fingers. Called also *collateral digital arteries* and *proper volar digital arteries*.
arte′riae digita′les planta′res commu′nes [TA] common plantar digital arteries: *origin*, plantar metatarsal arteries; *branches*, proper plantar digital arteries; *distribution*, toes.
arte′riae digita′les planta′res pro′priae [TA] proper plantar digital arteries: *origin*, common plantar digital arteries; *branches*, none; *distribution*, toes.
a. dorsa′lis clito′ridis [TA] dorsal artery of clitoris: *origin*, internal pudendal artery; *branches*, none; *distribution*, clitoris.
a. dorsa′lis na′si [TA] dorsal nasal artery: *origin*, ophthalmic artery; *branches*, branch to nasolacrimal sac and branch anastomosing with terminal part of facial artery; *distribution*, skin of nose. Called also *external nasal artery*.

a. dorsa′lis pe′dis [TA] dorsal artery of foot: *origin*, continuation of anterior tibial artery; *branches*, lateral and medial tarsal, arcuate, and deep plantar arteries; *distribution*, foot, toes.

a. dorsa′lis pe′nis [TA] dorsal artery of penis: *origin*, internal pudendal artery; *branches*, none; *distribution*, glans, corona, and prepuce of penis.

a. dorsa′lis sca′pulae dorsal scapular artery: 1. [TA] *origin*, second or third part of subclavian artery; *branches*, none; *distribution*, rhomboid, latissimus dorsi, and trapezius muscles. 2. TA alternative for the same artery when it occurs as the deep branch of the transverse cervical artery (ramus profundus arteriae transversae colli).

a. duc′tus deferen′tis [TA] artery of ductus deferens: *origin*, umbilical artery; *branches*, ureteral artery; *distribution*, ureter, ductus deferens, seminal vesicles, testes. Called also *deferential artery*.

a. epigas′trica infe′rior [TA] inferior epigastric artery: *origin*, external iliac artery; *branches*, pubic branch, cremasteric artery, artery of round ligament of uterus; *distribution*, abdominal wall.

a. epigas′trica superficia′lis [TA] superficial epigastric artery: *origin*, femoral artery; *branches*, none; *distribution*, abdominal wall, groin.

a. epigas′trica supe′rior [TA] superior epigastric artery: *origin*, internal thoracic artery; *branches*, none; *distribution*, abdominal wall, diaphragm.

arte′riae episclera′les [TA] episcleral arteries: *origin*, anterior ciliary arteries; *branches*, none; *distribution*, iris, ciliary processes.

a. ethmoida′lis ante′rior [TA] anterior ethmoidal artery: *origin*, ophthalmic artery; *branches*, anterior meningeal, anterior septal, and anterior lateral nasal branches; *distribution*, dura mater, nose, frontal sinus, anterior ethmoidal cells.

a. ethmoida′lis poste′rior [TA] posterior ethmoidal artery: *origin*, ophthalmic artery; *branches*, meningeal and septal and lateral nasal branches; *distribution*, posterior ethmoidal cells, dura mater, nose.

a. facia′lis [TA] facial artery: *origin*, external carotid artery; *branches*, ascending palatine, tonsillar, submental, inferior labial, superior labial, septal, lateral nasal, angular, glandular; *distribution*, face, tonsil, palate, submandibular gland. Called also *external maxillary artery*.

a. femora′lis [TA] femoral artery: *origin*, continuation of external iliac; *branches*, superficial epigastric, superficial circumflex iliac, external pudendal, deep femoral, descending genicular; *distribution*, lower abdominal wall, external genitalia, lower extremity. NOTE: Vascular surgeons refer to the portion of the femoral artery proximal to the branching of the deep femoral as the *common femoral a.*, and to its continuation as the *superficial femoral a.* In this classification, the descending genicular artery is a branch of the superficial femoral artery.

a. fibula′ris [TA] peroneal artery: *origin*, posterior tibial artery; *branches*, perforating, communicating, calcaneal, and lateral and medial malleolar branches, and calcaneal rete; *distribution*, outside and back of ankle, deep calf muscles. Called also *a. peronea* [TA alternative].

a. frontobasa′lis latera′lis [TA] lateral frontobasal artery: *origin*, superior terminal branch of middle cerebral artery: *branches*, none; *distribution*, cortex of lateroinferior frontal lobe. Called also *a. orbitofrontalis lateralis* [TA alternative] and *orbitofrontal artery*.

a. frontobasa′lis media′lis [TA] medial frontobasal artery: *origin*, postcommunicating part of anterior cerebral artery; *branches*, none; *distribution*, cortex of medioinferior frontal lobe. Called also *a. orbitofrontalis medialis* [TA alternative] and *medial orbitofrontal artery*.

arte′riae gas′tricae bre′ves [TA] short gastric arteries: *origin*, splenic artery; *branches*, none; *distribution*, upper part of stomach.

a. gas′trica dex′tra [TA] right gastric artery: *origin*, common hepatic artery; *branches*, none; *distribution*, lesser curvature of stomach. Called also *pyloric artery*.

a. gas′trica poste′rior [TA] posterior gastric artery: *origin*, splenic artery; *branches*, none; *distribution*, posterior gastric wall.

a. gas′trica sinis′tra [TA] left gastric artery: *origin*, celiac trunk; *branches*, esophageal branches; *distribution*, esophagus, lesser curvature of stomach. Called also *left coronary artery of stomach*.

a. gastroduodena′lis [TA] gastroduodenal artery: *origin*, common hepatic artery; *branches*, supraduodenal and posterior superior pancreaticoduodenal arteries; *distribution*, stomach, duodenum, pancreas, greater omentum.

a. gastroomenta′lis dex′tra [TA] right gastro-omental artery: *origin*, gastroduodenal artery; *branches*, gastric, omental branches; *distribution*, stomach, greater omentum. Called also *right inferior gastric artery*.

a. gastroomenta′lis sinis′tra [TA] left gastro-omental artery: *origin*, splenic artery; *branches*, gastric, omental branches; *distribution*, stomach, greater omentum. Called also *left inferior gastric artery*.

a. glu′tea infe′rior [TA] inferior gluteal artery: *origin*, internal iliac artery; *branches*, sciatic artery; *distribution*, buttock, back of thigh.

a. glu′tea supe′rior [TA] superior gluteal artery: *origin*, internal iliac artery; *branches*, superficial and deep branches; *distribution*, buttocks.

a. gy′ri angula′ris ramus gyri angularis arteriae cerebri mediae.

arte′riae helici′nae pe′nis [TA] helicine arteries of penis: helicine arteries arising from the vessels of the penis, whose engorgement causes erection of the organ. Called also *arteries of Mueller*.

a. hepa′tica commu′nis [TA] common hepatic artery: *origin*, celiac trunk; *branches*, right gastric and gastroduodenal arteries and hepatic artery proper; *distribution*, stomach, pancreas, duodenum, liver, gallbladder, greater omentum.

a. hepa′tica pro′pria [TA] hepatic artery proper: *origin*, common hepatic artery; *branches*, right and left branches; *distribution*, liver, gallbladder.

a. hyaloi′dea [TA] hyaloid artery: a fetal vessel that continues forward from the central artery of retina through the vitreous body to supply the lens; it normally is not present after birth.

a. hypophysia′lis infe′rior [TA] inferior hypophysial artery: a small branch from the cavernous part of the internal carotid artery that supplies the pituitary gland.

a. hypophysia′lis supe′rior [TA] superior hypophysial artery: a small branch from the cerebral part of the internal carotid artery that supplies the pituitary gland.

arte′riae ilea′les [TA] ileal arteries: *origin*, superior mesenteric artery; *branches*, none; *distribution*, ileum. See illustration at *arteria mesenterica superior*.

a. ileoco′lica [TA] ileocolic artery: *origin*, superior mesenteric artery; *branches*, anterior and posterior cecal and appendicular arteries and colic (ascending) and ileal branches; *distribution*, ileum, cecum, vermiform appendix, ascending colon. Called also *inferior right colic artery*. See illustration at *arteria mesenterica superior*.

a. ili′aca commu′nis [TA] common iliac artery: *origin*, abdominal aorta; *branches*, internal and external iliac arteries; *distribution*, pelvis, abdominal wall, lower limb.

a. ili′aca exter′na [TA] external iliac artery: *origin*, common iliac; *branches*, inferior epigastric, deep circumflex iliac arteries; *distribution*, abdominal wall, external genitalia, lower limb. Called also *anterior iliac artery*.

a. ili′aca inter′na [TA] internal iliac artery: *origin*, continuation of common iliac artery; *branches*, iliolumbar, obturator, superior gluteal, inferior gluteal, umbilical, inferior vesical, uterine, middle rectal, and internal pudendal arteries; *distribution*, wall and viscera of pelvis, buttock, reproductive organs, medial aspect of thigh. Called also *hypogastric artery* and *posterior pelvic artery*.

a. iliolumba′lis [TA] iliolumbar artery: *origin*, posterior trunk of internal iliac artery; *branches*, iliac, spinal, and lumbar branches; *distribution*, pelvic muscles and bones, fifth lumbar segment, sacrum. Called also *small iliac artery*.

a. infe′rior ante′rior cerebel′li [TA] anterior inferior cerebellar artery: *origin*, basilar artery; *branches*, labyrinthine artery (usually); *distribution*, anterolateral inferior part of cerebellum, lower and lateral parts of pons, and sometimes upper part of medulla oblongata.

a. infe′rior latera′lis ge′nus [TA] lateral inferior artery of knee: *origin*, popliteal artery; *branches*, none; *distribution*, knee joint. Called also *lateral inferior genicular artery*.

a. infe′rior media′lis ge′nus [TA] medial inferior artery of knee: *origin*, popliteal artery; *branches*, none; *distribution*, knee joint. Called also *medial inferior genicular artery*.

a. infe′rior poste′rior cerebel′li [TA] posterior inferior cerebellar artery: *origin*, vertebral artery; *branches*, medial, lateral and cerebellar tonsillar branches, choroidal branch to fourth ventricle, posterior spinal artery; *distribution*, lower and medial cerebellum, medulla.

a. infraorbita′lis [TA] infraorbital artery: *origin*, maxillary artery; *branches*, anterior superior alveolar arteries; *distribution*, maxilla, maxillary sinus, upper teeth, lower eyelid, cheek, nose.

arte′riae insula′res [TA] insular arteries: *origin*, insular part of middle cerebral artery; *branches*, none; *distribution*, cortex of insula.

arte′riae intercosta′les posterio′res [TA] posterior intercostal arteries: for the first two, see *a. intercostalis posterior prima* and *a. intercostalis posterior secunda;* there are nine other pairs (III–XI): *origin*,

thoracic aorta; *branches*, dorsal, collateral, muscular, and lateral cutaneous; *distribution*, thoracic wall.
a. intercosta'lis poste'rior pri'ma [TA] first posterior intercostal artery: *origin*, supreme intercostal artery; *branches*, dorsal and spinal branches; *distribution*, upper thoracic wall.
a. intercosta'lis poste'rior secun'da [TA] second posterior intercostal artery: *origin*, supreme intercostal artery; *branches*, dorsal and spinal branches; *distribution*, upper thoracic wall.
a. intercosta'lis supre'ma [TA] supreme intercostal artery: *origin*, costocervical trunk; *branches*, first and second posterior intercostal arteries; *distribution*, upper thoracic wall. Called also *superior intercostal artery*.
arte'riae interloba'res re'nis [TA] interlobar arteries of kidney: *origin*, lobar branches of segmental arteries; *branches*, arcuate arteries; *distribution*, parenchyma of kidney.
arte'riae interlobula'res he'patis [TA] interlobular arteries of liver: arteries originating from the right or left branch of the hepatic artery proper, forming a plexus outside each hepatic lobule and supplying the walls of the interlobular veins and the accompanying bile ducts.
arte'riae interlobula'res re'nis TA alternative for *arteriae corticales radiatae*.
a. interos'sea ante'rior [TA] anterior interosseous artery: *origin*, posterior or common interosseous artery; *branches*, median artery; *distribution*, deep parts of front of forearm. Called also *volar interosseous artery*.
a. interos'sea commu'nis [TA] common interosseous artery: *origin*, ulnar artery; *branches*, anterior and posterior interosseous arteries; *distribution*, antecubital fossa.
a. interos'sea poste'rior [TA] posterior interosseous artery: *origin*, common interosseous artery; *branches*, recurrent interosseous artery; *distribution*, deep parts of back of forearm. Called also *dorsal interosseous artery*.
a. interos'sea recur'rens [TA] recurrent interosseous artery: *origin*, posterior interosseous or common interosseous artery; *branches*, none; *distribution*, back of elbow joint.
arte'riae intrarena'les [TA] intrarenal arteries: the arteries within the kidney, including the interlobar, arcuate, and cortical radiate (interlobular) arteries, and the arteriolae rectae.
arte'riae jejuna'les [TA] jejunal arteries: *origin*, superior mesenteric; *branches*, none; *distribution*, jejunum. See illustration at *arteria mesenterica superior*.
a. juxtaco'lica TA alternative for *a. marginalis coli*.
a. labia'lis infe'rior [TA] inferior labial artery: *origin*, facial artery; *branches*, none; *distribution*, lower lip.
a. labia'lis supe'rior [TA] superior labial artery: *origin*, facial artery; *branches*, septal and alar; *distribution*, upper lip, nose.
a. labyrin'thi [TA] labyrinthine artery: *origin*, anterior inferior cerebellar or basilar artery; *branches*, anterior vestibular and common cochlear arteries; *distribution*, through the internal acoustic meatus to the internal ear. Called also *internal auditory artery*.
a. lacrima'lis [TA] lacrimal artery: *origin*, ophthalmic artery; *branches*, lateral palpebral arteries and anastomotic branch with middle meningeal artery; *distribution*, lacrimal gland, upper and lower eyelids, conjunctiva.
a. laryn'gea infe'rior [TA] inferior laryngeal artery: *origin*, inferior thyroid artery; *branches*, none; *distribution*, larynx, trachea, esophagus.
a. laryn'gea supe'rior [TA] superior laryngeal artery: *origin*, superior thyroid artery; *branches*, none; *distribution*, larynx.
a. liena'lis TA alternative for *a. splenica*.
a. ligamen'ti te'retis u'teri [TA] artery of round ligament of uterus: *origin*, inferior epigastric artery; *branches*, none; *distribution*, round ligament of uterus.
a. lingua'lis [TA] lingual artery: *origin*, external carotid artery; *branches*, suprahyoid, sublingual, dorsal lingual, deep lingual; *distribution*, tongue, sublingual gland, tonsil, epiglottis.
a. lingula'ris [TA] lingular artery: a branch of the left pulmonary artery to the superior lobe of the left lung, consisting almost entirely of the superior and inferior lingular arteries and supplying the lingular segments. Called also *lingular segmental artery*.
a. lingula'ris infe'rior [TA] inferior lingular artery: a branch of the lingular artery, supplying the inferior lingular segment of the superior lobe of the left lung. Called also *inferior lingular segmental artery*.
a. lingula'ris supe'rior [TA] superior lingular artery: a branch of the lingular artery, supplying the superior lingular segment of the superior lobe of the left lung. Called also *superior lingular segmental artery*.
arte'riae loba'res inferio'res pulmo'nis dex'tri [TA] inferior lobar arteries of right lung: the branches of the right pulmonary artery that supply the inferior lobe of the right lung, consisting of the superior, anterior basal, lateral basal, medial basal, and posterior basal segmental arteries.
arte'riae loba'res inferio'res pulmo'nis sinis'tri [TA] inferior lobar arteries of left lung: the branches of the left pulmonary artery that supply the inferior lobe of the left lung, consisting of the superior, anterior basal, lateral basal, medial basal, and posterior basal segmental arteries.
a. loba'ris me'dia pulmo'nis dex'tri [TA] middle lobar artery of right lung: the branch of the right pulmonary artery that carries blood to the middle lobe of the right lung, giving rise to the lateral and medial segmental arteries.
arte'riae loba'res superio'res pulmo'nis dex'tri [TA] superior lobar arteries of right lung: the branches of the right pulmonary artery that carry blood to the superior lobe of the right lung, consisting of the apical, anterior, and posterior segmental arteries.
arte'riae loba'res superio'res pulmo'nis sinis'tri [TA] superior lobar arteries of left lung: the branches of the left pulmonary artery that carry blood to the superior lobe of the left lung, consisting of the apical, anterior, and posterior segmental arteries.
a. lo'bi cauda'ti [TA] artery of caudate lobe: either of two branches, one from the right and one from the left branch of the hepatic artery proper, supplying twigs to the caudate lobe of the liver.
arte'riae lumba'les [TA] lumbar arteries: *origin*, abdominal aorta; *branches*, dorsal and spinal branches; *distribution*, posterior abdominal wall, renal capsule.
arte'riae lumba'les i'mae [TA] lowest lumbar arteries: *origin*, median sacral artery; *branches*, none; *distribution*, sacrum, gluteus maximus muscle. Called also *fifth lumbar arteries*.
a. luso'ria an abnormally situated retroesophageal vessel, usually the subclavian artery from the aortic arch, which may cause symptoms by compression of the esophagus, the trachea, or a nerve.
a. malleola'ris ante'rior latera'lis [TA] lateral anterior malleolar artery: *origin*, anterior tibial artery; *branches*, none; *distribution*, ankle joint.
a. malleola'ris ante'rior media'lis [TA] medial anterior malleolar artery: *origin*, anterior tibial artery; *branches*, none; *distribution*, ankle joint.
arte'riae mammilla'res [TA] mammillary arteries: *origin*, posterior communicating artery; *branches*, none; *distribution*, mammillary bodies.
a. margina'lis co'li [TA] marginal artery of colon; a continuous vessel running along the inner perimeter of the large intestine from the ileocolic junction to the rectum, formed by branches from the superior and inferior mesenteric arteries and giving rise to straight arteries that supply the intestinal wall. Called also *a. juxtacolica* and *arcus marginalis coli* [TA alternatives], *juxtacolic artery*, *marginal artery of Drummond*, and *marginal arcade*.
a. massete'rica [TA] masseteric artery: *origin*, maxillary artery; *branches*, none; *distribution*, masseter muscle.
a. maxilla'ris [TA] maxillary artery: *origin*, external carotid artery; *branches*, deep auricular, anterior tympanic, inferior alveolar, middle meningeal, pterygomeningeal, masseteric, anterior and posterior deep temporal, buccal, posterior superior alveolar, infraorbital, descending palatine, and sphenopalatine arteries, and artery of pterygoid canal; *distribution*, both jaws, teeth, muscles of mastication, ear, meninges, nose, paranasal sinuses, palate. Called also *internal maxillary artery*.
a. me'dia ge'nus [TA] middle artery of knee: *origin*, popliteal artery; *branches*, none; *distribution*, knee joint, cruciate ligaments, patellar synovial and alar folds. Called also *middle genicular artery*.
a. medulla'ris segmenta'lis [TA] segmental medullary artery: one of the spinal branches of the vertebral artery, of the dorsal branch of a posterior intercostal artery, or of a lumbar artery; it supplies the root of a particular spinal nerve and, unlike a radicular artery, extends to anastomose with the anterior and posterior spinal arteries and the arterial vasocorona.
arte'riae mem'bri inferio'ris [TA] arteries of lower limb: the arteries supplying the thigh, leg, and foot, including the external iliac, femoral, deep femoral, popliteal, anterior and posterior tibial, dorsalis pedis, medial and lateral plantar, and peroneal arteries.

arte′riae mem′bri superio′ris [TA] arteries of upper limb: the arteries supplying the arm, forearm, and hand, including the axillary, brachial, radial, and ulnar arteries.

a. menin′gea me′dia [TA] middle meningeal artery: *origin*, maxillary artery; *branches*, frontal, parietal, and lacrimal anastomotic, accessory meningeal, and petrosal rami, and superior tympanic artery; *distribution*, cranial bones, dura mater.

a. menin′gea poste′rior [TA] posterior meningeal artery: *origin*, ascending pharyngeal artery; *branches*, none; *distribution*, bones and dura mater of posterior cranial fossa.

arte′riae mesencepha′licae [TA] mesencephalic arteries: *origin*, basilar artery; *branches*, none; *distribution*, cerebral peduncle.

a. mesente′rica infe′rior [TA] inferior mesenteric artery: *origin*, abdominal aorta; *branches*, left colic, sigmoid, and superior rectal arteries; *distribution*, descending colon, rectum.

a. mesente′rica supe′rior [TA] superior mesenteric artery: *origin*, abdominal aorta; *branches*, inferior pancreaticoduodenal, jejunal, ileal, ileocolic, right colic, and middle colic arteries; *distribution*, small intestine, proximal half of colon. See illustration.

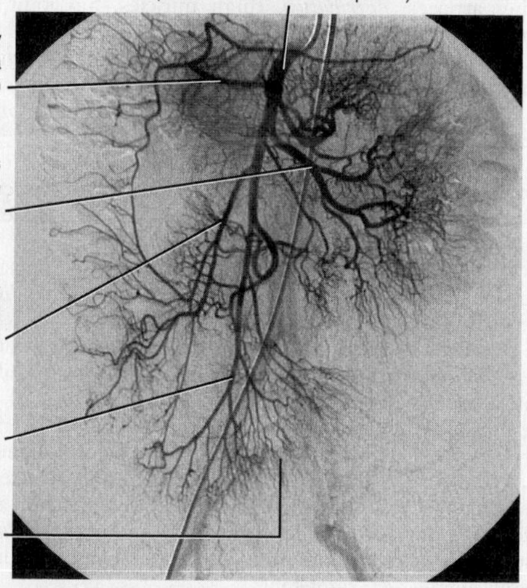

■ Digital subtraction angiography of the superior mesenteric artery (arteria mesenterica superior) and its branches.

arte′riae metacarpa′les dorsa′les [TA] dorsal metacarpal arteries: *origin*, dorsal carpal rete and radial artery; *branches*, dorsal digital arteries; *distribution*, dorsum of fingers.

arte′riae metacarpa′les palma′res [TA] palmar metacarpal arteries: *origin*, deep palmar arch; *branches*, none; *distribution*, deep parts of metacarpus. Called also *volar metacarpal* or *palmar intermetacarpal arteries*.

arte′riae metatarsa′les dorsa′les [TA] dorsal metatarsal arteries: *origin*, arcuate artery of foot; *branches*, dorsal digital arteries; *distribution*, dorsum of foot, including toes.

arte′riae metatarsa′les planta′res [TA] plantar metatarsal arteries: *origin*, plantar arch; *branches*, perforating branches, common and proper plantar digital arteries; *distribution*, toes. Called also *common digital arteries of foot*.

arte′riae muscula′res [TA] muscular arteries: branches of the ophthalmic artery consisting of a superior group and an inferior group; the inferior group gives origin to the anterior ciliary arteries.

a. musculophre′nica [TA] musculophrenic artery: *origin*, internal thoracic artery; *branches*, none; *distribution*, diaphragm, abdominal and thoracic walls.

arte′riae nasa′les posterio′res latera′les [TA] posterior lateral nasal arteries: *origin*, sphenopalatine artery; *branches*, none; *distribution*, frontal, maxillary, ethmoidal, and sphenoidal sinuses.

a. nutri′cia [TA] nutrient artery: any artery that supplies the marrow of a long bone; called also *a. nutriens* [TA alternative] and *medullary artery*. See also *nutrient vessels*, under *vessel*.

arte′riae nutri′ciae fe′moris [TA] nutrient arteries of femur: *origin*, third perforating artery; *branches*, none; *distribution*, femur. Called also *arteriae nutrientes femoris* [TA alternative].

a. nutri′cia fi′bulae [TA] nutrient artery of fibula: *origin*, peroneal artery; *branches*, none; *distribution*, fibula. Called also *a. nutriens fibulae* [TA alternative].

arte′riae nutri′ciae hu′meri [TA] nutrient arteries of humerus: *origin*, brachial and profunda brachii arteries; *branches*, none; *distribution*, humerus. Called also *arteriae nutrientes humeri* [TA alternative].

a. nutri′cia ti′biae [TA] nutrient tibial artery: *origin*, posterior tibial artery; *branches*, none; *distribution*, tibia. Called also *nutrient artery of tibia* and *a. nutriens tibiae* [TA alternative].

a. nu′triens TA alternative for *a. nutricia*.

arte′riae nutrien′tes fe′moris TA alternative for *arteriae nutriciae femoris*.

a. nu′triens fi′bulae TA alternative for *a. nutricia fibulae*.

arte′riae nutrien′tes hu′meri TA alternative for *arteriae nutriciae humeri*.

a. nu′triens ti′biae TA alternative for *a. nutricia tibiae*.

a. obturato′ria [TA] obturator artery: *origin*, internal iliac artery; *branches*, pubic, acetabular, anterior, and posterior branches; *distribution*, pelvic muscles, hip joint.

a. obturato′ria accesso′ria [TA] accessory obturator artery: a name given to the obturator artery when it arises from the inferior epigastric instead of the internal iliac artery.

a. occipita′lis [TA] occipital artery: *origin*, external carotid artery; *branches*, auricular, meningeal, mastoid, descending, occipital, and sternocleidomastoid branches; *distribution*, muscles of neck and scalp, meninges, mastoid cells.

a. occipita′lis latera′lis [TA] lateral occipital artery: *origin*, third segment of posterior cerebral artery; *branches*, anterior temporal, intermediate temporal, and posterior temporal branches; *distribution*, cortex of anterior, middle, and posterior parts of temporal lobe.

a. occipita′lis media′lis [TA] medial occipital artery: *origin*, fourth segment of posterior cerebral artery; *branches*, parietal, parieto-occipital, calcarine, and occipitotemporal branches, and branch to dorsal corpus callosum; *distribution*, dorsum of corpus callosum, precuneus, cuneus, lingual gyrus, and posterior part of lateral surface of occipital lobe.

a. ophthal′mica [TA] ophthalmic artery: *origin*, cerebral part of internal carotid artery; *branches*, lacrimal and supraorbital arteries, central artery of retina, ciliary, muscular, posterior and anterior ethmoidal, palpebral, supratrochlear, and dorsal nasal arteries, and recurrent meningeal branch; *distribution*, eye, orbit, adjacent facial structures.

a. orbitofronta′lis latera′lis TA alternative for *a. frontobasalis lateralis*.

a. orbitofronta′lis media′lis TA alternative for *a. frontobasalis medialis*.

a. ova′rica [TA] ovarian artery: *origin*, abdominal aorta; *branches*, ureteral, tubal; *distribution*, ureter, ovary, uterine tube. Called also *tubo-ovarian artery* or *aortic uterine artery*.

a. palati′na ascen′dens [TA] ascending palatine artery: *origin*, facial artery; *branches*, none; *distribution*, soft palate, wall of pharynx, tonsil, auditory tube.

a. palati′na descen′dens [TA] descending palatine artery: *origin*, maxillary artery; *branches*, greater and lesser palatine arteries; *distribution*, soft palate, hard palate, tonsil.

a. palati′na ma′jor [TA] greater palatine artery: *origin*, descending palatine artery; *branches*, none; *distribution*, hard palate.

arte′riae palati′nae mino′res [TA] lesser palatine arteries: *origin*, descending palatine artery; *branches*, none; *distribution*, soft palate, tonsil.

arte′riae palpebra′les latera′les [TA] lateral palpebral arteries: *origin*, lacrimal artery; *branches*, none; *distribution*, eyelids, conjunctiva.

arte′riae palpebra′les media′les [TA] two arteries, superior and inferior medial palpebral arteries: *origin*, ophthalmic artery; *branches*, posterior conjunctival arteries and superior and inferior palpebral arches; *distribution*, eyelids.

a. pancrea′tica dorsa′lis [TA] dorsal pancreatic artery: *origin*, splenic artery; *branches*, inferior pancreatic artery; *distribution*, neck and body of pancreas.

a. pancrea′tica infe′rior [TA] inferior pancreatic artery: *origin*, dorsal pancreatic artery; *branches*, none; *distribution*, body and tail of pancreas.

Arteria *Continued*

a. pancrea′tica mag′na [TA] great pancreatic artery: *origin,* splenic artery; *branches and distribution,* right and left branches anastomose with other pancreatic arteries.

a. pancreaticoduodena′lis infe′rior [TA] inferior pancreaticoduodenal artery: *origin,* superior mesenteric artery; *branches,* anterior, posterior; *distribution,* pancreas, duodenum.

a. pancreaticoduodena′lis supe′rior ante′rior [TA] anterior superior pancreaticoduodenal artery: *origin,* gastroduodenal artery; *branches,* pancreatic and duodenal; *distribution,* pancreas and duodenum.

a. pancreaticoduodena′lis supe′rior poste′rior [TA] posterior superior pancreaticoduodenal artery: *origin,* gastroduodenal artery; *branches,* pancreatic and duodenal; *distribution,* pancreas, duodenum.

a. parieta′lis ante′rior [TA] anterior parietal artery: *origin,* superior terminal branch of middle cerebral artery; *branches,* none; *distribution,* anterior parietal lobe.

a. parieta′lis poste′rior [TA] posterior parietal artery: *origin,* superior terminal branch of middle cerebral artery; *branches,* none; *distribution,* posterior parietal lobe.

arte′riae perforan′tes [TA] perforating arteries: *origin,* branches (usually three) of the deep femoral artery that perforate the insertion of the adductor magnus to reach the back of the thigh; *branches,* nutrient arteries; *distribution,* adductor, hamstring, and gluteal muscles, and femur.

arte′riae perforan′tes anterio′res [TA] anterior perforating arteries: *origin,* precommunicating part of anterior cerebral artery; *branches,* none; *distribution,* enter anterior perforated substance.

arte′riae perforan′tes radia′tae [TA] perforating radiate arteries: small arteries that are continuations of the cortical radiate arteries and perforate the renal capsule.

a. pericallo′sa [TA] pericallosal artery: *origin,* postcommunicating part of anterior cerebral artery, distal to the origin of the callosomarginal artery; *branches,* precuneal and parietooccipital branches; *distribution,* runs along corpus callosum, supplying cerebral cortex.

a. pericardiacophre′nica [TA] pericardiacophrenic artery: *origin,* internal thoracic artery; *branches,* none; *distribution,* pericardium, diaphragm, pleura.

a. perinea′lis [TA] perineal artery: *origin,* internal pudendal artery; *branches,* none; *distribution,* perineum, skin of external genitalia.

a. perone′a TA alternative for *a. fibularis.*

a. pharyn′gea ascen′dens [TA] ascending pharyngeal artery: *origin,* external carotid artery; *branches,* posterior meningeal, pharyngeal, and inferior tympanic; *distribution,* pharynx, soft palate, ear, meninges.

a. phre′nica infe′rior [TA] inferior phrenic artery: *origin,* abdominal aorta; *branches,* superior suprarenal arteries; *distribution,* diaphragm, suprarenal gland. Called also *great phrenic artery.*

arte′riae phre′nicae superio′res [TA] superior phrenic arteries: *origin,* thoracic aorta; *branches,* none; *distribution,* upper surface of vertebral portion of diaphragm.

a. planta′ris latera′lis [TA] lateral plantar artery: *origin,* posterior tibial artery; *branches,* plantar arch and plantar metatarsal arteries; *distribution,* sole of foot and toes. Called also *external plantar artery.*

a. planta′ris media′lis [TA] medial plantar artery: *origin,* posterior tibial artery; *branches,* deep and superficial branches; *distribution,* sole of the foot and toes.

a. planta′ris profun′da [TA] deep plantar artery: *origin,* dorsalis pedis artery; *branches,* none; *distribution,* sole of foot to help form plantar arch.

a. pola′ris fronta′lis [TA] polar frontal artery: *origin,* postcommunicating part of anterior cerebral artery; *branches,* none; *distribution,* frontal pole of cerebral hemisphere. Called also *frontopolar artery.*

a. pola′ris tempora′lis [TA] polar temporal artery: *origin,* sphenoid part of middle cerebral artery; *branches,* none; *distribution,* temporal pole of cerebral hemisphere.

arte′riae pon′tis [TA] pontine arteries: *origin,* basilar artery; *branches,* none; *distribution,* pons and adjacent areas of brain. There are shorter (rami mediales pontis) and longer (rami laterales pontis) pontine arteries.

a. popli′tea [TA] popliteal artery: *origin,* continuation of femoral artery; *branches,* lateral and medial superior genicular, middle genicular, sural, lateral and medial inferior genicular, anterior and posterior tibial arteries, and the genicular articular and the patellar retes; *distribution,* knee, calf.

a. prefronta′lis [TA] prefrontal artery: *origin,* superior terminal branch of middle cerebral artery; *branches,* none; *distribution,* prefrontal area of cerebrum.

arte′riae preop′ticae [TA] preoptic arteries: *origin,* precommunicating part of anterior cerebral artery; *branches,* none; *distribution,* preoptic region.

a. prepancrea′tica [TA] prepancreatic artery: an arterial arch between the neck and uncinate process of the pancreas, formed by the right branch of the dorsal ramus of the splenic artery and a branch from the anterior superior pancreaticoduodenal artery.

a. prin′ceps pol′licis [TA] princeps pollicis artery: *origin,* radial artery; *branches,* radialis indicis artery of index finger; *distribution,* each side and palmar aspect of thumb.

a. profun′da bra′chii [TA] profunda brachii artery: *origin,* brachial artery; *branches,* deltoid branch, nutrient of humerus and middle and radial collateral arteries; *distribution,* humerus, muscles and skin of arm. Called also *deep artery of arm.*

a. profun′da clito′ridis [TA] deep artery of clitoris: *origin,* internal pudendal artery; *branches,* none; *distribution,* clitoris.

a. profun′da fe′moris [TA] deep femoral artery: *origin,* femoral artery; *branches,* medial and lateral circumflex arteries of thigh, perforating arteries; *distribution,* thigh muscles, hip joint, gluteal muscles, femur.

a. profun′da lin′guae [TA] deep lingual artery: *origin,* lingual artery; *branches,* none; *distribution,* tongue. Called also *ranine artery.*

a. profun′da pe′nis [TA] deep artery of penis: *origin,* internal pudendal artery; *branches,* none; *distribution,* corpus cavernosum penis.

a. puden′da exter′na profun′da [TA] deep external pudendal artery: *origin,* femoral artery; *branches,* anterior scrotal or anterior labial branches, inguinal branches; *distribution,* external genitalia, upper medial thigh.

a. puden′da exter′na superficia′lis [TA] superficial external pudendal artery: *origin,* femoral artery; *branches,* none; *distribution,* external genitalia.

a. puden′da inter′na [TA] internal pudendal artery: *origin,* internal iliac artery; *branches,* posterior scrotal or posterior labial branches and inferior rectal, perineal, urethral arteries, artery of bulb of penis or vestibule, deep artery of penis or clitoris, dorsal artery of penis or clitoris; *distribution,* external genitalia, anal canal, perineum.

a. pulmona′lis dex′tra [TA] right pulmonary artery: *origin,* pulmonary trunk; *branches, of superior lobe:* apical, anterior ascending and descending, posterior ascending and descending, *of medial lobe:* medial and lateral, *of inferior lobe:* anterior basal, lateral basal, medial basal; posterior basal; *distribution,* right lung.

a. pulmona′lis sinis′tra [TA] left pulmonary artery: *origin,* pulmonary trunk; *branches, of superior lobe:* apical, ascending and descending, posterior, lingular (inferior and superior), *of inferior lobe:* superior, anterior basal, lateral basal, medial basal, posterior basal; *distribution,* left lung.

a. quadrigemina′lis TA alternative for *a. collicularis.*

a. radia′lis [TA] radial artery: *origin,* brachial artery; *branches,* palmar carpal, superficial palmar and dorsal carpal rami, recurrent radial artery, princeps pollicis artery, deep palmar arch; *distribution,* forearm, wrist, hand.

a. radia′lis in′dicis [TA] radialis indicis artery: *origin,* princeps pollicis artery; *branches,* none; *distribution,* index finger.

a. radicula′ris ante′rior [TA] anterior radicular artery: one of the spinal branches of the dorsal branch of a posterior intercostal artery; it is the branch supplying the anterior root of a particular spinal nerve.

a. radicula′ris mag′na artery of Adamkiewicz.

a. radicula′ris poste′rior [TA] posterior radicular artery: one of the spinal branches of the dorsal branch of a posterior intercostal artery; it is the branch supplying the posterior root of a particular spinal nerve.

a. recta′lis infe′rior [TA] inferior rectal artery: *origin,* internal pudendal artery; *branches,* none; *distribution,* rectum, anal canal. Called also *inferior hemorrhoidal artery.*

a. recta′lis me′dia [TA] middle rectal artery: *origin,* internal iliac artery; *branches,* vaginal; *distribution,* rectum, prostate, seminal vesicles, vagina. Called also *middle hemorrhoidal artery.*

a. recta′lis supe′rior [TA] superior rectal artery: *origin,* inferior mesenteric artery; *branches,* none; *distribution,* rectum. Called also *superior hemorrhoidal artery.*

a. recur′rens radia′lis [TA] radial recurrent artery: *origin,* radial artery; *branches,* none; *distribution,* brachioradialis, brachialis, elbow region.
a. recur′rens tibia′lis ante′rior [TA] anterior tibial recurrent artery: *origin,* anterior tibial artery; *branches,* none; *distribution,* tibialis anterior, extensor digitorum longus, knee joint, contiguous fascia and skin.
a. recur′rens tibia′lis poste′rior [TA] posterior tibial recurrent artery: *origin,* anterior tibial artery; *branches,* none; *distribution,* knee.
a. recur′rens ulna′ris [TA] ulnar recurrent artery: *origin,* ulnar artery; *branches,* anterior and posterior; *distribution,* elbow joint region.
a. rena′lis [TA] renal artery: *origin,* abdominal aorta; *branches,* ureteral branches, inferior suprarenal artery; *distribution,* kidney, suprarenal gland, ureter.
arte′riae retroduodena′les [TA] retroduodenal arteries: *origin,* first branch of gastroduodenal artery; *branches,* none; *distribution,* bile duct, duodenum, head of pancreas.
arte′riae sacra′les latera′les [TA] lateral sacral arteries: usually two, a superior and an inferior, on each side; *origin,* posterior trunk of internal iliac artery; *branches,* spinal branches; *distribution,* structures about coccyx and sacrum.
a. sacra′lis media′na [TA] median sacral artery: *origin,* continuation of abdominal aorta; *branches,* lowest lumbar artery; *distribution,* sacrum, coccyx, rectum. Called also *caudal, coccygeal,* or *sacrococcygeal artery.*
a. segmenta′lis ante′rior pulmo′nis dex′tri [TA] anterior segmental artery of right lung: one of the branches of the right pulmonary artery to the superior lobe of the right lung, supplying its anterior segment; it gives rise to ascending and descending branches.
a. segmenta′lis ante′rior pulmo′nis sinis′tri [TA] anterior segmental artery of left lung: one of the branches of the left pulmonary artery to the superior lobe of the left lung, supplying its anterior segment; it gives rise to ascending and descending branches.
a. segmenta′lis apica′lis pulmo′nis dex′tri [TA] apical segmental artery of right lung: one of the branches to the superior lobe, supplying its apical segment.
a. segmenta′lis apica′lis pulmo′nis sinis′tri [TA] apical segmental artery of left lung: one of the branches to the superior lobe, supplying its apical segment.
a. segmenta′lis basa′lis ante′rior pulmo′nis dex′tri [TA] anterior basal segmental artery of right lung: one of the branches to the inferior lobe, supplying the anterior basal segment.
a. segmenta′lis basa′lis ante′rior pulmo′nis sinis′tri [TA] anterior basal segmental artery of left lung: one of the branches to the inferior lobe, supplying its anterior basal segment.
a. segmenta′lis basa′lis latera′lis pulmo′nis dex′tri [TA] lateral basal segmental artery of right lung: one of the branches to the inferior lobe, supplying the lateral basal segment.
a. segmenta′lis basa′lis latera′lis pulmo′nis sinis′tri [TA] lateral basal segmental artery of left lung: one of the branches to the inferior lobe, supplying its lateral basal segment.
a. segmenta′lis basa′lis media′lis pulmo′nis dex′tri [TA] medial basal segmental artery of right lung: one of the branches to the inferior lobe, supplying the medial basal segment.
a. segmenta′lis basa′lis media′lis pulmo′nis sinis′tri [TA] medial basal segmental artery of left lung: one of the branches to the inferior lobe, supplying its medial basal segment.
a. segmenta′lis basa′lis poste′rior pulmo′nis dex′tri [TA] posterior basal segmental artery of right lung: one of the branches to the inferior lobe, supplying the posterior basal segment.
a. segmenta′lis basa′lis poste′rior pulmo′nis sinis′tri [TA] posterior basal segmental artery of left lung: one of the branches to the inferior lobe, supplying its posterior basal segment.
a. segmenta′lis latera′lis pulmo′nis dex′tri [TA] lateral segmental artery of right lung: one of the two branches to the middle lobe, supplying its lateral segment.
a. segmenta′lis media′lis pulmo′nis dex′tri [TA] medial segmental artery of right lung: one of the two branches to the middle lobe, supplying its medial segment.
a. segmenta′lis poste′rior pulmo′nis dex′tri [TA] posterior segmental artery of right lung: one of the branches of the right pulmonary artery to the superior lobe of the right lung, supplying its posterior segment; it gives rise to ascending and descending branches.
a. segmenta′lis poste′rior pulmo′nis sinis′tri [TA] posterior segmental artery of left lung: one of the branches of the left pulmonary artery to the superior lobe of the left lung, supplying its posterior segment; it gives rise to ascending and descending branches.
a. segmenta′lis supe′rior pulmo′nis dex′tri [TA] superior segmental artery of right lung: one of the branches of the right pulmonary artery to the inferior lobe, supplying its superior segment.
a. segmenta′lis supe′rior pulmo′nis sinis′tri [TA] superior segmental artery of left lung: one of the branches of the left pulmonary artery to the inferior lobe, supplying its superior segment.
a. segmen′ti anterio′ris hepa′tici [TA] anterior segmental artery of liver: *origin,* right branch of hepatic artery proper; *branches,* none; *distribution,* anterior segment of right liver (see table at *segmentum*).
a. segmen′ti anterio′ris inferio′ris rena′lis [TA] anterior inferior segmental artery of kidney: *origin,* anterior branch of renal artery; *branches,* none; *distribution,* anterior inferior segment of kidney.
a. segmen′ti anterio′ris superio′ris rena′lis [TA] anterior superior segmental artery of kidney: *origin,* anterior branch of renal artery; *branches,* none; *distribution,* anterior superior segment of kidney.
a. segmen′ti inferio′ris rena′lis [TA] inferior segmental artery of kidney: *origin,* anterior branch of renal artery; *branches,* none; *distribution,* inferior segment of kidney.
a. segmen′ti latera′lis hepa′tici [TA] lateral segmental artery of liver: *origin,* left branch of hepatic artery proper; *branches,* none; *distribution,* lateral segment of left liver (see table at *segmentum*).
a. segmen′ti media′lis hepa′tici [TA] medial segmental artery of liver: *origin,* left branch of hepatic artery proper; *branches,* none; *distribution,* medial segment of left liver (see table at *segmentum*).
a. segmen′ti posterio′ris hepa′tici [TA] posterior segmental artery of liver: *origin,* right branch of hepatic artery proper; *branches,* none; *distribution,* posterior segment of right liver (see table at *segmentum*).
a. segmen′ti posterio′ris rena′lis [TA] posterior segmental artery of kidney: *origin,* posterior branch of renal artery; *branches,* none; *distribution,* posterior segment of kidney.
a. segmen′ti superio′ris rena′lis [TA] superior segmental artery of kidney: *origin,* anterior branch of renal artery; *branches,* none; *distribution,* superior segment of kidney.
arte′riae sigmoi′deae [TA] sigmoid arteries: *origin,* inferior mesenteric artery; *branches,* none; *distribution,* sigmoid colon.
a. sphenopalati′na [TA] sphenopalatine artery: *origin,* maxillary artery; *branches,* posterior lateral nasal artery and posterior septal branches; *distribution,* structures adjoining nasal cavity, the nasopharynx. Called also *nasopalatine artery.*
a. spina′lis ante′rior [TA] anterior spinal artery: *origin,* intracranial part of vertebral artery; *branches,* none; *distribution,* the two branches, one from each vertebral artery, unite to form a single vessel, which descends on the anterior midline of the spinal cord, supplying the anterior region of the cord.
a. spina′lis poste′rior [TA] posterior spinal artery: *origin,* posterior inferior cerebellar artery (usually) or vertebral artery; *branches,* none; *distribution,* posterior column nuclei and posterior region of spinal cord.
a. spira′lis modio′li [TA] spiral modiolar artery: *origin,* common cochlear artery; *branches,* none; *distribution,* internal auditory meatus, running a spiral course around the auditory nerve.
a. sple′nica [TA] splenic artery: *origin,* celiac trunk; *branches,* pancreatic and splenic branches, prepancreatic, left gastro-omental, and short gastric arteries; *distribution,* spleen, pancreas, stomach, greater omentum. Called also *a. lienalis* [TA alternative].
a. stria′ta media′lis dista′lis [TA] distal medial striate artery: *origin,* postcommunicating part of anterior cerebral artery; *branches,* none; *distribution,* anterior part of head of caudate nucleus and adjacent regions of putamen and internal capsule.
arte′riae stria′tae media′les proxima′les [TA] proximal medial striate arteries: *origin,* precommunicating part of anterior cerebral artery; *branches,* none; *distribution,* anterior part of head of caudate nucleus and adjacent regions of putamen and internal capsule.
a. stylomastoi′dea [TA] stylomastoid artery: *origin,* posterior auricular artery; *branches,* mastoid and stapedial branches, posterior tympanic artery; *distribution,* tympanic cavity walls, mastoid cells, stapedius muscle.
a. subcla′via [TA] subclavian artery: *origin,* brachiocephalic trunk (right), arch of aorta (left); *branches,* vertebral, internal thoracic arteries,

thyrocervical and costocervical trunks; *distribution*, neck, thoracic wall, spinal cord, brain, meninges, upper limb.

a. subcosta′lis [TA] subcostal artery: *origin*, thoracic aorta; *branches*, dorsal and spinal branches; *distribution*, upper posterior abdominal wall.

a. sublingua′lis [TA] sublingual artery: *origin*, lingual artery; *branches*, none; *distribution*, sublingual gland.

a. submenta′lis [TA] submental artery: *origin*, facial artery; *branches*, none; *distribution*, tissues under chin.

a. subscapula′ris [TA] subscapular artery: *origin*, axillary artery; *branches*, thoracodorsal and circumflex scapular arteries; *distribution*, scapular and shoulder region.

a. sul′ci centra′lis [TA] artery of central sulcus: *origin*, superior terminal branch of middle cerebral artery; *branches*, none; *distribution*, cortex on either side of central sulcus.

a. sul′ci postcentra′lis [TA] artery of postcentral sulcus: *origin*, superior terminal branch of middle cerebral artery; *branches*, none; *distribution*, cortex on either side of postcentral sulcus.

a. sul′ci precentra′lis [TA] artery of precentral sulcus: *origin*, superior terminal branch of middle cerebral artery; *branches*, none; *distribution*, cortex on either side of precentral sulcus.

a. supe′rior cerebel′li [TA] superior cerebellar artery: *origin*, basilar artery; *branches*, lateral and medial branches; *distribution*, upper cerebellum, midbrain, pineal body, choroid plexus of third ventricle.

a. supe′rior latera′lis ge′nus [TA] lateral superior artery of knee: *origin*, popliteal artery; *branches*, none; *distribution*, knee joint, femur, patella, contiguous muscles. Called also *lateral superior genicular artery*.

a. supe′rior media′lis ge′nus [TA] medial superior artery of knee: *origin*, popliteal artery; *branches*, none; *distribution*, knee joint, femur, patella, contiguous muscles. Called also *medial superior genicular artery*.

a. suprachiasma′tica [TA] suprachiasmatic artery: *origin*, anterior communicating artery; *branches*, none; *distribution*, optic chiasm.

a. supraduodena′lis [TA] supraduodenal artery: *origin*, gastroduodenal artery; *branches*, duodenal branch; *distribution*, superior part of duodenum.

a. supraop′tica [TA] supraoptic artery: *origin*, precommunicating part of anterior cerebral artery; *branches*, none; *distribution*, superior surface of optic nerve and optic chiasm.

a. supraorbita′lis [TA] supraorbital artery: *origin*, ophthalmic artery; *branches*, superficial, deep, diploic; *distribution*, forehead, upper muscles of orbit, upper eyelid, frontal sinus.

a. suprarena′lis infe′rior [TA] inferior suprarenal artery: *origin*, renal artery; *branches*, none; *distribution*, suprarenal gland. Called also *inferior capsular artery*.

a. suprarena′lis me′dia [TA] middle suprarenal artery: *origin*, abdominal aorta; *branches*, none; *distribution*, suprarenal gland. Called also *middle capsular artery*, and *aortic suprarenal artery*.

arte′riae suprarena′les superio′res [TA] superior suprarenal arteries: *origin*, inferior phrenic artery; *branches*, none; *distribution*, suprarenal gland.

a. suprascapula′ris [TA] suprascapular artery: *origin*, thyrocervical trunk; *branches*, acromial branch; *distribution*, clavicular, deltoid, and scapular regions. Called also *transverse scapular artery*.

a. supratrochlea′ris [TA] supratrochlear artery: *origin*, ophthalmic artery; *branches*, none; *distribution*, anterior scalp. Called also *frontal artery*.

arte′riae sura′les [TA] sural arteries: *origin*, popliteal artery; *branches*, none; *distribution*, popliteal space, calf.

a. tarsa′lis latera′lis [TA] lateral tarsal artery: *origin*, dorsalis pedis artery; *branches*, none; *distribution*, tarsus.

arte′riae tarsa′les media′les [TA] medial tarsal arteries: *origin*, dorsalis pedis artery; *branches*, none; *distribution*, side of foot.

a. tempora′lis ante′rior [TA] anterior temporal artery: *origin*, sphenoid part of middle cerebral artery; *branches*, none; *distribution*, cortex of anterior temporal lobe. Called also *anterior temporal artery*.

a. tempora′lis me′dia [TA] 1. [TA] middle temporal artery: *origin*, superficial temporal artery; *branches*, none; *distribution* temporal region. 2. ramus temporalis medius arteriae cerebri mediae.

a. tempora′lis profun′da ante′rior [TA] anterior deep temporal artery: *origin*, maxillary artery; *branches*, to zygomatic bone and greater wing of sphenoid bone; *distribution*, temporalis muscle, and anastomoses with middle temporal artery.

a. tempora′lis profun′da poste′rior [TA] posterior deep temporal artery: *origin*, maxillary artery; *branches*, none; *distribution*, temporal muscle, and anastomoses with middle temporal artery.

a. tempora′lis superficia′lis [TA] superficial temporal artery: *origin*, external carotid artery; *branches*, parotid, auricular, and occipital rami, transverse facial, zygomatico-orbital, and middle temporal arteries; *distribution*, parotid and temporal regions.

a. testicula′ris [TA] testicular artery: *origin*, abdominal aorta; *branches*, ureteral, epididymal; *distribution*, ureter, epididymis, testis. Called also *funicular artery*.

a. thalamogenicula′ta [TA] thalamogeniculate artery: *origin*, postcommunicating part of posterior cerebral artery; *branches*, none; *distribution*, caudal thalamus.

a. thalamotubera′lis [TA] thalamotuberal artery: *origin*, posterior communicating artery; *branches*, none; *distribution*, premammillary area. Called also *premammillary artery*.

a. tha′lami per′forans [TA] thalamoperforating artery: *origin*, precommunicating part of posterior cerebral artery; *branches*, none; *distribution*, penetrates posterior perforating substance to supply the thalamus and midbrain.

a. thora′cica inter′na [TA] internal thoracic artery: *origin*, subclavian artery; *branches*, mediastinal, thymic, bronchial, tracheal, sternal, perforating, medial mammary, lateral costal, and anterior intercostal branches, pericardiacophrenic, musculophrenic, and superior epigastric arteries; *distribution*, anterior thoracic wall, mediastinal structures, diaphragm. Called also *internal mammary artery*.

a. thora′cica latera′lis [TA] lateral thoracic artery: *origin*, axillary artery; *branches*, mammary branches; *distribution*, pectoral muscles, mammary gland. Called also *external mammary artery*.

a. thora′cica supe′rior [TA] superior thoracic artery: *origin*, axillary artery; *branches*, none; *distribution*, axillary aspect of chest wall. Called also *highest thoracic artery*.

a. thoracoacromia′lis [TA] thoracoacromial artery: *origin*, axillary artery; *branches*, clavicular, pectoral, deltoid, acromial rami; *distribution*, deltoid, clavicular, and thoracic regions. Called also *acromiothoracic artery*, *thoracicoacromial artery*, and *thoracic axis*.

a. thoracodorsa′lis [TA] thoracodorsal artery: *origin*, subscapular artery; *branches*, none; *distribution*, subscapularis and teres muscles.

a. thyroi′dea i′ma [TA] lowest thyroid artery: *origin*, arch of aorta, brachiocephalic trunk, or right common carotid, internal mammary, subclavian, or inferior thyroid arteries; *branches*, none; *distribution*, thyroid gland. Called also *Neubauer artery*.

a. thyroi′dea infe′rior [TA] inferior thyroid artery: *origin*, thyrocervical trunk; *branches*, pharyngeal, esophageal, and tracheal rami, inferior laryngeal and ascending cervical arteries; *distribution*, thyroid gland and adjacent structures.

a. thyroi′dea supe′rior [TA] superior thyroid artery: *origin*, external carotid artery; *branches*, hyoid, sternocleidomastoid, superior laryngeal, cricothyroid, muscular, and anterior, posterior, and lateral glandular branches; *distribution*, thyroid gland and adjacent structures.

a. tibia′lis ante′rior [TA] anterior tibial artery: *origin*, popliteal artery; *branches*, posterior and anterior tibial recurrent, and lateral and medial anterior malleolar arteries, lateral and medial malleolar retia; *distribution*, leg, ankle, foot.

a. tibia′lis poste′rior [TA] posterior tibial artery: *origin*, popliteal artery; *branches*, fibular circumflex branch, peroneal, medial plantar, and lateral plantar arteries; *distribution*, leg, foot.

a. transver′sa cer′vicis [TA] transverse artery of neck: *origin*, subclavian artery; *branches*, deep and superficial branches; *distribution*, root of neck, muscles of scapula. Called also *transverse cervical artery* and *a. transversa colli* [TA alternative].

a. transver′sa col′li TA alternative for *a. transversa cervicis*.

a. transver′sa facie′i [TA] transverse facial artery: *origin*, superficial temporal artery; *branches*, none; *distribution*, parotid region.

a. tu′beris cine′rei [TA] artery of tuber cinereum: *origin*, posterior communicating artery; *branches*, medial and lateral rami; *distribution*, tuber cinereum.

a. tympa′nica ante′rior [TA] anterior tympanic artery: *origin*, maxillary artery; *branches*, none; *distribution*, tympanic cavity.

a. tympa′nica infe′rior [TA] inferior tympanic artery: *origin*, ascending pharyngeal artery; *branches*, none; *distribution*, tympanic cavity.

a. tympa′nica poste′rior [TA] posterior tympanic artery: *origin*, stylomastoid artery; *branches*, none; *distribution*, tympanic cavity.

a. tympa′nica supe′rior [TA] superior tympanic artery: *origin*, middle meningeal artery; *branches*, none; *distribution*, tympanic cavity.

Arteria *Continued*

a. ulna′ris [TA] ulnar artery: *origin,* brachial artery; *branches,* palmar carpal, dorsal carpal, and deep palmar rami, ulnar recurrent and common interosseous arteries, superficial palmar arch; *distribution,* forearm, wrist, hand.

a. umbilica′lis [TA] umbilical artery: *origin,* internal iliac artery; *branches,* artery of ductus deferens and superior vesical arteries; *distribution,* ductus deferens, seminal vesicles, testes, urinary bladder, ureter. In the fetus, there is also a distal segment of the artery that passes upward along the urinary bladder into the umbilical cord; it is obliterated after birth, becoming the medial umbilical ligament.

a. unca′lis [TA] uncal artery: a branch of the internal carotid, or rarely the middle cerebral, artery; it supplies the uncus.

a. urethra′lis [TA] urethral artery: *origin,* internal pudendal artery; *branches,* none; *distribution,* urethra.

a. uteri′na [TA] uterine artery: *origin,* internal iliac artery; *branches,* ovarian and tubal rami, vaginal artery; *distribution,* uterus, vagina, round ligament of uterus, uterine tube, ovary. Called also *fallopian artery.*

a. vagina′lis [TA] vaginal artery: *origin,* uterine artery; *branches,* none; *distribution,* vagina, fundus of bladder.

a. ver′mis supe′rior [TA] superior vermian branch of superior cerebellar artery: a branch from the medial branch of the superior cerebellar artery that supplies the superior vermis of the cerebellum. Called also *superior vermian artery.*

a. vertebra′lis [TA] vertebral artery: divided into four parts: the *first* or *prevertebral part (pars prevertebralis),* the *second* or *cervical part (pars transversaria),* the *third* or *atlantal part (pars atlantica),* and the *fourth* or *intracranial part (pars intracranialis); origin,* subclavian artery; *branches,* (cervical part) spinal and muscular branches; (intracranial part) anterior spinal artery and posterior inferior cerebellar artery and its branches, meningeal branches, and lateral and medial medullary branches; *distribution,* muscles of neck, vertebrae, spinal cord, cerebellum, medulla oblongata. The artery is also described as being subdivided into four segments, V1–V4, corresponding to the four parts, respectively. See also illustration at *arteria carotis communis.*

a. vesica′lis infe′rior [TA] inferior vesical artery: *origin,* internal iliac artery; *branches,* prostatic branches; *distribution,* bladder, prostate, seminal vesicles, lower ureter.

arte′riae vesica′les superio′res [TA] superior vesical arteries: *origin,* umbilical artery; *branches,* none; *distribution,* bladder, urachus, ureter.

a. vestibula′ris ante′rior [TA] anterior vestibular artery: *origin,* labyrinthine artery; *branches,* none; *distribution,* vestibular nerves, utricle, part of the cristae and semicircular canals. Called also *a. vestibuli* [TA alternative].

a. vestibulocochlea′ris [TA] vestibulocochlear artery: *origin,* common cochlear artery; *branches,* cochlear and posterior vestibular branches; *distribution,* cochlea, saccule, semicircular canals.

a. vesti′buli TA alternative for *a. vestibularis anterior.*

a. zygomaticoorbita′lis [TA] zygomatico-orbital artery: *origin,* superficial temporal artery; *branches,* none; *distribution,* lateral side of orbit.

---

ar•te•ri•ae (ahr-te′re-e) [L.] plural of *arteria.*

ar•te•ri•al•i•za•tion (ahr-te″re-əl-ĭ-za′shən) surgical alteration of a vein so that it functions as an artery.

ar•te•ri•ec•ta•sia (ahr″tə-re-ek-ta′zhə) arteriectasis.

ar•te•ri•ec•ta•sis (ahr-tēr″e-ek′tə-sis) [*arteri-* + *ectasis*] dilatation and, usually, lengthening of an artery.

ar•te•ri•ec•to•my (ahr-tēr″e-ek′tə-me) [*arteri-* + *-ectomy*] excision of a portion of an artery.

ar•te•ri•ec•to•pia (ahr-tēr″e-ek-to′pe-ə) [*arteri-* + *ectopia*] displacement of an artery from its normal location.

arteri(o)- [L. *arteria,* q.v.] a combining form denoting relationship to an artery or arteries.

ar•te•rio•cap•il•lary (ahr-tēr″e-o-kap′ĭ-lar″e) pertaining to the arteries and the capillaries.

ar•te•rio•di•lat•ing (ahr-tēr″e-o-di′lāt-ing) increasing the caliber of the arteries, particularly of arterioles.

ar•te•rio•gen•e•sis (ahr-tēr″e-o-jen′ə-sis) the formation of arteries. Cf. *vascularization.*

ar•te•rio•gram (ahr-tēr′e-o-gram) [*arterio-* + *-gram*] a radiograph of an artery taken during arteriography.

ar•te•rio•graph (ahr-tēr′e-o-graf) a film produced by arteriography.

ar•te•ri•og•ra•phy (ahr″tēr-e-og′rə-fe) [*arterio-* + *-graphy*] angiography of arteries.

catheter a. radiography of vessels after introduction of contrast material through a catheter inserted into an artery.

coronary a. angiography of the coronary arteries, in which a cardiac catheter is inserted into an artery, usually the femoral or brachial artery, advanced under fluoroscopic guidance, and used to inject contrast medium directly into the coronary orifices. It is most often used in evaluations of patients with angina pectoris, prior to coronary artery surgery or percutaneous transluminal coronary angioplasty.

selective a. radiography of a specific vessel which is opacified by a medium introduced directly into it, usually via a catheter.

ar•te•rio•he•pat•ic (ahr-tēr″e-o-hə-pat′ik) pertaining to or affecting the liver and an artery or arteries.

ar•te•ri•o•la (ahr-tēr″e-o′lə) pl. *arterio′lae* [L., dim. of *arteria*] [TA] arteriole: a minute arterial branch, especially one just proximal to a capillary.

a. glomerula′ris af′ferens [TA] afferent glomerular arteriole: a branch of an interlobular artery that goes to a renal glomerulus; called also *afferent artery of glomerulus* and *afferent vessel of glomerulus.*

a. glomerula′ris ef′ferens [TA] efferent glomerular arteriole: an arteriole that arises from a renal glomerulus and breaks up into capillaries to supply renal tubules. Called also *efferent artery of glomerulus* and *efferent vessel of glomerulus.*

a. macula′ris infe′rior [TA] inferior macular arteriole: the inferior arteriole supplying the macula lutea.

a. macula′ris me′dia [TA] medial arteriole of retina: the small branch supplying blood to the central region of the retina.

a. macula′ris supe′rior [TA] superior macular arteriole: the superior arteriole supplying the macula lutea.

a. nasa′lis re′tinae infe′rior [TA] inferior nasal retinal arteriole: a small branch of the central artery of the retina, supplying the inferior nasal region of the retina.

a. nasa′lis re′tinae supe′rior [TA] superior nasal retinal arteriole: a small branch of the central artery of the retina, supplying the superior nasal region of the retina.

arterio′lae rec′tae re′nis [TA] straight arterioles of kidney: branches of the arcuate arteries of the kidney arising from the efferent glomerular arterioles and passing down to the renal pyramids; called also *straight arteries of kidney* and *vasa recta renis* [TA alternative]. Also sometimes

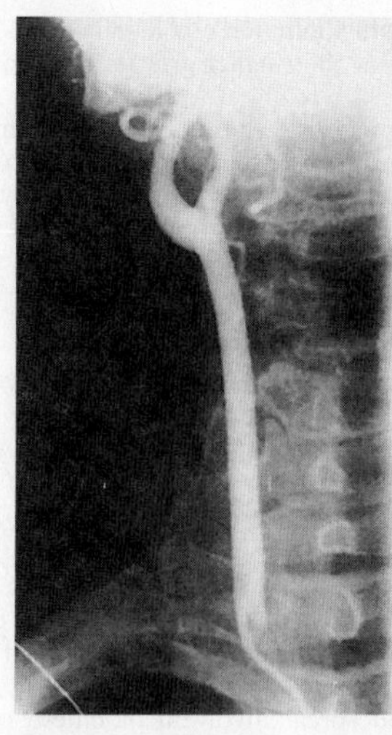

■ Arteriography of the right common carotid artery and its bifurcation into internal and external carotid arteries, shown in an anteroposterior (AP) projection.

called *arteriolae rectae spuriae* or *false straight arterioles of the kidney* to distinguish them from straight direct branches from the arcuate and interlobular arteries that are called *arteriolae rectae verae* or *true straight arterioles of the kidney*.

arterio′lae rec′tae spu′riae see *arteriolae rectae renis.*

arterio′lae rec′tae ve′rae see *arteriolae rectae renis.*

a. tempora′lis re′tinae infe′rior [TA] inferior temporal arteriole of retina: a branch of the central artery of the retina, supplying the inferior temporal region of the retina.

a. tempora′lis re′tinae supe′rior [TA] superior temporal arteriole of retina: a branch of the central artery of the retina, supplying the superior temporal region of the retina.

ar•te•ri•o•lae (ahr-tēr″e-o′le) [L.] genitive and plural of *arteriola.*

ar•te•ri•ole (ahr-tēr′e-ōl) [L. *arteriola*] arteriola. **arterio′lar** *adj*

afferent glomerular a. arteriola glomerularis afferens.

efferent glomerular a. arteriola glomerularis efferens.

ellipsoid a's sheathed arteries.

Isaacs-Ludwig a. an arteriolar twig that sometimes branches from the afferent glomerular arteriole of the kidney to communicate directly with the tubular capillary plexus.

macular a., inferior arteriola macularis inferior.

macular a., superior arteriola macularis superior.

medial a. of retina arteriola medialis retinae.

nasal a. of retina, inferior arteriola nasalis retinae inferior.

nasal a. of retina, superior arteriola nasalis retinae superior.

nasal retinal a., inferior arteriola nasalis retinae inferior.

nasal retinal a., superior arteriola nasalis retinae superior.

postglomerular a. arteriola glomerularis efferens.

precapillary a. arterial capillaries.

preglomerular a. arteriola glomerularis afferens.

sheathed a's see under *artery.*

straight a's of kidney arteriolae rectae renis.

straight a's of kidney, false see *arteriolae rectae renis.*

straight a's of kidney, true see *arteriolae rectae renis.*

temporal a. of retina, inferior arteriola temporalis retinae inferior.

temporal a. of retina, superior arteriola temporalis retinae superior.

ar•te•rio•lith (ahr-tēr′e-o-lith″) [*arterio-* + *-lith*] a chalky concretion in an artery.

ar•te•rio•li•tis (ahr-tēr″e-o-li′tis) inflammation of the arterioles.

hyperplastic a. onionskin lesion (def. 2).

necrotizing a. fibrinoid necrosis.

arteriol(o)- [L. *arteriola*, dim. of *arteria* artery] a combining form denoting relationship to one or more arterioles.

ar•te•ri•ol•o•gy (ahr-tēr″e-ol′ə-je) [*arterio-* + *-logy*] the sum of what is known regarding the arteries; the science or study of the arteries.

ar•te•rio•lo•ne•cro•sis (ahr-tēr″e-o″lo-nə-kro′sis) necrosis of arterioles, as may be seen in nephrosclerosis; called also *arteriolar necrosis.*

ar•te•ri•o•lop•a•thy (ahr-tēr″e-o-lop′ə-the) any disease of the arterioles.

calcific uremic a. a syndrome of unknown etiology, characterized by calcification of the tunica media of the subcutaneous arterioles accompanied by livedo reticularis and necrosis of the skin. It is seen most often in patients with end-stage renal disease, but also occurs with primary hyperparathyroidism, alcoholic cirrhosis, and metastatic breast cancer. Mortality is high and death most often results from sepsis. Called also *calciphylaxis.*

ar•te•rio•lo•scle•ro•sis (ahr-tēr″e-o″lo-sklə-ro′sis) sclerosis and thickening of the walls of the smaller arteries (arterioles). **arterioloscle-rot′ic** *adj*

hyaline a. arteriolosclerosis characterized by homogeneous pink hyaline thickening of vessel walls, associated with benign nephrosclerosis.

hyperplastic a. arteriolosclerosis characterized by concentrated thickening with progressive narrowing of the lumina, sometimes associated with malignant hypertension, nephrosclerosis, and scleroderma.

ar•te•rio•mo•tor (ahr-tēr″e-o-mo′tər) pertaining to or causing change in the caliber of an artery.

ar•te•rio•ne•cro•sis (ahr-tēr″e-o-nə-kro′sis) necrosis of an artery or of arteries.

ar•te•ri•op•a•thy (ahr-tēr″e-op′ə-the) [*arterio-* + *-pathy*] any arterial disease.

cerebral autosomal dominant a. see *CADASIL syndrome*, under *syndrome.*

cyclosporine-associated a. a manifestation of chronic cyclosporine-induced nephrotoxicity, consisting of hyaline degeneration of the tunica media and mucoid thickening of the intima of the arterioles of the peripheral vascular tree.

hypertensive a. widespread involvement, chiefly of arterioles and small arteries, associated with arterial hypertension and characterized primarily by hypertrophy and thickening of the media.

plexogenic a., plexogenic pulmonary a. hypertrophy of arterial walls in part of the pulmonary vasculature, which may become obstructed, leading to plexiform thin-walled vessels distally; seen in some cases of pulmonary hypertension. Cf. *Ayerza syndrome.*

ar•te•rio•plas•ty (ahr-tēr′e-o-plas″te) [*arterio-* + *-plasty*] surgical repair or reconstruction of an artery. **arterioplas′tic** *adj*

ar•te•rio•pres•sor (ahr-tēr″e-o-pres′ər) hypertensive (def. 2).

ar•te•rio•re•nal (ahr-tēr″e-o-re′nəl) pertaining to the arteries of the kidney.

ar•te•ri•or•rha•phy (ahr-tēr″e-or′ə-fe) [*arterio-* + *-rrhaphy*] suture of an artery.

ar•te•ri•or•rhex•is (ahr-tēr″e-o-rek′sis) [*arterio-* + *-rrhexis*] rupture of an artery.

ar•te•rio•scle•ro•sis (ahr-tēr″e-o-sklə-ro′sis) [*arterio-* + *sclerosis*] any of a group of diseases characterized by thickening and loss of elasticity of arterial walls; there are three distinct forms: *atherosclerosis, Mönckeberg arteriosclerosis*, and *arteriolosclerosis*. Called also *arterial sclerosis* and *vascular sclerosis.* **arteriosclerot′ic** *adj*

cerebral a. arteriosclerosis of the arteries of the brain.

coronary a. arteriosclerosis or atherosclerosis of the coronary arteries.

hyaline a. see under *arteriolosclerosis.*

hypertensive a. arteriosclerosis intensified by hypertension.

infantile a. see under *arteritis.*

intimal a. arteriosclerosis in which the major changes affect the intima of the arteries.

medial a. 1. a condition of large and medium-sized arteries, with primary destruction of the muscle and elastic fibers of the medial coat, which are replaced by fibrous tissue; when there are deposits of calcium it is called *Mönckeberg arteriosclerosis.* 2. Mönckeberg a.

Mönckeberg a. medial arteriosclerosis with extensive deposits of calcium in the media of the artery; called also *Mönckeberg calcification, degeneration, mesarteritis*, or *sclerosis; medial a.*; and *medial calcific sclerosis.*

a. obli′terans arteriosclerosis in which proliferation of the intima of small vessels has caused obliteration of the lumen. See also *endarteritis obliterans.*

peripheral a. arteriosclerosis of the extremities.

presenile a. idiopathic arteriosclerosis occurring at an unusually early age.

senile a. arteriosclerosis occurring in old age.

ar•te•rio•spasm (ahr-tēr′e-o-spaz″əm) spasm of an artery. **arterio-spas′tic** *adj*

ar•te•rio•ste•no•sis (ahr-tēr″e-o-stə-no′sis) [*arterio-* + *stenosis*] the narrowing or diminution of the caliber of an artery.

ar•te•ri•os•teo•gen•e•sis (ahr-tēr″e-os′te-o-jen′ə-sis) [*arteri-* + *osteogenesis*] calcification of an artery.

ar•te•ri•os•to•sis (ahr-tēr″e-os-to′sis) [*arteri-* + *ostosis*] arteriosteogenesis.

ar•te•ri•ot•o•my (ahr-tēr″e-ot′ə-me) [*arterio-* + *-tomy*] incision of an artery.

ar•te•rio•ve•nous (ahr-tēr″e-o-ve′nəs) both arterial and venous; pertaining to or affecting an artery and a vein.

ar•ter•i•tis (ahr″tə-ri′tis) pl. *arteri′tides* [*arteri-* + *-itis*] inflammation of an artery.

aortic arch a. Takayasu a.

brachiocephalic a., a. brachiocepha′lica Takayasu a.

coronary a. inflammation of the coronary arteries.

cranial a. giant cell a.

equine viral a. a frequently fatal disease of horses, caused by the equine arteritis virus, affecting especially the smaller arteries, with hemorrhagic enteritis, abdominal pain and diarrhea, and pulmonary edema. Abortion is common in affected mares.

giant cell a. a chronic vascular disease in the elderly, of unknown origin, often associated with polymyalgia rheumatica, seen usually in the external carotid arteries but sometimes in other arteries. Characteristics include proliferative inflammation, often with giant cells and granulomas; headache; pain with chewing; weight loss; fever; sometimes ocular symptoms; and increased erythrocyte sedimentation rate. Called also *cranial, granulomatous*, or *temporal a.* and *Horton a., disease*, or *syndrome.*

granulomatous a., Horton a. giant cell a.

infantile a. diffuse arteritis in infants and children, rarely with atherosclerotic processes.

infectious a. arteritis secondary to an infectious disorder, caused by direct invasion by, or less commonly, hematogenous spread of, infectious organisms.

localized visceral a. hypersensitivity vasculitis.

necrotizing a. polyarteritis nodosa

a. obli′terans endarteritis obliterans.

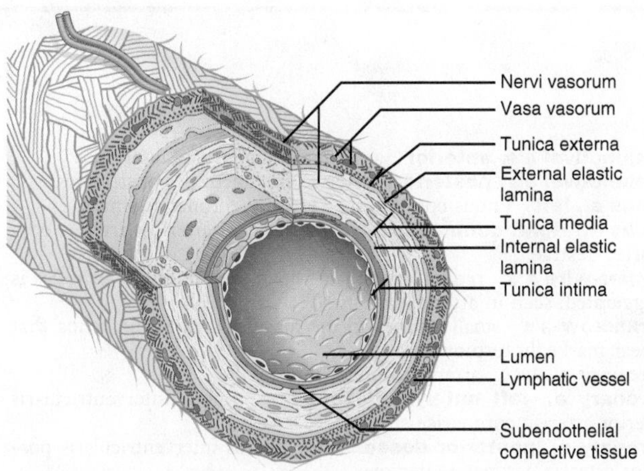

■ Diagrammatic representation of the principal structural features of a large muscular artery.

rheumatic a. generalized inflammation of arterioles and arterial capillaries occurring in rheumatic fever.

syphilitic a. a late manifestation of syphilis characterized by intimal proliferation and degeneration of the arterial tunica media, usually in the ascending aorta, aortic arch, and pulmonary artery, sometimes leading to aneurysm.

Takayasu a. progressive obliteration of the brachiocephalic trunk and the subclavian and common carotid arteries above their origin in the aortic arch, leading to loss of pulse in both arms and carotids. This may be followed by symptoms associated with ischemia of the brain (such as syncope or transient hemiplegia), of the eyes (such as transient blindness or retinal atrophy), of the face (such as muscular atrophy), of the arms (such as claudication), or of the kidneys. Called also *aortic arch a.*, *brachiocephalic a.* or *ischemia*, *Martorell syndrome*, *pulseless disease*, *reversed coarctation*, and *Takayasu disease* or *syndrome.*

temporal a. giant cell a.

tuberculous a. endarteritis obliterans in those arteries intimately involved in a tubercular focus.

a. umbilica'lis septic inflammation of the umbilical artery in newborn infants.

verminous mesenteric a. verminous aneurysm.

Ar·te·ri·vi·ri·dae (ahr-tēr″ĭ-vir′ĭ-de) the arteriviruses; a family of RNA viruses having a virion 60 nm in diameter consisting of a lipid envelope with 12–15 ringlike surface structures surrounding an isometric nucleocapsid about 35 nm in diameter. The genome consists of a single molecule of linear positive-sense RNA (size about 13 kb). Viruses contain at least four major structural proteins. Replication is similar to that of the Coronaviridae. Host range is narrow and transmission is horizontal. There is a single genus, *Arterivirus.*

Ar·te·ri·vi·rus (ahr-tēr′ĭ-vi″rəs) [*arteritis* + *virus*] a genus of viruses of the family Arteriviridae. Species include equine arteritis virus and swine infertility and respiratory syndrome virus.

ar·te·ri·vi·rus (ahr-tēr′ĭ-vi″rəs) any virus belonging to the family Arteriviridae.

ar·te·ry (ahr′tə-re) [Gr. *artēria* q.v.] a vessel through which the blood passes away from the heart to the various parts of the body. The wall of an artery consists typically of an outer coat (tunica externa), a middle coat (tunica media), and an inner coat (tunica intima). Called also *arteria* [TA]. **arte′rial** *adj*

Artery

For names and descriptions of specific arteries, see under *arteria.*

accompanying a. of median nerve arteria comitans nervi mediani.
accompanying a. of sciatic nerve arteria comitans nervi ischiadici.
acetabular a. 1. ramus acetabularis arteriae circumflexae femoris medialis. 2. ramus acetabularis arteriae obturatoriae.
acromiothoracic a. arteria thoracoacromialis.
a. of Adamkiewicz an unusually large anterior segmental medullary artery arising from an intersegmental branch of the aorta, varying from the lower thoracic to the upper lumbar level, and traveling posteriorly to supply the spinal cord by anastomosing with the anterior spinal artery. It may be the main supply to as much as the lower two-thirds of the spinal cord. Called also *arteria radicularis magna.*
adipose a's of kidney rami capsulares arteriae renalis.
adrenal a., middle arteria suprarenalis media.
afferent a. of glomerulus arteriola glomerularis afferens.
alveolar a's, anterior superior arteriae alveolares superiores anteriores.
alveolar a., inferior arteria alveolaris inferior.
alveolar a., posterior superior arteria alveolaris superior posterior.
anastomotic atrial a. ramus atrialis anastomoticus rami circumflexi arteriae coronariae sinistrae.
angular a. arteria angularis.
a. of angular gyrus ramus gyri angularis arteriae cerebri mediae.
appendicular a. arteria appendicularis.
arcuate a. of foot arteria arcuata pedis.
arcuate a's of kidney arteriae arcuatae renis.
arcuate a's of uterus branches of the uterine artery that run circumferentially in the uterine wall as anterior and posterior groups, anastomosing across the midline both anteriorly and posteriorly, and giving rise to radial arteries that supply deeper layers.
ascending a. arteria ascendens.
atrial anastomotic a. ramus atrialis anastomoticus rami circumflexi arteriae coronariae sinistrae.
atrioventricular nodal a. ramus nodi atrioventricularis arteriae coronariae dextrae.
auditory a., internal arteria labyrinthi.
auricular a's, anterior rami auriculares anteriores arteriae temporalis superficialis.
auricular a., deep arteria auricularis profunda.
auricular a., left arteria coronaria sinistra.
auricular a., posterior arteria auricularis posterior.
auricular a., right arteria coronaria dextra.
axillary a. arteria axillaris.
azygos a's of vagina rami vaginales arteriae uterinae.
basilar a. arteria basilaris.
brachial a. arteria brachialis.
brachial a., superficial arteria brachialis superficialis.
brachiocephalic a. truncus brachiocephalicus.
bronchial a's rami bronchiales partis thoracicae aortae.
bronchial a's, anterior rami bronchiales arteriae thoracicae internae.
buccal a., buccinator a. arteria buccalis.
bulbourethral a., a. of bulb of penis arteria bulbi penis.
a. of bulb of vestibule arteria bulbi vestibuli.
callosal a., median arteria callosa mediana.
callosomarginal a. arteria callosomarginalis.
capsular a's rami capsulares arteriae renalis.
capsular a., inferior arteria suprarenalis inferior.
capsular a., middle arteria suprarenalis media.
caroticotympanic a's arteriae caroticotympanicae.
carotid a., common arteria carotis communis.
carotid a., external arteria carotis externa.
carotid a., internal arteria carotis interna.
caudal a. arteria sacralis mediana.
cecal a., anterior arteria caecalis anterior.
cecal a., posterior arteria caecalis posterior.
celiac a. see under *trunk.*
central a's, anterolateral arteriae centrales anterolaterales.
central a's, anteromedial arteriae centrales anteromediales.
central a., long arteria striata medialis distalis.
central a's, posterolateral arteriae centrales posterolaterales.
central a's, posteromedial, of posterior cerebral a. arteriae centrales posteromediales arteriae cerebri posterioris.
central a's, posteromedial, of posterior communicating a. arteriae centrales posteromediales arteriae communicantis posterioris.

Artery *Continued*

central a's, short the anteromedial central arteries, excepting the long central artery (distal medial striate artery).
central a. of retina arteria centralis retinae.
central a's of spleen branches of the splenic artery after they leave the trabeculae; their tunica adventitia is replaced by a cylindrical lymphoid sheath and they pass through the aggregations of lymphatic nodules and branch out to terminate as splenic penicilli.
a. of central sulcus arteria sulci centralis.
cerebellar a., anterior inferior arteria inferior anterior cerebelli.
cerebellar a., lateral superior ramus lateralis arteriae superioris cerebelli.
cerebellar a., medial superior ramus medialis arteriae superioris cerebelli.
cerebellar a., posterior inferior arteria inferior posterior cerebelli.
cerebellar a., superior arteria superior cerebelli.
cerebral a's the arteries supplying the cerebral hemispheres, derived from the internal carotid artery (anterior choroid, anterior cerebral, middle cerebral, and posterior communicating arteries and the circle of Willis) or from the basilar artery (posterior cerebral artery).
cerebral a., anterior arteria cerebri anterior.
cerebral a., middle arteria cerebri media.
cerebral a., posterior arteria cerebri posterior.
a. of cerebral hemorrhage one of the larger lateral striate branches of the middle cerebral artery, which is a common site of cerebral hemorrhage.
cervical a., ascending arteria cervicalis ascendens.
cervical a., deep arteria cervicalis profunda.
cervical a., deep descending the deep branch of the descending branch of the occipital artery; see *ramus descendens arteriae occipitalis.*
cervical a., superficial ramus superficialis arteriae transversae colli.
cervical a., transverse arteria transversa cervicis.
choroidal a., anterior arteria choroidea anterior.
ciliary a's, anterior arteriae ciliares anteriores.
ciliary a's, long, ciliary a's, long posterior arteriae ciliares posteriores longae.
ciliary a's, short, ciliary a's, short posterior arteriae ciliares posteriores breves.
circumflex a. ramus circumflexus arteriae coronariae sinistrae.
circumflex a., internal deep ramus profundus arteriae circumflexae femoris medialis.
circumflex femoral a., lateral arteria circumflexa femoris lateralis.
circumflex femoral a., medial arteria circumflexa femoris medialis.
circumflex fibular a. ramus circumflexus fibularis arteriae tibialis posterioris.
circumflex humeral a., anterior arteria circumflexa humeri anterior.
circumflex humeral a., posterior arteria circumflexa humeri posterior.
circumflex iliac a., deep arteria circumflexa ilium profunda.
circumflex iliac a., superficial arteria circumflexa ilium superficialis.
circumflex a. of scapula arteria circumflexa scapulae.
coccygeal a. arteria sacralis mediana.
cochlear a. arteria cochlearis propria.
cochlear a., common arteria cochlearis communis.
cochlear a., proper arteria cochlearis propria.
colic a., accessory superior arteria colica media.
colic a., inferior right arteria ileocolica.
colic a., left arteria colica sinistra.
colic a., middle arteria colica media.
colic a., right arteria colica dextra.
collateral a., inferior ulnar arteria collateralis ulnaris inferior.
collateral a., middle arteria collateralis media.
collateral a., radial arteria collateralis radialis.
collateral a., superior ulnar arteria collateralis ulnaris superior.
collicular a. arteria collicularis.
commissural a., median arteria commissuralis mediana.
communicating a., anterior arteria communicans anterior.
communicating a., posterior arteria communicans posterior.
conal a. 1. ramus coni arteriosi arteriae coronariae dextrae. 2. ramus coni arteriosi arteriae coronariae sinistrae.
conducting a's arterial trunks characterized by large size and elasticity, such as the aorta, subclavian artery, common carotid artery, brachiocephalic trunk, and pulmonary trunk. Called also *elastic a's.*
conjunctival a's, anterior arteriae conjunctivales anteriores.
conjunctival a's, posterior arteriae conjunctivales posteriores.
conus a., left ramus coni arteriosi arteriae coronariae sinistrae.
conus a., right, conus a., third ramus coni arteriosi arteriae coronariae dextrae.
copper-wire a's retinal arteries on which the bright line of reflex is exaggerated; seen in arteriosclerosis.
corkscrew a's small arteries in the macular area of the retina that appear markedly tortuous.
coronary a., left arteria coronaria sinistra.
coronary a., left anterior descending ramus interventricularis anterior arteriae coronariae sinistrae.
coronary a., posterior descending ramus interventricularis posterior arteriae coronariae dextrae.
coronary a., right arteria coronaria dextra.
coronary a. of stomach, left arteria gastrica sinistra.
cortical radiate a's arteriae corticales radiatae.
cremasteric a. arteria cremasterica.
cricothyroid a. ramus cricothyroideus arteriae thyroideae superioris.
cystic a. arteria cystica.
deep a. of arm arteria profunda brachii.
deep a. of clitoris arteria profunda clitoridis.
deep a. of penis arteria profunda penis.
deep a. of thigh arteria profunda femoris.
deferential a. arteria ductus deferentis.
dental a's, anterior arteriae alveolares superiores anteriores.
dental a., inferior arteria alveolaris inferior.
dental a., posterior arteria alveolaris superior posterior.
diagonal a. an inconstant artery, occasionally duplicated, arising from the trunk of the left coronary artery and crossing the anterior aspect of the left ventricle diagonally, toward the left margin.
digital a's, collateral arteriae digitales palmares propriae.
digital a's, common palmar arteriae digitales palmares communes.
digital a's, common plantar arteriae digitales plantares communes.
digital a's, common volar arteriae digitales palmares communes.
digital a's, proper palmar arteriae digitales palmares propriae.
digital a's, proper plantar arteriae digitales plantares propriae.
digital a's, proper volar arteriae digitales palmares propriae.
digital a's of foot, common arteriae metatarsales plantares.
digital a's of foot, dorsal arteriae digitales dorsales pedis.
digital a's of hand, dorsal arteriae digitales dorsales manus.
distributing a's most of the arteries except the conducting arteries; of muscular type, they extend from the large vessels to the arterioles. Called also *muscular a's.*
dorsal a. of clitoris arteria dorsalis clitoridis.
dorsal a. of foot arteria dorsalis pedis.
dorsal a. of nose arteria dorsalis nasi.
dorsal a. of penis arteria dorsalis penis.
dorsal a. of tongue see *rami dorsales linguae arteriae lingualis.*
dorsalis pedis a. arteria dorsalis pedis.
a. of ductus deferens arteria ductus deferentis.
efferent a. of glomerulus arteriola glomerularis efferens.
elastic a's conducting a's.
end a. an artery which undergoes progressive branching without development of channels connecting with other arteries, so that if occluded it cannot supply sufficient blood to the tissue depending on it.
epigastric a., inferior arteria epigastrica inferior.
epigastric a., superficial arteria epigastrica superficialis.
epigastric a., superior arteria epigastrica superior.
episcleral a's arteriae episclerales.
esophageal a. the esophageal branch of an artery; see terms starting with *rami oesophageales,* under *ramus.*
esophageal a's, inferior rami oesophageales arteriae gastricae sinistrae.
ethmoidal a., anterior arteria ethmoidalis anterior.
ethmoidal a., posterior arteria ethmoidalis posterior.
facial a. arteria facialis.
facial a., transverse arteria transversa faciei.
fallopian a. arteria uterina.
femoral a. arteria femoralis.
femoral a., common see *arteria femoralis.*
femoral a., deep arteria profunda femoris.
femoral a., superficial see *arteria femoralis.*
fibular a. arteria fibularis.

frontal a. arteria supratrochlearis.
frontobasal a., lateral arteria frontobasalis lateralis.
frontobasal a., medial arteria frontobasalis medialis.
frontopolar a. arteria polaris frontalis.
funicular a. arteria testicularis.
gastric a., left arteria gastrica sinistra.
gastric a., left inferior arteria gastroomentalis sinistra.
gastric a., posterior arteria gastrica posterior.
gastric a., right arteria gastrica dextra.
gastric a., right inferior arteria gastroomentalis dextra.
gastric a's, short arteriae gastricae breves.
gastroduodenal a. arteria gastroduodenalis.
gastroepiploic a., left arteria gastroomentalis sinistra.
gastroepiploic a., right arteria gastroomentalis dextra.
gastro-omental a., left arteria gastroomentalis sinistra.
gastro-omental a., right arteria gastroomentalis dextra.
genicular a., descending arteria descendens genus.
genicular a., lateral inferior arteria inferior lateralis genus.
genicular a., lateral superior arteria superior lateralis genus.
genicular a., medial inferior arteria inferior medialis genus.
genicular a., medial superior arteria superior medialis genus.
genicular a., middle arteria media genus.
gluteal a., inferior arteria glutea inferior.
gluteal a., superior arteria glutea superior.
gonadal a's the ovarian arteries or the testicular arteries.
helicine a's 1. small arteries that for their entire length have a band of thickened intima on one side, in which longitudinal muscle fibers are embedded. They follow a convoluted or curled course and open directly into cavernous sinuses instead of capillaries; they play a dominant role in erection of erectile tissue. 2. arteriae helicinae penis. 3. rami helicinae arteriae uterinae.
hemorrhoidal a., inferior arteria rectalis inferior.
hemorrhoidal a., middle arteria rectalis media.
hemorrhoidal a., superior arteria rectalis superior.
hepatic a., common arteria hepatica communis.
hepatic a. proper arteria hepatica propria.
hyaloid a. arteria hyaloidea.
a's of hybrid type a term denoting the short transitional regions where arteries of the mixed or elastic (conducting) type pass into arteries of the muscular (distributing) type.
hypogastric a. arteria iliaca interna.
hypophysial a., inferior arteria hypophysialis inferior.
hypophysial a., superior arteria hypophysialis superior.
ileal a's arteriae ileales.
ileocolic a. arteria ileocolica.
ileocolic a., ascending ramus colicus arteriae ileocolicae.
iliac a., anterior arteria iliaca externa.
iliac a., common arteria iliaca communis.
iliac a., external arteria iliaca externa.
iliac a., internal arteria iliaca interna.
iliac a., small arteria iliolumbalis.
iliolumbar a. arteria iliolumbalis.
infracostal a. ramus costalis lateralis arteriae thoracicae internae.
infraorbital a. arteria infraorbitalis.
inguinal a's rami inguinales arteriae pudendae externae profundae.
innominate a. truncus brachiocephalicus.
insular a's arteriae insulares.
intercostal a's, anterior rami intercostales anteriores arteriae thoracicae internae.
intercostal a., first posterior arteria intercostalis posterior prima.
intercostal a., highest arteria intercostalis suprema.
intercostal a's, posterior arteriae intercostales posteriores.
intercostal a., second posterior arteria intercostalis posterior secunda.
intercostal a., superior arteria intercostalis suprema.
intercostal a., supreme arteria intercostalis suprema.
interlobar a's of kidney arteriae interlobares renis.
interlobular a's of kidney arteriae corticales radiatae.
interlobular a's of liver arteriae interlobulares hepatis.
intermediate atrial a., left ramus atrialis intermedius rami circumflexi arteriae coronariae sinistrae.
intermediate atrial a., right ramus atrialis intermedius arteriae coronariae dextrae.
intermetacarpal a's, palmar arteriae metacarpales palmares.
interosseous a., anterior arteria interossea anterior.
interosseous a., common arteria interossea communis.
interosseous a., dorsal arteria interossea posterior.
interosseous a., posterior arteria interossea posterior.
interosseous a., recurrent arteria interossea recurrens.
interosseous a., volar arteria interossea anterior.
intersegmental a's paired dorsal branches of the embryonic aorta, originally going to the spinal cord but later mainly to the neck, back, and body wall.
interventricular a., anterior ramus interventricularis anterior arteriae coronariae sinistrae.
interventricular septal a's, anterior rami interventriculares septales arteriae coronariae sinistrae.
interventricular septal a's, posterior rami interventriculares septales arteriae coronariae dextrae.
intestinal a's the arteries arising from the superior mesenteric, and supplying the intestines, including the pancreaticoduodenal, jejunal, ileal, ileocolic, and colic arteries.
intrarenal a's arteriae intrarenales.
jejunal a's arteriae jejunales.
juxtacolic a. arteria marginalis coli.
a's of kidney arteriae intrarenales.
labial a., inferior arteria labialis inferior.
labial a., superior arteria labialis superior.
labial a's of vulva, anterior rami labiales anteriores arteriae pudendae externae profundae.
labial a's of vulva, posterior rami labiales posteriores arteriae pudendae internae.
labyrinthine a. arteria labyrinthi.
lacrimal a. arteria lacrimalis.
laryngeal a., inferior arteria laryngea inferior.
laryngeal a., superior arteria laryngea superior.
lateral inferior a. of knee arteria inferior lateralis genus.
lateral superior a. of knee arteria superior lateralis genus.
lenticulostriate a's arteriae centrales anterolaterales.
lingual a. arteria lingualis.
lingual a., deep arteria profunda linguae.
lingular a. arteria lingularis.
lingular a., inferior arteria lingularis inferior.
lingular a., superior arteria lingularis superior.
lobar a's of left lung, inferior arteriae lobares inferiores pulmonis sinistri.
lobar a's of left lung, superior arteriae lobares superiores pulmonis sinistri.
lobar a's of right lung, inferior arteriae lobares pulmonis dextri.
lobar a. of right lung, middle arteria lobaris media pulmonis dextri.
lobar a's of right lung, superior arteriae lobares superiores pulmonis dextri.
a's of lower limb arteriae membri inferioris.
lumbar a's arteriae lumbales.
lumbar a's, fifth, lumbar a's, lowest arteriae lumbales imae.
malleolar a., lateral anterior arteria malleolaris anterior lateralis.
malleolar a., medial anterior arteria malleolaris anterior medialis.
mammary a., external arteria thoracica lateralis.
mammary a., internal arteria thoracica interna.
mammillary a's mammillary arteries.
mandibular a. arteria alveolaris inferior.
marginal a., left ramus marginalis sinister rami circumflexi arteriae coronariae sinistrae.
marginal a., right ramus marginalis dexter arteriae coronariae dextrae.
marginal a. of colon, marginal a. of Drummond arteria marginalis coli.
masseteric a. arteria masseterica.
mastoid a. ramus mastoideus arteriae occipitalis.
maxillary a. arteria maxillaris.
maxillary a., external arteria facialis.
maxillary a., internal arteria maxillaris.
meandering mesenteric a. Riolan arch.
medial a. of foot, superficial ramus superficialis arteriae plantaris medialis.
medial inferior a. of knee arteria inferior medialis genus.
medial superior a. of knee arteria superior medialis genus.
median a. arteria comitans nervi mediani.

mediastinal a's, anterior rami mediastinales arteriae thoracicae internae.
mediastinal a's, posterior rami mediastinales partis thoracicae aortae.
medullary a. arteria nutricia.
medullary a., great anterior a. of Adamkiewicz.
meningeal a., accessory ramus accessorius arteriae meningeae mediae.
meningeal a., anterior ramus meningeus anterior arteriae ethmoidalis anterioris.
meningeal a., middle arteria meningea media.
meningeal a., posterior arteria meningea posterior.
mental a. ramus mentalis arteriae alveolaris inferioris.
mesencephalic a's arteriae mesencephalicae.
mesenteric a., inferior arteria mesenterica inferior.
mesenteric a., superior arteria mesenterica superior.
metacarpal a., deep volar ramus palmaris profundus arteriae ulnaris.
metacarpal a's, dorsal arteriae metacarpales dorsales.
metacarpal a's, palmar arteriae metacarpales palmares.
metacarpal a's, ulnar arteriae digitales palmares communes.
metacarpal a's, volar arteriae metacarpales palmares.
metatarsal a's, dorsal arteriae metatarsales dorsales.
metatarsal a's, plantar arteriae metatarsales plantares.
a's of mixed type arteries having both elastic (conducting) and muscular (distributing) elements.
a's of Mueller arteriae helicinae penis.
muscular a's 1. distributing a's. 2. arteriae musculares.
musculophrenic a. arteria musculophrenica.
mylohyoid a. ramus mylohyoideus arteriae alveolaris inferioris.
myomastoid a. ramus occipitalis arteriae auricularis posterioris.
nasal a., dorsal, nasal a., external arteria dorsalis nasi.
nasal a's, posterior lateral arteriae nasales posteriores laterales.
nasopalatine a. arteria sphenopalatina.
Neubauer a. arteria thyroidea ima.
nodal a. see *ramus nodi atrioventricularis arteriae coronariae dextrae* and *ramus nodi sinuatrialis arteriae coronariae dextrae.*
nutrient a. arteria nutricia.
nutrient a's of femur arteriae nutriciae femoris.
nutrient a. of fibula arteria nutricia fibulae.
nutrient a's of humerus arteriae nutriciae humeri.
nutrient a. of tibia arteria nutricia tibiae.
obturator a. arteria obturatoria.
obturator a., accessory arteria obturatoria accessoria.
occipital a. arteria occipitalis.
occipital a., lateral arteria occipitalis lateralis.
occipital a., medial arteria occipitalis medialis.
ophthalmic a. arteria ophthalmica.
orbitofrontal a., lateral arteria frontobasalis lateralis.
orbitofrontal a., medial arteria frontobasalis medialis.
ovarian a. arteria ovarica.
palatine a., ascending arteria palatina ascendens.
palatine a., descending arteria palatina descendens.
palatine a., greater arteria palatina major.
palatine a's, lesser arteriae palatinae minores.
palpebral a's, lateral arteriae palpebrales laterales.
palpebral a's, medial arteriae palpebrales mediales.
pancreatic a., caudal arteria caudae pancreatis.
pancreatic a., dorsal arteria pancreatica dorsalis.
pancreatic a., great arteria pancreatica magna.
pancreatic a., inferior arteria pancreatica inferior.
pancreaticoduodenal a., anterior superior arteria pancreaticoduodenalis superior anterior.
pancreaticoduodenal a., inferior arteria pancreaticoduodenalis inferior.
pancreaticoduodenal a., posterior superior arteria pancreaticoduodenalis superior posterior.
paracentral a. rami paracentrales arteriae callosomarginalis.
paramedian a's arteriae centrales posteromediales arteriae cerebri posterioris.
parietal a., anterior arteria parietalis anterior.
parietal a., posterior arteria parietalis posterior.
pelvic a., posterior arteria iliaca interna.
perforating a's arteriae perforantes.
perforating a's, anterior arteriae perforantes anteriores.
perforating radiate a's arteriae perforantes radiatae.
pericallosal a. arteria pericallosa.
pericardiac a's, posterior rami pericardiaci partis thoracicae aortae.
pericardiacophrenic a. arteria pericardiacophrenica.
perineal a. arteria perinealis.
perirenal a's rami capsulares arteriae renalis.
peroneal a. arteria fibularis.
peroneal a., perforating ramus perforans arteriae fibularis.
pharyngeal a., ascending arteria pharyngea ascendens.
phrenic a., great, phrenic a., inferior arteria phrenica inferior.
phrenic a's, superior arteriae phrenicae superiores.
plantar a., deep arteria plantaris profunda.
plantar a., external arteria plantaris lateralis.
plantar a., lateral arteria plantaris lateralis.
plantar a., medial arteria plantaris medialis.
polar frontal a. arteria polaris frontalis.
pontine a's arteriae pontis.
popliteal a. arteria poplitea.
a. of postcentral sulcus arteria sulci postcentralis.
a. of precentral sulcus arteria sulci precentralis.
precuneal a's rami precuneales arteriae pericallosae.
prefrontal a. arteria prefrontalis.
premammillary a. arteria thalamotuberalis.
preoptic a's arteriae preopticae.
prepancreatic a. arteria prepancreatica.
princeps pollicis a., principal a. of thumb arteria princeps pollicis.
profunda brachii a. arteria profunda brachii.
pterygoid a's rami pterygoidei arteriae maxillaris.
a. of pterygoid canal arteria canalis pterygoidei.
pubic a. ramus pubicus arteriae epigastricae inferioris.
pudendal a., deep external arteria pudenda externa profunda.
pudendal a., internal arteria pudenda interna.
pudendal a., superficial external arteria pudenda externa superficialis.
pulmonary a. truncus pulmonalis.
pulmonary a., left arteria pulmonalis sinistra.
pulmonary a., right arteria pulmonalis dextra.
a. of the pulp a name given the first portion of one of the penicilli arteriae splenicae (see under *penicillus*).
pyloric a. arteria gastrica dextra.
quadriceps a. of femur ramus descendens arteriae circumflexae femoris lateralis.
quadrigeminal a. arteria collicularis.
radial a. arteria radialis.
radial a., collateral arteria collateralis radialis.
radialis indicis a. arteria radialis indicis.
radial a's of uterus branches of the uterine arcuate arteries that supply the deeper layers of the myometrium and penetrate the endometrium, giving rise to the spiral arteries.
radiate a's of kidney arteriae corticales radiatae.
radicular a., anterior arteria radicularis anterior.
radicular a., great a. of Adamkiewicz.
radicular a., posterior arteria radicularis posterior.
ranine a. arteria profunda linguae.
rectal a., inferior arteria rectalis inferior.
rectal a., middle arteria rectalis media.
rectal a., superior arteria rectalis superior.
recurrent a., anterior tibial arteria recurrens tibialis anterior.
recurrent a., posterior tibial arteria recurrens tibialis posterior.
recurrent a., radial arteria recurrens radialis.
recurrent a., ulnar arteria recurrens ulnaris.
recurrent a. of Heubner arteria striata medialis distalis.
renal a. 1. arteria renalis. 2. *(in the pl.)* arteriae intrarenales.
retinal a., central arteria centralis retinae.
retrocostal a. ramus costalis lateralis arteriae thoracicae internae.
retroduodenal a's arteriae retroduodenales.
a. of round ligament of uterus arteria ligamenti teretis uteri.
sacral a's, lateral arteriae sacrales laterales.
sacral a., median arteria sacralis mediana.
sacrococcygeal a. arteria sacralis mediana.
scapular a., descending, scapular a., dorsal arteria dorsalis scapulae.

Artery *Continued*

scapular a., transverse arteria suprascapularis.
sciatic a., a. to sciatic nerve arteria comitans nervi ischiadici.
scrotal a's, anterior rami scrotales anteriores arteriae pudendae externae profundae.
scrotal a's, posterior rami scrotales posteriores arteriae pudendae internae.
segmental a., inferior lingular arteria lingularis inferior.
segmental a., lingular arteria lingularis.
segmental a., superior lingular arteria lingularis superior.
segmental a. of kidney, anterior inferior arteria segmenti anterioris inferioris renalis.
segmental a. of kidney, anterior superior arteria segmenti anterioris superioris renalis.
segmental a. of kidney, inferior arteria segmenti inferioris renalis.
segmental a. of kidney, posterior arteria segmenti posterioris renalis.
segmental a. of kidney, superior arteria segmenti superioris renalis.
segmental a. of left lung, anterior arteria segmentalis anterior pulmonis sinistri.
segmental a. of left lung, anterior ascending ramus ascendens arteriae segmentalis anterioris pulmonis sinistri.
segmental a. of left lung, anterior basal arteria segmentalis basalis anterior pulmonis sinistri.
segmental a. of left lung, anterior descending ramus descendens arteriae segmentalis anterioris pulmonis sinistri.
segmental a. of left lung, apical arteria segmentalis apicalis pulmonis sinistri.
segmental a. of left lung, lateral basal arteria segmentalis basalis lateralis pulmonis sinistri.
segmental a. of left lung, medial basal arteria segmentalis basalis medialis pulmonis sinistri.
segmental a. of left lung, posterior arteria segmentalis posterior pulmonis sinistri.
segmental a. of left lung, posterior ascending ramus ascendens arteriae segmentalis posterioris pulmonis sinistri.
segmental a. of left lung, posterior basal arteria segmentalis basalis posterior pulmonis sinistri.
segmental a. of left lung, posterior descending ramus descendens arteriae segmentalis posterioris pulmonis sinistri.
segmental a. of left lung, superior arteria segmentalis superior pulmonis sinistri.
segmental a. of liver, anterior arteria segmenti anterioris hepatici.
segmental a. of liver, lateral arteria segmenti lateralis hepatici.
segmental a. of liver, medial arteria segmenti medialis hepatici.
segmental a. of liver, posterior arteria segmenti posterioris hepatici.
segmental medullary a. arteria medullaris segmentalis .
segmental medullary a., great anterior a. of Adamkiewicz.
segmental a. of right lung, anterior arteria segmentalis anterior pulmonis dextri.
segmental a. of right lung, anterior ascending ramus ascendens arteriae segmentalis anterioris pulmonis dextri.
segmental a. of right lung, anterior basal arteria segmentalis basalis anterior pulmonis dextri.
segmental a. of right lung, anterior descending ramus descendens arteriae segmentalis anterioris pulmonis dextri.
segmental a. of right lung, apical arteria segmentalis apicalis pulmonis dextri.
segmental a. of right lung, lateral arteria segmentalis lateralis pulmonis dextri.
segmental a. of right lung, lateral basal arteria segmentalis basalis lateralis pulmonis dextri.
segmental a. of right lung, medial arteria segmentalis medialis pulmonis dextri.
segmental a. of right lung, medial basal arteria segmentalis basalis medialis pulmonis dextri.
segmental a. of right lung, posterior arteria segmentalis posterior pulmonis dextri.
segmental a. of right lung, posterior ascending ramus posterior ascendens arteriae pulmonalis dextrae.
segmental a. of right lung, posterior basal arteria segmentalis basalis posterior pulmonis dextri.
segmental a. of right lung, posterior descending ramus descendens arteriae segmentalis posterioris pulmonis dextri.
segmental a. of right lung, superior arteria segmentalis superior pulmonis dextri.
segmental spinal a. any artery that supplies, or that provides a branch supplying, one or more segments of the spinal cord, including the vertebral, ascending cervical, posterior intercostal, subcostal, iliolumbar, lumbar, and lateral sacral arteries.
septal a's, anterior rami interventriculares septales arteriae coronariae sinistrae.
septal a's, posterior rami interventriculares septales arteriae coronariae dextrae.
sheathed a's arterial branches having spindle-shaped thickenings in their walls (Schweigger-Seidel sheaths) and forming the penicilli of the spleen; called also *ellipsoid* or *sheathed arterioles.*
short circumferential a's arteriae circumferentiales breves.
sigmoid a's arteriae sigmoideae.
sinoatrial nodal a., sinuatrial nodal a., sinus node a. ramus nodi sinuatrialis arteriae coronariae dextrae.
spermatic a., external arteria cremasterica.
spermatic a., internal arteria testicularis.
sphenopalatine a. arteria sphenopalatina.
spinal a. any artery supplying the spinal cord, including the segmental spinal arteries and the anterior and posterior spinal arteries.
spinal a., anterior arteria spinalis anterior.
spinal a., posterior arteria spinalis posterior.
spiral a's, spiral endometrial a's tightly coiled branches of the uterine radial arteries, which supply the endometrium and in pregnancy supply blood to the intervillous space. During the secretory phase of the menstrual cycle they become more prominent; if pregnancy does not occur, they become constricted, with consequent necrosis of the endometrial tissues that results in menstruation.
spiral modiolar a. arteria spiralis modioli.
splenic a. arteria splenica.
sternal a's, posterior rami sternales arteriae thoracicae internae.
sternocleidomastoid a's see *rami sternocleidomastoidei arteriae occipitalis.*
sternocleidomastoid a., superior ramus sternocleidomastoideus arteriae thyroideae superioris.
straight a's of kidney arteriolae rectae renis.
striate a., distal medial arteria striata medialis distalis.
striate a's, lateral arteriae centrales anterolaterales.
striate a's, proximal medial arteriae striatae mediales proximales.
stylomastoid a. arteria stylomastoidea.
subclavian a. arteria subclavia.
subcostal a. arteria subcostalis.
sublingual a. arteria sublingualis.
submental a. arteria submentalis.
subscapular a. arteria subscapularis.
superior a. of cerebellum arteria superior cerebelli.
suprachiasmatic a. arteria suprachiasmatica.
supraduodenal a. arteria supraduodenalis.
suprahyoid a. ramus suprahyoideus arteriae lingualis.
supraoptic a. arteria supraoptica.
supraorbital a. arteria supraorbitalis.
suprarenal a., aortic arteria suprarenalis media.
suprarenal a., inferior arteria suprarenalis inferior.
suprarenal a., middle arteria suprarenalis media.
suprarenal a's, superior arteriae suprarenales superiores.
suprascapular a. arteria suprascapularis.
supratrochlear a. arteria supratrochlearis.
sural a's arteriae surales.
sylvian a. arteria cerebri media.
a. to tail of pancreas arteria caudae pancreatis.
tarsal a., lateral arteria tarsalis lateralis.
tarsal a's, medial arteriae tarsales mediales.
temporal a., anterior 1. arteria temporalis anterior. 2. ramus temporalis anterior arteriae cerebri mediae.
temporal a., anterior deep arteria temporalis profunda anterior.
temporal a's, deep see *arteria temporalis profunda anterior* and *arteria temporalis profunda posterior.*
temporal a., intermediate ramus temporalis medius arteriae cerebri mediae.

Artery *Continued*

temporal a., middle 1. arteria temporalis media (def. 1). 2. ramus temporalis medius arteriae cerebri mediae.
temporal a., polar arteria polaris temporalis.
temporal a., posterior ramus temporalis posterior arteriae cerebri mediae.
temporal a., posterior deep arteria temporalis profunda posterior.
temporal a., superficial arteria temporalis superficialis.
terminal a. 1. end a. 2. an artery that does not divide into branches but is directly continuous with capillaries. Called also *telangion.*
testicular a. arteria testicularis.
thalamogeniculate a. arteria thalamogeniculata.
thalamoperforating a. arteria thalami perforans.
thalamostriate a's, anterolateral arteriae centrales anterolaterales.
thalamostriate a's, anteromedial arteriae centrales anteromediales.
thalamotuberal a. arteria thalamotuberalis.
thoracic a., highest arteria thoracica superior.
thoracic a., internal arteria thoracica interna.
thoracic a., lateral arteria thoracica lateralis.
thoracic a., superior arteria thoracica superior.
thoracicoacromial a., thoracoacromial a. arteria thoracoacromialis.
thoracodorsal a. arteria thoracodorsalis.
thymic a's rami thymici arteriae thoracicae internae.
thyroid a., inferior arteria thyroidea inferior.
thyroid a. of Cruveilhier, inferior ramus cricothyroideus arteriae thyroideae superioris.
thyroid a., lowest arteria thyroidea ima.
thyroid a., superior arteria thyroidea superior.
tibial a., anterior arteria tibialis anterior.
tibial a., posterior arteria tibialis posterior.
tonsillar a. ramus tonsillaris arteriae facialis.
transverse cervical a. arteria transversa cervicis.
transverse a. of face arteria transversa faciei.
transverse a. of neck arteria transversa cervicis.
a. of tuber cinereum arteria tuberis cinerei.
tubo-ovarian a. arteria ovarica.
tympanic a., anterior arteria tympanica anterior.
tympanic a., inferior arteria tympanica inferior.
tympanic a., posterior arteria tympanica posterior.
tympanic a., superior arteria tympanica superior.
ulnar a. arteria ulnaris.
ulnar collateral a., inferior arteria collateralis ulnaris inferior.
ulnar collateral a., superior arteria collateralis ulnaris superior.
umbilical a. arteria umbilicalis.
uncal a. arteria uncalis.
a's of upper limb arteriae membri superioris.
urethral a. arteria urethralis.
uterine a. arteria uterina.
uterine a., aortic arteria ovarica.
vaginal a. arteria vaginalis.
venous a's venae pulmonales.
vermian a., superior arteria vermis superior.
vermiform a. arteria appendicularis.
vertebral a. arteria vertebralis.
vesical a., inferior arteria vesicalis inferior.
vesical a's, superior arteriae vesicales superiores.
vestibular a., anterior arteria vestibularis anterior.
vestibular a., posterior ramus vestibularis posterior arteriae vestibulocochlearis.
vestibulocochlear a. arteria vestibulocochlearis.
vidian a. arteria canalis pterygoidei.
a. of Zinn arteria centralis retinae.
zygomatico-orbital a. arteria zygomaticoorbitalis.

ar·tes·u·nate (ahr-tes′ə-nāt) a derivative of artemisinin, used in combination with amodiaquine or sulfadoxine-pyrimethamine in the treatment of malaria; administered orally, intravenously, or rectally.

ar·thral (ahr′thrəl) articular.

ar·thral·gia (ahr-thral′jə) [*arthr-* + *-algia*] pain in a joint; called also *arthrodynia.* **arthral′gic** *adj*

ar·threc·to·my (ahr-threk′tə-me) [*arthr-* + *-ectomy*] the excision of a joint.

ar·threm·py·e·sis (ahr″threm-pi-e′sis) [*arthr-* + *empyesis*] arthropyosis.

ar·thres·the·sia (ahr″thres-the′zhə) [*arthr-* + *esthesia*] joint sensibility; the perception of joint motions.

ar·thrit·ic (ahr-thrit′ik) 1. pertaining to or affected with arthritis. 2. a person affected with arthritis.

ar·thri·tis (ahr-thri′tis) pl. *arthri′tides* [*arthr-* + *-itis*] inflammation of a joint; see also *rheumatism.*
acute a. arthritis marked by pain, heat, redness, and swelling, due to inflammation, infection, or trauma.
acute rheumatic a. joint tenderness and swelling due to rheumatic fever.
acute suppurative a. septic a.
apatite-associated destructive a. Milwaukee shoulder syndrome.
bacterial a. septic a.
Bekhterev (Bechterew) a. ankylosing spondylitis.
bypass a. arthritis in a person who has undergone an intestinal bypass; it is usually polyarticular and symmetric.
caprine a.-encephalitis see under *encephalitis.*
chronic inflammatory a. inflammation of joints in chronic disorders such as rheumatoid arthritis.
climacteric a. menopausal a.
cricoarytenoid a. inflammation of the cricoarytenoid joint in rheumatoid arthritis; it may cause laryngeal dysfunction and rarely stridor.
crystal a., crystal-induced a. arthritis due to the deposition of inorganic crystalline material within the joints; see *gout* and see *calcium pyrophosphate deposition disease,* under *disease.* Called also *crystal* or *crystal-induced arthropathy.*
a. defor′mans severe destruction of joints, seen in disorders such as rheumatoid arthritis.
degenerative a. osteoarthritis.
enteropathic a. arthritis associated with inflammatory bowel disease or following bacterial infection of the bowel.
exudative a. arthritis with exudate into or about the joint.
facet a., facet joint a. see under *osteoarthritis.*
fungal a., a. fungo′sa mycotic a.
gonococcal a., gonorrheal a. bacterial arthritis occurring secondary to gonorrhea; it is often characterized by migratory polyarthritis associated with erythematous skin lesions and tenosynovitis. It may progress to septic arthritis if untreated.
gouty a. arthritis due to gout.
hemophilic a. bleeding into the joint cavities.
hypertrophic a. osteoarthritis.
infectious a., infective a. arthritis caused by bacteria, rickettsiae, mycoplasmas, viruses, fungi, or parasites. Cf. *septic a.*
Jaccoud a. see under *arthropathy.*
juvenile a. any arthritic condition affecting children under 18 years of age, most commonly juvenile idiopathic arthritis.
juvenile chronic a., juvenile idiopathic a. (JIA), juvenile rheumatoid a. (JRA) rheumatoid arthritis in children, with swelling, tenderness, and pain in one or more joints, which may lead to impaired growth and development, limitation of movement, ankylosis, and flexion contractures. See also *systemic onset juvenile rheumatoid a.*
Lyme a. see under *disease.*
menopausal a. a condition sometimes seen in women at menopause, due to ovarian hormonal deficiency and marked by pain in the small joints, shoulders, elbows, or knees; called also *climacteric a.*
a. mu′tilans a severe deforming polyarthritis with gross bone and cartilage destruction, usually an atypical variant of rheumatoid arthritis.
mycoplasmal a. see under *polyarthritis.*
mycotic a. infectious arthritis secondary to any invasive mycosis, such as coccidioidomycosis, blastomycosis, histoplasmosis, actinomycosis, candidiasis, and sporotrichosis, usually by extension from adjacent bone, and having manifestations similar to those of tuberculous arthritis. Called also *fungal a.* and *a. fungosa.*
navicular a. inflammation of the navicular bursa and the cartilage covering the navicular bone of the foot of a horse.
neuropathic a. neuropathic arthropathy.

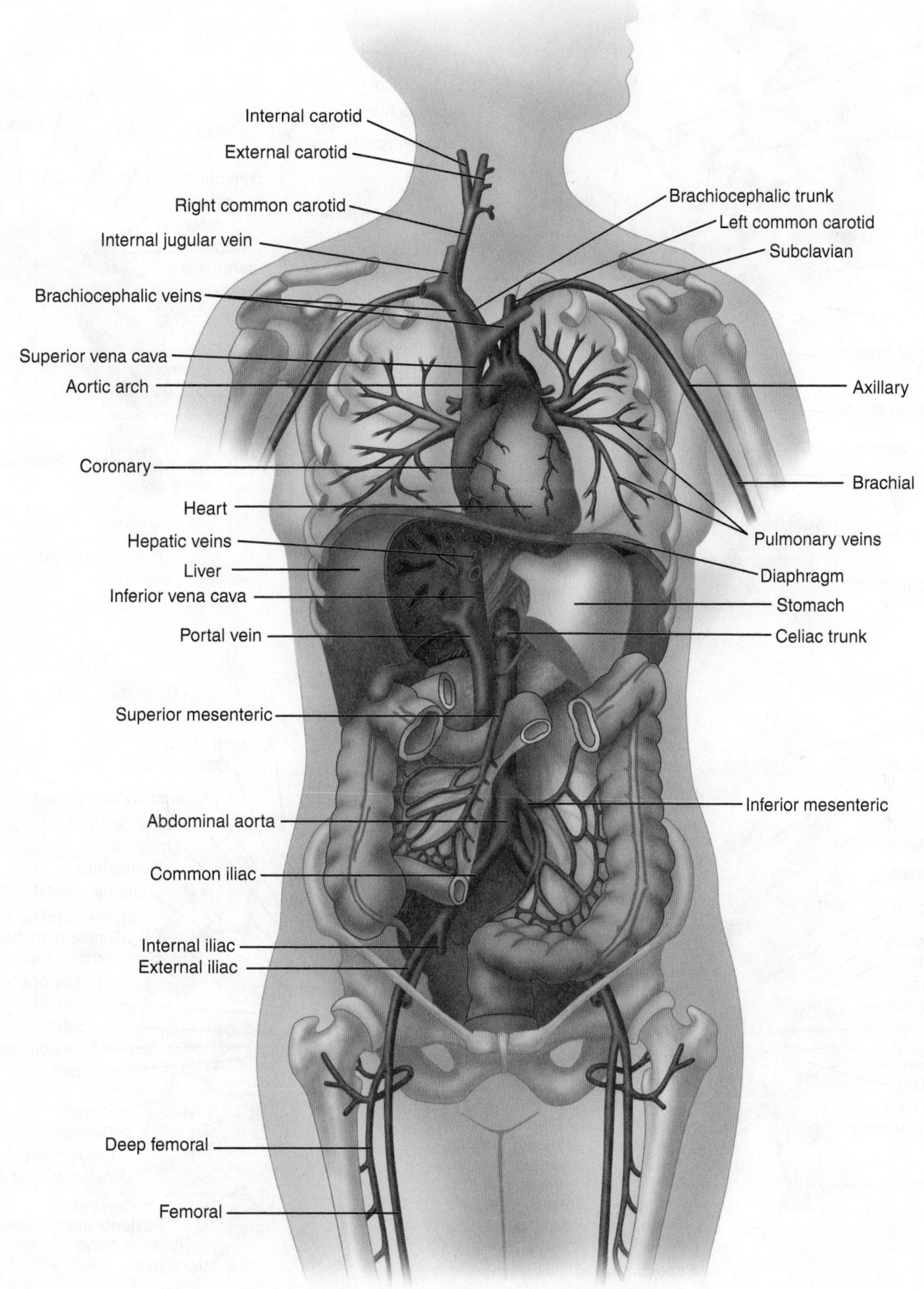

■ **PLATE 1**—PRINCIPAL ARTERIES OF THE BODY AND THE PULMONARY VEINS

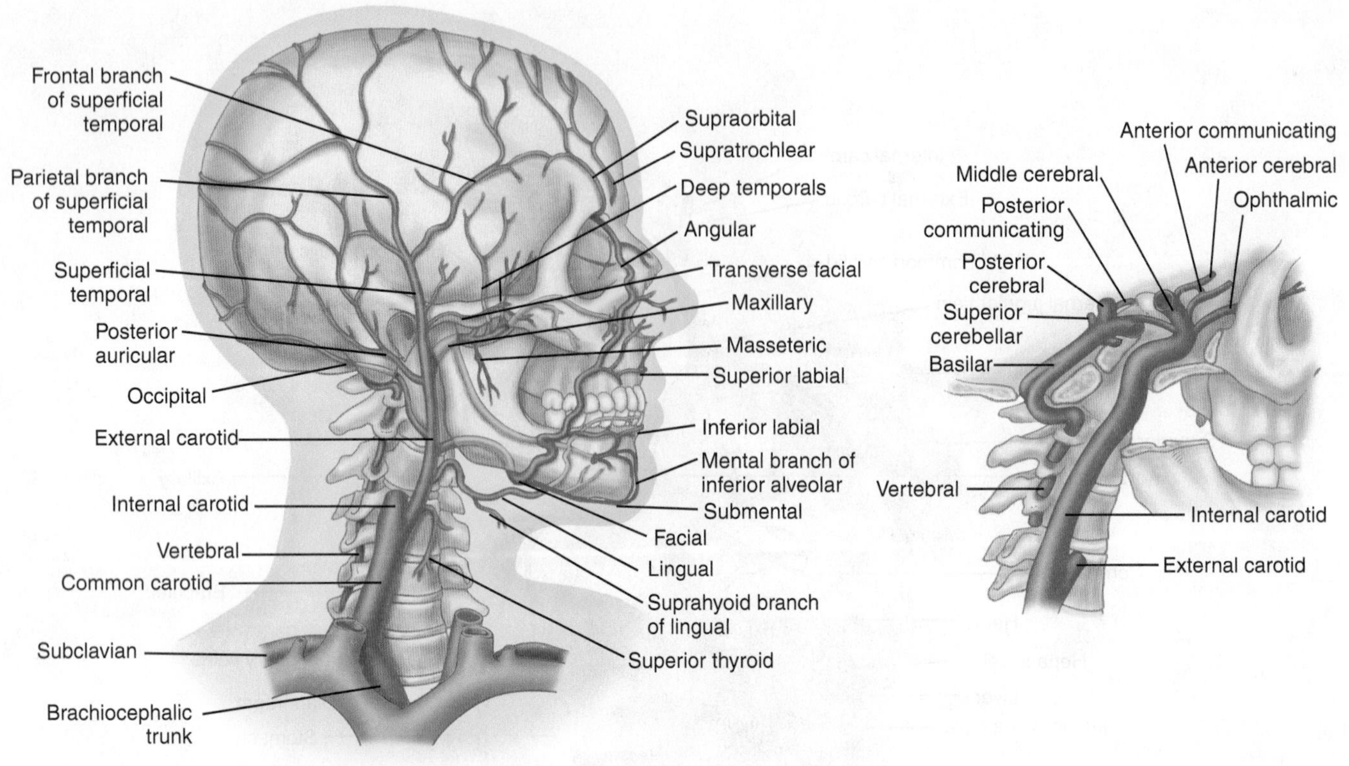

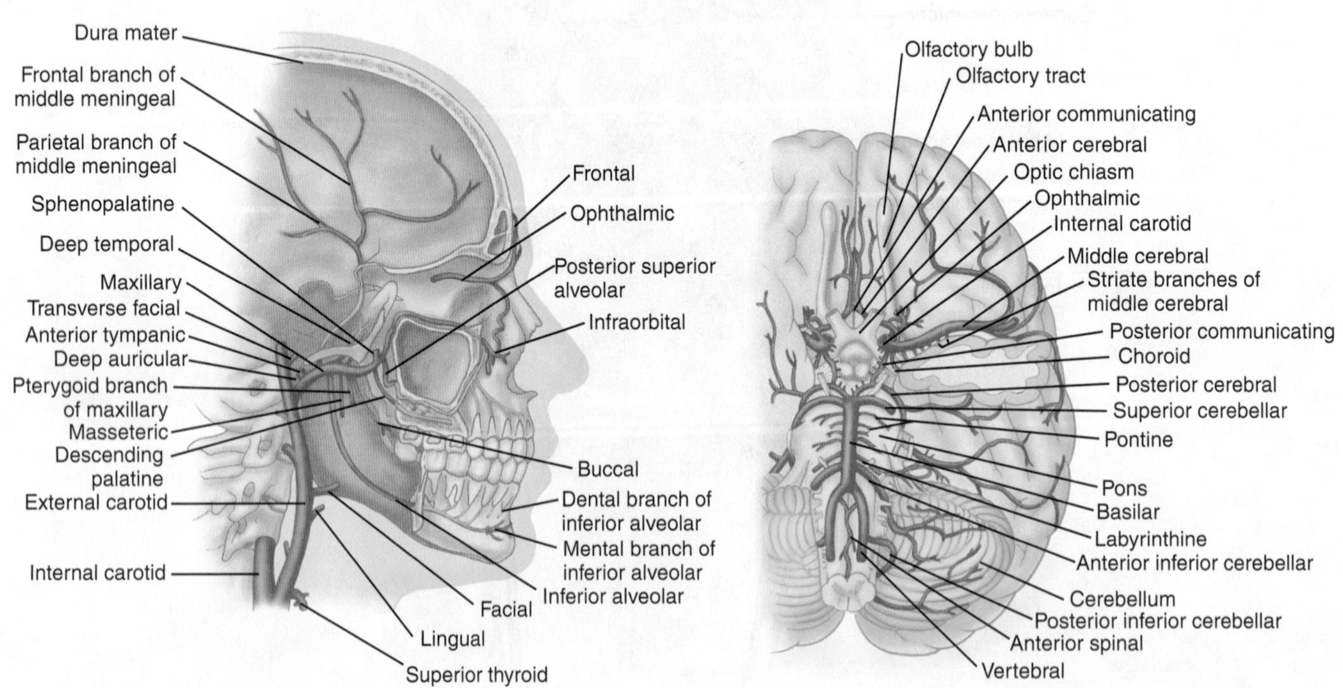

■ **PLATE 2**—ARTERIES OF THE HEAD, NECK, AND BASE OF THE BRAIN

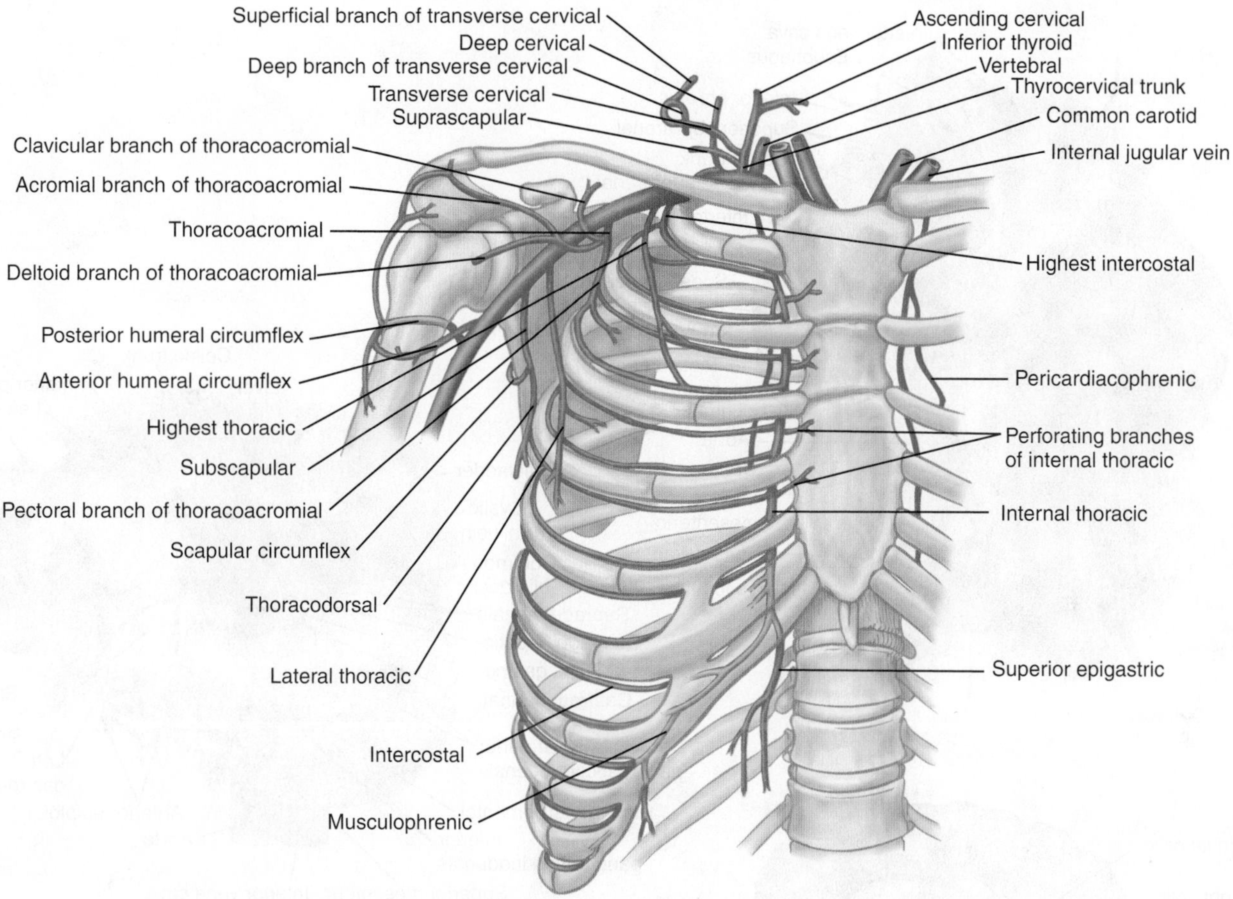

Superficial branch of transverse cervical
Deep cervical
Deep branch of transverse cervical
Transverse cervical
Suprascapular
Clavicular branch of thoracoacromial
Acromial branch of thoracoacromial
Thoracoacromial
Deltoid branch of thoracoacromial
Posterior humeral circumflex
Anterior humeral circumflex
Highest thoracic
Subscapular
Pectoral branch of thoracoacromial
Scapular circumflex
Thoracodorsal
Lateral thoracic
Intercostal
Musculophrenic
Ascending cervical
Inferior thyroid
Vertebral
Thyrocervical trunk
Common carotid
Internal jugular vein
Highest intercostal
Pericardiacophrenic
Perforating branches of internal thoracic
Internal thoracic
Superior epigastric

Ascending cervical
Inferior thyroid
Thyrocervical trunk
Vertebral
Common carotids
Internal jugular vein
Subclavian
Brachiocephalic
Internal thoracic
Brachiocephalic veins
Superior vena cava
Pulmonary
Right coronary
Left coronary
Heart
Aorta
Inferior vena cava
Deep cervical
Suprascapular
Transverse cervical
Deep branch of transverse cervical
Subclavian
Highest intercostal
Thoracoacromial
Highest thoracic
Lateral thoracic
Axillary
Subscapular
Anterior circumflex humeral
Posterior circumflex humeral
Scapular circumflex
Brachial
Intercostal

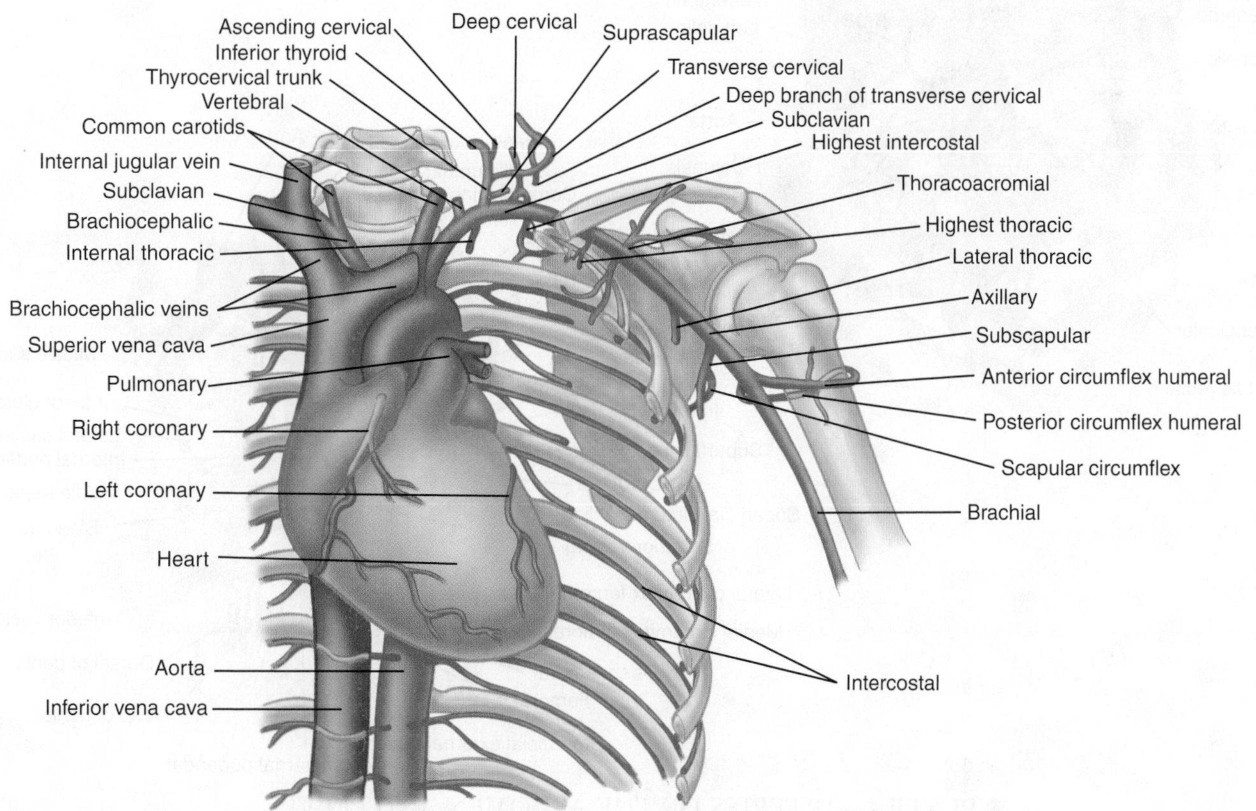

■ **PLATE 3**—ARTERIES OF THE THORAX AND AXILLA

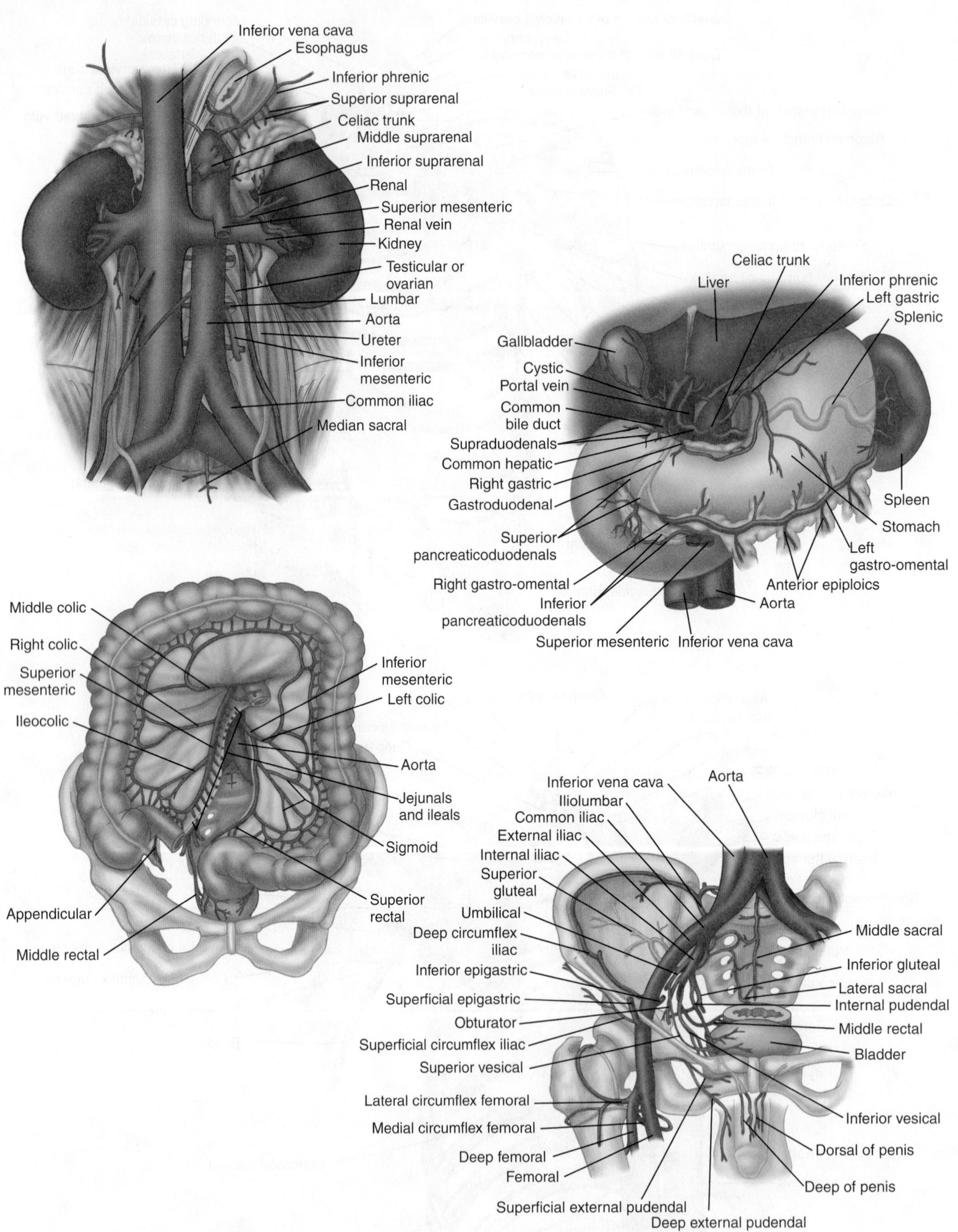

■ **PLATE 4**—ARTERIES OF THE ABDOMEN AND PELVIS

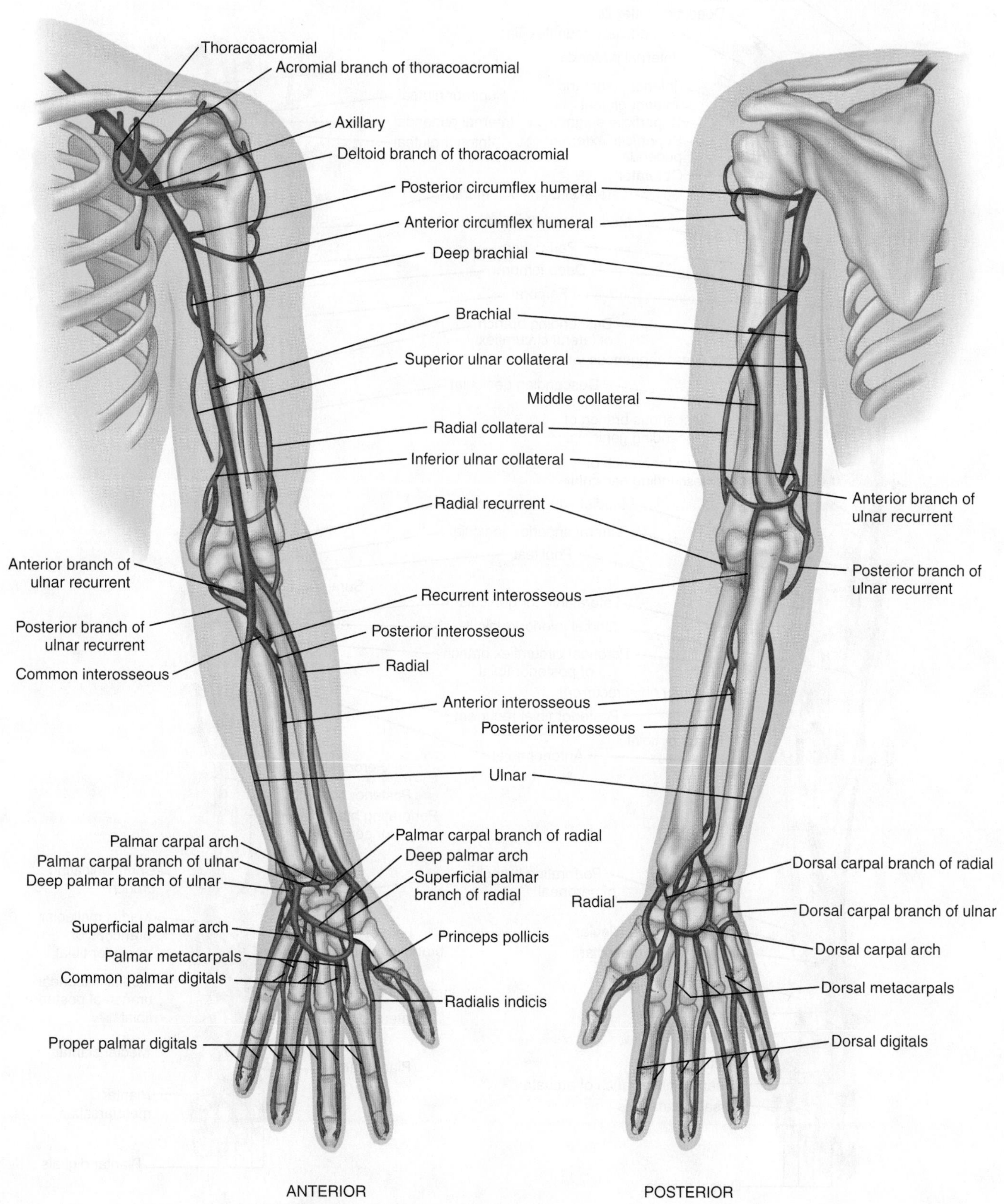

■ **PLATE 5**—ARTERIES OF THE UPPER LIMB

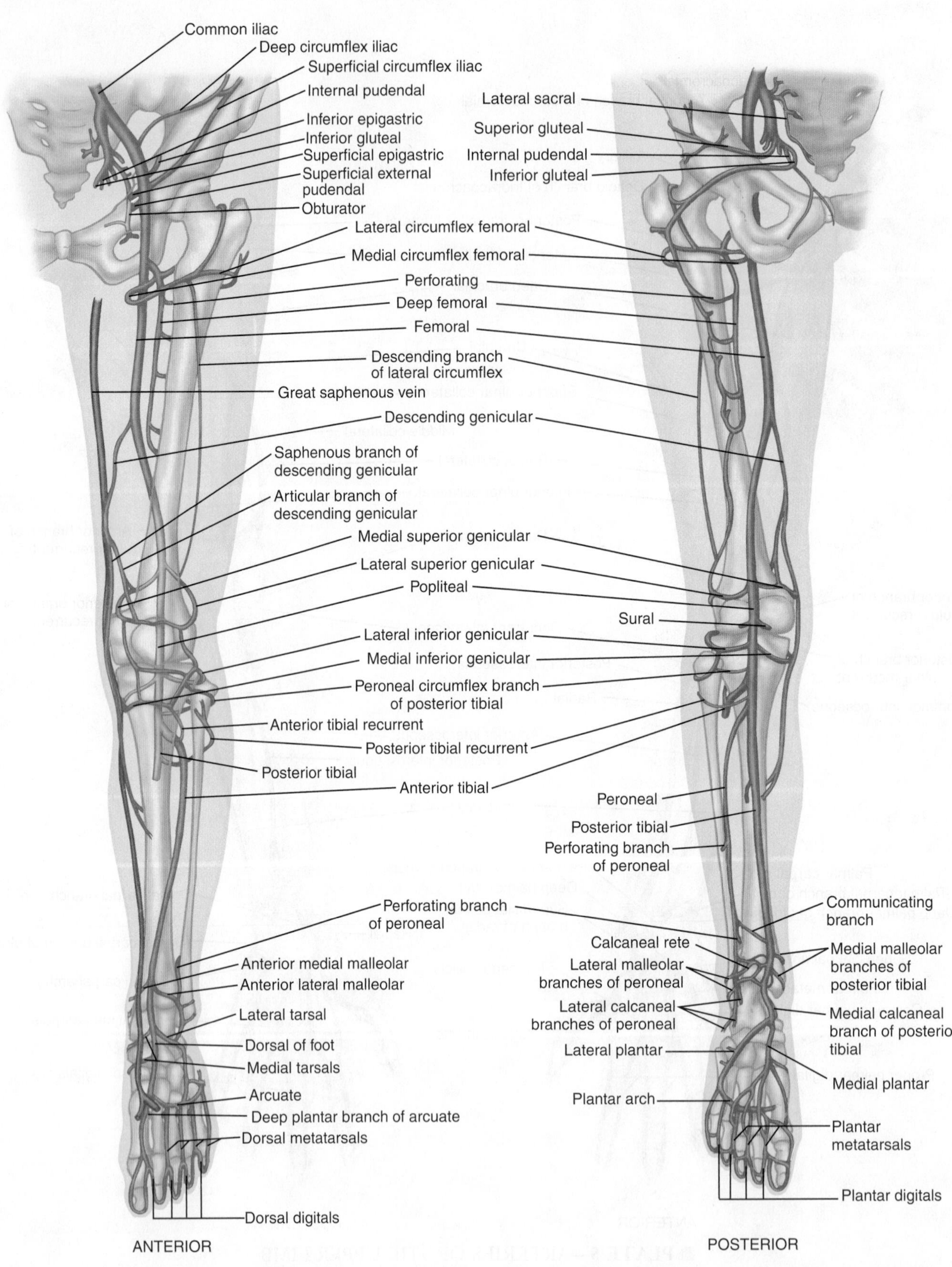

■ **PLATE 6**—ARTERIES OF THE LOWER LIMB

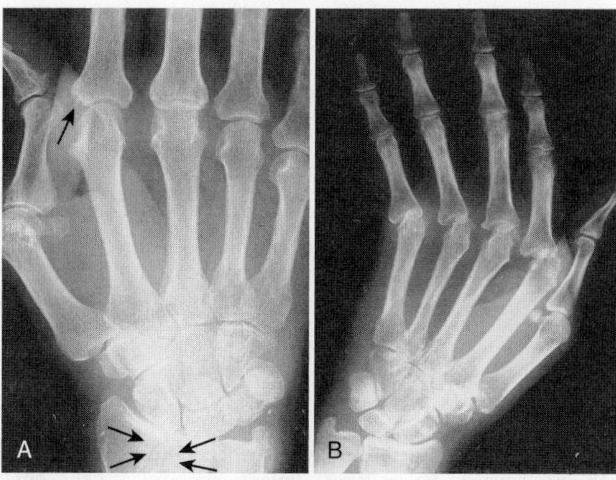

■ Rheumatoid arthritis. *(A)*, Classic findings including narrowing of the carpal joint with subchondral cyst formation *(bottom arrows)* and periarticular erosions of the metacarpophalangeal joints *(top arrow)*. *(B)*, Subluxation and ulnar deviation at the metacarpophalangeal joint, characteristic late changes.

pauciarticular juvenile idiopathic a., pauciarticular juvenile rheumatoid a. juvenile idiopathic arthritis in just a few joints; cf. *oligoarthritis.*

peripheral a. rheumatoid arthritis in the limbs; cf. *spondylarthritis.*

proliferative a. inflammation of joints with proliferation of the synovium, seen in rheumatoid arthritis.

psoriatic a. a syndrome of psoriasis in association with arthritis; rheumatoid factor is usually not present in the serum of affected individuals. Called also *arthritic psoriasis, psoriasis arthropathica,* and *psoriatic arthropathy.*

pyogenic a. septic a.

reactive a. acute aseptic arthritis occurring after bacterial infection of the gastrointestinal or genital tracts or other distant site; it is often characterized by lower limb involvement, psoriasiform lesions of skin and mucous membranes, and eye lesions, but the defining factor is the temporal relation to infection. It usually affects young adults and runs a self-limited but relapsing course. Most patients have increased levels of the histocompatibility antigen HLA-B27. It may represent an abnormal immune response to infection, perhaps with a hereditary susceptibility. Cf. *Reiter syndrome.*

rheumatoid a. a chronic systemic disease primarily of the joints, usually polyarticular, marked by inflammatory changes in the synovial membranes and articular structures and by muscle atrophy and rarefaction of the bones. In late stages deformity and ankylosis develop. The cause is unknown, but autoimmune mechanisms and virus infection have been postulated.

septic a. a type of infectious arthritis, usually acute, characterized by inflammation of synovial membranes with purulent effusion into a joint or joints. It is most often due to *Staphylococcus aureus, Streptococcus pyogenes, S. pneumoniae,* or *Neisseria gonorrhoeae,* usually caused by hematogenous spread from a primary site of infection although joints may also become infected by direct inoculation or local extension. Called also *bacterial, pyogenic,* or *suppurative a.*

spinal a. spondylarthritis.

suppurative a. septic a.

syphilitic a. a rare form of bacterial arthritis occurring as a manifestation of primary, secondary, or tertiary syphilis; types include *neuropathic arthropathy, Clutton joint,* and *Parrot pseudoparalysis.*

systemic onset juvenile idiopathic a., systemic onset juvenile rheumatoid a. a form of juvenile idiopathic arthritis accompanied by systemic manifestations such as spiking fever, transient rash on the trunk and limbs, hepatosplenomegaly, generalized lymphadenopathy, and anemia. Called also *Still disease.*

tuberculous a. bacterial arthritis occurring secondary to tuberculosis; it usually affects a single joint and is characterized by chronic inflammation with effusion and destruction of contiguous bone.

a. urethri′tica, venereal a. Reiter syndrome.

vertebral a. inflammation involving the intervertebral disks.

viral a. infectious arthritis, usually polyarticular and self-limited, associated with a viral disease, such as rubella, mumps, infectious mononucleosis, varicella, hepatitis B, and arboviral or adenoviral infection.

arthr(o)- [Gr. *arthron* joint] a combining form denoting some relationship to a joint or joints.

Ar·thro·bo·trys (ahr″thro-bo′trəs) a genus of Fungi Imperfecti of the form-family Moniliaceae, some of which infect and destroy nematodes.

Ar·thro·bac·ter (ahr′thro-bak″tər) [*arthro-* + *-bacter*] a genus of bacteria of the family Micrococcaceae, consisting of gram-positive, rod-shaped or coccoid cells that may exhibit branching; organisms are obligately aerobic and chemo-organotrophic. Several species have been isolated from clinical specimens and can cause septicemia in immunocompromised persons.

ar·thro·cen·te·sis (ahr″thro-sen-te′sis) puncture and aspiration of a joint.

ar·thro·cha·la·sis (ahr″thro-kal′ə-sis) [*arthro-* + Gr. *chalasis* relaxation] abnormal relaxation or flaccidity of a joint.

a. mul′tiplex conge′nita the arthrochalasis type of Ehlers-Danlos syndrome.

ar·thro·chon·dri·tis (ahr″thro-kon-dri′tis) [*arthro-* + *chondritis*] inflammation of the cartilage of a joint.

ar·thro·cla·sia (ahr″thro-kla′zhə) [*arthro-* + Gr. *klaein* to break] the surgical breaking down of an ankylosis in order to secure free movement in a joint.

ar·thro·co·nid·ium (ahr″thro-kə-nid′e-əm) arthrospore.

Ar·thro·der·ma (ahr″thro-dur′mə) a genus of fungi of the family Gymnoascaceae; the hyphae around the gymnothecium are dichotomously branched, and cells have deep constrictions to give them a dumbbell shape. It has been found to be identical to the former genus *Nannizzia.* This genus contains the perfect (sexual) stages of fungi of genera *Microsporum* and *Trichophyton. A. cajeta′ni* is the sexual stage of *M. cookei* and *A. persi′color* is the sexual stage of *M. persicolor.*

ar·thro·de·sia (ahr″thro-de′zhə) arthrodesis.

ar·thro·de·sis (ahr″thro-de′sis) [*arthro-* + *-desis*] the surgical fixation of a joint by a procedure designed to accomplish fusion of the joint surfaces by promoting the proliferation of bone cells; called also *artificial ankylosis.*

Moberg a. fusion of a finger joint with a small squared bone peg.

triple a. fusion of the subtalar, calcaneocuboid, and talonavicular joints, to provide lateral stability to the paralyzed foot.

ar·thro·dia (ahr-thro′de-ə) [Gr. *arthrōdia* a particular kind of articulation] articulatio plana.

ar·thro·di·al (ahr-thro′de-əl) of the nature of an arthrodia.

ar·thro·dyn·ia (ahr″thro-din′e-ə) [*arthro-* + *-odynia*] arthralgia.

ar·thro·dys·pla·sia (ahr″thro-dis-pla′zhə) [*arthro-* + *dysplasia*] a hereditary condition marked by deformity of various joints.

ar·thro·em·py·e·sis (ahr″thro-em″pi-e′sis) [*arthro-* + *empyesis*] arthropyosis.

ar·thro·en·dos·co·py (ahr″thro-en-dos′ko-pe) arthroscopy.

ar·thro·erei·sis (ahr″thro-ə-ri′sis) [*arthro-* + Gr. *ereisis* a raising up] operative limiting of the motion in a joint that is abnormally mobile from paralysis.

ar·throg·e·nous (ahr-throj′ə-nəs) [*arthro-* + *-genous*] formed as a separate joint, as an arthrogenous spore.

ar·thro·gram (ahr′thro-gram) a radiographic record obtained after introduction of opaque contrast material into a joint.

Ar·thro·graph·is (ahr″thro-graf′is) a genus of Fungi Imperfecti of the form-class Hyphomycetes, form-family Dematiaceae. Some species cause dermatomycosis, and *A. kal′rae* has been found chronically in the sputum of patients with lung disease.

ar·throg·ra·phy (ahr-throg′rə-fe) [*arthro-* + *-graphy*] radiography of a joint after injection of opaque contrast material.

air a. pneumarthrography.

ar·thro·gry·po·sis (ahr″thro-grə-po′sis) [*arthro-* + *gryposis*] persistent flexure or contracture of a joint.

congenital a. congenital articular rigidity.

congenital multiple a., a. mul′tiplex conge′nita a syndrome characterized by congenital immobility of most of the joints, fixed in various postures, with lack of muscle development and growth.

distal a. a clinically and genetically heterogeneous, autosomal dominant condition characterized by contractures of the of the hands and feet, causing severe deformity, with variable involvement of more proximal joints. It may occur alone or in combination with other anomalies, which form the basis for its classification into a number of types. *Type 1,* caused by mutation in the *TPM2* gene (locus: 9p13.2-p13.1), which encodes the β isoform of tropomyosin, is the condition without other anomalies. *Type 2A* is Freeman-Sheldon syndrome; *type 2B* is Sheldon-Hall syndrome; *type 3* is Gordon syndrome (def. 2); *type 7* is trismus-pseudocamptodactyly syndrome; *type 8* is autosomal dominant multiple pterygium syndrome; *type 9* is congenital contractural arachnodactyly.

ar·thro·ka·tad·y·sis (ahr″thro-kə-tad′ə-sis) [*arthro-* + Gr. *katadysis* a falling down] protrusio acetabuli.

ar·thro·lith (ahr′thro-lith) [*arthro-* + *-lith*] a calculous deposit in a joint; cf. *arthrophyte* and *joint mouse.*

ar·thro·li·thi·a·sis (ahr″thro-lĭ-thi′ə-sis) gout.

ar•throl•o•gy (ahr-throl′ə-je) [*arthro-* + *-logy*] the scientific study of the joints and ligaments; also applied to the body of knowledge relating thereto. Called also *syndesmology.*

ar•throl•y•sis (ahr-throl′ə-sis) [*arthro-* + *-lysis*] the operative loosening of adhesions in an ankylosed joint.

ar•thro•men•in•gi•tis (ahr″thro-men″in-ji′tis) synovitis.

ar•throm•e•ter (ahr-throm′ə-tər) [*arthro-* + *-meter*] goniometer.

ar•throm•e•try (ahr-throm′ə-tre) goniometry.

ar•thron•cus (ahr-throng′kəs) [*arthro-* + Gr. *onkos* mass] swelling of a joint.

ar•thro•neu•ral•gia (ahr″thro-nŏŏ-ral′jə) [*arthro-* + *neuralgia*] pain arising in or around a joint.

ar•thro-ony•cho•dys•pla•sia (ahr″thro-on″ə-ko-dis-pla′zhə) onycho-osteodysplasia.

ar•thro-oph•thal•mop•a•thy (ahr″thro-of-thəl-mop′ə-the) an association of degenerative joint disease and eye disease.

hereditary progressive a. an autosomal dominant disorder consisting of myopia progressing to retinal detachment and blindness, and premature degenerative changes in the joints; sensorineural deafness may also occur. Called also *Stickler syndrome.*

ar•thro•pa•thol•o•gy (ahr″thro-pə-thol′ə-je) [*arthro-* + *pathology*] the study of the structural and functional changes produced in the joints by disease.

ar•throp•a•thy (ahr-throp′ə-the) [*arthro-* + *-pathy*] any joint disease. **arthropath′ic** *adj*

calcium pyrophosphate a. calcium pyrophosphate deposition disease.

Charcot a. neuropathic a.

chondrocalcific a. progressive polyarthritis with joint swelling and bony enlargement, most commonly in the small joints of the hand but also affecting other joints, characterized radiographically by narrowing of the joint space with subchondral erosions and sclerosis and frequently chondrocalcinosis.

crystal a., crystal-induced a. see under *arthritis.*

facet a., facet joint a. see under *osteoarthritis.*

hemophilic a. chronic arthropathy in hemophiliacs due to bleeding into a joint followed by inflammation and thickening of the synovial membrane.

inflammatory a. a disease of a joint of inflammatory origin.

Jaccoud a. chronic arthritis occurring after rheumatic fever, usually after repeated attacks, and characterized by fibrous changes in the joint capsules and tendons, leading to deformities that may resemble rheumatoid arthritis (especially ulnar deviation of fingers); the joints may be painful and rheumatic nodules are often present, but erosion of bone does not take place. Called also *Jaccoud arthritis* or *syndrome.*

neurogenic a. neuropathic a.

neuropathic a. chronic progressive degeneration of the stress-bearing portion of a joint, with bizarre hypertrophic changes at the periphery; it is usually a complication of a neurologic disorder such as tabes dorsalis, syringomyelia, or diabetic neuropathy. Loss of sensation leads to relaxation of supporting structures and chronic instability of the joint. Called also *Charcot a., neurogenic a., Charcot disease* or *joint,* and *neuropathic arthritis.*

osteopulmonary a. clubbing of the fingers and toes, enlargement and swelling of the ends of the long bones associated with cardiac and pulmonary disease.

psoriatic a. see under *arthritis.*

pyrophosphate a. calcium pyrophosphate deposition disease (q.v.), particularly the structural joint changes that occur in the disease.

static a. a disturbance in a joint of the extremity secondary to a disturbance in some other joint of the same extremity, as one in the knee joint secondary to one in the hip joint.

syphilitic a. see under *arthritis.*

tabetic a. neuropathic arthropathy (q.v.) occurring in patients with tabes dorsalis.

ar•thro•phy•ma (ahr″thro-fi′mə) [*arthro-* + *phyma*] the swelling of a joint.

ar•thro•phyte (ahr′thro-fit) [*arthro-* + *-phyte*] an abnormal growth in a joint cavity; cf. *arthrolith* and *joint mouse.*

ar•thro•plas•ty (ahr′thro-plas″te) [*arthro-* + *-plasty*] plastic surgery of a joint or of joints; the formation of movable joints. Called also *joint replacement.* **arthroplas′tic** *adj*

abrasion a. arthroplasty with eburnation of one surface with a bur, which induces bleeding and fibrocartilaginous repair tissue to form a new articular surface, done in patients who cannot tolerate other arthroplasty procedures, such as after a first procedure has failed.

Austin Moore a. total hip arthroplasty using an Austin Moore prosthesis.

capsular a. correction of dislocation or deformation of the hip by soft tissue manipulation, curetting of the acetabulum, and muscle transfer but without osteotomy.

Charnley hip a. total hip arthroplasty with insertion of a Charnley prosthesis to form a low-friction joint.

interposition a. surgical correction of ankylosis of the temporomandibular joint by separating the immobile fragment from the mobilized fragment and interposing a substance, such as fascia, cartilage, metal, or plastic, between them.

intracapsular temporomandibular joint a. operative recontouring of the articular surface of the mandibular condyle without the removal of the articular disk.

Thompson a. total hip arthroplasty using a Thompson prosthesis.

total elbow a. arthroplasty of both sides of the elbow joint, with humeral and ulnar components.

total hip a. (THA) arthroplasty of both sides of the hip joint, with acetabular and femoral components.

total joint a. (TJA) arthroplasty in which both sides of a joint are removed and replaced by artificial implants anchored to the bones; the most common joints treated are the hip, knee, elbow, and shoulder. Called also *total joint replacement.*

total knee a. (TKA) arthroplasty of both sides of the knee joint, with tibial, patellar, and femoral components.

ar•thro•pod (ahr′thro-pod) an animal belonging to the Arthropoda. **arthrop′odal, arthrop′odous** *adj*

Ar•throp•o•da (ahr-throp′ə-də) [*arthro-* + Gr. *pous* foot] a phylum of the animal kingdom composed of organisms having a hard, jointed exoskeleton and paired, jointed legs, and including, among other classes, the Arachnida and Insecta. Many species are important medically as parasites or as vectors for disease-causing organisms.

ar•throp•o•dan (ahr-throp′ə-dən) arthropodous.

ar•thro•po•dic (ahr″thro-po′dic) arthropodous.

ar•thro•py•o•sis (ahr″thro-pi-o′sis) [*arthro-* + *pyo-* + *-sis*] the formation of pus in a joint cavity. Called also *arthrempyesis* and *arthroempyesis.*

ar•thro•ri•sis (ahr″thro-ri′sis) arthroereisis.

ar•thro•scle•ro•sis (ahr″thro-sklə-ro′sis) [*arthro-* + *sclerosis* hardening] stiffening or hardening of the joints.

ar•thro•scope (ahr′thro-skōp) [*arthro-* + *-scope*] an endoscope for examining the interior of a joint and for carrying out diagnostic and therapeutic procedures within the joint.

ar•thros•copy (ahr-thros′kə-pe) examination of the interior of a joint with an arthroscope.

ar•thro•sis[1] (ahr-thro′sis) [Gr. *arthrōsis* a jointing] joint; see also *articulatio.*

ar•thro•sis[2] (ahr-thro′sis) [*arthr-* + *-osis*] arthropathy.

ar•thro•spore (ahr′thro-spor) [*arthro-* + *spore*] an asexual fungal spore formed by hyphal segmentation. Called also *arthroconidium.*

ar•thros•to•my (ahr-thros′tə-me) [*arthro-* + *-stomy*] surgical creation of an opening into a joint, as for the purpose of drainage.

ar•thro•syn•o•vi•tis (ahr″thro-sin″o-vi′tis) [*arthro-* + *synovitis*] inflammation of the synovial membrane of a joint.

Ar•thro•tec (ahr′thro-tek) trademark for a combination preparation of diclofenac sodium and misoprostol.

ar•thro•tome (ahr′thro-tōm) [*arthro-* + *-tome*] a knife for incising a joint.

arth•ro•to•mog•ra•phy (ahr″thro-to-mog′rə-fe) tomographic examination of a joint.

ar•throt•o•my (ahr-throt′ə-me) [*arthro-* + *-tomy*] surgical incision of a joint.

ar•thro•tro•pic (ahr″thro-tro′pik) [*arthro-* + *-tropic*] having an affinity for or tending to settle in the joints.

ar•throx•e•sis (ahr-throk′sə-sis) [*arthro-* + Gr. *xesis* scraping] the scraping of diseased tissue from an articular surface.

Ar•thus reaction (phenomenon) (ahr-tūs′) [Nicolas-Maurice *Arthus,* French physiologist, 1862–1945] see under *reaction.*

Ar•thus-type reaction (ahr-tūs′) [N.-M. *Arthus.*] see under *reaction.*

ar•ti•caine hy•dro•chlo•ride (ahr′tĭ-kān″) a local anesthetic used in conjunction with epinephrine in dental procedures or oral surgery to produce infiltration anesthesia or nerve block.

ar•ti•choke (ahr′tĭ-chōk″) [Ar. *al-kharshūf* "the artichoke"] 1. *Cynara scolymus* or its edible immature flower. 2. a preparation of the leaves of *C. scolymus,* having choleretic and diuretic properties, used for dyspepsia and hyperlipidemia.

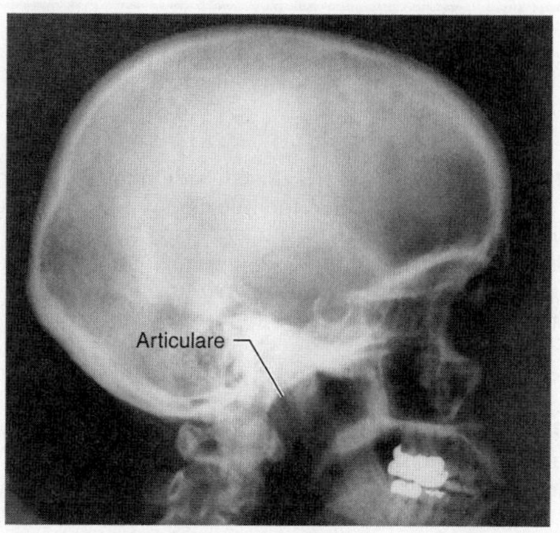

ar•ti•cle (ahr′tĭ-kəl) [L. *articulus* a little joint] an interarticular segment; one of the portions or segments forming a jointed series.

ar•tic•u•lar (ahr-tik′u-lər) [L. *articularis*] of or pertaining to a joint.

ar•tic•u•la•re (ahr-tik″u-lar′e) a craniometric landmark used in radiographic cephalometry, being the point of intersection of the posterior margin of the ascending ramus of the mandible and the shadow of the cranial base, as seen on the lateral x-ray of the head. Called also *point Ar.*

ar•tic•u•late[1] (ahr-tik′u-lāt) [L. *articulatus* jointed] 1. to pronounce clearly and distinctly. 2. to make speech sounds by manipulation of the vocal organs. 3. to express in coherent verbal form. 4. to divide into or to unite so as to form a joint. 5. in dentistry, to adjust or place the teeth in their proper relation to each other in making an artificial denture.

ar•tic•u•late[2] (ahr-tik′u-lət) 1. divided into distinct, meaningful syllables or words. 2. endowed with the power of speech. 3. characterized by the use of clear, meaningful language. 4. divided into or united by joints.

ar•tic•u•lat•ed (ahr-tik′u-lāt″əd) connected by movable joints; consisting of separate segments so joined as to be movable on each other.

ar•tic•u•la•tio (ahr-tik″u-la′she-o) pl. *articulatio′nes* [L.] 1. joint. 2. TA alternative for *junctura synovialis.*

Articulatio

Descriptions of articulations are given on TA terms, and include anglicized names of specific articulations.

a. acromioclavicula′ris [TA] acromioclavicular joint: the joint formed by the acromion of the scapula and the acromial extremity of the clavicle; called also *scapuloclavicular joint.*

a. atlantoaxia′lis latera′lis [TA] lateral atlantoaxial joint: either of a pair of joints, one on each side of the body, formed by the inferior articular surface of the atlas and the superior surface of the axis.

a. atlantoaxia′lis media′na [TA] median atlantoaxial joint: a single joint formed by the two articular facets of the dens of the axis, one in relation with the articular facet on the anterior arch of the atlas, the other in relation with the transverse ligament of the atlas.

a. atlantooccipita′lis [TA] atlanto-occipital joint: either of two joints, each formed by a superior articular pit of the atlas and a condyle of the occipital bone; called also *craniovertebral, occipitoatlantal,* or *Cruveilhier joint.*

a. bicondyla′ris [TA] bicondylar joint: a condylar joint with a meniscus between the articular surfaces, such as the temporomandibular joint.

a. calcaneocuboi′dea [TA] calcaneocuboid joint: one formed between the cuboidal articular surface of the calcaneus and the cuboid bone, forming part of the transverse tarsal joint.

a. ca′pitis cos′tae [TA] joint of head of rib: the junction of the head of the rib with the bodies of two vertebrae, one of the two types of joints between ribs and vertebrae. Called also *capitular* or *costocentral joint.* Cf. *a. costotransversaria.*

articulatio′nes car′pi [TA] carpal joints: any of the joints that connect the carpal bones together, comprising the joints between bones in a given row, distal and proximal; the joint between the distal and proximal rows *(a. mediocarpalis)*; and the joint formed by the pisiform and triquetral bones *(a. ossis pisiformis).* Called also *articulationes intercarpales* [TA alternative] and *intercarpal joints.*

articulatio′nes carpometacarpa′les [TA] carpometacarpal joints: joints formed by the trapezial, trapezoid, capitate, and hamate bones together with the bases of the four medial metacarpal bones.

a. carpometacarpa′lis pol′licis [TA] carpometacarpal joint of thumb: the joint formed by the first metacarpal and the trapezial bones; called also *first carpometacarpal joint.*

articulatio′nes cin′guli mem′bri superio′ris TA alternative for *articulationes cinguli pectoralis.*

articulatio′nes cin′guli pectora′lis [TA] synovial joints of pectoral girdle: the subset of the joints of the pectoral girdle that are specifically synovial, including the acromioclavicular and sternoclavicular joints. Called also *articulationes cinguli membri superioris* [TA alternative].

articulatio′nes colum′nae vertebra′lis [TA] synovial joints of vertebral column: those joints of the vertebral column that are synovial, including the zygapophyseal, lumbosacral, sacrococcygeal, and lateral and median atlantoaxial joints.

a. compo′sita [TA] composite joint: a synovial joint in which more than two bones are involved; called also *compound joint.*

articulatio′nes costochondra′les [TA] costochondral joints: joints between the lateral extremity of each costal cartilage and the sternal ends of the ribs.

a. costotransversa′ria [TA] costotransverse joint: one of the two types of joints between the ribs and vertebrae, being that of the tubercle of the rib with the transverse process of a vertebra. It is lacking for the eleventh and twelfth ribs. Called also *joint of tubercle of rib.* Cf. *a. capitis costae.*

articulatio′nes costovertebra′les [TA] costovertebral joints: the joints between the ribs and vertebrae, of which there are two types: *a. capitis costae* and *a. costotransversaria.*

a. coty′lica [TA] cotyloid joint: a type of ball-and-socket joint.

a. cox′ae [TA] hip joint: the joint formed between the head of the femur and the acetabulum of the hip bone; called also *a. coxofemoralis* [TA alternative], and *coxal, femoral,* or *iliofemoral joint.* Sometimes loosely called *hip* or *coxa.*

a. coxofemora′lis TA alternative for *a. coxae.*

articulatio′nes cra′nii [TA] cranial synovial joints: the temporomandibular joint and the atlanto-occipital joint considered together.

a. cricoarytenoi′dea [TA] cricoarytenoid joint: the synovial joint between the upper border of the cricoid cartilage and the base of the arytenoid cartilage.

a. cricothyroi′dea [TA] cricothyroid joint: the articulation between the lateral aspect of the cricoid cartilage and the inferior horn of the thyroid cartilage.

a. cu′biti [TA] cubital joint: the joint at the elbow where the arm and forearm come together, comprising the humeroulnar, humeroradial, and proximal radioulnar joints; called also *elbow joint.*

a. cuneonavicula′ris [TA] cuneonavicular joint: the joint between the anterior surface of the navicular bone and the proximal ends of the three cuneiform bones.

a. ellipsoi′dea [TA] ellipsoidal joint: a modification of the ball-and-socket joint in which the articular surfaces are ellipsoid rather than spheroid; because of the arrangement of the muscles and ligaments around the joint, all movements are permitted except rotation about a vertical axis. Called also *condylar* or *condyloid joint.*

a. ge′nus [TA] knee joint: the compound joint at the knee, formed between the articular surface of the patella, the condyles and patellar surface of the femur, and the superior articular surface of the tibia.

a. glenohumera′lis TA alternative for *a. humeri.*

Articulatio *Continued*

a. hu′meri [TA] shoulder joint: the joint formed by the head of the humerus and the glenoid cavity of the scapula; called also *a. glenohumeralis* [TA alternative], and *glenohumeral* or *humeral joint.*
a. humeroradia′lis [TA] humeroradial joint: the joint in the elbow region where the capitulum of the humerus meets the radius; called also *brachioradial* or *radiocapitellar joint.*
a. humeroulna′ris [TA] humeroulnar joint: the joint in the elbow region where the humerus meets the ulna.
a. incudomallea′ris [TA] incudomallear joint: the junction of the incus and the malleus; called also *incudomalleolar joint.*
a. incudostapedia′lis [TA] incudostapedial joint: the junction of the incus and the stapes.
articulatio′nes intercarpa′les TA alternative for *articulationes carpi.*
articulatio′nes interchondra′les [TA] interchondral joints: the unions, on either side, between the costal cartilages of the upper false ribs, usually ribs seven through ten; called also *intercostal joints.*
articulatio′nes intercuneifor′mes [TA] intercuneiform joints: the synovial joints between the cuneiform bones.
articulatio′nes intermetacarpa′les [TA] intermetacarpal joints: the joints formed between the adjoining bases of the second, third, fourth, and fifth metacarpal bones.
articulatio′nes intermetatarsa′les [TA] intermetatarsal joints: the joints formed between the adjoining bases of the five metatarsal bones.
articulatio′nes interphalan′geae ma′nus [TA] interphalangeal joints of hand: the hinge joints of the fingers; called also *digital* or *phalangeal joints of hand.*
articulatio′nes interphalan′geae pe′dis [TA] interphalangeal joints of foot: the hinge joints of the toes; called also *digital* or *phalangeal joints of foot.*
a. lumbosacra′lis [TA] lumbosacral joint: the articulation between the sacrum and the lumbar vertebrae; called also *lumbosacral junction.*
articulatio′nes ma′nus [TA] joints of hand: the wrist joint considered together with the carpal, intermetacarpal, interphalangeal, carpometacarpal, and metacarpophalangeal joints.
a. mediocarpa′lis [TA] mediocarpal joint: the joint between distal and proximal rows of carpal bones. Called also *midcarpal joint.*
articulatio′nes mem′bri inferio′ris li′beri [TA] synovial joints of free lower limb: the synovial joints of the thigh, leg, and foot.
articulatio′nes mem′bri superio′ris li′beri [TA] synovial joints of free upper limb: the synovial joints of the arm, forearm, and hand.
articulatio′nes metacarpophalan′geae [TA] metacarpophalangeal joints: joints formed between the heads of the five metacarpal bones and the bases of the corresponding proximal phalanges.
articulatio′nes metatarsophalan′geae [TA] metatarsophalangeal joints: the joints formed between the heads of the five metatarsal bones and the proximal ends of the corresponding phalanges.
articulatio′nes ossiculo′rum audi′tus [TA] joints of auditory ossicles: the incudomallear and incudostapedial joints considered together.
articulatio′nes ossiculo′rum auditorio′rum TA alternative for *articulationes ossiculorum auditus.*
a. os′sis pisifor′mis [TA] joint of pisiform bone: the carpal joint formed by the pisiform and triquetral bones; called also *pisotriquetral joint.*
articulatio′nes pe′dis [TA] joints of foot: the ankle (talocrural) joint considered together with the subtalar, transverse tarsal, cuneonavicular, intercuneiform, tarsometatarsal, intermetatarsal, metatarsophalangeal, and interphalangeal joints.
a. pla′na [TA] plane joint: a type of synovial joint in which the opposed surfaces are flat or only slightly curved; it permits only simple gliding movement, in any direction, within narrow limits imposed by ligaments. Called also *arthrodia* and *arthrodial* or *gliding joint.*
a. radiocarpa′lis [TA] radiocarpal joint: a condylar joint formed by the radius and the articular disk with the scaphoid, lunate, and triquetral bones; called also *wrist joint* or sometimes *wrist.*
a. radioulna′ris dista′lis [TA] distal radioulnar joint: the joint formed by the head of the ulna and the ulnar notch of the radius; called also *inferior radioulnar joint.*
a. radioulna′ris proxima′lis [TA] proximal radioulnar joint: the proximal of the two joints between the radius and the ulna; it enters into pronation and supination of the forearm. Called also *superior radioulnar joint.*
a. sacrococcy′gea [TA] sacrococcygeal joint: the articulation between the coccyx and sacrum.
a. sacroili′aca [TA] sacroiliac joint: the joint formed between the auricular surfaces of the sacrum and ilium; called also *iliosacral joint.*
a. sella′ris [TA] sellar or saddle joint: a type of synovial joint in which the articular surface of one bone is concave in one direction and convex in the direction at right angles to the first (concavoconvex), and the articular surface of the second bone is reciprocally convexoconcave; movement is possible along two main axes at right angles to each other. Called also *ovoid joint.*
a. sim′plex [TA] simple joint: a synovial joint in which only two bones are involved.
a. spheroi′dea [TA] spheroidal joint: a type of synovial joint in which a spheroidal surface on one bone ("ball") moves within a concavity ("socket") on the other bone; it is the most movable type of joint. Called also *ball-and-socket, enarthrodial, multiaxial,* or *polyaxial joint.*
a. sternoclavicula′ris [TA] sternoclavicular joint: the joint formed by the sternal extremity of the clavicle, the clavicular notch of the manubrium of the sternum, and the first costal cartilage.
articulatio′nes sternocosta′les [TA] sternocostal joints: the joints between the costal notches of the sternum and the medial ends of the costal cartilages of the upper seven ribs; called also *costosternal* or *chondrosternal joints.*
a. subtala′ris [TA] subtalar joint: the joint formed between the posterior calcaneal articular surface of the talus and the posterior articular surface of the calcaneus; called also *a. talocalcanea* [TA alternative] and *talocalcaneal joint.*
a. synovia′lis junctura synovialis.
a. talocalca′nea TA alternative for *a. subtalaris.*
a. talocalcaneonavicula′ris [TA] talocalcaneonavicular joint: a joint formed by the head of the talus, the anterior articular surface of the calcaneus, the plantar calcaneonavicular ligament, and the posterior surface of the navicular bone. It forms part of the transverse tarsal joint.
a. talocrura′lis [TA] talocrural joint: the joint formed by the inferior articular and malleolar articular surfaces of the tibia, the malleolar articular surface of the fibula, and the medial malleolar, lateral malleolar, and superior surfaces of the talus. Called also *ankle joint.*
a. tar′si transver′sa [TA] transverse tarsal joint: a joint running across the middle of the foot, comprising the calcaneocuboid and talocalcaneonavicular joints. Called also *Chopart joint.*
articulatio′nes tarsometatarsa′les [TA] tarsometatarsal joints: joints formed by the cuneiform and cuboid bones together with the bases of the metatarsal bones; called also *Lisfranc joints.*
a. temporomandibula′ris [TA] temporomandibular joint: a bicondylar joint formed by the head of the mandible and the mandibular fossa, and the articular tubercle of the temporal bone; called also *mandibular joint.*
articulatio′nes tho′racis [TA] thoracic synovial joints: the costovertebral, sternocostal, costochondral, and interchondral joints.
a. tibiofibula′ris [TA] tibiofibular joint: a plane joint between the lateral condyle of the tibia and the head of the fibula. Called also *proximal* or *superior tibiofibular joint*
a. trochoi′dea [TA] trochoid joint: a type of synovial joint that allows a rotary motion in just one plane; a pivotlike process turns within a ring, or a ring turns on a pivot. Called also *pivot joint.*
articulatio′nes vertebra′les articulationes columnae vertebralis.
articulatio′nes zygapophysia′les [TA] zygapophyseal joints: the articulations between the articular processes of the vertebrae (zygapophyses); called also *facet joints.*

ar•tic•u•la•tion (ahr-tik″u-la′shən) [L. *articulatio*] 1. joint; see also *articulatio*. 2. a place of junction between two different parts or objects. 3. the forming of speech sounds. 4. in dentistry: *(a)* the contact relationship of the occlusal surfaces of the teeth while in action; *(b)* the arrangement of artificial teeth so as to accommodate the various positions of the mouth and to serve the purpose of the natural teeth that they are to replace.

articulator a. the use of a mechanical device that simulates the movements of the temporomandibular joint, permitting the orientation of casts in a manner duplicating or simulating various positions or movements of the mandible.

balanced a. the simultaneous contact between the upper and lower teeth as they glide over each other when the mandible is moved from centric relation to the various eccentric relations and back to centric relation again.

confluent a. a manner of speaking in which the syllables are run together.

ar•tic•u•la•ti•o•nes (ahr-tik″u-la″she-o′nēz) [L.] plural of *articulatio*.

ar•tic•u•la•tor (ahr-tik′u-la″tər) 1. a device for effecting a jointlike union. 2. dental a.

adjustable a. 1. a dental articulator that can be adjusted to permit movement of the casts into recorded eccentric relationships. 2. a dental articulator capable of adjustment to more than one eccentric position.

dental a. a mechanical device that represents the temporomandibular joint and jaws and simulates jaw movements, and to which maxillary and mandibular dental casts may be attached. It is used for the mounting of dental casts for diagnosis, treatment planning, and patient presentation; fabrications of occlusal surfaces for dental restorations; and arrangement of teeth for complete and partial dentures.

semiadjustable a. a dental articulator that can be adjusted so that one movement conforms with a mandibular movement.

ar•tic•u•la•to•ry (ahr-tik′u-lə″to-re) pertaining to utterance.

ar•tic•u•lo (ahr-tik′u-lo) [L., ablative of *articulus*, q.v.] at the moment or crisis of.

a. mor′tis at the moment or point of death.

ar•tic•u•lus (ahr-tik′u-ləs) pl. *artic′uli* [L.] joint.

ar•ti•fact (ahr′tĭ-fakt″) [L. *ars* art + *factum* made] 1. any artificial product. In histology or microscopy, any structure or feature that has been introduced by processing a tissue. In radiology, a substance or structure not naturally present in living tissue, but of which an authentic image appears in a radiograph. 2. distortion or fuzziness of an image caused by manipulation, such as during compression of a digital file.

aliasing a. aliasing (def. 3).

wraparound a. aliasing (def. 3).

ar•ti•fac•ti•tious (ahr′tĭ-fak-tish′əs) having the character of an artifact.

ar•ti•fi•cial (ahr″tĭ-fish′əl) [L. *ars* art + *facere* to make] made by art; not natural or pathological.

Ar•tio•dac•ty•la (ahr″te-o-dak′tə-lə) [Gr. *artios* even + *daktylos* finger] an order of mammals, the ungulates with an even number of toes, including ruminants, pigs, deer, and antelopes. Cf. *Perissodactyla*.

ar•tio•dac•ty•lous (ahr″te-o-dak′tə-ləs) 1. having an even number of digits on the hands or feet. 2. pertaining to Artiodactyla.

Ar•ty•fech•i•nos•to•mum (ahr-tə-fek″ĭ-nos′tə-məm) *Paryphostomum*.

ARVO Association for Research in Vision and Ophthalmology.

ary•ep•i•glot•tic (ar″e-ep″ĭ-glot′ik) arytenoepiglottic.

ary•ep•i•glot•ti•cus (ar″e-ep″ĭ-glot′ĭ-kəs) see under *musculus*.

ary•ep•i•glot•tid•e•an (ar″e-ep″ĭ-glŏ-tid′e-ən) arytenoepiglottic.

aryl (ar′əl) a radical derived from an aromatic compound by removal of a hydrogen atom from the ring. The term can also be used as a prefix.

ar•yl•amine (ar″əl-ə-mēn′) any of a group of amines in which one or more of the hydrogen atoms are replaced by aromatic groups. Some are poisonous or carcinogenic, such as *p*-aminobiphenyl, the anilines, benzidine, and naphthylamine.

ar•yl•di•al•kyl•phos•pha•tase (ar″əl-di-al″kəl-fos′fə-tās) [EC 3.1.8.1] an enzyme of the hydrolase class that catalyzes the hydrolytic cleavage of the phosphoric acid ester from organophosphorus compounds; it is important in the detoxification of organophosphorus insecticides. Called also *paraoxonase*.

ar•yl•es•ter•ase (ar″əl-es′tər-ās) [EC 3.1.1.2] an enzyme of the hydrolase class that catalyzes the hydrolytic cleavage of the ester group from a variety of esterified phenols. The enzyme occurs in normal serum.

ar•yl•for•mam•i•dase (ar″əl-for-mam′ĭ-dās) [EC 3.5.1.9] an enzyme of the hydrolase class that catalyzes the cleavage of formylkynurenine to formate and kynurenine, a step in the catabolism of tryptophan. The enzyme also acts on other formyl aromatic amines.

ar•yl•sul•fa•tase (ar″əl-sul′fə-tās) [EC 3.1.6.1] any of a group of enzymes of the hydrolase class that catalyze the cleavage of sulfate residues from sulfate esters; physiological substrates are generally sulfolipids or sulfated polysaccharides, while in vitro substrates include aryl or alkyl sulfates. Called also *sulfatase*.

a. A cerebroside-sulfatase.

a. B *N*-acetylgalactosamine-4-sulfatase.

a. C an arylsulfatase believed to be identical to steryl-sulfatase.

ar•yl•sul•fa•tase A de•fi•cien•cy (ar″əl-sul′fə-tās) metachromatic leukodystrophy.

ar•yl•sul•fa•tase B de•fi•cien•cy (ar″əl-sul′fə-tās) Maroteaux-Lamy syndrome.

ar•y•te•no•ep•i•glot•tic (ar-it″ə-no-ep″ĭ-glot′ik) [Gr. *arytaina* ladle + *epiglottis*] pertaining to the arytenoid cartilage and to the epiglottis.

ar•y•te•noid (ar″ə-te′noid) [Gr. *arytaina* ladle + *-oid*] shaped like a jug or pitcher, as arytenoid cartilage.

ar•y•te•noid•ec•to•my (ar″ə-te″noid-ek′tə-me) [*arytenoid* + *-ectomy*] surgical removal of an arytenoid cartilage.

ar•y•te•noi•de•us (ar″ə-te-noi′de-əs) [L.] see *musculus arytenoideus obliquus* and *transversus*.

ar•y•te•noi•di•tis (ar-ə-te″noi-di′tis) inflammation of the arytenoid cartilage or muscles.

ar•y•te•noi•do•pexy (ar″ə-te-noi′do-pek″se) [*arytenoid* + *-pexy*] surgical fixation of arytenoid cartilage or muscle.

AS[1] [L.] au′ris sinis′tra (left ear).

AS[2] aortic stenosis; arteriosclerosis.

As arsenic; astigmatism.

ASA acetylsalicylic acid; American Society of Anesthesiologists; American Standards Association; American Surgical Association; American Society on Aging; argininosuccinic acid; antisperm antibody.

5-ASA 5-aminosalicylic acid; see *mesalamine*.

asac•cha•ro•lyt•ic (a-sak″ə-ro-lit′ik) unable to metabolize carbohydrates; microorganisms with this quality have to get energy from non-carbohydrate sources of carbon.

Asa•col (a′ə-kol) trademark for a preparation of mesalamine.

asa•cria (ə-sa′kre-ə) congenital absence of the sacrum.

as•a•fet•i•da (as″ə-fet′ĭ-də) the oily gum-resin obtained from the roots of *Ferula asafoetida* L. and other related species of Umbelliferae; the main odorous principle is isobutylpropanyldisulfide. In parts of Asia it is used as a condiment and food flavoring; former uses include application to animal bandages to prevent bandage chewing, and as a carminative, expectorant, and antispasmodic.

asa•na (ə-sah′nə) [Sanskrit] any of the postures used in hatha yoga for the purpose of achieving balance, promoting physical health, and attaining mental relaxation.

As•a•rum (as′ə-rəm) [Gr. *asaron*] the snakeroots, a genus of herbs found in temperate regions of the Northern Hemisphere.

A. europae′um a species native to Europe and western Siberia; the dried roots are used for bronchitis, bronchial spasms, and bronchial asthma.

ASAS American Society of Abdominal Surgeons.

ASAT aspartate aminotransferase; see *aspartate transaminase*.

ASB American Society of Bacteriologists.

as•bes•ti•form (as-bes′tĭ-form) having a fibrous structure that is or looks like that of asbestos; said of asbestos and substances that resemble it.

as•bes•tos (as-bes′təs) [Gr. *asbestos* unquenchable] any of several fibrous, incombustible materials, forms of magnesium and calcium silicate, used as thermal insulation; the two major types are *amphibole a.* and *serpentine a.* Its dust causes asbestosis and acts as an epigenetic carcinogen for pleural mesothelioma and possibly bronchogenic carcinoma.

amphibole a. one of the two major classes of asbestos, characterized by fibers too brittle to be spun but more resistant to chemicals and heat than the serpentine form. It is less widely used than serpentine asbestos and is thought to be much more carcinogenic. The group includes amosite and crocidolite.

blue a. crocidolite.

brown a. amosite.

chrysotile a. chrysotile.

crocidolite a. crocidolite.

serpentine a. one of the two major classes of asbestos, characterized by strong, flexible fibers that can be spun; it includes chrysotile.

white a. chrysotile.

as•bes•to•sis (as″bes-to′sis) [*asbestos* + *-osis*] a form of pneumoconiosis (silicatosis) caused by inhaling fibers of asbestos, marked by interstitial

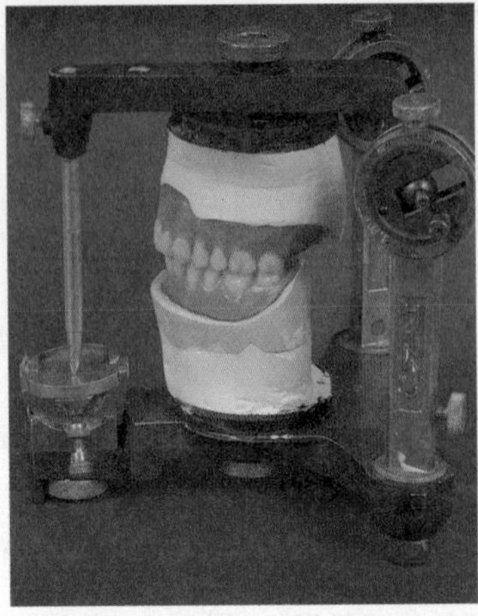

■ Dental articulator with wax-up of dentures.

fibrosis of the lung varying in extent from minor involvement of the basal areas to extensive scarring; it is associated with pleural mesothelioma and bronchogenic carcinoma.

A-scan see under *scan*.

as•ca•ri•a•sis (as″kə-ri′ə-sis) [*ascaris* + *-iasis*] 1. infection by the roundworm *Ascaris lumbricoides*, which is found in the small intestine, causing colicky pains and diarrhea, especially in children. On ingestion, the larvae migrate from the intestine to the lungs, where they cause a pneumonitis, and then to the trachea, esophagus, and intestine, where they mature. If adult worms are present in sufficient number, they may cause intestinal obstruction. 2. infection by any member of the family Ascarididae, usually seen in the intestine, liver, or lungs, .

pulmonary a. *Ascaris* pneumonitis.

as•car•i•cid•al (as-kar″ĭ-si′dəl) destructive to intestinal parasites of the genus *Ascaris*.

as•car•i•cide (as-kar′ĭ-sīd″) [*ascaris* + *-cide*] an agent that destroys worms of the genus *Ascaris*.

as•ca•rid (as′kə-rid) any member of the superfamily Ascaridoidea.

as•car•i•des (as-kar′ĭ-dēz) plural of *ascaris*.

As•ca•rid•ia (as″kə-rid′e-ə) a genus of nematode parasites of the superfamily Ascaridoidea. *A. gal′li* is parasitic in the large intestines of chickens and other birds, causing enteritis and diarrhea. *A. linea′ta* is a common roundworm parasitizing the small intestines of birds in the United States.

as•ca•ri•di•a•sis (as″kə-rĭ-di′ə-sis) ascariasis.

As•ca•ri•di•dae (as-kə-rid′ĭ-de) a family of nematodes that includes the genera *Ascaris*, *Parascaris*, *Toxascaris*, and *Toxocara*. Many species are intestinal parasites in mammals.

As•ca•ri•doi•dea (as″kə-rĭ-doi′de-ə) a superfamily of phasmid nematodes, including the families Ascarididae and Heterakidae.

as•ca•ri•do•sis (as″kə-rĭ-do′sis) ascariasis.

As•ca•ris (as′kə-ris) [L., from Gr. *askaris*] a genus of large intestinal nematode parasites of the family Ascarididae.

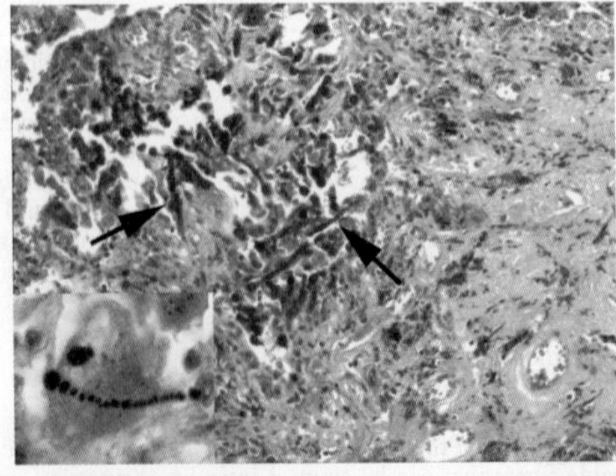

■ Asbestosis specimen showing asbestos fibers *(arrows)* coated with iron to form ferruginous bodies. Alveolar walls demonstrate fibrotic thickening and parenchymal scarring (H & E stain). *(Inset)*, Beaded ferruginous body within a macrophage (Prussian blue stain).

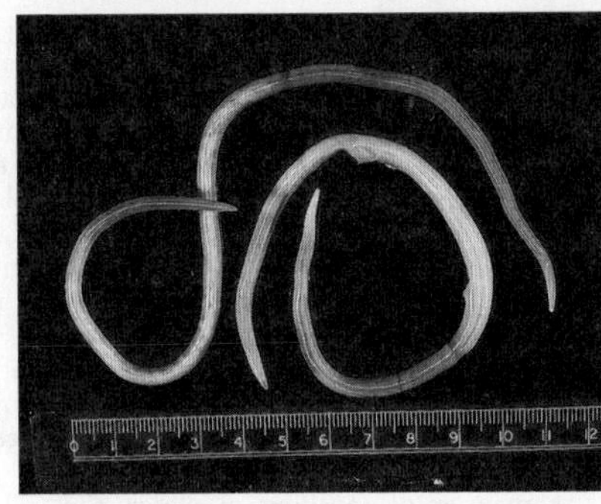

■ *Ascaris lumbricoides*. Adult males are thinner and 15–30 cm long; adult females are thicker and 20–35 cm long.

A. e′qui, **A. equo′rum** *Parascaris equorum*.

A. lumbricoi′des a species parasitic in the intestines and lungs of humans and occasionally pigs. See also *ascariasis* and *Ascaris pneumonitis*.

A. megaloce′phala *Parascaris equorum*.

A. o′vis *A. lumbricoides*.

A. su′is, **A. suil′la**, **A. su′um** a species closely related to *A. lumbricoides*, found in pigs and occasionally humans.

A. vermicula′ris see *Enterobius vermicularis*.

A. vitulo′rum a species found in cattle and the Indian buffalo.

as•ca•ris (as′kə-ris) pl. *asca′rides*. A worm of the genus *Ascaris*.

As•ca•rops (as′kə-rops) a genus of parasitic nematodes of the family Spirocercidae. *A. strongyli′na* is a small red blood-sucking species found in the stomachs of pigs.

as•cend•ing (ə-send′ing) having an upward course.

as•cer•tain•ment (ă″sər-tān′mənt) in genetic studies, the method by which persons with a trait or disease are selected or found by an investigator.

complete a. the method in which families for study are selected through affected parents, and all their offspring are included.

incomplete a. ascertainment in which only those sibships with at least one affected sib are identified; this is far more common than complete ascertainment.

multiple a. a type of incomplete ascertainment in which some sibships are counted more than once because they have more than one affected member; multiplex families (those with more than one affected member) have a higher chance of being ascertained than simplex families.

single a. a type of incomplete ascertainment in which there is no chance that any one sibship will be ascertained more than once; thus there is only one proband in each sibship, and the chance that a sibship will be ascertained is proportional to the number of its affected members.

truncate a. a type of incomplete ascertainment in which any sibship in which there is no affected member is not ascertained.

as•cet•i•cism (ə-set′ĭ-siz-əm) a way of life or character trait described by the elimination of pleasurable effects associated with experiences and characterized by renunciation, self-denial, withdrawal from society, and sometimes dedication to an unattainable ideal or to eradication of some specific evil.

ASCH American Society of Clinical Hypnosis.

Asch forceps, operation, splint (ash) [Morris Joseph *Asch*, American laryngologist, 1833–1902] see under *forceps*, *operation*, and *splint*.

asc•hel•minth (ask′həl-minth) any worm of the phylum Aschelminthes.

Asc•hel•min•thes (ask″həl-minth′ēz) a phylum of unsegmented, bilaterally symmetrical, pseudocoelomate, mostly wormlike animals whose bodies are almost entirely covered with a cuticle; they and possess a complete digestive tract that lacks definite muscular walls. The phylum includes the classes Gastrotricha, Kinorhyncha, Nematoda, Nematomorpha, and Rotifera.

Asch•er syndrome (ahsh′ər) [Karl Wolfgang *Ascher*, Czech-born American ophthalmologist, 1887–1971] see under *syndrome*.

Asch•er•son membrane (ahsh′ər-sən) [Ferdinand Moritz *Ascherson*, German physician, 1798–1879] see under *membrane*.

Asch•ner reflex (phenomenon) (ahsh′nər) [Bernhard *Aschner*, Austrian gynecologist, 1883–1960] oculocardiac reflex.

Asch•off bodies (nodules), cell, node (ahsh′of) [Karl Albert Ludwig *Aschoff*, German pathologist, 1866–1942] see under *body* and *cell*, and see *nodus atrioventricularis*.

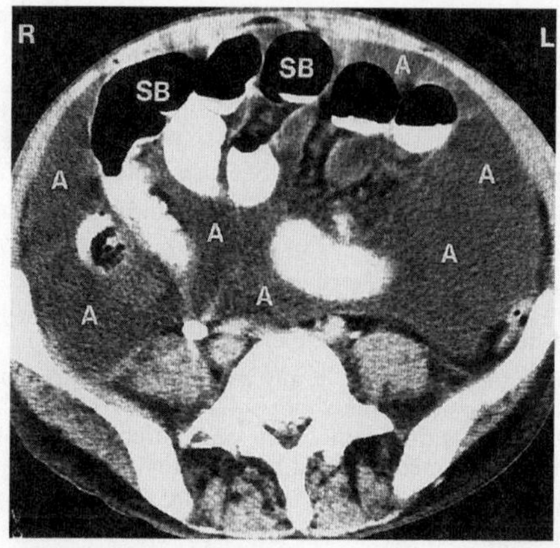

■ Ascites. Transverse CT scan of the abdomen shows the air- and contrast-filled small bowel *(SB)* floating in the ascitic fluid *(A)*.

Asch·off-Ta·wa·ra node (ahsh′of tah-wah′rah) [K.A.L. *Aschoff;* K. Sunao *Tawara,* Japanese pathologist, 1873–1938] nodus atrioventricularis.

ASCI American Society for Clinical Investigation.

as·ci (as′i) plural of *ascus.*

as·ci·tes (ə-si′tēz) [L., from Gr. *askitēs,* from *askos* bag] effusion and accumulation of serous fluid in the abdominal cavity. **ascit′ic** *adj*

bile a., biliary a. choleperitoneum.

bloody a. hemorrhagic a.

chyliform a., a. chylo′sus chylous ascites

chylous a. the presence of chyle in the peritoneal cavity as a result of anomalies, injuries, or obstruction of the thoracic duct. Called also *chyloperitoneum.*

exudative a. low albumin gradient ascites.

fatty a. chylous a.

gelatinous a. pseudomyxoma peritonei.

hemorrhagic a. ascites in which the fluid is mixed with blood.

high albumin gradient a. ascites in which the serum-ascites albumin gradient is equal to or greater than 1.1 g/dL; called also *transudative ascites.*

low albumin gradient a. ascites in which the serum-ascites albumin gradient is less than 1.1 g/dL; called also *exudative ascites.*

milky a. chylous a.

a. prae′cox ascites (usually chylous) that develops prior to edema in constrictive pericarditis.

preagonal a. a flow of serum into the peritoneal cavity just before death.

pseudochylous a. ascites in which the fluid resembles chyle but does not contain fatty matter.

transudative a. high albumin gradient ascites.

as·ci·tog·e·nous (as″ĭ-toj′ə-nəs) causing ascites.

as·cle·pi·a·din (as″klə-pi′ə-din) a toxic bitter principle found in species of *Asclepias.*

As·cle·pi·as (as-kle′pe-əs) [L.] the milkweeds or swallow-worts, a genus of herbs of the family Umbelliferae. Most species are poisonous to animals, containing asclepiadin, volatile oils, cardiac glycosides, or toxic resins.

ASCLS American Society for Clinical Laboratory Science.

ASCO American Society of Clinical Oncology; American Society of Contemporary Ophthalmology.

As·co·bo·la·ceae (as″ko-bo-la′se-e) a family of coprophilic fungi of the order Pezizales; it includes the genus *Ascobolus.*

As·cob·o·lus (as-kob′ə-lus) [*ascus* + *bolus*] a genus of fungi of the family Ascobolaceae that eject their sporangia forcefully; used in genetic studies of crossing over.

as·co·carp (as′ko-kahrp) [Gr. *askos* bag + *carp*] the fruiting body of an ascomycetous fungus, including the asci and ascospores. Types include *apothecium, cleistothecium, gymnothecium,* and *perithecium.* Called also *ascoma.*

as·cog·en·ous (as-koj′ə-nəs) producing asci; said of hyphae.

as·co·go·ni·um (as″ko-go′ne-əm) the receiving (female) organ in ascomycetous fungi which, after fertilization, gives rise to ascogenous hyphae and later to asci and ascospores. Called also *carpogonium* and, in British usage, *archicarp.*

as·co·ma (as-ko′mə) pl. *asco′mata* [Gr. *askōma* the leather padding that protected the opening for the oar] ascocarp.

as·co·my·cete (as″ko-mi′sēt) any individual fungus of the Ascomycotina. **ascomyce′tous** *adj*

As·co·my·ce·tes (as″ko-mi-se′tēz) name given to Ascomycotina when it is considered a class and placed within the phylum Eumycota.

As·co·my·co·ta (as″ko-mi-ko′tə) name given to Ascomycotina when it is considered a separate phylum.

As·co·my·co·ti·na (as″ko-mi″ko-ti′nə) [Gr. *askos* bag + *mykēs* fungus] the sac fungi, a subphylum of perfect fungi variously grouped under either Dikaryomycota or Eumycota, characterized by the formation of an ascus in which sexual spores (ascospores) are produced; it includes the yeasts, mildews, and cheese, jelly, and fruit molds. Some authorities consider this group a class and call it Ascomycetes, whereas others consider it a separate phylum and call it Ascomycota. A number of different classifications of fungi within this group have been proposed.

ascor·bate (ə-skor′bāt) a compound or derivative of ascorbic acid.

as·cor·be·mia (as″kor-be′me-ə) the presence of ascorbic acid in the blood.

ascor·bic ac·id (ə-skor′bik) 1. vitamin C; a water-soluble vitamin found in many fruits and vegetables. Ascorbic acid is required for the optimal function of a number of enzymes; deficiency causes scurvy and poor wound repair. Called also *cevitamic acid.* 2. [USP] a preparation of ascorbic acid used as an antiscorbutic and nutritional supplement, as an adjunct to improve absorption in the treatment of iron deficiency anemia and to improve chelation during deferoxamine therapy for chronic iron toxicity, and for the treatment of methemoglobinemia; administered orally or by intravenous or intramuscular injection. Ascorbic acid is also used as an adjunct in the sodium chromate Cr 51 labeling of red blood cells.

as·corb·uria (as″korb-u′re-ə) the presence of ascorbic acid in the urine.

ascor·byl pal·mi·tate (ə-skor′bəl) [NF] an antioxidant used as a preservative in pharmaceutical preparations.

as·co·spore (as′ko-spor) [Gr. *askos* bag + *spore*] a sexual spore formed within a special sac, or ascus, as in ascomycetous fungi.

ASCP American Society of Clinical Pathologists.

ASCT autologous stem cell transplantation.

as·cus (as′kəs) pl. *as′ci* [Gr. *askos* bag] the sporangium or spore case of certain lichens and fungi, consisting of a single terminal cell. See *Ascomycotina.*

bitunicate a. a cylindrical ascus whose wall has two layers; at maturity, the outer layer splits and the inner layer expands during expulsion of spores. See also *Bitunicatae.*

prototunicate a. a type of ascus that is more or less spherical (as opposed to cylindrical) and has a thin wall that ruptures or disintegrates at maturity to release spores. See also *Prototunicatae.*

unitunicate a. a cylindrical ascus whose wall has a single layer. There are two types: the *operculate* type has a small cap at the end of the ascus, which pops open when the mature organism is ready to eject its spores; and the *inoperculate* type has no cap and ejects its spores through a pore or slit that momentarily opens. See also *Unitunicatae.*

ASCVD arteriosclerotic cardiovascular disease.

-ase a word termination used in forming the names of enzymes, ordinarily affixed to a stem that indicates the substrate, the type of reaction catalyzed, or a combination of these factors.

ase·cre·to·ry (a-se′krə-tor″e) without secretion.

Asel·li pancreas (glands) (ə-sel′e) [Gasparo *Aselli* (or Gaspare Asellio, or Gaspar Asellius), Italian anatomist, 1581–1626] see under *pancreas.*

as·e·ma·sia (as″ə-ma′zhə) [*a-*[1] + Gr. *sēmasia* the giving of a signal] asemia.

ase·mia (a-se′me-ə) [*a-*[1] + Gr. *sēma* sign + *-ia*] aphasia with inability to employ or to understand either speech or signs. Called also *asemasia* and *asymbolia.*

Asen·din (ə-sen′din) trademark for a preparation of amoxapine.

asep·sis (a-sep′sis) [*a-*[1] + *sepsis*] 1. freedom from infection. 2. prevention of contact with microorganisms; see also *aseptic technique,* under *technique.* Called also *sterility.*

asep·tic (a-sep′tik) [*a-*[1] + Gr. *sēpsis* decay] free from infection or septic material; called also *sterile.*

a.-antiseptic both aseptic and antiseptic.

asep·ti·cism (a-sep′tĭ-siz-əm) the principles and practices of aseptic techniques.

as·e·ta·ke (as″e-tak′e) any of various poisonous Japanese mushrooms of the genus *Hebeloma.*

asex·u·al (a-sek′shoo-əl) having no sex; not sexual; not pertaining to sex. Called also *agamous.*

asex•u•al•i•ty (a″seks-u-al′ĭ-te) the state of being asexual; absence of sexual interests.

ASF a synthetic resin composed of aniline, formaldehyde, and sulfur, used for mounting microscopic objects.

ASGE American Society for Gastrointestinal Endoscopy.

ASH American Society of Hematology; asymmetrical septal hypertrophy.

ash (ash) 1. the incombustible residue remaining after any process of incineration. 2. any tree of the genus *Fraxinus*.

ASHA American School Health Association; American Speech and Hearing Association.

ASHD arteriosclerotic heart disease; see *ischemic heart disease*, under *disease*.

Ash•er•man syndrome (ash′ər-mən) [Joseph G. *Asherman*, Czechoslovakian-born physician in Israel, 20th century] see under *syndrome*.

Ash•er•son syndrome (ash′ər-sən) [Nehemiah *Asherson*, English otorhinolaryngologist, 1897–1989] see under *syndrome*.

ASHP American Society of Hospital Pharmacists.

ash•wa•gan•dha (ahsh″wah-gahn′də) 1. *Withania somnifera*. 2. a preparation of the roots of *W. somnifera*, used in ayurveda as a rejuvenative and sedative.

ASI Addiction Severity Index.

ASIA American Spinal Injury Association.

asi•a•lia (a″si-a′le-ə) [*a-*[1] + Gr. *sialon* spittle] aptyalism.

asi•a•lo (a-si″ə-lo) [*a-*[1] + *sialo*] lacking a sialic acid group, as do certain sphingolipids.

asi•at•i•co•side (a″zhe-at′ĭ-ko-sīd″) the active principle of the umbelliferous plant *Centella asiatica* L., which has been used for various dermatological conditions, including wounds and burns.

asid•er•o•sis (a″sid-ər-o′sis) [*a-*[1] + *sider-* + *-sis*] abnormal decrease of the iron reserve of the body.

ASII American Science Information Institute.

ASIM American Society of Internal Medicine.

Asim•i•na (ə-sim′ĭ-nə) [L., from Algonquian] a genus of North American trees and shrubs of the family Annonaceae. *A. trilo′ba* (L.) Dunal is the papaw or pawpaw.

asim•i•nine (ə-sim′ĭ-nin) an alkaloid from the seeds of *Asimina triloba*.

-asis [Gr.] a word termination denoting an action, process, or condition; see also *-sis*.

asit•ia (ə-sish′e-ə) [*a-*[1] + *sit-* + *-ia*] anorexia.

As•ka•na•zy cells (as′kə-nah″ze) [Max *Askanazy*, German pathologist, 1865–1940] see under *cell*.

As•kin tumor (as′kin) [Frederic Barton *Askin*, American pathologist, 20th century] see under *tumor*.

As•kle•pi•os (as-kle′pe-əs) [Gr.] see *Aesculapius*.

Ask-Up•mark kidney (ahsk′-up′mahrk) [Erik *Ask-Upmark*, Swedish physician, 1901–1985] see under *kidney*.

ASL antistreptolysin.

ASM American Society for Microbiology.

ASN American Society of Nephrology.

Asn asparagine.

ASO arteriosclerosis obliterans.

aso•ma (a-so′mə) pl. *aso′mata* [*a-*[1] + *soma*] a fetus with an imperfect head and the merest rudiments of a trunk.

aso•ma•tog•no•sia (ə-so″mə-tog-no′zhə) lack of awareness of the condition of all or part of one's body; lack of somatognosis. Cf. *amorphosynthesis* and *anosognosia*.

aso•ma•to•phyte (a-so′mə-to-fīt″) [*a-*[1] + *somato-* + *-phyte*] a plant in which there is no distinction between body and reproductive cells.

Aso•pia (ə-so′pe-ə) a genus of pyralid moths. *A. farina′lis* is a meal moth that acts as the intermediate host of the tapeworm *Hymenolepis diminuta*.

ASP American Society of Parasitologists.

Asp aspartic acid.

as•pal•a•so•ma (as″pal-ə-so′mə) [Gr. *aspalax* mole + *soma*] a fetus with lateral or median abdominal eventration and other deformities.

as•par•a•gin•ase (as-par′ə-jin-ās″) 1. [EC 3.5.1.1] an enzyme of the hydrolase class that catalyzes the hydrolytic deamination of asparagine to form aspartate, a step in the degradation of asparagine. 2. a preparation of this enzyme isolated from *Escherichia coli* and used in the treatment of acute lymphoblastic leukemia, primarily in pediatric patients, to reduce availability of asparagine to tumor cells; administered intravenously or intramuscularly.

as•par•a•gine (ə-spar′ə-jēn, ə-spar′ə-jin) [Gr. *asparagos* asparagus] a nonessential amino acid that is the β-amide of aspartic acid. It is found in most plants, and has diuretic properties. It is used as a culture medium for certain bacteria. Symbols Asn and N. See also table at *amino acid*.

as•par•a•gin•yl (as-par′ə-jin″əl) the acyl radical of asparagine.

As•par•a•gus (ə-spar′ə-gəs) a genus of perennial Old World herbs of the family Liliaceae having erect, many-branched stems, scalelike leaves, and small flowers; the shoots of *A. officina′lis* are used for food and its roots, rhizome, and herb are used medicinally.

as•par•a•gus (ə-spar′ə-gəs) 1. any plant of the genus *Asparagus*, especially *A. officinalis* or its edible shoots. 2. a preparation of *A. officinalis*, particularly the root and rhizome, used as a diuretic; the root is also used in traditional Chinese medicine and homeopathy.

as•par•tame (ə-spahr′tām, as′pahr-tām″) [NF] an artificial sweetener about 200 times as sweet as sucrose and used as a low-calorie sweetener.

as•par•tate (ə-spahr′tāt) a salt of aspartic acid, or aspartic acid in dissociated form.

as•par•tate ami•no•trans•fer•ase (ə-spahr′tāt ə-me″no-trans′fər-ās) aspartate transaminase.

as•par•tate car•bam•o•yl•trans•fer•ase (ə-spahr′tāt kahr-bam″o-əl-trans′fər-ās) [EC 2.1.3.2] an enzyme activity of the trifunctional CAD protein; it is a transferase that catalyzes the formation of carbamoylaspartate from carbamoyl phosphate and aspartate in the first committed step in pyrimidine biosynthesis. Called also *aspartate transcarbamoylase*.

as•par•tate trans•am•i•nase (AST, ASAT) (ə-spahr′tāt trans-am′ĭ-nās) [EC 2.6.1.1] an enzyme of the transferase class that catalyzes the reversible transfer of an amino group from aspartate to α-ketoglutarate to form glutamate and oxaloacetate, with pyridoxal phosphate required as a cofactor. The enzyme is present in most eukaryotic cells, occurring as distinct isozymes in mitochondria and cytosol. Both isozymes participate in the malate-aspartate shuttle, and in the liver the reaction transfers excess metabolic nitrogen into aspartate for disposal via the urea cycle. The serum level of aspartate transaminase (SGOT) and that of other transaminases are frequently elevated in a variety of disorders causing tissue damage (e.g., myocardial infarction). Called also *aspartate aminotransferase* and *glutamic-oxaloacetic transaminase (GOT)*.

as•par•tate trans•car•bam•oyl•ase (ə-spahr′tāt trans″kahr-bam′o-əl-ās) aspartate carbamoyltransferase.

as•par•thi•one (ə-spahr′thi-ōn″) a tripeptide analogous to glutathione but containing aspartic acid in place of glutamic acid.

as•par•tic ac•id (ə-spahr′tik) 1. a nonessential amino acid, aminosuccinic acid, occurring in proteins; it is also an excitatory neurotransmitter in the central nervous system. Symbols Asp and D. See also table at *amino acid*. 2. [USP] a preparation of aspartic acid used as a dietary supplement.

as•par•tic en•do•pep•ti•dase (ə-spahr′tik en″do-pep′tĭ-dās) [EC 3.4.23] any member of the group of endopeptidases that have an acidic residue involved in the catalytic process and so have a pH optimum below 5.

as•par•tyl (ə-spahr′təl) the acyl radical of aspartic acid.

as•par•tyl•glu•co•sa•mine (ə-spahr″təl-gloo-kōs′ə-mēn) *N*-acetylglucosamine in *N*-glycosidic linkage with the amino group of asparagine; it is an intermediate in the degradation of glycoproteins and accumulates abnormally in aspartylglycosaminuria.

as•par•tyl•glu•co•sa•min•i•dase (ə-spahr″təl-gloo-kōs″ə-min′ĭ-dās) a lysosomal enzyme of the hydrolase class that catalyzes the cleavage of *N*-glycosidic linkages between *N*-acetylglucosamine and asparagine in glycoproteins, a step in the degradation of glycoproteins. Deficiency of the enzyme, an autosomal recessive trait, causes aspartylglycosaminuria. In official nomenclature, called *N^4-(β-N-acetylglucosaminyl)-L--asparaginase* [EC 3.5.1.26].

as•par•tyl•glu•co•sa•min•uria (ə-spahr″təl-gloo″kōs-am″in-u′re-ə) a severe autosomal recessive lysosomal storage disease caused mutations in the *AGA* gene (locus: 4q32-q33), which encodes aspartylglucosaminidase. The disorder is preceded by diarrhea and frequent infections in infancy, with later onset of severe mental retardation, coarsening of features, lens opacity, and skeletal dysplasia, as well as storage and urinary excretion of abnormal levels of aspartylglucosamine and related glycopeptides. Called also *aspartylglycosaminuria*.

as•par•tyl•gly•cos•amin•i•dase (ə-spahr″təl-gli-kōs″ə-min′ĭ-dās) N^4-(β-*N*-acetylglucosaminyl)-L-asparaginase; see *aspartylglucosaminidase*.

as•par•tyl•gly•cos•a•mi•nu•ria (ə-spahr′təl-gli′kōs-ə-min-u′re-ə) aspartylglucosaminuria.

aspe•cif•ic (a″spə-sif′ik) nonspecific.

as•pect (as′pekt) [L. *aspectus*, from *aspicere* to look toward] 1. that part of a surface facing in some designated direction. 2. the look or appearance.

anterior a. the surface of a body viewed from the front; in humans this is a synonym of *ventral aspect.*

anterior a. of cranium norma facialis.

dorsal a. in humans, the posterior aspect. In quadrupeds, the surface viewed from a superior direction.

facial a. of cranium, frontal a. of cranium norma facialis.

inferior a. of cranium norma inferior.

lateral a. of cranium norma lateralis.

occipital a. of cranium norma occipitalis.

posterior a. the surface of a body viewed from the back; in humans this is a synonym of *dorsal aspect.*

sagittal a. of cranium norma sagittalis.

superior a. of cranium norma superior.

temporal a. of cranium norma lateralis.

ventral a. in humans, the anterior aspect. In quadrupeds, the surface viewed from an inferior direction.

vertical a. of cranium norma superior.

As•per•ger syndrome (ahs′pər-gər) [Hans *Asperger*, Austrian psychiatrist, 1906–1980] see under *syndrome.*

as•per•gil•lar (as″pər-jil′ər) pertaining to or caused by *Aspergillus.*

as•per•gil•li (as″pər-jil′i) plural of *aspergillus.*

as•per•gil•lo•ma (as″pər-jil-o′mə) the most common kind of fungus ball, formed by colonization of *Aspergillus* in a bronchus or lung cavity.

as•per•gil•lo•my•co•sis (as″pər-jil″o-mi-ko′sis) aspergillosis.

as•per•gil•lo•sis (as″pər-jil-o′sis) infection by species of *Aspergillus*, marked by inflammatory granulomatous lesions in the skin, ear, orbit, nasal sinuses, lungs, and sometimes the bones and meninges; called also *aspergillomycosis.*

allergic a. an allergic reaction to *Aspergillus* in body passages or orifices, such as the bronchi and lungs in atopic asthma. Species commonly implicated include *A. clava′tus, A. fla′vus, A. fumiga′tus, A. ni′dulans, A. ni′ger*, and *A. ter′reus.* See also *malt worker's lung*, under *lung.*

allergic bronchopulmonary a. bronchopulmonary a. accompanied by allergic (immunologic) symptoms in the bronchi, often with expectoration of yellow or brown bronchial plugs composed of eosinophils and fungal hyphae. It is frequently seen in patients with asthma or cystic fibrosis and may progress to bronchiectasis or bronchocentric granulomatosis.

aural a. *Aspergillus* otomycosis.

bronchopneumonic a., bronchopulmonary a. infection of the bronchi and lungs by species of *Aspergillus*; subtypes include *allergic bronchopulmonary a., chronic necrotizing a., invasive a.*, and *aspergilloma.* Called also *bronchoaspergillosis.*

cerebral a. invasion of the central nervous system by a species of *Aspergillus*, seen most often in immunocompromised persons; symptoms include delirium and seizures. Called also *neuroaspergillosis.*

chronic necrotizing a. a slowly progressive invasive type of aspergillosis seen in patients with severe lung disease such as chronic obstructive pulmonary disease, often in diabetics or the immunocompromised. Characteristics include cavitary infiltration that may extend into the pleura and sometimes fungus balls in the cavities.

invasive a. a frequently fatal type of bronchopulmonary aspergillosis seen in immunocompromised or debilitated patients, characterized by fungal invasion of the tissues. In lung involvement, there is pneumonia with dyspnea, coughing, and hemoptysis. Invasion of blood vessels can lead to infarction of tissues supplied by the vessels. Less often, the fungus invades the central nervous system and may cause seizures.

pulmonary a. infection of the lungs with *Aspergillus*; an acute invasive form is sometimes seen in immunocompromised patients, characterized by pulmonary infiltration and often pulmonary vascular involvement, necrosis, cavitation, areas of hemorrhagic pulmonary infarction, and sometimes aspergillomas that may impede air flow. Cf. *Aspergillus pneumonia.*

as•per•gil•lo•tox•i•co•sis (as″pər-jil″o-tok″sĭ-ko′sis) any mycotoxicosis caused by *Aspergillus* species, such as those containing aflatoxin, citrinin, ochratoxin A, patulin, or sterigmatocystin. Called also *aspergillustoxicosis.*

As•per•gil•lus (as″pər-jil′əs) [L. *aspergere* to scatter] a genus of Fungi Imperfecti of the form-class Hyphomycetes, form-family Moniliaceae. When found, the perfect, or sexual, stage is classified with the ascomycetous fungi in the family Trichocomaceae. This genus includes several common molds and some that are opportunistic pathogens and is characterized by elongated conidiophores thickly set with chains of basipetally formed conidia. See also illustration at *mold.*

A. amsteloda′mi a species with blue to green conidial heads, found in nasal and occasionally cerebral infections.

A. clava′tus a species with blue or green conidial heads, found in soils and manure; inhalation of its spores in contaminated barley dust causes malt worker's lung. Its cultures produce the toxic antibacterial substance patulin.

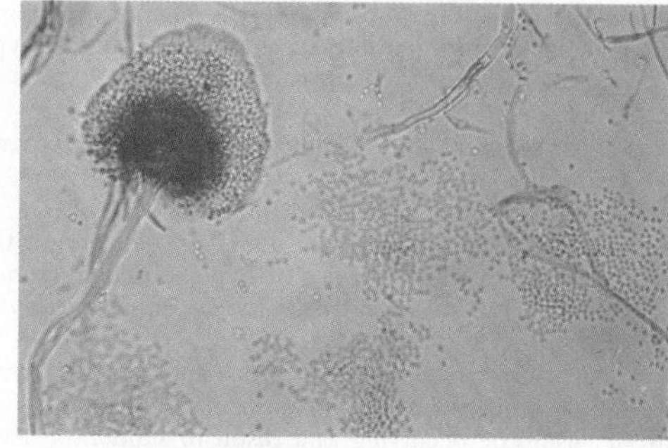

■ *Aspergillus.* Hyphae and a conidiophore.

A. fische′ri a thermophilic soil fungus, occasionally found in ear or lung infections.

A. fla′vus a species with yellow or yellow-green conidial heads, usually found on corn, peanuts, or grain; it contains aflatoxin and causes aflatoxicosis. It can also cause allergic aspergillosis, eumycotic mycetoma, and lung disease, and in weak or immunocompromised patients it can cause disseminated forms of aspergillosis.

A. fumiga′tus a thermotolerant species with blue or green conidial heads, usually found growing in soils and manure. It can cause infections of the ear, nose, lungs and other organs, and in birds it can cause brooder pneumonia. Inhalation of its spores in contaminated barley dust causes malt worker's lung. Its cultures produce various antibiotics, such as gliotoxin.

A. gigan′teus a species that contains the carcinogenic mycotoxin patulin.

A. glau′cus a group of species of bluish molds common on dry and decaying vegetation and sometimes found in otomycosis or infections of the nasal passages, lungs, or other parts of the body.

A. ni′dulans a species common in soil and sometimes isolated from onychomycosis, maduromycosis, eumycotic mycetoma, and other disease processes.

A. ni′ger a species common in soil, sometimes causing severe or persistent otomycosis or allergic aspergillosis.

A. ni′veus a species that contains the mycotoxin citrinin and sometimes contaminates grain, causing fatal renal failure in rats and occasionally human infection.

A. ochra′ceus a species with yellow conidial heads, important economically because it ferments the coffee berry and produces the characteristic and desirable odor; it contains ochratoxin and sometimes contaminates cereals, causing ochratoxicosis in animals. In humans it has been implicated in nasal and orbital infections and allergic aspergillosis.

A. ory′zae a species with yellow-green conidial heads that change to brown with age, closely related to *A. flavus;* it is commonly found in soil and manure and can cause aspergillosis.

A. parasi′ticus a mold found on peanut seedlings that elaborates aflatoxin.

A. re′pens a species that is the perfect stage of *Eurotium repens* and is sometimes found in the external auditory canal or lungs.

A. restric′tus a species with blue to green conidial heads, found in pulmonary and occasionally disseminated infections.

A. ter′reus a species associated with infection of the bronchi and lungs (see *aspergilloma* and *allergic aspergillosis*), and occasionally with other infections such as of the orbit or central nervous system. It contains the mycotoxin patulin.

A. versi′color a species with yellow to green conidial heads, a common soil saprobe; it has been found in infections of the lungs, bronchi, and occasionally the central nervous system.

as•per•gil•lus (as″pər-jil′əs) pl. *aspergil′li.* An individual of the genus *Aspergillus.*

as•per•gil•lus•tox•i•co•sis (as″pər-jil″əs-tok″sĭ-ko′sis) aspergillotoxicosis.

asper•ma•tism (ə-spur′mə-tiz-əm) 1. aspermatogenesis. 2. anejaculation.

as•per•ma•to•gen•e•sis (a-spur″mə-to-jen′ə-sis) failure in a male of production of spermatozoa; cf. *azoospermia.*

asper•mia (ə-spur′me-ə) [*a-*[1] + *sperm-* + *-ia*] 1. permatogenesis. 2. anejaculation.

ASPET American Society for Pharmacology and Experimental Therapeutics.

as•phyg•mia (as-fig′me-ə) temporary disappearance of the pulse.

as·phyx·ia (as-fik′se-ə) [Gr. "a stopping of the pulse"] pathological changes caused by lack of oxygen in respired air, resulting in hypoxia and hypercapnia; see also *respiration.* **asphyx′ial** *adj*

birth a. perinatal a.

fetal a. asphyxia in utero due to hypoxia; see also *fetal hypoxia,* under *hypoxia.*

a. neonato′rum perinatal asphyxia in the newborn.

perinatal a. asphyxia in the infant during labor, delivery, or the immediate postnatal period, a common cause of hypoxic-ischemic encephalopathy. See also *neonatal respiratory distress syndrome,* under *syndrome.* Called also *birth a.*

secondary a. asphyxia recurring after apparent recovery from suffocation.

traumatic a. asphyxia occurring as a result of sudden or severe compression of the thorax or upper abdomen, or both. See also under *apnea.*

as·phyx·i·ant (as-fik′se-ənt) a substance capable of producing asphyxia.

as·phyx·i·ate (as-fik′se-āt) to put into a state of asphyxia.

as·phyx·i·a·tion (as-fik″se-a′shən) the causing of or state of asphyxia. Called also *suffocation.*

As·pid·i·um (as-pid′e-əm) [L., from Gr. *aspidion* little shield] *Dryopteris.*

as·pid·i·um (as-pid′e-əm) a fern of the genus *Dryopteris (Aspidium),* particularly *D. filix-mas.*

as·pi·rate (as′pĭ-rāt) 1. to treat by aspiration. 2. the substance or material obtained by aspiration. 3. a consonantal speech sound in which part of the respiratory tract is constricted, the nasal cavity shut off, and the breath makes a whistling noise; an example is *h.*

as·pi·ra·tion (as″pĭ-ra′shən) [L. *ad-* to + *spirare* to breathe] 1. the drawing of a foreign substance, such as the gastric contents, into the respiratory tract during inhalation. 2. removal by suction, using an aspirator, as of excess fluid or gas from a body cavity or of a specimen for biopsy.

fine-needle a. see under *biopsy.*

meconium a. aspiration of meconium by the fetus or newborn, which may result in atelectasis, emphysema, pneumothorax, or pneumonia.

microsurgical epididymal sperm a. (MESA) retrieval of sperm from the epididymis using microsurgical techniques, done in men with obstructive azoospermia.

percutaneous epididymal sperm a. retrieval of sperm from the epididymis using fine-needle aspiration, done in men with obstructive azoospermia.

percutaneous testicular sperm a. testicular fine-needle a.

suction a. vacuum curettage.

testicular fine-needle a. a type of testicular sperm extraction in which sperm is retrieved from the testicle by fine-needle aspiration, done in men with obstructive azoospermia.

vacuum a. vacuum curettage.

as·pi·ra·tor (as″pĭ-ra′tər) an apparatus used for removal by suction of fluids or gases contained within a cavity.

as·pi·rin (as′pĭ-rin) [USP] acetylsalicylic acid, a drug having antiinflammatory, analgesic, and antipyretic effects; it is the prototype of the nonsteroidal antiinflammatory drugs whose mechanism of action is inhibition of prostaglandin synthesis; used for relief of pain, fever, and inflammation and for treatment of arthritis, osteoarthritis, and rheumatic fever. Because it is a platelet inhibitor, it is also used to reduce the risk of recurrent transient ischemic attacks, stroke syndrome, thromboembolism following certain surgical procedures, and initial or recurrent myocardial infarction. Administered orally or rectally.

asple·nia (a-sple′ne-ə) [*a-*^{1} + *splen-* + *-ia*] absence of the spleen. **asplen′ic** *adj*

functional a. impaired reticuloendothelial function of the spleen, as in children with sickle cell anemia.

aspo·ro·gen·ic (as″po-ro-jen′ik) [*a-*^{1} + *sporogenic*] 1. not producing spores. 2. not reproduced by spores.

as·po·rog·e·nous (as″po-roj′ə-nəs) asporogenic.

aspor·ous (ə-spor′əs) [*a-*^{1} + Gr. *sporos* seed] having no true spores; applied to microorganisms.

asRNA antisense RNA.

ASRT American Society of Radiologic Technologists.

ASS anterior superior spine (of ilium); see *spina iliaca anterior superior.*

as·say (as′a) determination of the amount of a particular constituent of a mixture, or determination of the biological or pharmacological potency of a drug.

antigen capture a. a method for identifying minute quantities of antigen in solution: large quantities of antibody against the desired antigen are fixed to a solid support matrix, over which the solution is passed. The antigen is retained by the matrix and can be identified by reaction with labeled antibody.

biological a. bioassay.

blastogenesis a. see *lymphocyte proliferation test,* under *test.*

cancer antigen 125 (CA 125) a. determination of the level of CA 125 in serum by radioimmunoassay after reaction with a specific murine monoclonal antibody; it is used in the evaluation of women with suspected, diagnosed, or treated primary epithelial ovarian cancer to aid diagnosis, assess prognosis, or predict recurrence.

cell-mediated lympholysis a. (CML assay) see under *lympholysis.*

CH50 a. a functional assay of total complement activity that measures the capacity of serial dilutions of serum to lyse a standard preparation of sheep red blood cells coated with antisheep erythrocyte antibody. The reciprocal of the dilution of serum that lyses 50 per cent of the erythrocytes is reported as the whole complement titer in CH50 units per milliliter of serum. Called also *hemolytic, total,* or *whole complement a.*

Clauss a. see under *method.*

CML a. cell-mediated lympholysis a.; see under *lympholysis.*

comet a. single-cell gel electrophoresis.

competitive protein-binding a. a radioimmunoassay in which labeled and unlabeled ligands compete for sites on a carrier that has the same avidity for both; the concentration of unlabeled ligand is inversely proportional to the amount of labeled ligand bound.

D-dimer a. an immunoassay for the fibrin degradation product D dimer. Levels are elevated in deep venous thrombosis, acute myocardial infarction, pulmonary embolism, unstable angina, and disseminated intravascular coagulation (DIC). Called also *D-dimer test.*

EAC rosette a. an assay for human B lymphocytes using complement receptors, a B cell marker. Peripheral blood cells are mixed with ox red blood cells, IgM antierythrocyte antibody, and complement deficient in C5 (to prevent red cell lysis). The antibody-and-complement-coated erythrocytes (EAC) form rosettes with B cells, which are counted using a hemocytometer.

electrophoretic mobility shift a. gel retardation a.

enzyme-linked immunosorbent a. see *ELISA.*

E rosette a. an assay for human T lymphocytes based on the existence of a specific receptor on T cells for a sheep red blood cell membrane antigen. Peripheral blood lymphocytes are incubated with sheep red cells. T cells are surrounded by a ring of erythrocytes (an E rosette) and are counted using a hemacytometer.

fibrinogen a. an assay for the level of fibrinogen in a plasma sample; a thrombin reagent is added to the diluted sample and the time needed to form clots is compared with that for a reference containing a known amount of fibrinogen.

footprinting a. footprinting.

four-point a. an assay based on a mixture of two doses of test material and two doses of standard material.

gel retardation a. an assay used to determine whether a specific protein binds to DNA or to determine some characteristics of such binding; protein is incubated with or without nucleic acid under various conditions and the electrophoretic mobilities of the samples are compared. In a nondenaturing type of gel electrophoresis, a decreased rate of migration relative to an unbound control is indicative of binding.

HeLa cell adherence a. a test for adherence of HeLa cells to strains of *Escherichia coli;* strains with positive adherence are more likely to cause diarrhea.

hemagglutination inhibition (HI, HAI) a. see under *test.*

hemizona a. an in vitro test of sperm function: a human zona pellucida is divided in half; one half is incubated with sperm from a donor known to be normal, and the other half with sperm from the patient being tested. The number of sperm bound to each half is calculated and that from the patient's sperm is divided by that from the donor's sperm. A figure of less than 0.60 indicates abnormal patient sperm.

hemolytic complement a. CH50 a.

hemolytic plaque a. a quantitative assay that counts antibody-producing cells. Lymphocytes sensitized against sheep erythrocytes (SRBCs) are plated in agar with SRBCs. After incubation complement is added; this lyses SRBCs, leaving a clear circular plaque around each cell that produced antibody against SRBC. The plaques are counted and reported as the number of plaque-forming cells (PFCs, pfcs). Called also *Jerne plaque a.*

immune a. immunoassay.

immune adherence hemagglutination a. (IAHA) see *immune adherence,* under *adherence.*

immunobead a. an assay for any of various types of antibodies or antigens, using immunobeads coated with a corresponding antigen or antibody that aggregates or agglutinates in the presence of the one in question.

immunofluorescence a. (IFA) fluorescence immunoassay.

immunoradiometric a. (IRMA) a variant of radioimmunoassay in which the antigen being measured reacts directly with radiolabeled antibody.

Jerne plaque a. hemolytic plaque a.

lymphocyte proliferation a. see under *test.*
microbiological a. assay by the use of microorganisms.
microcytotoxicity a. the standard method of typing serologically defined human leukocyte antigens (HLA) as HLA-A, -B, and -C antigens. Multiple typing sera are placed in wells of a microtiter plate, and peripheral blood lymphocytes and complement are added to each well. The pattern of lysed cells indicates the HLA phenotype.
microhemagglutination a.–*Treponema pallidum* (MHA-TP) a type of *Treponema pallidum* hemagglutination assay that uses microtechniques in testing for syphilis.
mixed lymphocyte culture a., MLC a. see under *culture.*
radioimmunoprecipitation a. (RIPA) immunoprecipitation conducted with radiolabeled antibody or antigen.
radioligand a. any assay procedure that uses radioisotopic labeling and biologically specific binding of reagents, such as a radioimmunoassay, competitive protein-binding assay, or radioreceptor assay.
radioreceptor a. a radioligand assay in which a radiolabeled hormone is used to measure the concentration of specific cellular receptors for the hormone in tissue specimens, an example being radioassay of estrogen receptors in breast tissue.
Raji cell a. an assay for immune complexes using the Raji lymphoblastoid cell line (see *Raji cell,* under *cell*).
sandwich a. sandwich technique (def. 1).
serum free light chain a. a nephelometric assay that measures the amounts of free κ and λ chains in serum in order to test for plasma cell dyscrasias.
sperm penetration a. (SPA) a test for the ability of spermatozoa to penetrate oocytes in vitro: hamster oocytes that lack the zona pellucida are exposed to the spermatozoa in question; such zona-free oocytes can undergo heterologous membrane fusion with the membranes of spermatozoa that have undergone the acrosome reaction. An assessment is then made of the proportion of oocytes that have been successfully penetrated.
stem cell a. a test for determining the effectiveness of particular drugs against human cancer, in which human tumor cell suspensions are first incubated with various drugs and then suspended in agar and plated over a layer of agar at the bottom of the plate. Effectiveness of the drugs is determined by counting the number of colonies that grow in comparison with the number of colonies on control plates.
target detection a. an assay using randomized oligonucleotides in conjunction with the polymerase chain reaction in order to determine which amino acids of a nucleic acid–binding protein are responsible for the recognition of specific nucleic acid sequences.
thyroid-stimulating hormone a. thyroid-stimulating hormone test.
time-kill a. a method of assessing the rate of killing of bacteria by an antimicrobial agent, done by measuring the number of viable bacteria left at various times after exposure to the agent.
total complement a. CH50 a.
***Treponema pallidum* hemagglutination a. (TPHA)** a serologic test for syphilis that measures specific treponemal antibodies. It combines nonhuman red blood cells sensitized with antigen from a strain of *Treponema pallidum* with patient serum absorbed with an extract of other treponemes for removal of nonspecific antibodies; hemagglutination denotes a positive result.
whole complement a. CH50 a.

as•sess•ment (ə-ses′mənt) an evaluation or appraisal.
Fugl-Meyer a. a standardized assessment of motor function of a part after neurological damage.
functional a. an objective evaluation of a patient's functional level, including ability to perform activities of daily living, done to prescribe or evaluate rehabilitation measures.
Subjective Global A. a method of rating a patient's nutritional status, with subjective observations being given values on an ordinal scale; factors assessed include weight change, appetite or anorexia, subcutaneous tissue and muscle, gastrointestinal symptoms, and others.

As•sé•zat triangle (ah-sa-zah′) [Jules *Assézat,* French anthropologist, 1832–1876] facial triangle.

as•si•dent (as′ĭ-dənt) generally but not always accompanying a disease.

as•sim•i•la•ble (ə-sim′ĭ-lə-bəl) capable of being assimilated.

as•sim•i•la•tion (ə-sim″ĭ-la′shən) [L. *assimilatio,* from *ad* to + *similare* to make like] 1. in psychology, the absorption of new experiences into the existing psychological make-up. Called also *integration.* 2. anabolism.

as•sis•tant (ə-sis′tənt) one who aids or helps another; an auxiliary.
physician a. see under *physician.*

Ass•mann focus (tuberculous infiltrate) (ahs′mahn) [Herbert *Assmann,* German internist, 1882–1950] see under *focus.*

as•so•ci•at•ed (ə-so′she-āt″əd) connected; accompanying; joined with another or others.

as•so•ci•a•tion (ə-so″se-a′shən) [L. *associatio,* from *ad* to + *socius* a fellow] 1. a state in which two attributes occur together either more or less often than expected by chance. 2. in neurology, a term applied to those regions of the brain that link the primary motor and sensory cortices; see *association areas,* under *area.* 3. in genetics, the occurrence together of two or more phenotypic characteristics more often than would be expected by chance. To be distinguished from linkage (q.v.). 4. in psychiatry, a connection between ideas or feelings, especially between conscious thoughts and elements of the unconscious, or the formation of such a connection.
CHARGE a. see under *syndrome.*
clang a. see *clanging.*
dream a's emotions or thoughts associated with previous dreams, as developed by the patient in psychoanalysis.
free a. a psychoanalytical method in which the patient is encouraged to describe the association of thoughts and emotions as they arise spontaneously during the analysis.
genetic a. association (def. 3).
VACTERL a. a nonrandom association of congenital anomalies similar to the VATER association but also including *c*ardiac and *l*imb anomalies; the etiology is unknown.
VATER a. a nonrandom association of congenital anomalies consisting of *v*ertebral defects, imperforate *a*nus, *t*racheo*e*sophageal fistula, and *r*adial and *r*enal dysplasia. Called also *VATER complex.*

as•sor•ta•tive (ə-sor′tə-tiv) characterized by or pertaining to selection on the basis of likeness or kind.

as•sor•tive (ə-sor′tiv) assortative.

as•sort•ment (ə-sort′mənt) the random distribution of different combinations of the parental chromosomes to the gametes, each gamete therefore containing one chromosome of each homologous pair, but randomly receiving the maternal versus paternal homologue for any pair.
independent a. 1. the independent behavior of alleles of different, unlinked genes in gametogenesis, a consequence of the random distribution of the chromosomal homologues. 2. assortment.

AST aspartate transaminase.

Ast. astigmatism.

asta•sia (as-ta′zhə) [*a-*[1] + Gr. *stasis* stand] motor incoordination with inability to stand; cf. *dysstasia* and *posture.* **astat′ic** *adj*
a.-aba′sia motor incoordination with an inability to stand or walk despite normal ability to move the lower limbs when sitting or lying down, a form of hysterical ataxia. Called also *abasia-astasia.*

as•ta•tine (At) (as′tə-tēn) [Gr. *astatos* unstable] the radioactive element of atomic number 85, atomic weight 210. It is prepared by alpha particle bombardment of bismuth on the cyclotron. It has a half-life of 75 hours and may be of use in the treatment of hyperthyroidism.

aste•a•to•des (as″te-ə-to′dēz) asteatosis.

aste•a•to•sis (as″te-ə-to′sis) [*a-*[1] + *stear-* + *-osis*] any condition characterized by persistent, fine, dry scaling of the skin that suggests scantiness or absence of the sebaceous secretion, such as in asteatotic eczema.

As•te•lin (as′tə-lin) trademark for a preparation of azelastine hydrochloride.

as•tem•i•zole (ə-stem′ĭ-zōl) [USP] an H_1-receptor antagonist formerly used in the treatment of chronic urticaria and seasonal allergic rhinitis (hay fever); it has been withdrawn in many countries because of interactions with other drugs and with food (grapefruit juice) and potentially serious adverse effects.

as•ter (as′tər) [L., from Gr. *astēr* star] a structure seen in a cell during mitosis, composed of a system of microtubules arranged in starlike rays around each pair of centrioles.

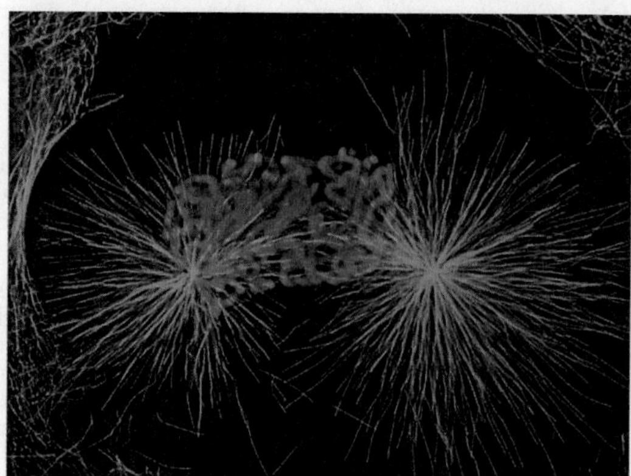

■ Asters in an immunofluorescent image of a cell in the prometaphase stage of mitosis; spindle microtubules are green and chromosomes are blue.

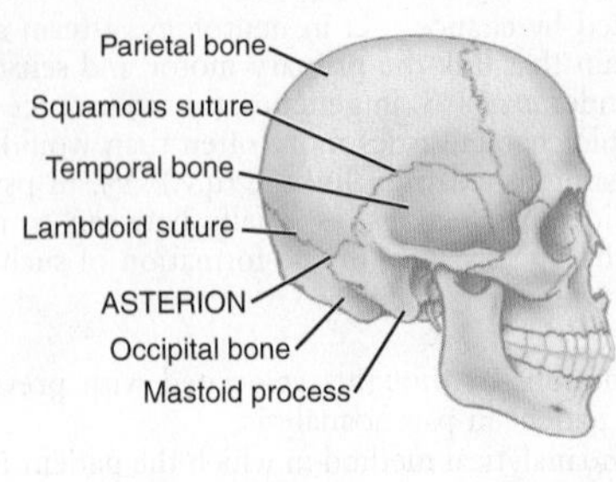

■ Asterion.

sperm a. the centriole, with astral microtubules, that precedes the male pronucleus during fertilization.

As•ter•a•ce•ae (as″tər-a′se-e) Compositae.

aste•reo•cog•no•sy (ə-stēr″e-o-kog′nə-se) astereognosis.

aste•re•og•no•sis (ə-ster″e-og-no′sis) [*a-*[1] + Gr. *stereo-* + *gnōsis*] loss or lack of the ability to understand the form and nature of objects that are touched (stereognosis), a form of tactile agnosia; called also *astereocognosy, stereoagnosis,* and *tactile amnesia.*

as•te•ri•on (as-te′re-on) pl. *aste′ria* [Gr. "starred"] [TA] the point on the surface of the skull where the lambdoid, parietomastoid, and occipitomastoid sutures meet.

as•ter•ix•is (as″tər-ik′sis) [*a-*[1] + Gr. *stērixis* a fixed position] a motor disturbance marked by intermittent lapse of an assumed posture, as a result of intermittency of the sustained contraction of groups of muscles, a characteristic of hepatic coma but observed also in numerous other conditions; called also *liver flap* and *flapping tremor.*

aster•nal (a-stur′nəl) 1. not joined to the sternum. 2. pertaining to asternia; lacking a sternum.

aster•nia (a-stur′ne-ə) [*a-*[1] + *stern-* + *-ia*] congenital absence of the sternum.

as•ter•oid (as′tər-oid) [*aster* + *-oid*] star-shaped; resembling the aster.

Asth. asthenopia.

as•the•nia (as-the′ne-ə) [*asthen-* + *-ia*] lack or loss of strength and energy; weakness. **asthen′ic** *adj*

cutaneous a. a disease of domestic and farm animals, similar to human Ehlers-Danlos syndrome; the skin is fragile and easily torn. It is due to an abnormally low activity of the enzyme procollagen *N*-endopeptidase. Called also *dermatosparaxis.*

myalgic a. any condition characterized by a sensation of general fatigue and muscular pains.

neurocirculatory a. a syndrome characterized by palpitations, dyspnea, a sense of fatigue, fear of effort, and discomfort brought on by exercise or even slight effort; considered by most authorities to be a particular presentation of an anxiety disorder, the physical symptoms being attributed to autonomic responses to anxiety or to hyperventilation. Called also *Da Costa* or *effort syndrome.*

periodic a. a condition marked by periodically recurring attacks of marked asthenia.

tropical anhidrotic a. a rare condition seen under conditions of heat stress; miliaria profunda causes extensive occlusion of the sweat ducts, producing anhidrosis and heat retention that may lead to heat exhaustion (see under *exhaustion*). Called also *sweat retention syndrome* and *thermogenic anhidrosis.*

asthen(o)- [Gr. *asthenēs* weak, from *a-*[1] + *sthenos* strength] a combining form denoting lack of strength or weakness.

as•the•no•bi•o•sis (as-the″no-bi-o′sis) [*asthen-* + *biosis*] a condition of reduced biologic activity resembling hibernation or estivation but not directly related to or dependent on temperature or humidity.

as•the•no•co•ria (as″thə-no-kor′e-ə) [*astheno-* + *cor-* + *-ia*] sluggishness of the pupillary reflex, as seen in hypoadrenalism. Called also *Arroyo sign.*

as•the•nope (as′then-ōp) a person affected with asthenopia.

as•the•no•pia (as″thə-no′pe-ə) [*asthen-* + *-opia*] weakness or easy fatigue of the visual organs, attended by pain in the eyes, headache, dimness of vision, etc. Previously a diagnostic term; now used mainly as a descriptive term. **asthenop′ic** *adj*

accommodative a. asthenopia due to strain of the ciliary muscle.

muscular a. asthenopia due to weakness of the external ocular muscles.

nervous a. 1. asthenopia due to a functional disorder. 2. asthenopia due to organic nervous disease.

tarsal a. asthenopia due to irregular astigmatism produced by the pressure of the lids on the cornea.

as•the•no•sper•mia (as″thə-no-spur′me-ə) [*astheno-* + *sperm-* + *-ia*] asthenozoospermia.

as•the•no•ter•a•to•sper•mia (as″thə-no-ter″ə-to-spur′me-ə) [*astheno-spermia* + *teratospermia*] a condition in which some spermatozoa have decreased motility and others are malformed.

as•the•nox•ia (as″then-ok′shə) [*astheno-* + *oxygen*] lack of power to oxidize waste products.

as•the•no•zo•o•sper•mia (as″thə-no-zo″o-spur′me-ə) [*astheno-* + *zoospermia*] reduced motility or vitality of spermatozoa; called also *asthenospermia.*

as•thma (az′mə) [Gr. *asthma* panting] recurrent attacks of paroxysmal dyspnea, with airway inflammation and wheezing due to spasmodic contraction of the bronchi. Some cases are allergic manifestations in sensitized persons *(allergic a.);* others are provoked by factors such as vigorous exercise, irritant particles, psychologic stresses, and others. Called also *bronchial a.* and *spasmodic a.* **asthmat′ic** *adj*

allergic a. atopic a.

atopic a. asthma due to atopy (atopic allergy). Called also *allergic a.* and *extrinsic a.*

bakers' a. a usually mild form of occupational asthma seen in bakery workers, caused by the inhalation of flour; some cases are due to contaminants such as mites in the flour.

bronchial a. asthma.

bronchitic a. asthmatic disorder accompanying bronchitis; see also *asthmatic bronchitis,* under *bronchitis.*

cardiac a. paroxysmal nocturnal dyspnea that occurs in association with heart disease, such as left ventricular failure.

cat a. atopic asthma brought on by inhalation of cat dander by a sensitized person.

catarrhal a. bronchitic a.

colophony a. a type of occupational asthma in workers in electronics industries caused by inhalation of fumes of colophony (rosin), which is used to solder parts together.

cotton-dust a. byssinosis.

cough variant a. asthma characterized by minimal wheezing and a nonproductive, often severe, cough lasting from a few hours to days.

cryptogenic a. intrinsic a.

diisocyanate a. isocyanate a.

dust a. atopic asthma caused by inhalation of dust; many cases are caused by presence in the dust of the house dust mite (*Dermatophagoides pteronyssinus*), and some other cases are caused by allergies to animal dander.

exercise-induced a. asthma due to a narrowing of the airways occurring in moderate to heavy exercise; called also *exercise-induced bronchoconstriction* or *bronchospasm.*

extrinsic a. 1. asthma caused by some factor in the environment, usually atopic asthma. Onset is usually in childhood and almost always before age 30. Cf. *intrinsic a.* 2. atopic a.

food a. atopic asthma brought on by ingestion of certain foods to which the person is allergic.

horse a. atopic asthma caused by an allergy to horses or horse products.

intrinsic a. asthma attributed to pathophysiologic disturbances and not to environmental factors; usually seen in adults. Called also *cryptogenic a.*

isocyanate a. asthma, usually occupational, caused by allergy to toluene diisocyanate and similar materials.

millers' a. occupational asthma in millers, caused by the inhalation of cereal dusts.

nasal a. asthma caused by a disease of the nose.

occupational a. asthma, sometimes atopic in nature, caused by inhalation of an irritant in the workplace.

reflex a. asthma attributed to a reflex reaction to another condition.

Rostan a. cardiac a.

spasmodic a. asthma.

steam-fitters' a. occupational asthma in steam-fitters, associated with asbestosis.

stripper's a. byssinosis.

western red cedar a. occupational asthma in sawmill workers, carpenters, and other susceptible persons who work with western red cedar *(Thuja plicata);* plicatic acid in the wood is the probably cause.

asth•mat•i•form (az-mat′ĭ-form) resembling asthma.

asth•mo•gen•ic (az″mo-jen′ik) causing asthma.

astig•ma•graph (ə-stig′mə-graf) [*astigma* tism + *-graph*] an instrument for demonstrating astigmatism.

astig•ma•tism (ə-stig′mə-tiz-əm) [*a-*[1] + Gr. *stigma* point] an error of refraction caused by unequal curvature of the refractive surfaces of the eye, so that a point source of light cannot be brought to a point focus on the retina but is spread over a more or less diffuse area. This results from the radius of curvature in one plane being longer or shorter than the radius at right angles to it. **astigmat′ic, astigmic** *adj*

acquired a. astigmatism caused by disease or injury of the eye.

■ Astigmatism: the appearance of lines as seen by *(A)* the normal eye and *(B)* the astigmatic eye.

a. against the rule astigmatism in which the greatest refraction takes place along the horizontal meridian; called also *inverse a.*

compound a. astigmatism that is complicated in all meridians by hypermetropia or myopia.

compound hyperopic a. astigmatism in which all meridians are hyperopic, both principal meridians having their foci behind the retina.

corneal a. astigmatism due to irregularity in the curvature or refracting power of the cornea.

direct a. a. with the rule.

hypermetropic a., hyperopic a. astigmatism that complicates hyperopia.

inverse a. a. against the rule.

irregular a. astigmatism in which the curvature in different parts of the same meridian of the eye varies or in which successive meridians differ irregularly in refraction, the image produced being an irregular area.

lenticular a. astigmatism that is due to an irregularity or abnormality of the lens.

mixed a. astigmatism in which one principal meridian is myopic and the other hyperopic.

myopic a. astigmatism that complicates myopia.

myopic a., compound astigmatism in which all meridians are myopic, both principal meridians having their foci in front of the retina; vertical lines are usually more distinct.

myopic a., simple astigmatism in which the focus of one meridian is situated on the retina, while that of the other lies in front of the retina; vertical lines appear distinct.

oblique a. astigmatism in which the direction of the principal meridians approaches 45° and 135°.

physiological a. the slight astigmatism possessed by nearly all eyes and causing the twinkling sensation when distant points of light are viewed.

regular a. astigmatism in which the refractive power of the eye shows a uniform increase or decrease from one meridian to the other, being practically constant in each meridian; the image produced is regular in shape, either a line, an oval, or a circle. See also *Sturm conoid*, under *conoid.*

simple hyperopic a. astigmatism in which one meridian, usually the vertical, is emmetropic and the horizontal meridian is hyperopic. The focus of the vertical meridian is not in the retina; that of the horizontal is behind the retina; horizontal lines appear distinct.

a. with the rule astigmatism in which the greatest refraction takes place in a vertical or nearly vertical meridian; called also *direct a.*

astig·ma·tom·e·ter (ə-stig″mə-tom′ə-tər) [*astigmatism* + *-meter*] an instrument used in measuring astigmatism.

astig·ma·tom·e·try (ə-stig″mə-tom′ə-tre) [*astigmatism* + *-metry*] the measurement of astigmatism; the use of the astigmatometer. Called also *astigmometry.*

as·tig·mato·scope (as″tig-mat′ə-skōp) [*astigmatism* + *-scope*] an instrument for discovering and measuring astigmatism.

as·tig·ma·tos·co·py (ə-stig″mə-tos′kə-pe) the use of the astigmatoscope.

astig·mia (ə-stig′me-ə) [*a-*[1] + Gr. *stigma* a point + *ia*] astigmatism.

as·tig·mom·e·ter (as″tig-mom′ə-tər) astigmatometer.

as·tig·mom·e·try (as″tig-mom′ə-tre) astigmatometry.

as·tig·mo·scope (ə-stig′mo-skōp) astigmatoscope.

as·tig·mos·co·py (as″tig-mos′kə-pe) astigmatoscopy.

astom·a·tous (ə-stom′ə-təs) [*a-*[1] + *stomat-* + *-ous*] having no mouth, such as certain ciliates.

asto·mia (ə-sto′me-ə) [*a-*[1] + *stom-* + *-ia*] congenital absence of the mouth.

asto·mus (ə-sto′məs) a fetus without a mouth.

as·trag·a·lec·to·my (as″trag-ə-lek′tə-me) [*astragalus* + *-ectomy*] excision of the astragalus (talus).

as·trag·a·lo·cal·ca·ne·an (as-trag″ə-lo-kal-ka′ne-ən) talocalcaneal.

as·trag·a·lo·cru·ral (as-trag″ə-lo-kroo͞r′əl) talocrural.

as·trag·a·lo·scaph·oid (as-trag″ə-lo-skaf′oid) talonavicular.

as·trag·a·lo·tib·i·al (as-trag″ə-lo-tib′e-əl) talotibial.

As·trag·a·lus (as-trag′ə-ləs) a genus of plants of the family Leguminosae, having many species, some poisonous and others medicinal. *A. gum′mifer* and other Asian species are sources of tragacanth. *A. mollis′simus* and at least seven other North American species are types of *locoweed* and have a mydriatic active principle. Six other species grow preferentially in seleniferous soil and may accumulate large quantities of selenium, causing selenium poisoning in livestock. Preparations of the root of *A. membrana′ceus* and other species are used for the treatment of colds and mild infections and in traditional Chinese medicine for a variety of indications.

as·trag·a·lus (as-trag′ə-ləs) [L., from Gr. *astragalos* ball of the ankle joint] talus (def. 1). **astrag′alar** *adj*

as·tral (as′trəl) of or relating to an aster.

As·tra·morph/PF (as′trə-morf″) trademark for a preparation of morphine sulfate.

as·tra·pho·bia (as″trə-fo′be-ə) [Gr. *astrapē* lightning + *-phobia*] irrational fear of thunder and lightning.

as·tra·po·pho·bia (as″trə-po-fo′be-ə) astraphobia.

astric·tion (ə-strik′shən) [L. *astringere* to constrict] the action of an astringent.

astringe (ə-strinj′) to act as an astringent.

astrin·gen·cy (ə-strin′jən-se) the quality of being astringent.

astrin·gent (ə-strin′jənt) [L. *astringens*, from *ad* to + *stringere* to bind] 1. causing contraction, usually locally after topical application. 2. an agent that causes contraction; see also *styptic.*

astr(o)- [Gr. *astron* star] a combining form denoting relationship to a star, or to an aster.

as·tro·blast (as′tro-blast) [*astro-* + *-blast*] an embryonic cell that develops into an astrocyte.

as·tro·blas·to·ma (as″tro-blas-to′mə) an astrocytoma of Grade II; its cells resemble astroblasts, with abundant cytoplasm and two or three nuclei.

as·tro·cyte (as′tro-sīt) [*astro-* + *-cyte*] a neuroglial cell of ectodermal origin, characterized by fibrous, protoplasmic, or plasmatofibrous processes. Collectively, such cells are called *astroglia.*

Alzheimer type II a. a type of giant astrocyte with a large, prominent nucleus, found in the brain in liver conditions such as hepatic encephalopathy, hepatolenticular degeneration, and hepatic coma.

fibrillary a's, fibrous a's astrocytes found mainly in the white matter of the brain, having long, thin, infrequently branched cytoplasmic processes containing numerous fibrillar structures.

gemistocytic a. gemistocyte.

plasmatofibrous a's astrocytes found at the junction of the gray and white matter of the brain; the cytoplasmic processes extending into the white matter are fibrous and those extending into the gray matter are protoplasmic.

protoplasmic a's astrocytes found mainly in the gray matter of the brain, having many branching, thick cytoplasmic processes.

as·tro·cy·to·ma (as″tro-si-to′mə) a tumor composed of astrocytes; it is the most common type of primary brain tumor and is also found throughout the central nervous system. One classification groups astrocytomas according to their histologic appearance and distinguishes *pilocytic, protoplasmic, gemistocytic,* and *fibrillary* types. Another classification groups them in order of increasing malignancy as *Grade I, Grade II, Grade III,* and *Grade IV* types. Called also *astrocytic glioma.*

anaplastic a. a malignant to highly malignant form of astrocytoma that often degenerates into a glioblastoma; variously classified as a Grade II or a Grade III astrocytoma.

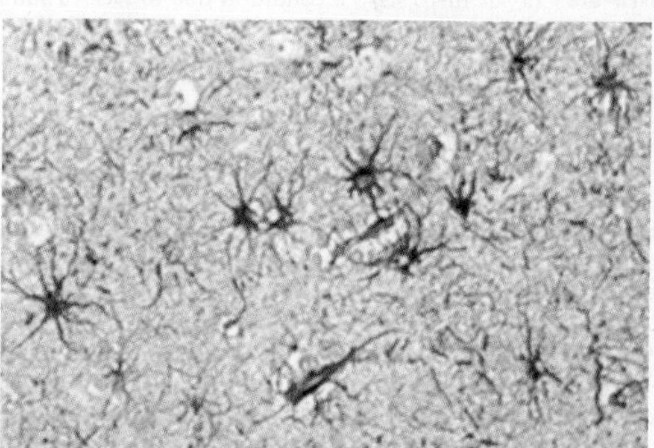

■ Astrocytes with well-developed processes demonstrated by immunohistochemical staining for glial fibrillary acidic protein *(brown).*

cerebellar a. an astrocytoma in the cerebellum; the most common kind, the *juvenile pilocytic a.*, has a low grade of malignancy, but a second variety, the *diffuse cerebellar a.*, is of a higher grade.

diffuse cerebellar a. a cerebellar astrocytoma that is solid, dense, and infiltrative and resembles a fibrillary astrocytoma; it occurs more frequently in adults and has a higher grade of malignant potential than a pilocytic astrocytoma.

a. fibrilla′re, fibrillary a. an astrocytoma whose cells resemble fibrous astrocytes, usually a Grade I or Grade II astrocytoma found in the cerebrum of an adult, but occasionally occurring in the brainstem or cerebellum. A minority are malignant and undergo anaplastic changes.

gemistocytic a. an astrocytoma whose cells resemble gemistocytes; their cytoplasm is swollen, homogeneously hyaline, and acidophilic in appearance. Their tendency to undergo malignant transformation is variable.

Grade I a's a group of generally slow-growing astrocytomas, including most fibrillary and pilocytic astrocytomas.

Grade II a's astrocytomas with slightly more malignant potential than those of Grade I, including astroblastomas and some fibrillary and pilocytic astrocytomas. One classification system includes some anaplastic astrocytomas in this group.

Grade III a's moderately malignant astrocytomas, including most anaplastic astrocytomas.

Grade IV a's astrocytomas that are highly malignant; this group includes only glioblastoma.

juvenile pilocytic a. a pilocytic astrocytoma found in the cerebellum in children, one of the most common juvenile brain tumors; it grows slowly and has a low grade of malignancy.

malignant a. an astrocytoma of Grade III or Grade IV; see *anaplastic a.* and *glioblastoma.*

pilocytic a. an astrocytoma resembling the fibrillary type but with its fibrils arranged in parallel rows; its grade of malignancy is low. The most common kind is the cerebellar *juvenile pilocytic a.* In adults the pilocytic type is usually found in the cerebrum.

piloid a. 1. pilocytic a. 2. polar spongioblastoma.

protoplasmic a., a. protoplasma′ticum a tumor composed of protoplasmic astrocytes. The distinction between this type and fibrillary astrocytoma has been questioned.

subependymal giant cell a. a rare, usually slow-growing astrocytoma found in the wall of the lateral ventricle; it is sometimes associated with tuberous sclerosis complex.

as•tro•cy•to•sis (as″tro-si-to′sis) proliferation of astrocytes owing to the destruction of nearby neurons during a hypoxic or hypoglycemic episode. See also *gliosis.*

as•trog•lia (as-trog′le-ə) [*astro-* + *neuroglia*] 1. astrocytes. 2. the astrocytes considered as tissue; see *macroglia.*

as•trog•li•o•sis (as-trog″le-o′sis) gliosis.

as•tro•pyle (as″tro-pīl) [*astro-* + *pyle*] the main opening in the capsular membrane of certain marine planktonic protozoa.

As•tro•vi•ri•dae (as″tro-vir′ĭ-de) the astroviruses; a family of RNA viruses having a nonenveloped spherical virion 28–30 nm in diameter with a characteristic star-shaped outline. The genome consists of a single molecule of polyadenylated positive-sense single-stranded RNA (size 6.8–7.9 kb). Viruses contain four structural proteins and are chloroform-resistant. Infection is host restricted and transmission is by the fecal-oral route. There is a single genus, *Astrovirus.*

As•tro•vi•rus (as′tro-vi″rəs) [*astro-* + *virus*] the sole genus of the family Astroviridae. At least seven serotypes of human viruses have been identified. Infection causes gastroenteritis.

as•tro•vi•rus (as′tro-vi″rəs) any virus belonging to the family *Astroviridae.* **astrovi′ral** *adj*

asul•fu•ro•sis (a-sul″fu-ro′sis) a condition due to lack of sulfur in the body.

asyl•la•bia (ă″sə-la′be-ə) a type of alexia in which a person can recognize letters but cannot form them into syllables.

asy•lum (ə-si′ləm) [L.] a place of refuge and shelter, as an institution of the past for the support and care of helpless and deprived individuals, such as the mentally deficient, emotionally disturbed, or the blind.

asym•bo•lia (ă-sim-bo′le-ə) [*a-*[1] + *symbolia*] 1. loss of power to comprehend the symbolic meaning of things such as words, figures, gestures, and signs; cf. *dyssymbolia.* 2. asemia.

pain a. absence of psychic reaction to pain sensations; it may be congenital or result from a brain lesion, particularly of the supramarginal gyrus of the dominant parietal lobe.

asym•bo•ly (ə-sim′bo-le) 1. asymbolia (def. 1). 2. asemia.

asym•me•try (a-sim′ə-tre) [*a-*[1] + *symmetry*] 1. lack or absence of symmetry; dissimilarity in corresponding parts or organs on opposite sides of the body which are normally alike. 2. in chemistry, lack of symmetry in the special arrangements of the atoms and radicals within the molecule or crystal. **asymmet′ric, asymmet′rical** *adj*

chromatic a. difference in color in the irides of the two eyes.

encephalic a. a condition in which the two sides of the brain are not the same size.

asym•phy•tous (ə-sim′fə-təs) separate or distinct; not grown together.

asymp•to•mat•ic (a″simp-to-mat′ik) showing or causing no symptoms.

asyn•ap•sis (a-sĭ-nap′sis) [*a-*[1] + *synapsis*] the failure of homologous chromosomes to pair during meiosis.

asyn•chro•nism (a-sing′krə-niz-əm) asynchrony.

asyn•chro•ny (a-sing′krə-ne) [*a-*[1] + *synchrony*] the occurrence at distinct times of events normally synchronous; disturbance of coordination; called also *asynchronism* and *dyssynchrony.* See also *heterochrony.* **asyn′chronous** *adj*

asyn•cli•tism (ə-sin′klĭ-tiz-əm) [*a-*[1] + *synclitism*] 1. lateral deflection of the fetal head in labor so that the sagittal suture is deflected anteriorly toward the symphysis or posteriorly toward the sacrum. 2. dyserythropoiesis.

anterior a. Nägele obliquity.

posterior a. Litzmann obliquity.

asyn•de•sis (ə-sin′də-sis) [*a-*[1] + *syn-* + *-desis*] a pattern of language in which words and phrases are juxtaposed without grammatical linkage; seen in schizophrenic and other mental disorders.

asyn•ech•ia (a″sin-ek′e-ə) [*a-*[1] + Gr. *synecheia* continuity] absence of continuity of structure.

asyn•er•gia (a″sin-ur′je-ə) asynergy.

asyn•er•gy (a-sin′ər-je) [*a-*[1] + *synergy*] lack of coordination among parts or organs normally acting in harmony. See also *ataxia* and *dyssynergia.* **asyner′gic** *adj*

asy•no•via (a″sə-no′ve-ə) deficiency of the synovial secretion.

asyn•tax•ia (a″sin-tak′se-ə) [Gr. "want of arrangement"] lack of proper and orderly embryonic development.

a. dorsa′lis failure of the neural groove to close in the developing embryo.

asys•to•le (a-sis′to-le) [*a-*[1] + *systole*] absence of a heartbeat; see *cardiac arrest,* under *arrest.* **asystol′ic** *adj*

asys•to•lia (a″sis-to′le-ə) asystole.

AT atrial tachycardia.

At astatine.

ATA alimentary toxic aleukia.

Ata•brine (at′ə-brēn) trademark for a preparation of quinacrine hydrochloride.

At•a•cand (at′ə-kand) trademark for a preparation of candesartan cilexetil.

atac•tic (ə-tak′tik) [Gr. *ataktos* irregular] lacking coordination; irregular; pertaining to or characterized by ataxia.

atac•ti•form (ə-tak′tĭ-form) resembling ataxia.

Ata•met (at′ə-met) trademark for a combination of carbidopa and levodopa.

at•a•rac•tic (at″ə-rak′tik) [Gr. *ataraktos* without disturbance; quiet] 1. pertaining to or capable of producing ataraxia. 2. tranquilizer.

At•a•rax (at′ə-raks) trademark for preparations of hydroxyzine hydrochloride.

at•a•rax•ia (at″ə-rak′se-ə) [Gr. "impassiveness," "calmness"] serenity, calmness, peace of mind.

at•a•rax•ic (at″ə-rak′sik) ataractic.

at•a•vic (at′ə-vik) atavistic.

at•a•vism (at′ə-viz-əm) [L. *atavus* grandfather] the apparent inheritance of a characteristic from remote rather than from immediate ancestors, which may be due to recessive or complementary recessive genes, chance recombination of genes, or unusual environmental conditions favoring expression. **atavis′tic** *adj*

atax•ia (ə-tak′se-ə) [Gr., from *a-*[1] + *taxis* order] failure of muscular coordination; irregularity of muscular action. Cf. *asynergy* and *dystaxia.*

acute a. ataxia of sudden onset.

acute cerebellar a. a usually unilateral type of cerebellar ataxia that may be associated with infectious disease, tumor, or trauma, and results in marked hypotonia of muscles on the affected side, with asynergy and assumption of a characteristic posture.

Bruns frontal a. gait apraxia.

cerebellar a. ataxia due to disease of the cerebellum. See also *acute cerebellar a.* and *spinocerebellar a.*

cerebral a. ataxia due to disease of the cerebrum.

childhood a. with central nervous system hypomyelination vanishing white matter disease.

enzootic a. congenital ataxia of lambs, with cerebral demyelination, sometimes proceeding to paralysis, blindness, and death; the cause is thought to be a copper deficiency. Called also *swayback*.

episodic a. either of two autosomal dominant syndromes characterized by transient episodes of ataxia. *Type 1* is caused by a mutation in the potassium channel gene on chromosome 12p13, and is characterized by tetanic contractions between the attacks of ataxia. *Type 2* is caused by a mutation in the calcium channel gene on chromosome 19p and is characterized by cerebellar abnormalities.

equine sensory a. wobbler syndrome (def. 2).

feline a. panleukopenia.

Friedreich a. an autosomal recessive disorder, usually beginning before adolescence, with sclerosis of the posterior and lateral columns of the spinal cord. It is attended by ataxia, speech impairment, lateral curvature of the vertebral column, and peculiar swaying and irregular movements, with paralysis of the muscles, especially of the lower limbs, and a high-arched foot. It is often associated with hypertrophic cardiomyopathy. In most cases, it is a triplet repeat disorder associated with amplification of a GAA triplet repeat sequence in the first intron of the *FXN* gene (locus: 9q13), which encodes frataxin. Called also *hereditary a.*

frontal a., gait a. gait apraxia.

gluten a. cerebellar ataxia owing to brain damage complicating celiac disease.

hereditary a. 1. Friedreich a. 2. an autosomal recessive disease of fox terrier and Jack Russell terrier dogs in which demyelination of the ventromedial and dorsolateral columns of the spinal cord begins before age 6 months and progresses at varying rates until the animals cannot walk.

hysterical a. ataxia that is part of a conversion disorder; see also *astasia-abasia*, under *astasia*.

intrapsychic a. the separation of ideas and affect seen in schizophrenic disorders; inappropriateness of affect.

kinetic a. motor a.

limb a. ataxia limited to the lower limbs, usually owing to a cerebellar lesion.

locomotor a. tabes dorsalis.

motor a. inability to coordinate the movements of the muscles; called also *kinetic a.*

ocular a. nystagmus.

proprioceptive a., sensory a. ataxia due to loss of joint position sense, characterized by poorly judged movements, loss of vibration sense, and Romberg sign; the incoordination becomes aggravated when the eyes are closed.

spinal a. ataxia due to disease of the spinal cord.

spinocerebellar a. any of a group of hereditary disorders, some of autosomal dominant and others of autosomal recessive inheritance, characterized by progressive degeneration of the cerebellum, brainstem, spinal cord, peripheral nerves, and sometimes other regions of the brain, with neuronal loss from affected areas and secondary degeneration of white matter tracts. The autosomal dominant disorders are triplet repeat disorders; in most, expansion of a CAG triplet repeat leads to large polyglutamine tracts in the affected protein, although the disorders differ in many other details, such as the gene affected and the threshold for clinical disease.

a.-telangiectasia an autosomal recessive disorder caused by mutations in the *ATM* gene (locus: 11q22.3), which is involved in a number of biological functions, including DNA repair and cell cycle control. It is characterized by cerebellar ataxia and nystagmus, oculocutaneous telangiectasia, variable degrees of humoral and cellular immunodeficiency, recurrent bacterial infections of the respiratory tract from sinuses to lungs, and an increased incidence of lymphoreticular malignancies. There is an increased sensitivity to ionizing radiation. Gonadal hypoplasia, insulin resistance and hyperglycemia, liver function abnormalities, and elevated levels of alpha-fetoprotein and carcinoembryonic antigen are also seen in some patients. Called also *Louis-Bar syndrome.*

thermal a. ataxia accompanied by great and paradoxic fluctuations of the temperature of the body.

truncal a. ataxia affecting the muscles of the trunk.

vestibular a. ataxia with vertigo, nystagmus, nausea, and vomiting, caused by a lesion in the brainstem, vestibular nuclei, or vestibulocochlear nerve.

atax·ia·gram (ə-tak′se-ə-gram″) a tracing drawn by an ataxic patient; also the record made by an ataxiagraph.

atax·ia·graph (ə-tak′se-ə-graf″) [*ataxia* + *-graph*] an apparatus used to assess the extent of ataxia by measuring the amount of swaying of the body when standing erect with eyes closed.

atax·i·am·e·ter (ə-tak″se-am′ə-tər) [*ataxia* + *-meter*] ataxiagraph.

ataxi·apha·sia (ə-tak″se-ə-fa′zhə) [*ataxia* + *aphasia*] syntactical aphasia.

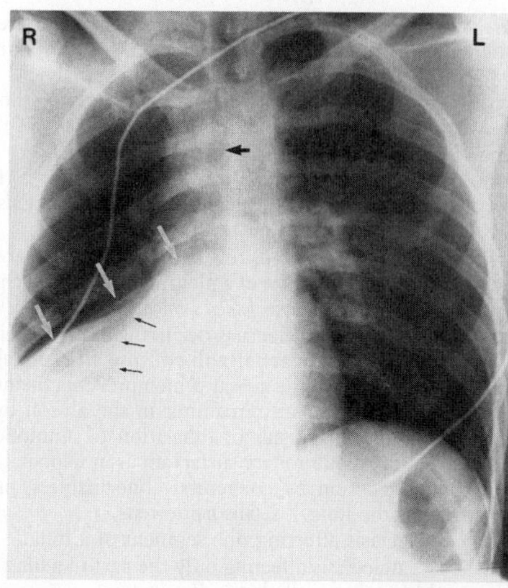

■ Right lower lobe atelectasis. Complete collapse of the right lower lobe with volume loss evidenced by shift of the trachea and cardiac border to the right side *(black arrows)*. Air in the right lower lobe has been resorbed, resulting in a diffuse infiltrate *(white arrows)*.

atax·ic (ə-tak′sik) atactic.

atax·in (ə-tak′sin) an abnormal protein found in the cerebrospinal fluid in some types of spinocerebellar ataxia.

atax·io·phe·mia (ə-tak″se-o-fe′me-ə) dysarthria.

atax·io·pho·bia (ə-tak″se-o-fo′be-ə) ataxophobia.

ataxo·phe·mia (ə-tak″so-fe′me-ə) dysarthria.

ataxo·pho·bia (ə-tak″so-fo′be-ə) [Gr. *ataxia* disorder + *-phobia*] irrational dread of disorder or untidiness.

ataxy (ə-tak′se) ataxia.

at·a·zan·a·vir sul·fate (at″ə-zan′ə-vir) an inhibitor of human immunodeficiency virus-1 (HIV-1) protease, used in the treatment of HIV-1 infection; administered orally.

ATCC American Type Culture Collection.

-ate[1] [L. *-atus*, past participial ending of verbs ending in *-are*] a word termination forming a participial noun, as the object of the process indicated by the root to which it is affixed, e.g., *hemolysate*, something hemolyzed; *homogenate*, something homogenized; *injectate*, something injected. Also forming adjectives, signifying possession of the quality indicated by the root, e.g., *dentate* and *corticate;* and verbs, signifying performance of the action indicated by the root, e.g., *decussate* and *pulsate*.

-ate[2] [L. *-atus*, past participial ending of verbs ending in *-are*] in chemistry, a suffix replacing the suffix *-ic* and the word *acid* in forming the names of anions, salts, and esters, e.g., acetate ion, sodium acetate, methyl acetate from acetic acid. Cf. *-ite*.

at·e·lec·ta·sis (at″ə-lek′tə-sis) [*atel-* + *-ectasis*] 1. incomplete expansion of a lung or a portion of a lung; it may be a primary (congenital), secondary, or otherwise acquired condition. 2. airlessness or collapse of a lung that had once been expanded. 3. absence of air in a normally air-filled space such as the middle ear. **atelectat′ic** *adj*

absorption a., acquired a. atelectasis produced by any factor (such as secretions, foreign body, tumor, or abnormal external pressure) that completely obstructs the airway, prevents intake of air into the alveolar sacs, and permits absorption of air into the bloodstream. Called also *obstructive a.*, *resorption a.*, and *secondary a.*

adhesive a. alveolar collapse with patent airways, often related to absence or inactivation of surfactant, such as in respiratory distress syndrome of newborn or radiation pneumonitis.

cicatrization a. loss of lung volume due to fibrosis and the resultant cicatrization.

compression a. acquired atelectasis due to abnormal external pressure on the lung, such as from a large pleural effusion.

initial a. primary a.

lobar a. atelectasis affecting one lobe of the lung; see also *middle lobe syndrome*, under *syndrome*.

lobular a. atelectasis affecting a lobule of the lung; called also *patchy a.*

obstructive a. absorption a.

passive a. relaxation a.

patchy a. lobular a.

platelike a. subsegmental a.

primary a. congenital atelectasis, common among premature infants, in which there is failure of initial alveolar expansion, due to pulmonary immaturity or to inadequacy of respiratory effort that may be a result of weakness of respiratory muscles, severe illness, softness of thoracic cage, brain damage with injury to the respiratory center, or oversedation. Called also *anectasis* and *initial a.*

relaxation a. atelectasis caused by large amounts of air or fluid in the pleural cavity, as in pneumothorax or pleural effusion. Called also *passive a.*

resorption a. absorption a.

round a., rounded a. a localized, reversible form in subjacent peripheral tissue, often following resorption of a pleural effusion and characterized by focal pleural scarring. Called also *folded lung syndrome.*

secondary a. 1. absorption atelectasis occurring at birth or in the newborn period, in which the pulmonary alveoli collapse after initial expansion by air; it is due to obstruction of the airway which prevents further entrance of air or to prevention of air from remaining in the alveoli by increased surfaces forces, occurring as a result of inhalation of amniotic debris or mucous plugs, deficiency of pulmonary surfactant as in neonatal respiratory distress syndrome, obstruction by congenital abnormalities; or abnormal external pressure upon the lung. 2. absorption a.

segmental a. atelectasis affecting one segment of a lung.

subsegmental a. atelectasis affecting only the part of a lung distal to an occluded segmental bronchus; called also *platelike a.*

tympanic membrane a. a complication of chronic serous otitis media in which the middle ear contains a viscous fluid and the tympanic membrane has become thin, atrophic, retracted, and adherent to middle ear structures; there is usually conductive hearing loss. Called also *adhesive* or *atelectatic otitis media.*

atel•en•ce•pha•lia (ə-tel″en-sə-fa′le-ə) [*atel-* + *encephal-* + *-ia*] congenital imperfect development of the brain.

ate•lia (ə-te′le-ə) [Gr. *ateleia* incompleteness] imperfect or incomplete development. **ateliot′ic** *adj*

atel(o)- [Gr. *atelēs* incomplete] a combining form meaning imperfect or incomplete.

at•e•lo•car•dia (at″ə-lo-kahr′de-ə) [*atelo-* + Gr. *kardia* heart] congenitally incomplete development of the heart.

at•e•lo•ceph•a•lous (at″ə-lo-sef′ə-ləs) [*atelo-* + Gr. *kephalē* head] having an incomplete head.

at•e•lo•ceph•a•ly (at″ə-lo-sef′ə-le) congenitally incomplete development of the cranium.

at•e•lo•chei•lia (at″ə-lo-ki′le-ə) [*atelo-* + *cheil-* + *-ia*] congenitally incomplete development of a lip.

at•e•lo•chei•ria (at″ə-lo-ki′re-ə) [*atelo-* + *cheir-* + *-ia*] congenitally incomplete development of the hand.

at•e•lo•en•ce•pha•lia (at″ə-lo-en″sə-fa′le-ə) atelencephalia.

at•e•lo•glos•sia (at″ə-lo-glos′e-ə) [*atelo-* + *gloss-* + *-ia*] congenitally incomplete development of the tongue.

at•e•log•na•thia (at″ə-log-na′the-ə) [*atelo-* + *gnath-* + *-ia*] congenitally incomplete development of the jaw.

at•e•lo•my•elia (at″ə-lo-mi-e′le-ə) [*atelo-* + *myel-* + *-ia*] congenitally incomplete development of the spinal cord.

atel•op•id•tox•in (a-təl-op′id-tok″sin) a potent dialyzable toxin derived from the skin of frogs of the genus *Atelopus*, of Central and South America. The LD_{50} in mice is 16 μg/kg. Its chemical and pharmacological nature has not been fully defined.

at•e•lo•po•dia (at″ə-lo-po′de-ə) [*atelo-* + *pod-* + *-ia*] congenitally incomplete development of the foot.

at•e•lo•pro•so•pia (at″ə-lo-pro-so′pe-ə) [*atelo-* + *prosop-* + *-ia*] congenitally incomplete development of the face.

at•e•lo•ra•chid•ia (at″ə-lo-ra-kid′e-ə) [*atelo-* + *rhachi-* + *-ia*] congenitally incomplete development of the vertebral column.

at•e•lo•sto•mia (at″ə-lo-sto′me-ə) [*atelo-* + *stom-* + *-ia*] congenitally incomplete development of the mouth.

aten•o•lol (ə-ten′ə-lol) [USP] a cardioselective β_1-adrenergic blocking agent used in the treatment of hypertension and chronic angina pectoris and the prophylaxis and treatment of myocardial infarction and cardiac arrhythmias; administered orally or intravenously.

ATG antithymocyte globulin.

At•gam (at′gam) trademark for preparations of antilymphocyte globulin and antithymocyte globulin (equine).

athe•lia (ə-the′le-ə) [*a-*[1] + *thel-* + *-ia*] congenital absence of the nipple(s).

ath•er•ec•to•my (ath″ər-ek′tə-me) [*ather-* + *ectomy*] the removal of atherosclerotic plaque from an artery using a rotary cutter inside a special catheter guided radiographically; it does not extend to the tunica intima as endarterectomy does.

directional a. atherectomy performed using a directional atherectomy catheter.

rotational a. rotablation.

transluminal a. see under *endarterectomy.*

ather•man•cy (ə-thur′mən-se) the state of being athermanous.

ather•ma•nous (ə-thur′mə-nəs) [*a-*[1] + *thermic*] absorbing heat rays and not permitting them to pass.

ather•mic (a-thur′mik) afebrile.

ather•mo•sys•tal•tic (ə-thur″mo-sis-tal′tik) [*a-*[1] + *thermo-* + *systaltic*] not contracting under the action of cold or heat; said of skeletal muscle.

ather(o)- [Gr. *athērē* gruel] a combining form denoting fatty degeneration, or relationship to an atheroma.

ath•ero•em•bo•lism (ath″ər-o-em′bo-liz-əm) [*athero-* + *embolism*] embolism due to blockage of a blood vessel by an atheroembolus.

ath•ero•em•bo•lus (ath″ər-o-em′bo-ləs) pl. *atheroem′boli* [*athero-* + *embolus*] an embolus composed of cholesterol or its esters or of fragments of atheromatous plaques, typically lodging in small arteries.

ath•ero•gen•e•sis (ath″ər-o-jen′ə-sis) [*athero-* + *genesis*] the formation of atheromatous lesions in the arterial intima.

ath•ero•gen•ic (ath″ər-o-jen′ik) conducive to or causing atherogenesis.

ath•er•o•ma (ath″ər-o′mə) [Gr. *athērōma* a tumor filled with gruellike matter, from *athērē* gruel] a mass of plaque of degenerated, thickened arterial intima occurring in atherosclerosis; called also *atherosis* and *atheromatous degeneration.*

ath•er•o•ma•to•sis (ath″ər-o″mə-to′sis) a diffuse atheromatous disease of the arteries.

ath•er•o•ma•tous (ath″ər-o′mə-təs) affected with or of the nature of atheroma.

ath•ero•scle•ro•sis (ath″ər-o-sklə-ro′sis) [*athero-* + *sclerosis*] a common form of arteriosclerosis with formation of deposits of yellowish plaques (atheromas) containing cholesterol, lipoid material, and lipophages in the intima and inner media of large and medium-sized arteries. **atherosclerot′ic** *adj*

a. obli′terans arteriosclerosis obliterans.

ath•er•o•sis (ath″ər-o′sis) atheroma.

ath•ero•throm•bo•sis (ath″ər-o-throm-bo′sis) thrombus formation as a complication of atherosclerosis.

ath•e•toid (ath′ə-toid) [Gr. *athetos* not fixed + *-oid* form] resembling or affected with athetosis.

ath•e•to•sic (ath″ə-to′sik) athetotic.

ath•e•to•sis (ath″ə-to′sis) [Gr. *athetos* not fixed + *-osis*] a form of dyskinesia marked by ceaseless occurrence of slow, sinuous, writhing movements, especially severe in the hands, and performed involuntarily; it may occur after hemiplegia, and is then known as *posthemiplegic chorea.* Called also *mobile spasm.* **athetot′ic** *adj*

double a., double congenital a. congenital bilateral athetosis due to birth trauma, which may occur in association with spastic paraplegia, as in *Vogt syndrome* and *Little disease.*

pupillary a. hippus.

athi•a•mi•no•sis (a-thi″ə-mĭ-no′sis) thiamine deficiency.

athrep•sia (ə-threp′se-ə) [*a-*[1] + Gr. *threpsis* nutrition] marasmus. **athrep′tic** *adj*

ath•rep•sy (ə-threp′se) athrepsia.

ath•ro•phago•cy•to•sis (ath″ro-fa″go-si-to′sis) non-nutritive phagocytosis; phagocytosis of inert particles, such as the removal of injected carbon particles.

athym•ia[1] (ə-thīm′e-ə) [*a-*[1] + *thymus*] athymism.

athym•ia[2] (ə-thīm′e-ə) [Gr. "lack of spirit"] name formerly given to absence of feeling or emotion, as seen in depression or the dysthymic disorder.

athym•ism (ə-thīm′iz-əm) 1. absence of the thymus. 2. the condition resulting from absence of the thymus; if it is congenital or the result of neonatal thymectomy, it will be accompanied by a lack of T lymphocytes with some degree of immunodeficiency. Called also *athymia.*

athy•rea (ə-thi′re-ə) 1. hypothyroidism. 2. athyria (def. 2).

athy•re•o•sis (ə-thi″re-o′sis) 1. hypothyroidism. 2. athyria (def. 2).

athy•re•ot•ic (ə-thi″re-ot′ik) 1. hypothyroid. 2. athyrotic (def. 2).

athy•ria (ə-thi′re-ə) 1. hypothyroidism. 2. complete absence of thyroid function; the concept has largely been replaced by severe hypothyroidism. **athyrot′ic** *adj*

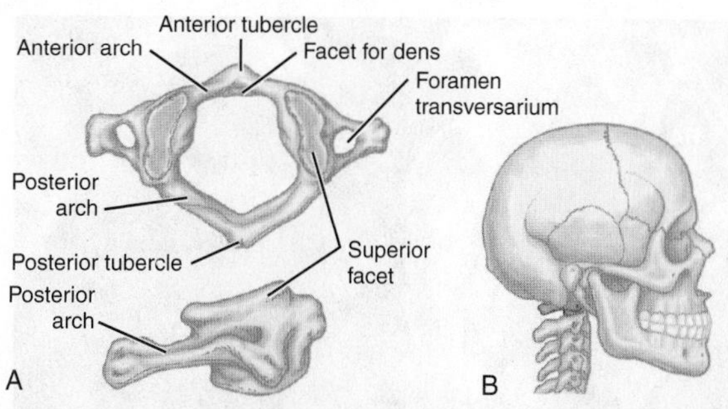

■ Atlas. *(A)*, *(Top)* superior aspect; *(bottom)* transverse aspect. Note the absence of the body and spinous process. *(B)*, Position.

athy·roid (a-thi′roid) athyrotic.

athy·roid·emia (a-thi″roi-de′me-ə) [*a-*[1] + *thyroid* + *-emia*] absence of thyroid hormone from the blood.

athy·roid·ism (a-thi′roid-iz-əm) 1. hypothyroidism. 2. athyria (def. 2).

athy·roi·do·sis (a-thi″roi-do′sis) 1. hypothyroidism. 2. athyria (def. 2).

athy·ro·sis (a″thi-ro′sis) 1. hypothyroidism. 2. athyria (def. 2).

Athys·a·nus (ə-this′ə-nəs) a genus of blood-sucking flies of Algeria.

At·i·van (at′ĭ-van) trademark for preparations of lorazepam.

ATL adult T-cell leukemia/lymphoma; see under *leukemia*.

atlant(o)- [Gr. *atlas*, q.v., gen. *atlantos*] a combining form denoting relationship to the atlas; also *atl(o)-*.

at·lan·tad (at-lan′tad) toward the atlas.

at·lan·to·ax·i·al (at-lan″to-ak′se-əl) pertaining to the atlas and the axis.

at·lan·to·did·y·mus (at-lan″to-did′ə-məs) dicephalus.

at·lan·to·mas·toid (at-lan″to-mas′toid) pertaining to the atlas and the mastoid process.

at·lan·to·oc·cip·i·tal (at-lan″to-ok-sip′ĭ-təl) pertaining to the atlas and the occipital bone.

at·lan·to·odon·toid (at-lan″to-o-don′toid) pertaining to the atlas and the odontoid process of the axis.

at·las (at′ləs) [Gr. *Atlas* the Greek god who bears up the pillars of Heaven] 1. [TA] the first cervical vertebra, which articulates above with the occipital bone and below with the axis. 2. a collection of related illustrations. atlan′tal *adj*

stereotactic a. a group of maps of the areas of the cerebrum, usually stressing physiologic functions, for use in stereotactic surgery.

atl(o)- see *atlant(o)-*.

at·lo·ax·oid (at″lo-ak′soid) pertaining to the atlas and the axis.

at·lo·did·y·mus (at″lo-did′ə-mus) [*atlo-* + Gr. *didymos* twin] dicephalus.

at·loid (at′loid) atlantal.

at·loi·do·oc·cip·i·tal (at-loi″do-ok-sip′ĭ-təl) pertaining to the atlas and the occiput.

atm atmosphere (def. 3).

atm(o)- [Gr. *atmos* steam or vapor] a combining form denoting relationship to steam or vapor.

at·mol·y·sis (at-mol′ə-sis) [*atmo-* + *-lysis*] 1. the separation of mixed gases by passing through a porous plate, the more diffusible passing through first. 2. the disintegration of organic tissue by the fumes of toxic volatile fluids.

at·mom·e·ter (at-mom′ə-tər) [*atmo-* + *-meter*] an instrument for measuring exhaled vapors, or the amount of water exhaled by evaporation in a given time, in order to ascertain the humidity of the atmosphere.

at·mos·phere (at′məs-fēr) [*atmo-* + *sphere*] 1. the entire gaseous envelope surrounding the earth and subject to the earth's gravitational field. 2. the air or climate in a particular place. 3. a unit of pressure, being that exerted by the earth's atmosphere at sea level; equal to 1.01325×10^5 pascals (approximately 760 mm Hg). Abbreviated atm. atmospher′ic *adj*

at no atomic number.

ato·cia (a-to′shə) [*a-*[1] + *toc-* + *-ia*] 1. nulliparity. 2. sterility in the female.

at·om (at′əm) [Gr. *atomos* indivisible] any one of the ultimate particles of a molecule or of any matter. An atom is the smallest particle of an element that is capable of entering into a chemical reaction. The atom consists of a minute central nucleus, in which practically all of the mass of the atom is concentrated, and of surrounding electrons. The nucleus is positively charged; the amount of the charge corresponds to the atomic number of the atom. See Appendix 5. In a neutral atom the surrounding negative electrons are equal in number to the positive charges on the nucleus. The number and arrangement of these electrons determine all the properties of the atom except its atomic weight and its radioactivity. atom′ic *adj*

activated a. 1. an ionized atom. 2. an atom in which some of the orbital electrons have been driven out into larger and less stable orbits; the atom is thus prepared to release its stored energy as these electrons return to their normal and stable orbits. Called also *excited a.*

asymmetric carbon a. a carbon atom with four different substituents. Such a molecule does not have a mirror plane passing through the asymmetric atom, and thus may be optically active.

Bohr a. the conception of a nuclear atom in which the orbital electrons are able to occupy only certain orbits, these orbits being determined by quantum limitations.

chiral carbon a. asymmetric carbon a.

excited a. activated a.

ionized a. an atom from which one or more of the outer or valence electrons have been removed, or to which one or more electrons have been added (hence positive and negative ions).

nuclear a. the conception or theory of the atom as composed of a small central nucleus surrounded by orbital electrons; called also *Rutherford a.*

recoil a., rest a. the portion of an atom from which an alpha particle or other subatomic particle has been given off; this remaining part recoils with a velocity inversely proportional to its mass.

Rutherford a. nuclear a.

stripped a. an atom from which the orbital electrons have been more or less completely removed.

tagged a. an atom that has been made radioactive, so that its course in the body may be checked; see *radioactive tracer*, under *tracer*.

at·om·i·za·tion (at″əm-ĭ-za′shən) nebulization.

at·om·iz·er (at′əm-i″zər) nebulizer.

at·om·ox·e·tine hy·dro·chlo·ride (at″ə-mok′sə-tēn) a selective norepinephrine reuptake inhibitor used in the treatment of attention-deficit/hyperactivity disorder, administered orally.

ato·nia (ə-to′ne-ə) atony.

choreatic a. the deficient muscular tonicity seen in chorea.

at·o·nic·i·ty (at″ə-nis′ĭ-te) atony.

at·o·ny (at′ə-ne) [L. *atonia*, from *a-*[1] + Gr. *tonos* tension] lack of normal tone or strength, such as in a muscle deprived of its innervation. Called also *atonia* and *atonicity*. aton′ic *adj*

abomasal a. inadequate tone in the abomasal muscles, often seen in postparturient cows and a contributing factor to right and left displacement of the abomasum (see under *displacement*).

at·o·pen (at′ə-pen) the allergen involved in an atopic disorder.

atop·ic (a-top′ik, ə-top′ik) [*a-*[1] + *top-* + *-ic*] 1. ectopic. 2. pertaining to an atopen or to atopy. 3. allergic.

Ato·po·bi·um (at″ə-po′be-əm) [*a-*[1] + Gr. *topos* place + *bios* life] a genus of gram-positive bacteria of the family Coriobacteriaceae, consisting of anaerobic, non–spore-forming, lactic acid–producing cocci or coccobacilli that occur singly or in short chains. Organisms can be isolated from the gingival crevice and vagina and cause soft tissue infections. The type species is *A. minu′tum.*

A. vagi′nae a species that is a cause of bacterial vaginosis.

atop·og·no·sia (ə-top″og-no′zhə) [*a-*[1] + *topo-* + *gnōsis* knowledge + *-ia*] loss of the power of topesthesia; called also *atopognosis, topagnosia*, and *topoanesthesia*.

atop·og·no·sis (ə-top″og-no′sis) atopognosia.

at·o·py (at′ə-pe) [Gr. *atopos* out of place] a genetic predisposition toward the development of immediate (type I) hypersensitivity reactions against common environmental antigens (atopic allergy). The most common clinical manifestation is allergic rhinitis; bronchial asthma, atopic dermatitis, and food allergy occur less frequently.

ator·va·stat·in cal·ci·um (ə-tor′və-stat″in) a synthetic HMG-CoA reductase inhibitor that acts as an antihyperlipidemic by inhibiting cholesterol synthesis; used in treatment of hypercholesterolemia and other forms of dyslipidemia, administered orally.

ato·va·quone (ə-to′və-kwōn″) an inhibitor of parasite mitochondrial transport, effective as an antimalarial against the erythrocytic and exoerythrocytic stages of *Plasmodium* spp., used in the prophylaxis and treatment of falciparum malaria; administered orally. It is also effective against *Pneumocystis jiroveci* and is used in the treatment of mild to moderate cases of pneumocystis pneumonia, administered orally.

atox·ic (a-tok′sik) [*a-*[1] + *toxic*] not poisonous; not due to a poison.

atox·i·gen·ic (a-tok″sĭ-jen′ik) not producing or elaborating toxins.

ATP adenosine triphosphate.

ATP·ase (a-te-pe′ās) adenosinetriphosphatase.

ATP cit·rate ly·ase (sit′rāt li′ās) an enzyme of the lyase class that catalyzes the ATP-dependent cleavage of citrate to form oxaloacetate and acetate, the latter then condensing with coenzyme A to form acetyl coenzyme A. The reaction is part of the mechanism by which acetyl coenzyme A produced in the mitochondria from pyruvate can be transported to the cytosol to be used in fatty acid synthesis. In EC nomenclature, called *ATP citrate* (pro-S) *lyase* [EC 4.1.3.8]. Called also *citrate cleavage enzyme.*

ATP syn·thase (sin′thās) H^+-transporting ATP synthase.

Atrac·tas·pis (ə-trak-tas′pis) a genus of African vipers with a toxic bite.

atra·cu·rium bes·y·late (at″rə-kūr′e-əm) a nondepolarizing neuromuscular blocking agent of intermediate duration, administered intravenously as an adjunct to general anesthesia to induce skeletal muscle relaxation during surgery and facilitate mechanical ventilation.

atrans·fer·ri·ne·mia (a-trans″fer-ĭ-ne′me-ə) absence of iron-binding transferrin from the circulating blood.

atrau·mat·ic (a″traw-mat′ik) [*a-*[1] + *traumatic*] not inflicting or causing damage or injury.

Atrax (a′traks) the funnel-web spiders, a tarantulalike genus found in Australia, of the family Dipluridae. *A. formida′bilis* is the tree funnel-web spider. This and other species have a venomous bite. *A. robus′tus* has caused human deaths.

at·rep·sy (at′rep-se) [*a-*[1] + Gr. *threpsis* nutrition] athrepsia (def. 1).

atrep·tic (ə-trep′tik) athreptic.

atre·sia (ə-tre′zhə) [*a-*[1] + Gr. *trēsis* a hole + *-ia*] congenital absence or closure of a normal body orifice or tubular organ.

anal a., a. a′ni imperforate anus.

aortic a. absence or closure of the aortic orifice of the heart, a rare congenital anomaly in which the left ventricle is hypoplastic, oxygenated blood passing from the left into the right atrium through an atrial septal defect, and the mixed venous and arterial blood passing from the pulmonary artery to the aorta by way of a patent ductus arteriosus.

aural a. obstruction of the external acoustic meatus; it may be either congenital or acquired through trauma or disease.

biliary a. obliteration or hypoplasia of one or more components of the bile ducts due to arrested fetal development, resulting in persistent jaundice and liver damage ranging from biliary stasis to biliary cirrhosis. As portal hypertension progresses, infants develop splenomegaly.

bronchial a. atresia of a lobar or segmental bronchus, usually in the left upper lobe; the affected lung segment is often hyperinflated due to leakage of air through the alveolar pores.

choanal a. congenital bony or membranous occlusion of one or both choanae, due to failure of the embryonic bucconasal membrane to rupture. Cf. *atretorrhinia.*

duodenal a. atresia of a portion of the duodenum, a type of intestinal atresia; infants have vomiting a few hours after birth, cessation of bowel movements after one to three days, and usually distention of the epigastrium. The condition is often associated with Down syndrome.

esophageal a. congenital lack of continuity of the esophagus, commonly associated with tracheoesophageal fistula and characterized by excessive salivation, gagging, vomiting when fed, cyanosis, and dyspnea.

follicular a., a. folli′culi degeneration and resorption of the ovarian follicles in a given menstrual cycle that began maturing but did not become the dominant follicle. See *atretic ovarian follicle,* under *follicle.*

ileal a. atresia of the ileum, the most common type of intestinal atresia.

intestinal a. congenital obstruction of the intestine at any level; symptoms vary with the site of obstruction. The most common type is ileal atresia. See also *duodenal a.* and *jejunal a.*

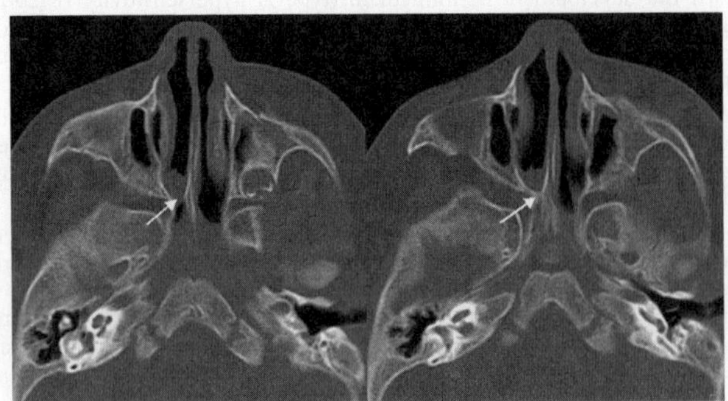

■ Unilateral right-sided choanal atresia in a child with chronic nasal discharge. Axial CT scan shows bony narrowing of the posterior right choana down to a bony bridging bar *(arrows)* and pooling of secretions proximally.

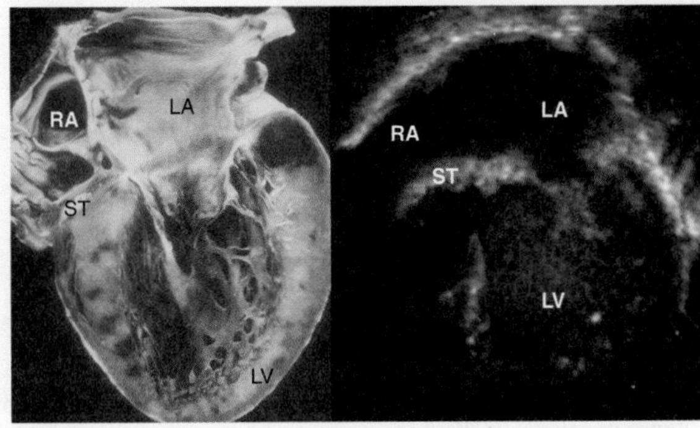

■ Tricuspid atresia, in a clinical specimen *(left)* and apical four chamber view *(right)*. There is a notable wedge of sulcus tissue *(ST)* in the floor of the right atrium *(RA)*. *LA,* left atrium; *LV,* left ventricle.

a. i′ridis closure of the pupillary opening.

jejunal a. atresia of the jejunum, a type of intestinal atresia.

jejunoileal a. intestinal atresia involving the jejunum and ileum.

lacrimal duct a. blockage of a lacrimal duct, as in congenital imperforation or with scar tissue.

laryngeal a. congenital lack of the normal opening into the larynx. See also *laryngeal web.*

mitral a. congenital obliteration of the mitral orifice of the heart; it is associated with hypoplastic left heart syndrome or transposition of great vessels.

prepyloric a. congenital obstruction of the pyloric orifice of the stomach by an antral or pyloric membrane; infants vomit gastric contents only. Called also *pyloric a.*

pulmonary a. congenital severe narrowing or obstruction of the pulmonary orifice of the heart, characterized by cardiomegaly, reduced pulmonary vascularity, and right ventricular atrophy. It is usually associated with tetralogy of Fallot, transposition of great vessels, or other cardiovascular anomalies.

pyloric a. prepyloric a.

tricuspid a. absence of the tricuspid orifice of the heart; circulation is made possible only by the presence of an atrial septal defect, with blood passing from the right to the left atrium and thence to the left ventricle and aorta. Classification by type is made according to the presence or absence of pulmonary stenosis and of transposition of great vessels.

urethral a. congenital imperforation of the urethra.

atre·sic (ə-tre′zik) atretic.

atret·ic (ə-tret′ik) [*atret-* + *-ic*] without an opening; pertaining to or characterized by atresia.

atret(o)- [Gr. *atrētos* not perforated] a combining form denoting absence of a normal opening; imperforate or closed.

atre·to·ble·pha·ria (ə-tre″to-blə-far′e-ə) [*atreto-* + *blepharo-* + *-ia*] symblepharon.

atre·to·ceph·a·lus (ə-tre″to-sef′ə-ləs) [*atreto-* + Gr. *-cephalus*] a fetus lacking the orifices normally present in the head.

atre·to·cor·mus (ə-tre″to-kor′məs) [*atreto-* + Gr. *kormos* trunk] a fetus or infant having one of the body openings imperforate.

atre·to·gas·tria (ə-tre″to-gas′tre-ə) [*atreto-* + *gastr-* + *-ia*] lack of one of the normal openings of the stomach.

atre·top·sia (ă″tre-top′se-ə) atresia iridis; see under *atresia.*

atre·tor·rhi·nia (ə-tre″to-ri′ne-ə) [*atreto-* + *rhin-* + *-ia*] absence of the external opening into the nose. Cf. *choanal atresia,* under *atresia.*

atre·to·sto·mia (ə-tre″to-sto′me-ə) [*atreto-* + *stom-* + *-ia*] lack of the normal opening into the oral cavity.

atria (a′tre-ə) [L.] plural of *atrium.*

atrich·ia (ə-trik′e-ə) alopecia.

at·ri·cho·sis (at″rĭ-ko′sis) alopecia.

atrich·ous (ə-trik′əs) 1. having no flagella; said of bacteria. 2. bald.

Atri·dox (at′rĭ-doks) trademark for an extended-release preparation of doxycycline hyclate for periodontal use.

atri(o)- [L. *atrium,* q.v.] a combining form denoting relationship to an atrium of the heart.

atrio·com·mis·su·ro·pexy (a″tre-o-kom″ĭ-su′ro-pek″se) [*atrio-* + *commissure* + *-pexy*] repair of the mitral valve with sutures passed from the ventricle through the valve cusps and the atrial wall, for correction of mitral insufficiency.

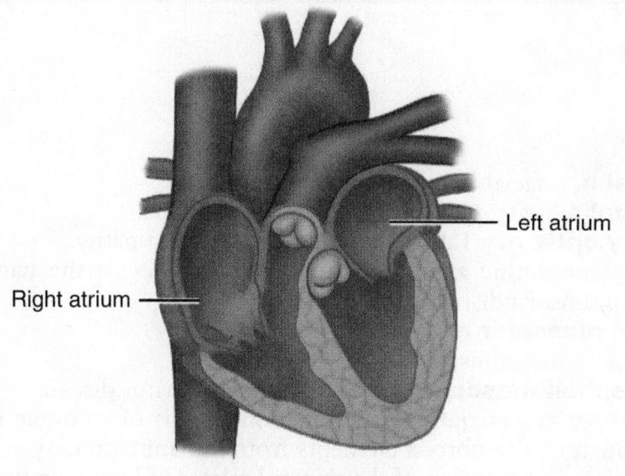

■ Atria of the heart.

atrio•his•i•an (a″tre-o-his′e-ən) connecting the atrium and the bundle of His.

atrio•meg•a•ly (a″tre-o-meg′ə-le) [*atrio-* + *-megaly*] abnormal dilatation or enlargement of an atrium of the heart.

atri•o•pep•tin (a″tre-o-pep′tin) atrial natriuretic peptide.

atrio•sep•to•pexy (a″tre-o-sep′to-pek″se) [*atrio-* + *septo-* + *-pexy*] a closed technique for surgical repair of a defect in the interatrial septum by suturing together part of the atrial wall to obstruct the defect.

atrio•sep•to•plas•ty (a″tre-o-sep′to-plas″te) [*atrio-* + *septo-* + *-plasty*] plastic repair of the interatrial septum.

atri•ot•o•my (a″tre-ot′ə-me) [*atrio-* + *-tomy*] surgical incision of an atrium of the heart.

atrio•ven•tric•u•lar (a″tre-o-ven-trik′u-lər) pertaining to both an atrium and a ventricle of the heart.

atri•o•ven•tric•u•la•ris com•mu•nis (a″tre-o-ven-trik″u-la′ris kə-mu′nis) a congenital cardiac anomaly in which the endocardial cushions fail to fuse, the ostium primum persists (producing a low-lying atrial septal defect), sometimes a single atrioventricular valve occurs which has anterior and posterior cusps, and there is commonly a defect of the membranous interventricular septum. Called also *persistent common atrioventricular canal.*

Atrip•la (ə-trip′lə) trademark for a combination preparation of efavirenz, emtricitabine, and tenofovir disoproxil fumarate.

Atrip•lex (ə-trip′leks) a genus of herbs and shrubs. *A. littora′lis* and other species are commonly fed to livestock, but in selenium-rich soils they may absorb large amounts of selenium and be a cause of atriplicism, a form of selenium poisoning.

atrip•li•cism (ə-trip′lĭ-siz-əm) selenium poisoning in livestock produced by eating *Atriplex littoralis* or other species grown in selenium-rich soil.

atri•um (a′tre-əm) pl. *a′tria* [L., from Gr. *atrion* hall] a chamber; used in anatomy to designate a chamber affording entrance to another structure or organ. Usually used alone to designate an atrium of the heart *(a. cordis).* **a′trial** *adj*

common a. a congenital anomaly caused by failure of formation of the interatrial septum, the heart having one atrium and two ventricles; called also *cor triloculare biventriculare.*

a. cor′dis dex′trum [TA] right atrium of heart: the atrium of the right side of the heart; it receives blood from the superior and the inferior venae cavae, and delivers it to the right ventricle.

a. cor′dis sinis′trum [TA] left atrium of heart: the atrium of the left side of the heart; it receives blood from the pulmonary veins, and delivers it to the left ventricle.

a. of lateral ventricle a. ventriculi lateralis.

left a. of heart a. cordis sinistrum.

a. mea′tus me′dii [TA] atrium of middle meatus: a depression in front of the middle nasal meatus, between the agger nasi and the middle nasal concha.

right a. of heart a. cordis dextrum.

a. ventri′culi latera′lis [TA] atrium of lateral ventricle: the expansion of the lateral ventricle marking the meeting of the body (pars centralis) and the occipital (cornu occipitale) and temporal horns (cornu temporale).

At•ro•mid-S (at′ro-mid) trademark for a preparation of clofibrate.

At•ro•pa (at′ro-pə) [Gr. *Atropos* "undeviating," one of the Fates] a genus of plants of the family Solanaceae, many of which contain alkaloids such as atropine, hyoscyamine, and scopolamine. *A. belladon′na* is deadly nightshade or belladonna (q.v.).

atroph•e•de•ma (ə-trof″ə-de′mə) angioedema.

atro•phia (ə-tro′fe-ə) [L., from Gr., from *a-*[1] + Gr. *trophē* nourishment] atrophy.

a. choroi′deae et re′tinae atrophy of the choroid and retina, formerly associated with night blindness.

a. cu′tis atrophoderma.

a. cu′tis seni′lis senile atrophy of skin.

a. doloro′sa atrophy of the eyeball accompanied by violent attacks of pain.

a. maculo′sa anetoderma.

a. musculo′rum lipomato′sa pseudohypertrophic muscular dystrophy.

a. seni′lis senile atrophy.

atro•phie (ah-tro-fe′) [Fr.] atrophy.

a. blanche (blahnsh) ["white atrophy"] a late stage of livedoid vasculitis characterized by white, smooth, atrophic scar tissue with telangiectasia within a hyperpigmented areola, usually seen on the ankles of middle-aged women. Called also *white atrophy.*

at•ro•phied (at′ro-fēd) marked by atrophy; shrunken.

atroph(o)- [Gr. *atrophia* want of nourishment] a combining form pertaining to atrophy.

at•ro•pho•der•ma (at″ro-fo-dur′mə) [*atropho-* + *derma*] atrophy of the skin or of any part of it. Called also *atrophia cutis* and *atrophodermia.* See also *anetoderma.*

idiopathic a. of Pasini and Pierini see *a. of Pasini and Pierini.*

a. macula′tum anetoderma.

a. neuri′ticum a condition following nerve injury, usually in a limb, in which the skin becomes erythematous and then gray, shiny, and ivory-like; it may be associated with alopecia, skin fissuring, and ulceration.

Pasini-Pierini a., a. of Pasini and Pierini a condition most often seen on the backs of young women, characterized by soft, blue, brown, or violet atrophic plaques with central induration, resembling lesions of the late stages of morphea. The etiology is unknown, and it usually resolves spontaneously in a few months to years. Two types have been distinguished: one idiopathic and the other closely related to morphea.

a. reticula′tum symme′tricum facie′i folliculitis ulerythematosa reticulata.

senile a. senile atrophy of skin.

a. vermicula′ris, a. vermicula′tum any of a group of autosomal recessive skin disorders, usually seen in children or young adults, characterized by inflammation followed by a reticulated honeycomblike or wormlike follicular atrophy, often with erythema and follicular plugging. The lesions are usually confined to the cheeks *(folliculitis ulerythematosa reticulata),* but may appear first on the forehead or eyebrow region *(ulerythema ophryogenes)* and spread to the scalp. Called also *atrophodermia vermiculata.*

at•ro•pho•der•ma•to•sis (at-ro″fo-dur″mə-to′sis) any skin disease having atrophoderma as a prominent symptom.

at•ro•pho•der•mia (at″ro-fo-dur′me-ə) atrophoderma.

a. vermicula′ta atrophoderma vermiculatum.

at•ro•phy (at′rə-fe) [Gr. *atrophia*] 1. a wasting away; a diminution in the size of a cell, tissue, organ, or part. See also *atrophia* and *atrophie.* 2. to undergo this process. **atroph′ic** *adj*

Atrophy

a. of aging senile a.

Aran-Duchenne muscular a. spinal muscular a.

arthritic a. wasting of the muscles and bone that surround a joint, due to injury or to constitutional disease.

bone a. resorption of bone evident both in external form and in internal density. Cf. *osteoporosis.*

brown a. atrophy in which an organ or part becomes brown due to intracellular accumulation of lipofuscin, seen chiefly in the heart, liver, and spleen of the elderly.

bulbospinal muscular a. spinobulbar muscular a.

Charcot-Marie a., Charcot-Marie-Tooth a. Charcot-Marie-Tooth disease.

Atrophy *Continued*

circumscribed cerebral a. Pick disease (def. 1).
compensatory a. atrophy, particularly of an endocrine organ, caused by negative feedback mechanisms when its paired organ or another structure releases large amounts of a regulator similar to or identical with the gland's product.
compression a. atrophy of a part due to constant pressure.
concentric a. atrophy of a hollow organ in which its cavity is contracted.
congenital microvillus a. a rare intestinal disorder, thought to be hereditary and autosomal recessive; infants have severe watery diarrhea with malabsorption of nutrients owing to atrophy of intestinal villi in the neonatal period. The condition is fatal unless the infant is given total parenteral nutrition. Cf. *microvillus inclusion disease*, under *disease*.
corticostriatospinal a. Creutzfeldt-Jakob disease.
Cruveilhier a. spinal muscular a.
degenerative a. the wasting of a part due to a degeneration of its cells.
Dejerine-Sottas a. progressive hypertrophic neuropathy.
Dejerine-Thomas a. olivopontocerebellar a.
denervated muscle a. neuropathic a.
dentatorubral a. dyssynergia cerebellaris progressiva.
dentatorubral-pallidoluysian a. (DRPLA) an autosomal dominant neurodegenerative syndrome of myoclonic epilepsy, dementia, ataxia, and choreoathetosis, with combined degeneration of the dentatorubral and pallidoluysian systems. Onset is usually in early adulthood, and it has been found mainly in Japan. It is a triplet repeat disorder associated with expansion of the triplet sequence CAG in the *DRPLA* gene (locus: 12p13.31), which encodes the atrophin-1 protein, and hence of glutamine residues in the protein, with an inverse correlation between the age of onset and the size of the expansion. Cf. *Haw River syndrome*.
disuse a., a. of disuse wasting caused by lack of normal exercise of a part.
Duchenne-Aran muscular a. spinal muscular a.
eccentric a. atrophy of a hollow organ in which the size of the cavity is increased.
Eichhorst a. the femorotibial form of progressive muscular atrophy with contraction of the toes.
endocrine a. atrophy in organs that are dependent upon endocrine stimulation for the maintenance of their normal structure, occurring when their tropic hormone stimulation diminishes or is absent.
endometrial a. atrophy of the endometrium, occurring physiologically at menopause or pathologically before menopause and accompanied by absence of menstrual flow and shrinkage of the uterus.
Erb a. 1. Duchenne muscular dystrophy. 2. limb-girdle muscular dystrophy; see under *dystrophy*.
essential a. of iris a progressive disease of unknown etiology, marked by patchy degeneration and disappearance of the iris stroma followed by loss of epithelium and formation of holes in the iris; it is associated with severe glaucoma.
exhaustion a. atrophy of an endocrine organ from prolonged overwork of it.
facial a. facial hemiatrophy.
facioscapulohumeral muscular a. see under *dystrophy*.
fatty a. fatty infiltration following atrophy of a tissue or organ.
Fazio-Londe a. progressive bulbar palsy of childhood.
gastric a. marked reduction in thickness of the mucosa of the stomach, with complete or almost complete disappearance of gastric glands and pyloric glands, which are replaced by simple mucus-secreting epithelium; this is often accompanied by intestinal metaplasia.
geographic retinal a. a pattern of well-demarcated epithelial atrophy of retinal pigment, leading to vision loss, most often associated with age-related macular degeneration.
gray a. secondary optic a.
gyrate a. of choroid and retina an autosomal recessive form of tapetoretinal degeneration, caused by mutations in the *OAT* gene (locus: 10q26) that result in ornithine aminotransferase deficiency and hyperornithinemia. It is marked by ring-shaped areas of thinning in the periphery of the fundus that enlarge and become confluent, resulting in tunnel vision; night blindness and other disturbances of vision follow.
hemifacial a. facial hemiatrophy.
hemilingual a. atrophy of one side of the tongue.
hereditary optic a. Leber hereditary optic neuropathy.
Hunt a. neuropathic atrophy of the small muscles of the hand unattended by sensory disturbance.
idiopathic muscular a. spinal muscular a.
infantile a. marasmus.
infantile spinal muscular a. Werdnig-Hoffmann disease.
inflammatory a. atrophy of the functioning part of an organ caused by overgrowth of the fibrous elements from inflammation.
interstitial a. absorption of the mineral matter of bones, so that only the reticulated portion remains.
ischemic muscular a. Volkmann contracture.
juvenile muscular a., juvenile spinal muscular a. Kugelberg-Welander syndrome.
lactation a. hyperinvolution of the uterus, which occasionally follows prolonged lactation.
Landouzy-Dejerine a. facioscapulohumeral muscular dystrophy.
leaping a. progressive muscular atrophy that begins in the hand and extends to the shoulder without affecting the muscles of the arm.
Leber hereditary optic a., Leber optic a. see under *neuropathy*.
linear a. striae distensae.
lobar a. Pick disease (def. 1).
macular a. anetoderma.
multiple system a. (MSA), multisystem a. a progressive neurodegenerative disorder characterized by striatonigral and olivopontocerebellar degeneration with formation of Papp-Lantos bodies and exhibiting varying combinations of parkinsonism, cerebellar ataxia, autonomic failure, urogenital dysfunction, and corticospinal disorders. It is divided into two categories, MSA with predominant parkinsonism (MSA-P) and MSA with predominant cerebellar ataxia (MSA-C), and includes several conditions formerly classified as separate diseases (olivopontocerebellar atrophy, striatonigral degeneration, and Shy-Drager syndrome).
muscular a. a wasting of muscle tissue; there are many kinds and causes. See also *spinal muscular a.*
myelopathic muscular a. muscular atrophy due to lesion of the spinal cord, as in spinal muscular atrophy.
myopathic a. muscular atrophy due to disease of the muscle tissue.
neural a. neuropathic a.
neuritic muscular a. neuropathic a.
neuropathic a. atrophy of muscular tissue due to disease of the peripheral nervous system; called also *neural a.*
neurotrophic a. atrophy attributed to destruction of the peripheral neurons that innervate a particular tissue.
olivopontocerebellar a. a form of multiple system atrophy in which neurodegeneration occurs in the cerebellar cortex, middle peduncles, ventral pontine surface, and olivary nuclei. It occurs in young to middle-aged persons and is characterized by ataxia, dysarthria, and parkinsonism. Both autosomal dominant and autosomal recessive types have been distinguished. Called also *olivopontocerebellar degeneration* and *Dejerine-Thomas syndrome*.
optic a. atrophy of the optic disk resulting from degeneration of the nerve fibers of the optic nerve and optic tract.
pallidal a. juvenile paralysis agitans (of Hunt); see under *paralysis*.
Parrot a. of the newborn primary marasmus.
pathologic a. a decrease in the size of tissues or organs beyond the range of normal variability.
periodontal a. reduction of the size of the alveolar process, associated with recession of the gingiva with subsequent exposure of the root surface.
peroneal a., peroneal muscular a. Charcot-Marie-Tooth disease.
physiologic a. atrophy caused by normal physiologic processes, such as pregnancy or aging.
pigmentary a. wasting marked by the deposit of pigment in the atrophied cells, as in brown atrophy.
postmenopausal a. atrophy of tissues such as the genital mucosa after menopause.
posttraumatic a. of bone posttraumatic osteoporosis.
pressure a. decrease in the size of a tissue cell caused by excessive pressure.
primary optic a. optic atrophy in which the optic disk is characterized by sharp margins, enlarged physiologic cup, enhanced visibility of the lamina cribrosa, and a white color.

Atrophy *Continued*

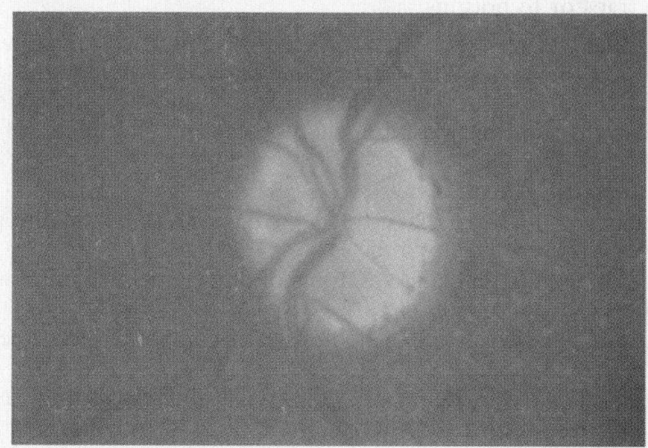

■ Severe primary optic atrophy secondary to multiple episodes of optic neuritis.

progressive choroidal a. choroideremia.
progressive hemifacial a. facial hemiatrophy.
progressive muscular a. spinal muscular a.
progressive neural muscular a., progressive neuromuscular a. Charcot-Marie-Tooth disease.
progressive retinal a. any of a group of hereditary retinal diseases of dogs characterized by progressive dysplasia or degeneration of the retinal rods or cones. Affected animals first have night blindness and then increasingly lose their daytime vision; some develop cataracts.
progressive spinal muscular a. spinal muscular a.
proximal spinal muscular a. Kugelberg-Welander syndrome.
pseudohypertrophic muscular a. pseudohypertrophic muscular dystrophy.
pulp a. a degenerative process of the dental pulp, characterized by a diminution in size and wasting away of pulpal cells, usually associated with an interference with nutrition. Called also *atrophic pulp degeneration.*
rheumatic a. atrophy of muscles after an attack of rheumatism.
secondary optic a. optic atrophy in which the optic disk is characterized by blurred margins, poor visibility of the lamina cribrosa, filling-in of the physiologic cup, and gray-white glial tissue on its surface and along its blood vessels; called also *gray a.*
segmental sensory dissociation with brachial muscular a. see *syringomyelia.*
senile a. the natural atrophy of tissues and organs occurring with advancing age. Called also *atrophy of aging.* Cf. *senile degeneration.*
senile a. of skin the mild atrophic changes in the epidermis and dermis that occur naturally with aging. Called also *atrophia cutis senilis.*
serous a. atrophy with the effusion of a serous fluid into the wasted tissues; wasting of fat.
simple a. atrophy due to a shrinkage in size of individual cells.
spinal muscular a. any of several hereditary, progressive, degenerative diseases of the motor cells of the spinal cord. Beginning usually in the small muscles of the hands, but in some cases (scapulohumeral type) in those of the upper arms and shoulders, the atrophy progresses to the muscles of the lower limbs. *Type I* is *Werdnig-Hoffmann disease,* the most severe type, usually fatal in infancy. *Type II* is an intermediate type seen in babies that is not always fatal. *Type III* is *Kugelberg-Welander syndrome,* the least severe type. Called also *Aran-Duchenne disease* or *muscular a., Duchenne-Aran disease* or *muscular a., Cruveilhier a.* or *paralysis,* and *progressive spinal muscular a.*
spinobulbar muscular a. (SBMA) an X-linked, adult-onset disorder with degeneration of lower motor neurons in the brainstem and spinal cord, characterized by distal limb amyotrophy and bulbar signs such as atrophy and fasciculations of the tongue and dysphagia, as well as androgen insensitivity with gynecomastia, testicular atrophy, and oligospermia. It is a triplet repeat disorder with expansion of CAG repeats in the *AR* gene (locus: Xq11-q12), which encodes the androgen receptor. Called also *Kennedy disease.*
Sudeck a. posttraumatic osteoporosis.
Tooth a. Charcot-Marie-Tooth disease.
trophoneurotic a. atrophy due to disease of the nerves or of a center supplying a part.
vascular a. progressive loss of substance in cells and organs when the blood supply to that organ or tissue becomes reduced below a critical level.
white a. 1. atrophy of a nerve, leaving only white connective tissue. 2. atrophie blanche.
yellow a. massive hepatic necrosis.
Zimmerlin a. Duchenne muscular dystrophy.

at•ro•pine (at′ro-pēn) [USP] an alkaloid derived from species of belladonna, hyoscyamus, or stramonium, or produced synthetically. It is an anticholinergic and antimuscarinic, used as an antispasmodic to relax smooth muscles and to increase and regulate the heart rate by blocking the vagus nerve. It also serves as an antidote for various toxic and anticholinesterase agents and as an antisecretory, mydriatic, and cycloplegic. Ingestion of excessive amounts causes atropinism.

a. methonitrate, a. methylnitrate methylatropine nitrate.

a. sulfate [USP] the sulfate salt of atropine, having the same actions as the base; administered parenterally and orally as an anticholinergic and antispasmodic, antidote to cholinesterase inhibitors or toxins, antiarrhythmic, cholinergic adjunct during surgery, and preanesthetic antisialagogue; also applied topically to the conjunctiva as a cycloplegic and mydriatic.

at•ro•pin•ic (at″ro-pin′ik) having actions similar to atropine, that is, antagonizing the muscarinic effects of acetylcholine.

at•ro•pin•ism (at′ro-pin-iz-əm) poisoning caused by ingestion of atropine or belladonna or parts or preparations of any of the plants from which the drugs are derived; the symptoms include excessive dryness of the mouth and throat, dilation of the pupils, fever, rapid pulse, flushing of the face, confusion, mania, and hallucinations, and sometimes a rash.

at•ro•pin•i•za•tion (at-ro″pin-ĭ-za′shən) subjection to the influence of atropine.

at•ro•pism (at′ro-piz-əm) atropinism.

At•ro•pi•sol (at′ro-pĭ-sol″) trademark for preparations of atropine sulfate.

At•ro•vent (at′ro-vent) trademark for preparations of ipratropium bromide.

ATS American Thoracic Society; antitetanic serum.

ATSDR Agency for Toxic Substances and Diseases Registry, an agency of the United States Public Health Service.

at•tach•ment (ə-tach′mənt) 1. a connection by which one thing is fixed to another. 2. a device for retention and stabilization of a dental prosthesis. 3. the initial stage of imfection of a cell by a virus, in which the viral envelope finds a suitable receptor on the cell surface, enabling the virus to enter. Called also *adsorption.*

edgewise a. see under *appliance.*

epithelial a. (of Gottlieb) a band or wedge of epithelium whose external surface adheres to the tooth crown and whose internal surface adheres to the lamina propria of the free gingiva, forming a peripheral cuff that seals the periodontal tissue and protects it from foreign material in the oral cavity.

extracoronal a. a precision attachment in which the retaining mechanism is outside the crown of an abutment tooth or restoration.

friction a., internal a. intracoronal a.

intracoronal a., key-and-keyway a. a precision attachment with a slotlike unit (female part) built entirely into the crown and an insert or flange (male part) extending from the prosthesis proper and fitting into the slot when the denture is attached to the crown; the flange may be retained by friction alone or by augmenting mechanical locks, screws, or adjustable latches. Called also *friction a., internal a., parallel a., precision a.,* and *slotted a.*

orthodontic a. see *bracket* (def. 2).

parallel a. intracoronal a.

precision a. 1. a device using a precision rest (q.v.) to attach fixed or removable partial dentures to the crown of an abutment tooth or a restoration; the two primary types are the intracoronal attachment and the extracoronal attachment. Called also *precision anchorage.* See also *extracoronal a., intracoronal a.,* and *semiprecision a.* 2. intracoronal a.

semiprecision a. attachment of a denture to an abutment tooth or a restoration by a semiprecision rest (q.v.), sometimes supplemented by a spring-loaded plunger or clip, fitting into a rest seat on the lateral surface of a crown, which is especially deepened to provide added retention.

slotted a. intracoronal a.

at·tack (ə-tak′) an episode or onset of illness.

Adams-Stokes a. an episode of syncope in Adams-Stokes syndrome.

anxiety a. panic a.

drop a. sudden loss of balance without loss of consciousness, usually seen in elderly women; various causes are hypothesized.

heart a. 1. popular term for myocardial infarction. 2. any of various types of acute episodes of ischemic heart disease.

panic a. [DSM-IV] an episode of acute intense anxiety, with symptoms such as racing or pounding heart, sweating, trembling, chest pains, nausea, dizziness, faintness, chills or hot flashes, and feelings of choking or smothering. It is the essential feature of panic disorder (q.v.) but may also occur in agoraphobia and other anxiety disorders, as well as in other psychiatric disorders such as schizophrenic disorders or mood disorders. Called also *anxiety a.*

short-lasting unilateral neuralgiform headache a's with conjunctival injection and tearing (SUNCT) a type of trigeminal autonomic cephalalgia marked by unilateral, stabbing or pulsating, orbital, supraorbital or temporal pain, a few seconds to a few minutes in duration, accompanied by conjunctival injection and lacrimation affecting the ipsilateral eye. As many as 200 attacks can occur in a single day; intervals between attacks are pain-free.

Stokes-Adams a. Adams-Stokes a.

transient ischemic a. (TIA) a brief attack (from a few minutes to an hour) of cerebral dysfunction of vascular origin, with no persistent neurological deficit; TIAs are most commonly associated with occlusive vascular disease, especially in the distribution of the carotid and vertebral-basilar systems.

vagal a., vasovagal a. vasovagal syncope.

at·ta·pul·gite (at″ə-pul′jīt) [*Attapulgus*, a town in Georgia near which it is found] a hydrated aluminum silicate containing magnesium, which is the chief ingredient of fuller's earth (q.v.).

activated a. [USP] attapulgite that has been heat treated to increase its adsorbency; used as an adjunct to adsorb bacteria and toxins in the treatment of diarrhea; administered orally.

at·tar (at′ar) [Persian "essence"] any essential or volatile oil of vegetable origin.

a. of roses rose oil.

at·tend·ing (ə-ten′ding) 1. attending physician. 2. being or pertaining to such a physician.

at·ten·tion (ə-ten′shən) 1. selective awareness of a part or aspect of the environment. 2. selective responsiveness to one class of stimuli.

at·ten·u·ant (ə-ten′u-ənt) 1. causing thinness, as of the blood. 2. an agent or means that thins or dilutes, particularly one that thins the blood.

at·ten·u·ate (ə-ten′u-āt) [L. *attenuare* to thin] 1. to render thin. 2. to render less virulent; see *attenuation* (def. 2).

at·ten·u·a·tion (ə-ten″u-a′shən) [L. *attenuatio*, from *ad-* to + *tenuis* thin] 1. the act of thinning or weakening. 2. reduction in virulence of a pathogenic organism, usually by adaptation to another host or a different culture medium. 3. reduction in energy of a beam of radiation when it passes through tissue or other material. Cf. *radiation absorption.*

At·ten·u·vax (ə-ten′u-vaks) trademark for a preparation of measles virus vaccine live.

at·tic (at′ik) [L. *atticus*] recessus epitympanicus.

at·ti·co·an·trot·o·my (at″ĭ-ko-an-trot′ə-me) the operation of opening the mastoid antrum and the attic of the middle ear; called also *antroatticotomy.*

at·ti·co·mas·toid (at″ĭ-ko-mas′toid) pertaining to the recessus epitympanicus (attic) and the mastoid process.

at·ti·cot·o·my (at″ĭ-kot′ə-me) [*attic* + *-tomy*] the surgical opening of the attic.

transmeatal a. removal through the external auditory meatus of the outer wall of the attic.

at·ti·tude (at′ĭ-to͞od) [L. *attitudo* posture] 1. habitus; the term is particularly used in obstetrics to refer to the relation of the parts of the fetal body to one another, with the normal attitude being one of moderate flexion of all the joints, back curved forward, head slightly bent on chest, and all four limbs free to move in all natural directions. 2. a tendency to respond positively or negatively to other individuals, institutions, or programs of activity.

a. of combat [Fr. *attitude de combat*] the stiff defensive position with flexion of the elbows, knees, fingers, and neck, like those of a boxer, seen in burned corpses.

discobolus a. a position resembling that of a discus thrower, caused by stimulation of the semicircular canals.

forced a. an abnormal position or attitude due to some disease, such as is seen in meningitis or as the result of contractures.

military a. the condition early in labor in which the fetal neck is deflexed and the cervical spine is in extension.

atto- [Danish *atten* eighteen] a prefix used in naming units of measurement to indicate one quintillionth (10^{-18}) of the unit designated by the root with which it is combined. Symbol a.

at·trac·tant (ə-trak′tənt) [L. *attrahere* to draw toward] a substance that exerts an attracting influence, such as one used to attract insect or animal pests to traps or to poisons.

at·trac·tion (ə-trak′shən) [L. *attractus* past part. of *attrahere* to draw together] 1. the process of drawing one body toward another. 2. a condition in which the teeth or other maxillary and mandibular structures are higher than normal position, thereby causing shortening of the face. Cf. *abstraction* (def. 2).

a. of affinity chemical a.

capillary a. the force that attracts the particles of a fluid into and along the caliber of a very narrow tube.

chemical a. the tendency of atoms of one element to unite with those of another; called also *a. of affinity.*

electric a. the tendency of bodies bearing opposite electric charges to move toward each other.

magnetic a. the tendency of bodies possessing circulating electric currents to move toward each other.

at·tri·tion (ə-trish′ən) [L. *attritio* a rubbing against] the physiologic wearing away of a substance or structure (such as the teeth) in the course of normal use.

at vol atomic volume.

at wt atomic weight.

atyp·ia (a-tip′e-ə) the condition of being irregular or not conforming to type.

koilocytotic a. an abnormal condition of cells of the stratified squamous epithelium of the uterine cervix, characterized by vacuolation and nuclear abnormalities; it may be a premalignant condition.

atyp·i·cal (a-tip′ĭ-kəl) [a-[1] + *typical*] irregular; not conforming to type; in microbiology, applied specifically to strains of unusual type.

atyp·ism (a-tip′iz-əm) atypia.

AU [L.] au′res uni′tas (both ears together); au′ris uter′que (each ear).

Au Australia antigen (see *hepatitis B surface antigen*, under *antigen*); gold (L. *au′rum*).

AUA American Urological Association.

Aub-Du·bois table (awb′ doo-bois′) [Joseph Charles *Aub*, American physician, 1890–1973; Eugene Floyd *Dubois*, American physician, 1882–1959] see under *table.*

Au·ber·ger blood group (o-bār-zha′) [*Auberger*, surname of the French propositus first reported on in 1961] see under *blood group.*

Au·bert phenomenon (ou-bert′) [Hermann *Aubert*, German physiologist, 1826–1892] see under *phenomenon.*

AUC area under the curve.

Auch·mero·my·ia (awk″mər-o-mi′yə) a genus of flies of the family Calliphoridae. The species *A. lute′ola* and *A. senegalen′sis* have larvae called Congo floor maggots that parasitize humans and pigs in Nigeria and Central Africa.

au·dile (aw′dīl) pertaining to hearing; understanding or recalling most readily what has been heard. Cf. *visile.*

audi(o)- [L. *audire* to hear] a combining form denoting relationship to hearing.

au·dio·an·al·ge·sia (aw″de-o-an″al-je′ze-ə) reduction or abolition of the perception of pain by listening through a head set to recorded music to which a background of "white noise" has been added.

au·dio·gen·ic (aw″de-o-jen′ik) produced by sound.

au·dio·gram (aw′de-o-gram″) [*audio-* + *-gram*] a record of the thresholds of hearing of an individual for various sound frequencies.

cortical a. a graphic representation of the result of cortical audiometry.

au·di·ol·o·gist (aw″de-ol′ə-jist) a person skilled in audiology, including diagnostic testing and the rehabilitation of those whose impaired hearing cannot be improved by medical or surgical means.

au·di·ol·o·gy (aw″de-ol′ə-je) [*audio-* + *-logy*] the science of hearing, particularly diagnostic testing and the study of impaired hearing that cannot be improved by medication or surgical therapy.

au·di·om·e·ter (aw″de-om′ə-tər) [*audio-* + *-meter*] an electronic device that produces acoustic stimuli of known frequency and intensity for the measurement of hearing.

evoked potential a. an instrument that detects response to sound stimuli by changes in the electroencephalogram.

au·dio·met·ric (aw″de-o-met′rik) pertaining to the measurement of hearing, as by means of an audiometer.

au•dio•me•tri•cian (aw″de-o-mə-trish′ən) a technician specializing in the measurement of hearing ability (audiometry).

au•di•om•e•try (aw″de-om′ə-tre) measurement of hearing, as by means of an audiometer.

Békésy a. audiometry in which the patient, by pressing a signal button, traces monaural thresholds for pure tones: the intensity of the tone decreases as long as the button is depressed and increases when it is released. Both continuous and interrupted tones are used.

cortical a. a method of determining auditory acuity by recording and averaging auditory evoked potentials from the cortex of the brain in response to pure tones.

electrocochleographic a. electrocochleography.

electrodermal a. audiometry in which the subject is conditioned to pure tones by harmless electric shock; thereafter when a pure tone is heard a shock is anticipated, resulting in a brief electrodermal response, which is recorded. The lowest intensity at which the response is elicited is taken to be the subject's hearing threshold.

localization a. a technique for measuring the capacity to locate the source of a pure tone received binaurally in a sound field.

pure tone a. audiometry utilizing pure tones that are relatively free of noise and overtones.

speech a. audiometry that measures speech reception threshold in decibels and speech discrimination (ability to understand).

au•dio•scope (aw′de-o-skōp) an instrument for the detection of hearing impairment consisting of an otoscope combined with an audiometer.

au•di•tion (aw-dish′ən) [L. *auditio*] 1. hearing. 2. the act of hearing.

chromatic a. color hearing.

gustatory a. a synesthesia in which certain sounds call up a sensation of taste.

au•di•tive (aw′dĭ-tiv) a person in whom the prime sense is hearing.

au•di•tog•no•sis (aw″dĭ-tog-no′sis) [L. *auditio* hearing + Gr. *gnōsis* knowledge] the sense by which sounds are understood and interpreted.

au•di•to•ry (aw′dĭ-tor″e) [L. *auditorius*] pertaining to the sense of hearing; called also *aural.*

Au•en•brug•ger sign (ou″en-broog′ər) [Leopold Joseph Elder von *Auenbrugger*, Austrian physician, 1722–1809] see under *sign.*

Au•er bodies (rods) (ou′ər) [John *Auer*, American physician, 1875–1948] see under *body.*

Au•er•bach ganglion, plexus (ou′ər-bahk) [Leopold *Auerbach*, German anatomist, 1828–1897] see under *ganglion*, and see *plexus myentericus.*

aug•men•ta•tion (awg″men-ta′shən) an adding on, or the resulting condition.

bladder a. augmentation cystoplasty.

breast a. popular name for augmentation mammaplasty.

Aug•men•tin (awg-men′tin) trademark for combination preparations of amoxicillin and clavulanate potassium.

aug•men•tor (awg-men′tər) 1. increasing; a term applied to nerves or nerve cells concerned in increasing the size and force of heart contractions. 2. a substance supposed to increase the action of an auxetic.

aug•na•thus (awg-na′thəs) dignathus.

Au•jesz•ky disease (ou-yes′ke) [Aladár *Aujeszky*, Hungarian physician, 1869–1933] pseudorabies.

AUL acute undifferentiated leukemia.

au•la (aw′lə) [L., from Gr. *aulē* hall] the red erythematous areola formed about the periphery of the vesicle of the vaccination lesion.

au•ra (aw′rə) pl. *auras* or *au′rae* [L. "breath"] a subjective sensation or motor phenomenon that precedes and marks the onset of an episode of a neurological condition, particularly an epileptic seizure *(epileptic a.)* or a migraine *(migraine a.)*. Cf. *prodrome.*

a. asthma′tica premonitory symptoms preceding an attack of asthma.

auditory a. a simple partial seizure marked by auditory sensations.

electric a. the tingling sensation experienced on the receipt of a discharge of static electricity through the air.

epigastric a. a simple partial seizure with autonomic manifestations, causing an uncomfortable sensation in the epigastrium.

epileptic a. a subjective sensation or motor phenomenon that sometimes gives warning of an approaching generalized or complex partial seizure. Formerly considered part of the prodrome of a seizure, it is now known to be itself a type of simple partial seizure and may occur without progression to a more serious attack.

a. hyste′rica an aura like that preceding an epileptic attack, sometimes experienced by hysterical patients.

intellectual a. a simple partial seizure with psychic manifestations, causing a dreamy mental condition; called also *reminiscent a.*

kinesthetic a. 1. a sensation of movement of some part of the body, with or without such actual movement. 2. focal motor seizure.

migraine a. visual, motor, or psychic disturbances, paresthesias, and other neurologic abnormalities that accompany a migraine; see also *migraine with aura, migraine without aura*, and *migraine a. without headache.*

migraine a. without headache symptoms such as teichopsia that fit the definition of migraine aura but occur without headache or brain lesions; called also *migraine equivalent.*

motor a. an epileptic aura that is a focal motor seizure.

reminiscent a. intellectual a.

vertiginous a. a sensory seizure affecting the vestibular sense, causing a feeling of vertigo. See also *vertiginous epilepsy.*

au•ral[1] (aw′rəl) [L. *auris* ear] 1. auditory. 2. otic.

au•ral[2] (aw′rəl) [L. *aura*] pertaining to or of the nature of an aura.

Au•ral•gan (aw-ral′gan) trademark for a preparation of antipyrine and benzocaine otic solution.

au•ra•mine O (aw′rə-mēn) a yellow fluorescent dye used to stain acid-fast bacteria and DNA and as a component of the Truant auramine-rhodamine stain for tubercle bacilli.

au•ran•o•fin (aw-ran′ə-fin) a gold-containing compound used as a disease-modifying antirheumatic drug in treatment of active rheumatoid arthritis, usually that not adequately controlled by nonsteroidal antiinflammatory drugs, or nondrug therapy such as physical therapy; administered orally.

au•ran•tia (aw-ran′shə) an orange coal tar stain, the ammonium salt of hexanitrodiphenylamine; used in staining mitochondria.

Au•re•lia (aw-rel′e-ə) a genus of large discophorous jellyfish found in oceans throughout the world; nematocysts of many of the larger forms can penetrate the human skin and produce intense pain.

Au•reo•ba•sid•i•um (aw″re-o-bə-sid′e-əm) a genus of Fungi Imperfecti of the form-class Hyphomycetes, form-family Dematiaceae, which produce black yeastlike cells; inhalation of sawdust contaminated with the spores causes sequoiosis. *A. pul′lulans* is a common soil organism and contaminant.

au•re•o•lin (aw-re′o-lin) a yellow dye.

au•res (aw′rēz) [L.] plural of *auris.*

aur(i)- [L. *auris* ear] a combining form denoting relationship to the ear.

au•ri•a•sis (aw-ri′ə-sis) chrysiasis (def. 1).

au•ric (aw′rik) pertaining to or containing gold.

au•ri•cle (aw′rĭ-kəl) [L. *auricula*, q.v.] 1. auricula. 2. auricula atrii. 3. formerly, one of the atria of the heart.

cervical a. a flap of skin and yellow cartilage sometimes seen on the side of the neck at the external opening of a persistent branchial cleft (pharyngeal groove).

left a. of heart auricula atrii sinistra.

right a. of heart auricula atrii dextra.

au•ric•u•la (aw-rik′u-lə) pl. *auri′culae* [L., dim of *auris*] 1. [TA] auricle: the portion of the external ear not contained within the head; the flap of the ear. Called also *pinna.* 2. auricula atrii. 3. formerly, either of the atria of the heart.

atrial a., a. a′trii [TA] the ear-shaped appendage of either atrium of the heart; called also *atrial appendage.*

a. a′trii dex′tra [TA] right auricle of heart: the ear-shaped appendage of the right atrium of the heart.

a. a′trii sinis′tra [TA] left auricle of heart: the ear-shaped appendage of the left atrium of the heart.

au•ric•u•lar (aw-rik′u-lər) 1. pertaining to an auricle. 2. pertaining to the ear.

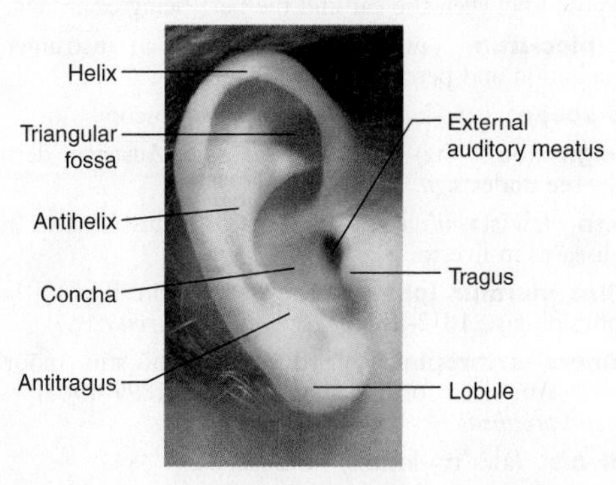

■ Auricula (auricle).

au•ric•u•la•re (aw-rik″u-lar′e) [L. *auricularis* pertaining to the ear] a craniometric point at the top of the opening of the external auditory meatus.

au•ric•u•la•ris (aw-rik″u-lar′is) [L.] pertaining to the ear; auricular.

au•ric•u•lec•to•my (aw-rik″u-lek′tə-me) removal of the auricle of the ear.

au•ric•u•lo•cra•ni•al (aw-rik″u-lo-kra′ne-əl) pertaining to an ear and the cranium.

au•ric•u•lo•tem•po•ral (aw-rik″u-lo-tem′pə-rəl) pertaining to an ear and the temporal region.

au•ric•u•lo•ther•a•py (aw-rik″u-lo-ther′ə-pe) electrical stimulation of the outer ear for the relief of pain.

au•ri•form (aw′rĭ-form) ear-shaped.

au•rin (aw′rin) a triphenylmethane derivative occurring as deep red masses with a greenish metallic luster; used as an indicator and dye intermediate. Called also *corallin.*

auri•na•ri•um (aw″rĭ-nar′e-əm) a medicated suppository for insertion into the external auditory meatus.

au•ri•na•sal (aw″rĭ-na′zəl) pertaining to the ear and the nose.

au•ri•pig•ment (aw″rĭ-pig′mənt) arsenic trisulfide.

au•ris (aw′ris) pl. *au′res* [L.] [TA] ear.

a. exter′na [TA] external ear: the portion of the auditory organ comprising the auricle and the external acoustic meatus.

a. inter′na [TA] internal ear: the labyrinth, comprising the vestibule, cochlea, and semicircular canals; called also *inner ear.*

a. me′dia [TA] middle ear: the cavity in the temporal bone comprising the cavitas tympani, auditory ossicles, and tuba auditiva.

au•ri•scope (aw′rĭ-skōp) [*auri-* + *-scope*] otoscope.

au•ro•chro•mo•der•ma (aw″ro-kro″mo-dur′mə) [L. *aurum* gold + *chromo-* + *derma*] a permanent greenish-blue staining of the skin due to injection of certain gold compounds.

Au•ro•ra ki•nase (ə-ro′rə ki′nās) [the aurora locus of *Drosophila*] any of a family of protein kinases that catalyze phosphorylation of serine and threonine and are key regulators of mitosis; they are involved in centrosome separation and maturation, spindle assembly and stability, chromosome segregation, and cytokinesis. There are three mammalian Aurora kinases, designated A, B, and C; overexpression occurs in a number of malignancies and they can be used as markers of tumor progression and prognosis. Written also *aurora kinase.*

au•ro•ther•a•py (aw″ro-ther′ə-pe) chrysotherapy.

au•ro•thio•glu•cose (aw″ro-thi″o-gloo′kōs) [USP] a monovalent gold salt used in the treatment of early active rheumatoid arthritis (both adult and juvenile types) not controlled by nonsteroidal antiinflammatory drugs, rest, and physical therapy; administered intramuscularly.

aus•cult (aws-kult′) auscultate.

aus•cul•tate (aws′kəl-tāt) [L. *auscultare* to listen to] to examine by listening, usually to the sounds of the thoracic or abdominal viscera, with or without a stethoscope. **aus′cultator** *n* **auscul′tatory** *adj*

aus•cul•ta•tion (aws″kəl-ta′shən) the act of listening for sounds within the body, chiefly for ascertaining the condition of the lungs, heart, pleura, abdomen and other organs, and for the detection of pregnancy or monitoring fetal heart sounds.

direct a., immediate a. auscultation performed without the stethoscope.

Korányi a. auscultatory percussion done by tapping with one forefinger the second joint of the other forefinger applied perpendicularly to the part; called also *Korányi percussion.*

mediate a. auscultation performed by the aid of an instrument (stethoscope) interposed between the ear and the part being examined.

aus•cul•to•plec•trum (aws-kul″to-plek′trəm) an instrument for use in both auscultation and percussion.

aus•cul•to•scope (aws-kul′tə-skōp) phonendoscope.

Au•spitz sign (ou′shpitz) [Heinrich *Auspitz*, Austrian dermatologist, 1835–1886] see under *sign.*

Au•ste•ni•na (aw″stə-ni′nə) a subgenus of genus *Glossina* (tsetse flies) that cause diseases in livestock.

Aus•tin Flint murmur (phenomenon) (aw′stin flint′) [*Austin Flint*, American physiologist, 1812–1886] see under *murmur.*

Aus•tin Moore arthroplasty, prosthesis (aw′stin mo͞or′) [*Austin* Talley *Moore*, American orthopedic surgeon, 1899–1963] see under *arthroplasty* and *prosthesis.*

Aus•tra•lor•bis (aws″trə-lor′bis) *Biomphalaria.*

au•ta•coid (aw′tə-koid) [*aut-* + Gr. *akos* remedy] local hormone.

■ Autoagglutination of erythrocytes.

au•techo•scope (aw-tek′o-skōp) [*aut-* + *echo* + *-scope*] an instrument for auscultating one's own body.

au•te•cic (aw-te′sik) autoecious.

au•te•cious (aw-te′shəs) autoecious.

au•te•col•o•gy (aw″tə-kol′ə-je) [*aut-* + *ecology*] the ecology of an organism as an individual; cf. *synecology.*

au•tism (aw′tiz-əm) [*aut-* + *-ism*] 1. autistic disorder. 2. autistic thinking.

infantile a. autistic disorder.

au•tis•tic (aw-tis′tik) characterized by self-absorption, impairment in social interaction and communication, and a restricted range of activities and interests.

aut(o)- [Gr. *autos* self] a prefix denoting relationship to self.

au•to•ac•ti•va•tion (aw″to-ak″tĭ-va′shən) the activation of a cell by its own secretory products.

au•to•ag•glu•ti•na•tion (aw″to-ə-gloo″tĭ-na′shən) 1. clumping or agglutination of an individual's cells by their own serum, as in autohemagglutination. 2. nonspecific clumping or agglutination of particulate antigens (e.g., bacteria) that does not involve antibody; an important cause of error in bacterial agglutination tests.

au•to•ag•glu•ti•nin (aw″to-ə-gloo′tĭ-nin) an autologous serum factor with the property of agglutinating the individual's own cellular elements.

au•to•ag•gres•sive (aw″to-ə-gres′iv) attacking constituents of the body's own tissues.

au•to•al•ler•gy (aw′to-al′ər-je) autoimmunity. **autoaller′gic** *adj*

au•to•am•pu•ta•tion (aw″to-am″pu-ta′shən) the spontaneous detachment from the body and elimination of an appendage or of an abnormal growth, such as a polyp.

au•to•anal•y•sis (aw″to-ə-nal′ə-sis) self-analysis.

au•to•an•ti•body (aw″to-an′tĭ-bod″e) an antibody formed in response to, and reacting against, a self antigen (i.e., one of the individual's own normal tissue constituents).

anti-islet a's islet cell a's.

antineutrophil cytoplasmic a. (ANCA) an autoantibody to cytoplasmic constituents of monocytes and neutrophils, found in increased amounts in some types of vasculitis. There are several different subtypes, each characterized serologically by reactivity against particular cellular antigens; some are specific to given disease states. Called also *antineutrophil cytoplasmic antibody.*

islet a's, islet cell a's autoantibodies against the islet cells, seen in some persons with type 1 diabetes mellitus; called also *anti-islet a's.*

thyroid a's autoantibodies against thyroid peroxidase, thyroglobulin, and thyroid-stimulating hormone receptors, seen in autoimmune thyroiditis.

au•to•an•ti•com•ple•ment (aw″to-an″ti-kom′plə-mənt) an anticomplement formed in the body against its own complement.

au•to•an•ti•gen (aw″to-an′tĭ-jen) an antigen that, despite being a normal tissue constituent, is the target of a humoral or cell-mediated immune response, as in autoimmune disease. Called also *self-antigen.*

au•to•an•ti•tox•in (aw″to-an″te-, aw″to-an″ti-tok′sin) [*auto-* + *antitoxin*] antitoxin produced by the animal itself, as opposed to exogenous antitoxin.

au•to•body (aw′to-bod″e) an antibody that both carries an idiotypic determinant that is stereochemically similar to the epitope on the antigen against which the antibody was originally directed and at the same time expresses a binding site for the antigen; autobodies therefore have the potential for self-aggregation.

au·to·ca·tal·y·sis (aw″to-kə-tal′ə-sis) a catalytic reaction that gradually accelerates in velocity because some of the products of the reaction themselves act as catalytic agents. **autocatalyt′ic** *adj*

au·to·cat·a·lyst (aw″to-kat′ə-list) an element participating in autocatalysis.

au·to·ca·thar·sis (aw″to-kə-thahr′sis) a form of psychiatric treatment in which the patient writes down thoughts, feelings, and experiences in order to release disturbing emotions associated with them.

au·toch·tho·nous (aw-tok′thə-nəs) [Gr. *autochthōn* sprung from the land itself] 1. found in the place of formation; not removed to a new site. 2. denoting a tissue graft to a new site on the same individual.

au·to·ci·ne·sis (aw″to-si-ne′sis) [*auto-* + Gr. *kinēsis* motion] autokinesis.

au·toc·la·sis (aw-tok′lə-sis) [*auto-* + Gr. *klasis* breaking] destruction of a part due to conditions within the part.

au·to·clave (aw′to-klāv) [*auto-* + L. *clavis* key] an apparatus for effecting sterilization by steam under pressure; it is fitted with a gauge that automatically regulates the pressure and therefore the degree of heat to which the contents are subjected.

Au·to·clip (aw′to-klip) trademark for a stainless steel surgical clip for wound closing inserted by means of a mechanical applicator that automatically feeds a series of clips.

Au·to·plex T (aw′to-pleks) trademark for a preparation of antiinhibitor coagulant complex.

au·to·coid (aw′to-koid) local hormone.

au·to·crine (aw′to-krin) denoting a mode of hormone action in which a hormone binds to receptors on and affects the function of the cell type that produced it.

au·to·cys·to·plas·ty (aw″to-sis′tə-plas″te) a plastic operation on the bladder using grafts from the patient's body.

au·to·cy·tol·y·sin (aw″to-si-tol′ĭ-sin) autolysin.

au·to·cy·tol·y·sis (aw″to-si-tol′ĭ-sis) autolysis.

au·to·cy·to·lyt·ic (aw″to-si″to-lit′ik) autolytic.

au·to·cy·to·tox·in (aw″to-si′to-tok″sin) a cytotoxin for the cells of the body in which it is formed.

au·to·der·mic (aw″to-dur′mik) [*auto-* + *derma*] pertaining to or created from the patient's own skin; a term applied to skin grafts. See *dermatoautoplasty* and *autograft.*

au·to·di·ges·tion (aw″to-di-jes′chən) autolysis.

pancreatic a. premature breakdown of pancreatic zymogens into digestive enzymes that digest pancreatic tissue, causing acute pancreatitis.

au·to·drain·age (aw″to-drān′əj) removal of fluid from an abscess or cavity by diversion into a newly formed channel or into a viscus within the patient's own body; this may be accomplished by surgery or may occur spontaneously.

au·to·echo·la·lia (aw″to-ek″o-la′le-ə) [*auto-* + *echolalia*] parrot-like repetition of words and phrases initially uttered by the patient himself; seen in catatonic schizophrenia and in certain cerebral degenerative disorders.

au·toe·cic (aw-te′sik) [*auto-* + Gr. *oikos* house] autoecious.

au·toe·cious (aw-te′shəs) [*auto-* + Gr. *oikos* house] characterized by a developmental cycle spent on the same host, as opposed to *heteroecious;* said of parasitic fungi. Called also *autecious* and *autoecic.*

au·to·ec·zem·a·ti·za·tion (aw″to-ek-zem″ə-tĭ-za′shən) an id reaction involving spread, at first locally, and later more generally, of lesions from an originally circumscribed focus of eczema.

au·to·erot·i·cism (aw″to-ə-rot′ĭ-siz-əm) 1. sexual self-gratification or arousal without the participation of another person, such as masturbation. 2. in psychoanalytic theory, the most primitive stage in the development of object relations, preceding the narcissistic stage. Cf. *heteroeroticism, alloeroticism.* **autoerot′ic** *adj*

au·to·eryth·ro·phago·cy·to·sis (aw″to-ə-rith″ro-fa″go-si-to′sis) [*auto* + *erythro*cyte + *phagocytosis*] phagocytosis of erythrocytes by autologous neutrophils or monocytes.

au·to·flu·o·res·cence (aw″to-flə-res′ens) fluorescence in tissues produced by substances normally present in the tissues. Cf. *secondary fluorescence,* under *fluorescence.* **autofluores′cent** *adj*

au·to·flu·o·ro·scope (aw″to-floor′o-skōp″) a type of scintillation camera that utilizes in its detector sodium iodide crystals packed in an array, each connected to specific photomultiplier tubes by individual light pipes.

au·to·fun·do·scope (aw″to-fun′do-skōp) [*auto-* + *fundus* + *-scope*] an instrument that makes use of the fact that by observing an illuminated blank space through a pin-perforated card, one can see faint images of the retinal vessels of one's own eyes.

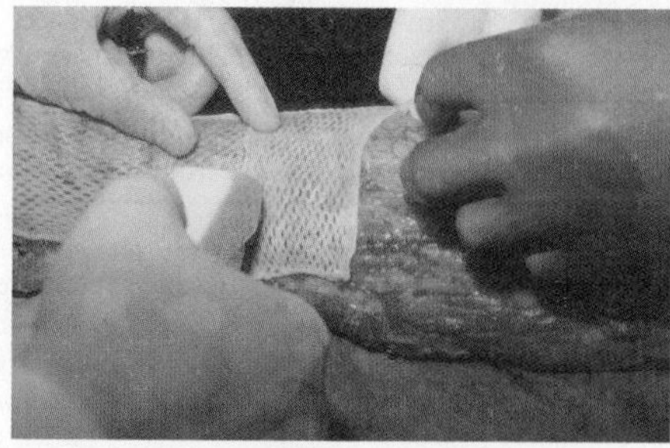

■ Meshed autograft being applied to the recipient site.

au·to·fun·dos·co·py (aw″to-fun-dos′kə-pe) examination with the autofundoscope.

au·tog·a·my (aw-tog′ə-me) [*auto-* + Gr. *gamos* marriage] a form of self-fertilization; fertilization within a cell by union of two gametic nuclei from the same micronucleus, as in certain ciliate protozoa and plants. Cf. *endogamy* (def. 1) and *exogamy.* **autog′amous** *adj*

au·to·gen·e·ic (aw″to-jen-e′ik) autologous.

au·to·gen·e·sis (aw″to-jen′ə-sis) [*auto-* + *-genesis*] self-generation; origination within the organism. **autogenet′ic** *adj*

au·tog·e·nous (aw-toj′ə-nəs) [*auto-* + *-genous*] autologous.

au·to·graft (aw′to-graft) a graft of tissue derived from another site in or on the body of the organism receiving it; called also *autologous* or *autochthonous graft.*

au·to·graft·ing (aw″to-graft′ing) autotransplantation.

au·to·gram (aw′to-gram) [*auto-* + *-gram*] a mark forming on the skin following pressure by a blunt instrument.

au·to·gyne·phil·ia (aw″to-gi″nə-fil′e-ə) a type of gender dysphoria in which a man is sexually aroused by the thought or image of himself as a woman.

au·to·he·mag·glu·ti·na·tion (aw″to-he″mə-gloo″tĭ-na′shən) hemagglutination of the subject's own erythrocytes.

au·to·he·mag·glu·ti·nin (aw″to-he″mə-gloo′tĭ-nin) a hemagglutinin that causes the clumping or agglutination of the subject's own erythrocytes.

au·to·he·mol·y·sin (aw″to-he-mol′ĭ-sin) a hemolysin that causes complement-dependent hemolysis of the patient's own erythrocytes.

au·to·he·mol·y·sis (aw″to-he-mol′ĭ-sis) hemolysis of the blood cells of a person by his own serum. **autohemolyt′ic** *adj*

au·to·he·mo·ther·a·py (aw″to-he″mo-ther′ə-pe) [*auto-* + *hemo-* + *therapy*] therapy using an autotransfusion.

au·to·he·mo·trans·fu·sion (aw″to-he″mo-trans-fu′zhən) autotransfusion.

au·to·his·to·ra·dio·graph (aw″to-his″to-ra′de-o-graf) autoradiograph.

au·to·hyp·no·sis (aw″to-hip-no′sis) the act or process of hypnotizing oneself. **autohypnot′ic** *adj*

au·to·im·mune (aw″to-ĭ-mūn′) characterized by a specific humoral or cell-mediated immune response against constituents of the body's own tissues (self antigens or autoantigens). **autoimmu′nity** *n*

au·to·im·mu·ni·za·tion (aw″to-im″u-nĭ-za′shən) the induction in an individual of an immune response to its own tissue constituents, which may lead to pathological sequelae such as autoimmune disease. Called also *autosensitization.* See also *autoantibody.*

au·to·in·fec·tion (aw″to-in-fek′shən) [*auto-* + *infection*] infection by an agent already present in the body, such as the transferral of a pathogen from one part of the body to another.

au·to·in·flam·ma·to·ry (aw-to-in-flam′ə-tor″e) characterized by a disorder of the body's innate immunity, with inflammation that is not caused by an external irritant such as infection.

au·to·in·fu·sion (aw″to-in-fu′zhən) [*auto-* + *infusion*] the forcing of the blood toward the heart by bandaging the extremities, compression of the abdominal aorta, etc.

au·to·in·oc·u·la·ble (aw″to-in-ok′u-lə-bəl) susceptible to autoinoculation.

au·to·in·oc·u·la·tion (aw″to-in-ok′u-la″shən) [*auto-* + *inoculation*] inoculation with microorganisms from one's own body.

au·to·in·ter·fer·ence (aw″to-in″tər-fēr′əns) interference with the replication of a virus by an intact, attenuated, or inactivated virus of the same kind.

au·to·isol·y·sin (aw″to-i-sol′ĭ-sin) autoantibody that causes complement-dependent lysis of cells in the individual from which it was obtained and in others of the same species.

au·to·ker·a·to·plas·ty (aw″to-ker′ə-to-plas″te) [*auto-* + *keratoplasty*] corneal transplantation of tissue from one of the patient's eyes to the other one.

au·to·ki·ne·sis (aw″to-kĭ-ne′sis) [*auto-* + *-kinesis*] voluntary motion.
visible light a. see *autokinetic visible light phenomenon,* under *phenomenon.*

au·to·ki·net·ic (aw″to-kĭ-net′ik) having the power of voluntary motion.

au·to·le·sion (aw″to-le′zhən) a self-inflicted injury.

au·to·leu·ko·ag·glu·ti·nin (aw″to-loo″ko-ə-gloo′tĭ-nin) an antibody capable of agglutinating leukocytes of the same individual in which it is generated.

au·tol·o·gous (aw-tol′ə-gəs) [*auto-* + *log-* + *-ous*] related to self; originating within an organism itself, as an autograft or autotransfusion. Called also *autogeneic* and *autogenous.*

au·tol·y·sate (aw-tol′ĭ-sāt) a substance or substances produced by autolysis.

au·tol·y·sin (aw-tol′ĭ-sin) autoantibody causing complement-dependent lysis of autologous cells; called also *autocytolysin.*

au·tol·y·sis (aw-tol′ĭ-sis) [*auto-* + *-lysis*] digestion of cellular components by endogenous hydrolases released from lysosomes following cell death, seen as a postmortem change and in certain pathological conditions.
postmortem a. enzymatic self-digestion of cells or tissues after death.

au·to·ly·so·some (aw″to-li′so-sōm) an organelle, formed by the fusion of an autophagosome with a primary lysosome, in which digestion of intracellular elements occurs in autophagy. Called also *autophagolysosome.*

au·to·lyt·ic (aw-to-lit′ik) pertaining to or causing autolysis; autocytolytic.

au·to·lyze (aw′to-līz) to undergo or to cause to undergo autolysis.

au·to·mat·ic (aw″to-mat′ik) [Gr. *automatos* self-acting] 1. spontaneous or involuntary; done by no act of the will. 2. self-moving; self-regulating.

au·to·ma·ti·ci·ty (aw″to-mə-tis′ĭ-te) 1. the state or quality of being automatic. 2. the capacity of a cell to initiate an impulse, such as depolarization, without an external stimulus.
triggered a. pacemaker activity occurring as a result of a propagated or stimulated action potential, such as an afterdepolarization, in cells or tissues not normally displaying a spontaneous automaticity.

au·tom·a·tism (aw-tom′ə-tiz-əm) [Gr. *automatismos* self-action] aimless and apparently undirected behavior that is not under conscious control and is performed without conscious knowledge; seen in psychomotor epilepsy, catatonic schizophrenia, dissociative fugue, and other conditions. Called also *automatic behavior.*
ambulatory a. a condition in which the patient walks about and performs acts mechanically and without consciousness of what they are doing.
command a. the performance of suggested acts without exercise of critical judgment; seen in catatonic schizophrenia and in the hypnotic state.

au·to·mato·graph (aw″to-mat′o-graf) [Gr. *automatismos* self-action + *-graph*] an instrument for recording involuntary movements.

Au·tom·e·ris (aw-tom′ə-ris) a genus of moths. *A. i′o* is the io moth, whose larva has irritant hairs that produce moth dermatitis.

au·to·my·so·pho·bia (aw″to-mi″so-fo′be-ə) [*auto-* + *mysophobia*] irrational fear of being unclean or smelling bad.

au·to·ne·phrec·to·my (aw″to-nə-frek′tə-me) [*auto-* + *nephr-* + *-ectomy*] obliteration of a kidney as the result of disease.

au·to·nom·ic (aw″tə-nom′ik) self-controlling; functionally independent. See *autonomic nervous system,* under *system.*

au·to·nomo·tro·pic (aw″to-nom-o-tro′pik) [*autonomic* + *-tropic*] having an affinity for the autonomic nervous system.

au·ton·o·my (aw-ton′ə-me) [*auto-* + Gr. *nomos* law] the state of functioning independently, without extraneous influence. **auton′omous** *adj*

au·to-oph·thal·mo·scope (aw″to-of-thal′mə-skōp) [*auto-* + *ophthalmoscope*] an ophthalmoscope for examining one's own eyes.

au·to-oph·thal·mos·co·py (aw″to-of-thəl-mos′kə-pe) the use of the auto-ophthalmoscope.

au·to-ox·i·da·tion (aw″to-ok″sĭ-da′shən) spontaneous direct combination, at ordinary temperatures, of a substance with molecular oxygen.

auto-ox·i·di·za·ble (aw″to-ok″sĭ-di′zə-bəl) capable of spontaneous combination with oxygen.

au·to·pa·thog·ra·phy (aw″to-pə-thog′rə-fe) [*auto-* + *patho-* + *-graphy*] a written description of one's own disease.

au·to·pha·gia (aw″to-fa′jə) [*auto-* + *-phagia*] 1. the biting or eating of one's own flesh. 2. nutrition of the body by the consumption of its own tissues. 3. autophagy.

au·to·pha·gic (aw″to-fa′jik) pertaining to or characterized by autophagia or autophagy.

au·to·phago·ly·so·some (aw″to-fag″ə-li′sə-sōm) autolysosome.

au·to·phago·some (aw″to-fag′ə-sōm) [*auto-* + *phagosome*] an intracytoplasmic vacuole containing elements of the cell's own cytoplasm, formed by macroautophagy; it fuses with a primary lysosome to form an autolysosome, subjecting its contents to enzymatic digestion. Called also *cytolysosome* and *autophagic vacuole.*

au·toph·a·gy (aw-tof′ə-je) 1. the segregation and digestion of part of the cell's own cytoplasmic material within lysosomes. See also macroautophagy and microautophagy. Cf. *heterophagy.* 2. autophagia.

au·to·phar·ma·col·o·gy (aw″to-fahr″mə-kol′ə-je) the chemical regulation of bodily function by the natural constituents of the body tissues, such as hormones. **autopharmacolog′ic** *adj*

au·to·phe·re·sis (aw-to-fĕ-re′sis) [*auto-* + *pheresis*] withdrawal of lymphocytes from a patient followed by in vitro incubation with autologous or heterologous tumor antigens and reinfusion into the original patient; the cells have increased cytotoxicity to the antigens in vivo.

au·to·pho·bia (aw″to-fo′be-ə) [*auto-* + *-phobia*] irrational dread of oneself, of being alone.

au·to·pho·nom·e·try (aw″to-fo-nom′ə-tre) [*auto-* + *phono-* + *-metry*] the application of a vibrating tuning fork to the body of a patient for the purpose of having him describe the sensations that it produces.

au·toph·o·ny (aw-tof′ə-ne) [*auto-* + Gr. *phōnē* voice] abnormal hearing of one's own voice and respiratory sounds, usually as a result of a patulous eustachian tube.

au·toph·thal·mo·scope (aw″tof-thal′mə-skōp) auto-ophthalmoscope.

au·to·phyte (aw′to-fīt) [*auto-* + *-phyte*] a plant that does not depend on organized food material, but derives its nourishment directly from inorganic matter. Cf. *saprophyte.*

au·to·plast (aw′to-plast) autograft.

au·to·plas·tic (aw″to-plas′tik) 1. autologous. 2. pertaining to autoplasty.

au·to·plas·ty (aw′to-plas″te) [*auto-* + *-plasty*] 1. autotransplantation. 2. in psychoanalytic theory, adaptation by changing oneself (autoplastic change) rather than changing the external environment. Cf. *alloplasty.*

au·to·po·di·um (aw″to-po′de-əm) the fourth, or most distal, part of an embryonic limb; see *limb* (def. 1).

au·to·poi·son·ous (aw″to-poi′zən-əs) poisonous to the organism by which it is formed.

au·to·pol·y·mer (aw″to-pol′ĭ-mər) a material that polymerizes without the use of heat, but on the addition of an activator and a catalyst.

au·to·po·lym·er·iza·tion (aw″to-pə-lim″ər-ĭ-za′shən) polymerization occurring without the use of heat but as a chemical reaction following the addition of an activator and a catalyst.

au·to·pro·te·ol·y·sis (aw″to-pro-te-ol′ĭ-sis) autolysis.

au·to·pro·tol·y·sis (aw″to-pro-tol′ĭ-sis) proton transfer from one molecule to another of the same substance.

au·top·sy (aw′top-se) [*auto-* + Gr. *opsis* view] the postmortem examination of a body, including the internal organs and structures after dissection, so as to determine the cause of death or the nature of pathological changes. Called also *necropsy.*

au·to·psy·chic (aw″to-si′kik) [*auto-* + *psychic*] pertaining to one's own mind or to self-consciousness.

au·to·ra·dio·gram (aw″to-ra′de-o-gram) an autoradiograph.

au·to·ra·dio·graph (aw″to-ra′de-o-graf) a radiograph of an object or tissue made by recording the radiation emitted by radioactive material within it, especially after the purposeful introduction of radioactive material.

au·to·ra·di·og·ra·phy (aw″to-ra″de-og′rə-fe) the making of a radiograph by introducing a radioactive tracer into a specimen and recording the radiation distribution on a photographic film or emulsion placed on or close to the specimen.

au·to·re·ac·tive (aw″to-re-ak′tiv) reacting with autoantigens; said of B and T lymphocytes.

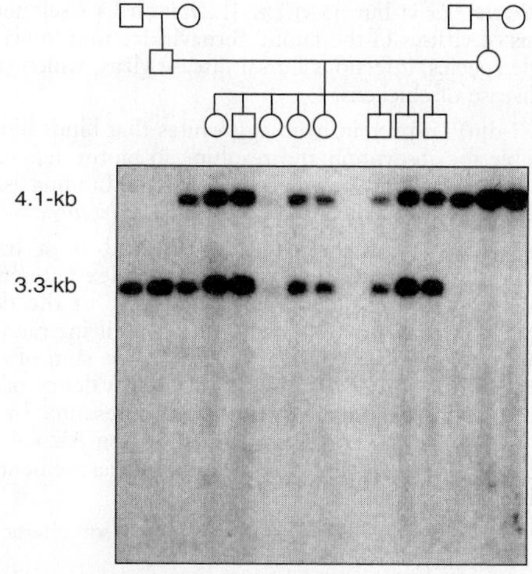

■ Autoradiograph, showing the results of hybridization of radiolabeled DNA to DNA fragments that have been separated by size electrophoretically; each lane represents DNA from the member of the family whose pedigree is shown above the autoradiogram, revealing restriction fragment length polymorphisms.

au·to·reg·u·la·tion (aw″to-reg″u-la′shən) 1. the process occurring when some mechanism within a biological system detects and adjusts for changes within the system; exercised by negative feedback. 2. in circulatory physiology, the intrinsic tendency of an organ or tissue to maintain constant blood flow despite changes in arterial pressure, or the adjustment of blood flow through an organ in order to provide for its metabolic needs.

heterometric a. intrinsic mechanisms controlling the strength of ventricular contractions that depend on the length of myocardial fibers at the end of diastole.

homeometric a. 1. intrinsic mechanisms controlling the strength of ventricular contractions that are independent of the length of myocardial fibers at the end of diastole. 2. Anrep effect.

au·to·re·in·fu·sion (aw″to-re″in-fu′zhən) intravenous infusion of a patient's own blood or serum that has escaped into the pleural or peritoneal cavities, usually because of trauma or spontaneous rupture of a major vessel.

au·to·sen·si·ti·za·tion (aw″to-sen″sĭ-tĭ-za′shən) sensitization toward one's own tissues; see *autoimmunization.*

erythrocyte a. autoerythrocyte sensitization.

au·to·sen·si·tized (aw″to-sen′sĭ-tīzd) rendered hypersensitive to one's own serum or tissues; see *autoimmunization.*

au·to·sep·ti·ce·mia (aw″to-sep″tĭ-se′me-ə) septicemia arising from microorganisms within the body; endosepsis.

au·to·se·rum (aw″to-sēr′əm) [*auto-* + *serum*] a serum administered to the patient from whom it was derived. **autose′rous** *adj*

au·to·sex·ing (aw″to-seks′ing) the deliberate breeding of an early-appearing sex-linked phenotype to distinguish male from female organisms prior to the appearance of sexually dimorphic traits; used particularly for domestic fowl production.

au·to·site (aw′to-sīt) [*auto-* + *site*] the larger, more nearly normal component of asymmetrical conjoined twins, to which the parasite is attached as a dependent growth. **autosit′ic** *adj*

au·tos·mia (aw-tos′me-ə) [*auto-* + *osm-*[1] + *-ia*] the smelling of one's own body odor.

au·to·so·ma·tog·no·sis (aw″to-so″mə-tog-no′sis) [*auto-* + *somato-* + *gnōsis* recognition] the feeling that a part of the body that has been removed, as by amputation, is still present. See *phantom limb*, under *limb.* **autosomatognos′tic** *adj*

au·to·some (aw′to-sōm) [*auto-* + *-some*] any of the chromosomes other than the pair of sex chromosomes; in humans there are 22 pairs of autosomes. **autoso′mal** *adj*

au·to·sper·mo·tox·in (aw″to-spur′mo-tok″sin) a substance capable of agglutinating the spermatozoa of the animal in which they are formed.

au·to·sple·nec·to·my (aw″to-sple-nek′tə-me) the almost complete disappearance of the spleen through progressive fibrosis and shrinkage, such as may occur in sickle cell anemia.

au·to·spray (aw′to-spra) an apparatus for spraying, to be used by the patient.

au·to·stim·u·la·tion (aw″to-stim″u-la′shən) stimulation of an animal with antigenic material originating from its own tissues.

au·to·sug·ges·ti·bil·i·ty (aw″to-səg-jes″tĭ-bil′ĭ-te) the state of being readily amenable to autosuggestion.

au·to·sug·ges·tion (aw″to-səg-jes′chən) [*auto-* + *suggestion*] self-suggestion; the process of inducing in oneself the uncritical acceptance of an idea, belief, or opinion, as by self-hypnosis.

au·to·ther·a·py (aw″to-ther′ə-pe) [*auto-* + *therapy*] 1. the spontaneous cure of disease. 2. self-cure. 3. treatment of disease by filtrates from the patient's own secretions.

au·to·throm·bo·ag·glu·ti·nin (aw″to-throm″bo-ə-gloo′tĭ-nin) a platelet autoagglutinin.

au·to·to·mog·ra·phy (aw″to-to-mog′rə-fe) a method of tomography involving movement of the patient instead of the x-ray source. **autotomograph′ic** *adj*

au·tot·o·my (aw-tot′ə-me) [*auto-* + *-tomy*] the spontaneous shedding of an appendage, as in some invertebrates.

au·to·top·ag·no·sia (aw″to-top″ag-no′zhə) [*auto-* + *topo-* + *agnosia*] agnosia affecting the posture sense, characterized by inability to localize or orient correctly different parts of the body; the cause is usually a lesion in the parietal part of the posterior thalamic radiations. Called also *body-image agnosia* and *somatotopagnosia.*

au·to·trans·fu·sion (aw″to-trans-fu′zhən) reinfusion of blood or blood products derived from the patient's own circulation. Called also *autologous transfusion.*

intraoperative a. the collection, processing, and reinfusion of a patient's blood shed from a wound or body cavity during surgery.

postoperative a. the collection, processing, and reinfusion of the patient's blood shed from the mediastinum following open heart or chest surgery or from the chest following traumatic hemothorax.

au·to·trans·plant (aw″to-trans′plant) autograft.

au·to·trans·plan·ta·tion (aw″to-trans″plan-ta′shən) transplantation of an autograft.

au·to·trep·a·na·tion (aw″to-trep″ə-na′shən) erosion of the skull by a brain tumor.

au·to·troph (aw′to-trōf) an autotrophic organism.

facultative a. an organism, especially a bacterium, having a metabolism that is either autotrophic or heterotrophic and thus is capable of growth on either inorganic or organic media.

obligate a. a microorganism that can exist only by autotrophic means.

au·to·tro·phic (aw″to-tro′fik) [*auto-* + *-trophic*] self-sustaining; said of a type of nutrition in which organisms are capable of synthesizing organic molecules as nutritive substances. Cf. *heterotrophic.*

au·tot·ro·phy (aw-tot′rə-fe) the state of being autotrophic; autotrophic nutrition.

au·to·vac·ci·na·tion (aw″to-vak″sĭ-na′shən) 1. treatment of a patient with autovaccine. 2. treatment of a patient by causing liberation of antigenic products from some invading microorganism or diseased tissue and thus bringing about the formation of antibodies.

au·to·vac·cine (aw″to-vak-sēn′) a bacterial vaccine prepared from cultures of organisms isolated from the patient's own secretions or tissues.

au·to·vac·cin·ia (aw″to-vak-sin′e-ə) [*auto-* + *vaccinia*] a vaccinial reaction appearing on an area of the body other than at the primary site of smallpox vaccination as a result of transference of vaccinia virus by scratching.

au·to·vac·ci·no·ther·a·py (aw″to-vak″sĭ-no-ther′ə-pe) autovaccination.

au·tox·i·da·tion (aw″tok-sĭ-da′shən) auto-oxidation.

au·to·zy·gous (aw″to-zi′gəs) homozygous at a locus by virtue of descent of the alleles from a common ancestor.

aux·ano·gram (awk-san′ə-gram) the plate culture in auxanography.

aux·an·og·ra·phy (awk″san-og′rə-fe) [Gr. *auxanein* to increase + *-graphy*] determination of the most suitable medium for a microbe by placing drops of various solutions on a plate containing a poor medium; the microbe will develop the strongest colonies on the spot that contains the best medium. **auxanograph′ic** *adj*

aux·e·sis (awk-se′sis) [Gr. *auxēsis*] increase in the size of an organism; often used specifically to designate increase in volume of an organism as a result of growth of its individual cells, without increase in their number.

aux·et·ic (awk-set′ik) [Gr. *auxētikos* growing] 1. pertaining to auxesis. 2. a substance that stimulates auxesis.

aux·il·i·a·ry (awg-zil′yə-re) [L. *auxiliaris*] 1. affording aid. 2. that which affords aid.

torquing a. an accessory arch wire used to apply torsion on a tooth in any of the three planes of space; used in orthodontic therapy.

aux·il·io·mo·tor (awk-sil″e-o-mo′tər) aiding or stimulating motion.

aux·i·lyt·ic (awk-sĭ-lit′ik) [Gr. *auxein* to increase + *-lytic*] increasing the lytic or destructive power.

aux·i·om·e·ter (awk″se-om′ə-tər) [Gr. *auxein* to increase + *-meter*] an apparatus for measuring the magnifying powers of lenses; called also *auxometer.*

aux(o)- [Gr. *auxē* increase] a combining form denoting relationship to growth, or to stimulation or acceleration.

auxo·chrome (awk′so-krōm) [*auxo-* + *-chrome*] a chemical group which, if introduced into a chromogen, will convert the latter into a dye. auxochro′mous *adj*

auxo·drome (awk′so-drōm) [*auxo-* + Gr. *dromos* a course] the course of growth as plotted on a Wetzel grid.

auxo·flore (awk′so-flor) an atom or group that increases the intensity of fluorescence of a compound in which it occurs; cf. *bathoflore.*

aux·om·e·ter (awk-som′ə-tər) auxiometer.

aux·om·e·try (awk-som′ə-tre) [*auxo-* + *-metry*] measurement of rate of growth. auxomet′ric *adj*

auxo·ton·ic (awk″so-ton′ik) [*auxo-* + *tonic*] contracting against increasing resistance.

auxo·tox (awk′so-toks) a chemical group that causes a compound to be toxic.

auxo·troph (awk′so-trōf) an auxotrophic organism.

auxo·tro·phic (awk″so-tro′fik) [*auxo-* + *-trophic*] 1. requiring a growth factor that is not required by the parental or prototype strain; said of microbial mutants. 2. requiring specific organic growth factors in addition to the carbon source present in a minimal medium.

auxo·type (awk′so-tīp) [*auxo-* + *type*] the type of an individual strain of *Neisseria gonorrhoeae* as determined by its nutritional requirements.

AV, A-V atrioventricular; arteriovenous.

av avoirdupois; see *avoirdupois weight,* under *weight.*

AVA anthrax vaccine adsorbed.

aval·vu·lar (a-val′vu-lər) having no valves.

Avan·da·met (ə-van′də-met) trademark for a preparation of rosiglitazone maleate and metformin hydrochloride.

Avan·dia (ə-van′de-ə) trademark for a preparation of rosiglitazone maleate.

Ava·pro (av′ə-pro) trademark for a preparation of irbesartan.

avas·cu·lar (a-vas′ku-lər) [*a-*[1] + *vascular*] not supplied with blood vessels.

avas·cu·lar·i·za·tion (a-vas″ku-lər-ĭ-za′shən) the diversion of blood from tissues; it may be accomplished by ligating vessels or by applying tight elastic bandages.

Avas·tin (ə-vas′tin) trademark for a preparation of bevacizumab.

AVC trademark for preparations of sulfanilamide.

Av·el·lis syndrome (paralysis) (ah-vel′is) [Georg *Avellis,* German laryngologist, 1864–1916] see under *syndrome.*

Ave·lox (a′və-loks) trademark for a preparation of moxifloxacin hydrochloride.

Ave·na (ə-ve′nə) [L.] a genus of grasses (family Gramineae). *A. sati′va* is the oat plant, whose seeds are the edible cereal called *oats.*

ave·nin (ə-ve′nin) any of a group of closely related proteins present in oats *(Avena sativa),* which may be harmful to patients with celiac disease.

Aven·tyl (ə-ven′təl) trademark for a preparation of nortriptyline hydrochloride.

av·er·ag·ing (av′ər-əj-ing) 1. the finding of a mean value in a population. 2. reducing to or taking a typical example of the group under consideration.

signal a. a method for minimizing noise interference in a periodic signal; the relative constancy of the signal intensity over time versus the randomness of noise is exploited by averaging the waveforms over a number of periods.

av·er·mec·tin (av″ər-mek′tin) any of a group of lactones that are potent anthelmintics and insecticides.

aver·sive (ə-vur′siv) characterized by or giving rise to avoidance; noxious. Cf. *appetitive.*

Avi·ad·e·no·vi·rus (a″ve-ad′ə-no-vi″rəs) [L. *avis* bird + *adenovirus*] adenoviruses of birds; a genus of viruses of the family Adenoviridae that infect many bird species, causing a wide variety of diseases; infection by some viral species is asymptomatic. Species names are abbreviated by a prefix derived from the host genus and a number designating the serotype, e.g., DAdV-2 for duck adenovirus 2.

avi·an (a′ve-ən) [L. *avis* bird] of or pertaining to birds. Cf. *gallid.*

Av·i·ane (av′e-ahn) trademark for a combination preparation of levonorgestrel and ethinyl estradiol.

Avi·bir·na·vi·rus (a″vĭ-bur′nə-vi″rəs) [L. *avis* bird + *bi*segmented *RNA* + *virus*] a genus of viruses of the family Birnaviridae that infect birds, containing a single species, infectious bursal disease virus, which causes infectious bursal disease of chickens.

av·i·din (av′ĭ-din) a protein from egg whites that binds biotin, rendering it unavailable for absorption and resulting in biotin deficiency if large quantities of raw egg whites are ingested. Because binding is strong and specific, it has been used in biochemical assays (see *biotinylation*).

avid·i·ty (ə-vid′ĭ-te) 1. the strength of an acid or a base. 2. the strength of binding between antibody and a complex antigen. Since the antigen has more than one determinant and many of the determinants differ from one another, avidity expresses the overall interaction between antigen and antibody; it is, however, greater than the sum of the affinities for the single determinants, since the effective multivalency of the antigen gives rise to a cooperative "bonus" effect. Often represented by constant K_a (the value of the association constant for the reaction Ab + Ag $\rightleftarrows$ AbAg). Avidity is a function of the techniques used in its measurement and can be expressed only in arbitrary units. Cf. *affinity.*

avi·fau·na (a″vĭ-faw′nə) the bird life present in or characteristic of a given region or locality.

Avi·hep·ad·na·vi·rus (a″vĭ-hep-ad′nə-vi″rəs) [L. *avis* bird + *hepadnavirus*] a genus of viruses of the family Hepadnaviridae containing hepatitis B viruses that infect birds.

Avi·pox·vi·rus (a′vĭ-poks″vi-rəs) [L. *avis* bird + *poxvirus*] avipoxviruses; a genus of viruses of the subfamily Chordopoxvirinae (family Poxviridae) with antigenic cross-reactivity, comprising the fowlpox and related viruses.

avi·pox·vi·rus (a′vĭ-poks″vi-rəs) any virus of the genus *Avipoxvirus.*

avir·u·lence (a-vir′u-ləns) lack of virulence; lack of competence of an infectious agent to produce pathologic effects.

avir·u·lent (a-vir′u-lənt) not virulent.

Avi·ta (ə-ve′tə) trademark for preparations of tretinoin.

avi·ta·min·o·sis (a-vi″tə-mĭ-no′sis) hypovitaminosis. avitaminot′ic *adj*

Avin·za (ə-vin′zə) trademark for a preparation of morphine hydrochloride.

Av·lo·sul·fon (av-lo-sul′fon) trademark for a preparation of dapsone.

AVMA American Veterinary Medical Association.

AVN atrioventricular node.

av·o·ben·zone (av″o-ben′zōn) [USP] a sunscreen that absorbs light in the UVA range.

Avo·dart (av′o-dahrt) trademark for a preparation of dutasteride.

Avo·gad·ro's law, number (constant) (ah-vo-gahd′rōz) [Amedeo *Avogadro,* Italian physicist, 1776–1856] see under *law* and *number.*

avo·gram (av′o-gram) one septillionth (10^{-24}) of a gram, or one picopicogram (ppg); so named from Avogadro number, 6.0233×10^{23}. The mass of a molecule in avograms is therefore 1.66 times its conventional molecular weight.

avoid·ance (ə-void′əns) a conscious or unconscious defense mechanism consisting of refusal to encounter situations, activities, or objects that would produce anxiety or conflict.

avoid·ant (ə-void′ənt) moving away from; negatively oriented.

av·oir·du·pois (av″ər-də-poiz′, av-wahr″doo-pwah′) see under *weight.*

Av·o·nex (av′ə-neks) trademark for a preparation of interferon beta-1a.

AVP arginine vasopressin.

AVRT atrioventricular reciprocating tachycardia.

Avu·la·vi·rus (a′vu-lə-vi″rəs) a genus of viruses of the family Paramyxoviridae, subfamily Paramyxovirinae; it includes Newcastle disease virus.

avul·sion (ə-vul′shən) [L. *avulsio,* from *a-*[2] + *vellere* to pull] the ripping or tearing away of a part either accidentally or surgically.

nerve a. the operation of tearing a nerve by traction.

aware·ness (ə-wār′nəs) consciousness; the possession of knowledge gained through perception.

a. through movement see *Feldenkrais method,* under *method.*

awu atomic weight unit; see *atomic mass unit,* under *unit.*

ax. axis.

Ax·en·feld anomaly, syndrome (ahk′sən-felt″) [Theodor *Axenfeld,* German ophthalmologist, 1867–1930] see under *anomaly* and *syndrome.*

axen·ic (a-zen′ik) [*a-*[1] + *xen-* + *-ic*] not contaminated by or associated with any foreign organisms; used in reference to pure cultures of microorganisms or to germ-free animals. Cf. *gnotobiotic.*

Ax·ert (aks′ərt) trademark for a preparation of almotriptan malate.

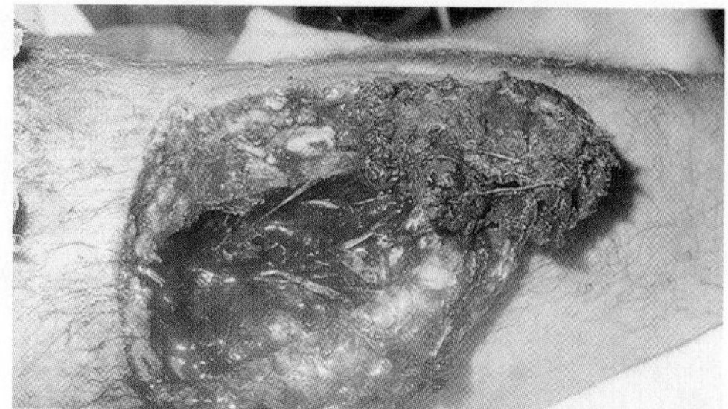

■ Deep avulsion of the leg.

ax•es (ak′sēz) [L.] plural of *axis.*

ax•e•til (ak′sə-til″) USAN contraction for 1-acetoxyethyl.

ax•i•al (ak′se-əl) of or pertaining to the axis of a structure or part, as the long axis of a tooth.

ax•i•a•lis (ak″se-a′lis) [L., from *axis,* q.v.] [TA] axial; a general term denoting relationship to an axis or location near the long axis or central part of the body.

ax•i•a•tion (ak″se-a′shən) the establishment of an axis, or the development of polarity, as in an embryo, organ, or other body structure.

Ax•id (ak′sid) trademark for preparations of nizatidine.

ax•if•u•gal (ak-sif′u-gəl) [*axi-* + *-fugal*[2]] directed away from an axon or axis.

ax•i•lem•ma (ak″sĭ-lem′ə) [*axi-* + *-lemma*] axolemma.

ax•il•la (ak-sil′ə) gen. and pl. *axil′lae* [L.] [TA] the pyramidal region between the upper thoracic wall and the upper limb, its base formed by the skin and apex bounded by the approximation of the clavicle, coracoid process, and first rib; it contains axillary vessels, the brachial plexus of nerves, many lymph nodes and vessels, and loose adipose areolar tissue. Cf. *armpit.* **ax′illary** *adj*

ax•il•lo•bi•fem•o•ral (ak-sil″o-bi-fem′ə-rəl) pertaining to the axillary artery and both femoral arteries.

ax•il•lo•fem•o•ral (ak-sil″o-fem′ə-rəl) pertaining to the axillary and femoral arteries.

ax•il•lo•pop•lit•e•al (ak-sil″o-pop-lit′e-əl) pertaining to the axillary and popliteal arteries.

axi(o)- [L. *axis,* q.v.] a combining form denoting relationship to an axis. In dentistry, it is used in special reference to the long axis of a tooth, as in the names of cavity angles. See specific terms.

ax•io•buc•cal (ak″se-o-buk′əl) pertaining to or formed by the axial and buccal walls of a tooth cavity.

ax•io•buc•co•cer•vi•cal (ak″se-o-buk″o-sur′vĭ-kəl) pertaining to or formed by the axial, buccal, and cervical walls of a tooth cavity.

ax•io•buc•co•gin•gi•val (ak″se-o-buk″o-jin′jĭ-vəl) pertaining to or formed by the axial, buccal, and gingival walls of a tooth cavity.

ax•io•buc•co•lin•gual (ak″se-o-buk″o-ling′gwəl) pertaining to the long axis and the buccal and lingual surfaces of a posterior tooth.

ax•io•cer•vi•cal (ak″se-o-sur′vĭ-kəl) pertaining to or formed by the axial and cervical walls of a tooth cavity.

ax•io•dis•tal (ak″se-o-dis′təl) pertaining to or formed by the axial and distal walls of a tooth cavity.

ax•io•dis•to•cer•vi•cal (ak″se-o-dis″to-sur′vĭ-kəl) pertaining to or formed by the axial, distal, and cervical walls of a tooth cavity.

ax•io•dis•to•gin•gi•val (ak″se-o-dis″to-jin′jĭ-vəl) pertaining to or formed by the axial, distal, and gingival walls of a tooth cavity.

ax•io•dis•to•in•ci•sal (ak″se-o-dis″to-in-si′zəl) pertaining to or formed by the axial, distal, and incisal walls of a tooth cavity.

ax•io•dis•to•oc•clu•sal (ak″se-o-dis″to-ə-kloo′zəl) pertaining to or formed by the axial, distal, and occlusal walls of a tooth cavity.

ax•io•gin•gi•val (ak″se-o-jin′jĭ-vəl) pertaining to or formed by the axial and gingival walls of a tooth cavity.

ax•io•in•ci•sal (ak″se-o-in-si′zəl) pertaining to or formed by the axial and incisal walls of a tooth cavity.

ax•io•la•bi•al (ak″se-o-la′be-əl) pertaining to or formed by the axial and labial walls of a tooth cavity.

ax•io•la•bio•gin•gi•val (ak″se-o-la″be-o-jin′jĭ-vəl) pertaining to or formed by the axial, labial, and gingival walls of a tooth cavity.

ax•io•la•bio•lin•gual (ax″se-o-la″be-o-ling′gwəl) pertaining to the long axis and the labial and lingual surfaces of an anterior tooth.

ax•io•lin•gual (ak″se-o-ling′gwəl) pertaining to or formed by the axial and lingual walls of a tooth cavity.

ax•io•lin•guo•cer•vi•cal (ak″se-o-ling″gwo-sur′vĭ-kəl) pertaining to or formed by the axial, lingual, and cervical walls of a tooth cavity.

ax•io•lin•guo•gin•gi•val (ak″se-o-ling″gwo-jin′jĭ-vəl) pertaining to or formed by the axial, lingual, and gingival walls of a tooth cavity.

ax•io•lin•guo•oc•clu•sal (ak″se-o-ling″gwo-ə-kloo′zəl) pertaining to or formed by the axial, lingual, and occlusal walls of a tooth cavity.

ax•io•me•si•al (ak″se-o-me′zhəl) pertaining to or formed by the axial and mesial walls of a tooth cavity.

ax•io•me•sio•cer•vi•cal (ak″se-o-me″ze-o-sur′vĭ-kəl) pertaining to or formed by the axial, mesial, and cervical walls of a tooth cavity.

ax•io•me•sio•dis•tal (ak″se-o-me″ze-o-dis′təl) pertaining to the long axis and the mesial and distal surfaces of a tooth.

ax•io•me•sio•gin•gi•val (ak″se-o-me″ze-o-jin′jĭ-vəl) pertaining to or formed by the axial, mesial, and gingival walls of a tooth cavity.

ax•io•me•sio•in•ci•sal (ak″se-o-me″ze-o-in-si′zəl) pertaining to or formed by the axial, mesial, and incisal walls of a tooth cavity.

ax•io•me•sio•oc•clu•sal (ak″se-o-me″ze-o-ə-kloo′zəl) pertaining to or formed by the axial, mesial, and occlusal walls of a tooth cavity.

ax•io•oc•clu•sal (ak″se-o-ə-kloo′zəl) pertaining to or formed by the axial and occlusal walls of a tooth cavity.

ax•io•po•di•um (ak″se-o-po′de-əm) axopodium.

ax•io•pul•pal (ak″se-o-pul′pəl) pertaining to or formed by the axial and pulpal walls of a tooth cavity.

ax•ip•e•tal (ak-sip′ə-təl) [*axi-* + *-petal*] directed toward an axon or axis.

ax•is (ak′sis) pl. *ax′es* [L., from Gr. *axōn* axle] 1. a line about which a revolving body turns or about which a structure would turn if it did revolve. 2. a line around which specified parts of the body are arranged. 3. [TA] the second cervical vertebra; called also *epistropheus.* 4. one of the reference lines in a coordinate system. In a two-dimensional coordinate system there are two axes, one horizontal (designated the *x*-axis), and the other intersecting it (designated the *y*-axis). Cf. *abscissa* and *ordinate.*

basibregmatic a. a vertical line from the basion to the bregma; the maximum height of the cranium.

basicranial a. a line from the basion to the gonion.

basifacial a. a line joining the gonion and the subnasal point; called also *facial a.*

binauricular a. a line joining the two auricular points.

celiac a. truncus coeliacus.

cell a. an imaginary line connecting the proximal and distal sides of a cell or passing through the centrosome and nucleus of a cell.

cephalocaudal a. the long axis of the body.

condylar a. an imaginary line passing through the two mandibular condyles around which the mandible may rotate during a part of the opening movement of the jaw; called also *condyle chord.*

costocervical arterial a. truncus costocervicalis.

craniofacial a. the axis of the bones at the base of the skull, including the mesethmoid, presphenoid, basisphenoid, and basioccipital bones.

dorsoventral a. any line in the median plane at right angles to the long axis of the body.

Downs Y a. Y a.

electrical a. of heart the resultant of the electromotive forces within the heart at any instant. See also *axis deviation,* under *deviation.*

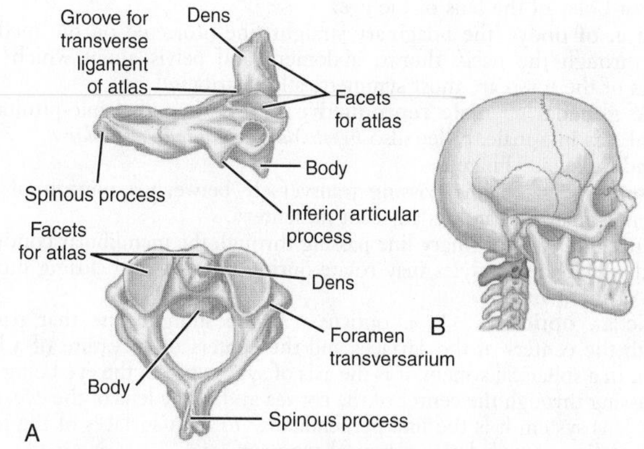

■ Axis. *(A), (Top)* transverse aspect; *(bottom)* superior aspect. *(B),* Position.

embryonic a. an imaginary line from the head end to the tail end of an embryo or, before that, the line of elongation of the primitive streak and groove.

external a. of eye, a. exter′nus bul′bi o′culi [TA] an imaginary line that passes from the anterior to the posterior pole of the eyeball.

facial a. basifacial a.

female gonadal a., female reproductive a. hypothalamic-pituitary-ovarian a.

frontal a. an imaginary line running from right to left through the center of the eyeball.

a. of heart an imaginary line passing through the center of the base of the heart and the apex.

hinge a. the imaginary line connecting the mandibular condyles around which the mandible can rotate without translatory movement; called also *mandibular a.*

HPA a. hypothalamic-pituitary-adrenal a.

HPG a. hypothalamic-pituitary-gonadal a.

HPT a. hypothalamic-pituitary-thyroid a.

hypothalamic-pituitary a. the interrelationships between the hypothalamus and the adenohypophysis, both endocrine and neural, including stimulation of the adenohypophysis by neurosecretory neurons, production of releasing and inhibiting hormones in the hypothalamus, reception of the hormones at sites on pituitary acidophils and basophils, production of hormones by acidophils and basophils, and negative feedback mechanisms by which high levels of circulating hormones act on the hypothalamus and adenohypophysis to inhibit secretion of anterior pituitary hormones. Called also *hypothalamus-pituitary a.*

hypothalamic-pituitary-adrenal a. the interrelationships between the endocrine structures and functions of the hypothalamus and adenohypophysis (the *hypothalamic-pituitary axis*) and the adrenal cortex, including production of corticotropin, its reception at sites in the adrenal cortex, and negative feedback mechanisms by which high levels of circulating glucocorticoids such as cortisol act on the hypothalamus and adenohypophysis to inhibit secretion of corticotropin. Called also *HPA a.* and *hypothalamus-pituitary-adrenal a.*

hypothalamic-pituitary-gonadal a. the interrelationships between the hypothalamic-pituitary axis and the gonads, including production of gonadotropins, their reception at sites in the testis or ovary, and negative feedback mechanisms by which high levels of circulating estrogens or androgens act on the hypothalamus and adenohypophysis to inhibit secretion of gonadotropins. It is sometimes called the *hypothalamic-pituitary-testicular axis* in males and the *hypothalamic-pituitary-ovarian axis* in females. Called also *HPG a.* and *hypothalamus-pituitary-gonad a.*

hypothalamic-pituitary-ovarian a. the hypothalamic-pituitary-gonadal axis in a female; called also *female gonadal* or *female reproductive a.*

hypothalamic-pituitary-testicular a. the hypothalamic-pituitary-gonadal axis in a male; called also *male gonadal* or *reproductive a.*

hypothalamic-pituitary-thyroid a. the interrelationships between the hypothalamic pituitary axis and the thyroid gland, including production of thyrotropin, its reception at sites in the thyroid gland, and negative feedback mechanisms by which high levels of circulating thyroid hormones act on the hypothalamus and adenohypophysis to inhibit secretion of thyrotropin. Called also *HPT a.*

hypothalamus-pituitary a. hypothalamic-pituitary a.

hypothalamus-pituitary-adrenal a. hypothalamic-pituitary-adrenal a.

hypothalamus-pituitary-gonad a. hypothalamic-pituitary-gonadal a.

hypothalamus-pituitary-thyroid a. hypothalamic-pituitary-thyroid a.

internal a. of eye, a. inter′nus bul′bi o′culi [TA] an imaginary line in the eyeball, passing from the anterior pole to a point on the anterior surface of the retina just deep to the posterior pole.

a. len′tis [TA] axis of lens: an imaginary line joining the anterior and posterior poles of the lens of the eye.

long a. of body the imaginary straight line projected on the median plane through the neck, thorax, abdomen, and pelvis about which the weights of the torso are most symmetrically distributed.

male gonadal a., male reproductive a. the hypothalamic-pituitary-gonadal axis in a male; called also *hypothalamic-pituitary-testicular a.*

mandibular a. hinge a.

mesenteric a. a line passing transversely between a portion of the gastrointestinal tract and its adjacent mesentery.

opening a. an imaginary line passing through the mandibular condyles around which the condyles may rotate during opening and closing movements of the mandible.

optic a., optical a. 1. a. opticus. 2. the straight line that passes through the centers of the surfaces and the centers of curvature of a lens system. In a spherical system, it is the axis of symmetry, in the eye being the line passing through the center of the cornea and of the lens of the eye; in a simple lens system it is the line perpendicular to both surfaces of the lens, the lens being regarded as a spherical segment.

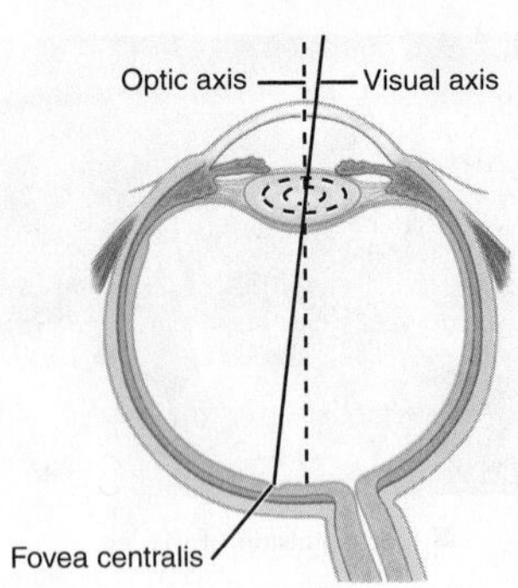

■ Axes of the eye.

a. op′ticus [TA] optic axis: a line connecting the center of the anterior curvature of the cornea (anterior pole) with that of the posterior curvature of the sclera (posterior pole).

a. pel′vis [TA] axis of pelvis: an imaginary curved line through the lesser pelvis at right angles to the plane of the superior aperture, the plane of the cavity, and the plane of the inferior aperture at their central points.

a. of preparation the path taken by a dental restoration as it slides on or off the preparation.

principal a. optic a.

pupillary a. the imaginary line perpendicular to the cornea that passes through the center of the pupil of entrance.

renal a. an imaginary straight line extending through the upper and lower poles of the kidney or, radiographically, through the most inferior and superior calices of the kidney; when projected superiorly, it intersects the thoracic spine.

renin-aldosterone a., renin-angiotensin a. renin-angiotensin-aldosterone system.

secondary a. an imaginary line passing through the optical center of a lens.

spinal a. the vertebral column and spinal cord considered as a unit; sometimes the term also includes the skull.

thoracic a. arteria thoracoacromialis.

thyroid a. truncus thyrocervicalis.

vertical a. of eye an imaginary line connecting the extreme upper and lower points of the eyeball.

visual a. the line between the fovea centralis retinae and the point of fixation, intersecting the optic axis as it passes through the nodal point; it is sometimes defined as the line extending from the fovea to the nodal point and then continuing anteriorly through the cornea.

Y a. the angle of an imaginary line connecting the sella turcica and the gnathion related to the Frankfort horizontal plane; it is an indicator of downward and forward growth of the mandible.

ax(o)- [Gr. *axōn* axle, axis] a combining form denoting relationship to an axis, or to an axon.

axo•ax•on•ic (ak″so-ak-son′ik) [*axo-* + *axon*] referring to a synapse between the axon of one neuron and the axon of another.

Axo•cet (ak′so-set) trademark for a combination preparation of butalbital and acetaminophen.

axo•den•drit•ic (ak″so-den-drit′ik) [*axo-* + *dendritic*] referring to a synapse between the axon of one neuron and dendrites of another; see *synapse.*

ax•of•u•gal (ak-sof′u-gəl) axifugal.

ax•o•graph (ak′so-graf) an apparatus for recording axes in kymographic tracings.

ax•oid (ak′soid) pertaining to the axis (second cervical vertebra).

ax•oi•de•an (ak-soi′de-ən) axoid.

axo•lem•ma (ak-so-lem′ə) [*axo-* + *lemma*] the plasma membrane of an axon; called also *Mauthner membrane* or *sheath.*

ax•o•lotl (ak′so-lot-əl) [Nahuatl] a larval salamander of the genus *Ambystoma;* used in experiments with thyroid feeding.

ax•ol•ysis (ak-sol′ĭ-sis) [*axo-* + *-lysis*] degeneration and breaking up of the axon of a nerve cell.

ax•om•e•ter (ak-som′ə-tər) [*axo-* + *-meter*] an instrument for measuring an axis, especially an instrument for adjusting a pair of spectacles with respect to the optic axes of the eyes.

ax•on (ak′son) [Gr. *axōn* axle, axis] 1. the process of a neuron by which impulses travel away from the cell body; at the terminal arborization of the axon, the impulses are transmitted to other nerve cells or to effector organs.

The larger axons are surrounded by a myelin sheath (see under *sheath*). Called also *axone*. See also *neurofibra*. 2. columna vertebralis. **ax′onal** *adj*

fusimotor a. see under *fiber*.

giant a. an axon of certain invertebrates, e.g., the squid, whose size (500 to 700 microns) has facilitated physiological studies of cell membrane excitation.

myelinated a. an axon with a myelin sheath.

naked a. an axon which has no myelin sheath.

unmyelinated a. naked a.

ax•on•aprax•ia (ak″son-ə-prak′se-ə) neurapraxia.

ax•one (ak′sōn) axon (def. 1).

ax•o•neme (ak′so-nēm) [*axo-* + Gr. *nēma* thread] the central core of a cilium or flagellum, consisting of a central pair of microtubules surrounded by nine other microtubule pairs; called also *axial filament*.

ax•o•nom•e•ter (ak″so-nom′ə-tər) axometer.

axo•nop•a•thy (ak″sə-nop′ə-the) [*axon* + *-pathy*] a disorder disrupting the normal functioning of the axons.

distal a. the more common kind of axonopathy, in which the disease process starts centrally and proceeds towards the periphery; cf. *wallerian degeneration*.

proximal a. axonopathy in which the disease process starts at the periphery and proceeds towards the center; cf. *dying-back*.

ax•on•ot•me•sis (ak″son-ot-me′sis) [*axo-* + Gr. *tmēsis* a cutting apart] nerve injury characterized by disruption of the axon and myelin sheath but with preservation of the connective tissue fragments, resulting in degeneration of the axon distal to the injury site; regeneration of the axon is spontaneous and of good quality. Cf. *neurapraxia* and *neurotmesis*.

ax•op•e•tal (ak-sop′ə-təl) axipetal.

axo•phage (ak′so-fāj) [*axo-* + *-phage*] a neuroglial cell occurring in excavations in the myelin in myelitis.

axo•plasm (ak′so-plaz″əm) [*axo-* + *plasma*] the cytoplasm of an axon. **axoplas′mic** *adj*

axo•po•di•um (ak″so-po′de-əm) pl. *axopo′dia* [*axo-* + Gr. *pous* foot] a long and slender, semipermanent type of locomotor pseudopodium that has a central axial filament composed of a bundle of microtubules; cf. *filopodium*, *lobopodium*, and *reticulopodium*. Called also *axiopodium*.

axo•so•mat•ic (ak″so-so-mat′ik) [*axo-* + *somatic*] referring to a synapse between the axon of one neuron and the cell body of another.

axo•style (ak′so-stīl) [*axo-* + Gr. *stylos* pillar] a filamentous or hyaline-supporting structure passing through the longitudinal axis of certain flagellate protozoa, such as trichomonads, and sometimes extending beyond the posterior end of the organism. Its enlarged capitulum may give rise to or be covered by a pelta.

ax•ot•o•my (ak-sot′ə-me) transection or severing of an axon.

aya•pa•na (ah″yah-pah′nah) 1. *Eupatorium ayapana*. 2. the leaves of *E. ayapana*, which are used in South America as an aromatic, stomachic, diaphoretic, stimulant, and household remedy for many conditions.

Ayer-To•bey test (a′yər to′be) [James Bourne *Ayer*, American neurologist, 1882–1963; George L. *Tobey*, Jr., American otolaryngologist, 1881–1947] Tobey-Ayer test.

Ayer•za disease, syndrome (ah-yār′sah) [Abel *Ayerza*, Argentine physician, 1861–1918] see under *disease* and *syndrome*.

Ay•ges•tin (a-jes′tin) trademark for a preparation of norethindrone acetate.

ayur•ve•da (i-yur′ved-ə, i″yər-va′də) [Sanskrit "science of life" or "knowledge of living," from *ayur* life + *veda* science] the classical system of medicine founded in the Indus valley civilization as oral tradition 5000 years ago and currently practiced in India. It is distinguished by its emphasis on balance with the environment and interpersonal communication and is based on the principles that humans are microcosmic representations of the entire universe and that health is the natural end of living in harmony with the environment. Disease results from disharmony between the person and the environment, and each case of disease is a manifestation of a unique state in a unique individual. Because no two cases of disease are exactly the same, no two cures are exactly alike. The goal of the practitioner is to maintain or restore the balance of the doshas. Therapy includes diet; herbal, color, and sound therapies; aromatherapy; application of medicated oils to the skin and massage; and meditation. Written also *Ayurveda*. **ayurve′dic** *adj*

Az azote.

aza•ci•ti•dine (a″zə-si′tĭ-dēn) INN for *5-azacytidine*.

Azac•tam (a-zak′tam) trademark for preparations of aztreonam.

5-aza•cy•ti•dine (a″zə-si′tĭ-dēn) a cytidine analogue that can be incorporated into RNA and DNA; unlike cytidine, it cannot be 5-methylated, a process that is important in gene regulation and post-transcriptional processing of RNA. Used in treatment of myelodysplastic syndromes; administered by subcutaneous injection.

Az•a•di•rach•ta (az″ə-dĭ-rak′tə) [Persian *azad dirakht* noble tree] a genus of trees (family Meliaceae) native to India and Southeast Asia, closely related to and formerly included in the genus *Melia*. *A. in′dica* is neem (q.v.).

az•a•guan•ine (az″ə-gwahn′ēn) a mitotic poison that resembles the purine guanine but is actually incorporated into nucleic acids and acts to block nucleic acid synthesis by competitive inhibition.

Aza•lea (ə-za′le-ə) a former genus of shrubs and trees now classified as part of the genus *Rhododendron*; they contain andromedotoxin and have caused poisoning in sheep.

az•a•lide (az′ə-līd) a subclass of the macrolide antibiotics to which the antibacterial azithromycin belongs.

aza•per•one (a″zə-per′ōn) [USP] a butyrophenone antipsychotic used as a tranquilizer in veterinary medicine.

aza•pro•pa•zone (a″zə-pro′pə-zōn) apazone.

azat•a•dine mal•e•ate (ə-zat′ə-dēn) [USP] an antihistamine (H_1 receptor antagonist) with sedative and anticholinergic effects; used in the treatment of allergic rhinitis, allergic conjunctivitis, and cutaneous manifestations of allergic reactions, and as an ingredient in some cough and cold preparations, administered orally.

aza•thio•prine (az″ə-thi′o-prēn) [USP] the imidazolyl derivative of 6-mercaptopurine, its active metabolite; used as an immunosuppressive agent for prevention of transplant rejection in organ transplantation; as a disease-modifying antirheumatic drug for treatment of severe, progressive rheumatoid arthritis unresponsive to other agents; and in treatment of a number of autoimmune disorders, such as systemic lupus erythematosus, autoimmune hemolytic anemia, or inflammatory bowel disease; administered orally.

a. sodium [USP] the sodium salt of azathioprine, used to prevent transplant rejection in organ transplantation; administered intravenously.

azed•a•rach (ə-zed′ə-rak″) *Melia azedarach*.

az•e•la•ic ac•id (az″ə-la′ik) a dicarboxylic acid occurring in whole grains and animal products; it has antibacterial effects on both aerobic and anaerobic organisms, particularly *Propionibacterium acnes* and *Staphylococcus epidermidis*, normalizes keratinization, and has a cytotoxic effect on malignant or hyperactive melanocytes; applied topically in the treatment of acne vulgaris.

azel•as•tine hy•dro•chlo•ride (ə-zel′ə-stēn) an antihistamine (H_1 receptor antagonist) administered intranasally in the treatment of seasonal allergic rhinitis (hay fever) and topically to the conjunctiva in the treatment of allergic conjunctivitis.

Az•e•lex (az′ə-leks) trademark for a preparation of azelaic acid.

azeo•trope (a′ze-o-trōp″) [*a-*[1] + Gr. *zein* to boil + *tropē* a turn, or turning] a mixture of two substances that has a constant boiling point and cannot be separated by fractional distillation. **azeotrop′ic** *adj*

aze•ot•ro•py (a″ze-ot′rə-pe) having the characteristics of an azeotrope; the absence of any change in the composition of a mixture of substances when it is boiled under a given pressure, the vapor having the same characteristics as the liquid.

az•ide (az′īd) a compound that contains the group $—N_3$.

3′-az•i•do-3′-de•oxy•thy•mi•dine (az″ĭ-do″de-ok″se-thi′mĭ-dēn) zidovudine.

az•i•do•thy•mi•dine (az″ĭ-do-thi′mĭ-dēn) zidovudine.

Az•i•lect (az′ĭ-lekt) trademark for a preparation of rasagiline mesylate.

azir•i•dine (ə-zir′ĭ-dēn) ethylenimine.

az•ith•ro•my•cin (az-ith″ro-mi′sin) [USP] an azalide antibiotic, derived from erythromycin, that inhibits bacterial protein synthesis, effective against a wide range of gram-positive, gram-negative, and anaerobic bacteria; used in the treatment of mild to moderate infections caused by susceptible organisms, administered orally and intravenously.

Az•lin (az′lin) trademark for a preparation of azlocillin sodium.

az•lo•cil•lin (az″lo-sil′in) a broad-spectrum penicillin of the ureidopenicillin group, effective against a wide variety of gram-positive and gram-negative organisms but used primarily in the treatment of *Pseudomonas aeruginosa* infections; its bactericidal activity results from interference with cell wall synthesis.

a. sodium the monosodium salt of azlocillin, administered intravenously by infusion or injection.

Az•ma•cort (az′mə-kort) trademark for a preparation of triamcinolone acetonide.

azo- a prefix indicating the presence of the group —N═N—, as in azobenzene.

azo·ben·zene (az″o-ben′zēn) [*azo-* + *benzene*] an orange-red crystalline product, of the reduction of nitrobenzene; it is the parent substance of azo dyes and some pH indicators and is carcinogenic. Called also *diphenyldiimide.*

azo·bil·i·ru·bin (a″zo-bil′ĭ-roo″bin) bilirubin that has been diazotized by exposure to Ehrlich diazo reagent during the Jendrassik-Grof method of bilirubin measurement.

azo·car·mine (az″o-kahr′min) either azocarmine G or azocarmine B, red basic dyes used in certain staining procedures.

azo·ic (a-zo′ik) [*a-*[1] + Gr. *zōe* life] 1. devoid of living organisms. 2. a protoplasmic poison, hydrazoic acid, N_3H, resembling hydrocyanic acid in its action, made by heating hydrogen chloride with sodium nitrate. It is highly explosive. Called also *triazoic acid* and *hydronitric acid.*

az·ole (az′ōl) 1. any of a group of organic compounds containing a five-membered heterocyclic ring, the ring having one or more nitrogen atoms and often also other atoms such as oxygen or sulfur. See also under *antifungal.* 2. pyrrole.

azo·lit·min (az″o-lit′min) a coloring principle, from litmus; it is used as a pH indicator, being red at a pH of 4.5 and blue at 8.3.

AZOOR acute zonal occult outer retinopathy.

azoo·sper·mia (a-zo″ə-spur′me-ə) [*a-*[1] + *zoospermia*] lack of live spermatozoa in the semen; see also *aspermatogenesis.*

  nonobstructive a. azoospermia that is not due to obstruction of any passageway but rather to a cause such as infection, aspermatogenesis, or retrograde ejaculation.

  obstructive a. azoospermia due to obstruction of tubules or ducts.

azo·pig·ment (a″zo-pig′mənt) a purple derivative of bile pigment containing an azo (—N═N—) linkage; formed by reacting bile pigments with diazotizing agents.

azo·pro·tein (az″o-pro′tēn) a protein some constituents of which have been diazotized.

Azopt (a′zopt) trademark for a preparation of brinzolamide.

Azor·e·an disease (a-zor′e-ən) [*Azores* Islands, because it occurs in families of Portuguese-Azorean descent] Machado-Joseph disease; see under *disease.*

Azo-Stan·dard (a′zo-stan′dərd) trademark for a preparation of phenazopyridine hydrochloride.

azo·sul·fa·mide (az″o-sul′fə-mīd) an antibacterial compound; it was one of the forerunners of the sulfonamide drugs.

az·ote (az′ōt) [Fr., from *a-*[1] + Gr. *zōe* life] nitrogen; used only in France. It is the basis of the prefix *azo-* and occurs as a stem in such words as *azotemia.*

az·o·te·mia (az″o-te′me-ə) [*azote* + *-emia*] an excess of urea or other nitrogenous compounds in the blood; called also *uremia.* **azote′mic** *adj*

  extrarenal a. azotemia due to a condition or process outside the kidney; see *prerenal a.* and *postrenal a.*

  intrarenal a. azotemia due to a reduced glomerular filtration rate resulting from acute or chronic disease of the renal parenchyma; see also *acute renal failure,* under *failure.* Called also *renal a.*

  postrenal a. azotemia due to obstruction of the urinary tract, as seen with postrenal acute renal failure (see under *failure*).

  prerenal a. azotemia resulting from inadequate perfusion of the kidneys, as in prerenal acute renal failure (see under *failure*).

  renal a. intrarenal a.

az·o·tom·e·ter (az″o-tom′ə-tər) [*azote* + *-meter*] an instrument for measuring the proportion of nitrogen compounds in a solution.

azo·to·my·cin (ə-zo″to-mi′sin) an antibiotic substance with antineoplastic properties produced by *Streptomyces ambofaciens.*

az·o·tor·rhea (az″o-tə-re′ə) [*azote* + *-rrhea*] excessive loss of nitrogen in the feces.

az·o·tu·ria (az″o-tu′re-ə) [*azote* + *-uria*] 1. an excess of urea or other nitrogen compounds in the urine. 2. a type of exertional rhabdomyolysis in horses marked by sudden perspiration and paralysis of the hind quarters and by the passing of light red to dark brown urine. It occurs in animals that, after being engaged in continuous work, are given a long rest (such as a weekend for work horses) with continuation of the high-protein diet and then return to work. Called also *cording-up, set-fast, tying up, tying-up syndrome, Monday morning disease,* and *paralytic myoglobinuria.* **azotu′ric** *adj*

az·oxy (az-ok′se) the group:

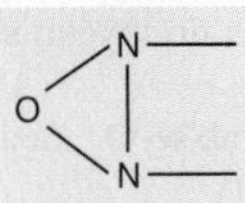

az·oxy·ben·zene (az-ok″se-ben′zēn) a pale yellow product, $C_6H_5{\bullet}N{\bullet}({\bullet}O)N{\bullet}C_6H_5$, of the reduction of nitrobenzene.

AZQ diaziquone.

AZT zidovudine.

az·tre·o·nam (az′tre-o-nam″) [USP] a narrow-range monobactam antibiotic effective against aerobic gram-negative bacteria; used for the treatment of infections caused by susceptible organisms. Administered intravenously or intramuscularly.

Azul·fi·dine (a-zul′fĭ-dēn) trademark for a preparation of sulfasalazine.

az·ure (azh′ər) any of the partially methylated homologues of the series of basic dyes extending from thionine to methylene blue or to certain mixtures of members of this series. They are metachromatic and are used in many important staining procedures.

  a. I a. B.

  a. II a mixture of equal parts of azure I and methylene blue.

  a. A asymmetrical dimethylthionine, $(CH_3)_2N{\bullet}C_6H_3(SN)C_6H_3{\bullet}NH_2{\bullet}Cl$.

  a. B trimethylthionine chloride; a dye used as a biological stain; it is a component of polychrome methylene blue.

  a. C monomethylthionine chloride, $(CH_3)N{\bullet}C_6H_3(SN)C_6H_3NH_2{\bullet}Cl$.

  methylene a. a. B.

az·u·ro·phil (azh′u-ro-fil) [*azure* + *-phil*] 1. an element or cell that stains well with blue aniline dyes. 2. azurophilic.

az·u·ro·phile (azh′u-ro-fīl) 1. azurophil. 2. azurophilic.

az·u·ro·phil·ia (azh″u-ro-fil′e-ə) 1. the quality of staining well with blue aniline dyes. 2. the presence of azurophil granules, as in many lymphocytes.

az·u·ro·phil·ic (azh″u-ro-fil′ik) 1. easily stained with blue aniline dyes. 2. pertaining to or characterized by azurophilia. Called also *azurophil* and *azurophile.*

azyg(o)- [Gr. *azygos* unpaired, from *a-*[1] + *zygon* yoke] a combining form denoting something unpaired, or relationship to the azygous vein.

az·y·go·esoph·a·ge·al (az″ĭ-go-e-sof″ə-je′əl) pertaining to or located between the azygos vein and the esophagus.

az·y·go·gram (az′ĭ-go-gram) the radiographic record obtained by azygography.

az·y·gog·raphy (az″ĭ-gog′rə-fe) radiography of the azygos venous system following its opacification with contrast material; usually employed for evaluation of abnormal tumor masses in the mediastinum, as evidenced by extrinsic pressure upon, or complete obstruction of, the visualized azygos vein.

az·y·go·me·di·as·ti·nal (az″ĭ-go-me″de-ə-sti′nəl) pertaining to or located between the azygos vein and the mediastinum.

az·y·gos (az′ĭ-gəs, ə-zi′gəs) [Gr., from *a-*[1] + Gr. *zygon* yoke] 1. unpaired. 2. any unpaired part, such as the azygos vein.

azy·go·sperm (ə-zi′go-sperm″) [*a-*[1] + *zygosperm*] azygospore.

azy·go·spore (ə-zi′go-spor″) [*a-*[1] + *zygospore*] a spore developed directly from a gamete without conjugation; called also *azygosperm.*

az·y·gous (az′ĭ-gəs, ə-zi′gəs) [Gr. *azygos,* q.v.] having no fellow; unpaired.

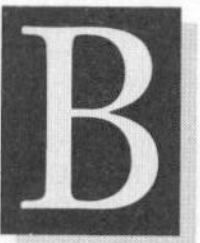

B bel; boron.

B magnetic flux density.

b barn; base (def. 5), used in designating lengths of nucleic acid sequence, e.g., 50 b, a sequence of 50 bases (50 nucleotides long); born.

β beta, the second letter of the Greek alphabet; symbol for the β chain of hemoglobin and the probability of *Type II error*.

β- a prefix designating (1) the second carbon atom of a chain starting with that adjacent to the principal functional group, e.g., β-hydroxybutyric acid (see α-); (2) the specific rotation of an optically active substance, e.g., β-D-glucose; (3) the orientation of an exocyclic atom or group, e.g., cholest-5-en-3-β-ol (cholesterol); (4) a plasma protein migrating with the β band (subdivided into β_1 and β_2 bands) in protein electrophoresis, e.g., β-lipoprotein; (5) one in a series of related chemical compounds, particularly a series of stereoisomeric, isomeric, polymeric, or allotropic forms, e.g., β-carotene; and (6) one in a group of related entities, e.g., β-ray. For compounds prefixed with the symbol β-, see the unprefixed form.

BA Bachelor of Arts.

Ba barium.

Baas·trup disease (syndrome) (bah′stroop) [Christian Ingerslev *Baastrup*, Danish physician, 1885–1950] kissing spines; see under *spine*.

Ba·bès nodules (nodes, tubercles) (bah′besh) [Victor *Babeş*, Romanian bacteriologist, 1854–1926] see under *nodule*.

Ba·be·sia (bə-be′ze-ə) [V. *Babeş*] a genus of protozoa of the order Piroplasmida, occurring as single or paired parasites within the erythrocytes of various vertebrates, causing babesiosis and other diseases; they are transmitted by ticks, in which a sexual multiplicative cycle occurs.

B. argenti′na an etiologic agent of bovine babesiosis in Central and South America and Australia; the vector is *Boophilus microplus* or sometimes *Boophilus australis*.

B. bige′mina an etiologic agent of bovine babesiosis in Central and South America, the West Indies, and certain regions of Europe and Africa; it is transmitted by various ticks, especially *Boophilus* species.

B. bo′vis a species found in some of the same regions as *B. bigemina;* this is the major cause of bovine babesiosis in Europe and northern Asia. Ticks of genus *Boophilus* are usually the vectors, but in some areas *Ixodes* ticks are vectors.

B. cabal′li a species causing equine babesiosis in Africa and some parts of Asia, transmitted by ticks of the genera *Anocentor*, *Dermacentor*, *Hyalomma*, and *Rhipicephalus*.

B. ca′nis an etiologic agent of canine babesiosis, found around the world; its vectors are ixodid ticks such as *Rhipicephalus sanguineus*, *Haemaphysalis leachi*, *Hyalomma plumbeum*, and *Dermacentor* species.

B. ca′ti an etiologic agent of feline babesiosis in Asia; the vector is unknown.

B. diver′gens an etiologic agent of bovine and human babesiosis in temperate regions of Europe and perhaps Asia, transmitted by the ticks *Ixodes ricinus* and *Haemaphysalis punctata*.

B. e′qui a species causing equine babesiosis in various parts of Asia, Africa, and the Americas, transmitted by ticks of the genera *Dermacentor*, *Rhipicephalus*, and *Hyalomma*.

B. fe′lis an etiologic agent of feline babesiosis in various parts of Africa; the vector is unknown.

B. gibso′ni an etiologic agent of canine babesiosis found in East Asia and adjacent islands, as well as the United States, transmitted by the ticks *Haemaphysalis bispinosa* and *Rhipicephalus sanguineus*.

B. ma′jor an etiologic agent of bovine babesiosis, transmitted by the tick *Boophilus calcaratus*, and occurring in North Africa, Europe, and the former Soviet Union.

B. micro′ti a parasite normally found in rodents in North America, but also causing human babesiosis; the usual vector is the tick *Ixodes scapularis*, although transmission by means of blood transfusion has been reported.

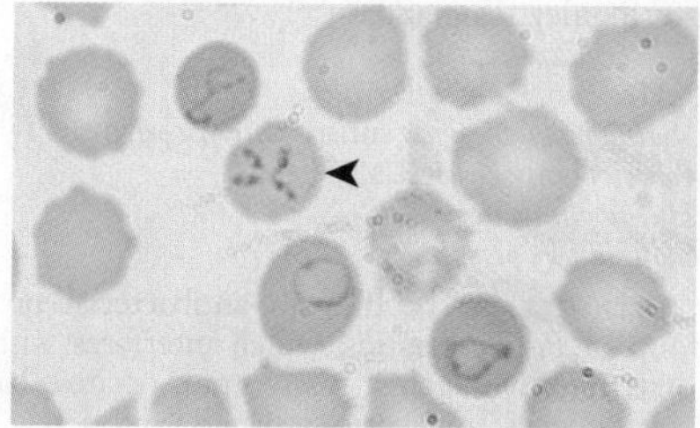

■ *Babesia*; some erythrocytes contain multiple parasites, and in one the organisms are arranged in a characteristic Maltese cross shape *(arrow)*.

B. mota′si a species causing ovine babesiosis in parts of Europe, the Middle East, and Asia; the vector is usually a tick of species *Rhipicephalus bursa*, *Dermacentor sylvarum*, or *Haemaphysalis punctata*.

B. o′vis a species causing ovine babesiosis in the tropics and in southern Europe, the former Soviet Union, and the Middle East, transmitted by the ticks *Rhipicephalus bursa* and *Ixodes persulcatus*.

B. perronci′toi a species causing swine babesiosis in Africa; the vector is unknown.

B. trautman′ni a species causing swine babesiosis in Europe, Asia, Africa, and Central and South America; transmitted by the tick *Rhipicephalus sanguineus*.

B. voge′li an etiologic agent of canine babesiosis in the domestic dog, transmitted by the tick *Rhipicephalus sanguineus*, and occurring in Asia and Africa.

ba·be·si·a·sis (bă″be-zi′ə-sis) babesiosis.

ba·be·si·o·sis (bə-be″ze-o′sis) any of various tickborne diseases due to infection with protozoa of the genus *Babesia*, occurring in wild and domestic mammals and as a zoonosis in humans. Called also *babesiasis* and *piroplasmosis*.

bovine b. infection of cattle by *Babesia;* the acute phase is manifested by fever, hemoglobinuria, anemia, icterus, and splenomegaly. The variety that was once endemic in the southern United States, infection with *B. bigemina*, has been largely eliminated by eradication of its tick vector. Other species of *Babesia* still cause the disease in various parts of the world. Called also *redwater*, *redwater fever*, *Texas fever*, and *Texas cattle fever*.

canine b. infection of dogs or other canines with any of various species of *Babesia*. The acute phase, which may be fatal, is characterized by depression, weakness, loss of appetite, pallor of the mucous membranes, icterus, fever, and splenomegaly.

equine b. infection of horses or other equines with *Babesia caballi* or *B. equi;* characteristics include high fever, immobility, icterus, gastrointestinal disturbances, rapid emaciation, and dependent edema.

feline b. infection of cats or other felines with any of various species of *Babesia*, characterized by loss of appetite, lethargy, weakness, rough coat, and pale mucous membranes.

human b. human infection with species of *Babesia*, particularly *B. divergens* or *B. microti*, a classic type of zoonosis occurring after exposure to infected animals. Characteristics include anemia, hemoglobinemia, hemoglobinuria, and a malarialike fever with chills, sweats, myalgia, nausea and vomiting, hemolytic anemia, and splenomegaly. In asplenic or immunocompromised patients, the infection may be fulminant and even fatal.

ovine b. infection in sheep and goats with *Babesia motasi* or *B. ovis;* symptoms include jaundice and hematuria. The *B. motasi* form is usually more severe than the *B. ovis* form.

porcine b., swine b. infection of swine with any of several species of *Babesia*.

Ba·bin·ski reflex, sign, syndrome (bə-bin′ske) [Joseph François Félix *Babinski*, French physician, 1857–1932] see under *reflex*, *sign*, and *syndrome*.

Ba·bin·ski-Fröh·lich syndrome (bə-bin′ske frur′lik) [J.F.F. *Babinski;* Alfred *Fröhlich*, Austrian-born neurologist in United States, 1871–1953] adiposogenital dystrophy.

Ba·bin·ski-Na·geotte syndrome (bə-bin′ske nah-zhot′) [J.F.F. *Babinski;* Jean *Nageotte*, French pathologist, 1866–1948] see under *syndrome*.

Ba·bin·ski-Va·quez syndrome (bə-bin′ske vah-ka′) [J.F.F. *Babinski;* Louis Henri *Vaquez*, French physician, 1860–1936] Babinski syndrome.

ba·by (ba′be) infant.

blue b. an infant born with cyanosis due to a congenital heart lesion.

blueberry muffin b. an infant whose skin has numerous erythematous to blue nodules and papules, resembling blueberries in a muffin, owing to extramedullary hematogenesis.

collodion b. an infant born encased in a tight membrane resembling collodion or parchment, which is subsequently shed. This usually leaves fissures in the baby's skin and is a primary manifestation of some form of ichthyosis, most often the lamellar type. Occasionally shedding of the membrane leaves relatively normal skin; see *lamellar exfoliation of newborn*.

test tube b. popular term for an embryo or fetus conceived by in vitro fertilization.

BAC bacterial artificial chromosome.

ba·cam·pi·cil·lin hy·dro·chlo·ride (bə-kam″pĭ-sil′in) [USP] a semisynthetic penicillin of the aminopenicillin group, which is hydrolyzed to ampicillin during absorption from the gastrointestinal tract and has the same actions and uses as ampicillin. Administered orally.

bac·cate (bak′āt) resembling a berry.

Bac·cel·li sign (bə-chel′e) [Guido *Baccelli*, Italian physician, 1832–1916] aphonic pectoriloquy.

bac·ci·form (bak′sĭ-form) [L. *bacca* berry + *form*] berry-shaped.

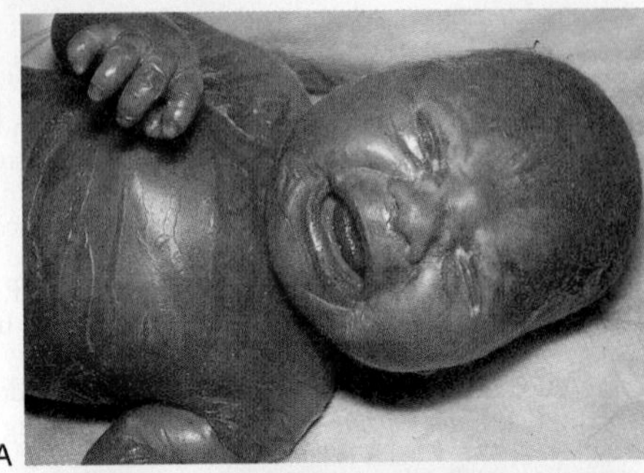

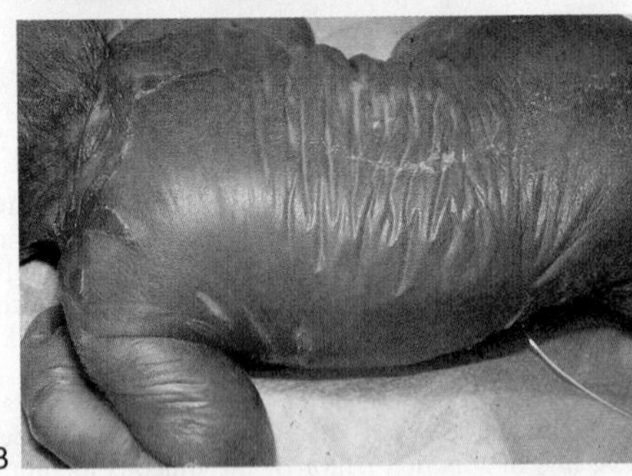

■ Collodion baby, with ectropion and eversion and fissuring of the eyelid margins and lips. A shiny transparent membrane covered the infant at birth; she later developed lamellar ichthyosis.

Bach remedies (flower remedies) (bahk) [Edward *Bach*, English homeopath, 1886–1936] see *Bach remedies*, under *remedy*.

Bach•mann bundle (bahk′mən) [Jean George *Bachmann*, American physiologist, 1877–1959] see under *bundle*.

Ba•cil•la•ceae (bas″ĭ-la′se-e) a family of bacteria of the order Bacillales made up of endospore-forming rods and cocci. The mostly gram-positive organisms are usually soil saprophytes, but a few are insect or animal parasites and may produce disease. Medically important organisms are included in the genus *Bacillus*.

Ba•cil•la•les (bas″ĭ-la′lēz) an order of gram-positive, endospore-forming bacteria of the class Bacilli; medically important organisms are included in the families Bacillaceae, Listeriaceae, Paenibacillaceae, Planococcaceae, Staphylococcaceae, and Thermoactinomycetaceae.

bac•il•lary (bas′ĭ-lar″e) 1. rod-shaped. 2. consisting of small rods or rodlike structures. 3. pertaining to, caused by, or resembling bacilli.

ba•cille (bah-sēl′) [Fr.] bacillus.

b. Calmette-Guérin (BCG) an organism of the strain *Mycobacterium bovis*, rendered completely avirulent by cultivation for many years on bile-glycerol-potato medium. The strain, commonly called BCG, is used for immunization against tuberculosis and in cancer chemotherapy. See also *BCG vaccine*, under *vaccine*.

bac•il•le•mia (bas″ĭ-le′me-ə) [*bacill-* + *-emia*] the presence of bacilli in the blood.

Ba•cil•li (bə-sil′i) a class of bacteria of the phylum Firmicutes, containing the orders Bacillales and Lactobacillales.

ba•cil•li (bə-sil′i) [L.] plural of *bacillus*.

bacilli- [L. *bacillus*, q.v.] a combining form denoting relationship to a bacillus or to bacilli. Also *bacill(o)-*.

ba•cil•lif•er•ous (bă″sĭ-lif′ər-əs) bearing or carrying bacilli.

ba•cil•li•form (bə-sil′ĭ-form) [*bacilli-* + *form*] having the appearance of a bacillus; rod-shaped.

ba•cil•lin (bə-sil′in) an antibiotic substance isolated from strains of *Bacillus subtilis*.

bacill(o)- see *bacilli-*.

ba•cil•lu•ria (bas″ĭ-lu′re-ə) [*bacill-* + *-uria*] bacteriuria with bacilli in the urine.

Ba•cil•lus (bə-sil′əs) [L. "little rod"] a genus of bacteria of the family Bacillaceae, including large aerobic or facultatively anaerobic, spore-forming, rod-shaped cells, the great majority of which are gram-positive and motile. Most species are saprophytic soil forms; three are pathogenic or potentially pathogenic. Many organisms historically called *Bacillus* are now classified in other genera.

B. al′vei *Paenibacillus alvei.*

B. an′thracis the cause of anthrax; its virulence is associated with the production of capsules and a potent exotoxin.

B. bre′vis see *Brevibacillus*.

B. ce′reus a sometimes motile, aerobic or facultatively anaerobic spore-forming species that is a common soil saprophyte. It causes food poisoning by the formation of an enterotoxin in contaminated foods.

B. cir′culans a species that can cause meningitis, endocarditis, and other types of infections.

B. fusifor′mis former name for *Fusobacterium nucleatum*.

B. lar′vae *Paenibacillus larvae.*

B. lichenifor′mis a species that can cause bacteremia and food poisoning.

B. megate′rium a species that is a widely distributed saprophyte in soil and commonly occurs as a laboratory contaminant; it has also been found in persons with meningitis, bacteremia, and other infections.

B. polymyx′a former name for *Paenibacillus polymyxa*.

B. pumi′lus a species that can cause bacteremia, meningitis, and other types of infections.

B. sphae′ricus a species that can cause bacteremia, meningitis, and other types of infections.

B. stearothermo′philus former name for *Geobacillus stearothermophilus*.

B. sub′tilis a species that is a common saprophyte in soil and water, often a laboratory contaminant, and can cause conjunctivitis. It also produces the antibiotic bacitracin.

ba•cil•lus (bə-sil′əs) pl. *bacil′li* [L.] 1. an organism of the genus *Bacillus*. 2. any rod-shaped bacterium.

anthrax b. *Bacillus anthracis.*

Bang b. *Brucella abortus.*

Battey b. *Mycobacterium intracellulare.*

Bordet-Gengou b. *Bordetella pertussis.*

butter b. *Clostridium butyricum.*

b. Calmette-Guérin (BCG), Calmette-Guérin b. bacille Calmette-Guérin.

coliform bacilli gram-negative bacilli found in the intestinal tract that resemble *Escherichia coli*, particularly in the fermentation of lactose with gas. The term generally is used to refer to the genera *Citrobacter*, *Escherichia*, *Edwardsiella*, *Enterobacter*, *Klebsiella*, and *Serratia*.

diphtheria b. *Corynebacterium diphtheriae.*

Döderlein b. one of the gram-positive rods commonly found in vaginal secretions that may consist of mixtures of *Lactobacillus acidophilus*, *L. casei*, *L. cellobiosisus*, *L. fermentum*, or *Leuconostoc mesenteroides*. Said by some to be identical with *L. acidophilus*.

Ducrey b. *Haemophilus ducreyi.*

dysentery bacilli a group that causes bacillary dysentery; see *Shigella*.

enteric b. a bacillus belonging to the family Enterobacteriaceae.

Escherich b. *Escherichia coli.*

Flexner b. *Shigella flexneri.*

fusiform b. fusobacterium.

Ghon-Sachs b. *Clostridium septicum.*

glanders b. *Burkholderia mallei.*

Hansen b. *Mycobacterium leprae.*

Hofmann b. *Corynebacterium pseudodiphtheriticum.*

hog cholera b. *Salmonella enterica* subsp. *enterica* serovar choleraesuis.

Johne b. *Mycobacterium avium* subsp. *paratuberculosis*.

Klebs-Löffler b. *Corynebacterium diphtheriae.*

Koch b. *Mycobacterium tuberculosis.*

Koch-Weeks b. *Haemophilus aegyptius.*

lepra b., leprosy b. *Mycobacterium leprae.*

Morax-Axenfeld b. *Moraxella (Moraxella) lacunata.*

paracolon bacilli microorganisms commonly found in the intestinal flora, distinguished by delayed (5–21 days) fermentation of lactose. Organisms of this type belong to the genera *Escherichia*, *Citrobacter*, or *Klebsiella*.

Preisz-Nocard b. *Corynebacterium pseudotuberculosis.*

rhinoscleroma b. *Klebsiella pneumoniae rhinoscleromatis.*

Shiga b. *Shigella dysenteriae* 1.

smegma b. *Mycobacterium smegmatis.*

Stanley b. a serovar of *Salmonella enterica* isolated from patients with food poisoning in Stanley, England.

tetanus b. *Clostridium tetani.*

tubercle b. *Mycobacterium tuberculosis.*

typhoid b. *Salmonella enterica* subsp. *enterica* serovar Typhi.

vole b. *Mycobacterium microti.*

Weeks b. *Haemophilus aegyptius.*

Welch b. *Clostridium perfringens.*

bac•i•tra•cin (bas″ĭ-tra′sin) [USP] an antibacterial produced by the *licheniformin* group of *Bacillus subtilis*, which interferes with bacterial cell wall synthesis. It is effective against many gram-positive bacteria, such as staphylococci, streptococci, and various bacilli, and a few gram-negative bacteria, including *Neisseria*, *Haemophilus influenzae*, and *Treponema pallidum*. It is applied topically to the skin or conjunctiva in the prophylaxis and treatment of infections. It is also administered orally in the treatment of antibiotic-associated pseudomembranous enterocolitis caused by toxins A and B of *Clostridium difficile*.

b. zinc [USP] the zinc salt of bacitracin, having actions and uses similar to the base.

back (bak) the posterior part of the trunk from the neck to the pelvis; called also *dorsum* [TA].

angry b. excited skin syndrome.

flat b. a back that appears flat as a result of a decrease of normal lumbar lordosis and normal thoracic kyphosis.

functional b. a condition of fatigue and defective balance marked by more or less continuous lumbar or dorsal pain.

hollow b. see *lordosis.*

hump b., hunch b. kyphosis.

kinky b. a type of developmental spondylolisthesis in chickens in which the sixth thoracic vertebra is deformed and downwardly rotated; pressure on the spinal cord can cause posterior paralysis.

poker b. ankylosing spondylitis.

saddle b. see *lordosis.*

back•bone (back′bōn) columna vertebralis.

back-cal•cu•la•tion (bak-kal″ku-la′shən) a statistical method that uses the current incidence and the length of incubation of a disease to estimate the cumulative incidence of the disease and project the number of cases that will occur in the future.

back•cross (bak′kros) in experimental genetics, a cross between an offspring and one of its parents, or an organism genetically identical to one of its parents. Written also *back cross.*

double b. a backcross that gives information about linkage between two genes by examining the effects of the cross on two separate loci.

back•fil•tra•tion (bak″fil-tra′shən) passage of fluids and solutes in the reverse direction across a hemodialyzer membrane, from the dialysate back into the blood, contaminating nondialyzed blood that may reenter the patient's body.

back•flow (bak′flo) reflux or regurgitation (def. 1).

intrarenal b. see under *reflux.*

pyelointerstitial b. backflow of fluid from the renal pelvis into interstitial tissue under certain conditions of back pressure.

pyelosinus b. backflow of fluid from the renal pelvis into the renal sinus under certain conditions of back pressure.

pyelovenous b. backflow of fluid from the renal pelvis into the venous system under certain conditions of back pressure.

back•ing (bak′ing) in dentistry, the piece of metal that supports a porcelain or resin facing on a fixed or removable partial denture.

back•knee (bak′ne) genu recurvatum.

back-rak•ing (bak-rāk′ing) see under *raking.*

back•scat•ter (bak′skat-ər) in radiology, radiation deflected by scattering processes at angles greater than 90 degrees to the original direction of the beam of radiation; see *scatter,* and see also *scattered radiation.*

bac•lo•fen (bak′lo-fen″) [USP] an analogue of γ-aminobutyric acid administered orally or intrathecally as a muscle relaxant and antispastic in the treatment of spasticity of spinal origin, including multiple sclerosis and spinal cord injury. It is also used intrathecally to treat spasticity of cerebral origin, including as trauma to the brain or cerebral palsy.

BACOP a cancer chemotherapy regimen consisting of bleomycin, Adriamycin (doxorubicin), cyclophosphamide, Oncovin (vincristine), and prednisone.

-bacter [L. *bacterium,* q.v.] a word termination denoting a bacterium.

bac•ter•as•ci•tes (bak″tər-ə-si′tēz) [*bacterium* + *ascites*] bacterial infection of ascitic fluid.

monomicrobial non-neutrocytic b. spontaneous bacterial peritonitis caused by a single organism; the ascitic fluid neutrophil count is less than 250 cells/mm^3.

polymicrobial b. an iatrogenic infection of ascitic fluid caused by needle perforation of the bowel during paracentesis and characterized by the presence of several species of bacteria.

bac•ter•e•mia (bak″tər-e′me-ə) [*bacter-* + *-emia*] the presence of bacteria in the blood.

enterococcal b. the presence of enterococci in the blood; called also *enterococcemia.*

Bac•te•ria (bak-tēr′e-ə) in the three-domain system of classification, one of the two large divisions into which prokaryotes are grouped, genetically distinct from the Archaea and comprising a large number of unicellular microorganisms that commonly multiply by cell division (fission) and whose cell is typically contained within a cell wall. Cf. *Archaea* and see *bacterium.*

bac•te•ria (bak-tēr′e-ə) [L.] plural of *bacterium.*

bac•te•ri•ci•dal (bak-tēr″ĭ-si′dəl) [*bacteri-* + L. *caedere* to kill] destructive to bacteria; cf. *antibacterial.*

bac•te•ri•cide (bak-tēr′ĭ-sīd) an agent that destroys bacteria; cf. *antibacterial.*

specific b. bacteriolysin.

bac•te•ri•ci•din (bak-tēr″ĭ-si′din) 1. an antibody that destroys bacteria. 2. any of various bactericidal, nonantibody components found in the serum.

bac•ter•id (bak′tər-id) [*bacteri-* + *-id*] an id reaction associated with a bacterial infection.

pustular b. see under *psoriasis.*

bac•ter•i•form (bak-tēr′ĭ-form) resembling a bacterium in form.

bac•ter•in (bak′tər-in) bacterial vaccine.

***Bordetella bronchiseptica* b.** a suspension of inactivated and adsorbed *Bordetella bronchiseptica,* used for prevention of atrophic rhinitis of swine.

***Clostridium chauvoei-septicum* b.** see under *bacterin-toxoid.*

***Clostridium haemolyticum* b.** a chemically killed culture of *Clostridium haemolyticum,* used for prevention of bacillary hemoglobinuria in cattle, sheep, and goats.

***Erysipelothrix rhusiopathiae* b.** a formalin-killed, adsorbed culture of *Erysipelothrix rhusiopathiae,* used for immunization of swine against erysipelas.

***Haemophilus paragallinarum* b.** a chemically inactivated and adsorbed suspension of *Haemophilus paragallinarum,* used for immunization of chickens against infectious coryza.

***Leptospira canicola-grippotyphosa-hardjo-icterohaemorrhagiae-pomona* b.** chemically inactivated, adsorbed whole cultures of *Leptospira canicola, L. grippotyphosa, L. hardjo, L. icterohaemorrhagiae,* and *L. pomona,* used for immunization of cattle against leptospirosis.

***Pasteurella haemolytica-multocida* b.** an inactivated and adsorbed whole culture of *Mannheimia haemolytica* and *Pasteurella multocida,* used for prevention of pasteurellosis in cattle and sheep.

***Pasteurella multocida* b.** 1. chemically killed, adsorbed whole culture of *Pasteurella multocida* bovine and porcine isolates, used for prevention of pasteurellosis in cattle, sheep, goats, and swine. 2. chemically killed, emulsified whole culture of *Pasteurella multocida* avian isolates, used for prevention of fowl cholera in chickens and turkeys.

***Salmonella dublin-typhimurium* b.** a formalin-inactivated, adsorbed suspension of the *Salmonella enterica* subsp. *enterica* serovars Dublin and Typhimurium, used for prevention of salmonellosis in cattle.

***Staphylococcus aureus* b.** a formalin-inactivated, adsorbed lysed culture of *Staphylococcus aureus,* used for prevention of *S. aureus* infection in cattle.

***Streptococcus equi* b.** a chemically killed, adsorbed suspension of *Streptococcus equi,* used for prevention of strangles in horses.

***Vibrio fetus* b.** a chemically inactivated, adsorbed whole culture of *Campylobacter fetus,* used for immunization of cows (*C. fetus* subspecies *fetus*) or of ewes (*C. fetus* subspecies *intestinalis* or *jejuni*) for prevention of bovine or ovine genital campylobacteriosis.

bac•ter•in-tox•oid (bak′tər-in-tok′soid) an active immunizing agent prepared from chemically inactivated bacterial cultures containing both killed bacteria and inactivated toxin.

***Clostridium botulinum* type C b.-t.** a chemically killed, alum-adsorbed culture of *Clostridium botulinum,* type C, used for prevention of type C botulism in mink.

***Clostridium chauvoei-septicum* b.-t.** a chemically killed culture of *Clostridium chauvoei* and *C. septicum,* used for prevention of blackleg and malignant edema in cattle, horses, sheep, and goats.

***Clostridium novyi-sordelli* b.-t.** a chemically inactivated suspension of *Clostridium novyi* and *C. sordelli,* used for immunization of cattle and sheep against diseases caused by these organisms (e.g., black disease, bighead).

***Clostridium perfringens* b.-t.** a chemically killed culture of *Clostridium perfringens* type C and/or type D organisms, used for prevention of enterotoxemia caused by these strains in sheep and cattle.

bacter(i)(o)- [L. *bacterium,* q.v.] a combining form denoting relationship to bacteria.

bac•te•rio•chlo•ro•phyll (bak-tēr″e-o-klor′ə-fil) any of a group of pigments (designated bacteriochlorophyll *a, b, c, d,* or *e*) occurring in bacteria and functioning in anaerobic photosynthesis.

bac•te•rio•ci•dal (bak-tēr″e-o-si′dəl) bactericidal.

bac•te•rio•ci•din (bak-tēr″e-o-si′din) bactericidin.

bac•te•rio•cin (bak-tēr′e-o″sin) a protein substance, e.g., colicin or staphylococcin, released by certain bacteria that kills but does not lyse closely related strains of bacteria. Specific bacteriocins attach to specific receptors on cell walls and induce specific metabolic block, e.g., cessation of nucleic acid or protein synthesis of oxidative phosphorylation.

bac•te•ri•o•cin•o•gen (bak-tēr″e-o-sin′ə-jen) a bacterial plasmid that controls the synthesis of bacteriocin.

bac•te•ri•o•cin•o•gen•ic (bak-tēr″e-o-sin″ə-jen′ik) giving rise to bacteriocin.

bac•te•ri•oc•la•sis (bak-tēr″e-ok′lə-sis) [*bacterio-* + Gr. *klasis* breaking] bacteriolysis.

bac•te•rio•flu•o•res•cin (bak-tēr″e-o-floo-res′in) a fluorescent dye produced by *Pseudomonas aeruginosa.*

bac•te•ri•o•gen•ic (bak-tēr″e-o-jen′ik) caused by bacteria.

bac•te•ri•og•e•nous (bak-tēr″e-oj′ə-nəs) bacteriogenic.

bac•te•ri•oid (bak-tēr′e-oid) [*bacteri-* + *-oid*] 1. resembling the bacteria. 2. a structure resembling a bacterium.

bac•te•ri•ol•o•gist (bak-tēr″e-ol′ə-jist) a specialist in bacteriology.

bac•te•ri•ol•o•gy (bak-tēr″e-ol′ə-je) [*bacterio-* + *-logy*] the science that treats of bacteria. Cf. *microbiology.* **bacteriolog′ic, bacteriolog′ical** *adj*

systematic b. the branch of bacteriology that deals with the classification and relationship of bacteria (taxonomy).

bac•te•ri•ol•y•sin (bak-tēr″e-ol′ĭ-sin) an antibacterial antibody that produces lysis of bacterial cells.

bac•te•ri•ol•y•sis (bak-tēr″e-ol′ĭ-sis) [*bacterio-* + *-lysis*] disruption of the structural integrity of a bacterial cell resulting in release of the cell contents. Cf. *bacteriophagia.*

bac•te•rio•lyt•ic (bak-tēr″e-o-lit′ik) 1. pertaining to, characterized by, or promoting bacteriolysis. 2. bactericidal.

bac•te•ri•o•op•so•nin (bak-tēr″e-o-op′sə-nin) bacteriopsonin.

bac•te•rio•phage (bak-tēr′e-o-fāj″) [*bacterio-* + *-phage*] a virus that lyses bacteria; see *bacterial virus,* under *virus,* and see *phage typing,* under *typing.* Called also *phage.* **bacteriopha′gic** *adj*

temperate b. a bacteriophage whose genetic material (prophage) becomes an intimate part of the bacterial cell, persisting through many cell division cycles. The affected bacterial cell is known as a *lysogenic bacterium* (q.v.).

bac•te•rio•pha•gia (bak-tēr″e-o-fa′jə) bacteriolysis by a bacteriophage.

bac•te•rio•pha•gol•o•gy (bak-tēr″e-o-fə-gol′ə-je) the study of bacteriophage.

bac•te•ri•oph•a•gy (bak-tēr″e-of′ə-je) bacteriophagia.

bac•te•rio•plas•min (bak-tēr″e-o-plaz′min) plasmin produced by bacteria.

bac•te•rio•pre•cip•i•tin (bak-tēr″e-o-pre-sip′ĭ-tin) a precipitin formed in the body in response to bacterial antigens.

bac•te•rio•pro•tein (bak-tēr″e-o-pro′tēn) any protein of bacterial origin.

bac•te•ri•op•son•ic (bak-tēr″e-op-son′ik) exerting an opsonic effect on bacteria.

bac•te•ri•op•so•nin (bak-tēr″e-op′so-nin) an opsonizing antibody that interacts with bacteria to render them more susceptible to ingestion by phagocytic cells than they otherwise would be.

bac•te•rio•pur•pu•rin (bak-tēr″e-o-pur′pu-rin) [*bacterio-* + L. *purpur* purple] a light purple pigment produced by certain bacteria.

bac•te•ri•o•sis (bak-tēr″e-o′sis) any bacterial disease.

bac•te•rio•sper•mia (bak-tēr″e-o-spur′me-ə) the presence of bacteria in the semen.

bac•te•rio•sta•sis (bak-tēr″e-o-sta′sis) [*bacterio-* + *stasis*] the inhibition of growth, but not the killing, of bacteria by chemicals or biologic materials.

bac•te•rio•stat (bak-tēr′e-o-stat″) an agent that inhibits growth of bacteria; cf. *antibacterial.*

bac•te•rio•stat•ic (bak-tēr″e-o-stat′ik) 1. inhibiting growth of bacteria; cf. *antibacterial.* 2. bacteriostat.

bac•te•rio•ther•a•py (bak-tēr″e-o-ther′ə-pe) [*bacterio-* + *therapy*] treatment of disease by the introduction of bacteria into the system.

bac•te•rio•tox•ic (bak-tēr′e-o-tok″sik) toxic to bacteria.

bac•te•rio•tox•in (bak-tēr′e-o-tok″sin) [*bacterio-* + *toxin*] 1. bacterial toxin. 2. a substance toxic to bacteria.

bac•te•ri•o•tro•pic (bak-tēr″e-o-tro′pik) [*bacterio-* + *-tropic*] 1. turning toward or changing bacteria. 2. bacteriopsonic.

bac•te•ri•ot•ro•pin (bak-tēr″e-ot′ro-pin) bacteriopsonin.

bac•te•ri•um (bak-tēr′e-əm) pl. *bacte′ria* [L., from Gr. *baktērion* little rod] in general, any of the unicellular prokaryotic microorganisms that commonly multiply by cell division (fission) and whose cell is typically contained within a cell wall. They may be aerobic or anaerobic, motile or nonmotile, and may be free-living, saprophytic, parasitic, or even pathogenic, the last causing disease in plants or animals. See Plate 7 and see also *Bacteria.* **bacter′ial** *adj*

acid-fast b. a bacterium that retains stains by dyes (e.g., carbolfuchsin or auramine) so tenaciously that it is not decolorized by 5 per cent mineral acids, especially *Mycobacterium* species and *Nocardia.*

autotrophic b. a bacterium that has no organic nutritional requirements; none of these are pathogenic.

beaded b. a bacterium that has deeply staining granules equally spaced along its rod.

bifid b. a bacterium that has a branched rod- or cleft-shaped cell, especially *Bifidobacterium.*

blue-green bacteria see *Cyanobacteria.*

chemoautotrophic b. a bacterium that is autotrophic and obtains energy by the oxidation of inorganic compounds of iron, nitrogen, sulfur, or hydrogen; none of these are pathogenic.

chemoheterotrophic b. a bacterium that is heterotrophic and obtains energy by the oxidation of organic compounds by mechanisms similar to those existing in higher animals.

chromo b., chromogenic b. a bacterium that produces pigment.

coliform b. one of the facultative gram-negative, rod-shaped bacteria that are normal inhabitants of the intestinal tract. See *Citrobacter, Edwardsiella, Enterobacter, Escherichia, Klebsiella,* and *Serratia.*

coryneform bacteria a group of bacteria that are morphologically similar to those of the genus *Corynebacterium;* see also *corynebacterium* (def. 2). Called also *coryneform group.*

denitrifying b. a bacterium that is able to reduce nitrates to nitrites, ammonia, or nitrogen gas.

flesh-eating bacteria popular name for bacteria causing necrotizing fasciitis, because of their rapid and aggressive action; the term is sometimes used specifically for *Streptococcus pyogenes.*

gram-negative b. see *gram-negative,* under *G.*

gram-positive b. see *gram-positive,* under *G.*

hemophilic b. a bacterium that has a nutritional affinity for constituents of blood or whose growth is stimulated by blood-enriched media.

heterotrophic b. a bacterium that requires organic compounds of carbon and nitrogen as sources of energy or as essential parts of the cell.

higher bacteria a term used to denote filamentous bacteria (e.g., Actinomycetales) that seem to be intermediate between bacteria and fungi.

hydrogen b. a facultative chemoautotrophic bacterium that respires by the oxidation of hydrogen to water, using various organic compounds as carbon and energy sources. Hydrogen bacteria are included in the genera *Pseudomonas (P. facilis, P. ruhlandii, P. saccharophila), Alcaligenes (A. eutrophus, A. paradoxus),* and *Nocardia (N. opaca).*

lactic acid bacteria the group of gram-positive rods and cocci that produce lactic acid as an endproduct of carbohydrate formation; included are streptococci and lactobacilli.

lysogenic b. a bacterium that harbors in its genome the genetic material (prophage) of a temperate bacteriophage and thus reproduces the bacteriophage in cell division; occasionally the prophage develops into the mature form, replicates, lyses the bacterial cell, and is free to infect other cells.

mesophilic b. a bacterium whose optimal temperature for growth is in a middle range (30° to 45°C); some of these can grow in the human body.

parasitic b. a bacterium that is dependent on a living host for its nutrition.

pathogenic b. any bacterium that can cause disease.

photoautotrophic b. an autotrophic bacterium capable of deriving energy from light.

photoheterotrophic b. a heterotrophic bacterium capable of deriving energy from light.

photosynthetic b. a bacterium that contains pigments such as bacteriochlorophylls and carotenoids, which enable it to conduct photosynthesis and assimilate carbon dioxide, with or without the production of oxygen. The process depends on the presence of oxidizable electron donors such as water and reduced sulfur compounds. See also *Cyanobacteria.*

psychrophilic b. a bacterium whose optimum temperature for growth is 15° to 20°C.

purple b. a photosynthetic bacterium that reduces CO_2 in the presence of sulfur compounds; there are two types: the *purple sulfur bacteria* and the *purple nonsulfur bacteria.*

purple nonsulfur b. a photosynthetic, heterotrophic, microaerophilic bacterium of the family Rhodospirillaceae. Purple nonsulfur bacteria reduce CO_2 and oxidize sulfide or thiosulfate but not elemental sulfur in the presence of the pigment bacteriochlorophyll *a.*

purple sulfur b. a photosynthetic, autotrophic, anaerobic bacterium of the family Chromatiaceae. Purple sulfur bacteria reduce carbon dioxide and oxidize sulfides and elemental sulfur in the presence of the pigment bacteriochlorophyll *a* or *b.*

pyogenic bacteria bacteria, most commonly *Staphylococcus* and *Streptococcus,* that cause suppuration when they infect tissue.

pyrogenetic b. a bacterium that causes fever when it infects an organism.

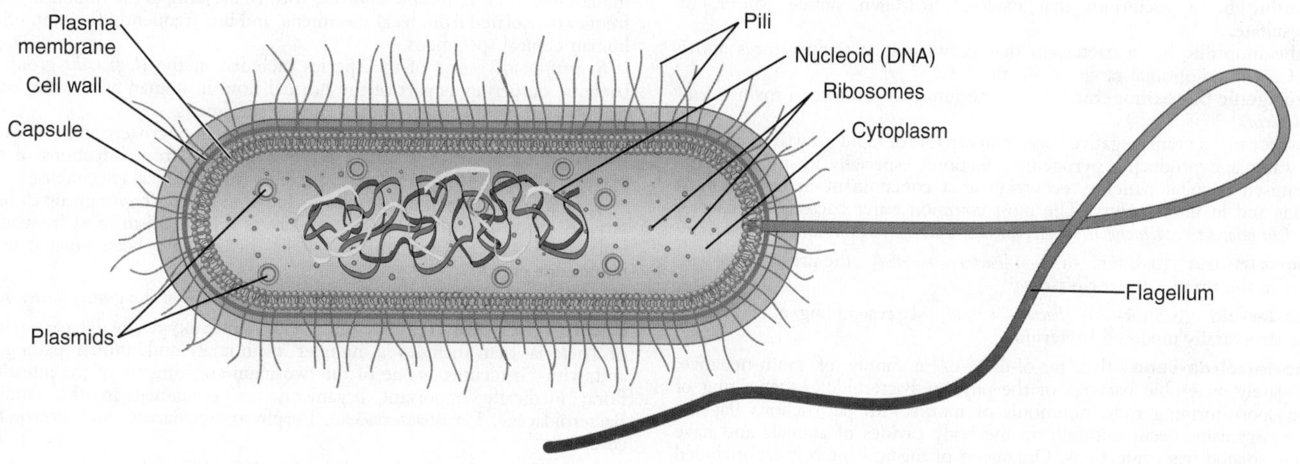

Generalized structure of a monotrichous bacterium (Not all structures occur in all cells)

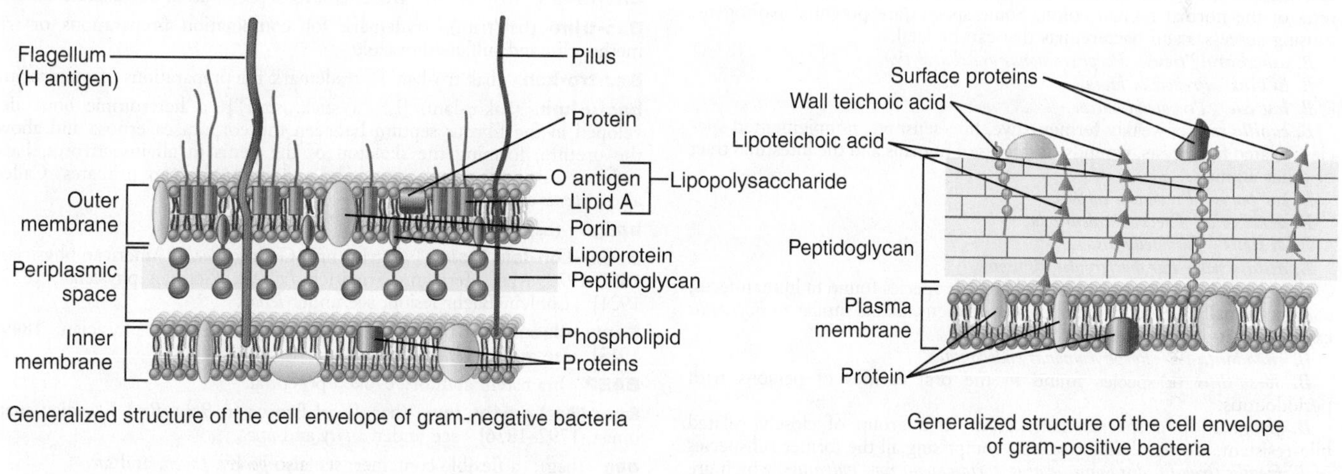

Generalized structure of the cell envelope of gram-negative bacteria

Generalized structure of the cell envelope of gram-positive bacteria

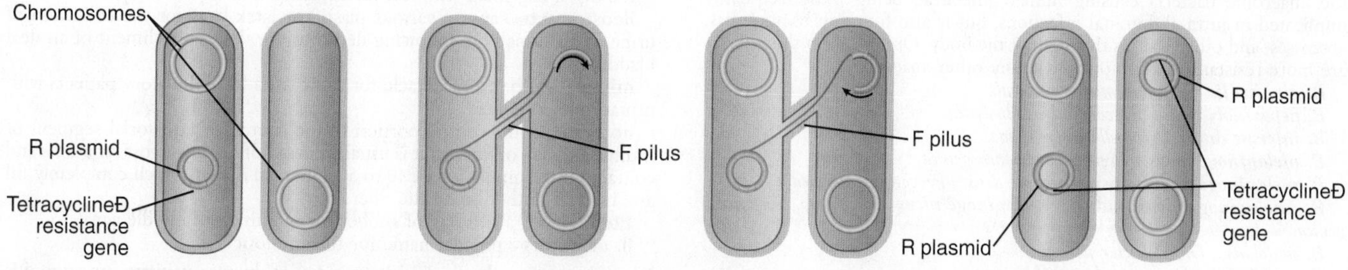

Transfer of drug resistance, in this case to tetracycline, between bacteria by transfer of the R plasmid during conjugation

■ **PLATE 7—GENERALIZED STRUCTURES OF TYPICAL BACTERIAL CELLS AND TRANSFER OF A PLASMID BETWEEN BACTERIAL CELLS VIA CONJUGATION**

rough b. a variant form of a bacterium characterized by dry, wrinkled colonies on solid media. See *smooth-rough variation,* under *variation.*

saprophytic b. a bacterium that lives in decaying organic matter.

smooth b. a bacterium that forms smooth, glossy colonies on solid media. See *smooth-rough variation,* under *variation.*

sulfur b. a bacterium that oxidizes hydrogen sulfide, sulfur, or thiosulfate.

thermophilic b. a bacterium that grows best at temperatures above 40°C, with an optimal range of 50° to 70°C.

toxigenic b., toxinogenic b. a bacterium that produces a toxin *(bacterial toxin).*

water b. a gram-negative bacterium capable of rapid growth in all types of water and producing pyrogenic infections, especially in immunocompromised hospital patients, occurring as a contaminant in hemodialysis fluids and in flood waters. The most common water bacteria are species of *Achromobacter, Acinetobacter, Aeromonas, Flavobacterium,* and *Pseudomonas.*

bac•te•ri•uria (bak-tēr″e-u′re-ə) [*bacteri-* + *-uria*] the presence of bacteria in the urine. **bacteriu′ric** *adj*

bac•ter•oid (bak′tər-oid) [*bacter-* + *-oid*] 1. resembling a bacterium. 2. a structurally modified bacterium.

Bac•te•roi•da•ceae (bak″tər-oi-da′se-e) a family of gram-negative, obligately anaerobic bacteria of the phylum Bacteroidetes, consisting of non–spore-forming rods, nonmotile or motile with peritrichous flagella. The organisms occur naturally in the body cavities of animals and have been isolated from infections. Organisms of medical interest are included in the genera *Bacteroides* and *Parabacteroides.*

Bac•te•roi•des (bak″tər-oi′dēz) [*bacterio-* + *-oid*] a genus of gram-negative, anaerobic, non–spore-forming, rod-shaped bacteria of the family Bacteroidaceae, made up of organisms that are nonmotile or motile with peritrichous flagella. They are normal inhabitants of oral, respiratory, intestinal, and urogenital cavities, and may constitute the predominant bacteria of the normal human colon. Some species are potential pathogens, causing abscesses and bacteremias that can be fatal.

B. asaccharoly′ticus *Porphyromonas asaccharolytica.*

B. bi′vius *Prevotella bivia.*

B. buc′cae *Prevotella buccae.*

B. capillo′sus a weakly fermentative, bile-sensitive, nonpigmented species isolated from cysts, wounds, and feces of humans and the intestinal tract of other animals.

B. cor′poris *Prevotella corporis.*

B. denti′cola *Prevotella denticola.*

B. di′siens *Prevotella disiens.*

B. distaso′nis *Parabacteroides distasonis.*

B. egger′thii a bile-resistant saccharolytic species found in human feces, and occasionally isolated from clinical specimens, that is similar to *B. fragilis* except that it does not ferment sucrose.

B. endodonta′lis *Porphyromonas endodontalis.*

B. forsy′thus a species found in the oral cavities of persons with periodontitis.

B. fra′gilis 1. a species name given to a group of closely related bile-resistant, saccharolytic organisms comprising all the former subspecies of *B. fragilis (fragilis, distasonis, ovatus, thetaiotaomicron, vulgatus),* which are now considered to be separate species, along with a few other species, such as *B. uniformis.* Collectively, the organisms constitute the numerically dominant species found in the human intestine and are the most commonly encountered anaerobic bacteria in clinical specimens. They are also present normally in the mouth, throat, and vaginal tract. 2. one of the species included in the *B. fragilis* group of bacteria. It is the most important of the anaerobic bacteria causing human infection, being most frequently implicated in intra-abdominal infections, but is also found in bacteremias, abscesses, and other lesions throughout the body. Organisms in this species are more resistant to antibiotics than any other anaerobe.

B. gingiva′lis *Porphyromonas gingivalis.*

B. heparinoly′ticus *Prevotella heparinolytica.*

B. interme′dius *Prevotella intermedia.*

B. melaninoge′nicus *Prevotella melaninogenica.*

B. melaninoge′nicus* subsp. *interme′dius *Prevotella intermedia.*

B. melaninoge′nicus* subsp. *melaninoge′nicus *Prevotella melaninogenica.*

B. nodo′sus *Dichelobacter nodosus.*

B. ochra′ceus *Capnocytophaga ochraceus.*

B. ora′lis *Prevotella oralis.*

B. o′ris *Prevotella oris.*

B. ova′tus one of the species included in the *B. fragilis* group of bacteria, isolated from normal human feces and occasionally from clinical specimens.

B. praeacu′tus *Tissierella praeacutus.*

B. putre′dinis a bile-sensitive, nonpigmented, nonfermentative species isolated from abdominal and rectal abscesses and from feces of humans, from soil, and from sheep foot rot.

B. rumini′cola *Prevotella ruminicola.*

B. splanch′nicus a bile-resistant, saccharolytic species isolated from human feces, the vagina, and occasionally from abdominal infections, which is similar to *B. fragilis* except that it does not ferment sucrose.

B. thetaiotao′micron one of the species included in the *B. fragilis* group of bacteria. Except for *B. fragilis,* it is the most important anaerobe causing human infection. *B. thetaiotaomicron,* with *B. vulgatus,* is the organism most frequently isolated from fecal specimens, and it is frequently found in other human clinical specimens.

B. unifor′mis one of the species included in the *B. fragilis* group of bacteria, occurring as part of the normal flora in human and swine feces, and isolated from various human clinical specimens.

B. ureoly′ticus a bile-sensitive, nonpigmented, microaerophilic, nonfermentative species that is urease positive, isolated from infections of the respiratory and intestinal tracts and from various clinical specimens.

B. vulga′tus one of the species included in the *B. fragilis* group of bacteria. *B. vulgatus,* with *B. thetaiotaomicron,* is the organism most frequently isolated from fecal specimens, and it has occasionally been isolated from human infections.

bac•te•roi•des (bak″tər-oi′dēz) any bacterium of the genus *Bacteroides.*

Bac•te•roi•de•tes (bak″tər-oid′ə-tēz) a phenotypically diverse phylum of bacteria that includes a number of human and animal pathogens and, with Firmicutes, is one of the two main constituents of the intestinal flora; medically important organisms are contained in the families Bacteroidaceae, Flavobacteriaceae, Porphyromonadaceae, and Prevotellaceae.

bac•te•roi•do•sis (bak″tər-oi-do′sis) infection with organisms of the genus *Bacteroides.*

bac•ter•uria (bak″tēr-u′re-ə) bacteriuria.

bac•ti•bil•ia (bak″tĭ-bil′e-ə) bacteria in the bile, such as from bile duct obstruction with infection.

Bac•to•cill (bak′to-sil) trademark for a preparation of oxacillin sodium.

Bac•trim (bak′trim) trademark for combination preparations of trimethoprim and sulfamethoxazole.

Bac•tro•ban (bak′tro-ban″) trademark for preparations of mupirocin.

bac•u•lum (bak′u-ləm) [L. "a stick, staff"] a heterotopic bone developed in the fibrous septum between the corpora cavernosa and above the urethra, forming the skeleton of the penis in all insectivores, bats, rodents, carnivores, and pinnipeds, and in nonhuman primates. Called also *os penis* and *os priapi.*

badge (baj) see *film badge.*

Baehr-Löh•lein lesion (bār lur′līn) [George *Baehr,* American physician, 1887–1978; Max Hermann Friedrich *Löhlein,* German physician, 1877–1921] Löhlein-Baehr lesion; see under *lesion.*

Baelz disease (bālts) [Erwin von *Baelz,* German physician, 1849–1913] see *cheilitis glandularis.*

BAEP brainstem auditory evoked potential.

Baer (Ber) cavity, law (bār) [Karl Ernst von *Baer (Ber),* Estonian anatomist, 1792–1876] see under *cavity* and *law.*

bag (bag) a flexible container; see also *pocket, pouch,* and *sac.*

Bunyan b. a bag of light waterproof material for covering wet dressings.

colostomy b. a receptacle worn over the stoma to receive the fecal discharge from a colostomy.

Douglas b. a receptacle for the collection of exhaled air, permitting measurement of respiratory gases.

ice b. a bag filled with ice, for applying cold to the body.

ileostomy b. any of various plastic or latex bags for the collection of urine or fecal material following ileostomy or the establishment of an ileal bladder.

micturition b. a receptacle for urine used by ambulatory patients with urinary incontinence.

nuclear b. the central portion of the central or equatorial segment of intrafusal fibers of muscle; it is usually devoid of obvious cross striations and contains an accumulation of 40 to 50 spherical nuclei, which completely fill and often slightly distend the fiber.

Politzer b. a soft bag of rubber for inflating the middle ear.

b. of waters popular name for the amniotic sac.

bag•as•so•sis (bag″ə-so′sis) a type of hypersensitivity pneumonitis caused by inhalation of the dust of bagasse, the waste of sugar cane after the sugar has been extracted.

BAHA (bah′hah) trademark for a bone-anchored hearing aid.

Bail•lar•ger bands, etc. (bi-yahr-zha′) [Jules Gabriel François *Baillarger,* French psychiatrist, 1809–1890] see *stria laminae granularis internae* and *stria laminae pyramidalis internae,* and see under *sign.*

Bain•bridge reflex (bān′brij) [Francis Arthur *Bainbridge,* English physiologist, 1874–1921] see under *reflex.*

Bairns·dale ulcer (bānz′dāl) [*Bairnsdale*, Australia, where early cases were observed] Buruli ulcer; see under *ulcer*.

bake (bāk) to expose to high temperature at low humidity, as in the processing of porcelain.

Ba·ker cyst (ba′kər) [William Morrant *Baker*, British surgeon, 1839–1896] see under *cyst*.

BAL British antilewisite (see *dimercaprol*); biphenotypic acute leukemia.

Bal·a·mu·thia (bal″ə-moo′the-ə) a genus of ramicristate amebae of the order Leptomyxida. *B. mandrilla′ris* can cause granulomatous amebic encephalitis.

bal·a·mu·thi·a·sis (bal″ə-moo-thi′ə-sis) granulomatous amebic encephalitis as a result of infection with *Balamuthia mandrillaris*.

bal·ance (bal′əns) [L. *bilanx*] 1. an instrument for weighing. 2. the harmonious adjustment of parts; the harmonious performance of functions. 3. equilibrium.

acid-base b. a condition in which the net rate of acid or alkali production by the body is balanced by the net rate of acid or alkali excretion from the body, resulting in a stable concentration of H^+ (hydrogen ions) in the body fluids.

analytical b. a balance used in the laboratory, sensitive to variations of the order of 0.05 to 0.1 mg.

calcium b. the balance between the calcium intake and its output through the body excretions.

fluid b. the state of the body in relation to ingestion and excretion of water and electrolytes; called also *water b.*

genic b. the ratio of sex chromosomes to autosomes as the determiner of sex, as in *Drosophila*.

glomerulotubular b. the balance between reabsorption of solutes in the proximal renal tubules and glomerular filtration, which must be maintained as constant as possible; if the glomerular filtration rate rises or falls, the rate of tubular reabsorption must rise or fall proportionally. Balance is maintained by neural, hormonal, and other mechanisms.

metabolic b. the balance between intake from potential sources of energy and expenditure of energy by any living system.

microchemical b. a balance used in the laboratory, sensitive to variations of the order of 0.001 mg.

negative b. a state in which the amount of water or an electrolyte excreted from the body is greater than that ingested.

nitrogen b. the state of the body in regard to ingestion and excretion of nitrogen. In *negative nitrogen balance* the amount of nitrogen excreted is greater than the quantity ingested; in *positive nitrogen balance* the amount excreted is smaller than the amount ingested.

occlusal b. balanced occlusion.

positive b. a state in which the amount of water or an electrolyte excreted from the body is less than that ingested.

semimicro b. a balance used in the laboratory, sensitive to variations of 0.01 mg.

torsion b. 1. a balance used in the laboratory, having a scale beam supported by metallic ribbons that act by torsion. 2. an electrometer that acts by the twisting of a single fiber of the web of a silkworm.

water b. fluid b.

zero b. a state in which the amount of water or an electrolyte excreted from the body is exactly equal to that ingested; see *equilibrium*.

bal·anced (bal′ənst) existing in or maintaining an equilibrium.

ba·lan·ic (bə-lan′ik) pertaining to the glans penis or glans clitoridis.

bal·a·ni·tis (bal″ə-ni′tis) [*balan-* + *-itis*] inflammation of the glans penis; it is usually associated with phimosis.

amebic b. balanitis caused by *Entamoeba histolytica*.

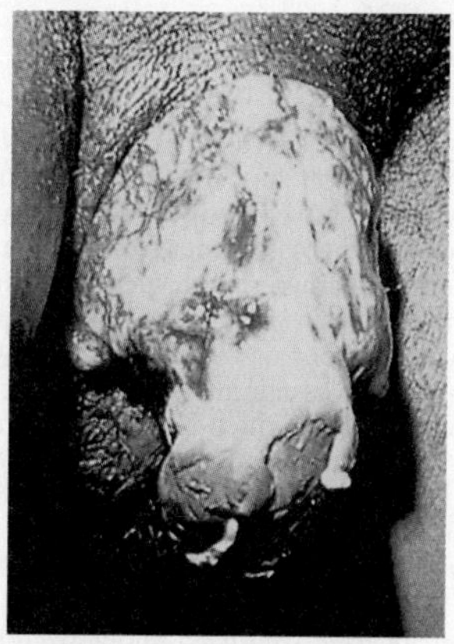

■ Amebic balanitis.

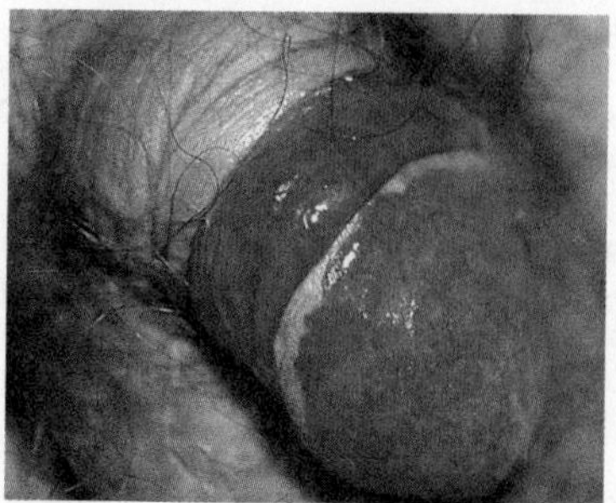

■ Zoon balanitis.

b. circina′ta, circinate b. a shallow, painless ulcer with a gray border, seen on the glans penis in some patients with Reiter syndrome.

b. circumscrip′ta plasmacellula′ris Zoon b.

erosive b. balanitis due to mixed microbial infection that progresses to gangrenous ulcerations of the penis similar to the lesions seen in noma of oral tissues.

plasma cell b., b. plasmacellula′ris Zoon b..

pseudoepitheliomatous keratotic and micaceous b. a rare type of white, plaquelike, hyperkeratotic lesion of the glans penis that may be premalignant and progress to a verrucous type of carcinoma.

b. xero′tica obli′terans lichen sclerosus in males; see under *lichen*.

Zoon b., Zoon plasma cell b. a benign erythroplasia of the inner surface of the prepuce or the glans penis, characterized histologically by plasma cell infiltration of the dermis, and clinically by a moist, erythematous lesion. Plasma cell vulvitis is a corresponding condition in females. Called also *b. circumscripta plasmacellularis, plasma cell b., b. plasmacellularis,* and *Zoon erythroplasia*.

balan(o)- [Gr. *balanos* acorn] a combining form indicating relationship to the glans penis.

bal·a·no·plas·ty (bal′ə-no-plas″te) [*balano-* + *-plasty*] plastic surgery of the glans penis.

bal·a·no·pos·thi·tis (bal″ə-no-pos-thi′tis) [*balano-* + *posth-* + *-itis*] inflammation of the glans penis and prepuce.

chronic circumscribed plasmocytic b., b. chro′nica circumscrip′ta plasmocellula′ris Zoon balanitis.

enzootic b. a disease of castrated male sheep in Australia and New Zealand, marked by spreading ulceration of the glans penis and prepuce and severe swelling and distention of the sheath; the cause is infection by *Corynebacterium renale* of animals fed a high protein diet so that their urine is high in urea. Called also *enzootic posthitis, pizzle rot,* and *sheath rot*.

infectious pustular b. a venereal infection of bulls, caused by bovine herpesvirus 1 and characterized by small pustules on the penis and prepuce; it can also be spread through artificial insemination. It is the male counterpart of infectious pustular vulvovaginitis.

bal·a·no·pre·pu·ti·al (bal″ə-no-pre-poo′shəl) pertaining to the glans penis and the prepuce.

bal·an·ti·di·a·sis (bal″an-tĭ-di′ə-sis) infection by protozoa of the genus *Balantidium*, most often by *B. coli*; symptoms include diarrhea and dysentery, sometimes with ulceration of colonic mucous membranes.

bal·an·tid·i·o·sis (bal″an-tid-e-o′sis) balantidiasis.

Bal·an·tid·i·um (bal″an-tid′e-əm) [Gr. *balantidion* little bag] a genus of ciliate protozoa of the order Trichostomatida, including many species found in the intestines of animals.

B. co′li the largest protozoan and the only ciliate parasite of humans (see *balantidiasis*), which is also found in pigs and monkeys; it may measure 30 to 150 μm long by 25 to 120 μm wide.

B. su′is a nonpathogenic species found in pigs, considered by some to be identical with *B. coli* and by others to be a separate species.

bal·an·ti·do·sis (bal″an-tĭ-do′sis) balantidiasis.

bal·a·nus (bal′ə-nəs) glans penis.

Bal·bi·a·ni nucleus (body), ring (bahl-be-ah′ne) [Edouard Gérard *Balbiani*, French embryologist, 1823–1899] yolk nucleus; see under *nucleus*, and see under *ring*.

bald (bawld) having no hair; see *alopecia*.

bald·ness (bawld′nis) alopecia, especially of the scalp.

common b. androgenetic alopecia.

female pattern b. the female pattern of androgenetic alopecia; see under *alopecia*.

male pattern b. the male pattern of androgenetic alopecia; see under *alopecia*.

Bal·dy operation (bawl′de) [John Montgomery *Baldy,* American gynecologist, 1860–1934] Webster operation; see under *operation.*

Bal·dy-Web·ster operation (bawl′de web′stər) [J.M. *Baldy;* John Clarence *Webster,* American gynecologist, 1863–1950] Webster operation; see under *operation.*

Bal·int syndrome (bah-lēnt′) [Rezsoe *Balint,* Hungarian neurologist and psychiatrist, 1874–1929] see under *syndrome.*

Bal·kan frame, splint (bawl′kən) [*Balkan* countries, where first used] see under *frame* and *splint.*

ball (bawl) a more or less spherical mass. Cf. *sphere.*
 chondrin b. one of the ball-like masses in hyaline cartilage, consisting of cells surrounded by a capsule of basophilic matrix.
 food b. phytobezoar.
 fungus b. a tumorlike mass formed by colonization of a fungus in a body cavity, usually a bronchus or pulmonary cavity but occasionally the nasal cavity or urinary tract, with spread through the bloodstream to the brain, heart, or kidneys. The most common type is the aspergilloma. Called also *fungal bezoar* and *fungoma.*
 hair b. trichobezoar.
 Marchi b's ellipsoid or ovoid segments of myelin produced by degeneration, staining brown by Marchi methods.
 oat hair b. a trichobezoar formed in the stomach of the horse from the fine hairs within the outer husk of the oat grain and other materials.
 pleural fibrin b's fibrin bodies of pleura.
 wool b. a trichobezoar containing wool fibers and other substances.

Bal·lance sign (bal′əns) [Sir Charles Alfred *Ballance,* English surgeon, 1857–1936] see under *sign.*

Bal·lard score (bal′ərd) [Jeanne L. *Ballard,* American pediatrician, late 20th century] see under *score.*

Bal·ler-Ger·old syndrome (bah′lər ga′rōlt) [Friedrich *Baller,* German physician, 20th century; M. *Gerold,* German physician, 20th century] see under *syndrome.*

Bal·let sign (bah-la′) [Louis Gilbert *Ballet,* French neurologist, 1853–1916] see under *sign.*

bal·lism (bal′iz-əm) ballismus.

bal·lis·mus (bə-liz′məs) [Gr. *ballismos* a jumping about, dancing] violent flinging dyskinetic movements caused by contractions of the proximal limb muscles as a result of destruction of the subthalamic nucleus or its fiber connections, sometimes affecting only one side of the body *(hemiballismus).* Called also *ballism.*

bal·lis·tic (bə-lis′tik) 1. jerking or twitching; pertaining to or characterized by ballismus. 2. pertaining to or caused by projectiles.

bal·lis·tics (bə-lis′tiks) [Gr. *ballein* to throw] the scientific study of the motion of projectiles in flight.
 wound b. the scientific study of the speed and direction of missiles (bullets and other projectiles) in relation to the injuries they produce.

bal·lis·to·car·dio·gram (BCG) (bə-lis″to-kahr′de-o-gram″) the tracing made by a ballistocardiograph.

bal·lis·to·car·di·o·graph (bə-lis″to-kahr′de-o-graf″) an apparatus for recording the movements of the body caused by cardiac contractions and associated blood flow; it has been used to determine cardiac output and other aspects of cardiac function.

bal·lis·to·car·di·og·ra·phy (bə-lis″to-kahr″de-og′rə-fe) the graphic recording, by means of a ballistocardiograph, of the recoil movements of the body which result from motion of the heart and blood.

bal·lis·to·spore (bə-lis′to-spor) a fungal spore that is forcibly discharged upon maturity; seen in some basidiomycetes.

bal·loon (bə-lo͞on′) 1. a sac that can be distended with gas or fluid, such as after insertion into a body cavity or tube. 2. to distend with air, gas, or fluid.
 Shea-Anthony antral b., sinus b. a balloon expandable with liquid or air to support depressed fractures of the walls of the maxillary sinus; a Foley catheter may also be used.

bal·loon·ing (bə-lo͞on′ing) distending any cavity of the body with air, gas, or fluid; it may be pathological such as with an aneurysm or done for therapeutic purposes. Cf. *inflation.*

bal·lotte·ment (bə-lot′mənt) [Fr. "a tossing about"] 1. a palpatory maneuver to test for a floating object. 2. a maneuver used to monitor pregnancy by pushing on the cervix during vaginal examination, which may cause the floating fetus to rise and then rebound to its original position.
 abdominal b., indirect b. ballottement done by a finger applied to the abdominal wall.
 renal b. palpation of a floating kidney by pressing one hand into the abdominal wall while the other hand makes quick thrusts forward from behind so as to throw the kidney against the anterior hand.

balm (bahm) [Fr. *baume*] 1. a healing or soothing medicine. 2. a plant of the genus *Melissa,* especially *M. officinalis;* it is carminative and aromatic. 3. balsam.
 blue b. *lemon b.*
 b. of Gilead 1. the balsam poplar tree *Populus candicans,* whose buds contain volatile oils and resins and are used as a stimulating expectorant in cough syrups and in the topical treatment of various skin disorders. 2. any of various trees of the genus *Commiphora,* especially *C. opobalsamum* or *C. meccanensis.* 3. Mecca balsam. 4. incorrect term for *Canada balsam.*
 lemon b. 1. *Melissa officinalis,* a shrub native to the Mediterranean region and Asia. 2. a preparation of the fresh or dried herb of *M. officinalis,* or the volatile oil, used for nervousness and insomnia and as a homeopathic preparation for menstrual irregularities; it has a wide variety of uses in folk medicine.
 mountain b. *Eriodictyon.*
 sweet b. *lemon b.*

Balme cough (bahlm) [Paul Jean *Balme,* French physician, late 19th century] see under *cough.*

bal·neo·ther·a·py (bal″ne-o-ther′ə-pe) [L. *balneum* bath + *therapy*] the treatment of disease by baths.

Bal·ne·tar (bal′nə-tahr) trademark for a preparation of coal tar.

Ba·ló disease (concentric sclerosis) (bah-lo′) [Jozsef Matthius *Baló,* Hungarian-born physician in the United States, 1895–1979] see under *disease.*

bal·sal·a·zide di·so·di·um (bal-sal′ə-zīd) a prodrug of mesalamine, to which it is converted by enzymatic action in the colon, used as an anti-inflammatory in the treatment of ulcerative colitis; administered orally.

bal·sam (bawl′səm) [L. *balsamum;* Gr. *balsamon*] 1. a semifluid, resinous, and fragrant liquid of vegetable origin, usually from trees, often composed chiefly of resins, volatile oils, and various esters. 2. balm.
 Canada b. a liquid oleoresin from *Abies balsamea,* which contains volatile oils, chiefly *l*-pinene, and over 70 per cent resins; a microscopic medium that was formerly used medicinally. Sometimes incorrectly called *balm of Gilead.*
 b. of Gilead see under *balm.*
 Mecca b. the resinous juice of *Commiphora opobalsamum,* a light-colored viscid liquid with an aromatic aroma used in medicines and cosmetics in northeastern Africa and southern and southwestern Asia. Called also *balm of Gilead.*
 b. of Peru, peruvian b. a dark brown viscid liquid obtained from *Myroxilon pereirae* Klotzsch, used as a local skin protectant and rubefacient; applied topically.
 tolu b. [USP] a balsam obtained from *Myroxilon balsamum,* used as an ingredient of compound benzoin tincture and as an expectorant.

Bam·ber·ger disease, sign (bahm′bər-gər) [Heinrich von *Bamberger,* Austrian physician, 1822–1888] see under *disease* and *sign.*

Bam·ber·ger-Ma·rie disease (bahm′bər-gər mah-re′) [Eugen *Bamberger,* Austrian physician, 1858–1921; Pierre *Marie,* French physician, 1853–1940] hypertrophic pulmonary osteoarthropathy.

bam·ber·my·cins (bam″bər-mi′sinz) an antibacterial antibiotic complex containing at least four components, with two (the A and C components) predominating; produced by various species of *Streptomyces,* as well as synthetically; used as a feed additive or food supplement for pigs, poultry, and calves. Called also *moenomycins.*

BAN British Approved Name.

Ban·cap (ban′kap) trademark for a combination preparation of butalbital and acetaminophen.

ban·crof·ti·an (bang-krof′te-ən) named for Joseph *Bancroft,* English physician in Australia, 1836–1894.

ban·crof·to·sis (ban″krof-to′sis) bancroftian filariasis.

band (band) 1. a strip that holds together or binds two or more separate objects or parts; for anatomical structures, see *frenulum, taenia, trabecula,* and *vinculum.* 2. an object or appliance that confines or restricts while allowing a limited degree of movement. 3. an elongated area with parallel or roughly parallel borders that is distinct from the surrounding surface by its color, texture, or other characteristics, such as a chromosome band. See also *layer, stria,* and *stripe.* 4. in dentistry, a thin metal hoop that horizontally encircles the crown or root of a natural tooth.
 A b. [*a*nisotropic] the dark-staining zone of a sarcomere, whose center is traversed by the paler H band, which in turn contains the darker M band; called also *A disk, Q disk, anisotropic disk,* and *transverse disk.*
 absorption b's dark bands in the spectrum due to absorption of light by the medium (a solid, a liquid, or a gas) through which the light has passed. Cf. *absorption lines,* under *line.*
 amniotic b. an abnormal fibrous band passing from a fetus to the amnion. See also *amniotic band syndrome,* under *syndrome.*
 anchor b. orthodontic b.

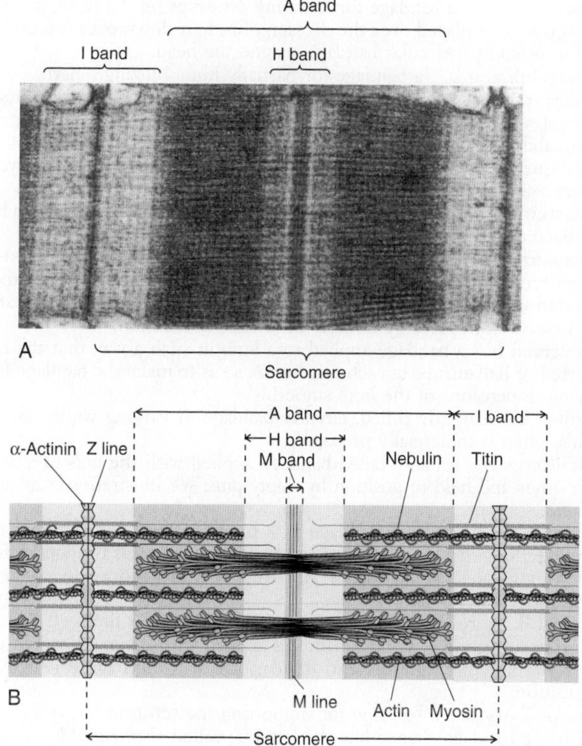

■ Electron micrograph *(A)* and diagrammatic representation *(B)* of a sarcomere, showing the arrangement of the A, H, I, M, and Z bands in the thick and thin filaments of striated muscle.

anogenital b. the primordium of the embryonic perineum.

atrioventricular b. bundle of His.

axis b. primitive streak.

Baillarger external b. stria laminae granularis internae.

Baillarger inner b., Baillarger internal b. stria laminae pyramidalis internae.

Baillarger outer b. stria laminae granularis internae.

b. of Broca, Broca diagonal b. stria diagonalis.

Büngner b's bands of syncytium formed by the union of sheath cells during the regeneration of peripheral nerves; called also *Ledbänder.*

C b. a type of chromosome band (q.v.); see also *C banding,* under *banding.*

chromosome b. any of the alternating dark and light or fluorescent transverse bands produced on chromosomes by differential staining; named according to the procedure used, i.e., C band, G band, Q band, and R band. See *chromosome banding,* under *banding.*

Clado b. the suspensory ligament of the ovary covered with peritoneum.

clamp b. an orthodontic band held in place with a screw nut.

constriction b. amniotic b.

contoured b. an orthodontic band shaped to the contour of the tooth.

contraction b. one of the bands seen by light microscopy in fully contracted muscle on either side of the Z band, caused by distortion of the ends of the myosin filaments by the Z band.

coronary b. a band of vascular tissue at the upper edge of the wall of the hoof, concerned in secretion of the wall. Called also *coronary cushion, coronary ring, coronet,* and *cutidure.*

dentate b. gyrus dentatus (def. 1).

diagonal b., diagonal b. of Broca stria diagonalis.

elastic b. elastic (def. 2).

external b. of Baillarger stria laminae granularis internae.

furrowed b. a strip of cortex that connects the tonsil of the hemisphere of the cerebellum to the uvula of the vermis.

G b. a type of chromosome band (q.v.); see also *G banding,* under *banding.*

b. of Gennari see under *line.*

Giacomini b. the grayish band constituting the anterior extension of the gyrus dentatus of the hippocampus over the inferior surface of the uncus.

H b. [*H*enson's disk] a relatively pale zone sometimes seen traversing the center of the A band of fibrils of striated muscle; called also *Hensen* or *Engelmann disk.*

Henle b. fibers from the anterior aponeurosis of the transversus abdominis muscle extending posterior to the rectus abdominis muscle and inferior to the arcuate line.

His b. see under *bundle.*

Hunter-Schreger b's the dark and light lines visible under reflected light in a ground section of a tooth, which terminate at the dentinoenamel junctions, coinciding with the enamel prism curvatures. The dark bands are known as *diazones,* and the light ones as *parazones.*

I b. [*i*sotropic] the band or disk within a striated muscle fibril that appears as a light region under the light microscope and as a dark region under polarized light; it contains the proteins actin, troponin, and tropomyosin. Called also *isotropic disk* and *J disk.*

iliotibial b. tractus iliotibialis.

inner b. of Baillarger, internal b. of Baillarger stria laminae pyramidalis internae.

Ladd b's bands of peritoneum that attach the cecum to the right lateral abdominal wall, becoming visible in Ladd syndrome (see under *syndrome*).

Lane b's adhesions between tight loops of the terminal ileum, sometimes extending as ligamentous bands to the right iliac fossa.

limbic b's a superior and an inferior muscular band developed in the right atrium of the fetal heart that become the basis of the intervenous or Lower tubercle.

M b. [*m*esophragma] the narrow dark band in the center of the H band of the sarcomere; called also *M disk, Hensen line,* and *mesophragma.* Cf. *Z b.*

Maissiat b. tractus iliotibialis.

matrix b. a cylindrical stainless steel or copper band or short tube with a special clamp or holder; it is filled with a softened impression compound and seated over a tooth, so that the compound flows into the prepared cavity and an impression of a single tooth can be obtained. Also used in the placement and contouring of restorative materials such as resin or glass ionomer cement, and to form the fourth wall of a class II cavity preparation during the condensation of an amalgam restoration.

Meckel b. a part of the anterior ligament fastening the malleus to the wall of the tympanum. Called also *Meckel ligament.*

moderator b. trabecula septomarginalis.

molar b. an orthodontic band applied to a molar tooth; a bracket is attached to the band to hold the arch wire of the appliance.

oligoclonal b's discrete bands of immunoglobulins with decreased electrophoretic mobility; their appearance in electrophoretograms of cerebrospinal fluid when absent in the serum is a sign of possible multiple sclerosis or other diseases of the central nervous system.

orthodontic b. a band fitted over a tooth to anchor a fixed orthodontic appliance. Called also *anchor b.*

outer b. of Baillarger stria laminae granularis internae.

Parham b. a metallic ribbon used to fix a fractured long bone by encircling the bone at the site of the fracture.

perioplic b. the band of secretor cells at the upper border of the hoof of animals; it secretes the periople.

periosteal b. see under *collar.*

Q b. a type of chromosome band (q.v.); see also *Q banding,* under *banding.*

R b. a type of chromosome band (q.v.); see also *R banding,* under *banding.*

b. of Reil trabecula septomarginalis.

Schreger b's Hunter-Schreger b's.

Simonart b. 1. Simonart thread. 2. a weblike band of tissue that sometimes joins the medial and lateral parts of a cleft lip.

Soret b. the absorption band of porphyrins at 400–410 nm.

Vicq d'Azyr b. Kaes-Bekhterev layer.

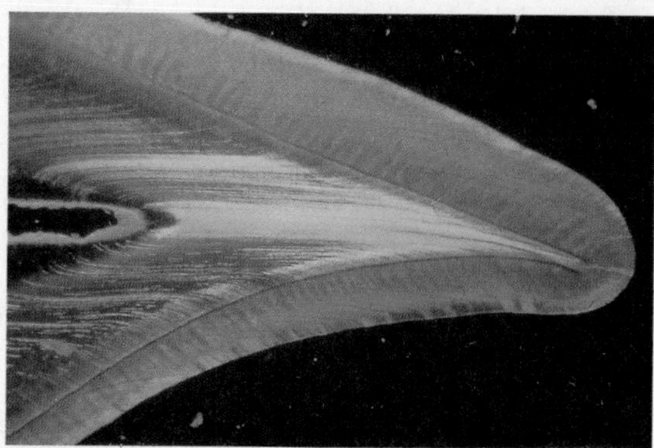

■ Hunter-Schreger bands in reflected light in a longitudinal section of enamel.

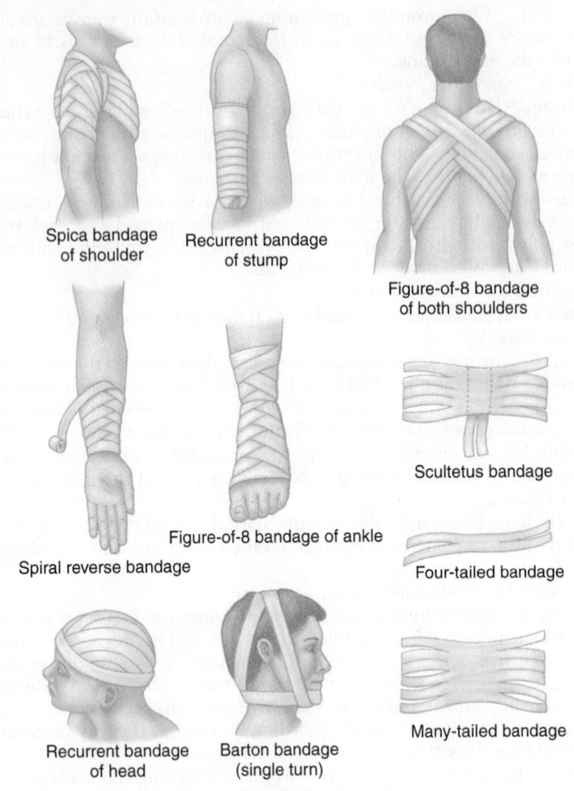

■ Various types of bandages.

Z b. [Ger. *Zwischenscheibe* between-disk] a thin membrane seen on longitudinal section as a dark line in the center of the I band; the distance between successive Z bands serves to delimit the sarcomeres of striated muscle. Called also *Z disk* or *line* and *Dobie line.* See also *inophragma* and *M b.*

zonular b. zona orbicularis articulationis coxae.

ban•dage (ban′dəj) 1. a strip or roll of gauze or other material for wrapping or binding any part of the body. 2. to cover by wrapping with a strip of gauze or other material. See also *dressing* and *strapping.*

Ace b. trademark for a bandage of woven elastic material.

adhesive b. [USP] a sterile compress of layers of gauze or other material, affixed to a fabric or film coated with a pressure-sensitive adhesive.

Barton b. a figure-of-8 bandage supporting the lower jaw below and in front. See illustration.

Borsch b. an eye bandage covering both the diseased and the healthy eye.

Buller b. see under *shield.*

capeline b. a bandage applied like a cap or hood to the head or shoulder or to an amputation stump.

circular b. a bandage applied in circular turns, usually about a limb.

compression b. a bandage by which pressure is applied to a limb to prevent edema.

crucial b. T b.

demigauntlet b. a bandage that covers the hand but leaves the fingers exposed.

Desault b. a bandage binding the elbow to the side, with a pad in the axilla, for fractured clavicle; called also *Desault apparatus.*

elastic b. a bandage of elastic material applied to an area to exert continuous pressure upon it.

Esmarch b. a type of roller bandage applied around a limb from distal to proximal in order to expel blood from it; the limb is often elevated as the elastic pressure is applied. Called also *Esmarch tourniquet.*

figure-of-eight b. a bandage in which the turns cross each other like the figure eight (8), used especially over joints. See illustration.

four-tailed b. a bandage with each end cut into two strips of equal width, which are used to secure the center portion over a prominence, e.g., tied over the head to support the jaw. See illustration.

gauntlet b. a bandage that covers the hand and fingers like a glove.

gauze b. [USP] Type I absorbent gauze containing no dyes or additives; it may be sterilized.

Gibney b. strips of adhesive about 1 cm wide, overlapped along the sides and back of the foot and leg to hold the foot in slight varus position and leave the dorsum of the foot and anterior aspect of the leg exposed; called also *Gibney strapping.*

hammock b. a bandage for retaining dressings on the head; it consists of a broad strip placed over the dressing, brought down over the ears, and held in place by a circular bandage around the head.

immobilizing b. a bandage for partially immobilizing a part.

many-tailed b. a wide bandage with each end cut into several strips of equal width which may be overlapped as the bandage is applied, usually to the abdomen or chest. See *Scultetus b.*

oblique b. a bandage applied obliquely up a limb without reverses. Cf. *reversed b.*

plaster b. a bandage stiffened with a paste of plaster of Paris, which sets and becomes very hard.

pressure b. a bandage for applying pressure.

recurrent b. a bandage used on a distal part, such as a finger, toe, or amputation stump, that is turned lengthwise to cover the end of the stump and is secured in place by circular turns. See illustration.

reversed b. a bandage applied to a limb in such a way that the roll is inverted or half-turned at each revolution, so as to make the bandage fit the varying dimensions of the limb smoothly.

roller b. a tightly rolled, circular bandage of varying widths and materials, often commercially prepared.

Scultetus b. a many-tailed bandage applied with the tails overlapping each other and held in position by safety pins; see illustration. Called also *scultetus.*

spica b. a figure-of-8 bandage with turns that cross one another regularly like the letter V, usually applied to anatomical areas of quite different dimensions, such as the pelvis and thigh or the thorax and arm. See illustration.

spiral b. a roller bandage applied spirally around a limb.

spiral reverse b. a spiral bandage applied with reverse turns in order to fit the varying contours and dimensions of a limb more snugly. See illustration.

suspensory b. a bandage for supporting the scrotum.

T b. a bandage shaped like the letter T; called also *crucial b.*

triangular b. a triangle of cloth used as a sling or bandage.

Velpeau b. a bandage to support the upper limb and provide immobilization of the elbow and shoulder; it is useful in supporting the limb in severe injuries involving the shoulder girdle and upper end of humerus.

Y b. a bandage shaped like the letter Y.

ban•da•let•ta (ban″də-let′ə) [L., from Fr. *bandelette* (q.v.)] 1. a small band. 2. a small bandlike anatomical structure.

b. diagona′lis stria diagonalis.

ban•de•lette (ban″də-let′) [Fr., dim. of *bande* band] a small band.

ban•di•coot (ban′dĭ-ko͞ot) [Teluga *bantikoku*] 1. *Nesokia bengalensis,* a large rodent found in India and Sri Lanka that is a reservoir of *Spirillum minus,* which causes rat-bite fever. 2. any member of the family Paramelidae, small marsupials found in Australia and nearby islands; they are hosts to the bandicoot tick *(Haemaphysalis humerosa),* which is a vector of *Coxiella burnetii,* the cause of Q fever.

band•ing (band′ing) 1. the act of encircling and binding with a thin strip of material. 2. chromosome b.

C b., centromeric b. differential staining of chromosomes to elicit chromosome bands, using a method that specifically stains the regions of the chromosomes that contain constitutive heterochromatin (C bands), particularly the pericentromeric areas, secondary constrictions of chromosomes 1, 9, and 16, and the distal segment of the long arm of the Y chromosome; the method consists of a denaturation and renaturation technique involving treatment of the chromosomes with acid, alkali, or heat before Giemsa staining.

adjustable gastric b. a laparoscopic procedure for the treatment of morbid obesity, in which a saline-filled silicone band is placed around the proximal stomach to create a small gastric pouch and stoma. The circumference of the band can be changed by altering the amount of saline in the bladder through a subcutaneous port.

chromosome b. the use of various physical and cytochemical preparations with differential staining techniques, which allows visualization of differentially stained regions of a chromosome as a continuous series of light and dark bands specific for the chromosome and species; this has permitted definitive identification and delineation of all the chromosomes and chromosomal segments of many different species. Named according to the staining technique used, see *C b., G b., Q b.,* and *R b.*

G b. differential staining of chromosomes to elicit chromosome bands (G bands), consisting of pretreatment with a salt solution or with proteolytic enzymes (usually trypsin or pronase) before staining with Giemsa solution. Such bands are AT-rich, replicate late in S phase, and are relatively inactive in transcription. The same banding pattern may be obtained with other agents.

gastric b. see *adjustable gastric b.*

Giemsa b. G b.

GTG b. G banding in which trypsin is used as the pretreatment to Giemsa stain.

high-resolution b. a banding technique in which cultured cells are blocked in the S phase of the cell cycle; the block is then released, and the culture is harvested when the greatest number of cells are in late prophase or prometaphase, revealing 800–1400 bands rather than the 400–600 seen in metaphase preparations. Used to detect precise breakpoints or small structural alterations. Called also *prophase b.*

laparoscopic gastric b. (LGB) gastric banding performed through a laparoscope.

prophase b. high-resolution b.

pulmonary artery b. an operation to provide constriction of the pulmonary artery with a band to reduce pulmonary blood flow and relieve congestive heart failure in children with congenital heart defects that produce left to right shunts between ventricles or the great arteries.

Q b., quinacrine b. differential staining of chromosomes to elicit chromosome bands (Q bands), consisting of examination of the chromosomes by fluorescence microscopy after they have been stained with quinacrine mustard or related compounds, the degree of fluorescence varying from one chromosome segment to another and the resultant fluorescent patterns characteristic for each chromosome. The bright (intense) Q bands correspond almost exactly with the dark bands of G banding (q.v.).

R b., reverse b. differential staining of chromosomes to elicit chromosome bands (R bands), consisting of pretreatment with hot alkali before staining; the banding pattern obtained is the reverse of that of G and Q banding—darkly stained R bands are light in G and Q banding and vice versa. The dark R bands are GC-rich and show transcriptional activity.

tooth b. the technique of cementing stainless steel bands to the teeth to hold orthodontic attachments in position.

Ban•dl ring (bahn′dəl) [Ludwig *Bandl*, German obstetrician in Austria, 1842–1892] pathologic retraction ring; see *retraction ring*, under *ring*.

band•pass (band′pas) the range of frequencies passed by a filter, or the range of wavelengths used by a spectrophotometer or colorimeter; equal to the range in which the transmittance is equal to or greater than one-half the peak transmittance.

band•width (band′width) bandpass.

bane (bān) poison.

leopard's b. 1. *Arnica.* 2. arnica.

bane•wort (bān′wort) belladonna (def. 1).

Ban•flex (ban′fleks) trademark for a preparation of orphenadrine citrate.

Bang bacillus, disease, test (bahng) [Bernhard Laurits Frederik *Bang*, Danish physician, 1848–1932] see *Brucella abortus*, and under *disease* and *test*.

ban•ian (ban′yən) *Ficus bengalensis.*

Ban•is•te•ria (ban″is-te′re-ə) a genus of plants of the family Malpighiaceae. *B. caa′pi* Spruce is a South American woody vine whose seeds contain the hallucinogens harmine and harmaline.

ban•is•ter•ine (ban-is′tər-ēn) harmine.

bank (bangk) a stored supply of human material or tissues for future use by other individuals, such as a *blood bank, bone bank, eye bank, human-milk bank, skin bank*, or *sperm bank*.

blood b. an organization that collects, processes, and stores blood in preparation for transfusions.

eye b. an agency that collects and stores eye tissue and then prepares it and supplies it for transplantation.

Ban•na•yan-Zo•na•na syndrome (ban′ə-yən zo-nă′nə) [George A. *Bannayan*, American physician, 20th century; Jonathan *Zonana*, American physician, 20th century] see under *syndrome*.

Ban•nis•ter disease (ban′is-tər) [Henry Martyn *Bannister*, American physician, 1844–1920] angioedema.

Bann•warth syndrome (bahn′vahrt) [Alfred *Bannwarth*, German neurologist, 1903–1970] see under *syndrome*.

Ban•thine (ban′thēn) trademark for preparations of methantheline bromide.

Ban•ti disease (bahn′te) [Guido *Banti*, Italian pathologist, 1852–1925] congestive splenomegaly.

ban•yan (ban′yən) *Ficus bengalensis.*

BAO basal acid output.

Bap•tis•ia (bap-tiz′e-ə) [L., from Gr. *baptizein* to dip in or under water] a genus of plants of the family Leguminosae. *B. leucan′tha* is the wild indigo, which contains quinolizidine alkaloids and may cause poisoning of horses and cattle.

bar (bahr) 1. a structure having greater length than width, and often some degree of rigidity. 2. a metal segment of greater length than width that serves to connect two or more parts of a removable partial denture. 3. tarsal coalition; for this and its various types, see under *coalition*. 4. a unit of pressure, being a pressure of 10^6 dyne per square cm; equal to 0.987 atm or 10^5 Pa. 5. the upper part of the gums of a horse, between the grinders and the tusks, which bears no teeth. 6. that portion of the wall of a horse's hoof reflected posteriorly at an acute angle. Called also *spine, stay*, and *frog stay*.

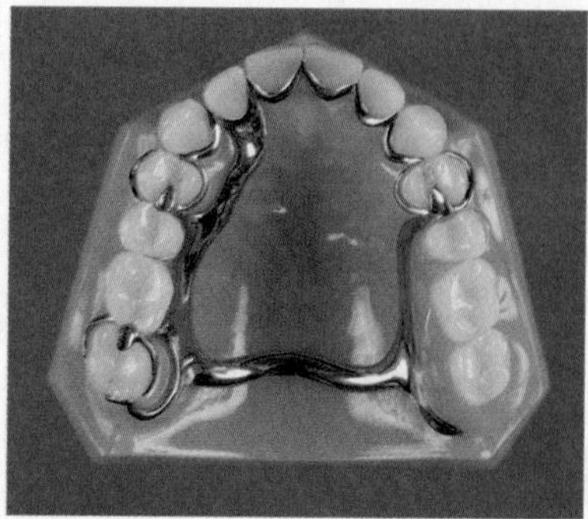

■ Connector bars in a maxillary removable partial denture.

arch b. any of several types of heavy wire bars shaped to the outer circumference of the dental arch and extending from one side to the other so that intervening teeth may be attached to it; used for treatment of fractures of the jaws and for stabilization of injured teeth.

Bill b. crista verticalis meatus acustici interni.

b. of bladder plica interureterica.

chromatoid b. see under *body*.

connector b. a connector unit of a removable partial denture that is fabricated as parallel-, round-, or oval-sided bars and serves to connect parts of dentures, splint or connect abutments, connect and splint crowns, or splint teeth that have received root therapy. Called also *connecting b.* and *minor connector*. Cf. *major connector*.

Dolder b. an attachment designed to secure and stabilize an overlay denture; it consists of a bar transected by several screw holes, which are used to attach it to the jaw, and is ovoid to allow some rotational movement of the denture.

Erich arch b. an arch bar made of soft, readily contoured metal, used for intermaxillary fixation.

hyoid b's a pair of cartilaginous plates forming the second pharyngeal (branchial) arch, from which a part of the hyoid bone is developed.

Kazanjian T b. an appliance used in reconstruction of the lip and jaw; it is fixed with an acrylic prosthesis to provide soft tissue support during reconstruction.

Kennedy b. 1. a metal bar, usually resting on the lingual surfaces of teeth, that aids in their stabilization and acts as an indirect retainer. 2. continuous clasp.

labial b. a major connector located labial to the dental arch, and joining two or more bilateral parts of a mandibular removable partial denture.

lingual b. continuous clasp.

Mercier b. plica interureterica.

occlusal rest b. a minor connector used to attach an occlusal rest to a major part of a removable partial denture.

palatal b. a major connector that extends across the palate and joins two or more parts of a maxillary removable partial denture.

Passavant b. crista palatopharyngea.

sternal b. one of the paired cartilaginous bars in the embryo that unite to form the sternum.

tarsal b. see under *coalition*.

terminal b's zones where epithelial cells contact one another, once thought to represent an accumulation of dense cementing substance, but with the electron microscope shown to be a junctional complex (see under *complex*).

Bar•a•clude (bar′ə-klo͞od) trademark for preparations of entecavir.

bar•ag•no•sis (bar″ag-no′sis) [*bar-* + *a-*[1] + Gr. *gnosis* knowledge] lack or loss of the faculty of barognosis; called also *abarognosis* and *baroagnosis*.

Ba•ra•lyme (bar′ə-līm″) trademark for barium hydroxide lime.

Bá•rá•ny symptom (sign, test), pointing test (bah′rah-ne) [Robert *Bárány*, Austrian physician in Sweden and Nobel prize winner, 1876–1936] see under *symptom* and *test*.

bar•ba (bahr′bə) [L.] [TA] beard.

bar•ba ama•ri•lla (ah-mah-re′yah) [Sp. "yellow beard"] *Bothrops atrox*, a large venomous pit viper found in Central and South America; it is sometimes erroneously called *fer-de-lance*.

bar•bal•o•in (bahr-bal′o-in) an anthraquinone pentoside found in various species of *Aloe* and mainly responsible for their cathartic properties.

bar·ban (bahr′ban) an herbicide chemically related to the carbamate group, which in heavy doses causes a condition similar to carbamate poisoning.

bar·bar·a·la·lia (bahr″bər-ə-la′le-ə) a form of paralalia that is shown when speaking a foreign language.

bar·bas·co (bahr-bas′ko) either of two tropical plants, *Jacquinia paramensis* and *Paullinia pinnata,* used as fish poisons.

bar·bei·ro (bahr-ba′ro) [Port.] Brazilian name for *Panstrongylus megistus.*

Bar·ber psoriasis (bahr′bər) [Harold Wordsworth *Barber,* English dermatologist, 1886–1955] localized pustular psoriasis.

bar·ber·ry (bahr′bər-e) 1. the shrub *Berberis vulgaris,* which contains resins and berberine; the bark of its stems and roots is used as a bitter tonic. 2. the berry of *B. vulgaris,* which is the source of a yellow dye and is used as a preservative.

bar·bi·tur·ate (bahr-bich′ər-ət) any of a class of sedative-hypnotic agents derived from barbituric acid or thiobarbituric acid and classified into long-, intermediate-, short-, and ultrashort-acting classes. The ultrashort-acting barbiturates, e.g., thiopental, are used as intravenous anesthetics. The long-acting barbiturate phenobarbital is an important anticonvulsant used in the treatment of epilepsy. Many other barbiturates were widely used as sedatives or hypnotics, but benzodiazepines have replaced them in most uses. Some of these have a high potential for abuse.

bar·bi·tur·ic ac·id (bahr-bĭ-tūr′ik) the parent compound of the barbiturates, 2,4,6-trioxohexahydropyrimidine. It is not itself a central nervous system depressant; the presence of alkyl or aryl groups at position 5 gives its derivatives their sedative and hypnotic effects.

bar·bo·tage (bahr″bo-tahzh′) [Fr. *barboter* to dabble] repeated injection and withdrawal of fluid, as in the administration of an anesthetic into the subarachnoid space by alternate injection of a small amount of the anesthetic and withdrawal of a small quantity of cerebrospinal fluid into the syringe, until the anesthetic is completely administered.

bar·bu·la (bahr′bu-lə) [L.] a little beard.

b. hir′ci tufts of hair in the ears.

Bard sign (bahrd) [Louis *Bard,* French physician, 1857–1930] see under *sign.*

Bar·det-Biedl syndrome (bahr-da′ be′dəl) [Georges *Bardet,* French physician, 20th century; Artur *Biedl,* Austrian physician, 1869–1933] see under *syndrome.*

bar·es·the·sia (bar″es-the′zhə) [*bar-* + *esthesia*] pressure sense.

bar·es·the·si·om·e·ter (bar″əs-the″ze-om′ə-tər) [*bar-* + *esthesio-* + *-meter*] an instrument for determining sensitivity to weight or pressure.

bar·i·at·ric (bar″e-at′rik) [*bar-* + *-iatric*] pertaining to obesity.

bar·i·at·rics (bar″e-at′riks) [*bar-* + *-iatrics*] the study of obesity, its causes, prevention, and treatment.

bar·ite (bar′īt) 1. barium oxide. 2. barium sulfate.

bar·i·to·sis (bar-ĭ-to′sis) a benign pneumoconiosis due to inhalation of the dust of barium or barite. Called also *barytosis.*

bar·ium (Ba) (bar′e-əm) [L., from Gr. *baros* weight] a pale, yellowish, metallic element belonging to the alkaline earths; atomic number 56, atomic weight 137.34. Its acid-soluble salts are poisonous; see *barium poisoning,* under *poisoning.*

b. hydrate, b. hydroxide $Ba(OH)_2$, a crystalline soluble base employed as a test for sulfates.

b. oxide BaO_2, a white or light yellow powder used for drying gases; called also *barite, baryta,* and *baryte.*

b. sulfate [USP] $BaSO_4$, an odorless fine white powder used as a contrast medium in radiography of the digestive tract. Called also *barite, baryta,* and *baryte.*

bark (bahrk) [Old Norse *börkr*] the rind or outer cortical cover of the woody parts of a plant, tree, or shrub; called also *cascara.*

bearberry b. cascara sagrada.

buckthorn b. the dried bark of *Rhamnus frangula,* a cathartic.

calisaya b. cinchona (def. 2).

casca b. the bark of *Erythrophloeum guineense,* an ordeal poison used in western Africa; called also *Mancona b.*

chittem b. cascara sagrada.

cinchona b. cinchona (def. 2).

cramp b. the dried bark of *Viburnum opulus,* the high bush or cranberry tree; it has been used as an antispasmodic, uterine sedative, and antiscorbutic.

cuprea b. the bark of *Remijia pedunculata,* which contains cupreine and has been used as an antimalarial.

elm b. slippery elm b.

Jesuit b. cinchona (def. 2).

Mancona b. casca b.

Peruvian b. cinchona (def. 2).

Purshiana b. cascara sagrada.

quillay b. quillaia.

sacred b. cascara sagrada.

slippery elm b. the dried inner bark of the slippery elm, *Ulmus rubra,* which is mucilaginous and demulcent; the official preparation [USP] is *elm.* Called also *elm b.*

soap b., soap tree b. quillaia.

white willow b. a preparation of the bark of various *Salix* species native to central and southern Europe and collectively known as white willow, containing salicin, a precursor of salicylic acid, to which it is converted metabolically; used as an antiinflammatory and antipyretic.

wild black cherry b. wild cherry (def. 2).

yohimbe b. a preparation of the bark of *Pausinystalia yohimbe,* used for the same indications as yohimbine hydrochloride; it has also been used traditionally as an aphrodisiac and for skin diseases and obesity.

Bar·kan operation (bahr′kən) [Otto *Barkan,* American ophthalmologist, 1887–1958] goniotomy.

bark·er (bahr′kər) a foal with neonatal maladjustment syndrome.

Bar·low disease (bahr′lo) [Sir Thomas *Barlow,* British physician, 1845–1945] infantile scurvy; see under *scurvy.*

Bar·low syndrome (bahr′lo) [John Brereton *Barlow,* South African cardiologist, born 1924] mitral valve prolapse syndrome; see under *syndrome.*

barn (bahrn) [jocular "big as a barn"] a unit of area equal to 10^{-24} square centimeter, used in measuring nuclear scattering cross sections. Symbol b.

Barnes curve (bahrnz) [Robert *Barnes,* English obstetrician, 1817–1907] see under *curve.*

bar(o)- [Gr. *baros* weight] a combining form denoting relationship to weight or pressure.

baro·ag·no·sis (bar″o-ag-no′sis) baragnosis.

baro·cep·tor (bar″o-sep′tər) baroreceptor.

baro·don·tal·gia (bar″o-don-tal′jə) pain in an otherwise asymptomatic tooth caused by a change in barometric pressure, as during high-altitude flight or scuba diving. Called also *aerodontalgia.*

bar·og·no·sis (bar″og-no′sis) [*baro-* + Gr. *gnosis* knowledge] conscious perception of weight; the faculty by which weight is recognized, such as when an object is placed in the hand. Cf. *baragnosis.*

baro·pac·er (bar′o-pās″ər) an electronic unit implanted in the necks of dogs for continuous stimulation of the carotid sinuses.

baro·phil·ic (bar″o-fil′ik) [*baro-* + *-philic*] growing best under high atmospheric pressure; said of bacterial cells.

baro·re·cep·tor (bar″o-re-sep′tər) a type of interoceptor that is stimulated by changes in pressure, particularly one located in the wall of a blood vessel; see also under *reflex.* Called also *baroceptor* and *pressoreceptor.*

baro·re·flex (bar′o-re″fleks) baroreceptor reflex.

baro·si·nus·itis (bar″o-si″nəs-i′tis) inflammation and pain of one or more paranasal sinuses (usually the frontal sinus) due to difference in pressure between the surrounding atmosphere and the air within the sinus cavity; it occurs on ascent to or descent from a high altitude, such as in an airplane, when the opening into the sinus is obstructed. Called also *aerosinusitis* and *sinus barotrauma.*

baro·tax·is (bar″o-tak′sis) [*baro-* + *taxis*] stimulation of living matter by change of the pressure relations under which it exists; see also *barotropism.*

bar·oti·tis (bar″o-ti′tis) a morbid condition of the ear produced by exposure to differing atmospheric pressures. Called also *aerotitis.*

b. me′dia traumatic inflammation of the middle ear caused by a difference in pressure between the surrounding atmosphere and the air in the middle ear space, marked by otalgia, tinnitus, hearing loss, and sometimes vertigo. It occurs in rapid descent in altitude, such as in an aircraft or in diving. Called also *aerotitis media, aviator's ear, aviation otitis,* and *middle ear* or *otitic barotrauma.*

baro·trau·ma (bar″o-traw′mə) [*baro-* + *trauma*] injury caused by pressure, especially to enclosed cavities of the body such as the eustachian tube, middle ear, paranasal sinuses, or lung. See also *barotitis media.*

middle ear b., otitic b. barotitis media.

pulmonary b. traumatic damage to the lung as a result of pressure changes, such as in divers, usually characterized by peribronchial rupture and pneumomediastinum.

sinus b. barosinusitis.

bar·ot·ro·pism (bar-ot′rə-piz-əm) [*baro-* + *tropism*] a relatively stereotyped response, often a movement, to pressure stimuli.

Barr body (bahr) [Murray Llewellyn *Barr,* Canadian anatomist, 1908–1995] sex chromatin.

bar·ra·cu·da (bar″ə-koo′də) any of various carnivorous marine fish of the genus *Sphyraena*, found in tropical waters; they are often eaten by humans but sometimes contain ciguatoxin and cause ciguatera.

Bar·ra·quer disease (bah-rah-kār′) [José Luis Antonio Roviralta *Barraquer*, Spanish physician, 1855–1928] partial lipodystrophy; see under *lipodystrophy*.

Bar·ra·quer method, operation (bah-rah-kār′) [Ignacio *Barraquer*, Spanish ophthalmologist, 1884–1965] phacoerysis.

Bar·ra·quer-Si·mons syndrome (bah-rah-kār′ se′monz) [J.L.A.R. *Barraquer*; Arthur *Simons*, German physician, 1879–1942] partial lipodystrophy; see under *lipodystrophy*.

Bar·ré sign (bah-ra′) [Jean Alexandre *Barré*, French neurologist, 1880–1971] see under *sign*.

bar·ren (bar′ən) see *sterile* (def. 1).

Bar·rett epithelium, syndrome (esophagus), ulcer (bar′ət) [Norman Rupert *Barrett*, English surgeon, 1903–1979] see under *epithelium*, *syndrome*, and *ulcer*.

bar·ri·er (bar′e-ər) an obstruction.

alveolar b., alveolar-capillary b., alveolocapillary b. alveolocapillary membrane.

blood-air b. alveolocapillary membrane.

blood-aqueous b. the anatomical mechanism that prevents exchange of materials between the chambers of the eye and the blood.

blood-brain b., blood-cerebral b. the barrier system separating the blood from the parenchyma of the central nervous system. Its anatomical component consists of unique endothelial cells in the brain capillaries, having tight junctions without fenestrations and with few microvilli and few vesicles for fluid transport. Its physiologic component in part consists of enzymes unique to the brain endothelia and of active transport via carrier proteins.

blood–cerebrospinal fluid b. blood-brain b.

blood-gas b. alveolocapillary membrane.

blood-retinal b. a transport barrier for certain substances, between the retinal capillaries and retinal tissue, consisting of specialized nonfenestrated, tightly joined endothelial cells.

blood-testis b. a barrier separating the blood from the seminiferous tubules, consisting of special junctional complexes between adjacent Sertoli cells near the base of the seminiferous epithelium.

blood-thymus b. a barrier in the thymus that excludes certain substances, possibly constituted by the interposition of a sheet of epithelial cell processes around the periphery of the lobules and between the lymphocytes and the perivascular connective tissue.

filtration b. the structures in the visceral layer of the glomerular capsule of the kidney that separate the blood in the glomerular capillaries from the urinary space, consisting of the glomerular capillary membrane and the layer of podocytes, pedicels, and slit pores.

gastric mucosal b. a physiological property of the gastric mucosa rendering the epithelium relatively impermeable to ions. Its function is impaired by aspirin, organic acids, and bile salts, and in patients subjected to severe trauma or shock. Back diffusion of acid from the gastric lumen may cause mucosal erosion or ulceration.

gut b. impermeability of the intestinal mucosa to intraluminal bacteria and endotoxins; failure of barrier function can result in sepsis and multiple organ failure.

hematoencephalic b. blood-brain b.

histohematic connective tissue b. the barrier between the blood and the dependent parenchymal tissue through which diffusion of nutrients and gases takes place.

placental b. the placental separation of fetal from maternal blood and bloodborne materials of greater than molecular size; in humans the term placental membrane is preferred, because it is not a barrier to most substances in the maternal blood, such as drugs and viruses.

protective b. an intervening shield of radiation-absorbing material such as lead, concrete, or plastic whose atomic number and thickness are specifically sufficient to give adequate body protection against ionizing radiation of various types.

protective b's, primary barriers sufficient to reduce a primary beam of radiation to a permissible exposure rate.

protective b's, secondary barriers sufficient to reduce stray or scattered radiation to a permissible exposure rate.

radiation b. protective b.

Bar·ron ligation, ligature (bar′ən) [J. *Barron*, American proctologist, 20th century] see *rubber band ligation*, under *ligation*, and *rubber band ligature*, under *ligature*.

bar·sati (bahr-saht′e) [Hindi "of the rainy season"] 1. cutaneous habronemiasis. 2. pythiosis.

Bart syndrome (bahrt) [Bruce Joseph *Bart*, American dermatologist, born 1936] see under *syndrome*.

Barth hernia (bahrt) [Jean Baptiste Philippe *Barth*, French physician, 1806–1877] see under *hernia*.

Bar·thel index (bahr-tel′) [D.W. *Barthel*, American physiatrist, 20th century] see under *index*.

Bar·tho·lin abscess, adenitis, etc. (bahr′to-lin) [Caspar Thomèson *Bartholin*, Jr., Danish anatomist, 1655–1738] see under *abscess*, *adenitis*, and *cyst*, and see *ductus sublingualis major* and *glandula vestibularis major*.

bar·tho·lin·i·an (bahr″to-lin′e-ən) named for Caspar T. *Bartholin*.

bar·tho·lin·itis (bahr″to-lin-i′tis) inflammation of Bartholin glands.

Bar·ton bandage, fracture, operation (bahr′tən) [John Rhea *Barton*, American surgeon, 1794–1871] see under *bandage*, *fracture*, and *operation*.

Bar·to·nel·la (bahr″tə-nel′ə) [Alberto Leopoldo *Barton*, Peruvian microbiologist, 1871–1950] a genus of bacteria of the family Bartonellaceae, order Rhizobiales, consisting of gram-negative, aerobic, slightly curved rods characteristically occurring in chains, found in tissue cells and erythrocytes. The organism occurs in humans, sometimes asymptomatically, and in arthropod vectors. The type species is *B. bacillifor′mis*.

B. bacillifor′mis a species transmitted by the sandfly *Phlebotomus verrucarum;* it is the etiologic agent of Carrión disease (see *bartonellosis*, def. 2).

B. clarrid′geiae a species that is normally found in cats and can cause cat-scratch disease in humans.

B. elizabe′thae a species that is a cause of bacterial endocarditis and *neuroretinitis*.

B. hen′selae a species that is the etiologic agent of cat-scratch disease and is the primary cause of bacillary angiomatosis and bacillary peliosis; it also is a cause of bacteremia in immunocompromised patients and of bacterial endocarditis. Cats are the reservoir and transmission is by a cat bite or scratch. Formerly called *Rochalimaea henselae*.

B. koeh′lerae a species that is a cause of bacterial endocarditis.

B. quinta′na the etiologic agent of trench fever, transmitted by the body louse *Pediculus humanus*. It is also a cause of bacterial endocarditis and of bacillary angiomatosis and peliosis. Formerly called *Rochalimaea quintana*.

B. vinso′nii a species that is a cause of bacterial endocarditis.

Bar·to·nel·la·ceae (bahr″tə-nel-a′se-e) a family of bacteria of the order Rhizobiales, consisting of small rod-shaped, coccoid, or ring- or disk-shaped, filamentous and beaded organisms, having a diameter of usually less than 3 μm; these are pathogenic and are transmitted by arthropods. The family has a single genus, *Bartonella*.

bar·to·nel·li·a·sis (bahr″to-nel-i′ə-sis) bartonellosis.

bar·to·nel·lo·sis (bahr-tə-nel-o′sis) 1. infection with any organism of the genus *Bartonella*. 2. infection by *Bartonella bacilliformis*, transmitted by sandflies in mountain valleys of Peru, Ecuador, and Colombia. Besides humans, it also affects dogs and rodents, especially after splenectomy. There are two stages: the first or acute stage is a highly fatal fever called *Oroya fever;* the second or chronic stage is a benign skin eruption called *verruga peruana*. Called also *Carrión disease*.

Bart·ter syndrome (bahr′tər) [Frederic Crosby *Bartter*, American internist, 1914–1983] see under *syndrome*.

bar·u·ria (bar-u′re-ə) [*bar-* + *uria*] the passage of urine of a high specific gravity.

bary·es·the·sia (bar″e-es-the′zhə) baresthesia.

bary·la·lia (bar″ĭ-la′le-ə) [Gr. *barys* heavy + *lal-* + *-ia*] thick, indistinct speech due to imperfect articulation.

ba·ry·ta (bə-ri′tə) 1. barium oxide. 2. barium sulfate.

bar·yte (bar′īt) 1. barium oxide. 2. barium sulfate.

bar·y·to·sis (bar″ĭ-to′sis) baritosis.

ba·sad (ba′sad) toward a base or basal aspect.

ba·sal (ba′səl) pertaining to or situated near a base.

ba·sal·i·o·ma (ba-sal″e-o′mə) basal cell carcinoma.

ba·sa·lis (ba-sa′lis) [L., from Gr. *basis* base] [TA] basal; a general term denoting relationship to or location near a base.

ba·sa·loid (ba′sə-loid) resembling basal cells of the skin; see under *carcinoma*.

ba·sa·lo·ma (ba″sə-lo′mə) basal cell carcinoma.

bas·cule (bas′kūl) [Fr. "seesaw"] a device working on the principle of the seesaw, so that when one end is lowered the other is raised.

cecal b. a form of volvulus in which the cecum becomes folded anteriorly and medially over bands or adhesions that run across the ascending colon.

base (bās) [L., Gr., *basis*] 1. the lowest part or foundation of anything; see also *basis*. 2. the main ingredient of a compound. 3. in chemistry, the nonacid part of a salt; a substance that combines with acids to form salts; a substance that dissociates to give hydroxide ions in aqueous solutions; a substance whose molecule or ion can combine with a proton (hydrogen ion); a substance capable of donating a pair of electrons (to an acid) for the formation of a coordinate covalent bond. 4. a unit of a removable prosthesis that supports the supplied tooth and any intermediary material and in turn receives support from the tissue of the basal seat. 5. in genetics, a nucleotide, particularly one in a nucleic acid sequence. See also *base pair,* under *pair.* **ba′sal, basa′lis** *adj*

acidifiable b. a chemical substance that will unite with water to form an acid.

acrylic resin b. a denture base made of an acrylic resin.

apical b. the portion of the jaws that supports the teeth; called also *basal arch.*

b. of bladder fundus vesicae urinariae.

b. of brain the inferior surface of the brain, including the undersurfaces of the cerebrum, cerebellum, and brainstem.

buffer b. the sum of all the buffer anions in the blood (bicarbonate, hemoglobin, proteins, and phosphate), determined by titrating the blood with a strong acid; it is used as an index of the degree of metabolic disturbance in the acid-base balance.

cement b. a layer of dental cement placed in the deep portions of a cavity preparation to protect the pulp; a base may be placed to protect the pulp from postoperative sensitivity and damage, to insulate and protect the tooth from thermal shock, or to act as a sedative for the pulp.

b. of cerebral peduncle basis pedunculi cerebri.

conjugate b. a chemical species that is formed from its conjugate acid by removal of a proton; e.g., acetate (CH_3COO^-) is the conjugate base of acetic acid (CH_3COOH).

cranial b. basis cranii.

denture b. the part of a denture, made of metal or resin or a combination of the two, that supports the supplied teeth and receives support from the abutment teeth, the residual alveolar ridge, or both. See also *denture base saddle,* under *saddle.*

b. of dorsal horn of spinal cord basis cornus posterioris medullae spinalis.

external b. of skull basis cranii externa.

film b. a thin, flexible, transparent sheet of cellulose acetate or similar material which carries the radiation and light-sensitive emulsion of x-ray or photographic films.

b. of gastric gland the main part of a gastric gland, interior to the neck.

b. of heart basis cordis.

internal b. of skull basis cranii interna.

Lewis b. an electron-pair donor, e.g., ammonia and halide ion.

b. of lung basis pulmonis.

metal b. a metallic portion of a denture base forming a part or all of the basal surface of the denture, which serves as the attachment for the plastic (resin) part of the denture base and the teeth.

nitrogenous b. an aromatic, nitrogen-containing molecule that serves as a proton acceptor, e.g., purine or pyrimidine.

b. of nose apertura piriformis.

ointment b. a vehicle for the medicinal substances carried in an ointment. Ointment bases are divided into hydrocarbon bases, which are oleaginous; absorption bases, which include both anhydrous and water-in-oil emulsions and are able to incorporate aqueous solutions; water-removable (or water-washable) bases, which are oil-in-water emulsions; and water-soluble bases.

plastic b. a denture or baseplate made of a plastic material.

b. of posterior horn of spinal cord basis cornus posterioris medullae spinalis.

b. of prostate basis prostatae.

purine b's a group of chemical compounds of which purine is the base, including 6-oxypurine (hypoxanthine); 2,6-dioxypurine (xanthine); 6-aminopurine (adenine); 2-amino-6-oxypurine (guanine); 2,6,8-trioxypurine (uric acid); and 3,7-dimethyl xanthine (theobromine). Called also *xanthine b's.* See illustration.

pyrimidine b's a group of chemical compounds of which pyrimidine is the base, including 2,4-dioxypyrimidine (uracil), 2,4-dioxy-5-methylpyrimidine (thymine), and 2-oxy-4-aminopyrimidine (cytosine), which are common constituents of nucleic acids. See illustration.

record b. baseplate.

b. of renal pyramid the part of a renal pyramid that is directed away from the renal sinus.

Schiff b. any of a class of compounds having the general formula R—CH═N—R′, formed by condensation of primary amines with ketones or aldehydes.

shellac b's resinous materials adapted to maxillary or mandibular edentulous casts to form baseplates for the construction of dentures.

b. of skull basis cranii.

b. of stapes basis stapedis.

temporary b. baseplate.

tooth-borne b. the base of a partial denture which is supported by the abutment teeth and not by the tissues beneath it.

trial b. baseplate.

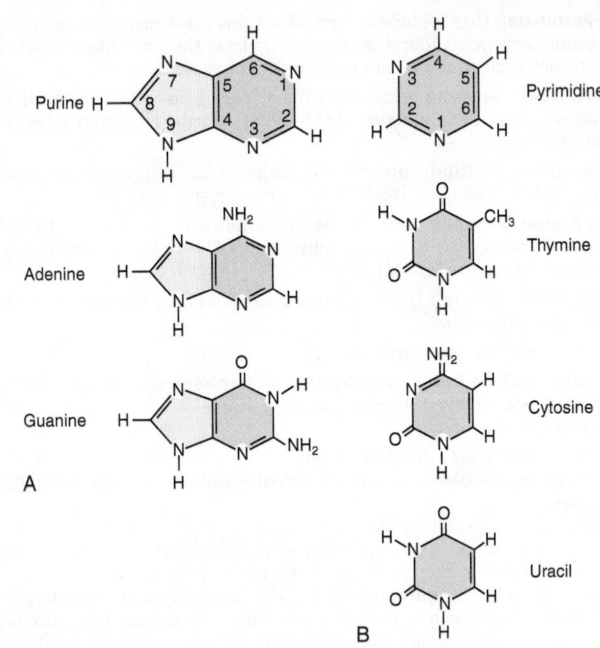

■ Purine and pyrimidine bases. *(A),* Purine and some substituted purine bases occurring in nucleic acids; *(B),* pyrimidine and some substituted pyrimidine bases occurring in nucleic acids.

b. of urinary bladder fundus vesicae urinariae.

xanthine b's purine b's.

bas·e·doid (baz′ə-doid) a condition resembling Graves (Basedow) disease, but without thyrotoxicosis.

Ba·se·dow disease, goiter, paraplegia (bah′zə-do) [Karl Adolf von *Basedow,* German physician, 1799–1854] see under *goiter* and *paraplegia,* and see *Graves disease,* under *disease.*

bas·e·dow·i·form (baz″ə-do′ĭ-form) resembling Graves (Basedow) disease.

base·line (bās′līn) an observation or value that represents the normal background level, or an initial level, of a measurable quantity; used for comparison with values representing response to experimental intervention or an environmental stimulus, usually implying that the baseline and response values refer to the same individual or system.

base·plate (bās′plāt) 1. a temporary preformed shape made of shellac, wax, or acrylic resin, representing the base of a denture and used for making maxillomandibular relation records, for arranging artificial teeth, or for trial placement in the mouth. Called also *record base, temporary base,* and *trial base.* Written also *base plate.* 2. the tissue circumferential to and somewhat eccentric to the internal urethral orifice, thought to act as a floor during the filling of the bladder and to assume a cone shape during micturition so that the proximal urethra can fill.

stabilized b. a baseplate lined with a plastic or other suitable material to improve its adaptation and stability.

ba·ses (ba′sēz) [L.] plural of *basis.*

bas-fond (bah-fawn′) [Fr.] fundus vesicae urinariae.

ba·si·al·ve·o·lar (ba″se-al-ve′ə-lər) extending from the basion to the alveolar point.

ba·sic (ba′sik) 1. pertaining to or having the properties of a base. 2. capable of neutralizing acids.

ba·sic·i·ty (bə-sis′ĭ-te) 1. the quality of being a base, or basic. 2. the combining power of an acid; it is measured by the number of hydrogen atoms replaceable by a base.

ba·si·cra·ni·al (ba″sĭ-kra′ne-əl) pertaining to the cranial base (basis cranii).

ba·si·cra·ni·um (ba″sĭ-kra′ne-əm) [*basi-* + *cranium*] basis cranii.

ba·sid·ia (bə-sid′e-ə) plural of *basidium.*

Ba·sid·i·ob·o·la·ceae (bə-sid″e-ob″o-la′se-e) a family of fungi of the order Entomophthorales, consisting of widespread saprobes; one genus, *Basidiobolus,* contains organisms pathogenic for humans and horses.

ba·sid·i·ob·o·lo·my·co·sis (bə-sid″e-ob″ə-lo-mi-ko′sis) a chronic type of emtomophthoromycosis caused by *Basidiobolus ranarum,* with formation of gradually enlarging granulomas in the subcutaneous tissues of the upper limbs, chest, and trunk. Multiple purulent ulcers may also develop. It occurs in Indonesia, central Africa, and India, affecting chiefly children and adolescents. Unlike the other zygomycoses, it is not associated with any apparent predisposing factors. Called also *subcutaneous phycomycosis* and *subcutaneous zygomycosis.*

Ba·sid·i·ob·o·lus (bə-sid″e-ob′ə-ləs) [*basidium,* old name for conidiophore + Gr. *bolos* a throw] a mainly saprobic genus of fungi of the family Basidiobolaceae, which produces zygospores, chlamydospores, and conidia that carry along a piece of the conidiophore when they are ejected. *B. haptospo′rus,* **B. meristospo′rus** *B. ranarum.*

B. rana′rum a species that causes basidiobolomycosis in humans and horses.

ba·sid·io·carp (bə-sid′e-o-kahrp″) [*basidium* + *carp*] the large fruiting body characteristic of the majority of fungi of the subphylum Basidiomycotina; it is composed of masses of intertwined hyphal elements and produces basidia. Mushrooms and toadstools are common examples.

ba·sid·io·my·cete (bə-sid″e-o-mi′sēt) an individual fungus of the Basidiomycotina. **basidiomyce′tous** *adj*

Ba·sid·io·my·ce·tes (bə-sid″e-o-mi-se′tēz) name given to Basidiomycotina when it is considered a class and placed within the phylum Eumycota.

Ba·sid·i·o·my·co·ta (bə-sid″e-o-mi-ko′tə) name given to Basidiomycotina when it is considered a separate phylum.

Ba·sid·io·my·co·ti·na (bə-sid″e-o-mi″ko-ti′nə) [*basidium* + Gr. *mykēs* fungus] the club fungi, a subphylum of perfect fungi variously grouped under either Dikaryomycota or Eumycota. Spores (basidiospores) are borne on club-shaped organs (basidia). Some authorities consider this group a class and call it Basidiomycetes, whereas others consider it a separate phylum and call it Basidiomycota. Several different systems have been proposed for classifying the taxa above family within this group.

ba·sid·io·spore (bə-sid′e-o-spor) a type of sexual spore that forms on a basidium.

ba·sid·i·um (bə-sid′e-əm) pl. *basid′ia* [Gr. *basis* base] the clublike organ of the fungal class Basidiomycotina which, following karyogamy and meiosis, bears the basidiospore.

ba·si·fa·cial (ba-sĭ-fa′shəl) [*basi-* + *facial*] pertaining to the inferior part of the face.

ba·sig·e·nous (bə-sij′ə-nəs) capable of forming a chemical base.

ba·si·hy·al (ba″sĭ-hi′əl) basihyoid.

ba·si·hy·oid (ba″sĭ-hi′oid) the body of the hyoid bone (corpus ossis hyoidei [TA]); in certain animals other than humans, either of the two lateral bones that are its homologues.

bas·i·lad (bas′ĭ-lad) toward the basilar aspect.

bas·i·lar (bas′ĭ-lər) [L. *basilaris,* q.v.] pertaining to a base or basal part.

bas·i·la·ris (bas″ĭ-lar′is) [L., from Gr. *basis* base] [TA] basilar; a general term denoting relationship to a base or location at a base.

ba·si·lat·er·al (ba″sĭ-lat′ər-əl) both basilar and lateral.

ba·si·lem·ma (ba″sĭ-lem′ə) [*basi-* + *lemma*] basement membrane.

ba·sil·ic (bə-sil′ik) [L. *basilicus;* Gr. *basilikos* royal] important or prominent.

bas·i·lix·i·mab (bas″ĭ-liks′ĭ-mab) an interleukin-2 receptor antagonist produced by recombinant technology as a chimeric mouse/human monoclonal antibody; it is used as an immunosuppressant for prophylaxis of acute organ rejection after renal transplantation as part of a regimen that also includes cyclosporine and corticosteroids. Administered by intravenous injection.

ba·si·na·si·al (ba″sĭ-na′ze-əl) pertaining to the basion and the nasion.

basi(o)- [Gr. *basis*] a combining form denoting relationship to a base or foundation, to the basion, or to a chemical base.

ba·si·oc·cip·i·tal (ba″se-ok-sip′ĭ-təl) pertaining to the basilar part of the occipital bone.

ba·sio·glos·sus (ba″se-o-glos′əs) [*basio-* + Gr. *glōssa* tongue] the part of the hyoglossus muscle that is attached to the base of the hyoid bone.

ba·si·on (ba′se-on) [Gr. *basis* base] [TA] a craniometric landmark located at the midpoint of the anterior border of the foramen magnum, at the base of the clivus. Called also *point Ba.* ba′sial, basialis *adj*

ba·si·ot·ic (ba″se-ot′ik) [*basi-* + *otic*] see under *bone.*

ba·sip·e·tal (bə-sip′ə-təl) [*basi-* + *-petal*] descending toward the base; developing in the direction of the base, as a spore.

ba·si·phil·ic (ba″sĭ-fil′ik) basophilic.

ba·si·rhi·nal (ba″sĭ-ri′nəl) [*basi-* + *rhinal*] pertaining to the base of the brain and to the nose.

ba·sis (ba′sis) pl. *ba′ses* [L., from Gr.] base: the lowest or fundamental part of a structure or organ, or the part opposite to or distinguished from the apex.

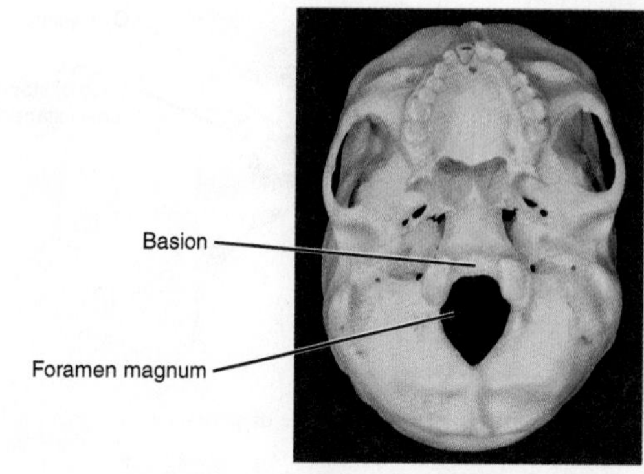

■ Basion, in an inferior view of the skull.

b. cartila′ginis arytenoi′deae [TA] base of arytenoid cartilage: the triangular inferior part of the arytenoid cartilage, which bears the articular surface.

b. coch′leae [TA] base of cochlea: the posterior of the cochlea, which rests upon the internal acoustic meatus.

b. cor′dis [TA] base of heart: a poorly delimited region of the heart, formed, in general, by the atria and the area occupied by the roots of the great vessels. It lies opposite the middle thoracic vertebrae, its exact position varying with heart action, and is directed superiorly, posteriorly, and to the right.

b. cor′nus posterio′ris medul′lae spina′lis [TA] base of posterior horn of spinal cord: the portion of the posterior horn of gray substance in the spinal cord that is adjacent to the intermediate zone (Rexed lamina VII); it corresponds approximately to lamina VI. Called also *base of dorsal horn of spinal cord.*

b. cra′nii [TA] cranial base: a composite of the numerous bones which serve the brain as a supportive floor and form the axis of the skull, comprising the *basis cranii externa* and *basis cranii interna.* Called also *basicranium.*

b. cra′nii exter′na [TA] external surface of cranial base: the outer surface of the inferior aspect of the skull; called also *norma ventralis, external base of skull,* and *scaphion.*

b. cra′nii inter′na [TA] internal surface of cranial base: the inner surface of the inferior region of the skull, constituting the floor of the cranial cavity. Called also *internal base of skull.*

b. mandi′bulae [TA] base of mandible: the lower margin of the body of the mandible; called also *inferior border of mandible.*

b. modi′oli [TA] base of modiolus: the broad part of the modiolus situated near the lateral part of the internal acoustic meatus.

b. os′sis metacar′pi [TA] the base of a metacarpal bone, being the proximal end of each metacarpal, which articulates with a carpal(s) and with adjacent metacarpals.

b. os′sis metatar′si [TA] the base of the metatarsal bone, being the wedge-shaped proximal end of each metatarsal, which articulates with bone(s) of the tarsus and with adjacent metatarsals.

b. os′sis sa′cri [TA] base of sacral bone: the cranial surface of the sacrum; its lateral portions consist of the alae of the sacrum, and its middle portion is the upper surface of the body of the first sacral vertebra, which articulates with the fifth lumbar vertebra.

b. patel′lae [TA] base of patella: the superior border of the patella, to which the tendon of the quadriceps femoris muscle is attached; called also *superior border of patella.*

b. pedun′culi ce′rebri [TA] base of cerebral peduncle: the part of the midbrain consisting of the crus cerebri and the substantia nigra; some authorities do not include the latter.

b. phalan′gis ma′nus [TA] base of phalanx of hand: the proximal end of each phalanx of the fingers.

b. phalan′gis pe′dis [TA] base of phalanx of foot: the proximal end of each phalanx of the toes.

b. pro′statae [TA] base of prostate: the broad upper part of the prostate, in contact with the lower surface of the urinary bladder.

b. pulmo′nis [TA] base of lung: the portion of each lung that is directed toward the diaphragm.

b. stape′dis [TA] base of stapes: the flat oval plate of bone on the stapes that fits into the fenestra vestibuli (oval window) on the medial wall of the middle ear. Called also *footplate* and *stapedial footplate.*

ba·si·sphe·noid (ba″sĭ-sfe′noid) 1. postsphenoid. 2. basisphenoid bone.

ba·si·tem·po·ral (ba″sĭ-tem′po-rəl) [*basi-* + *temporal*] pertaining to the lower part of the temporal bone.

ba·si·ver·te·bral (ba″sĭ-vur′tə-brəl) [*basi-* + *vertebral*] pertaining to the body of a vertebra.

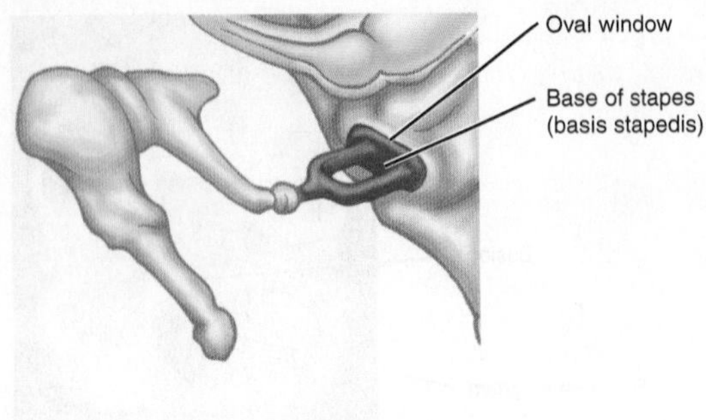

■ Basis stapedis (base of stapes).

bas•ket (bas′kət) 1. a container made of material woven together. 2. something resembling such a container. 3. basket cell.

Dormia b. a common type of stone basket.

fiber b's fine fibers extending from the external limiting membrane of the retina to surround the adjacent portions of the rods and cones.

nuclear b. a structure of the nuclear pore complex, formed by the fibrils extending from the nucleoplasmic ring into the nucleoplasm, and the terminal ring that connects them; it is believed to mediate transport from the nucleus to the cytoplasm.

stone b., stone retrieval b. a tiny apparatus consisting of several wires that can be advanced through an endoscope into a body cavity or tube, manipulated to trap a calculus or other object, and withdrawn.

Basle No•mi•na Ana•to•mi•ca (BNA) (bah′zəl no′mĭ-nə an-ə-tom′ĭ-kə) the official body of anatomical nomenclature prepared by a group of German anatomists with some help from anatomists in other countries, and presented for final criticism at the annual meeting of the German Anatomic Society held in Basle, Switzerland in 1895. It has been superseded by *Terminologia Anatomica* (TA) (1998).

bas(o)- see *basi(o)-*.

ba•so•ca•ten•u•late (ba″so-kə-ten′u-lāt) [*baso-* + *catenulate*] characterized by a chain of conidia in which the youngest cells are at the base away from the apex. Cf. *blastocatenulate*.

ba•so•lat•er•al (ba″so-lat′ər-əl) pertaining to the base and sides.

ba•so•meta•chro•mo•phil (ba″so-met″ə-kro′mo-fil) [*baso-* + *metachromophil*] staining with basic dyes to a color different from that of surrounding substances.

Ba•som•ma•toph•o•ra (ba″som-ə-tof′o-rə) a suborder of snails of the order Pulmonata, including mostly fresh water snails; two families of medical importance are Planorbidae and Lymnaeidae.

ba•so•phil (ba′so-fil) [*baso-* + *-phil*] 1. a structure, cell, or other histologic element that stains readily with basic dyes. 2. a granular leukocyte with an irregularly shaped, pale-staining nucleus that is partially constricted into two lobes, and with cytoplasm that contains coarse, bluish-black granules of variable size. Basophils contain vasoactive amines such as histamine and serotonin, which are released on appropriate stimulation. Called also *basophilic leukocyte*. 3. one of the hormone-producing basophilic cells of the

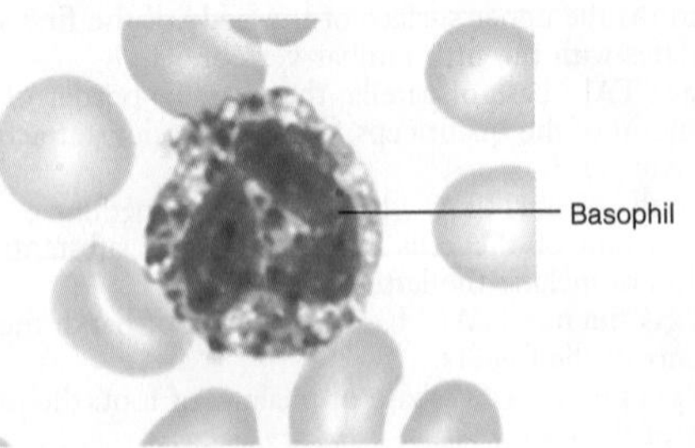

adenohypophysis; types include *gonadotrophs* and *thyrotrophs*. Called also *beta cell* and *B cell*. 4. basophilic.

beta b. thyrotroph.

Crooke-Russell b's the basophils in Crooke hyaline degeneration; see under *degeneration*.

delta b. gonadotroph (def. 1).

ba•so•phile (ba′so-fil) 1. basophilic. 2. basophil (def. 3).

ba•so•phil•ia (ba″so-fil′e-ə) 1. an abnormal increase of basophils in the blood, as seen in myxedema, hypothyroid conditions, ulcerative colitis, certain types of anemia, and other conditions. Called also *basophilism* and *basophilic leukocytosis*. 2. the reaction of immature erythrocytes to basic dyes so that they become stippled; there are two varieties, *diffuse b.* and *punctate b.*

diffuse b. basophilia in which erythrocytes are blue-gray and not stippled.

punctate b. basophilic stippling.

ba•so•phil•ic (ba-so-fil′ik) 1. pertaining to basophils. 2. staining readily with basic dyes; called also *basophil*, *basophile*, and *basophilous*.

ba•soph•i•lism (ba-sof′ĭ-liz-əm) basophilia (def. 1).

Cushing b., pituitary b. Cushing syndrome (def. 1); see under *syndrome*.

ba•so•phil•o•pe•nia (ba″so-fil″o-pe′ne-ə) abnormal reduction in the number of basophils in the blood; seen in hypothyroidism, stress, and a few other conditions. Called also *basophilic leukopenia*.

ba•soph•i•lous (ba-sof′ĭ-ləs) basophilic.

ba•so•plasm (ba′so-plaz″əm) cytoplasm that stains with basic dyes.

Bas•sen-Korn•zweig syndrome (bas′ən korn′zwīg) [Frank Albert *Bassen*, American physician, 20th century; Abraham Leon *Kornzweig*, American ophthalmologist, 1900–1982] abetalipoproteinemia; see *familial lipoprotein deficiency*, under *deficiency*.

Bas•set operation (bah-sa′) [Antoine *Basset*, French surgeon, 1882–1951] see under *operation*.

Bas•si•ni repair (operation) (bə-se′ne) [Edoardo *Bassini*, Italian surgeon, 1847–1924] see under *repair*.

Bas•ti•an-Bruns law (sign) (bas′chən broonz′) [Henry Charlton *Bastian*, English neurologist, 1837–1915; Ludwig *Bruns*, German neurologist, 1858–1916] see under *law*.

bat (bat) any member of the order Chiroptera, small flying mammals.

leaf-nosed b. any bat of the family Phyllostomatidae.

vampire b. a member of genera *Desmodus*, *Diaemus*, or *Diphylla*, found in tropical parts of the Americas, which subsist on the blood of warm-blooded animals. Some are reservoirs of rabies virus while others are reservoirs of *Trypanosoma cruzi*.

bath (bath) 1. a conductive or convective medium, as water, vapor, sand, or mud, with which the body is washed or scrubbed or in which the body is wholly or partly immersed for therapeutic or cleansing purposes. 2. the application of a conductive or convective medium to the body for therapeutic or cleansing purposes. 3. a piece of equipment or scientific apparatus in which a body or object may be immersed.

acid b. a bath of water medicated with a mineral acid.

air b. therapeutic exposure of the body to warm air.

alcohol b. the washing of the body with dilute alcohol; it is defervescent and stimulant.

alkaline b. the washing of a patient in a weak solution of an alkaline carbonate; useful in skin diseases.

cabinet b. a hot-air bath or a radiant heat bath in which the patient is enclosed in a special cabinet.

cold b. a bath in which cold water is used at a temperature of less than 18°C.

colloid b. a bath containing gelatin, oatmeal, starch, or similar substances, used for its soothing or antipruritic effects.

contrast b. immersion of a part of the body alternately in hot and in cold water.

cool b. a bath in water from 18° to 24°C.

douche b. the application of water to the body from a jet spray.

emollient b. a bath in a solution of an emollient substance, used in the treatment of pruritic conditions and other dermatoses.

hip b. sitz b.

hot b. a bath in water above body temperature (37°C).

immersion b. a bath in which the body of the patient is immersed.

kinetotherapeutic b. a bath providing facilities for underwater exercise.

light b. exposure of the body to light rays; see *phototherapy*.

lukewarm b. warm b.

needle b. a shower bath in which the water is projected in a fine, needle-like spray.

oatmeal b. a colloid bath containing oatmeal, used for its soothing or antipruritic effects in some dermatoses.

paraffin b. 1. wax b. 2. application of heated liquid paraffin to a part of the body and allowing it to solidify, used to promote relaxation and relieve pain; called also *wax b*. Cf. *thermotherapy*.

sand b. the immersion of the body in dry, heated sand.

sauna b. a sweat bath given in an enclosed room, usually followed by a cold shower.

sitz b. a bath in which the patient sits in the tub, the hips and buttocks being immersed; called also *hip b*.

sponge b. a bath in which the patient's body is not immersed in water but is rubbed with a wet cloth or sponge.

sweat b. any bath given to promote sweating.

tepid b. a bath in water from 24° to 33°C.

vapor b. exposure of the body to steam.

warm b. a bath in water from 33° to 36°C.
water b. a container of water for immersing bodies or for immersing liquid-containing vessels that are to be heated or cooled, or are to be held at a given temperature.
wax b. paraffin b.
whirlpool b. a variously sized tank in which the body or an extremity can be submerged as the heated water is mechanically agitated.

bath·es·the·sia (bath″es-the′zhə) [*bath-* + *esthesia*] deep sensibility.

bath·mo·tro·pic (bath″mo-tro′pik) [*bathmo-* + *-tropic*] influencing the response of muscle tissue to stimuli.
negatively b. lessening response of muscle tissue to stimuli.
positively b. increasing response of muscle tissue to stimuli.

bath·mot·ro·pism (bath-mot′ro-piz-əm) influence on the excitability of muscular tissue.

bath(o)- [Gr. *bathos* depth] a combining form meaning deep or denoting relationship to depth; cf. *bathy-*.

batho·chrome (bath′o-krōm) [*batho-* + *-chrome*] an atom or group whose introduction into a compound shifts the compound's absorption peak to a longer wavelength; cf. *hypsochrome*.

batho·chro·my (bath″o-kro′me) a shift of the absorption band toward lower frequencies (longer wavelengths) with deepening of color from yellow to red to black.

batho·flore (bath′o-flor) [*batho-* + *fluorescence*] an atom or group that decreases the intensity of fluorescence of a compound in which it occurs; cf. *auxoflore*.

batho·rho·dop·sin (bath″o-ro-dop′sin) a transient intermediate produced upon irradiation of rhodopsin in the visual cycle; see illustration at *visual cycle*, under *cycle*.

bath·ro·ceph·a·ly (bath″ro-sef′ə-le) [Gr. *bathron* a step + *-cephaly*] a developmental anomaly characterized by a steplike posterior projection of the skull, caused by excessive bone formation at the lambdoid suture.

bathy- [Gr. *bathys* deep, *bathos* depth] a combining form meaning deep or denoting relationship to depth; cf. *bath(o)-*.

bathy·an·es·the·sia (bath″e-an″es-the′zhə) [*bathy-* + *anesthesia*] loss of deep sensibility (bathyesthesia).

bathy·car·dia (bath″ĭ-kahr′de-ə) [*bathy-* + Gr. *kardia* heart] a fixed low position of the heart due to anatomical conditions and not to disease.

bathy·es·the·sia (bath″e-es-the′zhə) [*bathy-* + *esthesia*] deep sensibility.

bathy·hy·per·es·the·sia (bath″e-hi″pər-es-the′zhə) [*bathy-* + *hyperesthesia*] increased sensitiveness of deep structures of the body. Cf. *deep sensibility*, under *sensibility*.

bathy·hyp·es·the·sia (bath″e-hip″es-the′zhə) [*bathy-* + *hypesthesia*] decreased deep sensibility.

bath·yp·nea (bath″ip-ne′ə) [*bathy-* + *-pnea*] deep breathing.

BATO a boronic acid adduct of a technetium oxime; as a class they are neutral lipid-soluble agents some of which have been used as radioactive tracers for diagnostic imaging, including siboroxime and teboroxime.

Bat·son plexus (bat′sən) [Oscar Vivian *Batson*, American otolaryngologist, 1894–1979] see under *plexus*.

Bat·ten disease (bat′ən) [Frederick Eustace *Batten*, English ophthalmologist, 1865–1918] see under *disease*.

Bat·ten-Ma·you disease (bat′ən ma-yoo′) [F.E. *Batten;* Marmaduke Stephen *Mayou*, English ophthalmologist, 1876–1934] Batten disease; see under *disease*.

bat·te·ry (bat′ər-e) 1. a set or series of cells that yield an electric current. 2. any set, series, or grouping of similar things, as a battery of tests.

Bat·tey ba·cil·li (bat′e) [*Battey*, a tuberculosis hospital in Rome, Georgia, where many strains of these mycobacteria were first recognized] see under *bacillus*.

bat·tey·in (bat′e-in) [*Battey* bacillus] a product prepared from Battey bacilli (Group III of the unclassified mycobacteria), comparable to tuberculin, used in a cutaneous test of hypersensitivity.

Bat·tle incision, sign (bat′əl) [William Henry *Battle*, English surgeon, 1855–1936] see under *sign* and see *Kammerer-Battle incision*, under *incision*.

Bat·tle-Ja·la·guier-Kam·mer·er incision (bat′əl zhah-lah-gya′ kam′ər-ər) [W.H. *Battle;* Adolphe *Jalaguier*, French surgeon, 1853–1924; Frederic *Kammerer*, American surgeon, 1856–1928] see *Kammerer-Battle incision*, under *incision*.

Bau·de·locque diameter (line) (bo-də-lōk′) [Jean Louis *Baudelocque*, French obstetrician, 1746–1810] conjugata externa pelvis.

Bau·hin gland, valve (bo-ă′) [Gaspard (Caspar) *Bauhin*, Swiss anatomist, 1560–1624] see *anterior lingual glands*, under *gland*, and see *ileocecal valve*, under *valve*.

Bau·mé scale (bo-ma′) [Antoine *Baumé*, French chemist, 1728–1804] see under *scale*.

baux·ite (bawk′sīt) [Les *Baux*, France, site of the first bauxite mines] an impure mixture of aluminum hydroxides, clay, and other metal oxides, the primary natural source of aluminum. See also *bauxite pneumoconiosis*.

Bax·ter nerve (baks′tər) [Donald E. *Baxter*, American orthopedic surgeon, 21st century] see under *nerve*.

bay (ba) a recess or inlet.
lacrimal b. lacus lacrimalis.

Bay·col (ba′kol) trademark for a preparation of cerivastatin sodium.

Bayes theorem (bāz) [Thomas *Bayes*, English mathematician, 1702–1761] see under *theorem*.

bayes·ian (ba′ze-ən) named for Thomas *Bayes*, as *bayesian statistics*.

Bay·Gam (ba′gam) trademark for a preparation of immune globulin.

Bay·Hep B (ba-hep′) trademark for a preparation of hepatitis B immune globulin.

Bayle disease (bāl) [Antoine Laurent Jesse *Bayle*, French physician, 1799–1858] paralytic dementia.

Bay·ley Scales of Infant Development (ba′le) [Nancy *Bayley*, American psychologist, 1899–1994] see under *scale*.

Bay·lis·as·car·is (ba″lis-as′kə-ris) a genus of nematodes of the family Ascaridae. *B. columna′ris* infests the central nervous system of dogs. *B. procy′onis* is usually found in raccoons and rodents, but fecal contamination from those animals can cause spread to domestic animals and humans, resulting in nervous system infection or larva migrans.

Bay·liss effect (ba′lis) [Sir William Maddock *Bayliss*, British physician, 1860–1924] see under *effect*.

Bay·Rab (ba-rab′) trademark for a preparation of rabies immune globulin.

Bay·Rho-D (ba′ro-de) trademark for a preparation of $Rh_0(D)$ immune globulin.

Bay·Tet (ba-tet′) trademark for a preparation of tetanus immune globulin.

Ba·zex syndrome (bah-zeks′) [J. *Bazex*, French dermatologist, 20th century] see under *syndrome*.

Ba·zin disease (bah-ză′) [Antoine Pierre Ernest *Bazin*, French dermatologist, 1807–1878] see under *disease*.

BBB blood-brain barrier; bundle branch block.

BBBB bilateral bundle branch block.

BBT basal body temperature.

BC bone conduction.

BCAA branched-chain amino acids.

B-CAVe a cancer chemotherapy regimen consisting of bleomycin, CCNU (lomustine), Adriamycin (doxorubicin), and vinblastine.

BCDF B cell differentiation factors.

BCF basophil chemotactic factor.

BCG bacille Calmette-Guérin; bicolor guaiac test; ballistocardiogram.

BCGF B cell growth factors.

BCNU carmustine.

b.d. [L.] bis di′e (twice a day).

BDA British Dental Association.

Bdel·la (del′ə) [Gr. "leech"] a genus of mites. *B. cardina′lis* is parasitic on other insects.

BDNF brain-derived neurotrophic factor.

B-DNA see under *DNA*.

BDS Bachelor of Dental Surgery.

BDSc Bachelor of Dental Science.

B-E, BE below-elbow; see under *amputation*.

Be beryllium.

bead (bēd) a small spherical structure or mass.
rachitic b's a series of palpable or visible prominences at the points where the ribs join their cartilages; seen in certain cases of rickets.
scorbutic b's a series of visible prominences at the costochondral joints, sometimes seen in children with scurvy.

bead·ed (bēd′əd) having the appearance of beads or a string of beads.

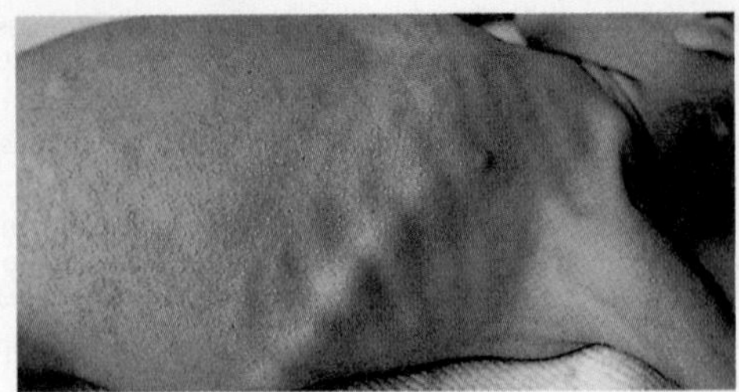

■ Rachitic beads.

bead·ing (bēd′ing) alternate local constriction and dilatation of a blood vessel so that on an angiograph it resembles a string of beads.
 venous b. localized increases in diameter of retinal veins so that they appear like strings of beads; seen in diabetic retinopathy.

beak (bēk) [Fr. *bec*] 1. the forward-projecting jaws of a bird, along with their leathery or horny covering. 2. something shaped like the beak of a bird. See also *rostrum.*

Beale ganglion cells (bēl) [Lionel Smith *Beale*, British physician, 1828–1906] see under *cell.*

Beals syndrome (bēlz) [Rodney Kenneth *Beals*, American orthopedic surgeon, born 1931] congenital contractural arachnodactyly; see under *arachnodactyly.*

BEAM a cancer chemotherapy regimen consisting of BCNU (carmustine), etoposide, ara-C (cytarabine), and melphalan.

beam (bēm) 1. a unidirectional, or approximately unidirectional, emission of electromagnetic radiation or particles. 2. any slender structure of a denture or orthodontic appliance designed to provide support to the structure and subjected to lateral stresses, such as a dental bar or an orthodontic arch wire whose curvature changes under load.
 cantilever b. a beam that is supported by one fixed support at only one of its ends.
 continuous b. a beam that continues over three or more supports, those supports not at the beam ends being equally free supports.
 primary b. useful b.
 restrained b. a beam that has two or more supports, at least one of which permits some freedom of rotation to the point of support.
 simple b. a straight beam that has two supports, one at either end.
 useful b. in radiology, that part of the primary radiation that is permitted to emerge from the tubehead assembly of an x-ray machine, as limited by the tubehead aperture or port and accessory collimating devices.

Bean syndrome (bēn) [William Bennett *Bean*, American hepatologist, 1909–1989] blue rubber bleb nevus syndrome; see under *syndrome.*

bean (bēn) 1. any of various leguminous plants of the pea family. 2. the seed of such a plant.
 broad b. 1. *Vicia faba.* 2. the seed of *V. faba.*
 cacao b's cacao (def. 2).
 Calabar b. 1. *Physostigma venenosum.* 2. the poisonous seed of *P. venenosum*, which contains physostigmine and has been used by native peoples in ordeal trials. Called also *ordeal b.*
 carob b. 1. *Ceratonia siliqua.* 2. carob (def. 2).
 castor b. 1. *Ricinus communis.* 2. the seed of *R. communis*, which yields castor oil but is also toxic.
 cocoa b's cacao (def. 2).
 djenkol b. 1. *Pithecolobium lobatum.* 2. the seed of *P. lobatum*, a broad round reddish bean eaten as a delicacy in Indonesia and nearby areas, sometimes causing djenkol bean poisoning. Called also *jering b.*
 fava b. 1. *Vicia faba.* 2. the seed of *V. faba.*
 jack b. any of various edible beans of the genus *Canavalia.*
 jequirity b. 1. *Abrus precatorius.* 2. the toxic seed of *A. precatorius*, which is used as a decorative bead but contains abrin. Called also *crab's eye* and *rosary pea.*
 jering b. djenkol b.
 locust b. 1. *Ceratonia siliqua.* 2. carob (def. 2).
 mescal b. *Sophora secundiflora.*
 ordeal b. Calabar b.
 St. Ignatius b. the poisonous seed of the tropical tree *Strychnos ignatii;* it contains strychnine and brucine.
 tonka b. 1. *Dipteryx odorata.* 2. the seed of *D. odorata*, which has been used as a flavoring agent and contains coumarin.
 vanilla b. vanilla (def. 2).

bear·ber·ry (ber′ber-e) 1. *Arctostaphylos uva-ursi.* 2. the fruit of *A. uva-ursi.* 3. *Rhamnus purshiana.*

beard (bērd) heavy hair growing on the lower part of the face, normally a secondary sex character after puberty in males. Called also *barba* [TA].

bear·ing (bar′ing) a supporting surface or point.
 central b. application of forces between the maxillae and mandible at a single point as near as possible to the center of the supporting areas of the upper and lower jaws, for the purpose of distributing closing forces evenly throughout the areas of the supporting structures during the registration and recording of maxillomandibular (jaw) relations and during the correction of occlusal errors.

bear·ing down (bār′ing doun′) 1. a feeling of weight in the pelvis occurring in certain diseases. 2. the expulsive effort of a woman in labor.

Bearn-Kun·kel syndrome (bərn′ kung′kəl) [Alexander Gordon *Bearn*, English-born American physician, 1923–1983; Henry George *Kunkel*, American physician, 1916–1983] chronic active hepatitis.

Bearn-Kun·kel-Sla·ter syndrome (bərn′ kung′kəl sla′tər) [A.G. *Bearn;* H.G. *Kunkel;* Robert James *Slater*, Canadian-born American pediatrician, born 1923] chronic active hepatitis.

bear·wood (bār′wood) cascara sagrada.

beat (bēt) a throb or pulsation, as of the heart or of an artery; see also *pulse.*
 apex b. the most inferolateral point of visible or palpable pulsation of the chest wall due to movement of the apex of the heart, normally medial and superior to the intersection of the left midclavicular line and the fifth left intercostal space. Generally it corresponds roughly to the position of the apex of the heart and is often the point of maximal impulse.
 atrial b. an ectopic beat originating within the atria; it occurs when the sinus node does not fire or fires ineffectively.
 atrial premature b. (APB) see under *complex.*
 atrioventricular (AV) junctional escape b. a depolarization initiated in the atrioventricular junction when one or more impulses from the sinus node are nonexistent or ineffective.
 atrioventricular (AV) junctional premature b. see under *complex.*
 capture b's in atrioventricular dissociation, occasional ventricular responses to a sinus impulse that reaches the atrioventricular node in a nonrefractory phase.
 ciliary b. the rhythmic, coordinated contraction of cilia of cells in a two-step process involving intraciliary excitation followed by interciliary conduction. The beat may be divided into two parts, the *effective stroke* and the *recovery stroke.* The rhythm may be either *isochronous* (all cilia beating simultaneously) or *metachronous* (beats moving along the cilia in waves).
 dropped b. absence of a single ventricular contraction.
 echo b. reciprocal b.
 ectopic b. a heart beat originating at some point other than the sinus node.
 escape b., escaped b. an ectopic beat that follows an abnormally long pause between impulses propagated by the sinoatrial node; name for the escape of impulse propagation from normal control.
 forced b. an extrasystole produced by artificial stimulation of the heart.
 fusion b. in electrocardiography, the complex resulting when an ectopic ventricular beat coincides with normal conduction to the ventricle; the complex has features of both the normal and the ectopic beat.
 heart b. heartbeat.
 interpolated b. a contraction occurring exactly between two normal heart beats without altering the sinus rhythm.
 interpolated ventricular premature b. see under *complex.*
 junctional escape b. atrioventricular junctional escape b.
 junctional premature b. atrioventricular junctional premature complex.
 nodal b. atrioventricular junctional escape b.
 postectopic b. the normal beat following an ectopic beat.
 premature b. extrasystole.
 pseudofusion b. an ineffective pacing stimulus delivered during the absolute refractory period following a spontaneous depolarization but

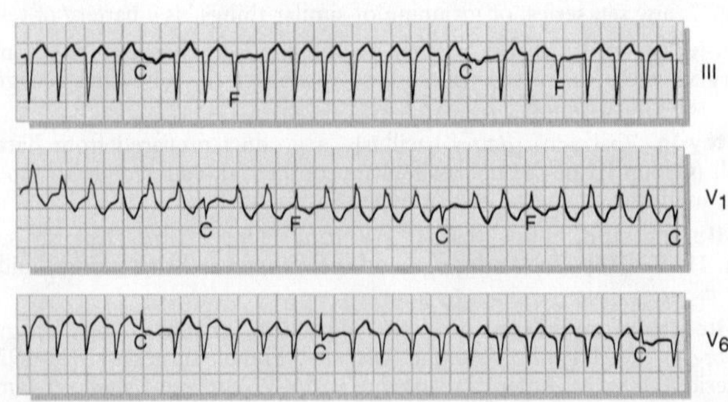

■ Intermittent capture *(C)* and fusion *(F)* beats during ventricular tachycardia. The QRS complex is prolonged and the R–R interval is regular except for occasional capture beats that have abnormal contour and are slightly premature.

before sufficient charge accumulates to prevent pacemaker discharge; on the electrocardiogram the pacemaker impulse spike is superimposed on the QRS complex of the spontaneous complex.

reciprocal b. a cardiac impulse that in one cycle causes ventricular contraction, travels back toward the atria, then reexcites the ventricles; a series of such beats constitutes a reciprocal rhythm.

reentrant b. any of the characteristic beats of a reentrant circuit.

retrograde b. a beat occurring as a result of impulse conduction backward relative to the normal atrioventricular direction.

sinus b. a natural pulsation of the heart, originating in the sinus node.

ventricular escape b. an ectopic beat of ventricular origin occurring in the absence of supraventricular impulse generation or conduction; it is characterized by a bizarre, usually wide QRS complex and lack of an ectopic P wave.

ventricular premature b. (VPB) see under *complex.*

Beau lines (bo) [Joseph Honoré Simon *Beau*, French physician, 1806–1865] see under *line.*

Beau·ver·ia (bo-vēr′e-ə) a genus of Fungi Imperfecti of the form-class Hyphomycetes, form-family Moniliaceae. *B. bassia′na* causes muscardine in silkworms, and *B. tenel′la* causes a disease of the larvae of beetles; formerly called *Botrytis bassiana* and *B. tenella*, respectively.

Be·bu·lin VH (be′bu-lin) trademark for a preparation of factor IX complex.

be·cap·ler·min (bə-kap′lər-min) human platelet-derived growth factor produced by recombinant DNA technology; it is similar in action to endogenous platelet-derived growth factor and is applied topically for the treatment of neuropathic diabetic ulcers of the lower extremity that extend into or beyond the subcutaneous tissue.

Bech·te·rew see *Bekhterev.*

Beck (Bek) disease (bek) [E.V. *Beck* (or *Bek*), Russian physician, early 20th century] Kashin-Bek disease.

Beck triad (bek) [Claude Schaeffer *Beck*, American surgeon, 1894–1971] see under *triad.*

Beck·er disease (bek′ər) [Peter Emil *Becker*, German geneticist, 1908–2000] the autosomal recessive form of myotonia congenita (q.v.).

Beck·er muscular dystrophy (bek′ər) [P.E. *Becker*] see under *dystrophy.*

Beck·er nevus (melanosis) (bek′ər) [Samuel William *Becker*, American physician, 1894–1964] see under *nevus.*

Beck·er phenomenon (sign), test (bek′ər) [Otto Heinrich Enoch *Becker*, German oculist, 1828–1890] see under *phenomenon* and *test.*

Beck·with syndrome (bek′with) [John Bruce *Beckwith*, American pediatric pathologist, born 1933] Beckwith-Wiedemann syndrome; see under *syndrome.*

Beck·with-Wie·de·mann syndrome (bek′with ve′də-mahn) [J.B. *Beckwith;* Hans Rudolf *Wiedemann*, German pediatrician, 1915–2006] see under *syndrome.*

Bé·clard amputation, etc. (ba-klahr′) [Pierre Augustin *Béclard*, French anatomist, 1785–1825] see under *amputation*, *hernia*, *nucleus*, *sign*, and *triangle.*

bec·lo·meth·a·sone di·pro·pi·o·nate (bek″lo-meth′ə-sōn) [USP] a synthetic glucocorticoid administered by inhalation for the chronic treatment of bronchial asthma and intranasally for seasonal and nonseasonal allergic rhinitis or other allergic or inflammmatory nasal conditions, and to prevent recurrence of nasal polyps after surgical removal; also used topically for relief of inflammation and pruritus in corticosteroid-responsive dermatoses.

Bec·lo·vent (bek′lo-vent″) trademark for a preparation of beclomethasone dipropionate.

Bec·on·ase (bek′ə-nāz″) trademark for preparations of beclomethasone dipropionate.

bec·que·rel (Bq) (bek″ə-rel′) [Antoine Henri *Becquerel*, French physicist and Nobel prize winner, 1852–1908] a unit of radioactivity, defined as that of quantity of a radioactive nuclide whose rate of spontaneous nuclear transformation is one decay per second ($1\ s^{-1}$); 1 curie equals 3.7×10^{10} becquerels; 1 microcurie equals 37 kilobecquerels.

bed (bed) 1. a supporting structure or tissue. 2. a couch or support for the body during sleep.

air b. an airtight, inflatable mattress.

capillary b. the total combined mass of capillaries forming a large reservoir which may be more or less completely filled with blood. See illustration at *capillary.*

CircOlectric b. trademark for a revolving circular bed which induces constant pressure alteration.

flotation b. a mattress filled with water or air for prevention of decubitus ulcers; see also *water b.*

fracture b. a bed for the use of patients with broken bones.

Gatch b. a bed fitted with joints beneath the hips and knees, allowing patient to be raised to a half-sitting position and so maintained by elevation of the knees to prevent sliding toward the footboard.

hydrostatic b. water b.

metabolic b. a bed so arranged that all the feces and urine of the patient are saved; the amount of excreta compared with the intake gives an indication of the metabolism in the body.

nail b. matrix unguis.

rocking b. a bed mounted on a rocking apparatus, moving between the head-up and head-down positions to promote movement of the diaphragm and thus breathing, particularly for patients who are quadriplegic or have paralysis of the diaphragm.

Sanders b. a rocking bed used to improve circulation in the treatment of chronic occlusive arterial disease.

vascular b. the sum of the blood vessels supplying an organ or region.

water b. a type of flotation bed that is filled with water.

bed·bug (bed′bug) 1. any bug of the genus *Cimex.* 2. any of various other biting insects that infest human bedding.

Mexican b. any of various biting reduviid bugs of the genus *Triatoma* found in the southern United States and Mexico.

Bed·nar aphthae (bed′nahr) [Alois *Bednar*, Austrian physician, 1816–1888] see under *aphtha.*

bed·pan (bed′pan) a vessel for receiving the urinary and fecal discharges of a patient unable to leave the bed.

bed·sore (bed′sor″) decubitus ulcer.

bee (be) any of several flying insects of the family Apidae. See *Apis* and *Bombus.*

Beer's law (bār) [August *Beer*, German physicist, 1825–1863] see under *law.*

bees·wax (bēz′waks) wax derived from the honeycomb of *Apis mellifera;* see *yellow wax*, under *wax.*

bleached b. see *white wax*, under *wax.*

unbleached b. see *yellow wax*, under *wax.*

beet (bēt) 1. any plant of the genus *Beta.* 2. the enlarged root of such a plant.

bee·tle (be′təl) an insect of the order Coleoptera.

blister b. any beetle of the family Meloidae; their dried bodies raise blisters when rubbed on human skin and are sometimes used as counterirritants.

coconut b. any beetle of the genus *Sessinia.*

grain b. a beetle of the genus *Tenebrio;* its larva is the mealworm.

rove b. any beetle of the family Staphylinidae.

Bee·vor sign (be′vər) [Charles Edward *Beevor*, British neurologist, 1854–1908] see under *sign.*

Begg appliance, technique (beg) [Percy Raymond *Begg*, Australian orthodontist, 1898–1983] see under *appliance* and *technique.*

beg·ma (beg′mə) [Gr.] phlegm.

Bé·guez Cé·sar disease (ba′gās sa′sahr) [Antonio *Béguez César*, Cuban pediatrician, 20th century] Chédiak-Higashi syndrome.

be·hav·ior (be-hāv′yər) deportment or conduct; any or all of a person's total activity, especially that which can be externally observed. **behav′ioral** *adj*

automatic b. automatism.

invariable b. activity whose character is determined by innate structure, such as reflex action.

operant b. see under *conditioning.*

respondent b. see *conditioning.*

variable b. behavior that is modifiable by individual experience.

be·hav·ior·ism (be-hāv′yər-iz-əm) a school of psychology founded by John B. Watson that regards as the subject matter of psychology only overt actions capable of direct observation and measurement and ignores unobservable mental events such as ideas and emotions.

be·hav·ior·ist (be-hāv′yər-ist) a psychologist who is a disciple of behaviorism.

Beh·çet syndrome (bĕ-chet′) [Hulûsi *Behçet*, Turkish dermatologist, 1889–1948] see under *syndrome.*

be·hen·ate (bə-hen′āt) a salt (soap), ester, or anionic form of behenic acid.

be·hen·ic ac·id (bə-hen′ik) a saturated 22-carbon fatty acid present in oil of mustard and other plant seed oils. See table accompanying *fatty acid.*

Behr pupil (bār) [Carl *Behr*, German ophthalmologist, 1874–1943] see under *pupil.*

Beh·ring's law (ba′ringz) [Emil Adolf von *Behring*,. German physician, bacteriologist, and Nobel prize winner, 1854–1917] see under *law.*

Bei•gel disease (bi'gəl) [Hermann *Beigel*, German physician, 1830–1879] white piedra.

bej•el (bej'əl) [Ar. *bajlah*] endemic syphilis.

Bé•ké•sy audiometry (ba'ka-she) [Georg von *Békésy* Hungarian-born American physicist and Nobel prize winner, 1899–1972] see under *audiometry*.

Bekh•te•rev (Bech•te•rew) layer, nucleus, reaction, etc. (bek-ter'yev) [Vladimir Mikhailovich *Bekhterev* (or *Bechterew*), Russian neurologist, 1857–1927] see under *nucleus, reaction, reflex, sign,* and *test*; see *rheumatoid spondylitis*, under *spondylitis;* and see *Kaes-Bekhterev layer*, under *layer*.

Bekh•te•rev-Men•del reflex (bek-ter'yev men'del) [V.M. *Bekhterev; Kurt Mendel*, German neurologist, 1874–1946] Mendel-Bekhterev reflex.

bel (B) (bel) [Alexander Graham *Bell*, American inventor, 1847–1922] a unit of relative power intensity used for acoustic or electric power, defined as the base 10 logarithm of the ratio of the measured power to some reference power level. A change of one bel is a tenfold power increase. Measurements are usually expressed in decibels (q.v.).

belch•ing (belch'ing) eructation.

Bell muscle (bel) [John *Bell*, Scottish surgeon and anatomist, 1763–1820] see under *muscle*.

Bell nerve, palsy (paralysis), phenomenon (bel) [Sir Charles *Bell*, Scottish physiologist in London, 1774–1842] see *nervus thoracicus longus*, and see under *palsy* and *phenomenon*.

bel•la•don•na (bel"ə-don'ə) [Ital. "fair lady"] 1. *Atropa belladonna*, a perennial plant indigenous to central and southern Europe and cultivated in North America; it contains various anticholinergic alkaloids, including atropine, hyoscyamine, and scopolamine, which are used medicinally. Ingestion of belladonna or its alkaloids can cause anticholinergic poisoning (q.v.). Called also *banewort, deadly nightshade, death's herb,* and *dwale*. 2. belladonna leaf.

Bel•ler•gal-S (bel'ər-gal") trademark for a combination preparation of ergotamine tartrate, belladonna alkaloids, and phenobarbital sodium.

Bel•li•ni duct, ligament (bel-e'ne) [Lorenzo *Bellini*, Italian anatomist, 1643–1704] see *papillary duct*, under *duct*, and see under *ligament*.

bel•ly (bel'e) 1. abdomen. 2. the fleshy contractile part of a muscle (venter [TA]).

anterior b. of digastric muscle venter anterior musculi digastrici.

drum b. tympanites.

frontal b. of occipitofrontal muscle venter frontalis musculi occipitofrontalis.

inferior b. of omohyoid muscle venter inferior musculi omohyoidei.

occipital b. of occipitofrontal muscle venter occipitalis musculi occipitofrontalis.

posterior b. of digastric muscle venter posterior musculi digastrici.

prune b. see under *syndrome*.

superior b. of omohyoid muscle venter superior musculi omohyoidei.

bel•o•ne•pho•bia (bel"o-nə-fo'be-ə) [Gr. *belonē* needle + *-phobia*] irrational fear of pins, needles, and other sharp objects.

bel•o•noid (bel'o-noid) [Gr. *belonē* needle + *-oid*] needle-shaped; styloid.

Bel•sey Mark IV operation (fundoplication) (bel'se) [Ronald Herbert Robert *Belsey*, English surgeon, 20th century] see under *operation*.

Ben•a•dryl (ben'ə-drəl) trademark for preparations of diphenhydramine hydrochloride.

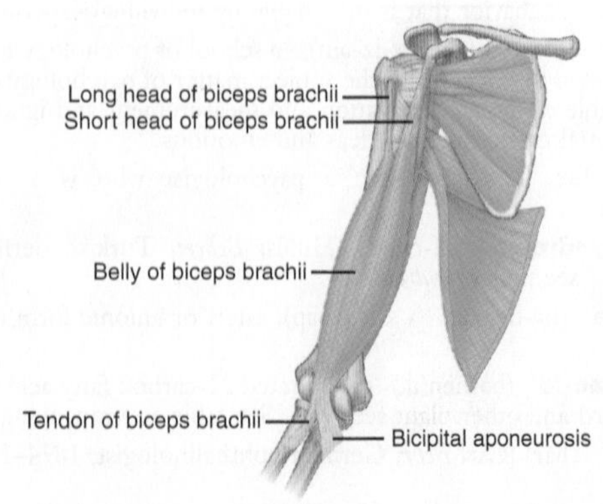

■ Belly of biceps brachii muscle.

ben•a•ze•pril hy•dro•chlo•ride (ben-a'zə-pril) [USP] an angiotensin-converting enzyme inhibitor administered orally, alone or in combination with a thiazide diuretic, for treatment of hypertension.

Bence Jones protein, etc. (bens' jōnz') [Henry *Bence Jones*, English physician, 1814–1873] see under *cylinder, protein, proteinuria,* and *reaction*.

bend (bend) a flexure or curve; a flexed or curved part.

first order b's adjustments made in a labial arch wire, incorporating offsets in the horizontal plane, which are usually made in the areas of the cuspids and premolar and molar teeth, accommodating differences in thickness in the labiolingual or buccolingual diameters of the teeth.

head b., neck b. cervical flexure.

second order b's bends in the vertical plane of an arch wire.

third order b's bends in an arch wire to maintain or produce torsion of a tooth.

V b's V-shaped bends incorporated in an arch wire, usually placed mesial or distal to the cuspids to improve the axial relationship of teeth.

varolian b. the third cerebral flexure in the developing fetus.

Ben•der Vis•u•al-Mo•tor Ges•talt test (ben'dər) [Lauretta *Bender*, American psychiatrist, 1897–1987] see under *test*.

ben•dro•flu•a•zide (ben"dro-floo'ə-zīd) bendroflumethiazide.

ben•dro•flu•me•thi•a•zide (ben"dro-floo"mə-thi'ə-zīd) [USP] a thiazide diuretic used for treatment of hypertension and edema; administered orally.

bends (bendz) pain in the limbs and abdomen occurring as a result of rapid reduction of air pressure; see *decompression sickness*, under *sickness*.

be•ne (ben'a) [L.] well.

Ben•e•dict solution, test (ben'ə-dikt) [Stanley Rossiter *Benedict*, American physiological chemist, 1884–1936] see under *solution* and *test*.

Ben•e•dikt syndrome (ben'ə-dikt) [Moritz *Benedikt*, Austrian physician, 1835–1920] see under *syndrome*.

Bene•Fix (ben'ə-fiks") trademark for a preparation of coagulation factor IX (recombinant).

Ben•e•mid (ben'ə-mid) trademark for a preparation of probenecid.

Ben•i•car (ben'ĭ-kahr) trademark for a preparation of olmesartan medoxomil.

be•nign (bə-nīn') [L. *benignus*] not malignant; not recurrent; favorable for recovery.

be•nig•nan•cy (bə-nig'nan-se") the quality of being benign.

Ben•nett fracture (ben'ət) [Edward Hallaran *Bennett*, Irish surgeon, 1837–1907] see under *fracture*.

Ben•o•quin (ben'o-kwin) trademark for preparations of monobenzone.

ben•ox•i•nate hy•dro•chlo•ride (ben-ok'sĭ-nāt) [USP] a benzoic acid ester related to procaine, used as a topical anesthetic in ophthalmology; applied topically to the conjunctiva to produce anesthesia of short duration.

ben•ser•a•zide (ben-ser'ə-zīd) an inhibitor of the decarboxylation of peripheral levodopa to dopamine, having actions similar to those of carbidopa. When given with levodopa, benserazide produces higher brain concentrations of dopamine with lower doses of levodopa, thus lessening the side effects seen with higher doses. It is used orally, in conjunction with levodopa, as an antiparkinsonian agent.

Ben•son disease (ben'sən) [Alfred Hugh *Benson*, Irish ophthalmologist, 1852–1912] asteroid hyalosis.

ben•thos (ben'thos) [Gr. *benthos* bottom of the sea] the flora and fauna of the bottom of oceans.

ben•tir•o•mide (ben-tēr'o-mīd) a compound containing *p*-aminobenzoic acid, used in a noninvasive pancreatic function test; see *bentiromide test*, under *test*.

ben•ton•ite (ben'ton-īt) [Fort *Benton*, Montana, after which the geological formation where it was found was named] [NF] a colloidal hydrated aluminum silicate, which on the addition of water swells to produce a slippery paste; its chief pharmaceutical use is as a suspending agent.

ben•to•qua•tam (ben'to-kwah"tam) a topical skin protectant used to prevent or reduce allergic contact dermatitis resulting from contact with urushiol-containing plants such as poison ivy, poison oak, or poison sumac.

Ben•tyl (ben'təl) trademark for preparations of dicyclomine hydrochloride.

Ben•za•Clin (ben'zə-klin) trademark for a combination preparation of clindamycin phosphate and benzoyl peroxide.

Ben•za•gel (ben'zə-jel) trademark for preparations of benzoyl peroxide.

ben•zal•de•hyde (ben-zal'də-hīd) [NF] an aldehyde derivative of benzene, occurring in the kernels of bitter almonds or produced synthetically; used as a pharmaceutical flavoring agent in place of almond oil.

ben·za·lin (ben′zə-lin) nigrosin.

ben·zal·ko·ni·um chlo·ride (ben″zal-ko′ne-əm) [NF] a quaternary ammonium compound, being a mixture of alkylbenzyl dimethylammonium chlorides; a rapidly acting surface disinfectant and detergent active against both gram-negative and gram-positive bacteria and certain viruses, fungi, yeasts, and protozoa; applied topically to the skin and mucous membranes and to wounds as an antiseptic and used intravaginally as a spermicide. It is also used as a preservative for pharmaceuticals and a disinfectant for surgical instruments.

Ben·za·my·cin (ben″zə-mi′sin) trademark for a combination preparation of erythromycin and benzoyl peroxide.

ben·zan·thra·cene (ben-zan′thrə-sēn) one of a group of aromatic hydrocarbons consisting of anthracene with one benzene substitution; some of them have carcinogenic properties.

ben·zaz·o·line hy·dro·chlo·ride (ben-zaz′o-lēn) tolazoline hydrochloride.

benz·bro·ma·rone (benz-bro′mə-rōn) a potent uricosuric agent that blocks tubular reabsorption of uric acid; used in the treatment of hyperuricemia of gout.

Ben·ze·drex (ben′zə-dreks) trademark for propylhexedrine.

ben·zene (ben′zēn) a colorless volatile liquid hydrocarbon, C_6H_6, obtained as a byproduct in the destructive distillation of coal. It is harmful by transdermal absorption and acutely toxic by ingestion or inhalation, causing mucous membrane irritation, neurological symptoms, and death due to respiratory failure; chronic exposure may result in bone marrow depression and aplasia and leukemia. Benzene is a known carcinogen. See illustration under *ring.* Called also *benzol.*

dimethyl b. xylene.

b. hexachloride (BHC) a chlorinated hydrocarbon, $C_6H_6Cl_6$, occurring in numerous isomeric forms; the gamma isomer is lindane (q.v.), a powerful insecticide. Called also *hexachlorocyclohexane.*

methyl b. toluene.

1,2-ben·zene·di·car·box·yl·ic ac·id (ben″zēn-di-kahr″bok-sil′ik) see *phthalic acid.*

ben·zene·meth·a·nol (ben″zēn-meth′ə-nol) benzyl alcohol.

ben·ze·noid (ben′zə-noid) a compound having a structure related to benzene or other compounds of aromatic character.

ben·ze·tho·ni·um chlo·ride (ben″zə-tho′ne-əm) [USP] a synthetic quaternary ammonium compound with detergent, emulsifying, antibacterial (gram-positive and some gram-negative bacteria), some antiviral, and some antifungal activity; applied topically to skin, mucous membranes, and wounds as an antiseptic, and used as a preservative in pharmaceutical preparations and cosmetics. It is also used to control algal growth in swimming pools.

benz·hex·ol hy·dro·chlo·ride (benz-hek′sol) BAN for *trihexyphenidyl hydrochloride.*

ben·zi·dine (ben′zĭ-dēn) a colorless, crystalline arylamine compound formed by the action of acids on hydrazobenzene; once widely used in testing for occult blood, its use is now limited because it is a carcinogen and is toxic if absorbed through the skin, ingested, or inhaled. Called also p-*diaminodiphenyl.*

ben·zil·o·ni·um bro·mide (ben″zil-o′ne-əm) an anticholinergic used in the treatment of peptic ulcer and functional gastrointestinal disorders.

ben·zi·mid·a·zole (ben″zĭ-mid′ə-zōl) a dicyclic compound comprising a benzene ring and an imidazole ring, occurring as part of the nucleotide portion of vitamin B_{12}. Substituted benzimidazoles inhibit the action of H^+/K^+-ATPase at the secretory surface of the parietal cells, thus blocking the final step of gastric acid production, and are used as inhibitors of gastric acid secretion. Several benzimidazoles are used as anthelmintics.

ben·zin (ben′zin) petroleum benzin; see under *petroleum.*

petroleum b. see under *petroleum.*

ben·zine (ben′zēn) petroleum benzin; see under *petroleum.*

ben·zi·sox·a·zole (ben″zi-sok′səzōl) 1. the parent compound of the benzisoxazole derivatives, a class of antipsychotic agents. 2. any of a family of drugs that have a substituted benzene ring bound to a ring that contains nitrogen and oxygen atoms.

benz(o)- a combining form denoting *(a)* fusion of a benzene ring to a cyclic organic molecule or *(b)* derivation from benzene or benzoic acid.

ben·zo·ate (ben′zo-āt) a salt of benzoic acid.

ben·zo·at·ed (ben′zo-āt-əd) containing or combined with benzoic acid.

ben·zo·caine (ben′zo-kān) [USP] a local anesthetic, applied topically to the skin and mucous membranes; it is also used to suppress the gag reflex in dental procedures, endoscopy, and intubation.

ben·zo·di·az·e·pine (ben″zo-di-az′ə-pēn) any of a group of compounds having a common molecular structure and acting similarly as depressants of the central nervous system, their actions including antianxiety, sedative, hypnotic, amnestic, anticonvulsant, and muscle relaxing effects.

ben·zo·ic ac·id (ben-zo′ik) [USP] benzenecarboxylic acid, a fungistatic compound used as a pharmaceutical and food preservative; it is conjugated to glycine in the liver and excreted as hippuric acid. See also *benzoic and salicylic acids ointment,* under *ointment.*

ben·zo·ic al·de·hyde (ben-zo′ik) benzaldehyde.

ben·zo·in (ben′zo-in) 1. [USP] a balsamic resin with an aromatic odor and taste, obtained from certain species of *Styrax;* it is used as a topical skin protectant, topical antiseptic, irritant expectorant, and inhalant in respiratory tract inflammation. Called also *gum benjamin* and *gum benzoin.* 2. a highly toxic crystalline compound, $C_{14}H_{12}O_2$, prepared by the condensation of benzaldehyde in an alkaline cyanide solution, used in organic synthesis.

ben·zol (ben′zol) benzene.

ben·zo·na·tate (ben-zo′nə-tāt) [USP] a peripherally acting antitussive that reduces the cough reflex by anesthetizing the stretch receptors in the respiratory passages, lungs, and pleura; administered orally.

ben·zo·phen·one (ben″zo-fen′ōn) an aromatic ketone that is a component of various drugs and cosmetics.

ben·zo·pur·pu·rine (ben′zo-pur′pu-rin) any of a series of red azo dyes, used especially as a contrast stain with hematoxylin and other blue stains.

b. 4B a compound used as an analytical reagent, as a biological stain, and as an indicator with a pH range of 1.2 (violet) to 4.0 (red).

ben·zo[*a*]py·rene (ben″zo-pi′rēn) 3,4-benzpyrene; a highly carcinogenic polycyclic aromatic hydrocarbon occurring as a product of incomplete combustion of carbonaceous materials. It is a procarcinogen that requires metabolic activation to exert a mutagenic effect.

ben·zo·qui·none (ben″zo-kwin′ōn) 1. a substituted benzene ring containing two carbonyl groups, usually in the *para* (1,4) position. *p*-Benzoquinone is used in the manufacture of dyes and hydroquinone, and in fungicides; it is toxic by inhalation and is an irritant to skin and mucous membranes. Called also *quinone.*

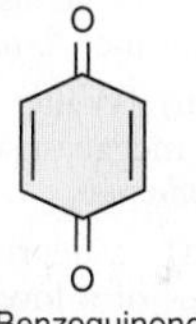

p-Benzoquinone

2. any of a subclass of quinones that are derived from or contain this structure, such as those involved in the electron transport chain of respiration.

ben·zo·thi·a·di·a·zide (ben″zo-thi″ə-di′ə-zīd) thiazide.

ben·zo·thi·a·di·a·zine (ben″zo-thi″ə-di′ə-zēn) thiazide.

ben·zo·yl (ben′zo-əl) the radical, C_6H_5CO—, of benzoic acid and of an extensive series of compounds.

b. peroxide, hydrous b. peroxide [USP] a topical antibacterial used in the treatment of acne vulgaris; it also has keratolytic, drying, and desquamative actions which promote evacuation of comedones. It is also used as an oxidizing agent in the treatment of decubital and stasis ulcers.

ben·zo·yl·ec·go·nine (ben″zo-əl-ek′go-nēn) the major metabolite of cocaine, produced by hydrolysis of the drug by plasma esterases and detectable in the blood by laboratory testing.

ben·zo·yl·gly·cine (ben″zo-əl-gli′sēn) hippuric acid.

ben·zo·yl·phen·yl·car·bi·nol (ben″zo-əl-fen″əl-kahr′bĭ-nol) benzoin (def. 2).

benz·phet·amine hy·dro·chlo·ride (benz-fet′ə-mēn) a sympathomimetic amine, related to amphetamine, used as an oral anorectic in the control of exogenous obesity.

3,4-benz·py·rene (benz-pi′rēn) benzo[*a*]pyrene.

benz·tro·pine mes·y·late (benz′tro-pēn) [USP] an antidyskinetic believed to act by partially blocking central cholinergic receptors, so that cholinergic and dopaminergic activity in the basal ganglia is more balanced; used in the treatment of parkinsonism and for the control of drug-induced extrapyramidal reactions (except tardive dyskinesia); administered orally, intramuscularly, and intravenously.

ben·zyl (ben′zəl) the hydrocarbon radical, C_7H_7 or $C_6H_5CH_2$—, of benzyl alcohol and various other compounds.

b. benzoate [USP] a clear, colorless, oily liquid, one of the active substances in peruvian and tolu balsams, and produced synthetically; applied topically as a scabicide.

b. bromide a war gas causing lacrimation and irritation of the skin; called also *cylite*.

b. carbinol phenylethyl alcohol.

ben·zyl·i·dene (ben-zil′ĭ-dēn) a hydrocarbon radical, $C_6H_5CH=$.

***p*-ben·zyl·oxy·phe·nol** (ben″zəl-ok″se-fe′nol) monobenzone.

ben·zyl·pen·i·cil·lin (ben″zəl-pen″ĭ-sil′in) INN and BAN for *penicillin G.*

ben·zyl·pen·i·cil·lo·yl poly·ly·sine (ben″zəl-pen″ĭ-sil′o-əl) a skin test antigen composed of a benzylpenicilloyl moiety (a major antigenic determinant of benzylpenicillin) conjugated to poly-L-lysine as a carrier, used in assessing hypersensitivity to penicillin by scratch test or intradermal test.

bep·ri·dil hy·dro·chlo·ride (bep′rĭ-dil) a calcium channel blocking agent that inhibits influx of calcium ions; it is nonselective, affecting both cardiac and smooth muscle and also inhibiting fast sodium inward currents; administered orally in the treatment of chronic angina pectoris.

ber·ac·tant (bər-ak′tənt) a modified bovine lung extract containing chiefly phospholipids that mimics the action of pulmonary surfactant, used in the prevention and treatment of neonatal respiratory distress syndrome; administered by endotracheal instillation.

Be·rar·di·nel·li-Seip syndrome (bə-rahr″dĭ-nel′e sīp′) [Waldemar *Berardinelli*, Argentine physician, 1903–1956; Martin Fredrik *Seip*, Norwegian pediatrician, born 1921] total lipodystrophy.

Bé·rard ligament (ba-rahr′) [Auguste *Bérard*, French surgeon, 1802–1846] see under *ligament.*

Bé·raud valve (ba-ro′) [Bruno Jean Jacques *Béraud*, French surgeon, 1823–1865] see under *valve.*

Ber·ber·i·da·ceae (bur″bər-ĭ-da′se-e) a family of herbs and shrubs, many of which have berries. Genera include *Berberis*, *Caulophyllum*, *Jeffersonia*, and *Podophyllum.*

ber·ber·ine (bur′bər-ēn) an alkaloid obtained from species of *Berberis* and other plants of the family Berberidaceae, as well as from *Hydrastis canadensis;* it has antimicrobial activity and has been used in treatment of various infections, as well as in ulcer dressings.

Ber·ber·is (bur′bər-is) [L.] a genus of shrubs of the family Berberidaceae that contain berberine. *B. vulga′ris* is the barberry (q.v.).

Ber·don syndrome (bur′dən) [Walter E. *Berdon*, American pediatric radiologist, late 20th century] megacystis-microcolon–intestinal hypoperistalsis syndrome; see under *syndrome.*

be·reave·ment (bə-rēv′mənt) a deprivation causing grief and desolation, especially the death or loss of a loved one. The period of grief and mourning following a bereavement often resembles clinical depression, but is a normal response. See also *mourning.*

Be·reit·schafts·po·ten·tial (bə-rīt″shahfts-pə-ten′shəl) [Ger.] readiness potential.

ber·ga·mot (bur′gə-mot) [L. *bergamium*] 1. *Citrus bergamia.* 2. the orangelike fruit of *C. bergamia;* its rind is a source of bergamot oil, which is used in perfumes. 3. any of various fragrant labiate plants, such as *Mentha citrata* and *Monarda fistulosa.*

Ber·ger disease (bār-zha′) [Jean *Berger*, French nephrologist, born 1930] IgA nephropathy.

Ber·ger operation (bār-zha′) [Paul *Berger*, French surgeon, 1845–1908] see under *operation.*

Ber·ger rhythm (bur′gər) [Hans *Berger*, German neurologist, 1873–1941] alpha rhythm; see under *rhythm.*

Ber·ger sign (bur′gər) [Emil *Berger*, Austrian ophthalmologist, 1855–1926] see under *sign.*

Ber·gey classification (bur′ge) [David Hendricks *Bergey*, American bacteriologist, 1860–1937] see under *classification.*

Ber·gey·el·la (bur′ge-el″ə) a genus of bacteria of the family Flavobacteriaceae, consisting of gram-negative rods; species are found most often in mammals other than humans.

B. zoohel′cum a species that is part of the normal flora in the mouths of dogs and cats but can cause cat-scratch in humans who are bitten by such animals.

Berg·man sign (bərg′mən) [Harry *Bergman*, American urologist, 1912–1998] see under *sign.*

Berg·mann cells, fibers (berg′mahn) [Gottlieb Heinrich *Bergmann*, German physician, 1781–1861] see under *cell* and *fiber.*

Ber·go·nié-Tri·bon·deau law (bār-go-nya′ tre-bon-do′) [Jean Alban *Bergonié*, French physician, 1857–1925; Louis *Tribondeau*, French naval physician, 1872–1918] see under *law.*

beri·beri (ber″e-ber′e) [Singhalese, "I cannot," signifying that the person is too ill to do anything] a disease caused by a deficiency of thiamine (vitamin B_1) and characterized by polyneuritis, cardiac pathology, and edema. The epidemic form is found primarily in areas in which white (polished) rice is the staple food, as in Japan, China, the Philippines, India, and other countries of Southeast Asia. Called also *rice disease*, *dietetic neuritis*, *neuritis multiplex endemica*, and *endemic polyneuritis*. See also *nutritional polyneuropathy*. **beriber′ic** *adj*

atrophic b. dry b.

cerebral b. Wernicke-Korsakoff syndrome.

dry b. a form of beriberi in which flaccid paralysis, muscular atrophy, and areflexia are the prominent signs; cardiac enlargement and tachycardia may be present. Called also *atrophic b.* and *paralytic b.*

infantile b. a disease of breast-fed infants whose mothers have thiamine deficiency; it is characterized by diminished urine secretion, progressive edema, and often by acute cardiac failure, which may terminate in sudden death. Vomiting, aphonia, opisthotonos, and convulsions may occur.

paralytic b. dry b.

wet b. beriberi marked by cardiac failure and edema, but without extensive nervous system involvement.

Berke operation (bərk) [Raynold Nathaniel *Berke*, American ophthalmologist, 1901–1986] see under *operation.*

berke·li·um (Bk) (burk′le-əm) [*Berkeley*, California, where it was produced] an element of atomic number 97, atomic weight 247, produced by bombardment of the isotope of americium of atomic weight 241 by helium ions; half-life $4\frac{1}{2}$ hours.

Ber·lin edema (bər-lin′) [Rudolf *Berlin*, German oculist, 1833–1897] commotio retinae.

Ber·nard puncture, syndrome (bār-nahr′) [Claude *Bernard*, French physiologist, 1813–1878] see under *puncture* and *syndrome.*

Ber·nard-Hor·ner syndrome (bār-nahr′ hor′nər) [C. *Bernard;* Johann Friedrich *Horner*, Swiss ophthalmologist, 1831–1886] Horner syndrome; see under *syndrome.*

Ber·nard-Sou·lier syndrome (bār-nahr′ sōō l-ya′) [Jean Alfred *Bernard*, French hematologist, 1907–2006; Jean-Pierre *Soulier*, French hematologist, 1915–2003] see under *syndrome.*

Ber·nays sponge (bur′nāz) [Augustus Charles *Bernays*, American surgeon, 1854–1907] see under *sponge.*

Bern·hardt disease, paresthesia (bern′hahrt) [Martin *Bernhardt*, German neurologist, 1844–1915] meralgia paresthetica.

Bern·hardt-Roth disease, syndrome (bern′hahrt rōt′) [M. *Bernhardt;* Vladimir Karlovich *Roth*, Russian neurologist, 1848–1916] meralgia paresthetica.

Bern·heim syndrome (bārn′hīm) [P. *Bernheim*, French physician, early 20th century] see under *syndrome.*

Ber·noul·li distribution, theorem, trial (bər-noo′le, bār-noo-e′) [Jakob *Bernoulli*, Swiss mathematician, 1654–1705] see under *distribution*, *theorem*, and *trial.*

Bern·stein test (bərn′stīn) [Lionel M. *Bernstein*, American internist, born 1923] see under *test.*

Ber·o·tec (ber′o-tek) trademark for a preparation of fenoterol hydrobromide.

Ber·ry ligament (ber′e) [Sir James *Berry*, Canadian surgeon, 1860–1946] ligamentum thyroideum laterale.

ber·ry (ber′e) a small fruit with a succulent pericarp.

bear b. bearberry.

chaste b., chaste tree b. the fruit of the chaste tree, which is used medicinally.

buckthorn b. *Rhamnus cathartica.*

horse nettle b. *Solanum carolinense.*

Ber·the·lot reaction (reagent) (bār-tə-lo′) [Pierre Eugène Marcellin *Berthelot*, French chemist, 1827–1907] see under *reaction.*

Ber·ti·el·la (bur″te-el′ə) a genus of tapeworms of the family Anoplocephalidae. *B. sa′tyri* (or *B. stu′deri*) is found in humans and other primates in India, Africa, the West Indies, the Philippines, and various islands in the Indian Ocean.

ber·ti·el·li·a·sis (bur″te-ə-li′ə-sis) infection with *Bertiella.*

Ber·tin bone (ossicle), columns (septa), ligament (bār-tă′) [Exupère Joseph *Bertin*, French anatomist, 1712–1781] see *concha sphenoidalis*, *columnae renales*, and *ligamentum iliofemorale.*

Ber·to·lot·ti syndrome (bār-to-lot′ē) [Mario *Bertolotti*, Italian physician, 20th century] see under *syndrome.*

Be·ru·bi·gen (bə-roo′bĭ-jen) trademark for preparations of cyanocobalamin.

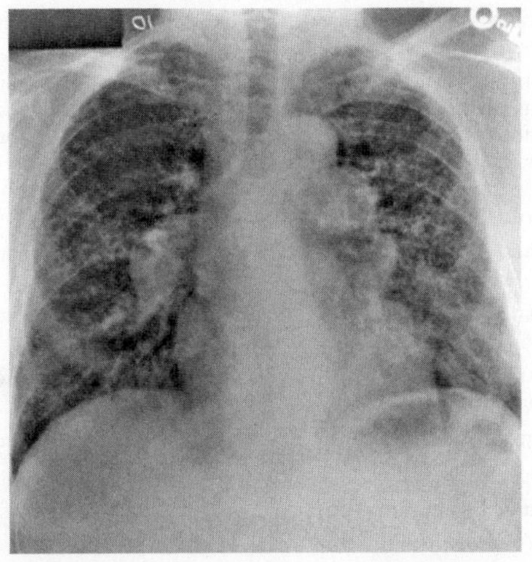

■ Beryllioisis. Posteroanterior chest radiograph demonstrates hilar adenopathy and extensive infiltrates.

be•ryl•li•o•sis (bə-ril″e-o′sis) [*beryllium* + *-osis*] a hypersensitivity response to beryllium, usually involving the lungs and less often the skin, subcutaneous tissues, lymph nodes, liver, or other structures. Beryllium fumes, its oxide and salts, and finely divided dust all may cause a tissue reaction when inhaled or implanted in the skin. Two varieties are distinguished: *acute b.* and *chronic b.* Called also *beryllium poisoning*.

acute b. an often fulminating reaction to inhalation of beryllium, characterized by a toxic or allergic pneumonitis, sometimes with rhinitis, pharyngitis, and tracheobronchitis. Symptoms may last for weeks, and serious cases can be fatal.

chronic b. the usual form of berylliosis, characterized by beryllium granulomas (q.v.), a diffuse inflammatory reaction that may be indistinguishable from sarcoidosis, and sometimes dyspnea and hypertrophic pulmonary osteoarthropathy. In time the granulomas may combine to form pulmonary nodules with fibrosis.

be•ryl•li•um (Be) (bə-ril′e-əm) [Gr. *bēryllos* beryl] a metallic element of atomic number 4, atomic weight 9.012. It is often found mixed with coal, and has many uses both in alloys and in pure form. Inhalation of its fumes causes berylliosis.

bes•i•clom•e•ter (bes″i-klom′ə-tər) [Fr. *besides* spectacles + *-meter*] an instrument for measuring the forehead to ascertain the proper width of spectacle frames.

Bes•nier prurigo (ba-nya′) [Ernest *Besnier*, French dermatologist, 1831–1909] see *atopic dermatitis*, under *dermatitis*, and see *prurigo gestationis*.

Bes•nier-Boeck disease (ba-nya′ bek′) [E. *Besnier;* Caesar Peter Moller *Boeck*, Norwegian dermatologist and syphilologist, 1845–1917] sarcoidosis.

Bes•noi•tia (bes-noi′te-ə) a genus of coccidian protozoa of the order Eucoccidiida whose oocysts resemble those of *Toxoplasma;* various species cause besnoitiosis in mammals. *B. bennet′ti* infects horses; *B. besnoi′ti* infects cattle; and *B. jelliso′ni* and *B. walla′cei* infect rodents.

bes•noi•ti•o•sis (bes-noi″te-o′sis) infection of herbivores with protozoa of the genus *Besnoitia*, transmitted mechanically by biting flies or by ingestion of oocysts shed in the feces of the cat, the definitive host. The organisms localize in the skin, blood vessels, mucous membranes of the upper respiratory tract, and subcutaneous and other tissues, where they eventually form characteristic thick-walled cysts. Other symptoms include fever, anasarca, loss of appetite, photophobia, rhinitis, sclerodermatitis, and alopecia of varying severity.

Best disease (macular degeneration) (best) [Franz *Best*, German ophthalmologist, 1878–1920] see under *disease*.

bes•ti•al•i•ty (bes-te-al′ĭ-te) [L. *bestia* beast] sexual connection with an animal. See also *zoophilia*.

bes•y•late (bes′ə-lāt) USAN contraction for benzenesulfonate.

Be•ta (be′tə) [L.] the beets, a genus of herbaceous plants of the family Chenopodiaceae. *B. vulga′ris* L. is the sugar beet, a commercial source of sucrose. The leafy tops of beets are rich in oxalates and can cause oxalate poisoning in animals that eat them in large amounts.

be•ta (ba′tə) [B, β] the second letter of the Greek alphabet. See also β-.

be•ta•car•o•tene (ba″tə-kar′ə-tēn) see under *carotene*.

be•ta•cho•les•ta•nol (ba″tə-ko-les′tə-nol) see under *cholestanol*.

be•ta•cism (ba′tə-siz-əm) [*beta*] a speech disorder involving excessive use of the *b* sound.

be•ta•dex (ba′tə-deks) [NF] β-cyclodextrin, a sequestrant used as a pharmaceutic aid; it has also been used as a carrier molecule for drug delivery. Called also *beta cyclodextrin*.

Be•ta•dine (ba′tə-dīn) trademark for preparations of povidone-iodine.

Be•ta•gan (ba′tə-gan) trademark for a preparation of levobunolol hydrochloride.

be•ta glob•u•lin (ba″tə-glob′u-lin) see *β-globulins*, under *globulin*.

pregnancy-specific b. g. a beta globulin secreted by the placenta; its function is unknown.

Be•ta•her•pes•vi•ri•nae (ba″tə-hur″pēz-vir-i′ne) the cytomegalovirus group: a subfamily of viruses of the family Herpesviridae; genera causing human infection include *Cytomegalovirus* and *Roseolovirus*. A number of species have not yet been assigned to a genus. See *cytomegalovirus*.

be•ta•his•tine hy•dro•chlo•ride (ba″tə-his′tēn) a histamine analogue used as a vasodilator to reduce the frequency of attacks of vertigo in Meniere disease, especially in patients having a high frequency of such attacks; administered orally.

be•ta•ine (be′tə-ēn) an oxidation product of choline that is a transmethylating intermediate in metabolism and has been shown to have lipotropic activity. It was found first in the sugar beet and later in many other plants, as well as in animals. It is produced synthetically, and is used in the treatment of homocystinuria. The term has also been used to designate any of a class of trimethyl derivatives of amino acids, such as carnitine, or more generally, the internal salts of quaternary ammonium bases. Called also *lycine* and *oxyneurine*.

b. hydrochloride [USP] the hydrochloride salt of betaine, which on hydrolysis yields hydrochloric acid; used as a gastric acidifier.

Be•ta•lin (ba′tə-lin) trademark for preparations containing components of the vitamin B complex. *Betalin Complex* is a sterile solution of synthetic B complex factors in sterile distilled water. *Betalin Complex F.C.* consists of synthetic vitamin B factors and synthetic ascorbic acid in sterile distilled water. *Betalin S* is a synthetic preparation of thiamine hydrochloride. *Betalin 12 crystalline* is a sterile isotonic solution of crystalline cyanocobalamin.

be•ta•ly•sin (ba″tə-li′sin) [so-called to distinguish it from antibodies, "alpha lysins"] a heat-stable cationic protein released by platelets during coagulation that is bactericidal for gram-positive bacteria with the exception of streptococci. Written also *beta lysin*.

be•ta•meth•a•sone (ba″tə-meth′ə-sōn) [USP] a synthetic glucocorticoid, the most active of the antiinflammatory steroids; used topically as an antiinflammatory and administered orally in replacement therapy for adrenal insufficiency and as an antiinflammatory and immunosuppressant in a wide variety of disorders.

b. acetate [USP] the acetate ester of betamethasone, having the same actions as the base; administered parenterally in combination with betamethasone sodium phosphate as an antiinflammatory and immunosuppressant.

b. benzoate [USP] the 17-benzoate ester of betamethasone, having the same actions as the base; used topically for the relief of inflammation and pruritus in corticosteroid-responsive dermatoses.

b. dipropionate [USP] the 17,21-dipropionate ester of betamethasone, having the same actions as the base; used topically for the relief of inflammation and pruritus in corticosteroid-responsive dermatoses.

b. sodium phosphate [USP] the disodium salt of the 21-phosphate ester of betamethasone, having the same actions as the base; used intramuscularly in the treatment of adrenocortical insufficiency and parenterally, alone or in combination with betamethasone acetate, as an antiinflammatory and immunosuppressant; also applied topically to the conjunctiva and ear canal and given as a retention enema as an antiinflammatory.

b. valerate [USP] the 17-valerate ester of betamethasone, used topically for the relief of inflammation and pruritus in corticosteroid-responsive dermatoses.

be•ta•naph•thol•sul•fon•ic ac•id (ba″tə-naf″thol-sul-fon′ik) white pearly scales tinged with red, $OH•C_{10}H_6SO_2•OH$, used as a test for albumin in the urine; it is a toxic drug that causes profound narcotism and symptoms resembling diabetic coma and is not used as a medication.

be•ta•nin (be′tə-nin) the red pigment of the root of the beet.

Be•ta•pace (ba′tə-pās″) trademark for preparations of sotalol hydrochloride.

Be•ta•pap•il•lo•ma•vi•rus (ba″tə-pap″ĭ-lo′mə-vi″rəs) a genus of viruses of the family Papillomaviridae that contains several of the human papillomaviruses.

Be•ta•par (ba′tə-pahr) trademark for a preparation of meprednisone.

Be•ta•prone (ba′tə-prōn) trademark for a preparation of propiolactone.

be•ta•pro•pio•lac•tone (ba″tə-pro″pe-o-lak′tōn) propiolactone.

Be•ta•pro•teo•bac•te•ria (ba″tə-pro″te-o-bak-tēr′e-ə) [*beta* the second letter of the Greek alphabet + *Proteobacteria*] a class of bacteria of the Proteobacteria, grouped together on the basis 16S rRNA sequence analysis; organisms of medical interest are included in the orders Burkholderiales, Comamonadaceae, Neisseriales, and Nitrosomonadales.

be•ta•qui•nine (ba″tə-kwi′nīn) quinidine.

Be•ta•ret•ro•vi•rus (ba″tə-ret′ro-vi″rəs) a genus of the family Retroviridae, with species that infect sheep, mice, and Old World primates. The viruses have a characteristic dense core 40–60 nm in diameter that is enclosed by a membranous envelope 90–120 nm in diameter with prominent surface spikes; capsid assembly occurs in the cytoplasm prior to budding from the plasma membrane. It contains the species mouse mammary tumor virus. **betaretrovi′ral** *adj*

Be•ta•ser•on (ba″tə-sēr′on) trademark for a preparation of interferon beta-1b.

Be•ta•trex (ba″tə-treks′) trademark for preparations of betamethasone valerate.

be•ta•tron (ba′tə-tron) an apparatus for accelerating electrons to millions of electron volts by means of magnetic induction.

Beta-Val (ba′tə-val″) trademark for preparations of betamethasone valerate.

be•tax•o•lol hy•dro•chlo•ride (ba-tak′sə-lol) [USP] a cardioselective beta-adrenergic blocking agent that acts at β_1-adrenergic receptors; used as an oral antihypertensive and also as an ophthalmic preparation to treat ocular hypertension and glaucoma.

Be•tax•on (ba-tak′son) trademark for a preparation of levobetaxolol hydrochloride.

bête (bet) [Fr.] beast; a nonhuman animal.
 b. rouge (rōōzh) ["red beast"] chigger.

be•tel (be′təl) [Tamil *vettilei*] 1. a plant of the species *Piper betle*, or the dried leaf of this plant (betel leaf). 2. a plant of the species *Areca catechu*, or the dried ripe seed of this plant (areca, also called betel nut). 3. a masticatory used in India and Southeast Asia, consisting of a piece of areca (betel nut) rolled up with lime in a betel leaf; it is tonic, astringent, and stimulant, but can be toxic (see *betel cancer*, under *cancer*).

be•than•e•chol chlo•ride (bə-than′ə-kol) [USP] a cholinergic agonist having primarily muscarinic, prokinetic effects; used to stimulate smooth muscle contraction of the urinary bladder in the treatment of postoperative, postpartum, or neurogenic atony of the bladder with retention. Administered orally or subcutaneously.

Be•thea sign (method) (bə-tha′ə) [Oscar Walter *Bethea*, American physician, 1878–1963] see under *sign*.

Be•thes•da Sys•tem (bə-thez′də) [*Bethesda*, Maryland, location of the National Cancer Institute, which sponsored its development] see under *system*.

Bet•i•mol (bet′ĭ-mol) trademark for preparations of timolol.

Be•top•tic (ba-top′tik) trademark for preparations of betaxolol hydrochloride.

Bet•u•la (bet′u-lə) [L.] the birches, a genus of deciduous trees of the family Betulaceae, native to the Northern Hemisphere. *B. al′ba* L. is the white birch, whose bark yields birch tar oil. *B. len′ta* is the black birch, whose bark is a source of methyl salicylate.

Betz cells, cell area (bets) [Vladimir Aleksandrovich *Betz*, Russian anatomist, 1834–1894] see under *cell*, and see *primary somatomotor area*, under *area*.

BeV, Bev billion electron volts; the term is now largely replaced by the term *gigaelectron volt* (GeV).

bev•a•ciz•u•mab (bev″ə-siz′u-mab) a monoclonal antibody that interferes with tumor blood supply by inhibiting vascular endothelial growth factor, used in combination with standard chemotherapeutic agents for the treatment of metastatic colorectal cancer; administered intravenously.

Bev•an incision (bev′ən) [Arthur Dean *Bevan*, American surgeon, 1861–1943] see under *incision*.

bev•el (bev′əl) 1. a slanting edge. 2. to produce a slanting of the enamel margins of a tooth cavity.

Bev•i•dox (bev′ĭ-doks) trademark for a solution of vitamin B_{12}; see *cyanocobalamin*.

bex•ar•o•tene (bek-sar′ə-tēn) a retinoid that modulates transcription and expression of genes involved in cellular differentiation and proliferation; used as an antineoplastic in the treatment of cutaneous T-cell lymphoma, administered orally. It is also applied topically in the treatment of cutaneous lesions of T-cell lymphomas and Kaposi sarcoma.

Bex•tra (beks′trə) trademark for a preparation of valdecoxib.

Bex•xar (beks′ər) trademark for a preparation of tositumomab.

be•za•fi•brate (be″zə-fi′brāt) a fibric acid derivative used in the treatment of hyperlipoproteinemia, administered orally

be•zoar (be′zor) [Farsi *pādzohr* antidote to poison] a concretion of foreign material found in the gastrointestinal tract or urinary tract; types include trichobezoar (hair), phytobezoar (fruit and vegetable fibers), trichophytobezoar (hair mixed with plant fibers), and fungus ball.
 fungal b. fungus ball.
 medication b. pharmacobezoar.

Be•zold abscess, etc. (bāt′sōlt) [Friedrich *Bezold*, German otologist, 1842–1908] see under *abscess*, *mastoiditis*, *perforation*, *sign*, and *triad*.

Be•zold ganglion, reflex (bāt′sōlt) [Albert von *Bezold*, German physiologist, 1836–1868] see under *ganglion* and *reflex*.

Be•zold-Jar•isch reflex (bāt′sōlt yah′rish) [A. von *Bezold*; Adolf *Jarisch*, Austrian dermatologist, 1850–1902] Bezold reflex.

BF blastogenic factor; see *lymphocyte mitogenic factor*, under *factor*.

BFP biologic false-positive.

BFU-E burst-forming unit–erythroid.

BH4, BH_4 tetrahydrobiopterin.

BHA butylated hydroxyanisole.

BHC benzene hexachloride.

BHCDA Bureau of Health Care Delivery and Assistance, an agency of the Health Resources and Services Administration.

BHPR Bureau of Health Professions, an agency of the Health Resources and Services Administration.

BHRD Bureau of Health Resources Development, an agency of the Health Resources and Services Administration.

BHT butylated hydroxytoluene.

Bi bismuth.

bi- [L. *bi-*, from *bis* twice] a prefix meaning two, twice, or double. In chemistry, it denotes the presence of a component in twice the proportion of the other component or in twice the usual proportion, or a double radical, except that in bicarbonate, bisulfate, and bitartrate, the prefix *di-* is preferred. Before vowels it appears as *bin-*.

bi-acro•mi•al (bi-ə-kro′me-əl) between the two acromia.

Bi•al reagent, test (be′əl) [Manfred *Bial*, German physician, 1870–1908] see under *reagent* and *test*.

bi•ar•tic•u•lar (bi″ahr-tik′u-lər) diarthric.

bi•ar•tic•u•late (bi″ahr-tik′u-lāt) pertaining to or having two joints.

bi•as (bi′əs) 1. (in a measurement process) systematic error. 2. (of a statistical estimator) the difference between the expected value of the estimator and the true parameter value.
 ascertainment b. systematic error causing failure to represent equally all groups of cases or persons that should be represented in a sample.
 conservative b. a bias in study design that makes it less likely to find a true difference than it would be with an unbiased study.
 lead-time b. systematic error introduced when monitoring of all groups or individuals does not begin at precisely the same time, such as an illusion of longer survival that is really due to earlier diagnosis of the disease.
 measurement b. bias due to systematic error in measurement during data collection.
 misclassification b. see *misclassification*.
 recall b. systematic error due to differential recall across subjects, particularly a tendency for cases to remember more events from the study period than do controls.
 selection b. systematic error in the manner in which cases and controls are chosen for a study or for allocation to groups.
 surveillance b. increased detection of signs or symptoms, many of which would otherwise go unnoticed, caused by increased frequency and intensity of surveillance, as that of subjects under treatment in a study.

bi•as•ter•ic (bi″əs-ter′ik) pertaining to the two asteria, especially to the shortest distance between them (biasteric width).

bi•au•ric•u•lar (bi″aw-rik′u-lər) [*bi-* + *auricular*] pertaining to the two auricles of the ears. Called also *binauricular*.

Bi•ax•in (bi-ak′sin) trademark for a preparation of clarithromycin.

Bib. [L.] bi′be (drink).

bib (bib) the remaining fragment of an erythrocyte in which the crescentic gametocyte of *Plasmodium falciparum* is developing in malaria.

bi•ba•sic (bi-ba′sik) doubly basic; having two hydrogen atoms that may react with bases. Cf. *dibasic*.

bi•ba•si•lar (bi-bas′ĭ-lər) pertaining to or affecting the bases of both of a pair of structures or organs.

bi•bev•eled (bi-bev′əld) having a slanting surface on two sides, as some dental instruments; hatchet-edged.

bib•lio•ther•a•py (bib″le-o-ther′ə-pe) [Gr. *biblion* book + *therapy*] the reading of selected books as part of the treatment of mental disorders or for mental health; see also *poetry therapy*, under *therapy*.

bib•u•lous (bib′u-ləs) [L. *bibulus*, from *bibere* to drink] 1. absorbent or spongy. 2. having the property of absorbing moisture. Cf. *hygroscopic*.

bi•ca•lu•ta•mide (bi″kə-loo′tə-mīd) an antiandrogen used as a treatment adjunct, in combination with measures to lower testosterone levels, such as administration of a luteinizing hormone–releasing hormone analogue, in the treatment of prostatic carcinoma; administered orally.

bi•cam•er•al (bi-kam′ər-əl) [*bi-* + *camera*] having two chambers.

bi•cap•su•lar (bi-kap′su-lər) [*bi-* + *capsular*] having two capsules, as an articular capsule.

bi•car•bo•nate (bi-kahr′bə-nāt) any salt containing the HCO_3^- anion.
blood b., plasma b. the bicarbonate of the blood, an index of the alkali reserve.
b. of soda sodium bicarbonate.
standard b. the plasma bicarbonate concentration in blood equilibrated with a gas mixture having a P_{CO_2} of 40 mm Hg and a P_{O_2} over 100 mm Hg at 37°C.

bi•car•bo•na•te•mia (bi-kahr″bə-na-te′me-ə) hyperbicarbonatemia.

bi•car•bo•na•tu•ria (bi-kahr″bə-na-tu′re-ə) excretion of excessive amounts of bicarbonates in the urine, as seen in proximal renal tubular acidosis.

bi•cau•dal (bi-kaw′dəl) [*bi-* + *caudal*] having two tails.

bi•cau•date (bi-kaw′dāt) bicaudal.

bi•cel•lu•lar (bi-sel′u-lər) made up of two cells, or having two cells.

bi•ceph•a•lus (bi-sef′ə-ləs) dicephalus.

bi•ceps (bi′seps) [*bi-* + L. *caput* head] a muscle having two heads.
b. bra′chii see under *musculus*.
b. fem′oris see under *musculus*.

Bi•chat fissure, ligament, etc. (be-shah′) [Marie François Xavier *Bichat*, French anatomist and physiologist, 1771–1802, founder of scientific histology and pathological anatomy] see under *ligament*, see *fenestrated membrane* under *membrane*, and see *fissura transversa cerebri*.

bi•chlo•ride (bi-klor′īd) any chloride that contains two equivalents of chlorine.

bi•chro•mate (bi-kro′māt) dichromate.

Bi•cil•lin C-R (bi-sil′in) trademark for combination preparations of penicillin G benzathine and penicillin G procaine.

Bi•cil•lin L-A (bi-sil′in) trademark for preparations of penicillin G benzathine.

bi•cip•i•tal (bi-sip′ĭ-təl) 1. having two heads. 2. pertaining to a biceps muscle.

bi•cir•o•mab (bi-sir′o-mab) mouse anti-human monoclonal antibody to fibrin; used in the radioactive form (complexed with technetium 99m) in the diagnosis of deep vein thrombosis. See table at *technetium*.

bi•cis•ate (bi-sis′āt) a lipophilic amine having the ability to cross the blood-brain barrier and localize in the brain; complexed with technetium 99m, it is used in imaging of the cerebrovascular system, giving a static image of regional cerebral blood flow. See table at *technetium*. Called also *ethyl cysteinate dimer (ECD)*.

bi•cis•tron•ic (bi-sis-tron′ik) pertaining to or having two cistrons; said of uncommon messenger RNAs that contain information for two proteins.

Bic•ker•staff migraine (bik′ər-staf) [Edwin Robert *Bickerstaff*, British physician, born 1920] basilar migraine.

BiCNU (bik′noo) trademark for preparations of carmustine.

bi•col•lis (bi-kol′is) [L., from *bi-* + *collum*] having a double cervix; see *uterus bicornis bicollis*, under *uterus*.

bi•con•cave (bi″kon-kāv′) [*bi-* + *concave*] having two concave surfaces, as the opposite sides of a structure.

bi•con•vex (bi″kon-veks′) having two convex surfaces, as the opposite sides of a structure.

bi•cor•nate (bi-kor′nāt) bicornuate.

bi•cor•nu•ate (bi-kor′nu-āt) [*bi-* + *cornuate*] having two horns or horn-shaped branches, such as the uterus of most mammals.

bi•cor•o•nal (bi-kor′ə-nəl) 1. pertaining to the two coronae radiatae, one radiating from each internal capsule of the brain. 2. pertaining to or performed through both coronal sutures.

bi•cor•po•rate (bi-kor′pə-rət) [*bi-* + *corpora* + *-ate*] having two bodies.

bi•cris•tal (bi-kris′təl) [*bi-* + L. *crista* crest] pertaining to two crests.

bi•cu•cul•line (bi-koo′kə-lēn″) an alkaloid neurotoxin found in species of *Corydalis*, *Dicentra*, and other plants; it is a convulsant and acts as an antagonist to the inhibitory neurotransmitter γ-aminobutyric acid.

bi•cus•pid (bi-kus′pid) [*bi-* + *cuspid*] 1. having two cusps or points. 2. (pl.) premolar teeth.

bi•cus•pi•dal (bi-kus′pĭ-dəl) bicuspid (def. 1).

b.i.d. [L.] bis in di′e (twice a day).

Bid•der ganglia, organ (bid′ər) [Heinrich Friedrich *Bidder*, Estonian anatomist, 1810–1894] see under *ganglion* and *organ*.

bi•den•tal (bi-den′təl) [*bi-* + *dental*] having, pertaining to, or affecting two teeth.

bi•den•tate (bi-den′tāt) having two teeth or toothlike structures.

bi•der•mal (bi-dur′məl) made up of two of the three germ cell layers; said of tumors.

bi•der•mo•ma (bi″dər-mo′mə) didermoma.

Bi•Dil (bi′dil) trademark for a preparation of isosorbide dinitrate.

Biedl disease, syndrome (be′dəl) [Artur *Biedl*, Austrian physician, 1869–1933] Bardet-Biedl syndrome.

Biels•chow•sky head tilting test (byels-chov′ske) [Alfred *Bielschowsky*, German ophthalmologist, 1871–1940] see under *test*.

Biels•chow•sky method (byels-chov′ske) [Max *Bielschowsky*, German neuropathologist, 1869–1940] see *Stains and Staining Methods*, under *stain*.

Biels•chow•sky-Jan•ský disease (byels-chov′ske yahn′ske) [A. *Bielschowsky*; Jan *Janský*, Czech psychiatrist, 1873–1921] Janský-Bielschowsky disease; see under *disease*.

Bie•mond syndrome (be-maw′) [Arie *Biemond*, Dutch neurologist, 1902–1973] see under *syndrome*.

Bier amputation (operation), block (anesthesia) (byār) [August Karl Gustav *Bier*, German surgeon, 1861–1949] see under *amputation* and *block*.

Bier•nac•ki sign (byer-naht′ske) [Edmund Adolfevich *Biernacki*, Polish physician, 1866–1912] see under *sign*.

Bie•sia•dec•ki fossa (byĕ-syah-det′ske) [Alfred von *Biesiadecki*, Polish physician, 1839–1888] iliacosubfascial fossa.

Biett collarette (byet) [Laurent Théodore *Biett*, French dermatologist, 1781–1840] see under *collarette*.

bi•fas•cic•u•lar (bi″fə-sik′u-lər) pertaining to two bundles, or fasciculi.

bi•fe•ri•ens (bi-fer′e-ənz) [L.] bisferious.

bi•fer•i•ous (bi-fer′e-əs) [*bi-* + L. *ferire* to beat] bisferious.

bi•fid (bi′fid) [L. *bifidus* divided into two parts] cleft into two parts or branches.

bi•fid•i•ty (bĭ-fid-ĭ-te) the quality of being bifid, either from a birth defect or as an iatrogenic deformity such as after rhinoplasty.

Bi•fi•do•bac•te•ri•a•ceae (bi″fid-o-bak-tēr″e-a′se-e) a family of bacteria of the order Bifidobacteriales, grouped together on the basis of 16S rRNA sequence analysis and including the genera *Bifidobacterium* and *Gardnerella*.

Bi•fi•do•bac•te•ri•a•les (bi″fid-o-bak-tēr″e-a′lēz) an order of bacteria of the subclass Actinobacteridae (class Actinobacteria), containing the single family Bifidobacteriaceae.

Bi•fid•o•bac•te•ri•um (bi″fid-o-bak-tēr′e-əm) [*bifidus* + *bacterium*] a genus of gram-positive, anaerobic bacteria of the family Bifidobacteriaceae, occurring as irregularly staining rods of bifurcated Y and V forms and club or spatulate shapes.
B. adolescen′tis a species isolated from human feces, the appendix, the vagina, dental caries, and abscesses.
B. bi′fidum a species found in the alimentary tract and in the stools of breast- and bottle-fed infants and in human adults.
B. infan′tis a species that is the predominant bifidobacterium found in the feces of breast-fed infants.

bi•fid•o•bac•te•ri•um (bi″fid-o-bak-tēr′e-əm) pl. *bifidobacte′ria*. Any bacterium of the genus *Bifidobacterium*.

bif•i•dus (bif′ĭ-dəs) bifid.

bi•fo•cal (bi-fo′kəl, bi′fo-kəl) 1. having two foci. 2. containing one part for near vision and another part for distant vision; see under *lens*.

bi•fo•cals (bi′fo-kəlz) bifocal glasses.

bi•fo•rate (bi-for′āt) [*bi-* + L. *fora* opening] having two foramina or openings.

bi•for•myl (bi-for′məl) glyoxal.

bi•fur•cate (bi-fur′kāt) [L. *bifurcatus*, from *bi-* + *furca* fork] forked; divided into two branches.

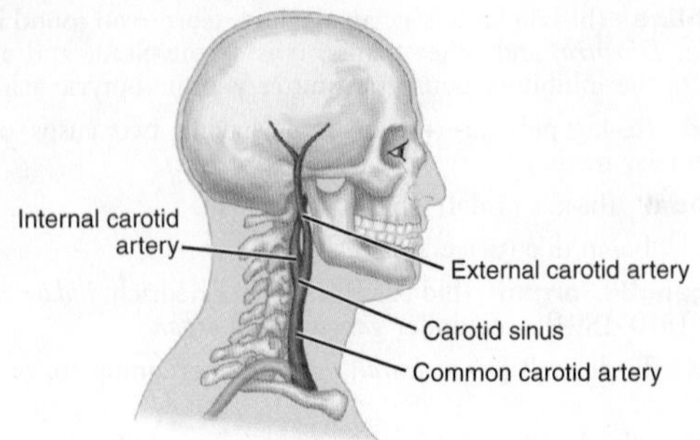

■ Bifurcatio carotidis (carotid bifurcation).

bi•fur•ca•tio (bi″fər-ka′she-o) pl. *bifurcatio′nes* [L.] bifurcation; the site where a single structure divides into two, as in blood vessels or teeth.

b. aor′tae [TA] bifurcation of aorta: the site on the left side of the body of the fourth lumbar vertebra, where the abdominal aorta divides into the right and left common iliac arteries.

b. caro′tidis [TA] carotid bifurcation: the site where the common carotid artery divides into the external carotid artery and internal carotid artery, usually marked by a dilatation, the carotid sinus.

b. tra′cheae [TA] tracheal bifurcation: the site of division of the trachea into the right and left main bronchi.

b. trun′ci pulmona′lis [TA] bifurcation of pulmonary trunk: the site of the division of the pulmonary trunk into right and left pulmonary arteries.

bi•fur•ca•tion (bi″fər-ka′shən) [L. *bifurcatio,* from *bi-* + *furca* fork] 1. division into two branches. 2. bifurcatio.

b. of aorta bifurcatio aortae.

carotid b. bifurcatio carotidis.

b. of pulmonary trunk bifurcatio trunci pulmonalis.

b. of trachea, tracheal b. bifurcatio tracheae.

bi•fur•ca•ti•o•nes (bi″fər-ka″she-o′nēz) [L.] plural of *bifurcatio.*

Big•e•low ligament, operation (big′ə-lo) [Henry Jacob *Bigelow,* American surgeon, 1818–1890] see *ligamentum iliofemorale,* see *litholapaxy.*

bi•gem•i•na (bi-jem′ĭ-nə) 1. plural of *bigeminum.* 2. bigeminal pulse.

bi•gem•i•num (bi-jem′ĭ-nəm) pl. *bigem′ina* [L. "twin"] either of the corpora bigemina; see under *corpus.*

bi•gem•i•ny (bi-jem′ĭ-ne) [*bi-* + *geminus*] 1. occurring in pairs. 2. the occurrence of a bigeminal pulse. **bigem′inal** *adj*

atrial b. an arrhythmia consisting of the repetitive sequence of one atrial premature complex followed by one normal sinus impulse.

atrioventricular nodal b. an arrhythmia in which an atrioventricular extrasystole is followed by a normal sinus impulse in repetitive sequence.

nodal b. atrioventricular nodal b.

ventricular b. an arrhythmia consisting of the repeated sequence of one ventricular premature complex followed by one normal beat.

bi•ger•mi•nal (bi-jur′mĭ-nəl) pertaining to two germs, oocytes, or ova.

big•head (big′hed) 1. bulging of the skull bones of an animal, due to osteomalacia. 2. acute infection of young rams by *Clostridium novyi,* which enters the tissues through head wounds acquired in fighting; it is characterized by intense edematous swelling of the head, face, and neck. Called also *swellhead* and *swelled head.* 3. photosensitization in white-faced sheep after ingestion of certain plants, characterized by thickening and pendulous swelling of the face and ears. 4. hydrocephalus in mink. 5. nutritional secondary hyperparathyroidism.

bi•gly•can (bi-gli′kan) a small (150–240kD) leucine-rich repeat protein of the extracellular matrix, consisting of two glycosaminoglycan chains and associated oligosaccharides.

bi•go•ni•al (bi-go′ne-əl) connecting the two gonions.

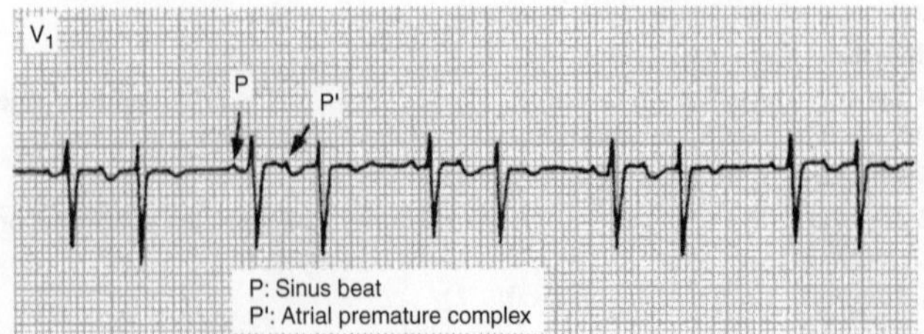

■ Atrial bigeminy; each sinus beat is followed by an atrial premature complex.

bi•gua•nide (bi-gwah′nīd) 1. a base:

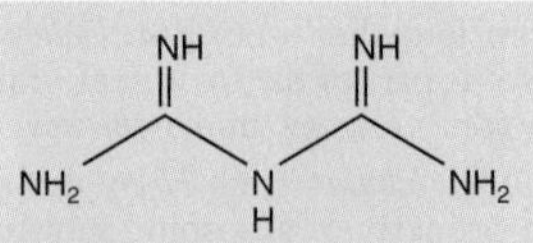

2. any of a group of substituted derivatives of biguanide, which are used as oral antihyperglycemic agents; they increase insulin action in peripheral tissues and by inhibiting gluconeogenesis decrease hepatic glucose production.

bi•labe (bi′lāb) [*bi-* + *labium*] an instrument for taking small calculi from the bladder through the urethra.

bi•la•bi•al (bi-la′be-əl) a consonantal speech sound produced using the two lips, such as *b, p,* or *m.* Called also *labial.*

bi•lam•i•nar (bi-lam′ĭ-nər) [*bi-* + *laminar*] having or pertaining to two layers, as the basement membrane that comprises the basal lamina and the reticular lamina.

Bil•ar•cil (bil-ahr′sil) trademark for preparations of trichlorphon.

bi•lat•er•al (bi-lat′ər-əl) [*bi-* + *lateral*] having two sides, or pertaining to both sides.

bi•lat•er•al•ism (bi-lat′ər-əl-iz-əm) bilateral symmetry.

bi•lay•er (bi′la-ər) a membrane consisting of two molecular layers, such as the cell membrane or the envelope of some viruses.

lipid b., phospholipid b. the structure common to all biological membranes, consisting of two layers of phospholipids with their hydrophilic head groups exposed to the aqueous medium and hydrophobic tails directed inward.

bil•ber•ry (bil′ber-e) 1. any of various shrubs of the genus *Vaccinium* having edible blue to blue-black fruit. 2. the leaves and fruit of *V. myrtillus,* having astringent and antidiarrheal effects, used topically for local inflammation, burns, and skin diseases, and orally for gout, arthritis, dermatitis, and gastrointestinal, urinary tract, and kidney disorders, and for the prevention and treatment of diabetes mellitus.

bile (bīl) [L. *bilis*] a fluid secreted by the liver and drained into the small intestine via the bile ducts. Important constituents are conjugated bile salts, cholesterol, phospholipids, bilirubin diglucuronide, and electrolytes. Bile is alkaline due to its bicarbonate content, is golden brown to greenish yellow in color, and has a bitter taste. After it is secreted by the liver (see *C bile*), it is concentrated in the gallbladder (see *B bile*). Its formation depends on active secretion by hepatic cells into the bile canaliculi. Excretion of bile salts by hepatic cells and secretion of bicarbonate-rich fluid by ductular cells in response to secretin are the major factors that normally determine the volume of secretion. Conjugated bile salts and phospholipids normally dissolve cholesterol in a mixed micellar solution. In the upper small intestine, bile is in part responsible for alkalinizing the intestinal contents, and conjugated bile salts play an essential role in fat absorption by dissolving the products of fat digestion (fatty acids and monoglycerides) in water-soluble micelles. Called also *gall.*

A b. bile from the common bile duct; samples are obtained by use of a duodenal tube before gallbladder stimulation. It usually contains 20–200 mg of bilirubin per 100 mL.

B b. bile from the gallbladder; samples are obtained by use of a duodenal tube after gallbladder contraction stimulation, usually with magnesium sulfate. It may occur despite absence of the gallbladder and contains up to 1 gram of bilirubin per 100 mL.

C b. bile from the liver; samples are obtained from a duodenal drainage tube after the gallbladder has been emptied.

limy b. milk of calcium b.

milk of calcium b. bile containing an increased amount of calcium, usually as the carbonate but sometimes as the phosphate or bilirubinate. It varies in consistency from a thick, milky fluid to a putty, gel, or solid, and is usually suspended in a thin, more watery bile. Called also *limy b.*

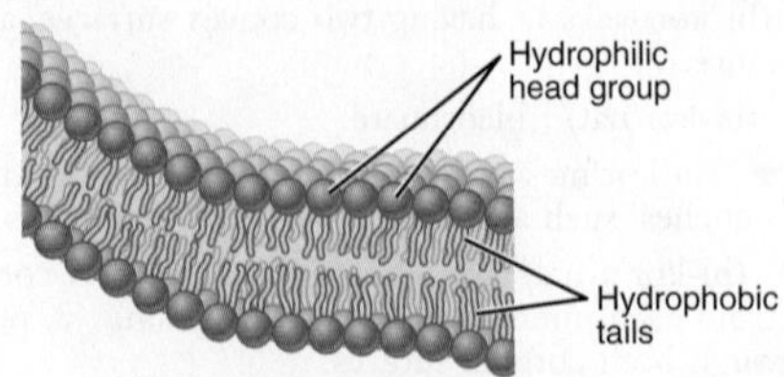

■ Lipid bilayer, a fluid barrier to permeability, with polar head groups exposed and hydrophobic tails sequestered.

white b. a colorless liquid containing mucoproteins and calcium salts but no bile pigments, sometimes found in the gallbladder in obstructions above the entrance of the cystic duct.

bile ac·id (bīl) any of the steroid carboxylic acids derived from cholesterol. The *primary bile acids,* cholic and chenodeoxycholic acids, are formed in the liver and conjugated to glycine or taurine, forming bile salts (e.g., cholylglycine), which are secreted in the bile and aid in the digestion of fats. *Secondary bile acids,* deoxycholic, lithocholic, and ursodeoxycholic acids, are formed from the primary bile acids by the action of intestinal bacteria, either as bile salts or as deconjugated bile acids. Most of the bile acids are reabsorbed and returned to the liver via enterohepatic circulation, where, after free acids are reconjugated, they are again excreted. Because the lithocolyl conjugates are relatively insoluble they are excreted mostly in the form of sulfate esters (sulfolithocholylglycine and sulfolithocholyltaurine) produced by the liver.

Bil·har·zia (bil-hahr′ze-ə) [Theodor Maximilian *Bilharz,* German physician, 1825–1862] *Schistosoma.*

bil·har·zi·al (bil-hahr′ze-əl) schistosomal.

bil·har·zi·a·sis (bil″hahr-zi′ə-sis) schistosomiasis.

bil·har·zic (bil-hahr′zik) schistosomal.

bil·har·zi·o·ma (bil-hahr″ze-o′mə) a tumor in the skin or mucous membrane caused by a schistosome. Cf. *schistosomal bladder carcinoma.*

bil·har·zi·o·sis (bil-hahr″ze-o′sis) schistosomiasis.

bil·he·mia (bil-he′me-ə) a rare condition in which bile enters the bloodstream, usually via the portal circulation, owing to trauma to the liver or a complication of surgery.

bil(i)- [L. *bilis* bile] a combining form denoting relationship to the bile.

bil·i·ary (bil′e-ar-e) pertaining to the bile, bile ducts, or gallbladder. See also *bilious.*

bil·i·cy·a·nin (bil″ĭ-si′ə-nin) [*bili-* + L. *cyaneus* blue] a blue bile pigment, derivable from biliverdin by oxidation and found in gallstones.

bil·i·fus·cin (bil″ĭ-fus′in) [*bili-* + L. *fuscus* brown] a brown bile pigment found in bile and gallstones.

bil·i·gen·e·sis (bil″ĭ-jen′ə-sis) the production of bile. **biligenet′ic,** biligen′ic *adj*

bil·i·hu·min (bil″ĭ-hu′min) [*bili-* + L. *humus* earth] a dark, insoluble bile pigment found in gallstones.

bi·lin (bi′lin) [L. *bilis* bile] collective name for yellow bile pigments, including urobilin and stercobilin, formed by spontaneous oxidation of the central methylidene group of corresponding bilinogen; they are generated in the final steps of bilirubin catabolism.

bi·lin·o·gen (bĭ-lin′ə-jen) a colorless bile pigment, which can be oxidized to form a bilin.

bil·i·o·en·ter·ic (bil″-e-o-en-ter′ik) pertaining to or connecting a biliary duct and the small intestine.

bil·ious (bil′yəs) [L. *biliosus*] 1. characterized by an excess of bile or by biliousness. 2. biliary.

bil·ious·ness (bil′yəs-nis) a symptom complex formerly attributed to excessive secretion of bile, consisting of nausea, abdominal discomfort, headache, and constipation.

bil·i·pra·sin (bil″ĭ-pra′sin) [*bili-* + Gr. *prasinos* green] a green bile pigment found in gallstones.

bil·i·ra·chia (bil″ĭ-ra′ke-ə) [*bili-* + *rachi-* + *-ia*] the presence of bile pigments in the spinal fluid.

bil·i·ru·bin (bil″ĭ-roo′bin) [*bili-* + *ruber*] a yellow bile pigment that is a breakdown product of heme mainly formed from the degradation of erythrocyte hemoglobin in reticuloendothelial cells; it is also formed by breakdown of other heme pigments, such as cytochromes. Bilirubin normally circulates in plasma as a complex with albumin, and is taken up by the liver cells and conjugated to form water-soluble bilirubin diglucuronide for excretion in the bile. In patients with cholestasis, this latter form accumulates in the blood and tissues and is excreted in the urine. (Unconjugated bilirubin is not excreted in the urine.) High concentrations of bilirubin may result in jaundice. **bilirubin′ic** *adj*

conjugated b. bilirubin that has been taken up by the liver cells and conjugated to form the water-soluble compound bilirubin diglucuronide, which can be excreted in the bile.

b. diglucuronide a conjugated water-soluble form of bilirubin, formed in the liver by esterification of two molecules of glucuronide to the bilirubin molecule; this is the usual form in which bilirubin is found in the bile.

direct b. conjugated b.

indirect b. unconjugated b.

unconjugated b. the lipid-soluble form of bilirubin that circulates in loose association with the plasma proteins; called also *indirect b.*

bil·i·ru·bi·nate (bil″ĭ-roo′bĭ-nāt) a salt of bilirubin.

bil·i·ru·bin·emia (bil″ĭ-roo″bĭ-ne′me-ə) the presence of bilirubin in the blood; see *hyperbilirubinemia.*

bil·i·ru·bin·uria (bil″ĭ-roo″bĭ-nu′re-ə) presence of bilirubin in the urine, a sign of hepatic disease or obstruction of bile ducts.

bil·i·uria (bil″ĭ-u′re-ə) [*bili-* + *-uria*] choluria.

bil·i·ver·din (bil″ĭ-vur′din) [*bili-* + L. *viridis* green] a green bile pigment, the initial one formed from catabolism of hemoglobin; it is converted to bilirubin by reduction of a methene bridge. It may also arise from air oxidation of bilirubin. Called also *dehydrobilirubin.*

bil·i·ver·di·nate (bil″ĭ-vur′dĭ-nāt) a salt of biliverdin.

bil·i·ver·din re·duc·tase (bil″ĭ-vur′din re-duk′tās) [EC 1.3.1.24] an enzyme of the oxidoreductase class that catalyzes the reduction of biliverdin to bilirubin, using NADH or NADPH as an electron donor; the reaction is a step in heme catabolism.

Bill·roth cords, disease, operation (gastrectomy, gastroenterostomy) (bil′rōt) [Christian Albert Theodor *Billroth,* German surgeon in Austria, 1829–1894] see *red pulp cords* under *cord* and *traumatic meningocele* under *meningocele,* and see under *operation.*

bi·lo·bate (bi-lo′bāt) [*bi-* + *lobate*] having two lobes.

bi·lob·u·lar (bi-lob′u-lər) having two lobules.

bi·lob·u·late (bi-lob′u-lāt) bilobular.

bi·loc·u·lar (bi-lok′u-lər) [*bi-* + *locular*] having two compartments.

bi·loc·u·late (bi-lok′u-lāt) bilocular.

bi·lo·ma (bi-lo′mə) an encapsulated collection of bile in the peritoneal cavity.

Bi·lo·phi·la (bi-lof′ĭ-lə) [L. *bilis* bile + Gr. *philos* loving] a genus of gram-negative, anaerobic, bile-tolerant, nonmotile, rod-shaped bacteria of the family Desulfovibrionaceae, isolated from gastrointestinal, genital, and oral cavities of humans and dogs; unlike most members of the Desulfovibrionales, these bacteria cannot use sulfate as an electron acceptor. The type species is *B. wadswor′thia.*

B. wadswor′thia a β-lactamase species that causes intra-abdominal infections; it has also been isolated in other infections, including brain abscesses, pericarditis, breast abscesses, empyema, gingivitis, osteomyelitis, and soft tissue infection.

bi·loph·odont (bi-lof′ə-dont) [*bi-* + Gr. *lophos* ridge + *odous* tooth] having molariform teeth with two ridges on them; applied to certain mammals, e.g., the kangaroo.

Bil·tri·cide (bil′trĭ-sīd) trademark for a preparation of praziquantel.

Bim·a·na (bim′ə-nə) [*bi-* + L. *manus* hand] a name sometimes applied to a group of mammals distinguished by having hands of character different from that of the feet; humans are the only species in the group.

bi·man·u·al (bi-man′u-əl) [*bi-* + *manual*] with both hands; performed by both hands.

bi·mas·toid (bi-mas′toid) pertaining to both mastoid processes.

bi·mat·o·prost (bĭ-mat′o-prost) a synthetic prostaglandin analogue that acts as an ocular hypotensive; applied topically to the conjunctiva in the treatment of open-angle glaucoma and ocular hypertension.

bi·max·il·lary (bi-mak′sĭ-lar″e) pertaining to or affecting both jaws.

Bim·ler appliance (bim′lər) [H.P. *Bimler,* German orthodontist, 20th century] see under *appliance.*

bi·mo·dal (bi-mo′dəl) having two modes; of a graph, having two maxima.

bi·mo·lec·u·lar (bi″mo-lek′u-lər) relating to or formed from two molecules.

bin- see *bi-*.

bin·an·gle (bin′ang-gəl) having two angles; a dental instrument having two angulations in the shank connecting the handle, or shaft, with the working portion of the instrument, known as the blade, or nib.

bi·na·ry (bi′nə-re) [L. *binarius* of two] 1. made up of two elements. 2. denoting a number system with a base of two.

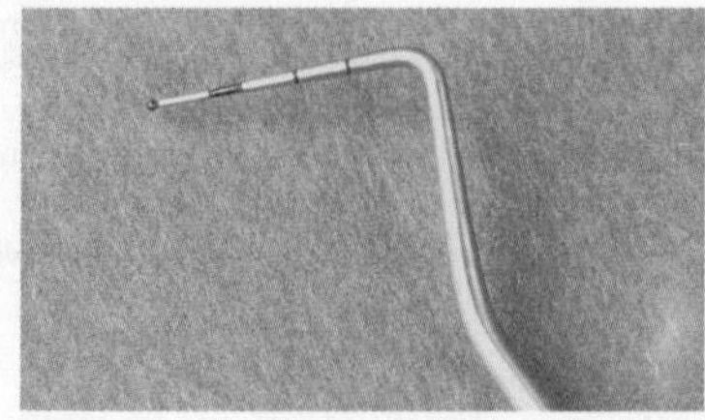

■ Binangle.

bi•nau•ral (bi-naw′rəl) [*bin-* + *aural*] pertaining to both ears; called also *binotic.*

bi•nau•ric•u•lar (bi″naw-rik′u-lər) [*bin-* + *auricular*] biauricular.

bind (bīnd) 1. to wrap with a binder or bandage. 2. to form a weak, reversible chemical bond, e.g., antigen to antibody or hormone to receptor. 3. a predicament or dilemma.

double b. a situation in which one person receives conflicting messages from another and in which response to either message, recognition of the conflict, or withdrawal is met with rejection or disapproval; thought to be a characteristic mode of interaction in some families of schizophrenics and in other dysfunctional families.

nail b. foot pain and lameness in a horse due to a horseshoe nail having been driven close to, but not into, the soft tissue. If a nail penetrates soft tissue, the condition is called *pricked foot* or *nail prick.*

bind•er (bīnd′ər) 1. an abdominal girdle or bandage, especially one applied after childbirth to support the relaxed abdominal walls. 2. a substance that attaches to another, such as to facilitate its removal from the body; see *bind* (def. 2).

phosphate b. a substance such as aluminum hydroxide, calcium acetate, or calcium carbonate that binds phosphate in the blood, removing it from the circulation; used in treatment of hyperphosphatemia, as in patients with end-stage renal disease or hypoparathyroidism.

bi•neg•a•tive (bi-neg′ə-tiv) having two negative charges, especially in ions such as SO_4^{2-}.

binge (binj) 1. a period of uncontrolled or excessive self-indulgent activity, particularly of eating or drinking. 2. to engage in such activity. See also under *eating.*

binge•ing (binj′ing) engaging in a binge, particularly of eating; see also *binge eating,* under *eating.*

Bi•net test (be-na′) [Alfred *Binet,* French psychologist, 1857–1911] see under *test.*

Bi•net-Si•mon test (be-na′ se-maw′) [A. *Binet;* Théodore *Simon,* French physician, 1873–1961] Binet test.

Bing test (bing) [Albert *Bing,* German otologist, 1844–1922] see under *test.*

Bing-Neel syndrome (bing′ nāl′) [Jens *Bing,* Danish physician, 1906–1980; Axel Valdemar *Neel,* Danish physician, 1878–1952] see under *syndrome.*

bin•oc•u•lar (bĭ-nok′u-lər) [*bin-* + *ocular*] 1. pertaining to both eyes. 2. having two eyepieces, as in a microscope.

bi•no•mi•al (bi-no′me-əl) [*bi-* + L. *nomen* name] 1. composed of two names, as the scientific names of organisms formed by combination of genus and species names (binomial nomenclature). 2. a mathematical expression obtained by taking powers of the sums or differences of two terms; see *binomial coefficient* and *distribution,* under *coefficient* and *distribution.*

bin•oph•thal•mo•scope (bin″of-thal′mə-skōp) [*bin-* + *ophthalmoscope*] an ophthalmoscope for examining both fundi of the patient at one time.

bino•scope (bin′o-skōp) [L. *bini* two + *-scope*] an instrument for inducing binocular vision in squint by presenting one object in the central part of the field of vision, the peripheral parts of the field being screened out.

bin•ot•ic (bin-ot′ik) [*bin-* + *otic*] binaural.

bin•ov•u•lar (bin-ov′u-lər) [*bin-* + *ovular*] pertaining to or derived from two distinct oocytes or ova.

Bins•wang•er disease (dementia, encephalitis) (bin′swahng-ər) [Otto *Binswanger,* German neurologist, 1852–1929] see under *disease.*

bi•nu•cle•ar (bi-noo′kle-ər) [*bi-* + *nuclear*] having two nuclei.

bi•nu•cle•ate (bi-noo′kle-āt) binuclear.

bi•nu•cle•a•tion (bi″noo-kle-a′shən) the formation of two nuclei within a cell by division of the nucleus without division of the cytoplasm.

bi•nu•cleo•late (bi-noo-kle′o-lāt) [*bi-* + L. *nucleolus*] having two nucleoli.

bi(o)- [Gr. *bios* life] a combining form denoting relationship to life, or to living organisms.

bio•ac•cu•mu•la•tion (bi″o-ə-ku″mu-la′shən) an increase over time in the amount of a substance in a living organism because intake of the substance exceeds the organism's ability to excrete it. It may be either more or less than the amount of the substance in the environment. Cf. *bioconcentration* and *biomagnification.*

bio•acous•tics (bi″o-ə-koo′stiks) the science dealing with the communicating sounds made by animals.

bio•ac•tive (bi″o-ak′tiv) having an effect on or eliciting a response from living tissue.

bio•amine (bi′o-ə-mēn″) biogenic amine.

bio•am•in•er•gic (bi″o-am″in-ur′jik) of or pertaining to neurons that secrete biogenic amines.

bio•ar•ti•fi•cial (bi″o-ahr″tĭ-fĭ′shəl) pertaining to a biological product, such as an organ or group of cells, that has been removed from the person or animal of origin and artificially processed in vitro for later insertion into a diseased or malfunctioning body part as a therapeutic measure.

bio•as•say (bi″o-as′a) [*bio-* + *assay*] determination of the active power of a sample of a drug by noting its effect on a live animal or an isolated organ preparation, as compared with the effect of a standard preparation; called also *biological assay.*

bio•as•tro•nau•tics (bi″o-as″trə-nawt′iks) the science concerned with study of the effects of space and interplanetary travel on living organisms.

bio•avail•a•bil•i•ty (bi″o-ə-vāl″ə-bil′ĭ-te) the degree to which a drug or other substance becomes available to the target tissue after administration.

Bio•brane (bi″o-brān′) trademark for a type of synthetic wound dressing containing nylon and porcine collagen, used in treatment of burns.

bio•cat•a•lyst (bi″o-kat′ə-list) enzyme.

bio•ce•no•sis (bi″o-se-no′sis) [*bio-* + *ceno-*[3] + *-sis*] the relation of diverse organisms that live in association.

bio•ce•not•ic (bi″o-se-not′ik) characterized by biocenosis.

bio•chem•is•try (bi″o-kem′is-tre) [*bio-* + *chemistry*] the chemistry of living organisms and of vital processes; called also *physiological chemistry.* biochem′ical *adj*

bio•che•mor•phic (bi″o-ke-mor′fik) pertaining to biochemorphology.

bio•che•mor•phol•o•gy (bi″o-ke-mor-fol′ə-je) the study of the relationship between chemical constitution and biological action.

bio•che•mo•ther•a•py (bi″o-ke″mo-ther′ə-pe) chemotherapy combined with biological therapy.

bio•cide (bi′o-sīd) an agent that kills living organisms. Cf. *antibiotic.* bioci′dal *adj*

Bio•clate (bi′o-klāt) trademark for a preparation of antihemophilic factor (recombinant).

bio•cli•mat•ics (bi″o-kli-mat′iks) bioclimatology.

bio•cli•ma•tol•o•gist (bi″o-kli″mə-tol′ə-jist) a specialist in bioclimatology.

bio•cli•ma•tol•o•gy (bi″o-kli″mə-tol′ə-je) [*bio-* + *climatology*] the science devoted to the study of effects on living organisms of conditions of the natural environment (rainfall, daylight, temperature, humidity, air movement) prevailing in specific regions of the earth. See also *biometeorology.*

bio•coe•no•sis (bi″o-se-no′sis) biocenosis.

bio•col•loid (bi″o-kol′oid) [*bio-* + *colloid*] a colloid from animal, plant, or microbial tissue.

bio•com•pat•i•bil•i•ty (bi″o-kom-pat″ĭ-bil′ĭ-te) the quality of being biocompatible.

bio•com•pat•i•ble (bi″o-kom-pat′ĭ-bəl) being harmonious with life; not having toxic or injurious effects on biological function.

bio•con•cen•tra•tion (bi″o-kon″sən-tra′shən) the concentration within an organism, through a process of bioaccumulation, of quantities of a chemical that are greater than those in the surrounding environment.

bio•cy•ber•net•ics (bi″o-si″bər-net′iks) the science of communications and control in animals.

bio•cy•cle (bi″o-si′kəl) [*bio-* + *cycle*] the rhythmic repetition of certain phenomena observed in living organisms.

bio•cy•tin (bi″o-si′tin) biotin in amide linkage with the ε-amino group of lysine, as occurs in the holoenzymes for which biotin is the coenzyme.

bio•de•grad•a•ble (bi″o-de-grād′ə-bəl) susceptible to decomposition by natural biological processes, such as by the action of bacteria, plants, or animals.

bio•deg•ra•da•tion (bi″o-deg″rə-da′shən) the series of processes by which living systems render chemicals less noxious to the environment.

bio•de•tri•tus (bi″o-de-tri′təs) detritus derived from the disintegration and decomposition of once-living organisms; further designated as phytodetritus or zoodetritus, depending on whether the original organism was vegetal or animal.

bio•dy•nam•ics (bi″o-di-nam′iks) [*bio-* + *dynamics*] the scientific study of the nature and determinants of all organismic (including human) behavior.

bio•elec•tric•i•ty (bi″o-e″lek-tris′ĭ-te) the electrical phenomena that appear in living tissues, as that generated by muscle and nerve tissue.

bio·elec·tron·ics (bi″o-e″lek-tron′iks) the study of the role of intermolecular transfer of electrons in biological regulation and defense.

bio·el·e·ment (bi″o-el′ə-mənt) any chemical element that is a component of living tissue.

bio·en·er·get·ics (bi″o-en″ər-jet′iks) the study of the energy transformations in living organisms.

bio·en·gi·neer·ing (bi″o-en″jĭ-nēr′ing) biomedical engineering.

bio·equiv·a·lent (bi″o-e-kwiv′ə-lənt) having the same strength and similar bioavailability in the same dosage form as another specimen of a given drug substance. **bioequiv′alence** *n*

bio·eth·ics (bi″o-eth′iks) obligations of a moral nature relating to biological research and its applications.

bio·feed·back (bi″o-fēd′bak) the process of furnishing an individual information, usually in an auditory or visual mode, on the state of one or more physiological variables such as heart rate, blood pressure, or skin temperature; such a procedure often enables the individual to gain some voluntary control over the physiological variable being sampled.

alpha b. a procedure in which a person is presented with continuous information, usually auditory, on the state of his brain-wave pattern, with the intent of increasing the percentage of alpha activity; this is done with the expectation that it will be associated with a state of relaxation and peaceful wakefulness. Called also *alpha feedback*.

breathing b. the monitoring of breathing rate, volume, rhythm, and location by sensors placed on the chest and abdomen, used in the treatment of asthma, hyperventilation, and anxiety. The feedback is displayed to the patient visually and is used by the patient to learn to breathe more slowly, deeply, and rhythmically using the abdominal muscles.

electrodermal response b. see *electrodermal activity therapy*, under *therapy*.

electromyographic b. a method of muscle retraining for patients with neurological deficits; for treatment of conditions, such as headache, associated with muscle tension; and for general relaxation. Electrical activity of the muscle or area is recorded by electromyography and displayed on a video screen in front of the patient, accompanied by a variable audible signal, which allows the patient to monitor muscle movements .

thermal b. the monitoring of skin temperature as an index of blood flow changes due to the dilatation and constriction of blood vessels, the feedback being displayed to the patient on a video monitor, accompanied by an audible signal; used for stress management and in the treatment of Raynaud disease, hypertension, and migraine.

bio·film (bi′o-film″) a thin layer of microorganisms adhering to the surface of a structure, which may be organic or inorganic, together with the polymers that they secrete.

bio·fla·vo·noid (bi″o-fla′və-noid) any of the flavonoids (q.v.) with biological activity in mammals; despite being reported to decrease capillary fragility, they have not been shown to be essential or to have any medical or nutritional value.

bi·o·gen·ic (bi″o-jen′ik) having origins in biological processes, as a biogenic amine.

bi·og·e·nous (bi-oj′ə-nəs) originating from life or producing life.

bio·ge·og·ra·phy (bi″o-je-og′rə-fe) the scientific study of geographic distribution of living organisms.

bio·group (bi′o-gro͞op) biovar.

bio·haz·ard (bi′o-haz″ərd) a potentially dangerous infectious agent such as may be found in a clinical microbiology laboratory or used in experimental studies on genetic recombination.

Bio·hist (bi′o-hist″) trademark for a combination preparation of chlorpheniramine maleate and pseudoephedrine hydrochloride.

bio·hy·drau·lic (bi″o-hi-draw′lik) [*bio-* + Gr. *hydōr* water] pertaining to the action of water and solutions in living tissue.

bio·im·ped·ance (bi″o-im-pēd′əns) the impedance of a section of tissue to passage of an electric current; see also *bioimpedance analysis*, under *analysis*.

bio·im·plant (bi″o-im′plant) a prosthesis made of a biomaterial.

bio·in·com·pat·i·ble (bi″o-in″kəm-pat′ə-bəl) being inharmonious with life; having toxic or injurious effects on biological function.

bio·in·for·mat·ics (bi″o-in″for-mat′iks) the organization and use of biological information, particularly computer-driven storage, processing, and analysis of data and databases in the fields of molecular biology and genetics.

bio·ki·net·ics (bi″o-kĭ-net′iks) [*bio-* + Gr. *kinētikos* of or for putting in motion] 1. the science of the movements within organisms. 2. the application of therapeutic exercise in rehabilitative treatment or performance enhancement.

bi·o·log·i·cal (bi-o-loj′ĭ-kəl) 1. pertaining to biology. 2. a medicinal preparation made from living organisms and their products, including serums, vaccines, antigens, antitoxins, etc.

bi·ol·o·gist (bi-ol′ə-jist) a specialist in biology.

cell b. a specialist in cell biology.

bi·ol·o·gy (bi-ol′ə-je) [*bio-* + *-logy*] the science that deals with the phenomena of life and living organisms in general. **biolog′ic** *adj*

cell b. the study of the origin, structure, function, behavior, growth, and reproduction of cells and their components. Called also *cytobiology* and *cytology*.

developmental b. embryology.

molecular b. the study of molecular structures and events underlying biological processes, including the relation between genes and the functional characteristics they determine.

radiation b. the scientific study of effects of ionizing radiation on living organisms.

bio·lu·mi·nes·cence (bi″o-loo″mĭ-nes′əns) chemoluminescence occurring in living cells, especially the emission of light as a result of cellular oxidation of a heat-stable substrate (luciferin) in the presence of a heat-sensitive enzyme (luciferase).

bi·ol·y·sis (bi-ol′ĭ-sis) chemical decomposition of organic matter by the action of living organisms.

bio·lyt·ic (bi-o-lit′ik) [*bio-* + *-lytic*] 1. pertaining to or characterized by biolysis. 2. destructive to life.

bio·mag·ni·fi·ca·tion (bi″o-mag″nĭ-fĭ-ka′shən) the concentration of chemicals in increased quantities within animals, through a process of bioaccumulation, by being passed through a food chain.

bio·mark·er (bi′o-mahr″kər) 1. a biological molecule used as a marker for the substance or process of interest. 2. tumor marker.

bio·mass (bi′o-mas″) the entire assemblage of living organisms, both animal and vegetable, of a particular region, considered collectively.

bio·ma·te·ri·al (bi″o-mə-tēr-e-əl) any substance, synthetic or natural (other than a drug), that can be used as a system or part of a system to treat, augment, or replace a tissue, organ, or function of the body.

bio·math·e·mat·ics (bi″o-math″ə-mat′iks) [*bio-* + *mathematics*] the application of mathematics to biology and medicine.

bi·ome (bi′ōm) [Gr. *bios* life + *-ome* (-oma) mass] the recognizable community unit of a given region, produced by interaction of climatic factors, biota, and substrate, usually designated according to the characteristic adult or climax vegetation, such as tundra, coniferous forest or taiga, deciduous forest, or grassland.

bio·me·chan·ics (bi″o-mə-kan′iks) [*bio-* + *mechanics*] the application of mechanical laws to living structures, as to a locomotor system. See also *kinesiology* and *bionics*. **biomechan′ical** *adj*

dental b. the relationship between the biologic behavior of oral structures and the physical influence of a dental restoration or appliance. Called also *dental biophysics*.

bio·med·i·cine (bi″o-med′ĭ-sin) medicine based on the principles of the natural sciences (biology, biochemistry, biophysics, etc.). **biomed′ical** *adj*

bio·mem·brane (bi″o-mem′brān) the lipid bilayer, together with integral and peripheral proteins, that surrounds cells and organelles. **biomem′branous** *adj*

bio·me·te·or·ol·o·gist (bi″o-me″te-or-ol′ə-jist) a specialist in biometeorology.

bio·me·te·or·ol·o·gy (bi″o-me″te-or-ol′ə-je) [*bio-* + *meteorology*] the branch of ecology that deals with the effects on living organisms of the extraorganic aspects of the physical environment (such as temperature, humidity, barometric pressure, rate of air flow, and air ionization). It considers not only the natural atmosphere but also artificially created atmospheres such as those to be found in buildings and shelters, and in closed ecological systems, such as satellites and submarines.

bi·om·e·ter (bi-om′ə-tər) [*bio-* + *-meter*] an apparatus by which extremely minute quantities of carbon dioxide can be measured; used in measuring the carbon dioxide given off from functioning tissue.

bio·me·tri·cian (bi″o-mə-trish′ən) a specialist in biometry.

bio·met·rics (bi″o-met′riks) biometry.

bi·om·e·try (bi-om′ə-tre) [*bio-* + *-metry*] 1. the science of the application of statistics in biology and medicine. 2. in life insurance, the calculation of the expectation of life.

fetal b. the use of statistics to study numerical data about fetuses.

bio·mi·cro·scope (bi″o-mi′krə-skōp) a microscope for examining living tissue in the body.

slit-lamp b. see *slit lamp*, under *lamp*.

bio•mi•cros•co•py (bi″o-mi-kros′kə-pe) [*bio-* + *microscopy*] 1. microscopic examination of living tissue in the body. 2. examination of the cornea or the lens by a combination of slit lamp and corneal microscopes.

bio•mi•met•ic (bi″o-mĭ-met′ik) imitating something that exists in nature; said of a synthetic product or process.

bio•mod•u•la•tion (bi″o-mod″u-la′shən) reactive or associative adjustment of the biochemical or cellular status of an organism.

bio•mod•u•la•tor (bi″o-mod′u-la″tər) biologic response modifier.

bio•mol•e•cule (bi″o-mol′ə-kūl) a molecule produced by a living cell, as a protein, carbohydrate, or lipid.

Bi•om•pha•la•ria (bi-om″fə-lar′e-ə) a genus of snails of the family Planorbidae; some species are intermediate hosts of *Schistosoma mansoni.* Called also *Australorbis.*

bi•on (bi′on) [Gr. *bioun* a living being] an individual living organism.

bio•ne•cro•sis (bi″o-nə-kro′sis) necrobiosis.

bi•on•ics (bi-on′iks) the science concerned with study of the functions, characteristics, and phenomena found in the living world and application of the knowledge gained to new devices and techniques in the world of machines. See also *biomechanics.*

bi•o•nom•ics (bi″o-nom′iks) [*bio-* + Gr. *nomos* law] the study of the relations of organisms to their environment; ecology.

bi•on•o•my (bi-on′ə-me) [*bio-* + Gr. *nomos* law] the sum of knowledge regarding the laws of life.

bio•nu•cle•on•ics (bi″o-noo″kle-on′iks) the study of the biological applications of radioactive and rare stable isotopes.

bio•os•mot•ic (bi″o-oz-mot′ik) [*bio-* + *osmotic*] a term applied to osmotic pressure phenomena in living organisms.

bi•oph•a•gism (bi-of′ə-jiz-əm) [*bio-* + *phag-* + *-ism*] the eating or absorption of living matter.

bi•oph•a•gous (bi-of′ə-gəs) feeding on living matter.

bi•oph•a•gy (bi-of′ə-je) biophagism.

bio•phys•ics (bi-o-fiz′iks) [*bio-* + *physics*] the science dealing with the application of physical methods and theories to biological problems. biophys′ical *adj*

dental b. see under *biomechanics.*

bio•phys•i•og•ra•phy (bi″o-fiz-e-og′rə-fe) [*bio-* + *physiography*] structural or descriptive biology.

bio•phys•i•ol•o•gy (bi″o-fiz-e-ol′ə-je) [*bio-* + *physiology*] the part of biology that includes organogeny, morphology, and physiology.

bio•pla•sia (bi″o-pla′zhə) [*bio-* + *-plasia*] the storing up of food energy in the form of growth.

bio•poi•e•sis (bi″o-poi-e′sis) [*bio-* + *-poiesis*] the origin of life from inorganic matter.

bio•poly•mer (bi″o-pol′ĭ-mər) a polymer formed in a living organism, as a polypeptide formed from amino acids (monomers).

bio•pros•the•sis (bi″o-pros-the′sis) [*bio-* + *prosthesis*] a prosthesis that contains biological material.

bi•o•pros•thet•ic (bi″o-pros-thet′ik) pertaining to a bioprosthesis; see under *valve.*

bi•op•sy (bi′op-se) [*bio-* + Gr. *opsis* vision] the removal and examination, usually microscopic, of tissue from the living body, performed to establish precise diagnosis.

aspiration b. biopsy in which the tissue is obtained by the application of suction through a needle attached to a syringe.

bite b. the instrumental removal of a fragment of tissue.

blastomere b. a technique for preimplantation genetic diagnosis, in which a blastomere is removed from a 6- or 8-cell embryo and tested for genetic abnormalities.

brush b. biopsy in which the sample is obtained by manipulating tiny brushes against it, such as through a bronchoscope.

chorionic villus b. see under *sampling.*

cone b. conization.

core b., core needle b. needle biopsy with a large hollow needle that extracts a core of tissue.

cytologic b. removal of cells for pathological examination; any of various methods can be used, such as brush biopsy or irrigation of hollow viscera.

endomyocardial b. sampling of the endomyocardial tissue with a bioptome inserted percutaneously and advanced via the femoral or internal jugular vein to the right heart or via the femoral artery to the left heart; used to assess cardiac transplant rejection or anthracycline-induced cardiotoxicity, and sometimes in diagnosing myocarditis, cardiomyopathy, or infiltrative diseases.

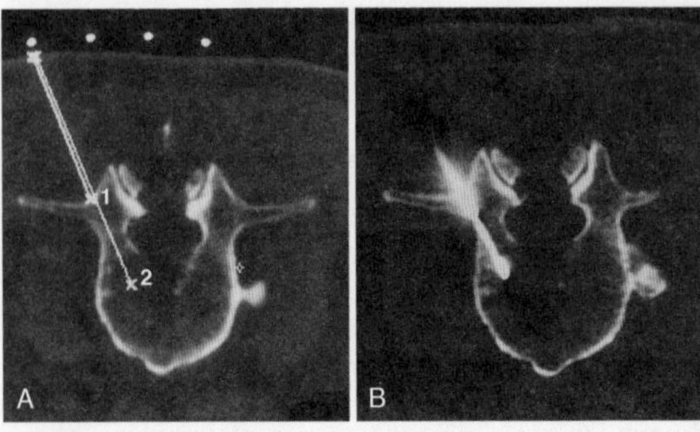

■ CT-guided needle biopsy of multiple myeloma lesion in vertebral body. *(A)*, Patient is prone with grid placed on the skin to localize needle entry point; measurements are made of needle depth from the skin surface to the posterior elements *(1)* and to the center of the lesion *(2)*. *(B)*, CT confirmation of biopsy needle position within the destructive lesion.

endoscopic b. removal of tissue by appropriate instruments introduced through an endoscope.

excisional b. biopsy of tissue removed by excision; biopsy of an entire lesion, including a significant margin of contiguous normal-appearing tissue. Cf. *lumpectomy.*

exploratory b. exploration combined with biopsy to determine the type and extent of neoplasms, both deep and superficial.

fine-needle aspiration b. aspiration biopsy using a fine needle; for superficial tissue such as the thyroid, breast, or prostate the needle is unguided but for deep tissue it must be guided radiologically.

incisional b. biopsy of a selected portion of a lesion and, if possible, of adjacent normal-appearing tissue.

laparoscopic b. biopsy of the abdominal organs using instruments introduced through a laparoscope for the removal of tissue.

needle b. biopsy in which tissue from deep within the body is obtained by insertion through the skin of a specifically designed needle that detaches tissue with an inner needle so that the tissue can be brought to the surface in the needle's lumen. Called also *percutaneous b.*

optical b. any technique that uses the interaction of light and tissue to provide information about the tissue.

percutaneous b. needle b.

punch b. biopsy in which tissue is obtained by a specifically designed round knife biopsy punch.

sentinel node b. biopsy of a sentinel node to assess for malignancy; if it does not contain malignant cells, this usually eliminates the need for removal of more distal nodes. Called also *intraoperative lymphatic mapping.*

shave b. biopsy of a skin lesion in which the sample is excised using a cut parallel to the surface of the surrounding skin.

stereotactic b. biopsy performed using a stereotactic technique to locate the biopsy site.

sternal b. biopsy of bone marrow of the sternum; done by puncture or trephination.

surface b. biopsy of cells scraped from the surface of suspicious or obvious lesions, usually done in examination for cancer of the cervix.

transbronchial lung b. biopsy of the lung through a bronchofiberscope (or rigid bronchoscope in small children) positioned under fluoroscopic guidance.

transrectal ultrasound-guided b. biopsy of the prostate using an endoscope inserted transrectally.

bio•psy•chic (bi″o-si′kik) pertaining to mental phenomena in their relation to the living organism.

bio•psy•chol•o•gy (bi″o-si-kol′ə-je) psychobiology (def. 1).

bi•op•ter•in (bi-op′tər-in) an oxidized degradation product of tetrahydrobiopterin; the term is also used to denote the class of related compounds.

bi•op•tic (bi-op′tik) pertaining to or dependent on biopsy.

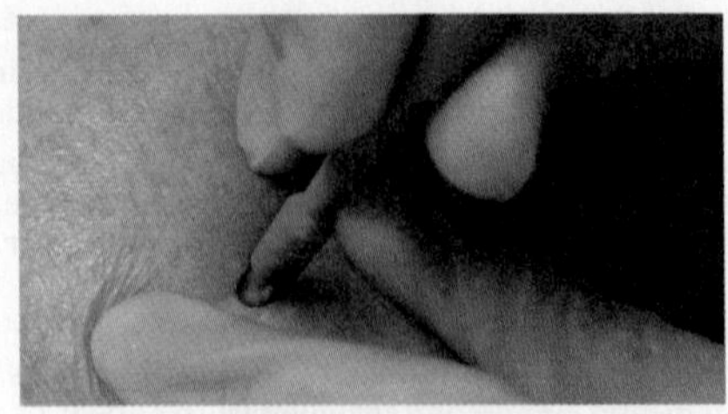

■ Punch biopsy.

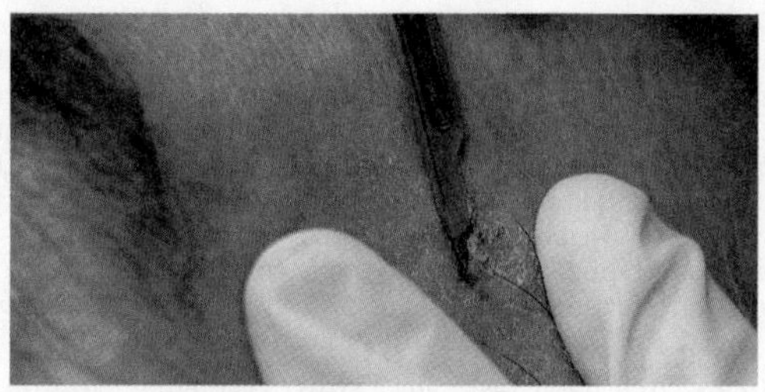

■ Shave biopsy.

bi·op·tome (bi′op-tōm″) a cutting instrument introduced through a cardiac catheter for taking endomyocardial biopsy specimens.

bio·ra·tion·al (bi″o-rash′ə-nəl) based on biological principles; having an effect by natural means; said, for example, of such pesticidal agents as viruses, bacteria, protozoa, fungi, or naturally occurring biochemicals.

bi·or·bi·tal (bi-or′bĭ-təl) pertaining to both orbits.

bio·re·ver·si·ble (bi″o-re-vur′sĭ-bəl) capable of being changed back to the original biologically active chemical form by processes within the organism; said of drugs.

bi·or·gan (bi′or-gən) a physiological organ, as distinguished from a morphological organ, or *idorgan.*

bio·rhe·ol·o·gy (bi″o-re-ol′ə-je) the study of the deformation and flow of matter in living systems and in materials directly derived from them.

bio·rhythm (bi′o-rith-əm) the established regularity with which certain phenomena recur in living organisms, such as a circadian rhythm. Called also *biologic rhythm.*

bio·safe·ty (bi″o-sāf′te) procedures used to reduce or limit the risks to laboratory and other workers, as well as the general public, from exposure to biotechnology and its products.

bio·sci·ence (bi″o-si′ens) the study of biology wherein all the sciences (physics, chemistry, etc.) are applied.

bio·sen·sor (bi′o-sen″sər) a sensor that incorporates biologic or biotic elements such as enzymes, antibodies, cell receptors, or organelles.

bi·o·sis (bi-o′sis) [Gr. *bios* life] vitality, or life.

bi·os·mo·sis (bi″os-mo′sis) osmosis through a living membrane.

bio·so·cial (bi″o-so′shul) pertaining to interrelationships between biological and social phenomena.

bio·spec·tros·co·py (bi″o-spek-tros′kə-pe) examination of living tissue with the spectroscope.

bio·stat·ics (bi″o-stat′iks) [*bio-* + *statics*] the science of the structure of organisms in relation to their function.

bio·stat·is·ti·cian (bi″o-stat″is-tish′ən) a specialist in biostatistics.

bio·sta·tis·tics (bi″o-stə-tis′tiks) biometry.

bio·ste·reo·met·rics (bi″o-ster-e-o-met′riks) analysis of the spatial and spatial-temporal characteristics of biological form and function by means of three-dimensional mapping of the body.

bio·syn·the·sis (bi″o-sin′thə-sis) the building up of a chemical compound in the physiologic processes of a living organism. biosynthet′ic *adj*

Biot respiration (breathing, sign) (byo) [Camille *Biot,* French physician, 19th century] see under *respiration.*

bi·o·ta (bi-o′tə) [Gr. *bios* life] all the living organisms of a particular area; the combined flora and fauna of a region.

bio·tax·is (bi″o-tak′sis) [*bio-* + *taxis*] the selecting and arranging powers of living cells.

bio·taxy (bi″o-tak′se) 1. biotaxis. 2. taxonomy.

bio·tech·nol·o·gy (bi″o-tek-nol′ə-je) any application of technology that uses biological systems, organisms, or their derivatives, to create new products or processes or modify existing ones. Broadly used, the term includes processes traditional to agriculture and food production, but it may be used more narrowly to encompass only new DNA techniques, molecular biology, and reproductive technological applications, such as gene manipulation and transfer, or cloning.

bio·te·lem·e·try (bi″o-tə-lem′ə-tre) the use of telemetry to record and measure certain vital phenomena of living organisms.

bio·ther·a·py (bi″o-ther′ə-pe) [*bio-* + *-therapy*] biological therapy.

bio·the·si·om·e·ter (bi″o-the″ze-om′ə-tər) an instrument for measuring the vibratory-perception threshold.

Bio·Thrax (bi′o-thraks) trademark for a preparation of anthrax vaccine adsorbed.

bi·ot·ic (bi-ot′ik) 1. pertaining to life or living matter. 2. pertaining to the biota.

bi·ot·ics (bi-ot′iks) [Gr. *biōtikos* living] the functions and qualities peculiar to living organisms, or the sum of knowledge regarding these qualities.

bio·tin (bi′o-tin) 1. a water-soluble dicyclic monocarboxylic acid considered to be part of the vitamin B complex; it is an essential cofactor for several carboxylases, plays a role in the metabolism of fatty acids and the deamination of certain amino acids, and is also used in vitro in biochemical assays based on biotinylation (q.v.) of various molecules. Deficiencies in humans have occurred only after prolonged total parenteral nutrition not supplemented with biotin or on ingestion of large quantities of raw egg whites (see *avidin*); manifestations have included dermatologic, neurologic, and ocular disorders. In some animals, deficiency has resulted in graying and loss of hair. 2. [USP] a preparation of biotin, used as a nutritional supplement.

bi·o·tin·i·dase (bi″o-tin′ĭ-dās) [EC 3.5.1.12] an enzyme of the hydrolase class essential for the recycling of biotin; it catalyzes the cleavage of biocytin or of biotin in amide linkage with peptide fragments, freeing biotin for reuse. Deficiency of the enzyme, an autosomal recessive trait, results in multiple carboxylase deficiency.

bi·o·tin·i·dase de·fi·cien·cy (bi″o-tin′ĭ-dās) a biotin-responsive, autosomal recessive aminoacidopathy caused by mutations in the *BTD* gene (locus: 21q22.1), which encodes biotinidase, leading to deficiency of activity of the biotin-containing carboxylases. Features include ketoacidosis, alopecia, skin rash, hypotonia, developmental delay, ataxia, conjunctivitis, visual abnormalities, hearing loss, hepatosplenomegaly, and coma. There may be mild hyperammonemia, and the urine contains organic acids characteristic of each individual carboxylase deficiency. Called also *juvenile* or *late-onset multiple carboxylase deficiency.*

bi·o·tin·yl (bi″o-tin′əl) the acyl radical of biotin.

bi·o·tin·yl·a·tion (bi″o-tin″ə-la′shən) the incorporation of biotinyl groups into molecules, either that catalyzed by holocarboxylase synthetase during enzyme biosynthesis or that undertaken in vitro to visualize specific substrates by incubating them with biotin-labeled probes and avidin that has been linked to any of a variety of substances amenable to biochemical assay. **biotinylat′ed** *adj*

bi·ot·o·my (bi-ot′ə-me) [*bio-* + *-tomy*] 1. the study of animal and plant structure by dissection. 2. vivisection.

bio·tox·i·ca·tion (bi″o-tok″sĭ-ka′shən) an intoxication resulting from a plant or animal poison (biotoxin).

bio·tox·i·col·o·gy (bi″o-tok″sĭ-kol′ə-je) [*bio-* + *toxicology*] the science of poisons produced by living things, their cause, detection, and their effects, and of the treatment of conditions produced by them.

bio·tox·in (bi′o-tok″sin) any poisonous substance produced by and derived from a living organism, either plant or animal.

bio·trans·for·ma·tion (bi″o-trans″for-ma′shən) the series of chemical alterations of a compound (e.g., a drug) that take place within the body, such as by enzymatic activity.

bio·trau·ma (bi″o-traw′mə) an inflammatory response in the lung, seen in patients on mechanical ventilation, resulting from alveolar overdistention or rupture, alveolar hypoperfusion, and repetitive shear stresses across alveolar walls.

bio·type (bi′o-tīp) 1. a group of individuals possessing the same genotype. 2. biovar.

bio·ty·pol·o·gy (bi″o-ti-pol′ə-je) the study of anthropological types with their constitutional variations, inadequacies, etc.

bio·var (bi′o-vahr, bi′o-var) a variant strain of a bacterial species, differentiated by identifiable biochemical or physiologic characteristics. Called also *biotype.*

bi·ov·u·lar (bi-ov′u-lər) binovular.

bi·para·sit·ic (bi″par-ə-sit′ik) hyperparasitic.

bi·par·en·tal (bi″pə-ren′təl) derived from two parents, male and female.

bi·pa·ri·e·tal (bi″pə-ri′ə-təl) pertaining to the two parietal eminences or bones.

bip·a·rous (bip′ə-rəs) [*bi-* + *-parous*] producing two offspring or eggs at one time.

bi·par·tite (bi-pahr′tīt) [L. *bipartitus*] having two parts or divisions.

bi·ped (bi′ped) [*bi-* + L. *pes* foot] 1. an animal with two feet. 2. bipedal.

bip·e·dal (bip′ə-dəl) [*bi-* + *pedal*] having or pertaining to both feet.

bi·pen·ni·form (bi-pen′ĭ-form) doubly feather-shaped; said of muscles whose fibers are arranged on each side of a tendon, like the barbs on the shaft of a feather.

bi·per·fo·rate (bi-pur′fə-rāt) [*bi-* + L. *perforatus* bored through] having two perforations.

bi·per·i·den (bi-per′ĭ-den) [USP] a synthetic anticholinergic agent having antisecretory, spasmolytic, and mydriatic activity, used in the form of its salts as an antidyskinetic.

b. hydrochloride [USP] the hydrochloride salt of biperiden, used in the treatment of parkinsonism and drug-induced extrapyramidal reactions; administered orally.

b. lactate [USP] the lactate salt of biperiden, used in the treatment of severe drug-induced extrapyramidal reactions; administered intramuscularly or intravenously.

bi·pha·sic (bi-fa′zik) 1. having two phases. 2. in histopathology, consisting of two morphologically distinct components, as in a biphasic tumor.

bi·phe·no·typ·ic (bi″fe-no-tip′ik) characterized by expression in a single cell of markers characteristic of more than one cell lineage; said of certain acute leukemias.

bi·phen·yl (bi-fen′əl) diphenyl.

polybrominated b. (PBB) any of various brominated derivatives of biphenyl; uses and toxic hazards are similar to those of polychlorinated biphenyls. They typically are deposited in body fat stores and are rarely mobilized except through lactation.

polychlorinated b. (PCB) any of a group of substances in which chlorine replaces hydrogen in biphenyls, used as heat-transfer agents and as insulators in electrical equipment. They are chemically very stable and accumulate in animal tissues, causing a variety of toxic effects including carcinogenesis.

***p*-bi·phen·yl·amine** (bi-fen″əl-am′ēn) *p*-aminobiphenyl.

bi·po·lar (bi-po′lər) 1. having two poles or pertaining to both poles. 2. describing neurons that have processes at both ends. 3. denoting bacterial staining confined to the poles of the organism. 4. pertaining to mood disorders in which both major depressive episodes and manic or hypomanic episodes occur.

Bi·po·la·ris (bi-po-lar′is) a genus of Fungi Imperfecti of the form-class Hyphomycetes, form-family Dematiaceae, closely related to *Drechslera* and *Exserohilum*. *B. australien′sis*, *B. hawaiien′sis*, and *B. spici′fera* have been isolated from humans with fatal encephalitis or meningoencephalitis, as well as those with nasal polyps and sinusitis. The perfect (sexual) stage of *Bipolaris* species is in genus *Cochliobolus*.

bi·pos·i·tive (bi-poz′ĭ-tiv) having two positive charges, as in Ca^{2+}.

bi·po·ten·tial (bi″po-ten′shəl) pertaining to or characterized by bipotentiality.

bi·po·ten·ti·al·i·ty (bi″po-ten″she-al′ĭ-te) [*bi-* + L. *potentia* power] possession of the power of developing or acting in either of two possible ways.

b. of the gonad the capability of an undifferentiated gonad to develop into either an ovary or a testis.

bi·pus (bi′pəs) dipodial.

bi·ra·mous (bi-ra′məs) [*bi-* + L. *ramus* branch] consisting of or possessing two branches.

birch (burch) any tree of the genus *Betula*.

bi·re·frac·tive (bi″re-frak′tiv) doubly refractive.

bi·re·frin·gence (bi″re-frin′jəns) the quality of transmitting light unequally in different directions, so that an incident ray is split into two refracted rays that travel at different velocities; double refraction. birefrin′gent *adj*

crystalline b. birefringence occurring in systems in which the bonds between molecules or ions have a regular asymmetrical arrangement; it is independent of the refractive index of the medium.

flow b. birefringence exhibited only when the substance is in solution and flowing; e.g., it is seen in solutions of long thin molecules, such as nucleoproteins.

form b. birefringence produced by regular orientation of submicroscopic asymmetrical particles in a substance or object, differing in refractive index from the surrounding medium; it is the most common form occurring in organisms.

intrinsic b. crystalline b.

strain b. birefringence observed occasionally in isotropic structures when subjected to tension or pressure; it occurs in muscle and in embryonic tissues.

streaming b. flow b.

Bir·kett hernia (bur′kət) [John *Birkett*, English surgeon, 1815–1904] synovial hernia.

Bir·na·vi·ri·dae (bur′nə-vir″ĭ-de) [*bi*segmented *RNA* + *virus*] the two-segmented double-stranded RNA viruses: a family of RNA viruses having a nonenveloped icosahedral virion 60 nm in diameter with 92 capsomers in a T = 9 arrangement. The genome consists of two segments of linear double-stranded RNA (MW 2.2–2.5 × 10^6 and 2.4–2.6 × 10^6, size of total genome about 6 kbp). Viruses contain five major structural polypeptides and are resistant to light and ultraviolet radiation, heat, lipid solvents, and trypsin. Replication and assembly occur in the cytoplasm; it includes *Aquabirnavirus* (infecting fish, mollusks, and crustaceans), *Avibirnavirus* (infecting birds), and *Entomobirnavirus* (infecting insects).

bir·na·vi·rus (bur′nə-vi″rəs) any virus belonging to the family Birnaviridae.

Birt-Hogg-Dube syndrome (bərt′ hog′ dūb′) [Arthur R. *Birt*, Canadian dermatologist, late 20th century; Georgina R. *Hogg*, Canadian dermatologist, late 20th century; W. James *Dube*, Canadian dermatologist, late 20th century] see under *syndrome*.

birth (burth) the act or process of being born.

multiple b. the birth of two or more offspring produced in the same gestation period, the frequency of birth of viable offspring after such multiple pregnancy having been computed as follows: twins, 1 in 80; triplets, 1 in 6400 (80 × 80); quadruplets, 1 in 512,000 (80 × 80 × 80); etc. (Hellin's law).

postterm b. birth of an infant at or after 42 completed weeks (294 days) of gestation.

premature b., preterm b. birth of an infant before 37 completed weeks (259 days) of gestation.

birth·mark (burth′mahrk) any congenital blemish or spot on the skin, usually visible at birth or shortly after, such as a nevus or mole.

vascular b. hemangioma.

bis- [L. *bis* twice] a prefix meaning two or twice.

bis·ac·o·dyl (bis-ak′ə-dəl, bis″ə-ko′dəl) [USP] a contact laxative used for short-term relief of constipation and for bowel evacuation prior to radiography, endoscopy, and elective colon surgery; administered orally or rectally.

b. tannex a water-soluble complex of bisacodyl and tannic acid, having similar actions and uses as the base.

bis·acro·mi·al (bis-ə-kro′me-əl) pertaining to the two acromial processes.

bis·ax·il·lary (bis-ak′sĭ-lar″e) pertaining to both axillae.

bis(chlo·ro·meth·yl)ether (bis-klor″o-meth′əl-e′thər) an alkylating agent used as a chemical intermediate in industry; it is irritating to eyes and mucous membranes and carcinogenic. Called also sym-*dichloromethyl ether*.

Bis·chof myelotomy (bish′of) [W. *Bischof*, German neurosurgeon, 20th century] see under *myelotomy*.

bis·cuit (bis′kət) dental porcelain that has undergone the first firing and has assumed a surface texture like that of a cookie. Called also *bisque*.

bis·cuit·ing (bis′kət-ing) the first baking of porcelain paste, by which biscuit is formed.

bi·sec·tion (bi-sek′shən) [*bi-* + *section*] division into two parts by cutting.

bi·seg·men·tec·to·my (bi″seg-men-tek′tə-me) resection of two segments (i.e., one lobe) of the liver; hepatic lobectomy.

bi·sep·tate (bi-sep′tāt) [*bi-* + *septate*] divided into two parts by a septum.

bi·sex·u·al (bi-sek′shoo-əl) [*bi-* + *sexual*] 1. of or pertaining to bisexuality. 2. an individual exhibiting bisexuality. 3. hermaphroditic. 4. androgynous.

bi·sex·u·al·i·ty (bi-sek″shoo-al′ĭ-te) 1. sexual attraction to persons of both sexes; exhibition of both homosexual and heterosexual behavior. 2. true hermaphroditism. 3. androgyny (def. 1).

bis·fe·ri·ens (bis-fe′re-ənz) [L.] bisferious.

bis·fe·ri·ous (bis-fe′re-əs) [*bis-* + L. *ferire* to beat] having two beats, said of a type of pulse; see *pulsus bisferiens*. Called also *biferiens* and *biferious*.

BIS-GMA dimethacrylate.

bis·il·i·ac (bis-il′e-ak) [*bis* + *iliac*] pertaining to both iliac bones or to any two corresponding points on the two iliac bones.

bis in die (b.d., b.i.d.) (bis in de′a) [L.] twice a day.

bis·muth (Bi) (biz′məth) a silver-white metal, atomic number 83, atomic weight 208.980. Its salts have astringent, antacid, and mildly germicidal properties and are used to treat diarrhea, nausea, indigestion, and other gastrointestinal conditions; they were formerly used in the treatment of syphilis but have been superseded by antibiotics. Excessive ingestion can cause bismuth poisoning; see under *poisoning*.

basic b. carbonate, b. subcarbonate [USP] a salt of bismuth that has been used as an antacid and mild astringent in relief of inflammatory diseases of the stomach and intestines, and also as a topical skin protectant.

b. subgallate [USP] a salt of bismuth that has been used similarly to bismuth subcarbonate.

b. subnitrate [USP] a basic salt, used as a pharmaceutic necessity in the preparation of compound resorcinol ointment.

b. subsalicylate [USP] a bismuth salt of salicylic acid, administered orally in the treatment of diarrhea and gastric distress, including nausea, indigestion, and heartburn.

bis•muth•ism (biz′məth-iz-əm) bismuth poisoning.

bis•mu•tho•sis (biz″mə-tho′sis) bismuth poisoning.

bis•o•pro•lol fu•ma•rate (bis″o-pro′lol) [USP] a beta-adrenergic blocking agent selective for β_1-adrenergic receptors; administered orally in the treatment of hypertension.

1,3-bis•phos•pho•glyc•er•ate (bis″fos-fo-glis′ər-āt) an anion of the form of bisphosphoglyceric acid phosphorylated at the 1 and 3 carbons; it is an intermediate in gluconeogenesis and glycolysis, and a precursor to 2,3-bisphosphoglycerate.

2,3-bis•phos•pho•glyc•er•ate (bis-fos″fo-glis′ər-āt) a salt or ester of bisphosphoglyceric acid; it is contained in red blood cells, where it plays a role in liberating oxygen from hemoglobin in the peripheral circulation. It is also an intermediate in the conversion of 3-phosphoglycerate to 2-phosphoglycerate. Called also *2,3-diphosphoglycerate.*

bis•phos•pho•glyc•er•ate mu•tase (bis-fos″fo-glis′ər-āt mu′tās) [EC 5.4.2.4] an enzyme of the isomerase class that catalyzes the interconversion of 1,3-bisphosphoglycerate and 2,3-bisphosphoglycerate; it requires Mg^{2+} as a cofactor and is more active in the presence of 3-phosphoglycerate. The reaction produces 2,3-bisphosphoglycerate necessary for glucose catabolism and for erythrocytic regulation of hemoglobin oxygen affinity. Deficient enzyme activity, an autosomal recessive trait, results in a form of hemolytic anemia.

bis•phos•pho•glyc•er•ate phos•pha•tase (bis-fos″fo-glis′ər-āt fos′fə-tās) [EC 3.1.3.13] an enzyme of the hydrolase class that catalyzes the hydrolysis of 2,3-bisphosphoglycerate to form 3-phosphoglycerate. The reaction is one of the control mechanisms regulating the affinity of hemoglobin for oxygen.

bis•phos•pho•gly•cer•ic ac•id (bis″fos-fo-glĭ-sĕr′ik) glyceric acid esterified with phosphate at two positions.

bis•phos•pho•glyc•ero•mu•tase (bis-fos″fo-glis″ər-o-mu′tās) bisphosphoglycerate mutase.

bis•phos•pho•nate (bis-fos′fə-nāt) diphosphonate.

bisque (bisk) [Fr.] biscuit.

bi•ste•phan•ic (bi-stə-fan′ik) pertaining to the two stephanions, especially to the shortest distance between them (bistephanic width).

Bis•ton (bis′tən) a genus of moths. *B. betula′ria* is the peppered moth, a species demonstrating industrial melanism.

bis•tou•ry (bis′to͞o-re) [Fr. *bistouri*] a long, narrow surgical knife, straight or curved, used for incising abscesses and enlarging sinuses, fistulas, etc.

bi•stra•tal (bi-stra′təl) [*bi-* + *stratum*] disposed in two layers.

bi•sul•fate (bi-sul′fāt) an acid sulfate (not to be confused with *disulfate*).

bi•sul•fide (bi-sul′fīd) disulfide.

bi•sul•fite (bi-sul′fīt) an acid sulfite.

bi•tar•trate (bi-tahr′trāt) any salt containing the anion $C_4H_5O_6^-$ derived from the diacid tartaric acid ($C_4H_6O_6$).

bite (bīt) 1. the forcible closure of the lower against the upper teeth. 2. the measure of force exerted in the closure of the teeth. 3. a record of the relationship of upper and lower teeth, in occlusion, obtained by biting into a mass of modeling substance. 4. the part of an artificial tooth on the lingual side between the shoulder and the incisal edge of the tooth. 5. a wound or puncture made by the teeth or other parts of the mouth. 6. a morsel of food.

balanced b. balanced occlusion.

check b. a thin sheet of wax or a modeling compound placed between the teeth in centric, eccentric, lateral, or protrusive occlusion, and pressed to their buccal or labial surfaces after the jaws have been closed; used to check dental occlusion in the articulator in properly aligning study models. Written also *check-bite.*

closed b. malocclusion with decreased occlusal vertical dimension and an abnormal overbite in which the mandible protrudes. Called also *deep b., closed-bite malocclusion,* and *deep overbite.*

cross b. crossbite.

deep b. closed b.

edge-to-edge b., end-to-end b. see under *occlusion.*

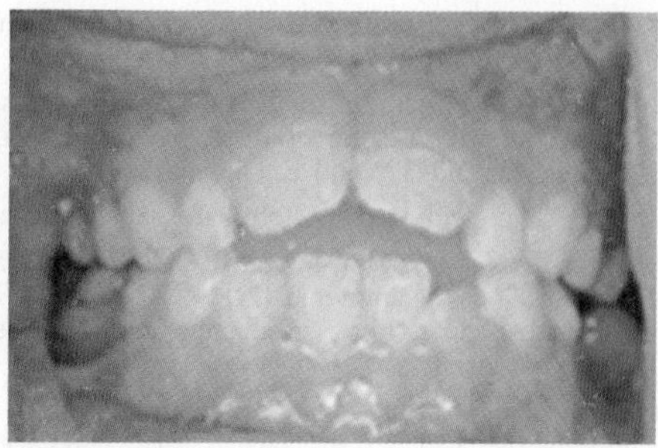

■ Open bite resulting from prolonged thumb sucking.

open b. a condition marked by failure of certain opposing teeth to establish occlusal contact when the jaws are closed. Called also *apertognathia* and *nonocclusion.*

over b. vertical overlap (def. 1).

overshot b. veterinary term for *retrognathism.*

scissors b. total lingual crossbite of the mandible, with the mandibular teeth completely contained within the maxillary dental arch in habitual occlusion.

stork b. popular term for a salmon patch on the nape of the neck of a neonate.

underhung b. a characteristic of mandibular prognathism in which the incisal edges of the mandibular anterior teeth extend labially to the incisal edges of the maxillary anterior teeth when the jaws are in habitual occlusion.

undershot b. veterinary term for *prognathism;* it is normal in animals such as boxers and bulldogs.

wax b. a simultaneous impression of both the upper and the lower jaw, made by having the subject bite on a double layer of soft baseplate wax.

X-b. crossbite.

bite-block (bīt′blok) occlusion rim.

bite•gage (bīt′gāj) a device used in prosthetic dentistry as an aid in securing proper occlusion of the maxillary and mandibular teeth.

bite•lock (bīt′lok) occlusion rim.

bi•tem•po•ral (bi-tem′pə-rəl) pertaining to both temples or temporal bones.

bite•plane (bīt′plān) an orthodontic removable appliance, made of acrylic resin, covering all the maxillary teeth, and kept in place by orthodontic wrought-wire clasps and labial wires; used in the diagnosis and treatment of pain of the temporomandibular joint and adjacent muscles. Written also *bite plane.*

bite•plate (bīt′plāt) bite plate; see under *plate.*

bi•ter•mi•nal (bi-tur′mĭ-nəl) performed by using two terminals of an alternating current.

bite-wing (bīt′wing) a central tab or wing of a dental x-ray film, which is held between the upper and lower teeth during radiography of oral structures. See also under *film* and *radiograph.*

Bi•thyn•ia (bĭ-thin′e-ə) *Bulimus.*

Bi•tis (bi′tis) a genus of venomous snakes of the family Viperidae. *B. arie′tans* is the puff adder; *B. gabo′nica* is the Gaboon viper; and *B. nasicor′nis* is the rhinoceros viper. See table at *snake.*

bi•tol•ter•ol mes•y•late (bi-tol′tər-ol) a β-adrenergic agonist, selective for β_2-adrenergic receptors; administered by inhalation as a bronchodilator in the treatment of asthma-associated bronchospasm, and the prophylaxis and treatment of reversible bronchospasm associated with chronic obstructive airway disease, including bronchitis and pulmonary emphysema. Bitolterol is an inactive prodrug that is hydrolyzed to the active drug colterol by blood and tissue esterases.

Bi•tot spots (patches) (be-to′) [Pierre A. *Bitot,* French physician, 1822–1888] see under *spot.*

bi•tro•chan•ter•ic (bi″tro-kan-ter′ik) pertaining to both trochanters on one femur or to both greater trochanters.

bit•ter (bit′ər) having an unpalatable taste, such as that of quinine.

bit•ters (bit′ərz) a medicinal agent that has a bitter taste; used as a tonic, alterative, or appetizer.

aromatic b. bitter vegetable drugs that have an aromatic quality.

bit•ter•wood (bit′ər-wood) *Picrasma excelsa.*

Bitt•ner virus (bit′nər) [John Joseph *Bittner,* American pathologist, 1904–1961] see *mouse mammary tumor virus,* under *virus.*

Bit•torf reaction (bit′orf) [Alexander *Bittorf,* German physician, 1876–1949] see under *reaction.*

bi•tu•mi•no•sis (bi-too″mĭ-no′sis) a mild type of pneumoconiosis caused by inhalation of the dust from soft (bituminous) coal.

Bi•tu•ni•ca•tae (bi-too″nĭ-ka′te) in fungal taxonomy, a series of the subphylum Ascomycotina, consisting of those having a bitunicate ascus. It includes the orders Dothideales and Erysiphales.

bi•urate (bi′u-rāt) an acid urate; a monobasic salt of uric acid.

bi•u•ret (bi′u-rət) [*bis-* + *urea*] a derivative of urea, equivalent to two molecules of urea less one of ammonia ($NH_2CONHCONH_2$); it forms a colored chelate with copper sulfate in alkaline solution. See also under *reaction.* Called also *allophanamide.*

bi•va•lence (bi-va′ləns) the property of being bivalent.

bi•va•lent (bi-va′lənt) 1. having a valence of two; divalent. 2. the structure formed by a pair of homologous chromosomes joined by synapsis along their length during the zygotene and pachytene stages of the first meiotic prophase. After each of the paired chromosomes separates into two sister chromatids during the pachytene, this structure is called a *tetrad.* 3. effective against two different entities, as diseases or strains of a pathogen.

bi•val•i•ru•din (bi-val′ĭ-roo-din) a type of direct thrombin inhibitor used in conjunction with aspirin as an anticoagulant in patients with unstable angina pectoris who are undergoing percutaneous transluminal coronary angioplasty; administered intravenously.

bi•valve (bi′valv) [*bi-* + *valve*] having two valves, as the shells of such mollusks as clams.

Bi•val•via (bi-val′ve-ə) [*bi-* + *valva* + *-ia*] Pelecypoda.

Bi•val•vu•li•da (bi″val-vu′lĭ-də) [*bi-* + *valve*] an order of parasitic protozoa (class Myxosporea, phylum Myxozoa), the spores of which have two valves.

bi•ven•ter (bi-ven′tər) [*bi-* + *venter*] a part or organ (as a muscle) with two bellies.

bi•ven•tral (bi-ven′trəl) 1. having two bellies. 2. musculus digastricus.

bi•ven•tric•u•lar (bi″ven-trik′u-lər) pertaining to or affecting both ventricles of the heart.

bi•vi•tel•line (bi″vĭ-tel′in) having two yolks.

bi•zy•go•mat•ic (bi″zi-go-mat′ik) [*bi-* + *zygoma*] pertaining to the two most prominent points on the two zygomatic arches. See also *bizygomatic breadth*, under *breadth.*

Bjer•rum scotoma (sign) (byer′oom) [Jannik Petersen *Bjerrum*, Danish ophthalmologist, 1851–1920] see under *scotoma.*

Bjer•rum screen (byer′oom) [J. *Bjerrum*, Danish ophthalmologist, 1827–1892] tangent screen.

Björn•stad syndrome (byorn′stahd) [R. *Björnstad*, Swedish dermatologist, 20th century] see under *syndrome.*

B-K, BK below-knee; see *transtibial amputation*, under *amputation.*

Bk berkelium.

Black classification (blak) [Greene Vardiman *Black*, American dentist, 1836–1915] see under *classification.*

black (blak) 1. reflecting no light or true color; of the darkest hue. 2. a dye or stain with this color.

animal b., bone-b. animal charcoal.

fat b. HB Sudan b. B.

indulin b. nigrosin.

ivory b. animal charcoal.

lamp b. finely divided carbon deposited from the smoky flame of burning oils, rosin, and other substances.

Paris b. animal charcoal.

solvent b. 3, Sudan b. B a black, fat-soluble diazo dye, used as a stain for fats.

black•ber•ry (blak′ber-e) 1. any of various plants of the genus *Rubus;* some have medicinal root bark. 2. the fruit of one of these plants.

Black•fan-Di•a•mond anemia (syndrome) (blak′fan di′mənd) [Kenneth D. *Blackfan*, American pediatrician, 1883–1941; Louis Klein *Diamond*, American pediatrician, 1902–1999] see *congenital hypoplastic anemia*, under *anemia.*

black haw (blak haw) *Viburnum prunifolium.*

black•head (blak′hed) 1. open comedo. 2. histomoniasis.

black•leg (blak′leg) an acute anaerobic bacterial disease of cattle and sheep caused by *Clostridium chauvoei;* symptoms include crepitant swelling in the musculature and a high fever, often leading to death within a day. Called also *symptomatic anthrax, blackquarter*, and *quarter evil* or *ill.* Spelled also *black leg.*

black•out (blak′out) a condition characterized by failure of vision and momentary unconsciousness, due to diminished circulation to the brain.

alcoholic b. anterograde amnesia experienced by alcoholics during episodes of drinking, even when not fully intoxicated; indicative of early but still reversible brain damage.

black•quar•ter (blak-kwor′tər) blackleg.

black•snake (blak′snāk) 1. *Pseudechis porphyriacus*, a large venomous semiaquatic Australian snake whose body is black on top and red underneath. 2. *Coluber constrictor*, a nonvenomous snake found in North America; called also *black racer.* See table at *snake.*

black•tongue (blak′tung″) black tongue (def. 2).

blad•der (blad′ər) [L. *vesica*, *cystis;* Gr. *kystis*] 1. a membranous sac, such as one serving as receptacle for a secretion. Called also *vesica.* 2. vesica urinaria.

allantoic b. a membranous sac formed in amphibians as an outgrowth of the cloaca for the storage of urine.

areflexic b. autonomous b.

atonic b., atonic neurogenic b. neurogenic bladder due to destruction of the sensory nerve fibers from the bladder to the spinal cord, marked by absence of control of bladder functions and of desire to urinate, bladder overdistention, and an abnormal amount of residual urine; it is most often associated with tabes dorsalis *(tabetic b.)* or pernicious anemia, and less often with other diseases. Called also *paralytic b.* and *sensory paralytic b.*

automatic b. neurogenic bladder due to complete transection of the spinal cord above the sacral segments, marked by complete loss of micturition reflexes and bladder sensation, violent involuntary voiding, and an abnormal amount of residual urine. Called also *cord, reflex*, or *spastic b.*

autonomic b., autonomous b. neurogenic bladder due to a lesion in the sacral portion of the spinal cord that interrupts the reflex arc controlling the bladder; the lesion may be in the cauda equina, conus medullaris, sacral roots, or pelvic nerve. Symptoms include loss of normal bladder sensation and reflex activity, inability to initiate urination normally, and incontinence. Called also *areflexic b., denervated b.*, and *nonreflex b.*

chyle b. cisterna chyli.

cord b. automatic b.

denervated b. autonomous b.

double b. a rare anomaly in which the urinary bladder is doubled, often along with the urethra.

fasciculated b. trabeculated b.

gall b. vesica biliaris.

ileal b. a neobladder made from a section of ileum.

irritable b. a urinary bladder marked by increased frequency of contraction with associated urge incontinence. Called also *overactive, spasmodic*, or *unstable b.*

motor paralytic b. neurogenic bladder due to impairment of the lower motoneurons or nerves controlling the bladder. The *acute* form is marked by painful distention and inability to initiate urination; the *chronic* form is marked by difficult initiation of urination, straining, interruption or decreased size and force of the stream, and recurrent urinary tract infections.

neurogenic b., neuropathic b. any condition of dysfunction of the urinary bladder caused by a lesion of the central or peripheral nervous system, such as *atonic neurogenic b., automatic b., autonomous b., motor paralytic b.*, or *uninhibited neurogenic b.*

nonneurogenic neurogenic b. Hinman syndrome.

nonreflex b. autonomous b.

overactive b. irritable b.

paralytic b. atonic neurogenic b.

pear-shaped b. a urinary bladder with widening of the inferior section, seen in conditions including pelvic lipomatosis, perivesical hematoma or urinoma, lymphoma or lymphocyst, and others.

reflex b. automatic b.

sacculated b. a urinary bladder with pouches between hypertrophied muscle fibers.

sensory paralytic b. atonic neurogenic b.

spasmodic b. irritable b.

spastic b. automatic b.

tabetic b. see *atonic neurogenic b.*

trabeculated b. a urinary bladder ridged on its inner surface due to hypertrophy of the muscular coat, usually due to obstruction of the urethra. Called also *fasciculated b.*

uninhibited neurogenic b. neurogenic bladder due to a lesion in the region of the upper motoneurons with subtotal interruption of the corticospinal pathways, marked by frequent urgency and incontinence.

unstable b. irritable b.

urinary b. vesica urinaria.

Blain•ville ears (blă-vēl′) [Henri Marie Ducrotay de *Blainville*, French zoologist, 1777–1850] see under *ear.*

Blake disk (blāk) [Clarence John *Blake*, American otologist, 1843–1919] see under *disk.*

Bla•lock-Han•lon operation (bla′lok han′lən) [Alfred *Blalock*, American surgeon, 1899–1964; C. Rollins *Hanlon*, American surgeon, born 1915] see under *operation.*

Bla•lock-Taus•sig operation (shunt) (bla′lok taw′sig) [A. *Blalock;* Helen Brooke *Taussig*, American pediatrician, 1898–1986] see under *operation.*

Blanc•o•phor (blank′o-for) trademark for a type of blankophore.

bland (bland) [L. *blandus*] mild or soothing.

Blan•din glands (blah-dă′) [Philippe Frédéric *Blandin*, French surgeon, 1798–1849] anterior lingual glands, see under *gland.*

Blan•din and Nuhn's glands (blah-dă′ nōōn′) [P.F. *Blandin;* Anton *Nuhn*, German anatomist, 1814–1889] anterior lingual glands, see under *gland.*

blank•o•phore (blank′o-for) any of a group of optical whitening agents chemically related to the sulfonamides, added to detergents, paper, and textiles; they may produce phototoxic dermatitis or allergic contact dermatitis.

Blasch•ko lines (blahsh′ko) [Alfred *Blaschko*, Austrian dermatologist, 1858–1922] see under *line.*

Blas•ko•vics operation (blahs′ko-vitz) [Laszlo de Blaskovics, Hungarian ophthalmologist, 1869–1938] see under *operation.*

blast[1] (blast) [Gr. *blastos* germ] 1. an immature stage in cellular development before appearance of the definitive characteristics of the cell; used also as a word termination (see *-blast*). 2. blast cell (def. 2).

blast[2] (blast) [A.S. *blaest*, blast] the wave of air pressure *(air concussion)* produced by the detonation of a high-explosive bomb shell or other explosion. A wave of high-pressure velocity (shock wave) is created and this is followed by one of negative decreased velocity, exerting a suction-like action. Blast causes pulmonary concussion and hemorrhage *(lung blast, blast chest)*, laceration of other thoracic and abdominal viscera, ruptured ear drums, and minor effects in the central nervous system.

-blast [Gr. *blastos* germ] a word termination denoting a type of blast[1]. See also *blast(o)-.*

blas•te•ma (blas-te′mə) [Gr. *blastēma* shoot] 1. in species with asexual reproduction, a group of cells that give rise to a new individual. 2. in other species, a group of cells with little or no differentiation that gives rise to an organ or part in either normal development or regeneration. blaste′mic *adj*

metanephric b. a mass of intermediate mesodermal cells around the distal end of the ureteric bud that gives rise to nephrons in the permanent kidney; called also *metanephric cap* or *mass.*

blas•tic (blas′tik) pertaining to or characterized by conidiogenesis in which new growth of a conidium takes place by a process of enlargement before delimitation by a septa.

blast(o)- [Gr. *blastos* shoot, germ] a combining form denoting relationship to a bud or budding, particularly to an early embryonic stage, as to a primitive or formative element, cell, or layer.

blas•to•cat•e•nate (blas″to-kat′ə-nāt) [*blasto-* + L. *catena* chain] characterized by a chain of conidia in which the youngest cells are at the apex. Cf. *basocatenulate.*

blas•to•cele (blas′to-sēl) blastocoele.

blas•to•ce•lic (blas″to-se′lik) blastocoelic.

blas•to•chyle (blas′to-kīl) [*blasto-* + Gr. *chylos* juice] the fluid contained in the blastocoele.

blas•to•coele (blas′to-sēl) [*blasto-* + *-coele*] the fluid-filled cavity of the mass of cells (blastula) produced by cleavage of a zygote. Sometimes spelled *blastocoel.* Called also *cleavage*, or *segmentation, cavity.* **blastoce′lic, blastocoe′lic** *adj*

blas•to•co•nid•i•um (blas″to-kə-nid′e-əm) blastospore.

Blas•to•cri•thid•ia (blas″to-krĭ-thid′e-ə) [*blasto-* + Gr. *krithē* barleycorn] a genus of protozoa of the order Kinetoplastida, phylum Euglenozoa, parasitic in arthropods and other invertebrates; they are monogenetic and the epimastigote form is dominant in the life cycle, although amastigotes may be produced as flagellar cysts.

blas•to•cyst (blas′to-sist) [*blasto-* + Gr. *kystis* bladder] the mammalian conceptus in the postmorula stage; it is like a blastula in having a fluid-filled cavity, but unlike it in having the surface layer not exclusively embryoblast but mainly or entirely trophoblast, in having an eccentric embryoblast, and in not being limited to one germ layer. The human blastocyst consists of an embryoblast (inner cell mass) and a thin trophoblast layer enclosing the blastocyst cavity.

Blas•to•cys•tis (blas″to-sis′tis) a genus of yeasts of the family Entomophthoraceae. *B. ho′minis* is a species frequently found in human feces that causes blastocystosis.

blas•to•cys•to•sis (blas″to-sis-to′sis) intestinal infection with *Blastocystis hominis;* it is often subclinical, but sometimes causes diarrhea, flatulence, and abdominal cramps.

blas•to•cyte (blas′to-sīt) [*blasto-* + *-cyte*] an undifferentiated embryonic cell.

blas•to•derm (blas′to-dərm) [*blasto-* + *-derm*] collectively, the mass of cells produced by cleavage of a zygote, forming the hollow sphere of the blastula, or the cellular cap above a floor of segmented yolk in the discoblastula of telolecithal eggs. Called also *germinal membrane*, or *membrana germinativa.* **blastoder′mal, blastoder′mic** *adj*

bilaminar b. the stage of development in which the embryo is represented by two primary layers: the ectoderm and the endoderm. See *gastrula.*

embryonic b. the region of the blastoderm forming the embryo proper.

extraembryonic b. the region of the blastoderm forming membranes rather than the embryo proper.

trilaminar b. the stage of development in which the embryo is represented by the three primary layers: the ectoderm, the mesoderm, and the endoderm.

blas•to•disc (blas′to-disk) [*blasto-* + Gr. *diskos* disk] the convex structure formed by the blastomeres at the animal pole of an ovum undergoing incomplete cleavage, as the telolecithal egg of a bird or fish.

blas•to•gen•e•sis (blas″to-jen′ə-sis) 1. the development of an individual from a blastema, that is, by asexual reproduction. 2. the morphological transformation of small lymphocytes into larger cells resembling blast cells, occurring on exposure to phytohemagglutinin or to antigens to which the donor is immunized. **blastogenet′ic, blastogen′ic** *adj*

blas•tog•e•ny (blas-toj′ə-ne) [*blasto-* + *-geny*] the germ history of an organism or species.

blas•to•ki•nin (blas″to-ki′nin) uteroglobin.

blas•tol•y•sis (blas-tol′ĭ-sis) [*blasto-* + *-lysis*] dissolution or destruction of the blastocyst or blast cells. **blastolyt′ic** *adj*

blas•to•ma (blas-to′mə) pl. *blastomas, blasto′mata* [*blast-* + *-oma*] a neoplasm composed of embryonic cells derived from the blastema of an organ or tissue. **blasto′matous** *adj*

pulmonary b. a rare malignant pulmonary neoplasm whose cells resemble those of the fetal pulmonary blastema; it is usually large, develops in the peripheral portions of the lungs, and may invade the bronchi.

blas•to•ma•toid (blas-to′mə-toid) [*blastoma* + *-oid*] resembling blastomas.

blas•to•mere (blas′to-mēr) [*blasto-* + *-mere*] one of the cells produced by cleavage of a zygote; called also *cleavage cell.*

blas•to•mo•gen•ic (blas″to-mo-jen′ik) producing or tending to produce blastomas.

blas•to•mog•e•nous (blas″to-moj′ə-nəs) blastomogenic.

Blas•to•my•ces (blas″to-mi′sēz) [*blasto-* + Gr. *mykēs* fungus] a genus of thermal dimorphic Fungi Imperfecti of the form-class Hyphomycetes; species grow as mycelial forms at room temperature and as yeastlike forms at body temperature. It includes several yeasts that are pathogenic.

B. brasilien′sis *Paracoccidioides brasiliensis.*

B. dermati′tidis a species endemic in the midwestern United States and adjacent parts of Canada, the etiologic agent of North American blastomycosis; its perfect (sexual) stage is *Ajellomyces dermatitidis.*

blas•to•my•ces (blas″to-mi′sēz) pl. *blastomyce′tes.* A fungus of the genus *Blastomyces.* Called also *blastomycete.*

blas•to•my•cete (blas″to-mi′sēt) 1. blastomyces. 2. any yeastlike organism.

Blas•to•my•ce•tes (blas″to-mi-se′tēz) a form-class of Fungi Imperfecti (subphylum Deuteromycotina), comprising the yeasts. Most members of the group do not have known teleomorphs; those that do are classified under Ascomycotina or Basidiomycotina. The form-family Cryptococcaceae is sometimes classified here and sometimes in Hyphomycetes.

blas•to•my•cin (blas″to-mi′sin) a skin test antigen prepared from *Blastomyces dermatitidis* organisms, formerly used in diagnosis of blastomycosis but found to be unreliable.

blas•to•my•co•sis (blas″to-mi-ko′sis) 1. an infection caused by *Blastomyces dermatitidis*, usually acquired through the lungs. There may be suppurating skin lesions *(cutaneous b.)* or lesions in the lungs, bones, subcutaneous tissues, liver, spleen, and kidneys *(systemic b.).* It runs a fulminant, sometimes fatal, course in immunocompromised patients. Called also *North American b.* and *Gilchrist disease.* 2. a general term for any infection caused by a yeastlike organism.

Brazilian b. paracoccidioidomycosis.

cutaneous b. the cutaneous manifestations of blastomycosis, consisting of verrucous or ulcerating skin lesions that may form plaques; occasionally

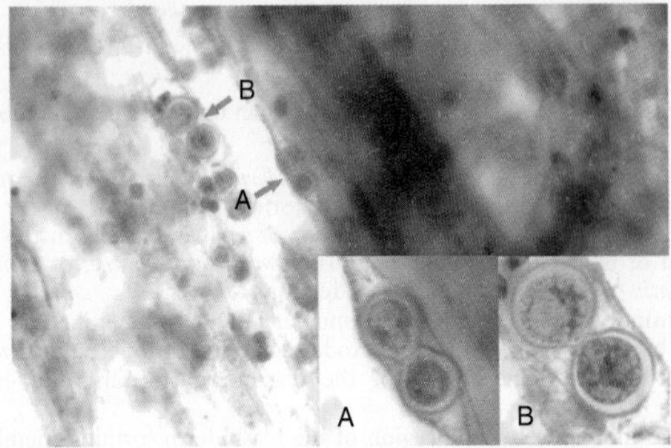

■ Blastomycosis, showing multiple large yeast with equal-sized single budding admixed with acute inflammatory cells in a sputum smear. *(Insets A, B)*, Higher magnification highlighting the equal-sized budding (Papanicolaou stain).

these cause more serious necrosis of areas of skin. Called also *blastomycetic dermatitis.*

European b. cryptococcosis.

keloidal b. lacaziosis.

North American b. blastomycosis (def. 1).

pulmonary b. blastomycosis affecting primarily the lungs and bronchi; it often resolves with fibrosis or takes an indolent course, sometimes with cavitation and eventual spread to other organs. In some patients there is an acute onset of symptoms with acute respiratory distress syndrome that can be fatal.

South American b. paracoccidioidomycosis.

systemic b. see *blastomycosis* (def. 1).

blas•to•neu•ro•pore (blas″to-noor′o-por) [*blasto-* + *neuro-* + *pore*] in certain embryos, a temporary aperture formed by the coalescence of the blastopore and neuropore.

blas•to•phyl•lum (blas″to-fil′əm) [*blasto-* + Gr. *phyllon* leaf] a primordial germ layer.

blas•toph•y•ly (blas-tof′ə-le) [*blasto-* + Gr. *phylē* tribe] the tribal history, or arrangement, of organisms.

blas•to•pore (blas′to-por) [*blasto-* + *pore*] the opening of the archenteron to the exterior of the embryo at the gastrula stage; called also *archistome, protostoma,* and *anus of Rusconi.*

Blas•to•schiz•o•my•ces (blas″to-skiz″o-mi′sēz) a genus of Fungi Imperfecti of the form-class Hyphomycetes.

B. capita′tus a species that sometimes causes fatal opportunistic infections; formerly called *Trichosporon capitatum.*

blas•to•sphere (blas′to-sfēr) [*blasto-* + *sphere*] blastula.

blas•to•spore (blas′to-spor) [*blasto-* + *spore*] a spore formed by budding, as in yeast. Called also *blastoconidium.*

blas•to•zo•oid (blas″to-zo′oid) [*blasto-* + *zooid*] an individual developed as a result of asexual reproduction. Cf. *oozooid.*

blas•tu•la (blas′tu-lə) pl. *blas′tulae* [L.] the usually spherical structure produced by cleavage of a zygote, consisting of a single layer of cells (blastoderm) surrounding a fluid-filled cavity (blastocoele); called also *blastosphere.* See also *discoblastula.* **blas′tular** *adj*

blas•tu•lae (blas′tu-le) [L.] plural of *blastula.*

blas•tu•la•tion (blas″tu-la′shən) conversion of a morula to a blastula or blastocyst by the development of a central cavity (the blastocoele, blastocystic cavity, or cleavage cavity).

Blat•ta (blat′ə) [L.] a genus of cockroaches of the family Blattidae. Their dried, crushed bodies were formerly administered medically as diuretics. They may act as intermediate hosts of *Raillietina madagascariensis* and *Gongylonema pulchrum. B. orienta′lis* is the Oriental cockroach.

Blat•tar•ia (blă-tar′e-ə) the cockroaches, an order of crawling winged insects with flat oval bodies; many are household pests or reservoirs of disease. See also *cockroach.*

Blat•tel•la (blă-tel′ə) a genus of cockroaches of the family Blattidae. *B. germa′nica* is the German cockroach.

Blat•ti•dae (blat′ĭ-de) a family of cockroaches (order Blattaria); genera include *Blatta* and *Blattella.*

Blau syndrome (blou) [Edward B. *Blau,* American pediatrician, late 20th century] see under *syndrome.*

BLB mask [Walter Meredith *Boothby,* American medical researcher, 1880–1953; William R. *Lovelace,* American surgeon, 1907–1965; Arthur H. *Bulbulian,* Turkish-born American medical researcher, 20th century] see under *mask.*

bleach•ing (blēch′ing) the act or process of removing stains or color by chemical means.

coronal b. the use of a chemical agent, usually but not necessarily in combination with heat, to remove discolorations from the crown of a pulpless tooth.

bleb (bleb) bulla (def. 1).

bleed•er (blēd′ər) 1. popular term for a person who tends to bleed too easily, usually because of a deficiency of one of the coagulation factors, such as in hemophilia. 2. any blood vessel cut during a surgical procedure that requires clamping, cautery, or ligature.

bleed•ing (blēd′ing) 1. the escape of blood from an injured vessel; see also *hemorrhage.* 2. phlebotomy.

breakthrough b. a light type of dysfunctional uterine bleeding sometimes seen in women during the first few cycles of usage of an oral contraceptive.

dysfunctional uterine b. (DUB) bleeding from the uterus when no organic uterine lesions are present.

implantation b. bleeding in the uterus at the time of implantation of the blastocyst in the decidua, owing to leakage of blood into the uterine lumen from disrupted blood vessels about the implantation site.

obscure gastrointestinal b. persistent or recurrent gastrointestinal bleeding when a standard endoscopic evaluation is negative; it may be either overt, with melena or hematochezia, or occult, with anemia or a positive test for occult blood.

occult b. escape of such a small amount of blood that it can be detected only by chemical test or by examination with the microscope or spectroscope. See also *occult blood,* under *blood.*

summer b. dermatorrhagia parasitica.

blen•ad•e•ni•tis (blen″ad-ə-ni′tis) [*blenn-* + *adeno-* + *-itis*] myxadenitis.

blen•em•e•sis (blen-em′ə-sis) [*blenn-* + *emesis*] the vomiting of mucus.

blenn(o)- [Gr. *blenna* mucus] a combining form denoting relationship to mucus.

blen•no•gen•ic (blen-o-jen′ik) [*blenno-* + *-genic*] muciparous.

blen•nog•e•nous (blen-oj′ə-nəs) muciparous.

blen•noid (blen′oid) [*blenn-* + *-oid*] mucoid (def. 1).

blen•nor•rha•gia (blen″o-ra′jə) blennorrhea.

blen•nor•rhea (blen″o-re′ə) [*blenno-* + *-rrhea*] a free discharge from the mucous surfaces, especially a gonorrheal discharge from the urethra or vagina. Called also *blennorrhagia.* **blennorrhag′ic, blennorrhe′al** *adj*

Stoerk b. blennorrhea with profuse chronic suppuration producing hypertrophy of the mucosa of the nose, pharynx, and larynx.

blen•no•stat•ic (blen″o-stat′ik) [*blenno-* + *-static*] mucostatic (def. 1).

blen•no•tho•rax (blen″o-thor′aks) [*blenno-* + *thorax*] a pleural effusion consisting of mucus.

blen•nu•ria (blen-u′re-ə) [*blenn-* + *-uria*] excretion of mucus in the urine.

Blen•ox•ane (blen-ok′sān) trademark for a preparation of bleomycin sulfate.

ble•o•my•cin (ble″o-mi′sin) any of a mixture of glycopeptide antibiotics produced by a strain of *Streptomyces verticillus,* designated A_1 to A_6, A_2', and B_1 to B_6, that bind to DNA causing chain scission and removal of purine and pyrimidine bases, resulting in inhibition of DNA synthesis and, to a lesser extent, RNA and protein synthesis and also accumulation of cells in the G_2 phase of the cell cycle. The drug used clinically is a mixture consisting primarily of bleomycins A_2 and B_2.

b. sulfate [USP] a mixture of the sulfate salts of the components of bleomycin, especially that of bleomycin A_2, used alone or in conjunction with other chemotherapeutic agents as an antineoplastic, particularly to treat testicular carcinoma, lymphomas, and various squamous cell carcinomas; administered intravenously, intramuscularly, intra-arterially, or subcutaneously.

Bleph (blef) trademark for preparations of sulfacetamide sodium.

Bleph•a•mide (blef′ə-mīd) trademark for a combination preparation of sulfacetamide sodium and prednisolone acetate.

bleph•a•rad•e•ni•tis (blef″ə-rad″ə-ni′tis) [*blephar-* + *aden-* + *-itis*] inflammation of the meibomian glands; called also *blepharoadenitis.*

bleph•a•ral (blef′ə-ral) palpebral.

bleph•a•rec•to•my (blef″ə-rek′tə-me) [*blephar-* + *-ectomy*] excision of a lesion of the eyelids.

bleph•a•rel•o•sis (blef″ə-rel-o′sis) entropion (def. 2).

bleph•a•rism (blef′ə-riz″əm) palpebration (def. 2).

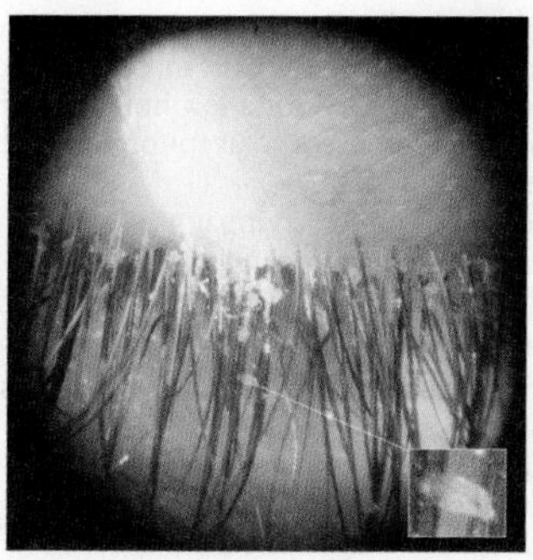

■ Seborrheic blepharitis, with typical translucent scales which are easily removed.

bleph·a·ri·tis (blef″ə-ri′tis) [*blephar-* + *-itis*] inflammation of the eyelids; called also *palpebritis.*

angular b., b. angula′ris blepharitis ulcerosa affecting the medial commissure (angle) and blocking the punctum lacrimalis.

b. cilia′ris, marginal b., b. margina′lis a chronic inflammation of the hair follicles and sebaceous gland openings of the margins of the eyelids; called also *lippa* and *lippitude.*

nonulcerative b., seborrheic b., squamous b. blepharitis often associated with seborrhea of the scalp, brows, and skin behind the ears, marked by greasy scaling of the margins of the lids, scales around the lashes, hyperemia, and thickening.

b. ulcero′sa an ulcerous form of marginal blepharitis.

blephar(o)- [Gr. *blepharon* eyelid] a combining form denoting relationship to an eyelid.

bleph·a·ro·ad·e·ni·tis (blef″ə-ro-ad″ə-ni′tis) blepharadenitis.

bleph·a·ro·ad·e·no·ma (blef″ə-ro-ad″ə-no′mə) adenoma of the eyelid.

bleph·a·ro·ath·er·o·ma (blef″ə-ro-ath″ər-o′mə) an encysted tumor or sebaceous cyst of an eyelid.

bleph·a·ro·chal·a·sis (blef″ə-ro-kal′ə-sis) [*blepharo-* + Gr. *chalasis* relaxation] relaxation of the skin of the eyelid, due to atrophy of the intercellular tissue; called also *dermatolysis palpebrarum.*

bleph·a·roc·lo·nus (blef″ə-rok′lə-nəs) [*blepharo-* + *clonus*] clonic spasm of the orbicularis oculi muscle, appearing as an increased winking of the eye.

bleph·a·ro·con·junc·ti·vi·tis (blef″ə-ro-kən-junk″tĭ-vi′tis) inflammation of the eyelids and conjunctiva.

Bleph·a·ro·co·ryn·thi·na (blef″ə-ro-ko″rin-thi′nə) [*blepharo-* + Gr. *koryntheus* basket] a suborder of ciliate protozoa (order Trichostomatida, subclass Vestibuliferia) found in herbivorous mammals, especially horses, and characterized by a marked reduction in somatic ciliature and apically by a retractable oral area, prominent frontal lobe, and a distinctive corkscrew-like process.

bleph·a·ro·di·as·ta·sis (blef″ə-ro-di-as′tə-sis) [*blepharo-* + *diastasis*] excessive separation of the eyelids, or inability to close them completely, causing the fissure to be very wide.

bleph·a·ro·ker·a·to·con·junc·ti·vi·tis (blef″ə-ro-ker″ə-to-kən-junk-tĭ-vi′tis) inflammation of the eyelid, cornea, and conjunctiva.

bleph·a·ron·cus (blef″ə-rong′kəs) a tumor on the eyelid.

bleph·a·ro·pach·yn·sis (blef″ə-ro-pak-in′sis) [*blepharo-* + *pachynsis*] abnormal thickening of an eyelid.

bleph·a·ro·phi·mo·sis (blef″ə-ro-fĭ-mo′sis) [*blepharo-* + Gr. *phimōsis* a muzzling] abnormal narrowness of the palpebral fissures in the horizontal direction, caused by lateral displacement of the inner canthi.

bleph·a·ro·plast (blef′ə-ro-plast) basal body.

bleph·a·ro·plas·ty (blef′ə-ro-plas″te) plastic surgery of an eyelid; called also *tarsoplasty.* **blepharoplas′tic** *adj*

bleph·a·ro·ple·gia (blef″ə-ro-ple′jə) [*blepharo-* + *-plegia*] paralysis of an eyelid or of both muscles of the eyelid.

bleph·a·rop·to·sis (blef″ə-rop-to′sis, blef″ə-ro-to′sis) [*blepharo-* + *-ptosis*] drooping of an upper eyelid; ptosis (q.v.).

bleph·a·ro·py·or·rhea (blef″ə-ro-pi″ə-re′ə) purulent ophthalmia.

bleph·a·ror·rha·phy (blef″ə-ror′ə-fe) tarsorrhaphy.

bleph·a·ro·spasm (blef′ə-ro-spaz″əm) [*blepharo-* + *spasm*] tonic spasm of the orbicularis oculi muscle, producing more or less complete closure of the eyelids.

essential b. blepharospasm that is present when there is no abnormality of the eye or trigeminal (fifth cranial) nerve.

symptomatic b. blepharospasm occurring in association with a lesion of the eye or of the trigeminal (fifth cranial) nerve.

bleph·a·ro·sphinc·ter·ec·to·my (blef″ə-ro-sfingk″tər-ek′tə-me) [*blepharo-* + *sphincter* + *ectomy*] excision of some of the fibers of the orbicularis muscle, together with overlying skin, to relieve pressure of the eyelid on the cornea in blepharospasm.

bleph·a·ro·stat (blef′ə-ro-stat″) lid speculum.

bleph·a·ro·ste·no·sis (blef″ə-ro-stə-no′sis) blepharophimosis.

bleph·a·ro·syn·ech·ia (blef″ə-ro-sĭ-nek′e-ə) [*blepharo-* + *synechia*] the growing together or adhesion of the eyelids.

bleph·a·rot·o·my (blef″ə-rot′ə-me) surgical incision of an eyelid; tarsotomy.

Bles·sed Dementia Rating Scale (bles′əd) [G. *Blessed*, British psychiatrist, 20th century.] see under *scale*[1].

Bles·sig cysts (lacunae), groove (bles′ig) [Robert *Blessig*, German physician, 1830–1878] see under *cyst* and *groove.*

Blighia (bli′yə) a genus of evergreen trees of the family Sapindaceae, native to West Africa. *B. sa′pida* Kon. is the akee or ackee, whose aril is cooked and considered a delicacy in the West Indies but is poisonous if eaten raw. See *Jamaican vomiting sickness*, under *sickness.*

blind (blīnd) [A.S. *blind*] 1. not having the sense of sight; see *blindness.* 2. pertaining to a clinical trial or other experiment in which one or more of the groups receiving, administering, and evaluating the treatment are unaware of which treatment any particular subject is receiving. Some authorities prefer the term masked to avoid confusion with physical blindness. See *single blind*, *double blind*, and *triple blind.* Cf. *open.*

blind·ing (blīnd′ing) in clinical trials and other experiments, the process of making the participants blind; see *blind* (def. 2). Called also *masking.*

blind·ness (blīnd′nis) lack or loss of ability to see; lack of perception of visual stimuli, due to disorder of the organs of sight or to lesions in certain areas of the brain; see also *amaurosis.*

amnesic color b. a form of aphasia in which the patient sees a color correctly but cannot name it, due to a brain lesion.

blue b., blue-yellow b. popular names for inability to distinguish blue and yellow tints, such as in *tritanopia.*

color b. colloquial but misleading name for color vision deficiency.

complete color b. popular name for *monochromatic vision.*

concussion b. functional blindness due to a violent explosion, such as of a high explosive shell, or bomb.

congenital retinal b. Leber congenital amaurosis.

cortical b. blindness due to a lesion of one of the areas of the visual cortex.

day b. hemeralopia.

eclipse b. partial or total loss of central vision caused by a burn on the macula from direct fixation on the sun or from viewing a partial solar eclipse without proper protective lenses.

electric light b. temporary impairment of vision due to exposure to ultraviolet rays. Photophobia, blepharospasm, redness of the eye, and swelling of the conjunctiva are the symptoms, which usually occur several hours after exposure.

flight b. amaurosis fugax caused by high centrifugal forces encountered in aviation.

functional b. 1. any inability to see effectively, especially that owing to a defect not in the eye itself, such as in blepharoptosis or a disorder of the cortical visual pathways. 2. hysterical b.

green b. popular name for either *deuteranopia* or *protanopia.*

heather b. infectious ovine keratoconjunctivitis.

hysterical b. inability to see because of a conversion disorder rather than any disorder of the organs of sight.

legal b. blindness as defined by law; in most states of the United States, maximal visual acuity of the better eye, after correction, of 20/200 or less, with a total diameter of the visual field in that eye of 20 degrees or less.

letter b. alexia characterized by inability to recognize individual letters.

moon b. periodic ophthalmia.

music b. musical alexia.

night b. nyctalopia.

object b. visual agnosia.

psychic b. visual agnosia.

red b. popular name for *protanopia.*

red-green b., red-green color b. popular name for any imperfect perception of red and green tints, including all the most common types of color vision deficiency. See *deuteranomaly*, *deuteranopia*, *protanomaly*, and *protanopia.*

river b. blindness caused by onchocerciasis.

snow b. dimness of vision, usually temporary, due to the glare of the sun upon snow.

taste b. partial to complete ageusia; particularly used for the former, with some, but not all, substances producing no sensation of taste.

text b. alexia.

total b. complete absence of light perception.

total color b. popular name for *monochromatic vision.*

transient monocular b. an episode of total or partial loss of vision in one eye, due to ischemia of the eye and lasting several minutes or longer; the term is sometimes used synonymously with *amaurosis fugax* and sometimes to designate an episode of longer duration. Called also *transient monocular visual loss.*

word b. alexia.

yellow b. popular name for imperfect perception of yellow tints, such as in tritanopia.

blis·ter (blis′tər) [L. *vesicula*] 1. vesicle (def. 2). 2. bulla (def. 1).

blood b. a blister containing blood; it may be caused by a pinch, a bruise, or persistent friction.

fever b. herpes febrilis.

sucking b. a small blister on the center of the upper lip of an infant caused by friction during nursing.

water b. a blister with clear watery contents.

bloat (blōt) 1. indigestion with excessive formation of gas in one or more of the stomachs of a ruminant. 2. ruminal tympany. 3. enteritis in young rabbits, accompanied by gaseous distention of the abdomen.

abomasal b. bloat in calves or lambs on milk replacement diets, seen especially when the milk replacer is warm or contains insoluble ingredients or if the animals have not been fed for a few hours and drink too much. The distended abomasum may compress adjacent organs and vessels, resulting in fatal asphyxia or heart failure.

free gas b. secondary ruminal tympany.

frothy b. primary ruminal tympany.

leguminous b. primary ruminal tympany caused by a diet excessively high in legumes such as alfalfa or clover.

bloat·ing (blōt′ing) distention of the abdomen caused by swallowed air or by intestinal gas.

functional b. a recurrent sensation of abdominal distention, with or without measurable distention, that is not part of another functional bowel or gastroduodenal disorder.

Bloc·a·dren (blok′ə-dren) trademark for a preparation of timolol maleate.

Bloch-Sulz·ber·ger syndrome (blok′ sulz′bər-gər) [Bruno *Bloch*, Swiss dermatologist, 1878–1933; Marion Baldur *Sulzberger*, American dermatologist, 1895–1983] incontinentia pigmenti.

block (blok) 1. obstruction. 2. to obstruct. 3. regional anesthesia; see under *anesthesia.*

Block

adrenergic b. see under *blockade.*

air b. interference with the normal inflation and deflation of the lungs and with the pulmonary blood flow, produced by the leakage of air from the pulmonary alveoli into the interstitial tissue of the lung (interstitial emphysema) and into the mediastinum (mediastinal emphysema).

alveolar-capillary b. interference in the normal diffusion of gases across the membrane between the alveolar spaces and the pulmonary capillaries.

ankle b. regional anesthesia of the foot by the injection of a local anesthetic around the anterior and posterior tibial nerves at the level of the ankle.

anodal b. a conduction block resulting from hyperpolarization of the nerve cell membrane by an electric stimulus.

anterior fascicular b. left anterior hemiblock; see *hemiblock.* See also *fascicular b.*

atrioventricular b., AV b. impairment of conduction of cardiac impulses from the atria to the ventricles, usually due to a block in the atrioventricular junctional tissue (atrioventricular node, bundle of His, or bundle branches). It is generally subclassified as first, second, or third degree atrioventricular block. Cf. *heart b.*

2:1 AV b. second degree atrioventricular block in which conduction of every other impulse through the atrioventricular conduction system is prevented, resulting in a 2:1 ratio of atrial to ventricular depolarizations.

Bier b. regional anesthesia by intravenous injection, used for surgical procedures on the arm below the elbow or the leg below the knee; performed in a bloodless field maintained by a pneumatic tourniquet that also prevents the anesthetic from entering the systemic circulation. Called also *Bier local anesthesia, intravenous regional anesthesia,* and *intravenous b.*

bifascicular b. impairment of conduction in two of the three fascicles of the bundle branches (see *fascicular b.*), i.e., in the left bundle branch or in the right bundle branch plus either the anterior or posterior limb of the left bundle branch.

bilateral bundle branch b. (BBBB) interruption of conduction of cardiac impulses through both bundle branches, clinically indistinguishable from complete atrioventricular block.

brachial plexus b. regional anesthesia of the shoulder, arm, and hand by injection of a local anesthetic into the brachial plexus; called also *brachial plexus anesthesia.*

bundle branch b. (BBB) interruption of conduction in one of the main bundle branches, left or right; the sequence of ventricular depolarization is altered since the impulse reaches one ventricle and then travels to the other.

caudal b. regional anesthesia produced by injection of a local anesthetic into the caudal or sacral canal. Called also *caudal anesthesia.*

cervical plexus b. regional anesthesia of the neck by injection of a local anesthetic into the cervical plexus.

comparator b. see *comparator.*

complete atrioventricular b. third degree atrioventricular b.

complete heart b. third degree heart b.

conduction b. a blockage in a nerve that prevents impulses from being conducted across a given segment although the nerve is viable beyond that segment. Cf. *neurapraxia.*

congenital complete heart b. third degree atrioventricular block that presents in the fetal or neonatal period and is caused by defective development of the atrioventricular junctional tissue; it may be associated with other cardiac anomalies.

cryogenic b. local cooling of tissue.

depolarization b. failure of an excitable cell to respond to a stimulus, because the membrane is depolarized.

dynamic b. spinal subarachnoid b.

ear b. a type of barotrauma in which the auditory tube is closed and the tympanic membrane may rupture. See also *barotitis media.*

elbow b. regional anesthesia of the forearm and hand by injection of local anesthetic around the median, radial, and ulnar nerves at the elbow.

entrance b. in cardiology, a unidirectional impasse to conduction that prevents an impulse from entering a specific region of excitable tissue; it is part of the mechanism underlying parasystole.

epidural b. regional anesthesia produced by injection of the anesthetic agent into the epidural space. Injection may be between the vertebral spines, in the cervical, thoracic, or lumbar region, or into the sacral hiatus, which is also known as *caudal block* (q.v.) or *anesthesia.* See also *continuous epidural analgesia.* Called also *epidural anesthesia* and *peridural b.* or *anesthesia.*

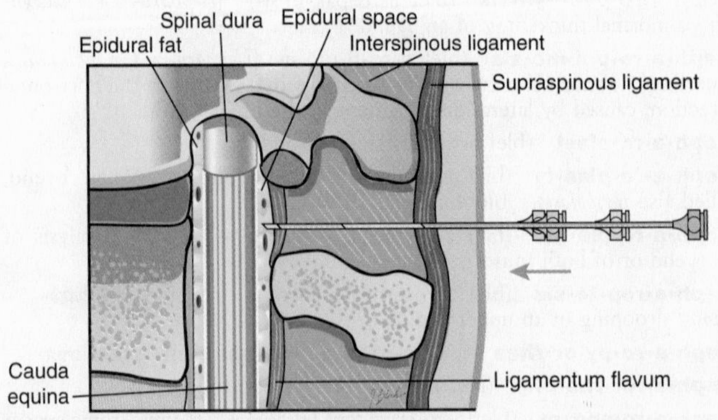

■ Production of epidural block by injection through the ligamentum flavum into the epidural space, the needle stopping just short of the dura.

Block *Continued*

exit b. in cardiology, delay or failure of an impulse to be conducted from a specific region to surrounding tissues; the region may be either a physiologic or artificial cardiac pacemaker.
fascicular b. any of a group of disorders of conduction localized within the bundle branches or their ramifications. The block may occur in any combination of the three fascicles of the bundle branches: the right bundle branch or the anterior or posterior limb of the left bundle branch. See also *unifascicular b.*, *bifascicular b.*, and *trifascicular b.*
femoral b. regional anesthesia of the posterior thigh and the leg below the knee by injection of a local anesthetic around the femoral nerve just below the inguinal ligament at the lateral border of the fossa ovalis.
field b. regional anesthesia achieved by blocking conduction in nerves with chemical or physical agents.
first degree atrioventricular b. a first degree heart block due to a block in the atrioventricular junctional tissue; the rate of conduction of impulses from the atria to the ventricles is slowed, resulting in regular electrocardiographic P–R intervals of greater than 0.21 second.
first degree heart b. the mildest form of heart block, in which conduction time is prolonged but all impulses are conducted; often used specifically for first degree atrioventricular block.
heart b. impairment of conduction of an impulse in heart excitation, either permanent or transient and due to anatomical or functional impairment. It is subclassified as first, second, or third degree heart block and is frequently used specifically to denote atrioventricular block.
high grade atrioventricular b. either second or third degree atrioventricular b.
incomplete heart b. heart block in which at least some impulses are conducted, i.e., first or second degree heart block.
intercostal b., intercostal nerve b. regional anesthesia produced by blocking intercostal nerves with a local anesthetic.
interventricular b. bundle branch b.
intra-Hisian b., intrahisian b. atrioventricular block located within the bundle of His.
intranasal b. local anesthesia produced by insertion into the nasal fossae of pledgets soaked in a solution of local anesthetic.
intraspinal b. spinal anesthesia (def. 1).
intravenous b. Bier b.
intraventricular b. impaired conduction within the ventricles due to absence of conduction within the bundle branches, their ramifications, or the ventricles.
IV b. Bier b.
joint b. regional anesthesia produced by injection of local anesthetic into a joint cavity; the most common sites for this are the zygapophyseal joints and the sacroiliac joint.
left anterior fascicular b. left anterior hemiblock; see *hemiblock.* See also *fascicular b.*
left bundle branch b. (LBBB) see *bundle branch b.*
left posterior fascicular b. left posterior hemiblock; see *hemiblock.* See also *fascicular b.*
lumbar plexus b. regional anesthesia of the anterior and medial aspects of the leg by injection of a local anesthetic into the lumbar plexus.
medial branch b. regional anesthesia of part of the cervical region of the back, produced by injection of a local anesthetic around a medial branch or branches of the posterior branch of a cervical nerve.
mental b. *blocking* (def. 2).
metabolic b. the blockade of a biosynthetic pathway caused by a genetic enzyme deficiency or by inhibition of an enzyme by a drug or other substance.
methadone b. see *narcotic blockade*, under *blockade*.
Mobitz type I b. Wenckebach b.
Mobitz type II b. a type of second degree atrioventricular block in which dropped beats occur periodically without previous lengthening of the P–R interval (cf. *Wenckebach b.*); it is due to a block within or below the bundle of His.
motor point b. interruption of impulses, by anesthesia or destruction of the nerve, at a motor point in order to relieve spasticity; a common method is *phenol motor point b.* Called also *intramuscular neurolysis.*
nerve b. 1. regional anesthesia achieved by making extraneural or paraneural injections of anesthetics next to the nerve whose conductivity is to be cut off. 2. neurolysis (def. 4).
neurolytic b. neurolysis (def. 4).
paracervical b. regional anesthesia of the inferior hypogastric plexus and ganglia produced by injection of the local anesthetic into the lateral fornices of the vagina; called also *uterosacral b.*
paraneural b. perineural b.
parasacral b. regional anesthesia produced by injection of a local anesthetic around the sacral nerves as they emerge from the sacral foramina.
paravertebral b. regional anesthesia produced by injection of a local anesthetic around the spinal nerves at their exit from the vertebral column, usually to cause anesthesia of the sympathetic trunk at a given level. Called also *paravertebral anesthesia.*
partial heart b. second degree heart b.
peridural b. epidural b.
periinfarction b. disturbance of intraventricular conduction after a myocardial infarction, due to delayed conduction in the infarct region.
perineural b. regional anesthesia produced by injection of the anesthetic agent close to the nerve; called also *paraneural b.* or *anesthesia.*
phenol b. 1. phenol neurolysis. 2. phenol motor point b.
phenol motor point b. the most common method of motor point block; a solution of 5 per cent phenol in water is injected at the motor point. Called also *phenol b.*
posterior fascicular b. left posterior hemiblock; see *hemiblock.* See also *fascicular b.*
presacral b. regional anesthesia produced by injection of the local anesthetic into the sacral nerves on the anterior aspect of the sacrum.
pudendal b. regional anesthesia produced by blocking the pudendal nerves, accomplished by injection of the local anesthetic into the region of the tuberosity of the ischium.
retrobulbar b. anesthetization and immobilization of the eye achieved by injection of a local anesthetic into the retrobulbar space.
right bundle branch b. (RBBB) see *bundle branch b.*
sacral b. regional anesthesia produced by injection of a local anesthetic into the extradural space of the sacral canal. Called also *transsacral anesthesia* or *transsacral b.*
saddle b. the production of spinal anesthesia in a region corresponding roughly with the areas of the buttocks, perineum, and inner aspects of the thighs that impinge on the saddle in riding, by introducing the anesthetic agent low in the dural sac.
sciatic b. regional anesthesia of the lower leg and foot by injection of a local anesthetic around the sciatic nerve.
second degree atrioventricular b. a second degree heart block due to partial impairment of impulse conduction through the atrioventricular junctional tissue; impulses intermittently fail to reach the ventricles (dropped beats). It occurs as two types: *type I* is Wenckebach or Mobitz type I block and *type II* is Mobitz type II block.
second degree heart b. the partial form of heart block, in which some impulses are not conducted; often used specifically for second degree atrioventricular block. Called also *partial heart b.*
sinoatrial b., sinoatrial exit b. a disturbance in which the atrial response is delayed or omitted because of partial or complete interference with the propagation of impulses from the sinoatrial node to the atria.
sinus b., sinus exit b. sinoatrial b.
spinal b. regional anesthesia produced by injection of a local anesthetic into the subarachnoid space around the spinal cord; cf. *epidural a.* Called also *intraspinal a.* or *block* and *subarachnoid a.* or *block.*
spinal subarachnoid b. a condition in which the flow of cerebrospinal fluid is interfered with by an obstruction in the spinal canal; called also *dynamic b.*
splanchnic b. regional anesthesia produced by blocking the splanchnic nerves and the celiac ganglia; it is accomplished by injection of the anesthetic agent into the retroperitoneal tissues in the immediate vicinity of the celiac plexuses.
stellate b., stellate ganglion b. regional anesthesia produced by blocking of the stellate (cervicothoracic) ganglion.
subarachnoid b. spinal anesthesia (def. 1).
sympathetic b. blocking of the sympathetic trunk by paravertebral infiltration with an anesthetic agent.
third degree atrioventricular b. a third degree heart block due to total cessation of impulse conduction through the atrioventricular junctional tissue; no correspondence exists between atrial and ventricular activity, and ventricular asystole and death occur unless a ventricular pacemaker is activated.
third degree heart b. the complete form of heart block, in which no impulses are conducted; often used specifically for third degree atrioventricular block. Called also *complete heart b.*
transsacral b. sacral block.

Block *Continued*

trifascicular b. impairment of conduction in all three fascicles of the bundle branches, i.e., the right bundle branch and both anterior and posterior limbs of the left bundle branch. It is a form of complete heart block. See also *fascicular b.*

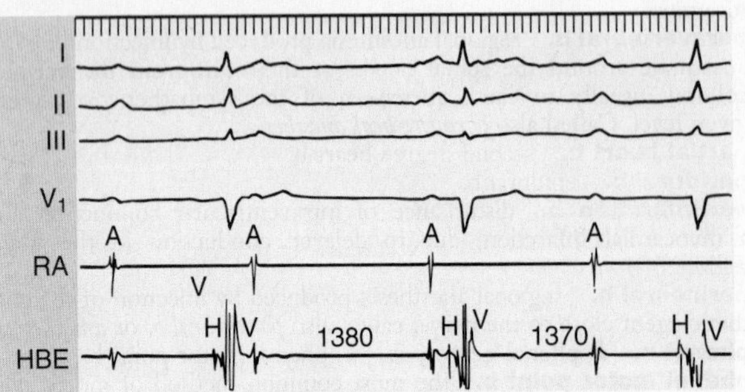

■ Congenital complete third degree atrioventricular (AV) block. No P wave is followed by a His bundle potential, whereas each ventricular depolarization is preceded by a His bundle potential. *HBE,* His bundle electrogram; *RA,* right atrium; *RV,* right ventricle.

unifascicular b. impairment of conduction in the right bundle branch or in either the anterior or posterior limb of the left bundle branch. See also *fascicular b.*

uterosacral b. paracervical b.

vagal b., vagus nerve b. regional anesthesia produced by blocking of vagal impulses by injection of a local anesthetic into the vagus nerve at its exit from the skull.

ventricular b. obstruction to the flow of cerebrospinal fluid within the ventricular system or through the exit foramina (foramina of Magendie and Luschka) by which the ventricles communicate with the subarachnoid space; it results in obstructive hydrocephalus.

Wenckebach b. a type of second degree atrioventricular block in which one or more dropped beats occur periodically after a series of steadily increasing P–R intervals (cf. *Mobitz type II b.*); it is usually due to a block within the atrioventricular node. Called also *Mobitz type I b.*

wrist b. regional anesthesia of the hand by injection of a local anesthetic around the median, radial, and ulnar nerves at the wrist.

---

block•ade (blok-ād′) 1. receptor blockade, the blocking of the effect of a hormone or neurotransmitter at a cell-surface receptor by a pharmacologic antagonist bound to the receptor. 2. in histochemistry, a chemical reaction that by modifying certain chemical groups blocks a specific staining method. 3. regional anesthesia.

adrenergic b. selective inhibition of the response to sympathetic impulses and to catecholamines and other adrenergic amines at either the alpha or beta receptor sites of the effector organ or at the postganglionic adrenergic neuron.

adrenergic neuron b. see *adrenergic b.*

alpha-adrenergic b., alpha-b. see *adrenergic b.*

beta-adrenergic b., beta-b. see *adrenergic b.*

cholinergic b. selective inhibition of cholinergic nerve impulses at autonomic ganglionic synapses, at postganglionic parasympathetic effectors, or at the neuromuscular junction.

combined androgen b., complete androgen b. treatment of prostate cancer by blocking both testicular and adrenal androgens, usually through orchiectomy followed by administration of an agent that blocks adrenal androgens. Called also *maximum androgen b.*

estrogen b. treatment of breast cancer by blocking the effects of estrogens in the body. Cf. *antiestrogen.*

ganglionic b. inhibition by drugs of nerve impulse transmission at autonomic ganglionic synapses. See also *ganglionic blocking agent,* under *agent.*

maximum androgen b. combined androgen b.

narcotic b. inhibition of the euphoric effects of narcotic drugs by the use of other drugs, such as methadone, in the treatment of addiction.

neuromuscular b. a failure in neuromuscular transmission that can be induced pharmacologically or may result from pathological disturbance at the myoneural junction.

renal b. obstructive uropathy with involvement of the genitourinary system distal to the collecting tubules; blockade of individual nephrons or nephron groups and the resultant anuria.

virus b. interference by a virus with the action of another virus; attenuated virus of a disease has been used to inhibit the multiplication of an active virus.

block•age (blok′əj) obstruction.

block•er (blok′ər) something that obstructs passage or activity. See also *antagonist,* and see *blocking agent,* under *agent.*

α-b. alpha-adrenergic blocking agent.

angiotensin receptor b., angiotensin II receptor b. see under *antagonist.*

β-b. beta-adrenergic blocking agent.

calcium channel b., calcium entry b. calcium channel blocking agent.

potassium channel b. potassium channel blocking agent.

sodium channel b. sodium channel blocking agent.

block•ing (blok′ing) 1. interfering with afferent nerve impulses; see *regional anesthesia,* under *anesthesia.* 2. sudden cessation of the train of thought or speech, such as may occur in a period of extreme emotion or when a repressed painful thought is approached. Called also *thought b.* or *deprivation.* 3. casting of tissue blocks in an embedding medium such as paraffin wax so that sections can be cut with a microtome.

adrenergic b. see under *blockade.*

thought b. *blocking* (def. 2).

block•out (blok′out) elimination in a master cast of undesirable undercut areas, including all areas that would offer interference to the placement of the denture framework and those not crossed by a rigid part of the denture, accomplished by filling in areas to be blocked out with suitable materials. See also *relief* (def. 4).

Blocq disease (blok) [Paul Oscar *Blocq,* French physician, 1860–1896] astasia-abasia.

Blom-Sing•er puncture (blom′ sing′ər) [Eric D. *Blom,* American speech pathologist, 20th century; Mark Irwin *Singer,* American otolaryngologist, born 1945] see *tracheoesophageal puncture,* under *puncture.*

blood (blud) [L. *sanguis, cruor;* Gr. *haima*] the fluid that circulates through the heart, arteries, capillaries, and veins, carrying nutriment and oxygen to the body cells. It consists of the *plasma,* a pale yellow liquid containing the microscopically visible formed elements of the blood: the *erythrocytes,* or red blood corpuscles; the *leukocytes,* or white blood corpuscles; and the *platelets,* or thrombocytes. Called also *haema* [TA], *hema,* and *sanguis* [TA alternative].

arterial b. oxygenated blood, found in the pulmonary veins, the left chambers of the heart, and the systemic arteries; it is bright red.

citrated b. blood treated with sodium citrate or citric acid to prevent its coagulation.

cord b. blood contained within the umbilical vessels at the time of delivery of the infant.

defibrinated b. whole blood from which fibrin was separated during the clotting process.

laky b. blood that has undergone laking and contains at least some lysed erythrocytes.

modified whole b. [USP] whole blood, drawn under aseptic conditions and preserved with citrate ion or heparin sodium, and from which antihemophilic factor has been removed.

occult b. blood present in such small quantities that it is not visible to the naked eye and can be detected only by chemical tests of suspected material, e.g., feces.

peripheral b. blood obtained from acral areas, or from the circulation remote from the heart, as from earlobe, fingertip, or heel pad (in a child), or from the antecubital vein; the blood in the systemic circulation.

predonated autologous b. blood donated prior to surgery or other invasive procedure for use in a possible autotransfusion.

sludged b. blood in which the red cells have become aggregated into masses; see *intravascular agglutination,* under *agglutination.*

venous b. deoxygenated blood, found in the systemic veins, the right chambers of the heart, and the pulmonary arteries; it is dark red.

whole b. 1. blood from which none of the elements have been removed. 2. [USP] blood that has been drawn from a selected donor under strict aseptic conditions, containing citrate ion or heparin sodium as an anticoagulant; used as a blood replenisher.

Human Blood Group Systems and Erythrocytic Antigenic Determinants

Blood Group System	Antigenic Determinants*
ABO	A [Subgroups A_1, A_2, A_3, A_m, A_o, A_x, A_{int}, A_{end}, A_{finn}, A_{e1}, A_{bantu}], B [Subgroups B_3, B_x, B_{el}]
Auberger	Au^a
Bg	Bg^a, Bg^b, Bg^c, DBG, Ho, Ho-like, Ot, Sto
Cartwright	Yt^a, Yt^b
Colton	Co^a, Co^b
Cost-Sterling	Cs^a, Yk^a
Diego	Di^a, Di^b
Dombrock	Do^a, Do^b
Duffy	Fy^a (Fyl), Fy^b (Fy2), Fy^{ab} (Fy3), Fy4, Fy5
Gerbich	Ge 1, Ge 2, Ge 3
H	H
Ii	I, I^D, I^F, I^T, i
Kell	K1 (K), K2 (k), K3 (Kp^a), K4 (Kp^b), K5 (Ku), K6 (Js^a), K7 (Js^b), K8 (kw), K9 (K1), K10 ($U1^a$), K11 (Côté), K12 (Bøk), K13 (Sgro), K14 (San), K15 (Kx), K16 (K-like), K17 (Wk^a), K18, K19, Kp^c
Kidd	Jk^a (Jk1), Jk^b (Jk2), Jk^{ab} (Jk3)
Lewis	Le^a (Le1), Le^b (Le2), Le^c (Le5), Le^d, Le^x (L^{ab}, Le3), Mag (Le4)
Lutheran	Lu^a (Lu1), Lu^b (Lu2), Lu^{ab} (Lu3), Lu4, Lu5, Lu6, Lu7, Lu8, Lu9, Lu10, Lu11, Lu12, Lu13, Lu14 (Sw^a)
MNSs	Cl^a, Far, He, Hill, Hu, M, M_1, M^A, M^c, M^e, M^g, M^k, M^r, M^v, M^z, Mi^a, Mt^a, Mur, N, N^A, N^a, N_2, Ny^a, Ri^a, S, S_2, S^B, s, Sj, St^a, Sul, Tm, U, U^B, Vr, Vw, Z
P	P1, P2 (Tj^a), P3 (P^k)
Rh	Rh1 (D, Rh_0), Rh2 (C, rh′), Rh3 (E, rh′), Rh4 (c, hr′), Rh5 (e, hr′), Rh6 (ce, f, hr), Rh7 (Ce, Rh_i), Rh8 (C^w, rh^{wl}), Rh9 (C^x, rh^x), Rh10 (V, ce^s, hr^v), Rh11 (E^w, rh^{w2}), Rh12 (G, rh^G), Rh13 (Rh^A), Rh14 (Rh^B), Rh15 (Rh^C), Rh16 (Rh^D), Rh17 (Hr_0), Rh18 (Hr), Rh19 (Hr^s), Rh20 (VS, e^s), Rh21 (C^G), Rh22 (CE), Rh23 (D^w), Rh24 (E^T), Rh25 (L^W), Rh26 (c-like), Rh27 (cE), Rh28 (hr^H), Rh29 (RH), Rh30 (D^{cor}), Rh31 (hr^B), Rh32, Rh33, Rh34 (Hr^B), Rh35, Rh36, Rh37, Rh38, Rh39, Rh40, Rh41, Rh42 (Ce^s)
Scianna	Sm (Sc1), Bu^a (Sc2)
Stolzfus	Sf^a
Vel	Vel 1, Vel 2
Wright	Wr^a, Wr^b
Xg	Xg^a

Antigenic Determinants That Depend on Gene Interactions

ABO/I	P/ABO	IP1, IP2 ($IT^a{}_j$), I^TP1, iP1	Fy5
P/I	Xor/Duffy	ILe^{bh}	Rh25 (L^W)
Lewis/I	Rh/L^W	A_1Le^b(Seidler)	
Lewis/ABO	Ih, IA, IB, iH	Luke	

Selected Antigenic Determinants Not Thus Far Associated with a Blood Group System

754, An^a, At^a, Be^a, Bec, Bi, Big Charles, Bp*a*, Bra, Bx*a*, By, Cad, Car, Chido (Gursha), Chr^a, Cip, Coates, Craig, Dahl, Donaviesky, Dp, Driver, Duch, E1, En^a, Evans, Evelyn, Fin, Fuerhart, Fuj, Gf^a, Gilbraith, Gn^a, Go^b, Good, Green, Gy^a, Hands, Hen, Heibel, Hill, Ht^a, Hy, Je^a, Jn^a, Jo^a, Job, Jr, Kam, Kelly, Ken, Knops (Kn^a), Kosis, Lan, Lev, Lw^a, McCall, McCoy (McC^a), Man, Mar, Mo^a, MZ443, Nij, Ola, Orr, Pea, Pt^a, Rd^a, Reid, Rogers (Rg^a), Savior, Sch, Sd^a, Simon, Skjelbred, Ters, Th^a, To^a, Todd, Tr^a, Ven, Vennera, Wb, Weeks, Wil, Winbourne, Wu, Yh^a, York (Yk^a), Za

*Symbols within parentheses are those of alternative nomenclatures. Antigenic determinants are systematized according to observed and assumed independent assortment of their responsible genes. Within many systems, alleles are responsible for differing combinations of antigenic determinants.

blood group (blud grōōp) 1. an allotype (or phenotype) of erythrocytes defined by one or more cell surface antigens that are under the control of allelic genes. Antigenic determinants irregularly incite allotypic and sometimes xenotypic immune responses. Human blood groups are identified by agglutination supported by specific human or animal antisera and by lectins extracted from certain plants. An abbreviated classification of human blood groups is given in the accompanying table. 2. any of certain other characteristics or traits of a cellular or fluid component of blood, considered as the expression (phenotype or allotype) of the actions and interactions of dominant genes; used in medicolegal and other studies of human inheritance. Such characteristics include the antigenic groupings of erythrocytes, leukocytes, platelets, and plasma proteins. Called also *blood type.*

ABO b. g. the major human blood group system, dependent on the presence or absence of A and B antigens, which are largely glycolipids on the cell membrane. The gene for A is responsible for synthesis of *N*-acetyl-α-D-galactosaminyl transferase, whereas that for B is responsible for α-D-galactosyl transferase. Either A or B is created when one of these hexasaccharides is positioned by a specific transferase in 1→3 linkage to the β-D-galactose of an H-active oligosaccharide. Type O occurs when neither transferase is present or, very rarely *(Bombay phenotype),* when H antigen does not exist. When both transferases are present, type AB results. Differences in degree of transferase activity are determined at the same locus: weak transferase gives rise to weak antigens (A_2, A_3A_x, B_3B_x). Similar oligosaccharides, especially in bacterial cell walls, immunize persons lacking A or B so that their serum contains anti-A or anti-B activity. A and B antigens are on the mucopolysaccharides of secretors; persons with dominant genes have H-active mucoids.

Auberger b. g. a blood group consisting of the erythrocytic antigen Au^a, related to the Lutheran blood group.

Bg b. g. a blood group consisting of the erythrocytic human leukocyte antigens Bg^a, Bg^b, Bg^c, DBG, Ho, Ho-like, Ot, and Sto.

Cartwright b. g. Yt b. g.

Chido-Rodgers b. g. a blood group consisting of antigens Ch^a and Rg^a, antigenic determinants of fragments of the C4 component of complement.

Colton b. g. a blood group consisting of erythrocytic antigens Co^a and Co^b.

Cromer b. g. a blood group consisting of erythrocytic antigens Cr^a, Tc^a, Tc^{ab}, Dr^a, Es^a, WES^b, UMC, and IFC, which are located on the membrane protein called *decay accelerating factor.*

Diego b. g. a blood group consisting of the erythrocytic antigens Di^a and Di^b, determined by allelic genes. Di^a is most frequent in South American Indians, Japanese, and Chinese.

Dombrock b. g. a blood group consisting of the erythrocytic antigens Do^a and Do^b, most common in people of European descent.

Duffy b. g. a blood group consisting principally of the erythrocytic antigens Fy^a and Fy^b, determined by allelic genes. Amorphic genes are common in individuals of African descent.

Gerbich b. g. a blood group consisting of the erythrocytic antigens Ge 1, Ge 2, and Ge 3; although rare in most parts of the world, it has been found often in Papua New Guinea.

H b. g. a blood group consisting of antigen H; see also *Bombay phenotype.*

high frequency b. g. a group containing over 99 per cent of individuals, who have a type of erythrocyte antigens called *public antigens.*

Ii b. g. a high frequency blood group involving receptors of most cold reactive hemagglutinins; it is expressed most strongly on cord blood cells.

Kell b. g. a blood group consisting of multiple erythrocytic antigens, especially three pairs of alternates, determined by complex genes at one locus, including an amorph; also regulated by the X chromosome, it is associated with sex-linked chronic granulomatous disease. One antigen, K6, is more frequent in people of African descent.

Kidd b. g. a blood group consisting principally of Jk^a and Jk^b antigens, determined by allelic genes; amorphic genes are most common in those of East Asian descent.

Knops b. g. a blood group consisting of antigens Kn[a], Kn[b], McC[a], Sl[a], and Yk[a], which are located on complement receptor type 1.

Lan b. g. a blood group consisting of the erythrocytic antigen Lan.

Lewis b. g. a blood group determined by plasma glycolipids that adhere to erythrocytic surfaces. It is based on dominant independent *Le* genes, but interacts with the H precursor oligosaccharides of A and B. Whereas *le/le* provides the "double negative" blood type Le(a−b−), *Le* without H gives rise to Le[a], i.e., blood type Le(a+b−), and that with H gives rise to Le[b]H, i.e., blood type Le(a−b+).

low frequency b. g. any small group that has erythrocytic antigens found in fewer than 1 per cent of the population *(private antigens)*.

Lutheran b. g. a complex blood group system consisting of antigens Lu[a] and Lu[b]; it somewhat resembles the Kell group in having pairs of alternative antigens and amorphic genes, but is also subject to a dominant independently segregating repressor.

MNSs b. g. a complex blood group system consisting principally of two pairs of antigens determined by closely linked genes (crossovers have been observed, but rarely). M and N, determined by allelic genes, depend on sialic (neuraminic) acid residues. S and s are also determined by allelic genes, and an amorphic gene is common in blacks when another antigen (U) is missing. The system also includes numerous low frequency antigens.

P b. g. a blood group system originally consisting of only P (now P1) antigen, but later found to include P2 (Tj[a]), a very high frequency antigen, and P3 (P[K]), a very low frequency antigen. P1 is most common in people of African descent (90 per cent), less so in those of European descent (75 per cent), and least in those of East Asian descent (30 per cent).

Rh b. g. the most complex of all human blood groups because the genes differ by determining different numbers of antigens *(Rh factors)* and do so with remarkably different quality; over 40 antigens have been described to date. People of African descent show the greatest degree of diversity and East Asians the least. The major antigen, *Rh1* (*Rh_0*, *D*, or *Rh_0D*), is highly immunogenic and before the development of passive immunization prophylaxis it was responsible for serious hemolytic disease of the newborn. Two other pairs of alternative antigens are inherited with or without Rh1; these are *Rh21* (*rh^G* or *C^G*) and *Rh4* (*hr′* or *c*), and *Rh3* (*rh′* or *E*) and *Rh5* (*hr′* or *e*). The most common groups of antigens are $R^{-1,-3,-21}$ (in Caucasians), $R^{1,-3,-21}$ (in blacks), $R^{1,-3,21}$ (in East Asians and Caucasians), and $R^{1,3,-21}$ (in East Asians and Caucasians). Another antigen Rh10 (hr[v], V) is common in blacks.

Scianna b. g. a blood group consisting of erythrocytic antigens Sc1 (formerly Sm) and Sc2 (formerly Bu[a]).

Sid b. g. a blood group consisting of those with extra amounts of the public erythrocytic antigen Sd[a], referred to as Sd(a++).

Vel b. g. a blood group consisting of the erythrocytic antigens Vel 1 and Vel 2.

Wright b. g. a blood group consisting of the erythrocytic antigens Wr[a] and Wr[b].

Xg b. g. a blood group consisting of erythrocytic antigen Xg[a], which is determined by a gene on the long arm of the X chromosome.

Yt b. g. a blood group consisting of the erythrocytic antigens Yt[a] and Yt[b]. Called also *Cartwright b. g.*

blood·less (blud′ləs) 1. deprived of blood; cf. *anemic.* Called also *exsanguinate.* 2. performed with little or no loss of blood.

blood·stream (blud′strēm) the blood flowing through the circulatory system in the living body. Written also *blood stream.*

Bloom syndrome (bloom) [David *Bloom*, American dermatologist, 20th century] see under *syndrome.*

bloom (bloom) 1. a surface texture on a colony of microorganisms that appears velvety or powdery owing to aerial projections of hyphae. 2. a film of cyanobacteria on the surface of water, often containing substances that are toxic.

blot (blot) 1. to transfer ionic solutes, such as DNA, RNA, or proteins, onto a membrane, filter, treated paper, or other immobilizing matrix for analysis, often after first using electrophoresis to separate fragments of different size. Transfer is often by capillary action, but may be expedited by application of electricity (electroblot) or a vacuum. 2. the matrix containing the transferred material.

dot b. a method for detecting and analyzing nucleic acids or proteins by hybridization, similar to the Southern, Northern, and Western blot methods, except that samples are spotted directly onto a membrane or paper substrate, rather than first being separated electrophoretically, before hybridization to the probe of interest.

Northern b. [by analogy to *Southern blot*] a method analogous to a Southern blot (q.v.), but performed on fragments of RNA instead of DNA; the probe may be either DNA or RNA.

Southern b. [E.M. *Southern*] a blot obtained by transferring denatured DNA fragments separated by agarose gel electrophoresis to a nitrocellulose or nylon membrane, followed by hybridization to a labeled DNA or RNA probe; used to detect and analyze specific DNA sequences.

Southwestern b. [combination of *Southern blot* and *Western blot*] a technique in which proteins are separated electrophoretically, transferred to a nitrocellulose filter, and probed with a labeled DNA fragment; used to detect expression of a specific DNA binding protein, such as a transcription factor.

Western b. [by analogy to *Southern blot*] a blot obtained by transferring proteins separated electrophoretically to a nitrocellulose membrane or other immobilizing matrix, followed by overlaying the matrix first with antibody against the protein of interest, then with labeled antibody against the first antibody; used for analysis and identification of specific proteins.

zoo b. a Southern blot used to determine whether a particular DNA sequence is present in more than one species by examining the ability of samples of DNA from several species to hybridize to a specific probe from one of the species.

blotch (bloch) a blemish or spot.

blot·ting (blot′ing) soaking up with or transferring to absorbent material. For specific techniques using blotting to analyze nucleic acids and proteins, see entries under *blot.*

Blount brace, disease (blunt) [Walter Putnam *Blount*, American orthopedic surgeon, 1900–1992] see under *brace* and see *tibia vara.*

blow·fly (blo′fli) blow fly.

blow·pipe (blo′pīp) a tube through which a current of air or other gas is forced upon a flame to concentrate and intensify the heat.

blue (bloo) 1. a color between green and indigo, produced by energy with wavelengths between 420 and 490 nm. 2. a dye or stain with this color.

alcian b. a copper-containing dye for staining acid mucopolysaccharides.

alizarin b. a blue dyestuff derived from anthracene.

aniline b., aniline b. WS a mixture of methyl blue and water blue, or either one individually; used as a counterstain, as a stain for collagen and for connective tissue, and as a component of bacteriological media.

Berlin b. Prussian b.

Borrel b. a silver oxide (Ag_2O) and methylene blue stain for spirochetes.

brilliant b. C, brilliant cresyl b. an oxazin dye, $C_{17}H_{20}N_3OCl$, used in staining blood cells; also used as a less toxic alternative to ethidium bromide in staining nucleic acids.

bromchlorphenol b. an indicator, dibromodichlorophenolsulfonphthalein, used in the determination of hydrogen ion concentration; yellow at pH 3.2 and blue at pH 4.8. Written also *bromochlorphenol b.*

bromphenol b. an indicator, tetrabromophenolsulfonphthalein, used in determining hydrogen ion concentration, being yellow at pH 3.0 and blue at pH 4.6. Written also *bromophenol b.*

bromthymol b. a dye, dibromothymolsulfonphthalein, used as an indicator in determining hydrogen ion concentration, being yellow at pH 6.0 and blue at pH 7.6. Written also *bromothymol b.*

china b. aniline b. WS.

Congo b. trypan b.

cyanol b. a bright blue acid coal tar dye related to triphenylmethane; used as a tracking dye in loading buffers for electrophoresis of nucleic acids.

Evans b. a dye in the form of a green, blue green, or brown powder, injected intravenously to determine blood volume and movement. Called also *T-1824.*

indigo b. indigotin.

Kühne methylene b. a mixture of methylene blue and dehydrated alcohol in phenol solution.

leukomethylene b. see *methylene b.*

Löffler methylene b. a mixture of methylene blue and absolute alcohol in aqueous solution of potassium hydroxide.

Luxol fast b. MBS, Luxol fast b. MBSN an alcohol-soluble dye used to stain myelinated nerve fibers. Called also *solvent b. 38.*

methyl b. a blue dye of the triarylmethane class, $C_{37}H_{27}N_3O_9S_3Na_2$; used, alone or in combination with water blue, as a biological stain; see *aniline b. WS.*

methylene b. [USP] methylthionine chloride; dark green crystals or crystalline powder having a bronzelike luster, readily reduced to colorless leukomethylene blue, which in turn is readily oxidized to methylene blue. Administered orally or intravenously in the treatment of congenital methemoglobinemia and intravenously in the treatment of toxic methemoglobinemia, and used as a bacteriological, biologic, and pathologic stain, as a colorimetric indicator for redox reactions, as a surgical marker, and as a diagnostic aid in the detection of the premature rupture of fetal membranes and to identify separate amniotic sacs in multiple pregnancies. Called also *Swiss b.*

Niagara b., Niagara b. 3B trypan b.

Nile b. A, Nile b. sulfate an oxazin dye used for staining lipids and for the differentiation of melanins and lipofuscins.

polychrome methylene b. a polychromatic mixture of several blue cationic thiazine dyes (including azures A, B, and C) and at least one uncharged dye, methylene violet Bernthsen; made by prolonged boiling of aqueous solutions of methylene blue, usually with alkali and sometimes with an oxidizing agent. It is commonly used as the cationic component of thiazine-eosinate stains.

Prussian b. an amorphous blue powder used as a dye; it is also administered orally in the treatment of known or suspected internal contamination with radioactive cesium and radioactive or nonradioactive thallium, to speed their elimination from the body. Called also *Berlin b.*

soluble b. 3M, soluble b. 2R aniline b. WS.

soluble indigo b. indigotindisulfonate sodium.

solvent b. 38 Luxol fast b. MBS.

Swiss b. methylene b.

thymol b. an indicator, thymolsulfonphthalein, with an acid pH range of 1.2 to 2.8, being red at 1.2 and yellow at 2.8, and an alkaline pH range of 8.0 to 9.6, being yellow at 8.0 and blue at 9.6.

toluidine b. O a basic blue dye related to methylene blue; used for both orthochromatic and metachromatic staining. It is used for staining histologic sections, in the Nissl method of staining, as a nuclear counterstain, for staining nucleic aicds during electrophoresis, and for staining proteoglycans. When used pharmaceutically, it is usually called *tolonium chloride* (q.v.).

trypan b. an acid azo dye used as a biologic stain. Called also *Niagara b. 3B.*

Unna alkaline methylene b. a strongly alkaline solution of methylene blue, used for staining plasma cells.

Victoria b. any of several related triphenylmethane dyes; used as a histologic and bacteriologic stain.

water b. a blue dye of the triarylmethane class, $C_{32}H_{25}N_3O_9S_3Na_2$; used, alone or in combination with methyl blue, as a biological stain; see *aniline b. WS.*

blue•grass (bloo′gras) any of various species of grasses of the genus *Poa* that have blue-green leaves. Some are commonly used as fodder for horses and cattle but can cause hay fever in susceptible persons.

blue•nose (bloo′nōz) photosensitization in horses in Great Britain, with cyanosis around the muzzle, after they eat fresh spring grass; in some cases edema becomes so severe that the condition resembles purpura hemorrhagica.

blue•tongue (bloo′tung″) a viral disease of sheep, cattle, goats, and wild ruminants, transmitted by biting flies of the genus *Culicoides;* the etiologic agent is an orbivirus. Characteristics include inflammation, ulceration, and necrosis of the tongue, lips, and dental pads, and fever.

Blum•berg sign (blum′bərg) [Jacob Moritz *Blumberg,* German-born surgeon and gynecologist in the United Kingdom, 1873–1955] see under *sign.*

Blu•me•nau nucleus (bloo′mə-nou) [Leonid Wassiljewitsch *Blumenau,* Russian neurologist, 1862–1932] nucleus cuneatus accessorius.

blunt (blunt) having a thick or dull edge or point; not sharp.

blunt•ing (blunt′ing) the condition of having dulled perception, understanding, or feeling.

emotional b. blunted affect.

blur (blər) indistinctness, clouding, or fogging.

spectacle b. the indistinct vision with spectacles occurring after removal of hard contact lenses, particularly non–gas permeable lenses; it is thought to result from chronic hypoxia of the cornea and attendant corneal edema.

blush (blush) sudden, brief erythema of the face and neck, resulting from vascular dilatation due to emotion or heat.

BMA British Medical Association.

BMI body mass index.

BMP bone morphogenetic protein.

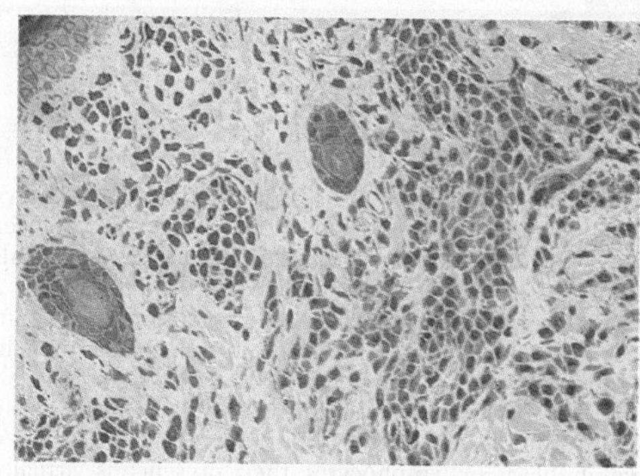

■ Toluidine blue O stain of skin biopsy showing diffuse cutaneous mastocytosis with extensive mast cell infiltration.

BMR basal metabolic rate.

BMS Bachelor of Medical Science.

BMT behavioral marital therapy; bone marrow transplantation.

BNA *Basle Nomina Anatomica.*

BNP brain natriuretic peptide; B-type natriuretic peptide.

BOA British Orthopaedic Association.

board (bord) 1. a long flat piece of wood or other solid material. 2. a group of administrators or experts serving a special function.

angle b. in dental radiology, a device used to facilitate the establishment of reproducible angular relationships between a patient's head and the plane of an x-ray film.

bed b. a rigid board put under the mattress of a bed for firm support of the patient.

Institutional Review B. (IRB) an official group associated with an institution performing medical research. The group reviews research studies being planned within the institution to ensure that the research is legal and ethical and to safeguard the safety, well-being, and rights of study subjects.

Bo•a•ri flap (bo-ah′re) [Achille *Boari,* Italian surgeon, late 19th century] see under *flap.*

Bo•as algesimeter, point (sign, test) (bo′ahs) [Ismar Isidor *Boas,* German physician, 1858–1938] see under *algesimeter* and *point.*

Bo•bath method (bo′baht) [Berta and Karel *Bobath,* German physical therapists in England, 20th century] see under *method.*

bob•bing (bob′ing) a quick, jerky, up-and-down movement.

ocular b. a jerky downward deviation of the eyes with slow return to the middle position, seen in comatose patients and thought to be due to a pontine lesion.

Boch•da•lek hernia, etc. (bok′dah-lek) [Vincent Alexander *Bochdalek,* Czech anatomist, 1801–1883] see *biatus pleuroperitonealis* and *plexus dentalis superior,* and see under *hernia* and *valve.*

Bock ganglion (bok) [August Carl *Bock,* German anatomist, 1782–1833] see *carotid ganglion,* under *ganglion.*

Bock•hart impetigo (bok′hahrt) [Max *Bockhart,* German physician, 1883–1921] see under *impetigo.*

Bo•dan•sky unit (bo-dan′ske) [Aaron *Bodansky,* American biochemist, 1887–1961] see under *unit.*

bo•den•plat•te (bo″dən-plah′tə) [Ger.] floor plate.

body (bod′e) 1. corpus. 2. any mass or collection of material. 3. a cadaver or corpse.

Body

For descriptions of specific anatomic structures not found here, see under *corpus.*

acetone b's ketone b's.

adrenal b. glandula suprarenalis.

Alder-Reilly b's coarse azurophil granules found in leukocytes in the Alder-Reilly anomaly.

Amato b's Döhle b's.

amygdaloid b. corpus amygdaloideum.

amylaceous b's, amyloid b's corpora amylacea.

anococcygeal b. corpus anococcygeum.

aortic b's corpora paraaortica.

apoptotic b's the membrane-bound cell fragments produced during apoptosis, containing organelles and sometimes fragments of the nucleus.

b's of Arantius noduli valvularum semilunarium valvae aortae.

asbestos b's, asbestosis b's golden yellow ferruginous bodies whose central core is asbestos.

Body *Continued*

Aschoff b's perivascular foci of inflammation in the interstitial tissues of the heart in rheumatic fever; the lesions consist of a central area of necrosis surrounded by a rosette of Anichkov cells. Called also *Aschoff nodules.*
asteroid b. an irregularly star-shaped inclusion body found in the giant cells in sarcoidosis and also found in numerous other diseases.
Auer b's finely granular lamellar bodies having acid phosphatase activity; they are found in the cytoplasm of myeloblasts, myelocytes, monoblasts, granular histiocytes, and occasionally plasma cells, but never lymphoblasts or lymphocytes; their presence is virtually pathognomonic of leukemia. Called also *Auer rods.*
Balbiani b. yolk nucleus.
Barr b. a chromatin mass in the nucleus of somatic cells of females of most species of mammals. It represents a single, inactive, condensed X chromosome. Called also *sex chromatin.* See also *Lyon hypothesis,* under *hypothesis.*
basal b. one of the cylindrical cytoplasmic bodies structurally resembling the centriole, from which it originates, located on the subsurface of flagellate protozoa and giving rise to the axoneme. Basal bodies are connected together in longitudinal rows by bundles of fibrils called kinetodesmata. Called also *basal granule, blepharoplast,* and *kinetosome.* See also *kinetoplast* and *parabasal b.*
b. of bladder corpus vesicae urinariae.
Bollinger b's inclusion bodies found in all tissue cells in fowlpox; they contain the fowlpox virus. Cf. *Borrel b's.*
Borrel b's minute virus-containing granules that aggregate to form Bollinger bodies.
Bracht-Wächter b's nonspecific inflammatory foci of lymphocytic and mononuclear cells in the myocardium, observed in bacterial endocarditis.
bull's eye b. dense b. (def. 2).
Cabot ring b's lines in the form of loops or figures of 8, possibly remnants of the nuclear membrane, seen in stained erythrocytes in severe anemias. Called also *Cabot rings.*
Cajal b's compact intranuclear structures, up to 10 per cell, about 1 μm in diameter and resembling balls of tangled thread on electron microscopy; they contain factors involved in messenger RNA processing and a number of nucleolar proteins and may be involved in regulation of some small nuclear RNA genes. Called also *coiled b's.*
Call-Exner b's the accumulations of densely staining material that appear among granulosa cells in maturing ovarian follicles; they may be intracellular precursors of follicular fluid. Also seen in ovarian tumors of granulosal origin.
carotid b. glomus caroticum.
b. of caudate nucleus corpus nuclei caudati.
cavernous b. of clitoris corpus cavernosum clitoridis.
cavernous b. of penis corpus cavernosum penis.
cell b. the portion of a cell that contains the nucleus, independent of projections such as an axon or dendrites.
central fibrous b. of heart trigonum fibrosum dextrum cordis.
b. of cerebellum corpus cerebelli.
chromaffin b. paraganglion.
chromatoid b. one of the dense accumulations of RNA found in the cysts of certain amebae (e.g., *Entamoeba* species), manifested as a deeply staining rodlike body. Called also *chromatoid bar.*
chromophilous b's Nissl b's.
ciliary b. corpus ciliare.
Civatte b's anuclear keratinocytes that have become incorporated into the papillary layer of the dermis; seen in lichen planus. Called also *colloid b's.*
coccygeal b. glomus coccygeum.
coiled b's Cajal b's.
colloid b's Civatte b's.
colostrum b's colostrum corpuscles.
conchoid b's Schaumann b's.
Councilman b's apoptotic bodies of hepatocellular origin seen in viral hepatitis, yellow fever, and other hepatic diseases.
Cowdry type I inclusion b's eosinophilic nuclear inclusions composed of nucleic acid and protein, seen in cells infected with herpes simplex or varicella-zoster virus.
Creola b's clumps of ciliated epithelial cells occasionally found in the sputum of persons with asthma.
cytoid b's 1. globular, shiny white structures resembling cell nuclei in size and shape, appearing in degenerated retinal nerve fibers; seen histologically in cotton-wool spots. 2. Civatte b's.
demilune b. achromocyte.
dense b. 1. any of the small regions of increased density in the sarcoplasm of skeletal muscles to which myofilaments seem to attach; cf. *attachment plaques,* under *plaque.* 2. an electron-dense granule occurring in blood platelets that stores and secretes adenosine nucleotides and serotonin. Called also *bull's eye b.* or *granule, dense granule,* and *platelet dense b.*
Döhle b's, Döhle inclusion b's round to oval blue-staining inclusions seen in the periphery of the cytoplasm of neutrophils, consisting mainly of RNA derived from rough endoplasmic reticulum; they are found in association with many infections, burns, aplastic anemia, uncomplicated pregnancy, and after administration of toxic agents. Similar structures, usually larger and more prominent, are present in granulocytes other than neutrophils in the May-Hegglin anomaly. Called also *Amato b's* and *leukocyte inclusions.*
Donné b's colostrum corpuscles.
Donovan b. 1. *Klebsiella granulomatis.* 2. amastigote.
Dutcher b. an intranuclear invagination of immunoglobulin-containing cytoplasm found in neoplastic plasmacytoid lymphocytes and plasma cells in both benign and malignant conditions.
elementary b. 1. inclusion b. 2. the infectious extracellular form of the *Chlamydiales,* consisting of electron-dense nuclear material and a few ribosomes surrounded by a rigid trilaminar wall. Elementary bodies are taken up into cells where they reorganize into reticulate bodies (q.v.); following reproduction, organisms are released from the cell as elementary bodies.
Elschnig b's clear grapelike clusters formed by proliferation of epithelial cells after extracapsular extraction of a cataractous lens; called also *Elschnig pearls.*
embryoid b's structures resembling embryos, seen in several types of germ cell tumors.
b. of epididymis corpus epididymidis.
epithelial b's parathyroid glands.
fat b. of ischioanal fossa corpus adiposum fossae ischioanalis.
ferruginous b's small masses of mineral matter of various shapes found in the lungs as a result of deposition of calcium salts, iron salts, and protein around a central core of foreign matter. See also *asbestos b's.*
fibrin b's of pleura movable or adherent, round, homogeneous, sharply demarcated opacities near the base of the pleural cavity, which may occur secondary to pleural effusion, pneumothorax, or hemopneumothorax; called also *pleural fibrin balls.*
foreign b. a mass or particle of material that is not normal to the place where it is found.
b. of fornix corpus fornicis.
fruiting b. a specialized structure that produces spores; see illustration at *mold* and see also *carp.*
fuchsin b's Russell b's.
b. of gallbladder corpus vesicae biliaris.
gastric b. corpus gastricum.
geniculate b., lateral corpus geniculatum laterale.
geniculate b., medial corpus geniculatum mediale.
Giannuzzi b's see under *crescent.*
glomus b. a specialized type of arteriovenous shunt that helps regulate blood flow and maintain or regulate body temperature; these are found most abundantly in the skin of the hands and feet (especially the digital pads and nail beds), the skin of the nose and ears, and along certain nerves and blood vessels. See also *glomus tumor,* under *tumor.*
Golgi b. see under *complex.*
Guarnieri b's inclusion bodies in the cells of the affected tissues in smallpox and vaccinia, regarded as caused by the reaction of the cell to the virus of the disease.
habenular b. habenula (def. 2).
Halberstaedter-Prowazek b's trachoma b's.
Harting b's deposits of calcium (calcospherites) in the cerebral capillaries.
Hassall b. Hassall corpuscles.
Heinz b's, Heinz-Ehrlich b's coccoid inclusion bodies resulting from oxidative injury to and precipitation of hemoglobin, seen in the presence of abnormal hemoglobins such as Hb H, Hb Köln, etc. and in erythrocytes with enzyme deficiencies. Refractile in fresh blood smears, they are not visible when stained with Romanowsky dyes but may be stained supravitally. See also *Heinz body anemias,* under *anemia.* Called also *Heinz granules.*

hematoxylin b. a dense, homogeneous, cyanophilous particle consisting of the denatured nuclear material of an injured cell together with a small amount of cytoplasm, occurring in systemic lupus erythematosus; lymphocytes that ingest such particles are known as LE cells. Called also *LE b.*
Henderson-Paterson b's molluscum b's.
Hensen b. a rounded modified Golgi net under the cuticle of an outer hair cell of the organ of Corti.
Herring b's hyaline or colloid masses scattered throughout the pars nervosa of the pituitary gland.
b. of Highmore mediastinum testis.
Hirano b's glassy, eosinophilic, rod-shaped inclusions, composed primarily of actin, seen in the cytoplasm of neurons of the central nervous system, chiefly the hippocampus, particularly in older persons; although they may occur in the absence of disease, they are more prevalent in patients with neurodegenerative disorders such as Alzheimer disease.
Howell b's, Howell-Jolly b's smooth, round remnants of nuclear chromatin seen in erythrocytes in megaloblastic anemia, hemolytic anemia, and after splenectomy. Called also *Jolly b's.*

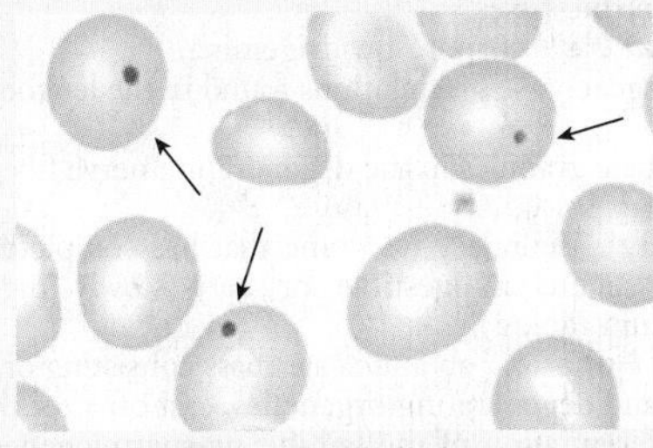

■ Howell-Jolly bodies.

HX b's Birbeck granules.
hyaline b's drusen.
hyaloid b. corpus vitreum.
b. of ilium corpus ossis ilii.
immune b. antibody.
inclusion b's round, oval, or irregular-shaped bodies occurring in the cytoplasm and nuclei of cells of the body, such as those seen in disease caused by viral infections (e.g., rabies and herpes). Called also *elementary b's* and *intranuclear inclusions.*
b. of incus corpus incudis.
infrapatellar fatty b. corpus adiposum infrapatellare.
infundibular b. neurohypophysis.
initial b. reticulate b.
interrenal b. an elongated organ that lies between the kidneys in elasmobranch fishes and that corresponds to the adrenal medulla in mammals.
b. of ischium corpus ossis ischii.
Jaworski b's see under *corpuscle.*
Joest b's intranuclear inclusion bodies found in the brain of animals with Borna disease.
Jolly b's Howell-Jolly b's.
jugulotympanic b. tympanic b.
juxtarestiform b. corpus juxtarestiforme.
ketone b's three substances that are produced by fatty acid and carbohydrate metabolism in the liver, being β-hydroxybutyric acid, acetoacetic acid, and acetone in approximately a 78:20:2 ratio. Acetoacetate is produced from acetyl-CoA; most is enzymatically converted to β-ketobutyrate, but a small amount is spontaneously decarboxylated to acetone. The ketone bodies can be used as fuels by muscle and brain tissue. In starvation and uncontrolled diabetes mellitus, large quantities are produced, causing metabolic acidosis and elevated blood and urine levels of all three ketone bodies.
Kurloff (Kurlov) b's bodies seen in the large mononuclear leukocytes of guinea pigs and related rodents. Observations with the electron microscope indicate that they probably result from intracellular secretion or from a sequestering and concentration of a serum molecular component.
Lafora b's intracytoplasmic inclusions consisting of a complex of glycoprotein and acid mucopolysaccharide; widespread deposits of these bodies are found in Lafora disease.
Lallemand b's, Lallemand-Trousseau b's Bence Jones cylinders.
lamellar b. one of the spherical granules that are formed in the upper spinous and granular layers of the skin, migrate into the cytoplasm, and then fuse with the plasma membrane to discharge their contents (bipolar phospholipids, glycoproteins, and acid phosphates) into the interior of the cell. The extruded material is thought to function as a barrier to penetration by foreign substances. Called also *keratinosome* and *lamellar granule.*
b. of lateral ventricle pars centralis ventriculi lateralis.
LCL b's minute coccoid bodies found in tissue infected with psittacosis; called also *Levinthal-Coles-Lillie b's.*
LE b. hematoxylin b.
Leishman-Donovan b. amastigote.
Levinthal-Coles-Lillie b's LCL b's.
Lewy b's concentrically laminated intracytoplasmic inclusion bodies consisting of α-synuclein, seen in neurodegenerative conditions such as Parkinson disease and multiple system atrophy.
Lindner initial b's cytoplasmic elementary bodies, resembling those in trachomatous epithelia, found in inclusion conjunctivitis of newborns.
Lipschütz b's intranuclear inclusion bodies found in the lesions of herpes simplex, both in the epithelial cells of the primary skin lesion (skin or cornea) and in the affected nerve cells.
Luschka b. glomus coccygeum.
Luys b. nucleus subthalamicus.
lyssa b's minute, red staining masses seen in rabies, somewhat resembling Negri bodies, but less sharply defined and with less internal structure.
Mallory b's hyaline cytoplasmic inclusions of cytokeratin, found in hepatocytes in steatohepatitis, alcoholic cirrhosis, and other liver disorders.
malpighian b's noduli lymphoidei splenici; see under *nodulus.*
mamillary b., mammillary b. corpus mammillare.
Marchal b's cell inclusion bodies observed in infectious ectromelia.
Masson b's the cellular components that fill the pulmonary alveoli and alveolar ducts in rheumatic pneumonia, thought to be modified Aschoff bodies.
medullary b. of cerebellum corpus medullare cerebelli.
medullary b. of vermis arbor vitae cerebelli.
melon seed b. any of a class of small fibrous masses sometimes occurring in the joints and in cysts of the tendon sheaths.
Michaelis-Gutmann b's bodies found in the lesion of malacoplakia of the urinary tract or kidney.
mitochondrial b. a fused colony of mitochondria found in the spermatids of insects.
molluscum b's large homogeneous intracytoplasmic inclusions found in the stratum granulosum and stratum corneum in molluscum contagiosum; they contain replicating virions and cellular debris.
Mott b's clear globules found in the cytoplasm of plasma cells *(Mott cells)* in multiple myeloma and certain other conditions.
multilamellar b. any of the osmiophilic, lipid-rich, layered bodies found in the type II alveolar cells of the lung; called also *cytosome.*
multivesicular b. a membrane-bound vacuole, derived from the early endosome, containing numerous small vesicles and tubules, along with lysosomal hydrolases delivered from the trans-Golgi network; it matures into a late endosome.
b. of nail corpus unguis.
Negri b's oval or round inclusion bodies, seen in the cytoplasm and sometimes the processes of certain nerve cells in rabies; these are pathognomonic for the disease.

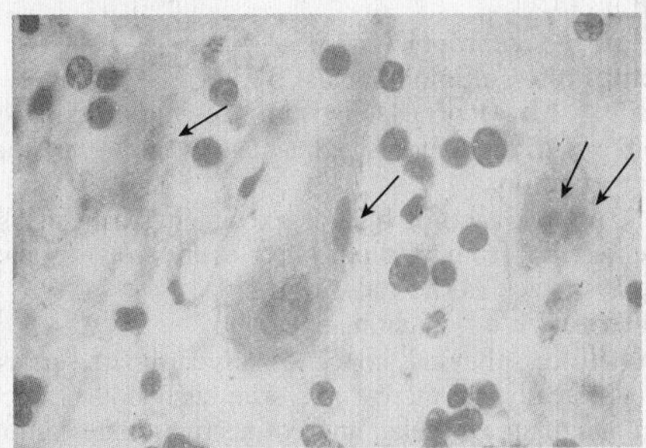

■ Negri bodies *(arrows)* in cerebellar Purkinje cells in rabies encephalitis.

nemaline b's small threadlike or rod-shaped bodies found scattered through muscle fibers in nemaline myopathy.
nigroid b. granula iridica.
Nissl b's large granular basophilic bodies found in the cytoplasm of neurons, composed of rough endoplasmic reticulum and free polyribosomes; called also *chromophilous b's, chromophilic* or *chromatic granules, tigroid b's* or *substance,* and *Nissl granules* or *substance.*
nuclear b's any of the particles, such as interchromatin granules, occurring in the interchromosomal domain of the cell nucleus.
Odland b. lamellar b.
Oken b. mesonephros.
olivary b. oliva.
orbital fat b. corpus adiposum orbitae.
oryzoid b's rice b's.
pacchionian b's granulationes arachnoideae.
pampiniform b. epoöphoron.
b. of pancreas corpus pancreatis.
Papp-Lantos b's glial cytoplasmic inclusion bodies composed of α-synuclein, found chiefly in the cytoplasm of oligodendrocytes, that are characteristic of multiple system atrophy.
Pappenheimer b's basophilic iron-containing granules observed in erythrocytes in sideroblastic anemia, sickle cell anemia, and certain other conditions.
para-aortic b's corpora paraaortica.
parabasal b. a cytoplasmic body of varying appearance, structure, and function closely associated with the nucleus, kinetoplast, and basal body in certain parasitic flagellate protozoa; it is usually connected to the basal body by a fibril or thread, which together are known as the *parabasal apparatus.* More than one such structure may be present in each organism. Some authorities consider the parabasal body to be the Golgi complex of these cells.
paranephric b. corpus adiposum pararenale.
paraphysial b. paraphysis (def. 1).
pararenal fat b. corpus adiposum pararenale.
paraterminal b. gyrus paraterminalis.
parathyroid b's parathyroid glands.
parietal b. epiphyseal eye.
parolivary b's accessory olivary nuclei; see *nucleus olivaris accessorius posterior* and *nucleus olivaris accessorius medialis.*
Paschen b's inclusion bodies in the cells of the tissues in variola and vaccinia; they are infective but whether they are the infective agents or mechanical carriers of the invisible virus is not known.
b. of penis corpus penis.
perineal b. corpus perineale.
pheochrome b. paraganglion.
Pick b's filamentous intracytoplasmic inclusions seen in neurons in Pick disease (def. 1).
pineal b. 1. glandula pinealis. 2. the posterior eyelike structure arising from the median of the dorsal wall of the thalamus in some lower vertebrates. See also *epiphyseal eye,* under *eye.*
pituitary b. hypophysis.
platelet dense b. dense b. (def. 2).
polar b's 1. small nonfunctional cells with a haploid chromosome complement, consisting of a small amount of cytoplasm and a nucleus, resulting from unequal division of the primary oocyte *(first polar b.)* and, if fertilization occurs, of the secondary oocyte *(second polar b.).* Called also *polar globules* and *polocytes.* 2. metachromatic granules located at one or both ends of a bacterial cell; called also *polar granules.*
polyglucosan b's corpora amylacea.
postbranchial b's ultimobranchial b's.
preepiglottic fat b. corpus adiposum pre-epiglotticum.
presegmenting b's malarial parasites *(Plasmodium)* before they undergo segmentation.
Prowazek b's 1. trachoma b's. 2. extremely small inclusion bodies found in the material from smallpox pustules and in cowpox vaccine and regarded by Prowazek as the cause of the disease.
Prowazek-Greeff b's trachoma b's.
psammoma b. a spherical, concentrically laminated mass of calcareous material, usually of microscopic size; such bodies occur in both benign and malignant epithelial and connective-tissue tumors, and are sometimes associated with chronic inflammation.

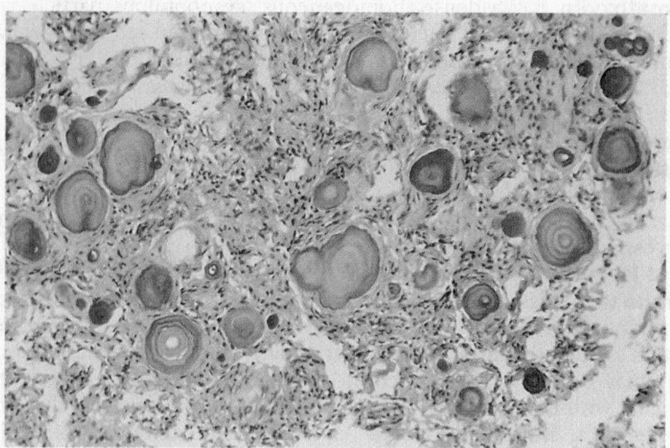
■ Psammoma bodies and a whorled pattern of cell growth in a meningioma.

purine b's purine bases.
quadrigeminal b's corpora quadrigemina.
Reilly b's large, coarse granulations found in the leukocytes in Hurler syndrome.
Renaut b's pale granules in the degenerating nerve fibers in muscular dystrophy.
residual b. 1. a secondary lysosome that has completed its digestive processes but retains indigestible or very slowly digestible material. 2. residuum (def. 2).
residual b. of Regaud an anucleate mass consisting of fine granules, lipid droplets, and degenerating organelles, cast off after the completion of regional differentiation of the tail during spermiogenesis.
restiform b. corpus restiforme.
reticulate b. the noninfectious intracellular form of the *Chlamydiales,* consisting of fibrillar nuclear material and more ribosomes than occur in elementary bodies (q.v.), surrounded by a thin trilaminar wall. Reticulate bodies reproduce within vacuoles in the host cell; following the reproductive cycle, reticulate bodies condense into elementary bodies, which are released from the cell. Called also *initial b.*
b. of Retzius a protoplasmic mass containing pigment granules at the lower end of an auditory hair cell of the organ of Corti.
b. of rib corpus costae.
rice b's small bodies resembling grains of rice which form in the tendons of joints and in the fluid of hygromas; called also *oryzoid b's* and *corpora oryzoidea.*
Russell b's globular plasma cell inclusions, mucoprotein in nature, containing surface gamma globulin, and representing aggregates of immunoglobulins synthesized by the cell; they are seen in both chronic inflammatory and malignant disorders. Called also *fuchsin b's.*
sand b's corpora arenacea.
Schaumann b's iron- and calcium-containing, red to brown, laminated inclusion bodies found in the cytoplasm of giant cells in sarcoidosis and other granulomatoses; called also *conchoid b's.*
Schiller-Duval b. a structure resembling a glomerulus seen in yolk sac tumors, composed of germ cells surrounding a central blood vessel and occurring within a space lined by germ cells.
Schmorl b. a portion of the nucleus pulposus that has protruded into an adjoining vertebra.
sclerotic b's a type of rounded cells surrounded by thick walls, characteristic of the dematiaceous fungi that cause chromoblastomycosis. Called also *muriform* or *sclerotic cells.*
semilunar b's Giannuzzi crescents.
spongy b. of male urethra, spongy b. of penis corpus spongiosum penis.
b. of sternum corpus sterni.
Stieda b. an ultrastructural organelle located at the polar region of the sporocyst of certain coccidia, appearing as a knoblike structure or representing a plug occluding a hole in the sporocyst, the breakdown of which allows excystation of the sporozoites.
b. of stomach corpus gastricum.
striate b. corpus striatum.
suprarenal b. glandula suprarenalis.
b. of sweat gland secretory coil.
Symington b. corpus anococcygeum.

Body *Continued*

telobranchial b's, telopharyngeal b's ultimobranchial b's.
thyroid b. glandula thyroidea.
tigroid b's Nissl b's.
Todd b's eosinophilic structures formed in the cytoplasm of the red cells of certain amphibians.
trachoma b's inclusion bodies found in clusters in the cytoplasm of the epithelial cells from the conjunctiva of a trachomatous eye; called also *Prowazek, Prowazek-Greeff,* or *Halberstaedter-Prowazek b's.*
trapezoid b. corpus trapezoideum.
Trousseau-Lallemand b's Bence Jones cylinders.
tympanic b. an ovoid body found in the adventitia of the upper part of the superior bulb of the internal jugular vein; its structure and presumably its function are similar to those of the glomus caroticum (carotid body). Called also *glomus jugulare, jugular glomus,* and *jugulotympanic b.* See also *glomus jugulare tumor,* under *tumor.*
ultimobranchial b's embryonic derivatives of the fourth pharyngeal pouches (sometimes described as a rudimentary fifth pouch); they migrate along with the parathyroid glands and are incorporated in the thyroid gland. In vertebrates other than mammals, these remain as discrete masses in the neck or mediastinum throughout adult life. The parafollicular cells of these bodies produce calcitonin. Called also *postbranchial* or *telobranchial b's.*
b. of urinary bladder corpus vesicae urinariae.
b. of uterus corpus uteri.
vagal b's corpora paraaortica.
Verocay b's small groups of fibrils surrounded by rows of palisaded nuclei, seen in schwannomas.
vertebral b. corpus vertebrae.
viral inclusion b's aggregates of viral structures, including replication complexes, transcriptional complexes, nucleocapsids, and virions, occurring in infected cells.
vitelline b. yolk nucleus.
vitreous b. corpus vitreum.
Weibel-Palade b's rod-shaped intracytoplasmic bundles of microtubules, believed derived from the Golgi complex; they are specific for vascular endothelial cells and are used as markers for benign or malignant endothelial cell neoplasms in electron microscopy.
wolffian b. mesonephros.
yellow b. of ovary corpus luteum.
zebra b. concentric, laminated, cytoplasmic inclusions of Schwann cells, occurring singly or in clusters, as a result of degeneration phenomena.
Zuckerkandl b's corpora paraaortica.

body•work (bod'e-wurk″) a general term for therapeutic methods that center on the body for the promotion of physical health and emotional and spiritual well-being, comprising a wide variety of techniques, including massage, various systems of touch and manipulation, relaxation techniques, and practices designed to affect the body's energy flow.

Boeck disease (sarcoid) (bərk) [Caesar Peter Moller *Boeck,* Norwegian dermatologist and syphilologist, 1845–1917] sarcoidosis.

Boer•haa•ve syndrome (boor'hah-vē) [Hermann *Boerhaave,* Dutch physician, 1668–1738] see under *syndrome.*

Boet•tcher see *Böttcher.*

Bo•gros space (bōg-ro') [Annet Jean *Bogros,* French anatomist, 1786–1823] see under *space.*

Bohr effect (bor) [Christian *Bohr,* Danish physiologist, 1855–1911] see under *effect.*

Bo•hun upas (bo'hən u'pəs) *Antiaris toxicaria.*

boil (boil) furuncle.
  Aleppo b., Baghdad b. Old World cutaneous leishmaniasis.
  blind b. a boil that does not develop a white or yellow "head" at its apex through which pus may be discharged; cf. *abscess.*
  gum b. parulis.
  shoe b. capped elbow in the horse.

Bol. [L.] bo'lus (pill).

Bol•bo•so•ma (bol″bo-so'mə) a parasitic genus of acanthocephalans that use crustaceans as their first intermediate hosts, fish as their second intermediate hosts, and sea mammals such as whales as their definitive or final hosts. Human intestinal infection has been reported from Japan, probably owing to the eating of raw fish.

bol•de•none un•dec•y•len•ate (bōl'də-nōn) an anabolic-androgenic steroid used in veterinary practice.

bol•dine (bol'dēn) an alkaloid from *Peumus (Boldu) boldus* Molina (Monimiaceae), which possesses diuretic properties.

bol•do (bol'do) the leaves and stems of *Peumus (Boldu) boldus* Molina (Monimiaceae), a Chilean evergreen shrub which contains over 15 alkaloids and is used variously as a choleretic, diuretic, stomachic, sedative, and anthelmintic.

bol•doa (bol'do-ə) boldo.

Bo•le•tus (bo-le'təs) [L. "mushroom"] a genus of fungi of the subphylum Basidiomycotina; some species are edible and others poisonous. *B. sata'nas* causes mycetismus gastrointestinalis.

Bol•lin•ger bodies (bol'in-gər) [Otto *Bollinger,* German pathologist, 1843–1909] see under *body.*

bo•lom•e•ter (bo-lom'ə-tər) [Gr. *bolē* a throw, a ray + *-meter*] an instrument for measuring minute changes in heat radiated by an object, such as a portion of the human body.

Boltz•mann constant (bōlts'mahn) [Ludwig Eduard *Boltzmann,* Austrian physicist, 1844–1906] see under *constant.*

bo•lus (bo'ləs) [L., from Gr. *bōlos* lump] 1. a rounded mass of food or a pharmaceutical preparation ready to swallow. 2. a concentrated mass of pharmaceutical preparation given intravenously for diagnostic purposes, e.g., an opaque contrast medium or radioactive isotope. 3. a mass of scattering material, such as wax, paraffin, bags of water, or a rice-flour mixture, placed between the radiation source and the skin so as to achieve precalculated isodose pattern in the tissue irradiated.
  alimentary b., food b. the mass of food in the oropharynx or the esophagus, comprising one swallow.

bomb (bom) a heavy metal-shielded apparatus containing a quantity of radium or other radioactive element for use in clinical teleradiation therapy.

bom•bard (bom-bahrd') to expose the whole body or a specific tissue target to the action of ionizing radiation.

Bom•bay phenotype (bom-ba') [*Bombay,* India, where it was first reported on in 1952] see under *phenotype.*

bom•be•sin (bom'bə-sin) a tetradecapeptide neurohormone and pressor substance with paracrine and autocrine effects; it was first isolated from the skin of frogs and is an important amphibian hormone, and it was later found in small amounts in normal human brain and intestinal tissue. Its amount is increased with certain tumors of the lung or thyroid gland. It is a potent mitogen, and its effects on gastrin and other hormones are attributed to increased cell numbers.

Bom•bi•na (bom-bi'nə) a genus of toads. *B. bombi'na* (the fire-bellied toad) and *B. variega'ta* are European species with colored bellies; their skin is toxic and contains serotonin with various amino acids.

Bom•bi•na•tor (bom'bĭ-na″tər) a genus of toads. *B. ig'neus* is the fire toad, whose venom contains the toxin phrynolysin.

Bom•bus (bom'bəs) a genus of bees of the family Apidae; the bumblebees. They are larger than honeybees (genus *Apis*), produce smaller amounts of honey, and can sting when bothered.

bom•by•kol (bom'bĭ-kol) a pheromone secreted by silkworms that serves as a sex attractant; it is a 16-carbon alcohol with two double bonds.

Bom•byx (bom'biks) a genus of moths of the family Bombycidae. *B. mo'ri* is the silkworm moth, a species native to Asia whose larva is the commercial silkworm and which is used extensively in experimental genetics.

bond (bond) 1. the linkage between two atoms or radicals of a chemical compound. 2. a mark used to indicate the number and attachment of the valences of an atom in constitutional formulas; it is represented by a pair of dots or a line between the atoms, e.g., H—O—H, H—C≡C—H or H:O:H, H:C:::C:H.
  coordinate covalent b. a covalent bond in which one of the bonded atoms furnishes both of the shared electrons.

covalent b. a chemical bond between two atoms or radicals formed by the sharing of a pair (single bond), two pairs (double bond), or three pairs of electrons (triple bond).

disulfide b. a strong covalent bond, —S—S—, important in linking polypeptide chains in proteins, the linkage arising as a result of the oxidation of the sulfhydryl (SH) groups of two molecules of cysteine; called also *disulfide bridge.*

energy rich b. high energy b.

glycosidic b's the bonds between the monosaccharide components of a polysaccharide.

high energy b. a chemical bond whose hydrolysis yields high levels of free energy; such bonds involve phosphate *(high energy phosphate b.)* or sulfur *(high energy sulfur b.)* or other mixed anhydride types of chemical structures.

high energy phosphate b. a high energy bond containing phosphate, occurring in ATP, phosphocreatine, phospho*enol*pyruvate, and other phosphate-containing high energy compounds; see *high energy compounds*, under *compound.* The energy released on hydrolysis of the bond can be transferred, stored, or used to drive metabolic processes such as the synthesis of glycogen from glucose.

high energy sulfur b. a high energy bond containing sulfur, occurring particularly in a variety of thioesters that are high energy compounds (q.v.); the most important such bond is that of the metabolic intermediate acetyl coenzyme A. The energy released by hydrolysis of a high energy sulfur bond can be transferred, stored, or used to drive metabolic processes such as the biosynthesis of fatty acids.

hydrogen b. a relatively weak, primarily electrostatic, bond between a hydrogen atom bound to a highly electronegative element (such as oxygen or nitrogen) in a given molecule, or part of a molecule, and a second highly electronegative atom in another molecule or in a different part of the same molecule. The hydrogen bond is generally represented by three dots, e.g., X—H•••Y, where X and Y are electronegative atoms.

hydrophobic b. a linkage resulting from the tendency of nonpolar molecules (or their side chains) to aggregate in an aqueous environment because of their mutual repulsion of solvent.

ionic b. a chemical bond in which electrons are transferred from one atom (e.g., sodium) to another (e.g., chlorine) so that one bears a positive and the other a negative charge, the attraction between these opposite charges forming the bond.

pair b. in ethology, the more or less permanent relationship between a male and a female for the purposes of mating and rearing the young.

peptide b. the —CO—NH— bond formed between the carboxyl group of one amino acid and the amino group of another; it is an amide linkage joining amino acids to form peptides.

van der Waals b. a weak electrostatic attraction arising from a nonspecific attractive force originating when two molecules are close to one another and the distribution of electrons is uneven, the locations lacking electrons attracting the locations with surplus electrons.

bond·ing (bond'ing) joining together securely with an adhesive substance, such as glue or cement.

dental b. the technique of fixing orthodontic brackets and other attachments directly to the enamel or dentin with orthodontic adhesives. Called also *tooth b.*

dentin b. dental bonding with establishment of a bond between cut dentin and the bonding agent.

enamel b. dental bonding with establishment of a bond between cut enamel and the bonding agent.

tooth b. dental b.

Bon·dy mastoidectomy (bon'de) [G. *Bondy*, German otologist, early 20th century] modified radical mastoidectomy.

bone (bōn) [L. *os;* Gr. *osteon*] 1. the hard form of connective tissue that constitutes the majority of the skeleton of most vertebrates; it consists of an organic component (the cells and matrix) and an inorganic, or mineral, component; the matrix contains a framework of collagenous fibers and is impregnated with the mineral component, chiefly calcium phosphate (85 per cent) and calcium carbonate (10 per cent), which imparts the quality of rigidity to bone. Called also *osseous tissue.* 2. any distinct piece of the osseous framework, or skeleton, of the body; called also *os.* See Plates 8 and 40.

Bone

accessory b. an occasionally occurring bone or ossicle adjoining one of the bones of the carpus or of the tarsus; recognized in the radiograph.
acetabular b. acetabulum.
acromial b. acromion.
alar b. os sphenoidale.
Albers-Schönberg marble b's osteopetrosis.
Albrecht b. basiotic b.
alisphenoid b. ala major ossis sphenoidalis.
alveolar b. the thin layer of bone making up the bony processes of the maxilla and mandible, and surrounding and containing the teeth; it is pierced by many small openings through which blood vessels, lymphatics, and nerve fibers pass. See also *alveolar process.*
ankle b. talus.
astragaloid b. talus.
astragaloscaphoid b. Pirie b.
back b. columna vertebralis.
basal b. the relatively fixed and unchangeable framework of the mandible and maxilla, which limits the extent to which teeth can be moved in the alveolar or supporting bone if the occlusion is to remain stable.
basihyal b. corpus ossis hyoidei.
basilar b., basioccipital b. a bone developing from a separate ossification center in the fetus, which becomes the basilar part of the occipital bone.
basiotic b. a small bone of the fetus between the basisphenoid and the basioccipital bones; called also *Albrecht b.*
basisphenoid b. a bone in the floor of the cranium of embryos of many different animal species. In humans, before birth it becomes part of the postsphenoidal part of the sphenoid bone (see under *part*); in most other animals it persists as a separate bone between the basioccipital bone and the presphenoidal bone.
Bertin b. concha sphenoidalis.
breast b. sternum.
bregmatic b. os parietale.
brittle b's osteogenesis imperfecta.
bundle b. one of the two types of bones composing the alveolar bone, so called because of the continuation into it of the principal fibers of the periodontal ligament. Large amounts of more calcified cementing substance render bundle bone more resistant to x-rays than surrounding bones; therefore it appears on dental radiographs as a thin radiopaque line (hence the synonym *lamina dura*). Called also *lamellated b.*
calcaneal b. calcaneus.
calf b. fibula.
cancellated b., cancellous b. substantia spongiosa ossium.
cannon b. a bone in the limb of hoofed animals, extending from the fetlock to the hock joint in the hind leg or the fetlock to the carpus in the foreleg; equivalent to a metacarpal or metatarsal in humans.
capitate b. os capitatum.
carpal b's ossa carpi; see under *os.*
carpal b., central os centrale.
carpal b., first os trapezium.
carpal b., fourth os hamatum.
carpal b., great os capitatum.
carpal b., intermediate os lunatum.
carpal b., radial os scaphoideum.
carpal b., second os trapezoideum.
carpal b., third os capitatum.
carpal b., ulnar os triquetrum.
cartilage b. any bone that develops within cartilage, in contrast to membrane bone, ossification taking place within a cartilage model; called also *endochondral b., replacement b.,* and *substitution b.*
cavalry b. rider's b.
central b. os centrale.
chalky b's osteopetrosis.
cheek b. os zygomaticum.
chevron b. the V-shaped hemal arches of the third, fourth, and fifth coccygeal vertebrae of dogs.
coccygeal b. os coccygis.
coffin b. the third or distal phalanx of the foot of a horse; called also *pedal b.* and *os pedis.*
collar b. clavicula.
compact b. substantia compacta ossium.
coronary b. small pastern bone; see *pastern b.*
cortical b. substantia corticalis ossium.
costal b. os costale.

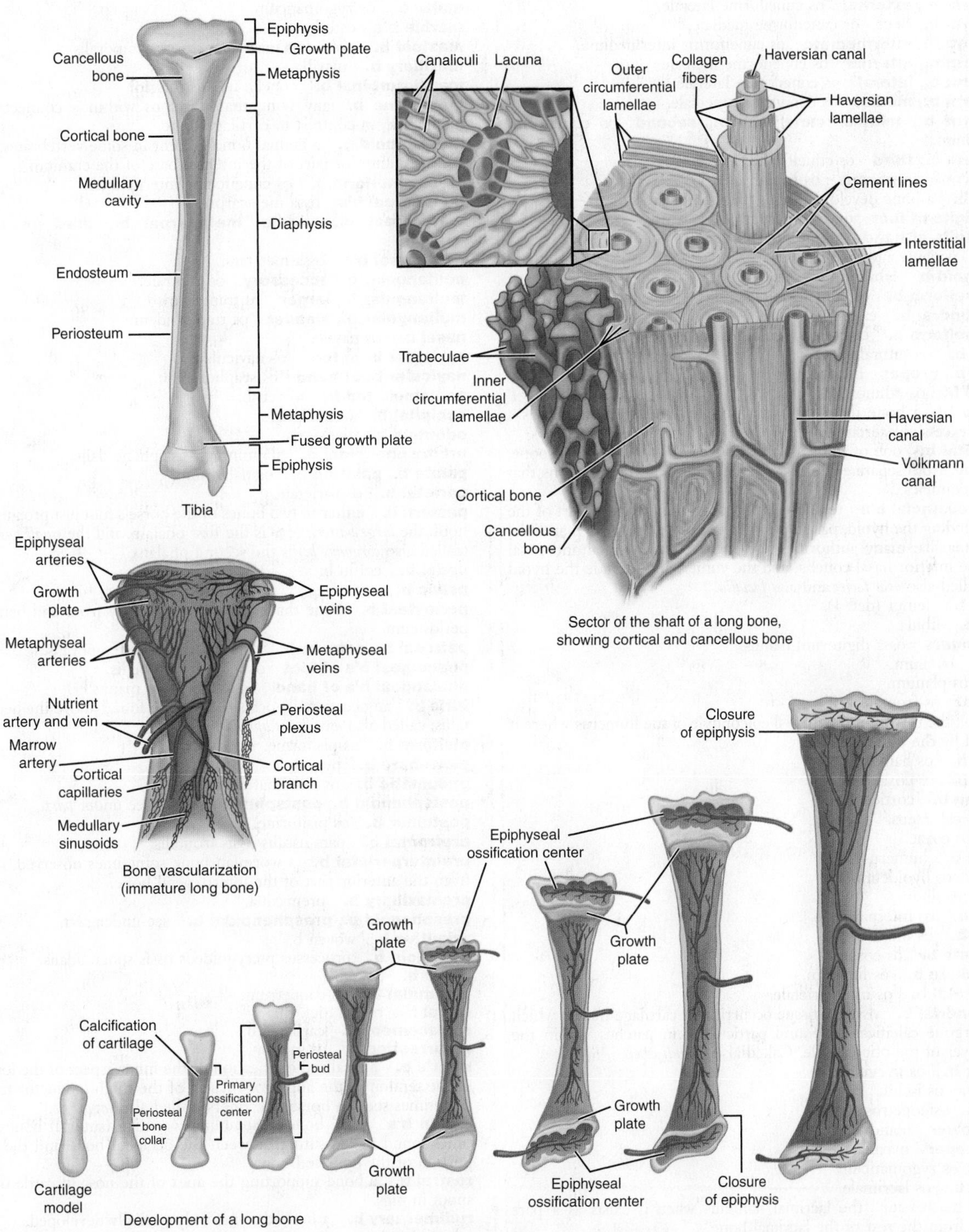

■ PLATE 8—STRUCTURE, VASCULARIZATION, AND DEVELOPMENT OF BONE

Bone *Continued*

cranial b's, b's of cranium ossa cranii.
cribriform b. os ethmoidale.
cuboid b. os cuboideum.
cuneiform b., external os cuneiforme laterale.
cuneiform b., first os cuneiforme mediale.
cuneiform b., intermediate os cuneiforme intermedium.
cuneiform b., internal os cuneiforme mediale.
cuneiform b., lateral os cuneiforme laterale.
cuneiform b., medial os cuneiforme mediale.
cuneiform b., middle, cuneiform b., second os cuneiforme intermedium.
cuneiform b., third os cuneiforme laterale.
cuneiform b. of carpus os triquetrum.
dermal b. a bone developed by ossification in the skin.
b's of digits of foot ossa digitorum pedis.
b's of digits of hand ossa digitorum manus.
ear b's ossicula auditus.
ectethmoid b. labyrinthus ethmoidalis.
ectocuneiform b. os cuneiforme laterale.
endochondral b. cartilage b.
entocuneiform b. os cuneiforme mediale.
epactal b. os suturale.
epactal b., proper os interparietale.
ethmoid b. os ethmoidale.
exercise b. a bone developed in a muscle, tendon, or fascia, as a result of excessive exercise.
exoccipital b. one of the two lateral portions of the occipital bone, developing, from separate centers of ossification, into the portions that bear the condyles.
b's of face, facial b's the bones that constitute the facial part of the skull, including the hyoid, palatine, and zygomatic bones, the mandible, and the maxilla; many authorities also include the lacrimal and nasal bones, the inferior nasal concha, and the vomer, and exclude the hyoid bone. Called also *ossa faciei* and *ossa facialia*.
femoral b. femur (def. 1).
fibular b. fibula.
b's of fingers ossa digitorum manus.
flank b. os ilium.
flat b. os planum.
frontal b. os frontale.
funny b. the region of the medial epicondyle of the humerus where it is crossed by the ulnar nerve.
hamate b. os hamatum.
haunch b. os coxae.
haversian b. cortical b.
heel b. calcaneus.
hip b. os coxae.
humeral b. humerus.
hyoid b. os hyoideum.
iliac b. os ilium.
incarial b. os interparietale.
incisive b. os incisivum.
innominate b. os coxae.
intermediate b. os lunatum.
interparietal b. os interparietale.
intrachondrial b. osseous tissue occurring in cartilage matrix which has undergone calcification; found particularly in patches within the middle layer of the otic capsule. Called also *globuli ossei*.
irregular b. os irregulare.
ischial b. os ischii.
ivory b's osteopetrosis.
jaw b., lower mandibula.
jaw b., upper maxilla.
jugal b. os zygomaticum.
lacrimal b. os lacrimale.
lacrimal b., lesser the lacrimal hamulus when it exists as a part separated from the rest of the lacrimal bone.
lamellar b. the normal type of adult bone, organized in layers (lamellae), which may be parallel (cancellous bone) or concentrically arranged (compact bone).
lamellated b. one of the two types of bone composing the alveolar bone, with some lamellae roughly parallel with the marrow spaces and others forming haversian systems. Cf. *bundle b.*
lenticular b. of hand, lentiform b. os pisiforme.
lingual b. os hyoideum.
long b. os longum.
lunate b. os lunatum.
malar b. os zygomaticum.
marble b's osteopetrosis.
mastoid b. processus mastoideus ossis temporalis.
maxillary b. maxilla.
maxilloturbinal b. concha nasalis inferior.
membrane b. any bone that develops within a connective tissue membrane, in contrast to cartilage bone.
mesethmoid b. a cranial bone present in some vertebrates, forming the most anterior part of the internal base of the cranium.
mesocuneiform b. os cuneiforme intermedium.
metacarpal b's ossa metacarpi.
metacarpal b., middle, metacarpal b., third os metacarpi tertium.
metatarsal b's ossa metatarsi.
multangular b., accessory os centrale.
multangular b., larger os trapezium.
multangular b., smaller os trapezoideum.
nasal b. os nasale.
navicular b. of foot os naviculare.
navicular b. of hand os scaphoideum.
nonlamellated b. woven b.
occipital b. os occipitale.
odontoid b. dens axis.
orbitosphenoidal b. ala minor ossis sphenoidalis.
palate b., palatine b. os palatinum.
parietal b. os parietale.
pastern b. either of two bones of the horse's foot just proximal to the hoof: the *large pastern bone* is the first phalanx and the *small pastern bone* (called also *coronary b.*) is the second phalanx.
pedal b. coffin b.
pelvic b. os coxae.
periosteal b. bone that is developed directly from and beneath the periosteum.
petrosal b., petrous b. pars petrosa ossis temporalis.
phalangeal b's of foot ossa digitorum pedis.
phalangeal b's of hand ossa digitorum manus.
Pirie b. an occasionally occurring ossicle found above the head of the talus; called also *astragaloscaphoid b.*
pisiform b. os pisiforme.
plowshare b. pygostyle.
pneumatic b. os pneumaticum.
postsphenoid b., postsphenoidal b. see under *part*.
postulnar b. os pisiforme.
prefrontal b. pars nasalis ossis frontalis.
preinterparietal b. a wormian bone sometimes observed, detached from the anterior part of the interparietal bone.
premaxillary b. premaxilla.
presphenoid b., presphenoidal b. see under *part*.
primitive b. woven b.
pterygoid b. processus pterygoideus ossis sphenoidalis.
pubic b. os pubis.
pyramidal b. os triquetrum.
radial b. radius (def. 2).
replacement b. cartilage b.
resurrection b. os sacrum.
rider's b. a localized ossification of the inner aspect of the lower end of the tendon of the adductor muscle of the thigh (adductor tubercle), sometimes seen in horseback riders; called also *cavalry b.*
Riolan b's small bones resembling wormian (sutural) bones, sometimes found in the suture between the occipital bone and the petrous portion of the temporal bone.
rostral b. a bone supporting the apex of the nose in cattle or of the snout in pigs.
rudimentary b. a bone that has only partially developed.
sacral b. os sacrum.
scaphoid b. os scaphoideum.
scaphoid b. of foot os naviculare.
scaphoid b. of hand os scaphoideum.
scapular b. scapula.
semilunar b. os lunatum.
sesamoid b's numerous ovoid nodular bones, often small, usually found embedded within a tendon or joint capsule, principally in the

Bone *Continued*

hands and feet (*ossa sesamoidea manus* and *ossa sesamoidea pedis*, respectively); two sesamoid bones, the fabella and patella, are associated with the knee.

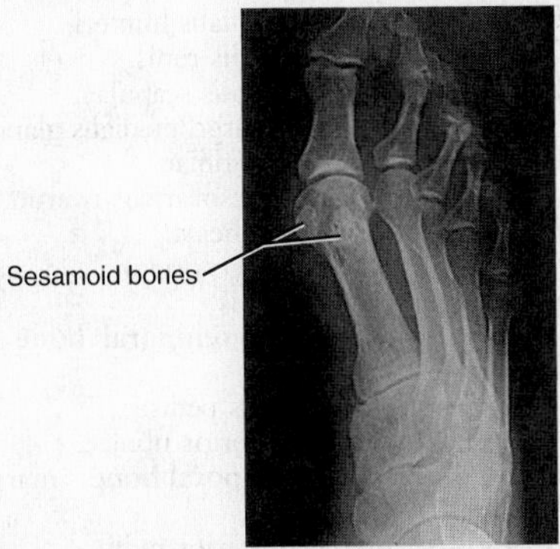

■ Sesamoid bones in a lateral oblique projection.

sesamoid b's of foot ossa sesamoidea pedis.
sesamoid b's of hand ossa sesamoidea manus.
shin b. tibia.
short b. os breve.
b's of skull ossa cranii.
solid b. substantia compacta ossium.
sphenoid b. os sphenoidale.
sphenoturbinal b. concha sphenoidalis.
splint b's the reduced second and fourth metacarpal and metatarsal bones of equines.
spongy b. substantia spongiosa ossium.
spongy b., inferior concha nasalis inferior.
spongy b., superior concha nasalis superior.
squamo-occipital b. the squamous portion of the fetal occipital bone, including the supraoccipital and interparietal bones.
squamous b. pars squamosa ossis temporalis.
stifle b. the patella of the horse.
stirrup b. stapes.
substitution b. cartilage b.
supernumerary b. a bone occurring in addition to the normal one, as a vertebra or a rib (cervical or lumbar rib).
suprainterparietal b. a wormian (sutural) bone sometimes occurring at the posterior part of the sagittal suture.
supraoccipital b. a bone developing from a separate ossification center in the fetus, which becomes the squamous part of the occipital bone below the superior nuchal line.
suprasternal b's ossa suprasternalia.
sutural b. os suturale.
tail b. os coccygis.
tarsal b's ossa tarsi.
tarsal b., first os cuneiforme mediale.
tarsal b., second os cuneiforme intermedium.
tarsal b., third os cuneiforme laterale.
temporal b. os temporale.
thigh b. femur (def. 1).
thoracic b's ossa thoracis.
b's of toes ossa digitorum pedis.
tongue b. os hyoideum.
trabecular b. substantia spongiosa ossium.
trapezium b. os trapezium.
trapezium b., lesser, trapezium b. of Lyser os trapezoideum.
trapezoid b. os trapezoideum.
trapezoid b. of Lyser os trapezium.
triangular b. os triquetrum.
triquetral b. os triquetrum.
turbinate b., highest concha nasalis suprema.
turbinate b., inferior concha nasalis inferior.
turbinate b., middle concha nasalis media.
turbinate b., superior concha nasalis superior.
turbinate b., supreme concha nasalis suprema.
tympanic b. pars tympanica ossis temporalis.
ulnar b. ulna.
unciform b., uncinate b. os hamatum.
vesalian b. os vesalianum pedis.
vomer b. vomer.
whettle b's vertebrae thoracicae.
wormian b. os suturale.
woven b. bony tissue found in the embryo and young children and in various pathologic conditions in adults, in which the bone fails to show the oriented arrangement of collagen fibers characteristic of lamellated bone; called also *nonlamellated b.* and *primitive b.*
xiphoid b. processus xiphoideus.
zygomatic b. os zygomaticum.

bone•let (bōn′lət) ossicle.

Bon•hoef•fer symptom (bon′hərf-ər) [Karl *Bonhoeffer*, German psychiatrist, 1868–1948] see under *symptom.*

Bo•nine (bo′nēn) trademark for preparations of meclizine hydrochloride.

Bo•ni•va (bo-ne′və) trademark for a preparation of ibandronate sodium.

Bon•net capsule, sign (bo-na′) [Amédée *Bonnet*, French surgeon, 1802–1858] see *vagina bulbi* and see under *sign.*

Bon•net-De•chaume-Blanc syndrome (bo-na′ də-shōm′ blah′) [Paul *Bonnet*, French physician, 1884–1959; Jean *Dechaume*, French physician, 1896–1968; Emile *Blanc*, French physician, 1901–1952] Wyburn-Mason syndrome.

Bon•tril (bon′tril) trademark for preparations of phendimetrazine tartrate.

Bon•will crown, triangle (bon′wil) [William Gibson Arlington *Bonwill*, American dentist, 1833–1899] see under *crown* and *triangle.*

book-lung (book′lung″) see under *lung.*

Böök syndrome (bo′ok) [Jan Arvid *Böök*, Swedish geneticist, 1915–1995] PHC syndrome.

boom•slang (bo͞om′slang) *Dispholidus typus*, a venomous, green to brownish black, arboreal snake found in southern Africa. See table at *snake.*

BOOP bronchiolitis obliterans with organizing pneumonia.

Bo•oph•i•lus (bo-of′ĭ-ləs) [Gr. *bous* ox + *philein* to love] a genus of blood-sucking ixodid cattle ticks comprising many species that are vectors of bovine anaplasmosis and babesiosis. *B. annula′tus* is a vector of *Babesia bigemina; B. mi′croplus* is a vector of *Babesia bovis; B. calcara′tus* is a vector of *Babesia major;* and *B. decolora′tus* is a vector of *Anaplasma marginale.*

Bo•op•o•nus (bo-op′ə-nəs) [Gr. *bous* ox + *ponos* pain] a genus of flies of the family Calliphoridae, found in the Philippines; the larvae of *B. inton′sus* (foot maggots) cause lameness in cattle and goats.

boost•er (bo͞ost′ər) see under *dose.*

Boost•rix (bo͞ost′riks) trademark for a preparation of tetanus toxoid, reduced diphtheria toxoid, and acellular pertussis vaccine, adsorbed (Tdap).

boot (bo͞ot) an encasement for the foot; a protective casing or sheath.
De Lorme b. quadriceps b.
Gibney b. an adhesive tape support used in treatment of sprains and other painful conditions of the ankle, the tape being applied in a basket-weave fashion with strips placed alternately under the sole of the foot and around the back of the lower leg.
quadriceps b. a metal plate that fits over the sole of a shoe and can be fitted with weights of various sizes for therapeutic exercise of the quadriceps muscles. Called also *De Lorme b.*
Unna b., Unna paste b. a dressing for varicose ulcers, consisting of a paste made from gelatin, zinc oxide, and glycerin, which is applied to the entire leg, then covered with a spiral bandage, this in turn being given a coat of the paste; the process is repeated until satisfactory rigidity is attained.

boot•strap (bo͞ot′strap) in statistics, a method for computing the distribution of values based on random resampling from the observed data.

bor•age (bor′ij) 1. *Borago officinalis.* 2. a preparation of the flowers, stems, and seeds of *B. officinalis*, used in folk medicine for a wide variety of disorders. See also under *oil.*

Bo•ra•go (bə-ra′go) [L.] a genus of herbs native to the Mediterranean region, including *B. officina′lis* or borage, a bristly, annual species with star-shaped blue or purplish flowers that is used medicinally.

bo•rate (bor′āt) any salt of boric acid.

bo•rat•ed (bor′at-əd) combined with or containing borax or boric acid.

bo•rax (bor′aks) [L., from Arabic *būraq*, from Persian *būrah*] sodium borate.

bor•bo•ryg•mus (bor″bə-rig′məs) pl. *borboryg′mi* [L.] a rumbling noise caused by the propulsion of gas through the intestines.

Bor•chardt triad (bor′chahrt) [Moritz *Borchardt*, German surgeon, 1868–1948] see under *triad*.

bor•der (bor′dər) a bounding line or edge; called also *margin* and *margo* [TA].

acetabular b. limbus acetabuli.
acute b. of heart inferior margin of heart.
alveolar b. of mandible arcus alveolaris mandibulae.
alveolar b. of maxilla arcus alveolaris maxillae.
anterior b. of body of pancreas margo anterior corporis pancreatis.
anterior b. of fibula margo anterior fibulae.
anterior b. of lung margo anterior pulmonis.
anterior b. of pancreas margo anterior corporis pancreatis.
anterior b. of radius margo anterior radii.
anterior b. of testis margo anterior testis.
anterior b. of tibia margo anterior tibiae.
anterior b. of ulna margo anterior ulnae.
brush b. a specialization of the free surface of certain cells, consisting of minute cylindrical processes (microvilli) that greatly increase the surface area; in vertebrates these are found especially on the cells of the proximal convoluted tubules of the kidney and on the intestinal epithelium.
corticomedullary b. the area where the renal medulla and cortex come together.
denture b. 1. the limit, boundary, or circumferential margin of a denture base. 2. the margin of the denture base at the junction of the polished surface with the impression (tissue) surface. 3. the extreme edges of a denture base at the buccolabial, lingual, and posterior limits. 4. the extreme margins of a denture base. Called also *denture edge*.
distal b. of nail margo liber unguis.
fibular b. of foot margo lateralis pedis.
free b. of nail margo liber unguis.
free b. of ovary margo liber ovarii.
frontal b. of parietal bone margo frontalis ossis parietalis.
hidden b. of nail margo occultus unguis.
inferior b. of body of pancreas margo inferior corporis pancreatis.
inferior b. of heart see under *margin*.
inferior b. of liver margo inferior hepatis.
inferior b. of lung margo inferior pulmonis.
inferior b. of mandible basis mandibulae.
inferior b. of pancreas margo inferior corporis pancreatis.
inferior b. of spleen margo inferior splenis.
interosseous b. of fibula margo interosseus fibulae.
interosseous b. of radius margo interosseus radii.
interosseous b. of tibia margo interosseus tibiae.
interosseous b. of ulna margo interosseus ulnae.
lambdoid b. of occipital bone margo lambdoideus ossis occipitalis.
lateral b. of foot margo lateralis pedis.
lateral b. of forearm margo radialis antebrachii.

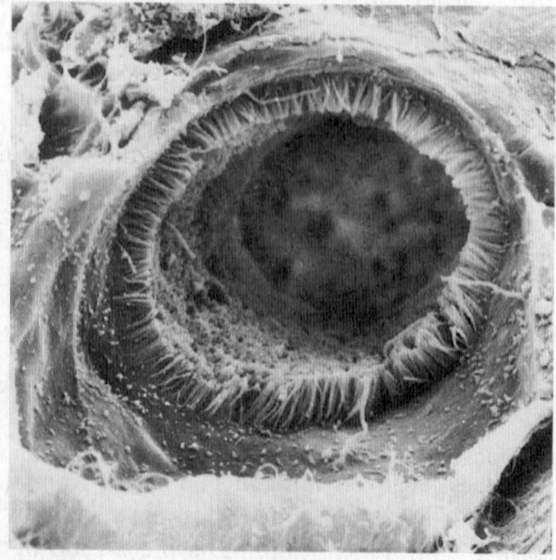

■ Brush border in a scanning electron micrograph of rat kidney proximal tubule, characterized by closely packed microvilli.

lateral b. of humerus margo lateralis humeri.
lateral b. of kidney margo lateralis renis.
lateral b. of nail margo lateralis unguis.
lateral b. of scapula margo lateralis scapulae.
left b. of heart see under *margin*.
mastoid b. of occipital bone margo mastoideus ossis occipitalis.
medial b. of adrenal gland margo medialis glandulae suprarenalis.
medial b. of foot margo medialis pedis.
medial b. of forearm margo ulnaris antebrachii.
medial b. of humerus margo medialis humeri.
medial b. of kidney margo medialis renis.
medial b. of scapula margo medialis scapulae.
medial b. of suprarenal gland margo medialis glandulae suprarenalis.
medial b. of tibia margo medialis tibiae.
mesovarian b. of ovary margo mesovaricus ovarii.
obtuse b. of heart left margin of heart.
occipital b. of parietal bone margo occipitalis ossis parietalis.
b. of oval fossa limbus fossae ovalis.
parietal b. of squamous part of temporal bone margo parietalis partis squamosae ossis temporalis.
peroneal b. of foot margo lateralis pedis.
posterior b. of fibula margo posterior fibulae.
posterior b. of petrous part of temporal bone margo posterior partis petrosae ossis temporalis.
posterior b. of radius margo posterior radii.
posterior b. of testis margo posterior testis.
posterior b. of ulna margo posterior ulnae.
proximal b. of nail margo occultus unguis.
radial b. of forearm margo radialis antebrachii.
right b. of heart margo dexter cordis.
sagittal b. of parietal bone margo sagittalis ossis parietalis.
sphenoidal b. of squamous part of temporal bone margo sphenoidalis partis squamosae ossis temporalis.
squamosal b. of parietal bone margo squamosus ossis parietalis.
superior b. of adrenal gland margo superior glandulae suprarenalis.
superior b. of body of pancreas, superior b. of pancreas margo superior corporis pancreatis.
superior b. of parietal bone margo sagittalis ossis parietalis.
superior b. of patella basis patellae.
superior b. of petrous part of temporal bone margo superior partis petrosae ossis temporalis.
superior b. of scapula margo superior scapulae.
superior b. of spleen margo superior splenis.
superior b. of suprarenal gland margo superior glandulae suprarenalis.
tibial b. of foot margo medialis pedis.
ulnar b. of forearm margo ulnaris antebrachii.
b. of uterus margo uteri.
vermilion b. the exposed red portion of the upper and lower lips.
vertebral b. of scapula margo medialis scapulae.

bor•der•line (bor′dər-līn) of a phenomenon, straddling the dividing line between two categories; see also *borderline personality disorder*, under *disorder*.

Bor•det-Gen•gou agar (culture medium), bacillus, phenomenon (reaction) (bor-da′ zhahn-goo′) [Jules Jean Baptiste Vincent *Bordet*, Belgian bacteriologist, serologist, and Nobel prize winner, 1870–1961; Octave *Gengou*, French bacteriologist, 1875–1957] see under *culture medium*, and see *Bordetella pertussis* and *complement fixation*.

Bor•de•tel•la (bor″də-tel′ə) [J.J.B.V. *Bordet*] a genus of gram-negative, aerobic, minute coccobacilli of the family Alcaligenaceae. It is made up of organisms that are parasites and pathogens of the respiratory tract and produce a toxin that causes necrosis of the skin.

B. bronchisep′tica a species resembling *B. pertussis* morphologically, culturally, and antigenically except that *B. bronchiseptica* is motile and grows sparsely on nutrient agar; it is a frequent cause of bronchopneumonia in many different species of mammals, and of canine infectious tracheobronchitis.

B. parapertus′sis a species that causes a reaction similar to that caused by *B. pertussis*, from which it can be distinguished by the readiness with which it grows on simple culture media. It causes parapertussis and occasionally classic pertussis.

B. pertus′sis the usual cause of pertussis (whooping cough), found only in the human respiratory tract. Virulent strains are encapsulated with smooth colonies (Phase I); prolonged laboratory culture produces loss of surface K antigens and altered colonial morphology (Phases II, III, and IV) progressing to obviously rough strains that are avirulent. Called also *Bordet-Gengou bacillus*.

bo•ric ac•id (bor′ik) [NF] a mild acid used as an acidifying agent and in buffer solutions; it is also a weak topical antiseptic used on intact skin and in ophthalmic solutions. It is used as a pesticide to kill ants and cockroaches.

Accidental ingestion may cause fatal poisoning (see *boron poisoning*, under *poisoning*).

Bör•je•son syndrome (bor'yə-sun) [Mats Gunnar *Börjeson*, Swedish physician, born 1922] see under *syndrome*.

Bor•na disease (bor'nə) [*Borna*, a district in Germany where an epidemic occurred] see under *disease*.

Bor•na•vir•i•dae (bor"nə-vir'ĭ-de) a family of RNA viruses having an enveloped virion containing a genome consisting of negative-sense single-stranded RNA (size 8.9 kb). Replication occurs within the nucleus. There is a single genus, *Bornavirus*.

Bor•na•vi•rus (bor'nə-vi"rəs) a genus of viruses of the family Bornaviridae, containing a single species, Borna disease virus.

Born•holm disease (born'hōm) [*Bornholm*, island in Denmark where some of the first documented cases occurred] epidemic pleurodynia.

bo•ron (B) (bor'on) [L. *borium*] a nonmetallic element occurring in the form of crystals and as a powder. It is the base of borax and boric acid; atomic number 5, specific gravity 2.54, atomic weight 10.811. See also *boron poisoning*, under *poisoning*.

b. carbide a compound, B_4C, slightly harder than silicon carbide (q.v.), obtained by heating boron at very high temperature to effect its union with carbon; used as a neutron absorber in nuclear reactors, and as an abrasive agent in industry and dentistry.

Bor•rel bodies (bo-rel') [Amédée *Borrel*, French bacteriologist, 1867–1936] see under *body*.

Bor•rel•ia (bə-rel'e-ə) [A. *Borrel*] a genus of bacteria of the family Spirochaetaceae, order Spirochaetales, made up of gram-negative, anaerobic, helical cells up to 1 µm wide by 20 µm long, with coarse, shallow, irregular coils surrounding a central fibrillar substance. The organisms are parasitic, living on mucous membranes, and are the cause of Lyme disease and relapsing fever.

B. afze'lii a genospecies, formerly classed as group 3 of *B. burgdorferi*, that is an agent of Lyme borreliosis in Europe and Asia.

B. anseri'na the etiologic agent of fowl spirochetosis, transmitted by species of the tick *Argas*, which occurs worldwide; it is not pathogenic for humans.

B. burgdor'feri the cause of acrodermatitis chronica atrophicans, erythema chronicum migrans, and Lyme disease, transmitted by various ticks of the genus *Ixodes*. See also *B. afzelii* and *B. garinii*.

B. cauca'sica an etiologic agent of tick-borne relapsing fever in the Caucasus area of southwestern Asia, transmitted by the tick *Ornithodoros verrucosus* from a reservoir of infection in field mice.

B. crocidu'rae an etiologic agent of tick-borne relapsing fever in North Africa, transmitted by the tick *Ornithodoros erraticus sonrai*, which is carried by small rodents.

B. dutto'nii an etiologic agent of tick-borne relapsing fever in Central and Southern Africa, carried by the tick *Ornithodoros moubata*, which transmits the microorganism from human to human in its saliva.

B. gari'nii a genospecies, formerly classed as group 2 of *B. burgdorferi*, that is an agent of Lyme borreliosis in Europe and Asia.

B. herm'sii an etiologic agent of tick-borne relapsing fever in western North America, transmitted by the tick *Ornithodoros hermsii*, which is transported by chipmunks and tree squirrels.

B. hispa'nica the etiologic agent of tick-borne relapsing fever in Spain, Portugal, and nearby areas of North Africa, transmitted by the large tick *Ornithodoros erraticus*, which is carried by rodents, reptiles, and amphibians.

B. latysche'wii the etiologic agent of tick-borne relapsing fever in Iran and nearby Central Asia, transmitted by the tick *Ornithodoros tartakovskyi*, which is carried by rodents and reptiles.

B. mazzot'tii the etiologic agent of tick-borne relapsing fever in the southern United States, Mexico, and Central and South America, transmitted by the tick *Ornithodoros talaje*, which is carried by rodents, armadillos, and monkeys.

B. neotropica'lis *B. venezuelensis*.

B. par'keri an etiologic agent of tick-borne relapsing fever in the western United States, spread by the tick vector *Ornithodoros parkeri*, which is carried by burrowing rodents such as ground squirrels.

B. per'sica an etiologic agent of tick-borne relapsing fever in Asia and Africa, spread by the tick vector *Ornithodoros tholozani*, which is carried by various rodents.

B. recurren'tis the cause of louse-borne relapsing fever, transmitted by the human body louse *(Pediculus humanus)*. The organism is spread by rubbing infected hemolymph of lice into the skin, as in scratching. The organism produces successive antigenic mutants that cause the clinical relapses.

B. theile'ri an etiologic agent of tick-borne spirochetosis in cattle, horses, and sheep in South Africa and Australia; tick vectors include species of *Rhipicephalus* and *Boophilus*.

B. turica'tae an etiologic agent of tick-borne relapsing fever in the southwestern United States and parts of Mexico, transmitted by the bite of the tick *Ornithodoros turicata*, which is carried by rodents and reptiles.

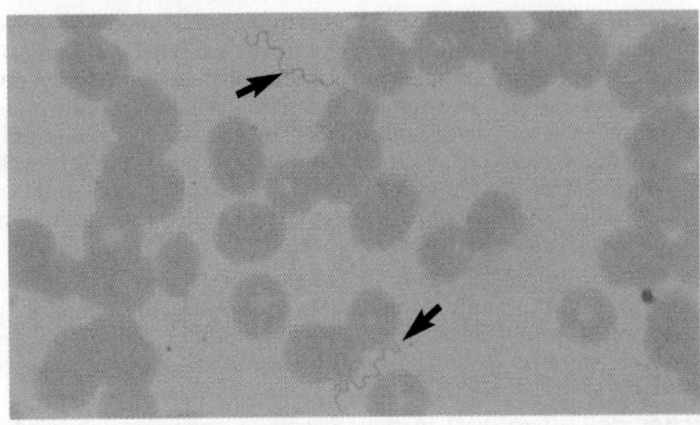

■ *Borrelia recurrentis* in blood (Giemsa stain).

B. venezuelen'sis an etiologic agent of tick-borne relapsing fever in Central and South America, transmitted by the tick *Ornithodoros rudis*, which is carried by monkeys and rodents. Called also *B. neotropicalis*.

bor•rel•i•o•sis (bə-rel"e-o'sis) infection with spirochetes of the genus *Borrelia*.

Lyme b. any of various diseases that are caused by *Borrelia burgdorferi* and have similar manifestations, including Lyme disease, acrodermatitis chronica atrophicans, Bannwarth syndrome, and erythema chronicum migrans.

Borr•mann classification (bor'mahn) [R. *Borrmann*, German surgeon and pathologist, 20th century] see under *classification*.

bor•tez•o•mib (bor-tez'ə-mib) a proteasome inhibitor with antineoplastic activity, used in treatment of multiple myeloma and mantle cell lymphoma; administered by intravenous injection.

bo•sen•tan (bo-sen'tən) an antagonist to endothelin-1 receptors, used in treatment of pulmonary arterial hypertension; administered orally.

boss (bos) a rounded eminence, as on the surface of a bone or tumor.

parietal b's sharp prominences on each side of the parietal bones.

Bos•ker implant (bos'kər) [Hans *Bosker*, Dutch surgeon, 20th century] see under *implant*.

bos•se•lat•ed (bos'ə-lāt-əd) [Fr. *bosseler*] marked or covered with bosses.

bos•se•la•tion (bos"ə-la'shən) 1. a small eminence; one of a set of bosses. 2. the condition or fact of being bosselated; the process of becoming bosselated.

Bos•ton sign (bos'tən) [L. Napoleon *Boston*, American physician, 1871–1931] see under *sign*.

bot (bot) the larva of a botfly, which may be parasitic in the stomach.

sheep nose b. the larva of *Oestrus ovis*.

Bo•tal•lo duct, foramen, ligament (bo-tah'lo) [Leonardo *Botallo*, Italian surgeon in Paris, 1530–1600] see *ductus arteriosus*, *foramen ovale cordis*, and *ligamentum arteriosum*.

bo•tan•ic (bo-tan'ik) 1. pertaining to or derived from plants; of the vegetable kingdom. 2. pertaining to botany.

bot•a•ny (bot'ə-ne) [L. *botanica*, from Gr. *botanē* herb] the science of plants or of the vegetable kingdom.

medical b. the botany of plants used in medicine.

bot•fly (bot'fli) an insect of the family Oestridae whose larvae (called *bots*) are parasitic, especially in horses and sheep. Genera include *Cuterebra*, *Dermatobia*, *Gasterophilus*, and *Oestrus*.

both•rid•i•um (both-rid'e-əm) one of the four leaf-like suckers symmetrically placed around the anterior end of the scolex of a tetraphyllidean cestode; called also *phyllidea*.

both•rio•ceph•a•li•a•sis (both"re-o-sef"ə-li'ə-sis) diphyllobothriasis.

Both•rio•ceph•a•lus (both"re-o-sef'ə-ləs) [Gr. *bothrion* pit + *-cephalus*] *Diphyllobothrium*.

both•ri•um (both're-əm) [Gr. *bothrion* pit] a sucker in the form of a groove such as is seen on either side of the head of *Diphyllobothrium latum*.

both•rop•ic (both-rop'ik) pertaining to, characteristic of, or derived from snakes of the genus *Bothrops*.

Both•rops (both'rops) [Gr. *bothros* pit + *ōps* eye] a genus of tropical and South American snakes of the family Crotalidae. *B. atrox'* is the barba amarilla, *B. jarara'ca* is the jararaca, and *B. lanceola'tus* of Martinique is the true fer-de-lance. See table at *snake*.

Bo•tox (bo'toks) trademark for a preparation of botulinum toxin type A.

bot•ry•oid (bot're-oid) [Gr. *botrys* bunch of grapes + *-oid*] resembling a bunch of grapes.

bot·ryo·my·co·sis (bot″re-o-mi-ko′sis) [Gr. *botrys* bunch of grapes + *mycosis* (because it was formerly thought to be caused by a fungus)] a rare, chronic, purulent, granulomatous bacterial infection usually caused by *Staphylococcus aureus*, characterized by lesions containing sulfur granules with a central mass of bacteria surrounded by a capsule; histologically, it resembles actinomycosis or mycetoma. Human infection is usually localized to the skin but may involve other organs such as the viscera and lymph nodes, especially in debilitated patients. Infection in domestic animals most often occurs as chronic, localized, or spreading skin abscesses.

Bo·try·tis (bo-tri′tis) a genus of Fungi Imperfecti of the form-class Hyphomycetes, form-family Moniliaceae; it includes the common gray mold and plant pathogens such as those that cause onion rot, peony blight, and turnip fire. *B. bassia′na* and *B. tenel′la* have been reclassified in genus *Beauveria*.

Böt·tcher cell (bərt′shər) [Arthur *Böttcher*, German anatomist, 1831–1889] see under *cell*.

bot·tle (bot′əl) a hollow narrow-necked vessel of glass or other material, used in laboratory procedures or for other purposes.

Castaneda b. a biphasic bottle containing both broth and a solid agar slant; used in the cultivation of fastidious organisms from blood.

Spritz b. a wash bottle for laboratory use.

wash b. 1. a flexible squeeze-bottle with delivery tube, or a bottle having two tubes through the cork, so arranged that blowing into one will force a stream of liquid from the other; used in washing chemical materials. 2. a bottle containing some washing fluid, through which gases are passed for the purpose of freeing them from impurities.

Woulfe b. a three-necked bottle used for washing gases or for saturating liquids with a gas.

bot·u·li·form (boch′u-lĭ-form) [L. *botulus* sausage + *form*] sausage-shaped.

bot·u·lin (boch′u-lin) [L. *botulus* sausage] botulinum toxin.

bot·u·li·nal (boch″u-li′nəl) 1. pertaining to *Clostridium botulinum*. 2. pertaining to botulinum toxin.

bot·u·lin·o·gen·ic (boch′u-lin″o-jen′ik) [*botulin* + *-genic*] producing or containing botulinum toxin.

bot·u·lism (boch′ə-liz-əm) [L. *botulus* sausage] 1. any poisoning caused by *Clostridium botulinum* in the body; it produces a neurotoxin called botulinum toxin. 2. specifically, in humans, food poisoning with neurotoxicity resulting from the eating of spoiled food contaminated with *Clostridium botulinum*. Characteristics include central nervous system symptoms with motor disturbances; visual and oculomotor difficulties; and disturbances of secretion such as dryness of the mouth and pharynx with coughing. It is usually due to ingestion of preformed toxin; sometimes (such as in *infant botulism*) the toxins can be produced in the gastrointestinal tract by ingested organisms. Called also *foodborne b.* See also *allantiasis*. 3. any of various neurotoxic syndromes in animals caused by ingestion of feed contaminated with *Clostridium botulinum*, such as moldy hay, grain, or silage. See *lamziekte*, *limberneck*, and *shaker foal syndrome*.

foodborne b. botulism (def. 2).

infant b. botulism affecting infants, typically 4 to 26 weeks of age, marked by constipation, lethargy, hypotonia, and feeding difficulty; it may lead to respiratory insufficiency. It results from toxin produced in the gut by ingested organisms, rather than from preformed toxins.

wound b. botulism resulting from infection of a wound with *Clostridium botulinum;* it is marked by the same symptoms as the foodborne form except for the absence of gastrointestinal symptoms.

bot·u·lis·mo·tox·in (boch″u-liz′mo-tok″sin) botulinum toxin.

Bou·chard disease, nodes (nodules) (boo-shahr′) [Charles Jacques *Bouchard*, French physician, 1837–1915] see under *disease* and *node*.

Bou·chut tubes (boo-shu′) [Jean Antoine Eugène *Bouchut*, French physician, 1818–1891] see under *tube*.

bou·fée dé·li·rante (boo-fa′ da-le-rahnt′) [Fr. "delirious outburst"] a reactive psychosis resembling schizophrenia but having a duration of less than three months and a favorable prognosis. It is roughly the French counterpart to schizophreniform disorder.

bou·gie (boo-zhe′) [Fr. "wax candle"] a slender, flexible, hollow or solid, cylindrical instrument for introduction into a tubular organ such as the urethra or esophagus, usually to calibrate or dilate constricted areas.

b. à boule (ah-bo͞ol′) [Fr.] bulbous b.

bulbous b. a bougie with a bulb-shaped tip; called also *b. à boule*.

dilating b. a bougie used for dilation; one type is the mercury dilators; another type has a screw that can be turned to increase the diameter. See *dilator*.

elastic b. a bougie made of rubber or other elastic material.

elbowed b. a bougie with an elbow or sharp bend near the tip.

filiform b. a bougie of very slender caliber; often used for the gentle exploration of strictures or sinus tracts of small diameter with multiple false passages.

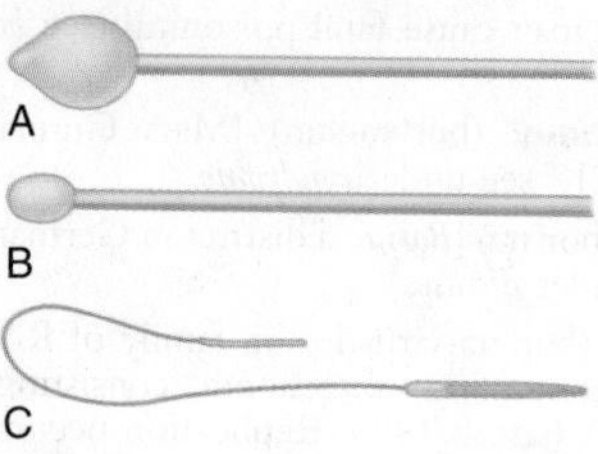

■ Bougies: *(A)*, Otis bougie à boule; *(B)*, olive-tipped bougie; *(C)*, filiform bougie.

Hurst b's a common type of mercury dilator system.

Maloney b's a common type of mercury dilator system.

mercury b's see under *dilator*.

olive-tipped b. a bulbous bougie with a tip shaped like an olive.

wax-tipped b. a long, slender, flexible bougie with a wax tip for passage into the ureter through the cystoscope to confirm the diagnosis of ureteral calculus.

whip b. a bougie with a filiform point and a stem of gradually increasing caliber.

bou·gie·nage (boo″zhe-nahzh′) the passage of a bougie through a tubular structure or organ, to increase its caliber, as in the treatment of stricture of the esophagus.

boug·i·nage (boo-zhe-nahzh′) bougienage.

Bouil·laud disease, sign, syndrome (boo-e-yo′) [Jean Baptiste *Bouillaud*, French physician, 1796–1881] see *rheumatic endocarditis*, under *endocarditis*, and see under *sign* and *syndrome*.

bouil·lon (boo-yaw′) [Fr.] a broth or soup prepared from the flesh of animals; used in food preparations and as a bacteriological culture medium. In the latter use, it is generally called *broth;* see under *culture medium* for specific broths.

Bou·in fluid (solution) (boo-ă′) [Pol André *Bouin*, French anatomist, 1870–1962] see under *fluid*.

bound (bound) 1. restrained or confined; not free. 2. held in chemical combination.

bou·quet (boo-ka′) [Fr.] a structure suggesting resemblance to a bunch of flowers, as a cluster of vessels, nerves, or fibers, or the polarized stage of synapsis at the start of meiosis.

Bour·gery ligament (bo͞or-zhə-re′) [Marc Jean *Bourgery*, French anatomist and surgeon, 1797–1849] ligamentum popliteum obliquum.

Bourne·ville disease (bo͞orn-vēl′) [Désiré-Magloire *Bourneville*, French neurologist, 1840–1909] tuberous sclerosis complex; see under *complex*.

Bourne·ville-Prin·gle syndrome (bo͞orn-vēl′ pring′gəl) [D.-M. *Bourneville;* John James *Pringle*, British dermatologist, 1855–1922] tuberous sclerosis complex; see under *complex*.

bout (bout) an attack or episode of illness.

bou·ton (boo-tahn′) [Fr. "button"] a buttonlike swelling on an axon where it has a synapse with another neuron.

b. de passage (pah-sahj′), b. en passant (pah-sahnt′) a buttonlike swelling on an axon at a synapse that is not at the end of the axon. Cf. *en passant synapse*.

synaptic b. b. terminal.

b. terminal (ter-mĭ-nahl′) pl. *boutons′ terminaux′* [Fr. "terminal button"] a buttonlike terminal enlargement of an axon that ends in relation to another neuron at a synapse; called also *terminal button*, *end-foot*, and *synaptic knob*.

Bou·ve·ret syndrome (boo-və-ra′) [Léon *Bouveret*, French physician, 1850–1929] see *paroxysmal supraventricular tachycardia*, under *tachycardia*, and see under *syndrome*.

bo·vine (bo′vīn) [L. *bos, bovis* ox, bullock, cow] pertaining to, characteristic of, or derived from cattle.

bow (bo) [A.S. *boga* bow, arch] an arched or curved appliance or device.

Logan b. an appliance used to prevent tension on sutures after surgical repair of cleft lip.

Bow·den cable (bo′dən) [Frank *Bowden*, British businessman and inventor, 1848–1921] see under *cable*.

Bow·ditch law, staircase phenomenon (bo′dich) [Henry Pickering *Bowditch*, American physiologist, 1840–1911] see *all or none*, under *A*, and see *treppe*.

bow·el (bou′əl) [Fr. *boyau*] intestinum.

Bo·wen disease (bo′ən) [John Templeton *Bowen*, American dermatologist, 1857–1941] see under *disease*.

Bow•en technique (bo'ən) [Thomas A. *Bowen*, Australian healer, 1916–1982] see under *technique*.

bow•en•oid (bo'ə-noid) pertaining to or resembling the lesions of Bowen disease.

bow•ie (bo'e) a disease resembling rickets that affects unweaned lambs in New Zealand.

bowl (bōl) [A.S. *bolla*] a rounded, more or less hemispherical open container, or a structure resembling such a container.

mastoid b., mastoidectomy b. the hollow bony defect in the temporal bone created by open mastoidectomy.

bow•leg (bo'leg) genu varum.

nonrachitic b. tibia vara.

Bow•man capsule, etc. (bo'mən) [Sir William *Bowman*, English physician, 1816–1892] see under *probe* and *tube; see capsular space*, under *space;* and see *capsula glomeruli, lamina limitans anterior corneae, musculus ciliaris,* and *glandulae olfactoriae*.

box (boks) a rectangular structure.

anatomical snuff-b. a triangular depression on the dorsum of the wrist at its radial border formed between the tendon of the extensor pollicis longus medially and the tendons of the extensor pollicis brevis and abductor pollicis longus laterally, formed when the thumb is abducted and extended.

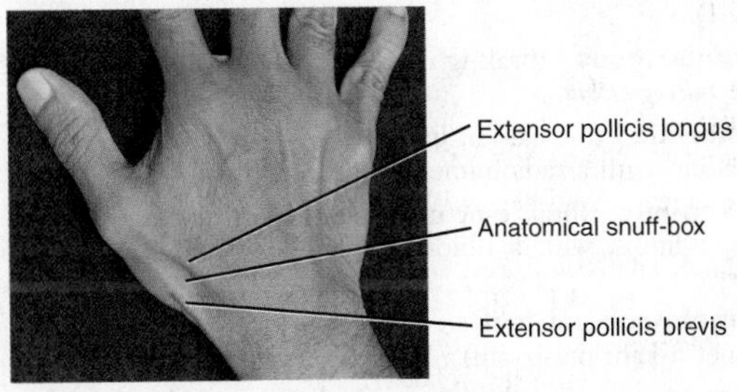

brain b. neurocranium.

CAAT b. a conserved noncoding DNA sequence approximating the consensus sequence 5′-GGCCAATCT-3′; it is located upstream from the site of transcription initiation in many eukaryotic genes and increases promoter activity.

GC b. a conserved noncoding DNA sequence approximating the consensus sequence 5′-GGGCGG-3′; it is located upstream from the site of transcription in some eukaryotic genes, particularly constitutively expressed housekeeping genes, and increases promoter activity.

Goldberg-Hogness b. TATA b.

HMG b. a DNA-binding motif of approximately 75 amino acids, occurring in pairs in HMG-1/2 (high mobility group) proteins, and also found in other transcription factors with varying specificities but having in common an ability to distort DNA and an affinity for binding distorted DNA.

Hogness b. TATA b.

Skinner b. an experimental enclosure for testing animal conditioning, in which the subject animal performs (e.g., presses a bar or lever) to obtain a reward.

T-b. a DNA-binding domain shared by a highly conserved family of genes (Tbx genes) that act as transcription factors involved in the regulation of various developmental processes.

TATA b. a conserved noncoding DNA sequence approximating the consensus sequence 5′-TATAAAA-3′; it occurs approximately 25 base pairs upstream from the site of transcription initiation in most eukaryotic genes, and binding to this site initiates the assembly of the active transcription complex. Called also *Goldberg-Hogness b.* and *Hogness b.*

Yerkes discrimination b. a maze with a series of doors, used in the laboratory in studies of visual discrimination in animals; opening of the proper door produces a reward, but opening of the wrong door produces an electric stimulus.

box•ing (bok'sing) in the fabrication of dental restorations and appliances, the building up of vertical walls of wax or other suitable material to form a box around a dental impression into which the freshly mixed plaster or stone is poured; done to produce the desired size and form of the base of the cast and to preserve certain landmarks of the impression.

box-note (boks'nōt) a hollow percussion sound heard in the chest of a person with emphysema.

Boyce sign (bois) [Frederick Fitzherbert *Boyce*, American physician, 1903–1993] see under *sign*.

Boy•den sphincter (boi'dən) [Edward A. *Boyden*, American anatomist, 1886–1976] musculus sphincter ductus choledochi.

Boy•er bursa, cyst (bwah-ya') [Alexis de *Boyer*, French surgeon, 1757–1833] see under *cyst* and see *retrohyoid bursa* under *bursa*.

Boyle's law (boilz) [Robert *Boyle*, English physicist, 1627–1691] see under *law*.

Boze•man position (bōz'mən) [Nathan *Bozeman*, American surgeon, 1825–1905] see under *position*.

Boz•zo•lo sign (bot-so'lo) [Camillo *Bozzolo*, Italian physician, 1845–1920] see under *sign*.

BP 1. blood pressure. 2. *British Pharmacopoeia*, a publication of the General Medical Council, describing and establishing standards for medicines, preparations, materials, and articles used in the practice of medicine, surgery, or midwifery.

bp base pair; boiling point.

BPA British Paediatric Association.

BPD bronchopulmonary dysplasia.

BPH benign prostatic hyperplasia.

B Ph British Pharmacopoeia.

BPI bactericidal permeability increasing protein.

BPIG bacterial polysaccharide immune globulin.

BPRS Brief Psychiatric Rating Scale.

BPV bovine papillomavirus.

Bq becquerel.

Br bromine.

Braasch bulb catheter (brahsh) [William F. *Braasch*, American urologist, 1878–1975] see under *catheter*.

brace (brās) 1. a device that holds parts together or in place. 2. an orthopedic appliance (orthosis) used to support, align, or hold parts of the body in correct position. 3. *(in the pl.)* orthodontic appliance.

back b. spinal orthosis.

Blount b. the original type of Milwaukee brace.

Boston b. a molded type of thoracolumbosacral orthosis that allows some lumbar flexion; used to treat scoliosis and arthritis of the lower spine.

carpal tunnel b. a static type of wrist-hand orthosis that limits motion of the wrist for treatment of carpal tunnel syndrome. Called also *carpal tunnel splint*.

CASH b. (cruciform *a*nterior *s*pinal *h*yperextension) a type of hyperextension orthosis that has bars and round pads in a cross arrangement on the front of the person's body for added support.

chairback b. any of several types of thoracolumbosacral or lumbosacral orthoses used to treat low back pain, having a pelvic band passing between the iliac crest and the greater trochanter and a thoracic band passing just below the angle of the scapula; steel upright bars connect the bands and provide rigidity.

Charleston bending b. a rigid, molded type of thoracolumbosacral orthosis that holds the patient in maximum side-bending correction; used at night in treatment of scoliosis.

collar b. cervical orthosis.

Fisher b. a type of thoracolumbosacral orthosis that has axillary holds and a corset front.

Goldthwait b. a type of thoracolumbosacral orthosis consisting of three padded, leather-covered metal strips, the uppermost fitting above the nipple line and the lowest encircling the pelvis.

hyperextension b. see under *orthosis*.

Jewett b. a type of hyperextension orthosis that has pads as corrective pressure points at the sternal notch, above the pubis, and in the lumbar lordosis.

Jones b. a type of thoracolumbosacral orthosis consisting of two vertical parallel bars that join a wider horizontal bar at the bottom, held in place by shoulder straps, an abdominal support, and groin straps, leaving the chest free.

Knight b. a type of chairback brace that has upper and lower bands and upright bars made of aluminum.

leg b. popular name for any orthosis of the lower limb, such as a hip-knee-ankle-foot orthosis or a knee-ankle-foot orthosis.

long leg b. popular term for an orthosis of the lower limb that has a knee component, such as a knee-ankle-foot or hip-knee-ankle-foot orthosis.

McKee b. a type of lumbosacral orthosis that has a lumbar pad and is used to support the lumbar spine and prevent flexion.

Milwaukee b. a type of spinal orthosis with a molded pelvic belt that fits above the upper edge of the iliac crest; it is joined to a turnbuckle that extends the length of the spine to an occipital hold with a throat mold; used in scoliosis and ankylosing spondylitis.

neck b. cervical orthosis.

short leg b. popular term for an orthosis of the lower limb that does not have a knee component, such as an ankle-foot orthosis.

Taylor b. a type of thoracolumbosacral orthosis that has steel rods for supporting the spine; used in cases of disease or mechanical derangement. Called also *Taylor apparatus* and *Taylor splint.*

brace·let (brās′let) 1. a small encircling band. 2. *(pl.)* transverse markings across the palmar surface of the skin of the wrists.

Nageotte b's bands covered with circular spines on the axons at the level of the nodes of Ranvier.

bra·chia (bra′ke-ə) [L.] plural of *brachium.*

bra·chi·al (bra′ke-əl) [L. *brachialis,* from *brachium* arm] pertaining to the upper limb.

bra·chi·al·gia (bra″ke-al′jə) [*brachi-* + *-algia*] pain in the upper limb.

b. sta′tica paresthe′tica painful paresthesias in the upper limb and hand during sleep due to compression of the blood vessels.

bra·chi·a·tion (bra″ke-a′shən) [*brachi-* + *-ation* suffix implying action] locomotion in a position of suspension by means of the hands and arms, as exhibited by monkeys when swinging from branch to branch.

brachi(o)- [L. *brachium,* q.v.] a combining form denoting arm.

bra·chio·ba·sil·ic (bra″ke-o-bə-sil′ik) pertaining to or connecting the brachial artery and the basilic vein.

bra·chio·ce·phal·ic (bra″ke-o-sə-fal′ik) [*brachio-* + *cephalic*] 1. pertaining to the upper limb and head. 2. pertaining to or connecting the brachial artery and the cephalic vein.

bra·chio·cru·ral (bra″ke-o-kroo′rəl) [*brachio-* + *crural*] pertaining to the upper limb and lower limb.

bra·chio·cu·bi·tal (bra″ke-o-ku′bĭ-təl) [*brachio-* + *cubital*] pertaining to the arm and elbow or forearm.

bra·chio·cyl·lo·sis (bra″ke-o-sə-lo′sis) [*brachio-* + Gr. *kyllōsis* a crooking] brachiocyrtosis.

bra·chio·cyr·to·sis (bra″ke-o-sər-to′sis) [*brachio-* + *cyrtosis*] crookedness of the upper limb.

bra·chio·fa·cio·lin·gual (bra″ke-o-fa″she-o-ling′gwəl) pertaining to or affecting the upper limb, face, and tongue.

Bra·chi·o·la (bra″ke-o′lə) a genus of parasitic protozoa (suborder Pansporoblastina, order Microsporida), usually found in insects. In immunocompromised persons, some species can cause microsporidiosis and myositis.

B. al′gerae a species that causes skin infections and myositis; formerly called *Nosema algerae.*

B. vesicula′rum a rare species that causes disseminated microsporidiosis in immunocompromised persons.

bra·chio·tho·ra·co·om·pha·lo·is·chi·op·a·gus (bra″ke-o-thor″ə-ko-om″fə-lo-is″ke-op′ə-gəs) conjoined twins joined from the forearms and shoulder to the pelvis.

b. bi′pus conjoined twins joined from the forearms and shoulder to the pelvis and having two feet.

bra·chi·um (bra′ke-əm) pl. *bra′chia* [L., from Gr. *brachiōn*] 1. [TA] arm: the part of the upper limb from shoulder to elbow. 2. an armlike process or structure.

b. colli′culi inferio′ris [TA] brachium of inferior colliculus: fibers from the lateral lemniscus that pass deep to the inferior colliculus and run forward to terminate in the medial geniculate body; they contain input from the lateral lemniscus and inferior colliculus.

b. colli′culi superio′ris [TA] brachium of superior colliculus: fibers diverging from the optic tract, coursing medially in a shallow groove between the pulvinar and the medial geniculate body to enter the superior colliculus of the mesencephalon and pretectal area; conveying fibers from the retina and the optic radiation to the superior colliculus.

b. conjunc′tivum usually, the superior cerebellar peduncle (pedunculus cerebellaris superior), although it can be used more specifically to denote only the large mass of cerebellar efferents of the peduncle, excluding the few afferents.

b. of inferior colliculus b. colliculi inferioris.

b. pon′tis pedunculus cerebellaris medius.

b. of superior colliculus b. colliculi superioris.

Brach·mann-de Lange syndrome (brahk′mahn da-lahng′ə) [W. *Brachmann,* German physician, early 20th century; Cornelia *de Lange,* Dutch pediatrician, 1871–1950] de Lange syndrome.

Bracht maneuver (brokt) [Erich Franz Eugen *Bracht,* German obstetrician and gynecologist, 1882–1969] see under *maneuver.*

Bracht-Wäch·ter lesion (brokt′ vek′tər) [E.F.E. *Bracht;* Hermann Julius Gustav *Wächter,* German physician, 20th century] see under *lesion.*

brachy- [Gr. *brachys* short] a combining form meaning short.

brachy·ba·sia (brak″e-ba′zhə) [*brachy-* + Gr. *basis* walking] a slow, shuffling, short-stepped gait, as seen in double hemiplegia.

brachy·ce·pha·lia (brak″e-sə-fā′le-ə) brachycephaly.

brachy·ce·phal·ic (brak″e-sə-fal′ik) pertaining to or characterized by brachycephaly. Called also *brachycephalous* and *eurycephalic.* See also *brachycranic.*

brachy·ceph·a·lous (brak″e-sef′ə-ləs) brachycephalic.

brachy·ceph·a·ly (brak″e-sef′ə-le) [*brachy-* + Gr. *-cephaly*] having a comparatively short head, with a cephalic index of 81.0 to 85.4, a characteristic of American Indians, Malayans, and Burmese.

brachy·chei·lia (brak″e-ki′le-ə) [*brachy-* + *cheil-* + *-ia*] abnormal shortness of the lip.

brachy·cne·mic (brak″e-ne′mik) brachyknemic.

brachy·cra·ni·al (brak″e-kra′ne-əl) brachycranic.

brachy·cra·nic (brak″e-kra′nik) [*brachy-* + Gr. *kranion* skull] having a comparatively short head, with a cranial index of 80.0 to 84.9. Called also *brachycranial* and *eurycranial.* See also *brachycephalic.*

brachy·dac·ty·ly (brak″e-dak′tə-le) [*brachy-* + Gr. *daktylos* finger] abnormal shortness of the fingers and toes.

brachy·esoph·a·gus (brak″e-ə-sof′ə-gəs) [*brachy-* + *esophagus*] abnormal shortness of the esophagus.

brachy·fa·cial (brak″e-fa′shəl) [*brachy-* + *facial*] having a comparatively low, broad face, with a facial index of 90 or less.

brach·yg·na·thia (brak″ig-na′the-ə) [*brachy-* + *gnath-* + *-ia*] micrognathia (def. 1).

brach·yg·na·thous (brak-ig′nə-thəs) having an unusually short mandible; see *micrognathia.*

brachy·ker·kic (brak″e-kur′kik) [*brachy-* + Gr. *kerkis* radius] having a short radius, with a radiohumeral index less than 75.

brachy·kne·mic (brak″e-ne′mik) [*brachy-* + Gr. *knēmē* shin] having short lower limbs, with a tibiofemoral index of 82 or less; also spelled *brachycnemic.*

brachy·meta·car·pal·ism (brak″e-met″ə-kahr′pəl-iz-əm) brachymetacarpia.

brachy·meta·car·pia (brak″e-met″ə-kahr′pe-ə) [*brachy-* + *metacarpus* + *-ia*] abnormal shortness of the metacarpal bones.

brachy·me·tap·o·dy (brak″e-mə-tap′o-de) [*brachy-* + *meta-* (2) + *pod-* + *-ia*] abnormal shortness of some of the metacarpal or metatarsal bones.

brachy·meta·tar·sia (brak″e-met″ə-tahr′se-ə) [*brachy-* + *metatarsus* + *-ia*] abnormal shortness of the metatarsal bones.

brachy·mor·phic (brak″e-mor′fik) [*brachy-* + *morph-* + *-ic*] built along lines that are shorter and broader than those of the normal figure; called also *brachytypical* and *brevilineal.*

bra·chy·o·nych·ia (bra″ke-o-nik′e-ə) [*brachy-* + *onych-* + *-ia*] abnormal shortness of the thumbnail.

brachy·pha·lan·gia (brak″e-fə-lan′jə) [*brachy-* + *phalanx*] abnormal shortness of one or more of the phalanges of a finger or toe.

brachy·ske·lous (brak″e-ske′ləs) [*brachy-* + Gr. *skelos* leg] abnormal shortness of one or both lower limbs.

Bra·chy·sp·ira (brak″e-spi′rə) [*brachy-* + Gr. *speira* coil] a genus of gram-negative bacteria of the family Serpulinaceae, consisting of helical cells that are motile by bipolar flagella; organisms are chemo-organotrophic, anaerobic or microaerophilic, and weakly fermentative. The type species is *B. aalbor′gi.*

B. hyodysente′riae a species that causes swine dysentery. Formerly called *Treponema hyodysenteriae.*

brachy·staph·y·line (brak″e-staf′ə-lēn) [*brachy-* + *staphyline*] pertaining to or characterized by a short, wide palate, with a palatal index of 85.0 or more.

brach·ys·ta·sis (brak-is′tə-sis) [*brachy-* + *stasis*] a state in which a muscle fiber is relatively decreased in length, and resists stretch; it contracts and relaxes, manifesting the same tension after contraction as before.

brachy·ther·a·py (brak″e-ther′ə-pe) in radiotherapy, treatment with ionizing radiation whose source is either implanted within the body, applied to the surface of the body, or located a short distance from the body area being treated; cf. *teletherapy.*

brachy·typ·i·cal (brak″e-tip′ĭ-kəl) brachymorphic.

brachy·uran·ic (brak″e-u-ran′ik) having a narrow maxilla, with a maxilloalveolar index of 115.0 or more.

brac·ing (brās′ing) 1. holding parts together or in place. 2. making something rigid or steady. 3. resistance to horizontal components of masticatory force.

brack·en (brak′ən) *Pteridium aquilinum,* a fern of worldwide distribution that causes bracken poisoning (q.v.) in many species of animals. Called also *bracken fern.*

brack·et (brak′ət) 1. a support projecting from the main structure. 2. orthodontic bracket; a small metal attachment soldered or welded to an orthodontic band or cemented directly to the teeth, serving to fasten the arch wire to the band or tooth. Called also *orthodontic attachment.* See also *orthodontic appliance*, under *appliance.*

bract (brakt) a small modified leaf in a flower cluster.

Brad·bury-Eg·gle·ston syndrome (brad′bə-re eg′əl-stən) [Samuel *Bradbury*, American physician, 1883–1947; Cary *Eggleston*, American physician, 1884–1966] see under *syndrome.*

Brad·ford frame (brad′fərd) [Edward Hickling *Bradford*, American orthopedic surgeon, 1848–1926] see under *frame.*

brad·shot (brad′shot) braxy.

brad·sot (brad′sot) braxy.

brady- [Gr. *bradys* slow] a combining form meaning slow.

brady·acu·sia (brad″e-ə-ku′zhə) [*brady-* + Gr. *akouein* to hear] dullness of hearing.

brady·ar·rhyth·mia (brad″e-ə-rith′me-ə) [*brady-* + *arrhythmia*] any disturbance in the heart rhythm in which the heart rate is abnormally slowed, usually to less than 60 beats per minute in an adult.

brady·ar·thria (brad″e-ahr′thre-ə) bradylalia.

brady·aux·e·sis (brad″e-awk-se′sis) [*brady-* + *auxesis*] a form of heterauxesis in which the part grows more slowly than the whole.

Brady·bae·na (brad″e-be′nə) a genus of land snails; they serve as hosts to the liver fluke *Dicrocoelium dentriticum* in Malaysia.

brady·car·dia (brad″e-kahr′de-ə) [*brady-* + Gr. *kardia* heart] slowness of the heartbeat, as evidenced by slowing of the pulse rate to less than 60.
 Branham b. see under *sign.*
 central b. bradycardia dependent on disease of the central nervous system.
 essential b. bradycardia occurring without discoverable cause.
 fetal b. a fetal heart rate of less than 120 beats per minute, generally associated with hypoxia and usually due to placental insufficiency; it may also result from placental transfer of local anesthetics or beta-adrenergic blocking agents, or occasionally from heart block associated with congenital heart disease or maternal collagen vascular disease.
 nodal b. bradycardia in which the stimulus of the heart's contraction arises in the atrioventricular node or common bundle.
 postinfective b. bradycardia occurring after infectious disease.
 sinoatrial b., sinus b. (SB) a slow sinus rhythm, with a heart rate of less than 60 beats per minute in an adult; it is common in young adults and in athletes but is also a manifestation of some disorders.
 vagal b. bradycardia due to increased vagal tone.

brady·car·di·ac (brad″e-kahr′de-ak) 1. pertaining to, characterized by, or causing bradycardia. 2. an agent that acts to slow the pulse.

brady·car·dic (brad″e-kahr′dik) bradycardiac.

brady·ci·ne·sia (brad″e-sĭ-ne′zhə) bradykinesia.

brady·crot·ic (brad″e-krot′ik) [*brady-* + Gr. *krotos* pulsation] pertaining to, characterized by, or inducing slowness of pulse.

brady·dys·rhyth·mia (brad″e-dis-rith′me-ə) [*brady-* + *dysrhythmia*] an abnormal heart rhythm with rate less than 60 beats per minute in an adult; the term *bradyarrhythmia* is usually used instead.

brady·es·the·sia (brad″e-es-the′zhə) [*brady-* + *esthesia*] slowness or dullness of perception; cf. *hypesthesia.*

brady·gas·tria (brad″e-gas′tre-ə) a dysrhythmia of the electric potentials in the stomach wall, with abnormally decreased frequency.

brady·gen·e·sis (brad″e-gen′ə-sis) [*brady-* + *-genesis*] the lengthening of certain stages in embryonic development.

brady·glos·sia (brad″e-glos′e-ə) [*brady-* + *gloss-* + *-ia*] slowness of speech due to impaired mobility of the tongue; cf. *bradylalia.*

brady·ki·ne·sia (brad″e-kĭ-ne′zhə) [*brady-* + *kinesi-* + *-ia*] abnormal slowness of muscular movement. Called also *bradycinesia* and *bradypragia.* Cf. *hypokinesia.*

brady·ki·net·ic (brad″e-kĭ-net′ik) 1. characterized by or performed with bradykinesia. 2. denoting a method of showing the details of motor action by motion pictures that are shown at reduced speed.

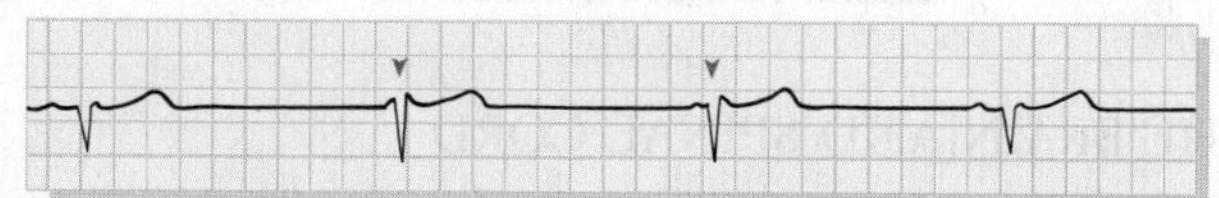

■ Sinus bradycardia. The second and third QRS complexes *(arrowheads)* represent atrioventricular junctional escape beats.

brady·ki·nin (brad″e-ki′nin) [*brady-* + Gr. *kinein* to move] a nonapeptide (Arg-Pro-Pro-Gly-Phe-Ser-Pro-Phe-Arg) produced by activation of the kinin system in a variety of inflammatory conditions. It is a potent vasodilator and also increases vascular permeability, stimulates pain receptors, and causes contraction of a variety of extravascular smooth muscles. The name refers to the slowly developing contraction produced in isolated guinea pig ileum. It is produced by the action of plasma kallikrein, trypsin, or plasmin on high-molecular-weight kininogen, a plasma α_2-globulin, and is destroyed by several kininases in the lungs and other tissues.
 lysyl-b. kallidin.

brady·la·lia (brad″e-la′le-ə) [*brady-* + *lal-* + *-ia*] abnormally slow utterance of words due to a brain lesion or mental disorder; called also *bradyarthria* and *bradyphasia.*

brady·lex·ia (brad″e-lek′se-ə) [*brady-* + Gr. *lexis* word] abnormal slowness in reading, due neither to defect of intelligence or of vision nor to ignorance of the alphabet.

brady·lo·gia (brad″e-lo′jə) bradylalia.

brady·pha·gia (brad″ĭ-fa′jə) [*brady-* + *-phagia*] abnormal slowness in eating.

brady·pha·sia (brad″ĭ-fa′zhə) bradylalia.

brady·phra·sia (brad″e-fra′zhə) 1. bradylalia. 2. bradyphrenia.

brady·phre·nia (brad″e-fre′ne-ə) [*brady-* + *phren-* + *-ia*] slowness of thought or fatigability of initiative, resulting from depression or central nervous system disease; called also *bradyphrasia.*

brady·pnea (brad″e-ne′ə, brad-ip′ne-ə) [*brady-* + *-pnea*] abnormal slowness of breathing. Cf. *hypopnea* and *hypoventilation.*

brady·pra·gia (brad″e-pra′je-ə) bradykinesia.

Brady·rhi·zo·bi·a·ceae (brad″e-ri-zo″be-a′se-e) a phenotypically diverse family of bacteria of the order Rhizobiales; it includes one genus, *Afipia*, that infects humans.

brady·rhyth·mia (brad″e-rith′me-ə) bradycardia.

brady·sper·ma·tism (brad″e-spur′mə-tiz-əm) [*brady-* + *spermatism*] abnormally slow ejaculation of semen.

brady·sphyg·mia (brad″e-sfig′me-ə) [*brady-* + *sphygm-* + *-ia*] abnormal slowness of the pulse, usually linked to bradycardia.

brady·tachy·car·dia (brad″e-tak″ĭ-kahr′de-ə) [*brady-* + *tachy-* + Gr. *kardia* heart] alternating attacks of bradycardia and tachycardia, as may occur in sick sinus syndrome.

brady·tel·eo·ci·ne·sia (brad″e-tel″e-o-si-ne′zə) bradyteleokinesis.

brady·tel·eo·ki·ne·sis (brad″e-tel″e-o-kĭ-ne′sis) [*brady-* + *teleo-* + *-kinesis*] a dyskinesia in which a movement is slowed or stopped prior to reaching its goal; called also *bradyteleocinesia.*

brady·tro·phia (brad″e-tro′fe-ə) a condition characterized by slow-acting nutritive processes.

brady·tro·phic (brad″e-tro′fik) [*brady-* + *-trophic*] having slow-acting nutritive processes.

brady·uria (brad″e-u′re-ə) [*brady-* + *-uria*] abnormally slow passage of urine.

brady·zo·ite (brad″e-zo′īt) [*brady-* + Gr. *zōon* animal] a small, comma-shaped form of *Toxoplasma gondii*, found in clusters enclosed by an irregular wall (pseudocyst) in the tissues, chiefly muscles and the brain, in chronic (latent) toxoplasmosis; considered to be the slow-growing form. Cf. *tachyzoite.*

Bra·gard sign (brah′gahrt) [Karl *Bragard*, German orthopedist, 20th century] see under *sign.*

braille (brāl) [Louis *Braille*, a French teacher of the blind, 1809–1852] a system of writing and printing for the blind by means of tangible points or dots.

Brain airway (brān) [A.I. *Brain*, British anesthesiologist, 20th century] see under *airway.*

Brain reflex (brān) [Walter Russell *Brain*, English neurologist, 1895–1966] see under *reflex.*

brain (brān) [A.S. *braegen*] that part of the central nervous system contained within the cranium, comprising the prosencephalon (forebrain: telencephalon plus diencephalon), mesencephalon (midbrain), and rhombencephalon (hindbrain: metencephalon plus myelencephalon). It is derived (developed) from the anterior part of the embryonic neural tube. Functions include muscle control and coordination, sensory reception and integration, speech production, memory storage, and the elaboration of thought and emotion. Called also *encephalon* [TA]. See Plates 9 and 10 and see also *cerebrum.*
 eloquent b. regions of the brain directly involved in speech, motor functions, sensory reception, and cranial nerve function (motor and

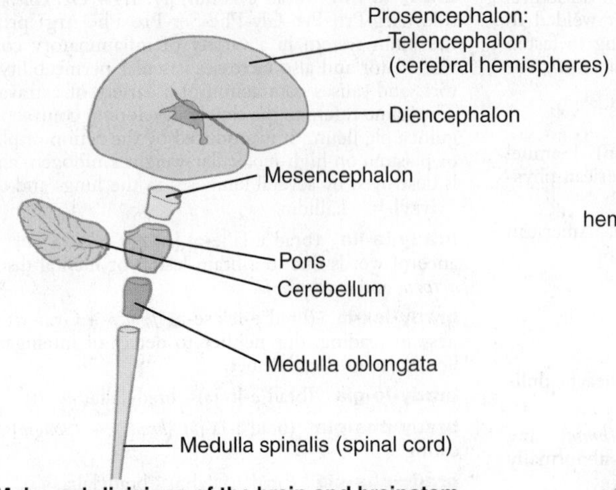

Prosencephalon:
Telencephalon
(cerebral hemispheres)
Diencephalon
Mesencephalon
Pons
Cerebellum
Medulla oblongata
Medulla spinalis (spinal cord)

Major subdivisions of the brain and brainstem

Parietal lobe
Cerebral hemispheres
Temporal lobe
Occipital lobe
Cerebellum
Cervical nerve I
Spinal cord
Cervical plexus
Thoracic nerve I
Brachial plexus
Lumbar nerve I
Lumbar plexus
Cauda equina
Femoral nerve
Sacral plexus
Sacral nerve I
Filum terminale
Coccygeal plexus
Coccygeal nerve
Sciatic nerve

Posterior view showing the posterior *(left)* and anterior *(right)* rami of the spinal nerves

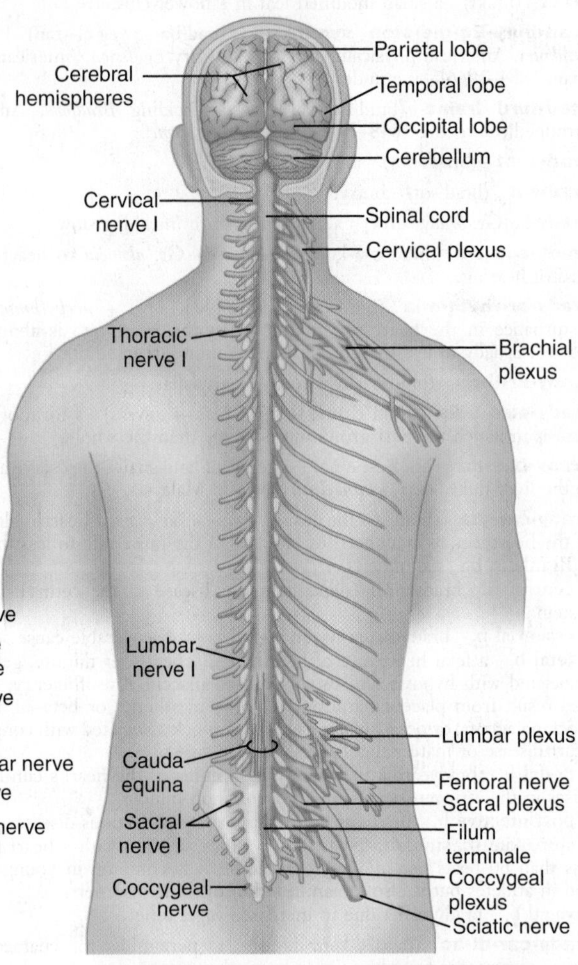

Longitudinal cerebral fissure
Cranial nerves
Frontal lobe
I Olfactory nerve
Temporal lobe
Optic chiasm
Pituitary gland
Hypothalamus
II Optic nerve
III Oculomotor nerve
IV Trochlear nerve
V Trigeminal nerve
Pons
VI Abducens nerve
Flocculus
VII Facial nerve
VIII Vestibulocochlear nerve
Medulla oblongata
XII Hypoglossal nerve
IX Glossopharyngeal nerve
Cerebellum
XI Spinal accessory nerve
Occipital lobe
X Vagus nerve

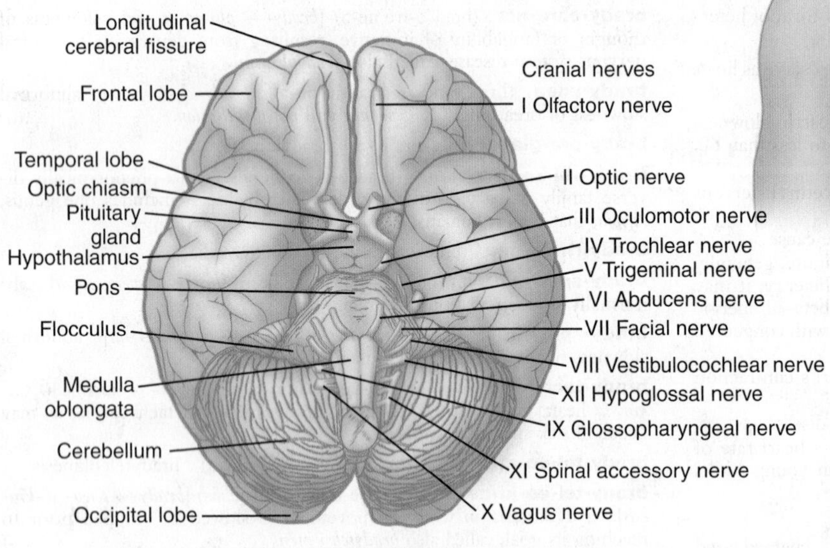

Basal view showing the brainstem and cranial nerves

Central sulcus
Postcentral gyrus
Precentral gyrus
Parietal lobe
Lateral ventricle
Lateral sulcus
(sylvian fissure)
Frontal lobe
Occipital lobe
Cerebellum
Thalamus
Temporal lobe
Pons
Medulla oblongata

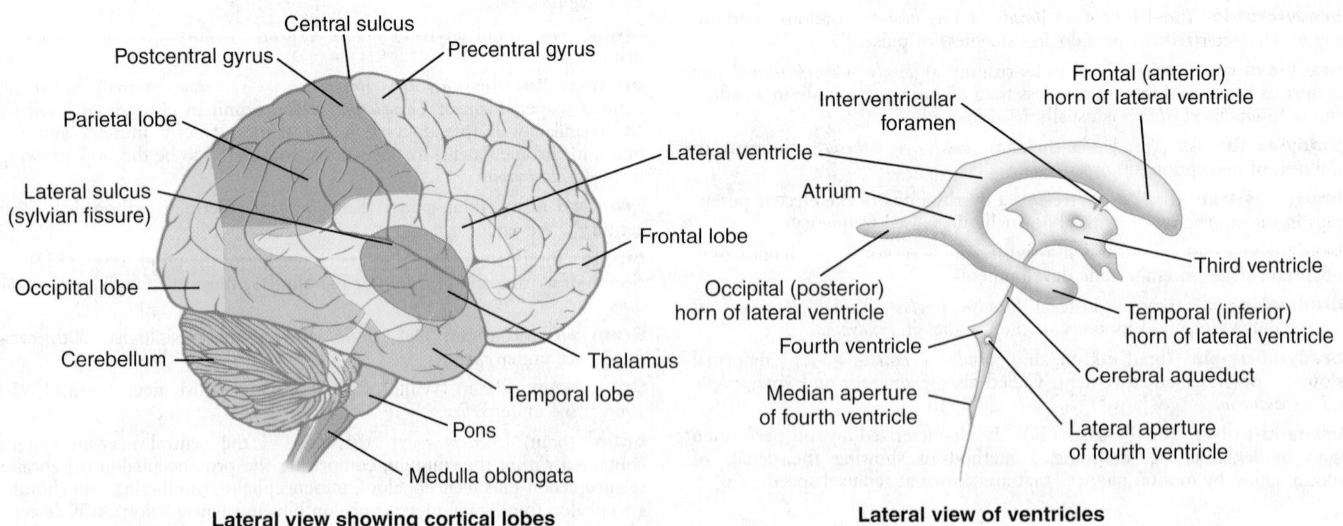

Lateral view showing cortical lobes

Frontal (anterior)
horn of lateral ventricle
Interventricular
foramen
Lateral ventricle
Atrium
Third ventricle
Occipital (posterior)
horn of lateral ventricle
Temporal (inferior)
horn of lateral ventricle
Fourth ventricle
Cerebral aqueduct
Median aperture
of fourth ventricle
Lateral aperture
of fourth ventricle

Lateral view of ventricles

■ PLATE 9—VARIOUS ASPECTS OF THE BRAIN AND SPINAL CORD

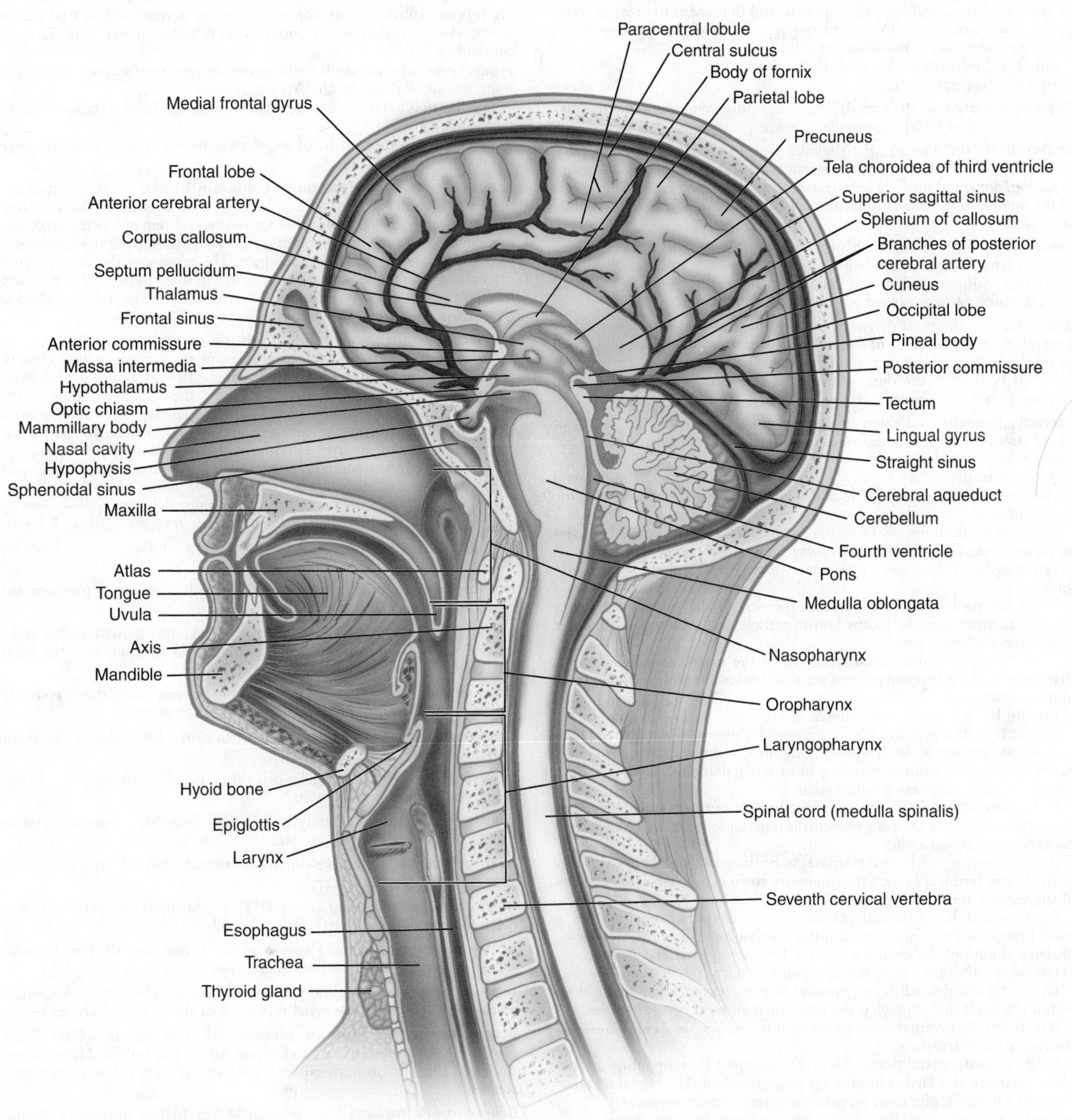

■ **PLATE 10**—HEMISECTION OF THE HEAD AND NECK, SHOWING VARIOUS PARTS OF THE BRAIN IN RELATION TO OTHER STRUCTURES

sensory); such regions are essential to localize in treating brain lesions. Called also *eloquent areas.*

olfactory b. rhinencephalon (def. 1).

respirator b. the congested, swollen brain of a patient who has been on a respirator longer than one day after suffering cerebral anoxia and ischemia; necrotic and autolytic changes begin to occur and the patient is comatose or brain dead.

split b. a brain in which connections between the hemispheres, mainly the corpus callosum, have been severed or otherwise disrupted; done surgically on experimental laboratory animals and in humans to provide access to the third ventricle or to control epilepsy. See also *split-brain syndrome,* under *syndrome,* and *corpuscallosotomy.*

smell b. rhinencephalon (def. 1).

wet b. cerebral edema.

Brai•nerd diarrhea (bra′nərd) [*Brainerd,* Minnesota, where the first outbreak occurred in 1983] see under *diarrhea.*

brain•stem (brān′stem) the stalklike portion of the brain connecting the cerebral hemispheres with the spinal cord and comprising the mesencephalon, pons, and medulla oblongata; the diencephalon is considered part of the brainstem by some. Called also *truncus encephalicus* [TA]. Also written *brain stem.*

brain•wash•ing (brān′wahsh″ing) any systematic effort aimed at instilling certain attitudes and beliefs against a person's will, usually beliefs in conflict with prior beliefs and knowledge. It initially referred to political indoctrination of prisoners of war and political prisoners.

bran (bran) the meal derived from the epidermis or outer covering of a cereal grain. It is a source of dietary fiber, which may be soluble (e.g., oats) or insoluble (e.g., wheat) depending on the type of grain.

wheat b. [USP] the outer covering of the cereal grain derived from various species of *Triticum.*

branch (branch) a division or offshoot from a main stem, especially of blood vessels, nerves, or lymphatics; for specific anatomical structures not found here, see under *ramus.*

anterior b. of axillary nerve a branch that winds around the humeral neck beneath the deltoid muscle and innervates both the muscle and the overlying skin.

anterior pulmonary b's of vagus nerve anterior bronchial branches of vagus nerve; see *rami bronchiales nervi vagi,* under *ramus.*

articular b. of deep peroneal nerve a twig that innervates the ankle joint.

b. to biceps brachii the muscular branch of the musculocutaneous nerve that innervates the biceps brachii muscle; see *rami musculares nervi musculocutanei,* under *ramus.*

b. to brachialis the muscular branch of the musculocutaneous nerve that innervates the brachial muscle; see *rami musculares nervi musculocutanei,* under *ramus.*

bundle b. a branch of the bundle of His.

circumferential pontine b's rami laterales pontis.

communicating b. with ciliary ganglion, communicating b. with nasociliary nerve, communicating b. of nasociliary nerve with ciliary ganglion radix sensoria ganglii ciliaris.

b. to coracobrachialis the muscular branch of the musculocutaneous nerve that innervates the coracobrachialis muscle; see *rami musculares nervi musculocutanei,* under *ramus.*

interosseous b's of lateral terminal b. of deep peroneal nerve twigs of the lateral terminal branch that innervate the metatarsophalangeal joints of the second, third, and fourth toes.

interosseous b. of medial terminal b. of deep peroneal nerve a small branch of the medial terminal branch that innervates the metatarsophalangeal joint of the great toe and the first dorsal interosseous space.

lateral pontine b's rami laterales pontis.

lateral terminal b. of deep peroneal nerve a branch beginning deep within the ankle and supplying the extensor digitorum brevis muscles.

left b. of atrioventricular bundle, left bundle b. crus sinistrum fasciculi atrioventricularis.

long circumferential pontine b's the group of lateral pontine arterial branches that travel farther around the pons, supplying the lateral tegmentum and substantia nigra; see *rami laterales pontis,* under *ramus.*

marginal b. of cingulate sulcus ramus marginalis sulci cinguli.

medial pontine b's rami mediales pontis.

medial terminal b. of deep peroneal nerve a branch beginning in the ankle and running along the dorsum of the foot to the first interosseous space, where it combines with the medial dorsal cutaneous nerve and then subdivides into the dorsal digital nerves of the great and second toes.

muscular b's of deep peroneal nerve rami musculares nervi fibularis profundi.

b. of oculomotor nerve to ciliary ganglion ramus parasympathica ganglii ciliaris.

paramedian pontine b's rami mediales pontis.

posterior b's of axillary nerve rami musculares nervi axillaris.

posterior pulmonary b's of vagus nerve posterior bronchial branches of vagus nerve; see *rami bronchiales nervi vagi,* under *ramus.*

right b. of atrioventricular bundle, right bundle b. crus dextrum fasciculi atrioventricularis.

short circumferential pontine b's the group of lateral pontine arterial branches that travel a short distance around the pons, supplying its anterolateral and posterolateral regions; see *rami laterales pontis,* under *ramus.*

b's to sternocleidomastoid deep branches of the cervical plexus that are proprioceptive sensory connectors to the sternocleidomastoid muscle.

superior vermian b. of superior cerebellar artery arteria vermis superior.

sural communicating b. with common peroneal nerve ramus communicans fibularis nervi fibularis communis.

zygomaticofacial b. of zygomatic nerve ramus zygomaticofacialis nervi zygomatici.

zygomaticotemporal b. of zygomatic nerve ramus zygomaticotemporalis nervi zygomatici.

branched-chain-ami•no-ac•id trans•am•i•nase (brancht-chān-ə-me′no-as′id trans-am′ĭ-nās) [EC 2.6.1.42] an enzyme of the transferase class that catalyzes the removal of the α-amino group of leucine, isoleucine, or valine to form the corresponding keto acid, transferring the amino group to α-ketoglutarate or a similar acceptor. The reaction is the first step in the catabolism of branched-chain amino acids. In some persons the enzyme for leucine and isoleucine is distinguishable from the one for valine. Called also *branched-chain-amino-acid aminotransferase.*

branched-chain α-ke•to ac•id de•hy•dro•gen•ase (brancht chān ke′to as′id de-hi′dro-jən-ās) an enzyme of the oxidoreductase class that is a component of the multienzyme branched-chain α-keto acid dehydrogenase complex (q.v.). The enzyme catalyzes the oxidative decarboxylation of the branched chain amino acids leucine, isoleucine, and valine, transferring the products formed to the lipoamide that is linked to the side chain of a lysine residue of another enzyme of the complex, dihydrolipoyllysine-residue (2-methylpropanoyl)transferase, using a thiamine pyrophosphate cofactor. See also *maple syrup urine disease,* under *disease.* Called also *α-ketoisovalerate dehydrogenase.* In official nomenclature, called *3-methyl-2-oxobutanoate dehydrogenase (2-methylpropanoyl-transferring)* [EC 1.2.4.4].

branch•er en•zyme (branch′ər en′zīm) 1,4-α-glucan branching enzyme.

branch•er en•zyme de•fi•cien•cy (branch′ər en′zīm) glycogen storage disease, type IV.

bran•chia (brang′ke-ə) [Gr. *branchia* gills] the gills of fishes and of others of the lower vertebrates; represented in the human fetus by the pharyngeal arches, separated by grooves or clefts.

bran•chi•al (brang′ke-əl) pertaining to or resembling the gills of a fish or the derivatives of homologous parts in other animals.

branch•ing en•zyme (branch′ing en′zīm) 1,4-α-glucan branching enzyme.

bran•chi•o•gen•ic (brang″ke-o-jen′ik) 1. gill-forming. 2. forming a pharyngeal or branchial arch.

bran•chi•og•e•nous (brang″ke-oj′ə-nəs) [*branchia* + *-genous*] formed from a pharyngeal arch or groove.

bran•chi•o•ma (brang″ke-o′mə) a tumor derived from branchial epithelium or branchial rests.

bran•chio•mere (brang′ke-o-mēr″) a segment of the splanchnic mesoderm from which the pharyngeal or branchial arches are developed.

bran•chio•mer•ic (brang″ke-o-mer′ik) pertaining to the branchiomeres or to pharyngeal or branchial arches.

bran•chi•om•er•ism (brang″ke-om′ər-iz-əm) [*branchia-* + *merism*] metamerism based on the serial repetition of the branchial arches.

Brandt-An•drews method (maneuver) (brahnt′ an′dro͞oz) [Thure *Brandt,* Swedish obstetrician and gynecologist, 1819–1895; Henry Russell *Andrews,* English obstetrician and gynecologist, 1871–1942] see under *method.*

Brå•ne•mark implant (brå′nə-mahrk) [Per-Ingmar *Brånemark,* Swedish physician, 20th century] see under *implant.*

Bran•ham sign (bradycardia) (bran′həm) [H.H. *Branham,* American surgeon, 19th century] see under *sign.*

Bran•ha•mel•la (bran″hə-mel′ə) [Sara Elizabeth *Branham,* American bacteriologist, 1888–1962] *Moraxella (Branhamella).*

B. catarrha′lis *Moraxella (Branhamella) catarrhalis.*

bran•ny (bran′e) resembling bran; rough, scaly, dry.

brash (brash) heartburn.

water b. heartburn with regurgitation into the mouth of fluid that may be sour or almost tasteless.

Bras•si•ca (bras'ĭ-kə) [L.] a genus of plants of the family Cruciferae, including cabbage, turnip, mustard, rape, and others. Species of medical interest include *B. na'pus*, the rape plant, and *B. ni'gra* (L.) Koch., black mustard.

Braun anastomosis (broun) [Heinrich *Braun*, German surgeon, 1847–1911] see under *anastomosis.*

Braun canal (broun) [Carl Ritter *Braun* von Fernwald, Austrian obstetrician, 1822–1891] neurenteric canal; see under *canal.*

Brau•ne muscle (brou'nə) [Christian Wilhelm *Braune*, German anatomist, 1831–1892] musculus puborectalis.

Braun•wald sign (broun'wahld) [Eugene *Braunwald*, American cardiologist, born 1929] see under *sign.*

Bra•vais-jack•so•ni•an epilepsy (brah-va' jak-so'ne-ən) [Louis François *Bravais*, French physician, early 19th century; John Hughlings *Jackson*, English neurologist, 1835–1911] jacksonian epilepsy.

Brax•ton Hicks contraction, version (brak'stən hiks') [John *Braxton Hicks*, English gynecologist, 1823–1897] see under *contraction* and *version.*

braxy (brak'se) a disease of sheep caused by *Clostridium septicum*, and marked by hemorrhagic abomasitis, with hemorrhage into the peritoneal cavity, by abdominal pain, and, usually, by diarrhea and high fever. Called also *bradshot*, *bransot*, and *malignant edema.*

braze (brāz) in dentistry, to solder with a relatively infusible alloy.

bra•zil•in (brə-zil'in) a yellow crystalline substance obtained from the bark of *Biancea sappan* and other redwood trees; it is very similar to hematoxylin and oxidizes to a bright red dye, brazilein.

BRCA see under *gene.*

BrdU 5-bromodeoxyuridine.

breadth (bredth) the distance measured horizontally from side to side; see also under *diameter.*

b. of accommodation range of accommodation.

bizygomatic b. the distance between the most laterally situated points (zygia) on the zygomatic arches.

break (brāk) 1. to interrupt the continuity, or an interruption in the continuity of a structure, especially a bone. See *fracture.* 2. the interruption of an electric circuit, as distinguished from the make.

break•down (brāk'doun) 1. the act or process of ceasing to function, or the resulting condition. 2. an often sudden collapse in health, physical or mental. 3. loss of self-control.

nervous b. a nonspecific, popular name for any type of mental disorder that interferes with the affected individual's normal activities, often implying a severe episode with sudden onset.

breast (brest) 1. the anterior aspect of the thorax. 2. mamma.

caked b. stagnation mastitis.

chicken b. pectus carinatum.

funnel b. pectus excavatum.

pigeon b. pectus carinatum.

shotty b. fibrocystic disease of the breast; see under *disease.*

breast•feed•ing (brest' fēd'ing) the feeding of an infant at the mother's breast; also written *breast feeding.*

breath (breth) [L. *spiritus halitus*] the air taken in and expelled during ventilation (q.v.).

bad b. halitosis.

lead b. the metallic odor of the breath in lead poisoning.

liver b. fetor hepaticus.

breath-hold•ing (breth' hōld'ing) cessation of breathing, either voluntarily or involuntarily, seen most often in young children. See *breath-holding spell*, under *spell.*

breath•ing (brēth'ing) ventilation (def. 2).

Biot b. see under *respiration.*

bronchial b. bronchial breath sounds; see under *sound.*

Cheyne-Stokes b. see under *respiration.*

frog b., glossopharyngeal b. respiration unaided by the primary or ordinary accessory muscles of respiration, the air being "swallowed" rapidly into the lungs by use of the tongue and muscles of the pharynx; used by patients with chronic muscle paralysis to augment their breathing.

intermittent positive pressure b. (IPPB) the active inflation of the lungs during inhalation under positive pressure from a cycling valve. Called also *intermittent positive pressure ventilation.*

mouth b. breathing through the mouth instead of the nose, usually because of some obstruction of the nasal passages.

periodic b. Cheyne-Stokes respiration.

pursed lip b. an abnormal breathing style in which the lips are pursed during exhalation, usually due to dyspnea in an effort to reduce respiratory muscle effort.

rescue b. any artificial respiration technique in which ventilation is supplied by exhaling into the patient's nose or throat, or into a laryngectomy site, airway, or special mask made for the purpose. Called also *expired air resuscitation* or *ventilation.*

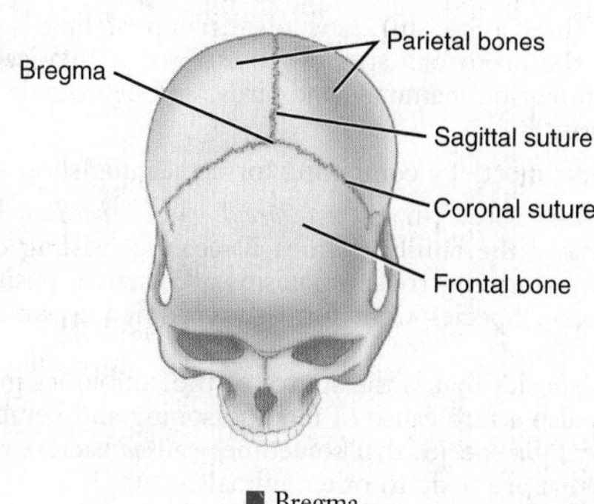

■ Bregma.

bre•douille•ment (brĕ"doo-e-maw') a speech defect in which only part of the word is pronounced, due to extreme rapidity of utterance.

breech (brēch) buttocks (nates [TA]).

breed•ing (brēd'ing) 1. the production of offspring or progeny. 2. the controlled propagation of animals or plants.

breg•ma (breg'mə) [Gr. "front of the head"] [TA] the point on the surface of the skull at the junction of the coronal and sagittal sutures; used as a craniometric landmark. **bregmat'ic** *adj*

breg•ma•to•dym•ia (breg"mə-to-dim'e-ə) [*bregma* + Gr. *didymos* twin + *-ia*] the state of conjoined twins fused at the bregmas.

brei (bri) [Ger. "pulp"] tissue that has been ground to a pulp; a homogenate.

Brei•sky disease (bri'ske) [August *Breisky*, Czechoslovakian gynecologist, 1832–1889] *lichen sclerosus* (q.v.) of the vulvar region.

brems•strah•lung (brem'strah-loong) [Ger. "braking radiation"] 1. the continuous spectrum of electromagnetic radiation produced by the rapid deceleration of a fast-moving charged particle (such as an electron or beta particle) in the electric field of another charged particle (usually a nucleus). Called also *braking radiation* and *continuous x-ray spectrum.* 2. the deceleration of a charged particle that produces this radiation.

Bren•ne•mann syndrome (bren'ə-mən) [Joseph *Brennemann*, American pediatrician, 1872–1944] see under *syndrome.*

Bren•ner tumor (bren'ər) [Fritz *Brenner*, German pathologist, 1877–1969] see under *tumor.*

breph•ic (bref'ik) [*breph-* + *-ic*] pertaining to an early stage of development.

breph(o)- [Gr. *brephos* embryo, newborn infant] a combining form denoting relationship to the embryo, fetus, or newborn infant.

brepho•plas•tic (bref"o-plas'tik) [*brepho-* + *plastic*] formed from embryonic tissue or during embryonic life.

brepho•tro•phic (bref"o-tro'fik) [*brepho-* + *-trophic*] pertaining to the nourishment of infants.

Bres•chet canals, sinus, veins (brə-sha') [Gilbert *Breschet*, French anatomist, 1783-1845] see *canales diploici*, *sinus sphenoparietalis*, and *venae diploicae.*

Bres•cia-Ci•mi•no fistula (bresh'e-ə sĭ-me'no) [Michael J. *Brescia*, American nephrologist, born 1933; James E. *Cimino*, American nephrologist, born 1928] see under *fistula.*

Bres•low thickness (bres'lo) [Alexander *Breslow*, American pathologist, 1928–1980] see under *thickness.*

Breth•aire (breth'ār) trademark for a preparation of terbutaline sulfate.

Breth•ine (breth'ēn) trademark for preparations of terbutaline sulfate.

Bret•y•late (bret'ə-lāt) trademark for a preparation of bretylium tosylate.

bre•tyl•i•um to•sy•late (brə-til'e-əm) [USP] an adrenergic blocking agent that also has direct myocardial effects; used as an antiarrhythmic in certain cases of ventricular tachycardia or fibrillation, administered intravenously or intramuscularly.

Bre•ty•lol (brĕ'tə-lol) trademark for a preparation of bretylium tosylate.

Breus mole (brois) [Karl *Breus*, Austrian obstetrician, 1852–1914] see under *mole.*

breve•tox•i•co•sis (brev"ə-tok"sĭ-ko'sis) neurotoxicity in marine mammals and birds caused by ingesting protozoa that contain brevetoxins.

breve·tox·in (brev′ə-tok″sin) any of a group of lipid-soluble neurotoxins found in the protozoan species *Karenia brevis;* they cause red tides, brevetoxicosis in marine mammals and birds, and neurotoxic shellfish poisoning in humans.

brevi- [L. *brevis* short] a combining form meaning short.

Bre·vi·ba·cil·lus (brev″ĭ-bə-sil′əs) [*brevi-* + L. *bacillus* little rod] a genus of bacteria of the family Paenibacillaceae, consisting of gram-positive, motile, spore-forming rods; organisms are catalase-positive and most are strictly aerobic. Species were formerly classified as strains of *Bacillus brevis.*

B. bre′vis a species that is the source of the antibiotics gramicidin and tyrocidine. It is also a rare cause of food poisoning and keratitis.

B. laterospo′rus a species that sometimes causes bacteremia in humans and has strains that are toxic to other animals.

Bre·vi·bac·te·ri·a·ceae (brev″ĭ-bak-tēr″e-a′se-e) a family of bacteria of the suborder Micrococcineae, order Actinomycetales, consisting of gram-positive, non–spore-forming, short unbranched rods. It includes the genus *Brevibacterium.*

Bre·vi·bac·te·ri·um (brev″ĭ-bak-tēr′e-əm) [*brevi-* + *bacterium*] a genus of bacteria of the family Brevibacteriaceae, consisting of short, unbranched rods found in salt and fresh water, dairy products, and decomposing material of many types. Organisms are opportunistic pathogens.

Brevi·bloc (brev′ĭ-blok″) trademark for a preparation of esmolol hydrochloride.

brevi·col·lis (brev″ĭ-kol′is) [*brevi-* + *collum*] shortness of the neck; see *dystrophia brevicollis.*

Brev·i·con (brev′ĭ-kon) trademark for a combination preparation of norethindrone and ethinyl estradiol.

brevi·flex·or (brev″ĭ-flek′sər) [*brevi-* + *flexor*] a short flexor muscle.

brevi·lin·e·al (brev″ĭ-lin′e-əl) brachymorphic.

brevi·ra·di·ate (brev″ĭ-ra′de-āt) having short processes; a term applied to one type of neuroglia cells.

Brev·i·tal (brev′ĭ-təl) trademark for a preparation of methohexital sodium.

Bre·vox·yl (brə-vok′səl) trademark for preparations of benzoyl peroxide.

Bre·vun·di·mo·nas (brev-un″dĭ-mo′nəs) [*brevi-* + L. *unda* wave + Gr. *monas* unit, from *monos* single] a genus of aerobic, gram-negative bacteria of the family Caulobacteraceae, consisting of non–spore-forming, rod-shaped to vibrioid cells that are chemo-organotrophic and oligotrophic; some species can form prosthecae and undergo a characteristic asymmetric fission in which one of the daughter cells is nonmotile and the other is flagellated and motile. The type species is *B. diminu′ta.*

B. diminu′ta a motile, rod-shaped species that does not form prosthecae or undergo asymmetric fission; it occurs in water and aqueous solutions and has been isolated from a variety of clinical specimens. Formerly called *Pseudomonas diminuta.*

B. vesicula′ris a motile, rod-shaped species that does not form prosthecae or undergo asymmetric fission, isolated from water and clinical specimens; it has been associated with genitourinary tract infections and is a rare cause of nosocomial central nervous system infection and bacteremia. Formerly called *Pseudomonas vesicularis.*

Brew·er infarcts (broo′ər) [George Emerson *Brewer*, American surgeon, 1861–1939] see under *infarct.*

Bric·a·nyl (brik′ə-nəl) trademark for preparations of terbutaline sulfate.

Brick·er procedure (operation, technique) (brik′ər) [Eugene M. *Bricker*, American surgeon, 1908–2000] see under *procedure.*

BrIDA mebrofenin.

bridge (brij) 1. a structure that connects two distant points, including parts of an organ. Called also *pons.* 2. fixed partial denture. 3. tarsal coalition. 4. intercellular b.

arteriolovenular b. the main and largest capillary connecting an arteriole and a venule; it retains some muscle elements and is rarely completely collapsed.

cantilever b. a fixed partial denture in which the pontic is cantilevered, i.e., retained only on one side by the abutment tooth. Called also *extension b.*

cell b's see *intercellular b.* and *protoplasmic b.*

conjugative b. in bacterial conjugation, a connection formed between two bacterial cells by the attachment of an F pilus from an F^+ cell to an F^- cell.

cytoplasmic b. 1. protoplasmic b. 2. see *intercellular b.*

dentin b. a scarlike deposit of reparative dentin or other calcific substance which reseals exposed pulp or which forms across the excised surface of pulp after pulpotomy.

disulfide b. see under *bond.*

extension b. cantilever b.

fixed b. fixed partial denture.

fixed-fixed b. fixed b. with rigid connectors.

fixed-movable b. fixed b. with rigid and nonrigid connectors.

fixed b. with rigid connectors a fixed partial denture in which all components are rigidly soldered or cast in one piece. Called also *fixed-fixed b.*

fixed b. with rigid and nonrigid connectors a fixed partial denture consisting of a major retainer attached to a pontic and supplied with a dovetail, and a minor retainer supplied with a slot into which the dovetail of the pontic fits; it provides some stress-breaking by allowing some movement. Called also *fixed-movable b.*

intercellular b. a structure seen especially in the prickle cell layer of the epidermis, formed by the meeting of short cytoplasmic projections from the cell surface of adjacent cells. It was formerly thought to constitute a bridge for cytoplasmic continuity between cells, but it is now known to be an artifact caused by dehydration during fixation, representing a desmosome in which are terminated the projections from each cell.

b. of the nose the upper portion of the external nose formed by the junction of the nasal bones.

protoplasmic b. a strand of protoplasm connecting two secondary spermatocytes, occurring as a result of incomplete cytokinesis; called also *cytoplasmic b.*

removable b. removable partial denture.

salt b. 1. an inverted-U–shaped tube filled with a gel, usually composed of agar, water, and potassium chloride, used to separate two chemically incompatible solutions in an electrochemical cell. 2. a chemical bond between a nitrogen atom, carrying a positive charge, and an oxygen atom, carrying a negative charge.

stationary b. fixed partial denture.

tarsal b. see under *coalition.*

ureteric b. Bell muscle.

bridge·work (brij′wərk) partial denture.

fixed b. fixed partial denture.

removable b. removable partial denture.

bridg·ing (brij′ing) the forming of a bridgelike structure.

myocardial b. anomalous formation by myocardial tissue of a bridge across part of a tunneling coronary artery (usually the left anterior descending coronary artery); this is usually asymptomatic, but in some persons the artery may become compressed, especially during systole.

bri·dle (bri′dəl) 1. a frenum. 2. a loop or filament that crosses the lumen of a passage or the surface of an ulcer.

bri·dou (bre-doo′) perlèche.

Bright disease (brīt) [Richard *Bright*, English physician, 1789–1858] see under *disease.*

Brill disease (bril) [Nathan Edwin *Brill*, American physician, 1860–1925] Brill-Zinsser disease.

Brill-Sym·mers disease (bril′ sim′ərz) [N.E. *Brill;* Douglas *Symmers*, American physician, 1879–1952] follicular lymphoma.

Brill-Zins·ser disease (bril′ zin′sər) [N.E. *Brill;* Hans *Zinsser*, American bacteriologist, 1878–1940] see under *disease.*

brim (brim) the upper edge of a basin.

pelvic b. apertura pelvis superior.

bri·mo·ni·dine tar·trate (brĭ-mo′nə-dēn) an α-adrenergic receptor agonist relatively selective for α_2-adrenergic receptors. It both reduces production of aqueous humor and increases aqueous outflow and is used in the treatment of open-angle glaucoma and ocular hypertension; administered topically to the conjunctiva.

Bri·nell hardness number (brĭ-nel′) [Johann August *Brinell*, Swedish engineer, 1849–1925] see under *number.*

Brin·ton disease (brin′ton) [William *Brinton*, English physician, 1823–1867] linitis plastica.

brin·zo·la·mide (brin-zo′lə-mīd) a carbonic anhydrase inhibitor that decreases secretion of aqueous humor; used in the treatment of open-angle glaucoma and ocular hypertension, administered topically to the conjunctiva.

Bri·quet syndrome (bre-ka′) [Paul *Briquet*, French physician, 1796–1881] see under *syndrome.*

brise·ment (brēz-maw′) [Fr. "breaking"] the breaking up or tearing of anything, as of an ankylosis.

b. forcé (for-sa′) ["forced breaking"] the forcible breaking up or tearing of a bony ankylosis.

bris·ket (bris′kət) the connective tissue and fat over the sternum of a ruminant, hanging down between the front legs.

Bris·saud reflex (bre-so′) [Edouard *Brissaud*, French physician, 1852–1909] see under *reflex.*

Bris•saud-Si•card syndrome (bre-so′ se-kahr′) [E. *Brissaud;* Jean Athanase *Sicard,* French neurologist, 1872–1929] see under *syndrome.*

Bris•towe syndrome (bris′to) [John Syer *Bristowe,* British physician, 1827–1895] see under *syndrome.*

brit•tle (brit′əl) [A.S. *britel*] 1. easily broken, snapped, or cracked, especially under slight pressure. 2. easily disrupted.

BRM biologic response modifier.

broach (brōch) 1. an elongated, tapered, and serrated cutting tool for shaping and enlarging holes. 2. barbed b.; root canal b.

barbed b. a thin, flexible, hand-operated or engine-driven endodontic instrument, usually tapered, with a series of sharply pointed barbs along the operative head; used for engaging and removing the dental pulp and other substances intact from the root canal or pulp chamber.

pathfinder b. root canal probe.

root canal b. a broach, usually barbed, used for removing the soft tissue contents of the root canal; see *barbed b.*

smooth b. root canal probe.

Broad•bent sign (brod′bent) [Sir William Henry *Broadbent,* English physician, 1835–1907] see under *sign.*

Bro•ca amnesia, motor speech area, etc. (bro-kah′) [Pierre Paul *Broca,* French anatomist, anthropologist, and surgeon, 1824–1880] see under *area, convolution,* and *fissure,* and see *expressive aphasia,* under *aphasia, visual plane,* under *plane,* and *stria diagonalis (Broca),* under *stria.*

Brock infundibulectomy, operation, syndrome (brok) [Sir Russell Claude *Brock,* British surgeon, 1903–1980] see under *infundibulectomy;* see *transventricular closed valvotomy,* under *valvotomy;* and see *middle lobe syndrome,* under *syndrome.*

Brock•en•brough sign (brok′en-bro) [Edwin C. *Brockenbrough,* American surgeon, born 1930] see under *sign.*

Brocq pseudopelade (brok) [Louis-Anne-Jean *Brocq,* French dermatologist, 1856–1928] pseudopelade.

Brö•del bloodless line (bra′dəl) [Max *Brödel,* American medical artist, 1870–1941] see under *line.*

Bro•ders index (classification) (bro′dərz) [Albert Compton *Broders,* American pathologist, 1885–1964] see under *index.*

Bro•die abscess, disease, knee (bro′de) [Sir Benjamin Collins *Brodie,* English surgeon, 1783–1862] see under *abscess, disease,* and *knee.*

Bro•die ligament (bro′de) [C. Gordon *Brodie,* British anatomist, 1786–1818] transverse humeral ligament.

bro•di•fa•coum (bro′dĭ-fə-ko͞om) a long-acting anticoagulant rodenticide.

Brod•mann areas (brod′mahn) [Korbinian *Brodmann,* German neurologist, 1868–1918] see under *area.*

bro•mat•ed (bro′māt-əd) brominated.

bro•ma•tol•o•gy (bro″mə-tol′ə-je) [Gr. *brōma* food + *-logy*] dietetics.

bro•ma•to•tox•in (bro′mə-to-tok″sin) [Gr. *brōma* food + *toxin*] a poison formed in food by fermentation.

bro•maz•e•pam (bro-maz′ə-pam″) a benzodiazepine used as an antianxiety agent in the treatment of anxiety disorders and anxiety associated with depression, and as a sedative and hypnotic in the treatment of insomnia; administered orally.

bro•me•lain (bro′mə-lān) any of several cysteine endopeptidases that catalyze the cleavage of proteins on the carboxyl side of alanine, glycine, lysine, and tyrosine bonds. Differing forms are derived from the fruit (fruit bromelain) and stem (stem bromelain) of the pineapple plant, *Ananas comosus.* The enzyme is administered orally (as *bromelains*) as an antiinflammatory agent and is also used in immunology to render red cells agglutinable by incomplete antibody. Called also *bromelin.*

bro•me•lains (bro′mə-lānz) a concentrate of proteolytic enzymes derived from pineapple plants (see *bromelain*); used to reduce inflammation and edema, and to accelerate tissue repair.

bro•mel•in (bro′mel-in) bromelain.

Brom•fed (brōm′fed) trademark for combination preparations of brompheniramine maleate and pseudoephedrine hydrochloride.

brom•hex•ine hy•dro•chlo•ride (brom-hek′sēn) an expectorant and mucolytic agent, administered orally and by inhalation in the treatment of respiratory disorders characterized by the production of excess or viscous mucus, and orally in the treatment of keratoconjunctivitis sicca in Sjögren syndrome.

brom•hi•dro•sis (bro″mĭ-dro′sis) [*brom-* (1) + *hidro-* + *-sis*] axillary (apocrine) sweat that has become foul smelling as a result of its bacterial decomposition. Called also *bromidrosis* and *osmidrosis.*

bro•mic (bro′mik) pertaining to or containing pentavalent bromine.

bro•mide (bro′mīd) any binary compound of bromine in which the bromine carries a negative charge (Br^-); specifically a salt (or organic ester) of hydrobromic acid (H^+Br^-). Bromides produce depression of the central nervous system, and were once widely used for their sedative effect. Because overdosage causes serious mental disturbances they are now seldom used, except occasionally in grand mal seizures. See also *bromism.*

bro•mi•dro•sis (bro″mĭ-dro′sis) bromhidrosis.

bro•mi•nat•ed (bro′mĭ-nāt″əd) combined with or containing bromine; called also *bromated* and *brominized.*

bro•mine (Br) (bro′mēn, bro′min) [Gr. *brōmos* stench] a reddish-brown liquid element, giving off suffocating vapors; atomic number 35, atomic weight 79.909. See also *bromide* and *bromism.*

bro•min•ism (bro′min-iz-əm) bromism.

bro•min•ized (bro′min-īzd) brominated.

bro•mism (bro′miz-əm) [*brom-* (2) + *-ism*] chronic bromide intoxication, caused by chronic ingestion of proprietary bromide preparations; it was once a common problem but is now rare. Characteristics include mental dullness, deficient memory, slurred speech, drowsiness, tremors, and ataxia. Skin eruptions of various forms are common. In most cases there is an accompanying mental disorder, which may be a delirium, a hallucinosis, or a transitory psychotic state resembling paranoid schizophrenia. Called also *brominism.*

bro•mi•za•tion (bro″mĭ-za′shən) impregnation with bromides or bromine; the administration of large doses of bromides.

bro•mized (bro′mīzd) under the influence of bromides.

brom(o)- [Gr. *brōmos* stench] 1. a combining form meaning foul-smelling. 2. in chemical terms, indicating the presence of bromine.

bro•mo•chlo•ro•tri•flu•o•ro•eth•ane (bro″mo-klor″o-tri-flo͞or″o-eth′ān) halothane.

bro•mo•crip•tine mes•y•late (bro″mo-krip′tēn) [USP] an ergot alkaloid that acts as a dopamine agonist; used to suppress prolactin secretion in the treatment of pituitary prolactinomas and of hyperprolactinemia-associated amenorrhea, galactorrhea, infertility, or male hypogonadism. It is also used as an antidyskinetic, usually in conjunction with levodopa, in the treatment of parkinsonism, and is used as a growth hormone suppressant in the treatment of acromegaly. Administered orally.

5-bro•mo•de•oxy•uri•dine (BrdU, BUdR) (bro″mo-de-ok-se-u′rĭ-din) a thymidine analogue that can be incorporated into DNA during replication and is used as a mutagen in genetic research; it causes breakage in chromosomal regions rich in heterochromatin and also alters the staining of chromatids. Written also *5-bromo-2-deoxyuridine.*

bro•mo•der•ma (bro″mo-dur′mə) [*brom-* (2) + *derma*] a halogenoderma resulting from ingestion of bromine or its compounds; see also *bromism.*

bro•mo•di•phen•hy•dra•mine hy•dro•chlo•ride (bro″mo-di″fen-hi′drə-mēn) [USP] a derivative of monoethanolamine, closely related to diphenhydramine; it is a sedating antihistamine (H_1 receptor antagonist) with anticholinergic effects, used in the treatment of allergic rhinitis, allergic conjunctivitis, and cutaneous manifestations of allergic reactions, and as an ingredient in some cough and cold preparations, administered orally.

bro•mo•men•or•rhea (bro″mo-men-o-re′ə) [*bromo-* (1) + *menorrhea*] the discharge of menses having a foul odor.

bro•mop•nea (bro-mop′ne-ə, bro″mo-ne′ə) [*bromo-* (1) + *-pnea*] halitosis.

5-bro•mo•ura•cil (bro″mo-u′rə-sil) a pyrimidine analogue with mutagenic properties.

brom•phen•ir•amine (brōm″fən-ir′ə-mēn) the bromine analogue of chlorpheniramine, an antihistamine (H_1 receptor antagonist) having anticholinergic and sedative effects.

b. maleate [USP] the maleate salt of brompheniramine, used in the treatment of allergic rhinitis, allergic conjunctivitis, and cutaneous manifestations of allergic reactions; administered orally or by intramuscular, intravenous, or subcutaneous injection. It is also an ingredient in some cold and cough preparations, administered orally.

brom•phe•nol (brōm-fe′nol) one of a series of brominized phenols, sometimes found in the precipitates of tested urine.

bro•mum (bro′məm) [L.] bromine.

brom•u•rat•ed (brōm′u-rāt″əd) containing bromine or bromine salts.

bronch•ad•e•ni•tis (brongk″ad-ə-ni′tis) [*bronch-* + *adenitis*] inflammation of the bronchial glands. Called also *bronchoadenitis.*

bron•chi (brong′ki) [L.] genitive and plural of *bronchus.*

bron•chia (brong′ke-ə) [L.] plural of *bronchium.*

bron•chi•ec•ta•sia (brong″ke-ek-ta′zhə) bronchiectasis.

bron•chi•ec•ta•sis (brong″ke-ek′tə-sis) [*bronchi-* + *ectasis*] chronic dilatation of the bronchi marked by fetid breath and paroxysmal coughing, with the expectoration of mucopurulent matter. Types are distinguished according to the nature of the dilatations. Called also *bronchiectasia*. **bronchiecta′sic, bronchiectat′ic** *adj*

capillary b. bronchiolectasis.

cylindrical b. bronchiectasis in which whole sections of the bronchi are uniformly widened.

cystic b. saccular b.

dry b. a rare variety of bronchiectasis, in which coughing is usually nonproductive but episodes of infection may be accompanied by hemoptysis.

follicular b. bronchiectasis in which the lymphoid tissue in the affected regions becomes greatly enlarged and, by projecting into the bronchial lumen, may seriously distort and partially obstruct the bronchus.

fusiform b. bronchiectasis in which the dilated tubes have terminal bulbous enlargements.

saccular b., sacculated b. bronchiectasis in which the bronchi terminate in enlarged blind sacs; called also *cystic b.*

varicose b. a condition similar to cylindrical bronchiectasis but having localized constrictions, so that the dilated bronchus has an irregular, tortuous shape.

bron•chil•o•quy (brong-kil′ə-kwe) [*bronchi-* + L. *loqui* to speak] bronchophony (def. 2).

bronchi(o)- a combining form denoting relationship to a bronchus. See also *bronch(o)-*.

bron•chio•cele (brong′ke-o-sēl) bronchocele.

bron•chio•gen•ic (brong″ke-o-jen′ik) bronchogenic.

bron•chi•ole (brong′ke-ōl) a subdivision of the branched bronchial tree 1 mm or less in diameter, differing from the bronchi in having cuboidal epithelial cells and lacking cartilage plates. Each bronchiole subdivides into several smaller terminal bronchioles. In official terminology, called *bronchiolus*.

alveolar b. respiratory b.

lobular b. bronchiole.

respiratory b. a short, thinner-walled branch of a terminal bronchiole; it is the first segment of the bronchiole that contains alveoli and in which gas exchange occurs. It further subdivides, subsequent branches becoming narrower in diameter and increasing in number of alveoli, with each branch terminating in an alveolar duct.

terminal b. a subdvision of a bronchiole, having a diameter 0.5 mm or less and itself subdividing into respiratory bronchioles. It is the terminus of the conducting portion of the respiratory system and does not contain alveoli.

bron•chio•lec•ta•sis (brong″ke-o-lek′tə-sis) [*bronchiol-* + *ectasis*] dilatation of the bronchioles. Called also *capillary bronchiectasis*.

bron•chi•o•li (brong-ki′o-li) [L.] genitive and plural of *bronchiolus*.

bron•chi•o•li•tis (brong″ke-o-li′tis) [*bronchiol-* + *-itis*] inflammation of the bronchioles, usually occurring in children less than 2 years old and resulting from a viral infection, particularly with respiratory syncytial virus. See also *bronchopneumonia*.

constrictive b. bronchiolitis fibrosa obliterans in which the fibrous tissue is between the muscularis mucosa layer and the epithelium.

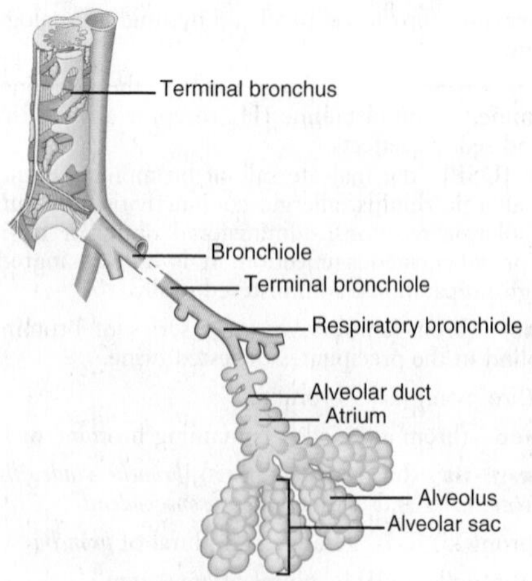

■ Bronchiole and subdivisions.

b. exudati′va, exudative b. bronchiolitis accompanied by exudation of Curschmann spirals and grayish, tenacious sputum; often associated with asthma.

b. fibro′sa obli′terans a usually chronic bronchiolitis with ingrowth of connective tissue from the wall of the terminal bronchi and occlusion of their lumina; it may be a complication of connective tissue disease or heart-lung transplant, and in children it may follow an acute attack of bronchiolitis or pneumonia. An acute form occurs in silo workers (silo filler's lung). Called also *b. obliterans* and *obliterative b.*

b. obli′terans b. fibrosa obliterans.

b. obliterans with organizing pneumonia (BOOP) an idiopathic disease combining organizing pneumonia with a condition resembling bronchiolitis fibrosa obliterans; terminal bronchioles and alveoli become occluded with masses of inflammatory cells and fibrotic tissue. Called also *cryptogenic organizing pneumonia*.

obliterative b. b. fibrosa obliterans.

proliferative b. bronchiolitis which the lumen of the bronchioles is obliterated by epithelial proliferation and exudate.

respiratory b. fibrosis in the respiratory bronchioles, seen mainly in cigarette smokers; see also *respiratory bronchiolitis–associated interstitial lung disease*.

bronchiol(o)- [L. *bronchiolus*, dim. of *bronchus*] a combining form denoting relationship to one or more bronchioles.

bron•chi•o•lus (brong-ki′o-ləs) pl. *bronchi′oli* [L., dim. of *bronchus*] [TA] a subdivision of the branched bronchial tree; see *bronchiole*.

bron•chio•spasm (brong′ke-o-spaz″əm) bronchospasm.

bron•chio•ste•no•sis (brong″ke-o-stə-no′sis) bronchostenosis.

bron•chis•mus (brong-kis′məs) bronchospasm.

bron•chi•tis (brong-ki′tis) [*bronch-* + *-itis*] inflammation of a bronchus or bronchi; there are both acute and chronic varieties. Symptoms usually include fever, coughing, and expectoration. Chronic forms may involve secondary changes to lung tissue. See also *chronic obstructive pulmonary disease*, under *disease*. **bronchit′ic** *adj*

acute b. a bronchitic attack with a short and more or less severe course; symptoms include fever and a productive cough. Repeated attacks may indicate chronic bronchitis.

arachidic b. bronchitis caused by the presence of a peanut kernel in a bronchus.

asthmatic b. bronchitis accompanying or just preceding asthma; see also *bronchitic asthma*, under *asthma*.

capillary b. bronchopneumonia.

Castellani b. hemorrhagic b.

chronic b. a type of chronic obstructive pulmonary disease in which there is bronchial irritation with increased secretions and a productive cough for at least three months, two years in succession; it is usually accompanied by pulmonary emphysema. The most common cause is long-term inhalation of irritants.

equine infectious b. equine influenza.

exudative b., fibrinous b. bronchitis with a violent cough, paroxysmal dyspnea, and expectoration of casts of the bronchi containing Charcot-Leyden crystals. Called also *fibrobronchitis*, *membranous b.*, *plastic b.*, and *pseudomembranous b.*

hemorrhagic b. chronic bronchitis with hemoptysis caused by a spirochetal infection. Called also *bronchospirochetosis* and *Castellani bronchitis* or *disease*.

infectious avian b. an acute, highly contagious, respiratory disease of chickens, caused by a coronavirus and characterized by tracheal rales, coughing, sneezing, nasal discharge, and a drop in egg production.

laryngotracheal b. laryngotracheobronchitis.

membranous b. fibrinous b.

b. obli′terans bronchitis in which the smaller bronchi become filled with nodules made up of fibrinous exudate.

parasitic b. verminous b.

plastic b., pseudomembranous b. fibrinous b.

putrid b. chronic bronchitis in which the sputum has an offensive smell; see also *Dittrich plugs*, under *plug*.

secondary b. bronchitis secondary to some other condition.

vanadium b. irritation of the bronchi in workers inhaling excessive amounts of vanadium pentoxide dust, usually accompanied by a green to black discoloration of the tongue. See also *vanadiumism*.

verminous b. a coughing and dyspnea in domestic animals due to presence in the bronchial tubes of nematode lungworms. In sheep, cattle, goats, and pigs it is called *hoose*; it also occurs in horses, donkeys, dogs, and cats. Called also *parasitic b.*

bron•chi•um (brong′ke-əm) pl. *bron′chia* [L.] a term sometimes used for one of the subdivisions of a bronchus larger than a bronchiole.

bronch(o)- [L. *bronchus*, q.v.] a combining form denoting relationship to a bronchus.

bron•cho•ad•e•ni•tis (brong″ko-ad″ə-ni′tis) bronchadenitis.

bron•cho•al•ve•o•lar (brong″ko-al-ve′ə-lər) pertaining to a bronchus and alveoli; called also *bronchovesicular.*

bron•cho•as•per•gil•lo•sis (brong″ko-as″pər-jil-o′sis) bronchopulmonary aspergillosis.

bron•cho•bil•i•ary (brong″ko-bil′e-ar-e) connecting a bronchus and a bile duct.

bron•cho•can•di•di•a•sis (brong″ko-kan″dĭ-di′ə-sis) bronchopulmonary candidiasis.

bron•cho•cav•ern•ous (brong″ko-kav′ər-nəs) having both bronchial and cavernous qualities, such as abnormal respiration.

bron•cho•cav•i•tary (brong″ko-kav′ĭ-tar-e) pertaining to or communicating between a bronchus and a cavity.

bron•cho•cele (brong′ko-sēl) [*broncho-* + *cele*[1]] a localized dilatation of a bronchus.

bron•cho•con•stric•tion (bron″ko-kən-strik′shən) constriction or narrowing of the lumina of the air passages of the lungs, typically as a result of bronchial smooth muscle contraction.

exercise-induced b. exercise-induced asthma.

bron•cho•con•stric•tor (brong″ko-kən-strik′tər) 1. constricting or narrowing the lumina of the air passages of the lungs. 2. an agent that causes narrowing of the lumina of the air passages of the lungs.

bron•cho•di•la•ta•tion (brong″ko-di-lə-ta′shən) 1. a dilated state of a bronchus. 2. a dilated area of a bronchus.

bron•cho•di•la•tion (brong″ko-di-la′shən) the act or process of increasing the caliber of a bronchus.

bron•cho•di•la•tor (brong″ko-di′la-tər, -di-la′tər) 1. dilating or expanding the lumina of air passages of the lungs. 2. an agent that causes expansion of the lumina of the air passages of the lungs.

bron•cho•egoph•o•ny (brong″ko-e-gof′ə-ne) egophony.

bron•cho•esoph•a•ge•al (brong″ko-ə-sof″ə-je′əl) pertaining to or communicating with a bronchus and the esophagus; called also *esophagobronchial.*

bron•cho•eso•pha•ge•us (brong″ko-e-so-fa′je-əs) [L.] bronchoesophageal; see under *musculus.*

bron•cho•esoph•a•gol•o•gy (brong″ko-ə-sof″ə-gol′ə-je) the branch of medicine that deals with the tracheobronchial tree and the esophagus.

bron•cho•esoph•a•gos•co•py (brong″ko-ə-sof″ə-gos′kə-pe) the instrumental examination of the bronchi and esophagus.

bron•cho•fi•ber•scope (brong″ko-fi′bər-skōp) a flexible bronchoscope that uses fiberoptics. Called also *fiberoptic bronchoscope.*

bron•cho•fi•ber•sco•py (brong″ko-fi-bur′skə-pe) bronchofibroscopy.

bron•cho•fi•bros•co•py (brong″ko-fi-bros′kə-pe) examination of the bronchi through a bronchofiberscope. Called also *bronchofiberscopy* and *fiberoptic bronchoscopy.*

bron•cho•gen•ic (brong-ko-jen′ik) originating in a bronchus.

bron•cho•gram (brong′ko-gram) the radiogram obtained by bronchography.

air b. a radiographic shadow of an air-filled bronchus running through an airless lung; applied also to any tapering, branching radiolucency in an opacified lung that corresponds in size and distribution to (and is assumed to be) a part of the bronchial tree.

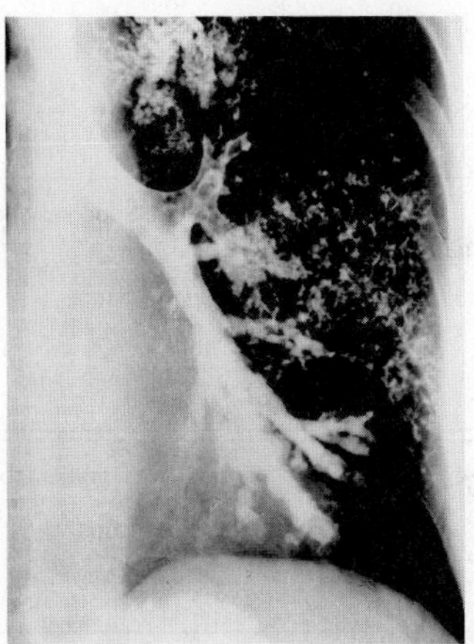

■ Fiberoptic bronchoscopic bronchogram of left lower lobe, showing gross dilatation of the airways typical of postinfective bronchiectasis.

bron•chog•ra•phy (brong-kog′rə-fe) [*broncho-* + *-graphy*] radiography of the lung after the instillation of an opaque medium in a bronchus. **bronchograph′ic** *adj*

bron•cho•lith (brong′ko-lith) [*broncho-* + *-lith*] a concretion in the bronchi, formed by accretion about an inorganic nucleus, or from calcified portions of lung tissue or adjacent lymph nodes; called also *bronchial calculus.*

bron•cho•li•thi•a•sis (brong″ko-lĭ-thi′ə-sis) the presence of broncholiths in the lumen of the tracheobronchial tree.

bron•chol•o•gy (brong-kol′ə-je) the study and treatment of diseases of the tracheobronchial tree. **broncholog′ic** *adj*

bron•cho•ma•la•cia (brong″ko-mə-la′shə) a deficiency in the cartilaginous wall of a bronchus, often accompanied by some degree of tracheomalacia, which may lead to atelectasis or obstructive emphysema; it may be congenital or acquired.

bron•cho•mo•tor (brong′ko-mo′tər) affecting the caliber of the bronchi.

bron•cho•mu•co•tro•pic (brong″ko-mu″ko-tro′pik) augmenting secretion by the respiratory mucosa.

bron•cho•my•co•sis (brong″ko-mi-ko′sis) [*broncho-* + *mycosis*] any infection of the bronchi or lungs by a fungus, particularly *Candida albicans;* see also *bronchopulmonary candidiasis.*

bron•cho•no•car•di•o•sis (brong″ko-no-kahr″de-o′sis) nocardiosis in the bronchi.

bron•cho•pan•cre•at•ic (brong″ko-pan″kre-at′ik) communicating between a bronchus and the pancreas.

bron•chop•a•thy (brong-kop′ə-the) [*broncho-* + *-pathy*] any disease of a bronchus.

bron•choph•o•ny (brong-kof′ə-ne) [*broncho-* + Gr. *phōnē* voice] 1. the normal voice sounds heard over a healthy large bronchus. 2. abnormal voice sounds heard over the lung, with the voice transmitted unusually clearly and with a high pitch; it is a type of pectoriloquy, indicating solidification of the lung tissue. Called also *bronchiloquy.*

whispered b. see under *pectoriloquy.*

bron•cho•plas•ty (brong′ko-plas″te) [*broncho-* + *-plasty*] plastic surgery of a bronchus. **bronchoplas′tic** *adj*

bron•cho•ple•gia (brong″ko-ple′jə) paralysis of the muscles of the walls of the bronchial tubes.

bron•cho•pleu•ral (brong″ko-ploor′əl) 1. pertaining to a bronchus and the pleura. 2. communicating with a bronchus and the pleural cavity, as a bronchopleural fistula.

bron•cho•pneu•mo•nia (brong″ko-nŏŏ-mo′nyə) [*broncho-* + *pneumonia*] an inflammation of the lungs that begins in the terminal bronchioles, which become clogged with a mucopurulent exudate forming consolidated patches in adjacent lobules. Called also *bronchial* or *lobular pneumonia, capillary bronchitis,* and *bronchopneumonitis.* **bronchopneumon′ic** *adj*

postoperative b. bronchopneumonia following surgical operations, particularly those on the abdomen. It may be due to the inhalation of irritant anesthesia or of infected material from the mouth or nose during the temporary depression of the cough reflex.

bron•cho•pneu•mo•ni•tis (brong″ko-noo″mə-ni′tis) bronchopneumonia.

bron•cho•pneu•mop•a•thy (brong″ko-nŏŏ-mop′ə-the) disease of the bronchi and lung tissue.

bron•cho•prov•o•ca•tion (brong″ko-prov″ə-ka′shən) bronchial challenge.

bron•cho•pul•mo•nary (brong″ko-pool′mə-nar″e) pertaining to the lungs and their air passages; both bronchial and pulmonary.

bron•cho•ra•di•og•ra•phy (brong″ko-ra-de-og′rə-fe) radiographic visualization of the bronchial tree.

bron•chor•rha•gia (brong″ko-ra′jə) [*broncho-* + *-rrhagia*] hemorrhage from the bronchi.

bron•chor•rha•phy (brong-kor′ə-fe) [*broncho-* + *-rrhaphy*] suture of a bronchus.

bron•chor•rhea (brong-ko-re′ə) [*broncho-* + *-rrhea*] excessive discharge of mucus from the bronchi.

bron•cho•scope (brong′ko-skōp) an instrument for inspecting the interior of the tracheobronchial tree and carrying out endobronchial diagnostic and therapeutic maneuvers, such as taking specimens for culture and biopsy and removing foreign bodies.

fiberoptic b. bronchofiberscope.

bron•cho•scop•ic (brong″ko-skop′ik) pertaining to bronchoscopy or to the bronchoscope.

bron•chos•co•py (brong-kos′kə-pe) [*broncho-* + *-scopy*] examination of the bronchi through a bronchoscope.

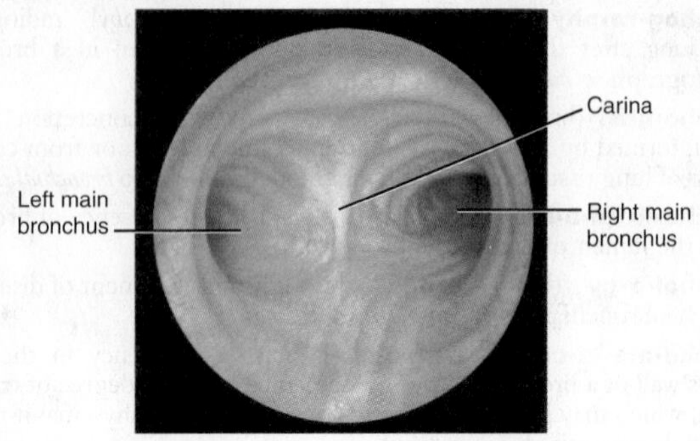

■ Bronchoscopy of the lower end of the trachea and its main branches.

fiberoptic b. bronchofibroscopy.

bron•cho•si•nus•itis (brong″ko-si″nəs-i′tis) coexisting infection of the paranasal sinuses and the lower respiratory passages.

bron•cho•spasm (brong′ko-spaz″əm) spasmodic contraction of the smooth muscle of the bronchi, as occurs in asthma. Called also *bronchial spasm.*

exercise-induced b. exercise-induced asthma.

bron•cho•spi•ro•che•to•sis (brong″ko-spi″ro-ke-to′sis) hemorrhagic bronchitis.

bron•cho•spi•rog•ra•phy (brong″ko-spi-rog′rə-fe) the recording of bronchospirometry results.

bron•cho•spi•rom•e•ter (brong″ko-spi-rom′ə-tər) an instrument used in bronchospirometry.

bron•cho•spi•rom•e•try (brong″ko-spi-rom′ə-tre) determination of the vital capacity, oxygen intake, and carbon dioxide excretion of a single lung, or simultaneous measurements of the function of each lung separately. Called also *bronchoscopic spirometry.*

differential b. measurement of the function of each lung separately.

bron•cho•stax•is (brong″ko-stak′sis) bronchorrhagia.

bron•cho•ste•no•sis (brong″ko-stə-no′sis) [*broncho-* + *stenosis*] narrowing of a bronchial tube by scarring or some other stricture.

bron•chos•to•my (brong-kos′tə-me) [*broncho-* + *-stomy*] the surgical creation of an opening into a bronchus.

bron•cho•tome (brong′ko-tōm) a cutting instrument used in performing bronchotomy.

bron•chot•o•my (brong-kot′ə-me) [*broncho-* + *-tomy*] surgical incision of a bronchus.

bron•cho•tra•che•al (brong″ko-tra′ke-əl) tracheobronchial.

bron•cho•ve•sic•u•lar (brong″ko-vĕ-sik′u-lər) 1. bronchoalveolar. 2. vesiculobronchial.

bron•chus (brong′kəs) pl. *bron′chi* [L., from Gr. *bronchos* windpipe] [TA] any of the larger air passages of the lungs, having an outer fibrous coat with irregularly placed plates of hyaline cartilage, an interlacing network of smooth muscle, and a mucous membrane of columnar ciliated epithelial cells. **bron′chial** *adj*

apical b. apical segmental b.

cardiac b. bronchus segmentalis basalis medialis; see table and illustration.

eparterial b. a name sometimes given to the superior lobar bronchus on the right, which arises above the level of the pulmonary artery; see table and illustration.

hyparterial bronchi a name sometimes given to the middle and inferior lobar bronchi on the right and the lobar bronchi on the left, all of which arise below the level of the pulmonary artery. See table and illustration.

lingular b., inferior bronchus lingularis inferior; see table and illustration.

lingular b., superior bronchus lingularis superior; see table and illustration.

bron′chi loba′res [TA] lobar bronchi: passages arising from the primary bronchi and passing to the lobes of the right and left lungs. There are three right and two left lobar bronchi, which divide into the segmental bronchi. See table and illustration, and see Plate 25.

main b., left b. principalis sinister.

main b., right b. principalis dexter.

primary b., left b. principalis sinister.

primary b., right b. principalis dexter.

b. principa′lis dex′ter [TA] right main bronchus: one of the two main branches into which the trachea divides, itself dividing into the superior, middle, and inferior lobar bronchi of the right lung. Called also *right primary b.*

b. principa′lis sinis′ter [TA] left main bronchus: one of the two main branches into which the trachea divides, itself dividing into the superior and inferior lobar bronchi of the left lung. Called also *left primary b.*

secondary bronchi subdivisions of the primary bronchi; see *bronchi lobares* and *bronchi segmentales.*

segmental bronchi bronchi segmentales.

segmental b., anteromedial basal the bronchus segmentalis basalis anterior and bronchus segmentalis basalis medialis of the left lung considered as a unit. See table and illustration.

segmental b., apical 1. bronchus segmentalis apicalis; see table and illustration. 2. the bronchus segmentalis superior of either the right or left inferior lobe. See table and illustration.

bron′chi segmenta′les [TA] segmental bronchi: air passages arising from the lobar bronchi and passing to the different segments of the two lungs, where they further subdivide into smaller and smaller passages (bronchioles). The segmental bronchi are designated by roman numerals, with the three right lobar bronchi divided into ten segmental bronchi and the two left lobar bronchi into eight or nine, depending on the system of classification. See accompanying table and illustration; see also table at *segmenta bronchopulmonalia* and Plate 25.

stem b. one of the two main bronchi; see *b. principalis dexter* and *b. principalis sinister.*

tracheal b. an ectopic or supernumerary bronchus, extending directly from the trachea to the apical segment of the upper lobe of the right lung, occurring normally in some animals but only as a congenital anomaly in humans.

bron•to•pho•bia (bron″to-fo′be-ə) [Gr. *brontē* thunder + *phobia*] irrational fear of thunder; astraphobia.

Brooke ileostomy (brook) [B.N. *Brooke*, British gastroenterologist, mid-20th century] see under *ileostomy.*

Brooke tumor (epithelioma) (brook) [Henry Ambrose Grundy *Brooke*, English dermatologist, 1854–1919] multiple trichoepithelioma.

Brooke-Spieg•ler syndrome (brook′ spēg′lər) [H.A.G. *Brooke;* Eduard *Spiegler*, Austrian dermatologist, 1860–1908] see under *syndrome.*

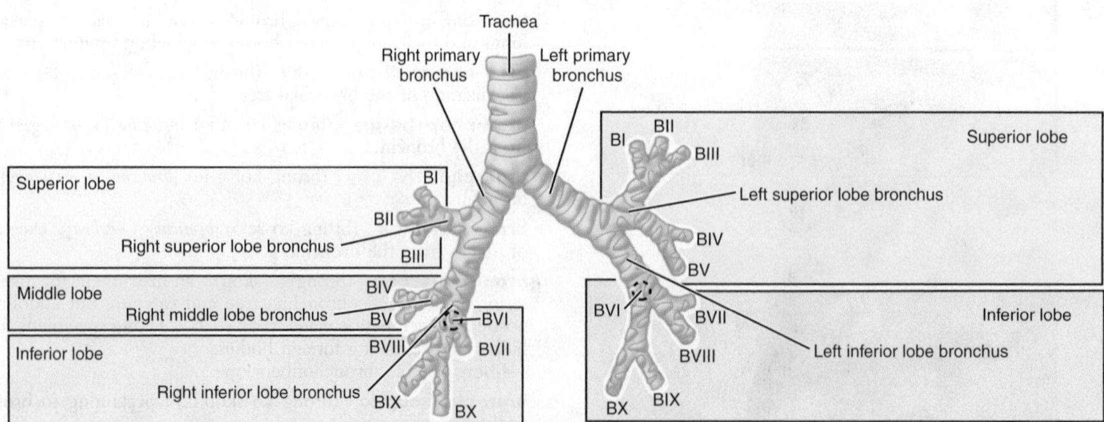

■ Bronchi, showing primary, lobar, and segmental bronchi, which connect to the bronchopulmonary segments (S I–X) of the right and left lungs. For correlation of the bronchopulmonary segments with subdivisions of the lungs, see Plate 27.

Bronchi Segmentales (Segmental Bronchi)

Terminologia Anatomica	Common Name
Bronchus lobaris superior dexter	Right superior lobar bronchus
Bronchus segmentalis apicalis [B I]	Apical segmental bronchus
Bronchus segmentalis posterior [B II]	Posterior segmental bronchus
Bronchus segmentalis anterior [B III]	Anterior segmental bronchus
Bronchus lobaris medius	Middle lobar bronchus
Bronchus segmentalis lateralis [B IV]	Lateral segmental bronchus
Bronchus segmentalis medialis [B V]	Medial segmental bronchus
Bronchus lobaris inferior dexter	Right inferior lobar bronchus
Bronchus segmentalis superior [B VI]	Superior segmental bronchus
Bronchus segmentalis basalis medialis [B VII] [B. cardiacus]*	Medial basal segmental bronchus (Cardiac bronchus)
Bronchus segmentalis basalis anterior [B VIII]	Anterior basal segmental bronchus
Bronchus segmentalis basalis lateralis [B IX]	Lateral basal segmental bronchus
Bronchus segmentalis basalis posterior [B X]	Posterior basal segmental bronchus
Bronchus lobaris superior sinister	Left superior lobar bronchus
Bronchus segmentalis apicoposterior [B I + II]	Apicoposterior segmental bronchus
Bronchus segmentalis anterior [B III]	Anterior segmental bronchus
Bronchus lingularis superior [B IV]	Superior lingular bronchus
Bronchus lingularis inferior [B V]	Inferior lingular bronchus
Bronchus lobaris inferior sinister	Left inferior lobar bronchus
Bronchus segmentalis superior [B VI]	Superior segmental bronchus
Bronchus segmentalis basalis medialis [B VII] [B. cardiacus]*	Medial basal segmental bronchus (Cardiac bronchus)
Bronchus segmentalis basalis anterior [B VIII]	Anterior basal segmental bronchus
Bronchus segmentalis basalis lateralis [B IX]	Lateral basal segmental bronchus
Bronchus segmentalis basalis posterior [B X]	Posterior basal segmental bronchus

*TA alternative.

broom (broom) any of various shrubs with long slender branches, such as *Cytisus scoparius*; see also *broom poisoning*, under *poisoning*.

butcher's b. (booch'ərz) 1. *Ruscus aculeatus*. 2. preparations of the rhizome *R. aculeatus*, used for symptomatic treatment of hemorrhoids and venous insufficiency.

brosse (bros) [Fr. *brush*] a brushlike organelle of cilia seen on the anterodorsal surface of certain ciliate protozoa, such as those of the suborder Prorodontina; its function is unknown.

broth (broth) 1. a thin soup prepared by boiling meat or vegetables. 2. a liquid culture medium for the cultivation of microorganisms; see under *culture medium* for specific broths.

Bro·vi·ac catheter (bro've-ak) [J.W. *Broviac*, American surgeon, 20th century] see under *catheter*.

brow (brou) forehead.

brown (broun) 1. a dusky, reddish yellow color. 2. a dye or stain with this color.

aniline b. Bismarck b. Y.

Bismarck b. R a dark brown solid, synthetically prepared, used as a leather and textile dye and as a biological stain.

Bismarck b. Y, Manchester b., phenylene b. a blackish brown powder, synthetically prepared, used as a textile dye and as a stain for demonstrating mucus in intestinal goblet cells and cartilage in the trachea and in embryonic tissue.

Brown-Ad·son forceps (broun' ad'sən) [James Barrett *Brown*, American plastic surgeon, 1899–1971; Alfred Washington *Adson*, American neurosurgeon, 1887–1951] see *Adson-Brown forceps*, under *forceps*.

Brown-Ro·berts-Wells apparatus, technique (broun' rob'ərts welz') [R.A. *Brown*, American neurosurgeon, 20th century; T.S. *Roberts*, American neurosurgeon, 20th century; T.H. *Wells*, Jr., American neurosurgeon, 20th century] see under *apparatus* and *technique*.

Brown-Sé·quard syndrome (broon'-sa-kahr') [Charles Edouard *Brown-Séquard*, French physiologist, 1817–1894] see under *syndrome*.

Brown-Sym·mers disease (broun' sim'ərz) [Charles Leonard *Brown*, American physician, 1899–1959; Douglas *Symmers*, American physician, 1879–1952] see under *disease*.

Brown-Vi·a·let·to-van Laere syndrome (broun' ve-ah-lĕ'to vahn lĕr') [C.H. *Brown*, American physician, late 19th century; E. *Vialetto*, Italian physician, 20th century; J. *van Laere*, Belgian physician, 20th century] see under *syndrome*.

Browne operation (broun) [Sir Denis John *Browne*, Australian-born pediatric surgeon in the United Kingdom, 1892–1967] see under *operation*.

brown·i·an (broun'e-ən) named for Robert *Brown*, English botanist, 1773–1858.

Brown·ing vein (broun'ing) [William *Browning*, American anatomist, 1855–1941] vena anastomotica inferior.

BRS British Roentgen Society.

Bruce tract (broos) [Alexander *Bruce*, Scottish anatomist, 1854–1911] fasciculus septomarginalis.

Bru·cea (broo'se-ə) a genus of evergreen shrubs of the family Simaroubaceae, found from Southeast Asia to Australia. *B. sumatra'na* Roxb. is the medicinal plant called *kosam*.

Bru·cel·la (broo-sel'ə) [Sir David *Bruce*, English physician, 1855–1931] a genus of gram-negative, aerobic coccobacilli of the family Brucellaceae, made up of nonmotile cells that require biotin, niacin, thiamine, and sometimes serum for growth; they are animal parasites and pathogens, causing brucellosis, and are transmissible to humans through contact with infected tissue or dairy products.

B. abor'tus the most common cause of brucellosis in humans; it causes infectious abortion in cattle, which are the animal reservoir of infection; called also *Bang bacillus*.

B. ca'nis a species that causes canine brucellosis in dogs and a respiratory tract infection in humans.

B. meliten'sis a species found in healthy and diseased goats and sheep and causing brucellosis in humans.

B. o'vis a species pathogenic for sheep, causing epididymitis in rams; not known to cause disease in humans.

B. su'is a species found primarily in pigs but also in rabbits and reindeer; it is highly pathogenic for humans, causing brucellosis.

bru·cel·la (broo-sel'ə) an individual organism of the genus *Brucella*. brucel'lar *adj*

Bru·cel·la·ceae (broo"sə-la'se-e) a family bacteria of the order Rhizobiales, grouped together on the basis of 16S rRNA sequence analysis and consisting of gram-negative, aerobic cocci and rod-shaped bacteria. Medically important organisms are included in the genera *Brucella* and *Ochrobactrum*.

bru·cel·lin (broo-sel'in) a preparation of antigenic material from several species of *Brucella*, used in the diagnosis of brucellosis.

bru·cel·lo·sis (broo"sə-lo'sis) infection caused by species of *Brucella*. In the natural animal reservoirs such as cattle, sheep, goats, pigs, deer, and rabbits, it may cause infertility or abortion. In humans coming in contact with such animals or their infected products or tissue, it is a generalized infection involving primarily the reticuloendothelial system, characterized by fever, sweating, weakness, malaise, and weight loss. Called also *Malta fever*, *Mediterranean fever*, and *undulant fever*.

canine b. infection of dogs by *Brucella canis*, characterized by lymphadenitis, splenitis, and infertility; fetal death or abortion in pregnant females; and epididymitis, scrotal dermatitis, and testicular atrophy in males.

Bruch glands, layer (membrane) (brook) [Karl Wilhelm Ludwig *Bruch*, German anatomist, 1819–1884] see under *gland*, and see *lamina basalis choroideae*.

bru•cine (broo′sēn) [from *Brucea*, a genus of shrubs named for J. *Bruce*, Scottish explorer, 1730–1794] a poisonous alkaloid, from *Strychnos ignatii* and *S. nux-vomica*, which resembles strychnine in its action, but is less poisonous. One of the principal constituents of nux vomica and ignatia, it was formerly used in the same manner as strychnine (q.v.).

Bruck disease (brook) [Alfred *Bruck*, German physician, late 19th century] see under *disease*.

Brü•cke lines, muscle (bre′kə) [Ernst Wilhelm von *Brücke*, Austrian physiologist, 1819–1892] see under *line* and *muscle*.

Bru•dzin•ski sign (reflex) (broo-jin′ske) [Józef *Brudzinski*, Polish physician, 1874–1917] see under *sign*.

Brue•ghel syndrome (broi′gəl) [Pieter *Brueghel* the Elder, Flemish painter, 1525–1569, whose painting *De Gaper* shows a person with this syndrome] Meige syndrome (def. 2).

Bru•ga•da syndrome (broo-gah′thah) [Josep *Brugada* and Pedro *Brugada*, Spanish cardiologists, late 20th century] see under *syndrome*.

Brug•ia (broo′je-ə) [S.L. *Brug*, Dutch parasitologist in Indonesia, early 20th century] a genus of parasitic filarial worms of the superfamily Filarioidea.

B. ma′layi a species causing filariasis and elephantiasis from eastern India through Southeast Asia to the China Sea area; it is similar to, and often found in association with, *Wuchereria bancrofti*. Called also *Wuchereria malayi*.

B. pahan′gi a species found in many species of mammals, including humans, in Malaysia; it may produce the symptoms of tropical eosinophilia.

B. ti′mori a species causing filariasis and elephantiasis in Timor and nearby Indonesian islands.

brug•i•an (brooj′e-ən) named for S.L. *Brug*; characterized by species of *Brugia*.

bruise (bro͞oz) 1. contusion. 2. to cause or develop a contusion.

stone b. a painful bruise, especially of the bare feet of children.

bruisse•ment (brwēs-maw′) [Fr.] a purring tremor; see under *tremor*.

bruit (brwe, bro͞ot) [Fr.] sound (def. 3).

aneurysmal b. a blowing sound heard over an aneurysm.

b. de canon (də kah-naw′) ["sound of cannon"] an abnormally loud first heart sound, heard intermittently in complete heart block when atrial contraction just precedes ventricular contraction.

b. de clapotement (də klah-pōt-maw′) ["sound of rippling"] a splashing sound indicative of dilatation of the stomach when pressure is put on the wall of the abdomen.

b. de claquement (də klahk-maw′) ["sound of clapping"] a snapping sound caused by the sudden contact of parts.

b. de craquement (də krak-maw′) ["a sound of crackling"] a crackling pericardial or pleural bruit.

b. de cuir neuf (də kwĕr′ noof′) ["sound of new leather"] a creaking noise; usually a sign of pericarditis or pleurisy.

b. de diable (də dyahbl′) ["sound of humming top"] venous hum.

false b. a bruit due to pressure by the stethoscope, or derived from the circulation in the ear of the auscultator.

b. de froissement (də frwahs-maw′) ["sound of clashing"] a clashing noise of varying origin.

b. de frolement (də frōl-maw′) ["sound of rustling"] a rustling murmur from a pericardial or pleural friction rub.

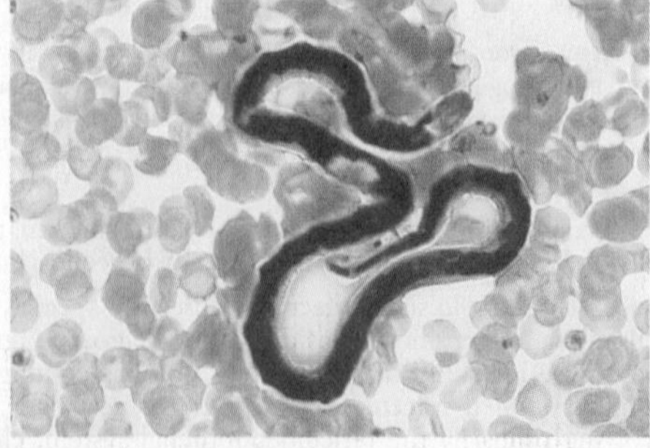

■ Sheathed microfilaria of *Brugia malayi*, showing two solitary cell nuclei in the tail tip (Giemsa stain).

b. de galop (də gah-lop′) ["sound of galloping"] gallop rhythm.

b. de lime (də lēm′) ["sound of a file"] a cardiac sound resembling filing.

b. de moulin (də moo-lă′) ["sound of a mill"] a splashing or water-wheel sound synchronous with systole, sometimes audible at some distance from the patient, variously attributed to cardiac, pericardiac, or mediastinal causes.

b. de parchemin (də parsh-mă′) ["sound of parchment"] a sound as of two pieces of parchment rubbed together, of valvular cardiac origin.

b. de piaulement (də pyōl-maw′) ["sound of whining"] a cardiac murmur like the mewing of a cat.

b. de pot fêlé (də po′ fĕ-la′) cracked-pot resonance.

b. de rape (də rahp′) ["sound of a grater"] a rasping cardiac valvular murmur.

b. de rappel (də rah-pel′) ["sound of a drum beating to arms"] a double sound as of two beats of a drum, describing splitting of the second heart sound or a second sound followed by an opening snap.

Roger b., b. de Roger (də ro-zha′) a loud long systolic murmur heard in the third interspace to the left of the sternum, characteristic of a small ventricular septal defect. Called also *Roger murmur*.

b. de scie (də se′) ["sound of a saw"] a cardiac murmur resembling the sound of a saw.

b. de soufflet (də soo-fla′) ["sound of a bellows"] see *souffle*.

systolic b. see under *murmur*.

b. de tabourka (də tah-bo͞or′kah) ["sound of drum"] timbre métallique.

b. de tambour (də tahm-bo͞or′) ["sound of drum"] a ringing sound heard in syphilitic aortic regurgitation.

Verstraeten b. an abnormal sound heard in auscultation over the lower border of the liver in cachectic patients.

Bru•na•ti sign (broo-nah′te) [M. *Brunati*, Italian physician, 20th century] see under *sign*.

bru•nes•cent (broo-nes′ənt) [A.S. *brūn* brown] brown; becoming brown.

Brunn membrane, epithelial nests (broon) [Albert von *Brunn*, German anatomist, 1849–1895] see under *membrane* and *nest*.

Brun•ner glands (broon′ər) [Johann Conrad *Brunner*, Swiss anatomist, 1653–1727] glandulae duodenales.

Brunn•strom method (brun′strəm) [Signe *Brunnstrom*, American physical therapist, 20th century] see under *method*.

Bruns apraxia (frontal ataxia), syndrome (sign) (broonz) [Ludwig *Bruns*, German neurologist, 1858–1916] see *gait apraxia*, under *apraxia*, and see under *syndrome*.

Bruns-Gar•land syndrome (broonz gahr′lənd) [L. *Bruns*; Hugh Gregory *Garland*, English neurologist, 1903–1967] see *diabetic amyotrophy*, under *amyotrophy*.

Brun•schwig operation (broon′shwig) [Alexander *Brunschwig*, American surgeon, 1901–1969] 1. pancreatoduodenectomy. 2. see under *operation*.

Brun•sting syndrome (brun′sting) [Louis A. *Brunsting*, Sr., American dermatologist, 1900–1980] see under *syndrome*.

Brun•sting-Per•ry syndrome (pemphigoid) (brun′sting per′e) [L.A. *Brunsting*, Sr.; H.O. *Perry*, American dermatologist, 20th century] see under *syndrome*.

brush (brush) tufts of bristles, hair, or other flexible materials set into a handle.

Haidinger b. two conical brushlike images with apexes touching, seen on looking through a Nicol prism; used in determining visual function.

Ruffini b. see under *ending*.

Brush•field spots (brush′fēld) [Thomas *Brushfield*, English physician, 1858–1937] see under *spot*.

Brush•field-Wy•att syndrome (brush′fēld wi′ət) [T. *Brushfield*; W. *Wyatt*, British physician, 20th century] see under *syndrome*.

brush•ite (brush′īt) a nearly colorless type of dibasic calcium phosphate, found in rock phosphates and sometimes as a component of human dental calculus or renal calculi.

Bru•ton agammaglobulinemia (disease), tyrosine kinase (broo′tən) [Col. Ogden Carr *Bruton*, American pediatrician, 1908–2003] see *X-linked agammaglobulinemia*, under *agammaglobulinemia*, and see *Bruton tyrosine kinase*.

Bru•ton ty•ro•sine ki•nase (BTK) (broo′tən ti′ro-sēn ki′nās) a nonreceptor tyrosine kinase (non-specific protein-tyrosine kinase, q.v.) that plays an important role in signaling in B-cell activation and differentiation; mutation has been linked to X-linked agammaglobulinemia.

brux (bruks) to grind the teeth rhythmically or spasmodically; cf. *bruxism*.

brux•ism (bruk′siz-əm) [Gr. *brychein* to gnash the teeth] involuntary, nonfunctional, rhythmic or spasmodic gnashing, grinding, and clenching of teeth (not including chewing movements of the mandible), usually during sleep, sometimes leading to occlusal trauma. Causes may be related to repressed aggression, emotional tension, anger, fear, and frustration. See also *bruxomania* and *clenching*.

centric b. bruxism characterized by clenching in centric occlusion. Called also *clamping habit* and *clenching habit*.

bruxo•ma•nia (bruk″so-ma′ne-ə) [Gr. *brychein* + *mania*] bruxism occurring in the daytime, usually performed unconsciously.

Bry•ant line, sign, traction, triangle (bri′ənt) [Sir Thomas *Bryant*, English surgeon, 1828–1914] see under *line*, *sign*, and *traction* and see *iliofemoral triangle* under *triangle*.

Bry•o•bia (bri-o′be-ə) a genus of mites of the family Tetranychidae. *B. praetio′sa* is the clover mite or spinning mite, a species found on clover and sometimes causing irritating dermatitis.

Bry•o•nia (bri-o′ne-ə) a genus of plants of the family Cucurbitaceae, all called *bryony*. They contain toxic glycosides including bryonidin, bryonin, and others, which cause diarrhea and sometimes convulsions. They were formerly used medicinally as strong cathartics.

bry•o•nia (bri-o′ne-ə) [L., from Gr. *bryōnia*] the air-dried root of *Bryonia alba* or related species, which was formerly used as a strong cathartic.

bry•o•ni•din (bri-o′nĭ-din) a toxic glycoside found in species of *Bryonia*, partially responsible for their cathartic effects.

bry•o•nin (bri′o-nin) a toxic glycoside found in species of *Bryonia*, partially responsible for their cathartic effects.

BS Bachelor of Surgery; Bachelor of Science; breath sounds; blood sugar.

BSA body surface area.

B-scan see under *scan*.

BSF B lymphocyte stimulatory factor.

BSS Bernard-Soulier syndrome.

BTK Bruton tyrosine kinase.

BTU British thermal unit.

bu•bo (bu′bo) [L., from Gr. *boubōn* groin] a tender, enlarged, and inflamed lymph node, particularly in the axilla or groin, due to such infections as plague, syphilis, gonorrhea, chancroid, lymphogranuloma venereum, and tuberculosis. **bubon′ic** *adj*

chancroidal b. a suppurating form accompanying or following chancroid.

climatic b. lymphogranuloma venereum.

inguinal b. a bubo in the groin area, commonly seen in bubonic plague, lymphogranuloma venereum, primary syphilis, and other conditions.

malignant b. the bubo of bubonic plague.

primary b. a bubo due to venereal exposure but not preceded by any visible lesion.

syphilitic b. nontender, nonfluctuant, firm regional lymphadenitis that follows the chancre of syphilis.

tropical b. lymphogranuloma venereum.

bu•bono•cele (bu-bon′o-sēl) indirect inguinal hernia.

bu•bon•u•lus (bu-bon′u-ləs) [L. "a small bubo"] a nodule or abscess along a lymphatic vessel, especially one on the dorsum of the penis.

buc•ca (buk′ə) [L.] [TA] cheek: the fleshy portion of the side of the face, constituting the lateral wall of the oral cavity. Called also *mala*.

buc•cal (buk′əl) [L. *buccalis*, from *bucca* cheek] pertaining to or directed toward the cheek. In dental anatomy, used to refer to the buccal surface of a tooth; see *buccal surface*, under *surface*. Cf. *labial*.

buc•cal•ly (buk′ə-le) toward the cheek.

buc•ci•na•tor (buk′sĭ-na″tər) [L. "trumpeter"] see under *musculus*.

bucc(o)- [L. *bucca* cheek] a combining form denoting relationship to the cheek.

buc•co•ax•i•al (buk″o-ak′se-əl) pertaining to or formed by the buccal and axial walls of a tooth cavity preparation.

buc•co•ax•io•cer•vi•cal (buk″o-ak″se-o-sur′vĭ-kəl) buccoaxiogingival.

buc•co•ax•io•gin•gi•val (buk″o-ak″se-o-jin′jĭ-vəl) pertaining to or formed by the buccal, axial, and gingival walls of a tooth cavity; called also *buccoaxiocervical*.

buc•co•cer•vi•cal (buk″o-sur′vi-kəl) 1. pertaining to the cheek and neck. 2. pertaining to the buccal surface of the neck of a posterior tooth. 3. buccogingival.

buc•co•clu•sal (buk″o-kloo′zəl) 1. pertaining to buccoclusion. 2. bucco-occlusal.

buc•co•clu•sion (buk″o-kloo′zhən) [*bucco-* + L. *cludere* to close] malocclusion in which the dental arch or a quadrant or group of teeth is buccal to the normal.

buc•co•dis•tal (buk″o-dis′təl) distobuccal.

buc•co•gin•gi•val (buk″o-jin′jĭ-vəl) 1. pertaining to the cheek and gingiva. 2. pertaining to or formed by the buccal and gingival walls of a tooth cavity preparation.

buc•co•glos•so•phar•yn•gi•tis (buk″o-glos′o-far″in-ji′tis) inflammation involving the cheek, tongue, and pharynx.

b. sic′ca inflammation and dryness of the buccal mucosa, tongue, and pharynx. Cf. *Sjögren syndrome*, under *syndrome*.

buc•co•la•bi•al (buk″o-la′be-əl) pertaining to the cheek and lip.

buc•co•lin•gual (buk″o-ling′gwəl) 1. pertaining to the cheek and tongue. 2. pertaining to the buccal and lingual surfaces of a posterior tooth.

buc•co•lin•gual•ly (buk″o-ling′gwə-le) from the cheek toward the tongue.

buc•co•max•il•lary (buk″o-mak′sĭ-lar″e) 1. pertaining to the cheek and maxilla. 2. communicating between the buccal cavity and the maxillary sinus.

buc•co•me•si•al (buk″o-me′ze-əl) pertaining to or formed by the buccal and mesial surfaces of a tooth, or the buccal and mesial walls of a tooth cavity.

buc•co-oc•clu•sal (buk″o-ə-kloo′zəl) pertaining to or formed by the buccal and occlusal surfaces of a tooth.

buc•co•pha•ryn•ge•al (buk″o-fə-rin′je-əl) pertaining to the mouth and pharynx.

buc•co•place•ment (buk′o-plās″ment) displacement of a tooth toward the cheek.

buc•co•pul•pal (buk″o-pul′pəl) pertaining to or formed by the buccal and pulpal walls of a tooth cavity.

buc•cos•to•my (buk-os′tə-me) an old method of treating cribbing in horses, consisting of the surgical creation of permanent buccal fistulae.

buc•co•ver•sion (buk″o-vur′zhən) the position of a tooth which lies buccally to the line of occlusion.

Bu•ceph•a•lus (bu-sef′ə-ləs) a genus of trematodes. *B. papillo′sus* is parasitic in the stomach and intestines of freshwater fish.

Buck extension, fascia, operation (buk) [Gurdon *Buck*, American surgeon, 1807–1877] see under *extension*, *fascia*, and *operation*.

buck•eye (buk′i) *Aesculus glabra* or any of several other plants of the same genus, whose fruit and seeds are toxic to livestock.

Buck•ley's syndrome (buk′le) [Rebecca H. *Buckley*, American physician, born 1933] hyperimmunoglobulinemia E syndrome.

buck•ling (buk′ling) the process or an instance of becoming crumpled or warped.

scleral b. a technique for repair of detachment of the retina, in which indentations or infoldings of the sclera are made over the tears in the retina so as to promote adherence of the retina to the choroid.

buck•thorn (buk′thorn) 1. any of various trees and shrubs of the genus *Rhamnus*. 2. *Karwinskia humboldtiana*. See also under *poisoning*.

alder b. *Rhamnus frangula*.

cascara b. *Rhamnus purshiana*.

common b. *Rhamnus cathartica*.

buck•wheat (buk′hwēt) *Fagopyrum esculentum*. See also *fagopyrism*.

bu•cli•zine hy•dro•chlo•ride (bu′klĭ-zēn) an antihistamine, used mainly as an antinauseant in the management of motion sickness; administered orally.

bu•cry•late (bu′krə-lāt) a compound, isobutyl 2-cyanoacrylate, used as a tissue adhesive.

bud (bud) 1. a structure on a plant, often round, that encloses an undeveloped flower or leaf. 2. any small part of the embryo or adult metazoon more or less resembling such a plant structure and presumed to have potential for growth and differentiation.

bronchial b. see *primary*, *secondary*, and *tertiary bronchial b's*.

end b. caudal eminence.

farcy b's small tubercular nodules on the skin seen in some cases of farcy.

gustatory b. caliculus gustatorius.

limb b. an ectodermally-covered mesenchymal swelling on the trunk of the embryo that becomes a limb.

liver b. hepatic diverticulum.

lobar b's secondary bronchial buds.

lung b. respiratory diverticulum.

metanephric b. ureteric b.

pancreatic b's two outgrowths, one dorsal and one ventral, from the endodermal lining of the caudal part of the embryonic foregut; they fuse and develop into the pancreas.

periosteal b. vascular connective tissue from the periosteum growing through apertures in the periosteal bone collar into the cartilaginous matrix of the primary center of ossification.

pineal b. in embryonic development, the median diverticulum from the caudal part of the roof of the diencephalon, which gives rise to the pineal gland.

primary bronchial b's two outgrowths from the respiratory diverticulum, which ultimately become the right and left primary bronchi and also give rise to the secondary bronchial buds.

secondary bronchial b's outgrowths of the primary bronchial buds, three on the right side and two on the left, which give rise to the lobes of the lungs and further branch to form the tertiary bronchial buds.

segmental b's tertiary bronchial buds.

tail b. 1. in animals having a tail, the primordium that forms it. 2. caudal eminence.

taste b. caliculus gustatorius.

tertiary bronchial b's outgrowths of the secondary bronchial buds which become the bronchopulmonary segments of the mature lung.

tongue b., distal lateral lingual swelling.

tongue b., median tuberculum impar.

tooth b. a knoblike tooth primordium developing into an enamel organ surrounded by a dental sac and encasing the dental papilla. See also *tooth germ*, under *germ*.

tracheal b. an intermediate stage between the respiratory diverticulum and the bronchial buds.

ureteric b. an outgrowth of the mesonephric duct that gives rise to all of the permanent kidney except the nephrons. Called also *metanephric b.* or *diverticulum*.

vascular b. an outgrowth of an existing vessel from which a new blood vessel arises.

wing b. a swelling on the trunk of an avian embryo that gives rise to a wing.

Budd-Chi•a•ri syndrome (disease) (bud′ ke-ah′re) [George *Budd*, English physician, 1808–1882; Hans *Chiari*, Austrian pathologist, 1851–1916] see under *syndrome*.

bud•ding (bud′ing) 1. a form of asexual reproduction in which a portion of the organism's body is thrust out and then becomes separated, forming a new individual. The larger part is considered the parent and the smaller one the bud. Called also *gemmation*. 2. the process by which a new blood vessel arises from a preexisting vessel. 3. a method of release of virus from a cell after replication has taken place. Viral protein associates itself with an area of cell membrane, which forms a coat or envelope around the virus; the enveloped virus then is released by pinching off.

bu•des•o•nide (bu-des′ə-nīd) an antiinflammatory glucocorticoid used by inhalation to treat asthma, intranasally to treat allergic rhinitis and other inflammatory nasal conditions, rectally to treat ulcerative colitis, and orally to treat Crohn disease.

Bud•ge center (bood′gē) [Julius Ludwig *Budge*, German physiologist, 1811–1888] 1. the ciliospinal center. 2. the genital center.

bud•ger•i•gar (buj′ər-ĭ-gahr″) [Australian aboriginal *gijirrigaa*] a species of parakeet, *Melopsittacus undulatus*, native to Australia, popular as a cage pet and used for experimental work in psittacosis. Called also *budgie*.

bud•gie (buj′e) budgerigar.

Bu•din joint, rule (boo-dă′) [Pierre-Constant *Budin*, French gynecologist, 1846–1907] see under *joint* and *rule*.

BUDR, BUdR 5-bromodeoxyuridine.

Buer•ger disease, symptom (bur′gər) [Leo *Buerger*, American physician, 1879–1943] see *thromboangiitis obliterans* and under *symptom*.

Buer•gi's theory (būr′gēz) [Emil *Buergi*, Swiss pharmacologist, 1872–1947] see under *theory*.

buf•fa•lo•pox (buf′ə-lo-poks) a disease resembling cowpox, seen in water buffaloes and humans having contact with infected animals, occurring in India and other nearby countries; the cause is a virus of the genus *Orthopoxvirus*.

buf•fer (buf′ər) 1. a chemical system that prevents change in the concentration of another chemical substance, e.g., proton donor and acceptor systems that prevent marked changes in hydrogen ion concentration (pH). 2. a physical or physiological system that tends to maintain constancy, e.g., reflexes regulating blood pressure.

bicarbonate b. a buffer system composed of bicarbonate ions and dissolved carbon dioxide. In the body, this system is an important factor in determining the pH of the blood; the concentration of bicarbonate ions is regulated by the kidneys and of carbon dioxide by the respiratory system.

cacodylate b. a buffer containing an organic arsenical salt, used in preparing fixatives for electron microscopy.

phosphate b. a buffer system composed of acid phosphate and sodium or potassium salts, e.g., monosodium and disodium acid phosphate; in the body, it is important in regulating the pH of the renal tubular fluids.

protein b. a buffer system involving proton donor and proton acceptor groups of the amino acid residues of proteins.

TRIS b. a buffer made using tromethamine; suitable for use from pH 7 to 9.

veronal b. a barbital buffer commonly used in the preparation of fixatives for electron microscopy.

buf•fer•ing (buf′ər-ing) the action produced by a buffer.

secondary b. chloride shift.

buf•fy (buf′e) the color of buff; light yellowish pink to yellow, including orange-yellow to yellow-brown.

bu•fil•con A (bu-fil′kon) a contact lens material (hydrophobic).

Bu•fo (bu′fo) [L. "toad"] a genus of toads, species of which have been extensively studied by population geneticists. Several species have alkaloids in their skins or secretions; see *bufotoxin*. *B. bu′fo bu′fo* contains bufotenin; *B. mari′nus* contains the cardiac poison marinobufagin; *B. val′liceps* contains the cardiac poison vallicepobufagin; and *B. vulga′ris* contains the toxin bufotalin.

bu•fo•tal•in (bu″fo-tal′in) a poisonous principle, $C_{26}H_{36}O_6$, present in the skin and saliva of the common European toad, *Bufo vulgaris*.

bu•fo•tox•in (bu′fo-tok″sin) any toxin derived from the skin of toads, such as bufotalin, bufotenin, marinobufagin, or vallicepobufagin.

bug (bug) 1. an insect of the order Hemiptera. 2. any of various other arthropods.

assassin b. 1. cone-nose b. (def. 1). 2. any of various other reduviids that have poisonous bites.

barley b. *Acarus hordei*.

blister b. *Lytta vesicatoria*.

blue b. *Argas persicus*.

cone-nose b. 1. any member of genus *Triatoma;* called also *triatome* and *triatomid*. 2. any of various other insects resembling this genus.

Croton b. German cockroach.

great black b. *Triatoma infestans*.

harvest b. chigger.

hematophagous b. a bug that lives on blood, such as the bedbug.

kissing b. 1. cone-nose b. (def. 1). 2. any of various other reduviid species that bite humans around the mouth.

Malay b. see *Reduviidae*.

miana b., Mianeh b. *Argas persicus*.

red b. chigger.

wheat b. *Pyemotes*.

Buhl disease (bo͞ol) [Ludwig von *Buhl*, German pathologist, 1816–1880] see under *disease*.

bu•iat•rics (bu″e-at′riks) [Gr. *bous* ox, cow + *-iatrics*] the treatment of diseases of cattle.

bulb (bulb) [L. *bulbus;* Gr. *bolbos*] a rounded mass, or enlargement. See also *bulbus*.

b. of aorta bulbus aortae.

duodenal b. ampulla duodeni.

end b. encapsulated nerve ending.

b. of eye bulbus oculi.

hair b., b. of hair bulbus pili.

b. of heart bulbus cordis.

b. of jugular vein, inferior bulbus inferior venae jugularis.

b. of jugular vein, superior bulbus superior venae jugularis.

b. of Krause Krause end-bulb.

b. of occipital horn of lateral ventricle bulbus cornus posterioris ventriculi lateralis.

olfactory b. bulbus olfactorius.

onion b. in neuropathology, a collection of overlapping Schwann cells resembling the bulb of an onion, encircling an axon that has become demyelinated; seen in progressive hypertrophic neuropathy and similar conditions that are characterized by repeated demyelination and remyelination.

b. of ovary a bulb formed by the interweaving of veins with the bundles of involuntary muscle within the mesovarium; called also *Rouget b.*

b. of penis bulbus penis.

b. of posterior horn of lateral ventricle bulbus cornus posterioris ventriculi lateralis.

b. of rhombencephalon myelencephalon; see *medulla oblongata*.

Rouget b. b. of ovary.

sinovaginal b. one of the pair of endodermal outgrowths of the urogenital sinus, which later fuse to form the lower part of the vagina.

terminal b. of Krause Krause end-bulb.

vaginal b. sinovaginal b.

b. of vestibule of vagina, vestibulovaginal b. bulbus vestibuli vaginae.

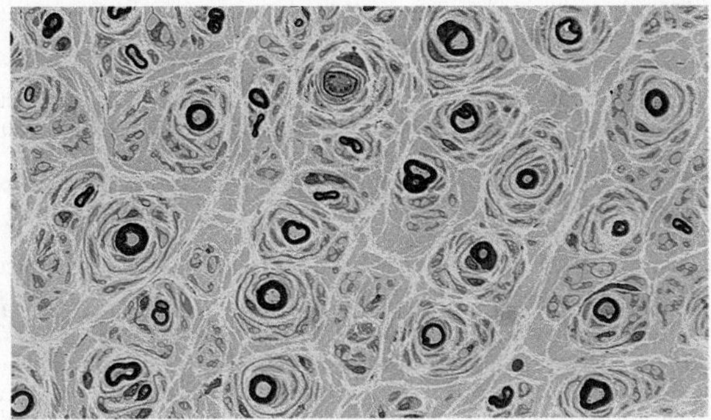

■ Onion bulbs in a cross-section of a sural nerve in a form of Charcot-Marie-Tooth disease.

bul·bar (bul′bər) 1. pertaining to a bulb; called also *bulbous*. 2. pertaining to or involving the medulla oblongata.

bul·bi (bul′bi) [L.] genitive and plural of *bulbus*.

bul·bi·form (bul′bĭ-form) bulb-shaped.

bul·bi·tis (bul-bi′tis) inflammation of the bulb of the penis.

bulb(o)- [L. *bulbus* bulb] a combining form denoting relationship to a bulb or bulbus.

bul·bo·atri·al (bul″bo-a′tre-əl) pertaining to the bulbus cordis and atrium of the heart of an embryo.

bul·bo·cap·nine (bul″bo-kap′nin) an alkaloid derived from various species of *Corydalis* and *Dicentra*, which inhibits the reflex and motor activities of striated muscle. It has been used in the treatment of muscular tremors and vestibular nystagmus. Ruminants eating such plants suffer neurotoxic effects with agitation, convulsions, and sometimes death.

bul·bo·cav·er·no·sus (bul″bo-kav″ər-no′səs) musculus bulbospongiosus.

bul·bo·cav·er·nous (bul″bo-kav′ər-nəs) pertaining to the bulb of the penis or to the bulbocavernous muscle.

bul·bo·gas·trone (bul″bo-gas′trōn) a polypeptide secreted by the duodenal bulb when the bulb is acidified; it inhibits gastric acid secretion in dogs.

bul·boid (bul′boid) shaped like a bulb; called also *bulbiform*.

bul·bo·pon·tine (bul″bo-pon′tīn) pertaining to the pons and the region of the medulla oblongata situated caudad to it.

bul·bo·spi·nal (bul″bo-spi′nəl) 1. spinobulbar (def. 1). 2. extending from the medulla oblongata to the spinal cord.

bul·bo·spi·ral (bul″bo-spi′rəl) pertaining to the root of the aorta (bulbus aortae) and having a spiral course; said of certain bundles of cardiac muscle fibers. See also under *fiber*.

bul·bo·spon·gi·o·sus (bul″bo-spon″je-o′səs) see under *musculus*.

bul·bo·ure·thral (bul″bo-u-re′thrəl) pertaining to the bulb of the penis.

bul·bous (bul′bəs) 1. bulbar. 2. bulboid. 3. bearing or arising from a bulb.

bul·bus (bul′bəs) gen. and pl. *bul′bi* [L.] bulb: a rounded mass or enlargement.

b. aor′tae [TA] bulb of aorta: the enlargement of the aorta at its point of origin from the heart, where the bulges of the aortic sinuses occur.

b. arterio′sus b. cordis.

b. cor′dis the foremost of the three parts of the primordial heart of the embryo; called also *bulb of heart* and *b. arteriosus*.

b. cor′nus occipita′lis ventri′culi latera′lis, b. cor′nus posterio′ris ventri′culi latera′lis [TA] bulb of occipital horn of lateral ventricle: an eminence in the upper part of the medial wall of the occipital horn of the lateral ventricle, above the calcar avis, produced by the splenial fibers of the forceps frontalis as they pass posteriorly into the occipital lobe; called also *bulb of posterior horn of lateral ventricle*.

b. duode′ni TA alternative for *ampulla duodeni*.

b. infe′rior ve′nae jugula′ris [TA] inferior bulb of jugular vein: a dilatation of the internal jugular vein just before it joins the brachiocephalic vein.

b. o′culi [TA] the eyeball or bulb of the eye; see Plate 15. Called also *globe*.

b. olfacto′rius [TA] olfactory bulb: the bulblike expansion of the olfactory tract on the undersurface of the frontal lobe of each cerebral hemisphere; the olfactory nerves enter it.

b. pe′nis [TA] bulb of penis: the enlarged proximal part of the corpus spongiosum found between the two crura of the penis.

b. pi′li hair bulb: the bulbous expansion at the proximal end of a hair, in which the hair shaft is generated. Called also *bulb of hair*.

b. rhombence′phali TA alternative for *myelencephalon;* see *medulla oblongata*.

b. supe′rior ve′nae jugula′ris [TA] superior bulb of jugular vein: a dilatation at the beginning of the internal jugular vein; called also *Heister diverticulum*.

b. vesti′buli vagi′nae [TA] bulb of vestibule of vagina: a body consisting of paired elongated masses of erectile tissue, one on either side of the vaginal opening, united anteriorly by a narrow median band, which then expands slightly to form the glans clitoridis.

bu·le·sis (bu-le′sis) [Gr. *boulēsis*] the will, or an act of the will.

bu·lim·ia (boo-le′me-ə) [L., from Gr. *bous* ox + *limos* hunger] episodic binge eating usually followed by behavior designed to negate the excessive caloric intake, most commonly purging behaviors such as self-induced vomiting or laxative abuse but sometimes other methods such as excessive exercise or fasting. While it is usually associated with *b. nervosa*, it may also occur in other disorders, such as *anorexia nervosa*. **bulim′ic** *adj*

b. nervo′sa [DSM-IV] an eating disorder occurring predominantly in females, with onset usually in adolescence or early adulthood and characterized by episodic binge eating followed by behaviors designed to prevent weight gain, including purging, fasting, and excessive exercise. Episodes of binge eating involve intake of quantifiably excessive quantities of food within a short, discrete period as well as a sense of loss of control over food intake during these periods. The person with bulimia nervosa has a preoccupying pathological fear of becoming overweight, feels an unusually strong tie between self-worth and body shape and size, is aware that the eating pattern is abnormal, and frequently experiences feelings of self-recrimination. In contrast to persons with *anorexia nervosa,* patients with bulimia nervosa tend to be somewhat older, more socially inclined, have less obsessive characteristics, and do not exhibit extreme weight loss; it is not diagnosed in the presence of anorexia nervosa.

Bu·lim·i·dae (bu-lim′ĭ-de) a family of fresh water snails of the subclass Streptoneura, order Mesogastropoda. It includes the genera *Bulimus, Oncomelania, Parafossarulus,* and *Pomatiopsis*.

Bu·lim·i·nae (bu-lim′ĭ-ne) a subfamily of snails of the family Hydrobiidae; medically important genera include *Bulimus* and *Parafossarulus*.

Bu·li·mus (bu-li′məs) a genus of small fresh water snails of the family Bulimidae; formerly called *Bithynia*.

B. fuchsia′nus the chief intermediate host of the human liver flukes *Clonorchis* and *Opisthorchis;* it is commonly found in southern China.

B. lea′chii a species found in northern Europe and the northwestern United States, which ingests the eggs of the liver fluke *Opisthorchis felineus* and in whose body the eggs hatch.

Bu·li·nus (bu-li′nəs) a genus of snails of the family Planorbidae. Several species are intermediate hosts of *Schistosoma haematobium* and *Opisthorchis*.

bulk·age (bulk′əj) material that will increase the mass (bulk) of the intestinal contents and consequently stimulate peristalsis.

Bull. [L.] bul′liat (let it boil).

bul·la (bul′ə) pl. *bul′lae* [L.] 1. a large blister; called also *bleb*. 2. in anatomy, a rounded, projecting structure. **bul′late, bul′lous** *adj*

emphysematous b. any space in a distended area of an emphysematous lung, ranging in size from one centimeter to most of a hemithorax.

ethmoidal b., b. ethmoida′lis [TA] a rounded projection of the ethmoid bone into the lateral wall of the middle nasal meatus just below the middle nasal concha, enclosing a large ethmoid air cell.

bul·lae (bul′e) plural of *bulla*.

bul·la·tion (bə-la′shən) bullosis.

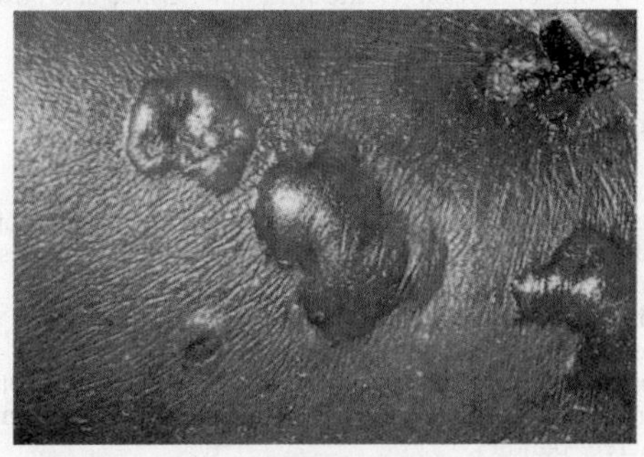

■ Bullae.

bul·lec·to·my (bə-lek′tə-me) [*bulla* + *-ectomy*] excision of a bulla, especially one of the giant ones seen in bullous emphysema in order to improve pulmonary function. See also *reduction pneumoplasty*.

Bul·ler shield (bandage) (bul′ər) [Frank *Buller*, Canadian ophthalmologic surgeon, 1844–1905] see under *shield*.

bull·neck (bool′nek) bull neck; see under *neck*.

bull·nose (bool′nōz) necrotic rhinitis.

bul·lo·sis (bul-o′sis) 1. the production of bullae. 2. a condition characterized by bullae.
diabetic b., b. diabetico′rum a condition in which bullae appear spontaneously, usually on the ankles and feet, in some uncontrolled diabetics.

bum·ble·foot (bum′bəl-foot) inflammation of the ball of the foot of fowls, usually caused by staphylococcus.

bu·met·a·nide (bu-met′ə-nīd) [USP] a loop diuretic used in treatment of edema associated with congestive heart failure or hepatic or renal disease, treatment of hypertension, usually in combination with other drugs, and as an adjunct in treatment of acute pulmonary edema; administered orally, intramuscularly, or intravenously.

Bu·mex (bu′meks) trademark for preparations of bumetanide.

Bu·mi·nate (bu′mĭ-nāt) trademark for a preparation of albumin human.

Bum·ke pupil (boom′kə) [Oswald Conrad Edward *Bumke*, German neurologist, 1877–1950] see under *pupil*.

bump (bump) 1. a blow or collision. 2. a small swelling. 3. (pl.) erythema nodosum sometimes seen in cases of primary coccidioidomycosis.
desert b's popular name for *coccidioidomycosis*.
pump b. popular term for retrocalcaneal bursitis.
razor b's, shave b's popular names for *pseudofolliculitis barbae*.

BUN blood urea nitrogen; see *urea nitrogen*, under *urea*.

bu·nam·i·dine hy·dro·chlo·ride (bu-nam′ĭ-dēn) an anthelmintic used in cats and dogs.

bun·dle (bun′dəl) a collection of muscle or nerve fibers; see also *fasciculus*, *fiber*, *lemniscus*, *tract*, and *tractus*.
aberrant b's collections of pyramidal fibers leaving the corticonuclear tract at successive levels of the brainstem, and giving off fibers to the motor nuclei of the cranial nerves.
atrioventricular b., AV b. b. of His.
Bachmann b. a group of fibers of the anterior internodal tract that penetrate the interatrial septum and diverge in the left atrium, connecting the atria.
comb b. nigrostriatal tract.
common b. truncus fasciculi atrioventricularis.
hair b. the organelle that contains the sensory receptors for hearing and equilibrium, found at the apex of a hair cell; it consists of about 100 stereocilia and usually one kinocilium.
b. of His a small band of atypical cardiac muscle fibers that originates in the atrioventricular node in the interatrial septum, passes through the atrioventricular junction, and then runs beneath the endocardium of the right ventricle on the membranous part of the interventricular septum. It divides at the upper end of the muscular part of the interventricular septum into right and left bundle branches which descend in the septal wall of the right and left ventricle, respectively, to be distributed to those two chambers. This bundle propagates the atrial contraction rhythm to the ventricles, and its interruption produces heart block. The term is often used to refer specifically to the trunk of the bundle *(truncus fasciculi atrioventricularis)* rather than the entire bundle. Called also *fasciculus atrioventricularis* [TA], *atrioventricular b.*, *AV b.*, and *Kent-His b.* See illustration at *nodus sinuatrialis*.
Kent b. a muscular bundle found normally in the hearts of certain mammalian species, forming a direct connection between the atrial and ventricular walls. In the human heart it is found only rarely, and may form an accessory pathway that allows the preexcitation of the ventricle found in the Wolff-Parkinson-White syndrome. Called also *atrioventricular pathway*.
Kent-His b. b. of His.
longitudinal medial b. fasciculus longitudinalis medialis.
medial forebrain b. fasciculus medialis telencephali.
Meynert b. tractus habenulointerpeduncularis.
Monakow b. tractus rubrospinalis.
muscle b. one of the primary longitudinal subdivisions of a muscle, made up of muscle fibers and separated from other bundles by fascial septa or perimysium.
olivocochlear b. of Rasmussen tractus olivocochlearis.
b. of Oort tractus olivocochlearis.
papillomacular b's an oval shaped arrangement of ganglion cell axons extending from the macula lutea to the optic disk, then entering the optic nerve as discrete bundles.
posterior longitudinal b. fasciculus longitudinalis medialis.
b. of Rasmussen tractus olivocochlearis.
Schütz b. fasciculus longitudinalis posterior.
solitary b. tractus solitarius medullae oblongatae.
Thorel b. a bundle of muscle fibers in the human heart, connecting the sinoatrial and atrioventricular nodes, and passing around the mouth of the inferior vena cava.
transverse b's of palmar aponeurosis fasciculi transversi aponeurosis palmaris; see under *fasciculus*.
Türck b. fibrae temporopontinae.
Weissmann b. the bundle of striated muscle fibers of a neuromuscular spindle.

bun·dle branch (bun′dəl branch) see under *branch*.

bun·ga·ro·tox·in (bung′gə-ro-tok″sin) a strong neurotoxin from the venom of kraits *(Bungarus)*; three electrophoretic fractions, α-, β-, and γ-bungarotoxin, have been identified. α-Bungarotoxin, the chief fraction, binds irreversibly with acetylcholine receptors, producing neuromuscular block.

Bun·ga·rus (bung′gə-rəs) the kraits, a genus of venomous snakes of the family Elapidae, found in the Indian subcontinent, Southeast Asia, and China. See table at *snake*.

Bun·ge amputation (boon′gə) [Richard *Bunge*, German surgeon, early 20th century] aperiosteal amputation.

bung·eye (bung′i) cutaneous habronemiasis around the eye.

Büng·ner bands (bēng′nər) [Otto von *Büngner*, German neurologist, 1858–1905] see under *band*.

bun·ion (bun′yən) [L. *bunio*; Gr. *bounion* turnip] abnormal prominence of the inner aspect of the first metatarsal head, accompanied by bursal formation and resulting in a lateral or valgus displacement of the great toe.
tailor's b. bunionette.

bun·ion·ec·to·my (bun″yən-ek′tə-me) [*bunion* + *-ectomy*] excision of an abnormal prominence on the mesial aspect of the first metatarsal head.

bun·ion·ette (bun″yən-et′) enlargement of the lateral aspect of the fifth metatarsal head; called also *tailor's bunion*.

Bun·nell suture (bə-nel′) [Sterling *Bunnell*, American surgeon, 1882–1957] see under *suture*.

bu·no·dont (bu′no-dont) [Gr. *bounos* hill + *odous* tooth] having cheek teeth with low rounded cusps on the occlusal surface of the crown, as in mammals with mixed diet, such as swine, many rodents, and humans.

bu·no·sto·mi·a·sis (bu″no-stə-mi′ə-sis) hookworm disease in ruminants caused by species of *Bunostomum*.

Bu·no·sto·mum (bu″no-sto′məm) a genus of hookworms of the family Ancylostomatidae that parasitize cattle, sheep, and other ruminants; called also *Monodontus*.

Bun·sen burner, coefficient (bun′sən) [Robert Wilhelm Eberhard *Bunsen*, German chemist, 1811–1899] see under *burner* and *coefficient*.

Bun·ya·vi·ri·dae (bun″yə-vir′ĭ-de) the bunyaviruses: a family of RNA viruses having a spherical or oval virion 80–120 nm in diameter consisting of a lipid bilayer envelope, with glycoprotein surface projections 5–10 nm long and 10–12 nm across in hexagonal arrangement, surrounding three loosely helical nucleocapsids. The genome consists of three molecules of circular negative-sense or ambisense single-stranded RNA, designated L, M, and S (total MW 4.8–8×10^6, size of total genome 11–20 kb).

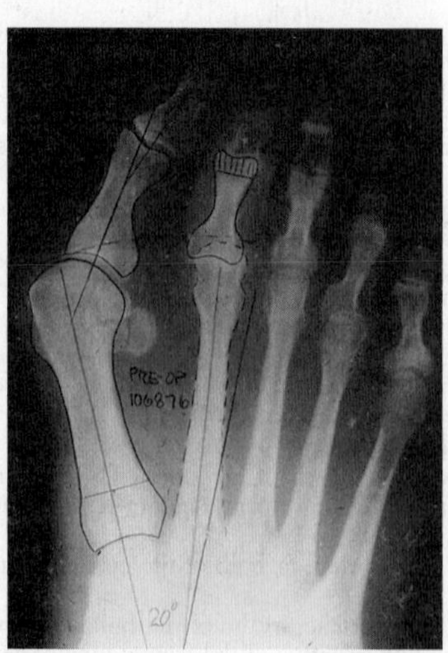

■ Bunion.

Viruses contain four major structural polypeptides, including a transcriptase, and are sensitive to lipid solvents and detergents. Replication occurs in the cytoplasm and assembly is by budding through the smooth membrane of the Golgi apparatus. Host ranges vary; transmission is generally by arthropod vectors, although transmission by aerosols and avian vectors sometimes occurs. Genera include *Orthobunyavirus*, *Hantavirus*, *Nairovirus*, *Phlebovirus*, and *Tospovirus*.

Bun•ya•vi•rus (bun′yə-vi″rəs) [*Bunyamwera*, town in Uganda where the type species was isolated] former name for *Orthobunyavirus*.

bun•ya•vi•rus (bun′yə-vi″rəs) any virus belonging to the family Bunyaviridae. **bunyavi′ral** *adj*

Bu•pap (bu′pap) trademark for a combination preparation of butalbital and acetaminophen.

Bu•phen•yl (bu-fen′əl) trademark for preparations of sodium phenylbutyrate.

buph•thal•mia (būf-thal′me-ə) 1. hydrophthalmos. 2. congenital glaucoma.

buph•thal•mos (būf-thal′mos) [Gr. *bous* ox + *ophthalmos* eye] 1. hydrophthalmos. 2. congenital glaucoma.

buph•thal•mus (būf-thal′məs) 1. hydrophthalmos. 2. congenital glaucoma.

bu•piv•a•caine hy•dro•chlo•ride (bu-piv′ə-kān) [USP] a homologue of mepivacaine, chemically related to lidocaine, used as a local anesthetic for infiltration, peripheral nerve block, retrobulbar block, subarachnoid block, sympathetic block, and caudal and epidural anesthesia.

Bu•pre•nex (būp′rə-neks) trademark for preparations of buprenorphine hydrochloride.

bu•pre•nor•phine hy•dro•chlo•ride (bu″prə-nor′fēn) [USP] a synthetic opioid agonist-antagonist derived from thebaine, used as an analgesic for moderate to severe pain and as an anesthesia adjunct; administered sublingually or by intramuscular or intravenous injection.

bu•pro•pi•on hy•dro•chlo•ride (bu-pro′pe-on) a monocyclic compound structurally similar to amphetamine, used as an antidepressant and as an aid in smoking cessation to reduce the symptoms of nicotine withdrawal; administered orally.

bur (bur) 1. a metal rotary dental instrument with cutting heads of various shapes, held and revolved in a handpiece; used to remove carious material from within decayed teeth, reduce decayed or fractured hard tissues, form the design of the cavity preparation, and finish and polish the teeth and restorations. Called also *drill*. 2. a type of surgical drill for making holes in bones. In both senses, also spelled *burr*.

bur•bu•lence (bur′bu-ləns″) a group of symptoms of intestinal origin, including a feeling of fullness, bloating or distention, borborygmus, and flatulence. Called also *gaseousness*.

Burch procedure (colposuspension) (burch) [John C. *Burch*, American surgeon, late 20th century] see under *procedure*.

Bur•dach fasciculus (column, fibers, tract), etc. (bo͞or′dahk) [Karl Friedrich *Burdach*, German physiologist, 1776–1847] see under *fissure*, and see *fasciculus cuneatus medullae spinalis*, and *nucleus cuneatus*.

bu•ret (bu-ret′) a graduated glass tube used in volumetric chemistry to deliver a measured amount of liquid.

bu•rette (bu-ret′) buret.

Bür•ger-Grütz syndrome (bēr′gər grētz′) [Max *Bürger*, German physician, 1885–1966; Otto *Grütz*, German dermatologist, 1886–1963] familial hyperlipoproteinemia, type I; see under *hyperlipoproteinemia*.

Bur•kitt lymphoma (bur′kit) [Denis Parsons *Burkitt*, Irish surgeon in Uganda, 1911–1993] see under *lymphoma*.

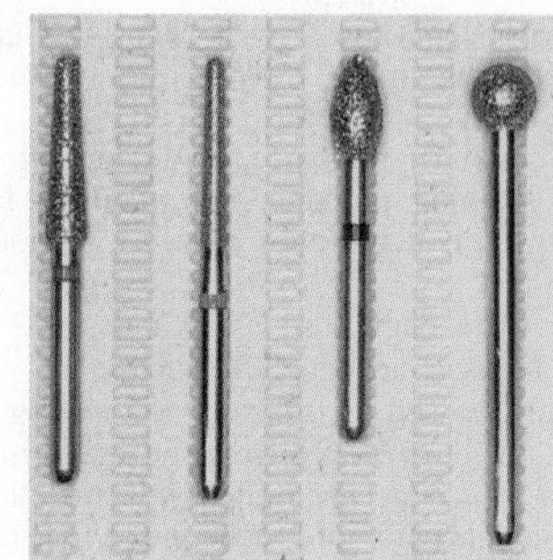

■ Diamond burs.

Burk•hol•de•ria (burk″hol-dēr′e-ə) a genus of gram-negative, rod-shaped bacteria of the family Burkholderiaceae, comprising animal and plant pathogens formerly classified in group II of the genus *Pseudomonas*.

B. cenocepa′cia a species isolated from the respiratory tracts of patients with cystic fibrosis.

B. cepa′cia the type species; a widespread species isolated from clinical specimens and hospital equipment and supplies that is an opportunistic pathogen and causes various nosocomial infections. It appears to be an important respiratory pathogen in children with cystic fibrosis. Formerly classified as *Pseudomonas cepacia*.

B. gladio′li a species that is a plant pathogen but has also been found in infections of immunocompromised persons.

B. mal′lei a nonmotile species that is pathogenic chiefly for horses, causing glanders; it may also infect other animals. Formerly classified as *Pseudomonas mallei*.

B. pseudomal′lei the species that causes melioidosis; it has been isolated from soil and water in tropical regions. Formerly classified as *Pseudomonas pseudomallei*.

Burk•hol•de•ri•a•ceae (burk″hol-dēr″e-a′se-e) a family of phenotypically, metabolically, and ecologically diverse bacteria of the order Burkholderiales, created on the basis of genetic sequence analysis; medically important organisms are included in the genera *Burkholderia* and *Ralstonia*.

Burk•hol•de•ri•a•les (burk″hol-dēr″e-a′les) an order of phenotypically, metabolically, and ecologically diverse bacteria of the class Betaproteobacteria, phylum Proteobacteria, created on the basis of genetic sequence analysis; medically important organisms are included in the families Alcaligenaceae and Burkholderiaceae.

burn (burn) injury to tissues caused by contact with dry heat (fire), moist heat (steam or hot liquid), chemicals (e.g., corrosive substances), electricity (current or lightning), friction, or radiant and electromagnetic energy. Burns are classified by the depth of injury as first-, second-, third-, or fourth-degree.

brush b. a skin wound caused by violent rubbing or friction, as by a rope pulled through the hands; called also *friction b.*

chemical b. irritant dermatitis caused by a caustic substance, such as an acid, disinfectant, or alkali.

contact b. a burn produced by direct contact with a chemical, hot object, or electric current.

deep partial-thickness b., deep second-degree b. see *second-degree b.*

electric b., electrical b. a thermal burn caused by the heat of an electric current; it may be either a flash burn or a contact burn.

first-degree b. a burn that affects the epidermis only, causing erythema and in some cases mild edema, without vesiculation.

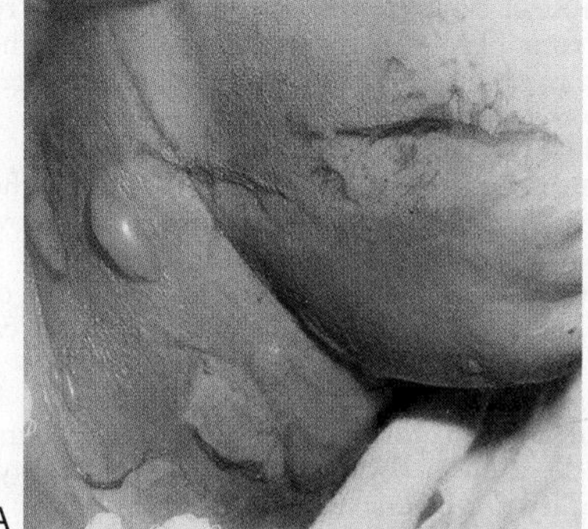

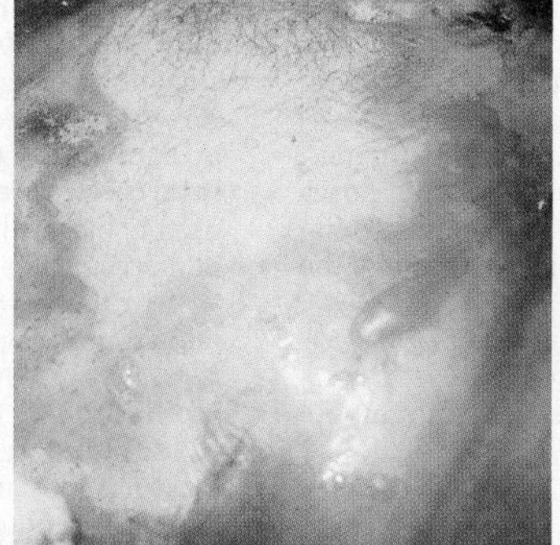

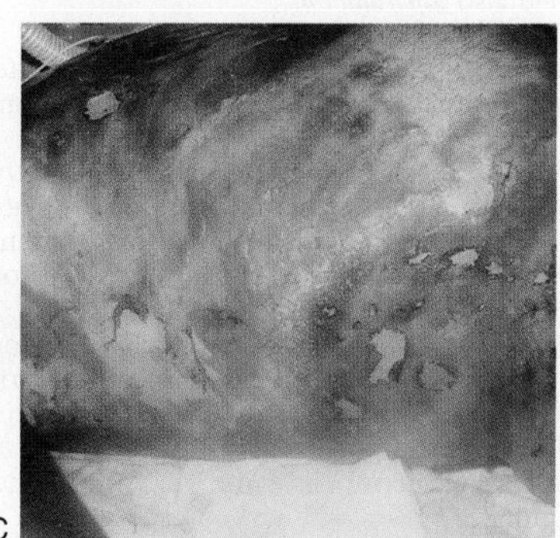

■ Burns. *(A)*, Superficial second-degree; *(B)*, deep second-degree; *(C)*, third-degree.

flash b. a thermal burn caused by a very brief exposure to radiant heat of high intensity, as in an explosion or a sudden discharge of electricity.

fourth-degree b. a burn that extends deeply into the subcutaneous tissue, completely destroying the skin, subcutaneous fat, and underlying tendons, and sometimes involving muscle, fascia, or bone.

friction b. brush b.

full-thickness b. third-degree b.

partial-thickness b. second-degree b.

radiation b. a burn caused by exposure to ionizing radiation.

second-degree b. a burn that affects the epidermis and the dermis, classified as *superficial* or *deep* according to the depth of injury. The superficial type involves the epidermis and the papillary dermis and is characterized by pain, edema, and the formation of blisters; it heals without scarring. The deep type extends into the reticular dermis, is pale and anesthetic, and results in scarring. Called also *partial thickness b.* See illustration.

sun b. sunburn.

superficial partial-thickness b., superficial second-degree b. see *second-degree b.*

thermal b. a burn caused by exposure to something of high temperature, such as a flame, a hot object, or electricity, as distinguished from a chemical burn.

third-degree b. a burn that destroys both the epidermis and the dermis, often also involving the subcutaneous tissue. Called also *full-thickness b.* See illustration.

wind b. windburn.

x-ray b. a type of radiation burn caused by exposure to x-rays.

burn·er (bur′nər) the part of a lamp, stove, or furnace from which the flame issues.

Argand b. a burner for oil or gas, with an inner tube for supplying air to the flame.

Bunsen b. a gas burner in which the gas is mixed with air before ignition, in order to give complete oxidation.

Bur·nett syndrome (bər-net′) [Charles Hoyt *Burnett*, American physician, 1913–1967] milk-alkali syndrome.

bur·nish·er (bur′nish-ər) a dental instrument with a blade or nib with a beveled edge used for smoothing out roughness at the margin of a restoration and the enamel.

bur·nish·ing (bur′nish-ing) 1. condensation and polishing under the sliding pressure of a smooth hard instrument, as in finishing the surface of a gold filling. 2. adaptation of a thin, annealed sheet metal by means of a burnisher, as in forming a band about a tooth root or in fitting a matrix for porcelain.

Burns ligament, space (bərnz) [Allan *Burns*, Scottish anatomist, 1781–1813] see *margo falciformis hiatus saphenus* and *spatium suprasternale*.

Bur·ow operation, solution, vein (boo′rov) [Karl August *Burow*, German surgeon, 1809–1874] see under *operation* and *vein*, and see *aluminum acetate topical solution*, under *solution*.

burr (bur) bur.

bur·sa (bur′sə) pl. *bur′sae* [L., from Gr. "a wine skin"] a sac or saclike cavity filled with a viscid fluid and situated at places in the tissues at which friction would otherwise develop. **bur′sal** *adj*

Bursa

Descriptions are given on TA terms, and include anglicized names of specific bursae.

b. of Achilles, b. of Achilles tendon b. tendinis calcanei.
acromial b. b. subdeltoidea.
adventitious b. an abnormal cyst due to friction or some other mechanical cause, and containing synovial fluid; called also *supernumerary b.*
anconeal b. b. subcutanea olecrani.
anconeal b. of triceps muscle b. subtendinea musculi tricipitis brachii.
b. anseri′na [TA], **anserine b.** a bursa between the tendons of the sartorius, gracilis, and semitendinosus muscles, and the tibial collateral ligament; called also *anterior genual b.*
bicipital b. 1. b. subtendinea musculi bicipitis femoris inferior. 2. intertubercular b..
bicipitofibular b. b. subtendinea musculi bicipitis femoris inferior.
bicipitoradial b., b. bicipitoradia′lis [TA] a bursa between the radial tuberosity and the biceps tendon.
Boyer b. b. retrohyoidea.
Brodie b. b. subtendinea musculi gastrocnemii medialis.
calcaneal b., b. of calcaneal tendon b. tendinis calcanei.
Calori b. a bursa situated between the trachea and the arch of the aorta.
b. copula′trix an appendage at the posterior end of the male of certain nematodes.
coracobrachial b. b. musculi coracobrachialis.
coracoid b. b. subtendinea musculi subscapularis.
b. cubita′lis interos′sea [TA], **cubitoradial b.** interosseous cubital bursa: a bursa between the ulna, the biceps tendon, and nearby muscles; called also *ulnoradial b.*
deltoid b. b. subacromialis.
external infracondyloid b. recessus subpopliteus.
external postgenual b. b. subtendinea musculi gastrocnemii lateralis.
b. of Fabricius a lymphoid organ of birds that, like the thymus, develops as an epithelial outpouching of the gut but near the cloaca rather than the foregut; it atrophies at 5 or 6 months of age, persisting as a fibrous remnant in sexually mature birds; before involution it is the site of maturation of B lymphocytes (q.v.).
fibular b. b. subtendinea musculi bicipitis femoris inferior.
Fleischmann b. a bursa located beneath the tongue.
gastrocnemiosemimembranous b. b. musculi semimembranosi.
genual b., anterior b. anserina.
genual b., external inferior b. subtendinea musculi bicipitis femoris inferior.
genual bursae, internal superior bursae subtendineae musculi sartorii.
genual b., posterior b. musculi semimembranosi.
gluteal b. a bursa situated beneath the gluteus maximus muscle.
gluteofascial bursae, gluteofemoral bursae bursae intermusculares musculorum gluteorum.
gluteotuberosal b. b. ischiadica musculi glutei maximi.
His b. the dilatation at the end of the archenteron.
humeral b. 1. b. subacromialis. 2. b. subtendinea musculi gastrocnemii lateralis.
hyoid b. b. subcutanea prominentiae laryngeae.
b. iliopecti′nea [TA], **iliopectineal b.** a bursa between the iliopsoas tendon and the iliopectineal eminence; called also *subiliac b.*
b. of iliopsoas muscle b. subtendinea iliaca.
infracardiac b. the cranial end of a coelomic recess of the embryo, extending upward between the esophagus and right primary bronchial bud; frequently persisting in the adult.
infragenual b. b. infrapatellaris profunda.
infrahyoid b., b. infrahyoi′dea [TA] a bursa sometimes present below the hyoid bone at the attachment of the sternohyoid muscle.
infrapatellar b. b. subtendinea prepatellaris.
infrapatellar b., deep b. infrapatellaris profunda.
infrapatellar b., subcutaneous b. subcutanea infrapatellaris.
infrapatellar b., superficial inferior b. subcutanea tuberositatis tibiae.
b. infrapatella′ris profun′da [TA] deep infrapatellar bursa: a bursa between the patellar ligament and the tibia; called also *infragenual b.*, *subpatellar b.*, and *subligamentous b.*
intermuscular gluteal bursae, bur′sae intermuscula′res musculo′rum gluteo′rum [TA] several sacs that surround the tendon attaching the gluteus maximus to the femur; called also *gluteofascial bursae* and *gluteofemoral bursae.*
interosseous cubital b. b. cubitalis interossea.
intertubercular b. on a quadruped, a bursa between the tendon of the biceps brachii muscle and the intertubercular groove of the humerus. Called also *bicipital b.*
b. intratendi′nea olec′rani [TA] intratendinous bursa of olecranon: a bursa within the triceps tendon near its insertion; called also *Monro b.*
ischiadic b. b. ischiadica musculi obturatorii interni.
b. ischia′dica mus′culi glu′tei max′imi [TA] sciatic bursa of gluteus maximus muscle: a bursa between the ischial tuberosity and the gluteus maximus; called also *gluteotuberosal b.*

Bursa *Continued*

b. ischia′dica mus′culi obturato′rii inter′ni [TA] sciatic bursa of obturator internus muscle: a bursa between the tendon of the obturator internus muscle and the lesser sciatic notch; called also *ischiadic b.* and *tuberoischiadic b.*
Luschka b. b. pharyngealis.
Monro b. b. intratendinea olecrani.
multilocular b. a bursa that is subdivided into several compartments.
b. mus′culi bici′pitis fe′moris supe′rior [TA] superior bursa of biceps femoris muscle: a bursa between the long head of the biceps, the semitendinosus, the tendon of the semimembranosus, and the ischial tuberosity; called also *subtendinous b.*
b. mus′culi coracobrachia′lis [TA] coracobrachial bursa: a bursa between the coracobrachialis and subscapularis muscles and the coracoid process; called also *subcoracoid b.*
b. mus′culi pirifor′mis [TA] bursa of piriformis muscle: a bursa between the piriformis tendon, the superior gemellus muscle, and the femur.
b. mus′culi semimembrano′si [TA] bursa of semimembranosus muscle: a bursa between the semimembranosus muscle and the medial head of the gastrocnemius. Called also *posterior genual b.*, *retrocondyloid b.*, and *semimembranosus b.*
b. mus′culi tenso′ris ve′li palati′ni [TA] bursa of tensor veli palatini muscle: a bursa between the hamular process of the sphenoid bone and the tendon of the tensor veli palatini.
omental b., b. omenta′lis [TA] a serous peritoneal cavity situated behind the stomach, the lesser omentum, and part of the liver and in front of the pancreas and duodenum. It communicates with the general peritoneal cavity (greater sac) through the epiploic foramen and sometimes is continuous with the cavity of the greater omentum. Called also *lesser peritoneal cavity* or *sac.*
patellar b., deep b. subtendinea prepatellaris.
patellar b., middle b. subfascialis prepatellaris.
patellar b., prespinous b. subcutanea tuberositatis tibiae.
patellar b., subcutaneous b. subcutanea prepatellaris.
pharyngeal b., b. pharyngea′lis [TA] an inconstant blind sac located above the pharyngeal tonsil in the midline of the posterior wall of the nasopharynx; it represents persistence of an embryonic communication between the anterior tip of the notochord and the roof of the pharynx. Called also *Luschka b.* and *Tornwaldt b.* or *cyst.*
b. of piriformis muscle b. musculi piriformis.
popliteal b. recessus subpopliteus.
postcalcaneal b. b. subcutanea calcanea.
postcalcaneal b., deep b. tendinis calcanei.
prepatellar b., middle b. subfascialis prepatellaris.
prepatellar b., subcutaneous b. subcutanea prepatellaris.
prepatellar b., subfascial b. subfascialis prepatellaris.
prepatellar b., subtendinous b. subtendinea prepatellaris.
pretibial b. b. subcutanea tuberositatis tibiae.
b. of quadratus femoris muscle b. subtendinea iliaca.
retrocalcaneal b. b. tendinis calcanei.
retrocondyloid b. b. musculi semimembranosi.
retrohyoid b., b. retrohyoi′dea [TA] a bursa sometimes present behind the hyoid bone at the attachment of the sternohyoid muscle.
retromammary b. a well-defined loose areolar tissue between the deep layer of superficial fascia on the posterior aspect of the breast, and the deep fascia covering the pectoralis major and other muscles of the chest wall.
sciatic b. of gluteus maximus muscle b. ischiadica musculi glutei maximi.
sciatic b. of obturator internus muscle b. ischiadica musculi obturatorii interni.
semimembranosogastrocnemial b., semimembranosus b. b. musculi semimembranosi.
semitendinous b. b. musculi bicipitis femoris superior.
sternohyoid b. either of two bursae located where the sternohyoid muscle attaches to the hyoid bone; see *b. infrahyoidea* and *b. retrohyoidea.*
subachilleal b. b. tendinis calcanei.
subacromial b., b. subacromia′lis [TA] a bursa located between the acromion and the insertion of the supraspinatus muscle, extending between the deltoid and the greater tubercle of the humerus; called also *deltoid b.* and *humeral b.*
subcalcaneal b. b. subcutanea calcanea.
subcoracoid b. 1. b. musculi coracobrachialis. 2. b. subtendinea musculi subscapularis.

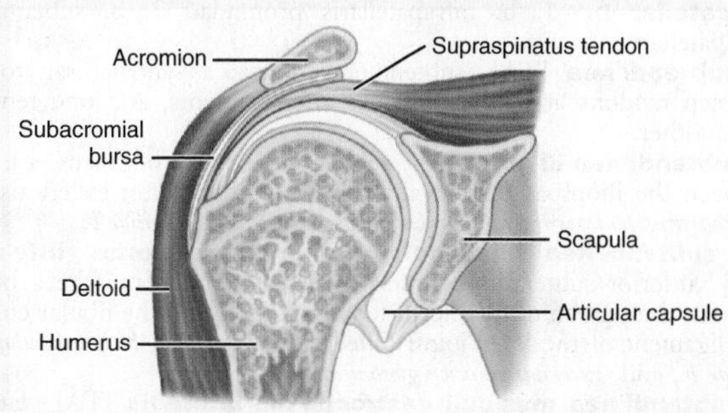

■ Bursa subacromialis (subacromial bursa), lying between the acromion and supraspinatus tendon and extending between the deltoid and greater tubercle.

subcrural b. b. suprapatellaris.
b. subcuta′nea [TA] subcutaneous bursa: a synovial sac found beneath the skin.
b. subcuta′nea acromia′lis [TA] subcutaneous acromial bursa: a bursa between the acromion and the overlying skin.
b. subcuta′nea calca′nea [TA] subcutaneous calcaneal bursa: a bursa between the calcaneus and the skin on the sole of the foot; called also *postcalcaneal b.* and *subcalcaneal b.*
b. subcuta′nea infrapatella′ris [TA] subcutaneous infrapatellar bursa: a bursa between the upper end of the patellar ligament and the skin; called also *subpatellar b.* and *superficial b. of knee.*
b. subcuta′nea malle′oli latera′lis [TA] subcutaneous bursa of lateral malleolus: a bursa between the lateral malleolus and the skin.
b. subcuta′nea malle′oli media′lis [TA] subcutaneous bursa of medial malleolus: a bursa between the medial malleolus and the skin.
b. subcuta′nea olec′rani [TA] subcutaneous bursa of olecranon: a bursa between the olecranon process and the skin; called also *anconeal b.* and *superficial b. of olecranon.*
b. subcuta′nea prepatella′ris [TA] subcutaneous prepatellar bursa: a bursa between the patella and the skin.
b. subcuta′nea prominen′tiae laryn′geae [TA] subcutaneous bursa of laryngeal prominence: a bursa anterior to the laryngeal prominence of the thyroid cartilage, under the skin; called also *hyoid b.*, *subhyoid b.*, and *thyrohyoid b.*
b. subcuta′nea trochante′rica [TA] subcutaneous trochanteric bursa: a bursa between the greater trochanter of the femur and the skin.
b. subcuta′nea tuberosita′tis ti′biae [TA] subcutaneous bursa of tuberosity of tibia: a bursa between the tibial tuberosity and the skin; called also *patellar b., prespinous, pretibial b.*, and *superficial inferior infrapatellar b.*
subcutaneous b. b. subcutanea.
subcutaneous acromial b. b. subcutanea acromialis.
subcutaneous calcaneal b. b. subcutanea calcanea.
subcutaneous b. of laryngeal prominence b. subcutanea prominentiae laryngeae.
subcutaneous b. of lateral malleolus b. subcutanea malleoli lateralis.
subcutaneous b. of medial malleolus b. subcutanea malleoli medialis.
subcutaneous b. of olecranon b. subcutanea olecrani.
subcutaneous trochanteric b. b. subcutanea trochanterica.
subcutaneous b. of tuberosity of tibia b. subcutanea tuberositatis tibiae.
subdeltoid b., b. subdeltoi′dea [TA] a bursa between the deltoid and the shoulder joint capsule, usually connected to the subacromial bursa; called also *acromial b.*
subfascial b., b. subfascia′lis [TA] a synovial sac found beneath a fascial layer.
b. subfascia′lis prepatella′ris [TA] subfascial prepatellar bursa: a bursa between the front of the patella and the investing fascia of the knee; called also *middle patellar* or *middle prepatellar b.*
subhyoid b. b. subcutanea prominentiae laryngeae.
subiliac b. 1. b. iliopectinea. 2. b. subtendinea iliaca.
subligamentous b. b. infrapatellaris profunda.
submuscular b., b. submuscula′ris [TA] a synovial sac found beneath a muscle.

Bursa *Continued*

subpatellar b. 1. b. infrapatellaris profunda. 2. b. subcutanea infrapatellaris.
b. subtendi′nea [TA] subtendinous bursa: a synovial sac found between tendons and bone, tendons and ligaments, and one tendon and another.
b. subtendi′nea ili′aca [TA] subtendinous bursa of iliacus: a bursa between the iliopsoas tendon and the lesser trochanter; called also *b. of quadratus femoris muscle*, *b. of iliopsoas muscle*, and *subiliac b.*
b. subtendi′nea mus′culi bici′pitis fe′moris infe′rior [TA] inferior subtendinous bursa of biceps femoris muscle: a bursa between the tendon of the biceps femoris muscle and the fibular collateral ligament of the knee joint; called also *bicipital b.*, *bicipitofibular b.*, *fibular b.*, and *external inferior genual b.*
b. subtendi′nea mus′culi gastrocne′mii latera′lis [TA] lateral subtendinous bursa of gastrocnemius muscle: a bursa between the tendon of the lateral head of the gastrocnemius muscle and the joint capsule; called also *humeral b.* and *external postgenual b.*
b. subtendi′nea mus′culi gastrocne′mii media′lis [TA] medial subtendinous bursa of gastrocnemius muscle: a bursa between the tendon of the medial head of the gastrocnemius, the condyle of the femur, and the joint capsule; called also *Brodie b.*, *internal supracondyloid b.*, and *medial supracondyloid b.*
b. subtendi′nea mus′culi infraspina′ti [TA] subtendinous bursa of infraspinatus muscle: a bursa between the tendon of the infraspinatus and the joint capsule or the greater tubercle.
b. subtendi′nea mus′culi latis′simi dor′si [TA] subtendinous bursa of latissimus dorsi muscle: a bursa between the tendons of the latissimus dorsi and teres major muscles.
b. subtendi′nea mus′culi obturato′rii inter′ni [TA] subtendinous bursa of obturator internus muscle: a bursa beneath the tendon of the obturator internus muscle.
bur′sae subtendi′neae mus′culi sarto′rii [TA] subtendinous bursae of sartorius muscle: bursae between the tendons of the sartorius, semitendinosus, and gracilis muscles; called also *internal superior genual bursae.*
b. subtendi′nea mus′culi subscapula′ris [TA] subtendinous bursa of subscapularis muscle: a bursa between the tendon of the subscapularis muscle and the glenoid border of the scapula; called also *coracoid b.* and *subcoracoid b.*
b. subtendi′nea mus′culi te′retis majo′ris [TA] subtendinous bursa of teres major muscle: a bursa deep to the tendon of insertion of the teres major muscle.
b. subtendi′nea mus′culi tibia′lis anterio′ris [TA] subtendinous bursa of tibialis anterior muscle: a bursa between the tibialis anterior and the medial surface of the medial cuneiform bone.
b. subtendi′nea mus′culi trape′zii [TA] subtendinous bursa of trapezius muscle: a bursa between the trapezius and the medial end of the spine of the scapula.
b. subtendi′nea mus′culi trici′pitis bra′chii [TA] subtendinous bursa of triceps brachii muscle: an inconstant sac between the triceps tendon, the olecranon, and the dorsal ligament of the elbow; called also *anconeal b. of triceps muscle.*
b. subtendi′nea prepatella′ris [TA] subtendinous prepatellar bursa: a bursa sometimes present between the quadriceps tendon and the patellar periosteum; called also *deep patellar b.*, *infrapatellar b.*, and *subcutaneous patellar b.*
subtendinous b. b. subtendinea.
subtendinous b. of biceps femoris muscle, inferior b. subtendinea musculi bicipitis femoris inferior.
subtendinous b. of gastrocnemius muscle, lateral b. subtendinea musculi gastrocnemii lateralis.
subtendinous b. of gastrocnemius muscle, medial b. subtendinea musculi gastrocnemii medialis.
subtendinous b. of iliacus b. subtendinea iliaca.
subtendinous b. of infraspinatus muscle b. subtendinea musculi infraspinati.
subtendinous b. of latissimus dorsi muscle b. subtendinea musculi latissimi dorsi.
subtendinous b. of obturator internus muscle b. subtendinea musculi obturatorii interni.
subtendinous bursae of sartorius muscle bursae subtendineae musculi sartorii.
subtendinous b. of subscapularis muscle b. subtendinea musculi subscapularis.
subtendinous b. of teres major muscle b. subtendinea musculi teretis majoris.
subtendinous b. of tibialis anterior muscle b. subtendinea musculi tibialis anterioris.
subtendinous b. of trapezius muscle b. subtendinea musculi trapezii.
subtendinous b. of triceps brachii muscle b. subtendinea musculi tricipitis brachii.
superficial b. of knee b. subcutanea infrapatellaris.
superficial b. of olecranon b. subcutanea olecrani.
superior b. of biceps femoris muscle b. musculi bicipitis femoris superior.
supernumerary b. adventitious b.
supracondyloid b., internal, supracondyloid b., medial b. subtendinea musculi gastrocnemii medialis.
supragenual b., suprapatellar b. b. suprapatellaris.
b. suprapatella′ris [TA] suprapatellar bursa: a bursa between the distal end of the femur and the quadriceps tendon; called also *supragenual b.* and *subcrural b.*
synovial b. b. synovialis.
b. synovia′lis [TA] synovial bursa: a closed synovial sac interposed between surfaces that glide upon each other; it may be simple or multilocular in structure, and subcutaneous, submuscular, subfascial, or subtendinous in location.
b. ten′dinis calca′nei [TA] bursa of tendo calcaneus: a bursa between the calcaneal tendon and the back of the calcaneus; called also *b. of calcaneal tendon*, *b. of Achilles*, *b. of Achilles tendon*, and *calcaneal*, *retrocalcaneal*, or *subachilleal b.*
b. of tensor veli palatini muscle b. musculi tensoris veli palatini.
Thornwaldt b. b. pharyngealis.
thyrohyoid b. b. subcutanea prominentiae laryngeae.
thyrohyoid b., anterior either of two bursae found below or behind the hyoid bone; see *b. infrahyoidea* and *b. retrohyoidea.*
Tornwaldt b. b. pharyngealis.
trochanteric b. of gluteus maximus muscle b. trochanterica musculi glutei maximi.
trochanteric bursae of gluteus medius muscle bursae trochantericae musculi glutei medii.
trochanteric b. of gluteus minimus muscle b. trochanterica musculi glutei minimi.
b. trochante′rica mus′culi glu′tei max′imi [TA] trochanteric bursa of gluteus maximus muscle: a bursa between the fascial tendon of the gluteus maximus, the posterolateral surface of the greater trochanter, and the vastus lateralis muscle.
bur′sae trochante′ricae mus′culi glu′tei me′dii [TA] trochanteric bursae of gluteus medius muscle: bursae between the gluteus medius and the lateral surface of the greater trochanter, and sometimes between the tendons of the gluteus medius and the piriformis.
b. trochante′rica mus′culi glu′tei mi′nimi [TA] trochanteric bursa of gluteus minimus muscle: a bursa between the edge of the gluteus minimus and the greater trochanter.
tuberoischiadic b. b. ischiadica musculi obturatorii interni.
ulnoradial b. b. cubitalis interossea.

bur•sae (bur′se) [L.] genitive and plural of *bursa.*

bur•sa-equiv•a•lent (bur′sə e-kwiv′ə-lent) analogous to the bursa of Fabricius; see *B lymphocyte*, under *lymphocyte*, and *bursa-equivalent tissue*, under *tissue.*

bur•sal•o•gy (bər-sal′ə-je) [*bursa* + *-logy*] the sum of knowledge regarding the bursae.

Bur•sa•ta (bər-sa′tə) a term sometimes used to designate those Nematoda which have a bursa copulatrix.

bur•sa•ti (bər-sah′te) [Hindi *barsati* of the rainy season] 1. pythiosis. 2. cutaneous habronemiasis. Spelled also *bursatti*, *bursattee*, and *bursautee.*

bur•sec•to•my (bər-sek′tə-me) [*bursa* + *-ectomy*] excision of a bursa.

bur•si•tis (bər-si′tis) inflammation of a bursa, occasionally accompanied by a calcific deposit in the underlying tendon; the most common site is the subdeltoid bursa.

Achilles b. retrocalcaneal b.

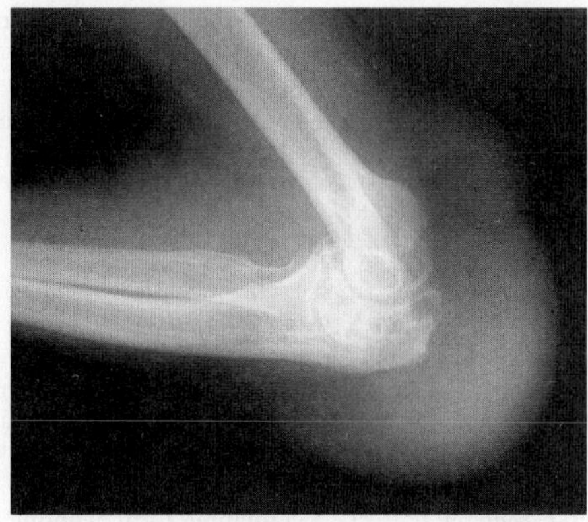

■ Olecranon bursitis associated with gout.

adhesive b. see under *capsulitis.*

anserine b. inflammation of the anserine bursa with pain on the medial side of the knee, sometimes seen after jogging or other heavy knee exercise and in heavy individuals with genu valgum.

bicipital b. inflammation of the intertubercular bursa in the forelimb of a horse, usually caused by trauma and resulting in lameness and stumbling. Called also *intertubercular b.*

calcific b. see under *tendinitis.*

intertubercular b. bicipital b.

ischiogluteal b. inflammation of the bursa over the ischial tuberosity, characterized by sudden onset of excruciating pain over the center of the buttock and down the back of the leg.

olecranon b. inflammation and enlargement of the bursa over the olecranon, caused by resting the weight of the body on the elbow, as in mining. Called also *miner's elbow.*

omental b. peritonitis localized to the omental bursa.

pharyngeal b. Tornwaldt b.

popliteal b. Baker cyst.

prepatellar b. inflammation of the bursa in front of the patella, with fluid accumulating within it; called also *carpet layer's* or *housemaid's knee.*

radiohumeral b. lateral epicondylitis.

retrocalcaneal b. inflammation and thickening of the bursae in front of the Achilles tendon. Called also *Achilles b., superficial calcaneal b.,* and *Haglund deformity* or *disease.*

scapulohumeral b. calcific tendinitis.

septic b. bursitis caused by infection, usually the result of bacterial inoculation due to trauma.

subacromial b. calcific tendinitis in the subacromial bursa.

subdeltoid b. calcific tendinitis in the subdeltoid bursa.

superficial calcaneal b. retrocalcaneal b.

Tornwaldt (Thornwaldt) b. chronic inflammation of the pharyngeal bursa, with formation of a pus-containing cyst, and nasopharyngeal stenosis; called also *pharyngeal b.* and *Tornwaldt disease.*

trochanteric b. inflammation of a trochanteric bursa with pain on the lateral part of the hip and thigh.

bur•so•lith (bur'so-lith) [*bursa* + *-lith*] a calculus or concretion in a bursa.

bur•sop•a•thy (bər-sop'ə-the) [*bursa* + *-pathy*] any disease of a bursa.

bur•sot•o•my (bər-sot'ə-me) [*bursa* + *-tomy*] incision of a bursa.

burst (bərst) 1. a sudden, intense increase in activity. 2. a small explosion. 3. on an electroencephalogram, any short waveform that has an abrupt onset and termination and differs from background activity.

metabolic b. respiratory b.

respiratory b. a sequence of four metabolic events that occur during oxidative killing of ingested microorganisms by granulocytes and mononuclear phagocytes, consisting of (1) an increase in oxygen consumption, (2) formation of superoxide anion, (3) formation of hydrogen peroxide, and (4) activation of the hexose monophosphate shunt. Molecular oxygen is converted to superoxide by NADPH oxidase and NADH oxidase. Superoxide is converted to hydrogen peroxide by superoxide dismutase. Hydrogen peroxide is utilized in myeloperoxidase-dependent bacterial killing, and both superoxide and hydrogen peroxide are spontaneously converted to other toxic metabolites, e.g., singlet oxygen and hydroxyl radicals. The hexose monophosphate shunt regenerates NADPH.

spider b. radiating lines of capillaries on the lower limb caused by venous dilatation but without distinct varicosity.

Bur•ton line (sign) (bur'tən) [Henry *Burton*, British physician, 1799–1849] see *lead line*, under *line.*

Bu•ru•li ulcer (boo'rə-le) [*Buruli* district in Uganda, where a large number of cases have occurred] see under *ulcer.*

Busch•ke disease, scleredema (boosh'kə) [Abraham *Buschke*, German dermatologist, 1868–1943] see *cryptococcosis* and *scleredema.*

Busch•ke-Lö•wen•stein tumor (boosh'kə lur'ven-shtīn) [A. *Buschke;* Ludwig W. *Löwenstein*, German-born American physician, 1885–1959] see under *tumor.*

Busch•ke-Ol•len•dorff syndrome (boosh'kə o'len-dorf) [A. *Buschke;* Helene *Ollendorff*, German dermatologist, 20th century] dermatofibrosis lenticularis disseminata.

Bu•sel•mei•er shunt (boo'səl-mi"ər) [T.J. *Buselmeier*, American nephrologist, 20th century] see under *shunt.*

bu•se•rel•in ace•tate (bu"sə-rel'in) a synthetic analogue of luteinizing hormone–releasing hormone, used in the palliative treatment of advanced prostatic carcinoma; administered intranasally.

bush•mas•ter (bush'mas-tər) *Lachesis mutus*, a large venomous pit viper of the Amazon region of South America. See table at *snake.* Called also *suruçucu.*

Bu•Spar (bu'spar) trademark for preparations of buspirone hydrochloride.

bu•spi•rone hy•dro•chlo•ride (bu-spi'rōn) [USP] an antianxiety agent used in the treatment of anxiety disorders and for short-term relief of anxiety symptoms; it is not related chemically or pharmacologically to the benzodiazepines, barbiturates, or other sedative/anxiolytic agents.

Bus•quet disease (bo͞os-ka') [Paul *Busquet*, French physician, 1866–1930] see under *disease.*

Buss disease (bus) [*Buss*, name of farmer whose animals were first observed with the disease] see under *disease.*

Bus•se-Busch•ke disease (boo'sə boosh'kə) [Otto Emil Franz Ulrich *Busse*, German physician, 1867–1922; Abraham *Buschke*, German dermatologist, 1868–1943] cryptococcosis.

bu•sul•fan (bu-sul'fan) [USP] a bifunctional cytotoxic alkylating agent, an antineoplastic agent unrelated to the nitrogen mustards; used primarily for the palliative treatment of chronic granulocytic leukemia and also for the treatment of myeloproliferative disorders including polycythemia vera and myeloid metaplasia; administered orally or intravenously. It is also used at high doses in lieu of whole body irradiation in bone marrow transplantation.

But. [L.] bu'tyrum (butter).

bu•ta•bar•bi•tal (bu-tə-bahr'bĭ-təl) [USP] an intermediate-acting barbiturate used for preoperative sedation as an adjunct to anesthesia; administered orally.

b. sodium [USP] the monosodium salt of butabarbital having the same actions and uses as the base.

bu•tal•bi•tal (bu-tal'bĭ-təl) [USP] a short- to intermediate-acting barbiturate, used as a sedative in combination with an analgesic in the treatment of tension or migraine headache; administered orally.

bu•tam•ben (bu-tam'bən) [USP] a local anesthetic applied topically to relieve pain and pruritus. Called also *butyl aminobenzoate.*

b. picrate the picrate salt of butamben, having actions and uses similar to those of the base.

bu•tam•i•sole hy•dro•chlo•ride (bu-tam'ĭ-sōl) a veterinary anthelmintic used to treat whipworm and hookworm infestations; administered parenterally or by subcutaneous injection.

bu•tane (bu'tān) [NF] *n*-butane; an aliphatic hydrocarbon of the methane series, C_4H_{10}, from petroleum, occurring as a colorless flammable gas with a characteristic odor, used in pharmacy as an aerosol propellant.

normal b. butane in straight line configuration, $CH_3(CH_2)_2CH_3$; cf. *isobutane* and see illustration at *isomerism.*

bu•ta•no•ic ac•id (bu"tə-no'ik) systematic name for n-*butyric acid.* See also table at *fatty acid.*

bu•ten•a•fine hy•dro•chlo•ride (bu-ten'ə-fēn) an antifungal that blocks the synthesis of ergosterol, a component of cell membranes in fungi; used topically in the treatment of tinea pedis, tinea corporis, and tinea cruris.

Bu•thi•dae (bu'thĭ-de) a family of scorpions (order Scorpionida) that contains most of the venomous genera, such as *Androctonus, Buthus, Centruroides, Leiurus,* and *Tityus.*

Bu•thus (bu'thəs) a genus of scorpions of the family Buthidae. *B. occita'nus* is a venomous species whose bite can be deadly, found in North Africa and the Middle East. *B. quinquestria'tus* has been reclassified as *Leiurus quinquestriatus.*

Bu•ti•sol (bu'tĭ-sol) trademark for preparations of butabarbital sodium.

But·ler-Al·bright syndrome (but′lər awl′brīt) [Alan Macy *Butler*, American physician, 20th century; Fuller *Albright*, American physician and endocrinologist, 1900–1969] see under *syndrome.*

bu·to·con·az·ole ni·trate (bu″to-kon′ə-zōl) [USP] an imidazole derivative used as a topical antifungal, applied intravaginally in the treatment of vulvovaginal candidiasis.

bu·to·nate (bu′tə-nāt) an insecticide and veterinary anthelmintic that is a potent cholinesterase inhibitor.

bu·tor·pha·nol (bu-tor′fə-nol) a synthetic opioid, having analgesic and antitussive properties.

b. tartrate [USP] the tartrate salt of butorphanol, administered intramuscularly, intravenously, or intranasally as an analgesic and intravenously as an adjunct to anesthesia.

butt (but) to bring the surfaces of two distinct objects squarely or directly into contact with each other.

but·ter (but′ər) [L. *butyrum*, from Gr. *boutyron*] 1. the oily mass procured by churning cream. 2. something resembling butter in consistency.

cacao b., cocoa b. [NF] the fat obtained from the roasted seed of *Theobroma cacao;* used in medicine as a suppository base and for softening and protecting the skin. Called also *theobroma oil.*

but·ter·fat (but′ər-fat″) the fat content of milk and the major component of butter; it is composed largely of glycerides of stearic, oleic, and palmitic acids and has high levels of saturated fats and cholesterol.

but·ter·fly (but′ər-fli) 1. any of numerous flying insects of the order Lepidoptera, or something resembling this insect. 2. a small piece of adhesive tape with broad, wing-shaped ends by means of which the edges of a superficial wound may be approximated. 3. butterfly rash.

but·tocks (but′əks) nates.

but·ton (but′ən) a knoblike elevation or structure.

bromide b. a verrucous cutaneous lesion occurring as a result of sensitivity to bromides.

dog b. nux vomica.

iodide b. a verrucous cutaneous lesion occurring as a result of sensitivity to iodides.

mescal b's transverse slices of the flowering heads of the Mexican dumpling cactus, *Lophophora williamsii*, whose major active principle is mescaline; used in divinatory and religious ceremonies in some North American Indian cultures.

peritoneal b. a short flanged glass tube for insertion between the peritoneal cavity and a subcutaneous pocket through which peritoneal transudate may be drained.

quaker b. nux vomica.

skin b. a connector or stretch of tubing covered with Dacron velour fabric, designed to encourage tissue ingrowth where it passes through the skin.

terminal b. bouton terminal; see under *bouton.*

but·ton·hole (but′ən-hōl) 1. a short straight incision into a cavity or organ. 2. an abnormal narrowing of the caliber of a structure.

mitral b. an advanced state of stenosis of the mitral orifice of the heart, adhesion and shortening of the cusps having produced a narrow slitlike orifice.

bu·tyl (bu′təl) a hydrocarbon radical, C_4H_9, being $CH_3(CH_2)_2CH_2$—, $(CH_3)_2CHCH_2$—, $CH_3CH_2CHCH_3$—, or $(CH_3)_3C$—.

b. acetate a liquid compound, used in the manufacture of lacquer, artificial leather, photographic film, plastics, and safety glass; it is an irritant which may cause conjunctivitis, and is narcotic in high concentrations.

b. aminobenzoate butamben.

b. formate an industrial solvent, the vapors of which are powerfully lacrimatory and suffocating.

bu·ty·lat·ed hy·droxy·an·isole (BHA) (bu′tə-la″təd hi-drok″se-an′ĭ-sōl) [NF] an antioxidant used in foods, cosmetics, and pharmaceuticals that contain fats or oils.

bu·ty·lat·ed hy·droxy·tol·u·ene (BHT) (bu′tə-la″təd hi-drok″se-tol′u-ēn) [NF] an antioxidant used in foods, cosmetics, pharmaceuticals, and petroleum products.

bu·ty·lene (bu′tə-lēn) a gaseous hydrocarbon, C_4H_8.

bu·tyl·par·a·ben (bu″təl-par′ə-ben) [NF] an antifungal compound, closely related to ethylparaben, methylparaben, and propylparaben; used as a preservative in pharmaceutic preparations.

bu·ty·ra·ceous (bu″tə-ra′shəs) of a buttery consistency.

bu·ty·rate (bu′tə-rāt) a salt, ester, or anionic form of butyric acid.

bu·ty·rate–CoA li·gase (bu′tə-rāt ko-a′ li′gās) [EC 6.2.1.2] an enzyme of the ligase class that catalyzes the formation of acyl coenzyme A from medium chain length fatty acids (4 to 12 carbons) and coenzyme A, using energy derived from ATP hydrolysis. The enzyme occurs in the mitochondrial matrix and acts on saturated and unsaturated fatty acids as well as on some hydroxy acids.

bu·tyr·ic ac·id (bu-tēr′ik) 1. any four-carbon carboxylic acid, either *n*-butyric acid or isobutyric acid. 2. *n*-butyric acid, a saturated four-carbon fatty acid occurring in butter, particularly rancid butter, and in much animal fat. Systematic name: *butanoic acid.*

bu·ty·rin (bu′tər-in) tributyrin.

bu·ty·rine (bu′tə-rēn) an amino acid derivative of butyric acid; it is α-amino butyric acid.

Bu·ty·ri·vib·rio (bu-tir″ĭ-vib′re-o) [L. *butyricus* butyric + *vibrio*] a genus of gram-negative, non–spore-forming, anaerobic bacteria of the family Lachnospiraceae, found in the rumen contents of animals, and consisting of motile curved rods that may be in chains or filaments. The type species is *B. fibrosol′vens.*

butyr(o)- [Gr. *boutyron* butter] a combining form denoting relationship to butter, or to butyric acid.

bu·ty·roid (bu′tə-roid) [*butyr-* + *-oid*] resembling or having the consistency of butter.

γ-bu·ty·ro·lac·tone (bu″tə-ro-lak′tōn) a prodrug of γ-hydroxybutyric acid, used as an industrial solvent; when consumed it has sedative and depressant qualities similar to those of γ-hydroxybutyric acid, so that it is a drug of abuse.

bu·ty·ro·phe·none (bu″tə-ro-fe′nōn) any of a class of structurally related antipsychotic agents; the prototype is haloperidol.

bu·ty·rous (bu′tə-rəs) like butter; having a butterlike appearance.

bu·ty·ryl (bu′tə-rəl) the radical of *n*-butyric acid.

bu·ty·ryl CoA syn·the·tase (bu′tə-rəl ko-a′ sin′thə-tās) butyrate–CoA ligase.

BVAD biventricular assist device.

By·et·ta (bi-a′tə) trademark for a preparation of exenatide.

By·ler disease (bi′lər) [*Byler*, name of the original Amish propositus family] progressive familial intrahepatic cholestasis; see under *cholestasis.*

by·pass (bi′pas) 1. an auxiliary channel, such as around a blocked segment in the circulatory system or alimentary tract; see also *shunt* (def. 2). 2. surgical creation of such a channel.

aortobifemoral b. aortofemoral bypass involving both femoral arteries.

aortocoronary b. coronary artery b.

aortofemoral b. insertion of a vascular prosthesis from the aorta to the femoral artery as a passage around atherosclerotic occlusions in the aorta and the iliac artery.

aortofemoral b., thoracic insertion of a vascular prosthesis from the thoracic aorta to the femoral artery, with femorofemoral bypass, as a passage around aortoiliac occlusion in patients in whom the abdominal aorta is unsuitable for grafting.

aortoiliac b. insertion of a vascular prosthesis from the abdominal aorta to the iliac artery as a passage around intervening atherosclerotic segments.

aortorenal b. a technique of renal revascularization involving insertion of a section of saphenous vein, hypogastric artery, or suitable substitute between the aorta and renal artery as a passage around occluded or stenotic segments.

aortosubclavian b. insertion of a vascular prosthesis from the aorta to a subclavian artery, serving as a passage around an occluded segment in or around their junction.

axillary-axillary b. insertion of a vascular prosthesis between the axillary arteries, passing over the sternum, serving as a passage around occluded or stenosed segments.

axillobifemoral b. an axillofemoral bypass combined with a femorofemoral bypass.

axillofemoral b. an extra-anatomic bypass consisting of a vascular prosthesis or section of saphenous vein extending from the axillary artery to the femoral artery on the same side; done to relieve lower limb ischemia in patients in whom normal anatomic placement of a graft is contraindicated, as by abdominal infection or aortic aneurysm.

axillopopliteal b. an extra-anatomic bypass consisting of a vascular prosthesis extending from the axillary artery to the popliteal artery to relieve lower limb ischemia in patients in whom the femoral artery is unsuitable for axillofemoral bypass.

biliopancreatic b. see under *diversion.*

cardiopulmonary b. diversion of the flow of blood to the heart directly to the aorta, via a pump-oxygenator, avoiding both the heart and the lungs; a form of extracorporeal circulation used in heart surgery.

carotid-carotid b. insertion of a vascular prosthesis from the left carotid to the right carotid artery, serving as a passage around an occluded or stenosed portion of the brachiocephalic trunk.

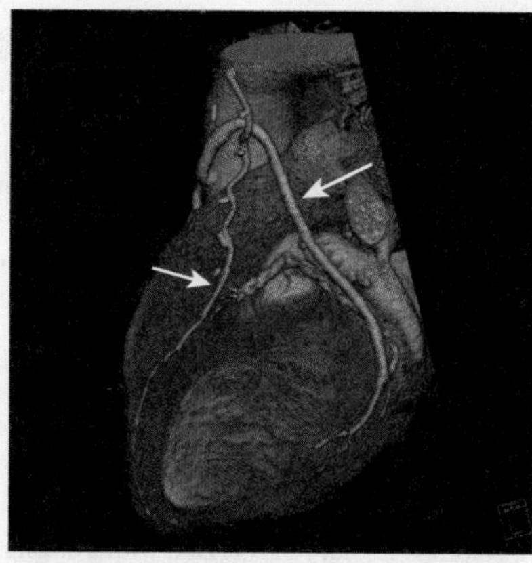

■ Coronary artery bypass. Three-dimensional reconstruction showing arterial bypass graft to the anterior interventricular branch of left coronary artery *(left arrow)* and venous graft to the circumflex branch of left coronary artery *(right arrow)*. A venous graft to the right coronary artery is not visible in this view.

carotid-subclavian b. insertion of a vascular prosthesis from the subclavian artery to the common carotid artery as a passage around occluded or stenotic segments of either artery.

coronary b., coronary artery b. a section of vein or other conduit grafted between the aorta and a coronary artery to circumvent an obstructive lesion in the coronary artery; called also *aortocoronary b.*

EC/IC b. extracranial/intracranial b.

extra-anatomic b. an arterial bypass that does not follow the normal anatomic pathway, such as an axillofemoral or axillopopliteal bypass.

extracranial/intracranial b. anastomosis of the superficial temporal artery to a branch of the middle cerebral artery on the brain surface to improve collateral blood flow that has been reduced by occlusion or stenosis of the internal carotid or middle cerebral artery. Called also *EC/IC b.*

femorofemoral b. insertion of a vascular prosthesis between the femoral arteries as a passage around an occluded or injured iliac artery.

femorofemoropopliteal b. insertion of a vascular prosthesis, or of a vascular prosthesis anastomosed to a section of saphenous vein, between the popliteal artery and the contralateral femoral artery as a passage around occluded, stenotic, or injured iliac and femoral arteries.

femoropopliteal b. insertion of a vascular prosthesis from the femoral to the popliteal artery as a passage around occluded, narrowed, or injured segments.

gastric b. a surgical treatment for morbid obesity consisting of gastrojejunostomy with partitioning of the stomach high on its body and joining of the proximal remnant to a loop of jejunum in end-to-side anastomosis.

hepatorenal b. a technique of renal revascularization involving insertion of a vascular prosthesis between the common hepatic artery and the renal artery, serving as a passage around an occluded segment of renal artery.

iliofemoral b. insertion of a vascular prosthesis from the iliac artery to the femoral artery, serving as a passage around an occluded or stenosed segment.

iliorenal b. a technique of renal revascularization involving insertion of a saphenous vein graft between an iliac artery and a renal artery to serve as a passage around an occluded segment of renal artery.

infrainguinal b. any of the bypass procedures connecting arteries of the lower limb, including femorofemoral, femoropopliteal, iliofemoral, and inframalleolar bypasses.

inframalleolar b. insertion of a vascular prosthesis in arteries of the foot to serve as a passage around an occluded or stenotic segment.

infrapopliteal b. a bypass procedure connecting arteries below the knee.

intestinal b. surgical treatment for morbid obesity consisting of rerouting of intestine, with anastomosis of a proximal to a distal portion, as in jejunoileal bypass or Roux-en-Y gastric bypass.

jejunal b., jejunoileal b. a formerly common type of intestinal bypass for morbid obesity, consisting of anastomosis of the proximal part of the jejunum to the distal part of the ileum so as to circumvent much of the small intestine and reduce intestinal absorption. Called also *jejunoileostomy.*

left heart b. diversion of the flow of blood from the pulmonary veins directly to the aorta, avoiding the left atrium and the left ventricle.

obturator b., obturator foramen b. an extra-anatomic type of iliofemoral bypass in which the graft passes through the obturator foramen; used when trauma or infection makes it necessary to avoid the femoral triangle.

partial b. the deviation of only a portion of blood flowing through an artery.

partial ileal b. a treatment for hyperlipidemia or morbid obesity, consisting of anastomosis of the proximal end of the transected ileum to the cecum; the bypass of the portion of the small intestine results in decreased intestinal absorption and increased fecal excretion of cholesterol.

right heart b. diversion of the flow of blood from the entrance of the right atrium directly to the pulmonary arteries, avoiding the right atrium and right ventricle.

Roux-en-Y gastric b. a treatment for morbid obesity consisting of surgical division of the small intestine to form two arms; the jejunum is attached to a stoma into a gastric pouch and the bypassed duodenum connects the pylorus with an end-to-side anastomosis into the lower jejunum.

splenorenal b. a technique of renal revascularization involving creation of a vascular prosthesis from the splenic artery to replace the occluded renal artery.

stomach b. gastric b.

by-prod·uct (by′prod′əkt) a secondary product obtained during the manufacture of a primary product.

bys·sa·ceous (bĭ-sa′shəs) [Gr. *byssos* flax] composed of fine flaxlike threads.

bys·si·no·sis (bis″ĭ-no′sis) [Gr. *byssos* flax + *-osis*] a pulmonary disease seen in cotton textile workers and preparers of flax and soft hemp, due to inhalation of textile dust. Two forms are distinguished, *acute* and *chronic b.* Called also *brown lung, cotton-dust asthma,* and *stripper's asthma.*

acute b. byssinosis occurring in those who return to work after a weekend or other time away, marked by tightness of the chest, wheezing, and cough. See also *mill fever*, under *fever.*

chronic b. byssinosis in workers who have had years of exposure to textile dust, marked by permanent dyspnea, probably due to smooth muscle contraction after histamine release induced by chemicals in the dust.

bys·si·not·ic (bis″ĭ-not′ik) 1. pertaining to byssinosis. 2. a person affected with byssinosis.

bys·soid (bis′oid) [Gr. *byssos* flax + *-oid*] made up of a fringe, the filaments of which are unequal in length.

by·stand·er (bi′stan-dər) that which is only incidentally involved in a process.

innocent b. a tissue cell that is lysed because it is in close proximity to the actual target of lysis, rather than itself being a target.

Bys·tol·ic (bis-tol′ik) trademark for a preparation of nebivolol.

Byth·nia (bith′ne-ah) *Bithynia.*

By·wa·ters syndrome (bi′wah-tərz) [Eric George Lapthorne *Bywaters*, British physician, 1910–2003] see under *syndrome.*

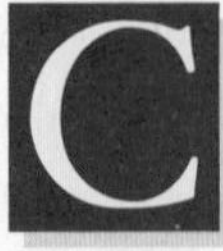

C canine (see under *tooth*); carbon (molecular carbon atoms are frequently designated C1, C2, C3, etc., or α-C, β-C, etc., beginning from one end or other standard reference point); large calorie; cathode; Celsius (see under *scale*); cervical vertebrae (C1 through C7); clonus; closure; complement (numbered C1 through C9, see *complement* for additional symbols); compliance (subscripts denote the structure, e.g., C_L lung compliance); contraction; coulomb; cylinder; cylindrical lens; cytidine or cytosine.

C capacitance; clearance (subscripts denote the substance, e.g., C_I or C_{In}, inulin clearance); heat capacity.

C_H see *constant region*, under *region*.

C_L see *constant region*, under *region*.

°C degree Celsius; see *Celsius scale*, under *scale*.

c small calorie; centi-.

c. [L.] ci′bus (food); cum (with).

c molar concentration; specific heat capacity; the velocity of light in a vacuum.

c̄ [L.] cum (with).

χ chi, the twenty-second letter of the Greek alphabet.

χ^2 chi-square; see under *distribution* and *test*.

CA cardiac arrest; chronologic age; cold agglutinin; coronary artery; croup-associated (virus).

CA1–4 four divisions of the cornu region of the hippocampus, CA1–3 composing the hippocampus proper and C4 adjacent to it, just within the dentate gyrus. See figure at *hippocampus*.

CA 125 cancer antigen 125.

Ca calcium.

ca [L.] cir′ca (about).

CA_2 a colloid antigen lacking iodine, the second most common antigen in thyroid colloid (the first being thyroglobulin); the presence in serum of antibodies against CA_2 is a sign of autoimmune disorders such as Hashimoto disease.

Ca^{2+}-ATP•ase (a-te-pe′ās) a membrane-bound enzyme that hydrolyzes ATP to provide the energy necessary to drive the cellular calcium pump (q.v.). See also *adenosinetriphosphatase*. In EC nomenclature, called *Ca^{2+}-transporting ATPase*.

ca•ber•go•line (kə-bur′go-lēn) a dopamine receptor agonist used in the treatment of disorders characterized by hyperprolactinemia; administered orally.

CABG coronary artery bypass graft; see under *bypass*.

ca•ble (ka′bəl) a strong rope usually made of steel, sometimes of braided wires.

Bowden c., control c. a thin cable enclosed in a casing, originally made for bicycles but now widely used in prosthetic and orthotic devices for the upper limb.

Cab•ot ring bodies (kab′ət) [Richard Clarke *Cabot*, American physician, 1868–1939] see under *body*.

cab•u•fo•con (kab″u-fo′kon) chemical name: cellulose acetate butanoate; either of two hydrophobic contact lens materials, designated A or B.

ca•cao (kə-ka′o) [Nahuatl *cacahuatl*] 1. *Theobroma cacao*. 2. the seeds of *T. cacao*, used in making chocolate, cocoa, and cocoa butter; called also *cocoa beans* and *cacao beans*.

Cac•chi-Ric•ci disease (kah′ke re′che) [Roberto *Cacchi*, Italian physician, 20th century; Vincenzo *Ricci*, Italian physician, 20th century] medullary sponge kidney; see under *kidney*.

ca•chet (kă-sha′) [Fr.] a disk-shaped wafer or capsule for enclosing a dose of medicine.

ca•chex•ia (kə-kek′se-ə) [*cac-* + Gr. *hexis* habit + *-ia*] a profound and marked state of constitutional disorder; general ill health and malnutrition. **cachec′tic** *adj*

cancer c. anorexia-cachexia syndrome in cancer patients.

cardiac c. emaciation due to heart disease, usually caused by a combination of increased caloric expenditure and decreased caloric intake or utilization.

hypophysial c. see *panhypopituitarism*.

c. hypophysiopri′va the train of symptoms resulting from total deprivation of function of the pituitary gland, including phthisis, loss of sexual function, atrophy of the pituitary target glands, bradycardia, hypothermia, apathy, and coma.

malarial c. a group of physical signs of a chronic nature that result from antecedent attacks of severe malaria; the principal signs are anemia, sallow skin, yellow sclera, splenomegaly, hepatomegaly, and, in children, retardation of body growth and puberty.

pituitary c. see *panhypopituitarism*.

rheumatoid c. loss of body cell mass, particularly in skeletal muscles, in persons with rheumatoid arthritis; it is masked in many patients because they may gain weight owing to decreased activity or other complications.

cach•in•na•tion (kak″ĭ-na′shən) [L. *cachinnare* to laugh aloud] immoderate, loud, and inappropriate laughter; commonly seen in disorganized schizophrenia.

cac(o)- [Gr. *kakos* bad] a combining form meaning bad, or ill.

caco•de•mono•ma•nia (kak″o-de″mon-o-ma′ne-ə) a condition marked by delusions of being possessed by evil spirits.

cac•o•dyl (kak′o-dəl) [*caco-* + Gr. *ozein* to smell + *hylē* matter] tetramethylbiarsine, a colorless liquid arsenic-containing compound, $(CH_3)_2As—As(CH_3)_2$, with an offensive odor; it gives off a poisonous vapor and is inflammable when exposed to air.

c. cyanide a white powder, $(CH_3)_2AsCN$, which, when exposed to air, gives off an extremely poisonous vapor.

c. hydride a colorless liquid, $(CH_3)_2AsH$, with a strong, garlicky odor; on exposure to air, it gives off a poisonous vapor and ignites spontaneously. Symptoms of poisoning are the same as those of arsenic poisoning.

cac•o•dyl•ate (kak′o-dəl-āt) a salt of cacodylic acid; the cacodylates were formerly used medicinally but release arsenic compounds when they metabolize, causing symptoms of arsenic poisoning.

cac•o•dyl•ic ac•id (kak″o-dil′ik) dimethylarsinic acid, a highly toxic herbicide.

caco•gen•e•sis (kak″o-jen′ə-sis) [*caco-* + *-genesis*] dysgenesis.

caco•geu•sia (kak″o-goo′zhə) [*caco-* + Gr. *geusis* taste + *-ia*] a parageusia consisting of bad taste not related to the ingestion of specific substances, or associated with gustatory stimuli usually considered to be pleasant.

caco•me•lia (kak″o-me′le-ə) dysmelia.

cac•os•mia (kak-oz′me-ə) [*caco-* + *osm-*[1] + *-ia*] a parosmia consisting of bad smell not related to exposure to a specific odor, or associated with olfactory stimuli usually considered to be pleasant.

CAD coronary artery disease; chronic actinic dermatitis.

ca•dav•er (kə-dav′ər) [L., from *cadere* to fall, to perish] a dead body; generally applied to a human body preserved for anatomical study. Cf. *corpse*. **cadav′eric** *adj*

ca•dav•er•ine (kə-dav′ər-in) [L. *cadaver* corpse] a foul-smelling nitrogenous base, pentamethylenediamine, produced by decarboxylation of lysine. It is produced in decaying protein material by the action of bacteria, particularly species of *Vibrio*.

ca•dav•er•ous (kə-dav′ər-əs) resembling a cadaver.

cad•dis (kad′is) see under *fly*.

cad•he•rin (kad-hēr′in) any of a family of over 80 calcium-dependent cell adhesion molecules, having in common the CAD domain of about 115 residues. Typically, they have 5 extracellular CAD domains (7 for protocadherins) connected to an intracellular C-terminal by a single hydrophobic sequence. Cell adhesion is by homophilic interaction.

cad•mi•o•sis (kad″me-o′sis) pneumoconiosis due to inhalation of and tissue reaction to cadmium dust. Cf. *cadmium lung*.

cad•mi•um (Cd) (kad′me-əm) [Gr. *kadmia* earth] a bivalent metal, similar to tin in appearance and properties; atomic number 48, atomic weight 112.40. Cadmium and its salts are poisonous; see *cadmium poisoning*, *cadmiosis*, and *cadmium lung*.

c. bromide $CdBr_2$, a compound used in photography, process engraving, and lithography; when swallowed it causes cadmium poisoning.

ca•du•ce•us (kə-doo′shəs) [L., from Gr. *karykeion*, herald's staff] the winged staff of Hermes or Mercury, the messenger of the gods, with two snakes winding around it. Used as a medical symbol and as the emblem of the Medical Corps, U.S. Army. The official symbol of the medical profession is the staff of Aesculapius.

ca•du•cous (kə-doo′kəs) [L. *cadere* to fall] falling off; deciduous.

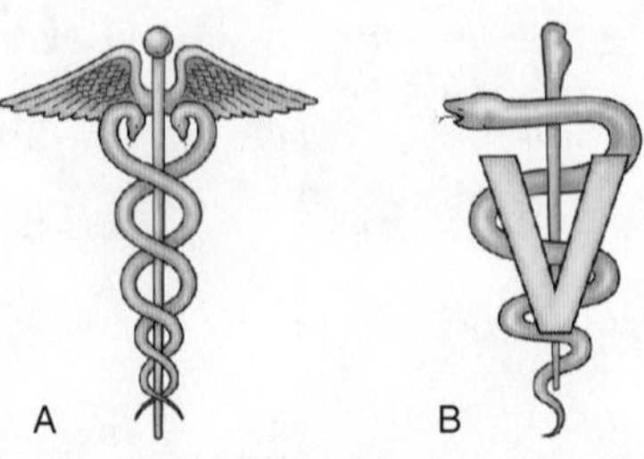

■ Caduceus. *(A)*, United States Army Medical Corps; *(B)*, American Veterinary Medicine Association.

Cad•u•et (kad′o͞o-ət) trademark for a combination preparation of amlodipine besylate and atorvastatin calcium.

cae- for words beginning thus, see those beginning *ce-*.

caec(o)- for words beginning thus, see also those beginning *cec(o)-*.

cae•cum (se′kəm) [L.] 1. a blind pouch or cul-de-sac. 2. [TA] the first part of the large intestine, forming a dilated pouch into which open the ileum, colon, and vermiform appendix. Spelled also *cecum.*

cupular c. of cochlear duct, c. cupula′re duc′tus cochlea′ris [TA] the closed blind apical end of the cochlear duct.

vestibular c. of cochlear duct, c. vestibula′re duc′tus cochlea′ris [TA] a small blind outpouching at the vestibular end of the cochlear duct.

cae•ru•le•us (sə-roo′le-əs) [L. "dark blue," "azure," probably from *caelum* sky] blue; azure; cerulean. Written also *ceruleus* and *coeruleus* (q.v.).

cae•sa•re•an (sə-za′re-ən) cesarean.

Caf•cit (kaf′sit) trademark for preparations of caffeine citrate.

Caf•er•got (kaf′ər-got) trademark for combination preparations of ergotamine tartrate and caffeine.

caf•feine (kă-fēn′, kaf′ēn) [Ger. *Kaffein,* from *Kaffee* coffee] [USP] one of the methylxanthines (q.v.), soluble in water and alcohol, and obtainable from coffee, tea, guarana, and maté. It stimulates the central nervous system, especially the cerebrum; has a diuretic effect on the kidneys; stimulates striated muscle; and has a group of effects on the cardiovascular system. It is used as a central nervous system stimulant, in combination with ergotamine in the treatment of vascular headache, as an adjunct to enhance pain relief in combination with analgesics, and as an adjunct in the treatment of neonatal apnea; administered orally. Ingestion of excessive amounts can cause caffeinism (q.v.). Called also *guaranine* and *methyltheobromine.*

c. benzoate a salt used as an accelerator for the conversion of unconjugated bilirubin to azobilirubin in the Jendrassik-Grof method for determining total bilirubin.

c. citrate, citrated c. a preparation of equal parts of caffeine and citric acid, used as a central nervous system stimulant and as an adjunct in the treatment of neonatal apnea; administered orally or intravenously.

caf•fein•ism (kaf′ēn-iz-əm) a morbid condition resulting from ingestion of excessive amounts of caffeine; characteristics include insomnia, restlessness, excitement, tachycardia, tremors, and diuresis.

Caf•fey disease (kaf′e) [John Patrick *Caffey,* American pediatrician, 1895–1978] infantile cortical hyperostosis.

cage (kāj) a box or enclosure.

rib c., thoracic c. skeleton thoracis.

CAH congenital adrenal hyperplasia.

cain(o)- see *cen(o)-¹*.

CAIS complete androgen insensitivity syndrome.

Ca•jal bodies, etc. (kah-hahl′) [Santiago Ramón y *Cajal,* Spanish physician, histologist, and Nobel prize winner, 1852–1934] see under *body* and *cell,* see *nucleus interstitialis,* and see *Stains and Staining Methods,* under *stain.*

caj•e•put (kaj′ə-poot) [Malay *kayu puteh* white tree] *Melaleuca leucadendron.*

caj•e•pu•tol (kaj′e-pu-tol) eucalyptol.

caj•u•put (kaj′ə-poot) *Melaleuca leucadendron.*

Cal large calorie (kilocalorie).

cal calorie.

Cal•a•bar bean, swellings (edema) (kal′ə-bahr) [*Calabar,* city and river in southeastern Nigeria] see under *bean* and *swelling.*

cal•a•mine (kal′ə-mīn) 1. [USP] a pink powder used as a mild astringent and skin protectant, consisting of zinc oxide with a small proportion of ferric oxide; applied topically. 2. a similar preparation containing zinc carbonate instead of zinc oxide.

cal•a•mus (kal′ə-məs) [L. "reed"] a reedlike structure.

c. scripto′rius the lowest portion of the floor of the fourth ventricle, shaped like a pen when viewed from the dorsal side and situated between the restiform bodies.

Cal•an (kal′an) trademark for preparations of verapamil hydrochloride.

cal•ca•ne•itis (kal-ka″ne-i′tis) inflammation of the calcaneus.

calcane(o)- [L. *calcaneus,* q.v.] a combining form denoting relationship to the calcaneus.

cal•ca•neo•apoph•y•si•tis (kal-ka″ne-o-ə-pof″ə-si′tis) an affection of the posterior part of the calcaneus marked by pain at the point of insertion of the Achilles tendon, with swelling of the soft parts.

cal•ca•neo•as•trag•a•loid (kal-ka″ne-o-ə-strag′ə-loid) talocalcaneal.

cal•ca•neo•ca•vus (kal-ka″ne-o-ka′vəs) see under *talipes.*

cal•ca•neo•cu•boid (kal-ka″ne-o-ku′boid) pertaining to the calcaneus and the cuboid bone.

cal•ca•ne•odyn•ia (kal-ka″ne-o-din′e-ə) pain in the heel, or calcaneus.

cal•ca•neo•fib•u•lar (kal-ka″ne-o-fib′u-lər) pertaining to the calcaneus and fibula.

cal•ca•neo•na•vic•u•lar (kal-ka″ne-o-nə-vik′u-lər) pertaining to the calcaneus and the navicular bone.

cal•ca•neo•plan•tar (kal-ka″ne-o-plan′tər) pertaining to the calcaneus and the sole of the foot.

cal•ca•neo•scaph•oid (kal-ka″ne-o-skaf′oid) calcaneonavicular.

cal•ca•neo•tib•i•al (kal-ka″ne-o-tib′e-əl) pertaining to the calcaneus and tibia; called also *tibiocalcanean.*

cal•ca•neo•val•go•ca•vus (kal-ka″ne-o-val″go-ka′vəs) clubfoot in which talipes calcaneus, talipes valgus, and talipes cavus are combined.

cal•ca•ne•um (kal-ka′ne-əm) pl. *calca′nea* [L.] calcaneus.

cal•ca•ne•us (kal-ka′ne-əs) pl. *calca′nei* [L., from *calx* heel] 1. [TA] the irregular quadrangular bone at the back of the tarsus; called also *calcaneal bone, calcaneum, heel bone, os calcis,* and *os tarsi fibulare.* 2. talipes calcaneus. calca′neal *adj*

cal•car (kal′kər) [L. "spur"] 1. spur. 2. a structure resembling a spur.

c. a′vis [TA] calcarine spur: an eminence on the medial wall of the occipital horn of the lateral ventricle, below the bulb of the occipital horn, produced by the impression of the calcarine sulcus on the ventricular wall.

c. femora′le the plate of strong tissue which strengthens the neck of the femur.

c. pe′dis heel.

c. scle′rae [TA] scleral spur: the posterior lip of the venous sinus of the sclera to which most of the fibers of the trabecular reticulum of the iridocorneal angle and the meridional fibers of the ciliary muscle are attached; called also *scleral roll.*

cal•car•e•ous (kal-kar′e-əs) [L. *calcarius*] pertaining to or containing lime or calcium; chalky.

cal•ca•rine (kal′kə-rīn) [L. *calcarinus* spur-shaped] 1. spur-shaped. 2. pertaining to a calcar.

cal•ca•ri•uria (kal-ka″re-u′re-ə) [L. *calcarius* containing lime + *-uria*] the presence of lime (calcium salts) in the urine; see *hypercalciuria.*

cal•ca•roid (kal′kə-roid) resembling calcium; a term given to certain deposits in cerebral tissue which resemble calcification but do not give a specific reaction for calcium.

cal•ce•mia (kal-se′me-ə) [*calci-* + *-emia*] hypercalcemia.

calc(i)- [L. *calx,* gen. *calcis* lime] a combining form denoting relationship to calcium or calcium salts.

cal•ci•bil•ia (kal″sĭ-bil′e-ə) the presence of calcium in the bile.

Cal•ci•bind (kal′sĭ-bīnd) trademark for a preparation of cellulose sodium phosphate.

cal•cic (kal′sik) of or pertaining to lime or to calcium.

cal•ci•co•sil•i•co•sis (kal″sĭ-ko-sil″ĭ-ko′sis) a type of mixed dust pneumoconiosis due to the inhalation of mineral dust containing silica and calcium-containing minerals such as lime, limestone, or marble.

cal•ci•co•sis (kal″sĭ-ko′sis) [*calci-* + *-osis*] pneumoconiosis resulting from the inhalation of dust containing calcium, such as from lime, limestone, or marble.

cal•ci•di•ol (kal″sĭ-di′ol) 25-hydroxycholecalciferol.

cal•cif•e•di•ol (kal″sif–ədi′ol) 1. 25-hydroxycholecalciferol. 2. [USP] a preparation of this compound, used in the treatment of hypocalcemia, hypophosphatemia, rickets, and osteodystrophy associated with various medical conditions including chronic renal failure and hypoparathyroidism; administered orally.

Cal•cif•er•ol (kal-sif′ər-ol) trademark for preparations of ergocalciferol.

cal•cif•er•ol (kal-sif′ər-ol) 1. a compound having vitamin D activity, e.g., cholecalciferol or ergocalciferol. 2. ergocalciferol.

cal•cif•ic (kal-sif′ik) forming lime.

cal•ci•fi•ca•tion (kal″sĭ-fĭ-ka′shən) [*calci-* + L. *facere* to make] the process by which organic tissue becomes hardened by a deposit of calcium salts within its substance. See also *calcinosis.*

dystrophic c. the deposition of calcium in abnormal locations, such as scar tissue or atherosclerotic plaques, but without abnormalities of blood calcium. See also *calcinosis.*

eggshell c. deposition of a thin layer of calcium around a thoracic lymph node, often seen in silicosis.

metastatic c. the deposition of calcium in vital tissues as a result of elevations in calcium and phosphate levels in the blood and tissue fluids.

Mönckeberg c. see under *arteriosclerosis.*

popcorn c. calcification that resembles a ball of popcorn, seen in cases of hamartomatous nodules of the lungs.

cal·cig·er·ous (kal-sij′ər-əs) [*calci-* + L. *gerere* to bear] producing or carrying calcium salts.

Cal·ci·jex (kal′sĭ-jeks) trademark for a preparation of calcitriol.

Cal·ci·mar (kal′sĭ-mahr) trademark for a preparation of calcitonin-salmon.

cal·ci·mi·met·ic (kal″se-mĭ-met′ik) 1. increasing the body's response to extracellular calcium, such as by increasing the ability of receptors in the parathyroid glands to respond to calcium. 2. an agent that increases the body's response to extracellular calcium.

cal·ci·na·tion (kal″sĭ-na′shən) [L. *calcinare* to char] the process of reducing to a dry powder by heat.

cal·cine (kal′sin) to reduce to a dry powder by heat.

cal·ci·neur·in (kal″sĭ-noor′in) a protein phosphatase that is specific for serine and threonine; it binds calmodulin and plays an important role in activation of T cells. See also *calcineurin inhibitor*, under *inhibitor.*

cal·ci·no·sis (kal″sĭ-no′sis) dystrophic calcification in various tissues of the body. Called also *Thibierge-Weissenbach syndrome.*

c. circumscrip′ta localized dystrophic calcifications with small nodules in subcutaneous tissues or muscle, seen in conditions such as systemic scleroderma or dermatomyositis.

c. cu′tis dystrophic calcifications in the skin in the form of nodules or plaques.

enzootic c. a chronic condition in ruminants caused by plant poisoning or mineral imbalance; symptoms include calcification of soft tissues, joint inflammation, diarrhea, and emaciation. Plants causing it include *Cestrum diurnum;* several species of *Solanum,* especially *S. malacoxylon;* and *Trisetum flavescens.* Called also *enteque* and *Manchester wasting disease.*

c. intervertebra′lis dystrophic calcifications in one or more intervertebral disks; called also *chondritis intervertebralis calcanea* and *Verse disease.*

tumoral c. development of large dystrophic calcifications around the joints of the shoulder, elbow, and hip, marked by symptoms such as sciatica due to pressure on adjacent nerves. It is of unknown etiology, with onset usually in the first or second decade of life.

c. universa′lis widespread dystrophic calcifications in the dermis, panniculus, and muscles, in the form of nodules or plaques, most often in young girls along with dermatomyositis.

cal·cio·ki·ne·sis (kal″se-o-kĭ-ne′sis) mobilization of calcium stored in the body. **calciokinet′ic** *adj*

cal·ci·or·rha·chia (kal″se-o-ra′ke-ə) [*calcio-* + *rhachi-* + *-ia*] the presence of calcium in the spinal fluid.

cal·ci·pe·nia (kal″sĭ-pe′ne-ə) [*calci-* + *-penia*] deficiency of calcium; called also *hypocalcia.* See also *hypocalcemia.* **calcipe′nic** *adj*

cal·ci·pex·is (kal″sĭ-pek′sis) calcipexy.

cal·ci·pexy (kal′sĭ-pek″se) [*calci-* + *-pexy*] fixation of calcium in the tissues of the organism. **calcipec′tic, calcipex′ic** *adj*

cal·ci·phil·ia (kal″sĭ-fil′e-ə) [*calci-* + *-philia*] a tendency to absorb calcium salts from the blood and thus to become calcified.

cal·ci·phy·lac·tic (kal″sĭ-fə-lak′tik) pertaining to or characterized by calciphylaxis.

cal·ci·phy·lax·is (kal″sĭ-fə-lak′sis) 1. a condition of induced hypersensitivity characterized by formation of calcified tissue in response to administration of a challenging agent. 2. calcific uremic arteriolopathy.

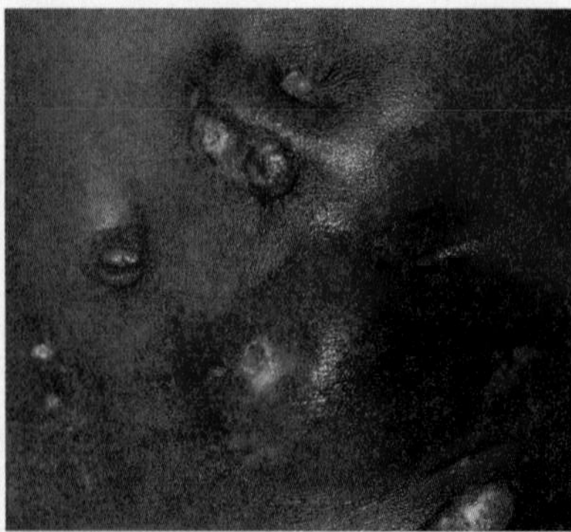

■ Calcinosis cutis on the abdomen of a child with dermatomyositis.

systemic c. a rare syndrome of rapidly progressive ischemic necrosis of skin and soft tissue secondary to calcific uremic arteriolopathy, seen in end-stage renal disease.

topical c. the formation of a circumscribed area of calcification in response to subcutaneous injection of the challenging agent.

cal·ci·po·tri·ene (kal″sĭ-po-tri′ēn) a synthetic derivative of vitamin D_3 (cholecalciferol), applied topically as an antipsoriatic.

cal·ci·po·tri·ol (kal-sĭ-po′tre-ol) INN and BAN for calcipotriene.

cal·ci·priv·ia (kal″sĭ-priv′e-ə) [*calci-* + L. *privus* without + *-ia*] deprivation or loss of calcium; see also *hypocalcemia.* **calcipri′vic** *adj*

Cal·ci·tite (kal′sĭ-tīt) trademark for hydroxylapatite.

cal·ci·to·nin (kal″sĭ-to′nin) a 32-amino-acid polypeptide hormone elaborated by the parafollicular cells of the thyroid gland in response to hypercalcemia; it lowers plasma calcium and phosphate levels, inhibits bone resorption, and acts as an antagonist to parathyroid hormone. It is secreted in lower vertebrates by the ultimobranchial bodies. Called also *thyrocalcitonin.*

c.-human, c. (human) a synthetic polypeptide having the same amino acid sequence as calcitonin naturally occurring in humans; administered by subcutaneous injection in the treatment of osteitis deformans and as an adjunct in the treatment of postmenopausal osteoporosis and hypercalcemia.

c.-salmon, c. (salmon) a polypeptide originally obtained from salmon but now also prepared synthetically, its amino acid sequence differing slightly from that of human origin; it has the same actions and uses as calcitonin-human, administered intranasally or by subcutaneous or intramuscular injection.

cal·ci·tri·ol (kal″sĭ-tri′ol) 1. 1,25-dihydroxycholecalciferol. 2. a preparation of this compound, used in the treatment of hypocalcemia, hypophosphatemia, rickets, and osteodystrophy associated with a variety of disorders, such as chronic renal failure and hypoparathyroidism. Administered orally or intravenously.

cal·ci·um (Ca) (kal′se-əm) [L. *calx* lime] a silvery yellow metal, the basic element of lime. Atomic number, 20; atomic weight, 40.08. It is found in nearly all organized tissues, being the most abundant mineral in the body. In combination with phosphorus it forms calcium phosphate, the dense, hard material of the teeth and bones. It is an essential dietary element, a constant blood calcium level being essential for the maintenance of the normal heartbeat, and for the normal functioning of nerves and muscles. It also plays a role in multiple phases of blood coagulation (in which it is called *coagulation factor IV*) and in many enzymatic processes.

c. 45 see *radiocalcium.*

c. 47 see *radiocalcium.*

c. acetate [USP] the calcium salt of acetic acid; administered orally as a source of calcium and as a phosphate binder. Also used as a pharmaceutical buffering agent.

c. ascorbate [USP] ascorbic acid calcium salt, used as a source of vitamin C (ascorbic acid) in nutritional supplements.

c. bilirubinate a salt consisting of calcium complexed with bilirubin, a major component of brown and black gallstones.

c. carbimide c. cyanamide.

c. carbonate 1. a compound, $CaCO_3$, occurring naturally in a variety of sources, including bones, shells, and limestone. It is used chiefly as an antacid and as a calcium supplement in its native form (see also *chalk*), and is also used in several purified forms; see *precipitated c. carbonate* and *prepared c. carbonate.* 2. [USP] official terminology for *precipitated c. carbonate.*

c. chloride [USP] a salt, $CaCl_2$, used as a calcium replenisher in the treatment of hypocalcemia and of electrolyte depletion, in the treatment of hyperkalemia, and as a treatment adjunct in cardiac arrest and in magnesium poisoning; administered intravenously.

c. citrate [USP] a calcium replenisher administered orally in the treatment and prophylaxis of hypocalcemia; also used in the treatment of hyperphosphatemia in renal osteodystrophy.

citrated c. carbimide a mixture containing calcium cyanamide (calcium carbimide) and citric acid; an antialcoholic. See also *c. cyanamide.*

c. cyanamide a compound, $CaCN_2$, which inhibits one or more of the enzymes required for oxidation of acetaldehyde formed from alcohol; used as a fertilizer, defoliant, herbicide, and pesticide. Drinking of alcohol after inhalation or ingestion of calcium cyanamide causes unpleasant symptoms (see *mal rouge*); thus it has been used to treat alcoholism, usually in a mixture with citric acid *(citrated c. carbimide).* Called also *c. carbimide* and *cyanamide.*

c. cyclamate cyclamate calcium; see *cyclamate.*

dibasic c. phosphate [USP] $CaHPO_4 \cdot 2H_2O$, used as a calcium supplement and as a base in preparation of tablets; it occurs in nature as brushite. Called also *dicalcium phosphate.*

c. disodium edathamil, c. disodium edetate edetate calcium disodium.

C. Disodium Versenate trademark for edetate calcium disodium.

c. EDTA edetate calcium disodium.

c. fluoride a compound, CaF_2, occurring in the bones and teeth.

c. glubionate [USP] a calcium replenisher, used as a nutritional supplement and for the treatment of hypocalcemia; administered orally.

c. gluceptate [USP] a calcium salt administered intramuscularly or intravenously in the treatment and prophylaxis of hypocalcemia and as an electrolyte replenisher.

c. gluconate [USP] a calcium salt of gluconic acid, administered intravenously or orally in the treatment and prophylaxis of hypocalcemia and as a nutritional supplement. It is also administered by injection as a treatment adjunct in cardiac arrest and in the treatment of hyperkalemia.

c. glycerophosphate a calcium salt administered intramuscularly or intravenously in conjunction with calcium lactate in the treatment and prophylaxis of hypocalcemia.

c. hydroxide [USP] a salt, $Ca(OH)_2$, used in solution as a topical astringent.

c. lactate [USP] a calcium replenisher, administered orally in the treatment and prophylaxis of hypocalcemia and as a nutritional supplement.

c. levulinate [USP] a calcium replenisher, administered orally or parenterally in the treatment of calcium deficiency.

c. oxalate CaC_2O_4, a salt of oxalic acid which, when formed in high concentrations in the urine, may lead to formation of an oxalate calculus (see under *calculus*). Natural forms include weddellite and whewellite.

c. oxide a corrosively alkaline and caustic earth, CaO, used for absorbing carbon dioxide from air, and industrially as a cheap alkali and as a base for mortar; called also *calx*, *lime*, and *quicklime*.

c. pantothenate [USP] the calcium salt of the dextrorotatory isomer of pantothenic acid, the B-complex vitamin; used, usually in combination with other B vitamins, as a nutritional supplement. See also *racemic c. pantothenate*.

c. phosphate any of three salts (monobasic, dibasic, and tribasic), containing calcium and the phosphate radical (PO_4); see *dibasic c. phosphate* and *tribasic c. phosphate*.

c. polycarbophil [USP] a calcium salt of a loosely cross-linked, hydrophilic resin of the polycarboxylic type; a bulk laxative.

precipitated c. carbonate a commercial form of calcium carbonate prepared by chemical means; used as an antacid, as a calcium supplement, and for the treatment of osteoporosis.

prepared c. carbonate native calcium carbonate freed from most of its impurities by elutriation; used as an antacid and calcium supplement.

c. propionate the calcium salt of propionic acid, which has antifungal properties; used alone or in combination with sodium propionate or other agents as a preservative to inhibit mold production in bakery and milk products, other foods, tobacco, and pharmaceuticals and as a topical antifungal in the treatment of various mycoses.

c. pyrophosphate the pyrophosphate salt of calcium, $Ca_2O_7P_2$, used as a polishing agent in dentifrices. Crystals of the dihydrate form occur in the joints in calcium pyrophosphate deposition disease.

racemic c. pantothenate [USP] a mixture of the calcium salts of the dextrorotatory and levorotatory isomers of pantothenic acid, with a physiological activity about half that of calcium pantothenate.

c. stearate [NF] a compound of calcium with organic acids obtained from fats, used as a tablet lubricant.

c. sulfate [NF] the sulfate salt of calcium, $CaSO_4$, found commonly in nature in the anhydrous form (anhydrite) and in a hydrated form known as *gypsum;* when gypsum is calcined it forms *plaster of Paris.* Dried calcium sulfate dihydrate is used as a tablet diluent.

tribasic c. phosphate 1. the compound $Ca_3(PO_4)_2$, true tribasic calcium phosphate, a rarely occurring form. It occurs in nature as whitlockite. 2. [NF] an amorphous variable mixture of calcium phosphates with approximate formula $(Ca_3(PO_4)_2)_3 \cdot Ca(OH)_2$ (see *hydroxyapatite*), used as a calcium supplement.

c. trisodium pentetate pentetate calcium trisodium.

c. undecylenate [USP] the calcium salt of undecylenic acid, applied topically in the treatment of infection by *Epidermophyton*, *Microsporum*, and *Trichophyton*.

c. urate see under *urate.*

cal·ci·um·ed·e·tate so·di·um (kal″se-əm-ed′ə-tāt) edetate calcium disodium.

cal·ci·ure·sis (kal″se-u-re′sis) excretion of calcium in the urine, especially in excessive amounts.

cal·ci·uret·ic (kal″se-u-ret′ik) 1. pertaining to or causing calciuresis. 2. an agent that promotes calciuresis.

cal·ci·uria (kal″se-u′re-ə) 1. the presence of calcium in the urine. 2. hypercalciuria.

calc(o)- see *calci-*.

cal·cu·li (kal′ku-li) plural of *calculus.*

cal·cu·lo·gen·e·sis (kal″ku-lo-jen′ə-sis) lithogenesis.

cal·cu·lo·sis (kal″ku-lo′sis) lithiasis.

cal·cu·lus (kal′ku-ləs) pl. *cal′culi* [L. "pebble"] an abnormal concretion in the body, usually composed of mineral salts. Called also *stone.* **cal′culous** *adj*

alternating c. a urinary calculus made up of successive layers of different composition; called also *combination c.*

apatite c. a urinary calculus composed of apatite.

articular c. a deposit in a joint; it is usually composed of sodium urate, sometimes of calcium urate. Called also *joint c.* and *chalk stone.*

bile duct c. choledocholith.

biliary c. gallstone.

bladder c. vesical c.

bronchial c. broncholith.

brushite c. a hard, light-colored phosphate calculus composed of brushite.

calcium oxalate c. oxalate c.

cholesterol c. a calculus composed of cholesterol, usually a gallstone.

combination c. alternating c.

cystine c. a soft variety of urinary calculus composed of cystine; seen in cystinuria.

decubitus c. a urinary calculus formed as a result of long immobilization.

dental c. a hard, stonelike concretion, varying in color from creamy yellow to black, that forms on the teeth or dental prostheses through calcification of dental plaque. According to location, there are two general types: *supragingival c.* and *subgingival c.* Called also *odontolith*, *tartar*, and *dental tophus.*

DHA c. a rare type of urinary calculus that contains 2,8-dihydroxyadenine (DHA), seen in adenine phosphoribosyltransferase deficiency.

encysted c. a vesical calculus enclosed in a sac developed from the wall of the bladder; called also *pocketed c.*

fibrin c. a urinary calculus formed largely from fibrinogen in blood.

gastric c. gastrolith.

gonecystic c. seminal vesicle c.

hemic c. a calculus in the bloodstream developed from organization of a blood clot.

hepatic c. hepatolith.

intestinal c. enterolith.

jackstone c. a urinary calculus with six spikes like those of the toy in the game of jacks.

joint c. articular c.

lacrimal c. dacryolith.

lacteal c. mammary c.

lung c. 1. pneumolith. 2. broncholith.

mammary c. a concretion in one of the lactiferous ducts; called also *lacteal c.*

matrix c. a white to light tan urinary calculus of a doughy consistency, containing calcium salts in an organic matrix of a mucoprotein and a sulfated mucopolysaccharide.

nasal c. rhinolith.

nephritic c. renal c.

oxalate c. a hard urinary calculus made of calcium oxalate, often in the form of weddellite or whewellite; some are covered with minute sharp spines that may abrade the renal pelvic epithelium, and others are smooth. Called also *calcium oxalate c.*

pancreatic c. a calculus that forms in the pancreatic duct from calcium carbonate, other salts, and organic materials. Called also *pancreatolith.*

phosphate c., phosphatic c. a urinary calculus composed of a phosphate such as brushite, struvite, or whitlockite; it may be hard, soft, or friable, and so large that it may fill the renal pelvis and calices.

pocketed c. encysted c.

preputial c. a concretion or calculus of the prepuce; called also *postholith.*

primary renal c. a calculus that forms in an apparently healthy urinary tract, usually an oxalate calculus or uric acid calculus.

prostatic c. a concretion formed in the prostate, chiefly of calcium carbonate and phosphate. Called also *prostatolith.*

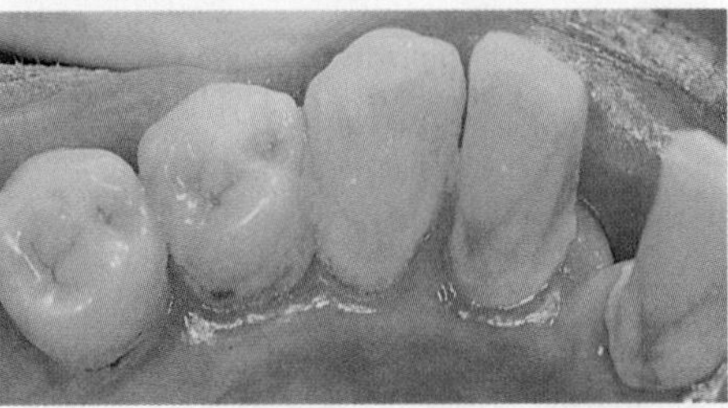

■ Dental calculus on the lingual surface of the lower anterior teeth.

renal c. a urinary calculus in the kidney; called also *nephritic c., nephrolith,* and *kidney stone.*
salivary c. 1. sialolith. 2. supragingival c.
secondary renal c. a calculus associated with infection and obstruction, usually composed of struvite (magnesium ammonium phosphate).
seminal vesicle c. a rare type of calculus found in a seminal vesicle, usually resulting from obstruction or infection. Called also *gonecystic c.*
serumal c. subgingival c., so called because it is supposed to result from exudation of serum.
staghorn c. a urinary calculus, usually struvite, found in the renal pelvis and shaped like the antlers of a stag because it extends into multiple calices.
struvite c. a urinary calculus composed of struvite, seen when the renal pelvis is infected with urea-splitting bacteria such as *Proteus.* Called also *infection stone.*
subgingival c. dental calculus located below the crest of the marginal gingiva, usually in periodontal pockets. Called also *serumal c.*
supragingival c. dental calculus that covers the coronal surface of the tooth to the crest of the gingival margin. Called also *salivary c.*
tonsillar c. tonsillolith.
triple phosphate c. struvite c.
urate c. uric acid c.
urethral c. a urinary calculus in the urethra; symptoms vary according to the patient's sex and the site of lodgment.
uric acid c. a hard, yellow or reddish-yellow urinary calculus formed from uric acid.
urinary c. a calculus in any part of the urinary tract; *vesical calculi* are those lodged in the bladder and *renal calculi* are those in the renal pelvis. Common types named for their primary components are *oxalate calculi, phosphate calculi,* and *uric acid calculi.* Called also *urolith.*
uterine c. an intrauterine concretion formed mainly by the calcification of a tumor.
vesical c. a urinary calculus found in the bladder. Called also *bladder c.* or *stone* and *cystolith.*
weddellite c. a common type of oxalate calculus, containing weddellite.
whewellite c. a common type of oxalate calculus, containing whewellite.
whitlockite c. a phosphate calculus composed of whitlockite.
xanthic c., xanthine c. a urinary calculus composed mainly of xanthine, seen in persons with xanthinuria.

Cal·da·ni ligament (kal-dah′ne) [Leopoldo Marcantonio *Caldani,* Italian anatomist, 1725–1813] see under *ligament.*

Cal·der·ol (kal′dər-ol) trademark for a preparation of calcifediol.

cal·des·mon (kal-dez′mən) a calcium-binding protein existing in two isoforms: a high molecular weight form found in smooth muscle and a low molecular weight form found in nonmuscle cells; it blocks the myosin binding site by binding to F-actin and plays a role in the calcium-dependent regulation of actin-myosin interaction.

Cald·well position, projection (kawld′wel) [Eugene Wilson *Caldwell,* American radiologist, 1870–1918] see under *position* and *projection.*

Cald·well-Luc operation (kawld′wel lūk′) [George W. *Caldwell,* American physician, 1834–1918; Henri *Luc,* French laryngologist, 1855–1925] see under *operation.*

Cald·well-Mo·loy classification (kawld′wel mə-loi′) [William Edgar *Caldwell,* American obstetrician, 1880–1943; Howard Carman *Moloy,* Canadian obstetrician, 1903–1953] see under *classification.*

Calef. [L.] calefac′tus (warmed); ca′lefac (make warm).

cal·e·fa·cient (kal″ə-fa′shənt) [L. *calidus* warm + *-facient*] 1. warming; causing a sensation of warmth. 2. an agent that causes a sensation of warmth.

Ca·len·du·la (kə-len′du-lə) [L.] a genus of composite-flowered plants (family Compositae). The dried florets of *C. officina′lis,* the pot marigold, have antimicrobial and antiinflammatory properties and are used topically for inflammatory lesions of the skin and mucous membranes and to promote healing of wounds and burns, as well as being used in homeopathy and folk medicine.

calf (kaf) [L. *sura*] 1. sura. 2. the young of a bovine. 3. the young of any of several other mammalian species.
baldy c. a calf with a lethal inherited condition characterized by alopecia, cracked and ulcerated skin, elongated feet, and hypersalivation.
bulldog c. a calf born with lethal skeletal defects including short limbs, a swollen cranium, and a cleft palate.

cal·fac·tant (kal-fak′tənt) a pulmonary surfactant from calf lung, which includes phospholipids, neutral lipids, and several surfactant-associated proteins; used in the prophylaxis and treatment of neonatal respiratory distress syndrome, instilled into the endotracheal tube for intratracheal administration.

cal·i·ber (kal′ĭ-bər) [Fr. *calibre* the bore of a gun] the diameter of a canal or tube.

cal·i·bra·tion (kal″ĭ-bra′shən) 1. determination of the accuracy of an instrument, usually by measurement of its variation from a standard, to ascertain necessary correction factors. 2. measurement of the caliber of a tube.

cal·i·ce·al (kal″ĭ-se′əl) calyceal.

cal·i·cec·ta·sis (kal″ĭ-sek′tə-sis) caliectasis.

cal·i·cec·to·my (kal″ĭ-sek′tə-me) excision of a renal calix.

ca·li·ces (ka′lĭ-sēz) [L.] plural of *calix.* In TA nomenclature, this plural is used with the singular *calyx.*

cal·i·cine (kal′ĭ-sēn) related to or resembling a calix.

Ca·li·ci·vi·ri·dae (kə-lis″ĭ-vir′ĭ-de) the caliciviruses: a family of RNA viruses having a nonenveloped virion 27–40 nm in diameter with 32 cuplike depressions in a t = 3 arrangement. The genome consists of a single molecule of positive-sense single-stranded polyadenylated RNA (MW 2.6–2.7 $\times 10^6$, size 7.4–7.7 kb). Viruses contain one major and two minor polypeptides and are resistant to chloroform, ether, mild detergents, and lipid solvents; some are inactivated by trypsin. Replication and assembly occur in the cytoplasm; virions are released by cell destruction. Host range is narrow and transmission is via infested food, by contact, or by airborne particles. It includes the genera *Lagovirus, Norovirus, Sapovirus,* and *Vesivirus.*

Ca·li·ci·vi·rus (kə-lis′ĭ-vi″rəs) [L. *calix,* gen. *calicis* cup + *virus*] a former genus of the family Caliciviridae whose species are now assigned to other genera.

ca·li·ci·vi·rus (kə-lis′ĭ-vi″rəs) any virus of the family Caliciviridae. **calicivi′ral** *adj*
feline c. a virus of the genus *Vesivirus,* transmitted by aerosol droplets and fomites, that causes respiratory disease in cats.
human c's a group of viruses of the genera *Norovirus* and *Sapovirus* that includes Norwalk virus and a number of other strains that cause acute, self-limited gastroenteritis in humans.

Cal·i·coph·o·ron (kal″ĭ-kof′ə-ron) a genus of trematodes of the family Paramphistomatidae that infest the rumen and intestines of ruminants, causing paramphistomiasis.

ca·lic·u·lus (kə-lik′u-ləs) pl. *cali′culi* [L., dim. of *calix*] a bud-shaped or cup-shaped structure.
c. gustato′rius [TA] taste bud: one of the minute, barrel-shaped terminal organs of the gustatory nerve, situated around the bases of the vallate, fungiform, and foliate papillae of the tongue. It contains several types of cells, including basal cells, taste cells, supporting cells, and some that are both supporting and taste cells. Called also *gustatory bud, Schwalbe corpuscle,* and *gemma gustatoria* [TA alternative].

ca·li·ec·ta·sis (ka″le-ek′tə-sis) [*calix* + *ectasis*] dilatation of a renal calyx; called also *calicectasis.*

cal·i·for·ni·um (Cf) (kal″ĭ-for′ne-əm) [*California* (University and state), where it was first produced] chemical element of atomic number 98, atomic weight 249, produced by irradiation of the isotope of curium of atomic weight 242 with helium ions; half-life 45 minutes.

cal·i·pers (kal′ĭ-pərz) [from *caliber*] compasses with bent or curved legs used for measuring the thickness or diameter of a solid.
skinfold c. calipers designed for measuring skinfolds (q.v.).

cal·is·then·ics (kal″is-then′iks) [Gr. *kalos* beautiful + *sthenic*] a system of light gymnastics for promoting strength and grace of carriage.

ca·lix (ka′liks) pl. *ca′lices* [L. "drinking cup"] calyx. NOTE: In official anatomical terminology, the preferred term is "calyx," but the preferred plural is "calices;" see also entries under *calyx.*
renal calices the recesses of the renal pelvis that enclose the renal pyramids; see *calices renales majores* and *calices renales minores.* Called also *calyces renales.*
renal calices, major calices renales majores.
renal calices, minor calices renales minores.
ca′lices rena′les majo′res [TA] major renal calices: the larger subdivisions of the renal pelvis, into which the minor calices open.
ca′lices rena′les mino′res [TA] minor renal calices: a variable number of smaller subdivisions of the renal pelvis that enclose the renal pyramids and open into the major calices. Called also *infundibula of kidney.*

Call-Ex·ner bodies (kahl′ eks′nər) [Friedrich von *Call,* Austrian physician, 1844–1917; Siegmund *Exner,* Austrian physiologist, 1846–1926] see under *body.*

CALLA common acute lymphoblastic leukemia antigen.

Cal·lan·der amputation (kal′ən-dər) [C. Latimer *Callander,* American surgeon, 1892–1947] see under *amputation.*

Cal·le·ja's islands (islets) (kahl-ya′hahz) [Julián *Calleja* y Sánchez, Spanish anatomist, 1836–1913] see under *island.*

Cal·liph·o·ra (kə-lif′o-rə) [Gr. *kallos* beauty + *phoros* bearing] a genus of scavenger flies of the family Calliphoridae, including the blow flies and bluebottle flies, which deposit their eggs in decaying matter, on wounds, or in the openings of the body. Several species lay eggs on wounds or wool, causing cutaneous myiasis. Species include *C. azu'rea*, *C. erythroce'phala*, *C. lionen'sis*, and *C. vomito'ria*.

C. vomito'ria the common bluebottle fly, whose larvae may invade the nasal fossae or produce intestinal myiasis.

cal·liph·o·rid (kə-lif'ə-rid) a member of the family Calliphoridae.

Cal·li·phor·i·dae (kal″ĭ-for'ĭ-de) a family of medium-sized to large flies of the order Diptera, including the genera *Auchmeromyia*, *Booponus*, *Calliphora* (type genus), *Cordylobia*, *Cochliomyia*, *Chrysomyia*, *Lucilia*, *Phaenicia*, and *Phormia;* all species may serve as vectors of pathogens and may also produce myiasis in humans; several are causes of cutaneous myiasis in domestic animals.

Cal·li·son fluid (kal'ĭ-sən) [James S. *Callison*, American physician, 20th century] see under *fluid.*

Cal·lis·ta (kə-lis'tə) a genus of shellfish. *C. brevisphona'ta* was the cause of callistin shellfish poisoning in Japan.

Cal·li·tro·ga (kal″ĭ-tro'gə) *Cochliomyia.*

cal·lo·sal (kə-lo'səl) pertaining to the corpus callosum.

Cal·lo·se·las·ma (kə-lo″sə-laz'mə) a genus of venomous snakes of the family Crotalidae. *C. rhodosto'ma* (formerly called *Agkistrodon rhodostoma*) is the Malayan pit viper, a species with a deadly bite that is found in Southeast Asia, Malaysia, and Indonesia.

cal·los·i·tas (kə-los'ĭ-təs) [L.] callus (def. 1).

cal·los·i·ty (kə-los'ĭ-te) [L. *callositas*, from *callus*] callus (def. 1).

cal·lo·so·mar·gin·al (kə-lo″so-mahr'jĭ-nəl) pertaining to the callosal and marginal gyri.

cal·lo·sot·o·my (kal″ə-sot'ə-me) corpuscallosotomy.

cal·lo·sum (kə-lo'səm) corpus callosum.

cal·lous (kal'əs) 1. hardened. 2. pertaining to or characterized by callus.

cal·lus (kal'əs) [L.] 1. localized hyperplasia of the stratum corneum due to pressure or friction. Called also *callosity*, *keratoma*, and *tyloma*. See also *hyperkeratosis* (def. 1) and *keratoderma*. 2. an unorganized meshwork of woven bone developed on the pattern of the original fibrin clot, which is formed following fracture of a bone and is normally ultimately replaced by hard adult bone; called also *bony c.* 3. a mass of plant tissue formed over a wound or at the base of a cutting.

bony c. see *callus* (def. 2).

central c. a provisional callus formed within the medullary cavity of a fractured bone; it arises from the cells covering the endosteal and trabecular surfaces near the fracture. Called also *inner c.*, *medullary c.*, and *myelogenous c.*

definitive c. the exudate formed between the fractured ends of the bone, which is permanent and becomes changed into true bone; called also *intermediate c.* and *permanent c.*

ensheathing c. provisional callus forming a sheath about the ends of the fragments of a fractured bone.

external c. the collar of callus formed by the periosteum in a long bone.

inner c. central c.

intermediate c. definitive c.

internal c., medullary c., myelogenous c. central c.

permanent c. definitive c.

provisional c., temporary c. callus formed within the medullary cavity and about the ends of a broken bone, and which is absorbed as the repair is completed.

sucking c. 1. a callus in the center of the upper lip of an infant, caused by friction during nursing. 2. a callus on a thumb or finger that a child sucks on excessively.

calm·a·tive (kahm'ə-tiv, kahl'mə-tiv) sedative.

Cal·mette test, vaccine (kahl-met') [Albert Léon Charles *Calmette*, French bacteriologist, 1863–1933] see *BCG vaccine*, under *vaccine*.

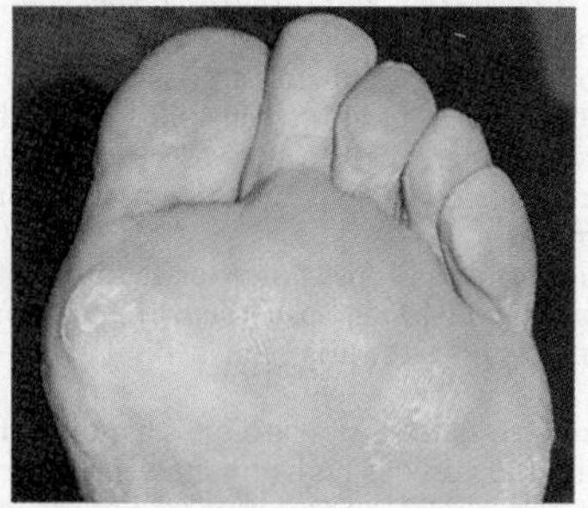

■ Calluses on the sole of the foot.

Cal·mette-Gué·rin bacillus (kahl-met' ga-ră') [A.L.C. *Calmette;* Camille *Guérin*, French bacteriologist, 1872–1961] see *bacille Calmette-Guérin.*

cal·mod·u·lin (kal-mod'u-lin) a ubiquitous calcium-binding protein of eukaryotic cells that mediates a variety of cellular responses to calcium. The calcium-calmodulin complex acts as a messenger, affecting the activity of many enzymes and nonenzyme proteins, including the calcium pump, numerous specific protein kinases and cyclic nucleotide phosphodiesterases, spectrin, histones, and tubulin.

cal·nex·in (kal-nek'sin) a 67-kD calcium-binding protein of the membrane of the endoplasmic reticulum that with calreticulin acts as a chaperone in the folding of newly synthesized proteins.

Ca·lo·ba·ta (kə-lo'bə-tə) a genus of South American flies whose larvae sometimes occur in the human intestine.

Cal·o·mys (kal'o-mis) the vesper mice, a genus of South American rodents of the family Muridae that are reservoirs for various disease-causing viruses. *C. callo'sus* is the reservoir for Machupo virus, and *C. musculi'nus* is the principal reservoir for Junin virus.

ca·lor (kal'or) [L.] heat; one of the cardinal signs of inflammation.

c. febri'lis the heat of fever.

c. fer'vens an intense heat.

c. inna'tus the normal or natural heat of the body.

c. inter'nus the heat of the interior of the body.

c. mor'dax, c. mor'dicans 1. biting or stinging heat. 2. the hot, burning, reddish-colored skin occurring in scarlet fever.

cal·o·ra·di·ance (kal″o-ra'de-əns) the radiation or rays which lie between 250 and 55,000 millimicrons, such as the rays from the sun, carbon arcs, incandescent rods and filaments, and hot black bodies.

cal·o·res·cence (kal″ə-res'əns) the conversion of nonluminous into luminous heat rays.

Ca·lo·ri bursa (kah-lo're) [Luigi *Calori*, Italian anatomist, 1807–1896] see under *bursa.*

calor(i)- [L. *calor*, gen. *caloris* heat] a combining form denoting relationship to heat.

ca·lo·ric (kə-lor'ik) pertaining to heat or to calories.

cal·o·ric·i·ty (kal″ə-ris'ĭ-te) the power of the animal body of developing and maintaining heat.

cal·o·rie (kal'ə-re) [Fr.; L. *calor* heat] any of several units of heat defined as the amount of heat required to raise the temperature of 1 kilogram of water 1 degree Celsius at a specified temperature. The calorie used in chemistry and biochemistry is equal to exactly 4.184 joules. Symbol cal. NOTE: There was formerly a distinction made between the "small calorie," defined above, and the "large calorie," written Calorie with a capital "C" and abbreviated Cal, which was equal to 1000 small calories or one kilocalorie. The use of the large calorie survives only in nutrition, where calorie, now usually written with a small "c," means kilocalorie when specifying the energy content of foods.

gram c. small c.

IT c., International Table c. a unit of heat, equivalent to 4.1868 joules.

large c. the calorie used in metabolic studies, being the amount of heat required to raise the temperature of 1 kilogram of water 1 degree Celsius, specifically from 14.5° to 15.5°C at a pressure of 1 atmosphere; abbreviated kg-cal. Called also *kilocalorie.* Also used to express the fuel or energy value of food.

mean c. one one-hundredth of the amount of heat required to raise the temperature of 1 gram of water from 0° to 100°C.

small c. the amount of heat required to raise the temperature of 1 gram of water 1 degree Celsius, specifically from 14.5° to 15.5°C at a pressure of 1 atmosphere; abbreviated g-cal. Called also *gram c.* and *standard c.*

standard c. small c.

thermochemical c. a unit of heat, equivalent to 4.184 joules.

ca·lor·i·fa·cient (kə-lor″ĭ-fa'shənt) [*calori-* + *-facient*] producing heat; said of certain foods.

cal·o·rif·ic (kal″ə-rif'ik) [*calori-* + L. *facere* to make] producing heat.

ca·lor·i·ge·net·ic (kə-lor″ĭ-jə-net'ik) calorigenic.

ca·lor·i·gen·ic (kə-lor″ĭ-jen'ik) [*calori-* + *-genic*] producing heat or energy; increasing heat or energy production; increasing the consumption of oxygen.

cal·o·rim·e·ter (kal″ə-rim'ə-tər) [*calori-* + *-meter*] an instrument for measuring the amount of heat exchanged in any system. In physiology, an apparatus for measuring the amount of heat produced by an individual.

bomb c. an apparatus for measuring the potential energy of food, a weighed amount of the food being placed on a platinum dish inside a hollow steel container (bomb) filled with pure oxygen. The heat produced by its combustion is absorbed by a known quantity of water in which the container is immersed, permitting its measurement.

compensating c. an apparatus in which the object to be tested, such as a developing chick in an egg, is placed at one junction of a thermocouple and an electrical resistance at the other. From the amount of current that must pass through the resistance to keep both junctions at the same temperature (as shown by lack of current in the thermocouple circuit), it is possible to calculate the amount of heat generated in the object being tested.

cal•o•rim•e•try (kal″ə-rim′ə-tre) [*calori-* + *-metry*] measurement of the amounts of heat absorbed or given out. **calorimet′ric** *adj*

direct c. measurement of the amount of heat produced by a subject enclosed within a small chamber.

indirect c. measurement of the amount of heat produced by a subject by determination of the amount of oxygen consumed and the quantity of nitrogen and carbon dioxide eliminated.

ca•lor•i•tro•pic (kə-lor″ĭ-tro′pik) [*calori-* + *-tropic*] thermotropic.

Ca•lot triangle (kah-lo′) [Jean-François *Calot*, French surgeon, 1861–1944] trigonum cystohepaticum.

ca•lotte (kə-lot′) [Fr. "cap"] 1. a part shaped like a skull cap. 2. in ophthalmology, a cap-shaped specimen removed from the eyeball for histopathologic examination. 3. in anatomy, the superior part of the calvaria.

cal•pain (kal′pān) any of a group of related calcium-activated proteases of eukaryotic cells, including calpain-1 [EC 3.4.22.52] and calpain 2 [EC 3.4.22.53]; they are implicated in cytoskeletal reorganization, membrane protein degradation, and apoptosis. Faulty regulation of calpain activity is associated with a number of disorders, including muscular dystrophy, cancer, Alzheimer disease, atherosclerosis, diabetes, and cataract formation.

cal•pa•stat•in (kal-pə-stat′in) an endogenous inhibitor of calpain, found in increased amounts in the blood in conditions of calpain deficiency; see *calpain*.

Cal•pho•san (kal′fo-san) trademark for a combination preparation of calcium glycerophosphate and calcium lactate.

cal•po•nin (kal-po′nin) a calcium-dependent actin-binding protein of smooth muscle, existing in three isoforms (acidic, neutral, and basic); it also binds calmodulin and tropomyosin. It is a regulator of smooth muscle contraction, which it inhibits when not phosphorylated.

cal•re•tic•u•lin (kal″rə-tik′u-lin) a 55–65 kDa high-affinity calcium-binding protein found in the sarcoplasmic reticulum and also in the endoplasmic reticulum of nonmuscle cells; its many functions include roles in protein folding, calcium homeostasis, control of viral RNA replication, lymphocyte activation, and cytotoxicity.

cal•ret•i•nin (kal-ret′ĭ-nin) a 29-kD calcium-binding protein expressed by a variety of mesothelial, epithelial, and stromal cells; it is used as an immunohistochemical marker to distinguish between mesothelioma and adenocarcinoma.

cal•se•ques•trin (kal″sə-kwes′trin) a calcium-binding protein rich in carboxylate side chains, occurring on the inner membrane surface of the sarcoplasmic reticulum; it serves to chelate and store calcium ions.

cal•va•ria (kal-var′e-ə) [L.] [TA] the domelike superior portion of the cranium, derived from the membranous neurocranium and consisting of the frontal and parietal bones and the squamous parts of the occipital and temporal bones. **calvar′ial** *adj*

cal•va•ri•um (kal-var′e-əm) incorrect term for *calvaria*.

Cal•vé-Per•thes disease (kahl-va′ per′təz) [Jacques *Calvé*, French orthopedist, 1875–1954; Georg Clemens *Perthes*, German surgeon, 1869–1927] Legg-Calvé-Perthes disease; see under *disease*.

Cal•vin cycle (kal′vin) [Melvin *Calvin*, American chemist, 1911–1997; winner of the Nobel prize in chemistry for 1961 for development of techniques to determine the chemical reactions of plant carbon dioxide assimilation] see under *cycle*.

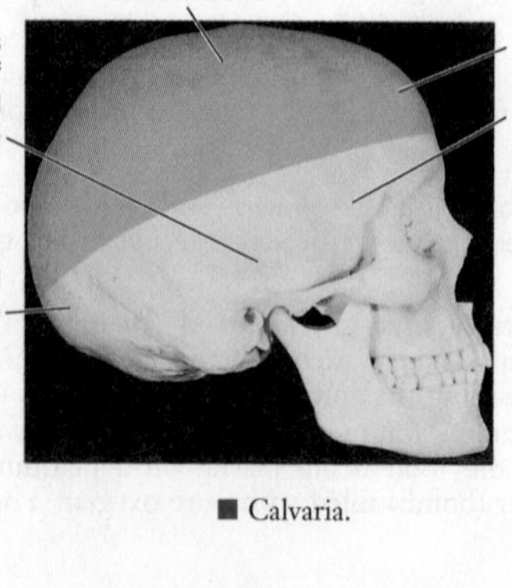

■ Calvaria.

cal•vi•ti•es (kal-vish′e-ēz) [L.] alopecia.

calx (kalks) [L.] 1. [TA] heel: the hindmost projection of the foot. 2. any residue obtained by calcination. 3. calcium oxide.

cal•y•ce•al (kal″ĭ-se′əl) pertaining to or affecting a calyx; spelled also *caliceal*.

ca•ly•ces (ka′lĭ-sēz) plural of *calyx*.

cal•y•cine (kal′ĭ-sĭn) calicine.

Ca•lym•ma•to•bac•te•ri•um (kə-lim″ə-to-bak-tēr′e-əm) [Gr. *kalymma* a hood or veil + *bacterium*] a former genus of bacteria whose members are now classified in the genus *Klebsiella* (q.v.).

C. granulo′matis former name for *Klebsiella granulomatis*.

ca•lyx (ka′liks) pl. *ca′lyces* [Gr. *kalyx* cup of a flower] a cup-shaped organ or cavity; also spelled *calix*. NOTE: In official anatomical terminology, the preferred term is "calyx," but the preferred plural is "calices;" see also entries under *calix*.

c. infe′rior re′nis [TA] inferior renal calyx: a major renal calyx that drains into the inferior part of a renal pelvis.

c. me′dius re′nis [TA] middle renal calyx: a major renal calyx that drains into the middle part of a renal pelvis.

renal calyces see under *calix*.

renal c., inferior c. inferior renis.

renal c., middle c. medius renis.

renal c., superior c. superior renis.

c. supe′rior re′nis [TA] superior renal calyx: a major renal calyx that drains into the superior part of a renal pelvis.

CAM cell adhesion molecules; complementary and alternative medicine.

Cam•al•la•nus (kam″ə-la′nəs) a genus of nematodes of the superfamily Spiruroidea, species of which are parasites in the intestines of fishes, reptiles, and amphibians.

Cam•ba•roi•des (kam″bə-roi′dēz) a genus of crayfish which harbor the metacercariae of *Paragonimus*.

cam•bi•um (kam′be-əm) [L. "exchange"] 1. the loose cellular inner layer of the periosteal tissue in the intramembranous ossification of bone. 2. a layer of cells beneath the bark of woody plants.

Ca•mel•lia (kə-mel′e-ə) a genus of flowering evergreen trees and shrubs of the family Theaceae, native to hot regions of Asia. *C. sinen′sis* (L.) Kuntze is the tea plant, whose leaves are dried to make the most common type of tea.

cam•el•pox (kam′əl-poks) an eruptive disease of camels caused by a species of *Orthopoxvirus*.

cam•era (kam′ə-rə) pl. *ca′merae*, *cameras* [L. "chamber"] 1. chamber: an enclosed space or ventricle. 2. a device for converting light or other energy from an object into a visible image.

Anger c. a device used to form an image of the distribution of a gamma ray–emitting radionuclide in a patient. The radiation is passed through a collimator to reduce scatter and interacts with a sodium iodide crystal, resulting in the production of pulses of light, which are detected and converted to amplified electrical signals by an array of photomultiplier tubes behind the crystal. A pulse height analyzer then discards all but those signals arising from the photopeak of the nuclide being imaged, and the remaining signals are used to form an image of the distribution of the radionuclide on a cathode ray tube. It was the original, and is by far the most commonly used, form of scintillation camera (or gamma camera), and the terms are often used interchangeably.

c. ante′rior bul′bi o′culi [TA] anterior chamber of eye: that portion of the aqueous humor–filled space between the cornea and the lens that is bounded in front by the cornea and part of the sclera, and behind by the iris, part of the ciliary body, and the part of the lens that presents through the pupil.

ca′merae bul′bi o′culi [TA] the chambers of the eye; see *c. anterior bulbi oculi*, *c. posterior bulbi oculi*, and *c. postrema bulbi oculi*.

gamma c. scintillation c.

c. lu′cida an optical device utilizing a prism or mirrors so arranged as to throw the reflected image of an object upon paper, thus permitting its outlines to be traced with a pencil.

c. obscu′ra a combined box, lens, and screen, used for viewing, tracing, or making photographs.

c. poste′rior bul′bi o′culi [TA] posterior chamber of eye: that portion of the aqueous humor–containing space between the cornea and the lens that is bounded in front by the iris, and behind by the lens and ciliary zonule.

c. post′rema bul′bi o′culi [TA] vitreous chamber of eye: the space in the eyeball enclosing the vitreous body, bounded anteriorly by the lens and ciliary body and posteriorly by the posterior wall of the eyeball. Called also *c. vitrea bulbi oculi* [TA alternative] and *postremal chamber of eye*.

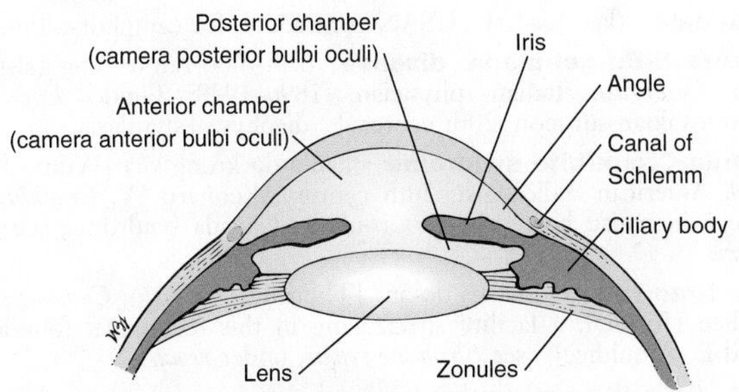

■ Camera anterior (anterior chamber) and camera posterior (posterior chamber) bulbi oculi in a cross-section of the anterior region of the eyeball.

recording c. photokymograph.

scintillation c. an electronic instrument that produces photographs or cathode-ray tube images of the gamma ray emissions from organs containing tracer compounds; the original and most commonly used type is the Anger camera (q.v.), with which the term is often equated, although other types, such as multicrystal versions, have also been used.

c. vi'trea bul'bi o'culi TA alternative for *c. postrema bulbi oculi.*

cam•erae (kam'ə-re) [L.] plural of *camera.*

Cam•er•er's law (kahm'ər-ərz) [Johann Friedrich Wilhelm *Camerer*, German pediatrician, 1842–1910] see under *law.*

Ca•mey neobladder (kah-ma') [Maurice *Camey*, French urologist, 20th century] see under *neobladder.*

Cam•mann stethoscope (kam'ən) [George Philip *Cammann*, American physician, 1804–1863] a binaural stethoscope.

Cam•path (kam'path) trademark for a preparation of alemtuzumab.

cAMP cyclic adenosine monophosphate.

Camp•bell ligament (kam'bəl) [William Francis *Campbell*, American surgeon, 1867–1926] the suspensory ligament of the axilla.

cAMP-de•pen•dent pro•tein ki•nase (de-pen'dənt pro'tēn ki'nās) [EC 2.7.11.11] any of a group of closely related protein-serine/threonine kinases that are activated by cyclic adenosine monophosphate (cAMP) and catalyze the activity of a variety of intracellular proteins via phosphorylation of specific serine and threonine moieties of other proteins. Called also *protein kinase A* and *cyclic AMP–dependent protein kinase.*

cam•pea•chy (kam-pe'che) *Haematoxylon campechianum.*

cam•phe•chlor (kam'fə-klor) toxaphene.

cam•phene (kam-fēn') a terpene found in many essential oils or prepared synthetically from pinene in the process of producing synthetic camphor; it is toxic by ingestion.

cam•phor (kam'for, kam'fər) [L. *camphora;* Gr. *kamphora*] [USP] a ketone with a characteristic penetrating odor and a pungent taste, obtained from the wood of *Cinnamomum camphora* or produced synthetically. It is applied topically to the skin as an antipruritic and antiinfective and is inhaled as a nasal decongestant; it is also used in folk medicine and in Indian medicine. Called also *gum c.*

cam•pho•ra•ceous (kam″fə-ra'shəs) having characteristics resembling those of camphor.

cam•pho•rat•ed (kam″fə-rāt'əd) [L. *camphoratus*] containing or tinctured with camphor.

cam•pim•e•ter (kam-pim'ə-tər) [L. *campus* field + *-meter*] an apparatus for mapping the central portion of the visual field on a flat surface.

cam•pim•e•try (kam-pim'ə-tre) the determination of the presence of defects in the central portion of the visual field by use of the campimeter.

cam•po•spasm (kam'po-spaz″əm) camptocormia.

cam•pot•o•my (kam-pot'ə-me) [L. *campi* fields (of Forel) + *-tomy*] the stereotaxic surgical technique of producing a lesion in the Forel fields, beneath the thalamus, for correction of tremor in Parkinson disease.

Cam•pral (kam'pral) trademark for a preparation of acamprosate calcium.

campt(o)- [Gr. *kamptos* bent] a combining form denoting a bending.

camp•to•cor•mia (kamp″to-kor'me-ə) [*campto-* + Gr. *kormos* trunk + *-ia*] a static deformity consisting of forward flexion of the trunk; called also *camptospasm.*

camp•to•cor•my (kamp″to-kor'me) camptocormia.

camp•to•dac•tyl•ia (kamp″to-dak-til'e-ə) camptodactyly.

camp•to•dac•tyl•ism (kamp″to-dak'tə-liz-əm) camptodactyly.

camp•to•dac•ty•ly (kamp″to-dak'tə-le) [*campto-* + Gr. *daktylos* finger] permanent and irreducible flexion of one or more fingers.

camp•to•me•lia (kamp″to-me'le-ə) [*campto-* + *-melia*] bending of the limbs, producing permanent bowing or curving of the affected part; see also *camptomelic syndrome*, under *syndrome.* **camptome'lic** *adj*

Camp•to•sar (kamp'to-sahr) trademark for a preparation of irinotecan hydrochloride.

camp•to•spasm (kamp'to-spaz″əm) camptocormia.

Camp•to•the•ca (kamp″to-the'kə) [Gr. *kamptos* bent + *thēkē* case] a genus of trees of the family Nyssaceae. *C. acuminata* is a species known as the happy tree, native to China and Tibet, and is the source of the alkaloid camptothecin.

camp•to•the•cin (kamp″to-the'sin) an alkaloid found in the tree *Camptotheca acuminata;* it has antitumor activity and has been chemically modified to form topoisomerase inhibitors.

Cam•py•lo•bac•ter (kam″pə-lo-bak'tər) [Gr. *kampylos* curved + *-bacter*] a genus of bacteria of the family Campylobacteraceae, consisting of gram-negative curved, S-shaped, or spiral rods. Organisms are microaerophilic to anaerobic, chemo-organotrophic, and motile by means of polar flagella; they are found in the oral cavity, intestinal tract, and reproductive organs. Some species are pathogenic. The type species is *C. fe'tus.*

C. cinae'di *Helicobacter cinaedi.*

C. co'li a species that causes diarrhea, septicemia, and occasionally abortion in humans. It may cause diarrhea in pigs and monkeys and is associated with hepatitis in certain bird species and proliferative enteritis in pigs. Called also *Vibrio coli.*

C. fennel'liae *Helicobacter fennelliae.*

C. fe'tus a microaerophilic species occurring as several subspecies.

C. fe'tus* subsp. *fe'tus a subspecies that causes abortion and infertility in cattle (bovine genital campylobacteriosis). It is an occasional human pathogen, capable of causing systemic infection in immunocompromised hosts.

C. fe'tus* subsp. *intestina'lis *C. fetus* subsp. *fetus.*

C. fe'tus* subsp. *jeju'ni *C. jejuni.*

C. fe'tus* subsp. *venera'lis a subspecies that causes abortion and infertility in cattle.

C. hyointestina'lis a species that can cause porcine proliferative enteritis in pigs and gastrointestinal infections and diarrhea in humans, as well as bacteremia in immunocompromised persons.

C. jeju'ni a species that is a common cause of enteric campylobacteriosis in humans, infectious abortion in sheep, and avian campylobacteriosis in fowls; it is also found as a commensal in swine, cattle, cats, and chickens. Called also *Vibrio jejuni.*

C. la'ri a species that sometimes causes gastrointestinal infections and diarrhea.

C. mucosa'lis a species commonly found in the intestinal mucosa and oral cavity of pigs; it is associated with gastrointestinal disease in pigs. Formerly called *Campylobacter sputorum* subsp. *mucosalis.*

C. pylo'ri *Helicobacter pylori.*

C. rec'tus a species associated with periodontal disease and isolated from dental root canal infections.

C. sputo'rum a usually nonpathogenic, microaerophilic to anaerobic species occurring as two subspecies.

C. sputo'rum* subsp. *bu'bulus a subspecies found in the genital tracts of sheep and cattle.

C. sputo'rum* subsp. *mucosa'lis *C. mucosalis.*

C. sputo'rum* subsp. *sputo'rum a subspecies found in the human oral cavity.

C. upsalien'sis a species that sometimes causes gastrointestinal infections and diarrhea, and can cause bacteremia in immunocompromised persons.

cam•py•lo•bac•ter (kam″pə-lo-bak'tər) a bacterium of the genus *Campylobacter.*

Cam•py•lo•bac•ter•a•ceae (kam″pə-lo-bak″tər-a'se-e) a family of bacteria of the order Campylobacterales, consisting of gram-negative, non–spore-forming, curved, S-shaped, or spiral rods; organisms are microaerophilic, chemo-organotrophic, and mainly motile, moving with a characteristic corkscrew motion. Pathogenic organisms are contained in the genera *Campylobacter* and *Arcobacter.*

Cam•py•lo•bac•ter•a•les (kam″pə-lo-bak″tər-a'lēz) a metabolically and ecologically diverse order of bacteria of the class Epsilonproteobacteria, phylum Proteobacteria, grouped together on the basis of 16S rRNA sequence analysis and consisting mainly of curved or spiral cells; many are human and animal pathogens. It includes the families Campylobacteraceae and Helicobacteraceae.

cam•py•lo•bac•te•ri•o•sis (kam″pə-lo-bak-tēr″e-o'sis) bacterial infection with *Campylobacter* species; symptoms vary between different species of animals. In humans it is usually an intestinal condition, acquired by eating inadequately cooked meat or through occupational exposure to infected animals. Other types of infections are particularly seen in immunocompromised persons.

avian c. infection of chickens and other birds by *Campylobacter jejuni*, with hepatitis of varying severity; symptoms range from the subclinical or a simple drop in egg production to weight loss, hemorrhage, depression, and death. Called also *vibrionic, avian vibrionic*, or *avian infectious hepatitis*.

bovine genital c. a venereal disease of cattle caused by *Campylobacter fetus* subsp. *fetus*; characterized by infertility and early embryonic death. Called also *bovine genital vibriosis*.

enteric c. *Campylobacter* enteritis.

ovine genital c. an infectious disease of sheep caused by *Campylobacter fetus* subsp. *fetus* and *C. jejuni*, characterized by abortion, and transmitted orally. Called also *ovine genital vibriosis*.

cam•sy•late (kam′sə-lāt) USAN contraction for camphorsulfonate.

Cam•u•ra•ti-En•gel•mann disease (kah-moo-rah′te eng′gəl-mahn) [Mario *Camurati*, Italian physician, 1896–1948; Guido *Engelmann*, Czechoslovakian surgeon, 20th century] diaphyseal dysplasia.

Can•a•da-Cronk•hite syndrome (kan′ə-də krong′kīt) [Wilma Jeanne *Canada*, American radiologist, 20th century; Leonard W. *Cronkhite*, Jr., American internist, born 1919] Cronkhite-Canada syndrome; see under *syndrome*.

Ca•na•di•an repair (kə-na′de-ən) [Thornhill, Ontario, *Canada*, site of Shouldice Hospital, a facility specializing in this technique, founded by Edward E. Shouldice] see *Shouldice repair*, under *repair*.

ca•nal (kə-nal′) a relatively narrow tubular passage or channel; see also *canalis*.

Canal

For descriptions of specific anatomic structures not found here, see under *canalis*.

abdominal c. canalis inguinalis.
accessory palatine c's canales palatini minores.
accessory root c. a lateral branching of the main root canal, usually occurring in the apical third of the root.
adductor c. canalis adductorius.
Alcock c. canalis pudendalis.
alimentary c. digestive tract.
alisphenoid c. a canal through the greater wing of the sphenoid bone of various animals, which transmits the internal carotid artery.
alveolar c's see *canalis mandibulae* and *canales alveolares corporis maxillae*.
alveolar c's of maxilla canales alveolares corporis maxillae.
anal c. canalis analis.
anterior alveolar c. an alveolar canal of the maxilla located anteriorly; see *canales alveolares corporis maxillae*.
anterior condyloid c. canalis nervi hypoglossi.
anterior ethmoidal c. foramen ethmoidale anterius.
anterior semicircular c. canalis semicircularis anterior.
archenteric c. neurenteric c.
Arnold c. 1. canaliculus mastoideus. 2. sulcus nervi petrosi minoris.
arterial c. ductus arteriosus.
atrioventricular c. the common canal connecting the primordial atrium and ventricle; it sometimes persists as a congenital anomaly as a result of failure of closure of the gap between the interatrial and interventricular septa due to arrest in development of the endocardial cushions.
c. for auditory tube semicanalis tubae auditivae.
basipharyngeal c. canalis vomerovaginalis.
birth c. the canal through which the fetus passes in birth, comprising the cervix uteri, vagina, and vulva; called also *obstetric c.* and *parturient c.*
blastoporic c. neurenteric c.
bony c's of ear canales semicirculares ossei.
bony semicircular c's canales semicirculares ossei.
Braun c. neurenteric c.
Breschet c's canales diploici.
calciferous c's canals containing lime salts in cartilage that is undergoing calcification.
caroticotympanic c's canaliculi caroticotympanici.
carotid c. canalis caroticus.
carpal c. canalis carpi.
c's of cartilage canals in an ossifying cartilage during its stage of vascularization.
central c. of modiolus see *canales longitudinales modioli*.
central c. of spinal cord canalis centralis medullae spinalis.
central c. of Stilling, central c. of vitreous canalis hyaloideus.
cerebrospinal c. the primordial cavity of the brain and spinal cord.
cervical c., cervical c. of uterus canalis cervicis uteri.
chordal c. notochordal c.
ciliary c's spatia anguli iridocornealis.
Civinini c. canaliculus chordae tympani.
Cloquet c. canalis hyaloideus.
cochlear c. canalis spiralis cochleae.
common atrioventricular c. atrioventricularis communis.
condylar c., condyloid c. canalis condylaris.
c. of Corti inner tunnel.
c. of Cotunnius the aqueductus vestibuli and canaliculus cochleae considered as a continuous passage.
craniopharyngeal c. an occasional passage through the sphenoid bone, opening into the sella turcica. Some authorities consider it a remnant of Rathke pouch.
crural c. canalis femoralis.
crural c. of Henle canalis adductorius.
dentinal c's dental canaliculi; see under *canaliculus*.
digestive c. see under *tract*.
diploic c's canales diploici.
Dorello c. an opening sometimes found in the temporal bone through which the abducent nerve and inferior petrosal sinus together enter the cavernous sinus.
c. of epididymis ductus epididymidis.
eustachian c. tuba auditiva.
external auditory c. meatus acusticus externus.
facial c., c. for facial nerve canalis nervi facialis.
fallopian c. canalis nervi facialis.
femoral c. canalis femoralis.
Ferrein c. rivus lacrimalis.
flexor c. canalis carpi.
Gartner c. ductus longitudinalis epoöphori.
gastric c. canalis gastricus.
genital c. any canal for the passage of ova or for copulatory use; called also *genital duct*.
greater palatine c. canalis palatinus major.
gubernacular c's four small openings in young crania, one behind each incisor tooth.
c. of Guidi canalis pterygoideus.
Guyon c. canalis ulnaris.
gynecophoral c., gynecophorous c. the ventral slot in which the male schistosome carries the female.
hair c. follicular infundibulum.
Hannover c. a potential space existing between the anterior and posterior portions of the suspensory ligament of the lens.
haversian c. canalis nutricius.
hemal c. the space within the hemal arch.
Hering c. cholangiole.
hernial c. an inguinal canal that contains an inguinal hernia.
Hirschfeld c's interdental c's.
horizontal semicircular c. canalis semicircularis lateralis.
c. of Hovius one of a series of connections between the venae vorticosae in certain mammals.
Huguier c. anterior canaliculus for chorda tympani.
Hunter c. canalis adductorius.
Huschke c. see under *foramen*.
hyaloid c. canalis hyaloideus.
hypoglossal c. canalis nervi hypoglossi.
iliac c. lacuna musculorum retroinguinalis.
incisive c's canales incisivi.
incisive c. of mandible an extension of the mandibular canal, leading forward to the symphysis inferiorly to the incisor teeth.
inferior dental c. canalis mandibulae.
infraorbital c. canalis infraorbitalis.
inguinal c. canalis inguinalis.
interdental c's channels in the alveolar process of the mandible, between the roots of the medial and lateral incisors, for the passage of anastomosing blood vessels between the sublingual and inferior dental arteries; called also *Hirschfeld c's*.

Canal *Continued*

interlobular biliary c's ductus biliferi interlobulares.
internal auditory c. meatus acusticus internus.
intralobular biliary c's ductuli biliferi.
Jacobson c., c. for Jacobson nerve canaliculus tympanicus.
Kovalevsky c. neurenteric c.
lacrimal c. canalis nasolacrimalis.
lateral inferior vomerobasilar c. canalis palatovaginalis.
lateral semicircular c. canalis semicircularis lateralis.
lateral superior vomerobasilar c. canalis vomerovaginalis.
Laurer c. a passage in trematode worms extending from the ovarian duct to the dorsal surface of the body.
lesser palatine c's canales palatini minores.
longitudinal c's of modiolus canales longitudinales modioli.
mandibular c. canalis mandibulae.
medullary c. 1. cavitas medullaris. 2. canalis vertebralis.
membranous semicircular c's ductus semicirculares.
mental c. an extension of the mandibular canal, leading superiorly to connect with the mental foramen.
c's of modiolus see *canalis spiralis modioli* and *canales longitudinales modioli.*
musculotubal c. canalis musculotubarius.
nasal c., nasolacrimal c. canalis nasolacrimalis.
nasopalatine c's canales incisivi.
neural c. canalis vertebralis.
neurenteric c. a passage, in the embryo, from the posterior part of the neural tube into the archenteron; called also *Braun, archenteric,* or *blastoporic c.*
notochordal c. a canal extending from the primitive pit into the notochordal process of the embryo; called also *chordal c.*
c. of Nuck a processus vaginalis peritonei (q.v.) in a female; it is usually obliterated after birth but may persist.
nutrient c. canalis nutricius.
obstetric c. birth c.
obturator c. canalis obturatorius.
olfactory c. the nasal fossae at an early stage of their embryonic development.
optic c. canalis opticus.
palatomaxillary c. canalis palatinus major.
palatovaginal c. canalis palatovaginalis.
parturient c. birth c.
pelvic c. the passage from the superior to the inferior aperture of the pelvis.
pericardioperitoneal c's a pair of passages in the embryo, connecting the primordial pericardial and peritoneal cavities.
perivascular c. a lymph space about a blood vessel.
persistent common atrioventricular c. atrioventricularis communis.
Petit c. spatia zonularia.
pharyngeal c. canalis palatovaginalis.
c. for pharyngotympanic tube semicanalis tubae auditivae.
pilary c. follicular infundibulum.
pleural c's pericardioperitoneal c's.
portal c. a space within Glisson capsule and the substance of the liver, containing branches of the portal vein, hepatic artery, and hepatic duct.
posterior alveolar c. an alveolar canal of the maxilla located posteriorly; see *canales alveolares corporis maxillae.*
posterior dental c's 1. canales alveolares corporis maxillae. 2. foramina alveolaria maxillae.
posterior ethmoidal c. foramen ethmoidale posterius.
posterior semicircular c. canalis semicircularis posterior.
pterygoid c. canalis pterygoideus.
pterygopalatine c. 1. canalis palatinus major. 2. canalis palatovaginalis.
pudendal c. canalis pudendalis.
pulp c. canalis radicis dentis.
pyloric c. canalis pyloricus.
c's of Recklinghausen small lymph spaces in the connective tissue.
recurrent c. canalis pterygoideus.
root c. canalis radicis dentis.
Rosenthal c. canalis spiralis modioli.
sacculocochlear c. ductus reuniens.
sacculoutricular c. ductus utriculosaccularis.
sacral c. canalis sacralis.
Santorini c. ductus pancreaticus accessorius.
Schlemm c. sinus venosus sclerae.
scleral c. the channel in the choroid and sclera of the eye through which the optic nerve passes.
semicircular c's canales semicirculares ossei.
serous c. a minute lymph space.
singular c. foramen singulare.
Sondermann c's conical extensions of the lumen of the Schlemm canal (venous sinus of the sclera) sometimes observed in the inner wall of the canal.
spermatic c. the canalis inguinalis in the male, providing for passage of the spermatic cord.
sphenopalatine c. 1. canalis palatovaginalis. 2. canalis palatinus major.
sphenopharyngeal c. canalis palatovaginalis.
spinal c. canalis vertebralis.
spiral c. of cochlea canalis spiralis cochleae.
spiral c. of modiolus canalis spiralis modioli.
Stensen c's canales incisivi.
c. of Stilling canalis hyaloideus.
c. of stomach canalis gastricus.
streak c. teat c.
subsartorial c. canalis adductorius.
Sucquet-Hoyer c. segmentum arteriale anastomosis arteriovenosae glomeriformis.
superior semicircular c. canalis semicircularis anterior.
supraciliary c. a small opening sometimes present near the supraorbital notch, which transmits a nutrient artery and a branch of the supraorbital nerve to the frontal sinus.
supraoptic c. a minute canal which is the anterior continuation of the optic recess above the optic chiasma.
tarsal c. sinus tarsi.
teat c. the canal leading from the lactiferous sinus to the exterior of the udder of an animal. Called also *streak c.*
c. for tensor tympani semicanalis musculi tensoris tympani.
Theile c. sinus transversus pericardii.
tubotympanic c. see under *recess.*
tympanic c. of cochlea scala tympani.
ulnar c. canalis ulnaris.
umbilical c. anulus umbilicalis.
urogenital c. see under *sinus.*
uterine c. cavitas uteri.
uterocervical c. canalis cervicis uteri.
utriculosaccular c. ductus utriculosaccularis.
vaginal c. the space within the vagina; called also *vulvouterine c.*
van Hoorne c. ductus thoracicus.
Velpeau c. canalis inguinalis.
ventricular c. canalis gastricus.
Verneuil c's collateral vessels of a venous trunk.
vertebral c. canalis vertebralis.
vestibular c. scala vestibuli.
vidian c. canalis pterygoideus.
Volkmann c's passages other than haversian canals (canales nutricii), for the passage of blood vessels through bone.
vomerine c. canalis vomerovaginalis.
vomerorostral c. canalis vomerorostralis.
vomerovaginal c. canalis vomerovaginalis.
vulvar c. vestibulum vaginae.
vulvouterine c. vaginal c.
zygomaticotemporal c. foramen zygomaticotemporale.

ca·na·les (kə-na'lēz) [L.] plural of *canalis.*

can·a·lic·u·li (kan″ə-lik'u-li) [L.] plural of *canaliculus.*

can·a·lic·u·li·tis (kan″ə-lik″u-li'tis) [L. *canaliculus,* from *canalis* channel + *-itis* inflammation] inflammation of the lacrimal ducts.

can·a·lic·u·li·za·tion (kan″ə-lik″u-lĭ-za'shən) the development of canaliculi, as in bone.

can·a·lic·u·lo·rhi·nos·to·my (kan″ə-lik″u-lo-ri-nos'tə-me) dacryocystorhinostomy.

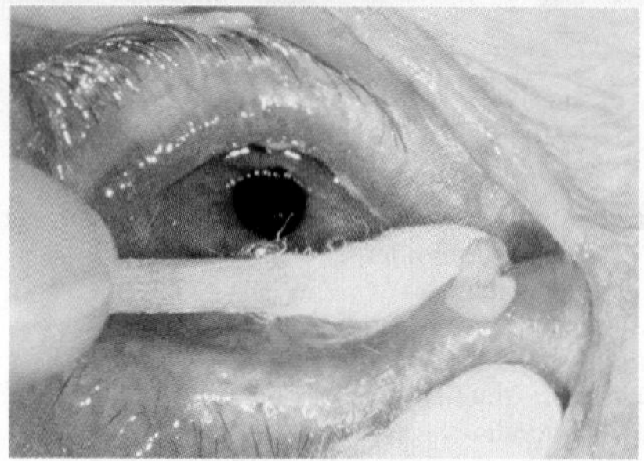

■ Canaliculitis, with conjunctivitis, inflamed punctum, and expressible discharge from the canaliculus.

can•a•lic•u•lus (kan″ə-lik′u-ləs) pl. *canalic′uli* [L. dim. of *canalis*] an extremely narrow tubular passage or channel. **canalic′ular** *adj*

anterior c. for chorda tympani an opening in the anterior part of the middle ear, at the medial end of the petrotympanic fissure, for exit of the chorda tympani nerve from the tympanic cavity; called also *Huguier canal.*

apical c. any of the numerous tubular invaginations arising from the clefts between the microvilli of the proximal convoluted tubule of the kidney and extending downward into the apical cytoplasm.

bile canaliculi, biliary canaliculi fine tubular canals running between liver cells throughout the parenchyma, usually occurring singly between each adjacent pair of cells, and forming a three-dimensional network of polyhedral meshes, with a single cell in each mesh. Called also *bile capillaries.*

bone canaliculi branching tubular passages radiating like wheel spokes from each bone lacuna to connect with the canaliculi of adjacent lacunae, and with the haversian canal.

caroticotympanic canaliculi, canali′culi caroticotympa′nici [TA] tiny passages in the temporal bone interconnecting the carotid canal and the tympanic cavity, and carrying communicating twigs between the internal carotid and tympanic plexuses.

c. for chorda tympani, c. chor′dae tym′pani [TA] a small canal that opens off the facial canal just before its termination, transmitting the chorda tympani nerve into the tympanic cavity; called also *Civinini canal.*

c. coch′leae [TA], **cochlear c.** a small canal in the petrous part of the temporal bone that interconnects the scala tympani of the internal ear with the subarachnoid space; it houses the perilymphatic duct and a small vein. Called also *aqueduct of Cotunnius.*

dental canaliculi minute channels in dentin, extending from the pulp cavity to the cementum and enamel. Called also *dental* or *dentinal tubules.*

haversian c. any of a system of minute channels in compact bone connected with each haversian canal.

innominate c., c. innomina′tus 1. sulcus nervi petrosi minoris. 2. foramen petrosum.

intercellular c. a tiny channel located between adjacent cells, such as one of the secretory capillaries (secretory canaliculi) of the gastric parietal cells.

intracellular canaliculi of parietal cells a system of canaliculi that seem to be intracellular, but are formed by deep invaginations of the surface of the gastric parietal cells rather than extending into the cytoplasm of the cell.

lacrimal c., c. lacrima′lis [TA] the short passage in an eyelid, beginning at the punctum, that leads from the lacrimal lake to the lacrimal sac; called also *lacrimal duct.*

mastoid c., c. mastoi′deus [TA] a minute passage beginning in the lateral wall of the jugular fossa of the temporal bone and passing into the temporal bone. The auricular branch of the vagus nerve passes through it to exit via the tympanomastoid fissure.

posterior c. for chorda tympani c. chordae tympani.

secretory c. see under *capillary.*

tympanic c., c. tympa′nicus [TA] a small opening on the inferior surface of the petrous part of the temporal bone in the floor of the petrosal fossa; it transmits the tympanic branch of the glossopharyngeal nerve and a small artery. Called also *Jacobson canal* and *canal for Jacobson nerve.*

c. vesti′buli [TA] vestibular canaliculus: a small canal extending from the vestibule of the internal ear to the posterior surface of the petrous part of the temporal bone; it houses the vestibular aqueduct.

ca•na•lis (kə-na′lis) pl. *cana′les* [L.] canal: a relatively narrow tubular passage or channel. Cf. *channel, tube,* and *tunnel.*

Canalis

Descriptions are given on TA terms, and include anglicized names of specific canals.

c. adducto′rius [TA] adductor canal: an intramuscular interval on the medial aspect of the middle third of the thigh, which contains the femoral vessels and the saphenous nerve. The lateral wall is formed by the vastus medialis, the posterior wall by the adductor longus and adductor magnus, the roof by a layer of fascia, and it is covered by the sartorius. Called also *crural canal of Henle, Hunter canal,* and *subsartorial canal.*

cana′les alveola′res cor′poris maxil′lae [TA] alveolar canals of maxilla: several canals in the maxilla for the passage of the posterior superior alveolar vessels and nerves, each canal beginning on the infratemporal surface of the maxilla at an alveolar foramen; called also *posterior dental canals.*

c. ana′lis [TA] anal canal: the terminal portion of the alimentary canal, about 4 cm long, extending from the anorectal junction to the anocutaneous line, containing the anus.

c. caro′ticus [TA] carotid canal: a passage in the petrous portion of the temporal bone, beginning on the inferior surface just anterior to the jugular foramen, and running anteromedially for about 2 cm; it is seen interiorly in the floor of the middle cranial fossa, where it meets the carotid sulcus on the body of the sphenoid bone. It houses the internal carotid artery.

c. car′pi [TA] carpal canal: an osseofibrous tunnel for passage of the tendons of the flexor muscles of the hand and digits, formed by the flexor retinaculum as it roofs over the concavity of the carpus on the palmar surface; called also *carpal tunnel* and *flexor canal.*

c. centra′lis medul′lae spina′lis [TA] central canal of spinal cord: a small canal extending throughout the length of the spinal cord, lined by ependymal cells. Above, it continues into the medulla oblongata, where it opens into the fourth ventricle.

c. cer′vicis u′teri [TA] cervical canal of uterus: the part of the uterine cavity that lies within the cervix.

c. condyla′ris [TA] condylar canal: an opening sometimes present in the floor of the condylar fossa for the transmission of a vein from the transverse sinus; called also *condyloid canal* and *posterior condyloid foramen.*

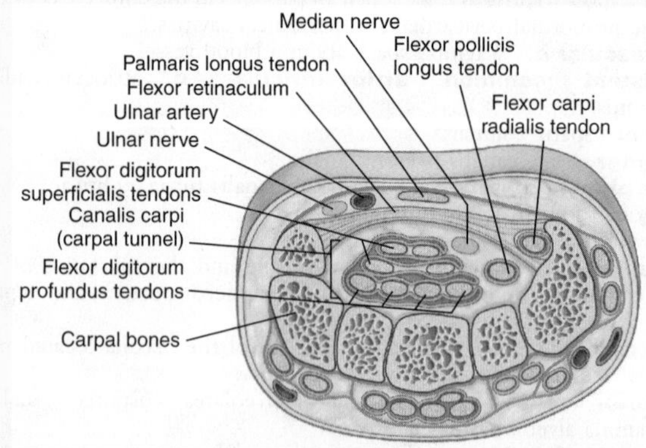

■ Canalis carpi (carpal tunnel), carrying the tendons of the flexor muscles.

cana′les diplo′ici [TA] diploic canals: bony canals in the cranial bones, located in the spongy bone between the compact tables and providing for passage of the veins of the diploë; called also *Breschet canals.*

c. femora′lis [TA] femoral canal: the cone-shaped medial part of the femoral sheath lateral to the base of the lacunar ligament; called also *crural canal.*

c. gas′tricus [TA] gastric canal: the longitudinal grooved channel formed by the more or less regular ridges along the lesser curvature of the stomach; called also *canal of stomach* and *ventricular canal.*

Canalis *Continued*

c. hyaloi′deus [TA] hyaloid canal: a passage running from in front of the optic disk to the lens of the eye; in the fetus it transmits the hyaloid artery. Called also *central canal of Stilling, central canal of vitreous,* and *Cloquet canal.*

cana′les incisi′vi [TA] incisive canals: the small canals opening into the incisive fossa of the hard palate, and transmitting small vessels and nerves from the floor of the nose into the front part of the roof of the mouth; called also *nasopalatine canals* and *Stensen canals.* See also *foramina incisiva,* under *foramen.*

c. infraorbita′lis [TA] infraorbital canal: a passage beneath the orbital surface of the maxilla, continuous posteriorly with the infraorbital sulcus, and opening anteriorly on the anterior surface of the body of the maxilla in the infraorbital foramen. It contains the infraorbital vessels and nerve.

c. inguina′lis [TA] inguinal canal: the passage superficial to the deep inguinal ring, transmitting the spermatic cord in the male and the round ligament in the female. Called also *abdominal canal* and *Velpeau canal.*

cana′les longitudina′les modi′oli [TA] longitudinal canals of modiolus: short tunnels in the modiolus that transmit blood vessels and nerves.

c. mandi′bulae [TA] mandibular canal: a canal that traverses the ramus and body of the mandible between the mandibular and mental foramina, transmitting the inferior alveolar vessels and nerve; beneath the first or second premolars it splits into the mental canal and the incisive canal. Called also *inferior dental canal.*

c. musculotuba′rius [TA] musculotubal canal: the combined canals for the pharyngotympanic tube and the tensor tympani muscle in the temporal bone.

c. nasolacrima′lis [TA] nasolacrimal canal: a canal formed by the downward continuation of the lacrimal groove, lacrimal bone, and inferior nasal concha; it lodges the nasolacrimal duct. Called also *lacrimal canal* and *nasal canal.*

c. ner′vi facia′lis [TA] facial canal: a canal in the temporal bone for the facial nerve, beginning in the internal acoustic meatus and passing anterolaterally dorsal to the vestibule of the internal ear for about 2 mm. Turning sharply backward at the genu of the facial canal, it runs along the medial wall of the tympanic cavity, then turns inferiorly and reaches the exterior of the petrous part of the temporal bone at the stylomastoid foramen. Called also *canal for facial nerve, fallopian aqueduct* or *canal,* and *aqueduct of Fallopius.*

c. ner′vi hypoglos′si [TA] hypoglossal canal: an opening in the lateral part of the occipital bone at the base of the condyle, which transmits the hypoglossal nerve and a branch of the posterior meningeal artery; called also *anterior condyloid canal* and *anterior condyloid foramen.*

c. nutri′cius [TA] nutrient canal of bone: one of the freely anastomosing channels of the haversian system of compact bone, which contain blood vessels, lymph vessels, and nerves; called also *c. nutriens* [TA alternative], *haversian canal,* and *haversian space.*

c. nu′triens TA alternative for *c. nutricius.*

c. obturato′rius [TA] obturator canal: an opening within the obturator membrane for the passage of the obturator vessels and nerve; its boundaries are the edge of the obturator membrane, together with the obturator groove of the pubic bone.

c. op′ticus [TA] optic canal: one of the paired openings in the sphenoid bone where the small wings are attached to the body of the bone at the apex of the orbit; each canal transmits one of the optic nerves and the ophthalmic artery of that side. Called also *foramen opticum ossis sphenoidalis* and *optic foramen of sphenoid bone.*

c. palati′nus ma′jor [TA] greater palatine canal: a passage in the sphenoid and palatine bones for the greater palatine vessels and nerve; it ends at the foramen palatinum majus. Called also *palatomaxillary canal, pterygopalatine canal,* and *sphenopalatine canal.*

cana′les palati′ni mino′res [TA] lesser palatine canals: openings in the palatine bone that branch off the great palatine canal to carry the lesser and middle palatine nerves and vessels to the roof of the mouth; they end at the foramina palatina minora. Called also *accessory palatine canals.*

c. palatovagina′lis [TA] palatovaginal canal: a narrow canal located in the roof of the nasal cavity between the inferior surface of the body of the sphenoid bone and the sphenoidal process of the palatine bone; it opens posteriorly into the nasal cavity and anteriorly into the pterygopalatine fossa. Called also *pharyngeal canal, pterygopalatine canal, sphenopalatine canal, sphenopharyngeal canal,* and *lateral inferior vomerobasilar canal.*

c. pterygoi′deus [TA] pterygoid canal: a horizontally running canal that passes forward through the base of the medial pterygoid plate of the sphenoid bone to open into the posterior wall of the pterygopalatine fossa just medial and inferior to the foramen rotundum; it transmits the pterygoid vessels and nerves. Called also *canal of Guidi, recurrent canal,* and *vidian canal.*

c. pudenda′lis [TA] pudendal canal: the tunnel in the special fascial sheath through which the pudendal vessels and nerve pass; it is intimately related to the obturator fascia. Called also *Alcock canal.*

c. pylo′ricus [TA] pyloric canal: the short, narrow part of the stomach extending from the gastroduodenal junction to the pyloric antrum.

c. ra′dicis den′tis [TA] root canal: the portion of the dental pulp cavity in the root of a tooth, extending from the pulp chamber to the apical foramen; more than one canal may be present in a single root, two commonly being present in the mesial root of the mandibular first molar. Called also *pulp canal.*

c. sacra′lis [TA] sacral canal: the continuation of the vertebral canal through the sacrum.

c. semicircula′ris ante′rior [TA] anterior semicircular canal: the anterior of the osseous semicircular canals, lodging the ductus semicircularis anterior of the membranous labyrinth. Called also *superior semicircular canal.*

c. semicircula′ris latera′lis [TA] lateral semicircular canal: the lateral of the osseous semicircular canals, lodging the ductus semicircularis lateralis of the membranous labyrinth; called also *horizontal semicircular canal.*

cana′les semicircula′res os′sei [TA] bony semicircular canals: three long canals of the bony labyrinth of the ear, forming loops and opening into the vestibule by five openings; they lodge the semicircular ducts. See *c. semicircularis anterior, c. semicircularis lateralis,* and *c. semicircularis posterior.* Called also *semicircular canals.*

c. semicircula′ris poste′rior [TA] posterior semicircular canal: the posterior of the semicircular canals, lodging the ductus semicircularis posterior of the membranous labyrinth.

c. spira′lis coch′leae [TA] spiral canal of cochlea: a winding tube that makes two and one-half turns about the modiolus of the cochlea; it is divided into two compartments, scala tympani and scala vestibuli, by the lamina spiralis.

c. spira′lis modi′oli [TA] spiral canal of modiolus: a canal following the course of the bony spiral lamina of the cochlea and containing the spiral ganglion of the cochlear division of the vestibulocochlear nerve. Called also *Rosenthal canal.*

c. ulna′ris [TA] ulnar canal: a small superficial canal at the base of the hypothenar bounded by the flexor retinaculum and the flexor carpi ulnaris muscle, which transmits blood vessels and the ulnar nerve from the forearm to the hand. Called also *Guyon canal* and *loge de Guyon.*

c. vertebra′lis [TA] vertebral canal: the canal formed by the foramina in the successive vertebrae, which encloses the spinal cord and meninges; called also *medullary canal, neural canal,* and *spinal canal.*

c. vomerorostra′lis [TA] vomerorostral canal: a canal located between the vomer and sphenoidal rostrum.

c. vomerovagina′lis [TA] vomerovaginal canal: an inconstant opening formed by the articulating margins of the ala of the vomer and the body of the sphenoid bone; called also *basipharyngeal canal, lateral superior vomerobasilar canal,* and *vomerine canal.*

---

can·a·lith (kan′ə-lith″) [*canal* + *-lith*] a free-floating particle within the endolymph of the semicircular canal; the presence of canaliths can cause benign paroxysmal positional vertigo.

can·a·li·za·tion (kan″ə-lĭ-za′shən) 1. formation of canals, natural or pathologic. 2. surgical establishment of canals for drainage. 3. recanalization. 4. in psychology, formation in the central nervous system of new pathways by repeated passage of nerve impulses.

ca·nalo·plas·ty (kan′ə-lo-plas″te) canalplasty.

ca·nal·plas·ty (kə-nal′plas-te) plastic reconstruction of a passage, as of the external auditory meatus.

ca·na·ry·pox (kə-na′re-poks) a type of fowlpox seen in canaries.

Can·a·sa (kan′ə-sə) trademark for a preparation of mesalamine.

Can·a·val·ia (kan″ə-val′yə) the jack bean, a genus of West Indian plants of the family Leguminosae, widely used as food. *C. ensifor′mis* D.C. and other species are the source of canavanine and concanavalin.

Can·a·van disease (kan′ə-vən) [Myrtelle May *Canavan*, American neurologist, 1879–1953] spongy degeneration of the central nervous system; see under *degeneration.*

Can·a·van-van Bo·gaert-Ber·trand disease (kan′ə-van vahn bo′gert bār-trahn′) [M.M. *Canavan;* Ludo *van Bogaert*, Belgian neurologist, 1897–1989; Ivan Georges *Bertrand*, French neurologist, 1893–1965] spongy degeneration of the central nervous system; see under *degeneration.*

can·av·a·nine (kə-nav′ə-nēn) an analogue of arginine found in alfalfa seeds and the jack bean; used in experimental medicine to study enzymes that usually act on arginine.

can·cel·lat·ed (kan′sə-lāt″əd) having a lattice-like structure; cancellous.

can·cel·lous (kan-səl′əs) of a reticular, spongy, or lattice-like structure; said mainly of bony tissue.

can·cel·lus (kan-səl′əs) pl. *cancel′li* [L. "a lattice"] any structure arranged like a lattice.

can·cer (kan′sər) [L. "crab," "malignant tumor"] a neoplastic disease the natural course of which is fatal. Cancer cells, unlike benign tumor cells, exhibit the properties of invasion and metastasis and are highly anaplastic. Cancer includes the two broad categories of carcinoma and sarcoma, but in normal usage it is often used synonymously with carcinoma. **can′cerous** *adj*

aniline c. cancer usually of the urinary bladder, occurring among those who work with aniline dyes; called also *dye workers' c.*

betel c. a type of squamous cell carcinoma of the cheek mucous membranes, seen in India and other Asian countries where betel nut, often mixed with tobacco, is held in the buccal vestibule for prolonged periods.

chimney sweeps' c. a type of squamous cell carcinoma of the skin of the scrotum that was formerly common in chimney sweeps owing to skin irritation by soot. Called also *soot c.*

colloid c. mucinous carcinoma.

contact c. cancer developing in a part of the body in contact with a previously existing cancer.

cystic c. see under *tumor.*

dendritic c. papillary carcinoma.

c. à deux [Fr. "cancer in two"] cancer attacking simultaneously or consecutively two persons who live together.

dye workers' c. aniline c.

endothelial c. endothelioma.

epithelial c. carcinoma.

glandular c. adenocarcinoma.

hereditary nonpolyposis colorectal c. (HNPCC) a group of hereditary, autosomal dominant cancers characterized by discrete adenomas of the colon and rectum without polyposis. Two types have been distinguished: in type 1, all affected persons have colorectal cancers; in type 2, some family members have cancer in other parts of the body, such as the female genital tract, stomach, brain, breast, or urinary tract. Both types are caused by mutations in mismatch repair genes, particularly *MSH2* (locus: 2p22-p21) and *MLH1* (locus: 3p21.3), and are characterized by microsatellite instability. Called also *Lynch syndrome.* Type 2 is also called *cancer family syndrome.*

latent c. cancer discovered, in the absence of any clinical manifestations, in the course of histological examination; cf. *occult c.*

mule spinners' c. one of the first types of skin cancer known to be caused by occupational exposure, affecting workers in the cotton spinning industry because of exposure to arsenic, tar, and carcinogenic oils; it was a form of squamous cell carcinoma.

nonmelanoma skin c's name given to a group of common skin cancers that do not metastasize, including basal cell carcinoma and squamous cell carcinoma.

occult c. a small cancer that may give rise to clinically evident distant metastases before it is itself clinically detectable; cf. *latent c.*

soot c. chimney sweeps' c.

swamp c. 1. pythiosis. 2. a general term for any of several syndromes in horses consisting of skin or mucosal lesions with ulcers and granulomatous tissue; they may be on the head, trunk, or legs. Included are *cutaneous habronemiasis, entomophthoromycosis,* and *pythiosis.*

tar c. squamous cell carcinoma caused by inflammatory irritation of fumes of tar or by the irritating effect of tar on the skin.

can·cer·emia (kan″sər-e′me-ə) the presence of cancer cells in the blood.

can·cer·i·ci·dal (kan″sər-ĭ-si′dəl) [*cancer* + L. *caedere* to kill] oncolytic.

can·cer·i·gen·ic (kan″sər-ĭ-jen′ik) giving rise to a malignant tumor; cf. *carcinogenic* and *sarcomagenic.* Called also *cancerogenic.*

can·cero·ci·dal (kan″sər-o-si′dəl) oncolytic.

can·cer·o·gen·ic (kan″sər-o-jen′ik) cancerigenic.

can·cero·pho·bia (kan″ser-o-fo′be-ə) cancerphobia.

can·cer·pho·bia (kan″sər-fo′be-ə) [*cancer* + *-phobia*] irrational fear of cancer.

Can·ci·das (kan-si′dəs) trademark for a preparation of caspofungin acetate.

can·cri·form (kang′krĭ-form) cancroid.

can·croid (kang′kroid) [L. *cancer*, gen. *cancri*, crab, malignant tumor + *-oid*] resembling cancer.

can·crum (kang′krəm) [L.] canker.

c. na′si gangrenous rhinitis of children.

c. o′ris noma (def. 1).

can·dela (cd) (kan-del′ə) [L. *candēla* candle] the base SI unit of luminous intensity, equal to the luminous intensity, in a given direction, of a source that emits a monochromatic radiation of frequency 540×10^{12} hertz and that has a radiant intensity in that direction of 1/683 watt per steradian. Called also *candle.*

Can·dep·tin (kan-dep′tin) trademark for preparations of candicidin.

can·de·sar·tan ci·lex·e·til (kan″də-sahr′tan) an angiotensin II receptor antagonist, used as an antihypertensive; administered orally.

can·di·ci·din (kan″dĭ-si′din) a polyene antifungal antibiotic produced by a strain of *Streptomyces griseus;* it is especially effective against *Candida albicans*, and is administered intravaginally in the treatment of vulvovaginal candidiasis.

Can·di·da (kan′dĭ-də) [L. *candidus* glowing white] a genus of yeastlike Fungi Imperfecti of the form-family Cryptococcaceae that produce yeast cells, mycelia, pseudomycelia, and blastospores. Some species are part of the normal flora of the skin and mucous membranes but can also cause infections. Formerly called *Monilia, Mycotoruloides,* and *Oidium.*

C. al′bicans a species that is part of the normal flora of the skin and mucous membranes and is the most frequent cause of candidiasis.

C. dublinien′sis a species that closely resembles *C. albicans* and causes infections particularly in immunocompromised persons.

C. glabra′ta *Torulopsis glabrata.*

C. guilliermon′dii a species that sometimes causes cutaneous candidiasis, onychomycosis, meningitis, and endocarditis.

C. kru′sei a species occasionally associated with candidiasis, esophagitis, endocarditis, and vaginitis.

C. lusita′niae a species that can cause opportunistic infections; its perfect (sexual) stage is *Clavispora lusitaniae.*

C. mesente′rica a species that causes fermentation in fruit acids; called also *Saccharomyces mesentericus.*

C. parapsilo′sis a species that sometimes causes endocarditis, paronychia, or otitis externa.

C. pseudotropica′lis a species that sometimes causes vulvovaginal candidiasis.

C. stellatoi′dea a species that sometimes causes vulvovaginal candidiasis or *Candida* endocarditis. Some authorities consider it a variant of *C. albicans.*

C. tropica′lis a species that sometimes causes *Candida* vaginitis, meningitis, onychomycosis, or bronchopulmonary infection.

C. vi′ni a species found in fermenting liquors and the urine of diabetics. Called also *Saccharomyces mycoderma.*

can·di·dal (kan′di-dəl) pertaining to or caused by *Candida.*

can·di·de·mia (kan″dĭ-de′me-ə) the presence in the blood of fungi of the genus *Candida*, usually resulting from *Candida* endocarditis or systemic candidiasis.

can·di·di·a·sis (kan″dĭ-di′ə-sis) infection with a fungus of the genus *Candida*, especially *C. albicans.* It is usually a superficial infection of the skin or mucous membranes, although sometimes it manifests as a systemic infection or endocarditis; any form can become more severe in immunocompromised patients. Called also *moniliasis* and *candidosis.*

acute pseudomembranous c. thrush (def. 1).

atrophic c. a type of oral c. (thrush) marked by erythematous, pebbled patches on the hard or soft palate, buccal mucosa, and dorsal surface of the tongue, a complication of numerous different conditions such as vitamin

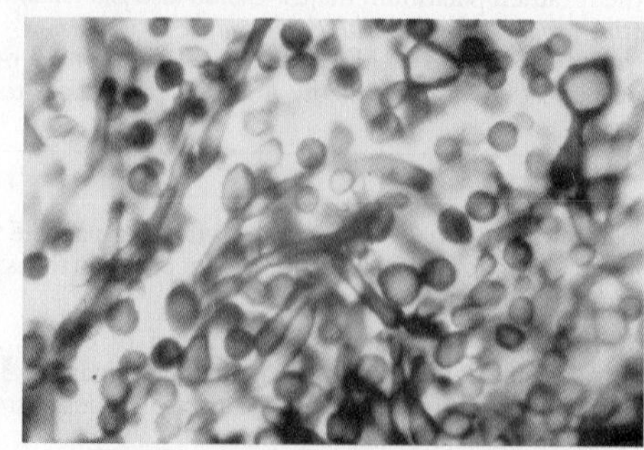

■ *Candida albicans* (methenamine silver stain).

deficiency, diabetes mellitus, or poorly-fitting dentures. There are acute forms and a chronic form called *denture stomatitis*.

bronchopulmonary c. candidiasis of the respiratory tract, either from colonization of the tracheobronchial tree in immunocompromised patients or those on antibiotics, or associated with pneumonia in the immunocompromised. It ranges from mild to severe and life-threatening. Called also *bronchocandidiasis*.

chronic mucocutaneous c. any of a diverse group of candidal infections of the oral mucosa, skin, nails, and vaginal mucosa; they are usually resistant to treatment, may be localized or diffuse, are sometimes familial, and may be associated with endocrinopathy or immunosuppression.

cutaneous c. candidiasis of the skin, which may be manifested as eczemalike lesions of the interdigital spaces, perlèche, or chronic paronychia.

endocardial c. *Candida* endocarditis.

oral c. thrush (def. 1).

pulmonary c. a type of fungal pneumonia caused by infection with *Candida* species, seen especially in immunocompromised patients or those with malignancies. Called also *Candida pneumonia*.

vaginal c., vulvovaginal c. candidal infection of the vagina, and usually also the vulva, commonly characterized by pruritus, creamy white discharge, vulvar erythema and swelling, and dyspareunia. Called also *Candida* or *candidal vaginitis* and *Candida* or *candidal vulvovaginitis*.

can·di·did (kan′dĭ-did) an id reaction expressing hypersensitivity to infection with *Candida* elsewhere on the body.

can·di·din (kan′dĭ-din) a skin test antigen derived from *Candida albicans*, used in testing for the development of delayed hypersensitivity to constituents of the microorganism.

can·di·do·sis (kan-dĭ-do′sis) candidiasis.

can·did·uria (kan″did-u′re-ə) the presence of *Candida* organisms in the urine.

can·din (kan′din) echinocandin.

can·dle (kan′dəl) 1. a mass of wax or similar substance, usually cylindrical in shape, with a wick for burning, to furnish illumination or heat. 2. a cylindrical mass of material used as a filter in microbiology. 3. candela.

cane (kān) a wooden stick or metal rod used for support in walking.

adjustable c. a cane whose length can be easily altered.

English c. forearm crutch.

quadripod c., quadruped c. a cane adapted for increased stability by forking to provide a four-legged rectangular base of support.

tripod c. a cane similar to a quadripod cane except that it has three legs to provide a triangular base of support.

ca·nes·cent (kə-nes′ənt) [L. *canus* gray] 1. becoming white or grayish. 2. in biology, having grayish or whitish hairs or down; hoary.

ca·nid (ka′nid, kan′id) any member of the family Canidae.

Ca·ni·dae (ka′nĭ-de) [L. *canis* dog + *-idae*] a family of carnivorous mammals that includes dogs, wolves, foxes, jackals, and coyotes.

ca·nine (ka′nīn) [L. *canis* dog] 1. of, pertaining to, or like that which belongs to a dog. 2. canine tooth. 3. pertaining to a canine tooth.

ca·ni·nus (ka-ni′nəs) musculus levator anguli oris.

ca·ni·ti·es (kə-nish′e-ēz) [L.] diffuse grayness or whiteness of the scalp hair, especially as associated with aging. Cf. *achromotrichia*, *leukotrichia*, and *poliosis*.

can·ker (kang′kər) 1. an ulceration, especially of the oral mucosa. 2. a disease of the keratogenous membrane in horses, usually in the hindlimb, with loss of function of horn-secreting cells and discharge of a serous exudate in place of the normal horny hoof; it begins at the frog and extends to the sole and wall. 3. otitis externa in a dog or cat.

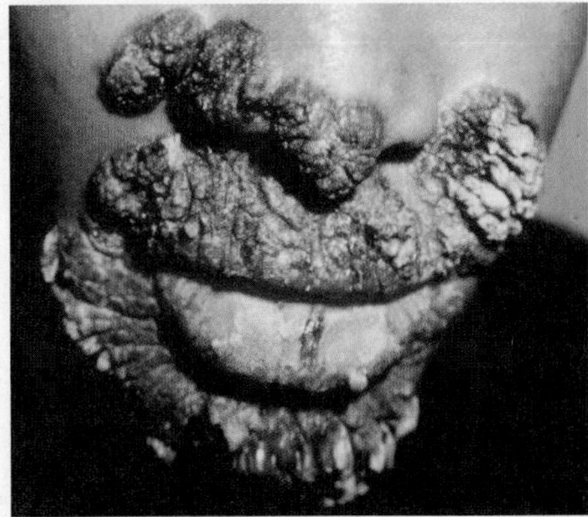

■ Chronic mucocutaneous candidiasis.

can·na·bi·di·ol (kan″ə-bĭ-di′ol) a nonpsychoactive diphenol isolated from cannabis.

can·nab·i·noid (kə-nab′ĭ-noid) any of the principles of cannabis, including tetrahydrocannabinol, cannabinol, and cannabidiol.

can·nab·i·nol (kə-nab′ĭ-nol) a nonpsychoactive constituent of resinous exudates of *Cannabis sativa* L.; its tetrahydro derivatives are active principles.

Can·na·bis (kan′ə-bis) a genus of flowering herbs. *C. sati′va* L. (Cannabaceae) is the hemp plant, widely used for fiber and rope; its dried leaves and flowers are called marijuana (q.v.) and contain tetrahydrocannabinol and other cannabinoids.

can·na·bis (kan′ə-bis) [Gr. *kannabis* hemp] the dried flowering tops of *Cannabis sativa*, which contain the euphoric principles Δ^1-3,4-*trans* and Δ^6-3,4-*trans* tetrahydrocannabinol, as well as cannabinol and cannabidiol. It is classified as hallucinogenic and is most commonly prepared as hashish or marijuana.

Can·niz·za·ro reaction (kahn″e-tsah′ro) [Stanislao *Cannizzaro*, Italian chemist, 1826–1910] see under *reaction*.

Can·non ring (point), theory (kan′ən) [Walter Bradford *Cannon*, American physiologist, 1871–1945] see under *ring* and see *emergency theory*, under *theory*.

Can·non-Bard theory (kan′ən bahrd′) [W.B. *Cannon;* Philip *Bard*, American psychologist, 1898–1977] emergency theory.

can·nu·la (kan′u-lə) [L. dim. of *canna* "reed"] a tube for insertion into a vessel, duct, or cavity; during insertion its lumen is usually occupied by a trocar. Cf. *catheter*.

nasal c. a cannula that fits into the nostrils for delivery of oxygen therapy. Called also *nasal prongs*.

perfusion c. a double tube for running a continuous flow of liquid into and out of an organ.

washout c. a cannula attached to a manometer and inserted into a blood vessel so that the connection between the artery and the manometer can be irrigated during long observations.

can·nu·late (kan′u-lāt) to introduce a cannula, which may be left in place.

can·nu·la·tion (kan″u-la′shən) the insertion of a cannula.

can·nu·li·za·tion (kan″u-lĭ-za′shən) cannulation.

can·ren·o·ate po·tas·si·um (kan-ren′o-āt) a potassium-sparing diuretic with actions and uses similar to those of spironolactone.

can·ren·one (kan-ren′ōn) an aldosterone antagonist, the active metabolite of canrenoate potassium and spironolactone, used as a potassium-sparing diuretic; administered orally.

cant (kant) an inclination or slope.

c. of mandible the angle formed by the intersection of the mandibular (gonion-gnathion) plane with the sella-nasion or Frankfort plane.

can·tha·ri·a·sis (kan″thə-ri′ə-sis) [Gr. *kantharos* beetle] infection by beetles as parasites, often after a person or other animal has accidentally ingested larval or adult forms and the beetles are living as endoparasites.

can·thar·i·dal (kan-thar′ĭ-dəl) containing or pertaining to cantharides.

can·thar·i·date (kan-thar′ĭ-dāt) any salt of cantharidic acid.

can·thar·i·des (kan-thar′ĭ-dēz) [L.] the dried body of *Lytta (Cantharis) vesicatoria*, containing the toxic active principle cantharidin (q.v.); it was formerly applied externally as a powerful rubefacient and blistering agent and given internally as a diuretic and aphrodisiac. Called also *Spanish fly*.

can·tha·rid·ic ac·id (kan″thə-rid′ik) a dibasic acid formed when cantharidin dissolves in water.

can·thar·i·din (kan-thar′ĭ-din) a bitter-tasting crystalline substance, the lactone of cantharidic acid and the most important active principle of cantharides; it is also found in the bodies of other beetles such as *Epicauta*. On human skin it produces blistering; consumption of the dead bodies of the beetles in hay or other feed can be lethal to farm animals.

can·thar·i·dism (kan-thar′ĭ-diz-əm) 1. a toxic reaction to the misuse of cantharides. 2. cantharidin poisoning.

Can·tha·ris (kan′thə-ris) [L., from Gr. *kantharos* beetle] *Lytta*.

C. vesicato′ria *Lytta vesicatoria*.

can·thec·to·my (kan-thek′tə-me) [*canth-* + *ectomy*] surgical removal of a canthus.

can·thi (kan′thi) [L.] plural of *canthus*.

can·thi·tis (kan-thi′tis) inflammation of a canthus or of the canthi.

canth(o)- [Gr. *kanthos*] a combining form denoting relationship to a canthus.

can·thol·y·sis (kan-thol′ĭ-sis) [*cantho-* + *-lysis*] surgical division of the canthus of an eye or of a canthal ligament.

can·tho·plas·ty (kan′tho-plas″te) [*cantho-* + *-plasty*] plastic surgery of the medial and/or lateral canthus, especially section of the lateral canthus to lengthen the palpebral fissure; also the surgical restoration of a defective canthus. **canthoplas′tic** *adj*

can·thor·rha·phy (kan-thor′ə-fe) [*cantho-* + *-rrhaphy*] the suturing of the palpebral fissure at either canthus.

can·thot·o·my (kan-thot′ə-me) [*cantho-* + *-tomy*] surgical division of the outer canthus.

can·thus (kan′thəs) pl. *can′thi* [L., from Gr. *kanthos*] the angle at either end of the fissure between the eyelids; see *angulus oculi lateralis* and *angulus oculi medialis.* **can′thal** *adj*

inner c., nasal c. angulus oculi medialis.

outer c., temporal c. angulus oculi lateralis.

Can·til (kan′til) trademark for a preparation of mepenzolate bromide.

can·ti·le·ver (kan′tĭ-le″vər) a projecting structure supported on only one end and carrying a load at the other end or along its length.

Cant·lie line (kant′le) [Sir James *Cantlie*, Scottish surgeon, 1851–1926] see under *line.*

Can·tor tube (kan′tər) [Meyer O. *Cantor*, American physician, 20th century] see under *tube.*

Can·trell pentalogy (kan-trel′) [James R. *Cantrell*, American physician, 20th century] see under *pentalogy.*

can·u·la (kan′u-lə) cannula.

cao gio (gou yaw) [Vietnamese] coin rubbing.

CAP College of American Pathologists; catabolite (gene) activator protein.

Cap. [L.] ca′piat (let him take).

cap (kap) 1. a protective covering for the head or for a similar structure. 2. colloquial term for an artificial crown.

5′ c. a structure consisting of a 7-methylguanosine (m^7G) residue attached backwards (i.e., 5′ to 5′) by a triphosphate linkage to the 5′ end of primary mRNA transcripts in eukaryotes; in addition, the first and, in some cases, second nucleotide of the mRNA are methylated at the 2′ position of the ribose residue. The 5′ cap protects the mRNA from attack by 5′ exonucleases and also functions in the recognition of the mRNA by ribosomes.

acrosomal c. acrosome.

cervical c. a contraceptive device similar to the diaphragm but smaller, consisting of a cup that fits directly over the cervix.

cradle c. crusta lactea.

duodenal c. ampulla duodeni.

enamel c., germinal c. a caplike structure of the enamel organ, developed during the third month of fetal development, and composed of an outer layer and an inner enamel layer; between the two layers are looser ectodermal cells that become the stellate reticulum.

head c. the double-layered caplike structure over the upper two-thirds of the acrosome of a spermatozoon, consisting of the collapsed acrosomal vesicle.

ink c., inky c. any mushroom of the genus *Coprinus.*

knee c. patella.

metanephric c. see under *blastema.*

phrygian c. the appearance of the gallbladder in cholecystography, showing kinking between the body and the fundus, with the fundus being fixed and folded.

polar c. a chromophilic, saclike organelle occurring beneath the spore wall in the polar region of microsporidian protozoa. Called also *polar capsule.*

postnuclear c. a broad band encircling the postacrosomal region of the nucleus of a spermatozoon.

root c. a thimble-shaped group of cells forming a protective covering over the apical meristem in the tip of a plant root.

c. of Zinn a prominence of the pulmonary arc in the left upper portion of the cardiac silhouette, usually seen in posteroanterior radiograms in cases of patent ductus arteriosus, and representing the dilated pulmonary artery.

ca·pac·i·tance (C) (kə-pas′ĭ-təns) 1. the property of being able to store an electric charge. 2. the ratio of the charge stored by a capacitor to the voltage across the capacitor. Formerly called *capacity.* The SI unit of capacitance is the farad.

membrane c. the electrical capacitance of a cell membrane; it is equal to the ratio of the net charge inside the cell to the membrane potential and is approximately 1 $\mu F/cm^2$.

ca·pac·i·ta·tion (kə-pas″ĭ-ta′shən) the process by which spermatozoa in the ampullary portion of a uterine tube become capable of going through the acrosomal reaction and fertilizing an oocyte.

ca·pac·i·tor (kə-pas′ĭ-tər) a device for holding and storing charges of electricity.

ca·pac·i·ty (kə-pas′ĭ-te) [L. *capacitas*, from *capere* to take] 1. power or ability to hold, retain, or contain, or the ability to absorb. 2. the volume or potential volume of material (solid, liquid, or gas) that can be held or contained. 3. capacitance. 4. mental ability to receive, accomplish, endure, or understand; sometimes specifically the cognitive ability to make informed medical decisions.

closing c. the volume of gas in the lungs at the time the airways close during respiration; the closing volume added to the residual volume, usually expressed as a percentage of total lung capacity.

cranial c. an expression of the amount of space within the cranium.

diffusing c., diffusion c. the ability of the alveolocapillary membrane to transfer gas: a reflection of the thinness and area of the alveolocapillary membrane. It is the amount of gas transferred per minute from the alveolar gas to the pulmonary capillary blood divided by the mean pressure gradient of the gas between the alveolar gas and the capillary blood; unit, mL/min/torr (or mm Hg). Symbol D.

forced vital c. (FVC) vital capacity measured when the patient is exhaling with maximum speed and effort.

functional residual c. the volume of gas remaining at the end of a normal quiet exhalation; abbreviated FRC. See illustration.

heat c. the amount of heat required to raise the temperature of a specific quantity of a substance by one degree Celsius. Symbol C (C_p at constant pressure, C_v at constant volume).

inspiratory c. the volume of gas that can be taken into the lungs on a full inhalation, starting from the functional residual capacity; it is equal to the tidal volume plus the inspiratory reserve volume. Abbreviated IC. See illustration.

iron-binding c. (IBC) the extent to which transferrin in the serum of a given patient can bind serum iron; see also *total iron-binding c.*

maximal breathing c. maximum voluntary ventilation.

maximal tubular excretory c. transport maximum; see under *maximum.*

molar heat c. heat capacity when the amount of the substance is expressed in moles.

specific heat c. specific heat. Symbol *c.*

thermal c. heat c.

total iron-binding c. (TIBC) a measure of the total amount of iron that can be bound by the transferrin in a serum sample, determined by saturating the transferrin with iron, then removing the unbound iron with an absorbent and measuring the iron in the filtrate; used in the evaluation of patients with iron deficiency or overload. See also *transferrin saturation*, under *saturation.*

total lung c. (TLC) the volume of gas contained in the lungs at the end of a maximal inhalation. See illustration.

virus neutralizing c. the ability of a serum to inhibit the infectivity of a virus.

vital c. (VC) the volume of gas that can be expelled from the lungs from a position of full inhalation, with no limit to the duration of exhalation; it is equal to the inspiratory capacity plus the expiratory reserve volume. See illustration.

Cap·a·stat (kap′ə-stat) trademark for a preparation of capreomycin sulfate.

CAPD continuous ambulatory peritoneal dialysis.

cap·e·ci·ta·bine (kap″ə-si′tə-bēn) an antineoplastic that is converted in vivo into 5-fluorouracil and is used in treatment of metastatic breast or colorectal carcinoma, administered orally.

cap·e·line (kap′ə-līn) [Fr.] a cap-shaped bandage for the head or for the stump of an amputated limb.

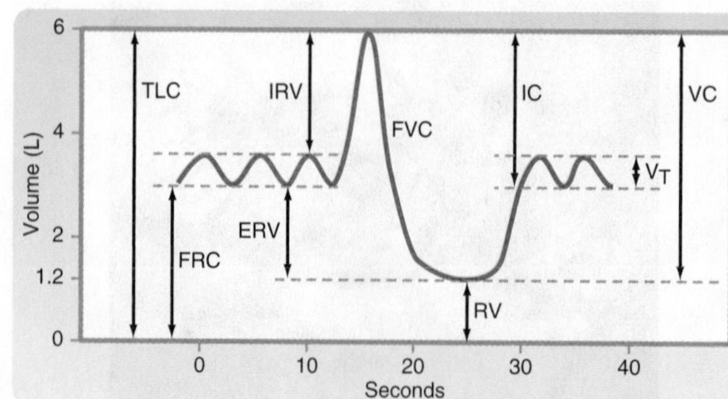

■ Diagram of lung volumes and capacities: *ERV*, expiratory reserve volume; *FRC*, functional residual capacity; *FVC*, forced vital capacity; *IC*, inspiratory capacity; *IRV*, inspiratory reserve volume; *RV*, residual volume; *TLC*, total lung capacity; *VC*, vital capacity; V_T, tidal volume.

Ca•pex (ka′peks) trademark for a preparation of fluocinolone acetonide.

Cap•gras syndrome (kahp-grah′) [Jean Marie Joseph *Capgras*, French psychiatrist, 1873–1950] see under *syndrome.*

cap•il•lar•ec•ta•sia (kap″ĭ-lar″ək-ta′zhə) [*capillary* + *ectasia*] dilatation of capillaries.

Ca•pil•la•ria (kap″ĭ-lar′e-ə) a genus of nematodes of the family Trichuridae, superfamily Trichuroidea.

C. contor′ta a species parasitic in domestic fowl.

C. hepa′tica a species parasitic in the liver of rats and many other mammals; a few human infections have been reported.

C. philippinen′sis a parasite of the human intestine in the Philippines and nearby areas, the primary cause of capillariasis in humans.

cap•il•la•ri•a•sis (kap″ĭ-lə-ri′ə-sis) infection with nematodes of the genus *Capillaria.* In humans this is most often intestinal infestation with *C. philippinensis,* with symptoms including severe diarrhea, malabsorption, malaise, and sometimes death. In birds the infecting species is *C. contorta,* and in many mammals (but only occasionally humans) it is *C. hepatica.*

cap•il•lar•io•mo•tor (kap″ĭ-lar″e-o-mo′tər) pertaining to the functional activity of the capillaries.

cap•il•lar•i•os•co•py (kap″ĭ-lar″e-os′kə-pe) capillaroscopy.

cap•il•lar•itis (kap″ĭ-lər-i′tis) inflammation of the capillaries, often with capillary fragility. Called also *telangiitis.*

cap•il•lar•i•ty (kap″ĭ-lar′ĭ-te) the action by which the surface of a liquid where it is in contact with a solid, as in capillary tubes, is elevated or depressed.

cap•il•la•rop•a•thy (kap″ĭ-lə-rop′ə-the) [*capillary* + *-pathy*] any disease of the capillaries; called also *telangiosis.*

cap•il•la•ros•co•py (kap″ĭ-lər-os′kə-pe) [*capillary* + *-scope*] diagnostic examination of the capillaries with the microscope. Called also *capillarioscopy* and *microangioscopy.*

cap•il•lary (kap′ĭ-lar″e) [L. *capillaris* hair-like] 1. pertaining to or resembling a hair. 2. any of the minute vessels that connect the arterioles and venules, forming a network in nearly all parts of the body. Their walls act as semipermeable membranes for the interchange of various substances, including fluids, between the blood and tissue fluid. The two principal types are *continuous* and *fenestrated capillaries.* Called also *vas capillare* [TA]. 3. vas lymphocapillare.

arterial c. a type of minute vessel lacking a continuous muscular coat, intermediate in structure and location between an arteriole and a capillary; called also *precapillary, precapillary arteriole,* and *metarteriole.*

bile c′s 1. bile canaliculi. 2. a term sometimes used to designate the cholangioles.

continuous c′s one of the two major types of capillaries, found in muscle, skin, lung, central nervous system, and other tissues, and characterized by an uninterrupted endothelium, a continuous basal lamina, fine filaments, and numerous pinocytotic vesicles. Cf. *fenestrated c′s.*

erythrocytic c′s capillaries of the bone marrow of early life which seem to produce erythrocytes.

fenestrated c′s one of the two major types of capillaries, found in the intestinal mucosa, renal glomeruli, pancreas, endocrine glands, and other tissues, and characterized by circular fenestrae or pores that penetrate the endothelium and may be closed by a very thin diaphragm. Cf. *continuous c′s.*

glomerular c. any of the capillaries of a renal glomerulus; see also *filtration barrier,* under *barrier.*

lymph c., lymphatic c. vas lymphocapillare.

Meigs c′s capillaries in the myocardium.

peritubular c. any of the capillaries around the proximal and distal convoluted tubules of the kidney.

secretory c. any of the extremely fine intercellular canaliculi situated between adjacent gland cells, such as the gastric parietal cells, being formed by the apposition of grooves in the surfaces of the cells, and opening into the gland's lumen.

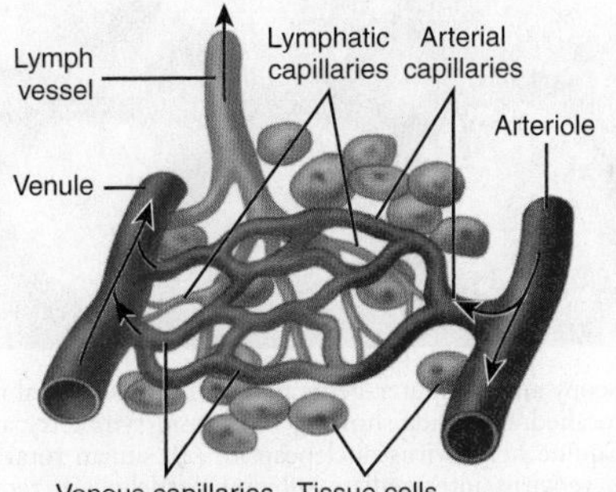

■ Capillary bed, showing the connection between the arterial and venous capillaries.

sheathed c′s see under *artery.*

sinusoidal c. vas sinusoideum.

venous c. a type of minute vessel lacking a muscular coat, intermediate in structure and location between a venule and a capillary. Called also *postcapillary* and *postcapillary venule.*

cap•il•li (kə-pil′i) (sing. *capil′lus*) [L.] [TA] the hairs of the scalp.

cap•il•li•ti•um (kap″ĭ-lish′e-əm) [L. "head of hair"] a filamentous structure that interlaces among the spores in the fruiting bodies of certain Gasteromycetes and Myxomycetes.

cap•il•lus (kə-pil′əs) [L.] singular of *capilli.*

cap•i•ta (kap′ĭ-tə) [L.] plural of *caput.*

cap•i•tal (kap′ĭ-təl) 1. of the highest importance; involving danger to life. 2. of or pertaining to the head of the femur.

cap•i•tate (kap′ĭ-tāt) [L. *caput* head] head-shaped.

cap•i•ta•tion (kap″ĭ-ta′shən) the annual fee paid to a physician or group of physicians by each participant in a health plan.

cap•i•ta•tum (kap″ĭ-ta′təm) [L. "having a head"] the capitate bone, or os capitatum [TA].

cap•i•tel•lo•con•dy•lar (kap″ĭ-tel″o-kon′də-lər) pertaining to a capitellum (especially the capitulum humeri) and a condyle, such as in reference to an elbow prosthesis.

cap•i•tel•lum (kap″ĭ-tel′əm) [L. dim. of *caput* head] capitulum humeri.

cap•i•ton•nage (kap″ĭ-to-nahzh′) [Fr.] the surgical closure of a cyst cavity by applying sutures in such a way as to cause approximation of the opposing surfaces.

cap•i•to•ped•al (kap″ĭ-to-ped′əl) pertaining to the head and foot.

Cap•i•trol (kap′ĭ-trol) trademark for a preparation of chloroxine.

ca•pit•u•la (kə-pit′u-lə) [L.] plural of *capitulum.*

ca•pit•u•lar (kə-pit′u-lər) pertaining to a capitulum or head of a bone.

ca•pit•u•lum (kə-pit′u-ləm) pl. *capit′ula* [L. dim. of *caput*] 1. a little head, or a small eminence on a bone by which it articulates with another bone. 2. a bulbous, knoblike, or enlarged terminal protuberance of a body or part, such as: *(a)* the movable head zone *(gnathosoma)* bearing the mouth parts of a tick or mite; *(b)* the end of an insect's antennae; or *(c)* the anterior end of the axostyle of certain zooflagellates, containing the nucleus of the organism.

c. hu′meri [TA], **c. of humerus** an eminence on the distal end of the lateral epicondyle of the humerus for articulation with the head of the radius; called also *capitellum* and *little* or *radial head of humerus.*

Cap•lan syndrome (kap′lən) [Anthony *Caplan*, British physician, 1907–1976] see under *syndrome.*

cap•ne•ic (kap′ne-ik) [*capno-* + *-ic*] under conditions of increased carbon dioxide in the atmosphere; said of the incubation of bacterial cultures.

capn(o)- [Gr. *kapnos* smoke] a combining form signifying a sooty or smoky appearance, or the presence of carbon dioxide.

Cap•no•cy•toph•a•ga (kap″no-si-tof′ə-gə) [*capno-* + Gr. *kytos* cell + *phagein* to eat] a genus of gram-negative, facultatively anaerobic, rod-shaped or fusiform bacteria of the family Flavobacteriaceae, which occur in normal and diseased sites of the human oral cavity. It has also been associated with systemic disease in debilitated persons. The type species is *C. ochra′cea.*

C. canimor′sus a species that is part of the normal oral flora of dogs and cats; when a human is bitten by an infected animal, an infection may follow that can be fatal, characterized by cellulitis, bacteremia, purulent meningitis, endocarditis, peripheral gangrene, malar purpura, and Waterhouse-Friderichsen syndrome. Infection is more severe in persons with asplenia, alcoholism, or a hematologic malignancy.

C. cynodeg′mi a species that is a normal inhabitant of the mouths of dogs but can cause infection in persons bitten by dogs.

C. gingiva′lis a species that is a normal inhabitant of the human oral cavity but has sometimes been implicated in cases of periodontitis, and occasionally causes sepsis or other infection, especially in immunocompromised patients.

C. ochra′cea a species that is a normal inhabitant of the human oral cavity but has sometimes been implicated in cases of periodontitis, and occasionally causes sepsis or other infection, especially in immunocompromised patients.

C. sputi′gena a species that is a normal inhabitant of the human oral cavity but has sometimes been implicated in cases of periodontitis, and occasionally causes sepsis or other infection, especially in immunocompromised patients.

cap•no•gram (kap′no-gram″) a real-time waveform record of the concentration of carbon dioxide in the respiratory gases.

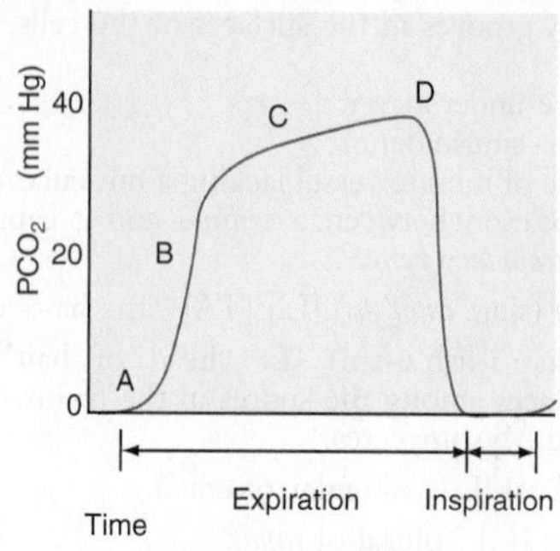

■ Normal capnogram. *(A)*, Carbon dioxide cleared from the anatomic dead space; *(B)*, dead space and alveolar carbon dioxide; *(C)*, alveolar plateau; *(D)*, end-tidal carbon dioxide tension ($P_{ET}CO_2$).

cap•no•graph (kap′no-graf″) [*capno-* + *-graph*] a system for monitoring the concentration of exhaled carbon dioxide, consisting of a sensor placed in the breathing circuit or a tube that carries part of the exhaled gases to the analyzing device, a mass spectrometer or an infrared spectrometer, and devices to provide continuous visual (cathode ray tube) and graphic (printer) displays.

cap•nog•ra•phy (kap-nog′rə-fe) [*capno-* + *-graphy*] monitoring of the concentration of exhaled carbon dioxide in order to assess the physiologic status of patients with acute respiratory problems or who are receiving mechanical ventilation and to determine the adequacy of ventilation in anesthetized patients.

cap•no•hep•a•tog•ra•phy (kap″no-hep″ə-tog′rə-fe) radiography of the liver after intravenous injection of carbon dioxide gas.

cap•nom•e•ter (kap-nom′ə-tər) a device for measuring the end-tidal partial pressure of carbon dioxide.

cap•nom•e•try (kap-nom′ə-tre) the determination of the end-tidal partial pressure of carbon dioxide.

cap•no•peri•to•ne•um (kap″no-per″ĭ-to-ne′əm) insufflation of carbon dioxide into the peritoneal cavity to achieve exposure during laparoscopic surgery.

cap•no•phil•ic (kap-no-fil′ik) [*capno-* + *-philic*] growing best in the presence of carbon dioxide; said of bacteria.

cap•o•ben•ate so•di•um (kap-o-ben′āt) the monosodium salt of capobenic acid, having cardiac depressant activity; used as an antiarrhythmic.

cap•o•ben•ic ac•id (kap-o-ben′ik) a vasodilator used in the treatment and prevention of myocardial infarction.

ca•pon (ka′pon) a castrated domestic fowl.

ca•pon•ize (ka′pon-īz) to castrate, especially male domestic fowl.

Cap•o•ten (kap′o-ten) trademark for a preparation of captopril.

Cap•o•zide (kap′o-zīd″) trademark for a combination preparation of captopril and hydrochlorothiazide.

capped (kapt) swollen with hygromas or fibrous degeneration due to prolonged pressure or repeated minor injuries, used particularly of joints of the legs of horses or cattle.

cap•pie (kap′e) double scalp.

cap•ping (kap′ing) 1. the provision of a protective or obstructive covering. 2. the movement of cell surface antigens into a small region (cap) on the cell surface owing to the cross-linking of antigens by specific antibody. 3. the attachment of a protein to the end of a linear polymer, such as actin, preventing the addition or loss of subunits at that end. 4. in restorative dental procedures: *(a)* covering of tooth cusps weakened by caries with a protective metal overlay; see *cusp restoration*, under *restoration; (b)* colloquial term for replacement of the crown of a natural tooth with an artificial crown (cap).
 pulp c. covering of an exposed or nearly exposed pulp with a dressing or cement to protect the pulp against further injury and to provide an environment for healing and repair processes. In *direct capping*, the dressing is placed directly over the pulp at the site of exposure. In *indirect capping*, it is placed over a thin partition of remaining dentin, which if removed, might expose the dental pulp.

cap•rate (kap′rāt) any salt, ester, or anionic form of capric acid.

cap•reo•my•cin (kap″re-o-mi′sin) a polypeptide antibiotic produced by *Streptomyces capreolus*, which is active against human strains of *Mycobacterium tuberculosis* and has four microbiologically active components.
 c. sulfate [USP] the disulfate salt of capreomycin; used as a tuberculostatic, administered intramuscularly.

cap•ric ac•id (kap′rik) a saturated ten-carbon fatty acid occurring as a minor constituent of numerous fats and oils. See also table accompanying *fatty acid.*

ca•pril•o•quism (kə-pril′o-kwiz″əm) [L. *caper* goat + *loqui* to speak] egophony.

cap•rine (kap′rin) [L. *caper* goat] 1. pertaining to or derived from a goat. 2. norleucine.

Cap•ri•pox•vi•rus (kap′rĭ-poks″vi-rəs) [L. *caper*, gen. *capri* goat + *poxvirus*] a genus of viruses of the subfamily Chordopoxvirinae (family Poxviridae) with serologic cross-reactivity, comprising the sheep pox, goatpox, and lumpy skin disease viruses.

cap•ri•zant (kap′rĭ-zənt) [L. *caprizans*, from *caper* a goat] bounding (like a goat); old term used to describe a strong pulse.

cap•ro•ate (kap′ro-āt) 1. a salt, anion, or ester of caproic acid. 2. USAN contraction for *hexanoate.*

ca•pro•ic ac•id (kə-pro′ik) a saturated six-carbon fatty acid occurring in butterfat and coconut and palm oils. Called also *hexanoic acid.* See also table accompanying *fatty acid.*

cap•ro•yl (kap-ro′əl) the acyl radical of caproic acid.

cap•ry•late (kap′rə-lāt) any salt, ester, or anionic form of caprylic acid.

ca•pryl•ic ac•id (kə-pril′ik) an eight-carbon saturated fatty acid occurring in butterfat and palm and coconut oils. Called also *octanoic acid.* See also table accompanying *fatty acid.*

cap•sa•i•cin (kap-sa′ĭ-sin) [USP] an alkaloid irritating to the skin and mucous membranes, the pungent active principle in capsicum, used as a topical counterirritant and analgesic.

Cap•si•cum (kap′sĭ-kəm) [L.] a genus of plants of the family Solanaceae, including types of hot peppers. *C. frutes′cens* is the African chili; *C. an′num* var. *conoi′dis* is the tabasco pepper; and *C. an′num* var. *lon′gum* is the Louisiana long pepper. See also *capsicum.*

cap•si•cum (kap′sĭ-kəm) 1. any plant of the genus *Capsicum.* 2. [USP] the dried fruit of certain species of *Capsicum*, containing the active principle capsaicin; used as a counterirritant and also in pepper gas and pepper spray. Called also *cayenne* or *red pepper.*

cap•sid (kap′sid) [L. *capsa* a box] the shell of protein that protects the nucleic acid of a virus; it may have helical or icosahedral symmetry and is composed of structural units, or capsomers. According to the number of subunits possessed by capsomers, they are called dimers (2), trimers (3), pentamers (5), or hexamers (6).

cap•so•mer (kap′so-mər) [L. *capsa* a box + Gr. *meros* part] the morphological unit of the capsid of a virus.

cap•so•mere (kap′so-mēr) capsomer.

cap•sot•o•my (kap-sot′ə-me) capsulotomy.

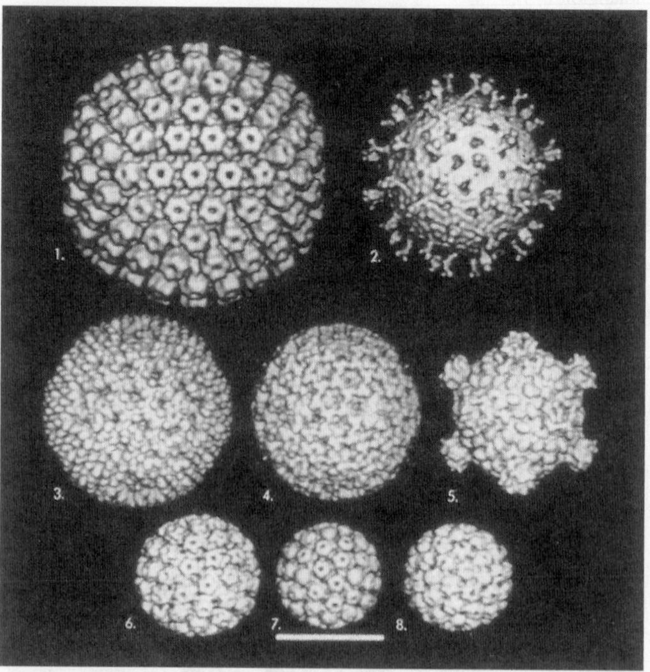

■ Electron microscopy and computer-generated three-dimensional image reconstructions of several icosahedral capsids showing the capsid symmetry and the individual capsomeres. *(1)*, Equine herpesvirus nucleocapsid; *(2)*, simian rotavirus; *(3)*, reovirus type 1 virion; *(4)*, reovirus intermediate subviral particle; *(5)*, reovirus core (inner capsid) particle; *(6)*, human papillomavirus type 19 (papovavirus); *(7)*, mouse polyomavirus (papovavirus); *(8)*, cauliflower mosaic virus. *(Bar equals 50 nm.)*

Capsul. [L.] cap′sula (capsule).

cap•su•la (kap′su-lə) pl. *cap′sulae* [L. "a small box"] capsule: a cartilaginous, fatty, fibrous, or membranous structure enveloping another structure, organ, or part.

c. adipo′sa re′nis [TA] adipose capsule of kidney: the investment of fat surrounding the fibrous capsule of the kidney and continuous at the hilum with the fat in the renal sinus; called also *fatty capsule of kidney* and *perinephric* or *perirenal fat.*

c. articula′ris [TA] articular capsule: the saclike envelope that encloses the cavity of a synovial joint by attaching to the circumference of the articular end of each involved bone; it consists of a fibrous membrane and a synovial membrane. Called also *joint capsule* and *synovial capsule.*

c. articula′ris cricoarytenoi′dea [TA] capsule of cricoarytenoid joint: the fibrous and synovial layers enclosing the cricoarytenoid joint.

c. articula′ris cricothyroi′dea [TA] the capsule enclosing the cricothyroid joint.

c. exter′na [TA] external capsule: the thin layer of white substance that separates the lateral part of the lentiform nucleus (putamen) from the claustrum.

c. extre′ma [TA] extreme capsule: the white matter between the claustrum and the cortex of the insula.

c. fibro′sa glan′dulae thyroi′deae [TA] fibrous capsule of thyroid gland: a connective tissue coat intimately adherent to the underlying gland.

c. fibro′sa perivascula′ris he′patis [TA] perivascular fibrous capsule of liver: the connective tissue sheath that accompanies the vessels and ducts through the hepatic portal; it is continuous with the fibrous coat. Called also *Glisson capsule* and *hepatobiliary capsule.*

c. fibro′sa re′nis [TA] fibrous capsule of kidney: the connective tissue investment of the kidney, which continues through the hilus to line the renal sinus.

c. gan′glii [TA] capsule of ganglion: the laminated connective tissue capsule surrounding a neural ganglion and continuous with epineurium of its associated nerve root.

c. glome′ruli capsule of glomerulus: the double-walled globular dilatation that forms the beginning of a renal tubule and surrounds the glomerulus; the inner wall is called the visceral layer and the outer wall is called the parietal layer. Called also *Bowman, glomerular, malpighian,* or *müllerian capsule.*

c. inter′na [TA] internal capsule: a fanlike mass of white fibers that separates the lentiform nucleus laterally from the head of the caudate nucleus, the dorsal thalamus, and the tail of the caudate nucleus medially; it consists of an anterior limb, a genu, and a posterior limb consisting of three parts, thalamolenticular, sublenticular, and retrolenticular. It carries corticofugal (efferent) fibers from the cerebral cortex to a wide range of targets and conveys afferent information to the cerebral cortex via input to the thalamus and thalamocortical connectiions.

c. len′tis [TA] lens capsule: the elastic envelope covering the lens of the eye and fusing with the fibers of the ciliary zonule; called also *crystalline capsule.*

c. no′di lymphoi′dei [TA] capsule of lymph node: the outer layer of a lymph node, composed mainly of collagen fibers with a few fibroblasts and elastin fibers.

c. prosta′tica [TA] capsule of prostate: the fibroelastic capsule that surrounds the prostate and contains an extensive plexus of veins.

c. sple′nica [TA] capsule of spleen: the fibroelastic coat of the spleen; called also *tunica fibrosa splenica* [TA alternative].

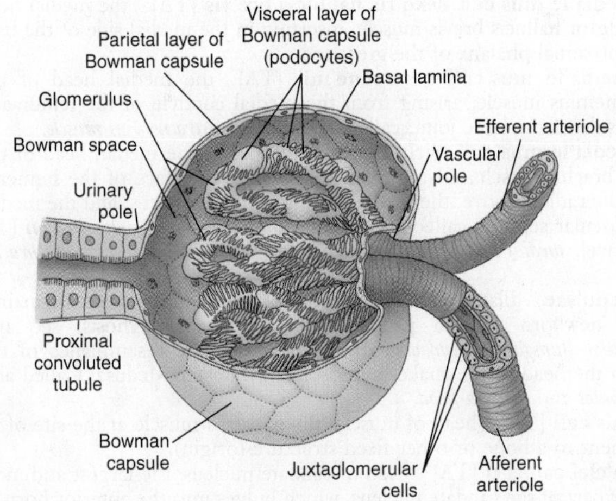

■ Capsula glomeruli (glomerular capsule), showing the double-walled cup shape invaginated by the glomerulus, which is closely approximated by the podocytes of the visceral layer of the capsule.

c. tonsilla′ris [TA] tonsillar capsule: a fibrous capsule covering the lateral surface of the palatine tonsils and separating them from the underlying connective tissue.

cap•su•lae (kap′su-le) [L.] plural of *capsula.*

cap•su•la•tion (kap″su-la′shən) the enclosure of a medicine in a capsule.

cap•sule (kap′səl) [L. *capsula* a little box] 1. a structure in which something is enclosed, such as a hard or a soft, soluble container of a suitable substance, for enclosing a dose of medicine. 2. an anatomical structure enclosing an organ or body part; see *capsula.* **cap′sular** *adj*

adherent c. an investing structure that is not readily separated from the organ or substance contained within it.

adipose c. a capsule consisting largely of fat.

adipose c. of kidney capsula adiposa renis.

articular c. capsula articularis.

auditory c. the cartilaginous capsule of the embryo that develops into the bony labyrinth of the internal ear.

bacterial c. an envelope of gel surrounding a bacterial cell, usually polysaccharide but sometimes polypeptide in nature, which is associated with the virulence of pathogenic bacteria.

biopsy c. a device that can be passed into the intestine to obtain specimens of the mucosa for examination.

Bonnet c. vagina bulbi.

Bowman c. capsula glomeruli.

brood c's capsular projections from the internal membrane of hydatid cysts, from which the scolices arise.

cartilage c. a basophilic zone of cartilage matrix bordering on a lacuna and its enclosed cartilage cell.

central c. a structure seen in certain protozoa of the superclass Actinopoda, such as radiolarians, that encloses the central nucleated core of cytoplasm and is surrounded by a membrane perforated to permit communication with the outer cortex *(calymma).*

c. of cricoarytenoid joint capsula articularis cricoarytenoidea.

c. of cricothyroid joint capsula articularis cricothyroidea.

Crosby c., Crosby-Kugler c. a type of biopsy capsule that contains a spring-activated knife triggered by suction.

crystalline c. capsula lentis.

external c. capsula externa.

extreme c. capsula extrema.

fatty c. of kidney capsula adiposa renis.

fibrous articular c. membrana fibrosa capsulae articularis.

fibrous c. of kidney capsula fibrosa renis.

fibrous c. of liver tunica fibrosa hepatis.

fibrous c. of spleen capsula splenica.

fibrous c. of testis tunica albuginea testis.

fibrous c. of thyroid gland capsula fibrosa glandulae thyroideae.

c. of ganglion capsula ganglii.

Gerota c. fascia renalis.

Glisson c. capsula fibrosa perivascularis hepatis.

glomerular c., c. of glomerulus capsula glomeruli.

c. of heart pericardium.

hepatobiliary c. capsula fibrosa perivascularis hepatis.

internal c. capsula interna.

joint c. capsula articularis.

lens c. capsula lentis.

c. of lymph node capsula nodi lymphoidei.

malpighian c., Müller c., müllerian c. capsula glomeruli.

ocular c. vagina bulbi.

optic c. the embryonic structure from which the sclera is developed.

otic c. the skeletal element enclosing the mechanism of the internal ear. In the human embryo, it develops as cartilage at various ossification centers and becomes completely bony and unified at about the twenty-third week of fetal life.

c. of pancreas, pancreatic c. a thin sheath of areolar tissue that invests the pancreas (but does not form a definite capsule); its septa extend into the pancreas and divide it into lobules.

perinephric c's renal capsules.

periotic c. the tissue surrounding the otic sac in the embryo.

perirenal fat c. capsula adiposa renis.

perivascular fibrous c. of liver capsula fibrosa perivascularis hepatis.

pH c. a telemetry device for monitoring esophageal or gastric pH, consisting of a small capsule with a means of fixing it at the desired level. The capsule is swallowed or inserted through a nasogastric tube and contains an electrode for measuring pH, a battery, and a transmitter that sends periodic pH measurements to a receiver.

polar c. 1. any of the thick-walled vesicles seen in the spores of certain protozoa and containing the polar filament. 2. see under *cap.*

c. of prostate capsula prostatica.

radiotelemetering c. telemetering c.

renal c's the fatty and fibrous capsules surrounding the kidney; see *capsula adiposa renis* and *capsula fibrosa renis.*

c. of spleen capsula splenica.
synovial c. capsula articularis.
telemetering c. a radio transmitter encased in a small capsule for use in telemetry to gain information about conditions within an organ, such as pressure, temperature, or pH. Called also *radiotelemetering c.* and *radio pill.*
c. of temporomandibular joint a ligamentous sac surrounding the temporomandibular joint.
Tenon c. vagina bulbi.
tonsillar c. capsula tonsillaris.

cap·su·lec·to·my (kap″su-lek′tə-me) [*capsule* + *-ectomy*] excision of a capsule, especially a joint capsule or the capsule of the lens; called also *decapsulation.*
renal c. see under *decapsulation.*

cap·su·li·tis (kap″su-li′tis) inflammation of a capsule, as that of the lens, joint, liver, or labyrinth.
adhesive c. adhesive inflammation between the joint capsule and the peripheral articular cartilage of the shoulder with obliteration of the subdeltoid bursa, characterized by shoulder pain of gradual onset, with increasing pain, stiffness, and limitation of motion. Called also *adhesive bursitis* and *frozen shoulder.*
hepatic c. perihepatitis.

cap·su·lo·len·tic·u·lar (kap″su-lo-len-tik′u-lər) pertaining to the lens of the eye and its capsule.

cap·su·lo·plas·ty (kap′su-lo-plas″te) [*capsule* + *-plasty*] a plastic operation on a joint capsule. **capsuloplas′tic** *adj*

cap·su·lor·rha·phy (kap″su-lor′ə-fe) [*capsule* + *-rrhaphy*] suturing of a capsule, especially a joint capsule.

cap·su·lor·rhex·is (kap″su-lo-rek′sis) [*capsule* + *-rrhexis*] the making of a continuous circular tear in the anterior part of the lens capsule during cataract surgery in order to allow expression or phacoemulsification of the nucleus of the lens.

cap·su·lo·tome (kap-su′lo-tōm) [*capsule* + *-tome*] a cutting instrument used for incising the lens capsule.

cap·su·lot·o·my (kap″su-lot′ə-me) [*capsule* + *-tomy*] the incision of a capsule, such as of the lens, the kidney, or a joint.
renal c. incision of a renal capsule.

cap·to·pril (kap′to-pril) [USP] an angiotensin-converting enzyme inhibitor used, alone or in combination with a thiazide diuretic, in the treatment of hypertension, congestive heart failure, and post–myocardial infarction left ventricular dysfunction. See also *captopril test,* under *test.*

cap·ture (kap′chər) 1. to seize or catch; to take control over. 2. the coalescence of an atomic nucleus and a subatomic particle, usually resulting in an unstable mass.
atrial c. depolarization of the atria in response to a stimulus either originating elsewhere in the heart or pacemaker-induced.
electron c. a type of radioactive decay in which the nucleus captures an orbital electron, with the emission of a neutrino and characteristic rays.
ventricular c. depolarization of the ventricles in response to an impulse originating either in the supraventricular region or in an artificial pacemaker.

cap·ut (kap′ət) pl. *cap′ita* [L.] 1. [TA] head: the superior extremity of the body, comprising the cranium and face, and containing the brain, the organs of special sense, and the first organs of the digestive system. 2. the expanded or chief extremity of an organ or part.
c. bre′ve mus′culi bicip′itis bra′chii [TA] the short head of the biceps brachii muscle, arising from the apex of the coracoid process; called also *medial head of biceps brachii muscle* and *coracoradialis.*
c. bre′ve mus′culi bicip′itis fem′oris [TA] the short head of the biceps femoris muscle, arising from the linea aspera of the femur.
c. cor′nus posterio′ris medul′lae spina′lis [TA] head of posterior horn of spinal cord: the oval or fusiform portion of the dorsal horn of gray substance in the spinal cord between the constricted portion (neck) and the apex of the horn.
c. cos′tae [TA] head of rib: the posterior end of a rib, articulating with the body of a vertebra.
c. epididy′midis [TA] head of epididymis: the upper part of the epididymis, in which are found the straight and coiled portions of the efferent ductules of the testis.
c. fe′moris [TA] head of femur: the proximal end of the femur, articulating with the acetabulum on the os coxae. Called also *femoral head.*
c. fi′bulae [TA] head of fibula: the proximal extremity of the fibula.
c. humera′le mus′culi extenso′ris car′pi ulna′ris [TA] the humeral head of the extensor carpi ulnaris muscle, arising from the lateral epicondyle of the humerus.
c. humera′le mus′culi flexo′ris car′pi ulna′ris [TA] the humeral head of the flexor carpi ulnaris muscle, arising from the medial epicondyle of the humerus.

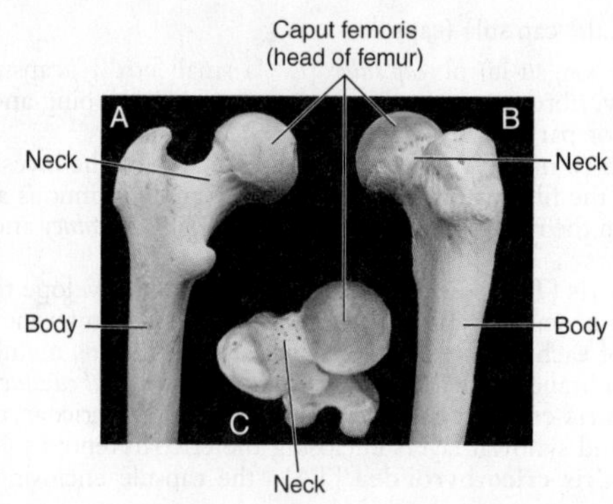

■ Caput femoris (head of femur) in posterior *(A);* lateral *(B);* and superior *(C)* views of the femur.

c. humera′le mus′culi pronato′ris tere′tis [TA] the humeral head of the pronator teres muscle, arising from the medial epicondyle of the humerus.
c. hu′meri [TA] head of humerus: the proximal end of the humerus, articulating with the glenoid cavity of the scapula.
c. humeroulna′re mus′culi flexo′ris digito′rum superficia′lis [TA] the humeroulnar head of the flexor digitorum superficialis muscle, arising from the medial epicondyle of the humerus and the coronoid process of the ulna.
c. infe′rius mus′culi pterygoi′dei latera′lis [TA] the lower head of the lateral pterygoid muscle, arising from the lateral surface of the lateral pterygoid plate. Called also *inferior head of lateral pterygoid muscle.*
c. latera′le mus′culi flexo′ris hal′lucis bre′vis [TA] the lateral head of the flexor hallucis brevis muscle, inserting in the lateral side of the base of the proximal phalanx of the great toe.
c. latera′le mus′culi gastrocne′mii [TA] the lateral head of the gastrocnemius muscle, arising from the lateral condyle and posterior surface of the femur, and the capsule of the knee joint; called also *lateral gastrocnemius muscle.*
c. latera′le mus′culi tricip′itis bra′chii [TA] the lateral head of the triceps brachii muscle, arising from the posterior surface of the humerus, the lateral border of the humerus, and the lateral intermuscular septum; called also *great* or *second head of triceps brachii muscle,* and *lateral* or *short anconeus muscle.*
c. lon′gum mus′culi bicip′itis bra′chii [TA] long head of biceps brachii muscle: the head that connects the muscle with the upper border of the glenoid cavity; called also *interarticular ligament of humeral joint.*
c. lon′gum mus′culi bicip′itis fem′oris [TA] long head of biceps femoris muscle: the head that connects the muscle with the ischial tuberosity.
c. lon′gum musculi tricip′itis bra′chii [TA] long head of triceps brachii muscle: the head that connects the muscle with the infraglenoid tubercle of the scapula; called also *first, middle,* or *scapular head of triceps brachii muscle.*
c. mal′lei [TA] head of malleus: the upper portion of the malleus, which includes the surface *(facet for incus)* that articulates with the incus.
c. mandi′bulae [TA] head of mandible: the articular surface of the condyloid process of the mandible; called also *head of condyloid process of mandible.*
c. media′le mus′culi flexo′ris hal′lucis bre′vis [TA] the medial head of the flexor hallucis brevis muscle, inserting in the medial side of the base of the proximal phalanx of the great toe.
c. media′le mus′culi gastrocne′mii [TA] the medial head of the gastrocnemius muscle, arising from the medial condyle of the femur and the capsule of the knee joint; called also *medial gastrocnemius muscle.*
c. media′le mus′culi tricip′itis bra′chii [TA] the medial head of the triceps brachii muscle, arising from the posterior surface of the humerus below the radial groove, the medial border of the humerus, and the medial intermuscular septum; called also *c. profundum musculi tricipitis brachii* [TA alternative], *medial anconeus muscle,* and *deep* or *short head of triceps brachii muscle.*
c. medu′sae dilated cutaneous veins around the umbilicus, seen mainly in the newborn and in patients suffering from cirrhosis; see also *Cruveilhier-Bumgarten syndrome.* It is named for the resemblance of the veins to the head of the snake-haired Greek monster Medusa. Called also *cirsomphalos* and *medusa head.*
c. mus′culi [TA] head of muscle: the end of a muscle at the site of its attachment to a bone or other fixed structure (origin).
c. nu′clei cauda′ti [TA] head of caudate nucleus: the largest and most anterior part of the caudate nucleus, which bulges into the anterior horn of the lateral ventricle.
c. obli′quum mus′culi adducto′ris hal′lucis [TA] the oblique head of adductor hallucis muscle: the head that connects the muscle with the bases of

the second, third, and fourth metatarsal bones, and the sheath of the peroneus longus muscle; called also *great* or *long head of adductor hallucis muscle.*

c. obli′quum mus′culi adducto′ris pol′licis [TA] the oblique head of adductor pollicis muscle: the head that connects the muscle with the capitate and trapezoid bones and the base of the second metacarpals.

c. os′sis metacar′pi [TA] head of metacarpal bone: the distal extremity of a metacarpal bone, which articulates with the base of a proximal digit.

c. os′sis metatar′si [TA] head of metatarsal bone: the distal extremity of a metatarsal bone, which articulates with the base of a digit.

c. pancre′atis [TA] head of pancreas: the discoidal mass forming the enlarged right extremity of the pancreas, lying in a flexure of the duodenum.

c. phalan′gis ma′nus [TA] head of phalanx of hand: the distal articular surface of each of the proximal and middle phalanges of the fingers.

c. phalan′gis pe′dis [TA] head of phalanx of foot: the distal articular extremity of each of the proximal and middle phalanges of the toes.

c. pla′num a flattened head occurring with osteochondritis deformans juvenilis.

c. profun′dum mus′culi flexo′ris pol′licis bre′vis [TA] the deep head of the flexor pollicis brevis muscle, arising from the trapezoid and capitate bones and from the palmar ligaments of the distal row of carpal bones. It varies in size and may be absent.

c. profun′dum mus′culi tricip′itis bra′chii TA alternative for *c. mediale musculi tricipitis brachii.*

c. quadra′tum a head deformity seen in rickets in which the eminences of the frontal and parietal bones form elevations separated by depressions marking the lines of the cranial sutures.

c. radia′le mus′culi flexo′ris digito′rum superficia′lis [TA] the radial head of the flexor digitorum superficialis muscle, arising from the oblique line and anterior border of the radius.

c. ra′dii [TA] head of radius: the disk on the proximal end of the radius that articulates with the capitulum of the humerus and the radial notch of the ulna.

c. rec′tum mus′culi rec′ti fe′moris [TA] straight head of rectus femoris muscle: the head of the rectus femoris that arises from anteroinferior iliac spine, which fuses with the reflected or posterior head and continues down into the belly of the muscle. Called also *anterior head of rectus femoris muscle.*

c. reflex′um mus′culi rec′ti fe′moris [TA] reflected head of rectus femoris muscle: the head of the rectus femoris that arises from a groove above the rim of the acetabulum, which fuses with the straight or anterior head and continues down into the belly of the muscle. Called also *posterior head of rectus femoris muscle.*

c. stape′dis [TA] head of stapes: the part that articulates with the incus.

c. succeda′neum edema occurring in and under the fetal scalp during labor.

c. superficia′le mus′culi flexo′ris pol′licis bre′vis [TA] the superficial head of the flexor pollicis brevis muscle, arising from the distal border of the flexor retinaculum and the distal part of the tubercle of the trapezium.

c. supe′rius mus′culi pterygoi′dei latera′lis [TA] the upper head of the lateral pterygoid muscle, arising from the infratemporal surface and infratemporal crest of the greater wing of the sphenoid bone. Called also *superior head of lateral pterygoid muscle.*

c. ta′li [TA] head of talus: the rounded anterior end of the talus; called also *head of astragalus.*

c. transver′sum mus′culi adducto′ris hal′lucis [TA] the transverse head of the adductor hallucis muscle, arising from the capsules of the metatarso-phalangeal joints of the third, fourth, and fifth toes.

c. transver′sum mus′culi adducto′ris pol′licis [TA] the transverse head of the adductor pollicis muscle arising from the lower two thirds of the anterior surface of the third metacarpal.

c. ul′nae [TA] head of ulna: the articular surface of the distal extremity of the ulna.

c. ulna′re mus′culi extenso′ris car′pi ulna′ris [TA] the ulnar head of the extensor carpi ulnaris muscle, arising from the posterior border of the ulna.

c. ulna′re mus′culi flexo′ris car′pi ulna′ris [TA] the ulnar head of the flexor carpi ulnaris muscle, arising from the olecranon, and the adjacent part of the ulna.

c. ulna′re mus′culi pronato′ris ter′etis [TA] the ulnar head of the pronator teres muscle, arising from the coronoid process of the ulna; called also *coronoid head of pronator teres muscle.*

CAR Canadian Association of Radiologists; cancer-associated retinopathy.

Ca•ra•bel•li cusp (tubercle) (kah-rə-bel′e) [Georg *Carabelli,* Hungarian dentist in Vienna, 1787–1842] see under *cusp.*

Car•ac (kar′ak) trademark for a preparation of fluorouracil.

Car•a•fate (kar′ə-fāt) trademark for preparations of sucralfate.

car•a•mel (kar′ə-məl, kahr′məl) [NF] a concentrated solution of the product obtained by heating sugar or glucose until the sweet taste is destroyed and a uniform dark brown mass results; used as a coloring agent for pharmaceuticals and foods.

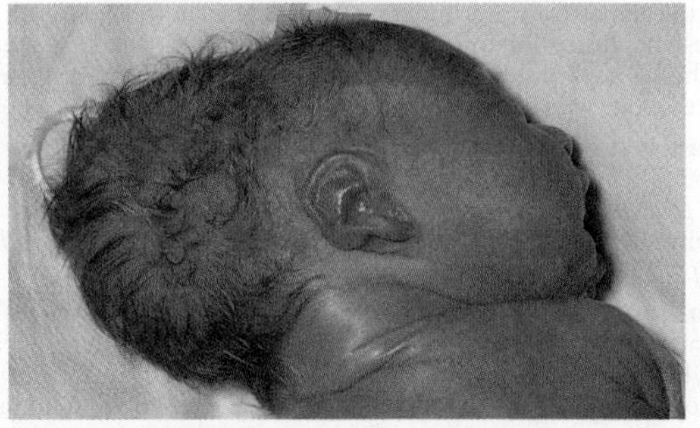

■ Caput succedaneum.

car•a•way (kar′ə-wa) [Ar. *karawyā,* from Gr. *karon*] 1. *Carum carvi.* 2. [NF] the dried ripe fruit of *C. carvi,* consisting of brown mericarps having an aromatic odor and taste; the source of caraway oil.

car•ba•ceph•em (kahr″bə-sef′əm) any of a class of β-lactam antibiotics closely related to the cephalosporins, having a methylene group substituted for the sulfur atom in the 7-aminocephalosporanic acid nucleus; carbacephems are chemically more stable than cephalosporins.

car•ba•chol (kahr′bə-kol) [USP] a cholinergic agonist, carbamylcholine chloride, that is not hydrolyzed by acetylcholinesterase or pseudocholinesterase; used as a miotic and to lower intraocular pressure in the treatment of glaucoma and following cataract surgery.

car•ba•dox (kahr′bə-doks) an antibacterial used in veterinary medicine.

car•ba•mate (kahr′bə-māt) 1. any ester of carbamic acid. 2. any of a group of insecticides and parasiticides that act by inhibiting cholinesterase; heavy exposure to some of them can cause carbamate poisoning (q.v.). See table.

car•ba•maz•e•pine (kahr″bə-maz′ə-pēn) [USP] an anticonvulsant and antineuralgic, used in the treatment of pain associated with trigeminal neuralgia and in epilepsy manifested by tonic-clonic and partial seizures; administered orally.

car•bam•ic ac•id (kahr-bam′ik) a compound, H_2NCOOH, that exists only in the form of salts or esters (carbamates), amides (carbamides), and other derivatives (its acyl radical, H_2NCO—, is carbamoyl).

car•ba•mide (kahr′bə-mīd) urea.

c. peroxide [USP] an equimolecular compound of urea and hydrogen peroxide used topically as a cerumen-softening agent and as a dental cleanser, bleaching agent, and antiinflammatory.

car•bam•i•no•he•mo•glo•bin (kahr-bam″ĭ-no-he′mo-glo″bin) a chemical combination of carbon dioxide with hemoglobin, CO_2HHb, being one of the forms in which carbon dioxide exists in the blood. Called also *carbhemoglobin* and *carbohemoglobin.*

car•bam•o•yl (kahr-bam′o-əl) the radical NH_2CO—. Called also *carbamyl.*

c. phosphate an important intermediate compound in the formation of pyrimidine and citrulline, the latter being an intermediate in urea formation.

car•bam•o•yl•as•par•tate (kahr-bam″o-əl-as-pahr′tāt) aspartate linked at the amino end to a carbamoyl moiety; it is an intermediate in pyrimidine biosynthesis.

car•bam•o•y•la•tion (kahr-bam″o-ə-la′shən) the transfer of a carbamoyl moiety to the amino group of an acceptor compound.

car•bam•o•yl-phos•phate syn•thase (am•mo•nia) (kahr-bam′o-əl-fos′fāt sin′thās ə-mo′ne-ə) [EC 6.3.4.16] an enzyme of the ligase class that catalyzes the synthesis of carbamoyl phosphate from ammonia and carbon dioxide, the first committed step in the urea cycle (see illustration at *urea cycle,* under *cycle*). The reaction occurs predominantly in liver mitochondria, requires *N*-acetylglutamate as a cofactor, and hydrolyzes two molecules of ATP. Decreased enzyme activity, an autosomal recessive trait, causes carbamoyl phosphate synthetase deficiency.

car•bam•o•yl-phos•phate syn•thase (glu•ta•mine-hy•dro•lyz•ing) (kahr-bam′o-əl-fos′fāt sin′thās gloo′tə-mēn hi′dro-li-zing) [EC 6.3.5.5]

Carbamate Insecticides

Aldicarb
Aminocarb
Carbaril
Carbofuran
Dimetilan
Methomyl
Propoxur

an enzyme activity of the trifunctional CAD protein (q.v.); it is a ligase that catalyzes the formation of carbamoyl phosphate as the first step in the biosynthesis of pyrimidine nucleotides. Glutamine is the nitrogen donor in the reaction, which is cytosolic and is inhibited by UTP.

car·bam·o·yl phos·phate syn·the·tase (CPS) (kahr-bam′o-əl fos′fāt sin′thə-tās) 1. carbamoyl-phosphate synthase (ammonia); called also *carbamoyl phosphate synthetase I* (CPSI). 2. carbamoyl-phosphate synthase (glutamine-hydrolyzing); called also *carbamoyl phosphate synthetase II* (CPSII).

car·bam·o·yl phos·phate syn·the·tase de·fi·cien·cy (kahr-bam′o-əl fos′fāt sin′thə-tās) an autosomal recessive aminoacidopathy caused by mutations in the *CPS1* gene (locus: 2q35), which encodes carbamoyl-phosphate synthase (ammonia); characteristic symptoms include pronounced hyperammonemia without oroticaciduria, protein intolerance, and neurologic disorders. Symptoms may begin in the neonatal period or appear later in infancy, with varying degrees of severity. Written also *carbamoyl phosphate synthetase I (CPSI) deficiency*.

car·bam·o·yl·trans·fer·ase (kahr-bam″o-əl-trans′fər-ās) a term used in the names of some of the enzymes of the sub-subclass carbamoyltransferases and carboxyltransferases [EC 2.1.3] to denote those that catalyze the transfer of a carbamoyl group from a donor compound to an acceptor compound. Called also *transcarbamoylase*.

car·ba·myl (kahr′bə-məl) carbamoyl.

car·bam·y·la·tion (kahr-bam″əl-a′shən) carbamoylation.

car·ba·myl·cho·line chlo·ride (kahr″bə-məl-ko′lēn klor′īd) carbachol.

car·ba·pen·ems (kahr″bə-pen′əmz) a class of broad-spectrum β-lactam antibiotics derived from thienamycin, including imipenem and meropenem.

car·ba·ril (kahr′bə-ril) a carbamate compound with cholinesterase-inhibiting activity, used as an insecticide. Excessive exposure can cause mild carbamate poisoning. Called also *carbaryl*.

car·ba·ryl (kahr′bə-rəl) carbaril.

Car·ba·trol (kahr′bə-trol) trademark for preparations of carbamazepine.

car·ba·zide (kahr′bə-zīd) a urea derivative, carbodihydrazide, $CO(NHNH_2)_2$, in which both the amide groups of urea have been replaced by hydrazine residues.

car·baz·o·tate (kahr-baz′o-tāt) any salt of picric acid; a picrate.

car·ben·i·cil·lin (kahr″bən-ĭ-sil′in) a semisynthetic penicillin, effective against gram-negative bacteria, such as susceptible strains of *Pseudomonas aeruginosa*, indole-positive *Proteus* species, certain strains of *Escherichia coli*, and *Haemophilus influenzae;* it also inhibits the growth of some gram-positive pathogens.

c. disodium [USP] the disodium salt of carbenicillin, having the same actions as the base; administered intramuscularly or intravenously in severe systemic infections and septicemia, urinary and genitourinary tract infections, acute and chronic respiratory infections, and soft tissue infections.

c. indanyl sodium [USP] the sodium salt of the indanyl ester of carbenicillin disodium, having the same actions as the base; administered orally in the treatment of upper and lower urinary tract infections and prostatitis due to susceptible organisms. Called also *carindacillin sodium*.

c. sodium c. disodium.

car·be·ta·pen·tane (kahr-ba″tə-pen′tān) an antitussive agent with mild atropine-like antisecretory activity; used in the treatment of cough associated with upper respiratory infections, administered orally; available as *c. tannate*.

carb·he·mo·glo·bin (kahrb″he-mo-glo′bin) carbaminohemoglobin.

car·bide (kahr′bīd) a compound of carbon with an element or radical.

metallic c. a compound of carbon with a transition metal, as in Fe_3C (as distinguished from a salt-like carbide, such as CaC_2).

car·bi·do·pa (kahr″bĭ-do′pə) [USP] an inhibitor of the decarboxylation of peripheral levodopa to dopamine, which does not penetrate the central nervous system. When given with levodopa, carbidopa produces higher brain concentrations of dopamine with lower doses of levodopa, thus lessening the side effects seen with higher doses. It is used orally, in conjunction with levodopa, as an antiparkinsonian agent.

car·bi·nol (kahr′bĭ-nol) 1. methyl alcohol. 2. any aromatic or fatty alcohol formed by substituting one, two, or three hydrocarbon groups for hydrogen in methyl alcohol.

acetylmethyl c. a keto-isomer of aldol, $CH_3{\cdot}CHOH{\cdot}CO{\cdot}CH_3$, which is formed from glucose by certain bacteria and which is detected in a broth culture of bacteria by the Voges-Proskauer reaction.

dimethyl c. isopropyl alcohol.

car·bi·nox·amine mal·e·ate (kahr″bin-ok′sə-mēn) [USP] an ethanolamine derivative that acts as an antihistamine (H_1 receptor antagonist) with sedative and anticholinergic effects; used in the treatment of allergic rhinitis, allergic conjunctivitis, and cutaneous manifestations of allergic reactions, and as an ingredient in some cough and cold preparations; administered orally.

carb(o)- [L. *carbo* charcoal] a combining form indicating the presence of carbon.

Car·bo·caine (kahr′bo-kān) trademark for preparations of mepivacaine hydrochloride.

car·bo·cho·line (kahr″bo-ko′lēn) carbachol.

car·bo·cy·clic (kahr″bo-sik′lik, -si′klik) having or pertaining to a closed chain or ring formation which includes only carbon atoms; said of chemical compounds.

car·bo·cys·te·ine (kahr″bo-sis′tēn) a mucolytic agent, administered orally and by inhalation in the treatment of respiratory disorders characterized by the production of excess or viscous mucus.

car·bo·di·im·ide (kahr″bo-di-im′id) a derivative of urea, NH:C:NH.

car·bo·gas·e·ous (kahr″bo-gas′e-əs) charged with carbon dioxide gas.

car·bo·gen (kahr′bo-jen) a mixture of oxygen with 5 per cent carbon dioxide.

car·bo·he·mo·glo·bin (kahr″bo-he″mo-glo′bin) carbaminohemoglobin.

car·bo·hy·drase (kahr″bo-hi′drās) any of a group of enzymes such as amylase that catalyze the hydrolysis of higher carbohydrates to lower forms.

car·bo·hy·drate (kahr″bo-hi′drāt) any of a class of aldehyde or ketone derivatives of polyhydric alcohols, particularly of the pentahydric and hexahydric alcohols. They are so named because the hydrogen and oxygen are usually in the proportion to form water, $C_n(H_2O)_n$; the most important include the small sugars as well as the large starches, glycogens, celluloses, and gums. See also *saccharide*.

C c. one of a group of polysaccharides found in cell walls of β-hemolytic streptococci and used for identification in the Lancefield classification (see under *classification*).

reserve c's carbohydrates that can be stored in the plant or animal in the form of high molecular weight, hydrolyzable compounds such as starch or glycogen.

car·bo·hy·dra·tu·ria (kahr″bo-hi″drət-u′re-ə) excess of carbohydrates in the urine, such as in fructosuria, galactosuria, glycosuria, lactosuria, or pentosuria.

car·bo·hy·dro·gen·ic (kahr″bo-hi″dro-jen′ik) producing carbohydrates.

car·bo·late (kahr′bo-lāt) 1. phenolate. 2. to charge with carbolic acid.

car·bol·fuch·sin (kahr″bol-fūk′sin) basic fuchsin treated with dilute phenol (carbolic acid); used in various staining methods for acid-fast bacteria. It is also used as a topical antifungal; see under *solution*.

Kinyoun c. a modification of Ziehl-Neelsen carbolfuchsin containing a higher concentration of phenol and basic fuchsin, eliminating the need for heating of the slide in staining. See *Kinyoun staining method*, at *Stains and Staining Methods*, under *stain*.

Ziehl-Neelsen c. a mixture of basic fuchsin and liquefied phenol in alcohol and purified water; used in the Ziehl-Neelsen staining method (see at *Stains and Staining Methods*, under *stain*).

car·bol·ic ac·id (kahr-bol′ik) phenol (def. 1).

car·bol·ism (kahr′bəl-iz-əm) phenol poisoning.

car·bol·ize (kahr′bəl-īz) to treat with phenol.

car·bol·uria (kahr″bol-u′re-ə) [*carbolic* acid + *-uria*] the presence of phenol in the urine.

car·bol·xy·lene (kahr″bol-zi′lēn) a mixture of 1 part carbolic acid and 3 parts xylene, used for clearing microscopical sections.

car·bo·mer (kahr′bo-mər) [NF] a polymer of acrylic acid, cross-linked with a polyfunctional agent, and occurring in various sizes; used as an emulsifying agent and as a suspending agent in pharmaceutical preparations.

car·bon (C) (kahr′bən) [L. *carbo* charcoal] a nonmetallic tetrad element, found nearly pure in the diamond, and approximately pure in charcoal, graphite, and anthracite; atomic number 6, atomic weight 12.011. The two naturally occurring, stable isotopes are ^{12}C (98.89 per cent) and ^{13}C (1.11 per cent).

c. 11 a radioactive isotope of carbon, atomic mass 11, having a half-life of 20.39 minutes; it decays by positron emission, with energy of 0.961 MeV, and is used as a tracer in positron emission tomography.

c. 13 a naturally occurring isotope of carbon, atomic mass 13, occurring 1.11 percent of the time. It is used as a tracer in liver function tests and a few metabolic tests.

c. 14 a radioactive isotope of carbon, atomic mass 14, having a half-life of 5730 years; it decays by beta emission, with energy of 0.156 MeV, and is used as a tracer in cancer and metabolic research.

c. dioxide 1. an odorless, colorless gas, CO_2, resulting from the oxidation of carbon. It is formed in the tissues and eliminated by the lungs. CO_2 and the carbonates assist in maintaining the neutrality of the tissues and fluids of the body. 2. [USP] a preparation of the gas, used in some pump-oxygenators to maintain the carbon dioxide tension in the blood. In solid form, carbon dioxide *(carbon dioxide snow* or *dry ice)* is used to freeze skin for local anesthesia, as an escharotic to destroy certain skin lesions, and as a peeling agent in chemabrasion.

c. disulfide a colorless, flammable, poisonous liquid, CS_2, used as a solvent, as a fruit preservative, and for numerous other industrial purposes. Excessive inhalation of its fumes causes carbon disulfide poisoning (q.v.).

c. monoxide a colorless poisonous gas, CO, formed by burning carbon or organic fuels with a scanty supply of oxygen; it causes asphyxiation by combining irreversibly with the blood hemoglobin. See also *carbon monoxide poisoning*, under *poisoning*.

c. monoxide C 11 [USP] carbon monoxide in which a portion of the molecules are labeled with ^{11}C; used to label erythrocytes for measurement of blood volume.

c. tetrachloride a clear, colorless, volatile liquid, CCl_4, used as a solvent in pharmaceutical preparations. Inhalation of its vapors can depress central nervous system activity and cause degeneration of the liver and kidneys. Called also *perchlormethane* and *tetrachlormethane*.

car•bon•ate (kahr′bə-nāt) any salt of carbonic acid.

car•bon•ate de•hy•dra•tase (kahr′bə-nāt de-hi′drə-tās) [EC 4.2.1.1] an enzyme of the lyase class that catalyzes the equilibration of dissolved carbon dioxide and carbonic acid, speeding the movement of carbon dioxide from tissues to blood to alveolar air. It is a zinc protein found in renal tubule cells and red blood cells. Called also *carbonic anhydrase*.

car•bon•ic ac•id (kahr-bon′ik) the chemical species H_2CO_3, which exists in chemical equilibrium with dissolved carbon dioxide in water; its dissociated forms are the bicarbonate (HCO_3^-) and carbonate (CO_3^{2-}) ions. In the blood the predominant species are HCO_3 and dissolved CO_2 in approximately a 20:1 ratio. The conversion of CO_2 to H_2CO_3 is catalyzed by the enzyme carbonate dehydratase.

car•bon•ic an•hy•drase (kahr-bon′ik an-hi′drās) carbonate dehydratase.

car•bon•ize (kahr′bon-īz) to char or to convert into charcoal.

car•bon•yl (kahr′bə-nəl) [*carbon* + Gr. *hylē* matter] the divalent group C=O, occurring in compounds such as aldehydes, ketones, carboxylic acids, and esters.

car•bo•pla•tin (kahr′bo-plat″in) [USP] a platinum coordination compound having the same mechanism of action as cisplatin, although its rate of action is slower and its spectrum of toxicity is different. Used in the treatment of ovarian carcinoma refractory to standard chemotherapy or in patients who cannot be safely treated with cisplatin; also used experimentally in the treatment of small and non–small cell lung carcinoma, head and neck carcinoma, testicular carcinoma, and seminoma. Administered intravenously.

car•bo•prost (kahr′bo-prost) a synthetic 15-methyl analogue of dinoprost, a prostaglandin of the F type; it has been used as an oxytocic for termination of pregnancy and missed abortion, administered intramuscularly.

c. methyl the methyl ester of carboprost, having the same actions and similar uses as the base; administered in vaginal suppositories or in an intravaginal device.

c. tromethamine an oxytocic compound of carboprost and 2-amino-2-(hydroxymethyl)-1,3-propanediol (1:1).

Car•bo•run•dum (kahr″bo-run′dəm) trademark for a preparation of silicon carbide.

Car•bo•wax (kahr′bo-waks) trademark for a series of polyethylene glycols; used in compounding water-soluble ointment vehicles.

car•box•a•mide (kahr-bok′sə-mīd″) 1. an amide of a carboxylic acid, having the general formula $RC(=O)NR_2$. 2. the group $-C(=O)NH_2$, including the carbon atom.

carboxy- a chemical prefix denoting the presence of a carboxyl group.

γ-car•boxy•glu•ta•mate (kahr-bok″se-gloo′tə-māt) a salt or dissociated form of γ-carboxyglutamic acid.

γ-car•boxy•glu•ta•mic ac•id (kahr-bok″se-gloo-tam′ik) an amino acid occurring in biologically active prothrombin and in noncollagen bone proteins; it is formed in the liver in the presence of vitamin K by carboxylation of glutamic acid residues.

car•boxy•he•mo•glo•bin (kahr-bok″se-he′mo-glo″bin) hemoglobin in which the sites usually bound to oxygen are bound to carbon monoxide, which has an affinity for hemoglobin over 200 times that of oxygen. See *carbon monoxide poisoning*, under *poisoning*.

car•boxy•he•mo•glo•bin•e•mia (kahr-bok″se-he″mo-glo″bin-e′me-ə) the presence of carboxyhemoglobin in the blood; see *carbon monoxide poisoning*, under *poisoning*.

car•box•yl (kahr-bok′səl) the monovalent radical, —COOH, occurring in those organic acids termed carboxylic acids.

car•box•y•lase (kahr-bok′sə-lās) an enzyme that catalyzes the addition of a molecule of carbon dioxide to another compound to form a carboxyl group. The carboxylases include some carboxy-lyases [EC 4.1.1] and those ligases, usually biotinyl-proteins, that cleave ATP to drive the reaction [EC 6.4.1].

amino acid c. an enzyme in many bacteria that catalyzes the removal of CO_2 from amino acids, thus producing amines.

multiple c. deficiency either of two autosomal recessive aminoacidopathies caused by mutations that lead to deficient activity of biotin-containing carboxylases. The *early-onset* (or *neonatal* or *infantile*) form results from holocarboxylase synthetase deficiency (q.v.); the *late-onset* (or *juvenile*) form results from biotinidase deficiency (q.v.)

car•box•y•late (kahr-bok′sə-lāt) any salt, ester, or conjugate base of a carboxylic acid.

car•box•y•la•tion (kahr-bok″sə-la′shən) the addition of a carboxyl group, as to pyruvate to form oxaloacetate.

car•box•yl•es•ter•ase (kahr-bok″səl-es′tər-ās) [EC 3.1.1.1] an enzyme of the hydrolase class that catalyzes cleavage of the ester bond in a carboxylic ester to form an alcohol and a carboxylic acid. It has wide specificity, usually acting on short-chain acids linked to monohydric alcohols, and also hydrolyzes esters of vitamin A.

car•box•yl•trans•fer•ase (kahr-bok″səl-trans′fər-ās) a term used in the names of some enzymes of the sub-subclass carbamoyltransferases and carboxyltransferases [EC 2.1.3] to denote those that catalyze transfer of a carboxyl group from a donor compound to an acceptor one. Called also *transcarboxylase*.

car•boxy•ly•ase (kahr-bok″se-li′ās) [EC 4.1.1] any member of a sub-subclass of enzymes of the lyase class that catalyze the nonhydrolytic addition or removal of a carboxyl group to or from a compound; it includes the carboxylases and decarboxylases.

car•boxy•meth•yl•cel•lu•lose (kahr-bok″se-meth″əl-sel′u-lōs) a semisynthetic substituted cellulose polymer of varying size, the molecular weight ranging from 21×10^3 to 50×10^4; used as a suspending agent, tablet excipient, and viscosity-increasing agent in pharmaceutical preparations. Called also *carmellose*.

c. calcium [NF] the calcium salt of carboxymethylcellulose; used as a tablet disintegrant in pharmaceutical preparations.

c. sodium [USP] the sodium salt of carboxymethylcellulose; used as a suspending agent, tablet excipient, and viscosity-increasing agent in pharmaceutical preparations, and administered orally as a laxative.

car•boxy•myo•glo•bin (kahr-bok″se-mi″o-glo′bin) a compound formed from myoglobin on exposure to carbon monoxide, with formation of a covalent bond with oxygen and without change of the charge of the ferrous state.

car•boxy•pen•i•cil•lin (kahr-bok″se-pen″ĭ-sil′in) any in a group of penicillin derivatives that have a carboxyl group attached.

car•boxy•pep•ti•dase (kahr-bok″se-pep′tĭ-dās) [EC 3.4.16–18] any exopeptidase that catalyzes the hydrolytic cleavage of the terminal or penultimate peptide bond at the C-terminal end of a peptide or polypeptide.

car•boxy•pep•ti•dase A (kahr-bok″se-pep′tĭ-dās) [EC 3.4.17.1] an enzyme of the hydrolase class that catalyzes the cleavage from aminopolypeptides of C-terminal acid residues other than arginine, lysine, or proline. It is a zinc metalloenzyme found in pancreatic juice.

car•boxy•pep•ti•dase B (kahr-bok″se-pep′tĭ-dās) [EC 3.4.17.2] an enzyme of the hydrolase class that catalyzes the cleavage of C-terminal arginine or lysine residues from polypeptides. It is a zinc metalloenzyme found in pancreatic juice.

lysosomal c. B cysteine-type carboxypeptidase (def. 2).

car•bun•cle (kahr′bəng-kəl) [L. *carbunculus* little coal] a necrotizing infection of skin and subcutaneous tissue composed of a cluster of boils (furuncles), usually due to *Staphylococcus aureus*, with multiple formed or incipient drainage sinuses.

malignant c. see under *pustule*.

renal c. a massive localized parenchymal suppuration consequent to bacterial metastasis, following localized vascular thrombosis or infarction of the kidney.

car•bun•cu•lar (kahr-bung′ku-lər) resembling or of the nature of a carbuncle.

car•bun•cu•lo•sis (kahr-bung″ku-lo′sis) a condition marked by the development of carbuncles.

car•bu•ta•mide (kahr-bu'tə-mīd) a sulfonylurea compound used as a hypoglycemic in the treatment of type 2 diabetes mellitus; administered orally.

car•cass (kahr'kəs) [Fr. *carcasse*] a dead body; generally applied to other than a human body.

car•cin•emia (kahr″sin-e'me-ə) [*carcin-* + *-emia*] canceremia.

carcin(o)- [Gk. *karkinos* a crab] a combining form meaning relationship to carcinoma.

car•ci•no•cy•the•mia (kahr″sĭ-no″si-the'me-ə) canceremia.

car•ci•no•em•bry•on•ic (kahr″sĭ-no-em″bre-on'ik) [*carcino-* + *embryonic*] occurring both in carcinoma and in embryonic tissue; see under *antigen.*

car•cin•o•gen (kahr-sin'ə-jen) any cancer-producing substance; often a distinction is made between *epigenetic* and *genotoxic carcinogens.*

epigenetic c. an agent that does not itself damage DNA but causes alterations such as hormonal derangements, immunosuppression, or chronic tissue injury that in turn predispose to cancer.

genotoxic c. a carcinogen that reacts directly with DNA or with macromolecules that then react with DNA.

car•ci•no•gen•e•sis (kahr″sĭ-no-jen'ə-sis) [*carcino-* + *-genesis*] the production of carcinoma.

car•cin•o•gen•ic (kahr″sin-o-jen'ik) 1. producing carcinoma; cf. *cancerigenic.* 2. pertaining to a carcinogen.

car•ci•no•ge•nic•i•ty (kahr″sĭ-no-jə-nis'ĭ-te) the ability or tendency to produce carcinoma; the quality of being carcinogenic.

car•ci•noid (kahr'sĭ-noid) carcinoid tumor.

ECL cell c., enterochromaffin-like cell c. a small, circumscribed, often polypoid tumor of the gastric fundus, consisting of enterochromaffin-like (ECL) cells and believed to be secondary to hypergastrinemia, which stimulates the proliferation of ECL cells; multiple tumors are usually present. Tumors may be classified into three types: *Type I,* associated with atrophic gastritis; *Type II,* associated with multiple endocrine neoplasia, type I; and *Type III,* which is sporadic.

thymic c. a type of APUDoma that arises from cells of foregut origin within the thymus and can be locally invasive or metastatic; some are found as part of multiple endocrine neoplasia type I or type II.

car•ci•nol•y•sin (kahr″si-nol'ə-sin) [*carcino-* + *lysin*] a ferment derived from a Chinese variety of pine called "haisung." It has been given subcutaneously or intramuscularly for cancer.

car•ci•nol•y•sis (kahr″sĭ-nol'ə-sis) destruction of carcinoma cells, as by perfusion of an antineoplastic agent through the vessels of the body segment in which the growth occurs. **carcinolyt'ic** *adj*

car•ci•no•ma (kahr″sĭ-no'mə) pl. *carcinomas* or *carcino'mata* [Gr. *karkinōma,* from *karkinos* crab, cancer] a malignant new growth made up of epithelial cells tending to infiltrate the surrounding tissues and give rise to metastases.

Carcinoma

acinar c., acinic cell c., acinous c. a slow-growing malignant tumor characterized by acinic cells arranged in small glandlike structures, usually occurring in the pancreas or salivary glands, particularly in females. Called also *acinar, acinic cell,* or *acinous adenocarcinoma* and *acinar cell* or *acinic cell tumor.*

adenocystic c. adenoid cystic c.

adenoid cystic c. carcinoma characterized by bands or cylinders of hyalinized or mucinous stroma separating or surrounded by nests or cords of small epithelial cells. It appears as one or more of three patterns: cribriform, solid, and tubular. The usual site is the salivary glands, but histologically similar tumors appear elsewhere. Malignant and invasive but slow-growing, it spreads by infiltrating the bloodstream and perineural spaces. Called also *adenocystic c., cribriform c.,* and *cylindroma.* NOTE: Certain unrelated tumors may have a cylindromatous or adenoid cystic pattern, e.g., ameloblastoma.

adenoid squamous cell c. adenoacanthoma.

adenosquamous c. 1. adenoacanthoma. 2. a diverse category of bronchogenic carcinoma with areas of glandular, squamous, and large-cell differentiation; in some cases inclusion of a tumor in this category rather than in one of the more specific categories of bronchogenic carcinoma has been questioned.

adnexal c's a large group of carcinomas arising from, or forming structures resembling, the skin appendages (or adnexa), particularly sweat glands or sebaceous glands.

c. of adrenal cortex, adrenocortical c. a malignant adrenal cortical tumor that can cause endocrine disorders such as Cushing syndrome or adrenogenital syndrome.

aldosterone-producing c., aldosterone-secreting c. a rare malignant form of aldosteronoma; it is larger than an aldosterone-producing adenoma.

alveolar c. bronchioloalveolar c.

alveolar basal cell c. cystic basal cell c.

alveolar cell c. bronchioloalveolar c.

ameloblastic c. a type of ameloblastoma in which malignant epithelial transformation has occurred; the metastatic lesions do not resemble the primary tumor histologically, instead usually resembling squamous cell carcinoma. Cf. *malignant ameloblastoma.*

ampullary c. a subset of periampullary carcinoma that comprises tumors arising in the immediate vicinity of the sphincter of Oddi.

anaplastic c. of thyroid gland, anaplastic thyroid c. a type of thyroid gland carcinoma with atypical cells of various types and patterns; it may be silent for years but then become highly malignant and locally invasive. It affects mainly the elderly and somewhat more women than men. Called also *undifferentiated c. of thyroid gland.*

apocrine c. 1. adnexal carcinoma arising in an apocrine gland. 2. a rare breast malignancy with a ductal or acinar growth pattern and apocrine secretions.

basal cell c. the most common form of skin cancer, consisting of an epithelial tumor of the skin originating from neoplastic differentiation of basal cells; many patients have histories of exposure to ionizing radiation, and less often of arsenic poisoning. These skin cancers are much more common in light-skinned individuals than in the darker-skinned, and in older than younger persons; they are rarely metastatic but usually locally invasive and aggressive. Several subtypes have been distinguished; the most common type is *nodular,* and other types include *cystic, infiltrating, morpheaform, pigmented,* and *superficial.*

basaloid c. 1. a nonspecific term referring to any of numerous carcinomas that resemble basal cell carcinoma. 2. a rare transitional cell carcinoma of the anus, resembling basal cell carcinoma of the skin. Called also *cloacogenic anal c.*

basosquamous c., basosquamous cell c. a type of carcinoma of the skin that has elements of both basal cell and squamous cell types.

bile duct c. 1. cholangiocarcinoma. 2. cholangiocellular c.

bilharzial c. schistosomal bladder c.

bronchioalveolar c., bronchiolar c., bronchioloalveolar c. a variant type of adenocarcinoma of the lung, with columnar to cuboidal epithelial cells lining the alveolar septa and projecting into alveolar spaces in branching papillary formations. Called also *alveolar c.* or *adenocarcinoma, alveolar cell c.* or *tumor, bronchiolar c.* or *adenocarcinoma, bronchoalveolar c.* or *adenocarcinoma,* and *bronchioalveolar adenocarcinoma.*

bronchoalveolar c., bronchoalveolar cell c. bronchioloalveolar c.

bronchogenic c. any of a large group of carcinomas of the lung, so called because they arise from the epithelium of the bronchial tree. Four primary subtypes are distinguished: *adenocarcinoma of the lung, large cell carcinoma, small cell carcinoma,* and *squamous cell carcinoma.*

cholangiocellular c. a rare type of hepatocellular carcinoma arising from the cholangioles, composed of tumor cells resembling the epithelial cells of the cholangioles arranged in cords consisting of two layers of cells surrounding a minute lumen. Called also *bile duct c., extrahepatic bile duct c.,* and *cholangiocarcinoma.*

chorionic c. choriocarcinoma.

choroid plexus c. an aggressive anaplastic tumor representing malignant transformation of a choroid plexus papilloma.

clear cell c. 1. see under *adenocarcinoma.* 2. renal cell c.

clinging c. of breast a rare form of ductal carcinoma in situ.

cloacogenic anal c. basaloid c. (def. 2).

colloid c. mucinous c.

comedo c. comedocarcinoma.

corpus c., c. of corpus uteri uterine corpus c.

cortisol-producing c. a type of carcinoma of the adrenal cortex that secretes cortisol, causing Cushing syndrome.

cribriform c. 1. adenoid cystic c. 2. an adenoid cystic carcinoma of the lactiferous ducts, one of the subtypes of ductal carcinoma in situ; many tumors have combined cribriform and micropapillary patterns.

Carcinoma *Continued*

cylindrical c., cylindrical cell c. carcinoma in which the cells are cylindrical (columnar) cells.
cystic basal cell c. a rare subtype of basal cell carcinoma that occurs as a cystic lesion formed by central degeneration, characterized histologically by edematous stroma rimmed by neoplastic cells.
duct c., ductal c. carcinoma of a duct, such as of the pancreas or breast; see also *ductal c. in situ.*
ductal c. in situ (DCIS) any of a large group of in situ carcinomas of the lactiferous ducts; subtypes distinguished by histology include comedocarcinoma, cribriform carcinoma, and micropapillary carcinoma, but many tumors include areas of more than one type. Called also *intraductal c.*
ductal c. of the prostate see under *adenocarcinoma.*
eccrine c. any of the adnexal carcinomas that originate in the eccrine sweat glands; see also *hidradenocarcinoma.*
embryonal c. a highly malignant germ cell tumor that is a primitive form of carcinoma, probably of primitive embryonal cell derivation; it may be found either in pure form or as part of a mixed germ cell tumor and has a histological appearance similar to that of a yolk sac tumor. In females, there is a median age of 15; in males the majority of patients are adolescents or older.
c. en cuirasse carcinoma of the skin manifest as thickening and induration over large areas of the chest, frequently as a result of metastasis from a primary breast lesion.
endometrial c. carcinoma of the endometrium of the corpus uteri, one of the most common gynecological cancers, mainly affecting postmenopausal women; a common symptom is abnormal vaginal bleeding. It includes types ranging in malignancy from locally invasive to metastasizing.
endometrioid c. carcinoma characterized by glandular patterns that resemble those of the endometrium, occurring in the uterine fundus and in the ovaries; see also under *adenocarcinoma.*
c. of endometrium endometrial c.
epidermoid c. squamous cell c. (def. 2).
epithelial c. a malignant epithelioma, such as of the respiratory tract or ovary.
c. erysipeloi′des a type of cutaneous metastasis that clinically resembles erysipelas, usually on the chest from carcinoma of the breast or an internal organ.
c. ex mixed tumor c. ex pleomorphic adenoma.
exophytic c. a malignant epithelial neoplasm with marked outward growth like a wart or papilloma.
c. ex pleomorphic adenoma a type of malignant pleomorphic adenoma that usually occurs in the salivary glands of older adults; an epithelial malignancy arises in a preexisting mixed tumor, with metastasis only of the malignant epithelial component. The term is sometimes used synonymously with *malignant mixed tumor.*
extrahepatic bile duct c. cholangiocellular c.
familial medullary thyroid c. (FMTC) a hereditary form of medullary thyroid carcinoma due to mutation in the *RET* oncogene and considered one of the subtypes of multiple endocrine neoplasia type 2 (q.v.), but occurring in the absence of adrenal or parathyroid involvement.
fibroepithelial basal cell c. premalignant fibroepithelioma.
fibrolamellar c. a rare variant of hepatocellular carcinoma in which there is a solitary mass, no evidence of cirrhosis, and no male predominance. It is characterized histologically by eosinophilic polygonal hepatocytes that contain swollen mitochondria, cytoplasmic bodies, and hyaline bodies and have prominent nucleoli; the cells are surrounded by a stroma of thin parallel collagen bands. Called also *fibrolamellar hepatoma.*
follicular c. of thyroid gland, follicular thyroid c. a type of thyroid gland carcinoma with many follicles, although it may have areas without follicles; it is more common in women and is more malignant than papillary carcinoma of thyroid gland.
gastric c. see under *adenocarcinoma.*
gelatiniform c., gelatinous c. mucinous c.
giant cell c. a poorly differentiated, highly malignant, epithelial neoplasm containing numerous very large, multinucleated tumor cells, such as occurs in the lungs.
giant cell c. of thyroid gland a type of anaplastic carcinoma of the thyroid gland, containing numerous giant cells, some of which are multinucleated.
c. gigantocellula′re giant cell c.
glandular c. adenocarcinoma.
granulosa cell c. a granulosa cell tumor that has undergone malignant transformation.
hepatocellular c. primary carcinoma of the liver cells; symptoms include hepatomegaly, abdominal pain, weight loss, jaundice, hemoperitoneum, and other symptoms of the presence of an abdominal mass. It is rare in North America and Western Europe but is one of the most common malignancies in parts of sub-Saharan Africa, Southeast Asia, East Asia, and elsewhere. A strong association seems to exist with chronic hepatitis B virus infection, and definite but less strong associations with some types of cirrhosis and hepatitis C virus infection. Called also *hepatoma, malignant hepatoma,* and *hepatocarcinoma.*
Hürthle cell c. a malignant Hürthle cell tumor.
hypernephroid c. renal cell c.
infantile embryonal c. yolk sac tumor.
infiltrating basal cell c. carcinoma in which strands of basal cells infiltrate between collagen bundles of the subcutaneous tissue.
infiltrating lobular c. invasive lobular c.
infiltrative basal cell c. infiltrating basal cell c.
inflammatory c. of breast a highly malignant carcinoma of the breast, presenting with pink to red skin discoloration, tenderness, edema, and rapid enlargement of the breast; it usually invades dermal lymphatic vessels.
c. in si′tu a neoplastic entity whose tumor cells are confined to the epithelium of origin, without invasion of the basement membrane; the likelihood of subsequent invasive growth is presumed to be high. See also *ductal c. in situ* and *lobular c. in situ.* Called also *noninfiltrating* or *preinvasive c.*
insular thyroid c., insular c. of thyroid gland a rare variant of papillary carcinoma of the thyroid gland, seen growing in nests or sheets.
intraductal c. 1. any carcinoma of the epithelium of a duct. 2. ductal c. in situ.
intraepidermal c. carcinoma confined within the epidermis, the basal layer of the epidermis not being penetrated by the proliferating cells, as in Bowen disease.
intraepidermal squamous cell c. Bowen disease.
intraepithelial c. c. in situ.
intrahepatic bile duct c. cholangiocarcinoma (def. 1).
invasive lobular c. an invasive type of carcinoma of the breast characterized by linear growth into desmoplastic stroma around the terminal part of the lobules of mammary glands; most cases develop from lobular carcinoma in situ.
juvenile embryonal c. yolk sac tumor.
Kulchitsky cell c. carcinoid tumor of the small or large intestine.
large cell c. a type of bronchogenic carcinoma of undifferentiated (anaplastic) cells of large size, a variety of squamous cell carcinoma that has undergone further dedifferentiation.
leptomeningeal c. meningeal c.
lobular c. 1. terminal duct c. 2. see *lobular c. in situ.*
lobular c. in situ (LCIS) a type of precancerous neoplasia found in the lobules of mammary glands, usually small and widely dispersed so that it is not palpable physically and is identified only on microscopic examination. It progresses slowly, sometimes developing into invasive lobular carcinoma 10 to 15 years after first being observed. Called also *lobular neoplasia.*
lymphoepithelial c. lymphoepithelioma.
c. medulla′re, medullary c. carcinoma composed mainly of epithelial elements with little or no stroma, found most often in the breast and thyroid gland.
medullary c. of thyroid gland, medullary thyroid c. a type of thyroid gland carcinoma that contains amyloid deposits and parafollicular cells and secretes calcitonin. See also *familial medullary thyroid c.*
melanotic c. malignant melanoma.
meningeal c. carcinomatous infiltration of the meninges, particularly the pia and arachnoid; it may be primary or secondary, especially metastatic from small-cell lung carcinoma or breast cancer. Called also *leptomeningeal c.* and *leptomeningeal* or *meningeal carcinomatosis.*
Merkel cell c. a rapidly growing malignant dermal or subcutaneous tumor occurring on sun-exposed areas in middle-aged or older adults and containing irregular anastomosing trabeculae and small dense granules typical of Merkel cells; whether these are the cells of origin is still under debate. Called also *neuroendocrine* or *trabecular c. of the skin* and *Merkel cell tumor.*
metatypical cell c. basosquamous cell c.

Carcinoma *Continued*

microcystic adnexal c. a rare type of adnexal carcinoma presenting as a hard, pale or flesh-colored plaque or nodule, usually on the face, especially the upper lip or paranasal area. It arises from sweat gland tissue, grows slowly, and remains local, without metastasis. Called also *sclerosing sweat duct c.*
micronodular basal cell c. a form of nodular basal cell carcinoma in which the nodules are particularly small and usually do not ulcerate.
micropapillary c. a type of ductal carcinoma in situ characterized by a regular pattern of small bulbous papillae; many tumors have combined micropapillary and cribriform patterns.
morpheaform basal cell c., morphealike basal cell c., morpheic basal cell c. carcinoma usually seen on the face or neck as white, scarlike, telangiectatic lesions with poorly defined borders, characterized histologically by strands of basal cells surrounded by dense hyalinized stroma, and usually spreading laterally. Called also *sclerosing basal cell c.*
mucinous c. an adenocarcinoma that produces mucin in significant amounts. Called also *colloid c.* or *cancer*
c. mucocellula′re Krukenberg tumor.
mucoepidermoid c. a malignant epithelial tumor of glandular tissue, especially the salivary glands, characterized by acini with mucus-producing cells and by the presence of malignant squamous elements; it may occur as a low, intermediate, or high grade malignancy.
multicentric basal cell c., multifocal basal cell c., multifocal superficial basal cell c. superficial basal cell c.
nasopharyngeal c. a malignant tumor arising in the epithelial lining of the nasopharynx, occurring with a high frequency in people of Chinese ancestry. Epstein-Barr virus has been implicated as a cause.
neuroendocrine c. of the skin Merkel cell c.
nodular basal cell c. the most common type of basal cell carcinoma, usually seen on the face as one or several small, waxy, translucent nodules with rolled edges around a central depression; these may be ulcerated, crusted, or bleeding and may spread laterally or invade deeply. Two subtypes are micronodular and noduloulcerative basal cell carcinoma.
noduloulcerative basal cell c. nodular basal cell carcinoma that has undergone ulceration.
noninfiltrating c. c. in situ.
non–small cell c., non–small cell lung c. (NSCLC) a general term comprising all lung carcinomas except small cell carcinoma, and including adenocarcinoma of the lung, large cell carcinoma, and squamous cell carcinoma.
oat cell c. a form of small cell carcinoma in which the cells are round or elongated and slightly larger than lymphocytes; they have scanty cytoplasm and clump poorly.
occult papillary thyroid c., occult papillary c. of thyroid gland papillary thyroid microcarcinoma.
c. ossi′ficans, osteoid c. carcinoma in which there is osteoid or osseous metaplasia of the stroma.
Paget c. Paget disease (def. 1).
papillary c. carcinoma in which there are papillary excrescences.
papillary c. of thyroid gland, papillary thyroid c. the most common thyroid gland carcinoma, occurring often before age 40 and much more in women than in men. It usually has both papillary and follicular elements, grows slowly, and may remain localized for years.
periampullary c. carcinoma arising in the immediate vicinity of the ampulla of Vater.

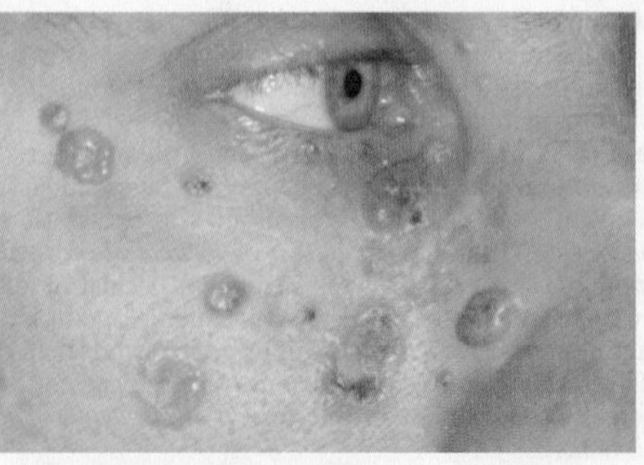

■ Noduloulcerative basal cell carcinoma.

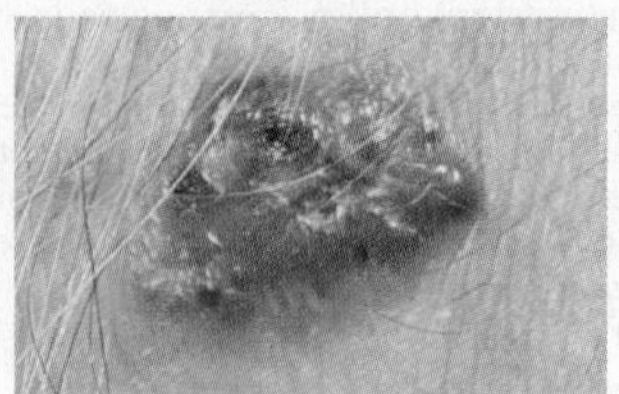

■ Pigmented basal cell carcinoma.

pigmented basal cell c. carcinoma whose lesions contain brown or black pigment; it grows slowly and is seen more often in darker-skinned individuals. Some cases are associated with chronic arsenic poisoning.
pilar c. a solitary, nodular, sometimes ulcerated lesion of the hair follicle, usually on the scalp of elderly women; it is frequently recurrent and metastasizes to regional lymph nodes.
planocellular c. squamous cell c.
preinvasive c. c. in situ.
prickle cell c. squamous cell c. (def. 1).
primary intraosseous c. a rare epithelial odontogenic malignancy occurring in the mandible and maxilla, particularly of male adults, and believed to arise from odontogenic epithelial remnants.
renal cell c. carcinoma of the renal parenchyma, usually occurring in middle age or later and composed of tubular cells in varying arrangements; symptoms depend on extent of invasion. Called also *adenocarcinoma of kidney*, *renal adenocarcinoma*, and *clear cell c.*
scar c. carcinoma associated with scarring, usually an adenocarcinoma of the lung; the scar may either precede the carcinoma or be a fibrotic response to it.
schistosomal bladder c. carcinoma of the wall of the urinary bladder, usually a squamous cell carcinoma, caused by chronic infection and irritation by *Schistosoma haematobium;* called also *bilharzial c.*
schneiderian c. a neoplasm of the mucosa of the nose and the paranasal sinuses.
scirrhous c. carcinoma with a hard structure owing to the formation of dense connective tissue in the stroma. Called also *fibrocarcinoma.*
sclerosing basal cell c. morpheaform basal cell c.
sclerosing sweat duct c. microcystic adnexal c.
sebaceous c., sebaceous gland c. adnexal carcinoma of the sebaceous glands, usually occurring as a slow-growing hard yellow nodule on the eyelid.
signet ring cell c. a type of highly malignant, mucus-secreting tumor usually found in the stomach or intestine; the mucus-secreting cells called *signet ring cells* are anaplastic.
c. sim′plex an undifferentiated carcinoma.
skin appendage c's adnexal c's.
small cell c., small cell lung c. (SCLC) a common, highly malignant form of bronchogenic carcinoma in the wall of a major bronchus, occurring mainly in middle-aged individuals with a history of tobacco smoking; it is radiosensitive and has small oval undifferentiated cells that are intensely hematoxyphilic. Metastasis to the hilum and to mediastinal lymph nodes is common.
spindle cell c. carcinoma, usually of the squamous cell type, marked by fusiform development of rapidly proliferating cells.
spinocellular c. squamous cell c. (def. 1).
squamous c., squamous cell c. 1. carcinoma developed from squamous epithelium, having cuboid cells and characterized by

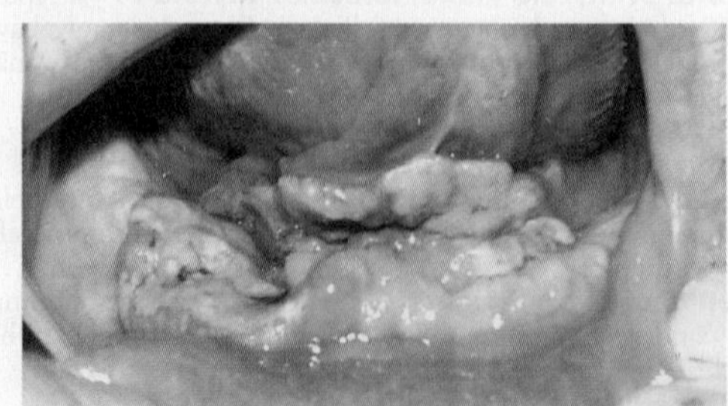

■ Squamous cell carcinoma of the anterior floor of the mouth.

Carcinoma *Continued*

keratinization and often by preservation of intercellular bridges. In the skin, it may originate in sun-damaged areas or other pre-existing lesions. Initially local and superficial, the lesion may later invade and metastasize. Called also *prickle cell* or *spinocellular c.* 2. one of the most common types of bronchogenic carcinoma, generally forming polypoid or sessile masses that obstruct the airways of the bronchi. It usually occurs in middle-aged individuals with a history of smoking. There is frequent invasion of blood and lymphatic vessels with metastasis to regional lymph nodes and other sites. Called also *epidermoid c.*

superficial basal cell c. carcinoma usually seen on the trunk as a plaque or plaques that are superficial, slowly spreading, erythematous, and scaly, and have threadlike, raised borders. Called also *multicentric* or *multifocal basal cell c.*

sweat gland c. hidradenocarcinoma.

syringomatous c. microcystic adnexal c.

c. telangiectoi´des a rare manifestation of breast cancer metastasis to the skin, presenting as red papules and telangiectasias.

terminal duct c. a slow-growing, locally invasive malignant neoplasm composed of myoepithelial and ductal elements, occurring in the minor salivary glands, particularly in the palate.

trabecular c. of the skin Merkel cell c.

transitional cell c. a malignant tumor arising from transitional epithelium, usually in the urinary bladder.

tubular c. 1. an adenocarcinoma in which the cells are arranged in the form of tubules. 2. a type of breast cancer in which small glandlike structures are formed and infiltrate the stroma; it usually develops from an earlier ductal carcinoma in situ and is rarely metastatic.

undifferentiated c. of thyroid gland, undifferentiated thyroid c. anaplastic c. of thyroid gland.

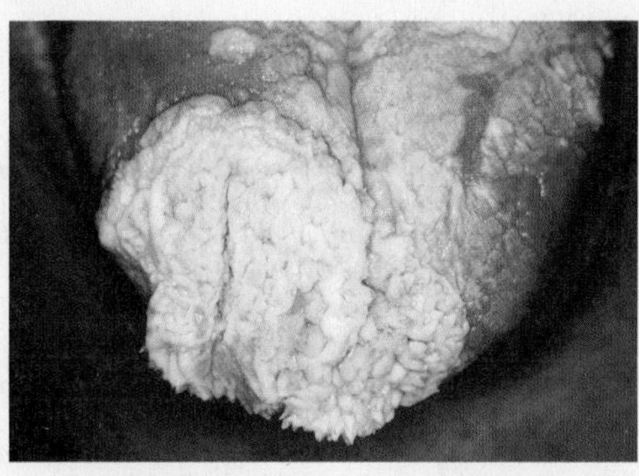

■ Verrucous carcinoma of the tongue.

uterine corpus c. carcinoma of the corpus uteri, usually endometrial carcinoma, one of the most common gynecological cancers; it ranges in malignancy from locally invasive to metastatic.

verrucous c. 1. a variety of squamous cell carcinoma that has a predilection for the buccal mucosa but also affects other oral soft tissue and the larynx. It is a slow-growing, somewhat invasive, exophytic neoplasm, either papillary or verrucous in appearance. 2. Buschke-Löwenstein tumor, so called because it is histologically similar to the oral lesion.

c. villo´sum, villous c. carcinoma in which the cells are arranged in a villous pattern, as papillary projections which are covered with neoplastic epithelium; usually seen in the gastrointestinal tract.

yolk sac c. see under *tumor.*

car·ci·no·ma·ta (kahr″sĭ-no´mə-tə) plural of *carcinoma.*

car·ci·nom·a·toid (kahr″sĭ-nom´ə-toid) resembling carcinoma.

car·ci·no·ma·to·pho·bia (kahr″sĭ-no″mə-to-fo´be-ə) cancerphobia.

car·ci·no·ma·to·sis (kahr″sĭ-no-mə-to´sis) the condition of widespread dissemination of cancer throughout the body.
 leptomeningeal c. meningeal carcinoma.
 meningeal c. see under *carcinoma.*

car·ci·nom·a·tous (kahr″sĭ-nom´ə-təs) pertaining to or of the nature of cancer; cf. *malignant.*

car·ci·no·pho·bia (kahr″sĭ-no-fo´be-ə) [*carcino-* + *phobia*] cancerphobia.

car·ci·no·sar·co·ma (kahr″sĭ-no-sahr-ko´mə) [*carcino-* + *sarcoma*] a malignant tumor composed of carcinomatous and sarcomatous tissues.
 embryonal c. Wilms tumor.

car·ci·no·stat·ic (kahr″sĭ-no-stat´ik) tending to check the growth of carcinoma.

car·da·mom (kahr´də-məm) [L. *cardamomum;* Gr. *kardamōmon*] 1. a plant of the species *Elettaria cardamomum.* 2. any of various other closely related plants that yield seeds similar to those of *E. cardamomum.* 3. the dried ripe seeds of *E. cardamomum* or related plants, used as a pharmaceutical flavoring agent; see also *cardamom oil,* under *oil.* Called also *cardamom seed* [NF]. 4. a preparation of the seeds of *E. cardamomum,* used for a variety of respiratory disorders and for disorders of the gastrointestinal tract, as well as in traditional Chinese medicine and ayurveda.

car·del·my·cin (kahr″dəl-mi´sin) novobiocin.

Car·den amputation (kahr´dən) [Henry Douglas *Carden,* English surgeon, died 1872] see under *amputation.*

Car·dene (kahr´dēn) trademark for a preparation of nicardipine hydrochloride.

car·dia (kahr´de-ə) [Gr. *kardia* heart] [TA] the part of the stomach immediately adjacent to and surrounding the cardiac opening where the esophagus connects to the stomach; it contains the cardiac glands, and does not have any parietal cells or chief cells. Called also *pars cardiaca gastrica* [TA alternative] and *cardiac part of stomach.*

car·di·ac (kahr´de-ak) [L. *cardiacus,* from Gr. *kardiakos*] 1. pertaining to the heart. 2. pertaining to the cardia of the stomach or the cardiac opening of the esophagus (ostium cardiacum). Called also *cardial.* 3. see note

car·dial (kahr´de-əl) cardiac (def. 2).

car·di·al·gia (kahr″de-al´jə) cardiodynia.

car·di·ec·ta·sis (kahr″de-ek´tə-sis) [*cardi-*(1) + *ectasis*] dilatation of the heart.

car·di·ec·to·mized (kahr″de-ek´tə-mīzd) having the heart removed, as a cardiectomized animal.

car·di·ec·to·my (kahr″de-ek´tə-me) [*cardi-* + *-ectomy*] 1. surgical removal of the heart, as during transplantation. 2. surgical removal of the cardia of the stomach.

car·di·nal (kahr´dĭ-nəl) [L. *cardinalis,* from *cardo* a hinge] 1. of primary or preeminent importance. 2. in embryology, pertaining to the main venous drainage.

cardi(o)- [Gr. *kardia* heart] a combining form denoting relationship (1) to the heart or (2) to the cardiac orifice or portion of the stomach.

car·dio·ac·cel·er·a·tor (kahr″de-o-ak-sel´ər-a-tər) 1. quickening the heart action. 2. an agent that accelerates the heart action.

car·dio·ac·tive (kahr″de-o-ak´tiv) having an effect upon the heart.

car·dio·an·gi·og·ra·phy (kahr″de-o-an″je-og´rə-fe) angiocardiography.

car·dio·an·gi·ol·o·gy (kahr″de-o-an″je-ol´ə-je) [*cardio-*(1) + *angio-* + *-logy*] the medical specialty which deals with the heart and blood vessels.

car·dio·ar·te·ri·al (kahr″de-o-ahr-tēr´e-əl) pertaining to the heart and the arteries.

Car·dio·bac·te·ri·a·ceae (kahr″de-o-bak-tēr″e-a´se-e) a family of bacteria of the order Cardiobacteriales, consisting of gram-negative, pleomorphic, straight rods and long filaments, occurring singly, in pairs or short chains, and in clusters; organisms are nonmotile, facultatively anaerobic, chemo-organotrophic, and catalase-negative. It contains the genera *Cardiobacterium, Dichelobacter,* and *Suttonella.*

Car·dio·bac·ter·i·a·les (kahr″de-o-bak-tēr″e-a´lēz) an order of bacteria of the class Gammaproteobacteria, phylum Proteobacteria, created on the basis of 16S rRNA sequence analysis, consisting of gram-negative, mainly aerobic, chemo-organotrophic rods; it contains the family Cardiobacteriaceae.

Car·dio·bac·te·ri·um (kahr″de-o-bak-tēr´e-əm) [*cardio-*(1) + *bacterium*] a genus of gram-negative, facultatively anaerobic, fermentative, rod-shaped bacteria of the family Cardiobacteriaceae; organisms are part of the normal flora of the nose and throat and are also isolated from blood. The type species is *C. ho´minis.*

C. ho′minis a species that is part of the normal flora of the nose and pharynx, and also an etiologic agent of endocarditis.

car·dio·cai·ro·graph (kahr″de-o-ki′ro-graf) [*cardio-*(1) + Gr. *kairos* time + *-graph*] a technique by means of which radiographs of the heart can be made at any chosen phase of its cycle.

car·dio·cele (kahr′de-o-sēl″) [*cardio-*(1) + *-cele*[1]] protrusion of the heart through a fissure of the diaphragm or through a wound.

car·dio·cen·te·sis (kahr″de-o-sen-te′sis) [*cardio-*(1) + *-centesis*] surgical puncture or incision of the heart.

car·dio·cha·la·sia (kahr″de-o-kə-la′zhə) [*cardio-*(2) + *chalasia*] esophageal achalasia.

car·dio·cir·cu·la·tory (kahr″de-o-sur′ku-lə-tor′e) pertaining to blood flow through the heart and cardiovascular system.

car·dio·cir·rho·sis (kahr″de-o-sĭ-ro′sis) cardiac cirrhosis.

car·dio·cyte (kahr′de-o-sīt″) [*cardio-*(1) + *-cyte*] myocyte.

car·dio·di·a·phrag·mat·ic (kahr″de-o-di″ə-frag-mat′ik) pertaining to the heart and the diaphragm.

car·dio·dy·nam·ics (kahr″de-o-di-nam′iks) [*cardio-*(1) + *dynamics*] the science of the motions and forces involved in the heart's action.

car·di·odyn·ia (kahr″de-o-din′e-ə) [*cardio-*(1) + *-odynia*] pain in the heart.

car·dio·esoph·a·ge·al (kahr″de-o-ə-sof″ə-je′əl) pertaining to or connecting the cardia of the stomach and the esophagus.

car·dio·gen·e·sis (kahr″de-o-jen′ə-sis) [*cardio-*(1) + *genesis*] the development of the heart in the embryo.

car·dio·gen·ic (kahr″de-o-jen′ik) [*cardio-*(1) + *-genic*] 1. originating in the heart; caused by normal or abnormal function of the heart. 2. pertaining to cardiogenesis.

car·dio·gram (kahr′de-o-gram″) [*cardio-*(1) + *-gram*] a tracing of a cardiac event made by means of the cardiograph.

apex c. apexcardiogram.

esophageal c. a tracing of the contractions of the left atrium made by registering the pulsations in the esophagus.

precordial c. kinetocardiogram.

vector c. vectorcardiogram.

car·dio·graph (kahr′de-o-graf″) [*cardio-*(1) + -graph] an instrument designed to record some element of the heartbeat.

car·di·og·ra·phy (kahr″de-og′rə-fe) [*cardio-*(1) + *-graphy*] the technique of graphically recording some physical or functional aspects of the heart. See also *apexcardiography*, *cardiokymography*, *echocardiography*, *electrocardiography*, *kinetocardiography*, *phonocardiography*, *telecardiography*, *vectorcardiography*, etc. **cardiograph′ic** *adj*

ultrasonic c. echocardiography.

car·dio·he·pat·ic (kahr″de-o-hə-pat′ik) pertaining to the heart and the liver.

car·dio·hep·a·to·meg·a·ly (kahr″de-o-hep″ə-to-meg′ə-le) enlargement of the heart and liver.

car·di·oid (kahr′de-oid) heartlike; resembling a heart.

car·dio·in·hib·i·tor (kahr″de-o-in-hib′ĭ-tər) an agent which restrains the heart's action.

car·dio·in·hib·i·to·ry (kahr″de-o-in-hib′ĭ-tor-e) restraining or inhibiting the movements of the heart.

car·dio·ki·net·ic (kahr″de-o-kĭ-net′ik) 1. stimulating the action of the heart. 2. an agent that stimulates action of the heart.

car·dio·ky·mog·ra·phy (kahr″de-o-ki-mog′rə-fe) the recording of the motion of the heart by means of the electrokymograph. **cardiokymograph′ic** *adj*

car·dio·lip·in (kahr″de-o-lip′in) [*cardio-*(1) + Gr. *lipos* fat] 1,3-diphosphatidylglycerol, a phospholipid occurring primarily in mitochondrial inner membranes and in bacterial plasma membranes. Cardiolipin is the main antigenic component of Wassermann-type antigens used in nontreponemal serologic tests for syphilis.

Car·dio·lite (kahr′de-o-līt″) trademark for a kit for the preparation of technetium Tc 99m sestamibi.

car·di·ol·o·gist (kahr″de-ol′ə-jist) a physician skilled in the prevention, diagnosis, and treatment of heart disease.

car·di·ol·o·gy (kahr″de-ol′ə-je) [*cardio-*(1) + *-logy*] the study of the heart and its functions.

invasive c. the theory and practice of diagnostic and therapeutic cardiac procedures that involve entry into the heart or central circulation, such as cardiac catheterization, coronary angioplasty, or electrophysiologic studies.

interventional c. the subspecialty of cardiology that uses catheter-based techniques to treat coronary artery, valvular, and congenital cardiac disease.

car·di·ol·y·sis (kahr″de-ol′ə-sis) [*cardio-*(1) + *lysis*] an operation of freeing the heart and pericardium in adhesive mediastinopericarditis; it is done by resecting the ribs and the sternum over the pericardium.

car·dio·ma·la·cia (kahr″de-o-mə-la′shə) [*cardio-*(1) + *malacia*] morbid softening of the muscular substance of the heart.

car·dio·me·ga·lia (kahr″de-o-mə-ga′le-ə) cardiomegaly.

c. glycoge′nica diffu′sa glycogen storage disease, type II; see under *disease*.

car·dio·meg·a·ly (kahr″de-o-meg′ə-le) [*cardio-*(1) + *-megaly*] abnormal enlargement of the heart from either hypertrophy or dilatation.

car·dio·mel·a·no·sis (kahr″de-o-mel″ə-no′sis) melanosis of the heart.

car·di·om·e·ter (kahr″de-om′ə-tər) [*cardio-*(1) + *-meter*] an instrument used in estimating the size of the heart or the force of its action.

car·di·om·e·try (kahr″de-om′ə-try) [*cardio-*(1) + *-metry*] the estimation of the size of the heart or the force of its action.

car·dio·mo·til·i·ty (kahr″de-o-mo-til′ĭ-te) [*cardio-*(1) + *motility*] the movements of the heart; the motility of the heart.

car·dio·myo·li·po·sis (kahr″de-o-mi″o-lĭ-po′sis) [*cardio-*(1) + *myo-* + *lipo-* + *-osis*] fatty degeneration of the heart muscle.

car·dio·my·op·a·thy (kahr″de-o-mi-op′ə-the) [*cardio-*(1) + *myopathy*] 1. a general diagnostic term designating primary noninflammatory disease of the heart muscle, often of obscure or unknown etiology and not the result of ischemic, hypertensive, congenital, valvular, or pericardial disease. It is usually subdivided into *dilated*, *hypertrophic*, and *restrictive c.* 2. In World Health Organization nomenclature, only those disorders in which the pathological process involves solely the myocardium and in which the cause is unknown and not part of a disease affecting other organs; called also *primary c.* Cf. *secondary c.*

alcoholic c. dilated cardiomyopathy occurring in patients with a history of chronic alcohol abuse; it is believed to be due to a direct toxic effect of alcohol or its metabolites.

beer-drinkers' c. cardiac dilatation and hypertrophy due to excessive beer consumption; in at least some cases it has been caused by addition of cobalt to the beer during manufacturing. See also *alcoholic c.*

congestive c. dilated c.

dilated c. a syndrome of ventricular dilatation, systolic contractile dysfunction, and often congestive heart failure; the course is usually progressive with a poor prognosis. It may be inherited, with age-related penetrance, or acquired. Inherited forms have been associated with numerous autosomal dominant mutations, most encoding proteins involved in muscle structure and assembly; causes of acquired cases include myocarditis, coronary artery disease, systemic diseases, and myocardial toxins.

dilated c. with ataxia 3-methylglutaconicaciduria type V.

hypertrophic c. (HCM) a condition, often of autosomal dominant inheritance, marked by ventricular hypertrophy, particularly of the left ventricle and often involving the interventricular septum, with diastolic dysfunction manifest as impaired ventricular filling; it is sometimes the cause of sudden cardiac death in athletes. See also *idiopathic hypertrophic subaortic stenosis*, under *stenosis*.

hypertrophic obstructive c. (HOCM) a form of hypertrophic cardiomyopathy in which the location of the septal hypertrophy causes obstructive interference with left ventricular outflow. Cf. *asymmetrical septal hypertrophy*.

idiopathic c. cardiomyopathy (def. 2).

infectious c. a chronic type seen following infection.

infiltrative c. restrictive cardiomyopathy characterized by deposition in the heart tissue of abnormal substances, as may occur in amyloidosis, hemochromatosis, and certain other conditions.

ischemic c. name given to heart failure with left ventricular dilatation resulting from ischemic heart disease; it does not meet the strict definition of a cardiomyopathy.

obliterative c. restrictive c.

obstructive hypertrophic c. hypertrophic obstructive c.

peripartum c. cardiac enlargement and congestive heart failure of unknown cause beginning in the last month of gestation or the first few months after delivery.

postpartum c. peripartum c.

primary c. cardiomyopathy (def. 2).

restrictive c. cardiomyopathy in which the ventricular walls are excessively rigid, impeding ventricular filling; it is marked by abnormal diastolic function sometimes with normal or nearly normal systolic function.

right ventricular c. a right-sided cardiomyopathy occurring predominantly in young males, characterized by dilatation of the right ventricle with partial to total replacement of its muscle by fibrous or adipose tissue, palpitations, syncope, and sometimes sudden death.

secondary c. cardiomyopathy that is due to another cardiovascular disorder (e.g., hypertension) or is a manifestation of systemic disease (e.g., sarcoidosis). See also *cardiomyopathy*.

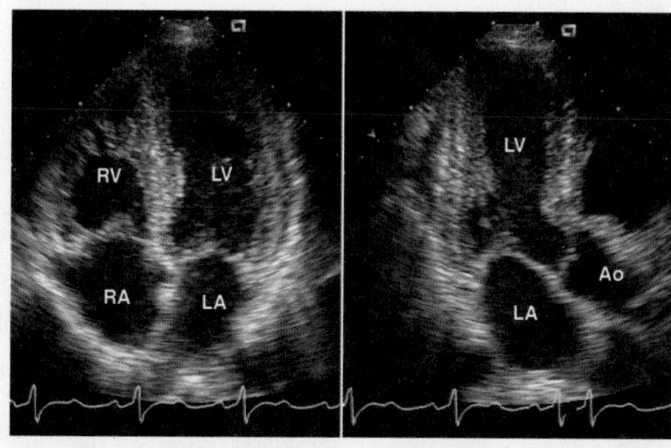

■ Restrictive cardiomyopathy in a patient with amyloidosis, in apical four-chamber *(left)* and apical two-chamber *(right)* echocardiographic images. There is biventricular hypertrophy, biatrial enlargement, mild valve thickening, and both systolic and diastolic dysfunction of the left ventricle *(LV)*. *Ao,* Aorta; *LA,* left atrium; *RA,* right atrium; *RV,* right ventricle.

toxic c. cardiomyopathy due to agents, such as alcohol or catecholamines, that cause toxic damage to the myocardium.

car•dio•my•ot•o•my (kahr″de-o-mi-ot′ə-me) [*cardio-*(1) + *myo-* + *-tomy*] esophagocardiomyotomy.

Heller c. esophagocardiomyotomy.

car•dio•neph•ric (kahr″de-o-nef′rik) pertaining to the heart and the kidney.

car•dio•neu•ral (kahr″de-o-noor′əl) pertaining to the heart and nervous system.

car•dio•path•ic (kahr″de-o-path′ik) pertaining to or marked by disease of the heart.

car•di•op•a•thy (kahr″de-op′ə-the) [*cardio-*(1) + *-pathy*] any disorder or disease of the heart.

infarctoid c. a heart condition with symptoms resembling those of myocardial infarction.

car•dio•peri•car•di•tis (kahr″de-o-per″ĭ-kahr-di′tis) [*cardio-*(1) + *pericarditis*] inflammation of both the heart and the pericardium.

car•dio•pho•bia (kahr″de-o-fo′be-ə) [*cardio-*(1) + *-phobia*] irrational dread of heart disease.

car•dio•plas•ty (kahr′de-o-plas″te) [*cardio-*(2) + *-plasty*] esophagogastroplasty. **cardioplas′tic** *adj*

car•dio•ple•gia (kahr″de-o-ple′jə) [*cardio-*(1) + Gr. *plēgē* stroke + *-ia*] arrest of contraction of the myocardium, as may be induced by the use of chemical compounds or of cold (cryocardioplegia) in the performance of surgery upon the heart. **cardiople′gic** *adj*

car•dio•pneu•mat•ic (kahr″de-o-noo-mat′ik) [*cardio-*(1) + *pneumatic*] of or pertaining to the heart and respiration.

car•dio•pro•tec•tant (kahr″de-o-pro-tek′tənt) 1. counteracting cardiotoxicity. 2. an agent that counteracts cardiotoxicity.

car•dio•pro•tec•tive (kahr″de-o-pro-tek′tiv) cardioprotectant.

car•di•op•to•sia (kahr″de-op-to′se-ə) cardioptosis.

car•di•op•to•sis (kahr″de-op-to′sis, kahr″de-o-to′sis) [*cardio-*(1) + *-ptosis*] downward displacement of the heart.

car•dio•pul•mo•nary (kahr″de-o-pool′mə-nar-e) pertaining to the heart and lungs. Called also *cardiorespiratory* and *pneumocardial.*

car•dio•py•lo•ric (kahr″de-o-pi-lor′ik) pertaining to the cardia of the stomach and the pylorus.

car•dio•re•nal (kahr″de-o-re′nəl) pertaining to the heart and the kidney. Called also *nephrocardiac.*

car•dio•res•pi•ra•to•ry (kahr″de-o-res′pĭ-rə-tor″e) cardiopulmonary.

car•di•or•rha•phy (kahr″de-or′ə-fe) [*cardio-*(1) + *-rrhaphy*] the operation of suturing the heart muscle.

car•di•or•rhex•is (kahr″de-o-rek′sis) [*cardio-*(1) + *-rrhexis*] rupture of the heart.

car•dio•scle•ro•sis (kahr″de-o-sklə-ro′sis) [*cardio-*(1) + *sclerosis*] fibrous induration of the heart.

car•dio•se•lec•tive (kahr″de-o-sə-lek′tiv) having greater activity on heart tissue than on other tissue.

car•dio•spasm (kahr′de-o-spaz″əm) esophageal achalasia.

car•dio•ta•chom•e•ter (kahr″de-o-tə-kom′ə-tər) [*cardio-*(1) + *tacho-* + *-meter*] the instrument used in cardiotachometry.

car•dio•ta•chom•e•try (kahr″de-o-tə-kom′ə-tre) [*cardio-*(1) + *tacho-* + *-metry*] continuous recording of the heart rate for long periods of time.

Car•dio•Tec (kahr′de-o-tek″) trademark for a kit for the preparation of technetium Tc 99m teboroxime.

car•dio•ther•a•py (kahr″de-o-ther′ə-pe) [*cardio-*(1) + *therapy*] the treatment of heart diseases.

car•dio•tho•rac•ic (kahr″de-o-thə-ras′ik) pertaining to the heart and the chest (thorax).

car•dio•thy•ro•tox•i•co•sis (kahr″de-o-thi″ro-tok″sĭ-ko′sis) hyperthyroidism with cardiac involvement.

car•dio•to•co•graph (kahr″de-o-to′ko-graf) the instrument used in cardiotocography.

car•dio•to•cog•ra•phy (kahr″de-o-to-kog′rə-fe) [*cardio-*(1) + *toco-* + *-graphy*] the monitoring of the fetal heart rate, as during delivery. Also spelled *cardiotokography.* See also *contraction stress test* and *nonstress test,* under *test.*

car•di•ot•o•my (kahr″de-ot′ə-me) [*cardio-* + *-tomy*] surgical incision of the heart for repair of cardiac defects.

car•dio•ton•ic (kahr″de-o-ton′ik) 1. having a tonic effect on the heart. 2. an agent that has a tonic effect on the heart.

car•dio•to•pom•e•try (kahr″de-o-tə-pom′ə-tre) [*cardio-*(1) + *topo-* + *-metry*] measurement of the area of superficial cardiac dullness observed in percussion of the chest.

car•dio•tox•ic (kahr′de-o-tok″sik) having a poisonous or deleterious effect upon the heart.

car•dio•tox•ic•i•ty (kahr″de-o-tok-sis′ĭ-te) the quality of being cardiotoxic.

car•dio•tro•pic (kahr″de-o-tro′pik) having a particular affinity for the heart or heart tissue.

car•dio•val•vu•lar (kahr″de-o-val′vu-lər) pertaining to the valves of the heart.

car•dio•val•vu•li•tis (kahr″de-o-val″vu-li′tis) [*cardio-*(1) + *valvulitis*] inflammation of the valves of the heart.

car•dio•val•vu•lo•tome (kahr″de-o-val′vu-lə-tōm″) [*cardio-*(1) + *valvula* + *-tome*] an instrument for performing cardiovalvulotomy.

car•di•o•val•vu•lot•o•my (kahr″de-o-val″vu-lot′ə-me) [*cardio-*(1) + *valvula* + *-tomy*] the operation of incising a cardiac valve, or of excising a portion of it, done for the relief of stenosis.

car•dio•vas•cu•lar (kahr″de-o-vas′ku-lər) pertaining to the heart and blood vessels.

car•dio•vas•cu•lar-re•nal (kahr″de-o-vas′ku-lər-re′nəl) pertaining to the heart, blood vessels, and kidney.

car•dio•ver•sion (kahr′de-o-vur″zhən) the restoration of normal rhythm of the heart by electrical shock.

car•dio•ver•ter (kahr′de-o-vur″tər) an energy-storage capacitor-discharge type of condenser which is discharged with an inductance; it delivers a direct-current shock which restores normal rhythm of the heart.

automatic implantable c.-defibrillator (AICD), implantable c.-defibrillator (ICD) an implantable device that detects sustained ventricular tachycardia or fibrillation and terminates it by a shock or shocks delivered directly to the myocardium.

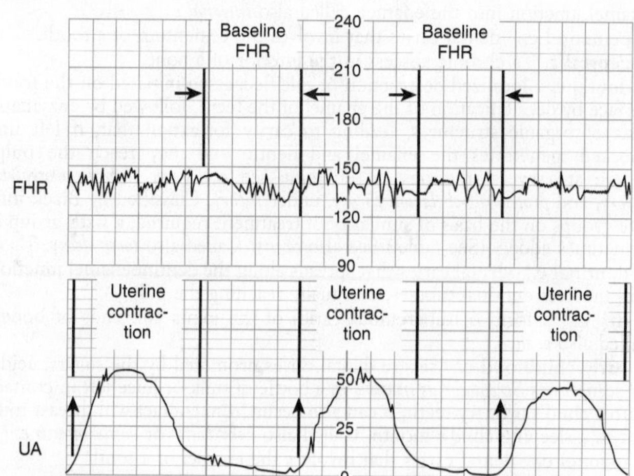

■ Cardiotocography tracing showing the interval between uterine contractions as the preferred time to assess baseline fetal heart rate. *FHR,* fetal heart rate; *UA,* uterine activity.

Car·dio·vi·rus (kahr′de-o-vi″rəs) [*cardio-*(1) + *virus*] a genus of viruses of the family Picornaviridae that cause encephalomyelitis and myocarditis; it contains two species, encephalomyocarditis virus and Theilovirus.

car·dio·vi·rus (kahr′de-o-vi″rus) any member of the genus *Cardiovirus.* **cardiovi′ral** *adj*

car·di·tis (kahr-di′tis) [*cardi-*(1) + *-itis*] inflammation of the heart.

Lyme c. cardiac involvement, generally transient, in Lyme disease; it usually manifests as some degree of atrioventricular block but ventricular tachycardia and left ventricular dysfunction may occur.

rheumatic c. cardiac involvement in rheumatic fever, which when severe may be manifested by congestive heart failure, progressive cardiac enlargement, pericarditis, and significant murmurs due to valvular dysfunction.

streptococcal c. carditis occurring as a result of streptococcal sore throat.

verrucous c. a nonbacterial endocarditis marked by a continuous chain of wartlike vegetations near the line of closure of the cusps of the mitral and tricuspid valves; seen in lupus erythematosus and occasionally in scleroderma, thrombotic purpura, and other collagen diseases.

Car·di·zem (kahr′dĭ-zem) trademark for preparations of diltiazem hydrochloride.

Car·dura (kahr-du′rə) trademark for preparations of doxazosin mesylate.

Car·mol (kahr′mol) trademark for preparations of hydrocortisone acetate.

care (kār) [A.S. *caru* anxiety] the services rendered by members of the health professions for the benefit of a patient. Called also *treatment.*

coronary c. see under *unit.*

critical c. intensive c.; see under *unit.*

intensive c. see under *unit.*

neurocritical c., neurointensive c. see under *unit.*

palliative c. see under *treatment.*

primary c. the care a patient receives at first contact with the health care system, usually involving coordination of care and continuity over time.

respiratory c. 1. the health care profession providing, under a physician's supervision, diagnostic evaluation, therapy, monitoring, and rehabilitation of patients with cardiopulmonary disorders. 2. a general term for the type of medical care provided by the members of this profession. 3. the diagnostic and therapeutic use of medical gases and their administering apparatus, environmental control systems, humidification, aerosols, medications, ventilatory support, bronchopulmonary drainage, pulmonary rehabilitation, cardiopulmonary resuscitation, and airway management. Called also *respiratory therapy.*

secondary c. treatment by specialists to whom a patient has been referred by primary care providers.

tertiary c. treatment given in a health care center that includes highly trained specialists and often advanced technology.

Car·i·ca (kar′ĭ-kə) a genus of trees of the family Caricaceae, native to tropical regions of the Americas. *C. papa′ya* L. is the papaya or papaw tree, source of the fruit called papaya and of the enzyme papain.

car·ies (kar′ēz, kar′e-ēz) [L. "rottenness"] 1. the molecular decay or death of a bone, in which it becomes softened, discolored, and porous. It produces a chronic inflammation of the periosteum and surrounding tissues, and forms a cold abscess filled with a cheesy, fetid, puslike liquid, which generally burrows through the soft parts until it opens externally by a sinus or fistula. 2. dental c.

baby bottle c., bottle mouth c. early childhood c.

backward c. dental caries that progresses backward from the dentinoenamel junction into the enamel; called also *internal c.*

cemental c. dental caries that involves the cementum of a tooth.

central c. a chronic abscess in the interior of a bone.

dental c. localized destruction of calcified tissue initiated on the tooth surface by decalcification of the enamel of the teeth, followed by enzymatic lysis of organic structures, leading to cavity formation that, if left unchecked, penetrates the enamel and dentin and may reach the pulp. There are several theories on etiology: see *acidogenic theory*, *proteolytic theory*, and *proteolysis-chelation theory*, under *theory*. Classified by Black into five groups on the basis of similarity of treatment required; a sixth group is sometimes added. (See table.) See also *cavity.* Called also *tooth decay.*

dentinal c. dental caries that spreads along the dentinoenamel junction and involves dentinal tubules, eventually reaching the pulp.

dry c. a form of tuberculous caries of the joints and ends of bones; called also *c. sicca.*

early childhood c. severe dental caries promoted by the sugars, acids, or sometimes *Streptococcus mutans* in a bottle of milk or juice left in contact with a child's primary teeth; it can also occur from contact with breast milk left in a sleeping child's mouth. Called also *baby bottle* or *bottle mouth c.*

enamel c. dental caries that involves the enamel of a tooth.

internal c. backward c.

lateral c. dental caries that extends laterally at the dentinoenamel junction.

necrotic c. a disease in which pieces of bone lie in a suppurating cavity.

Black Classification of Dental Caries

Class I	Cavities occurring in pit and fissure defects in occlusal surfaces of bicuspids and molars, lingual surfaces of upper incisors, and facial and lingual grooves sometimes found on occlusal surfaces of molar teeth.
Class II	Cavities in proximal surfaces of bicuspids and molars.
Class III	Cavities in proximal surfaces of incisors and cuspids not requiring removal of incisal angle.
Class IV	Cavities in proximal surfaces of incisors and cuspids that require removal of incisal angle.
Class V	Cavities in gingival third of labial, lingual, or buccal surfaces.
Class VI (not a true Black classification)	Cavities in incisal edges and smooth surfaces of teeth above the height of contour.

pit c. dental caries originating in pits or fissures, usually of the occlusal surfaces of molars and premolars or on the lingual surfaces of the maxillary incisors, typically occurring as a deep cavity with a narrow point of penetration.

primary dental c. dental caries in which the lesion constitutes the initial attack on the tooth surface.

rampant c., rampant dental c. dental caries involving several teeth, appearing suddenly, and often progressing rapidly.

recurrent c. dental caries beneath the margin of an existing tooth restoration.

secondary dental c. dental caries occurring around the edges and under restorations.

c. sic′ca dry c.

spinal c. tuberculotic osteitis of the vertebrae and of the intervertebral cartilages.

ca·ri·na (kə-ri′nə) pl. *cari′nae* [L. "keel"] a ridge or ridgelike structure.

c. for′nicis carina of fornix: a ridge on the undersurface of the fornix of the brain.

c. tra′cheae [TA] carina of trachea: a projection of the lowest tracheal cartilage, forming a prominent semilunar ridge running anteroposteriorly between the orifices of the two bronchi.

c. urethra′lis vagi′nae [TA] urethral carina of vagina: the column of rugae in the lower part of the anterior wall of the vagina, immediately beneath the urethra.

ca·ri·nae (kə-ri′ne) [L.] genitive and plural of *carina.*

car·i·nate (kar′ĭ-nāt) [L. *carina* a keel] keel-shaped; having a keellike process.

car·in·da·cil·lin so·di·um (kar″in-də-sil′in) carbenicillin indanyl sodium.

cari(o)- [L. *caries* rottenness] a combining form denoting relationship to caries.

car·io·gen·e·sis (kar″e-o-jen′ə-sis) development of caries.

car·io·gen·ic (kar″e-o-jen′ik) [*cario-* + *-genic*] conducive to the production of caries.

car·io·ge·nic·i·ty (kar″e-o-jə-nis′ĭ-te) the quality of being conducive to the production of caries.

car·i·ol·o·gy (kar″e-ol′ə-je) [*cario-* + *-logy*] the study of cariogenesis and its prevention.

car·i·os·i·ty (kar″e-os′ĭ-te) the quality of being carious.

ca·ri·ous (kar′e-əs) [L. *cariosus*] affected with or of the nature of caries.

car·iso·pro·dol (kar″i-so-pro′dol) a centrally acting skeletal muscle relaxant, for the symptomatic management of acute, painful musculoskeletal disorders, administered orally. Called also *isopropyl meprobamate.*

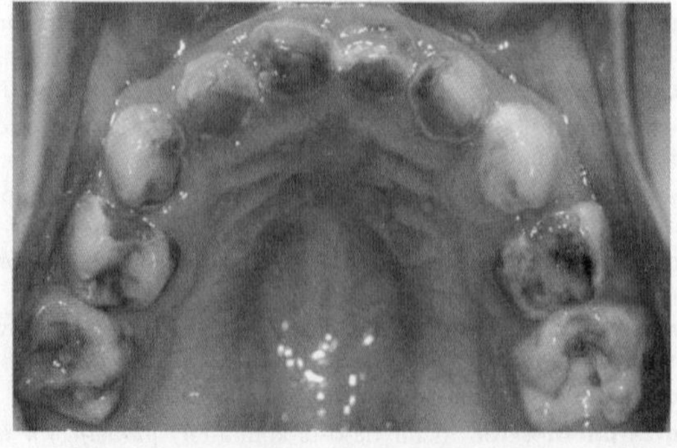

■ Early childhood caries on the primary teeth of a three-year-old child.

Car•lens tube (kahr′lənz) [Eric *Carlens,* Swedish physician, 1908–1990] see under *tube.*

car•mal•um (kahr-mal′əm) a stain composed of carmine, alum, and water.

Car•man sign (kahr′mən) [Russell Daniel *Carman,* American radiologist, 1875–1926] meniscus sign; see under *sign.*

Car•man-Kirk•lin sign (meniscus sign) (kahr′mən kərk′lin) [R.D. *Carman;* Byrl Raymond *Kirklin,* American radiologist, 1888–1957] meniscus sign; see under *sign.*

car•mel•lose (kahr′mə-lōs) carboxymethylcellulose.

car•min•a•tive (kahr-min′ə-tiv) [L. *carminare* to card, to cleanse, from *carmen,* a card for wool] 1. relieving flatulence. 2. a medicine that relieves flatulence and assuages pain.

car•mine (kahr′min) a red coloring matter derived from cochineal by the addition of alum and used as a histologic stain.
  alizarin c. sodium alizarinsulfonate.
  indigo c. indigotindisulfonate sodium.
  lithium c. a vital stain for macrophages.
  Schneider c. a saturated solution of carmine in concentrated acetic acid.

car•min•ic ac•id (kahr-min′ik) an aromatic acid that is the essential constituent of the dye carmine.

car•min•o•phil (kahr-min′ə-fil) [*carmine* + *-phil*] 1. easily stainable with carmine. 2. a cell or other element that readily takes a stain from carmine. 3. lactotroph.

car•mus•tine (kahr-mus′tēn) a cytotoxic alkylating agent of the nitrosourea (q.v.) group, used as an antineoplastic primarily against brain tumors, multiple myeloma, colorectal carcinoma, and Hodgkin disease and non-Hodgkin lymphomas; administered intravenously. It is also implanted into the surgical resection cavity to prolong survival in patients with recurrent glioblastoma. Called also *BCNU.*

car•nas•si•al (kahr-nas′e-əl) 1. adapted for shearing and tearing. 2. carnassial tooth.

car•nau•ba (kahr-naw′bə) *Copernicia cerifera,* the source of carnauba wax.

Car•ne•gie stages (kahr′nə-ge) [*Carnegie* Institution in Washington, D.C., where the stages were developed from research done between 1913 and 1920] see under *stage.*

car•ne•ous (kahr′ne-əs) [L. *carneus,* from *caro* flesh] fleshy.

Car•nett sign (kahr-net′) [J.B. *Carnett,* American physician, 20th century] see under *sign.*

Car•ney complex (syndrome), triad (kahr′ne) [J. Aidan *Carney,* American pathologist, 20th century] see under *complex* and *triad.*

car•ni•fi•ca•tion (kahr″nĭ-fĭ-ka′shən) [L. *caro,* gen. *carnis* flesh + *facere* to make] the change of tissue, such as that of the lungs, into a fleshy substance.

car•ni•tine (kahr′nĭ-tēn) a betaine derivative found in skeletal muscle and liver; it is required for mitochondrial beta oxidation of fatty acids, carrying the acyl groups (fatty acids) across the mitochondrial membrane to the matrix, where they are transferred back to coenzyme A prior to oxidation. It has been used as an investigational antithyroid and antiangina agent. Deficiency of carnitine leads to buildup of fatty acids in the body.

car•ni•tine ac•yl•trans•fer•ase (kahr′nĭ-tēn a″səl-trans′fər-ās) carnitine *O*-palmitoyltransferase.

car•ni•tine *O*-pal•mi•to•yl•trans•fer•ase (kahr′nĭ-tēn pahl″mĭ-to″əl-trans′fər-ās) [EC 2.3.1.21] an enzyme of the transferase class that catalyzes the transfer between coenzyme A and carnitine of long chain fatty acids. *Carnitine palmitoyltransferase I* transfers the fatty acid to carnitine; the acyl carnitine can then traverse the inner mitochondrial membrane. Once in the matrix, the fatty acid is transferred from carnitine back to coenzyme A by *carnitine palmitoyltransferase II;* the resultant acyl coenzyme A is a substrate for oxidation. Deficiency of the enzyme is a cause of defective fatty acid oxidation. Written also *carnitine palmityltransferase.*

car•ni•tine pal•mi•toyl•trans•fer•ase de•fi•cien•cy (kahr′nĭ-tēn pahl″mĭ-toil-trans′fər-ās) metabolic disorders of long-chain fatty acid oxidation caused by mutations in the genes encoding carnitine palmitoyltransferase.
  c. p. I d. a rare autosomal recessive disorder caused by mutations in the *CPT1A* gene (locus: 11q13), which encodes carnitine palmitoyltransferase IA. It is characterized by severe episodes of hypoketotic hypoglycemia, hepatomegaly, and encephalopathy, usually occurring after fasting or illness; onset is in infancy or early childhood.
  c. p. II d. an autosomal recessive disorder caused by mutations in the *CPT2* gene (locus: 1p32), which encodes carnitine palmitoyltransferase II; it occurs in 3 forms. The *lethal neonatal* and *infantile* forms are characterized by nonketotic hypoglycemia, cardiac and liver anomalies, and early death. The *late-onset* or *adult-onset* form is the most common and is marked by rhabdomyolysis following prolonged exercise, fasting, or febrile illness.

Car•ni•tor (kahr′nĭ-tor) trademark for preparations of levocarnitine.

Car•niv•o•ra (kahr-niv′ə-rə) [L. *caro* flesh + *vorare* to devour] an order of mammals that eat primarily flesh and have teeth adapted for that purpose, as well as a simple stomach and a short intestine. Included are the dog family, the cat family, bears, walruses, raccoons, and numerous others.

car•ni•vore (kahr′nĭ-vor) a flesh-eating animal, especially a member of the order Carnivora.

car•niv•o•rous (kahr-niv′ə-rəs) eating or subsisting on flesh.

car•no•sin•ase (kahr′no-sĭ-nās″) X-His dipeptidase.
  serum c. deficiency an autosomal recessive aminoacidopathy of carnosine metabolism, due to deficiency of the serum isozyme of X-His dipeptidase; it is characterized by urinary excretion of carnosine and accumulation of homocarnosine in the cerebrospinal fluid and may cause myoclonic seizures, severe mental retardation, and spasticity. See also *homocarnosinosis.*

car•no•sine (kahr′no-sēn) a dipeptide composed of β-alanine and histidine, found in skeletal muscle and in the brain, particularly in the primary olfactory pathways; it may play a role as a neurotransmitter.

car•no•si•ne•mia (kahr″no-sĭ-ne′me-ə) 1. accumulation of carnosine in the blood. 2. a rare autosomal recessive disorder associated with mutation at gene locus 18q21.3, characterized by deficiency of carnosinase (X-His dipeptidase), elevated levels of carnosine in the blood and urine, and in most cases neurologic and intellectual deficits.

car•no•sin•u•ria (kahr″no-sĭ-nu′re-ə) urinary excretion of high levels of carnosine, such as occurs after ingestion of meat or fowl or in serum carnosinase deficiency.

car•nos•i•ty (kahr-nos′ĭ-te) [L. *carnositas* fleshiness] any abnormal fleshy excrescence.

car•ob (kar′əb) [Ar. *al kharrubah*] 1. *Ceratonia siliqua.* 2. the finely pulverized meal of the dried ripe fruit of *Ceratonia siliqua;* it contains albuminous proteins, carbohydrates, and small amounts of fat and crude fiber, and is used in pharmaceutical formulations as an adsorbent and demulcent in treatment of diarrhea. Called also *algaroba* or *algarroba, carob bean,* and *locust bean.*

Ca•ro•li disease (kah-ro-le′) [Jacques *Caroli,* French physician, 1902–1979] see under *disease.*

car•o•tene (kar′ə-tēn) [L. *carota* carrot] one of four isomeric pigments (α-, β-, γ-, and δ-carotene), having colors from violet to red-yellow to yellow, found in many dark green, leafy, and yellow vegetables, as well as yellow fruits. They are fat-soluble, unsaturated aliphatic hydrocarbons that are converted to vitamin A in animals by an enzyme in the intestinal wall and the liver. β-Carotene is the major precursor (provitamin) of vitamin A in humans, although it is less well absorbed than is retinol. See also *retinol equivalent,* under *equivalent.*
  beta c. 1. the β isomer of carotene (q.v.). 2. [USP] a preparation of β-carotene, administered orally to prevent vitamin A deficiency and to reduce the severity of photosensitivity in patients with erythropoietic protoporphyria. Written also *β-carotene* and *betacarotene.*

β-car•o•tene 15,15′-mono•oxy•gen•ase (kar′o-tēn mon″o-ok′sĭ-jən-ās) [EC 1.14.99.36] an enzyme of the oxidoreductase class that catalyzes the oxidative cleavage of β-carotene in the intestinal mucosa, forming two molecules of all-*trans* retinal in a reaction requiring bile salts and iron.

car•o•ten•emia (kar″ə-tə-ne′me-ə) hypercarotenemia.

ca•rot•e•no•der•mia (kə-rot″ə-no-dur′me-ə) carotenosis.

ca•rot•e•noid (kə-rot′ə-noid) 1. any group of pigments, yellow to deep red in color, chemically consisting of tetraterpene (polyisoprene) hydrocarbons. Carotenoids are synthesized by prokaryotes and higher plants, and they concentrate in animal fat when eaten (where they are called *lipochromes*). Examples are β-carotene, cryptoxanthin, lycopene, and xanthophyll. 2. marked by a yellow color.
  provitamin A c′s carotenoids, particularly the carotenes and cryptoxanthin, that can be converted to vitamin A in the body; they are a major source of vitamin A in a normal diet.

car•o•te•no•sis (kar″o-tə-no′sis) the yellow discoloration of the skin occurring in hypercarotenemia. The palms, soles, and area behind the ears are most heavily pigmented, while the sclerae remain white.

ca•rot•i•co•tym•pan•ic (kə-rot″ĭ-ko-tim-pan′ik) pertaining to the carotid canal and the tympanum.

ca•rot•i•co•ver•te•bral (kə-rot″ĭ-ko-vur′tə-brəl) pertaining to or affecting the carotid and vertebral arteries.

ca•rot•id (kə-rot′id) [Gr. *karōtis,* from *karos* deep sleep] pertaining to the principal artery of the neck (arteria carotis communis).

ca•rot•i•dyn•ia (kə-rot″ĭ-din′e-ə) [contracted form from *carotid* + *-odynia*] episodic, usually unilateral neck pain with tenderness along the course of the common carotid artery.

ca•rot•odyn•ia (kə-rot″o-din′e-ə) carotidynia.

carp (kahrp) [Gr. *karpos* fruit] a fruiting body of a fungus; see also *ascocarp* and *basidiocarp.*

car·pal (kahr′pəl) [L. *carpalis*] of or pertaining to the carpus, or wrist.

car·pec·to·my (kahr-pek′tə-me) [*carpus* + Gr. *ektomē* excision] excision of a carpal bone.

Car·pen·ter syndrome (kahr′pən-tər) [George *Carpenter*, British physician, 1859–1910] see under *syndrome*.

car·phol·o·gy (kahr-fol′ə-je) [Gr. *karphologein* to pick bits of wool off a person's coat] floccillation.

car·pi·tis (kahr-pi′tis) inflammation of the synovial membranes of the knee (carpal joint) of the horse, with swelling, pain, and lameness. Called also *popped knee*.

car·po·car·pal (kahr″po-kahr′pəl) pertaining to two parts of the carpus, especially to the articulations between carpal bones.

Car·po·gly·phus (kahr″po-gli′fəs) a genus of mites of the family Acaridae. Some species infest dried fruit and cause dermatitis in those who handle the fruit.

car·po·go·ni·um (kahr″po-go′ne-əm) 1. the female sex organ (ascogonium) of members of the order Erysiphales. 2. the female sex organ of any of various algae. 3. ascogonium.

car·po·meta·car·pal (kahr″po-met″ə-kahr′pəl) pertaining to the carpus and metacarpus.

car·po·ped·al (kahr″po-ped′əl) [*carpus* + *pedal*] pertaining to or affecting the carpus and the foot, or the hand and the foot; as carpopedal spasm.

car·po·pha·lan·ge·al (kahr″po-fə-lan′je-əl) pertaining to the carpus and the phalanges.

car·pop·to·sis (kahr″pop-to′sis, kahr″po-to′sis) [*carpus* + *-ptosis*] wristdrop.

Car·pue operation, rhinoplasty (kahr′pu) [Joseph Constantine *Carpue*, English surgeon, 1764–1846] Indian rhinoplasty.

car·pus (kahr′pəs) [L., from Gr. *karpos*] 1. [TA] wrist: the joint between the forearm and hand, made up of eight bones (see *ossa carpi*, under *os*). See also *articulatio radiocarpalis*. 2. the region of the hand between the forearm and metacarpus. 3. the part of the forelimb of a quadruped that corresponds to this part in the human; called also *knee* and *wrist*.
c. cur′vus Madelung deformity.

car·ra·geen (kar′ə-gēn) [Irish *carraigin* little rock] 1. *Chondrus crispus*. 2. chondrus (def. 2).

car·ra·gee·nan (kar″ə-ge′nən) [*Carragheen*, village in southeastern Ireland] [NF] a colloidal extractive derived from certain red marine algae, such as of the genera *Chondrus*, *Eucheuma*, and *Gigartina*, composed of a mixture of sodium, potassium, calcium, and magnesium salts of an acid sulfate of a galactose-containing polysaccharide. Used chiefly as a suspending agent in foods, pharmaceuticals, and cosmetics. Spelled also *carrageenin*, *carragheenan*, and *carragheenin*.

car·ra·gee·nin (kar″ə-gee′nən) carrageenan.

car·ra·gheen (kar′ə-gēn) 1. *Chondrus crispus*. 2. chondrus (def. 2).

car·ra·ghee·nan (kar″ə-gee′nən) carrageenan.

car·ra·ghee·nin (kar″ə-gee′nən) carrageenan.

car·ri·er (kar′e-ər) 1. an instrument or apparatus for carrying something. 2. an individual who harbors the specific organisms of a disease without manifest symptoms and is capable of transmitting the infection. 3. a chemical substance that can accept one or more electrons and then donate them to another substance (being reduced and then reoxidized). Called also *electron carrier*. 4. in genetics, an individual who is heterozygous for a recessive gene and thus does not express the recessive phenotype but can transmit it to offspring. In humans, only females can be carriers of X-linked recessive traits. 5. a substance that carries a radioisotopic or other label, as in a tracer study. A second isotope mixed with a particular isotope is also referred to as a carrier; see *carrier-free*. 6. a transport protein that attaches to and carries a specific substance, particularly one that transports the substance across the cell membrane. 7. in immunology, a macromolecular substance to which a hapten is coupled in order to produce an immune response against the hapten, immune responses being usually produced only against large molecules capable of simultaneously binding both B cells and helper T cells. Called also *Schlepper*.
amalgam c. an instrument for carrying freshly mixed amalgam to the prepared cavity.
electron c. carrier (def. 3).
foil c. see under *passer*.
gametocyte c. in malaria, a person who has just gametocytes of *Plasmodium* species in the blood and so is not symptomatic; when such an individual is bitten by an *Anopheles* mosquito, malaria is transmitted.
obligate c. an individual who is known to possess a particular mutant allele, usually based on pedigree examination, but who is not necessarily clinically affected.
paste c. lentulo.

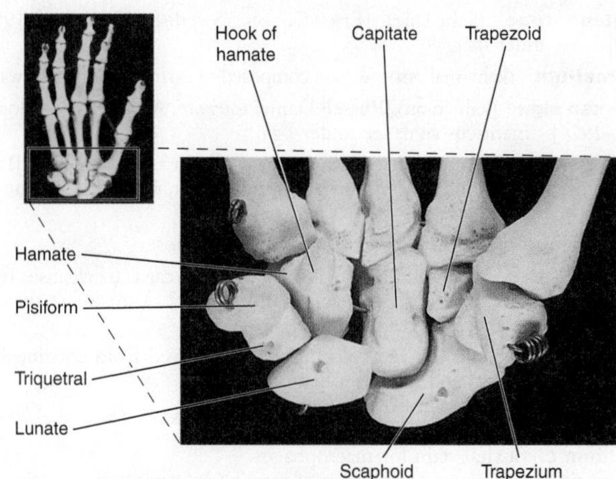

■ Carpus, viewed from the palmar aspect.

car·ri·er-free (kar′e-ər-fre′) a term denoting a radioisotope of an element in pure form, i.e., essentially undiluted with a stable isotope carrier.

Car·rión disease (kah-re-ōn′) [Daniel A. *Carrión*, 1850–1885, Peruvian physician who inoculated himself and died of the disease] bartonellosis (def. 2).

car·rot (kar′ət) [L. *carota*] 1. *Daucus carota*. 2. the orange or yellow root of *D. carota*, a food rich in vitamin A whose seed is diuretic and stimulant.

car·sick·ness (kahr′sik-nis) nausea and malaise produced by the motion of trains or automobiles or other vehicles. Written also *car sickness*.

cart (kahrt) a wheeled vehicle for conveying patients or equipment and supplies in a hospital.
crash c. resuscitation c.
dressing c. a cart containing all the supplies and equipment that may be necessary for changing dressings of surgical or injured patients.
resuscitation c. a cart containing all the equipment necessary for initiating emergency resuscitation.

car·te·o·lol hy·dro·chlo·ride (kahr′te-ə-lol) [USP] a beta-adrenergic blocking agent with intrinsic sympathetic activity, administered orally as an antihypertensive and applied topically to the conjunctiva in the treatment of glaucoma and ocular hypertension.

Car·tha·mus (kahr-tha′məs) a genus of herbs of the family Compositae, native to Europe and Asia, having brightly colored flowers. *C. tincto′rius* is the safflower, source of safflower oil.

car·ti·lage (kahr′tĭ-ləj) [L. *cartilago*] a specialized, fibrous connective tissue, forming most of the temporary skeleton of the embryo, providing a model in which most of the bones develop, and constituting an important part of the growth mechanism of the organism. It exists in several types, the most important of which are hyaline cartilage, elastic cartilage, and fibrocartilage. Also used as a general term to designate a mass of such tissue in a particular site in the body. See *cartilago*.

Cartilage

accessory c's of nose cartilagines nasi accessoriae.
c. of acoustic meatus cartilago meatus acustici.
alar c., major cartilago alaris major nasi.
alar c's, minor cartilagines alares minores nasi.
annular c. cartilago cricoidea.
aortic c. the second costal cartilage on the right side.
arthrodial c. articular c.
articular c. a thin layer of cartilage, usually hyaline, on the articular surface of bones in synovial joints. Called also *cartilago articularis* [TA], *arthrodial c.*, *diarthrodial c.*, *investing c.*, and *obducent c.*

Cartilage *Continued*

arytenoid c. cartilago arytenoidea.
c. of auditory tube cartilago tubae auditivae.
c. of auricle, auricular c. cartilago auricularis.
branchial c. pharyngeal c.
calcified c. cartilage in which granules of calcium phosphate and calcium carbonate have been deposited in the interstitial substance.
cariniform c. the cartilaginous prolongation at the anterior end of the sternum of a horse.
cellular c. cartilage composed almost entirely of cells, with little interstitial substance; called also *parenchymatous c.*
circumferential c. labrum glenoidale.
conchal c. the part of the auricular cartilage that is in the concha.
connecting c. cartilage connecting the surfaces of an immovable joint; called also *interosseous c.*
corniculate c. cartilago corniculata.
costal c. cartilago costalis.
costal c., interarticular ligamentum sternocostale intraarticulare.
cricoid c. cartilago cricoidea.
cuneiform c. cartilago cuneiformis.
dentinal c. the substance remaining after the lime salts of dentin have been dissolved in an acid.
diarthrodial c. articular c.
elastic c. a substance that is more opaque, flexible, and elastic than hyaline cartilage, and is further distinguished by its yellow color. The interstitial substance is penetrated in all directions by frequently branching fibers which give all the reactions for elastin. Called also *reticular c.* and *yellow c.*
ensiform c. processus xiphoideus.
epiglottic c. cartilago epiglottica.
epiphyseal c. cartilago epiphysialis.
eustachian c. cartilago tubae auditivae.
falciform c's see *meniscus lateralis articulationis genus* and *meniscus medialis articulationis genus.*
fibrous c. fibrocartilage.
first arch c., first pharyngeal arch c. Meckel c.
floating c. a detached piece of cartilage, usually from the articular surface of the medial condyle and femur, but also from the patella or lateral condyle of the femur.
gingival c. the tissue covering the loculus which contains an unerupted tooth.
hyaline c. a flexible, somewhat elastic, semitransparent substance with an opalescent bluish tint, composed of a basophilic, fibril-containing interstitial substance with cavities in which the chondrocytes occur; called also *chondroid.*
inferior c. of nose cartilago alaris major nasi.
innominate c. cartilago cricoidea.
interarticular c. 1. ligamentum longitudinale posterius. 2. an interarticular disk.
interarticular c. of little head of rib ligamentum capitis costae intraarticulare.
interosseous c. connecting c.
intervertebral c. discus intervertebralis.

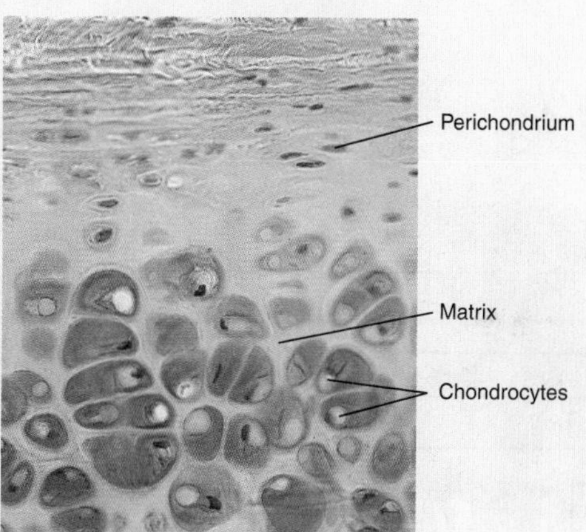

■ Hyaline cartilage, showing the chondrocytes in their lacunae and the surrounding matrix (light microscopy).

intrathyroid c. a cartilage connecting the alae of the thyroid cartilage in early life.
investing c. articular c.
Jacobson c. cartilago vomeronasalis.
laryngeal c's see *cartilagines et articulationes laryngis.*
lateral c's in the horse, the cartilages from the end of the third phalanx to the heel of the hoof.
lateral c. of nose cartilago nasi lateralis.
lower lateral c. cartilago alaris major nasi.
mandibular c. Meckel c.
meatal c. cartilago meatus acustici.
Meckel c. the cartilaginous bar (in the embryo) into which the mesenchymal core of the mandibular prominence of the first mandibular arch is converted; from it or its sheath, the sphenomandibular ligament, the anterior malleolar ligament, the malleus, and the incus develop. Called also *first arch c., mandibular c., tympanomandibular c.,* and *Meckel rod.*
nasal c's cartilagines nasi.
nasal c's, accessory cartilagines nasi accessoriae.
nasal c., inferior, nasal c., inferior lateral cartilago alaris major nasi.
nasal c., lateral cartilago nasi lateralis.
nasal c., lower lateral cartilago alaris major nasi.
nasal c., superior, nasal c., superior lateral cartilago nasi lateralis.
nasal c., upper lateral cartilago nasi lateralis.
c. of nasal septum cartilago septi nasi.
c's of nose cartilagines nasi.
obducent c. articular c.
ossifying c. temporary c.
parachordal c's the two cartilages at the sides of the occipital part of the notochord of the embryo.
parenchymatous c. cellular c.
periotic c. an oval mass on the upper surface of the fetal chondrocranium investing the internal ear.
permanent c. cartilage that does not normally become ossified.
pharyngeal c., pharyngeal arch c. one of the rods of cartilage in the mesenchyme of the pharyngeal arches of the embryo, from which the cartilaginous viscerocranium develops.
precursory c. temporary c.
pulmonary c. the third costal cartilage on the left side.
quadrilateral c. cartilago nasi lateralis.
Reichert c. cartilaginous bars in the lateral side of the embryonic tympanum from which develop the styloid processes, the stylohyoid ligaments, and the lesser horns of the hyoid bone. Called also *second arch c's.*
reticular c. elastic c.
Santorini c. cartilago corniculata.
second arch c's, second pharyngeal arch c's Reichert c.
semilunar c. of knee joint, external meniscus lateralis articulationis genus.
semilunar c. of knee joint, internal meniscus medialis articulationis genus.
septal c. of nose cartilago septi nasi.
sesamoid c. of cricopharyngeal ligament cartilago sesamoidea ligamenti cricopharyngei.
sesamoid c. of larynx cartilago sesamoidea ligamenti cricopharyngei.
sesamoid c's of nose cartilagines nasi accessoriae.
sigmoid c's see *meniscus lateralis articulationis genus* and *meniscus medialis articulationis genus.*
slipping rib c. loosening and deformity of the costal cartilages, causing painful symptoms.
sternal c. cartilago costalis.
stratified c. fibrocartilage.
subvomerine c. cartilago vomeronasalis.
supra-arytenoid c. cartilago corniculata.
temporary c. any cartilage that is being replaced by bone or that is normally destined to be replaced by bone; called also *ossifying c.* and *precursory c.*
tendon c. a form of embryonic cartilage by which tendons and bones are united.
thyroid c. cartilago thyroidea.
tip c. cartilago alaris major nasi.
tracheal c's cartilagines tracheales.
triangular c. of nose cartilago nasi lateralis.
triquetral c., triquetrous c. 1. cartilago arytenoidea. 2. discus articularis articulationis radioulnaris distalis.

Cartilage *Continued*

triradiate c. a secondary ossification center of the hip bone, occurring as a Y-shaped strip in the floor of the acetabulum.
triticeal c., triticeous c. cartilago triticea.
tubal c. cartilago tubae auditivae.
tympanomandibular c. Meckel c.
upper lateral c. cartilago nasi lateralis.
vomeronasal c. cartilago vomeronasalis.
Weitbrecht c. discus articularis articulationis acromioclavicularis.
Wrisberg c. cartilago cuneiformis.
xiphoid c. processus xiphoideus.
Y c. a Y-shaped cartilage in the acetabulum, joining the ilium, ischium, and pubes.
yellow c. elastic c.

car·ti·lag·i·nes (kahr″tĭ-laj′ĭ-nēz) [L.] plural of *cartilago.*

car·ti·la·gin·i·fi·ca·tion (kahr″tĭ-lə-jin′ĭ-fĭ-ka′shən) conversion into cartilage.

car·ti·la·gin·i·form (kahr″tĭ-lə-jin′ĭ-form) resembling cartilage; called also *cartilaginoid.*

car·ti·lag·i·noid (kahr″tĭ-laj′ĭ-noid) cartilaginiform.

car·ti·lag·i·nous (kahr″tĭ-laj′ĭ-nəs) consisting of or of the nature of cartilage.

car·ti·la·go (kahr″tĭ-lah′go) pl. *cartilag′ines* [L.] cartilage.

c. ala′ris ma′jor na′si [TA] major alar cartilage of nose: either of two thin, curved cartilages, one on either side at the apex of the nose, each of which possesses a lateral and a medial crus; called also *inferior cartilage of nose, inferior lateral* or *lower lateral nasal cartilage,* and *tip cartilage.*

cartila′gines ala′res mino′res na′si [TA] minor alar cartilages of nose: various small cartilages located in the fibrous tissue of the alae nasi posterior to a cartilago alaris major.

c. articula′ris articular cartilage: a thin layer of cartilage, usually hyaline, on the articular surface of bones in synovial joints; called also *arthrodial, diarthrodial, investing,* and *obducent cartilage.*

cartila′gines et articulatio′nes laryn′gis a general anatomical term grouping the various laryngeal cartilages together with the joints between them.

c. arytenoi′dea [TA] arytenoid cartilage: one of the paired, pitcher-shaped cartilages of the back of the larynx at the upper border of the cricoid cartilage; called also *triquetral* or *triquetrous cartilage.*

c. auri′culae [TA] auricular cartilage: the internal plate of elastic cartilage which is found in the external ear; called also *cartilage of auricle.*

c. cornicula′ta [TA] corniculate cartilage: a small nodule of cartilage at the apex of each arytenoid cartilage; called also *Santorini,* or *supra-arytenoid cartilage,* and *corniculum.*

c. costa′lis [TA] costal cartilage: a bar of hyaline cartilage by which the ventral extremity of a rib is attached to the sternum in the case of the true ribs, or to the superiorly adjacent ribs in the case of the upper false ribs; called also *sternal cartilage.*

c. cricoi′dea [TA] cricoid cartilage: a ringlike cartilage forming the lower and back part of the larynx; called also *annular* or *innominate cartilage.*

c. cuneifor′mis [TA] cuneiform cartilage: either of a pair of cartilages, one on the posterior border of each aryepiglottic fold; called also *Wrisberg cartilage.*

c. epiglot′tica [TA] epiglottic cartilage: the plate of cartilage that constitutes the central part of the epiglottis.

c. epiphysia′lis [TA] epiphyseal cartilage: the cartilage composing the epiphysis prior to ossification.

c. mea′tus acus′tici [TA] cartilage of acoustic meatus: the trough-shaped cartilage of the cartilaginous part of the external acoustic meatus; called also *meatal cartilage.*

cartila′gines na′si [TA] cartilages of nose: see *c. nasi lateralis, c. alaris major nasi, cartilagines alares minores nasi, c. septi nasi, c. vomeronasalis,* and *cartilagines nasi accessoriae.*

cartila′gines na′si accesso′riae [TA] accessory nasal cartilages: one or more small cartilages on either side of the nose between the greater alar and lateral nasal cartilages; called also *accessory* or *sesamoid cartilages of nose.*

c. na′si latera′lis lateral nasal cartilage: either of a pair of triangular cartilages extending laterally from the septal cartilages on either side of the nose, attached superiorly to the nasal bone and the frontal process of the maxilla. Called also *superior lateral* or *upper lateral nasal cartilage* and *triangular cartilage of nose.*

c. sep′ti na′si [TA] cartilage of nasal septum: the hyaline cartilage forming the framework of the cartilaginous part of the nasal septum, adjacent to and partly fused with the lateral nasal cartilages; called also *septal cartilage of nose* and *quadrilateral cartilage.*

c. sesamoi′dea ligamen′ti cricopharyn′gei [TA] sesamoid cartilage of cricopharyngeal ligament: a small cartilage occasionally found within the cricopharyngeal ligament.

c. thyroi′dea [TA] thyroid cartilage: the largest cartilage of the larynx, with two broad, posteriorly diverging laminae and two pairs of horns, superior and inferior, that extend from the posterior borders of the laminae.

cartila′gines trachea′les [TA] tracheal cartilages: the 16 to 20 incomplete rings which, held together and enclosed by a strong, elastic, fibrous membrane, constitute the wall of the trachea. Called also *annuli tracheae* and *tracheal rings.*

c. triti′cea [TA] triticeal cartilage: a small cartilage in the thyrohyoid ligament.

c. tu′bae auditi′vae [TA] cartilage of auditory tube: the cartilage on the inferomedial surface of the temporal bone that supports the walls of the cartilaginous portion of the auditory tube; called also *tubal* or *eustachian cartilage* and *c. tubae auditoriae* [TA alternative].

c. tu′bae audito′riae TA alternative for *c. tubae auditivae.*

c. vomeronasa′lis [TA] vomeronasal cartilage: either of the two narrow, longitudinal strips of cartilage, one lying on either side of the anterior portion of the lower margin of the septal cartilage; called also *Jacobson* or *subvomerine cartilage.*

Car·trol (kar′trol) trademark for a preparation of carteolol hydrochloride.

Cart·wright blood group (kahrt′rīt) [*Cartwright,* surname of the propositus first observed in 1956] Yt blood group.

ca·ru·bi·cin hy·dro·chlo·ride (kə-roo′bĭ-sin) an anthracycline antibiotic isolated from *Actinomadura carminata;* it has antineoplastic activity and has been used experimentally in the treatment of acute leukemias and some solid tumors.

Ca·ru·kia (kə-roo′ke-ə) a genus of jellyfish. *C. barne′si* Southcott is an Australian species whose sting causes Irukandji syndrome.

Ca·rum (kar′əm) a genus of plants of the family Umbelliferae. *C. car′vi* is caraway, a species native to Europe, the Middle East, and Central Asia; a source of caraway oil.

car·un·cle (kar′əng-kəl) caruncula.

hymenal c's carunculae hymenales.
lacrimal c. caruncula lacrimalis.
major c. of Santorini papilla duodeni major.
Morgagni c., morgagnian c. lobus medius prostatae.
sublingual c. caruncula sublingualis.
urethral c. a small, polypoid, sometimes painful deep red growth on the mucous membrane of the urinary meatus in women.

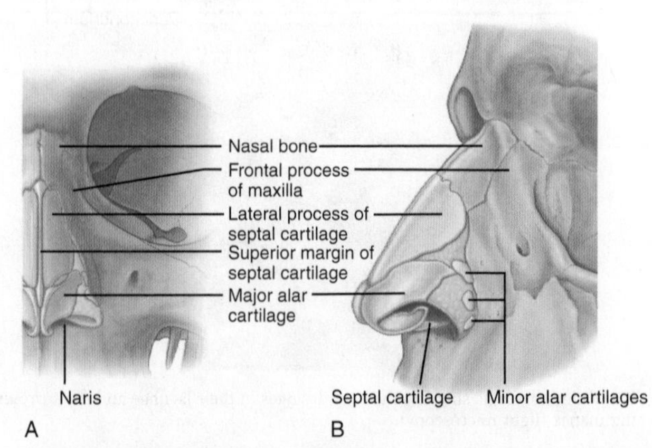

■ Cartilagines nasi (nasal cartilages). *(A),* Frontal view; *(B),* lateral view.

ca·run·cu·la (kə-rung′ku-lə) pl. *carun′culae* [L. dim. of *caro* flesh] caruncle: a small fleshy eminence, which may be normal or abnormal.

carun′culae hymena′les [TA] hymenal caruncles: small elevations of the mucous membrane encircling the vaginal orifice, being relics of the torn hymen; called also *carunculae myrtiformes.*

c. lacrima′lis [TA] lacrimal caruncle: the red eminence at the medial angle of the eye.

carun′culae myrtifor′mes carunculae hymenales.

c. sublingua′lis [TA] sublingual caruncle: an eminence on each side of the frenulum of the tongue, at the apex of which are the openings of the major sublingual duct and the submandibular duct.

Ca·rus curve (kah′rəs) [Karl Gustav *Carus,* German obstetrician, 1789–1869] see under *curve.*

Car·val·lo sign (kahr-vah′yo) [J.M. Rivero *Carvallo,* Mexican cardiologist, 20th century] see under *sign.*

car·ve·dil·ol (kahr′və-dil″ol) a beta-adrenergic blocking agent used in the treatment of essential hypertension and as an adjunct in the treatment of mild or moderate congestive heart failure; administered orally.

car·ver (kahr′vər) a knife or other instrument used for carving or fashioning an object by cutting, such as one used for shaping artificial teeth and dental restorations.

car·vone (kahr′vōn) a terpene ketone found in many volatile oils, such as caraway oil and spearmint oil.

cary(o)- for words beginning thus, see also words beginning *karyo-.*

caryo·chrome (kar′e-o-krōm″) karyochrome.

CASA computer-aided (or assisted) semen analysis.

Ca·sal necklace (collar) (kah-sahl′) [Gaspar *Casal,* Spanish physician, 1679–1759] see under *necklace.*

ca·san·thra·nol (kə-san′thrə-nol) [USP] a purified mixture of the anthranol glycosides derived from cascara sagrada; used as a laxative.

cas·ca·bel (kahs-kah-bel′) [Sp. "little round bell"] *Crotalus duris′sus terri′ficus,* a highly venomous rattlesnake found in South and Central America.

cas·cade (kas-kād′) a series of steps or stages (as of a physiological process) that once initiated continues to the final step by virtue of each step being triggered by the preceding one, sometimes with cumulative effect.

coagulation c. the series of steps beginning with activation of the intrinsic or extrinsic pathways of coagulation, or of one of the related alternative pathways, and proceeding through the common pathway of coagulation to the formation of the fibrin clot; each step involves zymogen activation, the activated zymogen catalyzing activation of the following step.

electron c. the electron transport chain (q.v.), emphasizing the passage of electrons from a large negative (reducing) potential to a positive (oxidizing) potential.

cas·ca·ra (kas-kah′rə) [Sp.] bark.

c. amar′ga [Sp. "bitter bark"] the bark of *Sweetia panamensis* Benth. (Leguminosae), a tree of tropical America; used as a bitter tonic.

c. sagra′da [Sp. "sacred bark"] [USP] the dried bark of *Rhamnus purshiana,* used as a cathartic; its laxative principles are glycosidal anthraquinones such as emodin and barbaloin. Called also *bearberry bark, bearwood, chittem bark, Purshiana bark,* and *sacred bark.*

case (kās) 1. a particular instance of disease, as a *case* of leukemia; sometimes used incorrectly to designate the patient with the disease. 2. a term sometimes used incorrectly in dentistry to designate a flask, denture, casting, or the like.

borderline c. an instance of a disease in which the symptoms resemble those of a recognized condition but are not typical of it.

index c. 1. the first case observed in a family or other defined group, which provides the stimulus for a genetic study; the affected individual is called the propositus. 2. in epidemiology of contagious disease, the first case of a disease, as opposed to subsequent cases.

trial c. a box containing convex and concave spherical, and convex and concave cylindrical lenses, arranged in pairs, a trial spectacle frame, and various other devices used in testing vision.

ca·se·a·tion (ka″se-a′shən) [L. *caseus* cheese] 1. the precipitation of casein. 2. necrosis in which the tissue becomes a soft, dry, crumbly mass resembling cheese, usually caused by mycobacterial infection. Called also *caseous* or *cheesy necrosis.*

case his·to·ry (kās′ his′tə-re) the collected data concerning an individual, his family, and environment, including his medical history and any other information that may be useful in analyzing and diagnosing his condition or for instructional purposes.

ca·sein (ka′sēn) [L. *caseus* cheese] a phosphoprotein, the principal protein of milk, the basis of curd and of cheese. It is precipitated from milk as a white amorphous substance by dilute acids, and redissolves on the addition of alkalis or of excess acid. Rennin (and other milk-clotting enzymes) influence the hydrolysis of casein to soluble paracasein, which in the presence of calcium (Ca^{2+}) is converted to an insoluble curd (insoluble paracasein or calcium paracaseinate). Casein, usually in the form of its calcium, potassium, or sodium salts, is added to other ingredients of the diet to increase its protein content. NOTE: In British nomenclature, casein is called *caseinogen,* and paracasein is called *casein.*

ca·sei·nate (ka′se-ə-nāt″, ka-se′nāt) 1. any salt of casein. 2. a combination of casein and a metal.

ca·sein·o·gen (ka-sēn′o-jen) [*casein* + *-gen*] the British term for casein.

ca·sein·og·e·nate (ka″se-noj′ə-nāt) a salt of caseinogen.

ca·se·og·e·nous (ka″se-oj′ə-nəs) producing caseation; conversion into cheese (casein).

ca·se·ous (ka′se-əs) resembling cheese or curd; cheesy.

ca·se·um (ka′se-əm) [L. "cheese"] cellular debris of a cheeselike consistency, produced as a result of caseation.

case·worm (kās′wərm) echinococcus.

cash·ew (kash′oo) 1. *Anacardium occidentale.* 2. the nut of this tree, used for food.

Cas·o·dex (kas′o-deks) trademark for a preparation of bicalutamide.

Ca·so·ni intradermal test (reaction) (kə-so′ne) [Tommaso *Casoni,* Italian physician, 1880–1933] see under *test.*

cas·pase (kas′pās) any of a group of cysteine endopeptidases that cleave proteins on the C-terminal side of aspartic acid residues as one of the final steps in apoptosis.

cas·po·fun·gin ac·e·tate (kas″po-fun′jin) an antifungal agent of the echinocandin class, acting by inhibiting the synthesis of a component of the cell wall of filamentous fungi; used in the treatment of invasive aspergillosis, administered intravenously.

cas·sa·va (kə-sah′və) [Sp., from Taino *casavi*] 1. a shrub of the genus *Manihot,* especially *M. esculenta.* 2. a starchy substance from the root of *Manihot,* used in many tropical regions in soups, breads, tapioca, and other foods, as well as in glue. The root contains hydrogen cyanide, which is removed during processing; if eaten raw, it causes cyanide poisoning. Called also *manioc.*

Cas·sel·ber·ry position (kas′əl-ber″e) [William Evans *Casselberry,* American laryngologist, 1858–1916] see under *position.*

Cas·ser fontanelle, ligament, muscle (kah′sər) [Giulio *Casserio* (L. *Casserius*), Italian anatomist, c. 1552–1616] see under *fontanelle, ligament,* and *muscle.*

cas·se·ri·an (kə-se′re-ən) named for Giulio *Casserio,* as *casserian fontanelle.*

cas·sette (kə-set′) [Fr. "a little box"] 1. a flat case for film or magnetic tape. 2. x-ray c.

x-ray c. a lightproof housing for x-ray film, containing front and back intensifying screens between which the film is placed; it is usually backed with lead to prevent backscatter.

Cas·sia (kash′e-ə) [L., from Gr. *kasia*] the sennas, a genus of tropical trees, shrubs, and herbs of the family Leguminosae.

C. acutifo′lia Del., a species native to Africa and cultivated in India that is the source of Alexandria senna; see *senna.*

C. angustifo′lia Vahl., a species native to Arabia that is the source of India or Tinnevelly senna; see *senna.*

C. obtusifo′lia *C. occidentalis.*

C. occidenta′lis coffee senna, a species whose seeds are often found as a contaminant in feed corn or soybeans; when eaten in excess by domestic animals, they cause muscle degeneration that can lead to fatal cardiomyopathy.

cast (kast) 1. a solid reproduction of an enclosed space such as a hollow organ (e.g., a renal tubule or bronchiole), formed of effused proteinaceous matter and extruded from the body. 2. an accurate reproduction of an object or part, made of plastic that has taken form in an impression or mold. 3. to form an object in a mold. 4. a rigid dressing, molded to the body while pliable, and hardening as it dries, to give firm support. 5. a positive reproduction of all or part of the maxillary or mandibular arch, made from an impression. Called also *model* and *dental c.* 6. strabismus.

bacterial c. a urinary cast that contains bacteria.

bilirubin c. a cast containing bilirubin, giving it a yellow-brown color, as seen with obstructive jaundice.

blood c. a urinary cast that contains blood cells; see *red blood cell c.* and *white blood cell c.*

bronchial c. a cylindrical solid or semisolid plug that blocks a bronchus and is sometimes expectorated.

decidual c. the mass of degenerating or necrotic decidua discharged from the uterus at the time of rupture of an ectopic pregnancy.

dental c. cast (def. 5).

diagnostic c. a dental cast of the maxillary and/or mandibular arches, usually made from gypsum, and used for study and treatment planning. Called also *preextraction c., preoperative c.,* and *study c.*

epithelial c. a urinary cast made up of cells of the epithelium of the tubules.

erythrocyte c. red blood cell c.

false c. pseudocast.

fatty c. a urinary cast made up of material loaded with fat globules derived from renal tubule cells, indicating tubular damage such as from the nephrotic syndrome.

fibrinous c. a urinary cast resembling a waxy cast, but having a darker yellow color, as seen in some types of nephritis.

gnathostatic c. a dental cast that has been trimmed so that the occlusal plane is in its normal position in the mouth when the cast is set on a plane surface; used in orthodontic diagnosis.

granular c. a dark colored urinary cast of a granular or cell-like substance, seen in a variety of renal diseases.

hair c. a small tubular structure on a hair shaft, white, shiny, and freely movable, usually near the scalp surface, formed by retention and desquamation of segments of the internal root sheath. Hair casts are sometimes mistaken for nits.

hanging c. a cast applied to the upper limb in fracture of the shaft of the humerus and suspended by a sling looped around the neck.

hemoglobin c. a granular cast that contains hemoglobin, such as in tubular bleeding or glomerulopathy.

hyaline c. a nearly transparent, slightly refractory urinary cast made up of homogeneous mucoprotein, seen transiently during exercise, fever, congestive heart failure, and diuretic therapy, and more continuously in some kidney diseases.

investment c. refractory c.

leukocyte c. white blood cell c.

master c. a facsimile of oral structures, including the prepared tooth surfaces, residual ridge areas, and/or other parts of the dental arch, reproduced from an impression from which a prosthesis is to be fabricated.

myeloma c. a urinary cast containing Bence Jones protein and desquamated cells of the tubular epithelium, seen with multiple myeloma in the condition known as myeloma kidney.

preextraction c., preoperative c. diagnostic c.

red blood cell c., red cell c. a hyaline cast that contains red blood cells, signifying bleeding in the renal glomerulus, such as occurs in glomerulonephritis.

refractory c. a dental cast made of heat-resistant materials that will withstand high temperatures without disintegrating and that, when used in partial denture casting, has expansion to compensate for metal shrinkage. Called also *investment c.*

renal c. urinary c.

study c. diagnostic c.

urinary c. a cast formed from gelled protein precipitated in the renal tubules and molded to the tubular lumen; pieces of these casts break off and are washed out with the urine. There are various different types, including *granular, hyaline, waxy,* and *epithelial.* Called also *renal c.* and *urinary cylinder.*

waxy c. a urinary cast made up of highly refractive, translucent, proteinaceous material, seen with chronic renal failure, graft rejection, and other advanced renal diseases.

white blood cell c., white cell c. a hyaline cast that contains white blood cells, such as in tubulointerstitial nephritis, pyelonephritis, or glomerulonephritis. Called also *leukocyte c.*

Cas·ta·nea (kas-ta′ne-ə) [L., from Gr. *kastanea*] the chestnuts, a genus of trees of the family Fagaceae. *C. denta′ta* (Marsh.) Borkh. is the American chestnut, which has an edible nut. Its wood and leaves contain tannin, and it has been used as an astringent and in pertussis. Its leaves and buds may be poisonous to livestock if consumed in large quantities.

Cas·tel·la·ni bronchitis (disease), paint (kahs-tə-lah′nē) [Marquis Aldo *Castellani,* Italian physican, 1879–1971] see *bronchospirochetosis,* and see under *paint.*

Cas·tel·la·ni-Low symptom (kahs-tə-lah′ne lo′) [A. *Castellani;* George Carmichael *Low,* British physician, 1872–1952] see under *symptom.*

cast·ing (kast′ing) 1. any object formed by the solidification of plastic material, such as a gypsum product or molten metal, poured into an impression or mold. 2. the act of forming such an object, e.g., the fabrication of a metallic dental restoration or appliance. 3. a metallic dental restoration or appliance fabricated by this process. 4. a metallic dental restoration made to fit a cavity preparation and retained to or luted into it with a cementing medium.

centrifugal c. the use of centrifugal force to cause a plastic material to flow into an impression or mold, a process commonly used in dental casting.

vacuum c. the pouring of plastic material into an impression or mold, under conditions of lowered atmospheric pressure; the end of the mold distal to the sprue is subjected to a vacuum, allowing atmospheric pressure to force the casting material into the mold.

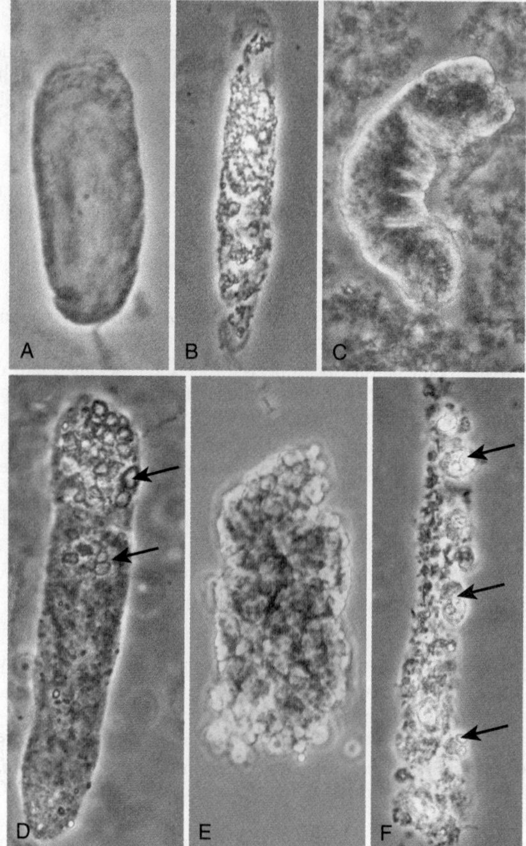

■ Urinary casts (phase contrast microscopy). *(A),* Hyaline cast; *(B),* hyaline-granular cast; *(C),* waxy cast; *(D),* erythrocyte cast, with erythrocytes *(arrows)* embedded in cast matrix; *(E),* hemoglobin cast; *(F),* leukocyte cast, showing large nuclei *(arrows)* characteristic of polymorphonuclear leukocytes.

Cas·tle factor (intrinsic factor) (kas′əl) [William Bosworth *Castle,* American physician, 1897–1990] intrinsic factor.

Cas·tle·man disease (kas′əl-mən) [Benjamin *Castleman,* American pathologist, 1906–1982] see under *disease.*

cas·trate (kas′trāt) 1. to deprive of the gonads, rendering the individual incapable of reproduction. Called *geld* for male horses, *emasculate* for any male, *spay* for female animals, and *oophorectomize* (if bilateral) for any female. Called also *neuter* (in veterinary medicine). 2. an individual that has been castrated, such as a *eunuch* (human being), or an *ox* or *gelding* (farm animals).

cas·tra·tion (kas-tra′shən) [L. *castratio*] 1. removal of the gonads; bilateral orchiectomy or bilateral oophorectomy. 2. destruction of the gonads, as by radiation.

female c. bilateral oophorectomy.

male c. bilateral orchiectomy; called also *emasculation.*

ca·su·al·ty (kazh′oo-əl-te) 1. an accident; an accidental wound; death or disablement from an accident; also the person so injured or killed. 2. in the armed forces, one missing from his unit as a result of death, injury, illness, capture, because his whereabouts are unknown, or other reasons.

cas·u·is·tics (kazh″u-is′tiks) the recording and study of cases of disease.

CAT computerized axial tomography.

cat (kat) any member of the family Felidae (lions, leopards, wildcats, etc.), especially the domesticated cat, *Felis catus.*

cata- [Gr. *kata* down] a prefix signifying down, lower, under, against, along with, very; see also words beginning *kata-*.

cata·ba·si·al (kat″ə-ba′zhəl) [*cata-* + *basial*] having the basion lower than the opisthion; said of certain skulls.

cata·bi·ot·ic (kat″ə-bi-ot′ik) dissipated or used up in the performance of function; said of the energy obtained from food.

ca·tab·o·lism (kə-tab′o-liz-əm) [Gr. *katabolē* a throwing down] any destructive metabolic process by which organisms convert substances into excreted compounds. **catabol′ic** *adj* antibody c. the rapid degradation (shortened half-life) of foreign gamma globulin in the body.

ca•tab•o•lite (kə-tab′o-līt) any product of catabolism.

ca•tab•o•lize (kə-tab′o-līz) to subject to catabolism; to undergo catabolism.

cata•crot•ic (kat″ə-krot′ik) 1. pertaining to the descending limb of a pulse tracing. 2. characterized by a notch (i.e., having two waveforms) in the descending limb of a pulse tracing.

ca•tac•ro•tism (kə-tak′ro-tiz-əm) [*cata-* + Gr. *krotos* beat] an anomaly of the pulse evidenced by appearance of a small additional wave or notch in the descending limb of the pulse tracing.

cata•di•crot•ic (kat″ə-di-krot′ik) on a pulse tracing, having two waveforms on the descending limb; see under *pulse.*

cata•di•cro•tism (kat″ə-di′kro-tiz-əm) [*cata-* + *di-* + *krotos* beat] presence of a catadicrotic pulse.

cata•did•y•mus (kat″ə-did′ĭ-məs) katadidymus.

cata•di•op•tric (kat″ə-di-op′trik) deflecting and reflecting light at the same time.

Cat•a•flam (kat′ə-flam) trademark for a preparation of diclofenac potassium.

cat•a•gen (kat′ə-jən) the brief second portion of the hair cycle in which growth (anagen) stops and resting (telogen) starts.

cat•a•lase (kat′ə-lās) [EC 1.11.1.6] a hemoprotein enzyme of the oxidoreductase class that catalyzes the conversion of hydrogen peroxide to water and oxygen, protecting cells. It is found in almost all animal cells except certain obligate anaerobic bacteria. Deficiency of the enzyme, an autosomal recessive trait, results in acatalasia. **catalat′ic** *adj*

cat•a•lep•sy (kat′ə-lep″se) [Gr. *katalēpsis*] indefinitely prolonged maintenance of a fixed body posture; seen in severe cases of catatonic schizophrenia. The term is sometimes used to denote *cerea flexibilitas.*

cat•a•lep•tic (kat″ə-lep′tik) 1. pertaining to, characterized by, or inducing catalepsy. 2. a person affected with catalepsy.

cat•a•lep•toid (kat″ə-lep′toid) resembling catalepsy.

ca•tal•y•sis (kə-tal′ə-sis) [Gr. *katalysis* dissolution] increase in the velocity of a chemical reaction or process produced by the presence of a substance that is not consumed in the net chemical reaction or process; *negative catalysis* denotes the slowing down or inhibition of a reaction or process by the presence of such a substance.

contact c., heterogeneous c. catalysis produced by the adsorbing power of contact surfaces; e.g., catalysis caused by colloidal platinum.

surface c. catalysis in which the reacting substances are adsorbed onto the surface of the catalyst and there react. Cf. *contact c.*

cat•a•lyst (kat′ə-list) any substance that brings about catalysis; called also *accelerant.*

negative c. a catalyst that retards the velocity of a reaction.

cat•a•lyt•ic (kat″ə-lit′ik) [Gr. *katalyein* to dissolve] causing or pertaining to an alterative effect; causing catalysis.

cat•a•ly•za•tor (kat″ə-lə-za′tər) catalyst.

cat•a•lyze (kat′ə-līz) to cause or produce catalysis.

cat•a•lyz•er (kat′ə-līz″ər) catalyst.

cat•a•me•ni•al (kat″ə-me′ne-əl) menstrual.

cat•am•ne•sis (kat″am-ne′sis) 1. the follow-up medical or psychiatric history of a patient after discharge from treatment or a hospital. 2. the history of a patient after the onset of medical or mental illness. **catamnes′tic** *adj*

cat•a•pasm (kat′ə-paz″əm) [Gr. *katapasma*] a dusting powder applied to an injured surface.

cata•pha•sia (kat″ə-fa′zhə) [*cata-* + *-phasia*] verbigeration.

cata•pho•re•sis (kat″ə-fə-re′sis) [*cata-* + *-phoresis*] the passage of charged particles toward the negative pole (cathode) in electrophoresis. **cataphoret′ic, cataphor′ic** *adj*

cata•pho•ria (kat″ə-for′e-ə) [*cata-* + Gr. *pherein* to bear] a type of heterophoria consisting of permanent downward turning of the visual axes of both eyes after the visual fusional stimuli have been eliminated.

cata•phy•lax•is (kat″ə-fə-lak′sis) [*cata-* + *phylaxis*] a breaking down of the body's natural defense to infection.

cat•a•plasm (kat′ə-plaz″əm) [L. *cataplasma;* Gr. *kataplasma*] a poultice or soft external application, often medicated.

kaolin c. a poultice prepared with kaolin, boric acid, and glycerin.

cat•a•plec•tic (kat″ə-plek′tik) 1. pertaining to or characterized by cataplexy. 2. coming on suddenly and overwhelmingly.

cat•a•plex•is (kat′ə-plek″sis) [Gr.] cataplexy.

cat•a•plexy (kat′ə-plek″se) a condition in which there are abrupt attacks of muscular weakness and hypotonia triggered by an emotional stimulus such as mirth, anger, fear, or surprise. It is often associated with narcolepsy.

Cat•a•pres (kat′ə-pres) trademark for preparations of clonidine hydrochloride.

cat•a•ract (kat′ə-rakt) [L. *cataracta,* from Gr. *katarraktēs* waterfall, portcullis (perhaps because an ocular opacity and a portcullis are obstructions)] a partial or complete opacity on or in the lens of the eye or its capsule, especially one impairing vision or causing blindness. Cataracts are classified by their morphology (size, shape, location) or etiology (cause or time of occurrence).

Cataract

after-c. a recurrent capsular cataract consisting of a membrane in the pupillary area after cataract removal.

age-related c. senile c.

aminoaciduria c. capsular thickening occurring in aminoaciduria, homocystinuria, and oculocerebrorenal syndrome.

atopic c. cataract sometimes occurring in the third decade or later in those with longstanding atopic dermatitis.

axial fusiform c. anterior and posterior polar cataracts joined with threadlike opacities extending axially through the lens; called also *spindle c.*

black c. a black or dark-colored opacity in the lens, occurring as part of a senile nuclear sclerotic cataract.

blue c., blue dot c. 1. a small, round developmental opacity that appears white, brown, or blue; it is common in the periphery of the cortex and occasionally moves into the axial zone of the lens; it rarely affects vision. Called also *cerulean c., punctate c.,* and *cataracta caerulea.* 2. coronary c.

brown c., brunescent c. a senile cataract in which the opacity is brown.

calcareous c. dystrophic calcium salt deposits in the subcapsular and cortical areas of the lens.

capsular c. capsular thickening occurring in heat cataracts and oculocerebrorenal syndrome.

cerulean c. 1. blue c. 2. coronary c.

complete c. total c.

complicated c. secondary c.

congenital c. 1. any of various usually bilateral opacities present at birth; they may be mild or severe and may or may not impair vision, depending upon their size, location, and density. Some have a hereditary, usually autosomal dominant cause; others result from intrauterine infection, drug-induced toxicity, ionizing radiation, trauma, prematurity, or chromosomal, endocrine, metabolic, or systemic disorders; and a sizable percentage are of unknown cause. Congenital cataracts are often associated with low birth weight, central nervous system abnormalities, mental retardation, convulsions, and cerebral palsy. 2. developmental c.

contusion c. a cataract due to shock or to injury of the eyeball.

coralliform c. a developmental, sutural opacity radiating axially forward and outward from the lens and ending in ampullae behind the capsule.

coronary c. 1. a white punctate or flakelike opacity around the periphery of the lens, forming a ring or crown. Coronary cataracts are transmitted by dominant inheritance and may be present in 25 per cent of the general population. 2. blue c.

cortical c. 1. developmental punctate opacity, white or light blue in color, commonly found in the cortex of the lens; this is present in most lenses and there are multiple ones as a person ages, but they rarely affect vision. 2. the most common type of senile cataract, consisting of white, wedgelike opacities distributed like spokes around the periphery of the cortex.

cuneiform c. cortical c. (def. 2).

Cataract *Continued*

cupuliform c. a posterior subcapsular cortical opacity seen as brown, saucer-shaped granules or cysts. It is centrally located and therefore seriously impairs vision very quickly. Cupuliform cataracts occur between the ages of 60 and 80, but earlier appearance may be an inherited trait.
dermatogenic c. syndermatotic c.
developmental c. a small, common opacity occurring in youth as a result of a congenitally caused defect such as heredity, malnutrition, toxicity, or inflammation. The number of developmental cataracts increases with age, but they rarely impair vision. Called also *evolutionary c.*
diabetic c. a rare, usually bilateral, opacity shaped like a snowflake, affecting the anterior and posterior cortices of young diabetics. Sometimes it can be reversed when the blood glucose is brought under control, but in most cases it progresses rapidly to a mature cataract.
duplication c. a disk-shaped cortical opacity forming in layers under capsular cataracts with clear zones between the layers.
electric c. a cataract occurring after an electric shock, especially to the head. Anterior subcapsular cataracts may form and develop within days after a severe shock; slowly developing or stationary opacities may follow a shock not on the head.
embryonal nuclear c. an opacity confined to the embryonic nucleus of the lens. It is an autosomal dominant trait, is often bilateral, has a powdery appearance, and seldom affects vision. Called also *cataracta centralis pulverulenta.*
embryopathic c. a congenital opacity caused by intrauterine infection, e.g., rubella, syphilis, or toxoplasmosis.
evolutionary c. developmental c.
galactosemic c. a cataract commonly observed in infants with galactosemia. The opacities look like oil droplets, are bilateral, and are zonular or nuclear.
glassblowers' c. heat c.
glaucomatous c. a patchy anterior subcapsular opacity following an attack of acute glaucoma; called also *glaukomflecken.*
heat c. posterior subcapsular opacity caused by chronic exposure to infrared radiation.
heterochromic c. a secondary, posterior cortical cataract symptomatic of heterochromic cyclitis; failing vision is often the first symptom.
hypermature c. a cataract with a swollen, milky cortex, the result of autolysis of the lens fibers of a mature cataract.
hypocalcemic c. punctate, sometimes cerulean, opacities, initially subcapsular, becoming lamellar, occurring with infantile tetany, hypoparathyroidism, or rickets.
immature c., incipient c. an incomplete cataract; the lens is only slightly opaque and the cortex clear.
intumescent c. a mature cataract that progresses; the lens becomes swollen from the osmotic effect of degenerated lens protein, and this may lead to secondary angle closure (acute) glaucoma.
juvenile c. a cataract in a child under nine years old; such cataracts are usually congenital or traumatic.
lamellar c. a concentric opacity, broad or narrow, usually consisting of powdery white dots, affecting one lamella or zonule of an otherwise clear lens. This is the most common type of congenital cataract, and causes include hypocalcemia, hypoglycemia, galactosemia, and rubella. Called also *zonular c.*
mature c. a cataract that produces swelling and opacity of the entire lens. Most cataracts are removed before maturity.

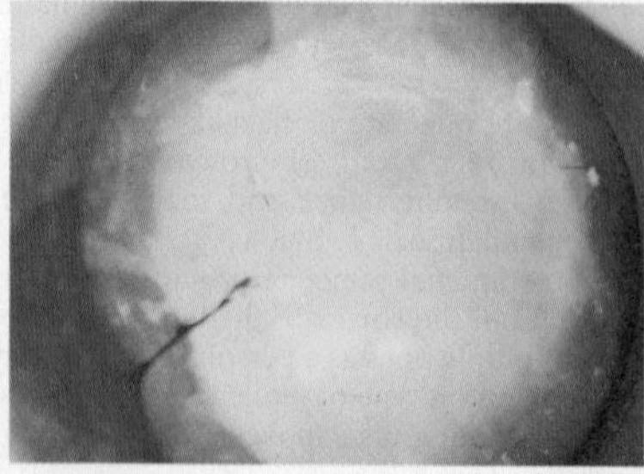

■ Total cataract, with no view of the red reflex or retina.

membranous c. a cataract formed of a collapsed, flattened capsule with little or no cortex or epithelium.
metabolic c. an opacity due to an endocrine or biochemical disorder.
morgagnian c. a mature cataract in which most of the cortex has become opaque and liquefied, so that the nucleus moves freely within the lens.
nuclear c. 1. embryonal nuclear c. 2. senile nuclear sclerotic c.
nutritional deficiency c. subcapsular opacity observed in patients with anorexia nervosa and in alcoholics.
overripe c. hypermature c.
polar c. a type of capsular cataract, usually disk-shaped; those in anterior locations are more common, and those in posterior locations reduce visual acuity more often.
postinflammatory c. a secondary cataract due to inflammation.
c's of prematurity clusters of vacuoles of unknown cause in the Y-shaped sutures of the lens in a premature infant; the condition usually disappears spontaneously within a month.
presenile c. a subcapsular senile cataract in a person under 40.
primary c. a cataract that develops independently of any other disease.
punctate c. 1. blue c. 2. coronary c.
pyramidal c. a conoid anterior polar cataract with its apex pointing forward.
radiation c. a subcapsular opacity caused by ionizing radiation such as x-rays, gamma rays, and neutrons, and by nonionizing radiation such as infrared rays (heat rays), ultraviolet rays, microwaves, and laser radiation.
ringform congenital c. a very rare opacity in which the nucleus of the lens is absent, and only a doughnut-shaped remnant of lens is left.
ripe c. mature c.
rubella c. a congenital nuclear cataract caused by maternal rubella during the first trimester of pregnancy.
secondary c. a cataract, usually posterior subcapsular, secondary to some other condition, such as disease (especially iridocyclitis), degeneration (such as chronic glaucoma or retinal detachment), or surgery (particularly glaucoma filtering or retinal reattachment). Called also *complicated c.*
senile c. the most common kind of cataract, painless and of unknown cause, developing without any traumatic, ocular, systemic, or congenital disorder. Senile cataracts are associated solely with aging, some degree of cataract being normal in persons over 50. Most form in the cortical area of the lens, but some form in the nuclear area and a few in the subcapsular area.
senile nuclear sclerotic c. an increasing hardening of the nucleus of the lens, with the opacity appearing brown or black and the lens becoming inelastic and unable to accommodate; the opacity is usually bilateral, begins between ages 50 and 60, and progresses slowly.
snowflake c., snowstorm c. the most common type of diabetic cataract, having the appearance of gray to bluish-white flaky opacities.
Soemmering ring c. see under *ring.*
spindle c. axial fusiform c.
subcapsular c. an opacity beneath the anterior or posterior lens capsule.
sunflower c. a brightly colored, usually red anterior capsular opacity with a sunflower pattern that occurs in patients with Wilson disease and hypercupremia; it has little effect on vision and clears after treatment with penicillamine.
supranuclear c. an opacity in the deep cortex of the lens, just above the nucleus.
sutural c. a congenital opacity of the lens affecting the Y-shaped sutures of the fetal membrane; it usually does not affect vision.
syndermatotic c. an inherited, usually bilateral opacity associated with cutaneous disease and occurring in youth; called also *dermatogenic c.*
thermal c. heat c.
total c. an opacity of all the fibers of the lens; called also *complete c.*
toxic c. an opacity caused by exposure to a drug or other toxic substance, such as a miotic, antimiotic, corticosteroid, metal, nitro compound, or substituted hydrocarbon.
traumatic c. a cataract resulting from injury to the eye, either immediately after injury (e.g., from perforation of the capsule) or years later (e.g., from concussion of the lens without a rupture of the capsule).
zonular c. lamellar c.

cat•a•rac•ta (kat″ə-rak′tə) [L.] cataract.
c. brunes′cens brown cataract.
c. caeru′lea blue cataract.
c. centra′lis pulverulen′ta embryonal nuclear cataract.
c. complica′ta secondary cataract.
c. ni′gra black cataract.

cat•a•rac•to•gen•e•sis (kat″ə-rak″to-jen′ə-sis) formation of a cataract.

cat•a•rac•to•gen•ic (kat″ə-rak″to-jen′ik) tending to cause formation of cataracts.

cat•a•rac•tous (kat″ə-rak′təs) of the nature of or affected with cataract.

ca•ta•ria (kə-tar′e-ə) [L. "catnip"] the leaves and tops of *Nepeta cataria* (catnip); used as a carminative and mild nerve stimulant.

ca•tarrh (kə-tahr′) [L. *catarrhus,* from Gr. *katarrhein* to flow down] inflammation of a mucous membrane, especially in the air passages of the head and throat, with a free discharge of mucus. catar′rhal *adj*
bovine malignant c. malignant catarrhal fever.
malignant c. of cattle, malignant head c. malignant catarrhal fever.
postnasal c. chronic rhinopharyngitis.
sinus c. a disorder of the lymph nodes characterized by dilatation of the sinuses accompanied by some proliferation of the littoral cells, which become swollen and detach themselves from the wall of the sinuses to lie free in the lumen.
vernal c. see under *conjunctivitis.*

cat•ar•rhine (kat′ə-rīn) [*cata-* + Gr. *rhis* nose] having nostrils that are close together and directed downward; said of certain primates, including humans. See *Cercopithecoidea.*

cat•a•stal•tic (kat″ə-stal′tik) [Gr. *katastaltikos*] 1. inhibitory; restraining. 2. an agent that tends to restrain or check any process.

ca•tas•tro•phiz•ing (kə-tas′trə-fi″zing) a maladaptive reaction to a negative or anxiety-producing situation, characterized by exaggeration of the negative response to the point that negative feelings far out of proportion to the situation are produced or a disastrous outcome is unreasonably expected.

cata•ther•mom•e•ter (kat″ə-thər-mom′ə-tər) katathermometer.

cata•thy•mia (kat″ə-thi′me-ə) the existence in the unconscious of elements sufficiently affect-laden to produce effects in consciousness. catathy′mic *adj*

cata•to•nia (kat″ə-to′ne-ə) [*cata-* + *ton-* + *-ia*] a wide group of motor abnormalities, most involving extreme under- or overactivity, occurring primarily in catatonic schizophrenia but also in other disorders; included are catalepsy, catatonic excitement, catatonic stupor, catatonic rigidity, bizarre posturing, unusual mannerisms, stereotypy, waxy flexibility, and negativism.

cata•ton•ic (kat″ə-ton′ik) 1. pertaining to catatonia or to catatonic schizophrenia. 2. an individual affected with catatonia or catatonic schizophrenia.

cata•tri•crot•ic (kat″ə-tri-krot′ik) on a pulse tracing, having three waveforms on the descending limb; see under *pulse.*

cata•tri•cro•tism (kat″ə-tri′kro-tiz-əm) [*cata-* + *tricrotism*] presence of a catatricrotic pulse.

cat•e•chin (kat′ə-kin) a crystalline principle from catechu; formerly used medicinally for its astringent qualities. Called also *catechol* and *catechuic acid.*

cat•e•chol (kat′ə-kol) 1. catechin. 2. pyrocatechol.

cat•e•chol•amine (kat″ə-kol′ə-mēn) one of a group of biogenic amines having a sympathomimetic action, the aromatic portion of whose molecule is catechol, and the aliphatic portion an amine; examples are dopamine, norepinephrine, and epinephrine.

cat•e•chol•am•in•er•gic (kat″ə-kol″ə-mĭ-nur′jik) activated by or secreting catecholamines.

cat•e•chol *O*-meth•yl•trans•fer•ase (kat′ə-kol meth″əl-trans′fər-ās) [EC 2.1.1.6] an enzyme of the transferase class that catalyzes the transfer of a methyl group from *S*-adenosylmethionine to a catechol or catecholamine such as dopa, dopamine, epinephrine, or norepinephrine. The enzyme occurs in the cytoplasm, particularly in the kidney, liver, and central nervous system.

cat•e•chol ox•i•dase (kat′ə-kol ok′sĭ-dās) [EC 1.10.3.1] any of a group of enzymes of the oxidoreductase class that catalyze the oxidation of catechols to 1,2-benzoquinones. They are copper-containing proteins that act also upon substituted catechols and many catalyze the reaction of monophenol monooxygenase. The group includes enzymes called also *diphenol oxidase* or *polyphenol oxidase*, based on their substrates. Cf. *monophenol monooxygenase.*

cat•e•chu (kat′ə-ku) 1. a powerfully astringent extract from the heartwood of *Acacia catechu;* its chief constituents are catechin, quercetin, and catechutannic acid; formerly used as an antidiarrheal agent. Called also *black c.* 2. gambir.
black c. catechu (def. 1).
pale c. gambir.

cat•e•chu•ic ac•id (kat″ə-ku′ik) catechin.

cat•elec•trot•o•nus (kat″ə-lek-trot′ə-nəs) [*cata-* + *electrotonus*] increase of irritability of a nerve or muscle near the cathode during passage of an electric current.

cat•e•nat•ing (kat′ə-nāt′ing) [L. *catena* a chain] forming part of a chain or complex of symptoms.

cat•e•nin (kat′ə-nin) any of a group of cytoplasmic proteins that serve to anchor cadherins to the cytoskeleton; β-catenin binds to the cytoplasmic tails of cadherins, and α-catenin links β-catenin to actin filaments.

cat•e•noid (kat′ə-noid) [L. *catena* chain] 1. resembling a chain. 2. arranged in a chain; called also *catenulate.*

ca•ten•u•late (kə-ten′u-lāt) catenoid (def. 2).

cat•er•pil•lar (kat′ər-pil″ər) the larva of an insect of the order Lepidoptera. Certain species have hairs that cause insect dermatitis.

cat•gut (kat′gut) surgical gut.
chromic c., chromicized c. see *chromic gut,* under *gut.*

Ca•tha (kath′ə) a genus of evergreen shrubs and trees of the family Celastracheae, native to East Africa. *C. e′dulis* Forsk. is a species whose leaves contain the central nervous system stimulant D-norpseudoephedrine and are chewed or made into a tea.

cath•a•rom•e•ter (kath″ə-rom′ə-tər) an instrument for measuring the thermal conductivity of air by the rate of heat loss from a heated platinum wire.

ca•thar•sis (kə-thahr′sis) [Gr. *katharsis* a cleansing] 1. evacuation. 2. in psychiatry, release of ideas, thoughts, and repressed material from the unconscious, accompanied by an emotional response and relief.

ca•thar•tic (kə-thahr′tik) 1. causing emptying of the bowels. 2. an agent that causes emptying of the bowels, such as by increasing bulk or stimulating peristaltic action. Called also *evacuant* and *purgative.* 3. producing emotional catharsis.
bulk c. an agent that stimulates evacuation of the bowels by increasing the bulk of the feces.
lubricant c. an agent that stimulates evacuation of the bowels by softening the feces and reducing friction between them and the intestinal wall.
saline c. an agent that increases fluidity of the intestinal contents by retention of water by osmotic forces and indirectly increases motor activity, thus stimulating evacuation. See *magnesium sulfate, sodium sulfate,* and *potassium sodium tartrate.*
stimulant c. an agent that causes evacuation of the bowels by directly increasing motor activity of the intestinal tract.

ca•the•li•ci•din (kə-the″lĭ-si′din) any of a family of mammalian cationic peptides that are expressed by leukocytes and epithelial cells and have a wide spectrum of antimicrobial activity, acting both directly and as multifunctional immunomodulators. Humans have a single cathelicidin; overexpression results in rosacea.

ca•the•mo•glo•bin (kə-the-mo-glo′bin) a substance produced by oxidizing hemochromogen; it consists of oxidized heme and denatured globin.

ca•thep•sin (kə-thep′sin) one of a number of enzymes of the hydrolase class that catalyze the hydrolysis of peptide bonds; most are lysosomal endopeptidases with an acidic optimum pH.
c. A a ubiquitous multifunctional enzyme with deamidase, esterase, and carboxypeptidase activities.
c. B [EC 3.4.22.1] a cysteine endopeptidase with specificity similar to that of papain; it occurs predominantly in lysosomes.
c. B_1 c. B.
c. B_2 cysteine-type carboxypeptidase (def. 2).
c. C dipeptidyl peptidase I.
c. D [EC 3.4.23.5] an aspartic endopeptidase of the hydrolase class with specificity resembling, but narrower than, that of pepsin A. The enzyme is optimally active at acidic pH and occurs in lysosomes.
c. G [EC 3.4.21.20] a serine endopeptidase with specificity similar to that of chymotrypsin; it is found in polymorphonuclear leukocyte lysosomes.

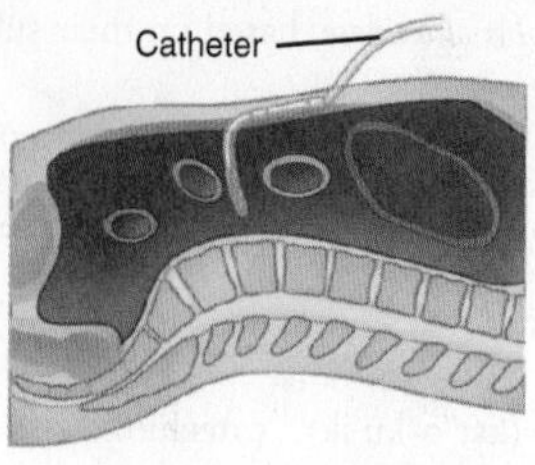

■ Catheter inserted into the abdomen.

c. H [EC 3.4.22.16] a cysteine endopeptidase that also catalyzes the removal of amino acids from the N-terminus of peptides with that end free; it is present in the lysosomes of most mammalian tissues.
c. K [EC 3.4.22.38] a cysteine endopeptidase that is expressed in osteoclasts and plays a key role in the degradation of bone.
c. L [EC 3.4.22.15] a cysteine endopeptidase of the lysosomes, structurally related to papain.

cath·e·ter (kath'ə-tər) [Gr. *kathetēr*] 1. a tubular, flexible, surgical instrument that is inserted into a cavity of the body to withdraw or introduce fluid. See also *cannula*. 2. urethral c.

Catheter

acorn-tipped c. a catheter used in ureteropyelography to occlude the ureteral orifice and prevent backflow from the ureter during and following the injection of an opaque medium.
Amplatz coronary c. a preformed J-shaped angiographic catheter used as an alternative to a Judkins coronary catheter in coronary arteriography.
angiographic c. a catheter through which a contrast medium is injected for visualization of the vascular system of an organ; it may have a preformed end to facilitate selective locating (as in a renal or coronary vessel) from a remote entry site. Different types may be named according to the site of entry and destination, such as *femoral-renal* or *brachial-coronary*.
arterial c. a catheter inserted into an artery, used as part of a catheter-transducer-monitor system to continuously observe the blood pressure of critically ill patients; it can also be used for x-ray studies of the arterial system and for delivery of chemotherapeutic agents directly into the arterial supply of malignant tumors.
atherectomy c. a catheter containing a rotating cutter and a collecting chamber for debris, used for atherectomy and endarterectomy; it is inserted percutaneously under radiographic guidance.
balloon c., balloon-tip c. a catheter whose tip is provided with an inflatable balloon that holds the catheter in place or is used to dilate the lumen of a vessel, such as in balloon angioplasty; common types are the *Gruentzig balloon c.* and the *Swan-Ganz c.*
bicoudate c., c. bicoudé an elbowed catheter with two bends.
biliary c. a catheter inserted via a skin incision through the liver and common bile duct into the duodenum in order to provide drainage of bile past obstructed ducts into the small intestine, where the bile can aid digestion.
Braasch bulb c. a bulb-tipped ureteral catheter used for dilation and determination of the inner diameter of the ureter.
Brockenbrough transseptal c. a specialized cardiac catheter with a curved steel inner needle that can puncture the interatrial septum; used to catheterize the left ventricle when the aortic valve cannot be crossed in a retrograde approach.
Broviac c. a type of central venous catheter similar to a Hickman catheter but with a smaller lumen.
butterfly c. a small-diameter venous catheter introduced through the lumen of a butterfly needle.
cardiac c. a long, fine catheter especially designed for passage, usually through a peripheral blood vessel, into the chambers of the heart under radiologic control; used to obtain blood samples and intracardiac pressures, in diagnosing cardiac abnormalities, and in therapeutic intervention.
cardiac c.-microphone phonocatheter.
Castillo c. a cardiac catheter similar to an Amplatz catheter in shape and use, but shorter and introduced via the brachial artery.
central venous c. a catheter introduced via a large vein, such as the femoral, internal jugular, or subclavian, into the superior vena cava or right atrium to administer parenteral fluids (as in hyperalimentation) or medications or to measure central venous pressure. This type of catheter can also be used for short-term hemodialysis.
closed end-hole c. a catheter that lacks a hole in its tip; used for rapid injection of large volumes of contrast solution. Cf. *end-hole c.*
condom c. an external urinary collection device that fits over the penis like a condom; used in the management of urinary incontinence.
conical c. a ureteral catheter that has a cone-shaped tip designed to dilate the lumen.
Cook c. a flexible catheter sometimes used in place of the Tenckhoff catheter in peritoneal dialysis.
Cope loop c. a type of nephrostomy catheter with a loop at the end to hold it in place.
c. coudé elbowed c.
Cournand c. a cardiac catheter with a single end hole; used for pressure measurement, usually in the right heart.
DeLee c. a catheter used to suction meconium and amniotic debris from the nasopharynx and oropharynx of neonates.
c. à demeure indwelling c.
de Pezzer c. a self-retaining urethral catheter having a bulbous extremity.
directional atherectomy c. a type of atherectomy catheter whose direction can be shifted to shave off additional plaque.
double-channel c., double-lumen c. a catheter having two channels, one for injection and one for removal of fluid. Called also *two-way c.*
Drew-Smythe c. an instrument used for the artificial rupture of the amniotic membranes to induce labor.
dual-lumen c. double-lumen c.
elbowed c. a urethral catheter with a sharp bend near the beak, used to get around an enlarged prostate. Called also *c. coudé* and *prostatic c.*
electrode c. a cardiac catheter containing one or more electrodes; it may be used to pace the heart or to deliver high-energy shocks.
end-hole c. a cardiac catheter with a hole in the tip, through which a guidewire may be passed or pressure monitored.
eustachian c. an instrument for inflating the eustachian tube for treatment of diseases of the middle ear.
female c. a short urethral catheter for passage through the female urethra.
femoral c. a central venous catheter inserted through the femoral vein.
filiform-tipped c. a small-caliber catheter whose tip has a lumenless filiform; used to dilate tight urethral strictures and to bypass obstructions due to angulations or calculi in the ureter.
fluid-filled c. an intravascular catheter connected by a saline-filled tube to an external pressure transducer; used to measure intravascular pressure.
Fogarty c. a type of balloon-tip catheter used to remove thrombi and emboli from blood vessels.
Foley c. an indwelling catheter that has a balloon filled with air or liquid to retain it in place in the bladder.
Gensini coronary c. a nonpreformed catheter used for coronary arteriography; it has an end-hole to accommodate a guidewire or monitor pressure as well as side holes for rapid injection of large volumes of contrast material.
Gouley c. a steel urethral catheter that is curved and grooved on its inferior surface so that it can be passed over a guide through a urethral stricture.
Groshong c. a modification of the Hickman catheter with a valve that is closed when the catheter is not in use, used for long-term administration of substances such as antibiotics, total parenteral nutrition, or chemotherapeutic agents.
Gruentzig balloon c. a flexible balloon catheter with a short guidewire fixed to the tip, used for dilation of arterial stenoses; the balloon is made of low-compliance plastic to reduce the risk of arterial rupture.
hemodialysis c. a catheter used on a temporary basis for vascular access for hemodialysis, usually some type of central venous catheter.

Catheter *Continued*

Hickman c. a type of central venous catheter used for long-term administration of substances such as antibiotics, total parenteral nutrition, or chemotherapeutic agents; it can be used for continuous or intermittent administration and may have either a single or a double lumen.
indwelling c. a urethral catheter that is held in position in the urethra.
internal jugular c. a central venous catheter inserted through the internal jugular vein.
Judkins coronary c. a preformed J-shaped angiographic catheter used in coronary arteriography to cannulate and deliver contrast material to one of the coronary arteries via a percutaneous femoral route. It is composed of polyurethane or polyethylene with a fine wire braid within its walls; right and left catheters are shaped specifically for use in the respective coronary arteries.
Judkins pigtail left ventriculography c. a specialized pigtail catheter used for left ventriculography.
left coronary c. a catheter designed for coronary arteriography of the left coronary artery.
Malecot c. a two- or four-winged female catheter.
manometer-tipped c. a catheter with a small pressure transducer on its tip; used in measuring intravascular or intracardiac pressure.
multipurpose c. 1. a catheter with several functions or applications. 2. a catheter for coronary angiography that is shaped so that it can be used in either coronary artery.
Nélaton c. a type of urethral catheter made of flexible rubber.
nephrostomy c. a catheter used with percutaneous nephrostomy, as for drainage.
NIH c. a nonpreformed catheter used for coronary arteriography; it has a closed end and several side holes for rapid injection of large volumes of contrast material.
olive-tip c. a ureteral catheter with an olive-shaped end, used to dilate a constricted ureteral orifice; larger sizes may also be used for dilating urethral strictures or calibrating stricture diameter.
pacing c. a cardiac catheter containing one or more electrodes on pacing wires; used as a temporary cardiac pacing lead.
percutaneous c. a catheter inserted through the skin rather than through an orifice, such as a central venous catheter or one used for hemodialysis or peritoneal dialysis.
peripherally inserted central c. (PICC) a long catheter introduced through a vein in the arm, then through the subclavian vein into the superior vena cava or right atrium to administer parenteral fluids (as in hyperalimentation) or medications or to measure central venous pressure.
Pezzer c. de Pezzer c.
pigtail c. an angiographic catheter ending in a tightly curled tip that resembles the tail of a pig.
preformed c. a preshaped catheter designed to require less operator manipulation but usually restricted to a single function.
prostatic c. elbowed c.
pulmonary artery c. any of various cardiac catheters for measuring pulmonary arterial pressures, introduced into the venous system through a large vein and guided by blood flow into the superior vena cava, the right atrium and ventricle, and into the pulmonary artery.
right coronary c. a catheter designed for coronary arteriography of the right coronary artery.
Robinson c. a straight urethral catheter with two to six openings to allow drainage, especially useful when there are blood clots that may occlude one or more openings.
self-retaining c. a urethral catheter constructed to be retained in the bladder and urethra; see *Foley c.* and *indwelling c.*
snare c. a catheter designed to remove catheter fragments introduced into the heart iatrogenically.
Sones coronary c. a woven Dacron or polyurethane catheter used in coronary arteriography to cannulate and deliver contrast material to the coronary arteries via the brachial artery. It is not preformed and may be used for several different tasks and with different approaches.
spiral-tip c. a type of filiform-tipped catheter with an off-center filiform.
subclavian c. a central venous catheter inserted through the subclavian vein.
Swan-Ganz c. a soft, flow-directed pulmonary artery catheter of the balloon-tip type; it is introduced into the venous system via an internal jugular or subclavian vein and is guided by blood flow into the superior vena cava, the right atrium and ventricle, and into the pulmonary artery.
swan neck c. a catheter used in peritoneal dialysis, having its end bent around almost to a U shape to impede catheter migration or extrusion.
Tenckhoff c. any of several types of catheter commonly used in peritoneal dialysis, consisting of a flexible silicone rubber tube with end and side holes and one or two extraperitoneal Dacron felt cuffs that help provide a bacteria-tight seal.
thermodilution c. a catheter used in thermodilution for introduction of the cold liquid indicator into the cardiovascular system.
toposcopic c. a miniature catheter that can pass through narrow, tortuous vessels to convey chemotherapy directly to specific sites.
tracheal c. an instrument for removing mucus from the trachea by application of suction.
transluminal endarterectomy c. a type of atherectomy catheter with a conical cutting window, inserted through the lumen of the vessel; debris is collected in a special vacuum bottle.
transtracheal c., transtracheal oxygen c. a catheter inserted into the trachea through a tracheostomy for patients who cannot tolerate a nasal or oral cannula.
tunneled c. a central venous catheter left in place for a long period so that scar tissue forms and anchors it in place.
two-way c. double-lumen c.
ureteral c. a catheter inserted into the ureter, either through the urethra and bladder or posteriorly via the kidney.
urethral c. a catheter for insertion through the urethra into the urinary bladder.
whistle-tip c. a urethral catheter with a terminal opening as well as a lateral one.
winged c. a urethral catheter that has winglike projections on the end to retain it in the bladder.

cath•e•ter•iza•tion (kath″ə-tur″ĭ-za′shən) 1. the insertion of a catheter. 2. the use of a catheter.
cardiac c. passage of a small catheter through a vein in an arm or leg or the neck and into the heart, permitting the securing of blood samples, determination of intracardiac pressure, detection of cardiac anomalies, planning of operative approaches, and determination, implementation, or evaluation of appropriate therapy.
hepatic vein c. passage of a cardiac catheter through an arm vein, right atrium, inferior vena cava, and hepatic vein, into a small hepatic venule, for recording of intrahepatic venous pressures.
retrograde c. passage of a cardiac catheter along an artery, usually the femoral artery, against the direction of blood flow and into the heart.
transseptal c. passage of a cardiac catheter through the right atrium and across the interatrial septum into the left atrium; used in cases of valve obstruction and in techniques such as balloon mitral valvuloplasty.

cath•e•ter•ize (kath′ə-tər-īz) to introduce a catheter within a body cavity.

cath•e•tero•stat (kath-e′tər-o-stat″) an apparatus for holding and sterilizing catheters.

cath•e•tom•e•ter (kath″ə-tom′ə-tər) an instrument for aiding in the reading of thermometers, burets, and other equipment.

ca•thex•is (kə-thek′sis) [Gr. *kathexis* a retaining] in psychiatry, conscious or unconscious investment of psychic energy in a person, idea, or any other object. **cathec′tic** *adj*

Cath•flo Ac•ti•vase (kath′flo ak′tĭ-vās) trademark for a preparation of alteplase.

cath•iso•pho•bia (kath″ĭ-so-fo′be-ə) [Gr. *kathizein* to sit down + *-phobia*] kathisophobia.

cath•ode (kath′ōd) [*cata-* + *hodos* way] 1. in an electrochemical cell, the electrode at which reduction occurs, i.e., the negative electrode in an electrolytic cell or a storage battery and the positive electrode in a voltaic cell that delivers current. 2. the negative electrode of devices such as electron tubes, x-ray tubes, and electrophoresis cells. Symbol C. Cf. *anode.* **cathod′ic** *adj*

cath•o•lyte (kath′o-līt) the portion of an electrolyte that adjoins the cathode.

Cath•o•my•cin (kath′o-mi″sin) trademark for preparations of novobiocin.

cat•ion (kat′i-on) [*cata-* + *ion*] an ion carrying a positive charge owing to a deficiency of electrons; in an electrolytic cell cations migrate toward the cathode, which is negatively charged. **cation′ic** *adj*

cat•i•on•o•gen (kat″i-on′ə-jən) a compound that may become or may liberate a cation in the body.

cat·lin (kat′lin) a long, straight, sharp-pointed, double-edged knife used in amputations.

cat·ling (kat′ling) catlin.

cat·nip (kat′nip) *Nepeta cataria.*

ca·top·tric (kə-top′trik) [Gr. *katoptrikos* in a mirror] pertaining to a reflected image, or to reflected light.

ca·top·trics (kə-top′triks) the branch of physics that deals with reflected light.

ca·top·tro·scope (kə-top′trə-skōp) [Gr. *katoptron* mirror + *-scope*] an instrument for examining objects by reflected light.

Ca^{2+}-trans·port·ing ATP·ase (trans-por′ting a-te-pe′ās) [EC 3.6.3.8] EC nomenclature for *Ca^{2+}-ATPase.*

cau·da (kaw′də) pl. *cau′dae* [L.] 1. a tail or taillike appendage. 2. an anatomical structure resembling such an appendage.

c. epididy′midis [TA] tail of epididymis: the lower part of the epididymis, where the ductus epididymidis is continuous with the ductus deferens.

c. equi′na [TA] the collection of spinal roots that descend from the lower part of the spinal cord and are located within the lumbar cistern of the caudal dural sac; their appearance resembles the tail of a horse.

c. he′licis [TA] tail of helix: the termination of the posterior margin of the cartilage of the helix.

c. nu′clei c.′ti [TA] tail of caudate nucleus: the part of the caudate nucleus that tapers off from the body, curves around in the roof of the inferior horn of the lateral ventricle, and extends rostrally as far as the amygdaloid nucleus.

c. pancre′atis [TA] tail of pancreas: the left extremity of the pancreas, usually in contact with the medial aspect of the spleen and the junction of the transverse colon and descending colon.

cau·dad (kaw′dad) directed toward the tail or the inferior end of the trunk, as opposed to *cephalad.* Called also *cephalocaudad.*

cau·dae (kaw′de) [L.] genitive and plural of *cauda.*

cau·dal (kaw′dəl) 1. pertaining to a cauda or tail. 2. in embryology and nonhuman anatomy, denoting a position more toward the cauda or tail; see also *posterior* (def. 2). 3. in human anatomy, a synonym of *inferior.*

cau·da·lis (kaw-da′lis) [TA] caudal.

cau·dal·ward (kaw′dəl-wərd) caudad.

Cau·da·ta (kaw-da′tə) an order of amphibians, including the salamanders (q.v.).

cau·date (kaw′dāt) [L. *caudatus*] having a tail.

cau·da·to·len·tic·u·lar (kaw-da″to-len-tik′u-lər) pertaining to the caudate and lenticular nuclei of the corpus striatum.

cau·dec·to·my (kaw-dek′tə-me) the surgical removal of all or part of the tail.

cau·do·ceph·a·lad (kaw″do-sef′ə-ləd) [*cauda* + *cephalad*] 1. proceeding in a direction from the tail toward the head. 2. cephalad. 3. in both a caudal and a cephalic direction.

caul (kawl) a piece of amnion that sometimes envelops a child's head at birth; called also *cowl, pileus,* and *veil.*

Cau·lo·bac·te·ra·ceae (kaw″lo-bak″tər-a′se-e) [L. *caulis* stalk + Gr. *baktron* rod] a family of anaerobic, oligotrophic and chemo-organotrophic bacteria of the order Caulobacterales, grouped together on the basis of 16S rRNA sequence analysis. Organisms of medical interest are contained in the genus *Brevundimonas.*

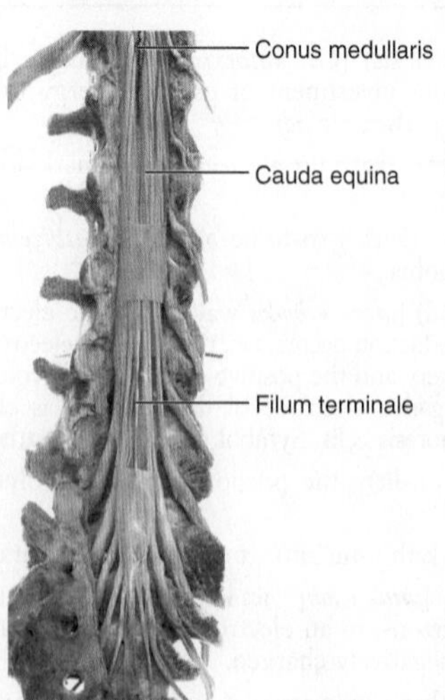

■ Cauda equina, descending from the conus medullaris of the spinal cord.

Cau·lo·bac·te·ra·les (kaw″lo-bak″tər-a′lēz) an order of aerobic, oligotrophic and chemo-organotrophic bacteria of the class Alphaproteobacteria, phylum Proteobacteria, grouped together on the basis of 16S rRNA sequence analysis. Organisms of medical interest are contained in the family Caulobacteraceae.

Cau·lo·phyl·lum (kaw″lo-fil′əm) [Gr. *kaulos* stem + *phyllon* leaf] a genus of herbs of the family Berberidaceae, having yellow flowers and blue berries and found in eastern Asia and the eastern United States; *C. thalictroi′des* (blue cohosh) is medicinal.

cau·mes·the·sia (kaw″mes-the′zhə) [Gr. *kauma* burn + *esthesia*] a condition in which, with a low temperature, the patient experiences a sense of burning heat.

cau·sal·gia (kaw-zal′jə) [Gr. *kausos* heat + *-algia*] complex regional pain syndrome type 2.

caus·a·tive (kawz′ə-tiv) effective or responsible as a cause or agent.

cause (kawz) [L. *causa*] that which brings about any condition or produces any effect. **caus′al** *adj*

constitutional c. a factor acting within the body that is not restricted to a specific site, but is systemic or has a genetic basis.

c. of death the injury or disease responsible for a death; cf. *manner of death,* under *manner.*

exciting c. a cause that leads directly to a specific condition.

immediate c. a cause that is operative at the beginning of the specific effect; called also *precipitating c.*

local c. a cause that is not general or constitutional, but is confined to the site where the effect is produced.

precipitating c. immediate c.

predisposing c. anything that renders a person more liable to a specific condition without actually producing it.

primary c. the principal factor contributing to the production of a specific result.

proximate c. a cause that immediately precedes and produces an effect.

remote c. any cause that does not immediately precede and produce a specific condition; a predisposing, secondary, or ultimate cause.

secondary c. a cause that is supplemental to the primary cause.

specific c. a factor that produces a special or specific effect.

ultimate c. the earliest factor, in point of time, that has contributed to production of a specific result.

caus·tic (kaws′tik) 1. corrosive. 2. having a burning taste.

lunar c. toughened silver nitrate.

cau·ter·ant (kaw′tər-ənt) an agent that cauterizes.

cau·ter·iza·tion (kaw″tər-ĭ-za′shən) destruction of tissue with a hot or cold instrument, electric current, caustic substance, or other agent. Called also *cautery.*

cau·ter·ize (kaw′tər-īz) to apply a cautery; to perform cauterization.

cau·tery (kaw′tər-e) [L. *cauterium;* Gr. *kautērion*] 1. a caustic substance or hot or cold instrument used in cauterization. 2. cauterization.

actual c. 1. an instrument that destroys tissue by burning rather than by chemical action. 2. the application of such an instrument.

chemical c. chemocautery.

cold c. cryocautery.

electric c., galvanic c. electrocautery.

gas c. cauterization by means of a specially controlled jet of burning gas.

potential c., virtual c. cauterization by an escharotic without applying heat.

ca·va (ka′və) [L.] 1. plural of *cavum.* 2. vena cava.

ca·val (ka′vəl) pertaining to a vena cava; called also *venacaval* or *vena caval.*

CAVB complete atrioventricular block.

cave (kāv) [L. *cavum*] cavum.

Meckel c. cavum trigeminale.

c. of septum pellucidum cavum septi pellucidi.

trigeminal c. cavum trigeminale.

ca·ve·o·la (ka-ve-o′lə) pl. *caveo′lae* [L.] a small (approximately 50 nm), flask-shaped invagination of the plasma membrane occurring in nearly all animal cells, coated with the membrane protein caveolin and rich in cholesterol and sphingolipids. Caveolae are a special form of lipid raft and are associated with endocytosis, budding from the plasma membrane to form pinosomes; they also concentrate signaling molecules and have been implicated in other processes, including the export of cholesterol to serum lipoproteins. Called also *plasmalemmal vesicle.*

ca·ve·o·lin (ka-ve-o′lin) any of a family of integral membrane proteins that are the principal components of caveola membranes and are believed to act as scaffolding for assembly of signaling complexes; they are approximately 20 kDa in size, form high molecular mass homo-oligomers, and have N- and C-terminal hydrophilic segments with a long central transmembrane domain. Currently, caveolin-1 (or VIP21), caveolin-2, and caveolin-3 (or M-caveolin) are known, with the last being specific to muscle. Mutations in the gene encoding caveolin-3 have been associated with an autosomal dominant subtype of limb-girdle muscular dystrophy and with a form of hyperCKemia lacking muscle weakness.

Cav•er•ject (kav′ər-jekt″) trademark for a preparation of alprostadil.

cav•ern (kav′ərn) a cavity, particularly one associated with pathology.

Schnabel c's a type of optic atrophy with marked loss of optic nerve substance, usually associated with severe glaucoma.

ca•ver•na (ka-vur′nə) pl. *caver′nae* [L.] a cavity or space.

caver′nae cor′porum cavernoso′rum pe′nis [TA] cavernous spaces of corpora cavernosa of penis: the dilatable spaces within the corpora cavernosa of the penis, which fill with blood and become distended with erection.

caver′nae cor′poris spongio′si pe′nis [TA] cavernous spaces of corpus spongiosum of penis: the dilatable spaces within the corpus spongiosum of the penis, which fill with blood and become distended with erection.

cav•er•nil•o•quy (kav″ər-nil′ə-kwe) [*caverna* + *loqui* to speak] cavernous voice.

cav•er•ni•tis (kav″ər-ni′tis) inflammation of the corpora cavernosa or corpus spongiosum of the penis.

fibrous c. Peyronie disease.

cav•er•no•ma (kav″ər-no′mə) cavernous hemangioma.

cav•er•no•sal (kav″ər-no′səl) 1. pertaining to a corpus cavernosum. 2. cavernous.

cav•er•no•si•tis (kav″ər-no-si′tis) cavernitis.

cav•er•no•sog•ra•phy (kav″ər-no-sog′rə-fe) radiographic visualization of the corpus cavernosum of the penis.

dynamic infusion c. radiographic imaging of the corporal bodies and associated vasculature following infusion of contrast medium or saline solution directly into the corpus cavernosum; used for detection of venous leaks.

cav•er•no•som•e•try (kav″ər-no-som′ə-tre) measurement of the vascular pressure in the corpus cavernosum.

dynamic infusion c. a graphic representation of intracorporal vascular pressure as a function of infused volume.

cav•er•nos•to•my (kav″ər-nos′tə-me) operative incision into a cavity.

cav•er•nous (kav′ər-nəs) [L. *cavernosus*] 1. containing caverns or hollow spaces. 2. having a characteristic low-pitched quality due to having a cavitary resonating chamber, said of certain auscultatory sounds.

Ca•via (ka′ve-ə) a genus of small South American rodents of the family Caviidae. *C. coba′ya* is the guinea pig.

cav•i•tary (kav′ĭ-tar″e) 1. characterized by the presence of a cavity or cavities. 2. any entozoon with a body space or alimentary canal.

cav•i•tas (kav′ĭ-təs) pl. *cavita′tes* [L., from *cavus* hollow] [TA] cavity: a hollow space or depression within the body. Called also *cavum*.

c. abdomina′lis TA alternative for *c. abdominis*.

c. abdo′minis [TA] abdominal cavity: the body cavity located inferior to the diaphragm and superior to the pelvis, forming the superior and major part of the abdominopelvic cavity.

c. abdo′minis et pel′vis [TA] abdominopelvic cavity: the space within the trunk between the diaphragm and the inferior boundary of the lesser pelvis; it is divided into the abdominal and pelvic cavities.

c. articula′ris [TA] articular cavity: the minute space of a synovial joint, enclosed by the synovial membrane and articular cartilages.

c. con′chae [TA] cavity of concha: the inferior part of the concha of the auricle, which leads into the external acoustic meatus; called also *cavum conchae* [TA alternative] and *innominate fossa of auricle*.

c. coro′nae [TA] pulp chamber: the portion of the dental (pulp) cavity located in the tooth crown, occupied by the dental pulp.

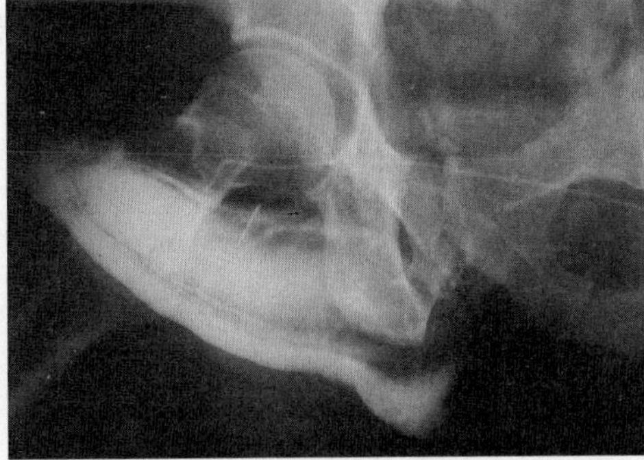

■ Cavernosography performed one year after penile fracture, showing a communication between the corpus cavernosum and corpus spongiosum.

c. cra′nii [TA] cranial cavity: the space enclosed by the bones of the cranium.

c. den′tis [TA] pulp cavity: the natural cavity in the central portion of a tooth occupied by the dental pulp, which is divided into the pulp chamber (*c. coronae*) and the root canal (*canalis radicis dentis*); called also *c. pulparis* [TA alternative], and *nerve cavity*.

c. glenoida′lis scapu′lae [TA] glenoid cavity of scapula: a depression in the lateral angle of the scapula for articulation with the humerus; called also *glenoid fossa of scapula*.

c. infraglot′tica [TA] infraglottic cavity: the most inferior part of the laryngeal cavity, extending from the rima glottidis above to the cavity of the trachea below. Called also *subglottis*.

c. laryn′gis [TA] laryngeal cavity: the space enclosed by the walls of the larynx.

c. medulla′ris [TA] medullary cavity: the space in the diaphysis of a long bone containing the marrow; called also *marrow cavity*, *medullary canal*, and *medullary space*.

c. nasa′lis os′sea [TA] bony nasal cavity: the part of the nasal cavity enclosed by the bony portion of the osteocartilaginous framework of the nose.

c. na′si [TA] nasal cavity: the portion of the passages of the respiratory system extending from the nares to the pharynx. It is divided into left and right halves by the nasal septum; its floor is the hard palate, which separates it from the oral cavity; and its lateral walls contain the nasal conchae and nasal meatus.

c. orbita′lis [TA] the space within the orbit.

c. o′ris [TA] oral cavity: the anterior or proximal opening of the alimentary canal, which is bounded externally by the lips and cheeks and internally by the oropharyngeal isthmus, and which also includes the palate, oral mucosa, teeth, tongue, and the glands whose ducts open into the cavity. It is subdivided into the oral vestibule (vestibulum oris) and the oral cavity proper (cavitas oris propria). Called also *mouth*.

c. o′ris pro′pria [TA] oral cavity proper: the part of the oral cavity internal to the teeth.

c. pelvi′na TA alternative for *c. pelvis*.

c. pel′vis [TA] pelvic cavity: the space within the walls of the pelvis, forming the inferior and lesser part of the abdominopelvic cavity. Called also *c. pelvina* [TA alternative].

c. pericardi′aca [TA] pericardial cavity: the potential space between the parietal layer and the visceral layer (epicardium) of the serous pericardium.

c. peritonea′lis [TA] peritoneal cavity: the potential space of capillary thinness between the parietal and the visceral peritoneum; it is normally empty except for a thin serous fluid that keeps the surfaces moist. Called also *greater peritoneal cavity*.

c. pharyn′gis [TA] pharyngeal cavity: the space enclosed by the walls of the pharynx.

c. pleura′lis [TA] pleural cavity: the potential space between the parietal and visceral pleurae. Called also *pleural space*.

c. pulpa′ris TA alternative for *c. dentis*.

c. thora′cica TA alternative for *c. thoracis*.

c. thora′cis [TA] thoracic cavity: the portion of the body cavity situated between the neck and the diaphragm; called also *c. thoracica* [TA alternative], *pectoral cavity*, and *thorax*.

c. tym′pani [TA] tympanic cavity: the major portion of the middle ear (auris media), consisting of a narrow air-filled cavity in the temporal bone that contains the auditory ossicles. It communicates with the mastoid air cells and the mastoid antrum via the aditus and with the nasopharynx via the auditory tube. The middle ear and the tympanic cavity were formerly regarded as being synonymous. Called also *tympanum*.

c. u′teri [TA] uterine cavity: the flattened space within the uterus, communicating on either side at the cornu with the uterine tubes and below with the vagina.

cav•i•ta•tes (kav″ĭ-ta′tēz) [L.] plural of *cavitas*.

cav•i•ta•tion (kav″ĭ-ta′shən) 1. the formation of pathological cavities, as in pulmonary tuberculosis. 2. a pathological cavity.

ca•vi•tis (ka-vi′tis) inflammation of the vena cava; called also *celophlebitis*.

cav•i•ty (kav′ĭ-te) [L. *cavitas*] 1. a hollow place or space, or a potential space, within the body or in one of its organs; it may be normal (called *cavitas* in anatomical nomenclature) or pathological (see *cavitation*). See also *pocket*, *pouch*, and *recess*. Called also *cave*, *cavern*, *caverna*, and *cavum*. 2. the lesion, or area of destruction in a tooth, produced by dental caries; classified as simple, compound, or complex, according to the number of surfaces involved. See also *dental caries*, under *caries*. 3. prepared c.

abdominal c. cavitas abdominis.

abdominopelvic c. *cavitas abdominis et pelvis*.

absorption c's cavities in developing compact bone due to osteoclastic erosion, usually occurring in the areas laid down first.

alveolar c. alveolus dentalis.

amniotic c. the closed sac between the embryo and the amnion, containing the amniotic fluid.

articular c. cavitas articularis.

Baer c. the cleavage cavity beneath the blastoderm.

blastocyst c., blastocystic c. the fluid-filled cavity developing in the morula as it becomes a blastocyst.
body c. a visceral cavity, such as the thoracic, abdominal, or pelvic cavity.
bony nasal c. cavitas nasalis ossea.
buccal c. 1. that portion of the oral cavity bounded on one side by the teeth and gingivae (or the residual alveolar ridges), and on the other by the cheeks. 2. a carious lesion beginning on the buccal surface of a posterior tooth. 3. cavitas oris. 4. a preoral chamber seen in higher ciliate protozoa, manifested as an indentation or pouch, containing compound ciliary organelles and leading to the cytostomal-cytopharyngeal complex. Called also *peristome.*
chorionic c. extraembryonic coelom.
cleavage c. blastocoele.
complex c. a carious lesion that involves three or more surfaces of a tooth in its prepared state.
compound c. a carious lesion that involves two surfaces of a tooth.
c. of concha cavitas conchae.
cotyloid c. acetabulum.
cranial c. cavitas cranii.
dental c. see *cavity* (def. 2), and see under *caries.*
distal c. a carious lesion beginning on the distal surface of a tooth.
epidural c. spatium epidurale.
exocoelomic c. the cavity surrounded by the exocoelomic membrane and roofed by the hypoblast during implantation and formation of the bilaminar embryonic disc in human embryonic development. The cavity and surrounding membrane will become the yolk sac.
fibrotic c's cavities of the lung composed of granulation tissue surrounded by scar tissue, as in idiopathic pulmonary fibrosis or tuberculosis; in tuberculosis they may be the source from which the disease spreads to other pulmonary segments.
fissure c. a carious lesion beginning in a fissure of a tooth. See *pit caries,* under *caries.*
gastrovascular c. the body cavity of a coelenterate, which opens to the outside at one end to form a mouth.
glandular c. a hollow sac formed by invagination of the epithelial sheath in the developing multicellular gland.
glenoid c. cavitas glenoidalis.
head c. modified somites that in lower vertebrates give rise to the extrinsic eye muscles.
hemal c. hemocoelom.
incisal c. a carious lesion beginning on the incisal surface of an anterior tooth.
infraglottic c. cavitas infraglottica.
ischioanal c., ischiorectal c. fossa ischioanalis.
labial c. a carious lesion beginning on the labial surface of an anterior tooth.
laryngeal c. cavitas laryngis.
laryngeal c., intermediate the smallest part of the laryngeal cavity, extending from the rima vestibuli to the rima glottidis.
laryngopharyngeal c. pars laryngea pharyngis.
lingual c. a carious lesion beginning on the lingual surface of a tooth.
lymph c's the larger lymph spaces and cisterns of the body.
marrow c. cavitas medullaris.
mastoid c. antrum mastoideum.
mediastinal c., anterior mediastinum anterius.
mediastinal c., middle mediastinum medium.
mediastinal c., posterior mediastinum posterius.
mediastinal c., superior mediastinum superius.
medullary c. cavitas medullaris.
mesial c. a carious lesion beginning on the mesial surface of a tooth.
nasal c. cavitas nasi.
nerve c. cavitas dentis.
occlusal c. a carious lesion beginning on the occlusal surface of a posterior tooth.
oral c. cavitas oris.
oral c., external vestibulum oris.
oral c., proper cavitas oris propria.
orbital c. cavitas orbitalis.
pectoral c. thoracic cavity (see *cavitas thoracis* [TA]).
pelvic c. cavitas pelvis.
pericardial c. cavitas pericardialis.
peritoneal c., peritoneal c., greater cavitas peritonealis.
peritoneal c., lesser bursa omentalis.
pharyngeal c. cavitas pharyngis.
pharyngolaryngeal c. pars laryngea pharyngis.
pharyngonasal c. pars nasalis pharyngis.
pharyngo-oral c. pars oralis pharyngis.
pit c. see *pit caries,* under *caries.*
pleural c. cavitas pleuralis.
pleuroperitoneal c. the temporarily continuous coelomic cavity in the embryo, which will later be partitioned by the developing diaphragm to become the pleural and peritoneal cavities.
popliteal c. fossa poplitea.
prepared c. a cavity that is produced in a tooth to support and retain the filling material and protect the tooth structure remaining after removal of all carious tissue. See also *cavity preparation,* under *preparation.*
proximal c. a carious lesion beginning on a proximal (the mesial or distal) surface of a tooth.
pulp c. cavitas dentis.
resorption c. the area excavated by the osteoclasts in the process of bone turnover.
Retzius c. spatium retropubicum.
Rosenmüller c. recessus pharyngeus.
segmentation c. blastocoele.
c. of septum pellucidum cavum septi pellucidi.
serous c. a coelomic cavity that does not communicate with the outside of the body and whose lining membrane secretes a serous fluid, such as the cavity enclosed by the pericardium, peritoneum, or pleura.
simple c. a carious lesion that involves only one surface of a tooth in its preparation, designated according to the surface involved as buccal, distal, incisal, labial, lingual, mesial, or occlusal.
somatic c. the intraembryonic portion of the coelom.
somite c. myocoele.
splanchnic c. visceral c.
tension c's cavities of the lung in which the air pressure is greater than that of the atmosphere, as in tension pneumothorax. Radiologically, they appear as large, spherical, thin-walled defects indicative of productive inflammatory reaction in the bronchus that drains the cavity or of partial stenosis due to peribronchial fibrosis.
thoracic c. cavitas thoracis.
trigeminal c. cavum trigeminale.
tympanic c. cavitas tympani.
uterine c. cavitas uteri.
visceral c. one of the cavities of the body containing organs, such as the thoracic, abdominal, or pelvic cavity; called also *splanchnic c.*
yolk c. the space between the embryonic disc and the yolk of the developing ovum of certain animals.

ca•vog•ra•phy (ka-vog′rə-fe) venacavography.

ca•vo•sur•face (ka′vo-sur″fəs) the surface of a cavity, as of a tooth.

ca•vo•val•gus (ka″vo-val′gəs) see under *talipes.*

ca•vo•va•rus (ka″vo-va′rəs) see under *talipes.*

ca•vum (ka′vəm) pl. *ca′va* [L.] cave: a type of cavity.
c. con′chae TA alternative for *cavitas conchae.*
c. epidura′le spatium epidurale.
c. sep′ti pellu′cidi [TA] cave of septum pellucidum: the median cleft between the two laminae of the septum pellucidum; called also *pseudoventricle, cavity of septum pellucidum, Duncan ventricle, fifth ventricle, ventricle of Sylvius,* or *Vieussens ventricle.*
c. trigemina′le [TA] trigeminal cave: the small outpocketing of the dura mater surrounding the ganglion and divisions of the trigeminal nerve at the end of the petrous portion of the temporal bone; it contains the trigeminal ganglion. Called also *Meckel space,* and *trigeminal cavity.*

ca•vus (ka′vəs) [L. "hollow"] see under *talipes.*

ca•vy (ka′ve) guinea pig.

cay•enne (ki-, ka-yen′) [Tupi *quiinia* hot pepper] capsicum.

CB [L.] Chirur′giae Baccalau′reus (Bachelor of Surgery).

CBC complete blood count.

CBF cerebral blood flow.

CBG corticosteroid-binding globulin; see *transcortin.*

Cbl cobalamin. A variety of defects in the intracellular utilization of cobalamin (vitamin B_{12}) and the synthesis of its coenzyme forms have been denoted *CblA–CblG.*

CC chief complaint.

cc cubic centimeter *(on the JCAHO "Do Not Use" List).*

CCA congenital contractural arachnodactyly.

CCAT conglutinating complement absorption test.

CCF crystal-induced chemotactic factor.

CCHS congenital central hypoventilation syndrome.

CCK cholecystokinin.

CCNU lomustine.
methyl CCNU semustine.

CCP complement control protein; cyclic citrullinated peptide.

CCPD continuous cycling peritoneal dialysis.

CCU coronary care unit; critical care unit.

CD cadaveric donor (see under *transplantation*); cluster designation (see under *antigen* and *system*); conjugata diagonalis; curative dose.

CD_{50} median curative dose.

Cd cadmium; caudal or coccygeal, used in vertebral formulas.

cd candela.

2-CdA cladribine.

CDC Centers for Disease Control and Prevention.

CDDP cisplatin (*cis*-diamminedichloroplatinum).

cdf cumulative distribution function.

CDG congenital disorder of glycosylation.

CDH congenital dislocation of the hip; see *developmental dysplasia of the hip*, under *dysplasia*.

CDK cyclin-dependent kinase.

cDNA complementary (or copy) DNA.

CDP cytidine diphosphate.

CDP-di•ac•yl•glyc•er•ol (di-a″səl-glis′ər-ol) cytidine diphosphate carrying a diacylglycerol moiety; it is a key intermediate in the synthesis and resynthesis of phospholipids.

CDP-di•ac•yl•glyc•er•ol–ino•si•tol 3-phos•pha•ti•dyl•trans•fer•ase (di-a″səl-glis′ər-ol in-o′sĭ-tol fos″fə-ti″dəl-trans′fər-ās) [EC 2.7.8.11] an enzyme of the transferase class that catalyzes the formation of phosphatidylinositol from *myo*-inositol and the diacylglycerol moiety of CDPdiacylglycerol.

CDR complementarity determining region.

Ce cerium.

CEA carcinoembryonic antigen.

ce•as•mic (se-as′mik) [Gr. *keasma* chip] characterized by the persistence after birth of embryonic fissures.

ce•bo•ceph•a•lus (se″bo-sef′ə-ləs) a fetus exhibiting cebocephaly.

ce•bo•ceph•a•ly (se″bo-sef′ə-le) [Gr. *kebos* monkey + *-cephaly*] a developmental anomaly characterized by a monkeylike head, the nose being defective and the eyes close together.

ce•ca (se′kə) [L.] plural of *cecum*.

ce•cal (se′kəl) [L. *caecalis*] 1. ending in a blind passage. 2. pertaining to a cecum (see also *caecum*).

ce•cec•to•my (se-sek′tə-me) [*ceco-* + *-ectomy*] surgical removal of the cecum.

Ce•cil operation (urethroplasty) (se′səl) [Arthur Bond *Cecil*, American surgeon, 1885–1967] see under *operation*.

ce•ci•tis (se-si′tis) inflammation of the cecum; called also *typhlitis*.

Cec•lor (se′klor) trademark for preparations of cefaclor.

cec(o)- [L. *cecum*, q.v.] a combining form denoting relation to the cecum.

ce•co•cele (se′ko-sēl) cecal hernia.

ce•co•cen•tral (se″ko-sen′trəl) centrocecal.

ce•co•col•ic (se″ko-kol′ik) pertaining to the cecum and the colon.

ce•co•co•lon (se″ko-ko′lən) the cecum and colon considered as a unit.

ce•co•co•lo•pexy (se″ko-ko′lə-pek″se) an operation for fixing the cecum and ascending colon to the abdominal wall.

ce•co•co•los•to•my (se″ko-kə-los′tə-me) 1. surgical creation of an anastomosis between the cecum and the colon; called also *colocecostomy*. 2. the anastomosis so created.

ce•co•cys•to•plas•ty (se″ko-sis′to-plas″te) augmentation cystoplasty using an isolated part of the cecum for the added segment.

ce•co•il•e•os•to•my (se″ko-il″e-os′tə-me) [*ceco-* + *ileostomy*] ileocecostomy.

ce•co•pexy (se′ko-pek″se) [*ceco-* + *-pexy*] fixation or suspension of the cecum to correct excessive mobility of the organ.

ce•co•pli•ca•tion (se″ko-plĭ-ka′shən) [*ceco-* + *plication*] plication of the cecal wall to correct ptosis or dilatation of the organ.

ce•cor•rha•phy (se-kor′ə-fe) [*ceco-* + *-rrhaphy*] suture or repair of the cecum.

ce•co•sig•moid•os•to•my (se″ko-sig″moi-dos′tə-me) 1. creation of an artificial opening between the cecum and sigmoid, usually surgically. 2. the opening so created.

ce•cos•to•my (se-kos′tə-me) [*ceco-* + *-stomy*] 1. surgical creation of an artificial opening or fistula into the cecum. 2. the opening so created.

ce•cot•o•my (se-kot′ə-me) [*ceco-* + *-tomy*] the operation of cutting into the cecum.

ce•co•ure•ter•o•cele (se″ko-u-re′tər-o-sēl) a ureterocele in which a blind pouch or cecum extends into the submucosa of the bladder or urethra.

ce•cum (se′kəm) [L. *caecum* blind, blind gut] 1. any blind pouch or cul-de-sac. 2. caecum.

gastric ceca outpocketings of the midgut, of uncertain function, seen in many insects.

high c. a cecum situated higher up in the abdomen than normal.

mobile c., c. mo′bile abnormal mobility of the cecum and lower portion of the ascending colon, caused by incomplete rotation or faulty fixation of the cecum in embryonic development.

ce•dar (se′dər) 1. one of the true cedars, evergreen trees of the genus *Cedrus*. 2. any of numerous coniferous evergreen trees resembling those of the genus *Cedrus*, especially from the genera *Juniperus* and *Thuja*.

red c. *Juniperus virginiana*.

western red c. *Thuja plicata*.

white c. *Thuja occidentalis*.

Ce•dax (se′daks) trademark for a preparation of ceftibuten.

Ce•de•cea (se-de′se-ə) [Centers for Disease Control and Prevention (CDC), q.v.] a genus of gram-negative, facultatively anaerobic, rod-shaped bacteria of the family Enterobacteriaceae, isolated primarily from clinical specimens of the human respiratory tract, and a possible opportunistic pathogen. The type species is *C. da′visae*.

Ce•dio•psyl•la (se″de-o-sil′ə) a genus of fleas, including some of the rabbit fleas.

CEE conjugated equine estrogens.

CeeNU (se′noo) trademark for preparations of lomustine.

cef•a•clor (sef′ə-klor) [USP] a semisynthetic, second-generation cephalosporin effective against a wide range of gram-positive and gram-negative bacteria, used in the treatment of infections of the urinary and respiratory tracts and of the skin and soft tissues; administered orally.

cef•a•drox•il (sef″ə-droks′il) [USP] a semisynthetic first-generation cephalosporin effective against a wide range of gram-positive and a very limited number of gram-negative bacteria; administered orally in the treatment of infections of the urinary and respiratory tracts and of the skin and soft tissues.

Cef•a•dyl (sef′ə-dəl) trademark for a preparation of cephapirin sodium.

cef•a•man•dole (sef″ə-man′dōl) a semisynthetic second-generation cephalosporin, having some resistance to β-lactamases.

c. nafate [USP] the sodium salt of cefamandole formyl ester, used in the treatment of infections of the skin and soft tissues and respiratory and urinary tracts; administered intravenously or intramuscularly.

cef•a•tri•zine (sef″ə-tri′zēn) a semisynthetic cephalosporin with actions and uses similar to those of cephalexin.

ce•faz•o•lin (sə-faz′o-lin) [USP] a first-generation cephalosporin, a semisynthetic analogue of the natural antibiotic cephalosporin C, effective against a wide range of gram-positive and a limited range of gram-negative bacteria.

c. sodium [USP] the monosodium salt of cefazolin, having the same actions as the base; used in the treatment of a wide variety of infections caused by sensitive pathogens; administered intramuscularly and intravenously.

cef•din•ir (sef′dĭ-nir) a semisynthetic, third-generation cephalosporin effective against a wide range of bacteria, used in the treatment of otitis media, bronchitis, pharyngitis, tonsillitis, sinusitis, bacterial pneumonia, and skin and soft tissue infections; administered orally.

cef•di•tor•en pi•vox•il (sef″dĭ-tor′ən) a third-generation cephalosporin antibiotic active against a wide range of bacteria, used for infections of the respiratory tract or skin.

cef•e•pime (sef′ə-pēm) a semisynthetic fourth-generation cephalosporin, having greater resistance to β-lactamases than do the third-generation cephalosporins.

c. hydrochloride the hydrochloride salt of cefepime, used in treatment of infections of the skin and soft tissues and of the respiratory and urinary tracts; administered intramuscularly or intravenously.

ce•fix•ime (sə-fik′sēm) [USP] a semisynthetic, third-generation cephalosporin effective against a wide range of bacteria, used in the treatment of otitis media, bronchitis, pharyngitis, tonsillitis, gonorrhea, and urinary tract infections; administered orally.

Cef•i•zox (sef′ĭ-zoks) trademark for a preparation of ceftizoxime sodium.

cef•men•ox•ime hy•dro•chlo•ride (sef″men-ok′sēm) [USP] a third-generation cephalosporin structurally related to cefotaxime and ceftizoxime, and having actions and uses similar to those of cefotaxime sodium; administered intramuscularly and intravenously.

cef•met•a•zole (sef-met′ə-zōl) [USP] a cephamycin antibiotic derived from cephamycin C and generally classified with the second-generation cephalosporins, having activity and uses similar to those of cefoxitin.

c. sodium [USP] the monosodium salt of cefmetazole, having the same actions and uses as the base.

Cef•o•bid (sef′o-bid) trademark for a preparation of cefoperazone sodium.

ce•fon•i•cid so•di•um (sə-fon′ĭ-sid) [USP] a semisynthetic, broad-spectrum, β-lactamase–resistant, second-generation cephalosporin effective against a wide range of gram-positive and gram-negative bacteria; administered parenterally.

cef•o•per•a•zone so•di•um (sef″o-per′ə-zōn) [USP] a semisynthetic, broad-spectrum, β-lactamase–resistant, third-generation cephalosporin effective against a wide range of aerobic and anaerobic gram-positive and gram-negative bacteria.

ce•for•a•nide (sə-for′ə-nīd) [USP] a semisynthetic second-generation cephalosporin with actions and uses similar to those of cefamandole; administered intramuscularly or intravenously.

Cef•o•tan (sef′o-tan) trademark for a preparation of cefotetan disodium.

cef•o•tax•ime so•di•um (sef″o-tak′sēm) [USP] a semisynthetic, broad-spectrum, β-lactamase–resistant, third-generation cephalosporin effective against a wide variety of gram-negative bacteria but less active against gram-positive cocci than are the first- and second-generation cephalosporins; administered intramuscularly or intravenously.

cef•o•te•tan (sef′o-te″tən) [USP] a semisynthetic cephamycin derived from cephamycin C and generally classified with the second-generation cephalosporins, effective against a wide range of gram-positive and gram-negative bacteria.

c. **disodium** [USP] the disodium salt of cefotetan, used for the treatment of a wide variety of infections caused by susceptible organisms; administered intravenously or intramuscularly.

cef•o•ti•am hy•dro•chlo•ride (sef″o-ti′əm) [USP] a cephalosporin having actions and uses similar to those of cefamandole; administered intramuscularly and intravenously.

ce•fox•i•tin (sə-fok′sĭ-tin) a cephamycin antibiotic derived from cephamycin C and generally classified with the second-generation cephalosporins, effective against a wide range of gram-positive and gram-negative organisms, with strong resistance to β-lactamases.

c. **sodium** [USP] the monosodium salt of cefoxitin, used to treat infections caused by susceptible organisms; administered intravenously.

cef•pir•a•mide (sef-pir′ə-mīd) [USP] a third-generation cephalosporin structurally related to cefoperazone, effective against *Pseudomonas aeruginosa*, staphylococci, and streptococci; administered by injection.

cef•po•dox•ime prox•e•til (sef″po-dok′sēm prok′sə-til) a broad-spectrum, β-lactamase–resistant, third-generation cephalosporin, effective against a wide range of gram-positive and gram-negative bacteria; administered orally.

cef•pro•zil (sef-pro′zil) [USP] a semisynthetic, broad-spectrum, second-generation cephalosporin effective against a wide range of gram-negative and gram-positive organisms, used in the treatment of otitis media and infections of the respiratory and oropharyngeal tracts, skin, and soft tissues; administered orally.

cef•ta•zi•dime (sef-taz′ĭ-dēm″) [USP] a semisynthetic, broad-spectrum, third-generation cephalosporin that acts by inhibiting enzymes responsible for cell-wall synthesis; effective against gram-positive and gram-negative bacteria; administered intravenously and intramuscularly.

cef•ti•bu•ten (sef-ti′bu-tən) a third-generation cephalosporin used in treatment of bronchitis, pharyngitis, tonsillitis, and acute otitis media; administered orally.

Cef•tin (sef′tin) trademark for a preparation of cefuroxime axetil.

cef•ti•o•fur so•di•um (sef-ti′o-foor) a semisynthetic cephalosporin used in cattle.

cef•ti•zox•ime so•di•um (sef″tĭ-zok′sēm) [USP] a semisynthetic, β-lactamase–resistant, third-generation cephalosporin effective against a wide range of aerobic and anaerobic gram-positive and gram-negative bacteria; administered intravenously or intramuscularly.

cef•tri•ax•one so•di•um (sef″tri-ak′sōn) [USP] a semisynthetic, β-lactamase–resistant, broad-spectrum, third-generation cephalosporin effective against a wide range of gram-positive and gram-negative bacteria; administered intravenously or intramuscularly.

cef•u•rox•ime (sef″u-rok′sēm) a semisynthetic, broad-spectrum, β-lactamase–resistant, second-generation cephalosporin effective against a wide range of gram-positive and gram-negative bacteria.

c. **axetil** [USP] an ester of cefuroxime with increased lipid solubility and better gastrointestinal absorption, for oral administration.

c. **sodium** [USP] the monosodium salt of cefuroxime, having similar actions and uses as the base; administered intramuscularly or intravenously.

Cef•zil (sef′zil) trademark for a preparation of cefprozil.

Ceg•ka sign (cheg′kah) [Josephus Joannes *Cegka*, Czech physician, 1812–1862] see under *sign*.

Cel Celsius; see *Celsius scale*, under *scale*.

cel (sel) a unit of velocity, being the velocity of 1 cm. per second.

-cele[1] [Gr. *kēlē* tumor, hernia] a word termination denoting relationship to a tumor or swelling.

-cele[2] [Gr. *koilos* hollow] a word termination denoting relationship to a cavity; see also words spelled *-coele*.

Cel•e•brex (sel′ə-breks) trademark for a preparation of celecoxib.

cel•e•cox•ib (sel″ə-kok′sib) a nonsteroidal antiinflammatory drug of the COX-2 inhibitors group, used for symptomatic treatment of osteoarthritis and rheumatoid arthritis; administered orally.

ce•len•ter•on (sə-len′tər-on) 1. archenteron. 2. gastrovascular cavity.

Ce•les•tone (sə-les′tōn) trademark for preparations of betamethasone.

Ce•lex•a (sə-lek′sə) trademark for a preparation of citalopram hydrobromide.

ce•li•ac (se′le-ak) abdominal.

ce•li•a•co•du•o•de•nal (se-li″ə-ko-doo-ə-de′nəl) pertaining to the celiac trunk and the duodenum.

celi(o)- [Gr. *koilia* belly] a combining form denoting relationship to the abdomen. For words beginning thus, see also words beginning *cel(o)-* and *coel(o)-*.

ce•lio•col•pot•o•my (se″le-o-kol-pot′ə-me) [*celio-* + *colpo-* + *-tomy*] incision into the abdomen through the vaginal wall.

ce•li•o•ma (se″le-o′mə) [*celio-* + *-oma*] a tumor of the abdomen, especially mesothelioma of the peritoneum.

ce•lio•scope (se′le-o-skōp″) laparoscope.

ce•li•os•co•py (se″le-os′kə-pe) laparoscopy.

ce•li•ot•o•my (se″le-ot′ə-me) laparotomy.

vaginal c. see under *laparotomy*.

ventral c. incision into the abdominal cavity through the abdominal wall.

ce•li•tis (se-li′tis) any abdominal inflammation.

cell (sel) [L. *cella* compartment] 1. the smallest living unit capable of independent function, consisting of cytoplasm containing various subcellular compartments (organelles and cytosol) and separated from the external environment by the plasma membrane. Eukaryotic cells also include a nucleus containing the genome and nucleolus; prokaryotic cells lack a nucleus and DNA is present as a naked chromosome. Cells may exist as independent organisms or, with specialization for specific functions, be subunits of more complex organisms. See Plates 11 and 12. 2. a small, more or less enclosed space; see also *cellula*.

Cell

A c. 1. alpha cell (def. 1). 2. acidophil (def. 2). 3. amacrine c.

accessory c. a type of cell, predominantly of the monocyte-macrophage lineage, that cooperates with B and T lymphocytes in the generation of the immune response.

acid c's parietal c's.

acinar c., acinic c., acinous c. any of the cells lining an acinus, especially applied to the zymogen-secreting cells of the pancreatic acini.

acoustic hair c's auditory hair c's.

adipose c. fat c.

adventitial c. pericyte.

agger nasi c's the cells of the anterior part of the ethmoidal crest of the maxilla, constituting the air-filled part of the lacrimal bone.

air c. 1. any minute bodily chamber filled with air, such as an alveolus of the lung. 2. a cavity containing air and surrounded by a bodily structure, usually one of the bones of the head, such as an ethmoidal air cell, mastoid air cell, or tubal air cell.

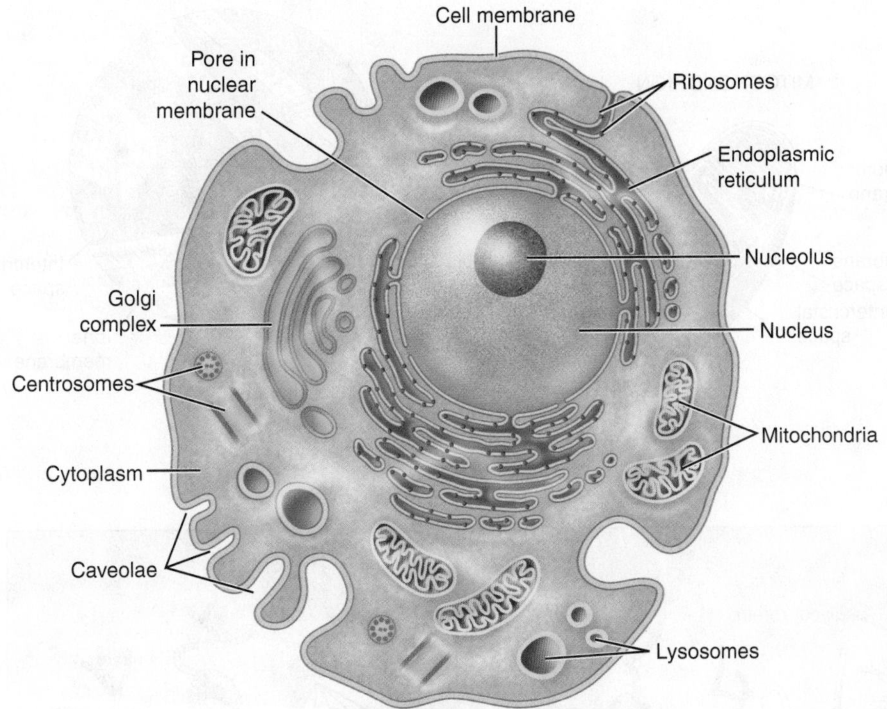

IDEALIZED ANIMAL CELL

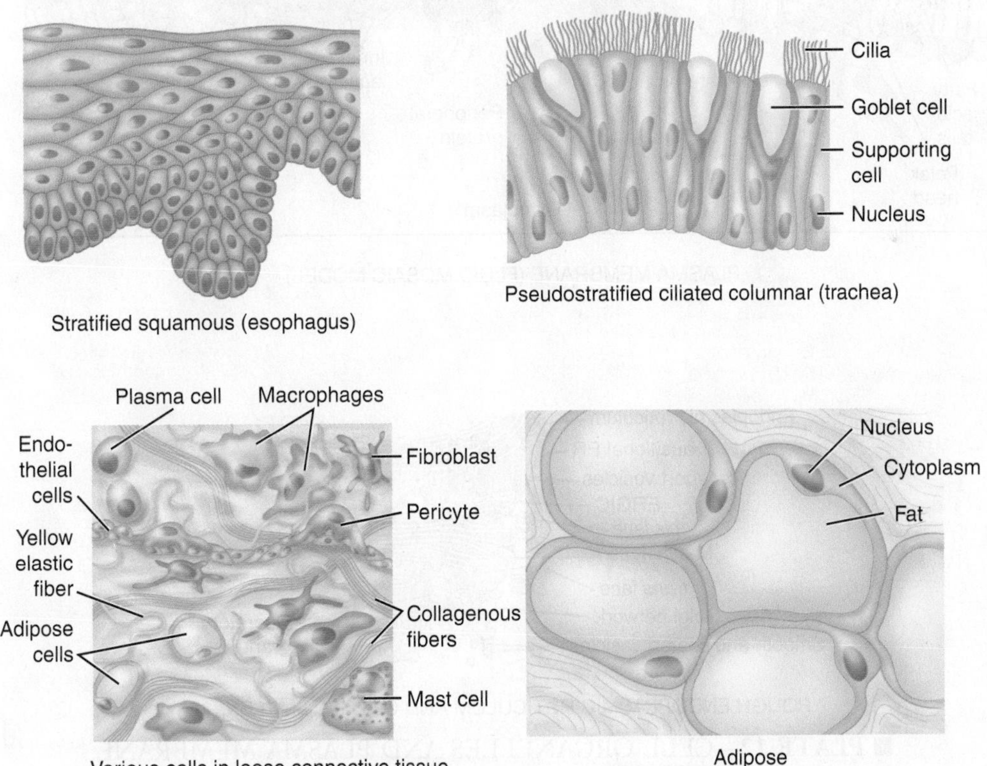

Stratified squamous (esophagus)

Pseudostratified ciliated columnar (trachea)

Various cells in loose connective tissue

Adipose

SEVERAL TYPES OF CELLS

■ **PLATE 11**—THE CELL: CELL STRUCTURES AND EPITHELIAL CELL TYPES

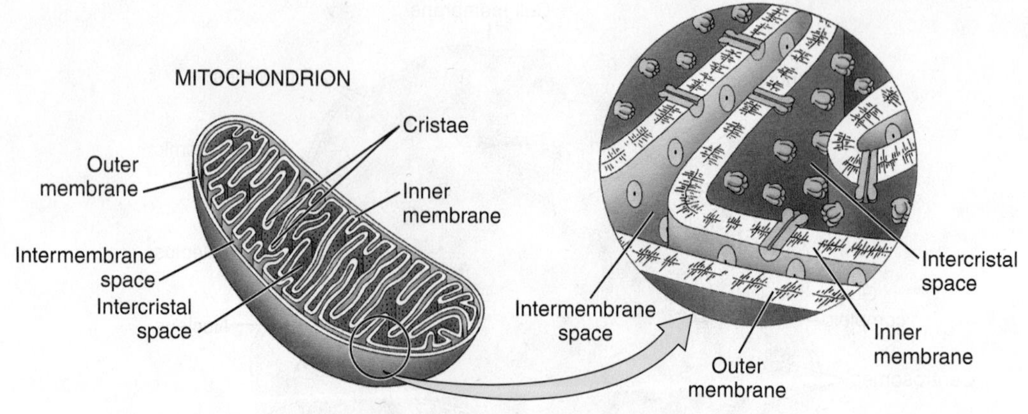

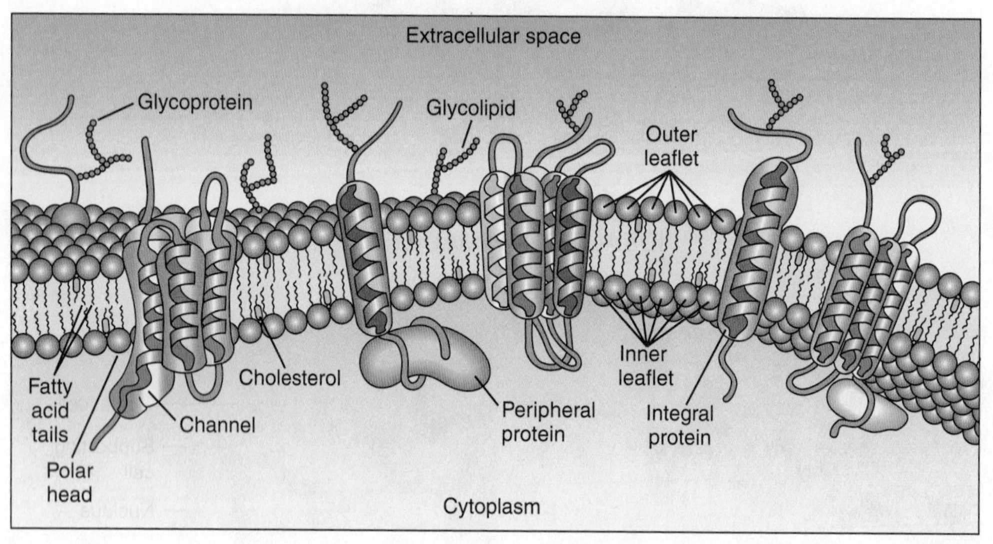

PLASMA MEMBRANE (FLUID MOSAIC MODEL)

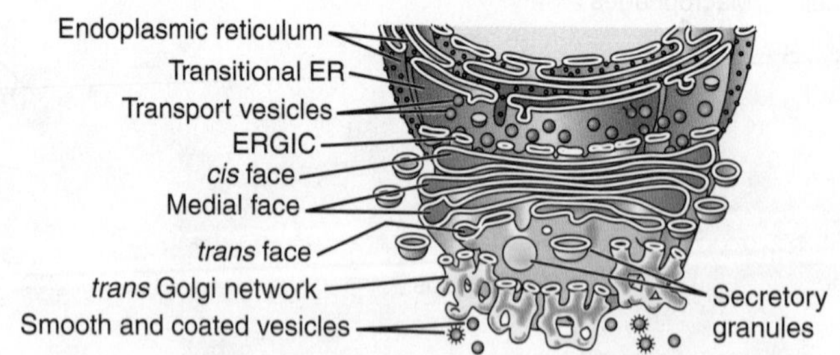

ROUGH ENDOPLASMIC RETICULUM AND GOLGI COMPLEX

■ PLATE 12—CELL ORGANELLES AND PLASMA MEMBRANE

air c's of auditory tube cellulae pneumaticae tubae auditivae.
albuminous c. serous c.
alpha c. 1. a type of islet cell that is found in the periphery of the pancreatic islets and secretes either somatostatin ($alpha_1$ cells) or glucagon ($alpha_2$ cells). 2. acidophil (def. 2).
alveolar c. any cell of the walls of the pulmonary alveoli; the term is often limited to alveolar epithelial cells (type I and type II alveolar cells) and alveolar macrophages. Called also *pneumocyte* and *pneumonocyte.*
alveolar epithelial c's the cells of the alveolar epithelium; see *type I alveolar c's* and *type II alveolar c's.*
Alzheimer c. Alzheimer type II astrocyte.
amacrine c. any of five types of retinal neurons that seem to lack large axons, having only processes that resemble dendrites. Called also *A c.*
ameboid c. any cell capable of ameboid movement; called also *amebocyte* and *wandering c.*
amine precursor uptake and decarboxylation c's APUD c's.
amphophilic c. a cell that stains readily with either acid or basic dyes; called also *amphocyte, amphophil, amphochromatophil,* and *amphochromophil.*
Anichkov (Anitschkow) c. a plump modified macrophage found in the Aschoff bodies, inflammatory lesions of the heart characteristic of rheumatic fever; they contain round to ovoid nuclei with a central, slender ribbon of chromatin. Called also *Anichkov myocyte, cardiac histiocyte,* and *caterpillar c.*
anterior horn c's motoneurons whose cell bodies are in the anterior horn of the spinal cord; see *alpha motoneurons* and *gamma motoneurons,* under *motoneuron.*
antigen-presenting c's cells that take part in antigen presentation (see under *presentation*); a group of dendritic cells that arise in the bone marrow and migrate to other body sites. They process antigens and put them on their surfaces to react with lymphocytes and induce an immune response. The group includes follicular dendritic cells in B-dependent areas of lymphoid tissues, interdigitating cells in T-dependent areas, Langerhans cells in the epidermis, and veil cells in lymphoid tissue.
antigen-reactive c's 1. T lymphocytes that rapidly proliferate in response to challenge by antigen. 2. antigen-sensitive c's.
antigen-sensitive c's small lymphocytes that when exposed to antigen can differentiate into antibody-producing cells. Called also *antigen-reactive c's.*
apocrine c's see *apocrine.*
apolar c. a neuron with no processes or poles.
APUD c's amine precursor uptake and decarboxylation cells: a diffuse group of cells, many originating in the neural crest, that share certain cytochemical and ultrastructural characteristics and are found scattered throughout the body; types include melanocytes, the cells of the chromaffin system, and cells in the hypothalamus, hypophysis, thyroid, parathyroids, lungs, gastrointestinal tract, and pancreas. They concentrate the amino acid precursors of certain amines and decarboxylate them, forming amines that function as regulators and neurotransmitters. They produce substances such as epinephrine, norepinephrine, dopamine, serotonin, enkephalin, somatostatin, neurotensin, and substance P, the actions of which may affect contiguous cells, nearby groups of cells, or distant cells, thus functioning as local or systemic hormones. See also *basal granular c's.*
arachnoid cap c. a type of epithelial cell in the arachnoid membrane; these are the cells of origin of some types of meningiomas.
argentaffin c's enterochromaffin cells whose granules stain readily with chromium and silver salts, located in the basilar portions of the glands of the gastrointestinal tract. Cf. *argyrophilic c's.* See also *argentaffinoma.*
argyrophilic c's enterochromaffin cells that require exposure to a reducing substance before their granules will react with silver; they are located in the fundic and pyloric glands between the basement lamina and zymogenic cells. Cf. *argentaffin c's.*
Arias-Stella c's cells in the endometrial epithelium which have hyperchromatic enlarged nuclei; they appear to be hypersecretory and associated with chorionic tissue in an intrauterine or extrauterine site.
Armanni-Ebstein c's vacuolated epithelial cells in the proximal straight tubules of the kidney, containing deposits of glycogen. See also *Armanni-Ebstein lesion,* under *lesion.*
Aschoff c. 1. Anichkov c. 2. sometimes restricted to the larger, multinucleate giant cell type of Anichkov cell.
Askanazy c's large granular eosinophilic cells, rich in mitochondria, found in the thyroid gland in autoimmune thyroiditis and Hürthle cell tumors. Called also *Hürthle c's, interfollicular c's, oxyphil c's,* and *oxyphils.*
auditory c's, auditory hair c's the hair cells in the organ of Corti whose cilia serve as sensory receptors for hearing. There are two types, inner hair cells and outer hair cells, having differing functions. Called also *acoustic* or *cochlear hair c.*
automatic c. pacemaker c.
B c. 1. beta c. (def. 1). 2. basophil (def. 3). 3. *(in the pl.)* see under *lymphocyte.*
balloon c. a type of unusual, swollen, degenerated cell with pale, almost clear, abundant cytoplasm; one variety is seen in the vesicles of herpes zoster and varicella and another is seen in a balloon cell nevus.
band c. a late metamyelocyte in which the nucleus is in the form of a curved or coiled band, not having acquired the typical multilobar shape of the mature polymorphonuclear neutrophil. Called also *band form* or *neutrophil, rod neutrophil,* and *stab c.* or *neutrophil.*
basal c. a type of keratinocyte found in the basal layer of the epidermis.
basal granular c's enteroendocrine c's.
basaloid c. a type of tumor cell that resembles a basal cell, seen in certain types of skin cancer. Cf. *basaloid carcinoma.*
basket c. 1. a cell of the cerebellar cortex whose axon gives off brushes of fibrils, forming a basketlike nest in which the body of each Purkinje cell rests. 2. myoepithelial c.
beaker c. goblet c.
Beale ganglion c's bipolar cells with one process coiled around the other; found in cardiac ganglia.
Bergmann c's peculiar glial cells in the molecular layer of the cerebellar cortex having dendrites that extend outward through that layer; called also *Bergmann glia.*
beta c. 1. the type of islet cell that makes up the bulk of the islets of Langerhans and secretes insulin. 2. basophil (def. 3).
Betz c's large pyramidal ganglion cells found in the internal pyramidal layer of the cerebral cortex; called also *giant pyramidal c's.*
bipolar c. a nerve cell with two processes.
bipolar retinal c's various types of bipolar neurons that are the second, intermediate, neurons in the vertical linkage of the retina and are analogous to the spinal ganglia. See also *visual c's.*
bladder c's swollen cells in the epidermis of the tips of the fingers and toes of the embryo. Called also *Zander c's.*
blast c. 1. blast[1] (def. 1). 2. in the monophyletic theory, the least differentiated, totipotential blood cell without commitment as to its particular series, from which all blood cells are derived, preceding a *stem cell.* Called also *blast, hematoblast, hematocytoblast, hemoblast,* and *hemocytoblast.*
blood c. one of the formed elements of the blood; a leukocyte, erythrocyte, or platelet. Called also *blood corpuscle, hemacyte, hematocyte,* and *hemocyte.*
bone c. a nucleated cell occupying a lacuna of bone; called also *osseous c.* and *bone corpuscle.*
border c's a row of columnar supporting cells that delimit the inner boundary of the organ of Corti.
Böttcher c's small groups of polyhedral cells interposed between Claudius cells and the basilar membrane of the cochlea.
bowenoid c's neoplastic cells derived from the epidermis, constituting lesions of Bowen disease.
breviradiate c's neuroglial cells that have short processes.
bristle c's auditory hair cells.
burr c. a spiculed erythrocyte that has multiple small projections evenly spaced over the cell circumference; observed in azotemia, gastric carcinoma, and bleeding peptic ulcer. Called also *burr erythrocyte, crenated erythrocyte, crenocyte,* and *echinocyte.*

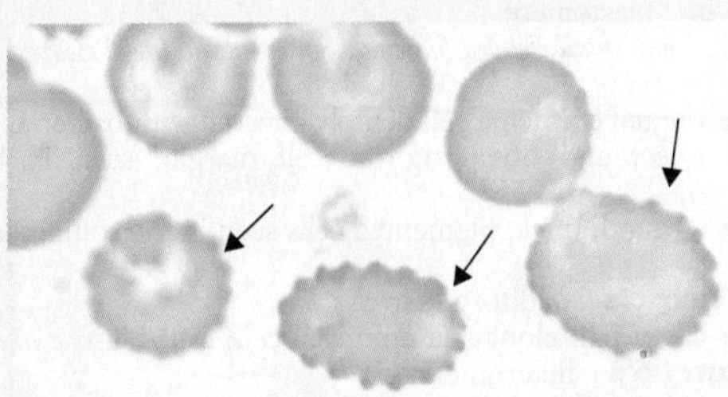

■ Burr cells *(arrows).*

C c's 1. parafollicular c's. 2. a type of cells that lack granules, such as are found in the pancreatic islets of guinea pigs. 3. chromophobe c's.
Cajal c. 1. astrocyte. 2. one of the neuroglial cells arranged horizontally in the molecular layer of the cerebral cortex; called also *horizontal c. of Cajal.*
caliciform c. goblet c.
capsule c's satellite c's (def. 1).
cartilage c. chondrocyte.
castration c's vacuolated basophil cells that develop in the anterior pituitary gland after castration.
caterpillar c. Anichkov c.
caudate c's neuroglial cells of the gray matter having several streaming prolongations like the tail of a comet.
caveolated c's epithelial cells with thick, short, apical microvilli containing bundles of filaments extending down into the cytoplasm and with irregular tubules (caveolae) passing as invaginations from the apical surface between microvilli; occasionally found in the small intestine and respiratory tract and thought to function as chemoreceptors.
CD4 c's, CD4$^+$ c's a major classification of T lymphocytes, referring to those that carry the CD4 antigen; most are helper cells. Called also *CD4 T lymphocytes.*
CD8 c's, CD8$^+$ c's a major classification of T lymphocytes, referring to those that carry the CD8 antigen; major subtypes are the cytotoxic T lymphocytes and the suppressor cells. Called also *CD8 T lymphocytes.*
cement c. cementocyte.
centroacinar c's the beginnings of the intralobular duct system of the pancreas within the pancreatic acini.
chalice c. goblet c.
chief c's 1. epithelial cells, either columnar or cuboidal, that line the lower portions of the gastric glands and secrete pepsin; called also *peptic c's.* 2. pinealocytes. 3. the most abundant cells of the parathyroid glands, being polygonal epithelial cells rich in glycogen, having granular cytoplasm and vesicular nuclei, and arranged in plates or cords. Called also *principal c's.* 4. the principal chromaffin cells of the paraganglia, each of which is surrounded by supporting cells. 5. chromophobe c's.
Chinese hamster ovary c's, CHO c's an established line of fibroblasts isolated from the ovary of a spontaneous aneuploid mutant Chinese hamster; used in a variety of biomedical applications.
chromaffin c's a type of APUD cells that stain readily with chromium salts, their cytoplasmic granules taking on a characteristic brown color; they are found especially in cells of the adrenal medulla and in paraganglia of the coccygeal gland and carotid gland, along the sympathetic nerves, and in various organs. They contain chromaffin granules. See also *enterochromaffin c's* and *argentaffin c's.* Called also *pheochrome cells* and *pheochromocytes.*
chromophobe c's, chromophobic c's small, faintly staining cells with scanty cytoplasm found often in clusters in the center of the cell cords in the adenohypophysis; their cytoplasm was formerly thought to be nongranular, but the granules are now known to be simply small and sparse. These cells are increased in chromophobic or null-cell adenomas. Called also *C c's, chief c's,* and *gamma c's of hypophysis.*
ciliated c. any cell with cilia.
Clara c's unciliated cells found in the epithelium of the respiratory and terminal bronchioles.
Clarke c's pigmented cells in the thoracic column of the spinal cord.
Claudius c's cuboidal cells found in the floor of the external spiral sulcus, external to the organ of Corti.
clear c's cells with empty-appearing cytoplasm, seen normally in the secretory coil of sweat glands, in the parathyroid glands, and in the lining of the renal collecting tubules and epididymis; they also occur pathologically in some neoplastic conditions.
cleavage c. blastomere.
cleaved c. see *small cleaved follicular center c.* and *large cleaved follicular center c.*
clue c. a vaginal epithelial cell densely covered with bacteria, creating a stippled effect and obscuring the cell margin; seen in bacterial vaginosis.
clump c's round, thick, pigmented cells seen in the sphincter muscle of the iris.
cochlear hair c's auditory hair c's.
columnar c. a tall, elongated epithelial cell; called also *cylindrical c.*
commissural c's heteromeral c's.
committed c. a lymphocyte which, after contact with antigen, is obligated to follow an individual course of development. In the bone marrow, these arise from pluripotential stem cells and themselves form precursor lines for various blood cells.
compound granule c. gitter c.
cone c. retinal cone.
conidiogenous c. a fungal cell that produces a conidium; see also *conidiogenesis.*
connective tissue c's any of the cellular elements of the fibrous and nonfibrous components of the various forms of connective tissue.
contractile fiber c's the spindle-shaped and nucleated cells which, collected into bundles, make up unstriated or smooth muscle.
contrasuppressor c's cells that augment the immune response by suppressing the activity of other suppressor cells, or by rendering the reactive cell unresponsive to suppression.
c's of Corti auditory hair c's.
corticotrope c., corticotroph c. corticotroph.
corticotroph-lipotroph c. corticotroph.
corticotropic c. corticotroph.
counting c. hemacytometer.
cover c. any cell that covers and protects other cells, especially any long epithelial cell of the outer layer of the taste buds; called also *encasing c.* and *incasing c.*
crescent c's Giannuzzi crescents.
Crooke c's the pituitary corticotrophs seen in Crooke hyalinization.
cuboid c., cuboidal c. an epithelial cell whose transverse and vertical diameters are approximately equal.
Custer c's cells with long delicate protoplasmic processes replacing the lymphoid tissue of lymph nodes in various lymphoproliferative disorders.
cylindric c., cylindrical c. columnar c.
cytotoxic T c's cytotoxic T lymphocytes.
cytotrophoblastic c. a type of polygonal, mononucleate cell resembling the cells of the cytotrophoblast, having prominent nucleoli and clear, eosinophilic or cyanophilous cytoplasm; one of the two cell types that compose a choriocarcinoma. Cf. *syncytiotrophoblastic c.*
D c. delta cell (def. 1).
dark c's intercalated c's.
daughter c. one of the two or more cells formed by the division of a mother cell.
Davidoff (Davidov) c's Paneth c's.
decidual c's cells of the uterine endometrium that become modified and specialized during pregnancy.
decoy c's a type of intranuclear viral inclusions found in immunocompromised patients with polyomavirus infections and detected when they are shed in the urine.
Deiters c's the outer phalangeal cells of the organ of Corti; they support the outer hair cells.
delta c. 1. a type of islet cell that secretes somatostatin. 2. gonadotroph.
demilune c's Giannuzzi crescents.
dendritic c's 1. a heterogeneous group of nonphagocytic lymph node constituents comprising follicular dendritic cells of the germinal centers, interdigitating cells of the deep cortex, and veil cells of the afferent lymphatic vessels and lymphatic sinuses; all such cells have an irregular shape with numerous branching processes and an inconspicuous complement of cell organelles. 2. follicular dendritic c's.
dense-core c. the smaller of the two morphological forms of bacteria of the family Anaplasmataceae, characterized by a dense condensation of chromatin strands, seen predominantly in cells propagated in vitro. Cf *reticulate c.*
dentin c. odontoblast.
dome c's the large cells that compose the epitrichium of the fetus.
Dorothy Reed c's Reed-Sternberg c's.
Downey c. any of several atypical lymphocytes seen in infectious mononucleosis. There are three types: *type I* cells are mature ones with a kidney-shaped or lobulated nucleus and vacuolated, basophilic, foamy cytoplasm; *type II* cells contain plasmacytoid nuclei with less vacuolated and basophilic cytoplasm; and *type III* cells have a finer chromatin pattern and one or two nucleoli.
dust c. alveolar macrophage.
ECL c. enterochromaffin-like c.
effector c. 1. a cell that becomes active in response to stimulation. 2. in immunology, a differentiated lymphocyte that carries out some part of the immune response, e.g., antibody production, lymphokine production, or helper, suppressor, or killer function. Cf. *memory c.*

electrochemical c. an apparatus consisting of two half-cells, each containing a solution in which an electrode is placed, connected by a salt bridge or semipermeable membrane. A voltaic cell is one in which chemical reactions occurring at the electrodes supply a voltage to an external circuit; an electrolytic cell is one in which an applied voltage drives the reactions occurring at the electrodes in the opposite direction from that in which they proceed spontaneously.
electrolytic c. an electrochemical cell (q.v.) to which voltage is applied to drive chemical reactions.
elementary c., embryonic c. blastomere.
embryonic stem c's totipotent stem cells derived from the embryoblast or inner cell mass of the blastocyst.
emigrated c. a leukocyte that has undergone diapedesis through the wall of a blood vessel and is in the neighboring tissue.
enamel c. ameloblast.
encasing c. cover c.
endocrine c's of the gut enteroendocrine c's.
endothelioid c. a large cell frequently seen in disease of the hematopoietic tissues; it is perhaps derived from the endothelial lining of blood vessels and lymph vessels.
enterochromaffin c's endocrine cells whose granules stain readily with silver and chromium salts, and which are sites of synthesis and storage of serotonin. They are distributed throughout the body but are most frequently identified in the intestinal and bronchial submucosa. Based upon their staining reactions with silver, these cells have been divided between those that reduce silver without pretreatment *(argentaffin cells)* and those that require prior exposure to a reducing substance *(argyrophilic cells)*.
enterochromaffin-like c. a paracrine cell of the fundic glands that controls the secretion of acid by releasing histamine in response to stimulation by gastrin. Called also *ECL c.*
enteroendocrine c's a group of APUD cells, which may be divided into a number of populations on the basis of polypeptide hormone and biogenic amine production, found scattered throughout the gastrointestinal epithelium, mainly at the base of the epithelium; their numerous small secretory granules are concentrated chiefly between the nucleus and the cell base. Their secretions affect gastrointestinal motility, pancreatic and biliary secretions, and gastrointestinal epithelial growth, as well as being regulators of other enteroendocrine products. Called also *basal granular c's* and *endocrine c's of the gut.*
ependymal c's the cells of the ependyma; called also *ependymocytes.*
epidermal c. a cell of the epidermis; the most common types are keratinocytes and melanocytes.
epithelial c. any of the cells that cover the surface of the body and line its cavities.
epithelioid c. 1. a large polyhedral cell of connective tissue origin. 2. a type of highly phagocytic, modified macrophage, resembling an epithelial cell, having a large, pale, vesicular nucleus with abundant, eosinophilic cytoplasm. Epithelioid cells are characteristic of granulomatous inflammation, and sometimes coalesce to form multinucleate giant cells. 3. pinealocyte.
erythroid c's blood cells of the erythrocytic series.
ethmoid c's, ethmoid air c's cellulae ethmoidales.
ethmoidal c's cellulae ethmoidales.
ethmoidal c's, anterior cellulae ethmoidales anteriores.
ethmoidal c's, middle cellulae ethmoidales mediae.

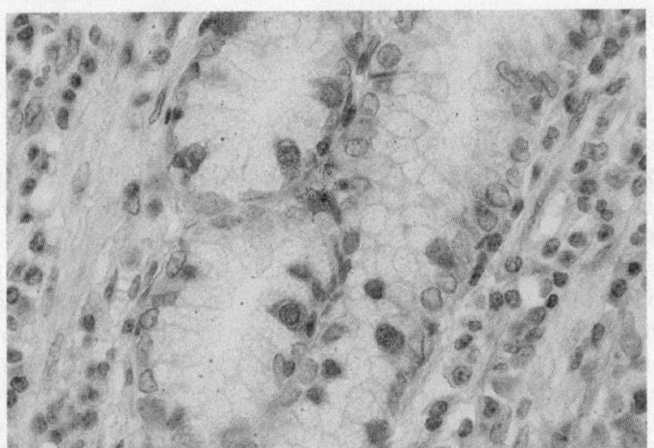

■ Scattered G cells *(pink)* in immunoperoxidase stain of pyloric glands.

ethmoidal c's, posterior cellulae ethmoidales posteriores.
ethmoidal air c's cellulae ethmoidales.
ethmoidal air c's, anterior cellulae ethmoidales anteriores.
ethmoidal air c's, middle cellulae ethmoidales mediae.
ethmoidal air c's, posterior cellulae ethmoidales posteriores.
eukaryotic c. a cell with a true nucleus; see *eukaryote.*
excitable c. a cell that can generate an action potential at its membrane in response to depolarization and may transmit an impulse along the membrane; most are nerve cells or muscle cells, although other kinds of cells have also been shown to be excitable.
F c. 1. in bacterial genetics, a cell with an inheritable mating type. The F^+ cell (male donor) carries the F (fertility) plasmid, while the F^- cell (female recipient) lacks this factor. 2. *(in the pl.)* PP c's.
Fañanás c. a type of neuroglial cell found in the molecular layer of the cerebellar cortex; called also *glia of Fañanás.*
fat c. a connective tissue cell specialized for the synthesis and storage of fat; such cells are bloated with globules of triglycerides, the nucleus being displaced to one side and the cytoplasm seen as a thin line around the fat droplet. Called also *adipose c., adipocyte,* and *lipocyte.*
fat-storing c. of liver hepatic stellate c.
fatty granule c. gitter c.
fiber c. any elongated and linear cell.
flagellate c. any cell having a flagellum or flagella.
flaming plasma c. an abnormal plasma cell that stains red to violet, probably because it contains immunoglobulins with a high carbohydrate content.
foam c. 1. a type of abnormal macrophage with a vacuolated appearance owing to the presence of complex lipids, seen in storage diseases, xanthomas, and certain other conditions. 2. a specific variety of this cell found in xanthomas; called also *xanthoma cell.* 3. Mikulicz c.
follicle c's, follicular c's cells located in the epithelium of follicles, such as thyroid follicular cells or the cells of ovarian follicles. Called also *follicular epithelial c's.*
follicular center c. any of a series of B lymphocytes occurring normally in the germinal center and pathologically in the neoplastic nodules of follicular center cell lymphoma; they are regarded as intermediate stages in the development of lymphoblasts and plasma cells from activated lymphocytes. They are distinguished according to size and presence or absence of folds or clefts on the nucleus; see *large cleaved, large noncleaved, small cleaved,* and *small noncleaved follicular center c.* Follicular center cells are thought to be the B memory cells.
follicular dendritic c's antigen-presenting cells found in the germinal centers of the lymph nodes, having the property of retaining for long periods of time antigen-antibody complexes in labyrinths of clefts bounded by their surface processes. Called also *dendritic c's.*
follicular epithelial c's follicle c's.
folliculostellate c. a stellate cell occurring in the adenohypophysis and forming networks with other cells of the same type via long processes; its function is uncertain.
foreign body giant c's giant cells that have clusters of nuclei scattered in an irregular pattern throughout the cytoplasm. They are formed by coalescence and fusion of macrophages, with only a rare internal nuclear division, and are characteristic of inflammation induced by inoculation or implantation of exogenous materials resistant to degradation.
formative c. a cell of the embryoblast of the conceptus, a blastomere destined to form a part of the embryo; as distinct from a cell of the trophoblast.
fusiform c. spindle c.
G c's granular enterochromaffin cells that are the primary source of gastrin and are found in the pyloric glands in the mucosa of the stomach.
galvanic c. voltaic c.
gametoid c's carcinoma cells resembling reproductive cells (gametes).
gamma c's of hypophysis chromophobic c's.
ganglion c. 1. a form of large nerve cell characteristic of ganglia; called also *gangliocyte.* 2. any of those retinal cells that are the third (last) neurons in the vertical linkage of the retina and are analogous to the relays in the spinal cord and brainstem. At least six types of ganglion cells have been classified according to their dendritic patterns. See also *visual cone,* under *cone.*
gastrin c's G c's.
Gaucher c. a large and distinctive cell characteristic of Gaucher disease, with one or more eccentrically placed nuclei and with fine wavy

kerasin fibrils running parallel to the long axis of the cell, imparting a wrinkled, tissue-paper appearance to the gray or bluish opaque cytoplasm.
Gegenbaur c. osteoblast.
germ c's the cells of an organism whose function it is to reproduce its kind, i.e., oocytes and spermatozoa and their immature stages. See also *gamete.* Called also *initial c's, sex c's,* and *sexual c's.*
germinal c. a cell capable of dividing and differentiating.
ghost c. 1. a keratinized anucleate cell with an unstained, shadowy center where the nucleus had been. Called also *shadow c.* 2. a degenerating or fragmented erythrocyte with no hemoglobin; cf. *achromocyte.* Called also *erythroclast* and *shadow c.*
Giannuzzi c's see under *crescent.*
giant c. 1. any very large cell; some are normal, such as the megakaryocytes of bone marrow, and some are abnormal, such as tumor cells. 2. any of the very large, multinucleate, modified macrophages that may be formed by coalescence of epithelioid cells or by nuclear division without cytoplasmic division of monocytes, such as those characteristic of granulomatous inflammation (Langhans giant cells) and those that form around large foreign bodies (foreign body giant cells).
giant pyramidal c's Betz c's.
Gierke c's small, deeply staining Golgi type II neurons that constitute the chief cells of Rolando gelatinous substance; cf. *Rolando c's.*
gitter c. a microglial cell that is globular and swollen after having phagocytized debris from cells destroyed pathologically in the central nervous system; called also *compound granule c.* and *compound granular corpuscle.*
glial c's neuroglial c's.
glitter c's polymorphonuclear leukocytes that stain a pale blue with gentian-violet-safranin and contain granules in the cytoplasm that exhibit brownian movement; their presence in urine may indicate pyelonephritis or other disease of the urinary tract.
globoid c. an abnormal large histiocyte found in large numbers in intracranial tissues in Krabbe disease.
glomerular c. glomus c. (def. 1).
glomus c. 1. any of the moderately large specific epithelioid cells (type I) of the carotid body (see *glomus caroticum*) containing abundant cytoplasm and membrane-bound, electron-dense granules and having a few dendritic processes; they are richly supplied with nerve endings and are surrounded by cells without cytoplasmic granules (type II). Called also *glomerular c.* 2. any of the modified smooth muscle cells with uniform nuclei, pale-staining cytoplasm, and indistinct margins that surround the arterial segment of a glomeriform arteriovenous anastomosis, which are richly innervated by fibers of the autonomic nervous system.
goblet c. a unicellular mucous gland found in the epithelium of various mucous membranes, especially that of the respiratory passages and intestines. Droplets of mucigen collect in the upper part of the cell and distend it, while the basal end remains slender, and the cell assumes the shape of a goblet. Called also *beaker c., caliciform c.,* and *chalice c.* See also *ptyocrinous.*
Golgi c's Golgi type I neurons or Golgi type II neurons; see under *neuron.*
gonadotrope c., gonadotroph c., gonadotropic c. gonadotroph.
Goormaghtigh c's lacis c's.
granular c. a keratinocyte in the stratum granulosum of the epidermis, when it has become flattened and rhomboid in shape and contains a dense collection of keratohyalin granules; it eventually dies and moves into the stratum corneum.

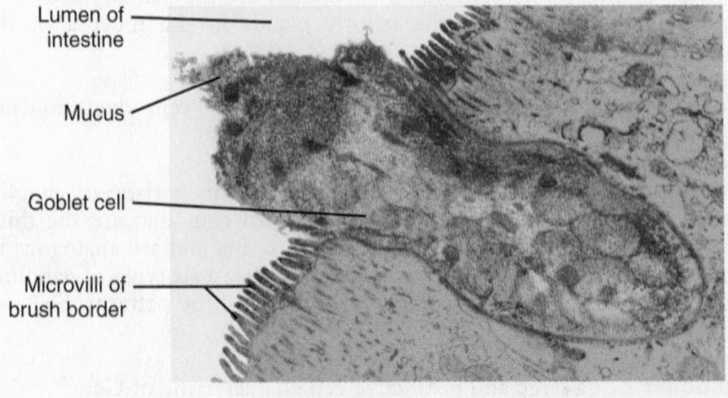

■ Jejunal goblet cell discharging mucus.

granule c's 1. diminutive stellate cells found chiefly in the granular layers of the cerebral and cerebellar cortices. 2. small nerve cells without axons, whose bodies are in the granular layer of the olfactory bulb; they have many dendrites that synapse with dendrites of mitral and tufted cells and probably act as dampers.
granulosa c's cells surrounding the vesicular ovarian follicle and forming the stratum granulosum and cumulus oophorus; after ovulation they are transformed into lutein cells.
granulosa-lutein c's lutein cells of the corpus luteum derived from granulosa cells.
great alveolar c's type II alveolar c's.
ground-glass c. a hepatocyte having finely granular, eosinophilic cytoplasm and staining positively for hepatitis B surface antigen, characteristic of chronic hepatitis B.
gustatory c's taste c's.
H c. horizontal c.
hair c's neuroepithelial cells with hairlike processes (kinocilia or stereocilia or both), found in the internal ear. Those in the organ of Corti are called auditory hair cells, are connected to fibers of the cochlear nerve, and control the sense of hearing. Those in the ampullary crest, utricle, and saccule are called auditory hair cells, are connected to fibers of the vestibular nerve, and control the sense of equilibrium.
hairy c. a type of abnormal large leukocyte, probably in the B lymphocyte lineage, found in the blood in hairy cell leukemia; it has numerous irregular cytoplasmic villi that give it a flagellated or hairy appearance, a round or oval nucleus, gray-blue cytoplasm, moderately clumped nuclear chromatin, and small to imperceptible nucleoli. Called also *tricholeukocyte.*
Hammar myoid c's myoid c's (def. 2).
heart disease c's, heart failure c's, heart lesion c's macrophages containing granules of iron, found in the pulmonary alveoli and sputum in congestive heart failure.
hecatomeral c's cells of gray matter of the spinal cord whose axis cylinder processes divide and send one branch into the white substance of the same side of the cord and another into the anterolateral columns of the other side.
HeLa c's cells of the first continuously cultured carcinoma strain, descended from a human cervical carcinoma; used in the study of life processes, including viruses, at the cell level.
helmet c. schistocyte.
helper c's, helper T c's differentiated T lymphocytes whose cooperation (help) is required for the production of antibody against most (T-dependent) antigens. Activation of B lymphocytes (B cells) requires recognition of the antigenic determinant against which specific antibody is produced by antigen receptors on a B cell, recognition of some other antigenic determinant by antigen receptors on a helper cell, and a signal passed from the helper cell to the B cell, probably requiring direct cell-to-cell contact. Murine helper cells are marked by the Ly-1 antigen, human helper cells by the CD4 antigen. See also *lymphocyte.*
hematopoietic progenitor c's, hematopoietic stem c's pluripotent blood cell progenitors that represent a slightly later stage than blast cells. They have the capacity for replication and differentiation and give rise to precursors of various blood cell lines, including the proerythroblast and myeloblast; neither of these cell types can self-replicate, and they must differentiate into more mature daughter cells. Called also *colony-forming unit–spleen.*
Hensen c's tall supporting cells arranged in rows adjacent to the last row of outer phalangeal cells, constituting the outer border of the organ of Corti.
hepatic c. one of the polyhedral epithelial cells that constitute the substance of a liver acinus; called also *hepatocyte, liver c.,* and *parenchymal hepatic c.*
hepatic stellate c. (HSC) a type of stellate cell found in the perisinusoidal spaces of the liver. These cells are the major site of vitamin A storage in the body and also synthesize collagen. They may be involved in hepatic tissue repair and be responsible for the excess collagen produced in cirrhosis. Called also *fat-storing c. of liver, Ito c.,* and *lipocyte.*
heteromeral c's, heteromeric c's nerve cells of the gray matter of the spinal cord whose axon processes pass to the white matter of the opposite side; called also *commissural c's.*
Hfr c's the sexual or donor (male) stage of bacteria having the F (fertility) factor in the chromosome, which enables them to transfer chromosomal material to recipient (female) bacteria not having this factor.

hilum c's groups of large epithelioid cells closely associated with vascular spaces and unmyelinated nerve fibers in the hilum of the ovary and the adjacent mesovarium.
Hodgkin c's Reed-Sternberg c's.
Hofbauer c's large, globular cells filled with vacuoles and large spherical nuclei, found in the connective tissue core of the chorionic villi of the placenta; they are probably macrophages.
homozygous typing c's (HTC) cells homozygous for a known HLA-D specificity; panels of HTC of all established HLA-D types are used to determine the HLA-D type of unknown cells using one-way mixed lymphocyte reactions.
horizontal c. a retinal neuron; there are two types, and their functions are unclear. Each cell has a multipolar soma in the internal nuclear layer and one long neurite and several short ones. All the neurites serve as both axons and dendrites, extending along and ramifying within the internal nuclear layer. The long neurites synapse in the outer plexiform layer with both pedicles and spherules; the short neurites synapse either with pedicles or with spherules. Called also *H c.*
horizontal c. of Cajal Cajal c. (def. 2).
horizontal c. of retina horizontal c.
horn c. 1. corneocyte. 2. any ganglion cell of the horns of the spinal cord.
Hortega c. microglial c.
Hürthle c's Askanazy c's.
hyperchromatic c. a cell that stains more intensely than is typical of its cell type.
I-c. an abnormal fibroblast containing a large number of dark inclusions that fill the central part of the cytoplasm except for the juxtanuclear zone; seen in mucolipidosis II.
immunologically competent c. immunocyte.
incasing c. cover c.
indifferent c. a cell that has no characteristic structure, or that is not an essential part of the tissue in which it is found.
inflammatory c. a cell that participates in the inflammatory response to a foreign substance; these include neutrophils, macrophages, and others.
initial c's germ c's.
inner hair c's a flask-shaped type of auditory hair cells, found in a single row on the medial side of the inner tunnel of the organ of Corti; they receive impulses from the outer hair cells and transform them into electrical signals that are given to the cochlear nerve for transmission to an auditory cortex in the brain. These cells are surrounded by supporting phalangeal cells.
integrator c. interneuron.
intercalary c's dark, rodlike structures between the other (secretory and nonsecretory) cells of the endosalpinx, which may be emptied secretory cells; called also *peg c's.*
intercalated c's dark-colored cells in the renal collecting tubules that are responsible for acidification of the urine. Called also *dark c's.*
intercapillary c's mesangial c's.
interdental c's cells found in the spiral limbus between the dentes acustici, which secrete the tectorial membrane of the cochlear duct.
interdigitating c's antigen-presenting cells found in the thymus-dependent (parafollicular) areas of the deep cortex of lymph nodes and spleen, having numerous surface processes that interdigitate with adjacent lymphocytes; the surface of these cells contains an Ia antigen of the major histocompatibility complex that causes T cells to cluster.
interfollicular c's Askanazy c's.
interstitial c's 1. Leydig c's (def. 1). 2. a type of cells found more often in other female mammals than in humans, consisting of masses of large epithelioid, lipid-containing cells in the ovarian stroma, believed to have a secretory function; they are derived from the theca interna of atretic ovarian follicles. In humans they are found in infant girls during the first year of life when atresia is proceeding rapidly, but in adult women few to none are present. In other mammals, such as rabbits, they are more prominent. See also *interstitial gland* (def. 2), under *gland.* 3. cells with elongated nuclei and long cytoplasmic processes, found in the perivascular areas and between the cords of pinealocytes in the pineal body, regarded by some to be glial elements. 4. hepatic stellate c's.
interstitial c's of Cajal (ICCs) pleomorphic cells with oval nuclei and long, branching cytoplasmic processes that interlace to form a network, occurring in the walls of the gastrointestinal tract. They are important in the regulation of gastrointestinal motility, transmitting impulses from enteric neurons to smooth muscle cells and serving as pacemakers. They are grouped into three functional types, each of which occurs in a specific location: in the plane of the myenteric plexus (ICC_{MY}), near the submucosal plexus (ICC_{SM}), and between the circular and longitudinal muscle layers (ICC_{IM}).

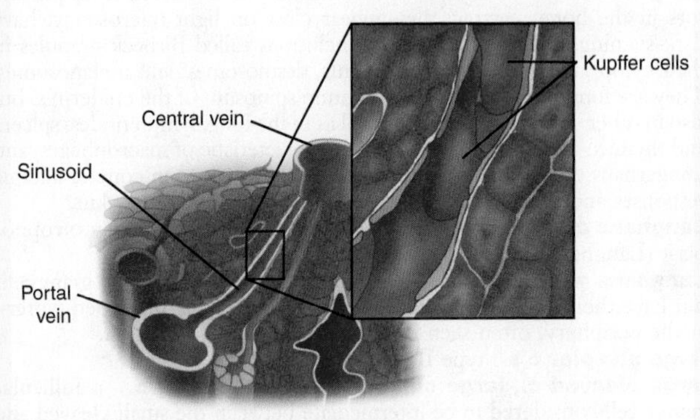

■ Kupffer cells lining a hepatic sinusoid.

interstitial c's of Leydig Leydig c's (def. 1).
intestinal absorptive c. one of the cells of the intestinal epithelium, having a brush border made up of many closely packed parallel microvilli, and believed to be associated with absorption, particularly of macromolecules.
islet c's cells composing the islets of Langerhans, including the *alpha cells, beta cells, delta cells,* and *PP cells.*
Ito c. hepatic stellate c.
juvenile c. metamyelocyte.
juxtaglomerular c's specialized smooth muscle cells found in the tunica media of the afferent glomerular arterioles, containing secretory granules. They are the major structural component responsible for the release of renin and play a major role in renal autoregulation and tubuloglomerular feedback.
K c's 1. cells mediating antibody-dependent cell-mediated cytotoxicity; they are large lymphocytes without T or B cell surface markers. K cells recognize IgG antibody coating the target cell by means of Fc receptors. Lysis of the target cell is extracellular, requires direct cell-to-cell contact, and does not involve complement. Called also *killer cells.* 2. a type of cells that are located primarily in the midzone of the duodenal and jejunal mucosa and synthesize gastric inhibitory polypeptide.
karyochrome c. karyochrome.
killer c's 1. K c's (def. 1). 2. cytotoxic T lymphocytes.
killer T c's cytotoxic T lymphocytes.
Kulchitsky c's argentaffin cells found between the cells that line the glands of Lieberkühn of the intestine.
Kupffer c's a type of stellate cell found in the sinusoids of the liver, having intense phagocytic activity and forming part of the reticuloendothelial system. Called also *von Kupffer c's.*
L c's 1. cells from a strain (C3H) of mouse fibroblasts grown in tissue culture for many years; employed for their ability to support replication of many types of viruses. 2. a type of argyrophilic cells with large cytoplasmic granules in the mucosa of the upper intestine; their ultrastructure resembles that of the alpha cells of the islets of Langerhans, and they secrete glicentin and glucagon-like peptides 1 and 2; called also *large granule c's.* 3. Langerhans c's. 4. Langhans c's. 5. null cells with natural killer or killer properties.
lacis c's lacelike cells in the pale-staining polkissen of the juxtaglomerular apparatus of the kidney; they have numerous processes to connect gap junctions and are thought to provide electrical coupling among themselves and to the mesangium and glomerular arterioles. Called also *Goormaghtigh c's* and *extraglomerular mesangium.*
lacrimoethmoid c's the ethmoidal cells situated under the lacrimal bone.
lactotrope c., lactotroph c., lactotropic c. lactotroph.
lacunar c. a variant of the Reed-Sternberg cell, typically having a single nucleus surrounded by an ample, pale-staining cytoplasm enclosed in a sharply defined cell membrane; it is primarily associated with nodular sclerosis type Hodgkin disease.
LAK c's lymphokine-activated killer c's.

Cell *Continued*

Langerhans c's a stellate type of dendritic cells derived from precursors in the bone marrow; they appear clear on light microscopy, have dark-staining, indented nuclei with inclusions called Birbeck granules in their cytoplasm, and lack tonofilaments, desmosomes, and melanosomes. They are found principally in the stratum spinosum of the epidermis, but also in other stratified epithelia as well as in the lung, lymph nodes, spleen, and thymus. Their surface markers are characteristic of macrophages, and Langerhans cells are antigen-presenting cells involved in contact allergic responses and other cell-mediated immune reactions in the skin.
Langhans c's polyhedral epithelial cells constituting the cytotrophoblast (Langhans layer).
Langhans giant c's giant cells that resemble foreign body giant cells but have their nuclei arranged in a circle or a horseshoe-shaped pattern at the periphery, often seen in granulomatous inflammation.
large alveolar c's type II alveolar c's.
large cleaved c., large cleaved follicular center c. a follicular center cell considered to be intermediate between the small cleaved and small noncleaved stages; it has a diameter of about 12 μm, a nucleus with deep folds or clefts and clumped chromatin, and cytoplasm that is not pyroninophilic but may have immunoglobulin inclusions.
large granule c's L c's (def. 2).
large noncleaved c., large noncleaved follicular center c., large uncleaved c. a follicular center cell considered to be the stage immediately preceding the development of the B lymphoblast and migration out of the follicle; it has a diameter of 15–20 μm, a nucleus without clefts that contains finely dispersed chromatin, and cytoplasm that is abundant and pyroninophilic.
LE c. a neutrophil or macrophage that has phagocytized the denatured nuclear material of an injured cell (LE or hematoxylin body); a characteristic of systemic lupus erythematosus, but also found in analogous disorders of connective tissue.
lepra c. a distinctive type of macrophage found in a leprous nodule, having been converted by the action of lepra bacilli into a sac containing degenerated protoplasm and bacilli. Called also *Virchow c.*
Leydig c's 1. clusters of epithelioid cells constituting the endocrine tissue of the testis, which elaborate androgens, chiefly testosterone; called also *interstitial c's* or *interstitial c's of Leydig* and *interstitial glands.* 2. mucous cells that do not pour their secretion out over the surface of the epithelium.
light c's parafollicular c's.
littoral c's flattened cells lining the walls of lymph or blood sinuses. Called also *rod* or *stave c's.*
liver c. hepatic c.
luteal c's, lutein c's the plump, pale-staining, polyhedral cells of the corpus luteum; they include the granulosa-lutein cells and the theca-lutein cells.
lymph c. lymphocyte.
lymphoid c's cells of the immune system that react specifically with antigen and elaborate specific cell products; they comprise the lymphocytes and plasma cells.
lymphokine-activated killer c's killer cells activated by interleukin-2 that have specificity towards tumors refractory to NK cells; they may represent a further activation state of the NK cell. Called also *LAK c's.*
M c's specialized cells of the epithelium, overlying the lymphoid nodules of the intestines, that bind antigens and transport them to the underlying lymphocytes; they may provide a continuous sampling of the intestinal contents to the immune system. Called also *microfold c's.*

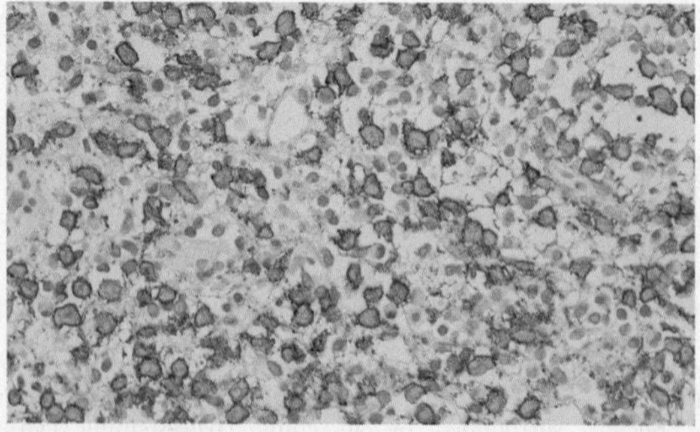

■ Langerhans cells identified in a jaw lesion. Immunohistochemical stain for CD1a antigen, specific to Langerhans cells, demonstrates large numbers of brown-staining Langerhans cells.

malpighian c. keratinocyte.
marginal c's Giannuzzi crescents.
marrow c. any of the immature blood cells that develop in the bone marrow, such as those involved in hematopoiesis. Called also *myeloid c.*
Martinotti c's fusiform cells with ascending axon processes in the layers of the cerebral cortex, especially in the multiform layer and also in the internal pyramidal layer.
mast c. a type of connective tissue cell whose specific physiologic function remains unknown; it can elaborate basophilic, metachromatic, cytoplasmic granules that contain histamine and heparin in humans and serotonin in species such as the rat and mouse. Called also *mastocyte* and *labrocyte.*
mastoid c's, mastoid air c's cellulae mastoideae.
matrix c's flat cells found in the lobules of sebaceous glands.
Mauthner c. a large cell in the metencephalon of fishes and amphibians that gives rise to the Mauthner fiber.
megaspore mother c. a type of diploid cell that develops in the megasporangium of plants and divides by meiosis to produce four haploid daughter cells called the megaspores; usually only one megaspore survives to become a megagametophyte (female gametophyte).
memory c's T and B lymphocytes that mediate immunologic memory (q.v.); believed to retain information that permits a subsequent challenge to be followed by a more rapid, efficient immune response on subsequent exposures to an antigen than occurred on first exposure.
Merkel c. a specialized cell at or near the dermal-epidermal junction, characterized by numerous membrane-bound granules with dense cores, some desmosomes, cytoplasmic microfilaments, intranuclear filaments bundled in parallel to form tiny rods, and spikelike processes that interdigitate with keratinocytes. Merkel cells are believed to act as tactile receptors by association with tactile menisci (flat, disklike endings of nerve fibers).
Merkel-Ranvier c. a type of clear cell found in the basal layer of the epidermis; it contains catecholamine granules and resembles a melanocyte.
Merkel tactile c. Merkel c.
mesangial c's phagocytic cells found in the mesangium of the glomerular capsule of the kidney, thought to aid in cleaning the filtration apparatus. Called also *intercapillary c's.*
mesenchymal c's the pluripotent cells constituting the mesenchyme.
mesothelial c's flattened epithelial cells of mesenchymal origin that line the serous cavities.
metallophil c's cells in which the cytoplasm has a great affinity for metal salts; these are cells of the reticuloendothelial system, and also a series of related cells that are not selectively stained by vital staining.
Mexican hat c. target c.
Meynert c's large solitary pyramidal cells in the cerebral cortex, found in a single row near the calcarine fissure; called also *solitary c's of Meynert.*
microfold c's M c's.
microglia c., microglial c. one of the small interstitial phagocytic cells of the microglia; see also *gitter c.* Called also *microgliocyte* and *Hortega c.*
microspore mother c. a type of diploid cell that develops in the microsporangium of plants, has a large nucleus, and divides by meiosis to produce four haploid microspores.
Mikulicz c. a type of cell found in rhinoscleroma, being the one containing the bacillus of the disease; called also *foam c.*
mitral c's neurons with pyramidal bodies located in the olfactory bulb, being the second stage in the pathway to the cortex; they receive impulses in the olfactory glomeruli from the olfactory cells and transmit impulses through the olfactory tracts to various areas of the cortex.
mononuclear c. a cell having a single nucleus, especially one in a group where some have multiple nuclei, such as a monocyte or a Sézary cell.
mossy c. 1. protoplasmic astrocyte. 2. any of the cells of the oligodendroglia or of the microglia.
mother c. a cell that divides so as to form new or daughter cells; called also *parent c.*
motor c. motoneuron.
Mott c. an abnormal plasma cell that contains Mott bodies or Russell bodies, seen in multiple myeloma and in the brain in late stages of African trypanosomiasis.
mouth c's squamous cells detached from the epithelium lining the oropharynx, found in the sputum.

mucoalbuminous c's, mucoserous c's trophochrome c's.
mucous c's cells that secrete mucus or mucin.
mucous neck c's cells found in the necks of gastric glands; they fill the spaces between the parietal cells and are filled with pale transparent granules.
mulberry c. a round cell with a centrally placed nucleus and coarse cytoplasmic vacuoles near the outer border; these develop at the periphery of a retrogressing corpus luteum.
c's of Müller see under *fiber.*
muriform c's sclerotic bodies.
muscle c. any contractile cell peculiar to muscle. Smooth muscle cells are elongated spindle-shaped cells containing a single nucleus and longitudinally arranged myofibrils. For cardiac and skeletal muscle cells, see *muscle fiber*, under *fiber*. Called also *myocyte.*
myeloid c. marrow c.
myeloma c. a cell found in bone marrow and occasionally in peripheral blood of patients with multiple myeloma. In the more anaplastic forms, the cell is large, has abundant blue-staining cytoplasm with no perinuclear pallor, and has one or more moderately large and vesicular nuclei that may be centrally or eccentrically placed and may contain nucleoli. In better differentiated tumors, the cell is smaller and, except for the finer chromatic structure, greatly resembles a plasmacyte.
myoepithelial c's modified smooth muscle cells, contractile in nature, believed to be of ectodermal origin, located around the secretory units of certain glands (salivary, mammary, sweat, and lacrimal glands) between the gland cells and basement membrane, having long dendritic interweaving cytoplasmic processes, and containing myofilaments. It is assumed that contraction of these cells functions to help express secretion from the gland. Called also *basket c's.*
myoepithelioid c's juxtaglomerular c's; so called because they appear to be highly modified smooth muscle cells.
myoid c's 1. cells found in the seminiferous tubules of common laboratory rodents, which cytologically resemble smooth muscle and are presumed to be contractile and to be responsible for the rhythmic shallow contractions of the seminiferous tubules of these species; called also *peritubular contractile c's.* 2. striated muscle cells found in the thymus of nonmammalian vertebrates, especially reptiles and birds, and rarely in mammals; called also *Hammar myoid c's.*
myointimal c. a smooth muscle cell found in the intima of an artery.
naive c. a lymphocyte that has not yet undergone activation (q.v.).
natural killer c's NK c's.
nerve c. neuron.
neuroendocrine c's the specialized neurons that secrete neurohormones.
neuroepithelial c's cells of the neuroepithelium.
neuroglia c's, neuroglial c's the cells of the supportive tissue of the central nervous system (neuroglia); these non-neural cells are of three kinds: astrocytes, oligodendrocytes (collectively termed macroglia), and microglia. See Plate 39.
neuromuscular c. a form of cell chiefly or always seen in the lower animals, of which the outer part receives stimuli and the inner part is contractile.
neurosecretory c. any cell with neuron-like properties that secretes a biologically active substance acting on another structure, often at a distant site; examples are the paraganglia and cells in the hypothalamus. See also *neuroendocrine c's.*
neutrophilic c. a cell, particularly a leukocyte, stainable by neutral dyes; called also *neutrophil.*
nevus c. a type of modified melanocyte, thought to be derived from an embryonal Schwann cell, found in clusters in the epidermis, and in the dermis after a kind of centripetal extrusion; these are the main constituents of melanocytic nevi.
Niemann-Pick c's round, oval, or polyhedral cells present in the bone marrow and spleen in Niemann-Pick disease; they have foamy, lipid-containing cytoplasm, in the form of sphingomyelin, which gives a positive reaction with Sudan III and other fat stains. Called also *Pick c's.*
NK c's natural killer cells; cells capable of mediating cytotoxic reactions without prior sensitization against the target. NK cells are small lymphocytes without B or T cell surface markers that originate in the bone marrow and develop fully in the absence of the thymus; their cytotoxic activity is not antibody-dependent. They can lyse a wide variety of tumor cells and other cell types and are probably important in natural resistance to tumors. Interferon augments their activity. See *lymphocyte.*
nodal c's P c's.
noncleaved c. see *small noncleaved follicular center c.* and *large noncleaved follicular center c.*
normal c. any cell found naturally in any part or organ free from disease.
nucleated c. any cell having a nucleus.
null c's lymphocytes that lack the surface markers for B or T cells; see *K c's* and *NK c's.*
nurse c's, nursing c's Sertoli c's.
oat c., oat-shaped c. a small round cell with little cytoplasm, resembling a grain of oats, seen in small cell lung carcinoma.
olfactory c's, olfactory receptor c's a set of specialized, fusiform nerve cells with large nuclei, embedded among the epithelial cells in the mucous membrane of the nose; they carry impulses from the olfactory receptors to the glomeruli in the olfactory bulb. Called also *Schultze c's.*
osseous c. a bone cell.
osteoprogenitor c's relatively undifferentiated cells found on or near all of the free surfaces of bone, which, under certain circumstances, undergo division and transform into osteoblasts or coalesce to give rise to osteoclasts.
outer hair c's a type of cylindrical auditory hair cell found in three rows on the lateral side of the Corti tunnel, supported by outer phalangeal cells; they receive sound waves and transmit them to the inner hair cells for transformation into electrical impulses that the cochlear nerve can receive and transmit towards the auditory cortex of the brain.
oval c. an epithelial cell, not seen in normal liver, that is activated in response to certain types of severe hepatic injury and serves as a progenitor cell in the regeneration of liver tissue.
oxyntic c's parietal c's.
oxyphil c's, oxyphilic c's 1. acidophilic cells found, along with the more numerous chief cells, in the parathyroid glands; they increase in number with age, have small dark nuclei and abundant finely granular cytoplasm, and are larger and have many more mitochondria than the chief cells. 2. any of various pathological acidophilic cells found in the thyroid gland. 3. Askanazy c's.
P c's poorly staining, pale, small cells almost devoid of myofibrils, mitochondria, or other organelles; they are clustered in the center of the sinoatrial node (where they are thought to be the source of impulse formation) as well as in the atrioventricular node.
pacemaker c. a myocardial cell demonstrating automaticity; i.e., one that initiates electrical activity in the absence of external stimuli. Called also *automatic c.*
packed red blood c's the remaining red blood cells of whole blood from which plasma has been removed; used therapeutically in blood transfusions. In official terminology, called *red blood c's* [USP].
Paget c., pagetoid c. a large, irregularly shaped, pale anaplastic tumor cell with vacuolated cytoplasm and a vesicular nucleus that is usually hyperchromatic and surrounded by a clear zone; cells occur singly or in small clusters in the epidermis in Paget disease of the breast and extramammary Paget disease.
palatine c's those parts of ethmoid cells that are extended into the palatine bone.
palisade c's a compact layer of cylindrical chloroplast-bearing cells located in the mesophyll layer of a leaf, and so arranged that their long axes are at right angles to the epidermal surface of the leaf.
Paneth c's narrow, pyramidal, or columnar epithelial cells with a round or oval nucleus close to the base, occurring in the fundus of the crypts of Lieberkühn; they contain large granules that secrete antimicrobial substances such as defensins. Called also *Davidoff c's.*
parabasal c. a type of cell found in the deeper part of the stratified squamous epithelium, being smaller in size and with a larger nucleus; these cells are less mature than those closer to the surface. See also *maturation index*, under *index.*
parafollicular c's ovoid cells with an irregular nucleus and many brown or black cytoplasmic granules, located in the follicular epithelium and interfollicular spaces along with the principal cells of the thyroid follicles, in the follicular epithelium and interfollicular spaces, and which elaborate calcitonin. They arise during embryonic life from the fifth pharyngeal pouches and are incorporated in the thyroid gland in mammals, but form discrete epithelial cell masses *(ultimobranchial bodies)* in submammalian vertebrates. Called also *C c's* and *light c's.*
paraluteal c's, paralutein c's theca-lutein c's.
parenchymal hepatic c. hepatic c.
parent c. mother c.

parietal c's large spheroidal or pyramidal cells that are the source of gastric hydrochloric acid and are the site of intrinsic factor production; they are found scattered along the walls of the gastric glands, with their tapered ends pushed between the chief cells. Called also *acid c's* and *oxyntic c's.*
pathologic c. any cell that results from a disease process or that belongs to or arises from a pathogenic microorganism.
pavement c's the flat cells composing pavement epithelium.
peg c's intercalary c's.
peptic c's a name sometimes given to the chief cells of the stomach.
pericapillary c. pericyte.
periglomerular c's nerve cells in the olfactory bulb that have synaptic connections with glomeruli, mitral cells, and tufted cells, and are thought to act as dampers.
peripheral blood progenitor c's (PBPC), peripheral blood stem c's stem cells found in the peripheral blood rather than the bone marrow; their numbers can be artificially increased by exposure to hematopoietic growth factors so that they can be extracted before myeloablative chemotherapy and later infused as an autologous bone marrow transplantation.
perithelial c. pericyte.
peritubular contractile c's myoid c's (def. 1).
perivascular c. pericyte.
pessary c. a hypochromic erythrocyte with the hemoglobin in a narrow circumferential rim; cf. *achromocyte.* Called also *pessary corpuscle.*
phalangeal c's elongated supporting cells of the organ of Corti with bases that rest on the basilar membrane adjacent to the pillar cells. *Inner phalangeal cells* are arranged in a row on the inner surface of the inner pillar cells and surround the inner hair cells; *outer phalangeal cells* (or *Deiters cells*) support the outer hair cells.
pheochrome c's chromaffin c's.
photoreceptor c's visual c's.
physaliferous c's, physaliphorous c's spheroidal nucleated cells, containing glycogen or mucin, causing them to appear vacuolated; they are characteristic of chordoma.
Pick c's Niemann-Pick c's.
pigment c. any cell containing pigment granules.
pillar c's elongated supporting cells found in the organ of Corti in a double row *(inner* and *outer pillar c's),* with their heads joined and their bases on the basilar membrane widely separated so as to form a tunnel *(inner tunnel* or *canal of Corti)* that extends the length of the cochlea. Called also *Corti rods.*
pineal c. pinealocyte.
plasma c. a terminally differentiated cell of the B lymphocyte lineage that produces antibodies; plasma cells are oval or round with extensive rough endoplasmic reticulum, a well-developed Golgi apparatus, and a round nucleus having a characteristic "cartwheel" heterochromatin pattern. Called also *plasmacyte.*
pneumatic c. air c. (def. 2).
PNH c's abnormal erythrocytes seen in paroxysmal nocturnal hemoglobinuria (PNH); they are classified in three groups: *PNH I cells,* which have normal or nearly normal sensitivity to complement; *PNH II cells,* which require about one fourth as much complement as normal cells for an equal amount of lysis; and *PNH III cells,* which require about one fifteenth as much complement as normal cells for an equal amount of lysis.

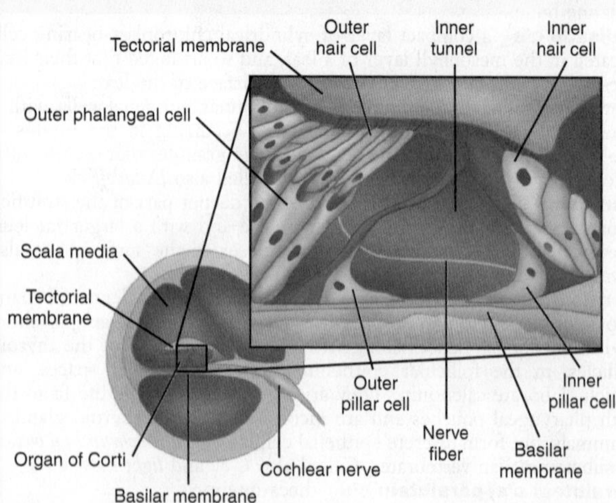

■ Pillar cells forming the inner tunnel in the organ of Corti in the internal ear.

polar c's polar bodies (def. 1).
polychromatic c's, polychromatophil c's immature erythrocytes staining with both acid and basic stains so that their color is a diffuse mixture of blue-gray and pink.
polyhedral c. a cell that is many-sided in form.
popcorn c. a variant of the Reed-Sternberg cell, having a multilobed nucleus that resembles an exploded popcorn kernel.
PP c's cells in the pancreatic islets, exocrine pancreas, and intestine that secrete pancreatic polypeptide. Called also *F c's.*
pre-B c's the earliest identifiable precursors of B lymphocytes: large, rapidly dividing cells found in the fetal liver and adult bone marrow that lack surface immunoglobulin but contain diffuse cytoplasmic immunoglobulin of the IgM type.
prefollicle c's cells encapsulating the primordial germ cells in the fetal ovary. Called also *primordial granulosa c's.*
pregnancy c. an altered chromophobe cell found in the adenohypophysis in pregnant women.
pre-T c. a T lymphocyte precursor before undergoing induction of the maturation process in the thymus; it lacks the characteristics of a mature T lymphocyte.
prickle c. one of the dividing keratinocytes present in the stratum spinosum of the epidermis; it contains many tonofilaments and has delicate radiating processes that connect with similar cells.
primordial germ c. the earliest recognizable precursor in the embryo of a germ cell; these originate extragonadally but migrate early in embryonic development to the gonads. Called also *gonocyte.*
primordial granulosa c's prefollicle c's.
primordial wandering c. a small mononuclear cell of the embryo that arises from the mesoderm and subsequently by differentiation gives rise to wandering cells of the body.
principal c's 1. chief c's (def. 3). 2. the fundamental cells of an organ, which usually have a specific function. 3. light-staining cells of the renal collecting tubules that transport water in response to antidiuretic hormone and sodium in response to aldosterone.
progenitor c. stem c.
prokaryotic c. a cell without a true nucleus; see *prokaryote.*
prolactin c. lactotroph.
pulmonary epithelial c's alveolar epithelial c's.
pulpar c's the typical cells of the spleen substance.
Purkinje c's 1. large neurons in the cerebellar cortex that have piriform cell bodies in the Purkinje layer (the *stratum purkinjense corticis cerebelli*) and large branching dendrite trees going through the outer (molecular) layer towards the surface. 2. cells of the Purkinje fibers of the heart; they are large, clear, tightly packed cells with many gap junctions between them and thus conduct impulses rapidly.
pus c's polymorphonuclear leukocytes, chiefly neutrophils, occurring in pus.
pyramidal c. one of the large multipolar pyramid-shaped cells of the cerebral cortex, having a single apical dendrite extending outward toward the surface and several dendrites extending inward; a few are inverted so that their apical dendrites extend inward. They vary in size from small to the giant Betz cells. Called also *pyramidal neuron.*
RA c. ragocyte.
racket c. a cell shaped like a tennis racket, with a swollen outer end, found in the racket hyphae of various dermatophytes.
radial c's of Müller Müller fibers.
Raji c's cells from a cultured human lymphoblastoid cell line, derived from a patient with Burkitt lymphoma, that have receptors for the C1q, C3b, and C3d complement components and can be used for detection of immune complexes.
red c., red blood c. erythrocyte.
red blood c's [USP] official terminology for *packed red blood c's.*
Reed c's, Reed-Sternberg c's giant histiocytic cells, typically multinucleate, most often binucleate with the two halves of the cell appearing as mirror-images of each other; the nuclei are enclosed in abundant amphophilic cytoplasm and contain prominent nucleoli. The presence of the cells is the common histiologic characteristic of Hodgkin disease. A variant form is the lacunar cell (q.v.). Called also *Dorothy Reed c's, Sternberg-Reed c's, Hodgkin c's,* and *Sternberg giant c's.*

Cell *Continued*

regulatory T c's a subset of $CD4^+$ T cells that can suppress activity of effector cells such as helper cells and suppressor cells, and inhibit autoimmune diseases. Called also *Treg* or *T-regulatory c's*.
Renshaw c's interneurons in the ventromedial region of the spinal cord that make inhibitory connections with the motoneurons.
reserve c's cells of the basal or germinal layer of the bronchial epithelium.
residential c. a cell that does not wander, especially one of the cells of the substantia propria of the cornea.
resting c. a cell that is not undergoing karyokinesis.
resting wandering c. fixed macrophage.
reticular c's the cells forming the reticular fibers of connective tissue; those forming the framework of lymph nodes, bone marrow, and spleen are part of the reticuloendothelial system and under appropriate stimulation may differentiate into macrophages.
reticulate c. the larger of the two morphological forms of bacteria of the family Anaplasmataceae, characterized by a homogeneous loose matrix of chromatin strands, seen predominantly in vivo. Cf *dense-core c.*
reticuloendothelial c. any of the cells of the reticuloendothelial system.
reticulum c's reticular c's.
Rieder c. a myeloblast seen in a type of acute myelogenous leukemia *(Rieder cell leukemia)*, as well as in chronic lymphocytic leukemia. It has a nucleus with wide and deep indentations suggesting lobulation, which may represent asynchronism of nuclear and cytoplasmic maturation. Called also *Rieder lymphocyte*.
rod c's 1. retinal rods. 2. an abnormality of microglial cells seen in chronic diseases of the cerebral cortex and in dementia paralytica; the cells become thin and their processes are confined mainly to the two ends. 3. littoral c's.
Rohon-Beard c's giant ganglion cells in the spinal cord of some vertebrates.
Rolando c's the ganglion cells of Rolando gelatinous substance; cf. *Gierke c's*.
root c's neurons whose axons form nerve roots.
Rouget c. pericyte.
round c. any cell having a spherical shape, especially a lymphocyte.
RS c's Reed-Sternberg c's.
S c's 1. mucoid cells of the adenohypophysis that contain a cysteine-rich protein. 2. enteroendocrine cells found predominantly in the duodenum, which have cytoplasmic granules that store and release secretin; called also *small granule c's*.
Sala c's star-shaped cells of connective tissue in the fibers that form the sensory nerve endings situated in the pericardium.
sarcogenic c's the cells that are developed into muscle fiber.
satellite c's 1. glial cells that cluster about a neuron. 2. free nuclei that accumulate around cells in certain diseases. 3. elongated cells that are closely associated with a muscle fiber; they either are flattened against the fiber or occupy shallow depressions in its surface.
scavenger c. a cell which absorbs and removes irritant products.
Schultze c's olfactory c's.
Schwann c. any of the large nucleated cells whose cell membrane spirally enwraps the axons of myelinated peripheral neurons and is the source of myelin; a single Schwann cell supplies the myelin sheath between two nodes of Ranvier.
sclerotic c's see under *body*.
segmented c. a mature granulocyte in which the nucleus is divided into definite lobes joined by a filamentous connection, as distinguished from a band cell. Called also *segmented granulocyte*.

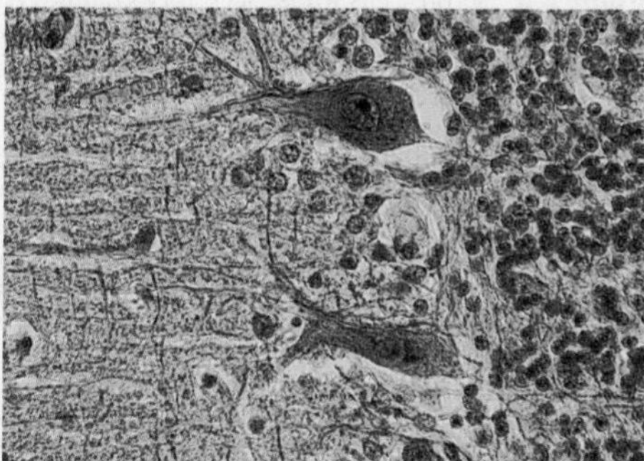

■ Purkinje cells (monkey cerebellum), with long, branching dendrites.

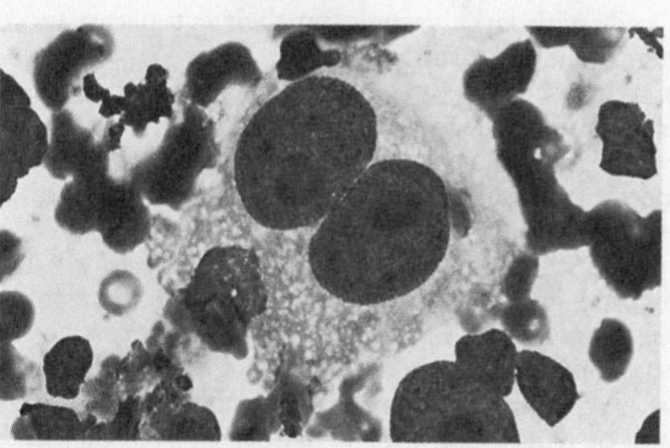

■ Intact classic Reed-Sternberg cell, with mirror-image macronuclei and macronucleoli, lies just above a mononuclear Reed-Sternberg cell that has been stripped of its cytoplasm (Romanowsky stain).

sensitized c. 1. a cell that has been primed (immunologically activated by an antigen). 2. an antibody-coated cell used in complement fixation tests.
sensory c. primary sensory neuron.
septal c's type II alveolar c's.
serous c. a cell concerned in the secretion of a watery fluid rich in protein, like the secretory cells of the parotid gland; called also *albuminous c.*
Sertoli c's elongated cells in the seminiferous tubules, to which the spermatids become attached; they provide support, protection, and possibly nutrition until the spermatids become transformed into mature spermatozoa. Called also *sustentacular c's*, *nurse* or *nursing c's*, and *trophocytes*.
sex c's, sexual c's germ c's.
Sézary c. an abnormal mononuclear T lymphocyte with a hyperchromic infolded cribriform nucleus and a narrow rim of cytoplasm that may contain vacuoles; it occurs in small and large cell variants and is a characteristic finding in certain types of cutaneous T-cell lymphoma, including mycosis fungoides and Sézary syndrome.
shadow c. ghost c..
sickle c. an erythrocyte shaped like a sickle or crescent owing to the presence of hemoglobin S; seen in sickle cell anemia and other sickle cell diseases (see under *disease*). Called also *drepanocyte*.
signet ring c. a cell in which the nucleus has been pressed to one side by an accumulation of intracytoplasmic mucin, as in signet ring cell carcinoma and Krukenberg tumor.
skeletogenous c. osteoblast.
small alveolar c's type I alveolar c's.
small cleaved c., small cleaved follicular center c. a follicular center cell considered to be the precursor of the other stages; it has a diameter of about 8 μm, a nucleus with a deep fold or cleft and clumped chromatin, and cytoplasm that is not pyroninophilic.
small granule c's S c's (def. 2).
small noncleaved c., small noncleaved follicular center c., small uncleaved c. a follicular center cell considered to be intermediate between the large cleaved and the large noncleaved stages; it has a diameter of about 12 μm, a nucleus without folds or clefts that contains finely dispersed chromatin, and cytoplasm that is pyroninophilic and basophilic.
smudge c. a disrupted leukocyte appearing during preparation of a peripheral blood smear.
solitary c's of Meynert Meynert c's.
somatic c's any of the cells of an organism other than the germ cells.
somatostatin c's endocrine cells that secrete somatostatin, found in oxyntic and pyloric glands.
somatotrope c., somatotroph c., somatotropic c. somatotroph.
sperm c. spermatozoon.
spermatogonial c. spermatogonium.
sphenoid c. see under *sinus*.
spider c. 1. astrocyte. 2. a cell occurring in rhabdomyoma; its nucleus, with a narrow rim of cytoplasm, is located in what appears to be a large vacuole, with thread-like processes radiating to the outer cell wall.
spindle c. any of various types of cells having a spindle shape; called also *fusiform c.*
spur c. acanthocyte.
squamous c. a flat, scalelike epithelial cell.
squamous alveolar c's type I alveolar c's.
stab c., staff c. band c.

star c's cells with large vacuoles in their cytoplasm and cytoplasmic bridges; seen in ameloblastoma.
stave c's littoral c's.
stellate c. any cell having a star-shaped appearance produced by numerous processes that extend in different directions, such as the Kupffer and hepatic stellate cells in the liver and astrocytes and granule cells in the cerebral and cerebellar cortices.
stem c's undifferentiated cells with the ability to divide and proliferate to provide precursor cells that can differentiate into specialized cells. See also *embryonic stem c's* and *hematopoietic stem c's*.
Sternberg giant c's, Sternberg-Reed c's Reed-Sternberg c's.
stippled c. an erythrocyte containing granules of varying size and shape, taking a basic or bluish stain with Wright stain, as in punctate basophilia.
strap c. a racquet-shaped rhabdomyoblast with an elongated cytoplasmic tail; called also *tadpole c.*
supporting c's cells that serve to provide support and protection and perhaps contribute to the nutrition of principal or other cells of certain organs; included are cells in the membranous labyrinth of the internal ear, olfactory epithelium, taste buds, and seminiferous tubules (Sertoli cells). Called also *sustentacular c's.*
suppressor c's, suppressor T c's differentiated T lymphocytes of the CD8 cells group that suppress antibody synthesis or cell-mediated immunity. They may be activated in response to antigen or to idiotypic determinants present on antibodies and T and B cell antigen receptors and may act either by suppressing activity of helper cells or by inhibiting the differentiation of activated lymphocytes into effector cells. Murine suppressor cells are marked by the Ly-2 and Ly-3 antigens, human suppressor cells by the CD5 and CD8 antigens. Cf. *contrasuppressor c's.*
sustentacular c's supporting c's.
sympathicotrophic c's large epithelioid cells occurring in groups and connected with bundles of nonmyelinated nerve fibers in the hilus of the ovary.
sympathochromaffin c's small round cells in the fetal suprarenal gland, the forerunners of the sympathetic neurons and cells of the medulla.
syncytial c. a cell whose cytoplasm is confluent with that of an adjacent cell.
syncytiotrophoblastic c. a type of large, multinucleate cell resembling a syncytiotrophoblast, having hyperchromatic nuclei and abundant eosinophilic, sometimes vacuolated, cytoplasm; one of the cell types that compose a choriocarcinoma. Cf. *cytotrophoblastic c.*
synovial c's fibroblasts lying between the cartilaginous fibers in the synovial membrane of joints.
T c's see under *lymphocyte.*
T_{DTH} c's activated T cells producing lymphokines mediating the delayed-type hypersensitivity reaction; most are in the population exhibiting the same surface markers as helper cells.
tactile c. see under *receptor.*
tadpole c. strap c.
target c. 1. an abnormally thin erythrocyte that when stained shows a dark center and a peripheral ring of hemoglobin, separated by a pale unstained ring containing less hemoglobin; seen in certain congenital and acquired anemias, thalassemia, certain hemoglobinopathies, liver disease, especially obstructive jaundice, and other disorders, and the postsplenectomy state. Called also *codocyte, leptocyte, Mexican hat c.* or *erythrocyte,* and *target erythrocyte.* 2. any cell selectively affected by a particular agent, such as a hormone or drug.
tart c. a macrophage or monocytoid reticuloendothelial cell that contains a phagocytized nucleus with well-preserved nuclear structure; the phagocytized nucleus, as distinguished from an LE cell inclusion, shows an intact chromatin pattern and chromatin that is more dense and tends to become vacuolated, and is frequently smaller than that in a true LE cell.

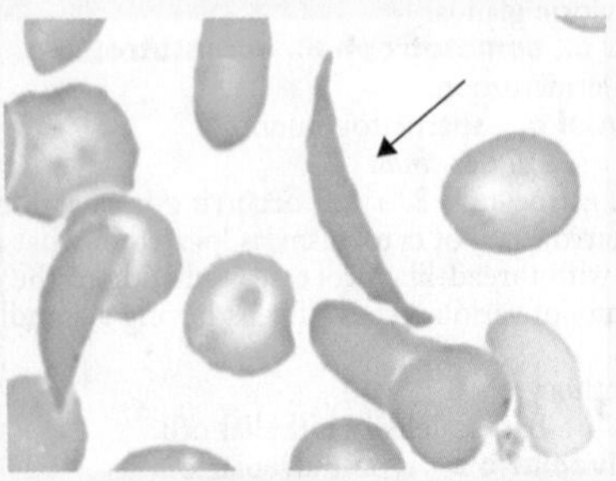

■ Sickle cell *(arrow).*

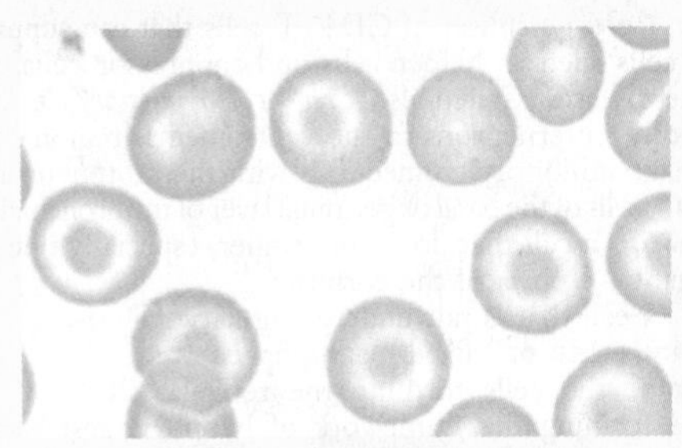

■ Target cells.

taste c's the cells in a taste bud that have gustatory receptors and are thus directly involved in taste; they undergo degeneration and replacement every few days. Called also *gustatory c's.*
tautomeral c's cells of the gray matter of the spinal cord whose axons pass into the white substance of the same side of the cord.
teardrop c. dacryocyte.
tegmental c's cells that cover any delicate structure.
tendon c's flattened tissue cells of connective tissue occurring in rows between the primary bundles of the tendons.
$T\gamma$ c's T lymphocytes that have Fc receptors for immunoglobulin M and have suppressor cell function.
theca c's, theca-lutein c's lutein cells derived from the theca interna; called also *paraluteal* or *paralutein c's.*
T-helper c's helper c's.
Thoma-Zeiss counting c. see under *chamber.*
thyroidectomy c's hypertrophied thyrotrophs found in the adenohypophysis after thyroidectomy and in severe thyroid hormone deficiency.
thyroid follicular c. an epithelial cell of a thyroid follicle; these produce thyroid hormones and become enlarged in some forms of goiter. Called also *thyrocyte.*
thyrotrope c., thyrotroph c., thyrotropic c. thyrotroph.
T-killer c's cytotoxic T lymphocytes.
$T\mu$ c's T lymphocytes that have Fc receptors for immunoglobulin M and have helper cell function.
totipotent c., totipotential c. an embryonic cell that is capable of developing into any variety of body cells.
touch c. tactile receptor.
Touton giant c. a large vacuolated cell with numerous nuclei surrounding a peripheral rim of foamy cytoplasm; characteristic of such diseases as xanthomas, juvenile xanthogranuloma, and histiocytosis X.
transformed c's cells that have undergone malignant transformation.
transitional c's 1. cells in the process of changing from one type to another, such as in transitional epithelium. 2. in the sinoatrial and atrioventricular nodes, small, slow-conducting, heterogeneous cells interposed between the P cells and Purkinje cells; they are thought to link the impulses generated by the P cells with the rest of the myocardium.
Treg c's, T-regulatory c's regulatory T c's.
trophochrome c's serous cells whose secretory granules give a staining reaction for mucus with mucicarmine; called also *mucoalbuminous c's* and *mucoserous c's.*
T-suppressor c's suppressor cells.
tubal air c's cellulae pneumaticae tubae auditivae.
tufted c. a type of cell in the olfactory bulb, smaller, more numerous, and more superficially located than a mitral cell but with similar functions and connections.
Türk c. a nongranular, mononuclear cell displaying morphologic characteristics of both an atypical lymphocyte and a plasma cell, observed in the peripheral blood during severe anemias, chronic infections, and leukemoid reactions.
tympanic c's, tympanic air c's cellulae tympanicae.
type I c's, type I alveolar c's the flattened cells of the alveolar epithelium, distinguished by their greatly attenuated cytoplasm and paucity of organelles; called also *membranous pneumonocytes* and *squamous alveolar* or *small alveolar c's.*

Cell *Continued*

type II c's, type II alveolar c's pleomorphic cells of the pulmonary alveolar epithelium that secrete surfactant and are distinguished by abundant cytoplasm containing numerous lipid-rich multilamellar bodies; called also *granular pneumonocytes* and *great* or *large alveolar c's.*
Tzanck c. a multinucleated giant cell, formed by the fusion of acantholytic keratinocytes, that occurs in the lesions of chickenpox, herpes simplex, herpes zoster, and pemphigus vulgaris; such cells are seen in the Tzanck test.
ultimobranchial c's parafollicular c's.
vacuolated c. a cell whose protoplasm contains vacuoles.
vasoformative c. angioblast (def. 2).
veil c's, veiled c's a type of antigen-presenting cells with numerous surface ruffles or veil-like processes, found in the afferent lymph and lymphatic sinuses; they may contain inclusions similar to the Birbeck granules characteristic of the Langerhans cells of the epidermis.
ventricular c. any of the columnar epithelial cells of the neural tube.
Vero c's a cell line derived from African green monkey kidney cells, used in the isolation of viruses.
vestibular hair c's hair cells found in the maculae of the utricle and saccule, serving as sensory receptors responsive to changes in position; they regulate the sense of equilibrium by sending impulses up the vestibular nerve to the brain. There are two types of these hair cells: *type I cells* are flask-shaped and *type 2 cells* are tubular.
veto c's a subset of suppressor cells that are passively recognized by autoreactive cytotoxic T cells that recognize major histocompatibility antigens on the veto cells; this one-way recognition results in the elimination of the autoreactive cytotoxic T cells.
Vignal c's embryonic connective tissue cells secreting myelin and associated with the formation of the axons of nerves in the fetus.
Virchow c. lepra c.
visceral epithelial c. podocyte.
visual c's the neuroepithelial photoreceptor portion of the retina, the first neurons of the vertical linkage of the retina, consisting of two kinds of cells: the *retinal cones* and *retinal rods* (see under *cone* and *rod*). Each rod or cone has an inner, axonal, process synapsing with one or more horizontal or bipolar retinal cells, has a soma in the outer nuclear layer, and has a photosensitive outer dendritic process that extends toward the pigment epithelium. See also *ganglion c.* Called also *photoreceptor c's.*
voltaic c. an electrochemical cell (q.v.) that serves as a voltage source. Called also *galvanic c.*
von Hansemann c's macrophages containing Michaelis-Gutmann bodies, occurring as sheets of cells in malacoplakia of the urinary tract or kidney. Called also *Hansemann macrophages.*
von Kupffer c's Kupffer c's.
wandering c. ameboid c.
Warthin-Finkeldey c. a type of multinucleate giant cell with intranuclear inclusions, of lymphoreticular origin, seen in various organs, including lymph nodes, tonsil, appendix, and thymus, just prior to or during the prodromal phase of measles.
wasserhelle c., water-clear c. a large clear cell found in the parathyroid gland; these cells have a ballooned appearance and are especially numerous in adenoma of the gland.
Wedl c's large swollen cells (bladder cells) formed by the capsular epithelium in cataract development.
white c., white blood c. leukocyte.
wing c's cells in the corneal epithelium with convex anterior surfaces and concave posterior surfaces.
xanthoma c. foam c. (def. 2).
Zander c's bladder c's.
zymogenic c's cells that contain zymogens and secrete enzymes; see *acinar c's* and *chief c's* (def. 1).

cel·lac·e·fate (sel-as′ə-fāt) [NF] a reduction product of phthalic anhydride and a partial acetate ester of cellulose; it is a free-flowing white powder used as a tablet-coating agent. Called also *cellulose acetate phthalate.*

Cel·lase 1000 (sel′ās) trademark for a preparation of cellulase, used as a digestant adjunct.

Cell·Cept (sel′sept) trademark for preparations of mycophenolate mofetil.

Cel·lia (sel′e-ə) [Angelo *Celli*, Italian physician, 1857–1914] a subgenus of mosquitoes of the genus *Anopheles*, vectors of malaria in Africa and Asia.

cel·lic·o·lous (sə-lik′ə-ləs) [*cella* + *colere* to dwell] inhabiting cells.

cel·li·form (sel′ĭ-form) cytoid.

cel·lo·bi·ose (sel″lo-bi′ōs) a disaccharide, two glucose moieties in β-(1,4) linkage, forming the basic repeating unit of cellulose and obtained by partial hydrolysis of the polysaccharide.

cel·lo·bi·uron·ic ac·id (sel″o-bi″u-ron′ik) a disaccharide consisting of glucose and glucuronic acid linked at positions 1 and 4, found in the capsular polysaccharides of *Streptococcus pneumoniae.* See also *pneumococcal polysaccharide*, under *polysaccharide.*

cel·loi·din (sə-loi′din) a concentrated preparation of pyroxylin, employed in microscopy for embedding specimens for section cutting.

cel·lo·phane (sel′o-fān) a transparent tissue of regenerated cellulose used as a dialysis membrane and for bandages, compresses, etc.

cel·lu·la (sel′u-lə) pl. *cel′lulae* [L., dim. of *cella*] 1. in anatomy, a small, more or less enclosed space. 2. in histology, a cell.

cel′lulae ethmoida′les [TA] ethmoidal cells: collective name for a type of paranasal sinus occurring in groups within the ethmoid bone and communicating with the ethmoidal infundibulum and bulla and the superior and highest meatuses. They are often subdivided into *cellulae ethmoidales anteriores, medii,* and *posteriores,* named according to the location of their openings into the nasal meatus. Called also *ethmoid* or *ethmoidal air cells* and *sinus ethmoidales.*

cel′lulae ethmoida′les anterio′res [TA] anterior ethmoidal cells: ethmoidal air cells that open into the middle nasal meatus; they are often grouped with adjacent middle and posterior ethmoidal cells and called simply *ethmoidal cells* or *sinuses.* Called also *sinus ethmoidales anteriores.*

cel′lulae ethmoida′les me′diae [TA] middle ethmoidal cells: ethmoidal air cells that open into the middle nasal meatus; they are often grouped with adjacent anterior and posterior ethmoidal sinuses and called simply *ethmoidal cells.* Called also *sinus ethmoidales medii.*

cel′lulae ethmoida′les posterio′res [TA] posterior ethmoidal cells: ethmoidal air cells that open into the superior nasal meatus; they are often grouped with adjacent middle and anterior ethmoidal sinuses and called simply *ethmoidal cells.* Called also *sinus ethmoidales posteriores.*

cel′lulae mastoi′deae [TA] mastoid cells: the air cells in the mastoid process of the temporal bone.

cel′lulae pneuma′ticae tu′bae auditi′vae [TA] air cells of auditory tube: air cells in the floor of the auditory tube close to the carotid canal, being similar to the air cells of the mastoid part of the temporal bone; called also *cellulae pneumaticae tubae auditoriae* [TA alternative] and *tubal air cells.*

cel′lulae pneuma′ticae tu′bae audito′riae TA alternative for *cellulae pneumaticae tubae auditivae.*

cel′lulae tympa′nicae [TA] tympanic cells: spaces in the tympanic cavity between the bony projections from the floor, or jugular wall; they sometimes communicate with the tubal air cells. Called also tympanic air cells.

cel·lu·lae (sel′u-le) [L.] plural of *cellula.*

cel·lu·lar (sel′u-lər) 1. pertaining to cells. 2. made up of cells.

cel·lu·lar·i·ty (sel″u-lar′ĭ-te) the state of a tissue or other mass as regards the number of constituent cells.

cel·lu·lase (sel′u-lās) [EC 3.2.1.4] an enzyme of the hydrolase class that catalyzes the cleavage of internal β-(1,4) glycosidic linkages, such as occur in cellulose. It occurs in various bacteria, fungi, plants, and more simple animals but is absent from higher animals.

cel·lule (sel′ūl) [L. *cellula*] cell, def. 2.

cel·lu·lic·i·dal (sel″u-lis′ĭ-dəl) [*cellula* + *-cide* + *-al*[1]] cytocidal.

cel·lu·lif·u·gal (sel″u-lif′ə-gəl) [*cellula* + *-fugal*[2]] directed away from a cell body.

cel·lu·lip·e·tal (cel″u-lip′ə-təl) [*cellula* + *-petal*] directed toward a cell body.

cel·lu·lite (sel′u-līt) a subcutaneous fat deposit that causes a dimpled condition of the skin, such as on the thigh or buttock.

cel·lu·li·tis (sel″u-li′tis) [*cellule* + *-itis*] an acute, diffuse, spreading, edematous, suppurative inflammation of the deep subcutaneous tissues and sometimes muscle, sometimes with abscess formation. It is usually caused by infection of a wound, burn, or other cutaneous lesion by bacteria, especially group A streptococci and *Staphylococcus aureus,* but it may also occur in immunocompromised hosts or following erysipelas (q.v.).

anaerobic c. cellulitis due to a necrotizing infection with anaerobic bacteria; the most common pathogen is *Clostridium perfringens,* but it can also be caused by species of *Bacteroides, Peptostreptococcus,* and *Prevotella,* or mixtures of different bacteria. It is usually in a contaminated wound or in otherwise compromised tissues; symptoms include a foul-smelling discharge, gas formation, and crepitus. The clinical findings are milder than those seen in true gas gangrene, but progressive tissue destruction may lead to fatal septicemia.

dissecting c. of scalp perifolliculitis capitis abscedens et suffodiens.

eosinophilic c. Wells syndrome.

facial c. cellulitis affecting the face, sometimes produced by spread of infection from nearby or distant foci. In children it is usually on just one cheek, and in adults it most often affects the neck; it may also occur around the eyes. It is tender, bluish in color, and poorly demarcated, with an edematous border, and patients often have fever, local pain, and bacteremia. *Haemophilus influenzae* type b, Group B streptococci, and *Streptococcus pneumoniae* are etiologic agents in young children. In adults and older children, *Staphylococcus aureus* and group A streptococci are the usual etiologic agents.

finger c. whitlow.

gangrenous c. 1. necrotizing fasciitis. 2. necrotic dermatitis.

indurated c. a hard, brawny induration of the skin, which may be painful and disabling; the usual site is the lower leg, generally proximal to the malleolus, although it can affect other areas and sometimes involves the entire circumference of the leg. The cause is low-grade inflammation with chronic venous insufficiency, such as in postphlebitic syndrome.

intermandibular c. pharyngeal phlegmon.

juvenile c. see under *pyoderma.*

necrotizing c. see under *fasciitis.*

orbital c. a type of facial cellulitis, usually secondary to sinusitis in children, characterized by proptosis, lid swelling, chemosis, and impaired ocular motility. In rare cases it may cause blindness and death.

pelvic c. parametritis.

periurethral c. an extensive fulminating cellulitis originating in and about the urethra; if left untreated, it may develop into gangrene of the genital and perigenital tissues.

phlegmonous c. an inflammatory reaction to infection with microaerophilic streptococci, forming a suppurative or gangrenous and undermining lesion that may extend into deep subcutaneous tissues and muscles.

preseptal c. facial cellulitis affecting the anterior part of the orbital septum, with edema of the eyelids; it may be caused by spread of infection from some other area or by trauma to the periorbital tissue.

synergistic necrotizing c. a variant of necrotizing fasciitis that particularly involves the skin and muscle, most often on a lower limb or in the perineal area.

ulcerative c. see under *lymphangitis.*

cel·lu·lo·fi·brous (sel″u-lo-fi′brəs) fibrocellular.

Cel·lu·lo·mo·na·da·ceae (sel″u-lo-mo″nə-da′se-e) [L. *cellulosa* cellulose + Gr. *monas* a unit, from *monos* single] a family of bacteria of the suborder Micrococcineae, order Actinomycetales, consisting of gram-positive, branching rods that do not produce mycelia. Pathogenic organisms are contained in the genera *Oerskovia* and *Tropheryma.*

cel·lu·lose (sel′u-lōs) the most abundant polysaccharide in nature, a rigid, colorless, unbranched, insoluble, long chain polymer, consisting of 3000 to 5000 glucose residues in β-(1,4) linkage and forming the skeleton of most plant structures and of plant cells; it can be enzymatically hydrolyzed to the disaccharide cellobiose, although humans lack the necessary enzyme, cellulase.

absorbable c. oxidized c.

c. acetate an acetylated cellulose used in membrane filters for a variety of functions; used as a hemodialyzer membrane, it has a greater permeability and higher ultrafiltration rate than cuprophane.

c. acetate phthalate cellacefate.

hydroxyethyl c. see under *H.*

hydroxypropyl c. see under *H.*

microcrystalline c. [NF] purified, partially depolymerized cellulose prepared by treating alpha cellulose, obtained as a pulp from fibrous plant material with mineral acids; used as a tablet and capsule diluent.

oxidized c. [USP] cellulose partially oxidized and with a varying content of carboxylic acid groups, which confers some solubility in dilute alkali; it is insoluble in water. Dried in a vacuum over phosphorus pentoxide, it is used as a local hemostatic. Called also *absorbable c.* and *absorbable cotton.*

c. sodium phosphate [USP] an insoluble, nonabsorbable cation exchange resin prepared by phosphorylation of cellulose; it exchanges sodium for calcium and when taken orally binds calcium, which is then excreted in the feces. Used to prevent the formation of calcium-containing renal calculi, as in absorptive hypercalciuria.

c. tetranitrate $(C_{12}H_{16}N_4O_{18})_n$, the principal constituent of pyroxylin.

cel·lu·lo·sic ac·id (sel″u-lo′sik) oxidized cellulose.

cel·lu·los·i·ty (sel″u-los′ĭ-te) the condition of being composed of cells.

cel(o)-[1] [Gr. *kēlē* tumor, hernia] a combining form denoting relationship to a tumor or swelling.

cel(o)-[2] [Gr. *koilos* hollow] see *coel(o)-.*

cel(o)-[3] [Gr. *koilia* belly] see *celi(o)-.*

ce·lom (se′ləm) coelom.

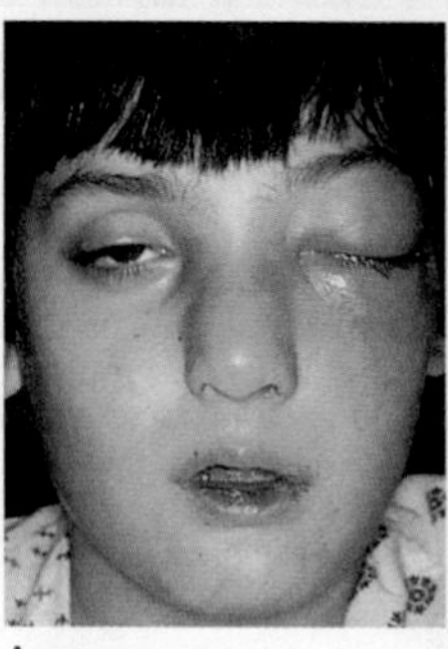

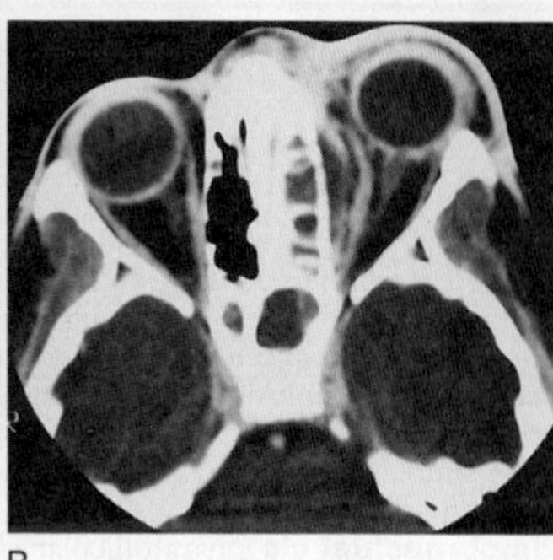

■ Orbital cellulitis. *(A)*, Clinical view; *(B)*, CT scan showing preseptal swelling, proptosis, and lateral displacement of globe and orbital contents by subperiosteal abscess.

ce·lom·ic (se-lom′ik) coelomic.

Ce·lon·tin (se-lon′tin) trademark for a preparation of methsuximide.

ce·lo·phle·bi·tis (se″lo-flə-bi′tis) [*celo-*[2] + *phlebitis*] cavitis.

ce·los·chi·sis (se-los′kĭ-sis) [*celo-*[3] + *-schisis*] abdominal fissure.

ce·los·co·py (sə-los′kə-pe) laparoscopy.

ce·lo·so·mia (se″lo-so′me-ə) [*celo-*[3] + *soma*] a developmental anomaly characterized by fissure or absence of the sternum and hernial protrusion of the viscera. Cf. *thoracogastroschisis.*

ce·lo·so·mus (se″lo-so′məs) a fetus with celosomia.

ce·lot·o·my (se-lot′ə-me) herniotomy.

Cel·si·us scale, thermometer (sel′se-əs) [Anders *Celsius,* Swedish astronomer, 1701–1744] see under *scale* and *thermometer.*

CEM contagious equine metritis.

ce·ment (sə-ment′) [L. *cementum*] 1. a substance that serves to produce solid union between two surfaces. 2. cementum. 3. dental c.

calcium hydroxide c. a dental cement that promotes the formation of a protective layer of secondary dentin, which is particularly beneficial in aiding healing of the pulp; used principally for pulp capping, as a thermal insulating base, and for protection from chemical insult.

dental c. any of various bonding substances that are placed in the mouth as a viscous liquid and set to a hard mass; used in restorative and orthodontic dental procedures as luting (cementing) agents, as protective, insulating, or sedative bases, and as restorative materials.

glass ionomer c. a dental cement produced by mixing a powder prepared from a calcium fluoroaluminosilicate glass and a liquid prepared from an aqueous solution of polyacrylic acid; used for small restorations on the proximal surfaces of anterior teeth, for restoration of eroded areas at the gingival margin, and as a luting agent for restorations and orthodontic bands.

glass ionomer c., hybrid resin-modified glass ionomer c.

glass ionomer c., resin-modified a type of glass ionomer cement with pendant methacrylate groups attached to polycarboxylic acid; it also may contain other water-soluble methacrylate monomers and complex vinyl-carboxylate monomers. Hardening occurs by acid-base reaction plus addition polymerization. Called also *hybrid glass ionomer c.*

intercellular c. a mucilaginous substance that holds cells, and especially epithelial cells, together.

muscle c. myoglia.

polycarboxylate c. a dental cement made by mixing a powder consisting chiefly of zinc oxide and an aqueous solution of polyacrylic acid; used as a luting agent for cementing restorations and as a cavity lining.

polymethacrylate c. a cement used in surgery and dentistry, consisting of an acrylic resin formed by the polymerization of methyl methacrylate monomers.

resin c. one of several polymer or monomer/polymer systems, usually containing finely divided inorganic filler particles, used as an insoluble dental luting agent in the cementation of orthodontic brackets, ceramic, resin, and metal restorations, and etched based metal extracoronal retainers to etched enamel.

root canal c. see under *sealer.*

silicate c. a dental cement that is translucent and porcelainlike when set; formerly used for esthetic temporary and semipermanent restorations of anterior teeth.

silicophosphate c. a mixture of silicate and zinc phosphate cements, formerly used as temporary filling material and for cementation of orthodontic bands, cast restorations, and porcelain jacket crowns; it has been replaced by resin cements and glass ionomer cements.

zinc oxide–eugenol c. a dental cement made by mixing zinc oxide powder with eugenol liquid and a small amount of water; used chiefly in temporary restorations, thermal insulating bases, and root canal fillings and as a temporary luting agent.

zinc phosphate c. a dental cement made by mixing a powder that consists chiefly of zinc oxide and magnesium oxide as a modifier with a liquid that is a mixture of phosphoric acid, water, and metallic salts that act as buffering agents; used primarily as a luting agent for fabricated restorations and secondarily in temporary restorations and as a thermal insulating agent.

ce•men•ta•tion (se″mən-ta′shən) the attachment of anything with cement, such as of restorative material to a natural tooth, or of bands to teeth.

ce•men•ti•cle (sə-men′tĭ-kəl) a small, discrete focus of calcified tissue that may or may not represent true cementum, found in the periodontal ligament.
adherent c., attached c. a cementicle that is firmly connected with the cementum.
free c., interstitial c. a cementicle that is completely surrounded by connective tissue of the periodontal ligament.

ce•men•ti•fi•ca•tion (sə-men″tĭ-fĭ-ka′shən) cementogenesis.

ce•men•tin (sə-men′tin) the material that sometimes unites the margins of squamous endothelial cells.

ce•men•ti•tis (se″mən-ti′tis) inflammation of the cementum of a tooth.

cement(o)- [L. *cementum*, q.v.] a combining form denoting relationship to the cementum.

ce•men•to•blast (sə-men′to-blast) [*cemento-* + *-blast*] a large cell ranging in shape from cuboidal to squamous with a large central nucleus and usually a single nucleolus, which is active in the formation of cementum (cementogenesis).

ce•men•to•blas•to•ma (sə-men″to-blas-to′mə) a rare, benign odontogenic tumor arising from the cementum and presenting as a proliferating mass contiguous with a tooth root, particularly that of a mandibular molar. Patients are generally asymptomatic, although cortical expansion and pain can occur.

ce•men•to•cla•sia (sə-men″to-kla′zhə) [*cemento-* + Gr. *klasis* breaking + *-ia*] dissolution and resorption of the cementum of a tooth; usually a complication of trauma or pathologic conditions.

ce•men•to•clast (sə-men′to-klast″) [*cemento-* + *-clast*] a cell, cytomorphologically the same as an osteoclast, involved in cementum resorption; the cavities produced by resorption are known as *resorption lacunae.* Called also *odontoclast.*

ce•men•to•cyte (sə-men′to-sīt) [*cemento-* + *-cyte*] a cell in the lacunae of cellular cementum, ranging in shape from round to oval or flattened, and exhibiting numerous protoplasmic processes extending from its free surface. Called also *cement cell.*

ce•men•to•enam•el (sə-men″to-ə-nam′əl) pertaining to the cementum and the dental enamel.

ce•men•to•gen•e•sis (sə-men″to-jen′ə-sis) [*cemento-* + *-genesis*] the development of the cementum on the root dentin of a tooth; called also *cementification.*

ce•men•toid (sə-men′toid) [*cement* + *-oid*] the surface uncalcified layer of the cementum in areas of intact periodontal tissue. Called also *precementum* and *uncalcified cementum.*

ce•men•to•ma (se″mən-to′mə) any of a variety of benign cementum-producing odontogenic tumors, including cementoblastoma, cementifying fibroma, florid osseous dysplasia, and periapical cemental dysplasia.
gigantiform c. florid osseous dysplasia.
true c. cementoblastoma.

ce•men•to•path•ia (sə-men′to-path′e-ə) periodontitis or periodontosis resulting from disease or defect of the cementum.

ce•men•to•peri•os•ti•tis (sə-men″to-per″e-os-ti′tis) periodontitis.

ce•men•to•sis (se″mən-to′sis) hypercementosis.

ce•men•tum (sə-men′təm) [L. *caementum* rough stone] [TA] the bone-like, rigid connective tissue covering the root of a tooth from the cementoenamel junction to the apex and lining the apex of the root canal; it also serves as an attachment structure for the periodontal ligament, thus assisting in tooth support. Called also *substantia ossea dentis.*
acellular c. the cementum without cellular components that covers one third to a half of the tooth root adjacent to the cementoenamel junction; it is usually apposed by a layer of cellular cementum.

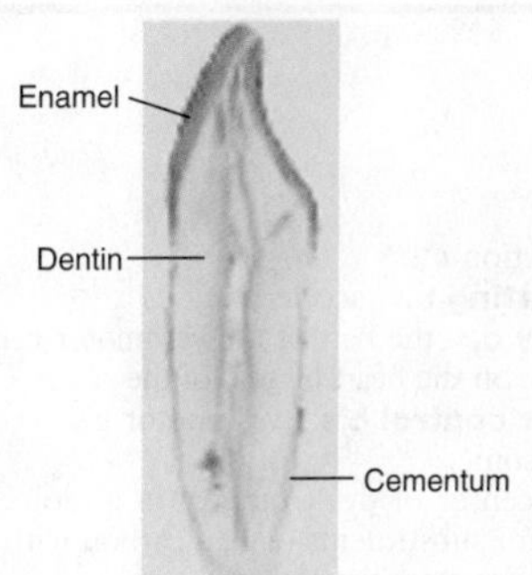

■ Cementum covering the anatomical root, thickening toward the apical region, in a ground longitudinal section of a tooth. The dental pulp has been lost in preparation.

afibrillar c. a layer of cementum, containing acid mucopolysaccharides and possibly nonfibrillar collagen, that sometimes extends onto the enamel of a tooth at the cementoenamel junction.
cellular c. the cementum covering the apical half to two thirds of the tooth root; it contains cementocytes embedded in the calcified matrix and is usually apposed by a layer of acellular cementum.
uncalcified c. cementoid.

ce•na•del•phus (se″nə-del′fəs) [*cen-*[2] + *-adelphus*] symmetrical conjoined twins.

ce•nes•the•sia (se″nes-the′zhə) [*cen-*[2] + *esthesia*] somatognosis. **cenesthe′sic, cenesthe′tic** *adj*

ce•nes•the•si•op•a•thy (se″nəs-the″ze-op′ə-the) [*cenesthesia* + *-pathy*] cenesthopathy.

ce•nes•thop•a•thy (se″nəs-thop′ə-the) a general feeling of discomfort, unease, and lack of wellness not referable to any particular part of the body.

Cen•es•tin (sĕ-nes′tin) trademark for preparations of conjugated estrogens.

cen(o)-[1] [Gr. *kainos* new, fresh] a combining form meaning new; written also *cain(o)-* and *kain(o)-.*

cen(o)-[2] [Gr. *koinos* shared in common] a combining form denoting relationship to a common feature or characteristic; written also *coen(o)-*, *coin(o)-*, and *koin(o)-.*

ce•no•bi•um (sə-no′be-əm) [Gr. *koinobios* living in communion with others] a colony of independent cells or organisms held together by a common investment.

ce•no•cyte (se′no-sīt) coenocyte.

ce•no•site (se′no-sīt) coinosite.

ce•no•type (se′no-tīp) [*ceno-*[2] + *type*] the original type from which all forms have arisen.

cen•sor (sen′sər) a term used by Freud to refer to the mental faculty that guards the border between the unconscious and preconscious, preventing unconscious thoughts and wishes from coming into consciousness unless disguised, as in dreams. In Freud's later theory, the actions of the censor (displacement, condensation, symbolism, and repression) are considered defense mechanisms of the ego and superego.

Cen•tau•rea (sen-taw′re-ə) a genus of plants with yellow flowers, found mainly in the western United States and Australia; when eaten by horses they cause nigropallidal encephalomalacia. *C. re′pens* is the Russian knapweed and *C. solstitia′lis* is the yellow star thistle.

Cen•tel•la (sen-tel′ə) a widespread genus of small, creeping, umbelliferous plants with shovel-shaped leaves, including *C. asia′ticus* or gotu kola, which grows in swampy areas in India, Sri Lanka, Madagascar, and South Africa, and is used medicinally.

cen•ter (sen′tər) [L. *centrum*, from Gr. *kentron*] 1. the middle point of a body. 2. a collection of neurons in the central nervous system concerned with performance of a particular function; see also *area.*

Center

accelerating c. the part of the vasomotor center involved in acceleration of the heart; called also *cardioaccelerating c.*
anospinal c's the centers for contracting the sphincter ani, for relaxing it (defecation center), and for the anal reflex; all are in the lumbar enlargement.
apneustic c. the neurons in the brainstem that control normal respiration; not a true center.
auditopsychic c. auditory association area.
auditory word c. Wernicke area.
Broca c. Broca motor speech area.

Center *Continued*

Budge c. erection c.
cardioaccelerating c. accelerating c.
cardioinhibitory c. the part of the vasomotor center that exerts an inhibitory influence on the heart by way of the vagus. Called also *Kronecker c.*
cardiovascular control c's vasomotor c's.
cell c. centrosome.
chiral c. the center of dyssymmetry in a molecule, usually an atom with four different substituents (e.g., a carbon with four single bonds or the nitrogen of a quaternary amine).
c's of chondrification dense aggregations of embryonic mesenchymal cells at sites of future cartilage formation; called also *protochondral tissue.*
ciliospinal c. a center in the lower cervical and upper thoracic portions of the spinal cord, connected with the dilatation of the pupil.
community mental health c. (CMHC) a mental health facility or group of affiliated agencies that provide various psychotherapeutic services to a designated catchment area.
coordination c. a nerve center serving the function of coordination.
coughing c. a center in the medulla oblongata that is above the respiratory centers and controls the act of coughing.
defecation c. see *anospinal c's.*
deglutition c. a nerve center in the medulla oblongata that controls the function of swallowing; called also *swallowing c.*
dentary c. an ossification center of the mandible, giving origin to the lower border and outer plate.
C's for Disease Control and Prevention (CDC) an agency of the U.S. Department of Health and Human Services, with headquarters in Atlanta, Georgia, concerned with all phases of control of communicable, vector-borne, and occupational diseases and with the prevention of disease, injury, and disability. The CDC's responsibilities include epidemiology, surveillance, detection, laboratory science, ecologic investigations, training, disease control methods, chronic disease prevention, health promotion, and injury prevention and control. Formerly called *Communicable Disease Center* (1946), *Center for Disease Control* (1970), and *Centers for Disease Control* (1980).
ejaculation c. the reflex center in the lumbar spinal cord that regulates ejaculation of semen during sexual stimulation.
epiotic c. the center of ossification that forms the mastoid process.
erection c. a reflex center in the sacral spinal cord that regulates erection of the penis or clitoris. Called also *Budge* or *genital c.*
eupraxic c. premotor area.
feeding c. a group of cells in the lateral hypothalamus that when stimulated cause a sensation of hunger; called also *hunger c.*
Flemming c. germinal c.
gaze c's centers in the brain that control eye coordination and gaze; a *vertical gaze center* is thought to be located in the midbrain and a *lateral gaze center* is thought to be located in the pons.
genital c., genitospinal c. erection c.
germinal c. the spherical area in the center of a secondary lymphoid nodule containing mainly aggregations of actively proliferating B lymphocytes, developing in a primary lymphoid nodule in response to antigenic stimulation.
glossokinesthetic c. motor speech area.
health c. 1. a community health organization for creating health work and coordinating the efforts of all health agencies. 2. an educational complex consisting of a medical school and various allied health professional schools.
heat-regulating c's thermoregulatory c's.
hunger c. feeding c.
Kerckring (Kerkring) c. an ossification center sometimes present in the posterior margin of the foramen magnum at about the sixteenth week of fetal life; it unites with the other squamous parts prior to birth. Called also *Kerckring ossicle.*
Kronecker c. cardioinhibitory c.
Lumsden c. pneumotaxic c.
medullary c. 1. medullary c. of cerebellum. 2. medullary respiratory c.
medullary c. of cerebellum corpus medullare cerebelli.
medullary respiratory c. the part of the respiratory centers that is in the medulla oblongata, divided between the *dorsal respiratory group* and the *ventral respiratory group.*
microtubule organizing c. (MTOC) general term for a region of cytoplasm from which microtubules radiate and which regulates their number and organization; in animal cells, the centrosome is the primary microtubule organizing center.
micturition c's centers in the brain and spinal cord that control functioning of the bladder and urethra in micturition; see *pontine micturition c.* and *sacral micturition c.*
nerve c. center (def. 2).
optic c. that point in a lens, or combination of lenses, where all rays that help to form a clear image cross the principal axis; in the eye, about 2 mm behind the cornea.
ossification c. centrum ossificationis.
ossification c., primary centrum ossificationis primarium.
ossification c., secondary centrum ossificationis secundarium.
panting c. polypneic c.
phrenic c. centrum tendineum diaphragmatis.
pneumotaxic c. a center in the upper part of the pons that rhythmically inhibits inhalation independently of the vagus nerve; called also *Lumsden c.*
polypneic c. a center in the tuber cinereum that accelerates the respiration rate.
pontine micturition c. a group of neurons in the dorsolateral pontine tegmentum that project to spinal nuclei and coordinate urethral sphincter relaxation and detrusor contraction to facilitate urination. Called also *Barrington nucleus.*
pteriotic c. a center of ossification in the fetus and infant, from which are developed the tegmen tympani and the covering of the lateral semicircular canal.
reaction c. germinal c.
rectovesical c. a reflex center in the spinal cord regulating reflexes of the rectum and urinary bladder.
reflex c. any center in the brain or spinal cord in which a sensory impression is changed into a motor impulse.
respiratory c's a series of centers in the medulla and pons which coordinate respiratory movements; they include the pneumotaxic center, the apneustic center, and the dorsal and ventral respiratory groups.
rotation c. the point or axis about which a body rotates.
sacral micturition c. a center in the sacral spinal cord that contributes to control of the bladder and inhibition of tension of the urethral sphincters.
satiety c. a group of cells in the ventromedial hypothalamus that when stimulated suppress the desire for food.
semioval c. centrum semiovale.
sensory c's primary receiving areas.
sex-behavior c. ventromedial nucleus of hypothalamus.
sphenotic c. a center of ossification in the fetal sphenoid bone for the lingula.
splenial c. one of the ossification centers of the mandible, forming a part of its inner plate.
sudorific c. sweat c.
swallowing c. deglutition c.
sweat c. 1. a center in the anterior hypothalamus controlling sweating. 2. any of several centers in the medulla oblongata or spinal cord that exercise parasympathetic control over sweating. Called also *sweat c.*
thermoregulatory c's hypothalamic centers regulating the conservation and dissipation of heat.
thirst c. a group of cells in the lateral hypothalamus that when stimulated cause a sensation of thirst.
vasoconstrictor c. a center in the medulla oblongata and lower pons that controls contraction of the blood vessels.
vasodilator c. a center in the medulla oblongata that causes dilation of blood vessels by repressing the activity of the vasoconstrictor center.
vasomotor c's centers in the medulla oblongata and the lower pons that regulate the caliber of the blood vessels and increase or decrease the heart rate and contractility. Called also *cardiovascular control c's;* see also *vasoconstrictor c.* and *vasodilator c.*
vesical c's, vesicospinal c's micturition c's.
vomiting c. a center in the lateral reticular formation of the medulla oblongata, stimulation of which causes vomiting. See also *chemoreceptor trigger zone,* under *zone.*

cen·tes·i·mal (sen-tes′ĭ-məl) [L. *centesimus* hundredth] divided into hundredths or based upon divisions into hundredths.

cen·te·sis (sen-te′sis) [Gr. *kentēsis*] perforation or tapping, as with an aspirator, trocar, or needle.

-centesis a word termination used to denote a perforation or tapping operation, with the part on which it is performed indicated by the root to which the suffix is affixed, e.g., *abdominocentesis* or *thoracocentesis.*

centi- [L. *centum* one hundred] a prefix denoting *(a)* one hundredth (10^{-2}) of the unit designated by the root with which it is combined (symbol c) as in centimeter (cm) or *(b)* one hundred, as in centipede.

cen·ti·grade (sen′tĭ-grād) [*centi-* + L. *gradus* a step] consisting of or having 100 gradations (steps or degrees); see under *scale.*

cen·ti·gray (cGy) (sen′tĭ-gra″) a unit of absorbed radiation dose equal to one hundredth (10^{-2}) of a gray, or 1 rad.

cen·ti·li·ter (cL) (sen′tĭ-le″tər) one hundredth (10^{-2}) of a liter.

cen·ti·me·ter (cm) (sen′tĭ-me″tər) a unit of length equal to one hundredth (10^{-2}) of a meter.

cubic c. (cm^3, cc) a unit of volume equal to that of a cube one centimeter on a side, equal to 1 mL or 10^{-6} m^3.

cen·ti·mor·gan (cM) (sen″tĭ-mor′gən) one-hundredth (10^{-2}) of a morgan; the unit of distance on a genetic map. The map distance between adjacent loci, expressed in centimorgans, is equal to the recombination frequency, expressed as a percentage; two loci are 1 cM apart if recombination is detected between them in one per cent of meioses. For nonadjacent loci the map distance can be greater than the recombination frequency, because recombination frequencies are not always additive. Called also *map unit.*

cen·ti·pede (sen′tĭ-pēd) any arthropod of the class Chilopoda.

cen·ti·poise (sen′tĭ-poiz, -pwahz) one hundredth (10^{-2}) of a poise.

cen·ti·unit (sen″tĭ-u′nit) one hundredth (10^{-2}) of a standard unit.

cen·tra (sen′trə) [L.] plural of *centrum.*

cen·trad[1] (sen′trad) [*centr-* + *-ad*] toward the center or a center, especially toward the center of the body.

cen·trad[2] (sen′trad) [L. *centum* hundred + *radian*] a measure of an angle of deviation, being 0.57 degree, or one one-hundredth part of a radian; called also *prism degree.*

cen·trage (sen′trāj) the condition in which the centers of the various refracting surfaces of the eye are in the same straight line.

cen·tral (sen′trəl) situated at or pertaining to a center; not peripheral.

cen·tra·lis (sən-tra′lis) [L.] [TA] a general term denoting a centrally located structure.

Cen·tra·moe·bi·da (sen″trə-me′bĭ-də) in newer systems of classification, an order of ramicristate amebae, protozoa of the class Lobosa, phylum Sarcomastigophora; it includes the genera *Acanthamoeba* and *Acanthopodina.*

cen·tra·phose (sen′trə-fōz) any aphose, or sensation of darkness, originating in the optic or visual centers.

cen·tra·tion (sən-tra′shən) the inability to pay attention to more than one salient feature at a time; it is a normal stage in human intellectual development.

cen·trax·o·ni·al (sen″trak-so′ne-əl) having the axis in a central median line.

cen·tre (sen′tər) center.

cen·tren·ce·phal·ic (sen″trən-sə-fal′ik) pertaining to the center of the encephalon; see under *system.*

centri- [L. *centrum* center, from Gr. *kentron* sharp point] a combining form denoting relationship to a center, or to a central location. Also, *centr(o)-.*

cen·tri·ac·i·nar (sen″trĭ-as′ĭ-nər) pertaining to the central portion of one or more acini.

cen·tric (sen′trik) 1. central. 2. having a center. 3. a term sometimes used as a noun to refer to *centric occlusion* or a *centric relation.*

power c. the position of the mandible during a forceful bite.

true c. centric relation.

cen·tric·i·put (sən-tris′ĭ-pət) [*centri-* + *caput*] the central part of the upper surface of the head, located between the occiput and sinciput.

cen·trif·u·gal (sen-trif′ə-gəl) [*centri-* + *-fugal*[2]] 1. efferent (def. 1). 2. corticifugal.

cen·trif·u·gate (sən-trif′u-gāt) material subjected to centrifugation.

cen·trif·u·ga·tion (sen-trif″u-ga′shən) the process of separating the lighter portions of a solution, mixture, or suspension from the heavier portions by centrifugal force.

density gradient c. ultracentrifugation in a liquid, such as cesium chloride solution, the density of which increases along the lines of centrifugal force, the substances under test or preparation seeking their level of density.

differential c. centrifugation based on the sedimentation coefficient of the substances under investigation; applied to homogenates to derive various subcellular fractions.

isopyknic c. centrifugation in which the solvent is of the same density as the substance to be isolated.

cen·tri·fuge (sen′trĭ-fūj) [*centri-* + *-fuge*] 1. a machine by which centrifugation is effected. 2. to subject to centrifugation.

microscope c. a high-speed centrifuge with a built-in microscope, permitting a specimen to be viewed under centrifugal force.

cen·tri·lob·u·lar (sen″trĭ-lob′u-lər) pertaining to the central portion of a lobule.

cen·tri·ole (sen′tre-ōl) either of the two cylindrical organelles located in the centrosome and containing nine triplets of microtubules arrayed around their edges; during cell division the centrioles are duplicated, with the resulting pairs migrating to opposite poles of the cell, where they serve to organize the spindles. They are capable of independent replication and of migrating to form basal bodies.

anterior c. proximal c.

distal c. that centriole of a spermatozoon which, after migrating to the cell surface and giving rise to a slender flagellum, returns to a position just caudal to the proximal centriole; called also *posterior c.*

posterior c. distal c.

proximal c. that centriole of a spermatozoon which migrates to a position in a depression in the wall of the posterior portion of the pronucleus, with its axis at right angles to the main axis of the spermatozoon, and from which the axoneme extends; called also *anterior c.*

ring c. a common misnomer for the anulus of the spermatozoon, which is not actually a centriole.

cen·trip·e·tal (sən-trip′ə-təl) [*centri-* + *-petal*] 1. afferent (def. 1). 2. corticipetal.

centr(o)- see *centri-.*

cen·tro·blast (sen′tro-blast″) [*centro-* + *-blast*] a general term encompassing both large noncleaved and small noncleaved follicular center cells.

cen·tro·ce·cal (sen″tro-se′kəl) pertaining to the central macular area and the blind spot; called also *cecocentral.*

Cen·tro·ces·tus (sen″tro-ses′təs) a genus of flukes. *C. cuspida′tus* is a species found in birds in Egypt and dogs in China and Taiwan.

cen·tro·cyte (sen′tro-sīt″) [*centro-* + *-cyte*] a general term encompassing both large cleaved and small cleaved follicular center cells.

cen·tro·des·mose (sen″tro-des′mōs) the connection between intranuclear centrioles during mitosis in certain protozoa; see *desmose.* Called also *centrodesmus.*

cen·tro·des·mus (sen″tro-des′məs) centrodesmose.

cen·tro·lec·i·thal (sen″tro-les′ĭ-thəl) [*centro-* + *lecithal*] having the yolk centrally located, surrounded by a peripheral layer of cytoplasm; such as the eggs of arthropods and insects.

cen·tro·lob·u·lar (sen″tro-lob′u-lər) centrilobular.

cen·tro·mere (sen′tro-mēr) [*centro-* + *-mere*] the region of the chromosome at which the sister chromatids are joined and by which the chromosome is attached to the spindle during cell division; it is required for normal segregation in mitosis and meiosis. According to its location, a centromere is said to be metacentric (central), submetacentric (off center), acrocentric (near one end), or telocentric (at one end). The last type does not occur in human chromosomes. **centromer′ic** *adj*

cen·tro·nu·cle·ar (sen″tro-noo′kle-ər) having or pertaining to a centrally located nucleus.

cen·tro·nu·cle·us (sen″tro-noo′kle-əs) amphinucleus.

cen·tro-os·teo·scle·ro·sis (sen″tro-os″te-o-sklə-ro′sis) centrosclerosis.

cen·tro·phose (sen′tro-fōz) any phose, or sensation of light, originating in the visual centers.

cen·tro·plast (sen′tro-plast) a central granule from which the axial filaments of the axopodia of certain heliozoa arise.

cen·tro·scle·ro·sis (sen″tro-sklə-ro′sis) [*centro-* + *osteosclerosis*] the filling of the marrow cavity of a bone with osseous material.

cen·tro·some (sen′tro-sōm) [*centro-* + *-some*] an organelle, located near the nucleus of animal cells, that contains the centrioles; it is the primary microtubule organizing center and directs the assembly of the spindle in mitosis. Called also *cell center* and *centrosphere.*

cen·tro·sphere (sen′tro-sfēr) [*centro-* + *sphere*] centrosome.

cen·trum (sen′trəm) pl. *cen′tra* [L., from Gr. *kentron*] 1. [TA] a center. 2. the large, central portion of the body of a vertebra, formed from the cranial and caudal portions of adjacent sclerotomes and ossified from a single center.

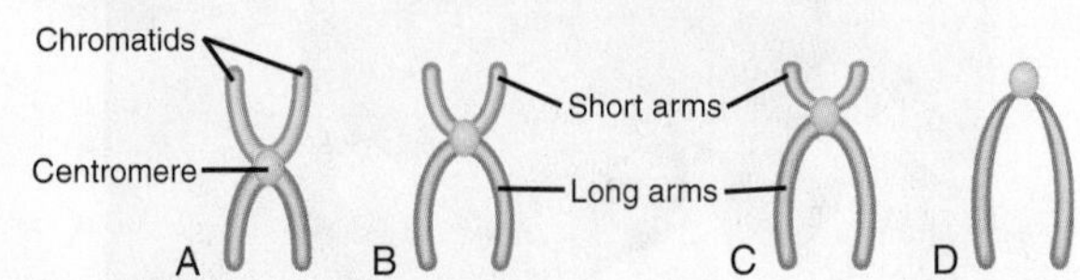

■ Position of the centromere in *(A)* metacentric; *(B)* submetacentric; *(C)* acrocentric; and *(D)* telocentric chromosomes.

c. ossificatio'nis [TA] ossification center: any point at which the process of ossification begins in bones; in a long bone there is a primary center for the diaphysis and a secondary center for the epiphysis. Called also *ossification point* and *punctum ossificationis.*

c. ossificatio'nis prima'rium primary ossification center: the first point at which a bone begins to ossify. Called also *primary ossification point* and *punctum ossificationis primarium.*

c. ossificatio'nis secunda'rium secondary ossification center: a point from which ossification proceeds that arises after a primary ossification center; it is concerned with progressive ossification toward the end of a bone. Called also *secondary ossification point* and *punctum ossificationis secundarium.*

c. perine'i TA alternative for *corpus perineale.*

c. semiova'le semioval center: the white matter of the cerebral hemispheres which underlies the cerebral cortex and which, in horizontal sections superior to the corpus callosum, has a semioval shape; it contains projection, commissural, and association fibers.

c. tendi'neum diaphrag'matis [TA] central tendon of diaphragm: the cloverleaf-shaped aponeurosis, immediately below the pericardium, onto which the diaphragmatic fibers converge to insert; called also *trefoil tendon, cordiform ligament of diaphragm,* and *phrenic center.*

c. of vertebra, vertebral c. centrum (def. 2).

Cen•tru•roi•des (sen″troo-roi'dēz) a genus of tropical and subtropical American scorpions of the family Buthidae, including several called bark scorpions. *C. exilicau'da* and *C. suffu'sus* are species found in desert areas of northern Mexico and the southwestern United States whose bites are poisonous.

CEP congenital erythropoietic porphyria.

Ceph•a•e•lis (sef″ə-e'lis) a genus of tropical shrubs and trees of the family Rubiaceae. *C. acumina'ta* and *C. ipecacua'nha* are sources of ipecac.

ceph•a•lad (sef'ə-lad) [*cephal-* + *-ad*] proceeding toward the head, as opposed to *caudad.* Called also *caudocephalad* and *craniad.*

ceph•a•lal•gia (sef″ə-lal'jə) [Gr. *kephalalgia*] headache.

histamine c. cluster headache.

pharyngotympanic c. glossopharyngeal neuralgia.

quadrantal c. headache affecting one quadrant of the head.

trigeminal autonomic c. (TAC) any of a group of primary headaches characterized by unilateral head pain accompanied by ipsilateral autonomic manifestations such as ptosis, conjunctival injection, lacrimation, rhinorrhea, nasal congestion, and Horner syndrome. Included here are cluster headache, chronic paroxysmal hemicrania, hemicrania continua, and short-lasting unilateral neuralgiform headache attacks with conjunctival injection and tearing (SUNCT).

ceph•al•ede•ma (sef″əl-ə-de'mə) [*cephal-* + *edema*] edema of the head.

ceph•a•lex•in (sef″ə-lek'sin) [USP] a semisynthetic first-generation cephalosporin, effective against a wide range of gram-positive and a limited range of gram-negative bacteria; administered orally in the treatment of tonsillitis, otitis media, and infections of the genitourinary tract, of bones and joints, and of skin and soft tissues.

c. hydrochloride [USP] the hydrochloride salt of cephalexin, having the same actions and uses as the base; administered orally.

ce•phal•gia (sə-fal'jə) headache.

ceph•al•he•mat•o•cele (sef″əl-he-mat'o-sēl) [*cephal-* + *hemato-* + *-cele*[1]] a bloody tumor under the pericranium, communicating with one or more sinuses of the dura through the cranial bones.

Stromeyer c. a subperiosteal cephalhematocele which communicates with veins and becomes filled with blood during strong expiratory efforts.

ceph•al•he•ma•to•ma (sef″əl-he″mə-to'mə) [*cephal-* + *hematoma*] a subperiosteal hemorrhage limited to the surface of one cranial bone, a usually benign condition seen frequently in the newborn as a result of bone trauma. Called also *cephalohematoma.*

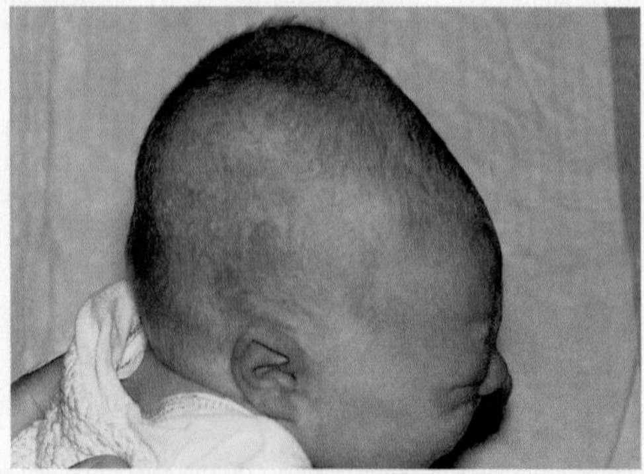

■ Bilateral cephalhematomas.

c. defor'mans a bulging of the anterior part of the skull due to hyperostosis, osteoporosis, and cavity formation in the bone.

ceph•al•hy•dro•cele (sef″əl-hi'dro-sēl) [*cephal-* + *hydrocele*] a serous or watery accumulation under the pericranium.

c. trauma'tica traumatic meningocele.

ce•phal•ic (sə-fal'ik) [Gr. *kephalikos*] 1. pertaining to the head. 2. cranial (def. 2).

ceph•a•li•za•tion (sef″ə-lĭ-za'shən) [Gr. *kephalē* head] 1. the concentration or initiation of the growth tendency at the head end of the embryo. 2. the development of a head; the concentration of nervous tissue and sense organs at the anterior end of the organism.

cephal(o)- [Gr. *kephalē* head] a combining form denoting relationship to the head.

ceph•a•lo•cau•dad (sef″ə-lo-kaw'dəd) 1. proceeding from the head toward the tail. 2. caudad. 3. in both a cephalic and caudal direction.

ceph•a•lo•cau•dal (sef″ə-lo-kaw'dəl) [*cephalo-* + *caudal*] pertaining to the long axis of the body, in a direction from head to tail.

ceph•a•lo•cele (sef'ə-lo-sēl″) [*cephalo-* + *-cele*[1]] encephalocele.

orbital c. protrusion of the cranial contents through a defect in the orbital wall, named according to its contents as meningocele, encephalocele, etc.

ceph•a•lo•cen•te•sis (sef″ə-lo-sen-te'sis) [*cephalo-* + *-centesis*] the surgical puncture of the skull.

ceph•a•lo•chord (sef'ə-lo-kord″) [*cephalo-* + *chord*] the intracranial portion of the embryonic notochord.

Ceph•a•lo•chor•da•ta (sef″ə-lo-kor-da'tə) a subphylum of primitive, small, fishlike chordates in which the notochord extends the entire length of the body; it includes the genus *Amphioxus.*

ceph•a•lo•chor•date (sef″ə-lo-kor'dāt) any member of the Cephalochordata.

ceph•a•lo•di•pros•o•pus (sef″ə-lo-di-pros'o-pəs) [*cephalo-* + *di-* + Gr. *prosopus* face] a fetus with a partially incomplete head attached to the head proper.

ceph•a•lo•dym•ia (sef″ə-lo-dim'e-ə) the condition of a cephalodymus.

ceph•a•lod•y•mus (sef″ə-lod'ə-məs) [*cephalo-* + *didymus* (2)] conjoined twins with a single or united head.

ceph•al•odyn•ia (sef″ə-lo-din'e-ə) [*cephal-* + *-odynia*] headache.

ceph•a•lo•gen•e•sis (sef″ə-lo-jen'ə-sis) [*cephalo-* + *-genesis*] the development of the head in the embryo.

ceph•a•lo•gram (sef'ə-lo-gram) [*cephalo-* + *-gram*] cephalometric radiograph.

ceph•a•log•ra•phy (sef″ə-log'rə-fe) [*cephalo* + *-graphy*] radiography of the head.

ceph•a•lo•gy•ric (sef″ə-lo-ji'rik) [*cephalo-* + *gyr-* + *-ic*] pertaining to turning motions of the head.

ceph•a•lo•hem•a•to•cele (sef″ə-lo-he-mat'o-sēl) cephalhematocele.

ceph•a•lo•he•ma•to•ma (sef″ə-lo-he″mə-to'mə) cephalhematoma.

ceph•a•lom•e•lus (sef″ə-lom'ə-ləs) [*cephalo-* + Gr. *melos* limb] a fetus with an accessory limb growing from the head.

ceph•a•lo•me•nia (sef″ə-lo-me'ne-ə) [*cephalo-* + *men-* + *-ia*] vicarious menstruation from the head, as in a nasal discharge at the menstrual period.

ceph•a•lom•e•ter (sef″ə-lom'ə-tər) [*cephalo-* + *-meter*] an instrument for measuring the head; an orienting device for positioning the head for radiographic examination and measurement.

ceph•a•lom•e•try (sef″ə-lom'ə-tre) scientific measurement of the dimensions of the head. In dentistry, certain combinations of linear and angular measurements developed from tracing the oriented lateral and frontal radiographic head film are used to assess craniofacial growth and development on a longitudinal basis and to determine the nature of orthodontic treatment response.

fetal c. measurement of the fetal skull in utero by means of x-ray films or by interpreting the echoes of ultrasonic radiation received from each side of the skull.

ceph•a•lo•mo•tor (sef″ə-lo-mo'tər) [*cephalo-* + *motor*] moving the head; pertaining to motions of the head.

ceph•a•lo•nia (sef″ə-lo'ne-ə) a condition in which the head is abnormally large with sclerotic hyperplasia of the brain.

ceph•a•lop•a•gus (sef″ə-lop'ə-gəs) craniopagus.

ceph•a•lop•a•thy (sef″ə-lop'ə-the) [*cephalo-* + *-pathy*] any disease of the head.

ceph•a•lo•pel•vic (sef″ə-lo-pel'vik) pertaining to the relationship of the fetal head to the maternal pelvis.

ceph•a•lo•pel•vim•e•try (sef″ə-lo-pəl-vim'ə-tre) pelvicephalometry.

ceph•a•lo•pha•ryn•ge•us (sef″ə-lo-fə-rin′je-əs) musculus constrictor pharyngis superior.

ceph•a•lo•ple•gia (sef″ə-lo-ple′jə) [*cephalo-* + *-plegia*] paralysis of the muscles about the head and face.

Ceph•a•lop•o•da (sef″ə-lop′ə-də) [*cephalo-* + Gr. *pous* foot] a class of large mollusks with elongated muscular arms; it includes the octopus, squid, cuttlefish, and nautilus.

ceph•a•lo•rha•chid•i•an (sef″ə-lo-rə-kid′e-ən) pertaining to the head and the vertebral column. Spelled also *cephalorachidian.*

ceph•a•lo•spo•rin (sef″ə-lo-spor′in) any of a group of broad-spectrum, relatively penicillinase-resistant antibiotics originally derived from a species of the fungus *Emericellopsis minimum,* a teleomorph of *Acremonium* (formerly called *Cephalosporium*). They are related to the penicillins in both structure and mode of action; their antibacterial activity results from inhibition of the cross-linking of peptidoglycan units in the cell wall. The cephalosporins available for medicinal use are semisynthetic derivatives of the natural antibiotic *cephalosporin C.* (The cephamycins cefmetazole, cefotetan, and cefoxitin and the β-lactam antibiotic moxalactam are included with the cephalosporins because of their close relationship to them.)

c. C the parent compound of the semisynthetic cephalosporin antibiotics, which are used in the treatment of a wide variety of infections due to sensitive gram-positive and gram-negative bacteria.

first-generation c. any of the group containing the first cephalosporins developed, comprising agents with a broad range of activity against gram-positive organisms but a narrow range of activity against gram-negative organisms and including cefadroxil, cefazolin, cephalexin, cephalothin, cephapirin, and cephradine.

fourth-generation c. a broad-spectrum cephalosporin having the greatest activity against gram-negative organisms of any of the cephalosporins. Cefepime is often so classified, although it is sometimes included with the third-generation cephalosporins.

second-generation c. any of a group containing cephalosporins that have greater resistance to β-lactamases and so are more active against gram-negative organisms, but are slightly less active against gram-positive organisms than are first-generation agents; it includes cefaclor, cefamandole, cefonicid, cefotetan, cefoxitin, cefprozil, ceftibuten, and cefuroxime. Cephamycins are usually classified as second-generation cephalosporins but have somewhat greater activity against anaerobes.

third-generation c. any of a group of β-lactamase–resistant cephalosporins that are more active against gram-negative organisms but less active against gram-positive organisms than are second-generation agents; it includes cefixime, cefoperazone, cefotaxime, cefpodoxime, ceftazidime, ceftizoxime, and ceftriaxone.

ceph•a•lo•spo•rin•ase (sef″ə-lo-spor′in-ās) a β-lactamase (q.v.) preferentially cleaving cephalosporins.

ceph•a•lo•spo•ri•o•sis (sef″ə-lo-spor″e-o′sis) acremoniosis.

Ceph•a•lo•spo•ri•um (sef″ə-lo-spor′e-əm) [*cephalo-* + Gr. *sporos* seed] former name for *Acremonium.*

ceph•a•lo•stat (sef′ə-lo-stat″) a head-positioning device used in dental radiology, facial photography, cephalometry, and other procedures requiring exact positioning of the head. See also *gnathostat.*

ceph•a•lo•style (sef′ə-lo-stīl″) the cranial end of the notochord.

ceph•a•lo•thin (sə-fal′o-thin) a semisynthetic first-generation cephalosporin, effective against a wide range of gram-positive and a limited range of gram-negative bacteria.

c. sodium [USP] the monosodium salt of cephalothin, used in the treatment of infections of the major organ and tissue systems due to sensitive pathogens; administered parenterally.

ceph•a•lo•tho•rac•ic (sef″ə-lo-thə-ras′ik) pertaining to the head and thorax.

ceph•a•lo•tho•ra•cop•a•gus (sef″ə-lo-thor″ə-kop′ə-gəs) conjoined twins united at the head, neck, and thorax.

c. disym′metros a cephalothoracopagus fused squarely in the frontal plane and presenting two broad anterior surfaces and two narrow posterior ones, with a common head bearing two faces, each being formed by the right and left halves of the different components.

c. monosym′metros a cephalothoracopagus with one complete face formed by a right and a left half of the two components, the other face being only rudimentary.

ceph•a•lo•tome (sef′ə-lo-tōm″) an instrument for cutting the fetal head.

ceph•a•lot•o•my (sef″ə-lot′ə-me) [*cephalo-* + *-tomy*] 1. the cutting up of the fetal head to facilitate delivery. 2. dissection of the fetal head.

ceph•a•lo•tro•pic (sef″ə-lo-tro′pik) [*cephalo-* + *-tropic*] having an affinity for brain tissue.

-cephalus [Gr. *kephalē* head] a word termination denoting *(a)* an abnormal condition of the head, the specific condition being indicated by the stem to which the ending is affixed, e.g., *hydrocephalus; (b)* an individual affected by an abnormal condition of the head, used especially of congenital anomalies in the fetus, e.g., *dicephalus; (c)* in taxonomy, having a head of a certain type.

-cephaly [Gr. *kephalē* head] a word termination denoting an abnormal condition of the head, the specific condition being indicated by the stem to which the ending is attached.

ceph•a•my•cin (sef″ə-mi′sin) any of a family of naturally occurring antibacterial antibiotics derived from various species of *Streptomyces* or produced semisynthetically, which are resistant to degradation by β-lactamase. Semisynthetic cephamycins, derived from cephamycin C, are generally classed as second-generation cephalosporins, but have greater activity against anaerobic bacteria.

ceph•a•pi•rin (sef-ə-pi′rin) a semisynthetic analogue of the natural antibiotic cephalosporin C, effective against a wide range of gram-positive bacteria and a few gram-negative species.

c. benzathine [USP] a salt of cephapirin having activity similar to that of the parent compound, used primarily for treatment of mastitis in cows.

c. sodium [USP] the monosodium salt of cephapirin, used in the treatment of infections of the respiratory and genitourinary tracts, skin, soft tissues, bones, joints, and blood due to sensitive pathogens; administered intramuscularly and intravenously.

ceph•ra•dine (sef′rə-dēn) [USP] a semisynthetic first-generation cephalosporin, effective against a wide range of gram-positive and a limited range of gram-negative bacteria; used in the treatment of otitis media and of infections of the genitourinary and respiratory tracts, skin, and soft tissues; administered orally, intramuscularly, or intravenously.

Ceph•u•lac (sef′u-lak) trademark for a preparation of lactulose.

Cep•taz (sep′taz) trademark for a preparation of ceftazidime.

-ceptor [shortened from *receptor*] a word termination denoting a receptor, with the root preceding it specifying the type.

ce•ra•ceous (sə-ra′shəs) [L. *cera* wax] waxlike in appearance.

ce•ram•ic (sə-ram′ik) 1. of or pertaining to ceramics. 2. a product, such as porcelain, produced by the action of heat on earthy materials, in which silicon and silicates occupy a predominant position. 3. a metal oxide.

castable c. a glass ceramic having a high compressive strength and hardness with translucency, and wear characteristics that approximate those of enamel; used in the casting of dental restorations.

glass c. any of a number of forms of partially crystallized glass having a variety of properties and uses, including the manufacture of dental restorations, formed by heating to the point of crystallization an amorphous glass matrix to which impurities have been added to provide nuclei for crystal formation.

metal c. a composite material made by mixing powdered metal with powdered ceramic and sintering the mixture. See also *cermet.*

metal-c. a dental restoration consisting of a cast metal substructure covered with an external fused ceramic veneer.

ce•ram•ics (sə-ram′iks) [Gr. *keramos* potters' clay] 1. the modeling and processing of objects made of clay or similar material. 2. objects made of ceramic material.

dental c. the employment of porcelain and similar materials in restorative dentistry.

cer•am•i•dase (sə-ram′ĭ-dās) [EC 3.5.1.23] an enzyme of the hydrolase class that catalyzes the cleavage of a ceramide (*N*-acylsphingosine) to form sphingosine and a fatty acid anion, a step in the degradation of sphingolipids. Acid, neutral, and alkaline isozymes occur; deficiency of the acid (lysosomal) enzyme, an autosomal recessive trait, results in accumulation of ceramides and gangliosides in Farber disease. Called also *acylsphingosine deacylase.*

cer•am•i•dase de•fi•cien•cy (sə-ram′ĭ-dās) Farber disease.

cer•a•mide (ser′ə-mīd) the basic unit of the sphingolipids; it is sphingosine, or a related base, attached via its amino group to a long chain fatty acyl group. Ceramides are accumulated abnormally in Farber disease. Called also *N-acylsphingosine.*

c. trihexoside any of a specific family of glycosphingolipids of composition galactose-galactose-glucose-ceramide; due to deficiency of α-galactosidase A activity, they accumulate abnormally in plasma and tissues in Fabry disease.

cer•a•mide cho•line•phos•pho•trans•fer•ase (ser′ə-mīd ko″lēn-fos″fo-trans′fər-ās) [EC 2.7.8.3] an enzyme of the transferase class that catalyzes the transfer of a phosphorylated choline group from CDPcholine to ceramide to form sphingomyelin.

cer•a•mide tri•hex•o•si•dase (ser′ə-mīd tri″hek-so′sĭ-dās) α-galactosidase A.

cer•a•mide tri•hex•o•si•dase de•fi•cien•cy (ser′ə-mīd tri″hek-so′sĭ-dās) Fabry disease.

Ce•ras•tes (sĕ-ras′tēz) a genus of venomous snakes of the family Viperidae. *C. ceras′tes* is the horned viper.

Ce•ra•ti•um (sə-ra′she-əm) [Gr. *keration,* dim. of *keras* horn] a genus of plantlike, marine and freshwater protozoa of the order Gonyaulacales, phylum Dinoflagellata; like other dinoflagellates, when present in vast numbers they produce red tide.

cerat(o)- for words beginning thus, see also those beginning *kerat(o)-*.

cer•a•to•cri•coid (ser″ə-to-kri′koid) pertaining to the inferior horn of the thyroid cartilage and the cricoid cartilage; see *musculus ceratocricoideus.*

cer•a•to•cri•coi•de•us (ser″ə-to-kri-koi′de-əs) ceratocricoid.

cer•a•to•hy•al (ser″ə-to-hi′əl) pertaining to a cornu minus of the hyoid bone.

Cer•a•to•nia (ser″ə-to′ne-ə) a genus of trees of the family Leguminosae. *C. sili′qua* L. is the carob (carob bean or locust bean) tree, native to the Mediterranean region, whose dried ripe fruit is the source of carob used in pharmaceutical preparations.

cer•a•to•pha•ryn•ge•us (ser″ə-to-fə-rin′je-əs) pertaining to the inferior horn of the thyroid cartilage and the pharynx; see under *musculus.*

Cer•a•to•phyl•lus (ser″ə-to-fil′əs) [Gr. *keras* horn + *phyllon* leaf] a genus of fleas, now including only bird fleas, but formerly including those of birds and small mammals.

C. acu′tus *Diamanus montanus.*
C. fascia′tus *Nosopsyllus fasciatus.*
C. galli′nae a species that attacks chickens and humans.
C. idahoen′sis *Oropsylla idahoensis.*
C. monta′nus *Diamanus montanus.*
C. punjaben′sis a rat flea of India.
C. silantie′wi *Oropsylla silantiewi.*
C. tesquo′rum a plague-transmitting flea of ground squirrels in the steppes of Central Asia.

Cer•a•to•po•gon•i•dae (ser″ə-to-po-gon′ĭ-de) Heleidae.

cer•ber•in (sur′bə-rin) a poisonous alkaloid from the Asian tree *Cerbera odallam;* it is cardiotonic.

cer•ca•ria (sər-kar′e-ə) pl. *cerca′riae* [Gr. *kerkos* tail] the final free-swimming larval stage of a trematode parasite, consisting of a body and tail. Some cercariae encyst on aquatic vegetation and penetrate the skin of a fish or the tissues of an aquatic arthropod to form encysted metacercariae. Cercariae of schistosomes penetrate directly into the skin of the definitive host without forming metacercariae.

cer•car•i•ci•dal (sər-kar″ĭ-si′dəl) destructive to cercariae.

cer•car•i•en•hul•len•re•ak•tion (sər-kar″e-ən-hul″ən-re-ak′shən) a test for *Schistosoma mansoni,* utilized in measuring the efficiency of chemotherapy against schistosomiasis. When cercariae of *S. mansoni* are placed in vitro in contact with sera of monkeys or humans infected with *S. mansoni,* a transparent envelope is formed around each cercaria.

cer•clage (ser-klahzh′) [Fr. "an encircling"] encircling of a part with a ring or loop, such as encirclement of the incompetent cervix uteri with suture material, or the binding together of the ends of a fractured bone with a metal ring or wire loop.

cerc(o)- [Gr. *kerkos* tail] a combining form denoting a relationship to a tail or to a tail-like structure.

cer•coid (sur′koid) the last stage in the development of a tapeworm.

Cer•co•pi•the•ci•dae (sər-ko-pĭ-thes′ĭ-de) the Old World monkeys, a family of the order Primates; genus *Macaca* includes species that are used as laboratory animals.

cer•co•pith•e•coid (sur″ko-pith′ə-koid) any member of the family Cercopithecidae.

Cer•co•pith•e•coi•dea (sur″ko-pith″ə-koid′e-ə) a superfamily of the order Primates, including the families Cercopithecidae (Old World monkeys) and Hominidae (human beings); they have nostrils that are close together and pointed downward, and if a tail is present it is not prehensile.

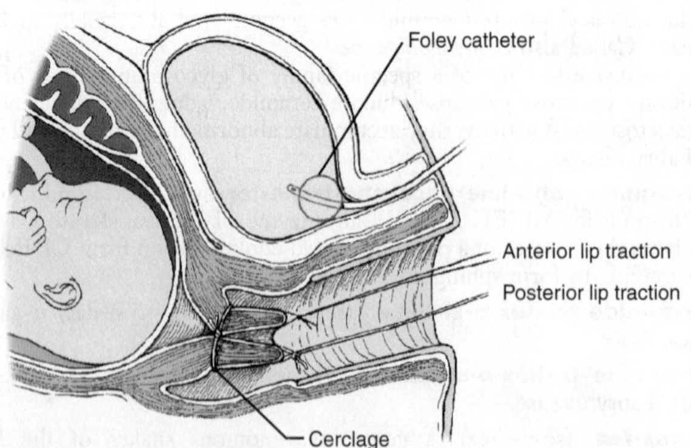

■ Cerclage used for reduction of bulging membranes at 23 weeks. Bladder was filled with saline, stay silk sutures on anterior and posterior cervical lips provided traction, and cerclage was placed distal to reduced membranes.

Cer•cos•po•ra (sər-kos′pə-rə) a genus of Fungi Imperfecti of the form-class Hyphomycetes. *C. a′pii* is a species that causes celery blight and occasionally hyphomycosis.

cer•cus (sur′kəs) pl. *cer′ci* [L., from Gr. *kerkos* tail] a rigid bristle-like appendage near the tail of most insects and some other arthropods, with varying functions including mechanoreception and copulation.

ce•rea flex•i•bil•i•tas (sēr′e-ə flek″sĭ-bil′ĭ-tas) [L. "waxy flexibility"] waxy flexibility.

ce•re•al (sēr′e-əl) [L. *cerealis*] 1. pertaining to edible grain. 2. any plant of the grass family (Gramineae) bearing an edible seed. 3. the seed or grain of such a plant.

cer•e•bel•la (ser″ə-bel′ə) [L.] plural of *cerebellum.*

cer•e•bel•lif•u•gal (ser″ə-bel-if′ə-gəl) [*cerebello-* + *-fugal*[2]] tending or proceeding from the cerebellum.

cer•e•bel•lip•e•tal (ser″ə-bel-ip′ə-təl) [*cerebello-* + *-petal*] tending or moving toward the cerebellum.

cer•e•bel•li•tis (ser″ə-bel-i′tis) inflammation of the cerebellum.

cerebell(o)- [L. *cerebellum,* q.v.] a combining form denoting relationship to the cerebellum.

cer•e•bel•lof•u•gal (ser″ə-bel-of′ə-gəl) cerebellifugal.

cer•e•bel•lo-ol•i•vary (ser″ə-bel″o-ol′i-var″e) conducting or proceeding from the cerebellum to the olivary body.

cer•e•bel•lo•pon•tile (ser″ə-bel″o-pon′tēl) cerebellopontine.

cer•e•bel•lo•pon•tine (ser″ə-bel″o-pon′tēn) conducting or proceeding from the cerebellum to the pons.

cer•e•bel•lo•ru•bral (ser″ə-bel″o-roo′brəl) conducting or proceeding from the cerebellum to the red nucleus.

cer•e•bel•lo•ru•bro•spi•nal (ser″ə-bel″o-roo″bro-spi′nəl) conducting or proceeding from the cerebellum, to the red nucleus, and then to the spinal cord.

cer•e•bel•lo•spi•nal (ser″ə-bel″o-spi′nəl) conducting or proceeding from the cerebellum to the spinal cord.

cer•e•bel•lum (ser″ə-bel′əm) [L. dim. of *cerebrum* brain] [TA] the part of the metencephalon that occupies the posterior cranial fossa behind the brainstem and is concerned in the coordination of movements. It is a fissured mass consisting of a body, comprising a narrow middle strip (the vermis) and two lateral lobes (the hemispheres), connected with the brainstem by three pairs (inferior, middle, and superior) of peduncles. The cerebellum is subdivided into an anterior lobe, which is separated from the posterior lobe by the primary fissure, which is in turn separated from the flocculonodular lobe by the posterolateral fissure. The lobes are further subdivided into lobules; those of the vermis are denoted I–X, with the corresponding hemisphere portion of each lobule denoted HII–X (with no HI in humans). Each lobule consists of a series of individual folia divided by deep transverse fissures, the deeper fissures demarcating the divisions into lobules. **cerebel′lar** *adj*

cer•e•bra (sə-re′brə, ser′e-brə) [L.] plural of *cerebrum.*

cer•e•bra•tion (ser″ə-bra′shən) [L. *cerebratio*] functional activity of the cerebrum; thinking; mental activity.

cerebri- see *cerebr(o)-.*

cer•e•bri•form (sə-re′brĭ-form) [*cerebri-* + *form*] resembling the surface of the cerebrum.

cer•e•brif•u•gal (ser″ə-brif′u-gəl) [*cerebri-* + *-fugal*[2]] conducting or proceeding away from the brain, or cerebrum.

cer•e•brip•e•tal (ser″ə-brip′ə-təl) [*cerebri-* + *-petal*] conducting or proceeding toward the brain, or cerebrum.

cer•e•bri•tis (ser″ə-bri′tis) [*cerebr-* + *-itis*] inflammation of the cerebrum.

lupus c. general term for the pathologic manifestations of systemic lupus erythematosus affecting the brain, most of which actually result from inflammation or thrombosis of the cerebral vasculature.

cerebr(o)- [L. *cerebrum,* q.v.] a combining form denoting relationship to the cerebrum; also *cerebri-.*

cer•e•bro•car•di•ac (ser″ə-bro-kahr′de-ak) [*cerebro-* + L. *cardia* heart] pertaining to the brain and heart.

cer•e•bro•cer•e•bel•lar (ser″ə-bro-ser″ə-bel′ər) pertaining to the cerebrum and the cerebellum.

cer•e•bro•cu•pre•in (ser″ə-bro-koo′prēn) a copper protein isolated from the human and bovine brain.

cer•e•broid (ser′ə-broid) resembling the cerebral substance.

cer•e•brol•o•gy (ser″ə-brol′ə-je) [*cerebro-* + *-logy*] the sum of knowledge regarding cerebral structure and function.

cer•e•bro•mac•u•lar (ser″ə-bro-mak′u-lər) pertaining to the cerebrum and the macula lutea; called also *maculocerebral.*

cer•e•bro•ma•la•cia (ser″ə-bro-mə-la′shə) [*cerebro-* + *malacia*] abnormal softening of the substance of the cerebrum.

cer•e•bro•me•nin•ge•al (ser″ə-bro-mə-nin′je-əl) pertaining to the cerebrum and its membranes.

cer•e•bro•men•in•gi•tis (ser″ə-bro-men″in-ji′tis) meningoencephalitis.

cer•e•bron•ic ac•id (ser″ə-bron′ik) a fatty acid, the 2-hydroxy derivative of lignoceric acid, found in cerebrosides such as phrenosine.

cer•e•bro•oc•u•lar (ser″ə-bro-ok′u-lər) pertaining to the cerebrum and the eye.

cer•e•bro•path•ia (ser″ə-bro-path′e-ə) [L.] cerebropathy.
 c. psy′chica toxe′mica Korsakoff psychosis.

cer•e•brop•a•thy (ser″ə-brop′ə-the) [*cerebro-* + *-pathy*] any disorder of the cerebrum; cf. *encephalopathy.*

cer•e•bro•phys•i•ol•o•gy (ser″ə-bro-fiz″e-ol′ə-je) the physiology of the cerebrum.

cer•e•bro•pon•tile (ser″ə-bro-pon′tīl) pertaining to the cerebrum and pons.

cer•e•bro•ra•chid•i•an (ser″ə-bro″rə-kid′e-ən) cerebrospinal.

cer•e•bro•scle•ro•sis (ser″ə-bro″sklə-ro′sis) encephalosclerosis.

cer•e•bro•side (sə-re′bro-sīd″) a sphingolipid in which the head group linked to ceramide is either of the monosaccharides glucose or galactose. Cerebrosides are abundant in cell membranes of brain and nervous tissue, especially the myelin sheath, but are also found in other tissues. See also *glucocerebroside* and *galactocerebroside.*
 c. sulfate sulfatide.

cer•e•bro•side-sul•fa•tase (sə-re′bro-sīd″ sul′fə-tās) [EC 3.1.6.8] an enzyme of the hydrolase class that catalyzes the cleavage of sulfate residues from sulfatides to form cerebrosides. Deficiency of the enzyme, an autosomal recessive trait, is one of the causes of metachromatic leukodystrophy. Called also *arylsulfatase A.*

cer•e•bro•si•do•sis (ser″ə-bro″sĭ-do′sis) a lipoidosis in which the fatty accumulation in the body consists largely of kerasin, as in Gaucher disease.

cer•e•bro•sis (ser″ə-bro′sis) cerebropathy.

cer•e•bro•spi•nal (ser″ə-bro-spi′nəl) pertaining to the brain and spinal cord; called also *encephalospinal* and *myeloencephalic.*

cer•e•bro•spi•nant (ser″ə-bro-spi′nənt) any medicine or agent that affects the brain and spinal cord.

cer•e•bros•to•my (ser″ə-bros′tə-me) [*cerebr-* + *ostomy*] the making of an artificial opening into the cerebrum.

cer•e•bro•ten•di•nous (ser″ə-bro-ten′dĭ-nəs) pertaining to the cerebrum and the tendons.

cer•e•brot•o•my (ser″ə-brot′ə-me) [*cerebr-* + *-otomy*] encephalotomy.

cer•e•bro•to•nia (ser″ə-bro-to′ne-ə) [*cerebro-* + *ton-* + *-ia*] a personality type associated with ectomorphy and characterized by love of privacy, introversion, emotional restraint, and intellectual intensity.

cer•e•bro•vas•cu•lar (ser″ə-bro-vas′ku-lər) pertaining to the blood vessels of the cerebrum, or brain.

cer•e•brum (sə-re′brəm, ser′ə-brəm) [L.] 1. the main portion of the brain, occupying the upper part of the cranial cavity; its two hemispheres (see *hemispherium cerebri*), united by the corpus callosum, form the largest part of the central nervous system in humans. It is derived (developed) from the telencephalon of the embryo. In official nomenclature, the term is considered an alternative to telencephalon [TA]. 2. a term sometimes applied to the postembryonic prosencephalon and mesencephalon together or to the entire brain. cere′bral *adj*

Cere•byx (ser′ə-biks) trademark for a preparation of fosphenytoin sodium.

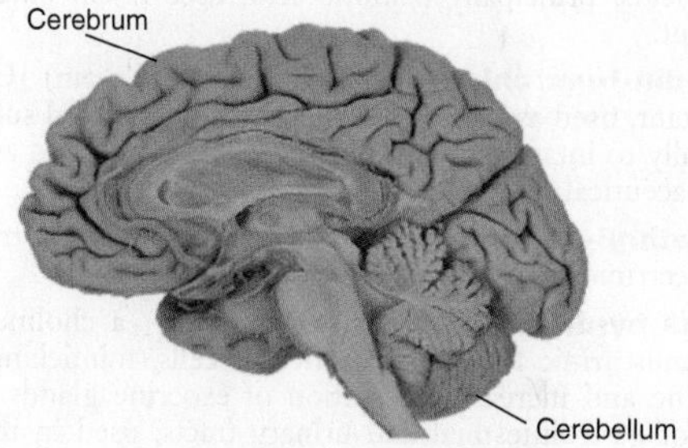

■ Cerebrum and cerebellum in a midline sagittal section.

cere•cloth (sēr′kloth) cloth impregnated with wax and made antiseptic; used in dressings.

Cer•e•dase (ser′ə-dās) trademark for a preparation of alglucerase.

Cer•en•kov radiation (chĕ′reng-kof) [Pavel Aleksandrovich *Cherenkov* (or *Cerenkov*), Russian physicist, 1904–1990] see under *radiation.*

Cer•e•tec (ser′ə-tek″) trademark for a kit for the preparation of technetium Tc 99m exametazime.

Cer•e•zyme (ser′ə-zīm″) trademark for a preparation of imiglucerase.

Cer•i•thid•ia (ser″ĭ-thid′e-ə) a genus of spiral-shelled snails of the family Cerithiidae, subclass Streptoneura, found in brackish water in tropical and subtropical areas. *C. cingula′ta* is a Japanese species that is the chief intermediate host for the trematode *Heterophyes heterophyes.*

ce•ri•um (Ce) (sēr′e-əm) [L.] a metallic element, atomic number 58, atomic weight 140.12.

ce•riv•a•stat•in so•di•um (sə-riv′ə-stat″in) a synthetic HMG-CoA reductase inhibitor, used as an adjunct to diet to lower blood lipid levels in the treatment of hypercholesterolemia and other forms of dyslipidemia; administered orally. Withdrawn in the United States because it is associated with an increased risk for rhabdomyolysis.

cer•met (sur′met) [*cer*amic *met*al] a type of metal ceramic that is a component of dental cements and heat-resistant solid materials.

cer•oid (ser′oid) an autofluorescent, waxy, yellow-brown pigment, similar to lipofuscin, that accumulates in cells in pathological conditions such as disease, malnutrition, or oxidative stress.

cer•ti•fi•a•ble (sur″tĭ-fi′ə-bəl) capable of being certified; said of infectious diseases, cases of which must by law be reported to public health officers.

cer•to•liz•u•mab peg•ol (ser-to-liz′u-mab) a tumor necrosis factor blocker used for reduction of signs and symptoms of Crohn disease; administered by subcutaneous injection.

Ce•ru•bi•dine (sə-roo′bĭ-dēn) trademark for a preparation of daunorubicin hydrochloride.

ce•ru•le•an (sə-ro͞ol′yən) [L. *caeruleus*] blue; azure.

ce•ru•le•in (sə-roo′le-in) a decapeptide amide isolated from the skin of frogs; it is a peptide analogue of cholecystokinin and gastrin; in mammals it is a powerful stimulant of gallbladder contraction.

ce•ru•le•us (sə-roo′le-əs) variant spelling of *caeruleus* (q.v.).

ce•ru•lo•plas•min (sə-roo″lo-plaz′min) a deep blue, copper-containing α_2-globulin with a single subunit, occurring in blood plasma. It is an acute phase protein, has ferroxidase activity, and binds 6 or 7 Cu^{2+} ions per molecule, functioning in transport and maintenance of tissue levels of copper. It can also oxidize other unsaturated compounds. Ceruloplasmin is absent in Wilson disease.

ce•ru•men (sə-roo′mən) [L., from *cera* wax] the waxlike secretion found within the external meatus of the ear; called also *earwax.* **ceru′minal, ceru′minous** *adj*
 impacted c. accumulated cerumen forming a solid mass that adheres to the wall of the external auditory canal.
 inspissated c. dried earwax in the external canal of the ear.

ce•ru•min•ol•y•sis (sə-roo″mĭ-nol′ə-sis) the solution or disintegration of cerumen in the external auditory meatus.

ce•ru•mi•no•ly•tic (sə-roo″mĭ-no-lit′ik) 1. pertaining to, characterized by, or promoting ceruminolysis. 2. an agent that dissolves cerumen in the external auditory canal.

ce•ru•mi•no•ma (sə-roo″mi-no′mə) a tumor of the ceruminous glands; there are both benign and malignant varieties.

ce•ru•mi•no•sis (sə-roo″mĭ-no′sis) excessive or disordered secretion of cerumen.

ce•ruse (se′ro͞os) [L. *cerussa*] the basic carbonate of lead; white lead.

cer•vi•cal (sur′vĭ-kəl) [L. *cervicalis*, from *cervix* neck] 1. pertaining to the neck. 2. pertaining to the neck or cervix of any organ or structure.

cer•vi•ca•lis (sur″vĭ-ka′lis) [L.] cervical.

cer•vi•cec•to•my (sur″vĭ-sek′tə-me) excision of the cervix uteri; called also *trachelectomy.*

cer•vi•ci•tis (sur″vĭ-si′tis) inflammation of the cervix uteri; called also *trachelitis.*
 granulomatous c. granulomatous infections of the cervix, including tuberculosis, syphilis, and granuloma inguinale.
 traumatic c. a nonspecific cervicitis resulting from such procedures as irradiation or cauterization.

cervic(o)- [L. *cervix* neck] a combining form denoting a neck or the cervix uteri.

cer•vi•co•ax•il•lary (sur″vĭ-ko-ak′sĭ-lar-e) pertaining to the neck and axilla.

cer•vi•co•bra•chi•al (sur″vĭ-ko-bra′ke-əl) pertaining to the neck and upper limb.

cer•vi•co•bra•chi•al•gia (sur″vĭ-ko-bra″ke-al′jə) pain in the neck radiating to the upper limb, due to compression of nerve roots of the cervical spinal cord.

cer•vi•co•buc•cal (sur″vĭ-ko-buk′əl) buccocervical.

cer•vi•co•col•pi•tis (sur″vĭ-ko-kol-pi′tis) cervicovaginitis.

cer•vi•co•dor•sal (sur″vĭ-ko-dor′səl) pertaining to the neck and back.

cer•vi•co•dyn•ia (sur″vĭ-ko-din′e-ə) [*cervico-* + *-odynia*] pain in the neck; called also *trachelodynia.*

cer•vi•co•fa•cial (sur″vĭ-ko-fa′shəl) pertaining to the neck and face.

cer•vi•co•la•bi•al (sur″vĭ-ko-la′be-əl) labiocervical.

cer•vi•co•lin•gual (sur″vĭ-ko-ling′gwəl) linguocervical.

cer•vi•co•med•ul•lary (sur″vĭ-ko-med′ə-lar″e) pertaining to or connecting the cervical spinal cord and the medulla oblongata.

cer•vi•co•oc•cip•i•tal (sur″vĭ-ko-ok-sip′ĭ-təl) pertaining to the neck and occiput.

cer•vi•co•pexy (sur′vĭ-ko-pek″se) [*cervico-* + *-pexy*] surgical fixation of the cervix uteri to some other part.

cer•vi•co•plas•ty (sur′vĭ-ko-plas″te) [*cervico-* + *-plasty*] 1. plastic surgery on the neck. 2. plastic surgery on the cervix uteri. **cervicoplas′tic** *adj*

cer•vi•co•scap•u•lar (sur″vĭ-ko-skap′u-lər) pertaining to the neck and scapula.

cer•vi•co•tho•rac•ic (sur″vĭ-ko-thə-ras′ik) pertaining to the neck and thorax.

cer•vi•cot•o•my (sə″vĭ-kot′ə-me) 1. an incision in the neck. 2. an incision of the cervix uteri.

cer•vi•co•uter•ine (sur″vĭ-ko-u′tər-in) of or pertaining to the uterine cervix.

cer•vi•co•vag•i•nal (sər″vĭ-ko-vaj′ĭ-nəl) pertaining to the cervix uteri and the vagina.

cer•vi•co•vag•i•ni•tis (sur″vĭ-ko-vaj″ĭ-ni′tis) inflammation involving both the cervix uteri and vagina.

cer•vi•co•ves•i•cal (sur″vĭ-ko-ves′ĭ-kəl) vesicocervical.

Cer•vi•dil (sur′vĭ-dil) trademark for a preparation of dinoprostone.

cer•vix (sur′viks) pl. *cer′vices* [L.] 1. TA alternative for *collum.* 2. a constricted portion of a body part or organ. 3. cervix uteri.

c. of axon a constricted part of an axon, before the beginning of the myelin sheath.

c. cor′nus dorsa′lis medul′lae spina′lis c. cornus posterioris medullae spinalis.

c. cor′nus posterio′ris medul′lae spina′lis [TA] neck of posterior horn of spinal cord: the constricted portion of the posterior horn of gray matter in the spinal cord between the base of the horn and the head. Called also *c. cornus dorsalis medullae spinalis* and *neck of dorsal horn of spinal cord.*

c. den′tis [TA] neck of tooth: the slightly constricted region of union of the crown and the root or roots of a tooth; called also *collum dentis* and *dental neck.*

c. glan′dis pe′nis collum glandis penis.

incompetent c. a cervix that is abnormally prone to dilate in the second trimester of pregnancy, resulting in premature expulsion of the fetus (middle trimester abortion).

strawberry c. colpitis macularis.

tapiroid c. a uterine cervix with a peculiarly elongated anterior lip.

c. u′teri [TA], **uterine c.** neck of uterus: the lower and narrow end of the uterus, between the isthmus and the ostium uteri.

c. vesi′cae urina′riae [TA] neck of urinary bladder: a constricted portion of the bladder, formed by the meeting of its inferolateral surfaces proximal to the internal urethral orifice. Called also *bladder neck* and *collum vesicae urinariae* [TA alternative].

ces central excitatory state.

ce•sar•e•an (sə-zar′e-ən) [L. *caesus,* from *caedere* to cut] see under *section.*

CESD cholesteryl ester storage disease.

ce•si•um (Cs) (se′ze-əm) [L. *caesium,* from *caesius* blue] a rare univalent metallic element with an alkaline oxide; atomic number 55, atomic weight 132.905.

Ces•tan syndrome (səs-tahn′) [Raymond J. *Cestan,* French neurologist, 1872–1934] Cestan-Chenais syndrome.

Ces•tan-Che•nais syndrome (səs-tahn′ shə-na′) [R.J. *Cestan;* Louis *Chenais,* French physician, 1872–1950] see under *syndrome.*

Ces•tan-Ray•mond syndrome (səs-tahn′ ra-maw′) [R.J. *Cestan;* Fulgence *Raymond,* French neurologist, 1844–1910] Raymond-Cestan syndrome.

ces•ti•ci•dal (ses″tĭ-si′dəl) destructive to cestodes.

Ces•to•da (səs-to′də) a subclass of Cestoidea comprising the true tapeworms, which have a head or scolex, and segments or proglottides. Adults are endoparasitic in the alimentary tract and associated ducts of various vertebrate hosts; their larval stages (cysticercus, coenurus, hydatid, sparganum) may be found in various organs or tissues. Of the eleven orders, two, Pseudophyllidea and Cyclophyllidea, contain parasitic species. Called also *Eucestoda.*

Ces•to•da•ria (ses″to-dar′e-ə) a subclass of tapeworms, the unsegmented tapeworms of the class Cestoidea, which are endoparasitic in the intestines and coelom of various primitive fishes and rarely in reptiles.

ces•tode (ses′tōd) [Gr. *kestos* girdle] 1. tapeworm (q.v.); either any member of the subclass Cestoda or any member of the class Cestoidea. 2. resembling a tapeworm.

ces•to•di•a•sis (ses″to-di′ə-sis) infection by cestodes.

ces•to•dol•o•gy (ses″to-dol′ə-je) the scientific study of cestodes.

ces•toid (ses′toid) cestode.

Ces•toi•dea (ses-toi′de-ə) a class of tapeworms (platyhelminths) characterized by the absence of a mouth and digestive tract and by the presence of a noncuticular layer covering their bodies. It comprises two subclasses: Cestodaria and Cestoda.

Ces•trum (ses′trum) a genus of tropical plants of the family Solanaceae. Several species cause hemorrhagic gastroenteritis and liver and kidney degeneration in animals. *C. diur′num,* the day jasmine, is a West Indian plant that causes enzootic calcinosis in farm animals and gastroenteritis in humans who eat its fruit.

Ceta•caine (se′tə-kān) trademark for combination preparations of benzocaine, butamben, and tetracaine hydrochloride.

cet•al•ko•ni•um chlo•ride (set″al-ko′ne-əm) a cationic quaternary ammonium surfactant, used as a topical antiinfective and disinfectant.

ce•ta•nol (se′tə-nol) cetyl alcohol.

ce•ti•e•dil cit•rate (sə-ti′ə-dil) a peripheral vasodilator, which has been used in the treatment of arteritis, Raynaud disease, and acrocyanosis.

ce•ti•ri•zine hy•dro•chlo•ride (sə-tir′ĭ-zēn) a nonsedating antihistamine (H_1-receptor antagonist) that is a metabolite of hydroxyzine, used in treatment of allergic rhinitis and chronic idiopathic urticaria, and as a treatment adjunct in asthma; administered orally.

CETP cholesteryl ester transfer protein.

Ce•tra•ria (sə-trar′e-ə) a genus of lichens occurring mainly in the high northern latitudes; *C. islan′dica,* or Iceland moss, is used medicinally.

ce•tri•mide (set′rĭ-mīd) a quaternary ammonium antiseptic and detergent composed of a mixture of tetradecyltrimethyl, dodecyltrimethyl, and hexadecyltrimethyl ammonium bromides, applied topically to the skin to cleanse wounds, as a preoperative disinfectant, and to treat seborrhea of the scalp; solutions are also used to cleanse utensils and store surgical instruments. Abbreviated CTBA.

cet•ri•mo•ni•um bro•mide (set″rĭ-mo′ne-əm) 1. hexadecyltrimethylammonium bromide, one of the ingredients of cetrimide. 2. former name for cetrimide.

cet•ro•rel•ix ac•e•tate (set″ro-rel′iks) a synthetic decapeptide that competes with natural gonadotropin-releasing hormone, thus controlling the release of luteinizing hormone and follicle-stimulating hormone; used to inhibit premature luteinizing hormone surges in women undergoing controlled ovarian hyperstimulation during infertility treatment; administered subcutaneously.

Cet•ro•tide (set′ro-tīd) trademark for a preparation of cetrorelix acetate.

ce•tux•i•mab (sə-tuk′sĭ-mab) a recombinant human-mouse monoclonal antibody that binds to the epidermal growth factor (EGF) receptor and inhibits the growth and survival of cells that overexpress the EGF receptor, used in the treatment of metastatic colorectal carcinoma, administered intravenously.

ce•tyl (se′təl) a univalent alcohol radical, $CH_3(CH_2)_{14}CH_2$—.

c. palmitate [NF] esters of cetyl alcohol and saturated high molecular weight fatty acids, principally palmitic acid; used as an emulsifying and stiffening agent.

ce•tyl•pyr•i•din•i•um chlo•ride (se″təl-pir″ĭ-din′e-əm) [USP] a cationic disinfectant, used as a local antiinfective administered sublingually or applied topically to intact skin and mucous membranes, and as a preservative in pharmaceutical preparations.

ce•tyl•tri•meth•yl•am•mo•ni•um bro•mide (se″təl-tri-meth″əl-ə-mo′ne-əm) cetrimonium bromide.

cev•i•mel•ine hy•dro•chlo•ride (sə-vim′ə-lēn) a cholinergic agonist that acts on muscarinic receptors of effector cells, mimicking the effects of acetylcholine and increasing secretion of exocrine glands and smooth muscle tone of gastrointestinal and urinary tracts; used in the treatment of xerostomia associated with Sjögren syndrome, administered orally.

ce•vi•tam•ic ac•id (se-vi-tam′ik) ascorbic acid.

Cey•lan•cy•clos•to•ma (se″lan-si-klos′to-mə) *Ancylostoma braziliense.*

CF carbolfuchsin; cardiac failure; Christmas factor; citrovorum factor.

Cf californium.

CFAP chronic functional abdominal pain.

CFC chlorofluorocarbon.

cff critical fusion frequency.

CFT complement fixation test; see under *fixation.*

CFTR cystic fibrosis transmembrane regulator.

CFU colony-forming unit (def. 2).

CFU-C colony-forming unit–culture.

CFU-E colony-forming unit–erythroid.

CFU-GM colony-forming unit–granulocyte-macrophage.

CFU-S colony-forming unit–spleen.

CGD chronic granulomatous disease.

CGH comparative genomic hybridization.

cGMP cyclic guanosine monophosphate.

CGS, cgs centimeter-gram-second system.

cGy centigray.

CH crown-heel; see under *length.*

CH50, CH_{50} total hemolytic complement; see *CH50 assay,* under *assay,* and *CH50 unit,* under *unit.*

Cha•ber•tia (shah-ber′te-ə) a genus of nematodes of the family Strongylidae. *C. ovi′na* is a bowel worm parasitic in the colon of sheep, goats, and cattle.

cha•ber•ti•a•sis (shah-bər-ti′ə-sis) infection by *Chabertia ovina,* which is clinically apparent mainly in sheep; characteristics include edema and small hemorrhages of the colon with passage of feces containing large amounts of mucus.

Chad•dock reflex (sign) (chad′ək) [Charles Gilbert *Chaddock,* American neurologist, 1861–1936] see under *reflex.*

Chad•wick sign (chad′wik) [James Read *Chadwick,* American gynecologist, 1844–1905] see under *sign.*

Chae•to•mi•um (ke-to′me-əm) a genus of fungi of the family Sordariaceae. *C. globo′sum* and other species have occasionally been found infecting human nails (onychomycosis) and skin (phaeohyphomycosis).

chafe (chāf) to irritate the skin, as by the rubbing together of opposing folds.

Cha•gas disease (chah′gəs) [Carlos Justiniano Ribeiro das *Chagas,* Brazilian physician, 1879–1934] see under *disease.*

Cha•gas•ia (chə-gās′e-ə) [C.J.R. das *Chagas*] a genus of mosquitoes of the tribe *Anophelini,* subfamily Anophelinae, native to Central and South America; they are sometimes vectors of disease.

cha•gas•ic (chə-gās′ik) pertaining to or due to Chagas disease.

cha•go•ma (chə-go′mə) an erythematous nodule appearing within a few days at the site of a bite by a reduviid bug carrying the parasite causing Chagas disease; lymphatic vessels draining the site may become blocked with scar tissue and produce edema of the area.

Cha•il•le•tia (ka-il-e′she-ə) a genus of tropical trees and shrubs. *C. toxica′ria* is a West African species with poisonous seeds and fruit. *C. cymo′sa* has been reclassified as *Dichapetalum cymosum.*

chain (chān) a collection of objects linked together in linear fashion, or end to end, as the assemblage of atoms or radicals in a chemical compound, or an assemblage of individual bacterial cells.

α c. a globin chain of 141 amino acids found in fetal hemoglobin and normal adult hemoglobin A.

β c. a globin chain of 146 amino acids found in normal adult hemoglobin A.

branched c. an open chain of atoms, usually carbon, with one or more side chains attached to it.

closed c. several atoms linked together so as to form a ring, which may be saturated, as in cyclopentane, or aromatic, as in benzene.

δ c. a globin chain of 146 amino acids, found in normal adult hemoglobin A_2.

ε c. a globin chain found in embryonic hemoglobin Gower and hemoglobin Portland.

electron transport c. the series of electron carriers in the inner mitochondrial membrane that pass electrons from reduced coenzymes (NADH, $FADH_2$) to molecular oxygen via sequential redox reactions coupled to vectorial transduction of protons across the membrane. The chain is the final common pathway of biological oxidation, using O_2 for fuel combustion; the energy produced is utilized for ATP synthesis, ion translocation, and protein synthesis. See illustration. Called also *respiratory c.* See also *oxidative phosphorylation.*

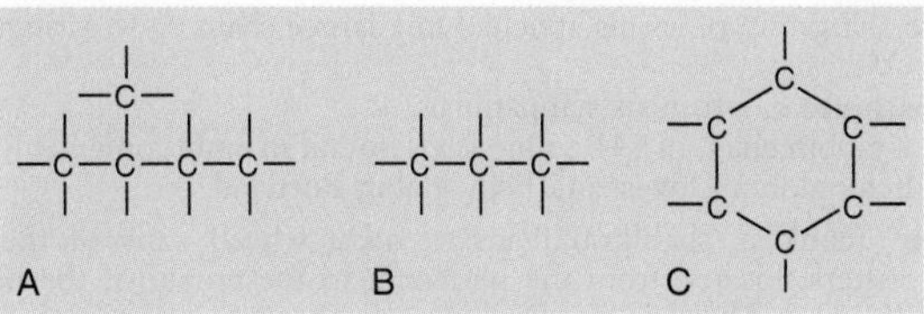

■ *(A),* Branched chain; *(B),* open chain; *(C),* closed chain.

food c. a sequence of organisms through which energy is transferred from its ultimate source in a plant; each organism eats the preceding and is eaten by the following member in the sequence.

free light c's light chains floating free in the serum, not bound to immunoglobulin molecules; see *serum free light chain assay,* under *assay.*

γ c. a globin chain of 146 amino acids, found in fetal hemoglobin and in small amounts in normal adult hemoglobin A.

globin c. the polypeptide chain that makes up a globin; those found in adults are *α, β, γ,* and *δ chains.*

H c., heavy c. any of the larger polypeptide chains of antibody molecules, two identical heavy chains occurring (with two identical light chains) in each immunoglobulin monomer. The heavy chains determine the immunoglobulin class and subclass and are designated accordingly: γ, α, μ, ε, and δ, the heavy chains of IgG, IgA, IgM, IgE, and IgD. The subclass may be designated by a number, e.g., γ1, the heavy chain of IgG1. Heavy chains have four homology regions of about 110 amino acid residues: one variable region (V_H) and three constant regions (C_H1, C_H2, C_H3) except for μ and ε chains which have an extra constant region (C_H4). See *immunoglobulin.*

J c. [for "joining"] a 15-kilodalton polypeptide occurring in all immunoglobulin polymers, a single J chain occurring in each IgM pentamer and in each IgA dimer, trimer, or tetramer.

κ c., kappa c. a type of light chain found in immunoglobulin molecules.

kinetic c. the series of body parts involved in a given movement, including muscles, ligaments, tendons, joints, and the accompanying motor and sensory nerves. See also *open kinetic chain exercises* and *closed kinetic chain exercises,* under *exercise.*

L c. light c.

λ c., lambda c. a type of light chain found in immunoglobulin molecules.

lateral c. side c.

light c. any of the smaller polypeptide chains of antibody molecules, two identical light chains occurring (with two identical heavy chains) in each immunoglobulin monomer. There are two types, designated κ and λ, both occurring in all immunoglobulin classes (in a ratio of about two κ chains to one λ chain in humans). Light chains have two homology regions of about 110 amino acid residues: one variable region (V_L) and one constant region (C_L). Called also *L c.* See *immunoglobulin.*

nuclear c. a longitudinal array of nuclei occurring on an intrafusal fiber of muscle.

open c. a series of atoms united in a straight line; compounds of this series are related to methane and are also called *aliphatic* or *acyclic compounds.*

ossicular c. ossicula auditus.

polypeptide c. the structural element of protein, consisting of a series of amino acid residues (peptides, q.v.) joined together by peptide bonds.

respiratory c. electron transport c.

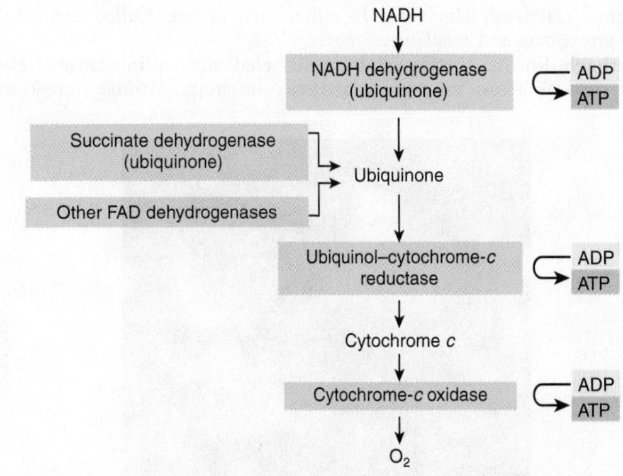

■ Electron transport chain showing the three sites of coupling with oxidative phosphorylation, generating adenosine triphosphate.

side c. a group of atoms attached to a larger chain or to a ring; called also *lateral c.*

sympathetic c. truncus sympathicus.

ζ c. a globin chain of 141 amino acids, found in embryonic hemoglobin such as hemoglobin Gower and hemoglobin Portland.

chak•ra (chuk′rə, shah′krə) [Sanskrit *cakra* wheel] any of the seven energy centers, located from the perineum to the crown of the head, of yoga philosophy. They are also used in some energy-based complementary medicine systems.

cha•la•sia (kə-la′zhə) [Gr. *chalasis* relaxation] relaxation of a bodily opening, such as the cardiac sphincter of the esophagus, a cause of vomiting in infants.

cha•la•za (kə-la′zə) [Gr. "lump"] a spiral band of albumin extending from either end of the yolk of a bird's egg to the shell.

cha•la•zi•on (kə-la′ze-on) pl. *chala′zia, chalazions* [Gr. "small lump"] an eyelid mass that results from chronic inflammation of a meibomian gland and shows a granulomatous reaction to liberated fat when subjected to histopathological examination; sometimes called *meibomian* or *tarsal cyst.*

cha•la•zo•der•mia (kə-la″zo-dur′me-ə) cutis laxa.

chal•ci•tis (kal-si′tis) chalkitis.

chal•co•sis (kal-ko′sis) [Gr. *chalkos* copper] the presence of copper deposits in the tissues.

c. cor′neae deposition of copper in the cornea resulting in a pigmented ring in the deeper layers.

chal•i•co•sis (kal-ĭ-ko′sis) [Gr. *chalix* gravel] pneumoconiosis in stonecutters due to the inhalation of stone dust. Called also *flint disease.*

chalk (chawk) [L. *calx*] 1. a natural calcium carbonate; the amorphous remains of minute marine organisms deposited on the sea bottom and decomposed by the action of acids and heat. Used as a polishing agent in dentistry and frequently as an ingredient in dentifrices. 2. any of various other substances physically resembling calcium carbonate.

chal•ki•tis (kal-ki′tis) [Gr. *chalkos* brass] inflammation of the eyes caused by rubbing them after the hands have been used on brass.

chal•lenge (chal′ənj) 1. to administer a chemical substance to a patient for observation of whether the normal physiological response occurs. 2. in immunology, to administer antigen to evoke an immune response in a previously sensitized individual. Called also *antigenic c.* 3. the administration of such a chemical or antigen in order to assess for a response. Called also *challenge test, provocative test,* and *provocation.*

antigenic c. challenge (def. 2).

bronchial c. 1. a challenge test in which a nonspecific agent such as histamine or methacholine is applied to the bronchi and they are assessed for a bronchoconstriction reaction. Called also *bronchoprovocation, bronchial provocation,* and *bronchial challenge test.* 2. inhalational c.

food c. a challenge test for determining food allergens; a small amount of a lyophilized preparation of the suspected allergen is administered orally and the patient is monitored for reactions such as rash, rhinorrhea, or diarrhea. Called also *food challenge test.*

histamine c. a type of bronchial challenge done to assess responsiveness of the mucosa: histamine is applied to the nose or mucous membrane and mucosal swelling is monitored; allergic or otherwise susceptible subjects have lowered thresholds of reactivity.

inhalational c. a type of challenge test done to determine reactivity to drugs or causative allergens in atopic or extrinsic asthma; a dilute concentrate of the suspected substance is inhaled and the patient is assessed for bronchial reactivity, which may be either early or late. Called also *inhalational provocation* and *inhalational challenge test.*

methacholine c. a type of bronchial challenge or inhalational challenge used as a test for airway reactivity or atopic asthma; aerosolized methacholine is applied to the airways and the patient is assessed for responsiveness or hyperresponsiveness.

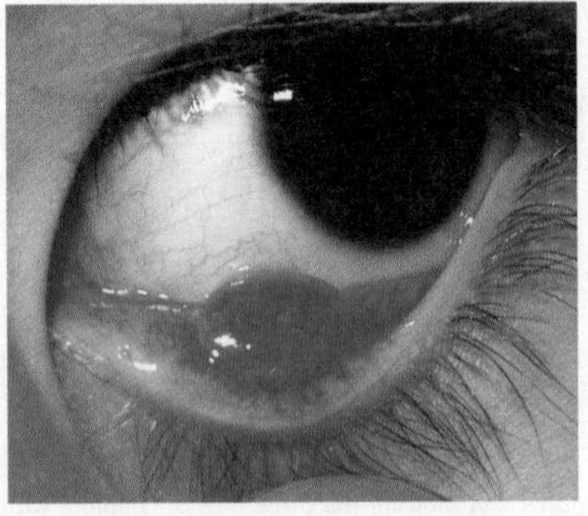

■ Chalazion.

chal•one (kal′ōn) [Gr. *chalan* to relax] a group of tissue-specific (but not species-specific) water-soluble proteins that are produced within a tissue and that inhibit mitosis of cells of that tissue and whose action is reversible. **chalon′ic** *adj*

cham•ae•ceph•a•ly (kam″e-sef′ə-le) [Gr. *chamai* low + *-cephaly*] the condition of having a low, flat head, that is, a cephalic index of 70 or less. **chamaecephal′ic** *adj*

Cha•mae•me•lum (kam″me-me′ləm) [Gr. *khamaimēlon*, from *khamai* on the ground + *mēlon* apple] a genus of herbs, including *C. nobile* (formerly *Anthemis nobilis*), Roman or English chamomile, a perennial medicinal herb native to Europe and North Africa.

cham•ae•pros•o•py (kam″e-pros′ə-pe) [Gr. *chamai* low + *prosōpon* face] the condition of having a low, broad face, i.e., a facial index of 90 or less. **chamaeproso′pic** *adj*

cham•ber (chām′bər) [L. *camera;* Gr. *kamara*] an enclosed space or antrum.

Abbe-Zeiss counting c. Thoma-Zeiss counting c.

acoustic c. a soundproof enclosure used in measuring hearing. See also *anechoic c.*

air-equivalent ionization c. in radiology, a chamber in which the materials of the wall and electrodes are such that ionizing radiations produce ionization essentially similar to that in a free-air ionization chamber.

altitude c. a vacuum chamber used to simulate the effects of high altitude and low atmospheric pressure.

anechoic c. an acoustic chamber that is echo-free. Called also *anechoic room.*

anterior c. of eye camera anterior bulbi oculi.

aqueous c. the part of the eyeball that is filled with aqueous humor; see *camera anterior bulbi oculi* and *camera posterior bulbi oculi.*

Boyden c. a device consisting of two compartments separated by a micropore filter, used in tests for chemotaxis. Cells are placed in the upper compartment and the chemotactic agent in the lower; if cells are attracted to the agent, they migrate through the pores of the filter. The filter is then stained so that cell migration can be measured.

counting c. hemacytometer.

diffusion c. an apparatus for separating a substance by means of a semipermeable membrane.

c's of eye the various spaces in the eyeball; see *camera anterior bulbi oculi, camera posterior bulbi oculi,* and *camera postrema bulbi oculi.*

Finn c. see under *test.*

free-air ionization c. an ionization chamber in which the ionization in an accurately defined volume of free air is measured.

c's of the heart the cavities of the atria and ventricles.

hyperbaric c. a compartment in which the air pressure may be raised to more than normal atmospheric pressure; used in treatment of gas gangrene and other anaerobic infections, or other conditions in which a high concentration of oxygen is desirable, and for studying the effects of pressure and decompression.

ionization c. a device for measuring ionizing radiation by the measurement of the ionization of the gas contained in the chamber.

lethal c. a chamber that may be filled with gas, for killing small animals.

posterior c. of eye camera posterior bulbi oculi.

postremal c. of eye camera postrema bulbi oculi.

pulp c. cavitas coronalis.

relief c. a recess in the impression surface of a denture to reduce or eliminate pressure or force from that area of the mouth. See also *relief,* defs. 3 and 4.

Storm van Leeuwen c. a room that can be kept free of airborne antigens for allergic patients.

thimble c. a small, thin-walled ionization chamber, usually with walls of organic material; used as a dosimeter.

Thoma-Zeiss counting c. a common kind of hemacytometer; called also *Abbe-Zeiss counting c.*

tissue-equivalent ionization c. an ionization chamber in which the walls, electrodes, and gas are selected to produce ionization essentially equivalent to that which would occur in the tissue under consideration.

vitreous c., vitreous c. of eye camera postrema bulbi oculi.

Zappert c. a type of hemacytometer.

Cham•ber•len forceps (chām′bər-lən) [Peter *Chamberlen*, English obstetrician, 1560–1631] see under *forceps.*

cham•e•ceph•a•ly (kam″e-sef′ə-le) chamaecephaly. **chamecephal′ic** *adj*

cham•e•pros•o•py (kam″e-pros′ə-pe) chamaeprosopy. **chameproso′pic** *adj*

cham•fer (cham′fər) 1. the flat surface made when the edge of a corner is cut off. 2. in dentistry, on an extracoronal cavity preparation, a more or less flat surface that curves around, resulting from planing or smoothing a sharply angled curve, and extending from an axial wall to the cavosurface.

cham•o•mile (kam′ə-mēl, -mīl) [Gr. *khamaimēlon*, from *khamai* on the ground + *mēlon* apple] 1. *Chamaemelum nobile*. 2. *Matricaria recutita* (formerly *M. chamomilla*). 3. [NF] the dried flower heads of *Matricaria recutita*, used topically as a counterirritant and as an antiinflammatory for the skin and mucous membranes and internally for inflammatory diseases of the gastrointestinal tract. Called also *German c.*

English c. Roman c.

German c. chamomile.

Roman c. the dried flowers of *Chamaemelum nobile* (formerly *Anthemis nobilis*), used as a homeopathic preparation and in folk medicine externally as a counterirritant and internally as a carminative. Called also *English c.*

Chance fracture (chans) [George Quentin *Chance*, British radiologist, 20th century] see under *fracture*.

chan•cre (shang′kər) [Fr. for "canker," a destructive sore, from L. *cancer* crab] 1. the usually painless primary lesion of syphilis, occurring at the site of entry of the infection, typically a small red papule or crusted erosion that breaks down to become round, hard, and elevated with an eroded surface that exudes serous fluid; it later gives rise to a bubo (regional lymphadenitis) and heals without scarring. Called also *hard c.* 2. any of various primary cutaneous lesions that are seen at the site of inoculation of infection in such diseases as herpes, sporotrichosis, trypanosomiasis, tuberculosis, and tularemia. **chan′crous** *adj*

hard c. chancre (def. 1).

mixed c. a skin lesion due to simultaneous infection with *Treponema pallidum* (primary syphilis) and *Haemophilus ducreyi* (chancroid).

monorecidive c., c. re′dux the reappearance of a chancre after partial healing as a result of insufficient treatment, accompanied by lymphadenopathy with numerous spirochetes at the site of the lesion.

soft c. chancroid.

true c. chancre (def. 1).

tuberculous c. a chancriform lesion seen with primary inoculation tuberculosis.

chan•cri•form (shang′krĭ-form) resembling a chancre.

chan•croid (shang′kroid) [*chancre* + *-oid*] a sexually transmitted disease caused by *Haemophilus ducreyi*, characterized by a painful primary ulcer at the site of inoculation, usually on the external genitalia, associated with regional lymphadenitis. See also *mixed chancre*, under *chancre*. Called also *soft chancre* and *soft ulcer*. **chancroi′dal** *adj*

phagedenic c. an advanced type in which there is sloughing of the tissues.

change (chānj) an alteration.

Armanni-Ebstein c. see under *lesion*.

Crooke c′s, Crooke-Russell c′s Crooke hyalinization.

fatty c. abnormal accumulation of fat within parenchymal cells; the term encompasses the older concepts defined as *fatty degeneration* and *fatty infiltration*.

harlequin color c. transient reddening of one half of the body longitudinally with simultaneous blanching of the other half; a temporary vasomotor disorder of the newborn.

hyaline c. a pale, eosinophilic, homogeneous glassy appearance seen in histologic specimens, especially of collagenous connective tissue and smooth muscle; it is a purely descriptive term and has a variety of causes.

hydropic c. hydropic degeneration.

personality c. due to a general medical condition [DSM-IV] persistent disturbance of personality due to the direct effects of a general medical condition and neither better accounted for by another mental disorder nor occurring exclusively during delirium.

ch′ang shan (chahng shahn) [Chinese] 1. *Dichroa febrifuga*. 2. the root of *D. febrifuga*, which contains the alkaloids dichroine, febrifugine, and isofebrifugine; used in Chinese medicine in the treatment of malaria because of its antiparasitic, emetic, and antipyretic properties.

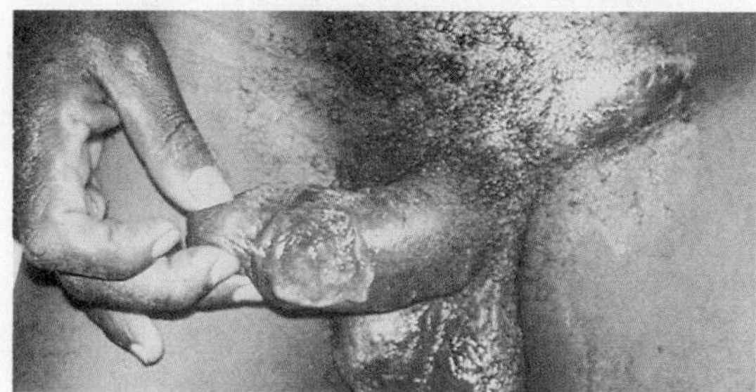

■ Chancroid of the penis, with draining buboes in the adjacent groin area.

chan•nel (chan′əl) [L. *canalis* a water pipe] 1. a passageway through which something flows; see also *canalis* and *groove*. 2. ion c.

acetylcholine c. a ligand-gated channel that is activated by acetylcholine; see *nicotinic receptors*, under *receptor*.

amiloride-sensitive sodium c. epithelial sodium c.

ATP-gated c′s a family of ligand-gated channels permeable to cations and widely expressed in nerves, muscles, and endocrine and exocrine glands, that open in response to extracellular ATP. Called also *P2X receptors*.

blood c′s narrow passages with indistinct walls, containing blood; they are found in fresh granulation tissue.

calcium c. a voltage-gated channel, very permeable to calcium ions and slightly permeable to sodium ions, that upon activation by membrane depolarization allows calcium to flow into the cell; channels are classified into six subtypes (L, N, P, Q, R, and T) on the basis of electrophysiologic and pharmacologic characteristics. Calcium channels contribute to membrane depolarization during action potentials and stimulate the contraction of cardiac and skeletal muscle and the secretion of neurotransmitters.

calcium-sodium c. calcium c.

chloride c. (ClC) any of a large family of ligand- and voltage-gated channels selective for chloride ions, important in membrane excitability, cell volume control, and epithelial transport. Mutations in the chloride channel genes cause several diseases, including cystic fibrosis and hereditary myotonias.

epithelial sodium c. (ENaC) a non-gated epithelial cell membrane channel through which sodium diffuses down its concentration gradient into the cell, leading to the absorption of water through water channels. Its functions include resorption of salt and water in renal collecting tubules and clearance of fluid from air spaces in the lungs. Called also *amiloride-sensitive sodium channel*.

fast c. an ion channel, such as a sodium channel, that becomes activated relatively quickly; a fast voltage-gated channel has a much lower activation potential than does the slow type. Cf. *slow c.*

gated c. an ion channel that is opened or closed by a conformational change in the channel protein in response to a stimulus, such as the binding of a ligand or a change in membrane potential.

inward rectifier potassium c′s a family of cell membrane channels selective for potassium that pass a large current of potassium ions into the cell in response to membrane hyperpolarization but only a small current outward above the resting potential. They help to maintain resting potential in many cells and to repolarize excitable cells.

ion c. a cell membrane protein with an ion-specific transmembrane pore, through which ions and small molecules pass into or out of a cell by diffusion downward along their electrochemical gradient; although some are always open, most open and close in response to a stimulus. Movement of ions through channels controls the electrical potential across the membrane and plays a vital role in depolarization and repolarization of nerve and muscle fibers. Called also *protein c.*

ligand-gated c. an ion channel that opens in response to the binding of a molecule (the ligand) to the channel protein, which causes a conformational change in the protein molecule. Cf. *voltage-gated c.*

lymph c′s the smaller lymph sinuses; irregular in and about the lymphatic glands and around lymphatic vessels.

mechanosensitive c. a channel that opens in response to stretching of the plasma membrane, allowing a large, nonspecific flux of cations; functions include protection of cells from osmotic shock and transduction of mechanical stimuli.

perineural c. a lymph channel that surrounds a nerve trunk.

potassium c. a voltage-gated channel selective for the passage of potassium ions, occurring in a wide variety of cells, including nerve, muscle, and secretory cells; its functions include regulation of cell membrane excitability, regulation of repetitive low frequency firing in some neurons, and recovery of the nerve fiber membrane at the end of the action potential.

protein c. ion c.

slow c. an ion channel, such as the calcium channel, that is slow to become activated; a slow voltage-gated channel has a much higher activation potential than does the fast type. Cf. *fast c.*

sodium c. a voltage-gated channel selective for the passage of sodium ions; sodium channels are activated by membrane depolarization and are the main causes of depolarization and repolarization of the nerve membrane during the propagation of action potentials.

thoroughfare c. a channel between terminal arterioles and venules, larger than a capillary.

voltage-gated c. an ion channel that opens or closes in response to changes in the electrical potential across the cell membrane. Cf. *ligand-gated c.*

water c. aquaporin.

chan•nel•op•a•thy (chan″əl-op′ə-the) a disorder of channels.

ion c. any of numerous hereditary conditions caused by mutations in genes encoding ion channels, resulting in abnormal function of the channels. Channelopathies are named for the ion channel affected, e.g., *sodium channelopathy*. Called also *ion channel disorders*.

Chan•tix (chan′tiks) trademark for a preparation of varenicline tartrate.

Cha·o·bor·us (ka″o-bor′əs) a genus of non–blood-sucking gnats of the family Culicidae; called also *Corethra. C. lacus′tris* is the Clear Lake gnat of California.

CHAOS congenital high airway obstruction syndrome.

cha·ot·ic (ka-ot′ik) [Gr. *chaos* primeval void] completely confused, disorganized, or irregular.

Cha·oul therapy, tube (shoul) [Henri *Chaoul,* Lebanese radiologist in Germany, 1887–1964] see under *therapy* and *tube.*

chap·er·one (shap′ər-ōn) someone or something that accompanies and oversees another.

molecular c. any of a diverse group of proteins that oversee the correct intracellular folding and assembly of polypeptides without being components of the final structure. The group includes nucleoplasmins, chaperonins, other heat shock proteins, and various other unrelated proteins.

chap·er·o·nin (shap″ər-o′nin) any of various heat shock proteins that act as molecular chaperones in bacteria, plasmids, mitochondria, and eukaryotic cytosol. They are large multi-subunit proteins with ring structures and act by enclosing unfolded proteins and preventing their nonspecific aggregation during assembly.

chapped (chapt) roughened and cracked, or split open by the cold or frequent wetting; said of skin.

char·ac·ter (kar′ak-tər) [Gr. *charaktēr* an engraved or impressed mark or stamp] 1. a quality or attribute indicative of the nature of an object or organism. 2. in genetics, the expression in the phenotype of a gene or group of genes; see also entries under *gene, trait,* and *inheritance.* 3. in psychiatry, a term used, especially in the psychoanalytic literature, in much the same way as personality (q.v.), particularly for those personality traits that are shaped by life experiences and developmental processes. See also *temperament.*

acquired c. a noninheritable modification produced in an animal as a result of its own activities or of environmental influences.

imvic c's four important characters in the classification of the coliform organisms: they are indole, methyl-red, Voges-Proskauer, and citrate.

primary sex c's those characters in the male or female that are directly involved in reproduction; the gonads and their accessory structures.

secondary sex c's those characters specific to the male or female but not directly involved in reproduction. See also *masculinization* and *feminization.*

char·ac·ter·is·tic (kar″ak-tər-is′tik) 1. character. 2. typical of an individual or other entity.

demand c's cues regarding the purpose of the study or the behavior expected that an experimental subject perceives and responds to.

char·ac·ter·ol·o·gy (kar″ak-tər-ol′ə-je) the study of character and personality.

Cha·rak Sam·hi·ta (chah′rə-kə sung′he-tah) [Sanskrit] the classic medical text of ayurveda, written about 1000 BCE by Charaka and composed of 120 chapters in 8 sections, summarizing the corpus of medical theory, ethics, diagnosis, treatment, and practice, originating from the sacred Indian texts known as the Vedas (approximately 3000 BCE).

char·coal (chahr′kōl) carbon prepared by charring wood or other organic material.

activated c. [USP] the residue from the destructive distillation of various organic materials, treated to increase its adsorptive powers; used as a general-purpose antidote.

animal c. charcoal prepared from bone; called also *animal, ivory,* or *Paris black,* and *bone-black.*

purified animal c. charcoal prepared from bone and purified by removal of materials dissolved by hot hydrochloric acid and water; adsorbent and decolorizer.

Char·cot arthropathy (disease, joint), etc. (shahr-ko′) [Jean Martin *Charcot,* French neurologist, 1825–1893] see under *foot, gait, sign,* and *triad;* see *neuropathic arthropathy,* under *arthropathy;* see *intermittent claudication,* under *claudication;* and see *intermittent hepatic fever,* under *fever.*

Char·cot-Bou·chard aneurysm (shahr-ko′ boo-shahr′) [J.M. *Charcot;* Charles Jacques *Bouchard,* French physician, 1837–1886] see under *aneurysm.*

Char·cot-Ley·den crystals (shahr-ko′ li′dən) [J.M. *Charcot;* Ernst Victor von *Leyden,* German physician, 1832–1910] see under *crystal.*

Char·cot-Ma·rie atrophy (syndrome) (shahr-ko′ mah-re′) [J.M. *Charcot;* Pierre *Marie,* French physician, 1853–1940] Charcot-Marie-Tooth disease.

Char·cot-Ma·rie-Tooth disease (atrophy) (shahr-ko′ mah-re′ to͞oth′) [J.M. *Charcot;* P. *Marie;* Howard Henry *Tooth,* English physician, 1856–1925] see under *disease.*

Char·cot-Weiss-Bak·er syndrome (shahr-ko′ wīs′ ba′kər) [J.M. *Charcot;* Soma *Weiss,* American physician, 1898–1942; James Porter *Baker,* American physician, 20th century] carotid sinus syndrome; see under *syndrome.*

charge (*Q, q*) (chahrj) a fundamental physical characteristic of elementary particles that determines the strength and nature of their interactions with the electromagnetic field. It is defined as positive or negative (or zero), existing only in integral numbers of charge quanta (e.g., proton, +1; electron, −1; neutron 0) each of which, symbolized *e,* is 1.602×10^{-19} coulomb. The charge of a body is the algebraic sum of the charges of its constituents. Called also *electric charge.*

Charles' law (shahrlz) [Jacques Alexandre César *Charles,* French physicist, 1746–1823] see under *law.*

char·ley horse (chahr′le hors) soreness and stiffness in a muscle caused by overstrain or contusion; the term is usually restricted to injuries of the quadriceps muscle.

Char·lin syndrome (chahr′lēn) [Carlos *Charlin,* Chilean ophthalmologist, 1886–1945] see under *syndrome.*

Charn·ley hip arthroplasty, prosthesis (charhn′le) [Sir John *Charnley,* British orthopedic surgeon, 1911–1988] see under *arthroplasty* and *prosthesis.*

Char·rière scale (shahr″e-ār′) [Joseph Frédéric Benoit *Charrière,* Swiss-born instrument maker in France, 1803–1876] see under *scale.*

Chart. [L.] char′ta (paper).

chart (chahrt) 1. a simplified graphic representation of the fluctuation of some variable, as of pulse, temperature, and respiration, or a record of all the clinical data of a particular case. 2. to record graphically the fluctuation of some variable, or to record the clinical data of a particular case.

alignment c. nomogram.

Amsler c's a set of charts showing various geometric patterns in black and white, e.g., grids or parallel lines, used for detecting defects of the central visual field.

growth c. a graphic representation of the normal progressive changes in selected measurements, such as weight, height, or head circumference, used as a tool for assessing growth in children; charts are composed of several percentile curves showing the distribution for the measurement of interest.

Guibor c. a chart containing outline pictures for orthoptic training.

Liley c. a chart that uses the spectrographic measurement of amniotic fluid bilirubin levels plotted against gestational age to estimate the severity of fetal hemolysis resulting from Rh isoimmunization. The chart is divided into three zones; a measurement falling in zone 1 indicates no disease or mild disease, while one falling in zone 3 indicates severe disease with impending fetal death.

Lund-Browder c. see under *classification.*

reading c. a chart bearing material printed in type of gradually increasing sizes; used in testing acuity of near vision.

Snellen c. a standardized chart imprinted with block letters (Snellen test type) in gradually decreasing sizes, identified according to distances at which they are ordinarily visible; used in testing visual acuity. See also *Snellen test type,* under *test type.*

Chas·sai·gnac tubercle (shahs″ən-yahk′) [Charles Marie Édouard *Chassaignac,* French surgeon, 1804–1879] *tuberculum caroticum.*

ChB [L.] Chirur′giae Baccalau′reus (Bachelor of Surgery).

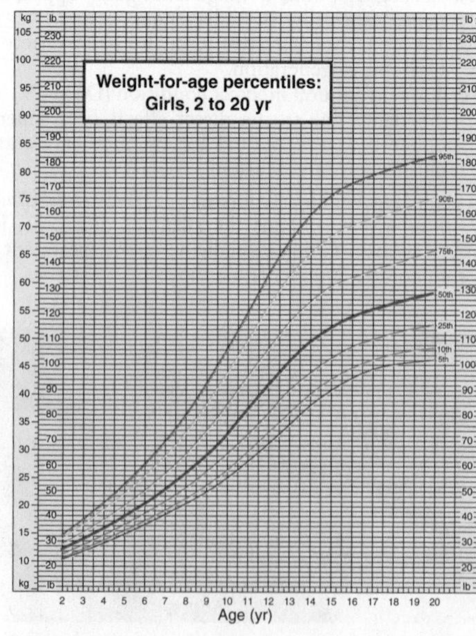

■ Growth chart showing percentile curves for weight by age for girls.

CHD congenital heart disease; coronary heart disease (see *ischemic heart disease*, under *disease*).

ChD [L.] Chirur′giae Doc′tor (Doctor of Surgery).

ChE cholinesterase.

check-bite (chek′bīt) check bite; see under *bite*.

chec•ker•board (chek′ər-bord) Punnett square.

check•point (chek′point″) in the cell cycle, any of a series of quality controls that monitor the status of the cell to ensure that required conditions, such as successful completion of a phase, are met before the cycle continues; checkpoints also detect damage to cellular components and block progression of the cycle until the damage is repaired. Faulty regulation of checkpoints is a cause of cancer.

Ché•di•ak-Hi•ga•shi syndrome (anomaly) (cha′de-ahk he-gah′she) [Moisés *Chédiak*, Cuban physician, 20th century; Otakata *Higashi*, Japanese physician, 20th century] see under *syndrome*.

Ché•di•ak-Stein•brinck-Hi•ga•shi anomaly (cha′de-ahk shtīn′bringk he-gah′she) [M. *Chédiak;* W. *Steinbrinck*, German physician, 20th century; O. *Higashi*] Chédiak-Higashi syndrome.

cheek (chēk) 1. bucca. 2. any fleshy protuberance resembling the cheek of the face.

cleft c. facial cleft caused by developmental failure of union between the maxillary and frontonasal prominences.

cheesy (che′ze) caseous.

Chei•lan•thes (ki-lan′thēz) a genus of ferns. *C. sei′beri* is the rock fern, an Australian species that causes poisoning in cattle similar to bracken poisoning. *C. sinna′ta* is the jimmy fern, a North American species poisonous to cattle, sheep, and goats, causing convulsions.

chei•lec•to•my (ki-lek′tə-me) [*cheil-* + *-ectomy*] 1. excision of a lip. 2. the operation of chiseling off the irregular bony edges of a joint cavity that interfere with motion.

chei•lec•tro•pi•on (ki″lek-tro′pe-on) [*cheil-* + *ectropion*] eversion of the lip.

chei•li•tis (ki-li′tis) [*cheil-* + *-itis*] inflammation affecting the lips. Spelled also *chilitis*. Cf. *cheilosis*.

actinic c. painful swelling of the lip(s) and development of scaly crust and erosions on the vermilion border after overexposure to sun rays; it may be acute or chronic. Called also *solar c.*

angular c. perlèche.

apostematous c. see *c. glandularis*.

commissural c. cheilitis affecting principally the angles (commissures) of the mouth. See also *perlèche*.

c. exfoliati′va, exfoliative c. persistent exfoliation of the lip caused by inflammation of the mucous membrane, a condition similar to dermatitis seborrheica of the lip.

c. glandula′ris a rare disease in which the lower lip becomes enlarged and later everted, exposing inflamed and dilated openings of accessory salivary glands; the glands themselves are enlarged and sometimes nodular. It may be associated with carcinoma of the lip. There are three types: the *simple type* is characterized by painless pinhead-sized lesions and may develop into one of the other types; the *superficial suppurative type* (called also *Baelz disease*) is characterized by painless swelling, induration, crusting, and ulcerations of the lip; and the *deep suppurative type* is a deep-seated infection with abscesses and fistulous tracts that eventually form scars. Called also *apostematous c., c. glandularis apostematosa*, and *myxadenitis labialis*.

c. glandula′ris apostemato′sa c. glandularis.

c. granulomato′sa, granulomatous c. orofacial granulomatosis localized to the lips, sometimes part of Melkersson-Rosenthal syndrome. Called also *Miescher granulomatous c.*

impetiginous c. impetigo of the lips.

Miescher granulomatous c. granulomatous c.

migrating c. perlèche.

solar c. actinic c.

c. venena′ta cheilitis caused by a toxic substance.

cheil(o)- [Gr. *cheilos* lip] a combining form denoting relationship to the lip, or to an edge.

chei•lo•an•gi•os•co•py (ki″lo-an″je-os′kə-pe) [*cheilo-* + *angioscopy*] microscopical observation of the circulation in the blood vessels of the lip.

chei•lo•car•ci•no•ma (ki″lo-kahr-sĭ-no′mə) carcinoma of the lip.

chei•lo•gnatho•pal•a•tos•chi•sis (ki″lo-na″tho-pal″ə-tos′kĭ-sis) cheilognathouranoschisis.

chei•lo•gnatho•pros•o•pos•chi•sis (ki″lo-na″tho-pros″o-pos′kĭ-sis) [*cheilo-* + *gnatho-* + *prosoposchisis*] a congenital anomaly consisting of an oblique facial cleft continuing into the lip and upper jaw.

chei•lo•gnath•os•chi•sis (ki″lo-na-thos′kĭ-sis) [*cheilo-* + *gnathoschisis*] a congenital anomaly consisting of a cleft lip and jaw.

chei•lo•gnatho•ura•nos•chi•sis (ki-″lo-na″tho-u-rə-nos′kĭ-sis) [*cheilo-* + *gnatho-* + *uranoschisis*] a congenital anomaly consisting of a cleft lip, upper jaw, and palate.

chei•lo•pha•gia (ki″lo-fa′jə) [*cheilo-* + *-phagia*] biting of the lips.

chei•lo•plas•ty (ki′lo-plas″te) [*cheilo-* + *-plasty*] plastic surgery of the lip; called also *labioplasty*. **cheiloplas′tic** *adj*

chei•lor•rha•phy (ki-lor′ə-fe) [*cheilo-* + *-rrhaphy*] the operation of suturing the lip, as in surgical repair of a congenitally cleft lip.

chei•los•chi•sis (ki-los′kĭ-sis) [*cheilo-* + Gr. *schisis* cleft] cleft lip.

chei•lo•sis (ki-lo′sis) [*cheil-* + *-osis*] a noninflammatory condition of the lips characterized by chapping and fissuring. Cf. *cheilitis*.

angular c. perlèche.

chei•lo•sto•ma•to•plas•ty (ki″lo-sto-mat′o-plas″te) [*cheilo-* + *stomato-* + *-plasty*] plastic restoration of the mouth and lips.

chei•lot•o•my (ki-lot′ə-me) [*cheilo-* + *-tomy*] incision into the lip.

Chei•ra•can•thi•um (ki″rə-kan′the-əm) *Chiracanthium*.

Chei•ra•can•thus (ki″rə-kan′thəs) *Gnathostoma*.

chei•ra•gra (ki-rag′rə) [*cheir-* + *agra*] gout of the hand, especially tophaceous gout with torsion of the fingers.

chei•ral•gia (ki-ral′jə) pain in the hand.

c. paresthe′tica a type of radial neuropathy owing to compression of the superficial ramus of the radial nerve, with pain and paresthesias.

cheir(o)- [Gr. *cheir* hand] a combining form denoting relationship to the hand. For words beginning thus, see also those beginning *chir(o)-*.

chei•ro•ar•throp•a•thy (ki″ro-ahr-throp′ə-the) a pathologic condition involving the joints of the hand and fingers.

diabetic c. a condition of tight skin on the fingers seen in diabetes mellitus, resembling that of scleredema, but without skin involvement; sometimes it may interfere with movement of the fingers.

chei•ro•cin•es•the•sia (ki″ro-sin″es-the′zhə) cheirokinesthesia.

chei•ro•kin•es•the•sia (ki″ro-kin″es-the′zhə) the subjective perception of the movements of the hand, especially in writing. **cheirokinesthet′ic** *adj*

chei•ro•meg•a•ly (ki-ro-meg′ə-le) megalocheiria.

chei•ro•plas•ty (ki′ro-plas″te) [*cheiro-* + *-plasty*] plastic surgery on the hand. **cheiroplas′tic** *adj*

chei•ro•po•dal•gia (ki″ro-po-dal′jə) [*cheiro-* + *podo-* + *-algia*] pain in the hands and feet.

chei•ro•pom•pho•lyx (ki″ro-pom′fo-liks) former name for *pompholyx*.

chei•ro•scope (ki′ro-skōp) [*cheiro-* + *-scope*] an instrument used in the training of binocular vision, by which the image of a test object seen reflected in a mirror by the sound eye is projected by the other eye to a drawing board, where it is traced with a pencil guided by the hand of the subject.

chei•ro•spasm (ki′ro-spaz″əm) [*cheiro-* + *spasm*] spasm of the muscles of the hand.

che•late (ke′lāt) [Gr. *chēlē* claw] 1. to combine with a metal in complexes in which the metal is part of a ring. 2. by extension, a chemical compound in which a metallic ion is sequestered and firmly bound into a ring within the chelating molecule. Chelates are used in chemotherapeutic treatments for metal poisoning.

che•la•tion (ke-la′shən) combination with a metal in complexes in which the metal is part of a ring.

che•la•tor (ke′la-tər) chelating agent.

che•lic•era (ke-lis′ər-ə) pl. *chelic′erae* [Gr. *chēlē* claw + *keras* horn] a pair of pincer-like head appendages of spiders, scorpions, and other arachnids. In certain arthropods, such as spiders, mites, and scorpions, anterior chelicerae serve as feeding appendages.

che•loid (ke′loid) keloid.

chem•abra•sion (kēm″ə-bra′zhən) superficial destruction and exfoliation of the epidermis and the upper layer of the dermis by application of a cauterant to the skin; done to remove lesions such as scars, tattoos, and pigmented nevi. Called also *chemexfoliation* and *chemical peel*.

Chem•et (kem′et) trademark for a preparation of succimer.

chem•ex•fo•li•a•tion (kēm″eks-fo″le-a′shən) chemabrasion.

chemi- see *chem(o)-*.

chem•i•cal (kem′ĭ-kəl) 1. of or pertaining to chemistry. 2. a substance composed of chemical elements, or obtained by chemical processes.

chemic(o)- see *chem(o)-*.

chem•i•co•bi•o•log•i•cal (kem″ĭ-ko-bi″o-loj′ĭ-kəl) biochemical.

chem•i•co•cau•tery (kem″ĭ-ko-kaw′tər-e) chemocautery.

chem•i•co•phys•i•cal (kem″ĭ-ko-fiz′ə-kəl) pertaining to chemistry and physics; pertaining to physical chemistry.

chem•i•co•phys•i•o•log•ic (kem″ĭ-ko-fiz″e-o-loj′ik) pertaining to physiology and chemistry.

chemi•lu•mi•nes•cence (kem″ĭ-loo″mĭ-nes′əns) luminescence produced by direct transformation of chemical energy into light energy.

chemi•os•mo•sis (kem″e-os-mo′sis) a mechanism by which the energy stored in a transmembrane electrochemical gradient is used to drive a process requiring energy, such as oxidative phosphorylation. Called also *chemiosmotic coupling*. **chemiosmot′ic** *adj*

chemi•sorp•tion (kem″ĭ-sorp′shən) the chemical adsorption of a gas or liquid onto the surface of a solid material, altering their molecular properties; in contrast to physical adsorption, which is characterized by weaker Van der Waals forces.

chem•ist (kem′ist) 1. a specialist in chemistry. 2. *(British)* pharmacist.

chem•is•try (kem′is-tre) [Gr. *chēmeia* alchemy] the science that deals with the elements and atomic relations of matter, and of the various compounds of the elements.

analytical c. chemistry that deals with analysis of different elements in a compound.

applied c. the application of chemistry to industry and the arts; called also *industrial c.*

biological c. biochemistry.

colloid c. chemistry dealing with the nature and composition of colloids.

ecological c. the study of those chemical compounds synthesized by plants that serve no metabolic purpose but which, by reason of their toxic effect on insects and higher animals, influence a community of interacting plants and animals.

forensic c. use of chemical knowledge in the solution of legal problems.

industrial c. applied c.

inorganic c. 1. the branch of chemistry which deals with all substances except for hydrocarbons and their derivatives. 2. originally, the branch of chemistry dealing with substances not associated with living organisms.

medical c. chemistry as it relates to medicine.

metabolic c. biochemistry.

mineral c. inorganic c.

organic c. 1. the branch of chemistry that deals with hydrocarbons and their derivatives. 2. originally, the branch of chemistry dealing with substances derived from living organisms.

pharmaceutical c. chemistry that deals with the composition and preparation of substances used in treatment of patients or diagnostic studies.

physical c. the branch of chemistry that uses a quantitative approach, applying the concepts and laws of physics, to describe and understand chemical properties.

physiological c. biochemistry.

surface c. the study of forces acting at the surfaces of gases, liquids, or solids, or the interfaces between two states.

synthetic c. the branch of chemistry that deals with the building up of chemical compounds from simpler substances or from the elements.

chem(o)- [Gr. *chēmeia* alchemy] a combining form denoting relationship to chemistry, or to a chemical. Also, *chemi-*, *chemic(o)-*.

che•mo•at•trac•tant (ke″mo-ə-trak′tənt) a substance that induces positive chemotaxis.

che•mo•au•to•troph (ke″mo-aw′to-trōf) a chemoautotrophic microorganism.

che•mo•au•to•tro•phic (ke″mo-aw″to-tro′fik) [*chemo-* + *autotrophic*] requiring for growth only inorganic compounds with carbon dioxide as the sole source of carbon (autotrophic), and oxidizing inorganic chemical compounds as the source of energy; said of certain bacteria and protozoa. Cf. *photoautotrophic*.

che•mo•bi•ot•ic (ke″mo-bi-ot′ik) the combination of a chemotherapeutic agent and an antibiotic, as of one or more of the sulfonamide compounds with penicillin.

che•mo•cau•tery (ke″mo-kaw′tər-e) destruction of tissue by application of a caustic chemical substance. Called also *chemical cautery*.

che•mo•co•ag•u•la•tion (ke″mo-ko-ag″u-la′shən) coagulation or destruction of tissue by the application of chemical agents.

che•mo•dec•to•ma (ke″mo-dek-to′mə) [*chemo-* + *dektos* to be received or accepted + *-oma*] any benign, chromaffin-negative tumor of the chemoreceptor system; the most common types are the *carotid body tumor*, the *glomus jugulare tumor*, and the *glomus vagale tumor*. Called also *nonchromaffin paraganglioma*.

che•mo•de•ner•va•tion (ke″mo-de″nər-va′shən) chemical interruption of nerves to treat a neurogenic condition such as spasticity, neurogenic bladder, or vagus-related conditions. Cf. *neurotomy* and *vagotomy*.

che•mo•dif•fer•en•ti•a•tion (ke″mo-dif″ər-en-she-a′shən) the invisible point of decision that precedes and controls actual differentiation of cells into rudimentary organs of the embryo.

che•mo•em•bo•li•za•tion (ke″mo-em″bo-lĭ-za′shən) percutaneous introduction of a substance to occlude a vessel in combination with a chemotherapeutic agent, used in the treatment of cancer to deliver sustained therapeutic levels of the agent to a tumor.

che•mo•en•do•crine (ke″mo-en′do-krin) [*chemo-* + *endocrine*] chemohormonal.

che•mo•het•ero•troph (ke″mo-het′ər-o-trōf″) a chemoheterotrophic organism.

che•mo•het•ero•tro•phic (ke″mo-het″ər-o-tro′fik) heterotrophic; requiring preformed organic compounds as a source of carbon and oxidizing organic compounds as a source of energy.

che•mo•hor•mo•nal (ke″mo-hor-mo′nəl) pertaining to drugs having hormone activity.

che•mo•kine (ke′mo-kīn) any of a family of low molecular weight (8–10 kD) cytokines that induce chemotaxis or chemokinesis in leukocytes (or in particular populations of leukocytes). They are classified into four groups, based on the structural arrangement of conserved cysteine: CXC or α, CC or β, C or γ, and CX_3C or δ, where C is cysteine and X is another amino acid. Chemokines are regulators of the immune system and may also play roles in the circulatory and central nervous systems.

che•mo•ki•ne•sis (ke″mo-kĭ-ne′sis) [*chemo-* + *-kinesis*] increased nondirectional activity of cells due to presence of a chemical substance. Cf. *chemotaxis*. **chemokinet′ic** *adj*

che•mo•litho•troph (ke″mo-lith′o-trōf) a chemolithotrophic organism.

che•mo•litho•tro•phic (ke″mo-lith″o-tro′fik) chemoautotrophic; utilizing carbon dioxide as the sole source of carbon and deriving energy from the oxidation of inorganic compounds.

che•mo•lu•mi•nes•cence (ke″mo-loo″mĭ-nes′əns) chemiluminescence.

che•mol•y•sis (ke-mol′ĭ-sis) [*chemo-* + *-lysis*] chemical decomposition.

che•mo•mor•pho•sis (ke″mo-mor-fo′sis) [*chemo-* + *morphosis*] change of form or developmental stage due to chemical action.

che•mo•nu•cle•ol•y•sis (ke″mo-noo″kle-ol′ə-sis) [*chemo-* + *nucleo-* + *lysis*] dissolution of the nucleus pulposus of an intervertebral disk by injection of a proteolytic agent such as chymopapain; used especially in the treatment of herniation of an intervertebral disk (see under *herniation*).

che•mo•or•ga•no•troph (ke″mo-or′gə-no-trōf″) a chemo-organotrophic organism.

che•mo•or•ga•no•tro•phic (ke″mo-or″gə-no-tro′fik) heterotrophic; requiring preformed organic compounds as a source of carbon and oxidizing organic compounds as a source of energy; said of bacteria.

che•mo•pal•li•dec•tomy (ke″mo-pal″ĭ-dek′tə-me) [*chemo-* + *pallidectomy*] destruction of a portion of the globus pallidus by the introduction of a chemical agent.

che•mo•pal•li•do•thal•a•mec•to•my (ke″mo-pal″ĭ-do-thal″ə-mek′tə-me) destruction of a portion of the globus pallidus and thalamus by the introduction of a chemical agent.

che•mo•phar•ma•co•dy•nam•ic (ke″mo-fahr″mə-ko-di-nam′ik) denoting the relationship between chemical constitution and biologic or pharmacologic activity.

che•mo•pre•ven•tion (ke″mo-pre-ven′shən) chemoprophylaxis.

che•mo•pro•phy•lax•is (ke″mo-pro″fə-lak′sis) [*chemo-* + *prophylaxis*] use of a chemotherapeutic agent as a means of preventing development of a specific disease. Called also *chemoprevention*, *chemical prophylaxis*, and *drug prophylaxis*.

primary c. prophylactic use of a chemotherapeutic agent before infection has occurred in an individual.

secondary c. prophylactic use of a chemotherapeutic agent in an individual after infection has occurred (with *Mycobacterium tuberculosis*, for example) but before disease has become manifest.

che•mo•pro•tec•tant (ke″mo-pro-tek′tənt) 1. providing protection against the toxic effects of chemotherapeutic agents. 2. an agent that has this effect.

che•mo•ra•dio•ther•a•py (ke″mo-ra″de-o-ther′ə-pe) [*chemo-* + *radiotherapy*] combined modality therapy using chemotherapy and radiotherapy, designed to reduce the need for surgery by maximizing the interaction between the radiation and the therapeutic agent or agents.

che•mo•re•cep•tion (ke″mo-re-sep′shən) the response of a sensory nerve or organ to chemical stimuli in the surrounding medium.

che•mo•re•cep•tor (ke″mo-re-sep′tər) [*chemo-* + *receptor*] 1. a sensory nerve terminal adapted for excitation by chemical substances, e.g., olfactory and gustatory receptors. 2. a sense organ such as the carotid body, the aortic bodies, or the glomus jugulare, which is sensitive to chemical changes in the blood stream, especially reduced oxygen content, and reflexively increases both respiration and blood pressure. See also *receptor* (def. 2) and *chemoreceptor system*, under *system*.

central c's chemoreceptors in the brain that monitor the pH of the cerebrospinal fluid; an increase in CO_2 causes increased respiration. Their location is thought to be on the ventral surface of the medulla oblongata.

peripheral c's chemoreceptors, located mainly in the carotid and aortic bodies, with a few associated with other arteries of the thorax and abdomen, that monitor oxygen, carbon dioxide, and hydrogen ion concentration and help to control respiration.

che•mo•re•pel•lent (ke″mo-re-pel′ənt) a substance that induces negative chemotaxis.

che•mo•re•sis•tance (ke″mo-re-zis′təns) specific resistance acquired by cells to the action of certain chemicals.

che•mo•sen•si•tive (ke″mo-sen′sĭ-tiv) sensitive to changes in chemical composition of the environment.

che•mo•sen•sory (ke″mo-sen′sər-e) relating to the perception of chemical substances, as in odor detection.

che•mo•sis (ke-mo′sis) [Gr. *chēmōsis*] excessive edema of the ocular conjunctiva. **chemot′ic** *adj*

che•mos•mo•sis (ke″mos-mo′sis) chemical action taking place through an intervening semipermeable membrane. **chemosmot′ic** *adj*

che•mo•sorp•tion (kem″o-sorp′shən) chemisorption.

che•mo•stat (ke′mo-stat) an apparatus in which the environment is so controlled that bacterial populations are maintained in a steady state of continuous cell division in a constant environment.

che•mo•ster•il•ant (ke″mo-ster′ĭ-lənt) a chemical compound the ingestion of which causes sterility of an organism; such compounds have been used as a means of controlling various insects and other pests by inducing sterility in the male.

che•mo•ster•il•iza•tion (ke″mo-ster″il-ĭ-za′shən) sterilization of an organism by means of a chemosterilant (q.v.).

che•mo•sur•gery (ke″mo-sur′jər-e) the destruction of tissue by chemical agents; originally applied to chemical fixation of malignant, gangrenous, or infected tissue, with the use of frozen sections to facilitate systematic microscopic control of the extent of ablation.

Mohs c. the original form of the Mohs technique, in which zinc chloride was applied to the tumor to fix it and isolate it in situ; this was later replaced by quick freezing of excised tumor.

che•mo•syn•the•sis (ke″mo-sin′thə-sis) [*chemo-* + *synthesis*] the synthesis of carbohydrate from carbon dioxide and water as a result of the energy derived from chemical reactions, rather than from absorbed light. Such synthesis is carried out by certain bacteria and algae. Cf. *photosynthesis*. **chemosynthet′ic** *adj*

che•mo•tax•in (ke″mo-tak′sin) chemotactic factor.

che•mo•tax•is (ke″mo-tak′sis) [*chemo-* + *-taxis*] directional movement of a cell or organism in response to a chemical concentration gradient. Cf *chemokinesis*. **chemotac′tic** *adj*

leukocyte c. the response of leukocytes to products formed during an immune response, wherein leukocytes are attracted to and accumulate at the site of the reaction; it is part of the inflammatory response. See also *inflammation*.

negative c. movement of a cell or organism from an area of higher concentration of a chemical to an area of lower concentration.

positive c. movement of a cell or organism from an area of lower concentration of a chemical to an area of higher concentration.

che•mo•thal•a•mec•to•my (ke″mo-thal″ə-mek′tə-me) destruction of a portion of the thalamus by the introduction of a chemical agent.

che•mo•ther•a•peu•tics (ke″mo-ther′ə-pu′tiks) chemotherapy.

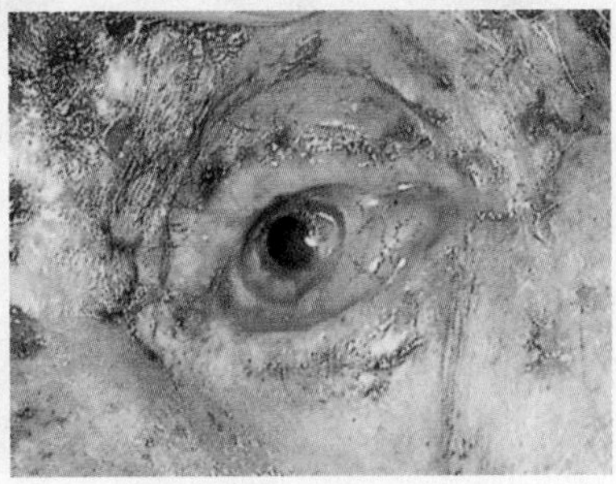

■ Chemosis.

che•mo•ther•a•py (ke″mo-ther′ə-pe) the treatment of disease by chemical agents; originally applied to use of chemicals that affect the causative organism unfavorably but do not harm the patient. Cf. *pharmacotherapy*. **chemotherapeu′tic** *adj*

adjuvant c. cancer chemotherapy employed after the primary tumor has been removed by some other method.

combination c. the use of several different agents at once in order to enhance effectiveness; seen particularly in cancer chemotherapy. Called also *polychemotherapy*.

consolidation c. a second round of cancer chemotherapy administered several months after the induction regimen in an effort to prolong or consolidate remission; it may be the same agents as in the induction regimen or different agents.

dose-dense c. cancer chemotherapy in which the dose per unit of time is increased, usually because the interval between cycles is shortened.

dose-intense c. cancer chemotherapy in which the total dose in one cycle period is increased.

induction c. chemotherapy as the initial treatment for cancer, especially as part of combined modality therapy.

neoadjuvant c. chemotherapy used as neoadjuvant therapy (q.v.) for cancer. Called also *preoperative c.*, *presurgical c.*, and *primary c.*

preoperative c., presurgical c. neoadjuvant c.

primary c. neoadjuvant c.

regional c. chemotherapy, especially for cancer, administered as a regional perfusion.

sequential c. chemotherapy in which several agents are administered one at a time rather than concurrently, in order to optimize dosage and increase patient tolerance.

che•mo•troph (ke′mo-trōf) a chemotrophic organism.

che•mo•tro•phic (ke″mo-tro′fik) deriving energy from the oxidation of organic (chemo-organotrophic) or inorganic (chemolithotrophic) compounds; said of bacteria. Cf. *phototrophic*.

che•mot•rop•ism (ke-mot′ro-piz-əm) [*chemo-* + *tropism*] tropism in response to a chemical stimulus. **chemotrop′ic** *adj*

chem•ur•gy (kem′ər-ge) [*chemo-* + Gr. *ergon* work] chemistry applied to the industrial use of raw organic products, especially agricultural products.

Che•nix (ke′niks) trademark for a preparation of chenodiol.

che•no•de•oxy•cho•late (ke″no-de-ok-se-ko′lāt) a salt or anionic form of chenodeoxycholic acid.

che•no•de•oxy•cho•lic ac•id (ke″no-de-ok″se-kol′ik) one of the primary bile acids, usually occurring conjugated with glycine or taurine; it facilitates fat absorption and cholesterol excretion. The pharmaceutical preparation is called *chenodiol*.

che•no•de•oxy•cho•lyl•gly•cine (ke″no-de-ok″se-ko″ləl-gli′sēn) a bile salt, the glycine conjugate of chenodeoxycholic acid. Called also *glycochenodeoxycholic acid*.

che•no•de•oxy•cho•lyl•tau•rine (ke″no-de-ok″se-ko″ləl-taw′rēn) a bile salt, the taurine conjugate of chenodeoxycholic acid. Called also *taurochenodeoxycholic acid*.

che•no•di•ol (ke″no-di′ol) chenodeoxycholic acid used as an anticholelithic to dissolve radiolucent, noncalcified gallstones; administered orally.

Che•no•po•di•um (ke″no-po′de-əm) a genus of herbs of the family Chenopodiaceae, native to temperate regions. *C. al′bum*, or white goosefoot, contains oxalates and nitrates and can cause oxalate poisoning and nitrite poisoning in ruminants.

cher•ry (cher′e) [L. *cerasus*] 1. any of various rosaceous trees and species of the genus *Prunus*. 2. the fruit of one of these trees; used as a flavoring. See also under *juice* and *syrup*. 3. any of certain other trees resembling the cherry trees of the genus *Prunus*.

Barbados c. acerola.

black c. wild c.

choke c. *Prunus virginiana*.

rum c. wild c.

sour c. *Prunus cerasus*.

wild c. 1. *Prunus serotina*. 2. the dried stem bark of *P. serotina*, used in wild cherry syrup. Called also *wild black cherry bark*.

cher•ub•ism (cher′əb-iz-əm) [*cherub* + *-ism*] hereditary and progressive bilateral swelling at the angle of the mandible, sometimes involving the entire jaw. The swelling imparts a cherubic look to the face, in some cases enhanced by upturning of the eyes. Called also *fibrous dysplasia of jaw* and *familial bilateral giant cell tumor*.

chest (chest) thorax.

alar c. flat c.

barrel c. a rounded, bulging chest with abnormal increase in the anteroposterior diameter, showing little movement on respiration; seen in emphysema and in kyphosis.

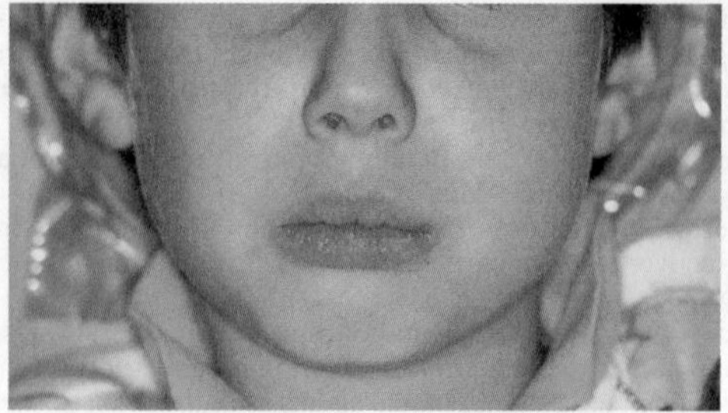
■ Cherubism resulting in fullness of the maxilla.

blast c. pulmonary concussion (q.v.) and hemorrhage occurring in blast injury (see under *injury*).

cobbler's c. a chest showing a sinking in at the lower end of the sternum.

flail c. paradoxical movement of the chest wall with respiration, owing to multiple fractures of the ribs.

flat c. deformity of the chest in which it is flattened from front to back; called also *alar c.* and *pterygoid c.*

foveated c., funnel c. pectus excavatum.

keeled c. pectus carinatum.

paralytic c. a long and narrow chest with emaciation so that the ribs stand out sharply under the skin.

pigeon c. pectus carinatum.

pterygoid c. flat c.

tetrahedron c. a chest that suggests a solid with four sides, each an equilateral triangle, the chest projecting in a peak between the nipples.

chest•nut (chest′nət) 1. *Castanea.* 2. the nut of any of various species of *Castanea.* 3. one of the masses of horn on the medial surface of the forearm or the distal part of the medial surface of the tarsus of horses.

horse c. 1. *Aesculus hippocastanum.* 2. a preparation of the medicinal parts of *A. hippocastanum;* the seeds have antiexudative, antiinflammatory, and immunomodulatory activity and are used in the treatment of chronic venous insufficiency. Horse chestnut preparations are also used in homeopathy and folk medicine.

Chey•le•ti•el•la (ki″lə-te-el′ə) a genus of nonburrowing mites of the family Cheyletiellidae. They are found most often on domestic animals, but some species cause dermatosis in humans. *C. bla′kei* infests cats; *C. parasito′vorax* infests rabbits; and *C. yas′guri* infests dogs.

Chey•le•ti•el•li•dae (ki″lə-te-el′ĭ-de) a family of mites that infest domestic mammals and occasionally humans. It includes the genus *Cheyletiella.*

chey•le•ti•el•lo•sis (ki″lə-te″el-o′sis) 1. infestation of a dog, cat, or rabbit with a species of *Cheyletiella*, characterized by a pruritic dermatitis. Called also *walking dandruff.* 2. pruritic dermatitis in humans caused by a species of *Cheyletiella.*

Cheyne-Stokes res•pi•ra•tion (breathing, sign) (chān′ stōks′) [John *Cheyne*, Scottish physician, 1777–1836; William *Stokes*, Irish physician, 1804–1878] see under *respiration.*

CHF congestive heart failure.

chi[1] (ki) [X, χ] the twenty-second letter of the Greek alphabet.

chi[2], **ch'i** (che) qi.

Chi•a•ri network (reticulum), malformation (deformity), syndrome (disease) (ke-ah′rē) [Hans *Chiari*, Austrian pathologist, 1851–1916] see under *network* and *malformation*, and see *Budd-Chiari syndrome*, under *syndrome.*

Chi•a•ri-Ar•nold syndrome (ke-ah′re ahr′nəld) [H. *Chiari;* Julius *Arnold*, German pathologist, 1835–1915] Arnold-Chiari malformation; see under *malformation.*

Chi•a•ri-From•mel syndrome (disease) (ke-ah′re from′əl) [Johann Baptist *Chiari*, German obstetrician, 1817–1854; Richard Julius Ernst *Frommel*, German gynecologist, 1854–1912] see under *syndrome.*

chi•asm (ki′az-əm) [L., Gr. *chiasma*] a decussation or X-shaped crossing; see *chiasma.*

c. of digits of hand chiasma tendinum digitorum manus.

optic c. chiasma opticum.

tendinous c. of fingers chiasma tendinum digitorum manus.

chi•as•ma (ki-az′mə) pl. *chias′mata* [L., from Gr. "a cross, crosspiece," from the shape of the letter *chi* (X)] 1. an anatomical term for a decussation or X-shaped crossing, such as of nerves. 2. a point where pairs of homologous chromatids remain in contact during late prophase to anaphase of meiosis I, indicating where an exchange of homologous segments has taken place between nonsister chromatids by recombination.

optic c., c. op′ticum [TA] optic chiasm: the part of the hypothalamus formed by the decussation, or crossing, of the fibers of the optic nerve from the medial half of each retina; called also *optic decussation.*

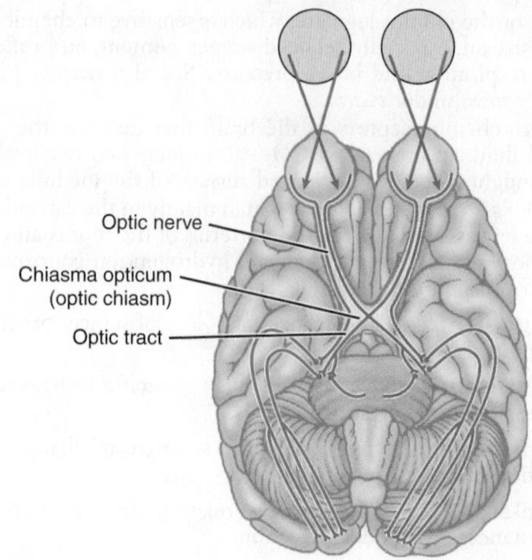

c. ten′dinum digito′rum ma′nus [TA] tendinous chiasm of fingers: the crossing of the tendons of the flexor digitorum profundus through the tendons of the flexor digitorum superficialis; called also *chiasm of digits of hand.*

chi•as•mal (ki-az′məl) chiasmatic.

chi•as•ma•ta (ki-az′mə-tə) [L.] plural of *chiasma.*

chi•as•mat•ic (ki-az-mat′ik) resembling a chiasm; crosswise.

chi•as•mic (ki-az′mik) chiasmatic.

chi•as•mom•e•ter (ki″az-mom′ə-tər) chiastometer.

chi•as•tom•e•ter (ki″az-tom′ə-tər) [Gr. *chiastos* crossed + *-meter*] an apparatus for measuring any deviation of the optic axes from their normal parallelism; called also *chiasmometer.*

Chi•ba needle (che′bə) [*Chiba* University in Japan, where it was developed] see under *needle.*

Chi•brox•in (ki-brok′sin) trademark for a preparation of norfloxacin.

Chick-Mar•tin test (method) (chik mahr′tin) [Harriette *Chick*, British physiologist, 20th century; Charles James *Martin*, British physiologist, 1866–1955] see under *test.*

chick•en•pox (chik′ən-poks) varicella: a highly contagious infectious disease caused by human herpesvirus 3, usually affecting children, spread by direct contact or the respiratory route via droplet nuclei, and characterized by the appearance on the skin and mucous membranes of successive crops of typical pruritic vesicular lesions that are easily broken and become scabbed; it is generally accompanied by mild constitutional symptoms. In most children it is relatively benign; a minority of adults may have complications of pneumonia or encephalitis. In immunocompromised or otherwise debilitated children or adults, it may spread to internal organs and sometimes prove fatal. See also *herpes zoster.*

chick•pea (chik′pe) 1. the leguminous plant *Cicer arietinum* of Southern Europe. 2. the edible seed of *C. arietinum*, widely used as food but toxic to certain individuals. Called also *garbanzo.*

Chi•do-Rod•gers blood group (che′do roj′ərz) [from the names of propositi first observed in the 1960s] see under *blood group.*

Chie•vitz layer, organ (che′vits) [Johan Henrik *Chievitz*, Danish anatomist, 1850–1901] see under *layer* and *organ.*

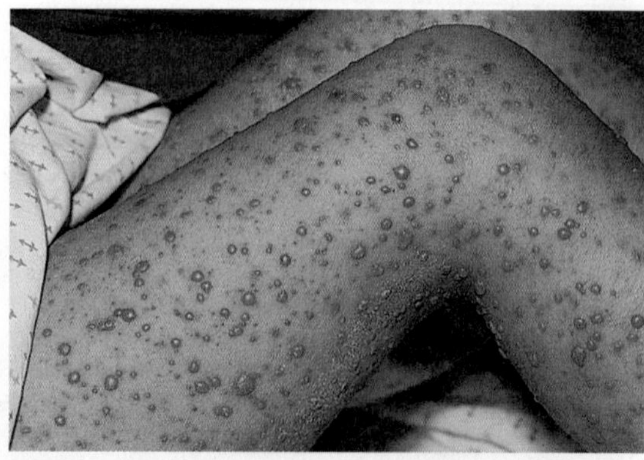
■ Lesions of chickenpox (varicella).

chig•ger (chig′ər) the six-legged red larva of a mite of the family Trombiculidae, which infests many types of vertebrates, especially mammals. Chiggers attach to the skin of their hosts and their bites produce a wheal, usually with severe itching and dermatitis *(trombiculiasis)*. Their habitat is tall grass and underbrush. *Eutrombicula alfreddugèsi* is the common chigger of the United States; *E. splendens* is found in the southeastern United States; and *Trombicula autumnalis* is a common European species. Some species in the East Asia–Pacific region are vectors of the rickettsiae of scrub typhus. The chigger is not the same as the *chigoe* (q.v.). Called also *bête rouge, harvest bug* or *mite, red bug* or *mite,* and *mower's mite.*

chigo (chig′o) chigoe.

chig•oe (chig′o) the flea *Tunga penetrans,* originally native to the West Indies but now found in hot climates around the world; it infests many different species of mammals. The pregnant female flea burrows into the skin of the feet, legs, or some other part of the body, causing intense irritation and ulceration that sometimes leads to spontaneous amputation of a digit. The chigoe is not the same as the *chigger* (q.v.). Spelled also *chigo.* Called also *burrowing flea, sand flea,* and *jigger.*

chik•un•gun•ya (chik″ən-gun′yə) [Makonde language of Tanzania and Mozambique, "that which bends up"] a self-limited disease resembling dengue, seen mainly in Africa and South and Southeast Asia, caused by an alphavirus transmitted chiefly by mosquitoes of genus *Aedes;* its most prominent symptoms are musculoskeletal and it has occasionally been associated with hemorrhagic fever.

Chi•lai•di•ti sign, syndrome (ke-lah-the′te) [Demetrios *Chilaiditi,* Austrian-born Turkish radiologist, 1883–1975] see under *sign* and *syndrome.*

chil•blain (chil′blān) [L. *pernio*] a recurrent localized erythema and doughy subcutaneous swelling caused by exposure to cold associated with dampness, and accompanied by pruritus and a burning sensation. In children it usually involves the hands, feet, ears, and face; in adults it more often involves the extremities. Called also *erythema pernio* and *pernio.*

Child-Pugh score (chīld′ pug′) [Charles G. *Child* III, American surgeon, 1908–1991; R.N.H. *Pugh,* British physician, 20th century] see under *score.*

Child-Tur•cotte-Pugh score (chīld′ tər-kot′ pug′) [C.G. *Child* III; Jeremiah G. *Turcotte,* American surgeon, 20th century; R.N.H. *Pugh*] Child-Pugh score; see under *score.*

child•birth (chīld′bərth) the act or process of giving birth to a child, including both *labor* and *delivery.* Called also *parturition.*

child•hood (chīld′hood) the period of life of the human young generally considered to extend from infancy to puberty.

chi•li•tis (ki-li′tis) cheilitis.

chill (chil) a shivering or shaking; an attack of involuntary contractions of the voluntary muscles, accompanied by a sense of cold and pallor of the skin.

creeping c. a chilly sensation, without any definite tremor or chattering of the teeth.

shaking c. a chill in which there is a definite tremor.

chil(o)- for words beginning thus, see also words beginning *cheil(o)-.*

Chi•lo•do•nel•la (ki″lə-də-nel′ə) a genus of ciliophoran protozoa that infect goldfish, guppies, and other common aquarium fish, causing weakness, incoordination, and loss of skin near the gills, which can be fatal.

Chi•log•na•tha (ki-log′nə-thə) an order of millipedes, arthropods of the class Diplopoda.

chi•lo•mas•ti•gi•a•sis (ki″lo-mas″tĭ-gi′ə-sis) infection with *Chilomastix.*

Chi•lo•mas•tix (ki″lo-mas′tiks) [*chilo-* + Gr. *mastix* whip] a genus of parasitic protozoa of the order Retortamonadida, having three flagella and a single nucleus with an adjacent cytostome; they inhabit the intestines of numerous different types of vertebrates. Species are normally nonpathogenic, but *C. mesni′li* occasionally causes watery diarrhea.

Chi•lop•o•da (ki-lop′ə-də) [Gr. *cheilos* lip + *pous* foot] the centipedes, a class of elongated arthropods of the superclass Myriapoda; they have one pair of legs to each body segment, with 15 to 173 pairs of legs. They paralyze and kill insects and small animals with their poison claws, which are modified legs of the first body segment. A few species of the genus *Scolopendra* are capable of penetrating human skin with a painful bite.

chi•mae•ra (ki-mēr′ə) chimera.

chi•me•ra (ki-mēr′ə) [Gr. *chimaira* a mythological fire-spouting monster with a lion's head, goat's body, and serpent's tail] 1. an individual organism whose body contains cell populations derived from different zygotes, of the same or of different species; it may occur spontaneously, as in twins (blood group chimeras), or be produced artificially, as an organism that develops from combined portions of different embryos, or one in which tissues or cells of another organism have been introduced. Cf. *mosaic.* 2. a substance created from proteins or genes of two species, as by genetic engineering. **chimer′ic** *adj*

heterologous c. a chimera whose cells or tissues are derived from organisms of two different species.

homologous c. a chimera whose cells or tissues are derived from organisms of the same species but of different genotypes.

isologous c. a chimera whose cells or tissues are derived from different organisms of the same genotype, such as identical twins.

radiation c. an organism that survives with immunologic characteristics of host and donor after a bone marrow graft from an antigenically different donor, the host having first been subjected to sublethal whole-body irradiation so that there is reduced or no immune response to foreign cells by the donor.

chi•mer•ism (ki-mēr′iz-əm) the quality of being a chimera; in genetics, the presence in an individual of cells of different origin, as of blood cells derived from a dizygotic co-twin. Cf. *mosaicism.*

chim•pan•zee (chim-pan-ze′, chim-pan′ze) [Kongo *chimpenzi* or *kimpenzi*] *Pan troglodytes,* an anthropoid ape that inhabits the tropical rain forests of Africa and is used for experimental purposes because of its susceptibility to some human diseases and in behavioral studies because of its high level of intelligence.

chin (chin) mentum.

galoche c. (gah-losh′) [Fr. "clog"] a chin that is long and pointed.

chi•na•ber•ry (chi′nə-ber″ry) *Melia azedarach.*

chin•a•crine (kin′ə-krēn) quinacrine; see *quinacrine hydrochloride.*

chin•cap (chin′kap) an extraoral orthodontic appliance consisting of a caplike device fitted over the chin, which is connected to the headgear by elastics for the purpose of exerting upward and backward force on the mandible in the treatment of prognathism.

chi•o•na•blep•sia (ki″o-nə-blep′se-ə) [Gr. *chiōn* snow + *ablepsia*] snow blindness.

chip (chip) a small piece, as of something broken off.

bone c's small pieces of bone, usually cancellous, generally used to fill in bony defects to facilitate recalcification.

Chi•ra•can•thi•um (ki″rə-kan′the-əm) a genus of venomous spiders. Two species, *C. inclu′sum* in California and *C. diver′sium* in Hawaii, have sometimes deadly bites.

chi•ral (ki′rəl) exhibiting chirality.

chi•ral•i•ty (ki-ral′ĭ-te) [Gr. *cheir* hand] the property of handedness, of not being superimposable on a mirror image; the handedness of an asymmetric molecule, as specified by its optical rotation or absolute configuration. Cf. *stereoisomerism.*

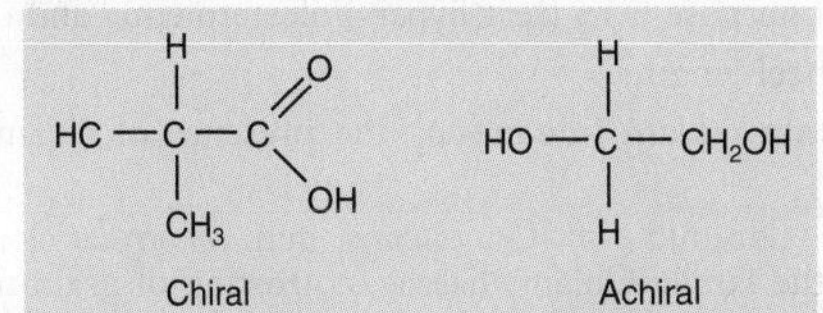

Chiral (Lactic acid) — Achiral (Ethylene glycol)

■ Lactic acid, its tetracoordinate carbon atom bearing four different substituents, is not superimposable on its mirror image. Ethylene glycol, with two identical substituents on its tetracoordinate carbon, can be superimposed on its mirror image.

chir(o)- [Gr. *cheir* hand] a combining form denoting relationship to the hand; for words beginning thus, see also those beginning *cheir(o)-.*

Chi•ro•caine (ki′ro-kān) trademark for a preparation of levobupivacaine hydrochloride.

chi•ro•meg•a•ly (ki″ro-meg′ə-le) megalocheiria.

Chi•ro•nex (ki′rə-neks) a genus of cubomedusan jellyfish. *C. flec′keri* Southcott is a species of sea wasp found along the coast of Australia whose sting is highly lethal and can cause death within 15 minutes.

Chi•ro•nom•i•dae (ki″ro-nom′ĭ-de) a family of insects of the suborder Nematocera, order Diptera, that comprises the true midges.

Chi•ron•o•mus (ki-ron′ə-məs) a genus of gnatlike flies with giant polytene chromosomes in some larval tissue nuclei, which have been useful in genetics studies.

chi•ro•plas•ty (ki′ro-plas″te) cheiroplasty.

chi•ro•po•dal•gia (ki″ro-po-dal′jə) cheiropodalgia.

chi•ro•pod•i•cal (ki″ro-pod′ĭ-kəl) podiatric.

chi•rop•o•dist (ki-rop′ə-dist) podiatrist.

chi•rop•o•dy (ki-rop′ə-de) podiatry.

chi•ro•prac•tic (ki″ro-prak′tik) [*chiro-* + Gr. *prassein* to do] a nonpharmaceutical, nonsurgical system of health care based on the self-healing capacity of the body and the primary importance of the proper function of the nervous system in the maintenance of health; therapy is aimed at removing irritants to the nervous system and restoring proper function. The most common method of treatment is by spinal manipulation and is primarily done for musculoskeletal complaints; other methods include lifestyle modification, nutritional therapy, and physiotherapy.

straight c. the practice of chiropractic in strict accordance with the principles of its founder, D.D. Palmer, without additions made by later practitioners. The original definition of subluxation (q.v.) as a vertebral displacement is adhered to, and chiropractic is considered to be nontherapeutic, its purpose being solely to contribute to health by the correction of vertebral subluxations.

chi•ro•prac•tor (ki′ro-prak″tər) a practitioner of chiropractic.

Chi•ro•psal•mus (ki″rə-sahl′məs) a genus of cubomedusan jellyfish. *C. quadra′tus* Haeckel is a species of sea wasp found in the Philippines whose sting can be deadly.

Chi•rop•te•ra (ki-rop′tə-rə) the bats, an order of flying mammals. The family Phyllostomatidae includes vampire bats.

chi•ro•scope (ki′ro-skōp) cheiroscope.

chi•ro•spasm (ki′ro-spaz″əm) cheirospasm.

chis•el (chis′əl) 1. a wedgelike instrument with a cutting edge at the end of the blade. 2. a dental instrument whose cutting edge is in line with the center of the handle; used for planing or smoothing a surface, as during cavity preparation.

periodontal c. a straight instrument that curves slightly as the blade extends from the shank, the straight cutting edge at the end of the instrument being beveled at a 45° angle. Used chiefly for scaling the proximal surfaces of teeth too closely spaced to permit the use of other scalers. Called also *chisel scaler.*

Wedelstaedt c. any of various periodontal chisels whose blade is continuous with the shank and at a curve from it.

chi-square (ki′skwār) see under *distribution* and *test.*

chi•tin (ki′tin) [Gr. *chitōn* tunic] a white, insoluble, linear homopolymer composed of *N*-acetylglucosamine residues in β-(1,4) linkage; it is widely distributed, forming the principal constituent of arthropod exoskeletons, and found in some plants, particularly fungi.

chi•tin•ous (ki′tin-əs) composed of or of the nature of chitin.

chi•to•bi•ose (ki″to-bi′ōs) a disaccharide, two *N*-acetylglucosamine moieties in β-(1,4) linkage, forming the basic repeating unit of chitin.

chi•to•san (ki′to-sən) a polysaccharide composed of repeating glucosamine units, obtained by deacetylation of chitin and used to absorb heavy metals in water treatment. It also binds lipids in vitro and is used in preparations whose purpose is to treat hypercholesterolemia and obesity.

CHL crown-heel length.

chla•my•de•mia (klam″ĭ-de′me-ə) the presence of chlamydiae in the blood.

Chla•my•dia (klə-mid′e-ə) [Gr. *chlamys,* gen. *chlamydos* cloak] a genus of bacteria of the family Chlamydiaceae, consisting of gram-negative, glycogen-producing, coccoid organisms that multiply only within a host cell and have a unique growth cycle (see *Chlamydiales*). They are common pathogens. Some former members of this genus are now classified in the genus *Chlamydophila.* The type species is *C. tracho′matis.*

C. pneumo′niae *Chlamydophila pneumoniae.*

C. psit′taci *Chlamydophila psittaci.*

C. su′is a species that is associated with conjunctivitis, enteritis, and pneumonia in pigs.

C. tracho′matis a species that causes trachoma, inclusion conjunctivitis, nonspecific urethritis, proctitis, mouse pneumonitis, lymphogranuloma venereum, and *Chlamydia trachomatis* pneumonia.

chla•myd•ia (klə-mid′e-ə) pl. *chlamyd′iae.* Any member of the phylum Chlamydiae.

Chla•myd•i•a•ceae (klə-mid″e-a′se-e) a family of bacteria of the order Chlamydiales, consisting of small coccoid microorganisms that are incapable of synthesizing ATP and multiply only within the cytoplasm of host cells by a unique developmental cycle (see *Chlamydiales*). Many are parasites of vertebrates and cause diseases. They have also been found in arthropods. The family contains the genera *Chlamydia* and *Chlamydophila.*

Chla•my•diae (klə-mid′e-e) 1. a phylum of gram-positive or gram-variable, nonmotile, obligately parasitic bacteria that multiply by means of a complex life cycle within cytoplasmic vacuoles of mammalian and avian host cells. It contains the single class Chlamydiae. 2. the sole class of this phylum, containing the single order Chlamydiales.

chla•myd•i•ae (klə-mid′e-e) plural of *chlamydia.*

chla•myd•i•al (klə-mid′e-əl) pertaining to or caused by organisms of the phylum Chlamydiae.

Chla•my•di•a•les (klə-mid′e-a″lēz) an order of bacteria of the class Chlamydiae, phylum Chlamydiae, consisting of coccoid, gram-negative, parasitic microorganisms that have a unique, obligately intracellular developmental cycle and are incapable of synthesizing ATP. Infection occurs when the small, rigid-walled extracellular form (elementary body) enters the cell and changes into a larger, thin-walled form (reticulate body) that divides by fission. The daughter cells thus formed reorganize and condense to become elementary bodies that are released and infect other cells. The organisms can produce disease in vertebrates and arthropods. Species of medical interest are in the families Chlamydiaceae, Parachlamydiaceae, and Simkaniaceae.

chla•myd•i•o•sis (klə-mid″e-o′sis) 1. any infection or disease caused by chlamydiae. 2. psittacosis (def. 1).

avian c. infection of birds by *Chlamydophila psittaci;* see *ornithosis* and *psittacosis.*

chlam•y•do•co•nid•i•um (klam″ĭ-do-kə-nid′e-əm) [Gr. *chlamys* cloak + *conidium*] a thick-walled intercalary or terminal asexual spore formed by the rounding up of a cell; it is not shed. See also *conidium.* Called also *chlamydospore.*

Chla•my•do•phi•la (klam″ĭ-dof′ĭ-lə) [Gr. *chlamys,* gen. *chlamydos* cloak + *phila* dear] a genus of bacteria of the family Chlamydiaceae, consisting of gram-negative, non–glycogen-producing coccoid organisms that multiply only within a host cell and have a unique growth cycle (see *Chlamydiales*). Organisms are pathogenic for numerous different animals, including humans. Several species formerly classified in the genus *Chlamydia* have been reclassified into this genus. The type species is *C. psit′taci.*

C. abor′tus a species that is enzootic in ruminants and can cause abortion.

C. fe′lis a species that causes rhinitis and conjunctivitis in cats.

C. peco′rum a species that infects mammals, including ruminants and swine, in which it causes abortion, conjunctivitis, encephalomyelitis, enteritis, pneumonia, and polyarthritis.

C. pneumo′niae a species, containing several biovars, that is primarily a respiratory pathogen and an important cause of pneumonia, bronchitis, and sinusitis. Formerly called *Chlamydia pneumoniae.* See also *Chlamydophila pneumoniae pneumonia,* under *pneumonia.*

C. psit′taci a species, various strains of which cause psittacosis in humans and birds and a variety of diseases in farm animals and other mammals. Formerly called *Chlamydia psittaci.*

chlam•y•do•spore (klam′ĭ-do-spor″) [Gr. *chlamys* cloak + *spore*] chlamydoconidium.

chlo•as•ma (klo-az′mə) [Gr. *chloazein* to be green] melasma.

chlor•a•ce•tic ac•id (klor″ə-se′tik) chloroacetic acid.

chlor•ac•ne (klor-ak′ne) acne caused by exposure to chlorine compounds; called also *chlorine acne.*

chlo•ral (klor′əl) [*chlor*ine + *-al*[3]] 1. a colorless, oily liquid with a pungent, irritating odor; used in the manufacture of chloral hydrate and DDT. 2. c. hydrate.

c. hydrate [USP] a hypnotic and sedative, now used predominantly as a preoperative adjunct to anesthesia and as a sedative for children undergoing medical and dental procedures; administered orally or rectally.

chlo•ra•lose (klor′ə-lōs) a compound of chloral and glucose, used as a rodenticide for mice and a bird repellent on grain. Called also *α-chloralose.*

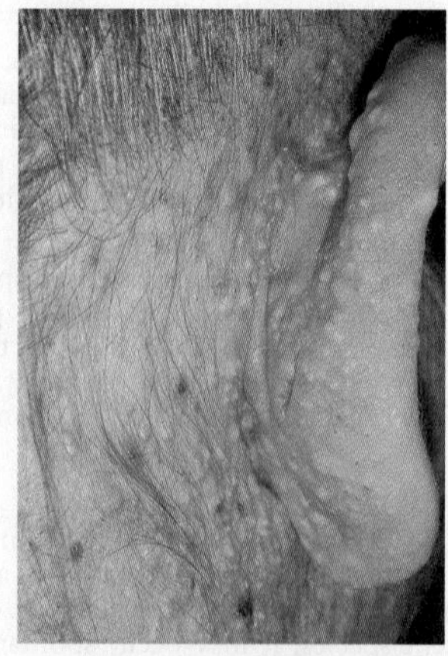

■ Chloracne. Typical heavy involvement of retroauricular skin, with comedones and cysts.

chlor·am·bu·cil (klor-am′bu-sil) [USP] an alkylating agent of the nitrogen mustard group, which acts both by cross-linking of DNA and RNA and by inhibiting of protein synthesis, used as an antineoplastic in the treatment of chronic lymphocytic leukemia, Hodgkin and non-Hodgkin lymphomas, Waldenström macroglobulinemia, and multiple myeloma; administered orally. It has also been used as an immunosuppressive in the treatment of steroid-resistant nephrotic syndrome.

chlo·ra·mine-T (klor′ə-mēn) a chlorine derivative used in solution as a topical antiseptic to irrigate and dress wounds, as a mouthwash, and for sterilization of drinking water.

chlor·am·phen·i·col (klor″əm-fen′ĭ-kol) [USP] a broad-spectrum antibiotic, originally derived from *Streptomyces venezuelae* and later shown to be elaborated by other spirochetes, and produced synthetically. It is effective against rickettsiae, gram-positive and gram-negative bacteria, and certain spirochetes, being used especially in the treatment of typhus and other rickettsial infections and in typhoid, shigellosis, and related enteric diseases; used as an antibacterial, administered orally or applied topically to the conjunctiva or ear, or as an antirickettsial, administered orally.
c. palmitate [USP] the monopalmitic ester of chloramphenicol, having the same actions and uses as the base; administered orally.
c. sodium succinate [USP] the sodium succinate derivative of chloramphenicol, having the same actions and uses as the base; administered intravenously.

chlo·rate (klor′āt) any salt of chloric acid.

chlor·bu·tol (klor-bu′tol) chlorobutanol.

chlor·dane (klor′dān) a toxic chlorinated hydrocarbon insecticide; poisoning may occur by percutaneous absorption, ingestion, or inhalation and consists of neurotoxic symptoms such as muscular spasms and seizures that can be fatal.

chlor·de·cone (klor′də-kōn) a polychlorinated ketone used as an insecticide; workers exposed to this nonbiodegradable compound have suffered neurologic symptoms, such as tremors and slurred speech.

chlor·di·az·ep·ox·ide (klor″di-az″ə-pok′sīd) [USP] a benzodiazepine used as an antianxiety agent in the treatment of anxiety disorders and for the short-term relief of anxiety symptoms, for the relief of acute alcohol withdrawal symptoms, and as an antitremor agent; administered orally.
c. hydrochloride [USP] the monohydrochloride salt of chlordiazepoxide, administered orally for the same indications as the base and intravenously or intramuscularly as an antianxiety agent in the treatment of anxiety and panic disorders, the short-term relief of anxiety symptoms and of preoperative anxiety, and the treatment of acute alcohol withdrawal symptoms.

Chlo·rel·la (klo-rel′ə) a genus of fresh-water green algae, easily cultured and often used in studies of photosynthesis.

chlor·emia (klor-e′me-ə) [*chlor-* + *-emia*] hyperchloremia.

Chlo·re·si·um (klo-re′ze-um) trademark for a preparation of chlorophyllin copper complex sodium.

chlor·gua·nide (klor-gwahn′īd) proguanil; see *proguanil hydrochloride.*

chlor·hex·i·dine (klor-heks′ĭ-dēn) an antibacterial, effective against a wide variety of gram-negative and gram-positive organisms.
c. acetate the diacetate salt of chlorhexidine, having the same actions as the base; used mainly as a preservative for eye drops.
c. gluconate [USP] the digluconate salt of chlorhexidine, used as a topical antiinfective for the skin and mucous membranes.
c. hydrochloride the dihydrochloride salt of chlorhexidine, having the same actions as the base; used as a topical antiinfective for the skin and mucous membranes.

chlor·hy·dria (klor-hi′dre-ə) hyperchlorhydria.

chlo·ric (klor′ik) [L. *chloricus*] derived from or containing pentavalent chlorine; a term used to distinguish those compounds which contain a smaller proportion of chlorine than the chlorous compounds, and forming salts known as chlorates.

chlo·ric ac·id (klor′ik) a strong oxidizing agent, $HClO_3 \cdot 7H_2O$, occurring only in aqueous solution; it is used as a catalyst and is strongly irritating to the skin and mucous membranes.

chlo·ride (klor′īd) a salt of hydrochloric acid; any binary compound of chlorine in which the latter is the negative element. For specific salts, see entries under the adjectival form, e.g., for *sodium chloride,* see under *sodium.*
acid c. a substance formed by substituting chlorine for hydroxyl in an acid molecule.

chlo·ri·dim·e·ter (klor″ĭ-dim′ə-tər) [*chloride* + *-meter*] an instrument for measuring the chloride content of the urine or other fluid.

chlo·ri·dim·e·try (klor″ĭ-dim′ə-tre) the determination of the chloride content of fluids.

chlo·rid·i·on (klor″id-i′on) negatively ionic chlorine, the anion of hydrochloric acid and the chlorides.

chlo·ri·dom·e·ter (klor″ĭ-dom′ə-tər) chloridimeter.

chlo·rid·or·rhea (klor″ĭ-də-re′ə) diarrhea with an excess of chlorides in the feces.
congenital c., familial c. congenital chloride diarrhea.

chlo·ri·du·ria (klor″ĭ-du′re-ə) chloruria.

chlo·ri·nat·ed (klor′ĭ-nāt″əd) treated or charged with chlorine.

chlo·rine (Cl) (klor′ēn) [Gr. *chlōros* green] a yellowish green, gaseous element, of suffocating odor; atomic number 17, atomic weight 35.453, specific gravity 1.56. It is a disinfectant, decolorant, and irritant poison. It is used for disinfecting, fumigating, and bleaching, either in an aqueous solution or in the form of chlorinated lime.
c. dioxide an oxidizing and germicidal agent, ClO_2, used in the purification of water and for bleaching.

chlor·io·dized (klor-i′o-dīzd) containing chlorine and iodine.

chlo·rite (klor′īt) any salt of chlorous acid.

chlor(o)- [Gr. *chlōros* green] a combining form meaning green, or denoting the presence of chlorine.

chlo·ro·ac·et·al·de·hyde (klor″o-as″et-al′də-hīd) a mutagenic metabolite produced by biotransformation of vinyl chloride in the liver.

chlo·ro·ace·tic ac·id (klor″o-ə-se′tik) a strong acid, $CH_2ClCOOH$, used as a laboratory reagent.

chlo·ro·ac·e·to·phe·none (CN) (klo″ro-as″ə-to-fe′nōn) a commonly used tear gas.

o-chlo·ro·ben·zyl·i·dene·mal·o·no·ni·trile (CS) (klo″ro-ben-zil″ĭ-dēn-mal″ə-no-ni′trīl) a commonly used tear gas.

chlo·ro·bu·ta·nol (klor″o-bu′tə-nol) [NF] colorless to white crystals with a camphoraceous odor and taste; used as an antimicrobial preservative in pharmaceutical solutions, especially injectables. Called also *chlorbutol.*

2-chlo·ro·de·oxy·aden·o·sine (klor″o-de-ok″se-ə-den′o-sēn) cladribine.

chlo·ro·eth·ane (klor″o-eth′ān) ethyl chloride.

chlo·ro·eth·y·lene (klor″o-eth′ə-lēn) vinyl chloride.
c. oxide a toxic metabolite produced by biotransformation of vinyl chloride in the liver.

chlo·ro·flu·o·ro·car·bon (CFC) (klo″ro-floo′o-ro-kahr″bən) any of a group of hydrocarbons in which some or all of the hydrogen atoms are replaced by chlorine or fluorine; some in this group were formerly widely used in aerosols, but their use is declining because of their destructive effect on stratospheric ozone.

chlo·ro·form (klor′ə-form) trichloromethane, $CHCl_3$, a colorless, volatile liquid with a strong ethereal odor and a sweetish, burning taste, a common laboratory solvent; it is hepatotoxic and nephrotoxic when ingested. It was once widely used as an inhalation anesthetic and analgesic, and as an antitussive, carminative, and counterirritant.
acetone c. chlorobutanol.

chlo·ro·gen·ic ac·id (klo′ro-jen″ik) a phenol compound important in plant metabolism, found in coffee beans and numerous other fruits and vegetables; it acts as an antioxidant and slows release of glucose into the bloodstream after a meal.

chlo·ro·gua·nide hy·dro·chlo·ride (klor″o-gwahn′īd) proguanil hydrochloride.

chlo·ro·hy·dro·car·bon (klor″o-hi″dro-kahr′bon) chlorinated hydrocarbon.

chlo·ro·leu·ke·mia (klor″o-loo-ke′me-ə) chloroma.

chlo·ro·ma (klor-o′mə) [*chlor-* + *-oma*] a malignant green-colored tumor arising from myeloid tissue, associated with myelogenous leukemia and occurring anywhere in the body. Besides containing green pigment, which has no clear metabolic role and is principally myeloperoxidase, chloroma tissue demonstrates a bright red fluorescence under ultraviolet light. Cf. *myeloblastoma.* Called also *chloroleukemia, chloromatous sarcoma,* and *granulocytic sarcoma.*

Chlo·ro·mag (klor′o-mag) trademark for a preparation of magnesium chloride.

p-chlo·ro·mer·cu·ri·ben·zo·ate (klor″o-mur″ku-re-ben′zo-āt) a univalent organic mercury compound that reacts with sulfhydryl groups on proteins, or other molecules, thereby often inhibiting their activities.

chlo·rom·e·try (klor-om′ə-tre) the quantitative determination of chlorine.

Chlo·ro·my·ce·tin (klor″o-mi-se′tin) trademark for preparations of chloramphenicol.

chlo·ro·naph·tha·lene (klor-o-naf′thə-lēn) chlorinated naphthalene.

chlo·ro·nych·ia (klor-o-nik′e-ə) green nail syndrome.

chlo·ro·phane (klor′o-fān) [*chloro-* + Gr. *phainein* to show] a greenish yellow pigment obtainable from the retina.

***p*-chlo•ro•phe•nol** (klor″o-fe′nol) parachlorophenol.

chlo•ro•phyll (klor′o-fil) [*chloro-* + Gr. *phyllon* leaf] any of a group of green magnesium-containing porphyrin derivatives occurring in all photosynthetic organisms. Chlorophylls act as respiratory pigments, converting light energy to reducing potential; the reduction of CO_2 is the first step in the synthesis of hexoses in photosynthetic organisms. Chlorophyll *a* occurs in all organisms exhibiting aerobic photosynthesis (green plants, algae, and cyanobacteria), chlorophyll *b* in higher plants, chlorophylls c_1 and c_2 in diatoms and brown algae, and chlorophyll *d* in red algae. Bacteriochlorophylls occur in bacteria exhibiting anaerobic photosynthesis. Preparations of water-soluble chlorophyll salts are used as deodorizers; see *chlorophyllin.*

chlo•ro•phyl•lin (klor′o-fil-in) any of the water-soluble salts obtained by alkaline hydrolysis of chlorophyll with replacement of the methyl and phytyl ester groups by sodium or potassium; preparations of the salts are applied topically for the deodorization of skin lesions and administered orally to deodorize ulcerative skin lesions and the urine and feces in colostomy, ileostomy, and incontinence.

c. copper complex a chlorophyllin in which copper has replaced the porphyrin magnesium; it is the most widely used form of chlorophyllin.

Chlo•ro•phyl•lum (klo-rof′ĭ-ləm) a genus of mushrooms of the family Agaricaceae. *C. molyb′dites* is similar in appearance to species of *Amanita* and contains small amounts of amatoxins, so that it occasionally causes mushroom poisoning (see under *poisoning*).

chlo•ro•pia (klor-ōp′e-ə) chloropsia.

Chlo•rop•i•dae (klor-op′ĭ-de) a family of small to minute flies (order Diptera); two medically important genera are *Hippelates* and *Siphunculina.*

chlo•ro•plast (klor′o-plast) [*chloro-* + *-plast*] any one of the chlorophyll-bearing bodies of plant cells.

chlo•ro•prene (klor′o-prēn) an organic compound used in the synthesis of neoprene rubber; it is toxic by inhalation, ingestion, and skin absorption, causes lung and liver cancer, and also affects the reproductive system.

chlo•ro•priv•ic (klor″o-priv′ik) [*chlorine* + L. *privare* to deprive] hypochloremic.

chlo•ro•pro•caine hy•dro•chlo•ride (klor″o-pro′kān) [USP] a local anesthetic used in minor and general surgery for infiltration anesthesia, field block, Bier block, regional nerve block, and caudal and lumbar epidural anesthesia; used also for infiltration and nerve block in dental procedures.

chlo•ro•pro•py•lene ox•ide (klo″ro-pro′pə-lēn) epichlorohydrin.

chlo•rop•sia (klor-op′se-ə) [*chloro-* + *-opsia*] a chromatopsia in which all objects seen appear to have a greenish tinge, a symptom of digitalis poisoning.

Chlor•op•tic (klor-op′tik) trademark for preparations of chloramphenicol.

chlo•ro•quine (klor′o-kwin) [USP] a 4-aminoquinoline compound with antiinflammatory and antiprotozoal properties, used for the suppression and treatment of malaria, for the treatment of giardiasis and extraintestinal amebiasis, for suppression of lupus erythematosus, and as an antiinflammatory in the treatment of rheumatoid arthritis; administered orally.

c. hydrochloride the dihydrochloride salt of chloroquine, used for suppression and treatment of malaria and as a second-line agent for treatment of extraintestinal amebiasis; administered intramuscularly.

c. phosphate [USP] the phosphate salt of chloroquine, used for suppression and treatment of malaria, for treatment of extraintestinal amebiasis, and as a lupus erythematosus suppressant; administered orally.

Chlo•ro•stig•ma (klor″o-stig′mə) a genus of plants of the family Asclepiadaceae. *C. stuckertia′num* is the source of the alkaloid chlorostigmine.

chlo•ro•stig•mine (klor″o-stig′mēn) an alkaloid from plants of the genus *Chlorostigma*, especially *C. stuckertia′num*, which has been used to stimulate secretion of milk in nursing mothers.

chlo•ro•thi•a•zide (klor″o-thi′ə-zīd) [USP] a thiazide diuretic, used for treatment of hypertension and edema; administered orally.

c. sodium [USP] the monosodium salt of chlorothiazide, having the same actions and uses as the base; administered intravenously.

chlo•rous (klor′əs) derived from or containing trivalent chlorine, as in chlorous acid, $HClO_2$; a term used to distinguish those compounds which contain a larger proportion of chlorine than the chloric compounds, and forming salts known as chlorites.

chlo•rous ac•id (klor′əs) a weak inorganic acid, $HClO_2$.

chlo•ro•vi•nyl•di•chlo•ro•ar•sine (klor″o-vīn″əl-di-klor″o-ahr′sin) lewisite.

chlo•rox•ine (klor-ok′sēn) a synthetic antibacterial, used in the topical treatment of dandruff and seborrheic dermatitis of the scalp.

chlo•ro•xy•le•nol (klor″o-zi′lə-nol) an antibacterial active chiefly against streptococci; used mainly as a skin disinfectant.

chlor•phen•ir•amine (klor″fən-ir′ə-mēn) an antihistamine (H_1 receptor antagonist) derived from pheniramine and having sedative and anticholinergic effects.

c. maleate [USP] the maleate salt of chlorpheniramine, used in the treatment of allergic rhinitis, allergic conjunctivitis, and cutaneous manifestations of allergic reactions, and as an ingredient in some cough and cold preparations; administered orally or by intramuscular, intravenous, or subcutaneous injection.

c. polistirex sulfonated styrene-divinylbenzene copolymer complex with chlorpheniramine, having the same actions as the base; used in cough and cold preparations, administered orally.

c. tannate the tannate salt of chlorpheniramine, having the same actions as the base; used in cough and cold preparations, administered orally.

chlor•pro•ma•zine (klor-pro′mə-zēn) [USP] a phenothiazine derivative, used as an antiemetic and tranquilizer, and for the management of severe behavior disorders in children; administered rectally.

c. hydrochloride [USP] the hydrochloride salt of chlorpromazine, used as an antipsychotic and antiemetic, to control presurgical apprehension, to control the manic phase of bipolar disorder, to treat intractable hiccups, acute intermittent porphyria, and tetanus, and for the management of severe behavior disorders in children.

chlor•pro•pa•mide (klor-pro′pə-mīd) [USP] a sulfonylurea compound used as a hypoglycemic in the treatment of type 2 diabetes mellitus; administered orally.

chlor•py•ri•fos (klor-pi′rĭ-fos) an organophosphorus insecticide used to disinfect plants; accidental overexposure can cause extrapyramidal effects such as salivation, tremors, dizziness, and eventually seizures, coma, and death.

chlor•tet•ra•cy•cline (klor″tet-rə-si′klēn) a broad-spectrum antibiotic, elaborated by *Streptomyces aureofaciens;* it was the first of the tetracycline group to be discovered.

c. hydrochloride [USP] the monohydrochloride salt of chlortetracycline, a broad-spectrum antibiotic used as an antibacterial and antiprotozoal; administered orally or intravenously, or applied topically to the skin or conjunctiva.

chlor•thal•i•done (klor-thal′ĭ-dōn) [USP] a sulfonamide derivative that has a different chemical structure from but the same actions as the thiazide diuretics, used in the treatment of hypertension and edema; administered orally.

Chlor-Tri•me•ton (klor-tri′mə-ton) trademark for preparations of chlorpheniramine maleate.

chlor•ure•sis (klor″u-re′sis) [*chlor-* + *-uresis*] excretion of excessive chlorides in the urine; called also *chloriduria* and *hyperchloriduria.*

chlor•uret•ic (klor″u-ret′ik) 1. promoting chloruresis. 2. an agent that promotes the excretion of chlorides in the urine.

chlor•uria (klor-u′re-ə) [*chlor-* + *-uria*] excess of chlorides in the urine.

chlor•zox•a•zone (klor-zok′sə-zōn) a skeletal muscle relaxant, used to relieve discomfort of painful musculoskeletal disorders, administered orally.

ChM [L.] Chirur′giae Magis′ter (Master of Surgery).

CHO Chinese hamster ovary; see under *cell.*

cho•a•na (ko′ə-nə) pl. *cho′anae* [L., from Gr. *choanē* funnel] 1. infundibulum. 2. [TA] one of the pair of openings between the nasal cavity and the nasopharynx; called also *posterior nasal aperture.*

primary c. the opening of the embryonic olfactory sac into the mouth.

secondary c. the definitive choana after the formation of the palate.

cho•a•nae (ko′ə-ne) [L.] genitive and plural of *choana.*

cho•a•nal (ko′ə-nəl) infundibular.

choan(o)- [L., Gr. *choanē* funnel] a combining form denoting a relationship to a funnel or to a funnellike structure.

cho•a•noid (ko′ə-noid) [*choan-* + *-oid*] infundibular (def. 2).

cho•a•no•mas•ti•gote (ko″ə-no-mas′tĭ-gōt) [*choano-* + Gr. *mastix* whip] a morphologic stage in the life cycle of some trypanosomatid protozoa; the kinetoplast and basal body are anterior to the nucleus and the flagellum emerges through a collarlike extension at the anterior end of the cell. Cf. *amastigote*, *epimastigote*, *opisthomastigote*, *promastigote*, and *trypomastigote.*

Cho•a•no•tae•nia (ko-a″no-te′ne-ə) [Gr. *choanē* funnel + *taenia* (def. 2)] a genus of tapeworms. *C. infundi′bulum* is a common but nonpathogenic parasite of chickens and turkeys.

choc•o•late (chok′ə-lət) [Nahuatl *xocolatl*] 1. [NF] in pharmacy, a powder prepared from roasted, cured ripe seeds of *Theobroma cacao*, which contains caffeine and theobromine; used as a flavor in pharmaceutical preparations (see also *chocolate syrup*, under *syrup*). 2. a confection made from the fermented, roasted, shelled, ground seeds of *T. cacao*; although widely consumed by humans, its theobromine content can poison dogs eating excessive amounts, leading to vomiting, diarrhea, muscle spasms, and coma.

choke (chōk) 1. to interrupt respiration by obstruction or compression. Called also *strangle.* 2. the condition resulting from interruption of respiration. Called also *strangulation.*

water c. laryngeal spasm caused by fluid entering the larynx and especially by getting between the true and false vocal cords.

chokes (chōks) a burning sensation experienced during decompression, beginning in the substernal region, with increasing uncontrollable urge to cough and a feeling of great apprehension, leading to vasovagal attack.

chol•a•gog•ic (ko″lə-goj′ik) stimulating the flow of bile to the duodenum.

chol•a•gogue (ko′lə-gog) [*chol-* + *-agogue*] an agent that stimulates the flow of bile into the duodenum.

cho•la•ic ac•id (ko-la′ik) cholyltaurine.

Cho•lan-DH (ko′lən) trademark for preparations of dehydrocholic acid.

cho•la•ner•e•sis (ko″lə-ner′ə-sis) increased output of bile acids or bile salts.

cho•lan•ge•itis (ko-lan″je-i′tis) cholangitis.

cho•lan•gi•ec•ta•sis (ko-lan″je-ek′tə-sis) dilatation of a bile duct.

cholangi(o)- [*chol-* + *angi(o)-*] a combining form denoting relationship to a bile duct.

cho•lan•gio•ad•e•no•ma (ko-lan″je-o-ad″ə-no′mə) bile duct adenoma.

cho•lan•gio•car•ci•no•ma (ko-lan″je-o-kahr″sĭ-no′mə) 1. an adenocarcinoma arising from the epithelium of the bile ducts, composed of eosinophilic cuboidal or columnar epithelial cells arranged in tubules or acini with abundant fibrous stroma; mucus may be secreted but not bile. 2. cholangiocellular carcinoma.

distal c. extrahepatic cholangiocarcinoma in the part of the bile ducts within the pancreas.

extrahepatic c. any cholangiocarcinoma arising in lower parts of the biliary tree.

hilar c. cholangiocarcinoma arising from the major intrahepatic bile ducts adjacent to the hilum; because it is near the hepatic portal vein, it may obstruct the vein as it grows. Called also *Klatskin tumor* and *perihilar c.*

intrahepatic c. 1. a rare type of cholangiocarcinoma that arises from small bile ducts within the liver; called also *peripheral c.* 2. any cholangiocarcinoma arising within the liver.

perihilar c. hilar c.

peripheral c. intrahepatic c.

cho•lan•gio•cel•lu•lar (ko-lan″je-o-sel′u-lər) of, resembling, or pertaining to cells of the cholangioles.

cho•lan•gio•cho•le•cys•to•cho•le•do•chec•to•my (ko-lan″je-o-ko″lə-sis″to-ko″lə-do-kek′tə-me) surgical removal of the hepatic duct, common bile duct, and gallbladder.

cho•lan•gio•cyte (ko-lan′je-o-sīt) [*cholangio-* + *-cyte*] one of the epithelial cells lining the bile ducts; those lining the intrahepatic ducts regulate salt and water secretion during bile formation.

cho•lan•gio•drain•age (kə-lan″je-o-drān′əj) [*cholangio-* + *drainage*] drainage of the bile ducts.

percutaneous transhepatic c. percutaneous transhepatic biliary drainage.

cho•lan•gio•en•ter•os•to•my (ko-lan″je-o-en″tər-os′tə-me) [*cholangio-* + *enterostomy*] surgical anastomosis of a bile duct to the intestine.

cho•lan•gio•gas•tros•to•my (ko-lan″je-o-gas-tros′tə-me) [*cholangio-* + *gastrostomy*] surgical anastomosis of a bile duct to the stomach.

cho•lan•gio•gram (ko-lan′je-o-gram″) a radiograph of the gallbladder and bile ducts.

cho•lan•gi•og•ra•phy (ko-lan″je-og′rə-fe) [*cholangio-* + *-graphy*] radiography of the biliary ducts after administration or injection of a contrast medium, orally, intravenously, or percutaneously.

fine needle transhepatic c. (FNTC) transhepatic cholangiography performed by means of a very fine, highly flexible steel needle (fine needle).

operative c. cholangiography performed during a surgical procedure on the gallbladder.

percutaneous transhepatic c. cholangiography after introduction of a radiopaque medium into the biliary system by percutaneous puncture of a bile duct. See also *endoscopic retrograde cholangiopancreatography*, under *cholangiopancreatography.*

retrograde c. cholangiography using retrograde injection of contrast medium into the bile ducts via a tube through the ampulla of Vater. See also *endoscopic retrograde cholangiopancreatography*, under *cholangiopancreatography.*

transhepatic c. percutaneous transhepatic c.

transjugular c. cholangiography after catheterization of a hepatic vein via the internal jugular vein in the neck and entry into a bile duct by percutaneous puncture across the wall of the hepatic vein.

cho•lan•gio•hep•a•ti•tis (ko-lan″je-o-hep″ə-ti′tis) severe inflammation of the bile passages in humans, ruminants, or horses, often associated with liver fluke infestation that causes obstruction of the bile ducts.

Oriental c. recurrent pyogenic cholangitis.

cho•lan•gio•hep•a•to•ma (ko-lan″je-o-hep″ə-to′mə) hepatocellular carcinoma of mixed liver cell and bile-duct cell origin; called also *hepatocholangiocarcinoma.*

cho•lan•gio•je•ju•nos•to•my (ko-lan″je-o-jə-joo-nos′tə-me) [*cholangio-* + *jejunostomy*] surgical anastomosis of a bile duct to the jejunum.

intrahepatic c. portoenterostomy.

cho•lan•gi•ole (ko-lan′je-ōl) [*cholangio-* + *-ole* diminutive suffix] one of the fine terminal elements of the bile duct system, leaving the portal canal, and pursuing a course at the periphery of a lobule of the liver; called also *bile* or *biliary ductule.* **cholangi′olar** *adj*

cho•lan•gi•o•li•tis (ko-lan″je-o-li′tis) inflammation of the cholangioles.

cho•lan•gi•o•ma (ko-lan″je-o′mə) [*cholangi-* + *-oma*] cholangiocellular carcinoma.

cho•lan•gio•pan•cre•a•tog•ra•phy (ko-lan″je-o-pan″kre-ə-tog′rə-fe) radiographic examination of the bile ducts and pancreas after administration of contrast medium.

endoscopic retrograde c. (ERCP) a combination of retrograde and transhepatic cholangiography, done to demonstrate all portions of the biliary tree; it is performed by cannulation of the common bile duct and pancreatic duct through the papilla of Vater using a flexible fiberoptic endoscope with retrograde injection of a radiopaque medium.

chol•an•gi•op•a•thy (ko-lan″je-op′ə-the) any disease of the bile ducts; see also *cholangitis.*

AIDS c. bile duct disease seen complicating the acquired immunodeficiency syndrome. The most common effect is primary sclerosing cholangitis; some patients also have sphincter of Oddi dysfunction (see under *dysfunction*).

autoimmune c. see under *cholangitis.*

cho•lan•gi•os•to•my (ko-lan″je-os′tə-me) [*cholangio-* + *-stomy*] surgical creation of an opening into a bile duct.

cho•lan•gi•ot•o•my (ko-lan″je-ot′ə-me) [*cholangio-* + *-tomy*] incision into a bile duct.

cho•lan•gi•tis (ko″lan-ji′tis) [*cholangi-* + *-itis*] inflammation of a bile duct or bile ducts.

autoimmune c. an autoimmune bile duct condition that may be a manifestation of autoimmune hepatitis; it closely resembles primary biliary cirrhosis, except that patients lack the antimitochondrial antibodies typical of that condition.

bacterial c. the most common type of cholangitis, caused by bacterial infection; if bacteria invade the liver they can enter the bloodstream and cause septicemia that can be fatal.

chronic nonsuppurative destructive c. primary biliary cirrhosis.

eosinophilic c. cholangitis occurring secondary to eosinophilic infiltration and characterized by multiple strictures in the bile ducts; the cause is unknown.

fibrous obliterative c. a condition sometimes seen in early stages of primary sclerosing cholangitis, consisting of fibrosis with obliteration of small bile ducts.

c. len′ta chronic infectious cholangitis without gallstones or biliary tract obstruction.

Oriental c. recurrent pyogenic c.

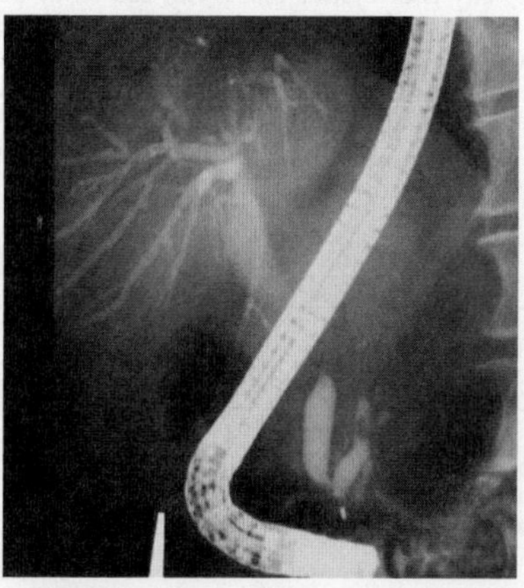

■ Endoscopic retrograde cholangiopancreatography radiograph demonstrating the biliary tree.

primary sclerosing c. a progressive chronic fibrosing inflammation of the bile ducts of unknown cause, occurring most commonly in young men and frequently in association with chronic ulcerative colitis; it also occurs as a complication of HIV infection.

progressive nonsuppurative c. primary biliary cirrhosis.

recurrent pyogenic c. recurrent attacks of cholangitis with brown pigment gallstones in the common bile duct (choledocholithiasis), ductal stenosis, fever, and jaundice; the highest instances are in eastern and southern Asia, and it is sometimes associated with dietary deficiencies (high carbohydrate, low protein diet) or parasite infections such as with *Ascaris* or *Clonorchis.* Called also *Oriental c.* and *Oriental cholangiohepatitis.*

sclerosing c. primary sclerosing c.

cho•lan•ic ac•id (ko-lan′ik) a steroidal acid, 5β-cholan-24-oic acid, which can be considered the parent compound of the bile acids.

cho•lano•poi•e•sis (ko″lə-no-poi-e′sis) the synthesis of bile acids or bile salts by the liver.

cho•lano•poi•et•ic (ko″lə-no-poi-et′ik) 1. pertaining to or promoting cholanopoiesis. 2. an agent that promotes cholanopoiesis.

cho•lan•threne (ko-lan′thrēn) a carcinogenic pentacyclic hydrocarbon; see also *3-methylcholanthrene.*

cho•late (ko′lāt) a salt, anion, or ester of cholic acid.

chole- a combining form denoting relationship to bile. Also, *chol(o)-.*

cho•le•cal•ci•fer•ol (ko″lə-kal-sif′ər-ol) 1. a hormone synthesized in the skin on irradiation of 7-dehydrocholesterol or obtained as a vitamin from dietary sources; it is activated when metabolized to 1,25-dihydroxycholecalciferol. See table. See also *ergocalciferol.* Called also *vitamin D_3.* 2. [USP] a preparation of this compound, derived from animal tissues and used in the prophylaxis and treatment of vitamin D deficiencies due to low intake, high requirement, or impaired absorption of the vitamin. It is also used in the treatment of hypocalcemic tetany and hypoparathyroidism.

cho•le•chro•mo•poi•e•sis (ko″lə-kro″mo-poi-e′sis) the synthesis of bile pigments.

cho•le•cyst (ko′lə-sist) vesica biliaris.

cho•le•cyst•a•gog•ic (ko″lə-sis″tə-goj′ik) cholecystokinetic.

cho•le•cyst•a•gogue (ko″lə-sis′tə-gog) a cholecystokinetic agent.

cho•le•cys•tal•gia (ko″lə-sis-tal′jə) [*cholecyst-* + *-algia*] 1. biliary colic. 2. pain due to inflammation of the gallbladder.

cho•le•cys•tat•o•ny (ko″lə-sis-tat′ə-ne) atony of the gallbladder.

cho•le•cys•tec•ta•sia (ko″lə-sis″tek-ta′zhə) [*cholecyst-* + *ectasia*] distention of the gallbladder.

cho•le•cys•tec•to•my (ko″lə-sis-tek′tə-me) [*cholecyst-* + *-ectomy*] surgical removal of the gallbladder.

cho•le•cys•ten•ter•ic (ko″lə-sis″ten-ter′ik) [*cholecyst-* + *enteric*] pertaining to communication between the gallbladder and intestine; called also *cholecystointestinal.*

cho•le•cyst•en•ter•or•rha•phy (ko″lə-sis-ten″tər-or′ə-fe) suture of the gallbladder to the small intestine.

cho•le•cyst•en•ter•os•to•my (ko″lə-sis″ten-tər-os′tə-me) cholecystoenterostomy.

cho•le•cys•tic (ko″lə-sis′tik) pertaining to the gallbladder.

cho•le•cys•tis (ko″lə-sis′tis) vesica biliaris.

cho•le•cys•ti•tis (ko″lə-sis-ti′tis) [*cholecyst-* + *-itis*] inflammation of the gallbladder; see *calculous c.* and *acalculous c.* Some types are named for other characteristics and may be either calculous or acalculous.

acalculous c. any cholecystitis that is not caused by gallstones. These types constitute not more than 10 per cent of cases but usually have a much more grave prognosis than calculous cholecystitis because there may be serious complications such as gangrene and perforation. Acalculous types are usually secondary to bile duct obstruction and biliary stasis, and many of the patients are already severely ill or injured from some other condition, such as a severe burn, sepsis, or other trauma.

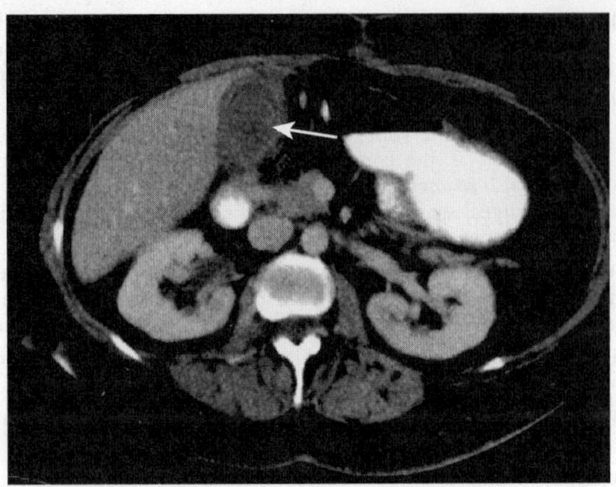

■ CT scan showing acute calculous cholecystitis with gallbladder wall thickening, pericholecystic fluid, and stones *(arrow)* in a 47-year-old woman.

acute c. a type of cholecystitis usually due to obstruction of the gallbladder outlet, with signs ranging from mild edema and congestion to severe infection with gangrene and perforation.

calculous c. cholecystitis accompanied by gallstones; most cases are of this type.

chronic c. cholecystitis with relatively mild symptoms persisting over a long period.

c. emphysemato′sa, emphysematous c. cholecystitis caused by gas-producing organisms, characterized by gas in the gallbladder lumen that frequently infiltrates into the wall of the gallbladder and surrounding tissues; it may be either calculous or acalculous. Called also *gaseous c.*

follicular c. cholecystitis in which there is conspicuous formation of lymphoid follicles that often contain germinal centers. It may be either calculous or acalculous.

gaseous c. emphysematous c.

c. glandula′ris proli′ferans a thickening of the wall of the chronically inflamed gallbladder, with formation of crypts which may develop into cysts.

hemorrhagic c. cholecystitis with hemorrhage into the gallbladder; it is usually acalculous, but sometimes there are gallstones. Called also *hemocholecystitis.*

xanthogranulomatous c. a type of chronic cholecystitis characterized by proliferative fibrosis and infiltration by lipid-laden macrophages; it is often accompanied by obstruction from gallstones.

cholecyst(o)- a combining form denoting relationship to the gallbladder.

cho•le•cys•to•cho•lan•gio•gram (ko″lə-sis″to-ko-lan′je-o-gram) radiograph of the gallbladder and bile ducts.

cho•le•cys•to•co•lon•ic (ko″lə-sis″to-ko-lon′ik) communicating between the gallbladder and colon.

cho•le•cys•to•co•los•to•my (ko″lə-sis″to-kə-los′tə-me) [*cholecysto-* + *colostomy*] surgical anastomosis of the gallbladder to the colon.

cho•le•cys•to•co•lot•o•my (ko″lə-sis″to-ko-lot′ə-me) surgical incision of the gallbladder and colon.

cho•le•cys•to•du•o•de•nal (ko″lə-sis-to-doo″o-de′nəl) [*cholecysto-* + *duodenal*] pertaining to communication between the gallbladder and duodenum.

cho•le•cys•to•du•o•de•nos•to•my (ko″lə-sis″to-doo″o-də-nos′tə-me) [*cholecysto-* + *duodenostomy*] surgical anastomosis of the gallbladder and the duodenum; called also *duodenocystostomy.*

cho•le•cys•to•en•ter•os•to•my (ko″lə-sis″to-en″tər-os′tə-me) [*cholecysto-* + *enterostomy*] surgical anastomosis of the gallbladder to the intestine; called also *cholecystenterostomy.*

cho•le•cys•to•gas•tric (ko″lə-sis″to-gas′trik) [*cholecysto-* + *gastric*] communicating between the gallbladder and stomach.

Cholecalciferol and Related Metabolites of Vitamin D

Systematic Name	Vitamin	Abbreviation
7-Dehydrocholesterol	Provitamin D_3	—
Cholecalciferol	Vitamin D_3	D_3
25-Hydroxycholecalciferol	25-Hydroxyvitamin D_3	$25(OH)D_3$
1,25-Dihydroxycholecalciferol	1,25-Dihydroxyvitamin D_3	$1,25(OH)_2D_3$
24,25-Dihydroxycholecalciferol	24,25-Dihydroxyvitamin D_3	$24,25(OH)_2D_3$

cho·le·cys·to·gas·tros·to·my (ko″lə-sis″to-gas-tros′tə-me) [*cholecysto-* + *gastrostomy*] surgical anastomosis between the gallbladder and the stomach.

cho·le·cys·to·gram (ko″lə-sis′to-gram) a radiograph of the gallbladder.

cho·le·cys·tog·ra·phy (ko″lə-sis-tog′rə-fe) [*cholecysto-* + *-graphy*] radiography of the gallbladder.

cho·le·cys·to·il·e·os·to·my (ko″lə-sis″to-il″e-os′tə-me) [*cholecysto-* + *ileostomy*] surgical anastomosis of the gallbladder and the ileum.

cho·le·cys·to·in·tes·ti·nal (ko″lə-sis″to-in-tes′tĭ-nəl) cholecystenteric.

cho·le·cys·to·je·ju·nos·to·my (ko″lə-sis″to-jə-joo-nos′tə-me) [*cholecysto-* + *jejunostomy*] surgical anastomosis of the gallbladder and the jejunum.

cho·le·cys·to·ki·net·ic (ko″lə-sis″to-kĭ-net′ik) [*cholecysto-* + *kinetic*] causing or promoting contraction of the gallbladder.

cho·le·cys·to·ki·nin (CCK) (ko″lə-sis″to-ki′nin) [*cholecysto-* + *kinin*] a polypeptide hormone secreted by the mucosa of the upper intestine and by the hypothalamus. It stimulates contraction of the gallbladder (with release of bile) and secretion of pancreatic enzymes; hypothalamic cholecystokinin is a neurotransmitter. Called also *pancreozymin*.

cho·le·cys·to·li·thi·a·sis (ko″lə-sis″to-lĭ-thi′ə-sis) [*cholecysto-* + *lithiasis*] the occurrence of gallstones (cholelithiasis) within the gallbladder. Called also *cholecystic* or *gallbladder lithiasis*.

cho·le·cys·to·li·thot·o·my (ko″lə-sis″to-lĭ-thot′ə-me) [*cholecysto-* + *lithotomy*] incision of the gallbladder for removal of gallstones.

cho·le·cys·to·litho·trip·sy (ko″lə-sis″to-lith′o-trip″se) [*cholecysto-* + *lithotripsy*] the fragmentation of gallstones within the gallbladder.

cho·le·cys·top·a·thy (ko″lə-sis-top′ə-the) [*cholecysto-* + *-pathy*] any gallbladder disease; see also *cholecystitis* and *cholecystosis*.

cho·le·cys·to·pexy (ko″lə-sis′to-pek″se) [*cholecysto-* + *-pexy*] suspension or fixation of the gallbladder by surgical means.

cho·le·cys·top·to·sis (ko″lə-sis″top-to′sis, ko″lə-sis″to-to′sis) [*cholecysto-* + *-ptosis*] downward displacement of the gallbladder; see also *wandering gallbladder*.

cho·le·cys·tor·rha·phy (ko″lə-sis-tor′ə-fe) [*cholecysto-* + *-rrhaphy*] suture or repair of the gallbladder.

cho·le·cys·to·sis (ko″lə-sis-to′sis) [*cholecyst-* + *-osis*] any noninflammatory disease of the gallbladder.

hyperplastic c. abnormal increase in cellular structure of the gallbladder.

cho·le·cys·tos·to·my (ko″lə-sis-tos′tə-me) [*cholecysto-* + *-stomy*] surgical creation of an opening into the gallbladder.

percutaneous c. insertion of a catheter into the gallbladder under radiologic guidance for drainage or for the removal of gallstones.

cho·le·cys·tot·o·my (ko″lə-sis-tot′ə-me) [*cholecysto-* + *-tomy*] surgical incision of the gallbladder; done for exploration, drainage (cholecystostomy), or removal of calculi.

cho·led·o·chal (ko-led′ə-kəl) pertaining to the common bile duct.

cho·le·do·chec·to·my (ko″lə-do-kek′tə-me) [*choledoch-* + *-ectomy*] excision of a portion of the common bile duct.

cho·le·do·chi·tis (ko″lə-do-ki′tis) inflammation of the common bile duct.

choledoch(o)- [*choledochus*] a combining form denoting relation to the common bile duct.

cho·led·o·cho·cele (ko-led′ə-ko-sēl) a rare form of congenital cystic dilatation of the common bile duct in which the dilated portion is within the wall of the duct.

cho·led·o·cho·chol·e·do·chos·to·my (ko-led″ə-ko-kol″ə-də-kos′tə-me) surgical formation of an anastomosis between two portions of the common bile duct.

cho·led·o·cho·du·o·de·nal (ko-led″ə-ko-doo″o-de′nəl) pertaining to or connecting the common bile duct and the duodenum.

cho·led·o·cho·du·o·de·nos·to·my (ko-led″ə-ko-doo″o-də-nos′tə-me) [*choledocho-* + *duodenostomy*] surgical anastomosis of the common bile duct to the duodenum.

cho·led·o·cho·en·ter·os·to·my (ko-led″ə-ko-en″tər-os′tə-me) [*choledocho-* + *enterostomy*] surgical anastomosis of the common bile duct to the intestine.

cho·led·o·cho·gas·tros·to·my (ko-led″ə-ko-gas-tros′tə-me) [*choledocho-* + *gastrostomy*] surgical anastomosis of the common bile duct and the stomach.

cho·led·o·cho·gram (ko-led′ə-ko-gram″) a radiograph of the common bile duct.

cho·led·o·chog·ra·phy (ko-led″ə-kog′rə-fe) [*choledocho-* + *-graphy*] radiography of the common bile duct after the administration of opaque material.

cho·led·o·cho·je·ju·nos·to·my (ko-led″ə-ko-jə-joo-nos′tə-me) [*choledocho-* + *jejunostomy*] surgical anastomosis of the common bile duct and the jejunum.

cho·led·o·cho·lith (ko-led′ə-ko-lith″) a gallstone or other calculus in the common bile duct. Called also *bile duct calculus*.

cho·led·o·cho·li·thi·a·sis (ko-led″ə-ko-lĭ-thi′ə-sis) the occurrence of calculi (cholelithiasis) in the common bile duct.

cho·led·o·cho·li·thot·o·my (ko-led″ə-ko-lĭ-thot′ə-me) [*choledocho-* + *lithotomy*] incision of the common bile duct for the removal of a calculus.

cho·led·o·cho·litho·trip·sy (ko-led″ə-ko-lith′o-trip″se) the crushing of a gallstone within the common bile duct.

cho·led·o·cho·plas·ty (ko-led′ə-ko-plas″te) [*choledocho-* + *-plasty*] the performance of a plastic operation on the common bile duct, such as plastic repair of it following injury.

cho·led·o·chor·rha·phy (ko-led″ə-kor′ə-fe) [*choledocho-* + *-rrhaphy*] suture or repair of the common bile duct.

cho·led·o·cho·scope (ko-led′ə-ko-skōp″) an endoscope for direct inspection of the interior of the common bile duct.

cho·led·o·chos·co·py (ko-led″ə-kos′kə-pe) visualization of the biliary tract with a choledochoscope.

cho·led·o·chos·to·my (ko-led″ə-kos′tə-me) [*choledocho-* + *-stomy*] surgical formation of an opening into the common bile duct and drainage by catheter or T-tube.

cho·led·o·chot·o·my (ko-led″ə-kot′ə-me) [*choledocho-* + *-tomy*] incision into the common bile duct for exploration or removal of a calculus.

cho·led·o·chus (ko-led′ə-kəs) [*chole-* + Gr. *dochos* receptacle] ductus choledochus.

Cho·le·dyl (ko′lə-dil″) trademark for preparations of oxtriphylline.

cho·le·glo·bin (ko″le-glo′bin) a compound of globin and an open-ring iron porphyrin, being an intermediate in the formation of bile pigment from the catabolism of hemoglobin.

cho·le·hem·a·tin (ko″lə-hem′ə-tin) phylloerythrin.

cho·le·ic (ko-le′ik) biliary.

cho·le·ic ac·id (ko-le′ik) any of the complexes formed between deoxycholic acid and a fatty acid or other lipid.

cho·le·lith (ko′lə-lith) gallstone.

cho·le·li·thi·a·sis (ko″lə-lĭ-thi′ə-sis) [*chole-* + *lithiasis*] the presence or formation of gallstones; they may be either in the gallbladder *(cholecystolithiasis)* or in the common bile duct *(choledocholithiasis)*.

cho·le·lith·ic (ko″lə-lith′ik) pertaining to or caused by gallstones.

cho·le·li·thot·o·my (ko″lə-lĭ-thot′ə-me) removal of gallstones through an incision in the gallbladder (cholecystolithotomy) or common bile duct (choledocholithotomy).

cho·le·litho·trip·sy (ko″lə-lith′o-trip-se) [*chole-* + *litho-* + *-tripsy*] the crushing of gallstones.

cho·lem·e·sis (ko-lem′ə-sis) [*chole-* + *emesis*] bilious vomiting.

cho·le·mia (ko-le′me-ə) [*chole-* + *-emia*] the presence of bile or bile pigments in the blood. **chole′mic** *adj*

familial c., Gilbert c. Gilbert syndrome.

cho·le·mim·e·try (ko″lə-mim′ə-tre) determination of the amount of bile pigment in the blood.

cho·le·peri·to·ne·um (ko″lə-per″ĭ-to-ne′əm) [*chole-* + *peritoneum*] the presence of bile in the peritoneum resulting from rupture of the bile passages; called also *bile* or *biliary ascites*, *bile* or *biliary peritonitis*, and *choleperitonitis*.

cho·le·peri·to·ni·tis (ko″lə-per″ĭ-tə-ni′tis) choleperitoneum.

cho·le·poi·e·sis (ko″lə-poi-e′sis) [*chole-* + *-poiesis*] the manufacture and secretion by the liver of bile constituents (other than water).

cho·le·poi·et·ic (ko″lə-poi-et′ik) 1. pertaining to or characterized by cholepoiesis. 2. increasing the secretion of bile without a fall in its specific gravity.

cho·le·pra·sin (ko″lə-pra′sin) a green bile pigment isolated from gallstones.

chol·era (kol′ər-ə) [Gr., from *cholē* bile] 1. an acute infectious, sometimes fulminant, enteritis endemic in India and Southeast Asia and periodically spreading in epidemics or pandemics to other warm regions of the world; it is spread by feces-contaminated water and food. The cause is a potent enterotoxin called a choleragen, elaborated by *Vibrio cholerae*, that acts on epithelial cells in the small intestine to cause copious secretion of isotonic fluid from the mucosal surface. Severe cases are marked by painless watery diarrhea called rice-water stools, which are diagnostic and result in massive fluid loss, saline depletion, acidosis, and shock that can be fatal. 2. any of several infections that resemble this disease, particularly in veterinary medicine, but are not caused by *Vibrio cholerae.* **cholera′ic** *adj*

Asiatic c. name sometimes given to cholera because it was originally from Asia.

dry c. c. sicca.

fowl c. an infection by *Pasteurella multocida,* seen in domestic and wild bird species around the world. There are both acute, often fatal, forms and chronic forms; symptoms include abdominal hyperemia with petechiae and hemorrhage, fever, anorexia, ruffled feathers, diarrhea, increased respiratory rate, and sometimes pneumonia.

hog c. an epizootic infectious disease of swine caused by a togavirus; marked by fever, loss of appetite, emaciation, ulceration of the intestines, diarrhea, and ecchymoses in the kidney and on the skin of the ventral surface of the body. Called also *swine fever.*

pancreatic c. Verner-Morrison syndrome.

c. sic′ca a rare type of cholera in which intestinal obstruction produces pooling of fluid in the colon, so that there is not diarrhea; called also *dry c.*

chol·er·a·gen (kol′ər-ə-jen) 1. the cholera enterotoxin, an extremely potent protein molecule elaborated by strains of *Vibrio cholerae* in the small intestine; it acts on the epithelial cells to cause hypersecretion of chloride and bicarbonate and an outpouring of large quantities of isotonic fluid from the mucosal surface. 2. cholera toxin.

chol·er·a·phage (kol′ər-ə-fāj) a bacteriophage that infects cholera bacilli.

cho·ler·e·sis (ko-ler′ə-sis) [*chole-* + Gr. *hairesis* a taking] the secretion of bile by the liver by either cholepoiesis or hydrocholeresis.

cho·ler·et·ic (ko″lər-et′ik) 1. stimulating the production of bile by the liver by either cholepoiesis or hydrocholeresis. 2. an agent that stimulates production of bile by the liver.

cho·ler·i·form (ko-ler′ĭ-form) resembling cholera.

chol·er·i·gen·ic (kol″ər-ĭ-jen′ik) causing cholera.

chol·er·oid (kol′ər-oid) choleriform.

cho·le·scin·ti·gram (ko″lə-sin′tĭ-gram) the two-dimensional images of the biliary system obtained by cholescintigraphy.

cho·le·scin·tig·ra·phy (ko″lə-sin-tig′rə-fe) scintigraphy of the biliary tract.

cho·les·tane (ko′ləs-tān) a saturated steroid hydrocarbon, with C-18 and C-19 methyl groups and an isooctyl side chain at C-17; obtained by reduction of cholesterol and other C_{27} steroids.

cho·les·tane·tri·ol (ko-les″tān-tri′ol) a triply hydroxylated intermediate formed in the biosynthesis of bile acids from cholesterol.

cho·les·tane·tri·ol 26-mono·oxy·ge·nase (ko-les″tān-tri′ol mon″o-ok′sə-jən-ās) [EC 1.14.13.15] an enzyme of the oxidoreductase class that hydroxylates 5β-cholestane-3α,7α,12α-triol (or any of several related intermediates) as a step in the major biosynthetic pathway of bile acids from cholesterol. Deficiency of the enzyme, an autosomal recessive trait, results in cerebrotendinous xanthomatosis. Called also *27-hydroxylase.*

cho·les·ta·nol (ko-les′tə-nol) a compound, $C_{27}H_{47}OH$, formed by the reduction of cholesterol.

beta-c. an isomer of coprosterol derived from cholesterol by bacterial action and found in the feces; called also *dihydrocholesterol.*

cho·le·sta·sia (ko″lə-sta′zhə) cholestasis.

cho·le·sta·sis (ko″lə-sta′sis) [*chole-* + *-stasis*] stoppage or suppression of the flow of bile. **cholestat′ic** *adj*

benign recurrent c., benign recurrent intrahepatic c. an autosomal recessive form of intrahepatic cholestasis characterized by intermittent episodes of elevated serum bile acids followed by jaundice and pruritus; there is usually complete resolution of symptoms between the attacks. Two types exist: *type 1* is caused by mutations in the *ATP8B1* gene (locus: 18q21), which encodes the FIC1 protein, which plays a role in bile synthesis; *type 2* is caused by mutations in the *ABCB11* gene (locus: 2q24), which encodes an ABC transporter involved in bile salt transport.

extrahepatic c. cholestasis occurring outside the liver, due to blockage of a bile duct or ducts; it may be due to a tumor or stricture, a gallstone or other damage in the duct, pancreatitis, or other causes.

intrahepatic c. cholestasis due to some condition, such as infection, sepsis, or cirrhosis, inside the liver.

intrahepatic c. of pregnancy a type of intrahepatic cholestasis sometimes seen during the third trimester of pregnancy, characterized by severe itching, hepatomegaly, and sometimes jaundice; it clears up after delivery. It occurs more frequently in certain ethnic groups, indicating that there may be a genetic basis.

progressive familial intrahepatic c. a genetically heterogeneous group of autosomal recessive disorders of bile acid transport, characterized by early onset of intrahepatic cholestasis that progresses to hepatic fibrosis, cirrhosis, and end-stage liver disease before adulthood. There are 3 types; type 1 is called also *Byler disease.*

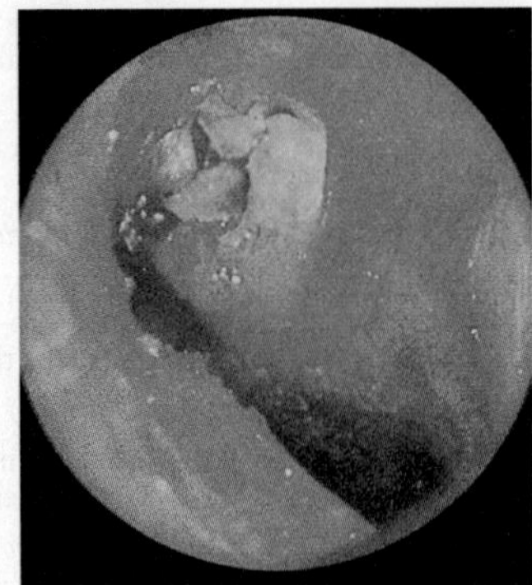

■ Cholesteatoma.

cho·le·ste·a·to·ma (ko″lə-ste″ə-to′mə) [*chole-* + *steatoma*] a cystlike mass or benign tumor lined with stratified squamous epithelium, usually keratinizing, and filled with desquamating debris often including cholesterol. Cholesteatomas are most common in the middle ear and mastoid region secondary to trauma or infection that heals improperly so that epithelium invaginates. A congenital variety (see *congenital c.*), resulting from embryonic inclusions, is less common.

congenital c. a benign tumor resulting from inclusion of epidermal elements at the time of closure of the neural groove; it may be in or near the ear but more often is in the form of an intracranial cholesteatoma.

intracranial c. a type of congenital cholesteatoma resembling an epidermal inclusion cyst, found in the skull, meninges, or brain; it grows slowly, often in the cisterns. Symptoms vary depending on what part of the brain is under pressure, but may become life-threatening.

c. tym′pani a type of cholesteatoma usually associated with chronic infection of the middle ear, formed of the outer desquamating layers of stratified squamous epithelium that have extended inward and upward to line the tympanum, epitympanum, and antrum.

cho·le·ste·a·to·ma·tous (ko″lə-ste″ə-to′mə-təs) relating to or of the nature of cholesteatoma.

cho·le·ste·a·to·sis (ko″lə-ste″ə-to′sis) fatty deposits of cholesterol esters in a tissue.

cho·les·ter·in (ko-les′tər-in) [Ger.] cholesterol.

cho·les·tero·gen·e·sis (ko-les″tər-o-jen′ə-sis) [*cholesterol* + *-genesis*] synthesis of cholesterol.

cho·les·tero·hy·dro·tho·rax (ko-les″tər-o-hi″dro-thor′aks) a chyliform effusion (q.v.) that is high in cholesterol.

cho·les·ter·ol (kə-les′tər-ol″) [*chole-* + *sterol*] 1. a eukaryotic sterol that in higher animals is the precursor of bile acids and steroid hormones and a key constituent of cell membranes, mediating their fluidity and permeability. Most is synthesized by the liver and other tissues, but some is absorbed from dietary sources, with each kind transported in plasma by specific lipoproteins. Cholesterol can accumulate or deposit abnormally, as in some gallstones and in atheromas. 2. [NF] a preparation of cholesterol used as an emulsifying agent in pharmaceuticals.

HDL c., high-density–lipoprotein c. (HDL-C) the serum cholesterol carried on high-density lipoproteins, approximately 20 to 30 per cent of the total serum cholesterol.

LDL c., low-density–lipoprotein c. (LDL-C) the serum cholesterol carried on low-density lipoproteins, approximately 60 to 70 per cent of the total serum cholesterol.

cho·les·ter·ol ac·yl·trans·fer·ase (kə-les′tər-ol a″səl-trans′fər-ās) sterol *O*-acyltransferase.

cho·les·ter·ol des·mo·lase (kə-les′tər-ol des′mol-ās) cholesterol monooxygenase (side-chain-cleaving).

cho·les·ter·ol·emia (kə-les″tər-ol-e′me-ə) hypercholesterolemia.

cho·les·ter·ol es·ter·ase (kə-les′tər-ol es′tər-ās) sterol esterase.

cho·les·ter·ol mono·oxy·gen·ase (side-chain-cleav·ing) (P_{450}SCC) (kə-les′tə-rol mon″o-ok′sə-jən-ās sīd chān klēv′ing) [EC 1.14.15.6] an enzyme of the oxidoreductase class that catalyzes the NADPH-dependent conversion of cholesterol to pregnenolone in a series of three reactions, successive hydroxylations of the 20 and 22 positions followed by cleavage of the side chain. The enzyme is a mitochondrial cytochrome P-450 acting as a terminal oxidase in an electron transport chain that also contains adrenodoxin and a flavoprotein. The reaction is the first step in the conversion of cholesterol to steroid hormones.

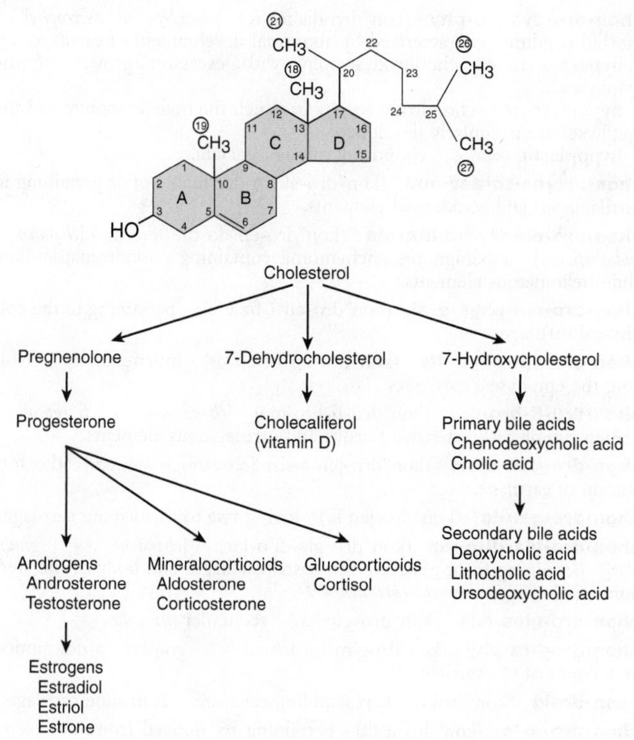

■ Structure and metabolism of cholesterol.

Deficiency of the enzyme, an autosomal recessive trait, causes lipoid adrenal hyperplasia, a type of congenital adrenal hyperplasia (type I). Called also *cholesterol desmolase* and *20,22-desmolase.*

cho•les•ter•olo•gen•e•sis (kə-les″tər-ol″o-jen′ə-sis) [*cholesterol* + *-genesis*] the synthesis of cholesterol by the liver; called also *cholesterolopoiesis.*

cho•les•ter•olo•poi•e•sis (kə-les″tər-ol″o-poi-e′sis) cholesterologenesis.

cho•les•ter•ol•o•sis (kə-les″tər-ol-o′sis) a condition in which cholesterol is deposited in tissues in abnormal quantities. Called also *cholesterosis.*

cho•les•ter•ol sul•fa•tase (kə-les′tər-ol sul′fə-tās) steryl-sulfatase.

cho•les•ter•ol•uria (kə-les″tər-ol-u′re-ə) the presence of cholesterol in the urine.

cho•les•ter•o•sis (kə-les″tər-o′sis) cholesterolosis.

cho•les•ter•yl (kə-les′tə-rəl″) the radical of cholesterol, formed by removal of the hydroxyl group.

cho•le•sty•ra•mine (ko″lə-sti′rə-mēn) see *cholestyramine resin,* under *resin.*

Cho•le•tec (ko′lə-tek″) trademark for a kit for the preparation of technetium Tc 99m mebrofenin.

cho•le•u•ria (ko″le-u′re-ə) choluria.

cho•lic ac•id (ko′lik) 1. one of the primary bile acids, usually occurring conjugated with glycine or taurine; it facilitates fat absorption and cholesterol excretion. 2. any of the substituted derivatives of cholic acid collectively constituting the bile acids.

cho•line (ko′lēn) a water-soluble compound derivable from many animal and some vegetable tissues and produced synthetically. Although it can be synthesized by humans, it is often included in the vitamin B complex (q.v.). It is the basic constituent of lecithin and prevents the deposition of fat in the liver; the acetic acid ester of choline (acetylcholine) is essential in synaptic transmission of nerve impulses. Choline is also oxidized to form betaine in methionine biosynthesis.

acetyl glyceryl ether phosphoryl c. platelet-activating factor; see under *factor.*

c. bitartrate [USP] the bitartrate salt of choline, used as a dietary supplement.

c. chloride [USP] the chloride salt of choline, used as a dietary supplement.

c. magnesium trisalicylate see under *trisalicylate.*

c. salicylate see under *salicylate.*

cho•line acet•y•lase (ko′lēn ə-set′ə-lās) choline *O*-acetyltransferase.

cho•line *O*-ac•e•tyl•trans•fer•ase (ko′lēn as″ə-tēl-trans′fər-ās) [EC 2.3.1.6] an enzyme of the transferase class that catalyzes the synthesis of acetylcholine, transferring the acetyl moiety from acetyl coenzyme A to choline. The enzyme occurs in synaptosomes of the autonomic nervous system and skeletal muscle, and in some regions of the central nervous system. Called also *choline acetyltransferase* and *choline acetylase.*

cho•line ac•e•tyl•trans•fer•ase de•fi•cien•cy (ko′lēn as″ə-tēl-trans′fər-ās) a congenital autosomal recessive disorder caused by mutation in the *CHAT* gene (locus: 10q11.2), which encodes choline *O*-acetyltransferase; it is characterized by generalized hypotonia that is present at birth, repeated episodes of life-threatening apnea, feeding difficulty, varying degrees of ophthalmoparesis, and occasionally arthrogryposis; symptoms often improve with age. Called also *familial infantile myasthenia gravis.*

cho•line es•ter•ase I (ko′lēn es′tər-ās) acetylcholinesterase.

cho•line es•ter•ase II (unspecific) (ko′lēn es′tər-ās un″spə-sif′ik) cholinesterase.

cho•lin•er•gic (ko″lin-ur′jik) 1. stimulated, activated, or transmitted by choline (acetylcholine): a term applied to the sympathetic and parasympathetic nerve fibers that liberate acetylcholine at a synapse when a nerve impulse passes. See also under *receptor.* 2. an agent that produces such effects. Called also *parasympathomimetic.* Cf. *adrenergic.*

cho•lin•es•ter•ase (CHS) (ko″lin-es′tər-ās) [EC 3.1.1.8] an enzyme of the hydrolase class that catalyzes the cleavage of the acyl group from various esters of choline, including acetylcholine, and some related compounds (cf. *acetylcholinesterase*). The enzyme occurs primarily in the serum, liver, and pancreas; determination of enzyme activity is used to test liver function, succinylcholine sensitivity, and whether organophosphate insecticide poisoning has occurred. Called also *choline esterase II (unspecific), pseudocholinesterase (PCE),* and *serum c. (SChE).*

serum c. (SChE) cholinesterase.

true c. acetylcholinesterase.

cho•li•no•cep•tive (ko″lin-o-sep′tiv) pertaining to the sites on effector organs that are acted upon by cholinergic transmitters.

cho•li•no•cep•tor (ko″lin-o-sep′tər) cholinergic receptor; see under *receptor.*

cho•li•no•lyt•ic (ko″lin-o-lit′ik) 1. blocking the action of acetylcholine, or of cholinergic agents. 2. an agent that blocks the action of acetylcholine in cholinergic areas, that is, organs supplied by parasympathetic nerves, and voluntary muscles.

cho•li•no•mi•met•ic (ko″lin-o-mi-met′ik) having an action similar to that of acetylcholine; parasympathomimetic.

chol(o)- [Gr. *cholē* bile] a combining form denoting relationship to bile. Also, *chole-.*

chol•o•ge•net•ic (kol″o-jə-net′ik) cholepoietic.

Cho•lo•gra•fin (ko″lo-gra′fin) trademark for preparations of iodipamide.

chol•o•he•mo•tho•rax (kol″o-he″mo-thor′aks) [*cholo-* + *hemothorax*] a pleural effusion containing bile and blood, usually due to a rupture in the intestinal wall.

chol•o•lith (kol′o-lith) cholelith.

chol•o•li•thi•a•sis (kol″o-lĭ-thi′ə-sis) cholelithiasis.

chol•o•poi•e•sis (kol″o-poi-e′sis) cholepoiesis.

chol•o•poi•et•ic (kol″o-poi-et′ik) cholepoietic.

chol•o•tho•rax (kol″o-thor′aks) [*cholo-* + *thorax*] a pleural effusion containing bile, usually due to a rupture in the intestinal wall. Cf. *cholohemothorax.*

chol•uria (kol-u′re-ə) [*chol-* + *-uria*] the presence of bile pigments or bile salts in the urine, such as in certain liver diseases or bile duct obstruction. Called also *biliuria.* **cholu′ric** *adj*

Cho•ly•bar (ko′le-bahr) trademark for a preparation of cholestyramine resin.

cho•lyl•gly•cine (ko″ləl-gli′sēn) a bile salt, the glycine conjugate of cholic acid, called also *glycocholic acid.*

cho•lyl•tau•rine (ko″ləl-taw′rēn) a bile salt, the taurine conjugate of cholic acid, called also *taurocholic acid* and *cholaic acid.*

Chon•do•den•dron (kon″do-den′dron) a genus of climbing shrubs of the family Menispermaceae. *C. tomento′sum* Ruiz et Pavon is one of the sources of curare (q.v.).

chon•dral (kon′drəl) pertaining to cartilage.

chon•dral•gia (kon-dral′jə) chondrodynia.

chon•dral•lo•pla•sia (kon″dral-o-pla′zhə) [*chondr-* + *allo-* + *-plasia*] dyschondroplasia.

chon•drec•to•my (kon-drek′tə-me) [*chondr-* + *-ectomy*] surgical removal of cartilage.

chon·drex (kon′dreks) a 40-kD major secretory protein of human chondrocytes and synovial fibroblasts; it may be useful as a serum marker of joint and cartilage disease.

chon·dric (kon′drik) cartilaginous; of or relating to cartilage.

Chon·drich·thy·es (kon-drik′the-ēz) [Gr. *chondros* cartilage + *ichthys* fish] a class of fishes with cartilaginous skeletons, including sharks, skates, and their allies. See also *elasmobranch.*

chon·dri·fi·ca·tion (kon″drĭ-fĭ-ka′shən) [*chondri-* + L. *facere* to make] the formation of cartilage; transformation into cartilage.

chondri(o)- [Gr. *chondrion* granule] a combining form denoting relationship to a granule.

chon·dri·ome (kon′dre-ōm) all of the mitochondria of a cell considered in aggregate.

chon·dri·tis (kon-dri′tis) [*chondr-* + *-itis*] inflammation of cartilage.
costal c. Tietze syndrome (def. 1).
c. intervertebra′lis calca′nea calcinosis intervertebralis.

chondr(o)- [Gr. *chondros* cartilage] a combining form denoting relationship to cartilage.

chon·dro·an·gi·o·ma (kon″dro-an″je-o′mə) [*chondro-* + *angioma*] a benign mesenchymoma containing chondromatous and angiomatous elements.

chon·dro·blast (kon′dro-blast) [*chondro-* + *-blast*] a cell that arises from the mesenchyma and forms cartilage; called also *chondroplast.*

chon·dro·blas·to·ma (kon″dro-blas-to′mə) [*chondroblast* + *-oma*] a usually benign tumor derived from immature cartilage cells, occurring primarily in the epiphyses of adolescents; it is characterized by fine, matrix-like calcifications arranged hexagonally, often resembling chicken wire, around closely packed cells.
benign c. chondroblastoma.
malignant c. clear cell chondrosarcoma.

chon·dro·cal·cif·ic (kon″dro-kal-sif′ik) characterized by deposition of calcium salts in the cartilaginous structures of one or more joints.

chon·dro·cal·ci·no·sis (kon″dro-kal″sĭ-no′sis) [*chondro-* + *calcinosis*] the presence of calcium salts, especially calcium pyrophosphate, in the cartilaginous structures of one or more joints. Cf. *calcium pyrophosphate deposition disease.*

chon·dro·clast (kon′dro-klast) [*chondro-* + *clast*] a giant cell of the class that is believed associated with the absorption of cartilage.

chon·dro·cos·tal (kon″dro-kos′təl) [*chondro-* + *costal*] of or pertaining to the ribs and costal cartilages.

chon·dro·cra·ni·um (kon″dro-kra′ne-əm) [*chondro-* + *cranium*] [TA] the part of the neurocranium formed by endochondral ossification and comprising the bones of the base of the cranium; called also *cartilaginous neurocranium.*

chon·dro·cyte (kon′dro-sīt) [*chondro-* + *-cyte*] a mature cell of cartilage, embedded in a lacuna within the cartilage matrix. Called also *cartilage cell.*
isogenous c's cartilage cells that make up a single group.

chon·dro·der·ma·ti·tis (kon″dro-dur″mə-ti′tis) an inflammatory process involving cartilage and skin.
c. nodula′ris chro′nica he′licis, c. nodula′ris he′licis a small, painful, scaly, nodular lesion on the helix of the ear, colored skin color, grayish, or translucent; it is seen most often in middle-aged men, and multiple lesions may occur on one ear. Called also *Winkler disease.*

chon·dro·dyn·ia (kon″dro-din′e-ə) [*chondr-* + *-odynia*] pain in a cartilage.

chon·dro·dys·pla·sia (kon″dro-dis-pla′zhə) [*chondro-* + *dysplasia*] any of a group of hereditary disorders of endochondral ossification that are characterized by disproportionate shortening of the limbs or trunk, so that affected individuals have either short limbs or short trunks. Severity ranges from mild short stature to malformations that are lethal in utero.
Grebe c. a severe form of acromesomelic dysplasia, caused by mutations in the *GDF5* gene (locus: 20q11.2), which encodes a growth factor of the TGF-β superfamily, characterized by profound shortening of the forearms, legs, and digits and severe abnormalities of the hands and feet. Inheritance is autosomal recessive. It is allelic with but more severe than Hunter-Thompson acromesomelic dysplasia.
metaphyseal c. see under *dysostosis.*
c. puncta′ta a heterogeneous group of bone dysplasias whose common characteristic is stippling of the epiphyses in infancy. There are a severe autosomal recessive form (rhizomelic dwarfism), an autosomal dominant form (Conradi-Hünermann syndrome), and a milder X-linked form. Called also *Conradi disease, dysplasia epiphysealis punctata, hypoplastic fetal chondrodystrophy,* and *stippled epiphyses.*

chon·dro·dys·tro·phia (kon″dro-dis-tro′fe-ə) chondrodystrophy.
c. calci′ficans conge′nita, c. conge′nita puncta′ta, c. feta′lis calci′ficans chondrodysplasia punctata.

chon·dro·dys·tro·phy (kon″dro-dis′trə-fe) [*chondro-* + *dystrophy*] a morbid condition characterized by abnormal development of cartilage.
hyperplastic c. chondrodystrophy with excessive growth of the epiphyses.
hypoplastic c. chondrodystrophy in which the bone is spongy and the epiphyses are irregularly developed.
hypoplastic fetal c. chondrodysplasia punctata.

chon·dro·ec·to·der·mal (kon″dro-ek″to-dur′məl) of or pertaining to cartilaginous and ectodermal elements.

chon·dro·en·do·the·li·o·ma (kon″dro-en″do-the″le-o′mə) [*chondro-* + *endothelioma*] a benign mesenchymoma containing chondromatous and endotheliomatous elements.

chon·dro·epi·phys·e·al (kon″dro-ep″ĭ-fiz′e-əl) pertaining to the epiphyseal cartilage.

chon·dro·epi·phys·itis (kon″dro-ep″ĭ-fiz-i′tis) inflammation involving the epiphyseal cartilages.

chon·dro·fi·bro·ma (kon″dro-fi-bro′mə) [*chondroma* + *fibroma*] a benign tumor with extensive fibrous and cartilaginous elements.

chon·dro·gen·e·sis (kon″dro-jen′ə-sis) [*chondro-* + *-genesis*] the formation of cartilage.

chon·dro·gen·ic (kon″dro-jen′ik) giving rise to or forming cartilage.

chon·dro·gla·di·o·lar (kon″dro-glə-di′o-lər) [*chondro-* + *gladiolus*] pertaining to or affecting the costal cartilages and body of the sternum (gladiolus); see *pectus carinatum.*

chon·dro·glos·sus (kon″dro-glos′əs) see under *musculus.*

chon·drog·ra·phy (kon-drog′rə-fe) [*chondro-* + *-graphy*] a description or account of the cartilages.

chon·droid (kon′droid) 1. resembling cartilage. 2. hyaline cartilage.

chon·dro·it·ic (kon″dro-it′ik) pertaining to, derived from, or resembling cartilage.

chon·dro·i·tin sul·fate (kon-dro′ĭ-tin) 1. a glycosaminoglycan that predominates in the ground substance of cartilage, bone, and blood vessels but also occurs in other connective tissues. It consists of repeating disaccharide units in specific linkage, each composed of a glucuronic acid residue linked to a sulfated *N*-acetylgalactosamine residue. There are two forms: chondroitin 4-sulfate *(chondroitin sulfate A)* and chondroitin 6-sulfate *(chondroitin sulfate C)*, named for the position of the sulfate group on the sugar. One or both types accumulate abnormally in several mucopolysaccharidoses. *Chondroitin sulfate B* is now called *dermatan sulfate.* 2. a preparation of chondroitin sulfate from bovine tracheal cartilage, administered orally for the treatment of osteoarthritis and joint pain.

chon·dro·li·po·ma (kon″dro-lĭ-po′mə) [*chondro-* + *lip-* + *-oma*] a benign mesenchymoma containing lipomatous and cartilaginous elements.

chon·drol·o·gy (kon-drol′ə-je) [*chondro-* + *-logy*] the sum of knowledge in regard to the cartilages.

chon·drol·y·sis (kon-drol′ĭ-sis) [*chondro-* + *-lysis*] the degeneration of cartilage cells that occurs in the process of intracartilaginous ossification.

chon·dro·ma (kon-dro′mə) pl. *chondromas, chondro′mata* [*chondr-* + *-oma*] a benign tumor or tumorlike growth of mature hyaline cartilage. It may remain centrally within the substance of a cartilage or bone *(enchondroma)* or may develop on the surface of a cartilage or bone *(juxtacortical chondroma)*, and usually occurs in adolescents or young adults in the small bones of the hands or feet, the femur, the humerus, or the ribs.
fibromyxoid c. chondromyxoid fibroma.
joint c. a mass of cartilage in the synovial membrane of a joint; see *synovial chondromatosis.*
juxtacortical c. an uncommon benign tumor of cartilage growing beneath the periosteum but external to the cortex of a bone, usually the small bones of the hands or feet. Called also *periosteal c.*
periosteal c. juxtacortical c.
synovial c. a cartilaginous body formed in a synovial membrane; see under *chondromatosis.*
true c. enchondroma.

chon·dro·ma·la·cia (kon″dro-mə-la′shə) [*chondro-* + *-malacia*] softening of the articular cartilage, most frequently in the patella.
cystic c. pseudocyst of auricle.
c. feta′lis a condition in which the limbs of the stillborn fetus are soft and pliable due to softening of the epiphyseal cartilage.
c. patel′lae pain and crepitus over the anterior aspect of the knee, particularly in flexion, with softening of the cartilage on the articular surface of the patella and, in later stages, effusion.

chon·dro·ma·nu·bri·al (kon″dro-mə-noo′bre-əl) [*chondro-* + *manubrium*] pertaining to or affecting the costal cartilages and manubrium; see *pectus carinatum.*

chon·dro·ma·to·sis (kon″dro-mə-to′sis) formation of multiple chondromas.

synovial c. formation of multiple intrasynovial nodules resembling osteochondromas, resulting from proliferative changes in the synovial linings of joints; as the disorder progresses, nodules increasingly forsake the intrasynovial areas for the joint cavities.

chon·dro·ma·tous (kon-dro′mə-təs) pertaining to or of the nature of cartilage.

chon·dro·mere (kon′dro-mēr) [*chondro-* + *-mere*] a cartilaginous vertebra of the fetal vertebral column.

chon·dro·meta·pla·sia (kon″dro-met″ə-pla′zhə) a condition characterized by metaplastic activity of the chondroblasts.
synovial c. synovial chondromatosis.
tenosynovial c. synovial chondromatosis affecting the sheath of a tendon.

chon·dro·mu·cin (kon″dro-mu′sin) chondromucoprotein.

chon·dro·mu·coid (kon″dro-mu′koid) chondromucoprotein.

chon·dro·mu·co·pro·tein (kon″dro-mu″ko-pro′tēn) the principal constituent of the ground substance of cartilage; it is a copolymer of a mucoprotein and chondroitin sulfates.

chon·dro·my·o·ma (kon″dro-mi-o′mə) [*chondro-* + *myoma*] a benign mesenchymoma containing myomatous and cartilaginous elements.

chon·dro·myx·oid (kon″dro-mik′soid) of, pertaining to, or characterized by chondroid and myxoid elements.

chon·dro·myx·o·ma (kon″dro-mik-so′mə) chondromyxoid fibroma.

chon·dro·myxo·sar·co·ma (kon″dro-mik″so-sahr-ko′mə) [*chondro-* + *myxo-* + *sarcoma*] a malignant mesenchymoma containing myxoid and cartilaginous elements.

chon·dro·ne·cro·sis (kon″dro-nə-kro′sis) necrosis of cartilage.

chon·dro-os·se·ous (kon″dro-os′e-əs) composed of cartilage and bone.

chon·dro·path·ia (kon″dro-path′e-ə) chondropathy.
c. tubero′sa Tietze syndrome.

chon·dro·pa·thol·o·gy (kon″dro-pə-thol′ə-je) the pathology of disease of cartilage.

chon·drop·a·thy (kon-drop′ə-the) [*chondro-* + *-pathy*] disease of a cartilage.

chon·dro·phyte (kon′dro-fit) [*chondro-* + *-phyte*] a cartilaginous growth at the articular extremity of a bone.

chon·dro·pla·sia (kon″dro-pla′zhə) the formation of cartilage by specialized cells (chondrocytes).
c. puncta′ta chondrodysplasia punctata.

chon·dro·plast (kon′dro-plast) [*chondro-* + *-plast*] chondroblast.

chon·dro·plas·ty (kon′dro-plas″te) [*chondro-* + *-plasty*] plastic surgery on cartilage; repair of lacerated or displaced cartilage. **chondroplas′tic** *adj*

chon·dro·po·ro·sis (kon″dro-po-ro′sis) [*chondro-* + *porosis* (2)] the formation of spaces or sinuses in the cartilages; it occurs normally during ossification.

chon·dro·sar·co·ma (kon″dro-sahr-ko′mə) [*chondro-* + *sarcoma*] a malignant tumor derived from cartilage cells or their precursors, but lacking direct osteoid formation; it occurs predominantly in the pelvis, femur, and shoulder girdle in middle-aged to older adults. It may be primary, arising from cartilage cells, or secondary to a pre-existing benign lesion. **chondrosarco′matous** *adj*
central c. a chondrosarcoma developing in the interior of a bone; it usually presents with dull pain, but a mass is rare.
clear cell c. a very rare form of chondrosarcoma characterized by swollen, glycogen-rich clear cells, occurring usually in the femur, tibia, vertebrae, or pubis in adults; it is slow-growing and metastasizes only after multiple local recurrences.
dedifferentiated c. a rare, fast-growing, very aggressive form of chondrosarcoma that contains additional malignant mesenchymal elements, such as areas of fibrosarcoma or spindle cells.
juxtacortical c. chondrosarcoma arising in relation to the cortex of the periosteum, occurring on the surface of the bone, particularly the femur or humerus, usually in adults.
mesenchymal c. a rare, aggressive, malignant neoplasm composed of a small cell stroma containing islands of cartilaginous elements; it occurs primarily in flat bones, but also in soft tissue, and particularly in adolescents and young adults.
myxoid c. chondromyxosarcoma.
periosteal c. juxtacortical c.
peripheral c. chondrosarcoma arising on the surface of a bone; it may be either primary or secondary to underlying neoplasms, which are usually benign cartilage tumors, and generally presents as a large mass.
spindle cell c. dedifferentiated c.

chon·dro·sar·co·ma·to·sis (kon″dro-sahr-ko″mə-to′sis) the formation of multiple chondrosarcomas.

chon·dro·sep·tum (kon″dro-sep′təm) [*chondro-* + *septum*] pars cartilaginea septi nasi.

chon·dro·sin (kon′dro-sin) the basic disaccharide unit of chondroitin sulfate, comprising a molecule each of glucuronic acid and sulfated *N*-acetylgalactosamine in specific linkage.

chon·dro·sis (kon-dro′sis) [*chondr-* + *-osis*] chondropathy.

chon·dro·skel·e·ton (kon″dro-skel′ə-tən) 1. a cartilaginous skeleton, as in certain fish. 2. the part of the skeleton that is composed of cartilage.

chon·dros·te·o·ma (kon-dros″te-o′mə) osteochondroma.

chon·dro·ster·nal (kon″dro-stur′nəl) pertaining to the costal cartilages and the sternum.

chon·dro·ster·no·plas·ty (kon″dro-stur′no-plas″te) surgical correction of funnel chest.

chon·dro·tome (kon′dro-tōm) an instrument for cutting cartilage.

chon·drot·o·my (kon-drot′ə-me) [*chondro-* + *-tomy*] the dissection or surgical division of cartilage.

chon·dro·tro·phic (kon″dro-tro′fik) [*chondro-* + *-trophic*] having an influence on the formation or growth of cartilage.

Chon·drus (kon′drəs) a genus of red algae. *C. cris′pus* (L.) Stackhouse is a source of carrageenan and chondrus.

chon·drus (kon′drəs) 1. any alga of the genus *Chondrus*. 2. dried and bleached algae, either *Chondrus crispus* or *Gigartina mammillosa*, which contain a polysaccharide widely used as a gel, thickening agent, emulsifier, and demulcent. Called also *carrageen*, *carragheen*, *killeen*, and *Irish*, *pearl*, or *salt rock moss*.

CHOP a cancer chemotherapy regimen consisting of cyclophosphamide, hydroxydaunomycin (doxorubicin), Oncovin (vincristine), and prednisone.

CHOP-BLEO a cancer chemotherapy regimen consisting of cyclophosphamide, hydroxydaunomycin (doxorubicin), Oncovin (vincristine), prednisone, and bleomycin.

Cho·part amputation (operation), joint (sho-pahr′) [François *Chopart*, French surgeon, 1743–1795] see under *amputation*, and see *articulatio tarsi transversa*.

cho·ran·gi·o·ma (ko-ran″je-o′mə) chorioangioma.

cho·ran·gi·o·sis (kor-an″je-o′sis) [*chorion* + *angi-* + *osis*] hypervascularity of the chorionic villi, a manifestation of idiopathic abnormal perfusion of the placenta.

chord (kord) 1. cord. 2. a line segment passing through two points on a curve.
condyle c. condylar axis.

chor·da (kor′də) gen. and pl. *chor′dae* [L., from Gr. *chordē* cord] a cord or sinew.
c. arte′riae umbilica′lis [TA] cord of umbilical artery: a fibrous cord that remains as the obliterated portion of each umbilical artery, extending upward on the abdomen along the urinary bladder, the two then converging in the median plane to reach the umbilicus; each is situated in and produces a medial umbilical fold. Called also *medial umbilical ligament*.
c. dorsa′lis notochord.
c. guberna′culum gubernacular cord: a portion of the gubernaculum testis or of the round ligament of the uterus that develops in the inguinal crest and adjoining body wall.
c. obli′qua membra′nae interos′seae antebra′chii [TA] a small ligamentous band extending from the lateral face of the tuberosity of the ulna to the radius a little distal to its tuberosity; called also *oblique cord of elbow joint*, and *Weitbrecht cord* or *ligament*.
chor′dae tendi′neae cor′dis [TA] the tendinous cords that connect each cusp of the two atrioventricular valves to appropriate papillary muscles

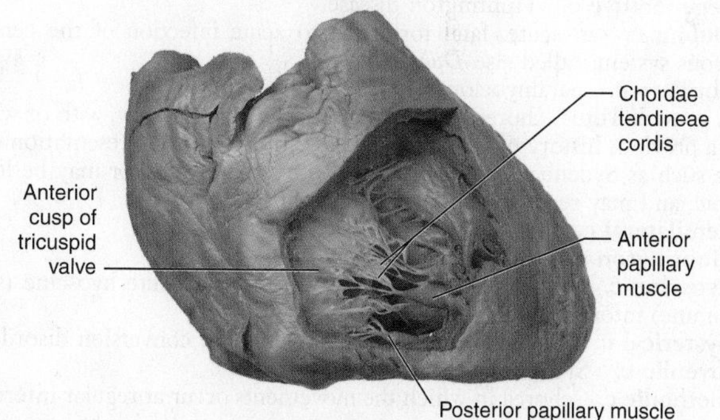

■ Chordae tendineae in a cutaway view of the right ventricle.

in the heart ventricles. The cords are of varying lengths and thicknesses and are frequently branched.

c. tym′pani [TA] a nerve originating from the facial nerve (nervus intermedius) and distributed to the submandibular, sublingual, and lingual glands and the anterior two-thirds of the tongue; modality: parasympathetic and special sensory. Called also *radix parasympathica ganglii submandibularis* [TA alternative] and *radix parasympathica ganglii sublingualis* [TA alternative].

c. voca′lis plica vocalis.

chor·dae (kor′de) [L.] genitive and plural of *chorda*.

chor·dal (kor′dəl) pertaining to any chorda (chiefly used of the notochord).

chor·da-meso·derm (kor″də-mes′o-dərm) tissue of the dorsal lip of the blastopore, which gives rise to both notochord and mesoderm.

Chor·da·ta (kor-da′tə) [L. *chordatus* having a cord] a phylum of the animal kingdom comprising all animals that have a notochord during some stage of their development. It includes the subphyla Cephalochordata, Urochordata, and Vertebrata.

chor·date (kor′dāt) 1. an animal belonging to the phylum Chordata. 2. having a notochord.

chor·dec·to·my (kor-dek′tə-me) [*chord-* + *-ectomy*] cordectomy.

chor·dee (kor′de, kor′da) [Fr. *cordée* corded] downward bowing of the penis as a result of congenital hypospadias or a urethral gonorrhea infection.

chor·di·tis (kor-di′tis) 1. inflammation of a vocal cord. 2. funiculitis (def. 1).

c. fibrino′sa acute laryngitis marked by the deposition of fibrin and the formation of erosions on the vocal cords.

c. nodo′sa c. tuberosa.

c. tubero′sa formation of small whitish nodules *(vocal cord nodules)* on one or both vocal cords, seen in persons who use their voices excessively; called also *c. nodosa*.

c. voca′lis inflammation of the vocal cords.

c. voca′lis infe′rior chronic subglottic laryngitis.

chord(o)- [L. *chorda*, q.v.] a combining form denoting relationship to a cord.

chor·do·car·ci·no·ma (kor″do-kahr″sĭ-no′mə) chordoma.

chor·do·epi·the·li·o·ma (kor″do-ep″ĭ-the″le-o′mə) chordoma.

chor·doid (kor′doid) resembling the notochord.

chor·do·ma (kor-do′mə) [*chord-* + *-oma*] a malignant tumor arising from the embryonic remains of the notochord, usually along the sella or in the sacrococcygeal region; called also *chordocarcinoma* and *chordoepithelioma*. Cf. *ecchondrosis physaliphora*.

chor·do·pexy (kor′do-pek″se) cordopexy.

Chor·do·pox·vi·ri·nae (kor″do-poks″vir-i′ne) poxviruses of vertebrates: a subfamily of viruses of the family Poxviridae, containing the poxviruses that infect vertebrates. It includes the genera *Avipoxvirus*, *Capripoxvirus*, *Leporipoxvirus*, *Orthopoxvirus*, *Parapoxvirus*, *Suipoxvirus*, *Molluscipoxvirus*, and *Yatapoxvirus*.

chor·do·sar·co·ma (kor″do-sahr-ko′mə) chordoma.

chor·do·skel·e·ton (kor″do-skel′ə-ton) [*chordo-* + *skeleton*] that portion of the bony skeleton which is formed around the notochord.

chor·dot·o·my (kor-dot′ə-me) [*chordo-* + *-tomy*] cordotomy.

cho·rea (kə-re′ə) [L., from Gr. *choreia* dance] the occurrence of a variety of continual, rapid, highly complex, jerky, dyskinetic movements that look well-coordinated but are actually involuntary. **chore′al, chore′ic** *adj*

acute c. Sydenham c.

chronic progressive nonhereditary c. senile c.

dancing c. saltatory c.

degenerative c. Huntington disease.

Dubini c. an acute, fatal form due to acute infection of the central nervous system; called also *Dubini disease*.

fibrillary c. paramyoclonus.

c. gravida′rum chorea in the early months of pregnancy, with or without a previous history of rheumatic disease; it may be the presentation of a type such as Sydenham chorea or some other acute type, or may be idiopathic, and may recur in subsequent pregnancies.

hemilateral c. hemichorea.

Huntington c. see under *disease*.

hyoscine c. chorealike movements occurring in acute hyoscine (scopolamine) intoxication.

hysterical c. choreiform movements owing to a conversion disorder.

juvenile c. Sydenham c.

methodic c. chorea in which the movements occur at regular intervals.

c. mi′nor Sydenham c.

c. noctur′na chorea in which the movements continue during sleep.

c. nu′tans 1. chorea with nodding head movements. 2. nodding spasm.

one-sided c. hemichorea.

paralytic c. chorea in which immobility replaces movement.

posthemiplegic c. chorea that affects the partially paralyzed muscles after hemiplegia; see *athetosis*.

saltatory c. any chorea, such as Sydenham chorea, that involves involuntary jumping or dancing movements. See also *saltatory spasm*, under *spasm*.

senile c. a benign, usually mild disorder of the elderly, marked by choreiform movements unassociated with mental disturbance.

simple c. Sydenham c.

Sydenham c. an acute, generally self-limited, neurological disorder seen most often in children between the ages of 5 and 15 years or in women during pregnancy; it is closely linked with rheumatic fever. It is characterized by involuntary movements that gradually become severe and affect all motor activities, including gait, arm movements, and speech. A mild psychic component is usually present. It may be limited to one side of the body (hemichorea) or may take the form of muscular rigidity (paralytic chorea). Called also *acute*, *juvenile*, or *simple c.*, *c. minor*, and *St. Vitus dance*.

cho·rea·bal·lism (kə-re′ə bal′iz-əm) a severe form of chorea in which the limbs are violently flung around.

cho·re·i·form (kə-re′ĭ-form) [*chorea* + *form*] resembling chorea.

chore(o)- [Gr. *choreia* dance] a combining form denoting relationship to chorea.

cho·reo·acan·tho·cy·to·sis (kor″e-o-ə-kan″tho-si-to′sis) [*choreo-* + *acanthocytosis*] an autosomal recessive syndrome caused by mutations in the *VPS13A* gene (locus: 9q21), which encodes a protein of unknown function; it is characterized by tics, chorea, and personality changes, with acanthocytes in the blood. Called also *neuroacanthocytosis*.

cho·reo·ath·e·toid (kor″e-o-ath′ə-toid) pertaining to or characterized by choreoathetosis.

cho·reo·ath·e·to·sis (kor″e-o-ath″ə-to′sis) a condition marked by choreic and athetoid movements.

familial paroxysmal c. Mount-Reback syndrome.

paroxysmal c. Mount-Reback syndrome.

paroxysmal kinesigenic c. an autosomal dominant type in which choreoathetotic movements are provoked by sudden movements or startling.

cho·re·oid (kor′e-oid) choreiform.

chori(o)- [Gr. *chorion* membrane] a combining form denoting relationship to a membrane.

cho·rio·ad·e·no·ma (kor″e-o-ad″ə-no′mə) [*chorio-* + *adenoma*] an adenomatous tumor of the chorion.

c. destru′ens a form of hydatidiform mole in which molar chorionic villi penetrate into the myometrium and/or parametrium or, rarely, are transported to distant sites, most often the lungs; called also *invasive* or *malignant mole*.

cho·rio·al·lan·to·is (kor″e-o-ə-lan′to-is) an extraembryonic structure derived from union of the chorion and allantois which by means of vessels in the associated mesoderm serves in gas exchange. In reptiles and birds, it is a membrane apposed to the egg shell; in many mammals, it forms the placenta. **chorioallanto′ic** *adj*

cho·rio·am·ni·o·ni·tis (kor″e-o-am″ne-o-ni′tis) inflammation of the chorion and amnion.

cho·rio·an·gio·fi·bro·ma (kor″e-o-an″je-o-fi-bro′mə) angiofibroma of the chorion.

cho·rio·an·gi·o·ma (kor″e-o-an″je-o′mə) an angiomatous tumor of the chorion.

cho·rio·blas·to·ma (kor″e-o-blas-to′mə) choriocarcinoma.

cho·rio·blas·to·sis (kor″e-o-blas-to′sis) overgrowth of the chorion.

cho·rio·cap·il·la·ris (kor″e-o-kap″ĭ-lar′is) lamina choroidocapillaris.

cho·rio·car·ci·no·ma (kor″e-o-kahr″sĭ-no′mə) [*chorio-* + *carcinoma*] an epithelial malignancy of trophoblastic cells, formed by the abnormal proliferation of cuboidal and syncytial cells of the placental epithelium, without the production of chorionic villi. Almost all cases arise in the uterus, developing from hydatidiform mole, following abortion, or during normal pregnancy. The remainder occur in ectopic pregnancies and genital (ovarian and testicular) and extragenital teratomas. Called also *chorioblastoma*, *chorioepithelioma*, *chorionic carcinoma* or *epithelioma*, and *syncytioma malignum*.

cho·rio·cele (kor′e-o-sēl″) [*chorio-* + *-cele*[1]] protrusion of the eye through an aperture in the choroid.

cho·rio·epi·the·li·o·ma (kor″e-o-ep″ĭ-the″le-o′mə) choriocarcinoma.

cho·rio·gen·e·sis (kor″e-o-jen′ə-sis) [*chorio-* + *-genesis*] the development of the chorion.

cho•rio•gon•a•do•tro•pin (kor″e-o-go′nə-do-tro″pin) chorionic gonadotropin.

c. alfa human chorionic gonadotropin (q.v.) produced by recombinant technology, used to induce ovulation and pregnancy in anovulatory women in whom the anovulation is secondary and not due to ovarian failure and to induce oocyte maturation in patients attempting conception using assisted reproductive technologies such as gamete intrafallopian transfer (GIFT) or in vitro fertilization; administered subcutaneously.

cho•ri•oid (kor′e-oid) choroid (def. 1).

cho•ri•oi•dea (kor″e-oi′de-ə) choroid (def. 1).

chorioid(o)- for words beginning thus, see those beginning *choroid(o)-*.

cho•ri•o•ma (kor″e-o′mə) [*chori-* + *-oma*] 1. any trophoblastic proliferation, benign or malignant. 2. choriocarcinoma.

cho•rio•mam•mo•tro•pin (ko″re-o-mam′o-tro″pin) human placental lactogen.

cho•rio•men•in•gi•tis (kor″e-o-men″in-ji′tis) cerebral meningitis with lymphocytic infiltration of the choroid plexuses.

lymphocytic c. (LCM) a form of meningitis caused by the lymphocytic choriomeningitis virus, usually occurring in adults 20 to 40 years of age during the late winter months. Infection results from contact with infected rodents and is usually asymptomatic or mild, although severe meningoencephalitis may occur.

cho•ri•on (kor′e-on) [Gr. "membrane"] 1. in human embryology, the cellular, outermost extraembryonic membrane, composed of trophoblast lined with mesoderm; it develops chorionic villi about 2 weeks after fertilization, is vascularized by allantoic vessels a week later, and gives rise to the fetal part of the placenta. 2. in mammalian embryology, the cellular, outer extraembryonic membrane, not necessarily developing villi. 3. in biology, the noncellular membrane covering eggs of various animals, including fish and insects. **cho′rial, chorion′ic** *adj*

bushy c., c. frondo′sum the region of the chorion that bears villi; called also *shaggy c.* or *villous c.*

c. lae′ve the smooth (nonvillous) and membranous part of the chorion. Called also *smooth c.*

primordial c. the chorion from its inception by addition of mesoderm to trophoblast through the stage in which it has many primordial villi.

shaggy c. c. frondosum.

smooth c. c. laeve.

villous c. c. frondosum.

cho•ri•on•epi•the•li•o•ma (kor″e-on-ep″ĭ-the″le-o′mə) choriocarcinoma.

cho•rio•pla•cen•tal (kor″e-o-plə-sen′təl) pertaining to the chorion and the placenta.

Cho•ri•op•tes (kor″e-op′tēz) a genus of parasitic mites of the family Psoroptidae, infesting the skin and hair of domestic animals and causing chorioptic mange.

cho•ri•op•tic (kor″e-op′tik) pertaining to or caused by *Chorioptes.*

cho•rio•ret•i•nal (kor″e-o-ret′ĭ-nəl) pertaining to the choroid and retina.

cho•rio•ret•i•ni•tis (kor″e-o-ret′ĭ-ni′tis) [*chorio-* + *retinitis*] inflammation of the choroid and retina; retinochoroiditis.

c. sclopeta′ria a concussive, nonpenetrating injury characterized by choroidal and retinal rupturing, hemorrhage, fibrosis, retinal destruction, and poor vision; caused by orbital injury from a missile such as a bullet.

toxoplasmic c. a unilateral or bilateral condition seen most often as a late sequel of congenital toxoplasmosis, with recurrent episodes of ocular pain and decreased vision with progressive visual loss; there are deep, heavily pigmented, necrotic lesions in both the macular and peripheral retina, as well as posterior uveitis. Called also *ocular toxoplasmosis* and *toxoplasmic retinochoroiditis.*

cho•rio•ret•i•nop•a•thy (kor″e-o-ret″ĭ-nop′ə-the) [*chorio-* + *retinopathy*] a noninflammatory process involving both choroid and retina.

cho•ris•to•blas•to•ma (kor-is″to-blas-to′mə) [*choristoma* + *blastoma*] choristoma.

cho•ris•to•ma (kor″is-to′mə) [Gr. *chōristos* separated + *-oma*] a mass of tissue histologically normal for an organ or part of the body other than the site at which it is located; called also *aberrant rest, choristoblastoma, heterotopia,* and *heterotopic tissue.*

cho•roid (kor′oid) [*chori-* + *-oid*] 1. the thin, pigmented, vascular coat of the eyeball extending from the ora serrata to the optic nerve; it furnishes blood supply to the retina and conducts arteries and nerves to the anterior structures. Called also *chorioid, choroidea* [TA], and *chorioidea.* 2. resembling the chorion.

cho•roid•al (kor-oid′əl) pertaining to the choroid (def. 1).

cho•roi•dea (kor-oid′e-ə) [TA] choroid (def. 1).

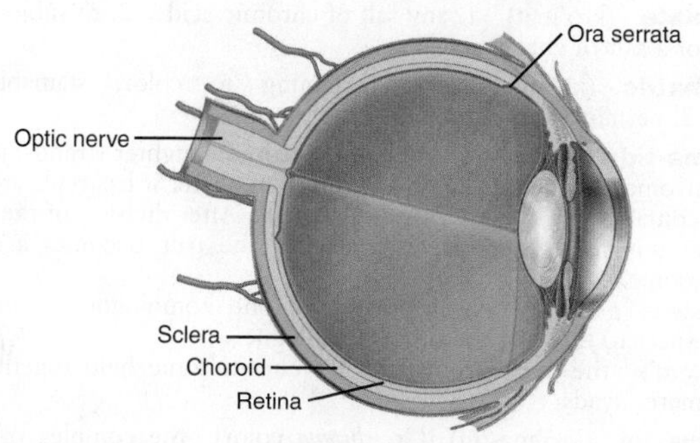

■ Choroid shown in relation to other coats and related structures of the eye.

cho•roid•ec•to•my (kor″oid-ek′tə-me) surgical removal or destruction of the choroid plexus of the lateral ventricles of the brain.

cho•roid•er•e•mia (kor″oid-ər-e′me-ə) [*choroid-* + Gr. *erēmia* destitution] hereditary primary choroidal degeneration, transmitted as an X-linked trait and beginning in the first decade of life. In males, the earliest symptom is usually night blindness, followed by constricted visual field and eventual blindness as the degeneration of the pigmented layer of the retina progresses to complete atrophy. In females, it is nonprogressive; usually there is normal vision and often an atypical pigmentary retinopathy. Called also *progressive tapetochoroidal dystrophy.*

cho•roid•itis (kor″oid-i′tis) [*choroido-* + *-itis*] uveitis affecting the choroid, the posterior portion of the uveal tract.

acute diffuse serous c. 1. a type of choroiditis having a sudden onset in adults, characterized by widespread, yellowish, fundal edema, by retinal detachment with loss of sight, and by later retinal reattachment with probable restoration of sight. 2. Vogt-Koyanagi-Harada syndrome.

areolar c., areolar central c. a type of choroiditis that starts around or near the macula lutea and progresses toward the periphery. Unlike in other types, lesions in this type first are pigmented but then lose their pigmentation. Called also *Förster c.* or *disease.*

Doyne familial honeycomb c., Doyne honeycomb c. Doyne honeycomb dystrophy.

exudative c. choroiditis characterized by scattered patches of an exudate.

Förster c. areolar c.

metastatic c. choroiditis due to metastasis, such as of pyemia or meningitis.

suppurative c. choroiditis that leads to the formation of pus.

choroid(o)- a combining form denoting relationship to the choroid.

cho•roi•do•cyc•li•tis (kor-oi″do-sik-li′tis) uveitis in the choroid and ciliary processes.

cho•roi•do•iri•tis (kor-oi″do-i-ri′tis) uveitis in the choroid coat and the iris.

cho•roid•op•a•thy (kor″oid-op′ə-the) choroiditis.

cho•roi•do•ret•i•ni•tis (kor-oi″do-ret″ĭ-ni′tis) chorioretinitis.

Chot•zen syndrome (kot′zən) [Fritz *Chotzen,* German psychiatrist, 1871–1937] see under *syndrome.*

chr chromosome.

Christ-Sie•mens-Tou•raine syndrome (krist′ se′mənz too-ren′) [Josef *Christ,* German dermatologist, 1871–1948; Hermann Werner *Siemens,* German dermatologist, 1891–1969; Henri *Touraine,* French dermatologist, 1883–1961] anhidrotic ectodermal dysplasia.

Chris•tian disease (syndrome) (kris′chən) [Henry Asbury *Christian,* American physician, 1876–1951] Hand-Schüller-Christian disease.

Chris•tian-We•ber disease (kris′chən va′bər) [H.A. *Christian;* Frederick Parkes *Weber,* English physician, 1863–1962] relapsing febrile nodular nonsuppurative panniculitis.

Christ•mas disease, factor (kris′məs) [Stephen *Christmas,* 20th century Englishman, the first patient with the disease who was studied in detail] see *hemophilia B* and see *factor IX* at *coagulation factors,* under *factor.*

chro•maf•fin (kro-maf′in) [*chromium-* + L. *affinis* having affinity for] taking up and staining strongly with chromium salts; see *chromaffin cells,* under *cell.* Called also *pheochrome.*

chro•maf•fin•i•ty (kro″mə-fin′ĭ-te) the property of staining strongly with chrome salts.

chro•maf•fi•no•ma (kro-maf″ĭ-no′mə) any tumor containing chromaffin cells, such as a pheochromocytoma.

medullary c. pheochromocytoma.

chro•maf•fi•nop•a•thy (kro-maf″ĭ-nop′ə-the) [*chromaffin* + *-pathy*] any disease of the chromaffin system.

chro•mate (kro′māt) 1. any salt of chromic acid. 2. to subject to the action of a salt of chromic acid.

chro•mat•ic (kro-mat′ik) 1. pertaining to color; stainable with dyes. 2. pertaining to chromatin.

chro•ma•tid (kro′mə-tid) one of the paired daughter strands, joined at the centromere, which make up a chromosome after it has replicated, each strand containing a single DNA double helix. After division of the centromere in mitosis or meiosis, each one of the pair becomes a separate chromosome.

nonsister c's the two chromatids of one homologous chromosome with respect to those of the other homologue.

sister c's the two chromatids of a chromosome held together by a centromere; dyads.

chro•ma•tin (kro′mə-tin) [Gr. *chrōma* color] the complex of nucleic acids (DNA and RNA) and proteins (primarily histones, but also nonhistone proteins) in the eukaryotic cell nucleus, comprising the chromosomes (q.v.). See also *euchromatin* and *heterochromatin*. **chromatin′ic** *adj*

sex c. Barr body.

chro•ma•tin-neg•a•tive (kro″mə-tin-neg′ə-tiv) lacking sex chromatin (Barr body); characteristic of the somatic cell nuclei of normal human males or other individuals with only one X chromosome.

chro•ma•tin-pos•i•tive (kro″mə-tin-poz′ĭ-tiv) containing sex chromatin (Barr body); characteristic of the somatic cell nuclei of normal human females or other individuals with two (or more) X chromosomes.

chro•ma•tism (kro′mə-tiz″əm) abnormal pigment deposits.

chro•ma•tize (kro′mə-tīz) to charge with some chromium compound.

chromat(o)- [Gr. *chrōma*, gen. *chrōmatos* color] a combining form denoting relationship to (1) color, or (2) chromatin.

chro•mato•blast (kro-mat′o-blast) [*chromato-* + *-blast*] a cell that can become a chromatophore, or bearer of pigment.

chro•ma•tog•e•nous (kro″mə-toj′ə-nəs) [*chromato-* + *-genous*] producing color or coloring matter.

chro•mato•gram (kro-mat′o-gram) [*chromato-* + *gram*] originally, the pattern of bands of substances separated by column chromatography, so called because the technique was first used to separate plant pigments producing a pattern of colored bands; by extension, a permanent record produced by any form of chromatography, e.g., in paper or thin-layer chromatography, a dried and stained filter paper or plate and, in gas or high-performance liquid chromatography, the chart recorder output.

chro•mato•graph (kro-mat′o-graf) 1. the apparatus used in chromatography. 2. to analyze by chromatography.

chro•ma•tog•ra•phy (kro″mə-tog′rə-fe) any of a diverse group of techniques used to separate mixtures of substances based on differences in the relative affinities of the substances for two different media, one (the mobile phase) a moving fluid and the other (the stationary phase or sorbent) a porous solid or gel or a liquid coated on a solid support; the speed at which each substance is carried along by the mobile phase depends on its solubility (in a liquid mobile phase) or vapor pressure (in a gas mobile phase) and on its affinity for the sorbent. **chromatograph′ic** *adj*

adsorption c. chromatography in which the stationary phase is a nonspecific adsorbent, such as silica gel, porous polymers, or charcoal.

affinity c. chromatography based on a highly specific biologic interaction such as that between antigen and antibody, enzyme and substrate, or receptor and ligand. Any of these substances, covalently linked to an insoluble support or immobilized in a gel, may serve as the sorbent allowing the interacting substance to be isolated from relatively impure samples; often a 1000-fold purification can be achieved in one step.

column c. a type of chromatography using a sorbent packed in a column. The sample, dissolved in a solvent, is poured in the top. Some components are retained in the column bound to the sorbent. They are then washed out (eluted) in successive aliquots of the same solvent (more strongly bound components being eluted later) or of different solvents.

exclusion c. gel filtration c.

gas c. (GC) an automated type of chromatography in which the sample, dissolved in a solvent, is vaporized and carried by an inert gas through a column packed with a sorbent to any of several types of detector. Each component of the sample, separated from the others by passage through the column, produces a separate peak in the detector output, which is graphed by a chart recorder. The sorbent may be an inert porous solid *(gas-solid c.)* or a nonvolatile liquid coated on a solid support *(gas-liquid c.)*.

gas-liquid c. (GLC) see *gas c.*

gas-solid c. (GSC) see *gas c.*

gel filtration c., gel permeation c. a type of chromatography in which the stationary phase consists of gel-forming hydrophilic beads containing pores of an accurately controlled size. As the sample is carried through the gel, small molecules are frequently trapped in the pores and delayed while larger molecules pass unimpeded. Sample components are thus separated on the basis of size and shape. Called also *molecular exclusion c.* and *molecular sieve c.*

high-performance liquid c., high-pressure liquid c. (HPLC) an automated type of chromatography in which the mobile phase is a liquid, which is forced under high pressure through a column packed with a sorbent. As in gas chromatography, a detector at the end of the column coupled to a chart recorder graphs the sample efflux. Various separation methods, including adsorption, gel filtration, ion exchange, and partition, are used.

ion exchange c. chromatography in which the stationary phase is an ion exchange resin. The mobile phase is an aqueous buffer solution that determines the degree of ionization of the sample components and thus their affinity for the stationary phase.

liquid-liquid c. partition c.

molecular exclusion c., molecular sieve c. gel filtration c.

paper c. a type of chromatography in which the stationary phase is a sheet of special-grade filter paper; it is in all other aspects similar to thin-layer chromatography (q.v.).

partition c. chromatography in which the stationary and mobile phases are immiscible liquids and the sample components are separated on the basis of their partition coefficients. Called also *liquid-liquid c.*

thin-layer c. (TLC) chromatography in which the stationary phase is a thin layer of an adsorbent, e.g., silica gel, coated on a rectangular plate and the mobile phase is a solvent mixture. The sample is applied to a small spot on the plate, and then the plate is stood on end with its lower edge in solvent. As the solvent rises by capillary action through the adsorbent, the components of the sample are carried along at different rates and can be visualized as a row of spots after the plate is dried and stained or viewed under ultraviolet light.

chro•ma•toid (kro′mə-toid) dying or staining like, or otherwise resembling, chromatin; see also under *body*.

chro•ma•tol•y•sis (kro″mə-tol′ə-sis) [*chromato-* + *-lysis*] disintegration of the Nissl (chromophil) bodies of a nerve cell as the result of injury, or of fatigue or exhaustion; a part of the axon reaction (q.v.).

chro•ma•tom•e•ter (kro″mə-tom′ə-tər) [*chromato-* + *-meter*] an instrument for measuring color or color perception; called also *chromatoptometer*, *chromometer*, and *chromoptometer*.

chro•ma•to•phil (kro-mat′o-fil″) a cell or element that stains easily.

chro•ma•to•phile (kro′mə-to-fīl″) 1. chromatophil. 2. chromatophilic.

chro•ma•to•phil•ia (kro″mə-to-fil′e-ə) [*chromato-* + *-philia*] the condition of staining easily.

chro•ma•to•phil•ic (kro″mə-to-fil′ik) staining easily.

chro•ma•toph•i•lous (kro″mə-tof′ĭ-ləs) chromatophilic.

chro•mato•phore (kro-mat′o-for″) [*chromato-* + *-phore*] 1. a pigment cell of the skin, such as a melanocyte or melanophore. 2. a color-producing plastid found in certain plants and protozoa.

chro•ma•to•pho•ro•tro•pic (kro″mə-to-for″o-tro′pik) having an influence or effect on chromatophores, such as the pigmentary effect of melanocyte-stimulating hormone.

chro•ma•top•sia (kro″mə-top′se-ə) [*chromato-* + *-opsia*] a visual defect in which colored objects appear unnaturally colored and colorless objects appear tinged with color. The chromatopsias are named for the colors seen: cyanopsia, blue; chloropsia, green; erythropsia, red; xanthopsia, yellow. Chromatopsia may be caused by drugs, disturbance of the optic centers, cataract extraction, or dazzling light.

chro•ma•top•tom•e•ter (kro″mə-top-tom′ə-tər) chromatometer.

chro•ma•top•tom•e•try (kro″mə-top-tom′ə-tre) the testing of the power of discriminating colors.

chro•mato•scope (kro-mat′o-skōp) [*chromato-* + *-scope*] an instrument used in chromatoscopy (def. 1).

chro•ma•tos•co•py (kro″mə-tos′kə-pe) [*chromato-* + *-scopy*] 1. the testing of color vision. 2. diagnosis of renal function by the color of the urine following the administration of dyes.

gastric c. diagnosis of gastric function by the color of the gastric contents; a test for achylia gastrica.

chro•ma•tot•ro•pism (kro″mə-tot′rə-piz-əm) [*chromato-* + *tropism*] an orienting response to a color.

chro•ma•tu•ria (kro″mə-tu′re-ə) [*chromato-* + *-uria*] abnormal coloration of the urine.

-chrome [Gr. *chroma* color] a word termination denoting relationship to color.

chro•mes•the•sia (kro″mes-the′zhə) [*chrom-* + *esthesia*] the association of imaginary sensations of color with actual sensations of hearing, taste, or smell; see *photism*.

chrom•hi•dro•sis (kro″mĭ-dro′sis) [*chrom-* + *hidro-* + *-sis*] a rare condition in which the sweat is colored because it contains pigments or other proteins. Called also *chromidrosis*.

chro•mic (kro′mik) of, pertaining to, or related to chromium; used particularly for compounds in which chromium is in the trivalent state or for the hexavalent acid.

c. chloride [USP] the trichloride salt of chromium, $CrCl_3$, used as a supplement for the treatment of chromium deficiency; administered intravenously.

c. phosphate P 32 [USP] the phosphate salt of chromium, labeled with radiophosphorus (^{32}P); a colloidal suspension administered intraperitoneally or intrapleurally in the treatment of intraperitoneal or intrapleural effusions resulting from metastatic disease and intrastitially in the treatment of certain ovarian and prostate carcinomas.

chro•mic ac•id (kro′mik) the common name for chromium trioxide (CrO_3), although the term strictly refers to the species H_2CrO_4, which exists only in aqueous solution. It is a highly toxic, corrosive, strong oxidizing agent.

chro•mi•cize (kro′mĭ-sīz) to treat with a chromium compound.

chro•mi•dro•sis (kro″mĭ-dro′sis) chromhidrosis.

chro•mist (kro′mist) an individual organism belonging to the Chromista.

Chro•mis•ta (kro′mis-tə) [Gr. *chrōma* color, by analogy with *Protista*] a eukaryotic taxon, classified by some authorities as a kingdom and by others as part of the Protista, consisting mainly of photosynthetic organisms that contain chlorophyll *c*. It comprises a wide variety of organisms, including diatoms, kelps, and a group of nonphotosynthetic organisms formerly classified among the fungi (the Oomycota, or water molds).

chro•mi•um (Cr) (kro′me-əm) [L., from Gr. *chrōma* color] a blue-white, brittle metal, atomic number 24, atomic weight 51.996, specific gravity 7.1; several of its compounds are pigments, and the metal itself is used for weather-resistant plating; it is also an important component of most base metal alloys used in dentistry. Chromium plays a role in glucose metabolism and is considered essential in trace amounts in nutrition. Hexavalent chromium is carcinogenic.

c. 51 a radioactive isotope of chromium, atomic mass 51, having a half-life of 27.7 days; it decays by electron capture, emitting gamma rays (0.32 MeV), and is used to label red blood cells for measurement of red cell mass or volume, survival time, and sequestration studies; for the diagnosis of gastrointestinal bleeding; and to label platelets to study their survival. It has also been used to label human serum albumin for measurements of gastrointestinal protein loss.

c. Cr 51 edetate [USP] a complex of chromium 51 with edetic acid, used in the measurement of the glomerular filtration rate.

c. picolinate [NF] a biologically active form of chromium, used as a nutritional supplement.

c. trioxide see *chromic acid.*

chrom(o)- [Gr. *chrōma* color] a combining form denoting relationship to color.

Chro•mo•bac•te•ri•um (kro″mo-bak-tēr′e-əm) [*chromo-* + *bacterium*] a genus of gram-negative, aerobic or facultatively anaerobic, usually nonpathogenic, rod-shaped bacteria of the family Neisseriaceae, found in soil and water in tropical countries, characteristically producing violet pigment that is soluble in alcohol but not in water or chloroform. The type species is *C. viola′ceum.*

C. viola′ceum a species that can cause abscesses, diarrhea, urinary tract infections, and systemic infections.

chro•mo•blast (kro′mo-blast) [*chromo-* + *-blast*] an embryonic cell that develops into a pigment cell.

chro•mo•blas•to•my•co•sis (kro″mo-blas″to-mi-ko′sis) [*chromo-* + *blasto-* + *mycosis*] a chronic fungal infection of the skin, usually beginning at the site of a puncture wound or other trauma and affecting one lower limb or foot (mossy foot) but sometimes involving other areas of the body, producing wartlike nodules or papillomas that may or may not ulcerate; microscopically, the lesions are characterized by round, brown bodies (sclerotic bodies) that reproduce by equatorial splitting and not by budding. It is usually caused by dematiaceous fungi such as *Phialophora verrucosa, Fonsecaea pedrosoi, F. compactum,* or *Cladosporium carrionii.* Called also *chromomycosis* and *verrucose* or *verrucous dermatitis.*

chro•mo•cen•ter (kro′mo-sen″tər) [*chromo-* + *center* (def. 1)] a fused, condensed mass of heterochromatin representing a point of attachment of polytene chromosomes.

chro•mo•cho•los•co•py (kro″mo-ko-los′kə-pe) [*chromo-* + *cholo-* + *-scopy*] testing the biliary function by a pigment excretion test (methylthionine chloride).

chro•mo•cys•tos•co•py (kro″mo-sis-tos′kə-pe) [*chromo-* + *cystoscopy*] examination of the interior of the bladder after administration of indigo carmine or other dye that is excreted in the urine, for identification and study of the activity of the ureteral orifices.

chro•mo•cyte (kro′mo-sīt) [*chromo-* + *-cyte*] any colored cell or pigmented corpuscle.

chro•mo•dac•ry•or•rhea (kro″mo-dak″re-o-re′ə) [*chromo-* + *dacryo-* + *-rrhea*] the shedding of bloody tears.

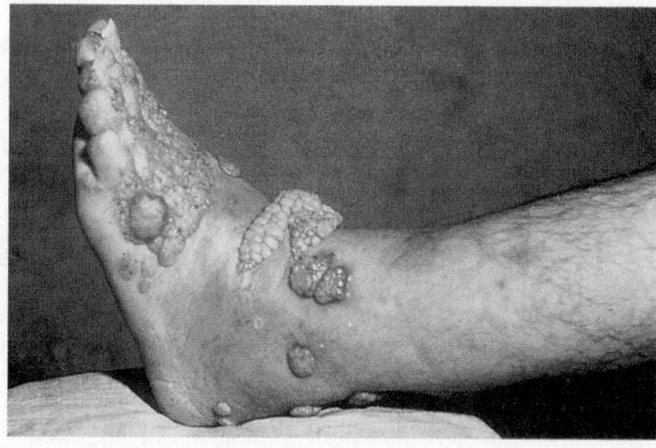

■ Chromoblastomycosis.

chro•mo•di•ag•no•sis (kro″mo-di″əg-no′sis) [*chromo-* + *diagnosis*] 1. diagnosis by change of color. 2. diagnosis of functional derangements by observing the rate at which coloring matters, such as methylthionine chloride, are excreted. 3. diagnostic examination made through colored glass or sheets of colored gelatin.

chro•mo•gen (kro′mo-jən) 1. a chemical compound, itself without color, that can be transformed into a colored compound or can react with another material to form a colored compound. 2. a microorganism that produces pigment, e.g., certain strains of *Mycobacterium* that produce yellow to red colonies.

Porter-Silber c. a 17-hydroxycorticosteroid with a dihydroxyacetone side chain; these react positively in the Porter-Silber reaction.

chro•mo•gen•e•sis (kro″mo-jen′ə-sis) [*chromo-* + *genesis*] the formation of pigments or colors, as by bacterial action.

chro•mo•gen•ic (kro″mo-jen′ik) producing a pigment or coloring matter.

chro•mo•gran•in (kro″mo-gran′in) any of a group of acidic polypeptides that are the major soluble protein constituents of the secretory granules of the chromaffin cells of the adrenal medulla; they are also widely distributed in endocrine tissues and tumor cells. Some are precursors of peptide hormones.

chro•mo•isom•er•ism (kro″mo-i-som′ər-iz-əm) [*chromo-* + *isomerism*] isomerism in which the isomers have different colors.

chro•mo•mere (kro′mo-mēr) [*chromo-* + *-mere*] 1. one of the series of beadlike granules occurring along eukaryotic chromosomes, representing localized coiling and condensation of the chromatin, as seen in the leptotene and zygotene stages of meiosis. The term is also used to denote such condensed chromatin regions at the base of loops in lampbrush chromosomes as well as condensed bands in polytene chromosomes. 2. granulomere.

chro•mom•e•ter (kro-mom′ə-tər) 1. chromatometer. 2. colorimeter.

chro•mo•my•co•sis (kro″mo-mi-ko′sis) chromoblastomycosis.

chro•mo•ne•ma (kro″mo-ne′mə) pl. *chromone′mata* [*chromo-* + *nema*] the coiled central thread of a chromatid, as opposed to the more densely coiled chromomere regions. **chromone′mal** *adj*

chro•mo•ne•ma•ta (kro″mo-ne′mə-tə) plural of *chromonema.*

chro•mo•neme (kro′mo-nēm) chromonema.

chro•mo•nych•ia (kro″mo-nik′e-ə) discoloration of the nails, such as in leukonychia or melanonychia.

chro•mo•pexy (kro′mo-pek″se) [*chromo-* + *-pexy*] the fixation of pigment, a term applied especially to the function of the liver in forming bilirubin. **chromopec′tic** *adj*

chro•mo•phane (kro′mo-fān) [*chromo-* + Gr. *phainein* to show] a retinal pigment found in some species of animals.

chro•mo•phil (kro′mo-fil) [*chromo-* + *-phil*] any easily stainable cell, structure, or tissue.

chro•mo•phile (kro′mo-fīl) 1. chromophil. 2. chromophilic.

chro•mo•phil•ic (kro-mo-fil′ik) readily or easily stained; said especially of certain leukocytes and other histologic elements.

chro•moph•i•lous (kro-mof′ĭ-ləs) chromophilic.

chro•mo•phobe (kro′mo-fōb) [*chromo-* + Gr. *phobos* fear] any cell, structure, or tissue that does not stain readily, such as the nonstaining cells of the adenohypophysis.

chro•mo•pho•bia (kro″mo-fo′be-ə) the quality of staining poorly with dyes.

chro•mo•phore (kro′mo-for) any chemical group whose presence gives a decided color to a compound and which unites with certain other groups (auxochromes) to form dyes; called also *color radical.*

chro•mo•phor•ic (kro″mo-for′ik) [*chromo-* + Gr. *pherein* to bear] 1. bearing color; said of chromogenic bacteria when the pigment is a component of the bacterial cell itself. 2. pertaining to a chromophore.

chro•moph•o•rous (kro-mof′ər-əs) chromophoric.

chro•mo•phose (kro′mo-fōs) [*chromo-* + *phose*] a subjective sensation of a spot of color in the eye.

chro•mo•plast (kro′mo-plast) chromoplastid.

chro•mo•plas•tid (kro″mo-plas′tid) [*chromo-* + *plastid*] any pigment-producing plastid other than a chloroplast.

chro•mo•pro•tein (kro″mo-pro′tēn) [*chromo-* + *protein*] a colored conjugated protein. Examples are the red hemoglobin of the higher animals, the blue hemocyanin of more primitive animals, and the red and blue pigments of seaweeds. Chromoproteins have respiratory functions and are closely related to the green chlorophyll of the higher plants.

chro•mop•sia (kro-mop′se-ə) chromatopsia.

chro•mop•tom•e•ter (kro″mop-tom′ə-tər) chromatoptometer.

chro•mo•ret•i•nog•ra•phy (kro″mo-ret″ĭ-nog′rə-fe) [*chromo-* + *retina* + *-graphy*] color photography of the retina.

chro•mo•rhi•nor•rhea (kro″mo-ri″no-re′ə) [*chromo-* + *rhinorrhea*] the discharge of a pigmented secretion from the nose.

chro•mo•scope (kro′mo-skōp) chromatoscope.

chro•mos•co•py (kro-mos′kə-pe) chromatoscopy.

chro•mo•some (chr) (kro′mə-sōm) [*chromo-* + *-some*] 1. in eukaryotic cells, a structure in the nucleus consisting of chromatin (q.v.) and carrying the genetic information for the cell. Each organism of a species is normally characterized by the same number of chromosomes in its somatic cells; 46 is the usual number in humans, including the two (XX or XY) that determine the sex of the organism. During cell division, the chromatin is compactly coiled and supercoiled, making the chromosome visible with appropriate staining and permitting its movement in the cell with minimal entanglement. The hierarchical levels of compaction begin with the DNA double helix, which is coiled into nucleosomes; the nucleosomes supercoil into 30-nm diameter chromatin fibers, and the chromatin fibers are packed into 100 kb loops attached to a nonhistone protein scaffold to form the condensed chromosome. 2. the analogous structure carrying the genetic material in prokaryotes, mitochondria, and chloroplasts; a closed circle of double-stranded DNA. **chromoso′mal** *adj*

Symbols Used in Chromosome Nomenclature

A–G	Chromosome groups
1–22	Autosome numbers
X, Y	Sex chromosomes
/	Diagonal line separating cell lines in descriptions of mosaicism
?	Identification of chromosome or chromosome structure questionable
+ –	When placed before the chromosome number, these denote addition or loss of a whole chromosome; when placed after the chromosome number, they denote an increase or decrease in length of a chromosome part.
:	Break with no reunion
::	Break with reunion
→	From ... to ...
ace	Acentric
cen	Centromere
del	Deletion
der	Derivative chromosome
dic	Dicentric
dup	Duplication
end	Endoreduplication
h	Secondary constriction or negatively staining region
I	Isochromosome
ins	Insertion
inv	Inversion
inv ins	Inverted insertion
mar	Marker chromosome
mat	Maternal origin
p	Short arm
pat	Paternal origin
q	Long arm
r	Ring chromosome
rep	Reciprocal translocation
rec	Recombinant chromosome
rob	Robertsonian translocation
s	Satellite
t	Translocation
ter	Terminal

Repeated symbols denote duplication of chromosome structure.
Symbols for rearrangements are placed before the chromosome number and the rearranged chromosomes are placed in parenthesis, e.g., t(14q21q), r(18).

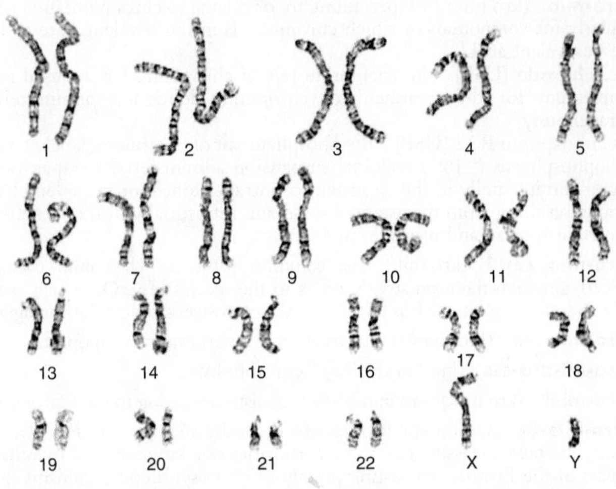

■ Human male chromosomes with GTG banding, arranged as a karyotype.

A c. a term used to denote one of the chromosomes normally present in an organism, as contrasted with a B chromosome.
accessory c's B c.
acentric c. a chromosome with no centromere.
acrocentric c. a chromosome with the centromere near one end. In humans such chromosomes have satellited short arms that carry hundreds of copies of genes for ribosomal RNA.
B c. one or more extra chromosomes found inconstantly in wild populations of certain species; they are not homologous to members of the regular set of chromosomes, are often heterochromatic and telocentric, have an irregular and nonmendelian pattern of inheritance, and exert little influence on the phenotype. Called also *accessory* or *B c.*
bacterial artificial c. (BAC) a genetically engineered cloning vector based on a bacterial plasmid; it can accept large (approximately 300 kb) inserts of foreign DNA and be introduced into and propagated in bacteria; used for cloning, mapping, and sequencing.
bivalent c. see *bivalent* (def. 2).
daughter c's the name for chromatids when they reach the poles of the cell in the anaphase stage of mitosis or the anaphase II stage of meiosis.
dicentric c. a structurally abnormal chromosome with two centromeres.
giant c. 1. polytene c. 2. lampbrush c.
homologous c's a matching pair of chromosomes, one from each parent, with the same gene loci in the same order.
lampbrush c. a giant chromosome with hundreds of paired loops extending laterally from the main axis, giving it a fuzzy, brushlike appearance at low magnification; most easily seen in primary oocytes of amphibians and used to study transcription.
m-c. mitochondrial genome.
metacentric c. a chromosome with its centromere in the center and arms of equal length.
mitochondrial c. see under *genome.*
Ph[1] **c., Philadelphia c.** an abnormality of chromosome 22 present in marrow cells of most patients with chronic granulocytic leukemia; it is generally a reciprocal translocation between chromosomes 9 and 22, involving breaks at 9q34 and 22q11. The translocation results in expression of a fusion gene (called *BCR-ABL*) that acts as an oncogene.
polytene c. a giant cablelike chromosome composed of numerous identical chromatids arranged in parallel, resulting from many rounds of DNA replication in the absence of chromatid separation and occurring especially in the salivary glands of some insects. Localized hypercoiling of the chromatids produces a characteristic banding pattern, perpendicular to the main axis, that has been used as a cytologic landmark.
recombinant c. a chromosome that results from recombination between two homologous chromosomes during meiosis; see *recombination* (def. 2).
ring c. (r) a chromosome in which both ends have been lost (deletion) and the two broken ends have reunited to form a ring. See illustration at *aberration.*
sex c's chromosomes that are associated with the determination of sex, in mammals constituting an unequal pair, the X and Y chromosomes.
somatic c. autosome.
submetacentric c. a chromosome with its centromere slightly off-center so that the arms are different in length.
supernumerary c. B c.
telocentric c. a chromosome with a terminal centromere; not normally found in humans.
W c. a sex chromosome of certain insects, birds, and fishes, in which the female is heterogametic (i.e., has a W and a Z chromosome) and the males are homogametic (having only Z chromosomes).

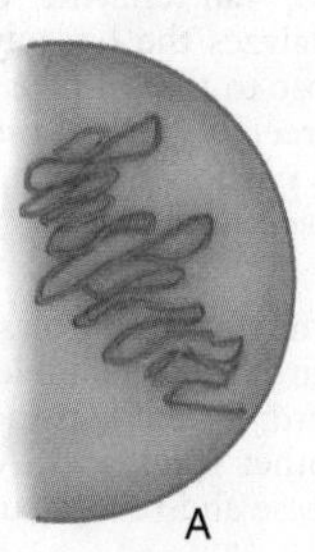
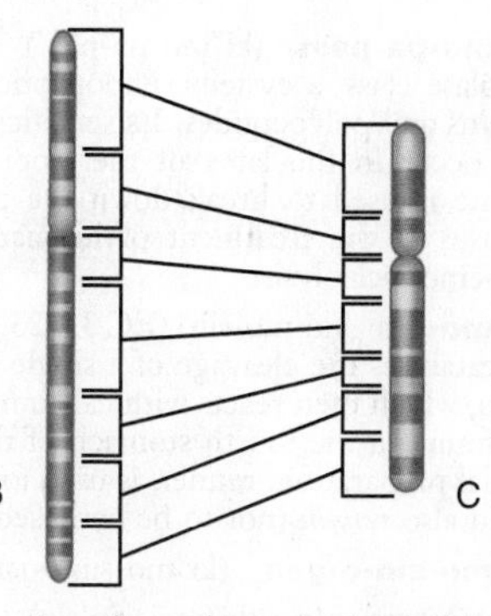

■ Chromosome. *(A)*, Long, threadlike interphase chromatin in nucleus. *(B)*, Giemsa-stained, partially condensed chromatid in late prophase. *(C)*, Giemsa-stained, fully condensed chromatid in metaphase; note that some of the sub-bands visible in late prophase have condensed into single bands. (In *B* and *C*, only one of a pair of sister chromatids is shown.)

X c. the sex chromosome present in two copies in female somatic cells of organisms in which the male is the heterogametic sex, as in humans; it is carried by half the male gametes and all female gametes.

Y c. the sex chromosome present in male somatic cells, but not female, of organisms in which the male is the heterogametic sex, as in humans; it is carried by half the male gametes and none of the female gametes.

yeast artificial c. (YAC) a genetically engineered chromosome that can be replicated in the yeast *Saccharomyces cerevisiae*, consisting of a foreign DNA segment inserted into a synthetic minichromosome that contains yeast elements including a centromere, fused telomeres, a replication origin, and marker genes; it allows the cloning and isolation of much larger DNA segments than is possible using conventional cloning vectors.

Z c. see *W c.*

chro•mo•ther•a•py (kro″mo-ther′ə-pe) color therapy.

chro•mo•tox•ic (kro′mo-tok″sik) [*chromo-* + *toxic*] destructive to hemoglobin or due to the destruction of hemoglobin.

chro•mo•trich•ia (kro″mo-trik′e-ə) [*chromo-* + *trich-* + *-ia*] the coloring of the hair.

chro•mo•trich•i•al (kro″mo-trik′e-əl) pertaining to hair color.

chro•mo•tro•pic (kro″mo-tro′pik) [*chromo-* + *-tropic*] turning to or attracting color or pigment.

chro•nax•ie (kro′nak-se) chronaxy.

chro•naxy (kro′nak-se) [*chron-* + Gr. *axios* fit] the minimum time an electric current must flow at a voltage twice the rheobase to cause a muscle to contract.

chron•ic (kron′ik) [L. *chronicus*, from Gr. *chronos* time] persisting over a long period of time.

chro•nic•i•ty (kro-nis′ĭ-te) the quality of being chronic.

chron(o)- [Gr. *chronos* time] a combining form denoting relationship to time.

chron•o•bi•o•log•ic (kron″o-bi″o-loj′ik) pertaining to chronobiology; relating to the effects of time and biologic rhythms on living systems. Written also *chronobiological.*

chron•o•bi•ol•o•gist (kron″o-bi-ol′ə-jist) a specialist in chronobiology.

chron•o•bi•ol•o•gy (kron″o-bi-ol′ə-je) [*chrono-* + *biology*] the scientific study of the effect of time on living systems.

chron•og•no•sis (kron″og-no′sis) [*chrono-* + Gr. *gnōsis* knowledge] the subjective appreciation of the passage of time.

chron•o•graph (kron′o-graf) [*chrono-* + *-graph*] an instrument for recording small intervals of time.

chro•nom•e•try (kro-nom′ə-tre) [*chrono-* + *-metry*] the measurement of time or intervals of time.

mental c. the measurement and study of the duration of mental processes.

chron•o•pho•bia (kron″o-fo′be-ə) [*chrono-* + *-phobia*] extreme, irrational fear of time; because it is so common in prisoners, it is sometimes called *prison neurosis* (q.v.).

chron•o•scope (kron′o-skōp) [*chrono-* + *-scope*] an instrument for measuring minute intervals of time.

chro•no•tar•ax•is (kron″o-tər-ak′sis) [*chrono-* + Gr. *taraxis* confusion] disorientation for time; observed as a transient symptom following thalamic or frontal lobe lesions.

chro•no•ther•a•py (kron′o-ther″ə-pe) treatment of certain sleep disorders by capitalizing on the natural phase delay in adults; the bedtime is successively advanced by one to several hours each day until the individual can retire, sleep, and arise at appropriate times.

chron•o•tro•pic (kron″o-tro′pik) [*chrono-* + *-tropic*] affecting the time or rate, as the rate of contraction of the heart.

chro•not•ro•pism (kro-not′ro-piz-əm) modulation of the regularity of a periodic movement, such as the heart beat.

chrys•a•lis (kris′ə-lis) [L.] the pupa of some insects, especially of a moth or butterfly.

Chry•san•the•mum (krĭ-san′thə-məm) a genus of perennial flowering herbs of the family Compositae, native to the Balkans and the Middle East, some of which were formerly classified in genus *Pyrethrum.* They are a common cause of allergic contact dermatitis, and their powdered flowers are insecticidal and scabicidal and a source of pyrethrins.

chry•sene (kri′sēn) a carcinogenic tetracyclic hydrocarbon derived from coal tar by distillation and used in organic synthesis.

Chrys•e•o•bac•te•ri•um (kris″e-o-bak-tēr′e-əm) a genus of gram-negative, aerobic or facultatively anaerobic bacteria of the family Flavobacteriaceae.

C. indolo′genes a species that can cause bacteremia and less often other conditions.

C. meningosep′ticum former name for *Elizabethkingia meningoseptica.*

chry•si•a•sis (krĭ-si′ə-sis) [*chrys-* + *-iasis*] 1. deposition of gold particles in the tissues as a result of prolonged or excessive parenteral chrysotherapy; common symptoms include dermatitis, stomatitis, and transient mild proteinuria; more serious toxicity involves the hematopoietic system, liver, kidney, eye (cornea, lens), and sometimes other vital organs. Called also *auriasis.* 2. chrysoderma.

chrys(o)- [Gr. *chrysos* gold] a combining form denoting relationship to gold.

chryso•der•ma (kris″o-dur′mə) [*chryso-* + *derma*] a manifestation of chrysiasis presenting as a permanent gray to light purple color on the face, eyelids, and other sun-exposed areas of the body. Called also *aurochromoderma.*

chryso•mo•nad (kris″o-mo′nad) [*chryso-* + *monad*] 1. a protozoan of the order Chrysomonadida. 2. a member of the class Chrysophyceae; these have been reclassified from the protozoa to the algae phylum Phaeophyta.

Chrys•o•mo•na•da (kris″o-mo′nə-də) name given to the class Chrysophyceae when it is considered protozoa.

Chryso•mo•nad•i•da (kris″o-mo-nad′ĭ-də) [*chryso-* + Gr. *monas* unit, from *monos* single] an order of free-swimming organisms now assigned to the algae class Chrysophyceae.

Chryso•my•ia (kris″o-mi′yə) [*chryso-* + Gr. *myia* fly] a genus of flies of the family Calliphoridae, found in Africa, Australia, and parts of Asia. Several species lay eggs on wounds or wool, causing cutaneous myiasis.

C. al′biceps a South African species whose larvae (wool maggots) live in the soiled wool of sheep, causing cutaneous blowfly myiasis.

C. bezzia′na a species widely distributed in Asia and Africa; its maggots are frequently found in wounds; it can cause cutaneous blowfly myiasis in sheep and a severe and disfiguring myiasis in humans. Called also *Cochliomyia bezziana.*

C. macella′ria *Cochliomyia hominivorax.*

Chrys•o•phy•ce•ae (kris″o-fi′se-e) a class of free-swimming, flagellate, ameboid, plantlike organisms, traditionally considered protozoa but now assigned to the algae phylum Phaeophyta. Species may live in either salt or fresh water and have two unequal flagella, sometimes brown chloroplasts, and a cyst wall that is typically siliceous.

Chrys•ops (kris′ops) [*chryso-* + Gr. *ōps* eye] a genus of small bloodsucking horseflies of the family Tabanidae, found in warm parts of the world.

C. cecu′tiens a species that bites near the eyes.

C. dimidia′ta a species of southwestern Africa that is an intermediate host of *Loa loa;* called also *mango* or *mangrove fly.*

C. disca′lis a common vector of tularemia in the western United States; called also *deer fly.*

C. sila′cea an intermediate host of *Loa loa.*

Chryso•spor•i•um (kris″o-spor′e-əm) a genus of Fungi Imperfecti of the form-class Hyphomycetes, keratinophilic soil fungi, related to the dermatophytes; some species have been isolated from dermatophytosis.

chryso•ther•a•py (kris″o-ther′ə-pe) [*chryso-* + *therapy*] treatment with gold salts; called also *aurotherapy.*

chryso•tile (kris′o-tīl) the most widely used form of asbestos, a gray-green magnesium silicate in the serpentine class of asbestos; inhalation of its dust may cause asbestosis and, rarely, forms of mesothelioma and other lung cancers.

CHS cholinesterase.

Churg-Strauss granuloma, syndrome (vasculitis) (chərg′ strous′) [Jacob *Churg*, Russian-born American pathologist, 1910–2005; Lotte *Strauss*, German-born American pathologist, 1913–1985] see *cutaneous extravascular necrotizing granuloma*, under *granuloma*, and see under *syndrome.*

Chvos•tek sign (kvos′tək) [Franz *Chvostek*, Austrian surgeon, 1835–1884] see under *sign.*

Chvos·tek-Weiss sign (kvos′tək vīs′) [F. *Chvostek;* Nathan *Weiss,* Austrian physician, 1851–1883] Chvostek sign.

chy·lan·gi·o·ma (ki-lan″je-o′mə) [*chyl-* + *angioma*] a tumor made up of intestinal lymph vessels.

chyl·aque·ous (ki-la′kwe-əs) [*chyl-* + *aqueous*] both chylous and watery. See *chylous hydrothorax,* under *hydrothorax.*

chyle (kīl) [G. *chylos* juice] 1. the milky fluid taken up by the lacteals from the food in the intestine during digestion, consisting of lymph and droplets of triglyceride fat (chylomicrons) in a stable emulsion. It passes into the veins by the thoracic duct, becoming mixed with the blood. 2. turbid, milky fluid resembling that produced during digestion. **chy′lous** *adj*

chy·le·mia (ki-le′me-ə) the presence of chyle in the blood.

chyli- see *chyl(o)-.*

chy·li·form (ki′lĭ-form) resembling chyle; cf. *pseudochylous.* Called also *chyloid.*

chyl(o)- [Gr. *chylos* juice] a combining form denoting relationship to chyle.

chy·lo·cele (ki′lo-sēl) elephantiasis scroti.

chy·lo·cyst (ki′lo-sist) cisterna chyli.

chy·lo·der·ma (ki″lo-dur′mə) elephantiasis.

chy·loid (ki′loid) chyliform.

chy·lo·me·di·as·ti·num (ki″lo-me″de-əs-ti′nəm) the presence of chyle in the mediastinum.

chy·lo·mi·cro·graph (ki″lo-mi′kro-graf) a curve plotted from counts of chylomicrons.

chy·lo·mi·cron (ki″lo-mi′kron) [*chylo-* + Gr. *mikros* small] a class of lipoproteins that transport exogenous (dietary) cholesterol and triglycerides from the small intestine to tissues after meals. Synthesized in the intestinal mucosa and carried via the intestinal lacteals and lymphatic system to the bloodstream, they are then degraded to chylomicron remnants (q.v.) in the capillaries of muscle and adipose tissue via cleavage of the majority of their triglycerides by endothelial lipoprotein lipase. These remnants are rapidly cleared by the liver via receptor-mediated endocytosis.

chy·lo·mi·cro·ne·mia (ki″lo-mi″kro-ne′me-ə) hyperchylomicronemia.

chy·lo·peri·car·di·tis (ki″lo-per″ĭ-kahr-di′tis) pericarditis due to effusion of chyle into the pericardial sac.

chy·lo·peri·car·di·um (ki″lo-per″ĭ-kahr′de-əm) the presence of effused chyle in the pericardium, usually due to trauma to the thoracic duct.

chy·lo·peri·to·ne·um (ki″lo-per″ĭ-to-ne′əm) chylous ascites.

chy·lo·pleu·ra (ki″lo-ploor′ə) chylothorax.

chy·lo·pneu·mo·tho·rax (ki″lo-noo″mo-thor′aks) the presence of chyle and air in the pleural cavity.

chy·lor·rhea (ki″lo-re′ə) [*chylo-* + *-rrhea*] discharge of chyle due to rupture of or injury to the thoracic duct.

chy·lo·tho·rax (ki″lo-thor′aks) [*chylo-* + *thorax*] a pleural effusion consisting of chyle or a chylelike fluid. There are two types: *chylous effusion,* due to leakage of chyle from the thoracic duct, and *chyliform* or *pseudochylous effusion,* consisting of chylelike fluid, the result of a chronic disease such as tuberculosis. Called also *chylopleura, chylous hydrothorax,* and *chylous pleurisy.*

congenital c. a chylous effusion due to some congenital defect of the thoracic duct; affected infants can die from malnutrition or systemic infection.

traumatic c. a chylous effusion resulting from traumatic damage to the thoracic duct; causes include surgery on thoracic organs or vessels and nonpenetrating trauma such as hyperextension of the spine.

chy·lu·ria (kīl-u′re-ə) [*chylo-* + *-uria*] the presence of chyle in the urine, giving it a milky appearance; this follows obstruction somewhere between the intestinal lymphatics and the thoracic duct, which causes rupture of renal lymphatics into the renal tubules. It also is seen as a result of obstruction of the retroperitoneal lymphatics in bancroftian filariasis. Called also *chylous urine.*

chy·lus (ki′ləs) [L.] chyle (def. 1).

chy·mase (ki′mās) [EC 3.4.21.39] an enzyme of the hydrolase class that catalyzes the hydrolysis of peptide bonds, with a specificity similar to that of chymotrypsin. It is a serine proteinase and is found in mast cell granules.

chyme (kīm) [Gr. *chymos* juice] the semifluid, homogeneous, creamy or gruellike material produced by digestion of food in the stomach; called also *chymus.* **chy′mous** *adj*

Chy·mex (ki′məks) trademark for a preparation of bentiromide.

chy·mi·fi·ca·tion (ki″mĭ-fĭ-ka′shən) [*chyme* + L. *facere* to make] gastric digestion.

chy·mo·pa·pain (ki″mo-pə-pān′) [EC 3.4.22.6] an enzyme of the hydrolase class, a cysteine endopeptidase, that catalyzes the hydrolysis of proteins and polypeptides. Its specificity is very close to that of papain and both occur in the latex of the tropical papaya tree, *Carica papaya.* The enzyme is used to break down the proteoglycan portion of the nucleus pulposus in the treatment of herniation of intervertebral (lumbar) disks by chemonucleolysis.

chy·mo·sin (ki′mo-sin) [EC 3.4.23.4] an enzyme of the hydrolase class that catalyzes the cleavage of a single bond in casein to form soluble paracasein, which then reacts with calcium to form a curd, insoluble paracasein. It is found in the fourth stomach of the calf and other ruminants. A commercial preparation, rennet, is used for making cheese and rennet custards. Called also *rennin* (not to be confused with *renin*).

chy·mo·sin·o·gen (ki″mo-sin′o-jən) prochymosin.

chy·mo·tryp·sin (ki″mo-trip′sin) 1. [EC 3.4.21.1] a serine endopeptidase that preferentially cleaves peptide bonds on the carboxyl side of amino acids with bulky hydrophobic residues, particularly tyrosine, tryptophan, phenylalanine, and leucine. It is secreted by the pancreas as the inactive proenzyme chymotrypsinogen. 2. [USP] a proteolytic enzyme preparation crystallized from an extract of ox pancreas, used for enzymatic zonulolysis in intracapsular lens extraction. It has also been used to debride necrotic lesions and to reduce inflammation and edema; administered orally, buccally, or intramuscularly.

chy·mo·tryp·sin·o·gen (ki″mo-trip-sin′o-jən) an inactive proenzyme secreted by the pancreas and cleaved by trypsin in the small intestine to yield the active enzyme chymotrypsin.

chy·mus (ki′məs) chyme.

CI cardiac index; Colour Index.

Ci curie.

Ciac·cio glands (chah′cho) [Giuseppe Vincenzo *Ciaccio,* Italian anatomist, 1824–1901] glandulae lacrimales accessoriae.

Ciac·cio method, stain (chah′cho) [Carmelo *Ciaccio,* Italian pathologist, 1877–1956] see under *method* and see *Stains and Staining Methods,* under *stain.*

Ci·al·is (se-al′is) trademark for a preparation of tadalafil.

cib. [L.] ci′bus (food).

cic·a·trec·to·my (sik″ə-trek′tə-me) excision of a cicatrix.

ci·ca·tri·ces (sĭ-ka′trĭ-sēz, sik″ə-tri′sēz) plural of *cicatrix.*

cic·a·tri·cial (sik″ə-trish′əl) pertaining to or of the nature of a scar (cicatrix).

cic·a·tri·cot·o·my (sik″ə-tri-kot′o-me) [*cicatrix* + *-tomy*] incision of a cicatrix.

cic·a·trix (sĭ-ka′triks, sik′ə-triks) pl. *cica′trices* [L.] scar (def. 1).

filtering c. a cicatrix following a glaucoma operation, through which the aqueous humor escapes.

hypertrophic c. a hard, rigid tumor formed by hypertrophy of the tissue of a cicatrix.

vicious c. a cicatrix that causes deformity or impairs the function of an extremity.

cic·at·ri·zant (sik-at′rĭ-zənt) an agent that promotes cicatrization.

cic·a·tri·za·tion (sik″ə-trĭ-za′shən) the formation of a cicatrix or scar; called also *scarring.*

cic·a·trize (sik′ə-trīz) to heal by the formation of a scar or cicatrix.

Ci·cer (si′sər) a genus of plants of the family Leguminosae, native to southern Europe and parts of Asia. *C. arieti′num* is the garbanzo or chickpea (q.v.).

ci·cles·o·nide (si-kles′o-nīd) a corticosteroid administered for maintenance treatment or prophylaxis of bronchial asthma or allergic rhinitis; administered by oral inhalation or nasal spray.

cic·lo·pir·ox ol·amine (si″klo-pēr′oks) [USP] a broad-spectrum antifungal with activity similar to that of the imidazoles, used in the treatment of cutaneous infections caused by susceptible organisms; applied topically.

Cic·u·ta (sik′u-tə) the water hemlocks, a genus of plants of the family Umbelliferae that contain the poisonous alcohol cicutoxin. *C. macula′ta* L. is the American water hemlock, which has cicutoxin in its roots. *C. viro′sa* is the European water hemlock.

cic·u·tox·in (sik′u-toks″in) a highly toxic unsaturated higher alcohol found in species of *Cicuta;* it causes hyperactivity of the central nervous system with convulsions and respiratory failure.

-cide [L. *-cida,* from *caedere* to kill] a word termination denoting a killer or a killing.

Ci·dex (si′dəks) trademark for a preparation of glutaraldehyde.

ci·dof·o·vir (sĭ-dof′o-vir) an antiviral nucleoside analogue that selectively inhibits viral DNA polymerase; used in the treatment of cytomegalovirus retinitis in patients with acquired immunodeficiency syndrome; administered by intravenous infusion.

CIDP chronic inflammatory demyelinating polyneuropathy.

CIDR Center for Inherited Disease Research, a division of the National Institutes of Health.

CIE counterimmunoelectrophoresis.

ci•gua•te•ra (se″gwə-ta′rə) [Sp. (orig. Taino) *cigua* a poisonous snail + *-era* Sp. noun suffix] a form of ichthyosarcotoxism, marked by gastrointestinal and neurologic symptoms, caused by ingestion of tropical or subtropical marine fish such as the grouper and snapper that have ciguatoxin in their tissues. The term was formerly applied to all types of fish poisoning in the West Indies.

ci•gua•tox•in (se′gwə-tok″sin) a heat-stable ichthyosarcotoxin secreted as a pretoxin by the dinoflagellate *Gambierdiscus toxicus* and biotransformed to the active form by certain marine fish. It becomes concentrated in the tissues of the fish, and when people eat the fish the toxin affects their sodium channels and causes ciguatera.

CIH Certificate in Industrial Health.

Ci-hr curie-hour.

cil•a•sta•tin so•di•um (si″lə-stat′in) a renal dipeptidase inhibitor that blocks the metabolism of imipenem; used in combination with imipenem to increase urinary levels of imipenem. The official preparation is *sterile cilastatin sodium* [USP].

cil•ia (sil′e-ə) (sing. *cil′ium*) [L.] 1. [TA] eyelashes: the hairs growing on the edges of the eyelids. 2. minute vibratile, hairlike processes that project from the free surface of a cell and are composed of nine pairs of microtubules arrayed around a central pair, anchored to the cellular cortex by the basal bodies. Dynein-powered sliding of the outer microtubules relative to one another causes the cilia to move in rhythmic beats *(ciliary beats)* that move the cell around in its environment or move fluid or mucous films over the cell surface. See also *flagellum* and *mucociliary clearance.*

cil•i•a•ris (sil″e-a′ris) [L., from *cilium*] see under *musculus.*

cil•i•ar•i•scope (sil″e-ar′ĭ-skōp) *[ciliary + -scope]* an instrument for examining the ciliary region of the eye.

cil•i•ar•ot•o•my (sil″e-ə-rot′ə-me) *[ciliary + -tomy]* surgical division of the ciliary zone for glaucoma.

cil•i•ary (sil′e-ar″e) [L. *ciliaris,* from *cilium*] 1. pertaining to or resembling a cilium. 2. pertaining to the eyelashes.

cil•i•ate (sil′e-āt) 1. having cilia. 2. any protozoan of the phylum Ciliophora; a ciliophoran.

cil•i•at•ed (sil′e-āt″əd) provided with cilia or with a fringe of hairs.

cil•i•ec•to•my (sil″e-ek′tə-me) *[cili- + -ectomy]* 1. excision of a portion of the ciliary body. 2. excision of a portion of the ciliary margin of the eyelid with the roots of the lashes.

cili(o)- [L. *cilium* eyelid, eyelash] a combining form denoting cilia or a ciliary structure.

cil•io•gen•e•sis (sil″e-o-jen′ə-sis) *[cilio- + genesis]* the formation or development of cilia, a multistep process in which centrioles are generated and migrate to the apical region of the cell, followed by the formation of basal body–associated structures and elongation of the cilia by polymerization of tubulin to form axonemes.

Cil•i•oph•o•ra (sil″e-of′ə-rə) *[cilio- +* Gr. *phoros* bearing] a phylum of protozoa characterized by the presence of cilia or compound ciliary structures as locomotor or food-gathering organelles at some time during their life cycle, a subpellicular infraciliature composed of ciliary basal bodies and kinetodesmata (even when cilia are absent), and two types of nuclei, a macronucleus and a micronucleus (with rare exceptions); a contractile vacuole is typically present. Sexuality involves conjugation, autogamy, and cytogamy. Most ciliophorans are free living, many are commensals of vertebrates and invertebrates, and some are parasites. The phylum comprises three classes: Kinetofragminophorea, Oligohymenophorea, and Polyhymenophorea. Cf. *Opalinata.*

cil•i•oph•o•ran (sil″e-of′ə-rən) any protozoan of the phylum Ciliophora; a ciliate.

cil•io•ret•i•nal (sil″e-o-ret′ĭ-nəl) pertaining to the retina and the ciliary body.

cil•io•scle•ral (sil″e-o-skler′əl) pertaining to the ciliary apparatus and to the sclera.

cil•io•spi•nal (sil″e-o-spi′nəl) *[cilio- + spinal]* pertaining to the ciliary body and the spinal cord; see under *center* and *reflex.*

cil•i•ot•o•my (sil″e-ot′ə-me) *[cilio- + tomy]* surgical division of the ciliary nerves.

cil•i•um (sil′e-əm) [L.] singular of *cilia.*
  olfactory cilia see under *hair.*

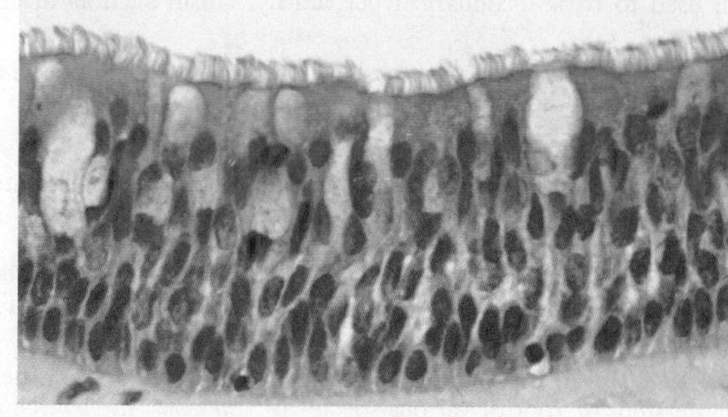

■ Electron micrograph of ciliated columnar pseudostratified epithelium in the respiratory tract.

cil•o•sta•zol (sĭ-lo′stə-zol) a quinolinone derivative that inhibits phosphodiesterase and degradation of cyclic adenosine monophosphate (cyclic AMP). It reversibly inhibits platelet aggregation and causes vasodilation, particularly in femoral beds; administered orally to produce symptomatic relief in the treatment of intermittent claudication.

Cil•ox•an (sĭ-lok′san) trademark for preparations of ciprofloxacin hydrochloride.

cim•bia (sim′be-ə) [L.] a white band running across the ventral surface of the crus cerebri.

ci•met•i•dine (si-met′ĭ-dēn) [USP] a histamine H_2 receptor antagonist; it inhibits gastric acid secretion and is used in the prophylaxis and treatment of peptic ulcer, the relief of symptoms associated with hyperacidity, and the treatment of gastroesophageal reflux disease, of upper gastrointestinal bleeding, and of pathologic gastric hypersecretion, as that associated with Zollinger-Ellison syndrome; administered orally.
  c. hydrochloride [USP] the monohydrochloride salt of cimetidine, having the same actions and uses as the base; administered orally, intravenously, or intramuscularly.

Ci•mex (si′məks) [L. "bug"] the bedbugs, a genus of bloodsucking insects of the family Cimicidae that often infest humans.
  C. boue′ti the tropical bedbug of West Africa and South America; called also *Leptocimex boueti.*
  C. hemip′terus *C. rotundatus.*
  C. lectula′rius the common bedbug of temperate regions of the world; called also *Acanthia lectularia.*
  C. rotunda′tus a flattened, oval, reddish bedbug found in tropical regions of the world; called also *C. hemipterus.*

ci•mex (si′məks) pl. *cim′ices* [L.] an individual of the genus *Cimex;* a bedbug.

ci•mi•cid (si′mĭ-sid) pertaining to insects of the family Cimicidae.

Ci•mic•i•dae (si-mis′ĭ-de) a family of wingless, blood-sucking, hemipterous insects of the suborder Heteroptera, including the bedbugs and related forms. *Cimex, Haematosiphon, Leptocimex,* and *Oeciacus* are medically important genera.

Cim•i•cif•u•ga (sim″ĭ-sif′u-gə) [L. *cimex* bug + *fugare* to put to flight] a genus of plants of the family Ranunculaceae. *C. racemo′sa* (L.) Nutt. is the black snakeroot or cohosh and has rootlets that are tonic and antispasmodic.

cim•i•co•sis (sim″ĭ-ko′sis) itching of the skin due to the bites of *Cimex lectularius* (bedbug).

Cim•zia (sim′ze-ə) trademark for a preparation of certolizumab pegol.

CIN cervical intraepithelial neoplasia.

cin•a•cal•cet hydrochloride (sin″ə-kal′set) a calcimimetic that increases the sensitivity of receptors in the parathyroid glands to extracellular

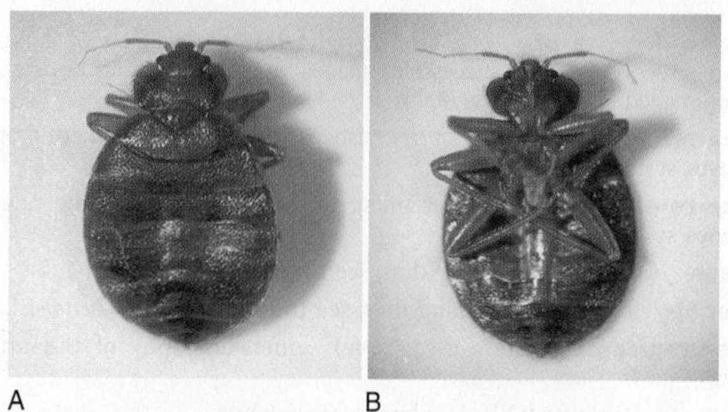

■ *Cimex lectularius* adult. *(A),* Dorsal and *(B),* ventral views.

calcium; used to treat secondary hyperparathyroidism such as in chronic renal failure.

cinch·ing (sinch'ing) [Sp. *cincha* girdle] surgical shortening of an ocular muscle by plicating.

cin·cho·caine (sin'ko-kān") INN and BAN for *dibucaine.*

Cin·cho·na (sin-ko'nə) [Francisca Henríquez de Ribera, Countess of *Chinchón,* 1576–1639] a genus of South American trees of the family Rubiaceae, the source of the medicinal bark called *cinchona.* The major species used are *C. succiru'bra* Pavon et Klotzsch and its hybrids (red cinchona), *C. calisa'ya* Weddell, and *C. ledgeria'na* (Howard) Moens et Trimen and its hybrids (yellow cinchona).

cin·cho·na (sin-ko'nə) 1. any tree of the genus *Cinchona.* 2. the dried bark of the stem or root of various species of *Cinchona,* the source of the medicinally important quinoline alkaloids quinine, quinidine, cinchonine, and cinchonidine; it was once widely used as an antimalarial but has been largely replaced by its alkaloids. Called also *calisaya bark, cinchona bark, Jesuit bark, Peruvian bark,* and *quinquina.*

cin·cho·ni·dine (sin-ko'nĭ-dēn) an alkaloid of cinchona, used as an antimalarial, chiefly in the form of the sulfate salt; administered orally.

cin·cho·nine (sin'ko-nēn) [L. *cinchonina*] an alkaloid of cinchona used as an antimalarial, chiefly in the form of the sulfate salt; administered orally.

cin·cho·nin·ic ac·id (sin"ko-nin'ik) quinoline 4-carboxylic acid, an oxidation product of cinchona alkaloids.

cin·cho·nism (sin'ko-niz"əm) poisoning by the injudicious use of cinchona bark or its alkaloids, characterized by nausea, vomiting, headache, tinnitus, deafness, symptoms of cerebral congestion, vertigo, and visual disturbances.

cine- [Gr. *kinēsis* movement] a combining form denoting relationship to movement. See also words beginning *kine-.*

cine·an·gio·car·diog·ra·phy (sin"ə-an"je-o-kahr"de-og'rə-fe) [*cine-* + *angiocardiography*] the photographic recording of fluoroscopic images of the heart and great vessels by motion picture techniques.

cine·an·gio·graph (sin"ə-an'je-o-graf) a motion picture camera for photographing fluoroscopic images.

cine·an·gi·og·ra·phy (sin"ə-an"je-og'rə-fe) [*cine-* + *angiography*] the photographic recording of fluoroscopic images of the blood vessels by motion picture techniques.

cine·def·e·cog·ra·phy (sin"ə-def"ə-kog'rə-fe) defecography.

cine·den·sig·ra·phy (sin"ə-dən-sig'rə-fe) the recording of movements of internal body structures by means of x-rays and radiosensitive cells.

cine·flu·o·rog·ra·phy (sin"ə-floo"or-og'rə-fe) cineradiography.

cin·e·mat·ics (sin"ə-mat'iks) kinematics.

cine·mi·crog·ra·phy (sin"ə-mi-krog'rə-fe) the making of moving pictures of a small object through the lens system of a microscope.

time-lapse c. the taking of motion pictures of a minute object through a microscope at a slower than normal speed, so that with projection at normal speed the movements of the object appear to occur more rapidly.

cin·e·ol (sin'e-ol) eucalyptol.

cin·e·paz·et mal·e·ate (sin"ə-paz'ət) a coronary vasodilator, which has been used in the treatment of angina of effort.

cine·phle·bog·ra·phy (sin"ə-flə-bog'rə-fe) cineradiography of the veins after administration of a contrast medium.

ascending functional c. cinephlebography in which the contrast medium is introduced into a vein in the foot and its progress is observed as it courses through the tibial, popliteal, femoral, and iliac veins.

cin·e·plas·ty (sin'ə-plas"te) kineplasty.

cine·ra·dio·flu·o·rog·ra·phy (sin"ə-ra"de-o-flo͞or-og'rə-fe) cineradiography.

cine·ra·di·og·ra·phy (sin"ə-ra"de-og'rə-fe) the making of a motion picture record of the successive images appearing on a fluoroscopic screen; called also *cinefluorography.*

ci·ne·rea (sĭ-nēr'e-ə) [L. *cinereus* ashen hued] the gray matter of the nervous system.

ci·ne·re·al (sĭ-nēr'e-əl) pertaining to the gray matter of the brain or nervous system.

cinesi- for words beginning thus, see those beginning *kinesi-.*

cinet(o)- for words beginning thus, see those beginning *kinet(o)-.*

cine·urog·ra·phy (sin"ə-u-rog'rə-fe) cineradiography of the urinary tract.

cin·gu·la (sing'gu-lə) [L.] plural of *cingulum.*

cin·gule (sing'gūl) cingulum.

cin·gu·lec·to·my (sing"gu-lek'tə-me) bilateral extirpation of the anterior half of the gyrus cinguli; cf. *cingulotomy.*

cin·gu·lot·o·my (sing"gu-lot'ə-me) the creation, by stereotaxic introduction of electrodes, of lesions in the gyrus cinguli for relief of intractable pain and in treatment of psychiatric disorders and addiction.

cin·gu·lum (sing'gu-ləm) pl. *cin'gula* [L. "girdle"] 1. an encircling structure or part; anything that encircles a body. Called also *cingule* and *girdle.* 2. [TA] a bundle of association fibers deep to the cingulate gyrus and partly encircling the corpus callosum not far from the median plane; the fibers interrelate the cingulate and hippocampal gyri. 3. the lingual lobe of an anterior tooth, making up the bulk of the cervical third of its lingual surface; called also *basal, linguocervical,* and *linguogingival ridge.* cin'gulate *adj*

c. mem'bri inferio'ris TA alternative for *c. pelvicum.*

c. mem'bri superio'ris TA alternative for *c. pectorale.*

c. pectora'le [TA] pectoral girdle: the encircling bony structure supporting the upper limbs, comprising the clavicles and scapulae, articulating with each other and with the sternum and vertebral column, respectively; called also *c. membri superioris* [TA alternative] and *shoulder girdle.*

c. pel'vicum [TA] pelvic girdle: the encircling bony structure supporting the lower limbs, comprising the two ossa coxae, articulating with each other and with the sacrum, to complete the essentially rigid bony ring; called also *c. membri inferioris* [TA alternative].

cin·gu·lum·ot·o·my (sing"gu-ləm-ot'ə-me) cingulotomy.

C1 INH C1 inhibitor.

cin·na·mal·de·hyde (sin"ə-mal'də-hīd) a yellowish oily liquid with a strong odor of cinnamon, a major constituent of cinnamon oil; used as a flavoring agent.

cin·na·mate (sin'ə-māt) 1. a salt or ester of cinnamic acid. 2. a chemical compound containing this structure; several are components of sunscreens.

cin·na·mene (cin'ə-mēn) styrene.

cin·nam·ic ac·id (sĭ-nam'ik) a phenyl-substituted, unsaturated, aliphatic carboxylic acid used as a flavoring agent.

cin·na·mol (cin'ə-mol) styrene.

Cin·na·mo·mum (sin"ə-mo'məm) a genus of evergreen trees of the family Lauraceae, native to Asia. The wood of *C. cam'phora* is the source of camphor, the bark of *C. lourei'rii* is true (or Saigon) cinnamon, and the bark of *C. cas'sia* (Chinese cinnamon) and *C. zeyla'nicum* (Ceylon cinnamon) are sources of cinnamon oil.

cin·na·mon (sin'ə-mən) [Gr. *kinnamon,* from Hebrew *quinnāmōn*] 1. the dried bark of any of several trees of the genus *Cinnamomum.* 2. the dried bark of *Cinnamomum loureirii,* containing, in each 100 g, not less than 2.5 mL of volatile oil; used as a flavor in pharmaceutical preparations.

Ceylon c. the dried bark of *Cinnamomum zeylanicum;* used as a flavor and as a source of cinnamon oil.

Chinese c. the dried bark of *Cinnamomum cassia;* used as a flavor and as a source of cinnamon oil.

Saigon c., true c. cinnamon (def. 2).

cin·nar·i·zine (sĭ-nahr'ĭ-zēn) an antihistamine, used chiefly in the treatment of nausea and vertigo associated with labyrinthine disorders and in the prevention and treatment of motion sickness.

Cin·o·bac (sin'o-bak) trademark for a preparation of cinoxacin.

cin·ox·a·cin (sin-ok'sə-sin) a broad-spectrum quinolone antibacterial agent, used in the treatment of urinary tract infections; administered orally.

cin·ox·ate (sin-ok'sāt) a cinnamate compound used as a topical sunscreen for protection from ultraviolet B.

Ci·o·nel·la (si"o-nəl'ə) a genus of land snails of the family Cionellidae; they serve as hosts of the liver fluke *Dicrocoelium dendriticum* in North America.

Ci·o·nel·li·dae (si"o-nel'ĭ-de) a family of garden snails of the suborder Stylommatophora, subclass Euthyneura; they often serve as hosts of the liver fluke *Dicrocoelium dendriticum.*

Cip·ro (sip'ro) trademark for preparations of ciprofloxacin hydrochloride.

ci·pro·fi·brate (si"pro-fi'brāt) a fibric acid derivative having actions similar to those of clofibrate, used as a hypolipidemic in the treatment of certain hyperlipoproteinemias; administered orally.

cip·ro·flox·a·cin (sip"ro-flok'sə-sin) [USP] a fluoroquinolone antibacterial effective against many gram-positive and gram-negative bacteria, including some strains resistant to penicillins, cephalosporins, and aminoglycosides.

c. hydrochloride [USP] the monohydrated hydrochloride salt of ciprofloxacin, having the same actions as the parent compound and used to treat a wide variety of bacterial infections; administered orally, intravenously, and topically to the conjunctiva.

cir•ca•di•an (sər-ka′de-ən) [L. *circa* about + *dies* a day] pertaining to a period of about 24 hours; applied especially to the rhythmic repetition of certain phenomena in living organisms at about the same time each day (circadian rhythm).

cir•can•nu•al (sər-kan′u-əl) [L. *circa* about + *annus* year] occurring every year; applied especially to the rhythmic repetition of certain phenomena (e.g., the flowering of plants) in living organisms at about the same time each year.

cir•cel•lus (sər-sel′əs) [L., dim. of *circulus*] a small ring, or circle.

cir•ci•nate (sur′sĭ-nāt) 1. circular. 2. annular.

cir•cle (sur′kəl) [L. *circulus*] a round figure, structure, or part. See also *anulus* and *ring*.

arterial c. circulus arteriosus.

arterial c. of iris, greater circulus arteriosus iridis major.

arterial c. of iris, lesser circulus arteriosus iridis minor.

arterial c. of Willis circulus arteriosus cerebri.

Berry c's charts with circles on them for testing stereoscopic vision.

cerebral arterial c. circulus arteriosus cerebri.

c. of confusion a disk representing the image of a theoretical point made by a lens.

c. of death an arterial formation sometimes encountered in surgery for inguinal hernias, with an aberrant branch of the obturator artery arising from the inferior epigastric or external iliac artery, crossing the pectineal ligament, and anastomosing with the obturator artery; this vessel can encircle the neck of a hernial sac and become damaged during surgery, causing hemorrhage.

defensive c. the coexistence of two conditions that tend to have an antagonistic or inhibitory effect on each other.

c. of dispersion, c. of dissipation the circular space on the retina within which the image of a luminous point is formed.

c. of Haller circulus vasculosus nervi optici.

c. of Hovius an intrascleral circular arrangement of anastomosing ciliary veins anterior to the vorticose veins, not far from the corneoscleral margin, occurring in mammals other than humans.

Huguier c. the circle formed about the junction of the cervix with the body of the uterus by the uterine arteries.

c. of iris, greater anulus iridis major.

c. of iris, lesser anulus iridis minor.

Latham c. a circle 5 cm in diameter covering the area of pericardial dullness and situated midway between the left nipple and the lower end of the sternum.

Minsky c's a series of circles used for the graphic recording of eye lesions.

Robinson c. an arterial circle formed by anastomoses between the abdominal aorta, common iliac, hypogastric, uterine, and ovarian arteries.

vascular c. circulus vasculosus.

vascular c. of optic nerve circulus vasculosus nervi optici.

Vieth-Müller c. see under *horopter*.

c. of Willis circulus arteriosus cerebri.

c. of Zinn circulus vasculosus nervi optici.

cir•clet (sur′klət) circellus.

cir•cling (sur′kling) walking in a circle, as that done by animals with listeriosis and other central nervous system disorders.

cir•cuit (sur′kət) [L. *circuitus*] the round or course traversed by an electrical current. The circuit is said to be *closed* when it is continuous, so that the current may pass through it; it is *open, broken,* or *interrupted* when it is not continuous and the current cannot pass through it.

gate c. gate.

macroreentrant c. a reentry pathway involving the bundle branches of the conduction system of the heart.

microreentrant c. a reentry pathway involving only a few myocardial cells.

open c. a circuit having some break in it so that current is not passing or cannot pass.

Papez c. a neuronal circuit in the limbic system, consisting of the hippocampus, fornix, mammillary body, anterior thalamic nuclei, and cingulate gyrus; postulated by Papez to be involved with the experiencing of emotions and responses to them.

reentrant c., reentry c. the circuit formed by the circulating impulse in reentry.

reflex c. see under *arc*.

reverberating c. a neuronal pathway arranged in a circle so that impulses are recycled to cause positive feedback or reverberation (q.v.).

reward c. a hypothesized pathway in the brain that receives stimuli and perceives them as pleasurable, especially stimuli from foods and drugs.

short c. an unwanted low-resistance connection between two points in an electric circuit.

cir•cu•lar (sur′ku-lər) [L. *circularis*] shaped like a circle or occurring in a circle. See also *annular*.

cir•cu•la•tion (sur″ku-la′shən) [L. *circulatio*] 1. movement of something through a circuitous course. 2. the movement of the blood through the heart and blood vessels.

allantoic c. fetal circulation through the allantoic vessels, the precursors to the umbilical vessels.

assisted c. pumping that aids the natural activity of the heart.

collateral c. circulation carried on through secondary channels after obstruction of the principal vessel supplying the part; called also *compensatory c.*

compensatory c. collateral c.

coronary c. circulation within the coronary vessels of the heart.

cross c. the circulation in a portion of the body of one animal of blood supplied from another animal.

dual c. the presence of two blood-carrying circuits, such as the pulmonary and systemic circuits, carrying deoxygenated and oxygenated blood respectively, or the hepatic and portal circuits in the liver.

enterohepatic c. the recurrent cycle in which bile salts and other substances excreted by the liver pass through the intestinal mucosa and become reabsorbed by the hepatic cells and re-excreted.

extracorporeal c. the circulation of blood outside the body, as through a heart-lung apparatus for carbon dioxide–oxygen exchange, or through an artificial kidney for removal of substances usually excreted in the urine.

fetal c. the circulation propelled by the fetal heart through the fetus, umbilical cord, and chorionic villi of the placenta, supplying oxygen and nutritive material and eliminating carbon dioxide and nitrogenous wastes.

first c. primordial c.

fourth c. the continuous movement of lymphocytes from their sources in all the hematopoietic and connective tissues to the blood passing through all the tissues and organs, then to the lymph nodes, then into the lymph of the thoracic duct, and into the blood again.

greater c. systemic c.

hepatic portal c. portal c. (def. 2).

hyperdynamic c. abnormally increased circulatory volume with low vascular resistance and often tachycardia, a condition sometimes accompanying septic shock, preeclampsia, and other conditions.

hypophysial portal c., hypophysioportal c. hypothalamo-hypophysial portal system.

intervillous c. the flow of maternal blood through the intervillous space of the placenta.

lesser c. pulmonary c.

lymph c. the passage of the lymph through lymph vessels and glands.

persistent fetal c. persistent pulmonary hypertension of the newborn.

placental c. 1. the circulation of blood through the placenta during prenatal life. 2. intervillous c.

portal c. 1. the circulation of blood from the capillaries of one organ through larger vessels to the capillaries of another organ, before returning through larger veins back to the heart. 2. the passage of the blood from capillaries of the gastrointestinal tract and spleen through capillaries of the

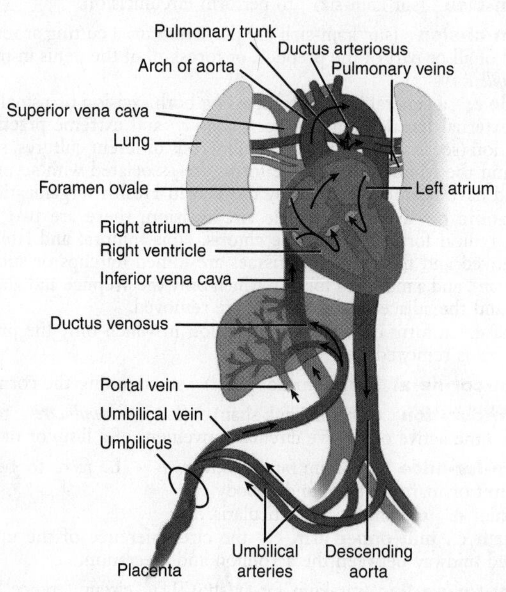

■ Schematic diagram of fetal circulation, with red indicating the highest level of oxygen saturation, blue the lowest, and purple an intermediate level.

liver before entering the hepatic vein. Called also *hepatic portal c.* 3. hypothalamo-hypophysial portal system.

primordial c. the earliest circulation by which nutriment material and oxygen are conveyed to the embryo; called also *first c.*

pulmonary c. the circulation that carries the venous blood from the right ventricle to the lungs, and returning oxygenated blood to the left atrium of the heart; called also *lesser c.*

sinusoidal c. the circulation of blood through the sinusoids.

systemic c. the general circulation, carrying oxygenated blood from the left ventricle to various tissues of the body, and returning the venous blood to the right atrium of the heart; called also *greater c.*

thebesian c. the circulation of blood through the venae cordis minimae (thebesian veins).

umbilical c. fetal circulation through the umbilical vessels.

vitelline c. the circulation through the blood vessels of the yolk sac.

cir•cu•la•to•ry (sur′ku-lə-tor″e) 1. pertaining to any circulation. 2. pertaining to the circulation of the blood. 3. containing blood; called also *sanguiferous.*

cir•cu•lus (sur′ku-ləs) pl. *cir′culi* [L. "a ring"] circle: in anatomy, a ringlike arrangement, usually of arteries or veins.

c. arterio′sus [TA] arterial circle: a complete or incomplete circle of anastomosing arteries.

c. arterio′sus ce′rebri [TA] cerebral arterial circle: the important polygonal anastomosis formed by the internal carotid, the anterior, middle, and posterior cerebral arteries, the anterior communicating artery, and the posterior communicating arteries; called also *arterial circle of Willis* and *circle of Willis.*

c. arterio′sus i′ridis ma′jor [TA] greater arterial circle of the iris: a circle of anastomosing arteries situated in the ciliary body along the ciliary margin of the iris.

c. arterio′sus i′ridis mi′nor [TA] lesser arterial circle of the iris: a circle of anastomosing arteries in the iris near the pupillary margin.

c. articula′ris vasculo′sus an arrangement of anastomosing vessels encircling a joint.

c. umbilica′lis an arterial plexus in the subperitoneal tissue surrounding the navel.

c. vasculo′sus [TA] vascular circle: a complete or incomplete circle of anastomosing blood vessels.

c. vasculo′sus ner′vi op′tici [TA] vascular circle of optic nerve: a circle of arteries in the sclera surrounding the site of entrance of the optic nerve; called also *circle of Haller* and *circle of Zinn.*

c. veno′sus hal′leri plexus venosus areolaris.

circum- [L.] a prefix signifying around or encircling.

cir•cum•anal (sur″kəm-a′nəl) surrounding the anus; cf. *perianal.*

cir•cum•ar•tic•u•lar (sur″kəm-ahr-tik′u-lər) surrounding a joint.

cir•cum•ax•il•lary (sur″kəm-ak′sĭ-lar″e) surrounding the axilla.

cir•cum•bul•bar (sur″kəm-bul′bər) surrounding the eyeball.

cir•cum•cal•lo•sal (sur″kəm-kə-lo′səl) surrounding the corpus callosum.

cir•cum•cise (sur′kəm-sīz) to perform circumcision.

cir•cum•ci•sion (sur″kəm-sizh′ən) [L. *circumcisio* a cutting around] the removal of all or part of the prepuce, or foreskin, of the penis in males; see also *female c.*

female c. a general term encompassing both excision of a small portion of the external female genitalia (see *Sunna c.*) and extreme practices with infibulation (see*pharaonic c.*), done in numerous different cultures, such as in Africa and the Middle East. Some forms are associated with severe health risks and have been condemned by the World Health Organization.

pharaonic c. a type of female circumcision; there are two different types: a radical form in which the clitoris, labia minora, and labia majora are removed and the remaining tissues are joined by clips or sutures (see *infibulation*), and a modified form in which only the prepuce and glans of the clitoris and the adjacent labia minora are removed.

Sunna c. a form of female circumcision in which only the prepuce of the clitoris is removed.

cir•cum•cor•ne•al (sur″kəm-kor′ne-əl) surrounding the cornea.

cir•cum•duc•tion (sur″kəm-duk′shən) [L. *circumducere* to draw around] the active or passive circular movement of a limb or of the eye.

cir•cum•fer•ence (sər-kum′fər-əns) [*circum-* + L. *ferre* to bear] the outer limit or margin of a rounded body.

articular c. circumferentia articularis.

midarm c., mid upper arm c. the circumference of the upper arm measured midway between the acromion and olecranon.

cir•cum•fer•en•tia (sər-kum″fər-en′shə) [L.] circumference.

c. articula′ris articular circumference: the rounded surface of a bone which is received into a depression of another bone with which it articulates.

c. articula′ris ca′pitis ra′dii [TA] articular circumference of head of radius: the rounded surface of the head or capitulum of the radius which articulates with the radial notch of the ulna.

c. articula′ris ca′pitis ul′nae [TA] articular circumference of head of ulna: the semilunar surface of the head of the ulna which articulates with the ulnar notch of the radius; called also *c. articularis capituli ulnae.*

c. articula′ris capi′tuli ul′nae c. articularis capitis ulnae.

cir•cum•fer•en•tial (sur″kəm-fər-en′shəl) pertaining to a circumference; encircling; peripheral.

cir•cum•flex (sur′kəm-fleks) [L. *circumflexus* bent about] curved like a bow.

cir•cum•flex•us (sur″kəm-flek′səs) [L.] bent about; circumflex.

cir•cum•gem•mal (sur″kəm-jem′əl) [*circum-* + *gemma* + *-al*] surrounding a bud; a term applied to that form of nerve ending in which an end-bud is surrounded by fibrils.

cir•cum•in•su•lar (sur″kəm-in′su-lər) [*circum-* + *insular*] surrounding or occurring near the insula.

cir•cum•in•tes•ti•nal (sur″kəm-in-tes′tĭ-nəl) surrounding the intestine.

cir•cum•len•tal (sur″kəm-len′təl) surrounding the lens.

cir•cum•nu•cle•ar (sur″kəm-noo′kle-ər) surrounding or occurring near a nucleus; perinuclear.

cir•cum•oc•u•lar (sur″kəm-ok′u-lər) surrounding or occurring around the eye.

cir•cum•oral (sur″kəm-or′əl) [*circum-* + *oral*] surrounding or occurring around the mouth; cf. *perioral.*

cir•cum•or•bi•tal (sur″kəm-or′bĭ-təl) surrounding or occurring near an orbit.

cir•cum•pul•pal (sur″kəm-pul′pəl) surrounding the pulp.

cir•cum•re•nal (sur″kəm-re′nəl) surrounding the kidney; cf. *perinephric.*

cir•cum•scribed (sur′kəm-skrībd″) [*circum-* + L. *scribere* to write] bounded or limited; confined to a limited space.

cir•cum•scrip•tus (sur″kəm-skrip′təs) [L.] circumscribed.

cir•cum•stan•ti•al•i•ty (sur″kəm-stan″she-al′ĭ-te) a disturbed pattern of speech or writing characterized by delay in getting to the point because of the interpolation of unnecessary details and irrelevant parenthetical remarks; seen in persons with schizophrenia and obsessive-compulsive disorders. Cf. *tangentiality.*

cir•cum•val•late (sur″kəm-val′āt) [*circum-* + *vallate*] surrounded by a trench or by a ridge; see *papillae vallatae*, under *papilla.*

cir•cum•vas•cu•lar (sur″kəm-vas′ku-lər) [*circum-* + *vascular*] around or encircling a vessel.

cir•cum•ven•tric•u•lar (sur″kəm-ven-trik′u-lər) surrounding a ventricle, particularly in the brain.

cir•cum•vo•lute (sur″kəm-vo′lūt) [*circum-* + *volute*] twisted about.

cir•rhog•e•nous (sĭ-roj′ə-nəs) producing cirrhosis or hardening.

cir•rhon•o•sus (sĭ-ron′ə-səs) [Gr. *kirrhos* orange yellow + *nosos* disease] a fetal disease characterized by a golden-yellow staining of the pleura and peritoneum.

cir•rho•sis (sĭ-ro′sis) [Gr. *kirrhos* orange-yellow] any of a group of chronic diseases of the liver characterized by loss of normal lobular architecture with fibrosis, and by destruction of parenchymal cells and their regeneration to form nodules. These diseases have long latent periods, usually followed by sudden abdominal swelling and pain, hematemesis, dependent edema, or jaundice. In advanced stages, prominent symptoms include ascites, jaundice, portal hypertension, and central nervous system disorders that may end in hepatic coma. Often informally called *c. of the liver*, but nowadays *all* cirrhosis is "of the liver." **cirrhot′ic** *adj*

acholangic biliary c. a type of cirrhosis seen in children up to 12 years old, due to complete or partial agenesis of the interlobular bile ducts, with manifestations similar to those in obstructive biliary cirrhosis.

acute juvenile c. chronic active hepatitis.

alcoholic c. cirrhosis in the alcoholic, attributed by some to associated nutritional deficiency and by others to chronic excessive exposure to alcohol as a hepatotoxin.

biliary c. cirrhosis caused by obstruction or infection of major extrahepatic or intrahepatic ducts, characterized by jaundice, abdominal pain, steatorrhea, hepatomegaly, and splenomegaly. NOTE: *primary biliary cirrhosis* is a different condition, not related to this.

cardiac c. congestive cirrhosis occurring in association with congestive heart failure, often following central hemorrhagic necrosis; it is characterized by scarring about the central veins of the hepatic lobules.

congestive c. cirrhosis caused by increased hepatic venous pressure or thrombosis; commonly due to congestive heart failure (cardiac cirrhosis) or to obstruction of the hepatic vein.

Cruveilhier-Baumgarten c. see under *syndrome.*
decompensated c. cirrhosis accompanied by ascites.
fatty c. cirrhosis accompanied by fatty change in the liver, usually caused by alcohol ingestion. See also *Laënnec c.*
Indian childhood c. a type of cirrhosis seen in children in India, characterized by insidious onset, stunting of growth, hepatomegaly, and a low inconstant fever; it may be due to a hereditary difficulty in copper metabolism and use of copper cooking utensils.
Laënnec c. a common type of alcoholic cirrhosis; in the early stages, liver enlargement may be due to fatty change (see *fatty cirrhosis*); this is followed by necrosis and inflammation due to acute alcohol injury, and fibrosis that progresses inward from portal areas.
c. of the liver popular name for *cirrhosis* (all types of cirrhosis are "of the liver").
macronodular c. cirrhosis in which regenerative nodules are more than 3 mm in diameter, seen most often following subacute hepatic necrosis due to toxic or viral hepatitis. The reticulin framework of normal lobules collapses and may be replaced by broad bands of fibrous tissue separating regenerative nodules of various sizes. Called also *multilobular c., periportal c., postnecrotic c.,* and *toxic c.*
metabolic c. cirrhosis associated with a metabolic disease such as hemochromatosis, Wilson disease, glycogen storage disease, galactosemia, or a disorder of amino acid metabolism.
micronodular c. cirrhosis in which the regenerative nodules are less than 3 mm in diameter; this is typical of alcoholic cirrhosis. Cf. *macronodular c.*
multilobular c., periportal c. macronodular c.
pigment c., pigmentary c. a type of cirrhosis marked by enlargement of the liver, diffuse nodules on its surface, and a brown color due to deposits of iron; this is the characteristic lesion of hemochromatosis.
pipestem c. a type of cirrhosis seen in hepatic schistosomiasis, characterized by fibrotic scars around the large portal vessels; the fibrosis surrounds parasites or ova trapped in branches of the portal vein.
portal c. Laënnec c.
posthepatitic c. cirrhosis, usually of the macronodular type, occurring as a sequela to acute hepatitis.
postnecrotic c. macronodular c.
primary biliary c. a type of cirrhosis with an unknown etiology, now known to be unrelated to biliary cirrhosis; it usually affects middle-aged to elderly women and involves destruction of small intrahepatic bile ducts while the major intrahepatic and extrahepatic ducts remain patent. Characteristics include chronic cholestasis with pruritus, jaundice, hypercholesterolemia, xanthomas, osteomalacia, and eventually portal hypertension and liver failure. Almost all patients have circulating antimitochondrial antibodies. Called also *chronic nonsuppurative destructive cholangitis* and *progressive nonsuppurative cholangitis.*
secondary biliary c. biliary cirrhosis resulting from chronic bile obstruction, such as with congenital atresia or stricture of bile ducts.
stasis c. cirrhosis due to obstruction of the outflow of the hepatic vein, as in cardiac cirrhosis or Budd-Chiari syndrome.
syphilitic c. cirrhosis due to congenital or tertiary syphilis.
toxic c. macronodular cirrhosis caused by a toxic agent.
viral c. cirrhosis resulting from a viral infection, most often hepatitis C.

cir•ri (sər'i) plural of *cirrus.*

cir•rus (sər'əs) pl. *cir'ri* [L. "curl"] 1. any of various slender, usually flexible, appendages, such as one of the organelles used for locomotion by certain peritrichous ciliate protozoa; an eversible penis seen in flatworms; a fingerlike projection of a polychete parapodium; a branch of the thoracic leg of a barnacle; a lateral appendage on the stalk or aboral base of a crinoid; or one of the short projections around the mouth of a cephalochordate that together form a sieve to prevent large particles from entering the mouth. 2. a coarse hair on an animal, longer than most body hair but less coarse than a tactile hair or a vibrissa.
c. ca'pitis one of the long hairs in the forelock of a horse.
c. cau'dae one of the long hairs in an animal's tail.

cirs(o)- [Gr. *kirsos* varix] a combining form denoting relationship to a varix. See also terms beginning with *varic(o)-.*

cir•soid (sur'soid) [*cirso-* + *-oid*] varicoid.

cir•som•pha•los (sər-som'fə-los) [*cirso-* + Gr. *omphalos* navel] caput medusae.

cir•soph•thal•mia (sur″sof-thal'me-ə) [*cirso-* + Gr. *ophthalmos* eye] a varicose state of the conjunctival vessels.

cis (sis) [L. "on this side"] 1. in organic chemistry, having certain atoms or radicals on the same side. 2. in genetics, denoting two or more loci, especially pseudoalleles, occurring on the same chromosome of a homologous pair. Cf. *trans.* See also *cis-trans test,* under *test.*

cis- [L. "on this side"] a prefix denoting on this side, on the same side, on the near side.

cis•a•pride (sis'ə-prīd) an agent that enhances the release of acetylcholine at the myenteric plexus, formerly used as a prokinetic agent to promote gastric emptying in the treatment of gastroesophageal reflux disease and gastroparesis; withdrawn because of its association with severe cardiac arrhythmias.

cis•at•ra•cu•ri•um bes•y•late (sis″at-rə-kūr'e-əm) a nondepolarizing neuromuscular blocking agent administered intravenously to facilitate endotracheal intubation and to induce skeletal muscle relaxation, either as an adjunct to general anesthesia during surgery or during mechanical ventilation.

cis•clo•mi•phene (sis-klo'mĭ-fēn) enclomiphene.

cis•plat•in (sis'plat-in) [USP] *cis*-diamminedichloroplatinum, a platinum coordination complex capable of producing inter- and intrastrand DNA crosslinks and having a broad spectrum of antitumor activity, used in the treatment of a wide variety of neoplasms, particularly metastatic ovarian and testicular carcinoma and advanced carcinoma of the bladder; administered intravenously. Called also *CDDP, cis-DDP,* and *DDP.*

Cis•sam•pe•los (sis-am'pə-los) [Gr. *kissos* ivy + *ampelos* vine] a genus of climbing vines of the family Menispermaceae. *C. capen'sis* of southern Africa is emetic and cathartic. *C. parei'ra* L. is the false pareira or velvetleaf, used in tropical parts of the Americas to treat snakebites and as a diuretic, expectorant, emmenagogue, and febrifuge.

cis•tern (sis'tərn) [L. *cisterna*] a closed space serving as a reservoir for fluid; see also *cisterna.*
ambient c. cisterna ambiens.
basal c. cisterna interpeduncularis.
cerebellomedullary c. see *cisterna cerebellomedullaris lateralis* and *cisterna cerebellomedullaris posterior;* sometimes used specifically to denote the latter.
chiasmatic c. cisterna chiasmatica.
crural c. the subarachnoid space between the crus cerebri of the midbrain and the parahippocampal gyrus; it contains the anterior choroidal and medial posterior choroidal arteries and the basal vein. Called also *cisterna cruralis.*
great c. cisterna cerebellomedullaris posterior.
c. of great cerebral vein cisterna quadrigeminalis.
interpeduncular c. cisterna interpeduncularis.
c. of lamina terminalis cisterna laminae terminalis.
lateral cerebellomedullary c. cisterna cerebellomedullaris lateralis.
c. of lateral cerebral fossa cisterna fossae lateralis cerebri.
lumbar c. cisterna lumbalis.
c. of Pecquet cisterna chyli.
pericallosal c. cisterna pericallosa.
perinuclear c. see under *space.*
pontine c., pontocerebellar c. cisterna pontocerebellaris.
posterior c., posterior cerebellomedullary c. cisterna cerebellomedullaris posterior.
premedullary c. a subarachnoid cistern sometimes recognized separately, lying ventral to the medulla oblongata and continuous caudally with the spinal subarachnoid space. It contains the terminal part of the vertebral artery, the anterior spinal artery, and the anterior medullary vein.
prepontine c. cisterna pontocerebellaris.
quadrigeminal c. cisterna quadrigeminalis.
subarachnoid c's cisternae subarachnoideae.
superior c. cisterna quadrigeminalis.
supracallosal c. cisterna pericallosa.
sylvian c. cisterna fossae lateralis cerebri.
terminal c's pairs of transversely oriented channels that are confluent with the sarcotubules, which together with an intermediate T tubule constitute a triad of skeletal muscle. See also *T system,* under *system; T tubule,* under *tubule;* and *triad of skeletal muscle.*

cis•ter•na (sis-tur'nə) gen. and pl. *cister'nae* [L.] 1. [TA] cistern: a closed space serving as a reservoir for lymph or other body fluid, especially one of the enlarged subarachnoid spaces containing cerebrospinal fluid. 2. an ultrastructural, membrane-lined space occurring in the endoplasmic reticulum and Golgi complex.
c. am'biens [TA] ambient cistern: a sheetlike curved layer of subarachnoid space extending from the cisterna quadrigeminalis and partially encircling the midbrain on each side, connecting with the cisterna interpeduncularis. The term is sometimes used to denote the combination of the sheetlike extensions and the cisterna quadrigeminalis.
c. basa'lis c. interpeduncularis.
c. cerebellomedulla'ris latera'lis [TA] lateral cerebellomedullary cistern: a narrow anterolateral expansion of the posterior cerebellomedullary cistern on each side of the medulla oblongata.
c. cerebellomedulla'ris poste'rior [TA] posterior cerebellomedullary cistern: the enlarged subarachnoid space between the inferior surface of the cerebellum and the posterior surface of the medulla oblongata, and continuous below with the spinal subarachnoid space. It can be tapped by means of a needle inserted through the posterior atlanto-occipital membrane (cisternal puncture). Called also *c. magna* [TA alternative] and *great* or *posterior cistern.*

c. chiasma'tica [TA] chiasmatic cistern: a subarachnoid cistern adjacent to the optic chiasm, related rostrally to the cisterna laminae terminalis and caudally to the cisterna interpeduncularis.

c. chy'li [TA] a dilated portion of the thoracic duct at its origin in the lumbar region; it receives several lymph-collecting vessels, including the intestinal, lumbar, and descending intercostal trunks. Called also *chylocyst, cistern of Pecquet, receptaculum chyli,* and *receptaculum Pecqueti.*

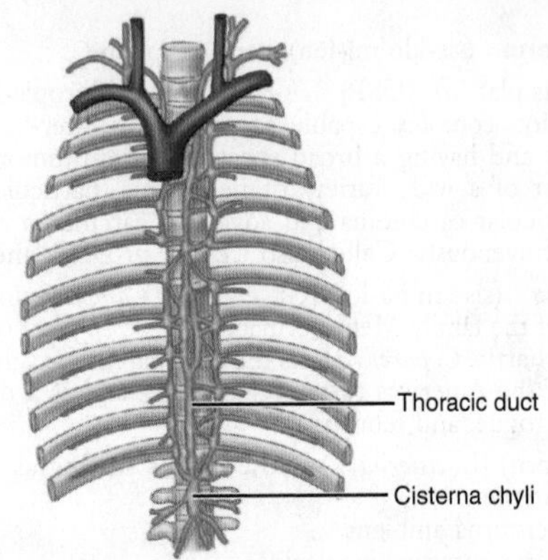

c. crura'lis crural cistern.

cylindrical confronting cisternae cytoplasmic structures often associated with tuboreticular structures in cells in a variety of pathological conditions including immunologic and neoplastic disorders, neurodegenerative diseases, and viral infections.

c. fos'sae latera'lis ce'rebri [TA] cistern of lateral cerebral fossa: the space between the arachnoid and the lateral cerebral fossa; it contains the middle cerebral artery. Called also *sylvian cistern.*

c. interpeduncula'ris [TA] interpeduncular cistern: a dilatation of the subarachnoid space between the cerebral peduncles; called also *basal cistern.*

c. la'minae termina'lis [TA] cistern of lamina terminalis: a subarachnoid cistern located posterosuperior to the optic chiasm, posteroinferior to the rostrum of the corpus callosum, and rostral to the lamina terminalis; it contains the anterior cerebral arteries.

c. lumba'lis [TA] lumbar cistern: the enlargement of the subarachnoid space caudal to the conus medullaris, containing the cauda equina, the pial part of the filum terminale, and cerebrospinal fluid; it is the site of lumbar puncture.

c. mag'na TA alternative for *c. cerebellomedullaris posterior.*

c. pericallo'sa [TA] pericallosal cistern: a subarachnoid cistern running longitudinally along the superior surface of the corpus callosum.

perinuclear c. see under *space.*

c. pon'tis, c. pontocerebella'ris [TA] pontine cistern: a large space ventral to the pons, continuous posteriorly with the cisterna magna and rostrally with the interpeduncular cistern; the basilar artery runs through it. It may be considered to be continuous caudally with the spinal subarachnoid space or with the premedullary cistern, when that cistern is recognized as distinct. Called also *pontocerebellar* or *prepontine cistern.*

c. quadrigemina'lis [TA] quadrigeminal cistern: the superior confluent of the subarachnoid space, lying in the angle between the splenium of the corpus callosum and the superior surfaces of the cerebellum and mesencephalon, and containing the great cerebral vein and the root of the trochlear nerve. Called also *c. venae magnae cerebri* [TA alternative], *cistern of great cerebral vein,* and *superior cistern.* See also *c. ambiens.*

cister'nae subarachnoi'deae [TA] subarachnoid cisterns: localized enlargements of the subarachnoid space, occurring in areas where the dura mater and arachnoid do not closely follow the contour of the brain with its covering pia mater, and serving as reservoirs of cerebrospinal fluid.

subsarcolemmal cisternae hollow swellings of the tubules of the sarcoplasmic reticulum; they participate in the coupling of the sarcoplasmic reticulum with the sarcolemma in cardiac muscle.

c. ve'nae mag'nae ce'rebri TA alternative for *c. quadrigeminalis.*

cis·ter·nae (sis-tur'ne) [L.] genitive and plural of *cisterna.*

cis·ter·nal (sis-tur'nəl) pertaining to a cistern, especially the cisterna cerebellomedullaris.

cis·ter·nog·ra·phy (sis″tər-nog'rə-fe) radiography of the basal cistern of the brain after subarachnoid injection of a contrast medium. **cisternograph'ic** *adj*

air c. visualization of the cisterns of the brain following administration of approximately 5 mL of air by lumbar puncture; used in the evaluation of masses in the cerebellopontine angle and for detecting small acoustic tumors in the internal acoustic meatus.

metrizamide c. visualization of the cisterns of the brain by computed tomography following intrathecal injection of metrizamide.

radionuclide c. imaging of the cisterns of the brain following the intrathecal injection of a radiopharmaceutical.

cis·tron (sis'tron) [L. *cis* on this side + *trans* on the other side + Gr. *on* neuter ending] originally, a unit of genetic material determined by a *cis-trans* test; it has been shown to be essentially equivalent to a gene (q.v.).

ci·tal·o·pram hy·dro·bro·mide (si-tal'o-pram) [USP] a selective serotonin reuptake inhibitor (SSRI), chemically unrelated to other SSRI's and consisting of a racemic mixture of two stereoisomers (*S-* and *R-*, the *S-*isomer being pharmaceutically active); used as an antidepressant, administered orally.

Ci·tel·li syndrome (che-tel'e) [Salvatore *Citelli,* Italian laryngologist, 1875–1947] see under *syndrome.*

cit·rate (sit'rāt) any anionic form, salt, or ester of citric acid. For specific salts, see entries under the adjectival form, e.g., for *ferric citrate,* see under *ferric.*

c. phosphate dextrose (CPD) anticoagulant citrate phosphate dextrose solution.

c. phosphate dextrose adenine (CPDA-1) anticoagulant citrate phosphate dextrose adenine solution.

cit·rate cleav·age en·zyme (sit'rāt kle'vij en'zīm) ATP citrate lyase.

cit·rat·ed (sit'rāt-əd) containing a citrate, especially potassium citrate.

cit·rate *(si)*-syn·thase (sit'rāt sin'thās) [EC 2.3.3.1] an enzyme of the transferase class that catalyzes the condensation of oxaloacetate and the acetyl group of acetyl coenzyme A to form citrate and coenzyme A. This is the initial reaction in the tricarboxylic acid cycle (see illustration under *cycle*).

ci·treo·vir·i·din (sĭ″tre-o-vir'ĭ-din) a mycotoxin found in the fungus *Penicillium citreoviride,* which sometimes contaminates rice and can cause cardiac damage.

cit·ric ac·id (sit'rik) 1. a compound from citrus fruits that is an intermediate in the tricarboxylic acid (Krebs) cycle (q.v.). It chelates calcium ions and prevents blood clotting. 2. [NF] anhydrous or monohydrated citric acid, used in the preparation of effervescent mixtures, as a synergist to enhance the action of antioxidants, and as an anticoagulant for stored whole blood and red cells and also for blood specimens.

Cit·ro·lith (sit'ro-lith) trademark for a combination preparation of potassium citrate and sodium citrate.

cit·ri·nin (sit'rĭ-nin) a mycotoxin produced by *Aspergillus ochraceus, Penicillium citrinum,* and related species, which contaminate grain; it causes mycotoxic nephropathy in livestock and has been implicated as a cause of Balkan nephropathy in humans.

Cit·ro·bac·ter (sit'ro-bak″tər) [L. *citrus* lemon + Gr. *baktron* a rod] a genus of gram-negative, facultatively anaerobic, rod-shaped bacteria of the family Enterobacteriaceae, consisting of motile organisms that are able to use citrate as a sole carbon source. The organisms occur in water, food, feces, and urine. They have been associated with diarrhea and secondary infections in debilitated persons, occasionally causing severe primary septicemia. The type species is *C. freun'dii.*

C. amalona'ticus a species found in feces, soil, water, sewage, and opportunistic infections.

C. braa'kii a species that has sometimes been found in human clinical specimens.

C. freun'dii the most commonly isolated species, found in soil, water, sewage, some normal clinical specimens, and some opportunistic infections.

C. ko'seri a species found in soil, water, sewage, food, some normal clinical specimens, and occasionally cases of neonatal meningitis.

cit·ro·nel·la (sit″rə-nel'ə) *Cymbopogon nardus,* the source of citronella oil.

cit·ro·phos·phate (sit″ro-fos'fāt) a compound of a citrate and a phosphate.

cit·rul·li·na·tion (sit-rul″ĭ-na'shən) a posttranslational modification of proteins in which peptidylarginine deiminase catalyzes the conversion of arginine residues to citrulline residues. It plays a role in differentiation of epidermis, regulation of gene expression, and apoptosis; it also occurs in a variety of inflammatory conditions. **citrul'linated** *adj*

cit·rul·line (sit'rə-lēn) an amino acid formed from ornithine and converted into arginine in the urea cycle.

cit·rul·lin·emia (sit-rul″in-e'me-ə) either of two clinically and genetically distinct autosomal recessive aminoacidopathies caused by deficient argininosuccinate synthase activity. Called also *argininosuccinate synthase deficiency* and *citrullinuria.*

classic c. citrullinemia type I.

c. type I a condition caused by mutations in the *ASS* gene (locus: 9q34.1), which encodes argininosuccinate synthase, marked elevation in plasma and urine levels of citrulline, with hyperammonemia and sometimes secondary oroticaciduria; mild to moderate mental deficiency is a common sequela. There are two forms. The *severe* or *neonatal form* appears in the first few days of life and is characterized by severe hyperammonemia. The *subacute form* appears after one year of age and is marked by failure to thrive, frequent vomiting, developmental delay, and dry, brittle hair.

c. type II a condition caused by mutations in the *SLC25A13* gene (locus: 7q21.3), which encodes a mitochondrial transport protein necessary for the conversion of citrulline to argininoscuccinic acid. It is seen almost exclusively in Japan and exists in two forms. The *neonatal form* is generally self-limited and characterized by fatty infiltration and moderate fibrosis of the liver, cholestatic jaundice, hyperbilirubinemia, hypoproteinemia, and clotting dysfunction; serum ammonia and citrulline levels are usually normal. The *adult-onset form* appears between 20 and 40 years of age and is manifested by neuropsychiatric symptoms, with moderate elevation of serum ammonia and citrulline.

Ci•trul•lus (sĭ-trul′əs) a genus of plants of the family Cucurbitaceae, originally native to Africa. *C. colocyn′this* is the colocynth. *C. vulga′ris* is the watermelon.

cit•rul•lin•uria (sit-rul″in-u′re-ə) 1. citrullinemia. 2. excretion of high levels of citrulline in the urine.

Cit•rus (sit′rəs) [L.] the citrus fruits, a genus of trees of the family Rutaceae, widely cultivated for their fruit. Several of the fruits are rich in vitamin C and are sources of flavorings; see specific fruits. *C. aurantifo′lia* is the lime; *C. auran′tium* L. is the bitter orange; *C. berga′mia* is the bergamot; *C. li′mon* is the lemon; and *C. sinen′sis* is the sweet orange.

Ci•vatte bodies, poikiloderma (se-vaht′) [Achille *Civatte*, French dermatologist, 1877–1956] see under *body* and *poikiloderma*.

Ci•vi•ni•ni ligament, process (che″ve-ne′ne) [Filippo *Civinini*, Italian anatomist, 1805–1844] see *ligamentum pterygospinale* and *processus pterygospinosus*.

CJD Creutzfeldt-Jakob disease.

CK creatine kinase.

CKD chronic kidney disease.

Cl chlorine.

clade (klād) [Gr. *klados* branch] 1. in taxonomy, a branch of a phylogenetic tree comprising all the organisms that share a particular common ancestor. 2. a group of organisms that share characteristics exclusive to the group members and distinguishing them from other organisms, such as genetic variants within a single species.

Cla•do anastomosis, band, ligament (klah-do′) [Spiro *Clado*, French gynecologist, 1862–1920] see under *anastomosis*, *band*, and *ligament*.

Clad•o•phi•a•loph•o•ra (klad″o-fi″ə-lof′ə-rə) a genus of chiefly saprobic Fungi Imperfecti of the form-class Hyphomycetes, form-family Dematiaceae, having mainly aseptate, acropetal conidia.

C. bantia′na a species that causes cerebral phaeohyphomycosis with thick-walled brain abscesses and sometimes meningitis that can be fatal. Formerly called *Cladosporium bantianum*.

C. carrio′nii a species that is an agent of chromoblastomycosis.

clad•o•spo•ri•o•sis (klad″o-spor″e-o′sis) infection with *Cladosporium;* common types include brain infections such as abscesses and meningitis, and skin infections such as chromoblastomycosis.

Clad•o•spo•ri•um (klad″o-spor′e-əm) [Gr. *klados* branch + *spores* seed] a genus of chiefly saprobic Fungi Imperfecti of the form-class Hyphomycetes, form-family Dematiaceae, having mainly aseptate, acropetal conidia.

C. bantia′num *Cladophialophora bantiana*.

C. carrio′nii *Cladophialophora carrionii*.

C. manso′nii former name for *Malassezia furfur*.

C. trichoi′des *Cladophialophora bantiana*.

clad•ri•bine (kla′drĭ-bēn) [USP] a purine antimetabolite used as an antineoplastic in the treatment of hairy cell leukemia; administered intravenously. Called also *2-chlorodeoxyadenosine*.

Claf•or•an (klaf′or-an) trademark for a preparation of cefotaxime sodium.

clair•voy•ance (klār-voi′əns) [Fr.] a form of extrasensory perception in which knowledge of objective events is acquired without the use of the senses. Cf. *telepathy*.

clamp (klamp) 1. any device used to grip, join, compress, or fasten parts. 2. a surgical instrument for effecting compression. See accompanying table and see also under *forceps*.

Selected Surgical Clamps

Abadie clamp	Gomco clamp
Allen clamp	Halstead mosquito clamp
Allis clamp	Kocher clamp
Best colon clamp	Mayo clamp
Carmel clamp	Pace-Potts clamp
curved Kelly clamp	Rumel clamp
DeBakey clamp	Satinsky clamp
deCourcy clamp	straight Kelly clamp
Dennis intestinal clamp	Von Petz clamp
Doyen clamp	Wangensteen clamp
Erhardt clamp	Zipser clamp
Fehland clamp	

Cope c. a crushing clamp with several hinged segments for use in surgery of the colon and rectum.

cotton roll rubber dam c. a rubber dam clamp with a buccal and lingual wing or flange to hold cotton rolls in position in the mouth; useful in the placement of direct gold or other restorative material in subgingival class V cavity preparations.

Crile c. a rubber-shod clamp to secure temporary hemostasis in suture of blood vessels.

Doyen c. a forceps with flexible blades for clamping tissues to control bleeding temporarily during operations on the gastrointestinal tract.

Gant c. a right-angled clamp used in operating on hemorrhoids.

gingival c. a clamp for retracting gingival tissues.

Goldblatt c. a clamp for the renal artery to produce experimental hypertension; see also *Goldblatt hypertension* under *hypertension* and *Goldblatt kidney*, under *kidney*.

Joseph c. a clamp used after a nasal operation to improve the alignment of the mobilized fragments of the bony framework of the nose.

Mikulicz c. a clamp used for crushing the septum between the proximal and distal segments of the colon after exteriorization.

mosquito c. a small hemostatic clamp.

patch c. a type of voltage clamp in which a patch electrode is pressed against an area of the plasma membrane of a cell, forming an electrically tight seal so that the flow of current through individual ion channels can be measured.

Payr c. a crushing clamp used in resections of the stomach, intestine, and colon.

Péan c. a curved or straight hemostatic clamp with serrations along the entire length of the jaw.

pedicle c. clamp forceps (def. 1); see under *forceps*.

Potts c. an atraumatic clamp used to grasp a blood vessel.

Rankin c. a three-bladed clamp for crushing the colon during resection.

rubber dam c. a device made of spring metal that is used to retain a rubber dam on a tooth; it has beveled jaws that contact the tooth and a bow that connects the jaws.

Sehrt c. a clamp for compressing the aorta or for compressing a limb to arrest hemorrhage; called also *Sehrt compressor*.

voltage c. an electronic technique employing the feedback principle to impose a fixed potential difference across a cell membrane; used in the study of ion channels. Voltage across the membrane is fixed at a set level and the current changes to counterbalance any induced flow of ions; the current change is a measure of the change in conductance of the membrane for one or more specific ions.

clamp•ing (klamp′ing) in the measurement of insulin secretion and action, the infusion of a glucose solution at a rate adjusted periodically to maintain a predetermined blood glucose concentration.

euglycemic c. clamping in which the blood glucose levels are maintained within the normal range.

clang•ing (klang′ing) a pattern of speech in which sound rather than sense governs word choice, and rhyming and punning *(clang association)* substitute for logic; commonly observed in schizophrenia and manic episodes.

clap (klap) popular name for gonorrhea.

clap•o•tage (klap″o-tahzh′) clapotement.

cla•pote•ment (klah-pawt-maw′) [Fr.] a splashing sound heard on succussion; called also *clapotage*.

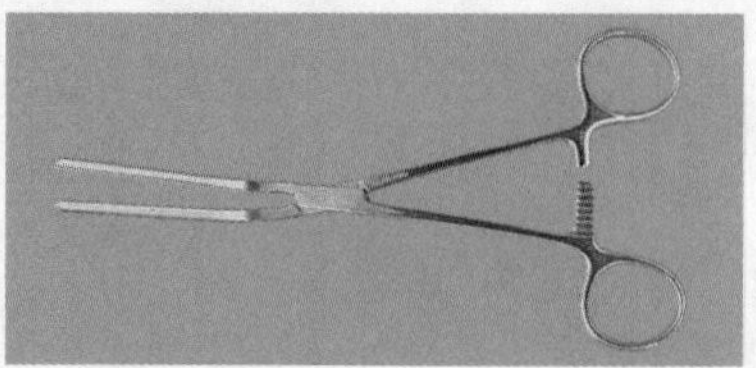

■ Clamp (DeBakey peripheral vascular).

Cla•ra cells (klah′rah) [Max *Clara*, Austrian anatomist, 1899–1966] see under *cell.*

clar•if•i•cant (klar-if′ĭ-kənt) an agent that clears liquids of turbidity.

clar•i•fi•ca•tion (klar″ĭ-fĭ-ka′shən) [L. *clarus* clear + *facere* to make] the clearing of a liquid from turbidity.

clar•i•fy (klar′ĭ-fi) [L. *clarificare* to render clear] to clear of turbidity or of suspended matter.

Clar•i•nex (klar″ĭ-neks′) trademark for preparations of desloratadine.

cla•rith•ro•my•cin (klə-rith″ro-mi′sin) [USP] a macrolide antibiotic effective against a wide spectrum of gram-positive and gram-negative bacteria, used in the treatment of respiratory tract infections and skin and soft tissue infections, and in conjunction with omeprazole in the treatment of duodenal ulcer associated with *Helicobacter pylori* infections; administered orally.

Clar•i•tin (klar′ĭ-tin) trademark for preparations of loratadine.

Clark-Col•lip method (klahrk′ kol′ip) [Earl Perry *Clark*, American biochemist, 20th century; James Bertram *Collip*, Canadian biochemist, 1892–1965] see under *method.*

Clarke cells, nucleus (column) (klahrk) [Jacob Augustus Lockhart *Clarke*, English anatomist and physician, 1817–1880] see under *cell*, and see *nucleus thoracicus posterior.*

Clarke-Had•field syndrome (klahrk′ had′fēld) [Cecil *Clarke*, British physician, 20th century; Geoffrey *Hadfield*, British physician, 1889–1968] see under *syndrome.*

clasp (klasp) 1. a device by which something is held. 2. in dentistry, a part of an extracoronal direct retainer that retains and stabilizes the denture by attaching to abutment teeth.

Adams c. a modified arrow clasp that utilizes buccal, mesial, and distal proximal undercuts of a tooth for retention. See illustration.

arrow c., arrowhead c. a clasp made by bending a piece of stainless steel wire in the shape of an arrowhead; used to stabilize an orthodontic appliance by holding the teeth in the interproximal areas.

bar c. a clasp whose arms are bar-type extensions from major connectors or from within the denture base; the arms approach the point of contact on the tooth in the cervico-occlusal direction.

circumferential c. a clasp that encircles more than 180° of a tooth, including opposite angles, and usually contacts the tooth throughout the extent of the clasp, at least one terminal being in the infrabulge area.

continuous c., continuous lingual c. a clasp made of two or more stainless steel lingual clasps joined to each other and then joined to a major connector by two or more minor connectors; used to brace lingual upper teeth. Called also *continuous bar retainer*, *Kennedy bar*, and *lingual bar.*

Crozat c. a metal attachment of a removable appliance adapted to the embrasure.

I-bar c., infrabulge c. a bar clasp arm that approaches the crown of the tooth from an apical direction, without crossing the survey line, crossing the tooth-tissue junction at right angles and continuing in a straight line to the unattached mucosa before turning to a horizontal position.

class (klas) 1. a taxonomic category subordinate to a phylum (or subphylum) and superior to an order. 2. in statistics, a subgroup of a population for which certain variables measured for individuals in the population fall within specific limits.

clas•sic (klas′ik) standard, typical, or traditional.

clas•si•cal (klas′ĭ-kəl) classic.

clas•si•fi•ca•tion (klas″ĭ-fĭ-ka′shən) the systematic arrangement of similar entities on the basis of certain differing characteristics.

adansonian c. numerical taxonomy.

Angle c. a classification of dental malocclusion based on the mesiodistal (anteroposterior) position of the mandibular dental arch and teeth relative to the maxillary dental arch and teeth; see also *malocclusion.*

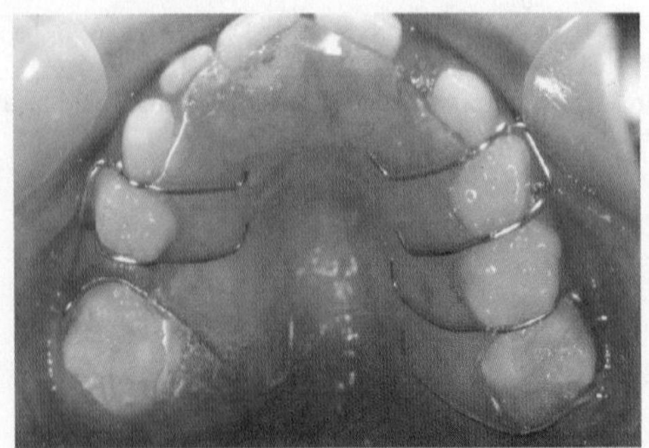

■ Removable appliance with multiple Adams clasps.

Arneth c. classification of neutrophils according to the number of lobes in their nuclei for calculating the Arneth count.

Bergey c. a system of classification of bacteria in which the organisms are grouped according to Gram reaction, metabolism, and morphology, with each group being further subdivided into orders, families, genera, and species.

Black c. a classification of dental caries into five groups on the basis of similarity of treatment required. See table at *caries.*

Borrmann c. a classification of gastric carcinoma as either polypoid, ulcerating, ulcerating-infiltrating, or infiltrating.

Broders c. see under *index.*

Caldwell-Moloy c. classification of female pelves as gynecoid, android, anthropoid, and platypelloid; see under *pelvis.*

Chicago c. the classification of human chromosomes adopted by geneticists in Chicago in 1966 for the identification of chromosomal bands and regions and for the location of structural chromosomal abnormalities. See also *Paris c.*

Child-Pugh c., Child-Turcotte-Pugh c. a classification of severity of cirrhosis (classes A, B, and C, in order of increasing severity), based on a composite score for five different parameters, each parameter being given a score of 1 to 3, with 3 being the most severe finding. The parameters are hepatic encephalopathy, ascites, total bilirubin, serum albumin, and prothrombin time.

Dukes c. a three-class staging system that classifies colorectal carcinoma from A to C based on the extent of the tumor: A, penetration into but not through the bowel wall; B, penetration through the bowel wall; C, lymph node involvement regardless of extent of bowel wall penetration. Many modifications of this classification exist.

FAB c. French-American-British c.

FIGO c. any of the classification systems established by the International Federation of Gynecology and Obstetrics for the staging of gynecological cancers. Cancers at any particular site are staged from 0 to IV with 0 being precancerous or in situ and IV being highly malignant or invasive; subdivisions using letters may also be used, as IA, IB, IIA, IIB, and so on.

Forrester c. a classification system for patients with suspected or overt heart failure, done after cardiac catheterization of the right heart and determination of cardiac index and pulmonary artery wedge pressure. Patients are divided into four classes according to severity (lower cardiac index and higher wedge pressure being severe). Those in class I were found to have no pulmonary congestion or peripheral vessel hypoperfusion, whereas those in class IV have both of these complications.

Frankel c. a classification dividing spinal cord injuries into five groups according to severity of deficit below the level of injury: *Group A*, complete interruption of all sensation and motor function; *Group B*, incomplete interruption, with some sensation but no motor function; *Group C*, incomplete interruption, with demonstrable voluntary motor function but at a minimal, nonuseful level; *Group D*, incomplete interruption, with some voluntary motor function that is useful to the patient; and *Group E*, recovery to normal functioning attained. Called also *ASIA scale.*

Fredrickson and Lees c. a scheme for subdividing the familial hyperlipoproteinemias on the basis of phenotypes, which are classified as I–V. See table at *hyperlipoproteinemia.*

French-American-British c. a classification of acute leukemia produced by a three-nation joint collaboration; acute lymphocytic leukemia is subdivided into three types and acute myelogenous leukemia is subdivided into eight types. Called also *FAB classification.*

Gell and Coombs c. a classification of immune mechanisms of tissue injury, called by Gell and Coombs "allergic reactions," comprising four types: *type I*, immediate hypersensitivity reactions, mediated by IgE antibody; *type II*, antibody-mediated hypersensitivity reactions, including complement-dependent lysis, antibody-dependent cell-mediated cytotoxicity (ADCC), and phagocytosis induced by opsonizing antibody; *type III*, immune complex–mediated hypersensitivity reactions, including serum sickness, Arthus reactions, and systemic lupus erythematosus; and *type IV*, cell-mediated hypersensitivity reactions, mediated by sensitized T lymphocytes either by release of lymphokines or by T-cell–mediated cytotoxicity, including contact dermatitis, allograft rejection, and graft-versus-host disease. Other authorities have added *type V*, antibody interference with the function of biologically active substances, including autoimmune diseases mediated by antireceptor antibodies and coagulation disorders mediated by antibodies to coagulation factors. The individual types I–IV are described under *hypersensitivity reaction*, under *reaction.*

Kauffman-White c. a scheme for the identification of serovars of *Salmonella* by classification of their reactions to O, H, and Vi antisera.

Keith-Wagener-Barker c. a classification of hypertension and arteriolosclerosis based on retinal changes. *Group 1*, essential benign hypertension indicated by moderate arteriolar attenuation. *Group 2*, constant high blood pressure but no apparent effect on health, indicated by more definite arteriolar attenuation with localized constriction. *Group 3*, hypertension with retinal, renal, cerebral, and other symptoms, indicated by marked attenuation of the arterioles, cotton-wool exudates, and hemorrhages. *Group 4*, severe hypertension with severe nervous system, visual, and other organ disturbances, indicated by ophthalmoscopic signs of Group 3, with papilledema.

Kennedy c. a classification of partially edentulous conditions and partial dentures, based on the location of the edentulous spaces in relation to the remaining teeth.

Kiel c. a classification of non-Hodgkin lymphomas, used primarily in Europe and based on morphologic and cytologic criteria. A later classification system is the Revised European-American Lymphoma (REAL) Classification. Called also *Lennert c.*

Killip c. a classification system for patients with suspected or overt heart failure, based on a physical examination to determine clinical manifestations. Patients are divided into four classes, with class I being no heart failure; class II being presence of the third heart sound or basal lung crepitation; class III being acute pulmonary edema; and class IV being presence of cardiogenic shock.

Lancefield c. a serologic classification of the hemolytic streptococci, based on extraction and examination by a precipitin technique of group-specific carbohydrate antigens called C carbohydrates in the cell wall. Groups A to O have been established, with groups A to G being the most common ones infecting humans.

Lennert c. Kiel c.

Lukes-Collins c. a classification of non-Hodgkin lymphomas based on their presumed cells of origin. It stresses the distinction between B-cell, T-cell, and lymphocytic lymphomas, with the B-cell and T-cell types having several subtypes that can be arranged by grade of malignancy. A later classification is the Revised European-American Lymphoma (REAL) Classification.

Lund-Browder c. a classification of burn severity, more accurate than the rule of nines and used especially for children; it attaches percentages to different body surface areas similarly to the rule of nines and is modified according to the age of the child.

McNeer c. Borrmann c.

New York Heart Association (NYHA) c. a functional and therapeutic classification for prescription of physical activity for cardiac patients; see table.

numerical c. see under *taxonomy*.

Nyhus c. a classification of inguinal hernias based on damage to the internal inguinal ring or the defect in Hesselbach triangle. See table at *inguinal hernia*, under *hernia*.

Paris c. a modification made in Paris in 1971 of the Chicago classification of human chromosomes, providing more detailed cytogenetic information.

Rappaport c. a classification of non-Hodgkin lymphomas based on histologic criteria; the categories it developed were *nodular lymphomas* and *diffuse lymphomas*. It was replaced by the Lukes-Collins classification and the Kiel classification.

REAL c., Revised European-American Lymphoma C. a classification of lymphomas based on histologic criteria, dividing them into three main categories: B-cell neoplasms, T- or NK-cell neoplasms, and Hodgkin disease.

Rome c. a set of symptom-based diagnostic criteria for the evaluation of functional gastrointestinal disorders.

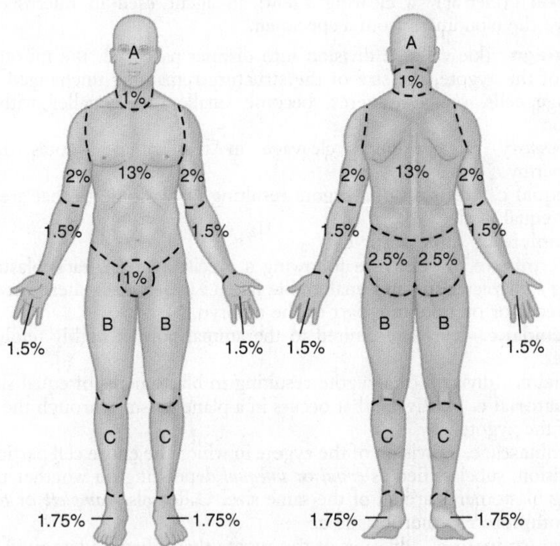

■ Lund-Browder classification; the percentages assigned to areas affected by growth are adjusted by age. *A* (Head) decreases in relative size from infancy to adulthood, while *B* (thigh) and *C* (leg) increase.

New York Heart Association Classification of Cardiac Patients

Class	Limitation of Activity	Symptoms
I(A)	None	None from ordinary activity
II(B)	Slight	On moderate or normal exertion
III(C)	Marked	On mild exertion
IV(D)	Complete	Even at rest, worsened by any exertion

Runyon c. a classification system that divides the nontuberculous mycobacteria (q.v.) into four groups on the basis of pigmentation and growth condition.

Rye c. a classification of Hodgkin disease on the basis of histology and pathology into the categories of lymphocyte predominance type, mixed cellularity type, lymphocyte depletion type, and nodular sclerosis type.

Skinner c. a method of classifying partially edentulous conditions and partial dentures, based on the location of the edentulous spaces in relation to the remaining teeth.

WHO c. of lymphoid neoplasms a classification of lymphomas, descended from the REAL classification, that divides them into three main categories (B-cell neoplasms, T-cell neoplasms, and Hodgkin lymphoma) based on morphology, immunophenotype, and genetic abnormalities.

-clast [Gr. *-klastēs* breaker, from *klan* to break] a word termination denoting that which breaks or destroys.

clas·tic (klas′tik) [Gr. *klastos* broken + *-ic*] 1. causing or undergoing a division into parts. 2. separable into parts, as an anatomic model.

clas·to·gen·ic (klas″to-jen′ik) [Gr. *klastos* broken + *-genic*] giving rise to or inducing disruption or breakages, as of chromosomes.

clas·to·thrix (klas′to-thriks) trichorrhexis nodosa.

clath·rate (klath′rāt) [L. *clathare* to provide with a lattice] 1. having the shape or appearance of a lattice. 2. clathrate compound. 3. pertaining to such a compound.

clath·rin (klath′rin) a protein consisting of three limbs, each composed of a heavy (180 kD) and a light (about 35 kD) chain, in a triskelion arrangement; it coats the cytoplasmic face of coated pits (q.v.) in receptor-mediated endocytosis. Clathrin-coated vesicles are also involved in retrieval of synaptic vesicle membrane following neurotransmitter release and in vesicle formation on the trans-Golgi network and endosomes. The coat depolymerizes after the vesicle buds from the membrane and the clathrin units are reused.

Claude hyperkinesis sign, syndrome (klōd) [Henri *Claude*, French psychiatrist, 1869–1945] see under *sign* and *syndrome*.

clau·di·cant (klaw′dĭ-kənt) 1. pertaining to claudication; called also *claudicatory*. 2. affected by claudication. 3. affected by intermittent claudication.

clau·di·ca·tion (klaw′dĭ-ka′shən) [L. *claudicatio*] limping or lameness.

intermittent c. a complex of symptoms characterized by pain, tension, and weakness in a limb when walking is begun, intensification of the condition until walking becomes impossible, and disappearance of the symptoms after a period of rest. It is caused by reversible muscle ischemia that occurs in occlusive arterial disease of the limbs. Called also *Charcot syndrome* and *angina cruris*.

jaw c. a complex of symptoms like those of intermittent claudication but seen in the muscles of mastication, occurring in giant cell arteritis.

neurogenic c. claudication accompanied by pain and paresthesias in the back, buttocks, and lower limbs, relieved by stooping or sitting; it is usually caused by lumbar spinal stenosis that may be a mechanical disturbance due to posture, and less often by ischemia of the cauda equina.

venous c. intermittent claudication caused by venous stasis.

clau·di·ca·tory (klaw′dĭ-kə-tor″e) claudicant (def. 1).

clau·din (klaw′din) any of a family of transmembrane proteins, connected with actin filaments of the cytoskeleton, that are the main sealing proteins of tight junctions.

Clau·di·us cells (klaw′de-əs) [Friedrich Matthias *Claudius*, German anatomist, 1822–1869] see under *cell*.

claus·tra (klaws′trə) [L.] plural of *claustrum*.

claus·tro·pho·bia (klaws″tro-fo′be-ə) [L. *claudere* to shut + *-phobia*] irrational fear of being shut in; fear of enclosed spaces, such as elevators and tunnels.

claus·trum (claws′trəm) pl. *claus′tra* [L. "a barrier"] [TA] the thin layer of gray matter lateral to the external capsule of the lentiform nucleus, separating the nucleus from the white substance of the insula; it is mainly composed of spindle cells. Called also *c. of insula.* **claus′tral** *adj*

cla•va (kla′və) [L. "stick"] tuberculum gracile.

cla•va•cin (kla′və-sin) patulin.

cla•val (kla′vəl) pertaining to the clava (tuberculum gracile [TA]).

cla•vate (kla′vāt) [L. *clavatus* club] 1. claval. 2. club-shaped.

Clav•i•ceps (klav′ĭ-seps) [L. *clava* club + *caput* head] a genus of parasitic fungi of the family Clavicipitaceae that infest the seeds of various plants; several species are sources of ergot. *C. purpu′rea* infests rye and is the most common source of ergotism in humans. *C. pas′pali* infests paspalum grasses and causes paspalum staggers in ruminants.

Clav•i•cip•i•ta•ceae (klav″ĭ-sip″ĭ-ta′se-e) a family of fungi of the order Clavicipitales, having long cylindrical asci and long filiform ascospores; it includes the genera *Claviceps* and *Cordyceps.*

Clav•i•cip•i•ta•les (klav″ĭ-sip″ĭ-ta′lēz) an order of perfect fungi of the subphylum Ascomycotina, series Unitunicatae, characterized by perithecia formed in well-developed stroma and inoperculate asci. Most species are parasitic on insects or fungi; some are plant parasites. It includes the family Clavicipitaceae.

clav•i•cle (klav′ĭ-kəl) clavicula. **clavic′ular** *adj*

clav•i•cot•o•my (klav″ĭ-kot′ə-me) [*clavicle* + Gr. *-tomy*] the operation of cutting or dividing the clavicle.

cla•vic•u•la (klə-vik′u-lə) [L. dim. of *clavis* key] [TA] the clavicle: a bone, curved like the letter *f,* that articulates with the sternum and scapula, forming the anterior portion of the shoulder girdle on either side; called also *collar bone.*

cla•vic•u•lec•to•my (klə-vik″u-lek′tə-me) [*clavicula* + *-ectomy*] excision of all or part of a clavicle.

cla•vic•u•lus (klə-vik′u-ləs) pl. *clavic′uli* [L. dim. of *clavus* nail] any one of Sharpey fibers (a set of fibers that hold together the laminae of a bone).

clav•i•pec•to•ral (klav″ĭ-pek′tə-rəl) [L. *clavis* clavicle + *pectoral*] pertaining to the clavicle and thorax.

Cla•vis•po•ra (klə-vis′pə-rə) a genus of fungi of the order Endomycetales. *C. lusita′niae* is the perfect (sexual) stage of *Candida lusitaniae.*

clav•u•la•nate po•tas•si•um (klav′u-lə-nāt) a β-lactamase inhibitor used in combination with penicillins in treating infections caused by β-lactamase–producing organisms.

cla•vus (kla′vəs) pl. *cla′vi* [L. "nail"] corn (def. 1).

c. du′rus hard corn.

c. hyste′ricus a sharp, painful sensation as if a nail were being driven into the head; usually regarded as a manifestation of conversion.

c. mol′lis soft corn.

claw (klaw) 1. a nail of an animal, particularly a carnivore, that is long and curved and has a sharp end. Called also *unguiculus.* 2. something resembling the claw of an animal.

cat's c. 1. *Uncaria tomentosa.* 2. a preparation of the root bark of *U. tomentosa,* having antiviral, immunostimulant, and antiinflammatory properties; used for a wide variety of indications in folk medicine.

devil's c. a perennial herb, *Harpagophytum procumbens,* native to southern Africa; its dried tubular secondary roots and lateral tubers are used for dyspepsia, loss of appetite, and rheumatism; it is also used in homeopathy for rheumatism and in folk medicine for a wide variety of disorders.

claw•foot (klaw′foot) gampsodactyly.

claw•hand (klaw′hand) flexion and atrophy of the hand and fingers; it occurs in lesions of the ulnar nerve, in leprosy, and in syringomyelia. Called also *main en griffe.*

cla•zu•ril (klaz′u-ril) a coccidiostat used in birds.

ClC chloride channel.

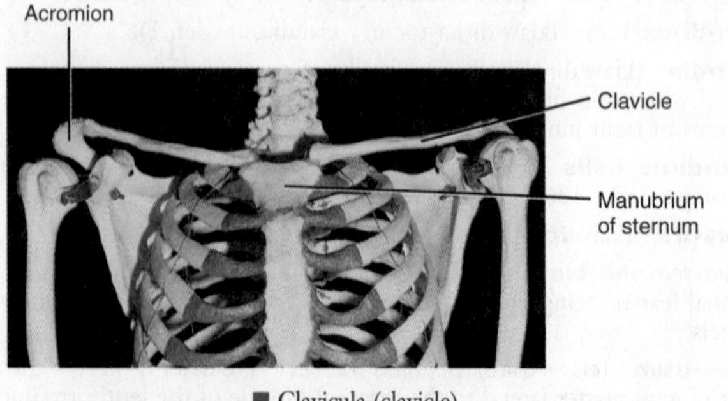

■ Clavicula (clavicle).

clear (klēr) 1. to remove cloudiness from microscopic specimens by the use of a clearing agent. 2. to remove a substance from the blood. 3. transparent; not cloudy, turbid, or opaque.

clear•ance (klēr′əns) 1. the process of removing a substance or an obstruction. 2. a quantitative measure of the rate at which a substance is removed from the blood by processes such as renal clearance, hepatic clearance, or hemodialysis; the volume of plasma that is completely cleared of the substance per unit time. Symbol *C.* 3. the space existing between opposed structures.

aerosol c. removal of particles that have been deposited in the respiratory tissues, done most often by ciliary transport, phagocytosis, dissolving the particle in tissue fluid, or encapsulation and immobilization in fibrous tissue.

***p*-aminohippurate c.** the renal clearance of exogenously administered *p*-aminohippuric acid, accepted as the most accurate measurement of effective renal plasma flow.

blood-urea c. urea c.

creatinine c. the renal clearance of endogenous creatinine, a commonly used clinical measurement that closely estimates the glomerular filtration rate.

free water c. the net amount of solute-free water moved from the blood to the urine; the difference between the urine volume and the osmolal clearance.

hepatic c. 1. the removal of a substance from the blood via the liver, as in liver function tests. 2. a measure of the rate of such removal.

immune c. immune elimination.

indocyanine green c. the hepatic clearance of indocyanine green, see *indocyanine green test,* under *test.*

interocclusal c. see under *distance.*

inulin c. the renal clearance of inulin maintained at a constant serum level by continuous infusion, accepted as the most accurate measurement and reference of the glomerular filtration rate.

mucociliary c. the clearance of mucus and other material from the airways by the cilia of the epithelial cells, which move mucus cephalad with every beat. See also *ciliary beat,* under *beat.*

occlusal c. a condition in which the opposing occlusal surfaces may glide over one another without any interfering projection.

osmolal c. the amount of water cleared from the plasma, resulting in urine having the same osmolality as plasma, calculated as urine volume × urine osmolality ÷ plasma osmolality.

plasma iron c. plasma iron clearance half-time.

renal c. 1. removal of a substance from the blood by the kidney. 2. a measure of the rate of such removal; given by the formula $C = V \times U/P$, where C is the clearance, V the urine volume in mL/min, U the urine concentration of the substance, and P the plasma concentration. See also clearances of specific substances such as *p-aminohippurate c., creatinine c., inulin c.,* and *urea c.*

total c., total body c. the total clearance of a substance via all the organs of the body. Cf. *hepatic c.* and *renal c.*

urea c. clearance of urea from the blood, by either renal clearance or hemodialysis; the efficiency, or fractional urea clearance, of one hemodialysis session is expressed by the formula *Kt/V* (q.v.). See also *urea kinetic modeling,* under *modeling.*

whole body c. total body c.

clear•er (klēr′ər) a clearing agent; an agent used in microscopy to remove the cloudiness from a specimen.

cleav•age (kle′vəj) 1. division into distinct parts. 2. the mitotic division of the zygote, the size of the structure remaining unchanged as the cleavage cells, or blastomeres, become smaller and smaller with each division.

accessory c. peripheral cleavage in telolecithal zygotes due to polyspermy.

adequal c. division of a zygote resulting in blastomeres that are practically equal in size.

complete c. holoblastic c.

determinate c. cleavage following a precise pattern, each blastomere having a characteristic and unalterable fate, i.e., each blastomere becoming the precursor of a definite part of the embryo.

discoidal c. cleavage limited to the animal pole of highly telolecithal zygotes.

equal c. division of a zygote resulting in blastomeres of equal size.

equatorial c. cleavage that occurs in a plane passing through the equator of the zygote.

holoblastic c. division of the zygote in which the entire cell participates in division; subclassified as *equal* or *unequal* depending on whether the resulting blastomeres are all of the same size. Called also *complete* or *total c.*

incomplete c. meroblastic c.

indeterminate c. division of the zygote that follows a less rigid cleavage pattern, the blastomeres having more developmental possibilities than they usually show, each of which, when isolated, being capable of developing into a normal embryo.

latitudinal c. cleavage in planes passing at right angles to the zygote axis.

meridional c. cleavage in planes passing through the zygote axis.

meroblastic c., partial c. division of the zygote in which only its protoplasmic portions participate, as occurs in fish, reptiles, and birds; called also *incomplete c.*

progressive c. in the formation of spores within a sporangium, the production of a series of cleavage planes in succession, resulting first in formation of protospores and later in formation of sporangiospores.

radial c. a cleavage pattern characteristic of vertebrates and echinoderms, in which the spindle axes are parallel or at right angles to the polar axis of the zygote.

spiral c. a cleavage pattern characteristic of such invertebrates as annelids and mollusks, in which the cleavage planes are oriented obliquely to the polar axis of the zygote.

superficial c. a form of cell division occurring in centrolecithal zygotes, in which only the surface region participates.

total c. holoblastic c.

unequal c. division of the zygote in which the blastomeres about the vegetal pole remain larger than those nearer the animal pole.

cleaved (klēvd) [A.S. *clēofan*] split or separated, as by cutting.

cleft (kleft) 1. a fissure or elongated opening, especially one occurring in the embryo. 2. a pathologic fissure derived from a failure of parts to fuse during embryonic development.

anal c. crena analis.

branchial c's 1. the slitlike openings in the gills of fishes, formed between the branchial arches. 2. pharyngeal grooves.

cholesterol c. a cleft in a section of tissue embedded in paraffin, due to the dissolving of cholesterol crystals.

clunial c. crena analis.

corneal c. see under *fissure.*

facial c. 1. any of the clefts between the embryonic prominences that normally unite to form the face. 2. failure of union of a facial cleft, which, depending on its site, causes such developmental defects as cleft cheek, cleft lip, cleft mandible, oblique facial cleft, and lateral facial cleft. Called also *prosoposchisis.*

genital c. a depression of the external genital region of the fetus, which develops into the male urethra or the female vestibule.

gingival c. an area of isolated gingival recession occurring over a dehiscence of the bone covering the root.

gluteal c. crena analis.

hyobranchial c. second pharyngeal groove; see *pharyngeal grooves,* under *groove.*

hyoid c., hyomandibular c. first pharyngeal groove; see *pharyngeal grooves,* under *groove.*

hyopharyngeal c. second pharyngeal groove; see *pharyngeal grooves,* under *groove.*

interdental c. diastema.

intergluteal c. crena analis.

intermammary c. sulcus intermammarius.

Lanterman c's Schmidt-Lanterman incisures.

Larrey c. trigonum sternocostale.

laryngotracheoesophageal c. a cleft between the larynx and the upper trachea resulting from incomplete separation of these structures during embryonic development, with respiratory manifestations including respiratory distress with feeding, flaccid aryepiglottic folds, chronic cough, and increased oral secretions, and frequently associated with other congenital anomalies of the respiratory system or gastrointestinal tract. Complications include failure to thrive and recurrent aspiration pneumonia.

lateral facial c. transverse facial cleft extending from the angle of the mouth toward the ear. See also *macrostomia.*

Maurer c's see under *dot.*

oblique facial c. a rare form of facial cleft extending from the lip to the inner canthus of the eye. It may be superficial but usually separates the underlying bone and is associated with cleft lip, cleft palate, or lateral facial cleft. Called also *meloschisis* and *prosopoanoschisis.*

natal c. crena analis.

posthyoidean c. second pharyngeal groove; see *pharyngeal grooves,* under *groove.*

primary synaptic c. synaptic trough.

pudendal c. rima pudendi.

Schmidt-Lanterman c's see under *incisure.*

secondary synaptic c's subneural c's.

sternal c. cleft sternum.

Stillman c. a small apostrophe-shaped or slitlike fissure of the gingiva extending from the gingival margin to a depth of up to 5 to 6 cm.

subneural c's evenly spaced lamella-like clefts within the primary synaptic cleft, formed by infoldings of the sarcolemma into the underlying sarcolemma of muscle; called also *subneural apparatus* and *secondary synaptic c's.*

synaptic c. 1. a narrow extracellular cleft between the presynaptic and postsynaptic membranes. 2. synaptic trough.

transverse facial c. lateral facial c.

visceral c. pharyngeal grooves.

vulval c. rima pudendi.

clei·dal (kli'dəl) pertaining to or affecting the clavicle.

cleid(o)- [Gr. *kleis,* gen. *kleidos,* key, clavicle] a combining form denoting relationship to the clavicle.

clei·do·cos·tal (kli″do-kos'təl) pertaining to the clavicle and the ribs.

clei·do·cra·ni·al (kli″do-kra'ne-əl) [*cleido-* + *cranium*] pertaining to the clavicle and the head.

clei·do·ic (kli-do'ik) [Gr. *kleidouchos* holding the keys] isolated from the environment, self-contained, such as the eggs of reptiles, birds, or primitive mammals; see under *egg.*

clei·do·mas·toid (kli″do-mas'toid) pertaining to the clavicle and the mastoid process.

clei·dot·o·my (kli-dot'ə-me) [*cleido-* + *-tomy*] surgical division of the clavicle of a dead fetus to facilitate passage of the shoulders through the birth canal.

-cleisis [Gr. *kleisis* a closing, from *kleiein* to enclose] a word termination denoting closure.

cleis·to·the·ci·um (klīs″to-the'se-əm) [Gr. *kleisis* a closing + *theca*] the fruiting body (ascocarp) produced by certain ascomycetes, in which there is no pore for the escape of ascospores, the spores being released by rupture or decay of the body. Cf. *apothecium, gymnothecium,* and *perithecium.*

clem·as·tine (klem'əs-tēn) an ethanolamine derivative used as an antihistamine (H_1 receptor antagonist) and having sedative and anticholinergic effects.

c. fumarate the fumarate salt of clemastine, used in the treatment of allergic rhinitis, allergic conjunctivitis, and cutaneous manifestations of allergic reactions, and as an ingredient in some cough and cold preparations; administered orally.

Clem·a·tis (klem'ə-tis) [Gr. *klēmatis*] a genus of flowering plants of the family Ranunculaceae. Most species contain ranunculin, which breaks down in the body to form the lethal toxin protoanemonin.

clem·i·zole (klem'ĭ-zōl) an antihistaminic compound which has also been used to produce a repository form of penicillin G.

c. hydrochloride the hydrochloride salt of clemizole, used as an antihistaminic in the treatment of skin allergies, food and cosmetic hypersensitivities, and serum sickness; administered orally.

clen·bu·ter·ol (klen-bu'tər-ol) a long-acting β_2-adrenergic agonist used to treat bronchospasms in the horse.

clench·ing (klench'ing) the clamping and pressing of the jaws and teeth together in centric occlusion, frequently associated with acute nervous tension or physical effort, such as pushing or lifting a heavy object or performing a difficult task. See also *bruxism.*

Cle·o·cin (kle'o-sin) trademark for preparations of clindamycin.

cle·oid (kle'oid) [Middle English *cle* claw + *-oid*] a claw-shaped nib used to carve amalgam restorations.

Clé·ram·bault see *de Clérambault.*

Cleth·ri·on·o·mys (kleth″re-on'ə-mis) a genus of voles, rodents of the family Muridae, reservoirs for viruses causing epidemic hemorrhagic fever and other diseases.

C. glare'olus the bank vole, a European species that is the natural host of Puumala virus.

click (klik) a brief sharp sound; see also *clicking.*

ejection c's see under *sound.*

midsystolic c. a high-frequency sound in mid-systole, often associated with prolapse of a floppy mitral valve; it may be accompanied by a late systolic murmur.

mitral c. mitral opening snap.

Mulder c. see under *sign.*

nonejection systolic c. midsystolic c.

Ortolani c. see under *sign.*

systolic c's short, dry, clicking heart sounds during systole; they are often indicative of various heart conditions associated with abnormal mitral or aortic valves but may have extracardiac causes. Their timing within systole may indicate the nature of the disorder; see *midsystolic c.* and *ejection sounds.*

click·ing (klik'ing) a series of clicks, such as the snapping, cracking, or crepitant noise evident on excursions of the mandibular condyle.

cli·din·i·um bro·mide (klĭ-din'e-əm) [USP] a quaternary ammonium anticholinergic with pronounced antispasmodic and antisecretory effects on the gastrointestinal tract; it has been used as adjunctive therapy in the treatment of peptic ulcer and other gastrointestinal disorders, administered orally.

clid(o)- for words beginning thus, see those beginning *cleid(o)-*.

cli·mac·ter·ic (kli-mak′tər-ik) [Gr. *klimaktēr* rung of ladder, critical point in human life] 1. the syndrome of endocrine, somatic, and psychic changes occurring at the time of menopause in women. 2. similar changes occurring in men; cf. *andropause.* Called also *climacterium.*

Cli·ma·ra (kli-mar′ə) trademark for a preparation of estradiol.

cli·mac·te·ri·um (kli″mak-tēr′e-əm) climacteric.

c. prae′cox premature menopause.

cli·ma·tol·o·gy (kli″mə-tol′ə-je) [Gr. *klima* the supposed slope of the earth from the equator to the pole + *-logy*] the science devoted to the study of the conditions of the natural environment (rainfall, daylight, temperature, humidity, air movement) prevailing in specific regions of the earth.

medical c. climatology that is concerned especially with the effect of climatic factors on human beings, on their functions, their health, and the treatment of disease.

cli·ma·to·ther·a·peu·tics (kli″mə-to-ther″ə-pu′tiks) climatotherapy.

cli·ma·to·ther·a·py (kli″mə-to-ther′ə-pe) [*climate* + *therapy*] the treatment of disease by means of a favorable climate.

cli·max (kli′maks) [Gr. *klimax* a ladder, staircase] the acme, or period of greatest intensity, as in the course of a disease (crisis), or in sexual excitement (orgasm).

Clin·ac BPO (klin′ak) trademark for a preparation of benzoyl peroxide.

clin·ar·thro·sis (klin″ahr-thro′sis) [*clin-* + *arthrosis*] abnormal deviation in the alignment of the bones at a joint.

Clin·da·gel (klin′də-jel) trademark for a preparation of clindamycin phosphate.

clin·da·my·cin (klin″də-mi′sin) a semisynthetic lincosamide antibiotic derived from lincomycin by chlorination; it is effective primarily against gram-positive bacteria.

c. hydrochloride [USP] the hydrated hydrochloride salt of clindamycin; used primarily in the treatment of penicillin-resistant gram-positive infections and in patients allergic to penicillin; administered orally.

c. palmitate hydrochloride [USP] a water-soluble hydrochloride salt of the ester of clindamycin and palmitic acid, having the same actions and uses as the hydrochloride salt; it is suitable for the preparation of solutions for oral administration.

c. phosphate [USP] a water-soluble ester of clindamycin and phosphoric acid, having the same actions and uses as the hydrochloride salt; administered intramuscularly or intravenously. It is also used topically in the treatment of acne vulgaris and vaginally in the treatment of bacterial vaginosis.

Clin·dets (klin-dets′) trademark for a preparation of clindamycin phosphate.

cline (klīn) [Gr. *klinein* to cause to slope] a continuous series of differences in structure or function exhibited by the members of a species along a line extending from one part of their range to another.

clin·ic (klin′ik) [Gr. *klinikos* pertaining to a bed] 1. an establishment where patients are admitted for special study and treatment by a group of physicians practicing medicine together. 2. a clinical lecture; examination of patients before a class of students; instruction at the bedside.

clin·i·cal (klin′ĭ-kəl) 1. pertaining to a clinic or to the bedside. 2. pertaining to or founded on actual observation and treatment of patients, as distinguished from theoretical or basic sciences.

cli·ni·cian (klĭ-nish′ən) an expert clinical physician and teacher.

nurse c. see under *nurse.*

clin·i·co·ge·net·ic (klin″ĭ-ko-jə-net′ik) pertaining to the clinical manifestations of a genetic abnormality.

clin·i·co·patho·log·ic (klin″ĭ-ko-path″ə-loj′ik) pertaining both to the symptoms of disease and to its pathology.

Clin·i·stix (klin′ĭ-stiks) trademark for an enzyme-impregnated strip of plastic used to test for sugar in the urine. The strip is dipped into the urine and positive or negative results are indicated by the color of the strip.

Clin·i·test (klin′ĭ-test) trademark for reagent tablets containing copper sulfate, used to test for the presence of sugar in the urine. Ten drops of water and 5 drops of urine are placed in a test tube. The tablet, which generates heat, is added and the solution is allowed to boil. After a few moments the color of the solution is compared to a color chart.

clin(o)- [Gr. *klinein* to cause to slope or bend] a combining form meaning sloping, leaning, or bent.

cli·no·ceph·a·ly (kli″no-sef′ə-le) [*clino-* + *-cephaly*] congenital flatness or concavity of the top of the head.

cli·no·dac·tyl·ism (kli″no-dak′təl-iz-əm) clinodactyly.

cli·no·dac·ty·ly (kli″no-dak′tə-le) [*clino-* + *daktylos* finger] permanent lateral or medial deviation or deflection of one or more fingers.

cli·nog·ra·phy (klĭ-nog′rə-fe) [Gr. *klinē* bed + *-graphy*] a system of graphic representations of the temperature, symptoms, and pathologic manifestations exhibited by a patient.

cli·noid (klī′noid) [Gr. *klinē* bed + *-oid*] resembling a bed; bed-shaped, as the clinoid processes (from their fancied resemblance to bedposts). See entries beginning *processus clinoideus.*

Clin·or·il (klin′ə-ril) trademark for a preparation of sulindac.

cli·no·stat·ic (klī″no-stat′ik) occurring when the patient lies down.

cli·no·stat·ism (kli′no-stat″iz-əm) [Gr. *klinē* bed + *stasis* position] a lying-down position of the body.

cli·no·ther·a·py (klī-no-ther′ə-pe) treatment by keeping the patient in bed.

cli·o·quin·ol (kli″o-kwin′ol) [USP] an antibacterial and antifungal agent with antieczematic and antipruritic properties; it was formerly used as a topical antiinfective in a wide range of dermatoses and was administered orally in the treatment of amebic dysentery; use has been discontinued because of associated neurotoxicity. Called also *iodochlorhydroxyquin.*

CLIP corticotropin-like intermediate lobe peptide.

clip (klip) a device for approximating the edges of a wound or for the prevention of bleeding from small individual blood vessels.

ligation c., silver c. a small V-shaped clip made from stainless steel, platinum, titanium, or an absorbable material, used to ligate bleeding vessels.

skin c., wound c. a heavy metal clip used to approximate the edges of a skin incision.

clis·e·om·e·ter (klis″e-om′ə-tər) [Gr. *klisis* inclination + *-meter*] an instrument for measuring the angle between the pelvic axis and the vertebral column.

cli·tel·lum (kli-tel′əm) [L. *clitellae* packsaddle] a saddle-like glandular segment in earthworms and leeches that secretes the cocoon in which the eggs are enclosed.

clit·i·on (klit′e-on) [Gr. *kleitys* slope, clivus] the midpoint of the anterior border of the clivus.

Cli·to·cy·be (kli-tos′ĭ-be) a genus of club fungi of the family Agaricaceae. Some species are poisonous and several contain muscarine. *C. nebula′ris* is the source of nebularine. Ingestion of *C. illu′dens,* the orange jack-o-lantern mushroom, causes mycetismus gastrointestinalis.

clit·o·rec·to·my (klit″ə-rek′tə-me) clitoridectomy.

clit·o·ri·dec·to·my (klit″ə-rĭ-dek′tə-me) [*clitoris* + *-ectomy*] excision of the clitoris; called also *clitorectomy.*

clit·o·ri·di·tis (klit″ə-rĭ-di′tis) clitoritis.

clit·o·ri·dot·o·my (klit″ə-rĭ-dot′ə-me) [*clitoris* + *-tomy*] incision of the clitoris.

clit·o·ri·meg·a·ly (klit″ə-rĭ-meg′ə-le) [*clitoris* + *-megaly*] clitoromegaly.

clit·o·ris (klit′ə-ris, kli′tə-ris, klĭ-tor′is) [Gr. *kleitoris*] [TA] a small, elongated, erectile body at the anterior angle of the rima pudendi in the female; it is homologous with the penis in the male. **clit′oral** *adj*

clit·o·rism (klit′ə-riz″əm, kli′tə-riz″əm) 1. clitoromegaly. 2. persistent and usually painful erection of the clitoris.

clit·o·ri·tis (klit″ə-ri′tis, kli″tə-ri′tis) inflammation of the clitoris.

clit·o·ro·meg·a·ly (klit″ə-ro-meg′ə-le) enlargement of the clitoris; called also *macroclitoris.*

clit·o·ro·plas·ty (klit′ə-ro-plas″te) plastic surgery of the clitoris. **clitoroplas′tic** *adj*

clit·o·rot·o·my (klit″ə-rot′ə-me) [*clitoris* + *-tomy*] surgical incision of the clitoris.

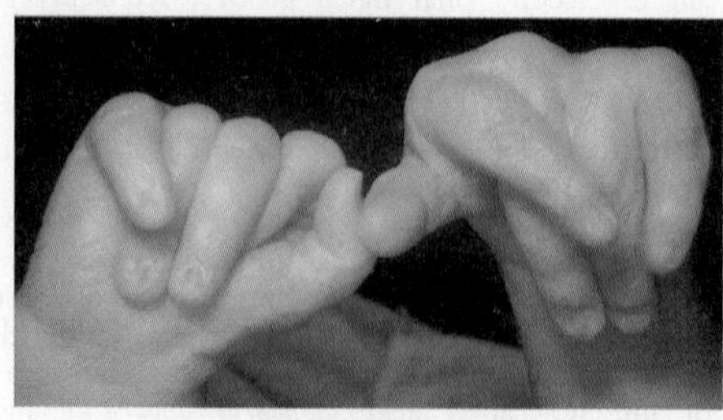

■ Clinodactyly.

cli•vog•ra•phy (kli-vog′rə-fe) radiographic visualization of the clivus, or posterior cranial fossa.

cli•vus (kli′vəs) [L. "slope"] [TA] a bony surface in the posterior cranial fossa, sloping superiorly from the foramen magnum to the dorsum sellae, the inferior part being formed by a portion of the basilar part of the occipital bone and the superior part by a surface of the body of the sphenoid bone. cli′val *adj*

clo (klo) a unit of measurement, being the insulation provided by normal everyday clothing and representing approximately the insulation provided by 0.25 inch thickness of wool.

clo•a•ca (klo-a′kə) pl. *cloa′cae* [L. "drain"] 1. a common passage for fecal, urinary, and reproductive discharge in monotremes, birds, and lower vertebrates. See also *cloacal aperture*, under *aperture*. 2. in mammalian embryology, the terminal end of the hindgut before division into rectum, bladder, and genital primordia (see *sinus urogenitalis*). Failure to divide properly during development may result in persistent cloaca (q.v.). 3. in pathology, an opening in the involucrum of a necrosed bone. cloa′cal *adj*

congenital c. persistent c.

ectodermal c. the portion of the embryonic cloaca originally external to the cloacal membrane.

endodermal c. the portion of the embryonic cloaca originally internal to the cloacal membrane.

persistent c. the congenital persistence of the cloaca, the common cavity into which the intestinal, urinary, and reproductive ducts open; called also *congenital c.*

clo•a•ci•tis (klo″ə-si′tis) inflammation of the cloaca of an animal.

clo•a•co•gen•ic (klo″ə-ko-jen′ik) originating from the cloaca or from persisting cloacal remnants.

clo•ba•zam (klo′bə-zəm) a benzodiazepine with anticonvulsant actions; administered orally as an adjunct in the treatment of epilepsy.

clo•be•ta•sol pro•pi•o•nate (klo-ba′tə-sol) [USP] a very high potency synthetic corticosteroid, an analogue of prednisolone; used topically for the relief of inflammation and pruritus in corticosteroid-responsive dermatoses.

clo•be•ta•sone bu•ty•rate (klo-ba′tə-sōn) a medium potency synthetic corticosteroid used topically for the relief of inflammation and pruritus in corticosteroid-responsive dermatoses.

Clo•be•vate (klo′bə-vāt) trademark for a preparation of clobetasol propionate.

clock (klok) a device by which time may be measured.

biological c. the physiologic mechanism that governs the rhythmic occurrence of certain biochemical, physiological, and behavioral phenomena in plants and animals.

clo•cor•to•lone piv•a•late (klo-kor′to-lōn) [USP] a low potency corticosteroid, used topically for the relief of inflammation and pruritus in corticosteroid-responsive dermatoses.

Clo•derm (klo′derm) trademark for a preparation of clocortolone pivalate.

clo•dro•nate disodium (klo-dro′nāt) the disodium salt of clodronic acid; a diphosphonate calcium-regulating agent that inhibits bone resorption and is used to treat osteitis deformans and hypercalcemia related to malignancy. Administered orally or intravenously.

clo•dron•ic ac•id (klo-dron′ik) a bone calcium regulator.

clo•far•a•bine (klo-far′ə-bēn) a purine nucleoside antimetabolite that inhibits DNA synthesis and repair; used for treatment of children and adolescents with acute lymphoblastic leukemia who have had at least two previous regimens. Administered by intravenous injection.

clo•faz•i•mine (klo-faz′ĭ-mēn) [USP] an antibacterial, having leprostatic and tuberculostatic actions.

clo•fen•am•ic ac•id (klo″fən-am′ik) a fenamate analgesic, antiinflammatory agent.

clo•fi•brate (klo-fi′brāt) [USP] a fibric acid derivative with antihyperlipidemic activity, used to reduce elevated serum lipids, administered orally.

Clo•lar (klo′lar) trademark for a preparation of clofarabine.

Clo•mid (klo′mid) trademark for a preparation of clomiphene citrate.

clo•mi•phene cit•rate (klo′mĭ-fēn) [USP] a synthetic gonad-stimulating principle consisting of a mixture of *cis-* and *trans-* isomers; used to induce ovulation in some types of female factor infertility due to anovulation; administered orally.

clo•mip•ra•mine hy•dro•chlo•ride (klo-mip′rə-mēn) a tricyclic antidepressant of the dibenzazepine class, also having anxiolytic activity. It is also used to relieve the symptoms of obsessive-compulsive disorder, panic disorder, bulimia nervosa, and cataplexy associated with narcolepsy, and to treat chronic, severe pain; administered orally.

clo•nal•i•ty (klo-nal′ĭ-te) the ability to be cloned.

clo•naz•e•pam (klo-naz′ə-pam) [USP] a benzodiazepine used as an anticonvulsant in the treatment of Lennox-Gastaut syndrome and of atonic and myoclonic seizures and as an antipanic agent in the treatment of panic disorders; administered orally.

clone (klōn) [Gr. *klōn* young shoot or twig] 1. one of a group of genetically identical (barring mutation) cells or organisms derived asexually from a single common ancestor. 2. a DNA population derived from a single molecule by recombinant DNA technology. 3. to establish such a progeny or population. clo′nal *adj*

forbidden c. see *clonal deletion theory*, under *theory*.

clo•nic•i•ty (klo-nis′ĭ-te) the condition of being clonic.

clon•i•co•ton•ic (klon″ĭ-ko-ton′ik) both clonic and tonic.

clo•ni•dine hy•dro•chlo•ride (klo′nĭ-dēn) [USP] an α_2-adrenergic agonist-antagonist (its major actions are agonistic, but it acts as an antagonist if the concentration of norepinephrine is high) administered orally or transdermally as an antihypertensive; orally for the prophylaxis of migraine and in the treatment of dysmenorrhea, anxiety, vasomotor symptoms of menopause, and opioid withdrawal; and epidurally, together with opiates, in the treatment of pain in cancer patients.

clon•ing (klōn′ing) the formation of a clone.

DNA c. in genetics, the production of many identical copies of a specific DNA fragment.

positional c. DNA cloning of a sequence based on its map position, without knowledge of the gene product produced; used to identify disease-causing genes.

subtraction c. a type of DNA cloning in which the sequences to be cloned are first isolated by removal of some or all undesirable sequences from a heterogenous DNA population. It is performed by hybridization of a nucleic acid population containing the differentially expressed sequences of interest to an excess of a complementary nucleic acid population that lacks these sequences, then removing hybridized molecules and so enriching for the specific sequences, repeating until all sequences common to both populations are removed; the nucleic acid of interest can then be used to prepare or screen a library.

clon•ism (klon′iz-əm) [Gr. *klonos* turmoil] a succession of clonic spasms.

clo•nis•mus (klo-niz′məs) clonism.

clo•no•gen•ic (klo″no-jen′ik) [*clone* + *-genic*] giving rise to a clone of cells.

clo•nor•chi•a•sis (klo″nor-ki′ə-sis) a type of opisthorchiasis seen in East and Southeast Asia, caused by infestation of biliary passages by the liver fluke *Opisthorchis sinensis (Clonorchis sinensis)*; it may lead to inflammation of the biliary tree, proliferation of the biliary epithelium, progressive portal fibrosis, and sometimes biliary duct carcinoma; extension into the liver parenchyma may lead to fatty change and cirrhosis. Called also *clonorchiosis.*

clo•nor•chi•o•sis (klo-nor″ki-o′sis) clonorchiasis.

Clo•nor•chis (klo-nor′kis) [Gr. *klōn* branch + *orchis* testicle] former name for a genus of trematodes, now considered identical to *Opisthorchis.*

clono•spasm (klon′o-spaz″əm) [*clonus* + *spasm*] clonic spasm.

clo•no•type (klo′no-tīp) [*clone* + *type*] a particular combination of immunoglobulin heavy and light chains, e.g., that produced by a single clone of plasma cells. A single organism produces a repertoire of about 10^7 to 10^8 clonotypes; a single antigenic determinant may react with 10^3 to 10^4 clonotypes.

clo•nus (klo′nəs) [Gr. *klonos* turmoil] 1. alternate muscular contraction and relaxation in rapid succession. 2. a continuous rhythmic reflex tremor initiated by the spinal cord below an area of spinal cord injury, set in motion by reflex testing. clon′ic *adj*

ankle c. a series of abnormal rhythmic reflex movements of the foot, induced by sudden dorsiflexion, which causes alternate contraction and relaxation of the triceps surae muscle (gastrocnemius and soleus muscles); called also *foot c.*

foot c. ankle c.

patellar c. rhythmic jerking movement of the patella produced by grasping it between the thumb and forefinger and pushing it suddenly and forcibly toward the foot; this is an abnormal reflex with alternate contraction and relaxation of the quadriceps muscle.

wrist c. spasmodic movement of the hand, induced by suddenly and forcibly extending the hand at the wrist.

clo•pa•mide (klo-pă′mīd) a diuretic used in treatment of edema and hypertension.

clo•pen•thix•ol (klo″pən-thik′səl) a compound with sedative, tranquilizing, antiemetic, antihistaminic, anticholinergic, and alpha-adrenergic blocking properties; it has been used as a tranquilizer in the treatment of schizophrenia.

clo·pid·o·grel bi·sul·fate (klo-pid′ə-grel) [USP] an inhibitor of platelet aggregation used as an antithrombotic for the prevention of myocardial infarction, stroke, and vascular death in patients with atherosclerosis; administered orally.

clo·pi·dol (klo′pĭ-dol) a coccidiostat for poultry.

clo·pros·te·nol so·di·um (klo-pros′tə-nol) a synthetic analogue of dinoprost, used as a luteolytic in veterinary medicine.

Clo·quet canal, node, etc. (klo-ka′) [Jules Germain *Cloquet*, French surgeon, 1790–1883] see *canalis hyaloideus, nodus lymphoideus inguinalis profundus proximalis, vestigium processus vaginalis,* and *septum femorale* and see *pectineal hernia,* under *hernia.*

Clo·quet ganglion (pseudoganglion) (klo-ka′) [Hippolyte *Cloquet*, French anatomist, 1787–1840] see under *ganglion.*

clor·az·e·pate di·po·tas·sium (klor-az′ə-pāt) [USP] a benzodiazepine used as an antianxiety agent for the treatment of anxiety disorders and the short-term relief of anxiety symptoms, as an anticonvulsant in the treatment of simple or complex partial seizures, and for the treatment of acute alcohol withdrawal symptoms; administered orally.

Clor·pac·tin XCB (klor-pak′tin) trademark for a preparation of oxychlorosene.

Clor·pres (klor′prez) trademark for combination preparations of clonidine hydrochloride and chlorthalidone.

clor·su·lon (klor′su-lon) [USP] a sulfonamide used as a fasciolicide.

clo·san·tel (klo′sən-təl) a salicylanilide anthelmintic used in cattle and sheep.

Clos·tri·dia (klos-trid′e-ə) a class of bacteria of the phylum Firmicutes, consisting of gram-positive or gram-negative, aerobic to anaerobic rods or cocci; some are thermophilic and a number are pathogenic. Medically important organisms are included in the order Clostridiales.

clos·trid·ia (klos-trid′e-ə) [L.] plural of *clostridium.*

Clos·tri·di·a·ceae (klos-trid″e-a′se-e) a family of bacteria of the order Clostridiales, consisting of anaerobic organisms that vary widely in morphology, physiology, and metabolism, grouped together on the basis of 16S rRNA sequence analysis. Organisms of medical interest are included in the genera *Acetivibrio, Clostridium,* and *Sarcina.*

clos·trid·i·al (klos-trid′e-əl) pertaining to or caused by clostridia.

Clos·tri·di·a·les (klos-trid″e-a′lēz) a phenotypically diverse order of bacteria of the class Clostridia that includes many medically important bacteria, which are contained in the families Acidaminococcaceae, Clostridiaceae, Eubacteriaceae, Lachnospiraceae, Peptococcaceae, and Peptostreptococcaceae.

clos·trid·i·o·sis (klos-trid″e-o′sis) any disease caused by infection with clostridia.

equine intestinal c. acute, usually fatal, diarrhea in horses due to infection with large numbers of *Clostridium perfringens* type A.

Clos·trid·i·um (klos-trid′e-əm) [Gr. *klōstēr* spindle] a genus of bacteria of the family Clostridiaceae, consisting of obligate anaerobic or microaerophilic, gram-positive, spore-forming, rod-shaped bacilli, with spores of greater diameter than the vegetative cells. The spores may be central, terminal, or subterminal. Nearly two hundred species have been differentiated on the basis of physiology, morphology, and toxin formation; pathogenic species produce destructive exotoxins or enzymes. Different species are found in soil, in water, and in the intestinal tracts of animals.

C. acetobuty′licum a species found widely distributed in agricultural soils but not found to be pathogenic.

C. bara′tii a species that sometimes causes botulism in infants.

C. bifermen′tans a species found widely distributed in nature, occurring commonly in feces, sewage, and soil; it is sometimes associated with cases of gas gangrene.

C. botuli′num the agent causing botulism in humans and waterfowl, as well as limberneck in fowl, certain forms of forage poisoning in cattle and horses in Australia, and lamziekte in cattle in South Africa. It produces a powerful exotoxin that is resistant to proteolytic digestion, and is divided into types A, B, C alpha and beta, D, E, F, and G on the basis of the immunologic specificity of the toxin.

C. buty′ricum a species isolated from the soil, fecal material, and dairy products.

C. cada′veris a species found in feces and infections.

C. chauvoe′i the principal cause of blackleg in cattle and sheep.

C. clostridiofor′me a weakly gram-positive species that is commonly isolated from clinical specimens.

C. diffi′cile a species that is part of the normal colon flora in infants and some adults; it produces a toxin that can cause pseudomembranous enterocolitis in patients receiving antibiotic therapy.

C. haemoly′ticum a species isolated from the blood and other tissues of cattle dying with bacillary hemoglobinuria, thought by some to be a type of *C. novyi.*

C. histoly′ticum a pathogenic species found in wounds and frequently associated with gas gangrene. It is commonly found in soil.

C. inno′cuum a species of uncertain pathogenicity, commonly isolated from gas gangrene and other anaerobic infections.

C. kluy′veri a species isolated from wetland soil of fresh and salt water, which has been used in studies of microbial synthesis and oxidation of fatty acids.

C. limo′sum a toxicogenic species found in soil and infections.

C. no′vyi a species that is an important cause of gas gangrene in humans and infections in other animals. Three immunologic types have been identified, designated A, B, and C.

C. paraputri′ficum a species found in soil and feces.

C. pasteuria′num an anaerobic microorganism in soil, the first nitrogen-fixing bacterium to be studied in pure culture.

C. perfrin′gens the most common etiologic agent of gas gangrene, distinguishable into types on the basis of the distribution of 12 different toxins: *type A* causes gas gangrene and necrotizing colitis, and is a major cause of food poisoning in humans; *type B* causes lamb dysentery; *type C* causes enteritis necroticans in humans and struck in sheep; *type D* causes pulpy kidney disease in sheep; *type E* causes enterotoxemia in lambs and calves.

C. pilifor′me a species that is the etiologic agent of Tyzzer disease.

C. ramo′sum a species found in infections and feces; it is one of the most common species in clinical specimens.

C. sep′ticum a toxicogenic species commonly found in animal intestines and soil, causing diseases such as braxy and malignant edema; in humans it is sometimes associated with gas gangrene. Six immunologic groups have been distinguished. Called also *Ghon-Sachs bacillus.*

C. sordel′lii a species of uncertain pathogenicity, found associated with infections.

C. sphenoi′des a species found in infected wounds.

C. sporo′genes a species widely distributed in nature; a harmless saprophyte in pure culture, it is reportedly associated with pathogenic anaerobes in gangrenous infections.

C. subtermina′le a species found in soil and wounds.

C. ter′tium a species found widely distributed in feces, sewage, and soil, and associated with gas gangrene.

C. te′tani a common inhabitant of soil and human and horse intestines, the cause of tetanus in humans and domestic animals; its potent exotoxin is made up of two components: the neurotoxin tetanospasmin and the hemolytic toxin tetanolysin.

clos·trid·i·um (klos-trid′e-əm) pl. *clostrid′ia.* A microorganism belonging to the genus *Clostridium.*

clo·sure (klo′zhər) 1. occlusion (def. 2). 2. obstruction.

delayed primary c. healing by third intention; see under *healing.*

flask c. the bringing together of the two halves or parts of a flask in which a denture base is formed. *Trial flask closure* is preliminary closure to eliminate excess material and ensure that the mold is completely filled. *Final flask closure* is the last closure before curing the denture base material packed in the mold.

vacuum-assisted c. wound closure by placing a sponge into or over the wound, covering it with an occlusive dressing, and inserting a suction tube with a pump to cause negative internal pressure.

velopharyngeal c. closure of nasal air escape by the elevation of the soft palate and contraction of the posterior pharyngeal wall. See also under *adequacy* and under *insufficiency.*

clo·sy·late (klo′sə-lāt) USAN contraction for *p*-chlorobenzenesulfonate.

clot (klot) 1. a semisolidified mass, as of blood or lymph; called also *coagulum.* 2. blood c. 3. coagulate.

adherent c. a clot that overlies the floor of a peptic ulcer and cannot be dislodged by irrigation.

agonal c., agony c. a type of antemortem clot formed in the process of dying.

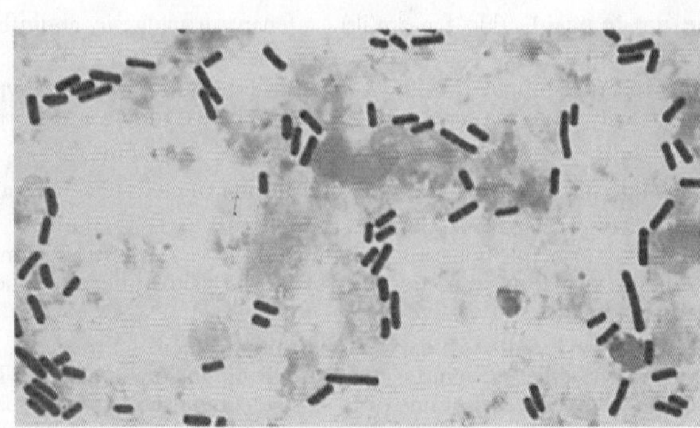

■ *Clostridium perfringens.*

antemortem c. a blood clot formed before death but found after death in the heart or in a large vessel.

blood c. a coagulum in the bloodstream formed of an aggregation of blood factors, primarily platelets, and fibrin with entrapment of cellular elements; see also *thrombus.* Some authorities differentiate thrombus formation from simple coagulation or clot formation. Called also *cruor.*

chicken fat c. a blood clot that appears yellow because of the settling out of the erythrocytes before clotting occurred, typically representing postmortem clotting.

currant jelly c. a blood clot of reddish color because of the presence of erythrocytes enmeshed in it.

distal c. a clot formed in a blood vessel distal to a ligature.

external c. a clot formed outside a blood vessel.

heart c. postmortem coagulation within the heart.

internal c. a blood clot formed within a blood vessel.

laminated c. a blood clot formed by successive deposits of fibrin and whole blood, giving it a layered appearance; post mortem, it indicates formation during life. Called also *stratified c.*

marantic c. a blood clot formed because of enfeebled circulation, general wasting, or thromboplastic substances released by cancers.

passive c. a clot formed in the sac of an aneurysm through which the blood has stopped circulating.

plastic c. a clot formed on the intima of an artery at the point of ligation, permanently obstructing the artery.

postmortem c. a blood clot formed in the heart or in a large blood vessel after death.

proximal c. a clot formed in a blood vessel proximal to a ligature.

sentinel c. a discrete protuberance within the crater of a peptic ulcer, usually representing a hemostatic clot in the vessel or a false aneurysm; pigmentation of the protuberance is often prognostic of rebleeding of the ulcer.

spiderweb c. the fine fibrin clot that forms when a sample of fluid from a subject with tuberculous meningitis is allowed to stand, especially when it is warmed to 37°C for a few hours.

stratified c. laminated c.

washed c., white c. a blood clot composed of fibrin and platelets; see also *white thrombus,* under *thrombus.*

clo·trim·a·zole (klo-trim′ə-zōl) [USP] an imidazole derivative used as a broad-spectrum antifungal agent, applied topically to the skin in the treatment of candidiasis and various forms of tinea, and administered intravaginally in the treatment of vulvovaginal candidiasis and orally in the prophylaxis and treatment of oropharyngeal candidiasis.

clot·ting (klot′ing) coagulation (def. 1).

cloud·ing (kloud′ing) loss of clarity.

c. of consciousness a lowered level of consciousness (q.v.) with loss of ability to respond properly to external stimuli. See also *levels of consciousness,* under *level.* Called also *mental fog.*

Cloud·man melanoma S91 (kloud′mən) [Arthur Mosher *Cloudman,* American zoologist, 20th century] see under *melanoma.*

cloudy (clou′de) [A.S. *clūd* cloud] 1. murky; turbid; not transparent. 2. marked by indistinct streaks.

Clou·ston syndrome (klou′ston) [H.R. *Clouston,* Canadian physician, 20th century] hidrotic ectodermal dysplasia.

clove (klōv) [L. *clavus* a nail or spike] 1. *Syzygium aromaticum.* 2. the dried flower bud of *Syzygium aromaticum,* used as an aromatic spice and flavoring and source of clove oil.

clo·ver (klo′vər) 1. any member of the genus *Trifolium;* called also *trefoil.* 2. any of various other members of the pea family, such as genus *Melilotus.*

red c. 1. *Trifolium pratense.* 2. a preparation of the flower heads of *T. pratense,* used internally for coughs and respiratory symptoms, and externally for chronic skin conditions such as psoriasis and eczema; it is also used in traditional Chinese medicine.

sweet c. any member of the genus *Melilotus;* see also *sweet clover disease,* under *disease.*

clox·a·cil·lin so·di·um (klok″sə-sil′in) [USP] a semisynthetic penicillinase-resistant isoxazolyl penicillin, used primarily in the treatment of infections due to penicillinase-producing staphylococci, administered orally or intravenously.

clo·za·pine (klo′zə-pēn) a sedative and antipsychotic agent, a dibenzodiazepine; used in the treatment of schizophrenia.

Cloz·aril (cloz′ə-ril) trademark for a preparation of clozapine.

club·bing (klub′ing) a digital deformity produced by proliferation of the soft tissues about the terminal phalanges of the fingers or toes, with no constant osseous changes; seen in various types of chronic disease of the thoracic organs. Cf. *clubbed finger.*

club·foot (klub′foot) talipes.

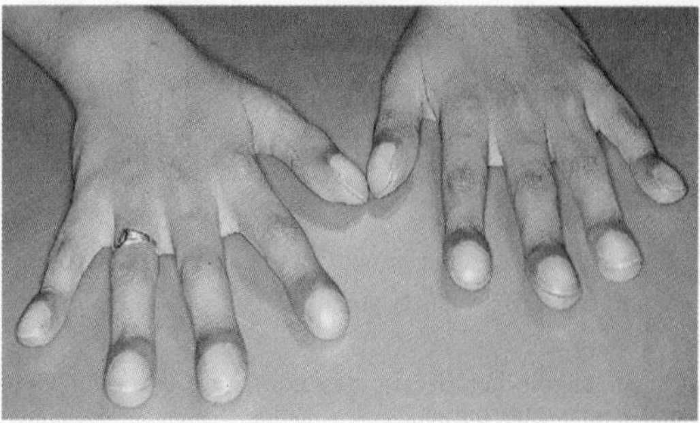

■ Clubbing of fingers in an adolescent with tetralogy of Fallot.

club·hand (klub′hand) a deformity of the hand due to congenital absence of the radius or ulna in which the hand is twisted out of shape or position; called also *talipomanus.*

radial c. the most common type of clubhand, with the hand deflected toward the radial side; if such a hand is in the anatomic position it is called *manus valga* and if it is in the opposite direction it is called *manus vara.* Called also *manus valga.* See also *Madelung deformity,* under *deformity.*

ulnar c. clubhand in which the hand is deflected toward the ulnar side; when the hand is held in the anatomic position it is known as *manus vara* and when it is held in the opposite direction as *manus valga.* Called also *manus vara.*

clump (klump) an aggregation as of bacteria caused by the action of agglutinins (agglutination).

clump·ing (klump′ing) the aggregation of particles, such as bacteria, into irregular masses.

clu·ne·al (kloo′ne-əl) gluteal; spelled also *clunial.*

clu·nes (kloo′nēz) (sing. *clu′nis*) [L.] TA alternative for *nates.*

clu·ni·al (kloo′ne-əl) cluneal; used especially of the nervi clunium.

clu·nis (kloo′nis) pl. *clu′nes* [L.] a buttock; see *nates.*

clus·ter (klus′tər) [A.S. *clyster*] a group of similar objects, events, or other elements in close proximity.

angiogenic cell c's angioblastic cords.

clus·ter·in (klus′tər-in) a multifunctional glycoprotein with roles in the metabolism and transport of lipids and membrane fragments, secretion of hormones, reproductive biology, inhibition of assembly of the membrane attack complex of complement activation, programmed cell death, and modulation of inter-cell interactions; its expression is enhanced in tissue injury and remodeling as well as in degenerative diseases such as Alzheimer disease and scrapie. Called also *SP-40,40.*

clut·ter·ing (klut′ər-ing) hurried nervous speech marked by the dropping of syllables, usually seen in children. Cf. *logorrhea.*

Clut·ton joint (klut′ən) [Henry Hugh *Clutton,* English surgeon, 1850–1909] see under *joint.*

cly·sis (kli′sis) [Gr. *klysis*] 1. administration other than by the oral route of a solution to replace lost body fluid, supply nutriment, or raise blood pressure. 2. the solution so administered.

clys·ma (kliz′mə) pl. *clys′mata* [Gr. *klysma*] enema.

clys·ter (klis′tər) [Gr. *klystēr* a syringe] enema.

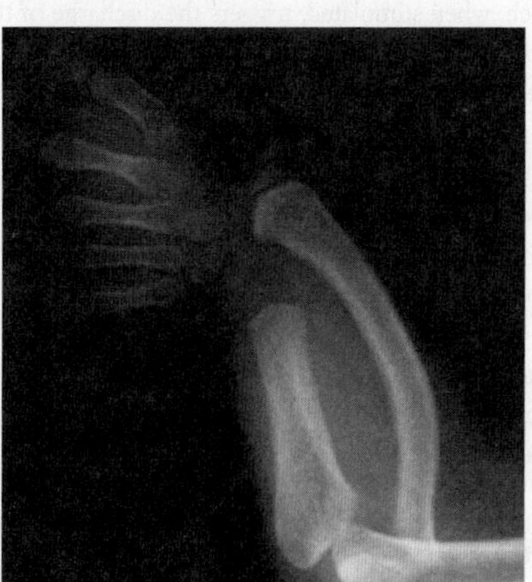

■ Ulnar clubhand with absent distal ulna and a bowed radius with an increased ulnar slope along its distal articular surface.

CM [L.] Chirur'giae Magis'ter (Master of Surgery).

Cm curium.

cM centimorgan.

cm centimeter.

cm^2 square centimeter.

cm^3 cubic centimeter.

CMA Canadian Medical Association; Certified Medical Assistant.

CMAP compound muscle action potential.

CMD cerebromacular degeneration.

CMF a cancer chemotherapy regimen consisting of cyclophosphamide, methotrexate, and 5-fluorouracil.

CMHC community mental health center.

cm H_2O centimeter of water, a unit of pressure equal to that exerted by a column of water at 4°C one millimeter high at mean sea level; officially defined as the pressure exerted by a 1 cm column of fluid with a density of 1 g/cm^3 in a gravitational field of 9.80665 m/s^2, which equals 9.80665 pascals.

CMI cell-mediated immunity.

CML cell-mediated lympholysis.

c mm cubic millimeter.

C-MOPP a cancer chemotherapy regimen consisting of cyclophosphamide, Oncovin (vincristine), procarbazine, and prednisone.

CMP cytidine monophosphate.

c.m.s. [L.] cras ma'ne sumen'dus (to be taken tomorrow morning).

CMT Charcot-Marie-Tooth disease; California mastitis test; Certified Medical Transcriptionist.

CMV cytomegalovirus.

CN chloroacetophenone.

c.n. [L.] cras noc'te (tomorrow night).

CNA Canadian Nurses Association.

CN-Cbl cyanocobalamin.

C3 NeF C3 nephritic factor.

cni•cin (ni'sin) an amaroid that is the main active constituent of blessed thistle.

Cni•cus (ni'kəs) [Gr. *knēkos* safflower] a genus of European herbs of the family Compositae; *C. benedic'tus* (blessed thistle) is medicinal.

Cni•da•ria (ni-dar'e-ə) [Gr. *knidē* a nettle] a phylum of marine invertebrates that includes three classes, Anthozoa, Hydrozoa, and Scyphozoa. It includes jellyfish, sea anemones, Portuguese men-of-war, and other animals that were formerly assigned to the phylum Coelenterata. Most members of the phylum have a radially symmetrical body with tentacles around the mouth. Numerous jellyfish and a few other species are venomous, some even deadly.

cni•dar•i•an (ni-dar'e-ən) 1. pertaining or belonging to the phylum Cnidaria. 2. an individual of the phylum Cnidaria; called also *coelenterate.*

cnid(o)- [Gr. *knidē* a nettle] a combining form denoting a relationship to a nettle or nettle-like structure.

cni•do•blast (ni'do-blast) [*cnido-* + *-blast*] the epidermal cells of coelenterates which contain the nematocysts, especially numerous on the tentacles.

cni•do•cil (ni'do-sil) [*cnido-* + *cil*ium] a bristle-like process at one end of a cnidoblast, which, when stimulated, triggers the discharge of the nematocyst.

Cni•do•spo•rid•ia (ni"do-spo-rid'e-ə) Microsporida.

CNM Certified Nurse-Midwife; see *nurse-midwife.*

CNS central nervous system.

c.n.s. [L.] cras noc'te sumen'dus (to be taken tomorrow night).

CNV contingent negative variation.

CO cardiac output; cervical orthosis.

Co cobalt; coccygeal (in vertebral formulas).

co- see *con-.*

COA Canadian Orthopaedic Association.

CoA coenzyme A.

co•ac•er•vate (ko-as'ər-vāt) [L. *coacervatus* heaped up] the viscous phase separating from a colloid-containing system in the phenomenon of coacervation.

co•ac•er•va•tion (ko-as"ər-va'shən) the separation of a mixture of two liquids, one or both of which are colloids, into two phases, one of which (the coacervate) contains the colloidal particles, the other being an aqueous solution, e.g., as when gum arabic is added to gelatin.

co•ac•ti•va•tor (ko-ak'tĭ-va"tər) a protein complex that serves as a bridge between a transcription factor and RNA polymerase to facilitate the transcription of a target gene.

co•ad•ap•ta•tion (ko-ad"ap-ta'shən) [*co-* + *adaptation*] the mutual, correlated, adaptive changes in two interdependent organs.

co•ad•u•na•tion (ko-ad"u-na'shən) [*co-* + *ad-* + L. *unus* one] union of dissimilar substances in one mass.

co•ad•u•ni•tion (ko-ad"u-nish'ən) coadunation.

co•ag•glu•ti•na•tion (ko"ə-gloo"tĭ-na'shən) the aggregation of particulate antigens combined with agglutinins of more than one specificity.

co•ag•u•la•bil•i•ty (ko-ag"u-lə-bil'ĭ-te) the state of being coagulable.

co•ag•u•la•ble (ko-ag'u-lə-bəl) capable of being formed into clots.

co•ag•u•lant (ko-ag'u-lənt) [L. *coagulans*] 1. promoting, accelerating, or making possible the coagulation of blood. 2. an agent that promotes or accelerates the coagulation of blood.

co•ag•u•lase (ko-ag'u-lās) a bacterial enzyme that reacts with a cofactor found in blood plasma to catalyze the formation of fibrin from fibrinogen. It is produced by *Staphylococcus aureus* and by *Yersinia pestis.*

co•ag•u•late (ko-ag'u-lāt) [L. *coagulare*] 1. to undergo coagulation; to *clot.* 2. to cause to undergo coagulation or clotting.

co•ag•u•la•tion (ko-ag"u-la'shən) [L. *coagulatio*] 1. formation of a clot; see also blood c. 2. in colloid chemistry, the solidification of a sol into a gelatinous mass; an alteration of a disperse phase or of a dissolved solid which causes the separation of the system into a liquid phase and an insoluble mass called the clot or curd; it is usually irreversible. 3. in surgery, the disruption of tissue by physical means to form an amorphous residuum, as in electrocoagulation and photocoagulation.

blood c. the sequential process by which the multiple coagulation factors of the blood interact in the coagulation cascade, ultimately resulting in the formation of an insoluble fibrin clot. See also *extrinsic, intrinsic,* and *common pathways of coagulation.*

diffuse intravascular c. (DIC), disseminated intravascular c. a bleeding disorder characterized by abnormal reduction in the elements involved in blood clotting due to their use in widespread intravascular clotting. It may be caused by any of numerous disorders; in the late stages, it is marked by profuse hemorrhaging. Called also *consumption coagulopathy, defibrination syndrome,* and *disseminated intravascular coagulation syndrome.*

massive c. coagulation of the spinal fluid so as to form an almost solid clot; a condition seen in some cases of Froin syndrome in meningomyelitis or tumor of the cord.

co•ag•u•la•tive (ko-ag'u-lə-tiv) associated with coagulation or promoting a process of coagulation; of the nature of coagulation.

co•ag•u•la•tor (ko-ag'u-la"tər) a surgical device that utilizes electrical current or light to stop bleeding.

argon beam c. (ABC) a device consisting of a needle electrode recessed inside a probe through which argon gas is passed; the energy from the electrode is carried by the jet of argon, which is directed at bleeding tissue to effect hemostasis.

co•ag•u•lo•gram (ko-ag'u-lo-gram") a term used colloquially in clinical hematology to denote a series of laboratory tests measuring the various parameters of hemostasis.

co•ag•u•lop•a•thy (ko-ag"u-lop'ə-the) any disorder of blood coagulation; called also *bleeding disorder.*

consumption c. diffuse intravascular coagulation.

co•ag•u•lum (ko-ag'u-ləm) pl. *coag'ula* [L.] clot (def. 1).

closing c. see under *plug.*

co•a•les•cence (ko"ə-les'əns) [L. *coalescere* to grow together] the fusion or blending of parts.

co•a•li•tion (ko"ə-lish'ən) [L. *coalescere* to grow together] the fusion of parts that are normally separate.

calcaneocuboid c. an often asymptomatic tarsal coalition involving the calcaneus and the cuboid bone.

calcaneonavicular c. one of the most common types of tarsal coalition, involving the calcaneus and the navicular bone.

cubonavicular c. tarsal coalition involving the cuboid and navicular bones.

naviculocuneiform c. tarsal coalition involving the navicular and cuneiform bones.

talocalcaneal c. one of the most common types of tarsal coalition, involving the talus and calcaneus.

talonavicular c. tarsal coalition involving the talus and the navicular bone.

tarsal c. the fibrous, cartilaginous, or bony fusion of two or more of the tarsal bones, often resulting in talipes planovalgus, although other deformities occur and some patients are asymptomatic; it may be congenital or acquired as a response to trauma, infection, or joint disease. Called also *tarsal bar* or *bridge*.

co·amil·o·zide (ko″ə-mil′ə-zīd) pharmacy equivalent name for a combination of amiloride hydrochloride and hydrochlorothiazide; used as a diuretic in the treatment of edema, hypertension, and hypokalemia.

co·amox·i·clav (ko″ə-mok′sĭ-klav) pharmacy equivalent name for a combination of amoxicillin, an antibiotic, and clavulanate potassium, a β-lactamase inhibitor; effective in infections caused by β-lactamase–producing organisms.

co·apt (ko-apt′) [L. *coaptare*] to join together, as the edges of a wound or the ends of a fractured bone.

co·ap·ta·tion (ko-ap-ta′shən) the process of approximating, or joining together.

co·arc·tate (ko-ahrk′tāt) 1. to press close together or contract. 2. pressed together or restrained.

co·arc·ta·tion (ko″ahrk-ta′shən) [L. *coarctatio*, from *cum* together + *arctare* to make tight] stenosis.

c. of aorta a localized malformation characterized by deformity of the aortic media, causing narrowing, usually severe, of the lumen of the vessel.

c. of aorta, adult type localized constriction at or below the insertion of the ductus arteriosus and distal to the aortic isthmus and left subclavian artery, with a closed ductus and absence of cyanosis.

c. of aorta, infantile type coarctation of the aorta in which there is cyanosis and diffuse involvement of the aortic isthmus; it is usually seen in infants and is associated with other anomalies such as a patent ductus.

reversed c. Takayasu arteritis.

coarse (kors) not fine; not microscopic.

co·ar·tic·u·la·tion (ko″ahr-tik″u-la′shən) [*co-* + *articulation*] a synarthrosis.

coast·ing (kōst′ing) continuation of neurotoxic symptoms, sometimes for several months, after exposure to a specific toxin has ended.

CoA-SH coenzyme A.

coat (kōt) [L. *cotta* tunic] 1. tunica. 2. the layer or layers of protective protein surrounding the nucleic acid in a virus. Cf. *capsid*.

adventitial c. tunica adventitia.

buffy c. the thin yellowish layer of leukocytes overlying the packed red cells in centrifuged blood; called also *buffy layer* and *leukocytic cream*.

dry c. anhidrosis (def. 2).

external c. of ureter tunica adventitia ureteris.

external c. of vessels tunica externa vasorum.

fibrous c. tunica fibrosa.

fibrous c. of ovary theca folliculi.

fibrous c. of testis tunica albuginea testis.

inner c. of vessels tunica intima vasorum.

middle c. of vessels tunica media vasorum.

mucous c. tunica mucosa.

muscular c. tunica muscularis.

muscular c. of colon tunica muscularis coli.

muscular c. of ductus deferens tunica muscularis ductus deferentis.

muscular c. of esophagus tunica muscularis oesophagi.

muscular c. of female urethra tunica muscularis urethrae femininae.

muscular c. of gallbladder tunica muscularis vesicae biliaris.

muscular c. of large intestine tunica muscularis intestini crassi.

muscular c. of membranous urethra tunica muscularis partis intermediae urethrae.

muscular c. of prostatic urethra tunica muscularis partis prostaticae urethrae.

muscular c. of rectum tunica muscularis recti.

muscular c. of renal pelvis tunica muscularis pelvis renalis.

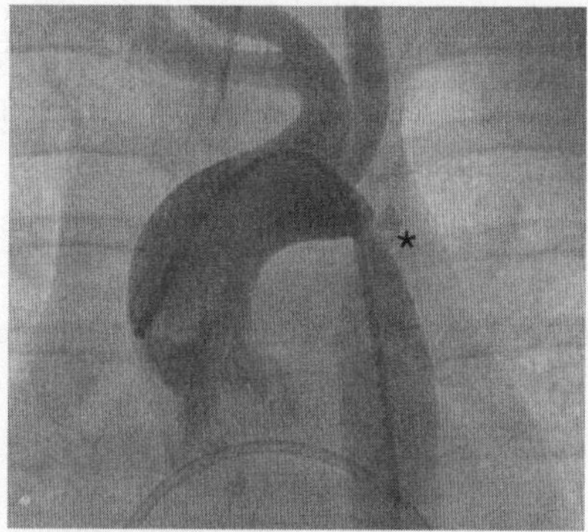

■ Angiography showing coarctation of aorta with reduced blood flow into the left subclavian artery *(asterisk)*.

muscular c. of seminal vesicle tunica muscularis glandulae vesiculosae.

muscular c. of small intestine tunica muscularis intestini tenuis.

muscular c. of spongy urethra tunica muscularis partis spongiosae urethrae.

muscular c. of stomach tunica muscularis gastrica.

muscular c. of ureter tunica muscularis ureteris.

muscular c. of urinary bladder tunica muscularis vesicae urinariae.

muscular c. of uterine tube tunica muscularis tubae uterinae.

muscular c. of vagina tunica muscularis vaginae.

outer c. of vessels tunica externa vasorum.

sclerotic c. the sclera.

serous c. tunica serosa.

serous c. of bladder tunica serosa vesicae urinariae.

serous c. of esophagus tunica serosa oesophagi.

serous c. of gallbladder tunica serosa vesicae biliaris.

serous c. of large intestine tunica serosa intestini crassi.

serous c. of liver tunica serosa hepatis.

serous c. of parietal pleura tunica serosa pleurae parietalis.

serous c. of pericardium tunica serosa pericardii.

serous c. of peritoneum tunica serosa peritonei.

serous c. of small intestine tunica serosa intestini tenuis.

serous c. of spleen tunica serosa splenica.

serous c. of stomach tunica serosa gastrica.

serous c. of testis tunica serosa testis

serous c. of urinary bladder tunica serosa vesicae urinariae.

serous c. of uterine tube tunica serosa tubae uterinae.

serous c. of uterus tunica serosa uteri.

serous c. of visceral pleura tunica serosa pleurae visceralis.

subserous c. tela subserosa.

uveal c. tunica vasculosa bulbi.

coat·o·mer (ko′to-mər) [*coat* + proto*mer*] one of the macromolecular protein complexes, composed of seven subunits (coat proteins or COPs) and present in the cytosol, that are assembled to form the coat of vesicles that transport proteins between cisternae of the Golgi complex and between the Golgi complex and the endoplasmic reticulum.

CoA-trans·fer·ase (ko′a trans′fər-ās) [EC 2.8.3.] one of a sub-subclass of enzymes of the transferase class that catalyze the transfer of coenzyme A from one molecule to another.

Coats disease (retinitis) (kōts) [George *Coats*, English ophthalmologist, 1876–1915] see under *disease*.

co·ax·i·al (ko-ak′se-əl) having a common axis; said of two tubes mounted with one inside the other. Cf. *concentric*.

co·bal·a·min (ko-bal′ə-min) 1. in chemical nomenclature, a compound comprising the substituted corrin ring and 5,6-dimethylbenzimidazole–containing nucleotide that are characteristic of vitamin B_{12}, but lacking a ligand at the 6 position of the cobalt. 2. a term used generically to denote any substituted derivative of this compound, including cyanocobalamin, particularly one with vitamin B_{12} activity.

co·b(I)al·a·min ad·e·no·syl·trans·fer·ase (ko-bal′ə-min ə-den″o-səl-trans′fər-ās) a mitochondrial enzyme of the transferase class that catalyzes the transfer of an adenosyl group to cobalamin from ATP, forming the coenzyme adenosylcobalamin. Deficiency of the enzyme, an autosomal recessive trait *(CblB)*, leads to deficiency of methylmalonyl-CoA mutase activity and results in methylmalonicacidemia. In official nomenclature, called *cob(I)yrinic acid a,c-diamide adenosyltransferase* [EC 2.5.1.17].

co·bal·amin re·duc·tase (ko-bal′ə-min re-duk′tās) either of two mitochondrial reductases that catalyze steps in the synthesis of adenosylcobalamin from hydroxocobalamin; deficiency of one or both is believed to be a cause of methylmalonicacidemia (q.v.).

co·bal·oph·i·lin (ko-bə-lof′ĭ-lin) R protein.

co·balt (Co) (ko′bawlt) [L. *cobaltum*] a metal, atomic number 27, atomic weight 58.9332; the metal is used in magnetic alloys, and the compounds afford pigments; inhalation of the dust can cause cobaltosis and exposure to the powder may cause dermatitis. See also *cobalt poisoning*, under *poisoning*. In animals, a deficiency of this element leads to anemia and an excess of normal dietary requirements leads to erythrocytosis. In humans, although cobalt has been used with limited transient effectiveness to treat the anemia of infection and renal disease, its sole physiologic function is probably as a constituent of vitamin B_{12}.

c. 57 a radioactive isotope of cobalt, atomic mass 57, having a half-life of 271.77 days and decaying in the form of electron capture and gamma rays (energy 0.122 MeV); used to label vitamin B_{12} for the Schilling and other tests of intestinal absorption.

c. 58 a radioactive isotope of cobalt, atomic mass 58, having a half-life of 71.92 days and decaying in the form of electron capture, positrons (energy 0.48 MeV), and gamma rays (energy 0.811 MeV); used together with ^{57}Co in a test of intestinal vitamin B_{12} absorption.

c. 60 a radioactive isotope of cobalt, atomic mass 60, having a half-life of 5.27 years and emitting beta particles (energy 0.318, 1.48 MeV) and gamma rays (energy 1.173, 1.332 MeV); used as a source of radiation in the treatment of malignancies. It has also been used to label vitamin B_{12} for the Schilling and other tests of intestinal absorption.

co•bal•to•sis (ko″bawl-to′sis) pneumoconiosis due to inhalation of and tissue reaction to cobalt dust.

co•bal•tous (ko-bawl′təs) pertaining to or containing cobalt in its bivalent state.

co•ba•mide (ko′bə-mīd) 1. in chemical nomenclature, a derivative of cobalamin lacking the 5,6-dimethylbenzimidazole moiety. 2. a term sometimes used generically for any substituted compound containing this structure, particularly any *cobalamin* (def. 2).

co•bra (ko′brə) [Port. *cobra de capello* snake with a hood, from L. *coluber* snake] any of several extremely poisonous elapid snakes of the large genus *Naja* and smaller genus *Ophiophagus,* commonly found in Africa, Asia, and India. They are capable of expanding the neck region to form a hood, and have two comparatively short, erect, deep grooved fangs. A serum obtained from animals inoculated with cobra venom is used in counteracting the effects of the venom. See table at *snake.*

Asian c. any member of the species *Naja naja,* whose subspecies are widely distributed throughout Asia and nearby islands including Indonesia and the Philippines; among the Asian cobras are the Indian cobra, *N. naja naja,* and a spitting cobra found in Southeast Asia and the Philippines, *N. naja sputatrix.*

black-necked c. *Naja nigricollis,* a type of spitting cobra found in southern Egypt, West Africa, and south through western Africa to South Africa.

Cape c. *Naja nivea,* a species found in southern Africa.

Egyptian c. *Naja haje,* a species found throughout Africa and the western part of the Arabian peninsula.

Indian c. *Naja naja naja,* a yellowish to dark brown cobra with black and white markings resembling a pair of spectacles on its hood; it sometimes attains a length of 2 meters. Called also *N. naja.*

king c. *Ophiophagus hannah,* a large cobra found from India to the Philippines, which may reach a length of 3.6 meters.

Mozambique c. *Naja mossambica,* a type of spitting cobra found in southeastern Africa.

spitting c. any of several cobras that have a venom canal opening forward in the fangs, so that the snake can eject a fine spray of venom over a distance of several meters ("spitting"). If the venom enters the eyes severe irritation results, and secondary infection may lead to blindness. The group includes the black-necked cobra, the Mozambique cobra, and *Naja naja sputatrix,* a subspecies of *N. naja.*

co•bra•ism (ko′brə-iz-əm) poisoning by cobra venom.

co•bral•y•sin (ko-bral′ĭ-sin) a hemolytic substance derived from the poison of the cobra.

COBS cesarean-obtained barrier-sustained; a term applied to animals delivered by cesarean section into a germ-free environment and maintained under the same conditions.

co•b(I)y•rin•ic (ko″bə-rin′ik as′id) a corrinoid with six carboxylic acid substituents on the methylene carbon atoms of the reduced pyrrole rings and a cobalt atom in the center of the macrocyclic ring. The carboxyl groups are designated by the locants a to g.

co•b(I)y•rin•ic ac•id *a,c*-di•a•mide ad•e•no•syl•trans•fer•ase (ko″bə-rin′ik as′id di-am′īd ə-den″o-səl-trans′fər-ās) [EC 2.5.1.17] official nomenclature for *cob(I)alamin adenosyltransferase.*

co-bu•caf•APAP (ko″bu-kaf′ə-pap) pharmacy equivalent name for a combination of butalbital, caffeine, and acetaminophen, an analgesic used in the treatment of tension and migraine headaches.

COC calcifying odontogenic cyst.

co•ca (ko′kə) 1. *Erythroxylon coca.* 2. the leaves of *E. coca,* widely used in parts of South America as a euphoriant masticatory. A central nervous system stimulant, it was once widely used medicinally and is a source of the crystalline extract cocaine.

co•caine (ko-kān′) [USP] a crystalline alkaloid, obtained from leaves of *Erythroxylon coca* (coca leaves) and other *Erythroxylon* species, or by synthesis from ecgonine or its derivatives; used as a local anesthetic and vasoconstrictor applied topically to mucous membranes. Abuse of cocaine or its salts leads to dependence.

crack c. a smokable form of cocaine prepared for illicit use, characterized by rapid absorption and onset of euphoric effects.

c. hydrochloride [USP] the hydrochloride salt of cocaine, used as a local anesthetic and vasoconstrictor, applied topically to mucous membranes.

co•cain•iza•tion (ko″kə-nĭ-za′shən) the act of putting under the influence of cocaine.

co•cain•ize (ko′kə-nīz) to put under the influence of cocaine.

co•car•cin•o•gen (ko-kahr-sin′ə-jən) promoter (def. 3).

co•car•ci•no•gen•e•sis (ko-kahr″sĭ-no-jen′ə-sis) the development, according to one theory, of cancer only in preconditioned cells and as a result of conditions favorable to its growth.

co-car•el•do•pa (ko″kar-əl-do′pə) pharmacy equivalent name for a combination of carbidopa and levodopa, an antiparkinsonian agent.

coc•ce•rin (kok′sə-rin) a wax from *Coccus,* the cochineal insect, being an ester of cocceryl alcohol and two acids, 13-keto-*n*-dotriacontanoic acid and *n*-triacontanoic acid; used as a biological stain.

coc•ci (kok′si) [L.] plural of *coccus.*

Coc•ci•dae (kok′sĭ-de) a family of insects of the order Hemiptera; it includes the genera *Coccus* and *Laccifer.*

Coc•cid•ia (kok-sid′e-ə) [Gr. *kokkos* berry] a subclass of parasitic protozoa (class Sporozoea, phylum Apicomplexa) found in many vertebrates and invertebrates, causing coccidiosis. Their life cycle involves merogony, gametogony, and sporogony, and gamonts are usually present, with mature gamonts being small and typically intracellular, without an epimerite or mucron. Syzygy does not usually occur, but if it does, it involves anisogamous gametes. The subclass comprises three orders: Agamococcidiida, Protococcidiida, and Eucoccidiida.

coc•cid•ia (kok-sid′e-ə) plural of *coccidium.*

coc•cid•i•al (kok-sid′e-əl) coccidian (def. 1).

coc•cid•i•an (kok-sid′e-ən) 1. pertaining to Coccidia. 2. any protozoan of the subclass Coccidia.

coc•cid•i•oi•dal (kok-sid″e-oi′dəl) pertaining to or caused by fungi of the genus *Coccidioides.*

Coc•cid•i•oi•des (kok-sid″e-oi′dēz) a pathogenic genus of Fungi Imperfecti of the form-class Hyphomycetes, form-family Moniliaceae. In soil it grows as a mycelium with arthrospores; in tissue it grows as a spherule with endospores.

C. im′mitis a species that is found primarily in the San Joaquin Valley of California and causes coccidioidomycosis and fungal pneumonia.

C. posada′sii a species that is found primarily in desert areas of the southwestern United States, as well as Central and South America, and causes coccidioidomycosis and fungal pneumonia.

coc•cid•i•oi•din (kok-sid″e-oi′din) [USP] a skin test antigen prepared from mycelial phase *Coccidioides immitis* organisms, used in the coccioidin test for coccidioidomycosis. Cf. *spherulin.*

coc•cid•i•oi•do•ma (kok-sid″e-oi-do′mə) a solid round focus of residual pulmonary granulomatous nodules, seen radiographically in coccidioidomycosis.

coc•cid•i•oi•do•my•co•sis (kok-sid″e-oi″do-mi-ko′sis) a fungal disease caused by infection with *Coccidioides immitis,* occurring in both primary and secondary forms. Called also *coccidioidosis, coccidioidal granuloma,* and *Posadas* or *Posadas-Wernicke disease.*

primary c. an acute, benign, self-limited respiratory infection due to inhalation of spores of *Coccidioides immitis,* seen primarily in the southwestern United States, northwestern Mexico, and parts of Central and South America. It varies in severity from a condition resembling a common cold to symptoms like those of influenza, sometimes with pneumonia, cavitation, high fever, and occasionally erythema nodosum *(bumps).* Called also *desert* or *valley fever, San Joaquin* or *San Joaquin Valley fever,* and *desert rheumatism.*

progressive c., secondary c. a virulent and severe chronic progressive granulomatous disease with involvement of the cutaneous and subcutaneous tissues, viscera, central nervous system, and lungs, with anemia, phlebitis, and a variety of allergic responses. It may be either a new infection or a reactivation of arrested primary disease, such as in immunocompromised patients.

coc•cid•i•oi•do•sis (kok-sid″e-oi-do′sis) coccidioidomycosis.

coc•cid•i•o•sis (kok″sid-e-o′sis) infection by coccidian protozoa. In humans it is often asymptomatic and found only upon testing of a stool sample, but occasionally it causes severe watery mucous diarrhea, especially in immunocompromised patients. In other mammals and birds, it may cause diarrhea, intestinal hemorrhage, emaciation, and sometimes fatal dysentery; young animals are especially vulnerable.

coc•cid•io•stat (kok-sid′ĭ-o-stat″) an agent that controls coccidiosis in animals; often administered as a feed additive or in drinking water. Called also *anticoccidial* and *coccidiostatic.*

coc•cid•io•stat•ic (kok-sid″ĭ-o-stat′ik) 1. inhibiting the growth of coccidia. 2. coccidiostat.

coc•cid•i•um (kok-sid′e-əm) pl. *coccid′ia.* Any protozoan of the subclass Coccidia.

coc•ci•gen•ic (kok″sĭ-jen′ik) caused by cocci.

coc•ci•nel•lin (kok″sĭ-nəl′in) [L. *coccinellinum*] carmine; the coloring principle of cochineal.

cocco- [Gr. *kokkos* berry] a word element denoting a resemblance to a berry.

coc·co·bac·il·lary (kok″o-bas′ĭ-lar″e) pertaining to or resembling a coccobacillus.

coc·co·ba·cil·li (kok″o-bə-sil′i) plural of *coccobacillus.*

coc·co·ba·cil·lus (kok″o-bə-sil′əs) pl. *coccobacil′li.* An oval bacterial cell intermediate between the coccus and bacillus forms.

coc·co·bac·te·ria (kok″o-bak-tēr′e-ə) [*cocco-* + *bacteria*] a common name for the spheroid bacteria, or for the various bacterial cocci.

coc·code (kok′ōd) a globular granule.

coc·co·gen·ic (kok″o-jen′ik) coccigenic.

coc·co·gen·ous (kok-oj′ə-nəs) [*cocco-* + *-genous*] coccigenic.

coc·coid (kok′oid) resembling a coccus; globose.

coc·cu·lus in·di·cus (kok′u-lus in′dĭ-kus) 1. *Anamirta cocculus.* 2. the seeds of *A. cocculus,* which contain picrotoxin.

Coc·cus (kok′əs) [L., from Gr. *kokkos* berry] a genus of hemipterous insects of the family Coccidae, order Hemiptera. *C. cac′ti* is a source of cochineal.

coc·cus (kok′əs) pl. *coc′ci* [L., from Gr. *kokkos* berry] a spherical bacterial cell, usually slightly less than 1 μm in diameter. **coc′cal** *adj*

coc·cy·al·gia (kok″se-al′jə) coccygodynia.

coc·cy·dyn·ia (kok″sə-din′e-ə) coccygodynia.

coc·cy·gal·gia (kok″sə-gal′jə) coccygodynia.

coc·cyg·e·al (kok-sij′e-əl) pertaining to or located in the region of the coccyx.

coc·cy·gec·to·my (kok″sĭ-jek′tə-me) [*coccyx* + *-ectomy*] excision of the coccyx.

coc·cy·ge·rec·tor (kok″sĭ-jə-rek′tər) the ventral sacrococcygeal muscle.

coc·cyg·e·us (kok-sij′e-əs) [L.] coccygeal.

coc·cy·go·dyn·ia (kok″sĭ-go-din′e-ə) [*coccyx* + *-odynia*] pain in the coccyx and neighboring region; called also *coccyalgia, coccydynia, coccygalgia,* and *coccyodynia.*

coc·cy·got·o·my (kok″sĭ-got′ə-me) [*coccyx* + *-tomy*] freeing the coccyx from its attachments.

coc·cy·odyn·ia (kok″se-o-din′e-ə) coccygodynia.

coc·cyx (kok′siks) [Gr. *kokkyx* cuckoo, whose bill it is said to resemble] TA alternative for *os coccygis.*

coch·i·neal (koch″ĭ-nēl′) the dried female insects, *Coccus cacti,* enclosing the young larvae; it is the source of carmine and carminic acid.

coch·lea (kok′le-ə) [L. "snail shell"] 1. anything of a spiral form. 2. [TA] a spirally wound tube, resembling a snail shell, which forms part of the internal ear. Its base lies against the lateral end of the internal acoustic meatus and its apex is directed anterolaterally. It consists of the modiolus, a bony canal, and the osseous spiral lamina, which partially divides the cochlea into the essential organs of hearing, the scala vestibuli and scala tympani; the scalae communicate through the helicotrema. **coch′lear** *adj*

membranous c. ductus cochlearis.

Mondini c. the misshapen cochlea seen in Mondini deformity.

Coch·le·a·ria (kok″le-ar′e-ə) [L.] a genus of plants of the family Cruciferae. *C. officina′lis* is scurvy grass, a species formerly used to treat scurvy. *C. armora′cia* is a former name for *Armoracia lapathifolia,* the horseradish plant.

coch·le·ar·i·form (kok″le-ar′ĭ-form) [L. *cochleare* spoon + *form*] shaped like a spoon.

coch·le·itis (kok″le-i′tis) inflammation of the cochlea.

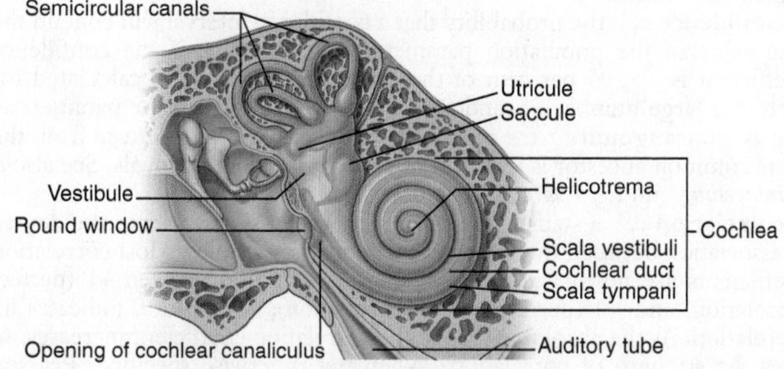

■ Cochlea and other structures of the bony labyrinth.

coch·leo·sac·cu·lot·o·my (kok″le-o-sak″u-lot′ə-me) creation of a fistula between the saccule and cochlear duct by means of a pick introduced through the round window, in order to relieve endolymphatic hydrops.

coch·leo·top·ic (kok″le-o-top′ik) relating to the organization of the auditory pathways and auditory area of the brain.

coch·leo·ves·tib·u·lar (kok″le-o-ves-tib′u-lər) pertaining to the cochlea and vestibule of the ear.

Coch·li·ob·o·lus (kok″le-ob′ə-ləs) a genus of fungi of the order Dothideales. It includes the perfect (sexual) stage of various species of *Bipolaris, Curvularia,* and *Drechslera.*

Coch·lio·my·ia (kok″le-o-mi′yə) [Gr. *kochlias* snail with a spiral shell + *myia* fly] a genus of flies of the family Calliphoridae.

C. america′na *C. hominivorax.*

C. bezzia′na *Chrysomyia bezziana.*

C. hominivo′rax the screw-worm fly, a bluish green fly that deposits its eggs during the warmest hours of the day on wounds of animals; the larvae, known as screw-worms, after hatching, burrow into the wound and feed on living tissue. Called also *C. americana* and *Chrysomyia macellaria.*

coch·li·tis (kok-li′tis) cochleitis.

co·ci·lla·na (ko″se-yah′nə) the bark of *Guarea rusbyi,* used as an emetic, expectorant, and cathartic.

Cock·ayne syndrome (kok-ān′) [Edward Alfred *Cockayne,* English physician, 1880–1956] see under *syndrome.*

Cock·croft-Gault formula (kok′kroft gawlt′) [Donald W. *Cockcroft,* Canadian physician, late 20th century; M. Henry *Gault,* Canadian physician, late 20th century] see under *formula.*

cock·le·burr (kok′əl-bər) any plant of the genus *Xanthium.*

cock·roach (kok′rōch) [Sp. *cucaracha*] any of various crawling winged insects of the order Blattaria, having flat oval bodies; many are household pests and reservoirs of disease. Common genera are *Blatta, Blattella,* and *Periplaneta.* Called also *roach.*

American c. *Periplaneta americana,* a common household pest in the Northern hemisphere.

Australian c. *Periplaneta australasiae,* a common household pest in warm regions of the world.

German c. *Blattella germanica,* a small light brown species found as a household pest in North America and Europe. Called also *Croton bug.*

Oriental c. *Blatta orientalis,* a black species originally seen in Asia but now found as a household pest in many parts of the world.

cock·tail (kok′tāl) a beverage concocted of various ingredients.

lytic c. a combination of meperidine, promethazine, and chlorpromazine which has been used for pediatric sedation and analgesia.

co·cli·ma·sone (ko-kli′mə-sōn) pharmacy equivalent name for a combination of clotrimazole, an antifungal, and betamethasone dipropionate, a corticosteroid; used as a topical antifungal in the treatment of tinea corporis, tinea cruris, and tinea pedis.

co·coa (ko′ko) 1. in pharmacy, former name for *chocolate.* 2. a powder made from fermented, roasted, shelled, ground cacao seeds from which at least some of the fat (cocoa butter) has been removed. It is widely consumed, often as a beverage, but poses the same risks to dogs as does chocolate (q.v.).

co·cod·APAP (ko-ko′də-pap) pharmacy equivalent name for a combination of codeine phosphate and acetaminophen, an analgesic.

co·co·da·prin (ko-ko′də-prin) pharmacy equivalent name for a combination of codeine phosphate and aspirin, an analgesic.

co·con·scious (ko-kon′shəs) 1. not in the field of the conscious yet capable under favorable circumstances of being remembered; preconscious. 2. characterized by or pertaining to coconsciousness.

co·con·scious·ness (ko-kon′shəs-nis) 1. a secondary consciousness coexisting with the main stream of consciousness, as in some dissociative disorders. 2. the edge of consciousness.

co·con·trac·tion (ko-kən-trak′shən) simultaneous contraction of agonist and antagonist muscles; this may happen normally in certain circumstances or abnormally to cause stiffness in conditions such as cerebral palsy. Also written *co-contraction.*

co·co·nut (ko′kə-nət) the fruit of *Cocos nucifera,* a palm tree whose nut is important as a food and a source of coconut oil.

Co·cos (ko′kōs) a genus of palm trees (family Palmae). *C. nuci′fera* is the coconut palm, the source of coconuts and coconut oil.

coct(o)- [L. *coctus,* past part. of *coquere* to cook] a combining form meaning boiling or boiled, or denoting modification by heating.

coc·to·an·ti·gen (kok″to-an′tĭ-jən) [*cocto-* + *antigen*] an antigen modified by heat treatment.

coc·to·im·mu·no·gen (kok″to-ĭ-mu′no-jən) coctoantigen.

coc·to·la·bile (kok″to-la′bəl, -la′bīl) [*cocto-* + *labile*] destroyed or altered by heating to the boiling point of water.

coc·to·pre·cip·i·tin (kok″to-pre-sip′ĭ-tin) [*cocto-* + *precipitin*] a precipitin produced by immunization with a coctoantigen.

coc·to·pro·tein (kok″to-pro′tēn) [*cocto-* + *protein*] a heated protein.

coc·to·sta·bile (kok″to-sta′bəl, -sta′bīl) [*cocto-* + *stabile*] not altered by heating to the temperature of boiling water.

coc·to·sta·ble (kok″to-sta′bəl) coctostabile.

co·cul·ti·va·tion (ko″kəl-tĭ-va′shən) the culturing of cells (e.g., normal uninfected human cells) with infected or latently infected cells of the same kind.

cod (kod) *Gadus morrhua.*

code (kōd) [L. *codex* something written] 1. a set of rules governing one's conduct. 2. a system by which information can be communicated.

degeneracy of c. see under *degeneracy.*

genetic c. the arrangement of consecutive nucleotide triplets (codons) in a nucleic acid that specifies the sequence of amino acids for synthesis of a protein (see accompanying table). See also *transcription* and *translation.*

The Genetic Code

UUU AAA phe	UCU AGA ser	UAU ATA tyr	UGU ACA cys
UUC GAA phe	UCC GGA ser	UAC GTA tyr	UGC GCA cys
UUA TAA leu	UCA TGA ser	UAA TTA *term*	UGA TGA *term*
UUG CAA leu	UCG CGA ser	UAG CTA *term*	UGG CCA trp
CUU AAG leu	CCU AGG pro	CAU ATG his	CGU ACG arg
CUC GAG leu	CCC GGG pro	CAC GTG his	CGC GCG arg
CUA TAG leu	CCA TGG pro	CAA TTG gln	CGA TCG arg
CUG CAG leu	CCG CGG pro	CAG CTG gln	CGG CCG arg
AUU AAT ile	ACU AGT thr	AAU ATT asn	AGU ACT ser
AUC GAT ile	ACC GGT thr	AAC GTT asn	AGC GCT ser
AUA TAT ile	ACA TGT thr	AAA TTT lys	AGA TCT arg
AUG CAT met (*init*)	ACG CGT thr	AAG CTT lys	AGG CCT arg
GUU AAC val	GCU AGC ala	GAU ATC asp	GGU ACC gly
GUC GAC val	GCC GGC ala	GAC GTC asp	GGC GCC gly
GUA TAC val	GCA TGC ala	GAA TTC glu	GGA TCC gly
GUG CAC val (*init*)	GCG CGC ala	GAG CTC glu	GGG CCC gly

Each grouping matches a messenger RNA codon (*top*), its complementary DNA codon (*middle*), and the amino acid they specify (*bottom*). U = uracil; C = cytosine; A = adenine; G = guanine; T = thymine; see *amino acid* for amino acid symbols. The codons marked *term* are chain termination codons. Those marked *init* are chain initiation codons which code for methionine (in the cytosol of eukaryotic cells) or *N*-formylmethionine (in mitochondria and prokaryotes) at the beginning of polypeptide chains and for the indicated amino acid (methionine or valine) within polypeptide chains. The genetic code for mitochondria differs slightly.

triplet c. the form taken by the genetic code, in which each amino acid or start or stop signal is encoded by a group of three nucleotides (codon).

co·deine (ko′dēn) [L. *codeina*] [USP] a narcotic alkaloid obtained from opium or prepared by methylating morphine. Called also *methylmorphine.*

c. phosphate [USP] the phosphate salt of codeine, administered orally as an opioid analgesic, antitussive, and antidiarrheal, and subcutaneously or intramuscularly as an opioid analgesic.

c. sulfate [USP] the sulfate salt of codeine, having the same actions and uses as the phosphate salt.

co·dex (ko′deks) pl. *cod′ices* [L.] an authorized medicinal formulary; especially the French Pharmacopoeia, *Codex medicamentarium.*

Cod·man sign, triangle (kod′mən) [Ernest Amory *Codman*, American surgeon, 1869–1940] see under *sign* and *triangle.*

co·do·cyte (ko′do-sīt) target cell.

co·dom·i·nance (ko-dom′ĭ-nəns) the full phenotypic expression in a heterozygote of both alleles of a pair, with each contributing to the phenotype, as in a person with blood group AB. **codom′inant** *adj*

co·don (ko′don) a set of three adjacent bases on an mRNA that specifies an amino acid to be added to the growing polypeptide chain, or directs chain initiation or termination. Of the 64 different possible codons, 61 direct the incorporation of a specific amino acid into a polypeptide chain, with several of those also sometimes signaling chain initiation, and three signal chain termination (see table at *genetic code*, under *code*).

initiation c. either of the codons AUG or GUG occurring at the beginning of mRNA sequences coding for polypeptide chains. There they are recognized by the initiator tRNA, which carries the amino acid methionine (in the cytosol of eukaryotes) or *N*-formylmethionine (in prokaryotes, mitochondria, and chloroplasts). In the middle of a polypeptide chain these codons are recognized by other tRNAs so that AUG directs the incorporation of methionine and GUG of valine.

nonsense c. termination c.

start c. initiation c.

stop c., termination c. any of the three codons UAA, UAG, and UGA that cause termination of the synthesis of a growing polypeptide chain and its release from the ribosome.

coe- for words beginning thus, see also words beginning *ce-*.

co·ef·fi·cient (ko″ə-fish′ənt) 1. a numerical factor multiplying a term in an algebraic equation. 2. a number preceding a formula in a chemical equation, indicating the relative number of molecules of that species entering the reaction. 3. a unitless constant characterizing a chemical or physical process. 4. a unitless statistical parameter indicating the amount of change in an outcome under given conditions.

absorption c. 1. absorptivity. 2. see *linear absorption c.* 3. see *mass absorption c.*

activity c. the ratio of the activity (of an electrolyte) as measured by some property, such as the depression of the freezing point of a solution, to the true concentration (molality). It is usually less than 1 and increases as the solution becomes more dilute, approaching unity at infinite dilution, when the attractive forces between oppositely charged ions become negligible.

binomial c. the number of different sets of size *k* that can be chosen from a set of *n* objects; denoted

$$\binom{n}{k}$$

or ${}_nC_k$, and equal to

$$\frac{n!}{k!(n-k)!}.$$

biological c. the amount of potential energy consumed by the body when at rest.

Bunsen c. (α) the number of milliliters of gas dissolved in a milliliter of liquid at atmospheric pressure (760 mm Hg) and a specified temperature. Called also *solubility c.*

confidence c. the probability that a confidence interval will contain the true value of the population parameter. For example, if the confidence coefficient is .95, 95 per cent of the confidence intervals so calculated for each of a large number of random samples would contain the parameter.

c. of consanguinity the probability that a single allele derived from the same common ancestor is identical by descent in two individuals. See also *c. of inbreeding* and *c.of relationship.*

correlation c. a statistical measure that when squared gives the degree of association between the values of two random variables. Most correlation coefficients are normalized so that they have values between +1 (perfect correlation) and −1 (perfect inverse correlation); a value of 0 indicates no correlation. As the absolute value of the correlation coefficient increases, so does the strength of correlation. When not otherwise specified, Pearson correlation coefficient is meant. The true theoretical correlation coefficient for a population is symbolized ρ; the sample correlation coefficient, computed from experimental data, estimates the theoretical and is symbolized *r*.

creatinine c. the figure obtained by dividing the total of milligrams of creatinine in the day's urine by the body weight expressed in kilograms.

cryoscopic c. the comparison of the freezing point depression of an electrolyte with that of an ideal nonelectrolyte of the same concentration (usually 1 molal of each).

c. of demineralization the proportion of mineral matter to the total dry residue of the urine; it averages 30 per cent.

diffusion c. the number of milliliters of a gas that will diffuse at a distance of 0.001 mm over a square centimeter surface per minute, at 1 atm of pressure. The diffusion coefficient for any given gas is proportional to the solubility and molecular weight of the gas.

dilution c. a number that expresses the effectiveness of a disinfectant for a given organism. It is calculated by the equation $tc^n = k$, where t is the time required for killing all organisms, c is the concentration of disinfectant, n is the dilution coefficient, and k is a constant. A low coefficient indicates the disinfectant is effective at a low concentration.

distribution c. partition c.

extinction c. absorptivity.

Hill c. a coefficient occurring in the Hill equation, indicating the degree of cooperativity of the enzyme being examined; a Hill coefficient of 1.0 indicates independent binding while greater and lesser values indicate positive and negative cooperativity, respectively. The value for hemoglobin is 2.8.

homogeneity c. in radiology, the ratio of the half-value layer to the second half-value layer; it is unity for radiation in which the photons all originate with the same energy.

c. of inbreeding (*F*) an expression of the probability that an individual has received both alleles of a pair from a single ancestor common to both parents, or of the proportion of loci at which he or she is homozygous. The inbreeding coefficient of an individual is the same as the coefficient of consanguinity of his or her parents. Called also *Wright inbreeding c.*

Kendall rank correlation c. a rank correlation coefficient used when both variables represent ordinal data in a limited number of grades, such as the categories none, mild, moderate, and severe, so that multiple samples can be assigned to each grade; called also *Kendall tau.* See also *Spearman rank correlation c.*

lethal c. dilution c.

linear absorption c. in radiation physics, the fraction of a beam of x-rays or gamma rays that is absorbed per unit thickness of the absorber.

linear attenuation c. (μ) in radiation physics, the fraction of a beam of x-rays or gamma rays that is absorbed or scattered per unit thickness of the absorber.

mass absorption c. in radiology, the linear absorption coefficient divided by the density of the absorber.

mass attenuation c. the linear attenuation coefficient divided by the density of the absorbing material.

mass transfer–area c. (MTAC) the permeability of a dialysis membrane multiplied by the available area of the membrane, calculated as the clearance rate by diffusion when there is no ultrafiltration and when there is not yet any solute in the dialysate.

molar absorption c., molar extinction c. molar absorptivity.

olfactory c. Proetz test.

osmotic c. a factor, ϕ, which corrects for the deviation in the behavior of a solute in question from ideal behavior defined by the ideal gas equation as applied to osmotic pressure.

partition c. the ratio in which a given substance distributes itself between two or more different phases; called also *distribution c.*

Pearson correlation c. the most common correlation coefficient; it is the covariance of two random variables divided by the product of their standard deviations. Called also *product-moment correlation c.* See also *correlation c.*

phenol c. a measure of the bactericidal activity of a chemical compound in relation to phenol. The test is standardized (Rideal-Walker method, U.S. Department of Agriculture method). The coefficient is calculated by dividing the concentration of the test compound at which it kills the test organism in 10 minutes, but not in 5 minutes, by the concentration of phenol that kills the organism under the same conditions. It can be determined in the absence of organic matter or in the presence of a standard amount of added organic matter.

product-moment correlation c. Pearson correlation c.

rank correlation c. the correlation coefficient of two variables calculated after ranks have been substituted for actual values. See also *Kendall rank correlation c.* and *Spearman rank correlation c.*

c. of relationship an expression of the probability that two persons have inherited a certain gene from a common ancestor; or the proportion of all their genes that have been inherited from common ancestors. Cf. *c. of inbreeding.*

Rideal-Walker c. see *phenol c.*

sample correlation c. see *correlation c.*

sedimentation c. the velocity at which a particle sediments in a centrifuge divided by the applied centrifugal field, the result having units of time (velocity divided by acceleration), usually expressed in Svedberg units (S), which equal 10^{-13} second. Sedimentation coefficients are used to characterize the size of macromolecules, e.g., 5.8S rRNA, 22S rRNA; they increase with increasing mass and density and are higher for globular than for fibrous particles. Called also *sedimentation constant.*

selection c. a measure of the relative disadvantage in contribution to the next generation of a given genotype as compared with that of another genotype, usually the most fit, in a population.

solubility c. Bunsen c.

Spearman rank correlation c. a rank correlation coefficient used when both variables represent ordinal data in an unlimited ranking, such as class standing, so that each sample is assigned a unique rank. Symbol r_s. Called also *Spearman rho.* Cf. *Kendall rank correlation c.*

temperature c. a number indicating the effect of temperature upon the velocity constant of a chemical reaction. Symbol Q_{10} because 10°C is the most commonly employed temperature change; see *van't Hoff rule,* under *rule.*

c. of thermal conductivity a number indicating the quantity of heat that passes in a unit of time through a unit thickness of a substance when the difference in temperature is 1°C.

c. of thermal expansion the change in volume per unit volume of a substance produced by a 1°C temperature increase.

ultrafiltration c. an expression of permeability to solutes of a membrane, such as a glomerular membrane or a high flux membrane.

c. of variation (CV) the standard deviation divided by the mean, sometimes multiplied by 100; a unitless quantity indicating the variability around the mean in relation to the size of the mean.

velocity c. a number expressing the rate of a reaction; the rate of transformation of a unit mass of a substance in a chemical reaction.

c. of viscosity the force necessary to slide tangentially a unit of area of smooth surface at unit velocity on another parallel surface separated from the first surface by a unit layer of viscous substance.

Wright inbreeding c. c. of inbreeding.

-coele [Gr. *koilia* cavity] a word termination denoting a cavity or space; sometimes spelled *-cele* and *-coel.*

Coe·len·ter·a·ta (se-len″tər-a′tə) [Gr. *koilos* hollow + *enteron* intestine] former name for a phylum of marine invertebrates that included sea anemones, hydras, jellyfish, and corals, which are now assigned to the phylum Cnidaria.

coe·len·ter·ate (se-len′tər-āt) cnidarian.

coe·li·ac (se′le-ak) abdominal.

coel(o)- [Gr. *koilos* hollow] a combining form denoting relationship to a cavity or space; sometimes spelled *cel(o)-.*

coe·lom (se′ləm) [Gr. *koilōma*] the body cavity. In higher invertebrates it persists throughout life (cf. *Eucoelomata*). In the mammalian embryo, it is situated between the somatopleure and the splanchnopleure and is both extraembryonic and intraembryonic. From the intraembryonic portion arise the principal cavities of the trunk. Also spelled *celom.* Called also *somatic cavity.* **coelom′ic** *adj*

extraembryonic c. the portion of the coelom external to the embryo, bordered by chorionic mesoderm and the mesoderm of the amnion and yolk sac; it communicates temporarily at the umbilicus with the intraembryonic coelom. Called also *chorionic cavity* and *exocoelom.*

intraembryonic c. a body cavity in the embryo that later develops into the pericardial and peritoneal cavities.

coe·lo·mate (sēl′o-māt) 1. having a coelom. 2. eucoelomate.

coe·lo·my·ar·i·an (se″lo-mi-ar′e-ən) designating a type of nematode musculature in which the muscle fibers are next to the hypodermis and perpendicular to it; myofibrils extend varying distances up the side of the muscle cell, partially enclosing the sarcoplasm.

coe·lo·my·cete (se″lo-mi-sēt′) any fungus of the form-class Coelomycetes. **coelomyce′tous** *adj*

Coe·lo·my·ce·tes (se″lo-mi-se′tēz) a form-class of Fungi Imperfecti whose members produce conidia in pycnidia or acervuli; many of its members are saprobes or parasites on plants, animals, or other organisms. There are several different systems for dividing this group into orders and families. Medically important genera include *Colletotrichum, Diplodia, Hendersonula, Phoma, Pyrenochaeta,* and *Scytalidium.*

coe·lo·thel (se′lo-thel) [*coelo-* + *thel*] mesothelium.

coe·lo·zo·ic (se″lo-zo′ik) [*coelo-* + *zoic*] inhabiting the intestinal cavities of the body; said of parasites.

coen(o)- see *cen(o)-²*.

coe·no·cyte (se′no-sīt″) [*coen(o)-* + *-cyte*] 1. a multinucleate plant cell enclosed within a hollow wall, examples of which are found within the fungi and algae. 2. a multinucleate bit of cytoplasm in which the nuclei are not separated by walls. 3. a multinucleate plant protoplast. Spelled also *cenocyte.* **coenocyt′ic** *adj*

coe·nu·ri·a·sis (se′nu-ri′ə-sis) 1. coenurosis (def. 1). 2. gid.

coe•nu•ro•sis (se″nu-ro′sis) 1. any infection by tapeworm larvae of the genus *Coenurus;* this is rare in humans, nearly always in the form of central nervous system cysts that obstruct the outflow of cerebrospinal fluid and cause a rise in intracranial pressure that can be fatal. Called also *coenuriasis.* 2. gid.

Coe•nu•rus (se-nu′rəs) [Gr. *koinos* common + *oura* tail] a genus of tapeworm larvae consisting of semitransparent fluid-filled organisms that contain multiple scoleces attached to the inner surface of the cavity wall; they do not form brood capsules. *C. cerebra′lis,* the larva of *Taenia multiceps,* is found in the brains of ruminants and occasionally humans.

coe•nu•rus (se-nu′rəs) a tapeworm larva of the genus *Coenurus;* cf. *cysticercus.* Called also *bladder worm.*

co•en•zyme (ko-en′zīm) an organic nonprotein molecule, frequently a phosphorylated derivative of a water-soluble vitamin, that binds with the protein molecule (apoenzyme) to form the active enzyme (holoenzyme).

c. A (CoA, CoA-SH) a coenzyme in which phosphorylated pantothenic acid is covalently linked to β-mercaptoethylamine and adenosine 3′,5′-bisphosphate. The terminal thiol group of the β-mercaptoethanolamine is enzymatically acylated to form high-energy thiol ester compounds such as the acetyl, acetoacetyl, and long chain fatty acid (acyl) compounds. These thiol esters play a central role in various metabolic reactions, such as the tricarboxylic acid cycle, the transfer of acetyl groups, and the oxidation of fatty acids. See also *acetoacetyl coenzyme A, acetyl coenzyme A, acyl coenzyme A,* and *succinyl coenzyme A.*

c. B_{12} adenosylcobalamin. See also *methylcobalamin.*

c. Q, c. Q_{10} ubiquinone.

coe•ru•le•us (sə-roo′le-əs) [L.] variant spelling of *caeruleus* (q.v.).

co•eryn•sul•fi•sox (ko″er-in-sul′fəzoks) pharmacy equivalent name for a combination of erythromycin ethylsuccinate and sulfisoxazole acetyl, an antibacterial.

coeur (kur) [Fr.] heart.

c. en sabot (ah să-bo′) ["wooden shoe–shaped heart"] a heart visible radiographically as having an increased transverse diameter, a convexity in the inferior line, and an elevation and rounded shape of the apex, so that its form suggests vaguely that of a wooden shoe; noted in tetralogy of Fallot.

co•fac•tor (ko′fak-tər) an element or principle, as a coenzyme, with which another must unite in order to function.

heparin c. II a member of the serpin group, a single-chain glycoprotein, M_r 65,000, that inhibits thrombin. It resembles antithrombin III in being markedly stimulated by heparin; it differs in that it binds and is activated by dermatan sulfate and in that it does not inhibit any other activated coagulation factors.

platelet c. I factor VIII; see under *coagulation factors,* at *factor.*

platelet c. II factor IX; see under *coagulation factors,* at *factor.*

Cof•fea (kaw′fe-ə) the coffee plants, a genus of small trees of the family Rubiaceae thought to have originated in Africa. Several species, particularly *C. ara′bica* L. and *C. cane′phora,* are cultivated in warm regions around the world as sources of coffee.

cof•fee (kof′e) [Ar. al-qahwah] 1. the dried, roasted seeds of *Coffea arabica* or *C. canephora.* 2. a stimulating drink made by decoction or infusion of these seeds. The active principles include caffeine (q.v.) in the seeds, coffee oil, sugars, protein, and numerous volatile flavoring oils.

Cof•fin-Low•ry syndrome (kof′in lou′re) [Grange S. *Coffin,* American pediatrician, born 1923; R. Brian *Lowry,* Irish-born Canadian physician, 20th century] see under *syndrome.*

Cof•fin-Sir•is syndrome (kof′in sir′is) [G.S. *Coffin;* Evelyn *Siris,* American radiologist, 1914–1987] see under *syndrome.*

Co•gan oc•u•lo•mo•tor aprax•ia, syndrome (ko′gən) [David Glendenning *Cogan,* American ophthalmologist, 1908–1993] see under *apraxia* and *syndrome.*

co•ge•ner (ko′jə-nər) congener.

Co•gen•tin (ko-jen′tin) trademark for preparations of benztropine mesylate.

Cog•nex (kog′neks) trademark for a preparation of tacrine hydrochloride.

cog•ni•tion (kog-nish′ən) [L. *cognitio,* from *cognoscere* to know] that operation of the mind by which one becomes aware of objects of thought or perception; it includes all aspects of perceiving, thinking, and remembering. **cog′nitive** *adj*

co•he•sin (ko-he′sin) a heterodimer that is assembled during DNA replication and mediates the cohesion of sister chromatids; it is cleaved by separase to trigger chromatid separation in anaphase.

co•he•sion (ko-he′zhən) [L. *cohaesio,* from *con* together + *haerere* to stick] the intermolecular attractive force that causes various particles of a single material to unite.

co•he•sive (ko-he′siv) uniting together, or characterized by cohesion.

Cohn•heim's areas (fields), theory (kōn′hīmz) [Julius Friedrich *Cohnheim,* German pathologist, 1839–1884] see under *area* and *theory.*

co•ho•ba (ko-ho′bə) [Sp.] parica.

co•hort (ko′hort) [L. *cohors* one of the ten units making up a Roman legion] 1. in epidemiology, a group of individuals who share a common characteristic, e.g., all of the individuals born in one year (a birth cohort) or a group of individuals entered in a prospective study or a clinical trial. The term always indicates observation of the individuals over time. 2. a taxonomic category approximately equivalent to a division, order, or suborder in various systems of classification.

co•hosh (ko-hosh′) [Algonquian] any of various North American medicinal plants.

black c. 1. *Cimicifuga racemosa.* 2. the fresh or dried root of *C. racemosa,* having estrogenic effects, used for symptomatic relief in menopause and premenstrual syndrome and for a wide variety of uses in folk medicine and traditional Chinese medicine.

blue c. 1. *Caulophyllum thalictroides.* 2. the fresh roots or the dried rhizome and roots of *C. thalictroides,* having weak estrogenic effects, used for menstrual disorders and as an antispasmodic and stimulant of uterine contractions during labor; in homeopathy it is used for disorders of menstruation and labor and for rheumatism of the fingers and toes.

co•hy•cod•APAP (ko″hi-ko′də-pap) pharmacy equivalent name for a combination of hydrocodone bitartrate and acetaminophen, an analgesic.

coil (koil) [Old Fr. *collier,* from L. *colligere* to gather together] 1. a winding structure. See also *spiral* and *helix.* 2. radiofrequency c.

body c. a type of receiver coil that has a large measurement field for imaging a wide area of the body.

detector c. receiver c.

Gianturco c. a small stainless steel coil inserted through a cardiac catheter to attract blood clots and occlude a patent ductus arteriosus.

gradient c's a group of radiofrequency coils oriented in different directions so that they generate a magnetic field gradient.

radiofrequency c. a loop of wire used in magnetic resonance imaging as an antenna for transmitting or receiving radio frequency data. Called also *RF c.*

random c. any protein secondary structure that does not have a regular repetitive pattern, such as an α-helix or a β sheet.

receiver c. a radiofrequency coil that can receive radio frequency transmissions. Called also *detector c.*

RF c. radiofrequency c.

secretory c. the coiled secretory part of a sweat gland, found in the deep part of the dermis; it secretes sweat that flows out through a sweat duct. Called also *body of sweat gland.*

shim c's radiofrequency coils that create additional weak magnetic fields in order to provide shim.

surface c. a receiver coil in magnetic resonance imaging that lies against the surface of the object being imaged.

transmitter c. a radiofrequency coil that can transmit radio frequency emissions.

co•in•fec•tion (ko′in-fek″shən) simultaneous infection by separate pathogens, as by hepatitis B and hepatitis D viruses.

coin(o)- see *cen(o)-*[2].

coi•no•site (koi′no-sīt) [*coino-* + *sitos* food] a facultative commensal organism; called also *cenosite.*

co•i•so•gen•ic (ko-i″so-jen′ik) of or relating to strains of inbred animals that are genetically identical except for a difference at a single genetic locus.

co•i•tion (ko-ish′ən) coitus.

co•i•to•pho•bia (ko″ĭ-to-fo′be-ə) [*coitus* + *-phobia*] irrational fear of coitus.

co•i•tus (ko′ĭ-təs) [L. *coitio* a coming together, meeting] sexual connection per vaginam between male and female. **co′ital** *adj*

c. incomple′tus, c. interrup′tus coitus in which the penis is withdrawn from the vagina before ejaculation; a widely used but unreliable method of contraception.

c. reserva′tus coitus in which ejaculation is intentionally suppressed.

Co•ke•ro•my•ces (ko″kə-ro-mi′sēz) a genus of fungi of the family Thamnidiaceae. *C. recurva′tus* has been isolated occasionally from cases of mucormycosis and cystitis.

col (kol) [Fr., from L. *collum* neck] a valley-like depression of the interdental gingiva, which connects the facial and lingual papillae and conforms to the shape of the interproximal contact area.

col- see *con-.*

Co•lace (ko′lās) trademark for a preparation of docusate sodium.

co•la•mine (ko′lə-min) monoethanolamine.

co·las·pase (kə-las′pās) BAN for asparaginase derived from *Escherichia coli* for use as an antineoplastic agent.

Colat. [L.] cola′tus (strained).

co·la·tion (ko-la′shən) [L. *colare* to strain] 1. the process of removing solids from liquids, by straining or filtration. 2. the product of such a process.

col·a·to·ri·um (kol″ə-tor′e-əm) [L. *colare* to strain] filter.

co·la·ture (ko′lə-chər) [L. *colatura*, from *colare* to strain] a liquid obtained by straining.

Col·a·zal (kawl′ə-zal) trademark for a preparation of balsalazide disodium.

Col·BEN·E·MID (kol-ben′ə-mid) trademark for a combination preparation of probenecid with colchicine.

col·chi·cine (kol′chĭ-sēn) [USP] an alkaloid obtained from species of *Colchicum*, used in the treatment of gouty arthritis and to prevent febrile attacks in familial Mediterranean fever. It binds to microtubules and is used in the laboratory to arrest cell division by disrupting the mitotic spindle. Its action in gout may be due to inhibition of granulocyte migration into areas of inflammation.

Col·chi·cum (kol′chi-kəm) a genus of plants of the family Liliaceae, native to Europe and Asia; their corms or dried ripe seeds are sources of colchicine. *C. autumna′le* is the meadow saffron; cattle eating excessive amounts of it may suffer a fatal enteritis.

COLD chronic obstructive lung disease.

cold (kōld) 1. low in temperature, physiologic activity, or in radioactivity. 2. a catarrhal disorder of the upper respiratory tract, which may be viral, a mixed infection, or an allergic reaction. It is marked by acute rhinitis, a slight rise in temperature, and chilly sensations. Called also *common c.*

  common c. see *cold* (def. 2).

Cole sign (kōl) [Lewis Gregory *Cole*, American radiologist, 1874–1954] see under *sign*.

co·lec·to·my (ko-lek′tə-me) [*col-* + *-ectomy*] excision of a portion of the colon *(partial c.)* or of the whole colon *(complete* or *total c.)*.

  left c. see under *hemicolectomy*.

  right c. see under *hemicolectomy*.

  sigmoid c. sigmoidectomy.

Col·e·op·tera (kol″e-op′tər-ə) [*coleo-* + Gr. *pteron* wing] the beetles, an order of insects having strong mouth parts for chewing and a pair of hard exterior wings that protect the body, are not used for flight, and cover the membranous flight wings.

co·le·sev·e·lam hy·dro·chlo·ride (ko″lə-sev′ə-lam) a hydrophilic, water-insoluble polymer that binds bile acids in the intestine and prevents them from being reabsorbed, resulting in decreased serum levels of total cholesterol, LDL cholesterol, and apolipoprotein B and increased levels of HDL cholesterol; administered orally as adjunctive therapy to reduce elevated LDL cholesterol levels in patients with primary hypercholesterolemia.

Co·les·tid (ko-les′tid) trademark for a preparation of colestipol hydrochloride.

co·les·ti·pol hy·dro·chlo·ride (ko-les′tĭ-pol) [USP] an insoluble, high-molecular-weight anion exchange resin that binds bile acids in the intestines to form a complex that is excreted in the feces; administered orally as an antihyperlipoproteinemic in the treatment of familial hyperlipoproteinemia, type IIa, pruritus associated with partial biliary obstruction, and diarrhea due to excess bile acids in the colon.

col·fos·ce·ril pal·mi·tate (kol-fos′ə-ril) a synthetic pulmonary surfactant used, in combination with cetyl alcohol and tyloxapol, in the prophylaxis and treatment of neonatal respiratory distress syndrome; instilled into the endotracheal tube for intratracheal administration.

coli- pertaining to *Escherichia coli.*

co·li·bac·il·lo·sis (ko″lĭ-bas-ĭ-lo′sis) [*coli-* + *bacill-* + *-osis*] infection with *Escherichia coli.*

  enteric c., enterotoxigenic c. coliform gastroenteritis.

  septicemic c. *Escherichia coli* septicemia.

co·li·bac·il·lu·ria (ko″lĭ-bas″ĭl-u′re-ə) [*coli-* + *bacilluria*] bacteriuria with *Escherichia coli* in the urine, seen with urinary tract infections. Called also *coliuria.*

co·li·bac·il·lus (ko″lĭ-bə-sil′əs) *Escherichia coli.*

co·lic[1] (ko′lik, kol′ik) [Gr. *kōlikos*] pertaining to the colon; colonic.

col·ic[2] (kol′ik) [L. *colica (passio)* (suffering) of the colon] acute abdominal pain, usually intermittent visceral pain with fluctuations that correspond to smooth muscle peristalsis. **col′icky** *adj*

  appendicular c. pain in the vermiform appendix from blockage and inflammation; called also *vermicular c.*

  biliary c. paroxysms of pain and other severe symptoms due to the passage of gallstones along the bile duct; called also *gallstone c., hepatic c.,* and *cholecystalgia.*

  copper c. colic due to copper poisoning.

  equine c. intestinal pain in horses; causes may include excessive gas; blockage by an impaction, foreign body, or twisting or other malposition; or infection or enteritis.

  flatulent c. tympanites.

  gallstone c. biliary c.

  hepatic c. biliary c.

  infantile c. benign paroxysmal abdominal pain during the first three months of life.

  intestinal c. colic in the small intestine, usually periumbilical in location.

  lead c. colic due to lead poisoning; called also *painters' c.*

  painters' c. lead c.

  pancreatic c. colic due to obstruction of the excretory duct of the pancreas.

  renal c. pain produced by thrombosis or dissection of the renal artery, renal infarction, intrarenal mass lesions, the passage of a stone within the collecting system, or thrombosis of the renal vein.

  sand c. chronic indigestion in horses and cattle due to the presence in the stomach or intestine of sand taken in with food or drink.

  tubal c. painful spasmodic contraction of the fallopian tube.

  ureteral c. colicky pains due to obstruction of the ureter.

  uterine c. hysteralgia.

  vermicular c. appendicular c.

  verminous c., worm c. colic due to the presence of intestinal worms.

  zinc c. colic due to chronic zinc poisoning.

col·i·cin (kol′ĭ-sin) [*coli* (from *Escherichia coli*) + *-cin* (adapted from L. *caedere* to kill)] a bacteriocin secreted by colicinogenic strains of *Escherichia coli* and *Shigella sonnei* that is lethal to closely related bacterial strains. Specific colicins attach to specific receptors on cell membranes and impair systems of electron transport, membrane function, molecular synthesis, or energy production.

col·i·cin·o·gen (kol″ĭ-sin′o-jən) bacteriocinogen; a plasmid in some strains of *Escherichia coli* that induces secretion of the corresponding colicin. Some colicinogens also serve as sex factors.

col·i·ci·nog·e·nic (kol″ĭ-sĭ-noj′ə-nik) elaborating colicin; said of strains of *Escherichia coli.*

col·i·ci·nog·e·ny (kol″ĭ-sin-oj′ə-ne) the production of colicin; see *colicinogen.*

co·li·cys·ti·tis (ko″lĭ-sis-ti′tis) [*coli-* + *cystitis*] cystitis due to infection with *Escherichia coli.*

co·li·cys·to·py·eli·tis (ko″lĭ-sis-to-pi″ə-li′tis) [*coli-* + *cystopyelitis*] pyelocystitis due to infection with *Escherichia coli.*

col·i·form (ko′lĭ-form) [L. *colum* a sieve] 1. a collective term denoting enteric, fermentative gram-negative rods, and sometimes restricted to the lactose-fermenting, gram-negative enteric bacilli, i.e., *Citrobacter, Edwardsiella, Enterobacter, Escherichia, Klebsiella,* and *Serratia.* 2. any organism of that group.

co·lin·e·ar·i·ty (ko″lin-e-ar′ĭ-te) the correspondence between the linear sequence of the nucleotide codons, the RNA, and the linear sequence of amino acids in the polypeptide coded for by that sequence; a concept implicit in the original Watson-Crick model of the DNA structure.

co·lip·ase (ko-li′pās) a cofactor of pancreatic lipase, secreted by pancreatic acinar cells as a proenzyme and activated via hydrolytic cleavage by trypsin.

col·i·phage (kol′ĭ-fāj) [*coli-* + *phage*] any bacteriophage that infects *Escherichia coli.*

co·li·sep·ti·ce·mia (ko″lĭ-sep″tĭ-se′me-ə) *Escherichia coli* septicemia.

co·lis·ti·meth·ate so·di·um (ko-lis″tĭ-meth′āt) [USP] chemical name: colistinmethanesulfonic acid pentasodium; the pentasodium salt of the methanesulfonate derivative of colistin, having actions and uses similar to those of the base (colistin); administered intramuscularly or intravenously.

co·lis·tin (ko-lis′tin) a polypeptide antibiotic of the polymyxin (q.v.) group, produced by the growth of the soil bacterium *Bacillus polymyxa* var. *colistinus*, specifically effective against many gram-negative bacteria, especially *Pseudomonas aeruginosa*, but also useful against others, including *Escherichia coli* and species of *Klebsiella, Shigella,* and *Brucella; Proteus* species are resistant.

  c. sulfate [USP] the sulfate salt of colistin, used in the treatment of various systemic, urinary tract, gastrointestinal, ophthalmic, and otic infections due to gram-negative bacteria; administered orally, parenterally, and topically.

co•li•tis (ko-li′tis) [*col-* + *-itis*] inflammation of the colon. See also *enterocolitis.*

amebic c. see under *dysentery.*

antibiotic-associated c. see under *enterocolitis.*

balantidial c. colitis due to infestation with *Balantidium coli.*

cathartic c. colitis due to chronic laxative abuse.

chemical c. colitis that is a reaction to a chemical instilled per rectum.

collagenous c. a type of colitis characterized by deposits of collagenous material beneath the epithelium of the colon, with crampy abdominal pain and marked reduction in fluid and electrolyte absorption, leading to watery diarrhea; there is no mucosal ulceration. The etiology is unknown.

Crohn c. see under *disease.*

c. cys′tica profun′da a rare condition marked by mucous retention cysts in the submucosa of the colon. The etiology is unknown; some cases may be postinflammatory changes, such as the healing of chronic lesions of bacillary dysentery.

c. cys′tica superficia′lis a rare cystic condition of the mucous membrane of the colon, sometimes seen in children with chronic debilitating diseases such as leukemia; it may be the result of malnutrition and vitamin deficiency.

cytomegalovirus c. colitis caused by activation of cytomegalovirus in the colon in immunocompromised individuals; characteristics include mucosal ulceration and watery diarrhea.

diversion c. inflammation of a segment of distal colon that has been defunctionalized by diversion of the fecal stream by subtotal colectomy; it may be asymptomatic or may be marked by tenesmus, anorectal pain, and bloody rectal discharge. It resolves following reanastomosis of the intestine.

equine ehrlichial c. equine monocytic ehrlichiosis.

granulomatous c. transmural colitis with formation of noncaseating granulomas.

hemorrhagic c. a usually afebrile diarrheal disease caused by *Escherichia coli* serovar O157:H57, characterized by abdominal cramping and watery diarrhea that progresses to bloody diarrhea after one or two days; it is generally self-limited but may be complicated by hemolytic-uremic syndrome.

infectious c. colitis caused by an infectious agent.

irradiation c. radiation c.

ischemic c. a type of colitis caused by acute vascular insufficiency of the colon, usually the part supplied by the inferior mesenteric artery; symptoms include pain at the left iliac fossa, bloody diarrhea, low-grade fever, abdominal distention and tenderness, and sometimes ulceration. Radiologically there is "thumbprinting" due to localized elevation of the mucosa by submucosal hemorrhage or edema.

lymphocytic c., microscopic c. a type of colitis similar to collagenous colitis but without deposits in the subepithelial region; marked reduction in fluid absorption is present, with chronic diarrhea and without ulceration.

mucous c. former term for *irritable bowel syndrome;* see under *syndrome.*

necrotizing amebic c. see under *pancolitis.*

neutropenic c. see under *enterocolitis.*

pseudomembranous c. see under *enterocolitis.*

radiation c. colitis resulting from radiation therapy to the abdominal region, marked by tenesmus, pain, rectal bleeding, diarrhea, and telangiectasis, which may progress to malabsorption, ulceration, and partial or complete obstruction. Called also *irradiation c.* and *radiation enteritis.*

regional c., segmental c. transmural or granulomatous inflammatory disease of the colon; regional enteritis involving the colon only. It may be associated with ulceration, strictures, or fistulas.

soap c. inflammation of the colon as a reaction to a soapsuds enema.

transmural c. inflammation of the full thickness of the intestinal wall, rather than just mucosa or submucosa, usually with formation of noncaseating granulomas. It may be confined to the colon, segmentally or diffusely, or extend into the small intestine *(regional enteritis).* Clinically, it may resemble ulcerative colitis, but the ulceration is often longitudinal or deep, and there are often strictures and fistulas, particularly in the perineum.

ulcerative c. one of the principal types of inflammatory bowel disease, consisting of chronic, recurrent ulceration in the colon, chiefly of the mucosa and submucosa, having an unknown cause. It is manifested clinically by cramping abdominal pain, rectal bleeding, and loose discharges of blood, pus, and mucus with scanty fecal particles. Complications include hemorrhoids, abscesses, fistulas, perforation of the colon, pseudopolyps, and carcinoma.

uremic c. colitis that results from the uremia of chronic renal failure.

col•i•tose (kol′ĭ-tōs) an unusual sugar found in the O-specific chains in the lipopolysaccharides of certain serovars of *Salmonella* and *Escherichia coli.*

co•li•tox•emia (ko″lĭ-tok-se′me-ə) [*coli-* + *toxemia*] toxemia due to infection with *Escherichia coli.*

co•li•tox•i•co•sis (ko″lĭ-tok″sĭ-ko′sis) [*coli-* + *toxicosis*] intoxication caused by *Escherichia coli.*

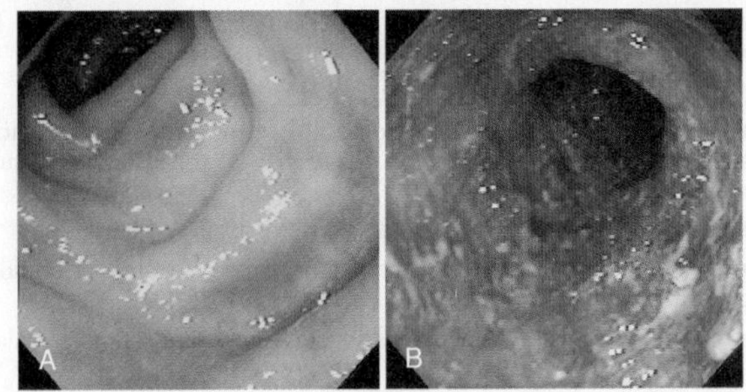

■ Colonoscopic findings in ulcerative colitis. *(A)*, Edema, loss of vascularity, and patchy subepithelial hemorrhage in mild disease; *(B)*, loss of vascularity, hemorrhage, friability of the mucosa, and mucopus in severe disease.

co•li•tox•in (ko′lĭ-tok″sin) [*coli-* + *toxin*] a substance contained in *Escherichia coli* that is the cause of colitoxicosis.

co•li•uria (ko″lĭ-u′re-ə) colibacilluria.

col•la (kol′ə) [L.] plural of *collum.*

col•la•cin (kol′ə-sin) degenerate collagenous tissue; collastin.

col•la•gen (kol′ə-jən) [Gr. *kolla* glue + *-gen*] any of a family of extracellular, closely related proteins occurring as a major component of connective tissue, giving it strength and flexibility. At least 25 types exist, each composed of tropocollagen (q.v.) units that share a common triple-helical shape but vary in composition between types, with the types being localized to different tissues, stages, or functions. In some types, including the most common, Type I, the tropocollagen rods associate to form fibrils or fibers; in other types the rods are not fibrillar but are associated with fibrillar collagens, while in others they form nonfibrillar, nonperiodic, but structured networks. Collagen is converted to gelatin by boiling. See also under *disease, fiber,* and *fibril.*

col•la•ge•nase (kə-laj′ə-nās) an enzyme that catalyzes the hydrolysis of peptide bonds in triple helical regions of collagen.

***Clostridium histolyticum* c.** any of several forms of microbial collagenase isolated from *Clostridium histolyticum* that catalyze the cleavage of collagen into small fragments, cleaving it in the triple helical region N-terminal to glycine residues. The extracellular Zn^{2+} enzyme degrades the collagen framework of muscles, facilitating the spread of gas gangrene by *C. histolyticum.*

interstitial c. [3.4.24.7] any of a group of enzymes of the hydrolase class that catalyze the cleavage of native collagen, usually at a glycine-leucine or glycine-isoleucine bond. The best studied are those that cleave the fibrillar collagens into a large N-terminal (75 per cent) and a small C-terminal fragment (25 per cent). The enzymes require zinc, occur widely in vertebrates, and are involved in the degradation of collagen during tissue repair or during embryonic and fetal development. Called also *vertebrate c.*

microbial c. [EC 3.4.24.3] any of various collagenases purified from a variety of microbes, particularly *Clostridium histolyticum* (see *C. histolyticum c.*); they preferentially cleave collagen on the N-terminal side of glycine residues and occur in several classes of differing specificity.

vertebrate c. interstitial c.

col•lag•e•na•tion (kə-laj″ə-na′shən) the appearance of collagen in developing cartilage.

col•la•gen•ic (kol″ə-jen′ik) 1. collagenous. 2. collagenogenic.

col•lag•e•no•blast (kə-laj′ə-no-blast) a cell that arises from a fibroblast and that as it matures is associated with the production of collagen; it may form cartilage and bone by metaplasia. Collagenoblasts proliferate at the site of chronic inflammation. Sometimes called also *fibroblast.*

col•lag•e•no•cyte (kə-laj′ə-no-sīt″) a mature collagen-producing cell; see *collagenoblast.*

col•la•gen•o•gen•ic (kə-laj″ə-no-jen′ik) pertaining to or characterized by the production of collagen; forming collagen or collagen fibers.

col•la•gen•ol•y•sis (kol″ə-jən-ol′ə-sis) dissolution or digestion of collagen.

col•lag•e•no•ly•tic (kə-laj″ə-no-lit′ik) effecting the digestion of collagen.

col•la•gen•o•ma (kol″ə-jĕ-no′mə) connective tissue nevus.

perforating verruciform c., verrucous perforating c. a rare, acquired form of reactive perforating collagenosis, occurring in response to severe skin trauma and characterized by verrucous papules resulting from the extrusion of collagen fibers through the epidermis.

col•la•gen•o•sis (kol″ə-jĕ-no′sis) collagen disease.

reactive perforating c. (RPC) a rare, usually familial type of acquired perforating dermatosis in which collagen fibers are extruded through the epidermis. It occurs at sites of frequent trauma (e.g., the knees and backs of the hands) and is characterized by skin-colored papules with a central area of umbilication containing keratinous material. Lesions grow to 5–8 mm in diameter and regress spontaneously; the Koebner phenomenon may occur. An acquired form, associated with diabetes and renal insufficiency, also occurs.

col·lag·e·nous (kə-laj′ə-nəs) pertaining to collagen; forming or producing collagen.

col·lapse (kə-laps′) [L. *collapsus*] 1. a state of extreme prostration and depression, with failure of circulation. 2. abnormal falling in of the walls of any part or organ.

circulatory c. shock (def. 2).

c. of the lung an airless or fetal state of all or a part of a lung, as seen in atelectasis from bronchial obstruction and in pneumothorax.

massive c. a condition in which an entire lung becomes airless, often due to obstruction of a main bronchus.

scapholunate advanced c. (SLAC) a common form of arthritic degeneration of the wrist, with gradual loss of ligamentous support due to chronic malalignment of the scaphoid bone, resulting in a rotational deformity.

col·lar (kol′ər) an encircling band, generally around the neck.

Casal c. see under *necklace.*

cervical c. cervical orthosis.

circumaortic venous c. a rare vascular anomaly in which the left renal vein encircles the inferior vena cava and constricts it. Called also *circumaortic venous ring.*

Cobb c. congenital stenosis of the bulbar urethra.

hair c. see *hair collar sign,* under *sign.*

periosteal bone c. a band of spongy bone that forms around the middle of the diaphysis of early bones.

Philadelphia c. a type of cervical orthosis that restricts anterior-posterior cervical motion to a great degree but allows some normal rotation and lateral bending.

c. of Stokes edematous thickening of the neck and soft parts of the thorax in the superior vena cava syndrome.

col·lar·ette (kol″ər-et′) 1. a narrow rim of loosened keratin overhanging the periphery of a circumscribed skin lesion, attached to the normal surrounding skin, such as in candidiasis or pityriasis rosea. 2. an irregular jagged line dividing the anterior surface of the iris into two regions, the ciliary zone and the pupillary zone. Called also *angular line.* 3. in mycology, a ring around the apex of a phialide resulting from rupture during release of the first phialospore.

Biett c. a papular syphilid in which the central papule is surrounded by a ring of scales.

col·las·tin (kŏ-las′tin) degenerate collagenous tissue that stains like normal elastic tissue.

col·lat·er·al (ko-lat′ər-əl) [*co-* + *lateral*] 1. secondary or accessory; not direct or immediate. 2. a small side branch, as of a blood vessel or nerve.

Schaffer c's branches of the axons of the stratum pyramidale of the hippocampus, some of which end on cells in the stratum oriens, but many of which pass into the stratum moleculare.

Col·les fascia, fracture, ligament, space (kol′ēz) [Abraham *Colles,* Irish surgeon, 1773–1843] see *ligamentum inguinale reflexum* and *membrana perinei,* and see under *fracture* and *space.*

Col·let syndrome (ko-la′) [Frédéric Justin *Collet,* French laryngologist, 1870–1966] see under *syndrome.*

Col·let-Si·card syndrome (ko-la′ se-kahr′) [F.J. *Collet;* Jean Athanase *Sicard,* French neurologist, 1872–1929] Collet syndrome.

Col·le·to·tri·chum (kol″ə-to-trī′kəm) a genus of Fungi Imperfecti of the form-class Coelomycetes. Some species have been isolated from cases of phaeohyphomycosis.

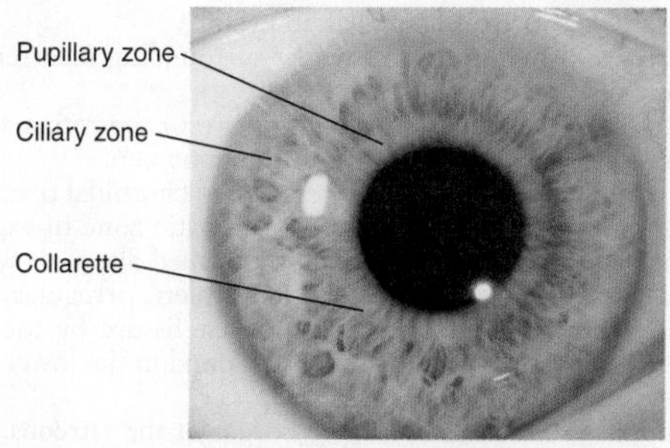

■ Collarette separating the ciliary and pupillary zones.

col·lic·u·lec·to·my (kə-lik″u-lek′tə-me) [*colliculus* + *-ectomy*] excision of the colliculus seminalis.

col·lic·u·li (kə-lik′u-li) [L.] genitive and plural of *colliculus.*

col·lic·u·lus (kə-lik′u-ləs) pl. *collic′uli* [L.] a small elevation or mound.

c. of arytenoid cartilage, c. cartila′ginis arytenoi′deae [TA] a small eminence on the anterior margin and anterolateral surface of the arytenoid cartilage.

caudal c., c. cauda′lis c. inferior.

c. cauda′tus nucleus caudatus.

c. facia′lis [TA] facial colliculus: an elevation of the medial eminence above the medullary striae in the rhomboid fossa, caused by the internal genu of the facial nerve as it loops around the abducent nucleus.

c. infe′rior [TA] inferior colliculus: either of the inferior (caudal) pair of rounded eminences symmetrically located in the tectum of the mesencephalon, containing reflex centers for auditory sensations; called also *caudal c.*

rostral c., c. rostra′lis c. superior.

seminal c., c. semina′lis [TA] a prominent portion of the urethral crest on which are the opening of the prostatic utricle and, on either side of it, the orifices of the ejaculatory ducts; called also *seminal hillock* and *verumontanum.*

c. supe′rior [TA] superior colliculus: either of the superior (rostral) pair of rounded eminences symmetrically located in the tectum of the mesencephalon, containing reflex centers for visual sensations; called also *rostral c.*

col·li·ga·tive (kol′ĭ-ga″tiv) in physical chemistry, depending on the number of molecules present in a given space, rather than on their size, molecular weight or chemical constitution. The colligative properties of solutions are osmotic pressure, boiling point elevation, freezing point depression, and vapor pressure lowering.

col·li·ma·tion (kol″ĭ-ma′shən) 1. in microscopy, the process of making light rays parallel; the process of aligning the optical axis of the optical system to the reference mechanical axes or surfaces of the instrument, or the adjustment of two or more optical axes with respect to each other. 2. in radiology, the elimination of the peripheral (more divergent) portion of an x-ray beam by means of metal tubes, cones, or diaphragms interposed in the path of the beam. 3. in nuclear medicine, the use of a perforated absorber to restrict the field of view of a detector and reduce scatter; the use of an absorber with converging or diverging perforations will also change the camera's angle of view.

col·li·ma·tor (kol′ĭ-ma″tər) a diaphragm or system of diaphragms made of an absorbing material, designed to define and restrict the dimensions and direction of a beam of radiation.

Col·lin·so·nia (kol″in-so′ne-ə) [Peter *Collinson,* 1694–1768] a genus of herbs of the family Labiatae. *C. canaden′sis,* the stoneroot or richweed, is tonic and diuretic.

col·liq·ua·tive (kə-lik′wə-tiv) [*co-* + L. *liquare* to melt] 1. characterized by an excessive fluid discharge. 2. marked by liquefaction of tissues.

col·li·sion (kə-lĭ′zhən) 1. in obstetrics, the contact in utero of any parts of one twin with those of the co-twin, so that engagement of either is prevented. 2. in nerve conduction studies, the meeting of two action potentials traveling toward each other along the same nerve; their refractory periods prevent propagation in either direction from the site of collision.

col·lo·chem·is·try (kol″o-kem′is-tre) the chemistry of colloids.

col·lo·di·a·phys·e·al (kol″o-di″ə-fiz′e-əl) [*collum* + *diaphyseal*] pertaining to the neck and shaft of a long bone, especially the femur.

col·lo·di·on (kə-lo′de-ən) [L. *collodium,* from Gr. *kollōdēs* glutinous] [USP] a clear or slightly opalescent, highly flammable, syrupy liquid compounded of pyroxylin, ether, and alcohol, which dries to a transparent, tenacious film; used as a topical protectant, applied to the skin to close small wounds, abrasions, and cuts, to hold surgical dressings in place, and to keep medications in contact with the skin.

flexible c. [USP] a preparation of camphor, castor oil, and collodion, used for the same purposes as collodion but providing a flexible, contracting film.

salicylic acid c. [USP] a preparation containing 9.5–11.5 per cent salicylic acid in flexible collodion; used as a topical keratolytic for warts and corns.

col·loid (kol′oid) [Gr. *kollōdēs* glutinous] 1. glutinous or resembling glue. 2. a substance comprising very small, insoluble particles, usually 1 to 1000 nm in diameter, that are uniformly dispersed or suspended in a finely divided state throughout a continuous dispersion medium, not settling readily; the phase may be solid, liquid, or gas. The particles are often called the *dispersed phase* and the dispersion medium the *continuous phase.* Colloid can refer specifically to the particles or to the system of particles plus dispersion medium. 3. thyroid c. **colloid′al** *adj*

antimony trisulfide c. antimony sulfide (Sb_2S_3), a pharmaceutic aid.

association c. a colloid in which the dispersed particles are each made up of many molecules.

dispersion c. colloid (def. 2); sometimes specifically an unstable colloid system.

emulsion c. 1. lyophilic c. 2. rarely, emulsion.

hydrophilic c. a lyophilic colloid in which the solvent is water.

hydrophobic c. a lyophobic colloid in which the solvent is water.

irreversible c. a colloid that once precipitated cannot be dispersed. Cf. *reversible c.*

lyophilic c. a stable colloid system in which the dispersed phase is relatively liquid, usually comprising highly complex organic substances, such as starch or glue, which readily absorb solvent, swell, and distribute uniformly through the medium.

lyophobic c. an unstable colloid system in which the dispersed phase particles tend to repel liquids, are easily precipitated, and cannot be dispersed with additional solvent.

lyotropic c. lyophilic c.

protective c. a hydrophilic colloid polymer that is able to prevent the precipitation of another colloid by acting as a stabilizer, suspending or thickening agent, or emulsifier.

reversible c. a colloid that can be dispersed after having been precipitated or a gel that can be converted into a sol.

stable c. reversible c.

stannous sulfur c. a sulfur colloid containing stannous ions, formed by reacting sodium thiosulfate with hydrochloric acid then adding stannous ions; complexed with technetium 99m it is used as a diagnostic aid (bone, liver, and spleen imaging).

suspension c. lyophobic c.

thyroid c. the colloid in the thyroid follicles; it contains several proteins, including thyroglobulin and CA_2. Called also *thyrocolloid.*

col•loi•din (ko-loid′in) a yellowish, translucent, jellylike product of colloid degeneration.

col•loid•oph•a•gy (kol″oi-dof′ə-je) [*colloid* + *-phagy*] resorption of colloid by macrophages under the influence of the thyroid-stimulating hormone.

col•lum (kol′əm) pl. *col′la* [L.] [TA] neck: the part of the body connecting the head and trunk; called also *cervix.*

c. anato′micum hu′meri [TA] anatomical neck of humerus: the somewhat constricted zone on the humerus just distal to the head, separating the articular surface from the tubercles.

c. chirur′gicum hu′meri [TA] surgical neck of humerus: the region on the humerus just below the tubercles, where the bone becomes constricted.

c. cos′tae [TA] neck of rib: the part of a rib extending from the head to the tubercle.

c. den′tis cervix dentis.

c. distor′tum torticollis.

c. fe′moris [TA] neck of femur: the heavy column of bone connecting the head of the femur and the shaft.

c. fi′bulae [TA] neck of fibula: the portion of the fibula between the head and shaft.

c. glan′dis pe′nis [TA] neck of the glans penis: the constricted portion between the corona of the glans penis and the corpora cavernosa; called also *cervix glandis penis.*

c. mal′lei [TA] neck of malleus: the constricted portion of the malleus below its head.

c. mandi′bulae [TA] neck of mandible: the narrow portion supporting the condyle of the mandible; called also *c. processus condyloidei mandibulae.*

c. os′sis fem′oris c. femoris.

c. pancre′atis [TA] neck of pancreas: a constricted portion marking the junction of the head and body of the pancreas.

c. proces′sus condyloi′dei mandi′bulae c. mandibulae.

c. ra′dii [TA] neck of radius: the somewhat constricted portion of the radius just distal to the head.

c. sca′pulae [TA] neck of scapula: the somewhat constricted part of the scapula that surrounds the lateral angle.

c. ta′li [TA] neck of talus: the constriction between the head and body of the talus.

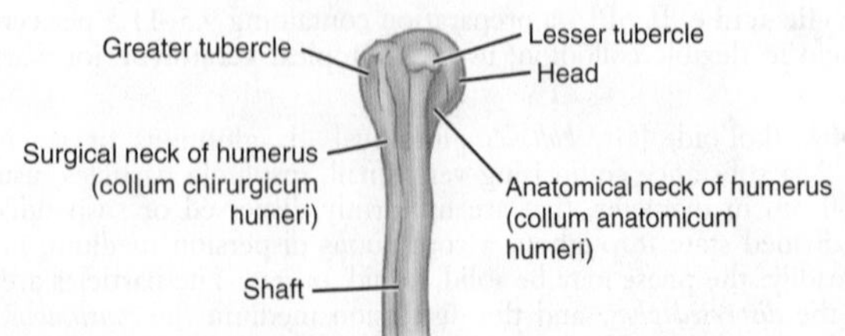

■ Anterior aspect of right humerus, showing the collum chirurgicum (surgical neck) and collum anatomicum (anatomical neck).

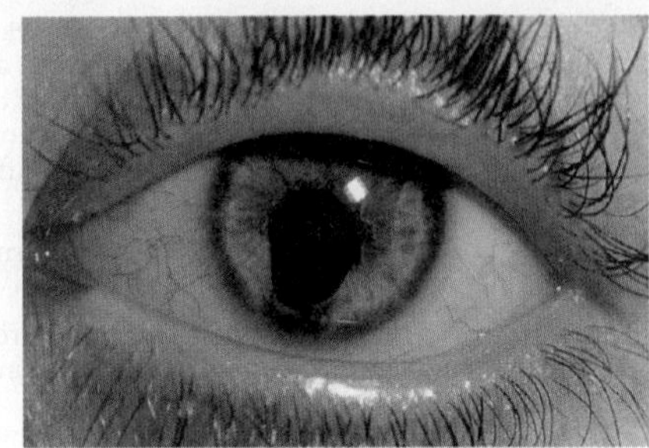

■ Coloboma of the iris.

c. vesi′cae bilia′ris [TA] neck of gallbladder: the upper constricted portion of the gallbladder, between the body and the cystic duct; called also *c. vesicae felleae* [TA alternative].

c. vesi′cae fel′leae TA alternative for *c. vesicae biliaris.*

c. vesi′cae urina′riae TA alternative for *cervix vesicae urinariae.*

col•lu•to•ry (kol′u-tor″e) [L. *collutorium*] a mouthwash or gargle.

Collyr. [L.] colly′rium (an eye wash).

Col•ly•ric•u•lum (kol″ə-rik′u-ləm) a genus of trematode parasites. *C. fa′ba* forms subcutaneous cysts in chickens, turkeys, and sparrows.

col•lyr•i•um (kə-lir′e-əm) pl. *colly′ria* [L., from Gr. *kollyrion* eye salve] a lotion for the eyes; an eye wash.

col(o)- [Gr. *kolon* colon] a combining form denoting the colon.

col•o•bo•ma (kol″o-bo′mə) pl. *colobomas, colobo′mata* [L., from Gr. *kolobōma* defect, from *koloboun* to mutilate] 1. an absence or defect of tissue. 2. particularly, a defect of ocular tissue, usually due to malclosure of the fetal intraocular fissure, or sometimes from trauma or disease. Such anomalies range from a small pit in the optic disk to extensive defects in the iris, ciliary body, choroid, retina, or optic disk. A scotoma is usually present, corresponding to the area of the coloboma.

atypical c′s a coloboma not originating from the embryonic cleft nor located in the inferonasal quadrant of the eye; it is usually unilateral.

bridge c. a narrow zone of normal fundus between a retinochoroidal coloboma and an optic nerve coloboma.

c. of choroid fissure in the choroid, causing a scotoma on the retina, and often associated with defects of the ciliary body and iris.

c. of ciliary body a white lesion surrounded by varying pigment and affecting the iris and lens. It is the most frequent congenital defect of the ciliary body and common in trisomy 13.

complete c. a typical coloboma when it extends from the pupillary margin to the posterior pole, therefore involving the iris, ciliary body, choroid, retina, and optic disk.

Fuchs c. a small conus or crescent on the choroid, at the lower edge of the optic disk.

c. of fundus retinochoroidal c.

c. i′ridis, c. of iris a keyhole-shaped notch in the inferonasal quadrant of the eye; it may also result from an iridectomy.

c. of lens, c. len′tis a cleft at the edge of the lens, extending down, with a defect in the ciliary zonule in the same area.

c. lo′buli fissure of the ear lobe, which may occur as a congenital defect, or be acquired.

c. of optic disk, c. of optic nerve 1. a coloboma, mild or severe, within or at the optic nerve head. A mild coloboma may be a separate, isolated entity, unilateral, and limited to minor cupping in the optic disk. A severe coloboma may be part of a bridge coloboma or part of a complete coloboma, or it may enlarge the optic disk two to four times and thus affect the adjacent retina and choroid. Nystagmus, strabismus, severe impairment of vision, microphthalmia, cyclopia, and anencephaly may be present. 2. a defect attributed to the incomplete closure of the fetal fissure of the optic stalk.

c. at optic nerve entrance a coloboma of the optic disk that affects only the optic nerve.

c. palpebra′le a vertical fissure of an eyelid.

peripapillary c. a chorioretinal defect surrounding or extending down from the optic disk.

c. of retina, c. re′tinae a congenital fissure of the retina attributed to incomplete closure of the fetal fissure in the optic cup.

retinochoroidal c. an absence of retinal and choroidal tissue, usually in the lower fundus, marked by a bright white ectatic zone of exposed sclera extending into and distorting the optic disk. Called also *c. of fundus.*

typical c. a defect resulting from incomplete, irregular, or lack of fusion of the lips of the embryonic intraocular fissure by the end of the sixth or seventh week. A typical coloboma is found in the lower nasal quadrant of the eye and is often bilateral.

c. of vitreous a notch in the lower border of the vitreous.

co•lo•ce•cos•to•my (ko″lo-se-kos′tə-me) cecocolostomy.

co•lo•cen•te•sis (ko″lo-sen-te′sis) [*colo-* + *-centesis*] surgical puncture of the colon for the withdrawal of fluid or gas; called also *colopuncture.*

co•loc•ly•sis (ko″lok′lĭ-sis) [*colo-* + *clysis*] irrigation of the colon.

co•lo•co•los•to•my (ko″lo-kə-los′tə-me) [*colon* + *colostomy*] surgical formation of an anastomosis between two portions of the colon.

Co•lo•cort (ko′lo-kort) trademark for a preparation of hydrocortisone.

co•lo•cu•ta•ne•ous (ko″lo-ku-ta′ne-əs) [*colo-* + *cutaneous*] pertaining to or communicating between the colon and the skin.

colo•cynth (kol′o-sinth) [L. *colocynthis;* Gr. *kolokynthē*] 1. *Citrullus colocynthus.* 2. the pulpy fruit of *C. colocynthus.* 3. the dried pulp of the full grown but unripe fruit of *C. colocynthus*, used as a drastic cathartic. Called also *bitter apple* and *bitter cucumber.*

colo•cyn•thi•dism (kol″o-sin′thĭ-diz-əm) poisoning by colocynth.

colo•cyn•thin (kol″o-sin′thin) a bitter, cathartic glycoside found in colocynth.

co•lo•cys•to•plas•ty (ko″lo-sis′to-plas″te) augmentation cystoplasty using an isolated section of colon.

co•lo•en•ter•itis (ko″lo-en″tər-i′tis) enterocolitis.

co•lo•fix•a•tion (ko″lo-fik-sa′shən) fixation or suspension of the colon.

Col•o•gel (kol′o-jəl) trademark for a preparation of methylcellulose.

co•log•ra•phy (kə-log′rə-fe) colonography.

co•lo•il•e•al (ko″lo-il′e-əl) ileocolic.

co•lon (ko′lən) [L., from Gr. *kolon*] [TA] the part of the large intestine extending from the cecum to the rectum; the term is sometimes used inaccurately as a synonym for the entire large intestine.

c. ascen′dens [TA], **ascending c.** the portion of the colon between the cecum and the right colic flexure.

congenital pouch c. a developmental anomaly of the colon in which part or all of it is replaced by a dilated pouch, accompanied by anorectal malformation and a fistula between the colon and the genitourinary tract.

c. descen′dens [TA], **descending c.** the portion of the colon between the left colic flexure and the sigmoid colon at the pelvic brim; the part of it that lies in the left part of the iliac fossa is sometimes called the *iliac colon.*

giant c. megacolon.

iliac c. the part of the descending colon lying in the left side of the iliac fossa just proximal to the sigmoid colon.

irritable c. irritable bowel syndrome.

lead pipe c. the radiologic appearance of a diseased colon that has become shortened, contracted, and rigid owing to inflammatory fibrosis, usually owing to chronic ulcerative or granulomatous colitis; the normal haustral pattern is lost and function may be impaired.

left c. the distal portion of the colon; it develops embryonically from the hindgut and functions in the storage and elimination of waste.

pelvic c. c. sigmoideum.

right c. the proximal portion of the colon (proximal to the left colic flexure); it develops embryonically from the terminal portion of the midgut and functions in absorption.

sigmoid c., c. sigmoi′deum [TA] the S-shaped part of the colon that lies in the pelvis, extending from the pelvic brim to the third segment of the sacrum; it is continuous above with the descending colon and below with the rectum. Called also *pelvic c.* and *sigmoid flexure.*

spastic c. irritable bowel syndrome.

transverse c., c. transver′sum [TA] the portion of the colon that runs transversely across the upper part of the abdomen, between the right and left colic flexures.

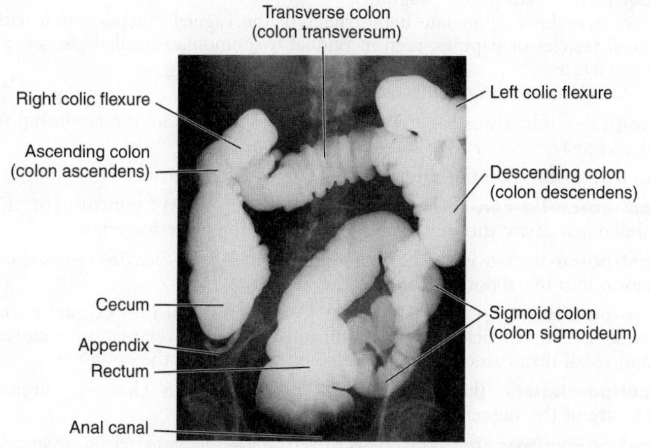

■ Colon, in a radiograph of the abdomen following a barium enema.

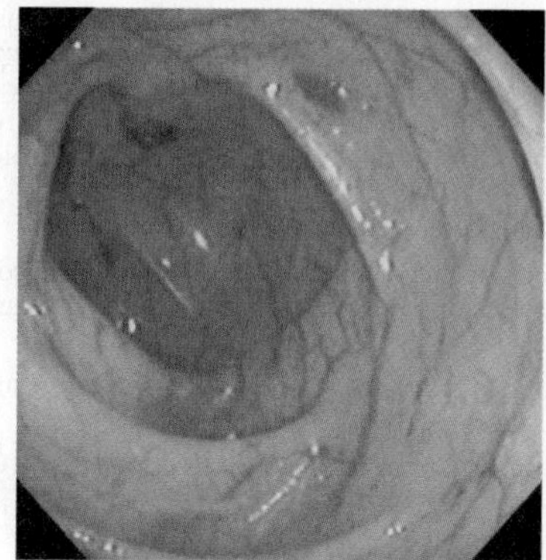

■ Colonoscopy showing a normal colon.

co•lon•al•gia (ko″lən-al′jə) [*colon* + *-algia*] pain in the colon.

co•lon•ic (ko-lon′ik) 1. pertaining to the colon; colic. 2. colon hydrotherapy.

col•o•ni•za•tion (kol″ə-nĭ-za′shən) 1. innidiation. 2. the establishment and growth of a new group of microorganisms on a host.

Co•lon•na operation (kŏ-lon′ah) [Paul *Colonna*, American orthopedic surgeon, 1892–1966] see under *operation.*

co•lon•o•fi•ber•scope (ko-lon″o-fi′bər-skōp) fiberoptic colonoscope.

co•lon•og•ra•phy (ko″lən-og′rə-fe) imaging of the colon, as by computed tomography or magnetic resonance imaging.

computed tomographic c., computed tomography c., CT c. virtual colonoscopy using computed tomography as the imaging technique.

magnetic resonance c. virtual colonoscopy using magnetic resonance imaging as the imaging technique.

virtual c. see under *colonoscopy.*

co•lon•op•a•thy (ko″lo-nop′ə-the) [*colon* + *-pathy*] any disease or disorder of the colon.

co•lono•scope (ko-lon′o-skōp) [*colon* + *-scope*] an elongated flexible endoscope for visual examination of the entire colon; called also *coloscope.*

fiberoptic c. a colonoscope that uses fiberoptic technology; called also *fibercolonoscope.*

co•lon•os•co•py (ko″lən-os′kə-pe) examination by means of the colonoscope. Called also *coloscopy.*

virtual c. an imaging technique, used for examination of the colon, in which cross-sectional images acquired by computed tomography or magnetic resonance imaging are processed by computer to reconstruct a three-dimensional display of the colonic lumen.

col•o•ny (kol′ə-ne) [L. *colonia*] a collection or group of bacteria in a culture derived from the increase of an isolated single organism or group of organisms.

checker c. a round, steeply elevated colony with a flat top, resembling the disk used in a game of checkers. It is frequently seen in cultures of *Streptococcus pneumoniae* on blood agar.

D c. dwarf c.

daisy-head c. a round gray or black colony with a narrow translucent scalloped border, typically produced by *Corynebacterium diphtheriae* on tellurite blood agar.

daughter c. a small bacterial colony formed as a papilla on the surface or in the margin of an older colony.

dwarf c. a bacterial colony smaller than normal and containing poorly developed forms; called also *D c.*

gregaloid c. a transient grouping of protozoa formed by union of previously independent organisms; seen in sarcodines and in the ameboid stages of certain other protozoa. Called also *gregaloid.*

H c. (*Hauch*, q.v.), a type of bacterial colony that spreads in a thin film over the culture medium. Cf. *O c.*

M c. mucoid c.

motile c. a colony that moves across the surface of the culture plate, leaving lines of bacterial cells on the paths of motion, typical of colonies of *Bacillus circulans.*

mucoid c. a colony that is large, dome-shaped, and shiny, containing large quantities of capsular polysaccharide material that may be drawn out in viscous strings by a needle; called also *M c.*

O c. (*ohne Hauch*, q.v.), a bacterial colony that is discrete and compact, as contrasted with an H colony.

R c., rough c. a colony that has a rough, wrinkled, granular, flattened surface. Cf. *smooth c.*

S c. smooth c.

satellite c. a bacterial colony that grows more vigorously in the immediate vicinity of a colony of some other organism, as *Haemophilus influenzae* near a colony of staphylococci; called also *bacterial satellite.*

smooth c. a colony that has a smooth, glistening, rounded, regular surface; this is the form normally shown by bacterial colonies. Cf. *rough c.* Called also *S c.*

co•lop•a•thy (ko-lop′ə-the) colonopathy.

portal hypertensive c. changes in the mucosa of the colon accompanying portal hypertension, sometimes with varices, telangiectasias, and bleeding.

co•lo•pexy (ko′lo-pek″se) [*colo-* + *-pexy*] fixation or suspension of the colon by surgical means.

co•loph•o•ny (ko-lof′ə-ne) [L. *colophonia;* Gr. *Kolophōn* (Colophon) a city of Asia Minor] rosin.

co•lo•pli•ca•tion (ko″lo-plĭ-ka′shən) [*colo-* + *plication*] the operation of infolding or taking tucks in the wall of the colon in cases of dilatation to shorten or decrease its lumen.

co•lo•proc•tec•to•my (ko″lo-prok-tek′tə-me) proctocolectomy.

co•lo•proc•ti•tis (ko″lo-prok-ti′tis) proctocolitis.

co•lo•proc•tos•to•my (ko″lo-prok-tos′tə-me) colorectostomy.

co•lop•to•sis (ko″lop-to′sis, ko″lo-to′sis) [*colo-* + *-ptosis*] downward displacement of the colon, a term based on the outmoded concept that variations in the position of abdominal organs are pathologic.

co•lo•punc•ture (ko′lo-pungk′chər) colocentesis.

col•or (kul′ər) [L. *color, colos*] 1. a property of a surface or substance resulting from absorption of certain of the incident light rays and reflection of others falling within the range of wavelengths (roughly 370–760 nm) adequate to excite the retinal receptors. 2. radiant energy within the range of adequate chromatic stimuli of the retina, that is, between the infrared and the ultraviolet. 3. a sensory impression of one of the rainbow hues, excited by stimulation of the retinal receptors, notably the cones, by radiant energy of the appropriate wavelength.

complementary c's two colors for which the sensory mechanisms are so linked that when they are mixed on the color wheel they cancel each other out, leaving neutral gray; they are also associated with each other in afterimage and contrast.

confusion c's different colors that are likely to be mistakenly matched by individuals with defective color vision (e.g., violet and blue with defect of vision for red); for this reason they are combined in the design on charts used for detecting different types of color vision defects.

contrast c. an illusory tinge of complementary hue or brightness induced by a vivid hue or luminance on the area surrounding it in the visual field.

incidental c. color seen as an afterimage.

metameric c's colors that appear identical to the normal eye, but which are the resultants of different combinations of chromatic stimuli or wavelengths.

Munsell c's a set of standardized colors, representing 40 hues in varying degrees of brightness and saturation, identifiable by a simple letter-number formula.

primary c's 1. a small number of fundamental colors; in visual science this refers to red, green, and blue, the colors specifically picked up by the retinal cones; mixtures of varying proportions of the primary colors will yield the 150 discriminable hues of normal human vision. 2. any of various other small groups of fundamental colors. For the painter and printer, blue, yellow, and red (or magenta); in the Newton theory, the seven rainbow hues of violet, indigo, blue, green, yellow, orange, and red; in the Helmholtzian theory (old school), red, green, and blue (or violet); and in the Hering theory, four paired complementary hues, red-green and blue-yellow, plus a black-white pair. There are other theories that list five to seven colors as primaries.

pseudoisochromatic c's colors that appear the same to an individual with defective color vision; see *confusion c's.*

pure c. a color whose stimulus consists of homogeneous wavelengths, with little or no admixture of other hues.

saturation c. a color that is high on the chroma or vividness scale, the farthest possible removed from gray.

col•or•a•tion (kul″ər-a′shən) the state of being colored; an arrangement of colors distinguishing a species.

protective c. coloration that blends with the background, making the organism less visible to predators.

warning c. brilliant, conspicuous coloration of poisonous or unpalatable animals, as a warning to potential predators.

co•lo•rec•tal (ko″lo-rek′təl) [*colo-* + *rectal*] pertaining to or affecting the colon and rectum.

co•lo•rec•ti•tis (ko″lo-rek-ti′tis) proctocolitis.

co•lo•rec•tos•to•my (ko″lo-rek-tos′tə-me) [*colo-* + *recto-* + *-stomy*] formation of an artificial opening between the colon and rectum; called also *coloproctostomy.*

co•lo•rec•tum (ko″lo-rek′təm) [*colo-* + *rectum*] the colon and rectum considered as a unit.

col•or•im•e•ter (kul″ər-im′ə-tər) [*color* + *-meter*] an instrument for measuring the color or color intensity of a solution. Cf. *spectrophotometer.* Called also *chromometer.*

co•lor•rha•phy (ko-lor′ə-fe) [*colo-* + *-rrhaphy*] suture or repair of the colon.

co•lo•scope (kol′o-skōp) colonoscope.

co•los•co•py (ko-los′ko-pe) colonoscopy.

co•lo•sig•moid•os•to•my (ko″lo-sig″moi-dos′tə-me) [*colo-* + *sigmoid* + *-stomy*] surgical creation of an artificial opening between the sigmoid and the proximal portion of the colon.

co•los•to•my (kə-los′tə-me) [*colo-* + *-stomy*] 1. surgical creation of an opening between the colon and the surface of the body. 2. the opening so created.

blow hole c. an operation sometimes done for toxic megacolon in which the distended walls have become thin and fragile; it consists of creation of a colostomy of the transverse colon for decompression, and is usually accompanied by creation of a loop ileostomy.

dry c. colostomy performed in the left half of the colon, the discharge from the stoma consisting of soft or formed fecal residue.

Hartmann c. see under *procedure.*

ileotransverse c. surgical anastomosis between the ileum and the transverse colon.

wet c. 1. colostomy in the right half of the colon, with drainage that is liquid in character. 2. colostomy in the left half of the colon following anastomosis of the ureters to the sigmoid or descending colon, so that urine and feces are both expelled through the stoma.

co•los•trum (kə-los′trəm) [L.] the thin, yellow, milky fluid secreted by the mammary gland before or after parturition. It contains up to 20 per cent protein, predominant among which are immunoglobulins, representing the antibodies found in maternal blood. It contains more minerals and less fat and carbohydrate than does milk. It also contains many colostrum corpuscles and usually will coagulate on boiling due to a large amount of lactalbumin. **colos′tral** *adj*

c. gravida′rum the colostrum secreted before parturition, and especially that secreted during the first few days following delivery.

co•lot•o•my (ko-lot′ə-me) [*colo-* + *-tomy*] incision into the colon, such as for removal of a foreign body, polyp, or other benign tumor.

co•lo•vag•i•nal (ko″lo-vaj′ĭ-nəl) pertaining to or communicating with both the colon and vagina.

co•lo•ves•i•cal (ko″lo-ves′ĭ-kəl) vesicocolonic.

col•pal•gia (kol-pal′jə) vaginodynia.

col•pa•tre•sia (kol″pə-tre′zhə) [*colp-* + *atresia*] atresia or occlusion of the vagina.

col•pec•ta•sia (kol″pek-ta′zhə) [*colp-* + *ectasia*] distention or dilatation of the vagina.

col•pec•ta•sis (kol-pek′tə-sis) colpectasia.

col•pec•to•my (kol-pek′tə-me) [*colp-* + *-ectomy*] excision of the vagina.

col•peu•ry•sis (kol-pu′rĭ-sis) [*colp-* + *eury-* + *-sis*] dilation of the vagina, particularly with a bag or sac.

col•pi•tis (kol-pi′tis) vaginitis.

c. macularis punctate hemorrhage of the vaginal mucosa, often with small vesicles or papules, seen in vaginal trichomoniasis; called also *strawberry cervix.*

c. myco′tica vaginomycosis.

colp(o)- [Gr. *kolpos* vagina] a combining form denoting relationship to the vagina.

col•po•cele (kol′po-sēl) [*colpo-* + *-cele*[1]] vaginal hernia.

col•po•ce•lio•cen•te•sis (kol″po-se″le-o-sen-te′sis) puncture of the abdominal cavity through the vagina, usually the posterior vault.

col•po•ce•li•ot•o•my (kol″po-se″le-ot′ə-me) [*colpo-* + *celio-* + *-tomy*] incision into the abdomen through the vaginal wall.

col•po•ceph•a•ly (kol″po-sef′ə-le) enlargement of the occipital horns of the lateral ventricles, often accompanied by mental retardation, seizures, and visual disturbances that result from hypoplasia of the optic nerve.

col•po•clei•sis (kol″po-kli′sis) [*colpo-* + Gr. *kleisis* closure] surgical closure of the vaginal canal.

col•po•cys•to•cele (kol″po-sis′to-sēl) [*colpo-* + *cystocele*] a cystocele into the vagina.

col·po·cys·tot·o·my (kol″po-sis-tot′ə-me) [*colpo-* + *cysto-* + *-tomy*] incision of the bladder through the vaginal wall.

col·po·cy·to·gram (kol″po-si′to-gram) a tabulation of the various types of cells observed in smears taken from the mucous membrane of the vagina.

col·po·cy·tol·o·gy (kol″po-si-tol′ə-je) the quantitative and differential study of cells exfoliated from the epithelium of the vagina.

Col·po·di·da (kol-po′dĭ-də) [Gr. *kolpos* a bosom or fold] an order of mostly free-living, commonly in the soil, ciliate, often reniform protozoa (subclass Vestibuliferia, class Kinetofragminophorea).

col·po·dyn·ia (kol″po-din′e-ə) vaginodynia.

col·po·hy·per·pla·sia (kol″po-hi″pər-pla′zhə) [*colpo-* + *hyperplasia*] excessive growth of the mucous membrane and wall of the vagina.

c. cys′tica colpohyperplasia characterized by the presence of cysts in the mucous membrane.

col·po·mi·cro·scope (kol″po-mi′kro-skōp) an instrument especially designed for the microscopic examination of tissues of the cervix in situ; it has higher powers of magnification than the colposcope.

col·po·mi·cro·scop·ic (kol″po-mi″kro-skop′ik) pertaining to the colpomicroscope, or to colpomicroscopy.

col·po·mi·cros·co·py (kol″po-mi-kros′kə-pe) examination of tissues of the cervix in situ with the colpomicroscope.

col·po·myo·mec·to·my (kol″po-mi″o-mek′tə-me) vaginal myomectomy.

col·po·per·i·neo·plas·ty (kol″po-per″ĭ-ne′o-plas″te) vaginoperineoplasty. **colpoperineoplas′tic** *adj*

col·po·per·i·ne·or·rha·phy (kol″po-per″ĭ-ne-or′ə-fe) vaginoperineorrhaphy.

col·po·pexy (kol′po-pek″se) [*colpo-* + *-pexy*] suture of the prolapsed vagina to a surrounding structure such as the abdominal wall; called also *vaginofixation*.

col·po·plas·ty (kol′po-plas″te) vaginoplasty. **colpoplas′tic** *adj*

col·po·poi·e·sis (kol″po-poi-e′sis) [*colpo-* + *-poiesis*] the creation of a vagina by plastic surgery.

col·pop·to·sis (kol″pop-to′sis, kol″po-to′sis) vaginocele (def. 2).

col·po·rec·to·pexy (kol″po-rek′to-pek″se) [*colpo-* + *recto-* + *-pexy*] suspension of a prolapsed rectum by suture to the vaginal wall.

col·por·rha·phy (kol-por′ə-fe) [*colpo-* + *-rrhaphy*] 1. the operation of suturing the vagina. 2. denudation and suturing of the vaginal wall in order to restructure the vagina.

col·por·rhex·is (kol″po-rek′sis) [*colpo-* + *-rrhexis*] laceration of the vagina.

col·po·scope (kol′po-skōp) [*colpo-* + *-scope*] 1. an instrument for examination of the tissues of the vagina and cervix by means of a magnifying lens. Cf. *colpomicroscope*. 2. vaginoscope.

col·po·scop·ic (kol″po-skop′ik) relating to the colposcope or to colposcopy.

col·pos·co·py (kol-pos′kə-pe) examination of the cervix and vagina by means of the colposcope.

col·po·spasm (kol′po-spaz″əm) [*colpo-* + *spasm*] a spasm in the vagina.

col·po·stat (kol′po-stat) [*colpo-* + *-stat*] an appliance for retaining something, such as radium, in the vagina.

col·po·ste·no·sis (kol″po-stə-no′sis) [*colpo-* + *-stenosis*] contraction or narrowing of the vagina.

col·po·ste·not·o·my (kol″po-stə-not′ə-me) [*colpo-* + *steno-* + *-tomy*] a cutting operation for stricture or atresia of the vagina.

col·po·sus·pen·sion (kol″po-səs-pen′shən) bladder neck suspension.

Burch c. see under *procedure*.

Pereyra c. see under *procedure*.

Stamey c. see under *procedure*.

col·pot·o·my (kol-pot′ə-me) [*colpo-* + *-tomy*] incision of the vagina with entry into the cul-de-sac; called also *vaginotomy*.

posterior c. culdotomy.

col·po·ure·ter·ot·o·my (kol″po-u-re″tər-ot′ə-me) incision of the ureter through the vagina, performed for the relief of ureteral stricture.

col·po·xe·ro·sis (kol″po-ze-ro′sis) [*colpo-* + *xerosis*] abnormal dryness of the vulva and vagina.

col·te·rol (kol′tə-rol) an adrenergic agonist, specific for β_2-adrenergic receptors, to which the prodrug bitolterol is converted.

Col·ti·vi·rus (kol′tĭ-vi″rəs) [*Col*orado *ti*ck fever + *virus*] a genus of viruses of the family Reoviridae, containing the Colorado tick fever virus and related viruses.

Col·ton blood group (kōl′tən) [*Colton*, surname of the Norwegian propositus first reported on in 1965] see under *blood group*.

Col·u·ber (kol′u-bər) a genus of nonvenomous snakes of the family Colubridae, found in northeastern Asia and North America. *C. constric′tor* is the American blacksnake.

col·u·brid (kol′u-brid) 1. any snake of the family Colubridae. 2. of or pertaining to the family Colubridae.

Col·u·bri·dae (kol-u′brĭ-de) [L. *coluber* serpent] a family of snakes found in North America and Africa; most genera are harmless. It includes the nonvenomous genus *Coluber* and the venomous southern African genus *Dispholidus*. See table at *snake*.

col·u·mel·la (kol″u-mel′ə) pl. *columel′lae* [L. "small column," dim. of *columna* column] 1. any of various columnlike anatomical structures. 2. in certain fungi and protozoa, a sterile invagination of the sporangiophore into the fertile area of the sporangium.

c. coch′leae modiolus.

nasal c., c. na′si the fleshy distal margin of the nasal septum.

col·u·mel·lae (kol″u-mel′e) [L.] genitive and plural of *columella*.

col·u·mel·late (kol″u-mel′āt) of certain protozoa and fungi, having columellae.

col·umn (kol′əm) [L. *columna*] an anatomical part in the form of a pillarlike structure, sometimes used specifically for the gray column of the spinal cord; see also *columna*.

c's of abdominal ring thickened fibers of the aponeurosis of the external oblique muscle around the superficial inguinal ring.

anal c's columnae anales.

anterior c. of fauces arcus palatoglossus.

anterior c. of spinal cord columna anterior medullae spinalis.

autonomic c. of spinal cord columna intermediolateralis medullae spinalis.

Bertin c's columnae renales.

Burdach c. fasciculus cuneatus medullae spinalis.

Clarke c. nucleus thoracicus posterior.

dorsal c. columna vertebralis.

dorsal funicular c., dorsal gray c. nucleus proprius.

dorsal c. of spinal cord columna posterior medullae spinalis.

enamel c's prismata adamantina.

c's of folds of tongue papillae foliatae.

c. of fornix columna fornicis.

fractionating c. an apparatus for separating the volatile constituents of a solution by distillation.

fundamental c. fasciculi proprii; see entries beginning thus under *fasciculus*.

Goll c. fasciculus gracilis medullae spinalis.

Gowers c. tractus spinocerebellaris anterior.

gray c's of spinal cord columnae griseae.

gray c. of spinal cord, anterior columna anterior medullae spinalis.

gray c. of spinal cord, lateral columna intermedia medullae spinalis.

gray c. of spinal cord, posterior columna posterior medullae spinalis.

intermediate c. of spinal cord columna intermedia medullae spinalis.

intermediolateral c. of spinal cord columna intermediolateralis medullae spinalis.

Kölliker c. sarcostyle (def. 2).

lateral c. of spinal cord columna intermedia medullae spinalis.

Lissauer c. tractus posterolateralis.

Morgagni c's columnae anales.

muscle c. sarcostyle (def. 2).

positive c. a pinkish stream of light seen when a current of high potential is passed through a tube from which the air has been partly exhausted.

posterior c. of fauces arcus palatopharyngeus.

posterior c. of spinal cord columna posterior medullae spinalis.

posteromedian c. of medulla oblongata fasciculus gracilis medullae oblongatae.

posteromedian c. of spinal cord fasciculus gracilis medullae spinalis.

Rathke c's two cartilages at the anterior end of the notochord.

rectal c's columnae anales.

renal c's, renal c's of Bertin columnae renales.

spinal c. columna vertebralis.

Spitzka-Lissauer c. tractus posterolateralis.

Stilling c. nucleus thoracicus posterior.

striomotor c. an efferent column of the anterior horn of the spinal cord supplying striated muscle.

thoracic c. nucleus thoracicus posterior.

Türck c. tractus corticospinalis anterior.

vaginal c's columnae rugarum vaginae.

vaginal c., anterior columna rugarum anterior vaginae.

vaginal c., posterior columna rugarum posterior vaginae.

ventral c. of spinal cord columna anterior medullae spinalis.

vertebral c. columna vertebralis.

white c's of spinal cord funiculi medullae spinalis.

co•lum•na (kə-lum′nə) gen. and pl. *colum′nae* [L.] [TA] column: in anatomical terminology, used to designate a pillarlike structure or part.

colum′nae ana′les [TA] anal columns: vertical ridges or folds of mucous membrane at the upper half of the anal canal; called also *Morgagni columns, rectal columns,* and *mucous folds of rectum.*

c. ante′rior medul′lae spina′lis [TA] anterior column of spinal cord: the anterior portion of the gray substance of the spinal cord (see *columnae griseae medullae spinalis*); it contains neurons that innervate the skeletal muscles of the neck, trunk, and limbs. In transverse section it is seen as a horn *(cornu anterius medullae spinalis)*. Called also *ventral column of spinal cord.*

c. for′nicis [TA] column of fornix: either of the two columnar masses of fibers diverging from the anterior end of the body of the fornix to descend into the diencephalon; called also *anterior pillar of fornix.*

colum′nae gri′seae medul′lae spina′lis [TA] gray columns of spinal cord: the three longitudinally oriented thickenings in the spinal cord *(columnae anterior, posterior,* and *intermedia medullae spinalis)*, composed of the gray substance, and containing the nerve cell bodies. The columns are commonly referred to as *cornua anterius, posterius,* and *laterale*, respectively, because in transverse sections of the spinal cord they have the appearance of horns.

c. interme′dia medul′lae spina′lis [TA] intermediate column of spinal cord: the lateral portion of the gray matter of the spinal cord (see *columnae griseae medullae spinalis*), extending from the second thoracic to the first lumbar segment of the spinal cord; in transverse section it is seen as a horn *(cornu laterale medullae spinalis)*. Called also *intermediate zone of spinal cord* and *lateral column of spinal cord.*

c. intermediolatera′lis medul′lae spina′lis intermediolateral column of spinal cord: the column of gray matter the cells of which (interomediolateral nucleus) form the intermediate column of the spinal cord; called also *autonomic column of spinal cord.*

c. poste′rior medul′lae spina′lis [TA] posterior column of spinal cord: the posterior portion of the gray substance of the spinal cord (see *columnae griseae medullae spinalis*); it contains groups of motoneurons that extend the length of the cord and two groups that are limited to the thoracic and upper lumbar segments. In transverse section it is seen as a horn *(cornu posterius medullae spinalis)*. Called also *dorsal column of spinal cord.*

colum′nae rena′les [TA] renal columns: inward extensions of the cortical structure of the kidney between the renal pyramids; called also *Bertin columns* or *septa.*

c. ruga′rum ante′rior vagi′nae [TA] anterior vaginal column: a well-marked longitudinal ridge on the anterior wall of the vagina.

c. ruga′rum poste′rior vagi′nae [TA] posterior vaginal column: a well-marked longitudinal ridge on the posterior wall of the vagina.

colum′nae ruga′rum vagi′nae [TA] vaginal columns: well-marked longitudinal ridges on either the anterior *(c. rugarum anterior vaginae)* or posterior *(c. rugarum posterior vaginae)* wall of the vagina.

c. vertebra′lis [TA] the columnar assemblage of the vertebrae from the cranium through the coccyx; called also *axon, backbone, spine,* and *vertebral, dorsal,* or *spinal column.*

co•lum•nae (ko-lum′ne) [L.] genitive and plural of *columna.*

col•um•ni•za•tion (kol″əm-nĭ-za′shən) the supporting of the prolapsed uterus with tampons.

Coly-My•cin M (kol′e-mi″sin) trademark for preparations of colistimethate sodium.

Coly-My•cin S Ot•ic (kol′e-mi″sin) trademark for a combination preparation of colistin sulfate, thonzonium bromide, neomycin sulfate, and hydrocorticone acetate.

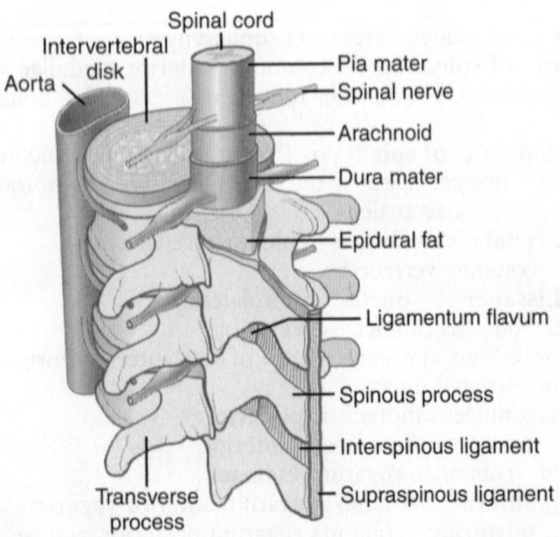

■ Columna vertebralis (spine) in an oblique view.

Co•lyte (ko′līt) trademark for combination preparations of polyethylene glycol 3350 and electrolytes (sodium sulfate, sodium bicarbonate, sodium chloride, and potassium chloride).

com- see *con-.*

co•ma (ko′mə) [L., from Gr. *kōma*] 1. a state of unconsciousness from which the patient cannot be aroused, even by powerful stimulation; called also *exanimation.* See also *consciousness.* 2. the optical aberration produced when an image is received upon a screen which is not exactly at right angles to the line of propagation of the incident light.

alcoholic c. coma accompanying severe alcoholic intoxication.

alpha c. coma in which there are electroencephalographic findings of dominant alpha-wave activity.

diabetic c. the coma of severe diabetic ketoacidosis, which is accompanied by Kussmaul respiration; called also *Kussmaul c.*

hepatic c., c. hepa′ticum coma accompanying hepatic encephalopathy.

hyperglycemic hyperosmolar c., hyperglycemic hyperosmolar nonketotic c., hyperosmolar hyperglycemic c. a type of diabetic coma without ketosis, seen as a severe complication of the hyperglycemic hyperosmolar state (see under *state*).

irreversible c. brain death; see under *death.*

Kussmaul c. diabetic c.

metabolic c. the coma accompanying metabolic encephalopathy.

myxedema c. an often fatal complication of long-term hypothyroidism in which the patient is comatose with hypothermia, depression of respiration, bradycardia, and hypotension; usually seen in elderly patients during cold weather.

nonketotic hyperglycemic c., nonketotic hyperosmolar c. hyperglycemic hyperosmolar c.

psychogenic c. a rare condition in which a person is in a comatose state without any physiologic cause.

uremic c. lethargic state due to uremia.

c. vigil locked-in syndrome.

Co•ma•mo•na•dac•eae (ko″mə-mo″nə-da′se-e) a family of gram-negative bacteria of the class Betaproteobacteria, phylum Proteobacteria, consisting of chemolithotrophic, non–spore-forming, straight or slightly curved rods or spirilla; most genera are motile by a single polar flagellum or bipolar tufts of flagella. Organisms of medical interest are contained in the genera *Comamonas* and *Delftia.*

Co•ma•mo•nas (ko″mə-mo′nəs) [L. *coma* lock of hair + Gr. *monas* unit, from *monos* single] a genus of gram-negative bacteria, commonly found in soil and water, of the family Comamonadaceae, consisting of straight or slightly curved, aerobic, chemo-organotrophic, oxidase- and catalase-positive rods or spirilla, occurring singly or in pairs; most species are motile by polar or bipolar tufts of flagella. *Comamonas* spp., particularly *C. testostero′ni* (formerly *Pseudomonas testosteroni*), are rare opportunistic pathogens. The type species is *C. terrige′na.*

com•a•tose (ko′mə-tōs) pertaining to or affected with coma.

Com•bi•Patch (kom′bĭ-patch) trademark for a combination preparation of estradiol and norethindrone acetate.

Com•bi•pres (kom′bĭ-pres) trademark for a combination preparation of clonidine hydrochloride and chlorthalidone.

Com•bi•vent (kom′bĭ-vent) trademark for a combination preparation of ipratropium bromide and albuterol sulfate.

Com•bi•vir (kom′bĭ-vir) trademark for a combination preparation of zidovudine and lamivudine.

Com•bu•nox (kom′bu-noks) trademark for a preparation of oxycodone hydrochloride and ibuprofen.

com•bus•tion (kəm-bus′chən) [L. *combustio*] rapid oxidation with emission of heat.

com•e•do (kom′ə-do) pl. *comedo′nes.* A noninflammatory lesion of acne vulgaris and a few other conditions, consisting of a plug of keratin and sebum within the dilated orifice of a hair follicle; it usually contains bacteria, especially *Propionibacterium acnes, Staphylococcus aureus,* or *Malassezia furfur.*

closed c. a comedo whose opening is not widely dilated, so that it appears as a small flesh-colored papule; because the keratin and sebum produced cannot escape, it may rupture and cause an inflammatory lesion in the dermis. Called also *whitehead.*

open c. a comedo whose orifice is widely dilated, so that the pigmented impaction is visible at the skin surface; called also *blackhead.*

com•e•do•car•ci•no•ma (kom″ə-do-kahr″sĭ-no′mə) [*comedo* + *carcinoma*] a type of ductal carcinoma in situ whose central cells are degenerated and easily expressed from the cut surface of the tumor.

com•e•do•gen•ic (kom″ə-do-jen′ik) producing comedones.

co•me•do•lyt•ic (kom″ə-do-lit′ik) serving to break down comedones.

com•e•do•mas•ti•tis (kom″ə-do-mas-ti′tis) mammary duct ectasia.

■ Closed comedones.

co•me•done (ko′mə-dōn) comedo.

co•me•do•nes (ko′mə-do′nēz) plural of *comedo.*

co•mes (ko′mēz) pl. *com′ites* [L. "companion"] an artery or vein that accompanies another artery, a vein, or a nerve trunk; see also terms beginning *arteria comitans* and *vena comitans.*

com•frey (kom′fre) 1. *Symphytum officinale.* 2. a preparation of the leaves and root of *S. officinale,* used topically for bruises and sprains and to promote bone healing; in folk medicine, it is used for rheumatism, pleuritis, and diarrhea.

com•i•tes (kom′ĭ-tēz) plural of *comes.*

com•men•sal (ko-men′səl) [*com-* + L. *mensa* table] 1. living on or within another organism, and deriving benefit without injuring or benefiting the other individual. 2. an organism living on or within another, but not causing injury to the host. See *symbiosis.*

com•men•sal•ism (ko-men′səl-iz″əm) symbiosis (q.v.) in which one population (or individual) gains from the association and the other is neither harmed nor benefited.

com•mi•nut•ed (kom′ĭ-nōōt′əd) [*com-* + L. *minuere* to diminish] broken or crushed into small pieces, as a comminuted fracture.

com•mi•nu•tion (kom″ĭ-noo′shən) [L. *comminutio*] the act of breaking, or condition of being broken, into small fragments, as of a fractured bone.

Com•miph•o•ra (kom-if′o-rə) a genus of trees of the family Burseraceae, native to Indonesia and Africa. *C. abyssi′nica* (Berg.) Engl. and other species yield myrrh. *C. opobal′samum* Engl. yields Mecca balsam.

com•mis•sion (kə-mish′ən) [L. *commissus,* past part. of *committere* to entrust] a group of people officially authorized to perform certain functions.

C. E a German interdisciplinary regulatory committee, whose function is to review herbal drugs and preparations from medicinal plants and evaluate and approve their safety and efficacy.

Enzyme C. (EC) the International Commission on Enzymes, a committee established in 1956 by the International Union of Biochemistry to standardize enzyme classification and nomenclature.

com•mis•su•ra (kom″ĭ-su′rə) gen. and pl. *commissu′rae* [L. "a joining together"] [TA] commissure: a site of union of corresponding parts; a general term used to designate such a junction of corresponding anatomical structures, frequently, but not always, across the median plane of the body.

c. al′ba ante′rior medul′lae spina′lis [TA] anterior white commissure of spinal cord: the aggregate of fibers crossing from one side of the spinal cord to the other, anterior to the gray commissure. Called also *ventral white commissure of spinal cord.*

c. al′ba poste′rior medul′lae spina′lis [TA] posterior white commissure of spinal cord: the group of transverse myelinated nerve fibers crossing from one side of the spinal cord to the other posterior to the central canal, permeating the gray commissure; called also *dorsal white commissure of spinal cord.*

c. ante′rior [TA] anterior commissure: a bundle of myelinated nerve fibers passing transversely through the lamina terminalis and connecting symmetrical parts of the two cerebral hemispheres; it consists of a smaller anterior part *(pars anterior commissurae anterioris)* and a larger posterior part *(pars posterior commissurae anterioris).* Called also *rostral commissure.* See illustration.

c. bulbo′rum vesti′buli [TA] commissure of bulbs of vestibule: a narrow median band spanning the vaginal orifice to unite the bulbs of the vestibule.

c. colli′culi inferio′ris [TA] commissure of inferior colliculus: a band of nerve fibers that connect the two inferior colliculi; called also *commissure of caudal colliculus.*

c. colli′culi superio′ris [TA] commissure of superior colliculus: a band of nerve fibers that connect the two superior colliculi; called also *commissure of rostral colliculus.*

c. epithala′mica TA alternative for *c. posterior.*

c. for′nicis [TA] commissure of fornix: a band of fibers connecting the hippocampi of the two sides through the body of the fornix; called also *hippocampal commissure.*

c. gri′sea ante′rior medul′lae spina′lis [TA] anterior gray commissure of spinal cord: the portion of the gray commissure anterior to the central canal. Called also *ventral gray commissure of spinal cord.*

c. gri′sea poste′rior medul′lae spina′lis [TA] posterior gray commissure of spinal cord: the portion of the gray commissure posterior to the central canal. Called also *dorsal gray commissure of spinal cord.*

c. habenula′rum [TA] habenular commissure: a band of fibers of the stria medullaris that pass through the habenula of each side to decussate and terminate in the habenula of the other side.

c. labio′rum ante′rior [TA] anterior commissure of labia: the junction of the two labia majora anteriorly, at the lower border of the pubic symphysis.

c. labio′rum o′ris [TA] commissure of lips of mouth: the junction of the upper and lower lips at either side of the mouth.

c. labio′rum poste′rior [TA] posterior commissure of labia: the apparent junction of the labia majora posteriorly, formed by the forward projection of the tendinous center of the perineum into the pudendal cleft.

c. latera′lis palpebra′rum [TA] lateral commissure of eyelids: the junction of the upper and lower eyelids on the lateral side. Called also *lateral palpebral commissure.*

c. media′lis palpebra′rum [TA] medial commissure of eyelids: the junction of the upper and lower eyelids on the medial side; called also *medial palpebral commissure.*

c. poste′rior [TA] posterior commissure: a large fiber bundle that crosses the midline of the epithalamus just dorsal to the point where the cerebral aqueduct opens into the third ventricle; called also *c. epithalamica* [TA alternative] and *commissure of epithalamus.* See illustration.

c. pro′statae TA alternative for isthmus prostatae.

c. supraop′tica dorsa′lis [TA] dorsal supraoptic commissure: the more dorsal fiber bundle that crosses the midline of the brain dorsal to the caudal border of the optic chiasm; see also *supraoptic commissures,* under *commissure.*

c. supraop′tica ventra′lis [TA] ventral supraoptic commissure: the more ventral fiber bundle that crosses the midline of the brain dorsal to the caudal border of the optic chiasm; see also *supraoptic commissures,* under *commissure.*

com•mis•su•rae (kom″ĭ-su′re) [L.] genitive and plural of *commissura.*

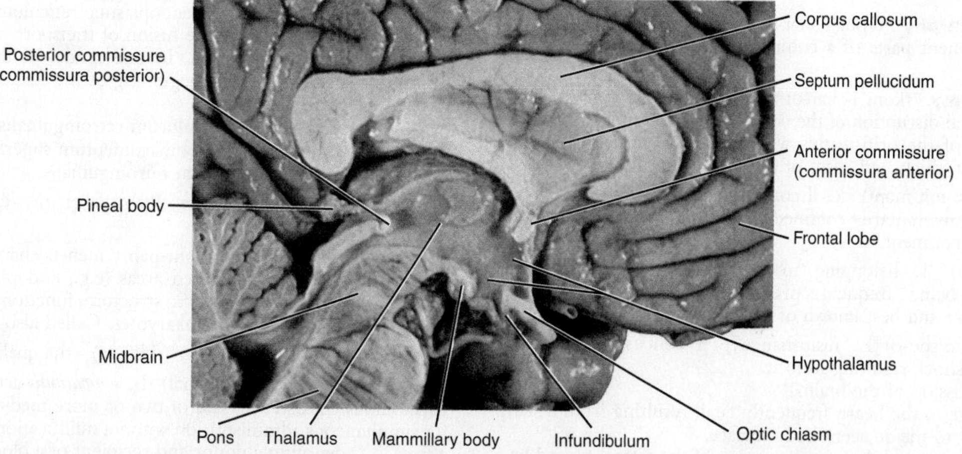

■ Midsagittal view of the diencephalon, showing the commissura anterior and commissura posterior (anterior and posterior commissures).

com·mis·su·ral (kə-mish′o͞o-rəl) pertaining to or acting as a commissure.

com·mis·sure (kom′ĭ-shər) 1. a site of union of corresponding parts; see also *commissura.* 2. the site of junction between adjacent cusps of a heart valve.
anterior c. commissura anterior.
c. of bulbs of vestibule commissura bulborum vestibuli.
c. of caudal colliculus commissura colliculi inferioris.
c. of epithalamus commissura posterior.
c. of fornix commissura fornicis.
Ganser c. the anterior supraoptic commissure; see *supraoptic c′s.*
gray c. substantia intermedia centralis medullae spinalis.
gray c. of spinal cord the transverse band of gray substance surrounding the central canal of the spinal cord external to the central gelatinous substance; it connects the intermediate, anterior, and posterior columns.
gray c. of spinal cord, anterior commissura grisea anterior medullae spinalis.
gray c. of spinal cord, dorsal commissura grisea posterior medullae spinalis.
gray c. of spinal cord, posterior commissura grisea posterior medullae spinalis.
gray c. of spinal cord, ventral commissura grisea anterior medullae spinalis.
Gudden c. the ventral, or inferior, supraoptic commissure; see *supraoptic c′s.*
c. of habenulae, habenular c. commissura habenularum.
hippocampal c. commissura fornicis.
c. of inferior colliculus commissura colliculi inferioris.
c. of labia, anterior commissura labiorum anterior.
c. of labia, posterior commissura labiorum posterior.
laryngeal c. the region of junction (anterior or posterior) of the two sides of the larynx.
lateral c. of eyelids, lateral palpebral c. commissura lateralis palpebrarum.
c. of lips of mouth commissura labiorum oris.
medial c. of eyelids, medial palpebral c. commissura medialis palpebrarum.
Meynert c. the dorsal, or superior, supraoptic commissure; see *supraoptic c′s.*
posterior c. commissura posterior.
c. of prostate isthmus prostatae.
rostral c. commissura anterior.
c. of rostral colliculus commissura colliculi superioris.
c. of superior colliculus commissura colliculi superioris.
supraoptic c′s at least three fiber bundles situated dorsal to the optic chiasm, which have been associated with the names of Gudden (ventral or inferior), Meynert (dorsal or superior), and Ganser (anterior), and which have been referred to as commissures but are probably decussations; their connections in humans are uncertain. Only the dorsal and ventral bundles are recognized in official anatomical nomenclature: see *commissura supraoptica dorsalis* and *commissura supraoptica ventralis.*
supraoptic c., dorsal commissura supraoptica dorsalis.
supraoptic c., ventral commissura supraoptica ventralis.
white c. of spinal cord, anterior commissura alba anterior medullae spinalis.
white c. of spinal cord, dorsal commissura alba posterior medullae spinalis.
white c. of spinal cord, posterior commissura alba posterior medullae spinalis.
white c. of spinal cord, ventral commissura alba anterior medullae spinalis.

com·mis·su·ror·rha·phy (kom″ĭ-shər-or′ə-fe) [*commissure* + *-rrhaphy*] suture of the component parts of a commissure, to decrease the size of the orifice.

com·mis·sur·ot·o·my (kom″ĭ-shər-ot′ə-me) [*commissure* + *-tomy*] surgical incision or digital disruption of the component parts of a commissure to increase the size of the orifice; this was formerly commonly done to separate the adherent, thickened cusps of a stenotic mitral valve.

com·mit·ment (kə-mit′mənt) civil commitment; the legal proceeding by which a person is involuntarily confined to a mental hospital or made to undergo outpatient treatment.

com·mon (kom′ən) 1. belonging to or shared by two or more entities. 2. usual; being frequent, prevalent, widespread, or habitual. 3. most frequent and best known of its kind.

com·mo·tio (kə-mo′she-o) [L. "disturbance"] 1. concussion. 2. a violent shaking, or the shock resulting from it.
c. ce′rebri concussion of the brain.
c. cor′dis damage to the heart, frequently fatal, resulting from a sharp nonpenetrating blow to the adjacent body surface.
c. re′tinae edema around the macular region of the retina, caused by a severe blow to the eyeball, and producing a permanent central scotoma as a result of destruction of the delicate cones in the fovea. Called also *Berlin edema,* and *concussion of the retina.*
c. spina′lis concussion of the spinal cord.

com·mu·ni·ca·ble (kə-mu′nĭ-kə-bəl) capable of being transmitted from one individual to another; contagious. Cf. *infectious.*

com·mu·ni·cans (kə-mu′nə-kanz) [L.] communicating; used in anatomical nomenclature to denote a communicating structure, as a nerve.

com·mu·ni·cat·ing (kə-mu′nə-ka″ting) 1. denoting spreading or transmission, as of a disease. 2. being connected, one with another.

com·mu·nis (kə-mu′nis) [L.] common: a general term denoting a structure serving several branches.

com·mu·ni·ty (kə-mu′nĭ-te) a body of individuals living in a defined area or having a common interest or organization.
biotic c. an assemblage of populations living in a defined area.
climax c. the final, stable, and mature community in a series that appears in succession, which is in equilibrium with the environmental conditions and is composed of a definite group of plant and animal species.
therapeutic c. a specially structured mental treatment center employing group and milieu therapy and encouraging the patient to function within social norms.

com·mu·ni·ty-ac·quired (kə-mu′nĭ-te-ə-kwīrd′) of an infectious disease, acquired in the general population, i.e., not arising in the hospital or as a result of other contact with the health-care system. Cf. *nosocomial.*

Com·ol·li sign (kom-ol′e) [Antonio *Comolli,* Italian pathologist, 20th century] see under *sign.*

co·mor·bid (ko-mor′bid) pertaining to a disease or other pathologic process that occurs simultaneously with another.

co·mor·bid·i·ty (ko″mor-bid′ĭ-te) 1. a comorbid disease or condition. 2. the state of being comorbid. 3. the extent to which two diseases or disorders occur together in a given population.

COMP 1. cartilage oligomeric matrix protein. 2. a cancer chemotherapy regimen consisting of cyclophosphamide, Oncovin (vincristine), methotrexate, and prednisone.

com·pact (kom′pakt, kəm-pakt′) dense; having a dense structure.

com·pac·tion (kəm-pak′shən) 1. a complication of labor in twin births in which there is simultaneous full engagement of the leading fetal poles of both twins, so that the lesser pelvis is filled and further descent is prevented. Cf. *interlocking.* 2. in embryology, the process during which blastomeres change their shape and align themselves tightly against each other to form a compact ball of cells (the morula).

com·par·a·scope (kəm-par′ə-skōp″) a device attached to a microscope for the purpose of comparing two slides.

com·par·a·tor (kəm-par′ə-tər) a simple colorimeter consisting of a block of wood with holes in which to place the test tubes to be compared, and transverse holes through which to view the colors; called also *comparator block.*

com·par·ti·men·tum (kəm-pahr″tĭ-men′təm) [L., from *compartiri* to share] [TA] compartment.
c. superficia′le perine′i [TA] superficial perineal compartment: the region between the perineal membrane and the superficial perineal fascia; called also *spatium superficiale perinei* [TA alternative] and *superficial perineal pouch* or *space.*

com·part·ment (kəm-pahrt′mənt) a small enclosure within a larger space.
endoplasmic reticulum–Golgi intermediate c. (ERGIC) a compartment of vesicles between the endoplasmic reticulum and the *cis* face of the Golgi complex, formed by the fusion of transport vesicles from the transitional endoplasmic reticulum. In one model of the Golgi complex, the fusion of vesicles marks the beginning of the formation of new Golgi cisternae. See Plate 12.
muscular c. lacuna musculorum retroinguinalis.
superficial perineal c. compartimentum superficiale perinei.
vascular c. lacuna vasorum retroinguinalis.

com·part·men·ta·li·za·tion (kəm-pahrt″men-tə-lĭ-za′shən) compartmentation.

com·part·men·ta·tion (kəm-pahrt″men-ta′shən) the internal division of cells into membrane-limited areas (e.g., endoplasmic reticulum, mitochondria), each having a specific structure, function, and biochemical composition; a characteristic of eukaryotes. Called also *compartmentalization.*

com·pat·i·bil·i·ty (kəm-pat″ĭ-bil′ĭ-te) the quality of being compatible.

com·pat·i·ble (kəm-pat′ĭ-bəl) [L. *compatibilis* accordant] 1. capable of harmonious coexistence; said of two or more medications that are suitable for simultaneous administration without nullification or aggravation of their effects. 2. denoting a donor and recipient of a blood transfusion in which there is no transfusion reaction. 3. histocompatible.

Com·pa·zine (kom′pə-zēn) trademark for preparations of prochlorperazine.

com·pen·sat·ed (kom′pən-sa″təd) counterbalanced; offset.

com·pen·sa·tion (kom″pən-sa′shən) [L. *compensatio*, from *cum* together + *pensare* to weigh] 1. the counterbalancing of any defect of structure or function. 2. a conscious process or, more frequently, an unconscious defense mechanism by which a person attempts to make up for real or imagined physical or psychological deficiencies. 3. in the presence of disease, the maintenance of an adequate blood flow without distressing symptoms, accomplished by such cardiac and circulatory adjustments as tachycardia, cardiac hypertrophy or dilation, and increase of blood volume by sodium and water retention.

dosage c. the mechanism that regulates the expression of sex-linked genes in the sex carrying two or more copies of the same chromosome in those species in which the genes differ in dose between males and females. See *Lyon hypothesis*, under *hypothesis*.

com·pen·sa·to·ry (kəm-pen′sə-tor″e) making good a defect or loss; restoring a lost balance.

com·pe·tence (kom′pə-təns) [L. *competens* sufficient] 1. the ability of an organ or part to perform adequately any function required of it. 2. in embryology, the ability of embryonic cells to differentiate into cell types determined by inductors.

embryonic c. the ability of embryonic tissue to respond normally to the influence of an inductor.

immunologic c. immunocompetence.

com·pe·ti·tion (kom″pə-tish′ən) the phenomenon in which two structurally similar molecules "compete" for a single binding site on a third molecule. See *competitive inhibition*, under *inhibition*.

antigenic c. an altered response to an immunogen resulting from the simultaneous or close administration of two immunogens: the response to one is normal, while the response to the second is suppressed or diminished.

com·plaint (kəm-plānt′) symptom.

chief c. presenting symptom.

com·ple·ment (kom′plə-mənt) [L. *complēre* to fill out or up] a term originally used to refer to the heat-labile factor in serum that causes immune cytolysis, the lysis of antibody-coated cells. It is now used to refer to the entire functionally related system comprising at least 20 distinct serum proteins, their cellular receptors, and related regulatory proteins that is the effector not only of immune cytolysis but also of other biologic functions including anaphylaxis, phagocytosis, opsonization, and hemolysis. Complement activation occurs by two different sequences, the classical and alternative pathways (qq.v.). All of the components of complement, designated C1 through C9, participate in the classical pathway; the alternative pathway lacks components C1, C2, and C4 but adds factors B and D and properdin. Regulatory proteins include factors H and I, clusterin, C3 nephritic factor, decay accelerating factor, homologous restriction factor, anaphylatoxin inactivator, C1 inhibitor, C4 binding protein, membrane cofactor protein, protectin, and vitronectin. Activation of the classical pathway triggers an enzymatic cascade involving C1, C4, C2, and C3; activation of the alternative pathway triggers a cascade involving C3 and factors B and D and properdin. Both result in the cleavage of C5 and the formation of the membrane attack complex, which in its final state creates a pore in the cell wall and causes cell lysis. See illustration. Complement activation also results in the formation of many biologically active complement fragments that act as anaphylatoxins, opsonins, or chemotactic factors. NOTE: Fragments resulting from proteolytic cleavage of complement proteins are designated with lower-case-letter suffixes, e.g., C3a. By convention, the smaller initial cleavage fragment is designated "a" and the larger "b," excepting the fragments C2a and C2b generated from C2, where the larger, active fragment has conventionally been designated C2a. Inactivated fragments are designated by the prefix "i," e.g., iC3b. Terminology of activated components or complexes with biologic activity is quite variable. A bar over the symbol is sometimes used, e.g., C$\overline{1}$ or C$\overline{4b, 2a}$, and in designating multicomponent complexes, commas may or may not be present between components, and the "a" and "b" designations may or may not be used. Thus, C4b,2a may also be written C$\overline{4b, 2a}$, C4b2a, C$\overline{4b2a}$, C42, or C$\overline{42}$. Some authors use the overbar for any activated component, while others reserve it specifically for those with enzymatic activity.

C1 the first component of the classical pathway of complement activation, a pentamolecular calcium-dependent complex comprising C1q and two molecules each of C1r and C1s.

C1q a six-subunit molecule, comprising 18 polypeptide chains, having the shape of six parallel rods flaring apart from each other at one end to terminate in a flower bunch arrangement, the globular head of each rod resembling a tulip; binding of the heads to IgM or IgG initiates the classical complement pathway, which continues by binding of two molecules each of C1r and C1s by C1q.

C1r a serine esterase component of C1 in the classical complement pathway, activated by cleavage of C1r bound to the stem of immunoglobulin-bound C1q; once activated, it can cleave and activate C1s. The activated state is sometimes specifically denoted by C$\overline{1r}$.

C1s an enzyme that cleaves C4 into C4a and C4b and C2 into C2a and C2b, activated by cleavage of a peptide bond when C1 interacts with activators of the classical pathway; it is inhibited by C1 inhibitor. Called also *C1 esterase*. The activated state is sometimes specifically denoted by C$\overline{1s}$.

C2 a component of the classical complement pathway that binds surface-bound C4b; cleavage of C2 by C1s releases a small C2b fragment and leaves C2a bound to C4b to form the classic pathway C3 convertase (C4b,2a).

C2a a constituent of the classical pathway C3 and C5 convertases (C4b,2a and C4b,2a,3b, respectively), generated by C1s-mediated cleavage of C2 bound to C4b. Because in most other cases the active fragment generated by cleavage of complement factors is designated the "b" fragment (e.g., C3b, C4b), some authors designate this active fragment as C2b, the small soluble fragment being thus C2a; in this case, the C3 and C5 convertases are designated C4b2b and C4b2b3b, respectively.

C3 a component of both the classical and alternative complement pathways; it can be cleaved spontaneously at low level (tickover) or by one of the C3 convertases (C4b,2a or C3b,Bb) to form C3a and C3b. Deficiency of C3 may be associated with repeated severe pyogenic bacterial infection.

C3a an anaphylatoxin generated, along with C3b, when C3 is cleaved by one of the C3 convertases.

C3b a constituent of the classical pathway C5 convertase and of the alternative pathway C3 and C5 convertases, generated by C3 convertases in both pathways and also continuously generated in the circulation in the small amounts required to initiate the alternative pathway (tickover); it is inactivated by variable combinations of factor H, factor I, membrane cofactor protein, decay accelerating factor, and complement receptor 1. C3b is also an opsonin having receptors on erythrocytes, B lymphocytes, granulocytes, monocytes, and macrophages.

C3b,Bb the alternative pathway C3 convertase, which splits C3 into C3a and C3b; it is generated by the interaction of factor B and factor D with C3b deposited on activators of the alternative pathway and thus protected from inactivation by factor I and factor H. It is unstable until the addition of properdin. See also note at *complement*.

C3b_n,Bb the alternative pathway C5 convertase, generated by addition of one or more C3b fragments to C3b,Bb; it is unstable until the addition of properdin. See also note at *complement*.

C3b,P,Bb a more stable form of the alternative pathway C3 convertase, generated by addition of properdin to C3b,Bb. See also note at *complement*.

C3b_n,P,Bb a more stable form of the alternative pathway C5 convertase, generated by addition of properdin to C3b_n,Bb. See also note at *complement*.

C3d a B cell growth factor generated by inactivation of C3b by factor I and various cofactors, including complement receptor 1, membrane

Defects in Complement Components and Selected Regulatory Proteins

Defective Protein	Pathway Affected	Clinically Associated Disorders
C1	Classical pathway	Autoimmune disorders; pyogenic infections
C2	Classical pathway	Autoimmune disorders; pyogenic infections
C3	Classical and alternative pathways	Autoimmune disorders; pyogenic infections
C4	Classical pathway	Autoimmune disorders
C5–C9	Membrane attack complex	Recurrent disseminated neisserial infection
Properdin	Alternative pathway	Neisserial and other pyogenic infections
Factor D	Alternative pathway	Neisserial and other pyogenic infections
C1 Inhibitor	Deregulation of classical pathway	Hereditary angioneurotic edema; some autoimmune disorders
Factor I	Deregulation of alternative pathway	Autoimmune disorders; pyogenic infections
Factor H	Deregulation of classical pathway	Glomerulonephritis

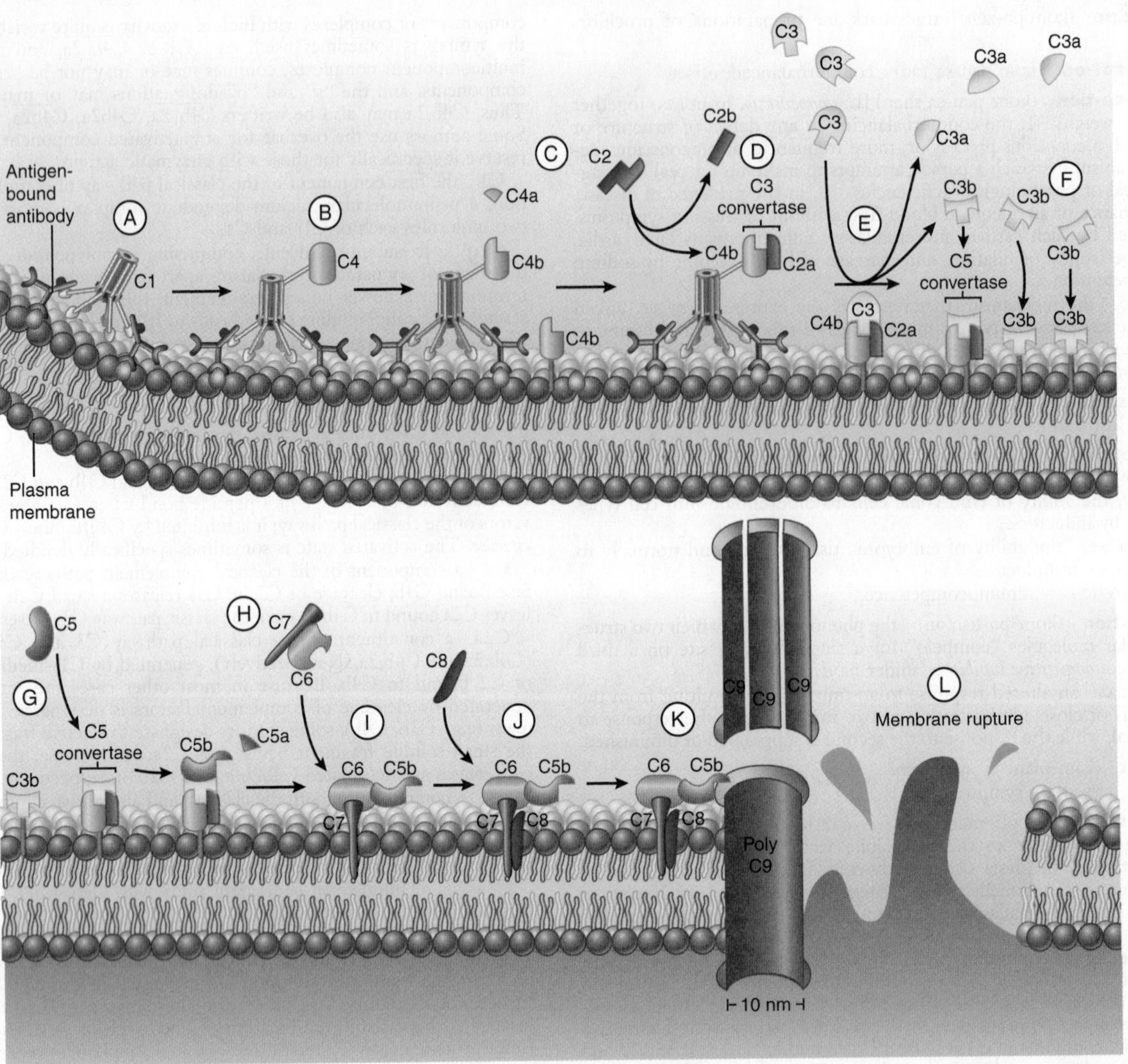

■ Schematic representation of the classical complement pathway. The pathway is initiated by binding of two antibody molecules to a multivalent antigen, followed by binding of complement protein C1q, and then by binding of two molecules each of C1r and C1s to C1q to form the active complex C1 *(A)*. C4 binds to the C1q portion of C1 *(B)*, and the esterolytic site on C1s activates C4 by splitting off C4b, which binds the antigen-antibody complex or the nearby cell surface *(C)*. The same site on C1s then cleaves and activates C2 which has bound to C4b, yielding a C4b2a complex (C3 convertase) *(D)*. The C3 convertase binds C3 and cleaves it to the active form C3b *(E)*, which binds to the cell surface and to the C3 convertase to form a C4b2a3b complex (C5 convertase) *(F)*. The late phase of complement activation begins when the C5 convertase cleaves C5 to the active form C5b *(G)*. C5b remains at the cell surface and binds first C6 then C7 *(H)*; the latter is hydrophobic and inserts into the plasma membrane *(I)*, where it is joined by C8 *(J)*. As many as 19 molecules of C9 then polymerize at C5678 to form pores in the plasma membrane *(K)*; this final complex is called the membrane attack complex (MAC). Entry of water through the pores into the cell causes osmotic swelling and cell rupture *(L)*.

cofactor protein, and factor H; it interacts with complement receptor 2 on B lymphocytes.

C4 a component of the classical complement pathway; it binds C1 and is cleaved by C1s to generate the small anaphylatoxin C4a and the larger active fragment C4b.

C4a a weak anaphylatoxin generated by cleavage of C4 by C1s in the classical complement pathway.

C4b a constituent of the classical pathway C3 convertase (C4b,2a), generated by cleavage of C4 by C1s; the active fragment C4b then binds C2 for cleavage of C2 by C1s. It is inactivated by factor I in the presence of C4 binding protein. C4b is also an opsonin that binds to the same receptors as C3b.

C4b,2a the classical pathway C3 convertase, which cleaves C3 to C3a and C3b, a complex of C4b and C2a formed on cell membrane surfaces in the presence of Mg^{2+}. See also notes at *C2a* and *complement.*

C4b,2a,3b the classical pathway C5 convertase, which cleaves C5 to C5a and C5b; the complex is formed by attachment of C3b to membrane-bound C4b,2a. See also notes at *C2a* and *complement.*

C4d a degradation product of complement factor C4 in the classical complement pathway; it binds covalently to endothelial cells and extracellular components of vascular basement membranes near the sites of C4 activation. Increased C4d in the urine of persons who have received kidney transplants is considered an early sign of humoral rejection of the transplant.

C5 a complement component that binds to the C3b component of both the classical and alternative pathway C5 convertases (C4b,2a,3b and $C3b_n$,P,Bb), being split by either convertase into the smaller anaphylatoxin C5a and the larger cell surface–bound C5b, the initial component of the membrane attack complex.

C5a an anaphylatoxin and chemotactic factor for basophils, neutrophils, mast cells, macrophages, and endothelium generated in the cleavage of C5 by C5 convertases. It is a potent local mediator of inflammation and also induces smooth muscle contraction.

C5b a constituent of the membrane attack complex generated by cleavage of C5 by the classical and alternative pathway C5 convertases; it can also be generated by the action of certain serum proteases, e.g., plasmin and trypsin.

C5b,6 the hydrophilic complex of C5b and C6 formed in the initial steps of formation of the membrane attack complex; it is loosely associated with the membrane until it is bound by C7.

C5b,6,7 a trimolecular complex of C5b, C6, and C7 that binds to cell membranes in the formation of the membrane attack complex; it can be inhibited by binding by vitronectin, which yields an inactivated complex unable to bind to membranes. C5b,6,7 is also a chemotactic factor for neutrophils. Sometimes abbreviated C5b–7.

C5b,6,7,8 a complex generated by binding of C8 to membrane-bound C5b,6,7; it causes a slow leakage of the cell membrane. Sometimes abbreviated C5b–8.

C5b,6,7,8,9 the complete membrane attack complex (cytolytic agent) of the complement system, generated by addition of multiple molecules of C9 to C5b,6,7,8; this complex has a hydrophilic center that allows the rapid passage of water and ions through the cell membrane, causing osmotic lysis of the cell. Sometimes abbreviated C5b–9 or $C5b–9_n$.

C6 a component of the membrane attack complex, bound by C5b to form C5b,6.

C7 a component of the membrane attack complex, bound by C5b,6 to form the lipophilic intermediate C5b,6,7.

C8 a component of the membrane attack complex, bound by membrane-bound C5b,6,7 to form C5b,6,7,8, which is anchored in the cell membrane by C8. C8 can then induce the polymerization of C9.

C9 a component of the membrane attack complex; multiple molecules are bound by a single C5b,6,7,8 complex to form the final membrane attack complex. Although as few as 3 to 4 molecules of C9 are sufficient for full lytic activity on many substrates, 12 to 15 are necessary to form the usual doughnut-shaped pore in the membrane. $C9_n$ is often used to denote the multiple molecules of C9 in the membrane attack complex.

total hemolytic c. (CH50, CH_{50}) see *CH50 assay*, under *assay*, and *CH50 unit*, under *unit*.

com·ple·men·tal (kom″plə-men′təl) complementary.

com·ple·men·ta·ry (kom″plə-men′tə-re) [L. *complēre* to fill out or up] 1. supplying a defect, or helping to do so; making complete; accessory. 2. in biochemistry, pertaining to the specific pairing between purine and pyrimidine bases in two nucleotide strands as a function of the base-pairing rules, so that the sequence of a strand defines the order of the strand that is complementary to it.

com·ple·men·ta·tion (kom″plə-men-ta′shən) [L. *complēre* to fill out or up] the interaction between two sets of genes introduced into the same cell, such that the cell can function even though each set of genes carries a mutated, nonfunctional gene; it indicates that the defects are not identical.

allelic c., interallelic c. intragenic c.

intergenic c. complementation in which there is full restoration of wild-type function, the two mutations being located in two different genes and the cells therefore producing normal versions of both gene products.

intragenic c. complementation in which there is restoration of function, sometimes partial, when the two mutations are located at different sites within the same gene; it usually occurs in genes that encode subunits of multimeric enzymes, the two mutant subunits combining to form an active enzyme.

com·plex (kom′pleks) [L. *complexus* woven together, encompassing] 1. the sum, combination, or collection of various things or related factors, like or unlike, e.g., a complex of symptoms. See also *syndrome*. 2. sequence (def. 2). 3. a group of interrelated ideas, mainly unconscious, that have a common emotional tone and strongly influence a person's attitudes and behavior. 4. the portion of an electrocardiographic tracing that represents the systole of an atrium or ventricle.

Complex

AIDS dementia c. HIV encephalopathy.

AIDS-related c. (ARC) term formerly used for a complex of signs and symptoms representing a less severe stage of human immunodeficiency virus (HIV) infection.

amniotic band disruption c. amniotic band syndrome.

amygdaloid c. corpus amygdaloideum.

amyotrophic lateral sclerosis–parkinsonism–dementia c. an autosomal dominant disorder caused by mutation in the *TRPM7* gene (locus: 15q21), which encodes a protein that functions as an ion channel and a kinase; it occurs among the Chamorro population of Guam and is characterized by gradually progressing parkinsonism associated with progressive dementia and amyotrophic lateral sclerosis.

anomalous c. in electrocardiography, an abnormal atrial or ventricular complex resulting from aberrant impulse conduction occurring over accessory conduction pathways.

antigen-antibody c. the complex formed by the noncovalent binding of an antibody and an antigen. Complexes of antibodies belonging to certain immunoglobulin classes may activate complement. Antigen-antibody complexes are mediators of Type III immune responses (Arthus reactions, serum sickness, and immune complex diseases). Called also *immune c.*, particularly in discussing disease processes.

anti-inhibitor coagulant c. (AICC) a concentrated fraction from pooled human plasma, which includes vitamin K–dependent coagulation factors (factors II, VII, IX, X), factors of the kinin-generating system, and factor VIII coagulant antigen. It is administered intravenously as an antihemorrhagic in hemophilic patients with factor VIII inhibitors; its mechanism of action has not been elucidated but may be due at least in part to its factor Xa content. Called also *activated prothrombin complex concentrate*.

apical c. an ultrastructural complex of apical organelles characteristic of certain protozoa *(apicocomplexan protozoa)* during some stage of their development, generally consisting of one or more polar ring(s), a conoid, micronemes, rhoptries, and subpellicular microtubules. It seems to function as a means of attachment to and penetration of host cells.

atrial c. the P wave of the electrocardiogram, representing electrical activation of the atria. Cf. *ventricular c.*

atrial premature c. (APC) a single ectopic atrial beat arising prematurely, manifest electrocardiographically as an abnormally shaped premature P wave, usually with a slightly increased PR interval. It occurs in normal hearts, sometimes associated with the use of stimulants, but may be associated with structural heart disease.

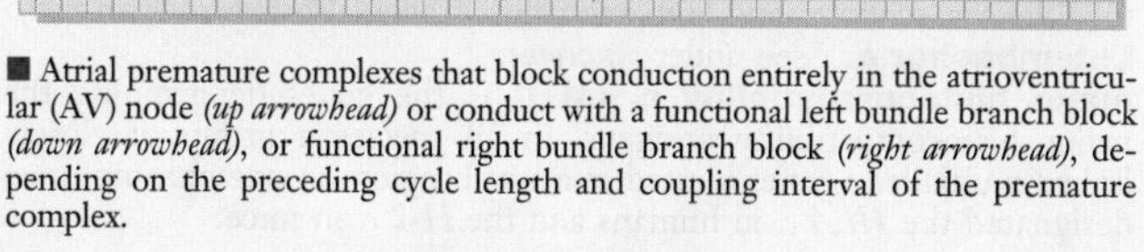

■ Atrial premature complexes that block conduction entirely in the atrioventricular (AV) node *(up arrowhead)* or conduct with a functional left bundle branch block *(down arrowhead)*, or functional right bundle branch block *(right arrowhead)*, depending on the preceding cycle length and coupling interval of the premature complex.

atrioventricular (AV) junctional escape c. see under *beat*.

atrioventricular (AV) junctional premature c. an ectopic beat arising prematurely in the atrioventricular junction and traveling toward both the atria and ventricles if unimpeded, causing the P wave to be premature and abnormal or absent and the QRS complex to be premature.

avian leukosis c. see *avian leukosis*, under *leukosis*.

avian sarcoma c. see under *sarcoma*.

avidin-biotin c. (ABC), **avidin-biotin peroxidase c.** a complex of avidin and biotinylated horseradish peroxidase that is added to a sample that has been treated with primary antibody specific for the antigen of interest and then with a biotinylated secondary antibody, which binds to an antigenic determinant on the primary antibody, so that several horseradish peroxidase molecules are localized to the site of the primary antigen. It is used in a number of immunocytochemical and immunohistochemical techniques.

Bötzinger c. neurons in the ventrolateral area of the medulla oblongata, ventral to the nucleus ambiguus, partially interspersed with the lateral reticular nucleus, and extending rostrally toward the facial nucleus; they provide essential rhythmic action potentials for respiratory function and constitute a respiratory center.

branched-chain α-keto acid dehydrogenase c. a multienzyme complex composed of 3-methyl-2-oxobutanoate dehydrogenase (2-methylpropanoyl-transferring) [EC 1.2.4.4] (more commonly called branched-chain α-keto acid dehydrogenase), dihydrolipoyllysine-residue (2-methylpropanoyl)transferase [EC 2.3.1.168], and dihydrolipoyl dehydrogenase [EC 1.8.1.4], with thiamine pyrophosphate, lipoic acid, NAD^+, FAD, and coenzyme A as cofactors. The integrated complex catalyzes the oxidative decarboxylation of the keto acid analogues of the branched-chain amino acids leucine, isoleucine, and valine. Deficiency of any enzyme of the complex causes maple syrup urine disease.

calcarine c. calcar avis.

Carney c. a genetically heterogeneous, autosomal dominant symptom complex consisting of myxomas of the soft tissues; spotty skin pigmentation; tumors of the adrenal gland, pituitary, and testicle; and schwannomas of peripheral nerves. Called also *Carney syndrome*.

castration c. in psychoanalytic theory, unconscious thoughts and motives stemming from fear of loss of genitals as punishment for forbidden sexual desires.

chlorophyllin copper c. sodium the sodium salt of copper-chelated chlorophyllin, applied topically for the deodorization of skin lesions and administered orally to deodorize the urine and feces in colostomy, ileostomy, or incontinence.

dystrophin-glycoprotein c. (DGC) a large oligomeric complex of proteins and glycoproteins of the sarcolemma that are critical to the stability of muscle fiber membranes and to the linking of the actin cytoskeleton to the extracellular matrix; it includes dystrophin, sarcoglycans, dystroglycans, sarcospan, syntrophins, and dystrobrevin. Abnormalities of the plasma membrane of the muscle fiber that destroy

Complex *Continued*

this complex have been associated with several types of muscular dystrophy and with cardiomyopathy.
EAHF c. the symptom complex of *e*czema, *a*sthma, and *h*ay *f*ever.
Eisenmenger c. a defect of the interventricular septum with severe pulmonary hypertension, hypertrophy of the right ventricle, and latent or overt cyanosis.
Electra c. the counterpart in females of the Oedipus complex, which was originally applied only to males, involving the daughter's love for her father and jealousy or resentment toward her mother; the term is now rarely used since *Oedipus c.* (q.v.) has come to be applied to both sexes.
eosinophilic granuloma c. any of several types of skin lesions in cats, of unknown etiology but apparently related to one another, characterized by lesions on the skin surface and eosinophilia of the dermis. There are three types: the mild *eosinophilic ulcer* on the lip; the circumscribed pruritic *eosinophilic plaque*, usually on the abdomen or groin; and the *linear granuloma*, usually on the thigh or near the mouth.
exstrophy-epispadias c. a group of congenital defects of the anterior abdominal wall, including exstrophy of the bladder, exstrophy of the cloaca, and epispadias, believed to be caused by failure of the cloacal membrane to be reinforced by ingrowth of mesoderm.
factor IX c. [USP] a sterile, freeze-dried powder consisting of partially purified factor IX fraction, as well as concentrated factor II, VII, and X fractions, of venous plasma from healthy human donors. It is used in the prophylaxis and treatment of bleeding in patients with hemophilia B, replacement of factor VII in patients deficient in that factor, and treatment of anticoagulant-induced hemorrhage. Cf. *coagulation factor IX (human)* and *coagulation factor IX (recombinant)*. Administered intravenously.
feline respiratory disease c. a group of contagious viral infections of the upper respiratory tract in cats, characterized by fever, sneezing and coughing, and discharges from the nose and eyes. The usual cause is infection with a herpesvirus (feline herpesvirus 1) or a calicivirus. See also *feline viral rhinotracheitis*. Called also *feline influenza*.
gene c. a DNA segment containing a number of genes coding for products with related functions, such as the human major histocompatibility complex.
Ghon c. primary c. (def. 1).
glucoamylase c. the two heat-stable maltases in humans, also known as α-glucosidases [EC 3.2.1.20] (q.v.); they are described as a complex because the two enzyme activities are formed as a single polypeptide which is cleaved to form a heterodimer active within the brush border of the intestinal mucosa; the enzyme activities catalyze the hydrolysis of α-1,4 linked glucose residues from the nonreducing ends of disaccharides and oligomers such as maltose, amylose, amylopectin, and glycogen.
β-glycosidase c. the enzyme complex comprising lactase and glycosylceramidase (phlorhizin hydrolase) activities, occurring in the brush border membrane of the intestinal mucosa and hydrolyzing lactose as well as cellobiose and cellotriose; it is a single polypeptide, processed from a larger precursor, with two catalytic sites for the two enzyme activities. See also *lactase deficiency*.
Golgi c. a complex intracellular compartment of eukaryotes, occupying the perinuclear region and consisting of a number of stacked, flattened sacs (cisternae) with associated tubules and vesicles. Its primary function is to process substances synthesized in the endoplasmic reticulum; in addition it synthesizes some carbohydrates, such as hyaluronan and chondroitin sulfate. Transport vesicles from the endoplasmic reticulum fuse with the Golgi complex at the *cis* face, their cargo is processed while passing through the cisternae, and the processed products are transported from the *trans* face to the *trans*-Golgi network for sorting and packaging. The mechanism by which cargo moves through the Golgi complex is not clear; one model proposes transport between cisternae by vesicular budding and fusion, while another proposes dynamic remodeling and recycling so that the cisternae themselves change in composition and move in a *cis*-to-*trans* direction. Called also *Golgi apparatus* and *Golgi body*. See illustration and see Plate 12.

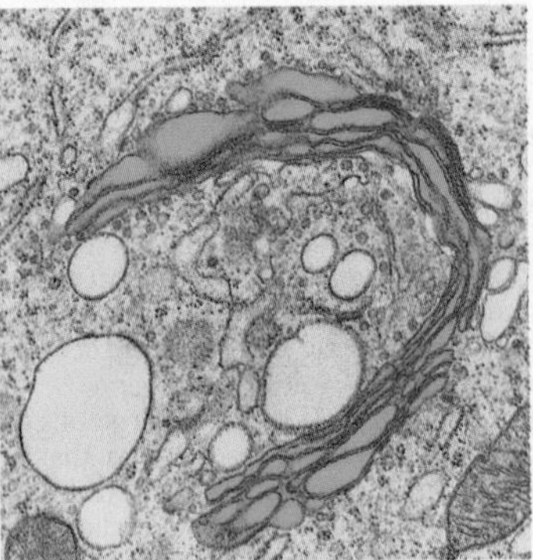

■ Golgi complex (color-highlighted transmission electron micrograph).

H-2 c. the murine major histocompatibility complex.
hapten-carrier c. the antigen formed by the coupling of a hapten and a carrier protein.
HLA c. the human major histocompatibility complex; see *human leukocyte antigens*, under *antigen*.
immune c. antigen-antibody c.
inclusion c. a compound in which molecules of one type are enclosed within cavities in the crystalline lattice of another substance.
inferiority c. unconscious feelings of inadequacy, producing timidity or, as a compensation, exaggerated aggressiveness and expression of superiority; based on Alfred Adler's concept that everyone is born with a feeling of inferiority stemming from real or imagined physical or psychological deficiency, with the manner in which the inferiority is handled determining behavior.
interdigestive migrating motor c. migrating motor c.
interpolated ventricular premature c. a ventricular premature complex that does not block conduction of the next sinus beat and thus is not associated with a compensatory pause.
jumped process c. dislocation of articular processes of spine.
junctional c. the intercellular arrangement between adjacent columnar epithelial cells, consisting of the zonula occludens, the zonula adherens, and the desmosome.
junctional premature c. atrioventricular junctional premature c.
juvenile nephronophthisis–medullary cystic disease c. a term preferred by some authorities to denote familial juvenile nephronophthisis (def. 1), on the grounds that although the various diseases have identical clinical manifestations, their modes of inheritance and ages of onset are different. Four variants are recognized: a sporadic form; familial juvenile nephronophthisis (def. 2), inherited recessively; Senior-Loken or renal-retinal syndrome, inherited recessively and associated with retinitis pigmentosa; and adult-onset medullary cystic disease (def. 2), inherited dominantly.
juxtaglomerular c. see under *apparatus*.
K c. a burst of high-voltage slow waves seen on the electroencephalogram during sleep; it may occur spontaneously or in response to a sensory (usually auditory) stimulus.
α-keto acid dehydrogenase c. any of the enzyme complexes catalyzing the oxidative decarboxylation of α-keto acids; see *branched-chain α-keto acid dehydrogenase c.*, *α-ketoglutarate dehydrogenase c.*, and *pyruvate dehydrogenase c.*
α-ketoglutarate dehydrogenase c. a multienzyme complex consisting of at least three distinct enzymes: oxoglutarate dehydrogenase (succinyl-transferring) [EC 1.2.4.2] (more commonly called α-ketoglutarate dehydrogenase), dihydrolipoyllysine-residue succinyltransferase [EC 2.3.1.61], and dihydrolipoyl dehydrogenase [EC 1.8.1.4]. The integrated enzyme complex catalyzes the overall reaction α-ketoglutarate + coenzyme A + NAD^+ = succinyl coenzyme A + NADH + CO_2. Thiamine pyrophosphate, lipoic acid, and FAD are required as cofactors. The reaction is a part of the tricarboxylic acid cycle. (See illustration under *cycle*.)
lactase–phlorhizin hydrolase c. β-glycosidase c.
LCMV-LASV c. a group of antigenically related arenaviruses; medically significant ones include the Lassa virus, cause of Lassa fever, and the lymphocytic choriomeningitis virus. Formerly called *Old World arenaviruses*.
limb–body wall c. a lethal sequence caused by early amnion rupture in utero, so that the fetus has abdominal wall defects with evisceration, neural tube defects, scoliosis, and limb anomalies. Called also *body stalk anomaly*.
Lutembacher c. see under *syndrome*.
major histocompatibility c. (MHC) the genes determining the major histocompatibility antigens, in all species a group of closely linked multiallelic genes located in a small region on one chromosome; designated the *HLA c.* in humans and the *H-2 c.* in mice.

Complex *Continued*

membrane attack c. (MAC) C5b,6,7,8,9; the pentamolecular complex that is the cytolytic agent of the complement system; see *C5b,6,7,8,9*, under *complement.*
Meyenburg c's groups of hamartomas in the bile ducts.
migrating motor c., migrating myoelectric c. a distinctive pattern of electromechanical activity in the gastrointestinal tract between meals, signifying motility of smooth muscles. There is a quiescent stage lasting 45 to 60 minutes, a time of gradually increasing peristaltic activity lasting about 30 minutes, a period of rapid, evenly spaced peristaltic waves for about 5 to 15 minutes, and a short period of transition back to the quiescent stage. Called also *interdigestive migrating motor c.*
***Mycobacterium avium-intracellulare* c.** a complex of *Mycobacterium avium* and *M. intracellulare* that causes tuberculosis in birds and swine and is associated with human pulmonary disease, lymphadenitis in children, and serious systemic disease in immunocompromised patients. See also *mycobacteriosis.*
nuclear pore c. a nuclear pore (q.v.) and its associated glycoproteins, which regulates transport between the nucleus and the cytoplasm. It has a diameter of approximately 80–100 nm and is composed of three stacked, octagonally symmetric, ringlike arrays of proteins (the cytoplasmic, middle, and nucleoplasmic rings), cytoplasmic fibers, a transporter, and a nuclear basket.
oculomotor nuclear c. nucleus nervi oculomotorius.
Oedipus c. in psychoanalytic theory, the feelings and conflicts occurring in a child during the phallic phase of psychosexual development that result from sexual attraction to the opposite-sex parent, including envious, aggressive feelings toward the same-sex parent.
olivary c., inferior complexus olivaris inferior.
olivary c., superior nucleus olivaris superior.
ostiomeatal c. the area of the nasal cavity between the middle and inferior nasal conchae, where the drainages from the frontal, ethmoid, and maxillary sinuses have their confluence.
perihypoglossal c., perihypoglossal nuclear c. nuclei perihypoglossales.
polysaccharide-iron c. ferric iron complexed to a low molecular weight polysaccharide prepared by extensive hydrolysis of starch; used as an oral hematinic.
posterior nuclear c. of thalamus nuclei posteriores thalami.
premature atrial c. (PAC) atrial premature c.
primary c. 1. the combination of a parenchymal pulmonary lesion *(Ghon focus* or *tubercle)* and a corresponding lymph node focus, occurring in primary tuberculosis, usually in children; it may undergo cellular necrosis and eventually calcify. Similar lesions may also be associated with other mycobacterial infections and with fungal infections such as histoplasmosis and coccidioidomycosis. Called also *Ghon c.* and *Ranke c.* 2. the primary cutaneous lesion at the site of an infection in the skin, such as a chancre in syphilis or cutaneous tuberculosis.
primary inoculation c., primary tuberculous c. primary inoculation tuberculosis.
pyruvate dehydrogenase c. a multienzyme complex consisting of multimers of the three distinct enzymes: pyruvate dehydrogenase (acetyl-transferring) [EC 1.2.4.1], dihydrolipoyllysine-residue acetyltransferase [EC 2.3.1.12], and dihydrolipoyl dehydrogenase [EC 1.8.1.4]. The integrated enzyme complex requires the cofactors thiamine pyrophosphate, lipoic acid, coenzyme A, FAD, and NAD^+. It catalyzes the formation of acetyl coenzyme A from pyruvate and coenzyme A, using NAD^+ as an electron acceptor; the acetyl coenzyme A is used in fatty acid synthesis, for acetylations, and for oxidation via the tricarboxylic acid cycle. Deficiency of any component of the complex results in lacticacidemia, ataxia, and psychomotor retardation.
QRS c. the portion of the electrocardiogram comprising the Q, R, and S waves, together representing ventricular depolarization. See also *electrocardiogram.*
QS c. in the electrocardiogram, a QRS complex in which the Q wave returns to baseline but does not produce a positive (R) wave; the entire ventricular complex is negative.
Ranke c. primary c. (def. 1).
RNA-induced silencing c. (RISC) a complex of proteins and small interfering RNA or microRNA that mediates the degradation of messenger RNA or the blocking of translation in RNA interference.
sicca c. primary Sjögren syndrome.
sling ring c. tracheal stenosis caused by pulmonary sling syndrome combined with a fixed complete cartilaginous ring.
stomatitis-pneumoenteritis c. peste des petits ruminants.
sucrase-isomaltase c. the enzyme complex comprising sucrase and α-dextrinase (isomaltase) activities, occurring in the brush border of the intestinal mucosa and hydrolyzing maltose as well as maltotriose and some other glycosidic bonds; the enzymes are synthesized as a single polypeptide and cleaved to form a heterodimer, each possessing a separate catalytic site. See also *sucrase-isomaltase deficiency*, under *deficiency.*
symptom c. a set of symptoms that occur together; the sum of signs of any morbid state; a syndrome.
synaptonemal c. a ladderlike structure consisting of two lateral elements connected to a central element by tranverse filaments that joins together homologous chromosomes in synapsis; it is formed during the zygotene and disintegrates during the early diplotene.
Tacaribe c. a group of antigenically related arenaviruses, nearly all found in South America; the medically significant ones are the Guanarito, Junin, Machupo, and Sabia viruses, which cause types of hemorrhagic fevers. Called also *New World arenaviruses.*
tuberous sclerosis c. an autosomal dominant disorder caused by mutation in either of two genes, the *TSC1* gene (locus: 9q34), which encodes hamartin, or the *TSC2* gene (locus: 16p13), which encodes tuberin; the two proteins are involved in tumor suppression; although hereditary, the majority of cases are due to de novo mutation. The disorder has variable manifestations, primarily neurologic and dermatologic; it is usually evident in childhood, although mild cases may not appear until later. The primary characteristics are hamartomas of the brain (tubers) that can cause seizures and mental retardation; and skin lesions such as periungual fibromas, patches of vitiligo or guttate leukoderma, shagreen patches, and café-au-lait spots; there may also be phakomas of the retina and hamartomas of the heart and kidney. Called also *tuberous sclerosis.*
ureterotrigonal c. ureterovesical junction.
VATER c. see under *association.*
ventral lateral c. of thalamus nuclei ventrales laterales thalami.
ventral medial c. of thalamus nuclei ventrales mediales thalami.
ventricular c. the combined QRS complex and T wave, together representing ventricular electrical activity. Cf. *atrial c.*
ventricular premature c. (VPC) an ectopic beat arising in the ventricles and stimulating the myocardium prematurely. It is characterized by an early, wide, oddly shaped QRS complex with an ST segment and T wave directed opposite to the QRS complex, usually without resetting of the sinus node, and with occasional fusion beats. It may occur in normal hearts but often is indicative of organic heart disease.
ventrobasal c. of thalamus nuclei ventrobasales thalami.
vertebral subluxation c. in chiropractic, malfunction of organs or tissues caused by impairment of nerve function that results from restriction of normal motion or from abnormal position of spinal segments.
vitamin B c. see under *vitamin.*

com·plex·ion (kəm-plek′shən) [L. *complexio* combination] the color and appearance of the skin of the face.

com·plex·us (kom-plek′səs) [L. "encompassing"] complex.

c. oliva′ris infe′rior [TA] inferior olivary complex: a folded band of gray matter that encloses a white core *(hilum nuclei olivaris inferioris)* and that produces the elevation called the *oliva* on the medulla oblongata. It is a nuclear complex that receives projections from the spinal cord, mesencephalon, cerebellar nuclei, and cerebral cortex and projects fibers via the contralateral inferior cerebellar peduncle to the cerebellar cortex and nuclei. Called also *nuclei olivares inferiores* [TA alternative], *inferior olivary nuclei*, and *caudal olivary nuclei.*

c. sti′mulans cor′dis [TA] conducting system of heart: a system of specialized muscle fibers that generate and rapidly transmit cardiac impulses and serve to coordinate contractions, comprising the sinoatrial node, atrioventricular node, bundle of His and its right and left bundle branches, and the subendocardial branches (rami subendocardiales) of Purkinje fibers. Called also *systema conducens cordis* [TA alternative].

com·pli·ance (kəm-pli′əns) 1. the quality of yielding to pressure or force without disruption. 2. an expression of the ability to yield to pressure without disruption, such as the distensibility of an air- or fluid-filled organ, e.g., the lung or urinary bladder, measured in terms of unit of volume change per unit of pressure change. Symbol C. It is the reciprocal of *elastance.*

dynamic c. compliance measured while an organ (such as the lung or bladder) is expanding or contracting; in the lung it is a measure of the change in volume per change in inflation pressure during air flow into or out of the lung. Cf. *static c.*

static c. compliance measured in the absence of any motion. Cf. *dynamic c.*

com·pli·cat·ed (kom′plĭ-kāt″əd) [L. *complicare* to infold] involved; associated with other injuries, lesions, or diseases.

com·pli·ca·tion (kom″plĭ-ka′shən) [L. *complicatio,* from *cum* together + *plicare* to fold] 1. a disease or diseases concurrent with another disease. 2. the concurrence of two or more diseases in the same patient.

com·po·mer (kom′pə-mər) a hybrid resin matrix composite filling material that contains components of glass ionomer but whose hardening occurs by polymerization of the resin matrix.

com·po·nent (kom-po′nənt) 1. a constituent element or part. 2. in neurology, a series of neurons forming a functional system for conducting the afferent and efferent impulses in the somatic and splanchnic (visceral) mechanisms of the body. 3. one part of a prosthesis system.

anterior c. Angle's term for "a forward propelling force which is the result of meshing and pounding of the occlusal inclined planes of the teeth and the mesial inclination of the teeth."

complement c's see *complement.*

group-specific c. vitamin D–binding protein, a serum protein of particular use in anthropological studies because of the great differences in gene frequency in different populations.

M c. [*M*yeloma or *M*acroglobulinemia] an abnormal monoclonal immunoglobulin with a characteristic electrophoretic pattern, occurring in the serum of patients with plasma cell dyscrasias and formed by the proliferating concentrations of immunoglobulin-producing cells. Called also *M protein.*

plasma thromboplastin c. (PTC) factor IX; see under *coagulation factors,* at *factor.*

secretory c. (SC) a 70,000 dalton glycopeptide occurring in secretory IgA; synthesized not by the plasma cell producing the IgA but added while the IgA is crossing the epithelium; it may protect secretory IgA from proteolytic attack after secretion, or it may play some role in the process of secretion. Secretory component deficiency has been seen in a few patients; there is complete lack of IgA in external secretions although serum IgA is normal. Called also *secretory piece.*

somatic motor c. the system of neurons that conduct impulses to the somatic effectors (skeletal muscle) of the body.

somatic sensory c. the system of neurons conducting impulses from the somatic receptors.

splanchnic motor c. the system of neurons conducting impulses to the splanchnic (visceral) effectors (cardiac muscle, smooth muscle, and glandular epithelium).

splanchnic sensory c. the system of neurons conducting impulses from the splanchnic (visceral) receptors.

visceral motor c. splanchnic motor c.

visceral sensory c. splanchnic sensory c.

Com·pos·i·tae (kəm-poz′ĭ-te) a large family of flowering herbs, shrubs, and trees having composite flower heads in which a number of small florets are on each head; many well-known genera such as *Chrysanthemum,* the sunflowers, and the dandelions are in this family. Called also *Asteraceae.*

com·pos·ite (kəm-poz′it) 1. made up of unlike parts. 2. resin matrix c.

resin matrix c. a synthetic resin, usually acrylic based, to which a high percentage (about 75 to 80 per cent) of an inert filler has been added (such as glass beads or rods, borosilicate glass powder, or natural silica); filler particles are coated with a coupling agent that binds them to the resin matrix. Used chiefly in dental restorative procedures. Called also *composite* and *composite resin.*

com·pos men·tis (kom′pəs men′tis) [L.] sound of mind; sane.

com·pound (kom′pound) [L. *componere* to place together] 1. made up of two or more parts or ingredients. 2. in chemistry, a substance that consists of two or more chemical elements in union. 3. to combine to form a whole; unite.

acyclic c. an open-chain compound; see *open chain,* under *chain.*

addition c. a compound formed by the union of two or more compounds or elements.

aliphatic c. an open-chain compound that does not contain multiple bonds; a saturated compound. See *open chain,* under *chain.*

APC c. a preparation of acetylsalicylic acid, phenacetin, and caffeine citrate.

aromatic c., benzene c. a closed-chain compound in which the ring contains several double bonds; see *closed chain,* under *chain.*

binary c. a compound whose molecule is composed of atoms of only two elements.

clathrate c. a type of inclusion complex in which molecules of one type are trapped within cavities of another substance, such as within a crystalline lattice structure or large molecule; called also *occlusion c.* and *clathrate.*

closed-chain c. see under *chain.*

condensation c. a compound that is formed by union of substances with the loss of one or more molecules, usually of low molecular weight, as water or ammonia.

cyclic c. a closed-chain compound; see *closed chain,* under *chain.*

diazo c. a compound containing the group $—N_2—$.

endothermic c. a compound whose formation takes place with absorption of heat from the environment.

energy-rich c's high-energy c's.

exothermic c. a compound whose formation is accompanied by loss of heat to the environment.

genetic c. a genotype in which there are two different mutant alleles at a locus, or a phenotype produced by such a genotype.

Grignard c. see under *reagent.*

heterocyclic c. a chemical substance that contains a ring-shaped nucleus composed of dissimilar elements.

high-energy c's compounds containing high-energy bonds (q.v.); because they yield high levels of free energy on hydrolysis, the compounds are basic to the energy supply of living organisms. Important classes include acid anhydrides (e.g., adenosine triphosphate, aminoacyl adenylates), enol phosphates (e.g., phospho*enol*pyruvate), thioesters (e.g., acetyl coenzyme A), and phosphagens (e.g., phosphocreatine). Called also *energy-rich c's.*

Hurler-Scheie c. see under *syndrome.*

inorganic c. a compound that contains no carbon, except for binary compounds such as carbon oxides and carbon disulfide; ternary compounds such as metallic cyanides, metallic carbonyls, and phosgene; and the metallic carbonates.

isocyclic c. a chemical substance that contains a ring-shaped nucleus composed of the same elements throughout.

low-energy c's compounds yielding relatively low levels of free energy on hydrolysis, such as adenosine monophosphate, glucose 1-phosphate, and glucose 6-phosphate. Cf. *high-energy c's.*

nonpolar c's compounds in which electrons are shared equally by the two atoms forming a bond and which therefore do not ionize in solution, e.g., the paraffins, olefins, and cyclic compounds.

occlusion c. clathrate c.

open-chain c. see under *chain.*

organic c. a compound containing carbon, except for certain binary and ternary carbon compounds and metallic carbonates; see also *inorganic c.*

organometallic c. a compound in which carbon is linked to a metal.

polar c's compounds in which the electrons are unequally shared by the two atoms forming the bond and which therefore may act as dipoles or, in some instances, completely ionize. They include the alcohols, water, and ammonia.

quaternary c. a compound composed of four elements.

quaternary ammonium c. an organic compound containing a quaternary ammonium group, a nitrogen atom carrying a single positive charge bonded to four carbon atoms, e.g., choline.

ring c. see *closed chain,* under *chain.*

saturated c. a compound in which the combining capacities of all the elements are satisfied.

substitution c. a compound formed by replacement of elements of a molecule by other elements.

ternary c., tertiary c. a compound composed of three elements.

unsaturated c. a compound in which the combining capacities of all the elements are not satisfied; see *unsaturated.*

com·press (kom′pres) [L. *compressus*] a pad or bolster of folded gauze or other material, applied with pressure; it is sometimes medicated, and may be wet or dry, hot or cold.

com·pres·si·bil·i·ty (kom-pres″ĭ-bil′ĭ-te) 1. the capability of a substance to be condensed or reduced in volume. 2. the volume decrease per unit of a substance produced by a unit increase in pressure.

com·pres·sion (kəm-presh′ən) [L. *compressio,* from *comprimere* to squeeze together] 1. the act of pressing together; an action exerted upon a body by an external force which tends to diminish its volume and augment its density. 2. in embryology, the shortening or omission of certain stages during development.

c. of the brain cerebral c.

cardiac c. see under *massage.*

cerebral c. any condition in which the brain is compressed, such as by a tumor or other mass, blood clot, or abscess. Called also *c. of the brain.*

cervicomedullary c. compression of the spinal cord at the cervicomedullary junction; this often occurs in children with achondroplasia.

digital c. compression of a blood vessel by the fingers for the purpose of checking hemorrhage.

instrumental c. compression of a blood vessel by instruments.

median nerve c. median neuropathy in which the nerve is compressed.

nerve c. entrapment of a nerve; cf. *entrapment neuropathy.*

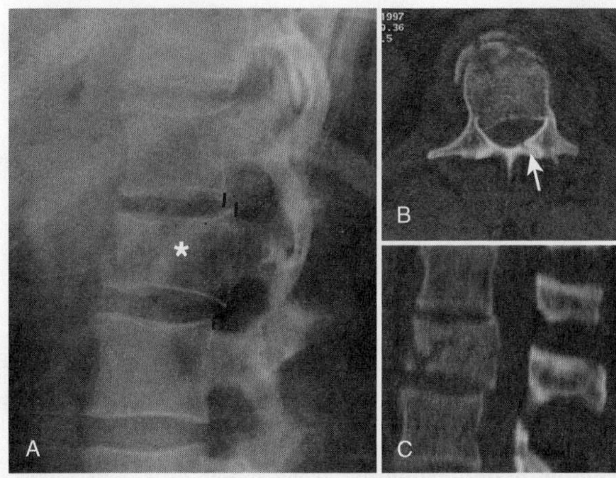

■ Spinal compression from traumatic compression fracture of the first lumbar vertebra (L1). *(A)*, Lateral x-ray of the thoracolumbar junction shows compression fracture of the vertebral body *(asterisk)* with decreased vertebra height and anterior inferior corner fracture; *(B)*, axial and *(C)*, sagittal reconstructed CT scans show the degree of canal narrowing secondary to the retropulsed fragment and reveal a left laminar fracture *(B, arrow)*.

spinal c., spinal cord c. a condition in which pressure is exerted on the spinal cord, as by a tumor, spinal fracture, etc.; its manifestations, which vary with location and degree of pressure, may include pain, paresthesias, and sensory and motor disturbances.

com•pres•sor (kəm-pres′ər) [L.] 1. an instrument that compresses a vessel. 2. a muscle that compresses or presses down on a part; see also *constrictor*.

Deschamps c. an instrument for the direct compression of an artery.

c. na′ris pars transversa musculi nasalis.

Sehrt c. see under *clamp*.

shot c. a forceps for compressing split shot applied to sutures; see also *shotted suture*, under *suture*.

c. ure′thrae musculus compressor urethrae.

c. vagi′nae the musculus bulbospongiosus in the female.

com•pres•so•ri•um (kom″pres-or′e-əm) pl. *compresso′ria* [L.] a device for applying graduated pressure upon objects under microscopic examination.

Com•pro (kom′pro) trademark for a preparation of prochlorperazine.

Comp•ton effect, scattering (komp′tən) [Arthur Holly *Compton*, American physicist, 1892–1962; winner of the Nobel prize in physics for 1927] see under *effect* and *scattering*.

com•pul•sion (kəm-pul′shən) 1. a persistent and irresistible impulse to perform an irrational, ritualistic, or apparently useless act. 2. a compulsive act or ritual; a repetitive and stereotyped action, such as hand-washing, touching, counting, or checking, that is engaged in for an unknown or unconscious purpose.

repetition c. in psychoanalytic theory, the impulse to reenact earlier emotional experiences or traumatic behavior.

com•pul•sive (kom-pul′siv) 1. pertaining to or characterized by compulsion. 2. perfectionistic, rigid, stubborn, indecisive, preoccupied with work; the personality traits of obsessive-compulsive personality disorder.

Com•tan (kom′tan) trademark for a preparation of entacapone.

Com•vax (kom′vaks) trademark for a combination preparation of *Haemophilus* b conjugate vaccine and hepatitis B vaccine (recombinant).

con- [L., from *cum* with] a prefix meaning with or together. It appears as *co-* before a vowel or *h; l* before another *l; m* before *b, m*, or *p;* and *r* before another *r*.

ConA concanavalin A.

co•nal (ko′nəl) pertaining to a conus, such as the conus arteriosus or conus medullaris.

con•al•bu•min (kon″al-bu′min) a glucoprotein, formed by the acidification of egg white to pH 3.9, containing 2.1 per cent of mannose and 0.7 per cent of galactose; the noncrystalline part of egg albumin.

co•na•tion (ko-na′shən) in psychology, the power that impels to effort of any kind; the conscious tendency to act.

con•a•tive (kon′ə-tiv) pertaining to the basic strivings of a person, as expressed by behavior and actions.

con•a•van•ine (kon″ə-van′in) a basic amino acid from soybean meal, α-amino-γ-guanidinoxybutyric acid.

c-*onc* (se′onk″) [cellular *onc*ogene] a proto-oncogene that has been activated within the host so that oncogenicity results. Cf. *v-onc*.

con•ca•nav•a•lin A (ConA) (kon″kə-nav′ə-lin) [*con-* + *canavalin*] a lectin isolated from the jack bean; it is a hemagglutinin that agglutinates mammalian erythrocytes and a mitogen that stimulates predominantly T lymphocytes.

con•cas•sa•tion (kon″kə-sa′shən) the act of breaking up roots or woods into small pieces in order that their active principles may be more easily extracted by solvents.

con•cat•e•nate (kən-kat′ə-nāt) [*con-* + L. *catena* chain] to fasten or link together, as in a chain.

con•cat•e•na•tion (kən-kat″ə-na′shən) a series of events or objects occurring together or in sequence.

Con•ca•to disease (kon-kah′tō) [Luigi Maria *Concato*, Italian physician, 1825–1882] see under *disease*.

con•cave (kon-kāv′) [L. *concavus*] having a rounded, somewhat depressed surface, resembling the hollowed inner surface of a segment of a sphere.

con•cav•i•ty (kon-kav′ĭ-te) [*con-* + *cavity*] a hollowed-out area on the surface of an organ or other structure.

con•ca•vo•con•cave (kən-ka″vo-kon′kāv) concave on each of two opposite surfaces.

con•ca•vo•con•vex (kən-ka″vo-kon′veks) concave on one surface and convex on the opposite one.

con•ceive (kən-sēv′) 1. to become pregnant. 2. to take in, grasp, or form in the mind.

con•cen•trate (kon′sən-trāt) [*con-* + *centrum*] 1. to bring to a common center; to gather together at one point. 2. to increase the strength by diminishing the bulk of, as of a liquid; to condense. 3. a drug or other preparation that has been strengthened by the evaporation of its nonactive parts.

activated prothrombin complex c. (APCC) anti-inhibitor coagulant complex.

lactulose c. [USP] a solution of sugars prepared from lactose, consisting principally of lactulose, with small quantities of lactose and galactose and traces of other related sugars and water. See also under *solution*.

plant protease c. bromelains.

prothrombin complex c. (PCC) factor IX complex.

con•cen•tra•tion (kon″sən-tra′shən) [L. *concentratio*] 1. increase in strength by evaporation. 2. the ratio of the mass or volume of a solute to the mass or volume of the solution or solvent. Cf. *molarity, molality, normality*, and *mole fraction*.

hydrogen ion c. the degree of concentration of hydrogen ions in a solution; it is inversely related to the pH of the solution by the equation $[H^+] = 10^{-pH}$.

ionic c. the number of moles of an ion that are contained in the unit volume of a solution or in the unit mass of solvent.

mass c. the mass of a constituent substance divided by the volume of the mixture, as milligrams per liter (mg/L), etc.

maximum cell (MC) c. the maximum number of microorganisms that can be produced in a given volume of culture medium.

maximum urinary c. (MUC) the highest attainable concentration of a solute or of the collective solutes of the urine, normally about 1200 mOsm/kg H_2O.

mean corpuscular hemoglobin c. (MCHC) the average hemoglobin concentration in erythrocytes, conventionally expressed in "per cent" meaning grams per deciliter of red cells, obtained by dividing the blood hemoglobin concentration (in g/dL) by the hematocrit (in L/L): MCHC = Hb/Hct.

minimal alveolar c. (MAC) the alveolar concentration of anesthetic that at a pressure of 1 atmosphere produces immobility in 50 per cent of subjects exposed to a noxious stimulus.

minimal bactericidal c. (MBC) the lowest concentration of a given antimicrobial agent required to kill almost all members of a given species of microorganism. Called also *minimal lethal c.*

minimal inhibitory c. (MIC) the lowest concentration of a given antimicrobial agent that inhibits the growth of almost all members of a given species of microorganism.

minimal lethal c. (MLC) minimal bactericidal c.

molar c. (*c*) the concentration of a substance expressed in terms of molarity. See *molar*[1].

mutant prevention c. the concentration of an antimicrobial agent that prevents mutation of a given bacteria that would lead to its developing resistance; this should be approximately equal to the minimal inhibitory concentration of the least susceptible of the mutants of the bacteria.

con•cen•tric (kən-sen′trik) [L. *concentricus*, from *con-* together + *centrum* center] having a common center; extending out equally in all directions from a common center.

con•cept (kon'sept) the image of a thing as held in the mind.

con•cep•tion (kən-sep'shən) [L. *conceptio*] 1. an imprecise term denoting the formation of a viable zygote. 2. concept.
 assisted c. assisted reproductive technology.

con•cep•tive (kən-sep'tiv) 1. pertaining to conception. 2. fertile (def. 1).

con•cep•tus (kən-sep'təs) [L.] the product of the union of oocyte and spermatozoon at any stage of development from fertilization until birth, including extraembryonic membranes as well as the embryo or fetus.

Con•cer•ta (kon-sur'tə) trademark for preparations of methylphenidate hydrochloride.

con•cha (kong'kə) pl. *con'chae* [L., from Gr. *konchē*] 1. a shell. 2. in anatomical nomenclature, a structure or part that resembles a sea shell in shape.
 c. auri'culae [TA], **c. auricula'ris** concha of auricle: the hollow of the auricle of the external ear, bounded anteriorly by the tragus and posteriorly by the antihelix.
 c. bullo'sa a cystic distention of the middle nasal concha, sometimes seen in chronic rhinitis.
 ethmoidal c., inferior c. nasi media.
 ethmoidal c., superior c. nasi superior.
 ethmoidal c., supreme c. nasi suprema.
 nasal c., inferior c. nasi inferior.
 nasal c., middle c. nasi media.
 nasal c., superior c. nasi superior.
 nasal c., supreme c. nasi suprema.
 c. nasa'lis infe'rior [TA] c. nasi inferior.
 c. nasa'lis me'dia [TA] c. nasi media.
 c. nasa'lis supe'rior [TA] c. nasi superior.
 c. nasa'lis supre'ma [TA] c. nasi suprema.
 c. na'si infe'rior [TA] inferior nasal concha: a thin bony plate with curved margins, articulating with the ethmoid, maxilla, and lacrimal and palatine bones, and forming the lower part of the lateral wall of the nasal cavity, and the mucous membrane covering the plate; called also *c. nasalis inferior* [TA], *inferior turbinate bone*, and *inferior turbinate*.
 c. na'si me'dia [TA] middle nasal concha: the lower of two bony plates projecting from the inner wall of the ethmoid labyrinth and separating the superior from the middle meatus of the nose, and the mucous membrane covering the plate; called also *c. nasalis media* [TA], *inferior ethmoidal c.*, *ethmoid cornu*, *middle turbinate bone*, and *middle turbinate*.
 c. na'si supe'rior [TA] superior nasal concha: the upper of two bony plates projecting from the inner wall of the ethmoid labyrinth and forming the upper boundary of the superior meatus of the nose, and the mucous membrane covering the plate. Called also *c. nasalis superior* [TA], *superior ethmoidal c.*, *superior turbinate bone*, and *superior turbinate*.
 c. na'si supre'ma [TA] supreme nasal concha: a thin bony plate occasionally found projecting from the inner wall of the ethmoid labyrinth above the bony superior nasal concha, and the mucous membrane covering the plate; called also *c. nasalis suprema* [TA], *highest* or *supreme turbinate bone*, *supreme ethmoidal c.*, and *supreme turbinate*.
 nasoturbinal c. agger nasi.
 c. sphenoida'lis [TA] sphenoidal concha: a thin curved plate of bone at the anterior and lower part of the body of the sphenoid bone, on either side, forming part of the roof of the nasal cavity; called also *sphenoturbinal bone* or *ossicle* and *Bertin bone* or *ossicle*.

con•chae (kong'ke) [L.] genitive and plural of *concha*.

con•chi•form (kong'kĭ-form) [*concha* + *form*] shaped like one half of a bivalve shell.

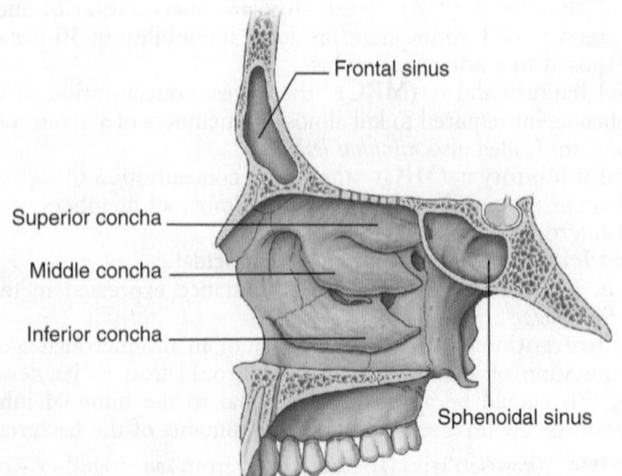

■ Nasal conchae; paramedian view of right nasal cavity.

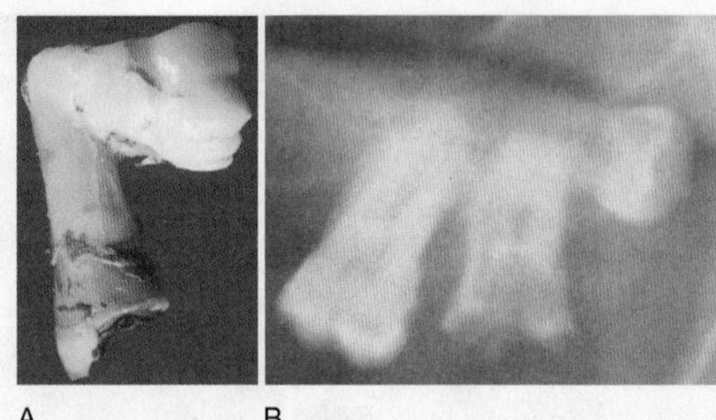

■ Concrescence in an area of cemental repair previously damaged by a periapical inflammatory lesion. Clinical specimen *(A)* and radiograph *(B)* show union by cementum of the maxillary second and third molars, with a large carious defect of the second molar.

con•chio•lin•os•teo•my•eli•tis (kong-ki″ə-lin-os″te-o-mi″ə-li'tis) a form of osteomyelitis occurring in pearl workers.

con•chi•tis (kong-ki'tis) an inflammation of a concha.

con•choi•dal (kong-koi'dəl) like a shell.

con•cho•scope (kong'ko-skōp) [*concha* + *-scope*] a speculum for examining the walls of the nasal cavity.

con•cho•tome (kong'ko-tōm) [*concha* + *-tome*] turbinotome.

con•chot•o•my (kong-kot'ə-me) turbinotomy.

Concis. [L.] conci'sus (cut).

con•cli•na•tion (kon″klĭ-na'shən) intorsion.

con•coc•tion (kən-kok'shən) [L. *concoctio*, from *con-* + *coquere* to cook] a mixture of medicinal substances usually prepared with the aid of heat.

con•com•i•tant (kən-kom'ĭ-tənt) [L. *concomitans*, from *cum* together + *comes* companion] accompanying; accessory; joined with another. Cf. *concurrent*.

con•cor•dance (kən-kor'dəns) [L. *concordare* to agree] in genetics, the occurrence of a given trait in both members of a twin pair, as opposed to discordance.

con•cor•dant (kən-kor'dənt) 1. exhibiting concordance. 2. belonging to closely related species; said of transplanted tissue. See under *xenograft*.

con•cre•ment (kon'krə-mənt) [L. *concrementum*, from *concrescere* to grow together] a concretion, especially a calcified tubercle or similar mass.

con•cres•cence (kən-kres'əns) [*con-* + L. *crescere* to grow] 1. a growing together; a union of parts originally separate. 2. in embryology, the flowing together and piling up of cells. 3. in dentistry, the union of the roots of two approximating teeth by a deposit of cementum.

con•cre•tio (kən-kre'she-o) [L.] concretion.
 c. cor'dis, c. pericar'dii a form of adhesive pericarditis in which the pericardial cavity is obliterated.

con•cre•tion (kən-kre'shən) [L. *concretio*, from *concrescere* to grow together] 1. a calculus or inorganic mass in a natural cavity or in tissue. 2. abnormal union of adjacent parts. 3. the process of becoming harder or more solid.
 conjunctival c's a condition marked by the formation of white, calcareous concretions in the acini of the meibomian glands; called also *lithiasis conjunctivae* and *conjunctival lithiasis*.
 preputial c. see under *calculus*.
 prostatic c's see under *calculus*.

con•cur•rent (kon-kur'ənt) happening at the same time; simultaneous. Cf. *concomitant*.

con•cus•sion (kən-kush'ən) [L. *concussio*] a violent jar or shock, or the condition which results from such an injury. **concus'sional, concus'sive** *adj*
 air c. see *blast*[2].
 c. of the brain loss of consciousness as the result of a blow to the head or sudden movement of the brain within the head as from violent shaking of the head. In *mild concussion* there is transient loss of consciousness with possible impairment of higher mental functions, such as retrograde amnesia and emotional lability. In *severe concussion* there is prolonged unconsciousness with impairment of the functions of the brainstem, such as transient loss of respiratory reflex, vasomotor activity, and dilatation of the pupils. Cf. *brain contusion*, under *contusion*.
 hydraulic abdominal c. abdominal injury produced in persons in the water by violent underwater explosions.
 c. of the labyrinth trauma to the labyrinth, usually from a blow on or explosion near the ear, resulting in tinnitus and deafness.
 pulmonary c. mechanical damage to the lungs produced by an explosion. See *blast chest*, under *chest* and *blast injury*, under *injury*.

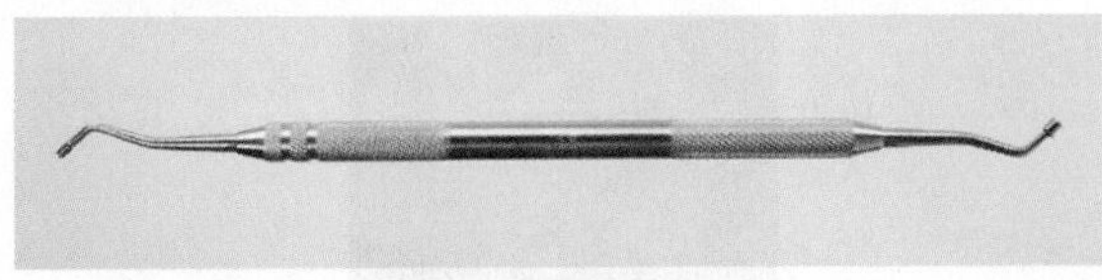

■ Condenser.

c. of the retina commotio retinae.

c. of the spinal cord transient spinal cord dysfunction due to mechanical injury.

con·den·sa·tion (kon″dən-sa′shən) [L. *condensare* to pack close together] 1. compression. 2. the packing of dental filling material into a prepared tooth cavity. 3. a mental process in which one symbol stands for a number of components and contains all the emotion associated with them. 4. conversion from the gaseous state to the liquid state (liquefaction) or solid state (solidification).

con·den·ser (kən-den′sər) [L. *condensare* to make thick, press close together] 1. a vessel or apparatus for condensing gases or vapors. 2. the lens in a microscope located just above the light source that aligns all available light into one beam. 3. an apparatus by which charges of electricity can be accumulated, consisting of two conducting surfaces separated by a nonconductor. 4. in dentistry, an instrument used to pack a plastic filling material into the prepared cavity of a tooth.

Abbe c. as originally designed, a two-lens condenser combination placed below the stage of a microscope.

automatic c. mechanical c.

back-action c. a condenser with a U-shaped shank so that the force applied is toward the operator. Called also *reverse c.*

cardioid c. a special type of condenser for illuminating a specimen in darkfield microscopy.

darkfield c. a condenser with a central stop, permitting production of a hollow cone of light having its apex in the plane of the specimen.

foot c. a condenser with a long, angled, foot-shaped nib.

gold c. a condenser for compacting gold filling material into the prepared cavity in dental restorations.

mechanical c. a condenser equipped with a spring-activated, pneumatic, or electronic mechanism for compacting the restorative material in a prepared tooth cavity through repeated blows. Called also *automatic c.*

paraboloid c. a special type of condenser for illuminating a specimen in darkfield microscopy.

reverse c. back-action c.

con·den·sin (kən-den′sin) a protein complex consisting of five polypeptides that binds to chromatin during mitosis, using the energy from ATP hydrolysis to produce supercoiling of DNA.

con·di·tion (kən-dish′ən) to train; to subject to conditioning.

con·di·tion·ing (kən-dish′ən-ing) 1. learning in which a stimulus initially incapable of evoking a certain response acquires the ability to do so by repeated pairing with another stimulus that does elicit the response. Called also *classical c., pavlovian c.,* and *respondent c.* 2. in physical medicine, improvement of physical condition with a program of exercises; called also *physical c.*

aversive c. learning in which punishment or other unpleasant stimulation is used to associate negative feelings with an undesirable response and so reduce the frequency of that response.

avoidance c. a form of operant conditioning in which an organism is trained to avoid certain responses or situations associated with negative consequences.

classical c. conditioning (def. 1).

instrumental c. learning in which the frequency of a particular voluntary response is altered by the application of positive or negative consequences; called also *operant c.*

operant c. instrumental c.

pavlovian c. conditioning (def. 1).

physical c. conditioning (def. 2).

respondent c. conditioning (def. 1).

con·dom (kon′dəm) [L. *condus* a receptacle; according to some authorities a corruption of *Condon,* the inventor] a sheath or cover worn over the penis during sexual activity to prevent impregnation or infection.

female c. a sheath worn inside the vagina, also extending outward to cover the vulva; used to prevent pregnancy or transmission of infection.

con·duc·tance (G) (kən-duk′təns) [L. *conducere* to lead together] capacity for conducting or ability to convey; the unit of electrical conductance is the siemens.

airway c. the reciprocal of airway resistance: the air flow divided by the mouth-to-alveoli pressure difference.

con·duc·tion (kən-duk′shən) the transfer of sound waves, heat, nervous impulses, or electricity; see also under *system.*

aberrant c. cardiac conduction through pathways not normally conducting cardiac impulses, particularly through ventricular tissue.

aerial c. air c.

aerotympanal c. the conduction of sound to the internal ear through the air and tympanum.

air c. the conduction of sound to the internal ear through the external auditory canal and middle ear.

anomalous c. conduction of the sinus impulse over accessory conducting pathways, thus avoiding the delay in passage through the normal atrioventricular node.

anterograde c. transmission of a cardiac impulse in the normal direction, from the sinus node to the ventricles; used particularly to describe forward conduction through the atrioventricular node.

antidromic c. the conduction of a nerve impulse in a direction contrary to the normal direction, as occurs in experimental conduction studies. It may occur naturally in some neurons of the dorsal roots of the spinal cord, although evidence suggests that the phenomenon may actually result from ephaptic transmission rather than backward transmission.

atrioventricular c., AV c. the normal conduction of atrial impulses in the heart, passing through the atrioventricular node and the His-Purkinje system to the ventricles.

avalanche c. the conduction of nerve impulses which takes place when the terminals of one neuron come in contact with the bodies of several neurons, resulting in widespread discharge following relatively little input.

bone c. the conduction of sound to the internal ear through the bones of the skull; called also *cranial c., osteotympanic c.,* and *tissue c.*

concealed c. incomplete penetration of a propagating impulse through the cardiac conducting system such that electrocardiograms reveal no evidence of transmission but the behavior of one or more subsequent impulses is somehow affected.

concealed retrograde c. retrograde conduction blocked in the atrioventricular node; it does not produce an extra P wave but leaves the node refractory to the next normal sinus beat, manifest as lengthening of the PR interval of that beat.

cranial c. bone c.

decremental c. the delay or failure of propagation of an impulse in the atrioventricular node resulting from progressive decrease in the rate of the rise and amplitude of the action potential as it spreads through the node.

delayed c. slowed cardiac impulse propagation resulting in an interval greater than 0.2 second between atrial and ventricular contractions, as occurs in first degree heart block.

direct bone c. the conduction of sound to to the internal ear from a hearing aid implanted into the skull.

ephaptic c. the conduction of a nerve impulse across an ephapse, as opposed to synaptic conduction.

osteotympanic c. bone c.

retrograde c. transmission of a cardiac impulse backward in the ventricular to atrial direction; particularly, conduction from the atrioventricular node into the atria.

saltatory c. the rapid passage of a potential from node (of Ranvier) to node of a myelinated nerve fiber, rather than along the full length of the membrane.

synaptic c. the conduction of a nerve impulse across a synapse.

tissue c. bone c.

ventriculoatrial c. retrograde conduction, specifically that in which the impulse is conducted from ventricles to atria.

volume c. in electromyography, the loss of measurable action potential because of spreading of current away from the source through conducting media such as extracellular fluid.

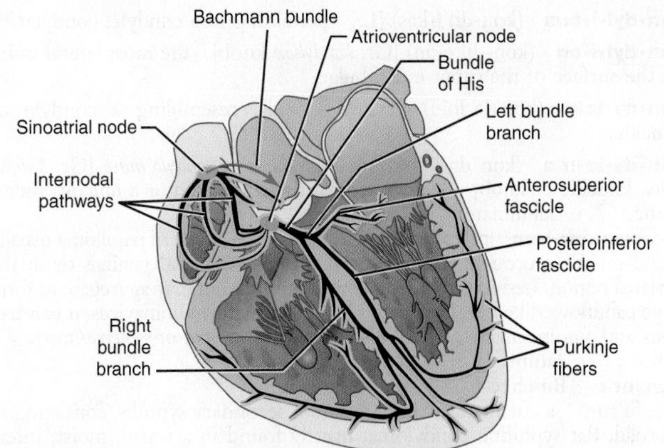

■ Diagrammatic view of the conducting system of the heart, showing the pathways of anterograde conduction of the cardiac impulse.

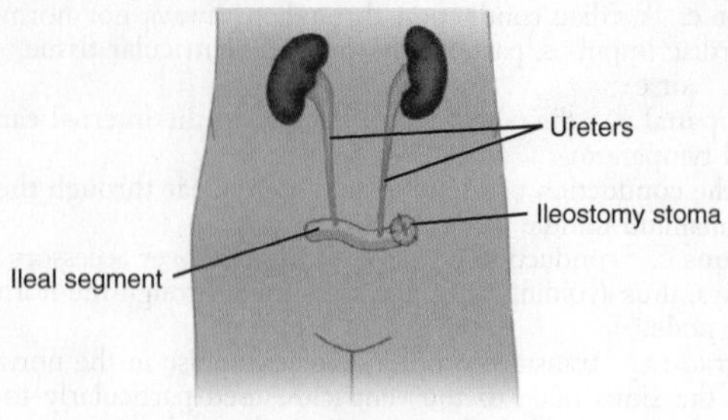

■ Ileal conduit.

con•duc•tiv•i•ty (kon″dək-tiv′ĭ-te) the capacity of a body to transmit a flow of electricity or heat; it is the conductance per unit area of the body. When expressed in figures, electrical conductivity is the reciprocal of resistivity.

con•duc•tor (kən-duk′tər) 1. a material that possesses conductivity; a substance that transmits electricity. 2. grooved director.

con•du•it (kon′doo-it) channel (def. 1).

ileal c., ureteroileal c. a type of urinary diversion consisting of surgical anastomosis of the ureters to one end of a detached segment of ileum, the other end being used to form a stoma on the abdominal wall (see *uretero-ileostomy*). Called also *ureteroileal anastomosis.*

con•du•pli•ca•to cor•po•re (kən-doo″plĭ-ka′to kor′por-e) [L. "with the body doubled up"] a doubled-up attitude of a fetus in shoulder presentation.

con•du•ran•gin (kon″du-rang′gin) either of two glycosides from condurango; in large amounts they are poisonous but in small amounts they are used as a bitter in homeopathy.

con•du•ran•go (kon″du-rang′go) [Spanish American] 1. *Marsdenia condurango.* 2. the bark of *Marsdenia condurango,* which contains condurangin and is normally poisonous but has been used as a bitter in homeopathy.

con•dy•lar•thro•sis (kon″dəl-ahr-thro′sis) [*condyle* + *arthrosis* (def. 1)] articulatio ellipsoidea.

con•dyle (kon′dīl) condylus. **con′dylar** *adj*

external c. of femur condylus lateralis femoris.
external c. of tibia condylus lateralis tibiae.
fibular c. of femur condylus lateralis femoris.
c. of humerus condylus humeri.
internal c. of femur condylus medialis femoris.
internal c. of tibia condylus medialis tibiae.
lateral c. of femur condylus lateralis femoris.
lateral c. of tibia condylus lateralis tibiae.
mandibular c. processus condylaris mandibulae.
medial c. of femur condylus medialis femoris.
medial c. of tibia condylus medialis tibiae.
occipital c. condylus occipitalis.
c. of scapula angulus lateralis scapulae.
tibial c. of femur condylus medialis femoris.

con•dy•lec•to•my (kon″dəl-ek′tə-me) [*condyle* + *-ectomy*] excision of a condyle.

con•dy•li (kon′də-li) [L.] genitive and plural of *condylus.*

con•dyl•i•cus (kon-dil′ĭ-kəs) [L.] pertaining to a condyle; condylar.

con•dyl•i•on (kon-dil′e-ən) [Gr. *kondylion* knob] the most lateral point on the surface of the caput mandibulae.

con•dy•loid (kon′də-loid) [*condyle* + *-oid*] resembling a condyle or knuckle.

con•dy•lo•ma (kon″də-lo′mə) pl. *condylomas* or *condylo′mata* [Gr. *kondylōma,* knuckle or knob] 1. a warty growth on the skin or a mucous membrane. 2. c. acuminatum.

c. acumina′tum pl. *condylo′mata acumina′ta.* a type of papilloma usually found on the mucous membrane or skin of the external genitals or in the perianal region. Lesions are usually few in number but may aggregate to form large cauliflowerlike masses. Caused by the human papillomavirus, it is infectious and autoinoculable. Called also *acuminate, genital,* or *venereal wart.*

flat c. c. latum.

giant c. Buschke-Löwenstein tumor.

c. la′tum a cutaneous manifestation of secondary syphilis, consisting of a broad, flat syphilitic condyloma, usually found in a warm, moist, intertriginous area, such as around the anus or external genitals. It may become hypertrophic and erode to form a soft, red mass with a moist, weeping surface. Called also *flat c.*

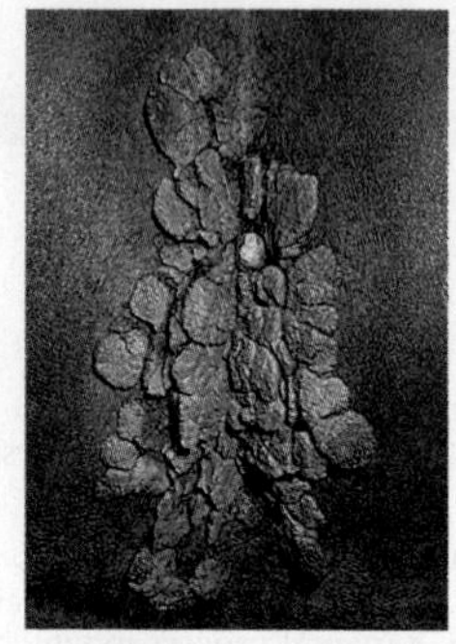
■ Condylomata acuminata in the perianal region.

pointed c. c. acuminatum.

con•dy•lo•ma•ta (kon″də-lo′mə-tə) [L.] plural of *condyloma.*

con•dy•lo•ma•toid (kon″də-lo′mə-toid) resembling a condyloma.

con•dy•lo•ma•to•sis (kon″də-lo″mə-to′sis) the presence of numerous condylomas.

con•dy•lom•a•tous (kon″də-lom′ə-təs) of the nature of a condyloma.

con•dy•lot•o•my (kon″də-lot′ə-me) [*condyle* + *-tomy*] surgical incision or division of a condyle or of condyles.

Con•dy•lox (kon′də-loks) trademark for preparations of podofilox.

con•dy•lus (kon′də-ləs) pl. *con′dyli* [L., from Gr. *kondylos* knuckle] [TA] condyle: a rounded projection on a bone, usually for articulation with another.

c. hu′meri [TA] condyle of humerus: the distal end of the humerus, including the various fossae as well as the trochlea and capitulum.

c. latera′lis fe′moris [TA] lateral condyle of femur: the lateral of the two surfaces at the distal end of the femur that articulate with the superior surfaces of the head of the tibia; called also *external* or *fibular condyle of femur.*

c. latera′lis ti′biae [TA] lateral condyle of tibia: the lateral articular eminence on the proximal end of the tibia; called also *external condyle of tibia.*

c. media′lis fe′moris [TA] medial condyle of femur: the medial of the two surfaces at the distal end of the femur that articulate with the superior surfaces of the head of the tibia; called also *internal* or *tibial condyle of femur.*

c. media′lis ti′biae [TA] medial condyle of tibia: the medial articular eminence on the proximal end of the tibia; called also *internal condyle of tibia.*

c. occipita′lis [TA] occipital condyle: one of two oval processes on the lateral portions of the occipital bone, on either side of the foramen magnum, for articulation with the atlas.

cone (kōn) [L. *conus,* from Gr. *konos*] 1. a solid figure or body with a circular base tapering to a point; called also *conus* [TA]. 2. retinal c. 3. in radiology, a conical or open-ended cylindrical structure formerly used as an aid in centering the radiation beam and as a guide to source-to-film distance. Cones were commonly attached to the x-ray tube prior to the use of the collimator. 4. in root canal therapy, a solid substance with a tapered form, usually made of gutta-percha or silver, fashioned to conform to the shape of a root canal. 5. a marine snail of the family Conidae.

arterial c. conus arteriosus.

attraction c. fertilization c.

bifurcation c. the cone-shaped structure at the bifurcation of a dendrite.

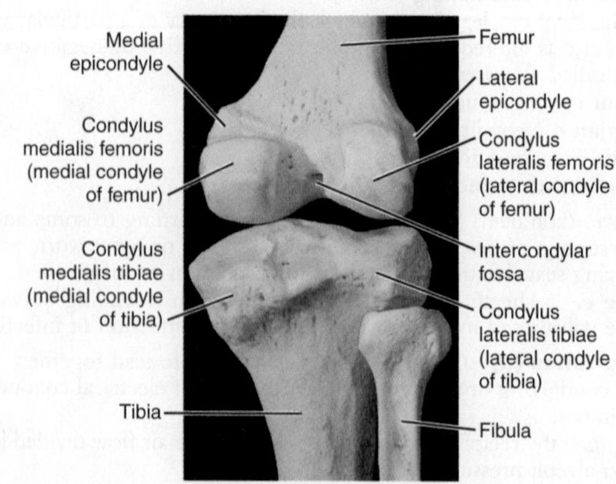

■ Posterior view of right knee, showing the medial and lateral condyles of the femur and tibia.

cerebellar pressure c. a deformity of the brain caused by increased intracranial pressure, which forces the cerebellar tonsils downward into the spinal canal.

ectoplacental c. the thickened trophoblast of the blastocyst in rodents that becomes the fetal portion of the placenta.

elastic c. conus elasticus.

ether c. an apparatus placed over the face for the administration of ether by inhalation.

fertilization c. a bulging of the cytoplasm in the oocyte at the site of contact of a spermatozoon, which gradually engulfs the spermatozoon and then retracts, carrying the spermatozoon inward; called also *attraction c.*

growth c. a bulbous enlargement of the growing tip of an axon.

gutta-percha c. in root canal therapy, a plastic radiopaque cone made from gutta-percha combined with other ingredients, available in standard sizes conforming to the dimensions of root canal reamers and files; used to fill and seal the canal in conjunction with sealer cements. Called also *gutta-percha point.*

implantation c. axon hillock.

c. of light the triangular reflection of light seen on the membrana tympani; called also *Politzer c.* and *light reflex.*

long c. in dental radiology, a tubular cone (see *cone*, def. 3) designed to establish an extended anode-to-skin distance, usually in a range of 10 to 25 cm or more.

medullary c. conus medullaris.

ocular c. a group of light rays in a cone shape within the eye, having its base on the cornea and its apex on the retina. Called also *visual c.*

Politzer c. c. of light.

pressure c. the area of compression exerted by a mass in the brain, as in uncal or transtentorial herniation.

retinal c. one of the two types of visual cells, along with retinal rods, having synapses internally with bipolar retinal cells. Cones serve light and color vision and visual acuity. Their synaptic terminals are broad, flattened pedicles. Those outside the fovea centralis have dendritic inner segments that are relatively short and squat with blunt, rounded tips; those within the fovea centralis have inner segments that are more elongated and narrow, so that these cones resemble rods. There are 6 million to 7 million cones, of which about 10 per cent are concentrated in the fovea centralis and the remainder are distributed fairly uniformly over the rest of the retina. Called also *cone* and *cone cell.*

sarcoplasmic c. the conical mass of sarcoplasm at each end of the nucleus of a smooth or cardiac muscle fiber.

short c. in dental radiology, a conical or tubular cone (see *cone*, def. 3) having as one of its functions the establishment of an anode-to-skin distance of up to 10 to 25 cm.

silver c. see under *point.*

terminal c. of spinal cord conus medullaris.

twin c's cone cells of the retina in which two cells are blended.

Tyndall c. the murky cone of scattered light seen when a colloid is viewed at right angles to the incident beam, due to the Tyndall effect; it distinguishes colloids from crystalloids.

visual c. 1. ocular c. 2. retinal c.

cone-nose (kōn′nōs″) cone-nose bug.

co•nex•us (kə-nek′səs) pl. *conex′us* [L. "connection," from *conectere* to join together] connexus.

co•ney (ko′ne) hyrax.

con•fab•u•la•tion (kon″fab-u-la′shən) [L. *confabulari* to converse together] unconscious filling in of gaps in memory with fabricated facts and experiences, most commonly associated with organic pathology. It differs from lying in that the patient has no intention to deceive and believes the fabricated memories to be real. Called also *fabrication* and *fabulation.*

con•fec•tion (kən-fek′shən) [L. *confectio*] electuary.

c. of senna a mild laxative containing powdered senna with other ingredients.

con•fer•tus (kən-fur′təs) [L.] close together; confluent.

con•fi•den•ti•al•i•ty (kon″fĭ-den″she-al′ĭ-te) the principle in medical ethics that the information a patient reveals to a health care provider is private and has limits on how and when it can be disclosed to a third party; usually the provider must obtain permission from the patient to make such a disclosure.

con•fig•u•ra•tion (kən-fig″u-ra′shən) 1. the arrangement of parts of a whole. 2. in chemistry, the spatial arrangement of atoms in a molecule, the property that distinguishes a compound from its stereoisomers. Cf. *constitution.*

***cis* c.** in genetics, arrangement of two or more loci, especially pseudoalleles, occurring on the same chromosome of a homologous pair. Cf. *trans c.*

***trans* c.** in genetics, arrangement of two or more loci, especially pseudoalleles, on opposite chromosomes of a homologous pair. Cf. *cis c.*

con•flict (kon′flikt) in psychiatry, a psychic struggle, often unconscious, arising from the clash of incompatible or opposing impulses, wishes, drives, or external demands.

approach-approach c. conflict resulting from two available goals which are desirable but incompatible.

approach-avoidance c. conflict resulting from a single goal having both desirable and undesirable consequences or qualities.

avoidance-avoidance c. conflict resulting from the desire to avoid two equally distasteful alternatives.

extrapsychic c. conflict between a person's wishes or needs and the expectations or desires of others.

intrapersonal c. intrapsychic c.

intrapsychic c. conflict between incompatible and often unconscious wishes, impulses, needs, thoughts, or demands within one's own mind. Called also *intrapersonal c.*

con•flu•ence (kon′floo-əns) [L. *confluens* running together] 1. a place of running together; the meeting of streams. 2. in embryology, the flowing of cells, a component process of gastrulation.

c. of sinuses confluens sinuum.

con•flu•ens (kon′floo-əns) [L., from *confluere* to run together] confluence.

c. si′nuum [TA] confluence of (venous) sinuses: the dilated point of confluence of the superior sagittal, straight, occipital, and two transverse sinuses of the dura mater, lodged in a depression at one side of the internal occipital protuberance; called also *torcular Herophili.*

con•flu•ent (kon′floo-ənt) [L. *confluens* running together] becoming merged; not discrete.

con•fo•cal (kon-fo′kəl) having the same focus.

con•for•ma•tion (kon″for-ma′shən) the particular shape of an entity. In chemistry, the spatial arrangement of atoms in a molecule produced by rotations about single bonds, the property that distinguishes different conformers (conformational isomers) from each other.

con•form•er (kən-for′mər) 1. any of the group of structures that are produced by rotations about single bonds in a molecule. 2. a device that covers the surface of a spherical eye implant, used following enucleation to preserve the shape of the conjunctival fornices prior to the fitting of a cosmetic prosthesis.

con•found•er (kən-foun′dər) a third variable that can indirectly distort the statistical relationship between two variables under manipulation or observation.

con•found•ing (kon-foun′ding) interference by a third variable so as to distort the association being studied between two other variables, because of a strong relationship with both of the other variables; a relationship between two causal factors such that their individual contributions cannot be separated.

con•fri•ca•tion (kon″frĭ-ka′shən) [L. *confricatio*] the rubbing of a drug to the consistency of a powder.

con•fron•ta•tion (kon″frən-ta′shən) [*con-* + *frons* face] the act of facing or being made to face one's own attitudes and shortcomings, the way one is perceived, and the consequences of one's behavior, or of causing another to face these things; a therapeutic technique which demonstrates where change must begin, but which also has destructive potential.

con•fu•sion (kən-fu′zhən) [L. *confusus*, past part. of *confundere* to mix together] disturbed orientation in regard to time, place, or person, sometimes accompanied by disordered consciousness. **confu′sional** *adj*

con•ge•la•tion (kon″jə-la′shən) [L. *congelatio*] 1. a process of freezing. 2. frostbite.

con•ge•ner (kon′jə-nər) [*con-* + *genus* race] 1. something closely related to another thing or derived from the same source or stock, such as a member of the same genus, a muscle having the same function as another, or a chemical compound closely related to another in composition and exerting similar or antagonistic effects. 2. a secondary product in alcohol fermentation that helps to determine the composition of the final product. **congener′ic, congen′erous** *adj*

con•gen•er•ous (kən-jen′ər-əs) [*con-* + *genus* race] having a common action or function; derived from the same source. See *congener.*

con•gen•ic (kən-jen′ik) [*con-* + L. *genus* race, kind] pertaining to two inbred strains of animals that are genetically identical except at a single locus or a small chromosomal segment. A congenic strain is produced by outbreeding an inbred strain and then eliminating the undesired background genes by many generations of backcrosses while maintaining the desired genetic differences by selection of progeny.

con•gen•i•tal (kən-jen′ĭ-təl) [L. *congenitus* born together] existing at, and usually before, birth; referring to conditions that are present at birth, regardless of their causation. Cf. *hereditary.*

con•gest•ed (kən-jest′əd) overloaded, as with blood; in a state of congestion.

con•ges•tin (kən-jes′tin) a toxic substance derived from the tentacles of sea anemones that, when injected into dogs, causes intense congestion of the splanchnic vessels, and hemorrhage; originally called *actinocongestin.*

con•ges•tion (kən-jes′chən) [L. *congestio*, from *congerere* to heap together] excessive or abnormal accumulation of fluid, as of blood in a part. Cf. *hyperemia.* **conges′tive** *adj*

active c. accumulation of blood in a part because of dilatation of the lumen of its supplying blood vessels.

chronic passive c. long-term passive congestion of the liver, most often due to right heart failure, giving it a swollen and mottled appearance *(nutmeg liver).*

functional c. increased vascularization and flow of blood to an organ during the performance of its function. Called also *physiologic c.*

hypostatic c. congestion of the lowest part of an organ simply from the effect of gravity when the circulation is weakened.

neurotonic c. congestion due to irritation of the vasodilator nerves.

passive c. congestion of a part due to obstruction to escape of blood from it; called also *venous c.*

physiologic c. functional c.

pulmonary c. engorgement of the pulmonary vessels, with transudation of fluid into the alveolar and interstitial spaces *(pulmonary edema)*; it occurs in cardiac disease, infections, and certain injuries.

venous c. passive c.

con•glo•bate (kon′glo-bāt) [L. *conglobatus*] forming a rounded mass or clump; said of certain glands and of a form of acne.

con•glo•ba•tion (kon″glo-ba′shən) the act of forming, or the state of being formed, into a rounded mass.

con•glom•er•ate (kən-glom′ər-āt) [L. *con-* together + *glomerare* to heap] heaped together.

con•glu•tin (kən-gloo′tin) a protein from almonds and from seeds of various leguminous plants.

con•glu•ti•nant (kən-gloo′tĭ-nənt) [L. *conglutinare* to glue together] promoting union, as of the edges of a wound.

con•glu•ti•na•tio (kən-gloo″tĭ-na′she-o) [L. *conglutinare* to glue together] conglutination (def. 2).

c. orifi′cii exter′ni a condition in labor in which the circular fibers around the cervical os will not relax, and the cervix does not dilate.

con•glu•ti•na•tion (kən-gloo″tĭ-na′shən) 1. agglutination by conglutinin or immunoconglutinin of bacteria or erythrocytes in the presence of specific antibody or complement components. 2. abnormal adhesion; see *adhesion* (def. 2).

con•glu•ti•nin (kən-gloo′tĭ-nin) a nonimmunoglobulin bovine serum protein that aggregates immune complexes with conglutinogen activity (inactivated C3b) in the presence of divalent cations. It has been used as an indicator system, replacing complement fixation, in serologic tests, and in the detection of immune complexes. Not to be confused with *immunoconglutinin.*

immune c. immunoconglutinin.

con•glu•ti•no•gen (kən-gloo′tĭ-no-jən) the capacity of certain immune complexes to react with conglutinin due to the fixation of the complement component C3 and the subsequent inactivation of C3b by factor I (formerly called *conglutinogen-activating factor*).

con•go•phil•ic (kon″go-fil′ik) [*Congo red* + *-philic*] staining with Congo red.

co•ni (ko′ni) [L.] genitive and plural of *conus.*

con•ic (kon′ik) conical.

con•i•cal (kon′ĭ-kəl) cone-shaped.

Co•ni•dae (kon′ĭ-de) the cones, a family of gastropods of the order Neogastropoda that live in warm ocean water. Some members of the genus *Conus* have a poisonous bite.

co•nid•ia (ko-nid′e-ə) [L.] plural of *conidium.*

co•nid•i•al (ko-nid′e-əl) 1. pertaining to or of the nature of conidia. 2. bearing conidia.

co•ni•dio•bo•lo•my•co•sis (kə-nid″e-o-bo″lo-mi-ko′sis) a type of entomophthoromycosis caused by *Conidiobolus coronatus*, usually involving the nose and paranasal sinuses *(rhinoentomophthoromycosis)*. Sometimes, especially in weak or immunocompromised patients, it can spread to the central nervous system and cause fatal rhinocerebral zygomycosis.

Co•ni•dio•bo•lus (ko-nid″e-ob′o-ləs) [*conidium* + Gr. *bolos* a throw] a genus of fungi of the family Entomophthoraceae, having few septa in the mycelium and producing few zygospores but many chlamydospores and a large number of conidia that are ejected from the conidiophores.

C. corona′tus a species that is usually a saprobe but sometimes causes conidiobolomycosis in humans and horses.

C. incon′gruus a species that has been isolated from cases of human conidiobolomycosis.

co•nid•io•gen•e•sis (ko-nid″e-o-jen′ə-sis) the development of conidia; the two principal types are *blastic c.* and *thallic c.*

blastic c. conidiogenesis in which a fertile hypha or conidiogenous cell enlarges or blows out to form a conidium before delimitation by a septa takes place; two types are distinguished, *holoblastic c.* and *enteroblastic c.*

enteroarthric c. thallic-arthric c. in which conidia are formed from only the inner part of the wall of the conidiogenous cell.

enteroblastic c. blastic c. in which only the inner part of the cell wall is used to form the conidium.

holoarthric c. thallic-arthric c. in which conidia are formed from both walls of the conidiogenous cell.

holoblastic c. blastic c. in which all of the cell wall is used to form the conidium.

holothallic c. thallic c. in which just one portion of the conidiogenous cell disarticulates to form a conidium.

thallic c. conidiogenesis in which an entire parent cell becomes a conidium with formation of a septum, without enlargement or new growth. Two types are distinguished: *holothallic c.* and *thallic-arthric c.*

thallic-arthric c. thallic c. in which several conidia form by separation at the septa; two types are distinguished: *enteroarthric c.* and *holoarthric c.*

co•nid•io•gen•ous (kə-nid″e-oj′ə-nəs) producing conidia.

co•ni•di•o•ma (kə-nid″e-o′mə) pl. *conidio′mata.* A specialized, polyhyphal structure bearing conidia.

co•nid•io•phore (ko-nid′e-o-for) [*conidium* + *-phore*] the branch of the mycelium of a fungus that bears conidia.

determinate c. a conidiophore whose growth does not continue after a conidium has started to form.

indeterminate c. a conidiophore that continues to lengthen as sporulation continues.

macronematous c. a conidiophore that is noticeably different morphologically from its hypha.

micronematous c. a conidiophore that is morphologically similar to its hypha.

co•nid•io•spore (ko-nid′e-o-spor) [Gr. *konidion* a particle of dust + *spore*] conidium.

co•nid•i•um (kə-nid′e-əm) pl. *conid′ia* [L., from Gr. *konidion* a particle of dust] An asexual fungal spore that is deciduous (shed at maturity) and formed by budding or splitting off from the summit of a conidiophore. Called also *conidiospore* and *exospore.* See also *aleurioconidium* and *chlamydoconidium.*

co•ni•ine (ko′ne-ēn) a poisonous alkaloid found in *Conium maculatum;* it causes gastrointestinal irritation and paralysis with respiratory failure.

coni(o)- [Gr. *konis* dust] a combining form denoting a relationship to dust.

co•nio•fi•bro•sis (ko″ne-o-fi-bro′sis) [*conio-* + *fibrosis*] a form of pneumoconiosis marked by an exuberant growth of connective tissue caused by a specific irritant, as in asbestosis, silicosis, and silicotuberculosis.

co•ni•ol•o•gy (ko-ne-ol′ə-je) [*conio-* + *-logy*] the scientific study of dust and its influence and its effects on plant and animal life.

co•nio•lymph•sta•sis (ko″ne-o-limf′stə-sis) a form of pneumoconiosis caused by dusts that act by blocking the lymphatics.

co•ni•om•e•ter (ko″ne-om′ə-tər) konimeter.

co•nio•phage (ko′ne-o-fāj″) [*conio-* + *-phage*] a macrophage that ingests dust particles.

co•ni•o•sis (ko″ne-o′sis) [Gr. *konis* dust] a disease state caused by the inhalation of dust, such as byssinosis or pneumoconiosis.

Co•nio•spor•i•um (ko″ne-o-spor′e-əm) *Cryptostroma.*

co•nio•spo•ro•sis (ko″ne-o-spə-ro′sis) maple bark disease.

co•ni•ot•o•my (ko″ne-ot′ə-me) cricothyrotomy.

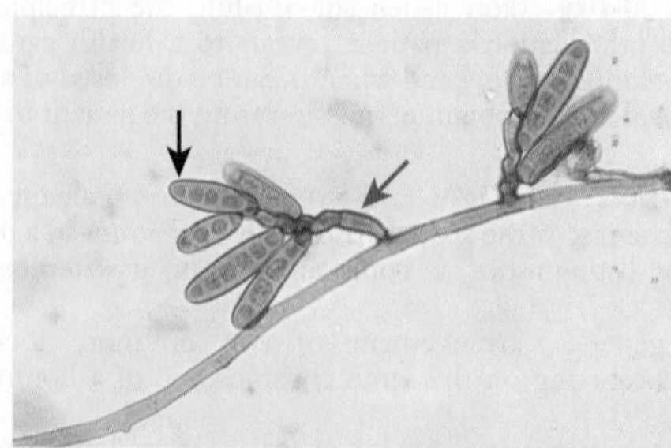

■ *Bipolaris* sp. conidia *(black arrow)* borne on geniculate conidiophores *(red arrow).*

co·nio·tox·i·co·sis (ko″ne-o-tok″sĭ-ko′sis) a form of pneumoconiosis in which the irritants affect the tissues directly.

Co·ni·um (ko-ni′əm) [L., from Gr. *kōneion*] a genus of plants of the family Umbelliferae. *C. macula′tum* L. is the poison hemlock (q.v.).

co·ni·vap·tan hydrochloride (ko″nĭ-vap′tan) an antagonist of arginine vasopressin, inhibiting its effects on receptors in the kidneys; administered intravenously in treatment of euvolemic hyponatremia.

con·iza·tion (kon″ĭ-za′shən) the removal of a cone of tissue, as in biopsy of the cervix uteri. Called also *cone biopsy*.

cold c. conization performed with a cold knife, as opposed to electrocautery.

con·joined (kən-joind′) joined together; united; see *conjoined twins*, under *twins*.

con·ju·gal (kon′jo͝o-gəl) [*con-* + *jugal*] pertaining to marriage.

con·ju·gant (kon′jo͝o-gənt) either individual of a pair of organisms or gametes during the process of conjugation; after separation, each is known as an *exconjugant*.

con·ju·ga·ta (kon″jə-ga′tə) 1. conjugate (def. 1). 2. conjugata vera pelvis.

c. anato′mica pel′vis [TA] c. vera pelvis.

c. diagona′lis pel′vis [TA] diagonal conjugate of pelvis: a diameter of the pelvic outlet; the distance from the posterior surface of the pubis to the tip of the sacral promontory. Called also *diagonal conjugate diameter*.

c. exter′na pel′vis [TA] external conjugate of pelvis: a diameter of the pelvic inlet; the distance from the depression under the last lumbar spine to the upper margin of the pubis. Called also *external conjugate diameter* and *Baudelocque diameter* or *line*.

c. media′na pel′vis [TA] median conjugate of pelvis: a diameter of the pelvic inlet; the anteroposterior diameter between the promontory of the sacrum and the upper posterior edge of the pubic symphysis.

c. rec′ta pel′vis [TA] straight conjugate of pelvis: a diameter of the pelvic outlet, the anteroposterior diameter between the tip of the coccyx and the lower edge of the pubic symphysis.

c. ve′ra pel′vis [TA] true conjugate of pelvis: a diameter of the pelvic outlet, the anteroposterior diameter measured between the superior margin of the symphysis pubis and the sacrovertebral angle; this is the shortest diameter that the fetal head must pass through in childbirth. Called also *anatomical*, *internal*, or *true conjugate diameter; conjugata anatomica pelvis;* and *anatomical* or *internal conjugate*.

con·ju·gate (kon′jə-gāt) [L. *conjugatus* yoked together] 1. paired, or equally coupled; working in unison. 2. the distance between two specified opposite points on the periphery of the pelvic inlet. Called also *conjugate diameter* and *pelvic c.* 3. conjugata vera pelvis. 4. the product of chemical conjugation.

anatomical c. of pelvis conjugata vera pelvis.
diagonal c. of pelvis conjugata diagonalis pelvis.
external c. of pelvis conjugata externa pelvis.
internal c. of pelvis conjugata vera pelvis.
median c. of pelvis conjugata mediana pelvis.
obstetric c. obstetric conjugate diameter.
pelvic c. conjugate (def. 1).
straight c. of pelvis conjugata recta pelvis.
true c. of pelvis conjugata vera pelvis.

con·ju·ga·tion (kon″jə-ga′shən) [L. *conjugatio* a blending] 1. the act of joining together or conjugating, or the state of being joined or conjugated. 2. a sexual process seen in bacteria, ciliate protozoa, and certain fungi in which nuclear material is exchanged during the temporary fusion of two cells (conjugants). In *bacterial genetics*, a form of sexual reproduction in which a donor bacterium (male) contributes some, or all, of its DNA (in the form of a replicated set) to a recipient (female), which then incorporates differing genetic information into its own chromosome by recombination and passes the recombined set on to its progeny by replication. In *ciliate protozoa*, two conjugants of separate mating types exchange micronuclear material and then separate, each now being a fertilized cell. In certain fungi, the process involves fusion of two gametes, resulting in union of their nuclei and formation of a zygote. 3. in chemistry, the joining together of two compounds to produce another compound, such as the combination of a toxic product with a substance in the body to form a detoxified product that can then be eliminated, or the binding of tumor-specific monoclonal antibodies to cytotoxic drugs in immunotherapy.

con·junc·ti·va (kən-junk′tĭ-və) pl. *conjunc′tivae* [L.] the delicate membrane that lines the eyelids and covers the exposed surface of the sclera, divided into the *palpebral c.* and the *bulbar* or *ocular c.* In official terminology, called *tunica conjunctiva* [TA]. **conjuncti′val** *adj*

bulbar c., ocular c. the portion of the tunica conjunctiva covering the cornea and front part of the sclera, appearing white because of the sclera behind it; in official terminology called *tunica conjunctiva bulbi* [TA].

palpebral c. the portion of the tunica conjunctiva lining the eyelids, appearing red because of its great vascularity. In official terminology called *tunica conjunctiva palpebrarum* [TA].

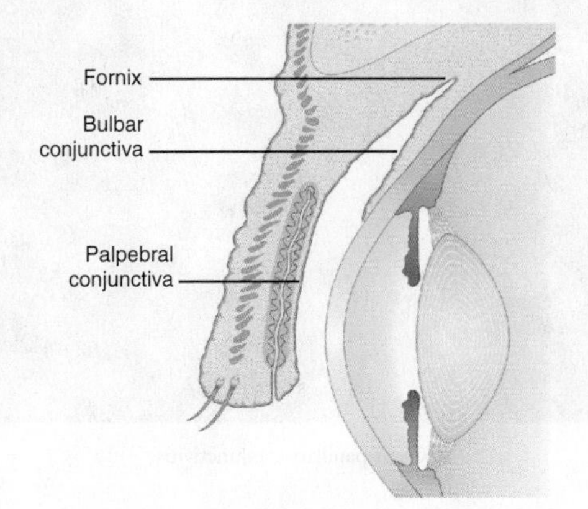

■ Divisions of the conjunctiva in a sagittal section.

con·junc·ti·vi·plas·ty (kən-junk′tĭ-vĭ-plas″te) conjunctivoplasty.

con·junc·ti·vi·tis (kən-junk″tĭ-vi′tis) pl. *conjunctivi′tides*. inflammation of the conjunctiva, generally consisting of conjunctival hyperemia associated with a discharge.

actinic c. conjunctivitis produced by ultraviolet rays (actinic rays), such as that of Klieg lights, therapeutic lamps, or acetylene torches. Called also *arc-flash* or *welder's c.*, *flash keratoconjunctivitis*, and *actinic ray, electric, flash*, or *ultraviolet ray ophthalmia*.

acute catarrhal c. an acute, infectious type of conjunctivitis with cold-like symptoms and hyperemia, edema, loss of translucence, and a mucous or mucopurulent discharge. Called also *mucopurulent c.*, *simple c.*, and *simple acute c.*

acute contagious c., acute epidemic c. a mucopurulent, epidemic type of conjunctivitis caused by *Haemophilus aegyptius*, occurring in the spring or fall, with the same symptoms as acute catarrhal conjunctivitis. Called also *pinkeye*.

acute hemorrhagic c. a highly contagious disease, certain epidemics of which have been associated etiologically with enteroviruses, characterized by subconjunctival hemorrhage varying from minute petechiae to confluent hemorrhages, and by sudden swelling of the eyelids and congestion, redness, and pain in the eye.

allergic c. conjunctival inflammation, itching, tearing, and redness caused by allergens; it includes vernal conjunctivitis, phlyctenular conjunctivitis, and that occurring in hay fever.

angular c. conjunctivitis with characteristic reddening at the canthi, usually due to Morax-Axenfeld bacillus or *Staphylococcus aureus;* called also *diplobacillary c.* and *Morax-Axenfeld c.*

arc-flash c. actinic c.

atopic c. allergic conjunctivitis of the immediate type, due to such airborne allergens as pollens, dusts, spores, and animal hair.

atropine c. a type of follicular conjunctivitis caused by continual use of atropine.

blennorrheal c. gonorrheal c.

chemical c. conjunctivitis due to exposure to a chemical irritant.

chronic catarrhal c. a mild, chronic type of conjunctivitis with only slight hyperemia and mucous discharge. It may be a sequel to acute catarrhal conjunctivitis, or the result of eyestrain, dust, glare, or ingrown lashes.

croupous c. pseudomembranous c.

diphtheritic c. membranous conjunctivitis occurring as a primary infection caused by *Corynebacterium diphtheriae* or secondarily to diphtheria of the respiratory tract.

diplobacillary c. angular c.
eczematous c. phlyctenular c.
epidemic c. acute contagious c.

follicular c. a type of conjunctivitis characterized by dense localized infiltrations of lymphoid tissue that occur as a response to irritation.

giant papillary c. chronic inflammation of the conjunctiva lining the upper eyelid, with formation of giant papillae on the tarsal conjunctiva, generally associated with contact lens wear but also occurring with ocular prostheses and protruding ocular sutures. There are mild itching, burning, tearing, and ocular discomfort with increased mucous discharge on awakening. Contact lens wear becomes increasingly uncomfortable and eventually inability to tolerate the lenses develops.

gonococcal c., gonorrheal c. severe conjunctivitis caused by infection with gonococci, marked by greatly swollen conjunctivae and eyelids and by a profuse purulent discharge. The infection is bilateral in newborns, who acquire it from an infected vaginal passage; it is usually unilateral in adults, who acquire it by autoinoculation into the eye of other gonococcal infections, e.g., gonococcal urethritis, either in themselves or in others. Called

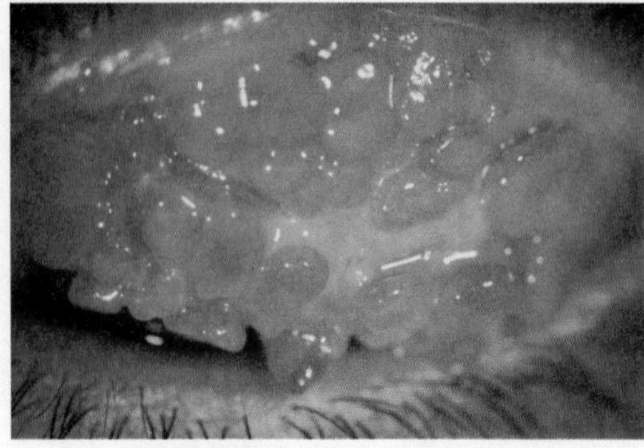

■ Giant papillary conjunctivitis.

also *blennorrheal c.* and *gonoblennorrhea.* Cf. *gonorrheal ophthalmia* and *ophthalmia neonatorum,* under *ophthalmia.*

granular c. trachoma.

inclusion c. conjunctivitis caused by *Chlamydia trachomatis;* it affects primarily newborn infants, beginning as an acute, purulent conjunctivitis that leads to papillary hypertrophy of the palpebral conjunctiva. Called also *swimming pool c.*

infantile purulent c. ophthalmia neonatorum.

Koch-Weeks c. acute contagious c.

larval c. myiasis of the conjunctiva.

lithiasis c. conjunctival concretions.

c. medicamento′sa conjunctivitis due to medication.

membranous c. severe conjunctivitis marked by the presence of a membrane on the inner surface of the lids formed by the profuse fibrinous exudation from the cul-de-sac, which on attempted removal leaves a raw, bleeding surface; it is caused by various bacteria, including *Corynebacterium diphtheriae,* streptococci, gonococci, and pneumococci. Cf. *pseudomembranous c.*

meningococcus c. conjunctivitis occurring as a complication of meningococcal meningitis.

molluscum c. conjunctivitis occurring as a complication of molluscum contagiosum.

Morax-Axenfeld c. angular c.

mucopurulent c. acute catarrhal c.

necrotic infectious c. a unilateral, purulent, necrotic type of conjunctivitis marked by small, diffuse, elevated, white spots in the palpebral conjunctiva and fornices, with ipsilateral swelling of the preauricular, parotid, and submaxillary lymph glands. Called also *Pascheff c.*

neonatal c. ophthalmia neonatorum.

c. nodo′sa, nodular c. ophthalmia nodosa.

Parinaud c. Parinaud oculoglandular syndrome.

Pascheff c. necrotic infectious c.

phlyctenular c. a type of conjunctivitis marked by small vesicles or ulcers, each surrounded by a reddened zone; called also *eczematous* or *scrofular c.* See also *phlyctenulosis.*

pseudomembranous c. a type of conjunctivitis that resembles membranous conjunctivitis except that the membrane can be removed without traumatizing the epithelium; also, in addition to being caused by bacterial infections, this type is sometimes caused by toxic and allergic factors or viral infections. Called also *croupous c.*

purulent c. acute conjunctivitis caused by bacteria or viruses, particularly gonococci, meningococci, pneumococci, and streptococci, characterized by severe inflammation of the conjunctiva and copious discharge of pus.

scrofular c. phlyctenular c.

shipyard c. epidemic keratoconjunctivitis.

simple c., simple acute c. acute catarrhal c.

spring c. vernal c.

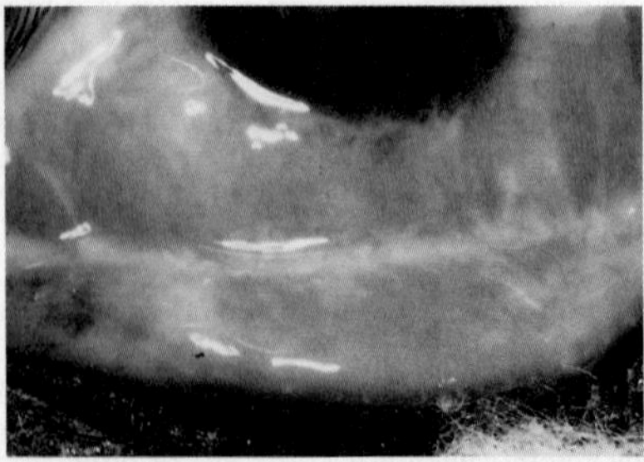

■ Gonococcal conjunctivitis caused by *Neisseria gonorrhoeae.*

swimming pool c. inclusion c.

trachomatous c. trachoma.

tularemic c. see *oculoglandular tularemia,* under *tularemia.*

vaccinial c. autovaccinia affecting the eye.

vernal c. a type of conjunctivitis that is seasonal, usually affects both eyes, has an unknown cause, and affects primarily children, especially boys. Flattened papules and a thick, gelatinous exudate develop on the conjunctivae on the inside of the upper lid; itching and photophobia are present. The condition is usually self-limiting, but it may become severe if corneal vascularization and ulceration develop. Called also *vernal catarrh* and *spring c.* or *ophthalmia.*

welder's c. actinic c.

Widmark c. congestion of the inferior tarsal conjunctiva, with occasional slight stippling of the cornea.

con•junc•ti•vo•dac•ryo•cys•tos•to•my (kən-junk″tĭ-vo-dak″re-o-sis-tos′tə-me) surgical connection of the lacrimal sac directly to the conjunctival sac.

con•junc•ti•vo•ma (kən-junk″tĭ-vo′mə) a tumor of the eyelid made up of conjunctival tissue.

con•junc•ti•vo•plas•ty (kən-junk′tĭ-vo-plas″te) [*conjunctiva* + *-plasty*] repair of a defect of the conjunctiva by plastic surgery. **conjunctivoplas′tic** *adj*

con•junc•ti•vo•rhi•nos•to•my (kən-junk″tĭ-vo-ri-nos′tə-me) surgical correction of total lacrimal canalicular obstruction: a dacryocystorhinostomy is done by suturing the posterior flaps, and the lacrimal caruncle is dissected out, preserving the conjunctiva.

Conn syndrome (kon) [Jerome W. *Conn,* American internist, 1907–1994] primary aldosteronism.

con•nec•tin (kə-nek′tin) titin.

con•nec•tion (kə-nek′shən) 1. something that joins other things together. 2. the act of joining or state of being joined together. 3. connector.

clamp c. a short tubular branch connecting one cell of a hypha to another, formed by fusion during cell division in certain basidiomycetous fungi, and serving in the transfer of the two daughter nuclei of the parent cell to a newly formed cell.

intertendinous c's connexus intertendinei.

Luer-Lok c. a connection between extracorporeal equipment for peritoneal dialysis and the intra-abdominal catheter, using two rigid tubes that screw together.

con•nec•tive (kə-nek′tiv) serving as a link or binding.

con•nec•tiv•i•ty (kə-nek-tiv′ĭ-te) the state or condition of being connected.

functional c. a parallel support mechanism in the brain for certain functions in cases where the primary area supporting a given function is resting or disabled; it is still under investigation which bodily functions have both a primary brain area and a parallel backup area.

con•nec•tol•o•gy (kə-nek-tol′ə-je) term coined to refer to the equipment and methods used to connect the dialysis apparatus outside the body to the intra-abdominal catheter.

con•nec•tor (kə-nek′tər) 1. anything serving as a link between two separate objects or units. 2. the part of a fixed partial denture that unites the retainer and the pontic; it may be rigid or nonrigid.

major c. a rigid unit of a removable partial denture, serving as its chassis, which joins the parts of the prosthesis on one side of the dental arch to those on the other side, and to which all other components are attached. Called also *saddle c.* Cf. *connector bar.*

minor c. a connecting link between the major connector or base of a partial denture and other units of the prosthesis, such as clasps, indirect retainers, and occlusal rests; called also *connector bar.*

saddle c. major c.

Con•nell suture (kon′əl) [Frank Gregory *Connell,* American surgeon, 1875–1968] see under *suture.*

con•nex•in (kə-nek′sin) one of the protein subunits of a connexon, six connexins in hexagonal array making up a connexon. Each connexin contains four transmembrane α-helices and numerous connexin subtypes exist.

c. 26 a connexin subtype encoded on chromosome 13q11-12; autosomal recessive mutation of the gene encoding it is the most common cause of congenital nonsyndromic hearing loss.

con•nex•on (kə-nek′son) the functional unit of a gap junction; it is the hexagonal array of membrane-spanning proteins, connexins, around a central lumen that connects with its counterpart in an adjacent cell to form the intercellular pore of the gap junction.

con•nex•us (kə-nek′səs) gen. and pl. *connex′us* [L., variant of *conexus,* q.v.] a connecting structure; written also *conexus.*

c. intertendi′nei [TA] intertendinous connections: narrow bands extending obliquely between the tendons of insertion of the extensor digitorum muscles on the dorsum of the hand. Called also *tendinous junctions.*

con(o)- [Gr. kōnos *cone*] a combining form denoting a relationship to a cone or to a conelike structure.

co•noid (ko′noid) [*cono-* + *-oid*] 1. resembling or shaped like a cone. 2. an electron-dense, protrusible, hollow region surrounded by polar rings and composed of spirally coiled microtubules that forms part of the apical complex of apicocomplexan protozoa.

Sturm c. the changing shapes of the diffusion images of a point in various forms of astigmatism; the image may be an ellipse, a circle, or a sharp line.

co•no•my•oi•din (ko″no-mi-oi′din) [*cono-* + *myoid*] a protoplasmic material within some retinal cones that expands and contracts under the influence of light, causing the cones to shift position.

con•oph•thal•mus (kon″of-thal′məs) staphyloma corneae (def. 1).

Co•no•po•di•na (ko″no-po-di′nə) [Gr. *kōnos* cone] a suborder of ramicristate amebae, characterized by fingerlike or nipplelike, blunt, normally unbranched subpseudopodia, most often produced from a broad hyaline lobe.

Co•no•rhi•nus (ko″no-ri′nəs) [*cono-* + Gr. *rhis* nose] a genus name formerly applied to insects of the family Reduviidae, now placed in the genera *Panstrongylus* and *Triatoma*.

co•no•trun•cal (ko″no-trun′kəl) pertaining to the conus arteriosus and a truncus arteriosus; said of congenital heart defects.

con•qui•nine (kon-kwin′in) quinidine.

Con•ra•di disease (syndrome) (kon-rah′de) [Erich *Conradi*, German physician, 20th century] see *chondrodysplasia punctata.*

Con•ra•di line (kon-rah′de) [Andreas Christian *Conradi*, Norwegian physician, 1809–1869] see under *line.*

Con•ra•di-Hün•er•mann syndrome (kon-rah′de hu′nər-mahn) [E. *Conradi;* Carl *Hünermann*, German physician, 20th century] see under *syndrome.*

Con•ray (kon′ra) trademark for preparations of iothalamate.

Cons. [L.] conser′va (keep).

con•san•guin•e•ous (kon″sang-gwin′e-əs) related by blood.

con•san•guin•i•ty (kon″sang-gwin′ĭ-te) [L. *consanguinitas*] kinship; relationship by blood.

con•science (kon′shəns) the nontechnical term for the moral faculty of the mind, corresponding roughly to the psychoanalytic concept of the superego (q.v.), although, unlike the ordinary conception of conscience, the actions of the superego are often unconscious.

con•scious (kon′shəs) [L. *conscius* aware] 1. having awareness of one's self, acts, and surroundings. 2. a state of awareness or alertness characterized by response to external stimuli. 3. the part of the mind that is constantly within awareness, one of the systems of Freud's topographic model of the mind. Cf. *preconscious* and *unconscious.*

con•scious•ness (kon′shəs-nəs) 1. the state of being conscious, fully alert, aware, oriented, and responsive to the environment; having a clear or intact sensorium. 2. subjective awareness of the aspects of cognitive processing and the content of the mind. 3. the current totality of experience of which an individual or group is aware at any time. 4. in psychoanalysis, the conscious.

con•sen•su•al (kən-sen′shoo-əl) excited by reflex stimulation; used especially to designate the similar reaction of both pupils to a stimulus applied to only one.

con•sent (kən-sent′) [L. *consentire* to agree] 1. to assent or approve; to grant permission. 2. the granting of permission or agreement; assent; approval.

informed c. voluntary permission given by a subject or guardian for participation in a study or investigation, or for medical care, after having been informed of the purpose, methods, procedures, benefits, and risks.

con•ser•va•tive (kən-sur′və-tiv) [L. *conservare* to preserve] designed to preserve health, restore function, and repair structures by nonradical methods, as conservative surgery. Cf. *radical.*

con•serve (kon′sərv) [L. *conserva*] electuary.

con•sis•ten•cy (kən-sis′tən-se) coherence among parts; reliability of successive events or results.

c. of an estimator the property of approaching the value of a population parameter as the sample size increases ad infinitum.

con•sol•i•dant (kən-sol′ĭ-dənt) [L. *consolidare* to make firm] 1. promoting the healing or union of parts. 2. an agent that promotes the healing or union of parts.

con•sol•i•da•tion (kən-sol″ĭ-da′shən) [L. *consolidatio*] solidification; the process of becoming or the condition of being solid, as when the lung becomes firm as air spaces are filled with exudate in pneumonia.

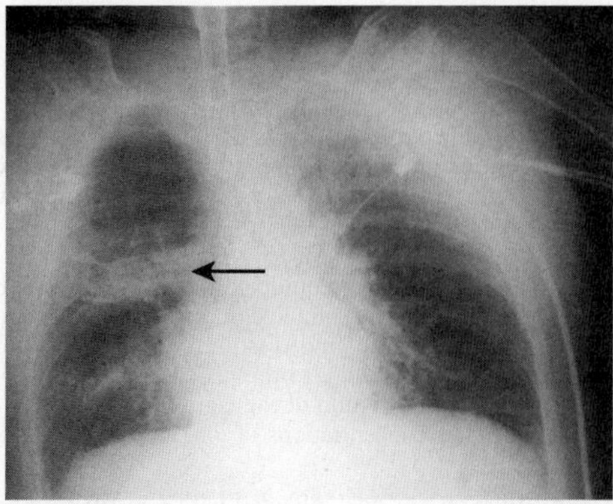

■ Areas of consolidation and atelectasis and increased interstitial markings *(arrow)* in a 20-year-old patient with chronic severe aspiration.

con•so•lute (kon′so-lo͞ot) perfectly miscible.

con•spe•cif•ic (kon″spə-sif′ik) 1. of or pertaining to the same species. 2. a member of the same species.

con•stan•cy (kon′stən-se) 1. the state of being constant. 2. stability.

object c. 1. the ability to perceive an object as unchanging even under different conditions of observation. 2. see under *permanence.*

con•stant (kon′stənt) [L. *constans* standing together] 1. not failing; remaining unaltered. 2. a datum, fact, or principle that is not subject to change.

absorption c. absorptivity.

acid dissociation c. the dissociation constant describing the ionization of an acid. Symbol K_a. For an acid HA,

$$K_a = \frac{[H^+][A^-]}{[HA]}.$$

association c. a measure of the extent of a reversible association between two molecular species; called also *binding c.*

Avogadro c. see under *number.*

base dissociation c. the dissociation constant describing the ionization of a base. Symbol K_b. For a base BOH,

$$K_b = \frac{[B^+][OH^-]}{[BOH]}.$$

binding c. association c.

Boltzmann c. the gas constant divided by Avogadro number; 1.38066 $\times 10^{-23}$ joule per kelvin. Symbol *k*.

decay c. (λ) the fraction of the number of atoms of a radionuclide which decay per unit time. Called also *disintegration c.* and *radioactive c.*

dielectric c. a measure of the capability of a unit volume of a material to store electrostatic energy on application of a unit voltage; the ability of that material to resist the formation of an electric field within it. It is the ratio of the capacitance of a capacitor having the material versus the same capacitor having only a vacuum as the dielectric. Symbol κ.

disintegration c. decay c.

dissociation c. an equilibrium constant, expressed in concentrations, describing the dissociation of a molecule or ion into its components. Symbol K_d. See also *acid dissociation c.* and *base dissociation c.* Called also *ionization c.*

equilibrium c. a constant, *K* (or K_{eq}), describing the amounts of reactants and products of a chemical reaction at equilibrium at constant temperature; technically defined by thermodynamic activities, it is usually approximated using concentrations (and sometimes therefore denoted K_c) and is defined by the equation for the reaction quotient (q.v.). For gases, it can be approximated by partial pressures rather than concentrations (and denoted K_p). See also *dissociation c.*

Faraday c. faraday.

gas c. (*R*) the proportionality constant in the ideal gas law (q.v.); 8.3144 joules per mole kelvin.

gravitational c. (*G*), **c. of gravitation** the constant of proportionality in the law of gravitation, equal to 6.67×10^{-11} N•m^2/kg^2.

ionization c. dissociation c.

Lapicque c. the figure 0.37, used for converting noninductive resistance into direct current equivalents.

Michaelis c. (K_M, K_m) a constant representing the substrate concentration at which the velocity of an enzyme-catalyzed reaction is half maximal. See also *Michaelis-Menten equation,* under *equation.*

newtonian c. of gravitation gravitational c.

Planck c., quantum c. a constant, h, which represents the ratio of the energy of any quantum of radiation to its frequency; the value of h is 6.626×10^{-34} joule second.

radioactive c. decay c.

rate c. a constant of proportionality, k, relating the rate of a single step of a reaction to the concentrations of the reactants, e.g., for a reaction $aA + bB \rightleftarrows yY + zZ$, the rate ($v$) = $k[A]^a[B]^b$. The rate constant for the forward reaction is k_f; for the reverse it is k_r.

sedimentation c. see under *coefficient.*

solubility product c. a derived equilibrium constant (K_{sp}) for the equilibrium existing between a slightly soluble compound and the solution it has saturated. Because so little compound dissolves, its concentration is considered constant and K_{sp} is equivalent to the product of K (equilibrium constant) times the original concentration of the compound; it is thus equivalent to the ion product. Higher concentrations of ions cause precipitation.

velocity c. rate c.

con·sti·pat·ed (kon′stĭ-pāt″əd) affected with constipation.

con·sti·pa·tion (kon″stĭ-pa′shən) [L. *constipatio* a crowding together] infrequent or difficult evacuation of the feces.

atonic c. constipation due to intestinal atony.

spastic c. constipation due to spastic constriction of the intestine.

con·sti·tu·tion (kon″stĭ-too′shən) [L. *constituere* to set up] 1. the make-up or functional habit of the body, determined by the genetic, biochemical, and physiologic endowment of the individual, and modified in great measure by environmental factors. Cf. *diathesis* and *genotype.* 2. in chemistry, the atoms making up a molecule and the way they are linked, the property that distinguishes a compound from its structural isomers. Cf. *configuration.*

con·sti·tu·tion·al (kon″stĭ-too′shən-əl) 1. affecting the whole constitution of the body; not local. 2. pertaining to the constitution.

con·sti·tu·tive (kon-stĭ-too′tiv, kon-stich′u-tiv) produced constantly or in fixed amounts, regardless of environmental conditions or demand; cf. *inducible.*

con·stric·tio (kən-strik′she-o) constriction.

c. bronchoaor′tica TA alternative for *c. partis thoracicae oesophagi.*

c. diaphragma′tica TA alternative for *c. phrenica.*

c. par′tis thora′cicae oeso′phagi [TA] thoracic constriction of esophagus: a narrowing of the thoracic esophagus where it is compressed by the aortic arch and the left main bronchus. Called also *c. bronchoaortica* [TA alternative].

c. pharyngooesophagea′lis [TA] pharyngoesophageal constriction: the narrowing where the pharynx ends and the cervical esophagus begins, the site of the pharyngoesophageal sphincter. Called also *pharyngoesophageal junction.*

c. phre′nica [TA] phrenic constriction: the narrowing in the esophagus where it crosses the diaphragm at the esophageal hiatus. Called also *c. diaphragmatica* [TA alternative] and *diaphragmatic constriction.*

con·stric·tion (kən-strik′shən) [L. *constringere,* past part. *constrictus,* to draw together] a narrowed part of an organ or other structure; see also *stenosis.*

bronchoaortic c. thoracic constriction of esophagus.

diaphragmatic c. constrictio phrenica.

duodenopyloric c. pyloric c.

pharyngoesophageal c. constrictio pharyngooesophagealis.

phrenic c. constrictio phrenica.

Pohl-Pinkus c. a limited thinning of the shaft of a hair, usually accompanied by interruption of the medulla; it is usually a sign of systemic disease, but may be due to trauma, coronary occlusion, skin disease, or the therapeutic administration of a single substantial dose of an antimetabolite such as methotrexate or cyclophosphamide. Called also *Pohl-Pinkus mark.*

primary c. term used to denote the centromere, because it is narrower than the surrounding regions in metaphase chromosomes.

pyloric c. the constriction at the distal end of the pylorus, overlying the pyloric orifice, marking the junction of the stomach and duodenum.

secondary c. 1. a narrowed heterochromatic area of the short arm of an acrocentric autosome by which a satellite is attached; it is the site of the nucleolar organizing region (NOR). 2. a region of constitutive heterochromatin occurring on the long arm of certain chromosomes, near the centromere. 3. a nonfunctional centromere in a dicentric chromosome.

thoracic c. of esophagus constrictio partis thoracicae oesophagi.

con·stric·tive (kən-strik′tiv) causing constriction or having a tendency to constriction.

con·stric·tor (kən-strik′tər) 1. an instrument that constricts a part or vessel. 2. a muscle that constricts a part; see terms beginning *musculus constrictor.* See also *compressor.*

c. na′ris pars transversa musculi nasalis.

c. ure′thrae musculus compressor urethrae.

c. vagi′nae compressor vaginae.

con·struc·tive (kən-struk′tiv) pertaining to any process of construction; in physiology, anabolic.

con·sult[1] (kən-sult′) [L. *consultus*] to confer with another physician about a case.

con·sult[2] (kon′sult) [L. *consultus*] consultation.

con·sul·tand (kən-sul′tand) [L. *consultare* to counsel] the individual who presents for genetic counseling and through whom a family is brought to the attention of a geneticist; it is not necessarily the affected individual.

con·sul·tant (kən-sul′tənt) [L. *consultare* to counsel] a physician called in for advice and counsel.

con·sul·ta·tion (kon″səl-ta′shən) [L. *consultatio*] a deliberation by two or more physicians with respect to the diagnosis or treatment in any particular case.

con·sump·tion (kən-sump′shən) [L. *consumptio* a wasting] 1. the act of consuming, or the process of being consumed. 2. a wasting away of the body.

oxygen c. the amount of oxygen consumed by the tissues of the body, usually measured as the oxygen uptake in the lung. The normal value is 250 mL/min (or 3.5 to 4.0 mL/kg/min), and it increases with increased metabolic rate.

Cont. [L.] contu′sus (bruised).

con·tact (kon′takt) [L. *contactus* a touching together] 1. a mutual touching of two bodies or persons. 2. an individual known to have been sufficiently near to an infected individual to have been exposed to the transfer of infectious material. 3. contactant.

balancing c. the contact between the upper and lower occlusal surfaces of the teeth (of the natural or artificial dentition) on the side opposite the working contact.

complete c. contact of the entire proximal surface of one tooth with the entire proximal surface of the adjacent tooth.

deflective c., deflective occlusal c. a form of occlusal interference in which the mandible is diverted from its normal path of closure to central jaw relation, or the denture slides or rotates on its basal seat. Called also *deflective c.* and *cuspal interference.*

direct c. transmission of infection from an infected host or reservoir to a susceptible individual by physical contact.

focal c. focal adhesion.

indirect c. transmission of infection to a susceptible host by means of fomites or a vector or through the air in dust or droplet nuclei.

initial c., initial occlusal c. the initial normal, noninterfering occlusal contact and intercuspation occurring when the mandibular and maxillary teeth are brought together. In ideal occlusion, it takes place in centric occlusion.

interceptive occlusal c. an initial contact of the teeth that stops or deviates from the normal movement of the mandible.

occlusal c. the contact between the upper and lower teeth when the jaws are closed in habitual occlusion. See *deflective occlusal c., initial occlusal c.,* and *interceptive occlusal c.*

premature c. an occlusal contact or interference that occurs before a balanced and stable jaw-to-jaw relationship is reached in either centric relation or centric occlusion, or in the area between the two positions.

proximal c., proximate c. touching of the proximal surfaces of two adjoining teeth.

weak c. contact in which the proximal surface of one tooth barely touches that of the adjacent tooth, enhancing the packing of food between the teeth.

working c. the contact between the upper and lower teeth (of the natural or artificial dentition) on the side toward which the mandible has been moved in mastication.

con·tac·tant (kən-tak′tənt) an allergen capable of inducing delayed contact-type hypersensitivity of the animal or human epidermis after one or more episodes of contact.

con·tac·tol·o·gist (kon″tak-tol′ə-jist) a specialist in contactology.

con·tac·tol·o·gy (kon″tak-tol′ə-je) the craft of making and fitting contact lenses.

con·ta·gion (kən-ta′jən) [L. *contagio* contact, infection] 1. the communication of disease from one individual to another. 2. a contagious disease.

psychic c. communication of psychological symptoms through mental influence.

con·ta·gious (kən-ta′jəs) [L. *contagiosus*] capable of being transmitted from one individual to another; communicable. Cf. *infectious.*

con·tam·i·nant (kən-tam′ĭ-nənt) something that causes contamination.

con·tam·i·na·tion (kən-tam″ĭ-na′shən) [L. *contaminatio,* from *con* together + *tangere* to touch] 1. the presence of any substance or organism that makes a preparation impure. 2. the soiling or pollution by inferior material, as by the introduction of organisms into a wound, or sewage into a stream. 3. the deposition of radioactive material where it is not desired, particularly where its presence may be harmful or constitute a radiation hazard.

con•tent (kon′tent) that which is contained within a thing.

latent c. in freudian theory, the hidden and unconscious true meaning of a symbolic representation, such as a dream or fantasy, as opposed to the manifest content.

manifest c. in freudian theory, the content of a dream or fantasy as it is experienced and remembered, and in which the latent content is disguised and distorted by displacement, condensation, symbolization, projection, and secondary elaboration.

con•tig (kon-tig′) one of a set of overlapping clones that span a segment of DNA; used in constructing a contig map (q.v.).

con•ti•gu•i•ty (kon″tĭ-gu′ĭ-te) [L. *contiguus* in contact] contact or close proximity; the quality of being contiguous.

con•tig•u•ous (kən-tig′u-əs) [L. *contiguus*] in contact or nearly so.

Contin. [L.] continue′tur (let it be continued).

con•ti•nence (kon′tĭ-nəns) [L. *continentia*] the ability to refrain from yielding to desire, as self-restraint with respect to sexual indulgence.

fecal c. the ability to retain the contents of the colon until conditions are proper for defecation.

urinary c. the ability to retain the contents of the bladder until conditions are proper for urination.

con•ti•nent (kon′tĭ-nənt) able to refrain from yielding to normal impulses, as sexual desire, or from the urge to defecate or urinate.

con•tin•ued (kən-tin′ūd) having no remission, intermission, or interruption.

con•ti•nu•i•ty (kon″tĭ-nu′ĭ-te) [L. *continuitas,* uninterrupted succession] the quality of being without interruption or separation.

con•tin•u•ous (kən-tin′u-əs) [L. *continuus*] not interrupted; having no interruption. See under *variable.*

con•tour (kon′to͞or) [Fr.] 1. the normal outline or configuration of the body or of a part. 2. to shape a solid along certain desired lines.

height of c. see under *height.*

con•toured (kon′to͞ord) having an irregularly undulating outline or surface; said of bacterial colonies.

con•tour•ing (kon′to͞or-ing) the process of forming a contour; shaping.

occlusal c. correction by grinding of gross disharmonies of the occlusal tooth forms. See also under *adjustment.*

contra- [L. *contra* against] a prefix signifying against, opposed.

con•tra-an•gle (kon″trə-ang′gəl) 1. an angulation by which the working point of a surgical or dental instrument is brought close to the long axis of its shaft; it may involve two, three, or four bends, or angles, in its shank. 2. see under *handpiece.*

con•tra•ap•er•ture (kon″trə-ap′ər-chər) [*contra-* + *aperture*] a second opening made in an abscess to facilitate the discharge of its contents.

con•tra•cep•tion (kon″trə-sep′shən) the prevention of conception or impregnation.

intrauterine c. prevention of conception by use of a device inserted into the uterus; see under *device.*

con•tra•cep•tive (kon″trə-sep′tiv) 1. diminishing the likelihood of, or preventing, conception. 2. an agent that diminishes the likelihood of or prevents conception.

barrier c. a contraceptive device, such as a condom or diaphragm, that physically prevents spermatozoa from entering the endometrial cavity and fallopian tubes.

chemical c. a spermicidal agent inserted into the vagina before intercourse to prevent pregnancy.

combined oral c. an oral contraceptive that includes both an estrogen and a progestagen, which may be administered in either two or three different phases during each menstrual cycle.

emergency c. postcoital c.

intrauterine c. see under *device.*

oral c. a compound, usually hormonal, taken orally in order to block ovulation and prevent the occurrence of pregnancy.

postcoital c. a contraceptive that blocks or terminates pregnancy after sexual intercourse. Called also *emergency c.*

progestagen-only c., progestin-only c., progestogen-only c. an oral contraceptive consisting only of a small dose of a progestational agent to be taken every day; called also *minipill.*

con•tract (kən-trakt′) [L. *contractus,* from *contrahere* to draw together] 1. to reduce in size or shorten. 2. in muscle physiology, to become activated and generate force; such a process does not necessarily result in the shortening of the muscle. See subentries under *contraction.* 3. to acquire or incur.

con•trac•tile (kən-trak′tīl) [*con-* + L. *trahere* to draw] having the power or tendency to contract in response to a suitable stimulus.

con•trac•til•i•ty (kon″trak-til′ĭ-te) capacity for contracting in response to a suitable stimulus.

cardiac c. the intrinsic property, belonging to cardiac cells and tissues, of contraction in response to an appropriate stimulus. Cardiac contractility is variable and under the control of the autonomic nervous system and is also affected by other factors such as loading conditions; changes in contractility give rise to changes in the strength of contraction of the heart. It may be estimated by the end-systolic pressure-volume relationship, the change in either pressure or volume over time. Called also *inotropic state.*

galvanic c. galvanocontractility.

idiomuscular c. a contractility peculiar to wasted or degenerated muscles.

neuromuscular c. normal, as distinguished from idiomuscular, contractility.

con•trac•tion (kən-trak′shən) [L. *contractus* drawn together] 1. a reduction in size or shrinkage. 2. in muscle, an increase in tension that may or may not shorten the muscle. 3. abnormal approximation of mandibular and maxillary structures to the median plane. See also *distraction* (def. 5).

atrial premature c. see under *complex.*

atrioventricular (AV) junctional premature c. see under *complex.*

automatic ventricular c. ventricular escape beat.

Braxton Hicks c's light, usually painless, irregular uterine contractions during pregnancy, gradually increasing in intensity and frequency and becoming more rhythmic during the late third trimester.

carpopedal c. chronic shortening of the muscles of the upper and lower limbs, including the fingers and toes, in tetany.

cicatricial c. wound c.

clonic c. clonus.

concentric c. shortening c.

Dupuytren c. Dupuytren contracture.

eccentric c. lengthening c.

escaped ventricular c. ventricular escape beat.

fibrillary c's abnormal spontaneous contractions occurring successively in different bundles of the fibers of a diseased muscle.

hourglass c. contraction of an organ (as the stomach or uterus) at or near the middle.

idiomuscular c. a contraction produced in a wasted or denervated muscle by direct electrical stimulation.

isometric c. muscle contraction without appreciable shortening or change in distance between its origin and insertion.

isotonic c. muscle contraction without appreciable change in the force of contraction; the distance between the muscle's origin and insertion becomes less.

isovolumetric c., isovolumic c. see under *period.*

junctional premature c. atrioventricular junctional premature complex.

lengthening c. a muscle contraction in which the ends of the muscle move farther apart, as when a limb is forcibly flexed. Called also *eccentric c.*

myotatic c. contraction or irritability of a muscle brought into play by sudden passive stretching or by tapping on its tendon. See also *stretch reflex* and *tendon reflex,* under *reflex.*

palmar c. Dupuytren contracture.

paradoxical c. the contraction of a muscle caused by the passive approximation of its extremities.

postural c. the state of muscular tension and contraction that is just sufficient to maintain the posture of the body.

premature c. extrasystole.

premature atrial c. atrial premature complex.

segmentation c. see under *movement.*

shortening c. a muscle contraction in which the ends of the muscle move closer together, as when a flexed limb is extended. Called also *concentric c.*

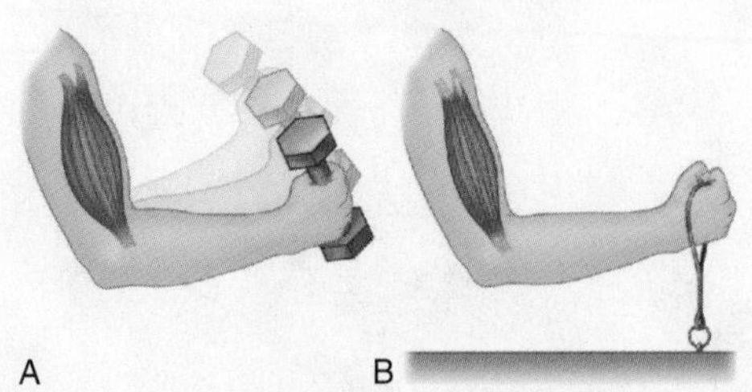

■ Isotonic *(A)* and isometric *(B)* contraction.

supraventricular premature c. an ectopic beat arising prematurely from a focus within the atria or atrioventricular junction, e.g., an atrial premature complex or atrioventricular junctional premature complex.

tetanic c. sustained contraction of a muscle without intervals of relaxation; see *tetanus* (def. 2). Called also *tonic c.*

tonic c. tetanus (def. 2).

twitch c. twitch.

uterine c's contractions of the uterus, as in menstruation and labor.

ventricular premature c. see under *complex.*

wound c. the shrinkage and spontaneous closure of open skin wounds. Called also *cicatricial c.*

con•trac•ture (kən-trak′chər) [L. *contractura*] a condition of fixed high resistance to passive stretch of a muscle, resulting from fibrosis of the tissues supporting the muscles or the joints, or from disorders of the muscle fibers.

Dupuytren c. 1. a usually autosomal dominant condition consisting of flexion contracture of a finger caused by shortening, thickening, and fibrosis of the palmar fascia; sometimes it is associated with longstanding epilepsy. Called also *Dupuytren disease.* 2. flexion deformity of a toe caused by involvement of the plantar fascia.

flexion c. a contracture that holds the joint in a position of flexion; called also *flexion deformity.*

ischemic c. contracture and degeneration of a muscle due to interference with the circulation from pressure, as by a tight bandage, or from injury or cold.

organic c. a contracture that is permanent and continuous.

postpoliomyelitic c. any distortion of a joint following an attack of poliomyelitis, due to partial or complete paralysis of one muscle or group of muscles, allowing overuse of an opposing muscle or group of muscles, such as flexion contracture of the knee and paralysis of the quadriceps muscle group.

Volkmann c. contracture of the fingers and sometimes the wrist after severe injury in or near the elbow or improper use of a tourniquet interferes with the blood supply to the muscles. A similar phenomenon may develop in the lower leg and foot after similar vascular damage to leg muscles. Called also *ischemic muscular atrophy* and *Volkmann syndrome.*

con•tra•fis•sure (kon″trə-fish′ər) a fracture in a part opposite the site of a blow.

con•tra•in•ci•sion (kon″trə-in-sizh′ən) counterincision to promote drainage.

con•tra•in•di•cant (kon″trə-in′dĭ-kənt) rendering any particular line of treatment undesirable or improper.

con•tra•in•di•ca•tion (kon″trə-in″dĭ-ka′shən) any condition, especially any condition of disease, which renders some particular line of treatment improper or undesirable.

con•tra•in•su•lar (kon″trə-in′su-lər) having an inhibiting influence on the secretion of pancreatic insulin.

con•tra•lat•er•al (kon″trə-lat′ər-əl) [*contra-* + *lateral*] situated on, pertaining to, or affecting the opposite side, as opposed to ipsilateral.

con•tra•sex•u•al (kon″trə-sek′shoo-əl) 1. a term used to describe the repressed side of an individual, embodying those characteristics normally occurring in the opposite sex. 2. showing secondary sex characters of the opposite sex; called also *heterosexual.*

con•trast (kon′trast) [*contra-* + L. *stare* to stand] 1. the degree to which light and dark areas of an image differ in brightness or in optical density. 2. in radiology, the difference in optical density in a radiograph that results from a difference in radiolucency or penetrability of the subject. Called also *radiocontrast.*

film c. contrast inherent in the film.

high c. short-scale c.

long-scale c., low c. an increased range of grays on a radiograph, which limits visual differentiation to those image densities produced by relatively disparate structural features.

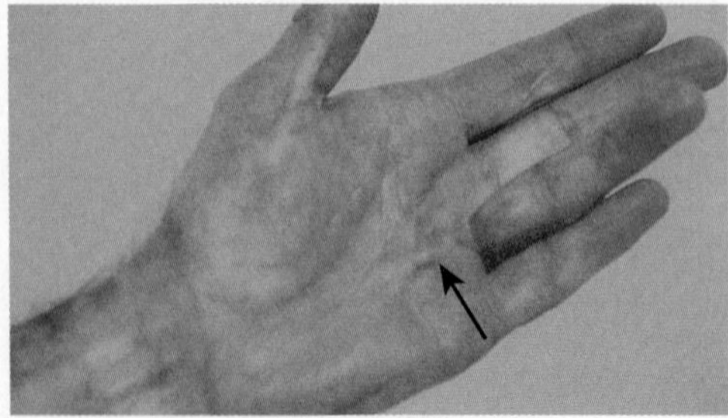

■ Dupuytren contracture.

short-scale c. a reduced range of grays on a radiograph, which favors visual differentiation of image densities produced by objects or object components with relatively comparable structural features.

subject c. contrast resulting from differences in absorption of radiation by various parts of the subject.

con•tra•stim•u•lant (kon″trə-stim′u-lənt) [*contra-* + *stimulant*] 1. counteracting or opposing stimulation. 2. a depressant medicine.

con•tra•stim•u•lus (kon″trə-stim′u-ləs) [*contra-* + *stimulus*] a remedy, force, or agent that opposes stimulation.

con•tre•coup (kōn″trə-koo′) [Fr. "counterblow"] injury resulting from a blow on another site, especially of the brain, such as a fracture by contrecoup of the skull or a contrecoup contusion.

con•trec•ta•tion (kon″trek-ta′shən) [L. *contrectare* to handle] the act of touching and fondling, especially in the sense of foreplay.

Cont. rem. [L.] continue′tur reme′dium (let the medicine be continued).

con•trol (kən-trōl′) [Fr. *contrôle* a register] 1. the governing or limitation of certain objects or events. 2. a standard against which experimental observations may be evaluated; see *negative c.* and *positive c.* 3. a patient or group differing from that under study (the treated or case group) by lacking the disease or by having a different or absent treatment or regimen; the controls and case or treated subjects usually otherwise have certain similarities to allow or enhance comparison between them. 4. in psychiatry, the process of consciously restraining and regulating impulses and suppressing instincts and affects.

aversive c. in behavior therapy, the use of unpleasant stimuli to change undesirable behavior.

birth c. deliberate limitation of childbearing by measures designed to control fertility and to prevent conception; see also *contraception.*

feedback c. a physiological control mechanism operating to regulate the metabolic processes of a cell and thus maintain a constant internal environment, in which the accumulation of the product of a reaction leads to a decrease in its rate of production, or a deficiency of the product leads to an increase in its rate of production.

idiodynamic c. nerve impulses from the cells of the ventral gray column and the motor nuclei of the brain that maintain the muscles in their normal trophic condition.

motor c. the systematic transmission of impulses from the motor cortex to motor units, resulting in coordinated muscular contractions.

negative c. a laboratory procedure identical in all respects to an experimental procedure except for the absence of the one factor being studied.

positive c. in an experimental study of a given substance, a sample of the substance with known values that can be used as a reference base.

reflex c. control of muscular activity by nerve impulses transmitted to the muscles by one of the reflex arcs by which reflex action is maintained.

Schick test c. [USP] heat-inactivated diphtheria toxin used as a control in the Schick test. Formerly called *inactivated diagnostic diphtheria toxin.*

sex c. regulation of the sex of future offspring by artificial means.

stimulus c. any influence exerted by the environment on behavior.

thought c. a delusion of control in which it is believed that one's thoughts are not one's own but come from another person or other outside source.

tonic c. nerve impulses transmitted to the final common pathway through the reflex arc for the maintenance of muscle tone.

vestibuloequilibratory c. nerve impulses from the semicircular canals, saccule, and utricle for the maintenance of body equilibrium.

volitional c., voluntary c. impulses from the motor area of the cerebral cortex that direct muscular action under the influence of the will.

Con•trolled Sub•stan•ces Act a federal law enacted in 1970 that regulates the prescribing and dispensing of psychoactive drugs, including narcotics, according to five schedules based on their abuse potential, medical acceptance, and ability to produce dependence; it also establishes a regulatory system for the manufacture, storage, and transport of the drugs in each schedule. Drugs covered by this act include opium and its derivatives, opiates, hallucinogens, depressants, and stimulants.

con•tund (kən-tund′) [L. *contundere*] to bruise.

con•tuse (kən-to͞oz′) to bruise.

con•tu•sion (kən-too′zhən) [L. *contusio*, from *contundere* to bruise] an injury of a part without a break in the skin and with a subcutaneous hemorrhage. Called also *bruise.*

brain c. contusion with loss of consciousness as a result of direct trauma to the head, usually associated with fracture of the skull. See also *concussion of the brain.*

cerebral c. a brain contusion affecting the cerebrum, usually after a head injury. It may cause an extradural or subdural hemorrhage, in which case the person may be left with neurologic defects or epilepsy. See also subdural hematoma.

contrecoup c. a contusion resulting from a blow on one side of the head with damage to the cerebral hemisphere on the opposite side by transmitted force.

myocardial c. contusion of the heart, most frequently due to impact against an automobile steering wheel or other blunt object; the trauma may cause arrhythmias, conduction disturbances, or clinical signs of infarction such as electrocardiographic abnormalities.

c. of spinal cord organic injury to the cord due to a blow to the vertebral column, with resultant transient or prolonged dysfunction below the level of the lesion. See also *concussion of spinal cord*.

con·tu·sive (kən-too′siv) producing a bruise.

con·u·lar (kon′u-lər) conical.

Co·nus (ko′nəs) a genus of marine snails (cones) of the family Conidae. *C. geogra′phicus* (the geographic cone) and *C. texti′le* (the textile cone) are carnivorous species that live in tropical oceans and kill fish by punching a hole with a proboscis and injecting poison; occasionally humans have been killed in the same manner.

co·nus (ko′nəs) gen. and pl. *co′ni* [L., from Gr. *kōnos*] 1. a structure resembling a cone in shape. 2. posterior staphyloma of the myopic eye.

c. arterio′sus [TA] arterial cone: the anterosuperior portion of the right ventricle of the heart, which is delimited from the rest of the ventricle by the supraventricular crest and which joins the pulmonary trunk, thus forming the outflow tract for blood in the right ventricle. Called also *infundibulum*.

distraction c. a crescentic white area at the temporal edge of the papilla of the optic nerve sometimes seen with the ophthalmoscope in myopic eyes.

c. elas′ticus 1. [TA] elastic cone: the paired lateral portion of the fibroelastic laryngeal membrane, which extends upward in parallel thickenings from the cricoid cartilage to the vocal ligaments. Called also *lateral cricothyroid ligament* and *cricothyroid* or *cricovocal membrane*. 2. cricothyroid ligament. 3. ligamentum cricothyroideum medianum.

co′ni epididy′midis TA alternative for *lobuli epididymidis*.

c. medulla′ris [TA] medullary cone: the cone-shaped lower end of the spinal cord, at the level of the upper lumbar vertebrae; called also *c. terminalis* and *terminal cone of spinal cord*.

myopic c. posterior staphyloma of the myopic eye.

supertraction c. a gray or yellowish ring on the nasal side of the optic papilla sometimes seen with the ophthalmoscope, especially in myopic eyes.

c. termina′lis c. medullaris.

co′ni vasculo′si lobuli epididymidis.

con·va·les·cence (kon″və-les′əns) [L. *convalescere* to become strong] the stage of recovery following an attack of disease, a surgical operation, or an injury.

con·va·les·cent (kon″və-les′ənt) 1. pertaining to or characterized by convalescence. 2. a patient who is recovering from a disease, surgical operation, or injury.

con·vec·tion (kən-vek′shən) [L. *convectio*, from *convehere* to convey] transmission of heat in liquids or gases by a circulation carried on by bulk movement of the heated particles to a cooler area. See also *convection current*, under *current*.

con·ver·gence (kən-vur′jəns) [L. *convergere* to lean together] 1. in evolution, the development of similar structures or organisms in unrelated taxa. 2. in embryology, the movement of cells from the periphery toward the midline during gastrulation. 3. in ophthalmic physiology, the coordinated inclination of the two lines of sight toward their common point of fixation, or the point of fixation itself. 4. in neurology, the exciting of a single sensory neuron by incoming impulses from multiple other neurons, particularly in the central nervous system.

accommodative c. the portion of convergence initiated by the stimulus to accommodation.

amplitude of c. see under *amplitude*.

far point of c. the point of intersection of the lines of sight at minimum convergence.

fusional c. convergence resulting from the attempt to keep the visual stimulus on the fovea of both eyes.

multimodal c., multisensory c. in neurology, convergence in which the incoming impulses are from neurons of different sensory modalities.

near point of c. the point of intersection of the lines of sight at maximum convergence.

negative c. outward vergence, or divergence, of the visual axes.

positive c. inward deviation of the visual axes.

proximal c. convergence induced by the sense of nearness of an object.

tonic c. the continuous convergence maintained by the tone of the medial rectus muscle in the primary position.

con·ver·gent (kən-vur′jənt) [*con-* + *vergere* to incline] meeting at or tending toward a common point.

con·ver·gi·om·e·ter (kən-vur″je-om′ə-tər) [*convergence* (def. 3) + *-meter*] an instrument for measuring latent strabismus.

Con·verse method (kon′vərs) [John Marquis *Converse*, American plastic surgeon, 1909–1981] see under *method*.

con·ver·sion (kən-vur′zhən) [*con-* + *version*] 1. a shift from one form or state to another. 2. a type of defense mechanism in which the anxiety coming from intrapsychic conflict is converted and expressed in a symbolic somatic manifestation; see *conversion disorder*, under *disorder*.

internal c. in decay of an isomer, transition between two nuclear energy states not characterized by emission of a photon because the energy is instead transferred to an inner orbital electron, which is ejected from the atom.

con·ver·tase (kən-vur′tās) an enzyme that releases an active protein from an inactive precursor, as in the activation of specific components of the complement system.

C3 c. an enzyme that splits the complement component C3 to C3a and C3b; the classical pathway C3 convertase is C4b,2a; the alternative pathway C3 convertases are C3b,Bb and C3b,P,Bb; see under *complement*.

C5 c. an enzyme that splits the complement component C5 to C5a and C5b; the classical pathway C5 convertase is C4b,2a,3b; the alternative pathway C5 convertases are $C3b_n$,Bb and $C3b_n$,P,Bb; see under *complement*.

con·ver·tin (kən-vur′tin) the activated form of factor VII; see *coagulation factors*, at *factor*.

con·vex (kon-veks′) [L. *convexus*] having a rounded, somewhat elevated surface, resembling a segment of the external surface of a sphere.

con·vex·i·ty (kon-vek′sĭ-te) [L. *convexitas*] 1. the condition of being convex. 2. a rounded, somewhat elevated area on the surface of an organ or other structure.

con·vexo·ba·sia (kon-vek″so-ba′zhə) [*convex* + *base* of the skull] a deformity of the occipital bone, which is bent forward by the spine; seen in osteitis deformans.

con·vexo·con·cave (kon-vek″so-kon′kāv) convex on one surface and concave on the other.

con·vexo·con·vex (kon-vek″so-kon′veks) convex on each of two opposite surfaces.

con·vo·lut·ed (kon″vo-lo͞ot′əd) [L. *convolutus*] rolled together or coiled.

con·vo·lu·tion (kon″vo-loo′shən) [L. *convolutus* rolled together] a tortuous irregularity or elevation caused by a structure being infolded upon itself; see *gyri cerebri*, under *gyrus*. **convolu′tional, convolu′tionary** *adj*

Broca c. the motor speech center, which in right-handed persons is the inferior frontal gyrus of the left hemisphere of the cerebrum; called also *Broca gyrus* or *region*.

c′s of cerebrum gyri cerebri.

Heschl c′s gyri temporales transversi; see under *gyrus*.

occipitotemporal c. either the gyrus occipitotemporalis lateralis or the gyrus occipitotemporalis medialis.

Zuckerkandl c. gyrus paraterminalis.

Con·vol·vu·la·ceae (kon-vol″vu-la′se-e) the morning glory family, a large family of plants that includes vines, herbs, shrubs, and trees, including the genera *Convolvulus* and *Ipomoea*.

Con·vol·vu·lus (kon-vol′vu-ləs) a genus of flowering plants of the family Convolvulaceae, native to Turkey and nearby areas of the Middle East. *C. scammo′nia* L. is scammony.

con·vul·sant (kən-vul′sənt) 1. producing or causing convulsions. 2. an agent that causes convulsions.

con·vul·si·bil·i·ty (kən-vul″sĭ-bil′ĭ-te) capability of being convulsed.

con·vul·sion (kən-vul′shən) [L. *convulsio*, from *convellere* to pull together] 1. a violent involuntary contraction or series of contractions of the voluntary muscles. 2. seizure (def. 2). **convul′sive** *adj*

central c. a convulsion not triggered by any external cause, but due to a lesion of the central nervous system.

clonic c. a convulsion marked by alternating contracting and relaxing of the muscles.

febrile c′s convulsions associated with high fever, usually seen in infants and children. Called also *febrile seizures*.

hysterical c. pseudoseizure.

puerperal c′s see under *seizure*.

salaam c′s infantile spasms.

tetanic c. a tonic spasm without loss of consciousness; see *tetanus* (def. 2) and *tetany* (def. 1).

tonic c. prolonged contraction of the muscles, as a result of an epileptic discharge.

uremic c. see under *seizure*.

con·vul·si·vant (kən-vul′sĭ-vənt) convulsant.

Coo·ley anemia, disease (koo′lē) [Thomas Benton *Cooley*, American pediatrician, 1871–1945] see *thalassemia*.

Coo·lidge tube (koo′lij) [William David *Coolidge*, American physicist, 1873–1977] see under *tube*.

cool•ing (ko͞ol′ing) the process of reducing the temperature, especially the body temperature of patients and experimental animals. See also *hypothermia.*

Coombs test (ko͞omz) [Robin Royston Amos *Coombs,* British immunologist, born 1921] see *antiglobulin test,* under *test.*

Coo•per fascia, etc. (koo′pər) [Sir Astley Paston *Cooper,* English surgeon, 1768–1841] see under *fascia, hernia,* and *ligament.*

co•op•er•a•tiv•i•ty (ko-op″ər-ə-tiv′ĭ-te) the phenomenon of alteration of binding of subsequent ligands upon binding of an initial ligand by an enzyme, receptor, or other molecule with multiple binding sites, such as frequently occurs in enzymes exhibiting allostery.

negative c. cooperativity in which the dissociation constant for each successive ligand bound is higher than for the one preceding it, so that the binding affinity is successively decreased.

positive c. cooperativity in which the dissociation constant for each successive ligand bound is lower than for the one preceding it, so that the binding affinity is successively increased.

Coo•pe•ria (koo-pe′re-ə) a genus of nematodes of the family Trichostrongylidae. *C. onco′phora, C. pectina′ta,* and *C. puncta′ta* are parasites found in the small intestines of cattle and other ruminants.

coo•pe•ri•a•sis (koo-pə-ri′ə-sis) infection of ruminants with nematodes of the genus *Cooperia.*

coo•per•id (koo′pər-id) a parasitic nematode of the genus *Cooperia.*

Coo•per•nail sign (koo′pər-nāl) [George Peter *Coopernail,* American physician, 1876–1962] see under *sign.*

co•or•di•nate (ko-or′dĭ-nət) one of a set of numbers that locate a point in space.

co•or•di•na•tion (ko-or″dĭ-na′shən) the harmonious functioning of interrelated organs and parts; applied especially to the process of the motor apparatus of the brain that provides for the coworking of particular groups of muscles for the performance of definite adaptive useful responses. Called also *integration.*

co•os•si•fi•ca•tion (ko-os″ĭ-fĭ-ka′shən) the action or state of being joined together by ossification.

co•os•si•fy (ko-os′ĭ-fi) to grow together by ossification.

co•oxy•cod•APAP (ko″ok-se-ko′də-pap) pharmacy equivalent name for a combination of oxycodone hydrochloride and acetaminophen, an analgesic.

COP 1. coat protein. 2. a cancer chemotherapy regimen consisting of cyclophosphamide, Oncovin (vincristine), and prednisone.

co•pal (ko-pal′) [Mex.] the commercial name of many resinous substances of extremely varied origin and character; the original copals came from trees of tropical America, chiefly of the leguminous species *Hymeaea courbaril* L. and various species of *Trachylobium.* It is used in various varnishes and cements and in dentistry for modeling compounds and varnishes for cavities.

Co•pax•one (ko-pak′sōn) trademark for a preparation of glatiramer acetate.

COP-BLAM a cancer chemotherapy regimen consisting of cyclophosphamide, Oncovin (vincristine), prednisone, bleomycin, Adriamycin (doxorubicin), and Matulane (procarbazine).

COPD chronic obstructive pulmonary disease.

Cope sign (kōp) [Sir Vincent *Cope,* English surgeon, 1881–1974] see under *sign.*

cope (kōp) 1. the upper half of a flask used in the casting art; applied in prosthetic dentistry to the upper or cavity side of a denture flask. 2. coping.

Co•peg•us (ko′peg-əs) trademark for a preparation of ribavirin.

co•pe•pod (ko′pə-pod) [Gr. *kōpē* oar + *pous* foot] any animal of the subclass Copepoda.

Co•pep•o•da (ko-pep′o-də) [Gr. *kōpē* oar + *pous* foot] a subclass of minute aquatic arthropods of the class Crustacea; some are intermediate hosts of the nematode *Diphyllobothrium* and others host the tapeworm *Dracunculus;* ingestion of copepods infected with the early larval stages of *Spirometra mansonoides* may cause human sparganosis.

Co•per•ni•cia (ko″pər-nish′e-ə) a genus of palms (family Palmae), native to the Americas. *C. ceri′fera* Mart. is the carnauba, a South American species that yields carnauba wax.

cop•ing (kōp′ing) a metal cap shaped like a truncated cone, which fits over the prepared natural tooth and serves as an abutment for dentures. Called also *cope* and *thimble.*

transfer c. a covering or cap of metal, acrylic resin, or other material, used to position a die in an impression.

copi•opia (kop″e-o′pe-ə) [Gr. *kopos* fatigue + *-opia*] eyestrain from overwork or improper use of the eyes.

Co•poly•mer 1 (ko-pol′ĭ-mər) trademark for a synthetic polypeptide consisting of alanine, glutamic acid, lysine, and tyrosine; it simulates myelin basic protein and is used experimentally in the treatment of relapsing and remitting multiple sclerosis, administered subcutaneously.

co•poly•mer (ko-pol′ĭ-mər) a polymer containing monomers of more than one kind.

ammonio methacrylate c. [NF] a copolymer of acrylic and methacrylic acid esters, used as a pharmaceutic aid.

COPP a cancer chemotherapy regimen consisting of cyclophosphamide, Oncovin (vincristine), procarbazine, and prednisone.

cop•per (Cu) (kop′ər) a reddish, malleable metal; atomic number 29, atomic weight 63.54; with poisonous salts. Copper is essential in nutrition, being a component of various proteins, including ceruloplasmin, erythrocuprein, cytochrome *c* oxidase, and tyrosinase. Deficiency, which is rare, may result in hypochromic microcytic anemia, neutropenia, and bone changes. Excessive accumulation in the body may lead to copper poisoning (see under *poisoning*).

c. 64 a radioactive isotope of copper, atomic mass 64, with a half-life of 12.70 hours, emitting positrons (energy 0.657 MeV), beta particles (energy 0.571 MeV), and gamma rays (energy 1.34 MeV); used in brain scanning.

c. 67 a radioisotope of copper, atomic mass 67, with a half-life of 2.58 days, emitting beta particles (energy 0.395, 0.484, 0.577 MeV) and gamma rays (energy 0.185, 0.092 MeV); used in radiotherapy as well as for imaging, tracer kinetic studies, and dosimetry.

c. acetoarsenite an emerald green powder derived by reaction of sodium arsenite, copper sulfate, and acetic acid; it is toxic by ingestion and is used as an insecticide and wood preservative. Called also *Paris green.*

c. gluconate [USP] a salt of copper used in the prophylaxis and treatment of copper deficiency.

c. sulfate cupric sulfate; see under *cupric.*

cop•per•as (kop′ər-əs) commercial ferrous sulfate, disinfectant and deodorizer. See also *ferrous sulfate,* under *ferrous.*

cop•per•head (kop′ər-hed) 1. *Agkistrodon contortrix,* a venomous snake of the United States that has a brown to copper-colored body with dark bands. Called also *highland moccasin.* 2. *Denisonia superba,* a highly venomous elapid snake found in Australia and the Solomon Islands. See table at *snake.*

co•pre•cip•i•tin (ko″pre-sip′ĭ-tin) a precipitin in the same serum with one or more other precipitins.

cop•rem•e•sis (kop-rem′ə-sis) fecal vomiting.

Co•pri•na•ceae (ko″prĭ-na′se-e) a family of mushrooms (order Agaricales); it includes the genus *Coprinus.*

co•prine (ko′prēn) a glutamic acid derivative found in the edible mushroom *Coprinus atramentarius;* its active metabolite is cyclopropanone hydrate.

Co•pri•nus (ko-pri′nəs) the ink caps or inky caps, a genus of mushrooms of the family Coprinaceae. *C. atramenta′rius* is an edible species that contains coprine and causes a disulfiram-like toxic response in the presence of alcohol.

copr(o)- [Gr. *kopros* dung] a combining form denoting relationship to feces.

cop•ro•an•ti•body (kop″ro-an′tĭ-bod″e) an antibody found in the feces, chiefly secretory IgA.

Cop•ro•coc•cus (kop″ro-kok′əs) [*copro-* + Gr. *kokkos* berry] a genus of bacteria, made up of gram-positive anaerobic cocci of the family Lachnospiraceae, occasionally isolated from human specimens.

cop•ro•dae•um (kop″ro-de′əm) [*copro-* + Gr. *hodiaos* on the way] the large dorsal passage in the proximal part of the cloaca in monotremes, into which the intestine opens.

cop•ro•de•um (kop″ro-de′əm) coprodaeum.

cop•ro•lag•nia (kop″ro-lag′ne-ə) [*copro-* + Gr. *lagneia* lust] sexual excitement occurring in association with feces or defecation.

cop•ro•la•lia (kop″ro-la′le-ə) [*copro-* + *lal-* + *-ia*] compulsive, stereotyped use of obscene, "filthy" language, particularly of words relating to feces; seen in some cases of schizophrenia and Gilles de la Tourette syndrome. Called also *coprophrasia.*

cop•ro•lith (kop′ro-lith) [*copro-* + *-lith*] fecalith.

cop•rol•o•gy (kop-rol′ə-je) [*copro-* + *-logy*] scatology (def. 1).

cop•ro•ma (kop-ro′mə) fecaloma.

cop•ro•pha•gia (kop″ro-fa′jə) [*copro-* + *-phagia*] ingestion of feces; called also *coprophagy.* **copropha′gic, coproph′agous** *adj*

cop•roph•a•gy (kop-rof′ə-je) coprophagia.

cop•ro•phil (kop′ro-fil) a coprophilous microorganism.

cop•ro•phile (kop′ro-fīl) 1. coprophil. 2. coprophilous.

cop•ro•phil•ia (kop″ro-fil′e-ə) [*copro-* + *-philia*] an absorbing interest in feces or filth, particularly a paraphilia in which sexual arousal or activity is linked to feces.

cop•ro•phil•i•ac (kop″ro-fil′e-ak) coprophilic (def. 1).

cop•ro•phil•ic (kop″ro-fil′ik) 1. pertaining to or characterized by coprophilia. 2. coprophilous.

cop•roph•i•lous (kop-rof′ĭ-ləs) living and growing on feces or in feces-polluted water; said of certain microorganisms and fungi. Called also *coprophilic.*

cop•ro•pho•bia (kop″ro-fo′be-ə) [*copro-* + *-phobia*] abnormal repugnance to defecation and to feces.

cop•ro•phra•sia (kop″ro-fra′zhə) coprolalia.

cop•ro•por•phy•ria (kop″ro-por-fir′e-ə) any of various types of porphyria characterized by elevated levels of coproporphyrin in the body.

erythropoietic c. a rare type of erythropoietic porphyria characterized by mild skin photosensitivity and elevated levels of erythrocyte coproporphyrin III.

hereditary c. (HCP) an autosomal dominant hepatic porphyria caused by mutations of the *CPOX* gene (locus: 3q12) that result in partial deficiency of coproporphyrinogen oxidase activity. It is characterized by recurrent attacks of gastroenterologic and neurologic dysfunction similar to those of acute intermittent porphyria, and sometimes by cutaneous photosensitivity. Coproporphyrin III is excreted constantly in the feces and intermittently, with δ-aminolevulinic acid and porphobilinogen, in the urine.

cop•ro•por•phy•rin (kop″ro-por′fə-rin) a porphyrin produced by oxidation of the methylene bridges in coproporphyrinogen. Four isomers are possible, but only two exist naturally. *Coproporphyrin III* is excreted in the feces and urine in hereditary coproporphyria and variegate porphyria, particularly during acute attacks. *Coproporphyrin I* is excreted in the feces and urine in congenital erythropoietic porphyria.

cop•ro•por•phy•rin•o•gen (kop″ro-por″fə-rin′o-jən) a porphyrinogen (q.v.) in which each pyrrole ring has one methyl side chain and one propionate side chain; it is formed by oxidative decarboxylation of uroporphyrinogen. Four isomers are possible but only two exist naturally, types I and III; the latter is a functional intermediate in heme biosynthesis while the former is produced in an abortive side reaction.

cop•ro•por•phy•rin•o•gen ox•i•dase (kop″ro-por″fə-rin′o-jən ok′sĭ-dās) [EC 1.3.3.3] an enzyme of the oxidoreductase class that catalyzes the conversion of coproporphyrinogen III to protoporphyrinogen IX. It occurs in mitochondria, and the reaction is a part of the pathway of heme biosynthesis. Deficiency of the enzyme, an autosomal dominant trait, results in hereditary coproporphyria.

cop•ro•por•phy•rin•uria (kop″ro-por″fə-rin-u′re-ə) the presence of coproporphyrin in the urine; see *coproporphyria.*

cop•ro•prax•ia (kop″ro-prak′se-ə) [*copro-* + Gr. *praxia* action, from *prassein* to perform] compulsive, stereotyped use of obscene movements or gestures, seen in some cases of Gilles de la Tourette syndrome.

cop•ros•ta•nol (kop-ros′tə-nol) a saturated sterol of the feces, formed by bacterial reduction of cholesterol in the intestines. Called also *coprosterol.*

cop•ros•ta•sis (kop-ros′tə-sis) [*copro-* + *-stasis*] fecal impaction.

cop•ros•ter•ol (kop-ros′tər-ol) coprostanol.

co-prox•APAP (ko-prok′sə-pap) pharmacy equivalent name for a combination of propoxyphene napsylate and acetaminophen, an analgesic.

cop•ro•zoa (kop″ro-zo′ə) [*copro-* + Gr. *zōon* animal] protozoa that are found in fecal matter outside the body but do not inhabit the intestine.

cop•ro•zo•ic (kop″ro-zo′ik) living in fecal material; found in fecal material.

cop•u•la (kop′u-lə) [L.] 1. any connecting part or structure. 2. c. linguae.

c. lin′guae a median ventral elevation on the embryonic tongue formed by union of the second pair of pharyngeal arches during the fourth week; it is overgrown by the hypopharyngeal eminence during the fifth and sixth weeks.

cop•u•la•tion (kop″u-la′shən) [L. *copulatio*] sexual union between male and female; the act transferring the sperm from male to female; used particularly for nonhuman animals.

Coq. [L.] co′que (boil).

Coq. in s. a. [L.] co′que in sufficien′te a′qua (boil in sufficient water).

Coq. s. a. [L.] co′que secun′dum ar′tem (boil properly).

co•quille (ko-kēl′) [Fr. "shell"] a glass or lens of uniform thickness shaped like a watch crystal.

Co•quil•let•tid•ia (ko-kwil′ə-tid′e-ə) a genus of large, mostly yellow, freshwater mosquitoes of the tribe Mansoniini, subfamily Culicini, that lay egg masses on stagnant water or weedy ponds and are vicious biters; some species have been implicated as vectors of disease.

C. juxtamanso′nia a species that is a vector of *Wuchereria bancrofti* in Brazil.

C. ochra′cea a species that is a vector of *Brugia malayi* in Southeast Asia.

C. pertur′bans a species that is a vector of eastern equine encephalitis in North America.

C. venezuelen′sis a South American species that is the vector of several arboviruses, including Oropouche virus.

cor (kor) gen. *cor′dis* [L.] [TA] the heart (q.v.): the muscular organ that maintains the circulation of the blood.

c. adipo′sum fatty heart (def. 2).

c. bilocula′re a congenital anomaly characterized by failure of formation of the interatrial and interventricular septa, the heart having only two chambers, a single atrium and a single ventricle, and a common atrioventricular valve.

c. bovi′num [L. "ox heart"] a greatly enlarged heart resulting from a hypertrophied or dilated left ventricle; called also *c. taurinum, bovine heart,* and *ox heart.*

c. dex′trum right heart.

c. pulmonale, acute acute overload of the right ventricle due to pulmonary hypertension, usually resulting from acute pulmonary embolism.

c. pulmonale, chronic heart disease characterized by hypertrophy and sometimes dilation of the right ventricle secondary to disease affecting the structure or function of the lungs, but excluding those pulmonary disorders resulting from congenital heart disease or from diseases primarily affecting the left side of the heart.

c. sinis′trum left heart.

c. tauri′num c. bovinum.

c. triatria′tum a congenital anomaly caused by failure of resorption of the embryonic common pulmonary vein, resulting in division of the left atrium by a fibromuscular diaphragm, the posterosuperior chamber receiving the pulmonary venous return and the anteroinferior chamber communicating with the left atrial appendage and mitral orifice. The orifice between the two compartments may be reduced or absent, producing pulmonary venous obstruction.

c. trilocula′re three-chambered heart.

c. trilocula′re biatria′tum common ventricle.

c. trilocula′re biventricula′re common atrium.

cor- see *con-.*

cor•a•cid•ia (kor″ə-sid′e-ə) [L.] plural of *coracidium.*

cor•a•cid•i•um (kor″ə-sid′e-əm) pl. *coracid′ia* [L.] The individual free-swimming or free-crawling, spherical, ciliated embryo of tapeworms of the order Pseudophyllidea.

cor•a•co•acro•mi•al (kor″ə-ko-ə-kro′me-əl) pertaining to the coracoid and acromion processes.

cor•a•co•cla•vic•u•lar (kor″ə-ko-klə-vik′u-lər) pertaining to the coracoid process and the clavicle.

cor•a•co•hu•mer•al (kor″ə-ko-hu′mər-əl) pertaining to the coracoid process and the humerus.

cor•a•coid (kor′ə-koid) [Gr. *korakoeidēs* crowlike] 1. like a raven's beak. 2. the coracoid process (processus coracoideus scapulae [TA]).

cor•a•coi•di•tis (kor″ə-koi-di′tis) a painful condition in the region of the scapula and the coracoid process, with deltoid atrophy; attributed to injury of the coracoid process.

cor•a•co•ra•di•a•lis (kor″ə-ko-ra″de-a′lis) caput breve musculi bicipitis brachii.

cor•a•co•ul•nar•is (kor″ə-ko-əl-nar′is) the fibers of the biceps muscle attached to the fascia of the forearm.

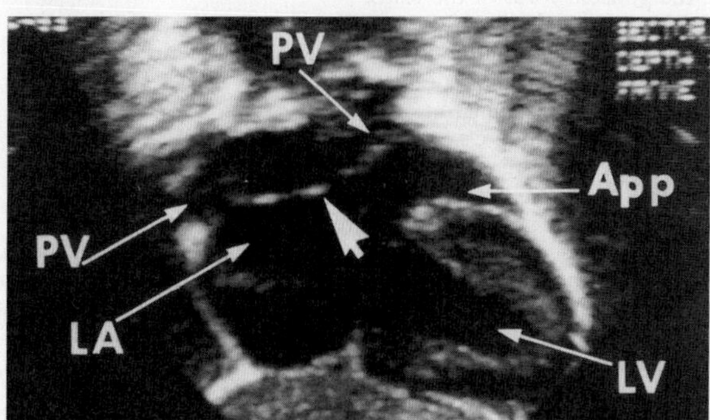

■ Echocardiogram (subxiphoid) of a young child with cor triatriatum. The membrane *(large arrow)* inserts proximal to the left atrial appendage *(App)* and distal to the pulmonary veins *(PV).(LA),* Left atrium; *(LV),* left ventricle.

co•ral•li•form (ko-ral′ĭ-form) [L. *corallum* coral + *form*] having the form of a coral; branching like a coral.

cor•al•lin (kor′ə-lin) aurin.

yellow c. the sodium salt of aurin, occurring as yellow masses with a greenish metallic luster, which turns red in solution; called also *corallin yellow*.

cor•al•loid (kor′ə-loid) coralliform.

cord (kord) [L. *chorda;* Gr. *chordē* string] any long, rounded, flexible structure; see also *chorda* and *funiculus*.

angioblastic c's cordlike masses of splanchnic mesenchymal cells ventral to the primordial coelom; they arrange themselves side by side to form the primordia of the endocardial heart tubes; called also *angiogenic cell clusters*.

Billroth c's red pulp c's.

cortical c's cellular cords concentrated in the cortical region of the early fetal ovary; the primordial germ cells are incorporated into them and they break up to form primordial ovarian follicles.

dental c. a cordlike mass of cells from which the enamel organ develops.

enamel c. a vertical extension of the enamel knot in a developing tooth, connecting the enamel knot with the outer dental epithelium, a temporary structure which disappears before enamel formation begins.

farcy c's enlarged lymphatic vessels seen in farcy; called also *farcy pipes*.

genital c. in the embryo, the midline fused caudal part of the two urogenital ridges, each containing a mesonephric and a paramesonephric duct.

germinal c's the precursors to the embryonic ovary or testis, derived from the gonadal cords.

gonadal c's epithelial cells derived from the coelomic epithelium that penetrate the underlying mesenchyme, where they form seminiferous cords.

gubernacular c. chorda gubernaculum.

hepatic c's, hepatic cell c's anastomosing plates of hepatic cells radiating outward from the central vein, composing the parenchyma of a hepatic lobule.

lateral c. of brachial plexus fasciculus lateralis plexus brachialis.

lymph c's medullary c's (def. 1).

medial c. of brachial plexus fasciculus medialis plexus brachialis.

medullary c's 1. strands of dense lymphoid tissue surrounded by the sinuses of the medulla of a lymph node; called also *lymph c's*. 2. rete c's.

nephrogenic c. a longitudinal cordlike part of the urogenital ridge, formed of fused or never separated nephrotome plates, that gives rise to the mesonephric tubules and part of the metanephric tubules.

oblique c. of elbow joint chorda obliqua membranae interosseae antebrachii.

ovigerous c's rete cords of the primordial ovary that resolve into eggs and their follicles.

posterior c. of brachial plexus fasciculus posterior plexus brachialis.

primordial sex c's gonadal c's.

red pulp c's the masses of red pulp of the spleen; called also *Billroth c's* and *splenic c's*.

rete c's strands of primordial cells in the medulla of the embryonic gonads that connect with some of the mesonephric tubules, and from which the rete ovarii or the rete testis develops; called also *medullary c's*.

retraction c. a cord impregnated with a chemical or medication, used in dental surgery for gingival retraction.

scirrhous c. chronic fibrous enlargement of the stump of the spermatic cord of a castrated horse caused by bacterial infection, with discharge of pus and sometimes formation of a tumorlike mass with numerous weeping sinuses.

seminiferous c's the primordia of the seminiferous tubules, derived from the gonadal cords of the testis.

sex c's germinal c's.

sexual c's the seminiferous tubules of the early fetus.

spermatic c. funiculus spermaticus.

spinal c. medulla spinalis.

splenic c's red pulp c's.

testis c's the germinal cords of the embryonic testis.

tethered c. see under *syndrome*.

umbilical c. the flexible structure connecting the umbilicus of the embryo and fetus with the placenta and giving passage to the umbilical arteries and vein. In the newborn it measures about 50 cm in length. First formed during the fifth embryonic week from the connecting stalk, it contains the omphaloenteric duct (yolk stalk) and the allantois.

c. of umbilical artery chorda arteriae umbilicalis.

vocal c., false plica vestibularis.

vocal c., true plica vocalis.

Weitbrecht c. chorda obliqua membranae interosseae antebrachii.

Willis c's numerous fibrous bands (dural trabeculae) that extend transversely across the inferior angle of the superior sagittal sinus.

cord•al (kor′dəl) pertaining to a cord; used specifically in referring to the vocal cord (*plica vocalis* [TA]).

Cor•da•rone (kor′də-rōn) trademark for preparations of amiodarone hydrochloride.

cor•date (kor′dāt) [L. *cor* heart] cordiform.

cor•dec•to•my (kor-dek′tə-me) [*cord-* + *-ectomy*] excision of all or part of a cord, such as a vocal cord or the spinal cord.

cor•di•form (kor′dĭ-form) [*cor* + *form*] heart-shaped.

cor•ding-up (kor″ding-up′) azoturia (def. 2).

cor•di•tis (kor-di′tis) 1. chorditis (def. 1). 2. funiculitis (def. 1).

cord(o)- see *chord(o)-*.

cor•do•cen•te•sis (kor″do-sen-te′sis) [*cordo-* + *-centesis*] percutaneous puncture of the umbilical vein under ultrasonographic guidance to obtain a fetal blood sample. Called also *percutaneous umbilical blood sampling*.

cor•do•pexy (kor′do-pek″se) [*cordo-* + *-pexy*] the operation of displacing outward the vocal cord for bilateral vocal cord paralysis.

cor•dot•o•my (kor-dot′ə-me) [*cordo-* + *-tomy*] 1. section of a vocal cord. 2. interruption of the lateral spinothalamic tract of the spinal cord, usually in the anterolateral quadrant, for relief of intractable pain. Also spelled *chordotomy*.

open c. cordotomy (def. 2) done through an open incision; now largely replaced by percutaneous cordotomy.

percutaneous c. cordotomy (def. 2) performed using percutaneous electrodes guided radiographically with stereotactic techniques; approaches used include lateral high cervical, posterior high cervical, and anterior low cervical.

Cor•dran (kor′dran) trademark for preparations of flurandrenolide.

Cor•dy•ceps (kor′dĭ-seps) a genus of fungi of the family Clavicipitaceae; certain species produce fatal disease of caterpillars.

C. sinen′sis a parasite of insect larvae; in Chinese medicine it is used as a drug coagulant.

Cor•dy•lo•bia (kor″də-lo′be-ə) a genus of flies of the family Calliphoridae.

C. anthropo′phaga the tumbu fly, a species found in Africa whose larvae (cayor worms) burrow under the skin and cause myiasis.

C. rodhai′ni the Lund fly, a species found in Africa whose larvae burrow under the skin and cause lesions in rodents, antelopes, and humans.

core (kor) 1. the central part of anything. 2. a bar of iron around which a wire is wound to form an induction coil or electromagnet. 3. the central part of a virion, consisting of nucleic acid and sometimes protein. 4. cast c.

cast c. a metal casting, usually with a post in the root canal, designed to support and retain an artificial crown.

core- [Gr. *korē* pupil] a combining form denoting relationship to the pupil of the eye; also, *chord(o)-* and *cor(o)-*. See also words beginning *irid(o)-*.

co•re•cep•tor (ko-re-sep′tər) a cell-surface molecule to which a ligand must bind, in addition to binding to a primary receptor, in order to initiate a biological process.

cor•ec•ta•sis (kor-ek′tə-sis) [*core-* + *ectasis*] dilatation of the pupil.

cor•ec•tome (kor-ek′tōm) a cutting instrument used in performing iridectomy (corectomy).

co•rec•to•me•di•al•y•sis (ko-rek″to-me″de-al′ə-sis) [*core-* + *ectomy* + *dialysis*] the operation of forming an artificial pupil by detaching the iris from the ciliary ligament.

co•rec•to•my (ko-rek′tə-me) [*cor-* + *ectomy*] iridectomy.

cor•ec•to•pia (kor″ek-to′pe-ə) [*core-* + *ectopia*] an abnormal location of the pupil.

core•di•al•y•sis (kor″ə-di-al′ə-sis) [*core-* + *dialysis*] the surgical separation of the external margin of the iris from the ciliary body.

core•di•as•ta•sis (kor″ə-di-as′tə-sis) [*core-* + Gr. *diastasis* distention] the dilatation or a dilated state of the pupil.

Co•reg (ko′reg) trademark for a preparation of carvedilol.

co•reg•o•nin (ko-reg′o-nin) a protamine obtained from the sperm of the whitefish.

co•rel•y•sis (kə-rel′ə-sis) [*core-* + *lysis*] operative destruction of the pupil; especially the surgical detachment of adhesions of the pupillary margin of the iris from the lens.

co•rem•i•um (kə-re′me-əm) synnema.

cor•e•mor•pho•sis (kor″ə-mor-fo′sis) [*core-* + *morphosis*] the surgical formation of an artificial pupil.

cor•en•cli•sis (kor″en-kli′sis) iridencleisis.

core(o)- see *core-*.

cor•e•om•e•ter (kor″e-om′ə-tər) pupillometer.

cor•e•om•e•try (kor″e-om′ə-tre) pupillometry.

cor•eo•plas•ty (kor′e-o-plas″te) [*coreo-* + *-plasty*] any plastic operation on the iris.

co•re•pres•sor (ko″re-pres′ər) a small molecule that combines with a protein aporepressor molecule to form an active substance, which then binds to an operator gene and inhibits the synthesis of an enzyme. The mechanism is a negative control in inducible enzyme systems.

cor•e•ste•no•ma (kor″e-stə-no′mə) [*core-* + Gr. *stenōma* contraction] an abnormally contracted state of the pupil.

  c. conge′nitum a congenital condition in which the pupil is partially occluded by excrescences which meet, leaving scattered small openings.

Co•re•thra (ko-re′thrə) *Chaoborus.*

co•re•to•me•di•al•y•sis (kor″ə-to″me-di-al′ə-sis) corectomedialysis.

co•ret•o•my (kor-et′ə-me) iridectomy.

Cor•gard (kor′gahrd) trademark for a preparation of nadolol.

Co•ri cycle, disease, ester (ko′re) [Carl Ferdinand *Cori* Czechoslovakian-born American physician and biochemist , 1896–1984, and Gerty Theresa Radnitz *Cori*, Czechoslovakian-born American physician and biochemist, 1896–1957, co-winners of the Nobel prize.] see under *cycle*, see *glycogen storage disease, type III*, under *disease*, and see *glucose 1-phosphate*.

co•ri•a•ceous (kor″e-a′shəs) [L. *corium* leather] resembling leather; leathery, tough; said of bacterial cultures.

co•ri•a•myr•tin (kor″e-ə-mur′tin) a toxic glycoside from *Coriaria* with neurostimulating activity, causing convulsions and sometimes death.

cor•i•an•der (kor″e-an′dər) [Gr. *koriandron*, variant of *koriannon*] 1. *Coriandrum sativum.* 2. the dried ripe fruit of *C. sativum*, used as a flavoring and source of coriander oil.

Co•ri•an•drum (ko″re-an′drəm) a genus of plants of the family Umbelliferae. *C. sati′vum* is coriander, used as a flavoring and source of coriander oil.

Co•ri•a•ria (kor″e-ar′e-ə) a genus of trees and shrubs of the family Coriariaceae, native to Europe and Asia. Most species contain the toxin coriamyrtin, which causes vomiting, convulsions, and death. Many of these plants are used for the dyes and tannins they contain.

Cor•id (kor′id) trademark for a preparation of amprolium.

co•ri•in (kor′e-in) a substance formed by treating fibrous connective tissue with alkalis.

Co•rio•bac•te•ri•a•ceae (kor″e-o-bak-tēr″e-a′se-e) a family of bacteria of the order Coriobacteriales, consisting of gram-positive, non–spore-forming, rod-shaped to coccoid cells; organisms of medical interest are contained in the genera *Atopobium* and *Eggerthella*.

Co•rio•bac•te•ri•a•les (kor″e-o-bak-tēr″e-a′lēz) an order of bacteria of the subclass Coriobacteridae, containing the single family Coriobacteriaceae.

Co•rio•bac•te•ri•dae (kor″e-o-bak-tēr′ĭ-de) a subclass of bacteria of the class Actinobacteria, containing the single order Coriobacteriales.

co•ri•um (kor′e-əm) [L. "hide"] TA alternative for *dermis*.

Cor•lo•pam (kor′lo-pam) trademark for a preparation of fenoldopam mesylate.

corm (korm) [L. *cormus*] a solid bulblike expansion of a plant stem below the surface of the ground.

Cor•max (kor′maks) trademark for preparations of clobetasol propionate.

corn (korn) [L. *cornu* horn] 1. a hardening and thickening of the stratum corneum of the skin of the toes, caused by friction and pressure from poorly fitting shoes or hose; it forms a conical mass pointing down into the dermis, producing pain and inflammation. There are two kinds, the *hard c.* and the *soft c.* Called also *clavus* and *heloma*. 2. *Zea mays.* 3. the seeds of certain cereal grains, especially *Zea mays*, used as both animal and human food. See also *corn oil*, under *oil*. 4. a bruise on the bottom of a horse's foot between the wall of the heel and the bar. 5. a circumscribed hyperkeratosis of the footpad of dogs, sensitive to pressure.

  hard c. a firm type of corn, usually found on the outside of the little toe or the upper surface of a toe; called also *clavus durus* and *heloma durum*.

  soft c. a type of corn found between the toes and kept soft by moisture; called also *clavus mollis* and *heloma molle*.

  squirrel c., turkey c. *Dicentra canadensis.*

corn cock•le (korn kok′əl) *Agrostemma githago.*

cor•nea (kor′ne-ə) [L. *corneus* horny] [TA] the transparent structure forming the anterior part of the sclera of the eye. It consists of five layers: (1) the anterior corneal epithelium, continuous with that of the conjunctiva; (2) the anterior limiting layer (Bowman membrane); (3) the substantia propria, or stroma; (4) the posterior limiting layer (Descemet membrane); and (5) the endothelium of the anterior chamber. **cor′neal** *adj*

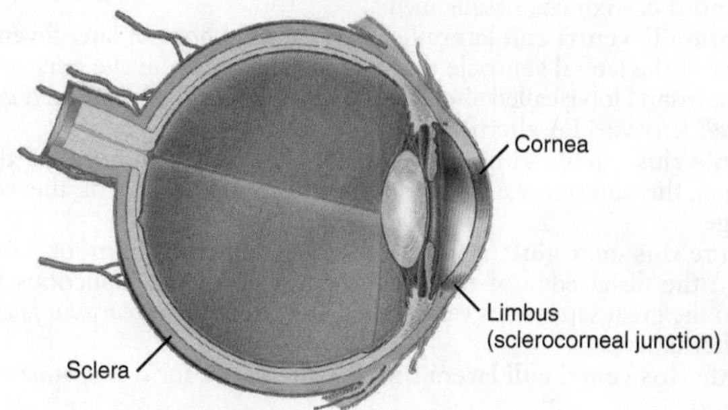

  conical c. keratoconus.

  c. farina′ta senile degeneration of the cornea marked by fine dustlike stippling.

  flat c. the configuration of the cornea when a shallow ocular chamber is present or when the eyeball is atrophic.

  c. globo′sa megalocornea.

  c. gutta′ta a degenerative condition of the cornea in which there are tiny spherical globules on its surface, owing to dystrophy of the endothelial cells.

  c. opa′ca the sclerotic coat of the eye.

  c. pla′na congenital flatness of the cornea.

  c. verticilla′ta Fleischer vortex.

cor•ne•itis (kor″ne-i′tis) keratitis.

Cor•ne•lia de Lange (kor-na′le-ah da lahng′ə) see *de Lange*.

cor•neo•bleph•a•ron (kor″ne-o-blef′ə-ron) [*cornea* + Gr. *blepharon* eyelid] adhesion between the eyelid and cornea.

cor•neo•cyte (kor′ne-o-sīt″) the remains of a keratinocyte in the stratum corneum ready to be shed.

cor•neo•des•mo•some (kor″ne-o-dez′mo-sōm) [*corneocyte* + *desmosome*] an intercellular junction that mediates adhesion between corneocytes; it is degraded by enzymatic action at the surface of the stratum corneum so that cells can be shed.

cor•neo•iri•tis (kor″ne-o-i-ri′tis) inflammation of the cornea and iris.

cor•neo•scle•ra (kor″ne-o-skler′ə) the cornea and sclera regarded as forming one organ.

cor•neo•scle•ral (kor″ne-o-skler′əl) affecting or pertaining to both the cornea and the sclera.

cor•ne•ous (kor′ne-əs) [L. *corneus*] 1. horny. 2. keratinous (def. 1).

cor•ner (kor′nər) corner tooth.

Cor•net forceps (kor′nət) [Georg *Cornet*, German bacteriologist, 1858–1915] a cover glass forceps.

cor•ne•um (kor′ne-əm) [L. "horny"] horny; see *stratum corneum*.

cor•nic•u•late (kor-nik′u-lāt) shaped like a small horn.

cor•nic•u•lum (kor-nik′u-ləm) [L. dim. of *cornu*] cartilago corniculata.

cor•ni•fi•ca•tion (kor″nĭ-fĭ-ka′shən) [*cornu* + L. *facere* to make] 1. conversion into horn. 2. keratinization. 3. conversion of epithelium to the stratified squamous type.

cor•ni•fied (kor′nĭ-fīd) 1. converted into horny tissue. 2. keratinized (see *keratinize*).

cor•noid (kor′noid) [*cornu* + *-oid*] abnormally hard or horny.

corn•starch (korn′stahrch) see *starch* (def. 2).

cor•nu (kor′noo) pl. *cor′nua* [L. "horn"] 1. horn (def. 1). 2. a structure resembling a horn in shape. **cor′nual, cor′nuate** *adj*

  c. ammo′nis [L. "horn of Ammon"] TA alternative for *hippocampus proprius*.

  c. ante′rius medul′lae spina′lis [TA] anterior horn of spinal cord: the horn-shaped configuration presented by the anterior column of the spinal cord in transverse section; called also *c. ventrale medullae spinalis* and *ventral horn of spinal cord*.

  c. ante′rius ventri′culi latera′lis TA alternative for *c. frontale ventriculi lateralis*.

  cor′nua cartila′ginis thyroi′deae the horns of the thyroid cartilage; see *c. inferius cartilaginis thyroideae* and *c. superius cartilaginis thyroideae*.

  c. coccygea′le c. coccygeum.

c. **coccy′geum** [TA], **c. of coccyx** coccygeal horn: either of the cranial pair of rudimentary articular processes of the coccyx that articulate with the cornua of the sacrum. Called also *c. coccygeale.*

c. **cuta′neum** cutaneous horn.

c. **dorsa′le medul′lae spina′lis** c. posterius medullae spinalis.

ethmoid c. concha nasalis media.

c. **fronta′le ventri′culi latera′lis** [TA] frontal horn of lateral ventricle: the part of the lateral ventricle that extends forward from the pars centralis into the frontal lobe; called also *anterior horn of lateral ventricle* and *c. anterius ventriculi lateralis* [TA alternative].

c. **infe′rius cartila′ginis thyroi′deae** [TA] inferior horn of thyroid cartilage: the inferior extension of the posterior border of the thyroid cartilage.

c. **infe′rius mar′ginis falcifor′mis** [TA] inferior horn of falciform margin: the distal edge of the falciform margin of the saphenous hiatus, deep to the great saphenous vein. Called also *crus inferius marginis falciformis* [TA alternative].

c. **infe′rius ventri′culi latera′lis** TA alternative for *c. temporale ventriculi lateralis.*

c. **latera′le medul′lae spina′lis** [TA] lateral horn of spinal cord: the horn-shaped configuration presented by the intermediate column of the spinal cord in transverse section. See also *columnae griseae* and *columna intermedia medullae spinalis.*

c. **ma′jus os′sis hyoi′dei** [TA] greater horn of hyoid bone: a bony projection passing posteriorly and superiorly from either side of the body of the hyoid bone.

c. **mi′nus os′sis hyoi′dei** [TA] lesser horn of hyoid bone: a small conical eminence projecting superiorly on either side of the hyoid bone at the angle of junction between the body and the greater horn.

c. **occipita′le ventri′culi latera′lis** [TA] occipital horn of lateral ventricle: the part of the lateral ventricle that extends backward from the atrium of the lateral ventricle into the occipital lobe; called also *c. posterius ventriculi lateralis* [TA alternative] and *posterior horn of lateral ventricle.*

cor′nua os′sis hyoi′dei the horns of the hyoid bone; see *c. majus ossis hyoidei* and *c. minus ossis hyoidei.*

c. **poste′rius medul′lae spina′lis** [TA] posterior horn of spinal cord: the horn-shaped configuration presented by the posterior gray matter of the spinal cord in transverse section; called also *c. dorsale medullae spinalis* and *dorsal horn of spinal cord.*

c. **poste′rius ventri′culi latera′lis** TA alternative for *c. occipitale ventriculi lateralis.*

sacral c., c. sacra′le [TA] sacral horn: either of the two hook-shaped processes extending downward from the arch of the last sacral vertebra.

cornua of spinal cord the horn-shaped structures seen in transverse section of the spinal cord; see *c. anterius medullae spinalis, c. laterale medullae spinalis,* and *c. posterius medullae spinalis.*

c. **supe′rius cartila′ginis thyroi′deae** [TA] superior horn of thyroid cartilage: the superior extension of the posterior border of the thyroid cartilage.

c. **supe′rius mar′ginis falcifor′mis** [TA] superior horn of falciform margin: the proximal end of the falciform margin of the saphenous hiatus; called also *crus superius marginis falciformis* [TA alternative] and *ligament of Scarpa.*

c. **tempora′le ventri′culi latera′lis** [TA] temporal horn of lateral ventricle: the part of the lateral ventricle that extends downward and forward from the atrium behind the thalamus and into the temporal lobe; called also *c. inferius ventriculi lateralis* [TA alternative] and *inferior horn of lateral ventricle.*

c. **u′teri** [TA] horn of uterus: either of the bluntly rounded superior lateral extremities of the body of the uterus that marks the entrance of the uterine tube.

c. **ventra′le medul′lae spina′lis** c. anterius medullae spinalis.

cor•nua (kor′noo-ə) [L.] plural of *cornu.*

cor•nu•com•mis•sur•al (kor″noo-ko-mis′u-rəl) pertaining to a cornu and to a commissure.

cor(o)- see *core-.*

co•ro•di•as•ta•sis (kor″o-di-as′tə-sis) corediastasis.

co•rol•la (ko-rol′ə) [L. "little crown"] the inner set of leaves of a floral envelope, the individual portions of which are called petals.

co•ro•na (kə-ro′nə) pl. *coronas, coro′nae* [L., from Gr. *korōnē*] a crown; used in anatomy to designate a crownlike eminence or encircling structure.

c. **cilia′ris** [TA] ciliary crown: the region on the anterior inner surface of the ciliary body of the eye from which radiate the ciliary processes; called also *pars plicata corporis ciliaris.*

c. **cli′nica** [TA] clinical crown: that portion of the tooth above the clinical root, i.e., the portion exposed beyond the gingiva, and thus visible in the oral cavity. Called also *extra-alveolar crown.*

dental c., c. den′tis [TA] crown of tooth: the upper part of the tooth, which joins the lower part, the root, at the cervix at the cementoenamel junction, and terminates as the grinding surface of molar or premolar teeth or the cutting edge of incisors. Called also *anatomical* or *dental crown.*

c. **glan′dis pe′nis** [TA] corona of glans penis: the rounded proximal border of the glans penis, separated from the corpora cavernosa penis by the neck of the glans.

c. **radia′ta** 1. [TA] the radiating crown of projection fibers which pass from the internal capsule to every part of the cerebral cortex. 2. an investing layer of radially elongated follicular cells surrounding the zona pellucida of a secondary oocyte.

c. **ve′neris** a ring of syphilitic sores around the forehead, sometimes deeply affecting the bones of the head.

Zinn c. circulus vasculosus nervi optici.

co•ro•nad (kor′ŏ-nad) toward the crown of the head or any corona.

co•ro•nae (kə-ro′ne) [L.] genitive and plural of *corona.*

cor•o•nal (kor′ə-nəl) [L. *coronalis*] 1. pertaining to the crown of the head, the crown of a tooth, or any other corona. 2. in the direction of the coronal suture; said of a longitudinal plane or section passing through the body at right angles to the median plane. See under *plane.* Called also *coronalis.*

co•ro•na•le (kor-o-na′le) 1. the point of the coronal suture at the end of the maximum frontal diameter. 2. os frontale.

co•ro•na•lis (kor″o-na′lis) [L.] [TA] coronal: general anatomical nomenclature denoting something situated in the direction of the coronal suture.

co•ro•na•rog•ra•phy (kəro″nərog′rəfe) [*coronary* + *-graphy*] coronary arteriography.

cor•o•nary (kor′ə-nar″e) [*corona*] encircling in the manner of a crown; a term applied to vessels, nerves, ligaments, etc. The term usually denotes the arteries that supply the heart muscle and, by extension, a pathologic involvement of them.

Co•ro•na•vi•ri•dae (kə-ro″nə-vir′ĭ-de) the coronaviruses and toroviruses: a family of RNA viruses having a pleomorphic virion 120–160 nm in diameter consisting of a lipid-containing membrane, with large peplomers, surrounding a helical (for coronaviruses) or tubular (for toroviruses) nucleocapsid. The genome consists of a single molecule of positive-sense single-stranded polyadenylated RNA (MW 5.5–6.1 × 10^6, size about 30 kb for coronaviruses and 25–30 kb for toroviruses). Viruses contain three major structural polypeptides and are resistant to trypsin but sensitive to lipid solvents, detergents, ultraviolet radiation, disinfectants, and heat. Replicating occurs in the cytoplasm and assembly is by budding, usually through intracytoplasmic membranes; virions are released by exocytosis or by cell destruction. Transmission is mechanical, including airborne particles, contaminated equipment, and contact with infected persons. Included here are the genera *Coronavirus* and *Torovirus.*

Co•ro•na•vi•rus (kə-ro′nə-vi″rus) [L. *corona* crown + *virus,* from the appearance of the virions on electron micrographs] coronaviruses; a genus of viruses of the family Coronaviridae that cause respiratory disease and possibly gastroenteritis in humans, and hepatitis, gastroenteritis, encephalitis, and respiratory disease in other animals. In newborn calves and lambs it causes neonatal diarrhea.

co•ro•na•vi•rus (kə-ro′nə-vi″rəs) any virus belonging to the family Coronaviridae. **coronavi′ral** *adj*

SARS-associated c. (SARS-CoV) a coronavirus that is the etiologic agent of severe acute respiratory syndrome (SARS).

co•ro•ne (kə-ro′ne) [L., from Gr. *korōnē* anything hooked or curved] the coronoid process of the mandible (processus coronoideus mandibulae [TA]).

cor•o•ner (kor′ə-nər) a public official, elected or appointed, who holds inquests in regard to violent, sudden, or unexplained deaths within a given jurisdiction. Coroners are not necessarily trained physicians. Cf. *medical examiner.*

cor•o•net (kor′ə-net) coronary band.

co•ro•ni•on (kə-ro′ne-on) the tip of the coronoid process of the mandible.

cor•o•ni•tis (kor-ə-ni′tis) inflammation of the coronary band or cushion, especially of the horse.

cor•o•noid (kor′ə-noid) [Gr. *korōnē* anything hooked or curved, a kind of crown + *-oid*] 1. shaped like a crow's beak. 2. crown-shaped.

cor•o•noi•dec•to•my (kor″ə-noi-dek′tə-me) surgical removal of the coronoid process of the mandible.

cor•o•noi•dot•o•my (kor″ə-noi-dot′ə-me) coronoidectomy.

coro•par•el•cy•sis (kor″o-pər-el′sə-sis) [*coro-* + Gr. *parelkein* to draw aside] the drawing aside of the pupil in partial corneal opacity in order to bring it under a transparent portion.

coro•plas•ty (kor′o-plas″te) coreoplasty.

co•rot•o•my (kə-rot′ə-me) iridectomy.

cor•pec•to•my (kor-pek′tə-me) [*corpus* + *-ectomy*] surgical removal of all or part of a vertebral body, performed for decompression of the spinal cord; the bone removed is replaced by a graft. Called also *corporectomy*.

cor•po•ra (kor′pə-rə) [L.] plural of *corpus*.

cor•po•ral (kor′pər-əl) corporeal.

cor•po•re•al (kor-por′e-əl) pertaining to the body.

cor•po•rec•to•my (kor″pə-rek′tə-me) corpectomy.

cor•por•ic (kor-por′ik) [*corpus*] affecting the body, or corpus, of an organ.

corps (kor) [Fr., from L. *corpus*] 1. an organized body, or group of individuals. 2. corpus.

medical c. the surgeon officers of the army or navy, comprising a surgeon general, medical directors, medical inspectors, surgeons, passed assistant surgeons, and assistant surgeons.

corpse (korps) [*corpus*] a dead body; used to refer specifically to a human body in the early period after death. Cf. *cadaver*.

cor•pu•len•cy (kor′pu-len″se) [L. *corpulentia*] obesity.

cor•pus (kor′pəs) gen. *cor′poris* pl. *cor′pora* [L. "body"] 1. the entire body of an organism. 2. the main portion of an anatomical part, structure, or organ. 3. a discrete mass of material, as of specialized tissue.

Corpus

Descriptions are given on TA terms, and include anglicized names of specific structures.

c. adipo′sum buc′cae [TA] buccal fat pad: an encapsulated mass of fat in the cheek, separated from the subcutaneous fascia by a facial cleft, and situated between the masseter and the external surface of the buccinator muscles; especially well developed in infants and said to aid in sucking. Called also *sucking cushion*, and *sucking* or *suctorial pad*.

c. adipo′sum fos′sae ischioana′lis [TA], **c. adipo′sum fos′sae ischiorecta′lis** fat body of the ischioanal fossa: a pad of fat found in the ischioanal fossa.

c. adipo′sum infrapatella′re [TA] infrapatellar fat pad: a mass of fibrous fatty tissue inferior to the patella, in the angle between the deep surface of the patellar ligament and the tibia. Called also *retropatellar fat pad*.

c. adipo′sum or′bitae [TA] orbital fat body: a mass of fatty tissue in the posterior part of the orbit, around the optic nerve, extraocular muscles, and vessels. Called also *retrobulbar fat*.

c. adipo′sum pararena′le [TA] pararenal fat body: a large mass of fat lying dorsal to the renal fascia; called also *paranephric body* and *paranephric* or *pararenal fat*.

c. adipo′sum preepiglot′ticum [TA] preepiglottic fat body: a mass of fatty tissue separating the lower anterior surface of the epiglottis from the thyroid cartilage and the thyrohyoid membrane.

c. al′bicans pl. *cor′pora albican′tia* [TA] white fibrous tissue that replaces the regressing corpus luteum in the human ovary in the latter half of pregnancy, or soon after ovulation when pregnancy does not supervene.

cor′pora alla′ta a set of small endocrine glands in the head of insects just behind the brain, which inhibit metamorphosis by secretion of juvenile hormone.

c. amygdaloi′deum [TA] amygdaloid body: a small, ovoid complex of nuclei partly covered by the pyriform cortex, within the tip of the temporal lobe, anterior to the inferior horn of the lateral ventricle of the brain; it is part of the limbic system. The amygdaloid body is divided into two main groups of nuclei, found in the basolateral and corticomedial parts, and in a poorly differentiated transitional region, the anterior amygdaloid area. It has olfactory connections, is reciprocally connected to the limbic cortex, and projects fibers to the hippocampus, the septum, the thalamus, and especially the hypothalamus. Called also *amygdala*, *amygdaloid complex*, and *nucleus amygdalae*.

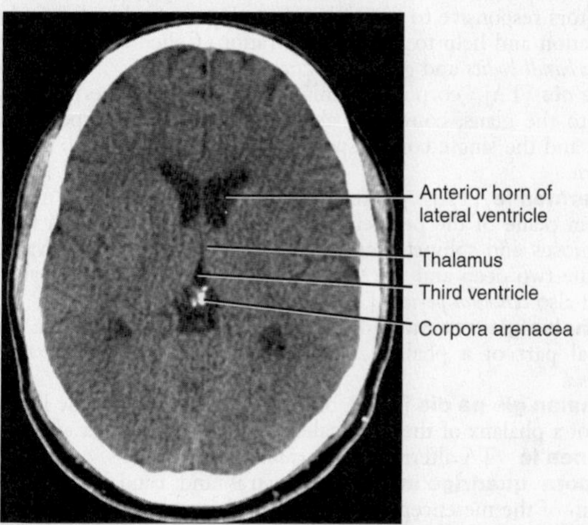

■ Axial CT scan showing corpora arenacea encircling the pineal gland.

cor′pora amyla′cea small basophilic, periodic acid–Schiff–positive, hyaline masses, 5–50 μm in diameter, derived from degenerate cells or inspissated secretions and consisting of a central nidus surrounded by concentric lamellae. They occur in the prostate, neuroglia, and pulmonary alveoli and become more numerous with advancing age; their significance is not known. Called also *amylaceous bodies* or *corpuscles*, *amyloid bodies* or *corpuscles*, and *colloid corpuscles*.

c. anococcy′geum [TA] anococcygeal ligament: a fibrous band connecting the posterior fibers of the sphincter of the anus to the coccyx.

cor′pora arena′cea gritty calcareous concretions deposited in concentric rings around an organic matrix in certain areas in the brain, particularly the extracellular matrix of the pineal body, and accumulating progressively with age; called also *brain sand*.

cor′pora atre′tica ovarian follicles that never mature, but undergo degeneration.

cor′pora bige′mina 1. two bodies in the brains of nonmammalian vertebrates that correspond to the superior colliculi of mammals; called also *optic lobes*. 2. two bodies in the brain of the human fetus that later split to become the corpora quadrigemina.

c. callo′sum [TA] an arched mass of white matter, found in the depths of the longitudinal fissure, composed of three layers of fibers, the central layer consisting primarily of transverse fibers connecting the cerebral hemispheres; its subsections, from anterior to posterior, are called the rostrum, genu, trunk (or body), and splenium.

c. caverno′sum clito′ridis [TA] cavernous body of clitoris: a column of erectile tissue on either side (right and left), the two fusing to form the body of the clitoris (c. clitoridis).

c. caverno′sum pe′nis [TA] cavernous body of penis: one of the columns of erectile tissue forming the dorsum and sides of the penis.

c. cerebel′li [TA] body of cerebellum: the main portion of the cerebellum, consisting of the two cerebellar hemispheres joined by a median strip, the vermis; see also *cerebellum*.

c. cilia′re [TA] ciliary body: the thickened part of the vascular tunic of the eye anterior to the ora serrata, connecting the choroid with the iris; it is composed of the corona ciliaris, ciliary processes and folds, ciliary orbiculus, the ciliary muscle, and a basal lamina. See illustration.

c. clavi′culae [TA] body of clavicle: the long curved central part of the clavicle, extending between the acromial and sternal extremities.

c. clito′ridis [TA] body of clitoris: the main part of the clitoris, formed by the two fused corpora cavernosa, which are embedded anteriorly in the floor of the vestibule of the vagina.

c. coccy′geum glomus coccygeum.

c. cos′tae [TA] body of rib: the part of a rib extending between its dorsally placed tubercle and its ventral extremity; called also *shaft of rib*.

c. epididy′midis [TA] body of epididymis: the middle part of the epididymis, formed by the convolutions of the ductus epididymidis.

c. fe′moris [TA] body of femur: the main part or shaft of the femur.

c. fibro′sum a mass of collagenous tissue that replaces an atretic ovarian follicle. Most corpora fibrosa eventually disappear.

c. fi′bulae [TA] body of fibula: the principal part or shaft of the fibula; called also *shaft of fibula*.

c. for′nicis [TA] body of fornix: the middle part of the fornix of the cerebrum, formed by fusion of the two lateral halves under the corpus callosum.

Corpus *Continued*

c. gas′tricum [TA] body of stomach: the part of the stomach between the fundus and the pyloric part; called also *gastric body.*
c. genicula′tum latera′le [TA] lateral geniculate body: an eminence of the metathalamus produced by the underlying lateral geniculate nucleus, just lateral to the medial geniculate body. It relays visual impulses from the optic tract to the calcarine cortex and links visual inputs to the nearby midbrain. Called also *optic thalamus.*
c. genicula′tum media′le [TA] medial geniculate body: an eminence of the metathalamus produced by the underlying medial geniculate nucleus, just lateral to the superior colliculus. It relays auditory impulses from the lateral lemniscus to the auditory cortex.
c. hemorrha′gicum a blood clot formed in the cavity left by the mature ovarian follicle after its rupture during ovulation.
c. hu′meri [TA] body of humerus: the long central part of the humerus; called also *shaft of humerus.*
c. incu′dis [TA] body of incus: the central part of the incus, which contains an excavation (facet for malleus) in which the head of the malleus articulates.
c. juxtarestifor′me [TA] juxtarestiform body: the smaller part of the inferior cerebellar peduncle, it joins the corpus restiforme as they enter the cerebellum and contains interconnections between vestibular structures and the cerebellar cortex and fastigial nucleus.
c. lin′guae [TA] the larger anterior part of the tongue, in the floor of the mouth.
c. lu′teum pl. *cor′pora lu′tea* [TA] yellow body of ovary: a yellow glandular mass in the ovary formed by an ovarian follicle that has matured and discharged its oocyte. If the oocyte has been fertilized, the corpus luteum increases in size and persists for several months *(true c. luteum, c. luteum of pregnancy, c. luteum graviditatis)*; if fertilization has not taken place, it degenerates and shrinks *(false c. luteum, c. luteum of menstruation, c. luteum menstruationis)*. The corpus luteum secretes progesterone. Cf. *c. albicans.*
c. mam′mae [TA] the essential mass of the mammary gland, exclusive of the glandular elements, which is thickest beneath the nipple and thinner toward the periphery; see illustration at *glandula mammaria.*
c. mammilla′re [TA] mammillary body: either of the pair of small spherical masses situated close together in the interpeduncular space rostral to the posterior perforated substance in the posterior hypothalamic region, consisting of two main nuclei, lateral and medial, and smaller associated aggregations of gray matter. It forms a portion of the *limbic system* (see under *system*).
c. mandi′bulae [TA] body of mandible: the horizontal horseshoe-shaped portion of the mandible.
c. maxil′lae [TA] body of maxilla: the large central portion of the maxilla, roughly pyramidal in shape, to which four major processes are connected; it contains the maxillary sinus.
c. medulla′re cerebel′li [TA] medullary body of cerebellum: the white substance of the cerebellum; called also *medullary center of cerebellum.*
c. nu′clei cauda′ti [TA] body of caudate nucleus: the part of the caudate nucleus lying in the lateral wall of the pars centralis of the lateral ventricle of the brain, extending posteriorly from the head of the caudate nucleus and continuous with the tail.

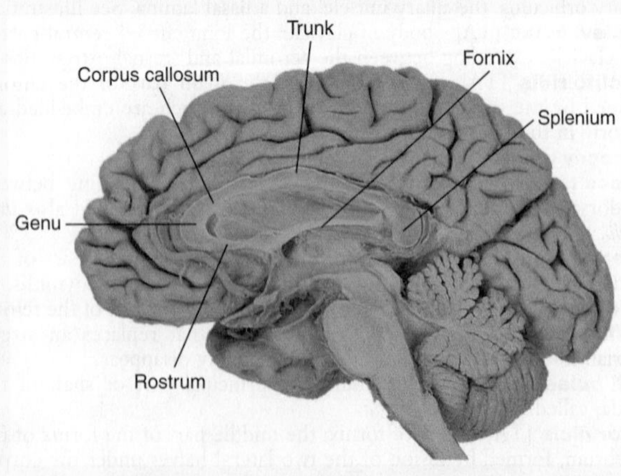

■ Corpus callosum in a midline sagittal section.

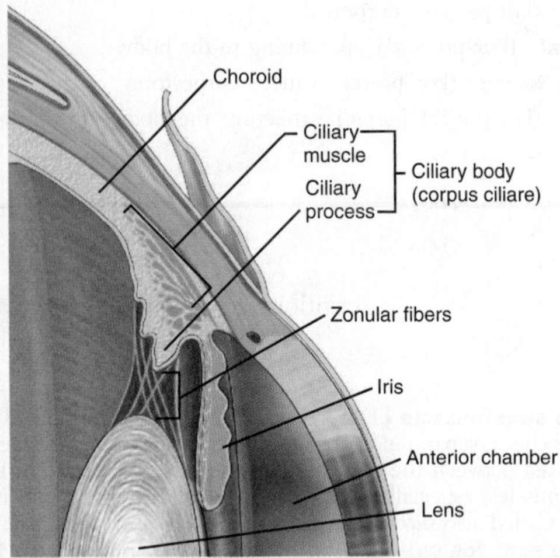

■ Corpus ciliare (ciliary body).

cor′pora oryzoi′dea (sing. *cor′pus oryzoi′deum*) rice bodies.
c. os′sis hyoi′dei [TA] body of hyoid bone: the central portion of the hyoid bone to which the large and small horns are attached; called also *basihyal* and *basihyoid.*
c. os′sis i′lii [TA] body of ilium: the inferior portion of the ilium, which forms roughly the superior two fifths of the acetabulum.
c. os′sis is′chii [TA] body of ischium: the thick, irregular, prismatic part of the ischium. Its superior end participates in the acetabulum, and from its inferior end the ramus of the ischium projects. It incorporates what was formerly called the superior ramus.
c. os′sis metacar′pi [TA] body of metacarpal bone: the long central part of a metacarpal bone. Called also *shaft of metacarpal bone.*
c. os′sis metatar′si [TA] body of metatarsal bone: the long central part of a metatarsal bone. Called also *shaft of metatarsal bone.*
c. os′sis pu′bis [TA] body of pubic bone: the irregular mass of the pubic bone that lies alongside the median plane, articulating with the similar portion of the opposite pubic bone. From it extend the superior and inferior rami of the pubic bone.
c. os′sis sphenoida′lis [TA] body of sphenoid bone: the central, cuboidal part of the sphenoid bone to which the greater wings, lesser wings, and pterygoid processes are attached; it contains the sphenoidal sinuses.
c. pancre′atis [TA] body of pancreas: the triangularly prismatic central portion of the pancreas, extending from the neck on the right to the tail on the left.
cor′pora paraaor′tica [TA] para-aortic bodies: exclaves of glandular cells of sympathetic origin (chromaffin cells) found near the sympathetic ganglia along the aorta in the abdominal cavity; they serve as chemoreceptors responsive to oxygen, carbon dioxide, and hydrogen ion concentration and help to control respiration. Called also *aortic, vagal,* or *Zuckerkandl bodies* and *glomera aortica.*
c. pe′nis [TA] corpus of penis: the free part of the penis from the root to the glans, consisting chiefly of the paired corpora cavernosa penis and the single corpus spongiosum penis; called also *body* or *shaft of penis.*
c. perinea′le [TA] perineal body: the fibromuscular mass in the median plane of the perineum where converge and attach the bulbospongiosus and sphincter ani externus muscles, the two levatores ani, and the two deep and the two superficial transverse perineal muscles; called also *centrum perinei* [TA alternative].
c. phalan′gis ma′nus [TA] body of phalanx of hand: the long central part of a phalanx of the hand; called also *shaft of phalanx of hand.*
c. phalan′gis pe′dis [TA] body of phalanx of foot: the long central part of a phalanx of the foot; called also *shaft of phalanx of foot.*
c. pinea′le TA alternative for *glandula pinealis.*
cor′pora quadrige′mina the rostral and caudal colliculi of the tectum of the mesencephalon considered together.
c. ra′dii [TA] body of radius: the long central part of the radius; called also *shaft of radius.*

Corpus *Continued*

c. restifor′me [TA] restiform body: the larger part of the inferior cerebellar peduncle, located on the dorsolateral aspect of the medulla oblongata and containing various cerebellar afferent fibers. It was formerly equated with the inferior cerebellar peduncle. Cf. *c. juxtarestiforme.*

c. spongio′sum pe′nis [TA] spongy body of penis: the column of erectile tissue that forms the urethral surface of the penis, and in which the urethra is found; its distal expansion forms the glans penis. Called also *spongy body of male urethra.*

c. ster′ni [TA] body of sternum: the second or principal portion of the sternum, located between the manubrium above and the xiphoid process (processus xiphoideus) below. Called also *gladiolus.*

c. stria′tum [TA] striate body: the main component of the basal nuclei; specifically, a subcortical mass of gray and white substance in front of and lateral to the thalamus in each cerebral hemisphere. The gray substance of this structure is arranged in two principal masses, the caudate nucleus and the lentiform nucleus; its name denotes the striate appearance on section of the area, produced by connecting bands of gray substance passing from one of these nuclei to the other through the anterior limb of the internal capsule.

c. ta′li [TA] body of talus: the roughly quadrilateral portion of the talus, which presents several surfaces for articulation with the calcaneus, tibia, and fibula.

c. ti′biae [TA] body of tibia: the long central part of the tibia; called also *shaft of tibia.*

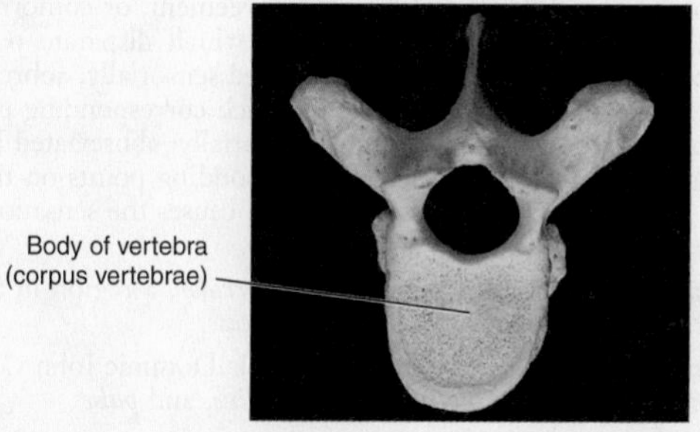

■ Corpus vertebrae in a superior view of a thoracic vertebra.

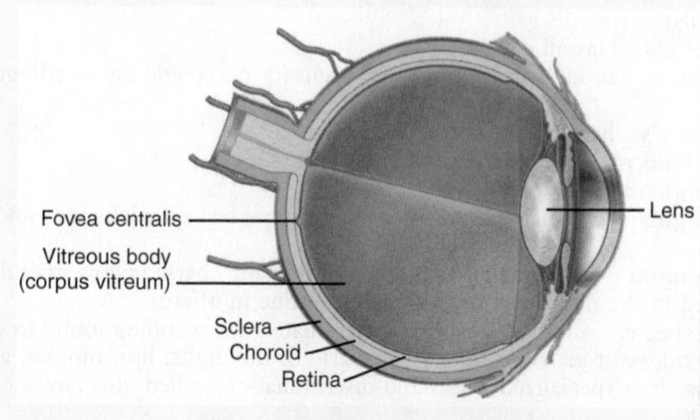

■ Corpus vitreum (vitreous body).

c. trapezoi′deum [TA] trapezoid body: a mass of transverse fibers extending through the central part of the caudal pons and forming a part of the path of the cochlear nerve.

c. ul′nae [TA] body of ulna: the long central part of the ulna; called also *shaft of ulna.*

c. un′guis [TA] body of nail: the large distal, exposed portion of the nail of a digit.

c. u′teri [TA] body of uterus: that part of the uterus above the isthmus and below the orifices of the uterine tubes.

c. ver′tebrae [TA] the body of a vertebra, consisting of the centrum, the ossified neurocentral joint and part of the vertebral arches, and the facets for the heads of the ribs. Called also *vertebral body.*

c. vesi′cae bilia′ris [TA] body of gallbladder: the central portion of the gallbladder, extending from the fundus to the neck; called also *c. vesicae felleae* [TA alternative].

c. vesi′cae fel′leae TA alternative for *c. vesicae biliaris.*

c. vesi′cae urina′riae [TA] body of urinary bladder: the central part of the bladder, between the apex and the fundus.

c. vi′treum [TA] vitreous body: the transparent, colorless, gelatinous substance that fills the inner portion of the eyeball between the lens, ciliary body, and retina; with increasing age it tends to become more fluid. Called also *hyaloid body.*

cor·pus·cal·lo·sot·o·my (kor′pəs-kal-ə-sot′ə-me) [*corpus callosum* + *-otomy*] surgical transection of the fibers in the corpus callosum, done to gain access to third ventricular structures; formerly used to treat intractable epilepsy. Written also *corpus callosotomy.* Called also *callosotomy.* Cf. *split brain.*

cor·pus·cle (kor′pəs-əl) any small mass or body; see also *corpusculum.* **corpus′cular** *adj*

amylaceous c's, amyloid c's corpora amylacea.

articular c. a type of lamellated corpuscle found within joints.

axile c., axis c. the central part of a tactile corpuscle.

blood c. see under *cell.*

blood c., red erythrocyte.

blood c., white leukocyte.

bone c. bone cell.

bulboid c. Krause end-bulb.

chromophil c's Nissl bodies.

chyle c. a lymphocyte found in chyle.

colloid c's corpora amylacea.

colostrum c's large rounded bodies in colostrum, containing droplets of fat and sometimes a nucleus; they apparently are phagocytic cells of the mammary gland, present for the first two weeks after parturition. Called also *Donné bodies* or *corpuscles.*

compound granular c. gitter cell.

concentric c's Hassall c's.

corneal c's star-shaped connective tissue cells within the corneal stroma; called also *Toynbee* and *Virchow c's.*

Dogiel c. genital c.

Donné c's colostrum c's.

dust c's hemoconia.

genital c. a type of lamellated corpuscle found in the genital mucous membranes and in the skin around the nipples.

Gierke c's Hassall c's.

Golgi c. Golgi tendon organ.

Golgi-Mazzoni c's tactile corpuscles found in the subcutaneous tissue of the fingertips, resembling pacinian corpuscles but possessing fewer lamellae and a relatively larger cone and having the contained nerve fibers more extensively branched.

Hassall c's spherical or ovoid bodies found in the medulla of the thymus, composed of concentric arrays of epithelial cells which contain keratohyalin and bundles of cytoplasmic filaments. Called also *Hassall bodies* and *concentric, Leber,* or *thymus c's.*

Herbst c's peculiar sensory end-organs in the skin of the bill and in the mucous membrane of the tongue of the duck.

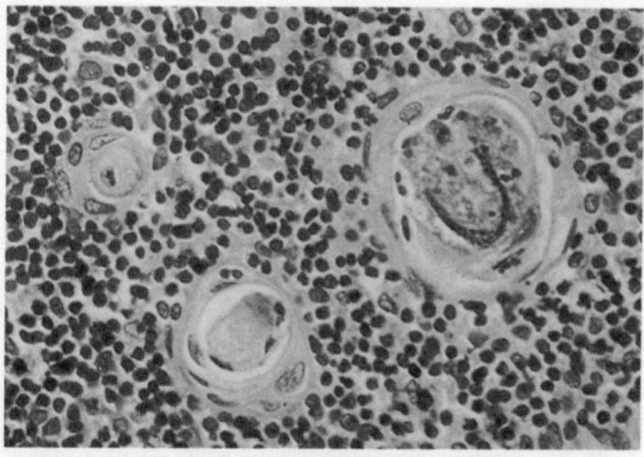

■ Medulla of neonatal thymus showing three Hassall corpuscles of varying degrees of maturity surrounded by closely packed lymphocytes.

Jaworski c's spiral mucous bodies seen in the secretion of the stomach in hyperchlorhydria.

Krause c. see under *end-bulb.*

lamellar c., lamellated c. an encapsulated nerve ending in which the connective tissue capsule takes the form of concentric layers of flattened cells; the term is sometimes used as a synonym of pacinian corpuscle, a type of lamellar corpuscle.

Leber c's Hassall c's.

lingual c. an encapsulated terminal sensory nerve ending in a lingual papilla.

lymph c's lymphocytes observed in lymph.

lymphoid c's lymphocytes observed in tissues.

malpighian c. of kidney renal c.

malpighian c's of spleen noduli lymphoidei splenici; see under *nodulus.*

meconium c's epithelial cells containing many coarse yellow granules, observed in the distal part of the small intestine in a fetus.

Meissner c. a rapidly adapting encapsulated nerve ending found in the dermal ridges of glabrous skin, particularly of the digits, lips, nipples, and genitalia. It is specialized for tactile discrimination; called also *tactile c. of Meissner.*

Merkel c. see under *cell.*

mucous c's bodies resembling leukocytes occurring in mucus.

Norris c's decolorized erythrocytes. See also *hypochromic erythrocyte,* under *erythrocyte.*

pacchionian c's granulationes arachnoideae.

Pacini c., pacinian c. a type of large, ovoid, rapidly adapting, encapsulated nerve ending sensitive to pressure, touch, and vibration. The most complicated of the nerve endings, its core contains the nonmyelinated nerve terminal and its Schwann cells, surrounded by concentric layers of modified fibroblasts, in cross-section resembling a sliced onion. It is found in the skin and deeper tissues, particularly in the palms, soles, digits of hands and feet, joints, external genitalia, and breasts. Called also *Vater-Pacini c.*

paciniform c's rapidly adapting lamellar nerve endings that are more elongated and have fewer laminae than pacinian corpuscles; found in the vibrissae and epidermis of the nose, in joint capsules, in aponeuroses, and at myotendinous junctions associated with Golgi tendon organs. They respond to muscle stretch and light pressure. Called also *paciniform receptors.*

pessary c. see under *cell.*

pus c's see under *cell.*

Rainey c. any of the uninucleate, crescentic trophozoites found in sarcocysts in sarcocystosis.

red c. erythrocyte.

renal c. a body that forms the beginning of a nephron, consisting of a glomerulus surrounded by the glomerular capsule (an expanded portion of the renal tubule). Called also *malpighian corpuscle of kidney.*

reticulated c. reticulocyte.

Röhl marginal c's small bodies seen in the margins of erythrocytes of animals after the administration of chemotherapeutic substances.

Ruffini c. see under *ending.*

salivary c. a white blood cell that has migrated through the oral epithelium and is mixed in the saliva.

Schwalbe c. caliculus gustatorius.

splenic c's noduli lymphoidei splenici; see under *nodulus.*

tactile c. see under *receptor.*

tactile c. of Meissner Meissner c.

taste c. caliculus gustatorius.

tendon c's flattened cells of connective tissue occurring in rows between the primary bundles of the tendons.

terminal nerve c. encapsulated nerve ending.

thymus c's Hassall c's.

Timofeew c. a specialized form of lamellated corpuscle found in the submucosa of the membranous and prostatic portions of the urethra.

touch c. tactile receptor.

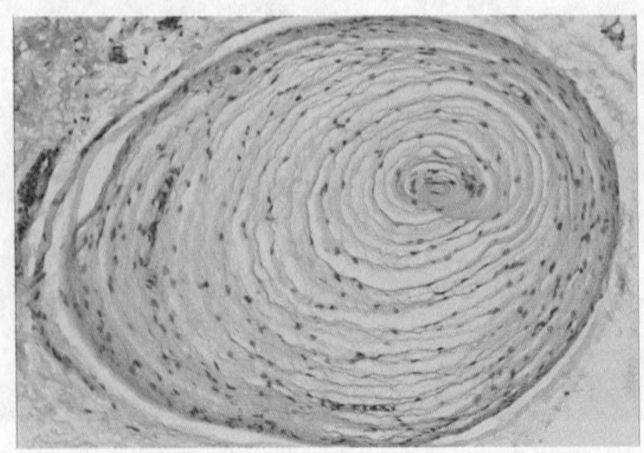

■ Pacinian corpuscle in dermis.

Toynbee c's corneal c's.

Tröltsch c's connective tissue spaces lined with flattened endothelial cells and appearing like corpuscular bodies among the radial fibers of the membrana tympani.

Valentin c's small amyloid bodies sometimes found in nerve tissue.

Vater-Pacini c. pacinian c.

Virchow c's corneal c's.

Weber c. utriculus prostaticus.

white c. leukocyte.

cor·pus·cu·la (kor-pus′ku-lə) [L.] plural of *corpusculum.*

cor·pus·cu·lum (kor-pus′ku-ləm) pl. *corpus′cula* [L. dim. of *corpus*] anatomical nomenclature for a discrete mass of specialized tissue; see *corpuscle.*

cor·rec·tion (kə-rek′shən) [L. *correctio* straightening out; amendment] a setting right, as the provision of specific lenses for the improvement of vision, or an arbitrary adjustment made in values or devices in performance of experimental procedures.

cor·rec·tor (kə-rek′tər) something that corrects or sets right.

function c. a removable orthodontic appliance utilizing oral and facial muscle forces to move teeth and possibly change the relationship of dental arches; called also *Fränkel appliance.*

cor·re·la·tion (kor″ə-la′shən) the degree to which one phenomenon or random variable is associated with or can be predicted from another. In statistics this usually refers to the degree to which a linear predictive relationship exists between random variables, as measured by a correlation coefficient (q.v.). Correlation is *positive* (never larger than 1) when both variables increase or decrease together; *negative* or *inverse* (never smaller than −1) when one variable increases when the other decreases; and defined as zero when a change in one variable does not affect the other.

cor·re·spon·dence (kor″ə-spon′dəns) [L. *correspondēre* to answer, to correspond] the condition of being in agreement, or conformity.

anomalous retinal c. a condition in which disparate points on the retinas of the two eyes come to be associated sensorially; abbreviated ARC.

normal retinal c. the condition in which corresponding points on the retinas of the two eyes are associated sensorially; abbreviated NRC.

retinal c. the relation between corresponding points on the retinas of the eyes such that simultaneous stimulation causes the sensation of a single object.

Cor·ri·dor disease (kor′ĭ-dor) [The *Corridor,* a region in South Africa where it was first reported] see under *disease.*

Cor·ri·gan disease, etc. (kor′ĭ-gən) [Sir Dominic John *Corrigan,* Irish physician, 1802–1880] see under *disease, line,* and *pulse.*

cor·ri·gent (kor′ĭ-jənt) [L. *corrigens* correcting] 1. amending or rendering milder. 2. any agent that favorably modifies the action of a drug which is too powerful or harsh, or that improves its taste.

cor·rin (kor′in) a tetrapyrrole ring system resembling the porphyrin ring system of hemoglobin, but in which a pair of the rings is joined directly rather than through a methylene bridge, with cobalt being bound to the inner four nitrogen atoms. The cobalamins contain a corrin ring system.

cor·rin·oid (kor′in-oid) a compound, such as a cobalamin, containing a corrin ring system.

cor·rode (kə-rōd′) [L. *corrodere* to gnaw] 1. to produce corrosion. 2. to undergo corrosion.

cor·ro·sion (kə-ro′zhən) 1. the gradual destruction of a metal or alloy by electrochemical reaction or of the body tissues by the action of a strong acid or alkali. 2. the product of a corrosive process.

cor·ro·sive (kə-ro′siv) 1. causing, or able to cause, corrosion. 2. an agent or substance that causes corrosion. Called also *caustic.* Cf. *escharotic.*

cor·ru·ga·tor (cor′ə-ga″tər) [*cor-* + *ruga*] that which wrinkles; a muscle that wrinkles.

cor·sair (kor′sār) any of various biting reduviid bugs of the genus *Melanolestes.*

cor·set (kor′sət) an orthopedic device that encircles and supports a part, particularly the trunk; see also *spinal orthosis,* under *orthosis.*

Cort. [L.] cor′tex (bark).

Cor·tane-B (kor′tān) trademark for combination preparations of chloroxylenol, pramoxine hydrochloride, and hydrocortisone.

Cor·tate (kor′tāt) trademark for preparations of desoxycorticosterone acetate.

Cort-Dome (kort′dōm) trademark for preparations of hydrocortisone.

Cor·tef (kor′təf) trademark for preparations of hydrocortisone.

Cor·ten·e·ma (kor-ten′ə-mə) trademark for a preparation of hydrocortisone.

cor•tex (kor′teks) gen. *cor′ticis,* pl. *cor′tices* [L. "bark, rind, shell"] 1. an external layer, as the bark of a tree or the rind of a fruit. 2. the outer layer of an organ or other body structure, as distinguished from the internal substance. 3. the region of the cytoplasm adjacent to the plasma membrane, containing a network of actin fibers.

adrenal c., c. of adrenal gland c. glandulae suprarenalis.

agranular c. a type of cortex occurring in some parts of the neocortex, having very thin granular layers; seen in the motor area of the precentral gyrus and elsewhere.

auditory c. two contiguous areas of the temporal lobe in the region of the anterior transverse temporal gyrus; Brodmann area 41 is called the *first* or *primary auditory cortex* and Brodmann area 42 is called the *second* or *secondary auditory cortex.*

cerebellar c., c. cerebel′li [TA] the superficial gray matter of the cerebellum; it consists of three layers, the stratum moleculare, stratum granulosum, and stratum purkinjense.

cerebral c., c. cere′bri [TA] the thin (about 3 mm) layer or mantle of gray substance covering the surface of each cerebral hemisphere, folded into gyri that are separated by sulci. It is responsible for the higher mental functions; for visceral functions; for motor and sensory functions; for perception and behavioral reactions; and for the association and integration of these functions. Many classifications have been suggested: it has been divided into *archicortex, paleocortex,* and *neocortex* according to supposed phylogenetic and ontogenetic differences; into functional areas such as *motor areas, primary receptive* or *receiving areas,* and *association areas;* and into areas according to the presence of six cell layers (the *isocortex*) or of variable numbers and arrangements of cell and fiber layers (the *allocortex*). Called also *pallium.* See also *layers of cerebral cortex.*

c. cor′ticis [TA] part of the renal cortex consisting of a narrow peripheral zone where the renal columns do not have visible renal corpuscles.

fetal adrenal c. fetal zone of adrenal cortex.

c. glan′dulae suprarena′lis [TA] cortex of adrenal or suprarenal gland: the outer, firm yellowish layer that comprises the larger part of the adrenal gland, consisting of the zona glomerulosa, the zona fasciculata, and the zona reticularis; it secretes, in response to release of corticotropin by the pulmonary gland, many steroid hormones. Called also *adrenal* or *suprarenal c.*

granular c. koniocortex.

hair c., c. of hair, c. of hair shaft the middle layer of a hair, constituting the bulk of the hair substance, surrounded by the hair cuticle and often enclosing a small hair medulla.

heterotypical c. allocortex.

homotypical c. isocortex.

insular c. insula (def. 2).

juxtamedullary c. the part of the renal cortex nearest to the medulla.

c. of kidney c. renalis.

c. of lens, c. len′tis [TA] the softer, external part of the lens of the eye.

mastoid c. name sometimes given to the platelike lateral surface of the mastoid process.

motor c. see under *area.*

c. no′di lympha′tici TA alternative for *c. nodi lymphoidei.*

c. no′di lymphoi′dei [TA] cortex of lymph node: the outer portion of the node, consisting mainly of dense lymphatic tissue and follicles; called also *c. nodi lymphatici* [TA alternative].

nonolfactory c. neocortex.

olfactory c. 1. see under *area.* 2. archicortex.

c. ova′rii [TA] cortex of ovary: the dense layer of compact stroma forming the peripheral zone around the medulla of the ovary, in which the ovarian follicles are embedded.

piriform c. the cortex of the piriform lobe or area.

provisional c. fetal zone of adrenal cortex.

renal c., c. rena′lis [TA], **c. re′nis** the outer part of the substance of the kidney, composed mainly of glomeruli and convoluted tubules.

somesthetic c. somatosensory area.

striate c. Brodmann area 17: the part of the occipital lobe of the cerebral cortex that receives the fibers of the optic radiation from the lateral geniculate body and is the primary receptive area for vision; so called because of the prominent broad line or stria of Gennari. Called also *striate area* or *first visual area.*

suprarenal c., c. of suprarenal gland c. glandulae suprarenalis.

tertiary c. thymus-dependent area.

c. thy′mi [TA], **c. of thymus** the outer part of each lobule of the thymus; it consists chiefly of closely packed lymphocytes (thymocytes) and surrounds the medulla.

visual c. the area of the occipital lobe of the cerebral cortex concerned with vision; it consists of the *first visual area* or *striate c.* (Brodmann area 17) and two other areas, the *second visual area* or *parastriate area* (Brodmann area 18), and the *third visual area* or *peristriate area* (Brodmann area 19).

cor•tex•one (kor-tek′sōn) 11-deoxycorticosterone.

Cor•ti arch, canal, cells, etc. (kor′te) [Alfonso *Corti,* Italian anatomist, 1822–1888] see under *arch, canal, cell, fiber, ganglion, rod,* and *tunnel,* and see *membrana tectoria ductus cochlearis* and *organum spirale.*

Cor•tic (kor′tik) trademark for a combination preparation of chloroxylenol, pramoxine hydrochloride, and hydrocortisone.

cor•ti•cal (kor′tĭ-kəl) [L. *corticalis*] pertaining to or of the nature of a cortex or bark.

cor•ti•cal•os•te•ot•o•my (kor″tĭ-kəl-os″te-ot′ə-me) osteotomy through the bone cortex at the base of the dentoalveolar segment, which serves to weaken the resistance of the bone to the application of orthodontic forces.

cor•ti•cate (kor′tĭ-kāt) possessing a cortex or bark.

cor•ti•cec•to•my (kor″tĭ-sek′tə-me) topectomy.

cor•ti•ces (kor′tĭ-sēz) [L.] plural of *cortex.*

cor•ti•cif•u•gal (kor″tĭ-sif′ə-gəl) [*cortex* + L. *fugere* to flee] proceeding or conducting away from the cerebral cortex. Cf. *efferent.*

cor•ti•cip•e•tal (kor″tĭ-sip′ə-təl) [*cortic-* + L. *-petal*] proceeding or conducting toward the cerebral cortex. Cf. *afferent.*

cortic(o)- [L. *cortex,* q.v.] a combining form denoting relationship to a cortex.

cor•ti•co•ad•re•nal (kor″tĭ-ko-ə-dre′nəl) adrenocortical.

cor•ti•co•af•fer•ent (kor″tĭ-ko-af′ər-ent) corticipetal.

cor•ti•co•au•to•nom•ic (kor″tĭ-ko-aw″to-nom′ik) denoting the relationship of autonomic function to definite areas in the cerebral cortex.

cor•ti•co•bul•bar (kor″tĭ-ko-bul′bər) [*cortico-* + *bulbar* (def. 2)] a term formerly used to denote fibers connecting the cerebral cortex with the medulla oblongata, pons, or midbrain; replaced by the broader term corticonuclear (q.v.).

cor•ti•co•can•cel•lous (kor″tĭ-ko-kan′sə-ləs) referring to bony tissue containing both cortical and cancellous elements.

cor•ti•co•di•en•ce•phal•ic (kor″tĭ-ko-di″en-sə-fal′ik) pertaining to or connecting the cerebral cortex and the diencephalon.

cor•ti•co•ef•fer•ent (kor″tĭ-ko-ef′ər-ent) corticifugal.

cor•ti•cof•u•gal (kor″tĭ-kof′u-gəl) corticifugal.

cor•ti•coid (kor′tĭ-koid) corticosteroid.

cor•ti•co•lipo•trope (kor″tĭ-ko-lip′o-trōp) corticotroph.

cor•ti•co•med•ul•lary (kor″tĭ-ko-med′u-lar-e) pertaining to the cortex and medulla of an organ.

cor•ti•co•mes•en•ce•phal•ic (kor″tĭ-ko-mes″en-sə-fal′ik) pertaining to or connecting the cerebral cortex and the mesencephalon.

cor•ti•co•nu•cle•ar (kor″tĭ-ko-noo′kle-ər) pertaining to fibers that connect the cerebral cortex and nuclei of one or more of the medulla oblongata, pons, and midbrain, or to the projections of the Purkinje cells to nuclei of the cerebellum.

cor•ti•co•pe•dun•cu•lar (kor″tĭ-ko-pə-dung′ku-lər) pertaining to the cortex and the peduncles of the brain.

cor•ti•cop•e•tal (kor″tĭ-kop′ə-təl) corticipetal.

cor•ti•co•pleu•ri•tis (kor″tĭ-ko-ploo̅-ri′tis) pulmonary pleurisy.

cor•ti•co•pon•tine (kor″tĭ-ko-pon′tīn) pertaining to or connecting the cerebral cortex and the pons.

cor•ti•co•rel•in ovine tri•flu•tate (kor″tĭ-ko-rel′in) an analogue of human corticotropin-releasing hormone; both stimulate release of adrenocorticotropic hormone (ACTH) from the anterior pituitary, which in turn stimulates cortisol production in the adrenal cortex. It is used as a diagnostic aid to distinguish between pituitary and ectopic production of ACTH in patients with ACTH hypersecretion; administered intravenously.

cor•ti•co•spi•nal (kor″tĭ-ko-spi′nəl) pertaining to or connecting the cortex of the brain and the spinal cord.

cor•ti•co•ster•oid (kor″tĭ-ko-ster′oid) any of the 21-carbon steroids elaborated by the adrenal cortex (excluding the sex hormones of adrenal origin) in response to corticotropin (ACTH) released by the pituitary gland or to angiotensin II. They are divided, according to their predominant biologic activity, into two major groups: *glucocorticoids,* chiefly influencing carbohydrate, fat, and protein metabolism, and *mineralocorticoids,* affecting the regulation of electrolyte and water balance. Some corticosteroids exhibit both types of activity in varying degrees, and others exert only one type of effect. They are used clinically for hormonal replacement therapy, for suppression of ACTH secretion by the anterior pituitary, as antineoplastic, antiallergic, and antiinflammatory agents, and to suppress immune responses. Called also *adrenocorticoid, corticoid, adrenal cortical* or *adrenocortical steroid,* and *adrenocortical* or *cortical hormone.*

cor•ti•cos•ter•one (kor″tĭ-kos′tər-ōn) a glucocorticoid with moderate activity, having life-maintaining properties in adrenalectomized animals and several other activities peculiar to the adrenal cortex. Its actions closely resemble those of cortisol, except that it is not antiinflammatory. It also shows some mineralocorticoid activity.

cor·ti·cos·ter·one meth·yl ox·i·dase (kor″tĭ-kos′tər-ōn meth′əl ok′sĭ-dās) corticosterone 18-monooxygenase.

cor·ti·cos·ter·one meth·yl ox·i·dase de·fi·cien·cy (kor″tĭ-kos′tər-ōn meth′əl ok′sĭ-dās) aldosterone synthase deficiency.

cor·ti·cos·ter·one 18-mono·oxy·ge·nase (kor″tĭ-kos′tər-ōn mon″o-ok′sə-jən-ās) [EC 1.14.15.5] an enzyme of the oxidoreductase class that catalyzes hydroxylation of corticosteroids at the 18 position followed by oxidation of the 18-hydroxy intermediates, steps in the biosynthesis of aldosterone. The two reactions are sometimes considered separately as I (hydroxylation) and II (oxidation); defects in each reaction have been described and called corticosterone methyl oxidase deficiency, types I and II. The enzyme may be an activity of steroid 11β-monooxygenase (q.v.)

cor·ti·co·ten·sin (kor″tĭ-ko-ten′sin) a low-molecular-weight polypeptide purified from kidney extract that exhibits a vasopressor effect when given intravenously.

cor·ti·co·tha·lam·ic (kor″tĭ-ko-thə-lam′ik) pertaining to or connecting the cerebral cortex and the thalamus.

cor·ti·co·ther·a·py (kor″tĭ-ko-ther′ə-pe) therapeutic administration of a corticosteroid.

cor·ti·co·trope (kor′ti-ko-trōp) corticotroph.

cor·ti·co·troph (kor′tĭ-ko-trōf″) a small, irregularly stellate, acidophilic cell of the adenohypophysis, having small, sparsely distributed secretory granules and secreting corticotropin and β-endorphin, which are cleaved from a large prohormone called *pro-opiomelanocortin.* Called also *corticotrope, corticotroph-lipotroph, corticolipotrope, corticotrope cell,* and *corticotroph cell.*

cor·ti·co·tro·phic (kor″tĭ-ko-tro′fik) adrenocorticotropic.

cor·ti·co·tro·phin (kor′tĭ-ko-tro″fin) corticotropin.

cor·ti·co·troph-li·po·troph (kor′tĭ-ko-trōf-lip′o-trōf) corticotroph.

cor·ti·co·tro·pic (kor″tĭ-ko-tro′pik) adrenocorticotropic.

cor·ti·co·tro·pin (kor′tĭ-ko-tro″pin) 1. a 39–amino-acid anterior pituitary hormone, one of the derivatives of pro-opiomelanocortin; it acts primarily on the adrenal cortex, stimulating its growth and the secretion of corticosteroids. Its production is increased during times of stress. 2. [USP] a preparation of the hormone derived from mammals used for food, administered intravenously for diagnostic testing of adrenocortical function. Called also *adrenocorticotropic hormone, ACTH, corticotrophin, adrenocorticotrophin,* and *adrenocorticotropin.*

repository c. see under *injection.*

cor·ti·co·tro·pi·no·ma (kor″tĭ-ko-tro″pĭ-no′mə) corticotroph adenoma.

Cor·ti·fair (kor′tĭ-fār) trademark for preparations of hydrocortisone.

Cor·ti·foam (kor′tĭ-fōm) trademark for a preparation of hydrocortisone acetate.

cor·ti·lymph (kor′tĭ-limf″) [organ of *Corti* + *lymph*] the fluid filling the intercellular spaces of the organ of Corti; it is similar in composition to perilymph.

Cor·ti·na·ri·a·ceae (kor″tĭ-nar-e-a′se-e) a family of mushrooms (order Agaricales). Some genera are edible, but genus *Galerina* contains amatoxins and can be deadly.

Cor·ti·na·ri·us (kor″tĭ-nar′e-əs) a large genus of mushrooms that includes many edible species; certain species found in Europe and Japan contain the toxins orelline and orellanine.

cor·ti·sol (kor′tĭ-sol) the major natural glucocorticoid synthesized in the zona fasciculata of the adrenal cortex; it affects the metabolism of glucose, protein, and fats and has appreciable mineralocorticoid activity. It also regulates the immune system and affects many other functions. When used as a pharmaceutical, it is usually referred to as hydrocortisone. For therapeutic uses, see *hydrocortisone.*

cor·ti·sone (kor′tĭ-sōn) a natural glucocorticoid that is metabolically convertible to cortisol. The human adrenal cortex secretes only minute amounts; most that is found in peripheral plasma is formed from cortisol by a reversible reaction. The synthetic hormone exerts its pharmaceutical effects through its metabolic conversion to cortisol.

c. acetate [USP] an ester of cortisone, having a slow onset but long duration of action, used in replacement therapy for adrenocortical insufficiency and as an antiinflammatory and immunosuppressant in a wide variety of disorders; administered orally and intramuscularly.

Cor·ti·spor·in (kor″tĭ-spor′in) trademark for combination preparations of polymyxin B, neomycin sulfate, hydrocortisone, and (in some preparations) bacitracin zinc.

Cor·tone (kor′tōn) trademark for preparations of cortisone acetate.

Cor·tril (kor′tril) trademark for preparations of hydrocortisone.

Cor·tro·syn (kor′tro-sin) trademark for a preparation of cosyntropin.

co·run·dum (ko-run′dəm) naturally occurring aluminum oxide; used in dentistry as an abrasive in grinding wheels and for points mounted on mandrels for the dental engine. See also *emery.*

cor·us·ca·tion (kor″əs-ka′shən) [L. *coruscatio* a flash] a glittering sensation, as of flashes of light before the eyes.

Cor·vert (kor′vərt) trademark for a preparation of ibutilide acetate.

Cor·vi·sart disease (kor″ve-sahr′) [Baron Jean Nicolas *Corvisart* des Marets, French physician, personal physician to Napoleon, 1755–1821] see under *disease.*

co·ryd·a·line (ko-rid′ə-lēn) an alkaloid from species of *Corydalis* and *Dicentra;* it is used as a diuretic and tonic in humans but can cause diarrhea and potentially fatal convulsions in other animals.

Co·ryd·a·lis (ko-rid′ə-lis) [L., from Gr. *korys* helmet] a large genus of herbs found in temperate climates. *C. bulbo′sa* (DC.), *C. ca′va* (L.) Schweigg. & Korte (Fumariaceae), and other species contain bulbocapnine and cause neurotoxicity in animals. It is used for a variety of indications in homeopathy.

co·ryd·a·lis (ko-rid′ə-lis) 1. any plant of the genus *Corydalis.* 2. the dried tuber of *Dicentra cucullaria* or *D. canadensis,* which contains bicuculline and several isoquinoline alkaloids, including corydaline, bulbocapnine, and corytuberine.

co·rym·bi·form (ko-rim′bĭ-form) [Gr. *korymbos* the cluster of ivy flower + *form*] clustered; said of lesions grouped around a single, usually larger, lesion, as in tinea versicolor or late secondary syphilis.

co·rym·bose (kor′im-bōs) corymbiform.

co·ry·ne·bac·te·ria (ko-ri″ne-bak-tēr′e-ə) plural of *corynebacterium.*

Co·ry·ne·bac·te·ri·a·ceae (ko-ri″ne-bak-tēr″e-a′se-e) a family of bacteria of the suborder Corynebacterineae, order Actinomycetales; it contains a single genus, *Corynebacterium.*

Co·ry·ne·bac·te·ri·neae (ko-ri″ne-bak-tər-in′e-e) a suborder of bacteria of the order Actinomycetales; medically important organisms are contained in the families Corynebacteriaceae, Gordoniaceae, Mycobacteriaceae, and Nocardiaceae.

Co·ry·ne·bac·te·ri·um (ko-ri″ne-bak-tēr′e-əm) [Gr. *korynē* club + *bacterium*] a genus of club-shaped bacteria of the family Corynebacteriaceae, consisting of gram-positive, nonsporulating, nonmotile, straight to slightly curved rods; organisms are catalase-positive, irregularly staining, sometimes granular, and sometimes arranged in angular and palisade groups. They are widely distributed in nature and include human and animal parasites and pathogens, plant pathogens, and nonpathogens. The type species is *C. diphthe′riae.*

C. acco′lens a species that colonizes the upper respiratory tract and occasionally causes septicemia or endocarditis.

C. afermen′tans a species that can cause septicemia in immunocompromised persons.

C. bo′vis a species that causes bovine mastitis in cows and a variety of infections in susceptible humans.

C. diphthe′riae the specific etiologic agent of diphtheria, which also causes skin infections. The organisms are separated according to cultural characteristics into three biovars: *mitis, intermedius,* and *gravis,* which apparently are not related to pathogenicity. Most strains produce a potent exotoxin. Called also *Klebs-Löffler bacillus.*

C. e′qui *Rhodococcus equi.*

C. flaves′cens an aerobic species occurring predominantly in dairy products and producing lactic acid without gas in carbohydrate fermentation.

C. glucuronoly′ticum a species that causes urinary tract infections and possibly prostatitis.

C. granulo′sum *Propionibacterium granulosum.*

C. jeikei′um a species closely related to *C. diphtheriae* that has been found on the skin of hospital patients and contaminating wounds, especially of immunocompromised persons.

C. kut′scheri 1. a species causing latent and overt infections in mice and rats. 2. a species found in the oral cavity of humans and other primates, particularly in dental calculus and plaque.

C. matrucho′tii a species found in the oral cavity of humans and other primates, particularly in dental calculus and plaque.

C. minutis′simum a species of uncertain affiliation that causes erythrasma in humans.

C. par′vum 1. *Propionibacterium acnes.* 2. a heat-killed and formaldehyde-treated preparation of *C. parvum (P. acnes)* administered orally or parenterally as an experimental cancer immunotherapeutic agent, usually in conjunction with conventional chemotherapy. It appears to act by activating macrophages and also seems to depress T cell function.

C. pseudodiphtheri′ticum a species normally present in the respiratory tract, which closely resembles *C. diphtheriae* but is nontoxigenic; it is sometimes an opportunistic pathogen. Called also *Hofmann bacillus.*

C. pseudotuberculo′sis a pathogenic toxin-producing species usually found in animals other than humans. It causes caseous lymphadenitis, abscesses, and chronic purulent infections, especially in sheep and goats, and contagious acne of horses. Occasional human disease may form from contact with infected animals or food. Called also *Preisz-Nocard bacillus.*

C. pyo'genes *Arcanobacterium pyogenes.*

C. rena'le a species that causes contagious bovine pyelonephritis in cattle and enzootic balanoposthitis in sheep.

C. rie'gelii a species that can cause urinary tract infections in women.

C. stria'tum a species found in various kinds of infections in immunocompromised persons.

C. tuberculostea'ricum a species that sometimes causes mastitis.

C. ul'cerans a toxigenic species of uncertain affiliation that causes nasopharyngeal infections in humans and acute mastitis in cattle.

C. urealy'ticum a species that causes urinary tract infections, especially in weak or immunocompromised persons.

C. xero'sis an opportunistic pathogenic species found in the conjunctival sac and on the skin and mucous membranes of humans.

co•ry•ne•bac•te•ri•um (ko-ri″ne-bak-tēr′e-əm) pl. *corynebacte'ria* [Gr. *korynē* club + *bacterium*] 1. any member of the family Corynebacteriaceae or of the genus *Corynebacterium.* 2. a bacterium that displays coryneform shape during some stage of its development on artificial media. See also *coryneform bacteria,* under *bacterium.*

co•ry•ne•form (ko-ri′nə-form) [Gr. *korynē* club + L. *forma*] club-shaped; see under *bacterium.*

Co•ry•nes•po•ra (kor″ĭ-nes′pə-rə) a widespread genus of imperfect fungi of the form-order Moniliales.

C. cassi'cola a species that is a cause of eumycotic mycetoma.

cor•y•tu•ber•ine (ko″re-too′bər-ēn) a crystalline alkaloid from commercial corydaline.

co•ry•za (ko-ri′zə) [L., from Gr. *koryza*] acute rhinitis.

c. foe'tida ozena.

infectious c., infectious avian c. an acute respiratory disease of chickens characterized by nasal discharge, sneezing, and edema of the face, and caused by *Haemophilus paragallinarum.* Infection of the lower respiratory tract sometimes occurs.

Cor•zide (kor′zīd) trademark for a combination preparation of nadolol and bendroflumethiazide.

COS Canadian Ophthalmological Society.

co•sen•si•tize (ko-sen′sĭ-tīz) to sensitize to two or more sensitizing agents.

Cos•me•gen (koz′mə-jən) trademark for a preparation of dactinomycin.

cos•me•ceu•ti•cal (koz″mə-soo′tĭ-kəl) 1. having both cosmetic benefits and pharmaceutical properties. 2. a compound having such effects.

cos•me•sis (koz-me′sis) [Gr. *kosmēsis* an arranging or adorning] 1. the preservation, restoration, or bestowing of bodily beauty. 2. the surgical correction of a disfiguring physical defect.

cos•met•ic (koz-met′ik) [Gr. *kosmētikos*] 1. pertaining to cosmesis. 2. a beautifying substance or preparation.

cos•mid (koz′mid) [*co*hesive end *s*ite + plas*mid*] a hybrid cloning vector constructed of plasmid DNA joined together with *cos* sites from a bacteriophage, having advantages of both types of vector and useful for cloning large (up to 50 kb) DNA fragments.

Co•sopt (ko′sopt) trademark for a combination preparation of dorzolamide hydrochloride and timolol maleate.

co•spir•o•no•zide (ko″spir-on′ə-zīd) pharmacy equivalent name for a combination of spironolactone and hydrochlorothiazide; used as a diuretic in the treatment of edema, hypertension, and hypokalemia.

cos•ta (kos′tə) gen. and pl. *cos'tae* [L. "rib"] 1. [TA] rib: one of the elastic arches of bone, found in pairs with twelve on either side *(costa I – costa XII),* extending from the thoracic vertebrae toward the median line on the anterior aspect of the trunk; they form the major part of the thoracic skeleton. The upper seven (I–VII) are called *costae verae* (true ribs) and are connected anteriorly with the sternum; the lower five (VIII–XII) are called *costae spuriae* (false ribs) and are not connected directly with the sternum. 2. the bony part of a rib. 3. a rodlike structure extending along the base of the undulating membrane in certain flagellate protozoa, such as trichomonads.

c. cervica'lis [TA] cervical rib: a supernumerary rib arising from a cervical vertebra, usually the seventh. See also *scalenus syndrome* and *cervical rib syndrome,* under *syndrome.*

cos'tae fluctuan'tes [TA], cos'tae fluitan'tes floating ribs: the lower two ribs on either side *(costa XI* and *costa XII),* which ordinarily have no ventral attachment; called also *vertebral ribs.*

c. pri'ma [TA] first rib: costa I, the superior rib on either side.

c. secun'da [TA] second rib: costa II, the rib just inferior to the costa prima on either side.

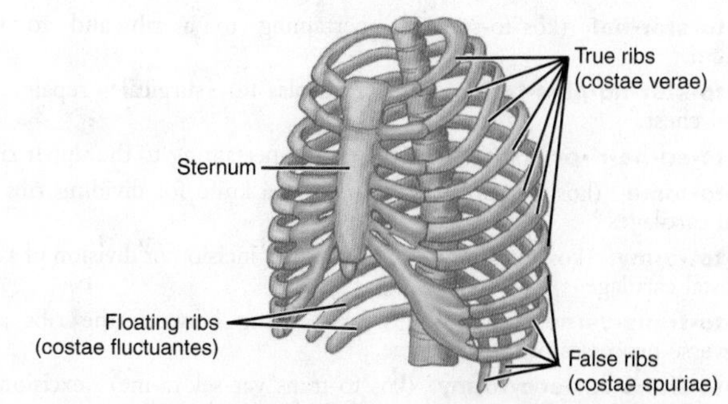

■ Costae (ribs), subdivided into the true (costae verae) and false ribs (costae spuriae); of the latter, the bottom two are also known as floating ribs (costae fluctuantes).

cos'tae spu'riae [TA] false ribs: the lower five ribs on either side (costa VIII to costa XII); the ventral tips of the upper three connect with the costal cartilages of the superiorly adjacent ribs, and the ventral tips of the lower two (costae XI and XII) ordinarily have no attachment.

cos'tae ve'rae [TA] true ribs: the upper seven ribs on either side (costa I to costa VII), which are connected to the sides of the sternum by their costal cartilages. Called also *sternal ribs* and *vertebrosternal ribs.*

cos•tae (kos′te) [L.] genitive and plural of *costa.*

cos•tal (kos′təl) [L. *costalis,* from *costa* rib] pertaining to a rib or ribs.

cos•tal•gia (kos-tal′jə) [*cost-* + *-algia*] 1. pain in the ribs. 2. pain in the costal muscles; called also *pleurodynia.*

cos•ta•lis (kos-ta′lis) [L.] costal; used in anatomical nomenclature to denote relationship to a rib.

cos•ta•tec•to•my (kos″tə-tek′tə-me) costectomy.

cos•tec•to•my (kos-tek′tə-me) [*cost-* + *-ectomy*] the operation of excising or resecting a rib.

Cos•ten syndrome (kos′tən) [James Bray *Costen,* American otolaryngologist, 1895–1962] see *temporomandibular disorder,* under *disorder.*

cos•ti•car•ti•lage (kos″tĭ-kahr′tĭ-ləj) [*cost-* + *cartilage*] the cartilage of a rib.

cos•tif•er•ous (kos-tif′ər-əs) [*cost-* + *-ferous*] bearing a rib, as the thoracic vertebrae of humans.

cos•ti•form (kos′tĭ-form) shaped like a rib.

co•stim•u•la•tor (ko″stim-u-la′shən) the action of a costimulator in activating helper T cells.

co•stim•u•la•tor (ko-stim′u-la″tər) a molecule expressed on the surface of an antigen-presenting cell that provides a stimulus that is required in addition to antigen for activation of helper T cells.

cos•ti•spi•nal (kos″tĭ-spi′nəl) pertaining to or connecting the ribs and spine.

cost(o)- [L. *costa* rib] a combining form denoting relationship to the ribs.

cos•to•cen•tral (kos″to-sen′trəl) pertaining to a rib and the centrum (body) of a vertebra.

cos•to•cer•vi•cal (kos″to-sur′vĭ-kəl) [*costo-* + *cervical*] pertaining to or connecting the ribs and the neck.

cos•to•cer•vi•ca•lis (kos″to-sur″vĭ-ka′lis) 1. costocervical. 2. musculus iliocostalis cervicis.

cos•to•chon•dral (kos″to-kon′drəl) pertaining to a rib and its cartilage.

cos•to•chon•dri•tis (kos″to-kon-dri′tis) inflammation of the cartilaginous junction between a rib or ribs and the sternum; called also *costosternal syndrome.*

cos•to•cla•vic•u•lar (kos″to-klə-vik′u-lər) pertaining to the ribs and clavicle.

cos•to•cor•a•coid (kos″to-kor′ə-koid) pertaining to the ribs and coracoid process.

cos•to•gen•ic (kos″to-jen′ik) [*costo-* + *-genic*] arising from a rib, especially from a defect of the marrow of the ribs.

cos•to•in•fe•ri•or (kos″to-in-fēr′e-ər) pertaining to the lower ribs.

cos•to•phren•ic (kos″to-fren′ik) pertaining to the ribs and diaphragm.

cos•to•pleu•ral (kos″to-ploor′əl) pertaining to the ribs and the pleura.

cos•to•scap•u•lar (kos″to-skap′u-lər) pertaining to the ribs and the scapula.

cos•to•scap•u•lar•is (kos″to-skap″u-lar′is) musculus serratus anterior.

cos·to·ster·nal (kos″to-stur′nəl) pertaining to a rib and to the sternum.

cos·to·ster·no·plas·ty (kos″to-stur′no-plas″te) surgical repair of funnel chest.

cos·to·su·pe·ri·or (kos″to-soo-pēr′e-ər) pertaining to the upper ribs.

cos·to·tome (kos′to-tōm) [*costo-* + *-tome*] a knife for dividing ribs or costal cartilages.

cos·tot·o·my (kos-tot′ə-me) [*costo-* + *-tomy*] incision or division of a rib or costal cartilage.

cos·to·trans·verse (kos″to-trans-vərs′) lying between the ribs and transverse processes of the vertebrae.

cos·to·trans·ver·sec·to·my (kos″to-trans″vər-sek′tə-me) excision of a part of a rib with the transverse process of a vertebra.

cos·to·ver·te·bral (kos″to-vur′tə-brəl) pertaining to a rib and a vertebra.

cos·to·xi·phoid (kos″to-zi′foid) connecting the ribs and the xiphoid process.

co·syn·tro·pin (ko″sin-tro′pin) a synthetic polypeptide identical with the first 24 amino acids of corticotropin, having the corticotropic activity of corticotropin but lacking its allergenicity; used in the diagnosis of adrenal insufficiency by plasma cortisol response following subcutaneous, intramuscular, or intravenous injection. Called also *tetracosactide.*

Co·tard syndrome (ko-tahr′) [Jules *Cotard,* French neurologist, 1840–1887] see under *syndrome.*

Cot·a·zym (kot′ə-zīm) trademark for preparations of pancrelipase.

co·ten·i·done (ko-ten′ĭ-dōn) pharmacy equivalent name for a combination of atenolol, a beta-adrenergic blocking agent, and chlorthalidone, a thiazide diuretic; used in the treatment of hypertension.

co·throm·bo·plas·tin (ko-throm″bo-plas′tin) factor VII; see under *coagulation factors,* at *factor.*

co·ti·nine (ko′tĭ-nēn) the major urinary metabolite of nicotine.

co·trans·duc·tion (ko″trans-duk′shən) simultaneous transduction of two or more genes, indicating close linkage of the genes on the transduced element.

co·trans·fec·tion (ko″trans-fek′shən) simultaneous transfection of two or more physically unlinked DNA fragments into eukaryotic target cells; generally one of the fragments contains a gene that is easily assayed and acts as a marker.

co·trans·for·ma·tion (ko″trans-for-ma′shən) 1. simultaneous transformation of a single cell by two or more bacterial genes. 2. cotransfection.

co·trans·la·tion·al (ko-trans-la′shən-əl) occurring in conjunction with translation (def. 2); see *cotranslational transport,* under *transport.*

co·trans·port (ko-trans′port) linking of the transport of two substances across a membrane, one substance being transported down its concentration gradient, which powers the movement of the other substance against its concentration gradient; movement in the same direction is termed *symport,* while movement in opposite directions is termed *antiport.* Cf. *countertransport.*

co·trans·port·er (ko″trans-port′ər) a cell membrane transport protein that couples the movement of an ion down its concentration gradient to the movement of another substance against its concentration gradient.

Co·trel-Du·bous·set instrumentation, rod (ko-trel′ du-boo-sa′) [Yves *Cotrel,* French orthopedic surgeon, 20th century; J. *Dubousset,* French orthopedic surgeon, 20th century] see under *instrumentation* and *rod.*

co·tri·am·ter·zide (ko″tri-am′tər-zīd) pharmacy equivalent name for a combination of triamterene and hydrochlorothiazide; used as a diuretic in the treatment of edema, hypertension, and hypokalemia.

Co·trim (ko′trim) trademark for combination preparations of trimethoprim and sulfamethoxazole.

co·tri·mox·a·zole (ko″tri-moks′ə-zol) pharmacy equivalent name for a combination of trimethoprim and sulfamethoxazole, an antibacterial and antiprotozoal used in the treatment of pneumocystis pneumonia, bronchitis, otitis media, enterocolitis due to *Shigella,* urinary tract infections, and traveler's diarrhea; administered orally or intravenously.

Cotte operation (kot) [Gaston *Cotte,* French surgeon, 1879–1951] see under *operation.*

cot·ton (kot′ən) [Ar. *al-qoton* or *al-qutn*] 1. a plant of the genus *Gossypium.* 2. a textile material derived from the hair of the seeds of one or more of the cultivated varieties of *Gossypium.*
  absorbable c. oxidized cellulose.
  absorbent c., purified c. [USP] cotton that has been purified, freed from fatty matter, bleached, and sterilized; used as a surgical dressing.
  styptic c. cotton impregnated with a styptic solution and dried.

cot·ton·mouth (kot′ən-mouth) water moccasin.

cot·ton·seed (kot′ən-sēd) the seeds of cultivated species of *Gossypium,* which are sources of cottonseed oil. They are commonly made into cakes and fed to livestock, but they must first be processed to remove the toxin gossypol, which could cause gossypol poisoning.

cot·ton-wool (kot′ən-wool) raw nonabsorbent cotton, especially the absorbent form prepared by removing the cottonseed oil.

Co·tu·gno disease (ko-toon′yō) [Domenico Felice Antonio *Cotugno,* Italian anatomist, 1736–1822] sciatica. See also *Cotunnius.*

Co·tun·ni·us aqueduct, canal, nerve (ko-tun′e-ə) [D.F.A. *Cotugno (Cotunnius)*] see under *aqueduct, canal,* and *nerve.*

co·tur·nism (ko-tōōr′niz-əm) food poisoning caused by ingestion of meat of the European migratory quail, genus *Coturnix,* and marked by such symptoms as difficult breathing, impaired speech, nausea, weakness and loss of feeling in the lower limbs, and partial paralysis, and sometimes resulting in death; the causative toxin, which occurs in only some of the quail, is unidentified.

Co·tur·nix (kə-tōōr′niks) a genus of birds of the family Phasianidae, including European migratory quails, whose meat can be poisonous; see *coturnism.*

co·twin (ko-twin) a twin; usually applied in twin studies to identify pairs of twins.

Cot·y·le·don (kot″ə-le′dən) a genus of herbaceous plants found in southern Africa; several species contain cotyledontoxin.

cot·y·le·don (kot″ə-le′don) [Gr. *kotylēdōn*] 1. the seed leaf of the embryo of a plant. 2. one of the subdivisions of the uterine surface of a discoidal placenta. 3. one of the tufted areas of a ruminant's placenta.

cot·y·le·do·no·sis (kot″ĭ-le″də-no′sis) krimpsiekte.

cot·y·le·don·tox·in (kot″ə-le′don-tok″sin) a toxic substance that is neutral, nonalkaloidal, nonglucosidal, non-nitrogenous, and amorphous and is found in several species of the genus *Cotyledon;* see also *krimpsiekte.*

Cot·y·lo·gon·i·mus (kot″ə-lo-gon′ĭ-məs) [Gr. *kotylē* cup + *gonimos* productive] *Heterophyes.*

cot·y·loid (kot′ə-loid) [Gr. *kotyloeides* cup shaped] 1. cup-shaped. 2. acetabular.

Co·ty·lo·pho·ron (kot″ə-lof′ə-ron) a genus of trematodes of the family Paramphistomatidae that infest the rumen and intestines of ruminants, causing paramphistomiasis.

cot·y·lo·sa·cral (kot″ə-lo-sa′krəl) pertaining to the acetabulum and the sacrum.

co·type (ko′tīp) any strain of microorganisms (of the same taxon), other than a holotype, from the collection of the bacteriologist who originally described the taxon.

cough (kawf) 1. a sudden noisy expulsion of air from the lungs, usually produced to keep the airways of the lungs free of foreign matter; see also under *reflex.* Called also *tussis.* 2. to produce such an expulsion of air.
  aneurysmal c. cough associated with aortic aneurysm, sometimes with paralysis of one vocal cord.
  Balme c. cough on lying down, seen in obstruction of the nasopharynx.
  barking c. a barklike cough of children, seen in croup and other conditions.
  brassy c. a cough with a metallic, barking quality due to inflammation of the trachea.
  dry c. a cough that is not accompanied by expectoration.
  ear c. a reflex cough caused by disease of the ear, when the auricular branch of the vagus nerve is stimulated.
  habit c. coughing, usually in children, that lacks a physical basis; it is a dry cough unaccompanied by other symptoms, seen only during waking hours, often lasting for weeks, and refractory to medication. Called also *psychogenic c.*
  hacking c. a short, frequent, shallow, and feeble cough. Called also *tussiculation.*
  kennel c. canine infectious tracheobronchitis.
  mechanical c. expulsion of air from the lungs produced by use of an exsufflator, with effects similar to those of a natural cough.
  privet c. an allergic cough noted in China and attributed to the pollen of privet.
  productive c. a cough that is effective in removing material from the respiratory tract. Called also *wet c.*
  psychogenic c. habit c.
  reflex c. a cough due to the irritation of some remote organ.
  trigeminal c. a cough due to irritation of the fibers of the trigeminal nerve distributed to the throat, nose, and external meatus of the ear.
  wet c. productive c.
  whooping c. pertussis.
  winter c. chronic bronchitis recurring in the winter.

Cou·i·naud segments (kwe-no′) [Claude *Couinaud*, French surgeon, 1922–2008] segmenta hepatis; see under *segmentum*.

cou·lomb (C) (koo′lom) [Charles Augustin de *Coulomb*, French physicist, 1736–1806] the SI unit of electric charge, defined as the charge carried across a surface by a steady current of 1 ampere in 1 second; it is equivalent to 6.25×10^{18} electrons.

Coul·ter counter (kōl′tər) [Wallace H. *Coulter*, American engineer, 20th century] see under *counter*.

Cou·ma·din (koo′mə-din) trademark for preparations of warfarin sodium.

cou·ma·rin (koo′mə-rin) 1. a principle with a bitter taste and an odor like that of vanilla beans, derived from tonka bean, sweet clover, and other plants, and also prepared synthetically. It contains a factor, dicumarol, that inhibits the hepatic synthesis of the vitamin K–dependent coagulation factors (prothrombin, factors VII, IX, and X), and a number of its derivatives are used widely as anticoagulants in the treatment of disorders in which there is excessive or undesirable clotting, such as thrombophlebitis, pulmonary embolism, and certain cardiac conditions. 2. any derivative of coumarin or any synthetic compound with coumarin-like actions.

Coun·cil·man bodies (koun′səl-mən) [William Thomas *Councilman*, American pathologist, 1854–1933] see under *body*.

coun·sel·ing (kown′səl-ing) provision of information, advice, and support.

genetic c. counseling provided to an individual, family, or group manifesting or at risk for developing or transmitting a genetic disorder, including risks, consequences, and methods of management.

count (kount) [L. *computare* to reckon] a numerical computation or indication.

absolute neutrophil c. the total number of neutrophils in a unit volume of blood, calculated from the leukocyte count using the combined percentages of mature neutrophils and band cells present.

Addis c. a formerly common method of determining the number of red blood cells, white blood cells, epithelial cells, and casts, as well as the protein content in an aliquot of a twelve-hour urine specimen, used in the diagnosis and management of kidney disease.

Arneth c. a method of determining what percentages of neutrophils in a population have each number of nuclear lobes or segments between one and five; normally over 75 per cent should have two or three lobes. An increase in the percentages with fewer lobes, called a *shift to the left*, is seen in bacterial infections, whereas an increased number with hypersegmentation of the nuclei, called a *shift to the right*, is seen in cobalamin and folate deficiency. Called also *neutrophil lobe c.*

blood c., blood cell c. determination of the number of formed elements in a cubic millimeter of blood; it may be a *complete blood count* or it may measure just one of the formed elements. Methods include manual counts with a hemacytometer and automated counts with a flow cytometer, a Coulter counter, or other means.

complete blood c. a series of tests of the peripheral blood, including the erythrocyte count, erythrocyte indices, leukocyte counts, and sometimes platelet count.

differential blood c., differential leukocyte c. a leukocyte count that calculates the percentages of different types of cells. Cf. *total leukocyte c.*

erythrocyte c. determination of the number of erythrocytes in a unit volume of blood that has been diluted in an isotonic solution, done with an automatic counter such as a flow cytometer. Called also *red blood cell c.* and *red cell c.*

filament-nonfilament c. in the differential leukocyte count, determination of the number of juvenile and mature leukocytes.

leukocyte c. determination of the number of leukocytes in a unit volume of blood, usually after the erythrocytes have been lysed and the blood has been diluted; it may be done either manually with a hemacytometer or electronically. See *total leukocyte c.* and *differential leukocyte c.* Called also *white blood cell c.* and *white cell c.*

neutrophil lobe c. Arneth c.

platelet c. determination of the number of platelets per cubic millimeter of blood; it may be either a *direct platelet count* with a hemacytometer and a microscope or an *indirect platelet count* in which the ratio of platelets to erythrocytes on a blood smear is determined and the number of platelets is computed from the erythrocyte count.

red blood cell c., red cell c. erythrocyte c.

reticulocyte c. a calculation of the number of reticulocytes in 1 mm^3 of peripheral blood, recorded as an absolute number or as the percentage of the erythrocyte count. It provides a means of assessing the erythropoietic activity of the bone marrow.

total leukocyte c. a leukocyte count measuring the total number of all the types in a given volume of blood. Cf. *differential leukocyte c.*

total lymphocyte c. a test that may be useful as an indicator of nutritional status and outcome.

white blood cell c., white cell c. leukocyte c.

coun·ter (koun′tər) an instrument or apparatus by which numerical value is computed; in radiology, a device for enumerating ionizing events.

Coulter c. an automated instrument for performing blood counts, based on the principle that cells are poor electrical conductors compared with saline solution.

Geiger c., Geiger-Müller c. a radiation counter that uses a gas-filled tube to indicate the presence of ionizing particles; the type and energy of a particle cannot be determined because the degree of ionization produced is independent of them. It is highly sensitive to beta particles but relatively insensitive to gamma rays and x-rays.

proportional c. a gas-filled radiation detection tube in which the pulse produced is proportional to the number of ions formed in the gas by the primary ionizing particle; thus it is possible to discriminate among radiations of different energies or types.

scintillation c. an instrument for indicating the emission of ionizing particles, making possible the determination of the concentration of radioactive isotopes in the body or other substance; the radiation is absorbed by a specific type of crystal or liquid that subsequently emits minute flashes of light, which are detected and amplified by a photomultiplier tube and counted if they fall within a preset window of energies characteristic of the radioisotope in question.

counter- [L. *contra* against] a prefix meaning *(a)* opposing, opposite or *(b)* complementary.

coun·ter·bal·ance (koun″tər-bal′əns) counterpoise; offset.

renal c. compensatory hypertrophy of a normal kidney or part of a kidney that has a diseased mate or part, with the latter remaining in a relatively atrophic state.

coun·ter·ca·thex·is (koun″tər-kə-thek′sis) anticathexis.

coun·ter·cur·rent (koun′tər-kur″ənt) 1. retrograde. 2. see *countercurrent multiplication*, under *multiplication*.

coun·ter·elec·tro·pho·re·sis (koun″tər-e-lek″tro-fə-re′sis) counterimmunoelectrophoresis.

coun·ter·ex·ten·sion (koun″tər-eks-ten′shən) countertraction.

coun·ter·im·mu·no·elec·tro·pho·re·sis (koun″tər-im″u-no-e-lek″tro-fə-re′sis) one-dimensional double electroimmunodiffusion; a technique in which antibody and antigen are placed in separate wells in an agar plate and driven toward each other by an applied electric field, because the gel is buffered at a pH between the isoelectric points of the antigen and antibody. It is more sensitive and faster than double immunodiffusion and is particularly useful for antigens that diffuse slowly in the gel. Abbreviated CIE. Called also *countercurrent immunoelectrophoresis* and *counterelectrophoresis*.

coun·ter·in·ci·sion (koun″tər-in-sĭ′zhən) a second incision usually made to promote drainage but occasionally to relieve tension on the edges of a clean wound during closure.

coun·ter·in·vest·ment (koun″tər-in-vest′mənt) anticathexis.

coun·ter·ir·ri·tant (koun″tər-ir′ĭ-tənt) 1. producing a counterirritation. 2. any agent that causes counterirritation.

coun·ter·ir·ri·ta·tion (koun″tər-ir″ĭ-ta′shən) a superficial irritation produced in one part of the body, intended to relieve an irritation in another part.

coun·ter·open·ing (koun″tər-o′pən-ing) a second incision made across an earlier one to promote drainage.

coun·ter·pho·bia (koun″tər-fo′be-ə) the state of seeking out situations or objects which one fears or has feared, consciously or unconsciously. **counterpho′bic** *adj*

coun·ter·poi·son (koun′tər-poi″zon) a poison given to counteract another poison.

coun·ter·pul·sa·tion (koun″tər-pəl-sa′shən) a technique for assisting the circulation and decreasing the work of the heart, by synchronizing the force of an external pumping device with cardiac systole and diastole.

intra-aortic balloon (IAB) c. circulatory support provided by a balloon inserted into the thoracic aorta, which is inflated during diastole (enhancing coronary perfusion pressure) and deflated during systole, resulting in a decrease in afterload and improvement in cardiac function.

coun·ter·punc·ture (koun″tər-punk′chər) counteropening.

coun·ter·shock (koun′tər-shok″) a high-intensity direct current shock delivered to the heart to interrupt ventricular fibrillation and restore synchronous electrical activity.

coun·ter·stain (koun′tər-stān″) a stain applied to render the effects of another stain more discernible.

coun·ter·trac·tion (koun″tər-trak′shən) traction opposed to another traction; employed in the reduction of fractures.

coun·ter·trans·fer·ence (koun″tər-trans-fur′əns) a transference reaction of a psychoanalyst or other psychotherapist to a patient, i.e., an emotional reaction that is generally a reflection of the analyst's own inner needs and conflicts but also may be a reaction to the client's behavior. See *transference*.

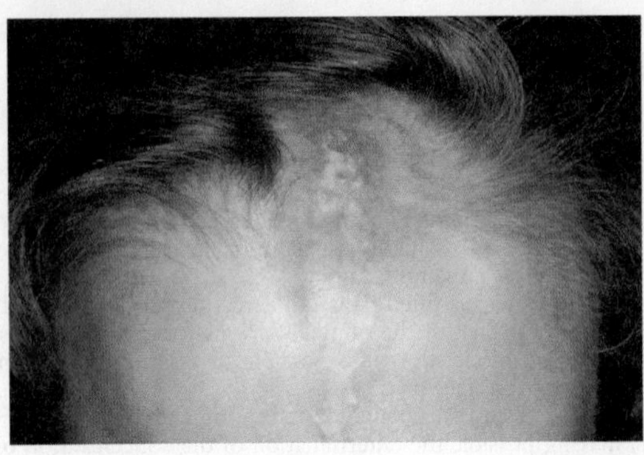

■ En coup de sabre.

coun•ter•trans•port (koun″tər-trans′port) the simultaneous transport of two substances across a membrane in opposite directions, either by the same carrier or by different carriers that are biochemically linked to each other. Cf. *antiport* and *cotransport.*

sodium-lithium c. a transport pathway by which sodium ions enter erythrocytes and lithium ions leave in order to maintain sodium balance in the cells and in the plasma.

count•ing (kount′ing) the act of making a count.

liquid scintillation c. determination of the concentration of radioisotopes in a body or sample by means of a scintillation counter (q.v.) that uses as a detector an organic liquid capable of emitting pulses of light when struck by radiation.

coup (koo) [Fr.] a blow or attack.

c. de fouet (də fwa′) ["strike of the whip"] rupture of the plantaris muscle accompanied by a sharp disabling pain.

c. de sabre (də sahb′), **en c. de sabre** (ah koo′ də sahb′) ["saber stroke"] a linear lesion of scleroderma involving the frontal or frontoparietal area of the forehead and scalp; it may also be associated with facial hemiatrophy.

c. de soleil (də so-la′) sunstroke.

c. sur coup (sur koo′) ["blow on blow"] the administration of a drug in small doses at short intervals, to secure rapid, complete, or continuous action; abbreviated CSC.

cou•ple (kup′əl) [L. *copula* a bond] 1. to link together; join; connect. 2. two equal forces operating on an object in parallel but opposite directions. 3. an area of contact between two dissimilar metals, producing a difference in electrical potential.

coup•let (kup′lət) pair (def. 2).

coup•ling (kup′ling) 1. the joining together of two things. 2. in genetics, the occurrence on the same chromosome in a double heterozygote of the two mutant alleles of interest. Cf. *repulsion.* 3. in cardiology, the serial occurrence of a normal heart beat followed closely by a premature beat.

chemiosmotic c. chemosmosis.

excitation-contraction c. the coupling of the action potential to muscle constriction by means of calcium ions which diffuse rapidly into the myofibrils and catalyze the chemical reactions that promote the contractile sliding of actin and myosin filaments.

fixed c. coupling in which the premature heart beats follow the preceding normal beats at identical intervals.

variable c. coupling in which the interval between extrasystoles and the sinus beats preceding them is not constant.

Cour•voi•si•er law, sign (koor-vwah″ze-a′) [Ludwig Georg *Courvoisier*, Swiss surgeon, 1843–1918] see under *law* and *sign.*

Cour•voi•si•er-Ter•rier syndrome (koor-vwah″sya′ ter-ya′) [L.G. *Courvoisier;* Louis Félix *Terrier*, French surgeon, 1837–1908] see under *syndrome.*

Cou•tard method (koo-tahr′) [Henri *Coutard*, French radiologist in United States, 1876–1950] see under *method.*

cou•vade (koo-vahd′) a custom of certain societies in which the husband feigns illness during his wife's parturient and puerperal periods.

cou•ver•cle (koo′vər-kəl) [Fr.] hematoma.

co•va•lence (ko-va′ləns) 1. the number of electron pairs an atom can share with other atoms. 2. one or more chemical bonds formed by sharing of electron pairs between atoms.

co•va•lent (ko′va-lənt) see under *bond.*

co•var•i•ance (ko-văr′e-əns) [*co-* + *variance*] in statistics, a measure of the tendency of two random variables to vary together: the expected value of the product of the deviations of corresponding values of the variables from their respective means. It may be positive, with both variables increasing or decreasing together; negative, with one variable decreasing as the other increases; or zero, with one variable unaffected by changes in the other.

co•va•ri•ate (ko-var′e-ət) a variable that is related to a second variable.

cov•er (kuv′ər) 1. to provide protection against, as by prophylaxis. 2. the prophylaxis so provided.

Co•ver•a-HS (ko-ver′ə) trademark for a preparation of verapamil hydrochloride.

cov•er•glass (kuv′ər-glas″) *cover glass;* see under *glass.*

cov•er•slip (kuv′ər-slip″) cover glass.

cow•age (kou′əj) 1. *Mucuna pruriens.* 2. the hairs of the pods of *M. pruriens,* used medicinally as a vermifuge, anthelmintic, and counterirritant mixed with such vehicles as honey; on the skin they can cause a type of allergic contact dermatitis. Also used as "itching powders" of joke-shop fame.

Cow•den disease (kou′dən) [*Cowden*, the family name of the first reported case] see under *disease.*

Cow•dria (kou′dre-ə) [Edmund Vincent *Cowdry*, American anatomist and zoologist, 1888–1975] a former genus of bacteria of the order Rickettsiales; organisms are now placed in genus *Ehrlichia.*

cow•dri•o•sis (kou″dre-o′sis) heartwater.

Cow•en sign (kou′ən) [J.P. *Cowen*, American ophthalmologist, 20th century] see under *sign.*

cowl (koul) caul (def. 1).

Cow•per cyst, gland, etc. (kou′pər) [William *Cowper*, English surgeon, 1666–1709] see under *syringocele;* see *ductus glandulae bulbourethralis, glandula bulbourethralis;* and see *pectineal fascia,* under *fascia.*

cow•pe•ri•an (kou-pēr′e-ən) named for William *Cowper*, as *cowperitis.*

cow•per•itis (kou″pər-i′tis) inflammation of the Cowper gland (glandula bulbourethralis).

cow•pox (kou′poks) 1. a mild, self-limited, eruptive skin disease of milk cows, principally confined to the udder and teats, caused by a poxvirus; milkers may spread the disease to uninfected animals. 2. human infection with the cowpox virus, as from milking an infected animal; the primary lesions are vesicles that usually appear on the fingers, may rupture and spread to the hands, and heal without scarring. Cowpox is not to be confused with *paravaccinia.* Cf. *vaccinia.* Edward Jenner first demonstrated vaccination in 1798 when he showed that inoculation with material from cowpox lesions conferred immunity against smallpox.

COX cyclooxygenase.

Cox proportional hazards model (koks) [David Roxbee *Cox*, British statistician, born 1924] see under *model.*

coxa (kok′sə) [L.] 1. [TA] hip (def. 1). 2. articulatio coxae.

c. adduc′ta, c. flex′a c. vara.

c. mag′na a condition marked by broadening of the head and neck of the femur.

c. pla′na Legg-Calvé-Perthes disease.

c. sal′tans snapping hip.

c. val′ga deformity of the hip in which the angle formed by the axis of the head and the neck of the femur and the axis of its shaft is materially increased.

c. va′ra deformity of the hip in which the angle formed by the axis of the head and neck of the femur and the axis of its shaft is materially decreased; called also *c. adducta* and *c. flexa.*

c. va′ra lux′ans fissure of the neck of the femur with dislocation of the head developing from coxa vara.

cox•al•gia (kok-sal′jə) [*coxa* + *-algia*] 1. hip-joint disease. 2. pain in the hip.

cox•ar•thria (kok-sahr′thre-ə) coxitis.

cox•ar•thri•tis (kok-sahr-thri′tis) coxitis.

cox•ar•throc•a•ce (kok″sahr-throk′ə-se) fungus disease of the hip joint.

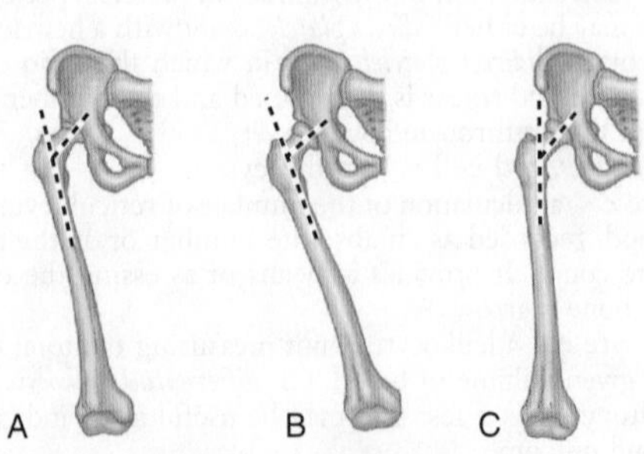

■ *(A)* Normal hip joint; *(B)* coxa vara; *(C)* coxa valga.

cox·ar·throp·a·thy (kok″sahr-throp′ə-the) [*coxa* + *arthro-* + *-pathy*] hip-joint disease.

cox·ar·thro·sis (kok″sahr-thro′sis) degenerative joint disease or osteoarthritis of the hip joint.

cox·ib (kok′sib) COX-2 inhibitor.

Cox·i·el·la (kok″se-el′ə) [Herald Rae *Cox*, American bacteriologist, 1907–1986] a genus of bacteria of the family Coxiellaceae, consisting of gram-negative rods without flagella or a capsule, occurring only in the vacuoles of host cells. The organisms are found worldwide in ticks and various vertebrates; infection is particularly prevalent in cattle, sheep, and goats. The type species is *Coxiella burne′tii*.

C. burne′tii the etiologic agent of Q fever, sometimes transmitted by ticks of the genera *Amblyomma*, *Dermacentor*, *Haemaphysalis*, and *Ixodes*. Human infection is most often not by way of a vector but by direct inhalation of infectious dust and aerosols from domestic livestock or from contaminated wool in textile plants.

Cox·i·el·la·ceae (kok″se-el-a′se-e) a family of bacteria of the order Legionellales grouped together on the basis of 16S rRNA sequence analysis and consisting of obligate intracellular parasites found only in cytoplasmic vacuoles of host cells. Medically important organisms are contained in the genus *Coxiella*.

cox·itis (kok-si′tis) inflammation of the hip joint; called also *coxarthritis*.

c. fu′gax transient synovitis.

cox·odyn·ia (kok″so-din′e-ə) coxalgia (def. 2).

coxo·fem·o·ral (kok″so-fem′o-rəl) [*coxa* + *femoral*] pertaining to the hip and thigh.

coxo·tu·ber·cu·lo·sis (kok″so-too-bur″ku-lo′sis) hip-joint disease.

cox·sack·ie·vi·rus (kok-sak′e-vi″rəs) [*Coxsackie*, New York, where it was first identified] any of a heterogeneous group of viruses of the genus *Enterovirus* that can cause a disease resembling poliomyelitis but without paralysis, as well as a disease with fever and rash. It is separable into two groups: A (23 serotypes, 1–22 and 24, with 23 being identical to echovirus 9), producing degenerative lesions of striated muscle, and B (6 serotypes), producing leptomeningitis in infant mice. A number of other serotypes have also been identified. Also written *Coxsackie virus*.

co·yo·ti·llo (koi-o-te′yo) [Mexican Spanish "little coyote"] *Karwinskia humboldtiana*.

Co·zaar (ko′zahr) trademark for a preparation of losartan potassium.

CP chemically pure (see *pure*); candle power.

cp centipoise.

CPAP continuous positive airway pressure.

CPC clinicopathological conference.

CPD citrate phosphate dextrose; see *anticoagulant citrate phosphate dextrose solution*, under *solution*.

CPDA-1 citrate phosphate dextrose adenine; see *anticoagulant citrate phosphate dextrose adenine solution*, under *solution*.

CPDD calcium pyrophosphate deposition disease.

C Ped Certified Pedorthist.

CPH Certificate in Public Health.

CPI California Personality Inventory; congenital palatopharyngeal incompetence.

CPK creatine phosphokinase; see *creatine kinase*.

CPM central pontine myelinolysis; cyclophosphamide.

cpm counts per minute, an expression of the rate of particle emission from a radioactive material.

CPP cerebral perfusion pressure.

CPPD calcium pyrophosphate dihydrate; see *calcium pyrophosphate deposition disease* under *disease*.

CPPS chronic pelvic pain syndrome.

CPR cardiopulmonary resuscitation.

CPS carbamoyl phosphate synthetase.

CPSI carbamoyl phosphate synthetase I; see *carbamoyl-phosphate synthase (ammonia)*.

CPSII carbamoyl phosphate synthetase II; see *carbamoyl-phosphate synthase (glutamine-hydrolyzing)*.

cps cycles per second; see *hertz*.

CR[1] complement receptor; conditioned response; crown-rump (see under *length*).

CR[2] dibenz(b,f)-1,4-oxazepine, a common tear gas.

CR3 complement receptor type 3; see *glycoprotein Mac-1*, under *glycoprotein*.

Cr chromium.

crab (krab) 1. any of various mollusks of the order Decapoda; see also *Potamon*. 2. a vernacular term for *Phthirus pubis*.

crack (krak) 1. an incomplete split, break, or fissure. 2. sand c.

hoof wall c. sand c.

quarter c. a sand crack on the quarter (medial aspect of the hoof).

sand c. a crack originating at the ground level in a horse's hoof, sometimes causing lameness. Two types are the *quarter c.* and the *toe c.* Called also *hoof wall c.*

toe c. a sand crack on the anterior part of the hoof.

crack·le (krak′əl) rale.

cra·dle (kra′dəl) a frame placed over the body of a bed patient for application of heat or cold or for protecting injured parts from contact with the bedclothes.

electric c., heat c. a tunnel- or hood-shaped cradle equipped with electric light bulbs, for application of heat to the body of a patient.

ice c. a device for lowering a patient's body temperature.

Crai·gia (kra′ge-ə) [Charles Franklin *Craig*, U. S. Army surgeon, 1872–1950] *Paramoeba*.

cramp (kramp) a painful spasmodic muscular contraction, especially a tonic spasm.

accessory c. spastic torticollis due to a lesion of the accessory nerve.

heat c. a form of heat exhaustion in which muscular spasm is attended by pains, dilated pupils, and weak pulse; seen in those who labor in intense heat (stokers, miners, cane-cutters) and lose much water and salt. Called also *Edsall disease*.

recumbency c's cramping of muscles in the lower limbs and feet while resting or during light sleep.

stoker's c. heat c.

writers' c. a muscle cramp in the hand, a type of focal dystonia caused by excessive use in writing; called also *graphospasm*, *writers' paralysis*, and *writers' spasm*.

Cramp·ton muscle (kramp′tən) [Sir Philip *Crampton*, Irish surgeon, 1777–1858] see under *muscle*.

Cramp·ton test (kramp′tən) [Charles Ward *Crampton*, American physician, 1877–1964] see under *test*.

cra·ni·ad (kra′ne-ad) [*crani-* + *-ad*[1]] cephalad.

cra·ni·al (kra′ne-əl) [L. *cranialis*] 1. pertaining to the cranium. 2. toward the head end of the body; a synonym of *superior* humans and other bipeds. In quadruped anatomy, *anterior* is sometimes used as a synonym. Called also *cephalic*.

cra·ni·a·lis (kra″ne-a′lis) [L.] [TA] cranial.

cra·ni·am·phit·o·my (kra″ne-am-fit′ə-me) [*crani-* + *amphi-* + *-tomy*] division of the entire circumference of the skull to secure decompression.

Cra·ni·a·ta (kra″ne-a′tə) the subphylum of the Chordata containing the species with a true skull and vertebral column; the vertebrates.

cra·ni·ec·to·my (kra″ne-ek′tə-me) [*crani-* + *-ectomy*] excision of a part of the skull.

cra·nii (kra′ne-i) genitive of *cranium*.

crani(o)- [L. *cranium*, q.v.] a combining form denoting relationship to the cranium or skull.

cra·nio·acro·mi·al (kra″ne-o-ə-kro′me-əl) pertaining to the cranium and acromion.

cra·nio·au·ral (kra″ne-o-aw′rəl) pertaining to the cranium and the ear.

cra·nio·buc·cal (kra″ne-o-buk′əl) pertaining to the cranium and the mouth.

cra·nio·cau·dal (kra″ne-o-kaw′dal) cephalocaudal.

cra·nio·cele (kra′ne-o-sēl″) [*cranio-* + *-cele*[1]] encephalocele.

cra·nio·cer·e·bral (kra″ne-o-ser′ə-brəl) pertaining to the cranium and the cerebrum.

cra·nio·cer·vi·cal (kra″ne-o-sur′vĭ-kəl) pertaining to the cranium and the neck.

cra·nio·did·y·mus (kra″ne-o-did′ĭ-məs) dicephalus.

cra·nio·fa·cial (kra″ne-o-fa′shəl) pertaining to the cranium and the face.

cra·nio·fe·nes·tria (kra″ne-o-fə-nes′tre-ə) [*cranio-* + L. *fenestra* an opening] defective development of the calvaria of the fetal cranium, with areas in which no bone is formed. Cf. *craniolacunia*.

cra·ni·og·no·my (kra-ne-og′nə-me) [*cranio-* + Gr. *gnōmōn* an interpreter or judge] the study of the shape of the head.

cra·nio·graph (kra′ne-o-graf″) [*cranio-* + *-graph*] an instrument for outlining the skull.

cra·ni·og·ra·phy (kra″ne-og′rə-fe) the study of the skull by means of photographs, charts, etc.

cra·nio·la·cu·nia (kra″ne-o-lə-koo′ne-ə) [*cranio-* + *lacuna* + *-ia*] defective development of the calvaria of the fetal cranium with depressed areas on the inner surfaces of the bones. Cf. *craniofenestria.* Called also *lückenschädel.*

cra·ni·ol·o·gy (kra″ne-ol′ə-je) [*cranio-* + *-logy*] the scientific study of skulls.

cra·nio·ma·la·cia (kra″ne-o-mə-la′shə) [*cranio-* + *-malacia*] abnormal softness of the skull.

cra·nio·me·nin·go·cele (kra″ne-o-mə-ning′go-sēl) cranial meningocele.

cra·ni·om·e·ter (kra″ne-om′ə-tər) [*cranio-* + *-meter*] an instrument for use in craniometry.

cra·ni·om·e·try (kra″ne-om′ə-tre) [*cranio-* + *-metry*] the scientific measurement of the dimensions of the bones of the skull and face. craniomet′ric *adj*

cra·ni·op·a·gus (kra″ne-op′ə-gəs) [*cranio-* + *-pagus*] conjoined twins united by the heads; called also *cephalopagus.*

c. occipita′lis craniopagus in which fusion is in the occipital region.

c. parasi′ticus craniopagus in which a parasitic head is attached to the head of the larger, more nearly normal twin.

c. parieta′lis craniopagus in which fusion is in the parietal region.

cra·ni·op·a·thy (kra″ne-op′ə-the) [*cranio-* + *-pathy*] any disease of the skull.

metabolic c. a condition characterized by lesions of the calvarium with multiple metabolic changes and marked by headache, obesity, and visual disturbances.

cra·nio·pha·ryn·ge·al (kra″ne-o-fə-rin′je-əl) pertaining to the cranium and the pharynx.

cra·nio·pha·ryn·gi·o·ma (kra″ne-o-fə-rin″je-o′mə) a tumor arising from cell rests derived from the hypophysial stalk or Rathke pouch, frequently associated with increased intracranial pressure, and showing calcium deposits in the capsule or in the tumor proper. Deficits of pituitary hormones may also occur. Called also *craniopharyngeal duct tumor*, *Rathke* or *Rathke pouch tumor*, *suprasellar cyst*, and *pituitary adamantinoma* or *ameloblastoma.*

cra·nio·phore (kra′ne-o-for) [*cranio-* + *-phore*] a device for holding a skull during measurement of its diameters and angles.

cra·nio·plas·ty (kra′ne-o-plas″te) [*cranio-* + *-plasty*] any plastic operation on the skull; surgical correction of defects of the skull. **cranioplas′tic** *adj*

cra·nio·punc·ture (kra′ne-o-punk″chər) [*cranio-* + *puncture*] cephalocentesis.

cra·nio·ra·chis·chi·sis (kra″ne-o-rə-kis′kĭ-sis) [*cranio-* + *rhachis* + *schisis* fissure] a developmental anomaly consisting of fissure of the cranium and vertebral column; see *cranium bifidum* and *spina bifida.*

cra·nio·sa·cral (kra″ne-o-sa′krəl) 1. pertaining to the skull and the sacrum. 2. pertaining to the parasympathetic nerves.

cra·ni·os·chi·sis (kra″ne-os′kĭ-sis) cranium bifidum.

cra·nio·scle·ro·sis (kra″ne-o-sklə-ro′sis) [*cranio-* + *sclerosis*] thickening of the bones of the skull.

cra·nio·spi·nal (kra″ne-o-spi′nəl) pertaining to the cranium and the vertebral column.

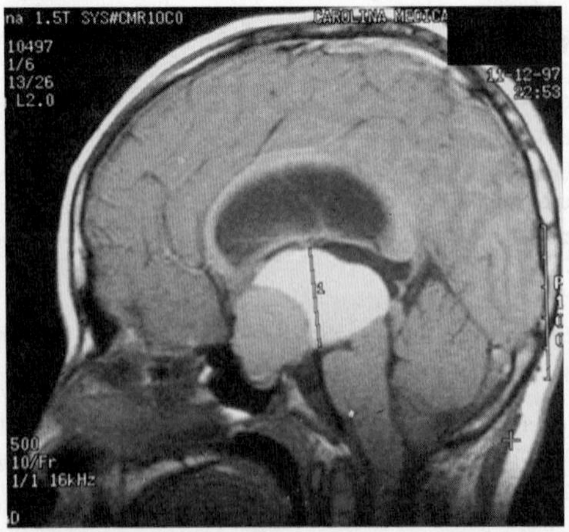

■ Craniopharyngioma; the heterogeneous densely enhancing suprasellar mass extends from the pituitary fossa into the hypothalamus and third ventricle.

cra·nio·ste·no·sis (kra″ne-o-stə-no′sis) [*cranio-* + *stenosis*] deformity of the skull caused by craniosynostosis, with consequent cessation of skull growth; the nature of the deformity depends on the sutures involved in the process.

cra·ni·os·to·sis (kra″ne-os-to′sis) craniosynostosis.

cra·nio·syn·os·to·sis (kra″ne-o-sin″os-to′sis) [*cranio-* + *syn-* + *ostosis*] premature closing of the sutures of the skull of an infant, causing deformities such as oxycephaly and scaphocephaly. Called also *craniostosis.*

cra·nio·ta·bes (kra″ne-o-ta′bēz) [*cranio-* + *tabes*] reduction in the mineralization of the skull, with abnormal softness of the bone, usually located in the occipital and parietal bones along the lambdoidal sutures.

cra·nio·tome (kra′ne-o-tōm″) [*cranio-* + *-tome*] an instrument for use in performing craniotomy.

cra·ni·ot·o·my (kra″ne-ot′ə-me) [*cranio-* + *-tomy*] any operation on the cranium; incision into the cranium.

bone flap c. craniotomy with a bone flap (see under *flap*).

cra·nio·try·pe·sis (kra″ne-o-trĭ-pe′sis) [*cranio-* + *trypesis*] trephination of the skull.

cra·nio·tym·pan·ic (kra″ne-o-tim-pan′ik) pertaining to the skull and the tympanum.

cra·ni·um (kra′ne-əm) gen. *cra′nii* pl. *cra′nia* [L., from Gr. *kranion* the upper part of the head] [TA] the large round superior part of the skull, enclosing the brain and made up of the cranial bones; see *ossa cranii*, under *os.*

c. bi′fidum incomplete formation of the calvaria, with defective development of the brain and often an encephalocele or meningocele. Called also *cranioschisis.*

c. bi′fidum occul′tum congenital cleft of the calvaria without associated abnormality of the brain or meninges, detectable only radiographically.

cerebral c., c. cerebra′le those portions of the bones of the head that contribute to the calvaria.

visceral c. viscerocranium.

crap·u·lent (krap′u-lənt) [L. *crapulentus* drunken] due to excess in eating or drinking; see *hyperalimentation.*

crap·u·lous (krap′u-ləs) crapulent.

-crasia [Gr. *krasis* mixture] a combining form denoting a mixture of different elements.

cras·sa·men·tum (kras″ə-men′təm) [L.] clot (def. 1).

Crast. [L.] cras′tinus (for tomorrow).

Cra·tae·gus (krə-te′gəs) [L., from Gr. *krataigos*] a genus of usually thorny shrubs or trees having shiny, often lobed, leaves, pink or white flowers, and small red fruits. *C. laeviga′ta*, *C. mono′gyna*, and *C. fo′lium* are used medicinally.

cra·ter (kra′tər) a circular area of depression surrounded by an elevated margin.

cra·ter·i·form (kra-ter′ĭ-form) [*crater* + *form*] depressed or hollowed, like a bowl.

cra·ter·iza·tion (kra″tər-ĭ-za′shən) the operation of excising a crater-like piece from a bone.

cra·vat (krə-vaht′) [Fr. *cravate*] a bandage made by folding a triangular piece of cloth from its apex toward the base.

craw (kraw) crop.

craz·ing (kra′zing) the appearance of minute cracks on the surface of artificial or natural teeth, porcelain, and resin denture bases.

cream (krēm) 1. the fatty part of milk from which butter is prepared, or a fluid mixture of similar consistency. 2. in pharmaceutical preparations, a semisolid dosage form being either an emulsion of oil and water or an aqueous microcrystalline dispersion of a long-chain fatty acid or alcohol.

cold c. a preparation of cetyl esters wax, white wax, mineral oil, sodium borate, and purified water, similar to rose water ointment but not subject to rancidity; used as a water-in-oil emulsion ointment base.

leukocytic c. buffy coat.

crease (krēs) a line or slight linear depression, such as a shallow skin furrow.

ear lobe c. a diagonal crease in the ear lobe associated with aging; when present in younger persons it may be a sign of coronary artery disease.

flexion c. any of the normal permanent skin furrows on flexor surfaces that accommodate flexion of a movable joint by separating folds of tissue.

inframammary c. see under *fold.*

palmar c. any of the flexion creases occurring on the palm. In certain congenital anomalies, there is only a single one; see *simian c.*

simian c. a single transverse palmar crease formed by fusion of the usual proximal and distal creases; frequently seen in congenital disorders

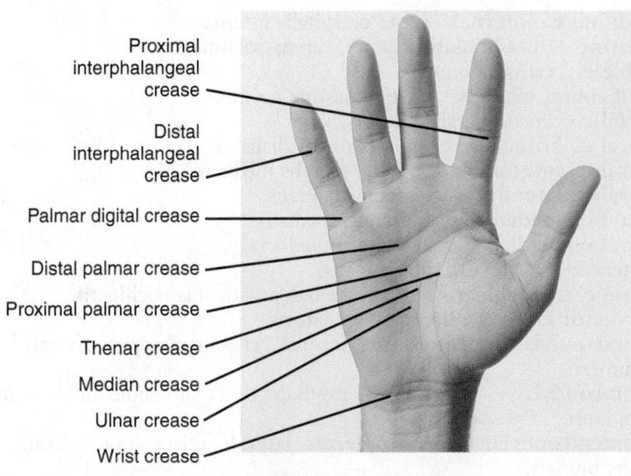

■ Flexion creases of the palmar surface of the hand and wrist.

such as Down syndrome and rarely in normal persons; called also *simian line.*

cre•at•i•nase (kre-at′ĭ-nās) [EC 3.5.3.3] an amidohydrolase that catalyzes the conversion of creatine to sarcosine and urea.

cre•a•tine (kre′ə-tin) [Gr. *kreas* flesh] an amino acid formed by methylation of guanidinoacetic acid, found in vertebrate tissues, particularly in muscle. Phosphorylated creatine (see *phosphocreatine*) is an important storage form of high energy phosphate, the energy source for muscle contraction.

c. **phosphate** phosphocreatine.

cre•a•tine ki•nase (CK) (kre′ə-tin ki′nās) [EC 2.7.3.2] an Mg^{2+}-activated enzyme of the transferase class that catalyzes the phosphorylation of creatine by ATP to form phosphocreatine. The reaction effectively stores the energy of ATP as phosphocreatine in muscle and brain tissue and holds the muscle concentration of ATP nearly constant during the initiation of exercise. It occurs as three isoenzymes, each having two components composed of M (muscle) and of B (brain) subunits. CK_1 (BB) is found primarily in brain, CK_2 (MB) primarily in cardiac muscle, and CK_3 (MM) primarily in skeletal muscle. Differential determination of isoenzymes is useful for clinical diagnoses.

cre•a•tin•emia (kre″ə-tĭ-ne′me-ə) excess of creatine in the blood.

cre•a•tine phos•pho•ki•nase (CPK) (kre′ə-tin fos″fo-ki′nāse) creatine kinase.

cre•a•ti•ni•nase (kre-at′ĭ-nin-ās) [EC 3.5.2.10] an amidohydrolase that catalyzes the conversion of creatinine to creatine.

cre•at•i•nine (kre-at′ĭ-nin) 1. the cyclic anhydride of creatine, produced as the final product of decomposition of phosphocreatine. It is excreted in the urine; measurements of excretion rates are used as diagnostic indicators of kidney function (see *creatinine clearance,* under *clearance*) and muscle mass and can be used to simplify other clinical assays. 2. [NF] a preparation of creatinine, used as a bulking agent in freeze-drying.

cre•a•tin•uria (kre″ə-tin-u′reə) increased concentration of creatine in the urine, as seen in muscular dystrophy, poliomyelitis, and various other conditions.

creat(o)- [Gr. *kreas,* gen. *kreatos* flesh] a combining form denoting relationship to meat or flesh.

cre•a•tor•rhea (kre″ə-to-re′ə) [*creato-* + *-rrhea*] the presence of undigested muscle fibers in the feces.

crèche (kresh) [Fr.] a day nursery for infants.

Cre•dé method (maneuver) (krə-da′) [Karl Sigmund Franz *Credé,* German gynecologist, 1819–1892] see under *method.*

creep (krēp) 1. a slow flow over time that occurs with materials under stress below their elastic limits, often due to warm temperature; it may occur with dental materials in the mouth. 2. the time-dependent strain in a tissue or body as a result of application and maintenance of a stress at a set level.

CREG cross-reactive group (of HLA antigens).

cre•mas•ter (kre-mas′tər) [L., from Gr. *kremasthai* to suspend] musculus cremaster.

internal c. of Henle fibers of the gubernaculum testis, inserted in elements of the fetal spermatic cord.

crem•as•ter•ic (krem″as-ter′ik) pertaining to the musculus cremaster.

cre•ma•tion (kre-ma′shən) [L. *crematio* a burning] the burning or incineration of dead bodies.

cre•ma•to•ri•um (kre″mə-tor′e-əm) an establishment for the burning of dead bodies.

Crem•o•phor (krem′o-for) trademark for a number of polyoxyl compounds used as lipid vehicles for solubilizing and emulsifying drugs.

cre•na (kre′nə) pl. *cre′nae* [L. "notch," from *crenare* to split] a notch or cleft.

c. **ana′lis** [TA] anal cleft: the cleft between the buttocks on which the anus opens. Called also *intergluteal, clunial, gluteal,* or *natal cleft, c. ani* or *c. interglutealis* [TA alternatives], and *rima ani.*

c. **a′ni,** c. **interglutea′lis** TA alternatives for *c. analis.*

cre•nate (kre′nāt) [L. *crenatus*] crenated.

cre•nat•ed (kre′nāt-əd) scalloped or notched; see *crenation.*

cre•na•tion (kre-na′shən) 1. the formation of abnormal notching in the edge of an erythrocyte; see *burr cell,* under *cell.* 2. the notched appearance of an erythrocyte caused by its shrinkage after suspension in a hypertonic solution. Cf. *echinosis.* Called also *crenulation.*

cren•il•a•brin (kren-il-a′brin) a protamine obtained from the sperm of the cunner (fish).

cre•no•cyte (kre′no-sīt) burr cell.

cre•no•cy•to•sis (kre″no-si-to′sis) the presence of burr cells (crenocytes) in the blood; called also *echinosis.*

Cre•no•so•ma (kre″no-so′mə) a genus of nematodes of the family Crenosomatidae. *C. vul′pis* is a lungworm of dogs and other carnivores.

Cre•no•so•mat•i•dae (kre″no-so-mat′ĭ-de) a family of nematodes that includes the genera *Crenosoma* and *Troglostrongylus.* Several species infect the lungs or bronchioles of dogs or cats.

cren•u•la•tion (kren″u-la′shən) crenation.

Cre•o•la bodies (kre-o′lə) [*Creola,* first name of a patient in whom they were observed] see under *body.*

Cre•on (kre′on) trademark for a preparation of pancrelipase.

cre•oph•a•gism (kre-of′ə-jiz-əm) [Gr. *kreas* flesh + *phagein* to eat] the eating of flesh (meat); see also *carnivore.*

cre•oph•a•gy (kre-of′ə-je) creophagism.

cre•o•sol (kre′o-sol) [*creosote* + L. *oleum* oil] a colorless oily liquid; one of the active constituents of creosote.

cre•o•sote (kre′o-sōt) an oily liquid obtained by distillation from coal tar, wood tar, or the resin from the creosote bush.

coal tar c. creosote obtained by high temperature carbonization of bituminous coal; it is a brown to black, oily liquid, a mixture of aromatic hydrocarbons, tar acids, and tar bases; mainly used as a wood preservative. It is toxic by skin contact, ingestion, or inhalation, and coal tar is a human carcinogen. Animals may suffer skin irritation or poisoning if they chew on recently treated wood.

wood c. creosote obtained by distilling wood tar, mainly from beech trees *(Fagus sylvatica);* it is a colorless to yellowish, oily, refractive liquid composed mainly of the phenol derivatives guaiacol and creosol. It was formerly used as an expectorant and external antiseptic but is now rarely used in the United States.

crep•i•tant (krep′ĭ-tənt) [L. *crepitare* to rattle or crackle] rattling or crackling. See under *rale.*

crep•i•ta•tion (krep″ĭ-ta′shən) 1. a sound like that made by throwing salt into a fire. See *crepitant rale,* under *rale.* 2. the noise made by rubbing together the ends of a fractured bone.

crep•i•tus (krep′ĭ-təs) [L.] 1. the discharge of flatus from the bowels. 2. crepitation. 3. crepitant rale.

articular c. joint c.

bony c. the crackling sound produced by the rubbing together of fragments of fractured bone.

false c. joint c.

c. **in′dux** a crepitant rale, or crackling sound, heard in pneumonia at the beginning of the process of solidification of the lung.

joint c. the grating sensation caused by the rubbing together of the dry synovial surfaces of joints; called also *articular c.*

c. **re′dux** crepitus heard in the resolving stage of pneumonia.

silken c. a sensation as of two pieces of silk rubbed between the fingers, felt on moving a joint affected with hydrarthrosis.

-crescence [L. *crescere* to grow] a word termination denoting relationship to growth.

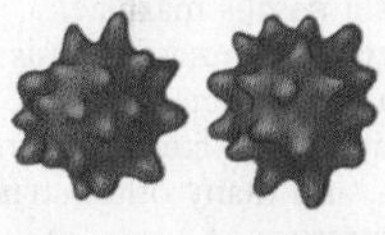

■ Crenated erythrocytes.

cres•cent (kres'ənt) [L. *crescens*] 1. shaped like a new moon. 2. something with this shape.

articular c. a crescent-shaped articular fibrocartilage.

epithelial c. a more or less crescentic mass of cells found between the tuft of a glomerulus and the inside of Bowman capsule in rapidly progressive glomerulonephritis.

Giannuzzi c's crescent-shaped patches of serous cells surrounding the mucous tubules in seromucous glands, and formed by the outnumbered albuminous cells pushed to the blind ends of the terminal portions or into saccular outpocketings. Called also *Heidenhain demilunes; Giannuzzi bodies* or *demilunes;* and *semilunar bodies.*

glomerular c. epithelial c.

gray c. an area on some amphibian eggs from which pigment retreats; it is dorsal and opposite to the point of sperm entry, giving the first visible sign of the dorsoventral axis.

malarial c's the gametocytes of *Plasmodium falciparum;* they may be male (microgametocytes) or female (macrogametocytes).

myopic c. a crescentic posterior staphyloma in the fundus of the eye in myopia.

sublingual c. the crescent-shaped area on the floor of the mouth, formed by the lingual wall of the mandible and the adjacent part of the floor of the mouth.

cres•cen•tic (krə-sen'tik) resembling a crescent.

cre•sol (kre'sol) a toxic liquid obtained from coal tar, containing phenol and ranging from colorless to yellow, brown, or pink. it is a corrosive mixture of three isomeric forms and is a more powerful disinfectant and antiseptic than phenol. Its primary use is for sterilizing items such as instruments, dishes, and utensils. Called also *cresylic acid* and *tricresol.*

cre•sol•phtha•lein (kre″sol-thal'ēn) an acid-base indicator that is colorless at pH 7.2 and red at 8.8.

crest (krest) [L. *crista*] a projection or projecting structure, or ridge, especially one surmounting a bone or its border; see also *crista* and *ridge.*

acoustic c. crista ampullaris.

alveolar c. the margin of compact bone on the coronal edge of a dental alveolus.

ampullar c., ampullary c. crista ampullaris.

anterior c. of tibia margo anterior tibiae.

arcuate c. of arytenoid cartilage crista arcuata cartilaginis arytenoideae.

basilar c. of cochlear duct crista basilaris ductus cochlearis.

c. of body of rib crista costae.

buccinator c. a ridge running from the base of the coronoid process of the mandible to a point near the last molar tooth, giving attachment to the buccinator muscle.

conchal c. of body of maxilla, conchal c. of maxilla crista conchalis corporis maxillae.

conchal c. of palatine bone crista conchalis ossis palatini.

dental c. the maxillary ridge passing along the alveolar processes of the fetal maxillary bones.

ethmoidal c. of maxilla crista ethmoidalis maxillae.

ethmoidal c. of palatine bone crista ethmoidalis ossis palatini.

frontal c., frontal c., internal crista frontalis.

gingival c. the coronal border of the gingiva.

gluteal c. tuberositas glutea.

c. of greater tubercle crista tuberculi majoris.

c. of head of rib crista capitis costae.

iliac c., c. of ilium crista iliaca.

infratemporal c. crista infratemporalis.

inguinal c. a prominence on the inguinal body wall in the embryo, participating in the formation of the gubernaculum testis.

interosseous c. of fibula margo interosseus fibulae.

interosseous c. of radius margo interosseus radii.

interosseous c. of tibia margo interosseus tibiae.

interosseous c. of ulna margo interosseus ulnae.

intertrochanteric c. crista intertrochanterica.

interureteric c. plica interureterica.

lacrimal c., anterior crista lacrimalis anterior.

lacrimal c., posterior crista lacrimalis posterior.

c. of lesser tubercle crista tuberculi minoris.

mammary c. see under *ridge.*

medial c. of fibula crista medialis fibulae.

mitochondrial c's see under *crista.*

c's of nail matrix cristae matricis unguis.

nasal c. of maxilla crista nasalis maxillae.

nasal c. of palatine bone crista nasalis ossis palatini.

c. of neck of rib crista colli costae.

neural c. a cellular band dorsolateral to the neural tube that gives origin to the spinal ganglia, and many other structures.

obturator c. crista obturatoria.

occipital c., external crista occipitalis externa.

occipital c., internal crista occipitalis interna.

palatine c., c. of palatine bone crista palatina.

pubic c. crista pubica.

c. of round window crista fenestrae cochleae.

sacral c. crista sacralis mediana.

sacral c., articular crista sacralis medialis.

sacral c., intermediate crista sacralis medialis.

sacral c., lateral crista sacralis lateralis.

sacral c., medial crista sacralis medialis.

sacral c., median crista sacralis mediana.

sphenoidal c. crista sphenoidalis.

spiral c. of cochlear duct crista basilaris ductus cochlearis.

supinator c. crista musculi supinatoris.

supracondylar c. of humerus, lateral crista supraepicondylaris lateralis humeri.

supracondylar c. of humerus, medial crista supraepicondylaris medialis humeri.

supraepicondylar c. of humerus, lateral crista supraepicondylaris lateralis humeri.

supraepicondylar c. of humerus, medial crista supraepicondylaris medialis humeri.

supramastoid c. crista supramastoidea.

supraventricular c. crista supraventricularis.

temporal c. of mandible crista temporalis mandibulae.

terminal c. of right atrium crista terminalis atrii dextri.

tibial c. margo anterior tibiae.

transverse c. of internal acoustic meatus crista transversa meatus acustici interni.

trigeminal c. the embryonic cell mass from which the trigeminal ganglion develops.

urethral c. of female urethra crista urethralis urethrae femininae.

urethral c. of male urethra crista urethralis urethrae masculinae.

vertical c. of internal acoustic meatus crista verticalis meatus acustici interni.

vestibular c. crista vestibuli.

vomerine c. of choana crista choanalis vomeris.

cres•to•my•cin sul•fate (kres-to-mi'sin) paromomycin sulfate.

Cres•tor (kres'tor) trademark for a preparation of rosuvastatin calcium.

cre•syl•ic ac•id (kre-sil'ik) cresol.

cre•tin•ism (kre'tin-iz-əm) a chronic condition due to congenital severe hypothyroidism; manifestations begin in late infancy and include arrested physical development (dwarfism), mental retardation, dystrophy of the bones and soft parts, and lowered basal metabolism.

athyreotic c., athyrotic c. cretinism due to thyroid aplasia or destruction of the thyroid of the fetus in utero; called also *sporadic nongoitrous c.*

endemic c. a type of cretinism seen in regions of severe endemic goiter; the two primary types are *neurologic cretinism* and *myxedematous cretinism.*

myxedematous c. an uncommon type of endemic cretinism with delayed growth of long bones, myxedema, and sometimes goiter but with fewer neurologic problems than are seen in neurologic cretinism.

neurologic c. the usual kind of endemic cretinism, characterized by delayed growth of long bones, neurologic complications such as deafness, mental retardation, and spasticity, sometimes with goiter, but usually without myxedema. Cf. *myxedematous c.*

spontaneous c., sporadic c. cretinism in a person not descended from cretins, and who has not lived in a region where goiter is endemic.

sporadic goitrous c. a genetically determined condition in which enlargement of the thyroid gland is associated with deficient biosynthesis of and a consequently reduced supply of circulating thyroid hormone.

sporadic nongoitrous c. athyrotic c.

cre•tin•is•tic (kre″tin-is'tik) cretinous.

cre•tin•oid (kre'tin-oid) resembling or suggestive of cretinism.

cre•tin•ous (kre'tin-əs) affected with cretinism.

Creutz•feldt-Ja•kob disease (kroits'felt yah'kōb) [Hans Gerhard *Creutzfeldt*, German psychiatrist, 1885–1964; Alfons Maria *Jakob*, German psychiatrist, 1884–1931] see under *disease.*

crev•ice (krev'is) [Fr. *crever* to split] fissure (def. 2).

gingival c. a shallow trough or fissure surrounding the anatomic crown of a tooth; considered by some authorities to be the same as the *gingival sulcus* and by others to be two separate and distinct entities. Called also *subgingival space.*

cre•vic•u•lar (krə-vik'u-lər) pertaining to a crevice, especially the gingival crevice.

CRF chronic renal failure.

CRH corticotropin-releasing hormone.

crib (krib) 1. any racklike structure. 2. a removable anchorage from an orthodontic appliance. 3. a habit-breaking orthodontic appliance.

clinical c. a crib in which an infant is placed for observation.
Jackson c. see under *appliance*.

crib·bing (krib′ing) a nervous habit of some horses consisting of grasping the manger or another object with the incisor teeth, arching the neck and making other peculiar head movements, and swallowing quantities of air; called also *crib-biting* and *windsucking*.

crib-bit·ing (krib′bīt-ing) cribbing.

crib·ral (krib′rəl) pertaining to a sievelike structure.

crib·rate (krib′rāt) cribriform.

crib·ra·tion (krib-ra′shən) 1. the quality of being cribrate. 2. the process or act of sifting or passing through a sieve, as a drug.

crib·ri·form (krib′rĭ-form) [L. *cribrum* sieve + *form*] perforated with small holes, like a sieve.

Cri·ce·tu·lus (kri-se′tu-ləs) a genus of rodents of the family Muridae, one of several genera of hamsters. *C. gri′seus* is the Chinese hamster.

Cri·ce·tus (kri-se′təs) a genus of rodents of the family Muridae, one of several genera of hamsters. *C. crice′tus* is the European hamster.

Crich·ton-Browne sign (kri′tən-broun′) [Sir James *Crichton-Browne*, Scottish physician, 1840–1938] see under *sign*.

cri·co·ar·y·te·noid (kri″ko-ahr″ĭ-te′noid) pertaining to or extending between the cricoid and arytenoid cartilages.

cri·coid (kri′koid) [Gr. *krikos* ring + *-oid*] 1. resembling a ring; ring-shaped. 2. the cricoid cartilage (cartilago cricoidea [TA]).

cri·coi·dec·to·my (kri″koi-dek′tə-me) excision of the cricoid cartilage.

cri·coi·dyn·ia (kri″koi-din′e-ə) [Gr. *krikos* ring + *-odynia*] pain in the cricoid cartilage.

cri·co·pha·ryn·ge·al (kri″ko-fə-rin′je-əl) pertaining to the cricoid cartilage and the pharynx.

cri·co·thy·roid (kri-ko-thi′roid) pertaining to or connecting the cricoid and thyroid cartilages.

cri·co·thy·roi·dot·o·my (kri″ko-thi″roi-dot′ə-me) cricothyrotomy.

cri·co·thy·rot·o·my (kri″ko-thi-rot′ə-me) tracheotomy involving incision through the skin and cricothyroid membrane to secure a patent airway for emergency relief of upper airway obstruction. Called also *inferior laryngotomy*, *intercricothyrotomy*, and *thyrocricotomy*.

cri·cot·o·my (kri-kot′ə-me) [Gr. *krikos* ring + *-tomy*] incision of the cricoid cartilage.

cri·co·tra·che·ot·o·my (kri″ko-tra″ke-ot′ə-me) tracheotomy with incision of the cricoid cartilage.

cri du chat (kre doo shah′) [Fr. "cat's cry"] see under *syndrome*.

Crig·ler-Naj·jar syndrome (krig′lər nah′jahr) [John Fielding *Crigler*, Jr., American pediatrician, born 1919; Victor Assad *Najjar*, Lebanese-born American microbiologist, 1914–2002] see under *syndrome*.

crim·i·nol·o·gy (krim″ĭ-nol′ə-je) [L. *crimen* crime + *-logy*] the scientific study of crime and criminals.

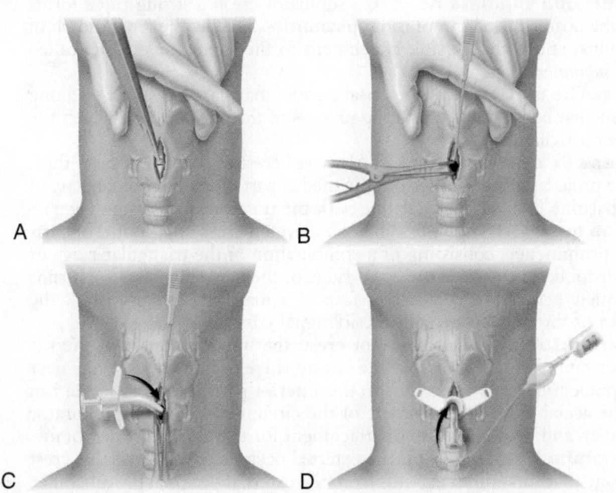

■ Cricothyrotomy. After immobilization of the larynx and creation of a vertical midline skin incision, the cricothyroid membrane is incised horizontally *(A)*. Upward traction is made with a traction hook and a bladed dilator is used to expand the tracheal incision vertically *(B)*. The tube is inserted through the blades of the dilator into the trachea *(C)*. The obturator is removed, the inner cannula is replaced, and the tube is inflated *(D)*.

cri·nis (kri′nis) pl. *cri′nes* [L.] hair.

Cri·none (crī′nōn) trademark for a preparation of progesterone.

crin·oph·a·gy (krin-of′ə-je) [Gr. *krinein* to separate + *-phagy*] fusion of a secretory granule with a lysosome, followed by digestion of its contents.

Cri·num (kri′nəm) a genus of plants of the family Amaryllidaceae. *C. asia′ticum* is an Indian species whose root has properties like those of squill.

cris·an·tas·pase (kris″ən-tas′pās) BAN for asparaginase derived from *Pectobacterium carotovorum (Erwinia carotovora)* for use as an antineoplastic agent.

cri·sis (kri′sis) pl. *cri′ses* [L., from Gr. *krisis*] 1. the turning point of a disease for better or worse; especially, a sudden change, usually for the better, in the course of an acute disease. A disease terminates by crisis when recovery is indicated by a sudden and definite decrease in the intensity of the symptoms. Cf. *lysis* (def. 4). 2. a sudden paroxysmal intensification of symptoms in the course of a disease.

addisonian c., adrenal c. acute onset of adrenocortical insufficiency or sudden worsening of Addison disease; manifestations include anorexia, vomiting, abdominal pain, apathy, confusion, extreme weakness, renal loss of sodium and water, and hypotension progressing to shock and, if untreated, death. Called also *acute adrenocortical insufficiency* and *Bernard-Sergent syndrome*.
anaphylactoid c. see under *reaction*.
aplastic c. the most common type of sickle cell crisis, a transient condition marked by sudden disappearance of erythroblasts from the bone marrow; it develops under various circumstances, including certain hemolytic states and infections.
blast c. a sudden, severe transformation of chronic myelogenous leukemia to a more aggressive course; the proportion of blast cells increases rapidly, and the clinical picture resembles that in acute myelogenous leukemia.
carcinoid c. a severe episodic attack of the carcinoid syndrome.
catathymic c. an isolated, nonrepetitive act of violence that develops as a result of intolerable tension.
celiac c. an attack of severe watery diarrhea and vomiting producing dehydration and acidosis, seen in celiac disease, particularly the infantile form.
cholinergic c. muscular weakness resulting from depolarization block due to overdosage of anticholinesterase agents used for myasthenia gravis; similar to but different from myasthenic crisis.
deglobulinization c. a condition observed in congenital spherocytic anemia, characterized clinically by the acute onset of fever, abdominal pain, and vomiting, associated with reticulocytopenia, leukopenia, thrombocytopenia, and erythroblastopenia.
Dietl c. a sudden severe attack of stomach and kidney pain, with chills, fever, nausea, vomiting, and then general collapse, due to obstruction of ureters.
false c. pseudocrisis.
febrile c. an attack of fever and chills, with sweating.
genital c. of newborn hyperplasia of the breasts of an infant, with estrinization of the vaginal mucosa and sometimes vaginal bleeding, under the influence of transplacentally acquired estrogens.
glaucomatocyclitic c. a rare, recurrent, unilateral form of secondary open-angle glaucoma, lasting one to two weeks, and rarely producing permanent damage to the optic disk or to the outflow facility. It is characterized by high intraocular pressure and marked depression of outflow facility, with minimal inflammatory signs and symptoms.
hemolytic c. a rare type of sickle cell crisis in which there is acute red cell destruction leading to jaundice.
hypertensive c. dangerously high blood pressure of acute onset.
identity c. a period in the psychosocial development of an individual, generally occurring during adolescence, usually manifested by a loss of the sense of the sameness and historical continuity of one's self, confusion over values, or an inability to accept the role the individual perceives as being expected of him by society.
megaloblastic c. megaloblastic anemia due to deficiency of folic acid, seen in some patients with hereditary spherocytosis after an aplastic crisis or during pregnancy.
myasthenic c. sudden development of dyspnea requiring respiratory support in myasthenia gravis; the crisis is usually transient, lasts several days, and is accompanied by fever.
nefast c. the peculiar onset of severe and unaccountable symptoms in experimental icterogenous spirochetosis.
ocular c. a sudden attack of intense pain in the eyes, with lacrimation, photophobia, and other symptoms.
oculogyric c. a crisis occurring in epidemic encephalitis, postencephalitic parkinsonism, or secondary to use of antipsychotic agents; the eyeballs become fixed in one position, typically upwardly rotated, for minutes or hours.
parkinsonian c. a condition sometimes observed in parkinsonism, superficially resembling akinetic mutism or coma vigil, the patient lying stiff and motionless, and making no spontaneous communication.
salt depletion c., salt-losing c. see under *syndrome*.

scleroderma renal c. acute renal failure with moderate to severe hypertension occurring in patients with scleroderma; the precise cause is unknown.
sickle cell c. a broad term used to describe several different acute conditions occurring with sickle cell disease, including aplastic crisis, hemolytic crisis, and vaso-occlusive crisis.
tabetic c. any of numerous types of painful paroxysms with functional disturbance occurring in the course of tabes dorsalis.
thyroid c., thyrotoxic c. a sudden and dangerous increase of the symptoms of thyrotoxicosis. Called also *thyroid* or *thyrotoxic storm.*
vasoocclusive c. a type of sickle cell crisis in which there is severe pain due to infarctions, which may be in the bones, joints, lungs, liver, spleen, kidney, eye, or central nervous system.

cris·pa·tion (kris-pa′shən) [L. *crispare* to curl] slight convulsive or spasmodic muscular contractions producing a creeping sensation.

cris·ta (kris′tə) gen. and pl. *cris′tae* [L.] 1. [TA] a projection or projecting structure, or ridge, especially one surmounting a bone or its border; called also *crest* and *ridge.* 2. see *mitochondrial cristae.*

Crista

Descriptions are given on TA terms, and include anglicized names of specific structures.

c. ampulla′ris [TA] ampullary crest: the most prominent part of a localized thickening of the membrane that lines the ampullae of the semicircular ducts, covered with neuroepithelium containing endings of the vestibular nerve; called also *acoustic crest.*
c. arcua′ta cartila′ginis arytenoi′deae [TA] arcuate crest of arytenoid cartilage: a ridge on the external surface of the arytenoid cartilage between the triangular pit and the oblong pit.
c. basila′ris duc′tus cochlea′ris [TA] basilar crest of cochlear duct: the triangular eminence on the spiral ligament of the cochlea, providing a site of attachment for the basilar membrane. Called also *c. spiralis ductus cochlearis* [TA alternative].
c. ca′pitis cos′tae [TA] crest of head of rib: a horizontal crest dividing the articular surface of the head of the rib into two facets, for articulation with the depression on the bodies of two adjacent vertebrae.
c. choana′lis vo′meris [TA] vomerine crest of choana: the concave crest on the posterior surface of the vomer, forming the medial border that separates the two choanae.
c. col′li cos′tae [TA] crest of neck of rib: a crest on the superior border of the neck of a rib, giving attachment to the anterior costotransverse ligament.
c. concha′lis cor′poris maxil′lae [TA] conchal crest of body of maxilla: an oblique ridge on the nasal surface of the body of the maxilla, just anterior to the lacrimal sulcus, which articulates with the inferior nasal concha.
c. concha′lis os′sis palati′ni [TA] conchal crest of palatine bone: a sharp transverse ridge, near the posterior edge of the palatine bone, which articulates with the inferior concha.
c. cos′tae [TA] crest of body of rib: the inferior margin of the body of a rib.
cris′tae cu′tis [TA] dermal ridges: ridges of the skin produced by the projecting papillae of the dermis on the palm or sole, such as to produce a fingerprint characteristic of the individual. Called also *skin* or *fingerprint ridges.*
c. divi′dens limbus foraminis ovalis.
c. ethmoida′lis maxil′lae [TA] ethmoidal crest of maxilla: a low, oblique ridge on the medial surface of the frontal process of the maxilla, which articulates with the middle nasal concha.
c. ethmoida′lis os′sis palati′ni [TA] ethmoidal crest of palatine bone: a ridge near the upper end of the medial surface of the palatine bone, which articulates with the middle concha.

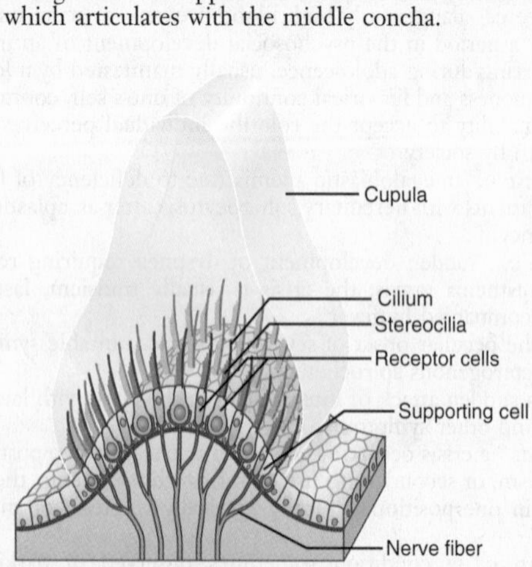

■ Crista ampullaris (ampullary crest) section.

c. fenes′trae coch′leae [TA] crest of round window: the ledge of bone that overhangs the round (cochlear) window of the middle ear.
c. fronta′lis [TA] frontal crest: a median ridge on the internal surface of the frontal bone, extending superiorly from the foramen cecum to unite with the sulcus for the superior sagittal sinus.
c. gal′li [TA] a thick triangular process projecting superiorly from the cribriform plate of the ethmoid bone; the falx cerebri attaches to it.
c. ili′aca [TA] iliac crest: the thickened, expanded upper border of the ilium; called also *crest of ilium.*
c. infratempora′lis [TA] infratemporal crest: a crest separating the temporal surface of the greater wing of the sphenoid bone into a superior temporal portion and an inferior infratemporal portion.
c. intertrochante′rica [TA] intertrochanteric crest: a prominent ridge running obliquely downward and medialward from the summit of the greater trochanter on the posterior surface of the neck of the femur to the lesser trochanter; called also *intertrochanteric ridge* and *posterior intertrochanteric line.*
c. lacrima′lis ante′rior [TA] anterior lacrimal crest: the lateral margin of the groove on the posterior border of the frontal process of the maxilla.
c. lacrima′lis poste′rior [TA] posterior lacrimal crest: a vertical ridge dividing the lateral or orbital surface of the lacrimal bone into two parts, and forming one margin of the fossa for the lacrimal sac.
c. margina′lis [TA] marginal ridge: a type of elevated, convex crest on a tooth; on posterior teeth they form the mesial and distal borders of the occlusal surface, and on anterior teeth they are toward the lingual side.
cris′tae ma′tricis un′guis crests of nail matrix: the vascular longitudinal ridges in the nail matrix.
c. media′lis fi′bulae [TA] medial crest of fibula: the long crest on the posterior surface of the body of the fibula, which separates the origin of the tibialis posterior muscle from that of the flexor hallucis longus muscle.
mitochondrial cristae, cris′tae mitochondria′les numerous narrow, transverse infoldings of the inner membrane of a mitochondrion.
c. mus′culi supinato′ris [TA] supinator crest: a strong ridge forming the posterior margin of the supinator fossa below the radial notch of the ulna, and with it giving attachment to the supinator muscle; called also *supinator ridge.*
c. nasa′lis maxil′lae [TA] nasal crest of maxilla: a ridge, raised along the medial border of the palatine process of the maxilla, with which the vomer articulates.
c. nasa′lis os′sis palati′ni [TA] nasal crest of palatine bone: a thick ridge projecting superiorly from the medial part of the horizontal plate of the palatine bone and articulating with the posterior part of the vomer.
c. obli′qua [TA] oblique ridge: an elevated crest on a tooth, of variable prominence, consisting of a combination of the triangular ridge of the distobuccal cusp and the distal ridge of the mesiolingual cusp; it runs obliquely across the occlusal surface of a maxillary molar to link the apices of the distobuccal and mesiolingual cusps.
c. obturato′ria [TA] obturator crest: the inferior border of the superior ramus of the pubic bone, a strong ridge of bone that begins near the pubic tubercle and extends to the anterior part of the gap in the rim of the acetabulum; it forms part of the circumference of the obturator foramen and provides a site of attachment for the obturator membrane.
c. occipita′lis exter′na [TA] external occipital crest: a variable crest of bone that sometimes extends from the external occipital protuberance toward the foramen magnum; called also *median* or *middle nuchal line.*
c. occipita′lis inter′na [TA] internal occipital crest: a median ridge on the internal surface of the occipital bone extending from the midpoint of the cruciform eminence toward the foramen magnum.

Crista *Continued*

c. palati′na os′sis palati′ni [TA] palatine crest: a transverse crest often seen on the inferior surface of the horizontal plate of the palatine bone a short distance anterior to the posterior border.
c. palatopharyn′gea [TA] palatopharyngeal ridge: a horizontal ridge that appears on the posterior wall of the pharynx during swallowing, produced by contraction of the palatopharyngeal sphincter; it also occurs during speech in persons with cleft palate. Called also *pharyngeal ridge* and *Passavant bar, cushion, pad,* or *ridge.*
c. pu′bica [TA] pubic crest: the thick, rough, anterior border of the body of the pubic bone.
c. sacra′lis latera′lis [TA] lateral sacral crest: either of two series of tubercles lateral to the dorsal sacral foramina, representing the transverse processes of the sacral vertebrae.
c. sacra′lis media′lis [TA] medial sacral crest: either of two indefinite crests just medial to the posterior sacral foramina, formed by fusion of the articular processes of the sacral vertebrae; called also *intermediate sacral crest.*
c. sacra′lis media′na [TA] median sacral crest: a median ridge on the dorsal surface of the sacrum, formed by the remnants of the spinous processes of the upper four sacral vertebrae.
c. sphenoida′lis [TA] sphenoidal crest: a median ridge on the anterior surface of the body of the sphenoid bone, articulating with the perpendicular plate of the ethmoid.
c. spira′lis duc′tus cochlea′ris TA alternative for *c. basilaris ductus cochlearis.*
c. supracondyla′ris latera′lis hu′meri TA alternative for *c. supraepicondylaris lateralis humeri.*
c. supracondyla′ris media′lis hu′meri TA alternative for *c. supraepicondylaris medialis humeri.*
c. supraepicondyla′ris latera′lis hu′meri [TA] lateral supraepicondylar ridge of humerus: a prominent curved ridge on the lateral surface of the humerus, giving attachment in front to the brachioradialis and extensor carpi radialis longus muscles; called also *c. supracondylaris lateralis humeri* [TA alternative] and *lateral supracondylar ridge of humerus.*
c. supraepicondyla′ris media′lis hu′meri [TA] medial supraepicondylar ridge of humerus: a prominent, curved ridge on the medial surface of the humerus, giving attachment to the brachialis muscle in front and to the medial head of the triceps behind; called also *c. supracondylaris medialis humeri* [TA alternative] and *medial supracondylar ridge of humerus.*
c. supramastoi′dea [TA] supramastoid crest: a ridge on the temporal bone that is a continuation of the superior border of the posterior root of the zygomatic process of the temporal bone.
c. supravalvula′ris aor′tae [TA] supravalvular ridge of aorta: a narrow fibromuscular ring projecting to a variable degree into the lumen of the aorta, superior to the aortic sinus.
c. supravalvularis trunci pulmonalis [TA] supravalvular ridge of pulmonary trunk: a narrow fibromuscular ring projecting to a variable degree into the lumen of the pulmonary trunk, superior to the pulmonic valve.
c. supraventricula′ris [TA] supraventricular crest: a ridge on the inner surface of the right ventricle of the heart, marking off the conus arteriosus or outflow tract from the remainder of the right ventricle, the inflow tract.
c. tempora′lis mandi′bulae [TA] temporal crest of mandible: a ridge on the medial aspect of the coronoid process, extending from near the apex of the coronoid process to the level of the last molar, that gives attachment to the temporalis muscle.
c. termina′lis a′trii dex′tri [TA] terminal crest of right atrium: a ridge on the internal surface of the right atrium of the heart, located to the right of the orifices of the superior and inferior venae cavae, and separating the sinus venarum cavarum from the atrium proper and auricle. The pectinate muscles of the right atrium are attached at this crest. It corresponds to a groove on the external surface, the sulcus terminalis.
c. transver′sa mea′tus acus′tici inter′ni [TA] transverse crest of internal acoustic meatus: a ridge of bone that divides the fundus of the internal acoustic meatus into a superior and an inferior fossa.
c. transversa′lis [TA] transverse ridge: an elevated crest on the occlusal surface of a mandibular premolar; it runs transversely across and links the apices of the buccal and lingual cusps. It includes the buccal and lingual cusps and may be an uninterrupted prominence or may be sharply divided by a groove across the middle.
c. triangula′ris [TA] triangular ridge: a ridge on the occlusal surface of a molar or premolar, descending from the tip of the tooth's cusp toward the center of the occlusal surface; so named because the slopes of each side of the ridge resemble two sides of a triangle.
c. tuber′culi majo′ris [TA] crest of greater tubercle: a projection on the greater tubercle of the humerus, forming one lip of the intertubercular groove; called also *labium laterale sulci intertubercularis* [TA alternative], *lateral lip of intertubercular sulcus, pectoral ridge,* and *external, outer,* or *posterior bicipital ridge.*
c. tuber′culi mino′ris [TA] crest of lesser tubercle: a projection on the lesser tubercle of the humerus, forming one lip of the intertubercular groove; called also *labium mediale sulci intertubercularis* [TA alternative], *medial lip of intertubercular sulcus,* and *anterior* or *internal bicipital ridge.*
c. urethra′lis ure′thrae femini′nae [TA] urethral crest of female urethra: a prominent longitudinal fold in the female urethra, consisting of mucosa bulging inward along the posterior wall of the urethra.
c. urethra′lis ure′thrae masculi′nae [TA] urethral crest of male urethra: a median elevation along the posterior wall of the male urethra, lying between the prostatic sinuses.
c. vertica′lis mea′tus acus′tici inter′ni [TA] a vertical bony crest in the internal acoustic meatus; superior to the transverse crest (crista transversa), it separates the facial canal from the superior vestibular area, and inferior to the transverse crest it separates the inferior vestibular area from the cochlear area.
c. vesti′buli [TA] vestibular crest: a ridge between the spherical and elliptical recesses of the vestibule of the bony labyrinth, dividing posteriorly to bound the cochlear recess.

cris•tae (kris′te) [L.] genitive and plural of *crista.*

cris•tal (kris′təl) pertaining to a crest or ridge.

cris•to•ba•lite (kris-to′bə-līt) a translucent crystalline form of silica used in casting investments because it has a high capacity for thermal expansion and is resistant to being broken down by heat.

cri•te•ri•on (kri-tēr′e-on) [Gr. *kritērion* a means for judging] a standard by which something may be judged.
Atlanta criteria a set of criteria for describing acute pancreatitis, consisting of four signs of organ failure (shock, pulmonary insufficiency, renal failure, and gastrointestinal bleeding), local complications in the pancreas (necrosis, abscess, or pseudocyst), and the results of the Ranson criteria and the APACHE score.
El Escorial criteria a group of criteria used for diagnosing amyotrophic lateral sclerosis, assessing the location and severity of motor neuron disease and assigning classifications of suspected, possible, probable, and definite disease.
Ranson criteria a set of eleven signs for the assessment of severity of acute pancreatitis; five are measured at admission to the hospital, and six are checked in the first 48 hours after admission. Three or more positive signs indicate that systemic complications are likely; four or more are associated with significantly increased mortality. See accompanying table.

crith (krith) [Gr. *krithē* barleycorn, the smallest weight] the unit of weight for gases, being the weight of a liter of hydrogen gas at 0°C and pressure equivalent to that of a column of mercury 760 mm high.

Ranson Criteria for Severity of Acute Pancreatitis

At Admission
- Age > 55 years
- White cell count > 16.0 × 10^9/L
- Blood glucose > 11 mmol/L
- Serum lactate dehydrogenase (LDH) > 350 IU/L
- Aspartate transaminase (SGOT) > 250 U/L

During Initial 48 Hours
- Hematocrit decrease > 10 percentage points
- Blood urea nitrogen (BUN) increase > 1.8 mmol/L as urea
- PaO_2 < 60 mm Hg
- Base deficit > 4 mEq/L
- Serum calcium < 2.0 mmol/L
- Fluid sequestration > 6 L

Cri•thid•ia (krĭ-thid′e-ə) [Gr. *krithē* barleycorn] a genus of parasitic protozoa of the order Kinetoplastida, phylum Euglenozoa, found in the digestive tract of arthropods. They are monogenetic, with the choanomastigote stage dominant in their life cycle.

cri•thid•ia (krĭ-thid′e-ə) any protozoan of the genus *Crithidia.*

cri•thid•i•al (krĭ-thid′e-əl) pertaining to the genus *Crithidia.*

crit•i•cal (krit′ĭ-kəl) 1. pertaining to or of the nature of a crisis. 2. pertaining to a disease or other morbid condition in which there is danger of death. 3. in sufficient quantity as to constitute a turning point, as a critical mass or critical concentration.

Crix•i•van (krik′sĭ-van) trademark for a preparation of indinavir sulfate.

CRL crown-rump length.

CRM cross-reacting material.

CRNA Certified Registered Nurse Anesthetist.

cRNA complementary RNA.

cro•cein (kro′sēn) any one of a series of bright red stains.

cro•che•tage (kro-sha-tazh′) [Fr.] a notch, as seen on an electrocardiogram.

cro•ci•dis•mus (kro″sĭ-diz′məs) [Gr. *krokē* a tuft of wool] floccillation.

cro•cid•o•lite (krə-sid′ə-līt) a sodium ferrosoferric silicate in the amphibole group of asbestos, bluish in color, used industrially but now restricted because it causes asbestosis and certain forms of cancer such as mesotheliomas. Called also *blue asbestos.*

Cro•Fab (kro′fab) trademark for a preparation of Crotalidae polyvalent immune Fab (ovine); see under *Fab.*

cro•fil•con A (kro-fil′kon) a contact lens material (hydrophobic).

Crohn disease (krōn) [Burrill Bernard *Crohn,* American physician, 1884–1983] see under *disease.*

cro•mo•gly•cate (kro″mo-gli′kāt) a salt of cromoglycic acid; the disodium salt, cromolyn sodium, is used in the treatment of bronchial asthma.

cro•mo•gly•cic ac•id (kro″mo-gli′sik) cromolyn.

cro•mo•lyn (kro′mə-lin) an inhibitor of the release of histamine and other mediators of immediate hypersensitivity from mast cells. Called also *cromoglycic acid.*

c. sodium [USP] the disodium salt of cromoglycic acid, having the same actions as the acid; administered by inhalation or intranasally for prophylaxis and treatment of allergic rhinitis and bronchial asthma associated with allergy, orally for treatment of mastocytosis, and topically to the conjunctiva for prevention and treatment of allergen-induced inflammation of the conjunctiva or cornea.

Cro•nin method (kro′nin) [Thomas Dillon *Cronin,* American plastic surgeon, 1906–1993] see under *method.*

Cron•khite-Can•a•da syndrome (krong′kīt kan′ə-də) [Leonard Wolsey *Cronkhite,* Jr., American internist, born 1919; Wilma Jeanne *Canada,* American radiologist, 20th century] see under *syndrome.*

Crooke cells, hyalinization (changes, hyaline degeneration) (krook) [Arthur Carleton *Crooke,* British pathologist, 1905–1990] see under *hyalinization.*

crop (krop) 1. in birds, a dilatation of the esophagus at the base of the neck where food is temporarily stored and softened by the uptake of water before digestion begins; it then is passed through the proventriculus and into the gizzard. Called also *craw* and *ingluvies.* 2. a similar organ of certain insects, earthworms, and other invertebrates.

Cross syndrome (kros) [Harold Eugene *Cross,* American physician, born 1937] see under *syndrome.*

cross (kros) [L. *crux*] 1. any figure or structure in the shape of a cross. 2. the production of progeny containing genetic information from two or more parents, as by mating between genetically different individuals, conjugation between microorganisms of different mating types, or recombination between viral particles of different genotypes. 3. the progeny derived from two or more parents of different genetic backgrounds.

back c. backcross.

phage c. the production of recombinant phage progeny, having genes from multiple parent phages that differ in one or more genes, as a result of their infection of a single bacterial cell followed by recombination.

Ranvier c's dark, cross-shaped markings at the nodes of Ranvier, seen on longitudinal section after staining with silver nitrate.

silver c's Ranvier c's.

test c. mating of an individual of unknown genotype but showing the dominant phenotype for a gene or genes to a tester that is homozygous recessive for the genes in question, as a means of revealing the unknown genotype.

two-factor c. recombination involving two genetic markers.

yellow c. dichlorodiethyl sulfide.

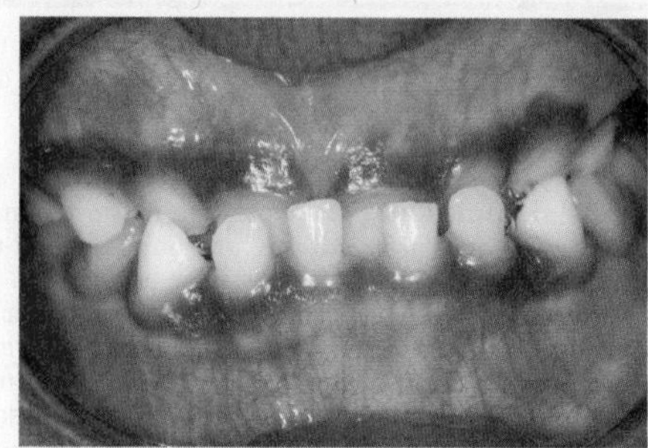

■ Anterior crossbite in a five-year-old child, caused by incisor interference and resultant anterior shift of the mandible on closure.

cross•bite (kros′bīt″) malocclusion in which the mandibular teeth are in buccal version (or in complete lingual version in posterior segments) to the maxillary teeth, bilaterally, unilaterally, or involving only a pair of opposing teeth, so that opposing occlusal surfaces are not in contact in habitual occlusion. Also written *cross bite* and *X-bite.*

anterior c. crossbite in which one or more primary or permanent maxillary incisors are lingual to the mandibular incisors.

buccal c. crossbite in which the maxillary molar is buccal to its mandibular antagonist.

lingual c. crossbite in which the maxillary or mandibular molar is lingual to its antagonist.

posterior c. crossbite in which one or more primary or permanent posterior teeth are locked in an abnormal relation with the opposing teeth of the opposite arch; it may be buccal or lingual crossbite and may be accompanied by a shift of the mandible.

scissors-bite c., telescoping c. crossbite in which the mandibular arch is entirely lingual to the maxillary arch.

cross•breed•ing (kros′brēd-ing) outbreeding.

cross-bridges (kros-brij′əz) in A bands of myofibrils, connections from the thick to the thin filaments formed by the heads of myosin molecules and appearing microscopically as dark striations; they provide the mechanical force that slides the thick and thin filaments past each other in muscle contraction.

cross-dress•ing (kros′dres-ing) the wearing of clothing specific to or characteristic of the opposite sex.

crossed (krost) shaped or arranged like a cross or the letter X.

cross-eye (kros′i) esotropia.

cross•foot (kros′foot) talipes varus.

cross•ing over (kros′ing o′vər) the reciprocal exchange of genetic material between homologous chromosomes, resulting in recombination; often specifically denoting exchange between nonsister chromatids of paired homologous chromosomes during the first meiotic division.

cross-link (kros′link″) a covalent bond formed between polymer chains, either between different chains or between different parts of the same chain.

cross-link•ing (kros′link″ing) establishment of covalent bonds between chains of molecules of a polymer or polymers, fastening the chains together. See also *cross-linked polymer,* under *polymer.*

cross•match (kros′mach) 1. a test of the compatibility of donor and recipient blood performed before transfusion: red cells of the donor are placed in serum of the recipient *(major crossmatch)* and red cells of the recipient in serum of the donor *(minor crossmatch)* and antiglobulin is added to increase reactivity; the presence of hemolysis or agglutination indicates incompatibility. 2. a test for the presence in the serum of a prospective transplant recipient of cytotoxic antibodies against donor tissue antigens: donor lymphocytes are placed in serum of the recipient; the presence of cytolysis indicates incompatibility and the likelihood of hyperacute graft rejection. Called also *pretransplant crossmatch* and *HLA crossmatch.* Written also *cross match* and *cross-match.*

cross•match•ing (kros′mach″ing) the performance of a crossmatch.

cross•over (kros′o-vər) 1. the result of the reciprocal exchange of genetic material between chromosomes; see *crossing over.* 2. see under *trial.*

cross-re•ac•ti•va•tion (kros″re-ak″tĭ-va′shən) the activation of an inactive virus particle by another active or inactive virus particle in the same cell.

cross re•ac•tiv•i•ty (kros″re-ak-tiv′ĭ-te) the degree to which an antibody or antigen participates in cross reactions (see under *reaction*).

cross-re•sis•tance (kros″re-zis′təns) multidrug resistance; see under *resistance.*

cross-sen•si•ti•za•tion (kros-sen″sĭ-tĭ-za′shən) sensitization to a substance induced by exposure to another substance having cross-reacting antigens.

cross•talk (kros′tawk) in cardiology, inappropriate detection of the atrial stimulus by the ventricular sensing mechanism, usually seen with dual-chamber pacemakers.

cross-tol•er•ance (kros′tol″ər-əns) extension of the tolerance for a substance to others of the same class, even those to which the body has not been exposed previously.

cross•way (kros′wa) the path by which something crosses; decussation.

Cro•ta•la•ria (kro″tə-lar′e-ə) [L. *crotalum* rattle or castanet] a large genus of leguminous herbs, most species of which grow in warm to tropical climates; many species contain pyrrolizidine alkaloids such as monocrotaline, which can cause crotalism in animals that consume them.

cro•ta•lid (kro′tə-lid) 1. any snake of the family Crotalidae; called also *pit viper*. 2. of or pertaining to the family Crotalidae.

Cro•tal•i•dae (kro-tal′ĭ-de) a family of venomous snakes, the pit vipers, characterized by front, movable, hollow fangs and a depression or pit between the nostril and the eye. Sometimes it is considered a subfamily of Viperidae and called Crotalinae. It includes the genera *Agkistrodon, Bothrops, Calloselasma, Crotalus, Lachesis, Sistrurus*, and *Trimeresurus*. See table at *snake*.

Cro•tal•i•nae (kro-tal′ĭ-ne) name given to the snake family Crotalidae when it is considered a subfamily under Viperidae.

cro•ta•line (kro′tə-lēn) crotalid.

cro•tal•ism (kro′təl-iz-əm) congestion and hemorrhage of the liver and spleen with emaciation, weakness, and stupor, seen in animals that consume plants of the genus *Crotalaria*, owing to poisonous pyrrolizidine alkaloids such as monocrotaline in the plants. Called also *bottom disease, Kimberley horse disease*, and *walkabout disease*.

cro•ta•lo•tox•in (kro′tə-lo-tok″sin) a poisonous substance from rattlesnake venom.

Cro•ta•lus (kro′tə-ləs) [L., from Gr. *krotalon* rattle] a genus of venomous rattlesnakes of the family Crotalidae; numerous species are found in North America. *C. adaman′teus* is the eastern diamondback rattlesnake; *C. atrox′* is the western diamondback rattlesnake; *C. ceras′tes* is the sidewinder; *C. duris′sus terri′ficus* is the cascabel of Central and South America; *C. hor′ridus* is the timber rattlesnake; and *C. scutula′tus scutula′tus* is the Mojave rattlesnake. *C. vi′ridis* has many subspecies in the western and southwestern United States, such as *C. vi′ridis vi′ridis*, the prairie rattlesnake. See *rattlesnake* and see table at *snake*.

cro•ta•mine (kro′tə-mēn) a toxic protein occurring in the venom of some *Crotalus* species.

cro•ta•mi•ton (kro″tə-mi′ton) [USP] a scabicide, occurring as a light yellow, oily liquid; applied topically to the skin.

cro•taph•i•on (kro-taf′e-on) [Gr. *krotaphos* the temple] a craniometric point at the tip of the great wing of the sphenoid.

cro•tin (kro′tin) a phytotoxin derived from the seeds of *Croton tiglium*, which causes crotonism.

Cro•ton (kro′tən) [L., from Gr. *krotōn* tick] a genus of shrubs of the family Euphorbiaceae, some of which are popular as ornamentals. Certain species are used medically in Mexico and South America, and others, such as *C. texen′sis* and *C. capita′tus*, are poisonous. *C. tig′lium* L., an Asian species, contains poisonous croton oil.

cro•ton•ic ac•id (kro-ton′ik) an unsaturated fatty acid, $CH_3CH{=}CHCOOH$, found in croton oil.

cro•ton•ism (kro′tən-iz-əm) poisoning by croton oil, characterized by a burning sensation in the mouth and sometimes vomiting, severe diarrhea, and intestinal cramps; this may be accompanied by headache, somnolence, vertigo, prostration, and collapse, with death from circulatory or respiratory failure.

cro•tox•in (kro-tok′sin) a crystalline neurotoxic principle from the venom of the rattlesnake, *Crotalus durissus terrificus*.

croup (kr o͞o p) a condition resulting from acute partial obstruction of the upper airway, seen mainly in infants and children; characteristics include resonant barking cough, hoarseness, and persistent stridor. It may be caused by a viral infection (usually a parainfluenza virus), a bacterial infection (usually *Staphylococcus aureus, Streptococcus pneumoniae*, or *Streptococcus pyogenes*), an allergy, a foreign body, or new growth. See also *laryngotracheobronchitis*. **croup′ous, croup′y** *adj*

bacterial c. see under *tracheitis*.
false c. laryngismus stridulus.
membranous c., pseudomembranous c. bacterial tracheitis.
spasmodic c. laryngismus stridulus.

croupy (kro͞op′e) affected with or resembling croup.

Crou•zon syndrome (kroo-zon′) [Octave *Crouzon*, French neurologist, 1874–1938] see under *syndrome*.

Crow-Fu•ka•se syndrome (kro′ foo-kah′se) [R.S. *Crow*, British physician, 20th century; Masaichi *Fukase*, Japanese physician, 20th century] POEMS syndrome; see under *syndrome*.

crowd•ing (kroud′ing) the condition in which the teeth are too close together and assume such altered positions as overlapping, displacement in various directions, and torsiversion.

Crowe sign (kro) [Frank W. *Crowe*, American physician, 20th century] see under *sign*.

crown (kroun) [L. *corona*] 1. the topmost part of an organ or other structure, such as the top of the head, or the upper part of a tooth (corona dentis [TA]); see *anatomical c.* and *physiological c.* 2. artificial c.

anatomical c. corona dentis.
artificial c. a restoration made of metal alone, metal with a veneer of porcelain or resin, or porcelain or resin alone that reproduces the entire surface anatomy of the clinical crown of a tooth; it may be attached to a prepared tooth stump, to one partially rebuilt by a cast metal core alone, or to a cast core and a post, or it may be cemented to the remaining tooth structure. Colloquially called *cap*.
basket c. an artificial gold crown fitted over a natural tooth with minimal removal of tissue, so-called because added retention is provided by a thin band of labial metal similar in shape to a basket handle.
bell c. a dental crown whose circumference at the occlusal surface is larger than usual in relation to the size of the circumference at the crown cervix.
Bonwill c. an artificial porcelain crown held to the tooth root by means of a threaded metal dowel extending through a hole in the porcelain, and upon which a nut is screwed.
cap c. shell c.
celluloid c. a temporary crown made of celluloid that facilitates the fabrication of a temporary crown during fixed prosthodontic procedures.
ciliary c. corona ciliaris.
clinical c. corona clinica.
collar c. an artificial crown attached by a metal ferrule to a natural tooth root.
complete c., complete veneer c. full c.
dental c. corona dentis.
dowel c. an artificial crown that replaces the entire coronal portion of a tooth and is retained by a dowel extending into a filled root canal.
extra-alveolar c. corona clinica.
full c., full veneer c. a dental restoration that completely reproduces the clinical crown of a natural tooth. Called also *complete c.* and *full veneer*.
half-cap c. open-face c.
jacket c. a porcelain or acrylic resin restoration of the clinical crown of a tooth that usually terminates under the gingiva.
open-face c. a gold crown that covers the labial or buccal cervical region in addition to the lingual, proximal, and occlusal surfaces, or the incisal edge of anterior teeth, the buccal or labial surface of the natural crown being left exposed through the opening. Called also *half-cap c.*
overlay c. a cast metal artificial crown fitted over a prepared natural crown to support the walls around an inlay that are not strong or thick enough to withstand occlusal stresses, while leaving exposed the labial surface of the natural crown for esthetic purposes.
partial veneer c. three-quarter c.
physiological c. the portion of a tooth that is exposed beyond the gingival crevice or the margin of the gum. It may involve all of the part of a tooth covered by enamel (dental c.; see *corona dentis* [TA]) or a portion of it (clinical crown; see *corona clinica* [TA]), and it may also involve a portion of the part not covered by enamel (anatomical root).
pinledge c. an artificial crown retained by means of pins that fit into prepared pinledges in a tooth.

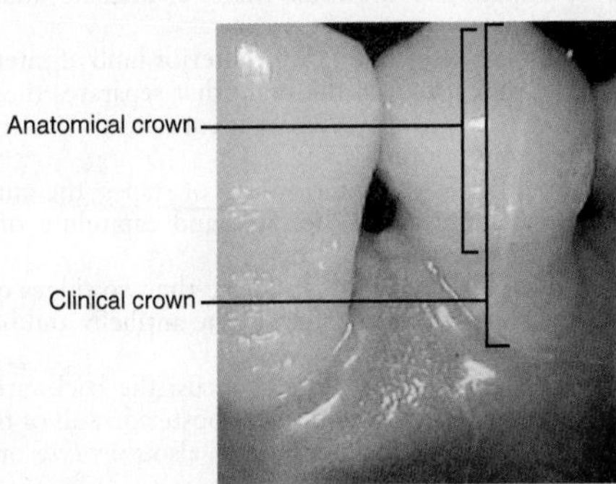

■ Anatomical and clinical crowns, demonstrating that the former are independent of the state of surrounding tissues while the latter depend on the height of the surrounding gingiva.

Richmond c. an artificial crown consisting of a metal base or cap, which fits the prepared face or a stump of a natural root and carries a post or pivot for insertion into the root canal, and a porcelain facing reinforced with metal backing.

shell c. an artificial crown applied like a shell or cap over the remaining natural crown of a tooth; the space between the crown and the shell is filled with cement. Called also *cap c.*

tapered c. an artificial crown seated over a tapered abutment so that it may be fitted in place and removed without obstruction.

three-quarter c. an artificial crown covering mainly three surfaces of anterior teeth (mesial, distal, and lingual) and four surfaces of posterior teeth (mesial, distal, lingual, and occlusal); used as a retainer for a bridge or as a single-unit restoration on a carious fractured tooth. Called also *partial veneer c.*

c. of tooth corona dentis.

veneered c., veneer metal c., window c. an artificial crown that bears a thin layer of resin or porcelain on the buccal or labial surface, attached to or bonded to the metal casting.

crown·ing (kroun′ing) that phase in the second stage of labor when a large segment of the fetal scalp is visible at the vaginal orifice, the perineum being distended.

Cro·zat appliance, clasp (kro′zat) [George B. *Crozat*, American dentist, early 20th century] see under *appliance* and *clasp.*

cro·zat (kro′zat) [G. B. *Crozat*] Crozat appliance.

CRP C-reactive protein.

CRPS complex regional pain syndrome.

CRRT continuous renal replacement therapy.

cru·ces (kroo′sēz) [L.] plural of *crux.*

cru·cial (kroo′shəl) [L. *crucialis*] severe and decisive.

cru·ci·ate (kroo′she-āt) cruciform.

cru·ci·ble (kroo′sĭ-bəl) [L. *crucibulum*] a vessel for melting refractory substances.

cru·ci·form (kroo′sĭ-form) [*crux* + *form*] shaped like a cross; called also *cruciate.*

crude (kro͞od) [L. *crudus* raw] raw or unrefined.

cru·fo·mate (kroo′fo-māt) a veterinary anthelmintic.

cru·or (kroo′or) pl. *cruo′res* [L.] blood clot.

cru·ra (kroo′rə) [L.] plural of *crus.*

cru·ral (kro͞or′əl) pertaining to the lower limb or to a leglike structure (crus).

cru·ral·gia (kroo-ral′jə) pain in a lower limb.

cru·re·us (kroo-re′əs) musculus vastus intermedius.

cru·ris (kroo′ris) genitive of *crus.*

cru·rot·o·my (kroo-rot′ə-me) surgical cutting of a crus of the stapes, usually the anterior crus.

crus (krus) gen. *cru′ris* pl. *cru′ra* [L.] 1. [TA] leg: the part of the lower limb from the knee to the ankle. 2. a leglike part.

ampullary bony crura crura ossea ampullaria.

ampullary membranous crura of semicircular duct crura membranacea ampullaria ductus semicircularis.

c. I of ansiform lobule lobulus semilunaris superior.

c. II of ansiform lobule lobulus semilunaris inferior.

anterior c. of external inguinal ring c. mediale anuli inguinalis superficialis.

anterior c. of internal capsule c. anterius capsulae internae.

anterior c. of stapes c. anterius stapedis.

anterior c. of superficial inguinal ring c. mediale anuli inguinalis superficialis.

c. ante′rius cap′sulae inter′nae [TA] anterior limb of internal capsule: the part of the internal capsule of the brain that separates the head of the caudate nucleus and the lentiform nucleus; it contains the anterior thalamic radiations and the frontopontine tract.

c. ante′rius stape′dis [TA] anterior crus of stapes: the anterior of the two bony limbs that connect the footplate and capitulum of the stapes; called also *anterior limb of stapes.*

cru′ra antihe′licis [TA] crura of antihelix: the two ridges on the external ear marking the superior termination of the antihelix and bounding the triangular fossa; called also *limbs of antihelix.*

c. bre′ve incu′dis [TA] short crus of incus: the backward-projecting process on the incus that is connected to the posterior wall of the tympanic cavity by the posterior incudal ligament; called also *short limb* or *short process of incus.*

c. ce′rebri the part of the basis pedunculi anterior to the substantia nigra; it is a large bundle of nerve fiber tracts consisting of the pyramidal tract, corticopontine tract, and corticoreticular fibers. Some authorities do not include the substantia nigra in the basis pedunculi and so use the terms crus cerebri and basis pedunculi synonymously to denote this fiber bundle.

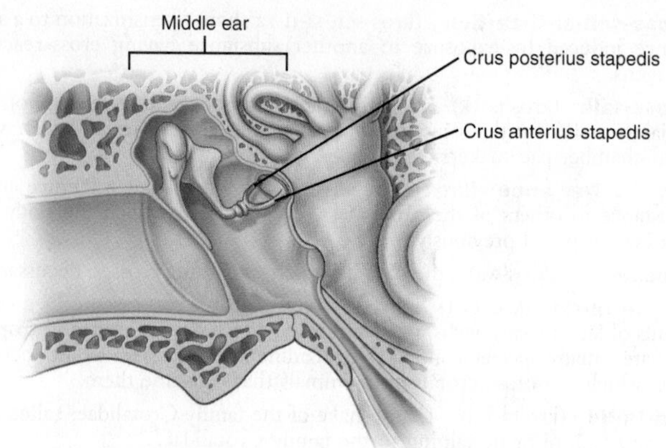

■ Close-up of middle ear, showing the two limbs (crura) of the stapes.

c. clito′ridis [TA] crus of clitoris: the continuation of each corpus cavernosum clitoridis, diverging posteriorly to be attached to the ischiopubic rami.

common bony c. c. osseum commune.

common membranous c. of semicircular duct c. membranaceum commune ductus semicircularis.

c. commu′ne cana′lis semicircula′ris c. osseum commune.

c. dex′trum diaphrag′matis [TA] right crus of diaphragm; a fibromuscular band arising from the superior three or four lumbar vertebrae, and ascending along with the left crus, to insert into the central tendon of the diaphragm.

c. dex′trum fascic′uli atrioventricula′ris [TA] right crus of atrioventricular bundle: a discrete group of fascicles arising from the trunk of the bundle at the superior end of the muscular part of the interventricular septum; it descends to be distributed to the right ventricle of the heart as a terminal network of Purkinje fibers that become continuous with the ventricular cardiac muscle fibers. Called also *right bundle branch* and *right branch of atrioventricular bundle.*

cru′ra diaphrag′matis see *c. dextrum diaphragmatis* and *c. sinistrum diaphragmatis.*

external c. of external inguinal ring, external c. of superficial inguinal ring c. laterale anuli inguinalis superficialis.

first c. of ansiform lobule lobulus semilunaris superior.

c. for′nicis [TA] crus of fornix: either of the two flattened bands of white substance of the brain that are in close contact with the splenium and that unite under the posterior part of the body of the corpus callosum to form the body of the fornix.

c. he′licis [TA] crus of helix: the anterior termination of the helix of the external ear located above the entrance to the external acoustic meatus.

crura of incus see *c. breve incudis* and *c. longum incudis.*

c. infe′rius mar′ginis falcifor′mis TA alternative for *cornu inferius marginis falciformis.*

internal c. of external inguinal ring c. mediale anuli inguinalis superficialis.

internal c. of greater alar cartilage c. mediale cartilaginis alaris majoris.

internal c. of superficial inguinal ring c. mediale anuli inguinalis superficialis.

lateral c. of external inguinal ring c. laterale anuli inguinalis superficialis.

lateral c. of greater alar cartilage c. laterale cartilaginis alaris majoris.

lateral c. of superficial inguinal ring, c. latera′le a′nuli inguina′lis superficia′lis [TA] the part of the superficial inguinal ring that blends with the inguinal ligament as it goes to the pubic tubercle; called also *external* or *posterior c. of external inguinal ring* and *external* or *posterior c. of superficial inguinal ring.*

c. latera′le cartila′ginis ala′ris majo′ris [TA] lateral crus of greater alar cartilage: the part of the greater alar cartilage that curves laterally around the naris and helps maintain its contour.

left c. of atrioventricular bundle c. sinistrum fasciculi atrioventricularis.

left c. of diaphragm c. sinistrum diaphragmatis.

long c. of incus, c. lon′gum incu′dis [TA] a process on the incus directed downward and inward, parallel with the manubrium of the malleus; called also *long limb* or *long process of incus.*

medial c. of external inguinal ring c. mediale anuli inguinalis superficialis.

medial c. of greater alar cartilage c. mediale cartilaginis alaris majoris.

medial c. of superficial inguinal ring, c. media′le a′nuli inguina′lis superficia′lis [TA] the part of the superficial inguinal ring that is attached to the symphysis and that blends with the fundiform ligament of the penis. Called also *anterior* or *internal c. of internal inguinal ring* and *anterior* or *internal c. of superficial inguinal ring.*

c. media′le cartila′ginis ala′ris majo′ris [TA] medial crus of greater alar cartilage: the part of the greater alar cartilage, loosely attached to its fellow of the opposite side, and helping to form the mobile septum of the nose; called also *internal c. of greater alar cartilage.*

cru′ra membrana′cea membranous crura: the two ends of each semicircular duct of the ear, both opening into the utricle. See *crura membranacea ampullaria ductus semicircularis, c. membranaceum commune ductus semicircularis,* and *c. membranaceum simplex ductus semicircularis.*

cru′ra membrana′cea ampulla′ria duc′tus semicircula′ris [TA] ampullary membranous crura of semicircular duct: the ends of the semicircular ducts of the ear, in which the membranous ampullae are situated.

c. membrana′ceum commu′ne duc′tus semicircula′ris [TA] common membranous crus of semicircular duct: an area consisting of the joined nonampullary ends of the anterior and posterior semicircular duct of the ear.

c. membrana′ceum sim′plex duc′tus semicircula′ris [TA] simple membranous crus of semicircular duct: the nonampullary end of the lateral semicircular duct of the ear, opening into the utricle.

membranous crura crura membranacea.

cru′ra os′sea osseous crura: those parts of the bony semicircular canals of the ear that lodge the correspondingly named parts of the membranous crura of the semicircular ducts; see *crura ossea ampullaria, c. osseum commune,* and *c. osseum simplex.*

cru′ra os′sea ampulla′ria [TA] ampullary bony crura: the parts of the bony semicircular canals of the ear that lodge the crura membranacea ampullaria ductus semicircularis.

c. os′seum commu′ne [TA] common bony crus: the part of a bony semicircular canal of the ear that lodges the crus membranaceum commune ductus semicircularis; called also *c. commune canalis semicircularis.*

c. os′seum sim′plex [TA] simple bony crus: that part of the lateral bony semicircular canal of the ear that lodges the crus membranaceum simplex ductus semicircularis; called also *c. simplex canalis semicircularis.*

c. pe′nis [TA] crus of penis: the continuation of each corpus cavernosum penis, diverging posteriorly to be attached to the pubic arch.

posterior c. of external inguinal ring c. laterale anuli inguinalis superficialis.

posterior c. of internal capsule c. posterius capsulae internae.

posterior c. of stapes c. posterius stapedis.

posterior c. of superficial inguinal ring c. laterale anuli inguinalis superficialis.

c. poste′rius cap′sulae inter′nae [TA] posterior limb of internal capsule: the part of the internal capsule of the brain that separates the thalamus from the lentiform nucleus; its main function is the conveyance of corticofugal fibers from the cerebral cortex such as corticospinal fibers, thalamocortical radiations, and other fiber projections.

c. poste′rius stape′dis [TA] posterior crus of stapes: the posterior of the two bony limbs that connect the footplate and capitulum of the stapes; called also *posterior limb of stapes.*

c. pri′mum lo′buli ansifor′mis TA alternative for *lobulus semilunaris superior.*

right c. of atrioventricular bundle c. dextrum fasciculi atrioventricularis.

right c. of diaphragm c. dextrum diaphragmatis.

second c. of ansiform lobule lobulus semilunaris inferior.

c. secun′dum lo′buli ansifor′mis TA alternative for *lobulus semilunaris inferior.*

short c. of incus c. breve incudis.

simple bony c. c. osseum simplex.

simple membranous c. of semicircular duct c. membranaceum simplex ductus semicircularis.

c. sim′plex cana′lis semicircula′ris c. osseum simplex.

c. sinis′trum diaphrag′matis [TA] left crus of diaphragm: a fibromuscular band arising from the superior two or three lumbar vertebrae, and ascending along with the right crus, to insert into the central tendon of the diaphragm.

c. sinis′trum fasci′culi atrioventricula′ris [TA] left crus of atrioventricular bundle: a dispersed array of fascicles arising from the trunk of the bundle at the superior end of the muscular part of the interventricular septum; they continue as a flattened sheet, generally diverging into anterior and posterior limbs, and descend to be distributed to the papillary muscles of the left ventricle of the heart as a terminal network of Purkinje fibers that become continuous with the ventricular cardiac muscle fibers. Called also *left bundle branch* and *left branch of atrioventricular bundle.*

crura of stapes see *c. anterius stapedis* and *c. posterius stapedis.*

c. supe′rius mar′ginis falcifor′mis TA alternative for *cornu superius marginis falciformis.*

crust (krust) [L. *crusta*] 1. a formed outer layer, especially an outer layer of solid matter formed by the drying of a bodily exudate or secretion. 2. scab (def. 1).

milk c. crusta lactea.

crus·ta (krus′tah) gen. and pl. *crus′tae* [L.] a crust.

c. lac′tea seborrhea of the scalp of nursing infants; called also *cradle cap* and *milk crust.*

Crus·ta·cea (krəs-ta′she-ə) [L., from *crusta* shell] a large class of arthropods including the lobsters, crabs, shrimps, wood lice, water fleas, and barnacles.

crus·tae (krus′te) [L.] genitive and plural of *crusta.*

crus·to·sus (krəs-to′səs) [L.] having a crust; said of skin lesions.

crutch (kruch) 1. a device of wood or metal, ordinarily long enough to reach from the armpit to the ground, with a concave surface fitting under the arm and a cross bar for the hand, used for supporting the weight of the body. 2. the perineal region, especially of a nonhuman animal.

axillary c. any of several types of crutches that have a long, rigid vertical structure, a short padded horizontal bar that fits under the axilla, and another short bar at waist level that is used as a hand grip.

Canadian c. triceps c.

forearm c. a crutch whose top is at the level of the forearm, with a hand bar as well as a cuff that goes around the forearm to increase stability.

Lofstrand c. the most common kind of forearm crutch, consisting of an aluminum tube that bends slightly posteriorly just above the hand grip.

Ortho c. trademark for a type of axillary crutch consisting of a long aluminum bar that bends at a right angle to fit under the axilla and has an adjustable hand grip bar.

triceps c. a crutch consisting of two uprights extending halfway between the elbow and shoulder, with a cross piece for the hand and a curved upper arm part against which the subject leans the upper arm.

Cru·veil·hier atrophy, disease, etc. (kroo-vāl-ya′) [Jean *Cruveilhier,* French pathologist, 1791–1874] see *spinal muscular atrophy* under *atrophy;* see *articulatio atlanto-occipitalis, tela subcutanea perinei, ligamenta palmaria articulationum interphalangealium manus,* and *ligamenta palmaria articulationum metacarpophalangealium;* and see under *disease.*

Cru·veil·hier-Baum·gar·ten syndrome (cirrhosis) (kroo-vāl-ya′ boum′gahr-tən) [J. *Cruveilhier;* Paul Clemens von *Baumgarten,* German pathologist, 1848–1928] see under *syndrome.*

crux (kruks) pl. *cru′ces* [L.] cross.

c. of heart the intersection of the walls separating the right and left sides and the atrial and ventricular chambers of the heart.

cru′ces pilo′rum [TA] crosslike figures formed by the pattern of hair growth, the hairs lying in opposite directions.

cry (kri) 1. a sudden loud, involuntary vocal sound. 2. to utter such a sound. 3. weep (def. 1).

arthritic c., articular c. night c.

cephalic c. a shrill, high-pitched penetrating cry of the newborn suggesting intracranial damage of some severity.

epileptic c. a loud scream that often occurs at the onset of an epileptic attack.

joint c. night c.

night c. a shrill cry uttered by a child in sleep, often heard in beginning joint disease; called also *arthritic, articular,* or *joint c.*

cry·al·ge·sia (kri″əl-je′ze-ə) [*cryo-* + *algesia*] pain due to the application of cold; cf. *psychroalgia.*

cry·an·es·the·sia (kri-an″es-the′zhə) [*cryo-* + *anesthesia*] loss of the power of perceiving cold; see *temperature sense,* under *sense.*

Cry·er's elevator (kri′ərz) [Matthew Henry *Cryer,* American surgeon, 1840–1921] see under *elevator.*

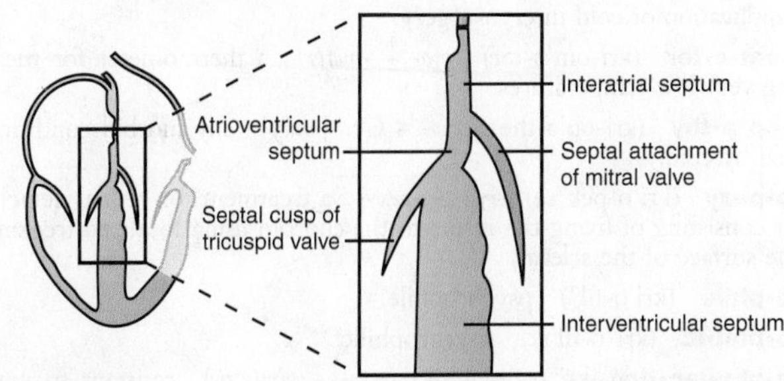

■ Diagram of the crux of the heart as it would be seen in an apical four-chamber view.

cry·es·the·sia (kri″es-the′zhə) [*cryo-* + *esthesia*] abnormal sensitiveness to cold.

cry(o)- [Gr. *kryos* cold] a combining form denoting relationship to cold.

cryo·ab·la·tion (kri″o-ab-la′shən) [*cryo-* + *ablation*] the removal of tissue by destroying it with extreme cold.

cryo·an·al·ge·sia (kri″o-an″əl-je′ze-ə) the relief of pain by application of cold by cryoprobe to peripheral nerves.

cryo·an·es·the·sia (kri″o-an″es-the′zhə) [*cryo-* + *anesthesia*] local anesthesia produced by chilling the part to near freezing temperature.

cryo·bank (kri′o-bank″) a facility for cryopreservation of tissue, organs, embryos, sperm, or other substances, such as while waiting for transplantation.

cryo·bi·ol·o·gy (kri″o-bi-ol′ə-je) [*cryo-* + *biology*] the science dealing with the effect of low temperatures on biological systems.

cryo·car·dio·ple·gia (kri″o-kahr″de-o-ple′jə) [*cryo-* + *cardioplegia*] cessation of contraction of the myocardium produced by cooling the heart during cardiac surgery.

cryo·cau·tery (kri″o-kaw′tər-e) [*cryo-* + *cautery*] cauterization by freezing, using a substance such as liquid nitrogen or carbon dioxide snow, or a very cold instrument. Called also *cold cautery.*

cryo·crit (kri′o-krit) [*cryo-* + Gr. *krinein* to separate] the volume of sedimented cryoglobulin after cold centrifugation of serum at 4° to 5°C.

cryo·dam·age (cri′o-dam″əj) damage to tissues, cells, or other biological substrates as a result of exposure to cold.

cryo·ex·trac·tion (kri″o-ek-strak′shən) the application of low temperature in the removal of a cataractous lens; it is accomplished with an instrument (cryoprobe) whose extremely cold tip forms an adhesion (iceball) with the lens, thus permitting removal of the lens.

cryo·ex·trac·tor (kri″o-ek-strak′tər) [*cryo-* + *extractor*] a cryoprobe used in cryoextraction.

cry·o·fi·brin·o·gen (kri″o-fi-brin′o-jən) [*cryo-* + *fibrinogen*] fibrinogen with the abnormal physical property of precipitating in the cold (4°C) and subsequently redissolving at 37°C.

cryo·fi·brin·o·gen·emia (kri″o-fi-brin″o-jə-ne′me-ə) the presence of cryofibrinogen in the blood.

cryo·gam·ma·glob·u·lin (kri″o-gam″ə-glob′u-lin) cryoglobulin.

cry·o·gen (kri′o-jən) [*cryo-* + *-gen*] a substance used for lowering temperatures.

cry·o·gen·ic (kri″o-jen′ik) pertaining to or causing the production of low temperatures.

cryo·glob·u·lin (kri″o-glob′u-lin) any of numerous immunoglobulins, not present in normal serum, that undergo reversible precipitation as serum cools. They are classified in three groups, *type I*, *type II*, and *type III*, on the basis of clonality. See also *cryoglobulinemia.*

cryo·glob·u·lin·emia (kri″o-glob″u-lĭ-ne′me-ə) the presence of cryoglobulin in the blood, associated with a variety of clinical manifestations including Raynaud phenomenon, vascular purpura, cold urticaria, necrosis of extremities, bleeding disorders, vasculitis, arthralgia, neurologic manifestations, hepatosplenomegaly, and glomerulonephritis.

essential mixed c. an idiopathic type of cryoglobulinemic vasculitis with immune deposits consisting of type II cryoglobulins, which induces cutaneous vasculitis, synovitis, and glomerulonephritis.

cryo·hy·drate (kri″o-hi′drāt) [*cryo-* + *hydrate*] 1. a salt containing water of crystallization at low temperatures. 2. a eutectic mixture, especially one having water as one of its constituents. 3. a crystal obtained by freezing a supersaturated solution and containing solute and solvent in the same ratio as occurred in solution.

cryo·hy·po·phys·ec·to·my (kri″o-hi″po-fiz-ek′tə-me) destruction of the hypophysis by the application of cold.

cryo·le·sion (kri′o-le″zhən) the area of tissue destruction caused by the application of cold in cryosurgery.

cry·om·e·ter (kri-om′ə-tər) [*cryo-* + *-meter*] a thermometer for measuring very low temperatures.

cry·op·a·thy (kri-op′ə-the) [*cryo-* + Gr. *-pathy*] any morbid condition caused by cold.

cryo·pexy (kri′o-pek″se) [*cryo-* + *-pexy*] a treatment for retinal detachment consisting of fixing the retina to the choroid using localized freezing of the surface of the sclera.

cryo·phile (kri′o-fīl″) psychrophile.

cryo·phil·ic (kri″o-fil′ik) psychrophilic.

cryo·phy·lac·tic (kri″o-fə-lak′tik) [*cryo-* + *phylactic*] resistant to very low temperatures; said of bacteria.

cryo·pre·cip·i·ta·bil·i·ty (kri″o-pre-sip″ĭ-tə-bil′ĭ-te) ability to undergo cryoprecipitation.

cryo·pre·cip·i·tate (kri″o-pre-sip′ĭ-tāt) [*cryo-* + *precipitate*] any precipitate that results from cooling; sometimes used specifically for the one rich in coagulation factor VIII obtained from cooling of blood plasma and used in the treatment of hemophilia A (cryoprecipitated antihemophilic factor).

cryo·pre·cip·i·ta·tion (kri″o-pre-sip″ĭ-ta′shən) precipitation of a substance in solution upon cooling, such as antihemophilic factor in blood plasma.

cryo·pres·er·va·tion (kri″o-prez″ər-va′shən) [*cryo-* + *preservation*] maintenance of the viability of excised tissue, organs, embryos, cells, or other substances, by storing them at very low temperatures.

cryo·probe (kri′o-prōb″) an instrument for applying extreme cold to tissue.

cryo·pro·tec·tion (kri″o-pro-tek′shən) protection, as of a tissue, cell, organism, or other substance, from cold-induced damage.

cryo·pro·tec·tive (kri″o-pro-tek′tiv) capable of protecting against injury due to freezing, as glycerol protects frozen red blood cells.

cryo·pro·tein (kri″o-pro′tēn) [*cryo-* + *protein*] any blood protein that precipitates on cooling, such as cryoglobulin or cryofibrinogen.

cryo·py·rin (kri″o-pi′rin) a complex protein containing a pyrin domain, a nucleotide binding site, and a leucine-rich repeat domain, found in inflammasomes. See also *cryopyrin-associated periodic syndrome.*

cryo·py·rin·op·a·thy (kri″o-pi″rĭ-nop′ə-the) cryopyrin-associated periodic syndrome.

cryo·scope (kri′o-skōp) an apparatus for performing cryoscopy.

cry·os·co·py (kri-os′kə-pe) [*cryo-* + *-scopy*] examination of liquids, based on the principle that the freezing point of solutions varies according to the amount and the nature of the solute. **cryoscop′ic** *adj*

cryo·stat (kri′o-stat″) [*cryo-* + *-stat*] 1. a device by which temperature can be maintained at a very low level. 2. in pathology and histology, a chamber containing a microtome for sectioning frozen tissue.

cryo·sur·gery (kri″o-sur′jər-e) [*cryo-* + *surgery*] destruction of tissue by the application of extreme cold, used in some forms of intracranial and cutaneous surgery.

cryo·sur·vi·val (kri″o-sər-vi′vəl) survival in a viable condition of tissue, organs, or anything else under cryopreservation.

cryo·thal·a·mec·to·my (kri″o-thal″ə-mek′tə-me) cryothalamotomy.

cryo·thal·a·mot·o·my (kri″o-thal″ə-mot′ə-me) destruction of a portion of the thalamus by application of extreme cold.

cryo·ther·a·py (kri″o-ther′ə-pe) [*cryo-* + *therapy*] the therapeutic use of cold. Called also *cold therapy.*

cryo·ther·mia (kri″o-ther′me-ə) [*cryo-* + Gr. *thermē* heat] the extreme cold used in cryosurgery.

cryo·tol·er·ant (kri″o-tol′ər-ənt) [*cryo-* + *tolerant*] able to withstand unusually low temperatures.

crypt (kript) [L. *crypta*, from Gr. *kryptos* hidden] a blind pit or tube on a free surface; see also *crypta* [TA].

anal c's sinus anales.

bony c. the crypt in the developing alveolar bone that becomes the socket of the developing tooth.

dental c. tooth c.

enamel c. a space bounded by the dental ledges on either side and usually by the enamel organ; it is filled with mesenchyma.

c's of Fuchs c's of iris.

c's of iris pitlike depressions found in the iris, in the region of the circulus arteriosus minor; called also *c's of Fuchs.*

c's of Lieberkühn glandulae intestinales.

Littre c's glandulae preputiales.

Luschka c's deep indentations of the gallbladder mucosa which penetrate into the muscular layer of the organ.

c. of Morgagni see *sinus anales.*

mucous c's of duodenum glandulae duodenales.

odoriferous c's of prepuce glandulae preputiales.

c's of palatine tonsil cryptae tonsillares tonsillae palatinae.

c's of pharyngeal tonsil cryptae tonsillares tonsillae pharyngealis.

synovial c. a pouch in the synovial membrane of a joint.

c's of tongue, tonsillar c's of lingual tonsil cryptae tonsillares tonsillae lingualis.

tonsillar c's of palatine tonsil cryptae tonsillares tonsillae palatinae.

tonsillar c's of pharyngeal tonsil cryptae tonsillares tonsillae pharyngealis.

tonsillar c's of tubal tonsil cryptae tonsillares tonsillae tubariae.

tooth c. the depression in the alveolar bone occupied by the tooth germ and the tooth follicle. Called also *dental c.*

Tyson c's glandulae preputiales.

cryp·ta (krip'tə) gen. and pl. *cryp'tae* [L.] crypt: a blind pit or tube opening on a free surface.

cryp'tae muco'sae see *mucous gland,* under *gland.*

cryp'tae tonsilla'res tonsil'lae lingua'lis [TA] tonsillar crypts of lingual tonsil: deep, irregular invaginations from the surface of the lingual tonsils.

cryp'tae tonsilla'res tonsil'lae palati'nae [TA] tonsillar crypts of palatine tonsil: crypts within a palatine tonsil, representing the blind ends of the tonsillar pits.

cryp'tae tonsilla'res tonsil'lae pharyngea'lis [TA] tonsillar crypts of pharyngeal tonsil: crypts found within a pharyngeal tonsil, representing the blind ends of the tonsillar pits.

cryp'tae tonsilla'res tonsil'lae tuba'riae [TA] tonsillar crypts of tubal tonsil: small invaginations extending into a tubal tonsil.

cryp·tae (krip'te) [L.] genitive and plural of *crypta.*

crypt·an·am·ne·sia (kript"an-am-ne'zhə) cryptomnesia.

cryp·tec·to·my (krip-tek'tə-me) [*crypt-* + *-ectomy*] excision or obliteration of a crypt.

cryp·tes·the·sia (krip"tes-the'zhə) [*crypt-* + *esthesia*] clairvoyance.

cryp·tic (krip'tik) [Gr. *kryptikos* hidden] concealed, hidden, larval.

cryp·ti·tis (krip-ti'tis) inflammation of a crypt.

anal c. inflammation of the anal crypts, with pain and tenderness (especially during bowel movements), pruritus, and spasm of the anal sphincter; it may progress to abscess of the crypt.

crypt(o)- [Gr. *kryptos* hidden] a combining form meaning hidden or concealed, or denoting relationship to a crypt.

Cryp·to·coc·ca·ceae (krip"to-kŏ-ka'se-e) a form-family of Fungi Imperfecti, usually classified in the form-class Blastomycetes, although some authorities place it in Hyphomycetes; its members are yeastlike throughout most or all of their life cycle. It includes a number of pathogenic genera, such as *Candida, Cryptococcus, Geotrichum, Malassezia, Rhodotorula,* and *Trichosporon.*

cryp·to·coc·cal (krip"to-kok'əl) pertaining to or caused by fungi of the genus *Cryptococcus.*

Cryp·to·coc·ca·les (krip"to-kok-a'lēz) in some systems of classification, a form-order of Fungi Imperfecti, usually classified in form-class Blastomycetes although some authorities consider it part of Hyphomycetes. It includes the form-family Cryptococcaceae.

cryp·to·coc·co·ma (krip"to-kok-o'mə) a fungus ball consisting of *Cryptococcus neoformans.* Those in the brain often cause symptoms, while those in the lungs may be quiescent.

cryp·to·coc·co·sis (krip"to-kŏ-ko'sis) infection by *Cryptococcus neoformans, Cryptococcus gattii,* or rarely other *Cryptococcus* species, most commonly seen in immunocompromised patients. It begins with a pulmonary infection, which may be asymptomatic, following inhalation of the organism. Disseminated disease may occur and can affect most other organs, but it has a predilection for the brain and meninges, where it causes meningoencephalitis that ranges from subacute to chronic; skin involvement is characterized by an acneiform rash. Called also *torulosis, European blastomycosis,* and *Buschke* or *Busse-Buschke disease.*

Cryp·to·coc·cus (krip"to-kok'əs) [*crypto-* + Gr. *kokkos* berry] a genus of yeastlike Fungi Imperfecti of the family Tremellaceae, which usually have a capsule and do not form pseudomycelia as do *Candida* species.

C. al'bidus a species that occasionally causes cryptococcosis; its perfect (sexual) stage is *Filobasidium floriforme.*

C. bacillispo'rus *C. gattii.*

C. gat'tii a species, closely related to *C. neoformans,* that causes cryptococcosis, chiefly in immunocompetent persons; it occurs mainly in subtropical and tropical regions but occasionally in more temperate areas. Its perfect (sexual) stage is *Filobasidiella gattii.* Called also *C. bacillisporus.*

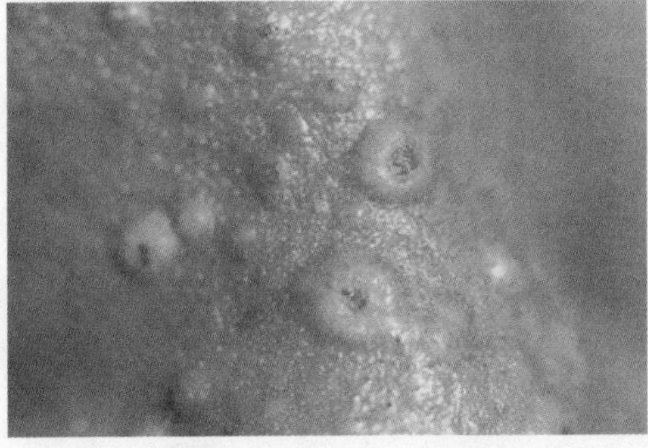

■ Skin lesions in disseminated cryptococcosis.

C. lauren'tii a psychrophilic species that occasionally causes cryptococcosis, almost exclusively in immunocompromised individuals; the perfect (sexual) stage has not been identified.

C. neofor'mans a species found worldwide in pigeon nests and droppings. It is the most common species causing human cryptococcosis, chiefly in immunocompromised persons, and it also infects other mammals. The perfect (sexual) stage is *Filobasidiella neoformans.*

cryp·to·crys·tal·line (krip"to-kris'tə-lēn) [*crypto-* + *crystalline*] composed of crystals of microscopic size.

cryp·to·de·ter·min·ant (krip"to-de-tur'mĭ-nənt) hidden determinant.

cryp·to·did·y·mus (krip"to-did'ə-məs) [*crypto-* + *-didymus*] endadelphos.

cryp·to·em·py·ema (krip"to-em"pi-e'mə) [*crypto-* + *empyema*] empyema that is difficult to aspirate, being loculated or interlobar.

cryp·to·gam (krip'to-gam) [*crypto-* + Gr. *gamos* marriage] any one of the lower plants that have no true flowers, but propagate by spores, such as fungi, algae, mosses, and ferns.

cryp·to·gam·ic (krip"to-gam'ik) pertaining to cryptogams; reproducing by spores.

cryp·to·ge·net·ic (krip"to-jə-net'ik) cryptogenic.

cryp·to·gen·ic (krip"to-jen'ik) [*crypto-* + *-genic*] idiopathic.

cryp·to·glan·du·lar (krip"to-glan'du-lər) [*crypto-* + *glandular*] pertaining to or arising from an anal gland and an anal crypt.

cryp·to·lith (krip'to-lith) [*crypto-* + *-lith*] a calculus or concretion in a crypt.

cryp·to·men·or·rhea (krip"to-men"o-re'ə) [*crypto-* + *menorrhea*] a condition in which the symptoms of menstruation are experienced but no external bleeding occurs, as in cases of imperforate hymen.

cryp·to·mere (krip'to-mēr) [*crypto-* + *-mere*] a cystic or saclike condition.

cryp·to·me·ro·ra·chis·chi·sis (krip"to-me"ro-rə-kis'kĭ-sis) [*crypto-* + *mero-*[1] + *rhachischisis*] spina bifida occulta.

cryp·tom·ne·sia (krip"tom-ne'zhə) [*crypto-* + Gr. *mnasthai* to be mindful] the recall of memories not recognized as such but thought to be original creations. cryptomne'sic *adj*

cryp·to·neu·rous (krip"to-noo'rəs) [*crypto-* + *neuro-* + *-ous*] having no definite or distinct nervous system.

cryp·toph·thal·mia (krip"tof-thal'me-ə) cryptophthalmos.

cryp·toph·thal·mos (krip"tof-thal'mos) [*crypto-* + Gr. *ophthalmos* eye] congenital absence of the palpebral fissure, the skin extending from the forehead to the cheek, with the eye malformed or rudimentary.

cryp·toph·thal·mus (krip"tof-thal'məs) cryptophthalmos.

cryp·to·pine (krip'to-pin) [*crypto-* + Gr. *opion* opium] a minor alkaloidal constituent of opium, of *Corydalis sempervirens* (L.) Pers., and of *Dicentra* spp. (Fumariaceae).

cryp·to·po·dia (krip"to-po'de-ə) [*crypto-* + Gr. *pous* foot] swelling of the lower part of the leg and dorsum of the foot that covers all but the soles of the feet.

cryp·to·py·ic (krip"to-pi'ik) [*crypto-* + *py-* + *-ic*] characterized by concealed suppuration.

cryp·tor·chic (krip-tor'kik) cryptorchid (def. 1).

cryp·tor·chid (krip-tor'kid) [*crypto-* + Gr. *orchis* testis] 1. pertaining to or characterized by cryptorchidism; called also *cryptorchic* and *cryptorchidic.* 2. an individual exhibiting cryptorchidism.

cryp·tor·chi·dec·to·my (krip"tor-kĭ-dek'tə-me) [*cryptorchid* + *-ectomy*] in veterinary medicine, excision of an undescended testis, most commonly done in horses.

cryp·tor·chid·ia (krip-tor-kid'e-ə) cryptorchidism.

cryp·tor·chid·ic (krip-tor-kid'ik) cryptorchid (def. 1).

cryp·tor·chi·dism (krip-tor'kĭ-diz"əm) a developmental defect characterized by failure of one or both of the testes to descend into the scrotum. Called also *cryptorchism* and *undescended testis.*

acquired c. ascending testis.

cryp·tor·chi·do·pexy (krip-tor"kĭ-do-pek'se) orchiopexy.

cryp·tor·chi·dy (krip-tor'kĭ-de) cryptorchidism.

cryp·tor·chism (krip-tor'kiz-əm) cryptorchidism.

cryp·tos·co·py (krip-tos'kə-pe) fluoroscopy.

cryp·to·spo·rid·i·o·sis (krip″to-spo-rid″e-o′sis) 1. infection of young farm animals with protozoa of the genus *Cryptosporidium*, which may be associated with or contribute to enteric disease. 2. human infection with protozoa of the genus *Cryptosporidium*, usually seen as a self-limited diarrhea in those who work with cattle; in immunocompromised patients it is much more serious, manifested as prolonged debilitating diarrhea, weight loss, fever, and abdominal pain, with occasional spread to the trachea and bronchial tree.

Cryp·to·spo·ri·di·um (krip″to-spo-rid′e-əm) [*crypto-* + *spore*] a genus of minute homoxenous coccidian protozoa (suborder Eimeriina, order Eucoccidiida), having oocysts with four sporozoites; they are parasitic in the intestinal tracts of many vertebrate species, causing cryptosporidiosis.

C. ca′nis a species seen mainly in dogs but causing opportunistic infections in immunocompromised persons.

C. fe′lis a species seen mainly in cats but causing opportunistic infections in immunocompromised persons.

C. ho′minis a species that causes opportunistic infections in immunocompromised persons.

C. melea′gridis a species seen in many species of birds and mammals and causing opportunistic infections in immunocompromised persons.

C. mu′ris a species seen in many species of mammals and causing opportunistic infections in immunocompromised persons.

C. parvum a species seen in many species of mammals and causing opportunistic infections in immunocompromised persons.

Cryp·to·stro·ma (krip″to-stro′mə) [*crypto-* + *stroma*] a genus of fungi of the form-class Hyphomycetes; called also *Coniosporium*. *C. cortica′le* grows under the bark of maple trees and inhalation of its spores causes maple bark disease in lumber workers.

cryp·to·tia (krip-to′she-ə) a rare anomaly in which the superior portion of the auricle is buried in the scalp.

cryp·to·tox·ic (krip′to-tok″sik) [*crypto-* + *toxic*] having hidden toxic properties; said of a solution normally nontoxic, but which may become toxic when the colloidal balance is disturbed.

cryp·to·xan·thin (krip″to-zan′thin) a yellow carotenoid widely distributed in nature (egg yolk, green grass, yellow corn, etc.), which can be converted into vitamin A in the body.

cryp·to·zo·ite (krip″to-zo′īt) [*crypto-* + Gr. *zōon* animal] a meront of certain sporozoan protozoa in the exoerythrocytic stage.

cryp·toz·y·gous (krip-toz′ə-gəs) [*crypto-* + Gr. *zygon* yoke] having the face no wider than the cranium, so that the zygomatic arches are concealed by the bulging of the cranium when the skull is viewed from above. Cf. *phenozygous*.

Crys. crystal.

crys·tal (kris′təl) [Gr. *krystallos* ice] a homogeneous angular solid formed from a chemical element, compound, or isomorphous mixture, having a definite form in which the ultimate units from which it is built up are systematically arranged.

asthma c's Charcot-Leyden c's.

blood c's hematoidin crystals in the blood.

calcium pyrophosphate dihydrate (CPPD) c's microscopic crystals of calcium pyrophosphate dihydrate occurring in the synovial fluid in calcium pyrophosphate deposition disease.

Charcot-Leyden c's elongated birefringent crystals in the form of two hexagonal pyramids joined base to base, formed by the action of lysophospholipase on the plasma membranes of disintegrating eosinophils; seen in the sputum in asthma, in the stool in some cases of intestinal parasitism, and in tissues infiltrated by eosinophils in a variety of disorders. Called also *asthma c's*.

coffin lid c's peculiar indented crystals of ammoniomagnesium phosphate from alkaline urine; called also *knife rest c's*.

CPPD c's calcium pyrophosphate dihydrate c's.

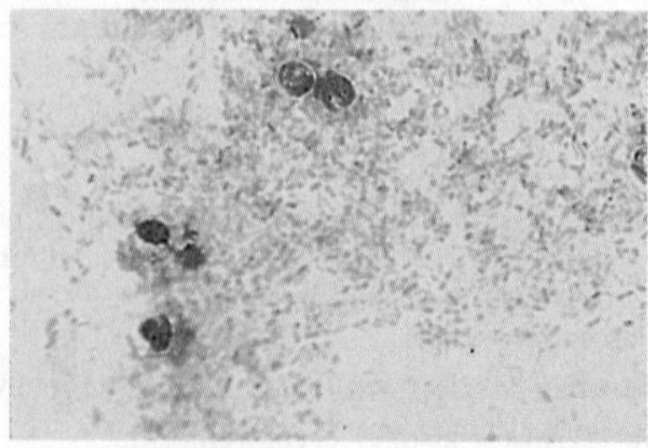

■ *Cryptosporidium* in feces, staining as bright red spheres (acid-fast stain).

dumbbell c's crystals of calcium oxalate occurring in the urine.

ear c. statoconium.

hedgehog c's a spiny form of uric acid concretions.

hydroxyapatite c. microscopic crystals of hydroxyapatite occurring in joints or bursae in a variety of connective tissue disorders. See also *apatite deposition disease*, under *disease*.

knife rest c's coffin lid c's.

liquid c's certain liquids which manifest some of the optical properties of crystals and the hydrodynamic properties of fluids, e.g., phosphatidylcholine.

c's of Reinke see under *crystalloid*.

rock c. quartz; a transparent form of silicon dioxide (silica), SiO_2; used for lenses.

scintillation c. a substance that emits a flash of light (scintillation) when contacted by high-energy particles, such as alpha, beta, or gamma rays, such as a sodium iodide crystal with a trace impurity of thallium used in the Anger camera to detect gamma radiation.

Teichmann c's crystals of hemin, seen in microscopic tests for the presence of blood.

thorn apple c's yellow or reddish brown spheres of ammonium urate which are covered with sharp spicules or prisms, as found in the urine.

Virchow c's yellow or orange crystals of hematoidin sometimes seen in extravasated blood.

whetstone c's crystals of xanthine sometimes seen in urine.

crys·tal·bu·min (kris″təl-bu′min) 1. an albuminous substance found in an aqueous extract of the crystalline lens. 2. a general term for crystallizable albumins of the type of egg albumin and serum albumin.

crys·tal·lin (kris-tal′in) a globulin existing in the crystalline lens of the eye. *Alpha c.* is precipitated by dilute acetic acid; *beta c.* is not.

crys·tal·line (kris′tə-lēn) 1. pertaining to crystals. 2. resembling a crystal in nature or clearness.

crys·tal·li·za·tion (kris″təl-ĭ-za′shən) the formation of crystals; conversion to a crystalline form.

fern-leaf c. crystallization of cervical mucus in a fernlike pattern, observable during the first half of the menstrual cycle and said to be most conspicuous at the time of ovulation.

crys·tal·log·ra·phy (kris″təl-og′rə-fe) [*crystal* + *-graphy*] the science dealing with the study of crystals.

x-ray c. the determination of the three-dimensional structure of molecules by means of diffraction patterns produced by x-rays of crystals of the molecules.

crys·tal·loid (kris′tə-loid) [*crystal* + *-oid*] 1. resembling a crystal. 2. a substance smaller than a colloid, in solution passing readily through semipermeable membranes, lowering the freezing point of the solvent containing it, and generally capable of being crystallized. Cf. *colloid* (def. 2).

Charcot-Böttcher c's slender spindle-shaped crystals 10 to 25 μm long, commonly found in Sertoli cells of the human testis but not in other species.

c's of Reinke conspicuous, variously shaped, crystal-like structures contained in Leydig cells.

crys·tal·lu·ria (kris″təl-u′re-ə) the excretion of crystals in the urine, producing renal irritation.

Crys·to·dig·in (kris″to-dij′in) trademark for preparations of digitoxin.

CS cesarean section; coronary sinus; conditioned stimulus; Cockayne syndrome; *o*-chlorobenzylidenemalononitrile.

Cs cesium.

CSAA Child Study Association of America.

CSC coup sur coup.

Csen·des procedure (chen′des) [Attila *Csendes* Juhasz, Hungarian-born Chilean gastroenterologist and surgeon, born 1941] see under *procedure*.

CSF cerebrospinal fluid; colony-stimulating factor.

CSF-1 macrophage colony-stimulating factor.

CSGBI Cardiac Society of Great Britain and Ireland.

CSII continuous subcutaneous insulin infusion; see *insulin pump*, under *pump*.

CSM cerebrospinal meningitis.

C-spine cervical spine.

CST contraction stress test.

CT computed tomography.

CTA Canadian Tuberculosis Association.

CTBA cetrimonium bromide.

ctei•no•phyte (ti′no-fīt) [Gr. *kteinein* to kill + *-phyte*] a fungus that has a destructive influence upon its host; limited to chemical rather than parasitic activity.

cteno- [Gr. *kteis*, gen. *ktenos* comb] a combining form denoting relationship to a comb or comblike structure.

Cte•no•ce•phal•i•des (te″no-sə-fal′ĭ-dēz) [*cteno-* + *cephalo-* + *eidos* form, shape] a genus of fleas often found parasitic on domestic animals.

C. ca′nis a species frequently found on dogs, which may transmit the dog tapeworm to humans.

C. fe′lis a species commonly found on cats that transmits cat flea typhus and murine typhus.

Cte•noph•thal•mus (te″nof-thal′məs) [*cteno-* + Gr. *ophthalmos* eye] a genus of fleas. *C. agry′tes* is the European mouse flea.

Cte•nus (te′nəs) a genus of spiders. *C. fe′rus* is the wandering spider of South America.

C-ter•mi•nal (tur′mĭ-nəl) the end of the peptide chain carrying the free alpha carboxyl group of the last amino acid, conventionally written to the right.

CTL cytotoxic T lymphocytes.

CTP cytidine triphosphate.

CTP syn•thase (sin′thās) [EC 6.3.4.2] an enzyme of the transferase class that catalyzes the transfer of an amino group to UTP to form CTP, using glutamine or ammonia as a donor. The reaction is part of pyrimidine nucleotide biosynthesis.

Cu copper (L. *cu′prum*).

cu•beb (ku′bəb) [L. *cubeba;* Arabic *kabāba*] 1. a plant of the species *Piper cubeba.* 2. the dried, unripe, almost fully grown fruit of *P. cubeba*, which contains 10 to 18 per cent volatile oil, cubebin, resins, fat, and wax. It has stimulant, local irritant, and mild urinary antiseptic properties. Ingestion of high dosages causes irritation of the kidneys and urinary tract, sometimes with nausea, vomiting, diarrhea, fever, skin eruptions, and other symptoms; in severe poisonings, death from respiratory failure may occur.

Cu•bi•cin (ku′bĭ-sin) trademark for a preparation of daptomycin.

cu•bi•cle (ku′bĭ-kəl) a compartment in a larger area, such as a dormitory or a ward, separated from similar adjoining compartments and from the rest of the room by low partitions.

cu•bi•tal (ku′bĭ-təl) 1. pertaining to the elbow. 2. pertaining to the ulna or to the forearm.

cu•bi•ta•lis (ku-bĭ-ta′lis) [L.] cubital.

cu•bi•to•car•pal (ku″bĭ-to-kahr′pəl) pertaining to the ulna and the carpus.

cu•bi•to•ra•di•al (ku″bĭ-to-ra′de-əl) pertaining to the ulna and the radius.

cu•bi•tus (ku′bĭ-təs) [L.] [TA] elbow: the bend in the upper limb between the arm and forearm.

c. val′gus deformity of the elbow in which the forearm (judged with the palm facing forward) deviates away from the midline of the body when extended.

c. va′rus deformity of the elbow, due to lateral angulation of the joint and accompanied by deviation of the forearm toward the midline of the body when the forearm is extended; called also *gun stock deformity.*

cu•boid (ku′boid) [Gr. *kyboeidēs*] 1. resembling a cube. 2. the cuboid bone (os cuboideum [TA]).

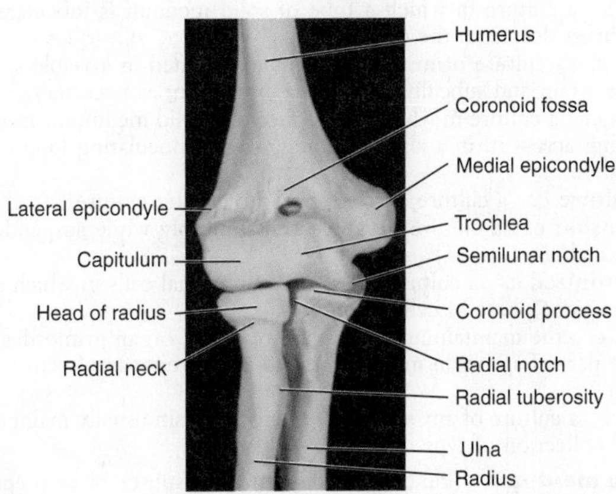

■ Cubitus (elbow) in an anterior view.

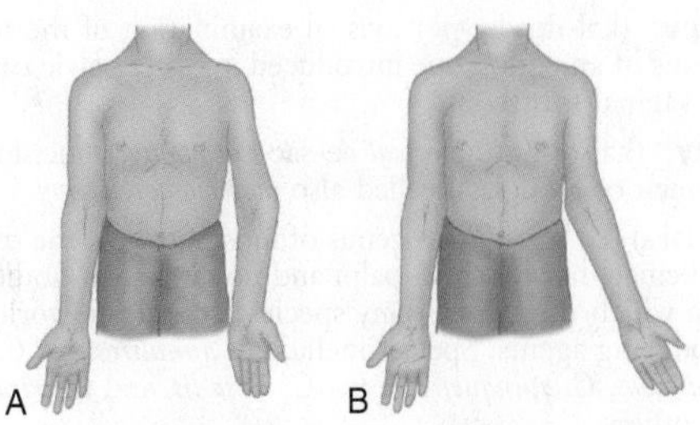

■ *(A)* Cubitus varus; *(B)* cubitus valgus.

cu•boi•dal (ku-boi′dəl) resembling a cube.

Cu•bo•me•du•sae (ku″bo-mə-doo′se) an order of jellyfish that have four-sided cup-shaped bodies; genera of medical importance include *Chironex* and *Chiropsalmus.*

cu•bo•me•du•san (ku″bo-mə-doo′sən) 1. pertaining to Cubomedusae. 2. a jellyfish of the order Cubomedusae.

cu•co•line (ku′ko-lēn) sinomenine.

cu•cul•la•ris (ku″ku-lar′is) [L. *cucullus* hood] musculus trapezius.

cu•cum•ber (ku′kəm-bər) [L. *cucumis*] 1. any of various species of the genus *Cucumis.* 2. the edible fruit of any of these species, chiefly *C. sativus;* their seeds are diuretic and their juice is astringent. 3. something resembling the fruit of the cucumber plant.

bitter c. colocynth.

sea c. any of several species of cylindrical echinoderms, especially those of the genus *Holothuria.* They are eaten as delicacies in Asia, but some species contain the hemotoxin holothurin.

Cu•cum•is (ku′kəm-is) a genus of plants of the family Curcurbitaceae. It includes several edible species and some that have medicinal properties, such as *C. sati′vus* L., the cucumber (q.v.).

Cu•cur•bi•ta (ku-kur′bĭ-tə) a genus of herbaceous vines of the family Cucurbitaceae, including the squashes, pumpkins, and some gourds, that produce fleshy, many-seeded fruits with thick, hard rinds. The seeds of *C. pe′po*, the pumpkin, are used medicinally.

cu•cur•bi•tol (ku-kur′bĭ-tol) a sterol, $C_{24}H_{40}O_4$, obtained from watermelon seeds.

cud (kud) the bolus of partially digested food that a ruminant casts back up from the rumen to be chewed a second time.

cud•bear (kud′bār) a red-brown powder, obtained from lichens, such as *Lecanora tartarea*, and used as a coloring matter in pharmacy.

cud•ding (kud′ing) rumination (def. 1).

cuff (kuf) a small bandlike structure encircling a part.

musculotendinous c. a cuff formed by intermingled muscle and tendon fibers; see *rotator c.*

rotator c. a musculotendinous structure about the capsule of the shoulder joint, formed by the inserting fibers of the supraspinatus, infraspinatus, teres minor, and subscapularis muscles, blending with the capsule, and providing mobility and strength to the shoulder joint.

vaginal c. the upper portion of the vagina, surrounding the vaginal portion of the cervix.

cuff•ing (kuf′ing) the formation of a cufflike surrounding border, such as collections of leukocytes surrounding blood vessels, noted in certain viral diseases and in multiple sclerosis. Called also *perivascular cuffing.*

cui•rass (kwe-rahs′) [Fr. *cuirasse* breastplate] a covering for the chest, such as the plastic shell or bubble used in a cuirass respirator (q.v.).

tabetic c. an area of diminished sense of touch encircling the chest of a patient with tabes dorsalis.

Cuj. [L.] cu′jus (of which).

cu•lard (ku-lahrd′) myofiber hyperplasia.

cul-de-sac (kul″də-sak′) [Fr. “dead-end street”] a blind pouch or cecum; a tubular cavity closed at one end, such as a diverticulum.

conjunctival c.-de-s. either of the conjunctival fornices; see *fornix conjunctivae inferior* and *fornix conjunctivae superior.*

Douglas c.-de-s., pelvic c.-de-s. excavatio rectouterina.

cul•do•cen•te•sis (kul″do-sen-te′sis) [*cul-de-*sac + *-centesis*] aspiration of fluid from the rectouterine space by puncture of the apex of the vaginal wall.

cul•do•scope (kul′do-skōp) an endoscope for performing culdoscopy.

cul·dos·co·py (kəl-dos′kə-pe) visual examination of the female pelvic viscera by means of an endoscope introduced into the pelvic cavity through the posterior vaginal fornix.

cul·dot·o·my (kəl-dot′ə-me) [*cul-de*-sac + *-tomy*] incision into the cul-de-sac (pouch of Douglas); called also *posterior colpotomy*.

Cu·lex (ku′ləks) [L. "gnat"] a genus of mosquitoes of the tribe Culicini, subfamily Culicinae, having short palpi and holding their bodies parallel to the surface on which they rest. Many species around the world are vectors of disease-producing agents. Species include *C. annuliros′tris, C. fa′tigans, C. moles′tus, C. pi′piens, C. quinquefascia′tus, C. tarsa′lis,* and *C. tritaeniorhyn′cus,* among many others.

cu·lic·i·cide (ku-lis′ĭ-sīd) culicide.

Cu·lic·i·dae (ku-lis′ĭ-de) the mosquitoes, a family of insects of the suborder Nematocerca, order Diptera. There are two subfamilies of particular medical interest: Anophelinae and Culicinae, containing tribes Anophelini, Aedini, Culicini, Mansoniini, and others.

cu·li·ci·dal (ku″lĭ-si′dəl) destructive to gnats and mosquitoes.

cu·li·cide (ku′lĭ-sīd) [*culex* + *-cide*] an agent destructive to gnats and mosquitoes.

cu·lic·i·fuge (ku-lis′ĭ-fūj) [*culex* + *-fuge*] a preparation that repels gnats and mosquitoes.

Cu·li·ci·nae (ku″lĭ-si′ne) a subfamily of mosquitoes of the family Culicidae; genera of medical interest include *Aedes, Culex,* and *Mansonia.*

cu·li·cine (ku′lĭ-sin, ku′lĭ-sīn) 1. a member of the genus *Culex* or the tribe Culicini. 2. pertaining to, involving, or affecting mosquitoes of the genus *Culex* or the tribe Culicini.

Cu·li·ci·ni (ku-lĭ-si′ni) a tribe of mosquitoes of the subfamily Culicinae; genera of medical importance include *Culex* and *Culiseta.*

Cu·li·coi·des (ku-lĭ-koi′dēz) a genus of biting flies of the family Heleidae; some are vectors for viral diseases such as bluetongue and African horse sickness. *C. aus′teni* and *C. gra′hami* are intermediate hosts of the parasitic roundworm *Mansonella perstans. C. fu′rens* and possibly other species are intermediate hosts of *M. ozzardi.*

Cu·li·se·ta (ku″lĭ-se′tə) a genus of mosquitoes of the subfamily Culicinae, some of whom transmit disease viruses; formerly called *Theobaldia. C. inora′ta* is a vector of the Cache Valley virus and *C. melanu′ra* is a vector of the eastern and western equine encephalomyelitis viruses.

Cul·len sign (kul′ən) [Thomas Stephen *Cullen,* American surgeon, 1868–1953] see under *sign.*

cull·ing (kul′ing) the process of selective removal. The term is applied to the removal from the circulation, by the spleen, of abnormal erythrocytes, such as those occurring in congenital spherocytosis, or to the selective separation of other elements or organisms.

cul·men (kul′mən) pl. *cul′mina* [L. "summit"] [TA] (IV and V): the portion of the anterior lobe of the cerebellum that lies medially between the central lobule and the primary fissure; it is divided into anterior (IV) and posterior (V) parts by the intraculminate fissure.

cul·mi·na (kul′mĭ-nə) [L.] plural of *culmen.*

Culp-DeWeerd pyeloplasty (kulp′ de-wērd′) [Ormond Skinner *Culp,* American surgeon, 1910–1977; James Henry *DeWeerd,* American surgeon, born 1914] see under *pyeloplasty.*

cult (kult) a system of treating disease based on some special and unscientific theory of disease causation.

cul·ti·va·tion (kul″tĭ-va′shən) [L. *cultivatio*] the propagation of living organisms, applied especially to the propagation of cells in artificial media.

cul·tur·a·ble (kul′chər-ə-bəl) capable of being cultured.

cul·tur·al (kul′chər-əl) pertaining to a culture.

cul·ture (kul′chər) [L. *cultura*] 1. the propagation of microorganisms or of living tissue cells in special media conducive to their growth. 2. a growth of microorganisms or other living cells. 3. to induce the propagation of microorganisms or living tissue cells in media conducive to their growth. See also *culture medium.*

asynchronous c. a culture in which cells are randomly distributed with respect to the phase of cell division, as in an ordinary culture of bacteria or animal cells.

attenuated c. a culture of pathogenic microorganisms whose virulence is weakened or abolished.

axenic c. a pure culture of microorganisms, i.e., one free from contaminating microorganisms or, in the case of parasites, without the presence of the host.

blood c. microbiologic examination of a blood sample to check for presence of microorganisms.

cell c. 1. the maintenance or growth of animal cells in vitro. 2. a culture of such cells.

chorioallantoic c. the cultivation of microorganisms, cells, or tissues on the chorioallantois of the developing chick.

continuous flow c. the cultivation of bacteria in a continuous flow of fresh medium to maintain bacterial growth in logarithmic phase.

direct c. a culture of microorganisms made by direct transfer from a natural source to an artificial medium.

enrichment c. a culture of microorganisms grown on a medium, usually liquid, that has been supplemented to encourage the growth of a given type of organism.

hanging-block c. a culture grown on a block of agar medium fastened to a coverglass, which is then inverted over a hollow slide.

hanging-drop c. a culture in which the material to be cultivated is inoculated into a drop of fluid attached to a coverglass, which is inverted over a hollow slide.

mixed c. a culture that contains two or more kinds of microorganisms.

mixed lymphocyte c. (MLC) a type of lymphocyte proliferation test (q.v.) in which lymphocytes from two individuals are cultured together and the proliferative response (mixed lymphocyte reaction) is measured by ^{3}H-labeled thymidine uptake. The test may be performed as a "two-way" MLC in which cells of both individuals can proliferate or as a "one-way" MLC in which the cells of one individual are prevented from responding by treatment with radiation or mitomycin. Three controls are used: cultures of syngeneic pairs, both untreated and radiation- or mitomycin-treated, and a culture of allogeneic irradiated or mitomycin-treated pairs. The primary clinical use of MLC is selection of compatible donors for bone marrow and living-related renal allotransplantation and for typing of HLA-D antigens; it is also used in diagnosis of immunodeficiency diseases.

needle c. stab c.

plate c. a culture grown on a medium, usually agar or gelatin, on a Petri dish.

primary c. a cell or tissue culture made by direct transfer from a natural source to an artificial medium.

pure c. a culture that contains only one kind of microorganism, without any contaminants.

radioisotopic c. a bacterial culture in a medium containing ^{14}C-labeled carbohydrate. Metabolism is detected by the release of $^{14}CO_2$, offering earlier detection of growth than do conventional methods.

roll-tube c. a culture made by inoculating a tube of molten agar medium and rotating it while it is solidifying, the medium being dispersed in a thin layer on the inner surface of the tube. The method is used for making colony counts, particularly of anaerobic bacteria.

secondary c. a culture derived from a primary culture.

selective c. a culture grown on a medium, usually solid, that has been supplemented to encourage the growth of a single species of microorganism. It may also include substances that inhibit the growth of other species.

sensitized c. bacterial cells that have been incubated with specific antiserum.

shake c. a culture made by inoculating warm liquid agar culture medium in a tube and shaking to distribute contents evenly. Incubation of the resolidified culture allows the development of separated colonies; especially applicable to obligate anaerobes.

slant c., slope c. a culture made on a slanting surface of a solidified medium in a tube, the tube being tilted to provide a greater surface area for growth.

stab c. a culture in which a tube of solid medium is inoculated by a needle thrust deep into the contents.

stock c. a culture of microorganisms maintained in a viable state as a reference strain and subcultured into fresh medium as necessary.

streak c. a culture in which the surface of a solid medium is inoculated by drawing across it, in a zigzag fashion, a wire inoculating loop carrying the inoculum.

subculture c. a culture derived from an existing culture.

suspension c. a culture in which cells multiply while suspended in a suitable medium.

synchronized c. a culture of bacterial or animal cells in which all cells are in the same phase of cell division.

tissue c. the maintaining or growing of tissue, organ primordia, or the whole or part of an organ in vitro so as to preserve its architecture and/or function.

type c. a culture of any species of microorganism usually maintained in a central collection of type cultures.

cul·ture me·di·um (kul′chər me′de-əm) any substance or preparation used for the cultivation of living cells.

Culture Medium

Abbreviations used in this table are: a. = agar, b. = broth, ba. = base, c. = culture medium, m. = medium.

agar c. m. a culture medium in which agar is used as the solidifying agent.
Amies transport medium an agar medium containing sodium thioglycolate, sodium and potassium chloride, phosphate buffer, calcium chloride, magnesium chloride, and neutral charcoal, used for transport of specimens for anaerobic culture.
antibiotic c. m. 3 FDA a broth medium containing peptone, yeast and beef extracts, sodium chloride, glucose, and potassium buffer, used for testing the activity of antibiotic agents against fungi.
antibiotic c. m. 12 FDA an agar medium containing peptone, yeast and beef extracts, sodium chloride, and glucose, used for agar dilution susceptibility tests with antifungal antibiotics. Called also *nystatin assay a.*
beef infusion c. m. see *infusion m.*
Bennett agar an agar medium containing casein digest, yeast extract, beef extract, and glucose, used as an isolation medium for *Nocardia* and *Streptomyces.*
BG agar brilliant green a.
B-G agar Bordet-Gengou a.
BHIA medium brain-heart infusion agar medium; see *brain-heart infusion medium.*
bile-esculin agar an agar medium containing beef extract, peptone, oxgall, ferric citrate, and esculin, sometimes supplemented with horse serum, used for the identification of group D streptococci.
birdseed agar Staib a.
bismuth-sulfite agar an agar culture medium containing beef extract, peptone, glucose, sodium sulfite, bismuth ammonium citrate, and brilliant green, used for samples of feces and other clinical specimens to isolate *Salmonella* species and serovars, especially *S. enterica* subsp. *enterica* serovar Typhi. Called also *BS agar* and *Wilson-Blair c. m.*
blood agar an agar medium containing heart infusion, peptone, and sodium chloride, autoclaved and enriched by the addition of sterile defibrinated blood, used for primary plating and subculturing, especially to determine bacterial hemolysis. The blood used may be sheep (for group A *Streptococcus*), rabbit, or horse.
Bordet-Gengou agar an agar base containing potato infusion, glycerol, and sodium chloride, enriched with blood, used for the isolation of *Bordetella pertussis* and *B. parapertussis.* Called also *B-G a.*
brain-heart infusion medium an agar medium containing calf brain and beef heart infusion, peptone, glucose, and phosphate buffer; sheep blood may also be added. It is used for the cultivation of bacteria, actinomycetes, and fungi. A broth medium without the agar is used for cultivating the pneumococcus for the bile solubility test. Called also *BHIA m.*
brilliant green agar a highly selective primary isolation medium containing yeast extract, peptone, lactose, sucrose, sodium chloride, phenol red, and brilliant green in an agar base, used for the culture of salmonellae other than the serovar causing typhoid fever. Called also *BG a.*
***Brucella* agar** an agar medium containing pancreatic digest of casein, peptic digest of animal tissue, yeast autolysate, and glucose, for the culture and isolation of *Brucella.* It may be supplemented by the addition of sheep blood and vitamin K_1 solution for the isolation of anaerobic bacteria.
BS agar bismuth sulfite a.
buffered glycerol-saline base (Sachs) a broth medium containing sodium chloride, phosphate buffer, phenol red, and glycerol, used to transport and preserve fecal specimen material.
***Campylobacter* medium** an agar medium containing pancreatic casein digest, peptic digest of animal tissues, yeast autolysate, glucose, sodium chloride, and sodium bisulfite, supplemented with sheep erythrocytes, vancomycin, trimethoprim, polymyxin, amphotericin, and cephalothin; used for isolating *Campylobacter* from specimens of fecal origin.
carbohydrate broth a broth medium that contains heart infusion or peptone, sodium chloride, and an indicator supplemented with a single carbohydrate, used to test the ability to ferment various sugars.
Cary-Blair transport medium an agar medium containing thioglycolate, phosphate, and sodium chloride, used for the collection and holding of clinical specimens containing gram-negative facultative organisms. The medium may be supplemented with calcium chloride, sodium bisulfite, and resazurin for culture of anaerobes.
casein agar a medium containing dehydrated skim milk and agar, used for differentiation of *Nocardia* and *Streptomyces.*
cefsulodin-irgasan-novobiocin agar a selective medium for *Yersinia.* Called also *CIN a.*
cetrimide agar an agar medium containing peptone, magnesium chloride, potassium sulfate, cetrimonium hydrochloride (cetrimide), and sometimes glycerol, used for the differentiation of strains of *Pseudomonas.*
charcoal agar a beef heart infusion–peptone culture medium containing soluble starch, yeast extract, and charcoal. The base medium is supplemented with sheep blood and cephalexin for the selective culture of *Bordetella pertussis.*
charcoal–yeast extract agar an agar medium containing activated charcoal, L-cysteine, ferric pyrophosphate, and yeast extract, used for the culture of *Legionella.* Called also *CYE a.*
charcoal–yeast extract diphasic blood c. m. a diphasic medium consisting of a lower solid slant containing charcoal and agar, partially covered with a liquid broth containing yeast extract, L-cysteine, and ferric nitrate. It is used for the culture of *Legionella.*
chlamydospore agar an inorganic salt medium containing polysaccharide, biotin, and trypan blue, for the identification of *Candida albicans* by favoring the formation of chlamydospores which are stained blue by the dye.
chocolate agar an agar medium containing casein digest, peptone, cornstarch, sodium chloride, and phosphate buffer; sterile hemoglobin or fresh blood is added and the medium heated until the color is chocolate brown. Other agar media may also be used as the base. It is used for the isolation of fastidious organisms, e.g., *Haemophilus influenzae* and *Neisseria* species.
chopped meat broth a liquid medium containing chopped meat treated with sodium hydroxide, casein digest, yeast extract, phosphate buffer, and cysteine; it may also include hemin, vitamin K_1, glucose, and resazurin. It is used for the cultivation of anaerobic bacteria, especially *Clostridium* species. Called also *CM b.*
Christensen urea agar an agar medium containing peptone or gelatin digest, sodium chloride, glucose, phenol red, urea, and phosphate buffer, used to detect urease production, especially in enteric bacteria such as species of *Proteus, Cryptococcus,* and aerobic actinomycetes. See also *urease test b.*
CIN agar cefsulodin-irgasan-novobiocin a.
citrate agar (Simmons) an agar medium containing sodium citrate, sodium chloride, magnesium sulfate, bromthymol blue, and phosphate buffer, used to determine the ability of gram-negative bacilli, particularly the Enterobacteriaceae, to utilize citrate as the sole carbon source.
CM broth chopped meat b.
CNA agar Columbia colistin–nalidixic acid a.
Columbia colistin–nalidixic acid agar an agar medium containing peptone, cornstarch, sodium chloride, colistin, nalidixic acid, and sheep blood, used for the selective culture of gram-positive cocci, especially *Proteus* species. Called also *CNA a.*
corn meal agar an agar medium containing corn meal infusion, used to stimulate sporulation in the identification of fungi. With the addition of Tween 80 it stimulates the production of chlamydospores by species of *Candida.* It may also be supplemented with glucose, sucrose, and yeast extract for the general culture of fungi.
cycloserine-cefoxitin-fructose–egg yolk agar an agar medium containing peptone, sodium chloride, magnesium sulfate, fructose, neutral red, and phosphate buffer, supplemented with cycloserine, cefoxitin, and egg yolk, used as a selective medium for *Clostridium difficile.*
CYE agar charcoal–yeast extract a.
cystine-heart agar an agar medium containing beef heart infusion, peptone, glucose, sodium chloride, and L-cystine. The medium is supplemented with hemoglobin for the in vitro conversion of dimorphic hyaline molds.
cystine-tellurite agar an agar medium containing meat infusion, potassium tellurite, cystine, and agar enriched with blood, used for the isolation of *Corynebacterium diphtheriae.*
cystine-trypticase agar an agar medium containing cystine, pancreatic digest of casein, sodium chloride, sodium sulfite, and phenol red, an aerobic differential medium for the general culture of pathogenic bacteria,

including fastidious organisms. It may be supplemented with specific sugars and used to test fermentation reactions in *Neisseria* species.

Czapek-Dox agar, **Czapek solution agar** an agar medium containing sucrose, sodium nitrate, magnesium sulfate, potassium chloride, ferrous sulfate, and potassium buffer, used for the culture of *Nocardia, Streptomyces,* and fungi. Called also *Czapek-Dox solution.*

decarboxylase broth a liquid culture medium containing beef extract, peptone, and glucose, to which is added an amino acid (commonly lysine, arginine, or ornithine), for the determination of the amino acid decarboxylase activity as a differential character of bacteria, especially Enterobacteriaceae.

deoxycholate citrate (Leifson) agar an agar medium containing meat infusion, peptone, lactose, sodium and ferric citrates, sodium deoxycholate, and neutral red, used for the primary culture and isolation of *Salmonella* and *Shigella.* Called also *LDC a.*

deoxycholate (Leifson) agar an agar medium containing peptone, lactose, sodium and ferric citrates, sodium chloride, sodium deoxycholate, neutral red, and potassium buffer, used for the isolation of Enterobacteriaceae and differentiation of lactose-fermenting and non–lactose-fermenting species. Called also *LD a.*

differential c. m. a culture medium, usually solid, that reveals the presence of two or more similar microorganisms by differences in the appearance of their colonies. Such a medium may or may not be selective also.

DNase test agar an agar medium containing deoxyribonucleic acid, peptone, sodium chloride, and toluidine blue, used for differentiating strains of *Serratia, Enterobacter,* and *Staphylococcus.*

egg yolk agar an agar medium containing peptone, phosphate buffer, sodium chloride, magnesium sulfate, glucose, and egg-yolk emulsion, used for the culture of *Bacillus anthracis.* When supplemented with hemin or yeast extract, it may be used for the culture of *Clostridium* and for the demonstration of lecithinase and lipase activity.

EMB agar eosin–methylene blue a.

enriched c. m. a basic medium to which specific nutrients, e.g., serum, blood, and vitamins, have been added to promote the growth of particular organisms.

eosin–methylene blue agar an agar medium containing peptone, lactose, eosin Y, methylene blue, and dipotassium phosphate; sucrose may be added. It is used for the primary isolation of species of Enterobacteriaceae. Called also *EMB a.*

esculin c. m. an agar medium containing heart infusion, peptone, sodium chloride, ferric citrate, and esculin, used to differentiate *Escherichia* from *Shigella.*

FDA medium 1. antibiotic c. m. 3 FDA. 2. antibiotic c. m. 12 FDA.

Feeley-Gorman agar an agar medium containing casein hydrolysate, beef extract, starch, L-cysteine, and ferric pyrophosphate, used for the culture of *Legionella.* A broth culture without the agar is also used for the same purpose. Called also *F-G a.*

fermentation medium a basal medium containing no carbohydrate to which is added a single sugar to be tested for fermentability.

F-G agar Feeley-Gorman a.

Fildes enrichment agar a sterile enzymatic digest of sheep blood added to liquid or solid culture media for the cultivation and isolation of *Haemophilus influenzae* and fastidious streptococci.

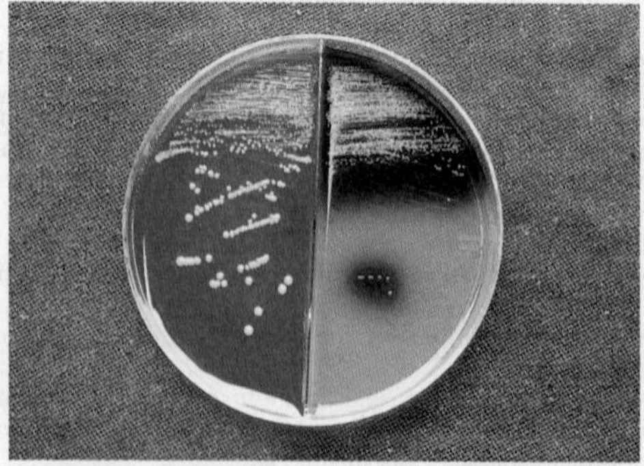

■ Selective culture medium. *Bacteroides fragilis* grows on bile-esculin agar; most aerobic and anaerobic bacteria are inhibited by bile and gentamicin in this medium, whereas *B. fragilis* is stimulated by bile, resistant to gentamicin, and able to hydrolyze esculin, producing a black precipitate.

Fletcher medium a liquid culture medium containing peptone, and beef extract enriched with 20 per cent fresh pooled rabbit serum, for the isolation, cultivation, and maintenance of *Leptospira.*

gelatin c. m. a medium containing extract or infusion broth solidified with 12 per cent gelatin, used to determine gelatinase activity in the identification of *Serratia* and *Clostridium.* The medium may be supplemented with thioglycolate for cultivation of *Clostridium* in an aerobic environment.

GN broth gram-negative b.

gram-negative broth a liquid medium containing peptone, glucose, D-mannitol, sodium citrate, sodium desoxycholate, sodium chloride, and phosphate buffer, used as an enrichment medium for the primary culture of salmonellae and shigellae in fecal specimens. Called also *GN b.*

HAT medium a tissue culture medium containing hypoxanthine, aminopterin, and thymidine, used in somatic cell fusion experiments. Aminopterin (an antifolate) blocks de novo synthesis of purine and thymine nucleotides, but these compounds can be produced from hypoxanthine and thymidine by normal cells possessing the enzymes hypoxanthine phosphoribosyltransferase (HPRT) and thymidine kinase (TK).

HE agar Hektoen enteric a.

heart infusion agar an agar medium containing beef heart infusion, peptone, and sodium chloride, used as a base for blood agar and esculin agar.

Hektoen enteric agar an agar medium containing peptone, bile salts, yeast extract, lactose, sucrose, salicin, sodium chloride, sodium thiosulfate, ferric ammonium citrate, acid fuchsin, and bromthymol blue. It is a selective medium used for the primary isolation and identification of enteric pathogens, especially coliform organisms, salmonellae, and shigellae. Called also *HE a.*

infusion medium a medium containing infusion of fresh meat (commonly veal or beef), peptone, and sodium chloride, used as a liquid medium (broth) or solidified with agar, used for the culture of fastidious bacteria and as a base for enriched media.

kanamycin-vancomycin blood agar an agar medium containing casein digest, soybean meal digest, sodium chloride, yeast extract, sheep blood, L-cystine, vitamin K_1, kanamycin, and vancomycin, used for selective isolation of anaerobes, particularly *Bacteroides.*

kanamycin-vancomycin–laked blood agar an agar medium having the same ingredients as kanamycin-vancomycin blood agar except that the blood is laked (hemolyzed) by freezing and thawing. It is used to isolate the *Bacteroides melaninogenicus* group. Called also *KVLB a.*

Kligler iron agar triple sugar iron agar.

KVLB agar kanamycin-vancomycin–laked blood a.

laked blood agar a solid culture medium containing blood that has been hemolyzed to release hemin. Called also *LB a.*

LB agar laked blood a.

LD agar deoxycholate (Leifson) a.

LDC agar deoxycholate citrate (Leifson) a.

litmus-milk c. m. milk culture medium containing sufficient litmus solution to give it a deep lavender color, used to determine lactose fermentation and production of gas in the identification of *Clostridium perfringens.*

Littman agar an agar medium containing peptone, oxgall, glucose, and crystal violet. Streptomycin may be added to inhibit bacteria, and the medium may be supplemented with birdseed extract. It is used for the isolation and culture of fungi.

Loeffler coagulated serum medium a culture medium containing veal infusion, beef serum, and glucose, solidified by coagulation of the serum, used for the isolation of *Corynebacterium diphtheriae.*

Löwenstein-Jensen c. m. a solid medium containing asparagine, potato flour, glycerol, magnesium sulfate, malachite green, magnesium citrate, and whole eggs, used for the primary isolation of mycobacteria; the medium is solidified by heat coagulation of the egg.

lysine-iron agar an agar medium containing peptone, yeast extract, glucose, L-lysine, ferric ammonium citrate, sodium thiosulfate, and bromcresol purple, used to determine lysine decarboxylase and lysine deaminase in the Enterobacteriaceae, especially for the genera *Proteus* and *Providencia.*

McBride *Listeria* medium an agar medium containing peptone, beef extract, sodium chloride, glycine anhydride, lithium chloride, and phenylethanol, used for the cultivation of *Listeria.*

MacConkey agar an agar medium containing peptone, lactose bile salts, sodium chloride, neutral red, and crystal violet, used to

Culture Medium *Continued*

differentiate lactose fermenters (coliforms) from non–lactose fermenters among the enteric bacilli. Called also *MC a.*
malt extract agar an agar medium containing malt extract, peptone, and glucose, used for the cultivation of yeasts and molds.
mannitol-salt agar an agar medium containing beef extract, peptone, mannitol, phenol red, and 7.5 per cent sodium chloride, used for the selective isolation of pathogenic staphylococci.
Martin-Lester agar, Martin-Lewis agar a modification of chocolate agar containing antibiotics, used for the transport and primary isolation of *Neisseria gonorrhoeae* and *N. meningitidis.*
MC agar MacConkey a.
meat extract medium a culture medium prepared with an extract from meat.
meat infusion medium see *infusion m.*
methylene blue–milk c. m. a liquid medium containing skim milk powder and methylene blue, used in the identification of *Streptococcus.*
methyl red–Voges-Proskauer broth a broth culture medium containing peptone, glucose, and phosphate, used for the culture of coliform bacteria and differentiation by the methyl red and Voges-Proskauer tests. Called also *MR-VP b.*
Middlebrook 7H10 agar a complex agar medium containing ammonium sulfate, D-glutamic acid, sodium citrate, ferric ammonium phosphate, magnesium sulfate, pyridoxine, biotin, malachite green, and phosphate buffer. OADC enrichment, containing oleic acid, albumin, glucose, and beef catalase, is added. The medium is used for the primary isolation of mycobacteria and for antimicrobial susceptibility testing.
milk c. m. fresh or dehydrated skim milk used as a culture medium. See also *litmus-milk c. m.* and *methylene blue–milk c. m.*
modified semisolid Rappaport-Vassiliadis medium a primary culture medium for *Salmonella.*
motility test medium a culture medium containing beef extract and peptone, partially solidified by the inclusion of 0.4 per cent agar, used for the detection of motility of Enterobacteriaceae. A medium containing pancreatic casein digest, yeast extract, sodium chloride, and 0.3 per cent agar is used to determine motility in nonfermenting gram-negative bacteria.
MR-VP broth methyl red–Voges-Proskauer b.
Mueller-Hinton medium an agar medium containing beef infusion, peptone, and starch, used for the primary isolation of *Neisseria gonorrhoeae* and *N. meningitidis,* and for antibiotic and sulfonamide susceptibility testing. A broth medium (MHB), prepared by omitting the agar, is used to determine antibiotic susceptibility by broth dilution testing.
Mueller-Hinton-IH agar an agar medium containing beef infusion, casein hydrolysate, starch, hemoglobin, and a complex enrichment supplement, used for the culture of *Legionella.*
***Mycoplasma* isolation c. m.** an agar medium containing beef heart infusion, peptone, sodium chloride, horse extract, yeast extract, and penicillin; thallium acetate and amphotericin B may also be added to reduce bacterial and fungal contamination. A broth culture is made by omitting the agar. It is used for the culture and isolation of mycoplasmas.
nitrate broth nutrient broth containing sodium nitrate, for testing for the bacterial reduction of nitrate to nitrite.
nutrient c. m. a bacterial culture medium containing beef extract and peptone, used as a liquid medium (nutrient broth) or solidified with agar (nutrient agar, plain agar) for the culture of nonfastidious organisms.
NYC medium [*N*ew *Y*ork *C*ity] an agar medium containing protease peptone, cornstarch, phosphate buffer, horse plasma, hemoglobin, glucose, yeast dialysate, vancomycin, colistin, nystatin or amphotericin, and trimethoprim lactate, used as a selective medium for *Neisseria.*
nystatin assay agar antibiotic c. m. 12 FDA.
oatmeal-tomato paste agar an agar medium containing strained oatmeal and tomato paste, used for the formation of ascospores in dermatophyte fungi.
OF medium oxidation-fermentation m.
oxidation-fermentation medium an agar medium containing peptone, sodium chloride, bromthymol blue, potassium buffers, and glucose; lactose, mannitol, or sucrose may be used instead of glucose. The medium is used to distinguish oxidative from fermentative utilization of carbohydrates, a characteristic used to differentiate *Acinetobacter, Alcaligenes,* and *Pseudomonas* from the Enterobacteriaceae. Called also *OF m.*
PEA blood agar phenylethyl alcohol–blood a.
peptone-yeast extract–glucose medium a liquid medium containing peptone, yeast extract, glucose, resazurin, L-cysteine, and salts, used as a transport medium for anaerobes. It may be supplemented with hemin and vitamin K_1, and used to prepare broth cultures of anaerobes for gas-liquid chromatography. Called also *PYG m.*
Petragnani c. m. a culture medium containing milk, potato flour, potato, whole egg and egg yolk, and malachite green, for the culture of tubercle bacilli; the medium is solidified by heat coagulation of the egg.
phenol red medium a liquid medium containing peptone, sodium chloride, and phenol red, used as a base medium supplemented with various sugars for determining fermentation reactions.
phenylalanine agar an agar medium containing yeast extract, DL-phenylalanine, disodium phosphate, and sodium chloride, used to test for phenylalanine deaminase activity by members of the Enterobacteriaceae, especially species of *Proteus* and *Providencia.*
phenylethyl alcohol–blood agar an agar medium containing pancreatic digest of casein, papain digest of soybean meal, sodium chloride, and phenylethyl alcohol. Defibrinated blood may be added. It is used for the isolation of gram-positive cocci, especially in a mixed culture containing *Proteus* or other gram-negative bacilli. Called also *PEA blood a.*
potato-blood agar Bordet-Gengou a.
potato-dextrose agar a culture medium containing potato infusion and glucose (dextrose), for culturing and inducing sporulation in molds.
PRAS medium prereduced and anaerobically sterilized media, used for the culture of anaerobes. See *Cary-Blair transport m.* and *peptone-yeast extract–glucose m.*
purple broth base a broth medium containing peptone, beef extract, sodium chloride, and bromcresol purple, used as a base to which is added a sugar supplement for use in fermentation studies.
PYG medium peptone–yeast extract–glucose m.
rice grain medium a medium containing water and polished white rice that is autoclaved; used for the differentiation of species of *Microspora* and other dermatophytes.
rice-Tween agar an agar medium containing cream of rice and Tween-80 (polysorbate 80), used for the development of chlamydospores in *Candida* and other fungi.
Rogosa selective *Lactobacillus* agar a selective culture medium containing tryptone, yeast extract, glucose, arabinose, sucrose, acetate, citrate, sorbitan monooleate, phosphate buffer, and agar, used in the culture and presumptive identification of lactobacilli. Called also *SL a.*
SAB agar Sabouraud dextrose a.
Sabhi agar [*Sab*ouraud dextrose and *b*rain *h*eart *i*nfusion] an agar medium containing brain infusion, heart infusion, gelatin digest, glucose, sodium chloride, peptone, and phosphate buffer; chloramphenicol may be added. It is used for isolating clinically important fungi.
Sabouraud dextrose agar an agar medium containing glucose, peptone, pancreatic digest of casein, and peptic digest of animal tissue; antibiotics may be added. Used for the cultivation and identification of fungi. Called also *SAB a.*
***Salmonella-Shigella* agar** a selective differential culture medium containing beef extract, peptone, lactose, bile salts, sodium and ferric citrates, thiosulfate neutral red, and brilliant green, used for the primary isolation of enteric bacilli, especially *Salmonella* and *Shigella.* Called also *SS a.*
selective c. m. a liquid or solid culture medium that contains inhibitory substances (antibiotics, dyes, tellurite, bile salts, etc.) that allow the growth of the desired microorganism while inhibiting the growth of contaminants.
selenite broth a liquid medium containing peptone, lactose, phosphate, and sodium selenite, used as an enrichment medium for the isolation of *Salmonella* and *Shigella.*
semisolid c. m. 1. a culture medium containing 0.3 to 0.5 per cent agar to give it a semisolid consistency; see *motility test medium.* 2. a culture medium containing agar or gelatin that is liquid in the warm state and solid when cooled.
Simmons citrate agar citrate a. (Simmons).
SL agar Rogosa selective *Lactobacillus* a.
sodium chloride (6.5 per cent) c. m. a broth medium containing beef heart infusion, peptone, and 6.5 per cent sodium chloride, used for the selective culture of enterococci (especially group D streptococci) and other salt-tolerant organisms. Nutrient broth or soybean-casein digest agar supplemented with 6.5 per cent sodium chloride is also used for *Pseudomonas* and other nonfermenting gram-negative bacteria.

Culture Medium *Continued*

soybean casein digest agar an agar medium containing pancreatic casein digest, papaic soybean meal digest, and sodium chloride; used as a general purpose primary isolation medium and as a base for blood agar.
SS agar *Salmonella-Shigella* a.
Staib agar an agar medium containing an extract of *Guizottia abyssinica* seeds, creatinine, glucose, chloramphenicol, and diphenyl, used for the identification of the yeast *Cryptococcus neoformans.* Called also *birdseed a.*
starch agar an agar medium containing peptone, beef extract, sodium chloride, and soluble starch, used for determining hydrolysis of starch. Bromcresol purple may be included for identification of *Haemophilus vaginalis.*
Stuart broth, modified a culture medium containing inorganic salts, asparagine, and glycerol, enriched with rabbit serum and used for the isolation and culture of *Leptospira.*
TCBS agar thiosulfate citrate–bile salts–sucrose a.
tellurite-taurocholate gelatin agar a selective agar medium containing sodium taurocholate, potassium tellurite, and sodium carbonate, used for the isolation of *Vibrio.*
tetrathionate broth a liquid medium containing peptone, bile salts, calcium carbonate, and sodium thiosulfate, which is converted to tetrathionate by the addition of iodine immediately before use, used as a selective medium for the isolation of *Salmonella* serovars other than the one causing typhoid fever.
Thayer-Martin agar chocolate agar enriched with vitamins and other supplements, to which is added antibiotic inhibitors (vancomycin, colistin, and nystatin), used for the transport and primary culture of *Neisseria gonorrhoeae* and *N. meningitidis.* Called also *TM a.*
THIO broth thioglycolate b.
thioglycolate broth a liquid medium containing peptone, glucose, sodium chloride, sodium thioglycolate, L-cystine, sodium sulfite, and 0.7 per cent agar, enriched with rabbit serum. It is used as a general utility medium for the growth of both aerobic and anaerobic bacteria. Methylene blue may be added as a redox indicator, and the medium may be enriched with yeast extract, vitamin K_1, and hemin. Called also *THIO b.* Spelled also *thioglycollate b.*
thiosulfate citrate–bile salts–sucrose agar a selective medium containing peptone, yeast extract, citrate, thiosulfate, oxgall, sodium cholate, sucrose, sodium chloride, ferric citrate bromthymol blue, and thymol blue, used for the isolation of *Vibrio cholerae* and *V. parahaemolyticus.* Called also *TCBS a.*
Tindale agar a base composed of proteose-peptone, sodium chloride, and agar to which is added an enrichment of bovine serum, L-cystine, sodium thiosulfate, and potassium tellurite; used to detect *Corynebacterium diphtheriae,* which form grayish-black colonies surrounded by a black halo.
TM agar Thayer-Martin a.
Todd-Hewitt broth a liquid medium containing beef heart infusion, peptone, glucose, sodium chloride, sodium bicarbonate, and phosphate buffer, used for growing streptococci for serological grouping.
transport medium a medium used for transport of clinical specimens for bacteriological examination. See *Amies transport m., buffered glycerol-saline ba. (Sachs), Cary-Blair transport m.,* and *peptone–yeast extract–glucose m.*
triple sugar–iron agar an agar medium containing peptone, lactose, sucrose, glucose, ferrous ammonium sulfate, sodium thiosulfate, sodium chloride, and phenol red, used for the preliminary screening of Enterobacteriaceae. Production of hydrogen sulfide causes the formation of black ferrous sulfide along the stab line, gas production causes bubbles in the agar, and fermentation of the sugars is indicated by the amount of acid produced. Called also *TSI a.*
trypticase soy broth with agar a medium containing a trypsin digest of soybean meal, peptone, sodium chloride, phosphate buffer, and glucose with 0.1 per cent agar, used for the primary culture of fastidious bacteria, including anaerobes.
TSI agar triple sugar–iron a.
tyrosine-xanthine agar an agar medium containing nutrient agar and tyrosine or xanthine, used for differentiation of species of aerobic actinomycetes.
urea agar of Christensen Christensen urea a.
urease test broth the medium used in the urease test (def. 2); a liquid medium containing yeast extract, urea, phenol red, and phosphate buffer. See also *Christensen urea a.*
veal infusion c. m. see *infusion m.*
Wilson-Blair c. m. bismuth sulfite a.
XLD agar xylose-lysine-deoxycholate a.
XLT4 agar xylose-lysine-Tergitol 4 a.
xylose-lysine-deoxycholate agar an agar medium containing xylose, L-lysine, lactose, sucrose, sodium chloride, yeast extract, phenol red, sodium desoxycholate, sodium thiosulfate, and ferric ammonium citrate, used for isolating intestinal pathogens, especially *Shigella* and *Salmonella.* Called also *XLD a.*
xylose-lysine-Tergitol 4 agar an agar medium containing xylose, L-lysine, and Tergitol 4 (sodium tetradecyl sulfate), used as a primary culture medium for *Salmonella.* Called also *XLT4 a.*
yeast extract agar an agar medium containing yeast extract and phosphate buffer, used for identification of *Histoplasma capsulatum, Blastomyces dermatitidis,* and *Coccidioides immitis.*

cu•mu•la•tive (ku'mu-lə-tiv) [L. *cumulus* heap] increasing by successive additions, the total being greater than the expected sum of its parts.

cu•mu•lus (ku'mu-ləs) pl. *cu'muli* [L.] a little mound, usually formed by a collection of cells.

c. oo'phorus, ovarian c. a solid mass of follicular cells surrounding the oocyte in the side of a developing vesicular ovarian follicle.

cu•ne•ate (ku'ne-āt) [*cuneus* + *-ate*] wedge-shaped.

cu•nei (ku'ne-i) [L.] genitive and plural of *cuneus.*

cu•ne•i•form (ku-ne'ĭ-form) [*cuneus* + *form*] shaped like a wedge.

cu•neo•cu•boid (ku"ne-o-ku'boid) pertaining to the cuneiform and cuboid bones.

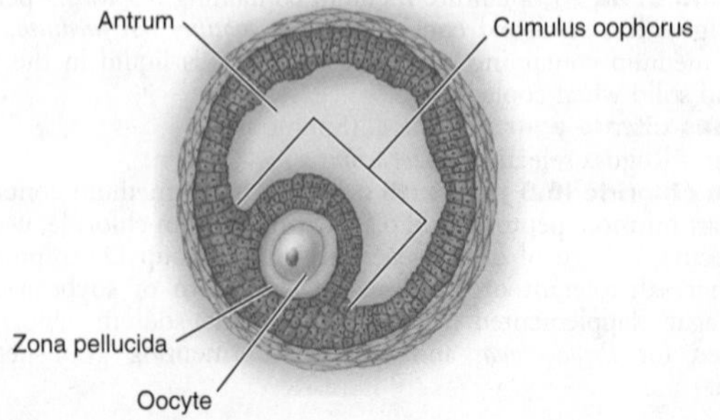

■ Ovarian follicle showing the cumulus oophorus surrounding the oocyte.

cu•neo•na•vic•u•lar (ku"ne-o-nə-vik'u-lər) pertaining to the cuneiform and navicular bones.

cu•neo•scaph•oid (ku"ne-o-skaf'oid) cuneonavicular.

cu•ne•us (ku'ne-əs) pl. *cu'nei* [L. "wedge"] [TA] a wedge-shaped lobule of the occipital lobe of the cerebrum on its medial aspect, between the parietooccipital and calcarine sulci.

cu•nic•u•li (ku-nik'u-li) [L.] genitive and plural of *cuniculus.*

Cu•nic•u•lus (ku-nik'u-ləs) a genus of burrowing rodents found in tropical parts of the Americas. *C. pa'ca* is the paca.

cu•nic•u•lus (ku-nik'u-ləs) pl. *cunic'uli* [L. "rabbit," "rabbit-burrow"] 1. a tunnel. 2. the burrow of an itch mite, *Sarcoptes scabiei,* in the skin.

cun•ni•linc•tus (kun"ĭ-link'təs) cunnilingus.

cun•ni•lin•gus (kun"ĭ-ling'əs) [*cunnus* + *lingere* to lick] oral stimulation of the female genitalia.

Cun•ning•ha•mel•la (kun"ing-ham-el'ə) a genus of fungi of the family Cunninghamellaceae, characterized by a lack of a sporangium and by conidia that arise from a vesicle. *C. bertholle'tiae* is a species that causes opportunistic mucormycosis of the lung in debilitated or immunocompromised patients, with progressive vascular invasion, thrombosis, and infarction.

Cun•ning•ha•mel•la•ceae (kun"ing-ham-əl-a'ce-e) a family of fungi of the order Mucorales, that lacks sporangia; it includes one pathogenic genus, *Cunninghamella.*

cup (kup) 1. a cupping glass. 2. a cup-shaped part or structure.

dry c. a cupping glass applied to the intact skin in order to induce a flow of blood to the area; no longer used.

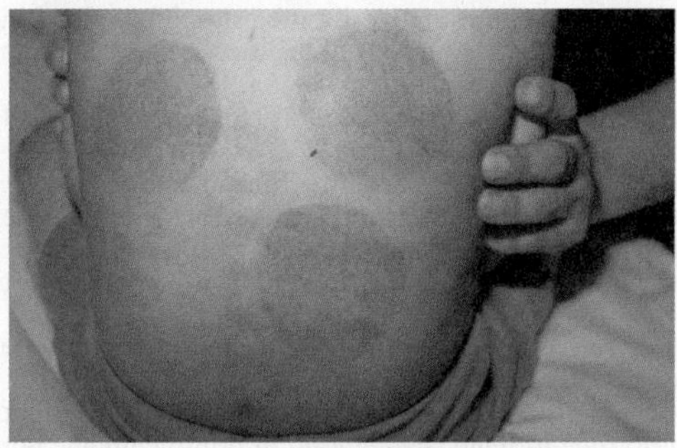

■ Cupping.

glaucomatous c. a type of depression of the optic disk seen in glaucoma.

optic c. 1. excavatio disci. 2. an indentation of the distal wall of the optic vesicle, brought about by rapid marginal growth and producing a double-layered cup, attached to the diencephalon by a tubular stalk.

physiologic c. excavatio disci.

wet c. a cupping glass applied to the incised skin in order to abstract blood; no longer used.

cu•po•la (koo'pə-lə) cupula.

cupped (kupt) hollowed out like a cup.

cup•ping (kup'ing) 1. the application of a small glass or bamboo cup to the skin, after exhausting the air from within it to create a vacuum, in order to draw blood and lymph to the surface of the body and increase local circulation; currently used in Chinese medicine. 2. the formation of a cup-shaped depression.

pathologic c. depression of the optic disk due to disease.

cu•pre•ine (ku'pre-ēn) an alkaloid from cuprea bark that is related to cinchonidine and has antimalarial properties.

cu•pre•mia (koo-pre'me-ə) [L. *cuprum* copper + *-emia*] the presence of copper in the blood. See also *hypercupremia.*

cu•pric (koo'prik) containing copper in its divalent form (=Cu), and yielding divalent ions (Cu^{2+}) in aqueous solution.

c. sulfate [USP] the pentahydrate sulfate salt of copper, $CuSO_4 \cdot 5H_2O$, a powerful emetic; used orally as an antidote to phosphorus poisoning. Topical application of a 1 per cent solution is used in the treatment of phosphorus burns of the skin. It is also used as a catalyst with iron in the treatment of iron deficiency anemia. In 1:1,000,000 concentration it is used to prevent growth of algae in ponds, reservoirs, and swimming pools. Called also *copper sulfate.*

Cu•pri•mine (koo'prĭ-mēn) trademark for a preparation of penicillamine.

cup•ri•myx•in (kup'rĭ-mik'sin) a veterinary antibacterial and antifungal.

cu•pri•uria (koo"pre-u're-ə) hypercupriuria.

cu•pro•phane (koo'pro-fān) a membranous substance made of regenerated cellulose, used in hemodialyzer membranes.

cu•prous (koo'prəs) containing copper in its monovalent form (Cu^+).

cu•pru•re•sis (koo"proo-re'sis) [L. *cuprum* copper + *-uresis*] hypercupriuria.

cu•pu•la (koo'pu-lə) pl. *cu'pulae* [L.] a small inverted cup or dome-shaped cap over some structure.

c. ampulla'ris [TA], **c. of ampullary crest** ampullary cupula: a cap of viscid, gelatinous fluid over the ampullary crest of the ear; in fixed material this cap stains slightly and is thus differentiated from the rest of the ampullar fluid. Called also *c. cristae ampullaris.*

c. coch'leae [TA] cupula of cochlea: the rounded or dome-shaped apex of the spiral cochlear duct.

c. cris'tae ampulla'ris c. ampullaris.

c. pleu'rae [TA], **c. pleura'lis** cupula of pleura: the domelike roof of the pleural cavity on either side, extending up through the superior aperture of the thorax.

cu•pu•li•form (koo'pu-lĭ-form") shaped like a small cup.

cu•pu•lo•gram (ku'pu-lo-gram") the record, in the form of a tracing, made during cupulometry.

cu•pu•lo•li•thi•a•sis (ku"pu-lo-lĭ-thi'ə-sis) the presence of calculi in the cupula of the posterior semicircular duct, a cause of benign paroxysmal positional vertigo.

cu•pu•lom•e•try (ku"pu-lom'ə-tre) an old method of testing vestibular function; subjects were accelerated and decelerated in a rotational chair and the duration of postrotational vertigo and nystagmus were plotted against angular deceleration.

cu•ran•de•ra (koo-rahn-da'rah) [Sp.] healer; a woman who practices curanderismo.

cu•ran•de•ris•mo (koo-ron"da-rēz'mo) [Sp. *curar* to heal] a traditional Mexican-American healing system, incorporating elements drawn from humoralism, from the practices of Spain and the Mediterranean basin, and from Native American cultural traditions of Mexico. According to curanderismo, disease may have not only natural but also spiritual causes, and healers *(curanderos)* treat a wide variety of physical, mental, social, and spiritual ailments; individual practictioners are considered to have gifts for certain types of healing.

cu•ran•de•ro (koo-rahn-da'ro) [Sp.] healer; a man who practices curanderismo.

cu•ra•re (koo-rah're) [South American Indian *Kurari*] a term applied to a wide variety of highly toxic extracts from numerous botanical sources, including various species of *Strychnos* and *Chondrodendron;* used originally as arrow poisons in South America. The most commonly used active principle of curare is tubocurarine (q.v.), obtained from *Chondodendron tomentosum.*

cu•ra•ri•form (koo-rah'rĭ-form) resembling curare.

cu•ra•ri•mi•met•ic (koo-rah"re-mi-met'ik) having an action similar to that of curare, or producing similar effects.

cu•rar•iza•tion (koo"rah-rĭ-za'shən) administration of curare until the physiologic effect of the drug is produced.

cur•a•tive (kūr'ə-tiv) [L. *curare* to take care of] tending to overcome disease and promote recovery.

curb (kərb) a thickening of the metatarsocalcaneal ligament of the horse, causing a swelling at the back of the hock joint and resulting in lameness.

Cur•cu•ma (kur'ku-mə) a genus of plants of the family Zingiberaceae, native to India, China, and the East Indies. *C. lon'ga* L. is turmeric, which yields the coloring agent and condiment also called turmeric.

cur•cu•min (kur'ku-min) an orange-yellow crystalline substance, the coloring principle of turmeric.

cure (kūr) [L. *curatio,* from *cura* care] 1. the course of treatment of any disease, or of a special case. 2. the successful treatment of a disease or wound. 3. a system of treating diseases. 4. a medicine effective in treating a disease. 5. the preservation of a product, such as tobacco, meat, or fish. 6. the hardening of a material by the process of curing. 7. a procedure for polymerization of resins such as those used in denture base materials. See also *curing.*

cu•ret (ku-ret') [Fr. *curette* scraper] 1. a spoon-shaped instrument for removing material from the wall of a cavity or other surface. Spelled also *curette.* 2. to remove growths or other material from the wall of a cavity or other surface with such an instrument.

Hartmann c. an instrument for removing adenoids.

cu•ret•tage (ku"rə-tahzh') [Fr.] the removal of growths or other material from the wall of a cavity or other surface, as with a curet; called also *curettement.*

apical c. periapical c.

gingival c. removal with a curet of the inflamed tissue wall of a periodontal pocket, including junctional and pocket epithelium and immediately underlying connective tissue. Called also *subgingival c.*

medical c. induction of bleeding from the endometrium by administration and withdrawal of a progestational agent.

periapical c. removal with a curet of diseased pathological soft tissues in the bony crypt surrounding a tooth root apex and smoothing of the apical surface of a tooth without excision of the tooth tip. Called also *apical c.*

subgingival c. 1. gingival curettage apical to the epithelial attachment to sever the connective tissue attachment down to the osseous crest without reflection of a flap. 2. gingival c.

suction c. vacuum c.

surgical c. a flap procedure to excise an inflamed periodontal pocket wall and the connective tissue attachment down to the osseous crest,

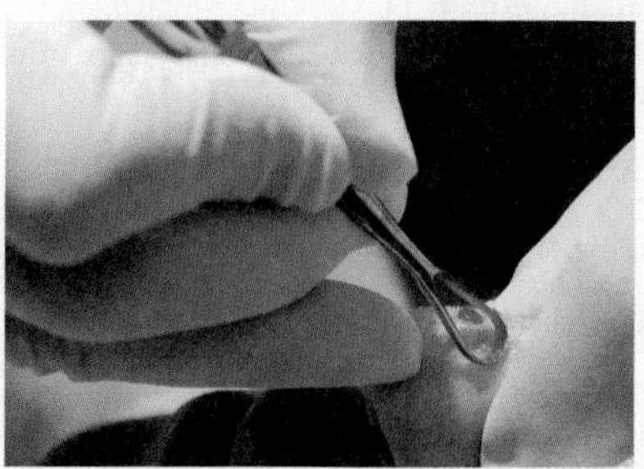

■ Curettage of a basal cell carcinoma.

followed by reattachment of the flap to the teeth. Called also *modified Widman flap.*

ultrasonic c. removal of inflamed tissue from the tooth surface and wall of the gingival crevice with an ultrasonic scaler.

vacuum c. removal of endometrial tissue or the entire contents of the uterus by means of a hollow curet introduced into the uterus through a dilated cervix, with suction through the curet; it may be done for diagnostic purposes or for an induced abortion. Called also *suction c.* or *aspiration* and *vacuum aspiration.*

cu•rette (ku-ret′) [Fr.] curet.

cu•rette•ment (ku-ret′ment) curettage.

physiologic c. enzymatic débridement.

Cu•rie's law (ku-rēz′) [Pierre *Curie,* French chemist, physicist, and Nobel prize winner, 1859–1906] see under *law.*

cu•rie (Ci) (ku′re) [Marie Sklodowska *Curie,* Polish-born chemist and physicist in France, 1867–1934, and Pierre *Curie,* French chemist and physicist, 1859–1906, Nobel prize winners] a unit of radioactivity, defined as the quantity of any radioactive nuclide in which the number of disintegrations per second is 3.700×10^{10}. Formerly abbreviated c.

cu•rie-hour (kūr′e our′) a unit of cumulated radioactivity equal to the presence of 1 curie for 1 hour. Abbreviated Ci-hr.

cu•rie•ther•a•py (ku″re-ther′ə-pe) originally, radium or radon therapy; but now applied to therapy given by emanations from any radioactive source.

cur•ing (kūr′ing) a method for promoting and accelerating hardening processes through the use of dampness, heat, cold, chemical agents, electromagnetic radiation, or other agents.

denture c. the process by which resinous denture base materials are polymerized; see also *resin.*

cu•ri•um (Cm) (kūr′e-əm) [Pierre and Marie *Curie*] the chemical element of atomic number 96, atomic weight 247, obtained by cyclotron bombardment of uranium and plutonium.

Cur•ling ulcer (kur′ling) [Thomas Blizard *Curling,* English physician, 1811–1888] see under *ulcer.*

curl•ing (kur′ling) helical or spiral.

Cu•ro•surf (ku′ro-surf″) trademark for a preparation of poractant alfa.

Cur•ra•ri•no syndrome (triad) (kur″ə-re′nō) [Guido *Currarino,* Italian-born American radiologist, born 1920] see under *syndrome.*

Cur•ra•ri•no-Sil•ver•man syndrome (kur″ə-re′no sil′vər-mən) [G. *Currarino;* Frederic Noah *Silverman,* American pediatrician, 1914–2006] see under *syndrome.*

cur•rent (kur′ənt) [L. *currens* running] 1. anything that flows. 2. electric c.

action c. the current generated in a cell membrane of a nerve or muscle by the action potential; it serves to depolarize adjacent membrane areas beyond the threshold, thus initiating a repetition of the action potential process along the nerve fiber. Called also *nerve-action c.*

alternating c. (AC) a current that periodically flows in opposite directions; its amplitude fluctuates as a sine wave.

ascending c. centripetal c.

axial c. the core of rapid flow *(laminar flow)* in the center of a channel, as in the lumen of a blood vessel, bordered or surrounded by a zone in which the elements move more slowly or do not move at all.

centrifugal c. an electric current in the body with the positive pole near the nerve center and the negative at the periphery; called also *descending c.*

centripetal c. an electric current passing through the body with the positive electrode on the nerve or at the periphery and the negative electrode near the nerve center: called also *ascending c.*

coagulating c. an electric current applied by a needle, ball, or other type of electrode to coagulate tissue.

convection c. a current caused by movement by convection of warmer fluid into an area of cooler fluid.

d'Arsonval c. a high-frequency, low-voltage current of comparatively high amperage. See also *high-frequency c.*

demarcation c. c. of injury.

descending c. centrifugal c.

direct c. (DC) a current that flows in one direction only; when modeled as a wave, its amplitude is constant. When used medically it is called *galvanic current.* This current has distinct and important polarity and marked secondary chemical effects.

electric c. the stream of electricity that moves along a conductor. Symbol *I.* An electric current is due to a difference of potential between two points, this difference being measured in *volts.* The volume of flow depends on the difference of potential and the resistance to be overcome and is measured in *amperes.* The quantity of current is measured in *coulombs.*

electrotonic c. a current induced in the sheath of a nerve by a current passing through the conducting part of that nerve, or by an action potential in an adjacent nerve.

fulguration c. the high-frequency current used in fulguration procedures.

galvanic c. a steady direct current, especially one produced chemically.

high-frequency c. an alternating current having a frequency of interruption or change of direction sufficiently high so that tetanic contractions are not set up when it is passed through living contractile tissues; see *d'Arsonval c.*

induced c. electricity in a circuit generated by proximity to another current, i.e., by induction.

c. of injury a flow of electric current to or from the injured region of an ischemic heart, due to regional alteration in transmembrane potential. See also *diastolic c. of injury* and *systolic c. of injury.*

c. of injury, diastolic net current flow from ischemic to normal cardiac tissue during diastole, due to more rapid repolarization of the injured region and thus a more positive transmembrane potential than in surrounding tissue. Cf. *systolic c. of injury.*

c. of injury, systolic net current flow from normal to ischemic cardiac tissue during systole, due to a decrease in the amplitude and duration of the action potential so that the transmembrane potential of the ischemic tissue is less negative than that of surrounding tissue. Cf. *diastolic c. of injury.*

nerve-action c. action c.

pacemaker c. the small net positive current flowing into certain cardiac cells, such as those of the sinoatrial node, causing them to depolarize.

saturation c. the amount of current in an x-ray tube when the voltage is sufficient to drive all the electrons produced from the cathode filament to the anode as fast as they are produced.

sinusoidal c. an alternating current whose form is that of a sine wave.

cur•ric•u•lum (kər-ik′u-ləm) pl. *curric′ula* [L.] a regular and established course of study.

Cursch•mann spirals (ko͞orsh′mahn) [Heinrich *Curschmann,* German physician, 1846–1910] see under *spiral.*

Cursch•mann-Bat•ten-Stei•nert syndrome (koorsh′mahn bat′ən shti′nərt) [Hans *Curschmann,* German physician, 1875–1950; Frederick Eustace *Batten,* English ophthalmologist, 1865–1918; Hans *Steinert,* German physician, early 20th century] myotonic dystrophy; see under *dystrophy.*

curse (kurs) an infliction thought to be invoked by a malevolent spirit.

Ondine c. primary alveolar hypoventilation.

Cur•ti•us syndrome (koor′te-us) [Friedrich *Curtius,* German internist, 1896–1975] see under *syndrome.*

cur•va•tu•ra (kur″və-tu′rə) gen. and pl. *curvatu′rae* [L.] curvature: a nonangular deviation from a straight course in a line or surface.

c. ma′jor gas′trica [TA] greater curvature of stomach: the left or lateral and inferior border of the stomach, marking the inferior junction of the anterior and posterior surfaces. Called also *greater gastric curvature.*

c. mi′nor gas′trica [TA] lesser curvature of stomach: the right or medial border of the stomach, marking the superior junction of the anterior and posterior surfaces. Called also *lesser gastric curvature.*

c. prima′ria colum′nae vertebra′lis [TA] primary curvature of vertebral column: a dorsally convex part of the spinal (vertebral) column; see *kyphosis thoracica* and *kyphosis sacralis.*

curvatu′rae secunda′riae colum′nae vertebra′lis [TA] secondary curvatures of vertebral column: dorsally concave sections of the spinal (vertebral) column; see *lordosis cervicis* and *lordosis lumbalis.*

cur•va•ture (kur′və-chər″) [L. *curvatura*] deviation from a rectilinear direction.

cervical c. lordosis cervicis.

compensating c. see under *curve.*

gastric c., greater curvatura major gastrica.

gastric c., lesser curvatura minor gastrica.

greater c. of stomach curvatura major gastrica.

lesser c. of stomach curvatura minor gastrica.

lumbar c. lordosis lumbalis.

occlusal c. curvea occlusalis.

pelvic c. kyphosis sacralis.

penile c. abnormal curving of the penis to one side when erect; called also *clubbed penis.*

Pott c. abnormal posterior curvature of the vertebral column caused by tuberculous caries.

primary c. of spinal column, primary c. of vertebral column curvatura primaria columnae vertebralis.

sacral c. kyphosis sacralis.

secondary c's of spinal column, secondary c's of vertebral column curvaturae secundariae columnae vertebralis.

Spee c., c. of Spee see under *curve.*

spinal c. 1. any of the normal primary or secondary curvatures of the vertebral column; see *curvatura primaria columnae vertebralis* and *curvaturae secundariae columnae vertebralis.* 2. deviation of the spine from its normal direction or position; see *kyphosis, lordosis,* and *scoliosis.*

thoracic c. kyphosis thoracica.

curve (kurv) [L. *curvum*] a nonangular deviation from a straight course in a line or surface.

alignment c. the dental curve determined by a line passing through the center of the teeth and paralleling the dental arch.

anti-Monson c. reverse c.

audibility c. a plotting of the relationship between frequency and the intensity of sound waves necessary to elicit a sensation.

Barnes c. the segment of a circle whose center is the promontory of the sacrum, the concavity being directed dorsally.

bell-shaped c. the curve of the probability density function of the normal distribution (q.v.).

Bragg c. a curve showing the increase in intensity of ionization produced by an ionizing particle as it loses velocity and energy; see also *Bragg peak*, under *peak.*

buccal c. the portion of the curve of occlusion from the mesial surface of the first premolar to the distal surface of the third molar.

cardiac output c. a graphic representation of cardiac output as a function of atrial pressure; it is a measure of the pumping ability of the heart under specific conditions. See also *Starling c.* and *venous return c.*

c. of Carus the normal axis of the pelvic outlet.

compensating c. the curve introduced in the construction of artificial dentures to compensate for the opening influence produced by the condylar and incisal guidances during lateral and protrusive mandibular excursive movements. Called also *compensating curvature.*

dental c. curvea occlusalis.

dissociation c. see *oxygen dissociation c.*

dose-effect c. a graphic representation of the effect (such as therapeutic response or the incidence of cancer) plotted against the dose of an agent (such as a drug or x-rays), showing the relationship of the effect to changes in the dose of the agent. See illustrations at *efficacy* and *potency.* Cf. *dose-frequency c.* and *dose-intensity c.*

dose-frequency c. a graphic representation of the relationship of the number of responses (such as cases of cancer) in a population to changes in the dose of an agent.

dose-intensity c. a graphic representation of the relationship of the intensity of effect (such as amount of vasodilation) in an individual to changes in the dose of an agent.

dose-response c. dose-effect c.

dromedary c. a temperature or other curve showing two phases of elevation separated by a phase of depression.

dye dilution c. an indicator dilution curve in which the indicator is a dye, usually indocyanine green; it is used in studies of cardiac output and other aspects of cardiovascular function.

force-displacement c. in structural testing of a given material, a graph showing the displacement in millimeters of a given material as different forces are applied, measured in newtons.

Frank-Starling c. Starling c.

gaussian c. bell-shaped c.

growth c. the curve obtained by plotting increase in size or numbers against the elapsed time, as a measure of the growth of a child, or the multiplication of microorganisms.

Harrison c. see under *groove.*

indicator dilution c. a graphic representation of the concentration of an indicator added in known quantity to the circulatory system and measured over time at a specific point in the system; the indicator is usually a dye (see *dye dilution c.*), radionuclide, or cold liquid (see *thermodilution*), and the curve is used in studies of cardiovascular function.

isodose c's diagrams delimiting body areas receiving equal quantities of radiation in radiotherapy.

isovolume pressure-flow c. a curve generated by plotting various values of pressures against the corresponding airflows at a single lung volume. At high lung volumes (approaching total lung capacity), the maximum flow or flow limitation is usually not reached. See illustration.

Kaplan-Meier survival c. a consistent estimate of the survival curve that can be computed from randomly censored data. At each patient death (or other endpoint) the conditional probability of survival during the interval since the last death is calculated as the number of patients observed to survive beyond that point (i.e., those who have not yet died and have not left the trial for other reasons) divided by the number at risk. The value of the survival curve at that point is calculated as the product of the conditional probabilities of survival for all of the intervals up to that point. Called also *product-limit estimate.*

labial c. the portion of the curve of occlusion between the distal surfaces of the two canine teeth in the dental arch.

Liley c. Liley chart.

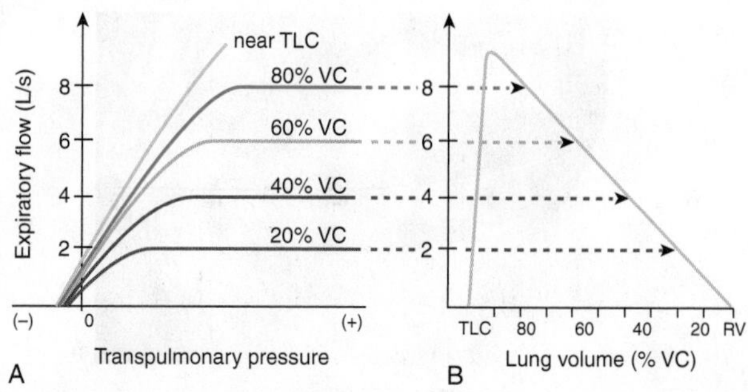

■ Series of isovolume pressure-flow curves *(A)*, from which can be constructed a maximal expiratory flow-volume curve *(B)*.

logistic c. an S-shaped curve that describes population growth under limiting conditions as a function of time; when the population is low, growth begins slowly, then becomes rapid and increases exponentially, finally slowing down and reaching equilibrium as the population reaches the maximum that the environment can support.

maximal expiratory flow–volume c. a curve generated during forced exhalation from total lung capacity to residual volume by plotting maximal expiratory flow against the corresponding lung volumes; it can also be constructed from a series of isovolume pressure-flow curves at different vital capacities. See illustration.

Monson c. a curve of occlusion conforming to a segment of the surface of a sphere 24.3 cm (8 in) in diameter, with its center in the region of the glabella. See also *compensating c.*

normal c., normal c. of distribution bell-shaped c.

occlusal c., c. of occlusion curvea occlusalis.

oxygen dissociation c. a graphic curve representing the normal variation in the amount of oxygen that combines with hemoglobin as a function of the partial pressure of oxygen. The curve is said to shift to the right *(the Bohr effect)* when less than a normal amount of oxygen is taken up by the blood at a given P_{O_2}, and to shift to the left *(the Haldane effect)* when more than a normal amount is taken up. Factors influencing the shape of the curve include changes in the blood pH, P_{CO_2}, and temperature, the presence of carbon monoxide, alterations in the constituents of the erythrocytes, and certain disease states. Called also *oxygen-hemoglobin dissociation c.*

oxygen-hemoglobin dissociation c., oxyhemoglobin dissociation c. oxygen dissociation c.

Price-Jones c. a frequency distribution curve of erythrocyte diameters, calculated electronically with a Coulter counter, a flow cytometer, or a similar instrument; it can detect conditions such as *macrocytic anemia* and *microcytic anemia.*

pulse c. sphygmogram.

receiver operating characteristic c. a curve that plots sensitivity versus [1 − specificity (or false-positive error rate)] to help determine the best cutoff point or points for demarcating dimensional data in diagnostic tests for disease, optimizing the balance between sensitivity and specificity.

regression c. a curve describing the relation between the average value of a dependent variable and the values of one or more independent variables; the regression curve of Y on X is the graph of the average value of Y associated with each value of X.

reverse c. in excessive wear of the teeth, obliteration of the cusps and formation of either flat or cupped-out occlusal surfaces, associated with reversal of the occlusal plane of the premolar and first and second molar teeth, so that the occlusal surfaces of the mandibular teeth slope facially instead of lingually, and those of the maxillary teeth incline lingually. Called also *anti-Monson c.*

ROC c. receiver operating characteristic c.

Spee c., c. of Spee anatomic curvature of the occlusal alignment of teeth, beginning at the tip of the lower canine, following the buccal cusps of the natural premolars and molars, and continuing to the anterior border of the ramus.

Starling c. a graphic representation of cardiac output, or other measure of ventricular performance, as a function of ventricular filling for a given level of contractility; as atrial pressure and venous return increase, cardiac output initially increases proportionately, then plateaus and decreases. Called also *ventricular function c.*

strength-duration c. a graphic representation of the relationship between the intensity of an electric stimulus at the motor point of a muscle and the length of time it must flow to elicit a minimal contraction; see also *chronaxy* and *rheobase.*

survival c. a graph of the probability of survival versus time, commonly used to present the results of clinical trials, e.g., a graph of the fraction of patients surviving (until death, relapse, or some other defined endpoint) at each time after a certain therapeutic procedure; see also *life table*, under *table.*

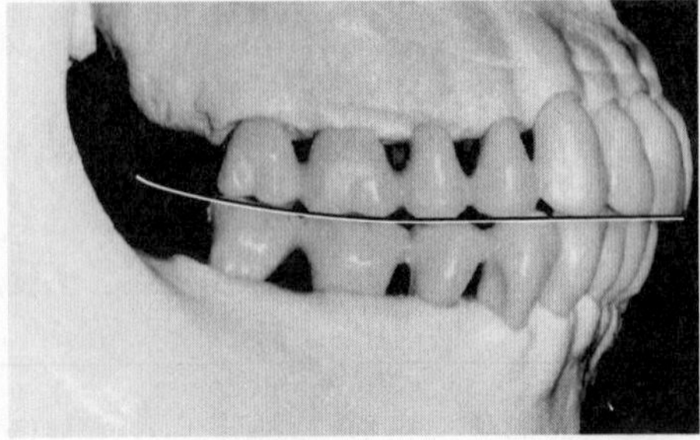

■ Curve of Spee.

temperature c. a graphic tracing showing variations in body temperature.

tension c's lines observed in the arrangement of the cancellous tissue of bones, depending on the directions of tension exerted on the bones.

thermal dilution c., thermodilution c. the graphic representation of results obtained with thermodilution.

venous return c. a graphic representation of venous return as a function of atrial pressure; it measures the contributions of peripheral factors that affect the flow of blood from the veins to the heart. Multiple curves generated under varying conditions are combined with similarly obtained cardiac output curves (q.v.) to analyze cardiac regulation.

ventricular function c. Starling c.

visibility c. a plotting of the relationship between wavelength and the intensity of light necessary to elicit a sensation.

c. of Wilson the curvature of the cusps of the teeth as projected on the frontal plane; that of the inferior dental arch is concave and that of the superior dental arch is convex.

Wunderlich c. the typical variation shown by the temperature in a patient with typhoid fever.

cur•vea (kur′ve-ə) curve.

c. occlusa′lis [TA] occlusal curve: the curve of a dentition on which the occlusal surfaces lie. Called also *curve of occlusion.*

Cur•vu•la•ria (kur″vu-lar′e-ə) a genus of Fungi Imperfecti of the form-class Hyphomycetes, form-family Dematiaceae, commonly found in soil and elsewhere. *C. genicula′ta, C. luna′ta, C. palles′cens,* and *C. senegalen′sis* have been isolated from human eumycotic mycetoma and other infections. The perfect (sexual) stage of *Curvularia* species is in genus *Cochliobolus.*

CUSA [Cavitron Ultrasonic Surgical Aspirator] trademark for an ultrasonic dissector and aspirator that is selective for tissue with high water and low collagen content.

cus•cam•i•dine (kəs-kam′ĭ-dēn) a cinchona alkaloid.

cus•cam•ine (kəs-kam′ēn) a cinchona alkaloid.

Cush•ing disease, response (phenomenon, reflex), etc. (koosh′ing) [Harvey Williams *Cushing,* American surgeon, 1869–1939] see under *disease, response, syndrome,* and *ulcer.* See also *equine Cushing disease,* under *disease.*

Cush•ing suture (koosh′ing) [Hayward W. *Cushing,* American surgeon, 1854–1934] see under *suture.*

Cush•ing-Ro•ki•tan•sky ul•cers (koosh′ing ro″kĭ-tahn′ske) [H.W. *Cushing;* Karl Freiherr von *Rokitansky,* Austrian pathologist, 1804–1878] Rokitansky-Cushing ulcers.

cush•ing•oid (koosh′ing-oid) resembling the features, symptoms, and signs associated with Cushing syndrome.

cush•ion (koosh′ən) a fleshy, padlike anatomical structure.

anal c's discrete masses of subepithelial tissue, located in the left lateral, right posterior, and right anterior quadrants of the anal canal and consisting of venous plexus, smooth muscle fibers, and elastic and connective tissue; they seal the anal canal and maintain continence.

coronary c. see under *band.*

digital c. a wedge-shaped mass of white and elastic fibers, containing fat and cartilage, overlying the frog of a horse's foot. Called also *plantar c.*

endocardial c's elevations of embryonic connective tissue covered by endothelium bulging into the atrioventricular canal of the embryonic heart, which later fuse with the free edge of the septum primum to separate the right and left atria.

eustachian c. torus tubarius.

intimal c's longitudinal thickenings of the intima of certain arteries, e.g., the penile arteries, formed by prominent local concentrations of smooth muscle fibers; they serve functionally as valves, controlling blood flow by occluding the lumen of the artery.

Passavant c. crista palatopharyngea.

plantar c. digital c.

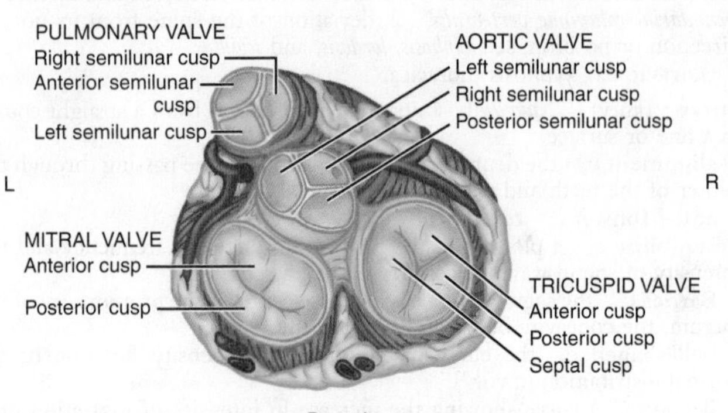

■ Cusps of the heart valves.

sucking c. corpus adiposum buccae.

cusp (kusp) [L. *cuspis* point] 1. a tapering projection; see *cuspis* and *valvula.* 2. cuspis dentis.

anterior c. of left atrioventricular valve, anterior c. of mitral valve cuspis anterior valvae atrioventricularis sinistrae.

anterior c. of pulmonary valve valvula semilunaris anterior valvae trunci pulmonalis.

anterior c. of right atrioventricular valve cuspis anterior valvae atrioventricularis dextrae.

anterior semilunar c. of pulmonary valve valvula semilunaris anterior valvae trunci pulmonalis.

anterior c. of tricuspid valve cuspis anterior valvae atrioventricularis dextrae.

Carabelli c. an accessory cusp on the lingual aspect of the mesiolingual cusp of an upper molar, which may be unilateral or bilateral and may vary considerably in size; it is common in Caucasians but quite rare in East Asians and certain other groups. Called also *Carabelli tubercle* and *tuberculum anomale dentis* [TA].

commissural c's cuspides commissurales.

dental c. cuspis dentis.

infundibular c. of tricuspid valve cuspis anterior valvae atrioventricularis dextrae.

left coronary c. of aortic valve valvula semilunaris sinistra valvae aortae; the name refers to its relation to the opening of the left coronary artery.

left c. of pulmonary valve valvula semilunaris sinistra valvae trunci pulmonalis.

left semilunar c. of aortic valve valvula semilunaris sinistra valvae aortae.

left semilunar c. of pulmonary valve valvula semilunaris sinistra valvae trunci pulmonalis.

marginal c. of tricuspid valve cuspis posterior valvae atrioventricularis dextrae.

medial c. of tricuspid valve cuspis septalis valvae atrioventricularis dextrae.

noncoronary c. of aortic valve valvula semilunaris posterior valvae aortae; the name denotes its distinction from the other two semilunar cusps of the aortic valve, which are marked by the openings of the coronary arteries.

paramolar c. cuspis paramolaris.

posterior c. of left atrioventricular valve, posterior c. of mitral valve cuspis posterior valvae atrioventricularis sinistrae.

posterior c. of right atrioventricular valve, posterior c. of tricuspid valve cuspis posterior valvae atrioventricularis dextrae.

posterior semilunar c. of aortic valve valvula semilunaris posterior valvae aortae.

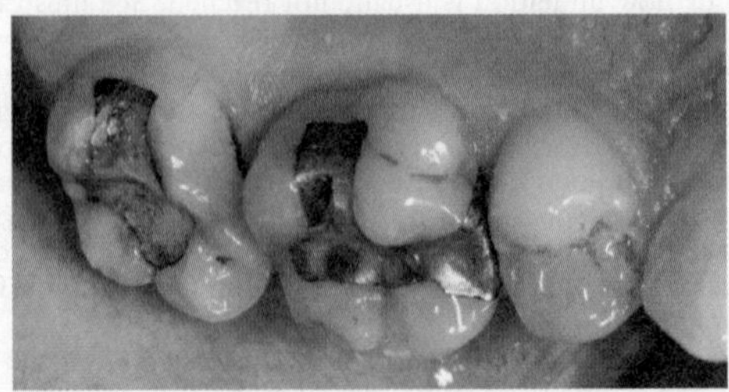

■ Carabelli cusp on the mesiolingual surface of the maxillary first molar.

right coronary c. of aortic valve valvula semilunaris dextra valvae aortae; the term refers to its relation to the opening of the right coronary artery.

right c. of pulmonary valve valvula semilunaris dextra valvae trunci pulmonalis.

right semilunar c. of aortic valve valvula semilunaris dextra valvae aortae.

right semilunar c. of pulmonary valve valvula semilunaris dextra valvae trunci pulmonalis.

semilunar c. any of the cusps surrounding the aortic and pulmonary valves; see entries beginning *vavlula semilunaris.*

septal c. of right atrioventricular valve, septal c. of tricuspid valve cuspis septalis valvae atrioventricularis dextrae.

talon c. a large accessory cusp on the lingual surface of a maxillary incisor, forming a T-shaped projection from the cingulum of the tooth and resembling the talon of an eagle.

c. of tooth cuspis dentis.

cus·pid (kus′pid) 1. having one cusp or point. 2. canine tooth.

cus·pi·date (kus′pĭ-dāt) [L. *cuspidatus*] having a cusp or cusps.

cus·pi·des (kus′pĭ-dēz) [L.] plural of *cuspis.*

cus·pis (kus′pis) pl. *cus′pides* [L.] 1. cusp; a tapering projection or structure. 2. [TA] one of the triangular segments of a cardiac valve; called also *leaflet.* See also *valvula.* 3. c. dentis.

c. ante′rior val′vae atrioventricula′ris dex′trae [TA] anterior cusp of tricuspid valve: the anterior of the three cusps of the tricuspid valve (valva atrioventricularis dextra). See illustration at *cusp.*

c. ante′rior val′vae atrioventricula′ris sinis′trae [TA] anterior cusp of mitral valve: the anterior of the two cusps of the mitral valve (valva atrioventricularis sinistra). See illustration at *cusp.*

cus′pides commissura′les [TA] commissural cusps: two small cusps that form the two outer of the three scallops constituting the posterior cusp of the left atrioventricular valve. See also *c. posterior valvae atrioventricularis sinistrae.*

c. den′tis [TA] cusp of tooth: an elevation or mound on the crown of a tooth making up part of the occlusal surface; they are named for the tooth surface they are adjacent to, such as *buccal, lingual, and palatal cusps.* Called also *dental cusp.* See also *tuberculum dentis.*

c. paramola′ris [TA] paramolar cusp: an accessory cusp on the mesiobuccal aspect of a molar; called also *tuberculum paramolare* [TA alternative].

c. poste′rior val′vae atrioventricula′ris dex′trae [TA] posterior cusp of tricuspid valve: the posterior of the three cusps of the tricuspid valve (valva atrioventricularis dextra). See illustration at *cusp.*

c. poste′rior val′vae atrioventricula′ris sinis′trae [TA] posterior cusp of mitral valve: the posterior of the two cusps of the mitral valve (valva atrioventricularis sinistra); the term is sometimes used to denote the entire three-scalloped region posterior to the anterior cusp of the mitral valve but at other times is restricted to the central scallop, with the two outer scallops called the *cuspides commissurales.* See illustration at *cusp.*

c. septa′lis val′vae atrioventricula′ris dex′trae [TA] septal cusp of tricuspid valve: the cusp of the tricuspid valve (valva atrioventricularis dextra) that is attached to the membranous interventricular septum. See illustration at *cusp.*

cut (kut) a narrow cleft or wound made by a sharp edge.

cu·ta·ne·ous (ku-ta′ne-əs) [L. *cutis* skin] pertaining to the skin; called also *dermal* and *dermic.*

cut·down (kut′doun) creation of a small incised opening over a vein to facilitate phlebotomy.

Cu·ter·e·bra (ku″tər-e′brə) a genus of botflies of the family Cuterebridae, whose larvae commonly infest rodents.

Cu·te·reb·ri·dae (ku″te-reb′rĭ-de) a family of New World botflies (order Diptera), whose larvae parasitize mammals. The one genus of medical interest is *Cuterebra.*

cu·ti·cle (ku′tĭ-kəl) [L. *cuticula,* from *cutis* skin] 1. a layer of more or less solid substance covering the free surface of an epithelial cell. 2. eponychium (def. 1).

dental c. cuticula dentis.

enamel c. primary c.

hair c., c. of hair, c. of hair shaft a layer of cells on the external surface of the hair shaft, interlocking with the cuticle of the root sheath.

primary c. a film on the enamel of unerupted teeth, considered to be the final product of degenerating ameloblasts after completion of enamel formation; electron microscopy shows it to consist primarily of ameloblasts of the reduced enamel epithelium attached to the enamel by a basal lamina. Called also *enamel c.* Cf. *cuticula dentis.*

c. of root sheath the innermost layer of cells of the inner root sheath of a hair follicle adjacent to the hair.

secondary c. cuticula dentis.

cu·tic·u·la (ku-tik′u-lə) pl. *cutic′ulae* [L. "little skin"] a horny secreted layer.

c. den′tis dental cuticle: a film occurring on some teeth on both the enamel and the cementum, external to the primary cuticle, with which it combines, being deposited by the epithelial attachment as it migrates along the tooth and separates from the crown and root. It is not present on cementum to which the periodontal ligament is not attached. Some authorities consider it to be a nonkeratinized product of the epithelial attachment cells, probably contributed by the gingival fluid and saliva; others consider it as a pathologic product of inflamed gingiva, or a conglutinate of erythrocytes. Called also *secondary cuticle* and *Nasmyth membrane.* Cf. *primary cuticle,* under *cuticle.*

cu·ti·dure (ku′tĭ-do͞or) coronary band.

cu·ti·du·ris (ku″tĭ-doo′ris) coronary band.

cu·tin (ku′tin) [*cutis*] a waxy substance that combines with cellulose to form the cuticle of plants.

cu·ti·re·ac·tion (ku″tĭ-re-ak′shən) [*cutis* + *reaction*] cutaneous reaction.

cu·tis (ku′tis) [L.] [TA] skin.

c. anseri′na a transitory localized change in the skin surface caused by elevation of the hair follicles as a result of contraction of the arrectores pilorum muscles, a reflection of sympathetic nerve discharge. Called also *goose flesh.*

c. hyperelas′tica Ehlers-Danlos syndrome.

c. lax′a a group of disorders of the elastic fiber network in which the skin lacks elasticity and resilience and hangs in loose, pendulous folds. Hereditary forms are genetically heterogeneous and vary in severity and may be present at birth or develop soon afterwards; there is also a rare acquired from. The *autosomal recessive form* can be caused by several mutations: in either of two fibulin genes (*FBLN4,* locus: 11q13; *FBLN5,* locus: 14q32.1); in the *ATP6V0A2* gene (locus: 12q24.3), which encodes a proton pump subunit; and in the *PYCR1* gene (locus: 17q25.3), which encodes pyrroline-5-carboxylate reductase. It is associated with severe complications, including pulmonary and cardiovascular anomalies, diverticula of the urinary and gastrointestinal tracts, and multiple hernias. The *autosomal dominant form* is caused by mutation in either the elastin gene (*ELN,* locus: 7q11.2) or the fibulin 5 gene *(FBLN5)* and is essentially benign and of only cosmetic significance. The *X-linked recessive form* is *occipital horn syndrome* (q.v.). The *acquired form,* which is often preceded by mild fever, usually presents after puberty and sometimes not until middle age or later. Individuals with cutis laxa have a prematurely aged appearance, hooked nose with everted nostrils, long upper lip, everted lower eyelids, and sagging cheeks. Called also *dermatochalasis, dermatomegaly, generalized elastolysis,* and *lax* or *loose skin.*

c. marmora′ta a transient form of livedo reticularis (q.v.) occurring as a normal response to cold. Called also *marble skin.*

c. marmora′ta telangiecta′tica conge′nita a rare congenital skin condition characterized by chronic cutis marmorata, telangiectasias, and phlebectasia, sometimes with ulceration and skin atrophy. The usual location is on a limb and often the adjacent area of the trunk. Called also *Van Lohuizen syndrome.*

c. rhomboida′lis nu′chae a type of actinic elastosis on the back of the neck, in which the skin of the nape of the neck becomes thickened, tough, leathery, and furrowed, with a rhomboidal pattern.

c. ver′ticis gyra′ta thickening of the skin of the scalp, usually at the vertex, so that it forms folds and furrows; this may occur alone or be characteristic of another condition, such as pachydermoperiostosis.

Cu·ti·vate (ku′tĭ-vāt″) trademark for preparations of fluticasone propionate.

cut·tle·bone (kut′əl-bōn) sepium.

cu·vette (ku-vet′) [Fr. dim. of *cuve* vat or tub] a container with specific dimensions (particularly thickness) and optical properties, used to examine colored or colorless solutions that are free of turbidity, as well as the light scattering of turbid suspensions, such as bacterial suspensions. Its efficacy depends on its chemical composition; e.g., one made of quartz is used for examination of materials in the ultraviolet region of the spectrum and one made of Pyrex is used for examination of materials in the visible region.

Cu·vier ducts (ku-vya′) [Georges Léopold Chrétien Frédéric Dagobert, Baron *Cuvier,* French naturalist, 1769–1832] see *common cardinal veins,* under *vein.*

CV cardiovascular; closing volume; coefficient of variation.

C.V. [L.] cras ves′pere (tomorrow evening); conjuga′ta ve′ra (true conjugate diameter of the pelvic inlet).

CVA cerebrovascular accident; costovertebral angle.

CVID common variable immunodeficiency.

CVP 1. central venous pressure. 2. a cancer chemotherapy regimen consisting of cyclophosphamide, vincristine, and prednisone.

CVS cardiovascular system; chorionic villus sampling.

CX circumflex artery.

Cx cervix; convex.

Cy cyanogen.

Cy·a·mop·sis (si″ə-mop′sis) a genus of plants of the family Leguminosae. *C. tetragonolo′bus* (L.) Taub. is the source of guar gum.

cy·an·al·co·hol (si″an-al′kə-hol) cyanohydrin.

cy·an·a·mide (si-an′ə-mīd) 1. carbamic acid nitril, N≡C—NH_2. 2. HN=C=NH, the anhydride of urea. 3. calcium cyanamide.

cy·an·he·mo·glo·bin (si″an-he′mo-glo″bin) a complex of cyanide and hemoglobin; see also *cyanmethemoglobin.*

cy·a·nide (si′ə-nīd) the CN^- anion or a salt containing this ion; all cyanides are extremely toxic; see *cyanide poisoning* under *poisoning.*

cy·an·met·he·mo·glo·bin (si″an-met-he′mo-glo″bin) a tightly bound complex of methemoglobin with the cyanide ion. The standard method of hemoglobinometry (measuring hemoglobin content) is determination of the amount of this compound via spectrophotometry; cyanmethemoglobin is produced quantitatively from oxyhemoglobin, deoxyhemoglobin, carboxyhemoglobin, and methemoglobin (but not sulfhemoglobin) by addition of Drabkin solution.

cy·an·met·myo·glo·bin (si″an-met-mi′o-glo″bin) a compound formed from metmyoglobin by addition of the cyanide ion to yield reduction to the ferrous state.

cyan(o)- [Gr. *kyanos* blue] a combining form denoting blue.

cy·a·no·ac·ry·late (si″ə-no-ak′rə-lāt) an acrylate monomer or polymer that has substitution with one or more cyano group(s); see also under *adhesive* and *resin.*

Cy·a·no·bac·te·ria (si″ə-no-bak-tēr′e-ə) [*cyano-* + *bacteria*] the blue-green bacteria (formerly called *blue-green algae*), a phylum of unicellular or filamentous phototrophic organisms of the domain Bacteria that use water as an electron donor and produce oxygen in the presence of light. Cells are enclosed by a rigid wall containing peptidoglycan, are generally motile, and reproduce by fission. Photopigments include chlorophyll *a* and phycobilin proteins. Cyanobacteria are the only organisms that fix both carbon dioxide (in the presence of light) and nitrogen. Most species are photosynthetic and many are strong nitrogen fixers. Several species are common causes of water pollution and are often used as indicators of eutrophication of lakes and streams; see *cyanobacteria poisoning*, under *poisoning.*

cy·a·no·bac·te·ria (si″ə-no-bak-te′re-ə) plural of *cyanobacterium.*

cy·a·no·bac·te·ri·um (si″ə-no-bak-te′re-um) an individual bacterium of the group *Cyanobacteria.*

cy·a·no·co·bal·a·min (si″ə-no″ko-bal′ə-min) 1. a cobalamin derivative in which the substituent is a cyanide ion; it is the form of vitamin B_{12} first isolated and hence is the form chemically defined as and the form used as a synonym of that vitamin, although it is actually an artifact of isolation. 2. [USP] a preparation of cyanocobalamin used to treat disorders caused by deficiencies of vitamin B_{12}, particularly to prevent and treat pernicious anemia and other megaloblastic anemias and associated neuropathy; administered subcutaneously or intramuscularly, intranasally, or, occasionally, orally. Abbreviated CN-Cbl. Called also *vitamin B_{12}.*

c. **Co 57** cyanocobalamin radioactively labeled with ^{57}Co; official preparations are *c. Co 57 capsules* [USP] and *c. Co 57 oral solution* [USP], in which a portion of the molecules is radioactively labeled. The preparations are used in the diagnosis of pernicious anemia and other disorders of vitamin B_{12} absorption. See also *Schilling test.*

c. **Co 58** cyanocobalamin labeled with ^{58}Co, used in the diagnosis of pernicious anemia and other disorders of vitamin B_{12} absorption. See also *Schilling test.*

c. **Co 60** cyanocobalamin in which a portion of the molecules is radioactively labeled with ^{60}Co, used in the diagnosis of pernicious anemia and other disorders of vitamin B_{12} absorption. See also *Schilling test*, under *test.*

cy·a·no·crys·tal·lin (si″ə-no-kris′tə-lin) a blue coloring matter from the integument of decapods.

cy·an·o·gen (si-an′o-jən) [*cyano-* + *-gen*] 1. the radical CN—; symbol Cy. 2. an extremely poisonous gas, NCCN; called also *ethanedinitrile.*

c. **bromide** a highly toxic lacrimatory war gas, BrCN.

c. **chloride** a gas, ClCN, used for fumigating houses, ships, etc. It is as lethal for rats and other vermin as hydrocyanic acid, but less dangerous to humans, as it also causes lacrimation, which makes it useful as a warning gas in fumigants.

cy·a·no·gen·e·sis (si″ə-no-jen′ə-sis) [*cyano-* + *-genesis*] the formation or production of cyanogen or hydrocyanic acid.

cy·a·no·ge·net·ic (si″ə-no-jə-net′ik) producing cyanogen or hydrocyanic acid.

cy·a·no·hy·drin (si″ə-no-hi′drin) a compound containing a cyano and a hydroxyl group; formed by the addition of hydrocyanic acid to an aldehyde group; called also *cyanalcohol.*

cy·a·no·phil (si-an′o-fil) 1. cyanophilous. 2. a cell or other histologic element readily stainable with blue.

cy·a·noph·i·lous (si″ə-nof′ĭ-ləs) [*cyano-* + Gr. *philein* to love] stainable with blue dyes.

cy·a·no·phor·ic (si″ə-no-for′ik) yielding hydrocyanic acid; e.g., the glycoside amygdalin yields HCN on hydrolysis.

cy·a·no·phose (si′ə-no-fōz) [*cyano-* + *phose*] a blue phose.

cy·a·nop·sia (si″ə-nop′se-ə) [*cyano-* + *-opsia*] a chromatopsia in which all objects appear to have a blue tinge.

cy·a·nop·sin (si″ə-nop′sin) [*cyano-* + *opsin*] a visual pigment of bluish tint found in the retinal cones of some animals and important for vision.

cy·a·nosed (si′ə-nōzd) cyanotic.

cy·a·no·sis (si″ə-no′sis) [Gr. *kyanos* blue] a bluish discoloration, especially of the skin and mucous membranes due to excessive concentration of deoxyhemoglobin in the blood. **cy′anosed, cyanot′ic** *adj*

autotoxic c. enterogenous c.

central c. cyanosis produced as a result of arterial unsaturation, the aortic blood carrying reduced hemoglobin.

enterogenous c. a syndrome due to absorption of nitrites and sulfides from the intestine, principally marked by methemoglobinemia and/or sulfhemoglobinemia associated with cyanosis. It is accompanied by severe enteritis, abdominal pain, constipation or diarrhea, headache, dyspnea, dizziness, syncope, anemia, and occasionally digital clubbing and indicanuria. Called also *autotoxic c., Stokvis-Talma syndrome,* and *van den Bergh disease.*

false c. cyanosis due to the presence of a pigment such as methemoglobin and not to deficient oxygenation of the blood.

hereditary methemoglobinemic c. cyanosis caused by a structural variant in the hemoglobin molecule, such as an M hemoglobin; see *methemoglobinemia.*

c. lie′nis passive congestion of the spleen.

peripheral c. cyanosis produced as a result of an excessive amount of reduced hemoglobin in the venous blood, caused by extensive oxygen extraction at the capillary level.

pulmonary c. central cyanosis caused by poor oxygenation of the blood in the lungs.

c. re′tinae distinct cyanosis of the retina, observable in some cases of cyanotic congenital heart disease, patent ductus arteriosus, and other congenital cardiac anomalies.

shunt c. central cyanosis caused by mixing of unoxygenated blood with the arterial blood in the heart or great vessels.

tardive c. cyanosis in congenital heart disease that appears only after heart failure has developed.

cy·an·uria (si″ən-u′re-ə) chromaturia in which the urine is blue.

cy·an·uric ac·id (si″ən-u′rik) a cyclic compound formed by heating urea.

cy·an·urin (si″ən-u′rin) [*cyan-* + *urine*] indigo blue found in the urine on the addition of a mineral acid to it.

Cyath. [L.] cy′athus (a glassful).

Cya·thos·to·ma (si″ə-thos′tə-mə) a genus of nematodes of the family Syngamidae that parasitizes the upper respiratory tract of birds.

cy·a·tho·sto·mi·a·sis (si″ə-tho-sto-mi′ə-sis) infection of the large intestines of horses with nematodes of the genus *Cyathostomum*; characteristics include anemia with diarrhea that can be fatal.

Cya·tho·sto·mum (si″ə-tho-sto′mum) a genus of small nematodes of the family Strongylidae, which parasitize the large intestines of horses, causing cyathostomiasis.

Cy·ber·Knife (si′bər-nīf) trademark for an apparatus used in stereotactic radiosurgery for the treatment of tumors anywhere in the body.

cy·ber·net·ics (si″bər-net′iks) [Gr. *kybernētēs* helmsman] the science of communication and control processes within systems. Control is based on communication both within the system and with the external environment and influences the actions of the system to bring it into some desired future state or to maintain homeostasis. Cybernetics includes the concepts of autoregulation and feedback (qq.v.), as well as the transmission and self-correction of information, and can be applied not only to machines like computers but also to living organisms, including humans, and to complex organizations and societies.

CYC cyclophosphamide.

cy·cad (si′kad) a palm tree of the genus *Cycas* or other closely related genera such as *Macrozamia* and *Zamia.* See also *zamia.*

Cy·cas (si′kəs) a genus of palms (family Palmae) found on Guam and other islands of the South Pacific. *C. circina′lis* L. and *C. revolu′tus* Thumb. have seeds that were formerly used as part of the diet on Guam and contain toxic glycosides such as cycasin and macrozamin. Cattle and sheep consuming the seeds may suffer fatal gastrointestinal and liver damage or the neurological condition known as *zamia staggers.*

cy·ca·sin (si′kə-sin) a toxic principle from the seeds of *Cycas revoluta* and *C. circinalis*. In humans it causes neoplastic lesions in the liver, kidneys, intestine, and lungs after hydrolysis by intestinal bacteria and yields the breakdown product methylazoxymethanol; in cattle it causes fatal gastrointestinal and liver damage.

cy·cla·cil·lin (si″klə-sil′in) an antibacterial agent effective against a wide range of gram-negative and gram-positive organisms.

cy·cla·mate (si′klə-māt) any salt of cyclamic acid. Cyclamate calcium and cyclamate sodium were once used widely as non-nutritive sweeteners, but because of an association with bladder tumors in animals they were banned as food additives in the United States in 1969.

Cyc·la·men (sik′lə-mən) [L.] a genus of plants of the family Primulaceae. *C. europae′um* L. is a common house plant in North America that has an acrid, cathartic root and contains the toxic alkaloid cyclamin.

cy·clam·ic ac·id (si-klam′ik) the free acid of cyclamate.

cyc·la·min (sik′lə-min) a toxic glycoside from *Cyclamen europaeum;* it is strongly cathartic and emetic.

Cy·cla·my·cin (si′klə-mi″sin) trademark for a preparation of troleandomycin.

cyc·lar·thro·sis (sik″lahr-thro′sis) [*cycl-* + *arthrosis*] a joint that permits rotation. **cyclarthro′dial** *adj*

cy·clase (si′klās) an enzyme that catalyzes the formation of a cyclic compound.

cy·cla·zo·cine (si″klə-zo′sēn) a narcotic antagonist which has been used as an analgesic and in the treatment of narcotic dependence.

cy·cle (si′kəl) [Gr. *kyklos* circle] a round or succession of observable phenomena, recurring usually at regular intervals and in the same sequence.

aberrant c. a cycle that in which there is variation in the interval or in the sequence of events.

anovulatory c. a sexual cycle in which no oocyte is discharged.

Calvin c. a dark reaction occurring in photosynthesis in plants in which carbon dioxide is affixed to a five-carbon sugar molecule and subsequently reduced to form other sugars.

carbon c. the steps by which carbon (in the form of carbon dioxide) is extracted from the atmosphere by living organisms and ultimately returned to the atmosphere. It comprises a series of interconversions of carbon compounds beginning with the production of carbohydrates by plants during photosynthesis, proceeding through animal consumption, and ending and beginning again in the decomposition of the animal or plant or in the exhalation of carbon dioxide by animals.

cardiac c. a complete cardiac movement or heart beat. The period from the beginning of one heart beat to the beginning of the next; the systolic and diastolic movement, with the interval between them. See illustration.

cell c. the cycle of biochemical and morphological events occurring in a reproducing cell population, divided into several phases: G_1 (with its subtype G_0), the longest and most variable phase; *S*, during which DNA is synthesized; G_2, during which the accuracy of DNA replication is checked; and *M*, consisting of the four phases of mitosis and followed by the return of the cell to the G_1 phase.

chewing c. masticating c.

citrate-pyruvate c. the mechanism by which acetyl groups and electrons are moved across the mitochondrial membrane during fatty acid synthesis.

citric acid c. tricarboxylic acid c.

Cori c. the mechanism by which lactate produced by muscles is carried to the liver, converted back to glucose via gluconeogenesis, and returned to the muscles.

cytoplasmic c. the stage in the life of a parasite during which it lives in cytoplasm of the cells of the host.

endogenous c. the portion of the life of a parasite spent within the body of its definitive host.

endometrial c. menstrual c.

estrous c. the type of sexual cycle seen in most adult female mammals, with recurring periods that include estrus and the correlated changes in the reproductive tract from one period to the next. The stages are *proestrus*, *estrus*, *metestrus*, and *diestrus* (the latter sometimes including *anestrus* of varying lengths of time). Cf. *ovarian c.* and *menstrual c.*

exogenous c. the part of the life of a parasite spent outside the body of its definitive host.

forced c. a cardiac cycle that is interrupted by a forced beat.

futile c. a combination of two or more biochemical reactions resulting only in the hydrolysis of ATP or other high-energy compounds; thermogenesis may result. Called also *substrate c.*

gait c. the series of movements of the leg and foot between one touch of the heel on the ground and the next time the same heel touches. See also *stance phase* and *swing phase*, under *phase*.

gastric c. rhythmic alterations in the shape of the stomach due to peristaltic waves.

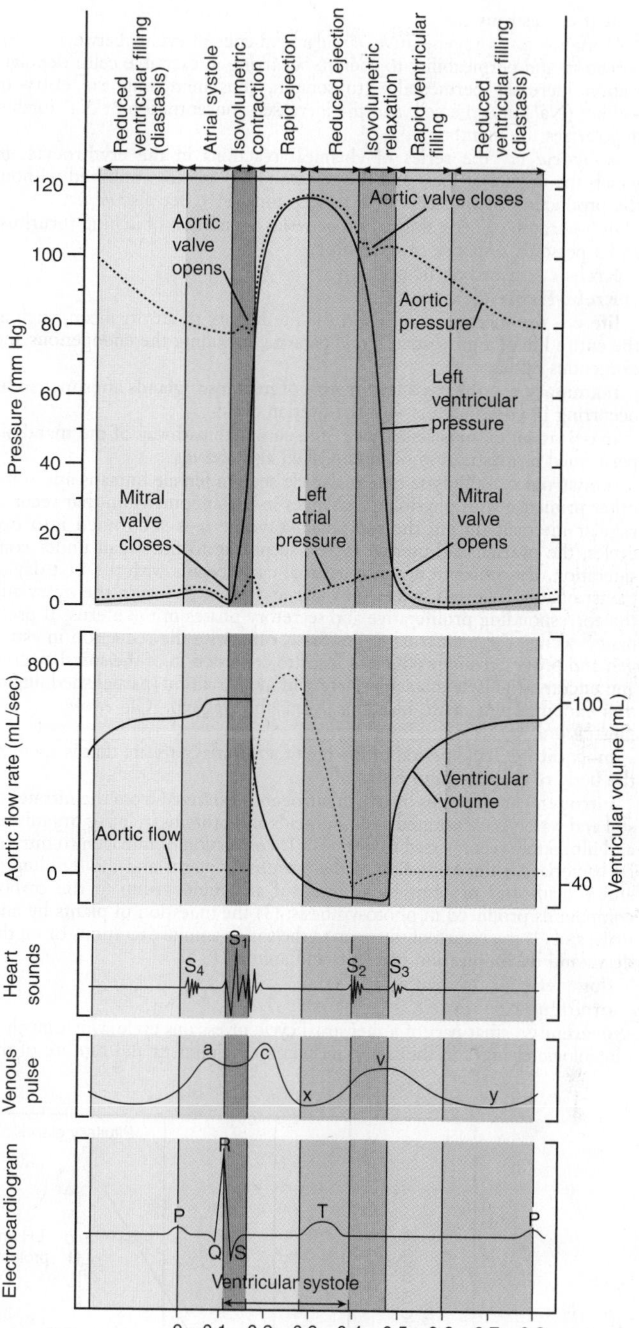

■ Events of the cardiac cycle. For the meaning of symbols, see individual entries and see illustrations at *electrocardiogram* and *venous pulse.*

glucose-lactate c. Cori c.

γ-glutamyl c. a metabolic cycle for transporting amino acids into cells. The reactions involve transfer of the γ-glutamyl group of glutathione to extracellular amino acids, enabling them to enter the cells; additional reactions recreate free amino acids and resynthesize glutathione.

glyoxylate c. a metabolic pathway by which certain microorganisms and plants convert fat to carbohydrate; its enzymes are contained in microbodies known as *glyoxysomes*. It is a modification of the tricarboxylic acid cycle but differs in that two auxiliary enzymes (isocitratase and malate synthetase) are used and two molecules of acetyl coenzyme A instead of one are required.

gonotrophic c. the interval in the life of an insect between the time of feeding to deposition of the ova.

hair c. the successive phases in the life of a hair from initiation of its growth to its loss from the follicle; the three phases are anagen, catagen, and telogen.

heat c. estrous c.

Hodgkin c. a regenerative, circular sequence of events between depolarization and permeability to sodium occurring in excitable cells: depolarization increases permeability to sodium, thus increasing the entry of sodium (Na^+) into the cell, and the increased concentration of Na^+ further depolarizes the membrane.

isohydric c. the series of chemical reactions in the erythrocyte, in which the uptake of CO_2 and the release of O_2 are accomplished without the production of an excess of hydrogen ions (H^+). See also *buffer.*

itch-scratch c. the alternation between a sensation of itching (pruritus) and a person's response of scratching.

Krebs c. tricarboxylic acid c.

Krebs-Henseleit c. urea c.

life c. the successive events in the life history of an organism, such as the entire life of a protozoan blood parasite, including the endogenous and exogenous cycles.

mammary c. the rhythmic growth of mammary glands after menarche occurring in coordination with the ovarian cycle.

masticating c., masticatory c. the complete pathway of the mandible performed in mastication of food. Called also *chewing c.*

menstrual c. the type of sexual cycle seen in female humans and some other primates, with physiologic changes in the endometrium that recur at regular intervals during the reproductive years; it is subdivided into two cycles, the ovarian and uterine cycles, according to the organ under consideration. By convention, the menstrual cycle begins with the first day of menstruation, followed by the follicular and luteal phases in the ovary and the corresponding proliferative and secretory phases in the uterus. If pregnancy occurs, the menstrual cycles cease, otherwise the reduction in estrogen and progesterone production leads to constriction of the spiral arteries and endometrial ischemia, culminating in menstruation (partial shedding of the endometrium with bleeding from the vagina). Cf. *estrous c.* See illustration.

mosquito c. the period of the life of a malarial parasite that is spent in the body of the mosquito host.

nitrogen c. the steps by which nitrogen is extracted from the nitrates of soil and water, incorporated as amino acids and proteins in living organisms, and ultimately reconverted to nitrates: (1) conversion of nitrogen to nitrates by bacteria; (2) the extraction of the nitrates by plants and the building of amino acids and proteins by addition of an amino group to the carbon compounds produced in photosynthesis; (3) the ingestion of plants by animals; and (4) the return of nitrogen to the soil in animal excretions or on the death and decomposition of plants and animals.

oogenetic c. ovarian c.

ornithine c. urea c.

ovarian c. that part of a menstrual cycle or estrous cycle which involves physiologic changes in the ovary, including development and rupture of the follicle, discharge of the oocyte, and corpus luteum formation and regression. It is divided into the follicular phase and the luteal phase. Called also *oogenetic c.*

reproductive c. the cycle of physiologic changes occurring in the female reproductive organs, from the time of fertilization of the oocyte through gestation and parturition.

restored c. a cardiac cycle following a returning cycle and taking up the normal rhythm.

returning c. a cardiac cycle that begins with an extrasystole.

sex c., sexual c. 1. a series of recurring physiologic changes in the genital organs of nonpregnant female mammals; they typically come at regular intervals. The two types are the *menstrual c.* and the *estrous c.* See also *ovarian c.* 2. the period of sexual reproduction in an organism that also reproduces asexually.

sporogenic c., sporogenous c. the sexual cycle in protozoa that is usually passed in another host, often an insect.

substrate c. futile c.

tricarboxylic acid c. the final common pathway for the oxidation to CO_2 of fuel molecules, most of which enter the cycle as acetyl coenzyme A; it also provides intermediates for biosynthetic reactions. The cycle occurs in mitochondria and generates ATP by providing electrons to the electron transport chain. See illustration. Called also *Krebs c.* and *citric acid c.*

urea c. a series of metabolic reactions, occurring in the liver, by which ammonia is converted to urea using cyclically regenerated ornithine as a carrier. See illustration.

uterine c. that part of a menstrual cycle or estrous cycle during which changes occur in the endometrium, preparing it for implantation of the blastocyst. It is divided into the proliferative phase and the secretory phase.

visual c. the cyclic association of 11-*cis* retinal with an opsin followed by photon-induced conformational changes in the compound protein (rhodopsin or an iodopsin) and dissociation of opsin and an all-*trans* isomeric form of retinal; the cycle is completed by direct or indirect reconversion of retinal to the 11-*cis* isomer. The conformational changes create an electric potential and initiate the cascade generating a sensory nerve impulse in vision. See illustration.

cyc•lec•to•my (sik-lek′tə-me) [*cycl-* + *-ectomy*] 1. excision of a piece of the ciliary body. 2. excision of a portion of the ciliary border of the eyelid.

cyc•len•ceph•a•lus (sik″len-sef′ə-ləs) [*cycl-* + *enkephalos* brain] a fetus with the cerebral hemispheres blended into one.

Cyc•les•sa (si-kles′ə) trademark for a therapeutic regimen of desogestrel and ethinyl estradiol.

cyc•lic (sik′lik, si′klik) 1. pertaining to or occurring in a cycle or cycles. 2. pertaining to a chemical compound that contains a ring of atoms in the nucleus; opposed to one that is aliphatic (q.v.). See also *closed chain,* under *chain.*

cyc•lic AMP cyclic adenosine monophosphate.

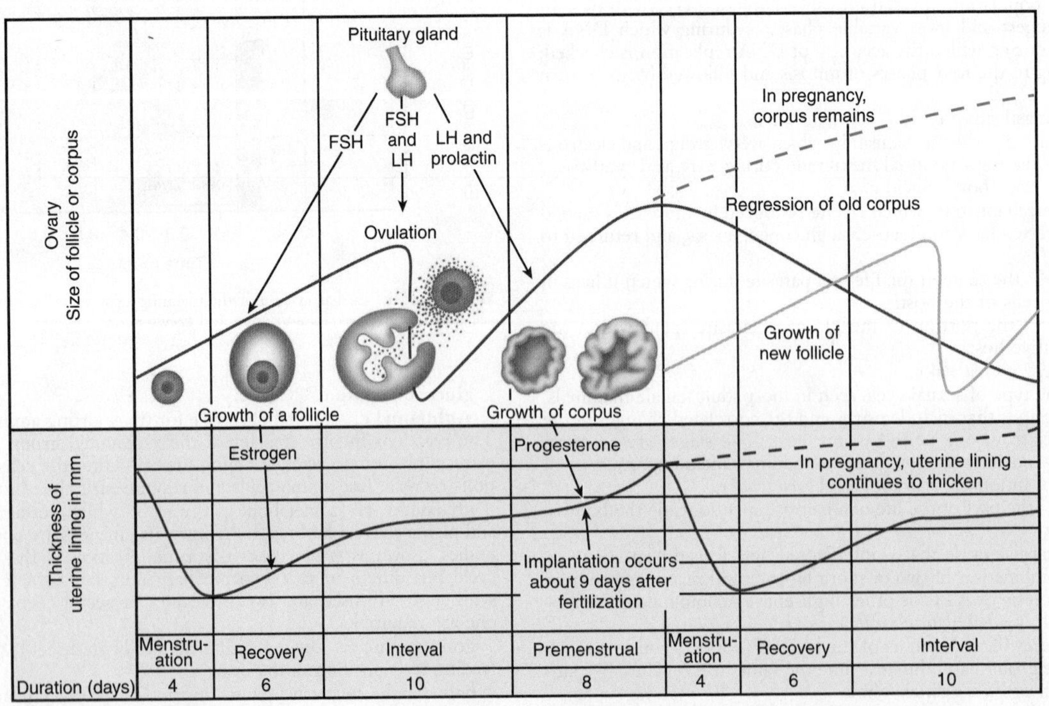

■ Changes in the menstrual cycle in the human female. Solid lines indicate the course of events when the oocyte is not fertilized; dotted lines indicate the course of events when fertilization occurs. Arrows indicate the actions of hormones of the pituitary and the ovary in regulating the cycle.

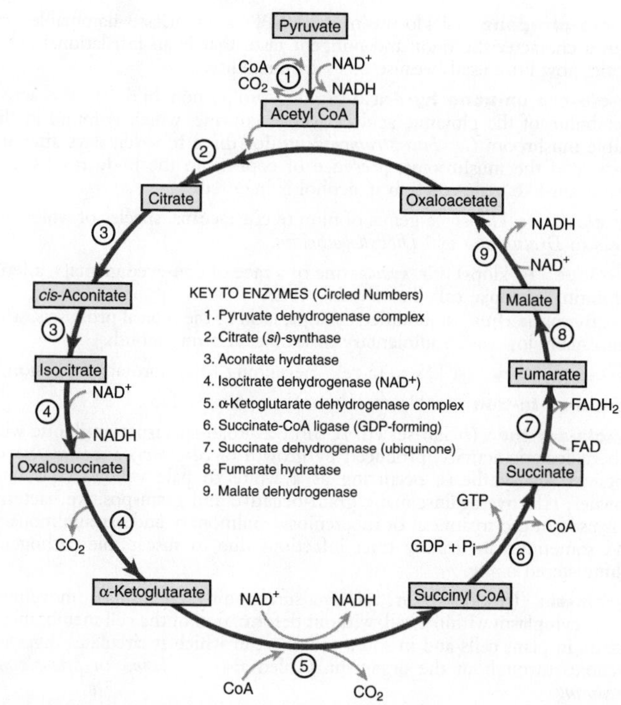

■ Tricarboxylic acid cycle. Diagrammatic representation of reactions by which carbon chains of sugars, fatty acids, and amino acids are metabolized to yield carbon dioxide. Water produced by the cycle and components of the high-energy phosphate pool generated by the associated electron chain are not shown.

cyc·lic AMP–de·pen·dent pro·tein ki·nase (si′klik de-pen′dent pro′tēn ki′nās) cAMP-dependent protein kinase.

cyc·lic GMP cyclic guanosine monophosphate.

3′,5′-cyc·lic-GMP phos·pho·di·es·ter·ase (si′klik fos″fo-di-es′tər-ās) [EC 3.1.4.35] an enzyme of the hydrolase class that catalyzes the cleavage of cyclic guanosine monophosphate to form guanosine monophosphate.

cy·clin (si′klin) any of a diverse group of proteins, ranging in size from 35 kD to 90 kD and having a similar core structure, that regulate various phases of the cell cycle by binding to and activating cyclin-dependent kinases and determining the protein to be phosphorylated.

cy·clin-de·pen·dent ki·nase (CDK) (si′klin de-pen′dənt ki′nās) [EC 2.7.11.22] any of a group of protein-serine/threonine kinases, active only when bound to a cyclin, that catalyze the phosphorylation of proteins determined by the associated cyclin in the regulation of the cell cycle.

cyc·ling (si′kling) the ending of an inspiratory phase of mechanical ventilation.

cyc·li·tis (sik-li′tis) [*cycl-* + *-itis*] inflammation of the ciliary body.

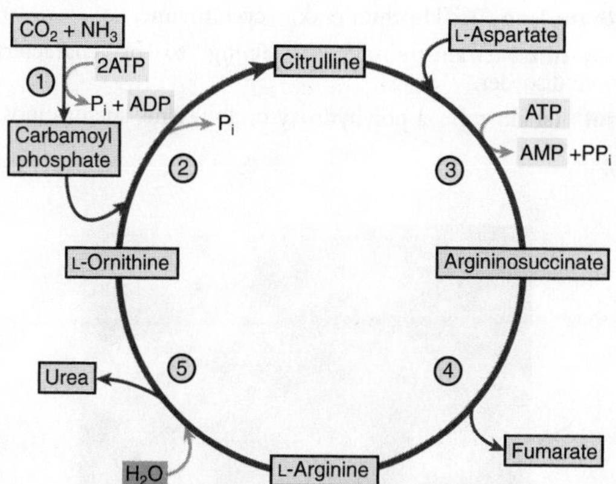

■ Urea cycle. Diagrammatic representation of reactions by which excess nitrogen in the form of ammonia is converted to soluble urea, using L-ornithine as a recyclable carrier. Enzymes involved are denoted by circled numerals: *(1)*, carbamoyl-phosphate synthase (ammonia); *(2)*, ornithine carbamoyltransferase; *(3)*, argininosuccinate synthase; *(4)*, argininosuccinate lyase; *(5)*, arginase.

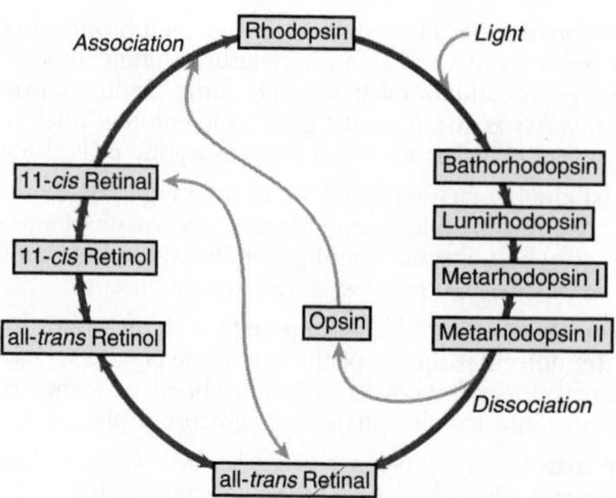

■ Visual cycle of retinal rod cells; an analogous cycle occurs with iodopsins in the cones.

heterochromic c. chronic cyclitis producing difference in the color of the two irides, the inflamed eye having the lighter iris.

plastic c. cyclitis with exudation of fibrinous matter into the anterior chamber.

pure c. inflammation of the ciliary body without involvement of the iris.

purulent c. suppuration in the ciliary body; it usually involves the entire uveal tract, constituting endophthalmitis.

serous c. simple inflammation of the ciliary body.

cycl(o)- [Gr. *kyklos* circle] a combining form denoting round or recurring; see *cyclic.* Often used with particular reference to the eye, or to the ciliary body of the eye.

cy·clo·ben·za·prine hy·dro·chlo·ride (si″klo-ben′zə-prēn) [USP] a compound structurally related to the tricyclic antidepressants, used as a skeletal muscle relaxant for relief of painful muscle spasms; administered orally.

cy·clo·ceph·a·lus (si″klo-sef′ə-ləs) [*cyclo-* + *-cephalus*] cyclops.

cy·clo·cer·a·ti·tis (si″klo-ser″ə-ti′tis) cyclokeratitis.

cy·clo·cho·roid·itis (si″klo-kor″oid-i′tis) [*cyclo-* + *choroid-* + *-itis*] inflammation of the choroid and ciliary body.

Cy·clo·cort (si′klo-kort″) trademark for preparations of amcinonide.

cy·clo·cryo·ther·a·py (si″klo-kri″o-ther′ə-pe) [*cyclo-* + *cryotherapy*] freezing of the ciliary body; done in the treatment of glaucoma.

cy·clo·da·mia (si″klo-da′me-ə) [*cyclo-* + Gr. *damazein* to subdue] subdued or suppressed accommodation of the eyes.

cy·clo·dex·trin (si″klo-dek′strin) any of a group of nonreducing cyclic compounds obtained by the enzymatic hydrolysis of starch, designated α-, β-, and γ-cyclodextrins; used as complexing agents and in the study of enzyme action.

β-c., beta c. betadex.

cy·clo·di·al·y·sis (si″klo-di-al′ə-sis) [*cyclo-* + *dialysis*] surgical creation of a communication between the anterior chamber of the eye and the perichoroidal space; done in the treatment of glaucoma.

cy·clo·di·a·ther·my (si″klo-di′ə-thur″me) [*cyclo-* + *diathermy*] destruction of a portion of the ciliary body by diathermy; employed as therapy in cases of glaucoma.

cy·clo·duc·tion (si″klo-duk′shən) [*cyclo-* + *duction*] the duction of the eyeball produced by the oblique muscle.

cy·clog·e·ny (si-kloj′ə-ne) [*cyclo-* + *-geny*] the developmental cycle of a microorganism.

Cy·clo·gyl (si′klo-jəl) trademark for a preparation of cyclopentolate hydrochloride.

cy·clo·hex·ane (si″klo-hek′sān) an alicyclic hydrocarbon, C_6H_{12}, existing in two forms, the "boat" and the "chair:"

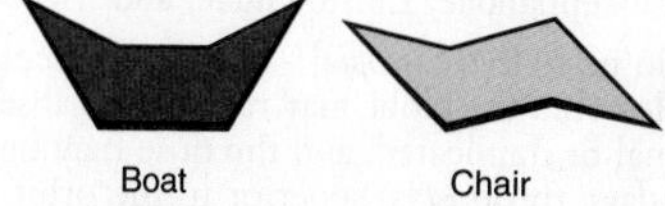

cy·clo·hex·ane·hex·ol (si″klo-heks″ān-heks′ol) inositol.

cy·clo·hex·ane·sul·fam·ic ac·id (si″klo-hek″sān-səl-fam′ik) cyclamic acid.

cy·clo·hex·a·nol (si″klo-hek′sə-nol) the monohydroxy derivative of cyclohexane; used as a solvent and blending agent.

cy·clo·hex·i·mide (si″klo-heks′ĭ-mīd) an antibiotic isolated from *Streptomyces griseus* and used as an agricultural fungicide and in selective media for fungi. It inhibits most saprobic fungi, while allowing dermatophytes and most systemic fungi to grow, and inhibits nuclear division of karyotic organisms but has no effect on prokaryotic cells (bacteria).

cy·cloid (si′kloid) characterized by alternating moods of elation and depression. The terms cycloid, cyclothymic, and manic-depressive overlap in meaning, although cycloid would generally be used for the least severe, and manic-depressive for the most severe conditions.

cy·clo·isom·er·ase (si″klo-i-som′ər-ās) a term used in the trivial names of intramolecular lipases of the isomerase class [EC 5.5.1] that catalyze certain rearrangements of a molecule to break or form a ring, e.g., the synthesis of *myo*-inositol phosphate from glucose 6-phosphate.

cy·clo·ker·a·ti·tis (si″klo-ker″ə-ti′tis) [*cyclo-* + *keratitis*] inflammation of the cornea and ciliary body; called also *Dalrymple disease.*

cy·clo·li·gase (si″klo-li′gās) [EC 6.3.3] one of a sub-subclass of enzymes of the ligase class that catalyze the formation of carbon-nitrogen bonds to produce a heterocyclic ring, driven by the hydrolysis of adenosine triphosphate.

cy·clo·mas·top·a·thy (si″klo-mas-top′ə-the) [*cyclo-* + *masto-* + *-pathy*] a disorder of the mammae, presenting excessive connective tissue overgrowth or epithelial proliferation or both in response to growth stimuli or as a manifestation of abnormal involution following normal response.

cy·clo·oxy·gen·ase (COX) (si″klo-ok′sə-jən-ās) an activity of prostaglandin-endoperoxide synthase (q.v.). There are two isoforms, called *cyclooxygenase-1 (COX-1)* and *cyclooxygenase-2 (COX-2).* COX-1 is involved in the synthesis of prostaglandins that maintain the integrity of the gastrointestinal mucosa. COX-2 is made primarily in response to injury or inflammation and is involved in the synthesis of prostaglandins involved in inflammation and the immune response. See also *COX-2 inhibitor,* under *inhibitor.*

cy·clo·pen·tane (si″klo-pen′tān) a hydrocarbon, C_5H_{10}, in which all five carbon atoms are in a single ring.

cy·clo·pen·ta·no·per·hy·dro·phen·an·threne (si″klo-pen″tə-no-pər-hi″dro-fə-nan′thrēn) the basic skeleton common to the steroids, consisting of a saturated phenanthrene ring (three fused six-member carbocyclic rings) joined to a cyclopentane.

cy·clo·pen·thi·a·zide (si″klo-pen-thi′ə-zīd) an orally effective diuretic, used in the treatment of edema associated with various disorders and in hypertension.

cy·clo·pen·to·late hy·dro·chlo·ride (si″klo-pen′to-lāt) [USP] an anticholinergic, used to produce cycloplegia and mydriasis by instillation into the eye.

cy·clo·pho·ria (si″klo-for′e-ə) [*cyclo-* + *phoria*] heterophoria in which there is deviation of the eye from the anteroposterior axis in the absence of visual fusional stimuli. See *excyclophoria* and *incyclophoria.* Cf. *cyclotropia.*
 accommodative c. cyclophoria due to oblique astigmatism.
 minus c. incyclophoria.
 plus c. excyclophoria.

cy·clo·pho·rom·e·ter (si″klo-for-om′ə-tər) [*cyclophoria* + *-meter*] an instrument for measuring cyclophoria.

cy·clo·phos·pha·mide (CPM, CYC) (si″klo-fos′fə-mīd) [USP] a cytotoxic alkylating agent of the nitrogen mustard group, used as an antineoplastic, often in combination with other agents, for a wide variety of conditions, including Hodgkin disease, lymphosarcoma, acute lymphocytic leukemia, Burkitt lymphoma, carcinoma of the breast, multiple myeloma, chronic lymphocytic leukemia, bronchogenic carcinoma, neuroblastoma, ovarian carcinoma, and carcinoma of the uterine cervix; also used as an immunosuppressive agent to prevent transplant rejection and in the treatment of certain diseases with abnormal immune function. Cyclophosphamide itself is pharmacologically inert; several active metabolites are produced by the microsomal enzyme systems in the liver.

Cy·clo·phyl·lid·ea (si″klo-fəl-id′e-ə) an order of tapeworms of the subclass Cestoda, class Cestoidea, comprising seven families that are habitually or accidentally parasitic: Taeniidae, Hymenolepididae, Dipylidiidae, Davaineidae, Anoplocephalidae, Linstowiidae, and Mesocestoididae.

cy·clo·pia (si-klo′pe-ə) [*cycl-* + *-opia*] any developmental anomaly characterized by a single orbit; the globe may range from absent or rudimentary to apparently normal or duplicated, and the nose may be absent or present as a tubular appendage (proboscis) superior to the orbit.

cy·clo·ple·gia (si″klo-ple′je-ə) [*cyclo-* + *-plegia*] paralysis of the ciliary muscles so as to prevent accommodation of the eye; called also *paralysis of accommodation.*

cy·clo·ple·gic (si″klo-ple′jik) 1. pertaining to, characterized by, or causing cycloplegia. 2. an agent that causes cycloplegia.

cy·clo·pro·pane (si″klo-pro′pān) [USP] a colorless, flammable gas with a characteristic odor and pungent taste that is an inhalational anesthetic; now little used because of its flammability.

cy·clo·pro·pa·none hy·drate (si″klo-pro′pə-nōn hi′drāt) the active metabolite of the glutamic acid derivative coprine, which is found in the edible mushroom *Coprinus atramentarius;* for three to seven days after ingestion of the mushrooms, presence of coprine in the body results in a disulfiram-like toxic reaction if alcohol is ingested.

Cy·clops (si′klops) a genus of minute crustaceans, species of which are hosts to *Dracunculus* and *Diphyllobothrium.*

cy·clops (si′klops) [Gr. *kyklōps* one of a race of one-eyed giants] a fetus exhibiting cyclopia; called also *cyclocephalus.*
 c. hypogna′thus a modified cyclops, lacking the typical proboscis, with abnormally low ears, rudimentary mandible, and tiny mouth.

cy·clo·ro·ta·ry (si″klo-ro′tə-re) pertaining to cyclorotation (torsion).

cy·clo·ro·ta·tion (si″klo-ro-ta′shən) torsion (def. 3).

cy·clo·ser·ine (si″klo-ser′ēn) [USP] a broad-spectrum antibiotic with tuberculostatic activity, produced by growth of *Streptomyces orchidaceus* or obtained by synthesis, occurring as a white to pale yellow, crystalline powder; effective against many gram-negative and gram-positive bacteria, it is used in the treatment of tuberculosis, pulmonary and extrapulmonary, and sometimes in urinary tract infections due to susceptible pathogens; administered orally.

cy·clo·sis (si-klo′sis) [Gr. *kyklōsis* a surrounding, enclosing] movement of the cytoplasm within a cell, without deformation of the cell membrane; it occurs in plant cells and in some protozoa, in which it circulates digestive vacuoles throughout the organism. Called also *cytoplasmic* or *protoplasmic streaming.*

cy·clo·spasm (si′klo-spaz″əm) spasm of accommodation of the eyes.

Cy·clo·spo·ra (si-klos′pə-rə) [*cyclo-* + Gr. *spora* seed] a genus of coccidian protozoa (suborder Eimeriina, order Eucoccidiida) that have two sporocysts in each oocyst (covered by a bivalve shell), and two sporozoites in each sporocyst. *C. cayetanen′sis* is the most common species, causing cyclosporiasis, and is spread by the fecal-oral route.

cy·clo·spo·ri·a·sis (si″klo-spə-ri′ə-sis) infection by protozoa of the genus *Cyclospora.* The most common species infecting humans is *C. cayetanensis,* primarily seen in immunocompromised patients; the predominant symptoms are recurrent gastrointestinal disease and watery diarrhea.

cy·clo·spor·in A (si″klo-spor′in) cyclosporine.

cy·clo·spor·ine (si″klo-spor′ēn) [USP] a macrolide immunosuppressant of the calcineurin inhibitor group, produced as a metabolite by the soil fungus *Tolypocladium inflatum Gams;* it acts by inhibiting activation of helper T lymphocytes. Administered orally or intravenously to prevent and treat rejection in organ transplant recipients, to treat severe psoriasis, and as a disease-modifying antirheumatic drug to treat rheumatoid arthritis; also administered topically to the conjunctiva in the treatment of chronic dry eye.

cy·clo·tate (si′klo-tāt) USAN contraction for 4-methylbicyclo-[2.2.2]oct-2-ene-1-carboxylate.

cy·clo·thyme (si′klo-thīm) an individual with a cyclothymic personality or exhibiting cyclothymic disorder.

cy·clo·thy·mia (si″klo-thi′me-ə) [*cyclo-* + *-thymia*] cyclothymic disorder.

cy·clo·thym·i·ac (si″klo-thim′e-ak) cyclothymic.

cy·clo·thy·mic (si″klo-thi′mik) pertaining to or characterized by cyclothymic disorder.

cy·clo·tol (si′klo-tol) a polyhydroxy cyclohexane, such as inositol.

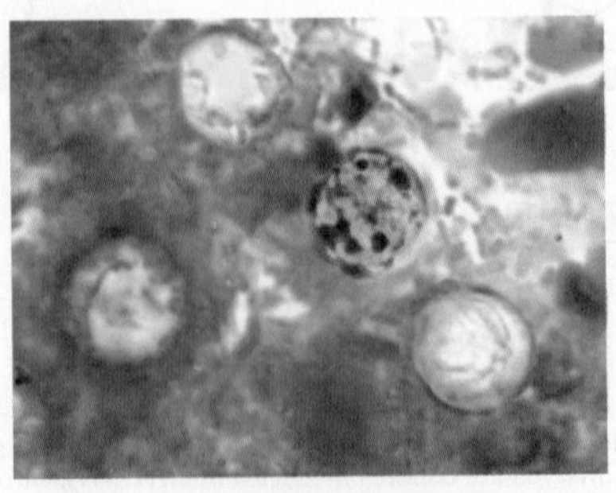

■ *Cyclospora* oocyst.

cy•clo•tome (si′klo-tōm) [*cyclo-* + *-tome*] a cutting instrument for use in cyclotomy or other operations upon the eye.

cy•clot•o•my (si-klot′ə-me) [*cyclo-* + *-tomy*] division of or incision of the ciliary muscle.

cy•clo•tron (si′klo-tron) an apparatus for accelerating charged particles (such as protons, deuterons, or ions) to high energies by a combination of a constant magnet and an oscillating electric field.

cy•clo•tro•pia (si″klo-tro′pe-ə) [*cyclo-* + *tropia*] a form of strabismus in which there is permanent cyclophoria of an eye around the anteroposterior axis even in the presence of visual fusional stimuli, resulting in diplopia. Cf. *excyclotropia* and *incyclotropia.*

cy•cri•mine hy•dro•chlo•ride (si′krĭ-mēn) an anticholinergic used in the treatment of parkinsonism, administered orally.

Cy•crin (si′krin) trademark for a preparation of medroxyprogesterone acetate.

-cyesis [Gr. *kyēsis,* pregnancy] a word termination denoting pregnancy.

cy•es•tein (si-es′tēn) a skinlike formation sometimes seen on the surface of urine of a pregnant woman.

cy•es•thein (si-es′thēn) cyestein.

Cy•klo•kap•ron (si″klo-kap′ron) trademark for preparations of tranexamic acid.

cyl cylinder; cylindrical lens.

Cy•lert (si′lərt) trademark for preparations of pemoline.

cyl•i•cot•o•my (sil″ĭ-kot′ə-me) cyclotomy.

cyl•in•der (sil′in-dər) [Gr. *kylindros* a roller] 1. a solid body shaped like a column. 2. cylindrical lens. **cylin′drical, cylin′driform** *adj*

axis c. axon (def. 1).

Bence Jones c's cylindrical gelatinous bodies forming the contents of the seminal vesicles; called also *Lallemand bodies.*

crossed c's two cylindrical lenses at right angles to each other.

Leydig c's bundles of muscular fibers separated by partitions of protoplasm.

Ruffini c. see under *ending.*

urinary c. see under *cast.*

cyl•in•drar•thro•sis (sil″in-drahr-thro′sis) [*cylinder* + *arthrosis*] a joint in which the articular surfaces are cylindrical, as in the proximal radioulnar joint or the odontoid process and atlas.

cyl•in•dro•car•ci•no•ma (sil″in-dro-kahr″sĭ-no′mə) [*cylinder* + *carcinoma*] a type of adnexal carcinoma with poorly differentiated cells, representing malignant transformation of a cylindroma.

Cy•lin•dro•car•pon (sə-lin″dro-kahr′pon) a genus of Fungi Imperfecti of the form-class Hyphomycetes. Several species have been isolated from human infections such as hyalohyphomycosis and eumycotic mycetomas.

cyl•in•dro•cel•lu•lar (sil″in-dro-sel′u-lər) composed of or containing cylindrical cells.

cyl•in•droid (sil′in-droid) [Gr. *kylindroeidēs* cylindrical] 1. resembling, or shaped like, a cylinder. 2. a urinary cast of irregular shape, resembling a hyaline cast but differing by having a slender tapering tail that may be twisted or curled upon itself.

cyl•in•dro•ma (sil″in-dro′mə) [*cylinder* + *-oma*] 1. a type of benign adnexal tumor, thought to be of sweat gland tissue, usually on the scalp (see *turban tumor*), but occasionally on the face or limbs. It consists of single or multiple nodules with cylindrical epithelial masses containing small basophilic and larger pale-staining cells surrounded by pink hyaline sheaths. Some authorities consider this a form of trichoepithelioma. 2. multiple trichoepithelioma. 3. adenoid cystic carcinoma. **cylindro′matous** *adj*

cyl•in•dro•ma•to•sis (sil″in-dro-mə-to′sis) 1. the presence of multiple cylindromas. 2. multiple trichoepithelioma.

familial c. Brooke-Spiegler syndrome.

Cy•lin•dro•tho•rax (sə-lin″dro-tho′raks) a genus of beetles. *C. melanoce′phala* is an African blister beetle that secretes cantharidin.

cyl•in•dru•ria (sil″in-droo′re-ə) [*cylindroid* + *uria*] the presence of casts in the urine; see *urinary cast,* under *cast.*

cy•lite (si′līt) benzyl bromide.

cyl•lo•so•ma (sil″o-so′mə) [Gr. *kyllos* lame + *soma*] a fetus with lower lateral abdominal eventration and absence or imperfect development of the lower limb on the side having the eventration.

cyl•lo•so•mus (sil″o-so′məs) cyllosoma.

cym•ba (sim′bə) pl. *cym′bae* [L., from Gr. *kymbē*] a boat-shaped structure.

c. con′chae auri′culae [TA], **c. concha′lis auri′culae** the upper part of the concha of the auricle.

Cym•bal•ta (sim-bawl′tə) trademark for a preparation of duloxetine hydrochloride.

cym•bi•form (sim′bĭ-form) [*cymbo-* + *form*] boat-shaped; scaphoid.

cymb(o)- [Gr. *kymbē,* boat] a combining form meaning boat-shaped.

cym•bo•ce•pha•lia (sim″bo-sə-fa′le-ə) scaphocephaly.

cym•bo•ce•phal•ic (sim″bo-sə-fal′ik) [*cymbo-* + *cephalic*] scaphocephalic.

cym•bo•ceph•a•lous (sim″bo-sef′ə-ləs) scaphocephalic.

cym•bo•ceph•a•ly (sim″bo-sef′ə-le) scaphocephaly.

Cym•bo•po•gon (sim″bə-po′gon) a genus of grasses found in warm regions of Europe, Africa, and Asia. *C. nar′dus* (L.) Rendle is citronella, a fragrant species that is the source of citronella oil.

cyme (sīm) a type of inflorescence composed of a flat-topped cluster of blossoms.

cy•nan•thro•py (sə-nan′thro-pe) [*cyn-* + Gr. *anthrōpos* man] a delusion in which the patient considers himself a dog or behaves like a dog.

Cy•na•ra (sin′ə-rə) [Gr. *kynara* artichoke] a genus of plants of the family Compositae having a tall stalk covered with spiny, pinnate leaves and ending in a large flower head; it includes *C. sco′lymus,* the artichoke, whose leaves are used medicinally.

cyn(o)- [Gr. *kyōn,* gen. *kynos* dog] a combining form denoting relationship to a dog, or doglike.

cy•no•ce•phal•ic (si″no-sə-fal′ik) [*cyno-* + *cephalic*] having a head shaped like that of a dog.

Cy•no•don (si′nə-don) a genus of grasses (family Gramineae). *C. dac′tylon* is Bermuda grass, whose pollen causes hay fever.

cy•no•dont (si′no-dont) [*cyno-* + Gr. *odous* tooth] a canine tooth.

cyn•o•mol•gus (sin″o-mol′gəs) *Macaca cynomolgus.*

Cy•no•my•ia (si″no-mi′yə) a genus of blue-bottle flies that deposit their ova in decaying meat and in wounds.

Cy•no•mys (si′no-mis) the prairie dogs, a genus of the family Sciuridae; some species harbor plague-transmitting fleas.

cy•no•pho•bia (si″no-fo′be-ə) [*cyno-* + *-phobia*] irrational fear of dogs.

Cy•on experiment, nerve (se′on) [Elie de *Cyon* (Il'ia Faddeevich Tsion), Russian physiologist, 1842–1912] see under *experiment* and *nerve.*

cy•ot•ro•phy (si-ot′rə-fe) [Gr. *kyos* fetus + *-trophy*] nutrition of the embryo or fetus.

Cy•pe•rus (si-pe′rəs) [L., from Gr. *kypeiros* rush] a genus of plants of the family Cyperaceae, grasslike sedges or rushes. *C. articula′tus* is adrue, whose root has medicinal uses.

cyph(o)- for words beginning thus, see those beginning *kyph(o)-.*

cyp•i•o•nate (sip′e-o-nāt) USAN contraction for cyclopentanepropionate.

cy•po•thrin (si′po-thrin) a veterinary anthelmintic.

cyp•ri•nin (sip′rĭ-nin) a toxic substance derived from the milt of the carp, *Cyprinus carpio.*

cy•pro•hep•ta•dine hy•dro•chlo•ride (si″pro-hep′tə-dēn) [USP] an antihistamine (H_1 receptor antagonist) with sedative, anticholinergic, serotonin-blocking, and calcium channel–blocking effects; used in the treatment of allergic rhinitis, allergic conjunctivitis, and cutaneous and systemic manifestations of allergic reactions, and the prophylaxis of migraine; administered orally.

cy•pro•quin•ate (si-pro-kwin′āt) a coccidiostat for poultry.

cy•pro•ter•one ac•e•tate (si-pro′tər-ōn) a synthetic antiandrogenic steroid used in the palliative treatment of advanced prostatic carcinoma; it has also been used in both men and women for its antiandrogenic hormonal effects, such as to treat female hirsutism.

Cyr•i•ax syndrome (sĭ′re-ak-sə) [Edward F. *Cyriax,* British orthopedic surgeon, early 20th century] see under *syndrome.*

cyr•to•sis (sir-to′sis) [Gr. *kyrtōsis*] 1. kyphosis. 2. distortion of the bones.

Cys cysteine.

Cys-Cys cystine.

cyst (sist) [Gr. *kystis* sac, bladder] 1. an abnormal closed cavity in the body, lined by epithelium and containing a liquid or semisolid material. Some cavities that are not lined by epithelium and should properly be called pseudocysts are commonly referred to as cysts; see *pseudocyst.* 2. a stage in the life cycle of certain parasites, during which they are enclosed within a protective wall; see, for example, *hydatid c., multilocular c.* (def. 2) and *pseudocyst* (def. 2). 3. vesica.

Cyst

adventitious c. pseudocyst (def. 1).
allantoic c. urachal c.
alveolar c. 1. dilatation of a pulmonary alveolus; several may fuse by breakdown of their septa to form large air cysts called *pneumatoceles.* 2. alveolar hydatid c.
alveolar hydatid c. a hydatid cyst with multiple loculi (small irregular cavities) that may contain scolices but generally little fluid; it is formed by larvae of *Echinococcus multilocularis* and tends to enlarge by budding since it has a poorly developed hyaline cuticle. Called also *multilocular hydatid c.* See *alveolar hydatid disease*, under *disease*.
amnionic c. cystlike processes containing amniotic fluid resulting from adhesion of amnionic folds.
aneurysmal bone c. a benign, rapidly growing, osteolytic lesion usually occurring in childhood or adolescence; it may be primary or secondary to an existing lesion and is characterized by blood-filled, often large, cystic spaces lined by bony or fibrous septa that contain osteoid and multinucleated giant cells.
angioblastic c. an ingrowth of the mesenchymal tissue having blood-forming power in an embryo.
apical c. an epithelium-lined cyst in the bone at the apex of a pulpless tooth.
arachnoid c. a fluid-filled cyst between the layers of the leptomeninges, lined with arachnoid membrane, most commonly occurring in the sylvian fissure; called also *leptomeningeal c.*
Baker c. a swelling behind the knee, caused by escape of synovial fluid which becomes enclosed in a membranous sac; called also *popliteal c.*
Bartholin c. a mucin-filled cyst resulting from obstruction of the duct of the greater vestibular gland (Bartholin gland).
Blessig c's cystic spaces that frequently appear at the periphery of the retina close to the ora serrata without significant effect on vision; called also *Blessig lacunae*, *cystoid degeneration*, and *Iwanoff c's.*
blue dome c. a benign retention cyst of the breast containing straw-colored fluid that shows a blue color when unopened; see *fibrocystic disease of breast*, under *disease.*
Boyer c. a painless and gradual enlargement of the subhyoid bursa.
branchial c., branchial cleft c. a cyst arising in the lateral aspect of the neck, from epithelial remnants of a branchial cleft (pharyngeal groove), usually between the second and third pharyngeal arches. Called also *cervical lymphoepithelial c.* and *lymphoepithelial c.*
branchiogenic c., branchiogenous c. branchial cleft c.
bronchial c. bronchogenic c.
bronchogenic c. a spherical congenital cyst arising from anomalous budding during the formation of the tracheobronchial tree; it is usually found in the mediastinum or the lung and is lined with bronchial epithelium that may contain secretory elements. It may contain air, and if it communicates with the trachea or a bronchus it may periodically evacuate fluid contents into the air passages, resulting in attacks of voluminous expectoration. Infection leads to mediastinal or pulmonary abscess. Called also *bronchial c.*
bronchopulmonary c. a bronchogenic cyst of the lung.
bursal c. a cyst derived from a serous bursa.
calcifying odontogenic c. a slow-growing benign neoplasm either in the mandible or in the gingiva, varying from solid to soft; the center contains a layer resembling stellate reticulum, with ghost cells, some of which have dystrophic calcification. Called also *Gorlin c.*
cervical c. a cyst in the neck; see *branchial c.* and *thyroglossal c.*
cervical lymphoepithelial c. branchial c.
chocolate c. a cyst whose contents are dark and syrupy, resulting from collection of hemosiderin following local hemorrhage, such as sometimes occurs after mastectomy or in the ovary in ovarian endometriosis (*endometrial c.*).
choledochal c., choledochus c. a congenital cystic dilatation of the lower end of the common bile duct, usually recognized during childhood. It may cause pain in the right upper quadrant, jaundice, fever, and vomiting, or it may be asymptomatic.
chyle c. an abnormal sac of the mesentery containing chyle.
colloid c. a cyst that contains jellylike material, particularly in the third ventricle.
compound c. multilocular c. (def. 1).
congenital preauricular c. a cyst resulting from imperfect fusion of the branchial arches in formation of the auricle, communicating with an ear pit (q.v.) on the surface. See also *congenital preauricular fistula*, under *fistula.*
corpus luteum c. a cyst of the ovary formed by a serous accumulation developed from a corpus luteum.
Cowper c. see under *syringocele.*
craniobuccal c's, craniopharyngeal c's Rathke c's.
cutaneous ciliated c. a type of solitary cyst found usually on the lower limbs of young women, located in the dermis and lined with cuboidal or columnar ciliated epithelium.
cutaneous myxoid c. digital mucous c.
daughter c. a small parasitic cyst developed from the wall of a larger one, such as a hydatid cyst. Called also *secondary c.*
dental c. one derived from some portion of the odontogenic apparatus.
dentigerous c. a fluid-containing odontogenic cyst surrounding the crown of an unerupted tooth, usually involving the crowns of normal permanent teeth.
dermoid c. 1. a type of epidermal cyst, usually present at birth along a line of embryonic fusion such as the middorsal, midventral, or branchial cleft; it represents a disorder of embryologic development, usually involves the head or neck (especially around the eyes), and is lined with stratified squamous epithelium containing cutaneous appendages, including hair. Called also *dermoid.* 2. a benign teratoma of the ovary, usually found in young women, presumably derived from ectodermal differentiation of totipotential cells, lined by apparent skin and its adnexal structures, usually filled with sebaceous, caseous material and hair. Called also *benign cystic*, *cystic*, or *mature teratoma* and *dermoid.*
digital mucous c. a nodular lesion usually over a distal finger joint, consisting of mucinous degeneration of the collagen of the dermis; it is not a true cyst, because it lacks an epithelial wall and does not communicate with the underlying area of the synovial capsule. Called also *myxoid c.*, *synovial c.*, and *synovial ganglion.*
dilatation c. a cyst formed by dilation of a previously existing cavity.
distention c. a collection of watery fluid in a normal, but distended cavity.
duplication c. a congenital cystic malformation of the alimentary tract, consisting of a duplication of the segment to which it is adjacent, occurring anywhere from the mouth to the anus but most frequently affecting the ileum and esophagus.
echinococcal c., echinococcus c. hydatid c.
endometrial c. 1. a chocolate cyst, particularly in the ovary, containing blood debris and endometrium. 2. endometrioma.
endometriotic c. endometrial c. (def. 1).
endothelial c. a cyst whose sac has an endothelial lining.
enteric c., enterogenous c. a cyst of the intestine arising or developing from a fold or pouch, often from a fold in the primitive foregut. Called also *enterocyst* and *enterocystoma.*
ependymal c. a circumscribed dilatation of some part of the ependyma.
epidermal c. a benign cyst derived from the epidermis or the epithelium of a hair follicle, formed by cystic enclosures of epithelium within the dermis, becoming filled with keratin and lipid-rich debris.

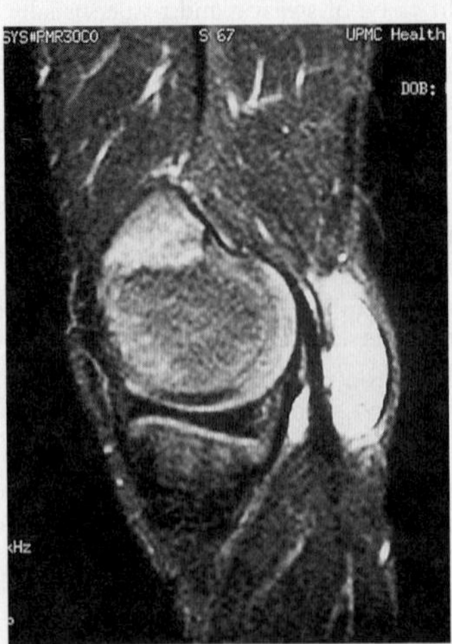

■ Sagittal plane MRI showing the posterior location of a Baker cyst.

Types include dermoid cyst, epidermal inclusion cyst, pilar cyst, milium, and steatocystoma. Called also *epidermoid* or *epithelial c.*

epidermal inclusion c. a type of epidermal cyst that is an inclusion cyst on the head, neck, or trunk; it is circumscribed and mobile and is formed by keratinizing squamous epithelium that has a granular layer and is similar to the normal epithelium of the follicular infundibulum. Called also *epidermoid c.*

epidermoid c. 1. epidermal c. 2. a benign tumor in the skull, meninges, or brain, formed by inclusion of epidermal elements, especially at the time of closure of the neural groove. It may grow gradually because of accumulations of desquamated debris and may become calcified. Called also *epidermoid, epidermoidoma,* and *epidermoid tumor.* 3. epidermal inclusion c.

epithelial c. 1. any cyst lined by keratinizing stratified squamous epithelium; see *epidermal c.* 2. epidermal c.

eruption c. a type of dentigerous cyst presenting as a dilatation of the follicular space about the crown of the erupting deciduous or permanent teeth in children, caused by the accumulation of tissue fluid or blood.

eruptive vellus hair c. a type of tiny papule that contains vellus hair, usually appearing in crops on the chest in men and ranging from flesh-colored to dark; this lesion is histologically similar and may be related to steatocystoma multiplex.

extravasation c. simple bone c.

exudation c. a cyst formed by an exudate collected in a closed cavity.

false c. pseudocyst (def.1).

fissural c. inclusion c. (def. 1).

follicular c. 1. a cyst that results from occlusion of the duct of a follicle or small gland. 2. a cyst formed by the enlargement of a graafian follicle as a result of accumulated transudate.

ganglionic c. subchondral c.

Gartner c., Gartner duct c., gartnerian c. a benign cystic vaginal tumor developed from remnants of either Gartner duct, the embryonic mesonephros, or the wolffian duct system.

gas c. a small cyst filled with gas, of bacterial origin.

gingival c. an odontogenic cyst of the soft tissue of either the free or attached gingiva, presenting as a small, well-circumscribed, painless swelling, sometimes resembling a superficial mucocele.

globulomaxillary c. an inclusion cyst of the maxillary bone, located in the globulomaxillary fissure, usually between the lateral incisor and cuspid teeth, which seldom presents any clinical manifestation.

Gorlin c. calcifying odontogenic c.

granddaughter c. a cyst occasionally seen within the daughter cyst of a hydatid cyst.

hemorrhagic c. simple bone c.

heterotopic oral gastrointestinal c. a cyst lined by gastric or intestinal mucosa but occurring in the oral cavity, usually in the tongue, floor of the mouth, or neck, or adjacent to the submaxillary gland.

hilar c. renal sinus c.

hydatid c. a cyst formed during the larval stage of tapeworms of species *Echinococcus;* it contains daughter cysts that contain many scoleces. There are two types, the *alveolar* or *multilocular hydatid cyst* and the *unilocular hydatid cyst.* Called also *echinococcal* or *echinococcus c.* and *hydatid.* See also *hydatid disease,* under *disease.*

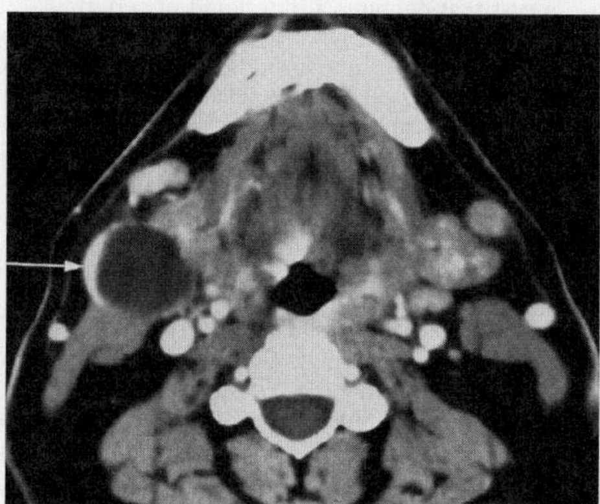

■ Branchial cleft cyst seen as a well-defined, low-density lesion in an axial contrast-enhanced CT scan through the midlevel of the tongue and base of the mandible. The lateral wall shows thick enhancement *(arrow),* indicating infection.

implantation c. epidermal inclusion c.

incisive canal c. median anterior maxillary c.

inclusion c. 1. a cyst formed by the inclusion of a small portion of epithelium or mesothelium within connective tissue along a line of fusion of embryonic processes; types found in the oral region are the median palatal cyst, median anterior maxillary cyst, globulomaxillary cyst, and nasoalveolar cyst. Called also *fissural c.* 2. epidermal inclusion c.

infundibular c. an epidermal cyst that arises from the follicular infundibulum.

intraluminal c's cysts that are duplications of part of the intestines, or retention cysts, and are sometimes the cause of intrinsic obstruction in the newborn.

intrapituitary c's Rathke c's.

involution c. mammary duct ectasia.

Iwanoff (Iwanow) c's Blessig c's.

keratinizing c., keratinous c. any cyst containing keratinous material, such as an epithelial cyst.

Klestadt c. nasoalveolar c.

lacteal c. a cyst of the breast due to obstruction of a lactiferous duct; called also *milk c.*

lateral periodontal c. a cyst of the lateral periodontal membrane of an erupted tooth, usually occurring in the bicuspid region of the mandible.

leptomeningeal c. arachnoid c.

lutein c. a cyst of the ovary developed from a corpus luteum.

lymphoepithelial c. branchial c.

median anterior maxillary c. a type of inclusion cyst of the maxilla found in or near an incisive canal, arising from proliferation of epithelial remnants of an embryonic duct. Called also *incisive canal c.* and *nasopalatine duct c.*

median mandibular c. a rare type of inclusion cyst found in the midline of the mandible, believed to be caused by inclusion of the epithelium trapped in the central groove of the mandibular process, or by cystic degeneration of a supernumerary tooth germ.

median palatal c. a type of inclusion cyst found in the midline of the hard palate between the lateral palatal processes.

median raphe c. a type of small solitary cyst found on the raphe of the penis, lined by stratified columnar epithelium.

mediastinal c. a congenital cyst arising in the mediastinum.

meibomian c. chalazion.

mesenteric c. a congenital thin-walled cyst of the abdomen between the leaves of the mesentery, which may be of wolffian or lymphatic duct origin; as it enlarges, it may cause obstruction and intestinal colic.

milk c. lacteal c.

morgagnian c. 1. appendix testis. 2. *(in the pl.)* appendices vesiculosae epoophori.

mother c. a cyst that encloses other cysts (the "daughter cysts"), such as sometimes occurs with hydatid cysts.

mucous c. a retention cyst containing mucus.

mucus retention c. a mucus-containing retention cyst caused by blockage of a salivary gland duct, visible as a small nodule on the oral mucosa. Called also *mucocele.* Cf. *mucus extravasation phenomenon,* under *phenomenon.*

multilocular c. 1. a cyst containing several loculi or spaces; cf. *unilocular c.* (def. 1). 2. multilocular hydatid c. 3. multilocular c. of kidney.

multilocular hydatid c. alveolar hydatid c.

multilocular c. of kidney a thick-walled cyst in the kidney, found in clusters and usually unilaterally. In children it contains blastema and may develop into a Wilms tumor. A variety in adults has more fibrous tissue than the juvenile variety. Called also *cystic* or *differentiated nephroblastoma, benign cystic* or *multilocular cystic nephroma,* and *multilocular cystic renal tumor.*

myxoid c. digital mucous c.

Naboth c's, nabothian c's Naboth follicles.

nasoalveolar c., nasolabial c. an inclusion cyst arising from epithelial remnants at the junction of the lateral nasal and maxillary processes; it may cause a swelling in the mucolabial fold and in the floor of the nose and superficial erosion of the outer surface of the maxilla.

nasopalatine duct c. median anterior maxillary c.

necrotic c. a cyst containing necrotic matter.

neural c. a cyst or cystlike structure occurring in the central nervous system, such as a soapsuds cyst or a porencephalic cyst.

neurenteric c. a type of mediastinal cyst found in the posterior mediastinum, containing tissues from the nervous system and other organs, and connecting with the spinal dura mater.
odontogenic c. a cyst in the jaw, derived from epithelium, usually containing fluid or semisolid material, developing during any of various stages of odontogenesis; nearly all are enclosed within bone. Types include dentigerous, gingival, periodontal, and primordial cysts.
oil c. a cyst that contains oily matter, due to fatty degeneration of the epithelial lining.
omental c. a cyst similar to a mesenteric cyst but confined to the omentum.
omphalomesenteric duct c. a cyst formed by failure of closure of part of the yolk stalk (omphalomesenteric duct); it may be at the umbilicus and visible on the skin, or more internally along the duct. Called also *umbilical* or *vitellointestinal c.*
oophoritic c. ovarian c..
osseous hydatid c. a type of hydatid cyst formed by the larvae of *Echinococcus granulosus*, and found in bone, which may become weakened and eroded by the exuberant growth.
ovarian c. a cyst of the ovary proper.
pancreatic c. a cyst in the pancreatic duct, usually a retention cyst. Cf. *pancreatic pseudocyst*.
parapelvic c., parapyelitic c. 1. renal sinus c. 2. peripelvic c. (def. 2).
parasitic c. a cyst formed by the larva of a parasite, such as a hydatid cyst.
parovarian c. a cyst of the epoöphoron.
pearl c. a cyst or a solid mass of epithelial cells in the iris caused by implantation of an eyelash, cotton, or other foreign particle.
periapical c. a periodontal cyst involving the apex of an erupted tooth, frequently a result of infection via the pulp chamber and root canal through carious involvement of the tooth. Called also *radicular c.*
pericardial c. a benign collection of clear fluid, usually found next to the pericardium; such cysts must be differentiated from the more serious mediastinal tumors.
perinephric c. urinoma.
perineurial c. an outpouching of the perineurial space on the extradural portion of the posterior sacral or coccygeal nerve roots at the junction of the root and ganglion; it may cause low back pain and sciatica.
periodontal c. a cyst in the periodontal ligament and adjacent structures, usually at the apex *(periapical c.)*, but sometimes along the lateral surfaces of the tooth *(lateral periodontal c.)*.
peripelvic c. 1. renal sinus c. 2. any cyst or pseudocyst adjacent to a renal pelvis; called also *parapelvic c.*
perirenal c. urinoma.
pilar c. a type of epidermal cyst, usually a firm, circumscribed, subepidermal nodule, especially on the scalp; it is formed by an outer wall of keratinizing epithelium without a granular layer, similar to the normal epithelium of the hair follicle near the sebaceous duct. Called also *sebaceous c.*, *trichilemmal c.*, and *wen.*
piliferous c., pilonidal c. pilonidal sinus.
placental c. a gray to white, disklike cyst of the placenta, resulting from degeneration of trophoblastic cells.
popliteal c. Baker c.

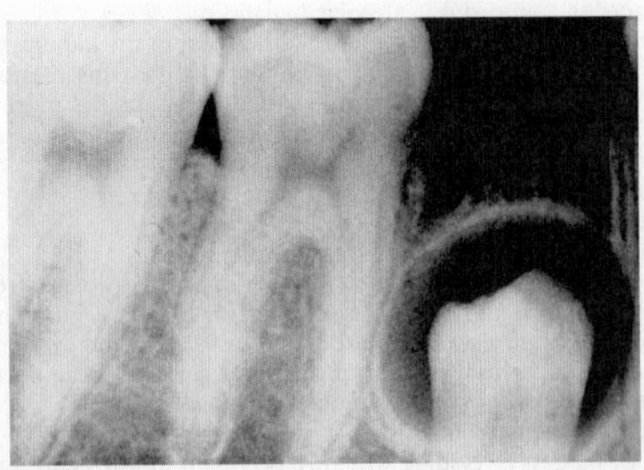

■ Dentigerous cyst around the crown of an unerupted bicuspid.

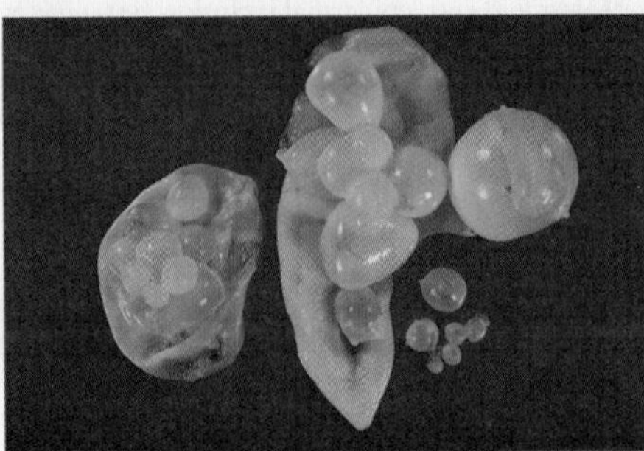

■ Hydatid cyst of liver.

porencephalic c. a cyst occurring in the brain substance in porencephaly.
primary c. mother c.
primordial c. a relatively uncommon type of odontogenic cyst that develops through cystic degeneration and liquefaction of the stellate reticulum in an enamel organ before any calcified enamel or dentin has been formed. Such cysts originate from supernumerary teeth, and are found in place of a tooth rather than being associated with one.
proliferating pilar c., proliferating trichilemmal c. see under *tumor.*
pseudomucinous c. mucinous cystadenoma.
pyelocaliceal c., pyelocalyceal c., pyelogenic renal c. calyceal diverticulum.
radicular c. periapical c.
Rathke c's, Rathke cleft c's groups of epithelial cells forming small colloid-filled cysts in the pars intermedia of the pituitary gland; they are vestiges of Rathke pouch and are closely related to craniopharyngiomas. Called also *craniobuccal c's* and *craniopharyngeal c's* .
renal sinus c. a cyst in a renal sinus, usually derived from aberrant lymphatic vessels, occurring either alone or in groups. Most appear after the fifth decade of life in association with inflammation, obstruction, or a calculus; they may be asymptomatic or may expand to cause pelvic compression and local deformity with pain, hematuria, infection, and pyuria. Called also *hilar c.*, *parapelvic c.*, and *peripelvic c.*
residual c. a periodontal cyst that remains after or develops subsequent to tooth extraction.
retention c. a cyst caused by blockage of the excretory duct of a gland, so that glandular secretions are retained; called also *secretory c.*
sarcosporidian c. sarcocyst (def. 2).
sebaceous c. pilar c.
secondary c. daughter c.
secretory c. retention c.
seminal vesicle c. a cyst in the wall of a seminal vesicle; it may be congenital and associated with other urinary tract anomalies, or acquired such as secondary to obstruction of the vesicle.
serous c. a cyst that contains a thin liquid or serum.
simple bone c. a unilocular, cystic, often asymptomatic bone lesion usually occurring in the long tubular bones of children and adolescents; it is hollow or fluid-filled, lacks an epithelial lining, and does not penetrate the cortex or extend into soft tissue. Its origin is debated, but it is postulated to occur secondary to traumatic hematoma formation. Called also *unicameral bone c.*
soapsuds c. a type of cyst found studding the cerebral cortex in cryptococcosis.
solitary bone c. simple bone c.
springwater c. pericardial c.
sterile c. acephalocyst.
subchondral c. a simple bone cyst within the fused epiphysis beneath the articular plate; it is lined with a membrane (probably modified synovia) that contains a mucinous material. Called also *ganglionic c.*
subepiglottic c. a congenital cyst in the subepiglottic mucosa of a horse, often associated with respiratory stridor.
sublingual c. ranula.
subsynovial c. a cyst caused by the accumulation of synovial or inflammatory fluid beneath the synovium.
suprasellar c. craniopharyngioma.

Cyst *Continued*

synovial c. digital mucous c.
Tarlov c. perineurial c.
tarry c. 1. a type of corpus luteum cyst resulting from hemorrhage into the corpus luteum. 2. a blood-filled cyst resulting from endometriosis.
tarsal c. chalazion.
thecal c. distention of a tendon sheath.
theca-lutein c. an ovarian cyst in which the cells lining the cystic cavity are theca-lutein cells.
thymic c. a rare congenital type of mediastinal cyst, arising in the upper anterior mediastinum, containing tissue resembling that of the thymus.
thyroglossal c., thyrolingual c. a cyst in the neck caused by persistence of portions of, or by lack of closure of, the primitive thyroglossal duct.
tissue c. see *cyst* (def. 2) and *pseudocyst* (def. 2).
Tornwaldt (Thornwaldt) c. bursa pharyngealis.

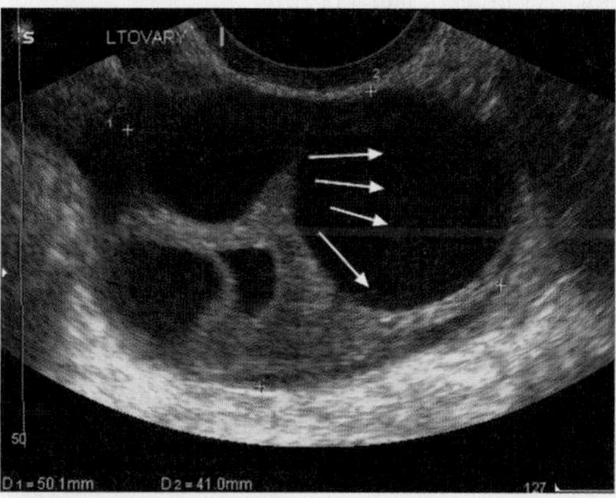

■ Endovaginal image of ovary containing several abnormally large cysts, including one with a fluid-filled level *(arrows)* indicating internal hemorrhage.

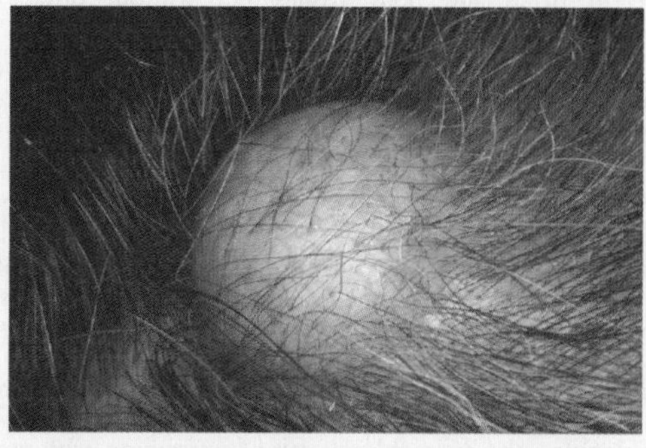

■ Pilar cyst.

traumatic bone c. simple bone c.
trichilemmal c. pilar c.
true c. any cyst that is not a normal structure and is not formed by the dilatation of a passage or cavity.
tubular c. tubulocyst.
umbilical c. omphalomesenteric c.
unicameral c. unilocular c. (def. 1).
unicameral bone c. simple bone c.
unilocular c. 1. a cyst containing but one cavity. Cf. *multilocular c.* (def. 1). 2. unilocular hydatid c.
unilocular hydatid c. the usual kind of hydatid cyst, having a single loculus or cavity, seen in infections with *Echinococcus granulosus* and *E. vogeli.*
urachal c., urachal remnant c. a congenital anomaly in which part of the urachus is dilated to form a cyst; it may contain mucinous fluid, cellular debris, or urine. Called also *allantoic c.*
urinary c. urinoma.
vellus hair c. eruptive vellus hair c.
vitellointestinal c. omphalomesenteric duct c.
wolffian c. a cyst of the remnants of the wolffian (mesonephric) duct.

cys·tad·e·no·car·ci·no·ma (sis-tad″ə-no-kahr″sĭ-no′mə) [*cyst-* + *adenocarcinoma*] adenocarcinoma characterized by tumor-lined cystic cavities; occurring usually in the ovaries but also in other sites such as the appendix, pancreas, or thyroid.

mucinous c. 1. cystadenocarcinoma in which epithelium-lined cystic masses produce a sticky, gelatinous, glycoprotein-rich fluid; it usually occurs in the ovary. 2. a malignant, usually bulky, exocrine pancreatic tumor, containing cystic epithelium; cf. *mucinous cystadenoma*, under *cystadenoma.*

papillary c. cystadenocarcinoma characterized by papillary projections into the cystic lumina, usually in the ovary.

pseudomucinous c. mucinous c.; the term was coined when the neoplasm was believed not to be truly mucinous.

serous c. cystadenocarcinoma in which epithelium-lined cystic neoplasms are filled with serous fluid, usually found in the ovaries, sometimes with papillary projections from, or masses or thickenings of, the cavity walls.

cys·tad·e·no·lym·pho·ma (sis-tad″ə-no-lim-fo′mə) adenolymphoma.

cys·tad·e·no·ma (sis″tad-ə-no′mə) [*cyst-* + *adenoma*] adenoma characterized by epithelium-lined cystic masses that contain secreted material, usually serous or mucinous; it generally occurs in the ovary, salivary glands, skin adnexa, or pancreas. Called also *adenocystoma.*

apocrine c. see under *hidrocystoma.*

bile duct c. a large multiloculated cystic tumor of the liver, usually in the right lobe and filled with clear or cloudy fluid.

eccrine c. see under *hidrocystoma.*

mucinous c. 1. a usually benign multilocular tumor with mucin-filled cavities, produced by the epithelial cells of the ovary. 2. a benign, usually bulky, exocrine pancreatic tumor, containing cystic epithelium; cf. *mucinous cystadenocarcinoma*, under *cystadenocarcinoma.*

papillary c. 1. any tumor producing patterns that are both papillary and cystic. 2. a type of adenoma in which the acini are distended by fluid or by outgrowths of tissue. Called also *papillary cystic adenoma.*

papillary c. lymphomatosum adenolymphoma.

papillary c. of thyroid a benign tumor of the thyroid gland with branching papillae and cystlike cavities; it may be an early stage of papillary carcinoma.

pseudomucinous c. mucinous c.; the term was coined when the contents were believed not to be truly mucinous.

serous c. a cystic tumor of the ovary, containing thin, clear, yellow serous fluid and varying amounts of solid tissue, with a malignant potential several times greater than that of mucinous cystadenoma.

Cys·ta·gon (sis′tə-gon) trademark for a preparation of cysteamine bitartrate.

cys·tal·gia (sis-tal′jə) [*cyst-* + *-algia*] pain in the urinary bladder; called also *cystodynia.*

γ-cys·ta·thi·o·nase (sis″tə-thi′o-nās) cystathionine γ-lyase.

cys·ta·thi·o·nine (sis″tə-thi′o-nēn) an unsymmetrical thio-ether of homocysteine and serine that serves as an intermediate in the transfer of a sulfur atom from methionine to cysteine.

cys·ta·thi·o·nine γ-ly·ase (sis″tə-thi′o-nēn li′ās) [EC 4.4.1.1] an enzyme of the lyase class that catalyzes the cleavage of cystathionine to cysteine, α-ketoglutarate, and ammonia as a step in the metabolism of methionine. It is a pyridoxal-phosphate protein and the reaction occurs in the liver. Deficiency of the enzyme, an autosomal recessive trait, results in cystathioninuria. Called also *γ-cystathionase.*

cys·ta·thi·o·nine β-syn·thase (sis″tə-thi′o-nēn sin′thās) [EC 4.2.1.22] an enzyme of the lyase class that catalyzes the condensation of serine and homocysteine to form cystathionine as a step in the catabolism of methionine. It is a pyridoxal-phosphate protein, found in the mammalian liver.

cys·ta·thi·o·nine β-syn·thase de·fi·cien·cy (sis″tə-thi′o-nēn sin′thās) an autosomal recessive aminoacidopathy caused by mutations in the *CBS* gene (locus: 21q22.3), which encodes cystathionine β-synthase, characterized by homocystinuria accompanied by hypermethioninemia. Clinical abnormalities occur primarily in the eye and the skeletal, nervous, and vascular systems; ectopia lentis, osteoporosis, mental retardation, and thrombosis are the most common manifestations. In older literature, the disorder is sometimes called homocystinuria (q.v.).

cys•ta•thi•o•nin•u•ria (sis″tə-thi″o-ne-nu′re-ə) a benign autosomal recessive aminoacidopathy caused by mutations in the *CTH* gene (locus: 1p31.1), which encodes cystathionine γ-lyase, characterized by excess of cystathionine in urine and body tissues but without other clinical manifestations.

cys•tat•in C (sis-tat′in) an inhibitor of cysteine endopeptidase, produced by most cells in the body and excreted into the bloodstream; it is freely filtered by the renal glomeruli and its rate of clearance can be used to calculate the glomerular filtration rate.

cys•ta•tro•phia (sis″tə-tro′fe-ə) [*cyst-* + *atrophia*] atrophy of the urinary bladder.

cys•te•amine (sis-te′ə-mēn″) a sulfhydryl amine that is part of coenzyme A; it reduces intracellular cystine levels and is used in treatment of nephropathic cystinosis; administered orally. Called also *β-mercaptoethylamine.*

c. bitartrate the bitartrate salt of cysteamine, with uses similar to those of the base.

c. hydrochloride the hydrochloride salt of cysteamine, with uses similar to those of the base.

cys•tec•ta•sia (sis″tek-ta′zhə) [*cyst-* +Gr. *ektasis* dilatation] slitting of the membranous portion of the urethra and dilation of the bladder neck for extraction of a calculus.

cys•tec•ta•sy (sis-tek′tə-se) cystectasia.

cys•tec•to•my (sis-tek′tə-me) [*cyst-* + *-ectomy*] 1. excision of a cyst. 2. resection of the bladder.

radical c. surgical treatment of invasive bladder cancer by removal of the bladder with its peritoneal covering, the lower ureters, pelvic lymph nodes, and surrounding organs and structures. In females it is a synonym of *anterior pelvic exenteration.* In males (called also *radical cystoprostatectomy*) the prostate, seminal vesicles, pelvic vas deferens and its ampulla, and sometimes part or all of the urethra are removed.

cys•te•ic ac•id (sis-te′ik) an intermediate formed by oxidation of the thiol group of cysteine to a sulfo group, and precursor of taurine.

cys•te•ine (sis′te-ēn) chemical name: 2-amino-3-mercaptopropanoic acid. A sulfur-containing nonessential amino acid produced by the enzymatic or acid hydrolysis of proteins. It is easily oxidized to cystine, is sometimes found in the urine, and has limited detoxification properties. Symbols Cys and C. See also table at *amino acid.*

c. hydrochloride [USP] the hydrochloride salt of cysteine; used as a dietary supplement.

cys•te•ine en•do•pep•ti•dase (sis′te-ēn en″do-pep′tĭ-dās) [EC 3.4.22] any of a group of endopeptidases containing at the active site a cysteine residue involved in catalysis; the group includes papain and several cathepsins. Called also *thiol endopeptidase.*

cys•te•ine-type car•boxy•pep•ti•dase (sis′te-ēn-tīp″ kahr-bok″se-pep′tĭ-dās) 1. [EC 3.4.18] any exopeptidase that contains a cysteine residue at the active site and catalyzes the thiol-dependent hydrolytic cleavage of the terminal or penultimate peptide bond at the C-terminal end of a peptide or polypeptide. 2. [EC 3.4.18.1] a lysosomal carboxypeptidase with broad specificity but not acting on C-terminal proline residues. Called also *lysosomal carboxypeptidase B* and *cathepsin* B_2.

cys•te•in•yl (sis-te′in-əl) the acyl radical of cysteine.

cys•tel•co•sis (sis″təl-ko′sis) [*cyst-* + *elcosis*] ulceration of the bladder.

cys•ten•ceph•a•lus (sis″tən-sef′ə-ləs) [*cyst-* + Gr. *enkephalos* brain] a fetus with a membranous sac in place of a brain.

cys•tic (sis′tik) 1. pertaining to a cyst. 2. pertaining to the urinary bladder or gallbladder. Cf. *vesical.*

cys•ti•cer•ci (sis″tĭ-sur′si) plural of *cysticercus.*

cys•ti•cer•coid (sis″tĭ-sur′koid) a form of larval tapeworm resembling *Cysticercus,* but having the cyst small, almost devoid of fluid, and provided with a caudal appendage, as in *Hymenolepis.*

cys•ti•cer•co•sis (sis″tĭ-sər-ko′sis) 1. human infection with cysticerci (larvae of tapeworms of genus *Taenia*). Those who ingest the eggs of *Taenia solium* (the pork tapeworm) in contaminated food or water may become infected with the larval stage called *Cysticercus cellulosae,* which penetrates the intestinal wall and invades the subcutaneous tissue, brain, eye, muscle, heart, liver, lung, peritoneum, and sometimes other sites. Brain involvement is called neurocysticercosis (q.v.). Those who eat incompletely cooked beef become infected with the adult form of *Taenia saginata* (the beef tapeworm), which can grow to a length of 3.5 to 8 meters in the intestine. Those who ingest the eggs of *T. saginata* apparently do not become infected with its larval stage called *Cysticercus bovis.* 2. infection of livestock with cysticerci; this usually occurs as cysts in striated muscles, causing no adverse symptoms. Depending on the animal, it is known as *beef measles, pork measles,* or *sheep measles.*

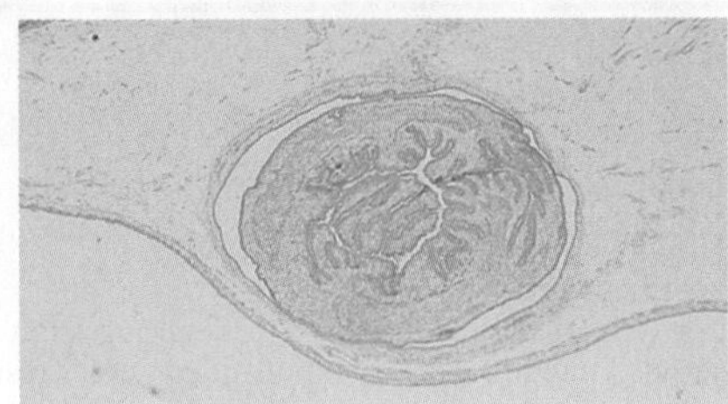

■ Cross-section of a cysticercus cyst.

Cys•ti•cer•cus (sis″tĭ-sur′kəs) [Gr. *kystis* bladder + *kerkos* tail] a former genus of larval forms of tapeworms of the genus *Taenia.*

C. bo′vis the larva of *Taenia saginata.*

C. cellulo′sae the larva of *Taenia solium;* see also *cysticercosis.*

C. o′vis the larva of *Taenia ovis.*

C. tenuicol′lis the larva of *Taenia hydatigena.*

cys•ti•cer•cus (sis″tĭ-sur′kəs) pl. *cysticer′ci.* A larval form of tapeworm, consisting of a single scolex enclosed in a bladderlike cyst; cf. *hydatid cyst,* under *cyst.* Called also *bladder worm.*

cys•ti•des (sis′tĭ-dēz) plural of *cystis.*

cys•tif•er•ous (sis-tif′ər-əs) cystigerous.

cys•ti•form (sis′tĭ-form) [*cysti-* + *form*] cystoid (def. 1).

cys•tig•er•ous (sis-tij′ər-əs) [*cysti-* + L. *gerere* to bear] containing cysts.

cys•tine (sis′tēn, sis′tin) chemical name: 3,3′-dithiobis(2-aminopropanoic acid). An amino acid produced by the digestion or acid hydrolysis of proteins. It is sometimes found in the urine and in the kidneys in the form of minute hexagonal crystals, frequently forming a cystine calculus in the bladder. Cystine is the chief sulfur-containing compound of the protein molecule and is readily reduced to two molecules of cysteine (hence, also called *dicysteine*).

cys•tin•emia (sis′tĭ-ne′me-ə) presence of cystine in the blood.

cys•tin•o•sin (sis-tĭ-no′sin) a lysosomal membrane protein, expressed strongly in the pancreas, kidney, and skeletal muscle and to a lesser degree in the placenta, heart, lungs, and liver, that transports cystine out of lysosomes.

cys•ti•no•sis (sis″tĭ-no′sis) a group of lysosomal storage diseases caused by mutations in the *CTNS* gene (locus: 17p13), which encodes cystinosin, characterized by widespread intralysosomal accumulation of cystine crystals and consequent cell and tissue destruction. Called also *cystine storage disease* and *Lignac-Fanconi syndrome.*

adolescent nephropathic c. late onset juvenile c.

adult nonnephropathic c., benign nonnephropathic c. cystinosis characterized by photophobia caused by deposition of cystine crystals in the cornea, without renal damage. Called also *ocular nonnephropathic c.*

early onset c. infantile nephropathic c.

infantile nephropathic c. the most common cause of Fanconi syndrome (def. 2), a type of cystinosis marked by vitamin D–resistant rickets, chronic acidosis, polyuria, and dehydration, all resulting from proximal renal tubular dysfunction, and by corneal opacities, growth failure, uremia, and chronic renal failure. Affected children formerly died before age 10, but with improved treatment, now some may live into adulthood. Called also *early onset c.*

late onset juvenile c. cystinosis with onset in the second decade of life, characterized by photophobia, mild proximal tubulopathy, and slowly progressive glomerulopathy that may progress to chronic renal failure. Called also *adolescent nephropathic c.*

nephropathic c. any of the types of cystinosis that involve kidney damage as well as ophthalmic symptoms; see *early onset c.* and *late onset juvenile c.*

ocular nonnephropathic c. adult nonnephropathic cystinosis.

cys•tin•uria (sis″tĭ-nu′re-ə) an autosomal recessive disorder of amino acid transport caused by mutations in the *SLC3A1* (locus: 2p16.3) and *SLC7A9* (locus: 19q13.1) genes, which encode amino acid transporter components, characterized by defective intestinal and renal tubular reabsorption of cystine and the dibasic amino acids ornithine, lysine, and arginine. The chief clinical manifestation is the formation of urinary cystine calculi. cystinu′ric *adj*

cys•ti•nyl ami•no•pep•ti•dase (sis′tĭ-nəl ə-me″no-pep′tĭ-dās) [EC 3.4.11.3] a zinc-containing enzyme released by the placenta that acts to break down oxytocin and vasopressin; called also *oxytocinase* and *vasopressinase.*

cys•tis (sis′tis) pl. *cys′tides* [Gr. *kystis*] 1. vesica. 2. cyst (def. 2).

cys•ti•stax•is (sis″tĭ-stak′sis) [*cysti-* + *staxis*] oozing of blood from the mucous membrane into the bladder.

cys·ti·tis (sis-ti′tis) pl. *cysti′tides.* inflammation of the urinary bladder; called also *urocystitis.*

allergic c. cystitis resulting from some unusual hypersensitivity, characterized by a large number of mononuclear leukocytes and eosinophils in the bladder mucosa and musculature, and in the urinary sediment.

bacterial c. bacterial infection of the bladder.

chemical c. allergic cystitis occurring in reaction to a chemical substance in the body; see also *drug-induced c.*

c. col′li bladder inflammation in the area of the bladder neck.

cystic c., c. cys′tica cystitis with formation of multiple submucosal cysts in the bladder wall.

drug-induced c. allergic cystitis occurring in reaction to a medication; see also *chemical c.*

c. emphysemato′sa, emphysematous c. a rare type of bladder inflammation with gas-filled vesicles and cysts in the bladder mucosa and musculature.

eosinophilic c. cystitis with large numbers of eosinophils in the urinary sediment.

c. follicula′ris cystitis in which the bladder mucosa has many nodules containing lymphoid follicles.

c. glandula′ris cystitis in which the mucosa contains mucin-secreting glands, seen most frequently in cases of exstrophy of bladder; it sometimes leads to malignant degeneration.

hemorrhagic c. cystitis accompanied by severe hemorrhage, seen as a dose-limiting toxic condition with administration of ifosfamide and cyclophosphamide and as a complication of bone marrow transplantation.

incrusted c. an intense cystitis characterized by deposition of phosphatic or other inorganic salts on the chronically inflamed bladder wall, generally at the site of ulcerations, granulations, or tumors.

interstitial c. an inflammatory condition of the bladder, seen mainly in women, whose lesion is a small patch of red to brown mucosa surrounded by a network of radiating vessels, usually in the vertex and involving the entire thickness of the wall. The lesions, known as *Hunner ulcers,* may heal superficially and be difficult to detect. Typically, there is urinary frequency and pain on bladder filling and at the end of urination. Called also *panmural c., submucous c.,* and *panmural fibrosis of the bladder.*

mechanical c. cystitis resulting from irritation by a calculus or other foreign body in the bladder, or from manipulation.

panmural c. interstitial c.

radiation c. acute or chronic inflammatory tissue changes in the urinary bladder caused by ionizing radiation; called also *radiocystitis.*

submucous c. interstitial c.

viral c. cystitis due to a viral infection, most often seen in immunocompromised persons infected with BK polyomavirus.

cys·tit·o·my (sis-tit′ə-me) [*cysti-* + *-tomy*] the surgical division of the capsule of the lens; capsulotomy.

cyst(o)- a combining form denoting a relationship to a sac, cyst, or bladder.

cys·to·ad·e·no·ma (sis″to-ad″ə-no′mə) cystadenoma.

cys·to·blast (sis′to-blast) [*cysto-* + *-blast*] the layer of cells that lines the amniotic cavity of the early embryo on the side of the enveloping layer.

Cys·to·cau·lus (sis″to-kaw′lus) a genus of parasitic nematodes of the family Protostrongylidae, several species of which are lungworms of sheep and goats.

cys·to·cele (sis′to-sēl) [*cysto-* + *cele*[1]] hernial protrusion of the urinary bladder, usually through the vaginal wall. Called also *vesicocele.*

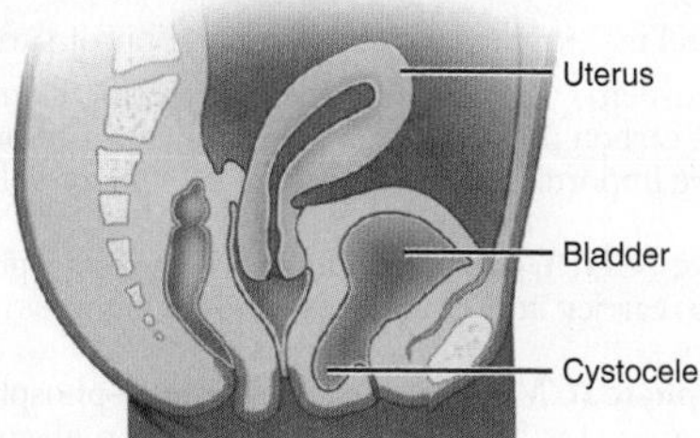

cys·to·chro·mos·co·py (sis″to-kro-mos′kə-pe) chromocystoscopy.

Cys·to-Con·ray (sis′to-kon″ra) trademark for preparations of iothalamate meglumine.

cys·to·di·a·pha·nos·co·py (sis″to-di″ə-fə-nos′kə-pe) [*cysto-* + *diaphanoscopy*] examination of the urinary bladder using transillumination (diaphanoscopy).

cys·to·du·o·de·nal (sis″to-doo″o-de′nəl, -doo-od′ə-nəl) 1. pertaining to a cyst and the duodenum. 2. pertaining to or connecting the gallbladder and the duodenum.

cys·to·du·od·e·nos·to·my (sis″to-du″o-də-nos′tə-me) internal drainage of an adjacent cyst or pancreatic pseudocyst into the duodenum.

cys·to·dyn·ia (sis″to-din′e-ə) [*cysto-* + *-odynia*] cystalgia.

cys·to·en·tero·cele (sis″to-en′tər-o-sēl) enterocystocele.

cys·to·en·ter·os·to·my (sis″to-en″ter-os′tə-me) internal drainage of an adjacent cyst or pancreatic pseudocyst into the intestine.

cys·to·epip·lo·cele (sis″to-e-pip′lo-sēl) hernia of a portion of the bladder and omentum.

cys·to·gas·tros·to·my (sis″to-gas-tros′tə-me) internal drainage of an adjacent cyst or pancreatic pseudocyst into the stomach.

cys·to·gen·e·sis (sis″to-jen′ə-sis) formation of a cyst.

cys·to·gram (sis′to-gram) a radiograph of the bladder.

cys·tog·ra·phy (sis-tog′rə-fe) [*cysto-* + *-graphy*] radiography of the bladder after injection of it with opaque solution.

delayed c. cystography in which film exposures are made at varying intervals up to 30 minutes or longer; useful in the study of urinary reflux.

voiding c. radiography of the bladder while the patient is urinating.

cys·toid (sis′toid) [*cysto-* + *-oid*] 1. resembling a cyst; called also *cystiform.* 2. a cystlike, circumscribed collection of softened material, differing from a true cyst in having no enclosing capsule.

Cys·to·i·sos·po·ra (sis″to-i-sos′pə-rə) a genus of coccidian protozoa that infects the intestines of mammals; formerly classified as part of *Isospora.* Infections may be subclinical or may lead to mild coccidiosis.

C. bel′li an intestinal parasite of humans that may cause coccidiosis, which is usually asymptomatic but may result in severe, watery, mucous diarrhea.

C. burrow′si a species that infects dogs.

C. ca′nis a species that infects dogs.

C. fe′lis a species that infects cats.

C. neorivol′ta a species that infects dogs.

C. ohioen′sis a species that infects dogs.

C. rivol′ta a species that infects cats.

C. su′is a species that infects pigs.

cys·to·isos·po·ri·a·sis (sis-to-i-sos″pə-ri′ə-sis) infection with protozoa of genus *Cystoisospora,* which produces diarrheal disease.

cys·to·je·ju·nos·to·my (sis″to-jə-joo-nos′tə-me) internal drainage of an adjacent cyst or pancreatic pseudocyst into the jejunum.

cys·to·lith (sis′to-lith) [*cysto-* + *-lith*] vesical calculus.

cys·to·li·thec·to·my (sis″to-lĭ-thek′tə-me) [*cysto-* + *lithectomy*] removal of a calculus from the urinary bladder; see *cystolithotomy.*

cys·to·li·thi·a·sis (sis″to-lĭ-thi′ə-sis) [*cysto-* + Gr. *lithos* stone] the development of calculi in the bladder; see *vesical calculus,* under *calculus.*

cys·to·lith·ic (sis″to-lith′ik) pertaining to a vesical calculus.

cys·to·li·thot·o·my (sis″to-lĭ-thot′ə-me) incision of the urinary bladder for removal of a calculus. The term has also been used erroneously for excision of a gallstone from the gallbladder (cholelithotomy).

cys·to·ma (sis-to′mə) cystic tumor.

cys·to·ma·tous (sis-to′mə-təs) relating to or containing cystoma.

cys·tom·e·ter (sis-tom′ə-tər) [*cysto-* + *-meter*] an instrument for studying the neuromuscular mechanism of the bladder by means of measurements of pressure and capacity.

cys·to·met·ro·gram (sis″to-met′ro-gram) the tracing recorded by cystometrography.

cys·to·me·trog·ra·phy (sis″to-mə-trog′rə-fe) the graphic recording of the pressure exerted at varying degrees of filling of the urinary bladder.

cys·tom·e·try (sis-tom′ə-tre) the study of bladder efficiency by means of the cystometer.

simple c. filling of the bladder to capacity through a urethral catheter, until an involuntary contraction of the detrusor muscle occurs.

cys·to·mor·phous (sis″to-mor′fəs) [*cysto-* + *morph-* + *-ous*] shaped like a cyst or bladder.

cys·to·pa·ral·y·sis (sis″to-pə-ral′ĭ-sis) cystoparesis.

cys·to·pa·re·sis (sis″to-pə-re′sis) paralysis of the urinary bladder; called also *cystoplegia.*

cys·top·a·thy (sis-top′ə-the) any disease of the urinary bladder.

diabetic c. bladder symptoms occurring as a complication of diabetes mellitus, usually resulting from autonomic neuropathy that decreases sensation in the bladder, so that it may become distended with urine but fail to cause discomfort to the patient.

cys·to·pexy (sis′to-pek″se) [*cysto-* + *-pexy*] fixation of the bladder to the abdominal wall in the treatment of cystocele; called also *vesicopexy.*

cys·toph·o·rous (sis-tof′ə-rəs) [*cysto-* + Gr. *phoros* bearing] containing cysts, such as in a parasitic infection.

cys•to•pho•tog•ra•phy (sis″to-fo-tog′rə-fe) the photographing of the inside of the bladder.

cys•to•plas•ty (sis′to-plas″te) [*cysto-* + *-plasty*] any plastic or reconstructive operation on the bladder, usually referring to augmentation cystoplasty. **cystoplas′tic** *adj*

augmentation c. enlargement or reconstruction of the bladder by grafting to it a detached segment of intestine *(enterocystoplasty)* or stomach *(gastrocystoplasty)*. Called also *bladder augmentation.*

sigmoid c. augmentation cystoplasty using a portion of the sigmoid colon for the added segment; called also *sigmoidocystoplasty.*

cys•to•ple•gia (sis″to-ple′jə) [*cysto-* + *-plegia*] cystoparesis.

cys•to•pros•ta•tec•to•my (sis″to-pros-tə-tek′tə-me) [*cysto-* + prostatectomy] surgical removal of the urinary bladder and prostate gland; called also *prostatocystectomy.*

radical c. radical cystectomy in a male.

cys•top•to•sis (sis″top-to′sis, sis″to-to′sis) [*cysto-* + *-ptosis*] prolapse of a part of the inner coat of the bladder into the urethra.

cys•to•py•eli•tis (sis″to-pi″ə-li′tis) pyelocystitis.

cys•to•py•elog•ra•phy (sis″to-pi″ə-log′rə-fe) radiography of the urinary bladder and renal pelvis.

cys•to•py•elo•ne•phri•tis (sis″to-pi″ə-lo-nə-fri′tis) [*cysto-* + *pyelonephritis*] combined cystitis and pyelonephritis.

cys•to•ra•di•og•ra•phy (sis″to-ra″de-og′rə-fe) [*cysto-* + *radiography*] radiography of the bladder.

cys•tor•rha•gia (sis″to-ra′jə) [*cysto-* + *-rrhagia*] hemorrhage from the bladder.

cys•tor•rha•phy (sis-tor′ə-fe) [*cysto-* + *-rrhaphy*] the operation of suturing the bladder.

cys•tor•rhea (sis″to-re′ə) [*cysto-* + *-rrhea*] discharge of mucus from the walls of the bladder.

cys•to•sar•co•ma (sis″to-sahr-ko′mə) phyllodes tumor.

c. phyllo′des phyllodes tumor.

cys•tos•chi•sis (sis-tos′kĭ-sis) [*cysto-* + *-schisis*] fissure of the bladder; see *exstrophy of bladder.*

cys•to•scle•ro•sis (sis″to-sklə-ro′sis) a cyst that has undergone sclerosis or fibrosis.

cys•to•scope (sis′to-skōp″) [*cysto-* + *-scope*] an endoscope for visual examination of the bladder.

cys•to•scop•ic (sis″to-skop′ik) 1. pertaining to cystoscopy. 2. performed with the cystoscope.

cys•tos•co•py (sis-tos′kə-pe) direct visual examination of the urinary tract with a cystoscope.

cys•tose (sis′tōs) 1. cystic (def. 1). 2. cystoid (def. 1).

cys•to•spasm (sis′to-spaz″əm) [*cysto-* + *spasm*] spasm of the bladder.

Cys•to•spaz (sis′to-spaz) trademark for preparations of hyoscyamine.

cys•to•sphinc•ter•om•e•try (sis-to-sfingk-tər-om′ə-tre) sphincterometry.

cys•to•stax•is (sis″to-stak′sis) cystistaxis.

cys•tos•to•my (sis-tos′tə-me) [*cysto-* + *-stomy*] the formation of an opening into the bladder, such as for urinary diversion. Called also *vesicostomy.*

suprapubic c. surgical diversion of the urethra to an opening in the skin above the symphysis pubis for bladder drainage in cases of urethral stricture.

tubeless c. cutaneous vesicostomy.

cys•tot•o•my (sis-tot′ə-me) surgical incision of the urinary bladder; called also *vesicotomy.*

suprapubic c. the operation of cutting into the bladder by an incision just above the pubic symphysis.

cys•to•ure•ter•itis (sis″to-u-re″tər-i′tis) inflammation involving the urinary bladder and ureters.

cys•to•ure•tero•gram (sis″to-u-re′tər-o-gram) a radiograph of the bladder and ureters.

cys•to•ure•ter•og•ra•phy (sis″to-u-re″tər-og′rə-fe) radiography of the bladder and ureter.

cys•to•ure•tero•py•eli•tis (sis″to-u-re″tər-o-pi″ə-li′tis) inflammation of the urinary bladder, ureter, and renal pelvis.

cys•to•ure•ter•o•py•elo•neph•ri•tis (sis″to-u-re″tər-o-pi″ə-lo-nə-fri-tis) combined inflammation of the bladder, ureter, renal pelvis, and renal pyramids.

cys•to•ure•thri•tis (sis″to-u″re-thri′tis) urethrocystitis.

cys•to•ure•thro•cele (sis″to-u-re′thro-sēl) prolapse of the urethra and bladder, usually seen in females.

cys•to•ure•thro•gram (sis″to-u-re′thro-gram) a radiograph of the urinary bladder and urethra.

voiding c. (VCUG) the radiograph made during voiding cystourethrography.

cys•to•ure•throg•ra•phy (sis″to-u″rə-throg′rə-fe) radiography of the urinary bladder and urethra.

chain c. cystourethrography in which a sterile beaded metal chain is introduced via a modified catheter into the bladder and urethra; used in evaluating anatomical relationships of the bladder and urethra.

voiding c. (VCU; VCUG) cystourethrography in which radiographs are made before, during, and after urination.

cys•to•ure•thro•pexy (sis″to-u-re′thro-pek″se) bladder neck suspension.

cys•to•ure•thro•scope (sis″to-u-re′thro-skōp″) an endoscope for examining the bladder and posterior urethra.

cys•to•ure•thros•co•py (sis″to-u″re-thros′kə-pe) examination of the urethra and bladder with a cystourethroscope.

cys•tous (sis′təs) 1. cystic (def. 1). 2. cystoid (def. 1).

cys•tyl (sis′təl) the divalent acyl radical of cystine.

Cy•ta•dren (si′tə-drən) trademark for a preparation of aminoglutethimide.

cyt•a•phe•re•sis (sīt″ə-fə-re′sis) [*cyt-* + *apheresis*] apheresis of blood cells; see *erythrocytapheresis, leukocytapheresis,* and *thrombocytapheresis.*

cy•tar•a•bine (ara-C) (si-tar′ə-bēn) [USP] a deoxycytidine analogue, cytosine arabinoside, that is metabolically activated to the triphosphate nucleotide (ara-CTP), which acts as a competitive inhibitor of DNA polymerase and produces S phase–specific cytotoxicity; used as an antineoplastic, generally as part of a combination chemotherapy regimen, in the treatment of acute lymphocytic and acute myelogenous leukemia and the blast phase of chronic myelogenous leukemia, administered intravenously and subcutaneously, and for the prophylaxis and treatment of meningitis associated with leukemia, administered intrathecally. Called also *arabinosylcytosine.*

liposomal c. a suspension of cytarabine molecules encapsulated in liposomes; it is a sustained-release preparation that is injected intrathecally in the treatment of meningitis associated with lymphoma.

cyt•ar•me (sit-ahr′me) [*cyt-* + *armē* union] flattening of rounded blastomeres at conclusion of cleavage.

Cy•taux•zo•on (si″tawk-zo′on) [*cyt-* + *aux-* + Gr. *zōon* animal] a genus of parasitic protozoa (order Piroplasmida, subclass Piroplasmia) found in African ungulates and in the domestic cat in North America. *C. fe′lis* causes fatal cytauxzoonosis in cats.

cy•taux•zoo•no•sis (si″tawk-zo″o-no′sis) a rapidly fatal disease due to infection with protozoa of the genus *Cytauxzoon,* occurring in African ungulates and in domestic cats. The feline infection is caused by *Cytauxzoon felis* and is seen chiefly in cats roaming the wooded areas of the Gulf Coast states of North America. It is clinically characterized by fever, anemia, icterus, anorexia, lethargy, dehydration, and depression, and microscopically by huge reticuloendothelial cells packed with schizonts in the peripheral blood that nearly occlude the lumens of the small and medium-sized veins of the lungs, spleen, and lymph nodes.

-cyte [Gr. *kytos* hollow vessel] a word termination denoting a cell, the type of which is designated by the root to which it is affixed, as *elliptocyte, erythrocyte, leukocyte.*

Cy•tel•lin (si-tel′in) trademark for a preparation of sitosterols.

cy•ti•dine (si′tĭ-dēn) a purine nucleoside, cytosine linked by its N9 nitrogen to the C1 carbon of ribose. It is a component of ribonucleic acid and its nucleotides are important in the synthesis of a variety of lipid derivatives. Symbol C.

c. diphosphate (CDP) a nucleotide, the 5′-pyrophosphate of cytidine, that serves as a carrier for choline and ethanolamine in phospholipid synthesis.

c. monophosphate (CMP) a nucleotide, the 5′-phosphate of cytidine, that serves as a carrier for *N*-acetylneuraminic acid in glycoprotein synthesis. Called also *cytidylic acid.*

c. triphosphate (CTP) a nucleotide, the 5′-triphosphate of cytidine; it is an activated precursor in the synthesis of ribonucleic acid and of CDP- and CMP-linked compounds.

cy•ti•dine de•am•i•nase (si′tĭ-dēn de-am′ĭ-nās) [EC 3.5.4.5] an enzyme of the hydrolase class that catalyzes the deamination of cytidine to form uridine. The reaction, occurring in animal tissues and bacteria, is part of the pyrimidine degradation pathway.

cy•ti•dyl•ate (si″tĭ-dil′āt) a dissociated form of cytidylic acid.

cy•ti•dyl•ate ki•nase (si″tĭ-dil′āt ki′nās) [EC 2.7.4.14] an enzyme of the transferase class that catalyzes the phosphorylation of CMP or dCMP to form the corresponding bisphosphate compound.

cy•ti•dyl•ic ac•id (si″tĭ-dil′ik) phosphorylated cytidine, usually cytidine monophosphate.

cy•ti•dyl•yl (si″tĭ-dil′əl) the radical formed by removal of OH from the phosphate group of cytidine monophosphate.

cyt•i•sine (sit′ĭ-sin) [Gr. *kytisos* laburnum] a highly toxic alkaloid from various members of the genus *Cytisus*, especially *C. laburnum;* it causes cytisism and was formerly used as an antiemetic and antitussive.

cyt•i•sism (sit′ĭ-siz-əm) poisoning by eating plants that contain cytisine, such as *Cytisus laburnum* or various members of the genus *Laburnum;* characteristics include burning in the mouth and pharynx, thirst, nausea, vomiting, diarrhea, prostration, an irregular pulse, and sometimes aphasia, visual disturbances, delirium, and unconsciousness with respiratory paralysis and death.

Cyt•i•sus (sit′ĭ-səs) a genus of trees of the family Leguminosae, native to Europe, northern Africa, and southern Asia. *C. scopa′rius* (L.) Link., or scotch broom, is the source of scoparin and scoparius and the cause of broom poisoning (q.v.). *C. labur′num* is a laburnum tree that contains cytisine and causes cytisism. Called also *Sarothamnus*.

cyt(o)- [Gr. *kytos* hollow vessel] a combining form denoting relationship to a cell.

cy•to•an•a•ly•zer (si″to-an′ə-li″zər) an electronic optical apparatus for the detection of malignant cells in smears.

cy•to•ar•chi•tec•ton•ic (si″to-ahr″kĭ-tek-ton′ik) pertaining to cytoarchitecture or to cytoarchitectonics.

cy•to•ar•chi•tec•ton•ics (si″to-ahr″kĭ-tek-ton′iks) 1. cytoarchitecture. 2. the study of cytoarchitecture.

cy•to•ar•chi•tec•tu•ral (si″to-ahr″kĭ-tek′chə-rəl) pertaining to cytoarchitecture.

cy•to•ar•chi•tec•ture (si″to-ahr′kĭ-tek′chər) the organization of cells in the structure of an organ or tissue such as the cerebral cortex.

cy•to•bi•ol•o•gy (si″to-bi-ol′ə-je) [*cyto-* + *biology*] cell biology.

cy•to•ce•ras•tic (si″to-sə-ras′tik) cytokerastic.

cy•to•chal•a•sin (si″to-kal′ə-sin) any of a group of fungal metabolites that interfere with the formation of microfilaments and thus disrupt the cellular processes dependent on those filaments.

c. B cytochalasin used to examine the role of microfilaments in the morphology and physiology of cells; it causes microfilaments to disappear by inhibiting the assembly of actin filaments, thus blocking numerous cell processes, e.g., cytokinesis, endocytosis, exocytosis, smooth muscle contraction, and cell migration.

cy•to•chem•is•try (si″to-kem′is-tre) [*cyto-* + *chemistry*] the study of the locations, structural relationships, and interactions of cellular constituents by means of methods such as electron microscopy, cell fractionation, and immunochemical techniques.

cy•to•chrome (si′to-krōm) [*cyto-* + *-chrome*] any electron transfer hemoprotein having a mode of action in which the transfer of a single electron is effected by a reversible valence change of the central iron atom of the heme prosthetic group between the +2 and +3 oxidation states; classified as cytochromes *a* when the heme contains a formyl side chain, cytochromes *b* when protoheme (or a closely similar heme) is not covalently bound to the protein, cytochromes *c* when protoheme or other heme is covalently bound to the protein, and cytochromes *d* when the iron-tetrapyrrole has fewer conjugated double bonds than the hemes have. Well-known cytochromes have been numbered consecutively within groups and are designated by subscripts (beginning with no subscript), e.g., cytochromes *c*, c_1, c_2, etc. New cytochromes are named according to the wavelength in nanometers of the absorption maximum of the α-band of the iron (II) form in pyridine, e.g., c-555.

c. aa_3 cytochrome-*c* oxidase.

c. *b* a cytochrome in the inner mitochondrial membrane that, with cytochrome c_1 and an iron-sulfur protein, acts as the electron carrier of the enzyme ubiquinol–cytochrome-*c* reductase.

c. b_5 a cytochrome occurring in the endoplasmic reticulum that acts as an intermediate electron carrier in some reactions catalyzed by mixed function oxidases, e.g., fatty acid desaturation; it activates molecular oxygen for an attack on the substrate.

c. *c* a cytochrome on the inner mitochondrial membrane that accepts electrons from ubiquinol–cytochrome-*c* reductase and transfers them to cytochrome-*c* oxidase, part of the electron transport chain (q.v.).

c. c_1 a cytochrome in the inner mitochondrial membrane that, with cytochrome *b* and an iron-sulfur protein, acts as the electron carrier of the enzyme ubiquinol–cytochrome-*c* reductase.

c. P-450, c. P_{450} trivial name (P for pigment, 450 nm for the absorption maximum of the carbon monoxide derivative) for a cytochrome occurring in most tissues and containing a protoheme IX prosthetic group. It serves as the oxygenating catalyst in a wide variety of reactions catalyzed by monooxygenases, e.g., hydroxylation of steroid hormones and oxidations involved in the detoxification of many drugs; cytochrome P-450 activates molecular oxygen for an attack on the substrate.

cy•to•chrome-b_5 re•duc•tase (si′to-krōm re-duk′tas) [EC 1.6.2.2] an enzyme of the endoplasmic reticulum and erythrocytes that catalyzes several series of redox reactions transferring electrons from NADH to an acceptor via the intermediate electron carrier cytochrome b_5. It is a flavoprotein (FAD). In the endoplasmic reticulum, the enzyme is composed of polar and hydrophobic segments and is membrane-bound; the reduced cytochrome b_5 carries electrons in several reactions of fatty acid desaturation and fatty acid elongation. In the erythrocytes, the enzyme comprises the polar segment only and is soluble; the reduced cytochrome b_5 transfers electrons to methemoglobin, reducing it to hemoglobin. Deficiency of the enzyme, an autosomal recessive trait, results in hereditary methemoglobinemia; deficiency in erythrocytes only is characterized by cyanosis whereas deficiency also in leukocytes, and sometimes brain and muscle, has been linked to both cyanosis and mental retardation. Called also *NADH cytochrome-b_5 reductase*, *NADH methemoglobin reductase*, and *methemoglobin reductase (NADH)*.

cy•to•chrome-c ox•i•dase (si′to-krōm ok′sĭ-dās) [EC 1.9.3.1] an enzyme complex of the inner mitochondrial membrane that catalyzes the transfer of electrons from cytochrome *c* to oxygen, oxidizing the former and reducing the latter in the final step of the electron transport chain (q.v.) by which oxygen is used for fuel combustion. The enzyme contains cytochromes *a* and a_3 and two copper atoms and is associated with proton translocation and the resultant synthesis of ATP. The Fe^{2+} in heme *a* has a strong affinity for CO; in the Fe^{3+} state it binds CN^-, S^{2-}, and N_3. The binding of these compounds inactivates the enzyme, a cause of their extreme toxicity for all aerobic organisms. Called also *cytochrome aa_3* and *cytochrome oxidase*.

cy•to•chrome-c ox•i•dase de•fi•cien•cy (si′to-krōm ok′sĭ-dās) a hereditary defect in the cytochrome-*c* oxidase complex that prevents the transfer of electrons from cytochrome *c* to molecular oxygen, ultimately halting the production of ATP. Manifestations are extremely variable and include myopathies, encephalopathies, ocular and cardiac defects, sensorineural deafness, Fanconi syndrome (def. 1), diabetes mellitus, and short stature. It can be caused by mutation in any of several nuclear or mitochondrial genes, and inheritance can be autosomal recessive, X-linked, or maternal (mitochondrial).

cy•to•chrome ox•i•dase (si′to-krōm ok′sĭ-dās) cytochrome-*c* oxidase.

cy•to•ci•dal (si″to-si′dəl) destructive to cells; cf. *cytolytic* and *cytotoxic*.

cy•to•cide (si′to-sīd) [*cyto-* + *-cide*] an agent that destroys cells; see also *cytolysin* and *cytotoxin*.

cy•toc•la•sis (si-tok′lə-sis) [*cyto-* + Gr. *klasis* a breaking] cytolysis.

cy•to•clas•tic (si″to-klas′tik) cytolytic.

cy•to•cu•prein (si″to-koo′prēn) superoxide dismutase.

cy•to•den•drite (si″to-den′drīt) [*cyto-* + *dendrite*] dendrite.

cy•to•des•ma (si″to-dez′mə) [*cyto-* + Gr. *desma* band] the lamellar or bridgelike tissues binding animal cells together (Studnicka).

cy•to•di•ag•no•sis (si″to-di″ag-no′sis) diagnosis based on examination of cells in an exudate or other body fluid. **cytodiagnos′tic** *adj*

cy•to•di•er•e•sis (si″to-di-er′ə-sis) [*cyto-* + *dieresis*] cytokinesis.

cy•to•dif•fer•en•ti•a•tion (si″to-dif″ə-ren″she-a′shən) development of specialized structures and functions in embryonic cells.

cy•to•dis•tal (si″to-dis′təl) [*cyto-* + *distal*] denoting that part of an axon remote from the cell of origin.

Cyto•Gam (si′to-gam″) trademark for a preparation of cytomegalovirus immune globulin.

cy•to•gen•e•sis (si″to-jen′ə-sis) [*cyto-* + *-genesis*] the origin and development of cells.

cy•to•ge•net•ic (si″to-jə-net′ik) 1. chromosomal. 2. pertaining to cytogenetics.

cy•to•ge•net•i•cal (si″to-jə-net′ĭ-kəl) cytogenetic.

cy•to•ge•net•i•cist (si″to-jə-net′ĭ-sist) a specialist in cytogenetics.

cy•to•ge•net•ics (si″to-jə-net′iks) the branch of genetics devoted to cellular constituents concerned in heredity, i.e., chromosomes.

clinical c. the scientific study of the relationship between chromosomal aberrations and pathological conditions.

cy•to•gen•ic (si-to-jen′ik) 1. pertaining to cytogenesis. 2. forming or producing cells.

cy•tog•e•nous (si-toj′ə-nəs) [*cyto-* + *-genous*] producing cells.

cy•to•glu•co•pe•nia (si″to-gloo″ko-pe′ne-ə) cytoglycopenia.

cy•to•gly•co•pe•nia (si″to-gli″ko-pe′ne-ə) [*cyto-* + *glyco-* + *-penia*] deficient glucose content of body or blood cells.

cy•tog•o•ny (si-tog′ə-ne) [*cyto-* + Gr. *gonos* seed] cytogenic reproduction.

cy•to•his•tol•o•gy (si″to-his-tol′ə-je) the combination of cytologic and histologic methods. **cytohistolog′ic** *adj*

cy•toid (si′toid) [*cyto-* + *-oid*] resembling a cell.

cy•to•kal•i•pe•nia (si″to-kal″ĭ-pēn′e-ə) [*cyto-* + *kalium* + *-penia*] deficient potassium content of body or blood cells.

cy•to•ke•ras•tic (si″to-kə-ras′tik) [*cyto-* + Gr. *kerastos* mixed] pertaining to the development of cells from a lower to a higher order.

cy•to•ker•a•tin (si″to-ker′ə-tin) one of the two types of keratin normally found in human tissue, constituting a group of proteins; these are normally found in keratin filaments. Called also *soft keratin.*

cy•to•kine (si′to-kīn) [*cyto-* + *kinesis*] a generic term for nonantibody proteins released by one cell population (e.g., primed T lymphocytes) on contact with specific antigen, which act as intercellular mediators, as in the generation of an immune response. Examples include lymphokines and monokines.

cy•to•ki•ne•sis (si″to-kĭ-ne′sis) [*cyto-* + *-kinesis*] the final stage of cell division, following telophase, during which an actin-myosin contractile ring forms at the equator of the cell; interaction between the actin and myosin filaments causes the cell to pinch in two, producing two daughter cells; the nucleolus appears during this stage.

cy•to•log•ic (si″to-loj′ik) pertaining to cell biology.

cy•tol•o•gist (si-tol′ə-jist) cell biologist.

cy•tol•o•gy (si-tol′ə-je) [*cyto-* + *-logy*] cell biology.

aspiration biopsy c. (ABC) the microscopic study of cells from superficial or internal lesions obtained by aspiration biopsy.

exfoliative c. the examination by a variety of techniques, such as microscopy and flow cytometry, of cells desquamated from a body surface or lesion, done for detection of malignancy, measurement of hormonal levels, and other purposes. The cells may be obtained by such procedures as aspiration, washing, smear, or scraping, and the technique may also be used for secretions such as sputum, urine, abdominal fluid, prostatic secretion, or vaginal secretions.

liquid-based c. a technique for collecting and preparing samples for cancer screening: cells obtained by biopsy are transferred to a liquid fixative, concentrated, and uniformly spread in a thin layer on slides for evaluation.

cy•tol•y•sin (si-tol′ə-sin) a substance or antibody that produces cytolysis (dissolution of cells); those with specific action for a certain type of cell are named accordingly, e.g., *bacteriolysin, hemolysin.*

cy•tol•y•sis (si-tol′ə-sis) [*cyto-* + Gr. *-lysis*] dissolution or destruction of a cell by rupture of the cell membrane with loss of cytoplasm; the type of cell involved may be designated by a prefix, e.g. hemolysis. **cytolyt′ic** *adj*

immune c. cell lysis produced by antibody with the participation of complement.

cy•to•ly•so•some (si″to-li′so-sōm) autophagosome.

cy•to•me•gal•ic (si″to-mə-gal′ik) pertaining to the greatly enlarged cells with intranuclear inclusions seen in cytomegalovirus infections.

cy•to•meg•a•lo•vi•ru•ria (si″to-meg″ə-lo-vi-roo′re-ə) presence in the urine of cytomegaloviruses.

Cy•to•meg•a•lo•vi•rus (si″to-meg′ə-lo-vi″rəs) [*cyto-* + *megalo-* + *virus,* from the appearance of infected cells] a genus of ubiquitous viruses of the subfamily Betaherpesvirinae (family Herpesviridae), containing the single species human herpesvirus 5, transmitted by multiple routes. It causes an infection that is usually mild or subclinical but may develop into cytomegalic inclusion disease.

cy•to•meg•a•lo•vi•rus (CMV) (si″to-meg′ə-lo-vi″rəs) any virus of the subfamily Betaherpesvirinae, highly host-specific herpesviruses that infect humans, monkeys, or rodents, with the production of unique large cells bearing intranuclear inclusions. Depending upon the age and the immune status of the host, cytomegaloviruses can cause a variety of clinical syndromes, collectively known as cytomegalic inclusion disease (see under *disease*), although the majority of infections are very mild or subclinical. Called also *salivary gland virus.* **cytomegalovi′ral** *adj*

cy•to•meg•a•ly (si″to-meg′ə-le) abnormal enlargement of a cell or group of cells.

adrenocortical c. abnormal enlargement of cells in the outer layer of the adrenal cortex.

Cy•to•mel (si′to-məl) trademark for a preparation of liothyronine sodium.

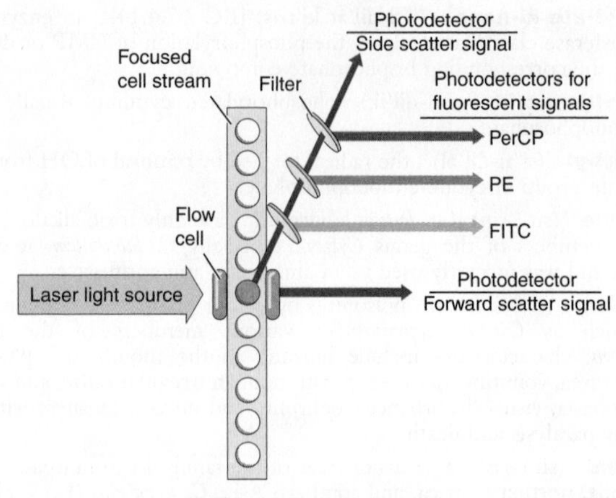

■ Flow cytometry schematic.

cy•to•mere (si′to-mēr) [*cyto-* + *-mere*] the multinucleate portion of the schizont of certain sporozoa that separates and gives rise to merozoites.

cy•tom•e•ter (si-tom′ə-tər) [*cyto-* + *-meter*] a device for counting cells, either visually, as a hemocytometer, or automatically, as a flow cytometer.

flow c. an instrument used to perform flow cytometry.

cy•tom•e•try (si-tom′ə-tre) the characterization and measurement of cells and cellular constituents.

flow c. a technique in which cells suspended in a fluid flow one at a time through a focus of exciting light, which is scattered in patterns characteristic to the cells and their components; they are often labeled with fluorescent markers so that light is first absorbed and then emitted at altered frequencies. A sensor detecting the scattered or emitted light measures the size and molecular characteristics of individual cells; tens of thousands of cells can be examined per minute and the data gathered are processed by computer.

image c. a technique in which histologically prepared cells are imaged using a scanning technique that divides the whole image into many smaller elements and aspects, which can then be analyzed by a computer and compared between many different cells in a series.

cy•to•mor•phol•o•gy (si″to-mor-fol′ə-je) the form and structure of cells or their components, or the study thereof.

cy•to•mor•pho•sis (si″to-mor-fo′sis) [*cyto-* + *morphosis*] the series of changes through which cells go in the process of formation, development, senescence, etc.

cy•to•ne•cro•sis (si″to-nə-kro′sis) death of individual cells.

cy•to•path•ic (si″to-path′ik) pertaining to or characterized by pathological changes in cells.

cy•to•patho•gen•e•sis (si″to-path″o-jen′ə-sis) the production of pathological changes in cells. **cytopathogenet′ic** *adj*

cy•to•path•o•gen•ic (si″to-path″o-jen′ik) capable of producing pathological changes in cells.

cy•to•patho•ge•nic•i•ty (si″to-path″o-jə-nis′ĭ-te) the quality of being capable of producing pathological changes in cells.

cy•to•patho•log•ic (si″to-path″o-loj′ik) 1. relating to cytopathology. 2. pertaining to the changes in cells in disease.

cy•to•patho•log•i•cal (si″to-path″o-loj′ĭ-kəl) cytopathologic.

cy•to•pa•thol•o•gist (si″to-pə-thol′ə-jist) a specialist in the study of cells in disease; a cellular pathologist.

cy•to•pa•thol•o•gy (si″to-pə-thol′ə-je) [*cyto-* + *patho-* + *-logy*] 1. the study of changes in cells in disease; called also *cellular pathology.* 2. the use of the techniques of exfoliative cytology in the diagnosis of disease.

cy•top•athy (si-top′ə-the) a disorder of a cell or of its constituents.

mitochondrial c's a diverse group of disorders characterized by decreased energy production by the mitochondria; they may be acquired or secondary to another disorder such as hyperthyroidism or result from heritable defects in the mitochondrial genome. Symptoms develop gradually and manifestations are extremely variable and often resemble those of other diseases, affecting the muscles, central and peripheral nervous systems, eyes, ears, heart, kidneys, liver, and pancreas.

cy•to•pe•nia (si″to-pe′ne-ə) [*cyto-* + *-penia*] deficiency in number of any of the cellular elements of the blood; called also *hemocytopenia.*

Cy•toph•aga (si-tof′ə-gə) a genus of gram-negative, aerobic or facultatively anaerobic, rod-shaped bacteria.

C. columna'ris *Flavobacterium columnare.*
C. psychro'phila *Flavobacterium psychrophilum.*

cy·to·phago·cy·to·sis (si″to-fa″go-si-to′sis) cytophagy.

cy·toph·a·gous (si-tof′ə-gəs) [*cyto-* + *phag-* + *-ous*] devouring or consuming cells; said of phagocytes.

cy·toph·a·gy (si-tof′ə-je) the ingestion of cells by phagocytes.

cy·to·phar·ynx (si″to-far′inks) [*cyto-* + *pharynx*] a nonciliated gullet-like canal between the cytostome and the endoplasm of ciliate and certain other protozoa. See also *cytopharyngeal apparatus*, under *apparatus*.

cy·to·phil (si′to-fil) an element or substance that has an affinity for cells.

cy·to·phil·ic (si-to-fil′ik) [*cyto-* + *-philic*] having an affinity for cells, as cytophilic antibodies.

cy·to·pho·tom·e·ter (si″to-fo-tom′ə-tər) a photometer for measuring localization of organic compounds within cells by measuring the light intensity through selected stained areas of cytoplasm.

cy·to·pho·tom·e·try (si″to-fo-tom′ə-tre) the study of organic compounds within cells by means of the cytophotometer. Called also *microfluorometry*. **cytophotomet′ric** *adj*

cy·to·phy·lac·tic (si″to-fə-lak′tik) cytoprotective.

cy·to·phy·lax·is (si″to-fə-lak′sis) [*cyto-* + *phylaxis*] cytoprotection (def. 2).

cy·to·phys·i·ol·o·gy (si″to-fiz-e-ol′ə-je) cell physiology.

cy·to·pi·pette (si″to-pi-pet′) a pipette for taking cytological smears.

cy·to·plasm (si′to-plaz″əm) [*cyto-* + *-plasm*] the protoplasm of a cell exclusive of that of the nucleus; it consists of a continuous aqueous solution (cytosol) and the organelles and inclusions suspended in it and is the site of most of the chemical activities of the cell. Cf. *nucleoplasm*. **cytoplas′mic** *adj*

cy·to·plast (si′to-plast) a cell from which the nucleus has been removed; cf *karyoplast*.

cy·to·prep·a·ra·tion (si″to-prep″ə-ra′shən) the preparation of a specimen for cytopathologic examination. **cytoprep′aratory** *adj*

cy·to·proct (si′to-prokt) [*cyto-* + Gr. *prōktos* anus] a permanent posterior pore seen in certain ciliates, through which waste egesta can be eliminated. Called also *cytopyge*.

cy·to·pro·tec·tant (si″to-pro-tek′tənt) cytoprotective.

cy·to·pro·tec·tion (si″to-pro-tek′shən) 1. enhancement of the ability of cells to resist injury. 2. the protection of cells; called also *cytophylaxis*.

cy·to·pro·tec·tive (si″to-pro-tek′tiv) 1. protecting cells from noxious chemicals or other stimuli. 2. an agent that so protects. Called also *cytoprotectant*.

cy·to·prox·i·mal (si″to-prok′sĭ-məl) [*cyto-* + *proximal*] denoting that part of an axon nearer to the cell of origin.

cy·to·pyge (si″to-pi′je) [*cyto-* + *pygē* rump] cytoproct.

cy·to·re·duc·tion (si″to-re-duk′shən) 1. decrease in the number of cells, such as in a tumor. 2. debulking.

cy·to·re·duc·tive (si″to-rə-duk′tiv) reducing the number of cells, as in surgery for a tumor; see *debulking*.

Cy·to·sar (si′to-sahr) trademark for preparations of cytarabine.

cy·to·sine (si′to-sēn) a pyrimidine base found in animal and plant cells, usually occurring condensed with ribose or deoxyribose to form the nucleosides cytidine and deoxycytidine, major constituents of nucleic acids. Symbol C. See also illustration of *purine and pyrimidine bases*, under *base*.
  c. arabinoside cytarabine.

cy·to·sine de·am·i·nase (si′to-sēn de-am′ĭ-nās) [EC 3.5.4.1] an enzyme of the hydrolase class that catalyzes the deamination of cytosine to form uracil, a step in the degradation of pyrimidine nucleotides.

cy·to·skel·e·ton (si″to-skel′ə-tən) a three-dimensional cytoplasmic network of protein polymers (microfilaments, intermediate filaments, and microtubules), occurring in eukaryotes, that supports and maintains the shape of the cell and provides motility (both of the whole cell and of organelles and vesicles within the cell). **cytoskel′etal** *adj*

cy·to·sol (si′to-sol) the liquid medium of the cytoplasm, i.e., cytoplasm minus organelles and nonmembranous insoluble components. **cytosol′ic** *adj*

cy·to·sol ami·no·pep·ti·dase (si′to-sol ə-me″no-pep′tĭ-dās) leucyl aminopeptidase.

cy·to·sol non·spe·cif·ic di·pep·ti·dase (si′to-sol non″spə-sif′ik di-pep′tĭ-dās) [EC 3.4.13.18] a dipeptidase that catylyzes the hydrolysis of dipeptides, preferentially hydrophobic dipeptides including prolyl amino acids. Called also *prolinase*, *prolyl dipeptidase*, and *pro-X dipeptidase*.

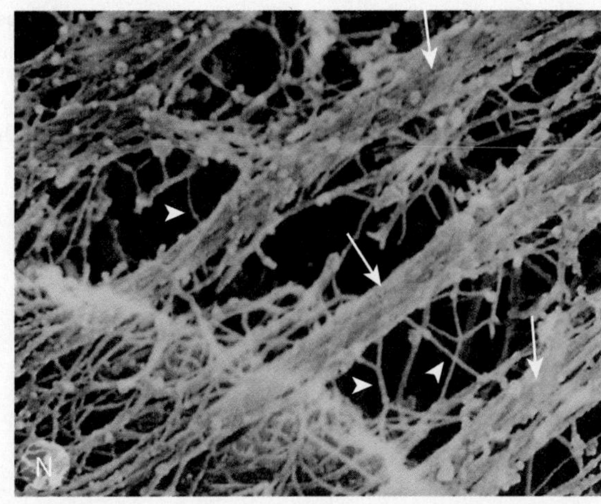

■ Cytoskeleton, shown in a color-enhanced electron micrograph. *N*, nucleus; *arrowheads*, intermediate filaments; *arrows*, microtubules.

cy·to·some (si′to-sōm) [*cyto-* + *-some*] multilamellar body.

cy·to·sta·sis (si″to-sta′sis) [*cyto-* + *-stasis*] the closure of capillaries by white blood corpuscles in the early stages of inflammation.

cy·to·stat·ic (si″to-stat′ik) [*cyto-* + *-static*] 1. suppressing the growth and multiplication of cells. 2. an agent that suppresses cell growth and multiplication.

cy·to·stome (si′to-stōm) [*cyto-* + *stoma*] the mouth opening of ciliates and certain other protozoa, which opens into the cytopharynx, which in turn opens into the endoplasm.

cy·to·tax·i·gen (si″to-taks′ĭ-jən) a substance that mediates chemotaxis of cells indirectly by inducing cytotaxin formation; thus antigen-antibody complexes are cytotaxigenic because when added to serum they fix complement, resulting in the liberation of chemotactic factors derived from complement.

cy·to·tax·in (si″to-taks′in) chemotactic factor.

cy·to·tax·is (si-to-tak′sis) [*cyto-* + *taxis*] the movement and arrangement of cells with respect to a specific source of stimulation. **cytotac′tic** *adj*

Cy·to·tec (si′to-tek) trademark for a preparation of misoprostol.

cy·to·tox·ic·i·ty (si″to-tok-sis′ĭ-te) the degree to which an agent possesses a specific destructive action on certain cells or the possession of such action; used particularly in referring to the lysis of cells by immune phenomena and to antineoplastic drugs that selectively kill dividing cells. **cy′totoxic** *adj*
  antibody-dependent cell-mediated c. (ADCC), antibody-dependent cellular c. lysis of target cells coated with antibody by effector cells with cytolytic activity and Fc receptors, including K cells, macrophages, and granulocytes; a form of type II hypersensitivity reaction. ADCC involves binding of the effector cell by means of Fc receptors which bind to the Fc portion of the IgG molecule. Lysis of the target cell is extracellular, requires direct cell-to-cell contact, and does not involve complement.
  cell-mediated c. cytolysis of a target cell by effector lymphocytes, such as cytotoxic T lymphocytes or NK cells; it may be antibody-dependent (see *antibody-dependent cell-mediated c.*) or independent, as in certain type IV hypersensitivity reactions (q.v.).

cy·to·tox·in (si′to-tok″sin) [*cyto-* + *toxin*] a toxin or antibody that has a specific toxic action on cells of special organs; cytotoxins are named according to the special variety of cell for which they are specific, as *nephrotoxin*.

cy·to·tropho·blast (si″to-trof′o-blast) [*cyto-* + *trophoblast*] 1. the cellular (inner) layer of the trophoblast; called also *Langhans layer*. 2. cytotrophoblastic cell. **cytotrophoblas′tic** *adj*

cy·to·tro·pic (si″to-tro′pik) [*cyto-* + *-tropic*] attracting cells; possessing an affinity for cells; said especially of antibodies that attach to cell surfaces. See also under *antibody*.

cy·to·tro·pism (si-tot′ro-piz-əm) 1. cell movement in response to external stimulation. 2. the ability, particularly of viruses, to localize in and affect specific cells of the body.

Cy·to·vene (si′to-vēn″) trademark for preparations of ganciclovir.

Cy·tox·an (si-tok′sən) trademark for preparations of cyclophosphamide.

cy·to·zo·ic (si″to-zo′ik) living within or attached to cells; said of parasites.

cy·tu·ria (si-tu′re-ə) [*cyt-* + *-uria*] the presence of excessive or unusual cells in the urine.

Cza·pek-Dox agar (solution) (chah′pek doks′) [Friedrich Johann Franz *Czapek*, Czech botanist, 1868–1921; Arthur Wayland *Dox*, American chemist, 20th century] see under *culture medium.*

Czer·mak spaces (lines) (cher′mahk) [Johann Nepomuk *Czermak*, Czech physician, 1828–1873] spatia interglobularia.

Czer·ny suture (cher′ne) [Vincenz *Czerny*, Czech surgeon in Germany, 1842–1916] see under *suture.*

Czer·ny-Lem·bert suture (cher′ne lahm-bār′) [V. *Czerny;* Antoine *Lembert*, French surgeon, 1802–1851] see under *suture.*

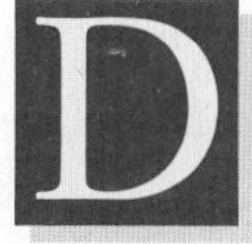

D diffusing capacity; dalton; deciduous (teeth; see under *tooth*); density; deuterium; died; diopter; distal; dorsal vertebrae (D1 through D12); dose; duration; *dwarf* (colony); decimal reduction time.

D. [L.] da (give); de′tur (let it be given); dex′ter (right); do′sis (dose).

D_{37} the dose necessary to reduce the surviving fraction, as of cells, to e^{-1} or 0.37, where the biological activity declines exponentially as a function of dose.

2,4-D a toxic chlorphenoxy herbicide (2,4-dichlorophenoxyacetic acid) that acts as a growth-regulating hormone, killing broadleaf plants by overstimulation.

D- a chemical prefix (small capital D) that specifies the relative configuration of an enantiomer, the mirror image configuration being specified as L-. Carbohydrates are designated as D or L depending on their configuration at the asymmetric carbon atom most distant from the carbonyl functional group; those with the same configuration as the D-glyceraldehyde (the arbitrarily chosen standard) are in the D (or D_g) configurational family. Amino acids are designated according to their configuration at the asymmetric carbon atom closest to the carbonyl group; D-serine is the standard and similarly configured amino acids are designated D or D_s. All of the α-amino acids occurring in proteins have the L configuration; a few D-amino acids occur in short peptides produced by bacteria. The symbols *R* and *S*, indicating absolute configuration, are preferable.

d day; deci-; deoxyribose (in specifying nucleosides and nucleotides, e.g., A is adenosine, dA is deoxyadenosine).

d. [L.] da (give); de′tur (let it be given); dex′ter (right); do′sis (dose).

d density; diameter.

***d*-** [abbreviation for *dextro* (right or clockwise)] a chemical prefix indicating an enantiomer that rotates the plane of polarization of a beam of light in the clockwise direction (dextrorotatory), the other enantiomer being specified as *l*- (for *levo*). NOTE: The prefixes *d*- and *l*- are now being replaced by (+)- and (−)-, respectively, especially when the prefixes D- and L- are also used, e.g., *l*-fructose is D-(−)-fructose.

Δ the Greek capital letter delta; symbol for an increment, e.g., ΔG (see *Gibbs free energy*, under *energy*); also used alone as an abbreviation for *change* (as in temperature).

Δ- a prefix designating the position of a double bond in a carbon chain, e.g., Δ^9- indicates a double bond between carbons 9 and 10.

δ delta, the fourth letter of the Greek alphabet; symbol for the heavy chain of IgD (see *immunoglobulin*) and the δ chain of hemoglobin.

δ- a prefix designating (1) the fourth carbon along a chain starting with that adjacent to the principal functional group, e.g., δ-aminolevulinic acid (see α-); (2) one in a series of related entities or chemical compounds, e.g., δ-carotene or δ-ray. For terms prefixed with the symbol δ-, see the unprefixed form.

DA developmental age; diphenylchlorarsine.

Da dalton.

da deca-.

Daae disease (dah′ə) [Anders *Daae*, Norwegian physician, 1838–1910] epidemic pleurodynia; see under *pleurodynia*.

da·boia (də-boi′ə) [Hindi "furtive mover"] Russell's viper.
  d. russel′li Russell's viper *(Vipera russelli)*.

Dab·ska tumor (dahb′skə) [Maria *Dabska*, Polish pathologist, born 1920] endovascular papillary angioendothelioma.

DAC decitabine.

da·car·ba·zine (DTIC) (də-kahr′bə-zēn) [USP] a cytotoxic alkylating agent used as an antineoplastic primarily for treatment of malignant melanoma and in combination chemotherapy for Hodgkin disease and sarcomas; administered intravenously.

da·cliz·u·mab (də-kliz′u-mab) an immunosuppressant used to prevent acute organ rejection in renal transplant patients; administered intravenously.

Dac·o·gen (dak′o-jen) trademark for a preparation of decitabine.

d'Acos·ta see *Acosta.*

Da Cos·ta syndrome (də kah′stə) [Jacob Mendes *Da Costa*, American physician, 1833–1900] neurocirculatory asthenia; see under *asthenia.*

Da·cron (da′kron) trademark for a polyethylene terephthalate fiber. In fiber form, it is used as a suture material; in fabric form, it is used for vascular grafts and prostheses and for vascular catheters.

dac·ry·ad·e·nal·gia (dak″re-ad″ə-nal′jə) dacryoadenalgia.

dac·ry·cys·tal·gia (dak″re-sis-tal′jə) dacryocystalgia.

dac·ry·cys·ti·tis (dak″re-sis-ti′tis) dacryocystitis.

dac·ry·el·co·sis (dak″re-əl-ko′sis) dacryohelcosis.

dacry(o)- [Gr. *dakryon* tear] a combining form denoting relationship to tears.

dac·ryo·ad·e·nal·gia (dak″re-o-ad″ə-nal′jə) [*dacryo-* + *aden-* + *-algia*] pain in a lacrimal gland.

dac·ryo·ad·e·nec·to·my (dak″re-o-ad″ə-nek′tə-me) [*dacryo-* + *aden-* + *ectomy*] excision of a lacrimal gland.

dac·ryo·ad·e·ni·tis (dak″re-o-ad″ə-ni′tis) inflammation of a lacrimal gland.

dac·ryo·blen·nor·rhea (dak″re-o-blen″o-re′ə) [*dacryo-* + *blennorrhea*] mucous discharge from the lacrimal ducts, as in chronic dacryocystitis.

dac·ryo·cana·lic·u·li·tis (dak″re-o-kan″ə-lik″u-li′tis) inflammation of the lacrimal ducts.

dac·ryo·cele (dak′re-o-sēl″) dacryocystocele.

dac·ryo·cyst (dak′re-o-sist″) [*dacryo-* + *cyst*] the lacrimal sac.

dac·ryo·cys·tal·gia (dak″re-o-sis-tal′jə) [*dacryocyst* + *-algia*] pain in a lacrimal sac.

dac·ryo·cys·tec·ta·sia (dak″re-o-sis″tek-ta′zhə) [*dacryocyst* + *ectasia*] dilatation of the lacrimal sac.

dac·ryo·cys·tec·to·my (dak″re-o-sis-tek′tə-me) [*dacryocyst* + *ectomy*] excision of the wall of the lacrimal sac.

dac·ryo·cys·tis (dak″re-o-sis′tis) [*dacryo-* + *cystis*] the lacrimal sac.

dac·ryo·cys·ti·tis (dak″re-o-sis-ti′tis) inflammation of the lacrimal sac.

dac·ryo·cys·ti·tome (dak″re-o-sis′tĭ-tōm) [*dacryocyst* + *-tome*] an instrument for incising strictures of the lacrimal duct.

dac·ryo·cys·to·blen·nor·rhea (dak″re-o-sis″to-blen″o-re′ə) [*dacryocyst* + *blennorrhea*] a chronic catarrhal inflammation of the lacrimal sac, with constriction of the lacrimal duct.

dac·ryo·cys·to·cele (dak″re-o-sis′to-sēl) [*dacryocyst* + *-cele*[1]] hernial protrusion of the lacrimal sac; called also *dacryocele.*

dac·ryo·cys·top·to·sis (dak″re-o-sis″top-to′sis, dak″re-o-sis″to-to′sis) [*dacryocyst* + *-ptosis*] prolapse or downward displacement of the lacrimal sac.

dac·ryo·cys·to·rhi·no·ste·no·sis (dak″re-o-sis″to-ri″no-stə-no′sis) narrowing of the duct leading from the lacrimal sac to the nasal cavity.

dac·ryo·cys·to·rhi·nos·to·my (dak″re-o-sis″to-ri-nos′tə-me) [*dacryocyst* + *rhino-* + *-stomy*] surgical creation of a communication between the lacrimal sac and the nasal cavity; called also *dacryorhinocystotomy.*

dac·ryo·cys·to·rhi·not·o·my (dak″re-o-sis″to-ri-not′ə-me) [*dacryocyst* + *rhino-* + *-tomy*] passage of a probe through the lacrimal sac into the nasal cavity.

dac·ryo·cys·to·ste·no·sis (dak″re-o-sis″to-stə-no′sis) narrowing of the lacrimal sac.

dac·ryo·cys·tos·to·my (dak″re-o-sis-tos′tə-me) [*dacryocyst* + *-stomy*] surgical creation of a new opening into the lacrimal sac.

dac·ryo·cys·to·tome (dak″re-o-sis′to-tōm) dacryocystitome.

dac·ryo·cys·tot·o·my (dak″re-o-sis-tot′ə-me) [*dacryocyst* + *-tomy*] incision of the lacrimal sac; called also *Ammon operation* (def. 2).

dac·ryo·cyte (dak′re-o-sīt) an abnormal erythrocyte shaped like a teardrop, seen in myelofibrosis and certain other myeloproliferative diseases. Called also *teardrop cell.*

dac·ry·o·gen·ic (dak″re-o-jen′ik) [*dacryo-* + *-genic*] promoting the secretion of tears.

dac·ryo·hel·co·sis (dak″re-o-həl-ko′sis) [*dacryo-* + *helcosis*] ulceration of the lacrimal sac or lacrimal duct.

dac·ryo·hem·or·rhea (dak″re-o-hem″o-re′ə) [*dacryo-* + *hemo-* + *-rrhea*] the discharge of tears mixed with blood.

dac·ryo·lith (dak′re-o-lith″) [*dacryo-* + *-lith*] a concretion in the lacrimal sac or duct; called also lacrimal calculus.

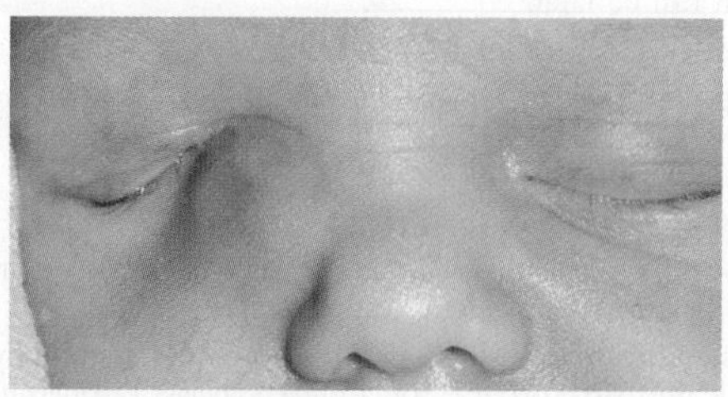

■ Dacryocystocele.

dac•ryo•li•thi•a•sis (dak″re-o-lĭ-thi′ə-sis) [*dacryo-* + *lithiasis*] the presence of calculi in the lacrimal sac or duct.

dac•ry•o•ma (dak″re-o′mə) a tumorlike swelling caused by obstruction of the lacrimal duct.

dac•ry•on (dak′re-on) [Gr. *dakryon* tear] a cranial point at the juncture of the lacrimal and frontal bones, and the maxilla.

dac•ry•ops (dak′re-ops) [*dacry-* + Gr. *ōps* eye] 1. a watery state of the eye. 2. distention of a lacrimal duct by contained fluid.

dac•ryo•py•or•rhea (dak″re-o-pi″o-re′ə) [*dacryo-* + *pyorrhea*] the discharge of tears mixed with pus.

dac•ryo•py•o•sis (dak″re-o-pi-o′sis) [*dacryo-* + *pyosis*] suppuration of the lacrimal sac and duct.

dac•ryo•rhi•no•cys•tot•o•my (dak″re-o-ri″no-sis-tot′ə-me) dacryocystorhinostomy.

dac•ry•or•rhea (dak″re-o-re′ə) [*dacryo-* + *-rrhea*] an overabundant flow of tears.

dac•ryo•scin•tig•ra•phy (dak″re-o-sin-tig′rə-fe) scintigraphy of the lacrimal ducts.

dac•ryo•si•nus•itis (dak″re-o-si″nəs-i′tis) inflammation of the lacrimal duct and ethmoid sinus.

dac•ryo•so•le•ni•tis (dak″re-o″so-lə-ni′tis) [*dacryo-* + *solen-* + *-itis*] inflammation of a lacrimal duct.

dac•ryo•ste•no•sis (dak″re-o-stə-no′sis) [*dacryo-* + *stenosis*] stricture or narrowing of a lacrimal duct.

dac•ryo•syr•inx (dak″re-o-sir′inks) [*dacryo-* + *syrinx*] 1. canaliculus lacrimalis. 2. a lacrimal fistula. 3. a syringe for irrigating the lacrimal ducts.

DACT dactinomycin.

dac•ti•no•my•cin (DACT) (dak″tĭ-no-mi′sin) [USP] an antineoplastic antibiotic (actinomycin D) produced by *Streptomyces parvulus;* it consists of a phenoxazone ring and two cyclic pentapeptide side chains and acts by binding to DNA with the ring intercalated between adjacent guanine-cytosine base pairs, resulting in blocking of transcription by RNA polymerase. It is used as an antineoplastic agent for treatment of rhabdomyosarcoma and Wilms tumor in children and is also effective against Ewing sarcoma, Kaposi sarcoma, osteogenic sarcoma and soft tissue sarcomas, testicular carcinoma, and choriocarcinoma; administered intravenously and by isolation-perfusion technique. Major side effects are nausea and vomiting, ulceration of the oral mucosa, and bone marrow depression.

dac•tyl (dak′təl) [Gr. *daktylos* a finger] digitus.

Dac•ty•la•ria (dak-tə-lār′e-ə) a genus of Fungi Imperfecti of the form-family Dematiaceae.

D. gallopa′va *Ochroconis gallopavum.*

dac•ty•late (dak′tə-lāt) digitate.

Dac•ty•lis (dak′tə-lis) a genus of grasses (family Gramineae). *D. glomera′ta* is orchard grass, whose pollen causes hay fever.

dac•ty•li•tis (dak″tə-li′tis) [*dactyl-* + *-itis*] inflammation of a finger or toe.

blistering distal d. localized infection of the fat pad at the end of a finger or less often a toe, with blister formation; the usual cause is bacterial infection with either *Staphylococcus aureus* or a β-hemolytic streptococcus.

dactyl(o)- [Gr. *daktylos* finger] a combining form denoting relationship to a digit, usually referring to the fingers but sometimes to the toes.

dac•ty•lo•camp•so•dyn•ia (dak″tə-lo-kamp″so-din′e-ə) [*dactylo-* + Gr. *kampsis* bend + *-odynia*] painful flexure of the fingers.

dac•tylo•gram (dak-til′o-gram) [*dactylo-* + *-gram*] a fingerprint taken for purposes of identification.

dac•ty•log•ra•phy (dak″tə-log′rə-fe) the study of fingerprints.

dac•ty•lo•gry•po•sis (dak″tə-lo-grĭ-po′sis) [*dactylo-* + *gryposis*] a permanent curving of the fingers.

Dac•ty•lo•gy•rus (dak″tə-lo-ji′rəs) a genus of trematodes that infect the skin and gills of aquarium fish, causing hyperactivity and breathing difficulty that can be fatal.

dac•ty•lol•o•gy (dak″tə-lol′ə-je) signing.

dac•ty•lol•y•sis (dak″tə-lol′ĭ-sis) [*dactylo-* + *-lysis*] loss or amputation of a digit.

d. sponta′nea ainhum.

dac•ty•lo•meg•a•ly (dak″tə-lo-meg′ə-le) megalodactyly.

dac•ty•los•co•py (dak″tə-los′kə-pe) [*dactylo-* + *-scopy*] examination of fingerprints for purposes of identification.

Dac•ty•lo•so•ma (dak″tə-lo-so′mə) [*dactylo-* + Gr. *soma* body] a genus of hematozoic protozoa (order Piroplasmida, subclass Piroplasmia) found in reptiles, amphibians, and fish.

dac•ty•lo•spasm (dak′tə-lo-spaz″əm) [*dactylo-* + *-spasm*] spasm or cramp of a finger or toe.

dac•ty•lus (dak′tə-ləs) [Gr. *daktylos* finger] digitus.

DAD delayed afterdepolarization.

dADP deoxyadenosine diphosphate.

DAEC diffusely adherent *Escherichia coli.*

DAF decay accelerating factor.

daf•fo•dil (daf′ə-dil) *Narcissus pseudonarcissus.*

DAG diacylglycerol.

dahl•ia (dahl′yə) the term for certain unspecified mixtures of methylated and ethylated pararosanilines and rosanilines; C.I.42530. Sometimes used as a basic dye for violet staining. Called also *Hofmann* or *iodine violet.*

Da•kin solution (da′kin) [Henry Drysdale *Dakin*, English chemist in the United States, 1880–1952] see under *solution.*

dak•ry•on (dak′re-on) dacryon.

Dal•a•lone (dal′ə-lōn″) trademark for a preparation of dexamethasone sodium phosphate.

Dal•a•lone D.P. (dal′ə-lōn″) trademark for a preparation of dexamethasone acetate.

Dal•a•lone L.A. (dal′ə-lōn″) trademark for a preparation of dexamethasone acetate.

Dale reaction (phenomenon) (dāl) [Sir Henry Hallett *Dale*, British physiologist, pharmacologist, and Nobel prize winner, 1875–1968] see under *reaction.*

dal•fo•pris•tin (dal-fo′pris-tin) a semisynthetic streptogramin antibacterial effective against a variety of gram-positive organisms, inhibiting the early phase of protein synthesis in the bacterial ribosome. It is used in conjunction with quinupristin in the treatment of serious bacteremia caused by vancomycin-resistant *Enterococcus faecium* and complicated skin and skin structure infections caused by *Streptococcus pyogenes* or methicillin-sensitive *Staphylococcus aureus;* administered intravenously.

Dal•gan (dal′gan) trademark for a preparation of dezocine.

Dal•mane (dal′mān) trademark for a preparation of flurazepam hydrochloride.

Dal•rym•ple disease, sign (dal′rim-pəl) [John *Dalrymple*, English oculist, 1804–1852] see *cyclokeratitis*, and see under *sign.*

dal•tep•a•rin so•di•um (dal-tep′ə-rin) an antithrombotic prepared from heparin sodium derived from porcine intestinal mucosa; it enhances the inhibition of factor Xa and thrombin by antithrombin. It is administered subcutaneously for the prevention of pulmonary thromboembolism and deep vein thrombosis in patients who are at risk for thromboembolism undergoing abdominal surgery.

Dal•ton's law (dawl′tənz) [John *Dalton*, English chemist and physicist, 1766–1844, the founder of the atomic theory] see under *law.*

Dal•ton-Hen•ry law (dawl′tən hen′re) [J. *Dalton;* Joseph *Henry*, American physicist, 1797–1878] see under *law.*

dal•ton (D, Da) (dawl′tən) [John *Dalton*] an arbitrary unit of mass, being $\frac{1}{12}$ the mass of the nuclide of carbon-12, equivalent to 1.657×10^{-24} g. Called also *atomic mass unit.*

dal•ton•ism (dawl′tən-iz-əm) [John *Dalton*] a name applied to defective perception of red and green; deuteranomaly or deuteranopia.

dam (dam) 1. a barrier to obstruct the flow of water or other fluid. 2. a thin sheet of latex used in surgical procedures to separate certain tissues or structures. 3. rubber d.

dental d., rubber d. a sheet of latex with punched-out holes that is placed over the teeth during dental procedures to isolate the operative field from the rest of the oral cavity.

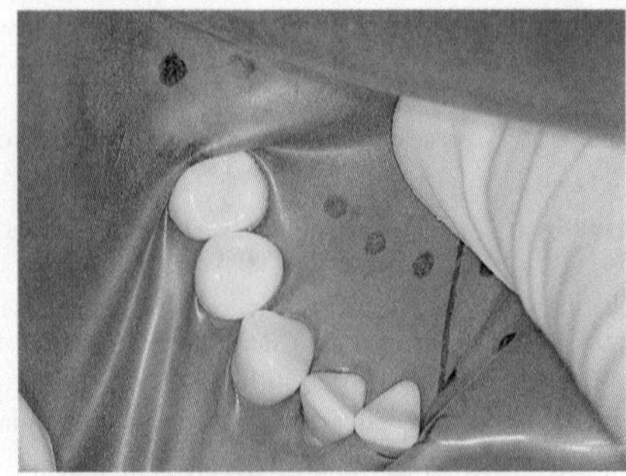

■ Rubber dam.

dam•age [Middle English, from L. *damnum* injury] injury or harm resulting in impairment or loss of function.
diffuse alveolar d. the nonspecific pathologic abnormalities seen in acute respiratory distress syndrome and acute lung injury.

Dam•a•lin•ia (dam″ə-lin′e-ə) a genus of parasitic biting lice (order Mallophaga); several species were formerly classified in the genus *Trichodectes*. *D. bo′vis* infests cattle; *D. e′qui* infests horses; *D. herm′si* and *D. o′vis* infest sheep; and *D. cap′rae*, *D. cras′sipes*, and *D. limba′ta* infest goats.

Dam•a•son-P (dam′ə-son) trademark for a combination preparation of aspirin and hydrocodone bitartrate.

D'Ama•to sign (dah-mah′to) [Luigi *D'Amato*, Italian physician, early 20th century] see under *sign*.

da•mi•a•na (dah″me-ah′nə) the leaves of the Mexican plants *Turnera aphrodisiaca (T. diffusa)* and *Haplopappus discoideus*, which are said to be tonic, analeptic, diuretic, and aphrodisiac. Called also *turnera*.

dam•mar (dam′ər) a transparent resin from tropical trees of the genera *Hopea*, *Shorea*, and others; used in varnishes, as a mounting medium in microscopy, and for the preservation of animal and vegetable specimens.

dAMP deoxyadenosine monophosphate.

damp (damp) [Middle Dutch "vapor"] foul air or noxious gas(es) in a mine.
after-d. a gaseous mixture formed in a mine by the explosion of fire damp or dust; it contains nitrogen, carbon dioxide, and usually carbon monoxide *(white d.)*.
black d., choke d. a nonrespirable atmosphere sometimes formed in a mine by the gradual absorption of the oxygen and the giving off of carbon dioxide by the coal.
cold d. foggy vapor charged with carbon dioxide.
fire d. light, explosive hydrocarbon gases, chiefly methane, CH_4, found in coal mines.
white d. carbon monoxide, occurring as a component of the after-damp.

damp•ing (damp′ing) the steady diminution of the amplitude of vibration of a specific form of energy, as of electricity or sound waves.

da•nap•a•roid so•di•um (də-nap′ə-roid) an antithrombotic used in the prophylaxis of pulmonary thromboembolism and deep vein thrombosis, administered subcutaneously. It is a depolymerized mixture of low-molecular-weight sulfated glycosaminoglycans, which inhibits coagulation factor Xa and thrombin and so prevents formation of fibrin in the coagulation cascade.

dan•a•zol (dan′ə-zol) [USP] an anterior pituitary suppressant used in the treatment of endometriosis, fibrocystic breast disease, and gynecomastia and the prophylaxis of attacks of hereditary angioedema; administered orally.

Dan•bolt-Closs syndrome (dahn′bōlt klos′) [Niels Christian *Danbolt*, Norwegian dermatologist, 1900–1984; Karl Philipp *Closs*, Belgian-born physician in Norway, 20th century] acrodermatitis enteropathica.

dance (dans) movement of a rhythmic type, or of an unusual or exaggerated type.
brachial d. writhing of tortuous brachial arteries under the skin, sometimes observed in elderly arteriosclerotic patients.
hilar d., hilus d. marked pulsations of the hilus shadows of both lungs on radiographic examination; seen in pulmonic regurgitation.
St. Anthony's d., St. Guy's d., St. John's d., St. Vitus' d. Sydenham chorea.

D and C dilatation and curettage.

dan•de•li•on (dan′də-li″ən) [Old Fr. *dentdelion*, from L. *dens leonis* lion's tooth (from the shape of its leaves)] a weedy Eurasian herb, *Taraxacum officinale*, widely naturalized in North America and having deeply notched leaves and brilliant yellow flowers; used for dyspepsia, loss of appetite, urinary tract infections, and liver and gallbladder complaints.

dan•der (dan′dər) small scales from the hair or feathers of animals, which may be the cause of allergy in sensitive persons.

dan•druff (dan′drəf) 1. dry scaly material desquamated from the scalp; the term is applied to that normally desquamated from the epidermis of the scalp as well as to the excessive scaly material associated with disease, as in seborrheic dermatitis. 2. seborrheic dermatitis of the scalp; called also *pityriasis sicca*.
walking d. cheyletiellosis (def. 1).

Dan•dy operation (dan′de) [Walter Edward *Dandy*, American surgeon, 1886–1946] see under *operation*.

Dan•dy-Walk•er malformation (deformity, syndrome) (dan′de wawk′ər) [W.E. *Dandy;* Arthur Earl *Walker*, American surgeon, 1907–1995] see under *malformation*.

Dane particle (dān) [David M.S. *Dane*, British virologist, 20th century] see under *particle*.

Dan•o•crine (dan′o-krin) trademark for a preparation of danazol.

DANS 5-dimethylamino-1-naphthalenesulfonic acid. See *dansyl chloride*.

dan•syl chlo•ride (dan′səl) [the acyl chloride of DANS] a fluorochrome that emits green fluorescence when excited by ultraviolet light; used as a fluorescent label in immunofluorescence methods and in amino acid analysis.

Dan•tri•um (dan′tre-əm) trademark for preparations of dantrolene sodium.

dan•tro•lene so•di•um (dan′tro-lēn) a skeletal muscle relaxant administered orally as an antispasmodic in conditions such as stroke, multiple sclerosis, and cerebral palsy; it is also used orally or intravenously in the prophylaxis and treatment of malignant hyperthermia.

Da•nysz phenomenon (effect) (dah′nish) [Jan *Danysz*, Polish pathologist in France, 1860–1928] see under *phenomenon*.

Daph•ne (daf′ne) [Gr. *daphnē* bay tree] a genus of trees and shrubs of the family Thymelaeaceae. *D. gni′dium* and *D. meze′reum* L. are medicinal species that contain daphnin and mezerein and are vesicatory and cathartic in small amounts but in larger amounts are poisonous, causing severe or even fatal irritation of the gastrointestinal tract.

daph•ne•tin (daf-ne′tin) 7,8-dihydroxycoumarin, the aglycon of daphnin.

Daph•nia (daf′ne-ə) a genus of fresh-water crustaceans, called water fleas, often used in biological research.

daph•nin (daf′nin) 7,8-dihydroxycoumarin-7-β-D-glucoside, a glycoside found in *Daphne mezereum*.

daph•nism (daf′niz-əm) poisoning by species of *Daphne;* symptoms include severe enteritis with diarrhea.

da•pip•ra•zole hy•dro•chlo•ride (də-pip′rə-zōl) an alpha-adrenergic blocking agent that blocks receptor binding in smooth muscle and affects the dilator muscle of the iris; used to reverse pharmacologically induced mydriasis, applied topically to the conjunctiva.

dap•sone (DDS) (dap′sōn) [USP] an antibacterial and antifungal, the parent compound of a group of sulfonamide-like sulfones, including acedapsone, acetosulfone sodium, glucosulfone sodium, sulfoxone sodium, and solapsone. Dapsone and its derivatives are bacteriostatic for a broad spectrum of gram-negative and gram-positive organisms, including *Mycobacterium tuberculosis* and *M. leprae*, and have suppressive action on *Plasmodium falciparum*. Dapsone is administered orally as a leprostatic, especially in tuberculoid and lepromatous leprosy, as a dermatitis herpetiformis suppressant; in the prophylaxis of falciparum malaria; and for the prophylaxis and treatment of pneumocystis pneumonia. Called also *diaminodiphenylsulfone* or *DDS*.

Dap•ta•cel (dap′tə-sel) trademark for a preparation of diphtheria and tetanus toxoids and acellular pertussis vaccine.

dap•to•my•cin (dap″to-mi′sin) a cyclic lipopeptide antibacterial derived from the fermentation of *Streptomyces roseosporus*, effective against gram-positive organisms; it acts by depolarizing the bacterial cell membrane, leading to inhibition of protein, DNA, and RNA synthesis. Used in the treatment of complicated skin and skin-structure infections, administered by intravenous infusion.

Dar•a•nide (dar′ə-nīd) trademark for a preparation of dichlorphenamide.

Dar•a•prim (dar′ə-prim) trademark for a preparation of pyrimethamine.

dar•be•poi•e•tin al•fa (dahr″be-poi′ə-tin al′fə) a protein closely related to erythropoietin, having similar erythropoiesis-stimulating activity; used for treatment of anemia associated with renal failure or certain types of cancer. Administered by intravenous or subcutaneous injection.

Dar•bid (dar′bid) trademark for a preparation of isopropamide iodide.

Dar es Sa•laam bacterium (dahr′ es sə-lahm′) [*Dar es Salaam*, now capital of Tanzania, where it was isolated in 1922] *Salmonella salamae*.

Dar•i•con (dar′ĭ-kon) trademark for a preparation of oxyphencyclimine hydrochloride.

Da•rier disease, sign (dah-re-a′) [Jean Ferdinand *Darier*, French dermatologist, 1856–1938] see under *disease* and *sign*.

Da•rier-Rous•sy sarcoid (dah-rya′ roo-se′) [J.F. *Darier;* Gustave *Roussy*, French pathologist and neurologist, 1874–1948] see under *sarcoid*.

Da•rier-White disease (dah-re-a′ hwīt′) [J.F. *Darier;* James Clarke *White*, American dermatologist, 1833–1916] see under *disease*.

dari•fen•a•cin (dar-ĭ-fen′ə-sin) a potent antagonist of muscarinic receptors, active against involuntary contractions of the detrusor muscle, used for treatment of urinary incontinence; administered orally.

Dark•she•vich nucleus (dahrk-sha′vich) [Liverij Osipovich *Darkshevich*, Russian neurologist, 1858–1925] see under *nucleus*.

Dar·ling disease (dahr′ling) [Samuel Taylor *Darling*, American physician, 1872–1925] histoplasmosis.

dar·nel (dahr′nəl) *Lolium temulentum.*

d'Ar·son·val current (dahr-saw-vahl′) [Jacques A. *d'Arsonval*, French physicist, 1851–1940] see under *current.*

dar·to·ic (dahr-to′ik) of the nature of a dartos; having a slow, involuntary contractility like that of the tunica dartos.

dar·toid (dahr′toid) dartoic.

dar·tos (dahr′tos) [Gr. "flayed"] dartos muscle.

Dar·vo·cet-N (dahr′vo-set) trademark for a combination preparation of propoxyphene napsylate and acetaminophen.

Dar·von (dahr′von) trademark for preparations containing propoxyphene.

Dar·win ear, tubercle (dahr′win) [Charles Robert *Darwin*, English biologist, 1809–1882] see under *ear* and see *tuberculum auriculare.*

dar·win·ian (dahr-win′e-ən) named for Charles Robert *Darwin*, as *darwinian theory.*

dar·win·ism (dahr′win-iz-əm) [C.R. *Darwin*] the theory of evolution stating that change in a species over time is partly the result of a process of natural selection, which enables the species to continually adapt to its changing environment. Called also *darwinian theory.*

da·sat·i·nib (də-să′tĭ-nib) a tyrosine kinase inhibitor used as an antineoplastic in treatment of chronic myeloid leukemia and certain types of acute lymphoblastic leukemia; administered orally.

das·sie (das′e) rock hyrax.

Das·y·proc·ta (das″e-prok′tə) a genus of large rodents of tropical America, including various species of agouti (q.v.).

DAT a cancer chemotherapy regimen consisting of daunorubicin, ara-C (cytarabine), and thioguanine.

da·ta (da′tə) [L., plural of *datum*] the material or collection of facts on which a discussion or an inference is based.

censored d. in statistics, observations whose final outcomes are not completely determined in a study, as, for example, data for patients who have not yet reached the study's endpoint (e.g., relapse or death) when the data are analyzed or who drop out of the study before reaching that endpoint.

dATP deoxyadenosine triphosphate.

Da·tu·ra (da-too′rə) a genus of plants of the family Solanaceae; several species contain the anticholinergic alkaloids hyoscyamine and scopolamine.

D. me′tel a species that is a source of scopolamine; its seeds sometimes contaminate animal feed, causing daturism.

D. stramo′nium the most common species of *Datura*; it is a source of hyoscyamine and scopolamine. Its seeds sometimes contaminate animal feed and cause daturism. Called also *Jimson weed, stramonium,* and *thorn apple.*

da·tu·rine (da-too′rin) hyoscyamine.

da·tu·rism (da-too′riz-əm) poisoning by plants of the genus *Datura*, which contain solanaceous alkaloids such as atropine, hyoscyamine, and scopolamine.

Dau·ben·ton angle, plane (line) (do-bon-ton′) [Louis Jean Marie *Daubenton*, French physician and naturalist, 1716–1800] see under *angle* and *plane.*

Dau·cus (daw′kəs) a genus of herbs of the family Umbelliferae, native to Europe and Asia. *D. caro′ta* is the carrot.

daugh·ter (daw′tər) decay product.

dau·no·my·cin (daw-no-mi′sin) daunorubicin.

dau·no·ru·bi·cin (daw″no-roo′bĭ-sin) an anthracycline (q.v.) antibiotic produced by *Streptomyces coeruleorubidus* or *S. peucetius* and used as an antineoplastic.

d. hydrochloride [USP] the hydrochloride salt of daunorubicin, having the same actions as the base; used in the treatment of acute lymphocytic leukemia, acute myelogenous leukemia, acute monocytic leukemia, erythroleukemia, and neuroblastoma, administered intravenously.

liposomal d. an aqueous solution of the citrate salt of daunorubicin, encapsulated within specifically constructed liposomes; the preparation shows enhanced selectivity for solid tumors in situ compared with that of the hydrochloride salt. It is administered intravenously in the treatment of advanced Kaposi sarcoma associated with acquired immunodeficiency syndrome (AIDS).

dau·no·sa·mine (daw-nōs′ə-mēn) a six-carbon amino sugar found in anthracycline antibiotics.

Dau·no·Xome (daw′nok-sōm) trademark for a preparation of liposomal daunorubicin.

Da·vai·nea (da-va′ne-ə) [Casimir Joseph *Davaine*, French physician, 1812–1882] a genus of tapeworms of the family Davaineidae. *D. proglotti′na* causes severe enteritis in fowls.

Da·vai·ne·i·dae (da″va-ne′ĭ-de) a family of small tapeworms of the order Cyclophyllidea, subclass Cestoda, which parasitize mammals and birds. *Davainea* and *Raillietina* are medically important genera.

Da·vid disease (dah-vēd′) [Jean Pierre *David*, French surgeon, 1737–1784] spinal tuberculosis.

Da·vid procedure (da′vid) [Tirone E. *David*, Brazilian-born Canadian cardiac surgeon, 20th century] see under *procedure.*

Da·vid·off (Da·vid·ov) cells (dah′vid-of) [M. von *Davidoff*, German histologist, died 1904] Paneth cells.

Da·vid·sohn differential absorption test (da′vid-sən) [Israel Davidsohn, American pathologist, 1895–1979] Paul-Bunnell-Davidsohn test.

Da·vi·el operation, spoon (dah-ve-el′) [Jacques *Daviel*, French oculist, 1696–1762, originator of treatment of cataract by extraction of the lens] see under *operation* and *spoon.*

Da·vis graft (da′vis) [John Staige *Davis*, American surgeon, 1872–1946] pinch graft; see under *graft.*

Da·vis ureterotomy (da′vis) [D.M. *Davis*, American surgeon, mid-20th century] see under *ureterotomy.*

Daw·barn sign (daw′bahrn) [Robert Hugh Mackay *Dawbarn*, American surgeon, 1860–1915] see under *sign.*

DAy Doctor of Ayurvedic Medicine.

Day·pro (da′pro) trademark for a preparation of oxaprozin.

dB, db decibel.

DBA dibenzanthracene.

DBS deep brain stimulation.

DC direct current; Doctor of Chiropractic.

D & C dilatation and curettage.

dC deoxycytidine.

DCA desoxycorticosterone acetate.

DCc double concave; see under *lens.*

dCDP deoxycytidine diphosphate.

DCF direct centrifugal flotation; see *Lane method*, under *method.*

DCH Diploma in Child Health.

DCIS ductal carcinoma in situ.

dCMP deoxycytidine monophosphate.

dCMP de·am·i·nase (de-am′in-ās) [EC 3.5.4.12] an enzyme of the hydrolase class that catalyzes the deamination of dCMP to form dUMP, a step in the synthesis of dTTP from CDP.

DCOG Diploma of the College of Obstetricians and Gynaecologists (British).

dCTP deoxycytidine triphosphate.

DCx double convex; see under *lens.*

d.d. [L.] de′tur ad (let it be given to).

DDAVP trademark for preparations of desmopressin.

ddC dideoxycytidine; see *zalcitabine.*

DDD TDE.

***o,p*′-DDD** mitotane.

DDH developmental dysplasia of the hip.

ddI dideoxyinosine; see *didanosine.*

DDP, *cis*-DDP cisplatin (*cis*-diamminedichloroplatinum).

DDS diaminodiphenylsulfone (see *dapsone*); Doctor of Dental Surgery.

DDSc Doctor of Dental Science.

DDT dichlorodiphenyltrichloroethane, a chlorinated hydrocarbon pesticide that is moderately toxic; it was formerly widely used but is now banned in the United States except for a few specialized purposes because of the ecological damage it causes.

de- [L. *de* away from, down from] a prefix often denoting negation or privation; it may signify down or away from, cessation, reversal, or removal. It sometimes has an intensive force.

de·ac·e·tyl·la·nat·o·side C (de-as″ə-tēl-lə-nat′o-sīd) deslanoside.

de·acid·i·fi·ca·tion (de″ə-sid″ĭ-fĭ-ka′shən) the act of correcting or destroying acidity or of neutralizing an acid.

de·ac·ti·va·tion (de-ak″tĭ-va′shən) the process of making or becoming inactive, as the removal or loss of radioactivity from a previously radioactive material.

de•acyl•ase (de-a′səl-ās) any enzyme of the hydrolase class that catalyzes the cleavage of an acyl group in ester or amide linkage.

dead (ded) 1. destitute of life; see also *death*. 2. anesthetic (def. 1).

deaf (def) lacking the sense of hearing or having profound hearing loss.

de•af•fer•en•ta•tion (de-af″ər-ən-ta′shən) the elimination or interruption of afferent nerve impulses, as by destruction of the afferent pathway.

deaf•ness (def′nis) hearing loss; lack or significant deficiency of the sense of hearing. For specific types, see under *hearing loss*.

Alexander d. congenital deafness due to cochlear aplasia, involving chiefly the organ of Corti and adjacent ganglion cells of the basal coil of the cochlea; a high-frequency hearing loss results. Called also *Alexander hearing loss*.

bass d. popular name for *low-frequency hearing loss*.

cortical d. central hearing loss due to a lesion of the subcortical pathways immediately below the auditory cortex of the hemisphere dominant for speech and language, or of the auditory cortex itself.

labyrinthine d. sensory hearing loss due to disease of the labyrinth of the internal ear.

Michel d. congenital deafness due to total lack of development of the internal ear (Michel aplasia).

midbrain d. central hearing loss due to injury of the fillet tract of the tegmentum.

Mondini d. congenital deafness due to dysgenesis of the organ of Corti, with partial aplasia of the bony and membranous labyrinth and a resultant flattened cochlea. See also *Mondini deformity*, under *deformity*.

music d. amusia.

nerve d., neural d. neural hearing loss.

pagetoid d. deafness occurring in osteitis deformans (Paget disease) of the bones of the skull.

Scheibe d. congenital deafness due to partial aplasia of the saccule and cochlear duct (Scheibe aplasia).

tone d. sensory amusia.

vascular d. deafness due to disease of blood vessels of the internal ear.

word d. auditory aphasia.

de•al•ba•tion (de″al-ba′shən) bleaching.

de•al•co•hol•iza•tion (de-al″ko-hol″ĭ-za′shən) the removal of alcohol from an object or substance.

de•al•ler•gi•za•tion (de-al″ər-jĭ-za′shən) the desensitization of an allergic individual to any particular allergen.

de•am•i•dase (de-am′ĭ-dās) amidohydrolase.

de•am•i•da•tion (de-am″ĭ-da′shən) deamidization.

de•am•i•di•za•tion (de-am″ĭ-dĭ-za′shən) the removal of an amido group from a molecule.

de•am•i•nase (de-am′ĭ-nās) a term used in the trivial names of some aminohydrolases (q.v.), usually restricted to those deaminating cyclic amidines; the enzymes are generally named for their substrates (e.g., adenosine deaminase).

de•am•i•na•tion (de-am″ĭ-na′shən) removal of the amino group, —NH_2, from a compound.

de•am•i•ni•za•tion (de-am″ĭ-nĭ-za′shən) deamination.

de•ar•te•ri•al•i•za•tion (de″ahr-te″re-əl-ĭ-za′shən) the occluding or cutting off of the arterial supply to a part, causing ischemia; sometimes done in a transient fashion as a treatment for liver cancer.

de•ar•tic•u•la•tion (de″ahr-tik″u-la′shən) dislocation of a joint.

death (deth) the cessation of life; permanent cessation of all vital bodily functions. For legal and medical purposes, the following definition of death has been proposed—the irreversible cessation of all of the following: (1) total cerebral function, (2) spontaneous function of the respiratory system, and (3) spontaneous function of the circulatory system.

activation-induced cell d. (AICD) recognition and deletion of T lymphocytes that have been induced to proliferate by receptor-mediated activation, preventing their overgrowth when responding to perception of a foreign agent. It is particularly important for regulation of lymphocytes that recognize self-antigens.

apparent d. a state of complete interruption of bodily processes from which the patient can be resuscitated.

black d. name formerly given to bubonic plague because affected tissues became black and gangrenous.

brain d. irreversible brain damage as manifested by absolute unresponsiveness to all stimuli and absence of all spontaneous muscle activity such as respiration and shivering, in patients who do not have hypothermia or intoxication by central nervous system depressants. Called also *irreversible coma* and *cerebral d.*

cell d. cessation of the cell's ability to carry out vital functions; cf. *apoptosis*, *necrosis*, and *programmed cell d.*.

cerebral d. brain d.

clinical d. the absence of heartbeat (no pulse being felt) and cessation of breathing.

cot d., crib d. sudden infant death syndrome.

fetal d. death in utero; failure of the product of conception to show evidence of respiration, heartbeat, or definite movement of a voluntary muscle after expulsion from the uterus, with no possibility of resuscitation. Called also *stillbirth*.

fetal d., early fetal death occurring during the first 20 weeks of gestation.

fetal d., intermediate fetal death occurring during the twenty-first to twenty-eighth weeks of gestation.

fetal d., late fetal death occurring after 28 weeks of gestation.

functional d. total, permanent destruction of cognition and related higher functions of the central nervous system, with vital functions being sustained by artificial means.

genetic d. the failure of a mutation to be passed on to the next generation because of the mutation's damaging phenotypic effects.

local d. death of a part of the body.

programmed cell d. the theory that particular cells are programmed to die at specific sites and during specific stages of development, often by the process of apoptosis. Although the two terms are often used synonymously, not all programmed cell death occurs by apoptosis.

somatic d. cessation of all vital cellular activity.

sudden cardiac d. unexpected natural death from cardiac causes, occurring rapidly after onset of acute symptoms in a patient with or without known preexisting heart disease; the cardiac dysfunction produces abrupt loss of cerebral blood flow. The interval between onset of symptoms and death may range from less than one hour to almost 24 hours.

vascular d. death caused by vascular pathology.

voodoo d. a phenomenon seen among certain cultural groups in which the affected individual dies after transgressing a taboo or becoming convinced that they are bewitched.

Dea•ver incision (de′vər) [John Blair *Deaver*, American surgeon, 1855–1931] see under *incision*.

De•Ba•key for•ceps (de-ba′ke) [Michael Ellis *DeBakey*, American surgeon, 1908–2008] see under *forceps*.

de•band•ing (de-band′ing) the removal of the bands of a fixed orthodontic appliance.

De•bary•o•my•ces (de″bar-e-o-mi′sēz) a genus of fungi of the family Saccharomycetaceae. *D. hanse′nii* changes sugars into oxalic acid and has occasionally been isolated from human infections.

de•bil•i•ty (də-bil′ĭ-te) asthenia.

dé•bouche•ment (da-bo͞osh-maw′) [Fr.] an opening out.

de•branch•er en•zyme (de-branch′ər en′zīm) see under *enzyme*.

de•branch•er en•zyme de•fi•cien•cy (de-branch′ər en′zīm) glycogen storage disease, type III.

de•branch•ing en•zyme (de-branch′ing en′zīm) see under *enzyme*.

De•bré-Sé•mé•laigne syndrome (də-bra′ sa-ma-len′yə) [Robert *Debré*, French pediatrician and bacteriologist, 1882–1978; Georges *Sémélaigne*, French pediatrician, 20th century] see under *syndrome*.

dé•bride (da-brēd′) to remove foreign material and contaminated or devitalized tissue, usually by sharp dissection.

dé•bride•ment (da-brēd-maw′) [Fr.] the removal of foreign material and devitalized or contaminated tissue from or adjacent to a traumatic or infected lesion until surrounding healthy tissue is exposed. Cf. *épluchage*.

enzymatic d. removal of fibrinous or purulent exudate by application of a nontoxic and nonirritating enzyme that is capable of lysing fibrin, denatured collagen, and elastin but does not destroy normal tissue.

surgical d. débridement by mechanical methods, usually sharp dissection.

de•bris (də-bre′) [Fr.] an accumulation of fragments of necrotic tissue or foreign material.

De•bri•san (də-bri′sən) trademark for dextranomer.

deb•ris•o•quine (deb-ris′o-kwin) INN and BAN for *debrisoquin*.

deb•ris•o•quin sul•fate (deb-ris′o-kwin) an antihypertensive agent having actions and uses similar to those of guanethidine; administered orally. Spelled also *debrisoquine*.

Deb. spis. [L.] deb′ita spissitu′dine (of the proper consistency).

debt (det) something owed.

oxygen d. the extra oxygen that must be used in the oxidative energy processes after a period of strenuous exercise to reconvert lactic acid to glucose, and decomposed ATP and creatine phosphate to their original states.

de•bulk•ing (de-bulk′ing) removal of a major portion of the material that composes a lesion, as the removal of most of a tumor so that there is less tumor load for subsequent treatment (e.g., by chemotherapy or radiotherapy). Called also *cytoreduction* and *cytoreductive surgery.*

Dec. [L.] decan′ta (pour off).

deca- [Gr. *deka* ten] a prefix designating ten; used in naming units of measurement to indicate a quantity ten (10^1) times the unit designated by the root with which it is combined. Symbol da.

Deca•derm (dek′ə-dərm″) trademark for a preparation of dexamethasone.

Deca•dron (dek′ə-dron″) trademark for preparations of dexamethasone.

Deca-Du•ra•bo•lin (dek″ə-dur″ə-bo′lin) trademark for a preparation of nandrolone decanoate.

Deca•ject (dek′ə-jekt″) trademark for a preparation of dexamethasone sodium phosphate.

Deca•ject-LA (dek′ə-jekt″) trademark for a preparation of dexamethasone acetate.

de•cal•ci•fi•ca•tion (de-kal″sĭ-fĭ-ka′shən) 1. the loss of calcium salts from a bone or tooth. 2. the process of removing calcareous matter.

de•cal•ci•fy (de-kal′sĭ-fi) [*de-* + *calcify*] to remove calcium salts.

dec•ane (dek′ān) a hydrocarbon, $C_{10}H_{22}$, from paraffin.

de•can•nu•la•tion (de-kan″u-la′shən) extubation, especially of a tracheostomy cannula.

dec•a•no•ate (dek″ə-no′āt) caprate.

dec•a•no•ic ac•id (dek″ə-no′ik) capric acid.

de•can•ta•tion (de″kan-ta′shən) [*de-* + L. *canthus* tire of a wheel] the pouring of a clear supernatant liquid from a sediment.

deca•pep•tide (dek″ə-pep′tīd) a peptide containing ten amino acids.

Deca•pep•tyl (dek″ə-pep′təl) trademark for a preparation of triptorelin pamoate.

de•cap•i•ta•tion (de-kap″ĭ-ta′shən) [*de-* + L. *caput* head] the removal of the head, as of an animal, a fetus, or a bone.

de•cap•i•ta•tor (de-kap′ĭ-ta″tər) an instrument for removing the head of a fetus in embryotomy.

De•ca•po•da (de-kə-po′də) [Gr. *deka* ten + *pous* foot] an order of Crustacea, including the crabs, lobsters, and shrimps, whose members have five pairs of legs attached to the thorax.

de•cap•su•la•tion (de-kap″su-la′shən) capsulectomy.

renal d. surgical removal of the capsule of the kidney; called also *renal capsulectomy.*

de•car•box•y•lase (de″kahr-bok′sə-lās) a term used in the recommended names of enzymes of the sub-subclass carboxy-lyase [EC 4.1.1]; they catalyze the nonhydrolytic removal of carbon dioxide from carboxylic acids.

de•car•box•y•la•tion (de″kahr-bok″sə-la′shən) removal of the carboxyl group from a molecule.

De•ca•spray (dek′ə-spra″) trademark for a preparation of dexamethasone.

Dec•a•vac (dek′ə-vak) trademark for a preparation of tetanus and diphtheria toxoids.

de•cay (de-ka′) [*de-* + L. *cadere* to fall] 1. the gradual decomposition of dead organic matter. 2. the process or stage of decline, as in aging.

alpha d. a form of radioactive decay in which an alpha particle (two neutrons plus two protons) is emitted, decreasing both the size and the charge of the nucleus and yielding a daughter product that is a different element. It often occurs serially.

beta d. disintegration of the nucleus of an unstable radionuclide in which the mass number is unchanged, but the atomic number is increased or decreased by 1, as result of emission of a negatively or positively charged (beta) particle and a neutrino.

free induction d. the signal analyzed in magnetic resonance imaging or spectroscopy; it results from the emission of energy by nuclei after they are excited by a pulse of radio frequency waves.

positron d. see under *emission.*

radioactive d. disintegration of the nucleus of an unstable nuclide by the spontaneous emission of charged particles and/or photons; called also *radioactive disintegration.*

tone d. the decrease in threshold sensitivity resulting from the presence of a barely audible continuous sound.

tooth d. dental caries.

de•ce•dent (də-se′dənt) a person who has recently died.

de•cel•er•a•tion (de-sel′ər-a″shən) decrease in speed or rate.

early d. in fetal heart rate monitoring, a transient decrease in heart rate that coincides with the onset of a uterine contraction.

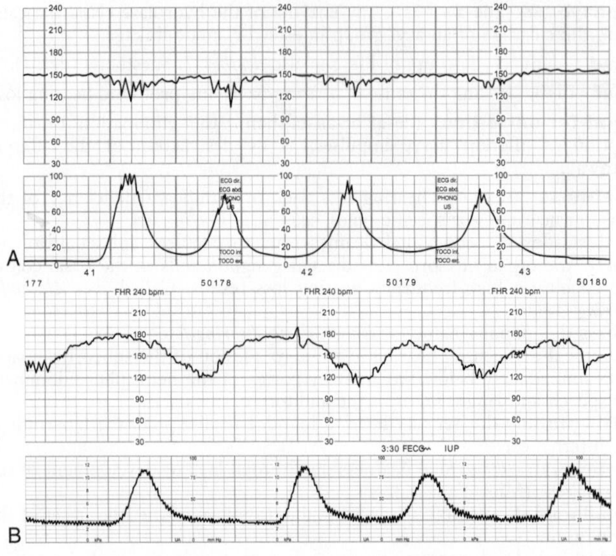

■ Tracings of early *(A)* and late *(B)* decelerations.

late d. in fetal heart rate monitoring, a transient decrease in heart rate occurring at or after the peak of a uterine contraction, which may result from fetal hypoxia.

variable d's in fetal heart rate monitoring, a transient series of decelerations in heart rate that vary in duration, intensity, and relation to uterine contractions; they are abrupt in onset and cessation and result from vagus nerve firing in response to stimuli such as umbilical cord compression in the first stage of labor.

de•cen•ter (de-sen′tər) [*de-* + *center*] in optics, to design or make a lens such that the visual axis does not pass through the optical center of the lens.

de•cen•tra•tion (de″sen-tra′shən) the act or process of removing from a center.

de•ce•ra•tion (de′sə-ra′shən) [*de-* + L. *cera* wax] the removal of paraffin from a tissue section prepared for the microscope.

de•cer•e•bel•la•tion (de-ser″ə-bəl-a′shən) removal of the cerebellum or elimination of its functions.

de•cer•e•brate[1] (de-ser′ə-brāt) in experimental animals, to eliminate cerebral function, as by removal of the brain, transection of the brainstem, or ligation of the common carotid arteries and the basilar artery.

de•cer•e•brate[2] (de-ser′ə-brət) 1. pertaining to an animal that has had cerebral function interrupted. 2. resulting from decerebration or, in humans, exhibiting neurologic characteristics similar to those of a decerebrated animal. See also *decerebrate rigidity*, under *rigidity.*

de•cer•e•bra•tion (de-ser″ə-bra′shən) the act of decerebrating.

de•chlo•ri•da•tion (de-klor″ĭ-da′shən) the removal of chloride, or salt.

De•cho•lin (de′ko-lin) trademark for preparations of dehydrocholic acid.

deci- [L. *decem* ten] a combining form designating one tenth; used in naming units of measurement to indicate one tenth (10^{-1}) of the unit designated by the root with which it is combined. Symbol d.

dec•i•bel (des′ĭ-bəl) a unit of relative power intensity equal to one tenth of a bel, used for electric or acoustic power measurements. The decibel level is ten times the base ten logarithm of the ratio of the measured power to some reference power level. A one decibel change is an increase in the power level by a factor of 1.26, approximately the smallest change in sound level detectable by human ears; a ten decibel (one bel) change multiplies the power by a factor of ten and approximately doubles the perceived sound level. In audiometry the reference power level (0 db) corresponds to a root-mean-square sound pressure level of 2×10^{-4} dyn/cm^2, which is approximately the threshold of hearing for healthy young persons. Symbol, dB.

de•cid•ua (də-sid′u-ə) [L., from *deciduus*, from *decidere* to fall off] the endometrium of the pregnant uterus, all of which, except the deepest layer, is shed at parturition. Called also *decidual* or *deciduous membrane.* **decid′ual** *adj*

d. basa′lis basal decidua: the portion of the decidua directly underlying the chorionic sac and attached to the myometrium; called also *d. serotina.*

d. capsula′ris capsular decidua: the portion of the decidua directly overlying the chorionic sac and facing the uterine cavity; called also *reflex d.* and *d. reflexa.*

menstrual d., d. menstrua´lis the hyperemic mucosa of the uterus that is shed during the menstrual period.

d. parieta´lis parietal decidua: the portion of the decidua lining the uterus elsewhere than at the site of attachment of the chorionic sac; called also *d. vera.*

reflex d., d. reflex´a d. capsularis.

d. seroti´na d. basalis.

d. subchoria´lis the maternal component of the tissue comprising the closing ring of Winkler-Waldeyer.

true d. d. parietalis.

d. tubero´sa papulo´sa decidual cast.

d. ve´ra d. parietalis.

de•cid•u•ate (də-sid´u-āt) characterized by shedding.

de•cid•u•itis (də-sid″u-i´tis) a bacterial disease leading to alterations in the decidua.

de•cid•u•o•ma (də-sid″u-o´mə) [*decidua* + *-oma*] an intrauterine mass containing decidual cells.

Loeb d. a tumorlike structure resembling the maternal placenta, produced in the uteri of guinea pigs by the action of progesterone.

d. malig´num choriocarcinoma.

de•cid•u•o•ma•to•sis (də-sid″u-o-mə-to´sis) formation of decidual tissue in the nonpregnant state.

de•cid•u•o•sis (də-sid″u-o´sis) the presence of decidual tissue or of tissue resembling the endometrium of pregnancy in an ectopic site.

de•cid•u•ous (də-sid´u-əs) [L. *deciduus*, from *decidere* to fall off] falling off or shed at maturity, as the teeth of the first dentition.

dec•ile (des´īl) [*deca-* + *-ile* (by analogy with *quartile*)] any of the nine values that divide the range of a probability distribution into ten equal parts of equal probability, i.e., the 1st, 2nd, 3rd, etc., deciles are the 10th, 20th, 30th, etc., percentiles.

dec•i•li•ter (dL) (des´ĭ-le″tər) one tenth (10^{-1}) of a liter; 100 milliliters.

de•cip•a•ra (də-sip´ə-rə) [*deca-* + *para*] a woman who has had ten pregnancies that resulted in viable offspring; also written *para X.*

de•ci•ta•bine (DAC) (de-si´tə-bēn″) an S-phase specific cytotoxic compound used as an antineoplastic in the treatment of acute leukemia; administered by intravenous infusion.

deck•platte (dek´plah-tə) [Ger.] roof plate; see under *plate.*

de•claw•ing (de-klaw´ing) onychectomy.

de Clé•ram•bault syndrome (də kla″rahm-bo´) [Gaetan Gatian *de Clérambault*, French psychiatrist, 1872–1934] see *erotomania.*

dec•li•na•tion (dek″lĭ-na´shən) [L. *declinare* to decline] deviation from a normally vertical position, as rotation of the eye about its anteroposterior axis so that its vertical meridian lies to the temporal *(positive d.)* or to the nasal side *(negative d.)* of its proper position. Cf. *extorsion* and *intorsion.*

dec•li•na•tor (dek´lĭ-na″tər) an instrument by which parts are retracted during an operation.

de•cline (de-klīn´) 1. the period or stage of the abatement of a disease or paroxysm. 2. a gradual deterioration or wasting away of the physical and mental faculties.

de•clive (de-kli´ve) [L. neuter of *declivis* sloping downward] [TA] (VI); the part of the vermis of the cerebellum just caudal to the primary fissure; it is part of the simple lobule (lobulus simplex).

de•cli•vis (de-kli´vis) [L.] declive.

Dec•lo•my•cin (dek´lo-mi″sin) trademark for preparations of demeclocycline hydrochloride.

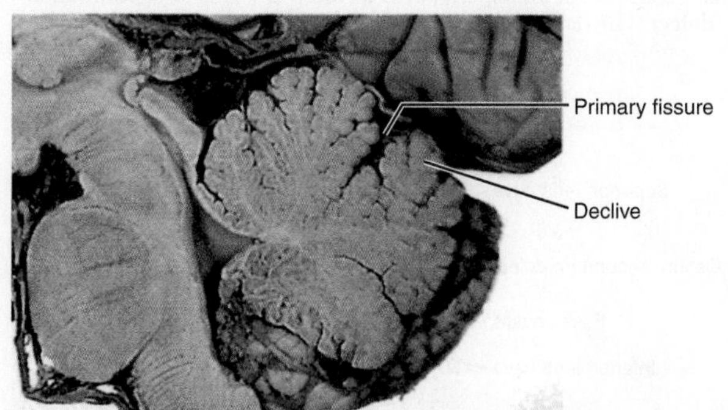

■ Median section of cerebellum, showing declive.

de•co•ag•u•lant (de″ko-ag´u-lənt) 1. reducing the amount of existing coagulants or procoagulants in the blood. 2. a substance that has this quality and inhibits coagulation of blood.

Decoct. [L.] decoc´tum (a decoction).

de•coc•tion (de-kok´shən) [L. *decoctum*, from *de* down + *coquere* to boil] 1. the act or process of boiling. 2. a medicine or other substance prepared by boiling.

de•col•la•tion (de″ko-la´shən) [*de-* + *collum*] decapitation, chiefly of a dead fetus.

de•col•or•a•tion (de-kul″ər-a´shən) 1. removal of color; bleaching. 2. lack or loss of color.

de•col•or•ize (de-kul´ər-īz) to free from color; to bleach.

de•com•pen•sat•ed (de-kom´pən-sāt″əd) characterized by decompensation.

de•com•pen•sa•tion (de-kom″pən-sa´shən) 1. failure of compensation; cardiac decompensation is marked by dyspnea, venous engorgement, and edema. 2. in psychiatry, failure of defense mechanisms resulting in progressive personality disintegration.

de•com•ple•men•tize (de-kom´plə-men″tīz) to remove complement from.

de•com•po•si•tion (de″kom-pə-zish´ən) [*de-* + L. *componere* to put together] the separation of compound bodies into their constituent principles by whatever process.

anaerobic d. the breakdown of organic compounds in the absence of oxygen. In animals, the process is known as *glycolysis;* in plants and microorganisms, *fermentation.*

d. of movement a form of ataxia characterized by irregularity in the successive flexion and extension of joints in performing a movement with the limb.

de•com•pres•sion (de″kom-presh´ən) 1. any removal of pressure. 2. the lessening of atmospheric pressure on deep-sea divers and caisson workers who return to normal pressure environments, or on persons ascending to great heights. If not controlled or artificially slowed, it can cause *decompression sickness.* 3. any technique for artificially controlling this process. 4. a surgical operation for the relief of pressure in a body compartment.

abdominal d. the removal of pressure from the abdomen during the first stage of labor.

cardiac d. d. of heart.

cerebral d. removal of a flap of the skull and incision of the dura mater for relief of intracranial pressure.

explosive d. decompression more rapid than that corresponding to a rate of ascent greater than 5000 feet per minute.

d. of heart pericardiotomy with evacuation of blood or fluid; called also *d. of pericardium.*

microvascular d. a microsurgical procedure for relief of trigeminal neuralgia; decompression of the sensory root of the trigeminal nerve is accomplished by insertion of a small nonabsorbable sponge to relieve pressure from small blood vessels where the root enters the pons. Called also *Jannetta procedure.*

nerve d. relief of pressure on a nerve by surgical removal of the constricting fibrous or bony tissue.

orbital d. removal of one or two of the walls of the orbit of the eye to relieve pressure, most often in persons with Graves orbitopathy.

d. of pericardium d. of heart.

d. of spinal cord relief of pressure on the spinal cord by means of surgery.

suboccipital d. cerebral decompression by occipital craniectomy and opening of the dura.

subtemporal d. cerebral decompression by removal of a portion of the temporal bone and opening of the dura.

de•con•di•tion•ing (de″kən-dish´ən-ing) a change in cardiovascular function after prolonged periods of weightlessness, probably related to a shift of a quantity of blood from the lower limbs to the thorax, resulting in reflex diuresis and a reduction of blood volume.

de•con•ges•tant (de″kən-jes´tənt) 1. tending to reduce congestion or swelling, such as of the nasal mucosa; called also *decongestive.* 2. an agent that reduces congestion or swelling.

de•con•ges•tive (de″kən-jes´tiv) decongestant (def. 1).

de•con•tam•i•na•tion (de″kən-tam″ĭ-na´shən) the freeing of a person or an object of some contaminating substance such as poisonous gas, radioactive material, etc.

de•con•vo•lu•tion (de-kon″və-loo´shən) in image processing, the algorithmic removal of the effects of blur to improve resolution.

de•co•quin•ate (de-ko-kwin´āt) [USP] a coccidiostat for poultry, effective against *Eimeria.*

dec•o•rin (dek′ə-rin) a small (90–140 kD) leucine-rich repeat protein of the extracellular matrix, expressed by connective tissue fibroblasts; it consists of a single glycosaminoglycan strand and associated oligosaccharides and binds and modifies the assembly of collagen fibrils.

de•cor•ti•cate (de-kor′tĭ-kāt) having brain damage such that functions of the cerebral cortex are eliminated.

de•cor•ti•ca•tion (de-kor″tĭ-ka′shən) [*de-* + *cortex*] 1. the removal of bark, hull, husk, or shell from a plant, seed, or root, as in pharmacy. 2. removal of portions of the cortex of a structure or organ, as of the brain, kidney, or lung.
chemical d., enzymatic d. removal of the cortex of a structure by chemical agents or enzymes.
d. of lung the removal of constricting visceral pleura to permit the lung to expand.

dec•re•ment (dek′rə-mənt) [L. *decrementum*] 1. subtraction, or decrease; the amount by which a quantity or value is decreased. 2. the stage of decline of a disease.

de•crep•i•tate (de-krep′ĭ-tāt) 1. to roast or calcine certain substances (salt, crystals, etc.) until crackling occurs, or until crackling ends. 2. to explode with a crackling noise upon heating, owing to the release of entrapped water as steam.

de•crep•i•ta•tion (de-krep″ĭ-ta′shən) the explosion or crackling of certain substances (salt, crystals, etc.) upon heating.

de•cru•des•cence (de″kroo-des′əns) diminution or abatement of the intensity of symptoms or physical signs.

de•crus•ta•tion (de″krəs-ta′shən) the detachment of a crust.

Decub. [L.] decu′bitus (lying down).

de•cu•bi•tal (de-ku′bĭ-təl) pertaining to decubitus or to a decubitus ulcer.

de•cu•bi•tus (de-ku′bĭ-təs) pl. *decu′bitus* [L. "a lying down"] 1. an act of lying down. 2. decubitus position. 3. decubitus ulcer.
dorsal d. lying in the supine position.
lateral d. lying on the side; used in radiologic examination, with the x-ray beam directed horizontally; designated *right lateral decubitus* when the subject lies on the right side and *left lateral decubitus* when on the left side.
ventral d. lying on the stomach.

de•cum•bin (de-kum′bin) a toxic substance obtained from *Penicillium decumbens*, which causes respiratory distress and hemorrhage; the oral LD_{50} for rats is about 275 mg/kg.

de•cur•rent (de-kur′ənt) [L. *decurrere* to run down] extending or moving from above downward.

de•cus•sate (de-kus′āt) [L. *decussare* to cross in the form of an X] 1. to cross or intersect in the form of the letter X. 2. crossing in the form of the letter X.

de•cus•sa•tio (de″kə-sa′she-o) pl. *decussatio′nes* [L.] [TA] decussation: anatomical terminology for the intercrossing of fellow parts or structures in the form of an X. See also *chiasma* and *commissura.*
d. fibra′rum nervo′rum trochlea′rium [TA] decussation of trochlear nerve fibers: the crossing of the fibers of the trochlear nerves in the most rostral portion of the superior medullary velum. Called also *trochlear decussation.*
d. lemnis′ci media′lis [TA] decussation of medial lemniscus: the region at the caudal end of the medulla oblongata in which the fibers from the nucleus cuneatus and the nucleus gracilis on each side intersect as they cross the midline before ascending as the medial lemniscus. Called also *sensory decussation.*
d. pedunculo′rum cerebella′rium superio′rum [TA] decussation of superior cerebellar peduncles: the crossing of the fibers of the peduncles within the tegmentum of the mesencephalon.
d. pyra′midum [TA] decussation of pyramids: the anterior part of the lower medulla oblongata in which most of the fibers of each pyramid intersect as they cross the midline and descend as the lateral corticospinal tracts. Called also *pyramidal* or *motor decussation.*
d.′nes tegmenta′les [TA] tegmental decussations: crossing fibers in the midbrain, including the decussatio tegmentalis anterior and the decussatio tegmentalis posterior.
d. tegmenta′lis ante′rior [TA] anterior tegmental decussation: fibers originating in the red nucleus, crossing the midline in the inferior portions of the midbrain tegmentum, and forming the rubrobulbar and rubrospinal tracts.
d. tegmenta′lis poste′rior [TA] posterior tegmental decussation: fibers originating in the quadrigeminal bodies, crossing the midline in superior portions of the midbrain tegmentum, and forming the tectobulbar and tectospinal tracts.
d. trochlea′ris d. fibrarum nervorum trochlearium.

de•cus•sa•tion (de″kə-sa′shən) a crossing over; see *decussatio.*
anterior tegmental d. decussatio tegmentalis anterior.
dorsal tegmental d. decussatio tegmentalis posterior.
Forel d. decussatio tegmentalis anterior.
fountain d. of Meynert decussatio tegmentalis posterior.
d. of medial lemniscus decussatio lemnisci medialis.
motor d. decussatio pyramidum.
optic d. chiasma opticum.
posterior tegmental d. decussatio tegmentalis posterior.
pyramidal d., d. of pyramids decussatio pyramidum.
rubrospinal d. decussatio tegmentalis anterior.
sensory d. decussatio lemnisci medialis.
d. of superior cerebellar peduncles decussatio pedunculorum cerebellarium superiorum.
tectospinal d. decussatio tegmentalis posterior.
tegmental d's, d's of tegmentum decussationes tegmentales.
trochlear d., d. of trochlear nerves, d. of trochlear nerve fibers decussatio fibrarum nervorum trochlearium.
ventral tegmental d. decussatio tegmentalis anterior.

de•cus•sa•ti•o•nes (de″kə-sa″she-o′nēz) [L.] plural of *decussatio.*

de•den•ti•tion (de″den-tish′ən) [*de-* + *dentition*] the shedding or loss of teeth.

de•dif•fer•en•ti•a•tion (de-dif″ər-en″she-a′shən) anaplasia.

de d. in d. [L.] de di′e in di′em (from day to day).

ded•o•la•tion (ded″o-la′shən) [L. *dedolare* to hew away] the removal of a thin piece of skin by an oblique cut.

de•ef•fer•en•ta•tion (de-ef″ər-ən-ta′shən) the elimination or interruption of efferent nerve impulses, as by destruction of the efferent pathway.

deep (dēp) situated far beneath the surface; not superficial.

de•epi•car•di•al•iza•tion (de-ep″ĭ-kahr″de-əl″ĭ-za′shən) a surgical procedure formerly used for the relief of intractable angina pectoris, in which epicardial tissue is destroyed by phenolization or the application of other caustic agents to promote the development of collateral circulation.

deer•fly (dēr′fli) *Chrysops discalis.*

DEET (dēt) diethyltoluamide.

DEF decayed, extracted, filled; see under *rate.*

de•fat•i•ga•tion (de-fat″ĭ-ga′shən) overstrain or fatigue of muscular or nervous tissue.

de•fat•ted (de-fat′əd) deprived of fat, as a food.

de•faun•ate (de-fawn′āt) [*de-* + *fauna*] to remove or destroy an animal population, especially parasites, such as by removing hookworms from the intestinal tract or delousing.

de•faun•a•tion (de-faw-na′shən) the process of defaunating; cf. *disinfestation.*

def•e•ca•tion (def″ə-ka′shən) [L. *defaecare* to deprive of dregs] 1. the removal of impurities, as chemical defecation. 2. the evacuation of feces from the rectum.

def•e•cog•ra•phy (def″ə-kog′rə-fe) [*defecation* + *-graphy*] the making of rapid-sequence radiographs or the recording of fluoroscopic images on videotape during defecation following the instillation of barium into the rectum; used in the evaluation of fecal incontinence.

de•fect (de′fekt) an imperfection, failure, or absence.
acquired d. a non-genetic imperfection arising secondarily, after birth.
aortic septal d., aorticopulmonary septal d. a congenital anomaly in which there is abnormal communication between the ascending aorta and pulmonary artery just above the semilunar valves; called also *aorticopulmonary fenestration* or *window.*
atrial septal d's, atrioseptal d's congenital cardiac anomalies in which there is persistent patency of the atrial septum due to failure of fusion between either the septum secundum or the septum primum and the endocardial cushions. In *ostium secundum d.* there is a rim of septum all around the defect. In *ostium primum d.*, which is an incomplete form of

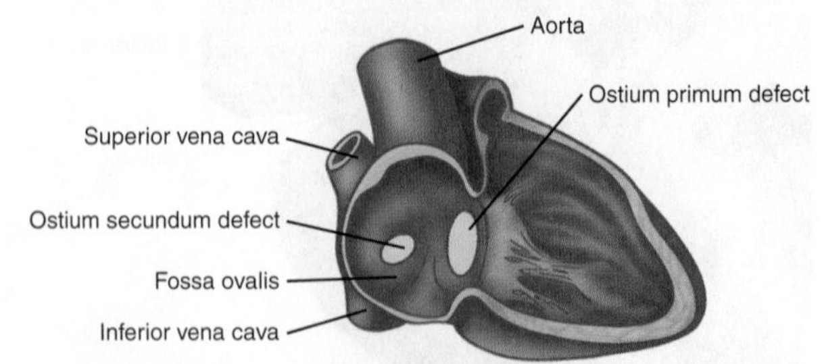

■ Atrial septal defects; cutaway composite view showing possible locations of ostium primum and secundum defects in the right atrium.

atrioventricularis communis, there is no septum at the base of the defect, between the mitral and tricuspid valves; it is usually associated with a cleft mitral cusp and occasionally with a cleft tricuspid valve or a ventricular septal defect.

birth d., congenital d. a defect present at birth; the term may refer to a morphological defect (dysmorphism) or to an inborn error of metabolism.

cortical d. a benign, symptomless, circumscribed rarefaction of cortical bone, detected radiographically.

endocardial cushion d's a spectrum of septal defects resulting from imperfect fusion of the endocardial cushions and ranging from persistent ostium primum to persistent complete common atrioventricular canal; see *atrial septal d's* and *atrioventricularis communis.*

fibrous cortical d. a small, asymptomatic, osteolytic, fibrous lesion occurring within the bone cortex, particularly in the metaphyseal region of long bones in childhood. When large and actively growing, it is generally termed *nonossifying fibroma*. Called also *metaphyseal fibrous d.*

filling d. any localized defect in the contour of the stomach, duodenum, or intestine, as seen in the radiograph after a barium enema, due to a wall lesion that projects into the lumen or to an object in the lumen.

genetic d. see under *disease.*

intercalary d. radial ray d.

junctional parenchymal d. on ultrasound of the kidney, an echogenic mass sometimes seen in the parenchyma, resembling a cortical scar but indicating only a benign collection of fat at the junction where two of the fetal lobes came together.

luteal phase d. inadequate secretory transformation of the endometrium during the luteal phase of the menstrual cycle, often with low levels of progesterone during this phase. Causes include poor follicle production, premature demise of the corpus luteum, and failure of the uterine lining to respond to normal levels of progesterone. It can cause infertility and habitual abortion. Called also *luteal phase deficiency.*

metaphyseal fibrous d. 1. fibrous cortical d. 2. nonossifying fibroma.

neural tube d. a developmental anomaly consisting of failure of closure of the neural tube, resulting in conditions such as cranium bifidum, encephalocele, spina bifida, and myelomeningocele. Called also *spinal dysraphism.*

ostium primum d. see *atrial septal d's.*

ostium secundum d. see *atrial septal d's.*

polytopic field d. a pattern of anomalies derived from the disturbance of a single developmental field.

radial ray d. pouce flottant associated with clubhand; called also intercalary d..

retention d. a defect in the power of recalling or remembering names, numbers, or events.

salt-losing d. see under *syndrome.*

septal d. a defect in one of the cardiac septa, resulting in an abnormal communication between the opposite chambers of the heart. See *atrial septal d's* and *ventricular septal d.*

ventricular septal d. a congenital cardiac anomaly in which there is persistent patency of the ventricular septum in either the muscular or fibrous (membranous) portions, most often due to failure of the bulbar septum to completely close the interventricular foramen.

de•fec•tive (de-fek′tiv) faulty; deficient; marked by subnormal function, structure, or behavior.

de•fem•i•ni•za•tion (de-fem″ĭ-nĭ-za′shən) loss of female secondary sex characters; see also *masculinization* (def. 2).

de•fense (de-fens′) the practice of, or measures taken to ensure, self-protection. See also under *mechanism.*

character d. any character trait, e.g., a mannerism, attitude, or affectation, which serves as a defense mechanism.

insanity d. a legal concept that a person cannot be convicted of a crime if they lacked criminal responsibility by reason of insanity at the time of commission. See *M'Naghten rule* and *Durham rule*, under *rule*, and *American Law Institute Formulation*, under *formulation.*

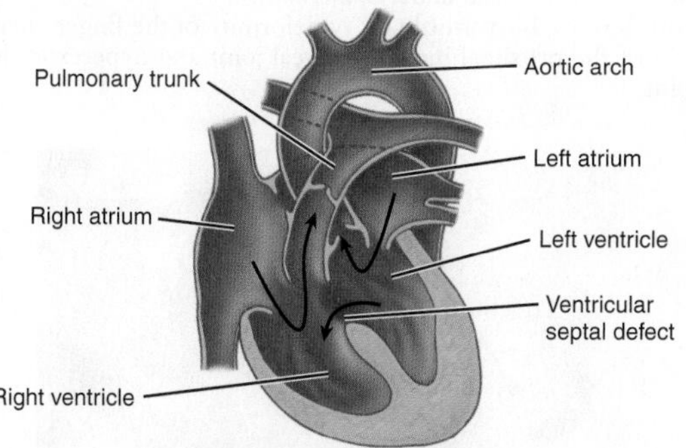

■ Abnormal communication between the ventricles in ventricular septal defect.

muscular d. the muscular tension and rigidity that accompanies a localized inflammation (as in appendicitis) or passage of a renal calculus.

de•fen•sin (de-fen′sin) any of a group of small antimicrobial cationic peptides occurring in neutrophils and macrophages; they act by binding fungal and bacterial membranes and increasing membrane permeability.

def•er•ens (def′ər-enz) [L.] deferent; see *ductus deferens.*

def•er•ent (def′ər-ənt) [L. *deferens* carrying away] conveying anything away, as from a center.

def•er•en•tial (def″ər-en′shəl) pertaining to the ductus deferens.

def•er•en•ti•tis (def″ər-ən-ti′tis) inflammation of the ductus deferens.

de•fer•ox•amine (de″fər-oks′ə-mēn) a chelating agent, isolated from *Streptomyces pilosus*, which binds with iron to form a soluble complex. Called also *desferrioxamine.*

d. mesylate [USP] the water-soluble mesylate salt of deferoxamine, having the same actions as the base; used as an antidote to iron poisoning, usually administered by intramuscular injection or by intravenous infusion.

def•er•ves•cence (def″ər-ves′əns) [L. *defervescere* to cease boiling] 1. the abatement of fever. 2. the period of abatement of fever.

def•er•ves•cent (def″ər-ves′ənt) 1. causing abatement of fever. 2. an agent that causes abatement of fever.

de•fib•ril•la•tion (de-fib″rĭ-la′shən) termination of atrial or ventricular fibrillation, usually by electroshock.

de•fib•ril•la•tor (de-fib″rĭ-la′tər) an electronic apparatus used to counteract atrial or ventricular fibrillation by the application of brief electroshock to the heart, either directly or through electrodes placed on the chest wall.

automatic external d. (AED) a portable defibrillator designed to be automated such that it can be used by persons without substantial medical training who are responding to a cardiac emergency.

automatic implantable cardioverter-d., implantable cardioverter-d. see under *cardioverter.*

de•fi•bri•nat•ed (de-fi′brĭ-nāt″əd) characterized by defibrination.

de•fi•bri•na•tion (de-fi″brĭ-na′shən) removal of fibrin from a blood sample to prevent clotting; it also occurs pathologically in diffuse intravascular coagulation.

de•fi•brino•gen•a•tion (de″fi-brin″ə-jə-na′shən) induced defibrination, such as that caused by ancrod in thrombolytic therapy.

de•fi•cien•cy (de-fish′ən-se) less than the normal amount of something; see also *defect.* For deficiencies of specific, individual enzymes, see under the enzyme name.

brancher d. glycogen storage disease, type IV.

cerebral folate d. decreased concentrations of 5-methyltetrahydrofolate in the cerebrospinal fluid while levels may be normal in the blood; the condition is usually congenital and seen in infants, and is characterized by progressive spasticity, speech difficulties, and sometimes dyskinesias and seizures. The etiology is unknown.

color vision d. any deviation from normal color vision; these conditions are popularly called by the misleading term *color blindness.* See *monochromatic vision, dichromatic vision, protanopia, deuteranopia, tritanopia,* and *tetartanopia.*

D-bifunctional protein d. 17β-hydroxysteroid dehydrogenase type 4 deficiency.

debrancher d. glycogen storage disease, type III.

disaccharidase d. less than normal activity of disaccharidases of the intestinal mucosa. It usually denotes a generalized deficiency of all such enzymes secondary to a disorder of the small intestine, which clinically may be manifest only as a deficiency of lactase activity; sometimes the term is used to denote deficiency of a single enzyme or enzyme complex, such as lactase, sucrase-isomaltase complex, or α,α-trehalase. See also individual enzyme deficiencies and see *disaccharide intolerance*, under *intolerance.*

factor XI d. an autosomal bleeding disorder caused by mutations in the *F11* gene (locus: 4q35), which encodes factor XI. It is characterized by reduced plasma factor XI levels, recurring episodes of minor bleeding and mild bruising, menorrhagia, severe prolonged postsurgical bleeding, and prolonged recalcification and partial thromboplastin times. It is seen predominantly in persons of Ashkenazi Jewish ancestry; inheritance can be dominant or recessive. Called also *plasma thromboplastin antecedent d., PTA d., hemophilia C,* and *Rosenthal syndrome.*

familial apo C-II d., familial apolipoprotein C-II d. an autosomal recessive disorder caused by mutations in the *APOC2* gene (locus: 19q13.2), leading to a lack of apo C-II, a necessary cofactor for lipoprotein lipase. It results in familial hyperchylomicronemia that is usually milder and of later onset than that caused by a defect in the enzyme itself. See also table at *hyperlipoproteinemia.*

familial high-density lipoprotein d. any of several inherited disorders of lipoprotein and lipid metabolism that result in decreased plasma levels of high-density lipoproteins, particularly Tangier disease.

familial lipoprotein d. any inherited disorder of lipoprotein metabolism resulting in deficiency of one or more plasma lipoproteins; see *abetalipoproteinemia, Tangier disease* under *disease*, and *hypobetalipoproteinemia.*
GM_2 activator d. GM_2 gangliosidosis, AB variant.
hepatic phosphorylase d. glycogen storage disease, type VI.
hexosaminidase activator d. GM_2 gangliosidosis, AB variant.
isolated IgA d., IgA d., selective selective IgA d.
immune d. immunodeficiency.
iron d. deficiency of iron in the system, usually caused by blood loss, low dietary levels of iron, or a disease condition that inhibits iron uptake. Three stages of severity are distinguished: *iron depletion, latent iron deficiency*, and *iron deficiency anemia.*
iron d., latent a moderate form of iron deficiency in which the serum iron level drops but the hematocrit is unchanged and there is no anemia.
iron d., prelatent iron depletion.
leukocyte adhesion d. (LAD) any of several autosomal recessive disorders characterized by abnormalities of leukocyte adhesion.
type I a disorder caused by mutations in the *ITGB2* gene (locus: 21q22.3), which encodes theβ subunit of β_2 integrins, leading to reduced or absent β_2 integrin expression and to integrin dysfunction. It is characterized by delayed umbilical cord separation, recurrent bacterial infections, impaired pus formation, poor wound healing, gingivitis, leukocytosis, and impairment of adhesion-dependent leukocyte functions. There are two phenotypes: *moderate*, resulting from dysfunction or partial expression, and *severe*, resulting from absence or near-absence of expression.
type II a disorder caused by mutations in the *SLC35C1* gene (locus: 11p11.2), which encodes a GDP-fucose transmembrane transporter located in the Golgi complex, leading to deficiency of fucose-dependent antigens. It is characterized by neutrophilia, recurrent infections, abnormal chemotaxis, mental retardation, short stature, distinctive facies, and the Bombay phenotype. Called also *congenital disorder of glycosylation type IIc.*
type III a disorder caused by mutations in the *FERMT3* gene (locus: 11q12), which encodes an intracellular protein necessary for integrin activation, resulting in β-integrin dysfunction on platelets and leukocytes. It is characterized by recurrent infections and severe bleeding tendencies resembling Glanzmann thrombasthenia.
luteal phase d. see under *defect.*
mental d. see under *retardation.*
molybdenum cofactor d. an autosomal recessive disorder in which mutations in any of three genes encoding enzymes necessary for the synthesis of molybdenum cofactor cause deficiency of the molybdoenzymes sulfite oxidase, xanthine dehydrogenase, and aldehyde oxidase, resulting in severe neurologic abnormalities, dislocated ocular lenses, mental retardation, xanthinuria, and early death. It is divided into three types according to the site of mutation: A (*MOCS1*, locus: 6p21.3), B (*MOCS2*, locus: 5q11), and C (*GPHN*, locus:14q24).
multiple acyl CoA dehydrogenation d. (MADD) glutaricaciduria, type II.
muscle phosphorylase d. glycogen storage disease, type V.
oxygen d. see *anoxia, hypoxia*, and *hypoxemia.*
plasma thromboplastin antecedent d., PTA d. factor XI deficiency.
selective IgA d. the most common immunodeficiency disorder: deficiency of IgA with normal levels of the other immunoglobulin classes and normal cellular immunity. It is marked by recurrent sinopulmonary infections and an increased incidence of allergy, gastrointestinal disease (celiac disease, ulcerative colitis, Crohn disease), and autoimmune diseases (rheumatoid arthritis, systemic lupus erythematosus). Many patients have anti-IgA antibodies that can cause severe transfusion reactions.
sphingomyelinase d. Niemann-Pick disease.
storage pool d. see under *disease.*
subclinical d. in orthomolecular medicine, deficiency of a nutrient sufficient to affect health but not severe enough to cause classic deficiency symptoms.
sucrase-isomaltase d. a disaccharidase deficiency caused by mutations in the *SI* gene (locus: 3q25-q26), which encodes the sucrase-isomaltase complex of the intestinal mucosa, leading to deficient activity of the complex with resulting malabsorption of sucrose and starch dextrins; it is characterized by watery, osmotic-fermentative diarrhea, sometimes leading to dehydration and malnutrition, manifest in infancy *(congenital sucrose intolerance).* While sucrase activity is always absent, α-dextrinase (isomaltase) activity may be either greatly reduced or relatively normal. See also *disaccharide intolerance*, under *intolerance.*
tetrahydrobiopterin d. any of several disorders in the synthesis or regeneration of the cofactor tetrahydrobiopterin; clinical presentation is usually similar to phenylketonuria but because the cofactor also functions in the synthesis of various monoamine neurotransmitters, the disorders are not responsive to dietary phenylalanine restriction unless the missing neurotransmitters can also be supplied. Causes include mutations in the genes encoding 6,7-dihydropteridine reductase, GTP cyclohydrolase I, 6-pyruvoyltetrahydropterin synthase, and pterin 4-α-carbinolamine dehydratase. There are also several variant forms not presenting with hyperphenylalaninemia, including dopa-responsive dystonia due to defects in GTP cyclohydrolase I and in sepiapterin reductase.
vitamin d. see specific vitamins.
vitamin E–selenium d. see under *syndrome.*

def·i·cit (def′ĭ-sit) a lack or deficiency.
oxygen d. see *anoxia, hypoxemia*, and *hypoxia.*
pulse d. the difference between the heart rate and the pulse rate in atrial fibrillation, resulting from failure of some of the ventricular contractions to produce peripheral pulse waves of sufficient magnitude to detect by palpation.
reversible ischemic neurologic d. (RIND) a type of cerebral infarction whose clinical course lasts longer than 24 hours but less than 72 hours; brain imaging usually reveals an infarct. Cf. *stroke in evolution.*
saturation d. the difference between the amount of water vapor a given volume of air could contain at a specific temperature and the amount it actually contains.

Def·i·nate (def′ĭ-nāt) trademark for a preparation of docusate sodium.

def·i·ni·tion (def″ĭ-nish′ən) the clear determination of the limits of anything, as of a disease process or a microscopic image. See also *resolution* (def. 2).

de·fin·i·tive (də-fin′ə-tiv) 1. established with certainty. 2. in embryology, denoting acquisition of final differentiation or character. 3. in parasitology, denoting the host in which a parasite reaches the sexual stage.

de·flec·tion (de-flek′shən) [L. *deflectere* to turn away] 1. deviation or movement from a straight line or given course. 2. in electrocardiography, any of the deviations from baseline, measured as the waves or complexes of the recording.
H d., His bundle d. in the His bundle electrogram, the deflection due to advance of the depolarizing impulse through the bundle of His. See also illustration at *electrogram.*
intrinsic d. the sharp reversal in polarity of surface electrical charge in a muscle, such as is registered in an electrode directly attached to muscle, as the dipole of an action potential passes the electrode during muscle activity.
intrinsicoid d. the sharp deflection occurring between the onset of the Q wave and the peak of the R wave in electrocardiography using indirect surface leads, such as unipolar precordial leads.

de·flo·res·cence (def″lo-res′əns) the disappearance of the eruption in any exanthematous disease.

de·flu·vi·um (de-floo′ve-əm) [L., from *defluere* to flow down] 1. a flowing down or shedding; cf. *effluvium* (def. 1). 2. a disappearance.
postpartum d. telogen effluvium in the mother after childbirth.
telogen d. see under *effluvium.*
d. un′guium onychomadesis.

de·flux·io (de-fluk′se-o) [L., from *defluere* flow down] defluvium.

de·flux·ion (de-fluk′shən) defluvium.

de·form·a·bil·i·ty (de-form″ə-bil′ĭ-te) the ability of cells to change shape as they pass through narrow spaces, such as erythrocytes passing through the microvasculature.

de·for·ma·tion (de″for-ma′shən) [L. *deformatio* a disfiguring] 1. in dysmorphology, a type of structural defect characterized by the abnormal form or position of a body part, caused by a nondisruptive mechanical force. 2. the process of adapting in shape or form, as the change in shape of erythrocytes as they pass through capillaries.
elastic d. temporary elongation of tissue when a prolonged force has been applied. See also *creep.*
plastic d. permanent elongation of tissue when a prolonged nondisruptive mechanical force has been applied. See also *creep.*

de·form·ing (de-form′ing) causing or producing deformity.

de·form·i·ty (də-for′mĭ-te) distortion of any part or general disfigurement of the body.
Åkerlund d. a deformity of the duodenal cap in the radiograph in duodenal ulcer, consisting of an indentation (incisura) in addition to the niche.
Arnold-Chiari d. see under *malformation.*
boutonnière d., buttonhole d. a deformity of the finger characterized by flexion of the proximal interphalangeal joint and hyperextension of the distal joint.

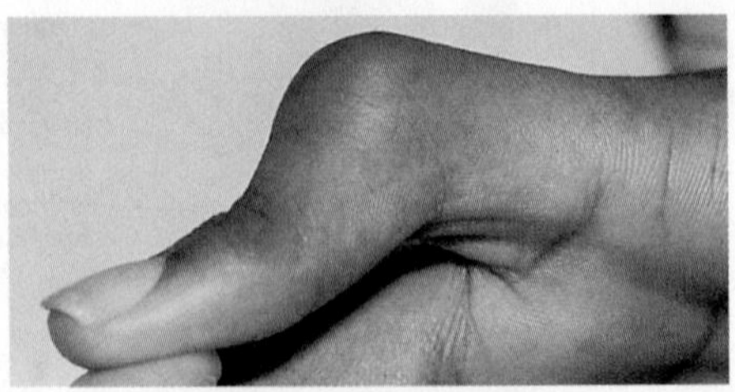

■ Boutonnière deformity.

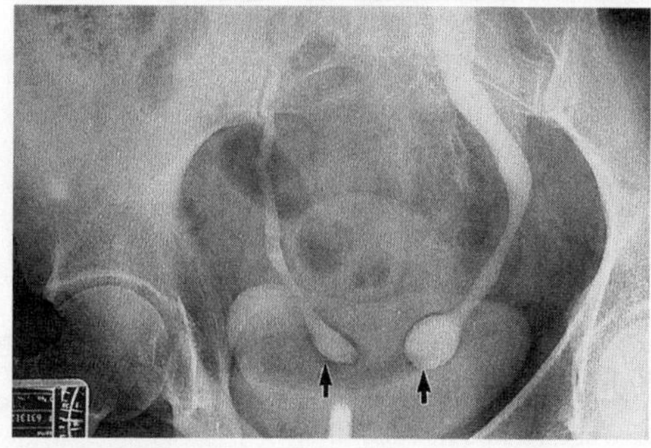

■ Cobrahead deformities *(arrows)* in an intravenous pyelogram of bilateral ureteroceles.

Chiari d. see under *malformation.*

Christmas tree d. a type of jejunoileal atresia in which the intestine coils around the superior mesenteric artery like tinsel around a Christmas tree.

cobrahead d. the appearance of a ureterocele in excretory urography, with the distal ureter slightly dilated and projecting into the bladder and an area of lesser density visible around it.

cock-up d. claw toe.

crossbar d. stiffening of a segment of the lesser curvature of the stomach, usually due to healing of a deep penetrating ulcer.

Dandy-Walker d. see under *malformation.*

flexion d. see under *contracture.*

gun stock d. cubitus varus.

Haglund d. retrocalcaneal bursitis.

Ilfeld-Holder d. prominent scapula with difficulty in raising the arm.

lobster claw d. cleft hand.

Madelung d. radial deviation of the hand secondary to overgrowth of the distal ulna or shortening of the radius; called also *carpus curvus.*

mitten d. the appearance the hand or foot can assume in pseudosyndacytyly or syndactyly when the epidermis encases it such that it resembles a mitten.

Mondini d. a misshapen cochlea with dysplasia or aplasia of the bony and membranous labyrinths, as seen in Mondini deafness. Called also *Mondini malformation.*

pincushion d. a complication of a transposition flap in which the graft fails to adhere to the underlying bed and bulges out to leave a pocket underneath. Called also *pincushioning* and *trapdoor d.*

pollybeak d. an iatrogenic bony deformity, occurring following rhinoplasty, in which the top of the nose is narrowed and the tip projects down over the lips, so that the nose resembles the beak of a parrot.

recurvatum d. a deformity of the proximal interphalangeal joint in which the joint extends when pressure is exerted between the thumb and middle finger.

reduction d. congenital absence of a portion or all of a body part, especially of the limbs.

rocker bottom d. see under *foot.*

rolled edge d. a highly characteristic deformity of the aortic valve cusps caused by syphilis.

saddle nose d. see under *nose.*

seal fin d. ulnar deviation of the fingers in rheumatoid arthritis.

silver fork d. the peculiar deformity seen in Colles fracture; see Plate 16. Called also *Velpeau d.*

spinning top d. see under *urethra.*

split foot d. cleft foot.

split hand d. cleft hand.

Sprengel d. congenital elevation of the scapula, due to failure of descent of the scapula to its normal thoracic position during fetal life.

swan neck d. a finger deformity in which the proximal interphalangeal joint is hyperextended and the distal interphalangeal joint is flexed.

thumb-in-palm d. adduction contracture of the thumb.

trapdoor d. pincushion d.

ulnar drift d. ulnar deviation.

Velpeau d. silver fork d.

windswept d. valgus deformity of one knee with varus deformity of the other.

Volkmann d. see under *disease.*

Deg degeneration; degree.

de•gas•sing (de-gas′ing) 1. treatment of a person or an object subjected to the fumes of gas. 2. the volatilization of foreign matter from the surface of a metal, as in the heat treatment of gold foil in rendering it cohesive; called also *annealing* (see *anneal,* def. 3).

de•gen•er•a•cy (de-jen′ər-ə-se) 1. the state of being degenerate. 2. the process of degenerating. 3. d. of code.

d. of code, code d. the presence in the genetic code of more than one codon encoding a specific amino acid and leading to its insertion into a growing polypeptide chain. See table at *genetic code,* under *code.*

de•gen•er•ate[1] (de-jen′er-āt) to change from a higher to a lower type or form.

de•gen•er•ate[2] (de-jen′er-ət) characterized by degeneration.

de•gen•er•a•tion (de-jen″ər-a′shən) [L. *degeneratio*] deterioration; change from a higher to a lower form; especially change of tissue to a less functionally active form. **degen′erative** *adj*

Degeneration

adipose d. fatty d.

adiposogenital d. see under *dystrophy.*

age-related macular d. (ARMD) a type of macular degeneration seen most often in persons over the age of 50, although retinal changes can be seen earlier; this is the leading cause of blindness in elderly persons. There are two main types, the more common *nonexudative (dry* or *involutional)* type and the less common *exudative (wet* or *neovascular)* type.

alcoholic cerebellar d. cerebellar cortical degeneration in alcoholics.

Alzheimer neurofibrillary d. neurofibrillary tangles.

amyloid d. degeneration with deposition of amyloid in the tissues; see also *amyloidosis.* Called also *waxy d.*

angiolithic d. degeneration with mineral deposits and hyaline changes in the coats of the vessels.

Armanni-Ebstein d. see under *lesion.*

ascending d. wallerian degeneration of centripetal nerve fibers that progresses toward the brain or spinal cord.

atheromatous d. atheroma.

atrophic pulp d. pulp atrophy.

axonal d. 1. axonal reaction. 2. wallerian d.

ballooning d. hydropic d.

Best macular d. Best disease.

calcareous d. degeneration with infiltration of calcareous materials into the tissues.

caseous d. caseation (def. 2).

cerebellar d. see *cerebellar cortical d., paraneoplastic cerebellar d.,* and *primary progressive cerebellar d.*

cerebellar cortical d. degeneration of the cerebellar cortex, especially around the vermis, with instability of muscles of the trunk and lower limbs; this is thought to be linked to thiamine deficiency and is seen in alcoholics and sometimes other malnourished individuals. Called also *cortical cerebellar d.*

cerebromacular d. (CMD), cerebroretinal d. 1. degeneration of brain cells and the macula luteae, as in Tay-Sachs disease. 2. any lipidosis with cerebral lesions and degeneration of the retinal macula. 3. any form of neuronal ceroid-lipofuscinosis.

cheesy d. caseation (def. 2).

colloid d. the assumption by the tissues of a gumlike or gelatinous character; called also *gelatiniform d.*

cortical cerebellar d. cerebellar cortical d.

corticobasal d. a neurologic condition similar to parkinsonism, with degeneration of the cerebral cortex and extrapyramidal structures; symptoms include progressive apraxia, rigidity, and alien limb syndrome.

corticostriatal-spinal d. Creutzfeldt-Jakob disease.

Crooke hyaline d. Crooke hyalinization.

cystic d. degeneration with formation of cysts.

cystoid d. Blessig cysts.

descending d. wallerian degeneration that progresses peripherally along nerve fibers.

Degeneration *Continued*

disciform macular d. a severe form of the exudative or wet type of age-related macular degeneration, characterized by hemorrhages between the Bruch membrane and the pigmented epithelium that produce a disclike area of sclerosis. Called also *macular disciform d., senile exudative macular d., senile disciform d.,* and *Kuhnt-Junius disease.*
Doyne colloid d., Doyne familial honeycomb d., Doyne honeycomb d. Doyne honeycomb dystrophy; see under *dystrophy.*
dry age-related macular d., dry macular d. nonexudative age-related macular d.
dystrophic d. degeneration arising from defective or faulty nutrition.
elastoid d. 1. hyaline degeneration of the elastic tissue of arteries. 2. elastosis (def. 2).
exudative age-related macular d., exudative macular d. a type of age-related macular degeneration characterized by growth of a neovascular membrane within or close to the macula, resulting in distorted or blurred vision; vision loss from this type is usually less severe than that from the more common nonexudative or dry type. Called also *neovascular* or *wet age-related macular d.*
familial colloid d. Doyne familial honeycombed choroiditis.
fascicular d. degeneration of paralyzed muscles due to lesion in the motor ganglion cells of the central tube of gray matter of the cord.
fatty d. deposit of fat globules in a tissue; an older term for a concept now included in *fatty change.*
fibrinous d. necrosis with deposit of fibrin within the cells of the tissue.
fibroid d. degeneration of a leiomyoma with subsequent fibrosis.
fibrous d. fibrosis.
gelatiniform d. colloid d.
glycogenic d. degeneration in which abnormal amounts of glycogen accumulate in the cells, as in glycogen storage disease.
granular d. hydropic d.
granulovacuolar d. neurodegeneration, most commonly occurring in the pyramidal cells of the hippocampus, in which the cytoplasm becomes filled with small vacuoles containing argyrophilic granules; it is a normal process in aging but is more pronounced in Alzheimer disease.
gray d. neurodegeneration involving the white matter of the spinal cord, in which it loses myelin and assumes a gray color.
hepatocerebral d. cirrhosis in combination with degenerative changes in the cerebrum; a congenital form is seen in Wilson disease and an acquired form sometimes follows hepatic coma or extensive portosystemic shunts. Symptoms may include tremor of the head and arms, asterixis, grimacing, chorea, gait ataxia, dysarthria, and mental deterioration.
hepatolenticular d. Wilson disease.
Holmes d. primary progressive cerebellar d.
Horn d. degeneration with nuclear proliferation in striated muscles.
hyaline d. a regressive cellular change in which the cytoplasm takes on a homogeneous, glassy, eosinophilic appearance. Also used loosely to describe the histologic appearance of tissues. Called also *vitreous d.* and *hyalinosis.*
hydropic d. swelling of cells caused by accumulation of intracellular water in response to cell injury; called also *ballooning d.* and *granular d.*
hypertrophic olivary d. a condition seen with damage to part of the Guillain-Mollaret triangle in the brain, characterized by palatal myoclonus and tremor of the limbs.
involutional macular d. nonexudative age-related macular d.
lattice d. of retina a pathologic condition of the retina, usually bilateral, benign, and asymptomatic. Characteristics include patches of fine gray or white lines that intersect at irregular intervals in the peripheral retina; there are usually numerous, round, punched-out areas of retinal thinning or retinal holes.
lipoidal d. a condition resembling fatty change but in which the extraneous material is lipoid.
macular d. degenerative changes in the macula lutea. *Age-related macular degeneration* (q.v.) is the most common cause of blindness in persons over age 65. Less common types that are congenital are *Best disease* and *Stargardt disease* (see under *disease*).
macular disciform d. disciform macular d.
Mönckeberg d. see under *arteriosclerosis.*
mucinoid d. a term used to include both mucoid and colloid degeneration; called also *mucinous d.*
mucinous d. mucous d.
mucoid d. degeneration accompanied by deposition of myelin and lecithin in the cells.
mucous d. degeneration in which mucus accumulates in epithelial tissues.
myofibrillar d. lysis of myofibrils with formation of vacuoles in the myocytes. It is nonspecific but can be associated with doxorubicin toxicity.
myxomatous d. degeneration in which mucoid material accumulates in connective tissues.
neovascular age-related macular d., neovascular macular d. exudative age-related macular d.
Nissl d. axonal reaction.
nonexudative age-related macular d., nonexudative macular d. the most common kind of age-related macular degeneration, characterized by gradual wearing out of the cells in the pigmented epithelium of the retina, resulting in a slow, progressive loss of central vision. Called also *dry* or *involutional macular d.*
olivopontocerebellar d. see under *atrophy.*
pallidal d. neurodegeneration involving the globus pallidus, as in juvenile paralysis agitans.
paraneoplastic cerebellar d., paraneoplastic subacute cerebellar d. the most common paraneoplastic syndrome affecting the brain, occurring most commonly with ovarian and breast carcinomas and Hodgkin disease, characterized pathologically by severe loss of Purkinje cells and clinically by insidious and progressive truncal and appendicular ataxia, dysarthria, nystagmus, and occasionally dementia. In some women with gynecologic or breast carcinoma, it is associated with an autoantibody (anti-Yo).
pigmental d., pigmentary d. degeneration in which cells of affected tissue become abnormally pigmented.
primary progressive cerebellar d. a familial disease in which neurodegeneration involves the cerebellum, causing motor disorders; it occurs most often in adults between the ages of 30 and 40 and progresses slowly to a fatal termination; called also *Holmes d.*
red d. degeneration of a uterine leiomyoma during pregnancy, marked by the formation of soft red areas due to necrosis and edema.
senile exudative macular d. disciform macular d.
retrograde d. axonal reaction.
sclerotic d. a variety of hyaline degeneration affecting connective tissue, especially the intima of arteries.
secondary d. wallerian d.
senile d. the widespread degenerative changes, principally fibrous and atheromatous, that occur in old age. Cf. *senile atrophy.*
senile disciform macular d., senile exudative macular d. disciform macular d.
spongy d. of central nervous system, spongy d. of white matter a rare, autosomal recessive form of leukodystrophy characterized by early onset, widespread demyelination and vacuolation of the cerebral white matter that gives rise to a spongy appearance, severe mental retardation, megalocephaly, atony of the neck muscles, spasticity of the arms and legs, and blindness, with death usually occurring at about 18 months of age. Called also *Canavan disease* and *Canavan-van Bogaert-Bertrand disease.*
Stargardt macular d. see under *disease.*
striatonigral d. a form of multiple system atrophy in which neurodegeneration occurs mainly in the region of the substantia nigra and the

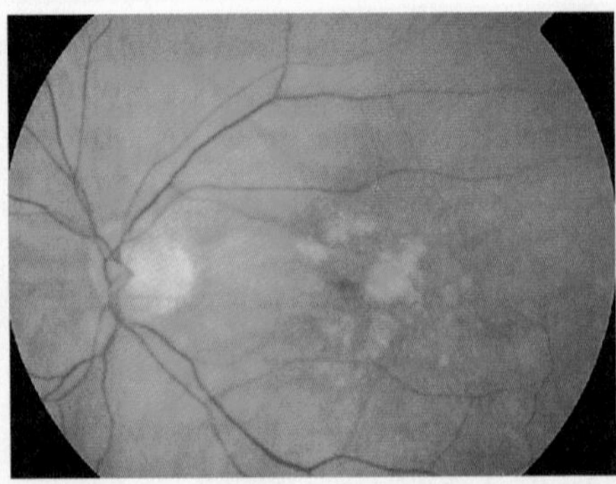

■ Nonexudative age-related macular degeneration with drusen and geographic atrophy.

Degeneration *Continued*

neostriatum. Symptoms are similar to those of parkinsonism, with rigidity, slowing of movements, poor balance, and mumbling speech, but parkinsonian tremor is absent.
subacute combined d. of spinal cord neurodegeneration involving both the posterior and lateral columns of the spinal cord, caused by vitamin B_{12} deficiency; a progressive disease, most often affecting persons over forty years of age, it is usually associated with pernicious anemia. The symptoms include paresthesias, ataxia, unsteadiness of gait, and sometimes emotional disorders. Called also *combined system disease, combined sclerosis, Lichtheim disease* or *syndrome, Putnam-Dana syndrome,* and *posterolateral sclerosis.*
tapetoretinal d. degeneration of the pigmented layer of the retina, as occurs in retinitis pigmentosa and other disorders.
transneuronal d. neurodegeneration involving neurons after interruption of afferent axons or death of other neurons to which they send their efferent output.
traumatic d. degeneration of a divided nerve up to the nearest node of Ranvier.
vacuolar d. the formation of vacuoles in the cells of a tissue.
vitelliform macular d., vitelline macular d. Best disease.
vitreous d. hyaline d.
wallerian d. a type of neurodegeneration consisting of fatty degeneration of a nerve fiber that has been severed from its nutritive centers; cf. *dying-back.* Called also *secondary d.*
waxy d. amyloid d.
wet age-related macular d., wet macular d. exudative age-related macular d.
Wilson d. see under *disease.*
Zenker d. necrosis and hyaline degeneration of striated muscle; called also *Zenker necrosis.*

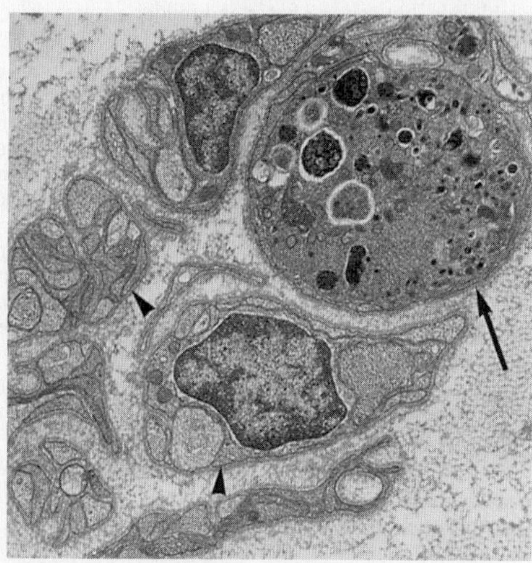

■ Wallerian degeneration. Electron micrograph of a markedly distended, degenerating axon *(arrow)*, containing numerous degenerating organelles and dense bodies, adjacent to intact, unmyelinated fibers *(arrowheads).*

de•germ (de-germ′) disinfect.

de•glov•ing (de-gluv′ing) intraoral surgical exposure of the bony mandibular structures, as by rolling the lower lip and vestibular soft tissue over the chin to expose the symphysis. The operation can also be performed in the posterior region if necessary.

Deglut. [L.] degluti′a′tur (let it be swallowed).

de•glu•ti•ble (de-gloo′tĭ-bəl) capable of being swallowed.

de•glu•ti•tion (deg″loo-tish′ən) [L. *deglutitio*] swallowing.

de•glu•ti•tive (de-gloo′tĭ-tiv) pertaining to or promoting swallowing; called also *deglutitory.*

de•glu•ti•to•ry (de-gloo′tĭ-tor″e) deglutitive.

de•glyc•er•ol•ize (de-glis′ər-ol-īz) to remove the glycerol cryopreservative medium from frozen red blood cells and replace it with an isotonic solution for transfusion.

De•gos acanthoma, disease (də-go′) [Robert *Degos,* French dermatologist, 1904–1987] see under *acanthoma,* and see *malignant atrophic papulosis,* under *papulosis.*

deg•ra•da•tion (deg″rə-da′shən) the reduction of a chemical compound to one less complex, as by splitting off one or more groups. Cf. *lysis.*

de•gran•u•la•tion (de-gran″u-la′shən) release of the contents of secretory granules from the cell by fusion with the plasma membrane.

de•gree (də-gre′) 1. a grade or rank within a series; especially, a rank awarded to scholars by a college or university. 2. a unit of measure of temperature. 3. a unit of measure of arcs and angles.
d's of freedom the number of ways the members of a sample can vary independently; a numerical index of a family of probability distributions that corresponds to the number of independent variables in the definition of each member, e.g., the chi-squared distribution with *n* degrees of freedom is the distribution of the sum of squares of *n* standard normal deviations. Symbol ν.
prism d. centrad (def. 2).

de•gus•ta•tion (de″gəs-ta′shən) [L. *degustatio*] taste.

de•hep•a•tized (de-hep′ə-tīzd) having the liver removed.

de•his•cence (de-his′əns) [L. *dehiscere* to gape] a splitting open.
Killian d. a triangular area in the wall of the pharynx between the inferior constrictor muscle and the cricopharyngeus muscle; it represents a potentially weak spot where a pharyngoesophageal diverticulum is more likely. Called also *Killian triangle.*
root d. an isolated area in which the root of a tooth is denuded of bone from the margin to near the apex; it occurs most often on anterior teeth, usually on the vestibular surface rather than the oral surface.
uterine d., d. of uterus rupture of the uterus following cesarean section, especially separation of the uterine scar prior to or during a subsequent labor.
wound d. separation of the layers of a surgical wound; it may be partial and superficial only, or complete, with disruption of all layers.

de•hu•mid•i•fi•er (de″hu-mid′ĭ-fi″ər) an apparatus by which the content of moisture in the air is reduced.

de•hy•drant (de-hi′drənt) 1. reducing hydration. 2. an agent that removes or reduces body water.

de•hy•drase (de-hi′drās) a term formerly applied to both the dehydrogenases and the dehydratases.

de•hy•dra•tase (de-hi′drə-tās) a term used in the usual recommended or trivial name for enzymes of the sub-subclass hydro-lyase (q.v.).

de•hy•drate (de-hi′drāt) to remove water from (a compound, the body, etc.).

de•hy•dra•tion (de″hi-dra′shən) [*de-* + *hydration*] 1. removal of water from a substance. 2. the condition that results from excessive loss of body water. Cf. *desiccation* and *xerosis.*
absolute d. water content below the normal or below a standard amount.
hypernatremic d. a condition in which electrolyte losses are disproportionately smaller than water losses.
relative d. dehydration resulting from increased osmotic pressure of the body fluids.
voluntary d. dehydration resulting when thirst does not stimulate sufficient replacement of water loss.

dehydro- a chemical prefix denoting the loss of two hydrogen atoms; in systematic nomenclature, *didehydro-* is used instead.

de•hy•dro•an•dros•ter•one (de-hi″dro-an-dros′tər-ōn) former name for *dehydroepiandrosterone.*

de•hy•dro•as•cor•bic ac•id (de-hi″dro-ə-skor′bik) the reversibly oxidized form of ascorbic acid, which has the same vitamin C activity as ascorbic acid when ingested.

de•hy•dro•bil•i•ru•bin (de-hi″dro-bil-ĭ-roo′bin) biliverdin.

de•hy•dro•cho•late (de-hi″dro-ko′lāt) a salt of dehydrocholic acid.

7-de•hy•dro•cho•les•ter•ol (de-hi″dro-kə-les′tər-ol) a sterol found in the skin; it is the provitamin of cholecalciferol, being converted to that compound upon irradiation by ultraviolet radiation.
7-d., activated cholecalciferol.

de•hy•dro•cho•lic ac•id (de-hi″dro-ko′lik) [USP] a synthetic bile acid that acts as a hydrocholeretic, increasing bile output to clear the increased bile acid load; bile pigment secretion is not increased. It has been used as a laxative and to produce choleresis after gallbladder surgery or in cholecystography.

11-de·hy·dro·cor·ti·cos·ter·one (de-hi″dro-kor″tĭ-kos′tər-ōn) an adrenocortical steroid made from, and convertible to, corticosterone; it is not directly active. Also produced synthetically, it is used like cortisone as a glucocorticoid and as an antiallergic agent.

de·hy·dro·em·e·tine (de-hi″dro-em′ə-tēn) an antiprotozoal used like emetine hydrochloride, but causing fewer and milder adverse effects; available as *dehydroemetine hydrochloride.*

de·hy·dro·epi·an·dros·ter·one (DHEA) (de-hi″dro-ep″e-an-dros′tər-ōn) a steroid secreted by the adrenal cortex, the major androgen precursor in females; it is often present in excessive amounts in body fluids of patients with adrenal virilism. During pregnancy it diffuses into the syncytiotrophoblasts and is metabolized to form estrogen; by the third trimester it metabolizes at nine times the rate seen in a nonpregnant woman. Because DHEA levels decrease dramatically with age, a link has been postulated between DHEA and the human aging process, and it has been used as an anti-aging supplement. Supplemental DHEA has also been used to treat or prevent heart disease and osteoporosis and to enhance immune function, cognitive function, mood, quality of life, and sexual function. Called also *dehydroisoandrosterone* and, formerly, *dehydroandrosterone.*

de·hy·dro·gen·ase (de-hi′dro-jən″ās) an enzyme of the oxidoreductase class [EC 1] that catalyzes the transfer of hydrogen or electrons from a donor, which becomes oxidized, to an acceptor compound, which becomes reduced. Dehydrogenases are usually designated according to the hydrogen donor.

de·hy·dro·gen·ate (de-hi′dro-jən-āt) to remove hydrogen from a molecule.

de·hy·dro·gen·a·tion (de-hi″dro-jə-na′shən) oxidation due to removal of hydrogen by the reaction of a hydrogen acceptor.

de·hy·dro·iso·an·dros·ter·one (de-hi″dro-i″so-an-dros′tər-ōn) dehydroepiandrosterone.

de·hy·dro·ret·i·nol (de-hi″dro-ret′ĭ-nol) a form of vitamin A, vitamin A_2, occurring with retinol in freshwater fish; it is similar in structure to retinol, but has an additional conjugated double bond and only approximately one third the biological activity.

de·hy·dro·sphin·ga·nine (de-hi″dro-sfing′gə-nēn) the product of the initial step in sphingolipid biosynthesis, which undergoes further processing to form sphinganine.

de·hyp·no·tize (de-hip′no-tīz) to arouse from the hypnotic state.

Dei·no·cer·i·tes (di″no-ser′ĭ-tēs) a genus of mosquitoes of the tribe Culicini, found in tropical parts of the Americas; several species are vectors of Venezualan equine encephalomyelitis.

de·io·din·a·tion (de-i″o-din-a′shən) the loss or removal of iodine from a compound.

de·ion·iza·tion (de-i″on-ĭ-za′shən) the production of a mineral-free state by the removal of ions, especially by use of ion exchange resins.

dei·ter·al (di′tər-əl) pertaining to Deiters nucleus.

Dei·ters cells, etc. (di′terz) [Otto Friedrich Karl *Deiters*, German anatomist, 1834–1863] see under *cell, frame, nucleus, phalanx, process,* and see *tractus vestibulospinalis.*

dé·jà en·ten·du (da′zhah on″ton-doo′) [Fr. "already heard"] the feeling that one has heard or perceived something previously although it is in fact new to one's experience. See also *déjà vu.*

dé·jà éprou·vé (da′zhah a″proo-va′) [Fr. "already tested"] a feeling that one has previously engaged in or experienced something when one has not. See also *déjà vu.*

dé·jà fait (da′zhah fa′) [Fr. "already done"] a feeling that what is happening has happened before. See also *déjà vu.*

dé·jà pen·sé (da′zhah pon-sa′) [Fr. "already thought"] a feeling that one has thought the same thoughts before. See also *déjà vu.*

dé·jà ra·con·té (da′zhah rah-kōn-ta′) [Fr. "already told"] 1. a feeling when telling someone about an experience that one had previously related the same experience either to them or to someone else, when in fact one had not. 2. a feeling that a long-forgotten event which is being recalled was told to one before, when it was not. See also *déjà vu.*

dé·jà vé·cu (da′zhah va-koo′) [Fr. "already lived"] a feeling that a new experience has been encountered before, in a previous existence. See also *déjà vu.*

dé·jà vou·lu (da′zhah voo-loo′) [Fr. "already desired"] a feeling that one has entertained the same desires before. See also *déjà vu.*

dé·jà vu (da′zhah voo′) [Fr. "already seen"] an illusion in which a new situation is incorrectly viewed as a repetition of a previous situation. The term is often used more generally to denote any sensation that appears to have already occurred or been perceived, e.g., thoughts, desires, or experiences.

De·jean syndrome (də-zhah′) [M.C. *Dejean*, French physician, 20th century] orbital floor syndrome.

de·jec·tion (de-jek′shən) [L. *dejectio*] a mental state marked by sadness; the lowered mood characteristic of depression.

De·je·rine disease, sign, syndrome (dĕ-zhĕ-rēn′) [Joseph Jules *Dejerine*, French neurologist, 1849–1917] see *progressive hypertrophic neuropathy*, under *neuropathy*, and see under *sign* and *syndrome.*

De·je·rine-Klump·ke paralysis, syndrome (dĕ-zhĕ-rēn′-kloomp′kə) [Augusta *Dejerine-Klumpke*, French neurologist, 1859–1927] Klumpke paralysis.

De·je·rine-Lan·dou·zy muscular dystrophy (dĕ-zhĕ-rēn′ lah-doo-ze′) [J.J. *Dejerine;* Louis Théophile Joseph *Landouzy*, French physician, 1845–1917] facioscapulohumeral muscular dystrophy.

De·je·rine-Licht·heim phenomenon (dĕ-zhĕ-rēn′ likt′hīm) [J.J. *Dejerine;* Ludwig *Lichtheim*, German physician, 1845–1928] Lichtheim sign.

De·je·rine-Rous·sy syndrome (dĕ-zhĕ-rēn′ roo-se′) [J.J. *Dejerine;* Gustav *Roussy*, French pathologist, 1874–1948] thalamic syndrome.

De·je·rine-Sot·tas atrophy, disease (dĕ-zhĕ-rēn′ so-tahz′) [J.J. *Dejerine;* Jules *Sottas*, French neurologist, 1866–1943] progressive hypertrophic neuropathy.

De·je·rine-Thom·as syndrome (dĕ-zhĕ-rēn′ to-mahs′) [J.J. *Dejerine;* André Antoine Henri *Thomas*, French neurologist, 1867–1963] olivopontocerebellar atrophy.

deka- deca-.

del deletion.

de·la·cri·ma·tion (de-lak″rĭ-ma′shən) [L. *delacrimatio* weeping] excessive and abnormal flow of tears.

Del·a·field hematoxylin (del′ə-fēld) [Francis *Delafield*, American pathologist, 1841–1915] see *Stains and Staining Methods*, under *stain.*

de·lam·i·na·tion (de-lam″ĭ-na′shən) [*de-* + *lamina*] separation into layers, as the separation of the inner cell mass or embryoblast into epiblast and hypoblast during early embryo development.

de Lange syndrome (da lahng′ə) [Cornelia *de Lange*, Dutch pediatrician, 1871–1950] see under *syndrome.*

Del·a·tes·tryl (del″ə-tes′trəl) trademark for a preparation of testosterone enanthate.

del·a·vir·dine mes·y·late (del″ə-vir′dēn) a nonnucleoside reverse transcriptase inhibitor, used in combination with other antiretroviral agents in the treatment of human immunodeficiency virus type 1 (HIV-1) infection; administered orally.

de·lay (de-la′) postponement to a later time.

atrioventricular d., AV d. see under *interval.*

constitutional growth d. a linear growth pattern, frequently familial, characterized by a decrease in growth velocity near the end of infancy, normal velocity in childhood, and accelerated growth near the end of adolescence ending in normal height; bone age is comparable to height age.

de·layed-re·lease (de-lād′ re-lēs′) releasing a drug at a time later than immediately following the administration of the drug.

Del·bet sign (del-ba′) [Pierre *Delbet*, French surgeon, 1861–1957] see under *sign.*

del Cas·ti·llo syndrome (dāl kahs-te′yo) [Enrique Benjamin *del Castillo*, Argentine endocrinologist, 1897–1969] Sertoli-cell–only syndrome; see under *syndrome.*

de-lead (de-led′) to remove lead from a tissue, as from the bones in lead poisoning by the administration of edetate disodium calcium. See also *deleading therapy*, under *therapy.*

De·Lee catheter, forceps (də-le′) [Joseph Bolivar *DeLee*, American obstetrician and gynecologist, 1869–1942] see under *catheter* and *forceps.*

DeLee-Hil·lis stethoscope (də-le′ hil′is) [J.B. *DeLee;* David S. *Hillis*, American obstetrician and gynecologist, 1873–1942] see under *stethoscope.*

Del·es·tro·gen (del-es′tro-jən) trademark for preparations of estradiol valerate.

del·e·te·ri·ous (del″ə-tēr′e-əs) [Gr. *dēlētērios*] hurtful; injurious.

de·le·tion (del) (də-le′shən) [L. *deletio* destruction] in genetics, the loss of any portion of the genetic material on a chromosome, ranging from loss of a single nucleotide within, which can throw the reading frame out of register and cause a frameshift mutation if it is within a coding sequence, to loss of part or all of a gene, to loss of a microscopically visible portion of the chromosome, possibly involving multiple genes.

antigenic d. loss or masking of antigenic determinants in daughter cells of cells whose parent tissue normally carries them; it may result from neoplastic or other mutational change in the parent tissue or may be due to loss or repression of genetic material from the cell.

interstitial d. loss of a segment within a chromosome arm. See illustration at *aberration.*

terminal d. loss of a segment from the end of a chromosome arm. See illustration at *aberration.*

Delf•tia (delf′te-ə) [*Delft,* Netherlands, where it was first isolated] a genus of aerobic, gram-negative bacteria of the family Comamonadaceae, consisting of non–spore-forming, catalase- and oxidase-positive, chemoorganotrophic, straight to slightly curved rods occurring singly or in pairs; organisms are motile by means of polar or bipolar tufts of flagella. The type species is *D. acido′vorans.*

D. acido′vorans a widespread species that is an occasional opportunistic pathogen. Formerly called *Pseudomonas acido′vorans.*

de•lim•i•ta•tion (de-lim″ĭ-ta′shən) [*de-* + *limitation*] 1. the process of limiting or of becoming limited. 2. ascertainment of the limits and extent of some diseased tissue or process, or the spread of a disease in a host or a community.

de•lin•quent (də-ling′kwənt) [L. *delinquens,* present participle of *delinquere,* to offend] 1. failing to do that which is required by law or obligation. 2. a person who neglects a legal obligation.

del•i•ques•cence (del″ĭ-kwes′əns) [L. *deliquescere* to grow moist] the condition of becoming moist or liquefied as a result of the absorption of water from the air.

del•i•ques•cent (del″ĭ-kwes′ənt) having a tendency to form an aqueous solution or become liquid by the absorption of moisture from the air.

de•lir•ia (də-lēr′e-ə) [L.] plural of *delirium.*

de•lir•i•ant (də-lēr′e-ənt) 1. capable of producing delirium. 2. a drug which may produce delirium. 3. a delirious person.

de•lir•i•fa•cient (də-lēr″ĭ-fa′shənt) [*delirium* + *-facient*] 1. capable of causing delirium. 2. a drug which may produce delirium.

de•lir•i•ous (de-lēr′e-əs) suffering from delirium.

de•lir•i•um (də-lēr′e-əm) pl. *delir′ia* [*de-* + L. *lira* furrow or track; i.e., "off the track"] [DSM-IV] an acute, transient disturbance of consciousness accompanied by a change in cognition and having a fluctuating course. Characteristics include reduced ability to maintain attention to external stimuli and disorganized thinking as manifested by rambling, irrelevant, or incoherent speech; there may also be a reduced level of consciousness, sensory misperceptions, disturbance of the sleep-wake cycle and level of psychomotor activity, disorientation to time, place, or person, and memory impairment. Delirium may be caused by a number of conditions that result in derangement of cerebral metabolism, including systemic infection, cerebral tumor, poisoning, drug intoxication or withdrawal, seizures or head trauma, and metabolic disturbances such as fluid, electrolyte, or acid-base imbalance, hypoxia, hypoglycemia, or hepatic or renal failure; specific types are named according to etiology, e.g., delirium due to hypoglycemia.

acute d. a suddenly appearing and severe delirium lasting only a short time.

alcohol withdrawal d. [DSM-IV] delirium caused by cessation or reduction in alcohol consumption, typically in alcoholics with 10 years or more of heavy drinking. Clinical manifestations include potentially life-threatening autonomic hyperactivity, such as tachycardia, sweating, and hypertension; a coarse, irregular tremor, and delusions, vivid hallucinations; and wild, agitated behavior. Seizures are possible. The onset is usually 2 or 3 days after cessation of drinking; the delirium and other withdrawal symptoms usually resolve in 3 or 4 days. Called also *d. tremens.*

febrile d. the delirium of fever.

low d. delirium marked by confusion of ideas and slowness of mental action rather than by excitement.

postcardiotomy d. postcardiotomy psychosis syndrome.

senile d. a form of senile dementia, usually of acute onset and characterized by disorientation, restlessness, insomnia, hallucinations, and aimless wandering.

substance-induced d. [DSM-IV] delirium associated with substance intoxication *(substance intoxication d.),* substance withdrawal *(substance withdrawal d.),* medication side effects, or exposure to toxins; individual cases are named for the specific substance involved, e.g., digitalis-induced delirium.

substance intoxication d. delirium that can occur during intoxication with any of a variety of substances, including alcohol, amphetamines and related substances, cannabis, cocaine, hallucinogens, inhalants, opioids, phencyclidine and related substances, and sedatives, hypnotics, and anxiolytics; specific disorders are named for the substance involved.

substance withdrawal d. delirium that can occur during withdrawal from any of a variety of substances, including alcohol and sedatives, hypnotics, and anxiolytics; specific disorders are named for the substance involved.

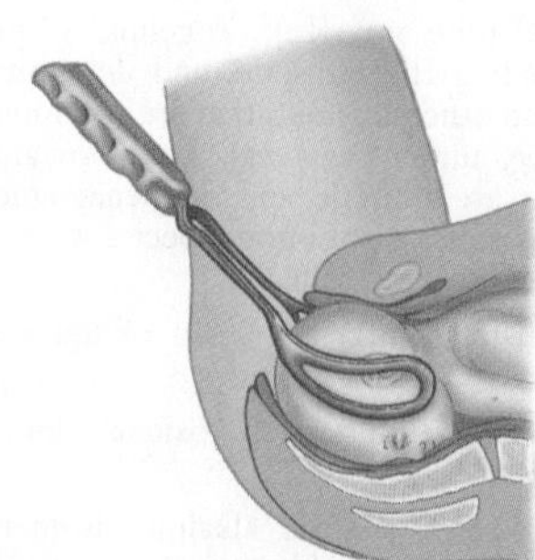

■ Forceps delivery.

toxic d. delirium caused by poisons.

traumatic d. delirium that follows severe head injury; superficially the patient is alert, but there is marked disorientation, memory defect, and confabulation.

d. tre′mens alcohol withdrawal d.

del•i•tes•cence (del″ĭ-tes′əns) [L. *delitescere* to lie hidden] 1. sudden disappearance of symptoms or of objective signs of a disease or of a lesion. 2. the period of latency or incubation of a poison or morbific agent.

de•liv•er (de-liv′ər) [Fr., from L. *deliberare* to set free] 1. to aid in the process of childbirth. 2. to remove, as the fetus or placenta, or the lens of the eye.

de•liv•ery (de-liv′ər-e) 1. the act of bringing or transporting something. 2. expulsion or extraction of the child and the afterbirth; see also *labor.* 3. removal of a part, as the lens of the eye.

abdominal d. cesarean section.

breech d. delivery of a fetus in breech presentation; see *breech extraction,* under *extraction.*

convection-enhanced d. a type of drug delivery system for gliomas in which the agent is injected directly into brain tissue near a tumor; used particularly for biologic response modifiers that have large molecules.

forceps d. extraction of a fetus from the maternal passages by application of forceps to the child's head.

forceps d., high forceps delivery in which the forceps is applied to the head before engagement has taken place.

forceps d., low forceps delivery in which the forceps is applied when the leading point of the fetal skull is at station equal to or greater than +2 centimeters but not on the pelvic floor, and rotation is necessary.

forceps d., outlet forceps delivery in which the forceps is applied when the scalp is or has been visible at the introitus without separating the labia and the skull has reached the pelvic floor, with the sagittal suture in the anteroposterior diameter of the pelvis; the fetus is in right or left occipitoanterior or occipitoposterior position.

midforceps d. the application of forceps when the fetal head is engaged but station is above +2 centimeters.

postmortem d. birth of a fetus after the death of the mother.

premature d. birth of a premature infant; see under *infant.*

spontaneous d. birth of an infant without any mechanical, pharmacologic, or medical assistance.

vaginal d. delivery of an infant through the normal openings of the uterus and vagina.

viral gene d. see under *transfer.*

dell (del′) a slight depression or dimple.

del•le (del′ə) the clear area in the center of a stained erythrocyte.

del•len (del′ən) [Ger. "dents"] Fuchs dimples.

dell•ing (del′ing) the formation of a slight depression; dimpling.

del•mad•i•none ac•e•tate (del-mad′ĭ-nōn) a veterinary progestin, antiandrogen, and antiestrogen; administered to male cats and dogs to control hypersexuality and other aggressive behavior and to treat prostatic hypertrophy and tumors, and to female cats as an estrus suppressant.

de•lo•mor•phic (del″o-mor′fik) delomorphous.

de•lo•mor•phous (del″o-mor′fəs) [Gr. *dēlos* evident + *morph-* + *-ous*] having definitely formed and well-defined limits, as a cell or tissue.

de•lous•ing (de-lous′ing) 1. the freeing of a human or animal from lice. 2. destruction of lice.

Del•phi•an node (del′fe-ən) [*Delphi,* a town in ancient Greece, site of a sanctuary and oracle of Apollo, because of the predictive nature of the node] see under *node.*

del•phine (del′fēn) delphinine.

del•phi•nine (del′fĭ-nēn) a poisonous alkaloid found in various species of *Delphinium,* causing larkspur poisoning in animals that eat the plants. Called also *delphine.*

Del·phin·i·um (del-fin′e-əm) [L.] a genus of plants of the family Ranunculaceae, including the larkspurs and delphinium, many of which contain delphinine and other alkaloids that are common causes of poisoning (see *larkspur poisoning*, under *poisoning*). *D. aja′cis* and *D. conso′lida* have poisonous seeds that are diuretic and emmenagogue. *D. staphisa′gria* is the lousewort or stavesacre, a poisonous species whose seeds, called staphisagria, were formerly used medicinally.

del·phin·i·um (del-fin′e-əm) any plant of the genus *Delphinium;* see also *larkspur.*

del·phi·noid·ine (del″fi-noid′in) a toxic alkaloid from the seeds of *Delphinium staphisagria.*

del·phi·sine (del′fi-sēn) a toxic alkaloid, isomeric with delphinine, from the seeds of *Delphinium staphisagria.*

del·ta (del′tə) [Δ, δ] 1. the fourth letter of the Greek alphabet. See also Δ- and δ-. 2. a triangular space.

d. mesosca′pulae the triangular area at the root of the spine of the scapula.

Del·ta-Cor·tef (del′tə-kor″təf) trademark for a preparation of prednisolone.

del·ta·meth·rin (del″tə-meth′rin) a pyrethroid insecticide applied topically to cattle and pigs.

Del·ta·pro·teo·bac·te·ria (del″tə-pro″te-o-bak-tēr′e-ə) [*delta* the fourth letter of the Greek alphabet + *Proteobacteria*] a class of bacteria of the Proteobacteria, grouped together on the basis of 16S rRNA sequence analysis; organisms of medical interest are included in the order Desulfovibrionales.

Del·ta·ret·ro·vi·rus (del″tə-ret′ro-vi″rəs) a genus of the family Retroviridae that includes bovine leukemia virus as well as the human T-lymphotropic viruses 1 and 2 that can cause B and T cell leukemia and lymphoma and neurologic disease. **deltaretrovi′ral** *adj*

Del·ta·sone (del′tə-sōn″) trademark for a preparation of prednisone.

Del·ta·vi·rus (del′tə-vi″rəs) [hepatitis *delta* + *virus*] a genus of satellite viruses that require helper hepatitis B viruses for their replication; an individual consists of spherical virion about 34 nm in diameter with an envelope derived from the helper virus surrounding a spherical core 18 nm in diameter; the genome consists of a single molecule of single-stranded, negative sense, circular RNA (size 1.7 kb). It contains a single species, hepatitis D virus.

del·toid (del′toid) [L. *deltoides* triangular] triangular in outline, as the deltoid muscle.

de·lu·sion (də-loo′zhən) [L. *delusio,* from *de* from + *ludus* a game] a false belief that is firmly maintained in spite of incontrovertible and obvious proof or evidence to the contrary and in spite of the fact that other members of the culture do not share the belief. **delu′sional** *adj*

d. of being controlled d. of control.

bizarre d. a delusion that is patently absurd and has no possible basis in fact, such as delusions of being controlled or thought broadcasting.

d. of control the delusion that one's thoughts, feelings, and actions are not one's own but are being imposed by someone else or by some external force.

depressive d. a delusion that is congruent with a predominant depressed mood, such as a delusion that one is being persecuted because of one's sinfulness or inadequacy, somatic delusions of serious illness, nihilistic delusions, or delusions of poverty.

encapsulated d. a delusion that has no significant effect on behavior.

erotomanic d. a delusional conviction associated with erotomania.

expansive d. d. of grandeur.

fragmentary d's unconnected delusions not organized around a coherent theme.

d. of grandeur, grandiose d. a delusion involving an exaggerated concept of one's importance, power, or knowledge or that one is, or has a special relationship with, a deity or a famous person; it is one of the subtypes of delusional disorder.

d. of jealousy a delusional belief that one's spouse or lover is unfaithful, based on erroneous inferences drawn from innocent events imagined to be evidence and often resulting in confrontation with the accused. It is one of the subtypes of delusional disorder.

d. of misidentification delusional misidentification.

mixed d. a delusion in which no central theme predominates; one of the subtypes of delusional disorder.

mood-congruent d. a delusion occurring as a manifestation of a mood disorder; see also *mood-congruent.*

mood-incongruent d. a delusion occurring as a manifestation of a psychotic disorder; see also *mood-incongruent.*

d. of negation, nihilistic d. a depressive delusion that the self or part of the self, part of the body, other persons, or the whole world has ceased to exist.

paranoid d's an older term denoting delusion of grandeur and delusion of persecution; its use is discouraged.

d. of persecution, persecutory d. a delusion that one is being attacked, harassed, cheated, persecuted, or conspired against; it is one of the subtypes of delusional disorder.

d. of poverty a delusion that one is, or soon will be, bereft of material possessions.

d. of reference a delusional conviction that ordinary events, objects, or behaviors of others have an unusual or peculiar meaning specifically for oneself. When less frequent or intense, or if not organized or systematized, such beliefs are called *ideas of reference.*

somatic d. a delusion that there is some alteration in a bodily organ or its function; it is one of the subtypes of delusional disorder.

systematized d's a group of delusions organized around a common theme.

De·ma·dex (de′mə-deks) trademark for preparations of torsemide.

De·man·sia (de-man′se-ə) a genus of venomous snakes of the family Elapidae, including the brown snake of Australia and New Guinea. See table at *snake.*

de·mar·ca·tion (de″mahr-ka′shən) [L. *demarcare* to limit] the marking off or ascertainment of boundaries.

surface d. any dividing line apparent on the surface of a solid body, such as the boundary between living and necrotic tissue.

De·mar·quay sign (də-mahr-ka′) [Jean Nicholas *Demarquay,* French surgeon, 1814–1875] see under *sign.*

de·mas·cu·lin·iza·tion (de-mas″ku-lin″ĭ-za′shən) the loss of normal male secondary sex characters; when hormonal in nature it may be accompanied by testicular atrophy and involution of the prostate. See also *feminization.*

De·mat·i·a·ceae (de-mat″ĭ-a′se-e) [Gr. *demation* little cord] in some systems of classification, a form-family of Fungi Imperfecti of the form-order Moniliales, producing simple conidiophores, and having dark brown or black conidia, spores, or hyphae. Genera of medical importance include *Acremoniella, Alternaria, Arthrographis, Aureobasidium, Bipolaris, Cladosporium, Curvularia, Dematium, Drechslera, Exophiala, Exserohilum, Fonsecaea, Madurella,* and *Phialophora.*

de·mat·i·a·ceous (de-mat″e-a′shəs) 1. dark brown to black in color; said of fungi. The color usually comes from pigment in the cell wall or other parts. 2. of or pertaining to a fungus of the family Dematiaceae.

De·ma·ti·um (de-ma′she-əm) a genus of soil and wood-rotting Fungi Imperfecti of the form-class Hyphomycetes, form-family Dematiaceae; some species have been reportedly isolated from human lesions.

deme (dēm) [Gk. *dēmos* common people] a population of very similar organisms randomly interbreeding in nature and occupying a circumscribed area.

dem·e·ca·ri·um bro·mide (dem″ə-kar′e-əm) [USP] an anticholinesterase agent applied topically to the conjunctiva to produce miosis, reduce intraocular pressure, and potentiate accommodation in the treatment of open-angle glaucoma and of closed-angle glaucoma after iridectomy, and in the management of accommodative esotropia.

dem·e·clo·cy·cline (dem″ə-klo-si′klēn) [USP] a broad-spectrum antibiotic of the tetracycline group, produced by a mutant strain of *Streptomyces aureofaciens* or semisynthetically. It also inhibits the effect of vasopressin on the renal tubules. Called also *demethylchlortetracycline.*

d. hydrochloride [USP] the monohydrochloride salt of demeclocycline, administered orally as an antibiotic. It is also used orally as a diuretic in the treatment of syndrome of inappropriate antidiuretic hormone (SIADH).

De·Mees·ter score (də-mēs′tər) [Tom R. *DeMeester,* American thoracic surgeon, born 1938] see under *score.*

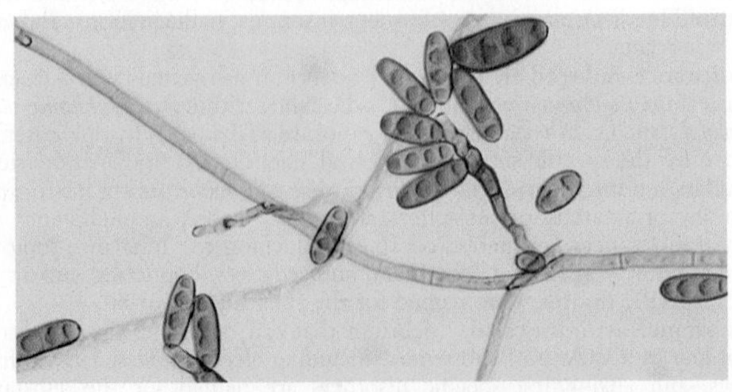

■ *Bipolaris* sp., a dematiaceous fungus, darkly pigmented by melanin in the cell walls.

de•ment•ed (də-men′təd) deprived of reason, mentally deteriorated; affected with dementia.

de•men•tia (də-men′shə) [*de-* + L. *mens* mind] [DSM-IV] a general loss of cognitive abilities, including impairment of memory as well as one or more of the following: aphasia, apraxia, agnosia, or disturbed planning, organizing, and abstract thinking abilities. It does not include loss of intellectual functioning caused by clouding of consciousness (as in delirium), depression, or other functional mental disorder (pseudodementia). Causes include a large number of conditions, some reversible and some progressive, that result in widespread cerebral damage or dysfunction. The most common cause is Alzheimer disease; others include cerebrovascular disease, central nervous system infection, brain trauma or tumors, vitamin deficiencies, anoxia, metabolic conditions, endocrine conditions, immune disorders, prion diseases, Wernicke-Korsakoff syndrome, normal-pressure hydrocephalus, Huntington chorea, multiple sclerosis, and Parkinson disease.

alcoholic d. Korsakoff syndrome.

Alzheimer d. see under *disease.*

d. of the Alzheimer type [DSM-IV] dementia occurring in Alzheimer disease, being of insidious onset and gradually progressive course, with histopathological changes characteristic of Alzheimer disease that are not due to other central nervous system, systemic, or substance-induced conditions known to cause dementia. It is characterized as *early onset* or *late onset* depending on whether or not it begins by the age of 65, and is subcategorized on the basis of accompanying features, including delirium, delusions, depressed mood, behavioral disturbances, or none (uncomplicated).

arteriosclerotic d. multi-infarct dementia as a result of cerebral arteriosclerosis.

Binswanger d. see under *disease.*

boxer's d. a syndrome more serious than chronic traumatic (boxer's) encephalopathy, the result of cumulative cerebral injuries in boxers; characterized by forgetfulness, slowness in thinking, dysarthric speech, and slow, uncertain movements, especially of the lower limbs. Called also *d. pugilistica.*

dialysis d. see under *encephalopathy.*

epileptic d. a progressive mental and intellectual deterioration that occurs in a small fraction of cases of epilepsy; it is thought by some to be caused by neuronal degeneration secondary to circulatory disturbances during seizures.

frontal d., frontal lobe d. any of various dementias caused by frontal lobe lesions, such as the dementia seen in Pick disease.

frontal-temporal d., frontotemporal d. any of several degenerative conditions of the frontal and anterior temporal lobes that cause personality and behavioral changes sometimes mistaken for those of Alzheimer disease; they may eventually progress to immobility and loss of speech. There is not the memory loss seen in Alzheimer disease, but there is often hyperorality.

Lewy body d., d. with Lewy bodies a type of dementia with similarities to both Parkinson disease and Alzheimer disease, with Lewy bodies in the cortical neurons; patients have decreased verbal fluency and visual-spatial awareness.

multi-infarct d. vascular d.

myoclonic d., d. myoclo′nica mental deterioration with myoclonus, as seen in disorders such as Alpers disease, Creutzfeldt-Jakob disease, subacute sclerosing panencephalitis, and Alzheimer disease.

paralytic d., d. paraly′tica general paresis.

posttraumatic d. dementia following head injury or other brain trauma; it may last from a few months to years. Cf. *boxer's d.* and *postconcussional syndrome.*

d. prae′cox original name for *schizophrenia,* when it was characterized as a psychosis with adolescent onset and a chronic course ending in deterioration.

presenile d. dementia in persons not classified as elderly, usually meaning those aged 65 or younger; since most cases are due to Alzheimer disease, the term is sometimes used as a synonym of *d. of the Alzheimer type, early onset,* and has also been used to denote *Alzheimer disease.*

primary degenerative d. severe loss of intellectual function of no discernible cause; the term generally denotes dementia of the Alzheimer type, but is sometimes used for dementia associated with Pick disease.

d. pugilis′tica boxer's d.

semantic d. a form of frontotemporal dementia characterized by profound loss of memory for the meanings of words and objects.

senile d. dementia in the elderly, usually meaning persons over the age of 65; since most cases are due to Alzheimer disease, the term is sometimes used as a synonym of *d. of the Alzheimer type, late onset.*

subcortical d. any of a group of dementias thought to be caused by lesions affecting subcortical brain structures (such as the centrum ovale, basal ganglia, or thalamus) more than cortical ones, and characterized by memory loss with slowness in processing information or making intellectual responses. Included are vascular dementia and dementias that accompany Huntington disease, Wilson disease, Parkinson disease, and thalamic atrophies.

substance-induced persisting d. [DSM-IV] dementia resulting from exposure to or use or abuse of a substance, such as alcohol, sedatives, anxiolytics, anticonvulsants, lead, mercury, carbon monoxide, and organophosphate insecticides, but persisting long after exposure to the substance ends, usually with permanent and worsening deficits. Individual cases are named for the specific substance involved.

toxic d. dementia caused by excessive exposure to a toxic substance.

vascular d. [DSM-IV] dementia with a stepwise deteriorating course (a series of small strokes) and a patchy distribution of neurologic deficits (affecting some functions and not others) caused by cerebrovascular disease. It may be classified as uncomplicated or as occurring with delusions, delirium, or depressed mood. Called also *multi-infarct d.*

Dem•er•ol (dem′ər-ol) trademark for preparations of meperidine hydrochloride.

de•meth•yl•a•tion (de-meth″əl-a′shən) the removal of a methyl group, —CH_3, from a compound.

de•meth•yl•chlor•tet•ra•cy•cline (de-meth″əl-klor-tet″rə-si′klēn) demeclocycline.

demi- [Fr. *demi* half, from L. *dimidius*] a prefix meaning half.

Dem•i•a•noff sign (dem″e-ah-nof′) [G.S. *Demianoff,* French physician, 20th century] see under *sign.*

demi•fac•et (dem″e-fas′ət) a small plane surface on either of two bones which both articulate with a third bone.

inferior d. for head of rib fovea costalis inferior.

superior d. for head of rib fovea costalis superior.

demi•gaunt•let (dem″e-gawnt′lət) demigauntlet bandage.

demi•lune (dem′e-lo͞on) crescent (def. 2).

Giannuzzi d's, Heidenhain d's Giannuzzi crescents.

demi•mon•stros•i•ty (dem″e-mon-stros′ĭ-te) malformation of a part which does not prevent the exercise of its function.

de•min•er•al•iza•tion (de-min″ər-əl-ĭ-za′shən) excessive elimination of mineral or inorganic salts, as in pulmonary tuberculosis, cancer, and osteomalacia.

demi•pen•ni•form (dem″e-pen′ĭ-form) feather-shaped as to one of the two margins; said of certain muscles.

Demi-Reg•ro•ton (dem′ĭ-reg′ro-ton) trademark for a combination preparation of chlorthalidone and reserpine.

dem•o•dec•tic (dem-o-dek′tik) pertaining to or caused by *Demodex.*

Dem•o•dex (dem′o-deks) [Gr. *dēmos* fat + *dēx* worm] a genus of acarid mites of the family Demodicidae, which cause demodectic mange. *D. bo′vis* affects cattle; *D. cap′ri,* goats; *D. ca′ti,* cats; *D. crice′ti,* hamsters; *D. o′vis,* sheep; and *D. phylloi′des,* pigs. *D. bre′vis* and *D. folliculo′rum* are hair follicle mites that infest humans.

Dem•o•dic•i•dae (dem″o-dis′ĭ-de) a family of minute follicular mites (order Acarina) that parasitize the skin of mammals. It includes the genus *Demodex.*

dem•o•dic•i•do•sis (dem″o-dis″ĭ-do′sis) 1. demodicosis (def. 1). 2. demodectic mange.

dem•o•di•co•sis (dem″ə-dĭ-ko′sis) 1. any infestation by species of *Demodex;* called also *demodicidosis.* 2. demodectic mange.

de•mo•gram (de′mo-gram) a graphic representation, in grid form, of the population of a given area according to the time period and the age and sex of the individuals constituting it.

de•mog•ra•phy (de-mog′rə-fe) [Gr. *dēmos* people + *-graphy*] the statistical study of a population or of populations, including characteristics such as geographical distribution, physical environment, disease, sex and age composition, and birth and death rates.

dynamic d. collective physiology of communities, with statistics of births, marriages, deaths, etc.

static d. collective anatomy of communities and study of their environment.

de•mo•ni•ac (de-mo′ne-ak) 1. frenzied. 2. possessed by demons, the medieval conception of insanity.

de•mono•pho•bia (de″mən-o-fo′be-ə) [Gr. *daimōn* demon + *-phobia*] irrational fear of demons.

dem•on•stra•tor (dem′ən-stra″tər) [L.] an instructor who teaches individuals or small groups by using dissections or other aids.

De Mor•gan spot (də mor′gən) [Campbell *De Morgan,* English physician, 1811–1876] cherry angioma.

de•mor•phin•iza•tion (de-mor″fin-ĭ-za′shən) treatment of morphine addiction by gradual withdrawal of the drug.

de Mor•si•er syndrome (də mor-se-a′) [Georges *de Morsier,* Swiss neurologist, 20th century] septo-optic dysplasia.

Dem•ser (dem′sər) trademark for a preparation of metyrosine.

de·mu·co·sa·tion (de-mu″ko-sa′shən) removal of the mucous membrane from a part.

de·mul·cent (de-mul′sənt) 1. soothing; bland; allaying the irritation of inflamed or abraded surfaces. 2. a soothing, mucilaginous, or oily medicine or application. Called also *lenitive.*

Dem·u·len (dem′u-lən) trademark for combination preparations of ethynodiol diacetate and ethinyl estradiol.

de Mus·set see *Musset.*

de·mus·tard·iza·tion (de-mus″tərd-ĭ-za′shən) 1. removal of mustard gas from a person. 2. treatment of a person subjected to the fumes of mustard gas.

de·mu·ti·za·tion (de-mu″tĭ-za′shən) [*de-* + L. *mutus* mute] the teaching of the deaf to communicate by lip reading or by dactylology.

de·my·elin·ate (de-mi′ə-lin′āt) to destroy or remove the myelin sheath of a nerve or nerves.

de·my·elin·a·tion (de-mi″ə-lĭn-a′shən) destruction, removal, or loss of the myelin sheath of a nerve or nerves. Called also *demyelinization and myelinolysis.*

osmotic d. see under *syndrome.*

segmental d. degeneration of the myelin sheath in segments between successive nodes of Ranvier, with preservation of the axon; seen in a variety of polyneuropathic conditions.

de·my·elin·iza·tion (de-mi″ə-lin-ĭ-za′shən) demyelination.

de·nar·co·tize (de-nahr′ko-tīz) 1. to deprive of a narcotic drug in the process of treating addiction. 2. to remove the narcotic element from an opiate.

de·na·sal·i·ty (de″na-zal′ĭ-te) hyponasality.

de·na·tal·i·ty (de″na-tal′ĭ-te) decrease in the number of births in proportion to the population.

de·na·to·ni·um ben·zo·ate (de″nə-to′ne-əm) [NF] an alcohol denaturant, used as a pharmaceutic aid.

de·na·tur·ant (de-na′chər-ənt) a denaturing agent.

de·na·tur·a·tion (de-na″chər-a′shən) the destruction of the usual nature of a substance, as the addition of methanol or acetone to alcohol to render it unfit for drinking, or the change in the physical properties of a substance, such as a protein or nucleic acid, caused by heat or certain chemicals that alter tertiary structure.

protein d. disruption of the configuration (tertiary structure) of a protein, as by heat, change in pH, or other physical or chemical means, resulting in alteration of the physical properties and loss of biological activity of the protein.

de·na·tured (de-na′chərd) having undergone denaturation.

Den·a·vir (den′ə-vir) trademark for a preparation of penciclovir.

den·dric (den′drik) 1. dendritic. 2. arborescent.

Den·drid (den′drid) trademark for a preparation of idoxuridine.

den·dri·form (den′drĭ-form) arborescent.

den·drite (den′drīt) [Gr. *dendron* tree] 1. one of the threadlike extensions of the cytoplasm of a neuron (q.v.), which typically branch into tree-like processes. In unipolar and bipolar neurons, there is a single dendrite, which proximally resembles an axon but branches distally; in multipolar neurons there are many short, branching dendrites. Dendrites compose most of the receptive surface of a neuron. Called also *dendron, neurodendrite,* and *neurodendron.* See illustration. 2. dendritic ulcer.

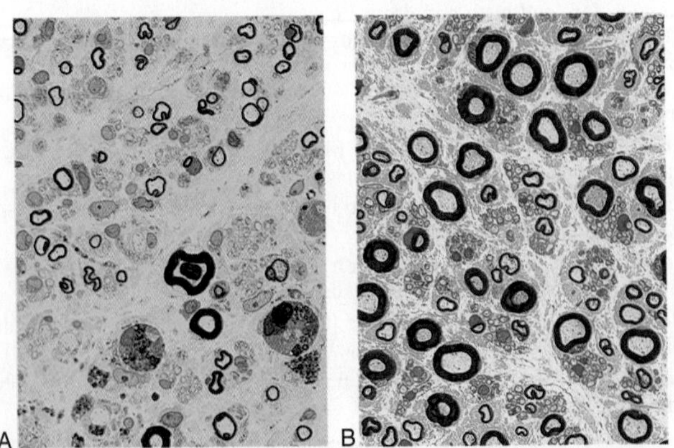

■ Cross-section of sural nerve in chronic inflammatory demyelination polyradiculoneuropathy. *(A),* Segmental demyelination; *(B),* relatively unaffected area.

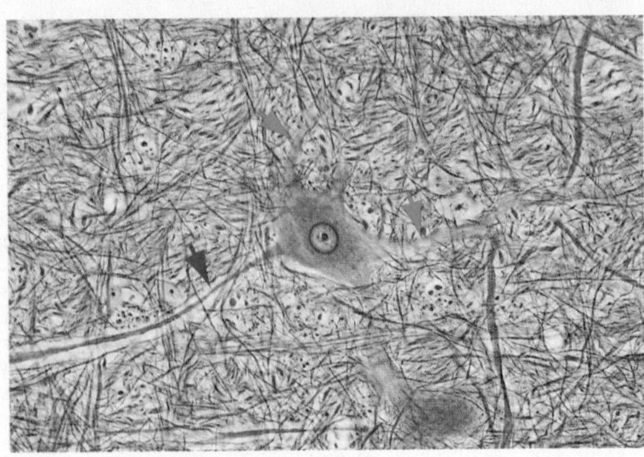

■ Dendrites *(green arrows)* and axon *(blue arrow)* of a motor neuron, with a dense surround of neuronal processes, in a preparation of spinal cord gray matter stained for neurofibrils.

apical d. a thick dendrite extending from the outer side of a pyramidal cell toward the surface of the cortex.

den·drit·ic (den-drit′ik) 1. pertaining to or possessing dendrites. 2. arborescent.

dendr(o)- [Gr. *dendron* tree] a combining form denoting relationship to a tree or treelike structure.

Den·dro·as·pis (den″dro-as′pis) a genus of extremely venomous African snakes of the family Elapidae, related to cobras but lacking a dilatable hood. *D. angus′ticeps* is the green mamba and *D. polyle′pis* is the black mamba. See table at *snake.*

den·dro·den·drit·ic (den″dro-den-drit′ik) referring to a synapse between dendrites of two neurons.

den·dro·do·chio·tox·i·co·sis (den-dro″do-ke-o-tok″sĭ-ko′sis) a form of mycotoxicosis caused by the fungus *Dendrodochium toxicum,* characterized by diarrhea and hemorrhagic gastroenterocolitis; seen in Russia and adjacent areas in horses and occasionally in humans.

Den·dro·do·chi·um (den-dro-do′ke-əm) a genus of Fungi Imperfecti of the family Stilbellaceae. *D. tox′icum* is the etiologic agent of dendrodochiotoxicosis.

Den·dro·hy·rax (den″dro-hi′raks) a genus of tree hyraxes that live in forested areas of Ethiopia and Kenya; they are common reservoirs for *Leishmania aethiopica.*

den·droid (den′droid) 1. branching like a tree or shrub. 2. arborescent.

den·dron (den′dron) dendrite.

den·dro·phago·cy·to·sis (den″dro-fa″go-si-to′sis) the absorption by microglia cells of broken portions of degenerating astrocytes or oligodendroglial cells.

de·ner·vate (de-nur′vāt) to deprive of a nerve supply.

de·ner·va·tion (de″nər-va′shən) resection or removal of the nerves to an organ or part.

chemical d. chemodenervation.

den·gue (deng′ge, Sp. dān′ga) [Swahili *ki-dinga*] an acute, self-limited disease, typically lasting 5 to 7 days, characterized by fever, prostration, severe muscle pains, headache, rash, lymphadenopathy, and leukopenia, caused by four antigenically related but distinct types of the dengue virus. It occurs epidemically and sporadically in warm to hot parts of the world, including West and Central Africa, parts of India, Southeast and East Asia, Indonesia, northeastern Australia, Polynesia, the Caribbean, and northern South America. It is transmitted by the bite of infected mosquitoes of the genus *Aedes.* Called also *breakbone, dandy,* or *dengue fever.*

hemorrhagic d. a severe form of dengue, characterized by hemorrhagic manifestations such as thrombocytopenia and hemoconcentration. The World Health Organization distinguishes four types according to severity: *grade I,* fever, constitutional symptoms, and positive tourniquet test; *grade II,* grade I plus spontaneous bleeding into skin, gums, gastrointestinal tract, and other sites; *grade III,* grade II plus circulatory failure and agitation; and *grade IV,* profound shock with undetectable blood pressure and pulse. Grades III and IV are also known as *dengue shock syndrome.* Called also *dengue hemorrhagic fever.*

de·ni·al (də-ni′əl) a type of defense mechanism in which the existence of unpleasant internal or external realities is kept out of conscious awareness; by being so disavowed they are prevented from causing anxiety.

den·i·da·tion (den″ĭ-da′shən) [*de-* + *nidation*] degeneration and expulsion of the endometrium (uterine mucous membrane) in the menstrual cycle.

den·i·leu·kin dif·ti·tox (den″ĭ-loo′kin dif′tĭ-toks) a fusion protein containing amino acid sequences for specific diphtheria toxin fragments linked to sequences for interleukin-2 (IL-2), so that the cytotoxic action of the diphtheria toxin is targeted to cells expressing a specific form of the IL-2 receptor, as in certain leukemias and lymphomas. It is used as an antineoplastic in the treatment of cutaneous T-cell lymphomas, administered intravenously.

Den·is Browne splint (den′is broun′) [Sir *Denis* John *Browne*, Australian-born English pediatric surgeon, 1892–1967] see under *splint.*

Den·i·so·nia (den″ĭ-so′ne-ə) a genus of highly venomous snakes of the family Elapidae; *D. super′ba* is the copperhead of Australia and nearby Pacific islands. See table at *snake.*

de·ni·tri·fi·ca·tion (de-ni″trĭ-fĭ-ka′shən) the setting free of gaseous nitrogen from nitrites and nitrates, as by certain soil bacteria, which results in depletion of nitrogen for plant growth. Denitrification carried out by aquatic bacteria can be beneficial in ridding waste waters of excess nitrates.

de·ni·tri·fi·er (de-ni′trĭ-fi″ər) a bacterium that causes denitrification.

de·ni·tri·fy (de-ni′trĭ-fi) to remove nitrogen from any substance; see *denitrification.*

de·ni·tro·ge·na·tion (de-ni″tro-jən-a′shən) removal of the dissolved nitrogen from the body, as a preventive of caisson disease, aeroembolism, etc.

Den·nie sign (den′e) [Charles Clayton *Dennie*, American dermatologist, 1883–1971] see *Morgan line*, under *line.*

Den·nie-Mar·fan syndrome (den′e mahr-fă′) [C.C. *Dennie;* Antoine Bernard Jean *Marfan*, French pediatrician, 1858–1947] see under *syndrome.*

De·non·vil·liers fascia, operation (dĕ-naw-ve-ya′) [Charles Pierre *Denonvilliers*, French surgeon, 1808–1872] see *fascia rectoprostatica* and see under *operation.*

dens (dens) pl. *den′tes* [L.] 1. [TA] tooth (q.v.): one of the small bone-like structures of the jaws. 2. d. axis. 3. a toothlike structure.

den′tes acus′tici [TA] auditory teeth: elevations along the free surface and margin of the labium limbi vestibulare; called also *auditory teeth of Huschke.*

d. acu′tus incisor tooth.

d. ax′is [TA] tooth of axis: the toothlike process that projects from the superior surface of the body of the axis, ascending to articulate with the atlas; called also *d. epistrophei, odontoid bone, odontoid apophysis, odontoid process of axis*, and *tooth of epistropheus.*

d. cani′nus [TA] canine tooth: the tooth immediately lateral to the lateral incisor; see under *tooth.*

den′tes deci′dui [TA] deciduous teeth: the teeth of the first dentition; see under *tooth.*

d. epistro′phei d. axis.

d. evagina′tus an anomalous tubercle protruding from the occlusal surface of a posterior tooth or the lingual surface of an anterior tooth. It contains a core of dentin surrounding an extension of the pulp and results from abnormal proliferation of the inner enamel epithelium into the stellate reticulum of the enamel organ during tooth development.

d. incisi′vus [TA] incisor tooth: either of the two most frontal teeth of each jaw; see under *tooth.*

d. in den′te a malformed tooth resulting from invagination of the crown before it is calcified; so named because severe invagination of enamel and dentin gives the appearance of a "tooth within a tooth." Called also *d. invaginatus* and *dilated odontoma.*

d. invagina′tus d. in dente.

d. mola′ris [TA] molar tooth: one of the grinding, double teeth at the back of each jaw. See under *tooth.*

d. mola′ris ter′tius [TA] third molar tooth: the last tooth on each side of each jaw. See under *tooth.*

den′tes permanen′tes [TA] permanent teeth: the teeth of the second dentition; see under *tooth.*

d. premola′ris [TA] premolar tooth: either of the two permanent teeth between the canine teeth and the molars. See under *tooth.*

d. sapien′tiae third molar tooth.

d. seroti′nus TA alternative for *d. molaris tertius;* see *third molar tooth*, under *tooth.*

den·si·fi·ca·tion (den″sĭ-fĭ-ka′shən) the increasing in density of a substance by decreasing its porousness, such as through thermal processing.

den·sim·e·ter (den-sim′ə-tər) densitometer (def. 1).

den·si·tom·e·ter (den″sĭ-tom′ə-tər) [L. *densus* dense + *-meter*] 1. an apparatus for determining the density of a liquid. Called also *densimeter.* 2. an instrument for determining the degree of darkening of developed photographic or x-ray film by means of a photocell which measures light transmission through a given area of the film. 3. an instrument for determining the density of deposits on electrophoresis strips and chromatographic plates by measuring light absorbancy.

gas d. an apparatus for measuring specific gravity of a gas.

den·si·tom·e·trist (den″sĭ-tom′ə-trist) a physician specializing in bone densitometry.

den·si·tom·e·try (den″sĭ-tom′ə-tre) determination of variations in density by comparison with that of another material, or with a certain standard.

bone d. the determination of bone mineral density, generally by dual energy x-ray absorptiometry (DEXA), used in the diagnosis and management of conditions such as osteogenesis imperfecta and osteoporosis.

dual energy d. bone densitometry using dual energy x-ray absorptiometry.

peripheral d. bone densitometry of an upper or lower limb.

den·si·ty (den′sĭ-te) [L. *densus* dense] 1. the quality of being compact or dense. 2. quantity per unit space, e.g., the mass of matter per unit volume. Symbol ρ or *d.* 3. the degree of darkening of exposed and processed photographic or x-ray film, expressed as the logarithm of the opacity of a given area of the film.

arciform d. a trough-shaped body separating the synaptic ribbon and the membrane of the cone pedicle or of the rod spherule in the retina.

background d. in radiography, the density of a processed film due to factors other than the radiation exposure received through the recorded objects or structures, e.g., inherent (film) density, scatter radiation, or fogging.

bone d., bone mineral d. a measurement of the mineral content of bone for indication of its structural strength and screening for osteoporosis.

fiber d. 1. the number of muscle or nerve fibers in a unit area of tissue. 2. after a number of recordings of single fiber electromyography to the same muscle, the mean number of muscle fiber action potentials found to be single fiber action potentials and therefore to belong to the same motor unit; it is usually between 1.5 and 1.8.

inherent d. the density of a processed film due to inherent factors such as the density of the film base, emulsion gelatin, etc.

ionization d. the number of ion pairs per unit volume.

magnetic flux d. (*B*) a vector quantity that measures the magnitude of a magnetic field, given by the equation $F = qvB$, where F is the force exerted by the magnetic field on a moving charged particle, q is the particle's charge, and v is the particle's velocity.

optical d. (OD) absorbance.

Dent disease (dent) [Charles Enrique *Dent*, British physician, 1911–1976] see under *disease.*

den·tag·ra (den-tag′rə, den′tə-grə) [*dent-* + *-agra*] 1. a forceps or key for extracting teeth. 2. toothache.

den·tal (den′təl) [L. *dentalis*] 1. pertaining to a tooth or teeth. 2. a speech sound such as *d, t,* or *th* that is made with the tongue against the front teeth; called also *linguodental.*

den·tal·gia (den-tal′jə) [*dent-* + *-algia*] toothache.

den·ta·ta (den-ta′tə) the second cervical vertebra or axis, so called from its toothlike process.

den·tate (den′tāt) [L. *dentatus*] having teeth or projections like saw teeth on the edges.

den·ta·to·ru·bral (den-ta″to-roo′brəl) 1. conducting or proceeding from the dentate to the red nucleus. 2. pertaining to or including the dentate and red nuclei.

den·ta·to·tha·lam·ic (den-ta″to-thə-lam′ik) pertaining to or connecting the dentate nucleus and the thalamus.

den·ta·tum (den-ta′təm) [L. "toothed"] the nucleus dentatus.

den·tes (den′tēz) [L.] plural of *dens.*

denti- see *dent(o)-.*

den·tia (den′shə) [L.] a condition relating to development or eruption of the teeth.

d. prae′cox 1. premature teeth. 2. predeciduous teeth.

d. tar′da delayed dentition.

-dentia a combining form denoting relationship to the teeth.

den·ti·buc·cal (den″tĭ-buk′əl) pertaining to the teeth and cheek.

den·ti·cle (den′tĭ-kəl) [L. *denticulus* a little tooth] 1. a small toothlike process. 2. a calcified concretion that develops in the dental pulp as part of the aging process; called also *pulp stone.* 3. in mycology, a small process on which a conidium develops.

adherent d., attached d. a calcified formation in a pulp chamber partially fused with the dentin.

embedded d. interstitial d.

false d. a calcified formation in the pulp chamber of a tooth that does not show the structure of true dentin.
free d. a calcified formation in a tooth completely surrounded by the dental pulp.
interstitial d. a calcified formation within a tooth, completely surrounded by dentin.
true d. a calcified formation in the pulp chamber of a tooth that consists of dentin and shows traces of dentinal tubules and odontoblasts.

den•tic•u•lat•ed (den-tik′u-lāt″əd) [L. *denticulatus*] having minute teeth.

den•ti•fi•ca•tion (den″tĭ-fĭ-ka′shən) dentinogenesis.

den•ti•form (den′tĭ-form) shaped like a tooth.

den•ti•frice (den′tĭ-fris) [L. *dentifricium*] a preparation, usually a paste, gel, or powder, used with a toothbrush for cleaning the accessible surfaces of the teeth.

den•tig•er•ous (den-tij′ər-əs) [*denti-* + L. *gerere* to carry] bearing or having teeth.

den•ti•la•bi•al (den″tĭ-la′be-əl) [*denti-* + *labial*] pertaining to the teeth and lips.

den•ti•lin•gual (den″tĭ-ling′wəl) [*denti-* + *lingual*] pertaining to the teeth and tongue.

den•tim•e•ter (den-tim′ə-tər) [*denti-* + *-meter*] an instrument for measuring teeth.

den•tin (den′tin) [L. *dens* tooth] the hard portion of the tooth surrounding the pulp, covered by enamel on the crown and cementum on the root, which is harder and denser than bone but softer than enamel. Called also *dentinum* [TA]. Sometimes spelled *dentine.* **den′tinal** *adj*
adventitious d. secondary irregular d.
calcified d. transparent d.
circumpulpal d. the inner portion of the dentin, adjacent to the pulp chamber, consisting of thinner fibrils. See also *predentin.*
cover d. mantle d.
functional d. secondary regular d.
hereditary opalescent d. the brown opalescent-appearing dentin observed in dentinogenesis imperfecta.
interglobular d. imperfectly calcified dentinal matrix situated between the calcified globules near the periphery of the dentin.
irregular d. secondary irregular d.
mantle d. the peripheral portion of the dentin adjacent to the enamel or cementum, consisting mostly of coarse fibers (Korff fibers). Called also *cover d.*
opalescent d. dentin giving an unusual translucent or opalescent appearance to the teeth, as in dentinogenesis imperfecta.
primary d. dentin formed subsequently to the time when the tooth takes its anatomic position in the oral cavity; it is separated from secondary dentin by a demarcation line, formed by a change in the directional path of the dentinal tubules.
reparative d. secondary irregular d.
sclerotic d. transparent d.
secondary d. dentin formed and deposited in response to a normal or slightly abnormal stimulus, after the complete formation of the tooth. See *secondary irregular d.* and *secondary regular d.*
secondary irregular d. dentin formed in response to stimuli associated with pathologic processes, such as caries or injury, or cavity preparation. Such dentin is usually irregular in nature, being composed of a few tubules that may be tortuous in appearance, and it often demonstrates cellular inclusions. Called also *adventitious d., irregular d., reparative d.,* and *tertiary d.*
secondary regular d. dentin formed in response to stimuli associated with normal body processes. Called also *functional d.*
tertiary d. secondary irregular d.
transparent d. dentin in which some dentinal tubules have become sclerotic or calcified (dental sclerosis), producing the appearance of translucency, usually resulting from injury, abrasion, or normal aging processes. Called also *calcified d.* and *sclerotic d.*

den•tine (den′tēn) dentin.

den•ti•no•blast (den′tĭ-no-blast) [*dentin* + *-blast*] a cell that forms dentin.

den•ti•no•ce•men•tal (den″tĭ-no-sə-men′təl) pertaining to the dentin and the cementum.

den•ti•no•enam•el (den″tĭ-no-ə-nam′əl) pertaining to the dentin and the enamel.

den•ti•no•gen•e•sis (den″tĭ-no-jen′ə-sis) [*dentin* + *-genesis*] the formation of dentin; called also *dentification.*
d. imperfec′ta an autosomal dominant disorder of tooth development characterized by opalescent dentin resulting in discoloration of the teeth, ranging from dusky blue to brownish. The dentin is poorly formed with an abnormally low mineral content; the pulp canal is obliterated, but the enamel is normal. The teeth usually wear down rapidly, leaving short, brown stumps. Called also *odontogenesis imperfecta.*

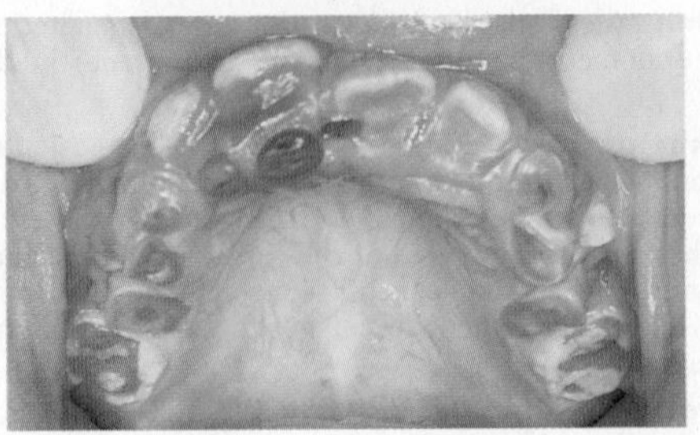
■ Dentinogenesis imperfecta.

den•ti•no•gen•ic (den″tĭ-no-jen′ik) forming or producing dentin.

den•ti•noid (den′tĭ-noid) 1. resembling dentin. 2. predentin.

den•ti•no•ma (den″tĭ-no′mə) an odontogenic tumor composed of immature connective tissue, odontogenic epithelium, and dysplastic dentin.

den•ti•nos•te•oid (den″tĭ-nos′te-oid) osteodentinoma.

den•ti•num (den-ti′nəm) [L.] [TA] dentin: the chief substance or tissue of the teeth. See *dentin.*

den•tip•a•rous (den-tip′ə-rəs) [*denti-* + *-parous*] bearing teeth.

den•tist (den′tist) a person who has received a degree from an accredited school of dentistry and is licensed to practice dentistry by a state board of dental examiners. Called also *odontologist.*
pediatric d. a specialist in pediatric dentistry (q.v.); called also *pedodontist.*

den•tis•try (den′tis-tre) 1. that department of the healing arts which is concerned with the teeth, oral cavity, and associated structures, including the diagnosis and treatment of their diseases and the restoration of defective and missing tissue. 2. the work done by dentists, such as the creation of restorations, crowns, and bridges, and surgical procedures performed in and about the oral cavity. Called also *odontoiatria, odontology,* and *oral medicine.*
cosmetic d., esthetic d. the aspect of dental practice concerned with the repair and restoration of carious, broken, or defective teeth in such a manner as to improve their appearance.
evidence-based d. the practice of dentistry in which the dentist finds, assesses, and implements methods of diagnosis and treatment on the basis of the best available, current research, their clinical expertise, and the needs and preferences of the patient. See also under *practice.*
forensic d. the branch of dentistry that deals with the application of the art and science of dentistry to the purposes of law. *Dental jurisprudence* and *forensic d.* are sometimes used synonymously, but some authorities consider dental jurisprudence a branch of law and forensic dentistry a branch of dentistry.
geriatric d. gerodontics.
holistic d. dental practice that takes into account the effects of dental treatment and materials on the overall health of the individual; especially important are the use of non-amalgam restorations and the replacement of existing amalgam with non–mercury-containing materials.
legal d. forensic d.
operative d. the branch of dentistry concerned with restoration of parts of the teeth that are defective through disease, trauma, or abnormal development to a state of normal function, health, and esthetics, including preventive, diagnostic, biological, mechanical, and therapeutic techniques, as well as material and instrument science and application.
pediatric d. the branch of dentistry concerned with the diagnosis and treatment of conditions of the teeth and mouth in children. Called also *pedodontia* and *pedodontics.*
preventive d. the branch of dentistry concerned with the preservation of healthy teeth and the maintenance of oral structures in a state of optimal health for the longest period of time possible.
prosthetic d. prosthodontics.
restorative d. the branch of dentistry concerned with the restoration of existing teeth that are defective through disease, trauma, or abnormal development to the state of normal function, health, and esthetics, including crown and bridgework. See also *restoration.*

den•ti•tion (den-tish′ən) [L. *dentitio*] the teeth in the dental arch; ordinarily used to designate the natural teeth in position in their alveoli.
artificial d. see *denture.*
deciduous d. deciduous teeth; see under *tooth.*
delayed d. eruption of the first deciduous teeth after the end of the thirteenth month of life or eruption of the first permanent teeth after the seventh year of life. Called also *retarded d., delayed eruption,* and *dentia tarda.*
first d. deciduous teeth; see under *tooth.*

mixed d. the complement of teeth in the jaws after eruption of some of the permanent teeth, before all of the deciduous teeth are shed; called also *transitional d.*

natural d. the natural teeth in the dental arch, considered collectively; it may comprise deciduous or permanent teeth, or a mixture of the two, present at one time.

permanent d. permanent teeth; see under *tooth.*

precocious d. premature teeth; see under *tooth.*

predeciduous d. see under *tooth.*

premature d. see under *tooth.*

primary d. deciduous teeth; see under *tooth.*

retarded d. delayed d.

secondary d. permanent teeth; see under *tooth.*

temporary d. deciduous teeth; see under *tooth.*

transitional d. mixed d.

dent(o)- [L. *dens* tooth] a combining form denoting relationship to a tooth or to the teeth. Also, *denti-*. Cf. *odont(o)-*.

den·to·al·ve·o·lar (den″to-al-ve′ə-lər) pertaining to a tooth and its alveolus.

den·to·al·ve·o·li·tis (den″to-al″ve-ə-li′tis) periodontal disease.

den·to·fa·cial (den″to-fa′shəl) of or pertaining to the teeth and alveolar process and the face.

den·tog·ra·phy (den-tog′rə-fe) odontography.

den·toid (den′toid) odontoid.

den·to·le·gal (den″to-le′gəl) pertaining to dental jurisprudence.

den·to·ma (den-to′mə) dentinoma.

den·to·me·chan·i·cal (den″to-mə-kan′ĭ-kəl) pertaining to the mechanics or to the biomechanics of dentistry.

den·ton·o·my (den-ton′ə-me) [*dent-* + Gr. *onoma* name] odontonomy.

den·to·sur·gi·cal (den″to-sur′jĭ-kəl) pertaining to or used in dentistry and oral surgery.

den·to·tro·pic (den″to-tro′pik) turning toward or having an affinity for tissues composing the teeth.

den·tu·lous (den′tu-ləs) possessing natural teeth.

den·ture (den′chər) [Fr., from L. *dens* tooth] 1. an artificial or prosthetic replacement for missing natural teeth and adjacent tissues, such as a bridge, restoration, or dental prosthesis. 2. any set of teeth.

cantilever fixed partial d. cantilever bridge.

clasp d. a removable partial denture retained with a clasp. See also *clasp* and *retainer.*

complete d. a dental prosthesis replacing all natural teeth and associated mandibular and maxillary structures; it is completely supported by the tissues. Called also *full d.*

conditioning d. a temporary denture used to condition the patient to wearing a denture. See also *interim d.*

distal extension partial d. a removable partial denture that is retained by natural teeth only at the anterior end of the base segments, with part of the functional load carried by the residual ridge.

fixed partial d. a prosthetic dental appliance that replaces lost teeth and is held in position by attachments to adjacent prepared natural teeth, roots, or implants. Called also *bridge* and *fixed bridge.*

full d. complete d.

immediate d., immediate-insertion d. a complete or removable partial denture made before all teeth are extracted, so constructed that it may be inserted immediately following the removal of the natural teeth.

implant d. an artificial denture retained and stabilized through the use of a subperiosteal, intraperiosteal, or intraosseous implant, consisting of the framework (substructure) implanted in contact with the bone, and the overlying structure (superstructure).

interim d. a denture to be used for a short interval of time for reasons of esthetics, mastication, occlusal support, convenience, or to condition the patient to the acceptance of an artificial substitute for missing natural teeth until more definitive prosthetic dental treatment can be provided. Called also *provisional d.* See also *conditioning d.* and *transitional d.*

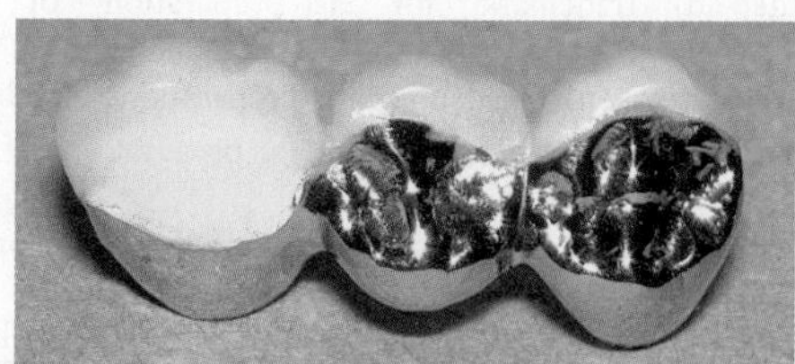

■ Fixed partial denture.

overlay d. a removable tooth-supported partial or complete denture whose built-in secondary copings overlay or telescope over the primary copings that fit over the prepared natural crowns, posts, or studs. Called *overdenture* and *telescopic d.*

partial d. a prosthetic appliance replacing a missing tooth or teeth in one jaw, and receiving its support and retention from the underlying tissues and/or some or all of the remaining teeth; see also *fixed partial d.* and *removable partial d.*

provisional d. interim d.

removable partial d. a denture replacing one or several of the natural teeth, made so that it can be readily removed from the mouth; it may be entirely supported by the residual teeth or supported by both the teeth and the tissue of the residual area. Called also *removable bridgework.*

telescopic d. overlay d.

temporary d. an artificial denture that serves for a short time in a temporary or emergency situation. See *conditioning d., interim d., transitional d.,* and *trial d.*

transitional d. a partial denture that serves temporarily, to which more teeth will be added later, and which will be replaced after postextraction tissue changes have occurred; it may become an interim denture when all the natural teeth have been removed from the dental arch.

trial d. a denture for placement in the mouth to verify its esthetic qualities, make a record, or do other procedures before completion of the final denture.

unilateral partial d. a partial denture for just one side of the dental arch.

den·tur·ism (den′chər-is-əm) the practice of fabrication and fitting of dentures by dental technologists without benefit of a dentist's expertise.

den·tur·ist (den′chər-ist) a dental technologist who fabricates and fits dentures for patients without benefit of a dentist's expertise. Denturists practice in parts of Canada and the United States, but in many states denturism is illegal.

De·nu·cé ligament (də-nu-sa′) [Jean Henri Maurice *Denucé*, French surgeon, 1859–1924] see under *ligament.*

de·nu·cle·at·ed (de-noo′kle-āt″əd) deprived of the nucleus.

de·nu·da·tion (den″u-da′shən) [L. *denudare* to make bare] 1. the act of laying bare. 2. removal of the epithelial covering from any surface, by surgery, trauma, or pathologic change.

Den·ys-Drash syndrome (den′is drash) [Joseph *Denys*, Belgian bacteriologist, 1857–1932; Allan Lee *Drash*, American pediatrician, born 1931] see under *syndrome.*

de·odor·ant (de-o′dər-ənt) [*de-* + *odorant*] 1. removing undesirable or offensive odors. 2. a substance that masks offensive odors. Called also *deodorizer.*

de·odor·ize (de-o′dər-īz) [*de-* + *odor* + *-ize*] to neutralize or absorb odor.

de·odor·iz·er (de-o′dər-īz″ər) deodorant (def. 2).

de·op·pi·lant (de-op′ĭ-lənt) removing obstructions.

de·op·pi·la·tion (de-op″ĭ-la′shən) [*de-* + L. *oppilatio* obstruction] the removal of obstructions.

de·or·sum·duc·tion (de-or″səm-duk′shən) infraduction.

de·or·sum·ver·gence (de-or″səm-vur′jəns) infravergence.

de·or·sum·ver·sion (de-or″səm-vur′zhən) infraversion (def. 3).

de·os·si·fi·ca·tion (de-os″ĭ-fĭ-ka′shən) [*de-* + *ossification*] loss of or removal of bone.

de·ox·i·da·tion (de-ok″sĭ-da′shən) [L. *de* from + *oxygen*] the removal of oxygen from a chemical compound.

de·ox·i·dize (de-ok′sĭ-dīz) to deprive of chemically combined oxygen.

deoxy- a prefix used in naming chemical compounds, to designate a compound containing one less atom of oxygen than the reference substance. For words beginning thus see also those beginning *desoxy-*.

de·oxy·aden·o·sine (de-ok″se-ə-den′o-sēn) a purine nucleoside, adenine linked by its N9 nitrogen to the C1 carbon of deoxyribose. Symbol dA.

d. diphosphate (dADP) a nucleotide, the 5′-pyrophosphate of deoxyadenosine.

d. monophosphate (dAMP) a nucleotide, the 5′-phosphate of deoxyadenosine, occurring in deoxyribonucleic acid.

d. triphosphate (dATP) a nucleotide, the 5′-triphosphate of deoxyadenosine; it is an activated precursor in DNA synthesis.

de·oxy·ad·e·no·syl (de-ok″se-ə-den′o-səl) the radical formed from deoxyadenosine on loss of an H or OH group.

de·oxy·ad·e·no·syl·co·bal·a·min (de-ok″se-ə-den″o-səl-ko-bal′ə-min) adenosylcobalamin.

de•oxy•aden•yl•ate (de-ok″se-ə-den′ə-lāt) a dissociated form of deoxyadenylic acid.

de•oxy•ad•e•nyl•ic ac•id (de-ok″se-ad″ə-nil′ik) deoxyadenosine monophosphate.

de•oxy•ad•e•nyl•yl (de-ok″se-ad″ə-nil′əl) the radical formed by removal of OH from the phosphate group of deoxyadenosine monophosphate.

de•ox•y•cho•lan•er•e•sis (de-ok″se-ko″lən-er′ə-sis) increase in the output of deoxycholic acid in the bile.

de•oxy•cho•late (de-ok″se-ko′lāt) a salt, ester, or anionic form of deoxycholic acid.

de•oxy•chol•ic ac•id (de-ok″se-ko′lik) a secondary bile acid formed by dehydroxylation of cholic acid in the intestine; it is a choleretic and is also used in biochemistry as a detergent.

de•oxy•chol•yl•gly•cine (de-ok″se-ko″ləl-gli′sēn) a bile salt, the glycine conjugate of deoxycholic acid.

de•oxy•chol•yl•tau•rine (de-ok″se-ko″ləl-taw′rēn) a bile salt, the taurine conjugate of deoxycholic acid.

11-de•oxy•cor•ti•co•ster•one (DOC) (de-ok″se-kor″tĭ-kos′tər-ōn) 21-hydroxypregn-4-ene-3,20-dione, a mineralocorticoid produced in small quantities by the human adrenal cortex, having about 3 per cent of the sodium-retaining activity of aldosterone. The acetate and pivalate salts are used for mineralocorticoid replacement therapy. Called also *cortexone, deoxycortone, desoxycorticosterone,* and *desoxycortone.*

11-d. acetate see under *desoxycorticosterone.*

11-d. pivalate see under *desoxycorticosterone.*

11-de•oxy•cor•ti•sol (de-ok″se-kor′tĭ-sol) an intermediate formed in the conversion of cholesterol to cortisol in steroidogenesis.

de•oxy•cor•tone (de-ok″se-kor′tōn) 11-deoxycorticosterone.

de•oxy•cy•ti•dine (de-ok″se-si′tĭ-dēn) a nucleoside, cytosine linked by its N1 nitrogen to the C1 carbon of deoxyribose. Symbol dC.

d. diphosphate (dCDP) a nucleotide, the 5′-pyrophosphate of deoxycytidine.

d. monophosphate (dCMP) a nucleotide, the 5′-phosphate of deoxycytidine, occurring in deoxyribonucleic acid.

d. triphosphate (dCTP) a nucleotide, the 5′-triphosphate of deoxycytidine; it is an activated precursor in the synthesis of DNA.

de•oxy•cy•ti•dyl•ate (de-ok″se-si-tĭ-dil′āt) a dissociated form of deoxycytidylic acid.

de•oxy•cy•ti•dyl•ic ac•id (de-ok″se-si″tĭ-dil′ik) deoxycytidine monophosphate.

de•oxy•cy•ti•dyl•yl (de-ok″se-si″tĭ-dil′əl) the radical formed by removal of OH from the phosphate group of deoxycytidine monophosphate.

de•ox•y•gen•a•tion (de-ok″sĭ-jən-a′shən) the act of depriving of oxygen.

de•oxy•guan•o•sine (de-ok″se-gwahn′o-sēn) a purine nucleoside, guanine linked by its N9 nitrogen to the C1 carbon of deoxyribose.

d. diphosphate (dGDP) a nucleotide, the 5′-pyrophosphate of deoxyguanosine.

d. monophosphate (dGMP) a nucleotide, the 5′-phosphate of deoxyguanosine, occurring in deoxyribonucleic acid.

d. triphosphate (dGTP) a nucleotide, the 5′-triphosphate of deoxyguanosine; it is an activated precursor in the synthesis of DNA.

de•oxy•guan•yl•ate (de-ok″se-gwahn′əl-āt) a dissociated form of deoxyguanylic acid.

de•oxy•guan•yl•ic ac•id (de-ok″se-gwah-nil′ik) deoxyguanosine monophosphate.

de•oxy•guan•yl•yl (de-ok″se-gwah-nil′əl) the radical formed by removal of OH from the phosphate group of deoxyguanosine monophosphate.

de•oxy•he•mo•glo•bin (de-ok″se-he′mo-glo″bin) hemoglobin not combined with oxygen, formed when oxyhemoglobin releases its oxygen; called also *deoxygenated* or *reduced hemoglobin.*

de•oxy•hex•ose (de-ok″se-hek′sōs) any deoxy sugar formed from a hexose; one in which the 6 carbon is reduced (6-deoxyhexose) is also called a *methylpentose.*

de•oxy•ni•val•e•nol (de-ok″se-nĭ-val′ə-nol) a trichothecene mycotoxin produced by species of *Fusarium,* causing fusariotoxicosis with vomiting and hemorrhaging in domestic animals. Called also *vomitoxin.*

de•oxy•pent•ose (de-ok″se-pen′tōs) any deoxy sugar formed from a pentose, e.g., deoxyribose.

de•oxy•ri•bo•nu•cle•ase (DNase) (de-ok″se-ri″bo-noo′kle-ās) any nuclease specifically catalyzing the cleavage of phosphate ester linkages in deoxyribonucleic acids; the deoxyribonucleases are grouped as those cleaving internal bonds (endodeoxyribonucleases) and those cleaving at termini (exodeoxyribonucleases).

d. I (DNase I) [EC 3.1.21.1] an endonuclease that produces di- and oligonucleotides with 5′-phosphate groups. The enzyme occurs in tissues such as the pancreas and thymus.

d. II (DNase II) [EC 3.1.22.1] an endonuclease that produces di- and oligonucleotides with 3′-phosphate groups. The enzyme occurs in tissues such as the pancreas, liver, thymus, and gastric mucosa.

de•oxy•ri•bo•nu•cle•ic ac•id (DNA) (de-ok″se-ri″bo-noo-kle′ik) the nucleic acid in which the sugar is deoxyribose, constituting the primary genetic material of all cellular organisms and the DNA viruses, and occurring predominantly in the nucleus. It is a linear or circular polymer with a backbone composed of deoxyribose moieties that are linked by phosphate groups attached to their 5′ and 3′ hydroxyls, with side chains composed of purine (adenine, guanine) and pyrimidine (cytosine, thymine) bases attached to the sugars. In double-stranded DNA (see illustration), the strands are twisted to form a double helix (q.v.) and are antiparallel. Adenine forms two hydrogen bonds with thymine, and cytosine forms three with guanine; these are complementary base pairs and thus each chain contains information completely specifying the other. The complementary base pairing provides the mechanism for DNA to duplicate itself by replication and also to serve as a template for synthesis of ribonucleic acid (transcription). For specific types of DNA, see under *DNA.*

de•oxy•ri•bo•nu•cleo•pro•tein (de-ok″se-ri″bo-noo″kle-o-pro′tēn) a nucleoprotein in which the nucleic acid sugar is D-2-deoxyribose.

de•oxy•ri•bo•nu•cleo•side (de-ok″se-ri″bo-noo′kle-o-sīd) a nucleoside having a purine or pyrimidine base bonded to deoxyribose.

de•oxy•ri•bo•nu•cleo•tide (de-ok″se-ri″bo-noo′kle-o-tīd) a nucleotide consisting of a purine or a pyrimidine base bonded to deoxyribose, which in turn is bound to a phosphate group.

de•oxy•ri•bose (de-ok″se-ri′bōs) a deoxypentose found in deoxyribonucleic acids (DNA), deoxyribonucleotides, and deoxyribonucleosides.

de•oxy•ri•bo•vi•rus (de-ok″se-ri′bo-vi″rəs) DNA virus.

de•oxy•thy•mi•dine (de-ok″se-thi′mĭ-dēn) a pyrimidine nucleoside, thymine linked by its N1 nitrogen to the C1 carbon of deoxyribose. Symbol dT. Often called *thymidine* (q.v.).

d. diphosphate (dTDP) a nucleotide, the 5′-pyrophosphate of deoxythymidine.

d. monophosphate (dTMP) a nucleotide, the 5′-phosphate of deoxythymidine, occurring in deoxyribonucleic acid.

d. triphosphate (dTTP) a nucleotide, the 5′-triphosphate of deoxythymidine; it is an activated precursor in the synthesis of deoxyribonucleic acid.

de•oxy•thy•mi•dyl•ate (de-ok″se-thi″mĭ-dil′āt) a dissociated form of deoxythymidylic acid.

de•oxy•thy•mi•dyl•ic ac•id (de-ok″se-thi″mĭ-dil′ik) deoxythymidine monophosphate.

de•oxy•thy•mi•dyl•yl (de-ok″se-thi″mĭ-dil′əl) the radical formed by removal of OH from the phosphate group of deoxythymidine monophosphate.

de•oxy•uri•dine (de-ok″se-ūr′ĭ-dēn) a pyrimidine nucleoside, uracil linked by its N1 nitrogen to the C1 carbon of deoxyribose. Symbol dU.

d. monophosphate (dUMP) a nucleotide, the 5′-phosphate of deoxyuridine; it is an intermediate in the synthesis of deoxythymidine triphosphate.

d. triphosphate (dUTP) a nucleotide, the 5′-triphosphate of deoxyuridine; it is an intermediate in the synthesis of deoxyribonucleotides.

de•oxy•uri•dyl•ate (de-ok″se-u″rĭ-dil′āt) a dissociated form of deoxyuridylic acid.

de•oxy•uri•dyl•ic ac•id (de-ok″se-u″rĭ-dil′ik) deoxyuridine monophosphate.

Dep. [L.] depura′tus (purified).

Dep•a•con (dep′ə-kon) trademark for a preparation of valproate sodium.

Dep•ade (dep′ād) trademark for a preparation of naltrexone hydrochloride.

Dep•a•kene (dep′ə-kēn) trademark for preparations of valproic acid.

Dep•a•kote (dep′ə-kōt) trademark for a preparation of divalproex sodium.

de•part•ment (də-pahrt′mənt) a specifically defined section of a larger agency or organization.

emergency d. (ED) an area of a hospital especially equipped and staffed for emergency medicine. Popularly called *emergency room.*

De•pen (dep′en) trademark for a preparation of penicillamine.

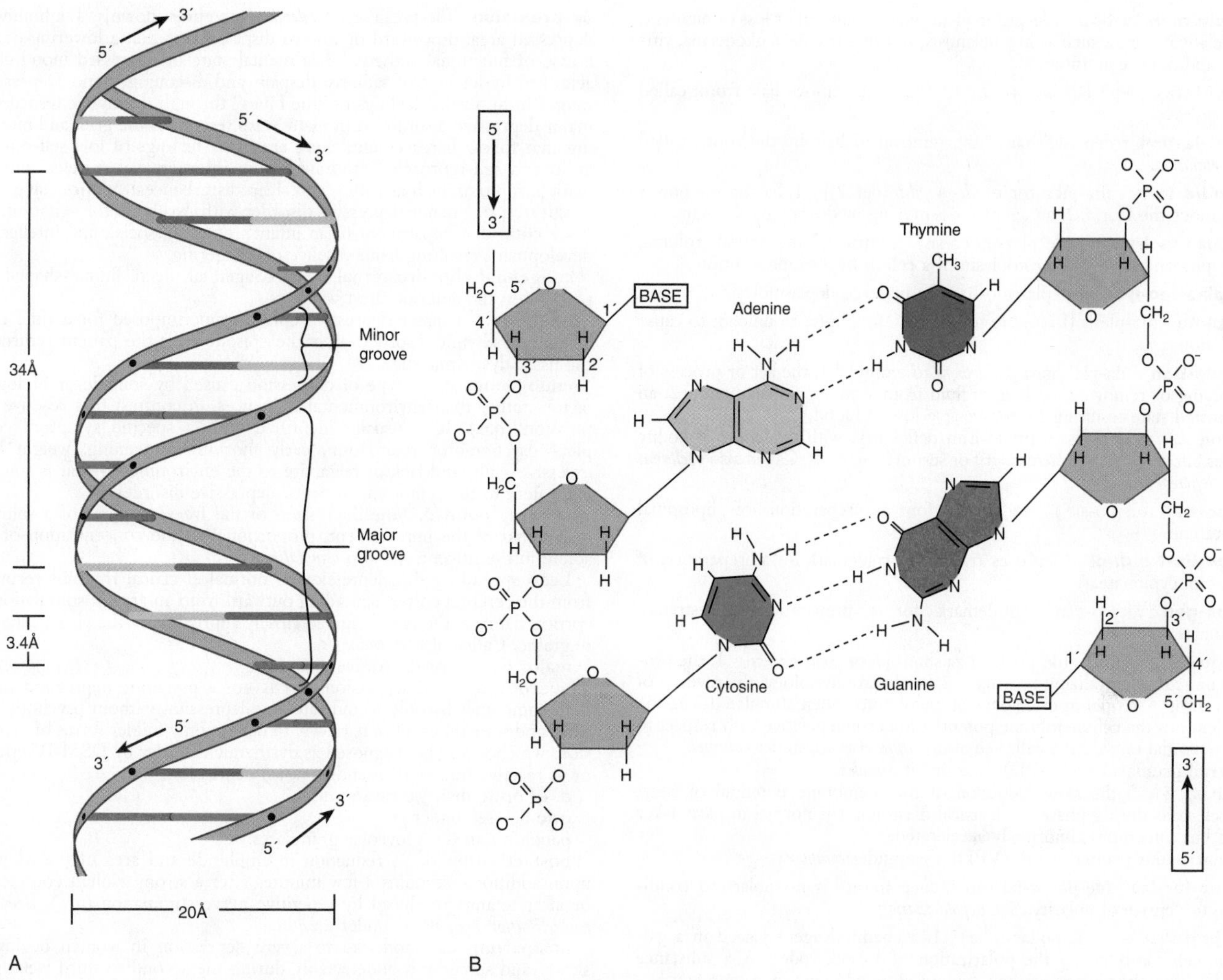

■ The DNA double helix. *A*, Diagrammatic model of the helical structure, showing its dimensions, the major and minor grooves, the periodicity of the bases, and the antiparallel orientation of the backbone chains (represented by ribbons). The base pairs (represented by rods) are perpendicular to the axis and lie stacked one on another. *B*, The chemical structure of the backbone and bases of DNA, showing the sugar phosphate linkages of the backbone and the hydrogen bonding between the base pairs. There are two hydrogen bonds between adenine and thymine, and three between cytosine and guanine.

de•pen•dence (de-pen′dəns) 1. a state of relying on or requiring the aid of something, particularly for support or maintenance. 2. a state in which there is a compulsive or chronic need, as for a drug; see *substance d.*

chemical d., drug d. substance d.

emotional d. psychological d.

physical d., physiological d. substance dependence in which there is evidence of tolerance, withdrawal, or both.

polysubstance d. [DSM-IV] substance dependence in which three or more substances, excluding nicotine and caffeine, are used repeatedly, with none of them predominating.

psychoactive substance d. substance d.

psychological d. substance dependence in which the drug is used to obtain relief from tension or emotional discomfort, rather than being associated with tolerance or withdrawal. Called also *emotional d.*

substance d. [DSM-IV] compulsive use of a substance despite significant problems resulting from such use. Although tolerance and withdrawal were previously defined as necessary and sufficient for dependence, they are currently only two of several possible criteria; others include taking the substance longer or in larger amounts than planned, repeatedly expressing a desire or attempting unsuccessfully to cut down or regulate use, and continuing use in the face of acknowledged substance-induced physical or mental problems. The term is sometimes used more narrowly to refer only to physiological dependence, and in this sense it may be considered to be a phenomenon distinct from tolerance. DSM-IV includes specific substance dependence disorders for alcohol, amphetamines or similarly acting sympathomimetics, cannabis, cocaine, hallucinogens, inhalants, nicotine, opioids, phencyclidines or similarly acting substances, and sedatives, hypnotics, or anxiolytics, as well as one for multiple substances (polysubstance). Called also *chemical d.* and *drug d.*

de•pen•den•cy (de-pen′dən-se) a state of relying on another for love, affection, mothering, comfort, security, food, warmth, shelter, protection, and the like—the so-called dependency needs.

de•pen•dent (de-pen′dənt) 1. exhibiting dependence or dependency. 2. hanging down.

De•pen•do•vi•rus (də-pen′do-vi″rəs) [L. *dependere* to depend on + *virus*] adeno-associated viruses; a genus of viruses of the subfamily Parvovirinae (family Parvoviridae) that require coinfection with an adenovirus or herpesvirus to provide helper functions for replication. If no helper virus is present, the genome can be integrated into the host cell DNA, resulting in latent infection. Asymptomatic infection is common.

de•per•son•al•iza•tion (de-pur″sən-əl-ĭ-za′shən) alteration in the perception of the self so that the usual sense of one's own reality is lost, manifested in a sense of unreality or self-estrangement, in changes of body image, or in a feeling that one does not control one's own actions and speech; seen in disorders such as depersonalization disorder, depression, dissociative states, hypochondriasis, temporal lobe epilepsy, schizophrenic disorders, and schizotypal personality disorder. Some do not draw a distinction between depersonalization and derealization, using depersonalization to include both.

de Pez•zer catheter (də pĕ-za′) [Oscar Michel Benvenuto *de Pezzer*, French surgeon, 1853–1917] see under *catheter.*

dep•Gyno•gen (dep″gi′no-jən) trademark for a preparation of estradiol cypionate.

de•phos•phor•y•la•tion (de-fos″for-ə-la′shən) removal of a phosphate group from an organic molecule.

de·pig·men·ta·tion (de-pig″mən-ta′shən) removal or loss of pigment, especially melanin, such as in amelanosis, achromotrichia, leukoderma, vitiligo, and other conditions.

dep·i·late (dep′ĭ-lāt) [*de-* + *pilus* (def. 2)] to remove hair from; called also *epilate.*

dep·i·la·tion (dep″ĭ-la′shən) the removal of hair by the roots; called also *epilation.*

de·pil·a·to·ry (də-pil′ə-tor″e) [*de-* + *pilus* (def. 2)] 1. having the power to remove the hair. 2. an agent for removing or destroying the hair.

de·plas·mol·y·sis (de″plaz-mol′ə-sis) return to the initial volume, after plasmolysis, of the protoplasm of a cell in hypertonic solution.

de·plas·mo·lyze (de-plaz′mo-līz) to undergo deplasmolysis.

de·plete (də-plēt′) [L. *deplere* to empty] to empty; to unload; to cause depletion.

de·ple·tion (də-ple′shən) [L. *deplere* to empty] 1. the act or process of emptying or removing, such as of fluid from a body compartment. 2. an exhausted state resulting from excessive loss of blood.

iron d. the mildest form of iron deficiency, with depletion of bodily stores but no change in hematocrit or serum iron levels. Called also *prelatent iron deficiency.*

Depo·Cyt (dep′o-sīt″) trademark for a preparation of liposomal cytarabine.

Depo-Es·tra·di·ol (dep″o-es″trə-di′ol) trademark for a preparation of estradiol cypionate.

Depo·gen (dep′o-gen″) trademark for a preparation of estradiol cypionate.

de·po·lar·iza·tion (de-po″lər-ĭ-za′shən) [*de-* + *polarization*] 1. the process or act of neutralizing polarity. 2. in electrophysiology, the reversal of the resting potential in excitable cell membranes when stimulated, i.e., the tendency of the cell membrane potential to become positive with respect to the potential outside the cell. See also *sodium channel,* under *channel.*

atrial premature d. (APD) see under *complex.*

phase 4 d. the slow reduction of the membrane potential of heart muscle cells during phase 4 (electrical diastole); it is normal in pacemaker cells but sometimes abnormally accelerated.

ventricular premature d. (VPD) see under *complex.*

de·po·lar·ize (de-po′lər-īz) to reduce toward a nonpolarized condition; to deprive of polarity. See *depolarization.*

de·po·lar·iz·er (de-po′lər-īz″ər) 1. a chemical agent placed in a galvanic cell for reducing the polarization of an electrode. 2. a substance that reduces the voltage across a biological membrane. 3. a muscle relaxant that produces striated muscle paralysis by altering the electrical state of the muscle receptor, thus blocking muscle response to nerve impulse.

de·po·lym·er·iza·tion (de″pə-lim″ər-ĭ-za′shən) the conversion of a polymer into its component monomers.

de·po·lym·er·ize (de″pə-lim′ər-īz) to cause to undergo depolymerization.

Depo-Med·rol (dep″o-med′rol) trademark for preparations of methylprednisolone acetate.

Depo-Pro·vera (dep″o-pro-ver′ə) trademark for a preparation of medroxyprogesterone acetate.

de·pos·it (de-poz′it) [*de-* + L. *ponere* to place] 1. sediment or dregs. 2. extraneous inorganic matter collected in the tissues or in a viscus or cavity. 3. tooth d.

immune d. an antigen-antibody complex (immune complex) that forms a solid in the bloodstream and precipitates out.

tooth d. a hard or soft material laid down on a tooth surface, such as dental calculus or plaque and materia alba.

de·pot (de′po, dep′o) [Fr. *dépôt,* from L. *depositum*] 1. a storehouse. 2. a body area in which a substance such as a medication can be accumulated, deposited, or stored and from which it can be distributed.

fat d. a site in the body in which large quantities of fat are stored, as in adipose tissue.

Depo-Tes·tos·ter·one (dep″o-tes-tos′tər-ōn) trademark for a preparation of testosterone cypionate.

L-de·pren·yl (dep′rə-nəl) selegiline.

de·pres·sant (de-pres′ənt) 1. diminishing functional activity. 2. an agent that reduces functional activity and the vital energies in general by producing muscular relaxation and diaphoresis.

cardiac d. an agent that depresses the rate or force of contraction of the heart.

de·pressed (de-prest′) 1. below the normal level. 2. associated with psychological depression.

de·pres·sion (de-presh′ən) [L. *deprimere* to press down] 1. a hollow or depressed area; downward or inward displacement. 2. a lowering or decrease of functional activity. 3. a mental state of depressed mood characterized by feelings of sadness, despair, and discouragement. Depression ranges from normal feelings of "the blues" through dysthymic disorder to major depressive disorder. It in many ways resembles the grief and mourning that follow bereavement; there are often feelings of low self-esteem, guilt, and self-reproach, withdrawal from interpersonal contact, and somatic symptoms such as eating and sleep disturbances. **depres′sive** *adj*

agitated d. major depressive disorder with psychomotor agitation.

anaclitic d. impairment of an infant's physical, social, and intellectual development resulting from absence of mothering.

congenital chondrosternal d. a congenital, deep, funnel-shaped depression in the anterior chest wall.

double d. a major depressive episode superimposed for a time on a chronic dysthymic disorder; after the episode ends the patient returns to the usual dysthymic state.

endogenous d. a type of depression caused by somatic or biological factors rather than environmental influences, in contrast to a reactive depression (q.v.). It is usually identified with a specific symptom complex—psychomotor retardation, early morning awakening, weight loss, excessive guilt, and lack of reactivity to the environment—that is roughly equivalent to the symptoms of major depressive disorder.

freezing point d. the depression of the freezing point of a solution below that of the pure solvent, proportional to the concentration of the solute in the solvent; see also *osmolality.*

Leão spreading d. depression of normal electrical rhythms recorded from the cerebral cortex, spreading outward from an area of stimulation or cortical damage; the rate of spread closely approximates the visual aura of a migraine. Called also *spreading d.*

major d. major depressive disorder.

neurotic d. any depression that is not a psychotic depression (q.v.); used sometimes broadly to indicate any depression without psychotic features and sometimes more narrowly to denote only milder forms of depression, which would be diagnosed as dysthymic disorder by DSM-IV criteria or as reactive (rather than endogenous) depression.

d. of optic disk excavatio disci.

otic d. see under *pit.*

pacchionian d's foveolae granulares.

postactivation d. a reduction in amplitude and area of the M wave upon additional stimulus a few minutes after a strong violent contraction or after tetanus produced by repetitive nerve stimulation (q.v.). See also *postactivation exhaustion,* under *exhaustion.*

postpartum d. moderate to severe depression in women beginning slowly and sometimes undetectably during the second to third week post partum, increasing steadily for weeks to months and usually resolving spontaneously within a year. Somatic complaints such as fatigue are common. It is intermediate in severity between the mood fluctuations experienced by the majority of new mothers and frank postpartum psychosis.

precordial d. epigastric fossa (def. 1).

psychotic d. major depressive disorder with psychotic features, such as hallucinations, delusions, mutism, or stupor. Cf. *neurotic d.*

pterygoid d. pterygoid fovea.

reactive d. a depression that is precipitated by a stressful life event or other environmental factor, in contrast to an endogenous depression, with an absence of significant vegetative disturbances; see also *neurotic d.* and *dysthymic disorder.*

retarded d. major depressive disorder with psychomotor retardation.

situational d. reactive d.

spreading d. Leão spreading d.

supratrochlear d. a slight depression on the anterior surface of the femur, above the trochlea.

tooth d. intrusion.

unipolar d. depression that is not accompanied by episodes of mania or hypomania, as in major depressive disorder or dysthymic disorder; the term is sometimes used to denote the former specifically.

ventricular d. the part of the venous pulse tracing that lies between the ventricular and atrial waves.

de·pres·so·mo·tor (de-pres″o-mo′tər) 1. retarding or abating motion. 2. an agent which lessens or depresses motor activity.

de·pres·sor (de-pres′ər) [L., from *deprimere* to press down] 1. that which causes depression, as a muscle, agent, instrument, or apparatus. 2. tending to decrease blood pressure; said of nerves and chemical substances. 3. depressor nerve.

d. an′guli o′ris see under *musculus.*

d. epiglot′tidis pars thyroepiglottica musculi thyroarytenoidei.

d. la′bii inferio′ris see under *musculus.*

tongue d. an instrument for pressing the tongue against the floor of the mouth, allowing better visualization of the oropharynx.

dep·ri·mens oc·u·li (dep′rĭ-mənz ok′u-le) [L.] musculus rectus inferior bulbi.

dep·ri·va·tion (dep″rĭ-va′shən) [*de-* + L. *privare* to remove] loss or absence of something, such as a part, organ, or capability.

androgen d. a treatment for prostate cancer consisting of blocking production of androgens, such as by orchiectomy or administration of antiandrogens. Called also *androgen ablation* and *androgen deprivation therapy*.

emotional d. deprivation of adequate and appropriate interpersonal or environmental experience in the early development years.

maternal d. the result of premature loss or absence of the mother or of lack of proper mothering; see also *maternal deprivation syndrome*, under *syndrome*.

sensory d. partial to total deprivation of visual, auditory, and tactile stimuli, such as may be produced experimentally or by solitary confinement, loss of sight or hearing, paralysis, or even hospital bed rest; it may result in some combination of anxiety, irritability, boredom, loss of ability to concentrate and organize thoughts, increased suggestibility, delusions, panic, and unpleasant vivid hallucinations.

thought d. blocking (def. 2).

water d. a method for testing the body's ability to concentrate urine when plasma osmolality is artificially increased; see *water deprivation test*, under *test*.

de·pro·tein·iza·tion (de-pro″tēn-ĭ-za′shən) removal of protein.

dep·side (dep′sīd) one of a class of compounds which are products of the condensation of two or more molecules of phenolic carboxylic acids, e.g., tannic acid.

depth (depth) an expression of the distance separating the upper and lower surfaces of an object.

focal d., d. of focus the measure of the power of a lens to yield clear images of objects at different distances from it. Called also *penetration*.

dep·u·rant (dep′u-rənt) 1. cleansing or purifying. 2. an agent that cleanses or purifies.

dep·u·rate (dep′u-rāt) [L. *depurare* to purify] to cleanse, refine, or purify.

dep·u·ra·tion (dep″u-ra′shən) cleansing, purification; especially placement of shellfish in clean water to allow them to cleanse themselves of bacteria.

dep·u·ra·tive (dep′u-ra″tiv) tending to purify or cleanse.

dep·u·ra·tor (dep′u-ra″tər) an agent that cleanses or purifies.

de Quer·vain disease, fracture, thyroiditis (də kār-vă′) [Fritz *de Quervain*, Swiss physician, 1868–1940] see under *disease* and *fracture* and see *subacute granulomatous thyroiditis*, under *thyroiditis*.

der·a·del·phus (der″ə-del′fəs) [*der-* + *-adelphus*] conjoined twins fused at or near the umbilicus and having only one head.

de·rail·ment (de-rāl′mənt) disordered thought or speech characteristic of schizophrenia and marked by constant jumping around from one topic to another before the first is fully realized, the topics often being clearly but obliquely related or unrelated. The term is sometimes used synonymously with *loosening of associations*.

der·an·en·ce·pha·lia (der-an″ən-sə-fa′le-ə) [*der-* + *an-*[1] + *encephal-* + *-ia*] anencephaly marked by defect of the brain and upper part of the spinal cord.

de·range·ment (de-rānj′mənt) disarrangement of a part or organ.

internal knee d. partial dislocation of the knee, marked by great pain and spasm of the muscles.

Der·cum disease (dur′kəm) [Francis Xavier *Dercum*, American physician, 1856–1931] adiposis dolorosa.

de·re·al·i·za·tion (de-re″əl-ĭ-za′shən) a loss of the sensation of the reality of one's surroundings; the feeling that something has happened, that the world has been changed and altered, that one is detached from one's environment. It is seen most frequently in schizophrenic disorders. See also *depersonalization*.

de·re·ism (de′re-iz-əm) [*de-* + *res* thing + *-ism*] dereistic thinking; see under *thinking*.

de·re·is·tic (de″re-is′tik) directed away from reality; not using normal logic; see *dereistic thinking*, under *thinking*.

der·en·ceph·a·lo·cele (der″en-sef′ə-lo-sēl) [*derencephalus* + *-cele*[1]] the brain substance that protrudes through the defect in the cervical vertebrae in a derencephalus.

der·en·ceph·a·lus (der″en-sef′ə-ləs) [*der-* + Gr. *enkephalos* brain] a fetus with rudimentary cranial bones and bifid cervical vertebrae, the brain resting in the bifurcation.

de·re·pres·sion (de″re-presh′ən) removal of repression of a gene or operon, leading to or enhancing gene expression. In prokaryotes, the mechanism involves inactivation of a repressor, as by inhibition of a corepressor or by the action of an inducer. In eukaryotes, the process appears to involve combinations of regulatory proteins and specific effectors.

De·ri·fil (der′ĭ-fil) trademark for a preparation of chlorophyllin copper complex sodium.

der·i·vant (der′ĭ-vənt) derivative.

de·riv·a·tive (də-riv′ə-tiv) a chemical substance produced from another substance either directly or by modification or partial substitution.

benzoporphyrin d. verteporfin.

hematoporphyrin d. a material prepared by an acetic acid–sulfuric acid treatment of hematoporphyrin that concentrates selectively in metabolically active tumor tissue; used in photodynamic therapy.

purified protein d. (PPD) see under *tuberculin*.

-derm [Gr. *derma* skin] a word termination denoting skin, or a germ layer.

der·ma (dur′mə) [Gr.] 1. skin. 2. dermis.

derma- see *dermat(o)-*.

Der·ma·bac·ter (dur′mə-bak″tər) a genus of gram-positive bacteria of the family Dermabacteraceae; organisms are facultatively anaerobic, non–spore-forming, non–acid-fast, and catalase-negative. The type species is *D. ho′minis*.

D. ho′minis a species that is a normal inhabitant of human skin. It is an opportunistic pathogen, causing bacteremia in immunocompromised persons and in patients undergoing long-term hospitalization or continuous ambulatory peritoneal dialysis.

Der·ma·bac·te·ra·ceae (dur″mə-bak-tər-a′se-e) [Gr. *derma* skin + *-bacter*] a family of gram-positive, facultatively anaerobic, non–spore-forming bacteria of the suborder Micrococcineae, order Actinomycetales. Pathogenic organisms are contained in the genus *Dermabacter*.

derm·abrad·er (dur″mə-brād′ər) any device used for dermabrasion.

derm·abra·sion (dur″mə-bra′zhən) planing of the skin by mechanical means, as by fine sandpaper or wire brushes. See *planing*.

Der·ma·cen·tor (dur″mə-sen′tər) [*derma-* + Gr. *kentein* to prick, stab] a genus of ticks of the family Ixodidae that are important as transmitters of disease.

D. albipic′tus the winter tick, a brown North American species parasitic on cattle, horses, deer, elk, and moose, a vector for the bacteria causing anaplasmosis and other diseases.

D. anderso′ni the Rocky Mountain wood tick, a reddish brown species that is a major vector for the organisms causing Rocky Mountain spotted fever, Colorado tick fever, and tularemia in humans and tick paralysis in various animal species. Its usual hosts include deer, elk, antelope, grizzly bears, porcupines, prairie dogs, and rabbits. Called also *D. venustus*.

D. hun′teri a brown tick found on Rocky Mountain sheep in the southwestern United States, transmitters of anaplasmosis and other diseases.

D. margina′tus a species found in northern Europe and Asia, transmitting Siberian tick typhus and tick-borne fever.

D. ni′tens *Anocentor nitens*.

D. nuttal′lii a species that feeds on horses and other large mammals in Asia and transmits Siberian tick typhus.

D. occidenta′lis the Pacific Coast tick, a brown species that feeds on cattle, horses, deer, dogs, and humans in the western United States and Canada and is a vector for Rocky Mountain spotted fever.

D. reticula′tus a tick that attacks numerous large mammals in Europe, Asia, and the Americas and is a vector of tularemia, tick-borne encephalitis, tick-borne fever, and canine babesiosis.

D. varia′bilis the American dog tick, a dark brown species found in North America across wide areas east of the Rocky Mountains and sometimes in California, usually on dogs but sometimes on cattle, horses, rabbits, and humans; it is the principal vector of Rocky Mountain spotted fever in these areas.

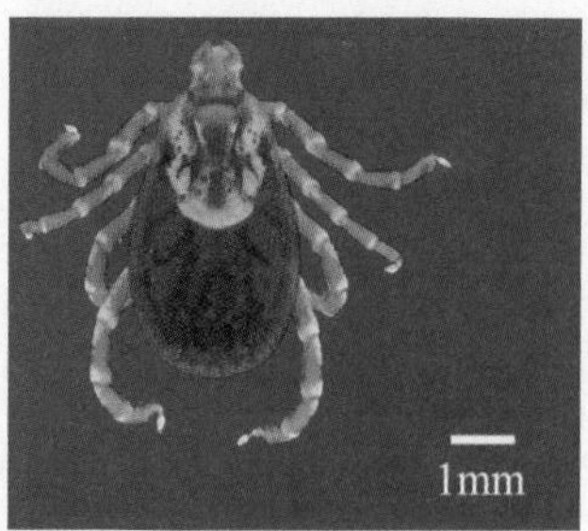

■ *Dermacentor variabilis* adult female.

D. venus'tus *D. andersoni.*

der•mad (dur′mad) toward the skin or other integument.

der•mal (dur′məl) 1. pertaining to the dermis; called also *dermic.* 2. cutaneous.

der•ma•my•ia•sis (dur″mə-mi-i′ə-sis) [*derma-* + *myiasis*] cutaneous myiasis.

Der•ma•nys•si•dae (dur″mə-nis′ĭ-de) a family of mites of the order Acarina, parasites of mammals, reptiles, and birds; their bites may cause a painful dermatitis. *Dermanyssus* is the type genus.

Der•ma•nys•sus (dur″mə-nis′əs) [*derma-* + Gr. *nyssein* to prick] a genus of mites of the family Dermanyssidae. *D. galli′nae,* the bird mite or chicken mite, infests poultry and sometimes humans.

der•ma•sand•ing (dur′mə-sand″ing) dermabrasion with a fine grade of silicon carbide sandpaper.

der•ma•skel•e•ton (dur″mə-skel′ə-tən) exoskeleton.

Der•ma-Smoothe/FS (dur′mə-smo͞oth) trademark for a preparation of fluocinolone acetonide.

der•ma•tan sul•fate (dur″mə-tan) a glycosaminoglycan found mostly in the skin but also in blood vessels, tendons, heart valves, and pulmonary connective tissues. It consists of repeating disaccharide units in specific linkage, each composed of a (C-4) sulfated *N*-acetylgalactosamine linked to a uronic acid, generally L-iduronic acid, which is sometimes sulfated. It is an accumulation product in several of the mucopolysaccharidoses.

der•ma•ti•tis (dur″mə-ti′tis) pl. *dermati′tides* [*dermat-* + *-itis*] inflammation of the skin.

Dermatitis

acral lick d. a psychogenic skin condition in dogs in which they lick excessively on a distal part of a limb until a thickened plaque or ulcer forms; the usual cause is boredom from enforced inactivity, but sometimes the licked area may be overlying a fracture, arthritic lesion, or area of nerve damage. Called also *acral lick granuloma.*
actinic d. photodamage with dermatitis resulting from exposure to actinic radiation, such as sunlight, ultraviolet rays, x-rays, or gamma rays. See also *chronic actinic d., phototoxic d.,* and *radiation d.* Called also *actinodermatitis.*
allergic d. 1. atopic d. 2. allergic contact d.
allergic contact d. contact dermatitis due to allergic sensitization to a substance, with an inflammatory reaction in the skin; this occurs primarily in persons who have acquired hypersensitivity to the allergen as a result of previous exposure to it. Called also *allergic d.* and *contact d.*. Cf. *irritant d.*
ammonia d. diaper d.
d. artefac′ta factitial d.
ashy d. erythema dyschromicum perstans.
asteatotic d. see under *eczema.*
atopic d. a common, chronic type of dermatitis, thought to be hereditary, sometimes associated with other allergic conditions such as allergic rhinitis, hay fever, or asthma. Severe pruritus leads to scratching, rubbing, and typical signs of eczema. In infants it usually occurs on the cheeks, whereas in older children and adults it is found chiefly on flexural surfaces. (See *infantile eczema* and *flexural eczema,* under *eczema.*) Called also *allergic d., allergic* or *atopic eczema,* and *Besnier prurigo.*
autosensitization d. id reaction.
berlock d., berloque d. (ber-lok′) [Fr. *berloque,* Ger. *Berlocke* pendant] photodermatitis on areas of the skin to which certain types of cologne, perfume, or other toilet articles have been applied; the original causative substance was bergamot oil in the toilet articles, but other substances can cause the same condition. Lesions are brown pigmented patches, often shaped like pendants. Called also *perfume d.*
blastomycetic d. cutaneous blastomycosis.
brown-tail moth d. a type of insect dermatitis produced by the hairs of the brown-tail moth, *Euproctis chrysorrhoea;* called also *brown-tail rash.*
d. bullo′sa stria′ta praten′sis meadow grass d.
d. calo′rica any dermatitis caused by heat or cold; see *erythema ab igne* and *cold erythema.*

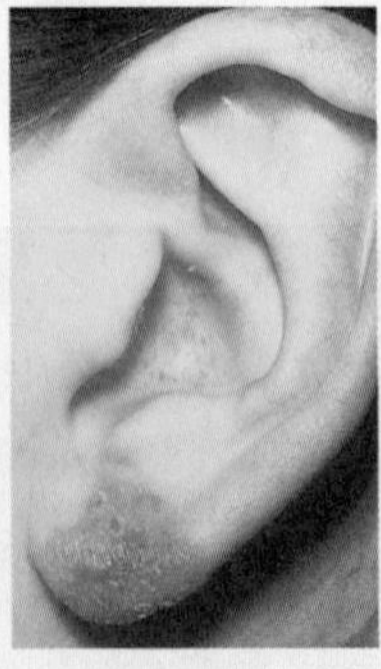

■ Allergic contact dermatitis due to nickel allergy.

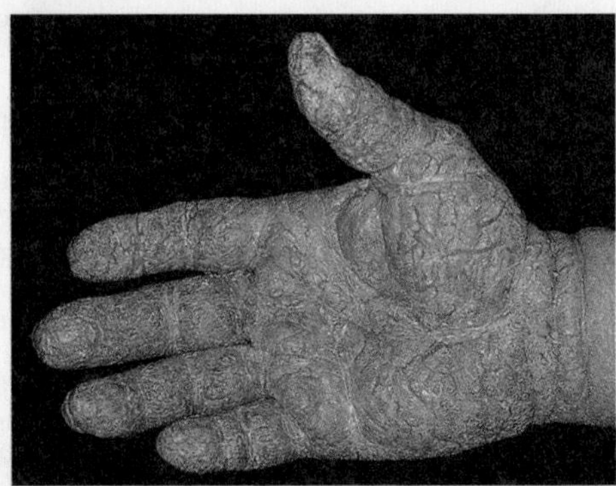

■ Severe chronic hand dermatitis in an adult with atopic dermatitis.

caterpillar d. insect dermatitis caused by caterpillar hairs. Called also *caterpillar rash* and *erucism.*
cercarial d. a pruritic papular eruption seen in persons who swim or wade in certain bodies of water (either fresh or salt), due to hypersensitivity to the cercariae of schistosomes in the water that penetrate the skin and die without gaining access to the circulation and deeper tissues. Called also *clam digger's* or *swimmer's itch, cutaneous schistosomiasis,* and *schistosomal, schistosome,* or *swimmers' d.*
chemical d. contact dermatitis caused by exposure of the skin to a chemical substance.
chigger d. dermatitis due to infestation with chiggers; see also *trombiculiasis.*
chronic actinic d. (CAD) a long-term form of photosensitivity dermatitis with an eczematous reaction to sunlight; the etiology is unknown, but in some patients it may be a continuation of photoallergic contact dermatitis after the allergen has been removed. Called also *actinic reticuloid, persistent light reactivity,* and *photosensitive eczema.*
contact d. acute or chronic dermatitis caused by substances coming in contact with the skin; it may involve either allergic or nonallergic mechanisms. See *allergic contact d.* and *irritant d.*
contagious pustular d. 1. contagious acne of horses. 2. contagious ecthyma.
cosmetic d. allergic contact dermatitis caused by an ingredient of a cosmetic preparation.
dhobie mark d. see under *itch.*
diaper d. irritant dermatitis in the area in contact with the diaper in infants, sparing the skinfold areas, caused by a reaction to prolonged contact with urine and feces; it may be aggravated by friction or maceration, or by presence of soaps or other topical preparations left on the skin. It is commonly associated with secondary bacterial and yeast infections, especially with *Candida albicans.* Popularly known as *diaper rash* and *napkin* or *nappy rash.* Called also *napkin* or *nappy d.*
drug-induced d. drug eruption.
eczematous d. eczema.
d. exfoliati′va exfoliative d.
d. exfoliati′va neonato′rum staphylococcal scalded skin syndrome.

exfoliative d. a scaly erythematous dermatitis over wide areas of the skin, sometimes with loss of hair and nails, hyperkeratosis of palms and soles, pruritus, or other severe, debilitating physiological effects. It may be a secondary or reactive process accompanying an underlying cutaneous disorder such as atopic dermatitis, psoriasis, scabies, or lichen planus; or it may be a primary or idiopathic disorder. Called also *erythroderma, generalized exfoliative d.*, and *pityriasis rubra.*
exudative discoid and lichenoid d. a rare type of neurodermatitis that was seen in older men of Jewish extraction in the United States, characterized by intense pruritus with exudative round patches over much of the body; it may be a form of nummular eczema. Called also *oid-oid disease* and *Sulzberger-Garbe syndrome.*
d. facti′tia, factitial d. dermatitis caused by self-inflicted trauma, such as by mechanical means, burning, or application of chemical irritants or caustics. Called also *d. artefacta.*
fiberglass d. irritant contact dermatitis from exposure to fiberglass.
filarial d. 1. stephanofilariasis. 2. elaeophoriasis.
d. gangreno′sa infan′tum a rare gangrenous skin disease of young children, usually seen on the lower back and buttocks, in which multiple small erosive and pustular lesions coalesce to form extensive areas of sloughing. It may occur as a primary condition or be secondary to varicella or some other exanthematous disease.
gangrenous d. necrotic d.
generalized exfoliative d. exfoliative d.
d. herpetifor′mis a chronic, relapsing multisystem disease whose primary manifestations are cutaneous, usually seen in light-skinned persons of Northern European extraction in association with celiac disease (q.v.). Characteristics include a symmetrical pruritic eruption with grouped erythematous, eczematous vesicles that upon healing may leave discoloration and sometimes scarring. The cause is unknown, but immunogenetic factors are thought to play a role. Called also *Duhring disease.*
d. hiema′lis asteatotic eczema.
hookworm d. ground itch.
industrial d. occupational d.
infectious eczematoid d., infectious eczematous d. a skin condition in which a primary lesion such as a boil, surgical wound, or draining ear or nose is the source of an infectious exudate that spreads by autoinoculation, tending to form circumscribed eczematous plaques that slowly enlarge, sometimes with vesicles or pustules.
insect d. localized or widespread dermatitis caused by the toxin-containing irritant hairs of certain insects, especially moths and caterpillars (see *moth d.* and *caterpillar d.*). Clinical manifestations vary according to the species and the intensity of exposure, and may include pain, conjunctivitis, pruritus, and burning sensations.
interdigital d. dermatitis of the interdigital skin of sheep, with exudate, varying amounts of necrotic skin, and lameness, due to infection with *Fusobacterium necrophorum, Corynebacterium pyogenes*, or *Bacteroides nodosus.* It is worse in cold or wet weather and may be a precursor of foot rot. Called also *scald* and *foot scald.*
interstitial granulomatous d. a skin condition seen in some patients with rheumatoid arthritis, consisting of red to violet indurated cords under the skin, most often on the thighs, axillae, or abdomen.
irritant d., irritant contact d. a nonallergic type of contact dermatitis due to exposure to a substance that damages the skin. Called also *primary irritant d.* Cf. *allergic contact d.*

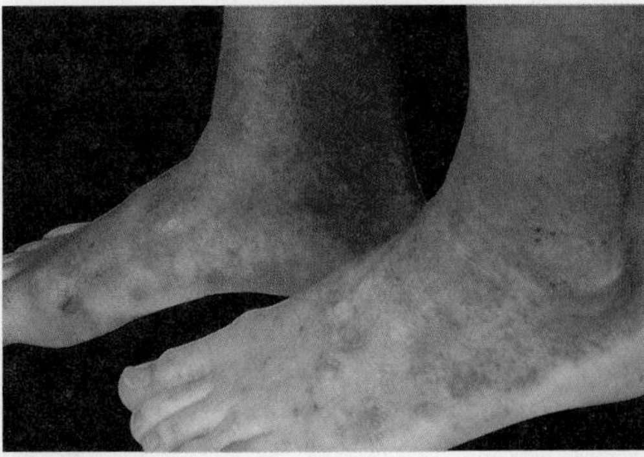

■ Bilateral irritant dermatitis from chronic use of occlusive footwear.

Jacquet d. diaper d.
livedoid d. Nicolau syndrome.
localized scratch d. irritation of skin by continual scratching; in some cases, the area has previously been affected by a condition such as contact dermatitis, but the person continues to scratch the area after the original condition has resolved.
mango d. a type of urushiol dermatitis caused by excessive contact with products of the tree *Mangifera indica* (skins of mangoes or leaves of the tree).
marine d. cercarial dermatitis after swimming in salt water.
meadow d., meadow grass d. a type of phytophotodermatitis caused by contact with meadow grass, usually *Agrimonia eupatoria.* Characteristics include vesicles and bullae in random linear or streaky arrangements on the skin when it is exposed to sunlight, later healing to leave intense melanoderma. Called also *d. bullosa striata pratensis*, and *d. striata pratensis bullosa.*
mechanical d., mechanical irritant d. irritant dermatitis caused by a mechanical irritant; the most common type is thorns and glochids from cactus plants.
d. medicamento′sa drug eruption.
moth d. insect dermatitis caused by moth hairs.
napkin d., nappy d. diaper d.
nasal solar d. actinic dermatitis of the nonpigmented parts of the nose of a dog, especially the bridge or the nasal plane; it is worse in the summer and may become inflamed or ulcerated. A similar but not identical condition occurs as part of some types of lupus in dogs. Called also *nasal eczema* and *collie nose.*
necrotic d. a contagious, usually fatal disease of young chickens in which there is gangrenous necrosis of the skin of the thighs and breast, caused by infection with *Clostridium septicum* or some other *Clostridium* species. Chickens suffering from infectious bursal disease are particularly susceptible. Called also *gangrenous cellulitis* and *gangrenous d.*
nickel d. allergic contact dermatitis caused by contact with nickel or a nickel-containing alloy.
nummular d., nummular eczematous d. see under *eczema.*
occupational d. contact dermatitis caused by substances found in the work place. Called also *industrial d.* and *industrial* or *occupational dermatosis.*
onion mite d. dermatitis affecting handlers of decaying onions, caused by the onion mite, *Acarus rhyzoglypticus hyacinthi.*
palisaded neutrophilic and granulomatous d. rheumatoid neutrophilic d.
d. papilla′ris capilli′tii acne keloidalis.
***Pelodera* d.** rhabditic d.
perfume d. berlock d.
periocular d. a variant of perioral dermatitis that has spread upward to the area around the eyes.
perioral d. a papular eruption on the face, of unknown etiology and seen most often in young women; papules and pustules develop slowly and progress to erythema and scaling. It is usually confined to the area about the mouth, but may also spread to involve the eyelids and forehead *(periocular d.).* See also *periorificial d.*
periorificial d. term used by some authorities to embrace both perioral dermatitis and periocular dermatitis.
photoallergic contact d., photocontact d. photodamage from photoallergy, consisting of a papulovesicular, eczematous, or exudative dermatitis, mainly on light-exposed areas of the skin.
photosensitivity d. any dermatitis occurring as a manifestation of photosensitivity, such as chronic actinic dermatitis, photoallergic contact dermatitis, or phototoxic dermatitis.
phototoxic d. a type of actinic dermatitis in which there is an exaggerated sunburnlike reaction on light-exposed areas of the skin, sometimes with blistering, hyperpigmentation, and desquamation; it is the cutaneous manifestation of phototoxicity. Called also *photodermatitis.*
phytophototoxic d. phytophotodermatitis.
pigmented purpuric d. chronic pigmented purpura.
pigmented purpuric lichenoid d. a type of chronic pigmented purpura seen most often in middle-aged men, chiefly on the legs, thighs, or lower trunk, characterized by tiny discolored, lichenoid papules that tend to fuse into plaques. Called also *Gougerot-Blum syndrome.*
d. planta′ris sic′ca juvenile plantar dermatosis.
poison ivy d., poison oak d., poison sumac d. see *rhus d.*
precancerous d. former name for *Bowen disease* when it was thought to be nonmalignant.

Dermatitis *Continued*

primary irritant d. irritant d.
proliferative d. dermatophilosis in sheep.
protein contact d. allergic contact dermatitis caused by proteins in food products, usually seen in professional food handlers.
radiation d. dermatitis resulting from exposure to ionizing radiation; called also *radiodermatitis.*
rat mite d. dermatitis resulting from the bite of the rat mite, *Ornithonyssus bacoti.*
d. re′pens acrodermatitis continua.
rhabditic d. a type of dermatitis found in domestic animals and occasionally spread to humans, due to invasion of a break in the skin by larvae of the nematode *Rhabditis strongyloides*, often as a result of sleeping in a damp, filthy bed. Called also *Pelodera d.*
rheumatoid neutrophilic d. an early cutaneous manifestation of rheumatoid arthritis, characterized by tender, erythematous papules (rheumatoid papules) surrounded by palisading histiocytes, usually on the limbs. Called also *palisaded neutrophilic and granulomatous d.*
rhus d. allergic contact dermatitis due to exposure to plants of the genus *Rhus* that contain the sensitizing agent urushiol; the most common plants are poison ivy, poison oak, and poison sumac.
roentgen ray d. x-ray d.
rosaceiform d. inflammation and worsening of rosacea occurring as a rare late reaction to drug treatment of rosacea.
sabra d. a type of mechanical irritant dermatitis resembling scabies, seen in Israel among persons who handle the fruit of *Opuntia ficus-indica*, the Indian fig or sabra, owing to penetration of glochids into the skin.
schistosomal d., schistosome d. cercarial d.
seborrheic d., d. seborrhe′ica chronic dermatitis with itching, erythema, dry, moist, or greasy scaling, and yellow crusted patches on the face, scalp, or elsewhere on the body; on the scalp the patches start out small but slowly spread and may become widespread, with exfoliation of many dry scales (dandruff). The etiology of this condition is unknown. Called also *seborrheic eczema.*
solar d. photodermatitis caused by exposure to sunlight.
stasis d. chronic, eczematous dermatitis caused by venous insufficiency in the lower limb, usually first involving the skin medially near the ankle and sometimes spreading over the entire lower limb; characteristics include edema, pigmentation, and often ulceration (see *venous ulcer*, under *ulcer*). Called also *congestion, gravitational, stasis,* or *varicose eczema.*

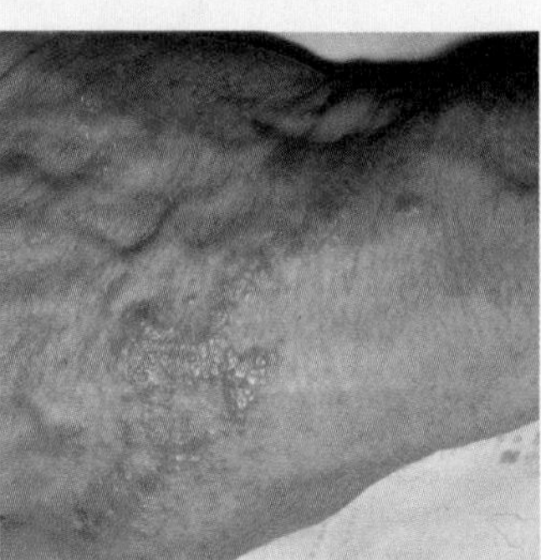
■ Classic linear distribution of rhus dermatitis.

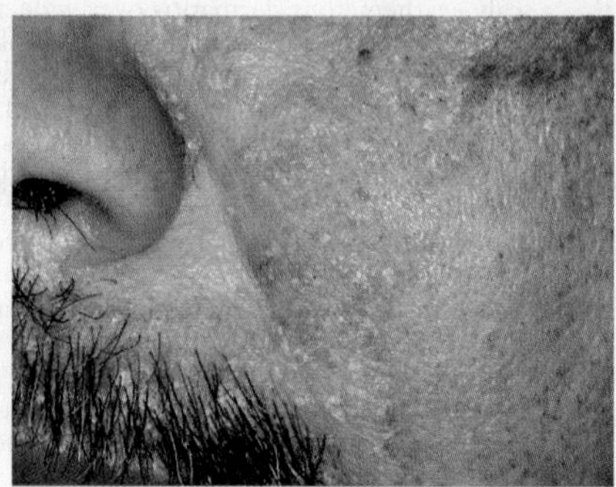
■ Seborrheic dermatitis.

d. stria′ta praten′sis bullo′sa meadow grass d.
swimmer's d. cercarial d.
trefoil d. a photosensitization condition seen in livestock that have eaten *Medicago polymorpha* (burr trefoil); it is similar to trifoliosis but without the liver damage.
uncinarial d. ground itch.
urushiol d. allergic contact dermatitis caused by contact with leaves, stems, or other parts of urushiol-containing plants; the most common urushiol-containing plants are in the family Anacardiaceae, such as in the genera *Rhus, Anacardium, Mangifera, Schinus,* and *Semecarpus.* See also *rhus d.* and *mango d.*
d. ve′getans the Hallopeau type of pemphigus vegetans.
d. venena′ta allergic contact d.
verminous d. stephanofilariasis.
verrucose d., verrucous d. 1. chromoblastomycosis. 2. a proliferative lesion of the skin of the legs in cattle, extending downward from the fetlock joint along the pastern, usually on the hind legs, with hyperkeratosis and papillomas forming cauliflowerlike lesions. It usually occurs in crowded unsanitary conditions as a result of a bacterial infection, such as with *Fusobacterium necrophorum.*
vesicular d. 1. dermatitis with vesicle formation. 2. a sometimes fatal disease of young poultry that range over unbroken prairie sod, believed to be a photosensitization after ingestion of certain plants and seeds; characteristics include formation of blisters and scabs on the feet and legs.
viral papular d. a type of dermatitis seen in horses in the United States, Great Britain, and Australia, characterized by formation of firm papules followed by a dry crust that detaches and leaves small areas of alopecia.
winter d., xerotic d. asteatotic eczema.
x-ray d. radiation dermatitis from exposure to x-rays.

dermat(o)- [Gr. *derma*, gen. *dermatos* skin] a combining form denoting relationship to the skin. Also, *derma-, derm(o)-.*

der·ma·to·ar·thri·tis (dur″mə-to-ahr-thri′tis) [*dermato-* + *arthritis*] skin disease associated with arthritis.
  lipid d., lipoid d. multicentric reticulohistiocytosis.

der·ma·to·au·to·plas·ty (dur″mə-to-aw′to-plas″te) [*dermato-* + *autoplasty*] skin grafting using skin taken from some other portion of the patient's own body.

Der·ma·to·bia (dur″mə-to′be-ə) [*dermato-* + Gr. *bios* life] a genus of botflies of the family Oestridae.
  D. ho′minis the human botfly of South America, the usual cause of dermatobiasis. Its larvae are parasitic in the skin of mammals, and birds; the eggs are deposited on the bodies of mosquitoes, flies, or ticks, which then transport them to the host.

der·ma·to·bi·a·sis (dur″mə-to-bi′ə-sis) infection with larvae of *Dermatobia*, usually on the skin as a form of cutaneous myiasis.

der·ma·to·chal·a·sia (dur″mə-to-kəl-a′zhə) cutis laxa.

der·ma·to·chal·a·sis (dur″mə-to-kal′ə-sis) cutis laxa.

der·ma·to·chal·a·zia (dur″mə-to-kəl-a′zhə) cutis laxa.

der·ma·to·con·junc·ti·vi·tis (dur″mə-to-kən-junk″tĭ-vi′tis) inflammation of the conjunctiva and of the skin around the eyes.

der·ma·to·dys·pla·sia (dur″mə-to-dis-pla′zhə) [*dermato-* + *dysplasia*] abnormal development of the skin.

der·ma·to·fi·bro·ma (dur″mə-to-fi-bro′mə) [*dermato-* + *fibroma*] a benign, circumscribed, red to brown nodule in the dermis, composed of macrophages that may differentiate to resemble fibroblasts, usually found on the lower legs of women, often after minor trauma. It is a form of benign fibrous histiocytoma, and the two terms are sometimes used synonymously. NOTE: Terminology is variable; several other lesions may be synonymous with or variants of dermatofibroma and benign fibrous histiocytoma, including *nodular subepidermal fibrosis* and *sclerosing hemangioma.*
  d. protu′berans see under *dermatofibrosarcoma.*

der·ma·to·fi·bro·sar·co·ma (dur″mə-to-fi″bro-sahr-ko′mə) [*dermato-* + *fibrosarcoma*] a fibrosarcoma of the skin.

d. protu′berans a bulky, protruding, nodular, fibrotic neoplasm in the dermis, usually on the trunk, often extending into the subcutaneous fat; it is locally aggressive and frequently recurs. It is sometimes classified as a type of malignant fibrous histiocytoma.

der•ma•to•fi•bro•sis (dur″mə-to-fi-bro′sis) a condition characterized by fibrotic changes in the skin.

d. lenticula′ris dissemina′ta connective tissue nevi of the elastic type, consisting of small, firm, skin-colored papules or plaques, found on the limbs and lower trunk in the Buschke-Ollendorff syndrome.

der•ma•to•glyph•ics (dur″mə-to-glif′iks) [*dermato-* + Gr. *glyphein* to carve] the study of fingerprints and similar patterns of skin ridges of the hands and feet; done in anthropology and law enforcement to establish identity, and in medicine, both clinically and as a genetic indicator, such as of chromosomal abnormalities.

der•ma•to•graph•ic (dur″mə-to-graf′ik) dermographic.

der•ma•tog•ra•phism (dur″mə-tog′rə-fiz″əm) dermographism.

der•ma•to•he•li•o•sis (dur″mə-to-he″le-o′sis) photodamage.

der•ma•to•het•ero•plas•ty (dur″mə-to-het′ər-o-plas″te) [*dermato-* + *heteroplasty*] the grafting of skin derived from a member of another species.

der•ma•to•log•ic (dur″mə-to-loj′ik) 1. pertaining to dermatology. 2. cutaneous.

der•ma•to•log•i•cal (dur″mə-to-loj′ĭ-kəl) dermatologic.

der•ma•tol•o•gist (dur″mə-tol′o-jist) a physician specializing in dermatology.

der•ma•tol•o•gy (dur″mə-tol′ə-je) the medical specialty concerned with the diagnosis and treatment of diseases of the skin and its appendages (hair and nails).

der•ma•to•lym•phan•gio•ad•e•ni•tis (dur″mə-to-lim-fan″je-o-ad″ə-ni′tis) a complication of obstructive peripheral lymphedema, characterized by local tenderness and erythema of the skin of the affected limb, often with red streaks along the distribution of the superficial lymphatics and lymph node enlargement. Systemic symptoms include fever, chills, and malaise.

der•ma•tol•y•sis (dur″mə-tol′ə-sis) [*dermato-* + *-lysis*] 1. loosening of the skin; called also *dermolysis.* 2. formerly, a synonym for *cutis laxa.*

d. palpebra′rum blepharochalasis.

der•ma•tome (dur′mə-tōm) [*derma-* + *-tome*] 1. an instrument for cutting thin skin slices for skin grafts. 2. the area of skin supplied with afferent nerve fibers by a single posterior spinal root; called also *dermatomic area.* 3. the lateral portion of a mesodermal somite; the cutis plate.

Brown d. an electric dermatome, the first to be developed, for cutting split-thickness skin grafts; it enables the surgeon to remove long strips of skin rapidly.

Castroviejo d. an electric dermatome used for cutting mucous membrane grafts for the treatment of eyelid and socket deformities and as an adjunct in the removal of tattoos after the initial excision has been done using either the Brown or Padgett dermatomes. It has a tiny cutting head with special blades and skims to control the thickness of the cut.

Padgett d. an instrument for rapid cutting of split-thickness skin grafts of any desired thickness.

Reese d. an instrument for cutting split-thickness skin grafts that permits careful calibration of the thickness of the graft.

der•ma•to•meg•a•ly (dur″mə-to-meg′ə-le) cutis laxa.

der•ma•to•mere (dur′mə-to-mēr″) [*dermato-* + *-mere*] any segment or metamere of the embryonic integument.

der•ma•tom•ic (dur″mə-tom′ik) pertaining to a dermatome (def. 2).

der•ma•to•my•co•sis (dur″mə-to-mi-ko′sis) [*dermato-* + *mycosis*] infection of the skin or its appendages by fungi, such as in dermatophytosis, various forms of tinea, and deeper fungal infections. Called also *epidermomycosis.*

d. furfura′cea tinea versicolor.

der•ma•to•my•ia•sis (dur″mə-to-mi-i′ə-sis) cutaneous myiasis.

der•ma•to•my•o•ma (dur″mə-to-mi-o′mə) [*dermato-* + *myoma*] leiomyoma cutis.

der•ma•to•myo•si•tis (dur″mə-to-mi″ə-si′tis) [*dermato-* + *myositis*] a type of polymyositis with characteristic inflammatory skin changes, including the Gottron sign (discolored papules, especially on extensor surfaces such as the knees, elbows, and knuckles); poikiloderma; discolored eyelids and edema of the eyelids and periorbital tissue; and an erythematous rash on the forehead, neck, trunk, and arms.

der•ma•to•neu•rol•o•gy (dur″mə-to-noo̅-rol′ə-je) [*dermato-* + *neurology*] the study of the nerves of the skin in health and disease.

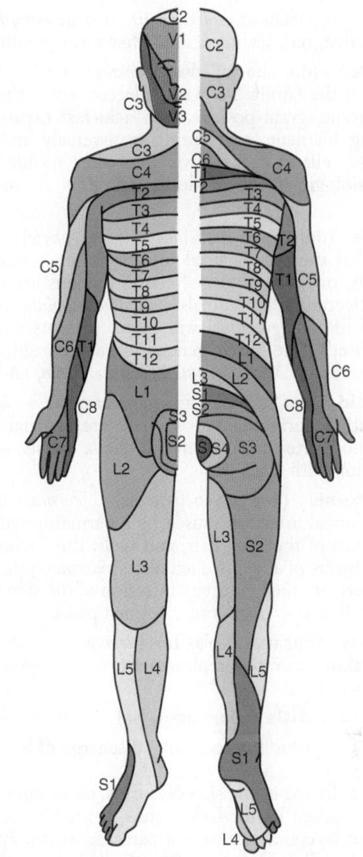

■ Anterior and posterior views of the dermatomes. Each segment is named for the principal spinal nerve serving it. *V,* trigeminal segments; *C,* cervical segments; *T,* thoracic segments; *L,* lumbar segments; *S,* sacral segments.

der•ma•to•oph•thal•mi•tis (dur″mə-to-of″thəl-mi′tis) inflammation of the skin and of the eye, such as the conjunctiva, cornea, and other structures.

Der•ma•top (dur′mə-top) trademark for preparations of prednicarbate.

der•ma•to•path•ia (dur″mə-to-path′e-ə) dermatosis.

d. pigmento′sa reticula′ris a rare autosomal dominant skin disorder caused by mutations in the *KRT14* gene (locus: 17q12-q21), which encodes keratin 14, a protein expressed in the basal layer of squamous strafied epithelium. It is characterized by generalized reticular hyperpigmentation, alopecia, and nail dystrophy.

der•ma•to•path•ic (dur″mə-to-path′ik) pertaining or attributable to disease of the skin; called also *dermopathic.*

der•ma•to•pa•thol•o•gy (dur″mə-to-pə-thol′ə-je) the pathology of the skin, including both anatomic pathology and pathologic histology.

der•ma•top•a•thy (dur″mə-top′ə-the) dermatosis.

Der•ma•toph•a•goi•des (dur″mə-tof″ə-goi′dēs) a genus of sarcoptiform mites, usually found on the skin of chickens.

D. fari′nae the house dust mite found in North America, which acts as an antigen and is a common cause of dust asthma.

D. pteronyssi′nus the house dust mite found in Europe, which acts as an antigen and is a common cause of dust asthma.

D. scheremetew′skyi a species that causes a mangelike inflammation.

der•ma•to•phar•ma•col•o•gy (dur″mə-to-fahr″mə-kol′ə-je) pharmacology as applied to dermatologic disorders.

Der•ma•to•phi•la•ceae (dur″mə-to-fi-la′se-e) a family of bacteria of the suborder Micrococcineae, order Actinomycetales, consisting of gram-positive aerobic microorganisms characterized by mycelial filaments or muriform thalli that divide transversely and in at least two longitudinal planes to form masses of coccoid or cuboid motile cells. Pathogenic organisms are included in the genera *Dermatophilus* and *Kytococcus.*

der•ma•to•phi•li•a•sis (dur″mə-to-fĭ-li′ə-sis) dermatophilosis.

der•ma•to•phi•lo•sis (dur″mə-to-fĭ-lo′sis) infection with *Dermatophilus congolensis,* seen in many different mammals. In humans it is characterized by nonpainful pustules on the hands and arms that later break down, forming shallow red ulcers that heal to leave scars. The sheep condition (also called *lumpy wool, proliferative dermatitis,* or *strawberry foot rot*) is characterized by exudative, red, scaling lesions that form pyramidal masses.

Der•ma•toph•i•lus (dur″mə-tof′ĭ-ləs) [*dermato-* + Gr. *philos* loving] a genus of bacteria of the family Dermatophilaceae, consisting of aerobic or facultatively anaerobic, gram-positive, non–acid-fast organisms that form mycelia containing filaments segmenting transversely and longitudinally to produce coccoid cells in packets, which become motile spores. *D. congolen′sis* is the etiologic agent of dermatophilosis in many species of mammals.

der•ma•to•phyte (dur′mə-to-fīt″) [*dermato-* + *-phyte*] any of various imperfect fungi that cause superficial infections on keratinized tissue of animals (skin, nails, or hair). Those affecting humans are called *anthropophilic,* and those affecting other animals are called *zoophilic.* Some fungi that are usually found in soil *(geophilic)* will infect patients who are weak or immunocompromised. The three genera usually considered to contain dermatophytic species are *Microsporum, Epidermophyton,* and *Trichophyton.*

der•ma•to•phy•tid (dur″mə-tof′ĭ-tid) [*dermatophyte* + *-id*] an id reaction associated with a dermatophytosis; these are associated with various types of lesions, most often vesicles on the hands, wrists, and sides of the fingers in association with tinea pedis.

der•ma•to•phy•to•sis (dur″mə-to-fi-to′sis) [*dermatophyte* + *-osis*] 1. any superficial fungal infection caused by a dermatophyte and involving the stratum corneum of the skin, hair, and nails; this includes onychomycosis and various forms of tinea. Called also *epidermomycosis* and *epidermophytosis.* 2. in veterinary medicine, any infection of the skin of an animal by a dermatophyte; called also *ringworm.* 3. tinea pedis.

der•ma•to•plas•ty (dur′mə-to-plas″te) [*dermato-* + *-plasty*] a plastic operation on the skin; operative replacement of destroyed or lost skin. dermatoplas′tic *adj*

der•ma•to•poly•neu•ri•tis (dur″mə-to-pol″e-noŏ-ri′tis) acrodynia.

der•ma•tor•rha•gia (dur″mə-to-ra′jə) discharge of blood into or from the skin.

d. parasi′tica a disease of the skin of horses, other equids, and cattle in Europe and Asia, marked by hard elevations formed by accumulations of blood between skin layers; the cause is a parasitic worm, *Parafilaria multipapillosa* (in equids) or *P. bovicola* (in cattle). Called also *summer bleeding.*

der•ma•tor•rhex•is (dur″mə-to-rek′sis) [*dermato-* + *-rrhexis*] rupture of the skin or its capillaries, as in Ehlers-Danlos syndrome.

der•ma•to•scle•ro•sis (dur″mə-to-sklə-ro′sis) scleroderma.

der•ma•tos•co•py (dur″mə-tos′kə-pe) epiluminescence microscopy.

der•ma•to•sis (dur″mə-to′sis) pl. *dermato′ses* [*dermat-* + *-osis*] any skin disease, especially one not characterized by inflammation.

acquired perforating d. general term for a group of dermatoses marked by umbilicated papules with a central keratotic plug, caused by the extrusion of connective tissue fibers through the epidermis. Most types occur in adults, especially in association with diabetes or renal insufficiency. Included are elastosis perforans serpiginosa, Kyrle disease, perforating folliculitis, and reactive perforating collagenosis.

acute febrile neutrophilic d. a type of neutrophilic dermatosis usually seen on the upper body of middle-aged women, characterized by one or more large, rapidly extending, erythematous, tender or painful plaques, with fever and dense infiltration of neutrophilic leukocytes in the upper and middle dermis. Called also *Sweet syndrome.*

arsenic d., arsenical d. the cutaneous manifestations of chronic arsenic poisoning, consisting of areas of hyperpigmentation and hypopigmentation, and arsenical keratosis that can progress to skin cancer.

ashy d. of Ramirez erythema dyschromicum perstans.

chronic bullous d. of childhood an autoimmune skin disorder seen in infants and children up to age 5, characterized by deposition of immunoglobulin A in lines along the dermoepidermal junction, forming vesicular bulbous lesions. See also *linear IgA d. of adulthood.* Called also *chronic bullous disease of childhood* and *linear IgA dermatosis of childhood.*

dermatolytic bullous d., dermolytic bullous d. epidermolysis bullosa dystrophica.

digitate d. small plaque parapsoriasis.

industrial d. occupational dermatitis.

juvenile plantar d. a skin condition seen in children, usually boys, consisting of inflammation of the sole of the foot and glazing of the skin, owing to friction and sweating inside shoes made of poorly ventilated synthetic material. Called also *dermatitis plantaris sicca.*

lichenoid d. any skin disorder characterized by lichenification, such as pigmented purpuric lichenoid dermatitis, lichen planus, or lichen sclerosus.

linear d. any skin disorder characterized by linear lesions, such as bullous pemphigoid, chronic bullous dermatosis of childhood, or linear IgA dermatosis of adulthood.

linear IgA d. see *linear IgA d. of adulthood* and *chronic bullous d. of childhood.*

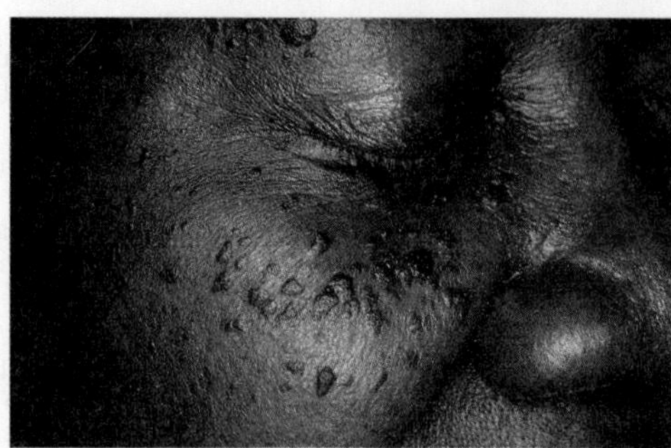

■ Dermatosis papulosa nigra.

linear IgA d. of adulthood an autoimmune skin disorder usually seen in adults over age 60, clinically resembling bullous pemphigoid. Characteristics include deposition of immunoglobulin A in lines along the dermoepidermal junction, forming vesicular bullous lesions. Cf. *chronic bullous dermatosis of childhood.*

linear IgA bullous d. see *linear IgA d. of adulthood* and *chronic bullous d. of childhood.*

linear IgA d. of childhood chronic bullous d. of childhood.

neutrophilic d's a group of skin disorders characterized by a neutrophilic infiltrate in the dermis without evidence of infection, with or without vasculitis. It includes acute febrile neutrophilic dermatosis, Behçet syndrome, bowel bypass syndrome, and pyoderma gangrenosum.

occupational d. see under *dermatitis.*

d. papulo′sa ni′gra a common, benign variant of seborrheic keratosis seen almost exclusively in persons of black African descent, characterized by small, pedunculated, pigmented papules on the cheeks or temples.

papulosquamous d's a group of skin conditions that are both papular and scaly, including psoriasis, parapsoriasis, lichen planus, pityriasis rosea, and seborrheic dermatitis.

pigmented purpuric d. chronic pigmented purpura.

pigmented purpuric lichenoid d. see under *dermatitis.*

precancerous d. any skin condition having a tendency to malignant change.

progressive pigmentary d., Schamberg d. Schamberg disease.

rheumatoid neutrophilic d. a rare type of neutrophilic dermatosis, seen in persons with severe rheumatoid arthritis, usually on the forearms or hands, consisting of erythematous urticarial papules and plaques that may ulcerate.

subcorneal pustular d. a superficial, pustular disorder with a chronic relapsing course, resembling dermatitis herpetiformis, and chiefly affecting women in middle life, with sterile pustular blebs in the subcorneal tissue of the epidermis on the trunk and in the major skin folds. Called also *Sneddon-Wilkinson disease.*

transient acantholytic d. a self-limited papulovesicular disease usually seen in middle-aged persons, most often on the trunk, with histologic changes resembling those of Darier disease or benign familial pemphigus. It is sometimes an epidermal reaction to actinic injury. Called also *Grover disease.*

ulcerative d. an infectious viral skin disease of sheep characterized by skin ulcers around the mouth, nose, external genitalia, and lower limbs; the genital ulcers are venereal in nature and may be so painful as to prevent copulation.

d. ve′getans a hereditary disease of young pigs characterized by raised skin lesions, abnormalities of the hooves, and pneumonitis.

der•ma•to•spa•rax•is (dur″mə-to-spə-rak′sis) [*dermato-* + Gr. *sparaxis* a tearing or mangling] 1. severe fragility of the skin, such as in the dermatosparaxis type of Ehlers-Danlos syndrome. 2. cutaneous asthenia (def. 1).

der•ma•to•ther•a•py (dur″mə-to-ther′ə-pe) [*dermato-* + *therapy*] treatment of the skin and its diseases.

der•ma•to•tro•pic (dur″mə-to-tro′pik) [*dermato-* + *-tropic*] preferentially infecting, infesting, or affecting the skin; said of certain microorganisms. Called also *dermotropic.*

der•ma•to•zo•on (dur″mə-to-zo′ən) [*dermato-* + Gr. *zōon* animal] any animal ectoparasite of the skin.

der•ma•to•zoo•no•sis (dur″mə-to-zo″o-no′sis) [*dermato-* + *zoonosis*] a skin disease caused by a dermatozoon.

der•mic (dur′mik) 1. cutaneous. 2. dermal (def. 1).

der•mis (dur′mis) [Gr. *derma* skin, hide] [TA] the layer of the skin deep to the epidermis, consisting of a dense bed of vascular connective tissue; it is divided into a papillary layer (TA, stratum papillare) and a reticular layer (TA, stratum reticulare). Called also *corium* [TA alternative].

papillary d. stratum papillare dermidis.

■ Dermographism.

reticular d. stratum reticulare dermidis.

derm(o)- see *dermat(o)-*.

der•mo•blast (dur′mo-blast) [*dermo-* + *-blast*] the part of the mesoblast that develops into the true skin or dermis.

der•mo•cy•ma (dur″mo-si′mə) endadelphos.

der•mo•cy•mus (dur″mo-si′məs) endadelphos.

der•mo•graph•ism (dur″mo-graf′iz-əm) a type of physical urticaria in which moderately firm stroking or scratching of the skin with a dull instrument produces a wheal with a red flare on each side. Called also *dermatographism.* dermograph′ic *adj*

black d. black or greenish streaking of the skin caused by deposit of fine metallic particles, such as those abraded from jewelry by dusting powders.

symptomatic d. a dermographic response in which wheals appear soon after stroking, mild scratching, or other friction.

white d. linear blanching of (usually erythematous) skin of persons with atopic dermatitis in response to firm stroking with a blunt instrument.

der•mo•hy•grom•e•ter (dur″mo-hi-grom′ə-tər) an instrument for measuring skin resistance without inducing a constant current into the skin.

der•moid (dur′moid) [*derm-* + *-oid*] 1. resembling skin. 2. dermoid cyst.

corneal d. a hairy tumorous growth on the cornea of certain mammals.

der•moid•ec•to•my (dur″moid-ek′tə-me) [*dermoid* + *-ectomy*] excision of a dermoid cyst.

der•mo•li•pec•to•my (dur″mo-lĭ-pek′tə-me) [*dermo* + *lipectomy*] resection of excess skin and fat, usually from the abdomen.

der•mo•li•po•ma (dur″mo-lĭ-po′mə) a congenital yellow fatty growth beneath the bulbar conjunctiva.

der•mol•y•sis (der-mol′ĭ-sis) dermatolysis.

transient bullous d. of newborn a rare form of dominant epidermolysis bullosa dystrophica that occurs in newborns but clears up around six months of age.

der•mom•e•ter (dər-mom′ə-tər) the instrument used in dermometry.

der•mom•e•try (dər-mom′ə-tre) [*dermo-* + *-metry*] the measurement of areas of skin resistance to a passage of direct electric current; these areas correspond to the areas of sensory loss.

der•mo•myo•tome (dur″mo-mi′o-tōm) [*dermo-* + *myo-* + *-tome*] all but the sclerotome of a mesodermal somite; the primordium of skeletal muscle and, perhaps, of dermis.

der•mo•ne•cro•sis (dur″mo-nə-kro′sis) necrosis of the skin, usually with sloughing. dermonecrot′ic *adj*

der•mo•path•ic (dur″mo-path′ik) dermatopathic.

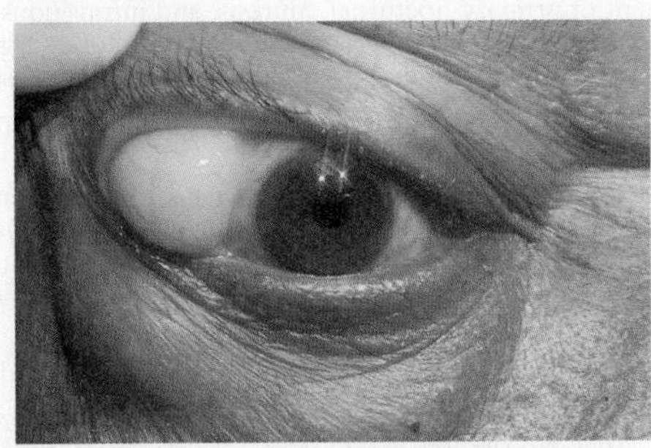

■ Dermolipoma.

der•mop•a•thy (dər-mop′ə-the) dermatosis.

diabetic d. cutaneous lesions on the shins, manifestations of diabetes mellitus, consisting of discolored, mildly ulcerated or cicatricial lesions; the cause is apparently a type of angiitis of small cutaneous blood vessels. Called also *shin spots.* The term is sometimes used more broadly to denote other cutaneous lesions of diabetes mellitus, such as bullosis diabeticorum and necrobiosis lipoidica diabeticorum.

Graves d., infiltrative d. pretibial myxedema.

nephrogenic fibrosing d. a fibrosing skin condition with nodules and plaques of induration, resembling scleroderma; most patients have renal insufficiency, but the exact etiology is unknown. Called also *nephrogenic systemic fibrosis.*

thyroid d. pretibial myxedema.

der•mo•plas•ty (dur′mo-plas″te) dermatoplasty.

der•mo•re•ac•tion (dur″mo-re-ak′shən) cutaneous reaction.

der•mos•co•py (dur-mos′kə-pe) epiluminescence microscopy.

der•mo•skel•e•ton (dur″mo-skel′ə-tən) exoskeleton.

der•mo•tox•in (dur′mo-tok″sin) a toxin produced by certain bacteria, especially staphylococci, which causes necrosis and other pathologic changes of the skin.

der•mo•tro•pic (dur″mo-tro′pik) dermatotropic.

der•mo•vas•cu•lar (dur″mo-vas′ku-lər) [*dermo-* + *vascular*] pertaining to the blood vessels of the skin.

der(o)- [Gr. *derē* neck] a combining form denoting relationship to the neck.

der•o•did•y•mus (der″o-did′ə-məs) dicephalus.

der•ren•ga•de•ra (da-rāng-gah-da′rah) [Sp. "crookedness" or "lameness"] murrina.

der•ren•gue (da-rāng′ga) [Sp., from *derrengar* to dislocate the hip] a fatal neuropathy of cattle seen in El Salvador following ingestion of the plant *Melochia pyramidata*, characterized by weakness and paralysis starting in the hindlimbs and progressing forward.

der•ri•en•gue (dar-yāng′ga) [Sp., from *derrengar* to dislocate the hip] a type of rabies, usually the paralytic form, transmitted by vampire bats in tropical parts of the Americas; it is usually seen in cattle, but infected bats may attack other domestic animals and even humans.

Der•ris (der′is) a genus of woody vines of the family Leguminosae, native to Australia and other islands of the southern Pacific. *D. ellip′tica* yields the toxic insecticide rotenone.

der•ris (der′is) 1. any plant of the genus *Derris.* 2. the dried roots and rhizomes of *Derris elliptica*, a source of the toxic insecticide rotenone.

DES diethylstilbestrol.

de•sal•i•na•tion (de-sal″ĭ-na′shən) [*de-* + *sal*] the removal of salt from a substance.

de•sal•i•va•tion (de-sal″ĭ-va′shən) the depriving of saliva.

des•am•i•do-NAD⁺ (des-ə-me′do) deaminated NAD⁺, an intermediate in the biosynthesis of NAD⁺. It is nicotinate ribonucleotide coupled in pyrophosphate linkage to adenosine monophosphate.

De Sanc•tis-Cac•chi•o•ne syndrome (da sahngk′tis kah″ke-o′na) [Carlo *De Sanctis*, Italian psychiatrist, 20th century; Aldo *Cacchione*, Italian psychiatrist, 20th century] see under *syndrome.*

de•sat•ur•ase (de-sach′ə-rās) an enzyme that, complexed with cytochrome b_5 reductase and cytochrome b_5, catalyzes the desaturation of fatty acids, e.g., stearoyl-CoA desaturase.

de•sat•u•ra•tion (de-sach″ə-ra′shən) the process of converting a saturated compound to one that is unsaturated, such as the introduction of a double bond between carbon atoms of a fatty acid.

De•sault bandage (apparatus), sign (də-so′) [Pierre Joseph *Desault*, French surgeon, 1744–1795] see under *bandage* and *sign.*

Des•cartes' law (da-kahrts′) [René *Descartes*, French mathematician and philosopher, 1596–1650] see under *law.*

Des•ce•met membrane (des-ə-ma′) [Jean *Descemet*, French anatomist, 1732–1810] see *lamina limitans posterior corneae.*

des•ce•me•ti•tis (des″ə-mə-ti′tis) inflammation of the Descemet membrane.

des•ce•me•to•cele (des″ə-met′o-sēl) [*Descemet membrane* + *-cele*[1]] herniation of the Descemet membrane.

des•cen•dens (de-sen′dənz) [L.] descending; a general term denoting a descending structure or part.

d. cervica′lis, d. cer′vicis radix inferior ansae cervicalis.

d. hypoglos′si radix superior ansae cervicalis.

des•cend•ing (de-send′ing) [L. *descendere* to go down] extending inferiorly.

des•cen•sus (de-sen′səs) pl. *descen′sus* [L.] the process of descending or falling.

d. tes′tis the descent of the testis from its fetal position in the abdominal cavity to the scrotum; the final descent normally occurs during the twenty-eighth week of fetal life and is essential to spermatogenesis.

d. u′teri uterine prolapse.

de•scent (də-sent′) [L. *descendere* to go down] the act or instance of descending.

perineal d. downward displacement of the perineum when a person is defecating.

x d. see under *wave.*

y d. see under *wave.*

Des•champs compressor, needle (da-shah′) [Joseph François Louis *Deschamps*, French surgeon, 1740–1824] see under *compressor* and *needle.*

de•sen•si•ti•za•tion (de-sen″sĭ-tĭ-za′shən) 1. the prevention or reduction of immediate hypersensitivity reactions by administration of graded doses of allergen; called also *hyposensitization* and *immunotherapy.* 2. in behavior therapy, the treatment of phobias and related disorders by intentionally exposing the patient, in imagination or in reality, to a hierarchy of emotionally distressing stimuli. Common forms of desensitization include flooding, implosion, and systematic desensitization (qq.v.).

systematic d. a form of desensitization therapy in which the patient is taught to relax and is then exposed, in imagination, to the mildest or least anxiety-provoking stimuli first; as treatment progresses she or he is exposed progressively to stronger anxiety-provoking stimuli until the most extreme stimuli can be tolerated.

de•sen•si•tize (de-sen′sĭ-tīz) 1. to deprive of sensation; paralysis of a sensory nerve by section or blocking. 2. to carry out desensitization.

de•ser•pi•dine (de-sur′pĭ-dēn) an alkaloid of *Rauwolfia canescens*, used as an antihypertensive, administered orally.

Des•fer•al (des′fər-əl) trademark for a preparation of deferoxamine mesylate.

des•fer•ri•ox•amine (des-fer″e-oks′ə-mēn) deferoxamine.

des•flu•rane (des-floo′rān) [USP] an inhalational anesthetic used for induction and maintenance of general anesthesia.

des•hy•dre•mia (des″hi-dre′me-ə) [*de-* + *hydremia*] deficiency of the watery element of the blood, with resultant hemoconcentration.

des•ic•cant (des′ĭ-kənt) 1. promoting dryness; causing to dry up. 2. an agent that promotes dryness. Called also *exsiccant.*

des•ic•cate (des′ĭ-kāt) [L. *desiccare* to dry up] to render thoroughly dry.

des•ic•ca•tion (des″ĭ-ka′shən) the act of drying; cf. *dehydration* and *xerosis.*

electric d. the treatment of a tumor or other disease by drying up the part by the application of a monopolar electric current (short spark) of high frequency and high tension.

des•ic•ca•tive (des′ĭ-ka″tiv) causing to dry up.

des•ic•ca•tor (des′ĭ-ka″tər) a closed vessel for containing apparatus or chemicals that are to be kept free from moisture.

de•sip•ra•mine hy•dro•chlo•ride (də-sip′rə-mēn) [USP] a metabolite of imipramine: a tricyclic antidepressant of the dibenzazepine class; used also in the treatment of anxiety, chronic pain, attention-deficit/hyperactivity disorder, cataplexy associated with narcolepsy, and bulimia nervosa. Administered orally.

-desis [Gr. *desis* "a binding together"] a word termination denoting a binding or fusion.

Des•jar•dins point (da″zhahr-dă′) [Abel *Desjardins*, French surgeon, early 20th century] see under *point.*

des•lan•o•side (des-lan′o-sīd) [USP] a digitalis glycoside derived from lanatoside C, having the same actions and uses as digitalis; administered intramuscularly or intravenously. Called also *deacetyllanatoside C.*

des•lor•at•a•dine (des″lə-rat′ə-dēn) a nonsedating antihistamine (H_1 receptor antagonist) used for the treatment of allergic rhinitis and chronic idiopathic urticaria, administered orally.

des•mal•gia (des-mal′jə) [*desmo-* + *-algia*] pain in a ligament; called also *desmodynia.*

des•mec•ta•sis (des-mek′tə-sis) [*desmo-* + *ektasis*] the stretching of a ligament.

des•mep•i•the•li•um (des-mep″ĭ-the′le-əm) [*desmo-* + *epithelium*] the endothelial lining of blood vessels, lymphatics, and synovial membranes.

des•mid (des′mid) unicellular, free-floating, aquatic algae characterized by symmetrical, curved, spiny or lacey bodies with a median constriction dividing the cell into two equal halves.

des•min (dez′min) a protein that polymerizes to form the intermediate filaments of muscle cells; it is used as an immunohistochemical marker of these cells. See also *desmin filaments.*

des•mi•og•nath•us (des″me-o-nath′əs) [Gr. *desmios* binding + *gnathos* jaw] a fetus with a parasitic head attached to its jaw or neck; called also *dicephalus parasiticus.*

des•mi•tis (des-mi′tis) [*desmo-* + *-itis*] inflammation of a ligament.

desm(o)- [Gr. *desmos* band, ligament] a combining form denoting relationship to a band, bond, or ligament.

des•mo•col•lin (dez″mo-kol′in) any of a family of cadherins found in desmosomes of epithelial and cardiac cells. Cf. *desmoglein.*

des•mo•cra•ni•um (des″mo-kra′ne-əm) [*desmo-* + *cranium*] [TA] the mass of mesoderm at the cranial end of the notochord in the early embryo, forming the earliest stage of the cranium.

des•mo•cyte (des′mo-sīt) [*desmo-* + *-cyte*] fibroblast.

des•mo•cy•to•ma (des″mo-si-to′mə) fibroma.

des•mo•don•ti•um (des″mo-don′she-əm) [*desmo-* + Gr. *odous* tooth] [TA] periodontal ligament.

Des•mo•dus (dez-mo′dəs) a genus of vampire bats of South America, Central America, Mexico, and the West Indies. *D. rotun′dus* is the most common species.

des•mo•dyn•ia (des″mo-din′e-ə) [*desm-* + *-odynia*] desmalgia.

des•mog•e•nous (des-moj′ə-nəs) [*desmo-* + *-genous*] of ligamentous origin.

des•mog•le•in (dez-mog′le-in) any of a family of cadherins found in desmosomes; they are the target of autoantibodies in pemphigus foliaceus and pemphigus vulgaris. Cf. *desmocollin.*

des•mog•ra•phy (des-mog′rə-fe) [*desmo-* + *-graphy*] a description of the ligaments.

des•mo•he•mo•blast (dez″mo-he′mo-blast) [*desmo-* + *hemoblast*] mesenchyme.

des•moid (dez′moid) [*desm-* + *-oid*] 1. fibrous or fibroid. 2. see under *tumor.*

periosteal d. a benign tumorlike fibrous proliferation of the periosteum, occurring particularly in the medial femoral condyle in adolescents, and often disappearing spontaneously.

des•mo•lase (dez′mo-lās) a nonspecific term for an enzyme that catalyzes the cleavage of a carbon-carbon bond in a substrate with formation of two products by a process other than hydrolysis, i.e., an oxidoreductase, a lyase, or a transferase. Used especially for enzymes involved in synthesis of steroid hormones.

17,20-d. 17α-hydroxyprogesterone aldolase.

20,22-d. cholesterol monooxygenase (side-chain-cleaving).

des•mol•o•gy (des-mol′ə-je) [*desmo-* + *-logy*] the study of ligaments, their structure and function.

des•mo•ma (dez-mo′mə) [*desm-* + *-oma*] desmoid tumor.

des•mop•a•thy (des-mop′ə-the) [*desmo-* + *-pathy*] any disease of the ligaments.

des•mo•plak•in (dez″mo-plak′in) any of a group of intracellular proteins that attach desmosomal cadherins to the intermediate filaments.

des•mo•pla•sia (des″mo-pla′zhə) the formation and development of fibrous tissue.

des•mo•plas•tic (des″mo-plas′tik) [*desmo-* + *-plastic*] characterized by or causing desmoplasia.

des•mo•pres•sin ace•tate (des″mo-pres′in) a potent synthetic analogue of vasopressin, used intranasally, orally, intramuscularly, or intravenously as an antidiuretic in the prophylaxis and treatment of central diabetes insipidus and in the treatment of temporary polyuria and polydipsia secondary to trauma to or surgery in the pituitary region, intranasally or orally in the treatment of primary nocturnal enuresis, and intravenously or intranasally to increase coagulation factor VIII activity before surgical procedures in patients with hemophilia A and von Willebrand disease.

des•mor•rhex•is (des″mo-rek′sis) [*desmo-* + *-rrhexis*] rupture of a ligament.

des•mose (des′mōs) [Gr. *desmos* band, ligament] a filament, fibril, or strand connecting intranuclear *(centrodesmose)* or extranuclear *(paradesmose)* basal bodies during mitosis; seen especially in certain protozoa (e.g., *Dientamoeba fragilis*). The terms *desmose, centrodesmose,* and *paradesmose* have been used synonymously by some authorities.

des•mo•sine (des′mo-sēn) one of two unusual amino acids found in elastin, the other being isodesmosine.

des•mo•sis (des-mo′sis) [*desm-* + *-osis*] a disease of the connective tissue.

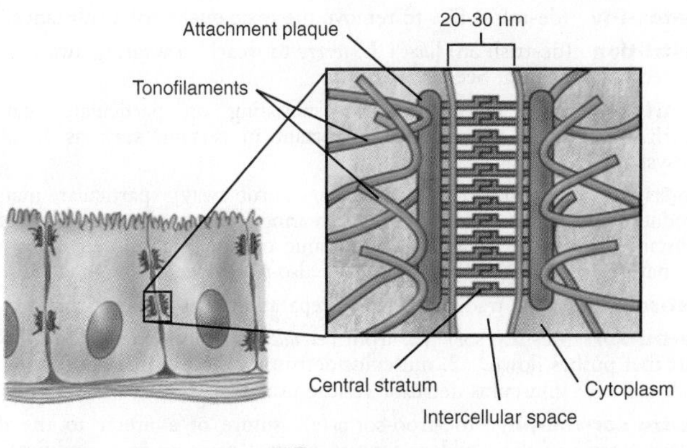

■ Desmosome.

des•mo•some (dez′mo-sōm) [*desmo-* + *-some*] a type of adhesive junction that links intermediate filaments and cell membranes within and between cells by homophilic interactions between cadherins (desmogleins and desmocollins); it is a small, discrete, circular, dense body abundant in epithelial cells but occurring also in other cell types. It consists of local differentiations of the apposing cell membranes, with a dense cytoplasmic plaque underlying each membrane, toward which numerous tonofilaments converge; a dense lamina may occur within the intercellular gap. Called also *macula adherens.* **desmoso′mal** *adj*

spot d. desmosome.

des•mos•ter•ol (des-mos′tər-ol) the immediate precursor of cholesterol in the biosynthetic pathway, 24-dehydrocholesterol; normally not present in the blood in amounts that can be detected by ordinary means.

des•mot•o•my (des-mot′o-me) [*desmo-* + *-tomy*] the cutting or division of ligaments.

Des•o•gen (des′o-jən) trademark for a combination preparation of desogestrel and ethinyl estradiol.

des•o•ges•trel (des″o-jes′trəl) a progestational agent having little androgenic activity; used in combination with an estrogen component as an oral contraceptive.

deso•leo•lec•i•thin (des-o″le-o-les′ĭ-thin) one of the components, the other being oleic acid, into which lecithin is split by the action of cobra venom.

des•o•nide (des′ə-nīd) a low potency synthetic corticosteroid used topically for the relief of inflammation and pruritus in corticosteroid-responsive dermatoses.

de•sorb (de-sorb′) to remove a substance from the state of absorption or adsorption.

de•sorp•tion (de-sorp′shən) the process of being desorbed.

Des•Owen (des-o′wən) trademark for preparations of desonide.

des•ox•i•met•a•sone (des-ok″sĭ-met′ə-sōn) [USP] a synthetic corticosteroid used topically for the relief of inflammation and pruritus in corticosteroid-responsive dermatoses.

desoxy- deoxy-.

des•oxy•cor•ti•cos•ter•one (des-ok″se-kor″tĭ-kos′tər-ōn) 11-deoxycorticosterone.

d. acetate [USP] the acetate salt of 11-deoxycorticosterone; used as replacement therapy to treat adrenocortical insufficiency; administered by intramuscular injection.

d. pivalate [USP] the pivalate salt of 11-deoxycorticosterone, used as replacement therapy to treat adrenocortical insufficiency; administered by intramuscular injection.

des•oxy•cor•tone (des-ok″se-kor′tōn) 11-deoxycorticosterone.

Des•ox•yn (des-ok′sən) trademark for preparations of methamphetamine hydrochloride.

de•spe•ci•ate (de-spe′she-āt) to undergo despeciation; to subject to (as by chemical treatment), or to undergo, loss of species antigenic characteristics.

de•spe•ci•a•tion (de-spe″she-a′shən) deviation from or loss of species characteristics.

de•spe•ci•fi•ca•tion (de-spes″ĭ-fĭ-ka′shən) the process of reducing the antigenicity of heterologous antisera used therapeutically, by treating them with enzymes such as pepsin to remove the antigenic Fc regions of the immunoglobulin molecules. This leaves $F(ab')_2$ fragments which contain both antigen binding regions of each immunoglobulin molecule.

d'Es•pine sign (des-pēn′) [Adolphe *d'Espine,* French physician, 1846–1930] see under *sign.*

de•squa•ma•tion (des″kwə-ma′shən) [*de-* + *squama*] the shedding (exfoliation) of epithelial elements, chiefly of the skin, in scales or sheets. **desquam′ative, desquam′atory** *adj*

furfuraceous d. desquamation in branlike scales.

lamellar d. of the newborn see under *exfoliation.*

dest. [L.] destil′la (distill); destilla′tus (distilled).

destil. [L.] destil′la (distill).

de•sulf•hy•drase (de″səlf-hi′drās) a term used in the recommended and trivial names of some carbon-sulfur lyases [EC 4.4], which catalyze the removal of hydrogen sulfide or substituted hydrogen sulfide from a compound.

De•sul•fo•mo•nas (de-sul″fo-mo′nəs) [*de-* + *sulfo-* + Gr. *monas* unit, from *monos* single] a former genus of bacteria whose members are now classified in *Desulfovibrio.*

De•sul•fo•vib•rio (de-sul″fo-vib′re-o) [*de-* + *sulfo-* + *vibrio*] a genus of gram-negative, non–spore-forming, anaerobic bacteria of the family Desulfovibrionaceae, consisting of actively motile curved rods that reduce sulfur compounds to hydrogen sulfide; they are found in animal intestines and feces, fresh and salt water, soil, and mud. The type species is *D. desulfu′ricans.*

D. pi′ger a species that is part of the normal flora of the oral cavity of many animals, as well as their respiratory, intestinal, and urogenital tracts. Formerly called *Desulfomonas pigra.*

De•sul•fo•vib•ri•o•na•ceae (de-sul″fo-vib″re-o-na′se-e) a family of mesophilic, rod-shaped, anaerobic bacteria of the order Desulfovibrionales; it includes the genera *Bilophila, Desulfovibrio,* and *Lawsonia.*

De•sul•fo•vib•ri•o•na•les (de-sul″fo-vib″re-o-na′lēz) an order of bacteria of the class Deltaproteobacteria, phylum Proteobacteria, consisting of anaerobic, chemo-organotrophic or chemolithotrophic, curved or rod-shaped cells, often motile; most species reduce sulfate to sulfide.

de•sul•fur•ase (de-sul′fər-ās) desulfhydrase.

des•ven•la•fax•ine suc•ci•nate (des″ven-lə-fak′sēn) a serotonin-norepinephrine reuptake inhibitor used as an antidepressant; administered orally.

de•syn•chro•ni•za•tion (de-sing″krə-nĭ-za′shən) a condition in which two or more rhythmic variables that were previously in synchronism with each other have lost that relationship.

de•syn•chro•ny (de-sing′krə-ne) a condition in which environmental cues and patterns, such as sleeping and eating, conflict with an individual's existing pattern; one type is jet lag. **desyn′chronous** *adj*

Des•yr•el (des′ir-əl) trademark for a preparation of trazodone hydrochloride.

DET diethyltryptamine.

Det. [L.] de′tur (let it be given).

de•tach•ment (de-tach′mənt) [Fr. *détacher* to unfasten; to separate] the condition of being unfastened, disconnected, or separated.

exudative retinal d. retinal detachment caused by pressure from fluid that has collected within the retina.

d. of retina, retinal d. separation of the inner (neural) layers of the retina from the pigmented layer; called also *amotio retinae.*

rhegmatogenous retinal d. retinal detachment caused by a hole or tear in the retina.

serous retinal d. retinal detachment with fluid between the separated layers.

traction retinal d. retinal detachment caused by traction exerted by a pathologic condition that alters the vitreous body or some other nearby structure, such as hemorrhage, inflammation, or trauma.

d. of vitreous, vitreous d. separation of the vitreous body from its attachments, especially from the retina.

de•tec•tion (de-tek′shən) discovery of the presence or existence of something.

coincidence d. in positron emission tomography, collimation in detection of ionization events, limiting recognition to simultaneous events occurring in opposite directions, which occurs when the emitted positron collides with an electron, simultaneously emitting two photons in opposing directions.

de•tec•tor (de-tek′tər) a device by which the presence of something, or the existence of a certain condition, is discovered.

lie d. polygraph.

radiation d. any device for converting radiant energy to a form more readily observable.

de•ter•gent (de-tur′jənt) [L. *detergere* to cleanse] 1. purifying, cleansing. 2. an agent which purifies or cleanses. 3. in biochemistry, any of a class of agents structurally consisting of a nonpolar hydrocarbon

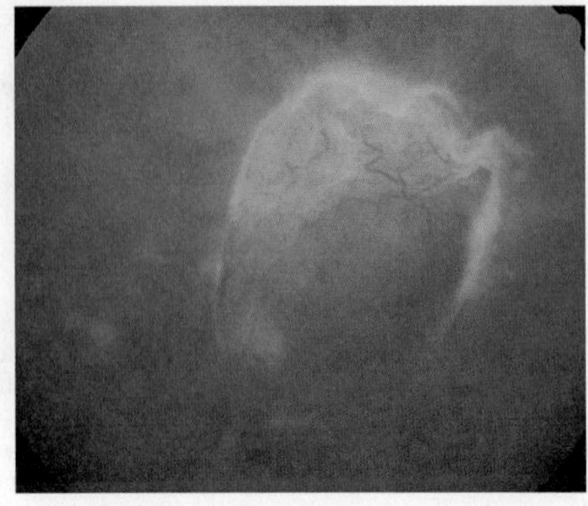

■ Severe tractional retinal detachment with vitreous hemorrhage secondary to proliferative diabetic retinopathy.

chain attached to a polar head group, which reduce the surface tension of water, emulsify, and aid in the solubilization of soil.

de·ter·mi·nant (de-tur′mĭ-nənt) [L. *determinare* to bound, limit, or fix] a factor that establishes the nature of an entity or event.

allotypic d. allotope.

antigenic d. a site on the surface of an antigen molecule to which a single antibody molecule binds; generally an antigen has several or many different antigenic determinants and reacts with antibodies of many different specificities. Called also *epitope*.

hidden d. an antigenic determinant located in an unexposed region of a molecule so that it is prevented from interacting with receptors on lymphocytes, or with antibody molecules, and is unable to induce an immune response unless exposed by conformational change or stereochemical alteration of the molecule. Such hidden determinants may appear following stereochemical alterations of molecular structure.

immunogenic d. the part of an immunogenic molecule that interacts with a helper T cell in triggering antibody production, as opposed to the antigenic determinant or hapten, which interacts with B cells.

sequential d. a polymeric antigenic determinant with antigenic specificity determined by monomer sequence rather than monomer composition.

de·ter·mi·na·tion (de-tur′mĭ-na′shən) establishment of the exact nature of an entity or event.

embryonic d. the loss of pluripotency in any part of an embryo and its start on the way toward an unalterable fate.

sex d. the process by which the sex of an organism is fixed; it is associated, in humans, with the SRY (sex-determining region Y) gene, located at Yp11.3, which when present acts as a switch to initiate the process of testis formation.

de·ter·min·er (de-tur′mĭ-nər) determinant.

de·ter·min·ism (de-tur′mĭ-niz-əm) the theory that all phenomena are the result of antecedent conditions, nothing occurs by chance, and there is no free will.

psychic d. the concept, originated by Freud, that mental events do not occur by chance but have their antecedent mental causes, that even accidents, slips of the tongue, or whims commonly felt to be inexplicable result from unconscious mental processes.

de To·ni-Fan·co·ni syndrome (da to′ne fahn-ko′ne) [Giovanni *de Toni*, Italian pediatrician, 1896–1973; Guido *Fanconi*, Swiss physician, 1892–1979] *Fanconi syndrome* (def. 2), see under *syndrome*.

Det. in dup., Det. in 2 plo. [L.] de′tur in du′plo (let twice as much be given).

de·to·mi·dine (de-to′mĭ-dēn) an analgesic and sedative used in horses.

de·tor·sion (de-tor′shən) 1. the correction of a twisting or deformity, as the reduction of torsion of the testis. 2. a deficiency in a normal twisting as may occur in the early development of the heart.

de·tox·i·cate (de-tok′sĭ-kāt) detoxify.

de·tox·i·ca·tion (de-tok″sĭ-ka′shən) detoxification.

de·tox·i·fi·ca·tion (de-tok″sĭ-fĭ-ka′shən) 1. reduction of the toxic properties of poisons. 2. treatment designed to free an addict from a drug habit. 3. in naturopathy, the elimination of toxic substances from the body, either by metabolic change or by excretion; the process may be assisted therapeutically by fasting, saunas, or hydrotherapy.

metabolic d. reduction of the toxic properties of a substance by chemical changes induced in the body, producing a compound which is less poisonous or is more readily eliminated.

de·tox·i·fy (de-tok′sĭ-fi) to remove the toxic quality of a substance.

de·tri·tion (de-trish′ən) [*de-* + L. *terere* to wear] a wearing away, as of the teeth, by friction. See also *abrasion*.

de·tri·tiv·o·rous (de″trĭ-tiv′ə-rəs) subsisting on particulate matter (detritus), a mode of existence important in certain, such as aquatic, ecosystems.

de·tri·tus (de-tri′təs) [L., from *deterere* to rub away] particulate matter produced by or remaining after the wearing away or disintegration of a substance or tissue; designated as organic or nonorganic, depending on the nature of the original material. See also *biodetritus*.

Det·rol (det′rol) trademark for a preparation of tolterodine tartrate.

de·tru·sor (de-troo′sər) [L., from *detrudere* to push down] 1. a body part that pushes down. 2. musculus detrusor vesicae urinariae.

d. uri′nae musculus detrusor vesicae urinariae.

de·tru·sor·rha·phy (de-troo-sor′ə-fe) suture of a ureter to the detrusor muscle of the bladder, done to prevent prolapse in a modification of the Lich-Gregoir technique.

D. et s. [L.] de′tur et signe′tur (let it be given and labeled).

de·tu·ba·tion (de″too-ba′shən) extubation.

de·tu·mes·cence (de″too-mes′əns) [*de-* + *tumescence*] the subsidence of swelling, or turgor.

Deur·sil (de-ur′sil) trademark for a preparation of ursodiol.

deu·tan (doo′tən) 1. pertaining to deuteranomaly or deuteranopia. 2. a person with deuteranomaly or deuteranopia.

deu·ter·anom·al (doo″tər-ə-nom′əl) a person with deuteranomaly.

deu·ter·anom·a·ly (doo″tər-ə-nom′ə-le) [*deuter-* + *anomaly*] a type of anomalous trichromatic vision in which the second, green-sensitive, cones have decreased sensitivity; therefore a greater than normal proportion of thallium green light to lithium red light is required to match a fixed sodium yellow light. Deuteranomaly is an X-linked trait, affects about 5 per cent of white males and 0.25 per cent of females, and is the most common color vision deficiency. **deuteranom′alous** *adj*

deu·ter·an·ope (doo′tər-ə-nōp″) an individual exhibiting deuteranopia.

deu·ter·an·o·pia (doo″tər-ə-no′pe-ə) [*deuter-* + *an-*[1] + *-opia*] a dichromasy characterized by retention of the sensory mechanism for two hues only (blue and yellow) of the normal 4-primary quota, and lacking that for red and green and their derivatives, without loss of luminance or shift or shortening of the spectrum. It is an X-linked trait occurring in about 1 per cent of males, but only rarely in females. **deuteranop′ic** *adj*

deu·ter·an·op·sia (doo″tər-ə-nop′se-ə) deuteranopia.

deu·te·ri·on (doo-te′re-on) deuteron.

deu·te·ri·um (D, ^{2}H) (doo-tēr′e-əm) [Gr. *deuteros* second] the mass two isotope of hydrogen (q.v.). It is available as a gas or as heavy water and has been used in metabolic studies; called also *heavy hydrogen*. Cf. *protium* and *tritium*.

d. oxide heavy water.

deuter(o)- [Gr. *deuteros* second] a combining form meaning second. Also, *deut(o)-*.

deu·tero·co·ni·di·um (doo″tər-o-ko-nid′e-əm) [*deutero-* + *conidium*] a reproductive element derived from a hemispore.

deu·tero·my·cete (doo″tər-o-mi′sēt) imperfect fungus.

Deu·tero·my·ce·tes (doo″tər-o-mi-se′tēz) name given to Deuteromycota when it is considered a class.

Deu·tero·my·co·ta (doo″tər-o-mi-ko′tə) the imperfect fungi (Fungi Imperfecti), a large, heterogeneous group ordinarily treated as a phylum, distinguished by having no known sexual stage; in many cases the sexual stage is later discovered and can be shown to be an ascomycete or basidiomycete. This group includes many pathogenic fungi. Deuteromycota are subclassified into form-classes, form-orders, and so on. For some fungi the name of the asexual stage is retained even though the sexual stage has been identified, so that the fungus has a different name for each stage of its life cycle; in such cases the name of the sexual stage is used to refer to the fungus in all its states. Some authorities consider this group a subphylum of the Eumycota and call it Deuteromycotina; others consider it a class and call it Deuteromycetes.

Deu·tero·my·co·ti·na (doo″tər-o-mi″ko-ti′nə) name given to Deuteromycota when it is considered a subphylum of Eumycota.

deu·ter·on (doo′tər-on) the nucleus of deuterium, or heavy hydrogen; deuterons are used as bombing particles for nuclear disintegration.

deu·tero·path·ic (doo″tər-o-path′ik) occurring secondarily to some other disease.

deu•ter•op•a•thy (doo″tər-op′ə-the) [*deutero-* + *-pathy*] a disease that is secondary to another disease.

deu•tero•pine (doo″tər-o′pēn) an alkaloid from opium.

deu•tero•plasm (doo′tər-o-plaz″əm) [*deutero-* + *-plasm*] the passive or inactive materials in protoplasm, especially reserve foodstuffs, such as yolk.

deu•tero•stome (doo′tər-o-stōm″) an animal belonging to the Deuterostomia.

Deu•tero•sto•mia (doo″tər-o-sto′me-ə) [*deutero-* + Gr. *stoma* mouth + *-ia*] a series of the Eucoelomata, including the echinoderms, hemichordates, and chordates, in all of which the site of the blastopore is posterior—far from the mouth, which forms a new structure unrelated to the blastopore. Cf. *Protostomia.*

deu•tero•to•cia (doo″tər-o-to′se-ə) [*deutero-* + Gr. *tokos* birth] asexual reproduction in which the female produces offspring of both sexes.

deu•ter•ot•o•ky (doo″tər-ot′ə-ke) deuterotocia.

deu•thy•alo•some (doo″thi-al′ə-sōm) [*deuto-* + *hyalo-* + *-some*] the matured nucleus of an oocyte.

deut(o)- see *deuter(o)-*.

deu•ton (doo′ton) deuteron.

deu•to•neph•ron (doo″to-nef′ron) [*deuto-* + Gr. *nephron*] mesonephros.

deu•to•plasm (doo′to-plaz″əm) deuteroplasm.

deu•to•plas•mol•y•sis (doo″to-plaz-mol′ə-sis) destruction or disintegration of deutoplasm.

Deutsch•län•der disease (doich′len-dər) [Karl Ernst Wilhelm *Deutschländer*, German surgeon, 1872–1942] 1. see under *disease.* 2. march foot.

de•val•u•a•tion (de-val″u-a′shən) a defense mechanism in which emotional conflict or stressors are faced by attributing exaggerated negative qualities to the self or to others.

de•vas•cu•lar•iza•tion (de-vas″ku-lər-ĭ-za′shən) interruption of the circulation of blood to a part caused by obstruction or destruction of the blood vessels supplying it. See also *ischemia.*

de•vel•op•ment (de-vel′əp-mənt) the process of growth and differentiation. **developmen′tal** *adj*

arrested d. cessation of the development process at some stage prior to its normal completion.

cognitive d. the development of intelligence, conscious thought, and problem solving ability that begins in infancy.

mosaic d. the development of an embryo in a fixed, unalterable way, local regions being independent portions of a mosaic whole.

psychosexual d. 1. a general term for the developing sexuality of the individual as affected by biological, cultural, and emotional influences from prenatal life onward through the life cycle. 2. in psychoanalysis, libidinal maturation from infancy through adulthood (in classic psychoanalysis including the oral, anal, and genital stages). One schema is Erikson's eight stages of development.

psychosocial d. the development of the personality, including the acquisition of social attitudes and skills, from infancy through maturity.

regulative d. the development of an embryo, the determination of the various organs and parts being gradually attained through the action of inductors.

de•vi•ant (de′ve-ənt) [L. *deviare* to turn aside] 1. varying from a determinable standard. 2. an individual with characteristics varying from what is considered normal or standard.

sexual d. an individual exhibiting sexual deviation.

de•vi•a•tion (de″ve-a′shən) [L. *deviare* to turn aside] 1. a turning away from the regular standard or course. 2. in ophthalmology, strabismus. 3. in statistics, the difference between a sample value and the mean.

animal d. the attracting of zoophilous mosquitos from human beings by the proximity of animals preferred by the insects.

axis d. alteration in the direction of the mean QRS complex vector, determined from the electrocardiogram; it may be due to alteration in the anatomical position of the heart or to any of a variety of disorders such as ventricular hypertrophy or bundle branch block. Relative to the hexaxial reference system (q.v.), a normal axis is −30° to 90°; right axis deviation is 90° to 180°; left axis deviation is −30° to −90°; and −90° to 180° is an indeterminate axis.

complement d. inhibition of complement fixation or complement-mediated immune hemolysis in the presence of excess antibody. Called also *Neisser-Wechsberg phenomenon.*

conjugate d. the deflection of two similar parts, as the eyes when turned in the same direction at the same time.

Hering-Hellebrand d. the amount of deviation between any point on the Vieth-Müller horopter and the frontoparallel plane passing through the point of fixation.

immune d. modification of the immune response to an antigen by previous inoculation of the same antigen.

latent d. heterophoria.

d. to the left shift to the left.

left axis d. (LAD) see *axis d.*

manifest d. strabismus.

minimum d. the smallest deflection of a ray of light that can be produced by a given prism.

population standard d. standard d.

primary d. deviation of the visual axis of the squinting eye in strabismus when the sound eye fixates.

radial d. a hand deformity sometimes seen in rheumatoid arthritis, in which the fingers are displaced to the radial side. Arthritic hands may be splinted into this position to counteract ulnar deviation. Called also *radial drift.*

d. to the right shift to the right.

right axis d. (RAD) see *axis d.*

sample standard d. an estimate of the population standard deviation, usually determined (from a sample of size n) by dividing the sum of the squared deviations from the sample mean by $n-1$ and taking the square root; $n-1$ is used (rather than n) in order to obtain an unbiased estimate of the population variance. Symbol s.

secondary d. deviation of the visual axis of the sound eye in strabismus when the squinting eye fixates.

sexual d. sexual behavior or fantasy outside that which is morally, biologically, or legally sanctioned, often specifically one of the paraphilias.

skew d. downward and inward rotation of the eye on the side of the cerebellar lesion and upward and outward deviation on the opposite side. Called also *Hertwig-Magendie phenomenon, Magendie sign,* and *Magendie-Hertwig sign.*

spiral d. of the penis corkscrew penis.

squint d. squint angle; see under *angle.*

standard d. (SD) in statistics a measure of the amount by which each value deviates from the mean; equal to the square root of the variance, i.e., the square root of the average of the squared deviations from the mean. It is the most commonly used measure of dispersion of statistical data. Called also *population standard d.*. Symbol σ. See figure at *normal distribution,* and see also *sample standard d.*

strabismic d. deviation of the visual axis of an eye in strabismus.

ulnar d. a hand deformity, seen in chronic rheumatoid arthritis and lupus erythematosus, in which the swelling of the metacarpophalangeal joints causes the fingers to become displaced to the ulnar side. Called also *ulnar drift* and *ulnar drift deformity.* Cf. *radial d.*

De•vic disease (də-vēk′) [Eugène *Devic*, French physician, 1869–1930] neuromyelitis optica.

de•vice (də-vīs′) something contrived for a specific purpose.

assistive listening d's devices other than hearing aids that help the deaf to hear.

biventricular assist d. (BVAD) a ventricular assist device with the combined functions of both left and right ventricular assist devices.

central-bearing d. a device that provides a central point of bearing, or support, between upper and lower occlusion rims, consisting of a contacting point attached to one occlusion rim and a plate that provides the surface on which the bearing point rests or moves.

central-bearing tracing d. a device for determining the central bearing or support between maxillary and mandibular occlusion rims or dentures.

contraceptive d. a device used to prevent conception, such as a barrier contraceptive, an intrauterine device, or a means of preventing ovulation (e.g., birth control pill).

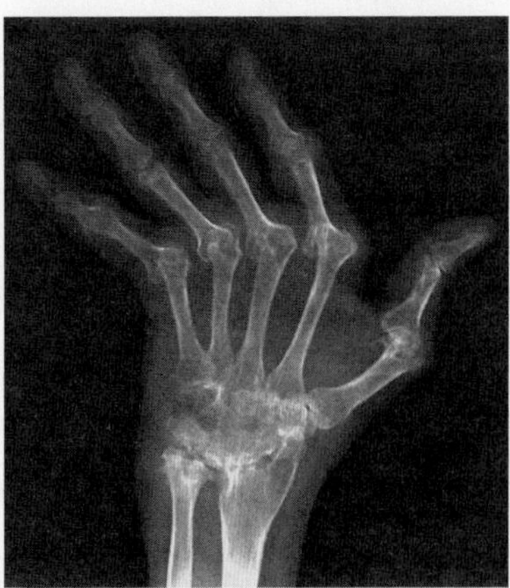

■ Ulnar deviation in rheumatoid arthritis.

halo d. a cervical orthosis that provides maximal rigidity of the cervical spine, consisting of a metal or plastic halo attached to the upper skull by tongs or pins and linked by upright bars to a rigid jacket on the chest. Called also *halo orthosis* or *ring*.

intrauterine d. (IUD), intrauterine contraceptive d. a plastic or metallic device inserted into the uterus to prevent pregnancy.

left ventricular assist d. (LVAD) a ventricular assist device capable of augmenting left ventricular function; its pump has an afferent conduit attached to the left atrium or left ventricular apex and an efferent conduit attached to the ascending aorta. Implanted systems are sometimes called *left ventricular assist systems*. Cf. *biventricular assist d.* and *right ventricular assist d.*

orthotic d. orthosis.

prosthetic d. prosthesis.

right ventricular assist d. (RVAD) a ventricular assist device capable of augmenting right ventricular function; its pump has an afferent conduit attached to the right atrium and an efferent conduit attached to the pulmonary artery. Cf. *biventricular assist d.* and *left ventricular assist d.*

terminal d. the end piece of a prosthesis for an upper or lower limb, which may have varying degrees of functionality; for the upper limb they may be hooktype mechanisms or cosmetic hands, and for the lower limb they may or may not resemble human feet.

ventricular assist d. (VAD) a device that aids circulation by augmenting function of the left ventricle, the right ventricle, or both; it consists of one or two implanted or extracorporeal pumps with afferent and efferent conduits attached so as to provide mechanically assisted pulsatile blood flow. See *left ventricular assist d.*, *right ventricular assist d.*, and *biventricular assist d.*

de•vi•om•e•ter (de″ve-om′ə-tər) strabismometer.

de•vis•cer•a•tion (de-vis″ər-a′shən) evisceration (def. 1).

de•vi•tal•iza•tion (de-vi″təl-ĭ-za′shən) the deprivation of vitality or life, as of a tissue.

pulp d. the destruction of vitality of the pulp of a tooth.

de•vi•tal•ize (de-vi′təl-īz) [*de-* + *vital* + *-ize*] to deprive of vitality or of life.

de•vit•ri•fi•ca•tion (de-vit″rĭ-fĭ-ka′shən) [*de-* + *vitrification*] the changing of a supercooled liquid such as glass into a crystalline state.

dew•claw (doo′klaw) a vestigial digit or claw, found in the feet of dogs, cats, and ruminants.

dew•lap (doo′lap) a heavy fold of skin on the ventral aspect of the neck in animals.

de•worm•ing (de-wərm′ing) the destruction and removal of worms from an infected person or animal; cf. *anthelmintic*.

DEXA dual energy x-ray absorptiometry.

Dex•a•cen (dek′sə-sen″) trademark for preparations of dexamethasone; *Dexacen-4* is dexamethasone sodium phosphate, and *Dexacen LA-8* is dexamethasone acetate.

dex•a•meth•a•sone (dek″sə-meth′ə-sōn) [USP] a synthetic glucocorticoid, 25 times as potent as cortisol; used topically on the skin and conjunctiva as an antiinflammatory and administered orally in replacement therapy for adrenocortical insufficiency, as an antiinflammatory and immunosuppressant in a wide variety of disorders, and as an antiemetic in cancer chemotherapy. It is also used as a diagnostic aid in the detection of Cushing syndrome in the high-dose and low-dose dexamethasone suppression tests (see under *test*).

d. acetate [USP] an ester of dexamethasone, having actions similar to those of the base and used as an antiinflammatory and immunosuppressant; administered by intra-arterial, intramuscular, intralesional, or soft-tissue injection.

d. sodium phosphate [USP] an ester of dexamethasone, having actions and uses similar to those of the base; administered by intra-articular, soft tissue, intravenous, or intramuscular injection, or applied topically to the skin or conjunctiva. It is also used as an antiinflammatory by topical application to the ear canal and intranasally.

Dex•a•sone (dek′sə-sōn″) trademark for preparations of dexamethasone.

dex•brom•phen•ir•a•mine (deks″brom-fən-ir′ə-mēn) the dextrorotatory isomer of brompheniramine, having similar actions as an antihistamine but approximately twice the activity by weight.

d. maleate [USP] the maleate salt of dexbrompheniramine, administered orally in the treatment of allergic rhinitis, allergic conjunctivitis, and cutaneous manifestations of allergic reactions. It is also an ingredient in some cold and cough preparations.

dex•chlor•phen•ir•a•mine (deks″klor-fən-ir′ə-mēn) the dextrorotatory isomer of chlorpheniramine, having similar actions as an antihistamine but approximately twice the activity by weight.

d. maleate [USP] the maleate salt of dexchlorpheniramine, administered orally in the treatment of allergic rhinitis, allergic conjunctivitis, and cutaneous manifestations of allergic reactions. It is also an ingredient in some cold and cough preparations.

Dex•e•drine (dek′sə-drēn) trademark for preparations of dextroamphetamine sulfate.

dex•et•i•mide (dek-set′ĭ-mīd) an anticholinergic which has been used as an antiparkinsonian agent.

Dex•Fer•rum (deks-fer′əm) trademark for a preparation of iron dextran.

dex•io•car•dia (dek″se-o-kahr′de-ə) dextrocardia.

dex•io•tro•pic (dek″se-o-tro′pik) [Gr. *dexios* on the right + *-tropic*] wound in a spiral from left to right, as a shell.

dex•lan•so•pra•zole (dex″lan-so′prə-zōl) a proton pump inhibitor used for the treatment of erosive esophagitis and heartburn associated with gastroesophageal reflux disease.

dex•med•e•to•mi•dine hy•dro•chlo•ride (deks″med-ə-to′mĭ-dēn) an imidazole derivative that is a selective α_2-adrenergic receptor agonist; administered intravenously as a sedative for patients in intensive care units.

dex•meth•yl•phen•i•date hy•dro•chlo•ride (deks″meth-əl-fen′ĭ-dāt) a central nervous system stimulant thought to block reuptake of norepinephrine and dopamine into the presynaptic neuron, increasing their release into the extraneuronal space; used in the treatment of attention-deficit/hyperactivity disorder, administered orally.

Dex•on (dek′son) trademark for a preparation of polyglycolic acid, a polymer used to make nonirritating absorbable sutures.

Dex•one (dek′sōn) trademark for preparations of dexamethasone.

Dex•pak (deks′pak) trademark for a preparation of dexamethasone.

dex•pan•the•nol (deks-pan′thə-nol) the D(+) form of panthenol (pantothenyl alcohol), the alcoholic analogue of pantothenic acid. It is claimed to be a precursor of coenzyme A, and is administered intravenously or intramuscularly to increase peristalsis in atony and paralysis of the lower intestine and orally to help relieve gas retention and abdominal distention in certain conditions. It is also applied topically to the skin to stimulate healing of various dermatologic lesions such as burns, infected wounds, eczema, diaper rash, etc.

dex•ra•zox•ane (deks″ra-zok′sān) a derivative of ethylenediaminetetraacetic acid (EDTA) used as a cardioprotectant in chemotherapy to counteract doxorubicin-induced cardiomyopathy; administered intravenously.

dex•ter (dek′stər) [L.] [TA] right: a term denoting the right-hand one of two similar structures, or the one situated on the right side of the body.

dex•trad (dek′strad) toward the right side.

dex•tral (dek′strəl) 1. pertaining to the right side. 2. right-handed.

dex•tral•i•ty (dek-stral′ĭ-te) [*dexter*] the preferential use, in voluntary motor acts, of the right member of the major paired organs of the body, as the right ear, eye, hand, or foot. See also *laterality* and *handedness*.

dex•tran (dek′strən) a high-molecular-weight polymer of D-glucose, produced by enzymes (glycosyltransferases) on the cell surface of certain lactic acid bacteria. Dextrans, formed from sucrose by bacteria in the mouth, adhere to the tooth surfaces and produce dental plaque, a major cause of dental caries. Uniform molecular weight dextrans from *Leuconostoc mesenteroides* preparations are used as plasma volume expanders. Specific preparations are designated, according to their average molecular weight in thousands, as *dextran 40 [USP]*, *dextran 70 [USP]*, and so on. Commercial preparations in bead form are also used in gel-filtration chromatography.

dex•trano•mer (dek-stran′o-mər) a preparation of highly hydrophilic dextran polymers occurring as small beads, used in débridement of secreting wounds, such as venous stasis ulcers; the sterilized beads are poured over secreting wounds to absorb wound exudates and prevent crust formation.

dex•trates (dek′strāts) a tablet binder and diluent, composed of a mixture of sugars (approximately 92 per cent dextrose monohydrate and 8 per cent high saccharides; dextrose equivalent is 95 to 97 per cent) resulting from the controlled enzymatic hydrolysis of starch.

dex•trin (dek′strin) [L. *dexter* right] 1. any one, or the mixture, of the intermediate polysaccharides formed during the hydrolysis of starch, which are dextrorotatory, soluble in water, and precipitable in alcohol. They may be linear or branched, and include the amylodextrins, erythrodextrins, and achroodextrins. 2. [NF] an official preparation, from starch by heating; used as a suspending and viscosity-increasing agent, tablet binder, and tablet and capsule diluent.

limit d. any of the small, nonreducing polymers remaining after exhaustive digestion of starch or glycogen with enzymes that catalyze the removal of terminal sugar residues but which cannot hydrolyze the linkages of branch points.

dex•trin•ase (dek′strin-ās) any enzyme that catalyzes the hydrolysis of dextrins.

α-dex•trin•ase (dek′strin-ās) an enzyme that catalyzes the hydrolysis of both α-1,6 and α-1,4 bonds in linear and branched oligoglucosides and maltose and isomaltose. It occurs on the brush border of the intestinal mucosa, completes the digestion of starch or glycogen to glucose, and is present as a complex with sucrase; absence of the enzyme complex activity, called sucrase-isomaltase deficiency, is a form of disaccharide intolerance. Called also *isomaltase* and *limit dextrinase*. In EC nomenclature called *oligo-1,6-glucosidase*.

dex•trin•ize (dek′strin-īz) to convert into dextrin.

dex•tri•no•sis (dek″strĭ-no′sis) accumulation in the tissues of an abnormal polysaccharide.

limit d. glycogen storage disease, type III.

dex•trin•uria (dek″strĭ-nu′re-ə) the presence of dextrin in the urine.

dextr(o)- [L. *dexter* right] 1. a combining form denoting relationship to the right. 2. chemical prefix used to designate the dextrorotatory enantiomorph of a substance; opposed to *levo-*. Symbol (+)- (formerly *d-*; sometimes Δ).

dex•tro•am•phet•amine (dek″stro-am-fet′ə-mēn) the dextrorotatory isomer of amphetamine, which has substantially more central nervous system–stimulating effect than the racemic form. Abuse of this drug may lead to dependence; see *amphetamine*.

d. sulfate [USP] the sulfate salt of dextroamphetamine, used orally in the treatment of narcolepsy and attention-deficit/hyperactivity disorder; formerly used as an anorectic in the treatment of obesity.

dex•tro•car•dia (dek″stro-kahr′de-ə) [*dextro-* + *cardia*] location of the heart in the right hemithorax, with the apex pointing to the right, occurring with transposition (situs inversus) of the abdominal viscera, or without such transposition.

isolated d. mirror-image transposition of the heart without accompanying alteration of the abdominal viscera.

mirror-image d. location of the heart in the right side of the chest, the atria being transposed and the right ventricle lying anteriorly and to the left of the left ventricle, usually associated with complete situs inversus.

secondary d. displacement of the heart to the right as a result of disease of the pleura, diaphragm, or lungs.

dex•tro•cer•e•bral (dek″stro-ser′ə-brəl) [*dextro-* + *cerebral*] pertaining to or situated in the right cerebral hemisphere.

dex•tro•cli•na•tion (dek″stro-klĭ-na′shən) [*dextro-* + L. *clinatus* leaning] rotation of the upper poles of the vertical meridians of the two eyes to the right; called also *dextrocycloduction* and *dextrotorsion*. Cf. *levoclination*.

dex•tro•com•pound (dek″stro-kom′pound) a dextrorotatory compound.

dex•troc•u•lar (dek-strok′u-lər) right eyed; affected with dextrocularity.

dex•troc•u•lar•i•ty (dek″strok-u-lar′ĭ-te) [*dextro-* + *oculus*] the condition of having greater visual power in the right eye and, therefore, using it more than the left.

dex•tro•cy•clo•duc•tion (dek″stro-si″klo-duk′shən) dextroclination.

dex•tro•duc•tion (dek″stro-duk′shən) [*dextro-* + *duction*] movement of either eye to the right.

dex•tro•gas•tria (dek″stro-gas′tre-ə) [*dextro-* + *gastr-* + *-ia*] displacement of the stomach to the right, either simple displacement or situs inversus.

dex•tro•gy•ral (dek″stro-ji′rəl) [*dextro-* + *gyrare* to turn] dextrorotatory.

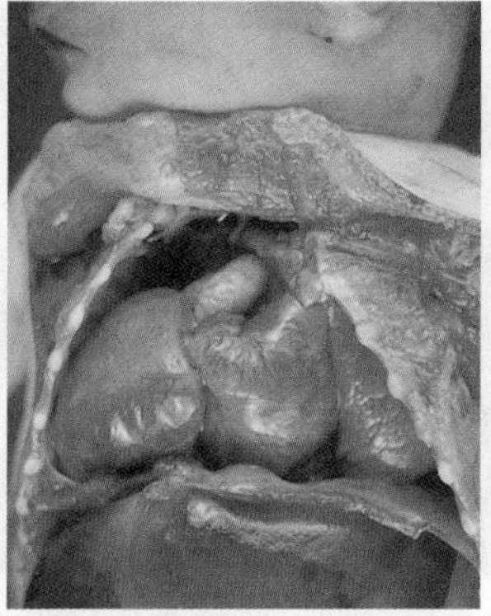

■ Dextrocardia in an infant.

dex•tro•gy•ra•tion (dek″stro-ji-ra′shən) [*dextro-* + *gyration*] a turning to the right or motion to the right; said of movements of the eye and of the plane of polarization.

dex•tro•man•u•al (dek″stro-man′u-əl) [*dextro-* + *manual*] right-handed.

dex•tro•meth•or•phan (dek″stro-məth-or′fan) [USP] a nonopioid, synthetic derivative of morphine that acts on the cough center to suppress the cough reflex, used as an antitussive; administered orally.

d. hydrobromide [USP] the monohydrated hydrobromide salt of dextromethorphan, having the same action and use as the base; administered orally.

d. polistirex sulfonated styrene-divinylbenzene copolymer complex with dextromethorphan, administered orally as an extended-release antitussive.

dex•trop•e•dal (dek-strop′ə-dəl) [*dextro-* + *pedal*] using the right foot in preference to the left.

dex•tro•po•si•tion (dek″stro-pə-zish′ən) displacement to the right.

dex•tro•pro•poxy•phene (dek″stro-pro-pok′sə-fēn) INN and BAN for *propoxyphene*.

dex•tro•ro•ta•ry (dek″stro-ro′tə-re) dextrorotatory.

dex•tro•ro•ta•to•ry (dek″stro-ro′tə-tor-e) [*dextro-* + *rotatory*] turning the plane of polarization, or rays of light, to the right; called also *dextrogyral*.

dex•trose (dek′strōs) chemical name: D-glucose monohydrate. A monosaccharide known as *glucose* (q.v.) in biochemistry and physiology. The official preparation [USP] is usually obtained by the hydrolysis of starch; it is used chiefly as a fluid and nutrient replenisher, usually administered by intravenous infusion. It is also used as a diuretic and alone or in combination with other agents for various other clinical purposes.

dex•tro•sin•is•tral (dek″stro-sin′is-trəl) [*dextro-* + *sinistral*] 1. extending from right to left. 2. a person naturally left-handed but trained to use the right hand in certain activities.

Dex•tro•stat (dek′stro-stat) trademark for a preparation of dextroamphetamine sulfate.

Dex•tro•stix (dek′stro-stiks) trademark for a reagent strip designed for determination of blood glucose levels with the use of fingertip venous blood.

dex•tros•uria (dek″strōs-u′re-ə) glycosuria.

dex•tro•tor•sion (dek″stro-tor′shən) dextroclination.

dex•tro•tro•pic (dek″stro-tro′pik) [*dextro-* + *-tropic*] turning to the right; see also *dexiotropic*.

dex•tro•ver•sion (dek″stro-vur′zhən) [*dextro-* + *version*] 1. version to the right side; especially movement of the eyes to the right. 2. location of the heart in the right hemithorax, the left ventricle remaining on the left as in the normal position, but lying anterior to the right ventricle.

dex•tro•vert•ed (dek″stro-vərt′əd) turned to the right.

dez•o•cine (dez′o-sēn) an opioid analgesic, having both agonist and antagonist activity, used for the short-term relief of pain; administered intramuscularly or intravenously.

DFDT a powerful insecticide, difluoro-diphenyl-trichloroethane.

DFP diisopropyl fluorophosphate.

DFT defibrillation threshold.

dG deoxyguanosine.

DGC dystrophin-glycoprotein complex.

dGDP deoxyguanosine diphosphate.

dGMP deoxyguanosine monophosphate.

dGTP deoxyguanosine triphosphate.

DH delayed hypersensitivity.

DHA docosahexaenoic acid; 2,8-dihydroxyadenine.

DHAD mitoxantrone hydrochloride (dihydroanthracenedione dihydrochloride).

DHAP a cancer chemotherapy regimen consisting of dexamethasone, ara-C (cytarabine), and Platinol (cisplatin).

dha•tu (thah′too) [Sanskrit "to support"] according to ayurveda, the seven physical interconnected body tissues that are produced from metabolism and energy and anchor mind and spirit: plasma, blood, muscle, fat, bone, marrow, and reproductive tissue. Each tissue, though separate, is formed from another and depends upon its predecessor for its health.

D.H.E. 45 trademark for a preparation of dihydroergotamine mesylate.

DHEA dehydroepiandrosterone.

d'He•relle phenomenon (də-rel′) [Félix Hubert *d'Herelle*, Canadian bacteriologist in France, 1873–1949] Twort-d'Herelle phenomenon; see under *phenomenon*.

DHF dihydrofolate or dihydrofolic acid.

DHFR dihydrofolate reductase.

DHg Doctor of Hygiene.

DHom Doctor of Homeopathic Medicine.

DHPG ganciclovir (9-[(1,3-dihydroxy-2-propoxy)methyl] guanine); 3,4-dihydroxyphenylglycol.

DHPR 6,7-dihydropteridine reductase.

DHS dehydrated hereditary stomatocytosis.

DHT[1] dihydrotestosterone.

DHT[2] trademark for preparations of dihydrotachysterol.

dhur·rin (doo′rin) a cyanogenetic glycoside from sorghum which hydrolyzes into glucose, a substituted benzaldehyde, and hydrocyanic acid.

DHy Doctor of Hygiene.

di- [Gr. *dis* twice] a prefix meaning twice. In chemical nomenclature, the use of *di-* is preferred to the use of *bi-* (q.v.).

dia- [Gr. *dia* through] a prefix meaning through, between, apart, across, or completely.

Dia·Be·ta (di-ə-ba′tə) trademark for a preparation of glyburide.

di·a·be·tes (di″ə-be′tēz) [Gr. *diabētēs* a siphon, from *dia* through + *bainein* to go] 1. any of various disorders characterized by polyuria. 2. d. mellitus.

adult-onset d. mellitus type 2 d. mellitus.

alloxan d. an animal model for diabetes mellitus; administration of alloxan produces selective destruction of the beta cells of the pancreas, causing hyperglycemia and ketoacidosis.

brittle d. type 1 diabetes mellitus that is characterized by wide, unpredictable fluctuations of blood glucose values and is difficult to control.

bronze d., bronzed d. hemochromatosis.

central d. insipidus diabetes insipidus due to injury of the neurohypophysial system, with a deficient quantity of vasopressin being released or produced, causing failure of renal tubular reabsorption of water. It may be inherited, acquired, or idiopathic. Called also *pituitary d. insipidus.*

chemical d. former name for *impaired glucose tolerance.*

gestational d., gestational d. mellitus (GDM) diabetes mellitus with onset or first recognition during pregnancy; it does not include diabetics who become pregnant or women who become lactosuric.

growth-onset d. mellitus type 1 d. mellitus.

d. insi′pidus any of several types of polyuria in which the volume of urine exceeds 3 liters per day, causing dehydration and great thirst, as well as sometimes emaciation and great hunger. The underlying cause may be hormonal *(central d. insipidus)* or renal *(nephrogenic d. insipidus).*

insulin-dependent d. mellitus (IDD, IDDM) type 1 d. mellitus.

juvenile d. mellitus, juvenile-onset d. mellitus type 1 d. mellitus.

ketosis-prone d. mellitus type 1 d. mellitus.

ketosis-resistant d. mellitus type 2 d. mellitus.

latent d. former name for *impaired glucose tolerance.*

lipoatrophic d. total lipodystrophy.

malnutrition-related d. mellitus (MRDM) a rare type of diabetes mellitus associated with chronic malnutrition and characterized by beta-cell failure, insulinopenia, insulin resistance, and moderate to severe hyperglycemia, but without ketosis. Called also *tropical* or *tropical pancreatic d. mellitus.*

maturity-onset d. mellitus type 2 d. mellitus.

maturity-onset d. of youth, maturity-onset d. of the young (MODY) an autosomal dominant variety of type 2 diabetes mellitus, classified into several types on the basis of the mutation involved, characterized by onset in late adolescence or early adulthood.

d. melli′tus (DM) a chronic syndrome of impaired carbohydrate, protein, and fat metabolism owing to insufficient secretion of insulin or to target tissue insulin resistance. It occurs in two major forms: *type 1 d. mellitus* and *type 2 d. mellitus,* which differ in etiology, pathology, genetics, age of onset, and treatment.

mitochondrial d. a rare form of maternally transmitted type 2 diabetes mellitus, often accompanied by sensorineural deafness, caused by any of several mutations in genes of mitochondrial DNA.

nephrogenic d. insipidus diabetes insipidus caused by failure of the renal tubules to reabsorb water in response to antidiuretic hormone, without disturbance in the renal filtration and solute excretion rates; characterized by polyuria, extreme thirst, growth retardation, and developmental delay. The condition does not respond to exogenous vasopressin. It may be inherited as an X-linked trait or be acquired as a result of drug therapy or systemic disease.

non–insulin-dependent d. mellitus (NIDDM, NIDD) type 2 d. mellitus.

pituitary d. insipidus central d. insipidus.

posttransplant d. glucose intolerance or overt hypoglycemia that first appears after an organ transplant; some cases are steroid diabetes caused by use of steroid immunosuppressive agents.

preclinical d. former name for *impaired glucose tolerance.*

puncture d. diabetes produced in an experimental animal by puncturing the floor of the fourth ventricle in the medulla oblongata; see *Bernard puncture,* under *puncture.*

renal d. see under *glycosuria.*

steroid d., steroidogenic d. glucose intolerance or overt hyperglycemia induced by glucocorticoids or estrogens; it is due in part to target tissue insulin resistance and is characterized by a relatively low incidence of microvascular sequelae.

subclinical d. former name for *impaired glucose tolerance.*

thiazide d. glucose intolerance or overt hyperglycemia induced by thiazide diuretics, which inhibit insulin secretion, possibly through thiazide-induced hypokalemia.

tropical d. mellitus, tropical pancreatic d. mellitus malnutrition-associated d. mellitus.

Type I d. mellitus type 1 d. mellitus.

type 1 d. mellitus (T1DM) one of the two major types of diabetes mellitus: an autoimmune disease that results in the destruction beta cells of the pancreas, leading to loss of the ability to secrete insulin. It is characterized by abrupt onset of symptoms, insulinopenia, and dependence on exogenous insulin to sustain life; peak age of onset is 12 years, although onset can be at any age. It is probably caused by a combination of factors, including viral infection and genetic and autoimmune factors; islet cell antibodies are usually detectable at diagnosis. When it is inadequately controlled, lack of insulin causes hyperglycemia, protein wasting, and production of ketone bodies owing to increased fat metabolism, and the hyperglycemia leads to overflow glycosuria, osmotic diuresis, hyperosmolarity, dehydration, and diabetic ketoacidosis. It is accompanied by angiopathy of blood vessels, particularly the small ones *(microangiopathy),* which affects the retinas, kidneys, and basement membrane of arterioles throughout the body. Other symptoms include polyuria, polydipsia, polyphagia, weight loss, paresthesias, blurred vision, and irritability; if untreated, diabetic ketoacidosis progresses to nausea and vomiting, stupor, and potentially fatal hyperosmolar coma (diabetic coma). Called also *insulin-dependent, juvenile, juvenile-onset,* and *Type I d. mellitus.*

Type II d. mellitus type 2 d. mellitus.

type 2 d. mellitus (T2DM) one of the two major types of diabetes mellitus, characterized by peak age of onset between 50 and 60 years, gradual onset with few symptoms of metabolic disturbance (glycosuria and its consequences), and no need for exogenous insulin; dietary control with or without oral hypoglycemic is usually effective. Obesity and genetic factors may also be present. Diagnosis is based on laboratory tests indicating glucose intolerance. Basal insulin secretion is maintained at normal or reduced levels, but insulin release in response to a glucose load is delayed or reduced. Defective glucose receptors on the beta cells of the pancreas may be involved. It is often accompanied by disease of various sizes of blood vessels, particularly the large ones, which leads to premature atherosclerosis with myocardial infarction or stroke syndrome. Called also *adult-onset, maturity-onset, non–insulin-dependent,* and *Type II d. mellitus.*

di·a·bet·ic (di″ə-bet′ik) 1. pertaining to or affected with diabetes. 2. a person with diabetes.

di·a·be·tid (di″ə-be′tid) diabetic dermopathy.

di·a·be·to·gen·ic (di″ə-bet″o-jen′ik) [*diabetes* + *-genic*] producing diabetes.

di·a·be·tog·e·nous (di″ə-be-toj′ə-nəs) produced by diabetes.

di·a·be·tol·o·gist (di″ə-be-tol′ə-jist) a specialist in diabetology.

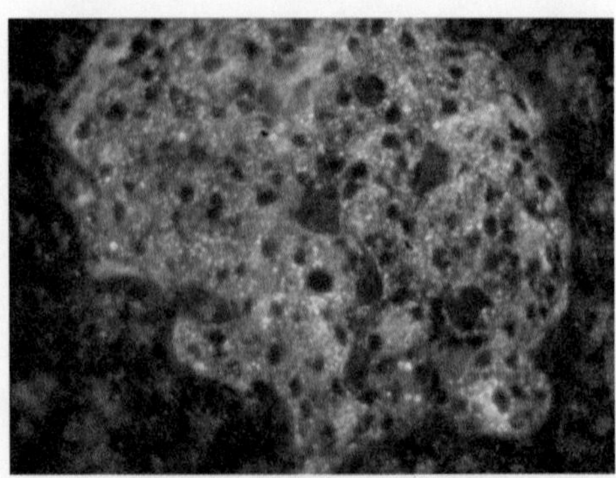

■ Fluorescein-labeled anti-islet autoantibodies in islet cells, characteristic of type 1 diabetes mellitus.

di·a·be·tol·o·gy (di″ə-be-tol′ə-je) the study of diabetes and its cause and control.

Di·ab·i·nese (di-ab′ĭ-nēs) trademark for a preparation of chlorpropamide.

di·a·bro·sis (di″ə-bro′sis) [*dia-* + Gr. *brōsis* eating] perforation resulting from a corrosive process, such as a perforating ulcer.

di·a·brot·ic (di″ə-brot′ik) [Gr. *diabrōtikos*] 1. ulcerative; caustic. 2. a corrosive or escharotic agent.

di·ac·e·tate (di-as′ə-tāt) acetoacetate.

di·ac·e·te·mia (di-as″ə-te′me-ə) the presence of acetoacetic acid (diacetic acid) in the blood.

di·a·ce·tic ac·id (di″ə-se′tik) acetoacetic acid.

di·ac·e·ton·uria (di-as″ə-to-nu′re-ə) diaceturia.

di·a·ce·tox·y·scir·pe·nol (di-as″ə-tok″se-sur′pə-nol) a trichothecene mycotoxin produced by species of *Fusarium* that contaminate grain and other foodstuffs, causing fusariotoxicosis and hemorrhaging in livestock.

di·ac·et·uria (di-as″ə-tu′re-ə) ketonuria involving the excretion of acetoacetic acid (diacetic acid) in the urine.

di·ac·e·tyl (di-as′ə-təl) a yellow liquid, 2,3-butane-dione, having the odor of butter.

d. peroxide acetyl peroxide.

di·ac·e·tyl·mor·phine (di″ə-se″təl-mor′fēn) heroin; a white, bitterish, crystalline powder, the diacetic acid ester of morphine, formerly used as an analgesic and narcotic. Because it is highly addictive, the importation of heroin and its salts into the United States, as well as its use in medicine, is illegal. Called also *acetomorphine* and *diamorphine*.

Di·a·chlo·rus (di-ə-klor′əs) a genus of South American biting flies of the family Tabanidae.

di·ac·id (di-as′id) [*di-* + *acid*] having two replaceable hydrogen atoms; a dibasic acid, having the acid activity of two molecules of a monobasic acid.

di·ac·la·sis (di-ak′lə-sis) [*dia-* + Gr. *klasis* fracture] osteoclasis.

di·ac·ri·nous (di-ak′rĭ-nəs) [Gr. *diakrinein* to separate] giving off secretion directly, as from a filter; said of gland cells, as those of the kidney. Opposed to *ptyocrinous*.

di·ac·ri·sis (di-ak′rĭ-sis) [Gr. *diakrisis* separation] 1. diagnosis. 2. a change in the character of secretions during an illness. 3. a disease marked by a morbid state of the secretions.

di·a·crit·ic (di″ə-krit′ik) [*dia-* + Gr. *krinein* to judge] distinguishing; diagnostic.

di·ac·tin·ic (di″ak-tin′ik) transmitting chemically active rays.

di·ac·tin·ism (di-ak′tin-izəm) [*dia-* + *actinism*] the property of transmitting chemically active rays.

di·acyl·glyc·er·ol (DAG) (di-a″səl-glis′ər-ol) a diester of glycerol in which two fatty acids are linked to its hydroxyl groups, usually at positions 1 and 2. Diacylglycerols are triglyceride and phospholipid degradation products and are second messengers in calcium-mediated responses to hormones, activating protein kinase C isozymes.

di·ac·yl·glyc·er·ol *O*-ac·yl·trans·fer·ase (di-a″səl-glis′ər-ol a″səl-trans′fər-ās) [EC 2.3.1.20] an enzyme of the transferase class that catalyzes the transfer of an acyl group from acyl CoA to a diglyceride, forming a triglyceride. Called also *diglyceride acyltransferase*.

di·ac·yl·glyc·er·ol ki·nase (di-a″səl-glis′ər-ol ki′nās) [EC 2.7.1.107] an enzyme of the transferase class that catalyzes the phosphorylation of a diacylglycerol to form a phosphatidate, using ATP as a phosphate donor. Called also *diglyceride kinase*.

Di·ad·e·ma (di″ade′ə) a genus of sea urchins. *D. seto′sum* is the black sea urchin, a venomous species.

di·ad·o·cho·ci·ne·sia (di-ad″ə-ko-sĭ-ne′zhə) diadochokinesia.

di·ad·o·cho·ki·ne·sia (di-ad″ə-ko-kĭ-ne′zhə) [Gr. *diadocha* in succession + *-kinesi-* + *-ia*] the function of arresting one motor impulse and substituting for it one that is diametrically opposite, to permit sequential alternating movements, as pronation and supination of the arm. Cf. *adiadochokinesia* and *dysdiadochokinesia*. Called also *diadochocinesia*. **diadochokinet′ic** *adj*

di·ad·o·cho·ki·ne·sis (di-ad″ə-ko-kĭ-ne′sis) diadochokinesia.

Di·ae·mus (di-e′mus) a rare genus of vampire bats of the family Phyllostomatidae, native to South America. *D. youn′gi* parasitizes wild and domesticated birds.

di·ag·nose (di′əg-nōs″) to make a diagnosis of; to recognize the nature of an attack of disease.

di·ag·no·sis (di″əg-no′sis) [*dia-* + Gr. *gnōsis* knowledge] 1. the determination of the nature of a case of disease. 2. the art of distinguishing one disease from another.

biological d. diagnosis by tests performed on animals.

clinical d. diagnosis based on signs, symptoms, and laboratory findings during life.

cytohistologic d. cytologic d.

cytologic d. the diagnosis of disease, both benign and malignant, by study of exfoliated cells; called also *cytohistologic d.*

differential d. the determination of which one of two or more diseases or conditions a patient is suffering from, by systematically comparing and contrasting their clinical findings.

direct d. pathologic diagnosis by observing structural lesions or pathognomonic symptoms.

d. by exclusion recognition of a disease by excluding all other known diseases.

d. ex juvan′tibus diagnosis based on the results of treatment.

laboratory d. diagnosis based on the findings of various laboratory examinations or measurements.

niveau d. [Fr. "level diagnosis"] localization of the exact level of a lesion; as, for instance, of an intervertebral tumor.

pathologic d. diagnosis by observing the structural lesions present.

physical d. determination of disease by inspection, palpation, percussion, and auscultation.

preimplantation genetic d. (PGD) in assisted reproductive technology, the determination of chromosomal abnormalities in the embryo before it is transferred to the uterus.

provocative d. the induction of a condition for the purpose of diagnosis, as the induction of a seizure in a doubtful case of epilepsy.

serum d. diagnosis by means of the analysis of serums; immunodiagnosis.

di·ag·nos·tic (di″əg-nos′tik) pertaining to or subserving diagnosis; distinctive of or serving as a criterion of a disease, as signs and symptoms.

Di·ag·nos·tic and Sta·tis·ti·cal Man·u·al of Men·tal Dis·or·ders (DSM) a system of classification of mental disorders, published by the American Psychiatric Association, that delineates objective criteria to be used in diagnosis. It is a categorical classification system, dividing the disorders into types on the basis of criteria sets, without assuming the disorders are completely discrete entities with absolute boundaries.

di·ag·nos·ti·cate (di″əg-nos′tĭ-kāt) diagnose.

di·ag·nos·ti·cian (di″əg-nos-tish′ən) an expert in diagnosis.

di·ag·nos·tics (di″əg-nos′tiks) the science and practice of diagnosis of disease.

di·a·gram (di′ə-gram) a graphic representation, in simplest form, of an object or concept, made up of lines and lacking entirely any pictorial elements. **diagrammat′ic** *adj*

ladder d. a diagrammatic representation of the routes of cardiac conduction as determined by electrocardiographic recording, used in diagnosing arrhythmias. Vectors describing the origins and paths of individual normal or ectopic impulses as well as points of blocks to conduction are drawn across a series of horizontal lines representing the atria, atrioventricular node, ventricles, and sometimes additional regions of the conduction system. See illustration. Called also *laddergram*.

scatter d. scatterplot.

vector d. a diagram representing the direction and magnitude of electromotive forces of the heart for one entire cycle, based on analysis of the scalar electrocardiogram.

Wiggers d. a graphic representation of the events of the cardiac cycle, showing the changes in a variety of physical variables over the period of a heartbeat; it includes depictions of the electrocardiogram, the pressure in the cardiac chambers and aorta, the ventricular volume, and the heart sounds, and sometimes of the aortic flow rate and the venous pulse. See illustration at *cardiac cycle*, under *cycle*.

di·a·graph (di′ə-graf) [*dia-* + *-graph*] an instrument for recording outlines; used in craniometry, etc.

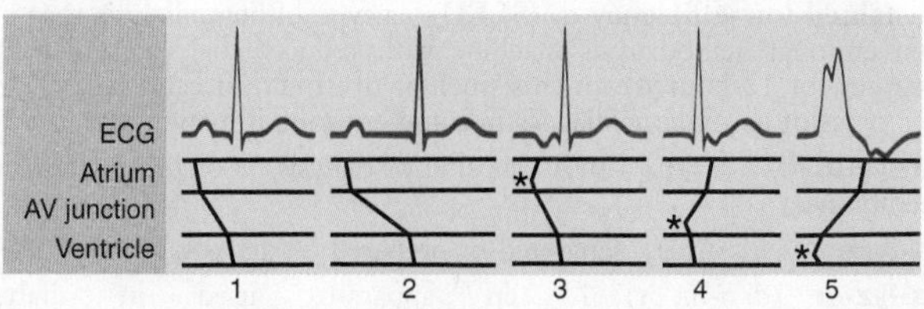

■ Ladder diagrams depicting different electrocardiographic *(ECG)* patterns. *(1)*, Normal beat; *(2)*, first degree atrioventricular block; *(3)*, atrial premature complex, with an inverted P wave on the ECG; *(4)*, ectopic impulse arising in the His bundle and conducting anterograde to the ventricle and retrograde through the AV node to the atrium; *(5)*, ventricular ectopic beat conducting retrograde through the His bundle and AV node to the atrium. A star marks the point of origin of each premature or ectopic impulse. *AV*, atrioventricular.

di•a•ki•ne•sis (di′ə-kĭ-ne′sis) [*dia-* + *-kinesis*] the fifth and final stage of prophase in meiosis I, during which the chromosomes condense and shorten, the nucleolus and nuclear envelope disappear, and the spindle fibers form.

di•al (di′əl) [L. *dialis* daily, from *dies* day] a circular area with graduations around the circumference and a centrally fixed pointer for indicating values of time, pressure, etc.

astigmatic d. a diagram arranged like the face of a watch, used to determine the presence and axis of astigmatism.

Di•a•lis•ter (di″ə-lis′tər) a genus of gram-negative, anaerobic bacteria of the family Acidaminococcaceae, consisting of small coccobacilli occurring singly, in pairs, or in short chains, found in human clinical samples; members of this genus are associated with oral infections. The type species is *D. pneumosin′tes*.

D. pneumosin′tes a species isolated from the nasopharynx, blood, and abscesses of the lung and brain.

di•al•lyl (di-al′əl) any compound containing two allyl molecules.

Di•a•lume (di′ə-loom) trademark for a preparation of dried aluminum hydroxide gel.

di•al•y•sance (di-al′ə-səns) [*dialysis* + *-ance* suffix denoting action or process] the minute rate of net exchange of a substance between blood and bath fluid, per unit blood-bath concentration gradient; a parameter in artificial kidney kinetics (nonfiltration) functionally equivalent to the renal clearance (q.v.) of the natural kidney.

di•al•y•sate (di-al′ə-sāt) 1. the fluid and solutes in a dialysis process that simply flow through the dialyzer and do not pass through the semipermeable membrane, being discarded along with removed toxic substances after they flow back out of the dialyzer. 2. diffusate (def. 2).

di•al•y•sis (di-al′ə-sis) [Gr. "dissolution"] 1. the process of separating macromolecules from ions and low-molecular-weight compounds in solution by the difference in their rates of diffusion through a semipermeable membrane, through which crystalloids can pass readily but colloids pass very slowly or not at all. Two distinct physical processes are involved, diffusion and ultrafiltration (qq.v.). 2. hemodialysis. **dialyt′ic** *adj*

continuous ambulatory peritoneal d. (CAPD) a common method of peritoneal dialysis, involving the continuous presence of dialysis solution in the peritoneal cavity; drainage of the cavity and replacement with fresh solution is done 3 or 4 times daily and can be performed by patients themselves at home.

continuous cycling peritoneal d. (CCPD) a procedure similar to continuous ambulatory peritoneal dialysis but taking place at night using a machine to make several fluid exchanges automatically; two liters of dialysate fluid are left in the peritoneal cavity during the daytime to facilitate one additional fluid exchange.

equilibrium d. a technique used to measure antibody-hapten affinities: solutions of pure antibody and hapten are placed in two cells separated by a semipermeable membrane, and the hapten diffuses across until the free hapten concentration is the same on both sides. From the known total amounts of antibody and hapten and the measured free hapten concentration, the concentrations of free antibody and antibody-hapten complex and the dissociation constant are calculated.

intermittent peritoneal d. (IPD) an older form of peritoneal dialysis in which dialysis solution is infused into the peritoneal cavity, allowed to equilibrate for 10 to 20 minutes, and then drained out; the process is repeated several times over a period of 24 hours at least twice a week.

kidney d. hemodialysis.

lymph d. removal of urea and other elements from lymph collected from the thoracic duct, treated outside the body, and later reinfused.

peritoneal d. hemodialysis through the peritoneum; the dialyzing solution is introduced into and removed from the peritoneal cavity, and solutes leave the blood because of a concentration gradient across the peritoneum. It may be done as either *continuous ambulatory*, *continuous cycling*, or *intermittent peritoneal dialysis*.

renal d. hemodialysis.

sustained low-efficiency d. (SLED) a type of hemodialysis that uses a conventional hemodialysis machine with reduced dialysate and blood flow rates for 12-hour treatments, such as overnight; it can substitute for other types of continuous dialysis in some critically ill patients.

di•a•lyz•able (di′ə-līz′ə-bəl) capable of dialysis or of passing through a membrane.

di•a•lyzed (di′ə-līzd) separated or prepared by dialysis.

di•a•lyz•er (di′ə-līz″ər) 1. an apparatus used in dialysis. 2. hemodialyzer.

Di•a•ma•nus (di″ə-ma′nəs) a genus of fleas. *D. monta′nus* infests rodents in the western United States and has been implicated in the transmission of sylvatic plague.

di•am•e•ter (di-am′ə-tər) the length of a straight line passing through the center of a circle and connecting opposite points on its circumference; hence the distance between two specified opposite points on the periphery of a structure such as the cranium or pelvis. Symbol *d.*

anteroposterior d. the distance between a point on the anterior aspect and one on the posterior aspect of a structure, such as the true conjugate diameter of the pelvis, or the occipitofrontal diameter of the skull.

anteroposterior d. of pelvis one of the pelvic diameters from the region of the coccyx to the midline of the pubic symphysis; see *conjugata recta pelvis* and *conjugata vera pelvis*.

anterotransverse d. (of the cranium), temporal d.

Baudelocque d. conjugata externa pelvis.

bicristal d. the greatest distance between the external margins of the iliac crests.

biischial d. transverse d. of pelvic outlet.

biparietal d. the distance between the two parietal eminences.

bisacromial d. the distance between the outermost points of the shoulder.

bisiliac d. the distance between the two most remote points of the iliac crests.

bispinous d. the distance between the opposite spines of the ischia.

bitemporal d. the distance between the two extremities of the coronal suture.

bitrochanteric d. the distance between the greater trochanters in the hips of a fetus.

buccolingual d. the distance from the buccal to the lingual surface of a tooth crown at its widest point or greatest curvature.

cervicobregmatic d. the distance between the center of the anterior fontanel and the junction of the neck with the floor of the mouth.

coccygeopubic d. the distance from the tip of the coccyx to the under margin of the symphysis pubis.

d. conjuga′ta pel′vis conjugata vera pelvis.

conjugate d. 1. conjugate (def. 1). 2. conjugata vera pelvis.

conjugate d., anatomical conjugata vera pelvis.

conjugate d., diagonal conjugata diagonalis pelvis.

conjugate d., external conjugata externa pelvis.

conjugate d., internal conjugata vera pelvis.

conjugate d., obstetric the shortest anteroposterior diameter of the pelvic inlet; the distance from a point 1 cm. below the top of the pubis to the tip of the sacral promontory, measuring 11 to 13 cm. in the normal pelvis. So called because it is intimately concerned in the process of labor. Called also *obstetric conjugate*.

conjugate d., true conjugata vera pelvis.

conjugate d. of pelvis 1. conjugata vera pelvis. 2. conjugate (def. 1).

cranial d., craniometric d. the distance between craniometric points on the skull; they include the *biparietal d.*, *bitemporal d.*, *cervicobregmatic d.*, *frontomental d.*, *occipitofrontal d.*, *occipitomental d.*, and *suboccipitobregmatic d.*

frontomental d. the distance from the forehead to the chin.

fronto-occipital d. occipitofrontal d.

intercristal d. distantia intercristalis.

interspinous d. distantia interspinosa.

intertuberal d. the distance between the sciatic notches.

longitudinal d., inferior the distance from the foramen cecum to the internal occipital protuberance.

mento-occipital d. occipitomental d.

mentoparietal d. the distance from the chin to the vertex of the skull.

d. obli′qua pel′vis [TA] oblique diameter of pelvis: the diagonal diameter across the pelvic inlet, measured from one sacroiliac joint to the iliopubic eminence of the other side. Designated right or left depending on which sacroiliac joint is used for reference; the left is uniformly 0.5 cm. shorter than the right.

occipitofrontal d. the distance from the external occipital protuberance to the most prominent midpoint of the frontal bone; called also *fronto-occipital d.*

occipitomental d. the distance from the external occipital protuberance to the most prominent midpoint of the chin; called also *mento-occipital d.*

parietal d. the distance between tuberosities of parietal bones; called also *posterotransverse d.*

pelvic d. any diameter of the pelvis.

posterotransverse d. parietal d.

pubosacral d. true conjugate d.

pubotuberous d. the distance from the tuberosity of the ischium to a point on the superior ramus of the pubis which is located directly perpendicular to the tuberosity.

sacropubic d. the distance from the tip of the sacrum or coccyx to the lower margin of the symphysis pubis.

sagittal d. the distance from the glabella to the external occipital protuberance.

suboccipitobregmatic d. the distance from the lowest posterior point of the occiput to the center of the anterior fontanel.

temporal d. the distance between the tips of the alae magnae; called also *anterotransverse d.*

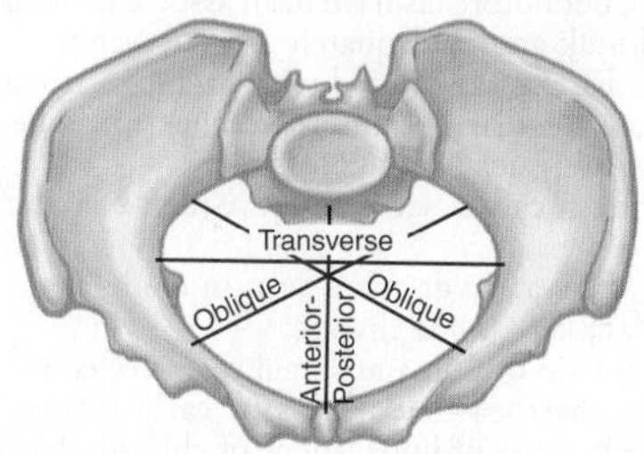

■ Diameters of pelvic inlet (see also *pelvic planes*).

d. transver′sa pel′vis [TA] transverse diameter of pelvis: the greatest distance from side to side across the pelvic inlet.

transverse d. the distance between two points located on the opposite sides of the body part being measured, such as the biparietal diameter of the head.

transverse d. of pelvic outlet the distance between the medial surfaces of the ischial tuberosities (average length 11 cm.); called also *biischial d.*

transverse d. of pelvis d. transversa pelvis.

vertebromammary d. the anteroposterior diameter of the chest.

vertical d. the distance between two points situated on the upper and lower aspects of the structure being measured, such as the distance between the occipital foramen and the vertex of the skull.

di•am•ide (di-am′īd) [*di-* + *amide*] a compound that contains two amido groups.

di•am•i•dine (di-am′ĭ-dēn) a compound that contains two amidine groups.

diamido- a prefix indicating the possession of two amido groups.

di•amine (di′ə-mēn″, -min″) [*di-* + *amine*] a compound that contains two amino groups, sometimes specifically hydrazine.

di•amine ox•i•dase (di′ə-mēn″ ok′sĭ-dās) amine oxidase (copper-containing).

***p*-di•ami•no•di•phen•yl** (di-ə-me″no-di-fen′əl) benzidine.

di•ami•no•di•phen•yl•sul•fone (DDS) (di-am″ĭ-no-di-fen″əl-sul′fōn) dapsone.

di•am•in•uria (di-am″ĭ-nu′re-ə) the presence of diamines in the urine.

***cis*-di•am•mine•di•chlor•o•plat•i•num** (di″ə-mēn-di-klor″o-plat′ĭ-nəm) cisplatin.

di•am•ni•on•ic (di″am-ne-on′ik) having or developing within separate amniotic cavities.

di•am•ni•ot•ic (di-am″ne-ot′ik) diamnionic.

Di•a•mond-Black•fan syndrome (di′ə-mond blak′fən) [Louis Klein *Diamond*, American pediatrician, 1902–1999; Kenneth D. *Blackfan*, American pediatrician, 1883–1941] see *congenital hypoplastic anemia*, under *anemia.*

di•a•monds (di′ə-məndz) the urticarial form of swine erysipelas.

dia•mor•phine (di″ə-mor′fēn) diacetylmorphine.

Di•a•mox (di′ə-moks) trademark for preparations of acetazolamide.

Di•an•a•bol (di-an′ə-bol) trademark for methandrostenolone.

di•an•hy•dro•an•ti•ar•i•gen•in (di″an-hi″dro-an″te-ahr′ĭ-jen″in) an aglycone from antiarin.

di•a•no•et•ic (di″ə-no-et′ik) [*dia-* + *noetic*] pertaining to the intellectual functions, especially to reasoning.

di•an•te•bra•chia (di″ən-tə-bra′ke-ə) a developmental anomaly characterized by duplication of a forearm.

Di•ap•a•rene (di-ap′ə-rēn) trademark for preparations of methylbenzethonium chloride.

di•a•pause (di′ə-pawz) [*dia-* + *pause*] a state of inactivity and arrested development accompanied by greatly decreased metabolism, as in many eggs, insect pupae, and plant seeds; it is a mechanism for surviving adverse winter conditions.

di•a•pe•de•sis (di″ə-pə-de′sis) [*dia-* + Gr. *pēdan* to leap] the outward passage through intact vessel walls of cellular elements of the blood (erythrocytes or leukocytes). Called also *migration* and *transmigration.* **diapedet′ic** *adj*

di•a•phane (di′ə-fān) [Gr. *diaphanēs* transparent] a minute electric lamp for use in transillumination.

di•a•pha•ne•i•ty (di″ə-fə-ne′ĭ-te) transparency.

di•aph•a•nog•ra•phy (di-af″ə-nog′rə-fe) transillumination of the breast, with photography of the transilluminated light on infrared-sensitive film.

di•aph•a•nom•e•ter (di-af″ə-nom′ə-tər) [*diaphane* + *-meter*] an instrument for testing urine and other fluids by means of transmitted light.

di•aph•a•nom•e•try (di-af″ə-nom′ə-tre) the measurement of the transparency of a fluid.

di•aph•a•no•scope (de-af′ə-no-skōp″) [*diaphane* + *-scope*] an instrument for illuminating a body cavity with transillumination.

di•aph•a•nos•co•py (di-af′ə-nos′kə-pe) transillumination.

di•aph•e•met•ric (di-af′ə-met′rik) [*dia-* + Gr. *haphē* touch + *-metric*] pertaining to measurement of the sense of touch.

di•aph•o•rase (di-af′o-rās) any flavoprotein catalyzing the oxidation of reduced nicotinamide adenine dinucleotide (NAD) or reduced nicotinamide adenine dinucleotide phosphate (NADP) using a nonphysiological compound such as methylene blue as electron acceptor, but not oxygen or cytochromes. The reaction is an artifact arising from removal of the enzyme from the complexes in which it occurs naturally.

di•a•pho•re•sis (di″ə-fə-re′sis) [Gr. *diaphorēsis*] sweating, sometimes specifically that induced artificially.

di•a•pho•ret•ic (di″ə-fo-ret′ik) [Gr. *diaphorētikos*] 1. pertaining to, characterized by, or promoting sweating. 2. an agent that promotes sweating. Called also *sudorific.*

di•a•phragm (di′ə-fram) 1. diaphragma (def. 1). 2. any separating membrane or structure. 3. a disk with one or more openings in it, or with an adjustable opening, mounted in relation to a lens or source of radiation by which part of the light or radiation may be excluded from the area. 4. a contraceptive device of molded rubber or other soft plastic material, fitted over the cervix uteri prior to intercourse to prevent the entrance of spermatozoa; for added efficacy, a spermicidal agent is usually placed within it. Called also *contraceptive d.* and *vaginal d.*

accessory d. urogenital d.

antral d. see under *membrane.*

contraceptive d. diaphragm (def. 4).

epithelial d. an epithelial structure, evolving from the root sheath (sheath of Hertwig), that narrows the opening into the pulp chamber, diminishing its caliber. It is in close contact with the bone forming the fundus of the developing alveolus, from which it is separated by the dental sac.

d. of mouth musculus mylohyoideus.

oral d. musculus mylohyoideus.

pelvic d., d. of pelvis diaphragma pelvis.

podocyte slit d. slit d.

polyarcuate d. abnormal scalloping of margins of the diaphragm on radiographic visualization.

Potter-Bucky d. see under *grid.*

pyloric d. see under *membrane.*

respiratory d. diaphragma (def. 1).

secondary d. urogenital d.

sellar d., d. of sella turcica diaphragma sellae.

slit d. a thin membrane that spans the slit pore of the renal glomerulus to form part of the glomerular filtration barrier. Called also *slit membrane, filtration slit membrane,* and *podocyte slit d.*

splinted d. inhibition of diaphragmatic movement, seen in a variety of disease processes. See also *paradoxical diaphragm phenomenon,* under *phenomenon.*

thoracic d. diaphragma (def. 1).

urogenital d. traditional but no longer valid concept that superior and inferior fascial layers enclose the sphincter urethrae and deep transverse perineal muscles and together form a musculomembranous sheet that extends between the ischiopubic rami. Called also *accessory* or *secondary d.* and *urogenital triangle* or *trigone.* See also *membrana perinei.*

vaginal d. diaphragm (def. 4).

di•a•phrag•ma (di″ə-frag′mə) pl. *diaphrag′mata* [Gr. "a partition-wall, barrier"] 1. [TA] diaphragm: the musculomembranous partition separating the abdominal and thoracic cavities, and serving as a major thoracic

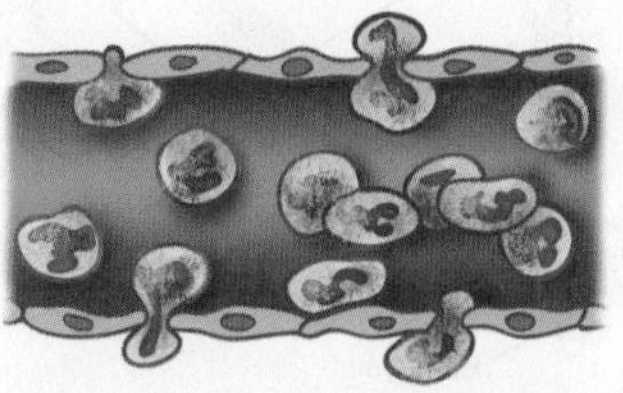
■ Diapedesis of leukocytes.

muscle. Called also *diaphragmatic muscle* and *thoracic* or *respiratory diaphragm.* 2. a separating structure.

d. pel'vis [TA] pelvic diaphragm: the portion of the floor of the pelvis that is formed by the coccygei (ischiococcygei) and levatores ani muscles and their fasciae.

d. sel'lae [TA] sellar diaphragm: a ring-shaped fold of dura mater covering the sella turcica and containing an aperture for passage of the infundibulum of the hypophysis.

d. urogenita'le urogenital diaphragm.

di•a•phrag•mal•gia (di″ə-frag-mal′jə) phrenalgia.

di•a•phrag•ma•ta (di″ə-frag′mə-tə) [Gr.] plural of *diaphragma.*

di•a•phrag•mat•ic (di″ə-frag-mat′ik) 1. pertaining to or of the nature of a diaphragm. 2. phrenic.

di•a•phrag•ma•ti•tis (di″ə-frag″mə-ti′tis) phrenitis.

di•a•phrag•mat•o•cele (di″ə-frag-mat′o-sēl) [*diaphragm* + *-cele*[1]] diaphragmatic hernia.

di•a•phrag•mi•tis (de″ə-frag-mi′tis) phrenitis.

di•aph•y•sary (di-af′ə-zar-e) diaphyseal.

di•a•phy•se•al (di″ə-fiz′e-əl) pertaining to or affecting the shaft of a long bone (diaphysis).

di•a•phys•ec•to•my (di″ə-fiz-ek′tə-me) [*diaphysis* + *-ectomy*] excision of a portion of the shaft of a long bone.

di•aph•y•ses (di-af′ə-sēz) [Gr.] plural of *diaphysis.*

di•a•phy•si•al (di″ə-fiz′e-əl) diaphyseal.

di•aph•y•sis (di-af′ə-sis) pl. *diaph′yses* [Gr. "the point of separation between stalk and branch"] 1. [TA] the elongated cylindrical portion of a long bone, between the ends or extremities (the epiphyses), which are usually articular and wider; it consists of a tube of compact bone that encloses the marrow cavity (cavitas medullaris). Called also *shaft.* 2. the portion of a long bone formed from a primary center of ossification.

di•a•phys•itis (di″ə-fiz-i′tis) inflammation of a diaphysis.

tuberculous d. inflammation involving intermediate segments of the shafts of long bones, caused by the tubercle bacillus.

di•a•pi•re•sis (di″ə-pi-re′sis) [Gr. *diapeirein* to drive through] diapedesis.

dia•pla•cen•tal (di″ə-plə-sen′təl) through the placenta.

di•a•poph•y•sis (di″ə-pof′ə-sis) [*dia-* + *apophysis*] the superior or articular part of a transverse process of a vertebra.

Di•ap•to•mus (di-ap′to-məs) a genus of copepod crustaceans, species of which act as hosts of the larvae of *Diphyllobothrium latum.*

di•a•py•e•sis (di″ə-pi-e′sis) suppuration.

di•a•py•et•ic (di″ə-pi-et′ik) promoting suppuration.

di•ar•rhea (di″ə-re′ə) [*dia-* + *-rrhea*] abnormal frequency and liquidity of fecal discharges. **diarrhe′al, diarrhe′ic, diarrhet′ic** *adj*

AIDS d., AIDS-related d. HIV-related d.

antibiotic-associated d. diarrhea accompanying treatment with antibiotics. It occurs as a component of antibiotic-associated enterocolitis and may also be caused by disturbance of intestinal microflora that break down carbohydrates and bile salts.

bacillary white d. pullorum disease.

bile acid d. diarrhea caused by malabsorption of bile acids in the colon, most often because of disease or resection of the ileum.

bovine viral d., bovine virus d. an infectious disease of cattle, caused by a virus of the genus *Pestivirus;* marked by ulceration and hemorrhage of the alimentary tract with diarrhea and dehydration. Called also *mucosal disease.*

Brainerd d. self-limited diarrhea of acute onset and a duration of more than four weeks (and sometimes a year or more), characterized by explosive, watery diarrhea, typically 10–20 episodes a day, often accompanied by gas, mild abdominal cramping, and fatigue; systemic symptoms are rare. The cause is unknown, but outbreaks have been associated with the consumption of unpasteurized milk and inadequately treated water.

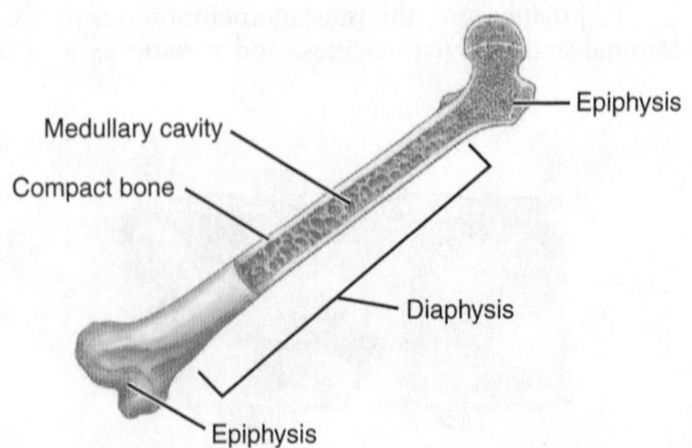

■ Diaphysis and epiphyses of a femur.

cachectic d. diarrhea associated with cachexia; it may be due to malabsorption, or both the diarrhea and the cachexia may be manifestations of an underlying disease, such as a neoplasm.

calf d. diarrhea in calves; see *neonatal d.* (def. 2) and *white scours.* Called also *calf scours.*

choleraic d. the watery diarrhea seen in cholera.

chronic bacillary d. Johne disease.

congenital chloride d. an autosomal recessive condition characterized by severe, watery diarrhea that begins in early infancy and contains an excess of chloride because of impairment of chloride-bicarbonate exchange in the lower colon. Affected infants have a distended abdomen, lethargy, and retarded growth and mental development. The condition is accompanied by alkalosis and hypokalemia, and is often associated with maternal hydramnios. Called also *congenital chloridorrhea.*

dientameba d. a mild though chronic diarrhea caused by infection with *Dientamoeba fragilis.*

dysenteric d. diarrhea with mucous and bloody feces, seen in dysentery,

epidemic d. of newborn a contagious diarrhea occurring in epidemics among newborn infants in hospitals; called also *neonatal d.*

factitious d. diarrhea induced by surreptitious ingestion of laxatives or diuretics.

familial chloride d. congenital chloride d.

fermentative d. diarrhea caused by fermentation due to microorganisms.

flagellate d. diarrhea containing flagellate organisms such as *Giardia.*

gastrogenic d. diarrhea due to a gastric disorder.

hill d. tropical sprue.

HIV d., HIV-related d. diarrhea in immunocompromised persons infected with the human immunodeficiency virus; it may result from opportunistic infection of the intestine by a fungus, protozoon, bacteria, or virus; from side effects of drug therapy, especially with antibiotics; or from disease processes such as HIV enteropathy.

infantile d. weanling d. (def. 1).

inflammatory d., irritative d. diarrhea due to inflammation or irritation of the intestine by improper food, poisons, cathartic medicines, bacteria, or other factors.

lienteric d. diarrhea containing undigested food.

morning d. diarrhea that occurs in the morning only.

mucous d. diarrhea containing mucus.

neonatal d. 1. epidemic d. of the newborn. 2. any diarrhea seen in newborn animals, such as white scours; the most common cause is infection with *Escherichia coli, Coronavirus,* or *Rotavirus.*

osmotic d. diarrhea resulting from the presence of osmotically active nonabsorbable solutes in the intestine, such as magnesium sulfate.

pancreatic d., d. pancrea′tica 1. Verner-Morrison syndrome. 2. the diarrhea that accompanies cystic disease of the pancreas or degeneration of its parenchyma.

pancreatogenous fatty d. diarrhea containing excessive fat owing to dysfunction of the pancreas.

parenteral d. diarrhea due to infections outside the gastrointestinal tract, such as tuberculosis or syphilis.

postweaning d. potentially fatal diarrhea in piglets just after they are weaned; causes may be allergies to ingredients of the new diet or intestinal infection, such as by a strain of *Escherichia coli* (see *coliform gastroenteritis*). Called also *weanling pig scours.*

putrefactive d. diarrhea due to putrefaction of the intestinal contents.

rotavirus d. diarrhea caused by a rotavirus; usually seen in children.

runner's d. diarrhea during or immediately after participation in a running exercise or event, especially one involving long-distance running; the cause is unknown, but contributing factors may be dehydration and the moving of blood flow away from the intestines to the heart and skeletal muscles.

secretory d. watery, voluminous diarrhea resulting from increased stimulation of ion and water secretion, inhibition of their absorption, or both; its osmolality approximates that of plasma, and diarrhea persists during fasting. Cf. *osmotic d.*

serous d. watery d.

summer d. a formerly common kind of diarrhea that occurred in children in the summertime.

toxigenic d. the watery, voluminous diarrhea caused by enterotoxins from enterotoxigenic bacteria such as *Vibrio cholerae* and ETEC strains of *Escherichia coli;* the enterotoxin is the primary pathogen and the bacteria do not invade the intestinal mucosa.

traveler's d. diarrhea occurring in travelers, particularly in those visiting tropical or subtropical areas where sanitation is inadequate; many different infectious agents can cause it, of which the most common is enterotoxigenic *Escherichia coli.* In Mexico, it is also called *turista.*

tropical d. see under *sprue.*

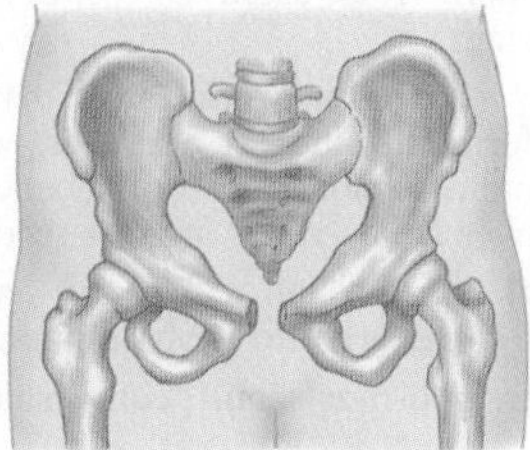

■ Diastasis of the pubic symphysis.

watery d. diarrhea with copious serous fluid; called also *serous d.*

weanling d. 1. diarrhea in an infant when put on food other than its mother's milk, usually due to inadequate sanitation and infection with an enterotoxigenic strain of *Escherichia coli* or a rotavirus. Called also *infantile d.* 2. postweaning d.

white d. pullorum disease.

di•ar•rhe•o•gen•ic (di″ə-re″o-jen′ik) [*diarrhea* + *-genic*] giving rise to diarrhea.

di•ar•thric (di-ahr′thrik) [*di-* + *arthr-* + *-ic*] pertaining to or affecting two different joints; called also *biarticular* and *diarticular.*

di•ar•thro•di•al (di″ahr-thro′de-əl) of the nature of a diarthrosis (junctura synovialis).

di•ar•thro•ses (di″ahr-thro′sēz) plural of *diarthrosis.*

di•ar•thro•sis (di″ahr-thro′sis) pl. *diarthro′ses* [Gr. *diarthrōsis* a movable articulation] TA alternative for *junctura synovialis.*

d. rotato′ria a joint characterized by mobility in a rotary direction.

di•ar•tic•u•lar (di″ahr-tik′u-lər) diarthric.

di•as•chi•sis (di-as′kĭ-sis) [*dia-* + *-schisis*] the loss of function and electrical activity caused by cerebral lesions in areas remote from the lesion but neuronally connected to it.

di•a•scope (di′ə-skōp) [*dia-* + *-scope*] a glass or clear plastic plate, usually a flat blade or microscope slide, pressed against the skin to cause blanching and permit observation of changes produced in the tissues.

di•as•co•py (di-as′kə-pe) examination with the diascope.

Di•a•sone (di′ə-sōn) trademark for a preparation of sulfoxone sodium.

di•a•stase (di′ə-stās) a mixture of amylases from malt, used to convert starch into simple sugars.

di•as•ta•sic (di″əs-ta′sik) diastatic.

di•as•ta•sis (di-as′tə-sis) [Gr. "separation"] 1. a form of dislocation in which there is separation of two bones normally attached to each other without the existence of a true joint; as in separation of the pubic symphysis. Also, separation beyond the normal between associated bones, as between the ribs, or the ulna and radius. 2. a relatively quiescent period of slow ventricular filling during the cardiac cycle; it occurs in mid-diastole, following the rapid filling phase and just prior to atrial systole. See illustration at *cardiac cycle*, under *cycle.*

iris d. iridodiastasis.

d. rec′ti abdo′minis separation of the rectus muscles of the abdominal wall; it may be present congenitally, and also may occur during pregnancy, especially in repeat pregnancies or pregnancies with multiple fetuses.

di•a•stas•uria (di″ə-stās-u′re-ə) amylasuria.

Di•a•stat (di′ə-stat) trademark for a preparation of diazepam.

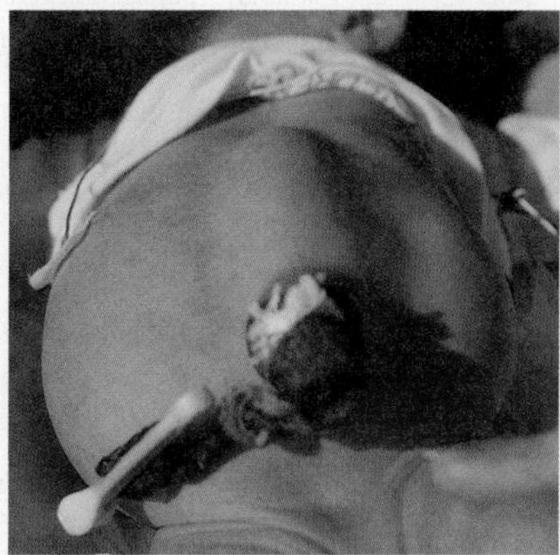

■ Diastasis recti abdominis in a newborn infant.

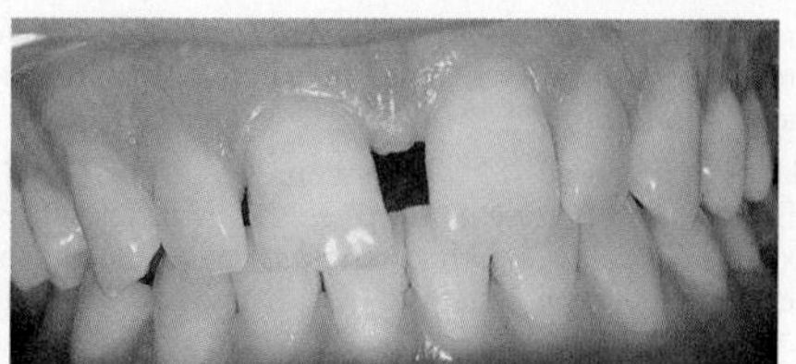

■ Anterior diastema produced by an enlarged labial frenulum.

di•a•stat•ic (di″ə-stat′ik) 1. pertaining to diastase. 2. pertaining to diastasis.

di•a•stem (di′ə-stem) diastema.

di•a•ste•ma (di″ə-ste′mə) pl. *diaste′mata* [Gr. *diastēma* an interval] 1. a space or cleft. 2. [TA] a space between two adjacent teeth in the same dental arch.

anterior d. a space between the incisor teeth, generally one between the maxillary central incisors.

di•a•stem•a•ta (di″ə-stem′ə-tə) [Gr.] plural of *diastema.*

di•a•stem•a•to•cra•nia (di″ə-stem″ə-to-kra′ne-ə) [*diastema* + *cranium*] congenital longitudinal fissure of the cranium.

di•a•stem•a•to•my•elia (di″ə-stem″ə-to-mi-e′le-ə) [*diastema* + *myelo-* + *-ia*] a congenital anomaly, often associated with spina bifida, in which the spinal cord is split into halves by a bony spicule or fibrous band, each half being surrounded by a dural sac. Cf. *myeloschisis.*

di•a•stem•a•to•py•elia (di″ə-stem″ə-to-pi-e′le-ə) [*diastema* + *pyelos* pelvis + *-ia*] congenital median fissure of the pelvis.

dia•ster•eo•iso•mer (di″ə-ster″e-o-i′so-mər) diastereomer.

dia•ster•eo•iso•mer•ic (di″ə-ster″e-o-i″so-mer′ik) exhibiting diastereoisomerism.

dia•ster•eo•isom•er•ism (di″ə-ster″e-o″i-som′ər-iz-əm) the relationship between two or more stereoisomers whose molecules are not mirror images of each other, e.g., glucose and galactose or *cis* and *trans* isomers.

dia•ster•eo•mer (di″ə-ster′e-o″mər) one of a group of compounds having a diastereoisomeric relationship.

Di•a•stix (di′ə-stiks) trademark for a reagent strip designed for the quantitative determination of glucose in urine.

di•as•to•le (di-as′to-le) [Gr. *diastolē* a drawing asunder; expansion] the dilatation, or period of dilatation, of the heart, especially of the ventricles; it coincides with the interval between the second and the first heart sounds. Cf. *systole* and see illustration at *cardiac cycle*, under *cycle.* **diastol′ic** *adj*

electrical d. the period of time during which the cell rests; it is represented by phase 4 of the action potential.

di•as•to•my•elia (di-as″to-mi-e′le-ə) diastematomyelia.

di•a•stroph•ic (di″ə-strof′ik) [Gr. *diastrephein* distortion] bent or curved; said of structures, such as bones, deformed in such manner.

di•atax•ia (di″ə-tak′se-ə) [*di-* + *ataxia*] ataxia affecting both sides of the body.

cerebral d., d. cerebra′lis infanti′lis cerebral palsy with ataxia.

di•a•ther•mal (di″ə-thur′məl) pertaining to diathermy; heated by high-frequency electromagnetic radiation.

di•a•ther•mic (di″ə-thur′mik) pertaining to diathermy; permeable to high-frequency electromagnetic radiation.

di•a•ther•my (di′ə-thur″me) [*dia-* + Gr. *thermē* heat] heating of the body tissues due to their resistance to the passage of high-frequency electromagnetic radiation, electric currents, or ultrasonic waves. Tissues may be either simply warmed *(medical d.)* or coagulated and destroyed *(surgical d.).*

medical d. application of currents of low tension and high amperage, which produce warmth in the deeper parts of the body; used particularly to promote muscle relaxation and to treat joint disorders including contractures. Called also *thermopenetration.*

microwave d. medical diathermy using electromagnetic radiation by microwaves; it heats to a greater tissue depth than short-wave diathermy and is particularly effective in heating tissues with high water content such as muscles, subcutaneous fat, and fluid-filled cavities.

short wave d. the therapeutic heating of the body tissues by means of an oscillating electromagnetic field of high frequency; the frequency varies from 10 million to 100 million cycles per second and the wavelength from 30 to 3 meters; it heats to a tissue depth of 2 to 3 cm and is used for heating large areas of body surface.

surgical d. electrosurgery.

ultrashort wave d. diathermy in which the wavelength used is less than 10 meters.

ultrasound d. medical diathermy using ultrasound; it heats to a tissue depth of 5 to 6 cm and is particularly used to warm areas around tissue interfaces such as joints.

di·ath·e·sis (di-ath'ə-sis) [Gr. "arrangement, disposition"] a constitution or condition of the body which makes the tissues react in special ways to certain extrinsic stimuli and thus tends to make the person more than usually susceptible to certain diseases. Cf. *constitution* (def. 1) and *type.* **diathet'ic** *adj*

d. of connective tissue a congenital condition of bone and ligamentous tissue that leads to such disorders as recurrent dislocation of the elbow.

exudative d. subcutaneous edema with surface exudation, seen in young pigs and chickens whose diet is deficient in selenium and vitamin E.

gouty d. predisposition to gout.

hemorrhagic d. a predisposition to abnormal hemostasis and hemorrhage.

di·a·tom (di'ə-tom) any of numerous unicellular microscopical forms of alga having a wall of silica; authorities disagree as to which phylum of kingdom Protista to put them in. Several species are toxic and can cause the ocean condition called red tide. The skeletal siliceous remains of many others are mined from deposits and used as filtering and abrasive agents. See also *infusorial earth*, under *earth*.

di·a·to·ma·ceous (di″ə-to-ma'shəs) composed of diatoms; see *infusorial earth*, under *earth*.

di·a·tom·ic (di″ə-tom'ik) [*di-* + *atomic*] 1. made up of two atoms. 2. dibasic. 3. diatomaceous.

di·at·o·mite (di-at'ə-mīt) infusorial earth (diatomaceous earth) in a dry, compacted, stony form; workers inhaling its dust may suffer from diatomite fibrosis.

dia·tri·zo·ate (di″ə-tri-zo'āt) the most commonly used water-soluble, iodinated radiopaque medium. The salts are used, alone or in combination, for a wide variety of diagnostic imaging methods, including angiography, urography, cholangiography, computed tomography, hysterosalpingography, and retrograde pyelography.

d. meglumine [USP] a radiopaque medium, available in solution, consisting of diatrizoate meglumine in water for injection or of diatrizoic acid in water for injection, prepared with the aid of meglumine.

d. sodium [USP] a radiopaque medium, available in solution, consisting of diatrizoate sodium in water for injection or of diatrizoic acid in water for injection, prepared with the aid of sodium hydroxide.

dia·tri·zo·ic ac·id (di″ə-tri-zo'ik) [USP] a compound used in the preparation of certain radiopaque media; see *diatrizoate.*

di·auch·e·nos (di-awk'ə-nos) a dicephalic fetus with two necks.

di·aux·ic (di-awk'sik) pertaining to or characterized by diauxie; implying two periods of growth separated by a lag period.

di·aux·ie (di-awk'se) [*di-* + Gr. *auxein* to increase in size] a phenomenon of bacterial growth in which an organism given a mixture of organic compounds first grows exclusively on one until that compound is exhausted, and then, after a lag during which it forms induced enzymes for utilizing the second compound, resumes growth on the latter.

dia·ver·i·dine (di″ə-ver'ĭ-dēn) an antibacterial and coccidiostat used in poultry, especially against *Eimeria.*

di·ax·on (di-ak'son) [*di-* + *axon*] bipolar cell.

di·az·e·pam (di-az'ə-pam) [USP] a benzodiazepine used as an antianxiety agent in the treatment of anxiety disorders and for short-term relief of anxiety symptoms, as a preoperative or preprocedural medication to relieve anxiety and tension, also as a skeletal muscle relaxant, anticonvulsant, antitremor agent, antipanic agent, and for treatment of symptoms of acute alcohol withdrawal; administered orally, rectally, intravenously, or intramuscularly.

di·a·zine (di-a'zēn) 1. any of a group of compounds derived from benzene by replacement of two carbon atoms by nitrogen atoms. 2. a suffix denoting a ring compound containing two nitrogen atoms.

di·a·zi·quone (AZQ) (di-a'zĭ-kwōn″) an alkylating agent that acts by cross-linking DNA, used as an antineoplastic in the treatment of primary brain malignancies, administered intravenously; it has also been used experimentally in the treatment of leukemia.

diaz(o)- a prefix indicating possession of the group —N═N—.

di·azo·ben·zene·sul·fon·ic ac·id (di-az″o-ben″zēn-səl-fon'ik) *p*-sulfobenzenediazonium hydroxide inner salt; white or slightly red crystals, prepared by the diazotization of sulfanilic acid and used in Ehrlich diazo reaction.

di·a·zo·ma (di″ə-zo'mə) [Gr. *diazōma* that which is put round] the diaphragm.

di·azo·meth·ane (di-az″o-meth'ān) an extremely poisonous yellow gas, N_2CH_2, used in organic synthesis.

di·a·zo·nal (di″ə-zo'nəl) 1. situated across or bridging two zones. 2. pertaining to a diazone.

di·a·zone (di'ə-zōn) one of the dark bands that alternate with light bands (parazones) to form the lines of Schreger, which are seen under reflected light in a ground section of a tooth; believed to be an area in which the enamel prisms have been cut in cross section.

di·azo·sul·fo·ben·zol (di-az″o-sul″fo-ben'zol) a substance which acts upon certain principles in the urine to form aniline colors.

di·az·o·ti·za·tion (di-az″o-tĭ-za'shən) conversion into a diazo compound.

di·az·o·tize (di-az'o-tīz) to introduce the diazo group into a compound.

di·az·ox·ide (di″ə-zok'sīd) an antihypertensive, structurally related to chlorothiazide but having no diuretic properties, administered intravenously in the treatment of acute hypertensive emergencies. Because it inhibits release of insulin, it is also administered orally in the treatment of hypoglycemia due to hyperinsulinism, particularly that associated with malignancy.

di·ba·sic (di-ba'sik) [*di-* + *basic*] containing two hydrogen atoms replaceable by bases, and thus yielding two series of salts, as H_2SO_4.

Di·ben·amine (di-ben'ə-mēn) trademark for a preparation of dibenzylchlorethamine.

di·ben·zan·thra·cene (di″ben-zan'thrə-sēn) a polycyclic aromatic hydrocarbon consisting of anthracene with two benzene substitutions; when injected into the body it may produce epithelial tumors. Abbreviated DBA.

di·ben·zaz·e·pine (di-ben-zaz'ə-pēn) any of a group of structurally related drugs including the tricyclic antidepressants clomipramine, desipramine, imipramine, and trimipramine.

di·ben·zo·cy·clo·hep·ta·di·ene (di-ben″zo-si″klo-hep″tə-di'ēn) any of a group of structurally related drugs including the tricyclic antidepressants amitriptyline, nortriptyline, and protriptyline.

di·ben·zo·di·az·e·pine (di-ben″zo-di-az'ə-pēn) any of a group of structurally related drugs including the antipsychotic agent clozapine.

di·ben·zo·thi·az·e·pine (di-ben″zo-thi-az'ə-pēn) any of a group of structurally related drugs including the antipsychotic agent quetiapine fumarate.

di·ben·zo·thi·a·zine (di-ben″zo-thi'ə-zēn) phenothiazine (def. 1).

di·ben·zox·az·e·pine (di-ben″zok-saz'ə-pēn) any of a class of structurally related heterocyclic drugs, including the antipsychotic loxapine and the antidepressant amoxapine.

di·benz(b,f)-1,4-ox·az·e·pine (di-ben″zoks-az'ə-pēn) CR^2.

di·ben·zox·e·pin (di-ben-zok'sə-pin) dibenzoxepine.

di·ben·zox·e·pine (di-ben-zok'sə-pēn) any of a group of structurally related drugs including the tricyclic antidepressant doxepin.

di·ben·zyl·chlo·reth·amine (di-ben″zəl-klor-eth'ə-mēn) an alpha-adrenergic blocking agent which has been used in the treatment of peripheral vascular disorders and in the diagnosis of pheochromocytoma.

Di·ben·zy·line (di-ben'zə-lēn) trademark for a preparation of phenoxybenzamine hydrochloride.

di·blas·tu·la (di-blas'tu-lə) [*di-* + *blastula*] a blastula in which the ectoderm and endoderm are both present.

di·both·rio·ceph·a·li·a·sis (di-both″re-o-sef″ə-li'ə-sis) diphyllobothriasis.

Di·both·rio·ceph·a·lus (di-both″re-o-sef'ə-ləs) *Diphyllobothrium.*

di·bra·chia (di-bra'ke-ə) [*di-* + *brachia*] duplication of an upper limb.

di·bra·chi·us (di-bra'ke-əs) conjoined twins having only two upper limbs.

di·bro·mide (di-bro'mīd) any bromide which combines two atoms of bromine with one of another element or radical.

di·bro·mo·chlo·ro·pro·pane (di-bro″mo-klor″o-pro'pān) a colorless halogenated hydrocarbon formerly used as a pesticide, soil fumigant, and nematocide; its use is now restricted because of its carcinogenicity.

di·bro·mo·dul·ci·tol (di-bro″mo-dul'sĭ-tol) mitolactol.

1,2-di·bro·mo·eth·ane (di-bro″mo-eth'ān) ethylene dibromide.

di·bro·mo·ke·tone (di-bro″mo-ke'tōn) methyl dibromoethyl ketone, a war gas.

di·bu·caine (di'bu-kān) [USP] a potent local anesthetic applied rectally or topically to the anorectal region for treatment of hemorrhoids and other anorectal disorders, and topically to the skin in the treatment of minor skin disorders. See also *dibucaine number*, under *number*.

di·bu·tyl (di-bu'təl) indicating the presence of two butyl groups.

DIC diffuse (or disseminated) intravascular coagulation.

di·cac·o·dyl (di-kak′o-dəl) cacodyl.

di·cal·cic (di-kal′sik) having in each molecule two atoms of calcium.

di·cal·ci·um phos·phate (di-kal′se-əm) dibasic calcium phosphate.

di·car·bon·ate (di-kahr′bon-āt) bicarbonate.

di·car·box·yl·ic (di″kahr-bok-sil′ik) containing two carboxyl groups; see under *acid.*

di·car·box·yl·ic·ac·id·uria (di″kahr-bok-sil″ik-as″id-u′re-ə) urinary excretion of high levels of dicarboxylic acids, as occurs in deficiencies of acyl-CoA dehydrogenase, when β-oxidation of fatty acids is blocked and ω-oxidation is predominant.

di·ce·lous (di-se′ləs) [*di-* + *cel(o)-*[2] + *-ous*] 1. amphicelous. 2. having two cavities.

Di·cen·tra (di-sen′trə) a genus of perennial herbs of north central North America that have white or cream-colored flowers. *D. canaden′sis* (DC.) Walp. (squirrel or turkey corn) and *D. cuculla′ria* (L.) Bernh. (Fumariaceae) (Dutchman's breeches) are sources of the dried tuber called *corydalis* and contain bicuculline, bulbocapnine, corydaline, corytuberine, and other alkaloids that are toxic to livestock.

di·cen·tric (di-sen′trik) [*di-* + *center*] in genetics, a structurally abnormal chromosome with two centromeres.

di·ceph·a·lous (di-sef′ə-ləs) having two heads.

di·ceph·a·lus (di-sef′ə-ləs) [*di-* + *-cephalus*] a fetus with two heads.

d. di′pus dibra′chius a fetus with two heads but only two feet and two upper limbs.

d. di′pus tetrabra′chius conjoined twins with only two lower limbs, but with varying degrees of fusion of the upper trunks, each component having a head and two upper limbs.

d. di′pus tribra′chius a fetus with two heads, two feet, and a median complete or rudimentary third upper limb.

d. dipy′gus anakatadidymus.

d. parasi′ticus desmiognathus.

d. tri′pus tribra′chius a fetus with a common trunk, but with two heads, three upper limbs, and three lower limbs, the third limbs being either rudimentary or complete.

di·ceph·a·ly (di-sef′ə-le) a developmental anomaly characterized by the presence of two heads.

Di·cha·pet·a·lum (di″kə-pet′ə-lum) a genus of southern African trees. *D. cymo′sum* contains fluoroacetate and can cause fatal fluoroacetate poisoning.

di·chei·lia (di-ki′le-ə) the appearance of a double lip, owing to folding of the oral mucosa.

di·chei·ria (di-ki′re-ə) [*di-* + *cheir-* + *-ia*] complete or incomplete duplication of a hand.

di·chei·rus (di-ki′rəs) an individual exhibiting dicheiria.

Di·che·lo·bac·ter (di-ke′lo-bak″tər) [Gr. *dichēlos* cloven-hoofed + *-bacter*] a genus of gram-negative, obligately anaerobic, nonmotile, nonspore-forming, rod-shaped bacteria of the family Cardiobacteraceae. The type species is *D. nodo′sus.*

D. nodo′sus a species that causes interdigital dermatitis and foot rot in sheep. Formerly called *Bacteroides nodosus.*

di·chlo·ral·phen·a·zone (di″klor-əl-fen′ə-zōn) [USP] a water-soluble complex of chloral hydrate and antipyrine (phenazone), into which it dissociates on administration; its properties are generally those of chloral hydrate, and it is used as a mild sedative and relaxant in combination with isometheptene mucate and acetaminophen in the treatment of migraine and tension headache.

di·chlo·ride (di-klor′id) a combination of a base or a metal with two atoms of chlorine.

carbonic d. phosgene.

di·chlo·ro·ace·tic ac·id (di-klor″o-ə-se′tik) acetic acid with two of its three hydrogen ions exchanged for chlorine atoms; it is a strong organic acid and is used as a protein precipitant in clinical chemistry.

o-di·chlo·ro·ben·zene (di-klor″o-ben′zēn) a solvent, fumigant, and insecticide, sometimes used as a spray; it is toxic if ingested or inhaled.

3,3-di·chlo·ro·ben·zi·dine (di-klor″o-ben′zĭ-dēn) a gray to purple crystalline solid used in the manufacture of dyes and plastics; it is carcinogenic.

di·chlo·ro·di·eth·yl sul·fide (di-klor″o-di-eth′əl) mustard gas, a vesicant gas once employed in war. It produces blistering and subsequent sloughing of the skin with involvement of the eyes and respiratory tract. Death results from bronchopneumonia. Called also *yellow cross* and *yperite.*

di·chlo·ro·di·flu·o·ro·meth·ane (di-klor″o-di-flōōr″o-meth′ān) [NF] a clear, colorless gas with a faint ethereal odor, CCl_2F_2, used as an aerosol propellant and also as a refrigerant.

1,1-di·chlo·ro·eth·ane (di-klor″o-eth′ān) ethylidene chloride.

1,2-di·chlo·ro·eth·ane (di-klor″o-eth′ān) ethylene dichloride.

di·chlo·ro·phen (di-klor′o-fən) an anthelmintic used to treat infestations of large tapeworms in dogs and cats.

2,4-di·chlo·ro·phen·oxy·ace·tic ac·id (di-klor″o-fən-ok″se-ə-se′tic) 2,4-D.

di·chlo·ro·tet·ra·flu·o·ro·eth·ane (di-klor″o-tet″rə-flōōr″o-eth′ān) [NF] a clear, colorless gas with a faint ethereal odor, $CClF_2$-$CClF_2$, used as an aerosol propellant.

di·chlor·phen·a·mide (di″klor-fen′ə-mīd) [USP] a carbonic anhydrase inhibitor used as an adjunct to reduce intraocular pressure in the treatment of glaucoma; administered orally.

di·chlor·vos (di-klor′vos) an organophosphorus insecticide, also used in veterinary medicine as an external parasiticide and anthelmintic.

di·chog·e·ny (di-koj′ə-ne) [Gr. *dicha* in two + *-geny*] development of tissues in different ways in accordance with changes in conditions affecting them.

di·cho·ri·al (di-kor′e-əl) dichorionic.

di·cho·ri·on·ic (di-kor″e-on′ik) having two distinct chorions; said of dizygotic twins.

di·chot·o·mi·za·tion (di-kot″ə-mĭ-za′shən) dichotomy.

di·chot·o·mous (di-kot′ə-məs) pertaining to or characterized by a dichotomy of parts or sections.

di·chot·o·my (di-kot′ə-me) [Gr. *dicha* in two + *-tomy*] 1. division into two parts. 2. the state of having two parts.

Di·chroa (di-kro′ə) a genus of plants of the family Saxifragaceae. *D. febrifu′ga* Lour. is a shrub found in China, India, Indonesia, and the Philippines, called *ch'ang shan* by the Chinese; its root, also called *ch'ang shan*, is used medicinally as a treatment for malaria.

di·chro·ic (di-kro′ik) exhibiting dichroism.

di·chro·ine (di-kro′ēn) an alkaloid from the plant *Dichroa febrifuga* (ch'ang shan); it has three isomeric forms: α-, β-, and γ-dichroine.

di·chro·ism (di′kro-iz-əm) [*di-* + Gr. *chroa* color] the quality or condition of presenting one color in reflected and another in transmitted light.

di·chro·ma·cy (di-kro′mə-se) dichromatic vision.

di·chro·mat (di′kro-mat) a person with dichromatic vision.

di·chro·mate (di-kro′māt) any salt containing the bivalent Cr_2O_7 radical.

di·chro·mat·ic (di″kro-mat′ik) [*di-* + Gr. *chrōma* color] able to see just two of the three primary colors of light; see *dichromatic vision.*

di·chro·ma·tism (di-kro′mə-tiz-əm) [*di-* + Gr. *chrōma* color] 1. the quality of existing in or exhibiting two different colors. 2. dichromatic vision.

di·chro·ma·top·sia (di″kro-mə-top′se-ə) dichromatic vision.

di·chro·mic (di-kro′mik) pertaining to two colors.

di·chro·mo·phil (di-kro′mo-fil) amphophilic; also, an amphophilic element.

di·chro·moph·i·lism (di″kro-mof′ĭ-liz-əm) capacity for double staining, that is, with both acid and basic dyes.

Dick test (reaction), toxin (dik) [George Frederick *Dick*, 1881–1967, and Gladys Rowena Henry *Dick*, 1881–1963, American physicians] see under *test*, and see *erythrogenic toxin*, under *toxin.*

di·clo·fen·ac (di-klo′fen-ak) a nonsteroidal antiinflammatory drug derived from phenylacetic acid.

d. epolamine a salt of diclofenac, used for local analgesia in the form of an impregnated patch applied to the skin of persons with sprains, strains, or contusions.

d. potassium the potassium salt of diclofenac, administered orally in the treatment of rheumatoid arthritis, osteoarthritis, and ankylosing spondylitis, a variety of nonrheumatic inflammatory conditions, pain, and dysmenorrhea.

d. sodium the sodium salt of diclofenac, administered orally in the treatment of rheumatoid arthritis, osteoarthritis, and ankylosing spondylitis and also for a variety of nonrheumatic inflammatory conditions. It is also applied topically to the conjunctiva to inhibit miosis during and to reduce ocular inflammation or photophobia after certain kinds of ophthalmic surgery and to the skin to treat actinic keratoses.

Di·co·did (di-ko′did) trademark for preparations of hydrocodone bitartrate.

di•coe•lous (di-se'ləs) [*di-* + *coelo-* + *-ous*] 1. hollowed on each of two sides. 2. having two cavities.

di•cot•y•le•don (di-kot"əl-e'don) [*di-* + *cotyledon*] a flowering plant with embryos having two seed leaves, or cotyledons.

dic•ro•ce•li•a•sis (dik"ro-sə-li'ə-sis) hepatic fascioliasis due to infection with *Dicrocoelium dendriticum.*

Dic•ro•coe•li•i•dae (dik"ro-se-li'ĭ-de) a family of trematodes that includes the genera *Dicrocoelium, Eurytrema,* and *Platynosomum.* They infect the liver, pancreas, and bile ducts of various animals and occasionally humans.

Dic•ro•coe•li•um (dik"ro-se'le-əm) [Gr. *dikroos* forked + *koilia* bowel] a genus of trematodes of the family Dicrocoeliidae.

D. dendri'ticum the lancet fluke, a species that infests the liver of cattle and sheep in Europe, North and South America, and northern Africa, the cause of dicroceliasis; it has also been found in human biliary passages. Called also *D. lanceolatum.*

D. hos'pes a species found in the gallbladder of cattle in the Sudan.

D. lanceola'tum *D. dendriticum.*

D. macrosto'mum a species found in the gallbladder of guinea fowl in Egypt.

di•crot•ic (di-krot'ik) [Gr. *dikrotos* double beating] pertaining to or characterized by dicrotism. See also *anadicrotic* and *catadicrotic.*

di•cro•tism (di'krŏ-tiz-əm) the presence of a dicrotic pulse.

dicty(o)- [Gr. *diktyon* net] a combining form denoting a relationship to a net or to a netlike structure.

Dic•tyo•cau•lus (dik"te-o-kaw'ləs) [*dictyo-* + Gr. *kaulos* stalk] a genus of nematode lungworms of the family Trichostrongylidae, parasitic in the bronchial tree of horses, sheep, goats, deer, and cattle. *D. arnfiel'di* can cause verminous bronchitis in horses and donkeys. *D. fila'ria* and *D. vivipa'rus* cause hoose in cattle, sheep, and other ungulates.

dic•tyo•co•nid•i•um (dik"te-o-kə-nid'e-əm) dictyospore.

dic•tyo•ki•ne•sis (dik"te-o-kĭ-ne'sis) [*dictyo-* + *kinesis*] the migration and distribution of the dictyosomes to the daughter cells in mitosis.

dic•ty•o•ma (dik"te-o'mə) [*dicty-* + *-oma*] diktyoma.

dic•tyo•spore (dik'te-o-spor) a spore that has both vertical and horizontal septa; called also *dictyoconidium.*

dic•tyo•tene (dik'te-o-tēn) [*dictyo-* + *-tene*] the protracted stage resembling suspended prophase in which the primary oocyte persists from late fetal life until discharged from the ovary at or after puberty.

di•cu•ma•rol (di-koo'mə-rol) 1. a coumarin anticoagulant found in spoiled sweet clover; animals eating the clover may develop the hemorrhagic condition known as *sweet clover disease.* 2. a synthetic preparation of the same substance, used as an oral anticoagulant; it acts by inhibiting the hepatic synthesis of vitamin K–dependent coagulation factors (prothrombin and factors VII, IX, and X) and proteins C and S.

di•cy•clic (di-sik'lik, -si'klik) 1. pertaining to or having two cycles. 2. in chemistry, having a molecular structure containing two rings.

di•cy•clo•mine hy•dro•chlo•ride (di-si'klo-mēn) [USP] an anticholinergic, used as an antispasmodic in the treatment of gastrointestinal disorders, administered orally or intramuscularly.

di•cy•clo•ver•ine hy•dro•chlo•ride (di-si"klo-ver'ēn) INN for *dicyclomine hydrochloride.*

di•cys•te•ine (di"sis-te'in) cystine.

di•dac•tic (di-dak'tik) [Gr. *didaktikos*] conveying instruction by lectures and books rather than by practice.

di•dac•tyl•ism (di-dak'təl-iz-əm) [*di-* + *daktyl-* + *-ism*] the condition of having only two digits on a hand or foot.

di•dac•ty•lous (di-dak'tə-ləs) having only two digits on a hand or foot.

di•dan•o•sine (di-dan'o-sēn) 2′3′-dideoxyinosine, a nucleoside analogue of 2′,3′-dideoxyadenosine; an antiretroviral agent that is converted intracellularly into the active metabolite dideoxyadenosine triphosphate, which inhibits viral replication both by incorporation into the viral genome and by interference with the action of reverse transcriptase; used for the treatment of advanced infection with human immunodeficiency virus-1 and acquired immunodeficiency syndrome; administered orally. Formerly called *dideoxyinosine (ddI).*

didehydro- in systematic chemical nomenclature, a prefix denoting the loss of two hydrogen atoms; cf. *dehydro-.*

di•del•phia (di-del'fe-ə) [*di-* + Gr. *delphys* uterus] uterus didelphys.

di•del•phic (di-del'fik) pertaining to or possessing a double uterus.

Di•del•phis (di-del'fis) [*di-* + Gr. *delphys* uterus] the opossums, a genus of marsupials; some species in South America are reservoirs of *Trypanosoma cruzi.*

2′,3′-di•de•oxy•aden•o•sine (di"de-ok"se-ə-den'o-sēn) a dideoxynucleoside in which the base is adenine, in plasma rapidly converted to 2′,3′-dideoxyinosine by the enzyme adenosine deaminase; it is used as an antiretroviral agent in the treatment of acquired immunodeficiency syndrome.

di•de•oxy•cy•ti•dine (di"de-ok"se-si'tĭ-dēn) former name for *zalcitabine.*

di•de•oxy•in•o•sine (ddI) (di"de-ok"se-in'o-sēn) didanosine.

di•de•oxy•nu•cleo•side (di"de-ok"se-noo'kle-o-sīd") any of a group of synthetic nucleoside analogues lacking two deoxy groups; several 2′,3′-dideoxynucleosides inhibit the enzyme reverse transcriptase and thus have antiretroviral activity.

di•der•mo•ma (di"dər-mo'mə) [*di-* + *derm-* + *-oma*] a teratoma composed of cells and tissues derived from two cell layers.

Di•di•ée projection (de-de-a') [J. *Didiée,* French radiologist, 20th century] see under *projection.*

Di•drex (di'dreks) trademark for a preparation of benzphetamine hydrochloride.

Di•dro•nel (di-dro'nəl) trademark for preparations of etidronate disodium.

did•y•mi•tis (did"ə-mi'tis) orchitis.

did•y•mo•spore (did'ĭ-mo-spor) a spore with two cells and one septa, as in certain imperfect fungi.

did•y•mous (did'ə-məs) occurring in pairs.

did•y•mus (did'ə-məs) [Gr. *didymos* double, twin] testis.

-didymus [Gr. *didymos* double, twin] a word termination denoting conjoined twins or duplication of body parts. See also *-pagus.*

die (di) 1. a form to be used in the construction of something. 2. a positive reproduction of the form of a prepared tooth in a suitable hard substance, such as a metal, resin, or plaster of Paris.

amalgam d. a model of a tooth made of amalgam; used in making dental prostheses.

electroformed d. a die formed by electroplating an impression, forming a metallic positive reproduction of a prepared tooth. Often incorrectly called *electroplated d.* or *plated d.*

electroplated d., plated d. incorrect terms for *electroformed d.*

waxing d. a die or model to which wax is adapted for the fabrication of a wax pattern.

Dieb. alt. [L.] die'bus alter'nis (on alternate days).

Dieb. tert. [L.] die'bus ter'tiis (every third day).

di•echo•scope (di-ek'o-skōp) [*di-* + *echo* + *-scope*] an instrument for the simultaneous perception of two different sounds in auscultation.

di•e•cious (di-e'shəs) [*di-* + Gr. *oikos* house] sexually distinct; denoting species in which male and female genitals do not occur in the same individual. In botany, having staminate and pistillate flowers on separate plants.

Dief•fen•bach operation (de'fən-bahk) [Johann Friedrich *Dieffenbach,* German surgeon, 1792–1847] see under *operation.*

Di•e•go blood group (de-a'go) [*Diego,* surname of the Venezuelan propositus first observed in 1955] see under *blood group.*

di•el•drin (di-el'drin) a chlorinated hydrocarbon insecticide closely related to aldrin, used against the sheep tick *Melophagus ovinus* and to control vectors of insect-borne diseases, especially mosquitoes. Inhalation, ingestion, or absorption through the skin may cause neurotoxic symptoms such as tremors and convulsions that can be fatal.

di•elec•tric (di"ə-lek'trik) 1. transmitting electric effects by induction, but not by conduction. 2. an insulating substance that transmits in this way, i.e., through or across which electric force is acting or may act, by induction without conduction.

di•elec•trol•y•sis (di"ə-lek-trol'ə-sis) [*dia-* + *electrolysis*] electrolysis of a drug, the current being passed through a diseased portion of the body, so that the drug passes through the part.

di•em•bry•ony (di-em'bre-on"e) [*di-* + *embryony*] the production of two embryos from a single zygote.

di•en•ceph•a•lo•hy•po•phys•i•al (di"ən-sef"ə-lo-hi"po-fiz'e-əl) pertaining to the diencephalon and the pituitary gland.

di•en•ceph•a•lon (di"ən-sef'ə-lon) [*dia-* + *encephalon*] 1. [TA] the caudal part of the prosencephalon, which largely bounds the third ventricle and connects the mesencephalon to the cerebral hemispheres; each lateral half is divided by the hypothalamic sulcus into a dorsal part, comprising the epithalamus, dorsal thalamus, and metathalamus, and a ventral part, comprising the ventral thalamus (subthalamus) and hypothalamus. Called also *interbrain.* See Plate 9. See also *brainstem.* 2. the posterior of the two brain vesicles formed by specialization of the prosencephalon in the developing embryo. **diencephal'ic** *adj*

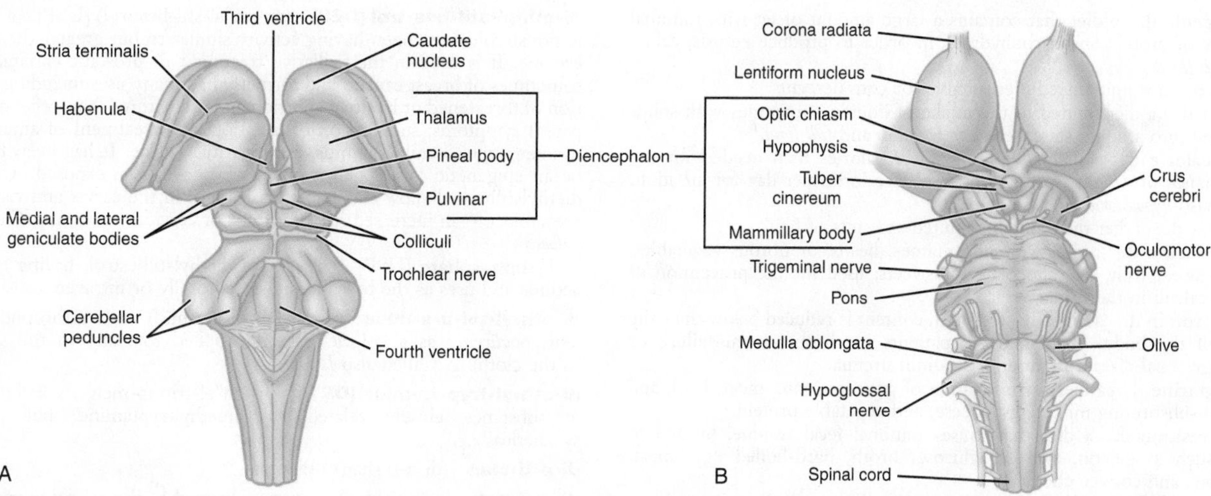

■ Diencephalon. Posterior (dorsal) *(A)* and anterior (inferior) *(B)* views of the base of the brain, showing the diencephalon in relation to the mesencephalon (midbrain) and rhombencephalon (hindbrain).

-diene a suffix used in chemistry to denote an unsaturated hydrocarbon containing two double bonds.

die•ner (de′nər) [Ger. "man-servant"] a technician or general auxiliary worker, usually in a gross laboratory.

di•en•es•trol (di″ən-es′trol) [USP] a synthetic estrogen administered intravaginally in the treatment of atrophic vaginitis and kraurosis vulvae.

Di•ent•amoe•ba (di″ent-ə-me′bə) [*di-* + *ent-* + *ameba*] a genus of small, highly active, usually nonpathogenic or mildly pathogenic ameboid protozoa (superorder Parabasalidea, order Trichomonadida) parasitic in the large intestine of humans and certain monkeys. They typically have two nuclei connected by a desmose, as well as an endosome formed by four to eight chromatin granules. *D. fra′gilis* has been associated with human infection, causing dientamoebiasis.

di•ent•amoe•bi•a•sis (di″ent-ə-me-bi′ə-sis) intestinal infection with *Dientamoeba fragilis,* characterized by diarrhea, abdominal pain, bloody, mucoid, or loose feces, and flatulence.

di•er•e•sis (di-er′ə-sis) [Gr. *diairesis* a taking] 1. the division or separation of parts normally united. 2. in surgery, the operative separation of parts by incision, electrosurgery, or cautery.

di•esoph•a•gus (di-ə-sof′ə-gəs) doubling of the esophagus.

di•es•ter (di-es′tər) a compound containing two ester groups.

di•es•trum (di-es′trəm) diestrus.

di•es•trus (di-es′trəs) 1. in female mammals that have estrous cycles, a period of sexual quiescence between metestrus and the next proestrus; it represents the phase of the mature corpus luteum. 2. anestrus (def. 2). Called also *diestrum.*

gestational d. the period of sexual inactivity occurring during gestation in female mammals.

lactational d. the period of sexual inactivity occurring during lactation in female mammals.

di•et (di′ət) [Gr. *diaita* way of living] the customary allowance of food and drink taken by any person from day to day, particularly one especially planned to meet specific requirements of the individual, and including or excluding certain items of food. **di′etary** *adj*

absolute d. fasting.

acid-ash d. a diet to produce acidification of the urine, consisting of meat, fish, eggs, and cereals, with little fruit and vegetables and no cheese or milk.

adequate d. a diet that enables an animal to grow, mature, and reproduce in a normal manner. Cf. *optimal d.*

alkali-ash d. a diet of fruit, vegetables, and milk with minimal meat, fish, eggs, and cereals, used to prevent some types of urinary calculi. Called also *basic d.*

Atkins d. a diet low in carbohydrates; used for weight reduction.

balanced d. a diet that contains all the nutritive factors in proper proportion for adequate nutrition.

basal d. a diet that is just sufficient to meet the caloric requirements of basal metabolism.

basic d. alkali-ash d.

bland d. a diet that is free from any irritating or stimulating foods.

challenge d. a diet to which foods suspected of causing sensitivity in the patient are added, usually one at a time, and the results assessed. Cf. *provocative d.*

clear liquid d. a temporary diet of clear liquids without residue; it is not nutritionally adequate, and is used in some acute illnesses and infections, in the postoperative period (especially after gastrointestinal surgery), and to reduce fecal matter in the colon.

DASH d. (Dietary Approach to Stop Hypertension) a diet high in fruits, vegetables, and low-fat dairy products; low in saturated and total fats; low in cholesterol; and high in fiber. Research studies support the hypothesis that this diet reduces blood pressure and may play a role in the prevention of high blood pressure.

diabetic d. a diet designed to prevent complications of diabetes mellitus by controlling the timing and amount of energy intake and minimizing the occurrence of ketosis or hypoglycemia; fat, carbohydrate, and protein ratios and amounts are controlled but specific diet plans vary.

elemental d. a diet consisting of a well-balanced, residue-free mixture of all essential and nonessential amino acids combined with simple sugars, electrolytes, trace elements, and vitamins.

elimination d. a procedure to identify food allergy in which foods are sequentially omitted in order to detect the one or ones responsible for symptoms.

Feingold d. a controversial diet for hyperactive children, which excludes artificial colors, artificial flavors, preservatives, and salicylates.

formula d. a diet in which one or more meals consist of or are supplemented by a processed drink formulated to contain defined levels of specific vitamins, nutrients, and caloric level; it is usually used in weight reduction.

full liquid d. a diet for patients who cannot eat solid food, consisting of any liquid such as milk or juice, as well as liquefied solids; this diet can be nutritionally adequate.

Gerson d. a detoxification diet, claimed to be useful in the treatment of cancer, allergies, and a wide variety of degenerative diseases, consisting of large quantities of organically grown fruits and vegetables, consumed mainly in the form of juice; often combined with other complementary therapies.

Giordano-Giovannetti d. a low protein diet given to alleviate gastrointestinal symptoms of chronic renal failure.

gluten-free d. a diet deficient in the cereal protein gluten; used as a specific treatment for celiac disease (gluten enteropathy).

Gonzalez d. an ovolactovegetarian diet with the addition of fish, used with pancreatic enzymes and other supplements and colonics; claimed to be effective against pancreatic cancer.

gouty d. a diet for mitigation of gout, restricting nitrogenous, especially high-purine foods, and substituting dairy products, with prohibition of wines and liquors. Cf. *low purine d.*

high calorie d. a diet that furnishes more calories than needed for the maintenance of weight, often more than 3500–4000 calories per day. Called also *hypercaloric d.*

high fat d. ketogenic d.

high fiber d. a diet relatively high in dietary fibers, which decreases transit time through the intestine and relieves constipation.

high protein d. a diet containing large amounts of protein, such as from meats, fish, milk, legumes, and nuts.

hypercaloric d. high calorie d.

hypocaloric d. low calorie d.

ketogenic d. a diet that contains a large amount of fat with minimal amounts of protein and carbohydrate, in order to produce ketosis; called also *high fat d.*

light d. a simple mixed diet suitable for convalescents.

liquid d. a diet limited to the intake of liquids, sometimes with solids processed into a liquid state; see *clear liquid d.* and *full liquid d.*

low calorie d. a diet containing fewer calories than needed for the maintenance of weight, e.g., less than 1200 calories per day for an adult. Called also *hypocaloric d.*

low fat d. a diet that contains limited amounts of fat.

low oxalate d. a diet with no potatoes, beans, or fibrous vegetables, and no sweet fruit, tea, chocolate, or sweets; used for the prevention of oxalate calculi in the urinary tract.

low protein d. a diet whose protein content is reduced below the daily needs of the body, prescribed for patients in chronic renal failure or end-stage renal disease in an effort to limit uremia.

low purine d. a diet for mitigation of gout, omitting meat, fowl, and fish and substituting milk, eggs, cheese, and vegetable protein.

low residue d. a diet that causes minimal fecal residue, limited to foods such as gelatin, sucrose, glucose, broth, hard-boiled egg, meat, liver, rice, and cottage cheese.

low salt d., low sodium d. a diet containing very little sodium chloride, sometimes prescribed for hypertension and for edematous states.

macrobiotic d. a diet theory based on a Japanese variation of the yin/yang principle and popularized in the United States; there are several different diets, ranging from a severe form that includes only cereal products to more moderate ones in which a wide variety of foods are kept balanced between those with "yin" energy and those with "yang" energy.

nutraceutical d. a diet containing functional foods (nutraceuticals).

optimal d. a diet that produces the most desirable growth, the most successful reproduction, and the maintenance of the best possible health; cf. *adequate d.*

Ornish d. a vegetarian diet containing 10 per cent of calories from fat and 5 mg cholesterol, used in combination with stress reduction techniques and moderate exercise for the prevention and treatment of cardiovascular disease.

protein-sparing d. a diet that consists only of liquid proteins or liquid mixtures of proteins, vitamins, and minerals, and containing no more than 600 calories; it is designed to maintain a favorable nitrogen balance.

provocative d. a diet designed to include the most common allergenic foods, from which they are eliminated one by one, as a means of determining the offending substances in cases of food allergy. Cf. *challenge d.*

purine-free d. see *low purine d.*

salt-free d. see *low salt d.*

Schemm d. a low-sodium, neutral, and acid-ash diet for patients with congestive heart failure.

Sippy d. a diet formerly widely used to treat peptic ulcers, consisting of milk, cream, and other supposedly bland foods; it was later proved ineffective.

smooth d. a diet that avoids the use of foods containing roughage.

subsistence d. a diet on which one can just live.

Taylor d. a preparation of egg whites, olive oil, and sugar, given when the urine is to be tested for chlorides.

test d. a diet designed to test allergy or sensitivity to certain foods by selectively omitting or including those foods, such as an elimination diet or provocative diet.

therapeutic d. a diet specifically formulated for use in the diagnosis or treatment of disease or deficiency.

very low calorie d. (VLCD) a diet providing 200 to 800 kilocalories per day, used for weight loss in markedly obese patients for whom other diet programs have been unsuccessful.

di·e·tet·ic (di″ə-tet′ik) [Gr. *diaitētikos*] 1. pertaining to diet. 2. pertaining to a diet that is restricted, such as for health reasons.

di·e·tet·ics (di″ə-tet′iks) the science or study and regulation of the diet.

di·eth·yl (di-eth′əl) a molecule having two ethyl groups.

d. ether, d. oxide ether (def. 2).

di·eth·yl·ene·di·amine (di-eth″əl-ēn-di′ə-mēn) piperazine.

1,4-di·eth·yl·ene di·ox·ide (di-eth′ə-lēn di-ok′sīd) dioxane.

di·eth·y·lene gly·col (di-eth′əl-ēn gli′kol) a sweet-tasting hygroscopic liquid used as a solvent in antifreeze, brake fluid, cigarettes, and dyes. Ingestion of excessive amounts may be toxic to the central nervous system, heart, respiratory system, liver, pancreas, and kidneys.

di·eth·yl·ene·tri·amine pen·ta·ace·tic ac·id (DTPA) (di-eth″əl-ēn-tri′ə-mēn pen″tə-ə-se′tik as′id) pentetic acid.

di·eth·yl·pro·pi·on hy·dro·chlo·ride (di-eth″əl-pro′pe-on) [USP] a sympathomimetic amine, related to amphetamine, used as an oral anorectic in the control of exogenous obesity.

di·eth·yl·stil·bes·trol (DES) (di-eth″əl-stil-bes′trol) [USP] a synthetic nonsteroidal estrogen having activity similar to but greater than that of estrone. It is used in the palliative treatment of prostatic carcinoma and sometimes of breast cancer, and formerly had many uses including prevention of threatened or habitual abortion and premature labor; relief of menopausal symptoms; suppression of lactation; and treatment of amenorrhea, dysmenorrhea, senile vaginitis, and pruritus vulvae. It has been found to be an epigenetic carcinogen; women who have been exposed in utero to diethylstilbestrol show characteristic changes in the cervix and vagina and are subject to an increased risk of vaginal or cervical carcinoma. Called also *stilbestrol.*

d. diphosphate [USP] an ester of diethylstilbestrol, having the same actions and uses as the base; administered orally or intravenously.

di·eth·yl·tol·u·a·mide (di-eth″əl-tol-u′ə-mīd) an arthropod repellent, occurring as a colorless liquid; applied topically to the skin and to the clothing. Called also *DEET.*

di·eth·yl·tryp·ta·mine (DET) (di-eth″əl-trip′tə-mēn) a hallucinogenic substance closely related to dimethyltryptamine, but prepared synthetically.

di·e·ti·cian (di″ə-tĭ′shən) dietitian.

di·e·ti·tian (di″ə-tish′ən) a person trained in the scientific use of diet in health and disease.

Die·tl crisis (de′təl) [Józef *Dietl*, Polish physician, 1804–1878] see under *crisis.*

di·e·to·ther·a·py (di″ə-to-ther′ə-pe) diet therapy.

Dieu·la·foy triad, lesion (ulcer, vascular malformation) (dyo͞o-lah-fwah′) [Paul Georges *Dieulafoy*, French physician, 1839–1911] see under *triad* and *lesion.*

di·fe·nox·in (di″fə-nok′sin) an antiperistaltic that is the active metabolite of diphenoxylate.

d. hydrochloride the hydrochloride salt of difenoxin, used as an antidiarrheal; administered orally.

dif·fer·ence (dif′ər-ens) the condition or magnitude of variation between two qualities or quantities.

arteriovenous oxygen d. the difference in the oxygen content of blood between the arterial and venous systems, usually expressed in mL/L of blood.

light d. the difference between the two eyes in their sensitivity to light; often abbreviated LD.

dif·fer·en·tial (dif″ər-en′shəl) [L. *differre* to carry apart] pertaining to a difference or differences.

dif·fer·en·ti·ate (dif″ər-en′she-āt) 1. to distinguish, on the basis of differences. 2. to develop specialized form, character, or function differing from that of surrounding cytoplasm, cells, or tissue or from the original type.

dif·fer·en·ti·a·tion (dif″ər-en″she-a′shən) 1. the distinguishing of one thing or disease from another. 2. the act or process of acquiring completely individual characters, as occurs in the progressive diversification of cells and tissues of the embryo. 3. increase in morphological or chemical heterogeneity.

correlative d., dependent d. differentiation caused by factors outside the tissue itself, as by an inductor.

functional d. differentiation that results from the functioning of the tissue of a part.

invisible d. the development toward a fixed fate, through chemodifferentiation, by cells that show no visible signs of this determination.

regional d. the appearance of regional differences within a field of development.

self d. self-differentiation.

sexual d. the process by which the male or female phenotype is produced; the entire developmental cascade initiated by the specific genotype.

Dif·fer·in (dif′ə-rin) trademark for a preparation of adapalene.

dif·flu·ence (dif′loo-əns) the act of becoming fluid or of flowing readily.

dif·flu·ent (dif′loo-ənt) [L. *diffluere* to flow off] 1. easily flowing away or dissolving. 2. deliquescent.

Diff-Quik (dif′kwik) trademark for a Giemsa-type stain.

dif·frac·tion (dĭ-frak′shən) [*dis-*[1] + L. *frangere* to break] the bending of waves around small obstacles and the spreading out of waves past openings that are small compared to the wavelengths. See also under *grating.*

x-ray d. a technique for studying the cell based on the diffraction of radiations when they encounter small obstacles; used especially in the study of inorganic and organic crystals, in which it is possible to determine the precise spatial relationships between the constituent atoms.

dif•fu•sate (dĭ-fu′zāt) 1. material that has passed through a membrane, as opposed to the retentate. 2. specifically, the solutes that pass out of the blood into the dialysate fluid in a dialyzer; sometimes also referred to as the *dialysate.*

dif•fuse[1] (dĭ-fūs′) [*dis-*[1] + *fundere* to pour] not definitely limited or localized; widely distributed.

dif•fuse[2] (dĭ-fūz′) [*dis-*[1] + *fundere* to pour] to pass through or to spread widely through a tissue or structure.

dif•fus•ible (dĭ-fūz′ĭ-bəl) susceptible of becoming widely spread.

dif•fu•si•om•e•ter (dĭ-fu″ze-om′ə-tər) an apparatus for measuring the speed of diffusion.

dif•fu•sion (dĭ-fu′zhən) 1. the process of becoming diffused, or widely spread. 2. the spontaneous movement of molecules or other particles in solution, owing to their random thermal motion, to reach a uniform concentration throughout the solvent, a process requiring no addition of energy to the system. 3. the movement of solutes down concentration gradients across a semipermeable membrane such as a hemodialyzer membrane; the movement is generally of urea and low molecular weight toxins from the blood to the dialysate and of bicarbonate and acetate from the dialysate to the blood. 4. immunodiffusion.

double d. immunodiffusion in which both the antigen and antibody diffuse through the medium toward each other.

double d. in one dimension double diffusion in which antiserum is placed in a test tube and overlaid with agar; the agar is allowed to solidify and antigen is layered over it. Precipitin lines form where the concentrations of each antigen and antibody are equivalent. Called also *Oakley-Fulthorpe technique.*

double d. in two dimensions double diffusion in which antigen and antiserum are placed in wells cut in an agar plate; antigen solutions to be compared are placed in wells equidistant from the antiserum well. Three principal types of reaction may occur, *reaction of identity, reaction of nonidentity,* and *reaction of partial identity* (see under *reaction*), each identified by a characteristic pattern of precipitin lines, indicating the extent to which the antigen samples a share antigenic determinants. Called also *Ouchterlony technique.*

exchange d. the process in which diffusion of a molecule across a membrane in one direction is balanced by diffusion of another molecule in the opposite direction.

facilitated d. diffusion across a plasma membrane or other biological membrane in which the molecules to be transported form complexes with specific transport proteins (uniporters) that shuttle them across the membrane down the concentration gradient and release them on the other side. Called also *uniport.*

free d. diffusion in which there is no obstacle such as a membrane.

gel d. immunodiffusion.

impeded d. diffusion in which the rate is slowed down by the difficulty of passing through a membrane.

single d. immunodiffusion in which either the antibody or antigen remains fixed and the other reactant diffuses through it.

single radial d. radial immunodiffusion.

thermal d. thermodiffusion.

di•flor•a•sone di•ac•e•tate (di-flor′ə-sōn) [USP] a synthetic corticosteroid used topically for the relief of inflammation and pruritus in corticosteroid-responsive dermatoses.

Di•flu•can (di′floo-kan) trademark for preparations of fluconazole.

di•flu•cor•to•lone va•ler•ate (di″floo-kor′tə-lōn″) a medium potency synthetic corticosteroid used topically for the relief of inflammation and pruritus in corticosteroid-responsive dermatoses.

di•flu•ni•sal (di-floo′nĭ-səl) [USP] a nonsteroidal antiinflammatory drug derived from salicylic acid, having analgesic activity but lacking antipyretic activity; used in the treatment of rheumatic disorders, acute attacks of gout or calcium pyrophosphate deposition disease, dysmenorrhea, and pain associated with various nonrheumatic inflammatory conditions or vascular headaches.

Dig. [L.] digera′tur (let it be digested).

di•gal•lic ac•id (di-gal′ik) an incorrect term for tannic acid.

di•ga•met•ic (di″gə-met′ik) 1. pertaining to or producing gametes (germ or sex cells) of two different types, female (oocytes) and male (spermatozoa). 2. heterogametic.

di•gas•tric (di-gas′trik) [*di-* + *gastric*] 1. having two bellies. 2. musculus digastricus.

di•gen•e•sis (di-jen′ə-sis) alternation of generations.

di•ge•net•ic (di″jə-net′ik) [*di-* + *genetic*] 1. having two stages of multiplication, one sexual in the mature forms, the other asexual in the larval stages; said of flukes and many other parasites. 2. heteroxenous.

Di•George syndrome (dĭ-jorj′) [Angelo Mario *DiGeorge,* American pediatrician, born 1921] see under *syndrome.*

di•ges•tant (di-jes′tənt) 1. assisting or stimulating digestion. 2. an agent that assists or stimulates digestion.

di•ges•tion (di-jes′chən) [L. *digestio,* from *dis-* apart + *gerere* to carry] 1. the process or act of converting food into chemical substances that can be absorbed and assimilated. 2. the subjection of a body to prolonged heat and moisture, so as to disintegrate and soften it.

artificial d. digestion that takes place outside the body.

biliary d. the digestive effect of bile upon food.

gastric d. digestion carried on in the stomach by aid of the gastric juice; called also *peptic d.* and *chymification.*

gastrointestinal d. gastric digestion and intestinal digestion considered together.

intercellular d. digestion carried on within an organ by secretions from the cells of the organ.

intestinal d. digestion that takes place in the intestine.

intracellular d. digestion carried on within a single cell.

lipolytic d. the splitting of fat into fatty acid and glycerol; cf. *lipolysis.*

pancreatic d. digestion by pancreatic juice in the duodenum.

parenteral d. digestion taking place somewhere else in the body than in the alimentary canal, as in the blood or under the skin.

peptic d. gastric d.

salivary d. the change of starch into maltose by the saliva.

self-d. 1. autophagy. 2. autolysis.

sludge d. the biochemical process by which organic matter in sludge is gasified, liquefied, mineralized, or converted into more stable organic matter.

di•ges•tive (di-jes′tiv) 1. pertaining to digestion. 2. digestant.

Dig•i•bind (dij′ĭ-bīnd″) trademark for a preparation of digoxin immune Fab (ovine).

dig•it (dij′it) [L. *digitus*] digitus.

dig•i•tal (dij′ĭ-təl) 1. of, pertaining to, or performed with, a finger. 2. resembling the imprint of a finger. 3. relating to data that are represented in the form of discrete numeric symbols.

dig•i•tal•in (dij″ĭ-tal′in) 1. a cardiac glycoside, $C_{36}H_{56}O_{14}$, from the seeds of *Digitalis purpurea.* 2. any of several mixtures of digitalis glycosides extracted from the leaves or seeds.

Dig•i•tal•is (dij″ĭ-tal′is) [L., from *digitus* finger, because of the fingerlike leaves of the corolla of its flowers] a genus of herbs of the family Scrophulariaceae, native to Europe and Asia. *D. purpu′rea* is the purple foxglove, whose leaves furnish digitalis. *D. lana′ta* is a Balkan species that yields digoxin and lanatoside.

dig•i•tal•is (dij″ĭ-tal′is) 1. [USP] the dried leaf of *Digitalis purpurea,* the purple foxglove, used to treat congestive heart failure, most supraventricular tachycardias, and cardiogenic shock. Digitalis and the digitalis glycosides act by increasing the force of myocardial contraction and by increasing the refractory period and decreasing the conduction rate of the atrioventricular node. When digitalis is prescribed, *powdered d.* (q.v.) is to be dispensed. 2. collectively, the digitalis glycosides or the cardiac glycosides. 3. fingerlike, or pertaining to a digit.

d. leaf digitalis (def. 1).

powdered d. [USP], **prepared d.** the standardized preparation to be dispensed when digitalis is prescribed; its actions and uses are as for digitalis; administered orally.

dig•i•tal•iza•tion (dij″ĭ-təl-ĭ-za′shən) the administration of digitalis or one of its glycosides in a dosage schedule designed to produce and then maintain optimal therapeutic concentrations of its cardiotonic glycosides.

dig•i•tal•oid (dij′ĭ-təl-oid) resembling or related to digitalis.

dig•i•tate (dij′ĭ-tāt) having fingerlike processes. Called also *dactylate.*

dig•i•ta•tio (dij″ĭ-ta′she-o) pl. *digitatio′nes* [L.] digitation: a fingerlike process.

digitatio′nes hippocam′pi [TA] pes hippocampi.

dig•i•ta•tion (dij″ĭ-ta′shən) 1. digitatio. 2. surgical creation of a functioning digit.

dig•i•ta•ti•o•nes (dij″ĭ-ta″she-o′nez) [L.] plural of *digitatio.*

Dig•i•tek (dij′ĭ-tek) trademark for preparations of digoxin.

dig•i•ti (dij′ĭ-ti) [L.] genitive and plural of *digitus.*

dig•i•ti•form (dij′ĭ-tĭ-form) resembling a finger; fingerlike.

dig•i•ti•grade (dij′ĭ-tĭ-grād″) [*digit-* + L. *gradi* to walk] characterized by standing or walking on the toes, with the posterior part of the foot being raised; said of quadrupeds such as cats and dogs. Cf. *plantigrade* and *unguligrade.*

digit(o)- [L. *digitus* finger, toe] a combining form denoting relationship to one or more fingers or toes.

dig•i•to•nin (dij″ĭ-to′nin) a saponin obtained from *Digitalis purpurea;* it possesses no cardiotonic action and is used as a reagent to precipitate free cholesterol.

dig•i•to•plan•tar (dij″ĭ-to-plan′tər) [*digito-* + *plantar*] pertaining to the toes and the sole of the foot.

di•gi•toxi•ge•nin (dij″ĭ-tok″sĭ-je′nin) the steroid nucleus that is the aglycone of digitoxin.

dig•i•tox•in (dij″ĭ-tok′sin) [USP] a cardiac glycoside obtained from *Digitalis purpurea*, *D. lanata*, and other *Digitalis* species, containing 3 molecules of digitoxose linked to digitoxigenin; it has the same actions and uses as digitalis; administered orally, intramuscularly, or intravenously.

dig•i•tox•ose (dij″ĭ-tok′sōs) a hexose sugar that forms the carbohydrate moiety of the cardiac glycosides obtained from *Digitalis*.

dig•i•tus (dij′ĭ-təs) pl. *dig′iti* [L.] digit: a finger or a toe; see also *ossa digitorum manus* and *ossa digitorum pedis*, under *os*[2].

d. anula′ris [TA] ring finger: the fourth digit of the hand. Called also *d. quartus (IV) manus* [TA alternative].

d. hippocra′ticus clubbed finger.

d. mal′leus mallet finger.

di′giti ma′nus [TA] the digits of the hand; the fingers. See *pollex*, *index* (def. 1), *d. medius*, *d. anularis*, and *d. minimus manus*.

d. me′dius [TA] middle finger: the third digit of the hand; called also *d. tertius (III) manus* [TA alternative].

d. mi′nimus ma′nus [TA] little finger: the fifth, and smallest, digit of the hand; called also *d. quintus (V) manus* [TA alternative].

d. mi′nimus pe′dis [TA] little toe: the fifth, and smallest, digit of the foot; called also *d. quintus (V) pedis* [TA alternative].

d. mor′tuus [L.] dead finger.

di′giti pe′dis [TA] the digits of the foot; the toes. See *hallux*, *d. secundus pedis*, *d. tertius pedis*, *d. quartus pedis*, and *d. minimus pedis*.

d. postmi′nimus an appendage ranging from a small round mass of fat and connective tissue to a longer mass containing bones and with a nail at its distal end, attached by a small pedicle to the soft tissue covering the lateral surface of the little finger or toe.

d. pri′mus (I) ma′nus TA alternative for *pollex*.

d. pri′mus (I) pe′dis TA alternative for *hallux*.

d. quar′tus (IV) ma′nus TA alternative for *d. anularis*.

d. quar′tus (IV) pe′dis [TA] the fourth digit of the foot.

d. quin′tus (V) ma′nus TA alternative for *d. minimus manus*.

d. quin′tus (V) pe′dis TA alternative for *d. minimus pedis*.

d. secun′dus (II) ma′nus TA alternative for *index*.

d. secun′dus (II) pe′dis [TA] the second digit of the foot.

d. ter′tius (III) ma′nus TA alternative for *d. medius*.

d. ter′tius (III) pe′dis [TA] the third digit of the foot.

d. val′gus deviation of a digit in the radial direction, or toward the digit of next lower number.

d. va′rus deviation of a digit in the ulnar direction, or toward the digit of next higher number.

di•glos•sia (di-glos′e-ə) [*di-* + *gloss-* + *-ia*] bifid tongue.

di•glu•cu•ro•nide (di-gloo′ku-rə-nīd) a compound containing two molecules of glucuronide.

di•glyc•er•ide (di-glis′ər-īd) diacylglycerol.

di•glyc•er•ide ac•yl•trans•fer•ase (di-glis′ər-īd a″səl-trans′fər-ās) diacylglycerol *O*-acyltransferase.

di•glyc•er•ide ki•nase (di-glis′ər-īd ki′nās) diacylglycerol kinase.

dig•na•thus (dig-na′thəs) [*di-* + Gr. *gnathos* jaw] a fetus with two lower jaws; see also *myognathus*.

di•goxi•ge•nin (dĭ-jok″sĭ-je′nin) the steroid nucleus that is the aglycone of digoxin.

di•gox•in (dĭ-jok′sin) [USP] a cardiac glycoside obtained from the leaves of *Digitalis lanata*, containing 3 molecules of digitoxose linked to digoxigenin, and having the same actions and uses as digitalis; administered orally, intramuscularly, or intravenously.

d. immune Fab (ovine) see under *Fab*.

Di•gram•ma brau•ni (di-gram′ə braw′ne) a larval tapeworm belonging to the family Diphyllobothriidae, found in humans in Romania.

Di Gu•gli•el•mo syndrome (de goo-lyel′mo) [Giovanni *Di Guglielmo*, Italian hematologist, 1886–1961] erythroleukemia.

di•het•ero•zy•gote (di-het″ər-o-zi′gōt) [*di-* + *heterozygote*] an individual heterozygous for two pairs of genes; called also *dihybrid*.

di huang (te″ hwahng′) *Rehmannia glutinosa*, a perennial herb native to China, Japan, and Korea; preparations of the root tuber are used in traditional Chinese medicine as a diuretic and for their effects on the heart, liver, and kidney meridians. The fresh and dried forms (*shu di huang* and *sheng di huang*, respectively), are used differently.

di•hy•brid (di-hi′brid) diheterozygote.

di•hy•drate (di-hi′drāt) [*di-* + *hydrate*] 1. any compound containing two hydroxyl groups. 2. any compound containing two molecules of water.

di•hy•drat•ed (di-hi′drāt-əd) compounded with two molecules of water.

di•hy•dric (di-hi′drik) having two hydrogen atoms in each molecule.

dihydro- a chemical prefix denoting the presence of two additional hydrogen atoms.

di•hy•dro•an•thra•cene•di•one di•hy•dro•chlo•ride (di-hi″dro-an″thrə-sēn-di′ōn) mitoxantrone hydrochloride.

di•hy•dro•bi•op•ter•in (di-hi″dro-bi-op′tər-in) a reduced pteridine derivative related to folic acid; its quinoid form is produced by oxidation of tetrahydrobiopterin in several biological hydroxylation reactions.

di•hy•dro•cho•les•ter•ol (di-hi″dro-kə-les′tər-ol) cholestanol.

di•hy•dro•co•deine (di-hi″dro-ko′dēn) an opioid analgesic related to codeine; it has also been used as an antitussive; called also *drocode*.

d. bitartrate [USP] the acid tartrate of dihydrocodeine, used for the relief of moderate to moderately severe pain; administered orally.

di•hy•dro•co•dei•none bi•tar•trate (di-hi″dro-ko′de-nōn) hydrocodone bitartrate.

di•hy•dro•cor•ti•sol (di-hi″dro-kor′tĭ-sol) either of two inactive metabolites of cortisol, 5α-dihydrocortisol and 5β-dihydrocortisol; the 5β form is predominant.

di•hy•dro•er•go•cor•nine (di-hi″dro-er″go-kor′nin) an ergot derivative that has sympatholytic and adrenolytic properties; see *ergoloid mesylates*.

di•hy•dro•er•go•cris•tine (di-hi″dro-er″go-kris′tin) an ergot derivative that has sympatholytic and adrenolytic properties; see *ergoloid mesylates*.

di•hy•dro•er•go•cryp•tine (di-hi″dro-er″go-krip′tin) an ergot derivative that has sympatholytic and adrenolytic properties; see *ergoloid mesylates*.

di•hy•dro•er•got•amine mes•y•late (di-hi″dro-ər-got′ə-mēn) [USP] an antiadrenergic produced by the catalytic hydrogenation of ergotamine; used as a vasoconstrictor in the treatment of migraine; administered intramuscularly, subcutaneously, intravenously, or intranasally.

di•hy•dro•fo•late (DHF) (di-hi″dro-fo′lāt) an ester or dissociated form of dihydrofolic acid.

di•hy•dro•fo•late re•duc•tase (di-hi″dro-fo′lāt re-duk′tās) [EC 1.5.1.3] an enzyme of the oxidoreductase class that catalyzes the reduction of dihydrofolate to tetrahydrofolate, using NADPH as an electron donor. The reaction produces reduced folate for amino acid metabolism, purine ring synthesis, and the formation of deoxythymidine monophosphate. Methotrexate and other folic acid antagonists used as chemotherapeutic drugs act by inhibiting this enzyme. Deficiency of the enzyme may be a cause of megaloblastic anemia responsive to therapy with reduced forms of folic acid. Abbreviated DHFR.

di•hy•dro•fol•ic ac•id (di-hi″dro-fo′lik) any of the folic acids in which the bicyclic pteridine structure is in the dihydro, partially reduced form; they are intermediates in folate metabolism and are reduced to their tetrahydro, reduced forms.

di•hy•dro•in•do•lone (di-hi″dro-in′do-lōn) any of a class of structurally related antipsychotic agents; the prototype is molindone.

di•hy•drol (di-hi′drol) the associated water molecule, $(H_2O)_2$.

di•hy•dro•lipo•am•ide (di-hi″dro-lip″o-am′īd) the reduced form of lipoamide, produced as an intermediate in the reactions in which lipoamide acts as a cofactor.

di•hy•dro•lip•o•yl (di-hi″dro-lip′o-əl) the acyl radical of dihydrolipoamide.

di•hy•dro•lip•o•yl de•hy•dro•gen•ase (di-hi″dro-lip′o-əl de-hi′drojən-ās) [EC 1.8.1.4] an enzyme of the oxidoreductase class that catalyzes the regeneration of lipoyl groups from dihydrolipoyl groups, reducing NAD^+. The enzyme contains FAD and is a component of several oxidative decarboxylation enzyme complexes, including the branched-chain α-keto acid dehydrogenase, α-ketoglutarate dehydrogenase, and pyruvate dehydrogenase complexes; deficiency of the enzyme, an autosomal recessive trait, is a cause of maple syrup urine disease.

di•hy•dro•lip•o•yl•lys•ine•res•i•due ac•e•tyl•trans•fer•ase (di-hi″dro-lip″o-əl-li′sēn rez′ĭ-doo as″ə-tēl-trans′fər-ās) [EC 2.3.1.12] an enzyme of the transferase class that is a component of the multienzyme pyruvate dehydrogenase complex (q.v.). The lipoyl group of this enzyme is reductively acetylated by pyruvate dehydrogenase (acetyl-transferring); the enzyme then catalyzes the transfer of acetyl from its lipoamide chain to coenzyme A to form acetyl CoA. Called also *dihydrolipoyl transacetylase*.

di•hy•dro•lip•o•yl•lys•ine•res•i•due (2-meth•yl•pro•pa•no•yl)-trans•fer•ase (di-hi″dro-lip″o-əl-li′sēn rez′ĭ-doo meth″əl-pro″pəno′əl trans′fər-ās) [EC 2.3.1.168] an enzyme of the transferase class that is a component of the multienzyme branched-chain α-keto acid dehydrogenase complex (q.v.). The enzyme catalyzes the transfer of the decarboxylated branched-chain acyl moiety to coenzyme A via its own lipoyl group.

di·hy·dro·lip·o·yl·lys·ine-res·i·due suc·cin·yl·trans·fer·ase (di-hi″dro-lip″o-əl-li′sēn rez′ĭ-doo suk″sin-əl-trans′fər-ās) [EC 2.3.1.61] an enzyme of the transferase class that is a component of the multienzyme α-ketoglutarate dehydrogenase complex (q.v.). The lipoyl group of this enzyme is reductively succinylated by α-ketoglutarate dehydrogenase and then catalyzes the transfer of succinyl from its lipoamide chain to coenzyme A to form succinyl coenzyme A. Called also *transsuccinylase.*

di·hy·dro·lip·o·yl trans·acet·y·lase (di-hi″dro-lip′o-əl trans″ə-set′ə-lās) dihydrolipoyllysine-residue acetyltransferase.

di·hy·dro·lu·ti·dine (di-hi″dro-loo′tĭ-dēn) an oily, poisonous, caustic base from rancid cod liver oil.

di·hy·dro·mor·phi·none hy·dro·chlo·ride (di-hi″dro-mor′fĭ-nōn) hydromorphone hydrochloride.

di·hy·dro·or·o·tase (di-hi″dro-or′o-tās) [EC 3.5.2.3] an enzyme activity of the trifunctional CAD protein (q.v.); it is a ligase that catalyzes the cyclization of carbamoylaspartate, creating the initial ring structure (dihydroorotate) in the biosynthesis of pyrimidine nucleotides.

di·hy·dro·or·o·tate (di-hi″dro-or′o-tāt) cyclized carbamoylaspartate, an intermediate in pyrimidine biosynthesis.

6,7-di·hy·dro·pter·i·dine re·duc·tase (DHPR) (di-hi″dro-ter′ĭ-dēn re-duk′tās) [EC 1.5.1.34] an enzyme of the oxidoreductase class that catalyzes the NAD(P)H-dependent reduction of dihydrobiopterin to regenerate tetrahydrobiopterin, the coenzyme essential to those enzymes that hydroxylate phenylalanine, tryptophan, and tyrosine, with subsequent formation of the corresponding neurotransmitters (e.g., dopamine). Deficiency of the enzyme, an autosomal recessive trait caused by mutation of the *QHPR* gene, which encodes the enzyme, is a form of tetrahydrobiopterin deficiency (q.v.).

di·hy·dro·py·rim·i·dine de·hy·dro·gen·ase (NADP⁺) (di-hi″dro-pə-rim′ĭ-dēn de-hi′dro-jən-ās) [EC 1.3.1.2] an enzyme of the oxidoreductase class that catalyzes the dehydrogenation of uracil and of thymine, using NADPH as an electron donor; the reaction is a step in the catabolism of pyrimidines. Deficiency of the enzyme, an autosomal recessive disorder, results in elevated pyrimidine levels in plasma, urine, and cerebrospinal fluid; it is manifest clinically in children by cerebral dysfunction and in adults by hypersensitivity to the drug 5-fluorouracil.

di·hy·dro·tach·ys·te·rol (di-hi″dro-tak-is′tə-rol) [USP] an analogue of ergocalciferol produced upon irradiation of ergosterol; it raises serum calcium levels via stimulation of intestinal absorption of calcium and mobilization of the mineral from bone in patients lacking renal function or parathyroid hormone. It is used in the treatment of chronic hypocalcemia, hypophosphatemia, rickets, and osteodystrophy associated with various medical conditions such as chronic renal failure and hypoparathyroidism, and the treatment and prophylaxis of postoperative and idiopathic tetany. Administered orally.

di·hy·dro·tes·tos·te·rone (DHT) (di-hi″dro-tes-tos′tə-rōn) 7β-hydroxy-5α-androstan-3-one, a powerful androgenic hormone, formed in peripheral tissue by the action of the enzyme 5α-reductase on testosterone; it is thought to be the essential androgen responsible for formation of primary sex characters in males during embryogenesis, for development of most male secondary sex characters at puberty, and for adult male sexual function. A semisynthetic analogue is called *stanolone.*

di·hy·dro·ura·cil de·hy·dro·gen·ase (NADP⁺) (di-hi″dro-ūr′ə-sĭl de-hi′dro-jən-ās) dihydropyrimidine dehydrogenase (NADP).

di·hy·droxy (di″hi-drok′se) a compound containing two molecules of the hydroxy (OH) radical; used also as a prefix (dihydroxy-) to denote such a compound.

di·hy·droxy·ac·e·tone (di″hi-drok″se-as″ə-tōn) [USP] the simplest ketose, a triose; it is an isomer of glyceraldehyde and is formally called *glycerone.* When applied to the skin it produces a brown pigmentation and is used to darken depigmented areas in vitiligo.

d. phosphate an intermediate in glycolysis, the glycerol phosphate shuttle, and the biosynthesis of carbohydrates and of lipids.

2,8-di·hy·droxy·ad·e·nine (DHA) (di″hi-drok″se-ad′ə-nēn) an insoluble purine produced in excess in deficiencies of the salvage pathway of adenine catalyzed by adenine phosphoribosyltransferase; accumulation can cause crystalluria and nephrolithiasis.

di·hy·droxy·alu·mi·num (di″hi-drok″se-ə-loo′mĭ-nəm) an aluminum compound having two hydroxyl groups in the molecule.

d. aminoacetate [USP] a basic aluminum salt of aminoacetic acid used as a gastric antacid. Called also *aluminum aminoacetate.*

di·hy·droxy·cho·le·cal·cif·e·rol (di″hi-drok″se-ko″lə-kal-sif′ə-rol) a group of active metabolites of cholecalciferol, numbered according to the carbon atoms on which a hydroxyl group is substituted. See also table at *cholecalciferol.* Called also *dihydroxyvitamin D_3.*

1,25-d. the most active metabolite of cholecalciferol, synthesized in the kidney from 25-hydroxycholecalciferol; it increases intestinal absorption of calcium and phosphate, enhances bone resorption, and prevents rickets. Because these activities occur at sites distant from its site of synthesis, it is considered a hormone. Called also *calcitriol* and *1,25-dihydroxyvitamin D_3.*

24,25-d. a metabolite of cholecalciferol with an uncertain physiological role.

di·hy·droxy·flu·o·rane (di″hi-drok″se-floor′ān) fluorescein.

3,4-di·hy·droxy·phen·yl·al·a·nine (di″hi-drok″se-fen″əl-al′ə-nēn) dopa.

3,4-di·hy·droxy·phen·yl·gly·col (DHPG) (di″hi-drok″se-fen″əl-gli′kol) a metabolite of norepinephrine; levels may be elevated in pheochromocytoma.

1,25-di·hy·droxy·vi·ta·min D (di″hi-drok″se-vi′tə-min) either 1,25-dihydroxycholecalciferol, the corresponding dihydroxy-derivative of ergocalciferol, or both collectively. See also table at *cholecalciferol.*

di·hy·droxy·vi·ta·min D_3 (di″hi-drok″se-vi′tə-min) dihydroxycholecalciferol.

1,25-d. D_3 1,25-dihydroxycholecalciferol.

24,25-d. D_3 24,25-dihydroxycholecalciferol.

di·io·dide (di-i′o-dīd) a combination of a base or a metal with two atoms of iodine.

diiodo- a chemical prefix denoting the presence of two iodine atoms.

di·io·do·hy·droxy·quin (di″i-o″do-hi-drok′sĭ-kwin) iodoquinol.

3,5-di·io·do·thy·ro·nine (di″i-o″do-thi′ro-nēn) an organic iodine-containing compound, used in the manufacture of thyroxine.

di·io·do·ty·ro·sine (di″i-o″do-ti′ro-sēn) an organic iodine-containing compound liberated from thyroglobulin in small amounts as a by-product of iodothyroglobulin hydrolysis. Called also *iodogorgoric acid.*

di·iso·cy·anate (di-i″so-si′ə-nāt) any of a group of compounds containing two isocyanate groups (—NCO), which are used in the manufacture of plastics and elastomers; diisocyanates can cause sensitization and are potent irritants of the eyes and respiratory system. See *isocyanate asthma,* under *asthma.*

di·iso·pro·pyl flu·o·ro·phos·phate (DFP) (di-i″so-pro′pəl flo͞or″o-fos′fāt) a potent irreversible acetylcholinesterase and pseudocholinesterase inhibitor, widely used in biochemistry in the study of serine proteases; radiolabeled $DF^{32}P$ has been used to label blood cells in kinetics studies. DFP is also used, as *isoflurophate,* as an ophthalmic cholinergic agent.

Di·karyo·my·co·ta (di-kar″e-o-mi-ko′tə) in some systems of classification, a phylum of perfect fungi characterized by an extended dikaryon in the life cycle; it includes two subphyla, Ascomycotina and Basidiomycotina (which are variously considered phyla or classes, and renamed, in other systems).

di·ka·ry·on (di-kar′e-on) [*di-* + *karyon*] a growth stage in the mycelium of fungi, especially Basidiomycetes, in which each cell has two haploid nuclei.

di·ka·ry·ot·ic (di″kar-e-ot′ik) pertaining to the dikaryon.

di·ke·tone (di-ke′tōn) a ketone containing two carbonyl groups.

di·ke·to·pi·per·a·zine (di-ke″to-pi-per′ə-zēn) a closed-ring compound produced by the condensation of two amino acids, the carboxyl group of each combining with the amino group of the other.

dik·ty·o·ma (dik″te-o′mə) a medulloepithelioma of the pars ciliaris retinae; written also *dictyoma.*

dil. [L.] dil′ue (dilute, dissolve).

di·lac·er·a·tion (di-las″ər-a′shən) [L. *dilaceratio*] 1. a tearing apart, as of a cataract; see *discission.* 2. in dentistry, a condition due to injury to a tooth during its developmental period and characterized by a crease or band at the junction of the crown and root, or by tortuous roots with abnormal curvatures.

Dil·a·cor-XR (dil′ə-kor″) trademark for a preparation of diltiazem hydrochloride.

Di·lan·tin (di-lan′tin) trademark for preparations of phenytoin.

dil·a·ta·tion (dil″ə-ta′shən) 1. the condition, as of an orifice or tubular structure, of being dilated or stretched beyond the normal dimensions. 2. dilation (def. 1).

d. and curettage (D & C) expanding of the ostium uteri to permit scraping of the walls of the uterus, a common technique used in induced abortion.

digital d. digital dilation.

gastric d. d. of the stomach.

gastric d.-volvulus see under *volvulus.*

d. of the heart enlargement of the cavities of the heart, with thinning of its walls.

idiopathic d. dilatation of a vessel or other channel, especially of the pulmonary artery, without a known cause.

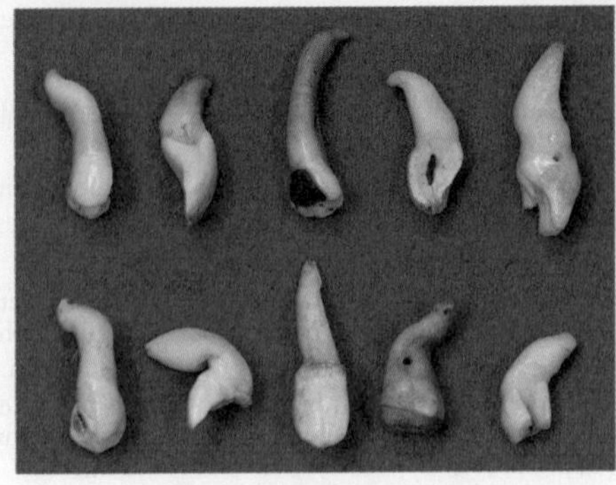
■ Dilaceration.

poststenotic d. dilatation of a vessel distal to a stenosed segment or valve, often seen in the pulmonary artery distal to valvular pulmonary stenosis.

segmental d. dilatation of a portion of a tubular structure, such as the intestine, the segments on either side of the dilatation being of normal caliber.

d. of the stomach distention of the stomach with retained secretions, food, or gas due to obstruction, ileus, or denervation; called also *gastric d.*

dil•a•ta•tor (dil″ə-ta′tər) [L.] 1. something that dilates. 2. in anatomical terminology, a structure (muscle) that dilates (musculus dilatator [TA]).

di•late (di′lāt) to stretch an opening or hollow structure beyond its normal dimensions; cf. *distend.*

di•la•tion (di-la′shən) 1. the act of dilating or stretching; it may be either a normal physiological process done by muscles or a therapeutic process done by dilators. 2. dilatation (def. 1).

digital d. the expansion or stretching of a cavity or orifice by means of a finger.

di•la•tor (di-la′tər, di′-la-tər) 1. an instrument used in enlarging a canal, orifice, tube, or vessel by stretching. 2. dilatator (def. 2).

anal d. an instrument for dilating or stretching the anal sphincter.

balloon d. an instrument that uses a balloon catheter to cause dilation.

esophageal d. a bougie or similar instrument for dilation of an esophageal stricture or the lower esophageal sphincter.

Hegar d's a series of bougies of varying sizes for dilating the ostium uteri.

Hurst d's see under *bougie.*

laryngeal d. 1. any of the muscles that serve to dilate the larynx. 2. a bougielike instrument used for distending a stenosed larynx.

Maloney d's see under *bougie.*

mercury d's, mercury-filled d's an esophageal dilator system consisting of a series of mercury-filled tubes of graded diameter for dilating the cardioesophageal sphincter. Called also *mercury bougies.*

d. naris pars alaris musculi nasalis.

pneumatic d. a dilator for esophageal strictures, consisting of a bougie leading to an inflatable bag that straddles the stricture.

d. pupillae musculus dilatator pupillae.

Di•la•trate (di′lə-trāt) trademark for preparations of isosorbide dinitrate.

Di•lau•did (di-law′did) trademark for preparations of hydromorphone hydrochloride.

Dil•e•pid•i•dae (dil″ə-pid′ĭ-de) Dipylidiidae.

dill (dil) *Anethum graveolens.*

Di•lor (di′lor) trademark for preparations of dyphylline.

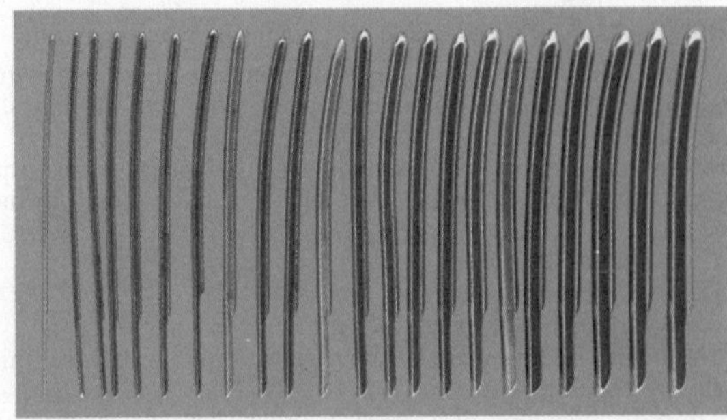
■ Hegar uterine dilators.

di•lox•a•nide fu•ro•ate (di-loks′ə-nīd) [USP] an antiprotozoal drug with amebicidal activity, used in treatment of intestinal amebiasis; administered orally.

dil•ti•a•zem hy•dro•chlo•ride (dil-ti′ə-zəm) [USP] a calcium channel blocking agent that acts as a vasodilator; administered orally in the treatment of angina pectoris and hypertension, and intravenously in the treatment of supraventricular tachycardia.

Diluc. [L.] dilu′culo (at daybreak).

dil•u•ent (dil′u-ənt) 1. causing dilution. 2. an agent that dilutes or renders less potent or irritant.

dilut. [L.] dilu′tus (diluted).

di•lute (di-lo͞ot′) [L. *diluere* to wash] to make something less concentrated, such as by adding fluid to a mixture or solution.

di•lu•tion (di-loo′shən) 1. the process of diluting or the state of being diluted. 2. a substance that has undergone dilution. 3. in homeopathy, the diffusion of a given quantity of a medicinal agent in ten or one hundred times the same quantity of water.

doubling d. a serial dilution in which the dilution in each tube is double that of the preceding tube.

nitrogen d. the addition of nitrogen to inhaled air to lower its oxygen tension, producing an alveolar oxygen tension equal to a desired oxygen pressure.

pigmentary d. mild hypopigmentation.

serial d. a set of dilutions in a mathematical sequence. In microbiological technique, serial dilutions are used to obtain a culture plate that yields a countable number of separate colonies. From this, a calculation of viable cells in the original suspension can be made, as a colony picked for pure culture.

dim. [L.] dimid′ius (one half).

Di•mas•tig•amoe•ba (di-mas″tig-ə-me′bə) *Naegleria.*

di•me•fil•con A (di″mə-fil′kon) a contact lens material (hydrophilic).

di•meg•lu•mine (di-meg′loo-mēn) any salt containing two meglumine molecules.

di•me•lia (di-me′le-ə) [*di-* + *-melia*] complete or incomplete duplication of a limb.

di•me•lus (di-me′ləs) a fetus exhibiting dimelia.

di•men•hy•dri•nate (di″mən-hi′drĭ-nāt) [USP] an antihistamine (H_1 receptor antagonist) with anticholinergic and significant sedative effects; used as an antiemetic and antivertigo agent, used in the prevention and treatment of motion sickness and other conditions in which nausea or vertigo may be a feature, administered orally, rectally, or by intramuscular or intravenous injection.

di•men•sion (dĭ-men′shən) a numerical expression, in appropriate units, of a linear measurement of an object, such as an organ or body part.

vertical d. the distance between two points, measured perpendicular to the horizontal. In prosthodontics, the length of the face determined by the distance of separation of the jaws. See *contact vertical d., postural vertical d.,* and *rest vertical d.*

vertical d., contact, vertical d., occlusal the lower face height with the teeth in centric occlusion.

vertical d., postural the vertical face height when the mandible is suspended in the postural resting position.

vertical d., rest the lower face height measured from a chin point just below the nose, with the mandible in the rest position.

di•men•sion•less (dĭ-men′shən-ləs) denoting a numerical constant or variable that has no units of measurement.

di•mer (di′mər) 1. a compound formed by combination of two identical simpler molecules. 2. a capsomer having two structural subunits.

D d. a fibrin degradation product containing a cross-link between two fibrin monomers; the cross-link does not occur in fibrinogen, so that tests for D-dimer are specific for fibrin. See *D-dimer assay,* under *assay.*

ethyl cysteinate d. (ECD) bicisate.

thymine d. two adjacent thymine residues linked together by a covalent bond along a single polynucleotide of DNA, which may lead to inactivation of the DNA molecule. It results from exposure to ultraviolet radiation and may be reversed by photoreactivation.

di•mer•cap•rol (di″mər-kap′rol) [USP] a metal complexing agent, used as an antidote to poisoning by arsenic, gold, mercury, and lead; administered intramuscularly. Called also *British antilewisite (BAL).*

di•mer•ic (di′mər-ik) exhibiting the characteristics of a dimer.

dim•er•ous (dim′ər-əs) [*di-* + *mero-*[1] + *-ous*] made up of two parts.

di•me•tal•lic (di″mə-tal′ik) containing two atoms or equivalents of a metallic element in the molecule.

Di•me•tane (di′mə-tān) trademark for preparations containing brompheniramine maleate.

di•me•thac•ry•late (di″mə-thak′rə-lāt) a common resin matrix material; called also *BIS-GMA.*

di•meth•i•cone (di-meth′ĭ-kōn) 1. a silicone oil, chemically polydimethylsiloxane, occurring in varying degrees of polymerization, with viscosities from 0.65 to 3,000,000 centistokes at 25°C. The term is used with a numeric suffix which indicates the approximate viscosity of the various grades in centistokes, e.g., the viscosity of dimethicone 200 in centistokes is 190 to 210. Dimethicones are used as ingredients of ointments and other preparations for topical application to protect the skin against water-soluble irritants. 2. occasionally, the mixture of dimethicone with silicon dioxide, more properly called *simethicone.*

d. 350 a grade of dimethicone having a viscosity of approximately 350 centistokes at 25°C, used as a prosthetic aid for soft tissues.

activated d. simethicone.

2,5-di•me•thoxy-4-meth•yl•am•phet•amine (DOM) (di″mə-thok″se-meth″əl-am-fet′ə-mēn) a hallucinogenic compound derived from amphetamine.

3,4-di•me•thoxy•phen•yl•eth•yl•amine (DMPE) (di″mə-thok″se-fen″əl-eth″əl-am′ən) a substance found in the urine of schizophrenics but not controls in some studies.

di•meth•yl•amine (di-meth″əl-am′ən) a gaseous and liquid ptomaine, isolated from decaying nitrogenous plant and animal sources, particularly fish, and synthesized for use in industrial and pharmaceutical processes; it is a skin irritant.

***p*-di•meth•yl•a•mi•no•azo•ben•zene** (di-meth″əl-ə-me″no-a″zo-ben′zēn) a dicyclic carcinogenic compound used as an indicator in tests for and in Ehrlich aldehyde reaction to detect urobilinogen. It has a pH range of 2.9 to 4, being red at 2.9 and yellow at 4. Called also *butter yellow* and *methyl yellow.*

di•meth•yl•ami•no•pro•pio•ni•trile (DMAPN) (di-meth″əl-ə-me″no-pro″pe-o-ni′tril) a colorless water-soluble liquid used in the manufacture of polyurethane foam; workers with excessive exposure to it are prone to urologic and neurologic disorders.

di•meth•yl•ar•sine (di-meth″əl-ahr′sēn) cacodyl hydride.

di•meth•yl•ar•sin•ic ac•id (di-meth″əl-ahr-sin′ik) cacodylic acid.

7,12-di•meth•yl•benz[*a*]an•thra•cene (di-meth″əl-benz-an′thrə-sēn) 9,10-dimethyl-1,2-benzanthracene; a highly carcinogenic polycyclic aromatic hydrocarbon produced during incomplete combustion of carbonaceous materials. It is a procarcinogen that requires metabolic activation to an epoxide intermediate to exert a mutagenic effect; it is widely used in research on chemical carcinogenesis. Abbreviated DMBA.

di•meth•yl•ben•zene (di-meth″əl-ben′zēn) xylene.

5,6-di•meth•yl•ben•zi•mid•az•ole (di″meth-əl-ben″zĭ-mid′ə-zōl) a derivative of benzimidazole doubly methylated on the benzene ring; it is an unusual base that together with a ribose 3′-phosphate moiety forms the nucleotide portion of the vitamin B_{12} molecule.

di•meth•yl•car•bam•yl chlo•ride (di-meth″əl-kahr′bə-məl) a colorless liquid used as a chemical intermediate in the manufacture of pharmaceuticals, dyes, and pesticides; it is lacrimatory and possibly carcinogenic.

di•meth•yl car•bate (di-meth′əl kahr′bāt) a clear oily liquid used as an insect repellent; it has neurotoxic effects if ingested or inhaled.

di•meth•yl•car•bi•nol (di-meth″əl-kahr′bĭ-nol) isopropyl alcohol.

di•meth•yl•eth•yl•pyr•role (di-meth″əl-eth″əl-pir′ōl) a substituted pyrrole obtained from bilirubin.

di•meth•yl•for•ma•mide (DMF) (di-meth″əl-for′mə-mīd) a solvent used in laboratories and in manufacturing acrylic resins; it is absorbed through the skin and by inhalation and is hepatotoxic.

***N,N*-di•meth•yl•gly•cine** (di-meth″əl-gli′sēn) an amino acid intermediate occurring as an immediate precursor of sarcosine in the metabolism of choline.

di•meth•yl•gly•cine de•hy•dro•gen•ase (di-meth″əl-gli′sēn de-hi′dro-jən-ās) [EC 1.5.99.2] a mitochondrial flavoprotein enzyme of the oxidoreductase class that catalyzes the oxidative demethylation of *N,N*-dimethylglycine to sarcosine in the metabolism of choline. It requires a folate cofactor and transfers electrons from its flavin moiety to electron transfer flavoprotein. The reaction occurs in the mitochondrial inner membrane in the liver and kidney.

di•meth•yl•gly•ox•ime (di-meth″il-gli-ok′sēm) a reagent for nickel and similar metals; see *dimethylglyoxime test,* under *test.*

di•meth•yl•ke•tone (di-meth″əl-ke′tōn) acetone.

di•meth•yl•ni•tro•sa•mine (di-meth″əl-ni-tro′sə-mēn) *N*-nitrosodimethylamine.

di•meth•yl•phe•nan•threne (di-meth″əl-fə-nan′thrēn) a carcinogenic and weakly estrogenic hydrocarbon.

di•meth•yl-*p*-phen•yl•ene•di•amine (di-meth″əl-fen″əl-ēn-di′ə-mēn) a reddish-violet, crystalline, substituted aniline derivative, toxic by ingestion or inhalation; used in reagents for various biochemical and microbiological assays.

di•meth•yl phthal•ate (di-meth′əl thal′āt) a clear, colorless, oily liquid, the normal methyl ester of phthalic acid; used as an insect repellent.

di•meth•yl sul•fate (di-meth′əl sul′fāt) a colorless liquid used in adhesives and as a methylating agent for organic chemicals; it is severely irritant to the skin and mucous membranes and is carcinogenic.

di•meth•yl sulf•ox•ide (DMSO) (di-meth′əl sul-fok′sīd) 1. a highly polar alkyl sulfoxide that is a powerful solvent and dissolves many organic and inorganic compounds; its biologic activities include the ability to penetrate plant and animal tissues and to preserve living cells during freezing. 2. [USP] a preparation instilled into the bladder for symptomatic relief of interstitial cystitis, and proposed as a topical analgesic and antiinflammatory agent and as a transcutaneous carrier, increasing penetrability of other substances. In veterinary medicine it is used as a topical antiinflammatory.

di•meth•yl•tryp•ta•mine (DMT) (di-meth″əl-trip′tə-mēn) a hallucinogenic substance derived from the apocynaceous plant *Prestonia amazonica* (Benth.) Macbride *(Haemadictyon amazonicum* Spruce and Benth.) which is native to parts of South America and the West Indies.

di•me•trid•a•zole (di″mə-tri′də-zōl) an antiprotozoal drug used against histomoniasis of turkeys.

di•min•a•zene ac•e•tu•rate (dĭ-min′ə-zēn) a veterinary antibacterial and antiprotozoal used against *Babesia* and *Trypanosoma.*

dim•i•nu•tion (dim″ĭ-noo′shən) reduction or decrease in size or substance.

Dim•mer keratitis (dim′ər) [Friedrich *Dimmer,* Austrian ophthalmologist, 1855–1926] keratitis nummularis.

di•mor•phic (di-mor′fik) dimorphous.

di•mor•phism (di-mor′fiz-əm) [*di-* + *morph-* + *-ism*] the property of having or existing in two forms, as fungi that can grow as molds or yeasts.

physical d. the property of certain solids of existing in two crystalline or allotropic forms.

sexual d. physical or behavioral differences associated with gender.

di•mor•pho•bi•ot•ic (di-mor″fo-bi-ot′ik) [*di-* + *morpho-* + *biotic*] showing alternation of generations and having a parasitic and a nonparasitic stage in the complete life history.

di•mor•phous (di-mor′fəs) [*di-* + *morpho-* + *-ous*] occurring in two distinct forms; having the property of dimorphism.

dim•ple (dim′pəl) 1. a slight depression, as in the flesh of the cheek, chin, or sacral region. 2. any of various other small pits that resemble the skin depression.

Fuchs d's saucer-shaped excavations at the periphery of the cornea, usually on the temporal side, probably caused by insufficiency of the limbal circulation; called also *dellen.*

postanal d. foveola coccygea.

dim•pling (dim′pling) the formation of slight depressions or dimples.

di•ner•ic (di-ner′ik) [*di-* + Gr. *nēros* liquid] denoting a solution made up of two immiscible solvents with a single solute soluble in each.

di•ni•trate (di-ni′trāt) a compound of a base or a metal with two nitrate groups, as in lead dinitrate, $Pb(NO_3)_2$.

di•ni•trat•ed (di-ni′trāt-əd) compounded with or containing two nitrate (NO_3) or nitro (NO_2) groups.

di•ni•tro•ami•no•phe•nol (di-ni″tro-ə-me″no-fe′nol) a phenol found in the blood after poisoning with trinitrophenol, forming red granules, free or in the leukocytes. Called also *aminodinitrophenol.*

di•ni•tro•ben•zene (di-ni″tro-ben′zēn) a poisonous substance, $C_6H_4(NO_2)_2$, whose fumes may cause breathlessness and finally asphyxia.

di•ni•tro•chlo•ro•ben•zene (di-ni″tro-klor″o-ben′zēn) a substance that produces a delayed-type hypersensitivity response (contact dermatitis) in sensitized individuals when applied to the skin; it is a commonly used sensitizing agent in laboratory immunology and has been used to test cellular immune function in evaluation of suspected immunodeficiency. Abbreviated DNCB.

di•ni•tro-o-cre•sol (DNOC) (di-ni″tro-kre′sol) a highly toxic pesticide and herbicide used in agriculture; symptoms of poisoning include convulsions, coma, disruption of energy-producing metabolic processes, and sometimes high fevers that can be fatal.

di•ni•tro•flu•o•ro•ben•zene (di-ni″tro-flŏŏr″o-ben′zēn) a substance that induces a delayed-type hypersensitivity reaction (contact dermatitis) in sensitized individuals when applied to the skin; a commonly used sensitizing agent and hapten in laboratory immunology. Abbreviated DNFB.

di•ni•tro•gen (di-ni′tro-jən) containing two nitrogen atoms.
  d. monoxide nitrous oxide.

di•ni•tro•phe•nol (di-ni″tro-fe′nol) any one of six isomeric compounds used in making dyes. 2,4-Dinitrophenol is highly toxic and is used as a reagent and indicator and frequently as a hapten.

di•ni•tro•re•sor•cin•ol (di-ni″tro-re-sor′sin-ol) a green coal tar derivative, $C_6H_2(NO_2)_2(OH)_2$, used in preparing degenerated nerve tissue for study.

di•ni•tro•tolu•ene (di-ni″tro-tol′u-ēn) a highly toxic crystalline compound existing as three isomers, used in organic synthesis and the manufacture of dyes and explosives; it is readily absorbed through the skin and is a potential carcinogen.

Di•nob•del•la (di″nob-del′ə) a genus of leeches of the family Gnathobdellidae, species of which attack the larynx of cattle in India when swallowed in drinking water.

Di•no•flag•el•la•ta (di″no-flaj″ə-la′tə) [Gr. *dinos* whirl + L. *flagellum* whip] a phylum of minute, plantlike, chiefly marine protozoa, an important component of plankton; most have transverse and longitudinal flagella in grooves, causing them to rotate as they advance, and have a cellulose covering and green, yellow, or brown chromatophores. The order Dinoflagellida contains the species causing red tides and some kinds of shellfish poisoning.

di•no•flag•el•late (di″no-flaj′ə-lāt) a protozoan of the phylum Dinoflagellata.

Di•no•fla•gel•li•da (di″no-flə-jel′ĭ-də) [Gr. *dinos* + L. *flagellum* whip] an order of plantlike protozoa of the phylum Dinoflagellata; when organisms are present in sea water in vast numbers (causing a discoloration known as red tide), they deplete the oxygen supply, causing marine animals and fish to die. Some species secrete saxitoxin; human consumption of shellfish that have ingested these species can result in neurotoxic or paralytic shellfish poisoning.

di•no•gun•el•lin (di″no-gun′ə-lin) the toxic lipoprotein found in the roe of the Japanese blenny *Stichaeus (Dinogunellus) grigorjewi.*

Di•noph•y•sis (di-nof′ə-sis) a genus of plantlike, marine and freshwater protozoa of the phylum Dinoflagellata; like other dinoflagellates, when present in vast numbers they can cause red tide. Certain species contain okadaic acid, and if shellfish ingest them, persons eating the contaminated shellfish get diarrhetic shellfish poisoning (see under *poisoning*).

di•no•prost (di′no-prost) name given to prostaglandin $F_{2\alpha}$ when used as a pharmaceutical; used as an oxytocic for induction of abortion, for evacuation of the uterus in management of missed abortion, and in treatment of hydatidiform mole.
  d. trometanol d. tromethamine.
  d. tromethamine [USP] the tromethamine salt of dinoprost, having the same actions as the base; used as an oxytocic for induction of labor, termination of pregnancy, missed abortion, fetal death, and hydatidiform mole. It is administered intravenously, extra-amniotically, or intra-amniotically. Called also *d. trometanol* and *prostaglandin $F_{2\alpha}$ tromethamine.*

di•no•prost•one (di″no-pros′tōn) name given to prostaglandin E_2 when used pharmaceutically; used as an oxytocic for induction of abortion and for the induction of labor, to evacuate the uterus in the management of missed abortion, to aid ripening of the cervix prior to the induction of labor, and in the treatment of hydatidiform mole; administered intravaginally or intracervically.

D. in p. aeq. [L.] divi′de in par′tes aequa′les (divide into equal parts).

din•sed (din′səd) a coccidiostat for use in poultry.

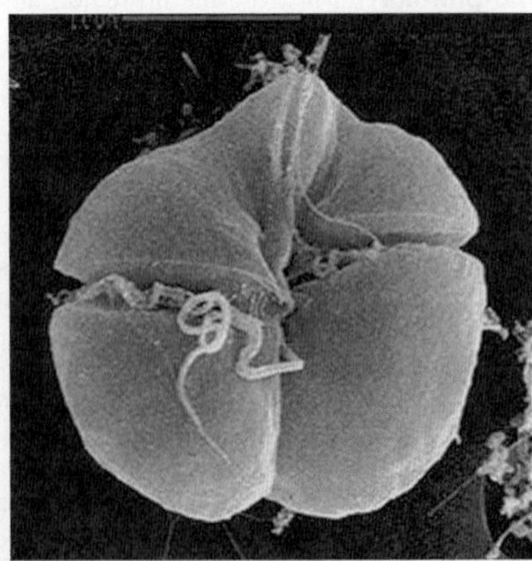

■ Electron micrograph of the dinoflagellate *Karenia brevis.*

di•nu•cleo•tide (di-noo′kle-o-tīd) one of the cleavage products into which a polynucleotide may be split; a dinucleotide itself may be split into two mononucleotides.

Di•oc•to•phy•ma (di-ok″to-fi′mə) a genus of nematodes of the family Dioctophymidae.
  D. rena′le the kidney worm, a red species that is the largest nematode known; males are 35 cm long and females 103 cm (1.03m). It is found in various mammals, but rarely in humans. The usual location is in the renal pelvis or free in the peritoneal cavity; it is highly destructive to kidney tissue and may cause death.

Di•oc•to•phy•mi•dae (di-ok″to-fi′mĭ-de) a family of nematodes found in the kidney and peritoneal cavity in mammals. It includes the single genus *Dioctophyma.*

Di•oc•to•phy•moi•dea (di-ok″to-fi″moi′de-ə) a superfamily of aphasmids, including the genus *Dioctophyma.*

di•oc•tyl cal•ci•um sul•fo•suc•ci•nate (di-ok′təl) docusate calcium.

di•oc•tyl so•di•um sul•fo•suc•ci•nate (di-ok′təl) docusate sodium.

Di•o•don (di′o-don) a genus of tetraodontiform fishes of the family Diodontidae; some species are poisonous when ingested.

di•oe•cious (di-e′shəs) diecious.

Di•on•o•sil (di-on′o-sil) trademark for preparations of propyliodone.

di•op•sim•e•ter (di″op-sim′ə-tər) [*dia-* Gr. *opsis* sight + *-meter*] a device for measuring the field of vision.

di•op•ter (di-op′tər) [Gr. *dioptra* optical instrument for measuring angles] a unit of refractive power of lenses: the reciprocal of the focal length in meters is the refractive power in diopters. Symbol D.
  prism d. a unit of prismatic deviation; deflection of one centimeter at a distance of one meter.

di•op•tom•e•ter (di″op-tom′ə-tər) [*dioptric* + *-meter*] an instrument for use in testing ocular refraction.

di•op•tom•e•try (di″op-tom′ə-tre) the measurement of refraction and accommodation of the eye.

di•op•tos•co•py (di″op-tos′kə-pe) [*dioptric* + *-scopy*] measurement of ocular refraction by means of the ophthalmoscope.

di•op•tre (di-op′tər) diopter.

di•op•tric (di-op′trik) pertaining to refraction or to transmitted and refracted light; refracting.

di•op•trics (di-op′triks) the science of refracted light.

di•op•trom•e•ter (di″op-trom′ə-tər) dioptometer.

di•op•trom•e•try (di″op-trom′ə-tre) dioptometry.

di•op•tros•co•py (di″op-tros′kə-pe) dioptoscopy.

di•op•try (di′op-tre) diopter.

di•os•cin (di-os′kin) a saponin from *Dioscorea tokoro* Mal.; see *diosgenin.*

Di•os•co•rea (di″os-kor′e-ə) the Mexican yams, a genus of plants of the family Dioscoreaceae. *D. mexica′na* is a source of the steroid botogenin. Several species, such as *D. villo′sa*, *D. floribun′da*, and *D. toko′ro*, are sources of diosgenin. *D. villo′sa* L. contains saponin and acrid resins and was formerly used for its diaphoretic, expectorant, and diuretic properties.

di•ose (di′ōs) any monosaccharide containing two carbon atoms; the only member of the class is glycoaldehyde (q.v.).

di•os•gen•in (di-os′jən-in) an aglycone of the saponin dioscin. Obtained from several species of *Dioscorea,* it is a precursor in the synthesis of pregnenolone, progesterone, and other medically useful steroids.

di•os•mec•tite (di-ōs-mek′tīt) a natural clay used for the treatment of diarrhea, especially in children.

Di•o•val (di′o-val) trademark for preparations of estradiol valerate.

Di•o•van (di′o-van) trademark for preparations of valsartan.

Di•o•van HCT (di′o-van) trademark for a combination preparation of valsartan and hydrochlorothiazide.

di•ov•u•la•to•ry (di-ov′u-lə-tor″e) discharging two oocytes in one ovarian cycle.

di•ox•ane (di-ok′sān) a colorless liquid prepared by treating ethylene glycol with sulfuric acid; used as a solvent for organic compounds and for dehydrating and clearing tissues prior to paraffin fixation. It is toxic if inhaled or absorbed through the skin and is carcinogenic. Called also *1,4-diethylene dioxide.*

di•ox•ide (di-ok′sīd) 1. a binary compound containing two oxide ions, such as silicon dioxide, SiO_2. 2. an oxide of a nonmetal with a valence of four, such as sulfur dioxide, SO_2.

di•ox•in (di-ok′sin) any of the heterocyclic hydrocarbons present as a trace contaminant in herbicides, especially the chlorinated dioxin

2,3,7,8-tetrachlorodibenzo-*p*-dioxin; many are teratogenic and carcinogenic.

di·oxy·ben·zone (di-ok″se-ben′zōn) [USP] a benzophenone compound used as a topical sunscreen.

di·oxy·gen (di-ok′sə-jən) the molecular form of oxygen, O_2.

di·oxy·gen·ase (di-ok′sə-jən-ās) a term used in the recommended names of oxygenases specifically catalyzing incorporation of both atoms of oxygen from O_2 into a single substrate [EC 1.13.11]. A C=C bond is frequently cleaved, and most of these enzymes require either iron or copper for activity.

DIP distal interphalangeal; see under *joint.*

di·pen·tene (di-pen′tēn) a liquid terpene found in various volatile oils.

Di·pen·tum (di-pen′təm) trademark for a preparation of olsalazine sodium.

di·pep·ti·dase (di-pep′tĭ-dās) [EC 3.4.13] any member of a sub-subclass of enzymes of the hydrolase class that catalyze the cleavage of the peptide linkage in a dipeptide.

di·pep·tide (di-pep′tīd) a peptide which on hydrolysis yields two amino acids.

di·pep·ti·dyl car·boxy·pep·ti·dase I (di-pep″tĭ-dəl kahr-bok″se-pep′tĭ-dās) peptidyl-dipeptidase A.

di·pep·ti·dyl-pep·ti·dase (di-pep″tĭ-dəl-pep′tĭ-dās) [EC 3.4.14] any member of a sub-subclass of enzymes of the hydrolase class that catalyze the cleavage of a dipeptide residue from a free N-terminal end of a peptide or polypeptide.

di·pep·ti·dyl-pep·ti·dase I (di-pep″tĭ-dəl-pep′tĭ-dās) [EC 3.4.14.1] an aminopeptidase that catalyzes the cleavage of a dipeptide from the N-terminus of a polypeptide. Called also *cathepsin C.*

di·per·o·don (di-per′o-don) a local anesthetic, applied topically to the skin for abrasions, irritations, and pruritus and intrarectally for relief of discomfort associated with hemorrhoids.

d. hydrochloride the monohydrochloride salt of diperodon, having the same actions and uses as the base.

Di·pet·a·lo·ne·ma (di-pet″ə-lo-ne′mə) a genus of nematodes of the superfamily Filarioidea. *D. recondi′tum* infests dogs. *D. per′stans* and *D. streptocer′ca* have been reclassified under genus *Mansonella.*

di·pet·a·lo·ne·mi·a·sis (di-pet″ə-lo-ne-mi′ə-sis) mansonellosis.

di·pha·ci·none (di-fa′sə-nōn) diphenadione.

di·phal·lia (di-fal′e-ə) diphallus.

di·phal·lus (di-fal′əs) complete or incomplete duplication of the penis; often associated with urogenital anomalies such as exstrophy of bladder; called also *bifid* or *double penis.*

di·pha·sic (di-fa′zik) [*di-* + Gr. *phasis* phase] occurring in two phases or stages. Cf. *monophasic* and *triphasic.*

di·phen·a·di·one (di-fen″ə-di′ōn) an anticoagulant rodenticide, causing fatal hemorrhaging in many mammals consuming sufficient doses. Called also *diphacinone.*

di·phen·hy·dra·mine (di″fen-hi′drə-mēn) a potent antihistamine (H_1 receptor antagonist) with anticholinergic, antitussive, antiemetic, antivertigo, antidyskinetic, and sedative actions.

d. citrate [USP] the citrate salt of diphenhydramine, used as a sedative and hypnotic; administered orally.

d. hydrochloride [USP] the hydrochloride salt of diphenhydramine, used for the symptomatic treatment of allergic symptoms, for the treatment of anaphylaxis, parkinsonism or drug-induced extrapyramidal disorders, and motion sickness or other causes of nausea, vomiting, or vertigo, as an antitussive, as a sedative and hypnotic, and as an ingredient in cough and cold preparations; administered orally, intramuscularly, and intravenously.

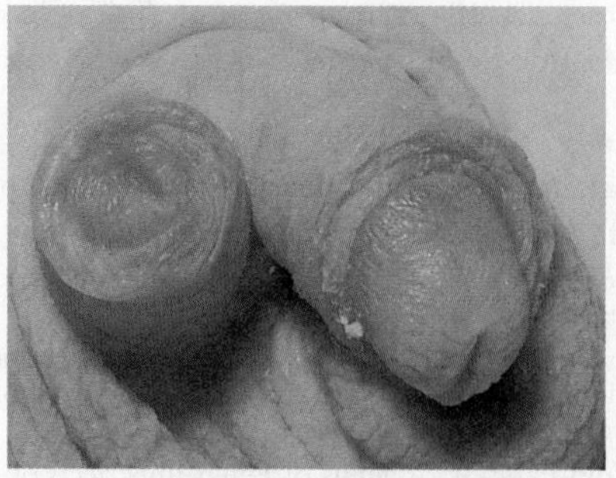

■ Diphallus.

di·phe·nol ox·i·dase (di-fe′nol ok′sĭ-dās) see *catechol oxidase.*

di·phen·ox·y·late hy·dro·chlo·ride (di″fə-nok′sə-lāt) [USP] an antiperistaltic derived from meperidine, used as an antidiarrheal; administered orally.

di·phen·yl (di-fen′əl) a colorless toxic compound, comprising two linked benzene rings, used as a fungistat in containers for shipping citrus fruit. Called also *biphenyl.*

diphenyl- a chemical prefix denoting the presence of two phenyl groups in a molecule.

di·phen·yl·amine (di-fen″əl-am′ēn) a compound comprising two benzene rings linked by a nitrogen atom; its uses include a test for oxidizing agents such as nitric acid and chlorine.

di·phen·yl·amine·chlor·ar·sine (DM) (di-fen′əl-ə-mēn″klor-ahr′sēn) phenarsazine chloride.

di·phen·yl·a·mi·no·azo·ben·zene (di-fen″əl-ə-me″no-a″zo-ben′zēn) an indicator with a pH range of 1.2 to 2.1.

di·phen·yl·bu·tyl·pi·per·i·dine (di-fen″əl-bu″təl-pi-per′ĭ-dēn) any of a class of structurally related antipsychotic agents that includes fluspirilene and pimozide.

di·phen·yl·chlor·ar·sine (di-fe″əl-klor-ahr′sin) sneezing gas, $(C_6H_5)_2AsCl$, a toxic war gas that causes sneezing, coughing, headache, salivation, and vomiting.

di·phen·yl·di·i·mide (di-fen″əl-di′ĭ-mīd) azobenzene.

di·phen·yl·hy·dan·to·in (di-fen″əl-hi-dan′to-in) phenytoin.

di·phen·yl·ni·tros·amine (di-fen″əl-ni-trōs′ə-mēn) *N*-nitrosodiphenylamine.

di·pho·nia (di-fo′ne-ə) [*di-* + *phon-* + *-ia*] the production of two different tones in speaking; called also *double voice.*

di·phos·gene (di-fos′jēn) a gas which is intensely irritating to the lungs, producing pulmonary edema.

di·phos·pha·ti·dyl·glyc·er·ol (di″fos-fə-ti″dəl-glis′ər-ol) glycerol linked to two molecules of phosphatidic acid; 1,3-diphosphatidylglycerol is cardiolipin.

2,3-di·phos·pho·glyc·er·ate (di-fos′fo-glis′ər-āt) 2,3-bisphosphoglycerate.

di·phos·pho·nate (di-fos′fə-nāt) 1. a salt, ester, or anion of diphosphonic acid. While structurally similar to pyrophosphate, its P—C—P bonds give it enhanced stability to enzymatic and chemical hydrolysis. 2. any of a group of such compounds, having affinity for sites of osteoid mineralization and used as sodium salts to inhibit bone resorption as well as complexed with technetium Tc 99m for bone imaging; the group includes alendronate, clodronate, etidronate, medronate, pamidronate, and zoledronic acid. Called also *bisphosphonate.*

methylene d. medronate.

di·phos·pho·nic ac·id (di″fos-fon′ik) a dimer of phosphonic acid; structurally it is similar to pyrophosphoric acid, but with an organic substituent replacing the central oxygen atom of that molecule.

di·phos·pho·trans·fer·ase (di-fos″fo-trans′fər-ās) [EC 2.7.6] any member of a sub-subclass of enzymes of the transferase class that catalyze the transfer of pyrophosphate (diphosphate) groups from one molecule to another. Called also *pyrophosphotransferase.*

diph·the·ria (dif-thēr′e-ə) [Gr. *diphthera* leather + *-ia*] an acute infectious disease caused by toxigenic strains of *Corynebacterium diphtheriae,* acquired by contact with an infected person or a carrier; it is usually confined to the upper respiratory tract. A prominent characteristic is formation of a tough false membrane that is attached firmly to the underlying tissue and bleeds if forcibly removed. In the most serious infections, the membrane begins in the pharyngeal area *(pharyngeal d.)* on the tonsils, then spreads to the uvula, soft palate, pharyngeal wall, larynx, trachea, and bronchial tree, where it may cause bronchial obstruction and death by hypoxia. Systemic effects, chiefly myocarditis and peripheral neuritis, are caused by the exotoxin produced by *C. diphtheriae.*

avian d. fowlpox.

calf d. a contagious disease of young calves caused by infection with *Fusobacterium necrophorum;* symptoms include gray patches in the mouth or throat, foul-smelling breath, fever, cough, and dyspnea, often ending fatally. In the throat it is called also *necrotic laryngitis,* and in the mouth it is called also *necrotic stomatitis.*

cutaneous d. a form of diphtheria involving the skin, occurring as a primary infection, usually seen in warm climates, characterized by a nonhealing, punched-out ulcer with a rolled border, surrounded by a zone of erythema, and sometimes covered by a hard, adherent membrane; or as a secondary infection of a preexisting lesion (burn, abrasion, cut, insect bite, etc.); or as a superinfection of various eczematous lesions.

faucial d. pharyngeal d.

fowl d. fowlpox.

laryngeal d., laryngotracheal d. diphtheria that has spread to the larynx.

nasal d. diphtheria localized to the nasal mucosa, usually one or both of the anterior nasal septa of infants; characteristics include a serosanguineous discharge that becomes mucopurulent and causes skin erosion below the nostrils, and presence of a whitish membrane. Constitutional symptoms may be absent or slight.

nasopharyngeal d. diphtheria that has spread to the nasopharynx.

pharyngeal d., respiratory d. diphtheria in the pharynx, the most common type; called also *faucial d.*

umbilical d. diphtheria in the umbilical stump of an infant.

diph•the•ri•al (dif-thēr′e-əl) diphtheritic.

diph•the•ric (dif-thĕr′ik) diphtheritic.

diph•the•rin (dif′the-rin) a polyvalent diphtheritic antigen for use in anaphylactic skin test.

diph•the•rit•ic (dif″the-rit′ik) pertaining to or resembling diphtheria or its characteristic false membrane. Called also *diphtherial* and *diphtheric.*

diph•the•roid (dif′thə-roid) 1. resembling diphtheria. 2. a bacterium resembling *Corynebacterium diphtheriae* but not causing diphtheria, such as one of the other species in the genus. 3. pseudodiphtheria.

diph•the•ro•tox•in (dif′thə-ro-tok″sin) see *diphtheria toxin,* under *toxin.*

diph•thon•gia (dif-thon′je-ə) [*di-* + Gr. *phthongos* sound] the production of double vocal sounds; called also *diplophonia.*

Di•phyl•la (di-fil′ə) a genus of vampire bats of South America, Central America, Mexico, and the West Indies. *D. ecauda′ta* is the most common species.

di•phyl•lo•both•ri•a•sis (di-fil″o-both-ri′ə-sis) infection with tapeworms of the genus *Diphyllobothrium,* seen most often in fish-eating mammals such as cats, dogs, and bears. Human infection usually follows the eating of inadequately cooked fish and may have a clinical picture like that of pernicious anemia.

Di•phyl•lo•both•ri•i•dae (di-fil″o-both-re′ĭ-de) a family of cestodes that are parasitic in humans and other fish-eating vertebrates. The genera *Diphyllobothrium* and *Spirometra* are of medical importance.

Di•phyl•lo•both•ri•um (di-fil″o-both′re-əm) [*di-* + Gr. *phyllon* leaf + *bothrion* pit] a genus of large tapeworms of the family Diphyllobothriidae; formerly called *Bothriocephalus* and *Dibothriocephalus.*

D. corda′tum the heart-headed tapeworm; a small species found in dogs, seals, and occasionally humans.

D. erina′cei a species found in the adult form in dogs and other carnivores; formerly called *D. mansoni.*

D. la′tum the broad tapeworm or fish tapeworm, a large species found in the intestines of mammals (including humans) that eat fish. It sometimes reaches a length of 9 meters, and its head has two grooves or suckers (bothria). It has two intermediate hosts, first a crustacean and then a fish. Called also *Dibothriocephalus latus.* See accompanying illustrations.

D. manso′ni *D. erinacei.*

D. mansonoi′des a species whose migrating larvae (spargana) are one of the causes of sparganosis.

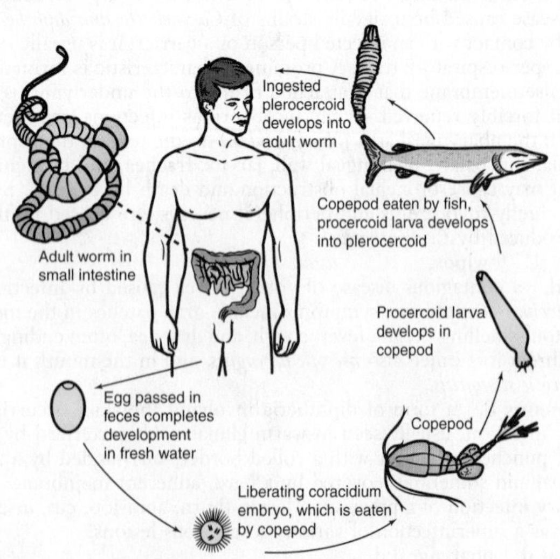

■ Life cycle of *Diphyllobothrium latum.*

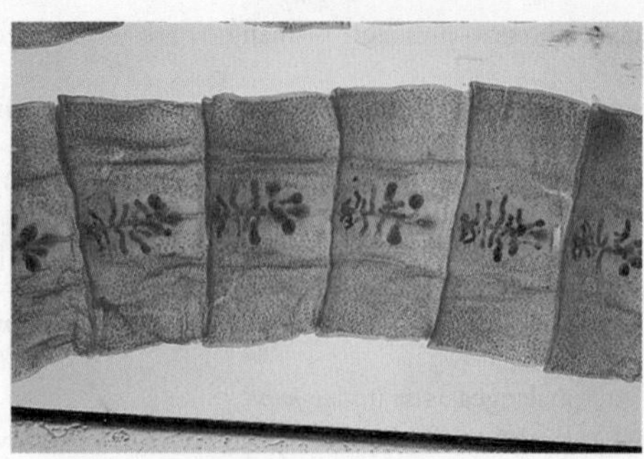

■ *Diphyllobothrium latum,* cross-section of gravid proglottids (acetocarmine stain).

di•phy•odont (di-fi′o-dont″) [*di-* + Gr. *phyein* to produce + *odous* tooth] having two dentitions, a deciduous and a permanent one, as humans do. Cf. *monophyodont* and *polyphyodont.*

di•piv•e•frin (di-piv′ə-frin) an ester and prodrug of epinephrine; it is converted by enzymatic hydrolysis in the eye to epinephrine, which lowers intraocular pressure by decreasing the production and increasing the outflow of aqueous humor.

d. hydrochloride [USP] the hydrochloride salt of dipivefrin, applied topically to the conjunctiva for the control of intraocular pressure in the treatment of open-angle glaucoma and secondary glaucoma.

dip•la•cu•sia (dip″lə-ku′zhə) diplacusis.

dip•la•cu•sis (dip″lə-koo′sis) [*diplo-* + *akousis* hearing] the perception of a single auditory stimulus as two sounds, as a result of cochlear pathology; called also *double disharmonic hearing.*

binaural d. different perception of a single auditory stimulus by the two ears; the difference may be in tone (disharmonic d.) or in timing (echo d.).

disharmonic d. diplacusis in which a given pure tone is heard differently in the two ears.

echo d. diplacusis in which a sound of brief duration is heard in the one ear a fraction of a second later than in the other ear.

monaural d., d. monaura′lis diplacusis in which a pure tone is heard in the same ear as a split tone of two frequencies.

di•ple•gia (di-ple′je-ə) [*di-* + *-plegia*] paralysis affecting like parts on both sides of the body; called also *bilateral paralysis.* **diple′gic** *adj*

atonic-astatic d. diplegic flaccid paralysis in infants; see *flaccid paralysis.* Called also *Förster d.* or *syndrome.*

brachial d. paralysis of both arms.

facial d. paralysis affecting both sides of the face.

facial d., congenital Möbius syndrome.

Förster d. atonic-astatic d.

infantile d. birth palsy.

masticatory d. paralysis of all the muscles which take part in mastication.

spastic d. 1. Little disease. 2. spastic paraplegia.

dipl(o)- [Gr. *diploos* double] a combining form meaning double, twin, twofold, or twice.

dip•lo•ba•cil•li (dip″lo-bə-sil′i) [L.] plural of *diplobacillus.*

dip•lo•ba•cil•lus (dip″lo-bə-sil′əs) pl. *diplobacil′li* [*diplo-* + *bacillus*] a short, rod-shaped bacterium occurring in pairs, joined end to end; diplobacterium.

Morax-Axenfeld d. *Moraxella lacunata.*

dip•lo•bac•te•ria (dip″lo-bak-tēr′e-ə) [L.] plural of *diplobacterium.*

dip•lo•bac•te•ri•um (dip″lo-bak-tēr′e-əm) pl. *diplobacte′ria* [*diplo-* + *bacterium*] a bacterial cell occurring as one of a pair of linked cells.

dip•lo•blas•tic (dip″lo-blas′tik) [*diplo-* + *blast-* + *-ic*] made up of two germ layers.

dip•lo•ceph•a•ly (dip″lo-sef′ə-le) dicephaly.

dip•lo•coc•cal (dip″lo-kok′əl) pertaining to or caused by diplococci.

dip•lo•coc•ci (dip″lo-kok′si) plural of *diplococcus.*

dip•lo•coc•coid (dip″lo-kok′oid) 1. resembling diplococci. 2. an organism that resembles a diplococcus.

dip•lo•coc•cus (dip″lo-kok′əs) pl. *diplococ′ci.* A spherical bacterium occurring predominantly in pairs as a consequence of incomplete separation following cell division in a single plane.

Dip•lo•dia (dip-lo′de-ə) a genus of Fungi Imperfecti of the form-class Coelomycetes. Certain species cause the dry rot or cornstalk disease of corn; contaminated feed is thought to be a cause of cornstalk disease in horses and diplodiosis in other animals.

dip·lo·di·a·tox·i·co·sis (dip″lo-di″ə-tok″sĭ-ko′sis) diplodiosis.

dip·lo·di·o·sis (dip″lo-de-o′sis) a form of mycotoxicosis with temporary paralysis, seen in farm animals that eat corn containing *Diplodia* fungi. Called also *diplodiatoxicosis.*

dip·loë (dip′lo-e) [Gr. *diploē* fold] [TA] the loose osseous tissue between the two tables of the cranial bones. **diploet′ic, diplo′ic** *adj*

Dip·lo·gas·ter (dip′lo-gas″tər) [*diplo-* + Gr. *gastēr* stomach] a genus of free-living coprozoic nematodes which may, in fecal examination, be confused with hookworms or *Strongyloides.*

dip·lo·gen·e·sis (dip″lo-jen′ə-sis) [*diplo-* + *-genesis*] the production of conjoined twins.

Dip·lo·go·nop·o·rus (dip″lo-go-nop′ə-rəs) [*diplo-* + Gr. *gonos* seed + *poros* passage] a genus of tapeworms of the family Diphyllobothriidae, having two sets of reproductive organs in each segment.

D. gran′dis a common parasite of whales that has been found in humans in Japan; it may be up to 10 meters long, and may cause diarrhea or constipation and secondary anemia.

dip·loid (dip′loid) [Gr. *diploos* twofold] having two sets of chromosomes, as normally found in the somatic cells of eukaryotes. In humans, the diploid number, $2n$, is 46. Cf. *haploid.*

dip·loi·dy (dip′loi-de) the state of being diploid.

dip·lo·mate (dip′lo-māt) a person who has received a diploma or certificate. In medicine the term refers particularly to a holder of a certificate of the National Board of Medical Examiners or of one of the American boards in the specialties.

dip·lo·mo·nad (dip″lo-mo′nad) [*diplo-* + Gr. *monas* unit, from *monos,* single] 1. pertaining to or caused by protozoa of the order Diplomonadida. 2. a protozoan of the order Diplomonadida.

Dip·lo·mo·nad·i·da (dip″lo-mo-nad′ĭ-də) [*diplo-* + Gr. *monas* unit, from *monos* single] an order of mostly parasitic, bilaterally symmetrical protozoa of the phylum Parabasalia, having one or two karyomastigonts, each with one to four flagella. Representative genera include *Enteromonas, Giardia, Hexamita,* and *Trepomonas.*

Dip·lo·mo·na·di·na (dip″lo-mo″nə-di′nə) a suborder of mostly parasitic protozoa of the order Diplomonadida, phylum Parabasalia, having two karyomastigonts, each containing four flagella.

dip·lo·my·elia (dip″lo-mi-e′le-ə) [*diplo-* + *myel-* + *-ia*] complete or incomplete duplication of the spinal cord; cf. *diastematomyelia.*

dip·lon (dip′lon) [Gr. *diploos* double] deuteron.

dip·lop·a·gus (dip-lop′ə-gəs) symmetrical conjoined twins.

dip·lo·pho·nia (dip″lo-fo′ne-ə) [*diplo-* + *phon-* + *-ia*] diphthongia.

di·plo·pia (dĭ-plo′pe-ə) [*diplo-* + *-opia*] the perception of two images of a single object; called also *ambiopia, double vision,* and *binocular polyopia.*

binocular d. double vision in which the images of an object are formed on noncorresponding points of the retinas.

crossed d. double vision in which the image belonging to the right eye is displaced to the left of the image belonging to the left eye, as occurs in exotropia (divergent squint). Called also *heteronymous d.*

direct d. double vision in which the image belonging to the right eye appears to the right of the image belonging to the left eye, as occurs in esotropia (convergent squint). Called also *homonymous d.* and *uncrossed d.*

heteronymous d. crossed d.

homonymous d. direct d.

horizontal d. diplopia in which the images lie in the same horizontal plane, being either crossed or direct.

monocular d. the perception by the same eye of two images of a single object, due to double pupil, early cataract, irregular astigmatism, or displacement of the lens.

paradoxical d. crossed d.

physiological d. diplopia in normal binocular vision; all objects not on the horopter of the fixated object are doubled through stimulation of disparate points of the retinae outside the corresponding retinal areas. For nearer objects, the diplopia is crossed; for farther objects, uncrossed. Called also *stereoscopic d.*

stereoscopic d. physiological d.

torsional d. double vision in which the upper pole of the vertical axis of one image is inclined toward or away from that of the other.

uncrossed d. direct d.

vertical d. double vision in which one image appears to be above the other.

di·plo·pi·om·e·ter (dĭ-plo″pe-om′ə-tər) [*diplopia* + *-meter*] an instrument for measuring diplopia.

Di·plop·o·da (di-plop′o-də) [*diplo-* + Gr. *pous* foot] the millipedes, a class of more or less cylindrical arthropods of the order Chilognatha, superclass Myriapoda, characterized by having two pairs of short legs on most of their body segments; they may have from 13 to almost 200 pairs of legs.

Dip·lo·py·lid·i·um (dip″lo-pi-lid′e-əm) a genus of small tapeworms of the family Dipylidiidae, species of which are parasites of birds and mammals.

dip·lo·scope (dip′lo-skōp) [*diplo-* + *-scope*] an apparatus for the study of binocular vision.

dip·lo·some (dip′lo-sōm) [*diplo-* + *-some*] the pair of centrioles in mammalian cells.

Dip·lo·sto·ma·ti·dae (dip″lo-sto-mat′ĭ-de) a family of trematodes that includes the genus *Alaria.*

dip·lo·tene (dip′lo-tēn) the fourth stage of prophase in meiosis I, during which the synaptonemal complex disintegrates and the homologous chromosomes separate (the sister chromatids remaining in association), held together only by chiasmata.

dip·lo·ter·a·tol·o·gy (dip″lo-ter″ə-tol′ə-je) [*diplo-* + *teratology*] the science concerned with the development of conjoined twins.

Dip·lur·i·dae (dip-loo′rĭ-de) a family of spiders of the suborder Orthognatha; genus *Atrax* has a poisonous bite.

di·po·dia (di-po′de-ə) [*di-* + *pod-* + *-ia*] 1. a developmental anomaly characterized by duplication of a foot. 2. dipodial symmelia.

di·po·di·al (di-po′de-əl) having symmelia with two feet present.

di·pole (di′pōl) 1. a molecule having charges of equal and opposite signs but in which the center of the positive charge does not coincide with that of the negative charge, a property which enables the molecule to be bound electrostatically by both positively and negatively charged groups. See *polar compounds,* under *compound.* 2. a pair of electric charges or magnetic poles separated by a short distance.

di·po·tas·si·um phos·phate (di″po-tas′e-əm) dibasic potassium phosphate; see under *potassium.*

dip·ping (dip′ing) 1. palpation of the liver by a quick depressing movement of the fingers with the hand flat across the abdomen. 2. the immersion of an animal in a large volume of dilute insecticide in order to kill external parasites.

Di·pri·van (di′prĭ-van) trademark for a preparation of propofol.

Di·pro·lene (di-pro′lene) trademark for preparations of betamethasone dipropionate.

Di·pro·sone (di-pro′sōn) trademark for preparations of betamethasone dipropionate.

di·pros·o·pus (di-pros′o-pəs) [*di-* + *prosopo-* + *-ous*] a fetus with a single trunk and normal limbs, but with varying degrees of duplication of the face.

d. tetrophthal′mus a fetus having two fused faces, the median eye of each being fused into a common orbit.

di·pro·tri·zo·ate (di″pro-tri′zo-āt) chemical name: 3,5-dipropionamido-2,4,6-triiodobenzoate; used as a contrast medium in radiography of the urinary tract.

dip·sia (dip′se-ə) thirst.

-dipsia a word termination denoting a relationship to thirst.

dip·so·gen (dip′so-jən) [Gr. *dipsa* thirst + *-gen*] an agent or measure that induces thirst and promotes ingestion of fluids.

dip·so·gen·ic (dip-so-jen′ik) causing thirst.

dip·so·ther·a·py (dip″so-ther′ə-pe) [Gr. *dipsa* thirst + *therapy*] treatment by strict limitation of the amount of water to be ingested.

dip·stick (dip′stik) a strip of cellulose chemically impregnated to render it sensitive to protein, glucose, or other substances in the urine.

Dip·tera (dip′tər-ə) [Gr. *dipteros* two winged] an order of insects including the flies, gnats, and mosquitoes.

dip·ter·ous (dip′tər-əs) 1. having two wings. 2. pertaining to insects of the order Diptera.

Dip·ter·yx (dip′tər-iks) a genus of tropical and subtropical American trees. *D. odora′ta* Willd. (Leguminosae) is the tonka bean, a North American species.

di·pus (di′pəs) [*di-* + Gr. *pous* foot] sympus dipus.

di·py·gus (di-pi′gəs) [*di-* + Gr. *pygē* rump] a fetus with a double pelvis.

d. parasi′ticus gastrothoracopagus dipygus.

dip·y·li·di·a·sis (dip″ə-lĭ-di′ə-sis) infection with *Dipylidium caninum,* usually seen in cats and dogs. Human infections are usually in children who have had close contact with infected pets, and are characterized by abdominal pain and diarrhea.

Dip·y·li·di·i·dae (dip″ə-lĭ-di′ĭ-de) a family of cestodes of the order Cyclophyllidea, which sometimes parasitize mammals, birds, and snakes. The genus *Dipylidium* is of medical interest. Formerly called Dilepididae.

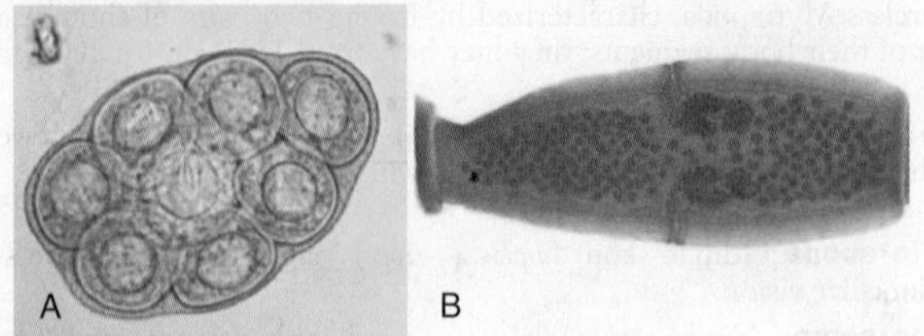

■ *Dipylidium caninum. (A),* Egg packet (wet mount); *(B),* proglottid with visible genital pores (carmine stain).

Dip·y·lid·i·um (dip″ə-lid′e-əm) [Gr. *dipylos* having two entrances] a genus of tapeworms of the family Dipylidiidae, usually found in cats and other small carnivores.

D. cani′num a common tapeworm of dogs and cats, the larval stage living in fleas *(Ctenocephalides canis)* and lice *(Trichodectes canis)* of dogs, as well as in *Pulex irritans,* which thus act as vectors; it has been found in humans. Called also *Taenia elliptica.*

di·py·rid·a·mole (di″pĭ-rid′ə-mōl) a platelet aggregation inhibitor and coronary vasodilator used to prevent thromboembolism associated with mechanical heart valves, in the treatment of transient ischemic attacks, as a prophylactic adjunct in the prevention of myocardial reinfarction, and as a diagnostic aid adjunct in myocardial perfusion imaging; administered orally or intravenously.

di·rect (dĭ-rekt′) [L. *directus*] 1. straight; in a straight line. 2. performed immediately and without the intervention of subsidiary means.

di·rec·tor (dĭ-rek′tər) [L. *dirigere* to direct] any person, thing, or device that guides or directs.

grooved d. a grooved instrument used to guide the direction and depth of a surgical incision.

di·rhi·nic (di-ri′nik) pertaining to both halves of the nasal cavity.

dir·i·go·mo·tor (dir″ĭ-go-mo′tər) [L. *dirigere* to direct + *motor*] controlling muscular activity.

di·rith·ro·my·cin (di-rith″ro-mi′sin) [USP] a macrolide antibiotic with activity similar to that of erythromycin, used in the treatment of bacterial infections of the respiratory tract, streptococcal pharyngitis, and skin and soft tissue infections; administered orally.

dir·lo·tap·ide (dir-lo′tə-pid) a selective inhibitor of microsomal triglyceride transfer protein; it blocks the assembly and release of lipoproteins into the bloodstream and is used in the treatment of obesity in dogs. It is believed to act both by reduction of fat absorption by cells lining the intestine and by early production of a satiety signal wich decreases food consumption.

Di·ro·fi·la·ria (di″ro-fĭ-lar′e-ə) a genus of nematodes of the superfamily Filarioidea; they have very long filiform bodies and striated cuticles.

D. immi′tis the heartworm, an important pathogen of dogs and other canids and occasionally humans, causing dirofilariasis.

D. magalhae′si *D. immitis.*

D. re′pens a species found in the subcutaneous connective tissues of dogs and occasionally humans.

di·ro·fil·a·ri·a·sis (di″ro-fil″ə-ri′ə-sis) infection with a nematode of genus *Dirofilaria;* it is common in dogs and has occurred in humans. Mosquitoes transmit the larvae, and adult worms are found in and may occlude the vessels of the heart, primarily the right ventricle and pulmonary artery, leading to symptoms such as cough, chest pain, and sometimes hemoptysis.

Dir. prop. [L.] directio′ne pro′pria (with proper direction).

DIS Diagnostic Interview Schedule.

dis-[1] [L.] a prefix denoting reversal or separation.

dis-[2] [Gr. *dis* twice] a prefix denoting duplication.

dis·a·bil·i·ty (dis″ə-bil′ĭ-te) 1. an incapacity or lack of the ability to function normally; it may be either physical or mental or both. 2. anything that causes such an incapacity. 3. as defined by the federal government: "inability to engage in any substantial gainful activity by reason of any medically determinable physical or mental impairment which can be expected to last or has lasted for a continuous period of not less than 12 months."

developmental d. any disorder in which developmental milestones are not reached on schedule, or may not be reached at all; e.g., mental retardation, autism, or cerebral palsy.

di·sac·cha·ri·dase (di-sak′ə-rĭ-dās″) an enzyme that hydrolyzes disaccharides. In humans, the disaccharidases, comprising the β-glycosidase (lactase–phlorhizin hydrolase) complex, sucrase-isomaltase complex; and trehalase, are located in the brush border membrane of the small intestine, hydrolyzing the oligo- and disaccharides produced after luminal digestion of starches and other dietary carbohydrates. See also under *deficiency* and see *disaccharide intolerance,* under *intolerance.*

di·sac·cha·ride (di-sak′ə-rīd) any of a class of sugars composed of two glycosidically linked monosaccharides; the term is most commonly used for those composed of hexoses, such as sucrose, lactose, and maltose.

reducing d's disaccharides that can reduce Fehling solution or other reagents, owing to the presence of a functional aldehyde group.

di·sac·cha·rid·uria (di-sak″ə-rīd-u′re-ə) presence of excessive levels of a disaccharide in the urine, as in disaccharide intolerance; types are named for the sugar in question, such as *lactosuria, maltosuria, sucrosuria,* and so on.

dis·ac·id·i·fy (dis″ə-sid′ĭ-fi) to remove an acid from, or to neutralize an acid in, a mixture.

Di·sal·cid (di-sal′sid) trademark for preparations of salsalate.

dis·ar·tic·u·la·tion (dis″ahr-tik″u-la′shən) [*dis-* + *articulation*] amputation or separation at a joint. Called also *exarticulation.*

ankle d. amputation of the foot at the ankle joint; see also *Syme amputation*

elbow d. amputation of the upper limb through the elbow joint.

hip d. amputation of the lower limb through the hip joint.

knee d. amputation of the lower limb through the knee joint.

shoulder d. amputation of the upper limb through the shoulder joint. Called also *Dupuytren amputation* or *operation* and *Lisfranc amputation* or *operation.*

wrist d. amputation of the hand through the wrist joint.

dis·as·sim·i·late (dis″ə-sim′ĭ-lāt) dissimilate.

dis·as·sim·i·la·tion (dis″ə-sim″ĭ-la′shən) [*dis-* + *assimilation*] dissimilation.

disc (disk) [*discus*] disk.

Bardeen primitive d., Bardeen primordial d. the embryonic structure that develops into the intervertebral ligament.

bilaminar d. embryonic d.

ectodermal d. an elongated plate of epithelial cells developed from the embryoblast in the human blastocyst about a week after fertilization.

embryonic d., germ d., germinal d. a flat area in a blastocyst in which the first traces of the embryo are seen, visible early in the second week in human development.

dis·cec·to·my (dis-kek′tə-me) diskectomy.

dis·charge (dis′chahrj) 1. a setting free, or liberation. 2. matter or force set free. 3. an excretion or evacuation. 4. release from a hospital or other course of care. 5. the passing of an action potential through a neuron, axon, or muscle fiber.

bizarre high-frequency d., bizarre repetitive d. complex repetitive d.

complex repetitive d. polyphasic or serrated formations seen on recordings of action potentials, having uniform amplitude and frequency and abrupt beginning and ending; seen in patients with muscular dystrophy and other motor unit diseases. Called also *bizarre high-frequency d., bizarre repetitive d.,* and *bizarre high-frequency potential.*

disruptive d. the passing of a current through an insulating medium due to the breakdown of the medium under the electrostatic stress.

double d. the repeated occurrence of two similar action potentials, separated by just a short interval, as part of a larger repeating pattern; called also *doublet.*

epileptic d. the pathological discharge of multiple neurons in the central nervous system, signaling an attack of epilepsy.

epileptiform d's see under *activity.*

grouped d. 1. on an electroencephalogram, the occurrence of several motor unit action potentials together. 2. repetitive d.

iterative d. repetitive d.

multiple d. the repeated occurrence of four or more similar action potentials separated by short intervals, as part of a larger repeating pattern; called also *multiplet.*

myokymic d. patterns of grouped or repetitive discharges of motor unit action potentials sometimes seen in myokymia. The most common type is groups of single units firing at a uniform rate interspersed with silent periods. A less common pattern is continuously recurring multiple discharges.

myotonic d. high frequency repetitive discharges seen in myotonia and evoked by insertion of a needle electrode, percussion of a muscle, or stimulation of a muscle or its motor nerve; characterized by waxing and waning of frequency and amplitude. There are two types: one with biphasic spike potentials resembling fibrillation potentials and one with waves resembling positive sharp waves.

nervous d., neural d. discharge (def. 5).

periodic lateralized epileptiform d. (PLED) a pattern of repetitive paroxysmal slow or sharp waves seen on an electroencephalogram from just one side of the brain.

repetitive d. multiple recurrences of an action potential in similar forms; examples are *double d.*, *triple d.*, *multiple d.*, *myokymic d.*, and *myotonic d.* Called also *iterative d.*

triple d. the repeated occurrence of three similar action potentials separated by short intervals, near each other as part of a larger repeating pattern; called also *triplet.*

dis•ci (dis′i) [L.] genitive and plural of *discus.*

dis•ci•form (dis′ĭ-form) [*disc-* + *form*] in the form of a disk.

dis•cis•sion (dĭ-sizh′ən) [L. *discissio; dis-* apart + *scindere* to cut] incision, or cutting into, as of a soft cataract.

d. of cataract an eye operation consisting of surgical rupturing of the lens capsule so that the aqueous humor may gain access to the lens.

posterior d. incision of the capsule of a cataract from behind.

dis•ci•tis (dis-ki′tis) diskitis.

dis•cli•na•tion (dis″klĭ-na′shən) extorsion.

disc(o)- [L. *discus*, q.v.] a combining form denoting relationship to a disk, or disk-shaped. See also words beginning *disk(o)-*.

dis•co•blas•tic (dis″ko-blas′tik) [*disco-* + *blast-* + *-ic*] pertaining to a discoblastula or to discoidal cleavage.

dis•co•blas•tu•la (dis″ko-blas′tu-lə) the specialized blastula formed by cleavage of a fertilized telolecithal egg, consisting of a cellular cap (the *embryonic disc* or *blastoderm*) separated by the blastocoele from a floor of uncleaved yolk.

dis•co•cyte (dis′ko-sīt) an erythrocyte of the normal discoid shape, as opposed to a poikilocyte or other irregular form.

dis•co•gas•tru•la (dis″ko-gas′troo-lə) a modified, flattened gastrula formed by discoidal cleavage of a highly telolecithal egg.

dis•co•ge•net•ic (dis″ko-jə-net′ik) discogenic.

dis•co•gen•ic (dis″ko-jen′ik) [*disco-* + *-genic*] caused by derangement of an intervertebral disk.

dis•co•gram (dis′ko-gram) diskogram.

dis•cog•ra•phy (dis-kog′rə-fe) diskography.

dis•coid (dis′koid) [*disc-* + *-oid*] 1. shaped like a disk. 2. a dental instrument with a circular blade around the entire periphery except where it meets the shank; used to carve dental restorations. 3. a disk-shaped dental excavator designed to remove the carious dentin of a decayed tooth.

dis•coid•ec•to•my (dis″koid-ek′tə-me) diskectomy.

dis•con•tin•u•ous (dis″kən-tin′u-əs) 1. interrupted; intermittent; marked by breaks. 2. discrete; separate. 3. lacking logical order or coherence.

dis•cop•a•thy (dis-kop′ə-the) [*disco-* + *-pathy*] disease of an intervertebral cartilage (disk).

traumatic d. herniation of an intervertebral disk due to trauma; see under *herniation.*

dis•coph•o•rous (dis-kof′ə-rəs) [*disco-* + Gr. *phoros* bearing] possessing a disklike organ or part.

dis•cord (dis′kord) [L. *discordia*] a simultaneous assemblage of two or more inharmonious sounds.

dis•cor•dance (dis-kor′dəns) in genetics, the occurrence of a given trait in only one member of a twin pair, as opposed to *concordance.*

dis•cor•dant (dis-kor′dənt) 1. exhibiting discordance. 2. belonging to divergent species; said of transplanted tissue. See under *xenograft.*

dis•co•ria (dis-kor′e-ə) dyscoria.

dis•co•spon•dy•li•tis (dis″ko-spon″də-li′tis) [*disco-* + *spondylitis*] inflammation of intervertebral disks in animals, often with osteomyelitis of adjacent vertebrae, caused by a bacterial infection or occasionally trauma. Resultant compression of the spinal cord can cause paralysis. It is most commonly seen in adult dogs but also affects pigs, horses, and cattle.

dis•crep•an•cy (dis-krep′ən-se) disagreement or inconsistency.

tooth size d. lack of harmony of size of individual or groups of teeth when related to those within the same arch or the opposing arch.

dis•crete (dis-krēt′) [L. *discretus; discernere* to separate] made up of separated parts or characterized by lesions which do not become blended.

dis•crim•i•na•tion (dis-krim″ĭ-na′shən) the making of a fine distinction.

speech d. ability to recognize spoken words, as measured by speech audiometry.

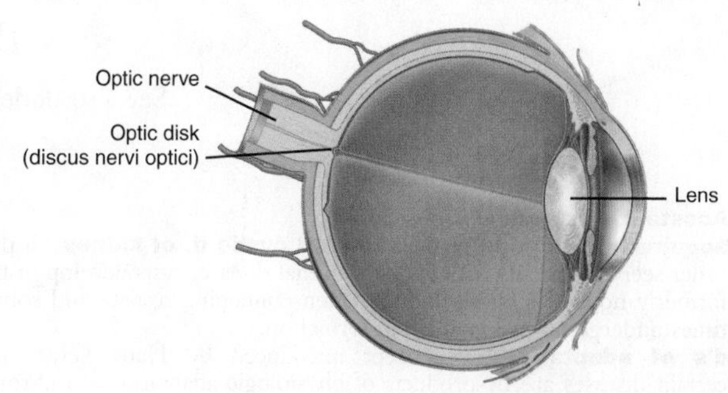

■ Discus nervi optici (optic disk).

dis•crim•i•na•tor (dis-krim′ĭ-na″tər) a circuit in which output is a function of how the input signal compares with one or more standard or reference signals.

dis•cus (dis′kəs) pl. *dis′ci* [L., from Gr. *diskos*] a circular or rounded flat plate; used as a general term in anatomical nomenclature to designate such a structure. Called also *disc* or *disk.*

d. articula′ris [TA] articular disk: a pad composed of fibrocartilage or dense fibrous tissue found in some synovial joints; it extends into the joint from a marginal attachment at the articular capsule and in some cases completely divides the joint cavity into two separate compartments. Called also *intra-articular disk.*

d. articula′ris articulatio′nis acromioclavicula′ris [TA] articular disk of acromioclavicular joint: a pad of fibrocartilage, sometimes present, commonly imperfect, within the articular cavity of the acromioclavicular joint. Called also *Weitbrecht cartilage* and *meniscus of acromioclavicular joint.*

d. articula′ris articulatio′nis radioulna′ris dista′lis [TA] articular disk of distal radioulnar joint: a triangular pad of fibrocartilage, attached at its base to the radius and at its apex to the base of the styloid process of the ulna; it usually separates the articular cavity of the distal radioulnar joint from that of the radiocarpal joint. Called also *meniscus of inferior radioulnar joint* and *triquetrous* or *triquetral cartilage.*

d. articula′ris articulatio′nis sternoclavicula′ris [TA] articular disk of sternoclavicular joint: a pad of fibrocartilage, the circumference of which is connected to the articular capsule of the sternoclavicular joint; it is attached superiorly to the clavicle and inferiorly to the first costal cartilage near its union with the sternum, and it divides the joint cavity into two parts. Called also *meniscus of sternoclavicular joint.*

d. articula′ris articulatio′nis temporomandibula′ris [TA] articular disk of temporomandibular joint: a plate of fibrocartilage or fibrous tissue that divides the temporomandibular joint into two separate cavities; its circumference is connected to the articular capsule. Called also *meniscus of temporomandibular joint.*

d. interpu′bicus [TA] interpubic disk: a midline plate of fibrocartilage interposed between the symphysial surfaces of the pubic bones, these surfaces being covered by a thin layer of hyaline cartilage.

d. intervertebra′lis [TA] intervertebral disk: a plate of fibrocartilage found between each of the bodies of adjacent vertebrae, from the axis to the sacrum, consisting of a fibrous ring (anulus fibrosus) enclosing a pulpy center (nucleus pulposus); called also *intervertebral cartilage.* See illustration at *intervertebral disk*, under *disk.*

d. ner′vi op′tici [TA] optic disk: the intraocular portion of the optic nerve formed by fibers converging from the retina and appearing as a pink to white disk; there are no sensory receptors in this region and hence no response to stimuli restricted to it. (See illustration.) Called also *blind spot*, *optic papilla*, and *papilla nervi optici.*

dis•cus•sive (dis-kus′iv) discutient.

dis•cu•ti•ent (dis-ku′shənt) [L. *discutere* to dissipate] 1. scattering; causing a disappearance. 2. an agent that scatters something or makes it disappear. Called also *discussive.*

dis•di•a•clast (dis-di′ə-klast) [*dis-*[2] + *dia-* + *-clast*] any of the doubly refracting elements of the contractile substance of muscle.

dis•di•ad•o•cho•ki•ne•sia (dis-di-ad″o-ko-kĭ-ne′zhə) dysdiadochokinesia.

dis•ease (dĭ-zēz′) [Fr. *dès* from + *aise* ease] any deviation from or interruption of the normal structure or function of a part, organ, or system of the body as manifested by characteristic symptoms and signs; the etiology, pathology, and prognosis may be known or unknown.

Disease

See also under *sickness* and *syndrome*.

Acosta d. acute mountain sickness.
acquired cystic kidney d., acquired cystic d. of kidney a disorder seen in patients with end-stage renal disease; cysts develop in the formerly noncystic failing kidney, often containing oxalate and sometimes undergoing malignant transformation.
d's of adaptation a concept introduced by Hans Selye that certain diseases are by-products of physiologic adaptations to chronic stress *(general adaptation syndrome)*; he included in this category rheumatoid arthritis, peptic ulcer, and essential hypertension.
Addison d. a chronic type of adrenocortical insufficiency, characterized by hypotension, weight loss, anorexia, weakness, and a bronzelike hyperpigmentation of the skin. It is due to tuberculosis- or autoimmune-induced destruction of the adrenal cortex, which results in deficiency of aldosterone and cortisol and is fatal in the absence of replacement therapy. See also *addisonian crisis*, under *crisis*. Called also *chronic adrenocortical insufficiency* and *primary adrenal* or *primary adrenocortical insufficiency*.
Addison-Schilder d. adrenoleukodystrophy.
Adema d. inherited parakeratosis.
adult celiac d. the adult form of *celiac disease* (q.v.).
aftermath d. fog fever.
airsac d. infectious sinusitis of turkeys.
Akabane virus d. the symptom complex seen in fetal sheep or calves after their mothers have been bitten by insects and infected with the Akabane virus; fetuses have encephalomyelitis or defective brains (sometimes hydranencephaly) and arthrogryposis. See also *congenital articular rigidity*, under *rigidity*.
akamushi d. scrub typhus.
Akureyri d. epidemic neuromyasthenia.
Åland eye d. Forsius-Eriksson syndrome.
Albers-Schönberg d. osteopetrosis.
Albert d. inflammation of the calcaneal bursa, which may be secondary to trauma or arthritis and is characterized by signs of inflammation in the retrocalcaneal space and by difficulty in walking. Called also *Swediaur d.*
Aleutian mink d. a chronic, progressive disease of mink, caused by a parvovirus, marked by inappetence, weight loss, lethargy, polydipsia, and hemorrhages; death may result from kidney failure.
Alexander d. an infantile form of leukodystrophy, characterized histologically by the presence of eosinophilic material at the surface of the brain and around its blood vessels, resulting in brain enlargement.
alkali d. chronic selenium poisoning; see under *poisoning*.
allogeneic d. graft-versus-host reaction occurring in immunosuppressed animals receiving injections of allogeneic lymphocytes.
Almeida d. paracoccidioidomycosis.
Alpers d. a rare disease of young children, caused by mutation of a nuclear gene (locus: 15q26) encoding a DNA polymerase responsible for mitochondrial DNA replication. It is characterized by progressive mental deterioration, motor disturbances, seizures, liver failure, and early death. There is neuronal loss in the cerebral cortex and deeper structures, with spongiform degeneration of the gray matter. Called also *progressive cerebral* or *progressive infantile poliodystrophy*.
alpha chain d., alpha heavy chain d. the most common heavy chain disease, occurring predominantly in young adults in the Mediterranean area, and characterized by plasma cell infiltration of the lamina propria of the small intestine resulting in malabsorption with diarrhea, abdominal pain, and weight loss, or, exceedingly rarely, by pulmonary involvement. The gastrointestinal form is called also *immunoproliferative small intestine d.*
altitude d. see under *sickness*.
alveolar hydatid d. a type of hydatid disease in which larval forms (hydatid cysts) of *Echinococcus multilocularis* invade and destroy tissues, undergoing endogenous budding to form an aggregate of small cysts that honeycomb the affected organ (usually the liver); in time the cysts may metastasize to other organs.
Alzheimer d. a progressive central neurodegenerative disorder; it may be inherited or sporadic, and inherited forms may show autosomal dominant or multifactorial inheritance. It is believed to be caused by defects in β-amyloid precursor protein metabolism, and is characterized by diffuse atrophy throughout the cerebral cortex with distinctive lesions called *senile plaques* and clumps of fibrils called *neurofibrillary tangles*. There is a loss of choline acetyltransferase activity in the cortex, and many of the degenerating neurons are cholinergic neurons of the hippocampus and other limbic areas. The plaques contain numerous proteins, including an altered form of Aβ amyloid and apolipoprotein E, and the tangles contain mainly hyperphosphorylated tau protein. The first signs of the disease are slight memory disturbance or changes in personality; deterioration progresses to profound dementia over 5 to 10 years on average. Women are affected twice as often as men, and onset may occur at any age; the disorder is currently divided into early-onset and late-onset forms, with the dividing age being approximately 65 years, but there is no clinical distinction between the two forms. Mutations associated with the early-onset autosomal dominant form have been identified in the β-amyloid precursor protein *(APP)*, presenilin 1 *(PSEN1)*, and presenilin 2 *(PSEN2)* genes, all of which lead to increased production of the altered form of Aβ amyloid. Both familial and sporadic late-onset forms have been associated with a particular allele (ε4) of the apolipoprotein E gene *(APOE)*.

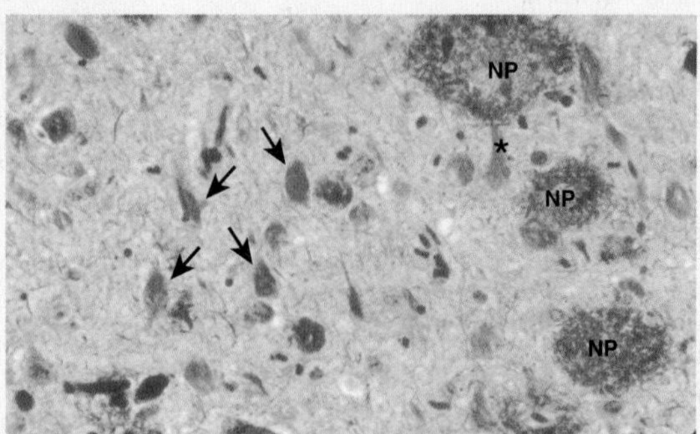

■ Neurofibrillary tangles *(arrows)* and neuritic plaques *(NP)* in the neuronal cytoplasm in Alzheimer disease (silver stain).

Anders d. adiposis dolorosa.
Andersen d. glycogen storage d., type IV.
Anderson d. chylomicron retention d.
Andes d. chronic mountain sickness.
anti-GBM d., anti–GBM antibody d., anti–glomerular basement membrane d. see under *nephritis*.
apatite deposition d. any acute or chronic connective tissue disorder marked by deposition of hydroxyapatite crystals in one or more joints or bursae; such deposition may be primary or it may be secondary to other disorders such as chronic renal failure. Called also *calcium hydroxyapatite deposition d.*
Aran-Duchenne d. spinal muscular atrophy.
arc welder's d. welder's lung.
Armstrong d. lymphocytic choriomeningitis.
arteriosclerotic cardiovascular d. (ASCVD) atherosclerotic involvement of arteries to the heart and to additional organs, resulting in debility or death; the term is sometimes used more narrowly as a synonym of ischemic heart disease.
arteriosclerotic heart d. (ASHD) ischemic heart d.
atopic d. atopy.
Aujeszky d. pseudorabies.
Australian X d. Murray Valley encephalitis.
autoimmune d. a disorder caused by an immune response directed against self antigens. The usual characteristics are demonstrable circulating autoantibodies or cell-mediated immunity against autoantigens, inflammatory lesions caused by immunologically competent cells or immune complexes in tissues containing the autoantigens, and clinical or experimental evidence that the autoimmune process is pathogenic and not secondary to other tissue damage. However, some diseases, such as systemic lupus erythematosus and rheumatoid arthritis are often classified as autoimmune diseases even though their pathogenesis is unclear.
autoinflammatory d's a group of hereditary conditions, usually rare and autosomal dominant, in which there are defects in genes that regulate the body's innate immunity; most are characterized by recurrent fevers and inflammation that may involve various different body systems. Called also *familial* or *hereditary periodic fevers* and *hereditary periodic fever syndromes*.

autosomal dominant polycystic kidney d. (ADPKD) see *polycystic kidney d.*
autosomal recessive polycystic kidney d. (ARPKD) see *polycystic kidney d.*
aviators' d. altitude sickness.
Ayerza d. a form of polycythemia vera associated with sclerosis of the pulmonary artery, marked by chronic cyanosis, dyspnea, bronchitis, bronchiectasis, enlargement of liver and spleen, and hyperplasia of bone marrow.
Azorean d. Machado-Joseph d.
Baastrup d. kissing spines.
baby pig d. neonatal hypoglycemia.
Baelz d. the superficial suppurative type of cheilitis glandularis.
Baló d. an atypical form of Schilder disease in which the demyelination is arranged in concentric rings around a central circle; called also *encephalitis periaxialis concentrica, leukoencephalitis periaxialis concentrica,* and *concentric sclerosis.*
Bamberger d. 1. saltatory spasm. 2. Concato d.
Bamberger-Marie d. hypertrophic pulmonary osteoarthropathy.
Bang d. infectious abortion (def. 1).
Bannister d. angioedema.
Banti d. congestive splenomegaly.
Barlow d. infantile scurvy.
barometer-maker's d. chronic mercurial poisoning in makers of barometers, due to the inhalation of the fumes of mercury.
Barraquer d. partial lipodystrophy.
Basedow d. Graves d.
Batten d., Batten-Mayou d. 1. Vogt-Spielmeyer d. 2. more generally, any or all of the group of disorders constituting neuronal ceroid-lipofuscinosis
bauxite workers' d. bauxite pneumoconiosis.
Bayle d. general paresis.
Bazin d. erythema induratum (def. 2).
Beck d. Kashin-Bek d.
Becker d. the autosomal recessive form of myotonia congenita (q.v.).
Béguez César d. Chédiak-Higashi syndrome.
Beigel d. white piedra.
Bekhterev (Bechterew) d. ankylosing spondylitis.
Benson d. asteroid hyalosis.
Berger d. IgA nephropathy.
Berlin d. commotio retinae.
Bernhardt d., Bernhardt-Roth d. meralgia paresthetica.
Besnier-Boeck d. sarcoidosis.
Best d. an autosomal dominant form of macular degeneration characterized by the presence of an orange cystlike lesion resembling an egg yolk; this form does not progress to blindness. Called also *Best macular degeneration* or *dystrophy* and *vitelliform macular degeneration.*
Bettlach May d. a fatal disease affecting adult honeybees, principally in Switzerland, marked by paralysis with inability to fly, caused by ingestion of the poisonous pollen of certain buttercups.
Biedl d. Bardet-Biedl syndrome.
Bielschowsky-Janský d. Janský-Bielschowsky d.
Bilderbeck d. acrodynia.
Billroth d. traumatic meningocele.
Binswanger d. a degenerative dementia of presenile onset caused by thinning of the subcortical white matter of the brain; some have attributed it to sclerotic changes in the blood vessels. Called also *Binswanger dementia* or *encephalitis, chronic subcortical encephalitis,* and *subcortical arteriosclerotic encephalopathy.*
Birdsville d. poisoning of horses after eating either of the herbs *Indigofera dominii* or *I. linnaea*; characteristics include abdominal pain, stiffness and incoordination, and discharges from the nose and eyes.
black d. infectious necrotic hepatitis.
Blocq d. astasia-abasia.
Blount d. tibia vara.
blue nose d. photosensitization of the face of a horse following ingestion of any of certain meadow plants; characteristics include blue discoloration of the muzzle, sloughing of nonpigmented skin, and frequently intense excitement.
Boeck d. sarcoidosis.
border d. of sheep a highly fatal disease caused by a togavirus, affecting sheep on the English-Welsh border, as well as in Australia and New Zealand (where it is called *hairy shaker d.*); it is manifested by increased hair in the fleece, slow growth, diminished stature, abnormal head shape, and a swaying gait.
Borna d. a fatal enzootic encephalitis of horses, cattle, and sheep, caused by the Borna disease virus; characteristics include tremor, lethargy, and flaccid paralysis. Called also *enzootic encephalitis of horses* and *equine encephalitis.*
Bornholm d. epidemic pleurodynia.
bottom d. crotalism.
Bouchard d. dilatation of the stomach from inefficiency of the gastric muscles.
Bouchet-Gsell d. swineherd's d.
Bourneville d. tuberous sclerosis complex.
Bowen d. a type of squamous cell carcinoma in situ, usually seen in elderly, light-skinned individuals after prolonged exposure to sunlight; a minority of cases have been caused by exposure to arsenic. It is characterized by one or more sharply defined, slightly thickened, erythematous, scaly plaques, on either sun-exposed skin or mucous membranes. A closely related lesion on the glans penis is that of penile intraepithelial neoplasia. Called also *intraepidermal squamous cell carcinoma.*
bran d. nutritional secondary hyperparathyroidism.
Breisky d. lichen sclerosus in women; see under *lichen.*
Bright d. term formerly often used for kidney disease with proteinuria, usually glomerulonephritis.
Brill d. Brill-Zinsser d.
Brill-Symmers d. follicular lymphoma.
Brill-Zinsser d. a recrudescence of epidemic typhus a few to many years after the initial infection, after the etiologic rickettsia has persisted inactively in the tissue of an infected person; compared with the original attack, this type is milder, with a lower fever, a less intense rash, and a much lower fatality rate. Called also *Brill d.* and *recrudescent typhus.*
Brinton d. linitis plastica.
brisket d. a disease seen in young cattle at altitudes above 7600 feet, resembling altitude sickness of humans and often progressing to fatal respiratory or cardiac failure; it is sometimes seen in sheep and has been produced experimentally in pigs.
brittle bone d. osteogenesis imperfecta.
broad beta d. familial dysbetalipoproteinemia; named for the electrophoretic mobility of the abnormal chylomicron and very-low-density lipoprotein remnants (β-VLDL) produced in this disorder.
Brodie d. 1. chronic synovitis, especially of the knee, with a pulpy degeneration of the parts affected. 2. hysterical pseudofracture of the spine.
Brody d. a rare muscular disorder characterized by painless cramping and exercise-induced impairment of muscle relaxation, due to a markedly reduced influx of calcium ions in the sarcoplasmic reticulum; both autosomal dominant and autosomal recessive forms have been recognized.
bronzed d. Addison d.
Brown-Symmers d. fatal acute serous encephalitis in children.
Bruck d. a condition marked by deformity of bones, multiple fractures, ankylosis of joints, and atrophy of muscles.
Bruton d. X-linked agammaglobulinemia.
Buerger d. thromboangiitis obliterans.
Buhl d. an acute sepsis affecting newborn infants, marked by hemorrhages into the skin, mucous membranes, and navel attended with cyanosis and jaundice; there are also hemorrhages in the intestinal organs.
Buschke d. cryptococcosis.
bush d. see under *sickness.*
Busquet d. exostoses on the dorsum of the foot due to osteoperiostitis of the metatarsal bones.
Buss d. encephalomyelitis with pleuritis affecting cattle in the United States, Japan, and parts of Europe, caused by infection with *Chlamydophila psittaci*; characteristics include fever, labored breathing, cough, diarrhea, and neurological signs such as a staggering gait; sometimes there is drooling or a nasal discharge. Called also *sporadic bovine encephalomyelitis.*
Busse-Buschke d. cryptococcosis.
Byler d. progressive familial intrahepatic cholestasis type 1.
Cacchi-Ricci d. medullary sponge kidney.
Caffey d. infantile cortical hyperostosis.
caisson d. decompression sickness.
calcium hydroxyapatite deposition d. apatite deposition d.

calcium pyrophosphate deposition d. (CPDD) an acute or chronic inflammatory arthropathy caused by deposition of calcium pyrophosphate dihydrate (CPPD) crystals in the joints and characterized by chondrocalcinosis and the presence of the crystals in synovial fluid (see also *chondrocalcinosis*). Clinically, it may resemble numerous connective tissue diseases, including osteoarthritis, rheumatoid arthritis, and gout, or it may be asymptomatic. While most commonly idiopathic, CPDD can also be hereditary or associated with a variety of metabolic diseases. Acute attacks are sometimes called *pseudogout.* Called also *CPPD d.*
California d. coccidioidomycosis.
Calvé-Perthes d. Legg-Calvé-Perthes disease.
Camurati-Engelmann d. diaphyseal dysplasia.
Canavan d., Canavan-van Bogaert-Bertrand d. spongy degeneration of the central nervous system; see under *degeneration.*
canine parvovirus d. an acute, often fatal gastroenteritis of dogs caused by a parvovirus related to the virus of feline panleukopenia or of mink enteritis.
Caroli d. congenital dilatation of the intrahepatic bile ducts.
Carrión d. bartonellosis (def. 2).
Castellani d. hemorrhagic bronchitis.
Castleman d. a condition resembling lymphoma but without recognizable malignant cells, occurring as isolated masses of lymphoid tissue and lymph node hyperplasia, usually in the abdominal or mediastinal area. There are two types, the *hyaline vascular type* and the *plasma cell type.* The former is much more common and is characterized by a large mass consisting of involuted germinal centers surrounded by concentric layers of lymphocytes, with hyalinization of the blood vessels entering the germinal centers; it is relatively benign and often asymptomatic. The second type, consisting of sheets of plasma cells, is more aggressive and often multicentric and may be premalignant; it is frequently accompanied by a variety of signs and symptoms that resolve when the lesion is excised. Called also *giant lymph node hyperplasia.*
cat-scratch d. a usually benign, self-limited infectious disease of the regional lymph nodes, caused by *Bartonella henselae* and chiefly characterized by subacute, painful regional lymphadenitis and mild fever of short duration. It is most often associated with close contact with a cat, the primary symptom being an isolated papule or pustule at the site of a cat scratch. Called also *benign lymphoreticulosis, cat-scratch fever,* and *regional lymphadenitis.*
celiac d. a malabsorption syndrome, thought to be hereditary, precipitated by ingestion of gluten-containing foods. It is characterized by degeneration of intestinal villi with loss of their absorptive function; diarrhea and steatorrhea; abdominal distention; flatulence; weight loss; asthenia; deficiency of vitamins B, D, and K; and electrolyte depletion. The *infantile form* (called also *Herter* or *Herter-Heubner disease*) has an insidious onset, with irritability, loss of appetite, weakness, extreme wasting, growth retardation, and celiac crisis. The *adult form* is marked by fatigue, dyspnea, clubbing of fingers, bone pain, muscle cramps, tetany, megacolon and abdominal distention, tympanitis, and skin pigmentation. The two forms were formerly considered different entities but are now believed to be the same. Called also *gluten* or *gluten sensitive enteropathy* and *celiac* or *nontropical sprue.*
central core d. an autosomal dominant form of myopathy characterized by dense, amorphous hyaline changes in the central portion of the myofibrils, which lack organelles. Onset is in infancy and causes delayed motor development, especially in the lower limbs. Called also *Shy-Magee syndrome.*
Chagas d. a form of trypanosomiasis seen widely in Central and South America, caused by *Trypanosoma cruzi,* and transmitted by the bites of reduviid bugs of the genera *Triatoma, Panstrongylus,* and *Rhodnius,* whose reservoir hosts are domestic and wild mammals. The *acute* form, prevalent in children, is characterized by an erythematous nodule (chagoma) at the site of inoculation, high fever, Romaña sign (swelling on one side of the face), regional lymphadenopathy, hepatosplenomegaly, and meningoencephalic irritation. If the child survives, the disease may resolve completely, or the subacute or chronic form may follow. The *subacute* form may last for several months or years and is characterized by mild fever, severe asthenia, and generalized lymphadenopathy. The *chronic* form, which may or may not be preceded by an acute episode, is characterized by cardiac manifestations such as myocarditis, as well as gastrointestinal manifestations such as megaesophagus and megacolon. Called also *American* or *South American trypanosomiasis.*
Charcot d. neuropathic arthropathy.
Charcot-Marie-Tooth d. (CMT) a group of hereditary conditions characterized by chronic motor and sensory polyneuropathy, of variable inheritance and including autosomal dominant, autosomal recessive, and X-linked forms. It is divided into two major types on the basis of nerve conduction velocities (NCV), each with subtypes: CMT1 is a demyelinating polyneuropathy with symmetrically slowed NCV, onion bulb formation, and segmental demyelination; CMT2 is an axonal neuropathy, with normal NCV but of decreased amplitude, axonal loss visible on biopsy, and no onion bulb formation or segmental demyelination. Both are characterized by progressive symmetric distal muscle weakness and atrophy starting in the feet and legs, gait disturbance, and absent stretch reflexes. A variety of causative mutations have been identified at different loci, all concerned with myelin in Schwann cells, with the majority of cases of autosomal dominant CMT1 caused by duplication of chromosomal region 17p12, containing a gene encoding a peripheral myelin protein *(PMP22).* Called also *Charcot-Marie atrophy* or *syndrome,* and *peroneal* or *peroneal muscular atrophy.*
cheese handler's d., cheese washer's d. see under *lung.*
Chester d. xanthomatosis of the long bones with spontaneous fractures.
Chiari-Frommel d. see under *syndrome.*
cholesteryl ester storage d. (CESD) a relatively mild lysosomal storage disease caused by deficiency of the lysosomal sterol esterase; hepatomegaly may be the only clinical abnormality; hyperbetalipoproteinemia is common, and there is often severe premature atherosclerosis; patients may survive past 40.
Christian d. Hand-Schüller-Christian d.
Christian-Weber d. relapsing febrile nodular nonsuppurative panniculitis.
Christmas d. hemophilia B.
chronic bullous d. of childhood see under *dermatosis.*
chronic granulomatous d. (CGD), chronic granulomatous d. of childhood any of a group of hereditary (X-linked or autosomal recessive) immunodeficiencies, caused by failure of the respiratory burst, resulting in deficient microbicidal ability. Patients have frequent, severe, prolonged bacterial and fungal infections of the skin, oral and intestinal mucosa, reticuloendothelial system, bones, lungs, and genitourinary tract. The course of the disease varies: symptoms may appear in the neonate, with death in childhood, or a patient may survive into middle age. There seem to be no physiologic differences between the X-linked and the autosomal recessive types.
chronic kidney d. (CKD) gradual loss of kidney function, with progressively more severe renal insufficiency; symptoms may include polyuria, anorexia or nausea, dehydration, and neurological symptoms. *Stage 1* involves a minimally decreased glomerular filtration rate (GFR). *Stage 2* has a GFR of 60 to 89. *Stage 3* has a moderately decreased GFR (30 to 59). *Stage 4* has a severely decreased GFR (15 to 29). *Stage 5* has a GFR below 15 (end-stage renal disease), and patients require dialysis. Called also *chronic renal failure.*
chronic obstructive lung d. (COLD), chronic obstructive pulmonary d. (COPD) 1. any disorder characterized by persistent or recurring obstruction of bronchial air flow, such as chronic bronchitis, asthma, or pulmonary emphysema. 2. heaves.
chronic respiratory d. of poultry a common respiratory disease of chickens caused by infection with *Mycoplasma gallisepticum* and marked by distressed breathing, swelling of the face, and nasal discharge. Abbreviated CRD.
chylomicron retention d. an autosomal recessive disorder of lipid metabolism consisting of inability of cells of the intestinal wall to secrete chylomicrons, so that a person has severe steatorrhea; affected children have diarrhea and growth retardation. Called also *Anderson d.*
circling d. listeriosis in domestic animals.
climatic d. any disease thought to be produced by a change of climate.
coast d. a type of enzootic marasmus seen in southeastern Australia, caused by cobalt and copper deficiencies.
Coats d. a type of retinopathy marked by masses of white to yellow exudate and blood debris from hemorrhage in the posterior part of the fundus oculi; if untreated, it can progress to destruction of the macula and blindness. Called also *exudative retinitis* or *retinopathy.*
coldwater d. infection of aquarium fish by *Flavobacterium psychrophilum;* symptoms include lumps or cottonlike lesions on the skin and gills with ulceration, necrosis, and hemorrhage. Called also *peduncle d.*

collagen d. any of a group of diseases that, although clinically distinct and not necessarily related etiologically, have in common widespread pathologic changes in the connective tissue; they include lupus erythematosus, dermatomyositis, scleroderma, polyarteritis nodosa, rheumatic fever, and rheumatoid arthritis. Collagen disease is not to be confused with *collagen disorder* (q.v.).
columnaris d. infection of warm-water fish by *Flavobacterium columnare*, with slimy or cottonlike skin lesions covering surface necrosis.
comb d. favus of fowl.
combined immunodeficiency d. 1. see under *immunodeficiency*. 2. an autosomal recessive disease of Arabian horses; foals lack their own cell-mediated immunity and seem normal only as long as they have passive immunity from the maternal blood acquired in utero. Soon after the age of two months, most die from uncontrollable infections, particularly respiratory.
combined system d. subacute combined degeneration of spinal cord; see under *degeneration*.
communicable d. an infectious disease transmitted from one individual to another, either by direct contact or indirectly by means of a vector or fomites. Called also *contagious d.*
complicating d. a disease that occurs as a complication in the course of some other disease.
compressed-air d. decompression sickness.
Concato d. progressive malignant polyserositis with large effusions into the pericardium, pleura, and peritoneum. Called also *Bamberger d.*
conformational d's a general term for a number of disorders, such as Alzheimer disease and Pick disease, caused by mutation in the structure of specific proteins, leading to the aggregation and deposition of abnormal proteins.
Conor and Bruch d. boutonneuse fever.
Conradi d. chondrodysplasia punctata.
constitutional d. a disease that involves a system of organs or is characterized by widespread symptoms.
contagious d. communicable d.
Cooley d. thalassemia major.
Cori d. glycogen storage d., type III.
cork handler's d. suberosis.
cornstalk d. moldy corn poisoning.
coronary artery d. (CAD) atherosclerosis of the coronary arteries, which may cause angina pectoris, myocardial infarction, and sudden death. Both genetically determined and avoidable risk factors contribute to the disease; they include hypercholesterolemia, hypertension, smoking, diabetes mellitus, and low levels of high density lipoproteins.
coronary heart d. (CHD) ischemic heart d.
Corridor d. a tick-borne protozoal disease caused by infection with *Theileria lawrencei;* it resembles East Coast fever but is less severe, and is highly pathogenic for cattle, with buffalo serving as a reservoir of infection.
Corrigan d. aortic regurgitation.
Corvisart d. 1. tetralogy of Fallot associated with right aortic arch. 2. formerly, chronic hypertrophic myocarditis.
Cotugno d. sciatica.
Cowden d. an autosomal dominant disorder caused by a mutation on chromosome 10q, comprising a combination of ectodermal, mesodermal, and endodermal anomalies; it is characterized by development of multiple hamartomatous lesions, especially in the skin, oral mucosa, breast, thyroid, colon, and intestines, and is associated with a high incidence of malignancies in the organs involved. Called also *multiple hamartoma syndrome.*
CPPD d. calcium pyrophosphate deposition d.
crazy chick d. 1. avian encephalomalacia. 2. avian encephalomyelitis.
creeping d. 1. see under *eruption*. 2. the cutaneous symptoms of gnathostomiasis.
Creutzfeldt-Jakob d. (CJD) a rare prion disease, associated with any of various mutations of the prion protein gene, existing in sporadic, familial (autosomal dominant), and infectious forms. Onset is usually in middle life, and there are a wide variety of clinical and pathological features. The most commonly seen are varying degrees of spongiform degeneration of neurons, neuronal loss, gliosis, and amyloid plaque formation, accompanied by rapidly progressive dementia, myoclonus, motor disturbances, and characteristic changes in the electroencephalogram. Death generally occurs within a year of onset, although longer courses of up to 5 years also occur. Sporadic cases account for 85–95 per cent of all occurrences. Infectious cases generally result from surgical procedures or injection of human growth hormone prepared from infected pituitary glands. Called also *Jakob d.* and *Jakob-Creutzfeldt d.*

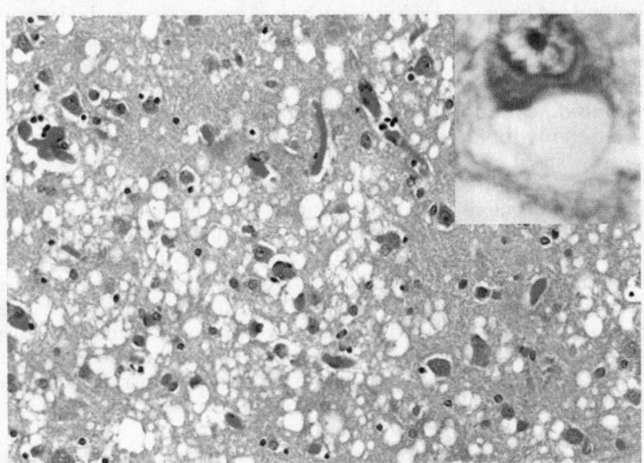

■ Creutzfeldt-Jakob disease, showing spongiform change in the cerebral cortex. *(Inset)*, High magnification of neuron with vacuoles.

Creutzfeldt-Jakob d., new variant (nvCJD) a variant of Creutzfeldt-Jakob disease occurring almost exclusively in the United Kingdom, having a younger age of onset than is seen in Creutzfeldt-Jakob disease, and caused by the same agent that causes bovine spongiform encephalopathy.
Crohn d. one of the principal forms of inflammatory bowel disease, a chronic granulomatous disease of the gastrointestinal tract of unknown etiology; it can involve any part of the tract, but most often is found in the terminal ileum. Characteristics include scarring and thickening of the bowel wall that frequently leads to intestinal obstruction, abscesses, and fistula formation. There is a high rate of recurrence after treatment. Called also *Crohn colitis* and *regional* or *segmental enteritis*. When confined to the ileum it is also called *regional* or *terminal ileitis*.
crooked calf d. a syndrome of congenital skeletal defects seen in calves in the western United States and Canada when their mothers have eaten certain species of *Lupinus* during pregnancy; characteristics include joint contractures, torticollis, and spinal deformities.
Cruveilhier d. spinal muscular atrophy.
Cushing d. 1. Cushing syndrome in which the hyperadrenocorticism is secondary to excessive anterior pituitary secretion of corticotropin by a pituitary adenoma or, rarely, as a result of corticotroph hyperplasia. 2. equine Cushing d.
cystic d. of breast fibrocystic d. of breast.
cystic kidney d., cystic d. of kidney see *acquired cystic kidney d.* and *polycystic kidney d.*

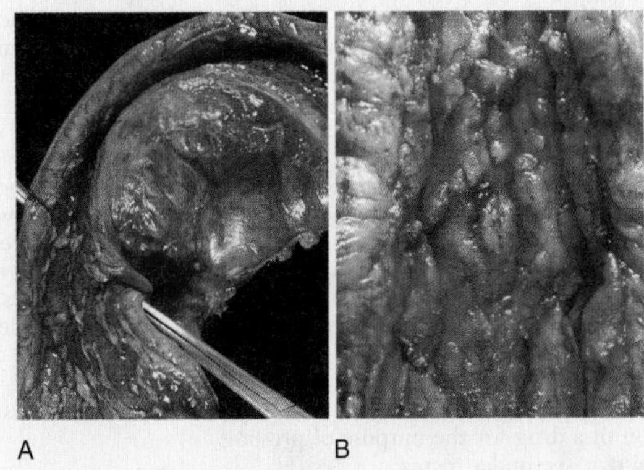

■ Crohn disease. *(A)*, Stricture of the small intestine; *(B)*, linear mucosal ulcers and thickened intestinal wall.

Disease *Continued*

cystic d. of lung a condition in which there are abnormally large air spaces in the lung parenchyma; the term is sometimes applied to cystic emphysema. Called also *pseudocysts of lung* and *pulmonary pseudocysts.*
cysticercus d. cysticercosis.
cystine d., cystine storage d. cystinosis.
cytomegalic inclusion d., cytomegalovirus d. any of a group of diseases caused by cytomegalovirus infection, marked by characteristic inclusion bodies in enlarged infected cells. They were formerly mainly congenital, acquired by a fetus in utero from the mother or during passage through the birth canal; most such infants are asymptomatic, but in some there may be hepatosplenomegaly, jaundice, chorioretinitis, purpura, and severe central nervous system sequelae. The incidence has gone up with the increase in immunodeficient states; the virus can be transmitted via respiratory droplets, tissue or blood donation, or sexual contact. Serious complications can occur in immunocompromised patients. The most common conditions are cytomegalovirus colitis, encephalitis, mononucleosis, pneumonia, and retinitis.
Czerny d. periodic hydrarthrosis of the knee.
Daae d. epidemic pleurodynia.
Dalrymple d. cyclokeratitis.
Darier d., Darier-White d. a slowly progressive, autosomal dominant disorder of keratinization caused by mutation in the *ATP2A2* gene (locus: 12q23-q24.1), which encodes a calcium-transporting ATPase of the sarcoplasmic reticulum. It is characterized by pink to tan or skin-colored papules on seborrheic areas of the body. The papules later coalesce to form plaques that may become crusted, infected, and foul-smelling; over time the lesions may become darker and fuse to form papillomatous or warty growths. Called also *follicular keratosis* and *keratosis follicularis.*
Darling d. histoplasmosis.
David d. spinal tuberculosis.
deficiency d. a condition caused by dietary or metabolic deficiency; the term includes all diseases caused by an insufficient supply of essential nutrients such as protein (or amino acids), vitamins, and minerals.
degenerative joint d. osteoarthritis.
Degos d. malignant atrophic papulosis; see under *papulosis.*
Dejerine d., Dejerine-Sottas d. progressive hypertrophic neuropathy.
demyelinating d. any condition characterized by destruction of the myelin sheaths of nerves. Cf. *multiple sclerosis.*
dense deposit d. type II membranoproliferative glomerulonephritis.
Dent d. tubulopathy of the proximal renal tubules with low molecular weight proteinuria, hypercalciuria, hypokalemia, nephrocalcinosis, rickets, and progressive renal failure.
deprivation d. deficiency d.
de Quervain d. overuse injury with painful tenosynovitis due to relative narrowness of the common tendon sheath of the abductor pollicis longus and extensor pollicis brevis.
Dercum d. adiposis dolorosa.
dermopathic herpesvirus d. a herpesvirus disease of cattle, characterized by ulcerative lesions in the skin; it resembles lumpy skin disease (q.v.).
Deutschländer d. 1. tumor of the metatarsal bones. 2. march foot.
Devic d. neuromyelitis optica.
diamond skin d. the urticarial form of swine erysipelas.
disappearing bone d. gradual, but often complete, resorption of a bone or group of bones, which may be associated with multiple hemangiomas; it usually occurs in children or young adults, sometimes following trauma, but its etiology is unknown.
diverticular d. a general term embracing the prediverticular state, diverticulosis, and diverticulitis.
Dowling-Degos d. a rare, autosomal dominant pigmentary genodermatosis caused by mutations in the *KRT5* gene (locus:12q13), which encodes keratin 5, characterized by brownish black macules in a reticular pattern in the axillary, inguinal, and submammary folds; the neck, scalp, trunk, and arms may be involved and pitted acneiform scars may occur at the angles of the mouth. Onset is usually in the fourth decade of life. Cf. *reticulate acropigmenation of Kitamura.*
drug d. 1. a morbid condition due to long-continued use of a drug. 2. in homeopathy, the group of symptoms seen after the administration of a drug for the purpose of proving.
Dubini d. see under *chorea.*
Dubois d. see under *abscess.*
Duchenne d. 1. spinal muscular atrophy. 2. bulbar paralysis. 3. tabes dorsalis. 4. Duchenne muscular dystrophy.
Duchenne-Aran d. spinal muscular atrophy.
Duchenne-Griesinger d. Duchenne muscular dystrophy.
Duhring d. dermatitis herpetiformis.
Dupuytren d. see under contracture.
Durand-Nicolas-Favre d. lymphogranuloma venereum.
Duroziez d. congenital mitral stenosis.
Eales d. a condition marked by recurrent hemorrhages into the retina and vitreous, affecting mainly males in the second and third decades of life.
Ebola d., Ebola virus d. an acute, often fatal, type of hemorrhagic fever seen in Central Africa, caused by the Ebola virus; symptoms include fever, prostration, hemorrhagic manifestations, pancreatitis, and hepatitis. The natural reservoir and mode of transmission of the virus are unknown, but secondary infection is by direct contact with infected blood and other body secretions and by airborne particles.
Ebstein d. see under *anomaly.*
echinococcus d. hydatid d.
Economo d. lethargic encephalitis.
edema d. enterotoxemia in recently weaned piglets caused by a strain of *Escherichia coli* that normally colonizes the small intestine; characteristics include edema in various parts of the body, with neurological signs such as circling and ataxia. See also *coliform gastroenteritis.* Called also *bowel edema, gut edema,* and E. coli *enterotoxemia.*
Edsall d. heat cramp.
elevator d. a type of pneumoconiosis affecting persons who work in grain elevators.
encephalomyocarditis virus d. a viral disease caused by a cardiovirus that usually occurs in rodents but is transmissible to other animals, especially pigs. It is often clinically inapparent but sometimes causes reproductive failure in young female pigs or encephalomyocarditis in various species, which can be fatal.
endemic d. a disease that is present or usually prevalent in a population or geographical area at all times; such diseases usually have low mortality. Called also *endemia.* See also *holoendemic d.* and *hyperendemic d.* Cf. *epidemic d.*
end-stage renal d. (ESRD) chronic renal failure that is irreversible; see under *failure.*
Engelmann d. diaphyseal dysplasia.
Engel-Recklinghausen d. osteitis fibrosa cystica.
eosinophilic endomyocardial d. Löffler endocarditis.
epidemic d. an infectious or other disease that suddenly affects individuals in a population or geographical area clearly in excess of the number of cases normally expected. Cf. *endemic d.*
Epstein d. pseudodiphtheria.
equine Cushing d. (ECD) a complex of symptoms associated with hyperadrenocorticism in horses, ponies, and donkeys, and caused by pituitary tumor of unknown origin; analogous to Cushing disease of humans, and characterized by polyuria, polydipsia, increased appetite, somnolence, laminitis, and hyperhidrosis associated with lack of cyclic shedding of hair.
Erb d. Duchenne muscular dystrophy.
Erb-Charcot d. Erb spastic paraplegia.
Erb-Goldflam d. myasthenia gravis.
Erdheim d. cystic medial necrosis.
Eulenburg d. paramyotonia congenita.
extensor process d. buttress foot.
Fabry d. an X-linked lysosomal storage disease of glycosphingolipid catabolism, resulting from a deficiency of α-galactosidase A, which causes an accumulation of ceramide trihexoside in the cardiovascular and renal systems. Clinical manifestations include telangiectases in the "bathing suit area," corneal opacities, burning pain in the palms, soles, and abdomen, chronic paresthesias of the hands and feet, cardiopulmonary involvement, edema of the legs, osteoporosis, retarded growth, and delayed puberty. Patients usually die of renal failure or cardiac or cerebrovascular disease. Called also *angiokeratoma corporis diffusum, diffuse angiokeratoma, α-galactosidase A deficiency,* and *ceramide trihexosidase deficiency.*
Fahr-Volhard d. malignant nephrosclerosis.
falling d. a condition seen in cattle with dietary copper deficiency, sometimes with molybdenum poisoning; affected animals suddenly throw up their heads, utter a loud cry, and usually quickly die. They

may show earlier signs of dietary deficiency such as diarrhea and depigmentation of the hair.
Farber d. a lysosomal storage disease of ceramide metabolism due to defective acid ceramidase and marked by painful swelling of joints, nodules over affected joints and over pressure points, hoarseness that may progress to aphonia, and feeding and respiratory problems, usually beginning during the first few months after birth and often leading to death within a few years. There is granulomatous infiltration of subcutaneous tissues, joints, and organs, including the liver, spleen, heart, and lung, and the neurons of the brain and spinal cord often show accumulation of ceramides and gangliosides. Called also *Farber lipogranulomatosis,* and *ceramidase deficiency.*
farmer's lung d. of cattle a disease in cattle similar to farmer's lung in humans, caused by hypersensitivity to moldy hay contaminated by *Saccharopolyspora rectivirgula* or *Thermoactinomyces vulgaris.*
fat-deficiency d. a condition characterized by cessation of growth and skin lesions that result when essential fatty acids (linolenic and linoleic acid) are absent from the diet.
fatty liver d. 1. fatty liver. 2. fat cow syndrome.
Fauchard d. marginal periodontitis.
Favre-Durand-Nicolas d. lymphogranuloma venereum.
Fazio-Londe d. progressive bulbar palsy of childhood.
Feer d. acrodynia.
fibrocystic d., fibrocystic breast d., fibrocystic d. of breast a form of mammary dysplasia with formation of cysts of varying sizes containing a semitransparent, turbid fluid that imparts a brown to blue color (blue dome cyst) to the unopened cysts; considered to be due to abnormal hyperplasia of the ductal epithelium and dilatation of the ducts of the mammary gland, occurring as a result of an exaggeration and distortion of the cyclic breast changes that normally occur in the menstrual cycle. Called also *chronic cystic mastitis, cystic d. of breast,* and *Schimmelbusch d.*
fibrocystic d. of the pancreas cystic fibrosis.
Fiedler d. Weil syndrome.
fifth d. erythema infectiosum.
file-cutters' d. lead poisoning from inhaling lead particles rising from the bed of lead used in file cutting.
fish eye d. a less severe form of lecithin–cholesterol acyltransferase deficiency due to a partial defect in the enzyme activity as a result of mutation in the *LCAT* gene (locus: 16q22.1); corneal opacities give the eye the appearance of the eye of a boiled fish, and lipoproteins show some abnormalities.
Flatau-Schilder d. Schilder d.
flax-dresser's d. byssinosis in flax-dressers.
Flegel d. hyperkeratosis lenticularis perstans.
Fleischner d. osteochondritis affecting the middle phalanges of the hand.
flint d. chalicosis.
floating beta d. familial dysbetalipoproteinemia.
fluke d. trematodiasis.
focal d. a disease that is localized at one or more foci.
Følling d. phenylketonuria.

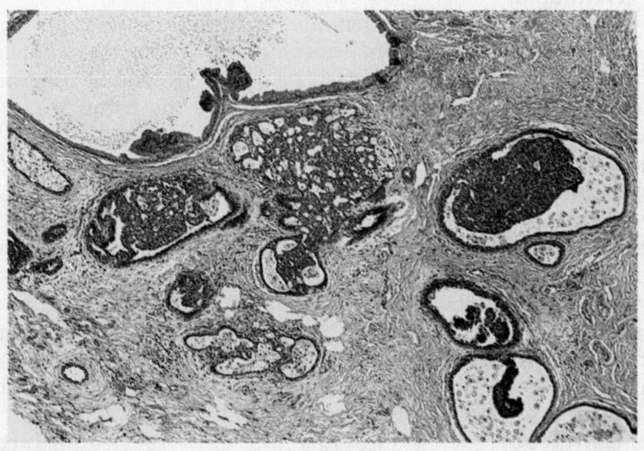

■ Fibrocystic disease of breast, with cystic dilatation, apocrine metaplasia, florid ductal hyperplasia, and fibrosis.

foot-and-mouth d. an acute, extremely contagious disease caused by a picornavirus, affecting wild and domestic animals, particularly ruminants and pigs; it is occasionally a zoonosis for humans. It is marked by an eruption of vesicles on the lips, buccal cavity, pharynx, legs, and feet; sometimes the skin of the udder or teats is involved. The animal condition is called also *epizootic aphthae* and *hoof-and-mouth d.*
foot process d. minimal change d.
Forbes d. glycogen storage d., type III.
Fordyce d. 1. see under *granule.* 2. Fox-Fordyce d.
Forestier d. diffuse idiopathic skeletal hyperostosis.
Förster d. areolar choroiditis.
Fournier d. see under *gangrene.*
Fox-Fordyce d. a chronic, usually pruritic disease seen chiefly in women, characterized by small follicular papular eruptions in apocrine gland–bearing areas such as the axillae and groin. It is caused by obstruction and rupture of the intraepidermal portion of the ducts of the glands, which results in alteration of the regional ductal epidermis, apocrine secretory tubule, and adjacent dermis. Called also *apocrine miliaria.*
Francis d. tularemia.
Freiberg d. Köhler bone disease (def. 2).
Friedländer d. endarteritis obliterans.
Friedreich d. paramyoclonus multiplex.
Frommel d. Chiari-Frommel syndrome.
functional d. see under *disorder.*
functional cardiovascular d. neurocirculatory asthenia.
Gaisböck d. stress polycythemia.
gamma chain d., gamma heavy chain d. a heavy chain disease occurring usually in elderly persons that clinically resembles a malignant lymphoma, with symptoms of lymphadenopathy, hepatosplenomegaly, and recurrent infections.
Gamna d. a form of splenomegaly, with thickening of the splenic capsule and the presence of small brownish areas (Gamna nodules), which are usually surrounded by a hematogenous zone; ferruginous pigment is deposited in the splenic pulp.
Gamstorp d. hyperkalemic periodic paralysis.
Gandy-Nanta d. siderotic splenomegaly.
Garré d. sclerosing nonsuppurative osteomyelitis.
gastroesophageal reflux d. (GERD) any condition noted clinically or histopathologically that results from gastroesophageal reflux, ranging in seriousness from mild to life-threatening; principal characteristics are heartburn and regurgitation. When there is damage to the esophageal epithelium, it is known as *reflux esophagitis.*
Gaucher d. a lysosomal storage disease characterized by glucocerebroside (glucosylceramide) accumulation in Gaucher cells, storage cells in the liver, spleen, lymph nodes, alveolar capillaries, and bone marrow; it is caused by mutations in either glucocerebrosidase (glucosylceramidase) or an activator protein associated with that enzyme, saposin C. There are three clinical types: *type 1,* called also chronic nonneuronopathic or "adult" type, may appear at any age and is associated with hypersplenism, thrombocytopenia, anemia, jaundice, and bone lesions; *type 2,* called also acute neuronopathic or "infantile" type, is associated with onset in infancy, hepatosplenomegaly, severe impairment of the central nervous system, and death usually within the first year; and *type 3,* called also subacute neuronopathic or "juvenile" type, is the most varied, having the same clinical features as types 1 and 2 but a longer course. Called also *glucosylceramide lipidosis.*
Gee d., Gee-Herter d., Gee-Herter-Heubner d. the infantile form of celiac disease.
Gee-Thaysen d. the adult form of celiac disease.
genetic d. a general term for any disorder caused by a genetic mechanism, comprising chromosome aberrations or anomalies, mendelian or monogenic or single-gene disorders, and multifactorial disorders.
Gerhardt d. erythromelalgia.
Gerlier d. an acute disease seen in farm workers and stable workers, characterized by vertigo, ptosis, and motor disorders; it is probably a form of vestibular neuronitis.
gestational trophoblastic d. see under *neoplasia.*
Gibney d. see under *perispondylitis.*
Gilchrist d. blastomycosis (def. 1).
Glanzmann d. see under *thrombasthenia.*
Glasser d. a disease of young pigs, caused by infection by *Haemophilus parasuis;* symptoms include swelling of the hocks or knee joints or both, accompanied by fever, lameness, and a disinclination to

move; in severe cases convulsions and death may occur. Called also *infectious porcine polyarthritis* and *porcine polyserositis.*
glycogen storage d. a group of rare inborn errors of metabolism caused by defects in specific enzymes or transporters involved in the metabolism of glycogen.

type 0 an autosomal recessive disorder due to mutation in the *GYS2* gene (locus: 12p12.2), which encodes the liver isozyme of glycogen synthase, resulting in decreased hepatic glycogen stores. Patients present in early infancy with early morning drowsiness and fatigue with hypoglycemia and hyperketonemia. An analogous autosomal recessive disorder due to mutation in the *GYS1* gene (locus: 19q13.3), which encodes the muscle isozyme of glycogen synthase, is sometimes also given this name; it is characterized by cardiomyopathy and exercise intolerance.

type I a severe autosomal recessive disorder due to mutation in the *G6PC* gene (locus: 17q21), which encodes the catalytic subunit of glucose-6-phosphatase, resulting in deficiency of the enzyme in liver, kidney, and intestinal mucosa. It is characterized by hepatomegaly, fasting hypoglycemia, hyperuricemia, hyperlacticacidemia, hyperlipidemia, xanthomas, bleeding, and adiposity.

type IA glycogen storage disease, type I.

type IB an autosomal recessive disorder due to mutation in the *G6PT1* gene (locus: 11q23), which encodes glucose-6-phosphatase translocase, resulting in a defect in the transport system for glucose 6-phosphate. Symptoms resemble those of the type IA disorder, but patients are additionally predisposed to infection related to neutropenia and to chronic inflammatory bowel disease.

type II an autosomal recessive disorder due to mutation in the *GAA* gene (locus: 17q25.2-q25.3), which encodes the lysosomal enzyme glucan 1,4-α-glucosidase (more commonly called acid maltase or acid alpha-glucosidase), resulting in generalized tissue accumulation of glycogen. In infants, it is characterized by mild hepatomegaly, mental and motor retardation, hypotonia, and cardiomegaly and cardiorespiratory failure resulting in death; the adult form is usually characterized primarily by a gradual skeletal myopathy that sometimes causes respiratory problems. Between the two extremes there is a heterogeneous juvenile-onset form with late onset myopathy and variable cardiac involvement.

type III an autosomal recessive disorder due to mutation in the *AGL* gene (locus: 1p21), which encodes the glycogen debranching enzyme (amylo-1,6-glucosidase); it usually affects both muscle and liver enzyme isoforms, but can affect the latter alone. Defects in the liver enzyme are characterized by hepatomegaly and hypoglycemia, while defects in the muscle enzyme are characterized by progressive muscle wasting and weakness. Heart and skeletal muscle are also frequently affected. Called also *debrancher deficiency.*

type IV an autosomal recessive disorder due to mutation in the *GBE1* gene (locus: 3p12), which encodes the glycogen branching enzyme (1,4-α-glucan branching enzyme), resulting in accumulation of long insoluble glycogen molecules with unbranched outer chains. The most severe abnormalities occur in the liver, with hepatosplenomegaly, early cirrhosis with portal hypertension, liver failure, and death in childhood; there are also neuromuscular abnormalities. Called also *brancher deficiency.*

type V an autosomal recessive disorder due to mutation in the *PYGM* gene (locus: 11q13), which encodes the skeletal muscle isozyme of glycogen phosphorylase (muscle phosphorylase); it is characterized by muscle cramps and fatigue during exercise.

type VI an autosomal recessive disorder due to mutation in the *PYGL* gene (locus: 14q21-q22), which encodes the hepatic isozyme of glycogen phosphorylase (liver phosphorylase); it is characterized by hepatomegaly, mild to moderate hypoglycemia, and mild ketosis.

type VII an autosomal recessive disorder due to mutation in the *PFKM* gene (locus: 12q13.3), which encodes the muscle isozyme of 6-phosphofructokinase; it is characterized by muscle weakness and cramping after exercise. Activity of the erythrocyte isozyme is also decreased, causing increased hemolysis and a mild compensated hemolytic anemia.

type VIII former name for *glycogen storage d., type IX.*

type IX glycogen storage disease caused by deficiency of phosphorylase kinase; it comprises at least six different subtypes, types IXa–IXf, which vary in their mode of inheritance (either X-linked or autosomal recessive) and in the tissues involved (liver, blood cells, muscle, heart, or some combination thereof). The genetic heterogeneity relates to the enzyme structure; its four subunits are encoded by separate genes and are differentially expressed in the tissues. The most common subtype, IXa, is an X-linked disorder due to mutation in the *PHKA2* gene (locus: Xp22.2-p22.1), which encodes the alpha subunit of hepatic phosphorylase kinase; it is characterized in affected males by hepatomegaly, occasional fasting hypoglycemia, and some growth retardation.

Goldflam d., Goldflam-Erb d. myasthenia gravis.
Goldstein d. hereditary hemorrhagic telangiectasia.
Gorham d., Gorham-Stout d. disappearing bone d.

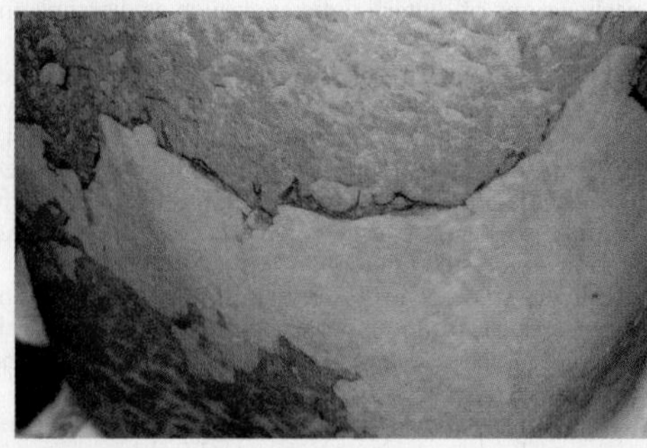

■ Graft-versus-host disease. Coalescence of bullae and epidermal necrosis leading to large areas of denudation after allogeneic bone marrow transplantation.

graft-versus-host d. (GVHD) disease caused by the immune response of histoincompatible, immunocompetent donor cells against the tissues of an immunoincompetent host; this can occur as a complication of bone marrow transplantation or as a result of maternal-fetal blood transfusion or therapeutic blood transfusion in which the recipient has a cellular immunodeficiency disease. Clinical manifestations include skin disease ranging from a maculopapular eruption to epidermal necrosis; intestinal disease with diarrhea, malabsorption, and abdominal pain; and liver dysfunction caused by cholestatic hepatitis or venoocclusive disease, marked by serum enzyme abnormalities. Called also *graft-versus-host reaction.*
grass d. see under *sickness.*
Graves d. a syndrome of diffuse hyperplasia of the thyroid, with a female predominance; it usually has an autoimmune etiology and has been linked to autoimmune thyroiditis. Characteristics include hyperthyroidism (q.v.), usually with goiter and ophthalmic symptoms *(Graves orbitopathy).* Most patients have circulating thyroid-stimulating immunoglobulins that cause excessive secretion of thyroid hormones by binding to TSH receptors on thyroid follicular cells. Called also *Basedow* or *Parry d.* and *diffuse toxic goiter.*
greasy pig d. seborrhea of piglets caused by infection of *Staphylococcus hyicus* through a cut or abrasion of the skin. Called also *exudative epidermitis.*
green muscle d. deep pectoral myopathy.
Greither d. a rare autosomal dominant type of diffuse palmoplantar keratoderma that slowly spreads to adjacent areas of the arms and legs and is accompanied by hyperhidrosis of the affected palms and soles.
Gross d. encysted rectum; saccular dilatation of anal wall with retained inspissated feces.
Grover d. transient acantholytic dermatosis.
guinea worm d. dracunculiasis.
Guinon d. Gilles de la Tourette syndrome.
Gull d. atrophy of the thyroid with myxedema.
Gumboro d. infectious bursal d.
Günther d. congenital erythropoietic porphyria.
GVH d. graft-versus-host d.
H d. Hartnup d.
Habermann d. pityriasis lichenoides et varioliformis acuta.
Haff d. rhabdomyolysis from consumption of fish that contained a toxin that was never identified, seen in the 1920s among fishermen of the Königsberg (or Frisches) Haff, a lagoon off the Baltic Sea.
Haglund d. retrocalcaneal bursitis.
Hagner d. hypertrophic pulmonary osteoarthropathy.
Hailey-Hailey d. benign familial pemphigus.
hairy shaker d. border d. of sheep.
Hallervorden-Spatz d. a hereditary disorder characterized by marked reduction in the number of myelin sheaths of the globus pallidus and substantia nigra, with accumulations of iron pigment, progressive rigidity beginning in the legs, choreoathetoid movements, dysarthria, and progressive mental deterioration. Transmitted as an autosomal recessive trait, it usually begins in the first or second decade, with death occurring before age 30.
Haltia-Santavuori d. a rare infantile form of neuronal ceroid-lipofuscinosis, beginning about one year of age, with excessive storage of lipofuscin, failure to thrive, myoclonic seizures, muscular hypotonia,

psychomotor developmental delay and deterioration, blindness with optic atrophy and cerebellar ataxia, and death within about 5 years.

Hamman d. pneumomediastinum.

Hammond d. athetosis.

Hand d. Hand-Schüller-Christian d.

hand-foot-and-mouth d. a usually mild and self-limited exanthematous eruption most often caused by coxsackievirus A16, primarily seen in preschool children, and characterized by vesicles on the buccal mucosa, tongue, soft palate, gingivae, and hands and feet, including the palms and soles.

Hand-Schüller-Christian d. a chronic, progressive form of multifocal Langerhans cell histiocytosis, sometimes with accumulation of cholesterol, characterized by the triad of calvarial bone defects, exophthalmos, and diabetes insipidus. Called also *chronic idiopathic xanthomatosis.*

Hansen d. leprosy.

Harada d. Vogt-Koyanagi-Harada syndrome.

hard metal d. a pneumoconiosis caused by inhalation of fine particles of cobalt, usually in conjunction with tungsten carbide. In early stages reversible hyperplasia and metaplasia of the bronchial epithelium are seen; later, subacute alveolitis and then chronic interstitial fibrosis develop. Called also *tungsten carbide d.* and *cobalt lung.*

hard pad d. canine distemper.

hardware d. 1. traumatic pericarditis (def. 2). 2. traumatic reticuloperitonitis.

Hartnup d. an inborn error of metabolism characterized by cerebellar ataxia, a pellagra-like condition of the skin, and massive aminoaciduria involving a group of neutral monoaminomonocarboxylic amino acids sharing a common renal reabsorption mechanism.

Hashimoto d. a progressive type of autoimmune thyroiditis with lymphocytic infiltration of the gland and circulating antithyroid antibodies; patients have goiter and gradually develop hypothyroidism. It has a familial predisposition, usually affects women, and sometimes precedes the onset of Graves disease or is manifested after the major symptoms subside. Called also *Hashimoto, chronic lymphadenoid,* or *chronic lymphocytic thyroiditis,* and *lymphadenoid goiter.*

heart d. any organic, mechanical, or functional abnormality of the heart, its structures, or the coronary arteries.

heavy chain d's a group of rare malignant neoplasms of lymphoplasmacytic cells that secrete an M component consisting of monoclonal immunoglobulin heavy chains or heavy chain fragments; they are classified according to heavy chain type. See also *alpha chain d., gamma chain d.,* and *mu chain d.*

Heberden d. 1. rheumatism of the smaller joints, accompanied by nodules in or about the distal interphalangeal joints. 2. angina pectoris.

Hebra d. erythema multiforme minus.

Heck d. focal epithelial hyperplasia.

Heckathorn d. a rare variant of hemophilia A in which the levels of coagulation factor VIII fluctuate; inherited as an X-linked recessive trait.

Heine-Medin d. the major illness of poliomyelitis; see *poliomyelitis.*

hemagglutinating encephalomyelitis virus d. of pigs vomiting and wasting d.

hemoglobin d. any of the hereditary conditions caused by the presence of abnormal hemoglobins in the blood, such as sickle cell anemia or various types of hemolytic anemia and thalassemia.

hemoglobin C d. the state of being homozygous for hemoglobin C, characterized by splenomegaly, mild to moderate hemolytic anemia, recurrent jaundice, and increased numbers of target cells and reticulocytes in the peripheral blood.

hemoglobin C–thalassemia d. a hereditary disorder involving simultaneous heterozygosity for hemoglobin C and thalassemia, manifested by mild hemolytic anemia and persistent splenomegaly; called also *hemoglobin C–thalassemia.*

hemoglobin D d. the state of being homozygous for hemoglobin D, characterized by mild hemolytic anemia with numerous target cells in the peripheral blood.

hemoglobin E d. the state of being homozygous for hemoglobin E; many patients are asymptomatic, but others have mild hemolytic anemia, usually without splenomegaly, and increased numbers of normochromic target cells in the peripheral blood.

hemoglobin E–thalassemia d. a hereditary condition involving simultaneous heterozygosity for hemoglobin E and thalassemia, manifested by mild hemolytic anemia and persistent splenomegaly; called also *hemoglobin E–thalassemia.*

hemoglobin H d. α-thalassemia in individuals heterozygous for hemoglobin H, characterized by chronic hemolytic anemia associated with splenomegaly; red blood cell hypochromia, anisocytosis, and poikilocytosis are accompanied by inclusion bodies detectable by supravital staining.

hemoglobin SC d. sickle cell–hemoglobin C d.

hemoglobin SD d. sickle cell–hemoglobin D d.

hemolytic d. of newborn erythroblastosis fetalis.

hemorrhagic d. of newborn a self-limited hemorrhagic disorder of the first days of life, caused by a deficiency of the vitamin K–dependent blood coagulation factors II, VII, IX, and X.

Henderson-Jones d. osteochondromatosis characterized by the presence of numerous cartilaginous foreign bodies in the joint cavity or in the bursa of a tendon sheath.

hepatic venoocclusive d. veno-occlusive d. of the liver.

hepatolenticular d. Wilson d.

hepatorenal glycogen storage d. glycogen storage d., type I.

hereditary d. a disease that is transmitted genetically from parents to children.

heredodegenerative d. any disease of the central nervous system characterized by specific loss of neural tissue due to hereditary influence.

Herlitz d. the Herlitz type of junctional epidermolysis bullosa.

Hers d. glycogen storage d., type VI.

Herter d., Herter-Heubner d. the infantile form of celiac disease.

Heubner d. syphilitic endarteritis of the cerebral vessels; called also *Heubner endarteritis.*

Heubner-Herter d. the infantile form of celiac disease.

hip-joint d. tuberculosis of the hip joint.

Hippel d. see *von Hippel d.*

Hippel-Lindau d. see *von Hippel-Lindau d.*

Hirschsprung d. congenital megacolon.

His d., His-Werner d. trench fever.

hock d. perosis.

Hodgkin d. a form of malignant lymphoma characterized by painless, progressive enlargement of the lymph nodes, spleen, and general lymphoid tissue; other symptoms may include anorexia, lassitude, weight loss, fever, pruritus, night sweats, and anemia. The characteristic histologic feature is presence of Reed-Sternberg cells. It affects twice as many males as females and is usually considered to be neoplastic in origin, although neither an infectious origin nor an immune response to Reed-Sternberg cells has been excluded. Four types have been distinguished according to histopathologic criteria, three with diffuse patterns *(lymphocyte predominance type, mixed cellularity type,* and *lymphocyte depletion type)* and one with a nodular pattern *(nodular sclerosis type).* Called also *Reed-Hodgkin d.* and *Hodgkin lymphoma.* See also *non-Hodgkin lymphoma,* under *lymphoma.*

Hodgkin d., lymphocyte depletion type a type of Hodgkin disease characterized by a low number of lymphocytes and an abundance of Reed-Sternberg cells with fibrosis; it is the most aggressive of the three diffuse types of Hodgkin disease. Called also *Hodgkin sarcoma.*

Hodgkin d., lymphocyte predominance type a type of Hodgkin disease characterized by a diffuse to slightly nodular infiltrate with abundant mature lymphocytes and varying numbers of benign histiocytes; there are few Reed-Sternberg cells and the degree of malignancy is low. Most patients are males under age 35. Called also *paragranuloma.*

Hodgkin d., mixed cellularity type a type of Hodgkin disease intermediate between the lymphocyte predominance and lymphocyte depletion types; Reed-Sternberg cells are plentiful and there are more

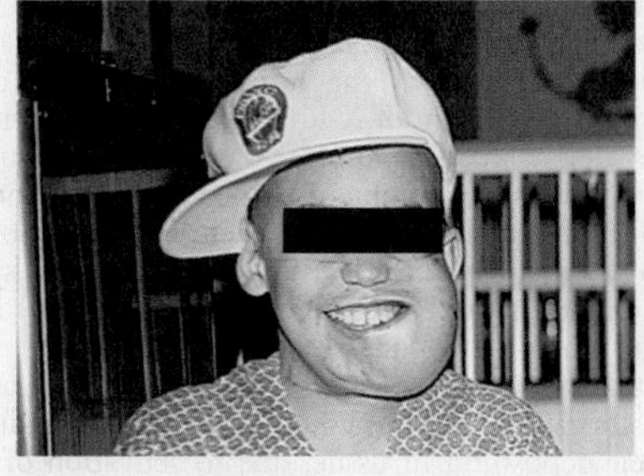

■ Hodgkin disease.

inflammatory cells, such as eosinophils and plasma cells, than in the lymphocyte predominance type.
Hodgkin d., nodular sclerosis type a type of Hodgkin disease in which Reed-Sternberg cells are in the form of lacunar cells and bands of collagen divide the lymphoid tissue into nodules; there are varying numbers of lymphocytes and inflammatory cells such as eosinophils and plasma cells. This type is most common in young women and often has a low grade of malignancy.
Hodgson d. an aneurysmal dilatation of the proximal part of the aorta, often accompanied by dilatation or hypertrophy of the heart.
Hoffa d. traumatic proliferation of fatty tissue (solitary lipoma) in the knee joint.
holoendemic d. an endemic disease occurring at a high level in a population so that most of the children are affected, the adults in the same population then being less so. Cf. *hyperendemic d.*
hoof-and-mouth d. foot-and-mouth disease in domestic animals.
hookworm d. 1. in humans, infection with hookworms of the genera *Ancylostoma* and *Necator*, seen in many hot, humid parts of the world. The larvae live in soil and gain entrance to the digestive tract indirectly through the skin of the feet or legs or directly in contaminated food or water. The skin infection is transitory and is known as *ground itch*. Parasites are then carried by the blood to the lungs, ascend the trachea, are swallowed, and settle in the small intestine, where they attach to the mucosa and ingest blood. Symptoms, varying with severity of infection, may include abdominal pain, diarrhea, and nausea, with anemia if infections are moderate or severe. See also *ancylostomiasis* and *necatoriasis*. 2. in mammals other than humans, infestation of the intestines with any of various hookworms. Dogs and cats are usually infested by *Ancylostoma* or *Uncinaria*, and cattle and sheep by *Bunostomum*. See also *ancylostomiasis, bunostomiasis,* and *uncinariasis*.
Horton d. 1. cluster headache. 2. giant cell arteritis.
Huchard d. continued arterial hypertension, thought to be a cause of arteriosclerosis.
hunger d., hungry d. excessive hunger accompanied by weakness and nervousness caused by the hypoglycemia of hyperinsulinism.
Huntington d. (HD) a triplet repeat disorder caused by expansion of CAG triplet repeats within the *HTT* gene (locus: 4p16.3), which encodes the protein huntingtin (q.v.), with autosomal dominant inheritance and anticipation, and characterized by chronic progressive chorea and mental deterioration terminating in dementia; the age of onset is variable but usually in the fourth decade of life, with death within 15 years. Called also *Huntington chorea*.
Hurler d. see under *syndrome*.
Hurst d. acute necrotizing hemorrhagic encephalomyelitis.
Hutchinson d. angioma serpiginosum.
Hutinel d. tuberculous pericarditis with cirrhosis of the liver in children.
hyaline membrane d. a type of neonatal respiratory distress syndrome in which there is formation of a hyalinelike membrane lining the terminal respiratory passages; extensive atelectasis is attributed to lack of surfactant.
hydatid d. an infection, usually of the liver or lungs, caused by larval forms (hydatid cysts) of tapeworms of the genus *Echinococcus*, and characterized by the development of expanding cysts. This can occur in humans, cattle, sheep, pigs, horses, and occasionally other mammals. The three types are *alveolar*, *polycystic*, and *unilocular hydatid disease* (qq.v.). Called also *hydatidosis*, *echinococcus d.*, and *echinococcosis*.
hydrocephaloid d. a condition similar to hydrocephalus, but marked by depression of the fontanels, due to diarrhea or some other wasting disease with dehydration.
hyperendemic d. an endemic disease equally prevalent in all age groups of a population. Cf. *holoendemic d.*
hypophosphatemic bone d. an autosomal dominant disorder clinically resembling a mild form of X-linked hypophosphatemia and similarly due to a defect in renal tubular function, but usually showing osteomalacia without radiographic evidence of rickets and responding to calcitriol without supplemental phosphate in at least some cases.
hypopigmentation-immunodeficiency d. Griscelli syndrome.
Iceland d. chronic fatigue syndrome.
I-cell d. mucolipidosis II alpha/beta.
immune complex d. any of a variety of local or systemic diseases caused by the formation of circulating antibody-antigen immune complexes and their deposition in tissue, due to activation of complement and to recruitment and activation of leukocytes; see also *type III hypersensitivity reaction*, under *hypersensitivity reaction* at *reaction*.
immunoproliferative small intestine d. (IPSID) the gastrointestinal form of alpha chain disease, characterized by diarrhea, malabsorption, abdominal pain, clubbing, plasma cell infiltration of the lamina propria of the small bowel, and presence of an abnormal alpha heavy chain fragment in the serum; it frequently evolves into primary malignant lymphoma. Called also *Mediterranean lymphoma*.
inborn lysosomal d. lysosomal storage d.
inclusion d. any disease in which cell inclusions are found.
infantile celiac d. see *celiac d.*
infectious d. a disease caused by a pathogenic microorganism, including bacteria, viruses, fungi, protozoa, and multicellular parasites; it may be transmitted from another host or arise from the host's indigenous microflora. See also *infection* and *communicable d.*
infectious bursal d. a highly contagious acute disease of chickens, caused by the infectious bursal disease virus, characterized by edema and swelling of the cloacal bursa, soiled wet feathers, whitish watery diarrhea, listlessness, and trembling, progressing to extreme kidney damage and damage of the bursa of Fabricius, with resulting immunosuppression that can be fatal. Called also *Gumboro d.* and *infectious avian nephrosis*.
inflammatory bowel d. (IBD) a general term for those inflammatory diseases of the intestines that have an unknown etiology, including Crohn disease and ulcerative colitis.
intercurrent d. a disease occurring during the course of another disease with which it has no connection.
interstitial d. a disease that affects mainly the stroma of an organ.
interstitial lung d. a heterogeneous group of noninfectious, nonmalignant disorders of the lower respiratory tract, affecting primarily the alveolar wall structures but also often involving the small airways and blood vessels of the lung parenchyma; slowly progressive loss of alveolar-capillary units may lead to respiratory insufficiency and death.
iron storage d. hemochromatosis.
ischemic bowel d. ischemic colitis.
ischemic heart d. (IHD) any of a group of acute or chronic cardiac disabilities resulting from insufficient supply of oxygenated blood to the heart; it may be due to increased oxygen demand, to diminished blood oxygen transport, or most commonly to reduction in coronary blood flow because of arterial narrowing or obstruction such as that caused by atherosclerosis. It may manifest as angina pectoris, myocardial infarction, ventricular fibrillation, or sudden cardiac death.
island d. scrub typhus.
Isle of Wight d. paralysis of muscles of flight in honeybees due to tracheal infestation by the mite *Acarapis woodi*.
itai-itai d. a type of cadmium poisoning seen in Japan, characterized by osteomalacia, osteoporosis, and tubulopathy.
Jaffe-Lichtenstein d. a form of polyostotic fibrous dysplasia characterized by an enlarged medullary cavity with a thin cortex, which is filled with fibrous tissue (fibroma). Called also *cystic osteofibromatosis*.
Jakob d., Jakob-Creutzfeldt d. Creutzfeldt-Jakob d.
Jansen d. metaphyseal dysostosis.
Janský-Bielschowsky d. the late infantile form of neuronal ceroid-lipofuscinosis, occurring between two and four years of age and characterized by abnormal accumulation of lipofuscin; it begins as myoclonic seizures and progresses to neurologic and retinal degeneration and death, usually by the age of 8 to 12 years.
Jensen d. retinochoroiditis juxtapapillaris.
Johne d. a usually fatal form of chronic enteritis due to *Mycobacterium avium* subsp. *paratuberculosis*, affecting chiefly cattle but also sheep, goats, and deer. It remotely resembles a tuberculous infection and is marked by intermittent or persistent diarrhea, progressive emaciation, anemia, and extreme weakness. Called also *chronic dysentery of cattle* and *paratuberculosis*.
Johnson-Stevens d. see *Stevens-Johnson syndrome*, under *syndrome*.
Joseph d. Machado-Joseph d.
jumping d. any of several culture-specific disorders characterized by exaggerated responses to small stimuli, muscle tics including jumping, automatic obedience even to dangerous suggestions, and sometimes coprolalia or echolalia. It is unclear whether they are neurogenic or psychogenic in origin. See also *latah*, *myriachit*, *jumping Frenchmen of Maine syndrome*, and *Gilles de la Tourette syndrome*.

Disease *Continued*

Kaiserstuhl d. a form of chronic arsenic poisoning that occurred prior to World War II among German workers in vineyards, due to arsenic-containing insecticides used on the grapes.
Kashin-Bek (Kaschin-Beck) d. a slowly progressive, chronic, disabling, degenerative disease of the peripheral joints and spine, which principally occurs in children and is endemic in eastern Siberia, northern China, and Korea. It is believed to be caused by the ingestion of cereal grains infected with *Fusarium sporotrichiella.* Called also *osteoarthritis deformans endemica.*
Katayama d. see under *fever.*
Kawasaki d. a syndrome of unknown etiology, usually affecting infants and young children, associated with vasculitis of the large coronary vessels and numerous other systemic signs, including fever, conjunctival injection, changes of the oropharyngeal mucosa, cervical lymphadenopathy, and maculoerythematous skin eruption that becomes confluent and bright red in a glove-and-sock distribution; the skin becomes indurated and edematous and often desquamates from the fingers and toes. Called also *mucocutaneous lymph node syndrome.*
Kennedy d. spinobulbar muscular atrophy.
Keshan d. a fatal, congestive cardiomyopathy caused by deficiency of essential trace elements in the diet; it primarily affects children and women of childbearing age and occurs in areas with low soil trace elements, such as parts of China, New Zealand, and Finland.
Kienböck d. slowly progressive osteochondrosis of the semilunar (carpal lunate) bone; it may affect other bones of the wrist. Called also *lunatomalacia.*
Kikuchi d., Kikuchi-Fujimoto d. see under *lymphadenitis.*
Kimberley horse d. crotalism.
Kimura d. a nodular skin disease considered by some authorities to be identical to angiolymphoid hyperplasia with eosinophilia, (q.v.) but differentiated by others because of differences in the nature of the proliferating vascular cells.
Kinnier Wilson d. Wilson d.
kissing d. popular term for infectious mononucleosis.
Köhler bone d. 1. osteochondrosis of the tarsal navicular bone in children; called also *tarsal scaphoiditis, epiphysitis juvenilis, osteoarthrosis juvenilis,* and *os naviculare pedis retardatum.* 2. a disease of the second metatarsal bone, with thickening of its shaft and changes about its articular head, characterized by pain in the second metatarsophalangeal joint on walking or standing. Called also *Köhler second d.,* and *juvenile deforming metatarsophalangeal osteochondritis.* See also *osteochondrosis.*
Köhler second d. Köhler bone d. (def. 2).
Köhler-Pellegrini-Stieda d. Pellegrini d.
Kohlmeier-Degos d. malignant atrophic papulosis.
Koshevnikoff (Koschewnikow, Kozhevnikov) d. epilepsia partialis continua.
Krabbe d. a lysosomal storage disease due to a deficiency of galactosylceramidase. It begins in infancy with irritability, fretfulness, and rigidity, followed by tonic seizures, convulsions, quadriplegia, blindness, deafness, dysphagia, and progressive mental deterioration. Pathologically, there is rapidly progressive cerebral demyelination and large globoid bodies in the white substance. Called also *galactosylceramide lipidosis* and *globoid cell* or *Krabbe leukodystrophy.*
Krishaber d. a syndrome characterized by tachycardia, insomnia, lightheadedness or vertigo, hyperesthesia, and a feeling of emptiness in the head; called also *cerebrocardiac syndrome.*
Kufs d. the adult form of neuronal ceroid-lipofuscinosis, beginning usually before the age of 40 and characterized by progressive neurologic degeneration, excessive storage of lipofuscin in the central nervous system, and shortened life expectancy. Unlike other forms of neuronal ceroid lipofuscinosis, it does not cause blindness.
Kuhnt-Junius d. disciform macular degeneration.
Kümmell d., Kümmell-Verneuil d. compression fracture of vertebra; a complex of symptoms coming on in a few weeks after spinal injury, and consisting of pain in the spine, intercostal neuralgia, motor disturbances of the legs, and a gibbus of the spine which is painful on pressure and easily reduced by extension. Called also *posttraumatic spondylitis.*
Kussmaul d., Kussmaul-Maier d. polyarteritis nodosa.
Kyasanur Forest d. a severe type of hemorrhagic fever seen in the Mysore State of India, caused by a flavivirus called the Kyasanur Forest disease virus. The usual animal reservoirs are monkeys and voles, and the vector for human infection is ticks of the genus *Haemaphysalis.* Besides the fever and hemorrhagic manifestations, there is also a rash.

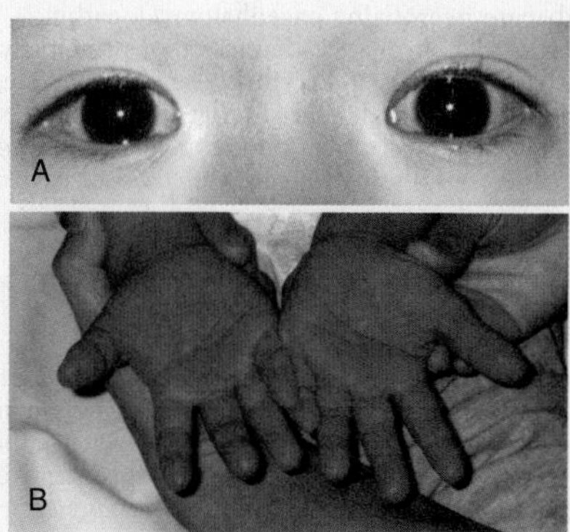

■ Kawasaki disease. *(A),* Bilateral nonexudative scleral injection with perilimbic sparing; *(B),* diffuse palmar erythema.

Kyrle d. a rare, chronic type of acquired perforating dermatosis characterized by papular eruptions containing plugs of keratin and cellular debris, often with a foreign body giant cell reaction and pain; the usually discrete lesions may coalesce to form patches and plaques. Called also *hyperkeratosis penetrans.*
Lafora d. a slowly progressive autosomal recessive disorder, a form of progressive myoclonic epilepsy, beginning in adolescence and characterized by attacks of intermittent or continuous myoclonus, resulting in difficulties in voluntary movement; there is mental deterioration, sometimes progressing to complete dementia, and the presence of Lafora bodies in various cells, including those of the nervous system, retina, heart, muscle, and liver. Called also *Lafora myoclonic epilepsy* and *progressive myoclonic epilepsy type 2 (EPM2).*
Lane d. chronic intestinal stasis; small bowel obstruction in chronic constipation.
Larsen d., Larsen-Johansson d. a type of overuse injury seen most often in children between the ages of 10 and 16, characterized by pain and tenderness over the lower pole of the patella, often with inflammation; there is radiographic evidence of a secondary ossification center in the lower pole of the patella.
Lauber d. fundus albipunctatus.
laughing d. kuru.
Leber d. Leber hereditary optic neuropathy.
Legg d., Legg-Calvé d. Legg-Calvé-Perthes d.
Legg-Calvé-Perthes d. osteochondrosis of the capitular epiphysis of the femur.
legionnaires' d. an acute, sometimes fatal, bacterial disease caused by infection with *Legionella pneumophila,* not spread by person-to-person contact; it is characterized by pneumonia, high fever, gastrointestinal pain, headache, and sometimes involvement of the kidneys, liver, or nervous system.

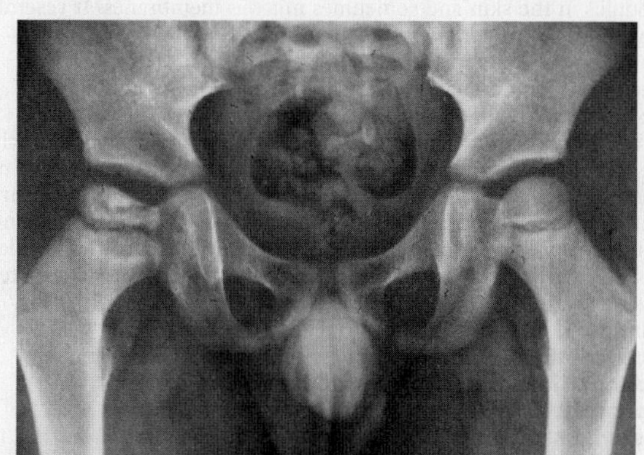
■ Legg-Calvé-Perthes disease affecting the right leg of a seven-year-old boy. Anteroposterior radiograph shows a flattened and fragmented right femoral epiphysis; the proximal femur is also displaced inferiorly and laterally.

Leigh d. subacute necrotizing encephalomyelopathy.
Leiner d. a disorder of infancy characterized principally by generalized seborrhealike dermatitis and erythroderma, intractable, severe diarrhea, recurrent infections, and failure to thrive. The cause is unclear, but familial cases associated with a dysfunction of the C5 component of complement, which results in decreased phagocytosis of the patient's serum (opsonic activity), have been reported. Called also *erythroderma desquamativum.*
Lenègre d. acquired complete heart block due to primary degeneration of the conduction system.
Leriche d. posttraumatic osteoporosis.
Letterer-Siwe d. a Langerhans cell histiocytosis of early childhood, of autosomal recessive inheritance, characterized by cutaneous lesions resembling seborrheic dermatitis, hemorrhagic tendency, hepatosplenomegaly with lymph node enlargement, and progressive anemia. If untreated it is rapidly fatal. Called also *L-S d.* and *acute disseminated Langerhans cell histiocytosis.*
Lev d. acquired complete heart block due to sclerosis of the cardiac skeleton.
Lewandowsky-Lutz d. epidermodysplasia verruciformis.
Libman-Sacks d. see under *endocarditis.*
Lichtheim d. subacute combined degeneration of the spinal cord; see under *degeneration.*
light chain deposition d. abnormal deposition of light chains in multiple organs; the most prominent symptoms are caused by glomerular deposition, which causes renal insufficiency, proteinuria, and the nephrotic syndrome. In some patients it is associated with multiple myeloma or lymphoproliferative disorders.
Lindau d., Lindau-von Hippel d. von Hippel-Lindau d.
linear IgA d., linear IgA bullous d. see *linear IgA dermatosis of adulthood* and *chronic bullous dermatosis of childhood.*
lipid storage d. lipidosis.
Lipschütz d. acute vulvar ulcer.
Little d. a type of cerebral palsy that usually dates from birth and is due to lack of development of the pyramidal tracts. Contributing causes may include birth trauma, fetal anoxia, or illness of the mother during pregnancy. Clinically, it is characterized by congenital spastic stiffness of the limbs, muscular weakness, walking difficulties, and, usually, by convulsions, bilateral athetosis, and mental deficiency. Called also *spastic diplegia.*
Lobo d. lacaziosis.
local d. a condition originating in and remaining in just one part of the body.
loco d., locoweed d. locoism.
Lou Gehrig d. amyotrophic lateral sclerosis.
Lowe d. oculocerebrorenal syndrome.
L-S d. Letterer-Siwe d.
Luft d. a hypermetabolic disorder of striated muscle caused by an abnormal quantity and type of mitochondria producing excessive cellular respiration; it is characterized by profuse perspiration, asthenia, progressive weakness, and an abnormally increased basal metabolic rate.
lumpy skin d. a highly infectious poxvirus disease in African cattle, which may result in permanent sterility or death, marked by formation of nodules in the skin and sometimes mucous membranes. It resembles dermopathic herpesvirus disease (q.v.).
lung fluke d. paragonimiasis.
lunger d. 1. pulmonary adenomatosis (def. 2). 2. fog fever.
Lutz-Splendore-Almeida d. paracoccidioidomycosis.
Lyme d. a recurrent, multisystemic disorder caused by the spirochete *Borrelia burgdorferi*; vectors for human infection are the ticks *Ixodes scapularis* and *I. pacificus.* It begins in most cases with erythema chronicum migrans (at least 5 cm in diameter), which is followed by highly variable manifestations that may include myalgia, arthritis of large joints, stiff neck, involvement of the nervous and cardiovascular systems, and systemic symptoms such as chills, fever, headache, malaise, and vomiting.
lymphocystic d. of fish, lymphocystis d. lymphocystis.
lymphoproliferative d's see under *disorder.*
lymphoreticular d's see under *disorder.*
lysosomal storage d. any inborn error of metabolism having four characteristics: (1) a defect in a specific lysosomal hydrolase; (2) intracellular accumulation of the unmetabolized substrate; (3) clinical progression affecting multiple tissues and organs; (4) considerable phenotypic variation within a disease. All but two of the lysosomal storage disorders are of autosomal recessive inheritance. The term comprises the *mucolipidoses, mucopolysaccharidoses, disorders of glycoprotein degradation, lipase deficiencies, ceramidase deficiency (Farber disease), α-galactosidase A deficiency (Fabry disease), lipidoses,* and *gangliosidoses.* Called also *lysosomal enzymopathy* and *inborn lysosomal d.* See also *inborn errors of metabolism,* under *error.*
lytico-bodig d. [*lytico-bodig,* a local name for the disease, formed from truncations of Sp. *paralitico* paralytic and *bodega* small store] amyotrophic lateral sclerosis–parkinsonism–dementia complex.
MAC d. *Mycobacterium avium* complex d.
McArdle d. glycogen storage d., type V.
Machado-Joseph d. (MJD) an autosomal dominant neurodegenerative disease first described in families of Portuguese-Azorean descent, having a variety of forms but characterized principally by ataxia, spasticity, distal muscular atrophy, and ocular movement abnormalities. It is a triplet repeat disorder associated with expansion of CAG triplet repeats in the *ATXN3* gene encoding the protein ataxin-3, on chromosome 14q, and has been shown to be a type of spinocerebellar ataxia (q.v.). Called also *Azorean d.* and *Joseph d.*.
MacLean-Maxwell d. a chronic condition of the calcaneus marked by enlargement of its posterior third and attended by pain on pressure.
mad cow d. bovine spongiform encephalopathy.
Madelung d. 1. see under *deformity.* 2. multiple symmetric lipomatosis.
Majocchi d. purpura annularis telangiectodes.
Manchester wasting d. enzootic calcinosis.
Manson d. see under *schistosomiasis.*
maple bark d., maple bark stripper's d. a type of hypersensitivity pneumonitis affecting logging and sawmill workers, caused by inhalation of the spores of the mold *Cryptostroma corticale,* which grows under the bark of maple logs.
maple syrup urine d. (MSUD) a genetically heterogeneous, autosomal recessive aminoacidopathy caused by mutation in genes that encode subunits of the branched-chain α-keto acid dehydrogenase complex. Branched-chain amino acids and their keto acid analogues accumulate in blood and urine, causing severe ketoacidosis, seizures, coma, physical and mental retardation, and a characteristic smell of maple syrup in the urine and on the body. The disease can be divided into four clinical phenotypes: *classic,* the most severe, with neonatal onset and usually rapid death; *intermediate,* of lessened severity and usually later onset; *intermittent,* with normal periods punctuated by periods of ataxia and ketoacidosis; and *thiamine-responsive,* caused by decreased affinity of the dehydrogenase complex for the cofactor thiamine pyrophosphate. Called also *branched-chain ketoaciduria.*
marble bone d. osteopetrosis.
Marburg d., Marburg virus d. a rare, acute, often fatal type of hemorrhagic fever caused by the Marburg virus; besides fever and hemorrhagic manifestations, it is also characterized by pancreatitis and hepatitis. It occurs most often in central and southern Africa, but attracted attention when laboratory workers in Germany fell ill after handling infected African green monkeys.
Marchiafava-Bignami d. progressive degeneration of the corpus callosum characterized by progressive intellectual deterioration, emotional disturbances, confusion, hallucinations, tremor, rigidity, and convulsions. It is a very rare disorder affecting chiefly middle-aged male alcoholics; also seen in patients with nutritional deficiency states.
Marek d. a lymphoproliferative disease of chickens, formerly included in the avian leukosis complex but now known to be caused by either of two viruses known as gallid herpesviruses 2 and 3. Lymphoid cell infiltrations are usually in the peripheral nerves and gonads but may also be found in visceral organs, skin, muscle, and the iris; there may be perivascular cuffing of blood vessels in the central nervous system. Where lesions are dictates the clinical signs, such as paralysis or blindness. When there are mainly neurological symptoms, it is called *fowl* or *range paralysis* or *neural lymphomatosis.* When there are mainly ocular symptoms, it is called *ocular lymphomatosis,* and with mainly skin symptoms it is called *skin leukosis.*
margarine d. name given to an outbreak of erythema multiforme in Germany and The Netherlands that was due to an emulsifier in margarine.
Marie-Bamberger d. hypertrophic pulmonary osteoarthropathy.
Marie-Strümpell d. ankylosing spondylitis.
Marie-Tooth d. Charcot-Marie-Tooth d.

Marion d. congenital obstruction of the posterior urethra due to muscular hypertrophy and stenosis of the bladder neck or absence of the plexiform dilator fibers in the urinary tract.
Marsh d. Graves d.
mast cell d. mastocytosis.
medullary cystic d., medullary cystic kidney d. 1. familial juvenile nephronophthisis. 2. according to some authorities, just one variant of the juvenile nephronophthisis–medullary cystic disease complex, of autosomal dominant inheritance with onset after age 30.
Meige d. lymphedema praecox.
Meleda d. mal de Meleda.
Ménétrier d. hypertrophic gastritis.
Meniere d. hearing loss, tinnitus, and vertigo resulting from nonsuppurative disease of the labyrinth with edema. Called also *endolymphatic hydrops, labyrinthine hydrops,* and *recurrent aural vertigo.*
Menkes d. an X-linked recessive disorder of copper metabolism caused by mutations in the *ATP7A* gene (locus: Xq12-q13), which encodes a copper transporter. Features result from dysfunction of copper-dependent enzymes and include sparse, brittle, twisted scalp hair; connective tissue abnormalities (loose skin, hyperextensible joints, bladder diverticula, and skeletal anomalies); and severe cerebral degeneration. Death occurs by 3 years of age in untreated patients. *Occipital horn syndrome* is a milder allelic variant. Called also *kinky hair syndrome, steely hair syndrome* and *trichopoliodystrophy.*
mental d. see under *disorder.*
Merzbacher-Pelizaeus d. Pelizaeus-Merzbacher d.
metabolic d. general term for diseases caused by disruption of a normal metabolic pathway because of a genetically determined enzyme defect.
metazoan d. a disease caused by metazoan parasites, such as nematodes, cestodes, trematodes, or arthropods.
Meyer d. adenoid vegetations of the pharynx.
Meyer-Betz d. a rare familial disease of unknown etiology, marked by attacks of myoglobinuria that may be precipitated by strenuous exertion or possibly by an infection, resulting in tenderness, swelling, and weakness of muscles of varying intensity. It may occur with or without diffuse chronic myopathy or dystrophy. Called also *idiopathic* or *familial myoglobinuria.*
microdrepanocytic d. sickle cell–thalassemia d.
microvillus inclusion d. a rare intestinal disorder, thought to be hereditary and autosomal recessive; infants have severe watery diarrhea with malabsorption of nutrients owing to incomplete development of intestinal villi. The condition is fatal unless the infant is given total parenteral nutrition. Cf. *congenital microvillus atrophy,* under *atrophy.*
Mikulicz d. former name for *benign lymphoepithelial lesion.* Cf. *Mikulicz syndrome.*
Miller d. osteomalacia.
miller's d. nutritional secondary hyperparathyroidism.
Milroy d. autosomal dominant primary lymphedema occurring at or soon after birth, caused by a mutation of chromosome locus 5q35.3; called also *Nonne-Milroy d.* and *Milroy l.*
Minamata d. symptoms of alkyl mercury poisoning that were seen between 1953 and 1958 among persons who ate seafood from a bay in Japan that was polluted with alkyl mercury compounds; it consisted of a severe neurologic disorder usually characterized by peripheral and circumoral paresthesia, ataxia, dysarthria, and loss of peripheral vision, which led to severe permanent neurologic and mental disabilities and sometimes death.
minimal change d. subtle alterations in kidney function demonstrable by clinical albuminuria and the presence of lipid droplets in cells of the proximal tubules; abnormalities of foot processes of the glomerular epithelial cells are present but too subtle to be seen with light microscopy. It is seen primarily in children under age 6 but sometimes in adults with the nephrotic syndrome, and it may or may not progress to glomerulosclerosis or glomerulonephritis. Called also *foot process d., nil d., minimal change glomerulopathy* or *nephropathy,* and *lipid* or *lipoid nephrosis.*
Minor d. hematomyelia involving the central parts of the spinal cord.
Mitchell d. erythromelalgia.
mitochondrial d's a diverse group of mainly multisystemic and maternally inherited disorders caused by mutations of mitochondrial DNA; some are sporadic and tissue-specific. They affect tissues having a high rate of oxidative metabolism, including the brain and peripheral nervous system, skeletal muscle, heart, liver, pancreas, kidneys, and endocrine system. Manifestations include encephalopathy, peripheral neuropathy, vision and hearing deficits, muscle pain and weakness, cardiac disease, renal tubular acidosis, liver failure, diabetes mellitus, short stature, and developmental delays.
mixed connective tissue d. a disorder combining features of scleroderma, myositis, systemic lupus erythematosus, and rheumatoid arthritis, and marked serologically by the presence of antibody against extractable nuclear antigen. Cf. *overlap syndrome.*
Möbius d. ophthalmoplegic migraine.
Moeller-Barlow d. subperiosteal hematoma in rickets.
molecular d. any disease in which the pathogenesis can be traced to a single molecule, usually a protein, which is either abnormal in structure or present in reduced amounts; the classic example is abnormal hemoglobin in sickle cell anemia.
Monday morning d. azoturia (def. 2).
Mondor d. phlebitis affecting the large subcutaneous veins normally crossing the lateral chest region and breast from the epigastric or hypochondriac region to the axilla. Called also *sclerosing periphlebitis.*
Monge d. chronic mountain sickness.
monoclonal immunoglobulin deposition d. light chain nephropathy.
monosymptomatic demyelinating d. acute occurrence of any one of a number of symptoms that suggest a diagnosis of multiple sclerosis; persons who have such an attack may or may not develop multiple sclerosis.
Morton d. see under *neuralgia.*
Moschcowitz d. thrombotic thrombocytopenic purpura.
motor neuron d. any disease of a motor neuron, including spinal muscular atrophy, progressive bulbar paralysis, amyotrophic lateral sclerosis, and lateral sclerosis.
motor system d. motor neuron d.
mountain d. see under *sickness.*
moyamoya d. [Japanese *moyamoya* foggy or smoky, from the angiographic appearance] cerebral ischemia due to occlusion of large arteries at the circle of Willis, with secondary proliferation of an abnormal network of vessels at the base of the brain, causing progressive neurologic disability; hemorrhage may occur from the abnormal vessels.
Mseleni joint d. a severe, progressive osteoarthropathy of unknown etiology, occurring in South Africa and seen predominantly in women. It begins in the hip joint, which is the most severely affected, and spreads to the knees and ankles and, less commonly, to the wrists, elbows, and shoulders. The ability to walk is severely compromised and is in some cases lost. Dwarfism occurs in some affected individuals.
Mucha d., Mucha-Habermann d. pityriasis lichenoides et varioliformis acuta.
mu chain d. the rarest heavy chain disease, found in patients with chronic lymphocytic leukemia, with symptoms of hepatomegaly and splenomegaly.
mucosal d. bovine virus diarrhea.
mu heavy chain d. mu chain d.
mulberry heart d. a form of vitamin E–selenium deficiency syndrome (q.v.) in pigs, characterized by subepicardial hemorrhaging, myocardial necrosis, and often death.
mule-spinners' d. warts or ulcers of the skin, especially of the scrotum, tending to become malignant (see *mule-spinners' cancer,* under *cancer*); so called because they were found among operators of spinning mules in cotton mills.
Münchmeyer d. fibrodysplasia ossificans progressiva.
Murray Valley d. see under *encephalitis.*
mushroom picker's d., mushroom worker's d. hypersensitivity pneumonitis in persons working with moldy compost prepared for growing mushrooms in closed areas, especially in those handling the dried material after harvesting, usually due to inhalation of spores of *Saccharopolyspora rectivirgula.*
mushy chick d. omphalitis of birds; see under *omphalitis.*
***Mycobacterium avium* complex d.** systemic disease caused by infection with organisms of the *Mycobacterium avium-intracellulare* complex in patients with human immunodeficiency virus infection. Manifestations include bacteremia, fever, chills, fatigue, night sweats, weight loss, abdominal pain, anemia, and elevated alkaline phosphatase. Called also *MAC d.*
myeloproliferative d's see under *disorder.*
mystery pig d. porcine epidemic abortion and respiratory syndrome.

Disease *Continued*

Nairobi sheep d. an infectious disease of sheep and goats in East Africa, marked by acute hemorrhagic gastroenteritis, green, watery diarrhea, mucopurulent nasal discharge, and breathing difficulty; it is caused by a bunyavirus transmitted by the ticks *Rhipicephalus appendiculatus* and *Amblyomma variegatum.*
Nasu-Hakola d. a rare autosomal recessive syndrome of bone cysts with presenile dementia.
navicular d. necrotic inflammation of the navicular bone in horses, causing intermittent lameness. Called also *podotrochlitis* and *podotrochlosis.*
Naxos d. a rare, autosomal recessive syndrome consisting of right ventricular cardiomyopathy, palmoplantar keratoderma, and woolly hair.
Nékam d. keratosis lichenoides chronica.
neonatal-onset multisystem inflammatory d. (NOMID) an autosomal dominant autoinflammatory disease (q.v.) in the cryopyrin-asociated periodic syndromes subgroup, characterized by urticaria, meningitis, and symmetrical arthropathy with overgrowth of the epiphyses of bones. Called also *CINCA syndrome.*
Newcastle d. an influenzalike, often fatal, disease of birds, including domestic fowl, caused by a virus of the genus *Avulavirus;* there are several different forms, characterized variously by pneumonia and other respiratory symptoms, gastrointestinal symptoms, and encephalitis. Humans having contact with infected birds may develop a mild infection characterized by malaise and conjunctivitis. Called also *avian pneumoencephalitis.*
new duck d. infectious avian serositis in ducklings.
Nicolas-Favre d. lymphogranuloma venereum.
Niemann d., Niemann-Pick d. a lysosomal storage disease due to a deficiency of sphingomyelin phosphodiesterase with sphingomyelin accumulation in the reticuloendothelial system. There are five types distinguished by age of onset and by the amount of CNS involvement and of sphingomyelin phosphodiesterase activity. *Type A* (acute neuronopathic) is the classic type, accounting for 85 per cent of patients; onset is in early infancy, CNS damage is severe, and death occurs by 4 years. *Type B* (chronic nonneuronopathic) has onset in early infancy but does not affect the CNS or intelligence, and a normal lifespan is possible. *Type C* (chronic neuronopathic) has variable ages of onset (at 2 years or older) and of death (from age 5 to adulthood) and variable CNS involvement. *Type D* (the Nova Scotia variant) resembles type C; *type E* (the adult, nonneuronopathic form) may be a late-onset variant of type C. Called also *sphingomyelin lipidosis* and *sphingomyelinase deficiency.*
nil d. minimal change d.
nodular worm d., nodule d. a disease of sheep, cattle, and pigs caused by intestinal infestation with species of *Oesophagostomum,* the nodular worm, which infest the intestines and become embedded in the mucous membrane, causing nodules of various sizes.
nonalcoholic fatty liver d. nonalcoholic steatohepatitis.
Nonne-Milroy d. Milroy d.
Norrie d. a congenital, X-linked disorder consisting of bilateral blindness from retinal detachment, hypoplasia, or dysplasia; and sometimes mental retardation and deafness developing later.
Norum-Gjone d. lecithin–cholesterol acyltransferase deficiency.
nosema d. a protozoal infection of bees caused by *Nosema apis,* characterized by dysentery and paralysis. Cf. *pébrine.*
notifiable d. a disease that is required to be reported to federal, state, or local health officials when diagnosed, because of infectiousness, severity, or frequency of occurrence; called also *reportable d.*
oasthouse urine d. methionine malabsorption syndrome.
obstructive small airways d. chronic bronchitis with irreversible narrowing of the bronchioles and small bronchi with hypoxia and often hypercapnia.
occupational d. a disease due to factors involved in one's employment, e.g., various forms of pneumoconiosis or dermatitis.
Ofuji d. eosinophilic pustular folliculitis.
Oguchi d. a form of congenital night blindness and fundus discoloration following light adaptation.
Ohara d. name used in Japan for *tularemia.*
oid-oid d. [from disc*oid* and lichen*oid*] exudative discoid and lichenoid dermatitis.
Ollier d. enchondromatosis, particularly when involvement is unilateral.
Opitz d. enlargement of the spleen due to thrombosis of the splenic vein; called also *thrombophlebitic splenomegaly.*

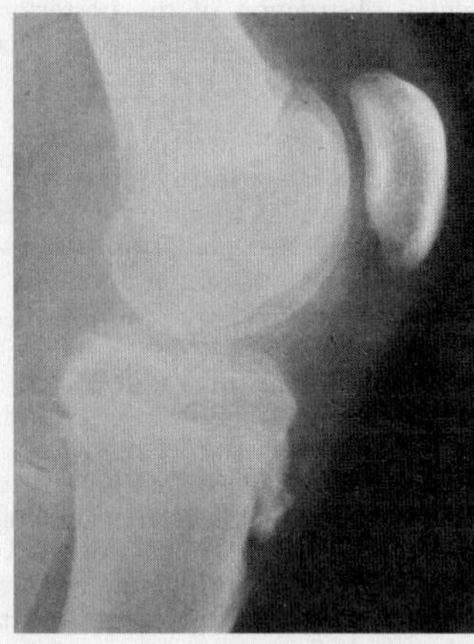

■ Osgood-Schlatter disease; radiography of a severe, long-standing case shows irregularity and fragmentation of the tibial tuberosity.

organic d. a disease associated with demonstrable change in a bodily organ or tissue.
Oriental lung fluke d. parasitic hemoptysis.
Ormond d. retroperitoneal fibrosis.
Osgood-Schlatter d. an overuse injury with osteochondrosis (q.v.) of the tuberosity of the tibia; seen most often in adolescent boys engaged in sports that involve jumping. Called also *Schlatter* or *Schlatter-Osgood d.*
Osler d. 1. polycythemia vera. 2. hereditary hemorrhagic telangiectasia.
Osler-Vaquez d. polycythemia vera.
Osler-Weber-Rendu d. hereditary hemorrhagic telangiectasia.
Otto d. protrusio acetabuli.
overeating d. pulpy kidney d.
Owren d. parahemophilia.
ox warble d. cutaneous larva migrans (def. 1).
Pacheco d. a highly fatal contagious disease of parrots caused by a herpesvirus; characteristics include hepatomegaly and diarrhea. Pigeons can get an almost identical disease, caused by a different herpesvirus.
Paget d. 1. intraductal carcinoma of the breast extending to involve the nipple and areola, characterized clinically by eczema-like inflammatory skin changes, and histologically by infiltration of the epidermis by malignant cells *(Paget cells).* 2. a neoplasm of the vulva and sometimes the perianal region histologically and clinically quite similar to Paget disease of the breast, but having less of a tendency to be associated with underlying invasive carcinoma. Called also *extramammary* or *vulvar Paget d.* 3. osteitis deformans.
Paget d., extramammary Paget d. (def. 2).
Paget d., juvenile hyperostosis corticalis deformans juvenilis.
Paget d., vulvar Paget d. (def. 2).
Paget d. of bone osteitis deformans.
Panner d. osteochondrosis of the capitellum of the humerus.
Parkinson d. a slowly progressive disorder affecting the basal ganglia, usually occurring in late life, with an average age of onset of 60 years;

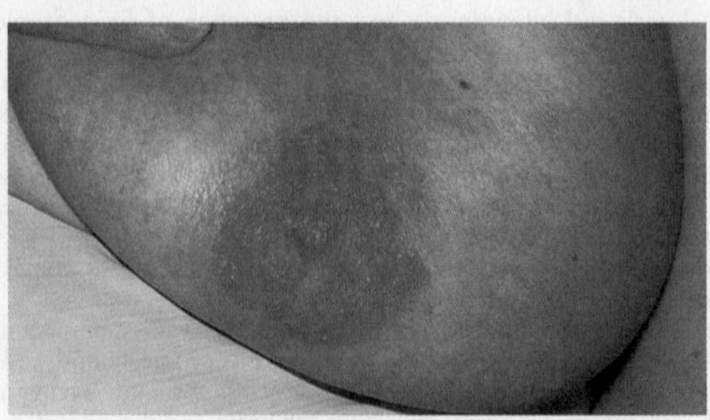

■ Paget disease of the breast.

however, a young-onset form diagnosed at or before 40 years of age is distinguished. It is characterized clinically by masklike facies, resting tremor, slowing of voluntary movements, festinating gait, flexed posture, and muscle weakness, sometimes with excessive sweating and feelings of heat. Pathologically, there is degeneration of dopaminergic neurones of the pars compacta of the substantia nigra, resulting in dramatic decrease in the levels of dopamine in the substantia nigra and corpus striatum.

parrot d. psittacosis.

Parry d. 1. Graves d. 2. toxic multinodular goiter.

Payr d. splenic flexure syndrome.

pearl d. bovine tuberculosis of the peritoneum and mesentery in which the tubercles are calcified and pearllike.

pearl-worker's d. recurrent inflammation of bone with hypertrophy, seen in persons who work in pearl dust.

peduncle d. coldwater d.

Pel-Ebstein d. see under *fever*.

Pelizaeus-Merzbacher d. an X-linked leukoencephalopathy caused by mutation of the *PLP1* gene (locus: Xq22) gene, which encodes proteolipid protein, occurring in early life and running a slowly progressive course into adolescence or adulthood. It is marked by nystagmus, ataxia, tremor, choreoathetoid movements, parkinsonian facies, dysarthria, and mental deterioration. Pathologically, there is diffuse demyelination in the white substance of the brain, which may involve the brainstem, cerebellum, and spinal cord. Called also *Merzbacher-Pelizaeus d.* and *Pelizaeus-Merzbacher sclerosis.*

Pellegrini d., Pellegrini-Stieda d. a condition characterized by a semilunar bony formation in the upper portion of the medial collateral ligament of the knee, due to trauma; called also *Köhler-Pellegrini-Stieda d.* and *Stieda d.*

pelvic inflammatory d. (PID) any pelvic infection involving the upper female genital tract beyond the cervix.

periodic d. any condition in which an otherwise healthy person has regularly recurring and intermittent episodes of fever, edema, arthralgia, or stomach pain and vomiting, continuing for years without further development.

periodontal d. any of a group of pathological conditions that affect the surrounding and supporting tissues of the teeth, generally classified as inflammatory (gingivitis and periodontitis), dystrophic (periodontal trauma and periodontosis), and anomalies. Called also *dentoalveolitis.*

Perthes d. Legg-Calvé-Perthes d.

Peyronie d. induration of the corpora cavernosa of the penis, producing a painful fibrous chordee and penile curvature. Called also *fibrous cavernitis, penile induration,* and *van Buren d.*

phytanic acid storage d. 1. Refsum d. 2. any of several disorders characterized by abnormal accumulation of phytanic acid in tissues.

Pick d. 1. [Arnold Pick] a rare progressive degenerative disease of the brain, similar in clinical manifestations and course to Alzheimer disease but having a distinctive histopathology; cortical atrophy is confined to the frontal and temporal lobes; degenerating neurons contain globular intracytoplasmic filamentous inclusions (Pick bodies). Called also *circumscribed cerebral atrophy.* 2. [Ludwig Pick] Niemann-Pick d.

Pictou d. a type of seneciosis in horses and cattle in Nova Scotia.

pink d. acrodynia.

plaster-of-Paris d. atrophy of a limb that has been enclosed in a plaster-of-Paris splint.

Plummer d. toxic multinodular goiter.

pneumatic hammer d. vibration d.

polycystic hydatid d. infection with the larval forms (hydatid cysts) of *Echinococcus vogeli,* in which the germinal membrane of the hydatid proliferates both inward into the original cyst to form septa that divide it into many sections, and outward to form new cysts. The condition is seen primarily in Central and South America.

polycystic kidney d. either of two unrelated heritable disorders marked by cysts scattered throughout both kidneys. *Autosomal dominant polycystic kidney disease* (ADPKD, formerly called the *adult form*) is the most common renal cystic condition, with deterioration of renal function that may not be detectable until the third or fourth decade of life; it runs a variable course, with only some cases progressing to renal failure. *Autosomal recessive polycystic kidney disease* (ARPKD, formerly called the *infantile form*) may be congenital or may appear at any time during childhood and has a high perinatal mortality rate; almost all cases lead to hypertension. In older children it may be associated with cystic and fibrotic disease of the liver. A similar acquired disease sometimes

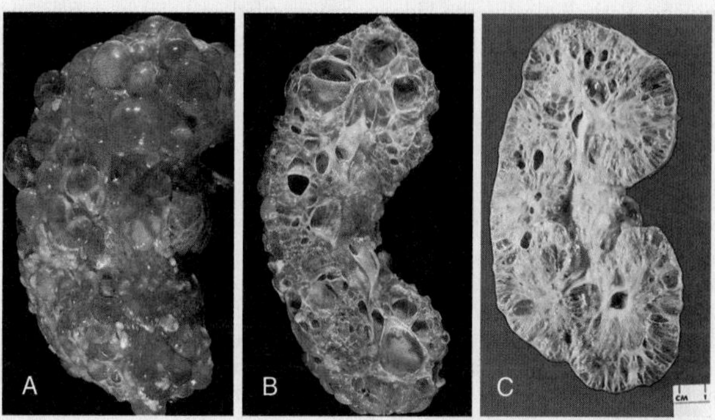

■ Autosomal dominant polycystic kidney disease viewed from the external surface *(A)* and bisected *(B)*, the kidney showing marked enlargement and numerous dilated cysts. *(C)*, Autosomal recessive polycystic kidney disease, characterized by smaller cysts and dilated channels at right angles to the cortical surface.

accompanies end-stage renal disease and is called *acquired cystic disease of kidney.* Called also *polycystic kidneys* and *polycystic renal d.*

polycystic liver d. any of several congenital conditions in which the liver develops cysts and sometimes Meyenburg complexes, often in association with polycystic kidney disease. An autosomal recessive type develops in childhood and can be rapidly fatal; an autosomal dominant type develops more gradually in adulthood and has a less grave prognosis.

polycystic ovary d. see under *syndrome.*

polycystic renal d. polycystic kidney d.

polyglutamine d's see under *disorder.*

Pompe d. glycogen storage d., type II.

Poncet d. tuberculous arthritis.

Portuguese-Azorean d. Machado-Joseph d.

Posadas d., Posadas-Wernicke d. coccidioidomycosis.

posttransplant lymphoproliferative d. a lymphoproliferative disorder seen after organ transplantation, characterized by presence of Epstein-Barr virus, lymphadenopathy with tonsillar enlargement, and development of lymphoma. Called also *posttransplant lymphoproliferative disorder.*

Pott d. tuberculosis of spine.

Preiser d. osteoporosis and atrophy of the carpal scaphoid due to trauma or a fracture which has not been kept immobilized.

primary electrical d. a condition characterized by serious ventricular tachycardia, and sometimes ventricular fibrillation, in the absence of recognizable structural heart disease.

Pringle d. adenoma sebaceum (def. 2).

prion d. any of a group of fatal, transmissible neurodegenerative diseases caused by abnormalities of prion protein metabolism, which may result from mutations in the prion protein gene or from infection with pathogenic isoforms of the protein (see *prion*). Characteristics include neuronal loss, gliosis, and extensive vacuolation of the cerebral cortex. Prion diseases may be sporadic, inherited as an autosomal dominant trait, or acquired. Human diseases include Creutzfeldt-Jakob disease, Gerstmann-Sträussler syndrome, fatal familial insomnia, and kuru; animal diseases include scrapie, bovine spongiform encephalopathy, and mink encephalopathy. Called also *transmissible neurodegenerative disease* and *subacute spongiform* or *transmissible spongiform encephalopathy.*

puff d. anhidrosis (def. 2).

pullorum d. an infectious disease of birds, including chickens, caused by *Salmonella enterica* subspecies *enterica* serovar Gallinarum. Birds have loss of appetite, dullness, diarrhea that leaves white lumps around the cloaca, reduced egg yield, and infertile eggs. It is sometimes fatal, with moribund and dead birds found at hatching time. Called also *white* or *bacillary white diarrhea.*

pulmonary venoocclusive d. an idiopathic form of primary pulmonary hypertension, usually seen in children or young adults, characterized by dyspnea and syncope, sometimes with intimal fibrosis, hemoptysis, paroxysmal nocturnal dyspnea, and orthopnea.

pulpy kidney d. a fatal enterotoxemia caused by *Clostridium perfringens* type B, usually seen in young animals, chiefly lambs, that are fed a high carbohydrate diet, although it may affect sheep, goats, and cattle of

any age. Pathologically, the kidneys are mottled and soft in consistency and the cortex is jelly-like or almost semifluid; the liver is severely congested with small hemorrhages diffusely scattered over its surface. Called also *overeating d.*
pulseless d. Takayasu arteritis.
Purtscher d. traumatic angiopathy of the retina with edema, hemorrhage, and exudation, usually following crush injuries of the chest; called also *Purtscher angiopathic retinopathy.*
Pyle d. metaphyseal dysplasia.
pyramidal d. buttress foot.
Quervain d. see *de Quervain d.*
Quincke d. angioedema.
rabbit hemorrhagic d. an acute infectious disease of wild and domestic rabbits and hares, caused by a calicivirus and characterized by necrotizing hepatitis and hemorrhagic lesions of many organs.
ragpicker's d. inhalational anthrax.
railroad d. transit tetany.
rat-bite d. see under *fever.*
Raynaud d. a primary or idiopathic vascular disorder characterized by bilateral attacks of Raynaud phenomenon; it affects females more often than males. Called also *Raynaud gangrene.*
reactive airways d. any of several conditions characterized by wheezing and allergic reactions; the most common ones are asthma, bronchiolitis, and chronic obstructive lung disease.
Recklinghausen d. 1. neurofibromatosis 1. 2. osteitis fibrosa cystica.
Recklinghausen-Applebaum d. hemochromatosis.
Recklinghausen d. of bone osteitis fibrosa cystica.
redwater d. bacillary hemoglobinuria.
Reed-Hodgkin d. Hodgkin d.
Refsum d. an autosomal recessive disorder of lipid metabolism in which deficiency of phytanic acid α-hydroxylase results in accumulation of phytanic acid; it is manifest chiefly by chronic polyneuritis, retinitis pigmentosa, cerebellar ataxia, and persistent elevation of protein in cerebrospinal fluid; there may also be ichthyosis, nerve deafness, and electrocardiographic abnormalities. Called also *phytanic acid storage d.*, and *heredopathia atactica polyneuritiformis.*
remnant removal d. familial dysbetalipoproteinemia.
reportable d. notifiable d.
respiratory bronchiolitis–associated interstitial lung d. a mild interstitial lung condition seen in cigarette smokers, characterized by patchy inflammation of bronchioles with filling of their lumina as well as adjacent alveoli and alveolar ducts by pigmented macrophages, resulting in dyspnea and a productive cough; it is usually a benign condition that will clear up upon cessation of smoking.
restrictive lung d. a general term comprising pulmonary diseases characterized by decreased total lung capacity, including those caused by disorders affecting the chest wall (e.g., poliomyelitis and scoliosis), and those caused by infiltrative interstitial diseases, such as adult respiratory distress syndrome.
reversible obstructive airway d. a condition characterized by bronchospasm reversible by intervention, as in asthma.
rheumatic heart d. the most important manifestation of and sequel to rheumatic fever, consisting chiefly of valvular deformities.
rheumatoid d. a systemic condition best known by its articular involvement (rheumatoid arthritis) but emphasizing nonarticular changes, e.g., pulmonary interstitial fibrosis, pleural effusion, and lung nodules.
Rh hemolytic d. a hemolytic reaction in the blood of a fetus or newborn to anti-Rh antibodies in the mother's blood, such as occurs in erythroblastosis fetalis.
rice d. beriberi.
Riedel d. see under *thyroiditis.*
Riga-Fede d. a small sublingual ulceration in infants with natal or neonatal teeth due to rubbing the lower central incisors; most often observed in whooping cough.
Riggs d. marginal periodontitis.
rippling muscle d. a rare, autosomal dominant condition characterized by myotonia and contractions of skeletal muscles, particularly in the lower limbs.
Ritter d. staphylococcal scalded skin syndrome.
Roger d. a ventricular septal defect; the term is usually restricted to small, asymptomatic defects.
rolling d. a disease of laboratory mice characterized by lateral rolling movements, neurolysis, and a polymorphonuclear leukocytic reaction in the brain; it is caused by a potent neurolytic exotoxin produced by *Mycoplasma neurolyticum.*
Romberg d. facial hemiatrophy.
Romney Marsh d. struck.
Rosai-Dorfman d. a rare syndrome, seen usually in children or adolescents, in which cervical lymph nodes (and sometimes other lymph nodes) are massively swollen and contain large numbers of histiocytes; extranodal disease is common, sometimes with fever, anemia, neutrophilia, elevated erythrocyte sedimentation rate, and hypergammaglobulinemia. Called also *sinus histiocytosis with massive lymphadenopathy.*
rose d. the urticarial form of swine erysipelas.
Roth (Rot) d., Roth-Bernhardt (Rot-Bernhardt) d. meralgia paresthetica.
Rougnon-Heberden d. angina pectoris.
round heart d. a fatal type of cardiopathy seen in inbred strains of turkeys; the right heart becomes greatly enlarged.
Rubarth d. infectious canine hepatitis.
runt d. graft-versus-host disease produced by injection of allogenic lymphocytes into immunologically immature experimental animals.
Rust d. tuberculous spondylitis of the cervical vertebrae.
Sachs d. Tay-Sachs d.
sacroiliac d. chronic tuberculous inflammation of the sacroiliac joint.
Salla d. an autosomal recessive disorder of sialic acid metabolism characterized by mental retardation, delayed motor development, ataxia, and sialuria, with onset in childhood and slow progression in early adulthood. Sialic acid accumulates in lysosomes; the disorder is believed to be due to a defect in the carrier transporting sialic acid across the lysosomal membrane.
Sanders d. epidemic keratoconjunctivitis.
Sandhoff d. a GM_2 gangliosidosis characterized by deficiency of both hexosaminidase A and B isozymes; it is caused by mutation in the *HEXB* gene, which encodes the β chain of the enzyme, common to both isozymes. Clinical features are very similar to Tay-Sachs disease, although it differs biochemically in accumulation of additional substances, such as globoside and *N*-acetylglucosamine-containing oligosaccharides. It occurs as several forms (infantile, juvenile, and adult), decreasing in severity with increasing age of onset.
sandworm d. cutaneous larva migrans.
San Joaquin Valley d. primary coccidioidomycosis.
Santavuori d., Santavuori-Haltia d. Haltia-Santavuori d.
Saunders d. a dangerous condition seen in infants that have digestive disturbances and are given a large percentage of carbohydrates; it is marked by vomiting, cerebral symptoms, and depression of circulation.
Schamberg d. a type of chronic pigmented purpura of the lower legs and feet of adolescent and young adult males, characterized by slightly discolored macules with red dots in the center (cayenne pepper spots). Called also *progressive pigmentary dermatosis* and *Schamberg dermatosis* or *purpura.*
Schanz d. traumatic inflammation of the Achilles tendon.
Schaumann d. sarcoidosis.
Scheuermann d. osteochondrosis of vertebral epiphyses in juveniles; see *osteochondrosis.*
Schilder d. a subacute or chronic form of leukoencephalopathy of children and adolescents, characterized by massive destruction of the white substance of the cerebral hemispheres with cavity formation and glial scarring. Clinical symptoms include blindness, deafness, bilateral spasticity, and progressive mental deterioration. The disease as a separate diagnostic entity has been disputed. It usually occurs sporadically, but a familial form has been reported. Called also *encephalitis periaxialis diffusa, Flatau-Schilder d.*, and *Schilder encephalitis.*
Schimmelbusch d. fibrocystic d. of breast.
Schlatter d., Schlatter-Osgood d. Osgood-Schlatter d.
Schmorl d. 1. herniation of the nucleus pulposus into an adjacent ventral body. 2. necrobacillosis in rabbits and rats, characterized by abscesses and areas of necrosis on the body, head, and interior of the mouth.
Schönlein d. see under *purpura.*
Schroeder d. a condition characterized by hypertrophic endometrium and excessive uterine bleeding.
Schüller d. 1. Hand-Schüller-Christian d. 2. osteoporosis circumscripta cranii.
Schüller-Christian d. Hand-Schüller-Christian d.
Schwediauer d. Swediaur d.; see *Albert d.*

secondary d. 1. a disease that occurs subsequent to or as a consequence of another disease. 2. a disease caused by introduction of incompatible immunologically competent cells into a host rendered incapable of rejecting them by heavy exposure to ionizing radiation; see also *graft-versus-host d.*
Seitelberger d. infantile neuroaxonal dystrophy.
self-limited d. a disease that by its very nature runs a limited and definite course.
Selter d. acrodynia.
senecio d. cirrhosis resulting from poisoning by the plant *Senecio.*
septic d. a disease caused by the presence of pyogenic or putrefactive organisms.
serum d. see under *sickness.*
Sever d. epiphysitis of the calcaneus.
severe combined immunodeficiency d. (SCID) see under *immunodeficiency.*
sexually transmitted d. (STD) an infection transmitted by sexual contact, either heterosexual or homosexual, caused by any of numerous biologically dissimilar pathogens; in some diseases (the classic venereal diseases) sexual transmission is the only important mode of spread, while in others (such as hepatitis, shigellosis, amebiasis, and giardiasis) infection can also be by nonsexual means. Called also *venereal d.*
Shaver d. bauxite pneumoconiosis.
sickle cell d. any of the diseases associated with the presence of hemoglobin S and sickle cells, including sickle cell anemia, sickle cell–hemoglobin C disease, sickle cell–hemoglobin D disease, and sickle cell–thalassemia disease.
sickle cell–hemoglobin C d. a genetically determined anemia in which the erythrocytes contain both hemoglobin S and hemoglobin C; symptoms are similar to but less severe than those of sickle cell anemia and may include abdominal and skeletal pain, splenomegaly, splenic infarction, and infarctions or deformities of bone. Called also *hemoglobin SC d.*
sickle cell–hemoglobin D d. a genetically determined anemia in which the erythrocytes contain both hemoglobin S and hemoglobin D, with symptoms like those of mild sickle cell anemia. Called also *hemoglobin SD d.*
sickle cell–thalassemia d. any of several hereditary anemias involving simultaneous heterozygosity for hemoglobin S and a thalassemia gene; symptoms resemble those of sickle cell anemia. Called also *microdrepanocytosis, microdrepanocytic d., hemoglobin S–thalassemia, sickle cell–thalassemia,* and *thalassemia–sickle cell d.*.
silo filler's d. see under *lung.*
Simmonds d. see *panhypopituitarism.*
Simons d. partial lipodystrophy.
Sinding-Larsen d., Sinding-Larsen–Johansson d. Larsen-Johansson d.
sixth d. exanthema subitum.
Skevas-Zerfus d. sponge diver's d.
slapped cheek d. erythema infectiosum.
sleepy foal d. a usually fatal type of equulosis affecting foals within the first three days of life, characterized by sudden onset and extreme prostration.
small airways d. chronic obstructive bronchitis with irreversible narrowing of the bronchioles and small bronchi. See also *obstructive small airways d.*
Smith-Strang d. methionine malabsorption syndrome.
Sneddon-Wilkinson d. subcorneal pustular dermatosis.
specific d. any disease caused by a specific agent.
specific heart muscle d. secondary cardiomyopathy.
Spielmeyer-Vogt d. Vogt-Spielmeyer d.
sponge diver's d. a condition seen in divers in the Mediterranean who are stung by tentacles of sea anemones attached to the base of sponges; it is marked by burning, itching, erythema, necrosis, and ulceration. Called also *Skevas-Zerfus d.*
Stargardt d. an autosomal recessive type of macular degeneration, usually occurring between the ages of six and twenty, marked by abnormal pigmentation and other changes in the macular area with rapid loss of visual acuity. Called also *Stargardt macular degeneration.*
startle d. hyperekplexia.
Steinert d. myotonic dystrophy.
sterility d. a deficiency disease observed in experimental animals and due to a lack of vitamin E in the diet.
Sticker d. erythema infectiosum.
Stieda d. Pellegrini d.
stiff lamb d. enzootic muscular dystrophy in lambs.
Still d. systemic onset juvenile idiopathic arthritis.
stone d. lithiasis.
storage d. a metabolic disorder in which some substance accumulates or is stored in certain cells in unusually large amounts; the stored substances may be lipids, proteins, carbohydrates, or other substances. See, for example, *glycogen storage d., mucopolysaccharidosis,* and *proteinosis.*
storage pool d. any of various types of coagulopathy due to defects in the dense bodies of platelets, so that the platelets fail to release ADP in response to aggregating agents such as collagen, epinephrine, exogenous ADP, and thrombin. It is characterized by mild bleeding episodes, prolonged bleeding time, and reduced aggregation response to collagen or thrombin. One type is a component of the autosomal recessive condition Hermansky-Pudlak syndrome. Called also *storage pool deficiency.*
structural d. any disease in which there are microscopic changes.
Strümpell d. a hereditary form of lateral sclerosis in which the spasticity is principally limited to the legs.
Strümpell-Leichtenstern d. hemorrhagic encephalitis.
Strümpell-Marie d. ankylosing spondylitis.
Stuttgart d. a type of canine leptospirosis without jaundice, primarily caused by *Leptospira interrogans* serovar *canicola*; called also *canicola fever* and *canine typhus.*
Sudeck d. posttraumatic osteoporosis.
Sutton d. 1. halo nevus. 2. periadenitis mucosa necrotica recurrens. 3. granuloma fissuratum.
Swediaur (Schwediauer) d. Albert d.
sweet clover d. a hemorrhagic disease of animals, especially cattle, caused by ingestion of spoiled *Melilotus* (sweet clover), which contains the anticoagulant dicumarol.
Swift d., Swift-Feer d. acrodynia.
swineherd's d. leptospirosis, manifested as a benign meningitis, caused by *Leptospira interrogans*, primarily serovars *pomona* and *tarassovi*, and affecting those who work with swine or pork or come in contact with the urine of carriers.
Sylvest d. epidemic pleurodynia.
Symmers d. follicular lymphoma.
systemic d. a disease affecting several different organs and tissues.
Takahara d. the symptomatic form of acatalasia (q.v.); it is characterized by oral ulcerations and gangrene.
Takayasu d. see under *arteritis.*
Talfan d. infectious porcine encephalomyelitis.
Tangier d. an autosomal recessive disorder of lipoprotein and lipid metabolism characterized by absence in plasma of normal high-density lipoproteins (HDL), deficiency of apolipoproteins A-I and A-II, low to normal low-density lipoproteins, and high triglycerides, and by accumulation in body tissues of cholesteryl esters. Clinical signs include enlargement and orange coloring of tonsils, pharyngeal mucosa, and rectal mucosa; recurrent peripheral neuropathy; splenomegaly; and corneal infiltration.
Tarui d. glycogen storage d., type VII.
Tay-Sachs d. (TSD) an autosomal recessive lysosomal storage disease, occurring particularly in Ashkenazi Jews; it is a GM_2 gangliosidosis characterized by deficiency of hexosaminidase A, and caused by mutation in the *HEXA* gene, which encodes the α subunit of that enzyme. The classic infantile form is characterized by infantile onset (3–6 months), doll-like facies, cherry-red macular spot (90+ per cent of the infants), early blindness, hyperacusis, macrocephaly, seizures, and hypotonia; the children die between 2 and 5 years of age. There are also juvenile and adult forms, with increased age of onset correlated with decreased severity and greater heterogeneity. See also *Sandhoff d.*
teart d. of cattle molybdenum poisoning (q.v.) in cattle that graze on teart, a type of English pasture in which the grass contains high levels of molybdenum.
Teschen d. infectious porcine encephalomyelitis.
thalassemia–sickle cell d. sickle cell–thalassemia d.
Thaysen d. celiac d.
Theiler d. a viral encephalomyelitis of mice caused by invasion of the central nervous system by Theilovirus, a picornavirus normally found in the intestinal tract; called also *mouse* or *murine encephalomyelitis, mouse* or *murine poliomyelitis,* and *Theiler mouse encephalomyelitis.*
Thiemann d. familial avascular necrosis of the phalangeal epiphysis, beginning in childhood or adolescence and resulting in deformity of the interphalangeal joints; called also *familial osteoarthropathy of fingers.*

Similar lesions may occur in the great toes and first tarsometatarsal joints, in which case the disorder is known as *osteochondritis ossis metacarpi et metatarsi.*

Thomsen d. the autosomal dominant form of myotonia congenita (q.v.).

Thomson d. an autosomal recessive skin disorder similar to Rothmund-Thomson syndrome except that saddle nose and cataract are not manifestations.

Thornwaldt d. Tornwaldt bursitis.

thyrocardiac d., thyrotoxic heart d. heart disease associated with hyperthyroidism, marked by atrial fibrillation, cardiac enlargement, and congestive heart failure.

Tillaux d. fibrocystic d. of breast.

Tommaselli d. pyrexia and hematuria due to excessive use of quinine.

Tooth d. Charcot-Marie-Tooth d.

Tornwaldt (Thornwaldt) d. see under *bursitis.*

transmissible neurodegenerative d. (TND) prion disease.

Traum d. brucellosis with abortion in swine.

Trevor d. dysplasia epiphysealis hemimelica.

trophoblastic d. gestational trophoblastic neoplasia.

tsutsugamushi d. scrub typhus.

tubotympanic d. inflammatory disease of the middle ear resulting from eustachian tube dysfunction and decreased pressure in the tympanic cavity.

tungsten carbide d. hard metal d.

tunnel d. decompression sickness.

twin-lamb d. pregnancy toxemia in ewes.

twist d. whirling d.

Tyzzer d. a disease caused by *Clostridium piliforme* and characterized by necrotic lesions of the liver and intestine; originally described in Japanese waltzing mice, it also affects rats, rabbits, gerbils, and dogs.

Tzaneen d. a tick-borne protozoal disease, seen in South Africa, due to *Theileria mutans,* and occurring in cattle and water buffalo, which may manifest as a mild febrile disease or may be severe and fatal.

Underwood d. sclerema.

unilocular hydatid d. infection with the larval forms (hydatid cysts) of *Echinococcus granulosus,* characterized by the formation of unilocular single or multiple expanding cysts; as the cysts expand they may give rise to symptoms of space-occupying lesions in the tissues or organs affected.

Unverricht d., Unverricht-Lundborg d. a slowly progressive autosomal recessive disorder, a form of progressive myoclonic epilepsy first seen in Finland. Onset is usually around the age of 10 and there are degenerative changes in the brain without presence of Lafora bodies. Myoclonic seizures are severe and continuous and tend to be triggered by movement, stress, and sensory stimuli, but mental deterioration is milder and survival is usually longer than in Lafora disease. It is associated with mutation in the gene encoding cystatin B, a cysteine protease inhibitor that blocks the actions of cathepsins; the mutation causes expansion of a minisatellite repeat sequence in the putative promoter region of the gene. Called also *Baltic myoclonic epilepsy* and *progressive myoclonic epilepsy type 1 (EPM1).*

Urbach-Wiethe d. lipoid proteinosis.

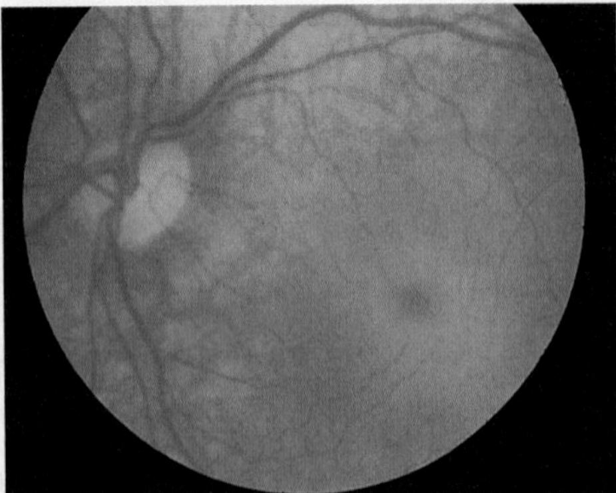

■ Tay-Sachs disease, showing characteristic cherry-red macular spot.

uremic bone d. renal osteodystrophy.

vagabond's d. discoloration of the skin due to longterm infestation with lice *(Pediculus humanus humanus).* Called also *parasitic melanoderma.*

van Buren d. Peyronie d.

van den Bergh d. enterogenous cyanosis.

vanishing white matter d. an autosomal recessive type of leukodystrophy, seen most often in young children, characterized by hypomyelination of variable severity; it usually develops slowly, although there may be rapid deterioration after an infection or head trauma. Affected children have spasticity and stiffness of the limbs; in severe cases there may be lethargy, optic atrophy, coma, and eventually death. Called also *childhood ataxia with central nervous system hypomyelination.*

Vaquez d., Vaquez-Osler d. polycythemia vera.

veld d., veldt d. heartwater.

venereal d. (VD) 1. sexually transmitted d. 2. a former classification of sexually transmitted diseases that included only gonorrhea, syphilis, chancroid, lymphogranuloma venereum, and granuloma inguinale.

venoocclusive d. of the liver symptomatic occlusion of the small hepatic venules, caused by ingestion of any of a variety of substances such as Senecio tea and certain chemotherapy agents (hepatotoxins) and by radiation. Many patients recover after withdrawal of the offending toxin; some progress to portal hypertension and liver failure, as in Budd-Chiari syndrome. Called also *hepatic venoocclusive d.*

vent d. rabbit syphilis.

Verneuil d. hidradenitis suppurativa.

Verse d. calcinosis intervertebralis.

vibration d. Raynaud phenomenon with osteoarthritic changes and diminished flexion in joints of the arms and hands, seen in those who use vibrating tools for long periods. Called also *pneumatic hammer d.*

Vilanova d. subacute nodular migratory panniculitis.

vinyl chloride d. acro-osteolysis resulting from exposure to vinyl chloride, characterized by Raynaud phenomenon, skin changes resembling scleroderma on the backs of the hands and on the forearms, and bony changes affecting the terminal phalanges of the fingers and toes, the styloid processes of the radius and ulna, the sacroiliac joints, and the patellae.

Vogt-Spielmeyer d. the juvenile form of neuronal ceroid-lipofuscinosis with onset between 5 and 10 years of age, characterized by rapid cerebroretinal degeneration, massive loss of brain substance, excessive neuronal storage of lipofuscin, and death within 10 to 15 years.

Volkmann d. a congenital deformity of the foot due to a tibiotarsal dislocation; called also *Volkmann deformity.*

Voltolini d. acute, painful inflammation of the internal ear followed by meningitis with deafness and unconsciousness.

vomiting and wasting d. a disease of pigs caused by infection with the hemagglutinating encephalomyelitis virus; the virus is endemic in many parts of the world and only occasionally causes symptoms. The disease varies from acute encephalomyelitis that can be fatal in a few days to anorexia, vomiting, and wasting that can last for two or three weeks without being fatal. Called also *Ontario encephalitis* and *hemagglutinating encephalomyelitis virus d. of pigs.*

von Economo d. lethargic encephalitis.

von Gierke d. glycogen storage d., type I.

von Hippel d. hemangiomatosis confined principally to the retina; when associated with hemangioblastoma of the cerebellum, it is known as *von Hippel-Lindau d.* Called also *retinal hemangioblastoma* and *Hippel d.*

von Hippel-Lindau d. hereditary phakomatosis characterized by hemangiomas of the retina and hemangioblastomas of the cerebellum; there may also be similar lesions of the spinal cord and cysts of the pancreas, kidneys, and other viscera. Neurologic symptoms, including seizures and mental retardation, may be present. Called also *cerebroretinal* or *retinocerebral angiomatosis, angiophakomatosis,* and *Lindau* or *Lindau-von Hippel d.*

von Recklinghausen d. 1. neurofibromatosis 1. 2. osteitis fibrosa cystica.

von Willebrand d. a congenital bleeding disorder, usually of autosomal dominant inheritance, characterized by deficiency of von Willebrand factor, with prolonged bleeding time and often impairment of adhesion of platelets on glass beads, associated with epistaxis and increased bleeding after trauma or surgery, menorrhagia, and postpartum bleeding. Several different types have been distinguished, ranging from mild to severe. Called also *angiohemophilia, pseudohemophilia, vascular hemophilia, Minot-von Willebrand syndrome,* and *Willebrand syndrome.*

Disease *Continued*

Vörner d. epidermolytic palmoplantar keratoderma.
Vrolik d. osteogenesis imperfecta, type II.
Waldenström d. Legg-Calvé-Perthes d.
walkabout d. crotalism.
Wartenberg d. cheiralgia paresthetica.
wasting d. any disease marked by wasting (q.v.), such as anorexia-cachexia syndrome or HIV wasting syndrome.
Weber d. Sturge-Weber syndrome.
Weber-Christian d. relapsing febrile nodular nonsuppurative panniculitis.
Weir Mitchell d. erythromelalgia.
Werdnig-Hoffmann d. Type I spinal muscular atrophy, an autosomal recessive condition caused by mutation or deletion in the telomeric copy of the *SMN1* gene (locus: 5q12.2-q13.3), which encodes a protein involved in RNA processing. It is usually seen in infancy and in siblings rather than in successive generations. It results from degeneration of the anterior horn cells of the spinal cord and is characterized by progressive hypotonia and wasting of the muscles with complete flaccid paralysis. Called also *infantile spinal muscular atrophy.*
Werlhof d. idiopathic thrombocytopenic purpura.
Werner Schultz d. agranulocytosis.
Wernicke d. see under *encephalopathy.*
Wesselsbron d. a viral disease of sheep and cattle in southern Africa, resembling Rift Valley fever but caused by a flavivirus. It causes death in newborn lambs and abortion in cows and ewes; human infection results in mild febrile illness.
Weston Hurst d. acute necrotizing hemorrhagic encephalomyelitis.
Westphal-Strümpell d. Wilson d.
wheat weevil d. miller's lung.
Whipple d. a malabsorption syndrome caused by infection with *Tropheryma whippelii,* characterized by diarrhea, steatorrhea, skin pigmentation, arthralgia and arthritis, lymphadenopathy, and sometimes central nervous system involvement with oculofacioskeletal or oculomasticatory myorhythmia. The intestinal mucosa is infiltrated with macrophages containing PAS-positive material that is the remnants of microorganisms that invaded the lamina propria. Called also *intestinal lipodystrophy* and *intestinal lipophagic granulomatosis.*
whirling d. a highly fatal protozoal disease of young salmonid fish caused by *Myxosoma cerebralis,* characterized chiefly by cartilaginous damage in the axial skeleton and granuloma formation involving the auditory-equilibrium apparatus of the fish, causing it to swim rapidly in a circular pattern. Called also *twist d.*
white heifer d. a congenital condition of heifers, most commonly white ones of the Shorthorn breed, in which there is a rubberlike sheet of fibrous tissue and membrane partially or completely covering the posterior part of the vagina. Called also *persistent hymen.*
white muscle d. enzootic muscular dystrophy.
white spot d. 1. guttate morphea. 2. a pustular eruption involving the skin, gills, and eyes of marine and freshwater fishes both in the wild and in aquaria, caused by the histophagous protozoan *Ichthyophthirius multifiliis,* and often leading to death, and sometimes to great economic loss. Called also *ich, ichthyophthiriasis,* and *ick.*
Whitmore d. melioidosis.
Whytt d. tuberculous meningitis causing acute hydrocephalus.
Wilson d. a rare, progressive, autosomal recessive disease due to a defect in metabolism of copper. Accumulation of copper in the liver, brain, kidney, cornea, and other tissues results in copper poisoning, with cirrhosis in the liver and degenerative changes in the brain, particularly the basal ganglia. Liver disease is the usual presenting symptom in children, and neurologic disease is most common in young adults. Another characteristic feature is the *Kayser-Fleischer ring,* a pigmented ring at the outer margin of the cornea. Called also *hepatolenticular d.* or *degeneration* and *Westphal-Strümpell d.*

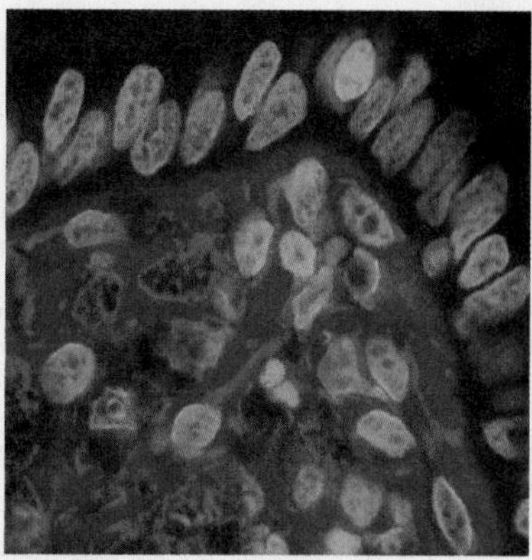

■ Whipple disease; confocal microscopy of a small intestine biopsy sample stains blue where a fluorescent probe for *Tropheryma whipplei* nucleic acid hybridizes to the bacteria. Human cell nuclei are stained fluorescent green and vimentin in human mesenchymal cells is stained red. Bacteria are localized to the lamina propria and are abundant in the extracellular spaces.

Winckel d. a fatal disease of newborn infants characterized by jaundice, hemoglobinuria, hemorrhage, bloody urine, cyanosis, polyuria, collapse, and convulsions.
Winiwarter-Buerger d. thromboangiitis obliterans.
Winkler d. chondrodermatitis nodularis chronica helicis.
winter vomiting d. gastroenteritis with vomiting caused by infection with Norovirus, seen primarily in cold weather in Europe.
Witkop d., Witkop-von Sallmann d. hereditary benign intraepithelial dyskeratosis.
Wolman d. a lysosomal storage disease caused by deficiency of the lysosomal sterol esterase, with onset in early infancy and death before one year of age. Clinical features include hepatosplenomegaly, steatorrhea, abdominal distention, anemia, inanition, and adrenal calcification. Called also *primary familial* or *Wolman xanthomatosis.*
woolsorter's d. inhalational anthrax.
Woringer-Kolopp d. pagetoid reticulosis.
x d. 1. aflatoxicosis. 2. former name for *hyperkeratosis* (def. 3).
X-linked lymphoproliferative d. see under *syndrome.*
yellow fat d. inflammation of adipose tissue in an animal whose diet is excessively high in unsaturated fats and low in vitamin E; it usually occurs in cats and mink fed certain kinds of fish. The body fat becomes hard, lumpy, and painful and the animal may be feverish or anorexic. Called also *steatitis* and *nutritional steatitis.*
Zahorsky d. exanthema subitum.

dis·en·gage·ment (dis″ən-gāj′mənt) emergence of the fetus from the vaginal canal.

dis·equi·lib·ri·um (dis-e″kwĭ-lib′re-əm) dysequilibrium.
 linkage d. the occurrence in a population of two linked alleles at a frequency higher than the expected equilibrium frequency (which is the product of the frequencies of the two alleles), suggesting a common mutation due to a founder effect.

dis·es·the·sia (dis″es-the′zhə) dysesthesia.

dis·ger·mi·no·ma (dis-jur″mĭ-no′mə) dysgerminoma.

DISH diffuse idiopathic skeletal hyperostosis.

dish (dish) a shallow vessel of glass or other material for laboratory work.
 culture d. a shallow glass vessel for making bacterial cultures.
 dappen d. a small, heavy, solid glass, octagonal dish with a shallow depression to hold a few drops of medicaments or filling material.
 evaporating d. a laboratory vessel, usually wide and shallow, in which material is evaporated by exposure to heat.
 Petri d. a round, shallow, flat-bottomed transparent glass or plastic dish with vertical sides and a similar but slightly larger dish that forms a cover; used for the culture of microorganisms on solid media and for tissue cell cultures.
 Stender d's vessels of various forms and sizes, used in preparing and staining histologic specimens.

dis·har·mo·ny (dis-hahr′mə-ne) lack of harmony; discord.
 occlusal d. a condition in which *(a)* contacts of opposing occlusal surfaces of teeth are not in harmony with other tooth contacts and with the anatomic and physiologic control of the mandible, or *(b)* occlusions do not coincide with their respective jaw relations.

dis·im·pac·tion (dis-im-pak′shən) removal of a fecal impaction, usually done digitally or with an enema.

DISIDA disofenin (diisopropyl iminodiacetic acid).

dis•in•fect (dis″in-fekt′) [*dis-*[1] + L. *inficere* to corrupt] to free from pathogenic organisms, or to render them inert; see also *disinfection.*

dis•in•fec•tant (dis″in-fek′tənt) 1. an agent that disinfects; applied particularly to agents used on inanimate objects. Cf. *antimicrobial* and *antiseptic.* 2. freeing from infection.

coal tar d. creosote.

dis•in•fec•tion (dis″in-fek′shən) the process of destroying pathogenic organisms, or of rendering them inert, especially as applied to the treatment of inanimate materials to reduce or eliminate infectious organisms. Cf. *antisepsis.*

concomitant d., concurrent d. immediate disinfection and disposal of discharges and infective matter all through the course of a disease.

terminal d. disinfection of a sick room and its contents at the termination of a disease.

dis•in•fes•ta•tion (dis″in-fəs-ta′shən) the extermination or destruction of insects, rodents, or other animal forms, especially those present on a person, an animal, or clothing; cf. *defaunation, delousing,* and *disparasitized.*

dis•in•hi•bi•tion (dis″in-hĭ-bish′ən) 1. removal of inhibitions, as reduction of the inhibitory function of the cerebral cortex by drugs such as ethyl alcohol or reduction in the severity of superego controls in psychotherapy. 2. in experimental psychology, the revival of an extinguished conditioned response by exposure to an unconditioned stimulus.

dis•in•sect•ed (dis″in-sek′təd) freed from unwanted insects.

dis•in•sec•tion (dis″in-sek′shən) disinsectization.

dis•in•sec•ti•za•tion (dis″in-sek″tĭ-za′shən) removal or extermination of unwanted insects.

dis•in•sec•tor (dis″in-sek′tər) an apparatus for the removal of insects or similar vermin from humans, animals, or clothing.

dis•in•ser•tion (dis″in-sur′shən) 1. rupture of a tendon from its insertion into a bone. 2. detachment of the retina at its periphery; retinodialysis.

dis•in•te•grant (dis-in′tə-grənt) disintegrator; an agent used in the pharmaceutical preparation of tablets, which causes them to disintegrate and release their medicinal substances on contact with moisture.

dis•in•te•gra•tion (dis-in″tə-gra′shən) [*dis-*[1] + L. *integer* entire] 1. the process of breaking up or decomposing. 2. disruption of integrative functions of personality in mental illness; disorganization of the psychic and behavioral processes.

radioactive d. see under *decay.*

dis•in•te•gra•tive (dis-in′tə-gra″tiv) 1. being reduced to components, particles, or fragments; losing cohesion or unity. 2. having disorganized psychic and behavioral processes.

dis•in•teg•rin (dis-in′tə-grin) any of a family of proteins occurring in snake venoms and interrupting the function of integrins by blocking their interaction with surface receptors. In very low concentrations, disintegrins also inhibit platelet aggregation.

dis•joint (dis-joint′) to disarticulate.

dis•junc•tion (dis-junk′shən) 1. the act or state of being disjoined. 2. in genetics, the moving apart of bivalent chromosomes at first anaphase of meiosis, or the moving apart of daughter chromatids at the second anaphase of meiosis or anaphase of mitosis.

craniofacial d. Le Fort III fracture; see under *fracture.*

disk (disk) [L. *discus* quoit, from Gr. *diskos*] a circular or rounded flat plate; spelled also *disc.* See also subentries under *disc.*

A d. A band.

abrasive d. dental d.

anangioid d. a retinal disk without blood vessels.

anisotropic d. A band.

articular d. 1. discus articularis. 2. meniscus articularis.

Blake d. a disk-shaped paper patch for a perforated tympanic membrane.

Bowman d's flat, disklike plates that make up striated muscle fibers.

Carborundum d. a dental disk with Carborundum (silicon carbide) as the abrasive material.

choked d. papilledema.

ciliary d. orbiculus ciliaris.

cloth d. rag wheel.

contained d. herniation of intervertebral disk (see under *herniation*) in which the anulus fibrosus remains intact. Cf. *noncontained d.*

cupped d. a pathologically depressed and enlarged optic disk, frequently seen in advanced glaucoma.

cutting d. a dental disk with abrasive material attached to its surfaces or edge, used for grinding or reducing teeth.

cuttlefish d. a dental disk with powdered cuttlefish bone bonded to its surface and edge.

dental d. a thin, flat, oval, or concave circular plate with abrasive materials bonded to its surface or edge; used to polish and finish cavity preparations and for cutting or polishing dental restorations. Called also *abrasive d.*

diamond d. a steel dental disk with diamond chips bonded to its surface or edge.

emery d. a paper or resin dental disk with emery powder attached to its surface.

Engelmann d. H band.

epiphyseal d. lamina epiphysialis.

extruded d. herniation of intervertebral disk (see under *herniation*) in which the nucleus pulposus protrudes through the anulus fibrosus and the nuclear material remains attached to the disk.

gelatin d. a disk or lamella of gelatin, variously medicated; used chiefly in eye diseases.

growth d. lamina epiphysialis.

hair d. a vascularized and innervated area of skin in the connective tissue sheath of a hair follicle, containing Merkel cells and acting as a mechanoreceptor.

Hensen d. H band.

herniated d. herniation of intervertebral disk.

I d. I band.

interarticular d. discus articularis.

intercalated d's dense bands running between myocardial cells both transversely and longitudinally, forming a stepped configuration. They contain intercellular junctions that link adjacent cells both electrically and mechanically; they are composed mainly of fascia adherens, but desmosomes and gap junctions are also present.

interpubic d. discus interpubicus.

intervertebral d. discus intervertebralis.

intra-articular d. discus articularis.

isotropic d., J d. I band.

M d. M band.

Merkel d. see under *cell.*

micrometer d. a glass disk, engraved with a scale, used in an ocular in making microscopical measurements.

Newton d. a disk divided into seven sectors, colored the seven primary colors of the spectrum; when rotated rapidly, the disk appears to be white.

noncontained d. herniation of intervertebral disk (see under *herniation*) in which there is rupture of the anulus fibrosus. Cf. *contained d.*

optic d. discus nervi optici.

Placido d. keratoscope.

polishing d. a dental disk with a very fine abrasive material, used for finishing and polishing of surfaces.

prolapsed d. herniation of intervertebral disk.

proligerous d. cumulus oophorus.

protruded d. herniation of intervertebral disk.

Q d. A band.

Ranvier tactile d's cup-shaped sensory nerve endings near the menisci tactus.

Rekoss d. the rotating device for quickly changing the lenses in the ophthalmoscope.

ruptured d. herniation of intervertebral disk.

sandpaper d. a dental disk with pulverized silica as the abrasive material.

sequestered d. a free fragment of the nucleus pulposus lying in the spinal canal outside of the annulus fibrosus and no longer attached to the intervertebral disk.

slipped d. popular name for *herniation of intervertebral disk.*

stenopeic d. an opaque disk having a narrow slit; used for testing for astigmatism.

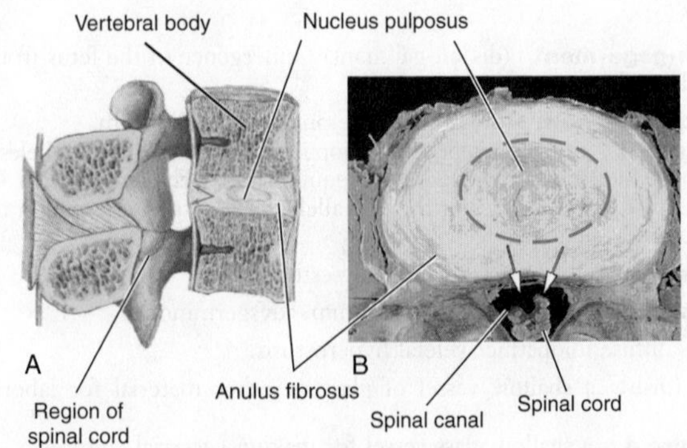

■ Intervertebral disk (discus intervertebralis) in *(A)*, sagittal section; *(B)*, cross-section, superior view.

stroboscopic d. a revolving disk with alternate open and closed sections that gives successive views of a moving object.
tactile d. see under *meniscus.*
transverse d. A band.
Z d. Z band.

dis•kec•to•my (dis-kek′tə-me) excision of an intervertebral disk; called also *discectomy.*

Disk•hal•er (disk′hāl-ər) trademark for a type of dry powder inhaler that can deliver multiple doses of medication.

dis•ki•tis (dis-ki′tis) inflammation of a disk, particularly of an intra-articular disk.

disk(o)- [Gr. *diskos* disk] a combining form denoting relationship to a disk, or disk-shaped. See also words beginning *disc(o)-.*

dis•ko•gram (dis′ko-gram) a radiograph of an intervertebral disk.

dis•kog•ra•phy (dis-kog′rə-fe) radiography of the spine for visualization of an intervertebral disk, after injection into the disk itself of an absorbable contrast medium.

dis•lo•ca•tion (dis″lo-ka′shən) [*dis-*[1] + L. *locare* to place] the displacement of any part, more especially of a bone; see Plate 13. Called also *luxation.*
Bell-Dally d. nontraumatic dislocation of the atlas.
closed d. simple d.
complete d. a dislocation that completely separates the surfaces of a joint.
complicated d. a dislocation that is associated with other important injuries.
compound d. a dislocation in which the joint communicates with the external air.
congenital d. a dislocation that exists from or before birth.
congenital d. of the hip (CDH) developmental dysplasia of the hip.
consecutive d. a dislocation in which the luxated bone has changed its position since its first displacement.
divergent d. a dislocation in which the ulna and radius are dislocated separately.
fracture d. dislocation complicated by fracture of, or adjacent to, a joint.
habitual d. a dislocation that often recurs after replacement.
incomplete d. a subluxation; a slight displacement. Called also *partial d.*
intrauterine d. a dislocation that occurs to the fetus in utero.
d. of the lens displacement of the crystalline lens of the eye.
Lisfranc d. dislocation of the forefoot at the tarsometatarsal joints.
Monteggia d. dislocation of the hip joint in which the head of the femur is near the anterosuperior spine of the ilium.
Nélaton d. dislocation of the ankle in which the talus is forced up between the end of the tibia and the fibula.
old d. a dislocation in which inflammatory or fibrotic changes have occurred.
open d. compound d.
partial d. incomplete d.
pathologic d. a dislocation that results from paralysis, synovitis, infection, or other disease.
primitive d. a dislocation in which the bones remain as originally displaced.
recent d. a dislocation in which there is no complicating inflammation.
simple d. a dislocation in which the joint is not penetrated by a wound.
Smith d. upward and backward dislocation of the metatarsals and the medial cuneiform bone.
subastragalar d. separation of the calcaneus and the navicular bone from the talus.
subcoracoid d. a type of dislocation of the head of the humerus. See Plate 13.
subglenoid d. a type of dislocation of the head of the humerus. See Plate 13.
subspinous d. dislocation of the head of the humerus into the space below the spine of the scapula.
traumatic d. a dislocation due to an injury or to violence.

dis•mem•ber•ment (dis-mem′bər-mənt) amputation of a limb or a portion of it.

dis•mu•ta•tion (dis″mu-ta′shən) a reaction or reactions involving two identical molecules in which one gains what the other loses. For example, one may be oxidized and the other reduced, or one may be phosphorylated and the other dephosphorylated.

dis•oc•clude (dis″ŏ-klo͞od′) to cause loss of contact between opposing teeth as a result of tooth guidance, occlusal interferences, or occlusal adjustment.

di•so•di•um (di-so′de-əm) having two atoms of sodium in each molecule.
d. cromoglycate cromolyn sodium.
d. edetate edetate disodium.

di•so•fen•in (DISIDA) (di″so-fen′in) a diisopropyl-substituted analogue of iminodiacetic acid (IDA); complexed with technetium Tc 99m it is used in hepatobiliary imaging. See also table at *technetium.*

di•so•mus (di-so′məs) [*di-* + *soma*] synencephalus.

di•so•my (di′so-me) the presence of two chromosomes of a homologous pair in a cell; in humans the normal state, with each pair usually comprising one chromosome from each parent.
uniparental d. the abnormal state in which both copies of a homologous pair of chromosomes are from the same parent, with none from the other parent.

di•so•pyr•a•mide (di″so-pir′ə-mīd) a cardiac depressant with anticholinergic properties, used as an antiarrhythmic.
d. phosphate [USP] the phosphate salt of disopyramide, having the same actions and uses as the base, administered orally.

dis•or•der (dis-or′dər) a derangement or abnormality of function; a morbid physical or mental state.

Disorder

acute stress d. [DSM-IV] an anxiety disorder characterized by development of anxiety and dissociative and other symptoms within one month following exposure to an extremely traumatic event; symptoms include reexperiencing the event, avoidance of trauma-related stimuli, anxiety or increased arousal, and some or all of the following: a subjective sense of diminished emotional responsiveness, numbing, or detachment, derealization, depersonalization, and amnesia for aspects of the event. If persistent, it may become *posttraumatic stress disorder.*

adjustment d. [DSM-IV] a maladaptive reaction to identifiable stressful life events, such as divorce, loss of job, physical illness, or natural disaster; this diagnosis assumes that the condition will remit when the stress ceases or when the patient adapts to the situation.

affective d's mood d's.

amnestic d's [DSM-IV] mental disorders characterized by acquired impairment in the ability to learn and recall new information, sometimes accompanied by inability to recall previously learned information, and not coupled to dementia or delirium. The disorders are subclassified on the basis of etiology as *amnestic disorder due to a general medical condition, substance-induced persisting amnestic disorder,* and *amnestic disorder not otherwise specified.* DSM-IV eliminates the distinction between this term and amnestic syndrome.

antisocial personality d. [DSM-IV] a personality disorder characterized by continuous and chronic antisocial behavior in which the rights of others or generally accepted social norms are violated; associated personality traits include impulsiveness, egocentricity, inability to tolerate boredom or frustration, irritability and aggressiveness, recklessness, disregard for truth, and inability to maintain consistent, responsible functioning at work, at school, or as a parent.

anxiety d's [DSM-IV] a group of mental disorders in which anxiety and avoidance behavior predominate. Included are panic disorder with and without agoraphobia, agoraphobia without history of panic disorder, specific phobia, social phobia, obsessive-compulsive disorder, posttraumatic stress disorder, acute stress disorder, generalized anxiety disorder, and substance-induced anxiety disorder.

attention-deficit/hyperactivity d. [DSM-IV] a childhood mental disorder characterized by inattention (such as distractibility, forgetfulness, not finishing tasks, and not appearing to listen), by hyperactivity and impulsivity (such as fidgeting and squirming, difficulty in remaining seated, excessive running or climbing, feelings of restlessness, difficulty awaiting one's turn, interrupting others, and excessive talking) or by both types of behavior. The disorder is subtyped as *predominantly hyperactive-impulsive type, predominantly inattentive type,* or *combined type,*

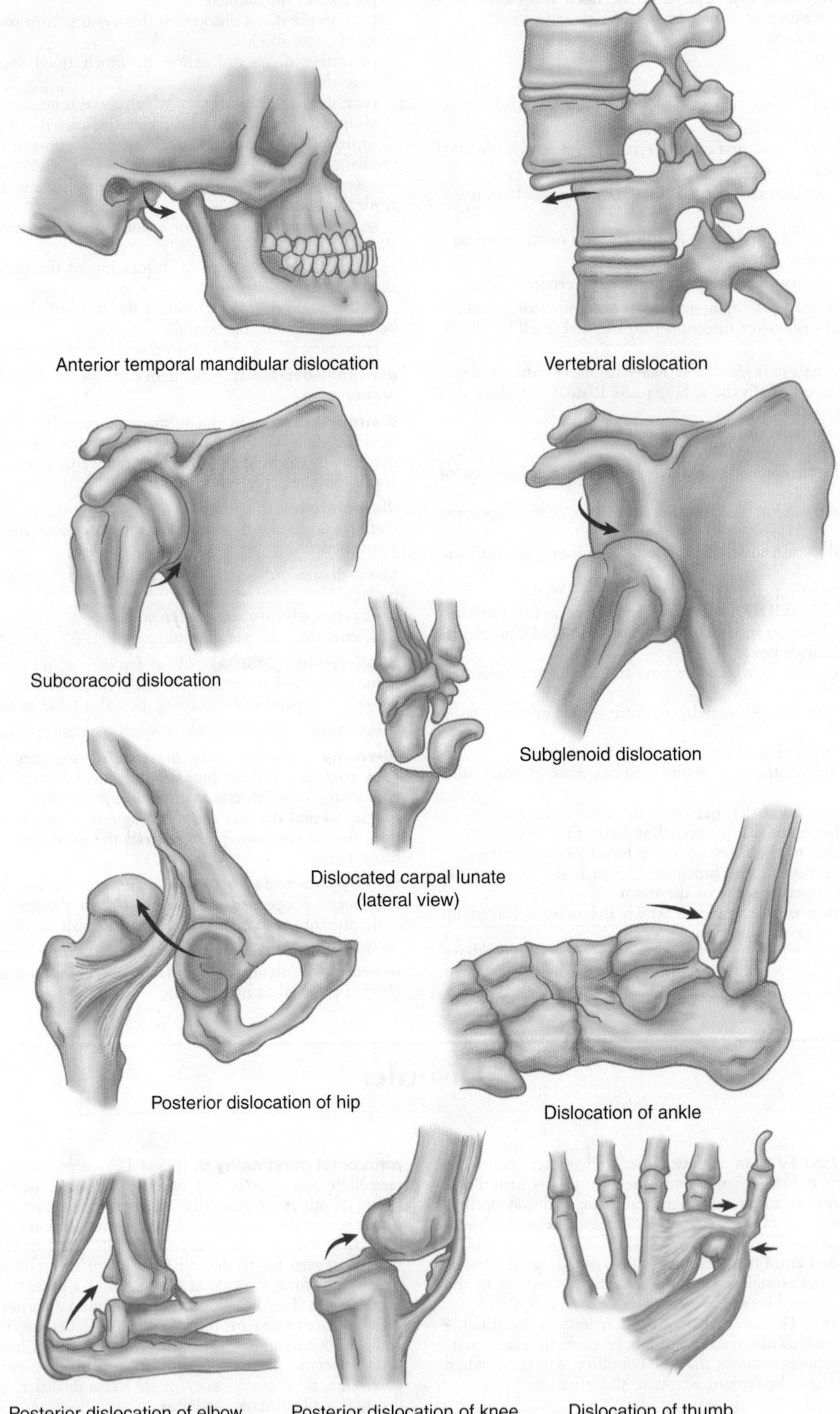

■ **PLATE 13—VARIOUS TYPES OF DISLOCATION**

depending on the criteria met. Behavior must interfere with academic, social, or work functioning, with impairment existing in at least two settings. Onset is before age seven but it can persist into adulthood.

autistic d. [DSM-IV] a severe pervasive developmental disorder with onset usually before three years of age and a biological basis related to neurologic or neurophysiologic factors; it is characterized by qualitative impairment in reciprocal social interaction (e.g., lack of awareness of the existence of feelings of others, failure to seek comfort at times of distress, lack of imitation), in verbal and nonverbal communication, and in capacity for symbolic play, and by restricted and unusual repertoire of activities and interests. Other characteristics sometimes include cognitive impairment, hyper- or hyporeactivity to certain stimuli, stereotypic behaviors, neurological abnormalities such as seizures or altered muscle tone, sleeping or eating pattern abnormalities, and severe behavioral problems. It is associated with several genetic conditions and pre- and perinatal risk factors. Called also *autism, infantile autism*, and *Kanner syndrome*.

autistic spectrum d's, autism spectrum d's pervasive developmental d's.

avoidant d. of childhood or adolescence former name for a disorder that would now be included under the diagnosis of social phobia (DSM-IV).

avoidant personality d. [DSM-IV] a personality disorder characterized by social discomfort, hypersensitivity to criticism, low self-esteem, and an aversion to activities that involve significant interpersonal contact; there is a proclivity to anxiety, an exaggeration of difficulties, a desire for affection and acceptance that is restrained for fear of rejection, and an avoidance of risks or new activities for fear of embarrassment.

behavior d. conduct d.

binge-eating d. an eating disorder characterized by repeated episodes of binge eating, as in bulimia nervosa, but not followed by inappropriate compensatory behavior such as purging, fasting, or excessive exercise.

bipolar d's 1. [DSM-IV] mood disorders characterized by a history of manic, mixed, or hypomanic episodes, usually with concurrent or previous history of one or more major depressive episodes, including *bipolar I disorder, bipolar II disorder*, and *cyclothymic disorder*. Cf. *depressive d's.* 2. a term sometimes used in the singular to denote either *bipolar I d.* or *bipolar II d.*, or both.

bipolar I d. [DSM-IV] a type of bipolar disorder characterized by one or more manic or mixed episodes, often with a history of one or more major depressive episodes.

bipolar II d. [DSM-IV] a type of bipolar disorder characterized by one or more major depressive episodes accompanied by at least one hypomanic episode but without any manic or mixed episodes.

bleeding d. coagulopathy.

body dysmorphic d. [DSM-IV] a mental disorder in which a normal-appearing person is either preoccupied with some imagined defect in appearance or is overly concerned about some very slight physical anomaly.

borderline personality d. [DSM-IV] a personality disorder marked by a pervasive instability of mood, self-image or sense of self, and interpersonal relationships; impulsive and self-damaging acts are common, as are uncontrolled anger, fears of abandonment, chronic feelings of emptiness, recurrent self-mutilating behavior and suicide threats, and transient, stress-induced periods of paranoia and dissociation.

breathing-related sleep d. [DSM-IV] any of several disorders characterized by sleep disruption due to some sleep-related breathing problem, resulting in excessive sleepiness or insomnia; included are central and obstructive sleep apnea syndromes (see *sleep apnea*, under *apnea*) and primary alveolar hypoventilation.

brief psychotic d. [DSM-IV] an episode of psychotic symptoms (incoherence, loosening of associations, delusions, hallucinations, disorganized or catatonic behavior) with sudden onset, lasting less than one month. If it occurs in response to a stressful life event, it may be called *brief reactive psychosis*.

catatonic d. [DSM-IV] catatonia due to the physiological effects of a general medical condition and neither better accounted for by another mental disorder nor occurring exclusively during delirium.

character d's personality d's. See also *character*.

childhood disintegrative d. [DSM-IV] pervasive developmental disorder characterized by marked regression in a variety of skills, including language, social skills or adaptive behavior, play, bowel or bladder control, and motor skills, after at least two, but less than ten, years of apparently normal development.

circadian rhythm sleep d. [DSM-IV] a sleep disorder of the dyssomnia group, consisting of a lack of synchrony between the schedule of sleeping and waking required by the external environment and that of a person's own circadian rhythm. It usually has an environmental cause such as rotating shift work or long-distance air travel, although some individuals simply have natural circadian rhythms sharply different from the predominant one of their society.

collagen d. any inborn error of metabolism involving abnormal structure or metabolism of collagen; the term includes Ehlers-Danlos syndrome, Marfan syndrome, cutis laxa, osteogenesis imperfecta, and epidermolysis bullosa. Collagen disorder is not to be confused with collagen disease (q.v.).

communication d's [DSM-IV] mental disorders characterized by difficulties in speech or language, severe enough to be a problem academically, occupationally, or socially; included are *expressive language disorder, mixed receptive-expressive language disorder, phonological disorder*, and *stuttering*.

conduct d. [DSM-IV] a type of disruptive behavior disorder of childhood and adolescence characterized by a persistent pattern of conduct in which rights of others or age-appropriate societal norms or rules are violated, with misconduct including aggression to people or animals, destruction of property, deceitfulness or theft, and serious violations of rules; it is classified as *childhood-onset* or *adolescent-onset* depending on whether the behavior begins before or after the age of ten.

congenital d's of glycosylation (CDG) a large, genetically heterogeneous group of autosomal recessive multisystemic diseases caused by defects in the synthesis and processing of the carbohydrate moiety of glycoproteins. Disorders are divided into two types: type I disorders result from defects in biosynthesis occurring in the endoplasmic reticulum; type II disorders result from defects in processing in the Golgi complex. Disorders whose molecular defect is not known are designated CDG-x.

type IIc leukocyte adhesion deficiency, type II.

d. of consciousness a state of disordered attention and apperception, e.g., confusion or delirium.

conversion d. [DSM-IV] a mental disorder characterized by conversion symptoms (loss or alteration of voluntary motor or sensory functioning suggesting physical illness, such as seizures, paralysis, dyskinesia, anesthesia, blindness, or aphonia) having no demonstrable physiological basis and whose psychological basis is suggested by (1) exacerbation of symptoms at times of psychological stress, (2) relief from tension or inner conflicts (primary gain) provided by the symptoms, or (3) secondary gains (support, attention, avoidance of unpleasant responsibilities) provided by the symptoms. Many patients exhibit "la belle indifférence," a lack of concern about the impairment caused by the symptoms; histrionic personality traits are also common. Symptoms are neither intentionally produced nor feigned, and are not limited to pain or sexual dysfunction.

cyclothymic d. [DSM-IV] a mood disorder characterized by numerous alternating short cycles of hypomanic and depressive periods with symptoms like those of manic and major depressive episodes but of lesser severity. Called also *cyclothymia*.

delusional d. [DSM-IV] a mental disorder marked by well-organized, logically consistent delusions but lacking other psychotic symptoms. Most functioning is not markedly impaired, the criteria for schizophrenia have never been satisfied, and symptoms of a major mood disorder have been present only briefly if at all. DSM-IV distinguishes six types on the basis of the predominant delusional theme: persecutory, jealous, erotomanic, somatic, grandiose, and mixed.

dependent personality d. [DSM-IV] a personality disorder marked by an excessive need to be taken care of, with submissiveness and clinging and preoccupation with fears of being abandoned; features include need for advice and reassurance in decision making, yielding of responsibility, initiative, and independence, avoidance of disagreement for fear of loss of support, voluntarily undertaking unpleasant tasks to ensure further care, and discomfort or helpless feelings when alone, with an indiscriminate rush to a new relationship.

depersonalization d. [DSM-IV] a dissociative disorder characterized by one or more severe episodes of depersonalization (feelings of unreality and strangeness in one's perception of the self or one's body image) not due to another mental disorder, such as schizophrenia. The perception of reality remains intact; patients are aware of their incapacitation. Episodes are usually accompanied by dizziness, anxiety, fears of going insane, and derealization.

depressive d's [DSM-IV] mood disorders in which depression is unaccompanied by manic or hypomanic episodes; e.g., major depressive disorder and dysthymic disorder. Cf. *bipolar d's.*

depressive personality d. a personality disorder characterized by a persistent and pervasive pattern of depressive cognitions and behaviors, such as chronic unhappiness, low self-esteem, pessimism, critical and derogatory attitudes toward oneself and others, feelings of guilt or remorse, and an inability to relax or feel enjoyment.

developmental d's see under *disability.*

developmental coordination d. [DSM-IV] problematic or delayed development of gross and fine motor coordination skills, not due to a neurological disorder or to general mental retardation; affected children appear to be clumsy rather than grossly impaired. It may persist into adulthood.

disruptive behavior d's [DSM-IV] a group of mental disorders of children and adolescents consisting of behavior that violates social norms, is disruptive, and may be illegal, often distressing others more than it does the person with the disorder. It includes *conduct disorder* and *oppositional defiant disorder* and is grouped with attention-deficit/hyperactivity disorder.

dissociative d's [DSM-IV] mental disorders characterized by sudden, temporary alterations in identity, memory, or consciousness, segregating normally integrated memories or parts of the personality from the dominant identity of the individual. This category includes *dissociative identity disorder, dissociative fugue, dissociative amnesia,* and *depersonalization disorder.*

dissociative identity d. [DSM-IV] a dissociative disorder characterized by the existence in an individual of two or more distinct personalities, each having unique memories, characteristic behavior, and social relationships. At least two of the personalities control the patient's behavior in turns, the transition often being abrupt. The host personality usually is totally unaware of the alternate personalities, experiencing only inexplicable gaps of time and inability to recall important personal information. Alternate personalities may or may not have awareness of the others. Called also *multiple personality d.*

dissociative trance d. a dissociative disorder characterized by an involuntary state of trance that is not a normal function of the person's cultural or religious practice and that causes impairment or distress.

dream anxiety d. nightmare d.

dysthymic d. [DSM-IV] a mood disorder characterized by depressed feeling (sad, blue, low), loss of interest or pleasure in one's usual activities, and by at least some of the following: altered appetite, disturbed sleep patterns, lack of energy, low self esteem, poor concentration or decision-making skills, and feelings of hopelessness. Symptoms have persisted for more than two years but are not severe enough to meet the criteria for major depressive disorder.

eating d. any of several disorders in which abnormal feeding habits are associated with psychological factors; in DSM-IV these include *anorexia nervosa, bulimia nervosa, pica,* and *rumination disorder.*

emotional d. see under *illness.*

expressive language d. [DSM-IV] a communication disorder occurring in children and characterized by problems with the expression of language, either oral or signed. It includes difficulties such as limited speech or vocabulary, vocabulary errors, difficulty or hesitation in word selection, oversimplification of grammatical or sentence structure, omission of parts of sentences, unusual word order, and slowed acquisition of language skills. Two types are recognized, *acquired* and *developmental.*

extrapyramidal d. see under *syndrome.*

factitious d. [DSM-IV] a mental disorder characterized by repeated, intentional simulation of physical or psychological signs and symptoms of illness for no apparent purpose other than obtaining treatment. It differs from malingering in that there is no recognizable motive for feigning illness. It is subtyped on the basis of whether the predominant signs and symptoms are physical (called also *Munchausen syndrome*), psychological, or both.

factitious d. by proxy a form of factitious disorder in which one person intentionally fabricates or induces signs and symptoms of one or more physical *(Munchausen syndrome by proxy)* or psychological disorders in another person under their care and subjects that person to needless and sometimes dangerous or disfiguring diagnostic procedures or treatment, without any external incentives for the behavior. The dyad is usually that of mother and child.

female orgasmic d. [DSM-IV] a sexual dysfunction characterized by consistently delayed or absent orgasm in a female, even after a normal phase of sexual excitement and accounting for her age and sexual experience and the amount of stimulation, and causing significant distress or interpersonal difficulty.

female sexual arousal d. [DSM-IV] a sexual dysfunction involving inability of a female either to attain or maintain the lubrication and swelling response of sexual excitement during sexual activity, after adequate stimulation, causing significant distress or interpersonal difficulty. Both physiological and psychological factors may be involved. Formerly called *frigidity.* Cf. *male erectile d.*

formal thought d. disturbance in the form, rather than the content, of thought; disruption in the flow of ideas or speech; inability to follow the normal semantic or syntactic rules in someone with adequate intelligence and education and the cultural background to do so.

functional d. a disorder of physiological function having no known organic basis. Although not strictly correct, the term is often used in psychiatry as roughly equivalent to "psychogenic disorder"; in other branches of medicine, to "idiopathic disorder."

gender identity d. [DSM-IV] a disturbance of gender identification in which the affected person has an overwhelming desire to change their anatomic sex or insists that they are of the opposite sex, with persistent discomfort about their assigned sex or about filling its usual gender role; the disorder may become apparent in childhood or not appear until adolescence or adulthood. Individuals may attempt to live as members of the opposite sex and may seek hormonal and surgical treatment to bring their anatomy into conformity with their belief. Cf. *transvestism.*

generalized anxiety d. (GAD) [DSM-IV] an anxiety disorder characterized by the presence of excessive, uncontrollable anxiety and worry about two or more life circumstances, for six months or longer, accompanied by some combination of restlessness, fatigue, muscle tension, irritability, disturbed concentration or sleep, and somatic symptoms.

genetic d. see under *disease.*

growth d. a condition in which growth is at one or the other statistical extreme, either below the 5th percentile or above the 95th percentile. See *gigantism* and *dwarfism.*

histrionic personality d. [DSM-IV] a personality disorder marked by excessive emotionality and attention-seeking behavior; there is overconcern with physical attractiveness, sexual seductiveness, intolerance of delayed gratification, and rapid shifting and shallow expression of emotions.

hypoactive sexual desire d. [DSM-IV] a sexual dysfunction consisting of persistently or recurrently low level or absence of sexual fantasies and desire for sexual activity, causing pronounced distress or interpersonal difficulties.

identity d. former name for a disorder of adolescence that was defined as severe subjective distress about inability to reconcile aspects of the self into a relatively coherent whole and acceptable sense of self, with uncertainty about many social, academic, career, and moral choices. Lacking in substantiation, the disorder is no longer officially recognized, but similar uncertainty on multiple issues may be labeled as identity problem.

immunosecretory d's a group of disorders characterized by monoclonal proliferation of immunoglobulin-producing cells that resemble lymphocytes or plasma cells; the group includes AL amyloidosis, cryoglobulinemia, heavy chain disease, benign monoclonal gammopathy, multiple myeloma, and plasma cell dyscrasias.

impulse control d's [DSM-IV] a group of mental disorders characterized by repeated failure to resist an impulse to perform some act harmful to oneself or to others. The person feels tension or an irresistible urge to perform the act which, even though ego-dystonic, gives pleasure or emotional release upon performance.

induced psychotic d. shared psychotic d.

intermittent explosive d. [DSM-IV] an impulse control disorder characterized by multiple discrete episodes of loss of control of aggressive impulses resulting in serious assault or destruction of property that are out of proportion to any precipitating stressors; behavior in between such episodes lacks impulsiveness or aggressiveness.

ion channel d's ion channelopathies.

isolated explosive d. a former classification used to denote a single violent catastrophic act performed for no apparent reason and not attributable to any other disorder.

language d. any disorder of normal language-based communication, whether psychogenic or neurogenic; see *communication d's* and *speech d.*
late luteal phase dysphoric d. former name for *premenstrual dysphoric d.*
LDL-receptor d. familial hypercholesterolemia.
learning d's [DSM-IV] a group of disorders characterized by academic functioning that is substantially below the level expected on the basis of the patient's age, intelligence, and education, interfering with academic achievement or other functioning. Included are *reading disorder, mathematics disorder,* and *disorder of written expression.*
lymphoproliferative d's a general term encompassing a variety of disorders characterized by abnormal proliferation of lymphocytes; they include both malignant and nonmalignant disease. Called also *lymphoproliferative diseases* or *syndromes.*
lymphoreticular d's a group of disorders of the lymphoreticular system, characterized by the proliferation of lymphocytes or lymphoid tissues; they may be either benign (e.g., lymphocytosis) or malignant (e.g., lymphocytic leukemias, multiple myeloma, or non-Hodgkin lymphomas). See also *lymphoproliferative d's.* Called also *lymphoreticular diseases* or *syndromes.*
major depressive d. [DSM-IV] a mood disorder characterized by the occurrence of one or more major depressive episodes (q.v.) and the absence of any history of manic, mixed, or hypomanic episodes.
major mood d's severe, full-blown mood disorders; e.g., major depressive disorder and bipolar I and II disorders.
male erectile d. [DSM-IV] a sexual dysfunction involving inability of a male to attain or maintain erection until completion of sexual relations, causing significant distress or interpersonal difficulty. Called also *psychogenic* pr *psychological impotence.* Cf. *female sexual arousal d.*
male orgasmic d. [DSM-IV] a sexual dysfunction characterized by consistently delayed or absent orgasm in a male, even after a normal phase of sexual excitement and stimulation that is adequate for his age in focus, duration, and intensity, and which causes significant distress or interpersonal difficulty.
manic-depressive d. former name for *bipolar d.*; see *bipolar d's* (def. 2).
mathematics d. [DSM-IV] a learning disorder (q.v.) in which the skill affected is mathematical calculation or reasoning.
mendelian d. a genetic disease, showing a mendelian pattern of inheritance, and caused by a single mutation in the structure of DNA, which causes a single basic defect that has some pathological consequence or consequences. Called also *monogenic* or *single-gene d.* See also *inborn error of metabolism,* under *error.*
mental d. [DSM-IV] any clinically significant behavioral or psychological syndrome characterized by the presence of distressing symptoms, impairment of functioning, or significantly increased risk of suffering death, pain, disability, or loss of freedom. Mental disorders are assumed to be the manifestation of a behavioral, psychological, or biological dysfunction in the individual. The concept does not include deviant behavior, disturbances that are essentially conflicts between the individual and society, or expected and culturally sanctioned responses to particular events.
minor depressive d. [DSM-IV] a mood disorder closely resembling major depressive disorder and dysthymic disorder but with symptoms intermediate in severity between the two and a course less protracted than that of dysthymic disorder.
mixed anxiety-depressive d. a mental disorder characterized by symptoms of depression and of anxiety, but not meeting the full criteria for either a depressive disorder or an anxiety disorder.
mixed receptive-expressive language d. [DSM-IV] a communication disorder involving both the expression and the comprehension of language, either spoken or signed. Patients have difficulties with language production, such as in the selection of words and the creation of appropriate sentences, and also have trouble understanding words, sentences, or specific types of words.
monogenic d. mendelian d.
mood d's [DSM-IV] mental disorders whose essential feature is a disturbance of mood manifested as one or more episodes of mania, hypomania, depression, or some combination. Functional mood disorders are subclassified as *bipolar disorders,* including bipolar I disorder, bipolar II disorder, and cyclothymic disorder; *depressive disorders,* including major depressive disorder and dysthymic disorder; *mood disorder due to a general medical condition*; and *substance-induced mood disorder.*
motor skills d. [DSM-IV] any disorder characterized by inadequate development of motor coordination severe enough to limit locomotion or restrict the ability to perform tasks, schoolwork, or other activities. Included is *developmental coordination d.*
movement d. any of numerous neurologic disorders characterized by disturbances of muscular movement, distinguished as either *hyperkinetic* (conditions such as chorea, dystonia, hemiballismus, myoclonus, stereotypy, tic, and tremor) or *hypokinetic* (conditions such as akinetic mutism, psychomotor retardation, and the stiff-man syndrome).
multifactorial d. a disorder caused by interaction of genetic factors and perhaps also nongenetic, environmental factors, e.g., some forms of birth defects and diabetes mellitus. See also *genetic disease,* under *disease.*
multiple personality d. dissociative identity d.
myeloproliferative d's a group of usually neoplastic diseases, which may be related histogenetically by a common multipotential stem cell, that includes among others acute and chronic granulocytic leukemias, acute and chronic myelomonocytic leukemias, polycythemia vera, and myelofibroerythroleukemia. An interrelationship with the lymphoproliferative disorders is thought to exist. Called also *myeloproliferative diseases* or *syndromes.*
narcissistic personality d. [DSM-IV] a personality disorder characterized by grandiosity (in fantasy or behavior), a lack of social empathy combined with a hypersensitivity to the judgment of others, interpersonal exploitiveness, enviousness, arrogance, a sense of entitlement, and a need for constant signs of admiration.
negativistic personality d. passive-aggressive personality d.
neuropsychologic d. any disorder in which brain dysfunction is manifested by disturbances in behavior or cognition.
neurotic d. neurosis.
nightmare d. [DSM-IV] a sleep disorder of the parasomnia group, consisting of repeated episodes of nightmares that awaken the sleeper, who rapidly becomes fully oriented and alert and can vividly recall the dreams. Onset is usually in childhood or adolescence, and children often outgrow the disorder. Called also *dream anxiety d.*
obsessive-compulsive d. (OCD) [DSM-IV] an anxiety disorder characterized by recurrent obsessions or compulsions that are severe enough to interfere significantly with personal or social functioning. Performing compulsive rituals may release tension temporarily, and resisting them causes increased tension. This disorder is not the same as *obsessive-compulsive personality disorder,* which is a personality disorder.
obsessive-compulsive personality d. [DSM-IV] a personality disorder characterized by an emotionally constricted manner that is unduly conventional, serious, rigid, stubborn, and stingy; by preoccupation with trivial details, rules, order, organization, schedules, and lists to the extent that the major point of an activity is lost or task completion is delayed; by reluctance to delegate tasks or work cooperatively unless everything is done one's own way; and by excessive devotion to work and productivity to the detriment of interpersonal relationships. This is not the same as *obsessive-compulsive disorder,* which is an anxiety disorder.
oppositional defiant d. [DSM-IV] a type of disruptive behavior disorder characterized by a recurrent pattern of defiant, hostile, disobedient, and negativistic behavior directed toward those in authority, including such actions as defying the requests or rules of adults, deliberately annoying others, arguing, spitefulness, and vindictiveness that occur much more frequently than would be expected on the basis of age and developmental stage.
organic anxiety d. see under *syndrome.*
organic mental d. a term formerly used to denote any mental disorder with a specifically known or presumed organic etiology; now discouraged because of the implication that other mental disorders do not have an organic basis. The term was also sometimes used to denote an organic mental syndrome (q.v.). Current classification divides these disorders into *delirium, dementia, and amnestic and other cognitive disorders; mental disorders due to a general medical condition;* and *substance-related disorders.*
organic personality d. see under *syndrome.*
orgasmic d's [DSM-IV] sexual dysfunctions characterized by inhibited or premature orgasm; see *female orgasmic d., male orgasmic d.,* and *premature ejaculation.*
overanxious d. former name for an anxiety disorder of childhood or adolescence, now subsumed by *generalized anxiety d.*
pain d. [DSM-IV] a somatoform disorder characterized by a chief complaint of severe chronic pain that causes substantial distress or impairment in functioning; the pain is neither feigned nor intentionally

produced, and psychological factors appear to play a major role in its onset, severity, exacerbation, or maintenance. It is subdivided into *pain d. associated with psychological factors* and *pain d. associated with both psychological factors and a general medical condition.* A third subtype, *pain d. associated with a general medical condition*, is not considered a mental disorder.

panic d. [DSM-IV] an anxiety disorder characterized by recurrent panic (anxiety) attacks, episodes of intense apprehension, fear, or terror associated with somatic symptoms such as dyspnea, hyperventilation, palpitations, dizziness, vertigo, faintness, or shakiness and with psychological symptoms such as feelings of unreality (depersonalization or derealization) or fears of dying, going insane, or losing control; there is usually chronic nervousness and tension between attacks. It is almost always associated with agoraphobia. (DSM-IV recognizes two types, *panic d. with agoraphobia* and *panic d. without agoraphobia.*) This disorder does not include panic attacks that may occur in phobias when the patient is exposed to the phobic stimulus.

paranoid d. delusional d.

paranoid personality d. [DSM-IV] a personality disorder marked by a view of other people as hostile, devious, and untrustworthy and a combative response to disappointments or to events experienced as rebuffs or humiliations. Notable are a questioning of the loyalty of friends, the bearing of grudges, a tendency to read threatening meanings into benign remarks, and unfounded suspicions of the fidelity of a partner. Unlike delusional disorder or paranoid schizophrenia, in which delusional or hallucinatory persecution occurs, it is not characterized by psychosis.

passive-aggressive personality d. a personality disorder characterized by an indirect resistance to demands for adequate social and occupational performance, such as by obstructionism, procrastination, or forgetfulness, and by negative, defeatist attitudes.

perforating d's acquired perforating dermatosis.

periodic leg movement d., periodic limb movement d. nocturnal myoclonus.

persistent genital arousal d. (PGAD) intense genital arousal occurring in the absence of subjective sexual interest or desire and persisting despite sexual activity or orgasm. Arousal is perceived as intrusive; it is usually only briefly diminished by orgasm and may even be exacerbated.

personality d's [DSM-IV] a category of mental disorders characterized by enduring, inflexible, and maladaptive personality traits that deviate markedly from cultural expectations, are self-perpetuating, pervade a broad range of situations, and either generate subjective distress or result in significant impairments in social, occupational, or other functioning. Onset is by adolescence or early adulthood.

pervasive developmental d's [DSM-IV] a group of disorders characterized by impairment of development in multiple areas, including the acquisition of reciprocal social interaction, verbal and nonverbal communication skills, and imaginative activity and by stereotyped interests and behaviors; included are *autistic disorder*, *Rett syndrome*, *childhood disintegrative disorder*, and *Asperger syndrome*.

phagocytic dysfunction d's a group of immunodeficiency conditions characterized by disordered phagocytic activity; disorders may be *extrinsic* (e.g., suppression of the number of phagocytes by immunosuppressive agents, or dysfunction caused by corticosteroids) or *intrinsic* (related to enzyme deficiencies). They are marked by bacterial or fungal infections that range from mild recurrent skin infection to fatal systemic infection. For a list of disorders of this type, see table at *immunodeficiency*.

phobic d's see *phobia*.

phonological d. [DSM-IV] a communication disorder of unknown etiology, characterized by failure to use age- and dialect-appropriate sounds in speaking, with errors occurring in the selection, production, or articulation of sounds. The most common errors are omissions, substitutions, and distortions of speech sounds.

plasma cell d's see under *dyscrasia*.

polyglutamine d's, polyQ d's any of the triplet repeat disorders in which a CAG triplet repeat sequence is expanded, yielding a large polyglutamine tract in the protein product. Although the affected protein differs, all have a toxic gain of function, the abnormal protein interfering with the normal protein, and causing damage to specific populations of neurons and neurotoxicity, with clinical onset in adulthood. Called also *polyglutamine diseases*.

postconcussional d. see under *syndrome*.

posttransplant lymphoproliferative d. see under *disease*.

posttraumatic stress d. (PTSD) [DSM-IV] an anxiety disorder caused by exposure to an intensely traumatic event; characterized by reexperiencing the traumatic event in recurrent intrusive recollections, nightmares, or flashbacks, by avoidance of trauma-associated stimuli, by generalized numbing of emotional responsiveness, and by hyperalertness and difficulty in sleeping, remembering, or concentrating. The onset of symptoms may be delayed for months to years after the event. Terms formerly used for disorders of this type include gross *stress reaction*, *shell shock*, and *combat*, *battle*, or *war exhaustion* or *fatigue*.

premenstrual dysphoric d. premenstrual syndrome viewed as a psychiatric disorder.

primary mental d. [DSM-IV] any of the mental disorders that are neither due to a general medical condition nor substance-induced.

psychoactive substance use d's substance use d's.

psychogenic pain d. pain d.

psychophysiologic d. psychosomatic d.

psychosexual d's sexual d's (def. 2).

psychosomatic d. a disorder in which the physical symptoms are caused or exacerbated by psychological factors, such as migraine headache, lower back pain, or irritable bowel syndrome. The synonym *psychophysiologic disorders*, used in previous official nomenclatures and defined as "physical disorders of presumably psychogenic origin," has been replaced in DSM-IV by the more neutral phrase *psychological factors affecting physical condition*, which may be applied to any physical condition judged to be adversely affected by one or more psychological or behavioral factors, and is subtyped on the basis of the specific factors involved.

psychotic d. [DSM-IV] psychosis (def. 1).

rapid eye movement sleep behavior d. REM sleep behavior d.

reactive attachment d. [DSM-IV] a mental disorder of infancy or early childhood, characterized by notably unusual and developmentally inappropriate social relatedness, usually associated with grossly pathological care. It may be the *inhibited type*, with failure to initiate or respond to social interactions, or the *disinhibited type*, with indiscriminate sociability or attachment.

reading d. [DSM-IV] a learning disorder (q.v.) in which the skill affected is reading ability, including accuracy, speed, and comprehension.

recurrent brief depressive d. short repeated episodes of depressive symptoms severe enough to qualify as major depressive episodes but of lesser duration, recurring at least once a month and not associated with the menstrual cycle.

REM sleep behavior d. (RBD) a sleep disorder of the parasomnia group characterized by abnormal electromyographic activity, altered dreams, and violent behaviors, often leading to self-injury, during REM sleep; it is often associated with α-synucleopathies.

rhythmic movement d. repetitive, rhythmic, stereotyped, large-muscle body or head movements occurring during the transition to sleep, such as in jactatio capitis nocturna; onset is usually in infancy and the disorder is usually outgrown by the age of five.

rumination d. [DSM-IV] an eating disorder seen in infants under one year of age; after a period of normal eating habits, the child begins excessive regurgitation and rechewing of food, which is then ejected from the mouth or reswallowed; if untreated, death from malnutrition may occur.

sadistic personality d. [DSM-IV] a pervasive pattern of cruel, demeaning, and aggressive behavior; satisfaction is gained in intimidating, coercing, humiliating, and inflicting pain and suffering on others.

schizoaffective d. [DSM-IV] a mental disorder in which a major depressive episode, manic episode, or mixed episode occurs along with prominent psychotic symptoms characteristic of schizophrenia, the symptoms of the mood disorder being present for a substantial portion of the illness, but not for its entirety, and the disturbance not being due to the effects of a psychoactive substance.

schizoid personality d. [DSM-IV] a personality disorder marked by detachment from social relationships and a restricted range of emotional experience and expression. Qualifying characteristics include lack of capacity for, or interest in, social relationships or family life, coldness, aloofness, consistent preference for solitary activities, lack of pleasure in activities, flattened affectivity, and indifference to praise, criticism, or the feelings of others.

schizophreniform d. [DSM-IV] a mental disorder with the signs and symptoms of schizophrenia but duration of less than 6 months.

Disorder *Continued*

schizotypal personality d. [DSM-IV] a personality disorder characterized by marked deficits in social and interpersonal competence and eccentricities in ideation, appearance, and behavior; ideas of reference are common, as are odd beliefs or magical thinking, cognitive or perceptual distortions, little capability or desire for close relationships, excessive social anxiety, suspiciousness, and occasional paranoid ideation. It differs from schizophrenia, to which it is related, in having only transient psychotic episodes, if any.
seasonal affective d. (SAD) a cyclically recurring mood disorder characterized by depression, extreme lethargy, increased need for sleep, hyperphagia, and carbohydrate craving; it intensifies in one or more specific seasons, most commonly the winter months, and is hypothesized to be related to melatonin levels. In DSM-IV terminology called *mood disorder with seasonal pattern*.
seasonal mood d. seasonal affective d.
self-defeating personality d. a persistent pattern of behavior detrimental to the self, including being drawn to problematic situations or relationships, failing to accomplish tasks crucial to life objectives, excessive self-sacrifice, inviting criticism and anger, undermining of pleasurable experiences, and inability to enjoy the rewards of success.
separation anxiety d. [DSM-IV] excessive, prolonged, developmentally inappropriate anxiety and apprehension in a child concerning removal from parents, home, or familiar surroundings.
sexual d's 1. any disorders involving sexual functioning, desire, or performance. 2. [DSM-IV] more specifically, any such disorders that are caused at least in part by psychological factors. Those characterized by decrease or other disturbance of sexual desire are called sexual dysfunctions, and those characterized by unusual or bizarre sexual fantasies, urges, or practices are called paraphilias. Called also *psychosexual d's*.
sexual arousal d's [DSM-IV] sexual dysfunctions characterized by alterations in sexual arousal; see *female sexual arousal d.* and *male erectile d.*
sexual aversion d. [DSM-IV] feelings of repugnance for and active avoidance of genital sexual contact with a partner, causing substantial distress or interpersonal difficulty.
sexual desire d's [DSM-IV] sexual dysfunctions characterized by alteration in sexual desire; see *hypoactive sexual desire d.* and *sexual aversion d.*
d. of sexual development (DSD) a congenital condition in which development of chromosomal, gonadal, or phenotypic sex is atypical.
sexual pain d's [DSM-IV] sexual dysfunctions characterized by pain associated with intercourse; they include dyspareunia and vaginismus not due to a general medical condition.
shared psychotic d. [DSM-IV] a delusional system that develops in one or more persons as a result of a close relationship with someone who already has a psychotic disorder with prominent delusions. Most commonly it involves two people and is called *folie à deux*. Involvement of three people would be *folie à trois* and so on.
simple deteriorative d. simple schizophrenia.
single-gene d. mendelian d.
sleep d's [DSM-IV] chronic disorders involving sleep. Primary sleep disorders comprise dyssomnias and parasomnias; causes of secondary sleep disorders may include a general medical condition, mental disorder, or psychoactive substance.
sleep terror d. [DSM-IV] a sleep disorder of the parasomnia group, consisting of repeated episodes of pavor nocturnus (sleep terrors).
sleep-wake schedule d. circadian rhythm sleep d.
sleepwalking d. [DSM-IV] a sleep disorder of the parasomnia group, consisting of repeated episodes of somnambulism.
social anxiety d. social phobia.
somatization d. [DSM-IV] a mental disorder characterized by multiple somatic complaints that cannot be fully explained by any known general medical condition or the direct effect of a substance, but are not intentionally feigned or produced, beginning before the age of 30 and occurring over several years. Complaints comprise a combination of at least multiple pain symptoms, multiple gastrointestinal symptoms, a sexual symptom, and a neurological symptom. They are often presented in a dramatic, vague, or exaggerated way, with involvement of numerous physicians, numerous diagnostic evaluations, and unnecessary medical treatment or surgery. Called also *Briquet syndrome*.
somatoform d's [DSM-IV] mental disorders characterized by symptoms suggesting a general medical condition but neither fully explained by a general medical condition, the direct effects of a psychoactive substance, or another mental disorder nor under voluntary control; this category includes *body dysmorphic disorder*, *conversion disorder*, *hypochondriasis*, *pain disorder*, *somatization disorder*, and *undifferentiated somatoform disorder*.
somatoform pain d. pain d.
speech d. defective ability to speak; it may be either psychogenic (see *communication d.*) or neurogenic. See also *language d.*.
stereotypic movement d. [DSM-IV] a mental disorder characterized by repetitive nonfunctional motor behavior, such as hand waving, rocking, head-banging, or self-biting, which often appears to be driven and can result in serious self-inflicted injuries.
substance-induced d's [DSM-IV] a subgroup of the substance-related disorders comprising a variety of behavioral or psychological anomalies resulting from ingestion of or exposure to a drug of abuse, medication, or toxin. Included are *substance intoxication*, *substance withdrawal*, *substance-induced delirium*, *substance-induced persisting dementia*, *substance-induced persisting amnestic disorder*, *substance-induced psychotic disorder*, *substance-induced mood disorder*, *substance-induced anxiety disorder*, *substance-induced sexual dysfunction*, and *substance-induced sleep disorder*. Specific disorders or groups are named on the basis of etiology, e.g., alcohol-induced disorders, alcohol intoxication. Cf. *substance use d's*.
substance-induced anxiety d. [DSM-IV] an anxiety disorder characterized by prominent anxiety, panic attacks, obsessions, or compulsions and directly due to the physiological effects of a psychogenic substance, including drugs of abuse, medications, and toxins. Individual cases are named for the specific substance involved.
substance-induced mood d. [DSM-IV] a prominent and lasting disturbance of mood, either manic, depressive, or both, due to direct physiological effects of a psychoactive substance, including medications, drugs of abuse, and toxins. Individual cases are named for the specific substance involved.
substance-induced persisting amnestic d. [DSM-IV] an amnestic disorder caused by the lasting effects of a drug of abuse, medication, or toxic substance, often remaining stable or even worsening long after exposure to the substance has ended. Individual cases are named for the specific substance involved.
substance-induced psychotic d. [DSM-IV] persistent delusions or hallucinations related to the use of a psychoactive substance, the patient being unaware of their etiology. Individual cases are named for the specific substance involved.
substance-induced sleep d. [DSM-IV] a disturbance of sleep due to the direct physiological effects of a psychoactive substance, including drugs of abuse, medications, and toxins; usually manifest as hypersomnia or insomnia but sometimes as a parasomnia or of mixed type. Individual disorders are named for the specific substance involved.
substance-related d's [DSM-IV] any of the mental disorders associated with excessive use of or exposure to psychoactive substances, including drugs of abuse, medications, and toxins. The group is divided into *substance use disorders* and *substance-induced disorders*, each of which is specified on the basis of etiology, e.g., alcohol use disorders. DSM-IV includes specific disorders for the classes alcohol, amphetamines or similarly acting sympathomimetics, caffeine, cannabis, cocaine, hallucinogens, inhalants, nicotine, opioids, PCP or similarly acting substances, and sedatives, hypnotics, or anxiolytics.
substance use d's [DSM-IV] a subgroup of the substance-related disorders (q.v.) in which psychoactive substance use or abuse repeatedly results in significantly adverse consequences. The group comprises *substance abuse* and *substance dependence*; specific disorders or groups of disorders are named on the basis of etiology, e.g., alcohol use disorders, alcohol abuse, and alcohol dependence.
temporomandibular d. (TMD), temporomandibular joint d. (TMJD) chronic facial pain associated with dysfunction of some combination of the temporomandibular joint, jaw muscles, and associated nerves. The most common symptoms include facial, neck, and shoulder pain, clicking or other sounds associated with jaw movement, limited jaw opening and locking of the jaw, headache, otalgia, neck and shoulder pain, and dizziness. TMD is often subdivided into *myogenous* and *arthrogenous* forms. The myogenous form is most often due to some combination of malocclusion, jaw clenching, bruxism, and physical and mental stress and anxiety. The arthrogenous form is usually caused by displacement of the articular disk, but may also be due to arthritis, ankylosis, dislocation, infection, neoplasia, or congenital anomaly. Called also *temporomandibular joint syndrome*.
thought d. a disturbance in the thought process that is most narrowly defined as disorganized thinking with altered associations, as is

Disorder *Continued*

characteristic of schizophrenia. The term is often used much more broadly to include any disturbance of thought, such as confusion, hallucinations, or delusions, which affects possession, quantity, or content of thought.

transient myeloproliferative d. usually transient leukocytosis associated with Down syndrome and generally diagnosed in the first few weeks of life, often with hepatosplenomegaly, pericardial and pleural effusions, hepatic disease, and a pustular rash. Although spontaneous remission occurs in most cases, some affected infants develop a myelodysplastic syndrome or acute leukemia. Called also *congenital leukemoid reaction* and *transient leukemia of infancy.*

trinucleotide repeat d's, triplet repeat d's disorders caused by unstable, dynamic mutations that result in expansion of triplet repeats within the affected gene, leading to abnormalities in gene expression and function. The disorders differ significantly in such factors as inheritance pattern; base sequence, size, and intragenic location of the affected repeat; and degree of expansion and of instability of the repeats; but the underlying mechanism appears to be slipped strand mispairing during DNA replication. The group includes Huntington disease, myotonic dystrophy, Friedreich ataxia, and fragile X syndrome.

undifferentiated somatoform d. [DSM-IV] one or more physical complaints, not intentionally produced or feigned and persisting for at least six months, that cannot be fully explained by a general medical condition or the direct effects of a substance; the category comprises persisting disorders that do not completely satisfy the criteria for other somatoform disorders.

unipolar d's depressive d's.

d. of written expression [DSM-IV] a learning disorder (q.v.) in which the affected skill is written communication, characterized by errors in spelling, grammar, or punctuation, by poor paragraph organization, or by poor story composition or thematic development.

---

dis•or•gan•iza•tion (dis-or″gən-ĭ-za′shən) the process of destruction of any organic tissue; any profound change in the tissues of an organ or structure which causes the loss of most or all of its proper characters.

dis•or•i•en•ta•tion (dis-or″e-ən-ta′shən) the loss of proper bearings, or a state of mental confusion as to time, place, or identity.

spatial d. a condition in which a pilot or other air crew member is unable to determine accurately his or her spatial attitude in relation to the surface of the Earth; it occurs only in conditions of poor visibility or when vision is otherwise restricted and results from vestibular illusions. Called also *pilot's vertigo.*

dis•ox•i•da•tion (dis″ok-sĭ-da′shən) deoxidation.

dis•par (dis′pahr) [L.] unequal.

dis•par•a•si•tized (dis-par′ə-sĭ-tīzd) freed from parasites. Cf. *disinfestation.*

dis•pa•rate (dis′pə-rāt) [L. *disparatus, dispar* unequal] not situated alike; not exactly paired; dissimilar in kind.

dis•pen•sa•ry (dis-pen′sə-re) [L. *dispensarium,* from *dispensare* to dispense] 1. a place where medical or dental skill, treatment, and remedies are provided for the indigent ambulant sick at little or no cost to them. 2. any place where drugs and medicines are actually dispensed.

dis•pen•sa•to•ry (dis-pen′sə-tor-e) [L. *dispensatorium*] a treatise on the qualities and composition of medicines.

D. of the United States of America a collection of monographs on unofficial drugs and drugs recognized by the United States Pharmacopoeia, the British Pharmacopoeia, and the National Formulary, and on general tests, processes, reagents, and solutions of the USP and NF, as well as drugs used in veterinary medicine.

dis•pense (dis-pens′) [L. *dispensare, dis-* out + *pensare* to weigh] to prepare and distribute medicines to those who are to use them.

Dis•per•Mox (dis′pər-moks) trademark for a preparation of amoxicillin.

di•sper•my (di′spər-me) the penetration of two spermatozoa into one oocyte.

dis•per•sate (dis′pər-sāt) a suspension of finely divided particles of a substance.

dis•perse (dis-purs′) [*dis-*[1] + L. *spargere* to scatter] 1. to scatter the component parts, as of a tumor or the fine particles in a colloid system. 2. the particles so scattered.

dis•per•si•ble (dis-pur′sĭ-bəl) capable of being dispersed.

dis•per•sion (dis-pur′zhən) [L. *dispersio*] 1. the act of scattering or separating; the condition of being scattered. 2. the incorporation of the particles of one substance into the body of another, comprising solutions, suspensions, and colloid systems. 3. a colloid system, particularly an unstable one.

colloid d. colloid system; see *colloid* (def. 2). Sometimes used specifically for an unstable colloid system.

molecular d. solution (def. 1).

temporal d. desynchronization of components of an evoked compound action potential as registered by the recording electrode, due to different rates of conduction of the fibers.

dis•per•si•ty (dis-pur′sĭ-te) the degree of dispersion of a colloid, i.e., the degree to which the dimensions of the dispersed particles have been reduced.

dis•per•sive (dis-pur′siv) 1. tending to become dispersed. 2. promoting dispersion.

dis•per•soid (dis-pur′soid) dispersion colloid.

dis•pert (dis′pərt) a medicinal preparation obtained from a vegetable drug or endocrine gland by extracting its therapeutic constituents in the cold and then reducing the product to a dry concentrated form.

Dis•phol•i•dus (dis-fol′ĭ-dəs) a genus of venomous snakes of the family Colubridae. *D. ty′pus* is the boomslang of South Africa. See table at *snake.*

dis•place•a•bil•i•ty (dis-plās″ə-bil′ĭ-te) the quality of being susceptible to movement from an initial position, or the degree to which such movement is possible.

dis•place•ment (dis-plās′mənt) 1. malposition. 2. percolation. 3. a defense mechanism in which emotions, ideas, wishes, or impulses are unconsciously shifted from their original object to a more acceptable, usually less threatening, substitute. 4. in dentistry, the malposition of the crown and root of one or more teeth from the normal line of occlusion; also the deflection of the mandible from its normal path of closure, i.e., posterior displacement. 5. in a chemical reaction, the replacement of one atom or group in a molecule by another.

character d. the adaptive characters that evolve and enable one species to exclude another from its ecological niche. See also *competitive exclusion,* under *exclusion.*

condylar d. an abnormal position of the head of the mandibular condyle in the fossa due to a deviation or shift of the mandible, which is often the result of malocclusion.

fetal d. a group of cells that becomes displaced from its normal relations during fetal development.

gallbladder d. wandering gallbladder.

left d. of the abomasum (LDA) displacement of the abomasum of a cow to the left, underneath the rumen, with abomasal atony, usually soon after birth of a calf. It may be due to previous pressure from the gravid uterus or to abomasal distention from a high-grain diet. Symptoms include anorexia, drop in milk production, and ketosis.

right d. of the abomasum (RDA) displacement of the abomasum of a cow to the right, with abomasal atony, usually soon after birth of a calf; it is sometimes due to obstruction of the pylorus. Symptoms include anorexia, drop in milk production, and a palpable fluid-filled organ on the right flank. It may progress to abomasal torsion, an emergency situation.

tissue d. change in the position of tissues as the result of pressure or other force.

di•spore (di′spor) in fungi, either of the spores of a two-spored basidium; cf. *tetraspore.*

di•spo•rous (di′spor-əs) having two spores, as the basidia of the higher fungi.

dis•po•si•tion (dis″pə-zĭsh′ən) 1. a tendency, physical or mental, toward a disease. 2. the prevailing temperament or character, giving a degree of predictability to the response to a situation or other stimulus.

dis•pro•por•tion (dis″pro-por′shən) a lack of the proper relationship between two elements or factors.

cephalopelvic d. a condition in which the head of the fetus is too large to permit passage through the pelvis of the mother.

dis•rup•tion (dis-rup′shən) [L. *diruptio* a bursting apart] a morphologic defect of an organ or larger region of the body, resulting from the extrinsic

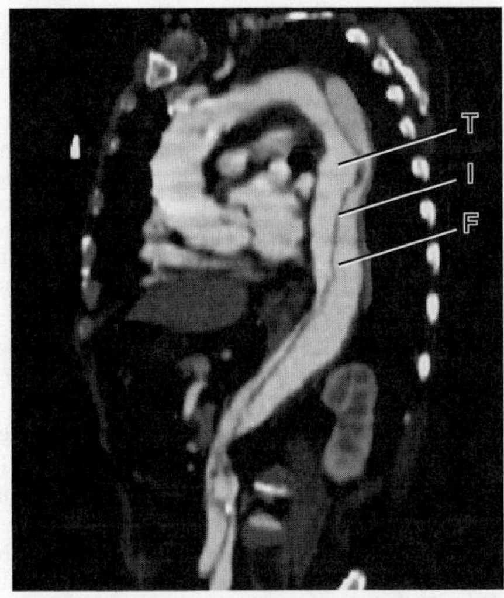

■ Aortic dissection of the descending thoracic aorta, in a reformatted left anterior oblique view of a contrast-enhanced CT angiogram. The intimal flap originates beyond the left subclavian artery and extends distally well into the abdominal aorta. The true lumen *(T)* and false lumen *(F)* are separated by the dark intimal flap *(I)*.

breakdown of, or interference with, an originally normal developmental process.

dis•rup•tive (dis-rup′tiv) 1. bursting apart; rending. 2. causing confusion or disorder.

Dis•se spaces (dis′ə) [Joseph *Disse*, German anatomist, 1852–1912] perisinusoidal spaces; see under *space.*

dis•sect (dĭ-sekt′, di-sekt′) [L. *dissecare* to cut up] 1. to cut apart or separate, as by surgery or trauma. 2. to expose structures of a cadaver for anatomical study.

dis•sec•tion (dĭ-sek′shən) [L. *dissectio*] 1. the act of dissecting. 2. a part or whole of an organism prepared by dissecting.

aortic d. dissecting aneurysm affecting the aorta, usually the thoracic aorta but sometimes the abdominal aorta.

axillary d., axillary lymph node d. surgical removal of axillary lymph nodes, done as part of radical mastectomy.

blunt d. dissection accomplished by separating tissues along natural cleavage lines, without cutting.

endoscopic submucosal d. a minimally invasive procedure for removal of polyps or tumors in the gastrointestinal tract, with excision down to the middle and deep layers of mucosa.

lymph node d. lymphadenectomy.

partial zona d. (PZD) an older micromanipulation technique used in male factor infertility; a cut is made into the zona pellucida and spermatozoa are inserted.

radical neck d. resection of a tumor in the neck along with an additional margin of at least 2 cm, as well as cervical lymphadenectomy.

sharp d. dissection accomplished by incising tissues with a sharp edge.

dis•sec•tor (dĭ-sek′tər) 1. one who dissects. 2. an instrument for dissecting. 3. a handbook used as a guide for the act of dissecting.

ultrasonic d. an instrument with a metal tip that vibrates at ultrasonic frequency and fragments parenchymal cells while leaving vessels intact. Cf. *CUSA.*

water-jet d. an instrument consisting of a nozzle that projects a fine stream of water under high pressure and a suction tube, used in hepatic resection to fragment liver parenchyma while sparing the hepatic vessels.

dis•sem•i•nat•ed (dĭ-sem′ĭ-nāt″əd) [*dis-* + *seminare* to sow] scattered; distributed over a considerable area.

dis•sep•i•ment (dĭ-sep′ĭ-mənt) partition; separation.

dis•sim•i•late (dĭ-sim′ĭ-lāt) [*dis-*[1] + *similare* to make alike] to decompose a substance into simpler compounds, for the production of energy or of materials that can be eliminated.

dis•sim•i•la•tion (dĭ-sim″ĭ-la′shən) the act or process of dissimilating (see *dissimilate*); the reverse of assimilation.

dis•so•ci•able (dĭ-so′shə-bəl) easily separable into component parts; separable from associations.

dis•so•ci•a•tion (dĭ-so″se-a′shən) [*dis-*[1] + *sociatio* union] 1. the act of separating or state of being separated. 2. the separation of a molecule into two or more fragments (atoms, molecules, ions, or free radicals) produced by the absorption of light or thermal energy or by solvation. 3. segregation of a group of mental processes from the rest of a person's usually integrated functions of consciousness, memory, perception, and sensory and motor behavior, as in the separation of the personality and aspects of memory or subpersonalities in the dissociative disorders (q.v.) or in the segregation of an idea or object from its emotional significance, as is sometimes seen in schizophrenia. **disso′ciative** *adj*

albuminocytologic d. increase of protein with normal cell count in the spinal fluid.

atrial d. independent beating of the left and right atria, each with normal rhythm or with various combinations of normal rhythm, atrial flutter, or atrial fibrillation.

atrioventricular d., AV d. control of the atria by one pacemaker and of the ventricles by another, independent pacemaker; it may be due to heart block, to severe slowing of the sinus rhythm with activation of an ectopic pacemaker, to acceleration of an ectopic pacemaker that usurps control of the ventricles, or to a combination of factors. See also *interference atrioventricular d.* and *isorhythmic atrioventricular d.*

bacterial d. the change, due to mutation and selection, in colonial morphology (usually from mucoid or smooth to rough) of bacteria in culture on laboratory media; called also *microbic d.* See also *smooth-rough variation*, under *variation.*

electromechanical d. pulseless electrical activity.

interference d., interference atrioventricular d. a form of atrioventricular dissociation in which an accelerated junctional or ventricular pacemaker usurps control of the ventricles and rapidly bombards the atrioventricular node from below, rendering the node refractory to supraventricular impulses.

isorhythmic atrioventricular d. a form of atrioventricular dissociation in which the atria and ventricles beat at similar rates, although independently; it usually results from severe sinus bradycardia in which the sinus node discharge rate drops just below that of the atrioventricular junctional tissue.

light-near d. an abnormality of pupillary reflexes in which the pupil constricts more with convergence on a near object than it does in response to light; see *tonic pupil*, under *pupil.*

microbic d. bacterial d.

syringomyelic d. loss of pain and temperature sense due to a lesion in the region of the central canal of the spinal cord implicating the spinothalamic fibers with preservation of other sensory modalities.

tabetic d. disturbance of the vibratory and muscle-tendon sensibility due to lesion of the dorsal columns.

dis•sog•e•ny (dĭ-soj′ə-ne) [Gr. *dissos* twofold + *-geny*] the state of having sexual maturity in both a larval and an adult stage.

dis•so•lu•tion (dis″o-loo′shən) [L. *dissolvere* to dissolve] 1. the process in which one substance is dissolved in another. 2. separation of a compound into its components by chemical action. 3. liquefaction. 4. the process of loosening or relaxing. 5. death.

dis•solve (dĭ-zolv′) 1. to cause a substance to pass into solution. 2. to pass into solution.

dis•sol•vent (dĭ-zol′vənt) 1. a solvent medium. 2. a medicine capable of dissolving concretions within the body. 3. solvent; capable of dissolving substances.

dis•so•nance (dis′o-nəns) discord or disagreement.

cognitive d. anxiety or other unpleasant feelings resulting from a lack of agreement between a person's established ideas, beliefs, and attitudes and some more recently acquired information or experience.

Dist. [L.] distil′la (distill).

dis•tad (dis′tad) in a distal direction.

dis•tal (D) (dis′təl) [L. *distans* distant] 1. remote; farther from any point of reference; opposed to proximal. 2. in dentistry, a position on the dental arch farther from the median line of the jaw.

dis•ta•lis (dis-ta′lis) [TA] distal; a term denoting remoteness from the point of origin or attachment of an organ or part.

dis•tal•ly (dis′tə-le) in a distal direction.

dis•tance (dis′təns) the measure of space intervening between two objects or two points of reference.

angular d. the aperture of the angle made at the eye by lines drawn from the eye to two objects.

focal d. the distance from the focal point to the optical center of a lens or the surface of a concave mirror.

infinite d. in ophthalmology, a distance of 20 feet or more: so called because rays entering the eye from an object at that distance are practically as parallel as if they came from a point at an infinite distance.

interarch d. 1. the vertical distance between the maxillary and mandibular arches (alveolar or residual) under certain conditions of vertical dimension that must be specified. 2. the vertical distance between the maxillary and mandibular ridges; called also *interridge d.*

interdomal d. the distance between the nasal domes over the major alar cartilages, often calculated for purposes of rhinoplasty.

interocclusal d. the distance between the occluding surfaces of the maxillary and mandibular teeth when the mandible is in physiologic rest position; called also *freeway space* and *interocclusal clearance*, *gap*, and *space*.

interocular d. the distance between the two eyes, usually used in reference to the interpupillary distance.

interpediculate d. the distance between the vertebral pedicles as measured on the radiograph.

interpupillary d. the distance between the centers of the pupils of the two eyes when the visual axes are parallel; in practice usually measured from the lateral margin of one pupil to the medial margin of the other.

interridge d. interarch d.

map d. the distance between two genetic loci on a linkage map, measured in centimorgans.

source-skin d. (SSD) the distance from the focal spot on the target of the x-ray tube to the skin of the subject, as measured along the central ray.

target-skin d. source-skin d.

working d. the distance between the front lens of a microscope and the object when the instrument is correctly focused.

dis•tan•tia (dis-tan′shə) distance.

d. intercrista′lis [TA] intercristal distance: the distance between the middle points of the iliac crests; called also *intercristal diameter*.

d. interspino′sa [TA] interspinous distance: the greatest width between the anterior superior iliac spines; called also *interspinous diameter*.

d. intertrochante′rica [TA] the distance across the pelvic region between the greater trochanters of the femurs.

dis•tem•per (dis-tem′pər) a name for several infectious diseases of animals, especially canine distemper.

canine d. an infectious respiratory and sometimes gastrointestinal disease of dogs, caused by a paramyxovirus and characterized by fever, dullness, loss of appetite, and a discharge from the eyes and nose. It is caused by a virus and it is also infectious for foxes and ferrets. Called also *hard pad disease*.

cat d. panleukopenia.

colt d., equine d. strangles (def. 1).

feline d. panleukopenia.

horse d. strangles (def. 1).

dis•tem•per•oid (dis-tem′pər-oid) an attenuated canine distemper virus that has been subjected to several passages in ferrets; called also *Green distemperoid*.

dis•tend (dis-tend′) to expand outward owing to pressure from within; cf. *dilate*.

dis•ten•si•bil•i•ty (dis-ten″sĭ-bil′ĭ-te) 1. capability of being distended. 2. elastance.

dis•ten•tion (dis-ten′shən) the state of being distended or enlarged; the act of distending.

dis•tich•ia (dis-tik′e-ə) distichiasis.

dis•ti•chi•a•sis (dis″tĭ-ki′ə-sis) [Gr. *distichia* a double line] the presence of a double row of eyelashes on an eyelid, one or both of which are turned in against the eyeball.

dis•ti•chous (dis′tĭ-kəs) arranged in two vertical rows; said of the arrangement of leaves where the leaf at one node is opposite to those just above and below it.

dis•till (dis-til′) [L. *destillare, from de* from + *stillare* to drop] to volatilize by heat and then cool and condense the evaporated matter, as to purify a substance or to separate a volatile substance from other less volatile substances.

dis•til•late (dis′til-āt) material that has been obtained by distillation.

dis•til•la•tion (dis″tĭ-la′shən) the process of vaporizing and condensing a substance to purify the substance or to separate a volatile substance from less volatile substances. Called also *vaporization*.

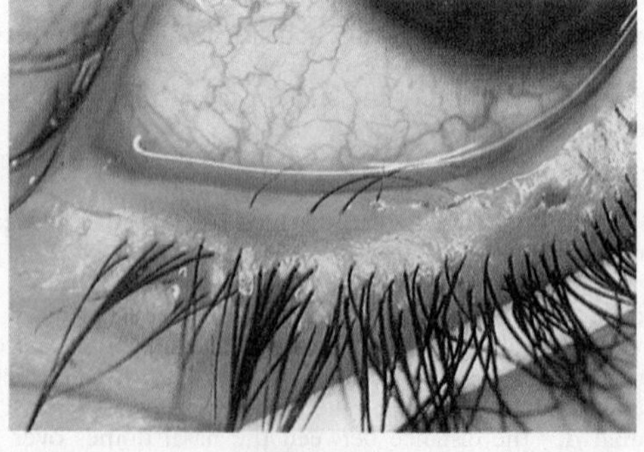

■ Distichiasis.

destructive d., dry d. decomposition of a solid by heating in the absence of air, which results in volatile liquid products.

fractional d. distillation in which volatilizable substances are separated in the order of their respective volatility.

molecular d. a process of purification applied to drugs and pharmaceuticals during which the crude material is evaporated under high vacuum of about one millionth of an atmosphere, and the condensate is caught on a cooled surface held close in front of the evaporating layer. The process is applied currently to vitamins A, D, and E, to animal and vegetable sterols and hormones, and to drugs and intermediates.

vacuum d. distillation under reduced pressure to avoid the decomposition which might occur at atmospheric pressure.

dis•to•ax•io•gin•gi•val (dis″to-ak″se-o-jin′jĭ-vəl) 1. pertaining to the line angle formed by the axial and gingival walls of a cavity preparation on the distal aspect of a tooth. 2. axiodistogingival.

dis•to•ax•io•in•ci•sal (dis″to-ak″se-o-in-si′zəl) pertaining to or formed by the distal, axial, and incisal walls of a tooth cavity preparation.

dis•to•ax•io•oc•clu•sal (dis″to-ak″se-o-ə-kloo′zəl) pertaining to or formed by the distal, axial, and occlusal walls of a tooth cavity preparation.

dis•to•buc•cal (dis″to-buk′əl) pertaining to or formed by the distal and buccal surfaces of a tooth, or by the distal and buccal walls of a tooth cavity preparation. Called also *buccodistal*.

dis•to•buc•co•oc•clu•sal (dis″to-buk″o-ə-kloo′zəl) pertaining to or formed by the distal, buccal, and occlusal surfaces of a tooth.

dis•to•buc•co•pul•pal (dis″to-buk″o-pul′pəl) pertaining to or formed by the distal, buccal, and pulpal walls of a tooth cavity preparation.

dis•to•cer•vi•cal (dis″to-sur′vĭ-kəl) 1. pertaining to the distal surface of the neck of a tooth. 2. distogingival.

dis•to•cli•na•tion (dis″to-klĭ-na′shən) deviation of a tooth from the vertical, in the direction of the tooth next distal (posterior) to it in the dental arch.

dis•to•clu•sal (dis″to-kloo′zəl) disto-occlusal.

dis•to•clu•sion (dis″to-kloo′zhən) [*distal* + L. *cludere* to close] malocclusion in which the mandibular arch is in a posterior (distal) position in relation to the maxillary arch. Generally considered identical with Class II in Angle classification of malocclusion (see *malocclusion*). Called also *disto-occlusion*, *posterior occlusion*, *posteroclusion*, and *retrusive occlusion*.

dis•to•gin•gi•val (dis″to-jin′jĭ-vəl) pertaining to or formed by the distal and gingival walls of a tooth cavity preparation; called also *distocervical*.

dis•to•la•bi•al (dis″to-la′be-əl) pertaining to or formed by the distal and labial surfaces of a tooth, or the distal and labial walls of a tooth cavity preparation.

dis•to•la•bio•in•ci•sal (dis″to-la″be-o-in-si′zəl) pertaining to or formed by the distal, labial, and incisal surfaces of a tooth.

dis•to•lin•gual (dis″to-ling′gwəl) pertaining to or formed by the distal and lingual surfaces of a tooth, or the distal and lingual walls of a tooth cavity preparation.

dis•to•lin•guo•in•ci•sal (dis″to-ling″gwo-in-si′zəl) pertaining to or formed by the distal, lingual, and incisal surfaces of a tooth.

dis•to•lin•guo•oc•clu•sal (dis″to-ling″gwo-o-kloo′zəl) pertaining to or formed by the distal, lingual, and occlusal surfaces of a tooth.

dis•to•lin•guo•pul•pal (dis″to-ling″gwo-pul′pəl) pertaining to or formed by the distal, lingual, and pulpal walls of a tooth cavity preparation.

di•sto•mia (di-sto′me-ə) the presence of two mouths.

dis•to•mi•a•sis (dis″to-mi′ə-sis) trematodiasis.

pulmonary d. paragonimiasis.

dis•to•mo•lar (dis″to-mo′lər) a supernumerary molar; any tooth found distal to a third molar.

di•sto•mus (di-sto′məs) [*di-* + *stoma*] a fetus having a double mouth.

dis•to•oc•clu•sal (dis″to-ə-kloo′zəl) pertaining to or formed by the distal and occlusal surfaces of a tooth, or the distal and occlusal walls of a tooth cavity preparation; called also *distoclusal*.

dis•to•oc•clu•sion (dis″to-ə-kloo′zhən) distoclusion.

dis•to•place•ment (dis″to-plās′mənt) displacement of a tooth distally.

dis•to•pul•pal (dis″to-pul′pəl) pertaining to or formed by the distal and pulpal walls of a tooth cavity preparation.

dis•to•pul•po•la•bi•al (dis″to-pul″po-la′be-əl) pertaining to or formed by the distal, pulpal, and labial walls of a tooth cavity preparation.

dis•to•pul•po•lin•gual (dis″to-pul″po-ling′gwəl) pertaining to or formed by the distal, pulpal, and lingual walls of a tooth cavity preparation.

dis•tor•tion (dis-tor′shən) [*dis-*[1] + *torsio* a twisting] 1. the state of being twisted out of a natural or normal shape or position. 2. in psychiatry, the process of altering or disguising unconscious ideas or impulses so that they become acceptable to the conscious mind. 3. in optics or radiology, deviation of an image from the true outline or shape of an object or structure.

barrel d. outward bowing of gridded straight lines in an image, resulting from lens distortion such that the lateral magnification at the center of the image is greater than that at the edges. Cf. *pincushion d.*

parataxic d. Harry Stack Sullivan's term for distortions in judgment and perception, particularly in interpersonal relations, based upon the perception of objects and relationships in accord with patterns from earlier experience.

pincushion d. inward bowing of gridded straight lines in an image as a result of lens distortion, the image of a square object thus resembling a pincushion or pillow. Cf. *barrel d.*

dis·tor·tor (dis-tor'tər) [L.] something that distorts.

d. o'ris musculus zygomaticus minor.

dis·to·ver·sion (dis″to-vur'zhən) the position of a tooth which is farther than normal from the median line of the face along the dental arch.

dis·trac·ti·bil·i·ty (dis-trak″tĭ-bil'ĭ-te) inability to focus one's attention on the task at hand; the attention is too frequently drawn to irrelevant and unimportant environmental stimuli.

dis·trac·tion (dis-trak'shən) [L. *distrahere* to draw apart] 1. a state in which the attention is diverted from the main portion of an experience or is divided among various portions of it. 2. a form of dislocation in which the joint surfaces have been separated without rupture of their binding ligaments and without displacement. 3. excessive space between fracture fragments due to interposed tissue or too forceful traction. 4. surgical separation of the two parts of a bone after the bone is transected. 5. unusual width of the dental arch; placement of the teeth or other maxillary or mandibular structures farther than normal from the median plane. See also *contraction* (def. 3).

dis·tress (dis-tres') [L. *distringere* to draw apart] physical or mental anguish or suffering.

idiopathic respiratory d. of newborn respiratory distress syndrome of newborn.

dis·tri·bu·tion (dis″trĭ-bu'shən) [L. *distributio*] 1. the specific location or arrangement of continuing or successive objects or events in space or time. 2. the extent of a ramifying structure such as an artery or nerve and its branches. 3. the geographical range of an organism or disease. 4. probability d. 5. in statistics, a synonym for *law;* for entries not found here, see under *law.*

Bernoulli d. binomial d.

binomial d. the probability distribution that describes the frequencies of the different possible combinations of two alternative outcomes in a series of n independent trials; it is given by expansion of the binomial $(p + q)^n$, where one of the two alternative outcomes has probability of p and the other of $q = 1 - p$.

χ^2 d., chi-square d. a theoretical probability distribution of the sum of the squares of a number (k) of normally distributed variables whose mean is 0 and standard deviation is 1; the parameter k is the number of degrees of freedom. Cf. *chi-square test.*

density d. frequency d.

dose d. in radiology, a representation of the variation of dose with position in any region of an irradiated object.

exponential d. a skewed probability distribution with right tail extending to infinity and having the density function

$$f(x) = \lambda e^{-\lambda x}$$

for $x \geq 0$ and $\lambda > 0$. The mean is $1/\lambda$ and the variance is $(1/\lambda)^2$. The mode is at zero and the larger the parameter λ, the more clustered the distribution toward zero. The exponential distribution arises in medicine and reliability as the time to mortality/morbidity or failure; λ is often interpreted as the force of mortality or failure.

F-d. the ratio of two independent chi-square distributions; the exact sampling distribution of the ratio of variances from two independent samples from identical normal distributions.

frequency d. a presentation, such as a table or graph, describing the relative frequency or theoretical probability of a random variable assuming any value in the range of possible values.

gaussian d. normal d.

log-normal d. a distribution of a random variable x such that $y = \ln x$ has a normal distribution; it is often used to model incubation times for diseases.

normal d. a symmetric, bell-shaped probability distribution having the density function

$$f(x) = \frac{1}{\sqrt{2\pi}\sigma} e^{-(x-\mu)^2/2\sigma^2}$$

where x is the abscissa, $f(x)$ is the ordinate, e is the base of natural logarithms (2.718), μ is the mean, and σ is the standard deviation. The normal distribution is entirely dependent on μ and σ; it is symmetric about the mean,

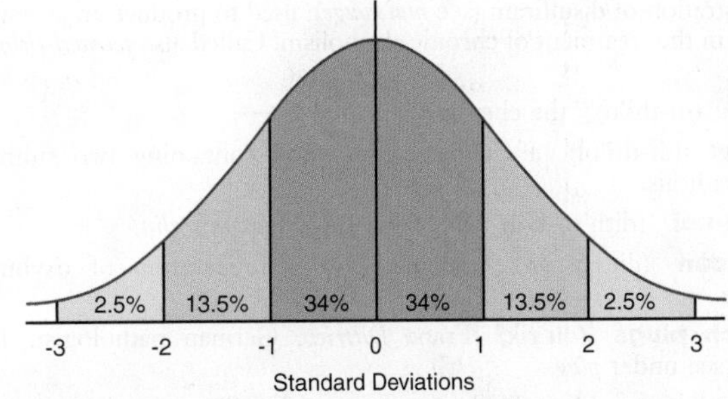

■ Normal distribution. The approximate percentage of the area (or frequency) lying under the curve between standard deviations is indicated.

with both tails extending to infinity; and the mean, the median, and the mode are identical. Roughly speaking, the normal distribution characterizes a random variable that is the sum of a large number of independent random effects. More precisely, it is typically the limiting distribution of a standardized sum of an infinite series of random variables with finite variance, each making a negligible contribution to the total variance (a fact known as the central limit theorem, q.v.). For this reason it is common statistical practice to assume that random sampling distributions of statistical measures are "approximately normal" and apply tests (e.g., *t*-test, analysis of variance) based on the normal distribution. See illustration. Called also *gaussian d.*

Poisson d. the probability distribution that describes counts of events randomly distributed in time or space, such as radioactive decay or blood cell counts. The probability of observing exactly k events in a fixed time period or region is

$$f(k) = \frac{\lambda^k e^{-\lambda}}{k!}$$

where λ is the average density of events in a period or region of that size and e is the base of natural logarithms (2.718). The mean and variance of the distribution are both equal to λ, thus the coefficient of variation for a Poisson distribution is

$$1/\sqrt{\lambda}$$

(the variability of the count is inversely proportional to the square root of the average count).

probability d. a mathematical function that assigns to each measurable event in a sample space the probability that the event will occur.

skew d. a frequency distribution that is asymmetric.

standard normal d. the normal distribution with mean 0 and standard deviation 1.

***t*-d.** the probability distribution of the statistic

$$t = \frac{\bar{X} - \mu}{s/\sqrt{n}},$$

where $\bar{X}$ and s are the mean and standard deviations of a sample of size n taken from a population with a normal distribution having mean μ; used in the *t*-test (q.v.). It is symmetric about zero and approaches the normal distribution as the sample size increases. Written also t *distribution.*

Weibull d. a skewed unimodal probability distribution for nonnegative variables, characterized by the parameters of shape and scale. It can be used for negatively skewed data; common uses include modeling lifespans of materials and modeling incubation times for diseases such as AIDS.

dis·tri·chi·a·sis (dis″trĭ-ki'ə-sis) [*dis*[2] + *trich-* + *-iasis*] a condition in which two hairs grow from a single follicle.

dis·tur·bance (dis-tur'bəns) a departure or divergence from that which is considered normal.

emotional d. see under *illness.*

transient situational d. acute stress reaction.

di·sub·sti·tut·ed (di-sub'stĭ-to͞ot″əd) having two atoms in each molecule replaced by other atoms or radicals.

di·sul·fate (di-sul'fāt) a compound containing two sulfate ions or radicals, as in titanium disulfate, $Ti(SO_4)_2$ (not to be confused with bisulfate).

di·sul·fide (di-sul'fīd) a compound of a base with two atoms of sulfur; see also under *bond.*

di·sul·fide isom·er·ase (di-sul'fīd i-som'ər-ās) protein disulfide-isomerase.

di·sul·fi·ram (di-sul'fĭ-ram) [USP] an antioxidant that inhibits the oxidation of the acetaldehyde metabolized from alcohol, resulting in high concentrations of acetaldehyde in the body. Extremely uncomfortable symptoms occur when alcohol is ingested subsequent to the oral administration of disulfiram (see *mal rouge*); used to produce an aversion to alcohol in the treatment of chronic alcoholism. Called also *tetraethylthiuram disulfide.*

di·thio (di-thi′o) the chemical group —S_2—.

di·thi·ol (di-thi′ol) a chemical compound containing two sulfhydryl (thiol) radicals.

dith·ra·nol (dith′rə-nol) INN and BAN for *anthralin.*

Dit·ro·pan (dit′ro-pan) trademark for a preparation of oxybutynin chloride.

Dit·trich plugs (dit′rik) [Franz *Dittrich*, German pathologist, 1815–1859] see under *plug.*

Dit·y·len·chus (dit″ə-len′kəs) a genus of small nematodes.

D. dip′saci the stem and bulb eelworm, a parasite of various grains, grasses, and bulbs, such as lilies, hyacinths, gladioli, narcissi, and onions; when ingested with the latter, it may be found as a pseudoparasite in the feces. Called also *Anguillulina putrefaciens.*

Di·u·car·din (di″u-kahr′din) trademark for a preparation of hydroflumethiazide.

Di·u·pres (di′u-prəs) trademark for combination preparations of chlorothiazide and reserpine.

di·ure·ide (di-u′re-īd) see *ureide.*

di·urese (di″u-rēs′) to bring about diuresis.

di·ure·sis (di″u-re′sis) pl. *diure′ses* [Gr. *diourein* to urinate, to pass in urine] increased excretion of urine. Cf. *polyuria.*

osmotic d. diuresis resulting from the presence of nonabsorbable or poorly absorbable, osmotically active substances (mannitol, urea, glucose, etc.) in the renal tubules.

pressure d. increased urinary excretion of water when there is an increase of arterial pressure, a compensatory mechanism to maintain blood pressure within the normal range. See also *pressure natriuresis*, under *natriuresis.*

di·uret·ic (di″u-ret′ik) [Gr. *diourētikos* promoting urine] 1. pertaining to or causing diuresis. 2. an agent that promotes diuresis.

high-ceiling d's, loop d's agents that inhibit the reabsorption of sodium and water in the thick ascending limb of the loop of Henle. They promote a high level of diuresis and their effect is not altered by acid-base imbalances or hypoalbuminemia. Used in the treatment of edema associated with congestive heart failure, acute pulmonary edema, or hepatic or renal disease and, alone or in combination with other drugs, in the treatment of hypertension.

osmotic d's diuretics such as mannitol that are filtered at the glomerulus and reabsorbed in the renal tubule only to a limited extent; they thus increase the amount of osmotically active solute in the urine with a corresponding increase in urine volume, and increase the osmolality of plasma. They also increase diffusion of water from the intraocular and cerebrospinal fluids and so are often used for reducing the pressure and volume of these fluids.

potassium-sparing d's a class of drugs that block the exchange of sodium for potassium and hydrogen ions in the distal tubule, causing an increase in the excretion of sodium and chloride with a negligible increase in potassium excretion; used in the treatment of edema and hypertension, usually as adjuncts to enhance the action and counteract the kaliuretic effects of thiazide and loop diuretics, and in the prophylaxis and treatment of hypokalemia.

thiazide d's a group of synthetic compounds that cause diuresis by altering electrolyte reabsorption at the distal tubules and increase urinary excretion of sodium and chloride in approximately equal amounts; they are used to treat edema, hypertension, and diabetes insipidus. The class of drugs is sometimes extended to include compounds which act like thiazide diuretics but are chemically dissimilar.

di·uria (di-u′re-ə) [L. *dies* day + *urine*] urinary frequency during the day.

Di·uril (di′u-ril) trademark for preparations of chlorothiazide.

di·ur·nal (di-ur′nəl) [L. *dies* day] occurring during the day.

Di·u·ten·sen-R (di″u-ten′sən) trademark for a combination preparation of methyclothiazide and reserpine.

Div. [L.] div′ide (divide).

di·va·ga·tion (di″və-ga′shən) rambling, incoherent speech and thought.

di·va·lent (di-va′lent) having a valence of two; bivalent.

di·val·pro·ex so·di·um (di-val′pro-eks) [USP] a coordination compound of valproate sodium and valproic acid in a 1:1 molar relationship, used in the treatment of manic episodes associated with bipolar disorder and epileptic seizures, particularly absence seizures, and the prophylaxis of migraine; administered orally.

di·var·i·ca·tion (di-var″ĭ-ka′shən) 1. divergence. 2. diastasis.

di·ver·gence (di-vur′jəns) a spreading or tending apart; in ophthalmology, the simultaneous abduction of both eyes.

negative vertical d. (–V.D.) the condition in which the visual line of the left eye deviates upward or the visual line of the right eye deviates downward.

positive vertical d. (+V.D.) the condition in which the visual line of the right eye deviates upward, or the visual line of the left eye deviates downward.

di·ver·gent (di-vur′jənt) [L. *divergens; dis-* apart + *vergere* to tend] tending apart; deviating or radiating away from a common point.

di·ver·sion (dĭ-vur′zhən) a turning aside.

antigenic d. the change in the antigenic structure of tumor cells or tissue to that normally found in different cells or tissue.

biliopancreatic d. a surgical treatment for morbid obesity consisting of resection of the distal two thirds of the stomach and attachment of the ileum to a stoma so that the entire duodenum and jejunum are bypassed; the duodenum and jejunum empty their secretions into the distal ileum through a new stoma. Called also *biliopancreatic bypass.*

continent urinary d. urinary diversion that preserves continence; examples include neobladders, ureterocolonic and ureterosigmoid anastomoses, the Indiana pouch, and the Mainz pouch.

partial external biliary d. a treatment for progressive familial intrahepatic cholestasis consisting of surgical placement of a tube connecting the gallbladder and the skin in order to drain off approximately half of the bile flow.

urinary d. surgical creation of an alternate route of flow for urine to replace an absent or diseased portion of the lower urinary tract in order to preserve renal function. See *ileal conduit*, under *conduit*, and see *continent urinary d.*

di·ver·tic·u·la (di″vər-tik′u-lə) [L.] plural of *diverticulum.*

di·ver·tic·u·lar·iza·tion (di″vər-tik″u-lər-ĭ-za′shən) the act of forming diverticula or pockets.

di·ver·tic·u·lec·to·my (di″vər-tik″u-lek′tə-me) [*diverticulum* + *-ectomy*] excision of a diverticulum.

di·ver·tic·u·li·tis (di″vər-tik″u-li′tis) inflammation of a diverticulum, especially inflammation related to colonic diverticula, which may undergo perforation with abscess formation. Sometimes called *left-sided appendicitis.*

di·ver·tic·u·lo·gram (di″vər-tik′u-lo-gram) [*diverticulum* + *-gram*] a radiograph of a diverticulum.

di·ver·tic·u·lo·pexy (di″vər-tik″u-lo-pek′se) surgical fixation of a diverticulum in a new position following its separation from the initial adjacent or adherent structures.

di·ver·tic·u·lo·sis (di″vər-tik″u-lo′sis) the presence of diverticula, particularly of colonic diverticula, in the absence of inflammation. Cf. *diverticulitis.*

di·ver·tic·u·lum (di″vər-tik′u-ləm) pl. *diverti′cula* [L. *divertere* to turn aside] a circumscribed pouch or sac of variable size occurring normally or created by herniation of the lining mucous membrane through a defect in the muscular coat of a tubular organ. **divertic′ular** *adj*

acquired d. any diverticulum produced secondarily, mechanically, or by disease.

allantoic d. the sausage-shaped endodermal sacculation that becomes the allantois; in humans it is an outpouching of the caudal wall of the yolk sac that becomes the urachus and remains throughout life as the median umbilical ligament. Called also *allantoic vesicle.*

diverti′cula ampul′lae duc′tus deferen′tis [TA] sacculations in the wall of the ampulla of the ductus deferens.

caliceal d., calyceal d. an epithelium-lined cavity adjacent to a renal calyx, often inflamed and filled with cloudy fluid or pus that in time may calcify into a calculus. Two types are distinguished: *type I* is more common, a bulbous diverticulum connected by a long thin neck to one pole of a calyx; *type II* is a rare type, a round diverticulum connected by a short neck to the central part of a calyx. Called also *pyelocalyceal d.*

cervical d. a diverticulum in the neck, such as in the pharynx or esophagus.

diverticula of colon, colonic diverticula acquired herniations of the mucosa of the colon through the muscular layers of its wall; they sometimes become inflamed (see *diverticulitis*).

cystic d. a ventral outgrowth at the base of the hepatic diverticulum in the embryo; it gives rise to the gallbladder and cystic duct.

endolymphatic d. see under *appendage.*

epiphrenic d. a diverticulum of the esophagus just above the diaphragm; called also *supradiaphragmatic d.*

false d. pseudodiverticulum.

functional d. a benign radiological entity, in which a diverticulum-like shadow is demonstrated by contrast medium, although subsequent laparotomy shows no sign of any corresponding anomaly.

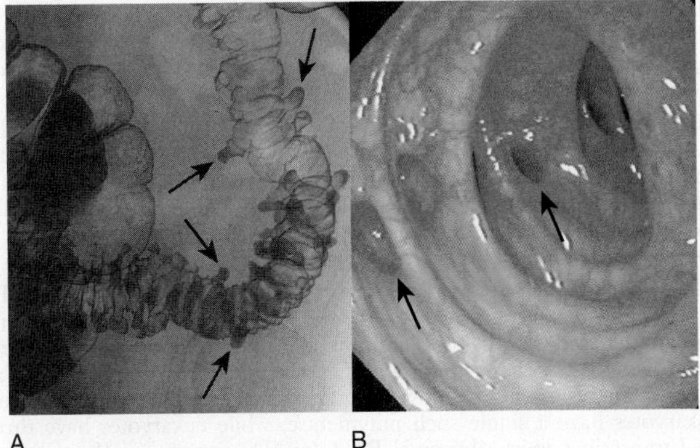

■ Colonic diverticula indicated by arrows in *(A)*, double-contrast enema (barium is black on this film) and *(B)*, colonoscopy.

gallbladder d. cystic d.
ganglion d. a hernial protrusion of the synovial membrane through a tendon sheath.
giant d. a large (6–29 cm) air-filled cyst formed following the perforation of a diverticulum as a complication of diverticulitis.
Graser d. a pseudodiverticulum of the sigmoid flexure.
Heister d. bulbus superior venae jugularis.
hepatic d. a pouch arising from the caudal part of the embryonic foregut and giving rise to the liver, gallbladder, and bile ducts.
Hutch d. herniation of bladder mucosa through a weak point in the wall near the ureterovesical junction, often caused by chronically high intravesical pressure.
ileal d., d. i'lei Meckel d.
intestinal d. a diverticulum in the wall of the intestine, with protrusion of mucous membrane through a defect in the muscular coat.
Kirchner d. a diverticulum of the eustachian tube.
laryngeal d. a diverticulum of the laryngeal mucous membrane.
Meckel d. an occasional sacculation or appendage of the ileum, derived from an unobliterated yolk stalk and sometimes attached to the umbilicus. If its mucosa includes gastric tissue, ulceration and bleeding may occur. Called also *ileal d.* and *d. ilei.*
metanephric d. ureteric bud.
neurohypophysial d. infundibulum (def. 3).
Nuck d. processus vaginalis peritonei.
pancreatic diverticula see under *bud.*
Pertik d. an unusually deep recessus pharyngeus.
pharyngoesophageal d. a diverticulum at the junction of the pharynx and esophagus, at the point of the Killian dehiscence; called also *Zenker d.*
pituitary d. Rathke pouch.
pressure d., pulsion d. a sac or pouch formed by hernial protrusion of the mucous membrane through the muscular coat (as of the colon or esophagus) as a result of pressure from within.
pyelocaliceal d., pyelocalyceal d. calyceal d.
respiratory d. a pouchlike evagination from the foregut that gives rise to the trachea, bronchi, and the branches that form the tracheobronchial tree.
Rokitansky d. traction d.
supradiaphragmatic d. epiphrenic d.
synovial d. a hernial protrusion of the synovial membrane of a joint or a tendon sheath.
thyroid d. an outpouching of the ventral floor of the embryonic pharynx that becomes the thyroid gland.
tracheal d. a blind pouch projecting from the trachea.
traction d. a localized distortion, angulation, or funnel-shaped bulging of the full thickness of the wall of the esophagus, caused by adhesions resulting from some external lesion. Called also *Rokitansky d.*
urachal d. a usually asymptomatic type of vesical diverticulum resulting from a urachus that has closed at the umbilical end but not at the bladder end; seen most often in children, those with prune-belly syndrome, and persons with a bladder outlet obstruction.
vesical d. a diverticulum of the urinary bladder.
Zenker d. pharyngoesophageal d.

di•vi•cine (di-vi'sin) a toxic pyrimidine aglycone produced by endogenous degradation of vicine by β-glucosidase in fava beans; it is believed to be important in the pathogenesis of favism.

divi-divi (div″e-div'e) the leguminous pods of *Caesalpinia coriaria* (Jacq.) Willd., plants of South America; the seeds contain tannin and gallic acid and have been used as an astringent and in tanning.

Divi•gel (div'ĭ-jel) trademark for a preparation of estradiol gel.

di•vi•nyl•ben•zene (di″vi″nəl-ben'zēn) a toxic liquid hydrocarbon, $C_6H_4(CH{=}CH_2)_2$, a monomer used in polymerization reactions.

di•vi•sio (dĭ-viz'e-o) pl. *divisio'nes* [L.] 1. the act or process of separating or sectioning into two or more parts. 2. a section or part of a larger structure.
divisio'nes anterio'res plex'us brachia'lis [TA] anterior divisions of brachial plexus: the three anterior divisions into which each of the three trunks (superior, medial, and inferior) of the brachial plexus splits (see also *divisiones posteriores plexus brachialis*). The anterior divisions of the superior and medial trunks unite to form the lateral fasciculus; and the anterior division of the inferior trunk forms the medial fasciculus of the plexus.
d. autono'mica systema'tis nervo'si periphe'rici [TA] official terminology for *autonomic nervous system.*
d. latera'lis mus'culi erecto'ris spi'nae lumbo'rum TA alternative for *pars lumbalis musculi iliocostalis lumborum.*
d. media'lis mus'culi erecto'ris spi'nae lumbo'rum TA alternative for *pars lumbalis musculi longissimus thoracis.*
divisio'nes posterio'res plex'us brachia'lis [TA] posterior divisions of brachial plexus: the three posterior divisions into which each of the three trunks (superior, medial, and inferior) of the brachial plexus splits (see also *divisiones anteriores plexus brachialis*). All three posterior divisions unite to form the posterior fasciculus of the plexus.

di•vi•sion (dĭ-vizh'ən) [L. *dividere* to separate] 1. the act or process of separation or sectioning into two or more parts. 2. a section or part of a larger structure. 3. in the taxonomy of plants, a primary grouping composed of classes; the equivalent of *phylum* in the animal kingdom. 4. in the taxonomy of fungi, former term for *phylum.*
anterior d's of brachial plexus divisiones anteriores plexus brachialis.
autonomic d. of peripheral nervous system autonomic nervous system.
cell d. fission of a cell; see *meiosis* and *mitosis.*
craniosacral d. parasympathetic nervous system.
dorsal d's of trunks of brachial plexus divisiones posteriores plexus brachialis.
equational d. meiosis II, so called because the sister chromatids are separated but the number of chromosomes remains the same.
lateral d. of lumbar erector spinae divisio lateralis musculi erectoris spinae lumborum.
mandibular d. nervus mandibularis.
maturation d. meiosis.
maxillary d. nervus maxillaris.
medial d. of lumbar erector spinae divisio medialis musculi erectoris spinae lumborum.
posterior d's of brachial plexus divisiones posteriores plexus brachialis.
reduction d., reductional d. meiosis I, so called because at this stage the chromosome number per cell is reduced from diploid to haploid.
thoracicolumbar d., thoracolumbar d. sympathetic nervous system.
ventral d's of trunks of brachial plexus divisiones anteriores plexus brachialis.

di•vi•si•o•nes (dĭ-viz″e-o'nēz) [L.] plural of *divisio.*

di•vulse (dĭ-vuls') [L. *divulsus,* past part. of *divellere* to tear in pieces] to pull apart forcibly.

di•vul•sion (dĭ-vul'shən) the act of forcibly separating or pulling apart.

di•vul•sor (dĭ-vul'sər) an instrument for dilating a tube such as the urethra.

Dix-Hall•pike maneuver (test) (diks' hawl'pīk) [Margaret R. *Dix,* British otologist, 20th century; Charles Skinner *Hallpike,* British otologist, 1900–1979] see under *maneuver.*

Dix•on Mann see *Mann.*

di•zy•got•ic (di″zi-got'ik) pertaining to or derived from two separate zygotes, as dizygotic (fraternal) twins.

di•zy•gous (di-zi'gəs) dizygotic.

diz•zi•ness (diz'e-nis) a disturbed sense of relationship to space; a sensation of unsteadiness with a feeling of movement within the head. See also *dysequilibrium* and *vertigo.*

DJD degenerative joint disease.

djen•kol•ic ac•id (jeng-kol'ik) a sulfur-containing amino acid found in djenkol beans, the cause of djenkol bean poisoning.

djen•kol•ism (jeng'kol-iz-əm) djenkol bean poisoning.

dk deca-.

DKA diabetic ketoacidosis.

D_L diffusing capacity of the lung; $D_{L_{O2}}$ denotes diffusing capacity for oxygen, $D_{L_{CO}}$, diffusing capacity for carbon monoxide, etc.

dL deciliter.

DL- chemical prefix (small capital D and L) used with the D and L convention to indicate a racemic mixture of enantiomers.

dl- chemical prefix used with the *d* and *l* convention to indicate a racemic mixture of enantiomers; the prefix (±)- is used with the same meaning.

DLE discoid lupus erythematosus.

DM diabetes mellitus; phenarsazine chloride (diphenylaminechlorarsine).

DMAPN dimethylaminopropionitrile.

DMARD disease-modifying antirheumatic drug.

DMBA 7,12-dimethylbenz[a]anthracene.

DMD Doctor of Dental Medicine.

DMF dimethylformamide; decayed, missing, filled (see *DMF rate).*

DMFO eflornithine hydrochloride.

DMPE 3,4-dimethoxyphenylethylamine.

DMRD Diploma in Medical Radio-Diagnosis (British).

DMRT Diploma in Medical Radio-Therapy (British).

DMSA succimer (*meso*-2,3-dimercaptosuccinic acid).

DMSO dimethyl sulfoxide.

DMT dimethyltryptamine.

DN dibucaine number.

DNA deoxyribonucleic acid.

A-DNA a double helical structure assumed by RNA-DNA and RNA-RNA chains, or sometimes formed by double-stranded DNA under dehydrating conditions, in which the two chains form a right-handed helix, but more compactly than in B-DNA; there are 11 bases per helical turn, and the stacked bases are tilted. Cf. *B-DNA* and *Z-DNA*.

B-DNA the usual double helical structure assumed by double-stranded DNA in vivo, in which the two chains coil together around an axis to form a right-handed helix, with a helical turn every 10 base pairs; see illustration at *deoxyribonucleic acid.* Cf. *A-DNA* and *Z-DNA*.

complementary DNA, copy DNA (cDNA) DNA transcribed from a specific RNA in vitro through the reaction of the enzyme reverse transcriptase.

genomic DNA the complete genome extracted from the nucleus, or a cloned copy of all or part of that DNA; it thus includes both coding and noncoding regions.

junk DNA selfish DNA.

DNA library see *library.*

linker DNA 1. linker. 2. the short stretch of DNA that connects two adjacent nucleosomes in eukaryotic chromatin.

microsatellite DNA see *microsatellite.*

minisatellite DNA see *minisatellite.*

mitochondrial DNA (mtDNA) the DNA of the mitochondrial genome (q.v.).

nuclear DNA (nDNA) the DNA of the chromosomes found in the nucleus of a eukaryotic cell.

parasitic DNA selfish DNA.

recombinant DNA a composite DNA molecule constructed in vitro by joining a fragment of foreign DNA with a vector DNA molecule capable of replicating in host cells.

repetitive DNA nucleotide sequences occurring multiply within a genome; they are characteristic of eukaryotes and generally do not encode polypeptides. Sequences may be clustered or dispersed, and repeated moderately (10 to 10^4 copies per genome) to highly ($\geq 10^6$ copies per genome). Moderately repetitive DNA sequences encode some structural genes for ribosomal RNA, transfer RNA, and histones; highly repetitive sequences are mostly satellite DNA. Cf. *single copy DNA.*

satellite DNA short, highly repeated DNA sequences found in eukaryotes, differing in base composition from that of the bulk of the DNA, usually occurring clustered in groups of many tandem repeats in constitutive heterochromatin and generally not transcribed.

selfish DNA term used for segments of eukaryotic DNA that are replicated with the rest of the chromosomal DNA but that have no apparent function; e.g., highly repetitive sequences or transposable elements. Called also *junk DNA.*

single copy DNA (scDNA) nucleotide sequences present once in the haploid genome, as are the majority of the gene sequences encoding polypeptides in eukaryotes.

spacer DNA nontranscribed DNA sequences occurring between functional gene regions in eukaryotic and some viral genomes; they may be long and may include many repetitive sequences.

unique DNA single copy DNA.

Z-DNA a double helical structure assumed by double-stranded DNA, in which the phosphate groups form a dinucleotide repeating unit zigzagging up a left-handed helix with a single, deep groove; it is particularly likely to occur in stretches of alternating purines and pyrimidines or under dehydrating conditions. Cf. *A-DNA* and *B-DNA.*

DNA (cy·to·sine-5-)-meth·yl·trans·fer·ase (si′to-sēn meth″əl-trans′fər-ās) [EC 2.1.1.37] official nomenclature for DNA methyltransferases (q.v.) that catalyze the transfer of a methyl group from *S*-adenosylmethionine to the C5 position of cytosine in DNA.

DNA-di·rect·ed DNA po·lym·er·ase (dĭ-rek′təd pə-lim′ər-ās) [EC 2.7.7.7] any of the enzymes of the transferase class that catalyze the template-directed, step-by-step addition of deoxyribonucleotides to the 3′ end of an RNA primer or growing DNA chain, using a single-stranded DNA template. The reaction is important in the replication and repair of deoxyribonucleic acids. Called also *DNA polymerase.*

DNA-di·rect·ed RNA po·lym·er·ase (dĭ-rek′təd pə-lim′ər-ās) [EC 2.7.7.6] any of the enzymes of the transferase class that catalyze the template-directed step-by-step addition of ribonucleotides to the 3′ end of a growing RNA chain, using a single-stranded DNA template. The reaction is important in the flow of information from DNA to proteins. Prokaryotes have a single such polymerase, while eukaryotes have three: *type I* transcribes most ribosomal RNA (rRNA) genes; *type II* synthesizes messenger (mRNA), some small nuclear (snRNA), and many small nucleolar RNA (snoRNA) molecules; and *type III* transcribes the genes for one species of rRNA, for transfer RNA (tRNA), and for various small RNA molecules. Called also *RNA polymerase.*

DNA gy·rase (ji′rās) DNA topoisomerase (ATP-hydrolyzing).

DNA li·gase (li′gās) an enzyme of the ligase class that catalyzes the energy-driven linkage of a double-stranded DNA chain with a free 3′ hydroxyl group to one with a 5′ phosphate group, forming a phosphodiester bond between them. The reaction is important in the repair of damaged DNA and in the joining of Okazaki fragments during DNA replication. In animals and bacteriophages, the enzyme uses ATP as an energy source and is officially called DNA ligase (ATP) [EC 6.5.1.1]. In bacteria, it uses NAD as the energy source and the enzyme is officially called DNA ligase (NAD) [EC 6.5.1.2]. Both are used in vitro in the formation of recombinant molecules.

DNA meth·yl·ase (meth′əl-ās) DNA methyltransferase.

DNA meth·yl·trans·fer·ase (meth″əl-trans′fər-ās) any of a group of enzymes that catalyze the transfer of a methyl group from *S*-adenosylmethionine to a specific nucleotide in a DNA molecule, with different enzymes specific for nucleotide and position of methylation. In eukaryotes, the methylated base is virtually always cytosine methylated at the C5 position, and the reaction is catalyzed by the methyltransferase officially called DNA (cytosine-5-)-methyltransferase. Different organisms have different methylation recognition sequences; in animal cells, methylation occurs specifically at 5′-CG-3′ sequences, and methylation is involved in gene expression. There are two types of DNA methyltransferases: those methylating unmethylated DNA, called de novo methyltransferases, and those that methylate the unmethylated strand of DNA produced upon replication of methylated DNA, called maintenance methyltransferases. See also *DNA methylation*, under *methylation.*

DNA nu·cleo·tid·yl·exo·trans·fer·ase (noo″kle-o-tīd′əl-ek″so-trans′fər-ās) [EC 2.7.7.31] an enzyme of the transferase class that acts as a DNA polymerase, specifically catalyzing the sequential addition of single deoxynucleotide residues, as nucleoside triphosphates, to the ends of nucleotide chains. The enzyme is often found in the blast cells of patients with acute lymphocytic leukemia; its presence is used in the differential diagnosis of this disease as well as to monitor response to treatment. Called also *terminal deoxynucleotidyl transferase.*

DNA nu·cleo·tid·yl·trans·fer·ase (noo″kle-o-tīd″əl-trans′fər-ās) DNA polymerase.

DNA po·lym·er·ase (pə-lim′ər-ās) 1. a general term denoting any enzyme catalyzing the template-directed incorporation of deoxyribonucleotides into a DNA chain; see *DNA-directed DNA polymerase* and *RNA-directed DNA polymerase.* 2. DNA-directed DNA polymerase.

DNase deoxyribonuclease.

DNA topo·isom·er·ase (to″po-i-som′ər-ās) [EC 5.99.1.2] an enzyme of the isomerase class that catalyzes the ATP-independent breakage, passage, and rejoining of a single strand of DNA, altering the topology of the molecule by single-step changes in linking number. The enzyme removes superhelical turns and interconverts other topoisomers, such as simple and knotted single-stranded rings. Called also *type I topoisomerase.*

DNA topo·isom·er·ase (ATP-hy·dro·lyz·ing) (to″po-i-som′ər-ās hi′dro-li-zing) [EC 5.99.1.3] an enzyme of the isomerase class that catalyzes the ATP-dependent breakage, passage, and rejoining of both strands of a DNA helix simultaneously, altering the topology of the molecule by changing the linking number in steps of two. The enzyme removes and introduces superhelical turns and in prokaryotes is believed to be important in replication, transcription, recombination, and other processes. Called also *type II topoisomerase* and *DNA gyrase.*

DNB dinitrobenzene; Diplomate of the National Board (of Medical Examiners).

DNCB dinitrochlorobenzene.

DNFB dinitrofluorobenzene.

DNOC dinitro-*o*-cresol.

DNR do not resuscitate.

DO Doctor of Osteopathy.

DOA dead on arrival.

Do·bie globule, layer (line) (do′be) [William Murray *Dobie*, English physician, 1828–1915] see under *globule*, and see *Z band*, under *band*.

Do·brin syndrome (do′brin) [Robert S. *Dobrin*, American pediatrician, 20th century] TINU syndrome; see under *syndrome*.

do·bu·ta·mine (do-bu′tə-mēn) a synthetic catecholamine having direct inotropic effects; it acts primarily on β_1-adrenergic receptors, increasing myocardial contractility and stroke volume and resulting in increased cardiac output.

d. hydrochloride the hydrochloride salt of dobutamine, having the same actions as the base; used in the treatment of cardiac decompensation in congestive heart failure or depressed contractility secondary to cardiac surgery; administered intravenously.

Do·bu·trex (do′bu-treks) trademark for a preparation of dobutamine hydrochloride.

DOC 11-deoxycorticosterone.

Do·ca (do′kə) trademark for desoxycorticosterone acetate.

do·ce·re (do-sēr′rə) [L. "to teach"] the physician as teacher, a principle of naturopathic medicine that states the importance of patient education in health care and emphasizes the respect that is to be shown to the patient as an individual.

do·ce·tax·el (do″sə-tak′səl) an antimitotic agent that inhibits cell division by promoting microtubule assembly and inhibiting disassembly; used as an antineoplastic agent, particularly in treatment of carcinoma of the breast and non–small cell lung carcinoma; administered by intravenous infusion.

Do·ci·bin (do′si-bin) trademark for a crystalline preparation of vitamin B_{12}; see *cyanocobalamin*.

dock (dok) to perform a caudectomy on an animal.

do·co·sa·hexa·eno·ic ac·id (do-ko″sə-hek″sə-e-no′ik) all *cis*-4,7,10,13,16,19-docosahexaenoic acid, an omega-3, polyunsaturated, 22-carbon fatty acid found almost exclusively in fish and marine animal oils; it is a substrate for cyclooxygenase. Abbreviated DHA. See also table accompanying *fatty acid*.

do·co·sa·nol (do-ko′sə-nol) *n*-docosanol, a saturated 22-carbon alcohol having antiviral activity against lipid-enveloped viruses, including herpes simplex virus, acting by inhibiting fusion between the human plasma cell membrane and the viral envelope; used topically in the treatment of recurrent herpes labialis.

doc·tor (dok′tər) [L. "teacher"] 1. a practitioner of the healing arts, one who has received a degree from a college of medicine, osteopathy, chiropractic, optometry, podiatry, pharmacy, dentistry, or veterinary medicine, licensed to practice by a state. 2. a holder of a diploma of the highest degree from a university, qualified as a specialist in a particular field of learning.

doc·trine (dok′trin) a theory supported by authorities and having general acceptance.

Arrhenius d. see under *theory*.

Monro-Kellie d. the central nervous system and its accompanying fluids are enclosed in a rigid container whose total volume tends to remain constant; an increase in volume of one component, e.g., brain, blood, or cerebrospinal fluid, will elevate pressure and decrease the volume of one of the other elements.

neuron d. the doctrine that the nervous system is entirely cellular, that its cells are distinctive as to morphological type and functional characteristics, and that its cells are not in protoplasmic continuity but are juxtaposed without a significant amount of intervening extracellular substance.

doc·u·sate (dok′u-sāt) any of a group of anionic surfactants widely used as emulsifying, wetting, and dispersing agents.

d. calcium [USP] an anionic surfactant used as a stool softener; administered orally.

d. potassium [USP] an anionic surfactant used as a stool softener; administered orally.

d. sodium [USP] an anionic surfactant used as a stool softener, administered orally or rectally; as a tablet disintegrant because of its solubilizing action; and as an emulsifier and dispersant in topical preparations.

do·de·ce·no·yl-CoA Δ-isom·er·ase (do″də-sə-no′əl-ko-a′ i-som′ər-ās) [EC 5.3.3.8] an enzyme of the isomerase class that catalyzes the shift of a *cis* double bond at C-2 of an unsaturated fatty acyl CoA to one *trans* at C-3; the reaction is necessary for oxidation of unsaturated fatty acids. Called also *enoyl CoA isomerase*.

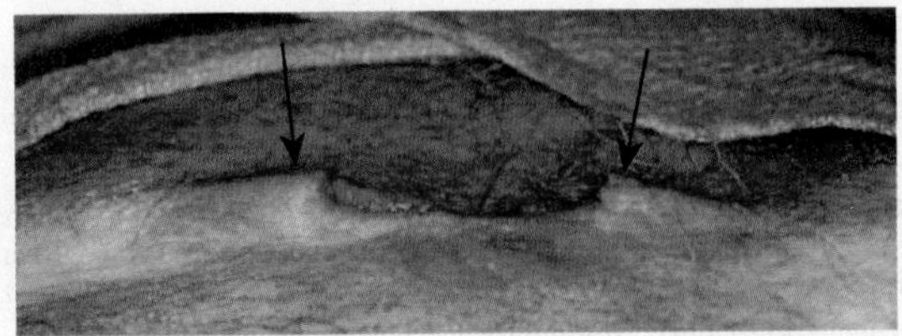

■ Dog-ears *(arrows)*.

Dö·der·lein bacillus (dur′dər-līn) [Albert Siegmund Gustav *Döderlein*, German obstetrician and gynecologist, 1860–1941] see under *bacillus*.

do·fet·i·lide (do-fet′ə-līd) an antiarrhythmic that prolongs the duration of the cardiac action potential and the effective refractory period without affecting conduction velocity; used in the treatment of atrial arrhythmias, administered orally.

dog·bane (dog′bān) any plant of the genus *Apocynum*.

dog·ear (dog′ēr) a redundancy of skin at the apical angle or along the side of a wound, forming a small protruding triangle of tissue with the appearance of a dog's ear.

Do·gi·el corpuscles (do′ge-el) [Alexander Stanislavovich *Dogiel*, Russian histologist, 1852–1922] see under *corpuscle*.

dog·ma (dog′mə) a belief or an opinion, or a system of beliefs or opinions, formally stated, defined, and held to be true.

Döh·le bodies (inclusion bodies) (dur′lə) [Karl Gottfried Paul *Döhle*, German pathologist, 1855–1928] see under *body*.

Döh·le-Hel·ler aortitis (dur′lə hel′ər) [K.G.P. *Döhle*; Arnold Ludwig Gotthilf *Heller*, German pathologist, 1840–1913] syphilitic aortitis.

Dohl·man procedure (dōl′mən) [Gosta *Dohlman*, Swedish otorhinolaryngologist, mid-20th century] see under *procedure*.

dol (dōl) [L. *dolor* pain] a unit of pain intensity.

do·lab·rate (do-lab′rāt) [L. *dolabra* ax] ax-shaped.

do·lab·ri·form (do-lab′rĭ-form) dolabrate.

do·las·e·tron mes·y·late (do-las′ə-tron) a selective serotonin receptor antagonist, used for the prevention of nausea and vomiting associated with chemotherapy and for the prevention and treatment of postoperative nausea and vomiting; administered orally and intravenously.

dolich(o)- [Gr. *dolichos* long] a combining form meaning long.

dol·i·cho·ce·pha·lia (dol″ĭ-ko-sə-fa′le-ə) dolichocephaly.

dol·i·cho·ce·phal·ic (dol″ĭ-ko-sə-fal′ik) [*dolicho-* + *cephalic*] long headed; having a cephalic index of 75.9 or less. Called also *mecocephalic*.

dol·i·cho·ceph·a·lous (dol″ĭ-ko-sef′ə-ləs) dolichocephalic.

dol·i·cho·ceph·a·ly (dol″ĭ-ko-sef′ə-le) the quality of being dolichocephalic.

dol·i·cho·co·lon (dol″ĭ-ko-ko′lən) [*dolicho-* + *colon*] an abnormally long colon.

dol·i·cho·cra·ni·al (dol″ĭ-ko-kra′ne-əl) having a cranial index of 74.9 or less.

dol·i·cho·der·us (dol″ĭ-ko-dēr′əs) [*dolicho-* + Gr. *dere* neck] an individual with a long neck.

dol·i·cho·fa·cial (dol″ĭ-ko-fa′shəl) having a long face.

dol·i·cho·hi·er·ic (dol″ĭ-ko-hi-er′ik) [*dolicho-* + Gr. *hieron* sacrum + *-ic*] having a long, narrow sacrum with a sacral index of less than 100.

dol·i·cho·ker·kic (dol″ĭ-ko-ker′kik) having a radiohumeral index above 80.

dol·i·cho·kne·mic (dol″ĭ-ko-ne′mik) having a tibiofemoral index of 83 or above.

dol·i·chol (dol′ĭ-kol) any of a group of polyisoprenoid lipids, containing 13–24 isoprene units and a terminal hydroxyl group, occurring in the endoplasmic reticulum. It is also the major lipid component of neuromelanin

d. phosphate a phosporylated form that serves a carrier for the oligosaccharide precursor (attached to the phosphate group) in *N*-linked glycosylation; transfer of the assembled precursor to the asparagine residue of the polypeptide chain is catalyzed by oligosaccharyltransferase.

dol·i·cho·mor·phic (dol″ĭ-ko-mor′fik) [*dolicho-* + Gr. *morphē* form] built along lines that tend toward the slender or longer type.

dol•i•cho•pel•lic (dol″ĭ-ko-pel′ik) [*dolicho-* + *pelvic*] having a pelvic index of 95 or above.

dol•i•cho•pel•vic (dol″ĭ-ko-pel′vik) dolichopellic.

dol•i•cho•pro•sop•ic (dol″ĭ-ko-pro-sop′ik) dolichofacial.

dol•i•cho•steno•me•lia (dol″ĭ-ko-sten″o-me′le-ə) [*dolicho-* + *steno-* + *-melia*] 1. the condition of having unusually long, thin extremities. 2. arachnodactyly.

Do•lo•bid (do′lo-bid) trademark for a preparation of diflunisal.

Do•lo•phine (do′lo-fēn) trademark for preparations of methadone hydrochloride.

do•lor (do′lor) pl. *dolo′res* [L.] pain; one of the cardinal signs of inflammation.

d. ca′pitis headache.

d. coxae coxalgia (def. 2).

Do•lo•rac (do′lə-rak) trademark for a preparation of capsaicin.

do•lo•res (do-lor′ēz) [L.] plural of *dolor*.

do•lor•if•ic (do″lor-if′ik) producing or causing pain.

do•lor•im•e•ter (do″lor-im′ə-tər) an instrument for measuring pain in dols; cf. *algesimeter*.

do•lor•im•e•try (do″lor-im′ə-tre) [*dolor* + *-metry*] the measurement of pain.

do•lor•o•gen•ic (do-lor″o-jen′ik) dolorific.

DOM 2,5-dimethoxy-4-methylamphetamine.

do•main (do-mān′) 1. an area or region that is defined or delimited in some way. 2. a compact globular structure composed of one section of a polypeptide chain that constitutes a recognizable unit of the tertiary structure of a protein. Domains may fold up independently and maintain their native conformation when the connecting sections of the chain are broken. 3. one of the three broad divisions into which all living organisms may be classified: the Archaea, the Bacteria, and the Eucarya; the first two consist of the prokaryotes, whereas the last contains the eukaryotes. This system is an alternative to the traditional five-kingdom classification (see *kingdom*).

apical d. see under *membrane*.

basolateral d. see under *membrane*.

chromatin d's subunits of condensed chromatin that make up the chromosomal territories of the cell nucleus.

immunoglobulin d's see *homology regions* under *region*.

interchromatin d., interchromosomal d. a compartment of the cell nucleus consisting of a network of channels separating and containing much less chromatin than the chromosome territories; most RNA transcription, processing, and transport are believed to occur in this domain.

kringle d. a cysteine-rich, triply disulfide-bonded sequence of amino acids folded into a characteristic shape resembling the looped Scandinavian pastry; such domains occur in plasminogen and contain the binding sites for fibrin. Similar domains are found in other proteins.

paired d., paired box d. [*paired*, the first *Drosophila* gene found to encode it] a conserved DNA-binding protein motif found in the transcription factors encoded by the PAX genes.

Dom•brock blood group (dom′brok) [*Dombrock*, surname of the propositus first observed in 1965] see under *blood group*.

dome (dōm) a vaulted roof having a more or less hemispherical shape.

nasal d. rounding of the tip of the nose over an alar cartilage.

Dome•boro (dōm′bor-o) trademark for preparations of aluminum subacetate.

dom•i•cil•i•ary (dom″ĭ-sil′e-ar″e) [L. *domus* house] pertaining to or carried on in the house or place of permanent residence, as domiciliary treatment.

dom•i•nance (dom′ĭ-nəns) [L. *dominari* to govern] 1. the state of being dominant. 2. in genetics, the phenotypic expression of a gene in both heterozygotes and homozygotes; see also *Mendel's laws*, under *law*. See also *codominance* and *quasidominance*. 3. in coronary artery anatomy, the state of supplying the posterior diaphragmatic part of the interventricular septum and the diaphragmatic surface of the left ventricle. In 85 percent of the population, the right coronary artery is dominant; in the remainder, the left coronary artery is dominant.

cerebral d. the dominance of one cerebral hemisphere over the other in cerebral functions, demonstrated by laterality in voluntary motor acts.

incomplete d. failure of one gene to be completely dominant, the heterozygotes showing a phenotype intermediate between the two parents; called also *partial d.* and *semidominance*.

lateral d. the preferential use, in voluntary motor acts, of ipsilateral members of the major paired organs of the body (arm, ear, eye, and leg). See *dextrality* and *sinistrality*.

ocular d. the preferential use of one eye over the other in vision.

one-sided d. lateral d.

partial d. incomplete d.

dom•i•nant (dom′ĭ-nənt) 1. exerting a ruling or controlling influence. 2. in genetics, capable of expression when carried by only one of a pair of homologous chromosomes. 3. in coronary artery anatomy, supplying the posterior diaphragmatic part of the interventricular septum and the diaphragmatic surface of the left ventricle; said of the right and left coronary arteries.

dom•o•ic ac•id (dom′o-ik) a neuroexcitatory, neurotoxic amino acid structurally similar to L-glutamic acid, occurring in the diatom *Nitzschia pungens* and other varieties of marine vegetation. Ingestion of mussels contaminated by it has resulted in amnesic shellfish poisoning (see under *poisoning*).

dom•per•i•done (dom-per′ĭ-dōn) an antiemetic and prokinetic agent; its actions are related to its peripheral dopamine receptor–blocking properties. It is used in the treatment of upper gastrointestinal motility disorders caused by chronic and subacute gastritis and diabetes and the prophylaxis of gastrointestinal symptoms caused by dopamine agonists used to treat parkinsonism.

Do•nath-Land•stein•er antibody, test (do′naht land′sti-nər) [Julius *Donath*, Austrian immunologist, 1870–1950; Karl *Landsteiner*, Austrian physician in United States, 1868–1943] see under *antibody* and *test*.

do•na•tion (do-na′shun) 1. a gift. 2. the act of giving.

oocyte d. a method of assisted reproductive technology in which an oocyte from a fertile woman is aspirated for incubation in the uterus of a woman who has female factor infertility, such as after oophorectomy or premature menopause. Fertilization may be either in vitro or in utero.

do•nax•ine (do-nak′sēn) gramine.

Don•ders' law (don′dərz) [Franciscus Cornelius *Donders*, Dutch physician and ophthalmologist, 1818–1889] see under *law*.

Donec alv. sol. fuerit [L.] do′nec al′vus solu′ta fu′erit (until the bowels are opened, i.e., until a bowel movement occurs).

do•nee (do-ne′) recipient; host (def. 2).

do•nep•e•zil hy•dro•chlo•ride (do-nep′ə-zil) a reversible acetylcholinesterase inhibitor used for the treatment of mild to moderate symptoms of dementia of the Alzheimer type; administered orally.

dong quai (doong kwa, -kwi) [Chinese *dāng* should + *guī* return (from the idea that it causes the blood to return where it should)] 1. the root of *Angelica sinensis*, used for gynecologic disorders. 2. *Angelica sinensis*.

Don Juan•ism (don hwahn′iz-əm) [*Don Juan*, legendary Spanish nobleman with this characteristic] hypersexuality in a man.

Don•nan equilibrium (effect) (don′ən) [Frederick George *Donnan*, English chemist, 1870–1956] see under *equilibrium*.

Don•na•tal (don′ə-tal) trademark for combination preparations of atropine sulfate, hyoscyamine sulfate, phenobarbital, and scopolamine hydrobromide.

Don•na•zyme (don′ə-zīm) trademark for a preparation of pancreatin.

Donné corpuscles (bodies) (do-na′) [Alfred *Donné*, French bacteriologist, 1801–1878] see *colostrum corpuscles*, under *corpuscle*.

Don•o•hue syndrome (don′ə-hu) [William Leslie *Donohue*, Canadian physician, 20th century] see under *syndrome*.

do•nor (do′nər) 1. an individual organism that supplies living tissue to be used in another body, as a person who furnishes blood for transfusion, or an organ for transplantation in a histocompatible recipient. Organs for donation usually come from cadavers (see *cadaveric donor transplantation*), although kidneys and certain other organs may be from living donors (see *living related donor transplantation* and *living unrelated donor transplantation*). 2. in chemistry, a substance or compound which contributes part of itself, as an atom or radical, to another substance (acceptor).

cadaveric d. an organ or tissue donor who has already died; see also *cadaveric donor transplantation*.

F d. in bacterial genetics, a cell that donates the F plasmid by means of bacterial conjugation.

hydrogen d. a substance or compound that gives up hydrogen to another substance (the hydrogen acceptor).

living nonrelated d. living unrelated d.

living related d. a donor who is a close biological relative of the recipient, such as a mother and child or a brother and sister; see also *living related donor transplantation*.

living unrelated d. a donor who is not a close blood relative of the recipient; see also *living unrelated donor transplantation*.

universal d. a person whose blood is type O in the ABO blood group system; such blood is sometimes used in emergency transfusion.

Don•o•van body (don′ə-vən) [Charles *Donovan*, Irish physician, 1863–1951] 1. *Klebsiella granulomatis*. 2. amastigote.

don•o•va•no•sis (don″ə-və-no′sis) granuloma inguinale.

do•pa (do′pə) 3,4-dihydroxyphenylalanine, an amino acid produced by oxidation of tyrosine by monophenol monooxygenase; it is the precursor of dopamine and an intermediate product in the biosynthesis of norepinephrine, epinephrine, and melanin. The naturally occurring form is L-dopa (see *levodopa*).

do•pa•mine (do′pə-mēn) 3,4-dihydroxyphenylethylamine, a catecholamine formed in the body by the decarboxylation of dopa; it is an intermediate product in the synthesis of norepinephrine, and acts as a neurotransmitter in the central nervous system. It is also produced peripherally and acts on peripheral receptors, e.g., in blood vessels. Called also *3-hydroxytyramine*.

d. hydrochloride the hydrochloride salt of dopamine, used to correct hemodynamic balance in the treatment of persons with acute hypotension as part of shock, and to improve cardiac function in the treatment of cardiac decompensation; administered intravenously.

do•pa•mine β-hy•drox•y•lase (do″pə-mēn hi-drok′sə-lās) dopamine β-monooxygenase.

do•pa•mine β-mono•oxy•gen•ase (do″pə-mēn mon″o-oks′ə-jən-ās) [EC 1.14.17.1] an enzyme of the oxidoreductase class that catalyzes the hydroxylation of dopamine to norepinephrine, simultaneously oxidizing ascorbate. It is a copper protein occurring in nervous tissue and the adrenal medulla. Called also *dopamine β-hydroxylase*.

do•pa•min•er•gic (do″pə-mēn-ur′jik) 1. activated or transmitted by dopamine. 2. pertaining to tissues or organs affected by dopamine. 3. pertaining to neurons that release dopamine and to the effects exerted by such release.

do•pant (do′pənt) an impurity purposely added, as to a laser crystal or a semiconductor, during manufacturing in order to create a desired characteristic. Called also *doping agent*.

do•pa•quin•one (do″pə-kwin′ōn) an oxidation product of dopa; it is an intermediate in the synthesis of melanin pigments from tyrosine.

Do•par (do′pahr) trademark for a preparation of levodopa.

doped (dōpt) having impurities (dopants) added purposely during manufacturing.

dop•ing (do′ping) 1. the addition of a dopant. 2. the administration of a substance, such as a performance-enhancing drug.

blood d. the administration of blood, red blood cells, or related blood products to an athlete in order to enhance performance, often preceded by the withdrawal of blood so that training continues in a blood-depleted state.

dop•pel•len•der (dop′əl-en″dər) myofiber hyperplasia.

Dop•pler (dop′lər) Doppler ultrasonography.

color D. color flow Doppler imaging.

Dop•pler effect (phenomenon, principle) (dop′lər) [Christian *Doppler*, Austrian physicist and mathematician, 1803–1853] see under *effect*.

Do•pram (do′prəm) trademark for a preparation of doxapram hydrochloride.

Dor•al (dor′al) trademark for a preparation of quazepam.

Do•rel•lo canal (do-rel′o) [Primo *Dorello*, Italian anatomist, 1872–1963] see under *canal*.

Dor•en•dorf sign (dor′ən-dorf) [Hans *Dorendorf*, German physician, 1866–1953] see under *sign*.

dor•man•cy (dor′mən-se) [L. *dormire* to sleep] 1. the state of being dormant. 2. in bacteriology, the property exhibited by some bacteria, and especially by bacterial spores, of remaining viable for an extended time with minimal physical or chemical change, often in response to unfavorable growth conditions.

dor•mant (dor′mənt) [L. *dormire* to sleep] sleeping, inactive, quiescent.

dor•mi•fa•cient (dor″mĭ-fa′shənt) [L. *dormire* to sleep + *-facient*] hypnotic (defs. 1 and 2).

dor•nase al•fa (dor′nāz al′fə) recombinant human deoxyribonuclease I (DNase I) used to reduce the viscosity of sputum in cystic fibrosis patients by hydrolysis of long extracellular DNA molecules to shorter fragments; administered by inhalation.

dor•sa (dor′sə) [L.] plural of *dorsum*.

dor•sad (dor′sad) toward the back or dorsal aspect.

dor•sal (dor′səl) [L. *dorsalis*, from *dorsum* back] 1. pertaining to the back or to any dorsum. 2. denoting a position more toward the back surface than some other object of reference; a synonym of *posterior* in human anatomy and of *superior* in the anatomy of quadrupeds.

dor•sal•gia (dor-sal′jə) [*dors-* + *-algia*] pain in the back; called also *notalgia*.

dor•sa•lis (dor-sa′lis) [L.] [TA] dorsal.

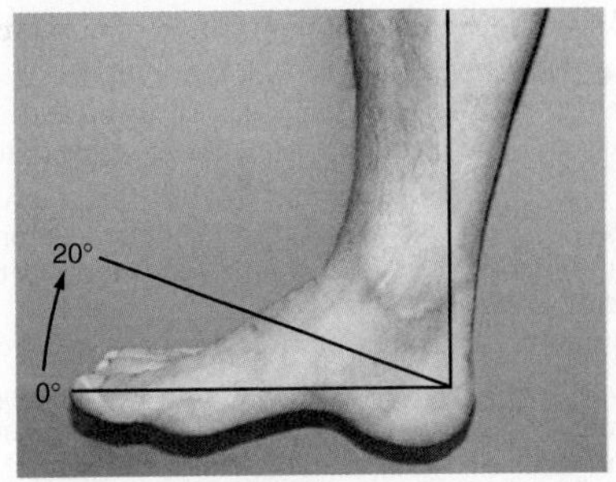

■ Dorsiflexion of foot.

dor•si (dor′si) genitive of *dorsum*.

dorsi- see *dors(o)-*.

dor•si•duct (dor′sĭ-dəkt) [*dorsi-* + *duct*] to draw toward the back or dorsum.

dor•si•flex•ion (dor″sĭ-flek′shən) [*dorsi-* + *flexion*] flexion or bending toward the extensor aspect of a limb, as of the hand or foot.

dor•si•mes•al (dor″sĭ-mes′əl) dorsomesial.

dor•si•spi•nal (dor″sĭ-spi′nəl) pertaining to the back and vertebral column.

dors(o)- [L. *dorsum* back] a combining form denoting relationship to a dorsum or to the back (posterior) aspect of the body. Also, *dorsi-*.

dor•so•an•te•ri•or (dor″so-an-tēr′e-ər) having the back of the fetus toward the front of the mother.

dor•so•ceph•a•lad (dor″so-sef′ə-lad) [*dorso-* + *cephalad*] directed toward the back of the head.

dor•so•in•ter•cos•tal (dor″so-in″tər-kos′təl) situated in the back and between the ribs.

dor•so•lat•er•al (dor″so-lat′ər-əl) pertaining to the back and the side.

dor•so•lum•bar (dor″so-lum′bər, -bahr) pertaining to the back and the loins, especially the region of the lower thoracic and upper lumbar vertebrae.

dor•so•me•di•an (dor″so-me′de-ən) the median line of the back.

dor•so•me•si•al (dor″so-me′se-əl) pertaining to the median line of the back.

dor•so•na•sal (dor″so-na′səl) pertaining to the dorsum of the nose or to the bridge of the nose.

dor•so•nu•chal (dor″so-noo′kəl) pertaining to the back of the neck.

dor•so•pos•te•ri•or (dor″so-pos-tēr′e-ər) having the back of the fetus directed toward the mother's back.

dor•so•ra•di•al (dor″so-ra′de-əl) pertaining to the radial or lateral side of the back of the forearm or hand.

dor•so•scap•u•lar (dor″so-skap′u-lər) pertaining to the posterior surface of the scapula.

dor•so•ven•trad (dor″so-ven′trəd) [*dorso-* + *ventrad*] directed from the dorsal toward the ventral aspect.

dor•so•ven•tral (dor″so-ven′trəl) 1. pertaining to the back and belly surfaces of the body. 2. passing from the back to the belly surface.

dor•sum (dor′səm) gen. *dor′si* pl. *dor′sa* [L.] [TA] 1. the back. 2. the aspect of an anatomical part or structure corresponding in position to the back; posterior, in the human.

d. of foot d. pedis.

d. of hand 1. d. manus. 2. regio dorsalis manus.

d. lin′guae [TA] dorsum of the tongue: the upper or posterosuperior surface of the tongue.

d. ma′nus [TA] back or dorsum of hand: the hand surface opposite the palm.

d. na′si [TA], **d. of nose** the part of the external surface of the nose formed by junction of the lateral surfaces.

d. pe′dis [TA] dorsum of foot: the upper surface of the foot; the surface opposite the sole. Called also *regio dorsalis pedis* [TA alternative].

d. pe′nis [TA], **d. of penis** the anterior, more extensive surface of the dependent penis, opposite the urethral surface.

d. of scapula facies posterior scapulae.

d. sel′lae [TA] the quadrilateral plate on the sphenoid bone that forms the posterior boundary of the sella turcica; the posterior clinoid processes project from its superior extremity, and it is continuous inferiorly with the clivus.

d. of testis margo posterior testis.

d. of tongue d. linguae.

Dor•yx (dor'iks) trademark for a preparation of doxycycline hyclate.

dor•zo•la•mide hy•dro•chlo•ride (dor-zo'lə-mīd) a carbonic acid anhydrase inhibitor, used as an antiglaucoma agent in the treatment of open-angle glaucoma and ocular hypertension; applied topically to the conjunctiva.

dos•age (do'səj) 1. the determination and regulation of the size, frequency, and number of doses. 2. the presence and relative representation of some factor or agent.

gene d. the number of copies of a specific gene in a genome.

dose (dōs) [*dosis*] 1. a quantity to be administered at one time, such as a specified amount of medication. 2. in radiology, the amount of energy absorbed per unit mass of tissue at a given site.

absorbed d. the amount of energy from ionizing radiation absorbed per unit mass of matter, expressed in rads.

air d. air exposure.

average d. the quantity of an agent that will usually produce the therapeutic effect for which it is administered.

booster d. a dose of an active immunizing agent, usually smaller than the initial dose, given to maintain immunity.

breakthrough d. the dose of an analgesic required for the relief of breakthrough pain; called also *rescue d.*

cumulative d., cumulative radiation d. the total dose resulting from repeated exposures to radiation.

curative d. (CD) a dose sufficient to restore normal health. See also *median curative d.*

daily d. the total amount of a drug or other agent administered in a 24-hour period.

depth d. the intensity of radiation at a given depth in an irradiated body, expressed as a percentage of that at the surface of the body nearest the portal of entry.

divided d. fractional d.

doubling d. the dose of ionizing radiation that will result in doubling of the rate of biological changes in a population, such as mutations or cancers.

effective d. (ED) the quantity of a drug or agent that will produce the effects for which it is administered. See also *median effective d.*

epilating d. the amount of radiation that causes temporary or permanent loss of hair.

equianalgesic d. the quantity of one analgesic that produces the same effect as a given quantity of another analgesic agent.

erythema d. (ED) the amount of ultraviolet radiation that causes temporary erythema on the skin; this is different for each individual.

exit d. the intensity of ionizing radiation that emerges from the body at the surface opposite the portal of entry.

exposure d. see *exposure* (def. 3).

fatal d. lethal d.

fractional d., fractionated d. a fraction of the total dose prescribed of a drug or therapeutic radiation; called also *divided d.*

infective d. (ID) the amount of a pathogenic agent that will cause infection in susceptible subjects. See also *median infective d.* and *median tissue culture infective d.*

infinitesimal d. see under *principle.*

integral d., integral absorbed d. the total amount of ionizing radiation absorbed by an individual or other biological object, expressed in gram-rads (100 ergs).

L+ d., L$_+$ d. (limes tod or death dose) in preparation of diphtheria toxoid, the smallest amount of diphtheria toxin that will kill a 250-g guinea pig within four days when mixed with one unit of diphtheria antitoxin before being injected subcutaneously. Cf. *lethal d.*

L0 d., L$_0$d. the limes nul or limes zero dose; in preparation of diphtheria toxoid, the largest amount of diphtheria toxin that when mixed with one standard unit of antitoxin produces no perceptible reaction when injected subcutaneously into a guinea pig.

lethal d. the amount of an agent, such as a toxin or radiation, that will or may be sufficient to cause death. See also *median lethal d.* and *minimum lethal d.* Called also *fatal d.* Cf. *L+ d.*

Lf d. (limes flocculating dose) in the Ramon flocculation test, the amount of diphtheria toxin that in the shortest time produces precipitation when mixed with one standard unit of antitoxin.

limes nul d., limes zero d. L0 d.

loading d. a dose of medication, often larger than subsequent doses, administered to establish a therapeutic level of the medication.

Lr d. (limes reacting dose) in preparation of diphtheria toxoid, the amount of diphtheria toxin that, when mixed with one standard unit of antitoxin, will produce a minimal skin reaction in a guinea pig.

maintenance d. a dose (often a daily dose or dosage regimen) sufficient to maintain at the desired level the influence of a drug achieved by earlier administration of larger amounts.

maximal d., maximum d. the largest quantity of an agent that may be safely administered to the average patient. Cf. *tolerance d.*

maximum permissible d. (MPD) the largest amount of ionizing radiation that can be received by a person in a specified period without expectation of appreciable bodily injury; this varies with age and other circumstances.

maximum tolerated d. (MTD) tolerance d.

median curative d. (CD$_{50}$) a dose that abolishes symptoms in half the test subjects.

median effective d. (ED$_{50}$) a dose that produces the desired effect in half of a population.

median immunizing d. the dose of vaccine or antigen sufficient to provide immunity in half the test subjects.

median infective d. (ID$_{50}$) the amount of pathogenic microorganisms that will produce demonstrable infection in half the test subjects.

median lethal d. (LD$_{50}$) the amount of pathogenic bacteria, bacterial toxin, or other poisonous substance required to kill half of a group of uniformly susceptible animals, or the amount of ionizing radiation that will kill half of a large group or population in a given time period.

median tissue culture infective d. (TCID$_{50}$) the quantity of a cytopathogenic agent (virus) that will produce a cytopathic effect in half of the cultures inoculated.

median toxic d. (TD$_{50}$) a dose producing a toxic effect in half the population.

minimal d. the smallest quantity of an agent that is likely to produce an appreciable effect.

minimal erythema d. (MED) the smallest amount of ionizing radiation that causes erythema in a given individual.

minimum d. minimal d.

minimum lethal d. (MLD) 1. the smallest amount of a toxic substance that can cause the death of a laboratory animal. 2. in preparing diphtheria toxoid, the smallest quantity of diphtheria toxin that will kill a guinea pig of 250 g weight in four to five days when injected subcutaneously.

optimal d., optimum d. the quantity of an agent that will produce the desired effect without other unfavorable effects.

organ tolerance d. (OTD) the amount of ionizing radiation that can be administered without appreciable damage to a normal organ.

permissible d. maximum permissible d.

priming d. a quantity several times larger than the maintenance dose, used at the initiation of therapy to rapidly establish the desired blood and tissue levels of the drug.

radiation absorbed d. see *absorbed d.* and *rad*[1].

reacting d. the second dose of sensitizing antigen administered to an animal; it is followed by an immediate hypersensitive (e.g., anaphylactic or allergic) response. Cf. *sensitizing d.*

reference d. an estimate of the daily exposure to a substance for humans that is assumed to be without appreciable risk; it is calculated using the no observed adverse effect level and is more conservative than the older margin of safety.

rescue d. breakthrough d.

sensitizing d. the first dose of sensitizing antigen (e.g., protein) administered to an animal in the induction of a hypersensitivity (e.g., anaphylactic or allergic) response; cf. *reacting d.*

skin d. (SD) 1. the air exposure of ionizing radiation at the skin surface, comprising primary radiation plus backscatter. 2. the absorbed dose in the skin.

therapeutic d. a dose several times larger than the maintenance dose, used in vitamin therapy when a marked deficiency exists.

threshold d. minimal d.

threshold erythema d. (TED) a single skin dose that within 30 days produces a faint but definite erythema in 80 percent of those tested, and causes no detectable reaction in the other 20 percent.

tissue d. the absorbed dose in a specific tissue or organ.

tolerance d. the largest quantity of an agent that can be administered without harm. Called also *maximum tolerated d.*

toxic d. the amount of an agent that causes toxic symptoms.

volume d. integral d.

dosha (dosh'ə) [Sanskrit *dus* fault] according to the principle of constitution of the physical body in ayurveda, one of the three vital bioenergies (vata, pitta, kapha) condensed from the five elements; the doshas are responsible for the physical and emotional tendencies in the mind and body, and along with the seven dhatus (tissues) and three malas (waste products) make up the human body. The attributes of the doshas and their specific combination within each individual help determine the individual's physical and mental characteristics, while imbalance among the doshas is the cause of disease.

do•sim•e•ter (do-sim'ə-tər) in radiology, an instrument used to detect and measure exposure to radiation of either personnel or radiotherapy patients. See also *film badge.* Called also *dosage meter.*

do•sim•e•trist (do-sim'ə-trist) a specialist who plans an optimum radiotherapy dosage pattern or establishes a summation isodose pattern for the radiotherapy by means of isodose curves or other data supplied by a radiation physicist.

do·sim·e·try (do-sim′ə-tre) [*dose* + *-metry*] the determination by scientific methods of the amount, rate, and distribution of radiation emitted from a source of ionizing radiation. **dosimet′ric** *adj*

biological d. determination of the level of exposure by measurement of radiation-induced changes such as cytogenetic abnormalities, lymphopenia, and agranulocytosis; the dose is estimated by comparison of the measurements under consideration to those observed in prior radiation accidents.

physical d. determination of the level of exposure by means of radiation measuring instruments such as environmental monitoring devices or individual dosimeters.

do·sis (do′sis) [L., Gr. "a giving"] dose.

dos·sier (dos′e-a) [Fr.] the accumulated records of a patient's case history.

Dos·ti·nex (dos′tĭ-neks) trademark for a preparation of cabergoline.

dot (dot) a small spot.

Gunn d's, Marcus Gunn d's white dots seen about the macula lutea of the normal eye on oblique illumination.

Maurer d's irregular dots, staining red with Leishman stain, seen in erythrocytes from malarial patients infected with *Plasmodium falciparum;* called also *Maurer clefts* or *spots.*

Mittendorf d. a congenital anomaly manifested as a small gray or white opacity just inferior and nasal to the posterior pole of the lens, representing the remains of the lenticular attachment of the hyaloid artery; it does not affect vision.

Schüffner d's minute granules observed in erythrocytes infected with *Plasmodium vivax* when stained by certain methods, such as Romanowsky stain or Wright stain.

Trantas d's small, white calcareous-looking dots in the limbus of the conjunctiva in vernal conjunctivitis.

Do·thi·de·a·les (do-thid″e-a′lēz) [Gr. *dothiēn* a boil] an order of perfect fungi of the subphylum Ascomycotina, series Bitunicatae, characterized by flasklike ascocarps in which the hymenium is exposed at maturity and by double-walled asci that develop in cavities in a preformed stroma. It is a large and varied order, and a number of different classifications have been proposed for it. It includes the family Piedraiaceae. Called also *Myriangiales.*

do·thi·e·pin hy·dro·chlo·ride (do-thi′ə-pin) a tricyclic antidepressant having actions and uses similar to those of amitriptyline; administered orally.

dou·ble blind (dub′əl blīnd) pertaining to a clinical trial or other experiment in which neither the subject nor the person administering treatment knows which treatment the subject is receiving. The term *double masked* is sometimes preferred to avoid confusion associated with the use of the term "blind."

dou·ble-con·trast (dub′əl kon′trast) pertaining to diagnostic imaging techniques in which two contrast media, such as a radiopaque medium with air or gas or iron oxide with a paramagnetic medium, are used in combination to enhance detail.

dou·ble masked (dub′əl maskt) double blind.

doub·let (dub′lət) [Middle English, from Old Fr. *double*] 1. a fixed combination of two lenses, as in a telescope or microscope, for reducing aberration and increasing power. 2. double discharge.

Wollaston d. a microscopical lens consisting of a combination of two planoconvex lenses for correcting chromatic aberration.

douche (do͞osh) [Fr.] a stream of water or gas directed against a part of the body or into a cavity.

air d. a current of air blown into a cavity, particularly into the tympanum for opening the eustachian tube.

Doug·las bag (dug′ləs) [Claude Gordon *Douglas,* English physiologist, 1882–1963] see under *bag.*

Doug·las septum, etc. (dug′ləs) [James *Douglas,* Scottish anatomist in London, 1675–1742] see under *septum,* and see *excavatio rectouterina, plica rectouterina,* and *linea arcuata vaginae musculi recti abdominis.*

doug·las·cele (dug′lə-sēl) posterior vaginal hernia.

doug·la·si·tis (dug″lə-si′tis) inflammation of Douglas pouch (excavatio rectouterina).

dou·la (doo′lə) [Gr. *doulē* maidservant] an aide, usually female, who gives continual physical and emotional support to a woman going through labor and childbirth; sometimes this extends to giving postpartum care.

dou·rine (doo-rēn′) [Fr.] a venereal type of trypanosomiasis seen in horses and asses in Africa, Asia, and certain regions of North and South America, caused by *Trypanosoma equiperdum;* characteristics include edematous swelling of the external genitalia, a mucopurulent discharge from the urethra or vagina, cutaneous plaques, and progressive emaciation and weakness. Called also *equine* or *horse syphilis.*

Do·vo·nex (do′və-neks) trademark for a preparation of calcipotriene.

dow·el (dou′əl) a rod or a pin, usually metal, fitted into a prepared posthole within the root canal and cemented in place, serving to retain a dental restoration, such as a crown. Called also *post.*

Dow·ling-De·gos disease (dou′ling də-go′) [Geoffrey Barrow *Dowling,* English dermatologist, 1892–1976; Robert *Degos,* French dermatologist, 1904–1987] see under *disease.*

Down syndrome (disease) (doun) [John Langdon Haydon *Down,* English physician, 1828–1896] see under *syndrome.*

down (doun) lanugo.

down·reg·u·la·tion (doun″reg-u-la′shən) controlled decrease, particularly the attenuation of expression of a gene in response to cellular or environmental factors, as by a decrease in transcription of the gene or by destabilization of mRNA, or the reduction in responsiveness of a cell to stimulatory factors after a first exposure, as by decrease in the number of receptors expressed on the cell surface.

Downs analysis, Y axis (dounz) [W.B. *Downs,* American orthodontist, 1899–1966] see under *analysis* and see *Y axis,* under *axis.*

down·stream (doun′strēm) in molecular biology, a term used to denote a region of DNA or RNA that is located to the 3′ side of a gene or region of interest.

dox·a·pram hy·dro·chlo·ride (dok′sə-pram) [USP] a respiratory stimulant used in the treatment of respiratory depression occurring after anesthesia or acute respiratory insufficiency associated with chronic obstructive pulmonary disease; administered intravenously.

dox·azo·sin mes·y·late (dok″sa′zo-sin) a quinazoline derivative that blocks α_1-adrenergic receptors and has a longer half life than that of prazosin; used in the treatment of hypertension and of benign prostatic hyperplasia, administered orally.

dox·e·pin hy·dro·chlo·ride (dok′sə-pin) [USP] a tricyclic antidepressant of the dibenzoxepine class, also having significant anxiolytic activity. It is administered orally to treat depression, chronic pain, peptic ulcer, pruritus, and idiopathic cold urticaria, and is used topically to treat pruritus.

dox·er·cal·cif·er·ol (dok″sər-kal-sif′ər-ol) a synthetic analogue of vitamin D_2, used to reduce levels of circulating parathyroid hormone in the treatment of secondary hyperparathyroidism associated with chronic renal failure; administered orally or intravenously.

Dox·il (dok′sil) trademark for a preparation of liposomal doxorubicin.

Dox·i·nate (dok′sĭ-nāt) trademark for a preparation of docusate sodium.

doxo·ru·bi·cin (dok″so-roo′bĭ-sin) an anthracycline (q.v.) antibiotic produced by *Streptomyces peucetius* var. *caesius* having one of the widest spectrums of antitumor activity of any antineoplastic agent.

d. hydrochloride [USP] the hydrochloride salt of doxorubicin, having the same actions as the base, used for the treatment of lymphomas, leukemias, soft tissue sarcomas, and a wide variety of carcinomas; administered intravenously.

liposomal d. doxorubicin hydrochloride encapsulated within liposomes; administered intravenously in the treatment of Kaposi sarcoma associated with acquired immunodeficiency syndrome (AIDS).

doxy·cy·cline (dok″se-si′klēn) [USP] a semisynthetic broad-spectrum antibacterial of the tetracycline group; administered orally.

d. calcium [USP] a complex prepared from doxycycline hyclate and calcium chloride, having the same actions as other tetracyclines and used in a wide variety of infections; administered orally.

d. hyclate [USP], **d. hydrochloride** a salt having the antibacterial effects of other tetracyclines; administered orally or intravenously. It is also used as an adjunct to scaling and root planing in the treatment of periodontitis; it promotes attachment level gain and reduces pocket depth, possibly by inhibiting collagenase activity.

dox·yl·amine suc·ci·nate (dok-sil′ə-mēn) [USP] an antihistamine (H_1 receptor antagonist) with sedative and anticholinergic effects; used in the treatment of allergic rhinitis, allergic conjunctivitis, and cutaneous manifestations of allergic reactions, as an ingredient in cough and cold preparations, and in the short-term treatment of insomnia; administered orally.

Doy·en clamp (dwah-yah′) [Eugène Louis *Doyen,* French surgeon, 1859–1916] see under *clamp.*

Doyne honeycomb dystrophy (choroiditis, degeneration) (doin) [Robert Walter *Doyne,* English ophthalmologist, 1857–1916] see under *dystrophy.*

DP Doctor of Pharmacy; Doctor of Podiatry.

D.P. [L.] directio′ne prop′ria (with proper direction).

DPH Diploma in Public Health.

DPM Diploma in Psychological Medicine; Doctor of Podiatric Medicine.

DPT diphtheria and tetanus toxoids and pertussis vaccine.

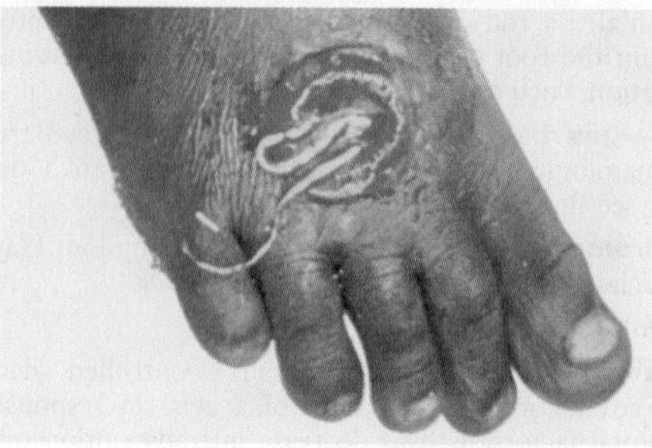

■ Dracunculiasis; guinea worm partially extruded from an ulcer on the dorsum of the foot.

DR reaction of degeneration.

dr dram.

drac·on·ti·a·sis (drak″ən-ti′ə-sis) [Gr. *drakontion* (little dragon) tapeworm] dracunculiasis.

dra·cun·cu·lar (drə-kung′ku-lər) pertaining to or caused by nematodes of the genus *Dracunculus.*

dra·cun·cu·li·a·sis (drə-kung″ku-li′ə-sis) infection with nematodes of the genus *Dracunculus;* characterized by pruritic skin vesicles that ulcerate, and nausea and vomiting that can be severe. Called also *dracontiasis, dracunculosis,* and *guinea worm disease.*

Dra·cun·cu·li·dae (drə-kəng-ku′lĭ-de) a family of nematodes that includes many parasitic species; it contains one genus of medical interest, *Dracunculus.*

Dra·cun·cu·loi·dea (drə-kung″ku-loi′de-ə) a superfamily of phasmid nematodes including the genus *Dracunculus.*

dra·cun·cu·lo·sis (drə-kung″ku-lo′sis) dracunculiasis.

Dra·cun·cu·lus (drə-kung′ku-ləs) [L. "little dragon"] a genus of nematode parasites of the family Dracunculidae.

D. insig′nis a species that parasitizes dogs, cats, raccoons, and other carnivores.

D. medinen′sis a threadlike worm 30 to 120 cm long that inhabits the subcutaneous and intermuscular tissues of humans and domestic animals from the Indian subcontinent across southern Asia to Africa, causing dracunculiasis. Its embryos are discharged through the skin upon contact with water; from the water they enter the body of a small crustacean, *Cyclops,* where they undergo larval development. Called also *dragon worm, guinea worm, Medina worm,* and *serpent worm.*

drag (drag) the lower or cast side of a denture flask to which the cope is fitted.

dra·gée (drah-zha′) [Fr. "sugar-plum"] a sugar-coated pill, or medicated confection.

drain (drān) any device by which a channel or open area may be established for the exit of fluids or purulent material from any cavity, wound, or infected area.

cigarette d. a drain made by drawing a strip of gauze or surgical sponge into the lumen of a rubber tube.

controlled d. a drain made by pressing a square of gauze into the wound and then packing with gauze strips, the ends of which, together with the corners of the square, are left projecting from the wound.

double-lumen d. a drain, such as a sump drain, consisting of two tubes, one inside the other.

Jackson-Pratt d. a closed wound drainage system comprising a drainage tube and collection vessel.

Mikulicz d. a drain formed by pushing a single layer of gauze into a wound or cavity, then packing with several thick wicks of gauze as the original layer is forced farther and farther into the defect.

Penrose d. a thin rubber tube, usually 0.5 to 1 inch in diameter.

stab wound d. drainage accomplished by bringing out the drain through a small separate wound adjacent to the major operative incision.

sump d. a double-lumen drain that allows air to enter the drained area through the smaller lumen and displace fluid into the larger lumen.

sump-Penrose d. a triple-lumen drain formed by placing a double-lumen tube within a Penrose drain.

triple-lumen d. a drain consisting of three tubes placed one inside another.

drain·age (drān′əj) the systematic withdrawal of fluids and discharges from a wound, sore, or cavity.

basal d. withdrawal of the cerebrospinal fluid from the basal subarachnoid space for the relief of intracranial pressure.

capillary d. drainage effected by strands of surgical gut, spun glass, or other material of tiny diameter that induces capillary attraction.

closed d. airtight drainage of a cavity carried out so that the entrance of air or contaminants is prevented.

manual lymph d. the application of light rhythmic strokes, similar to those used in effleurage, to the skin and superficial fascia in the direction of the heart in order to increase the drainage of lymph from the involved structures.

open d. drainage of a cavity through an opening into which one or more rubber drainage tubes are inserted, the opening not being sealed against the entrance of outside air.

percutaneous d. drainage of an abscess or collection of fluid by means of a catheter inserted through the skin and positioned under the guidance of computed tomography or ultrasonography.

percutaneous transhepatic biliary d. a treatment for extrahepatic cholestasis consisting of drainage through a catheter introduced through the liver and into the biliary tree under radiologic guidance. Called also *percutaneous transhepatic cholangiodrainage.*

postural d. removal of secretions in bronchiectasis and lung abscess by positioning the patient so that gravity helps to drain secretions from the affected region of the lung, often combined with other maneuvers such as chest percussion.

suction d. closed drainage of a cavity, with a suction apparatus attached to the drainage tube.

through d. drainage achieved by passing a perforated tube or other type of drain through a cavity, so that irrigation may be effected by injecting fluid into one aperture and letting it escape through another.

tidal d. drainage of the urinary bladder by an apparatus that first partially fills it and then empties it by a combination of siphonage and gravity flow.

dram (ʒ, dr) (dram) a unit of weight which, in the apothecaries' system, equals 60 grains, or $\frac{1}{8}$ ounce; in the avoirdupois system it equals 27.34 grains, or $\frac{1}{16}$ ounce.

fluid d. (fl dr) a unit of capacity (liquid measure) of the apothecaries' system, being 60 minims, or the equivalent of 3.697 mL. In Great Britain, it is the *imperial fluid dram* and is equivalent to 3.55 mL.

Dram·a·mine (dram′ə-mēn) trademark for preparations of dimenhydrinate or meclizine hydrochloride.

Dra·schia (drā′she-ə) a genus of nematodes of the family Habronematidae. *D. megasto′ma* (formerly called *Habronema megastoma*) infects the stomach of horses, and its larvae form nodules in the stomach walls (see *gastric habronemiasis*).

Drash syndrome (drash) [Allan Lee *Drash,* American pediatrician, born 1931] see under *syndrome.*

DRE digital rectal examination.

dream (drēm) 1. a mental phenomenon occurring during sleep in which images, emotions, and thoughts are experienced with a sense of reality. Dreaming occurs during REM sleep; typically there are four or five such periods a night having a total duration of about 90 minutes. Freud originated psychological interpretation of dreams, theorizing that dreams enable the conscious expression of repressed unconscious impulses and wishes. 2. to experience such a phenomenon.

day d. wishful, purposeless reveries, without regard to reality.

wet d. a slang term for *nocturnal emission.*

Drechs·le·ra (dreks′lə-rə) a genus of Fungi Imperfecti of the form-class Hyphomycetes, form-family Dematiaceae, closely related to *Bipolaris* and *Exserohilum. D. bisepta′ta* has been isolated from a human brain abscess. The perfect (sexual) stage of *Drechslera* species is in genus *Cochliobolus.*

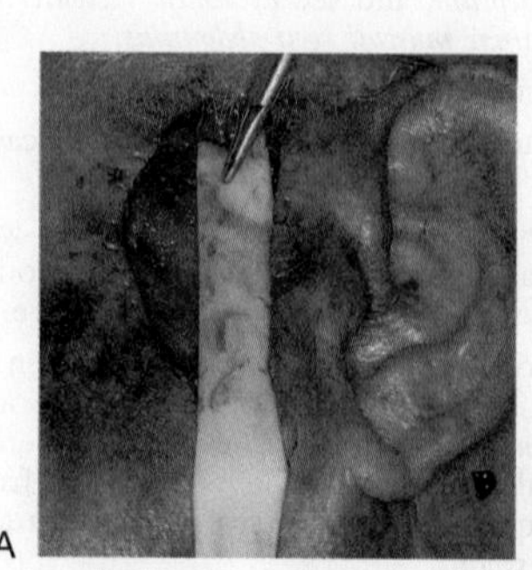

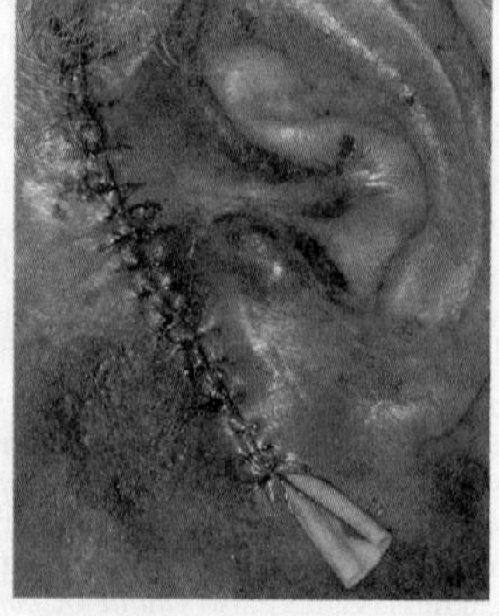

■ Placement of Penrose drain because of excessive bleeding.

drench (drench) a draft of medicine given to an animal by pouring it into its mouth.

Drep·a·nido·tae·nia (drep″ə-nid-o-te′ne-ə) former name for a genus of cestodes; now classified as part of *Hymenolepis.*

drep·a·no·cyte (drep′ə-no-sīt) [Gr. *drepanē* sickle + *-cyte*] sickle cell.

drep·a·no·cyt·ic (drep″ə-no-sit′ik) having or pertaining to sickle cells.

drep·a·no·cy·to·sis (drep″ə-no-si-to′sis) former name for *sickle cell anemia.*

Dres·bach syndrome (dres′bahk) [Melvin *Dresbach*, American physician, 1874–1946] hereditary elliptocytosis.

dress·ing (dres′ing) 1. any of various materials for covering and protecting a wound. See also *bandage.* 2. the putting on of clothing.

adhesive absorbent d. a sterile individual dressing consisting of a plain absorbent compress affixed to a film or fabric coated with a pressure-sensitive adhesive substance.

antiseptic d. a dressing of gauze impregnated with an antiseptic material.

bolus d. tie-over d.

cocoon d. a dressing of gauze affixed to the surrounding skin by collodion or other liquid adhesive in such a way that its elevated appearance resembles a cocoon.

cross d. cross-dressing.

dry d. dry gauze or absorbent cotton applied to a wound.

fixed d. a dressing impregnated with a stiffening agent such as plaster of Paris or starch, used to secure fixation of the part when the material dries.

occlusive d. a dressing that seals a wound from contact with air or bacteria.

pressure d. a dressing that exerts pressure on the area covered to prevent collection of fluids in underlying tissues; most commonly used after skin grafting and in treatment of burns.

protective d. a light dressing to prevent exposure to injury or infection.

rigid d. a rigid, socketlike cast, often made of plaster, worn over a stump after amputation to promote shrinkage.

stent d. a dressing in which is incorporated a mold or stent, to maintain position of a graft.

tie-over d. a dressing placed over a skin graft or other sutured wound and tied on by the sutures, which have been made of sufficient length for that purpose; called also *bolus d.*

Dress·ler syndrome (dres′lər) [William *Dressler*, Polish-born American physician, 1890–1969] postmyocardial infarction syndrome.

Drey·er and Ben·nett hypothesis (dri′ər ben′ət) [William J. *Dreyer*, American immunologist, born 1928; Joe Claude *Bennett*, American rheumatologist, born 1933] see *recombinational germline theory*, under *theory.*

DRG Diagnosis-Related Groups.

drift (drift) [A.S. *drifan* to drive] 1. slow movement away from the normal or original position. 2. a chance variation, as in gene frequency between populations; the smaller the population, the greater the chance of random variations. Called also *genetic d.* or *random genetic d.*

antigenic d. relatively minor changes in the antigenic structure of a virus strain, probably resulting from natural selection of virus variants circulating among an immune or partially immune population. Cf. *antigenic shift*, under *shift.*

genetic d. see *drift* (def. 2).

physiologic d. physiologic tooth migration.

radial d. see under *deviation.*

random genetic d. see *drift* (def. 2).

ulnar d. see under *deviation.*

drill (dril) [Ger. *drillen*] 1. a rotating cutting instrument for making holes in hard substances, such as bones or teeth. 2. bur (def. 1). 3. to bore or scoop out with such an instrument.

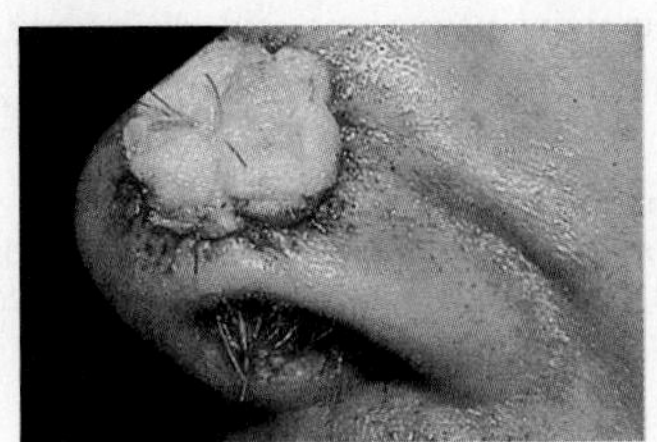

■ Tie-over dressing.

cannulated d. a drill with a hole through the center of its long axis, to be used over a guidewire.

drill·ing (dril′ing) the act or process of boring holes with a rotary instrument, such as in cavity preparation.

drink (drink) 1. a quantity of liquid taken in orally and swallowed. 2. to take in and swallow a liquid.

sham d. a drink, as by an esophagostomized dog, in which swallowed water fails to be ingested or retained in the stomach.

Drink·er respirator (dring′kər) [Philip *Drinker*, American public health engineer, 1894–1972] see under *respirator.*

drip (drip) the slow, drop by drop, infusion of a liquid.

intravenous d. continuous intravenous instillation, drop by drop, of saline or other solution.

nasal d. a method of giving fluid slowly to dehydrated infants through a catheter inserted into the nose and pushed down into the esophagus.

postnasal d. the dripping of discharges from the postnasal region into the pharynx due to hypersecretion of mucus in the nasal or nasopharyngeal mucosa or to chronic sinusitis.

Dris·dol (driz′dol) trademark for preparations of ergocalciferol.

Dritho·creme (drith′o-krēm″) trademark for preparations of anthralin.

Dritho-Scalp (drith′o-skalp″) trademark for a preparation of anthralin.

drive (drīv) 1. the force which activates human impulses. 2. to activate or cause to move.

aggressive d. death instinct.

sexual d. life instinct.

driv·en·ness (driv′ən-nis) hyperactivity (def. 1).

organic d. hyperactivity seen in brain-damaged individuals as a result of injury to and disorganization of cerebellar structures.

driv·ing (drīv′ing) an effect seen on an electroencephalogram, by which certain repetitive sensory stimuli cause changes in amplitude of brain waves. Cf. *following.*

photic d. driving in which alpha rhythms from the occipital cortex are altered when the eye is exposed to a rhythmically flashing light.

dro·car·bil (dro-kahr′bil) a mixture of acetarsone and arecoline, used as a veterinary anthelmintic.

dro·code (dro′kod) dihydrocodeine.

drom(o)- [Gr. *dromos* a course, race] a combining form denoting relationship to conduction, to running, or to speed.

dromo·graph (drom′o-graf) [*dromo-* + *-graph*] an instrument for recording conduction or flow.

drom·o·tro·pic (drom″o-tro′pik) affecting the conductivity of a nerve fiber.

dro·mot·ro·pism (dro-mot′ro-piz-əm) [*dromo-* + *tropism*] the quality or property of affecting the conductivity of a nerve fiber.

negative d. the property of diminishing the conductivity of a nerve.

positive d. the property of increasing the conductivity of a nerve.

dro·nab·i·nol (dro-nab′in-ol) [USP] Δ^9-tetrahydrocannabinol, one of the major active substances in cannabis; used to treat the nausea and vomiting associated with cancer chemotherapy and also anorexia with weight loss associated with acquired immunodeficiency syndrome. Because of its psychotomimetic activity, it is subject to abuse and its use is limited to patients resistant to more conventional agents.

Dron·cit (dron′cit) trademark for preparations of praziquantel.

drop (drop) [L. *gutta*] 1. a minute sphere of liquid as it hangs or falls. 2. to descend or cause to descend. 3. a descent or falling.

ear d's medicated oil or water to be dropped into the external auditory meatus.

enamel d. enameloma.

eye d's a medicated solution to be dropped into the conjunctival sac.

foot d. footdrop.

nose d's a medicated solution to be dropped into the nose.

wrist d. wristdrop.

dro·per·i·dol (dro-per′ĭ-dol) [USP] a drug of the butyrophenone series, used for its antianxiety, sedative, and antiemetic effects as a premedication prior to surgery and during induction and maintenance of anesthesia, for the prophylaxis of postoperative nausea and vomiting, and to produce conscious sedation; administered intravenously or intramuscularly. A combination of droperidol and fentanyl citrate is administered intramuscularly to produce neuroleptanalgesia.

drop·let (drop′lət) a tiny drop, such as one of the particles of moisture expelled from the mouth in coughing, sneezing, or speaking, which may carry infection to others through the air. See also under *nucleus.*

drop·per (drop′ər) a pipet or tube for dispensing liquid in drops.

drop·si·cal (drop′sĭ-kəl) edematous.

drop·sy (drop′se) [L. *hydrops*, from Gr. *hydōr* water] edema.
abdominal d. ascites.
articular d. hydrarthrosis.
d. of belly ascites.
d. of chest hydrothorax.
cutaneous d. edema.
epidemic d. a sometimes fatal condition seen in India, Fiji, South Africa, and elsewhere, characterized by edema of the extremities; dilatation of vessels of the skin, subcutaneous tissues, and uveal tract, resulting in glaucoma; cardiac insufficiency; and liver abnormalities. It is caused by contamination of cooking oil by argemone oil (q.v.), which contains the toxic glycoside sanguinarine.
peritoneal d. ascites.
salpingian d. hydrosalpinx.
wet d. beriberi.

drop·wort (drop′wort) any plant of the genus *Oenanthe.*

Dro·soph·i·la (dro-sof′ĭ-lə) [Gr. *drosos* dew + *philein* to love] a genus of flies; the pomace flies (often erroneously called fruit flies).
D. melanogas′ter a small fly often seen about decaying fruit; used extensively in experimental genetics.

dros·pi·re·none (dros-pi′rə-nōn) a spironolactone analogue with antimineralocorticoid activity; it acts as a progestational agent and is used in combination with an estrogen component as an oral contraceptive.

dro·tre·co·gin al·fa (dro″trə-ko′jin) recombinant human activated protein C, used for the reduction of mortality in severe sepsis in patients at high risk of death; administered intravenously.

drown·ing (droun′ing) suffocation and death resulting from filling of the lungs with water or other substance or fluid, so that gas exchange becomes impossible.
near d. survival for any length of time after submersion in water and temporary suffocation; it sometimes ends with secondary drowning.
secondary d. delayed death from drowning, due to such complications as pulmonary alveolar inflammation.

Drox·ia (drok′se-ə) trademark for a preparation of hydroxyurea.

drox·i·fil·con A (drok″sĭ-fil′kon) a hydrophilic contact lens material.

DrPH Doctor of Public Health.

DRPLA dentatorubral-pallidoluysian atrophy.

drug (drug) 1. a chemical substance that affects the processes of the mind or body. 2. any chemical compound that is administered as an aid in the diagnosis, treatment, or prevention of disease or other abnormal condition, for the relief of pain or suffering, or to control or improve any physiologic or pathologic condition. 3. recreational d. 4. to administer such a substance to someone.
antagonistic d. a drug that tends to counteract or neutralize the effect of another.
crude d. the whole drug with all its ingredients.
designer d. a new drug of abuse similar in action to an older abused drug, usually created by making a slight alteration in the chemical structure of the older one so that it is no longer a controlled substance.
disease-modifying antirheumatic d. (DMARD) a classification of antirheumatic agents referring to their ability to modify the course of disease, as opposed to simply treating symptoms such as inflammation and pain.
mind-altering d. a drug that produces an altered state of consciousness, usually referring to psychoactive substances that are used recreationally, such as mescaline and lysergic acid diethylamide (LSD).
nonsteroidal antiinflammatory d. (NSAID) any of a large, chemically heterogeneous group of drugs that inhibit cyclooxygenase activity, resulting in decreased synthesis of prostaglandin and thromboxane precursors from arachidonic acid. All NSAIDs have analgesic, antipyretic, and antiinflammatory actions. Called also *nonsteroidal antiinflammatory analgesic* or *agent.*
orphan d. a drug that has limited commercial appeal because of the rarity of the condition it is used to treat.
psychoactive d., psychotropic d. see under *substance.*
recreational d. a legal or illegal psychoactive substance that is used nonmedically for the satisfaction to be derived from it.

drug-fast (drug′fast″) drug-resistant.

drug·gist (drug′ist) pharmacist.

drug-re·sis·tant (drug′re-zis″tənt) resistant to the action of drugs; said of microorganisms. See also *drug resistance,* under *resistance.*

drum (drum) membrana tympanica.

drum·head (drum′hed) membrana tympanica.

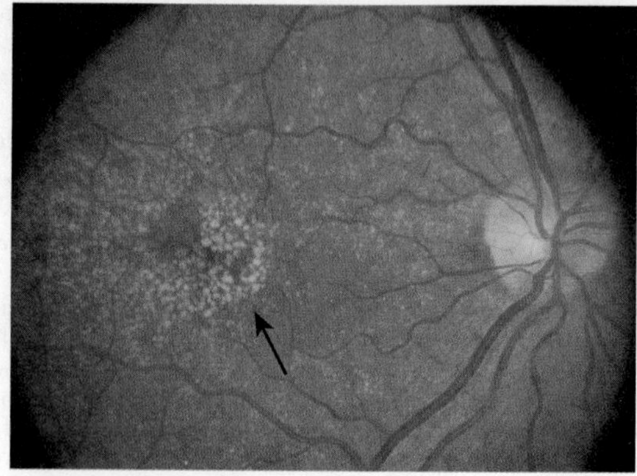

■ Extensive small or cuticular drusen in a 56-year-old man.

Drum·mond marginal artery, sign (drum′ənd) [Sir David *Drummond,* English physician, 1852–1932] see *arteria marginalis coli* and see under *sign.*

drum·stick (drum′stik) a nuclear lobule attached by a slender strand to the nucleus of a small proportion of polymorphonuclear leukocytes of normal females but not of normal males.

drunk·en·ness (drung′kən-nis) inebriation.
sleep d. a condition of prolonged transition from sleep to waking, with partial alertness, disorientation, drowsiness, and poor coordination; sometimes also characterized by excited or violent behavior.

drupe (dro͞op) [L. *drupa* an overripe olive] any of several stone fruits in which the outer part of the ovary wall forms a skin, the middle part becomes fleshy and juicy, and the inner part forms a hard pit or stone around the seed; e.g., peaches, plums, apricots.

dru·sen (droo′zən) (sing. *druse*) [Ger. "bumps"] 1. hyaline excrescences in the Bruch layer of the choroid; they usually result from aging, but sometimes occur with pathologic conditions. 2. sulfur granules.

Dry·op·te·ris (dri-op′tə-ris) a large genus of ferns of the family Polypodiaceae. *D. fi′lix-mas* is the male or male shield fern (filix mas), a poisonous species that yields oil of male fern, formerly used as an anthelmintic.

Dry·sol (dri′sol) trademark for a preparation of aluminum chloride.

DSH dyschromatosis symmetrica hereditaria.

DSC Doctor of Surgical Chiropody.

DSD disorder of sexual development.

dsDNA double-stranded DNA.

DSM *Diagnostic and Statistical Manual of Mental Disorders.*

dsRNA double-stranded RNA.

DT diphtheria and tetanus toxoids.

Dt duration tetany.

dT deoxythymidine.

DTaP diphtheria and tetanus toxoids and acellular pertussis vaccine.

D.T.D. [L.] da′tur ta′lis do′sis (give of such a dose).

dTDP deoxythymidine diphosphate.

DTH delayed-type hypersensitivity.

DTIC, Dtic dacarbazine.

DTIC-Dome (dōm) trademark for a preparation of dacarbazine.

dTMP deoxythymidine monophosphate.

dTMP ki·nase (ki′nās) [EC 2.7.4.9] an enzyme of the transferase class that catalyzes the phosphorylation of dTMP to form dTDP, a step in the synthesis of dTTP from dUMP.

DTP diphtheria and tetanus toxoids and pertussis vaccine.

DTPA diethylenetriamine pentaacetic acid; see *pentetic acid.*

dTTP deoxythymidine triphosphate.

dU deoxyuridine.

du·al·ism (doo′əl-iz-əm) [L. *duo* two] 1. dualistic theory; see under *theory.* 2. the theory that human beings are made up of two independent systems, mind and body, and that psychic and physical phenomena are fundamentally independent and different in nature.

dual-spec•i•fic•i•ty ki•nase (doo′əl spes″ĭ-fis′ĭ-te ki′nās) [EC 2.7.12] the group of protein kinases comprising those phosphophorylating both serine/threonine and tyrosine residues in proteins.

Duane syndrome (dwān) [Alexander *Duane*, American ophthalmologist, 1858–1926] see under *syndrome.*

DUB dysfunctional uterine bleeding.

Du•bin-John•son syndrome (doo′bən jon′sən) [Isidore Nathan *Dubin*, American pathologist, 1913–1981; Frank B. *Johnson*, American pathologist, born 1919] see under *syndrome.*

Du•bin-Sprinz syndrome (doo′bən shprintz′) [I.N. *Dubin;* Helmuth *Sprinz*, German-born American pathologist, 1911–1990] Dubin-Johnson syndrome.

Du•bi•ni chorea (disease) (doo-be′ne) [Angelo *Dubini*, Italian physician, 1813–1902] see under *chorea.*

Du•bois abscess (disease), sign (du-bwah′) [Paul *Dubois*, French obstetrician, 1795–1871] see under *abscess* and *sign.*

Du•boi•sia (doo-boi′se-ə) a genus of plants of the family Solanaceae. *D. myoporoi′des* is the corkwood tree, which contains hyoscyamine and scopolamine and can cause neurotoxicity in livestock.

Du•breu•ilh melanosis (du-broo͝′yə) [William *Dubreuilh*, French dermatologist, 1857–1935] lentigo maligna melanoma.

Du•breu•il-Cham•bar•del syndrome (du-broo-e′-shahm-bahr-del′) [Louis *Dubreuil-Chambardel*, French dentist, 1879–1927] see under *syndrome.*

-ducent [L. *ducens*, present part. of *ducere* to draw or lead] a word termination meaning leading or conducting.

Du•chenne disease, etc. (du-shen′) [Guillaume Benjamin Amand *Duchenne*, French neurologist, 1806–1875] see under *disease, paralysis,* and *sign*, see *pseudohypertrophic muscular dystrophy*, under *dystrophy*, and see *progressive bulbar palsy*, under *palsy.*

Du•chenne-Aran muscular atrophy (disease) (du-shen′ ah-rah′) [G.B.A. *Duchenne*; François Amilcar *Aran*, French physician, 1817–1861] spinal muscular atrophy; see under *atrophy.*

Du•chenne-Erb paralysis, syndrome (du-shen′ ār′) [G.B.A. *Duchenne;* Wilhelm Heinrich *Erb*, German internist, 1840–1921] Erb-Duchenne paralysis.

Du•chenne-Grie•sing•er disease (du-shen′ gre′sing-er) [G.B.A. *Duchenne;* Wilhelm *Griesinger*, German neurologist, 1817–1868] Duchenne muscular dystrophy.

Du•chenne-Lan•dou•zy muscular dystrophy (du-shen′ lahn-doo-ze′) [G.B.A. *Duchenne*; Louis Théophile Joseph *Landouzy*, French physician, 1845–1917] facioscapulohumeral muscular dystrophy.

Du•co•bee (doo′ko-be) trademark for preparations of vitamin B_{12}; see *cyanocobalamin.*

Du•crey bacillus (doo-kra′) [Augusto *Ducrey*, Italian dermatologist, 1860–1940] *Haemophilus ducreyi.*

duct (dukt) [L. *ductus*, from *ducere* to draw or lead] a passage with well-defined walls, especially such a channel for the passage of excretions or secretions. See also entries under *ductus* and *ductulus.* **duc′tal** *adj*

Duct

For descriptions of anatomic structures not found here, see under *ductus.*

aberrant d. 1. any duct that is not usually present or that takes an unusual course or direction, such as the ductulus aberrans superior. 2. *(in the pl.)* ductuli aberrantes.
accessory pancreatic d., accessory d. of Santorini ductus pancreaticus accessorius.
acoustic d. meatus acusticus externus.
adipose d. an elongated sac in the cellular tissue filled with fat.
allantoic d. see under *stalk.*
alveolar d's ductuli alveolares.
anterior semicircular d. ductus semicircularis anterior.
d. of Arantius ductus venosus.
archinephric d. pronephric d.
arterial d. ductus arteriosus.
Bartholin d. ductus sublingualis major.
Bellini d. papillary d.
bile d., biliary d. 1. any of the ducts that convey bile in and from the liver; see *ductus choledochus, ductus cysticus, ductus hepaticus dexter*, and *ductus hepaticus sinister.* 2. specifically, the ductus choledochus.
d. of Botallo ductus arteriosus.
branchial d's drawn-out branchial grooves 2, 3, and 4, which open into the temporary cervical sinus of the embryo.
d. of bulbourethral gland ductus glandulae bulbourethralis.
canalicular d's ductus lactiferi.
cervical d. the opening from the exterior into the temporary cervical sinus of the embryo.
choledochal d. ductus choledochus.
cloacal d. the cleft between the Douglas septum and the cloaca in the embryo.
cochlear d. ductus cochlearis.
collecting d. tubulus renalis colligens.
common bile d. ductus choledochus.
common hepatic d. ductus hepaticus communis.
cortical collecting d. see under *tubule.*
Cowper gland d. ductus glandulae bulbourethralis.
craniopharyngeal d. hypophysial d.
d's of Cuvier common cardinal veins.
cystic d. ductus cysticus.
deferent d. ductus deferens.
eccrine d., eccrine sweat d. the duct of an eccrine sweat gland.
efferent d. a duct that gives outlet to a glandular secretion.
ejaculatory d. ductus ejaculatorius.
endolymphatic d. ductus endolymphaticus.
d. of epididymis ductus epididymidis.
d. of epoöphoron ductus longitudinalis epoöphori.
excretory d. a duct that is merely conductive and not secretory.
excretory d. of seminal gland, excretory d. of seminal vesicle ductus excretorius glandulae vesiculosae.
frontonasal d. a duct in the lateral wall of the nasal cavity extending from the frontal sinus to the infundibulum of the ethmoid bone; called also *nasofrontal d.*
galactophorous d's ductus lactiferi.
gall d. bile d. (def. 1).
Gartner d. ductus longitudinalis epoöphori.
genital d. see under *canal.*
Haller aberrant d. ductulus aberrans inferior.
Hensen d. ductus reuniens.
hypophysial d. an embryonic structure composed of the elongated Rathke pouch joining the infundibulum of the embryonic hypophysis; called also *craniopharyngeal d.*
incisive d. ductus incisivus.
intercalated d. a slender initial portion of the duct system interposed between an acinus of a gland and a secretory duct.
interlobular d's 1. channels located between different lobules of a gland. 2. ductus biliferi interlobulares.
interlobular bile d's, interlobular biliary d's ductus biliferi interlobulares.
lacrimal d. canaliculus lacrimalis.
lacrimonasal d. ductus nasolacrimalis.
lactiferous d's ductus lactiferi.
lateral semicircular d. ductus semicircularis lateralis.
left d. of caudate lobe of liver ductus lobi caudati sinister hepatis.
left hepatic d. ductus hepaticus sinister.
left lymphatic d. ductus thoracicus.
longitudinal d. of epoöphoron ductus longitudinalis epoöphori.
Luschka d's tubular structures in the wall of the gallbladder, some connected with bile ducts but none connected with the lumen of the gallbladder; they may be aberrant bile ducts.
lymphatic d's the main lymph channels, the right lymphatic duct, thoracic duct, and cisterna chyli (when present), into which the converging lymph vessels drain, which in turn empty into the blood stream.
major sublingual d. ductus sublingualis major.
mammary d's, mammillary d's ductus lactiferi.
medullary collecting d. see under *tubule.*

Duct *Continued*

mesonephric d. an embryonic duct which, initiated in association with rudiments of the pronephric kidney, is taken over as an excretory duct by the mesonephros, and develops into the epididymis, the ductus deferens and its ampulla, the seminal vesicles, and the ejaculatory duct in the male and into vestigial structures in the female. Called also *wolffian d.* and *d. of Wolff.*
metanephric d. an embryonic duct that empties from the metanephros into the mesonephric duct and later develops into part of the ureter.
milk d's ductus lactiferi.
minor pancreatic d. ductus pancreaticus accessorius.
minor sublingual d's ductus sublinguales minores.
d. of Müller, müllerian d. paramesonephric d.
nasal d. ductus nasolacrimalis.
nasofrontal d. frontonasal d.
nasolacrimal d. ductus nasolacrimalis.
omphaloenteric d., omphalomesenteric d. yolk stalk.
ovarian d. tuba uterina.
pancreatic d. ductus pancreaticus.
papillary d. a wide terminal tubule in the renal pyramid, formed by the union of several straight collecting tubules and emptying into the renal pelvis in the area cribrosa. Called also *Bellini d.*
paramesonephric d. either of the paired embryonic ducts arising as a peritoneal pocket, extending caudally to join the urogenital sinus; in the female it develops into the uterine tubes and uterus and in the male it degenerates, leaving vestigial structures such as the appendix testis and utriculus prostaticus. Called also *d. of Müller, müllerian d.,* and *primordial d.*
paraurethral d's of female urethra ductus paraurethrales urethrae femininae.
paraurethral d's of male urethra ductus paraurethrales urethrae masculinae.
parotid d. ductus parotideus.
d. of Pecquet ductus thoracicus.
perilymphatic d. aqueductus cochleae.
persistent müllerian d. the persistence in otherwise normal males of müllerian structures that normally should regress in utero. See *persistent müllerian duct syndrome,* under *syndrome.*
posterior semicircular d. ductus semicircularis posterior.
primordial d. paramesonephric d.
pronephric d. the duct of the pronephros, which later serves as the mesonephric duct (ductus mesonephricus); called also *archinephric d.*
d's of prostate gland, prostatic d's ductuli prostatici.
Rathke d. the part of the ductus paramesonephricus lying between its main part and the sinus pocularis.
right d. of caudate lobe of liver ductus lobi caudati dexter hepatis.
right hepatic d. ductus hepaticus dexter.
right lymphatic d., right thoracic d. ductus lymphaticus dexter.
Rivinus d's ductus sublinguales minores.
saccular d. ductus saccularis.
sacculoutricular d. ductus utriculosaccularis.
salivary d's the ducts that convey the saliva: they are the ductus parotideus, ductus submandibularis, ductus sublingualis major, and ductus sublinguales minores.
d. of Santorini ductus pancreaticus accessorius.
secretory d. a smaller duct that is tributary to an excretory duct of a gland and that also has a secretory function.
semicircular d's ductus semicirculares.
seminal d's passages for the conveyance of spermatozoa and semen, including the ductus deferens, ductus excretorius glandulae vesiculosae, and ductus ejaculatorius.
Skene d's ductus paraurethrales urethrae femininae.
spermatic d. ductus deferens.
Stensen d. ductus parotideus.
sublingual d's the ducts of the sublingual salivary glands, including the ductus sublingualis major and ductus sublinguales minores.
submandibular d. ductus submandibularis.
sudoriferous d. sweat d.
superior semicircular d. ductus semicircularis anterior.
sweat d. the duct that leads from the body of a sweat gland to the surface of the skin.
tear d. ductus nasolacrimalis.
testicular d. ductus deferens.
thoracic d. ductus thoracicus.
thyroglossal d., thyrolingual d. ductus thyroglossalis.
umbilical d. yolk stalk.
urogenital d's the paramesonephric and mesonephric ducts.
utricular d. ductus utricularis.
utriculosaccular d. ductus utriculosaccularis.
vitelline d., vitellointestinal d. yolk stalk.
Wharton d. ductus submandibularis.
d. of Wirsung ductus pancreaticus.
d. of Wolff, wolffian d. mesonephric d.

duc•tile (duk′til) [L. *ductilis,* from *ducere* to draw, to lead] susceptible of being drawn out, as into a wire.

duc•tion (duk′shən) [L. *ductio,* from *ducere* to lead] in ophthalmology, the rotation of an eye by the extraocular muscles around its horizontal, vertical, or anteroposterior axis, the direction of the movement of the eye being indicated by prefixes. See *infraduction, supraduction, abduction, adduction,* and *cycloduction,* and see also *vergence* (def. 2) and *version* (def. 5).

duct•less (dukt′ləs) having no excretory duct.

duc•tog•ra•phy (duk-tog′rə-fe) the administering of craniocaudal and lateral mammograms after the mammary ducts have been injected with radiopaque medium, done to assess function of the ducts.

duc•to•pe•nia (duk″to-pe′nia) deficiency in the number of ducts, particularly bile ducts; it may be focal or generalized.

duct•ule (duk′tūl) a minute duct; called also *ductulus.*
  aberrant d's 1. ductules that are not usually present, or that follow an unusual course or direction. 2. ductuli aberrantes.
  alveolar d's ductuli alveolares.
  bile d's, biliary d's 1. ductuli biliferi. 2. cholangioles.
  efferent d's of testis ductuli efferentes testis.
  excretory d's of lacrimal gland ductuli excretorii glandulae lacrimalis.
  inferior aberrant d. ductulus aberrans inferior.
  interlobular d's ductus biliferi interlobulares.
  prostatic d's ductuli prostatici.
  superior aberrant d. ductulus aberrans superior.
  transverse d's of epoöphoron ductuli transversi epoöphori.

duc•tu•lus (duk′tu-ləs) gen. and pl. *duc′tuli* [L.] ductule: a minute duct; applied especially to branches of ducts nearest to the alveoli of a gland, or the smallest beginnings of the duct system of an organ.

  duc′tuli aberran′tes [TA] aberrant ductules: blind vestiges of mesonephric tubules near the epididymis; see *d. aberrans inferior* and *d. aberrans superior.*

  d. aber′rans infe′rior [TA] inferior aberrant ductule: a narrow, coiled tube often connected with the first part of the ductus deferens, or with the lower part of the duct of the epididymis.

  d. aber′rans supe′rior [TA] superior aberrant ductule: a narrow tube of variable length that lies in the epididymis and is connected with the rete testis; called also *ductus aberrans.*

  duc′tuli alveola′res alveolar ductules: small passages connecting the respiratory bronchioles and the alveolar sacs; see Plate 43. Called also *alveolar ducts.*

  duc′tuli bili′feri biliary ductules: the small channels that connect the interlobular ducts with the right and left hepatic ducts; called also *bile ductules* or *vessels.*

  duc′tuli efferen′tes tes′tis [TA] efferent ductules of testis: ductules entering the head of the epididymis from the rete testis.

  duc′tuli excreto′rii glan′dulae lacrima′lis [TA] excretory ductules of lacrimal gland: numerous ductules that traverse the palpebral part of the lacrimal gland and open into the superior fornix of the conjunctiva.

  duc′tuli prosta′tici [TA] prostatic ductules: minute ducts from the prostate gland that open on either side into or near the prostatic sinuses on the posterior wall of the urethra. Called also *ducts of prostate gland,* and *prostatic ducts.*

  duc′tuli transver′si epoö′phori [TA] transverse ductules of epoöphoron: the vestigial remains of the mesonephric ducts, which open into the longitudinal duct of the epoophoron.

duc•tus (duk′təs) gen. and pl. *duc′tus* [L.] duct; a passage with well-defined walls. see also *ductulus.*

Ductus

Descriptions of structures are given on TA terms, and include the anglicized names of specific ducts.

d. aberran′tes ductuli aberrantes.

d. arterio′sus [TA] arterial duct: a fetal blood vessel connecting the left pulmonary artery directly to the descending aorta; called also *arterial canal* and *duct of Botallo.*

d. bilia′ris TA alternative for *d. choledochus.*

d. bili′feri ductuli biliferi.

d. bili′feri interlobula′res [TA] interlobular bile ducts: small channels between the hepatic lobules, draining into the biliary ductules. Called also *interlobular biliary canals* and *interlobular ductules.*

d. chole′dochus [TA] bile duct: the duct formed by union of the common hepatic duct and the cystic duct; it empties into the duodenum at the major duodenal papilla, along with the pancreatic duct. Called also *d. biliaris* [TA alternative] and *biliary* or *common bile duct.*

d. cochlea′ris [TA] cochlear duct: a spirally arranged membranous tube in the bony canal of the cochlea along its outer wall, lying between the scala tympani below and the scala vestibuli above; called also *membranous cochlea, scala media,* and *scala of Löwenberg.*

d. cys′ticus [TA] cystic duct: the passage connecting the neck of the gallbladder and the common bile duct.

d. de′ferens [TA] the excretory duct of the testis, which unites with the excretory duct of the seminal vesicle to form the ejaculatory duct. It has been divided into four parts: scrotal, funicular, inguinal, and pelvic (see *pars scrotalis, pars funicularis, pars inguinalis,* and *pars pelvica ductus deferentis*). Called also *vas deferens, spermatic duct,* and *testicular duct.*

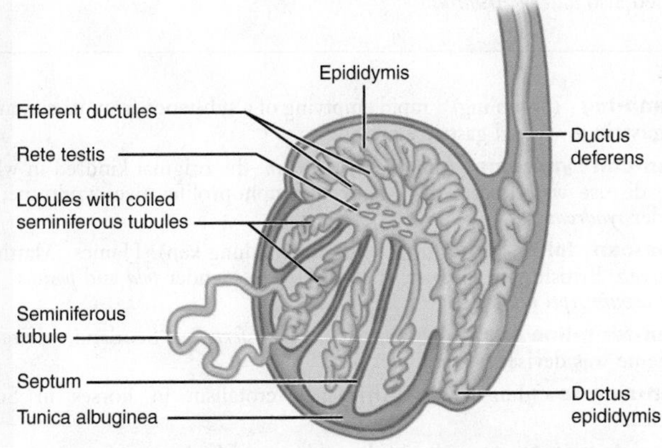

d. de′ferens vestigia′lis [TA] vestige of ductus deferens: the vestigial remnants of the mesonephric duct in the female.

d. ejaculato′rius [TA] ejaculatory duct: the canal formed by union of the ductus deferens and the excretory duct of the seminal gland; it enters the prostatic part of the urethra on the colliculus seminalis.

d. endolympha′ticus [TA] endolymphatic duct: the membranous tube connecting the utriculosaccular duct with the endolymphatic sac, located within the bony vestibular aqueduct.

d. epididy′midis [TA] duct of epididymis: the single tube into which the coiled ends of the efferent ductules of the testis open, the convolutions of which make up the greater part of the epididymis; called also *canal of epididymis.*

d. excreto′rius glan′dulae vesiculo′sae [TA] excretory duct of seminal gland: the duct that drains the seminal vesicle and unites with the ductus deferens to form the ejaculatory duct.

d. glan′dulae bulbourethra′lis [TA] duct of bulbourethral gland: a duct passing from the bulbourethral gland through the perineal membrane into the bulb of the penis, where it enters the spongy part of the urethra.

d. hepa′ticus commu′nis [TA] common hepatic duct: the duct formed by union of the right and left hepatic ducts, which in turn joins the cystic duct to form the common bile duct.

d. hepa′ticus dex′ter [TA] right hepatic duct: the duct that drains the right liver and part of the posterior liver (caudate lobe). It has anterior and posterior branches draining from specific segments of the liver; see table at *segmentum.*

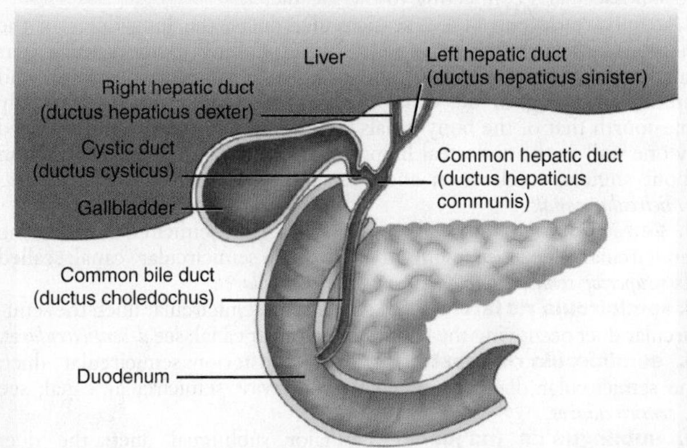

d. hepa′ticus sinis′ter [TA] left hepatic duct: the duct that drains the left liver and part of the posterior liver (caudate lobe). It has lateral and medial branches draining from specific segments of the liver; see table at *segmentum.*

d. inci′sivus [TA] incisive duct: a passage sometimes found in the incisive canal that interconnects the nasal and oral cavities during embryonic development; it occasionally fails to close.

d. lacti′feri [TA] lactiferous ducts: channels conveying the milk secreted by the lobes of the breast to and through the nipples; called also *lactiferous tubules* and *mammary ducts.*

d. lo′bi cauda′ti dex′ter he′patis [TA] the right duct draining the caudate lobe *(pars posterior hepatis).*

d. lo′bi cauda′ti sinis′ter he′patis [TA] the left duct draining the caudate lobe *(pars posterior hepatis).*

d. longitudina′lis epoö′phori [TA] longitudinal duct of epoöphoron: a closed rudimentary duct lying parallel to the uterine tube into which the transverse ducts of the epoöphoron open; it is a remnant of the part of the mesonephros that participates in formation of the reproductive organs. Called also *duct of epoöphoron* and *Gartner canal* or *duct.*

d. lympha′ticus dex′ter [TA] right lymphatic duct: a vessel draining the lymph from the upper right side of the body, typically formed by the right jugular, subclavian, and bronchomediastinal lymphatic trunks, any one of which may, however, end separately in the right brachiocephalic vein; when all three lymphatic vessels unite, a right lymphatic duct is formed, which empties directly into the junction of the internal jugular and subclavian veins. Called also *d. thoracicus dexter* [TA alternative] and *right thoracic duct*

d. nasolacrima′lis [TA] nasolacrimal duct: the passage that conveys the tears from the lacrimal sac into the inferior nasal meatus; called also *lacrimonasal, nasal,* or *tear duct.*

d. pancrea′ticus [TA] pancreatic duct: the main excretory duct of the pancreas, which usually unites with the common bile duct before entering the duodenum at the major duodenal papilla; called also *duct of Wirsung.*

d. pancrea′ticus accesso′rius [TA] accessory pancreatic duct: a small inconstant duct draining part of the head of the pancreas into the minor duodenal papilla; called also *minor pancreatic duct* and *duct of Santorini.*

d. paraurethra′les ure′thrae femini′nae [TA] paraurethral ducts of female urethra: inconstantly present ducts in the female, which drain a group of the urethral glands, the paraurethral glands, into the vestibule; called also *Skene ducts.*

d. paraurethra′les ure′thrae masculi′nae [TA] paraurethral ducts of male urethra: the ducts of the urethral glands situated in the spongy portion of the male urethra.

d. paroti′deus [TA] parotid duct: the duct that drains the parotid gland and empties into the oral cavity opposite the second superior molar; called also *Stensen duct.*

patent d. arteriosus (PDA) abnormal persistence of an open lumen in the ductus arteriosus after birth, the direction of flow being from the aorta to the pulmonary artery, resulting in recirculation of arterial blood through the lungs.

Ductus *Continued*

d. reu′niens [TA] a small canal leading from the saccule to the cochlear duct; called also *Hensen duct.*
d. saccula′ris [TA] saccular duct: the segment of the ductus utriculosaccularis connecting to the saccule.
d. semicircula′res [TA] semicircular ducts: the long ducts of the membranous labyrinth of the ear, corresponding to the semicircular canals of the bony labyrinth and designated anterior, posterior, and lateral, according to the canal they occupy. Their diameter is only one-fourth that of the bony canals containing them, and each is affixed by one wall to the endosteal lining of the canal. They give information about angular acceleration and deceleration. Called also *membranous semicircular canals.*
d. semicircula′ris ante′rior [TA] anterior semicircular duct: the semicircular duct occupying the anterior semicircular canal; called also *superior semicircular duct.* See *d. semicirculares.*
d. semicircula′ris latera′lis [TA] lateral semicircular duct: the semicircular duct occupying the lateral semicircular canal; see *d. semicirculares.*
d. semicircula′ris poste′rior [TA] posterior semicircular duct: the semicircular duct occupying the posterior semicircular canal; see *d. semicirculares.*
d. sublingua′lis ma′jor [TA] major sublingual duct: the duct that drains the sublingual gland and opens alongside the submandibular duct on the sublingual caruncle; called also *Bartholin duct.*
d. sublingua′les mino′res [TA] minor sublingual ducts: the ducts that drain the sublingual gland and open along the crest of the sublingual fold; called also *Rivinus ducts.*
d. submandibula′ris [TA] submandibular duct: the duct that drains the submandibular gland and opens at the sublingual caruncle; called also *Wharton duct.*
d. thora′cicus [TA] thoracic duct: the largest lymph channel in the body, which collects lymph from the portions of the body below the diaphragm and from the left side of the body above the diaphragm; it begins in the abdomen *(pars abdominalis)* at the junction of the intestinal, lumbar, and descending intercostal trunks (which consists of a plexus or the *cisterna chyli*) at about the level of the second lumbar vertebra, enters the thorax through the aortic hiatus of the diaphragm *(pars thoracica)*, ascends to cross the posterior mediastinum, and enters the neck *(pars cervicalis)*, where it forms a downward arch *(arcus ductus thoracici)* across the subclavian artery, and ends at the junction of the subclavian and internal jugular veins. Called also *duct of Pecquet, left lymphatic duct,* and *van Hoorne canal.*
d. thora′cicus dex′ter TA alternative for *d. lymphaticus dexter.*
d. thyroglossa′lis [TA] thyroglossal duct: a duct in the embryo extending between the thyroid primordium and the posterior part of the tongue, which opens as the foramen caecum; the distal part usually differentiates to form the pyramidal lobe of the thyroid and the remainder becomes obliterated, but occasionally persists into adult life, giving rise to cysts, fistulas, or sinuses. Called also *thyrolingual duct.*
d. utricula′ris [TA] utricular duct: the segment of the ductus utriculosaccularis connecting to the utricle.
d. utriculosaccula′ris [TA] utriculosaccular duct: a tiny Y-shaped duct in the membranous labyrinth connecting the utricle and saccule and joining with the endolymphatic duct (ductus endolymphaticus). Called also *sacculoutricular duct* or *canal* and *utriculosaccular canal.*
d. veno′sus a major blood channel that develops through the embryonic liver from the umbilical vein to the inferior vena cava; called also *duct of Arantius.*

Duf·fy blood group (duf′e) [*Duffy,* surname of the propositus first observed in 1950] see under *blood group.*

Du·gas test (sign) (doo-gahs′) [Louis Alexander *Dugas,* American physician, 1806–1884] see under *test.*

DUH dyschromatosis universalis hereditaria.

Du·ha·mel operation (du-ah-mel′) [Bernard Georges *Duhamel,* French surgeon, born 1917] see under *operation.*

Du·hot line (du-o′) [Robert *Duhot,* Belgian urologist and dermatologist, late 19th century] see under *line.*

Duh·ring disease (doo′ring) [Louis Adolphus *Duhring,* American dermatologist, 1845–1913] dermatitis herpetiformis.

Dührs·sen incisions, operation (dēr′sən) [Alfred *Dührssen,* German gynecologist, 1862–1933] see under *incision* and *operation.*

Duke test (method) (do͝ok) [William Waddell *Duke,* American pathologist, 1882–1946] see under *test.*

Dukes classification (do͝oks) [Cuthbert Esquire *Dukes,* English pathologist, 1890–1977] see under *classification.*

dul·ci·tol (dul′sĭ-tol) [L. *dulcis* sweet] galactitol.

dull (dul) not resonant on percussion.

dull·ness (dul′nis) diminished resonance on percussion; also a peculiar percussion sound which lacks the normal resonance.
Gerhardt d. see under *triangle.*
shifting d. dullness on abdominal percussion, the level of which shifts as the patient is rolled from side to side; indicative of free fluid in the abdominal cavity.
tympanitic d. resonance of a dull and diminished quality.

du·lox·e·tine hy·dro·chlo·ride (doo-lok′sə-tēn) a serotonin-norepinephrine reuptake inhibitor, used for the treatment of major depressive disorder and the relief of pain in diabetic neuropathy; administered orally.

dumb·bell (dum′bel″) a mass consisting of two spherical portions connected by a narrow isthmus.
d′s of Schäfer microscopic bodies found in striated muscular tissue.

Dum·dum fever (dum′dum) [*Dum Dum,* India, area of Calcutta where some of the first cases were observed in the early 20th century] visceral leishmaniasis.

dum·my (dum′e) 1. pontic. 2. placebo. 3. a foal with neonatal maladjustment syndrome.

dUMP deoxyuridine monophosphate.

dump·ing (dump′ing) rapid emptying of a substance from its container.
gastric d. rapid gastric emptying.

Dun·can syndrome (dung′kən) [*Duncan,* the original kindred in which the disease was described] X-linked lymphoproliferative syndrome; see under *syndrome.*

Dun·can folds, position, ventricle (dung′kən) [James Matthews *Duncan,* British gynecologist, 1826–1890] see under *fold* and *position,* and see *cavum septi pellucidi.*

Dun·ferm·line scale (dun′fərm-līn) [*Dunfermline,* Scotland, where the scheme was devised] see under *scale.*

dun·siek·te (dun-sēk′tə) [Afrikaans] crotalism in horses in South Africa.

du·o·de·nec·to·my (doo″o-də-nek′tə-me) [*duoden-* + *-ectomy*] excision of the duodenum, total or partial.

du·od·e·ni·tis (doo-od″ə-ni′tis) inflammation of the duodenal mucosa.

duoden(o)- [L. *duodeni* twelve at a time] a combining form denoting relationship to the duodenum.

du·o·de·no·cho·lan·ge·itis (doo″o-de′no-ko-lan″je-i′tis) inflammation of the duodenum and common bile duct.

du·o·de·no·cho·le·cys·tos·to·my (doo″o-de″no-ko″lə-sis-tos′tə-me) cholecystoduodenostomy.

du·o·de·no·cho·led·o·chot·o·my (doo″o-de″no-ko-led″ə-kot′ə-me) surgical incision of the duodenum and common bile duct.

du·o·de·no·col·ic (doo″o-de″no-kol′ik) 1. pertaining to the duodenum and colon. 2. proceeding from the duodenum to the colon.

du·o·de·no·cys·tos·to·my (doo″o-de″no-sis-tos′tə-me) cholecystoduodenostomy.

du·o·de·no·du·o·de·nos·to·my (doo″o-de″no-doo″o-də-nos′tə-me) anastomosis of the two portions of a divided duodenum.

du·o·de·no·en·ter·os·to·my (doo″o-de″no-en″tər-os′tə-me) surgical formation of a communication from the duodenum to another part of the small intestine.

du·o·de·no·gas·tric (doo″o-de′no-gas′trik) 1. proceeding from the duodenum to the stomach. 2. gastroduodenal.

du·o·de·no·gram (doo″o-de′no-gram) a radiograph of the duodenum.

du·o·de·nog·ra·phy (doo″o-də-nog′rə-fe) radiography of the duodenum using barium as a contrast medium.

du·o·de·no·he·pat·ic (doo″o-de″no-hə-pat′ik) pertaining to or connecting the duodenum and liver.

du·o·de·no·il·e·os·to·my (doo″o-de″no-il″e-os′tə-me) surgical formation of a communication between the duodenum and the ileum.

du·o·de·no·je·ju·nal (doo″o-de″no-jə-joo′nəl) pertaining to the duodenum and the jejunum.

du·o·de·no·je·ju·nos·to·my (doo″o-de″no-jĕ″joo-nos′tə-me) surgical formation of a new communication between the duodenum and the jejunum.

du·o·de·nol·y·sis (doo″o-də-nol′ə-sis) the operation of loosening the duodenum from adhesions.

du·o·de·no·pan·cre·a·tec·to·my (doo″o-de″no-pan″kre-ə-tek′tə-me) pancreatoduodenectomy.

du·o·de·nor·rha·phy (doo″o-də-nor′ə-fe) [*duodeno-* + *-rrhaphy*] the operation of suturing the duodenum.

du·o·de·no·scope (doo″o-de′no-skōp) a type of enteroscope for examining the duodenum.

du·o·de·nos·co·py (doo″o-də-nos′kə-pe) [*duodeno-* + *-scopy*] enteroscopy of the duodenum.

du·o·de·nos·to·my (doo″o-də-nos′tə-me) [*duodeno-* + *-stomy*] surgical formation of a permanent orifice into the duodenum.

du·o·de·not·o·my (doo″o-də-not′ə-me) [*duodeno-* + *-tomy*] incision of the duodenum.

du·o·de·num (doo″o-de′nəm, doo-od′ə-nəm) [L. *duodeni* twelve at a time] [TA] the first or proximal portion of the small intestine, much shorter than the following portions, extending from the pylorus to the jejunum; so called because its length is about 12 finger breadths. duode′nal *adj*

Duo·Neb (doo′o-neb) trademark for a combination preparation of ipratropium bromide and albuterol sulfate.

du·o·par·en·tal (doo″o-pə-ren′təl) biparental.

Du·pha·lac (doo′fə-lak) trademark for a preparation of lactulose.

Du·phas·ton (doo-fas′ton) trademark for a preparation of dydrogesterone.

du·pli·ca·tion (doo″plĭ-ka′shən) [L. *duplicatio* doubling] 1. the act or process of doubling, or the state of being doubled. 2. in genetics, the presence in the genome of additional genetic material (a chromosome or segment of one, a gene or part of one). See also *repeat.* 3. a doubling of parts, which may be connected at some point, the extra part may be a mirror image of the other. See also *conjoined twins*, under *twin.* Called also *duplicitas* and *reduplication.*
 incomplete d. of spinal cord diastematomyelia.
 gastric d. congenital duplication of all or part of the stomach, usually found along the greater curvature.
 incomplete d. of spinal cord diastematomyelia.
 ureteral d. double ureter.
 urethral d. double urethra.

du·pli·ci·tas (doo-plis′ĭ-təs) [L.] duplication (def. 3).
 d. ante′rior katadidymus.
 d. asym′metros heteropagus.
 d. comple′ta symmetrical conjoined twins.
 d. crucia′ta janiceps.
 d. incomple′ta asymmetrical conjoined twins.
 d. infe′rior anadidymus.
 d. me′dia thoracopagus.
 d. paralle′la conjoined twins consisting of two components united in a sagittal plane.
 d. poste′rior anadidymus.
 d. supe′rior katadidymus.
 d. sym′metros symmetrical conjoined twins.

dupp (dup) a syllable used to represent the second sound of the heart in auscultation; it is shorter and higher pitched than the first sound. See *lubb* and *lubb-dupp.*

Du·puy-Du·temps operation (du-pwe′-du-tah′) [Louis *Dupuy-Dutemps*, Paris ophthalmologist, 1871–1946] see under *operation.*

Du·puy·tren contracture (disease), fracture, etc. (du-pwe-trah′) [Baron Guillaume *Dupuytren*, French surgeon, 1777–1835] see under *contracture, fracture, hydrocele, sign,* and *suture;* see *shoulder disarticulation*, under *disarticulation;* and see *aponeurosis palmaris.*

du·ra (doo′rə) [L. "hard"] dura mater.

Du·rab·o·lin (doo-rab′o-lin) trademark for a preparation of nandrolone phenpropionate.

Du·ra·clon (dōōr′ə-klon) trademark for a preparation of clonidine hydrochloride.

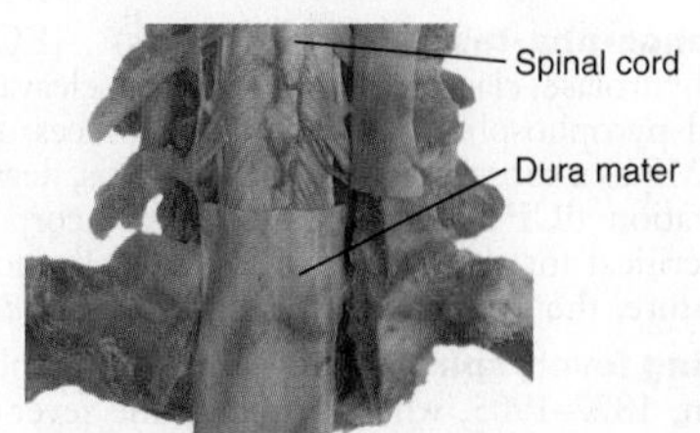

■ Cervical region, from behind.

Du·ra·ge·sic (doo″rə-je′zik) trademark for a preparation of fentanyl citrate.

du·ral (doo′rəl) pertaining to the dura mater.

du·ra ma·ter (doo′rə ma′tər) [L. "hard mother"] [TA] the outermost, toughest, and most fibrous of the three membranes (meninges) covering the brain and spinal cord; called also *pachymeninx.*
 d. m. of brain, d. m. crania′lis [TA] cranial dura mater: the dura mater covering the brain, composed of two mostly fused layers: an endosteal outer layer (endocranium) adherent to the inner aspect of the cranial bones, analogous to the periosteum of the bony skeleton, and an inner meningeal layer. Venous sinuses and the trigeminal ganglion are located between the layers. Called also *d. m. encephali* [TA alternative].
 d. m. ence′phali TA alternative for *d. m. cranialis.*
 d. m. of spinal cord, d. m. spina′lis [TA] spinal dura mater: the dura mater covering the spinal cord; it is separated from the periosteum of the enclosing vertebrae by an epidural space containing blood vessels and fibrous and areolar tissue.

Du·ra·morph (dōōr′ə-morf) trademark for a preparation of morphine sulfate.

Du·rand-Ni·co·las-Fa·vre disease (du-rah′ ne-ko-lah′ fahv′rə) [N. Joseph *Durand*, French physician, early 20th century; Joseph *Nicolas*, French physician, 1868–1960; Maurice Jules *Favre*, French physician, 1876–1954] lymphogranuloma venereum.

Du·ra·nest (doo′rə-nəst) trademark for preparations of etidocaine hydrochloride.

Du·ran-Rey·nals permeability factor (doo-rahn′-ra-nahlz′) [Francisco *Duran-Reynals*, American bacteriologist, 1899–1958] hyaluronidase.

dur·ap·a·tite (door-ap′ə-tīt) a crystalline form of the compound $(Ca_3(PO_4)_2)_3 \cdot Ca(OH)_2$ (see *hydroxyapatite*), used as a prosthetic aid.

du·ra·plas·ty (doo′rə-plas″te) [*dura* mater + *-plasty*] a plastic operation on the dura mater; graft of the dura.

du·ra·tion (doo-ra′shən) [L. *durare* to last or remain] 1. a period of time, such as the length of time an electrical stimulus is being applied. 2. the length of time covered by one waveform, usually measured from a point at which it leaves the baseline to the next point at which it returns to a corresponding position on the baseline.

Dur. dolor. [L.] duran′te dolo′re (while the pain lasts).

Du·ret hemorrhages (du-ra′) [Henri *Duret*, French neurological surgeon, 1849–1921] see under *hemorrhage.*

Dur·ham rule (dōōr′əm) [*Durham*, surname of an American felon judged to be criminally insane in 1954] see under *rule.*

Dur·ham tube[1] (dōōr′əm) [Arthur Edward *Durham*, English surgeon, 1834–1895.] see under *tube.*

Dur·ham tube[2] (dōōr′əm) [Herbert Edward *Durham*, English bacteriologist, 1866–1945] see under *tube.*

Du·ri·cef (door′ĭ-sef) trademark for preparations of cefadroxil.

du·ro·ar·ach·ni·tis (doo″ro-ar″ak-ni′tis) inflammation of the dura mater and arachnoid.

Du·ro·zi·ez disease, murmur (sign) (du-ro″ze-a′) [Paul Louis *Duroziez*, French physician, 1826–1897] see under *disease* and *murmur.*

dust (dust) fine, dry particles of earth or any other substance small enough to be blown by the wind. See also *coniosis* and *pneumoconiosis.*
 blood d. hemoconia.
 chromatin d. small red granules, smaller than Howell bodies, sometimes seen at the periphery of stained erythrocytes.

dust·borne (dust′born) spread through the air in dust particles, such as an infectious disease.

du·tas·ter·ide (doo-tas′tər-īd) an inhibitor of 5α-reductase, chemically related to finasteride; used in treatment of benign prostatic hyperplasia.

Dutch·er body (duch′er) [Thomas F. *Dutcher*, American pathologist, born 1923] see under *body.*

dUTP deoxyuridine triphosphate.

dUTP py·ro·phos·pha·tase (pi-ro-fos′fə-tās) [EC 3.6.1.23] an enzyme of the hydrolase class that catalyzes the cleavage of dUTP to form dUMP and pyrophosphate. It thus both reduces dUTP levels and also provides dUMP as a substrate dTTP biosynthesis, decreasing the intracellular concentration dUPT and so preventing incorporation of uracil into DNA; it is critical for the fidelity of DNA replication and repair. In official nomenclature, the preferred name is now *dUTP diphosphatase.*

Dut·ton relapsing fever, spirochete (dut′ən) [Joseph Everett *Dutton,* English physician, 1877–1905, who contracted the fever he was studying and died in Africa] see under *fever,* and see *Borrelia duttonii.*

Dut·to·nel·la (dut″o-nel′ə) [J. Everett *Dutton*] in some systems of classification a salivarian subgenus of genus *Trypanosoma,* including *T. uniforme* and *T. vivax.*

Du·ver·ney fracture, gland (du-vər-na′) [Joseph Guichard *Duverney,* French anatomist, 1648–1730] see under *fracture* and see *glandula bulbourethralis.*

Du·void (doo′void) trademark for preparations of bethanechol chloride.

dv double vibrations (a unit for the measurement of the frequency of sound waves).

DVA Department of Veterans Affairs (formerly the Veterans Administration).

DVM Doctor of Veterinary Medicine.

DVT deep vein thrombosis; deep venous thrombosis.

dwale (dwāl) belladonna (def. 1).

dwarf (dworf) [A.S. *dweorh*] 1. a person who is unusually short, particularly one of atypical proportions. Called also *nanus.* 2. an animal or plant that is small in size.

achondroplastic d. 1. a dwarf having a relatively large head with saddle nose and brachycephaly, short limbs, and usually lordosis; see also *achondroplasia.* 2. a calf with short legs, a wide head, a protruding mandible, and a malformed maxilla that partially obstructs the respiratory passages so that breathing is stertorous. Called also *snorter d.*

Amsterdam d. a dwarf with de Lange syndrome.

asexual d. an adult dwarf with deficient sexual development.

ateliotic d. a dwarf whose skeleton is infantile with persistent nonunion between epiphyses and diaphyses.

bird-headed d. a dwarf with Seckel syndrome; called also *nanocephalic d.* and *Seckel bird-headed d.*

cretin d. hypothyroid d.

diastrophic d. a dwarf with diastrophic dysplasia.

hypophysial d. pituitary d.

hypothyroid d. a dwarf with hypothyroidism, usually accompanied by cretinism. Called also *cretin d.*

Laron d. a dwarf whose skeletal growth retardation results from impaired ability to synthesize insulin-like growth factor I; see *Laron syndrome,* under *syndrome.*

micromelic d. a dwarf with very small limbs.

nanocephalic d. bird-headed d.

normal d. a person who is unusually short (more than 3 standard deviations below mean height for age in a child) but is not deformed. Called also *physiologic, primordial, pure,* or *true d.*

phocomelic d. a dwarf in whom the diaphyses of the long bones are abnormally short.

physiologic d. normal d.

pituitary d. a person with pituitary dwarfism. Called also *hypophysial d.*

primordial d., pure d. normal d.

rachitic d. a person dwarfed by rickets, having a high forehead with prominent bosses, bent long bones, and a Harrison groove on the thorax.

renal d. a person with renal dwarfism.

rhizomelic d. a dwarf with an autosomal recessive form of chondrodysplasia punctata, characterized by symmetric shortening of the limbs, cataracts, optic atrophy, mental retardation, fibrous joint contractures, and ichthyosis; it is lethal in early childhood.

Russell d. a dwarf with Silver-Russell syndrome.

Seckel bird-headed d. bird-headed d.

sexual d. a dwarf with normal sexual development.

Silver d. Russell d.

snorter d. achondroplastic d. (def. 2).

thanatophoric d. a micromelic dwarf having very short ribs and bones of the limbs, and vertebral bodies that are greatly reduced in height with wide intervertebral spaces; death usually occurs during the first few hours after birth. See also under *dysplasia.*

true d. normal d.

dwarfed (dworft) of unusually small size; characterized by dwarfism. Called also *nanoid.*

dwarf·ish (dwor′fish) pertaining to or like a dwarf; called also *nanoid* and *nanous.*

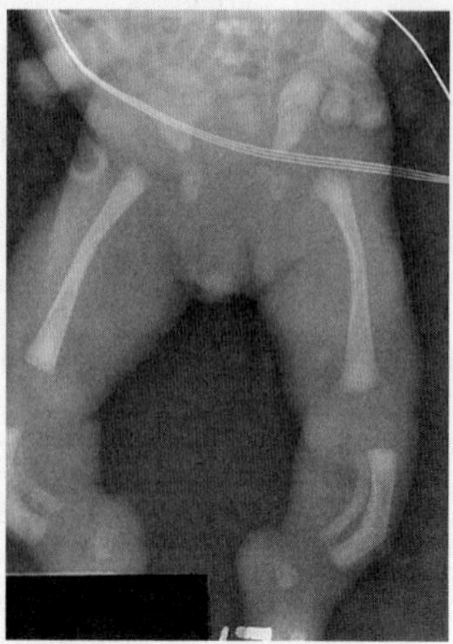
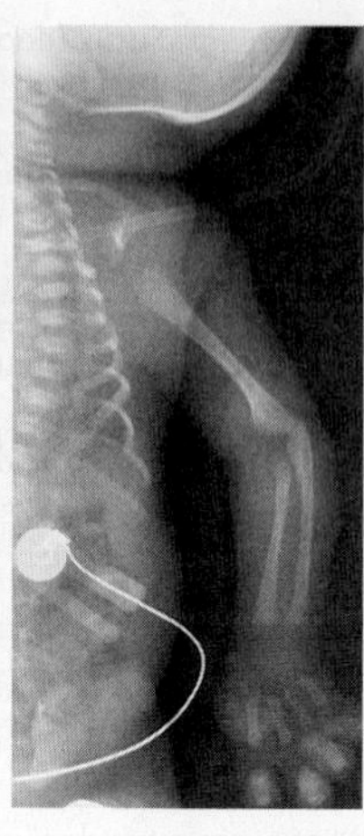

■ Camptomelic dwarfism, showing deformities of the distal long bones.

dwarf·ism (dworf′iz-əm) the state of being a dwarf; unusual shortness of the body. See also terms under *dwarf, infantilism,* and *stature.* Called also *microplasia, nanism,* and *nanosomia.*

bird-headed d. Seckel syndrome.

camptomelic d. dwarfism due to camptomelia of the lower limbs, often accompanied by cleft palate, retrognathia, and other abnormalities.

deprivation d. severe growth retardation in infants as a result of emotional deprivation, as in maternal deprivation syndrome. Called also *psychosocial d.* and *psychosocial short stature.*

hypophysial d. pituitary d.

Laron d. see under *syndrome.*

Lévi-Lorain d., Lorain-Lévi d. pituitary d.

pituitary d. a type of dwarfism with retention of infantile characteristics, due to undersecretion of growth hormone and gonadotropin deficiency. Called also *hypophysial* or *Lévi-Lorain d.*

psychosocial d. deprivation d.

renal d. dwarfism resulting from chronic renal failure such as that of renal osteodystrophy.

Robinow d. see under *syndrome.*

Russell d., Russell-Silver d., Silver-Russell d. Silver-Russell syndrome.

Seckel d. see under *syndrome.*

symptomatic d. dwarfism with defective ossification, dentition, and sexual development.

Walt Disney d. geroderma osteodysplasticum.

Dwy·er instrumentation (dwi′ər) [Allen Frederick *Dwyer,* American orthopedic surgeon, 1920–1975] see under *instrumentation.*

Dy dysprosium.

dy·ad (di′ad) [Gr. *dyas* the number two, from *dyo* two] a double chromosome resulting from the halving of a tetrad in the first meiotic division.

dy·clo·caine hy·dro·chlo·ride (di′klo-kān″) BAN for *dyclonine hydrochloride.*

Dy·a·zide (di′ə-zīd) trademark for preparations of triamterene with hydrochlorothiazide.

Dy·clone (di′klōn) trademark for preparations of dyclonine hydrochloride.

dy·clo·nine hy·dro·chlo·ride (di′klo-nēn) [USP] a local anesthetic having significant bactericidal and fungicidal activity, applied topically to the skin and mucous membranes to relieve the pain of anogenital, esophageal, vaginal, or perioral lesions and otorhinolaryngologic or dental procedures.

dy·dro·ges·ter·one (di″dro-jes′tər-ōn) an orally effective, synthetic progestin occurring as a white to pale yellow, crystalline powder; used mainly in the diagnosis and treatment of primary amenorrhea and severe dysmenorrhea, and in combination with estrogen in dysfunctional menorrhagia.

dye (di) any of various colored substances that contain auxochromes and thus are capable of coloring substances to which they are applied; used for staining and coloring, as test reagents, and as therapeutic agents in medicine.

acid d., acidic d. a dye which is acidic in reaction and usually unites with positively charged ions of the material acted upon; called also *anionic d.*

amphoteric d. a dye containing both reactive basic and reactive acidic groups, and staining both acidic and basic elements.

aniline d. a dye containing aniline; such dyes are an important cause of poisoning in the workplace (see *anilinism*).
anionic d. acid d.
azo d. any of a large group of synthetic dyes whose chromophore group is the structure —N═N—.
basic d., cationic d. a dye that is basic in reaction and unites with negatively charged ions of material acted upon.
metachromatic d. a dye that stains tissues two or more colors.
orthochromatic d. a dye that stains tissues a single color.
vital d. a dye that penetrates living cells and colors certain structures, without serious injury to the cells.

dy·ing (di′ing) a stage in life; the process of approaching death. It is sometimes divided into the stages of denial and disbelief, anger, bargaining, depression, and acceptance.

dy·ing-back (di′ing bak) degeneration of an axon beginning distally and progressing to more proximal areas. Cf. *wallerian degeneration.*

Dy·me·lor (di′mə-lor) trademark for a preparation of acetohexamide.

dyn dyne.

Dy·na·bac (di′nə-bak) trademark for a preparation of dirithromycin.

Dy·na·Circ (di′nə-sərk) trademark for a preparation of isradipine.

dy·nac·tin (di-nak′tin) a cytoplasmic protein complex that mediates the movement of vesicles and chromosomes along microtubules by binding dynein to vesicle membranes and kinetochores.

dy·nam·ic (di-nam′ik) [*dynam-* + *-ic*] 1. pertaining to or manifesting force. 2. of or relating to energy or to objects in motion. 3. characterized by or tending to produce change.

dy·nam·ics (di-nam′iks) that phase of mechanics which deals with the motions of material bodies taking place under different specific conditions.

dy·na·min (di′nə-min) a 100-kD protein with GTPase activity, targeted to coated pits; as the pits invaginate during endocytosis, it self-assembles into helical collarlike arrays around their necks and is instrumental in the pinching off of vesicles. In EC nomenclature, called *dynamin GTPase.*

dy·na·min GTP·ase (di′nə-min je-te-pe′ās) [EC 3.6.5.5] EC nomenclature for the GTP-hydrolyzing activity of dynamin.

dynam(o)- [Gr. *dynamis* power] a combining form denoting relationship to power or strength.

dy·na·mo·gen·e·sis (di″nə-mo-jen′ə-sis) [*dynamo-* + *genesis*] the development of energy or force, as in muscle or nerves.

dy·na·mo·gen·ic (di″nə-mo-jen′ik) [*dynamo-* + *-genic*] producing or favoring the development of power; pertaining to the development of power, as in muscle or nerves.

dy·na·mog·e·ny (di″nə-moj′ə-ne) dynamogenesis.

dy·namo·graph (di-nam′o-graf) [*dynamo-* + *-graph*] a self-registering dynamometer.

dy·na·mom·e·ter (di″nə-mom′ə-tər) [*dynamo-* + *-meter*] an instrument for measuring the force of muscular contraction.
grip d. squeeze d.
squeeze d. a dynamometer for measuring the grip of the hand.

dy·namo·path·ic (di-nam″o-path′ik) functional.

dy·namo·phore (di-nam′o-for) [*dynamo-* + *-phore*] food or any substance that supplies energy to the body.

dy·namo·scope (di-nam′o-skōp) [*dynamo-* + *-scope*] a device for performing dynamoscopy.

dy·na·mos·co·py (di″nə-mos′kə-pe) the observation of the performance of function by an organ or structure, as of muscle action or of kidney function by ureteral catheterization.

Dy·na·cin (di′nə-sin) trademark for preparations of minocycline hydrochloride.

dyne (dyn) (dīn) a unit of force, being the amount that when acting continuously upon a mass of 1 g will impart to it an acceleration of 1 cm per second per second. It is equal to 10^{-5} newton.

dy·nein (di′nēn) [Gr. *dynamis* power] any of a family of large cytoplasmic proteins with ATPase activity that move along microtubules toward the minus end by alternately forming and releasing cross-bridges between adjacent tubulin subunits. Dyneins are divided into two functional classes: *axonemal dynein* is attached to the microtubules of cilia and flagella and is responsible for their beating movement; *cytosolic dyneins* occur in the cytoplasm and produce dynactin-mediated movement of vesicles and chromosomes. Cf. *kinesin.* In EC nomenclature, called *dynein ATPase.*

dy·ne·in ATP·ase (di′nēn a-te-pe′ās) [EC 3.6.4.2] EC nomenclature for the ATP-hydrolyzing activity of dynein.

dy·nor·phin (di-nor′fin) [*dynamo-* + *morphine*] any of a family of opioid peptides found throughout the central and peripheral nervous systems; most are agonists at opioid receptor sites. Some are probably involved in pain regulation at the levels of the spinal cord and medulla and others may aid hypothalamic regulation of eating and drinking. See also *endorphin* and *enkephalin.*

dy·phyl·line (di′fəl-in) [USP] a theophylline derivative used as a bronchodilator in the treatment of bronchial asthma or bronchospasm associated with chronic bronchitis or emphysema; administered orally or intramuscularly.

Dy·ren·i·um (di-ren′e-əm) trademark for a preparation of triamterene.

dys- [Gr. "bad"] a combining form signifying difficult, painful, bad, disordered, abnormal; the opposite of *eu-*.

dys·acou·sia (dis″ə-koo′zhə) dysacusis.

dys·acou·sis (dis″ə-koo′sis) dysacusis.

dys·acous·ma (dis″ə-ko͞oz′mə) dysacusis.

dys·acu·sis (dis″ə-koo′sis) [*dys-* + Gr. *akousis* hearing] dysacousia; dysacousis. 1. a hearing impairment in which there is distortion of frequency or intensity. 2. a condition in which certain sounds produce discomfort; called also *auditory dysesthesia.*

dys·ad·ap·ta·tion (dis″ad-ap-ta′shən) dysaptation.

dys·adren·al·ism (dis″ə-dren′əl-iz-əm) adrenalism.

dys·al·li·log·na·thia (dis-al″ĭ-log-na′the-ə) disproportion of the maxilla and mandible.

dys·an·ag·no·sia (dis″an-ag-no′zhə) a form of dyslexia in which certain words cannot be recognized.

dys·an·ti·graph·ia (dis″an-tĭ-graf′e-ə) dysgraphia in which the ability to copy writing is lost.

dys·aphia (dis-a′fe-ə) [*dys-* + Gr. *haphē* touch] paraphia.

dys·ap·ta·tion (dis″ap-ta′shən) defective power of accommodation of the iris and retina to light variations.

dys·ar·te·ri·ot·o·ny (dis″ahr-tēr″e-ot′ə-ne) [*dys-* + *arteriotony*] abnormality of blood pressure.

dys·ar·thria (dis-ahr′thre-ə) [*dys-* + *arthr-*[2] + *-ia*] a speech disorder consisting of imperfect articulation due to loss of muscular control after damage to the central or peripheral nervous system. Cf. *anarthria* and *aphasia.* **dysar′thric** *adj*
ataxic d. dysarthria seen in patients with cerebellar lesions, characterized by slowness of speech, slurring, a monotonous tone, and scanning.
clumsy-hand d. a lacunar stroke characterized by facial weakness, dysarthria, dysphagia, and clumsiness of one hand. Called also *dysarthria–clumsy hand syndrome.*
flaccid d. lower motor neuron d.
hyperkinetic d. loud, harsh speech with peculiar stresses, seen in extrapyramidal diseases that involve hyperkinesia, such as myoclonus and chorea.
hypokinetic d. low-pitched, monotonous speech with slurred words and incomplete sentences, seen in parkinsonism and other extrapyramidal diseases that involve hypokinesia.
lower motor neuron d. dysarthria with severe lesions of motor nuclei of the lower pons or medulla oblongata that causes weakness or paralysis of the articulatory muscles; characteristics include a rasping, monotonous voice, and in advanced cases, shriveling and flaccidity of the tongue with laxness and tremulousness of the lips. Called also *flaccid d.*
spastic d. dysarthria accompanying paralysis of the tongue and facial muscles, usually with increased facial reflexes such as the jaw reflex; it occurs with bilateral lesions of the corticobulbar tracts.

dys·ar·thro·sis (dis″ahr-thro′sis) [*dys-* + *arthrosis*] deformity or malformation of a joint.

dys·au·to·no·mia (dis″aw-to-no′me-ə) [*dys-* + Gr. *autonomia* autonomy] malfunction of the autonomic nervous system.
familial d. an autosomal recessive disease of childhood caused by mutations in the *IKBKAP* gene (locus: 9q31), which encodes a protein involved in transcription and possibly other cell functions. It is characterized by defective lacrimation, skin blotching, emotional instability, motor incoordination, total absence of pain sensation, and hyporeflexia; seen almost exclusively in Ashkenazi Jews. Called also *familial autonomic dysfunction, Riley-Day syndrome,* and *hereditary sensory and autonomic neuropathy type III.*
feline d. a neurological disorder of cats, characterized by decreased numbers of neurons in autonomic and cranial nerve ganglia, resulting in mydriasis, dry mucous membranes, megaesophagus, bradycardia, and constipation. Called also *Key-Gaskell syndrome.*

dys·bar·ism (dis′bər-iz-əm) a general term applied to any clinical syndrome caused by difference between the surrounding atmospheric pressure and the total gas pressure in the various tissues, fluids, and cavities of the body, including such conditions as barotitis media, barosinusitis, or expansion of gases in the hollow viscera.

dys·ba·sia (dis-ba′zhə) [*dys-* + Gr. *basis* step] difficulty in walking, especially that due to a nervous lesion. Cf. *abasia.*

dys•be•ta•lipo•pro•tein•emia (dis-ba″tə-lip″o-pro″te-ne′me-ə) 1. the presence in the blood of abnormal β-lipoproteins. 2. familial d.

familial d. an inherited disorder of lipoprotein metabolism caused by mutations in the *APOE* gene (locus: 19q13.2), which encodes apolipoprotein E (apo E), that result in defective binding of apo E to lipoprotein receptors. It is characterized biochemically by accumulation of β-VLDL (chylomicron remnants and very-low-density lipoprotein remnants) enriched in mutant apo E, with equally elevated cholesterol and triglycerides; the phenotype is that of a type III hyperlipoproteinemia. Clinical manifestations include tuberous or planar xanthomas, particularly of the palmar crease (xanthoma striatum palmare), and premature coronary and peripheral atherosclerosis. The term is sometimes used for all patients with this mutant apo E, although the majority are normolipidemic and clinically normal. Inheritance is usually autosomal recessive, requiring interaction between the mutant apo E and genetic or environmental factors to cause hypertriglyceridemia, but rare autosomal dominant mutations occur. Called also *broad beta* or *floating beta disease.*

dys•bi•o•sis (dis″bi-o′sis) [*dys-* + *biosis*] variation from the normal composition of the microflora of the gut.

dys•bo•lism (dis′bo-liz-əm) [*dys-* + *metabolism*] a condition arising from an error in metabolism not necessarily of a disease nature, as in incomplete oxidation of tyrosine, giving a reddish color to the urine.

dys•cal•cu•lia (dis″kal-ku′le-ə) impairment of the ability to do mathematical problems because of brain injury or disease. Cf. *acalculia.*

dys•ceph•a•ly (dis-sef′ə-le) malformation of the cranial and facial bones.

mandibulo-oculofacial d. oculomandibulofacial syndrome.

dys•che•sia (dis-ke′shə) dyschezia.

dys•che•zia (dis-ke′zhə) [*dys-* + Gr. *chezein* to defecate + *-ia*] difficult or painful defecation.

dys•chi•a•sia (dis-ki-a′zhə) any disorder of sense localization.

dys•chi•ria (dis-ki′re-ə) [*dys-* + *chir-* + *-ia*] derangement of the power to tell which side of the body has been touched; see *allochiria* and *synchiria.*

dys•cho•lia (dis-ko′le-ə) [*dys-* + *chol-* + *-ia*] a disordered condition of the bile.

dys•chon•dro•pla•sia (dis″kon-dro-pla′zhə) [*dys-* + *chondroplasia*] enchondromatosis.

dys•chon•dros•te•o•sis (dis″kon-dros″te-o′sis) a form of dyschondroplasia that may produce micromelia.

Léri-Weill d. a dominantly inherited syndrome caused by mutations in pseudoautosomal region 1 (locus: Ypter-p11.2, Xpter-p22.32), characterized by short stature, mesomelic shortening, and Madelung deformity. Mutations affect the *SHOX* and *SHOXY* genes, which encode transcription factors important for skeletal growth. Called also *Léri-Weill syndrome.*

dys•chro•ma•sia (dis″kro-ma′zhə) dyschromatopsia.

dys•chro•ma•top•sia (dis-kro″mə-top′se-ə) [*dys-* + *chromat-* color + *-opsia*] disorder of color vision.

dys•chro•ma•to•sis (dis-kro″mə-to′sis) dyschromia.

d. symmet′rica heredita′ria (DSH) a rare, autosomal dominant pigmentary genodermatosis caused by mutations in the *ADAR* gene (locus:1q21.3), which encodes adenosine deaminase specific for double-stranded RNA, characterized by hyperpigmented and hypopigmented macules that appear on the skin of the face and the dorsal extremities in infancy and early childhood. It is seen primarily in Japan and China. Called also *reticulate acropigmentation of Dohi.*

d. universa′lis heredita′ria (DUH) a rare pigmentary genodermatosis, most often seen in Japan, characterized by hyperpigmented and hypopigmented macules on the trunk, extremities, and sometimes the face that appear in infancy or early childhood. Heredity is autosomal dominant or recessive, and sporadic cases occur. There are two forms, caused by mutations at different sites: DUH1, caused by mutation at 6q24.2-q25.2, and DUH2, caused by mutation at 12q21-q23.

dys•chro•mia (dis-kro′me-ə) [*dys-* + *chrom-* + *-ia*] any disorder of pigmentation of the skin or hair, such as hyperpigmentation or hypopigmentation. Called also *dyspigmentation.*

dys•chro•nism (dis-kro′niz-əm) [*dys-* + *chron-* + *-ism*] 1. separation in time. 2. desynchrony.

dys•chy•lia (dis-ki′le-ə) disordered formation of chyle.

dys•ci•ne•sia (dĭ-sĭ-ne′zhə) dyskinesia.

dys•con•trol (dis″kən-trōl′) inability to control one's behavior.

episodic d. dyscontrol syndrome.

dys•co•ria (dis-kor′e-ə) [*dys-* + *cor-* + *-ia*] abnormality of the form or shape of the pupil or in the reaction of the two pupils.

dys•cor•ti•cism (dis-kor′tĭ-siz-əm) disordered functioning of the adrenal cortex; see *hyperadrenocorticism* and *adrenocortical insufficiency.*

dys•cra•sia (dis-kra′zhə) [*dys-* + *-crasia*] a term formerly used to indicate an abnormal mixture of the four humors; in surviving usages it now is roughly synonymous with "disease" or "pathologic condition." **dyscra′sic** *adj*

blood d. a pathologic condition of the blood, usually referring to disorders of the cellular elements of the blood.

plasma cell d's a diverse group of neoplastic diseases involving proliferation of a single clone of cells producing a serum M component (a monoclonal immunoglobulin or immunoglobulin fragment); the cells usually have plasma cell morphology, but may have lymphocyte morphology or a combination of lymphocytic and plasma cellular. The group includes multiple myeloma, Waldenström macroglobulinemia, the heavy chain diseases, and benign monoclonal gammopathy. Called also *dysproteinemias, monoclonal gammopathies* or *immunoglobulinopathies,* and *paraproteinemias.*

dys•di•ad•o•cho•ci•ne•sia (dis″di-ad″o-ko″sĭ-ne′zhə) dysdiadochokinesia.

dys•di•ad•o•cho•ki•ne•sia (dis″di-ad″ŏ-ko-kĭ-ne′zhə) [*dys-* + *diadochokinesia*] a dyskinesia consisting of impaired ability to perform the rapid alternating movements of diadochokinesia. Called also *dysdiadochocinesia.* **dysdiadochokinet′ic** *adj*

dys•dip•sia (dis-dip′se-ə) [*dys-* + Gr. *dipsa* thirst] difficulty in drinking.

dys•ec•dy•sis (dis-ek′dĭ-sis) [*dys-* + *ecdysis*] incomplete or otherwise disordered shedding of the skin (ecdysis) by a reptile, such as due to malnutrition or an excessively dry or cold environment.

dys•eco•ia (dis″ə-koi′ə) dysacusis.

dys•ejac•u•la•tion (dis″e-jak″u-la′shən) 1. any failure of normal ejaculation of semen. 2. a painful, burning sensation in the groin during semen ejaculation.

dys•ei•det•ic (dis″i-det′ik) dyslexic regarding the sight or recognition of whole words.

dys•em•bry•o•ma (dis-em″bre-o′mə) teratoma.

dys•em•bryo•pla•sia (dis-em″bre-o-pla′zhə) [*dys-* + *embryo* + *-plasia*] an anomaly occurring during embryonic life.

dys•en•ce•pha•lia splanch•no•cys•ti•ca (dis-en″sə-fa′le-ə splank″no-sis′tĭ-kə) Meckel syndrome.

dys•en•ter•i•form (dis″ən-ter′ĭ-form) resembling dysentery.

dys•en•tery (dis′ən-ter″e) [L. *dysenteria,* from Gr. *dys-* + *enteron*] any of various disorders marked by inflammation of the intestines, especially of the colon, and attended by pain in the abdomen, tenesmus, and diarrhea or frequent defecation containing blood and mucus. Causes include chemical irritants, bacteria, protozoa, or parasitic worms. **dysenter′ic** *adj*

amebic d. dysentery due to intestinal ulceration caused by severe amebiasis; it may be associated with spread of the infection to the liver and other distant sites. Called also *amebic colitis* and *intestinal amebiasis.*

bacillary d. dysentery caused by infection with bacteria of the genus *Shigella,* marked by intestinal pain, tenesmus, diarrhea with mucus and blood in the feces, and often toxemia; it is especially prevalent in tropical countries, but frequently occurs elsewhere. Called also *Flexner d.* and *Shigella* or *shigella d.*

balantidial d. protozoal dysentery caused by the species *Balantidium coli,* with symptoms similar to those of amebic dysentery.

bilharzial d. schistosomal d.

chronic d. of cattle Johne disease.

ciliary d., ciliate d. protozoal dysentery caused by ciliate organisms; see *balantidial d.*

flagellate d. protozoal dysentery caused by a flagellate organism, such as *Giardia lamblia* or *Trichomonas.*

Flexner d. bacillary dysentery caused by *Shigella flexneri.*

fulminant d. dysentery having intense symptoms, with collapse, toxemia, and often death. Called also *malignant d.*

lamb d. a highly fatal form of enterotoxemia affecting young lambs, caused by *Clostridium perfringens* type B, and marked by ulcerative inflammation of the intestine and fetid diarrhea, sometimes tinged with blood. A similar condition is frequently seen in young foals and calves.

malarial d. dysentery occurring in malaria.

malignant d. fulminant d.

protozoal d. dysentery caused by protozoa; see *amebic d.* and *balantidial d.*

schistosomal d. dysentery accompanying intestinal schistosomiasis; called also *bilharzial d.*

***Shigella* d., shigella d.** bacillary d.

Sonne d. a type of bacillary dysentery seen in temperate regions, caused by *Shigella sonnei.*

swine d. a contagious form of enteritis in young swine, caused by *Brachyspira hyodysenteriae* and marked by grayish feces. Called also *bloody scours.*

viral d. a virus-caused dysentery occurring in epidemics and marked by acute watery diarrhea.

winter d. the black scours (q.v.) type of dysentery occurring in cattle when stabled for the winter. Called also *winter scours.*

dys•equi•lib•ri•um (dis″e-kwĭ-lib′re-əm) 1. any derangement of the sense of equilibrium (see under *sense*). See also *dizziness* and *vertigo.* 2. disturbance of a state of equilibrium.

dialysis d. dialysis dysequilibrium syndrome.

flow-volume d. the lower than normal solute content of blood that has just gone through dialysis, which tends to draw solutes out of other fluid-containing body compartments such as cells; urea rebound is one result.

dys•er•gia (dis-ur′jə) [*dys-* + *erg-* + *-ia*] motor incoordination due to defect of efferent nerve impulse.

dys•e•ryth•ro•poi•e•sis (dis-ə-rith″ro-poi-e′sis) [*dys-* + *erythropoiesis*] defective development of erythrocytes, such as *anisocytosis* and *poikilocytosis.* See also *congenital dyserythropoietic anemia*, under *anemia.*

dys•es•the•sia (dis″es-the′zhə) [*dys-* + *esthesia*] 1. distortion of any sense, especially of that of touch. See also *paraphia.* 2. an unpleasant abnormal sensation produced by normal stimuli. Cf. *paresthesia.* **dysesthet′ic** *adj*

auditory d. dysacusis (def. 2).

dys•fer•lin (dis-fur′lin) a protein expressed strongly in skeletal and cardiac muscle; mutation in the gene encoding it has been associated with a subtype of limb-girdle muscular dystrophy.

dys•fi•brin•o•ge•ne•mia (dis-fi-brin″o-jə-ne′me-ə) the presence in the blood of abnormal fibrinogen; both autosomal dominant and recessive forms are known.

dys•flu•en•cy (dis-floo′ən-se) the quality of being dysfluent; see also *stuttering* (def. 1).

dys•flu•ent (dis-floo′ənt) proceeding with difficulty; said of speech disorders such as stuttering.

dys•func•tion (dis-funk′shən) disturbance, impairment, or abnormality of the functioning of an organ.

autonomic d. dysautonomia.

constitutional hepatic d. Gilbert syndrome.

erectile d. (ED) impotence (def. 2).

familial autonomic d. familial dysautonomia.

minimal brain d. former name for *attention-deficit/hyperactivity disorder.*

sexual d. [DSM-IV] any of a group of sexual disorders characterized by disturbance either of sexual desire or of the psychophysiological changes that usually characterize sexual response. Included are sexual desire disorders, sexual arousal disorders, orgasmic disorders, sexual pain disorders, substance-induced sexual dysfunction, and sexual dysfunction due to a general medical condition.

sphincter of Oddi d. abdominal pain or jaundice with failure of the sphincter of Oddi to function properly; it may occur several years after cholecystectomy or owing to other unknown causes. Called also *biliary dyskinesia.*

substance-induced sexual d. [DSM-IV] any of various sexual dysfunctions, such as impaired desire, arousal, or orgasm, due to direct physiological effects of a psychoactive substance, including medications, drugs of abuse, and toxins. Individual cases are named for the specific substance and specific dysfunction involved.

d. of uterus inertia uteri.

dys•ga•lac•tia (dis″gə-lak′she-ə) [*dys-* + *galact-* + *-ia*] disordered milk secretion.

dys•gam•ma•glob•u•lin•emia (dis-gam″ə-glob″u-lin-e′me-ə) an immune deficiency state characterized by selective deficiencies of one or more, but not all, classes of immunoglobulins. See also *hypogammaglobulinemia.*

dys•gen•e•sis (dis-jen′ə-sis) defective development; see also *dysplasia* and *dyspoiesis.*

46,XY gonadal d. a complete androgen insensitivity syndrome in which a phenotypic female has a 46,XY karyotype with streak gonads, sexual infantilism, and primary amenorrhea; there are sporadic and X-linked types. Called also *Swyer syndrome.*

cerebral d. abnormal development of the telencephalon.

epiphyseal d. a condition in which epiphyseal centers may be irregularly formed or appear to be fragmented or stippled.

gonadal d. 1. defective development of the gonads. 2. Turner syndrome.

mixed gonadal d. a condition in which there is a testis on one side and a streak gonad on the other; those affected typically show some degree of virilization and ambiguous genitalia, and a uterus, vagina, and at least one fallopian tube are usually present. The most common karyotype is a mosaic, 45,XO/46,XY.

pure gonadal d. the gonadal lesions of Turner syndrome occurring without the somatic features.

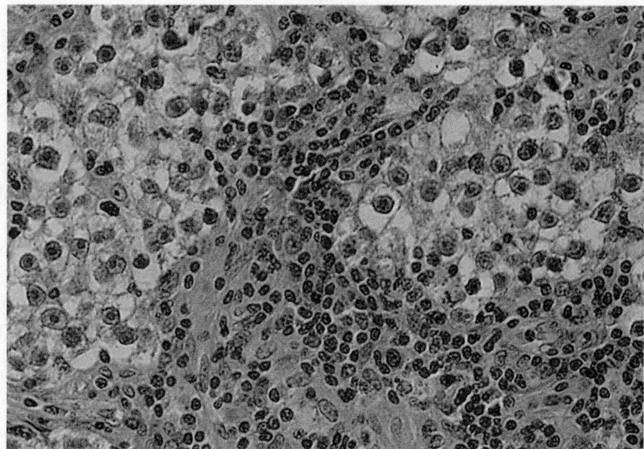

■ Dysgerminoma, showing polyhedral tumor cells with round nuclei and adjacent inflammation.

reticular d. the most severe form of severe combined immunodeficiency (q.v.), an autosomal recessive disorder caused by mutations in the *AK2* gene (locus: 1p34), which encodes the mitochondrial isozyme adenylate kinase 2, resulting in absence of granulocytes, macrophages, and lymphocytes due to defective lymphocyte differentiation.

seminiferous tubule d. Klinefelter syndrome.

dys•gen•ic (dis-jen′ik) considered to be detrimental to a race or tending to interfere with improvement of the race.

dys•gen•ics (dis-jen′iks) [*dys-* + Gr. *gennan* to produce] the study of racial deterioration. Cf. *eugenics.*

dys•gen•i•tal•ism (dis-jen′ĭ-təl-iz-əm) any abnormality of genital development.

dys•ger•mi•no•ma (dis″jər-mĭ-no′mə) [*dys-* + *germ* + *-oma*] the most common malignant ovarian germ cell tumor, composed of large round or polygonal glycogen-rich cells that are frequently radiosensitive and located bilaterally. It is the counterpart of the classical seminoma of the testis. The term *germinoma* is now used to encompass both the female and male neoplasms.

dys•geu•sia (dis-goo′zhə) [*dys-* + Gr. *geusis* taste + *-ia*] parageusia.

dys•glob•u•lin•emia (dis-glob″u-lin-e′me-ə) [*dys-* + *globulin* + *emia*] any disorder of the blood globulins; see also *hyperglobulinemia* and *dysgammaglobulinemia.*

dys•gly•ce•mia (dis″gli-se′me-ə) [*dys-* + *glyc-* + *-emia*] any derangement of the content of glucose in the blood; see *hyperglycemia* and *hypoglycemia.*

dys•gna•thia (dis-na′the-ə) [*dys-* + *gnath-* + *-ia*] an abnormality of the oral cavity and teeth that also involves the jaws. Cf. *eugnathia.* **dysgnath′ic** *adj*

dys•go•ne•sis (dis″go-ne′sis) [*dys-* + *gon-* + *-esis*] a functional disorder of the genital organs.

dys•gon•ic (dis-gon′ik) [*dys-* + *gon-* + *-ic*] seeding poorly; said of bacterial cultures, especially of species of *Mycobacterium*, that grow sparsely on culture media. Cf. *eugonic.*

Dys•go•no•mo•nas (dis-gon″o-mo′nəs) [*dysgonic* + Gr. *monas* unit, from *monos* single] a genus of gram-negative bacteria of the family Porphyromonadaceae, consisting of nonmotile, facultatively anaerobic, oxidase-negative, catalase-positive or -negative rods to coccobacilli. Organisms have been isolated from clinical specimens. The type species is *D. ga′dei.*

D. capnocytophagoi′des a catalase-negative species that is an opportunistic pathogen, causing diarrhea and bacteremia in immunocompromised patients.

dys•gram•ma•tism (dis-gram′ə-tiz-əm) 1. agrammatism. 2. dysphasia.

dys•graph•ia (dis-graf′e-ə) [*dys-* + *graph-* + *-ia*] difficulty in writing; cf. *agraphia.*

dys•he•ma•to•poi•e•sis (dis-he″mə-to″poi-e′sis) defective blood formation; called also *dyshemopoiesis.* **dyshematopoiet′ic** *adj*

dys•he•mo•poi•e•sis (dis-he″mo-poi-e′sis) dyshematopoiesis.

dys•he•mo•poi•et•ic (dis-he″mo-poi-et′ik) dyshematopoietic.

dys•he•sion (dis-he′zhən) [*dys-* + L. *haesio*, from *haerere* to stick] 1. disordered cell adherence. 2. loss of intercellular cohesion, a characteristic of malignancy, as determined by aspiration biopsy cytology.

dys•hi•dro•sis (dis″hĭ-dro′sis) [*dys-* + *hidro-* + *-sis*] 1. any disorder of the eccrine sweat glands. 2. former name for pompholyx, because of the misconception that that condition was a sweat retention disorder.

dys•hor•mo•no•gen•e•sis (dis-hor-mo″no-jen′ə-sis) defective or aberrant hormonogenesis; used especially in reference to the thyroid gland and thyroid hormones. **dyshormonogenet′ic** *adj*

dys•hy•dro•sis (dis″hī-dro′sis) dyshidrosis.

dys•junc•tion (dis-junk′shən) disjunction.

dys•kary•o•sis (dis-kar″e-o′sis) hyperchromatism and abnormal changes in the morphology of cell nuclei, indicative of premalignant or malignant conditions. **dyskaryot′ic** *adj*

dys•ker•a•to•ma (dis-ker″ə-to′mə) [*dys-* + *keratoma*] a tumor or other growth that is dyskeratotic.

warty d. a benign, usually solitary, pink to brown elevated papule with a depressed and crusted center containing a keratotic plug, occurring in association with the pilosebaceous unit; these are usually seen on the scalp, face, neck, or axilla of older men. Histologically, it resembles a lesion of Darier disease.

dys•ker•a•to•sis (dis-ker″ə-to′sis) abnormal, premature, or imperfect keratinization of the keratinocytes.

d. conge′nita, congenital d. a genetically and clinically heterogeneous, inherited disorder with onset in childhood, characterized by nail dystrophy, reticular hyperpigmentation of the skin, oral leukoplakia, and pancytopenia; additional features may occur and are highly variable. Autosomal dominant, autosomal recessive, and X-linked patterns of inheritance occur. Called also *Zinsser-Cole-Engman syndrome.*

hereditary benign intraepithelial d. an autosomal dominant disorder caused by mutation at 4q35, characterized by foamy gelatinous plaques on the conjunctiva and white thickenings resembling leukoplakia on the oral mucosa; photophobia is common in children, and blindness may occur. Called also *Witkop* or *Witkop-von Sallmann disease.*

dys•ker•a•tot•ic (dis-ker″ə-tot′ik) of, relating to, or affected by dyskeratosis.

dys•ki•ne•sia (dis″kĭ-ne′zhə) [Gr. *dyskinēsia* difficulty of moving] distortion or impairment of voluntary movement, as in tic, spasm, or myoclonus. **dyskinet′ic** *adj*

biliary d. sphincter of Oddi dysfunction.

d. intermit′tens disability of the limbs, coming on intermittently, and due to impairment of the circulation.

orofacial d. facial movements resembling those of tardive dyskinesia, seen in elderly patients who are edentulous and demented; cf. *Meige syndrome.*

paroxysmal kinesigenic d. brief episodes of dyskinesia caused by sudden movements, hyperventilation, or a sudden stimulus.

primary ciliary d. any of a group of hereditary syndromes characterized by delayed or absent mucociliary clearance from the airways; often there is also lack of motion of sperm. One variety is Kartagener syndrome. Called also *dyskinetic* or *immotile cilia syndrome.*

tardive d. an iatrogenic extrapyramidal disorder caused by long-term use of antipsychotic drugs; it is characterized by oral-lingual-buccal dyskinesias that usually resemble continual chewing motions with intermittent darting movements of the tongue; there may also be choreoathetoid movements of the extremities. It is more common in women than in men and in the elderly than in the young, and incidence is related to drug dosage and duration of treatment. In some patients symptoms disappear within a few months after the drugs are withdrawn; in others symptoms may persist indefinitely. Two minor variants are *withdrawal-emergent d.* and *tardive dystonia.*

withdrawal-emergent d. a variant of tardive dyskinesia in which symptoms appear after the drug has been withdrawn abruptly.

dys•la•lia (dis-la′le-ə) paralalia.

dys•lex•ia (dis-lek′se-ə) [*dys-* + *lexis* word + *-ia*] inability to read, spell, and write words, despite the ability to see and recognize letters; a familial disorder with autosomal dominant inheritance that occurs more frequently in males. Cf. *alexia.* **dyslex′ic** *adj*

dys•lip•id•e•mia (dis-lip″id-e′me-ə) [*dys-* + *lipid* + *-emia*] abnormality in, or abnormal amounts of, lipids and lipoproteins in the blood; see also *hyperlipidemia* and *hypolipemia.*

mixed d. mixed hyperlipemia.

dys•lip•i•do•sis (dis″lip-ĭ-do′sis) a disturbance of fat metabolism; it may be either localized or systemic.

dys•lip•oi•do•sis (dis-lip″oi-do′sis) dyslipidosis.

dys•lipo•pro•tein•emia (dis-lip″o-pro″te-ne′me-ə) the presence of abnormal concentrations of lipoproteins, or of abnormal lipoproteins, in the blood. See also *hyperlipoproteinemia* and *hypolipoproteinemia.*

dys•lo•chia (dis-lo′ke-ə) [*dys-* + *lochia*] disordered lochial discharge.

dys•lo•gia (dis-lo′jə) [*dys-* + *log-* + *-ia*] impairment of speech due to a mental disorder.

dys•ma•ture (dis″mə-chōōr′) showing disordered development; said of infants with the postmaturity syndrome.

dys•ma•tur•i•ty (dis-mə-chōōr′ĭ-te) 1. disordered development. 2. postmaturity syndrome.

pulmonary d. Wilson-Mikity syndrome.

dys•meg•a•lop•sia (dis-meg″ə-lop′se-ə) [*dys-* + *megal-* + *-opsia*] a disturbance of the visual appreciation of the size of objects, in which they appear larger than they are.

dys•me•lia (dis-me′le-ə) [*dys-* + *-melia*] anomaly of a limb or limbs resulting from a disturbance in embryonic development; the term includes defects of excessive development as well as reduction deformities. See also *amelia, meromelia,* and *phocomelia.*

dys•men•or•rhea (dis-men″ə-re′ə) [*dys-* + *menorrhea*] painful menstruation.

acquired d. secondary d.

congestive d. 1. secondary d. 2. primary dysmenorrhea characterized by premenstrual dull aching in the lower abdomen, sometimes accompanied by other symptoms including breast or ankle discomfort, lethargy, depression and irritability.

essential d. primary d.

d. intermenstrua′lis intermenstrual pain.

mechanical d. obstructive d.

membranous d. a type of dysmenorrhea characterized by membranous exfoliations derived from the uterus.

obstructive d. dysmenorrhea caused by mechanical obstruction to the discharge of the menstrual fluid.

ovarian d. neuralgic pain due to ovarian disease.

primary d. dysmenorrhea that begins near the time of menarche and onset of ovulatory cycles; it is not usually associated with pelvic pathology.

secondary d. dysmenorrhea that is associated with pelvic pathology, often arising some time after menarche.

spasmodic d. 1. primary d. 2. primary dysmenorrhea characterized by spasms of acute intermittent pain in the lower abdomen, low back or inner thighs beginning on the first day of menstruation.

tubal d. dysmenorrhea caused by disease of the uterine tube, such as chronic salpingitis.

uterine d. dysmenorrhea that arises from a uterine lesion.

dys•me•tab•o•lism (dis″mə-tab′o-liz-əm) defective metabolism.

dys•me•tria (dis-me′tre-ə) [*dys-* + Gr. *metron* measure] a condition in which there is improper estimation of distance in muscular acts, with disturbance of the power to control the range of muscular movement, often resulting in overreaching. See also *hypermetria* and *hypometria.*

ocular d. an error in ocular fixation consisting of overshooting the desired focus followed by oscillations of focus until fixation is achieved; the cause is a cerebellar lesion, usually of the vermis.

dys•met•rop•sia (dis″mə-trop′se-ə) [*dys-* + Gr. *metron* measure + *-opsia*] defect in the visual appreciation of the measure or size of objects.

dys•mne•sia (dis-ne′zhə) [*dys-* + Gr. *mnēmē* memory] impaired memory, as in the amnestic syndrome; cf. *paramnesia.*

dys•mne•sic (dis-ne′zik) characterized by impairment or disorder of memory.

dys•mor•phic (dis-mor′fik) 1. pertaining to dysmorphology. 2. characterized by dysmorphism (def. 1); malformed.

dys•mor•phism (dis-mor′fiz-əm) [*dys-* + *morph-* + *-ism*] 1. an abnormality in morphologic development, such as a malformation in an organ. 2. allomorphism. 3. ability to appear in different morphological forms.

dys•mor•phol•o•gist (dis″mor-fol′ə-jist) a specialist in dysmorphology.

dys•mor•phol•o•gy (dis″mor-fol′ə-je) [*dys-* + *morpho-* + *-logy*] a branch of clinical genetics concerned with the diagnosis and interpretation of patterns of the three types of structural defects—malformation, disruption, and deformation (qq.v.)

dys•mor•pho•pho•bia (dis-mor″fo-fo′be-ə) [*dys-* + *morpho-* + *-phobia*] body dysmorphic disorder.

dys•mor•phop•sia (dis″mor-fop′se-ə) [*dys-* + *morpho-* + *-opsia*] defective vision, with distortion of the shape of objects perceived.

dys•mor•pho•sis (dis″mor-fo′sis) malformation.

dys•mo•til•i•ty (dis-mo-til′ĭ-te) impaired or disordered motility, such as in the gastrointestinal tract.

dys•my•elin•a•tion (dis″mi-ə-lin-a′shən) breakdown or defective formation of a myelin sheath, usually involving biochemical abnormalities.

dys•my•elo•poi•e•sis (dis-mi″ə-lo-poi-e′sis) [*dys-* + *myelopoiesis*] myelodysplasia.

dys•myo•to•nia (dis″mi-o-to′ne-ə) [*dys-* + *myotonia*] dystonia.

dys•na•tre•mia (dis-nə-tre′me-ə) the presence of an abnormally low (hyponatremia) or high (hypernatremia) level of sodium in the blood. dysnatre′mic *adj*

dys•no•mia (dis-no′me-ə) anomic aphasia.

dys•odon•ti•a•sis (dis″o-don-ti′ə-sis) [*dys-* + *odonto-* + *-iasis*] imperfect or defective dentition; defective, delayed, or difficult eruption of the teeth.

dys•on•to•gen•e•sis (dis″on-to-jen′ə-sis) [*dys-* + *ontogenesis*] defective embryonic development. **dysontogenet′ic** *adj*

dys•opia (dis-o′pe-ə) [*dys-* + *-opia*] defective vision.

d. al′gera disturbances of vision due to pains in the eyes and head on looking at objects.

dys•op•sia (dis-op′se-ə) dysopia.

dys•orex•ia (dis″o-rek′se-ə) [*dys-* + Gr. *orexis* appetite] impaired or deranged appetite.

dys•or•gano•pla•sia (dis-or″gən-o-pla′shə) [*dys-* + *organo-* + *-plasia*] disordered development of an organ.

dys•os•mia (dis-oz′me-ə) [*dys-* + *osm-*[1] + *-ia*] parosmia.

dys•os•teo•gen•e•sis (dis-os″te-o-jen′ə-sis) defective bone formation; dysostosis.

dys•os•to•sis (dis″os-to′sis) [*dys-* + *ostosis*] defective ossification; defect in the normal ossification of fetal cartilages.

cleidocranial d. see under *dysplasia.*

craniofacial d. Crouzon syndrome.

d. enchondra′lis epiphysa′ria multiple epiphyseal dysplasia.

mandibulofacial d. a hereditary disorder occurring in two forms: the complete form (Franceschetti syndrome) is autosomal dominant and consists of antimongoloid slant of the palpebral fissures, coloboma of the lower lid, micrognathia, hypoplasia of the zygomatic arches, and microtia. The incomplete form (Treacher Collins syndrome) consists of the same anomalies in less pronounced degree; it occurs sporadically and autosomal dominance is suspected.

metaphyseal d. a skeletal abnormality in which the epiphyses are normal, or nearly so, and the metaphyseal tissues are replaced by masses of cartilage, producing interference with enchondral bone formation, and expansion and thinning of the metaphyseal cortices. Called also *Jansen disease* and *metaphyseal chondrodysplasia.*

d. mul′tiplex a term for the widespread skeletal manifestations typical of the mucopolysaccharidoses.

Nager acrofacial d. a congenital condition in which mandibulofacial dysostosis is associated with limb deformities consisting of absence of the radius, radioulnar synostosis, and hypoplasia or absence of the thumbs.

orodigitofacial d. oral-facial-digital syndrome.

postaxial acrofacial d. Miller syndrome.

dys•pa•reu•nia (dis″pə-roo′ne-ə) [Gr. *dyspareunos* badly mated] difficult or painful sexual intercourse.

dys•pep•sia (dis-pep′se-ə) [*dys-* + Gr. *peptein* to digest] impairment of the power or function of digestion; usually applied to epigastric discomfort following meals. **dyspep′tic** *adj*

acid d. epigastric discomfort associated with excessive acidity of the stomach.

appendicular d. symptoms of dyspepsia occurring in chronic appendicitis.

atonic d. functional d.

cholelithic d. the sudden dyspeptic attacks characteristic of gallbladder disturbance.

fermentative d. that characterized by the fermentation of ingested food.

flatulent d. dyspepsia associated with formation of gas in the stomach, upper abdominal discomfort, and frequent belching.

functional d. dyspepsia with no physical cause, usually resulting from nervousness or anxiety; it can have serious manifestations, resembling the symptoms of peptic ulcer, although no ulcer is detectable. Cf. *organic d.* Called also *atonic, nervous, nonorganic,* or *nonulcer d.*

gastric d. dyspepsia originating in the stomach.

intestinal d. dyspepsia originating in the intestines.

nervous d., nonorganic d., nonulcer d. functional d.

organic d. any type having a physical cause, as opposed to functional d.

dys•per•i•stal•sis (dis-per″ĭ-stawl′sis) [*dys-* + *peristalsis*] painful or abnormal peristalsis.

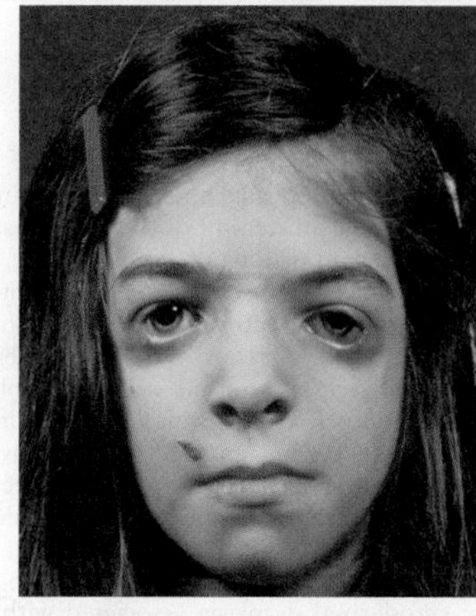

■ Mandibulofacial dysostosis.

dys•pha•gia (dis-fa′je-ə) [*dys-* + *phag-* + *-ia*] difficulty in swallowing.

contractile ring d. esophageal dysphagia due to an overactive interior esophageal sphincteric mechanism that gives rise to painful sticking sensations under the lower sternum.

esophageal d. dysphagia caused by an abnormality in the esophagus, such as a smooth muscle disorder that interferes with peristalsis or an obstruction from external compression or a stricture.

d. inflammato′ria, inflammatory d. dysphagia due to inflammation of the pharynx or esophagus.

d. luso′ria dysphagia resulting from compression of the esophagus caused by an anomalous right subclavian artery that arises from the descending aorta and passes behind the esophagus.

d. nervo′sa, neurogenic d. diffuse esophageal spasm.

oropharyngeal d. dysphagia caused by difficulty in initiating the swallowing process, so that solids and liquids cannot move out of the mouth properly.

paralytic d., d. paraly′tica dysphagia due to paralysis of the pharyngeal or esophageal muscles.

sideropenic d. Plummer-Vinson syndrome.

spastic d. diffuse esophageal spasm.

transfer d. oropharyngeal d.

vallecular d. dysphagia caused by the lodgment of food in the epiglottic valleculae.

dys•pha•gy (dis′fə-je) dysphagia.

dys•pha•sia (dis-fa′zhə) [*dys-* + *-phasia*] impairment of speech, consisting in lack of coordination and failure to arrange words in their proper order, due to a central lesion; called also *dysphrasia* and *dysgrammatism.* See also *aphasia* and *paraphasia.*

dys•phe•mia (dis-fe′me-ə) [*dys-* + *-phemia*] an old term for stuttering or other speech disorder of psychogenic origin.

dys•pho•nia (dis-fo′ne-ə) [*dys-* + *phon-* + *-ia*] any impairment of voice; a speech disorder or other difficulty in speaking. See also *aphonia, hyperphonia,* and *hypophonia.* **dysphon′ic** *adj*

d. clerico′rum clergyman's sore throat.

dysplastic d. chronic hoarseness due to malformation of the larynx.

d. pli′cae ventricula′ris a condition in which speech is accomplished with the false vocal cords.

d. pu′berum the harsh, irregular type of voice often observed around the age of puberty, due to the change of voice.

spasmodic d., spastic d., d. spas′tica difficulty in speaking due to excessively vigorous adduction of the vocal cords against each other (or occasionally abduction), so that the voice is hoarse, soft, and strained.

dys•pho•ret•ic (dis″for-et′ik) 1. dysphoric. 2. dysphoriant.

dys•pho•ria (dis-for′e-ə) [Gr. "excessive pain, anguish, agitation"] disquiet; restlessness; malaise. **dysphor′ic** *adj*

gender d. unhappiness with one's biological sex or its usual gender role, with the desire for the body and role of the opposite sex.

dys•pho•ri•ant (dis-for′e-ənt) 1. producing a condition of dysphoria. 2. an agent that produces dysphoria.

dys•phra•sia (dis-fra′zhə) dysphasia.

dys•pig•men•ta•tion (dis-pig″mən-ta′shən) dyschromia.

dys•pla•sia (dis-pla′zhə) [*dys-* + *-plasia*] 1. abnormality of development. 2. in pathology, alteration in size, shape, and organization of adult cells. See also *dysgenesis* and *dyspoiesis.*

Dysplasia

acromesomelic d. a genetically heterogenous, autosomal recessive condition characterized by shortening of the distal (hands and feet) and middle (forearms and legs) portions of the limbs.

Hunter-Thompson type a condition caused by mutations in the *GDF5* gene (locus: 20q11.2), which encodes a growth factor of the TGF-β superfamily, characterized by mildly shortened forearms and legs, extremely short metacarpals, absence of finger phalanges, and variable hypoplasia of the metatarsals and phalanges of the toes. It is allelic with Grebe chondrodysplasia.

Maroteaux type a syndrome caused by mutations of the *NPR2* gene (locus: 9p21-p12), which encodes a guanylyl cyclase (natriuretic peptide receptor B), characterized by distal shortness of limbs, largeness of the head with frontal prominence, and spinal abnormalities.

anhidrotic ectodermal d. a genetically heterogeneous disorder characterized by ectodermal dysplasia associated with aplasia or hypoplasia of the sweat glands, hypothermia, alopecia, missing or conical teeth, and typical facies (frontal bossing, midfacial hypoplasia, saddle nose, large chin, and thick lips). Inheritance is most commonly X-linked; it can also be autosomal recessive or autsomal dominant, and there is a distinct X-linked form with immune deficiency. Called also *Christ-Siemens-Touraine syndrome* and *hypohidrotic ectodermal d.*

anteroposterior facial d. defective development resulting in abnormal anteroposterior relationship of the maxilla and mandible to each other or to the cranial base with secondary malocclusion.

arrhythmogenic right ventricular d. a congenital cardiomyopathy in which transmural infiltration of adipose tissue results in weakness and aneurysmal bulging of the infundibulum, apex, and posterior basilar region of the right ventricle and leads to ventricular tachycardia arising in the right ventricle.

arteriohepatic d. Alagille syndrome.

autoimmune polyendocrinopathy-candidiasis–ectodermal d. (APECED) polyendocrine autoimmune syndrome, type I.

biliary d. biliary intraepithelial neoplasia.

bronchopulmonary d. chronic lung disease of premature infants that results from disruption of immature lung structures and necessitates the use of supplemental oxygen for at least 28 days after birth. It can be caused by oxygen toxicity and barotrauma during mechanical ventilation, resulting in squamous metaplasia and peribronchiolar fibrosis. It can also be caused by antenatal exposure to factors that interfere with development of normal lung structure, leading to a reduced surface area available for gas exchange.

canine hip d. a bone disorder seen in dogs, particularly in large breeds, in which it may be hereditary; the acetabulum is shallow, the femoral head may be deformed or small, and there is excessive movement at the hip joint, which eventually becomes inflamed and weakened.

cervical d., d. of cervix cellular deviations from the normal in the epithelium of the uterine cervix, which may begin as basal cell hyperplasia and progress through more disorderly epithelial changes toward anaplasia; it is considered a precursor to carcinoma.

chondroectodermal d. Ellis-van Creveld syndrome.

cleidocranial d. a rare autosomal dominant disorder caused by mutation in the *RUNX2* gene (locus: 6p21), which encodes an osteoblast-specific transcription factor. It is characterized by defective ossification of the cranial bones, with large fontanelles and delayed closing of the sutures; complete or partial absence of the clavicles, so that the shoulders may be brought together, or nearly together, in front; wide pubic symphysis; short middle phalanges of the fifth fingers; and dental and vertebral anomalies. An autosomal recessive form has also been observed. Called also *cleidocranial dysostosis.*

cortical d. dysplasia of the cerebral cortex, such as is seen in polymicrogyria and ulegyria.

craniocarpotarsal d. Freeman-Sheldon syndrome.

craniodiaphyseal d. an autosomal recessive condition in which progressive cranial and facial hyperostosis results in significant distortion of the shape of the head; the diaphyses of the long bones are expanded, and mental retardation usually occurs. An autosomal dominant form has also been reported.

craniometaphyseal d. metaphysial dysplasia associated with overgrowth of the head bones, leontiasis ossea, and hypertelorism.

cretinoid d. the abnormal development characteristic of cretinism, consisting of dwarfism, retarded ossification, and immaturity of the internal and sex organs.

cystic renal d. multicystic renal d.

dental d. dentoalveolar d.

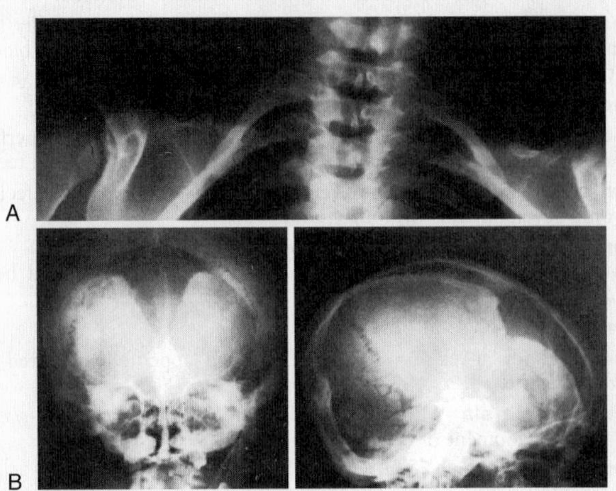

■ Cleidocranial dysplasia. *(A)*, Absent ossification of lateral portions of the clavicles, hypoplastic glenoid fossae, and dysraphism in the lower cervical spine. *(B)*, Wide fontanelles and suture with multiple wormian bones in the lambdoid suture.

dentinal d. an apparently hereditary disorder of dentin formation, marked by a normal appearance of coronal dentin associated with pulpal obliteration, faulty root formation, and a tendency for peripheral lesions without obvious cause. The teeth become loose and are exfoliated prematurely, probably because of the short pointed roots and periapical granulomas and cysts that are a common complication. Called also *rootless teeth.*

dentoalveolar d. abnormal development of two or more teeth within one or both jaws, producing disharmonious relationships between the teeth and their immediate supporting bone and periodontal structures, and resulting in malocclusion. Called also *dental d.*

developmental d. of the hip (DDH) instability of the hip joint leading to dislocation in the neonatal period; it may be associated with various neuromuscular disorders or occur in utero but occurs most commonly in neurologically normal infants and is multifactorial in origin. Formerly called *congenital dislocation of the hip.*

diaphyseal d. a condition characterized by thickening of the cortex of the mid-shaft area of the long bones, progressing toward the epiphyses, the thickening sometimes occurring also in the flat bones; excessive growth in length of bones of the extremities usually results in abnormal stature. Called also *diaphyseal sclerosis* and *Engelmann disease.*

diastrophic d. an autosomal recessive syndrome characterized by dwarfism with progressive structural deformities of the bones and joints, including scoliosis, bilateral clubfoot, deformity of the thumb, micromelia, joint contractures and subluxations, malformation of the pinna with calcification of the cartilage, premature calcification of the costal cartilages, and cleft palate.

ectodermal d. any of a group of hereditary disorders involving absence or deficiency of tissues and structures derived from the embryonic ectoderm, such as teeth, hair, nails, and certain glands; it is also a component of various syndromes, including anhidrotic and hidrotic ectodermal dysplasia and EEC syndrome.

encephalo-ophthalmic d. Krause syndrome.

epiphyseal d. faulty growth and ossification of the epiphyses, with radiographically apparent stippling and decreased stature, not associated with thyroid disease. See *d. epiphysealis hemimelica, multiple epiphyseal d.,* and *chondrodysplasia punctata.*

d. epiphysea′lis hemime′lica a rare condition characterized by swellings in the extremities, usually on the inner and outer aspects of the ankles and knees, made up of bone covered with epiphyseal cartilage, and leading to limitation of motion of the joints. Called also *tarsoepiphyseal aclasis* and *Trevor disease.*

d. epiphysea′lis mul′tiplex multiple epiphyseal d.

d. epiphysea′lis puncta′ta chondrodysplasia punctata.

faciogenital d. Aarskog syndrome.

familial white folded mucosal d. white sponge nevus.

fibromuscular d. dysplasia with fibrosis of the muscular layer of an artery wall, with collagen deposition and hyperplasia of smooth muscle,

Dysplasia *Continued*

causing stenosis and hypertension. It most commonly occurs in the renal arteries and is a major cause of renovascular hypertension. Several types have been distinguished, including *intimal fibroplasia*, *medial fibroplasia*, and *perimedial fibroplasia*. Called also *fibromuscular hyperplasia*.

fibrous d. of bone a disease of bone marked by thinning of the cortex and replacement of bone marrow by gritty fibrous tissue containing bony spicules, producing pain, disability, and gradually increasing deformity. Two types or stages are distinguished: *monostotic fibrous d.* and *polyostotic fibrous d.*

fibrous d. of jaw cherubism.

florid osseous d. an exuberant form of periapical cemental dysplasia that resembles diffuse sclerosing osteomyelitis but differs in being a dysplastic rather than inflammatory process: cysts are present and there is no inflammatory cell infiltrate. Patients are generally asymptomatic.

frontonasal d. median cleft facial syndrome.

geleophysic d. an autosomal recessive lysosomal storage disease caused by mutations in the *ADAMTSL2* gene (locus: 9q34.2), which encodes a protein that is believed to play a role in the regulation of transforming growth factor-β signaling. It is marked by a characteristic happy-appearing face, short stature, small hands and feet, thick skin, joint contractures, and progressive cardiac disease.

hidrotic ectodermal d. an autosomal dominant disorder caused by mutations in the *GJB6* gene (locus: 13q12), which encodes connexin 30. It is characterized by hypotrichosis; dystrophic, hypoplastic, or absent nails; hyperpigmentation of the skin over joints; hyperkeratosis of the palms and soles; normal dentition; and normal sweat gland function. Called also *Clouston syndrome*.

hypohidrotic ectodermal d. anhidrotic ectodermal d.

Kniest d. a rare autosomal dominant collagen disease caused by mutation in the *COL2A1* gene (locus: 12q13.11-q13.2), which encodes type II collagen; characteristics include short stature with skeletal abnormalities such as kyphoscoliosis, depressed nasal bridge, cleft palate, and widening of the epiphyses; hearing loss and ocular defects are frequent.

Langer mesomelic d. an autosomal recessive syndrome consisting of aplasia or hypoplasia of the ulna, the fibula, and sometimes the mandible, with displacement deformities of the hands and feet.

d. linguofacia'lis oral-facial-digital syndrome.

metaphyseal d. a disturbance in enchondral bone growth, failure of modeling causing the ends of the shafts to remain larger than normal in circumference; called also *Pyle disease*. See also *craniometaphyseal d.*

monostotic fibrous d. fibrous dysplasia of bone involving only one bone. Called also *osteitis fibrosa localisata*.

multicystic renal d. renal dysplasia with multiple cysts, usually unilateral and seen in children; the affected kidney is nonfunctional but often asymptomatic. If bilateral, the condition is fatal. See also *polycystic kidney disease*, under *disease*.

multiple epiphyseal d. an inherited developmental abnormality of various epiphyses, which appear late and are mottled, flattened, fragmented, and usually hypoplastic; the digits are short and thick, with blunt ends, and stature may be diminished owing to flattening deformities at the hips, knees, and ankles. It can be caused by any of several mutations; most forms are autosomal dominant, but at least one is autosomal recessive; one of the autosomal dominant forms is caused by mutation in the *COMP* gene and is allelic with pseudoachondroplasia (q.v.). Called also *d. epiphysealis multiplex*.

neuronal colonic d., neuronal intestinal d. a malformation of enteric plexuses resulting in neurons in abnormal locations, such as in intestinal smooth muscles or lamina propria. One complex of symptoms includes enterocolitis, diarrhea, and bloody defecation; another includes megacolon, decreased motility, constipation, and development of fecalomas. See also *congenital megacolon*, under *megacolon*.

oculoauriculovertebral (OAV) d. a congenital condition in which colobomas of the upper eyelid, epibulbar dermoids, bilateral accessory auricular appendages anterior to the ears, and vertebral anomalies are frequently associated with characteristic facies, consisting of asymmetry of the skull, prominent frontal bossing, low hairline, mandibular hypoplasia, low-set ears, and sometimes hemifacial microstomia. Called also *Goldenhar syndrome*.

oculodentodigital d. (ODDD), oculodento-osseous d. (ODOD) a rare hereditary condition caused by mutations in the *GJA1* gene (locus: 6q21-q23.2), which encodes connexin 43, characterized by bilateral microphthalmos, abnormally small nose with anteverted nostrils, hypotrichosis, dental anomalies, camptodactyly, syndactyly, and missing phalanges of the toes. Inheritance is mainly autosomal dominant, but a rare autosomal recessive form also exists. Called also *Meyer-Schwickerath and Weyers syndrome*, *oculodentodigital* or *oculodento-osseous syndrome*, and *ODD syndrome*.

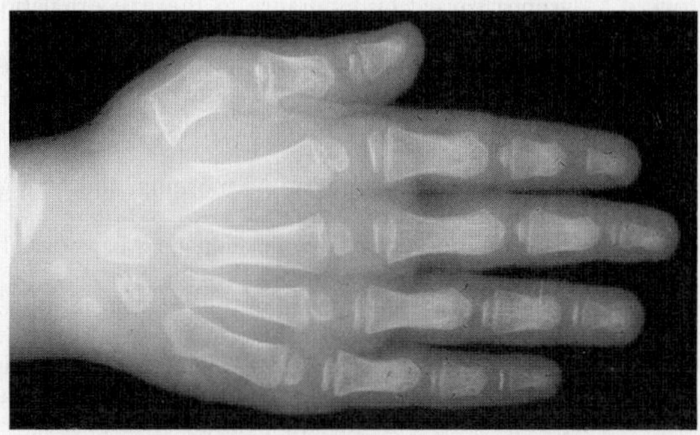

■ Multiple epiphyseal dysplasia. The radiograph shows delayed bone maturation with small carpal centers of ossification and flattened small and fragmented epiphyses.

periapical cemental d. a non-neoplastic condition characterized by the formation of areas of fibrous connective tissue, bone, and cementum around the apex of a tooth, particularly of a mandibular incisor. Patients are generally asymptomatic and affected teeth remain vital.

polyostotic fibrous d. a later stage of fibrous dysplasia of bone in which several or many bones are involved; when associated with skin and endocrine disorders, it is known as *Albright syndrome*. Called also *osteitis fibrosa disseminata*.

primary adrenocortical nodular d. nodular adrenal hyperplasia

progressive diaphyseal d. diaphyseal d.

pseudoachondroplastic spondyloepiphyseal d. pseudoachondroplasia.

renal d. a congenital disorder of the kidney, characterized by persistence of cartilage, undifferentiated mesenchyme, and immature collecting tubules and by abnormal lobar organization; it may be unilateral or bilateral, total or subtotal, and is nearly always cystic (see *multicystic renal d.*). Total bilateral dysplasia is rapidly fatal in the neonatal period, while milder disease may be asymptomatic.

renal-retinal d. Senior-Loken syndrome.

retinal d. 1. a general term for a congenital defect resulting from the abnormal growth and differentiation of a retina that fails to develop into functioning tissue and forms tubular, acinic rosettes. Further ocular defects, e.g. microphthalmos, may be present; syndromic abnormalities may accompany retinal changes. 2. amaurosis congenita. 3. a synonym for, or a conspicuous feature of, Krause syndrome and Patau syndrome.

septo-optic d. a syndrome of hypoplasia of the optic disk with other ocular abnormalities, absence of the septum pellucidum, and hypopituitarism leading to growth deficiency. Called also *de Morsier syndrome*.

spondyloepiphyseal d. a hereditary dysplasia of the vertebrae and extremities resulting in dwarfism of the short-trunk type, often with shortened limbs due to epiphyseal abnormalities. In the delayed onset form, the principal feature is precocious osteoarthritis. There are several forms, including autosomal dominant, autosomal recessive, and X-linked forms, the dominant form often being associated with such ocular anomalies as myopia and detached retina.

spondylothoracic d. Jarcho-Levin syndrome.

Streeter d. congenital ringlike concentric bands on the limbs or trunk.

thanatophoric d. a uniformly fatal type of skeletal dysplasia presenting as extreme shortening of limbs, thoracic cage deformity, and relative cephalomegaly. See also under *dwarf*.

ureteral neuromuscular d. megaureter.

dys·plas·tic (dis-plas′tik) marked by dysplasia.

dysp·nea (disp-ne′ə, disp′ne-ə) [*dys-* + *-pnea*] breathlessness or shortness of breath; difficult or labored respiration. **dyspne′ic** *adj*

cardiac d. dyspnea caused by heart disease.

exertional d. dyspnea provoked by physical effort or exertion.

expiratory d. dyspnea caused by hindrance to the free exhalation of air from the lungs.

functional d. dyspnea not attributable to organic disease, often associated with anxiety states.

inspiratory d. dyspnea caused by hindrance to the free inhalation of air into the lungs.

nocturnal d. dyspnea that is minimal in the morning, and may gradually progress until it becomes severe at night.

nonexpansional d. dyspnea caused by inadequate expansion of the chest.

orthostatic d. dyspnea experienced when in the erect position.

paroxysmal nocturnal d. episodes of respiratory distress that awaken patients from sleep and are related to posture (especially reclining at night), usually attributed to congestive heart failure with pulmonary edema but sometimes occurring in patients with chronic pulmonary diseases.

renal d. dyspnea attributable to anemia or volume overload associated with kidney disease.

dys·poi·e·sis (dis″poi-e′sis) 1. dysgenesis. 2. dyshematopoiesis.

dys·pon·der·al (dis-pon′dər-əl) [*dys-* + *ponderal*] pertaining to disorder of weight, either obesity or underweight.

dys·po·ne·sis (dis″po-ne′sis) [*dys-* + Gr. *ponēsis* toil, exertion] a reversible physiopathologic state consisting of unnoticed, misdirected neurophysiologic reactions to various agents (environmental events, bodily sensations, emotions, and thoughts) and the repercussions of these reactions throughout the organism. These errors in energy expenditure, which are capable of producing functional disorders, consist mainly of covert errors in action-potential output from the motor and premotor areas of the cortex and the consequences of that output. See also *hyperponesis* and *hypoponesis*.

dys·prax·ia (dis-prak′se-ə) [Gr. *dyspraxia* ill luck] partial loss of ability to perform coordinated acts. Cf. *apraxia*.

dys·pro·si·um (Dy) (dis-pro′se-əm) one of the rare earth elements, atomic number 66, atomic weight 162.50.

dys·pros·o·dy (dis-pros′o-de) [*dys-* + *prosody*] a rare speech disorder characterized by disturbance of stress, pitch, and rhythm of speech. See also *aprosody*, *hyperprosody*, and *hypoprosody*.

dys·pro·tein·emia (dis-pro″tēn-e′me-ə) [*dys-* + *protein* + *-emia*] 1. disorder of the protein content of the blood. 2. a plasma cell dyscrasia.

dys·ra·phia (dis-ra′fe-ə) dysraphism.

dys·ra·phism (dis-rāf′iz-əm) [*dys-* + *raphe* + *-ia*] incomplete closure of a raphe; called also *dysraphia*.

spinal d. neural tube defect.

dys·re·flex·ia (dis″re-flek′se-ə) disordered response to stimuli, as in *hyperreflexia* and *hyporeflexia*. Called also *parareflexia*.

autonomic d. a syndrome affecting persons with lesions of the spinal cord above the midthoracic level, characterized by paroxysmal hypertension, bradycardia, excessive sweating, facial flushing, nasal congestion, pilomotor responses, and headache. It is due to an exaggerated autonomic response to such stimuli as distention of the bladder or rectum.

dys·reg·u·la·tion (dis″reg-u-la′shən) failure of normal or expected regulation.

dys·rha·phism (dis′rə-fiz-əm) dysraphism.

dys·rhyth·mia (dis-rith′me-ə) [*dys-* + *rhythm* + *-ia*] disturbance of rhythm; in describing abnormal cardiac rhythms, the term *arrhythmia* is usually used, even for abnormal but regular heart rhythms (see subentries under *arrhythmia*).

cerebral d. disturbance or irregularity in the rhythm of the brain waves as recorded by electroencephalography; called also *electroencephalographic d.*

electroencephalographic d. cerebral d.

esophageal d. diffuse esophageal spasm.

d. pneumophra′sia abnormality of speech rhythm due to defective breath grouping.

d. proso′dia abnormality of speech rhythm due to defective placement of stress.

d. to′nia abnormality of speech rhythm due to defective inflection.

dys·se·ba·cea (dis″se-ba′shə) dyssebacia.

dys·se·ba·cia (dis″sə-ba′shə) [*dys-* + *sebum*] skin changes on the face and in the genital region resulting from ariboflavinosis, clinically resembling the lesions of seborrheic dermatitis.

dys·som·nia (dis-som′ne-ə) [*dys-* + *somn-* + *-ia*] [DSM-IV] a category of disorders consisting of disturbances in the quality, amount, or timing of sleep, due to abnormalities in the mechanisms generating the sleep/wake state or of the timing of sleep and wakefulness; included are primary insomnia, primary hypersomnia, narcolepsy, breathing-related sleep disorder, and circadian rhythm sleep disorder. Cf. *parasomnia*.

dys·sper·mia (dis-spur′me-ə) [*dys-* + *sperm-* + *-ia*] impairment of the spermatozoa, or of the semen.

dys·sta·sia (dis-sta′shə) [*dys-* + *-stasis*] difficulty in standing; called also *dystasia*. **dysstat′ic** *adj*

dys·sym·bo·lia (dis″sim-bo′le-ə) failure of conceptual thinking so that thoughts cannot be intelligently formulated in language; it may be a form of asymbolia or a sign of schizophrenia.

dys·sym·bo·ly (dis-sim′bo-le) dyssymbolia.

dys·sym·me·try (dis-sim′ə-tre) a condition characterized by absence of symmetry.

dys·syn·chro·ny (dis-sing′krə-ne) asynchrony.

dys·syn·er·gia (dis″sin-ur′je-ə) [*dys-* + *synergia*] disturbance of muscular coordination. See also *asynergy*.

biliary d. failure of coordinated action of the different parts of the biliary system. Cf. *biliary dyskinesia*.

bladder neck d. reduced opening of the bladder neck during urination due to dyssynergia of the smooth muscle, resulting in partial obstruction of urinary flow; seen primarily in young to middle-aged men. Called also *smooth sphincter d.*

d. cerebella′ris myoclo′nica dyssynergia cerebellaris progressiva associated with myoclonus epilepsy.

d. cerebella′ris progressi′va a condition marked by generalized intention tremors with disturbance of muscle tone and of muscular coordination; due to disorder of cerebellar function. Called also *Ramsay Hunt syndrome*.

detrusor–external sphincter d. detrusor-sphincter d.

detrusor-sphincter d., detrusor–striated sphincter d. contraction of the sphincter muscle of the urethra at the same time the detrusor muscle of the bladder is contracting, resulting in obstruction of normal urinary outflow; it may accompany detrusor hyperreflexia or detrusor instability. Called also *vesico-sphincter d.*

pelvic floor d. anismus.

smooth sphincter d. bladder neck d.

vesicosphincter d. detrusor-sphincter d.

dys·ta·sia (dis-ta′zhə) dysstasia.

hereditary areflexic d., Roussy-Lévy hereditary areflexic d. Roussy-Lévy syndrome.

dys·tax·ia (dis-tak′se-ə) [*dys-* + Gr. *taxis* arrangement] difficulty in controlling voluntary movements; partial ataxia.

dys·tec·tia (dis-tek′she-ə) [*dys-* + L. *tectum* roof] neural tube defect.

dys·te·le·ol·o·gy (dis-te″le-ol′ə-je) 1. the study of apparently useless organs or parts. 2. lack of purposefulness, or of contribution to the final result.

dys·thy·mia (dis-thi′me-ə) [*dys-* + Gr. *thymos* mind] dysthymic disorder.

dys·thy·mic (dis-thi′mik) characterized by symptoms of mild depression, as in dysthymic disorder.

dys·thy·re·o·sis (dis-thi″re-o′sis) dysthyroidism.

dys·thy·roid (dis-thi′roid) denoting defective functioning of the thyroid gland.

dys·thy·roid·al (dis″thi-roi′dəl) dysthyroid.

dys·thy·roid·ism (dis-thi′roid-iz-əm) imperfect development or function of the thyroid gland; see also *hyperthyroidism* and *hypothyroidism*.

dys·tith·ia (dis-tith′e-ə) [*dys-* + Gr. *tithēnē* a nurse + *-ia*] difficulty in breast feeding.

dys·to·cia (dis-to′shə) [*dys-* + *toc-* + *-ia*] abnormal or difficult labor.

cervical d. dystocia caused by mechanical obstruction at the ostium uteri.

constriction ring d., contraction ring d. dystocia caused by contraction of an area of circular muscle fibers, which may occur at various levels of the parturient uterus.

fetal d. dystocia due to the shape, size, or position of the fetus.

maternal d. dystocia due to some condition inherent in the mother.

placental d. difficulty in delivering the placenta.

shoulder d. dystocia caused by impaction of the fetal shoulder above the pubic symphysis after delivery of the head.

dys·to·nia (dis-to′ne-ə) [*dys-* + *ton-* + *-ia*] dyskinetic movements due to disordered tonicity of muscle; cf. *dyskinesia*. **dyston′ic** *adj*

action d. dystonia in which dyskinetic movements occur during voluntary action and are absent when the affected part is at rest.

cervical d. 1. a type of focal dystonia localized to the neck muscles, causing abnormal jerky turning of the head. 2. spasmodic torticollis.

d. defor′mans progressi′va d. musculorum deformans.

dopa-responsive d. an inherited, progressive type of dystonia characterized by gait disorder that usually presents in childhood and shows pronounced diurnal variation, improving during sleep; signs of parkinsonism may be concurrent or subsequent, and there is dramatic response to administration of L-dopa. It is believed to be due to abnormal functioning of the basal ganglia and is most commonly caused by a defect in either the *GCH1* gene (locus: 14q22.1-q22.2), which encodes GTP cyclohydrolase 1 (autosomal dominant inheritance), or the *TH* gene (locus: 11p15.5), which encodes tyrosine hydroxylase (autosomal recessive inheritance).

early childhood–onset d., early-onset d. early-onset torsion d.

early-onset torsion d. any of several forms of generalized dystonia resulting from a mutation in DYT genes that code for torsinA; the usual type is caused by mutations in the *DYT1* gene (locus: 9q34), is inherited as an autosomal dominant trait, and affects Ashkenazi Jews more commonly than other groups. It appears before the end of the third decade of life, often in childhood, beginning as an action dystonia in an arm or leg and spreading to affect the trunk and other limbs; when generalized, it results in severe disability. There are several other rare types that are apparently caused by mutations in other DYT genes. Called also *early-onset d.*, *early childhood–onset d.*, and *Oppenheim d.*

focal d. dystonia localized to just a few muscles.

generalized d. dystonia occurring in multiple muscles of the trunk and limbs, so that the body continually distorts and twists and the person has difficulty walking.

heredodegenerative d. any of a large group of neurodegenerative diseases in which dystonia is sometimes a prominent feature. Although most of these diseases are due to genetic abnormalities, some are idiopathic.

idiopathic cervical d. spasmodic torticollis.

idiopathic torsion d. former name for *early-onset torsion dystonia.*

jaw-opening d. oromandibular d.

laryngeal d. spasmodic dysphonia.

d. lenticula′ris dystonia due to a lesion of the lenticular nucleus.

d. musculo′rum defor′mans a rare hereditary type of generalized dystonia characterized by involuntary, irregular, clonic contortions of the muscles of the trunk and limbs, especially when the person is walking, which twist the body forward and sideways in a grotesque fashion. There are several types, including *early-onset torsion d.*. Called also *progressive torsion spasm* and *torsion d.*.

myoclonic d., myoclonus-d. dystonia with multifocal myoclonic jerks, generally of the proximal muscles; it may be accompanied by psychiatric disorders. It is genetically heterogeneous, most often caused by mutation in the *SGCE* gene (locus: 7q21), which encodes ε-sarcoglycan, and onset is in the first or second decade of life. The dystonia is mild and most often involves the neck and upper limbs, usually in the form of torticollis or writer's cramp. Symptoms can be relieved by alcohol consumption, which can lead to alcohol abuse.

nocturnal paroxysmal d. a type of parasomnia occurring during NREM sleep, characterized by paroxysms of dystonic movements; in some persons these may progress to epileptic seizures.

Oppenheim d. early-onset torsion d.

oromandibular d. a type of focal dystonia involving spasmodic contraction of mouth and jaw muscles, with involuntary movements of the mouth and lips; cf. *Meige syndrome.*

overflow d. dystonia in which action in other parts of the body can provoke dystonic movements in the affected part.

d.-plus any of several syndromes consisting of a combination of dystonia with other neurologic signs, such as myoclonus or parkinsonism, resulting from a genetic defect and not an underlying neurodegenerative process.

primary generalized d., primary torsion d. early-onset torsion d.

segmental d. focal dystonia in two or more muscles adjacent to each other.

tardive d. a variant of tardive dyskinesia in which there are dystonic rather than choreic movements.

task-specific d. action dystonia that occurs only during the performance of specific tasks, sparing other activities of the affected limb.

torsion d. d. musculorum deformans.

dys·to·pia (dis-to′pe-ə) [*dys-* + *top-* + *-ia*] malposition.

d. cantho′rum outward displacement of the inner canthi of the eyes.

dys·top·ic (dis-top′ik) misplaced; out of its normal place.

dys·to·py (dis′to-pe) dystopia.

dys·tro·brev·in (dis″tro-brev′in) any of several related proteins believed to have cellular scaffolding and signaling functions, each occurring as multiple isoforms: α-dystrobrevin occurs in muscle as part of the dystrophin-glycoprotein complex, and β-dystrobrevin occurs in brain and other tissues but not muscle and binds to dystrophin.

dys·tro·gly·can (dis″tro-gli′kan) a protein complex that plays a role as a link between cytoskeleton and extracellular matrix, binding dystrophin, utrophin, or both where present; it comprises α and β subunits, which are derived from a single transcript by posttranslational processing, and is widely expressed. In skeletal muscle, it occurs as a subcomplex of the dystrophin-glycoprotein complex, binding both dystrophin and laminin.

dys·tro·phia (dis-tro′fe-ə) [L., from *dys-* + Gr. *trophē* nutrition] dystrophy.

d. adipo′sa cor′neae primary fatty degeneration of the cornea; called also *xanthomatosis corneae.*

d. adiposogenita′lis adiposogenital dystrophy.

d. brevicol′lis a condition of dwarfism characterized especially by shortness of the neck.

d. epithelia′lis cor′neae Fuchs endothelial dystrophy.

d. media′na canalifor′mis median nail dystrophy.

d. mesoderma′lis conge′nita hyperplas′tica Weill-Marchesani syndrome.

d. myoto′nica myotonic dystrophy; see under *dystrophy.*

d. un′guis media′na canalifor′mis median nail dystrophy.

d. un′guium nail dystrophy.

d. un′gulae seedy toe.

dys·troph·in (dis′trə-fin) a protein found in skeletal and cardiac muscle, normally in a tightly bound complex with sarcolemmal glycoproteins; mutations in the gene encoding it have been associated with Duchenne muscular dystrophy, Becker muscular dystrophy, and occasionally also other types of skeletal muscle dysfunction. See also *dystrophin-glycoprotein complex*, under *complex.*

dys·trodot;phi·nop·a·thy (dis″trə-fĭ-nop′ə-the) any myopathic condition caused by an abnormality in dystrophin.

dys·tropho·neu·ro·sis (dis-trof″o-noo-ro′sis) [*dys-* + *tropho-* + *neurosis*] 1. any nervous disorder due to poor nutrition. 2. impairment of nutrition which is caused by nervous disorder.

dys·tro·phy (dis′trə-fe) [L. *dystrophia*, q.v.] 1. any disorder arising from defective or faulty nutrition. 2. muscular d. **dystroph′ic** *adj*

Dystrophy

adiposogenital d. a condition seen in adolescent boys characterized by fat distribution of the feminine type and genital hypoplasia associated with lesions of the hypothalamus or pituitary gland. Called also *adiposogenital degeneration* or *syndrome* and *Fröhlich* or *Babinski-Fröhlich syndrome.*

Albright d. see under *syndrome.*

anterior basement membrane d. a type of corneal dystrophy. Called also *epithelial basement membrane d.* and *map-dot-fingerprint d.*

asphyxiating thoracic d. (ATD) a genetically heterogeneous, autosomal recessive syndrome characterized by chondrodystrophy of the rib cage that usually causes asphyxia early in the newborn period, in association with defects of the phalanges and pelvis. It can be caused by mutation at any of three loci: 15q13, 3q24-q26 (the *IFT80* gene), and 11q13.5 (the *DYNC2H1* gene). Called also *Jeune syndrome* and *thoracic-pelvic-phalangeal dystrophy.*

autoimmune polyendocrinopathy-candidiasis–ectodermal d. (APECED) polyendocrine autoimmune syndrome, type I.

Becker muscular d., Becker type muscular d. a condition closely resembling Duchenne muscular dystrophy but having late onset and a slowly progressive course; it is transmitted as an X-linked trait and has been associated with mutations of the gene encoding the protein dystrophin.

Best macular d. see under *disease.*

Biber-Haab-Dimmer d. lattice d.

corneal d. see *granular corneal d.*, *lattice d.*, *macular corneal d.*, *Salzmann nodular corneal d.*, *cornea guttata*, *dystrophia epithelialis corneae*, and *dystrophia adiposa corneae.*

craniocarpotarsal d. Freeman-Sheldon syndrome.

Dejerine-Landouzy muscular d. facioscapulohumeral muscular d.

distal muscular d. see under *myopathy.*

Dystrophy *Continued*

Doyne honeycomb d., Doyne honeycomb retinal d. an autosomal dominant degenerative eye condition marked by light-colored patches near the optic disk and macula; called also *Doyne colloid degeneration* and *Doyne honeycomb choroiditis* or *degeneration.*
Duchenne d. Duchenne muscular d.
Duchenne muscular d., Duchenne type muscular d. the most common and severe type of pseudohypertrophic muscular dystrophy; chronic and progressive, it begins in early childhood. It is characterized by increasing weakness in the pelvic and shoulder girdles, with pseudohypertrophy of the muscles followed by atrophy, lordosis, and a peculiar swaying gait with the legs kept wide apart. It is transmitted as an X-linked trait and has been linked to mutations of the gene encoding the protein dystrophin. Affected individuals, predominantly males, rarely survive to maturity; death is usually due to respiratory weakness or heart failure. Called also *Duchenne* or *Duchenne-Griesinger disease, Erb muscular d.,* and *Zimmerlin atrophy.* Cf. *Becker muscular d.*
Duchenne-Landouzy muscular d. facioscapulohumeral muscular d.
Emery-Dreifuss muscular d. a rare type of muscular dystrophy that begins early in life and involves slowly progressive weakness of the upper arm and pelvic girdle muscles, with cardiomyopathy and flexion contractures of the elbows; muscles are not hypertrophied. The more common, X-linked, form is linked to mutations in the gene encoding the nuclear membrane protein emerin; the rarer autosomal dominant form is linked to mutations in the gene encoding lamins A and C. Called also *scapuloperoneal muscular d.*
enzootic muscular d. myodegeneration in calves, lambs, and colts caused by deficiency of selenium or vitamin E in the diet. Symptoms include dyspnea, cardiac arrhythmias, and difficulty walking. Called also *white muscle disease* and (in lambs) *stiff lamb disease.*
epithelial basement membrane d. anterior basement membrane d.
Erb d., Erb muscular d. 1. Duchenne muscular d. 2. limb-girdle muscular d.
facioscapulohumeral muscular d. a relatively benign autosomal dominant form of muscular dystrophy in which there is marked atrophy of the muscles of the face, shoulder girdle, and arm, producing a facial expression called myopathic face. Most patients enjoy a normal life-span. Called also *facioscapulohumeral muscular atrophy, Dejerine-Landouzy, Duchenne-Landouzy,* or *Landouzy-Dejerine muscular d.*
familial osseous d. Morquio syndrome.
Fuchs d., Fuchs corneal d., Fuchs endothelial d. dystrophy of the anterior epithelium (endothelium) of the cornea marked by small erosions known as Fuchs dimples. It is seen more commonly in women than in men, and usually from middle age onward.
Fukuyama type congenital muscular d. an autosomal recessive type of muscular dystrophy evident in infancy; muscle abnormalities resemble those of Duchenne muscular dystrophy, and patients are mentally retarded with polymicrogyria and other cerebral abnormalities. Called also *Fukuyama syndrome.*
granular corneal d. a dominantly transmitted form of corneal dystrophy occurring during the first decade and characterized by the presence of small opacities in the superficial layers of the cornea, which form a granular disk. Called also *Groenouw type I corneal d.*

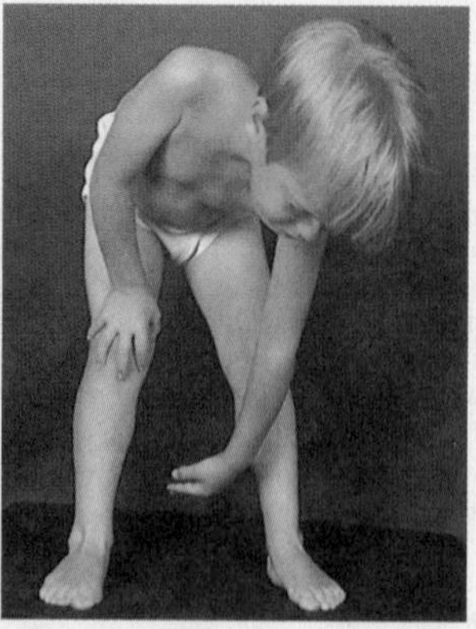

■ Duchenne muscular dystrophy. Earlier stage of characteristic and progressive difficulty in rising from the floor, requiring unilateral hand support on the knee.

Groenouw type I corneal d. granular corneal d.
Groenouw type II corneal d. macular corneal d.
hyperplastic d. squamous hyperplasia.
infantile neuroaxonal d. an autosomal recessive type of encephalopathy that is progressive and degenerative; symptoms begin in infancy with muscular hypotonia and arrested development, followed by dementia, blindness, spasticity, and ataxia. Pathologically it is characterized by widespread focal swellings and degeneration of the axons with scattered spheroids in the brain. One type is caused by a deficiency of α-*N*-acetylgalactosaminidase. Called also *Seitelberger disease.*
Landouzy muscular d., Landouzy-Dejerine muscular d. facioscapulohumeral muscular d.
lattice d., lattice corneal d. hereditary dystrophy of the cornea marked clinically by linear lesions having a filamentous interwoven appearance and histologically by fusiform areas of hyaline degeneration and dense deposits of hyalin between the epithelium and Bowman membrane; called also *Biber-Haab-Dimmer d.*
Leyden-Möbius muscular d. limb-girdle muscular d.
limb-girdle muscular d. a group of disorders characterized by progressive weakness and wasting in the pelvic girdle *(pelvifemoral muscular dystrophy)* or shoulder girdle *(scapulohumeral muscular dystrophy).* It occurs in various subtypes, some of which are of autosomal dominant and others of autosomal recessive inheritance; the latter usually have onset by early adulthood, while the former may have later onset. Progression ranges from rapid to very slow in different subtypes. The mutations causing many of the subtypes have been identified and include mutations in the genes encoding lamins A and C, calpain-3, myotilin, caveolin-3, dysferlin, telethonin, and several sarcoglycans. Called also *Leyden-Möbius muscular d.* or *syndrome.*
macular d. see under *degeneration.*
macular corneal d. a recessively transmitted form of corneal dystrophy occurring during the first or second decade, characterized by macular opacities with indistinct irregular borders, between which the stroma is cloudy. Called also *Groenouw type II corneal d.*
map-dot-fingerprint d. anterior basement membrane d.
median canaliform d., median nail d. a deep longitudinal split or canal in the nail plate, sometimes showing lateral branches. Called also *dystrophia mediana canaliformis, dystrophia unguis mediana canaliformis,* and *solenonychia.*
muscular d. a group of genetic degenerative myopathies characterized by weakness and atrophy of muscle without involvement of the nervous system. The three main types are called pseudohypertrophic, facioscapulohumeral, and limb-girdle.
myotonic d. a rare, slowly progressive, hereditary disease characterized by myotonia followed by atrophy of the muscles (especially those of the face and neck), cataracts, hypogonadism, frontal balding, and cardiac abnormalities. Called also *dystrophia myotonica, myotonia atrophica,* and *Steinert disease.*

type 1 the classic form, transmitted as an autosomal dominant trait with anticipation. It is a triplet repeat disorder associated with amplification of CTG triplet repeats in the 3′ untranslated region of the *DMPK* gene (locus: 19q13.2-q13.3), which encodes a protein kinase; clinical disease is associated with expansion of repeats above 50 in number, but there may be as many as 2000. Severe congenital cases are associated with the highest copy numbers, and are virtually always inherited from the mother.

type 2 a type caused by a CCTG repeat expansion in the *ZNF9* gene (locus: 3q13.3-q24), which encodes zinc finger protein 9; phenotypically it resembles type 1.

nail d. changes in the color, texture, and structure of the nails. Called also *dystrophia unguium* and *onychodystrophy.*
neuraxonal d., neuroaxonal d. 1. see *infantile neuroaxonal d.* 2. an inherited neurological disorder in sheep, dogs, and horses, characterized by ataxia and proprioceptive difficulties, usually with death at an early age.
oculocerebrorenal d. see under *syndrome.*
oculopharyngeal d., oculopharyngeal muscular d. an inherited disorder characterized by weakness of the external ocular and pharyngeal muscles that causes ptosis, ophthalmoplegia, and dysphagia; weakness of trunk and limb muscles may follow. Onset is in adulthood. It is a triplet repeat disorder associated with expansion of GCG triplet repeats in the *PABP2* gene (locus: 14q11.2-q13), which encodes a specific poly A–binding protein; the altered proteins form aggregates and appear to

Dystrophy *Continued*

be associated with accumulation of filamentous inclusions in muscle nuclei. Inheritance can be either autosomal dominant or recessive, differing as a function of the number of repeats. Called also *oculopharyngeal syndrome.*

pelvifemoral muscular d. limb-girdle muscular dystrophy affecting primarily the pelvic girdle.

progressive muscular d. muscular d.

progressive tapetochoroidal d. choroideremia.

pseudohypertrophic muscular d. a group of muscular dystrophies characterized by enlargement (pseudohypertrophy) of muscles. All are X-linked and affect mainly males. The most common types are *Duchenne muscular d.* and *Becker muscular d.*

reflex sympathetic d. complex regional pain syndrome type 1.

Salzmann nodular corneal d. a progressive hypertrophic degeneration of the epithelial layer of the cornea, Bowman membrane, and the outer portion of the corneal stroma.

scapulohumeral muscular d. limb-girdle muscular dystrophy affecting primarily the shoulder girdle.

scapuloperoneal muscular d. Emery-Dreifuss muscular d.

tapetochoroidal d. choroideremia.

thoracic-pelvic-phalangeal d. asphyxiating thoracic d.

twenty-nail d. trachyonychia.

wound d. a syndrome of defective protein metabolism (hypoproteinemia) that sometimes develops after severe injury.

dys•uria (dis-u′re-ə) [*dys-* + *uria*] 1. painful urination. 2. any difficulty of urination. **dysu′ric** *adj*

spastic d. difficult urination due to spasm of the bladder.

dys•vas•cu•lar (dis-vas′ku-lər) having a defective blood supply; cf. *ischemic.*

dys•vi•ta•min•o•sis (dis-vi″tə-min-o′sis) a disorder due to an excess or deficiency of a vitamin.

E

E enzyme; exa-.

E elastance; energy; expectancy; electromotive force; illumination; electric intensity; redox potential.

***E*-** [Ger. *entgegen* opposite] a stereodescriptor used to specify the absolute configuration of rigid compounds, such as those having double bonds. The substituents attached to the double-bonded carbons are ranked according to the Cahn-Ingold-Prelog sequence rules; then if the higher priority substituents are on the same side of the double bond the configuration is *Z*, otherwise *E*. In the simple case when both carbons have the same pair of substitutents, *Z*- is equivalent to *cis*-, *E*- to *trans*-.

E_1 estrone.

E_2 estradiol.

E_3 estriol.

E_4 estetrol.

E_h redox potential.

E° standard reduction potential.

e electron.

e- [L. *e* out of, away from] a prefix meaning away from, without, or outside.

e symbol for an elementary unit of electric charge (see *charge*) and for the base of natural logarithms (approximately 2.7182818285).

e^+ positron.

e^- electron.

ε epsilon, the fifth letter of the Greek alphabet; symbol for *molar absorptivity*, the heavy chain of IgE (see *immunoglobulin*), and the ε chain of hemoglobin.

ε- a prefix designating (1) the fifth carbon along a chain starting with that adjacent to the principal functional group, e.g., ε-aminocaproic acid (see α-); (2) one in a series of related entities or chemical compounds.

η eta, the seventh letter of the Greek alphabet; symbol for *absolute viscosity*.

EAC erythrocyte, antibody, and complement, sometimes used to denote complement complexes, e.g., EAC1 4b2a.

EACA ε-aminocaproic acid.

EAD early afterdepolarization.

ead. [L.] ea'dem (the same).

EAE experimental allergic encephalomyelitis.

EAEC enteroadherent *Escherichia coli*.

EAggEC enteroaggregative *Escherichia coli*.

Ea•gle effect (e'gəl) [Harry *Eagle*, American physician and pathologist, 1905–1992] paradoxical effect.

Ea•gle-Bar•rett syndrome (e'gəl bar'ət) [J.F. *Eagle*, Jr., American physician, 20th century; Norman Rupert *Barrett*, English surgeon, 1903–1979] see under *syndrome*.

EAHF [*e*czema, *a*sthma, *h*ay *f*ever] see under *complex*.

Eales disease (ēlz) [Henry *Eales*, British physician, 1852–1913] see under *disease*.

EAP epiallopregnanolone.

EAR expired air resuscitation.

Ea. R. [Ger.] Entartungs-Reaktion (reaction of degeneration).

ear (ēr) [L. *auris*; Gr. *ous*] the organ of hearing and of equilibrium, consisting of the external ear, the middle ear, and the internal ear; called also *auris* [TA]. See Plate 14.

aviator's e. barotitis media.

bat e. lop e.

beach e. otitis externa caused by irritation from ocean water and other beach conditions.

Blainville e's asymmetry of the two ears.

boxer's e. cauliflower e.

cat's e. an ear that is folded over on itself.

cauliflower e. a partially deformed auricle caused by injury and subsequent perichondritis; called also *boxer's* or *wrestler's e*.

cup e. a protruding, cup-shaped ear. Milder forms present with a poorly developed anthelical crus with deficient development of the superior helix and overdevelopment of its deep concave concha. In the severe forms, the ear is smaller than normal and the helical rim is shortened to such an extent that the helix margin cups forward over the scapha as a hood.

Darwin e. an ear having an eminence on the edge of the helix.

external e. auris externa.

glue e. a chronic condition marked by a collection of fluid of high viscosity in the middle ear, due to obstruction of the eustachian tube with or without tympanic membrane atelectasis (q.v.).

hairy e's hypertrichosis pinnae auris.

inner e., internal e. auris interna.

lop e. deformity of the external ear in which the conchal portion grows at a right angle to the head; called also *bat e*.

middle e. auris media.

Morel e. a deformed ear marked by abnormal development of the helix, antihelix, and scaphoid fossa, so that the folds of the ear seem obliterated, and the ear is smooth, large, and often prominent, with a thin edge.

Mozart e. congenital fusion of the crura of the antihelix and the helix.

outer e. auris externa.

prizefighter's e. cauliflower e.

satyr e. an ear with a pointed pinna.

scroll e. an ear in which the pinna is rolled up.

swimmer's e., tank e. acute otitis externa.

Wildermuth e. a deformed ear with prominent antihelix and poorly developed helix.

wrestler's e. cauliflower e.

ear•ache (ēr'āk) otalgia.

ear•drum (ēr'drəm) membrana tympanica.

ear•lobe (ēr'lōb) lobulus auriculae.

ear-mind•ed (ēr'mīnd-əd) audile.

earth (ərth) 1. the soil and other pulverulent substances forming the ground. 2. any amorphous, easily pulverizable mineral.

alkaline e. any oxide of the alkaline earth metals.

diatomaceous e. infusorial e.

fuller's e. an impure aluminum silicate, consisting mainly of attapulgite, having decolorizing and purifying properties. See also *fuller's earth pneumoconiosis*, under *pneumoconiosis*.

infusorial e. a silicon-rich earth composed mostly of fragments of diatoms; by boiling with dilute hydrochloric acid, washing, and calcining, it can be so purified as to be a very pure form of silica *(terra silicea purificata)*. It is often mixed with clay and used in various industries. See also *diatomite*. Called also *diatomaceous e*.

siliceous e., purified [NF] a form of silica *(infusorial e.)*, SiO_2, purified by boiling with acid, washing, and calcining; used as a pharmaceutical filtering agent.

ear•wax (ēr'waks) cerumen.

Eas•prin (ēz'prin) trademark for a preparation of aspirin.

eat•ing (ēt'ing) the act of ingestion.

binge e. uncontrolled ingestion of large quantities of food in a discrete interval, often with a sense of lack of control over the activity. It is sometimes followed by purging.

Ea•ton-Lam•bert syndrome (e'ton lam'bərt) [Lealdes McKendree *Eaton*, American neurologist, 1905–1958; Edward H. *Lambert*, American physiologist, 1915–2003] Lambert-Eaton myasthenic syndrome; see under *syndrome*.

EAV electroacupuncture after Voll.

EB elementary body.

E-Base (e-bās) trademark for a preparation of erythromycin.

EBCT electron beam computed tomography.

Eberth lines (a'bərt) [Karl Joseph *Eberth*, German pathologist, 1835–1926] see under *line*.

EBL enzootic bovine leukosis.

Eb•ner gland, line, reticulum (eb'nər) [Victor *Ebner* von Rofenstein, Austrian histologist, 1842–1925] see under *gland, line*, and *reticulum*.

Eb•o•la virus, virus disease (hemorrhagic fever) (eb'o-lə) [*Ebola* River in northern Zaïre, where the disease was first observed in 1976] see under *virus* and *disease*.

ebo•na•tion (e"bo-na'shən) [L. *e* out + *bone*] the removal of bone fragments from a wound.

ébranle•ment (a-brahn-lə-maw') [Fr.] removal of a polyp by twisting the pedicle of the tumor.

ebri•e•ty (e-bri'ə-te) inebriation.

Eb•stein angle, anomaly (disease) (eb'shtīn) [Wilhelm *Ebstein*, German physician, 1836–1912] see *cardiohepatic angle*, under *angle*, and see under *anomaly*.

eb•ul•li•tion (eb"u-lish'ən) [L. *ebullire* to boil] 1. the process or condition of boiling. 2. the motion of a boiling liquid.

ebur (e'bər) [L.] ivory.

e. den'tis dentin.

ebur•na•tion (e"bər-na'shən) [L. *ebur* ivory] 1. the conversion of a bone into an ivory-like mass. In osteoarthritis, the thinning and loss of the articular cartilage resulting in exposure of the subchondral bone,

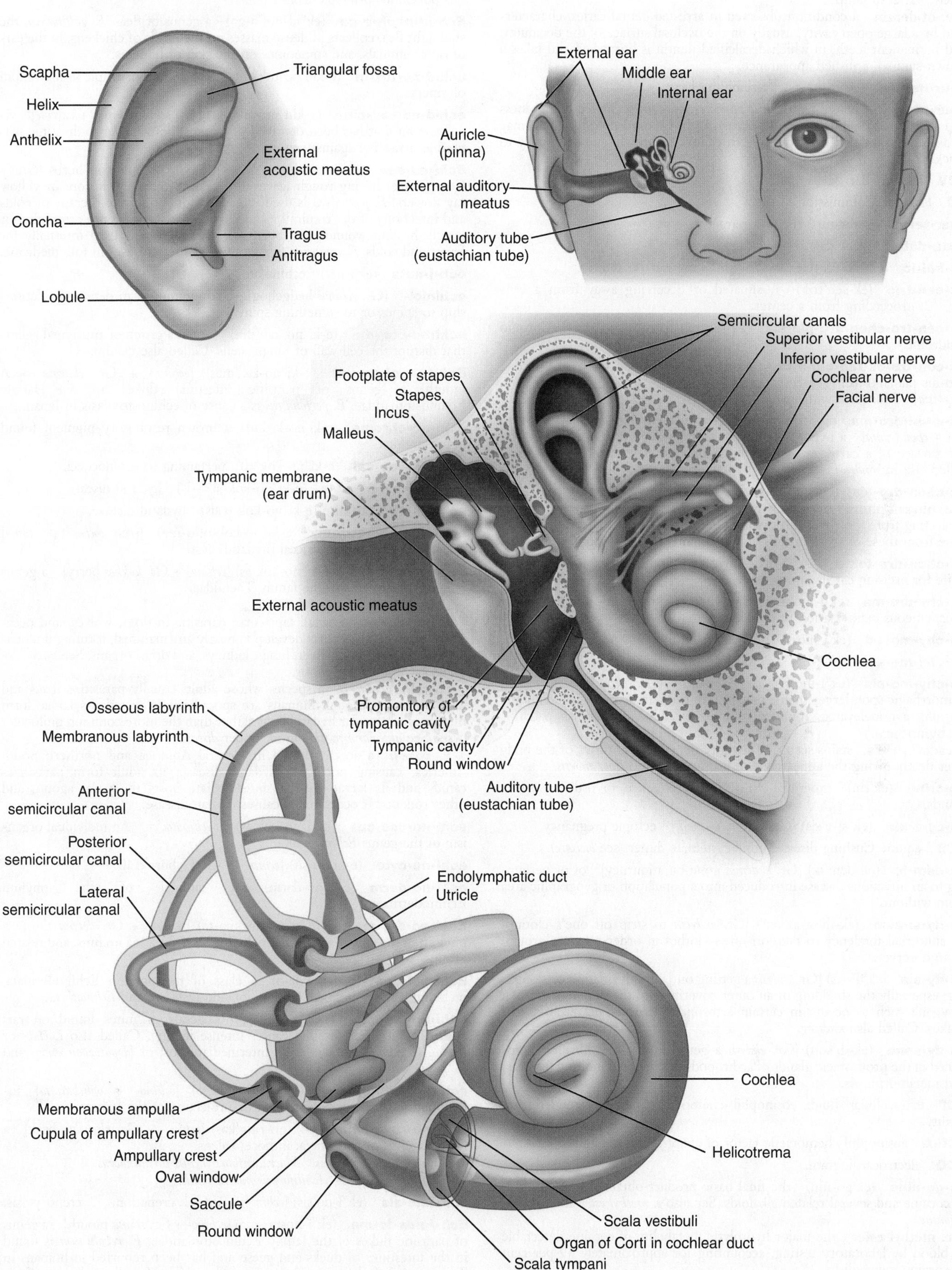

■ **PLATE 14**—EXTERNAL AND INTERNAL STRUCTURES OF THE EAR

which becomes denser and the surface of which becomes worn and polished. 2. e. of dentin.

e. of dentin a condition observed in arrested dental caries, characterized by a large open cavity, usually on the occlusal surface of the deciduous and permanent teeth, in which decalcified dentin is burnished and takes a brown-stained, polished appearance.

ebur•ne•ous (e-bur′ne-əs) resembling ivory.

ebur•ni•tis (e″bər-ni′tis) [L. *eburnus* of ivory + *-itis*] increased hardness and density of dentin, generally occurring in exposed dentin, which may also undergo gradual discoloration, to yellow, to brown, and eventually to black.

EBV Epstein-Barr virus.

EC Enzyme Commission.

écar•teur (a-kahr-tur′) [Fr.] a retractor.

ecau•date (e-kaw′dāt) [*e-* + *caudate*] acaudate.

ec•bol•ic (ek-bol′ik) [Gr. *ekbolikos* throwing out] oxytocic.

ec•cen•tric (ek-sen′trik) 1. situated or occurring away from a center. 2. proceeding from a center.

ec•cen•tro•chon•dro•pla•sia (ek-sen″tro-kon″dro-pla′zhə) Morquio syndrome.

ec•cen•tro•os•teo•chon•dro•dys•pla•sia (ek-sen″tro-os″te-o-kon″-dro-dis-pla′zhə) [Gr. *ekkentros* from the center + *osteo-* + *chondro-* + *dysplasia*] Morquio syndrome.

ec•chon•dro•ma (ek″on-dro′mə) pl. *ecchondromas, ecchondro′mata* [Gr. *ek* out + *chondroma*] a hyperplastic growth of cartilage tissue developing on the surface of a cartilage or projecting under the periosteum of a bone; called also *ecchondrosis.*

ec•chon•dro•sis (ek″on-dro′sis) ecchondroma.

e. physali′phora gelatinous nodules of heterotopic notochordal tissue projecting from the clivus or dorsum sellae. True tumors (chordomas) may arise from these or from intraosseous remnants of the notochord.

ec•chon•dro•tome (ə-kon′dro-tōm) [Gr. *ek* out + *chondro-* + *-tome*] a knife for excising cartilaginous tissue.

ec•chy•mo•ma (ek-ĭ-mo′mə) a swelling due to a bruise and formed by subcutaneous extravasation of blood.

ec•chy•mosed (ek′ĭ-mōzd) characterized by ecchymosis.

ec•chy•mo•ses (ek″ĭ-mo′sēz) [Gr.] plural of *ecchymosis.*

ec•chy•mo•sis (ek″ĭ-mo′sis) pl. *ecchymo′ses* [Gr. *ekchymōsis*] a small hemorrhagic spot, larger than a petechia, in the skin or mucous membrane forming a nonelevated, rounded or irregular, blue or purplish patch. ecchymot′ic *adj*

cadaveric e′s stains seen on the more dependent portions of the body after death, giving the appearance of bruises. See also *livor mortis.*

ec•crine (ek′rin) exocrine, with special reference to ordinary sweat glands.

ec•cy•e•sis (ek″si-e′sis) [Gr. *ek* out + *-cyesis*] ectopic pregnancy.

ECD equine Cushing disease; ethyl cysteinate dimer (see *bicisate).*

ec•dem•ic (ek-dem′ik) [Gr. *ekdēmos* gone on a journey] of or pertaining to an infectious disease introduced into a population or geographic area from without.

ec•dy•si•asm (ek-di′se-az″əm) [Gr. *ekdyein* to strip off one's clothes] an abnormal tendency to take off one's clothes in order to cause arousal in an observer.

ec•dy•sis (ek′dĭ-sis) [Gr. *ekdysis* a getting out] desquamation or sloughing; especially the shedding of an outer covering and the development of a new one such as occurs in certain arthropods, crustaceans, lizards, and snakes. Called also *molting.*

ec•dy•sone (ek-di′son) [Gr. *ekdysis* a getting out] the hormone produced in the prothoracic glands of arthropods that induces molting (ecdysis) and metamorphosis.

ECF extracellular fluid; eosinophil chemotactic factor; extended care facility.

ECF-A eosinophil chemotactic factor of anaphylaxis; see under *factor.*

ECG electrocardiogram.

ec•go•nine (ek′go-nin) the final basic product obtained by hydrolysis of cocaine and several related alkaloids. See also *e. methyl ester* and *benzoylecgonine.*

e. methyl ester the major hydrolytic metabolite of cocaine detectable in blood by laboratory testing, accounting for approximately 49 per cent of cocaine metabolism.

echid•nase (e-kid′nās) [Gr. *echidna* viper + *-ase*] an enzyme found in the venom of vipers.

echid•nin (e-kid′nin) [Gr. *echidna* viper] serpent venom, or a nitrogenous poisonous principle from it.

Ech•id•noph•a•ga (ek″id-nof′ə-gə) a genus of fleas. *E. gallina′cea,* the sticktight flea, collects in dense masses on the heads of chickens, in the ears of other animals, and sometimes on the skin of humans.

echid•no•tox•in (e-kid′no-tok″sin) a poisonous principle in the venom of vipers.

echid•no•vac•cine (e-kid″no-vak′sēn) [Gr. *echidna* viper + *vaccine*] viper venom that has been deprived of its poisonous power by heating; it is used as a vaccine against venom.

Echi•na•cea (ek″ĭ-na′shə) a genus of North American herbs (family Compositae) having rough leaves and pinkish-purple, crimson, or yellow ray flowers. *E. purpu′rea* is used internally for supportive therapy of colds and infections of the respiratory and lower urinary tract and externally for poorly healing wounds and burns. *E. pal′lida* root is used internally for fevers and colds. *E. angustifo′lia* has a wide variety of uses in folk medicine.

ech•i•nate (ek′ĭ-nāt) echinulate.

echin(o)- [Gr. *echinos* hedgehog] a combining form denoting relationship to spines or to something spiny.

echi•no•can•din (e-ki″no-kan′din) any in a group of antifungal agents that disrupt the cell wall of fungus cells. Called also candin.

Ech•i•no•chas•mus (e-ki″no-kaz′məs) [*echino-* + Gr. *chasma* open mouth] a genus of parasitic intestinal flukes of the family Echinostomatidae. *E. perfolia′tus* is a cause of echinostomiasis in Japan.

echi•no•chrome (e-ki′no-krōm) a brown respiratory pigment found in sea urchins.

echi•no•coc•cal (e-ki″no-kok′əl) pertaining to echinococci.

echi•no•coc•ci•a•sis (e-ki″no-kok-si′ə-sis) hydatid disease.

echi•no•coc•co•sis (e-ki″no-kok-o′sis) hydatid disease.

echi•no•coc•cot•o•my (e-ki″no-kok-ot′o-me) [*echinococcus* + *-tomy*] evacuation of an echinococcal (hydatid) cyst.

Echi•no•coc•cus (e-ki″no-kok′əs) [*echino-* + Gr. *kokkos* berry] a genus of small tapeworms of the family Taeniidae.

E. alveola′ris *E. multilocularis.*

E. granulo′sus a small tapeworm parasitic in dogs, wolves, and occasionally cats. Its larva may develop in nearly any mammal, forming unilocular hydatid cysts in the liver, lungs, kidneys, and other organs. See *unilocular hydatid disease,* under *disease.*

E. multilocula′ris a species whose adults usually parasitize foxes and wild rodents, although humans are sporadically infected. Its larvae form multilocular alveolar hydatid cysts rather than the more common unilocular cysts. See *alveolar hydatid disease,* under *disease.*

E. voge′li a species found in Central America and northern South America, causing polycystic hydatid disease; its adult form parasitizes canids and its larvae have as intermediate hosts the paca, agouti, and other rodents. It occasionally causes human disease.

echi•no•coc•cus (e-ki″no-kok′əs) pl. *echinococ′ci.* An individual organism of the genus *Echinococcus.*

echi•no•cyte (e-ki′no-sīt) [*echino-* + *-cyte*] burr cell.

echi•no•derm (e-ki′no-dərm) any animal of the phylum Echinodermata.

Echi•no•der•ma•ta (e-ki″no-dur′mə-tə) [*echino-* + Gr. *derma* skin] a phylum of the animal kingdom, including starfishes, sea urchins, and related groups.

Echi•noi•dea (e-ki-noi′de-ə) a class of the phylum Echinodermata, including the sea urchins. Genera include *Diadema* and *Echinothrix.*

Echi•no•lae•laps (e-ki″no-le′ləps) a genus of mites found on rats and in stable litter; its bite causes intense itching. Called also *Laelaps* or *Lelaps. E. echidni′nus* acts as an intermediate host of *Hepatozoon muris* and *H. perniciosum.*

echin•oph•thal•mia (e-kin″of-thal′me-ə) [*echino-* + *ophthalmia*] inflammation of the eyelids marked by projection of the lashes.

Echi•no•rhyn•chus (e-ki″no-ring′kəs) [*echino-* + Gr. *rhynchos* beak] a former genus of parasitic acanthocephalans.

E. gi′gas, E. ho′minis *Macracanthorhynchus hirudinaceus.*

E. monilifor′mis *Moniliformis moniliformis.*

ech•i•no•sis (ek″ĭ-no′sis) [*echin-* + *-osis*] 1. crenation. 2. crenocytosis.

Ech•i•nos•to•ma (ek″ĭ-nos′to-mə) [*echino-* + Gr. *stoma* mouth] a genus of parasitic flukes of the family Echinostomatidae. *E. revolu′tum* is found in the intestines of ducks and geese and has been reported in humans in Taiwan and Indonesia. *E. iloca′num* has been found in human feces in Indonesia and the Philippines. *E. lindoen′sis* occurs in Indonesia; *E. perfolia′tum* is found in Japan.

Echi•no•sto•mat•i•dae (ek″ĭ-no-sto-mat′ĭ-de) a family of trematodes, including the genera *Acanthoparyphium, Echinochasmus,* and *Echinostoma.*

echi•no•sto•mi•a•sis (e-kin″o-sto-mi′ə-sis) infection by flukes of the genus *Echinostoma* or a related genus.

Echi•no•thrix (e-ki′no-thriks) a venomous genus of sea urchins.

echin•u•late (e-kin′u-lāt) [L. *echinus* hedgehog] having small prickles or spines; applied in bacteriology to cultures showing toothed or pointed outgrowths.

Echis (e′kis) a genus of snakes of the family Viperidae, small venomous vipers found from India to northern Africa as far south as Ghana and Nigeria; *E. carina′tus* and *E. colora′tus* are both called *carpet viper* or *saw-scaled viper* and their bites are often deadly.

echo (ek′o) [Gr. *ēchō* a returned sound] 1. repetition of a sound as a result of reverberation of sound waves. 2. the reflection of ultrasonic, radio, or radar waves. 3. sometimes used in reference to any kind of repetition.

amphoric e. a resonant repetition of a sound heard on auscultation of the chest, occurring at an appreciable interval after the vocal sound.

metallic e. a peculiar ringing repetition of the heart sounds sometimes heard in patients with pneumopericardium and pneumothorax.

spin e. a signal generated by a previously magnetized substance a short time after the components of magnetization have been refocused or rephased by application of a pulse of radio frequency energy or by a rapid change in magnetic field gradient; it can then be received by a receiver coil for generating the images of magnetic resonance imaging.

echo•acou•sia (ek″o-ə-koo′zhə) [*echo* + Gr. *akousis* hearing + *-ia*] the subjective experience of hearing echoes after normally heard sounds.

echo•car•dio•gram (ek″o-kahr′de-o-gram″) the record produced by echocardiography.

echo•car•di•og•ra•phy (ek″o-kahr″de-og′rə-fe) a method of graphically recording the position and motion of the heart walls or the internal structures of the heart and neighboring tissue by the echo obtained from beams of ultrasonic waves directed through the chest wall. Called also *ultrasonic cardiography.*

color Doppler e. color flow Doppler imaging.

continuous wave Doppler e. echocardiography employing continuous wave Doppler ultrasonography to record the flow of blood through the cardiovascular system.

contrast e. echocardiography in which the ultrasonic beam detects tiny intravascular bubbles produced by intravascular injection of a liquid, such as the patient's blood, saline, or dextrose in water, or of small amounts of carbon dioxide gas; bubble movement can demonstrate abnormalities of blood flow.

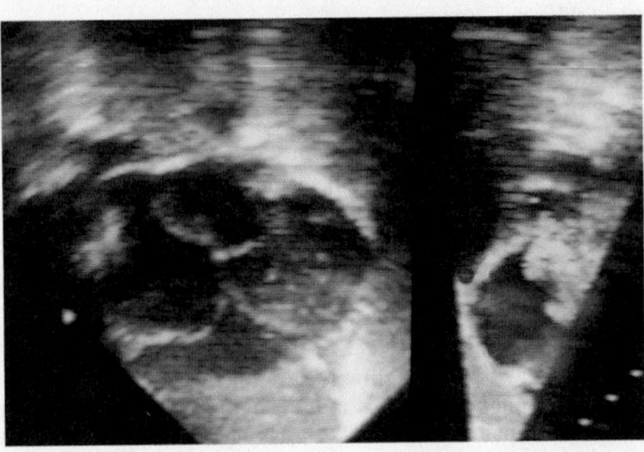

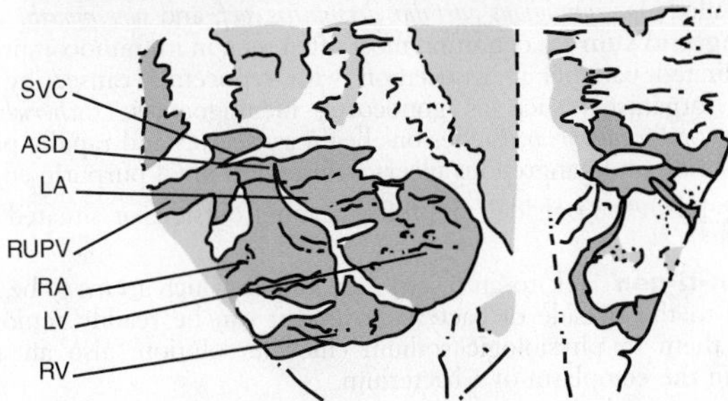

■ Echocardiography of sinus venosus type of atrial septal defect *(ASD).* Cross-sectional view *(left)* shows a defect in the posterosuperior portion of the atrial septum where the right upper pulmonary vein *(RUPV)* opens directly into the superior vena cava *(SVC).* Shunts from the anomalous drainage of RUPV and from the left atrium *LA* are shown in color flow imaging *(right). (LV),* Left ventricle; *(RA),* right atrium; *(RV),* right ventricle.

Doppler e. an echocardiographic technique that records the flow of red blood cells through the cardiovascular system by means of Doppler ultrasonography (q.v.).

M-mode e. echocardiography recording the amplitude and rate of motion (M) of a moving structure in real time by repeatedly measuring the distance of the structure from the single transducer at a given moment. It yields a monodimensional image often called an "icepick" view of the heart.

myocardial contrast e. (MCE) contrast echocardiography of the myocardium, used to assess myocardial perfusion and viability following acute myocardial infarction.

pulsed wave Doppler e. echocardiography employing pulsed wave Doppler ultrasonography to record the flow of blood through the cardiovascular system.

stress e. echocardiography performed while the patient is under stress, as during exercise.

three-dimensional e. a technique that creates a three-dimensional image of the heart, either by digital reconstruction from multiple stored two-dimensional echocardiograms or in real time by means of a transducer that generates a phased array of ultrasound beams from which a three-dimensional image is produced.

transesophageal e. (TEE) the introduction of a transducer attached to a fiberoptic endoscope into the esophagus to provide two-dimensional cardiographic images or Doppler information.

two-dimensional e. echocardiography performed by moving the ultrasonic beam in a sector, using multiple transducers or a rotating transducer; computer reconstruction yields a two-dimensional image of a specific plane of the heart.

echo•dense (ek′o-dens″) hyperechoic.

echo•gen•ic (ek″o-jen′ik) in ultrasonography, giving rise to reflections (echoes) of ultrasound waves.

echo•ge•nic•i•ty (ek″o-jen-is′ĭ-te) in ultrasonography, the extent to which a structure gives rise to reflections of ultrasound waves.

echo•gram (ek′o-gram) ultrasonogram.

echo•graph•ia (ek″o-graf′e-ə) [*echo* + *graph-* + *-ia*] a type of dysgraphia in which the patient can copy writing, but cannot write to express ideas. Called also *pseudoagraphia.*

echog•ra•phy (ə-kog′rə-fe) ultrasonography.

echo•ki•ne•sis (ek″o-kĭ-ne′sis) [*echo* + *-kinesis*] echopraxia.

echo•la•lia (ek″o-la′le-ə) [*echo* + *lal-* + *-ia*] stereotyped repetition of another person's words or phrases, seen in catatonic schizophrenia, Gilles de la Tourette syndrome, and neurological disorders such as transcortical aphasia. Called also *echophrasia.*

echo•lu•cent (ek″o-loo′sənt) permitting the passage of ultrasonic waves without giving rise to echoes, the representative areas appearing black on the sonogram.

echo•ma•tism (ĕ-ko′mə-tiz-əm) [*echo* + Gr. *matizein* to strive to do] echopraxia.

echo•mim•ia (ek″o-mim′e-ə) [*echo* + Gr. *mimos* actor, mime + *-ia*] echopraxia.

echop•a•thy (ĕ-kop′ə-the) [*echo* + *-pathy*] stereotyped repetition of the words or actions of others; echolalia or echopraxia.

echo•pho•no•car•di•og•ra•phy (ek″o-fo″no-kahr″de-og′rə-fe) the combined use of echocardiography and phonocardiography.

echoph•o•ny (ek-of′ə-ne) [*echo* + Gr. *phōnē* voice] an echolike sound heard immediately after a voice sound on auscultation of the chest.

echo•phot•o•ny (ek″o-fot′o-ne) [*echo* + *photo-* + *-tony*] the association of certain colors with certain sounds.

echo•phra•sia (ek″o-fra′zhə) echolalia.

echo•prax•ia (ek″o-prak′se-ə) [*echo* + Gr. *praxia* action, from *prassein* to perform] stereotyped imitation of the movements of another person; seen sometimes in catatonic schizophrenia and Gilles de la Tourette syndrome.

echo•prax•is (ek″o-prak′sis) echopraxia.

echo•rang•ing (ek″o-rānj′ing) in ultrasonography, the determining of the position or depth of a body structure on the basis of the time interval between the moment an ultrasonic pulse is transmitted and the moment its echo is received.

echo•tex•ture (ek′o-teks″chər) the general appearance of an ultrasonogram.

echo•thi•o•phate io•dide (ek″o-thi″o-fāt) [USP] an anticholinesterase agent applied topically to the conjunctiva to produce miosis, reduce intraocular pressure, and potentiate accommodation in the treatment of open-angle glaucoma, closed-angle glaucoma after iridectomy, and certain secondary types of glaucoma, and in the management of accommodative esotropia.

echo•vi•rus (ek′o-vi″rəs) [*e*nteric *c*ytopathic *h*uman *o*rphan + *virus*] any of numerous species and strains of the family Picornaviridae, some of which cause aseptic meningitis or a febrile rash; they have now been renamed and assigned to the genera *Enterovirus* and *Parechovirus*. **echovi′ral** *adj*

ECI electrocerebral inactivity.

Eck fistula (ek) [Nicolai Vladimirovich *Eck*, Russian physiologist, 1847–1908] see under *fistula*.

eclamp•sia (ə-klamp′se-ə) [Gr. *eklampein* to shine forth] 1. convulsions occurring in a pregnant or puerperal woman, associated with preeclampsia, i.e., with hypertension, proteinuria, or edema. 2. puerperal tetany. **eclamp′tic** *adj*

puerperal e. eclampsia occurring after childbirth.

uremic e. eclampsia with uremia.

eclamp•to•gen•ic (ə-klamp″to-jen′ik) causing convulsions.

eclipse (e-klips′) in virology, that period of the infective cycle during which infected bacterial cells contain no detectable infective bacteriophage.

ECLS extracorporeal life support.

ECM extracellular matrix.

ECMO extracorporeal membrane oxygenation; see *extracorporeal life support*, under *support*.

ec(o)- [Gr. *oikos* house] combining form denoting relationship to the environment.

eco•ge•net•ic (ek″o-jə-net′ik) pertaining to or characterized by the interaction of genetic and environmental factors.

eco•ge•net•ics (ek″o-jə-net′iks) [*eco-* + *genetics*] the study of genetically determined responses of organisms to the environment.

ecol•o•gist (e-kol′o-jist) a specialist in ecology.

ecol•o•gy (e-kol′ə-je) [*eco-* + *-logy*] the science of the relationship between organisms and their environments; the study of the effect of environment on the life history of organisms.

human e. application of the ecologic approach to the study of human societies.

econ•a•zole ni•trate (ə-kon′ə-zōl) [USP] an imidazole derivative used as a broad-spectrum antifungal agent, applied topically to the skin in the treatment of cutaneous candidiasis and various forms of tinea, and also applied intravaginally in the treatment of vulvovaginal candidiasis.

Econ•o•mo disease (encephalitis) (a-kon′o-mo) [Constantin von *Economo*, Austrian neurologist, 1876–1931] encephalitis lethargica.

econ•o•my (e-kon′ə-me) [Gr. *oikos* house + *nomos* law] the management of domestic affairs.

token e. a program of treatment in behavior therapy, usually conducted in a hospital setting, in which the patient may earn tokens by engaging in appropriate personal and social behavior, or lose tokens by inappropriate or antisocial behavior; tokens may be exchanged for tangible rewards (food snacks, clothing, etc.) or for special privileges (watching television, passes to leave the hospital, etc.).

écor•ché (a″kor-sha′) [Fr.] a painting or sculpture of a human or other animal exhibited as deprived of its skin, so that the muscles are exposed for study.

ecos•tate (e-kos′tāt) [*e-* without + *costa*] ribless; without ribs.

eco•sys•tem (e′ko-sis″təm) [*eco-* + *system*] the fundamental unit in ecology, comprising the living organisms and the nonliving elements interacting in a certain defined area. Called also *ecological system*.

eco•tax•is (ek′o-tak″sis) [Gr. *oikos* house + *taxis* arrangement] the "homing" of recirculating lymphocytes to specific compartments of peripheral lymphoid tissues, with B cells going to B-dependent areas and T cells to T-dependent areas.

eco•tone (ek′o-tōn) [*eco-* + Gr. *tonos* tension] a transition region where adjacent biomes blend, containing some organisms from each of the adjacent biomes plus some that are characteristic of, and perhaps restricted to, the ecotone; this region tends to have more species and to be more densely populated than either adjacent biome.

eco•tro•pic (e″ko-tro′pik) [Gr. *oikos* house + *-tropic*] pertaining to a virus that infects and replicates in cells from only the original host species. Cf. *xenotropic*.

écou•vil•lon (a-koo″ve-yaw′) [Fr.] a stiff brush or swab used for swabbing cavities and inflammatory lesions.

écou•vil•lo•nage (a-koo″ve-yo-nahzh′) [Fr.] the scrubbing of a cavity or an infected area.

écrase•ment (a-krahz-maw′) [Fr.] removal by means of an écraseur.

écra•seur (a-krah-zur′) [Fr. "crusher"] an instrument containing a chain or cord to be looped about a part and then tightened in order to transect the portion enclosed within the loop.

ECS electrocerebral silence; equine Cushing syndrome; see *equine Cushing disease*, under *disease*.

ec•so•mat•ics (ek″so-mat′iks) [Gr. *ek* out + *somatic*] the study by laboratory methods of the materials removed from the body.

Ec•sta•sy (ek′stə-se) popular name for *3,4-methylenedioxymethamphetamine*.

ec•sta•sy (ek′stə-se) [Gr. *ekstasis*] a state of rapture and trancelike elation. **ecstat′ic** *adj*

ECT electroconvulsive therapy.

ec•tad (ek′təd) [*ect-* + *-ad*[1]] outward; the reverse of inward.

ec•tal (ek′təl) [*ect-* + *-al*[1]] superficial or external.

ec•ta•sia (ek-ta′zhə) [Gr. *ektasis* dilatation + *-ia*] dilatation, expansion, or distention. **ectat′ic** *adj*

alveolar e. overdistention of the pulmonary alveoli.

annuloaortic e. dilatation of the proximal aorta and the fibrous ring of the heart at the aortic orifice, marked by aortic regurgitation and, when severe, by dissecting aneurysm; it is often associated with Marfan syndrome.

corneal e. keratectasia.

diffuse arterial e. racemose aneurysm.

gastric antral vascular e. (GAVE) a rare vascular anomaly of the gastric antrum, consisting of dilated and thrombosed capillaries and veins that form lines in the antrum that radiate toward the pylorus, resembling the stripes on a watermelon; seen most often in elderly women or patients with chronic liver disease. It may result in chronic blood loss and anemia. Called also *watermelon stomach*.

hypostatic e. dilatation of a blood vessel from the effect of gravity on the blood.

mammary duct e. a condition characterized chiefly by dilatation of the collecting ducts of the mammary gland, inspissation of breast secretion, intraductal inflammation, and marked periductal and interstitial chronic inflammatory reaction in which plasma cells are prominent; a benign process associated with atrophy of the duct epithelium, it generally occurs during or after the menopause.

papillary e. a circumscribed dilatation of the capillaries, forming a red spot on the skin.

precalyceal canalicular e. medullary sponge kidney.

scleral e. see under *staphyloma*.

tubular e. medullary sponge kidney.

vascular e. angiectasis.

ec•ta•sis (ek′tə-sis) ectasia.

ec•ta•sy (ek′tə-se) ectasia.

ec•ten•tal (ek-ten′təl) [*ect-* + *ental*] pertaining to the ectoderm and endoderm, and to their line of junction.

ec•teth•moid (ek-teth′moid) [*ect-* + *ethmoid*] labyrinthus ethmoidalis.

ec•thy•ma (ek-thi′mə) [Gr. *ekthyma*] an ulcerative pyoderma usually caused by infection with group A beta-hemolytic streptococci at the site of minor trauma; the usual site is on the shins or the backs of the feet, and it may or may not leave a scar upon healing.

contagious e. an endemic infectious disease of sheep and goats caused by a poxvirus, characterized by the development on non–wool-bearing areas, especially the lips and oral mucosa, of an erythematous vesiculopustular eruption, the lesions of which may coalesce and crust over, forming large scabs that fall off, followed by healing of the tissues without scarring. It can be transmitted to humans, as by milking, where it is usually characterized by a few painless pustules on a finger. If the infection becomes disseminated, there may be systematic symptoms such as lymphadenitis and fever. Called also *contagious pustular dermatitis*, *orf*, and *sore mouth*.

e. gangreno′sum a condition most often seen in immunocompromised or debilitated patients in association with septicemia caused by gram-negative organisms such as gonococci, meningococci, *Escherichia coli*, *Klebsiella*, or *Pseudomonas;* the lesions begin as vesicles and rapidly progress to pustulation and gangrenous ulcers with undermined purpuric edges.

ect(o)- [Gr. *ektos* outside] a prefix meaning outside, or situated on the outside.

ec•to•an•ti•gen (ek″to-an′tĭ-jən) an antigen which seems to be loosely attached to the outside of bacteria so that it can be readily removed by shaking them in physiologic sodium chloride solution; also an antigen formed in the ectoplasm of a bacterium.

ec•to•blast (ek′to-blast) [*ecto-* + *-blast*] ectoderm.

ec•to•car•dia (ek″to-kahr′de-ə) [*ecto-* + Gr. *kardia* heart] congenital displacement of the heart, either inside or outside the thorax.

ec•to•cer•vix (ek″to-sur′viks) portio vaginalis cervicis. **ectocer′vical** *adj*

ec•to•co•lon (ek″to-ko′lən) [*ectasia* + *colon*] dilatation of the colon.

ec·to·com·men·sal (ek″to-kə-men′səl) a commensal organism that lives outside the body of its symbiotic companion, but cannot be separated from it.

ec·to·con·dyle (ek″to-kon′dīl) the external condyle of a bone.

ec·to·cu·ne·i·form (ek″to-ku-ne′ĭ-form) the lateral cuneiform bone.

ec·to·cyst (ek′to-sist) the outer layer of a hydatid cyst.

ec·to·cy·tic (ek″to-si′tik) [*ecto-* + *cyt-* + *-ic*] outside the cell.

ec·to·derm (ek′to-dərm) [*ecto-* + *derm*] the outermost layer of cells of the three primary germ layers of the embryo. From it are developed the epidermis and the epidermal tissues, such as the nails, hair, enamel of teeth, and glands of the skin, the nervous system, the external sense organs such as the ear and eye, and the mucous membrane of the mouth and anus. Cf. *endoderm* and *mesoderm*. **ectoder′mal, ectoder′mic** *adj*

amniotic e. the inner layer of the amnion (and covering of the umbilical cord) that is continuous with body ectoderm.

basal e. trophoblast covering the eroded uterine tissue that faces the placental sinuses.

blastodermic e. the external layer of a blastula or blastodisc; called also *primordial e.*

chorionic e. trophoblast.

extraembryonic e. a derivative of epiblast or ectoderm located outside the body of the embryo.

neural e. neuroderm.

primitive e., primordial e. blastodermic e.

ec·to·der·ma·to·sis (ek″to-dur″mə-to′sis) ectodermosis.

ec·to·der·moid·al (ek″to-dər-moid′əl) of the nature of or resembling the ectoderm.

ec·to·der·mo·sis (ek″to-dər-mo′sis) a disorder based on congenital maldevelopment of the organs of ectodermal derivation, i.e., nervous system, retina, eyeball, and skin. Called also *ectodermatosis*. See also *phakomatosis*.

e. erosi′va pluriorificia′lis Stevens-Johnson syndrome.

ec·to·en·tad (ek″to-en′tad) from without inward.

ec·to·en·zyme (ek″to-en′zīm) exoenzyme.

ec·tog·e·nous (ek-toj′ə-nəs) exogenous.

ec·tog·lia (ek-tog′le-ə) [*ecto-* + *-glia*] the thin, external marginal layer of the early neural tube of the embryo.

ec·tog·o·ny (ek-tog′o-ne) the influence exerted on the mother by the developing embryo.

ec·to·hor·mone (ek″to-hor′mōn) a hormone secreted to the outside of the body, such as a pheromone.

ec·to·lec·i·thal (ek″to-les′ĭ-thəl) [*ecto-* + *lecithal*] having the yolk situated peripherally, as in flatworm eggs.

ec·to·mere (ek′to-mēr) [*ecto-* + *-mere*] any of the blastomeres which share in the formation of the ectoderm.

ec·to·mes·en·chyme (ec″to-mes′eng-kīm) mesenchyme originating from the ectoderm, particularly from the neural crest.

-ectomize [*-ectomy*, q.v.] a word termination meaning to surgically remove, used following a root designating the structure removed. By extension, used in terms to designate destruction or deprivation by other methods as well.

ec·to·morph (ek′to-morf) [*ectoderm* + Gr. *morphē* form] an individual having a type of body build in which tissues derived from the ectoderm predominate: there is a preponderance of linearity and fragility, with large surface area, thin muscles and subcutaneous tissue, and slightly developed digestive viscera, as contrasted with endomorph and mesomorph. **ectomor′phic** *adj*

ec·to·mor·phy (ek′to-mor″fe) the condition of being an ectomorph.

ec·to·my (ek′tə-me) [Gr. *ektomē* excision, from *ektemnein* to cut out] excision or resection.

-ectomy a word termination meaning surgical excision, used following a root designating the structure or organ removed. By extension, used in terms to designate destruction or deprivation by other methods as well.

ec·top·a·gus (ek-top′ə-gəs) [*ecto-* + *-pagus*] conjoined twins connected along the side of the body, so that the components are definitely right and left, the upper and/or lower limbs at the juncture being represented by single bilateral median limbs.

ec·to·par·a·site (ek″to-par′ə-sīt) [*ecto-* + *parasite*] a parasite that lives on the outside of the body of the host. Cf. *epiphyte* and *epizoon*.

ec·to·par·a·sit·i·cide (ek″to-par″ə-sit′ĭ-sīd) [*ectoparasite* + *-cide*] an agent destructive to ectoparasites.

ec·to·pec·to·ra·lis (ek″to-pek″to-ra′lis) musculus pectoralis major.

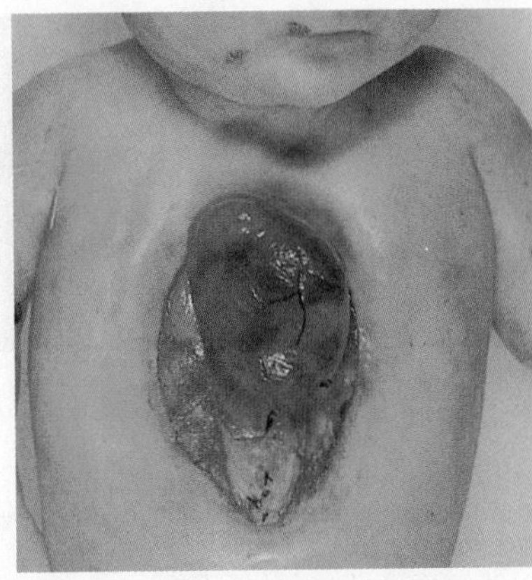

■ Ectopia cordis resulting from failure of closure of the superior abdominal wall.

ec·to·peri·to·ni·tis (ek″to-per″ĭ-to-ni′tis) [*ecto-* + *peritonitis*] inflammation of the external or abdominal side of the peritoneum.

ec·to·phyte (ek′to-fīt) epiphyte.

ec·to·pia (ek-to′pe-ə) [Gr. *ektopos* displaced + *-ia*] malposition, especially if congenital. Called also *ectopy* and *heterotopia*.

e. cloa′cae exstrophy of cloaca.

e. cor′dis congenital displacement of the heart outside the thoracic cavity because of maldevelopment of the pericardium and sternum.

e. cor′dis abdomina′lis a rare anomaly in which the heart is located in the abdominal cavity.

crossed renal e. displacement of one kidney to the opposite side of the body, so that its ureter crosses the midline; the two kidneys often form a fused kidney (see under *kidney*).

e. len′tis displacement of the crystalline lens of the eye.

pectoral e. cor′dis location of the heart outside the thoracic wall, through a cleft in the lower sternum.

e. pupil′lae conge′nita congenital displacement of the pupil.

renal e., e. re′nis displacement of the kidney, as in abdominal, lumbar, pelvic, and thoracic kidneys, nephroptosis, and crossed renal ectopia.

e. tes′tis malposition of a testis, such as an undescended testis.

e. vesi′cae exstrophy of bladder.

ec·top·ic (ek-top′ik) 1. pertaining to or characterized by ectopia. 2. located away from normal position, as in ectopic pregnancy. 3. arising in an abnormal site or tissue.

ec·to·pla·cen·ta (ek″to-plə-sen′tə) [*ecto-* + *placenta*] the actively growing trophoblast that becomes the placenta in rodents.

ec·to·plasm (ek′to-plaz″əm) [*ecto-* + *plasm*] the viscous, agranular part of the cytoplasm adjacent to the plasma membrane. **ectoplas′mic** *adj*

ec·to·py (ek′to-pe) ectopia.

ec·tos·co·py (ek-tos′ko-pe) [*ecto-* + *-scopy*] a diagnostic method based on observation of chest and abdominal movements, and said to be capable of determining the outlines of the lungs and of localized internal conditions.

ec·to·skel·e·ton (ek″to-skel′ə-ton) exoskeleton.

ec·tos·te·al (ek-tos′te-əl) pertaining to or situated on the outside of a bone.

ec·to·sto·sis (ek″to-sto′sis) [*ecto-* + *ostosis*] ossification beneath the perichondrium of a cartilage or the periosteum of a bone.

ec·to·sym·bi·ont (ek″to-sim′be-ont) a symbiont that lives outside the body of the organism with which it is biologically related.

ec·to·therm (ek′to-thərm) [*ecto-* + *therm*] 1. an animal that exhibits ectothermy. 2. poikilotherm.

ec·to·therm·ic (ek″to-thur′mik) 1. pertaining to or characterized by ectothermy. 2. poikilothermic.

ec·to·ther·my (ek″to-thur′me) 1. the regulation of body temperature by the external environment rather than by internal metabolism, with thermoregulation being accomplished by behavioral means; i.e., the animal seeks an appropriate environmental temperature. 2. poikilothermy.

ec·to·thrix (ek′to-thriks) [*ecto-* + *-thrix*] a fungus that grows inside the hair shaft and also produces a sheath of arthrospores on the outside of the hair.

large-spored e. an ectothrix that forms chains or sheaths of large spores; this type includes *Microsporum fulvum*, *M. gypseum*, *M. nanum*, *M. vanbreuseghemii*, and *Trichophyton gallinae*.

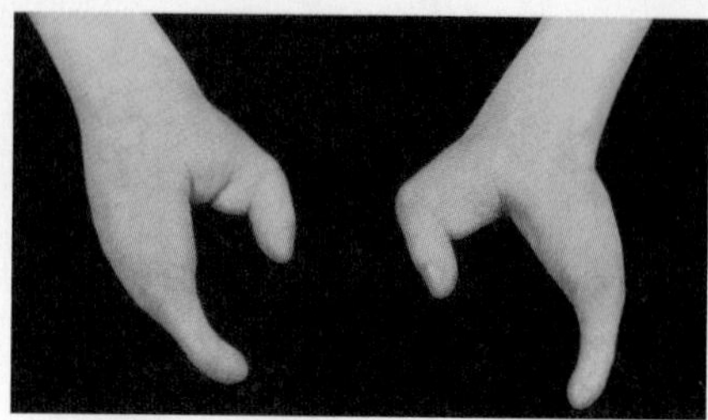

■ Ectrodactyly of the hands.

small-spored e. an ectothrix that forms small spores in sheaths, mosaic masses, or occasionally chains; this type includes *Microsporum audouinii, M. canis, M. ferrugineum,* and *Trichophyton mentagrophytes.*

ec•to•zo•on (ek″to-zo′on) pl. *ectozo′a.* Epizoon.

ectr(o)- [Gr. *ektrōsis* miscarriage] a combining form denoting congenital absence of a part.

ec•tro•dac•tyl•ia (ek′tro-dak-til′e-ə) ectrodactyly.

ec•tro•dac•ty•lism (ek′tro-dak′tə-liz-əm) ectrodactyly.

ec•tro•dac•ty•ly (ek″tro-dak′tə-le) [*ectro-* + *daktylos* finger] congenital absence of a digit or part of a digit; see also *EEC syndrome*, under *syndrome.*

ec•trog•e•ny (ek-troj′ə-ne) [*ectro-* + *-geny*] congenital absence or defect of a part. **ectrogen′ic** *adj*

ec•tro•me•lia (ek″tro-me′le-ə) [*ectro-* + *-melia*] gross hypoplasia or aplasia of one or more long bones of one or more limbs; the term includes amelia, hemimelia, and meromelia. **ectromel′ic** *adj*

infectious e. a disease of mice caused by a poxvirus and characterized by gangrene and often loss of one or more of the feet and sometimes of other external parts, and by necrotic areas in the liver, spleen, and other organs; called also *mousepox.*

ec•trom•e•lus (ek-trom′ə-ləs) [*ectros-* + *melos* limb] an individual exhibiting ectromelia.

ec•tro•meta•car•pia (ek″tro-met″ə-kahr′pe-ə) [*ectro-* + *metacarpus* + *-ia*] congenital absence of a metacarpal bone.

ec•tro•meta•tar•sia (ek″tro-met″ə-tahr′se-ə) [*ectro-* + *metatarsus* + *-ia*] congenital absence of a metatarsal bone.

ec•tro•pha•lan•gia (ek″tro-fə-lan′jə) congenital absence of one or more phalanges of a digit.

ec•tro•pi•on (ek-tro′pe-on) [Gr. "an everted eyelid"; *ektropē* a turning aside] 1. eversion (def. 1). 2. specifically, eversion of the eyelid, resulting in exposure of the palpebral conjunctiva.

atonic e. eversion due to loss of skin tone or of muscle tone, especially of the orbicularis oculi muscle.

cervical e. eversion of the cervical canal, with more columnar epithelium than normal outside the external os.

cicatricial e. eversion of the margin of an eyelid caused by contraction of scar tissue in the lid or by contraction of the skin.

flaccid e. ectropion of the lower lid resulting from reduced tone of the orbicularis oculi muscle.

paralytic e. eversion of the margin of the lower eyelid as a result of paralysis of the facial nerve, and loss of contractile power of the orbicularis oculi muscle.

e. of pigment layer proliferation of the cells in the posteriorly situated pigment layer of the iris, leading to their migration around the pupillary margin to encroach upon the anterior surface of the iris.

senile e. eversion of the lower eyelid associated with relaxation of the fibers of the palpebral portion of the orbicularis oculi muscle as a concomitant of age, or occurring as a result of atrophic changes in the skin.

spastic e. ectropion caused by tonic spasm of the orbicularis oculi muscle.

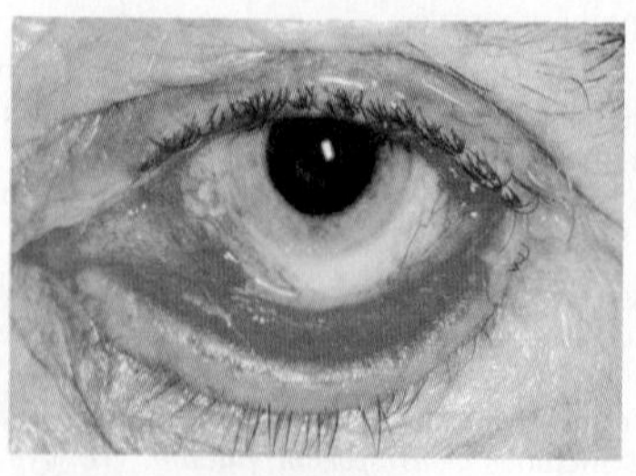

■ Ectropion.

e. u′veae eversion of the margin of the pupil, often congenital (*e. u′veae conge′nitum*), and frequently due to the presence of a newly formed membrane on the anterior layer of the iris, or to the formation of connective tissue in the stroma, particularly in diabetes. Called also *iridectropium.*

ec•tro•pi•um (ek-tro′pe-əm) ectropion.

ec•tro•sis (ek-tro′sis) [Gr. *ektrōsis*] 1. abortion. 2. treatment that arrests the development of disease.

ec•tro•syn•dac•tyl•ia (ek″tro-sin″dak-til′e-ə) ectrosyndactyly.

ec•tro•syn•dac•ty•ly (ek″tro-sin-dak′tə-le) [*ectro-* + *syndactyly*] a condition in which some of the digits are missing and those that remain are webbed, so that they are more or less attached.

ec•trot•ic (ek-trot′ik) 1. pertaining to or producing abortion. 2. arresting the development of a disease.

ecu•liz•u•mab (ĕ-ku-liz′oo-mab) a recombinant monoclonal antibody that binds to the terminal human complement protein C5 to prevent its cleavage; administered orally in treatment of paroxysmal nocturnal hemoglobinuria.

ec•ze•ma (ek′zə-mə) [Gr. *ekzein* to boil out] any of various pruritic, papulovesicular types of dermatitis occurring as reactions to endogenous or exogenous agents. In acute types there may be erythema, edema, inflammatory infiltrates in the dermis, vesiculation, crusting, and scaling. In chronic types there may be lichenification, skin thickening, signs of excoriation; and areas of hyperpigmentation or hypopigmentation. The most common type is atopic eczema (atopic dermatitis). Called also *eczematous dermatitis.*

allergic e. atopic dermatitis.

asteatotic e. a condition resulting from excessive dehydration of the skin, characterized by erythema, dry scaling, fine cracking, and pruritus; it occurs chiefly during cold weather when low humidity in heated rooms causes excessive water loss from the stratum corneum. Popularly known as *winter itch.* Called also *winter e.* or *dermatitis,* and *xerotic e.* or *dermatitis.*

atopic e. see under *dermatitis.*

congestion e. stasis dermatitis.

e. craquelé (krah-kĕ-la′) [Fr. "marred with cracks"] asteatotic e.

discoid e. nummular e.

dyshidrotic e. pompholyx.

facial e. of ruminants a type of hepatogenous photosensitization in ruminants, particularly in New Zealand, due to ingestion of grass or grain contaminated with the mold *Pithomyces chartarum,* which contains sporidesmin; it is often accompanied by hepatitis or biliary obstruction, which can be fatal. See also *pithomycotoxicosis.*

flexural e. the eczema accompanying atopic dermatitis in older children and adults, found chiefly on flexural surfaces such as the inside of the elbow and the back of the knee, and sometimes on the neck, eyelids, wrists, and elsewhere.

gravitational e. stasis dermatitis.

e. herpe′ticum Kaposi varicelliform eruption due to infection with the herpes simplex virus superimposed on a preexisting skin condition, usually atopic dermatitis. Cf. *e. vaccinatum.*

infantile e. the eczema seen in atopic dermatitis in infants, appearing first on the cheeks and sometimes spreading to other areas.

e. intertri′go intertrigo.

e. margina′tum tinea cruris.

nasal e. nasal solar dermatitis.

nummular e. eczema presenting in discrete, round (coin-shaped or annular) lesions that may coalesce to form large patches that ooze and crust over; the usual site is on the extensor limb surfaces or the chest, back, or buttocks. Called also *discoid e., exudative neurodermatitis,* and *nummular dermatitis* or *neurodermatitis.*

photosensitive e. chronic actinic dermatitis.

seborrheic e. see under *dermatitis.*

stasis e. see under *dermatitis.*

e. vaccina′tum Kaposi varicelliform eruption due to infection with the vaccinia virus superimposed upon a preexisting skin condition, usually atopic dermatitis. Cf. *e. herpeticum.*

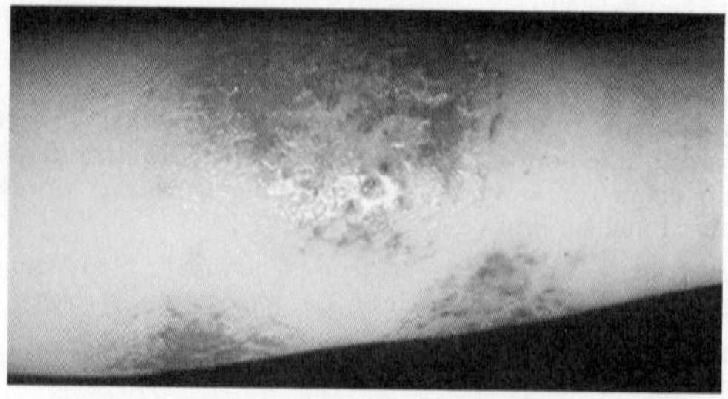

■ Nummular eczema.

varicose e. stasis dermatitis.
winter e., xerotic e. asteatotic e..

ec•zem•a•ti•za•tion (ek-zem″ə-tĭ-za′shən) persistent eczemalike lesions of the skin, usually due to the continued trauma of scratching.

ec•zem•a•to•gen•ic (ek-zem″ə-to-jen′ik) causing eczema.

ec•zem•a•toid (ek-zem′ə-toid) resembling eczema.

ec•zem•a•tous (ek-zem′ə-təs) affected with or of the nature of eczema.

ED effective dose; emergency department; erectile dysfunction; erythema dose.

ED_{50} median effective dose.

edath•a•mil (ə-dath′ə-mil) former name for *edetate*.

Ed•e•bohls position (ed′ə-bōlz) [George Michael *Edebohls*, New York surgeon, 1853–1908] see under *position*.

Edec•rin (ə-dek′rin) trademark for preparations of ethacrynic acid.

ede•ma (ə-de′mə) [Gr. *oidēma* swelling] the presence of abnormally large amounts of fluid in the intercellular tissue spaces of the body, usually referring to subcutaneous tissues. It may be localized (such as from venous obstruction, lymphatic obstruction, or increased vascular permeability) or systemic (such as from heart failure or renal disease). Edema is sometimes designated according to the site: *ascites* (peritoneal cavity), *hydrothorax* (pleural cavity), or *hydropericardium* (pericardial sac). Massive generalized edema is called *anasarca*. Called also *dropsy* and *hydrops*. **edem′atous** *adj*

acute hemorrhagic e. of infancy a rare type of small-vessel vasculitis with rapid onset, seen in young children, characterized by fever with tender, erythematous edema of the face, scrotum, hands, and feet.
alimentary e. nutritional e.
alveolar e. pulmonary edema in the alveoli, usually with hypoxemia and dyspnea.
angioneurotic e. angioedema.
Berlin e. commotio retinae.
bowel e. edema disease.
brain e. cerebral e.
brown e. pulmonary edema in which the fluid is a brown color, owing to chronic congestion.
e. bullo′sum vesi′cae, bullous e. of bladder a nonspecific inflammatory condition of the mucous lining of the bladder caused by irritation, marked by formation of clear vesicles with small white particles between them.
Calabar e. Calabar swellings.
e. ca′lidum inflammatory e.
cardiac e. a manifestation of congestive heart failure, caused by increased venous and capillary pressures and often associated with the retention of sodium by the kidneys.
cerebral e. excessive accumulation of fluid in the brain substance; causes include trauma, tumor, and increased permeability of capillaries as a result of anoxia or exposure to toxic substances. Called also *brain e.* and *wet brain*.
circumscribed e. angioedema.
cystoid macular e. thickening of the macula lutea with cystic changes, increased fluid within the sensory retina of the macula, and disruption of the blood–retinal barrier and consequent leakage on fluorescein angiography, with leaking capillaries in the posterior pole and around the optic disk; often secondary to cataract surgery.
cytotoxic e. cerebral edema caused by hypoxic injury to brain tissue and decreased functioning of the sodium pump, so that the cellular elements take in fluid and swell.
dependent e. edema affecting most seriously the lowest (most dependent) parts of the body.
diabetic macular e. a complication of diabetic retinopathy consisting of swelling of the retina due to leakage of fluid from adjacent blood vessels; the result is blurring in or next to the center of the visual field, which can progress to blindness.
famine e. nutritional e.
e. fri′gidum noninflammatory e.
e. fu′gax transient accumulation of fluid in a specific region.
gaseous e. edema accompanied with gas formation, as in gas bacillus infection and subcutaneous emphysema.
generalized e. edema that is caused by poor venous return and is not localized by the effects of gravity, in contrast to dependent edema.
gut e. edema disease.
hepatic e. edema due to faulty functioning of the liver.
hereditary angioneurotic e. (HANE) hereditary angioedema.
high-altitude pulmonary e. (HAPE) pulmonary edema caused by hypoxia from excessive physical exertion after ascending quickly to a high altitude without acclimatization. See also *high-altitude sickness*, under *sickness*.
hunger e. nutritional e.
hydremic e. edema in conditions marked by hydremia.
idiopathic e. edema of unknown cause, usually affecting women, occurring intermittently over a period of years, and worsening during the premenstrual period; it is associated with increased aldosterone secretion.
inflammatory e. edema resulting from inflammation, and accompanied by redness and pain.
insulin e. edema which sometimes follows the injection of insulin.
interstitial e. 1. an increase in interstitial fluid in the brain associated with hydrocephalus. 2. pulmonary edema in the interstitial tissues; there is dyspnea and sometimes hypoxemia.
intramyelinic e. edema within the white matter of the brain.
invisible e. the accumulation of a considerable amount of fluid in the subcutaneous tissues before it becomes demonstrable.
e. of lung pulmonary e.
lymphatic e. lymphedema.
macular e. edema of the macula lutea in the eye; see cystoid macular e. and diabetic macular e.
malignant e. 1. a severe manifestation of cutaneous anthrax in which massive spreading edema develops around the central necrotic eschar. 2. inflammatory edema in gas gangrene. 3. a usually fatal form of toxemia seen in farm animals, with fever, skin discoloration, and swelling around a wound contaminated by *Clostridium* species, especially *C. septicum*. Cf. *gas gangrene* and *blackleg*. 4. braxy.
mucous e. myxedema.
e. neonato′rum a disease of premature and feeble infants that resembles sclerema and is marked by spreading edema with cold, livid skin.
nephrotic e. edema secondary to volume overload associated with nephrosis or the nephrotic syndrome.
neuraxial e. a hereditary disease of calves in which they are unable to stand up and their legs and neck become vigorously extended upon certain types of stimulation.
noninflammatory e. edema without redness and pain, occurring from passive congestion or from lowered serum osmolarity.
nonpitting e. edema in which the tissues cannot be pitted by pressure.
nutritional e. a disorder of nutrition due to long-continued diet deficiency of protein and/or calories, and marked by anasarca and edema; called also *alimentary e.*, *famine e.*, *hunger e.*, and *war e.*
paroxysmal pulmonary e. pulmonary edema marked by attacks of difficult respiration, audible rales, wheezes, and cough, caused by acute left ventricular failure, usually associated with hypertensive or ischemic heart disease.
passive e. edema occurring because of obstruction to vascular or lymphatic drainage from the area.
periodic e. angioedema.
periretinal e. central serous retinopathy.
pitting e. edema in which the tissues show prolonged existence of the pits produced by pressure.
placental e. the presence of fluid in the villi of the placenta, the villi being club-shaped and irregularly swollen.
prehepatic e. edema occurring in prehepatic hypoproteinemia.
pulmonary e. abnormal, diffuse, extravascular accumulation of fluid in the pulmonary tissues and air spaces due to changes in hydrostatic forces in the capillaries or to increased capillary permeability; it is characterized clinically by intense dyspnea and, in the intra-alveolar form, by voluminous expectoration of frothy pink serous fluid and, if severe, by cyanosis. Called also *wet lung*.
purulent e. a swelling due to the effusion of a purulent fluid.
Quincke e. angioedema.
reexpansion pulmonary e. pulmonary edema in a lung that has been rapidly reinflated after a period of collapse such as that due to a pneumothorax or a pleural effusion.
Reinke e. inflammation and edema of the neck area called Reinke space after prolonged irritation, usually the result of chronic misuse of the voice, smoking, or excessive exposure to dry air or dust.
renal e. edema in or around the kidney; see *nephrotic e.*
rheumatismal e. painful red edematous swellings on the limbs in rheumatism, due to subcutaneous exudation.
salt e. edema produced by an increase of sodium chloride in the diet.
solid e. myxedema.
solid pulmonary e. a rubbery consistency and gelatinous appearance of the lungs sometimes associated with hypertensive left ventricular failure and uremia.
terminal e. pulmonary edema that develops just prior to death, from circulatory failure.
toxic e. edema caused by a poison.
vasogenic e. a type of cerebral edema seen in the area around tumors, largely confined to the white matter; it often results from increased permeability of capillary endothelial cells and less often is due to toxic injury to the vessels.
venous e. edema in which the effused liquid comes from the blood.

villous e. accumulation of fluid in the chorionic villi, resulting in compression of the blood vessels; reduced blood flow and gas exchange lead to fetal hypoxia.

war e. nutritional e.

ede•ma•gen (ə-de′mə-jen) an irritant that elicits edema by causing capillary damage but not the cellular response of true inflammation. Cf. *inflammagen.*

edem•a•tig•e•nous (ə-dem″ə-tij′ə-nəs) edematogenic.

edem•a•ti•za•tion (ə-dem″ə-tĭ-za′shən) the process of becoming or of making edematous.

edem•a•to•gen•ic (ə-dem″ə-to-jen′ik) producing or causing edema.

Eden•ta•ta (e″dən-ta′tə) an order of mammals including armadillos, tree sloths, and anteaters.

eden•tate (e-den′tāt) edentulous.

eden•tia (e-den′shə) [*e-* + *dentia*] anodontia.

eden•tu•late (e-den′tu-lāt) edentulous.

eden•tu•lism (e-den′tu-liz-əm) the condition of being without teeth.

eden•tu•lous (e-den′tu-ləs) without teeth; having lost some or all natural teeth. Called also *edentate* and *edentulate.*

ed•e•tate (ed′ə-tāt) USAN contraction for *ethylenediaminetetraacetate.*

e. calcium disodium [USP] a metal complexing agent, consisting of a mixture of the dihydrate and tetrahydrate calcium disodium salt of edetic acid, used intramuscularly or intravenously in the diagnosis and treatment of lead poisoning. Called also *calcium disodium edathamil.*

e. disodium [USP] a metal complexing agent, used as a chelating pharmaceutic aid. Because of its affinity for calcium, it is used in the treatment of hypercalcemia, administered intravenously, but is not used in the treatment of poisoning by lead or other heavy metals.

e. sodium the tetrasodium salt of edetic acid, used as a chelating agent.

e. trisodium the trisodium salt of edetic acid, sometimes used similarly to edetate disodium.

edet•ic ac•id (ə-det′ik) ethylenediaminetetraacetic acid (EDTA).

Edex (e′deks) trademark for a preparation of alprostadil.

edge (ej) a thin side; see also *border* and *margin.*

cutting e. the angle formed by the merging of two flat surfaces, by which something may be cut, such as the blade of a knife, or the incisal surface of an anterior tooth.

denture e. see under *border.*

distal e. of nail, free e. of nail margo liber unguis.

incisal e. the junction of the labial surface of an anterior tooth with a flattened linguoincisal surface created by occlusal wear.

lateral e. of nail margo lateralis unguis.

proximal e. of nail margo occultus unguis.

edge-strength (ej strength) the ability of fine edges to resist fracture or abrasion; applied especially to such resistance in dental restorations.

Ed•ing•er nuclei (ed′ing-gər) [Ludwig *Edinger,* German neurologist, 1855–1918] nuclei accessorii nervi oculomotorii.

Ed•ing•er-West•phal nuclei (ed′ing-gər vest′fahl) [L. *Edinger;* Carl Friedrich Otto *Westphal,* German neurologist, 1833–1890] nuclei accessorii nervi oculomotorii.

edis•y•late (ə-dis′ə-lāt) USAN contraction for 1,2-ethanedisulfonate.

EDR effective direct radiation; electrodermal response.

EDRF endothelium-derived relaxing factor.

ed•ro•pho•ni•um chlo•ride (ed″ro-fo′ne-əm) [USP] an anticholinesterase agent with a duration of action of approximately 10 minutes; used for differential diagnosis and evaluation of treatment requirements in myasthenia gravis and as an antagonist to nondepolarizing neuromuscular blocking agents (e.g., tubocurarine).

Ed•sall disease (ed′səl) [David Linn *Edsall,* American physician, 1869–1945] heat cramp.

EDTA ethylenediaminetetraacetic acid; European Dialysis and Transplant Association.

edul•co•rant (e-dul′ko-rənt) sweetening.

edul•co•rate (e-dul′ko-rāt) to sweeten.

EDV end-diastolic volume.

Ed•wards syndrome (ed′wərdz) [J.H. *Edwards,* British physician, 20th century] trisomy 18 syndrome.

Ed•ward•si•el•la (ed-wahrd″se-el′ə) [Philip R. *Edwards,* American bacteriologist, 1901–1966] a genus of gram-negative, facultatively anaerobic bacteria of the family Enterobacteriaceae, consisting of small rods that are mostly motile with peritrichous flagella. The organisms are pathogenic for aquatic animals and an occasional opportunistic pathogen for humans. The type species is *E. tar′da.*

E. tar′da an indole-producing species found in a wide variety of animals and occasionally isolated from the urine, blood, and feces of humans. It can cause acute gastroenteritis and serious septic infections.

EEE eastern equine encephalomyelitis.

EEG electroencephalogram.

EEJ electroejaculation.

eel•worm (ēl′wərm) nematode.

EENT eyes, ears, nose, and throat; see *otolaryngology.*

EERP extended endocardial resection procedure.

E.E.S. trademark for a preparation of erythromycin ethylsuccinate.

EFA essential fatty acid.

efa•liz•u•mab (ef″ə-liz′u-mab) a recombinant monoclonal antibody that binds to leukocytes, interferes with their binding to other cells, and thus acts as an immunosuppressant; administered by subcutaneous injection for treatment of psoriasis.

ef•a•vi•renz (ef′ə-vi″renz) a nonnucleoside reverse transcriptase inhibitor, used in combination with other antiretroviral agents in the treatment of human immunodeficiency virus type 1 (HIV-1) infection; administered orally.

ef•face•ment (ə-fās′mənt) the taking up or obliteration of the cervix in labor when it is so changed that only the thin external os remains.

ef•fect (ə-fekt′) the result produced by an action.

additive e. the combined effect produced by the action of two or more agents, being equal to the sum of their separate effects.

Anrep e. abrupt elevation of aortic pressure results in a positively inotropic inotropic effect (see *inotropic*) and augmented resistance to outflow in the heart. Called also *homeometric autoregulation* because it is independent of muscle length.

Bayliss e. increased perfusion pressure and subsequent stretch of vascular smooth muscle causes muscle contraction and increased resistance, which returns blood flow to normal in spite of the elevated perfusion pressure.

Blinks e′s brief enhancement in photosynthesis following shifts from a long wavelength to a shorter wavelength.

Bohr e. high concentrations of carbon dioxide and hydrogen ions, such as occur in the capillaries in metabolically active tissue, decrease the affinity of hemoglobin for oxygen, so that the oxygen dissociation curve shifts to the right. Cf. *Haldane e.*

Bruce e. the blocking of pregnancy in a newly impregnated female mouse by a pheromone (the odor of a strange male).

calorigenic e. obligatory thermogenesis.

clasp-knife e. see under *rigidity.*

Compton e. the change in the wavelength of gamma or x-rays due to interaction of an incident photon with an orbital electron of an atom, which produces a recoil electron and a scattered photon of reduced energy.

Crabtree e. the inhibition of oxygen consumption on the addition of glucose to tissues or microorganisms having a high rate of aerobic glycolysis; the converse of the Pasteur effect.

cumulative e. see under *action.*

cyclosporine e. perimyocytic fibrosis (with interstitial cellular infiltrates) occurring in transplanted hearts, due to the use of cyclosporine.

cytoprotective e. the enhancement of the ability of cells to resist injury.

Danysz e. see under *phenomenon.*

Deelman e. scarification of the skin in artificial carcinogenesis tends to localize the subsequent carcinomata at the scarified area.

Donnan e. see under *equilibrium.*

Doppler e. the relationship of the apparent frequency of waves, as of sound, light, and radio waves, to the relative motion of the source of the waves and the observer, the frequency increasing as the two approach each other and decreasing as they move apart.

Eagle e. paradoxical e.

Emerson e. the photosynthetic efficiency of a long wavelength of light is enhanced by simultaneous exposure of plant cells to shorter wavelengths of light.

experimenter e′s see *demand characteristics,* under *characteristic.*

extrapyramidal e′s the side effects caused by neuroleptic medications, including dystonias, parkinsonism, akathisia, and tardive dyskinesia.

Fahraeus-Lindqvist e. blood viscosity is lower in small vessels (diameter less than 1.5 mm) than in large vessels, the viscosity in capillaries being less than half that in large vessels; the effect is due to red cells moving together in single file through the small vessels.

founder e. an altered gene frequency in a particular derived population relative to the parental population, as a result of establishment of the derived population by a small number of founders carrying limited genetic diversity.

Gibbs-Donnan e. Donnan equilibrium.

Haldane e. high concentration of oxygen, such as occurs in the alveolar capillaries of the lungs, promotes the dissociation of carbon dioxide and hydrogen ions from hemoglobin, so that the oxygen dissociation curve shifts to the left. Cf. *Bohr e.*

Hallberg e. the crests and troughs of ultrashort standing-wave field have opposite electrical signs.

Hallwachs e. photoelectric e.

heel e. in radiology, variation in intensity through the cross-section of the useful beam due to differential attenuation of x-rays emerging at varying angles from beneath the focal spot; the intensity is greater on the cathode side.

isomorphic e. Koebner phenomenon.

McCollough e. an aftersensation of color; following exposure to vertical and horizontal lines of differing colors, a grid of vertical and horizontal black lines may be seen as edged with the previously seen colors.

Nagler e. gas-filled tubes, placed in high frequency fields, will act as rectifiers, causing a unidirectional current.

paradoxical e. a phenomenon seen in testing for the minimal bactericidal concentration of certain antimicrobial agents, in which higher concentrations of an agent kill fewer microorganisms; called also *Eagle effect.*

Pasteur e. the decrease in the rate of glucose utilization (glycolysis) and the suppression of lactate accumulation by tissues or microorganisms in the presence of oxygen. Cf. *Crabtree e.*

photechic e. Russell e.

photoelectric e. the ejection of electrons from matter when light of short wavelengths falls upon it; called also *Hallwachs e.*

placebo e. the sum total of all nonspecific effects, both good and adverse, of medical treatment, primarily psychological and psychophysiological effects associated with the physician-patient relationship and the patient's expectations and apprehensions concerning the treatment.

position e. in genetics, the change in expression of a gene as a function of a change in its position relative to that of other genes.

postantibiotic e. a period of continuing inhibition of bacterial growth after an antibiotic has been removed from a system; it may be short or long.

pressure e. the sum of the changes that are due to obstruction of tissue drainage by pressure.

proarrhythmic e. any new, more advanced form of arrhythmia caused by an antiarrhythmic agent, especially an effect producing hemodynamically important symptoms. These usually occur less than 30 days after initiation of treatment and do not include those caused by new events such as acute myocardial infarction or hypokalemia.

Purkinje e. see under *phenomenon.*

Raman e. when a substance is irradiated with monochromatic light, the spectrum which the substance scatters contains, in addition to a line of the same wavelength as the incident radiation, lines which are satellites of the primary line moving with it when the wavelength of the primary radiation is altered.

Russell e. the rendering of a photographic plate developable by agents other than light; called also *photechic e.*

side e. a consequence other than the one(s) for which an agent or measure is used, as the adverse effects produced by a drug, especially on a tissue or organ system other than the one sought to be benefited by its administration.

Somogyi e. see under *phenomenon.*

Soret e. when a solution is maintained for some time in a temperature gradient, a difference in concentration of one component develops along the temperature gradient.

specific dynamic e. former name for *obligatory thermogenesis.*

Staub-Traugott e. a second dose of glucose by mouth to a normal person one hour after a first dose does not elevate the blood glucose level. See also *Staub-Traugott phenomenon*, under *phenomenon.* Called also *Staub-Traugott test.*

thermic e. obligatory thermogenesis.

Tyndall e. a strong beam of light passes through a true solution invisibly but is clearly outlined passing through a colloidal solution because the light is reflected by the surfaces of the moving colloid particles. Called also *Tyndall phenomenon.*

Whitten e. initiation and synchronization of the estrous cycles and reduction of the frequency of reproductive abnormalities in female mice by the odor (pheromone) of a male mouse placed among them; when more than four female mice are placed together in a cage their estrous cycles become very erratic.

Wolff-Chaikoff e. inhibition of the synthesis of thyroid hormone by high concentrations of iodide.

Zeeman e. separation of a single line in the spectrum by suitable magnetic fields.

ef•fec•tive•ness (ə-fek′tiv-nəs) 1. the ability to produce a specific result or to exert a specific measurable influence. 2. the ability of an intervention to produce the desired beneficial effect in actual use; cf. *efficacy.*

relative biological e. (RBE) an expression of the effectiveness of other types of radiation in comparison with that of gamma or x-rays.

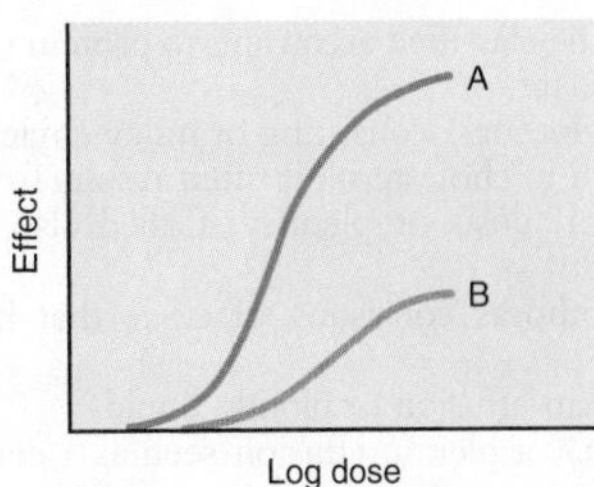

■ Dose-effect curve for two drugs of different efficacy: The efficacy of drug *A* is greater than that of drug *B.*

ef•fec•tor (ə-fek′tər) 1. an agent that mediates a specific effect, e.g., an allosteric effector or an effector cell. 2. an organ that produces an effect, e.g., contraction or secretion, in response to nerve stimulation. Called also *effector organ.*

allosteric e. an enzyme inhibitor or activator that has its effect at a site other than the catalytic site of the enzyme; see also under *site*, and see *allostery.*

ef•fem•i•na•tion (ə-fem″ĭ-na′shən) feminization (def. 2).

ef•fer•ent (ef′ər-ənt) [L. *ex* out + *ferre* to bear] 1. conveying away from a center; called also *centrifugal.* 2. something that so conducts; see under *fiber* and *nerve.* Cf. *corticifugal.*

ef•fer•en•tial (ef″ər-en′shəl) efferent.

ef•fer•ves•cent (ef″ər-ves′ənt) [L. *effervescens*] bubbling; sparkling; giving off gas bubbles.

Ef•fex•or (ə-fek′sor) trademark for preparations of venlafaxine hydrochloride.

ef•fi•ca•cy (ef′ĭ-kə-se) [L. *efficax* effectual] 1. the ability of an intervention to produce the desired beneficial effect in expert hands and under ideal circumstances. Cf. *effectiveness.* 2. in pharmacology, the ability of a drug to produce the desired therapeutic effect; it is independent of *potency*, which expresses the amount of the drug necessary to achieve the desired effect.

antiviral e. virologic e.

maximal e., maximum e. the greatest therapeutic effect that can be achieved with a given drug.

virologic e. the efficacy of a given antiviral regimen; called also *antiviral e.*

ef•fi•cien•cy (ə-fish′ən-se) 1. the ratio of the useful output of a system to the total input. 2. in statistics, the tendency of a procedure to make optimal use of the data.

Ef•fi•ent (ef′e-ənt) trademark for a preparation of prasugrel.

ef•fleu•rage (ef-lo͞o-rahzh′) [Fr.] stroking movement in massage; frottage.

ef•flo•res•cence (ef″lo-res′əns) [L. *efflorescere* to bloom] 1. the process of becoming powdery because of losing water of crystallization. 2. a skin eruption or rash.

ef•flo•res•cent (ef″lo-res′ənt) 1. becoming powdery; see *efflorescence.* 2. developing into a rash.

ef•flu•ent (ef′floo-ənt) [L. *ex-* + *fluere* to flow] something that flows out, especially a liquid discharge that carries waste products.

ef•fluve (ə-flo͞ov′) a conductive discharge of a high voltage current through a dielectric.

ef•flu•vi•um (ə-floo′ve-əm) pl. *efflu′via* [L. "a flowing out"] 1. a shedding, especially of the hair; cf. *alopecia.* 2. effluent.

anagen e. abnormal loss of hair during the anagen phase; it sometimes follows administration of certain cancer chemotherapeutic agents or exposure to certain chemicals, or in association with various other factors and diseases.

telogen e. the early, excessive, temporary loss of club hairs from normal resting follicles in the scalp as a result of traumatization by some stimulus (e.g., after surgery or childbirth; with starvation, side effects of drugs, traction on hair, high fever, or certain diseases; or with psychogenic stress). The normal hair cycle is changed and the anagen phase ends prematurely, moving into the catagen and telogen phases.

ef•frac•tion (ə-frak′shən) a breaking open; a weakening.

ef•fuse[1] (ə-fūs′) [L. *effusus*, from *ex* out + *fundere* to pour] spread out, profuse; said of bacterial growth that is thin, veillike, and unusually widespread.

ef•fuse[2] (ə-fūz′) to pour out and spread widely.

ef•fu•sion (ə-fu′zhən) [L. *effusio* a pouring out] 1. the escape of fluid into a part or tissue, as an exudation or a transudation. 2. an effused material, which may be classified according to protein or cellular content as an exudate or transudate.

chyliform e. chylothorax consisting of milky chylelike fluid that is low in fat but usually high in cholesterol; it often results from a chronic disease process such as tuberculosis or pleurisy. Called also *pseudochylous e.* and *pseudochylothorax.*

chylous e. chylothorax consisting of chyle that has leaked from the thoracic duct.

hemorrhagic e. an effusion of bloody liquid.

parapneumonic e. a pleural effusion seen as a complication of pneumonia.

pericardial e. the accumulation of more than 50 mL of pericardial fluid in the pericardium.

pleural e. the presence of fluid in the pleural space; types include *chylothorax, hemothorax, hydrothorax,* and *pyothorax (empyema).* See also *pleurisy with effusion.*

pseudochylous e. chyliform e.

tuberculous e., tuberculous pleural e. an exudative pleural effusion resulting from pulmonary tuberculosis.

ef·lor·ni·thine hy·dro·chlo·ride (ef-lor′nĭ-thēn″) an irreversible inhibitor of the enzyme ornithine decarboxylase applied topically to reduce growth of unwanted facial hair in females. It is also used in the treatment of African trypanosomiasis, administered intravenously. Called also *DMFO.*

e·for·mot·er·ol fu·mar·ate (e″for-mot′ə-rol) formoterol fumarate.

Ef·u·dex (ef′u-deks) trademark for preparations of fluorouracil.

EGD esophagogastroduodenoscopy.

eges·ta (e-jes′tə) excretion (def. 2).

eges·tion (e-jes′chən) excretion (def. 2).

EGF epidermal growth factor.

EGG electrogastrography.

egg (eg) [L. *ovum*] ovum.

cleidoic e. an egg (such as that of a reptile, bird, or primitive mammal) that has within itself enough nutritive material for production of a complete embryo, needing to absorb nothing from its environment except oxygen. Except for oxygen intake, it can develop, at the expense of the substances stored inside the egg itself, directly into miniature adults without passing through a larval stage.

egg-bound (eg′bound) 1. unable to discharge eggs in the normal manner; said of a hen or other egg-laying animal. 2. inability of an egg-laying animal to discharge eggs in the normal manner.

Eg·gers plate (eg′ərz) [George William Nordholtz *Eggers,* American orthopedic surgeon, 1896–1963] see under *plate.*

Eg·ger·thel·la (eg″ər-thel′ə) [Arnold H. *Eggerth,* American bacteriologist, 1889–1963] a genus of gram-positive bacteria of the family Coriobacteriaceae, consisting of obligately anaerobic, non–spore-forming, nonflagellated rods occurring singly and in pairs and short chains. The type species is *E. len′ta.*

E. len′ta a species isolated from various infections, including infected postoperative wounds and abscesses, and from human blood and feces. Formerly called *Eubacterium lentum.*

egland·u·lous (e-glan′du-ləs) [*e-* + *glandulous*] having no glands.

ego (e′go) [L. "I"] in modern psychoanalytic theory, the psychologic segment of the personality, dominated by the reality principle, comprising integrative and executive aspects that function to adapt the forces and pressures exerted by the impulses of the id, the demands of the superego, and the requirements of external reality through conscious perception, thought, reasoning, learning, and all other activities necessary to interact effectively with the world. Cf. *id*[1] and *superego.*

ego-ali·en (e″go-āl′e-ən) ego-dystonic.

ego·bron·choph·o·ny (e″go-brong-kof′ə-ne) [Gr. *aix* goat + *bronchophony*] egophony.

ego·cen·tric (e″go-sen′trik) [*ego* + *centric*] self-centered, conceited, egotistical; preoccupied with one's own interests and needs; lacking concern for others.

ego-dys·ton·ic (e″go-dis-ton′ik) denoting aspects of a person's thoughts, impulses, attitudes, and behavior that are felt to be repugnant, distressing, unacceptable, or inconsistent with the rest of their personality. Cf. *ego-syntonic.*

ego-ide·al (e′go-i′del) see under *ideal.*

ego·ism (e′go-iz-əm) 1. any of several ethical doctrines that morality is founded in self-interest or that self-interest is the appropriate motive for all conduct. 2. excessive preoccupation with oneself; self-interest with disregard for the needs of others. 3. egotism.

ego·ma·nia (e″go-ma′ne-ə) [*ego* + *mania*] extreme self-centeredness; extreme egotism.

egoph·o·ny (e-gof′ə-ne) [Gr. *aix* goat + *phōnē* voice] increased resonance of voice sounds, with a high-pitched nasal or bleating quality, heard especially over lung tissue that is compressed or consolidated by pleural effusion. Called also *bronchoegophony, egobronchophony, tragophonia, tragophony,* and *voix de Polichinelle.*

ego-syn·ton·ic (e″go-sin-ton′ik) denoting aspects of a person's thoughts, impulses, attitudes, and behavior that are felt to be acceptable and consistent with the rest of their personality. Cf. *ego-dystonic.*

ego·tism (e′go-tiz-əm) 1. conceit, selfishness, self-centeredness, with an inflated sense of one's importance. 2. egoism (def. 2).

EGTA egtazic acid; a tetracarboxylic acid chelator similar in structure and action to EDTA (ethylenediaminetetraacetic acid), but with a higher affinity for calcium than for magnesium. It is used in biochemical assays and as a pharmaceutic aid.

eg·ta·zic ac·id (əg-tāz′ik) ethylene glycol-bis(β-aminoethyl ether)-*N,N*-tetraacetic acid; see *EGTA.*

EHBF estimated hepatic blood flow.

EHDP etidronate (ethane-1-hydroxy-1,1-diphosphonate).

EHEC enterohemorrhagic *Escherichia coli* (former name for Shiga toxin–producing *Escherichia coli*).

Eh·lers-Dan·los syndrome (a′lərz dahn-los′) [Edvard *Ehlers,* Danish dermatologist, 1863–1937; Henri Alexandre *Danlos,* French dermatologist, 1844–1912] see under *syndrome.*

Ehr·en·rit·ter's ganglion (âr′ən-rit″ərz) [Johann *Ehrenritter,* Austrian anatomist, 18th century] ganglion superius nervi glossopharyngei.

Ehr·lich reaction, theory (âr′lik) [Paul *Ehrlich,* German physician, bacteriologist, and Nobel prize winner, 1854–1915] see under *reaction* and *theory.*

Ehr·lich-Heinz granules (âr′lik hīnts′) [P. *Ehrlich;* Robert *Heinz,* German pathologist, 1865–1924] Ehrlich granules.

Ehr·lich·ia (âr-lik′e-ə) [Paul *Ehrlich*] a genus of tick-borne bacteria of the family Anaplasmataceae, consisting of gram-negative, nonmotile coccoid to ellipsoidal cells; organisms are parasitic in mammalian endothelial and hematopoietic cells, occurring in cytoplasmic vacuoles and often forming inclusion bodies (morulae), and produce disease in dogs, cattle, sheep, and humans. The type species is *E. ca′nis.*

E. ca′nis a species causing canine ehrlichiosis, transmitted by the tick *Rhipicephalus sanguineus;* in humans it causes a condition similar to Rocky Mountain spotted fever.

E. chaffeen′sis a species, transmitted by the ticks *Amblyomma americanum* and *Dermacentor variabilis,* that causes human monocytic ehrlichiosis.

E. e′qui a former species now classified as a strain of *Anaplasma phagocytophilum.*

E. ewin′gii a species that causes canine and human granulocytic ehrlichiosis.

E. phagocyto′phila former name for *Anaplasma phagocytophilum.*

E. pla′tys former name for *Anaplasma platys.*

E. risti′cii former name for *Neorickettsia risticii.*

E. ruminan′tium the etiologic agent of heartwater (q.v.) of sheep, goats, and cattle; it is nonpathogenic for humans.

E. sennet′su former name for *Neorickettsia sennetsu.*

ehr·lich·ia (âr-lik′e-ə) an individual organism of the genus *Ehrlichia.*

ehr·lich·i·al (âr-lik′e-əl) pertaining to or caused by *Ehrlichia.*

ehr·lich·i·osis (âr-lik″e-o′sis) a type of tick-borne fever caused by infection with bacteria of the genus *Ehrlichia.* It is usually seen in domestic animals, but certain species can affect humans.

canine e. an often fatal febrile disease of dogs in warm regions of the world, caused by *Ehrlichia canis,* which is spread by the tick *Rhipicephalus sanguineus* and infects the circulating lymphocytes. The *acute phase* consists of fever, discharge from the eyes and nose, anorexia, dyspnea, lymphadenopathy, and central nervous system signs. In the *subclinical phase,* clinical signs disappear but antigenemia, thrombocytopenia, and anemia persist. In the *chronic phase,* dogs have depression, weight loss, abdominal tenderness, hemorrhage, ocular lesions, ataxia, paralysis, and cranial nerve deficits.

canine granulocytic e. a mild to moderate febrile disease of dogs, characterized by pancytopenia, polyarthritis, ataxia, and paresis, caused by *Ehrlichia ewingii;* it is transmitted by the ticks *Amblyomma americanum* and *Dermacentor variabilis.*

equine e. equine granulocytic anaplasmosis.

equine monocytic e. an often fatal infection of horses with *Neorickettsia risticii,* seen in the Middle Atlantic part of the United States, characterized by fever, diarrhea, and anorexia. Called also *Potomac horse fever.*

human granulocytic e. (HGE) 1. infection with *Ehrlichia ewingii,* affecting primarily granulocytes and resulting in mild to moderate febrile disease with pancytopenia. It is transmitted by the ticks *Amblyomma*

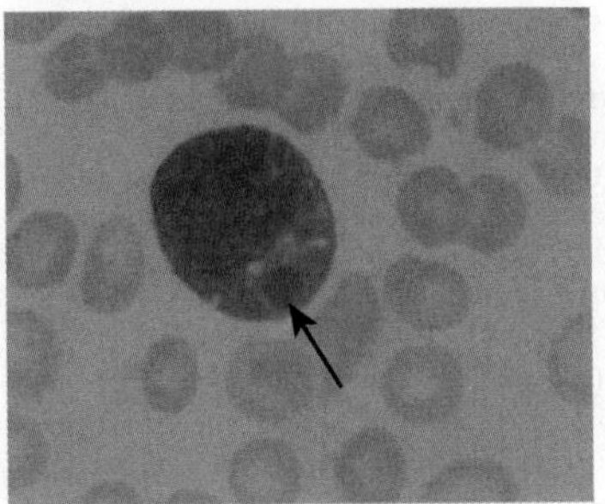

■ Morula containing *Ehrlichia chaffeensis (arrow)* in a monocyte in human monocytic ehrlichiosis.

americanum and *Dermacentor variabilis.* 2. former name for *human granulocytic anaplasmosis.*

human monocytic e. (HME) a type of ehrlichiosis in humans, seen in the United States, Europe, and Africa, caused by *Ehrlichia chaffeensis* and transmitted by the ticks *Amblyomma americanum* and *Dermacentor variabilis.* It involves predominantly fixed tissue mononuclear phagocytes and is characterized by flulike symptoms with leukopenia and thrombocytopenia, ranging in severity from asymptomatic to severe or occasionally fatal.

EI erythema infectiosum.

EIA enzyme immunoassay.

Eich•horst atrophy (īk′horst) [Hermann Ludwig *Eichhorst,* German physician in Switzerland, 1849–1921] see under *atrophy.*

Eic•ken method (i′kən) [Carl Otto von *Eicken,* German laryngologist and otologist, 1873–1960] see under *method.*

ei•co•nom•e•ter (i″kə-nom′ə-tər) eikonometer.

ei•co•sa•no•ate (i-ko″sə-no′āt) arachidate.

ei•co•sa•no•ic ac•id (i″ko-sə-no′ik) systematic name for *arachidic acid;* see table at *fatty acid.*

ei•co•sa•noid (i-ko′sə-noid) [Gr. *eikosa* twenty + *-oid*] any of the biologically active substances derived from arachidonic acid, including the prostaglandins and leukotrienes.

ei•co•sa•pen•ta•eno•ic ac•id (EPA) (i-ko″sə-pen″tə-e-no′ik) [Gr. *eikosa* twenty + *pentaene* + *-ic*] all *cis*-5,8,11,14,17-eicosapentaenoic acid, an omega-3, polyunsaturated, 20-carbon fatty acid found almost exclusively in fish and marine animal oils; it is a substrate for cyclooxygenase. See also table accompanying *fatty acid.*

ei•det•ic (i-det′ik) [Gr. *eidos* that which is seen; form or shape] 1. pertaining to or characterized by exact visualization of events or of objects previously seen. 2. an individual possessing such an ability.

ei•dop•tom•e•try (i″dop-tom′ə-tre) [Gr. *eidos* form + *opto-* + *-metry*] measurement of the acuteness of vision for the perception of form.

EIEC enteroinvasive *Escherichia coli.*

Ei•ken•el•la (i″kən-el′ə) [M. *Eiken,* Scandinavian biologist, 20th century] a genus of gram-negative, facultatively anaerobic, rod-shaped bacteria of the family Neisseriaceae. The organisms are part of the normal flora of the human oral cavity and upper respiratory tract but may cause infections of the head, neck, and abdominal area and general systemic disease. The single species is *E. corro′dens.*

ei•ko•nom•e•ter (i″kə-nom′ə-tər) [Gr. *eikōn* image + *-meter*] an instrument used in making an examination for aniseikonia.

ei•loid (i′loid) [Gr. *eilein* to roll up + *-oid*] having a coiled appearance.

Ei•me•ria (i-mēr′e-ə) [Gustav Heinrich Theodor *Eimer,* German zoologist, 1843–1898] a genus of homoxenous coccidian protozoa (suborder Eimeriina, order Eucoccidiida) found principally as parasites of the gastrointestinal tract of birds and herbivorous mammals. The organisms have four spores in each oocyst and two sporozoites in each spore, with oocysts being passed in the feces. Many species are of economic importance. Pathogenic species found in domestic animals include *E. bovis, E. ellipsoidalis,* and *E. zuernii* in cattle; *E. arloingi* A *(E. ovina), E. arloingi* B *(E. weybridgensis), E. ahsata, E. crandallis, E. gilruthi,* and *E. ovinoidalis* in sheep; *E. debliecki, E. scabra,* and *E. perminuta* in pigs; *E. leukarti* in horses and donkeys; *E. arloingi, E. caprina, E. faurei,* and *E. ninakohlyakimovae* in goats; *E. magna, E. stieda, E. sciurorum,* and *E. perforans* in rabbits; and *E. acervulina, E. maxima, E. meleagridis, E. necatrix,* and *E. tenella* in poultry. See also *coccidiosis.*

Ei•me•ri•i•na (i″me-ri′ī-nə) a suborder of homoxenous or heteroxenous protozoa (order Eucoccidiida, subclass Coccidia), usually parasitizing the gut epithelium of the host, in which the macrogamete and microgametocyte develop independently, syzygy does not occur, the microgametocyte gives rise to numerous biflagellated microgametes, and the sporozoites are typically enclosed in an oocyst. Representative genera include *Aggregata, Besnoitia, Cryptosporidium, Eimeria, Isospora, Sarcocystis, Toxoplasma,* and *Tyzzeria.*

ein•stei•ni•um (Es) (īn-sti′ne-əm) [Albert *Einstein,* theoretical physicist, born in Germany, became a naturalized citizen of Switzerland, then of the United States, 1879–1955; winner of the Nobel prize for physics in 1921] the chemical element of atomic number 99, atomic weight 254, originally discovered in debris from a thermonuclear explosion in 1952.

Ein•tho•ven galvanometer, law (formula), triangle (īn′to-vən) [Willem *Einthoven,* Dutch physiologist and Nobel prize winner, 1860–1927] see under *galvanometer, law,* and *triangle.*

Ei•se•nia (i-se′ne-ə) a genus of lumbricoid worms. *E. foe′tida* is a species reportedly found in human urine.

Ei•sen•men•ger complex, syndrome (i′sən-meng″ər) [Victor *Eisenmenger,* German physician, 1864–1932] see under *complex* and *syndrome.*

EIT erythrocyte iron turnover.

ejac•u•late[1] (e-jak′u-lāt) to expel suddenly, especially semen.

ejac•u•late[2] (e-jak′u-lət) the semen discharged in a single ejaculation in the male, consisting of the secretions of the Cowper gland, epididymis, ductus deferens, seminal vesicles, and prostate, and containing the spermatozoa. Called also *ejaculum.*

ejac•u•la•tio (e-jak″u-la′she-o) [L.] ejaculation.

e. defi′ciens a defective ejaculation; see also *anejaculation.*

e. prae′cox premature ejaculation.

e. retarda′ta male orgasmic disorder.

ejac•u•la•tion (e-jak″u-la′shən) [L. *ejaculatio*] a sudden act of expulsion, as of the semen. **ejac′ulatory** *adj*

premature e. ejaculation consistently occurring either prior to, upon, or immediately after penetration and before it is desired, taking into account factors such as age, novelty of the specific situation, and recent frequency of the sexual act. Used officially [DSM-IV], it denotes also significant resulting distress or interpersonal difficulty.

retarded e. male orgasmic disorder.

retrograde e. ejaculation in which semen travels up the urethra toward the bladder instead of to the outside of the body; seen with spinal cord injury, after prostatectomy or bladder neck surgery, and in other conditions.

ejac•u•la•tor (e-jak′u-la″tər) [L.] that which or one who ejaculates.

e. se′minis musculus bulbospongiosus.

ejac•u•lum (e-jak′u-ləm) ejaculate[2].

ejec•ta (e-jek′tə) discharge (def. 3).

ejec•tion (e-jek′shən) [L. *ejectus,* past part. of *ejicere* to cast out] 1. the act of casting out or the state of being cast out, as of excretions, secretions, or other bodily fluids. 2. something cast out; see *discharge* (def. 3). 3. the discharge of blood from the heart; see under *period.*

milk e. let-down reflex.

Ejusd. [L.] ejus′dem (of the same).

eka- [Sanskrit, "one" or "first"] a prefix added to the name of a known chemical element as a provisional designation of the unknown element which should occur next in the same group in the periodic system.

Ek•bom syndrome (ek′bom) [Karl-Axel *Ekbom,* Swedish neurologist, 1907–1977] restless legs syndrome.

EKG electrocardiogram.

eki•ri (ə-ke′re) an acute cerebral and cardiovascular disorder occurring in children with shigellosis in Japan.

Ek•man-Lob•stein syndrome (ek′mahn lōb′shtīn) [Olof Jacob *Ekman,* Swedish physician, 1764–1839; Johann Friedrich Georg Christian *Lobstein,* German physician, 1777–1835] osteogenesis imperfecta (type I).

EKY electrokymogram.

elab•o•rate (e-lab′o-rāt) [L. *elaborare* to work out] to produce complex substances out of simpler materials.

elab•o•ra•tion (e-lab″ə-ra′shən) 1. the process of producing complex substances out of simpler materials. 2. in psychiatry, an unconscious mental process of expansion and embellishment of detail, especially of a symbol or representation in a dream; called also *secondary eye.*

elae(o)- see *ele(o)-.*

El•ae•oph•ora (el″e-of′ə-rə) a genus of filariae of the family Onchocercidae. *E. schnei′deri* is found in the arteries of deer and sheep in the western United States, sometimes causing fatal brain disease (see *elaeophoriasis*).

elae•o•pho•ria•sis (el″e-of″ə-ri′ə-sis) infection of the arteries and facial and ocular capillaries of deer or sheep by microfilariae of *Elaeophora schneideri;* larvae are spread from animal to animal by the bites of *Tabanus* and *Hybomitra* horseflies. If the parasites spread to the leptomeningeal arteries they may cause necrosis of brain tissue, blindness, and death. Called also *elaeophorosis*, *filarial dermatitis*, and *sorehead*.

elae•o•pho•ro•sis (el″e-of″ə-ro′sis) elaeophoriasis.

elai(o)- see *ele(o)-*.

el•a•id•ate (el″ə-id′āt) a salt, ester, or anionic form of elaidic acid.

el•a•id•ic ac•id (el″ə-id′ik) the *trans* isomer of oleic acid; it does not occur naturally but can be synthesized from oleic acid.

elai•om•e•ter (e″la-om′ə-tər) eleometer.

el•a•pid (el′ə-pid) 1. any snake of the family Elapidae. 2. of or pertaining to the family Elapidae.

Elap•i•dae (e-lap′ĭ-de) a family of usually terrestrial, venomous snakes, which have cylindrical tails and front fangs that are short, stout, immovable, and grooved. It includes the genera *Acanthophis*, *Bungarus*, *Dendroaspis*, *Micruroides*, *Micrurus*, *Naja*, *Notechis*, and *Oxyuranus*. See table at *snake*.

Elaps (e′laps) *Micrurus*.

elas•mo•branch (e-las′mo-brank) [Gr. *elasmos* plate + *branchia*] 1. any cartilaginous fish having platelike gills, each gill slit opening independently on the body surface, such as sharks, skates, rays, and sawfish. See also *Chondrichthyes*. 2. of or pertaining to such fish.

elas•tance (e-las′təns) 1. the quality of recoiling without disruption upon removal of pressure. 2. an expression of the ability to recoil without disruption when pressure is removed, such as that of an air- or fluid-filled organ, e.g., the lung or urinary bladder, measured in terms of unit of pressure change per unit of volume change. Symbol *E*. It is the reciprocal of *compliance*.

elas•tase (e-las′tās) any of a group of serine endopeptidases secreted by neutrophils, macrophages, mast cells, the pancreas, and certain bacteria; they catalyze the cleavage of elastin and other proteins, preferentially cutting polypeptide chains at bonds involving the carbonyl groups of amino acids. Elastase activity is specifically inhibited by alpha$_1$-antitrypsin. See also *leukocyte elastase* and *pancreatic elastase II*.

elas•tic (e-las′tik) [L. *elasticus*] 1. able to resist and recover from stretching, compression, or distortion applied by a force. Cf. *resiliency*. 2. a ring-shaped strip that can do this, made of rubber or synthetic material, such as one used in orthodontic therapy. Called also *elastic band*.

intermaxillary e. an elastic band used to produce traction between the upper and lower teeth in orthodontic therapy.

intramaxillary e. an elastic band applied within the same dental arch to achieve space closure.

vertical e. an elastic band applied in a direction perpendicular to the occlusal plane, connecting one arch wire to the other, usually for approximating teeth to improve intercuspation.

elas•ti•ca (e-las′tĭ-kə) [L.] 1. elastic tissue. 2. either the internal or external elastic membrane.

elas•ti•cin (e-las′tĭ-sin) elastin.

elas•tic•i•ty (e″las-tis′ĭ-te) the quality or condition of being elastic.

physical e. of muscle the physical quality of muscle of being elastic, of yielding to passive physical stretch.

physiologic e. of muscle the biologic quality, unique to muscle, of being able to change and resume size under neuromuscular control.

total e. of muscle the combined effect of physical and physiologic elasticity of muscle.

elas•tin (e-las′tin) a scleroprotein that is the essential constituent of elastic connective tissue. It is arranged in fibers (see *elastic fibers*, under *fiber*) and discontinuous sheets in the extracellular matrix, particularly of the skin, lungs, and blood vessels.

elast(o)- [L. *elasticus* elastic, from Gr. *elastos*, beaten, ductile, from *elaunein* to beat out] a combining form denoting relationship to flexibility, to elastin, or to elastic tissue.

elas•to•fi•bro•ma (e-las″to-fi-bro′mə) [*elasto-* + *fibroma*] a rare, benign, firm, unencapsulated tumor consisting of abundant sclerotic collagen mixed with thick irregular elastic fibers, usually in the subscapular region of an older adult; these are often fibrous reactions to injury. Called also *e. dorsi*.

elas•toid (e-las′toid) a substance formed by the hyaline degeneration of the internal elastic lamina of blood vessels; seen in the vessels of the uterus after delivery.

elas•toi•do•sis (e-las″toi-do′sis) changes in the skin resembling those of elastosis.

nodular e. Favre-Racouchot syndrome.

elas•tol•y•sis (e″las-tol′ə-sis) [*elasto-* + *-lysis*] a defect in the elastic tissue, resulting in atrophy and laxity of the skin, seen in conditions such as anetoderma, atrophoderma, and cutis laxa.

generalized e. cutis laxa.

perifollicular e. a condition resembling anetoderma, seen around hair follicles and not preceded by folliculitis; it may be caused by an elastase-producing strain of *Staphylococcus epidermidis*, it may be drug induced, or endocrine factors may be involved.

postinflammatory e. a condition resembling anetoderma, usually seen in infants, characterized by round erythematous papules that enlarge to form plaques with a scaly collarette. It may appear anywhere on the body except on the palms and soles, but most often is on the face, ears, or neck. It is followed by skin laxity that clinically resembles that of cutis laxa.

elas•to•lyt•ic (e-las″to-lit′ik) 1. pertaining to or characterized by elastolysis. 2. capable of catalyzing the digestion of elastic tissue.

elas•to•ma (e″las-to′mə) [*elast-* + *-oma*] a localized tumorlike excess of elastic tissue fibers or abnormal collagen fibers of the skin.

juvenile e. connective tissue nevus.

elas•to•mer (e-las′to-mər) a synthetic rubber; any of various soft, elastic, rubber-like polymers; used in dentistry as an impression material and for maxillofacial extraoral prostheses.

elas•tom•e•ter (e″las-tom′ə-tər) [*elasto-* + *-meter*] an instrument for determining the elasticity of tissues, and thus measuring the degree of edema.

elas•tom•e•try (e″las-tom′ə-tre) [*elasto-* + *-metry*] the measurement of elasticity.

elas•top•a•thy (e″las-top′ə-the) [*elasto-* + *-pathy*] defect in elastic tissue content or composition.

elas•to•phag•o•cy•to•sis (e-las″to-fag″o-si-to′sis) phagocytosis of elastic fibers.

giant cell e. annular elastolytic giant cell granuloma.

Elas•to•plast (e-las′to-plast) trademark for an elastic bandage.

elas•tor•rhex•is (e-las″to-rek′sis) [*elasto-* + *-rrhexis*] 1. rupture of elastic fibers, such as in cutis laxa. 2. cutis laxa.

papular e. a rare skin disorder seen in adolescents, consisting of asymptomatic white papules on the trunk or limbs, similar to the lesions of Buschke-Ollendorff syndrome.

elas•to•sis (e″las-to′sis) 1. degeneration of elastic tissue. 2. elastoid degeneration; degenerative changes seen in the connective tissue of the skin or conjunctiva, in which collagen is replaced by a material that has the staining properties of elastin but is resistant to elastase.

actinic e. a type of photodamage to the skin seen especially in light-skinned individuals, marked by inelasticity, thinning (or sometimes thickening), wrinkling, dryness with fine scaling, and variable hyperpigmentation or other blemishes. Called also *farmers'* or *sailors' skin* and *senile* or *solar e.*

nodular e. Favre-Racouchot syndrome.

e. per′forans serpigino′sa, perforating e. a chronic type of acquired perforating dermatosis characterized by channels in the epidermis into which abnormal elastic tissue perforates and is extruded into the dermis. On the skin there are flesh-colored keratopapular eruptions and clustered arc-shaped serpiginous lesions. It usually occurs in young males, alone or with more widespread disease, on the sides and nape of the neck, or less often on the upper arms, face, trunk, or elsewhere.

senile e., solar e. actinic e.

solar e. actinic e.

elas•tot•ic (e″las-tot′ik) 1. pertaining to or characterized by elastosis. 2. resembling elastic tissue. 3. having the staining properties of elastin.

el•a•ter (el′ə-tər) a specialized structure of certain plants, such as liverworts and slime molds, which aids in the distribution of spores.

ela•tion (e-la′shən) emotional excitement marked by speeding up of mental and bodily activity, with extreme joy and an overly optimistic attitude even in the face of negative circumstances.

Elaut triangle (a-lo′) [Léon Josef Stephaan *Elaut*, Belgian anatomist, 1897–1978] see under *triangle*.

El•a•vil (el′ə-vil) trademark for preparations of amitriptyline hydrochloride.

el•bow (el′bo) [L. *cubitus*] 1. cubitus. 2. any angular bend.

capped e. a hygroma of the elbow or a hard, fibrous mass on the point of the elbow in horses or cattle; cf. *capped hock*. Called also *shoe boil*.

dropped e. radial paralysis (def. 2).

golfer's e. popular name for medial epicondylitis.

Little Leaguer's e. popular name for medial epicondylitis in children and adolescent ballplayers.

miner's e. popular name for *olecranon bursitis*.

nursemaid's e. pulled e.

pulled e. subluxation of the head of the radius distally under the annular ligament, produced by sudden traction on the hand with the elbow extended and the forearm pronated. Called also *nursemaid's e.*.

tennis e. popular name for lateral epicondylitis.

ELBW extremely low birth weight; see under *infant.*

El·de·pryl (el′də-prəl) trademark for a preparation of selegiline hydrochloride.

el·der (el′dər) any tree of the genus *Sambucus.*

El·do·paque (el′do-pāk) trademark for preparations of hydroquinone.

El·do·quin (el′do-kwin) trademark for a preparation of hydroquinone.

elec·tive (e-lek′tiv) 1. tending to combine with or act on one substance rather than another. 2. subject to the choice or decision of the patient or physician; applied to procedures that are advantageous to the patient but not urgent.

Elec·tra com·plex (e-lek′trə) [*Electra,* character in Greek legend who incited her brother to kill their mother and stepfather for having murdered their father] see under *complex.*

elec·tric (e-lek′trik) pertaining to or containing electricity.

elec·tri·cal (e-lek′trĭ-kəl) electric.

elec·tric·i·ty (e-lek-tris′ĭ-te) 1. a form of energy consisting of oppositely charged electrons and protons; it produces light, heat, magnetism, and chemical changes. 2. electric current.

electro- [Gr. *ēlektron* amber, because an electric charge can be produced in amber by rubbing] a combining form denoting relationship to electricity.

elec·tro·acous·tic (e-lek″tro-ə-ko͞os′tik) pertaining to the interaction or interconversion of electric and acoustic phenomena.

elec·tro·acu·punc·ture (e-lek″tro-ak″u-punk′chər) acupuncture in which the needles are stimulated electrically.

e. after Voll (EAV) a system of diagnosis and treatment based on the measurement of the electrical characteristics of acupoints, the results being used to determine a specific remedy.

elec·tro·af·fin·i·ty (e-lek″tro-ə-fin′ĭ-te) electronegativity.

elec·tro·an·al·ge·sia (e-lek″tro-an″əl-je′ze-ə) the reduction of pain by electrical stimulation of a peripheral nerve or the dorsal column of the spinal cord.

elec·tro·anal·y·sis (e-lek″tro-ə-nal′ə-sis) chemical analysis performed by the aid of the electric current.

elec·tro·an·es·the·sia (e-lek″tro-an″es-the′zhə) anesthesia, either local or general, induced by electricity.

elec·tro·bi·ol·o·gy (e-lek″tro-bi-ol′ə-je) [*electro-* + *biology*] the study of electric phenomena in living tissue.

elec·tro·bi·os·co·py (e-lek″tro-bi-os′ko-pe) [*electro-* + *bio-* + *-scopy*] the determination of the presence or absence of life by means of an electric current.

elec·tro·blot (e-lek′tro-blot″) a blot in which transfer of solutes from gel to membrane or other substrate is effected by electrophoresis rather than capillary action.

elec·tro·car·dio·gram (e-lek″tro-kahr′de-o-gram″) [*electro-* + *cardiogram*] a graphic tracing of the variations in electrical potential caused by the excitation of the heart muscle and detected at the body surface. The normal electrocardiogram is a scalar representation that shows deflections resulting from atrial and ventricular activity as changes in the magnitude of voltage and polarity (positive and negative) with time. The first deflection, the P wave, is due to excitation of the atria; the QRS complex of deflections, to excitation (depolarization) of the ventricles; and the T wave, to recovery of the ventricles (repolarization). Abbreviated ECG or EKG. See also *lead*[2] and see terms under *wave, complex,* and *interval.*

esophageal e. see under *electrogram.*

intracardiac e. see under *electrogram.*

scalar e. see *electrocardiogram.*

elec·tro·car·di·o·graph (e-lek″tro-kahr′de-o-graf″) an instrument for performing electrocardiography, i.e., for making electrocardiograms.

elec·tro·car·di·og·ra·phy (e-lek″tro-kahr″de-og′rə-fe) [*electro-* + *cardio-* + *-graphy*] the making of graphic records of the variations in electrical potential caused by electrical activity of the heart muscle and detected at the body surface, as a method for studying the action of the heart muscle; see also *electrocardiogram* and *electrogram.* **electrocardiograph′ic** *adj*

intracavitary e. electrocardiography in which electrodes are placed within the cardiac cavities.

12-lead e. electrocardiography performed using the twelve standard leads: the three standard bipolar limb leads, the three augmented unipolar limb leads (aV_F, aV_L, and aV_R), and the six standard precordial leads (V_1 to V_6).

precordial e. electrocardiography in which potentials over the chest wall near the surface of the heart are recorded; see *precordial leads,* under *lead*[2].

elec·tro·ca·tal·y·sis (e-lek″tro-kə-tal′ə-sis) the catalytic effect produced by electricity on the bodily processes.

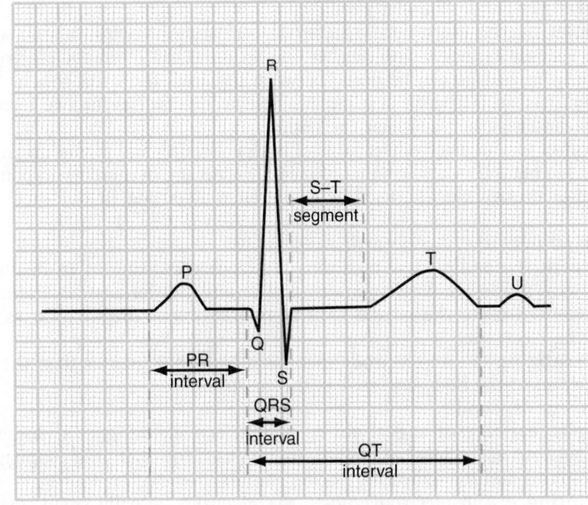

■ Normal electrocardiogram.

elec·tro·cau·ter·i·za·tion (e-lek″tro-kaw″tər-ĭ-za′shən) electrocautery (def. 2).

elec·tro·cau·tery (e-lek″tro-kaw′tər-e) 1. an apparatus for surgical dissection and hemostasis, using heat generated by a high-voltage, high-frequency alternating current passed through an electrode. 2. the cauterization of tissue using such an instrument; see also *electrocoagulation* and *electrohemostasis.* Called also *electrocauterization.*

bipolar e. an electrocautery in which both active and return electrodes are incorporated into a single handheld instrument, so that the current passes between the tips of the two electrodes and affects only a small amount of tissue.

monopolar e., unipolar e. an electrocautery in which current is applied through a handheld active electrode and travels back to the generator through a grounding pad and cable attached to the patient, so that the patient is part of the electrical circuit.

elec·tro·chem·i·cal (e-lek″tro-kem′ĭ-kəl) pertaining to interaction or interconversion of chemical and electrical energies, as in electrolysis.

elec·tro·chem·is·try (e-lek″tro-kem′is-tre) the study of relationships and transformations between chemical and electrical energy.

elec·tro·chro·ma·tog·ra·phy (e-lek″tro-kro″mə-tog′rə-fe) electrophoresis.

elec·tro·co·ag·u·la·tion (e-lek″tro-ko-ag″u-la′shən) coagulation of tissue usually by means of an electrocautery.

elec·tro·coch·leo·gram (e-lek″tro-kok′le-o-gram) the record obtained by electrocochleography.

elec·tro·coch·le·og·ra·phy (e-lek″tro-kok″le-og′rə-fe) measurement of electrical potentials (cochlear microphonics, summating potentials, and action potentials of the eighth cranial nerve) in response to acoustic stimuli measured by an electrode in the external acoustic canal, on the tympanic membrane, or through the tympanic membrane applied to the promontory or the round window. **electrococh′leographic** *adj*

elec·tro·con·trac·til·i·ty (e-lek″tro-kon″trak-til′ĭ-te) contractility in response to electric stimulation.

elec·tro·con·vul·sive (e-lek″tro-kən-vul′siv) inducing convulsions by means of electric shock; see under *therapy.*

elec·tro·cor·ti·co·gram (e-lek″tro-kor′tĭ-ko-gram″) the record obtained by electrocorticography.

elec·tro·cor·ti·cog·ra·phy (e-lek″tro-kor″tĭ-kog′rə-fe) electroencephalography with the electrodes applied directly to the cortex of the brain.

elec·tro·cu·tion (e-lek″tro-ku′shən) the taking of life by passage of electric current through the body.

elec·tro·cys·tog·ra·phy (e-lek″tro-sis-tog′rə-fe) the recording of changes of electric potential in the urinary bladder.

elec·trode (e-lek′trōd) [*electro-* + *hodos* way] 1. a medium used between an electric conductor and the object to which the current is to be applied. 2. in electrotherapy or electrosurgery, an instrument with a point or surface from which to transmit an electric current to the body of a patient or to another instrument. 3. in electrodiagnosis, a needle or metal plate used to stimulate or record the electrical activity of tissue; see also *lead*[2].

active e. 1. the electrode of an electrical therapeutic or surgical device through which electrical current is applied. 2. in electromyography, an exploring electrode.

bifilar needle e. bipolar needle e.
bipolar needle e. a needle electrode consisting of two insulated wires inside a single cylinder, with neither one acting as the reference electrode; variations in voltage can be noted between the areas the wires touch.
bipolar stimulating e. a stimulating electrode that has the two terminals attached together and near each other.
calomel e. an electrode capable of both collecting and giving up chloride ions in neutral or acidic aqueous media, consisting of mercury in contact with mercurous chloride; used as a reference electrode in pH measurements.
coaxial needle e. concentric needle e.
concentric needle e. a recording electrode consisting of an insulated metal wire inside a hollow stainless steel cannula; differences in potential are measured using the needle shaft as reference and the wire tip as the exploring electrode.
depolarizing e. an electrode that has a resistance greater than that of the portion of the body enclosed in the circuit.
earth e. ground e.
esophageal e., esophageal pill e. a pill electrode designed to lodge in the esophagus at the level of the atrium; it is used for obtaining esophageal electrograms and for delivering pacing stimuli.
exploring e. in electrodiagnosis, the electrode, usually small, placed nearest to the site of the bioelectric activity being recorded; it determines the potential in only that localized area.
ground e. an electrode that is connected to a ground; called also *earth e.*
inactive e. in an electrocautery, the electrode through which current distributed through the active electrode is returned to the generator.
indifferent e. reference e.
monopolar needle e. a needle electrode consisting of a single piece of stainless steel wire coated with insulating material except at the tip; it must be accompanied by another electrode as a reference.
monopolar stimulating e. a stimulating electrode that has the two terminals attached separately and relatively far apart.
multilead e. an electrode composed of a number of insulated wires inside a metal cannula, with their bare tips at apertures flush with the outer circumference of the cannula; used to determine the territory of a motor unit. Called also *multielectrode.*
needle e. a thin, cylindrical electrode with an outer shaft beveled to a sharp point, enclosing a wire or series of wires; needle electrodes are used to explore the activity of single motor or nerve units or stimulate them.
patch e. a tiny electrode with a blunt tip, used in studies of membrane potentials. See also *patch clamp* and *microelectrode.*
pill e. an electrode usually enclosed within a gelatin capsule and attached to a flexible slender wire so that it may be swallowed, such as an esophageal electrode.
recording e. an electrode used to measure electric potential change in body tissue; for recording, two electrodes must be used, the *exploring e.* and the *reference e.* (qq.v.).
reference e. an electrode whose placement is remote from the source of recorded activity, so that it is presumed to be at either a negligible or constant potential.
scalp e. an electrode placed on or just below the surface of the scalp; the most common type used in electroencephalography.
single fiber needle e. a needle electrode with a small recording surface for the recording of individual muscle fiber action potentials. See also *single fiber electromyography.*
stimulating e. an electrode used to apply electric current to tissue; it must include both a negative terminal and a positive terminal. See also *bipolar stimulating e.* and *monopolar stimulating e.*
surface e. an electrode placed on the skin surface and used to stimulate or record electrical activity in the underlying tissue.

elec·tro·der·mal (e-lek″tro-dur′məl) pertaining to the electrical properties of the skin, especially to changes in its resistance.

elec·tro·des·ic·ca·tion (e-lek″tro-des″ĭ-ka′shən) dehydration of tissue by the use of a high frequency electric current; see *fulguration.*

elec·tro·di·ag·no·sis (e-lek″tro-di″əg-no′sis) the use of electrical devices in the diagnosis of pathologic conditions.

elec·tro·di·ag·nos·tics (e-lek″tro-di″əg-nos′tiks) the science and practice of electrodiagnosis.

elec·tro·di·al·y·sis (e-lek″tro-di-al′ə-sis) dialysis done under the influence of an electric field.

elec·tro·di·a·ly·zer (e-lek″tro-di′ə-li″zər) a hemodialyzer that uses an applied electric field and semipermeable membranes for separating the colloids from the solution.

elec·tro·di·aph·a·ke (e-lek″tro-di-af′ə-ke) [*electro-* + *dia-* + Gr. *phakos* lentil] an instrument for removing the lens by diathermy.

elec·tro·ejac·u·la·tion (EEJ) (e-lek″tro-e-jak″u-la′shən) induction of ejaculation by application of a gradually increasing electrical current delivered through a probe inserted into the rectum, a technique originally used in veterinary medicine and now also used in humans for collection of sperm for insemination from men with spinal cord injuries and other conditions that prevent ejaculation.

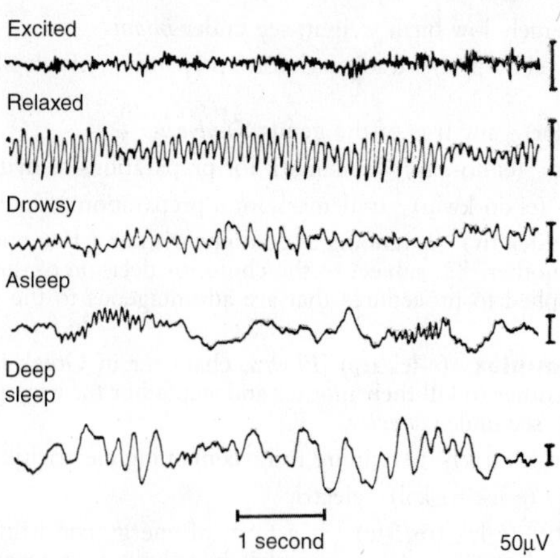

■ Electroencephalogram. Recordings made while the subject was excited, relaxed, and in various stages of sleep. During excitement the brain waves are rapid and of small amplitude, whereas in sleep they are much slower and of greater amplitude.

elec·tro·en·ceph·a·lo·gram (EEG) (e-lek″tro-en-sef′ə-lo-gram″) a recording of the potentials on the skull generated by currents emanating spontaneously from nerve cells in the brain. The normal dominant frequency of these potentials is about 8 to 10 cycles per second and the amplitude about 10 to 100 microvolts. Fluctuations in potential are seen in the form of waves, which correlate well with different neurologic conditions and so are used as diagnostic criteria. See also *brain waves,* under *wave.*
flat e., isoelectric e. an electroencephalogram in which no brain waves are recorded, indicating a complete lack of brain activity.

elec·tro·en·ceph·a·lo·graph (e-lek″tro-ən-sef′ə-lo-graf″) an instrument for performing electroencephalography.

elec·tro·en·ceph·a·log·ra·phy (e-lek″tro-ən-sef′ə-log′rə-fe) the recording of the electric currents developed in the brain, by means of electrodes applied to the scalp, to the surface of the brain *(intracranial e.),* or placed within the substance of the brain *(depth e.).* See *electroencephalogram.* **electroencephalograph′ic** *adj*

elec·tro·en·ceph·a·lo·scope (e-lek″tro-ən-sef′ə-lo-skōp) an instrument for detecting brain potentials at many different sections of the brain and displaying them on a cathode-ray tube.

elec·tro·en·dos·mo·sis (e-lek″tro-en″dos-mo′sis) 1. endosmosis under the influence of an electric field. 2. electro-osmosis.

elec·tro·ex·ci·sion (e-lek″tro-ek-sĭ′zhən) excision performed by electrosurgery.

elec·tro·fo·cus·ing (e-lek″tro-fo′kəs-ing) isoelectric focusing.

elec·tro·ful·gu·ra·tion (e-lek″tro-ful″gə-ra′shən) a type of electrosurgery used to produce superficial desiccation of tissue.

elec·tro·gas·tro·gram (e-lek″tro-gas′tro-gram) the graphic record obtained by electrogastrography.

elec·tro·gas·tro·graph (e-lek″tro-gas′tro-graf) an instrument for recording the electrical activity of the stomach by means of swallowed gastric electrodes.

elec·tro·gas·trog·ra·phy (EGG) (e-lek″tro-gas-trog′rə-fe) the recording of the electrical activity of the stomach as measured between its lumen and the surface of the body, used to evaluate gastric motor activity. **electrogastrograph′ic** *adj*

elec·tro·gen·ic (e-lek″tro-jen′ik) [*electro-* + *-genic*] pertaining to a process by which net charge is transferred to a different location so that hyperpolarization results, as in the pumping of ions across a membrane. See also under *pump.*

elec·tro·glot·tog·ra·phy (e-lek″tro-glŏ-tog′rəfe) glottography measuring the impedance of small electrical charges across the neck as a function of changes in apposition of the vocal cord folds during phonation or respiration.

elec·tro·go·ni·om·e·ter (e-lek″tro-go″ne-om′ə-tər) an electrical goniometer.

elec·tro·gram (e-lek′tro-gram) [*electro-* + *-gram*] any record produced by changes in electric potential, such as an electrocardiogram or electroencephalogram.
atrial e. see *intra-atrial e.* and *high right atrial e.*

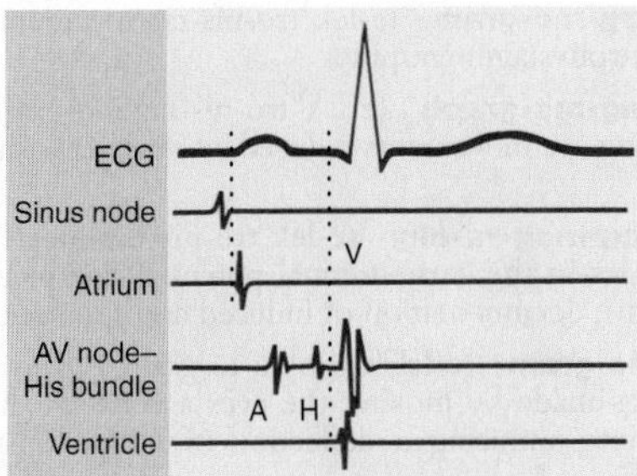

■ Intracardiac electrogram. Schematic illustration shows a single beat with accompanying intracardiac signals from the sinus node, right atrium, atrioventricular *(AV)* nodal and His bundle regions, and right ventricle, contrasted with a conventional body-surface electrocardiogram *(ECG)*. *A*, Atrial recording; *H*, His recording; *V*, ventricular recording.

coronary sinus (CS) e. an intracardiac electrogram that records electrical potentials within the coronary sinus; it is used for indirect monitoring of left atrial and left ventricular sites.

esophageal e. an electrogram recorded by an esophageal electrode; it is used for enhanced detection of P waves and elucidation of complex arrhythmias.

high right atrial (HRA) e. an intracardiac electrogram that records electrical potentials within the upper region of the right atrium, obtained by introduction of electrodes high in the atrium near the sinus node; used in localizing conduction blocks and diagnosing arrhythmias. See illustration.

His bundle e. (HBE) an intracardiac electrogram of potentials in the lower right atrium, atrioventricular node, and His-Purkinje system, obtained by positioning intracardiac electrodes near the tricuspid valve; it is used to pinpoint the site, extent, and mechanisms of arrhythmias and conduction defects. See illustration.

intra-atrial e. an intracardiac electrogram of potentials within the atrium; used particularly for monitoring P waves.

intracardiac e. a record of changes in the electric potentials of specific cardiac loci as measured by electrodes placed within the heart via cardiac catheters; it is used for loci that cannot be assessed by body surface electrodes, such as the bundle of His or other regions within the cardiac conducting system. See illustration.

right ventricular e. an intracardiac electrogram obtained by placing electrodes in the right ventricle; used to assess ventricular activity and response to stimuli.

right ventricular apical e. an intracardiac electrogram obtained by placing electrodes in the apex of the right ventricle; it is used in mapping ventricular arrhythmias.

sinus node e. an intracardiac electrogram obtained by placing electrodes near the sinus node; it is used in examining the time for impulse conduction from the node to the atrium.

elec•tro•graph (e-lek′tro-graf) electrogram.

elec•trog•ra•phy (e″lek-trog′rə-fe) [*electro-* + *-graphy*] the graphic recording of changes in electric potential, as in electrocardiography, electroencephalography, etc.

elec•tro•gus•tom•e•try (e-lek″tro-gəs-tom′ə-tre) the testing of the sense of taste by application of galvanic stimuli to the tongue.

elec•tro•he•mos•ta•sis (e-lek″tro-he-mos′tə-sis) [*electro-* + *hemostasis*] the arrest of hemorrhage by the application of a high frequency current to coagulate the bleeding point or surface.

elec•tro•hys•tero•gram (e-lek″tro-his′tər-o-gram) the graphic record obtained by electrohysterography.

elec•tro•hys•ter•og•ra•phy (e-lek″tro-his″tər-og′rə-fe) the recording of the changes in electric potential associated with contractions of the uterine muscle.

elec•tro•im•mu•no•dif•fu•sion (e-lek″tro-im″u-no-dĭ-fu′zhən) the combination of immunodiffusion with electrophoresis, using an applied electric field to speed up the migration of antigen and antibody. Two such techniques have achieved widespread use: *counterimmunoelectrophoresis* (one-dimensional double electroimmunodiffusion) and *Laurell rocket immunoelectrophoresis* (one-dimensional single electroimmunodiffusion).

elec•tro•ky•mo•gram (e-lek″tro-ki′mo-gram) the graphic record produced by electrokymography; abbreviated EKY.

elec•tro•ky•mo•graph (e-lek″tro-ki′mo-graf) an instrument for graphically recording motion of or changes in density of organs by recording variations in intensity of a small beam of x-rays. Its three essential parts are a fluoroscope, a pick-up unit, and a recording instrument; used especially for showing motion of the cardiac silhouette (see *cardiokymography*).

elec•tro•ky•mog•ra•phy (e-lek″tro-ki-mog′rə-fe) the photography on x-ray film of the motion of the heart or other structures using an electrokymograph.

elec•tro•lar•ynx (e-lek″tro-lar′inks) artificial larynx.

elec•tro•li•thot•ri•ty (e-lek″tro-lĭ-thot′rĭ-te) the disintegration of calculi by the application of electric current.

elec•trol•o•gist (e-lek-trol′o-jist) a specialist in electrolysis.

elec•trol•o•gy (e-lek-trol′ə-je) popular term for *electrolysis* (def. 2).

elec•trol•y•sis (e″lek-trol′ə-sis) [*electro-* + *-lysis*] 1. a chemical reaction caused by the passing of an electric current through a solution. 2. a plastic surgery technique whereby tissue such as unwanted hair is destroyed by exposing it to an electric current. **electrolyt′ic** *adj*

elec•tro•lyte (e-lek′tro-līt) [*electro-* + Gr. *lytos* that may be dissolved] a substance that dissociates into ions when fused or in solution, and thus becomes capable of conducting electricity; an ionic solute.

amphoteric e. a compound containing at least one group that can act as a base and at least one that can act as an acid; called also *ampholyte*.

colloidal e. an electrolyte in which one or more of the ionic components is of macromolecular dimensions.

elec•tro•mag•net (e-lek″tro-mag′nət) a temporary magnet made by passing an electric current through a coil of wire surrounding a core of soft iron or steel.

elec•tro•mag•net•ic (e-lek″tro-mag-net′ik) involving both electricity and magnetism.

elec•tro•mag•net•ism (e-lek″tro-mag′nə-tiz-əm) 1. magnetism produced by an electric current. 2. the branch of physics relating electricity and magnetism.

elec•tro•ma•nom•e•ter (e-lek″tro-man-om′ə-tər) an electronic instrument for measuring the pressure of gases or liquids.

elec•tro•me•chan•i•cal (e-lek″tro-mə-kan′ĭ-kəl) pertaining to interaction or interconversion of electrical and mechanical energies.

Types of Multiple Electrolytes Injection

Preparation	Ingredients
Multiple Electrolytes Injection Type 1	Sodium, potassium, magnesium, chloride May also contain acetate, acetate and gluconate, or acetate, gluconate, and phosphate
Multiple Electrolytes Injection Type 2	Sodium, potassium, magnesium, chloride May also contain either acetate and citrate or acetate and lactate
Multiple Electrolytes and Dextrose Injection Type 1	Dextrose, sodium, potassium, magnesium, calcium, chloride May also contain acetate, acetate and gluconate, acetate and phosphate, phosphate and lactate, or phosphate and sulfate
Multiple Electrolytes and Dextrose Injection Type 2	Dextrose, sodium, potassium, magnesium, chloride May also contain acetate, acetate and citrate, acetate and lactate, or gluconate and sulfate
Multiple Electrolytes and Dextrose Injection Type 3	Dextrose, sodium, potassium, chloride May also contain ammonium, acetate and phosphate, or phosphate and lactate
Multiple Electrolytes and Dextrose Injection Type 4	Dextrose, sodium, magnesium, calcium, chloride, gluconate, sulfate
Multiple Electrolytes and Invert Sugar Injection Type 1	Equal amounts of dextrose and sucrose*, sodium, potassium, magnesium, chloride, phosphate, lactate
Multiple Electrolytes and Invert Sugar Injection Type 2	Equal amounts of dextrose and sucrose*, sodium, potassium, magnesium, calcium, chloride, lactate
Multiple Electrolytes and Invert Sugar Injection Type 3	Equal amounts of dextrose and sucrose*, sodium, potassium, chloride, ammonium

*Or an equivalent solution produced by hydrolysis of sucrose.

elec•trom•e•ter (e″lek-trom′ə-tər) [*electro-* + *-meter*] an electrostatic instrument for measuring the difference in potential between two points. In radiology, it is used to measure changes in the potential of charged electrodes due to ionization occasioned by radiation.

elec•tro•mi•gra•to•ry (e-lek″tro-mi′grə-tor″e) moving under the influence of electric current.

elec•tro•mo•tive (e-lek″tro-mo′tiv) causing electric activity to be propagated along a conductor.

elec•tro•myo•gram (e-lek″tro-mi′o-gram) the record obtained by electromyography.

elec•tro•myo•graph (e-lek″tro-mi′o-graf) the instrument used in electromyography.

elec•tro•my•og•ra•phy (EMG) (e-lek″tro-mi-og′rə-fe) [*electro-* + *myography*] an electrodiagnostic technique for recording the extracellular activity (action potentials and evoked potentials) of skeletal muscles at rest, during voluntary contractions, and during electrical stimulation; performed using any of a variety of surface electrodes, needle electrodes, and devices for amplifying, transmitting, and recording the signals. **electromyograph′ic** *adj*

single fiber e. (SFEMG) electromyography using a needle electrode to record the action potential of one muscle fiber at a time.

ureteral e. electroureterography.

elec•tron (e-lek′tron) [Gr. *ēlektron* amber, because an electric charge can be produced in amber by rubbing] an elementary particle possessing the unit quantum of (negative) electric charge, 1.6×10^{-19} coulomb, with mass 1/1836 that of a proton, or 9.11×10^{-31} kilogram. Electrons can exist as atomic constituents or in the free state; flowing in a conductor they constitute an electric current; when ejected from a radioactive substance, they constitute beta rays; and when revolving about the nucleus of an atom they determine all of its physical and chemical properties except mass and radioactivity. Symbol e or e^-. See also *atom*.

Auger e. a low-energy electron emitted when an inner electron shell vacancy is created, such as by electron capture or internal conversion.

emission e. one of the electrons released from the atom during radioactive decay.

free e. an electron which is not bound to the nucleus of an atom but may move from one atom nucleus to another.

valence e. one of the electrons in the outermost shell of an atom and thus able to participate in chemical reactions and the formation of chemical bonds.

elec•tro•nar•co•sis (e-lek″tro-nahr-ko′sis) application of an electric current to the brain to alter the level of consciousness, without inducing convulsions; formerly used in the treatment of schizophrenia, but found to be both less effective and more likely to cause side effects than electroconvulsive therapy.

elec•tron-dense (e-lek′tron-dens″) in electron microscopy, having a density that prevents electrons from penetrating.

elec•tro•neg•a•tive (e-lek″tro-neg′ə-tiv) bearing a negative electric charge.

elec•tro•neg•a•tiv•i•ty (e-lek″tro-neg″ə-tiv′ĭ-te) the relative power of an atom or molecule to attract electrons.

elec•tro•neu•rog•ra•phy (e-lek″tro-noo͝-rog′rə-fe) the measurement of the conduction velocity and latency of peripheral nerves.

elec•tro•neu•rol•y•sis (ə-lek″tro-noo-rol′ə-sis) [*electro-* + *neuro-* + *-lysis*] destruction of nerve tissue with an electric needle or electric current.

elec•tro•neu•ro•my•og•ra•phy (e-lek″tro-noor″o-mi-og′rə-fe) electromyography in which the nerve of the muscle under study is stimulated by application of an electric current.

elec•tro•neu•ro•nog•ra•phy (e-lek″tro-noor″on-og′rə-fe) testing for the integrity of the facial nerve by applying an electrical stimulus to it near the stylomastoid foramen and measuring and recording its response.

elec•tron•ic (e″lek-tron′ik) 1. pertaining to electrons. 2. carrying electrons.

elec•tron•ics (e″lek-tron′iks) the science which treats of the conduction of electricity through gases, solids, or a vacuum.

elec•tron-mi•cro•scop•ic (e-lek′tron-mi-kro-skop′ik) visible under the electron microscope.

elec•trono•graph (e″lek-tron′o-graf) electron micrograph.

elec•tron trans•fer fla•vo•pro•tein:ubiq•ui•none ox•i•do•re•duc•tase (e-lek′tron trans′fər fla″vo-pro′tēn u-bik′wə-nōn ok″sĭ-do-re-duk′tās) [EC 1.5.5.1] a component of a side chain of redox reactions by which certain electrons are funneled to ubiquinone and hence to the electron transport chain; the oxidoreductase catalyzes the transfer of electrons from electron transfer flavoprotein (q.v.) to ubiquinone via its FAD prosthetic group and iron-sulfur center. Deficiency of the oxidoreductase, an autosomal recessive trait, causes glutaricaciduria, type II.

elec•tro•nys•tag•mo•gram (e-lek″tro-nis-tag′mo-gram) the record obtained by electronystagmography.

elec•tro•nys•tag•mo•graph (e-lek″tro-nis-tag′mo-graf) an instrument for recording eye movements induced by electrical stimulation; abbreviated ENG.

elec•tro•nys•tag•mog•ra•phy (e-lek″tro-nis″tag-mog′rə-fe) the recording of changes in the corneoretinal potential due to eye movements, providing objective documentation of induced and spontaneous nystagmus.

elec•tro•oc•u•lo•gram (e-lek″tro-ok′u-lo-gram″) the electroencephalographic tracings made by moving the eyes a constant distance between two fixation points, inducing a deflection of fairly constant amplitude; abbreviated EOG.

elec•tro•oc•u•log•ra•phy (e-lek″tro-ok″u-log′rə-fe) the production and interpretation of electro-oculograms.

elec•tro•ol•fac•to•gram (e-lek″tro-ol-fak′to-gram) a recording of electrical potential changes detected by an electrode placed on the surface of the olfactory mucosa as the mucosa is subjected to an odorous stimulus. Abbreviated EOG.

elec•tro•op•ti•cal (e-lek″tro-op′tĭ-kəl) said of devices that sense visual images and can turn them into electrical impulses.

elec•tro•os•mo•sis (e-lek″tro-os-mo′sis) the movement through a membrane of the solvent phase of a colloidal solution when an electric potential is applied by electrodes positioned on either side of the membrane; see also *iontophoresis*.

elec•tro•para•cen•te•sis (e-lek″tro-par″ə-sen-te′sis) puncture of the eyeball with a needle, using galvanic current and holding the needle in position until bubbles of hydrogen appear in the aqueous humor.

elec•tro•pa•thol•o•gy (e-lek″tro-pə-thol′ə-je) [*electro-* + *pathology*] the study of pathologic conditions of the body as revealed by electricity.

elec•tro•phar•ma•co•log•ic (e-lek″tro-fahr″mə-ko-loj′ik) pertaining to the effects of drugs upon conduction of electrical impulses in the body, such as in the heart.

elec•tro•phero•gram (e-lek″tro-fer′o-gram) electrophoretogram.

elec•tro•phile (e-lek′tro-fīl) an electron acceptor that is covalently bonded to a nucleophile.

elec•tro•phil•ic (e-lek″tro-fil′ik) having an affinity for electrons; serving as an electrophile.

elec•tro•pho•re•gram (e-lek″tro-fo′rə-gram) electrophoretogram.

elec•tro•pho•re•sis (e-lek″tro-fə-re′sis) [*electro-* + *phoresis*] the separation of ionic solutes based on differences in their rates of migration in an applied electric field. **electrophoret′ic** *adj*

agarose gel e. a type of gel electrophoresis with agarose as the support medium; used extensively to separate proteins, lipoproteins, nucleic acids, and other substances.

cellulose acetate e. a method of zone electrophoresis in which the support medium is a sheet of cellulose acetate; used mainly in clinical chemistry to analyze or purify serum proteins.

counter e. counterimmunoelectrophoresis.

disc e. a method of polyacrylamide gel electrophoresis involving discontinuous (hence the name) gel layers. A discontinuity in pore size and pH between the layers is used to prevent diffusion and maximize separation of the components.

gel e. a type of zone electrophoresis in which the support medium is a gel, in the form of tubes or a thin slab; it is usually composed of agarose, polyacrylamide, or starch and is so named. Specific types are used to separate certain classes of molecules on the basis of change, size, or both.

moving boundary e. the original method of electrophoresis, in which the movement of the solvent is unrestricted and all of the particles of a species move at the same rate, maintaining a sharp boundary which can be optically monitored.

paper e. an older method of zone electrophoresis in which the support medium is paper, mainly used to separate serum proteins.

polyacrylamide gel e. (PAGE) gel electrophoresis using a polymerized polyacrylamide matrix to separate molecules on the basis of size, charge, or both; usually used to separate proteins or sequence nucleic acids. Gels are usually discontinuous (see *disc e.*) but may be a single layer, and are either nondenaturing to examine native molecules or denaturing as in SDS-PAGE.

protein e. see *serum protein e.* and *urine protein e.*

pulsed-field e. a method of gel electrophoresis used to separate fragments of DNA as long as several million bases by subjecting the gel to an electrical current alternately delivered from two angles in timed intervals, which minimizes diffusion of large molecules.

SDS–polyacrylamide gel e. (SDS-PAGE) a type of polyacrylamide gel electrophoresis in which the anionic detergent sodium dodecyl sulfate (SDS) is used to denature the sample proteins into linear monomers, rendering their charge proportional to their length so that migration is a function of size.

serum protein e. an assay for presence of M component in the serum, indicative of plasma cell dyscrasias.

single-cell gel e. a type of gel electrophoresis used to detect the genotoxic potential of environmental hazards such as radiation, heavy metals, and toxic chemicals. Such agents may cause breaks in the nuclear DNA of cells. When such a cell is lysed and exposed to electrophoresis that denatures its DNA, the damaged DNA moves toward the electric field, making a formation like the tail of a comet. Called also *comet assay.*

starch gel e. an older form of gel electrophoresis using a hydrolyzed starch support matrix to separate macromolecules, particularly proteins.

two-dimensional gel e. a method of gel electrophoresis used for improved separation of complex mixtures of molecules by subjecting the support medium to electrophoresis in two directions, usually at right angles to each other, such as isoelectric focusing followed by SDS–polyacrylamide gel electrophoresis.

urine protein e. an assay for presence of M component in the urine, indicative of plasma cell dyscrasias.

zonal e., zone e. any of several methods of electrophoresis in which an inert support medium holds the molecules as they migrate in the conducting medium, thus preventing convection and diffusion.

elec•tro•pho•reto•gram (e-lek″tro-fə-ret′o-gram) the record produced on or in a supporting medium by bands of material which have been separated by the process of electrophoresis. Called also *electropherogram* and *electrophoregram.*

elec•troph•o•rus (e″lek-trof′o-rəs) [*electro-* + Gr. *phoros* bearing] an instrument for obtaining static electricity by means of induction.

elec•tro•pho•tom•e•ter (e-lek″tro-fo-tom′ə-tər) an instrument equipped with a photoelectric sensor for colorimetric determinations.

elec•tro•phren•ic (e-lek″tro-fren′ik) pertaining to electrical stimulation of the phrenic nerve or diaphragm; see under *respiration.*

elec•tro•phys•i•ol•o•gy (e-lek″tro-fiz″e-ol′ə-je) 1. the study of the mechanisms of production of electrical phenomena, particularly in the nervous system, and their consequences in the living organism. 2. the study of the effects electricity has on physiologic phenomena. **electrophysiolog′ic** *adj*

cardiac e., clinical cardiac e. the mechanisms, functions, and performance of the electrical activities of specific regions of the heart; the term is usually used in describing studies of such phenomena by invasive (intracardiac) recording of spontaneous activity as well as of cardiac responses to programmed stimuli. The studies are performed to assess complex arrhythmias, elucidate symptoms, evaluate abnormal electrocardiograms, assess risk, and design treatment; they increasingly include therapeutic methods in addition to diagnostic and prognostic procedures.

elec•tro•plat•ing (e-lek″tro-plāt′ing) plating or coating of an object with a layer of metal through the use of electrolytic processes. See also *electroplated die*, under *die.*

elec•tro•plexy (e-lek′tro-plek″se) [*electro-* + *-plexy*] electric shock.

elec•tro•po•ra•tion (e-lek″tro-pə-ra′shən) the application of an electric field to cause a reversible creation of porelike openings in the plasma membrane of a cell, through which nucleic acids may be introduced.

elec•tro•pos•i•tive (e-lek″tro-poz′ĭ-tiv) [*electro-* + *positive*] bearing a positive electric charge.

elec•tro•ra•di•om•e•ter (e-lek″tro-ra″de-om′ə-tər) an electroscope for measuring radiant energy.

elec•tro•re•sec•tion (e-lek″tro-re-sek′shən) excision performed by electrosurgery.

elec•tro•ret•i•no•gram (e-lek″tro-ret′ĭ-no-gram) the record obtained by electroretinography; abbreviated ERG.

elec•tro•ret•in•o•graph (e-lek″tro-ret′ĭ-no-graf) an instrument for measuring the electrical response of the retina to light stimulation; abbreviated ERG.

elec•tro•ret•i•nog•ra•phy (e-lek″tro-ret″ĭ-nog′rə-fe) the recording of the changes in electric potential in the retina after stimulation by light.

elec•tro•sa•li•vo•gram (e-lek″tro-sə-li′vo-gram) [*electro-* + *saliva* + *-gram*] a graphic record or curve showing the action potential of the salivary glands, obtained with an electrically operated instrument.

elec•tro•scis•sion (e-lek″tro-sizh′ən) the cutting of tissue by means of an electrocautery.

elec•tro•scope (e-lek′tro-skōp) [*electro-* + *-scope*] an instrument for measuring the intensity of radiation by detecting the motion imparted to charged strips suspended from a conductor.

elec•tro•sec•tion (e-lek″tro-sek′shən) an incision made by means of an electrocautery.

elec•tro•shock (e-lek′tro-shok) shock produced by application of electric current to the brain; see *electroconvulsive therapy*, under *therapy.*

elec•tro•sleep (e-lek′tro-slēp) the use of low-intensity electricity, below the threshold for inducing convulsions; formerly used in the treatment of insomnia, anxiety, and depression.

elec•tro•sol (e-lek′tro-sol) a colloidal solution of a metal obtained by passing electric sparks through distilled water between poles formed of the metal.

elec•tro•spec•tro•gram (e-lek″tro-spek′trə-gram) a record produced in electrospectrography.

elec•tro•spec•trog•ra•phy (e-lek″tro-spek-trog′rə-fe) the isolation and recording of the constituent wave systems that are merged in an electroencephalogram.

elec•tro•spi•no•gram (e-lek″tro-spi′no-gram) a tracing of the action potential of the spinal cord.

elec•tro•stat•ic (e-lek″tro-stat′ik) pertaining to static electricity.

elec•tro•ste•nol•y•sis (e-lek″tro-stə-nol′ə-sis) the oxidation and reduction which occur on opposite surfaces of a high resistance membrane in a solution when there is a steep electric potential gradient across the membrane, reduction occurring on the surface facing the anode.

elec•tro•stim•u•la•tion (e-lek″tro-stim″u-la′shən) electrical stimulation of tissues, as for therapeutic or experimental purposes.

elec•tro•stri•a•to•gram (e-lek″tro-stri-āt′o-gram) a record of waves derived by the bipolar technique from the several structures of the corpus striatum.

elec•tro•sur•gery (e-lek″tro-sur′jər-e) surgical procedures performed using an electrocautery; called also *surgical diathermy.*

elec•tro•syn•the•sis (e-lek″tro-sin′thə-sis) chemical reactions effected by means of electricity.

elec•tro•tax•is (e-lek″tro-tak′sis) [*electro-* + *-taxis*] the movement of organisms or cells under the influence of electric currents.

elec•tro•ther•a•pist (e-lek″tro-ther′ə-pist) a person trained in using electricity for therapeutic purposes.

elec•tro•ther•a•py (e-lek″tro-ther′ə-pe) treatment of disease by means of electricity.

cerebral e. electrosleep.

elec•tro•tome (e-lek′tro-tōm) [*electro-* + *-tome*] an electrical surgical cutting instrument.

elec•trot•o•my (e-lek-trot′ə-me) electroexcision with low current, high voltage, and high frequency; a procedure in which the tissues are not coagulated.

elec•tro•ton•ic (e-lek″tro-ton′ik) 1. pertaining to electrotonus. 2. denoting the direct spread of current in tissues by electrical conduction, without the generation of new current by action potentials.

elec•trot•o•nus (e-lek-trot′ə-nəs) the altered electrical state of a nerve or muscle cell when a constant electric current is passed through it.

elec•trot•ro•pism (e″lek-trot′ro-piz-əm) [*electro-* + *tropism*] the tendency of a cell or organism to react in a definite manner in response to an electric stimulus.

negative e. the tendency of a cell to be repelled by an electric stimulus.

positive e. the tendency of a cell to be attracted by an electric stimulus.

elec•tro•ul•tra•fil•tra•tion (e-lek″tro-ul″trə-fil-tra′shən) ultrafiltration in an electric field.

elec•tro•ure•tero•gram (e-lek″tro-u-re′tər-o-gram) the record obtained by electroureterography.

elec•tro•u•re•ter•og•ra•phy (e-lek″tro-u-re″tər-og′rə-fe) electromyography in which the action potentials produced by peristalsis of the ureter are recorded.

elec•tro•va•go•gram (e-lek″tro-va′go-gram) vagogram.

elec•tro•va•lence (e-lek″tro-va′ləns) 1. the number of charges an atom acquires by the gain or loss of electrons in forming an ionic bond. 2. the ionic bonding resulting from such a transfer of electrons.

elec•tro•va•lent (e-lek″tro-va′lənt) pertaining to electrovalence or to an ionic bond.

elec•tro•ver•sion (e-lek″tro-vur′zhən) the act of electrically terminating a cardiac dysrhythmia.

elec•tro•vi•bra•to•ry (e-lek″tro-vi′brə-tor″e) pertaining to electrically induced vibration.

elec•tu•ary (e-lek′tu-ar″e) [Gr. *ekleichein* to lick up] a medicinal preparation consisting of a powdered drug made into a paste with honey or syrup.

el•e•doi•sin (el-ə-doi′sin) an endecapeptide from the posterior salivary gland of a species of small octopus *(Eledone)*, which is a precursor of a large group of biologically active peptides. It has vasodilator, hypotensive, and extravascular smooth muscle stimulant properties.

el·e·i·din (el-e′ĭ-din) a protein chemically related to keratin, found in the cells of the stratum lucidum of the skin.

el·e·ment (el′ə-mənt) [L. *elementum*] 1. any of the constituent parts of which a more complex entity is composed. 2. in chemistry, a simple substance which cannot be decomposed by chemical means and which is made up of atoms which are alike in their peripheral electronic configurations and so in their chemical properties, and also in the number of protons in their nuclei, but which may differ in the number of neutrons in their nuclei and so in their atomic weight and in their radioactive properties. See Appendix 5. 3. in the philosophies underlying some complementary medicine systems, a member of a group of basic substances that give rise to everything that exists; see *five e's.*

anatomic e. morphologic e.

appendicular e's a set of cartilaginous rods attached to the chondral cranium of the embryo; from them are developed the auditory ossicles, the hyoid bone, and the styloid process.

electronegative e. any chemical element that adds electrons (or tends to add electrons) during chemical combination.

electropositive e. a chemical element that loses electrons (or tends to lose electrons) during chemical combination.

F e. see under *plasmid.*

five e's 1. see under *phase.* 2. in ayurvedic tradition, the basic entities (earth, air, fire, water, and space) whose interaction gives rise to material existence.

formed e's of the blood the blood cells; see under *cell.*

IS e. insertion sequence.

labile e. tissue cells which continue to multiply during the life of the individual.

mobile e. transposable e.

morphologic e. any cell, fiber, or other of the ultimate structures which go to make up tissues and organs.

radioactive e. a chemical element that spontaneously transmutes into another element with emission of corpuscular or electromagnetic radiations. The natural radioactive elements are all those with atomic numbers above 83, and certain other elements, such as potassium (at. no. 19) and rubidium (at. no. 37) are weakly radioactive.

rare earth e's elements of the lanthanum series, comprising elements with atomic numbers 57 to 71.

sarcous e. any of the elementary granules into which the primordial fibril of an elementary muscle fiber is divisible.

stable e. 1. a chemical element that does not spontaneously transmute into another element with emission of corpuscular or electromagnetic radiations; the stable elements are those with atomic number below 84, except for a few, such as potassium and rubidium, which are weakly radioactive. 2. a tissue cell of mature tissues which does not alter by mitosis.

tissue e. morphologic e.

trace e's chemical elements that are distributed throughout the tissues in very small amounts and are essential in nutrition, such as cobalt, copper, magnesium, manganese, selenium, and zinc; for optimal bioavailability they must be in a balanced mixture, and they may be harmful or toxic in excess.

transcalifornium e's the elements with atomic numbers higher than that of californium, and discovered subsequent to its discovery in 1950. They are einsteinium 99, fermium 100, mendelevium 101, nobelium 102, and lawrencium 103.

transposable e. a segment of DNA that can move from one genomic location to another. At its simplest, it encodes one or more enzymes necessary for transposition and is flanked by inverted repeats. Examples include insertion sequences, transposons, and some bacteriophages. The term, however, is sometimes used interchangeably with *transposon.*

transuranic e's, transuranium e's the elements with atomic numbers higher than that of uranium. Applied originally to neptunium 93, plutonium 94, americium 95, curium 96, berkelium 97, and californium 98, the term now, by definition, includes the transcalifornium elements as well.

el·e·men·ta·ry (el″ə-men′tə-re) not resolvable or divisible into simpler parts or components; see also under *particle.*

ele(o)- [Gr. *elaion* oil] a combining form denoting relationship to oil.

el·e·o·ma (el″e-o′mə) [*eleo-* + *-oma*] a tumor or swelling caused by the injection of oil into the tissues.

el·e·om·e·ter (el″e-om′ə-tər) [*eleo-* + *-meter*] an instrument for determining the percentage of oil in a mixture, or the specific gravity of oils.

el·e·op·tene (el″e-op′tēn) [*eleo-* + Gr. *ptēnos* volatile] the more volatile constituent of a volatile oil, as distinguished from its stearoptene.

el·eo·sac·cha·rum (el″e-o-sak′ə-rəm) oleosaccharum.

el·eo·ther·a·py (el″e-o-ther′ə-pe) [*eleo-* + *therapy*] oleotherapy.

el·e·phan·ti·a·sis (el″ə-fən-ti′ə-sis) [Gr. *elephas* elephant + *-iasis*] 1. lymphedema secondary to chronic obstruction of lymphatic vessels, with hypertrophy of the skin and subcutaneous tissues (pachyderma), usually of a lower limb or the scrotum. It is a filarial disease generally seen in the tropics due to infection of the lymphatics with any of the nematodes *Wuchereria bancrofti, Brugia malayi,* or *B. timori.* It begins with lymphangitis and enlargement of the part, along with chills and fever (elephantoid fever); this is followed by formation of ulcers and tubercles, with thickening, discoloration, and fissuring of the skin. See also *bancroftian filariasis* and *Malayan filariasis,* under *filariasis.* 2. hypertrophy and thickening of the tissues from any cause. **elephanti′asic** *adj*

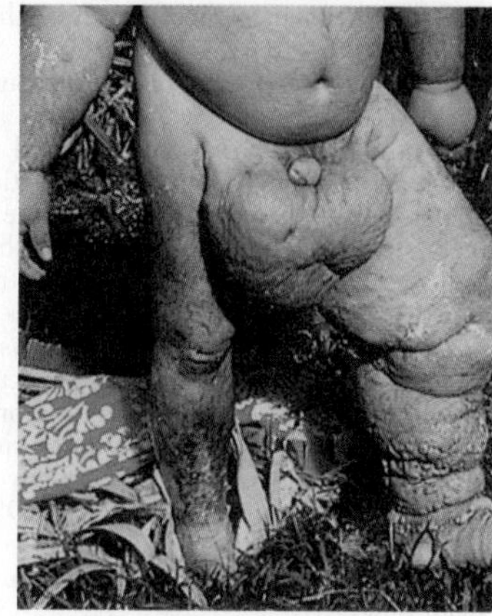

■ Elephantiasis of the leg and scrotum.

e. chirur′gica massive lymphedema of the arm after mastectomy.

congenital e. see under *lymphedema.*

e. gingi′vae fibromatosis gingivae.

lymphangiectatic e. the usual type of elephantiasis, caused by lymphangiectasis in the part.

e. neuromato′sa elephantiasis due to neurofibromatosis.

e. nos′tras lymphedema, usually on the lower limb, due to either chronic recurrent erysipelas or chronic recurrent cellulitis.

e. o′culi thickening and protrusion of the eyelids.

e. scro′ti elephantiasis in which the scrotum is the principal seat of the disease; called also *chylocele* and *lymph scrotum.*

el·e·phan·toid (el″ĕ-fan′toid) relating to or resembling elephantiasis.

El Es·co·ri·al criteria (el es″ko-re-ahl′) [*El Escorial,* Spain, location of a workshop in 1990 that drew up the original set of criteria] see under *criterion.*

el·e·trip·tan hy·dro·bro·mide (el″ə-trip′tan) a selective serotonin receptor agonist with actions similar to those of sumatriptan, used in the treatment of migraine; administered orally

El·et·ta·ria (el″ə-ta′re-ə) a genus of herbs of the family Zingiberaceae, native to Indonesia. *E. cardamo′mum* is cardamom, the usual source of the spice called cardamom (q.v.).

eleu·the·ro (ĕ-loo′thə-ro) [shortened from *Eleutherococcus*] Siberian ginseng.

Eleu·the·ro·coc·cus (ĕ-loo′thə-ro-kok″əs) a genus of shrubs native to northeastern Asia, including the species *E. sentico′sus,* the Siberian ginseng, whose root is used medicinally.

el·e·va·tion (el″ə-va′shən) a raised area, or point of greater height.

tactile e's toruli tactiles.

el·e·va·tor (el′ə-va″tər) [L. *elevare* to lift] an instrument for lifting tissues, removing bone fragments, or removing roots of teeth.

angular e. an elevator in which the blade angles from the shank to the right or to the left.

apical e. an instrument for removing fractured root tips retained in the apex of the tooth socket following tooth extraction; its shank has an angle to provide access within the socket and its tip has a barb for reaching a fractured root tip. Called also *apical pick* and *root pick.*

cross bar e. an elevator in which the handle is at a right angle to the shank. Called also T-*bar e.*

Cryer e. a dental instrument for removing the roots of molar teeth; furnished in pairs, one for mesial and one for distal roots, which are reversed for use on opposite sides of the jaw.

dental e. an instrument having a blade that engages the teeth or their roots and extracts teeth by elevating them from their alveoli through leverage applied to the handle.

malar e. an instrument used to elevate or reposition the zygomatic bone and/or arch.

periosteum e. a flat steel bar for separating the attachments of the periosteum to bone.

root e. a dental elevator for extracting a fractured root of a tooth; they may be designed in pairs, a right and a left, and as single, straight, mitered, or double ended.

screw e. a dental instrument designed to be screwed into a root canal for subsequent removal of the root, usually of the apical third.

straight e. an elevator in which the shank continues in a straight line with the handle.

T-bar e. cross bar e.

wedge e. an elevator used as a lever in tooth extraction, being placed in a hole drilled into the root of the tooth below the investing bony tissue to rework a tooth.

el•faz•e•pam (el-faz′ə-pəm) a benzodiazepine used as a veterinary appetite stimulant.

El•gi•loy (el′jĭ-loi) a corrosion-resistant alloy of cobalt and chromium, used in stents, prosthetic heart valves, and other devices placed inside the body.

El•i•del (el′ĭ-del) trademark for a preparation of pimecrolimus.

elim•i•nant (e-lim′ĭ-nənt) evacuant.

elim•i•na•tion (e-lim″ĭ-na′shən) [L. *eliminatio*, from *e* out + *limen* threshold] 1. the act of expulsion or of extrusion, especially of expulsion from the body. See *excretion*, *defecation*, *urination*, and *clearance*. 2. omission or exclusion, as in an elimination diet.

immune e. the period of accelerated degradation of antigen (e.g., foreign gamma globulin) as a result of its removal and destruction by antibodies. Also, a technique for determining antibody response by measuring the rate of removal of labeled antigen from the circulation of an immunized animal. Called also *immune clearance*.

El•i•mite (el′ĭ-mīt) trademark for a preparation of permethrin.

el•i•nin (el′ĭ-nin) a lipoprotein fraction of red cells containing the Rh and A and B factors.

ELISA (e-li′sə) [*e*nzyme-*l*inked *i*mmuno*s*orbent *a*ssay] any enzyme immunoassay utilizing an enzyme-labeled immunoreactant (antigen or antibody) and an immunosorbent (antigen or antibody bound to a solid support). A variety of methods (e.g., competitive binding between the labeled reactant and unlabeled unknown, or a sandwich technique in which the unknown binds both the immunosorbent and labeled antibody) may be used to measure the unknown concentration.

Eli•tek (el′ĭ-tek) trademark for a preparation of rasburicase.

elix•ir (e-lik′sər) [L., from Arabic] a clear, sweetened, alcohol-containing, usually hydroalcoholic liquid containing flavoring substances and sometimes active medicinal agents.

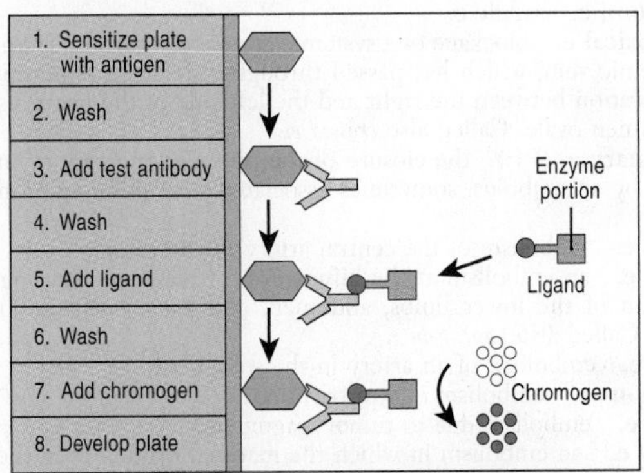

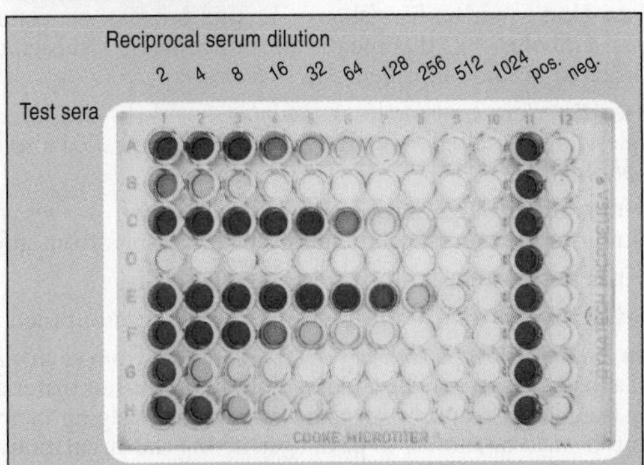

■ ELISA (enzyme-linked immunoassay) used to detect a test antibody, showing the technique *(top)* and a developed plate *(bottom)*. The results are quantitated by colorimetric scanning of the plate.

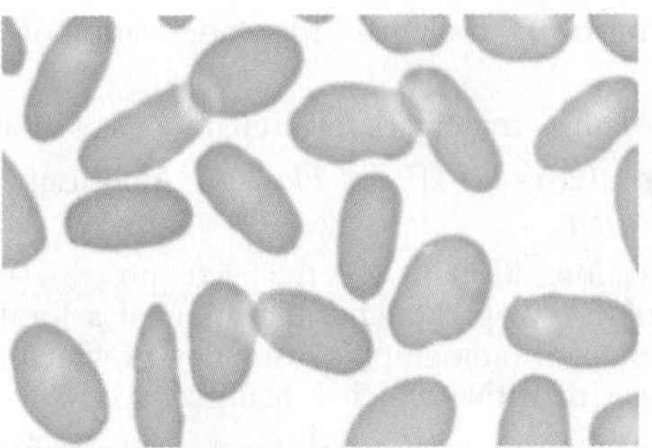

■ Elliptocytes.

aromatic e. [NF] an elixir prepared by filtration of a mixture of essential oils, such as orange, lemon, coriander, and anise oils, syrup, talc, alcohol, and purified water; used as a flavored vehicle for pharmaceutical preparations.

compound benzaldehyde e. [USP] a preparation of 0.05 per cent benzaldehyde, in a suitably flavored and sweetened hydroalcoholic liquid; used as a flavored vehicle for pharmaceutical preparations.

terpin hydrate e. [USP] a preparation containing, in each 100 mL, between 1.53 and 1.87 g of terpin hydrate, as well as sweet orange peel tincture, benzaldehyde, glycerin, alcohol, syrup, and purified water; used as an expectorant.

terpin hydrate and codeine e. [USP] a preparation containing, in 100 mL, between 1.53 and 1.87 g of terpin hydrate and between 180 and 220 mg of codeine, prepared by dissolving 2 g codeine in a sufficient quantity of terpin hydrate elixir to make 1000 mL; used as an expectorant and antitussive.

Elix•o•phyl•lin (e-lik″so-fil′in) trademark for preparations of theophylline.

Eli•za•beth•king•ia (e-liz″ə-beth-king′e-ə) [Elizabeth O. *King*, American bacteriologist, 20th century] a genus of gram-negative bacteria of the family Flavobacteriaceae, consisting of aerobic non–spore-forming, nonmotile, chemo-organotrophic, oxidase- and catalase-positive rods. The type species is *E. meningosep′tica*.

E. meningosep′tica a pathogenic species that is a major cause of nosocomial infections, producing meningitis and septicemia with a high fatality rate in premature and newborn infants. In adults, it causes a milder bacteremia. Formerly called *Flavobacterium meningosepticum*.

El•lence (ə-lens′) trademark for a preparation of epirubicin hydrochloride.

El•li•ot position (el′e-ət) [John Wheelock *Elliot*, American surgeon, 1852–1925] see under *position*.

El•li•ot sign (el′e-ət) [George T. *Elliot*, American dermatologist, 1851–1935] see under *sign*.

el•lip•sin (e-lip′sin) the insoluble constituents of cells which remain after the removal of the soluble proteins.

el•lip•soid (e-lip′soid) [Gr. *ellipēs (kyklos)*, defective (circle) + *-oid*] 1. any structure shaped like an oval or a spindle. 2. Schweigger-Seidel sheath. 3. in ophthalmology, the acidophilic outer region of the inner segment of the dendritic process of a retinal rod or cone, lying between the cilium and the myoid, and containing some glycogen and many mitochondria; called also *visual cell e.*

el•lip•to•cyte (e-lip′to-sīt) an abnormal oval-shaped erythrocyte, as seen in elliptocytosis. Called also *ovalocyte*. **elliptocyt′ic** *adj*

el•lip•to•cy•to•sis (e-lip″to-si-to′sis) presence of large numbers of elliptocytes in the blood; called also *ovalocytosis*.

hereditary e. any of a number of hereditary disorders in which 30 to 100 per cent of the erythrocytes are elliptocytes. In many patients there are no symptoms, but others show varying degrees of erythrocyte destruction and hemolytic anemia. Both autosomal dominant and recessive varieties are known. Called also *Dresbach syndrome* and *elliptocytic anemia*.

spherocytic e. a hereditary condition characterized by both elliptocytes and spherocytes that are osmotically and mechanically fragile; most patients have moderate hemolytic anemia and are at risk for aplastic crises.

El•lis-van Crev•eld syndrome (el′is vahn kre′veld) [Richard White Bernhard *Ellis*, Scottish pediatrician, 1902–1966; Simon *van Creveld*, Dutch pediatrician, 1894–1971] see *chondroectodermal dysplasia*, under *dysplasia*.

elm (elm) 1. any tree of the genus *Ulmus*. 2. [USP] slippery elm bark; the dried inner bark of the slippery elm *Ulmus rubra*, used as a demulcent.

slippery e. a deciduous tree of eastern North America, *Ulmus rubra* Muhlenberg (*U. fulva* Michaux), the source of elm [USP]; see also under *bark*.

El•mi•ron (el′mĭ-ron) trademark for a preparation of pentosan polysulfate sodium.

El•o•con (el′o-kon) trademark for preparations of mometasone furoate.

Eloes•ser flap (el-es′ər) [Leo *Eloesser*, American surgeon, 1881–1976] see under *flap*.

elon•ga•tion (e″long-a′shən) 1. the act, process, or condition of increasing in length. 2. pathologic migration of a tooth in the occlusal or incisal direction. 3. radiographic distortion in which the image is proportionately longer than that which is being x-rayed.

Elox•a•tin (e-lok′sə-tin) trademark for a preparation of oxaliplatin.

Els•berg test (els′bərg) [Charles Albert *Elsberg*, New York surgeon, 1871–1948] see under *test*.

Elsch•nig bodies (pearls) (elsh′nig) [Anton Philipp *Elschnig*, Austrian ophthalmologist, 1863–1939] see under *body*.

El•spar (el′spahr) trademark for a preparation of L-asparaginase derived from *Escherichia coli* for use as an antineoplastic agent.

El Tor vibrio (el tor′) [*El Tor* Quarantine Station on the Egyptian Sinai Peninsula, where it was first isolated in 1960] *Vibrio cholerae* biovar *eltor*.

el•u•ate (el′u-āt) the substance separated out by, or the product of, elution or elutriation.

elu•ent (e-loo′ənt) a solution used in elution.

elu•tion (e-loo′shən) [L. *e* out + *luere* to wash] in chemistry, the separation of material by washing, as in the freeing of an enzyme from its absorbent.

membrane e. a method of selecting cells in which a culture of cells is collected on a membrane filter and a fresh warm culture fluid is subsequently passed slowly over it, washing off excess cells and leaving only adsorbed cells at a particular developmental stage.

elu•tri•a•tion (e-loo″tre-a′shən) [L. *elutriare* to wash out] the operation of pulverizing substances and mixing them with water in order to separate the heavier constituents, which settle out in solution, from the lighter constituents.

counterflow centrifugal e. subjection of a cell population to elutriation and then centrifugation in order to separate particles according to sedimentation coefficients.

Ely test (sign) (e′li) [Leonard Wheeler *Ely*, American orthopedic surgeon, 1868–1944] see under *test*.

Em emmetropia.

em- see *en-*.

ema•ci•a•tion (e-ma″she-a′shən) [L. *emaciare* to make lean] excessive leanness; a wasted condition of the body.

EMACO a cancer chemotherapy regimen consisting of etoposide, methotrexate, actinomycin D, cyclophosphamide, and Oncovin (vincristine).

Ema•dine (em′ədēn) trademark for a preparation of emedastine hydrochloride.

em•an (em′ən) a unit for expressing the concentration of radium emanation in solution: it is the concentration present when one tenth of a millimicrocurie of radium emanation is dissolved in 1 liter of air or water, or 10^{-10} curie.

em•a•na•tion (em″ə-na′shən) [L. *e* out + *manare* to flow] that which is given off, such as a gaseous disintegration product given off from radioactive substances.

eman•ci•pa•tion (e-man″sĭ-pa′shən) [L. *emancipare* to release, give up] the establishment of local autonomy within restricted fields of a developing embryo.

emas•cu•late (e-mas′ku-lāt) to castrate a male.

emas•cu•la•tion (e-mas″ku-la′shən) [L. *emasculare* to castrate] bilateral orchiectomy.

EMB eosin–methylene blue (see under *agar*); ethambutol.

em•balm•ing (em-bahm′ing) the treatment of the dead body with antiseptics and preservatives, to prevent putrefaction.

em•bar•rass (əm-bar′əs) to impede the function of; to obstruct.

Emb•den es•ter (em′dən) [Gustav Georg *Embden*, German biochemist, 1874–1933] see under *ester*.

Emb•den-Mey•er•hof pathway (em′dən mi′ər-hof) [G.G. *Embden;* Otto Fritz *Meyerhof*, German physiologist, 1884–1951] see under *pathway*.

Emb•den-Mey•er•hof-Par•nas pathway (em′den mi′ər-hof pahr′nahs) [G.G. *Embden;* O.F. *Meyerhof;* Jakub Karol *Parnas*, Polish biochemist, 1884–1949] see *Embden-Meyerhof pathway*, under *pathway*.

em•bed•ding (əm-bed′ing) the fixation of a tissue specimen in a firm medium, in order to keep it intact during the cutting of thin sections.

Em•be•lia (em-be′le-ə) a genus of East Indian climbing plants of the family Myrsinaceae. *E. ri′bes* (called also *E. robus′ta*) is a species whose fruit has been used for its anthelminthic and cathartic principles.

em•bo•la•lia (em″bo-la′le-ə) embololalia.

em•bole (em′bə-le) [Gr. *embolē* a throwing in] 1. the reducing of a dislocated limb. 2. emboly.

em•bo•lec•to•my (em″bə-lek′tə-me) [*embolus* + *-ectomy*] surgical removal of an embolus.

em•bo•li (em′bə-li) [L.] plural of *embolus*.

em•bo•lia (em-bo′le-ə) embole.

e. cu′tis medicamento′sa Nicolau syndrome.

em•bol•ic (em-bol′ik) pertaining to an embolus or to embolism.

em•bol•i•form (em-bol′ĭ-form) resembling an embolus.

em•bo•lism (em′bə-liz-əm) [L. *embolus*, q.v.] the sudden blocking of an artery by a clot or foreign material which has been brought to its site of lodgment by the blood current.

air e. an embolism due to air bubbles entering the veins from trauma, surgical procedures, or severe decompression sickness. Called also *aeroembolism*.

amniotic fluid e. an embolism due to amniotic fluid in the maternal circulation.

artery-to-artery e. the breaking off of a piece of an embolus in a large artery and its subsequent occlusion of a smaller artery.

bacillary e. obstruction of a vessel by an aggregation of bacilli.

bland e. an embolism whose thrombotic plug is composed of nonseptic material.

bone marrow e. an embolism caused by material from a fractured long bone.

capillary e. blocking of the capillaries with bacteria.

cerebral e. embolism of a cerebral artery.

cholesterol e., cholesterol crystal e. an embolism resulting from fracture of a plaque of atherosclerosis.

coronary e. embolism of one of the coronary arteries.

crossed e. paradoxical e.

direct e. an embolism that travels in the direction of the bloodstream.

fat e. an embolism caused by fat that has entered the circulation, especially after fractures of long bones, or after corticosteroid administration. Called also *oil e.* See also *fat embolism syndrome*, under *syndrome*.

lymph e., lymphogenous e. embolism of a lymph vessel.

miliary e. embolism in which small emboli affect a number of small vessels at the same time.

multiple e. embolism by a number of small emboli.

oil e. fat e.

pantaloon e. saddle e.

paradoxical e. blockage of a systemic artery by a thrombus originating in a systemic vein, which has passed through a defect that permits direct communication between the right and the left side of the heart, usually an open foramen ovale. Called also *crossed e.*

pulmonary e. (PE) the closure of the pulmonary artery or one of its branches by an embolus, sometimes associated with pulmonary infarction (q.v.).

retinal e. embolism of the central artery of the retina.

saddle e. an embolism at the bifurcation of the aorta, causing sudden severe pain of the lower limbs, abdomen, and back, with numbing and coldness. Called also *pantaloon e.*

spinal e. embolism of an artery in the spinal cord.

trichinous e. embolism due to trichinae.

tumor e. embolism due to tumor fragments.

venous e. an embolism in which the material originates in the veins.

em•bo•li•za•tion (em″bə-lĭ-za′shən) 1. the process or condition of becoming an embolus. 2. therapeutic introduction of a substance into a vessel in order to occlude it; called also *embolotherapy*.

em•bo•lo•la•lia (em″bə-lo-la′le-ə) [*embolus* + *-lalia*] the interpolation of meaningless or unintelligible words into the speech; called also *embolalia* and *embolophrasia*.

em•bo•lo•my•cot•ic (em″bə-lo-mi-kot′ik) [*embolus* + *mycotic* (def. 3)] pertaining to or caused by an embolism that results from infection.

em•bo•lo•phra•sia (em″bə-lo-fra′zhə) embololalia.

em•bo•lo•ther•a•py (em″bo-lo-ther′ə-pe) embolization (def. 2).

em•bo•lus (em′bo-ləs) pl. *em′boli* [Gr. *embolos* plug, from *en* in + *ballein* to throw] 1. a mass, which may be a blood clot or some other material, that is brought by the bloodstream through the vasculature, lodging in a vessel or bifurcation too small to allow it to pass, obstructing the circulation. See also *embolism*. 2. nucleus emboliformis.

air e. an embolus composed of an air bubble; see also under *embolism*.

bullet e. migration of a bullet within a blood vessel; arterial emboli cause ischemia and possibly limb amputation and venous emboli may

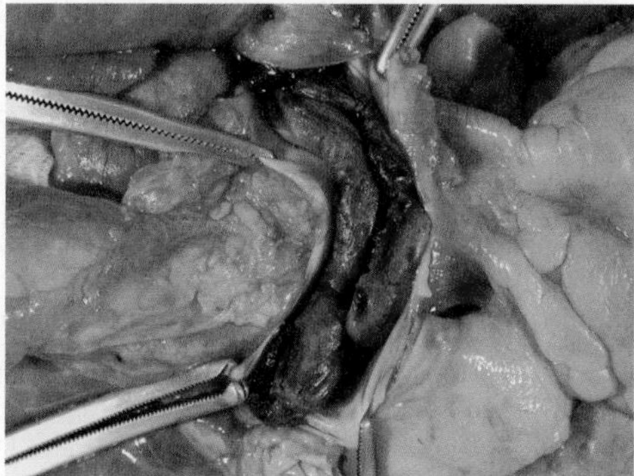

■ Saddle embolus at the bifurcation of the pulmonary artery.

travel to the pulmonary artery or heart, causing bacterial endocarditis, pericardial effusion, myocardiac irritability, or valve mechanism interference.

cancer e. tumor e.

fat e. an embolus composed of oil or fat. See also under *embolism.*

foam e. an embolus formed by a mixture of a gas and blood.

obturating e. an embolus that completely blocks a vessel.

riding e., saddle e., straddling e. an embolus at the bifurcation of an artery, blocking both branches. See illustration. See also *saddle embolism,* under *embolism.*

tumor e. an embolus composed of tumor cells; see also under *embolism.* Called also *cancer e.*

em•bo•ly (em′bə-le) [Gr. *embolē* a throwing in] the invagination of the blastula by which the gastrula is formed.

em•bouche•ment (ahm-bo͞osh-maw′) [Fr.] the opening of one vessel into another.

em•bra•sure (em-bra′zhər) a space continuous with an interproximal space, produced by curvatures of teeth in contact in the same arch, that provides a channel or passage through which food escapes from the occlusal surfaces of the teeth during mastication. Called also *spillway.*

buccal e. the embrasure opening out toward the cheek between molar and premolar teeth.

incisal e. occlusal e.

interdental e. the space formed by the interproximal contours of adjoining teeth, beginning at the contact area and extending lingually, facially, occlusally, and apically.

labial e. the embrasure that widens out from the area of contact toward the lips between the canine and incisor teeth.

lingual e. the embrasure that widens out from the area of contact toward the lingual sides of the teeth.

occlusal e. the space bounded by the marginal ridges as they join the cusps and incisal ridges. Called also *incisal e.*

em•bro•ca•tion (em″bro-ka′shən) [L. *embrocatio*] 1. the application of a liquid medicament to the surface of the body. 2. a liquid medicine for external use.

em•bry•ec•to•my (em″bre-ek′tə-me) [*embryo* + *-ectomy*] excision of the embryo in extrauterine pregnancy.

em•bryo (em′bre-o) [Gr. *embryon*] 1. in animals, those derivatives of the zygote that will eventually become the offspring, during their period of most rapid development, i.e., from the time the long axis appears until all major structures are represented. 2. in humans, the developing organism from fertilization to the end of the eighth week. Cf. *fetus.* 3. in plants, the element of the seed that develops into a new individual. **em′bryonal, embryon′ic** *adj*

hexacanth e. the six-hooked embryo, or onchosphere, characteristic of most tapeworms of humans and domestic animals.

Janošík e. a human embryo having three aortic arches and two pharyngeal pouches.

presomite e. the embryo at any stage prior to the appearance of the first pair of somites.

previllous e. the conceptus before the chorionic villi of the placenta develop.

somite e. the embryo at any stage between the appearances of the first and the last pairs of somites.

Spee e. a 1.5 mm human embryo, horizon IX, about 20 days old as described by Spee.

em•bryo•blast (em′bre-o-blast″) [*embryo* + *-blast*] an aggregation of cells at the embryonic pole of the blastocyst, destined to form the embryo proper. Called also *inner cell mass.*

em•bry•oc•to•ny (em″bre-ok′tə-ne) [*embryo* + Gr. *kteinein* to kill] the artificial destruction of the living embryo, or fetus.

em•bryo•gen•e•sis (em″bre-o-jen′ə-sis) [*embryo* + *genesis*] 1. the formation of an embryo. 2. the development of a new individual by means of sexual reproduction, that is, from a zygote; called also *embryogeny* and *embryony.*

em•bryo•ge•net•ic (em″bre-o-jə-net′ik) embryogenic.

em•bry•o•gen•ic (em″bre-o-jen′ik) 1. pertaining to the development of an embryo. 2. producing an embryo.

em•bry•og•e•ny (em″bre-oj′ə-ne) embryogenesis.

em•bryo•graph (em′bre-o-graf) [*embryo* + *-graph*] a combination of a microscope and a camera lucida, used to draw sketches of the embryo.

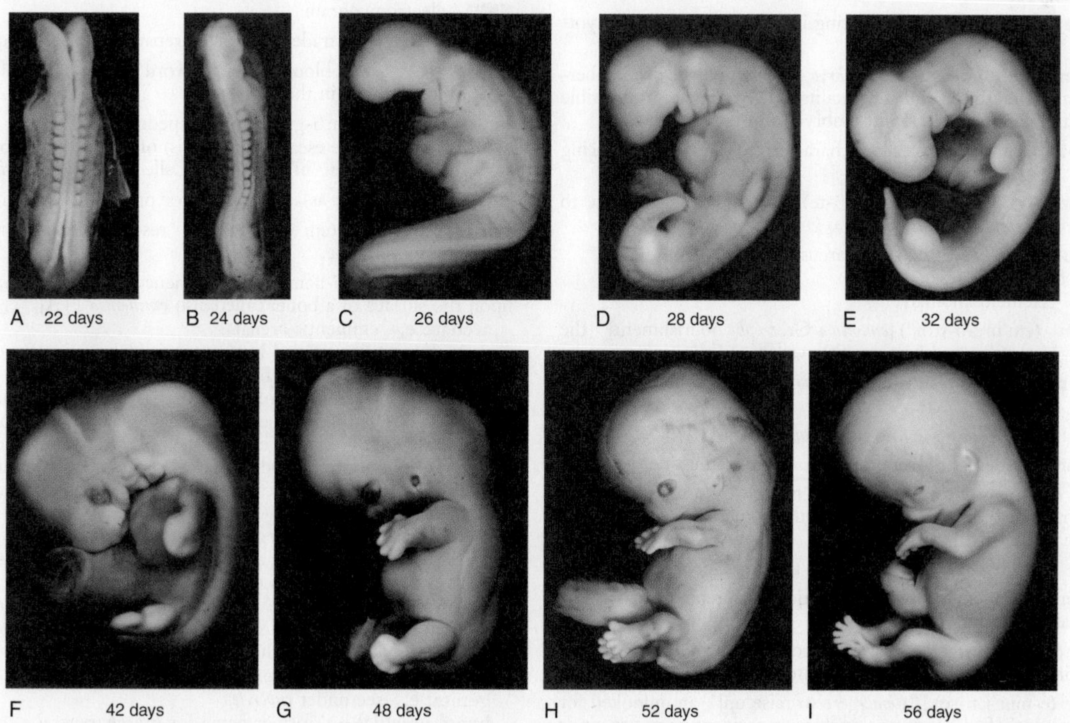

■ Human embryo at various stages of development. The relative size has been distorted to emphasize correspondence of parts, and the ages are approximate.

em•bry•og•ra•phy (em″bre-og′rə-fe) [*embryo* + *-graphy*] 1. a treatise or description of the embryo. 2. the sketching of an embryo by means of the embryograph.

em•bry•oid (em′bre-oid) [*embryo* + *-oid*] resembling an embryo.

em•bryo•le•thal•i•ty (em″bre-o-le-thal′ĭ-te) embryotoxicity that causes death of the embryo.

em•bry•ol•o•gist (em″bre-ol′ə-jist) a specialist in embryology.

em•bry•ol•o•gy (em″bre-ol′ə-je) [*embryo* + *-logy*] the science of the origin and development of the individual from fertilization of an oocyte to the end of the embryonic and fetal periods.
 causal e. experimental e.
 comparative e. embryology applied with a comparative view to various species studied with reference to their taxonomy and the principle that ontogeny recapitulates phylogeny.
 descriptive e. the study of embryos and fetuses and their components with reference to anatomical and chronological sequence so as to define stages and describe the course of development.
 experimental e. analysis of the factors and relations in development, obtained by subjecting embryos to experimental procedures; called also *causal e.*

em•bry•o•ma (em″bre-o′mə) any neoplasm thought to be derived from embryonic cells or tissues, such as a dermoid cyst, teratoma, primitive neuroectodermal tumor, embryonal carcinoma or sarcoma, nephroblastoma, or hepatoblastoma. Called also *embryonal tumor.*
 e. of kidney, renal e. Wilms tumor.

em•bryo•mor•phous (em″bre-o-mor′fəs) [*embryo* + *morph-* + *-ous*] having a form suggestive of an embryo; said of certain abnormal tissue elements supposed to be remnants of an embryo.

em•bry•o•nate (em′bre-o-nāt) 1. pertaining to or resembling an embryo. 2. containing an embryo. 3. impregnated; fecundated.

em•bry•o•ni•za•tion (em″bre-o′nĭ-za′shən) reversion to the embryonic form on the part of a tissue or cell.

em•bry•o•ny (em′bre-o-ne) embryogenesis.

em•bryo•pa•thol•o•gy (em″bre-o-pə-thol′ə-je) the study of abnormal embryos or of defective embryonic development.

em•bry•op•a•thy (em″bre-op′ə-the) [*embryo* + *-pathy*] a morbid condition of the embryo or a disorder resulting from abnormal embryonic development. Cf. *fetopathy.*
 rubella e. congenital rubella syndrome.

em•bryo•phore (em′bre-o-for) the inner egg shell surrounding the embryo, as seen in the eggs of *Taenia* found in the feces.

em•bryo•plas•tic (em″bre-o-plas′tik) embryogenic.

em•bryo•scope (em″bre-o-skōp) [*embryo* + *-scope*] an instrument for observing the embryo.

em•bryo•tome (em′bre-o-tōm) a cutting instrument used in embryotomy.

em•bry•ot•o•my (em″bre-ot′ə-me) [*embryo* + *-tomy*] 1. the dismemberment of a fetus in the uterus or vagina to facilitate delivery that is impossible by natural means. 2. the dissection of embryos and fetuses.

em•bry•o•tox•ic (em″bre-o-tok′sik) characterized by or producing embryotoxicity.

em•bryo•tox•ic•i•ty (em″bre-o-tok-sis′ĭ-te) developmental toxicity to an embryo. See also *embryolethality.*

em•bryo•tox•on (em″bre-o-tok′son) arcus corneae.
 anterior e. arcus corneae.
 posterior e. Axenfeld anomaly.

em•bryo•troph (em′bre-o-trōf″) [*embryo* + Gr. *trophē* nourishment] the total nutriment (histotroph and hemotroph) available to the embryo.

em•bry•ot•ro•phy (em″bre-ot′rə-fe) [*embryo* + *-trophy*] the nutrition of the embryo.

EMC encephalomyocarditis; see also under *virus.*

Em•cyt (em′sīt) trademark for a preparation of estramustine.

eme•das•tine di•fu•ma•rate (em″ə-das′tēn) [USP] an antihistamine (H_1-receptor antagonist) applied topically to the conjunctiva in the treatment of allergic conjunctivitis.

emed•ul•late (e-med′u-lāt) [*e-* + *medulla*] to extract bone marrow.

Emend (e′mend) trademark for a preparation of aprepitant or its prodrug fosaprepitant dimeglumine.

emer•gence (e-mur′jəns) the process of coming out of a former state, as the restoration to a normal physiological state of an anesthetized patient.

emer•gen•cy (e-mur′jən-se) [L. *emergere* to raise up] an unlooked for or sudden occurrence, often dangerous, such as an accident or an urgent or pressing need.

emer•gent (e-mur′jənt) 1. pertaining to an emergency. 2. coming into being through consecutive stages of development, as in emergent evolution.

Em•er•i•cel•la (em″ər-ĭ-sel′ə) a genus of fungi of the family Trichocomaceae. *E. ni′dulans* is the perfect (sexual) stage of *Aspergillus nidulans.*

Eme•ri•cel•lop•sis (em″ər-ĭ-sə-lop′sis) a teleomorph of *Acremonium*; *E. minimum* (formerly *Cephalosporium acremonium*) is the source of cephalosporin C.

em•er•in (em′ər-in) an integral membrane protein of the nuclear inner membrane; it binds to lamins A and C. Mutations in the emerin gene causing absence of emerin from cardiac and skeletal muscle have been shown to cause X-linked Emery-Dreifuss muscular dystrophy.

Em•ery-Drei•fuss muscular dystrophy (em′ə-re drī′fəs) [Alan Eglin Heathcote *Emery*, British geneticist, born 1928; Fritz Emanuel *Dreifuss*, German-born neurologist in the United Kingdom and the United States, 1926–1997] see under *dystrophy.*

em•ery (em′ər-e) impure crystalline corundum mixed with iron oxide; used as an abrasive.

eme•sia (ə-me′zhə) vomiting.

em•e•sis (em′ə-sis) vomiting.
 e. gravida′rum morning sickness.

-emesis [Gr. *emein* to vomit] a word termination denoting vomiting.

emet•ic (ə-met′ik) [Gr. *emetikos;* L. *emeticus*] 1. causing vomiting. 2. an agent that causes vomiting.
 central e. an emetic carried by the blood stream to the vomiting center, upon which it acts; called also *indirect e.* and *systemic e.*
 direct e. an emetic that acts directly on the stomach; called also *mechanical e.*
 indirect e. central e.
 mechanical e. direct e.
 systemic e. central e.

em•e•tine (em′ə-tēn) an alkaloid, obtained from ipecac or prepared by methylation of cephaeline.
 e. hydrochloride [USP] the dihydrochloride salt of emetine, used as an antiamebic, administered subcutaneously or intramuscularly.

em•e•to•ca•thar•tic (em″ə-to-kə-thahr′tik) 1. both emetic and cathartic. 2. an agent that is both emetic and cathartic.

em•e•to•gen•ic (em″ə-to-jen′ik) [Gr. *emetos* vomiting + *-genic*] emetic (def. 1).

em•e•to•ge•nic•i•ty (em″ə-to-jə-nis′ĭ-te) the degree of possibility that a given substance or other factor will cause nausea and vomiting.

EMF electromotive force.

EMG electromyogram.

Em•gel (em′jel) trademark for a preparation of erythromycin.

-emia [Gr. *haima* blood + *-ia*] a word termination denoting the presence of a substance in the blood.

em•i•gra•tion (em″ĭ-gra′shən) diapedesis.
 leukocyte e. the escape (diapedesis) of leukocytes through the walls of small blood vessels in inflammation. Called also *leukopedesis.*

Em•in•ase (em′in-ās) trademark for preparations of anistreplase.

em•i•nec•to•my (em″ĭ-nek′tə-me) resection of the articular eminence of the temporal bone.

em•i•nence (em′ĭ-nəns) a prominence or projection, especially one upon the surface of a bone; called also *eminentia* [TA].
 arcuate e. eminentia arcuata.
 articular e. of temporal bone tuberculum articulare ossis temporalis.
 canine e. a prominent bony ridge overlying the root of either canine tooth on the labial surface of both the maxilla and the mandible.
 caudal e. a taillike eminence produced by a proliferating mass of mesodermal cells at the caudal end of the early vertebrate embryo; it is the remnant of the primitive node and the precursor of hindgut, adjacent notochord and somites, and the caudal part of the spinal cord. Called also *end* or *tail bud.*
 collateral e. of lateral ventricle eminentia collateralis ventriculi lateralis.
 e. of concha eminentia conchae.
 cruciate e., cruciform e. of occipital bone eminentia cruciformis.
 deltoid e. tuberositas deltoidea.
 facial e. colliculus facialis.
 frontal e. tuber frontale.
 genital e. see under *tubercle.*
 hypobranchial e. former name for *hypopharyngeal e.*
 hypoglossal e. trigonum nervi hypoglossi.

hypopharyngeal e. 1. copula linguae. 2. a median ventral elevation on the embryonic tongue, caudal to the copula; formed by union of the third and fourth pairs of pharyngeal arches. It overgrows the copula during the fifth and sixth weeks and gives rise to the posterior third of the tongue.
hypothenar e. hypothenar (def. 1).
iliopectineal e., iliopubic e. eminentia iliopubica.
intercondylar e., intercondyloid e. eminentia intercondylaris.
maxillary e. tuber maxillae.
medial e. of rhomboid fossa eminentia medialis fossae rhomboideae.
median e. eminentia mediana.
occipital e. a ridge on the lateral ventricle of the embryonic brain, corresponding to the occipital fissure in the adult.
omental e. of pancreas tuber omentale pancreatis.
parietal e. tuber parietale.
pyramidal e. eminentia pyramidalis.
radial e. of wrist eminentia carpi radialis.
e. of scapha eminentia scaphae.
thenar e. thenar (def. 1).
thyroid e. prominentia laryngea.
e. of triangular fossa of auricle eminentia fossae triangularis auriculae.
ulnar e. of wrist eminentia carpi ulnaris.

em•i•nen•tia (em″ĭ-nen′shə) gen. and pl. *eminen′tiae* [L.] [TA] eminence: anatomical terminology for a prominence or projection, especially one on the surface of a bone.
e. arcua′ta [TA] arcuate eminence: an arched prominence on the internal surface of the petrous part of the temporal bone in the floor of the middle cranial fossa, marking the position of the superior semicircular canal. It is particularly prominent in young skulls.
e. car′pi radia′lis an eminence on the palmar surface of the radial side of the wrist, formed by the tubercles on the scaphoid and trapezium bones; called also *radial eminence of wrist.*
e. car′pi ulna′ris an eminence on the palmar surface of the ulnar side of the wrist, formed by the pisiform bone and the hook of the hamate bone; called also *ulnar eminence of wrist.*
e. collatera′lis ventri′culi latera′lis [TA] collateral eminence of lateral ventricle: an elevation in the lateral wall of the atrium and posterior horn of the lateral ventricle, produced by the collateral sulcus.
e. con′chae [TA] the projection on the medial surface of the auricle that corresponds to the concha on the lateral surface.
e. crucifor′mis [TA] cruciform eminence of occipital bone: the cross-shaped bony prominence on the internal surface of the squama of the occipital bone, at the intersection of the ridges associated with the sulci of the superior sagittal sinus and the transverse sinuses. Called also *cruciate line.*
e. fos′sae triangula′ris auri′culae [TA] the protuberance on the medial surface of the auricle of the ear that corresponds to the triangular fossa on the lateral surface.
e. fronta′lis TA alternative for *tuber frontale.*
e. hypothena′ris TA alternative for *hypothenar* (def. 1).
e. iliopu′bica [TA] iliopubic eminence: a diffuse enlargement just anterior to the acetabulum, marking the junction of the ilium with the superior ramus of the pubis; called also *iliopectineal eminence.*
e. intercondyla′ris [TA] intercondylar eminence: an eminence on the proximal extremity of the tibia, surmounted on either side by a prominent tubercle, on to the sides of which the articular facets are prolonged; called also *intercondyloid eminence.*
e. maxil′lae TA alternative for *tuber maxillae.*
e. media′lis fos′sae rhomboi′deae [TA] medial eminence of rhomboid fossa: an eminence in the medial part of the floor of the fourth ventricle, located immediately rostral to the facial colliculus.
e. media′na [TA] median eminence: the raised area on the infundibulum hypothalami at the floor of the third ventricle of the brain. Continuous below with the infundibular stem or stalk of the pituitary gland, it contains the primary capillary network of the hypophysial portal system. In some anatomical classification systems it is included as part of the neurohypophysis and in others as part of the tuber cinereum. See also *circumventricular organs,* under *organ.*
e. parieta′lis TA alternative for tuber parietale.
e. pyramida′lis [TA] pyramidal eminence: an elevation in the posterior wall of the middle ear, which contains the stapedius muscle.
e. sca′phae [TA] the prominence on the medial side of the auricle of the external ear that corresponds to the scapha on the lateral side.
e. thena′ris TA alternative for *thenar* (def. 1).

em•is•sary (em′ĭ-sar″e) [L. *emissarium* drain] 1. affording an outlet, as an emissary vein. 2. vena emissaria.

emis•sion (e-mish′ən) [L. *emissio,* a sending out] 1. discharge (def. 1). 2. an involuntary discharge of semen.
nocturnal e. reflex emission of the semen during sleep.

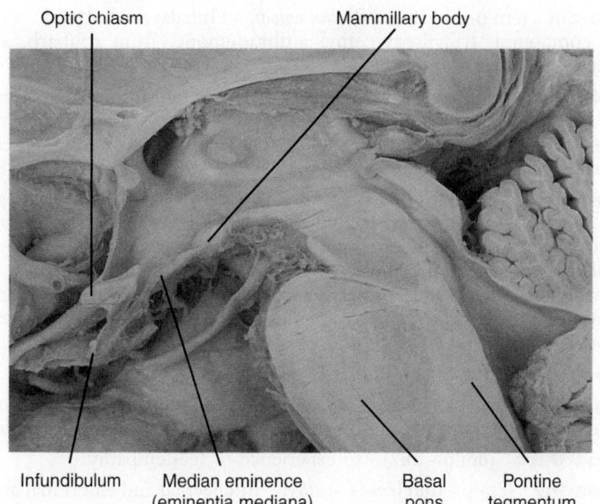

■ Eminentia mediana (median eminence) in the right half of a sagittally hemisected brain.

otoacoustic e's (OAE) subtle sounds produced by amplifying processes in the cochlea during normal hearing and transmitted through the middle ear to the external auditory canal.
positron e. a form of radioactive decay in which a positron (β^+) and neutrino are ejected from the nucleus as a proton is transformed into a neutron. Collision of the positron with an electron causes annihilation of both particles and conversion of their masses into energy in the form of two 0.511 MeV gamma rays.
thermionic e. the emission of electrons and ions by incandescent bodies.
transient evoked otoacoustic e's (TEOAE) sounds produced by the cochlea in response to sound stimuli, measured by a microphone placed in the external auditory canal; used to test the integrity of the cochlea in screening neonates for sensorineural hearing loss.

emis•siv•i•ty (e″mĭ-siv′ĭ-te) the ratio of emissive power (of radiant energy) of a surface to that of a black surface having the same temperature.

EMIT (e-mit′) [*e*nzyme-*m*ultiplied *i*mmunoassay *t*echnique] trademark for a homogeneous (single phase) enzyme immunoassay which utilizes the change in enzyme activity of an enzyme-labeled hapten that occurs on binding with antibody to determine the amount of unlabeled hapten (the unknown) present in a biologic specimen.

EMLA (em′lə) trademark for combination preparations of lidocaine and prilocaine.

em•men•a•gog•ic (ə-men″ə-goj′ik) inducing menstruation.

em•men•a•gogue (ə-men′ə-gog) [Gr. *emmēna* menses + *-agogue*] an agent or measure that induces menstruation.
direct e. an agent that induces menstruation by acting directly upon the reproductive organs.
indirect e. an agent or measure that acts to induce menstruation by relieving another condition of which amenorrhea is a secondary result.

em•me•nia (ə-men′e-ə) [Gr. *emmēna*] menses. **emmen′ic** *adj*

em•me•nol•o•gy (em″ə-nol′ə-je) [Gr. *emmēna* menses + *-logy*] the sum of knowledge regarding menstruation and its disorders.

Em•met operation, retractor (em′ət) [Thomas Addis *Emmet,* American gynecologist, 1828–1919] see under *operation* and *retractor.*

em•me•trope (em′ə-trōp) an individual who has no refractive error of vision.

em•me•tro•pia (em″ə-tro′pe-ə) [Gr. *emmetros* in proper measure + *-opia*] a state of proper correlation between the refractive system of the eye and the axial length of the eyeball, rays of light entering the eye parallel to the optic axis being brought to a focus exactly on the retina. **emmetrop′ic** *adj*

Em•mon•sia (ĕ-mon′se-ə) a genus of saprobic Fungi Imperfecti of the form-family Moniliaceae. Two species, *E. cres′cens* and *E. par′va,* cause adiaspiromycosis in rodents and humans. Called also *Haplosporangium.*

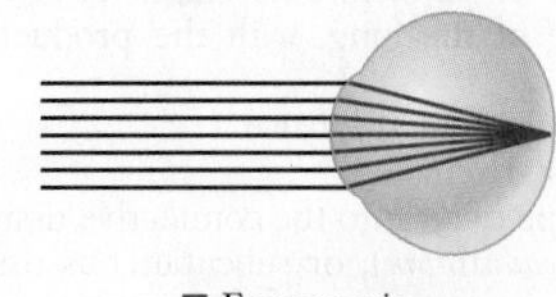
■ Emmetropia.

em•o•din (em′o-din) [from *Rheum emodi*, a Himalayan rhubarb] a cathartic compound, trihydroxymethyl anthraquinone, from rhubarb, aloes, senna, and cascara sagrada.

emol•li•ent (e-mol′e-ənt) [L. *emolliens* softening, from *e* out + *mollis* soft] 1. softening or soothing; called also *malactic.* 2. an agent which softens or soothes the skin, or soothes an irritated internal surface; called also *malagma.*

emo•tion (e-mo′shən) [L. *emovere* to disturb] a strong feeling state, such as excitement, distress, happiness, sadness, love, hate, fear, or anger, arising subjectively and directed toward a specific object, with physiological, somatic, and behavioral components. In psychoanalytic theory, it is a state of tension associated with an instinctual drive. The external manifestation of emotion is called *affect;* a pervasive and sustained emotional state is called a *mood.* **emo′tional** *adj*

Emp. [L.] emplas′trum (a plaster).

em•pa•cho (em-pah′cho) Mexican term for a gastrointestinal disorder characterized by constipation, bloating, lethargy, vomiting, and diarrhea.

em•pa•thize (em′pə-thīz) to experience or feel empathy.

em•pa•thy (em′pə-the) [*em-* + *-pathy*] intellectual and emotional awareness and understanding of another person's thoughts, feelings, and behavior, even those that are distressing and disturbing. *Empathy* emphasizes understanding, *sympathy* emphasizes sharing, of another person's feelings and experiences. **empath′ic** *adj*

Em•pe•do•bac•ter (em″pĕ-do-bak′tər) a genus of gram-negative, aerobic bacteria of the family Flavobacteriaceae.

E. bre′vis a species that has been found in various kinds of nosocomial infections.

em•phrax•is (em-frak′sis) [Gr.] a stoppage or obstruction.

em•phy•se•ma (em″fə-se′mə) [Gr. "an inflation"] 1. a pathological accumulation of air in tissues or organs. 2. pulmonary e. **emphysem′atous** *adj*

acute bovine pulmonary e., acute pulmonary e. of cattle fog fever.

alveolar duct e. distention of the alveolar ducts as seen in elderly individuals, often producing little or no functional disturbance.

atrophic e. senile e.

bullous e. single or multiple large cystic alveolar dilatations of lung tissue; see also *paraseptal e.* Called also *cystic e.*

centriacinar e., centrilobular e. one of the principal types of pulmonary emphysema, characterized by enlargement of air spaces in the proximal part of the acinus, primarily at the level of the respiratory bronchioles. See also *bronchiolectasis* and *coal workers' pneumoconiosis.*

chronic hypertrophic e. panacinar e.

compensating e., compensatory e. overdistention of lung tissue, which fills a void produced by contraction, atelectasis, surgical resection, fibrosis, or otherwise reduced volume of another part of the lung.

congenital lobar e. a condition characterized by overinflation, commonly affecting one of the upper lobes and causing respiratory distress in early life; called also *congenital lobar overinflation.*

cutaneous e. subcutaneous e.

cystic e. bullous e.

diffuse e. panacinar e.

distal acinar e. one of the principal types of pulmonary emphysema, limited to the distal ends of the alveoli along the interlobular septa and beneath the pleura, forming bullae; see also *bullous e.* Called also *interlobular* or *paraseptal e.*

ectatic e. panacinar e.

false e. deformity of the thoracic cage simulating that associated with pulmonary emphysema (increased anterior-posterior diameter, elevated rib angle, etc.); the lungs may or may not be normal. Called also *skeletal e.*

focal e., focal dust e. centriacinar emphysema associated with inhalation of environmental dusts, producing dilatation of the terminal and respiratory bronchioles.

gastric e. air or gas in the stomach wall owing to disruption of the wall by pressure, vomiting, or other usually mechanical processes; radiologically it resembles emphysematous gastritis but is much more benign.

generalized e. panacinar e.

glass blower's e. emphysema of the lungs attributed to overstrain in glass blowers.

hypoplastic e. pulmonary emphysema due to a developmental abnormality resulting in reduced number of alveoli, which are abnormally large; it may affect a pulmonary segment, lobe, or an entire lung.

idiopathic unilobar e. a syndrome characterized by emphysematous expansion of one lobe of the lung, with the production of dyspnea and cyanosis.

infantile lobar e. congenital lobar e.

interlobular e. distal acinar e.

interstitial e. escape of air into the connective tissue of the lung, mediastinum (see *pneumomediastinum*), or subcutaneous tissue (see *subcutaneous e.*); it results from a tear or rupture of the respiratory passages or alveoli, which may occur in association with bronchiolar obstruction, positive pressure ventilation, or a penetrating wound of the chest wall or lung.

intestinal e. pneumatosis cystoides intestinalis.

lobar e. emphysema involving fewer than all the lobes of the affected lung. Cf. *unilateral e.*

localized obstructive e. overinflation of a lobe or segment of lung, often due to partial bronchial obstruction; called also *obstructive pulmonary overinflation.*

e. of lungs pulmonary e.

mediastinal e. pneumomediastinum.

obstructive e. overinflation of the lungs associated with partial bronchial obstruction which interferes with exhalation.

panacinar e., panlobular e. one of the principal types of pulmonary emphysema, characterized by relatively uniform enlargement of air spaces throughout the acini. Called also *chronic hypertrophic, diffuse, ectatic, generalized,* or *vesicular e.*

paracicatricial e. alveolar distention occurring in the vicinity of pulmonary scars.

paraseptal e. distal acinar e.

pulmonary e. a condition of the lung characterized by an abnormal increase in the size of air spaces distal to the terminal bronchioles. Types named according to location of the damage include *centriacinar e., distal acinar e.,* and *panacinar e.*

pulmonary interstitial e. (PIE) a condition occurring mainly in premature infants, in which air leaks from the alveoli of the lungs into the interstitial spaces; it is often associated with underlying lung disease or with the use of mechanical ventilation.

senile e. pulmonary emphysema due to atrophic changes and dilatation of the alveoli occurring with age. Called also *atrophic e.*

skeletal e. false e.

small-lunged e. atrophic e.

subcutaneous e. interstitial emphysema with air in the subcutaneous tissue; it is usually caused by intrathoracic injury, generally associated with pneumothorax and pneumomediastinum. Called also *cutaneous e.*

surgical e. subcutaneous emphysema following a surgical procedure.

traumatic e. interstitial emphysema due to trauma.

unilateral e. emphysema affecting only one lung; it may be either congenital (such as from defects in circulation) or acquired *(Swyer-James syndrome).* Cf. *lobar e.* Called also *hyperlucent lung.*

vesicular e. panacinar e.

em•pir•ic (em-pir′ik) 1. empirical. 2. a practitioner whose skill is based on experience.

em•pir•i•cal (em-pir′ĭ-kəl) based on experience.

em•pir•i•cism (em-pir′ĭ-siz-əm) 1. reliance on mere experience; empirical practice. 2. quackery.

em•po•ri•at•rics (em-por″e-at′riks) [Gr. *emporos* a passenger on a ship + *-iatrics*] travel medicine.

em•pros•thot•o•nos (em″pros-thot′ə-nəs) [Gr. *emprosthen* forward + *tonos* tension] a form of tetanic spasm in which the head and feet are brought forward and the body is rendered tense; called also *episthotonos.*

em•pros•thot•o•nus (em″pros-thot′ə-nəs) emprosthotonos.

emp•ty•ing (emp′te-ing) evacuation.

delayed gastric e. failure of the stomach to evacuate partially digested food into the duodenum within an appropriate time, as in gastric stasis or gastroparesis; symptoms include early satiety and sometimes nausea and vomiting.

rapid gastric e. excessively rapid movement of partially digested food from the stomach into the jejunum; it occurs most often in patients who have had partial gastrectomy with gastrojejunostomy (see *dumping syndrome,* under *syndrome*). Called also *gastric dumping.*

em•py•e•ma (em″pi-e′mə) [Gr. *empyema*] 1. abscess. 2. a pleural effusion (q.v.) containing pus; called also *thoracic e., purulent* or *suppurative pleurisy,* and *pyothorax.*

e. benig′num latent e.

e. of the chest empyema (def. 2).

e. of gallbladder cholecystitis with purulent acute inflammation of the gallbladder.

interlobar e. thoracic empyema situated between two lobes of the lung.

latent e. thoracic empyema unaccompanied by any symptoms. Called also *e. benignum.*

loculated e. thoracic empyema in which the pus is trapped in an enclosed space.

mastoid e. suppurative inflammation of the mucous lining of the cavities of the mastoid process.

metapneumonic e. thoracic empyema developing some time after the subsidence of the pneumonia; cf. *synpneumonic e.*

e. necessita′tis thoracic empyema in which the pus can make a spontaneous escape toward the chest wall.

parapneumonic e. thoracic empyema occurring as a complication of pneumonia; cf. *metapneumonic e.* and *synpneumonic e.*

e. of pericardium purulent pericarditis.

pneumococcal e. thoracic empyema due to infection with *Streptococcus pneumoniae.*

pulsating e. thoracic empyema in which the movements of the heart produce a visible vibration of the chest wall.

putrid e. thoracic empyema in which the pus has become more or less decomposed.

streptococcal e. thoracic empyema due to infection with *Streptococcus pyogenes.*

subdural e. a collection of pus between the dura mater the arachnoid; most are intracranial, but a few are spinal.

synpneumonic e. thoracic empyema arising during the course of pulmonary inflammation. Cf. *metapneumonic e.*

thoracic e. empyema (def. 2).

tuberculous e. thoracic empyema due to infection with *Mycobacterium tuberculosis.*

em•py•emic (em″pi-e′mik) pertaining to or of the nature of empyema.

em•py•e•sis (em″pi-e′sis) [Gr. *empyēsis* suppuration] 1. a pustular eruption. 2. any disease characterized by phlegmonous vesicles becoming filled with purulent fluid.

em•pyo•cele (em′pi-o-sēl) [Gr. *empyein* to suppurate + *-cele*[1]] a collection of pus at the umbilicus.

em•py•reu•ma (em″pi-roo′mə) [Gr. *empyreuma* a live coal] the distinctive odor of animal or vegetable matter when charred in a closed vessel. **empyreumat′ic** *adj*

EMS Emergency Medical Service.

Em•sam (em′sam) trademark for a preparation of selegiline.

em•tri•ci•ta•bine (em″tri-si′tə-bēn) a synthetic nucleoside analogue of cytosine that is a reverse transcriptase inhibitor, used in the treatment of human immunodeficiency virus-1 infection; administered orally.

Em•tri•va (em′trĭ-və) trademark for a preparation of emtricitabine.

emul. [L.] emul′sum (emulsion).

emul•gent (e-mul′jənt) [L. *emulgere* to milk or drain out] causing a straining or purifying process.

emul•si•fi•er (e-mul′sĭ-fi″ər) an agent used to produce an emulsion.

emul•si•fy (e-mul′sĭ-fi) to convert or to be converted into an emulsion.

emul•sion (e-mul′shən) [L. *emulsio, emulsum*] a mixture of two immiscible liquids, one being distributed in small globules throughout the body of the second. It is a colloid system in which both the dispersed phase and the dispersion medium are liquids, the dispersed liquid being the discontinuous phase and the dispersion medium the continuous phase.

film e. a dehydrated gel emulsion of light- or radiation-sensitive silver halide that is applied to a suitable base.

mineral oil e. [USP] an emulsion of mineral oil, acacia, syrup, vanillin, and alcohol in purified water, used as a cathartic.

oil-in-water e. an emulsion in which oil is the dispersed liquid and an aqueous solution is the continuous phase; water can be used to dilute such an emulsion or to remove it, as from skin or clothing.

water-in-oil e. an emulsion in which water or aqueous solution is the dispersed phase and oil or oleaginous substance is the continuous phase.

emul•sive (e-mul′siv) 1. capable of emulsifying a substance. 2. susceptible of being emulsified. 3. affording an oil on pressure.

emul•soid (e-mul′soid) 1. lyophilic colloid. 2. rarely, emulsion.

emunc•to•ry (e-munk′tə-re) [L. *emungere* to cleanse] 1. excretory or depurant. 2. any excretory organ or duct.

en- [Gr. *en* in] a prefix meaning *in, within;* occurs as *em-* before *b, m,* or *p.*

E-My•cin (e-mi′sin) trademark for a preparation of erythromycin.

ENA extractable nuclear antigen.

en•ab•lex (en-a′bleks) trademark for a preparation of darifenacin.

ENaC epithelial sodium channel.

enal•a•pril (ə-nal′ə-pril) an angiotensin-converting enzyme inhibitor with antihypertensive and vasodilator actions. See also *enalaprilat.*

e. maleate [USP] the maleate salt of enalapril; used in the treatment of hypertension, alone or in combination with a thiazide diuretic, congestive heart failure, and asymptomatic left ventricular dysfunction.

enal•a•pril•at (ə-nal′ə-pril-at″) [USP] an angiotensin-converting enzyme inhibitor, the active metabolite of enalapril, administered intravenously in the treatment of hypertensive crisis or when oral administration of enalapril maleate is impractical.

enam•el (ə-nam′əl) [O.F. *esmail*] 1. the glazed surface of baked porcelain, metal, or pottery. 2. any hard, smooth, glossy coating. 3. dental e.

curled e. dental enamel in which the columns are bent and are wavy and intertwined with one another. Called also *gnarled e.* Cf. *straight e.*

dental e. a hard, thin, translucent layer of calcified substance that envelops and protects the dentin of the crown of the tooth; it is the hardest substance in the body and is almost entirely composed of calcium salts. Called also *adamantine layer, enamel, enamelum* [TA], and *substantia adamantina dentis.*

dwarfed e. nanoid e.

gnarled e. curled e.

hereditary brown e. amelogenesis imperfecta.

hypoplastic e. enamel hypoplasia.

mottled e. hypoplasia of the dental enamel caused by drinking water with a high fluoride content during the time of tooth formation. It is characterized by defective calcification that gives a white chalky appearance to the enamel, gradually changing to a brown discoloration. Called also *dental fluorosis* and *mottled teeth.*

nanoid e. imperfectly formed dental enamel that is thinner than normal. Called also *dwarfed e.*

straight e. dental enamel in which the rods are straight. Cf. *curled e.*

enam•elo•blast (ə-nam′əl-o-blast) ameloblast.

enam•elo•blas•to•ma (ə-nam″əl-o-blas-to′mə) ameloblastoma.

enam•el•o•ma (ə-nam″əl-o′mə) [*enamel* + *-oma*] a nonneoplastic excrescence sometimes found at the bifurcation of a multirooted tooth, at the end of an enamel spur, or on the root surface, which may be composed only of enamel, contain a small dentin nucleus, or contain a minute strand of dentin and pulp. Called also *enamel drop* and *enamel pearl.*

enam•e•lo•plas•ty (ə-nam′ə-lo-plas″te) contouring of the enamel surface of a tooth to remove superficial grooves and other defects. **enameloplas′tic** *adj*

enam•e•lum (ə-nam′əl-əm) [L.] [TA] dental enamel.

en•an•thate (ə-nan′thāt) the anionic form of enanthic acid; the term is used as a USAN contraction for *heptanoate.*

en•an•them (ə-nan′thəm) enanthema.

en•an•the•ma (en″ən-the′mə) pl. *enanthemas, enanthem′ata* [*en-* + *anthema* a blossoming] an eruption upon a mucous surface. **enanthem′atous** *adj*

enan•thic ac•id (ə-nan′thik) a saturated seven-carbon fatty acid, heptanoic acid, not definitely occurring in nature but producible by oxidation of fats.

en•an•tio•bio•sis (en-an″te-o-bi-o′sis) [Gr. *enantios* opposite + *biosis*] the condition in which organisms living together antagonize one another's development. Cf. *symbiosis* (def. 1).

en•an•tio•mer (en-an′te-o″mər) one of a pair of compounds having a mirror image relationship. Called also *enantiomorph.*

en•an•ti•om•er•ism (en-an″te-om′ər-iz-əm) [Gr. *enantios* opposite + *mero-* + *-ism*] the relationship between two stereoisomers having molecules that are mirror images of each other. Enantiomers have identical chemical and physical properties in an achiral environment. However, they form different products when reacted with other chiral molecules, and they exhibit optical activity. The enantiomer that rotates the plane of polarization of a beam of polarized light in the clockwise direction is indicated by the prefix (+)-, formerly *d-* or dextro-. The other enantiomer rotates the plane of polarization an equal amount in the counterclockwise direction and is indicated by the prefix (−)-, formerly *l-* or levo-. Two conventions are used to designate the actual configurations of enantiomers. The D, L system (see D-) is used to denote the configuration of carbohydrates relative to D-(+)-glyceraldehyde and of amino acids relative to L-(−)-serine. The *R,S* system (see *R-*) is a more general system used to specify the absolute configuration at every asymmetric carbon atom. An equimolar mixture of enantiomers (a racemic form or racemic modification) is optically inactive and is designated by the prefixes (±)-, DL-, or *dl-*.

en•an•tio•morph (en-an′te-o-morf″) enantiomer.

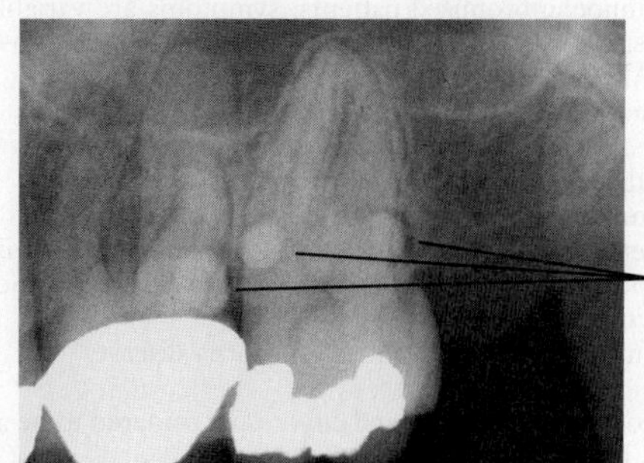

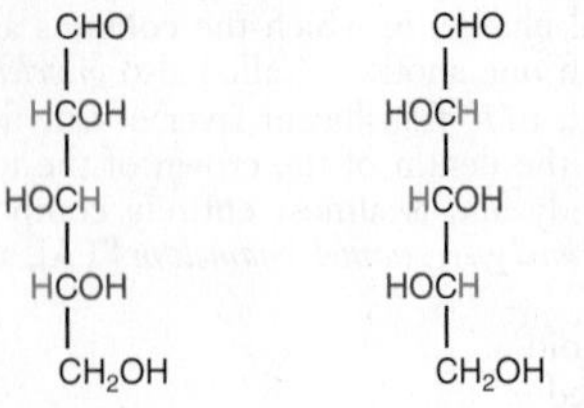

CHO CHO
HCOH HOCH
HOCH HCOH
HCOH HOCH
CH_2OH CH_2OH

■ Enantiomerism.

en·an·tio·mor·phism (en-an″te-o-mor′fiz-əm) enantiomerism.

en·ar·thri·tis (en″ahr-thri′tis) inflammation of an enarthrosis.

en·ar·thro·sis (en″ahr-thro′sis) [*en-* + *arthrosis*] articulatio spheroidea. **enarthro′dial** *adj*

en bloc (ahn blok′) [Fr.] in a lump; as a whole.

En·brel (en′brel) trademark for a preparation of etanercept.

en·cain·ide hy·dro·chlo·ride (en-ka′nīd) a sodium channel blocker that acts on the Purkinje fibers and myocardium, used in the treatment of life-threatening arrhythmias; administered orally.

en·can·this (en-kan′this) [Gr., from *en* in + *kanthos* the angle of the eye] a small red excrescence on the semilunar fold of the conjunctiva and inner lacrimal caruncle.

en·cap·su·lat·ed (en-kap′su-lāt-əd) [*en-* + L. *capsula* little box] enclosed within a capsule.

en·cap·su·la·tion (ən-kap″su-la′shən) 1. any act of inclosing in a capsule. 2. a physiologic process of inclosure in a sheath made up of a substance not normal to the part.

en·cap·suled (en-kap′səld) encapsulated.

en·car·di·tis (en″kahr-di′tis) endocarditis.

en·ceph·a·lal·gia (en-sef″ə-lal′jə) headache.

en·ceph·a·lat·ro·phy (en-sef″ə-lat′ro-fe) atrophy of the brain.

en·ce·phal·ic (en″sə-fal′ik) 1. pertaining to the encephalon. 2. within the skull.

en·ceph·a·li·tis (en-sef″ə-li′tis) pl. *encephali′tides* [*encephalo-* + *-itis*] inflammation of the brain. **encephalit′ic** *adj*

e. A lethargic e.

acute disseminated e. see under *encephalomyelitis.*

acute necrotizing e. encephalitis characterized by a particularly destructive reaction in the brain; cf. *herpes simplex e.* and *acute necrotizing hemorrhagic encephalomyelitis.*

Australian X e. Murray Valley e.

e. B Japanese B e.

benign myalgic e. epidemic neuromyasthenia.

Binswanger e. see under *disease.*

bovine e. Buss disease.

brainstem e. any of various symptoms caused by dysfunction of cranial nerves owing to a lesion in the brainstem, most often a paraneoplastic effect of lung or other types of cancer; symptoms may include oculomotor signs, hearing loss, dysarthria, dysphagia, and dyspnea.

e. C St. Louis e.

California e. a usually mild form of encephalitis caused by a bunyavirus and transmitted chiefly by the mosquito *Aedes melanimon;* it primarily affects children.

caprine arthritis-e. a disease of goats caused by a lentivirus. In kids it is characterized by encephalitis with paresis that is often fatal. In adults it takes the form of chronic arthritis with swollen carpal joints, giving it its nickname of *big knee.*

Central European e. the milder form of tick-borne encephalitis, first noted in Central Europe.

chronic subcortical e. Binswanger disease.

cytomegalovirus e. opportunistic infection of the brain by cytomegalovirus in immunocompromised patients; symptoms are variable and may include seizures, clouding of consciousness, and other symptoms similar to those of the AIDS dementia complex.

Dawson e. subacute sclerosing panencephalitis.

eastern equine e. see under *encephalomyelitis.*

Economo e. lethargic e.

enzootic e. of horses Borna disease.

epidemic e., e. epide′mica any viral encephalitis that occurs in epidemics; common types are *Japanese B e., St. Louis e.,* and *tick-borne e.* See also *equine encephalomyelitis.*

equine e. 1. equine encephalomyelitis. 2. Borna disease.

forest-spring e. tick-borne e.

fox e. a disease of foxes, raccoons, and coyotes, considered to be a form of infectious canine hepatitis.

granulomatous amebic e. a rare, chronic type of encephalitis seen most often in debilitated or immunocompromised persons, caused by infection with species of *Acanthamoeba* or the species *Balamuthia mandrillaris;* characteristics include focal granulomas, often with headaches, seizures, nausea, and vomiting.

hemorrhagic e. encephalitis in which there is inflammation of the brain with hemorrhagic foci and perivascular exudate; common types are herpes simplex encephalitis and acute necrotizing hemorrhagic encephalomyelitis.

herpes e., herpes simplex e., herpetic e. the most common form of acute encephalitis, caused by a herpesvirus and characterized by hemorrhagic necrosis of parts of the temporal and frontal lobes. Onset is over several days and involves fever, headache, seizures, stupor, and often coma, frequently ending in death.

HIV e. see under *encephalopathy.*

Ilheus e. a viral encephalitis transmitted by mosquitoes in Brazil. See also under *virus.*

influenzal e. encephalitis occurring as a complication of influenza.

Japanese e., Japanese B e. a form of epidemic encephalitis caused by a flavivirus and transmitted by the bites of infected mosquitoes, especially *Culex tritaeniorhyncus,* in eastern and southern Asia and nearby islands, chiefly in rural areas. It may occur as a symptomless subclinical infection or as an acute meningoencephalomyelitis with cortical damage and cord lesions resembling those of poliomyelitis. Called also *e. B* and *Russian autumnal e.* See also under *virus.*

La Crosse e. encephalitis caused by the La Crosse virus, transmitted by *Aedes triseriatus,* and occurring primarily in children, chiefly in the midwestern United States.

lead e. see under *encephalopathy.*

lethargic e., e. lethar′gica a form of epidemic encephalitis that was observed in various parts of the world between 1915 and 1926, characterized by increasing languor, apathy, and drowsiness, passing into lethargy. Called also *e. A* and *von Economo e.* or *disease.*

limbic e. encephalitis of the limbic system of the rhinencephalon, a type similar to herpes encephalitis, characterized by degenerative changes of the hippocampus and amygdaloid nuclei with memory loss, confusion, seizures, and progressive dementia. There is sometimes an association with tumors elsewhere in the body, although some authorities have linked it to chemotherapy or other tumor treatments.

microglial nodular e. a manifestation of cytomegalovirus encephalitis that appears earlier than cytomegalovirus ventriculoencephalitis and is characterized by acute onset with confusion and delirium.

Murray Valley e. a type of epidemic encephalitis seen in Australia and New Guinea, caused by a flavivirus with its reservoir in birds and mosquitoes; epidemics are infrequent, with children the most seriously affected.

Nipah e. a rapidly progressive, highly fatal encephalitis caused by the Nipah virus and characterized by fever, headache, dizziness, and vomiting and by signs of brainstem dysfunction; it occurs in Malaysia and is associated with contact with pigs.

Ontario e. vomiting and wasting disease.

e. periaxia′lis concen′trica Baló disease.

e. periaxia′lis diffu′sa Schilder disease.

postinfectious e., postvaccinal e. acute disseminated encephalomyelitis.

Powassan e. a rare form of tick-borne encephalitis seen in eastern Canada and the northeastern United States, caused by the Powassan virus and closely resembling Russian spring-summer encephalitis.

purulent e., pyogenic e. suppurative e.

rabies e. encephalitis caused by infection with rabies virus, characterized by agitation, delirium, muscle spasms, seizures, and usually death.

Rasmussen e. a rare type of encephalitis with a focal lesion of one hemisphere, characterized by chronic epilepsy and hemiparesis. The cause is believed to be infiltration of inflammatory cells into the cerebrospinal fluid with destruction of a local area of the cortex; it is usually seen in children and may be due to an autoimmune reaction. Called also *Rasmussen syndrome.*

Russian autumnal e. Japanese B e.

Russian spring-summer e., Russian tick-borne e. the severe form of tick-borne encephalitis, occurring mainly in the far eastern part of Russia.

St. Louis e. a form of epidemic encephalitis caused by a flavivirus; it is similar to western equine encephalomyelitis clinically, occurring in late summer and early fall and transmitted usually by mosquitoes of the genus *Culex.* It ranges from an abortive type of infection to severe disease and affects the elderly most often. Called also *e. C.*

Schilder e. see under *disease.*

Semliki Forest e. a viral encephalitis transmitted by mosquitoes in western Uganda. See also under *virus.*

spring-summer e. 1. Russian spring-summer e. 2. tick-borne e.

Strümpell-Leichtenstern e. hemorrhagic e.

subacute inclusion body e. subacute sclerosing panencephalitis.

e. subcortica′lis chron′ica Binswanger disease.

summer e. Japanese B e.

suppurative e. encephalitis accompanied by suppuration and abscess formation; called also *purulent e.* and *pyogenic e.*

tick-borne e. any of several types of epidemic encephalitis spread by the bites of ticks (usually species of *Ixodes*) that are infected with flaviviruses. They are most common during the spring and summer months, range from mild to fatal, and may affect organs outside the nervous system. Occasionally they may be spread via raw milk from goats, sheep, or cows infected with the virus. The most common and severe type is Russian spring-summer encephalitis; a rare, also serious type is Powassan encephalitis; a milder type is called Central European encephalitis. Called also *forest-spring* or *vernal e.*

toxoplasmic e. see under *meningoencephalitis.*

van Bogaert e. subacute sclerosing panencephalitis.

Venezuelan equine e. see under *encephalomyelitis.*

vernal e., vernoestival e. tick-borne e.

von Economo e. lethargic e.

western equine e. see under *encephalomyelitis.*

West Nile e. a mild, febrile, sporadic disease caused by the flavivirus West Nile virus, transmitted by *Culex* mosquitoes, occurring chiefly in the summer; frequently, infection does not lead to encephalitis. It may be of sudden onset, and symptoms may include drowsiness, severe frontal headache, maculopapular rash, abdominal pain, loss of appetite, nausea, and generalized lymphadenopathy. It was first reported in Uganda, but is widespread elsewhere in Africa and has now been reported in many other parts of the world.

woodcutter's e. tick-borne e.

en•ceph•a•lit•o•gen (en-sef″ə-lit′o-jen) any agent that causes encephalitis and related conditions; cf. *experimental allergic encephalomyelitis.*

en•ceph•a•lit•o•gen•ic (en-sef″ə-lit-o-jen′ik) [*encephalitis* + *-genic*] causing encephalitis.

En•ce•phal•i•to•zo•on (en″sə-fal″ĭ-to-zo′on) [*encephal-* + Gr. *zōon* animal] a genus of parasitic protozoa (suborder Apansporoblastina, order Microsporida), formerly thought to be identical with *Nosema*, first reported in the brains of rabbits.

E. cuni′culi a species causing encephalitozoonosis in many species of mammals; in humans it attacks mainly immunocompromised patients. It involves chiefly the brain and kidney but also such other organs as the liver and spleen. Called also *Nosema cuniculi.*

E. hel′lem a species causing encephalitozoonosis in immunocompromised patients, mainly causing eye infections.

E. intestina′lis a species causing encephalitozoonosis in immunocompromised patients, mainly causing gastrointestinal infections with severe diarrhea and wasting.

en•ce•phal•i•to•zoo•no•sis (en″sə-fal″ĭ-to-zo″o-no′sis) [*encephal-* + *zoonosis*] infection with protozoa of the genus *Encephalitozoon.* It was formerly seen more in other animals than in humans, and the most common infection was with *E. cuniculi*, but now other species are seen in opportunistic infections of immunocompromised persons. Different species cause different types of infections. Formerly called *nosematosis.*

en•ceph•a•li•za•tion (en-sef″ə-lĭ-za′shən) the developmental process by which the cerebral cortex has taken over the functions of the lower (spinal) centers.

encephal(o)- [L. *encephalon*, q.v.] a combining form denoting relationship to the brain.

en•ceph•a•lo•cele (en-sef′ə-lo-sēl″) [*encephalo-* + *cele*[1]] hernia of part of the brain and meninges through a cranial defect (cranium bifidum); it may be congenital, traumatic, or postoperative in origin. Called also *cephalocele, craniocele, encephalomeningocele*, and *meningoencephalocele.* Cf. *cranial meningocele* and *encephalocystocele.*

basal e. an encephalocele in the region of the base of the cranium.

frontal e. encephalocele in the region of the frontal bone; seen more commonly in Asia and Africa than in the Western Hemisphere.

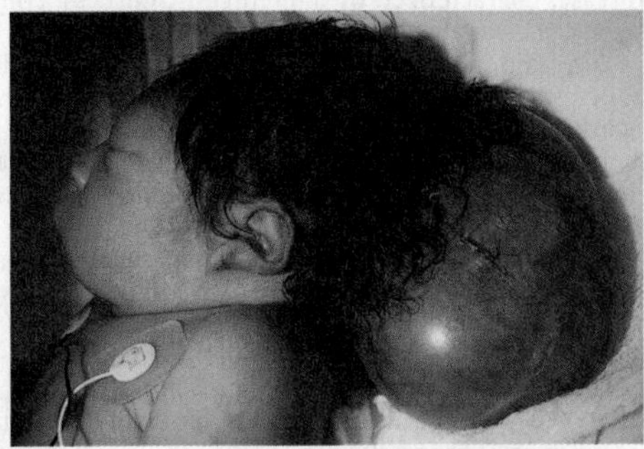

■ Encephalocele.

occipital e. an encephalocele in the occipital region, the most common kind seen in the Western Hemisphere.

en•ceph•a•lo•clas•tic (en-sef″ə-lo-klas′tik) [*encephalo-* + *clastic*] exhibiting the residues of a destructive lesion in the brain, such as porencephaly.

en•ceph•a•lo•cys•to•cele (en-sef″ə-lo-sis′to-sēl) [*encephalo-* + *cysto-* + *-cele*[1]] hydroencephalocele.

en•ceph•a•lo•di•al•y•sis (en-sef″ə-lo-di-al′ə-sis) encephalomalacia.

en•ceph•a•lo•du•ro•ar•te•ri•o•syn•an•gi•o•sis (en-sef″ə-lo-du″ro-ahr-te″re-o-sin-an-je-o′sis) a surgical treatment for moyamoya disease, consisting of transfer of a pedicle graft containing the superficial temporal artery onto the pia mater. In time, arterial linkages form between donor scalp artery branches and recipient brain surface artery branches to revascularize the cerebrum.

en•ceph•a•lo•dys•pla•sia (en-sef″ə-lo-dis-pla′zhə) any congenital anomaly of the brain.

en•ceph•a•log•ra•phy (en-sef″ə-log′rə-fe) [*encephalo-* + *-graphy*] radiography demonstrating the intracranial fluid-containing spaces after the withdrawal of cerebrospinal fluid and introduction of air or other gas; it includes pneumoencephalography and ventriculography.

en•ceph•a•loid (en-sef′ə-loid) [*encephalo-* + *-oid*] resembling the brain or brain substance.

en•ceph•a•lo•lith (en-sef′ə-lo-lith″) a brain calculus.

en•ceph•a•lo•ma (en-sef″ə-lo′mə) any swelling or tumor of the brain.

en•ceph•a•lo•ma•la•cia (en-sef″ə-lo-mə-la′shə) [*encephalo-* + *-malacia*] softening of the brain, especially that caused by an infarct.

avian e. a disease of young chickens due to vitamin E deficiency, in which there is ataxia, incoordination, paralysis, and severe encephalomalacia in several areas of the brain, especially the cerebellum. It must be differentiated from avian encephalomyelitis. Called also *crazy chick disease.*

nigropallidal e. neurotoxicity in horses that have spent an extended period grazing on *Centaurea repens* or *C. solstitialis*, which cause necrosis of the substantia nigra and globus pallidus; characteristics include wandering around in a confused manner and rigidity of facial muscles so that the animals cannot chew and may starve to death.

en•ceph•a•lo•men•in•gi•tis (en-sef″ə-lo-men″in-ji′tis) meningoencephalitis.

en•ceph•a•lo•me•nin•go•cele (en-sef″ə-lo-mə-ning′go-sēl) encephalocele.

en•ceph•a•lo•men•in•gop•a•thy (en-sef″ə-lo-men″in-gop′ə-the) meningoencephalopathy.

en•ceph•a•lo•mere (en-sef′ə-lo-mēr) [*encephalo-* + *-mere*] any one of the succession of segments which make up the embryonic brain.

en•ceph•a•lom•e•ter (en-sef″ə-lom′ə-tər) [*encephalo-* + *-meter*] an instrument used in locating certain of the regions of the brain.

en•ceph•a•lo•my•eli•tis (en-sef″ə-lo-mi″ə-li′tis) inflammation involving both the brain and the spinal cord. Called also *myeloencephalitis.*

acute disseminated e. an acute or subacute encephalomyelitis or myelitis characterized by perivascular lymphocyte and mononuclear cell infiltration and demyelination; it occurs most often after an acute viral infection, especially measles, but may occur without a recognizable antecedent. It is believed to be a manifestation of an autoimmune attack on the myelin of the central nervous system. Symptoms include fever, headache, and vomiting; sometimes tremor, seizures, and paralysis; and lethargy progressing to coma that can be fatal. Many survivors have residual neurologic deficits. Called also *acute perivascular myelinoclasis, postinfectious m., postvaccinal e.*, and *acute disseminated, postinfectious*, or *postvaccinal encephalitis.*

acute necrotizing hemorrhagic e. a rare, fatal postinfection or allergic demyelinating disease of the central nervous system, having a fulminating course and occurring mainly in young adults. It is characterized by destruction of the white matter to the point of liquefaction; widespread necrosis of blood vessel walls leading to the formation of multiple small hemorrhages in the involved areas and the exudation of fibrin into the surrounding tissue; and cellular infiltration of the necrotic areas. Onset is abrupt and marked by headache, stiff neck, and confusion; these are followed by focal seizures, paralysis, progressively deepening coma, and death.

autoimmune e. acute disseminated e.

avian e. a viral disease of chickens under six weeks old, caused by an enterovirus and marked by weakness of the legs followed by partial or complete paralysis of the legs, trembling of the head and neck, and degeneration of the neurons in the pons, medulla, and anterior horns of the spinal cord. Clinically, it resembles avian encephalomalacia and must be differentiated from that condition. Called also *crazy chick disease* and *epidemic tremor.*

benign myalgic e. chronic fatigue syndrome.

bovine e. Buss disease.

eastern equine e. (EEE) a form of equine encephalomyelitis that occurs in the eastern half of the United States and Canada, Mexico, and various other parts of the Americas. In humans it affects mainly children and the elderly; symptoms are fever, headache, and nausea followed by drowsiness, convulsions, and coma. Mortality is high in both humans and horses. Called also *eastern equine encephalitis.*

equine e. a type of encephalomyelitis in horses and mules, caused by an alphavirus and spread to humans by mosquitoes; it occurs in summer epizootics in various parts of the Americas. Three forms are recognized: *eastern equine e., western equine e.,* and *Venezuelan equine e.* Called also *equine encephalitis.* See also under *virus.*

experimental allergic e. (EAE) an animal model for acute disseminated encephalomyelitis in which the characteristic pathophysiology and clinical signs of this disease are produced by immunization of an animal with extracts of brain tissue or with myelin basic protein together with Freund adjuvant; it is transferable by adoptive transfer of lymphocytes but not by serum.

infectious porcine e. a type of encephalomyelitis of swine, seen primarily in Europe and caused by a picornavirus. It varies widely in severity; the severe form consists of a flaccid ascending paralysis similar to the paralysis of human poliomyelitis. Called also *porcine e., porcine poliomyelitis, Talfan disease,* and *Teschen disease.*

Mengo e. a type of encephalomyelitis seen in monkeys and mongooses in East Africa, caused by an encephalomyocarditis virus.

mouse e., murine e. Theiler disease.

myalgic e. chronic fatigue syndrome.

paraneoplastic e. inflammation of the central nervous system accompanying certain forms of cancer, most often small cell lung cancer; common symptoms include subacute sensory neuronopathy, limbic encephalitis, cerebellar degeneration, brainstem dysfunction, and myelopathy. In some patients neurologic complications precede the diagnosis of cancer.

porcine e., porcine viral e. infectious porcine e.

postinfectious e., postvaccinal e. acute disseminated e.

progressive e. with rigidity a syndrome resembling the stiff person syndrome, characterized by brainstem dysfunction, rigidity, and spinal myoclonus.

sporadic bovine e. Buss disease.

Theiler mouse e. Theiler disease.

toxoplasmic e. see under *meningoencephalitis.*

Venezuelan equine e. (VEE) a form of equine encephalomyelitis seen first in Colombia and Venezuela and later in Central America and the southwestern United States. The infection in humans resembles influenza, with only occasional central nervous system involvement; mortality is low. Called also *Venezuelan equine encephalitis.*

viral e., virus e. encephalomyelitis caused by a virus.

western equine e. (WEE) a form of equine encephalomyelitis seen in the western United States and Canada, and from Mexico to South America; it is less severe and has a lower mortality rate than the eastern type. In humans it usually affects young children; symptoms are fever, drowsiness, and convulsions. Called also *western equine encephalitis.*

en•ceph•a•lo•my•elo•cele (en-sef″ə-lo-mi-′ə-lo-sēl) [*encephalo-* + *myelo-* + *-cele*[1]] abnormality of the foramen magnum and absence of the laminae and spinous processes of the cervical vertebrae, with herniation of meninges, brain substance, and spinal cord.

en•ceph•a•lo•my•elo•neu•rop•a•thy (en-sef″ə-lo-mi″ə-lo-no͝o-rop′ə-the) disease involving the brain, spinal cord, and peripheral nerves.

en•ceph•a•lo•my•elop•a•thy (en-sef″ə-lo-mi″əl-op′ə-the) [*encephalo-* + *myelopathy*] any disease or diseased condition of the brain and spinal cord.

postinfection e. acute disseminated encephalomyelitis.

postvaccinial e. acute disseminated encephalomyelitis.

subacute necrotizing e. a type of encephalopathy of unclear clinical and pathological criteria, causing neuropathologic damage like that of the Wernicke-Korsakoff syndrome. It occurs in two forms: the *infantile form* is caused by mitochondrial energy metabolism protein mutations and pyruvate carboxylase complex mutations and is characterized by degeneration of gray matter with necrosis and capillary proliferation in the brainstem; hypotonia, seizures, and dementia; anorexia and vomiting; slow or arrested development; and ocular and respiratory disorders, with death usually before age 3. The *adult form* usually first manifests as bilateral optic atrophy with central scotoma and colorblindness, followed by a quiescent period of up to 30 years and then late symptoms such as ataxia, spastic paresis, clonic jerks, grand mal seizures, psychic lability, and mild dementia. Called also *subacute necrotizing encephalopathy* and *Leigh disease.*

en•ceph•a•lo•my•elo•ra•dic•u•li•tis (en-sef″ə-lo-mi″ə-lo-rə-dik″u-li-tis) inflammation of the brain, spinal cord, and spinal nerve roots.

en•ceph•a•lo•my•elo•ra•dic•u•lop•a•thy (en-sef″ə-lo-mi″ə-lo-rə-dik″u-lop′ə-the) disease involving the brain, spinal cord, and spinal nerve roots.

en•ceph•a•lo•myo•car•di•tis (en-sef″ə-lo-mi″o-kahr-di′tis) a viral disease of pigs and certain nonhuman primates, caused by a cardiovirus and characterized by degenerative and inflammatory changes in skeletal and cardiac muscle, and lesions of the central nervous system resembling those of poliomyelitis.

en•ceph•a•lo•my•op•a•thy (en-sef″ə-lo-mi-op′ə-the) any disease involving the brain and muscles.

mitochondrial e. any of a group of diseases characterized by abnormal mitochondrial function with involvement of the central nervous system and skeletal muscle and, in most cases, lactic acidosis. Diseases in this group, which includes subacute necrotizing encephalomyelitis, Leber hereditary optic neuropathy, MELAS syndrome, and MERRF syndrome, may also be classified as mitochondrial myopathies or mitochondrial encephalopathies.

mitochondrial neurogastrointestinal e. (MNGIE) a mitochondrial encephalomyopathy of autosomal recessive inheritance, having an onset between the second and fifth decades of life and characterized by intestinal dysmotility, ptosis, cachexia, ophthalmoplegia, peripheral neuropathy, and leukoencephalopathy.

en•ceph•a•lon (en-sef′ə-lon) [L., from Gr. *enkephalos,* from *en-* in + *kephalē* head] [TA] the brain: that part of the central nervous system contained within the cranium, comprising the prosencephalon, mesencephalon, and rhombencephalon; it is derived (developed) from the anterior part of the embryonic neural tube. See Plate 9. See also *cerebrum.*

en•ceph•a•lo•nar•co•sis (en-sef″ə-lo-nahr-ko′sis) [*encephalo-* + *narcosis*] stupor due to brain disease.

en•ceph•a•lo•path•ic (en-sef″ə-lo-path′ik) pertaining to encephalopathy.

en•ceph•a•lop•a•thy (en-sef″ə-lop′ə-the) [*encephalo-* + *-pathy*] any degenerative disease of the brain.

AIDS e. HIV e.

anoxic e. hypoxic e.

anoxic-ischemic e. hypoxic-ischemic e.

biliary e. kernicterus.

bilirubin e. kernicterus.

bovine spongiform e. a prion disease of adult cattle that is epizootic in Great Britain and Northern Ireland, characterized by apprehensive behavior, hyperesthesia, and ataxia. It is transmitted by feed containing protein in the form of meat and bone meal derived from infected animals. The etiologic agent is also the cause of new variant Creutzfeldt-Jakob disease. Called also *mad cow disease.*

boxer's e., boxer's traumatic e. chronic traumatic e.

chronic traumatic e. a syndrome due to cumulative head blows, such as in football or the boxing ring, characterized by general slowing of mental function, occasional bouts of confusion, and scattered memory loss. In time it may progress to the more serious *boxer's dementia.* Called also *boxer's, boxer's traumatic, punch drunk,* or *traumatic e.* Cf. *postconcussional syndrome.*

cytomegalovirus e. see under *encephalitis.*

demyelinating e. any encephalopathy accompanied by demyelination; see *Schilder disease,* under *disease.*

dialysis e. a degenerative disease of the brain formerly seen with long-term use of hemodialysis, due to aluminum poisoning (q.v.) caused by high levels of aluminum in the water used in the dialysis fluid or by aluminum-containing compounds given to control phosphorus levels. Symptoms include speech disorders, myoclonic jerks, and psychological changes progressing to global dementia. Called also *progressive dialysis e.* and *dialysis dementia.*

glycine e. a genetically heterogeneous, autosomal recessive aminoacidopathy caused by mutations that result in defects in enzymes of the glycine cleavage system, characterized by accumulation of glycine in body fluids, particularly the blood, urine, and cerebrospinal fluid. The *neonatal form* is the most common, with lethargy, absence of cerebral development, seizures, myoclonic jerks, and frequently coma and respiratory failure. *Infantile* and *late-onset* forms are milder. A *transient* form resembles the neonatal form, with glycine levels normalizing by 8 weeks of age; usually there are no neurologic deficits, although mild mental retardation sometimes occurs. Called also *nonketotic hyperglycinemia.*

Hashimoto e. a type of encephalopathy that occasionally accompanies Hashimoto disease, characterized by altered consciousness, confusion, and sometimes myoclonic seizures.

hepatic e. a condition usually seen secondary to advanced disease of the liver but also seen with other severe diseases and in patients with portacaval shunts. It is marked by disturbances of consciousness that may progress to deep coma (hepatic coma), psychiatric changes of varying degree, flapping tremor, and fetor hepaticus. Called also *portal-systemic, portasystemic,* or *portosystemic e.*

HIV e., HIV-related e. a progressive primary encephalopathy caused by infection with human immunodeficiency virus type 1; it involves principally the subcortical white matter and deep gray nuclei and is manifested by a variety of cognitive, motor, and behavioral abnormalities. Called also *AIDS dementia complex, AIDS e.,* and *HIV encephalitis.*

hyperammonemic e. the effects on the brain of hyperammonemia, often including seizures progressing to coma; the usual causes are liver disease (see *hepatic e.*) and disturbances in the urea cycle.

hypernatremic e. a severe hemorrhagic encephalopathy induced by the hyperosmolarity accompanying hypernatremia and dehydration.

hypertensive e. a complex of cerebral phenomena such as headache, convulsions, and coma that occur in the course of malignant hypertension.

hypoglycemic e. metabolic encephalopathy induced by severe hypoglycemia, as in glycogen storage disease, oversecretion or overdose of insulin, etc.

hyponatremic e. encephalopathy caused by influx of water into the brain in hyponatremia, with consequent swelling. Manifestations include lethargy, psychosis, and seizures. In severe cases, compression of the brainstem can result in pulmonary edema and hypoxemia; hypoxia can lead to brain damage and death.

hypoxic e. encephalopathy caused by hypoxia from either decreased rate of blood flow or decreased oxygen content of arterial blood; symptoms in mild cases include intellectual, visual, and motor disturbances. Severe cases, such as with cardiac arrest or blocking of the airways, can cause permanent damage within five minutes. Called also *anoxic e.*

hypoxic-ischemic e. encephalopathy resulting from asphyxia. In infants presumed to have suffered prenatal or perinatal asphyxia, common symptoms are lethargy, feeding difficulties, and convulsions; serious cases may involve necrosis of neurons in the brain with psychomotor retardation and spastic motor deficits such as cerebral palsy. In adults, syndromes range from cortical blindness to irreversible coma.

lead e. a condition caused by excessive ingestion of lead compounds, seen especially in young children. Pathological characteristics are edema and central demyelination; symptoms include vomiting and apathy followed by stupor, seizures, coma, and death. See also *lead poisoning*, under *poisoning*. Called also *lead encephalitis* and *saturnine e.*

metabolic e. neuropsychiatric disturbances due to metabolic brain disease; it may be primary, resulting from conditions such as hypoxia or ischemia that affect the brain directly, or it may be secondary to disease of other organs.

mink e. a type of prion disease seen in minks, characterized by locomotor incoordination that progresses to semicoma and death.

mitochondrial e. any of numerous encephalopathies associated with mitochondrial abnormalities, such as cytochrome-*c* oxidase deficiency.

multicystic e. the formation of large, multilocular cavities throughout the cerebral hemispheres, occurring in the perinatal period; causes include anoxia, necrotizing viral encephalitis (especially herpes simplex), and neonatal meningitis.

myoclonic e. of childhood a variant of opsoclonus-myoclonus syndrome seen in children, with onset between ages one and three, characterized by myoclonus of trunk and limbs and by opsoclonus, with ataxia of gait and intention tremor. The etiology is unknown, but some cases have been associated with occult neuroblastoma. Called also *Kinsbourne syndrome.*

pancreatic e. metabolic encephalopathy occurring as a complication of pancreatitis.

portal-systemic e., portasystemic e., portosystemic e. (PSE) hepatic e.

progressive dialysis e. dialysis e.

progressive subcortical e. Schilder disease; see under *disease.*

punch-drunk e. chronic traumatic e.

saturnine e. lead e.

sepsis-associated e., septic e. altered brain function owing to the presence of infectious agents in the blood, including the effects of fever; symptoms vary from mild to severe and may include confusion, myopathy with rigidity, and more serious conditions such as seizures and coma.

static e. an encephalopathy whose manifestations do not worsen over time.

subacute necrotizing e. see under *encephalomyelopathy.*

subacute spongiform e. prion disease.

subcortical arteriosclerotic e. Binswanger disease.

transmissible spongiform e. (TSE) prion disease.

traumatic e. 1. postconcussional syndrome. 2. chronic traumatic e.

uremic e. cerebral symptoms seen in patients with uremia, including lethargy, fatigue, inattentiveness, irritability, confusion, sensory disturbances, and sometimes seizures.

Wernicke e. a neurological disorder characterized by confusion, apathy, drowsiness, ataxia of gait, nystagmus, and ophthalmoplegia, now known to be due to thiamine deficiency, usually from chronic alcohol abuse. It is almost invariably accompanied by or followed by Korsakoff syndrome (organic amnesia) and frequently accompanied by other nutritional polyneuropathies. Called also *Wernicke disease.* See also *Wernicke-Korsakoff syndrome*, under *syndrome.*

en•ceph•a•lo•punc•ture (en-sef″ə-lo-pungk′chər) surgical puncture of the brain.

en•ceph•a•lo•py•o•sis (en-sef″ə-lo-pi-o′sis) [*encephalo-* + *pyo-* + *-sis*] suppuration or abscess of the brain.

en•ceph•a•lo•ra•dic•u•li•tis (en-sef″ə-lo-rə-dik′u-li″tis) inflammation of the roots of spinal nerves and of the brain.

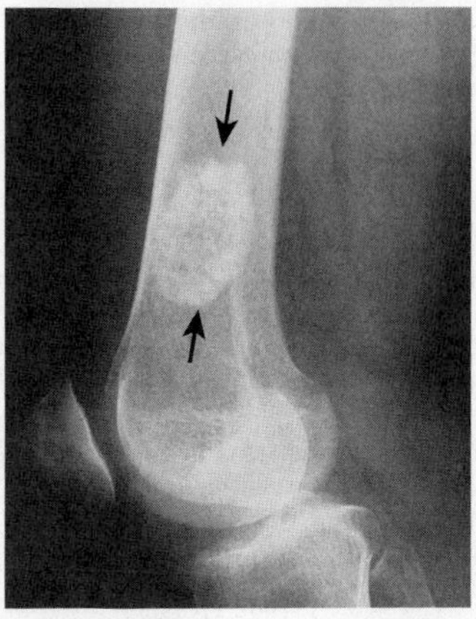

■ Enchondroma in a lateral view of the knee.

en•ceph•a•lor•rha•gia (en-sef″ə-lo-ra′jə) [*encephalo-* + *-rrhagia*] hemorrhage within the brain or from the brain, especially cerebral pericapillary hemorrhage.

pericapillary e. brain purpura.

en•ceph•a•lo•scle•ro•sis (en-sef″ə-lo-sklə-ro′sis) [*encephalo-* + *sclerosis*] hardening of the brain.

en•ceph•a•lo•scope (en-sef′ə-lə-skōp) an instrument for examining a cavity (such as an abscess cavity) in the brain.

en•ceph•a•los•co•py (en-sef″ə-los′kə-pe) [*encephalo-* + *-scopy*] inspection or examination of the brain.

en•ceph•a•lo•sep•sis (en-sef″ə-lo-sep′sis) [*encephalo-* + *sepsis*] gangrene of brain tissue.

en•ceph•a•lo•sis (en-sef″ə-lo′sis) encephalopathy.

en•ceph•a•lo•spi•nal (en-sef″ə-lo-spi′nəl) cerebrospinal.

en•ceph•a•lo•tome (en-sef′ə-lə-tōm) an instrument for performing encephalotomy.

en•ceph•a•lot•o•my (en-sef″ə-lot′ə-me) [*encephal-* + *-otomy*] incision of the brain; called also *cerebrotomy.*

en•chon•dral (en-kon′drəl) endochondral.

en•chon•dro•ma (en″kon-dro′mə) pl. *enchondromas, enchondromata* [*en-* + *chondroma*] a benign growth of cartilage arising in the metaphysis of a bone; called also *true chondroma.* **enchondro′matous** *adj*

multiple congenital e's enchondromatosis.

en•chon•dro•ma•to•sis (en-kon″dro-mə-to′sis) a condition characterized by hamartomatous proliferation of cartilage cells within the metaphysis of several bones, causing thinning of the overlying cortex and distortion of the growth in length; it may undergo malignant transformation, particularly to chondrosarcoma. Called also *multiple* or *skeletal e.* and *Ollier disease.* See also *Maffucci syndrome.*

en•chon•dro•sar•co•ma (en-kon″dro-sahr-ko′mə) central chondrosarcoma.

en•chon•dro•sis (en″kon-dro′sis) 1. an outgrowth from cartilage. 2. enchondroma.

en•chy•ma (en′kə-mə) [*en-* + Gr. *chymos* juice] the substance elaborated from absorbed nutritive materials; the formative juice of the tissues.

en•clave (en′klāv, ahn-klahv′) [Fr.] a tissue detached from its normal connection and enclosed within another organ or tissue.

en•clo•mi•phene (en-klo′mĭ-fēn) the *cis*-isomer of the gonad-stimulating principle clomiphene citrate; called also *cisclomiphene.* Cf *zuclomiphene.*

en•cod•ing (en-kōd′ing) the assigning of values to scientific data so that it can be stored as information.

frequency e. in magnetic resonance imaging, the sorting of radio frequencies that are detected and assigning values to them so that the image can be interpreted.

en•co•pre•sis (en-ko-pre′sis) fecal incontinence.

functional e. fecal incontinence that does not have an organic cause.

en•cra•ni•us (en-kra′ne-əs) [*en-* + Gr. *kranion* skull] in asymmetrical conjoined twins, a parasitic twin located within the cranium of the larger twin.

en•cyo•py•eli•tis (en-si″o-pi″ə-li′tis) [*encyesis* + *pyelitis*] dilatation of the ureters or renal pelvis or both during normal pregnancy with associated edema, but seldom with all the usual signs of inflammation.

en•cys•ta•tion (en″sis-ta′shən) in the life cycle of certain protozoa, such as species of *Amoeba*, *Entamoeba*, and *Toxoplasma*, the formation of cysts from trophozoites.

en•cyst•ed (en-sist′əd) [*en-* + Gr. *kystis* sac, bladder] enclosed in a sac, bladder, or cyst.

en•cyst•ment (en-sist′mənt) the process or condition of being or becoming encysted.

end (end) the farthest part of something with length; the outside or extreme edge.
acromial e. of clavicle extremitas acromialis claviculae.
sternal e. of clavicle extremitas sternalis claviculae.

end•a•del•phos (end″ə-del′fos) [*end-* + *-adelphus*] asymmetrical conjoined twins in which a parasitic fetus is enclosed within the body of or within a tumor in the larger twin. Cf. *fetus in fetu.*

end•an•gi•itis (end-an″je-i′tis) inflammation of the tunica intima; called also *endoangiitis*, *endovasculitis*, and *intimitis.*

end•aor•tic (en″da-or′tik) pertaining to the interior of the aorta.

end•aor•ti•tis (end″a-or-ti′tis) inflammation of the tunica intima of the aorta; called also *endoaortitis.*
bacterial e. the formation of bacterial vegetations on the endothelial surface of the aorta.

end•ar•ter•ec•to•my (end-ahr″tər-ek′tə-me) excision of the thickened, atheromatous tunica intima of an artery. See also *atherectomy.*
aortoiliac e. endarterectomy performed on the abdominal aorta and common iliac arteries, done for disease localized around their junctions.
carotid e. endarterectomy of the carotid artery, done for the prevention of stroke.
common femoral e. endarterectomy performed on the common femoral artery, done to relieve ischemia of the lower limb.
gas e. endarterectomy done with high-pressure carbon dioxide to remove plaque deposits from the coronary blood vessels in treatment of atherosclerosis.
renal e., renal artery e. endarterectomy of a renal artery, a technique of renal revascularization.
transluminal e. endarterectomy using a cutting device inside a catheter that is inserted through the lumen of a vessel; see *transluminal endarterectomy catheter*, under *catheter.* Called also *transluminal atherectomy.*
vertebral e. endarterectomy of the vertebral artery, done to treat some types of vertebrobasilar insufficiency.

end•ar•te•ri•al (end″ahr-tēr′e-əl) intra-arterial.

end•ar•ter•i•tis (end-ahr″tə-ri′tis) [*end-* + *arteritis*] inflammation of the tunica intima of an artery; intimitis. Cf. *arteritis* and *periarteritis.*
Heubner e. see under *disease.*
e. obli′terans endarteritis in which the lumina of the smaller vessels become narrowed or obliterated as a result of proliferation of the tissue of the intimal layer; called also *arteritis obliterans* and *Friedländer disease.* See also *arteriosclerosis obliterans.*
e. proli′ferans overgrowth of fibrous tissue in the internal layers of the aorta or some other artery.

end•ar•te•ri•um (end″ahr-tēr′e-əm) [*end-* + *arteria*] the tunica intima of an artery.

end•ar•ter•op•a•thy (end-ahr″tər-op′ə-the) a disorder of the tunica intima of an artery.
digital e. disorder of the tunica intima of the arteries of the digits, associated with Raynaud phenomenon and nutritional lesions of the pulp of the fingers.

end•au•ral (end-aw′rəl) intra-aural.

end•brain (end′brān) telencephalon.

end-brush (end′brush) telodendron.

end•bud (end′bud) caudal eminence.

end-bulb (end′bulb) encapsulated nerve ending.
e.-b. of Held an enlarged process at the end of an axon of a primary neuron of the cochlear nerve, synapsing with the body of a secondary neuron in the ventral cochlear nucleus.
Krause e.-b. a type of small, spherical, encapsulated nerve ending found particularly in the dermis, lips, mouth, and conjunctiva; thought to function as a rapidly adapting mechanoreceptor.

en•deic•tic (en-dīk′tik) [Gr. *endeixis* a pointing out] symptomatic.

en•de•mia (en-de′me-ə) endemic disease.

en•dem•ic (en-dem′ik) [Gr. *endēmos* dwelling in a place] present or usually prevalent in a population or geographical area at all times; said of a disease or agent. Cf. *epidemic.* See also *holoendemic* and *hyperendemic.*

en•de•mo•ep•i•dem•ic (en″də-mo-ep″ĭ-dem′ik) endemic, but occasionally becoming epidemic.

end•epi•der•mis (end″ep-ĭ-dur′mis) epithelium.

end•er•gon•ic (end″ər-gon′ik) [*end-* + Gr. *ergon* work] characterized by or accompanied by the absorption of energy; said of reactions, particularly biochemical reactions, that require energy in order to proceed, so that the products have a higher free energy than the reactants. Opposed to *exergonic.*

end-foot (end′foot) bouton terminal; see under *bouton.*

end•ing (end′ing) 1. a termination or finish. 2. nerve e.
annulospiral e's wide, ribbonlike sensory nerve endings wrapped around the center of intrafusal fibers of a muscle spindle; called also *primary e's.* See also *flower-spray e's.*
club e. of Bartelmez a type of nerve fiber ending in the vertebrate central nervous system, terminating abruptly on the dendrite of another neuron.
encapsulated nerve e. a sensory nerve ending characterized by a fibrous capsule of varying thickness that is continuous with the endoneurium.
epilemmal e's sensory nerve endings in striated muscle in which the nerve endings are in close contact with the muscle fibers.
flower-spray e's branched sensory nerve endings on intrafusal fibers of muscle spindles; their axons are more slender than those of annulospiral endings and they are at more peripheral locations or are confined to nuclear fibers. Called also *secondary e's.*
free nerve e. the type of neural receptor with the simplest form, in which the peripheral nerve fiber divides into fine branches that terminate freely in connective tissue or epithelium.
grape e's nerve endings in muscle which have the form of terminal swellings.
nerve e. any of the fine branchlike terminations of neurons. Sensory nerve endings are the beginnings of afferent pathways of myelinated fibers of pseudounipolar neurons; they are classified as either free or encapsulated. Motor nerve endings are the endings of axons and are called *motor end plates;* see under *end plate.*
nonencapsulated nerve e. free nerve e.
primary e's annulospiral e's.
Ruffini e. a type of lamellated corpuscle in the dermis that is a slowly adapting receptor for sensations of continuous pressure. Called also *Ruffini corpuscle.*
secondary e's flower-spray e's.

end•nu•cle•us (end-noo′kle-əs) terminal nucleus; see under *nucleus.*

end(o)- [Gr. *endon* within] prefix denoting an inward situation; within.

en•do•ab•dom•i•nal (en″do-ab-dom′ĭ-nəl) intra-abdominal.

en•do•am•y•lase (en″do-am′ə-lās) an amylase that catalyzes the cleavage of α-1,4-glucosidic bonds not necessarily at the nonreducing end of the polysaccharide. Cf. *exoamylase.*

en•do•an•eu•rys•mor•rha•phy (en″do-an″u-riz-mor′ə-fe) [*endo-* + *aneurysmorrhaphy*] a formerly common type of aneurysmoplasty done by opening the aneurysmal sac and narrowing the internal lumen by suture; called also *Matas operation.*

en•do•an•gi•itis (en″do-an-je-i′tis) endangiitis.

en•do•aor•ti•tis (en″do-a″or-ti′tis) endaortitis.

en•do•ap•pen•di•ci•tis (en″do-ə-pen″dĭ-si′tis) inflammation of the mucous membrane lining the vermiform appendix.

en•do•ar•ter•itis (en″do-ahr″tər-i′tis) endarteritis.

en•do•aus•cul•ta•tion (en″do-aws″kəl-ta′shən) auscultation of the stomach and thoracic organs by means of a tube passed into the stomach.

en•do•bac•il•lary (en″do-bas′ĭ-lar-e) contained within a bacillus.

en•do•bi•ot•ic (en″do-bi-ot′ik) [*endo-* + *biotic*] living parasitically within the tissues of the host.

en•do•blast (en′do-blast) [*endo-* + *-blast*] endoderm. **endoblas′tic** *adj*

en•do•bron•chi•al (en″do-brong′ke-əl) within a bronchus or bronchi.

en•do•bron•chi•tis (en″do-brong-ki′tis) inflammation of the epithelial lining of the bronchi.

en•do•can•nab•i•noid (en″do-kə-nab′ĭ-noid) any of a group of cannabinoids produced in the central nervous system under certain conditions, apparently acting as modulators of bodily responses to certain types of stimuli through effects on synaptic transmission.

en•do•car•di•op•a•thy (en″do-kahr″de-op′ə-the) [*endocardium* + *-pathy*] a disorder or disease of the endocardium.

en•do•car•di•o•sis (en″do-kahr″de-o′sis) a heart disease of dogs, consisting of chronic fibrosis of the atrioventricular valves, usually the mitral valve; it may lead to congestive heart failure.

en•do•car•di•tis (en″do-kahr-di′tis) [*endocardium* + *-itis*] exudative and proliferative inflammatory alterations of the endocardium, usually characterized by the presence of vegetations on the surface of the endocardium or in the endocardium itself, and most commonly involving a heart valve, but sometimes affecting the inner lining of the cardiac chambers or the endocardium elsewhere. It may occur as a primary disorder or as a complication of or in association with another disease. **endocardit′ic** *adj*

acute bacterial e. (ABE) see *infective e.*

atypical verrucous e. Libman-Sacks e.

bacterial e. infective endocarditis caused by any of various bacteria, such as streptococci, staphylococci, enterococci, gonococci, or gram-negative bacilli.

***Candida* e.** mycotic endocarditis caused by a species of *Candida;* called also *endocardial candidiasis.*

e. benig′na Libman-Sacks e.

e. chorda′lis endocarditis affecting particularly the chordae tendineae.

constrictive e. Löffler e.

fungal e. mycotic e.

infectious e., infective e. endocarditis caused by infection with microorganisms, especially bacteria and fungi, traditionally classified according to course as acute or subacute. The *acute* form is usually due to staphylococci, pneumococci, gonococci, or streptococci, involves a normal heart valve, and has a short history and rapid course. The *subacute* form usually is due to viridans or fecal streptococci or to fungi, affects damaged heart valves, and has a prolonged course. Because underlying causes and available therapies have changed, this category has largely been replaced by classification on the basis of etiology or underlying anatomy.

e. len′ta the subacute form of infective endocarditis.

Libman-Sacks e. a type of nonbacterial thrombotic endocarditis associated with systemic lupus erythematosus; the vegetations consist of necrotic debris, fibrinoid material, and trapped, disintegrating, fibroblastic and inflammatory cells, usually on the atrioventricular valves. Called also *Libman-Sacks disease* and *atypical verrucous* or *nonbacterial verrucous e.*

Löffler e., Löffler fibroplastic parietal e. endocarditis associated with eosinophilia, marked by fibroplastic thickening of the endocardium, and resulting in congestive heart failure, persistent tachycardia, hepatomegaly, splenomegaly, serous effusions into the pleural cavity, edema of the lower limbs, and edema and ascites of the upper limbs; called also *constrictive e.* and *eosinophilic endomyocardial disease.*

malignant e. infective endocarditis.

marantic e. nonbacterial thrombotic e.

mural e. endocarditis affecting the lining of the walls of the heart chambers, rather than the valvular, chordal, trabecular, or papillary tissue. Called also *parietal e.*

mycotic e. infective endocarditis, usually subacute, due to any of various fungi, most commonly *Candida* (especially *C. albicans*), *Aspergillus,* and *Histoplasma.* Called also *fungal e.*

native valve e. infective endocarditis involving one or more of the natural heart valves, in contrast to *prosthetic valve e.*

nonbacterial thrombotic e. (NBTE) endocarditis usually occurring in chronic debilitating disease, particularly malignancy; it is characterized by noninfected vegetations composed of fibrin and other blood elements, generally located on the line of closure of the mitral and aortic valves and susceptible to embolization.

nonbacterial verrucous e. Libman-Sacks e.

parietal e. mural e.

prosthetic valve e. infective endocarditis as a complication of implantation of a prosthetic heart valve; the vegetations usually occur along the line of suture.

rheumatic e. endocarditis associated with rheumatic fever. Involvement may be mural but is usually valvular and involves the entire valve; it is then more accurately termed rheumatic valvulitis (q.v.).

rickettsial e. infective endocarditis resulting from invasion of the heart valves with *Coxiella burnetii;* it is a sequela of Q fever, usually occurring in persons who have had rheumatic fever.

right-side e. infective endocarditis of the right side of the heart.

septic e. infective e.

staphylococcal e. infective endocarditis caused by staphylococcal invasion of the heart valves.

streptococcal e. infective endocarditis caused by streptococcal invasion of the heart valves.

subacute bacterial e. (SBE) see *infective e.*

syphilitic e. endocarditis resulting from extension of syphilitic infection from the aorta.

tuberculous e. a rare form of endocarditis in which the endocardium is involved by extension of a tuberculous perimyocarditis or of miliary tuberculosis.

ulcerative e. infective endocarditis characterized by rapid ulceration of the valvular lesions.

valvular e. endocarditis affecting the membrane over the valves of the heart, rather than the mural, chordal, trabecular, or papillary tissue.

vegetative e., verrucous e. endocarditis whose characteristic lesions are vegetations or verrucae on the endocardium; it may be either infective or some other type.

viridans e. a subacute form of infective endocarditis due to infection with viridans streptococci.

en·do·car·di·um (en″do-kahr′de-əm) [*endo* + Gr. *kardia* heart] [TA] the endothelial lining membrane of the cavities of the heart and the connective tissue bed on which it lies. This subendothelial connective tissue contains varying amounts of elastic and collagen fibers and smooth muscle cells. **endocar′dial** *adj*

en·do·ce·li·ac (en″do-se′le-ak) [*endo-* + Gr. *koilia* cavity] inside one of the body cavities.

en·do·cel·lu·lar (en″do-sel′u-lər) intracellular.

en·do·cer·vi·cal (en″do-sur′vĭ-kəl) pertaining to the interior of the cervix uteri.

en·do·cer·vi·ci·tis (en″do-sur″vĭ-si′tis) [*endo-* + *cervicitis*] inflammation of the mucous membrane of the cervix uteri.

en·do·cer·vix (en″do-sur′viks) 1. the mucous membrane lining the canal of the cervix uteri. 2. the region of the opening of the uterine cervix into the uterine cavity.

En·do·cet (en′do-set″) trademark for a combination preparation of oxycodone hydrochloride and acetaminophen.

en·do·chon·dral (en″do-kon′drəl) situated, formed, or occurring within cartilage.

en·do·cho·ri·on (en″do-kor′e-on) [*endo-* + *chorion*] the inner chorionic layer.

en·do·co·li·tis (en″do-ko-li′tis) inflammation of the mucous membrane of the colon.

en·do·com·men·sal (en″do-kə-men′səl) a commensal organism which lives inside the body of its symbiotic companion.

en·do·co·nid·io·tox·i·co·sis (en″do-ko-nĭd″e-o-tok″sĭ-ko′sis) mycotoxicosis from ingestion of fungi of the genus *Endoconidium;* see *darnel poisoning,* under *poisoning.*

En·do·co·ni·di·um (en″do-kə-nid′e-um) a genus of Fungi Imperfecti of the form-class Hyphomycetes. *E. temulen′tum* sometimes contaminates the grass *Lolium temulentum* and causes darnel poisoning.

en·do·cor·pus·cu·lar (en″do-kor-pus′ku-lər) intracorpuscular.

en·do·cra·ni·al (en″do-kra′ne-əl) intracranial.

en·do·cra·ni·o·sis (en″do-kra″ne-o′sis) hyperostosis frontalis interna.

en·do·cra·ni·tis (en″do-kra-ni′tis) inflammation of the endocranium.

en·do·cra·ni·um (en″do-kra′ne-əm) [*endo-* + Gr. *kranion* skull] the endosteal outer layer of the dura mater of the brain.

en·do·crine (en′do-krin, en′do-krīn) [*endo-* + Gr. *krinein* to separate] 1. secreting internally (as opposed to *exocrine*), applied to organs and structures that release their products into the blood or lymph, and to substances *(hormones)* that exert specific effects on other organs. See also under *system.* Called also *endosecretory.* 2. hormonal.

en·do·cri·nol·o·gist (en″do-krĭ-nol′ə-jist) a specialist in endocrinology.

en·do·cri·nol·o·gy (en″do-krĭ-nol′ə-je) [*endocrine* + *-logy*] 1. the study of hormones, the endocrine system, and their role in the physiology of the body. 2. a medical specialty concerned with the diagnosis and treatment of disorders of the endocrine system.

en·do·cri·nop·a·thy (en″do-krĭ-nop′ə-the) [*endocrine* + *-pathy*] any disease due to a disorder of the endocrine system (hormonal imbalance). Called also *endocrinosis.* **endocrinopath′ic** *adj*

en·do·cri·no·sis (en″do-krĭ-no′sis) endocrinopathy.

en·do·cri·no·ther·a·py (en″do-krĭ″no-ther′ə-pe) endocrine therapy.

en·do·cu·ti·cle (en″do-ku′tĭ-kəl) [*endo-* + L. *cuticula*] the inner layer of the procuticle in certain crustaceans and arthropods, which is almost entirely composed of protein and chitin.

en·do·cyc·lic (en″do-sik′lik, -si′klik) a term applied to cyclic compounds in which the bond occurs in the ring.

en·do·cyst (en′do-sist) the inner, germinative, or embryonic membrane of a hydatid cyst.

en·do·cy·to·sis (en″do-si-to′sis) [*endo-* + *cyt-* + *-osis*] the uptake by a cell of material from the environment by invagination of its plasma membrane; it includes both phagocytosis and pinocytosis.

En·do·dan (en′do-dan″) trademark for a combination preparation of oxycodone hydrochloride, oxycodone terephthalate, and aspirin.

en·do·de·oxy·ri·bo·nu·cle·ase (en″do-de-ok″se-ri″bo-noo′kle-ās) [EC 3.1.21–25] any member of several sub-subclasses of enzymes of the hydrolase class that catalyze the hydrolysis of interior bonds of deoxyribonucleic acids, producing oligonucleotides or polynucleotides.

en·do·derm (en′do-dərm) [*endo-* + *-derm*] the innermost of the three primary germ layers of the embryo; from it are derived the epithelium of the pharynx, respiratory tract (except the nose), digestive tract, bladder,

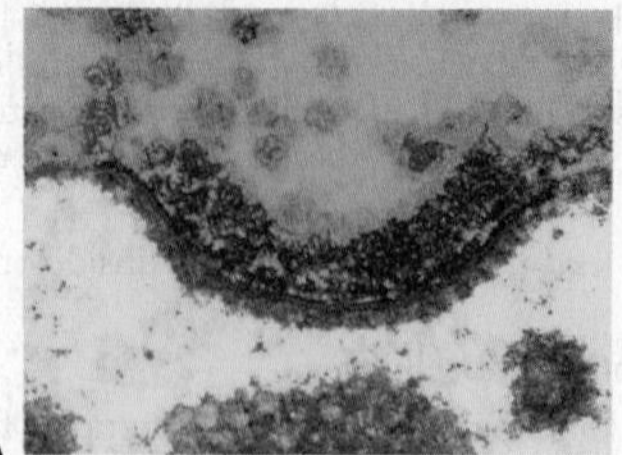

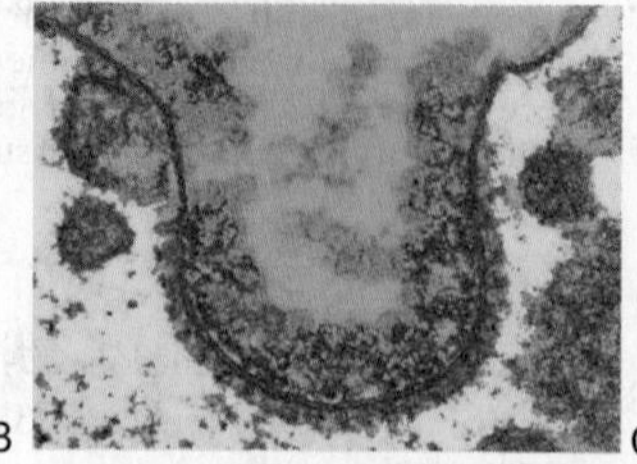

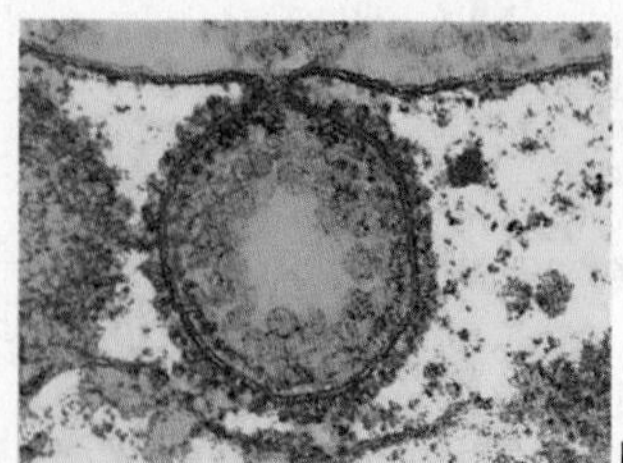

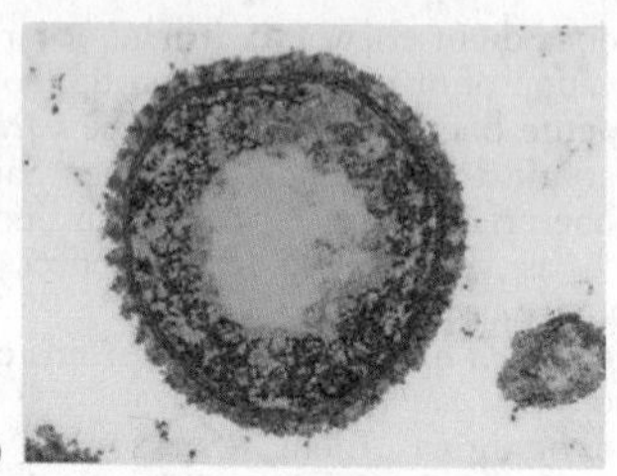

■ Endocytosis. *(A)*, Membrane receptors bind to specific molecules in the extracellular fluid; *(B)*, a portion of the plasma membrane is pulled inward by the cytoskeleton, forming a small pocket around the material to be moved into the cell; *(C)*, the edges of the pocket fuse to form a vesicle; *(D)*, the vesicle is pulled inward, away from the plasma membrane, by the cytoskeleton.

and urethra. Called also *entoderm, endoblast,* and *entoblast.* Cf. *ectoderm* and *mesoderm.*

primitive e., primordial e. the primary internal layer of the gastrula that becomes both gut and yolk sac.

yolk sac e. the epithelial lining of the yolk sac.

en•do•der•mal (en″do-dur′məl) 1. pertaining to the endoderm. 2. derived from endoderm.

en•do•don•tics (en″do-don′tiks) [*end-* + *odont-* + *-ics*] the branch of dentistry concerned with the etiology, prevention, diagnosis, and treatment of diseases and injuries affecting the dental pulp, tooth root, and periapical tissue. In current usage, this term has a more restrictive meaning than *endodontology,* which refers to study of the pulp in both health and disease, although sometimes the terms are used interchangeably.

surgical e. the treatment of diseases and injuries of the dental pulp through surgical means.

en•do•don•tist (en″do-don′tist) a dentist who specializes in endodontics; called also *endodontologist.*

en•do•don•ti•um (en″do-don′she-əm) pulpa dentis.

en•do•don•tol•o•gist (en″do-don-tol′ə-jist) endodontist.

en•do•don•tol•o•gy (en″do-don-tol′ə-je) [*end-* + *odont-* + *-logy*] the scientific study of the dental pulp and associated processes in health and disease. In current usage, this term has a broader sense than *endodontics,* which is restricted to the pulp in situations of injury or disease. Sometimes the terms are used interchangeably.

en•do•dy•og•e•ny (en″do-di-oj′ə-ne) reproduction by the formation of two daughter cells within the wall of the mother cell (internal budding), the progeny being released by rupture of the mother cell, as in the protozoan *Toxoplasma.*

en•do•ec•to•thrix (en″do-ek′to-thriks) a fungus that produces spores both on the interior and exterior of the hairs.

en•do•en•ter•itis (en″do-en″tə-ri′tis) inflammation of the mucous membrane of the intestine.

en•do•en•zyme (en″do-en′zīm) an enzyme that is retained in a cell and does not normally diffuse out of the cell into the surrounding medium; called also *intracellular enzyme.* Cf. *exoenzyme.*

en•do•er•gic (en″do-ur′jik) 1. endergonic. 2. endothermic.

en•do•esoph•a•gi•tis (en″do-e-sof″ə-gi′tis) inflammation of the lining membrane of the esophagus.

en•do•exo•ter•ic (en″do-ek″so-ter′ik) [*endo-* + *exoteric*] resulting from certain causes internal to the body, and from others of external origin.

en•do•far•a•dism (en″do-far′ə-diz-əm) the application of alternating current to an internal organ, as to the stomach.

en•do•gal•va•nism (en″do-gal′və-niz-əm) the application of direct current to an internal organ, as to the stomach.

en•dog•a•mous (ən-dog′ə-məs) characterized by endogamy.

en•dog•a•my (en-dog′ə-me) [*endo-* + Gr. *gamos* marriage] 1. fertilization by the union of separate cells having the same genetic ancestry. Cf. *autogamy* and *exogamy* (def. 1). 2. marriage within a community, range, or other group.

en•do•gas•tric (en″do-gas′trik) intragastric.

en•do•gas•tri•tis (en″do-gas-tri′tis) inflammation of the mucous membrane of the stomach.

en•do•ge•net•ic (en″do-jə-net′ik) endogenous.

en•do•gen•ic (en″do-jen′ik) endogenous.

en•do•geno•mor•phic (ən-doj″ən-o-mor′fik) of a condition, closely resembling an endogenous one but actually having an exogenous cause.

en•do•ge•note (en″do-je′nōt) in bacterial genetics, the recipient cell's own complement of genetic information, as opposed to the exogenote introduced by transduction.

en•dog•e•nous (en-doj′ə-nəs) [*endo-* + *-genous*] 1. growing from within. 2. developing or originating within the organism, or arising from causes within the organism. Called also *endogenic.*

en•do•glob•u•lar (en″do-glob′u-lər) intracorpuscular.

en•do•gna•thi•on (en″do-na′the-on) [*endo-* + *gnathion*] the inner segment of the incisive bone.

en•do•go•nid•i•um (en″do-go-nid′e-əm) a gonidium developed within a cell, especially in the algal component of a lichen.

en•do•in•tox•i•ca•tion (en″do-in-tok″sĭ-ka′shən) poisoning caused by an endogenous toxin.

en•do•la•ryn•ge•al (en″do-lə-rin′je-əl) [*endo-* + Gr. *larynx*] located or occurring within the larynx; called also *intralaryngeal.*

en•do•leak (en′do-leak″) the continued flow of blood into an aneurysmal sac after the aneurysm has been treated by an endoluminal graft, indicating a failed graft. Endoleaks are classified as types I–IV, depending on the cause.

En•do•li•max (en″do-li′maks) a genus of ameboid protozoa closely related to *Entamoeba. E. na′na* is a common inhabitant of the human intestine and occasionally may cause diarrhea in children or immunocompromised adults.

en•do•lu•mi•nal (en″do-loo′mĭ-nəl) intraluminal.

en•do•lymph (en′do-limf) endolympha. **endolymphat′ic** *adj*

en•do•lym•pha (en″do-lim′fə) [*endo-* + *lympha*] [TA] endolymph: the fluid contained in the membranous labyrinth of the ear; it is entirely separate from the perilymph. Called also *Scarpa fluid* and *liquor of Scarpa.*

en•dol•y•sin (en-dol′ĭ-sin) [*endo-* + *lysin*] a bactericidal substance existing in cells, acting directly on bacteria, e.g., leukin.

en•do•mas•toid•itis (en″do-mas″toi-di′tis) mastoiditis.

en•do•meso•derm (en″do-mes′o-dərm) [*endo-* + *mesoderm*] mesoderm originating from the endoderm of the two-layered blastodisc.

en•do•me•tria (en″do-me′tre-ə) [Gr.] plural of *endometrium.*

en•do•me•tri•oid (en″do-me′tre-oid) resembling endometrium.

en•do•me•tri•o•ma (en″do-me″tre-o′mə) a solitary, non-neoplastic mass containing endometrial tissue and blood.

en•do•me•tri•o•sis (en″do-me″tre-o′sis) [*endometrium* + *-osis*] a condition in which tissue containing typical endometrial granular and stromal elements occurs in locations outside the uterine cavity, chiefly on the ovaries and pelvic peritoneum; called also *adenomyosis externa* and *e. externa.* **endometriot′ic** *adj*

e. exter′na endometriosis.

e. inter′na adenomyosis.

ovarian e., e. ova′rii occurrence in the ovary of tissue resembling the uterine mucous membrane, either in the form of small superficial islands or in the form of endometrial ("chocolate") cysts of various sizes.

stromal e. adenomyosis in which nearly all of the tissue infiltrating the myometrium consists of stroma.

e. vesi′cae endometriosis involving the urinary bladder.

en•do•me•tri•tis (en″do-me-tri′tis) [*endometrium* + *-itis*] inflammation of the endometrium.

decidual e. inflammation of the decidua of pregnancy.

exfoliative e. endometritis with the casting off of portions of the membrane.

glandular e. endometritis of the uterine glands.

membranous e. endometritis with an exudate which forms a false membrane.

postpartum e., puerperal e. endometritis following childbirth, often a precursor of puerperal fever.

syncytial e. a post-pregnancy condition consisting of a benign tumor-like lesion with infiltration of the uterine wall by large syncytial trophoblastic cells; called also *syncytioma.*

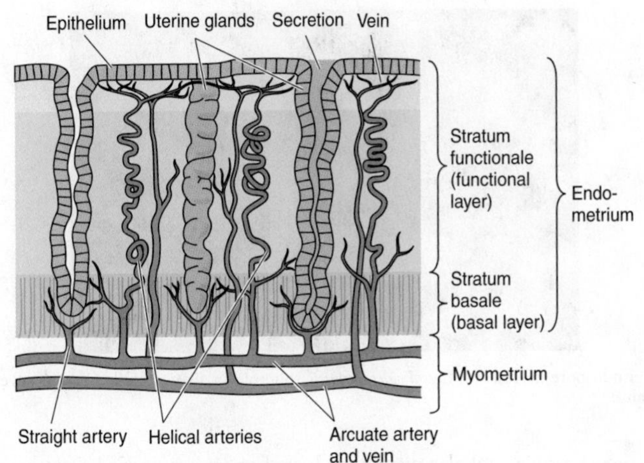

■ Endometrium, comprising the stratum functionale and stratum basale.

tuberculous e. inflammation of the endometrium due to infection by *Mycobacterium tuberculosis*, with the presence of tubercles; usually the uterine tubes are also involved.

en·do·me·tri·um (en″do-me′tre-əm) pl. *endome′tria* [L., from *endo-* + *metra*] TA alternative for *tunica mucosa uteri*. **endome′trial** *adj*

Swiss-cheese e. hyperplasia of the endometrium, under the influence of progesterone, in which the glands vary in size and shape, producing an appearance of small and large holes like those of Swiss cheese.

en·dom·e·try (en-dom′ə-tre) [*endo-* + *-metry*] the measurement of the capacity of a cavity.

en·do·mi·to·sis (en″do-mi-to′sis) reproduction of nuclear elements within an intact nuclear envelope, not followed by chromosome movements and cytoplasmic division; it results in endopolyploidy or in the formation of polytene chromosomes.

en·do·morph (en′do-morf) [*endo*derm + Gr. *morphē* form] an individual having a body build in which tissues derived from the endoderm predominate; there is relative preponderance of soft roundness throughout the body, with large digestive viscera and accumulations of fat, and with large trunk and thighs and tapering extremities, as contrasted with ectomorph and mesomorph. **endomor′phic** *adj*

en·do·mor·phy (en′do-mor″fe) the condition of being an endomorph.

En·do·my·ces (en″do-mi′sēz) [*endo-* + Gr. *mykēs* fungus] a genus of fungi of the order Endomycetales that includes a number of yeasts from soil, nectar, and decaying fruit.

En·do·my·ce·ta·les (en″do-mi″sə-ta′lēz) in some systems of classification, an order of perfect fungi (yeasts) of the subphylum Ascomycotina, mostly saprobes, in which the zygote results from fusion of two cells and immediately forms an ascus; it includes the family Saccharomycetaceae.

en·do·myo·car·di·al (en″do-mi″o-kahr′de-əl) pertaining to the endocardium and the myocardium.

en·do·myo·car·di·tis (en″do-mi″o-kahr-di′tis) [*endo-* + *myocarditis*] inflammation of the endocardium and myocardium.

en·do·mys·i·um (en″do-mis′e-əm) [*endo-* + Gr. *mys* muscle] [TA] the sheath of delicate reticular fibrils which surrounds each muscle fiber. **endomys′ial** *adj*

en·do·na·sal (en″do-na′zəl) intranasal.

en·do·neu·ral (en″do-noor′əl) within a nerve. Called also *intraneural*.

en·do·neu·ri·tis (en″do-nŏŏ-ri′tis) inflammation of the endoneurium.

en·do·neu·ri·um (en″do-noor′e-um) [*endo-* + Gr. *neuron* nerve] [TA] the innermost layer of connective tissue in a peripheral nerve, forming an interstitial layer around each individual fiber outside the neurilemma; called also *epilemma*, *Henle sheath*, and *sheath of Key and Retzius*. See also *epineurium* and *perineurium*. **endoneu′rial** *adj*

en·do·neu·rol·y·sis (en″do-nŏŏ-rol′ə-sis) [*endo-* + *neurolysis*] hersage.

en·do·nu·cle·ar (en″do-noo′kle-ər) within a cell nucleus.

en·do·nu·cle·ase (en″do-noo′kle-ās) any nuclease specifically catalyzing the hydrolysis of interior bonds of ribonucleotide or deoxyribonucleotide chains, producing poly- or oligonucleotides. Cf. *exonuclease*.

restriction e. an endonuclease that hydrolyzes deoxyribonucleic acid, cleaving it at an individual site of a specific base pattern. Thus, the enzyme degrades DNA foreign to a cell but spares the cell's own DNA, which is protected by methylation at the recognition site. Restriction endonucleases isolated from bacterial sources are used extensively for sequencing of DNA and recombinant technology.

en·do·par·a·site (en″do-par′ə-sīt) [*endo-* + *parasite*] a parasite that lives within the body of its host.

en·do·pel·vic (en″do-pel′vik) intrapelvic.

en·do·pep·ti·dase (en″do-pep′tĭ-dās) [EC 3.4.21–99] any peptidase that catalyzes the cleavage of internal peptide bonds in a polypeptide or protein; they are divided into subclasses on the basis of catalytic mechanism and comprise the serine endopeptidases, cysteine endopeptidases, aspartic endopeptidases, metalloendopeptidases, and other endopeptidases.

en·do·peri·car·di·al (en″do-per″ĭ-kahr′de-əl) pertaining to the endocardium and pericardium.

en·do·peri·car·di·tis (en″do-per″ĭ-kahr-di′tis) [*endo-* + *pericarditis*] inflammation involving both the endocardium and pericardium.

en·do·peri·myo·car·di·tis (en″do-per″ĭ-mi″o-kahr-di′tis) [*endo-* + *peri-* + *myocarditis*] inflammation of the endocardium, pericardium, and myocardium.

en·do·peri·neu·ri·tis (en″do-per″ĭ-noo-ri′tis) inflammation of the endoneurium and perineurium.

en·do·peri·to·ne·al (en″do-per″ĭ-to-ne′əl) intraperitoneal.

en·do·peri·to·ni·tis (en″do-per″ĭ-to-ni′tis) inflammation of the serous lining of the peritoneal cavity.

en·do·per·ox·ide (en″do-pə-rok′sīd) a peroxide in which the —O—O— group is attached as a bridge, joining two atoms within the molecule.

en·do·per·ox·ide-D-isom·er·ase (en″do-pə-rok′sīd i-som′ə-rās) prostaglandin-D synthase.

en·do·per·ox·ide-E-isom·er·ase (en″do-pə-rok′sīd i-som′ə-rās) prostaglandin-E synthase.

en·do·per·ox·ide re·duc·tase (en″do-pə-rok′sīd re-duk′tās) an enzyme of the oxidoreductase class that catalyzes the conversion of the intermediate prostaglandin H_2 (PGH_2) to prostaglandin $F_{2\alpha}$($PGF_{2\alpha}$). See also illustration at *prostaglandin*.

en·do·phle·bi·tis (en″do-flə-bi′tis) [*endo-* + *phlebitis*] inflammation of the intima of a vein; called also *endovenitis*.

e. hepa′tica obli′terans Budd-Chiari syndrome.

proliferative e. phlebosclerosis.

en·do·pho·to·co·ag·u·la·tion (en″do-fo″to-ko-ag′u-la-shən) photocoagulation performed within the vitreous, after vitrectomy, in the treatment of vitreous hemorrhage.

en·doph·thal·mi·tis (en″dof-thəl-mi′tis) [*end-* + *ophthalmitis*] inflammation involving the ocular cavities and their adjacent structures; called also *entophthalmia*.

phacoanaphylactic e. lens-induced uveitis.

en·do·phyte (en′do-fīt) [*endo-* + *-phyte*] a parasitic plant organism living within the body of its host.

en·do·phyt·ic (en″do-fit′ik) [*endo-* + Gr. *phyein* to grow] 1. pertaining to an endophyte. 2. growing inward; proliferating on the interior or inside of an organ or other structure, as a tumor.

en·do·plasm (en′do-plaz″əm) [*endo-* + *plasm*] the central portion of the cytoplasm of a cell. Cf. *ectoplasm*. **endoplas′mic** *adj*

en·do·poly·ploi·dy (en″do-pol″e-ploi′de) [*endo-* + *polyploidy*] the occurrence in a diploid individual of cells containing 4, 8, 16, 32, etc., times the haploid number of chromosomes as the result of endomitosis. **endopol′yploid** *adj*

en·do·pred·a·tor (en″do-pred′ə-tər) an individual or species that lives within the body of an organism of another species which it feeds upon and destroys.

en·do·pros·the·sis (en″do-pros-the′sis) [*endo-* + *prosthesis*] 1. a prosthesis placed entirely within the body, such as in arthroplasty. 2. a hollow stent, such as one inserted into a bile duct to allow biliary drainage across an obstruction.

en·do·py·elot·o·my (en″do-pi″ə-lot′ə-me) [*endo-* + *pyelotomy*] an incision procedure to correct a stenosed ureteropelvic junction by cutting from within using an instrument inserted through an endoscope.

en·do·ra·di·og·ra·phy (en″do-ra″de-og′rə-fe) the radiographic demonstration of the condition of internal organs and cavities by means of radiopaque materials.

en·do·ra·dio·sonde (en″do-ra″de-o-sond′) a small radio transmitter inserted into a body cavity or tube in a telemetering capsule (see under *capsule*).

en·do·rec·tal (en″do-rek′təl) inside the rectum.

en•do•re•du•pli•ca•tion (en″do-re-doo″plĭ-ka′shən) replication of the chromosomes without subsequent cell division, resulting in polyploidy.

end-or•gan (end-or′gən) one of the larger, encapsulated endings of the sensory nerves.

Ruffini e.-o. see under *ending.*

en•do•ri•bo•nu•cle•ase (en″do-ri″bo-noo′kle-ās) [EC 3.1.26–27] any member of two sub-subclasses of enzymes of the hydrolase class that catalyze the hydrolysis of interior bonds of ribonucleotides, producing oligonucleotides or polynucleotides.

en•dor•phin (en-dor′fin, en′dor-fin) [*endo*genous + mor*phine*] any of three neuropeptides, amino acid residues of β-lipotropin; they bind to opioid receptors in the brain and have potent analgesic activity. *β-Endorphin* is the C-terminal 30–amino acid residue and is found in the adenohypophysis, hypothalamus, and other sites in the brain; one function appears to be mediation of pain perception. *α-Endorphin* and *γ-endorphin* are the N-terminal 16 and 17 amino acid residues, respectively. See also *enkephalin* and *dynorphin.*

en•do•sal•pin•gi•tis (en″do-sal″pin-ji′tis) [*endosalpinx* + *-itis*] inflammation of the endosalpinx.

en•do•sal•pin•go•ma (en″do-sal″pin-go′mə) adenomyoma of the uterine tube.

en•do•sal•pinx (en″do-sal′pinks) [*endo-* + *salpinx*] tunica mucosa tubae uterinae.

en•do•scope (en′do-skōp) [*endo-* + *-scope*] an instrument for examination of the interior of a body cavity or hollow viscus; there are both rigid and flexible types. See also *fiberscope.*

fiberoptic e. fiberscope.

video e. videoendoscope.

en•do•scop•ic (en″do-skop′ik) 1. performed by means of an endoscope. 2. pertaining to endoscopy.

en•dos•co•py (en-dos′kə-pe) visual inspection of any cavity of the body by means of an endoscope.

capsule e. inspection of the digestive tract by means of a video camera enclosed in a pill-sized capsule. After the capsule is swallowed, the camera acquires images as it is propelled through the digestive system; the images are transmitted to a recording device worn on the belt and are later downloaded to a workstation for viewing. Called also *video capsule e.*, *wireless capsule e.*, and *capsule enteroscopy.*

fetal e. examination of a fetus with an endoscope.

peroral e. examination of organs accessible to observation through an endoscope passed through the mouth.

video capsule e. capsule e.

virtual e. an imaging technique in which cross-sectional images acquired by computed tomography or magnetic resonance imaging are processed by computer to reconstruct a three-dimensional display similar to that seen through an endoscope.

wireless capsule e. capsule e.

en•do•se•cre•to•ry (en″do-se′krə-tor-e) endocrine.

en•do•skel•e•tal (en″do-skel′ə-təl) 1. pertaining to the endoskeleton. 2. resembling an endoskeleton.

en•do•skel•e•ton (en″do-skel′ə-ton) [*endo-* + Gr. *skeleton*] the bony and cartilaginous skeleton of the body, exclusive of that part of the skeleton which is of dermal origin; called also *neuroskeleton.*

en•dos•mom•e•ter (en″dos-mom′ə-tər) [*endosmosis* + *-meter*] an instrument for determining the rate and extent of endosmosis.

en•dos•mo•sis (en″dos-mo′sis) [*end-* + *osmosis*] a movement in liquids separated by a membranous or porous septum, by which one fluid passes through the septum into the cavity which contains another fluid of a different density. Cf. *exosmosis.* **endosmot′ic** *adj*

en•do•some (en′do-sōm) [*endo-* + *-some*] 1. in endocytosis, a vesicle that has lost its coat of clathrin. Four classes of endosomes (early, recycling, and late endosomes and multivesicular bodies) are distinguishable; whether they are distinct organelles or functional subsets of a single compartment is uncertain. 2. a nucleolus-like, intranuclear, RNA-containing organelle of certain flagellate protozoa that persists during mitosis.

early e's tubulovesicular sorting compartments containing newly internalized proteins and their receptors and lying near the plasma membrane; their interior pH is approximately 6.0, which encourages the dissociation of receptors, which are transferred to recycling endosomes, and ligands, which are transferred to the Golgi complex by late endosomes.

late e's tubulovesicular compartments, derived from multivesicular bodies and having an internal pH of approximately 5.5, located in the cytoplasm near the Golgi complex; they prepare their contents for digestion by the lysosomes, with which they eventually fuse.

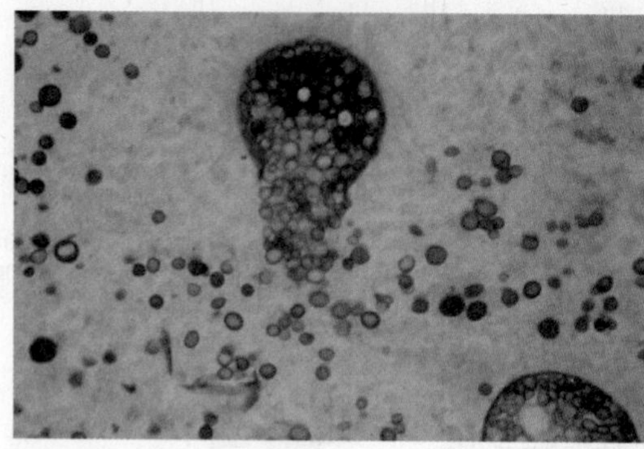

■ Endospore release by *Coccidioides immitis* spherule in tissue (methenamine silver stain).

recycling e's tubular membrane-bound structures derived from early endosomes, containing receptors and membrane proteins being returned to the cell surface.

sorting e's early e's.

en•do•so•nog•ra•phy (en″do-sə-nog′rə-fe) ultrasonography in which the ultrasound transducer is incorporated into the tip of a fiberoptic endoscope that is inserted into the lumen of a cavity or organ. See also *endoscopic ultrasonography.*

en•do•sperm (en′do-spərm) a substance containing reserve food materials, formed within the embryo sac of plants.

en•do•spore (en′do-spor) [*endo-* + *spore*] 1. a thick-walled body formed within the vegetative cells of certain bacteria (e.g., *Bacillus, Clostridium, Sarcina*) that is able to withstand adverse environmental conditions for prolonged periods; under favorable conditions it will germinate to form a vegetative bacterium. See also *spore.* 2. an asexual fungal spore produced within the hyphae or cell, as in a spherule of *Coccidioides immitis* or in a sporangium.

en•do•spor•i•um (en″do-spor′e-əm) the inner layer of the envelope of a spore.

en•dos•se•ous (en-dos′e-əs) endosteal (def. 2).

en•do•stat•in (en″do-stat′in) a protein produced in the body by proteolysis of collagen XVIII at its carboxyl terminal; it inhibits angiogenesis and tumor growth and is under study as an antineoplastic.

en•dos•te•al (en-dos′te-əl) 1. pertaining to the endosteum. 2. occurring or located within a bone.

en•dos•te•itis (en-dos″te-i′tis) inflammation of the endosteum.

en•dos•te•o•ma (en-dos″te-o′mə) [*endo-* + *oste-* + *-oma*] a tumor in the medullary cavity of a bone.

en•do•stetho•scope (en″do-steth′o-skōp) a stethoscope passed into the esophagus for auscultating the heart.

en•dos•te•um (en-dos′te-əm) [*endo-* + *osteon*] [TA] the tissue lining the medullary cavity of a bone.

en•dos•ti•tis (en″dos-ti′tis) endosteitis.

en•dos•to•ma (en″dos-to′mə) endosteoma.

en•do•sur•gery (en′do-sur″jər-e) endoscopic surgery.

en•do•sym•bi•ont (en″do-sim′be-ont) [*endo-* + *symbiont*] a symbiont which lives within the cells of its partner.

en•do•sym•bi•o•sis (en″do-sim″be-o′sis) the state achieved between a virus and its host cell in which cellular division is inhibited but the cell is not immediately destroyed.

en•do•ten•din•e•um (en″do-tən-din′e-əm) [*endo-* + L. *tendo, tendines*, after Gr. *tenōn*] the delicate connective tissue separating the secondary bundles (fascicles) of a tendon.

en•do•ten•on (en″do-ten′on) endotendineum.

en•do•the•lia (en″do-the′le-ə) [Gr.] plural of *endothelium.*

en•do•the•li•al•iza•tion (en″do-the″le-əl-ĭ-za′shən) the healing of the inner surfaces of vessels or grafts by endothelial cells.

en•do•the•li•itis (en″do-the-le-i′tis) inflammation of the endothelium.

en•do•the•lin (en″do-the′lin) any of three 21–amino acid polypeptides that are potent vasoconstrictors. Endothelin-1 was originally found as a product of endothelial cells and later in the brain, kidney, and lung; it is a contractile factor that may play a role in controlling blood pressure and may also function as a neurotransmitter. Endothelin-2 and endothelin-3 have been found in tissues such as the adrenal glands, kidneys, brain, and intestine.

en·do·the·lio·blas·to·ma (en″do-the″le-o-blas-to′mə) [*endothelium* + *blastoma*] a tumor derived from primitive vasoformative tissue with formation of usually small and slitlike vascular spaces lined by prominent endothelial cells; the term, which now includes hemangioendothelioma, angiosarcoma, lymphangioendothelioma, and lymphangiosarcoma, was applied formerly to such tumors arising from mesothelial tissue as well.

en·do·the·lio·cho·ri·al (en″do-the″le-o-kor′e-əl) [*endothelium* + *chorial*] denoting a type of placenta in which syncytial trophoblast embeds maternal vessels bared to their endothelial lining.

en·do·the·li·oid (en″do-the′le-oid) resembling endothelium.

en·do·the·li·ol·y·sin (en″do-the″le-ol′ə-sin) a cytolysin capable of lysing endothelial cells.

en·do·the·lio·lyt·ic (en″do-the″le-o-lit′ik) capable of destroying endothelial tissue.

en·do·the·li·o·ma (en″do-the″le-o′mə) [*endothelium* + *-oma*] any tumor, particularly a benign one, that originates from the endothelial linings of blood vessels *(hemangioendothelioma)* or lymphatics *(lymphangioendothelioma)*.

e. angiomato′sum angioma.

perithelial e. hemangiopericytoma.

en·do·the·li·o·ma·to·sis (en″do-the″le-o-mə-to′sis) the formation of multiple and diffuse endotheliomas in a tissue.

en·do·the·lio·sar·co·ma (en″do-the″le-o-sahr-ko′mə) Kaposi sarcoma.

en·do·the·li·o·sis (en″do-the″le-o′sis) proliferation of endothelium.

glomerular capillary e. a renal lesion typical of eclampsia; it is characterized by deposition of fibrous material in and beneath the cells of the grossly swollen glomerular capillary endothelium, resulting in near or total occlusion of the capillaries.

en·do·the·lio·tox·in (en″do-the′le-o-tok″sin) a specific toxin that acts on the endothelium of capillaries and small veins, producing hemorrhage. Cf. *hemorrhagin*.

en·do·the·li·um (en″do-the′le-əm) pl. *endothe′lia* [*endo-* + Gr. *thēlē* nipple] the layer of epithelial cells that lines the interior of structures such as the cavities of the heart, the lumina of blood and lymph vessels, and the serous cavities of the body; it originates from the mesoderm. **endothe′lial** *adj*

anterior e. of cornea, corneal e. epithelium posterius corneae.

extraembryonic e. endothelium that arises outside of the body of the embryo, such as that lining the vitelline vessels.

glomerular e. a layer of fenestrated epithelium lining the glomerular capillaries next to the visceral layer of the glomerular capsule, allowing solute-rich, nearly protein-free fluid to pass from the capillaries into the capsule.

en·do·therm (en′do-thərm″) [*endo-* + *therm*] homeotherm.

en·do·ther·mal (en″do-thur′məl) endothermic.

en·do·ther·mic (en″do-thur′mik) characterized by or accompanied by the absorption of heat, as a chemical reaction accompanied by absorption of heat and to which heat must be supplied if it is to proceed; storing up heat or energy in a potential form. Cf. *exothermic*.

en·do·ther·my (en″do-thur′me) diathermy.

en·do·tho·rac·ic (en″do-tho-ras′ik) within the thorax; situated internal to the ribs.

en·do·thrix (en′do-thriks) [*endo-* + *-thrix*] a dermatophyte whose growth and spore production are confined chiefly within the shaft of the hair, without formation of conspicuous external spores; such fungi include *Trichophyton tonsurans* and *T. violaceum*.

en·do·tox·e·mia (en″do-tok-se′me-ə) the presence of endotoxins in the blood, which may result in shock.

en·do·tox·ic (en′do-tok″sik) 1. pertaining to endotoxin. 2. possessing endotoxin.

en·do·tox·in (en′do-tok″sin) [*endo-* + *toxin*] a heat-stable toxin associated with the outer membranes of certain gram-negative bacteria, including the brucellae, the enterobacteria, neisseriae, and vibrios. Endotoxins are not secreted but are released only when the cells are disrupted; they are less potent and less specific than the exotoxins; and they do not form toxoids. They are composed of complex lipopolysaccharide molecules, of which the polysaccharide unit (somatic O antigen) is responsible for antigenicity, occurring in hundreds of variations, and the phospholipid moiety (lipid A) is the source of toxicity. When injected in large quantities the endotoxins produce hemorrhagic shock and severe diarrhea; smaller amounts cause fever, altered resistance to bacterial infection, leukopenia followed by leukocytosis, and numerous other biologic effects. Called also *bacterial pyrogen*. See also *toxin*.

en·do·tra·che·al (en″do-tra′ke-əl) [*endo-* + *tracheal*] 1. within or through the trachea. 2. performed by passage through the lumen of the trachea.

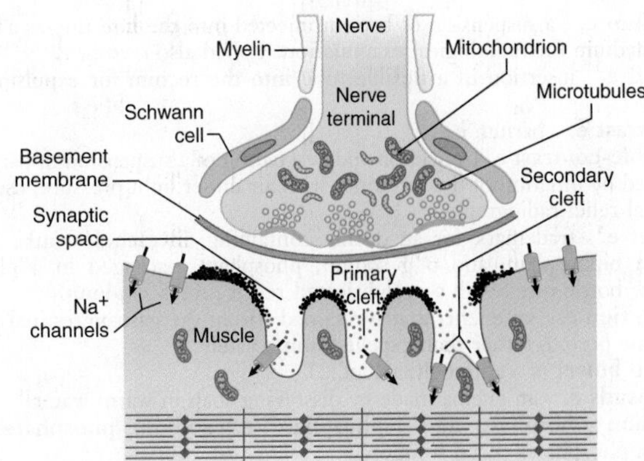

■ Schematic diagram of the motor end plate and its relation to the synaptic cleft and muscle.

en·do·ure·ter·al (en″do-u-re′tər-əl) intraureteral.

en·do·ure·ter·ic (en″do-u″re-ter′ik) intraureteral.

en·do·u·re·ter·ot·o·my (en″do-u-re″tər-ot′ə-me) treatment of a ureteral stricture by making an incision in the wall of the stenosed part, exposing periureteral fat; a stent may be put in place during healing.

en·do·ure·thral (en″do-u-re′thrəl) intraurethral.

en·do·urol·o·gy (en″do-u-rol′ə-je) [*endo-* + *urology*] the branch of urologic surgery concerned with closed procedures for visualizing or manipulating the urinary tract; it may refer to procedures involving any part of the urinary tract or may be limited to procedures involving only the kidney or ureter.

en·do·uter·ine (en″do-u′tər-in) intrauterine.

en·do·vac·ci·na·tion (en″do-vak″sĭ-na′shən) [*endo-* + *vaccination*] the administration of vaccines by mouth.

en·do·vas·cu·lar (en″do-vas′ku-lər) within a blood vessel; said of intraluminal diagnostic and therapeutic procedures, such as angioplasty, performed with a device inserted into the vascular tree remote from the site of the procedure.

en·do·vas·cu·li·tis (en″do-vas″ku-li′tis) endangiitis.

en·do·ve·ni·tis (en″do-ve-ni′tis) endophlebitis.

en·do·ve·nous (en″do-ve′nəs) intravenous.

en·do·ves·i·cal (en″do-ves′ĭ-kəl) intravesical.

En·dox·an (en-dok′sən) trademark for a preparation of cyclophosphamide.

en·do·zo·ite (en″do-zo′īt) tachyzoite.

end plate (end plāt) a flat termination. Spelled also *end-plate*.

motor e. p. the discoid expansion of a terminal branch of the axon of a motor nerve fiber, which apposes the subneural apparatus of a skeletal muscle fiber, forming the neuromuscular junction (q.v.).

end-plea·sure (end′plezh-ər) the pleasure produced by the sexual orgasm, as contrasted with the fore-pleasure that precedes it.

end point (end point) in titration, the highest dilution of a substance that produces a reaction with a given volume of another substance.

En·drate (en′drāt) trademark for preparations of edetate disodium.

en·drin (en′drin) a highly toxic chlorinated hydrocarbon insecticide; if ingested or absorbed through the skin by a human or other animal, it can cause potentially fatal neurotoxicity such as tremors and convulsions.

end-tidal (end-ti′dəl) pertaining to or occurring at the end of exhalation of a normal tidal volume.

En·du·ron (en′du-ron) trademark for a preparation of methyclothiazide.

En·dur·o·nyl (en-dūr′o-nəl) trademark for combination preparations of methyclothiazide and reserpine.

-ene a suffix used in chemistry to indicate an unsaturated hydrocarbon containing one double bond.

en·e·ma (en′ə-mə) [Gr.] 1. a liquid injected or to be injected into the rectum. 2. the injection of such a liquid.

air e. injection of air or gas into the rectum of a child for reduction of an intussusception.

antegrade colonic e., antegrade continence e. creation of a continent stoma in the right colon through which an irrigation fluid may be infused, used in the management of chronic evacuation disorders; called also *antegrade colonic irrigation*.

barium e. a suspension of barium injected into the intestine as a contrast medium for radiological examination. Called also *contrast e.*

blind e. insertion of a flexible tube into the rectum for expulsion of flatus.

contrast e. barium e.

double-contrast e. injection and evacuation of a suspension of barium, followed by inflation of the intestines with air under light pressure; used in mucosal relief radiography.

Fleet e. trademark for an enema containing, in each 100 mL, 16 g sodium biphosphate and 6 g sodium phosphate, packaged in a plastic squeeze bottle fitted with a prelubricated rectal tube 5 cm long.

retention e. an enema that is retained within the gastrointestinal tract for some period, rather than expelled immediately.

small bowel e. enteroclysis (def. 2).

soapsuds e. an enema made by dissolving soap in warm water.

sodium phosphate and biphosphate e., sodium phosphates e. sodium phosphates rectal solution.

en•e•ma•tor (en′ə-ma″tər) an apparatus for giving enemas.

en•er•get•ics (en″ər-jet′iks) the study of energy; the science of energy.

myocardial e. the study of energy usage and metabolism in cells of the myocardium.

en•er•gom•e•ter (en″ər-gom′ə-tər) an apparatus for studying the pulse.

en•er•gy (en′ər-je) [Gr. *energeia*] the capacity to operate or work; the capacity to produce motion, to overcome resistance, and to effect physical changes. Symbol *E.*

activation e. in a chemical reaction, the energy that must be supplied to the reactants in order to form an activated complex or transition state, which then breaks down to form the products.

atomic e. energy that can be liberated by changes in the nucleus of an atom (as by fission of a heavy nucleus or fusion of light nuclei into heavier ones with accompanying loss of mass).

binding e. the amount of energy that would be necessary to separate an atomic nucleus into its component protons and neutrons.

chemical e. energy evolved or absorbed by chemical reactions.

free e., Gibbs free e. (*G*) the thermodynamic function $G = H - TS$, where *H* is enthalpy, *T* absolute temperature, and *S* entropy. For chemical reactions occurring at a constant temperature and pressure, the free energy change $\Delta G = \Delta H - T\Delta S$ determines the direction in which a reaction proceeds; ΔG is negative for a spontaneous (exergonic) reaction; ΔG is positive for a nonspontaneous (endergonic) reaction. The free energy change can be determined from the equation $\Delta G = \Delta G^\circ + RT \ln Q$, where *R* is the gas constant, *Q* is the reaction quotient (q.v.), and ΔG° is the standard free energy change (the difference between the sum of the free energies of the products and the sum of the free energies of the reactants when all products and reactants are in their standard states; solids and liquids are pure substances; gases are at 1 atm pressure; the temperature is 25°C; and all solutions have a concentration of 1M). For a reaction at equilibrium, $\Delta G = 0$; thus $\Delta G^\circ = -RT \ln K$, where *K* is the equilibrium constant.

kinetic e. energy of motion; equal to one-half the mass of a body times the square of its velocity.

nuclear e. atomic e.

potential e. the energy that a body has due to its position, equal to the work required to move the body to that position from some reference position; e.g., a body has a gravitational potential energy equal to its mass times the acceleration due to gravity times its height above the reference position.

radiant e. the energy of electromagnetic waves.

vital e. see under *force.*

en•er•va•tion (en″ər-va′shən) [L. *enervatio*, from *ex* out + *nervus* nerve] 1. lack of nervous energy; languor. 2. neurectomy.

en•flag•el•la•tion (en-flaj″ə-la′shən) flagellation (def. 2).

en•flu•rane (en′floo-rān) [USP] a potent inhalational anesthetic agent, widely used for induction and maintenance of general anesthesia; it is nonflammable, induction and recovery are smooth and rapid, and the depth of anesthesia is rapidly altered; the incidence of arrhythmias and postoperative nausea and vomiting are somewhat less than with halothane or methoxyflurane. It is also used in low concentrations to provide analgesia during labor or painful procedures.

en•fu•vir•tide (en-fu′vər-tīd) an antiretroviral of the fusion inhibitor group, administered by subcutaneous injection as part of a medication cocktail for human immunodeficiency virus infection.

ENG electronystagmography.

en•gage•ment (en-gāj′mənt) in obstetrics, the entrance of the fetal head, or presenting part, into the superior pelvic aperture and beginning descent through the pelvic canal so that its biparietal plane is below the plane of the pelvic inlet.

en•gas•tri•us (en-gas′tre-əs) [*en-* + Gr. *gastēr* belly] asymmetrical conjoined twins with the parasitic twin contained within the abdomen of the larger twin.

En•gel-Reck•ling•hau•sen disease (eng′gəl rek′ling-hou″zən) [Gerhard *Engel*, German physician, 19th century; Friedrich Daniel von *Recklinghausen*, German pathologist, 1833–1910] osteitis fibrosa cystica; see under *osteitis.*

Eng•el•mann disease (eng′gəl-mahn) [Guido *Engelmann*, Austrian orthopedic surgeon, 1876–1959] diaphyseal dysplasia.

Eng•el•mann disk (eng′gəl-mahn) [Theodor Wilhelm *Engelmann*, German physiologist, 1843–1909] H band.

Eng•en orthosis (eng′en) [Thorkild Jensen *Engen*, American prosthetist, born 1924] see under *orthosis.*

En•ge•rix-B (en′jer-iks) trademark for a preparation of hepatitis B vaccine (recombinant).

en•gine (en′jin) a machine by which energy is converted into mechanical motion.

dental e. a machine operated by electricity, water, or compressed air that provides power for rotary dental instruments.

en•gi•neer•ing (en″jĭ-nēr′ing) the application of physical, mathematical, and mechanical principles to practical purposes.

biomedical e. the use of engineering in biomedical technology such as the analysis of movement of body parts or prosthetics. Called also *bioengineering.*

genetic e. the directed manipulation of the genome of a living organism for a variety of analytical, industrial, and medical applications; many of the methods involved utilize recombinant DNA technology (q.v.).

tissue e. a branch of regenerative medicine that applies the methods and principles of engineering to gain an understanding of the relationship between structure and function in normal and pathological tissue and to develop substitutes for pathological, damaged, or missing tissue. See also *biomaterial.*

en•globe (en-glōb′) phagocytose.

en•gorged (en-gorjd′) distended or swollen with fluids.

en•gorge•ment (en-gorj′mənt) 1. local congestion; excessive fullness of any organ, vessel, or tissue due to accumulation of fluids. 2. hyperemia.

en•graft•ment (ən-graft′mənt) incorporation of grafted tissue into the body of the host.

en•gram (en′gram) [*en-* + *-gram*] 1. a lasting mark or trace. 2. the permanent trace left by a stimulus in nerve tissue; see also *pattern generator.* 3. in psychology, the lasting trace left in the psyche by any experience; a latent memory picture.

en•hance•ment (en-hans′mənt) 1. an increase or promotion of something. 2. prolonged survival of tumor cells in animals previously immunized with antigens of the tumor owing to the presence of "enhancing" or "facilitating" antibodies that prevent an immune response against these antigens; called also *immunologic enhancement.*

edge e. a sharp increase in contrast on a xeroradiograph where there is an abrupt difference in the tissue densities of adjacent structures.

en•hanc•er (en-hans′ər) 1. something that promotes or augments. 2. a *cis*-acting regulatory sequence that increases the expression of one or more physically linked genes by binding specific proteins. It is tissue-specific, is position and orientation independent, and can occur upstream or downstream from the transcription start site or even within the coding region.

penetration e. a physical change performed on skin or a chemical applied to the skin that results in increased absorption of a topically applied drug.

En•hy•dri•na (en″hi-dri′nə) a genus of sea snakes (family Hydrophiidae). *E. schisto′sa* is a venomous species found in the Indian and southern Pacific Oceans.

En•kaid (en′kād) trademark for a preparation of encainide hydrochloride.

en•keph•a•lin (en-kef′ə-lin) either of two simple pentapeptides having the formula H_2N-Tyr-Gly-Gly-Phe-X, where X is leucine or methionine, referred to as *leu-enkephalin* and *met-enkephalin.* Although met-enkephalin is the N-terminal 5 residues of the endorphins and both enkephalins and endorphins bind to opioid receptors, the two groups derive from functionally and anatomically distinct groups of neurons. The enkephalins function as neurotransmitters or neuromodulators at many locations in the brain and spinal cord and play a part in pain perception, movement, mood, behavior, and neuroendocrine regulation; they are also found in nerve plexuses and exocrine glands of the gastrointestinal tract.

en•keph•a•lin•er•gic (en-kef″ə-lin-ur′jik) denoting synaptic transmission by enkephalin neurotransmitters.

en·large·ment (en-lahrj′mənt) 1. an increase in the size of an organ or part; see *hypertrophy* and *hyperplasia.* 2. in anatomy, a prominence or swelling; an intumescence.

atrial e. a term used in electrocardiography to denote increased size of one or both atria, due to hypertrophy, dilatation, or both; it is manifest in the morphology of the P waves. See also *P mitrale* and *P pulmonale.*

cardiac e. dilatation or hypertrophy of the heart, due to compensatory mechanisms or secondary to disease.

cervical e. intumescentia cervicalis.

choroidal e. glomus choroideum.

gingival e. hyperplastic enlargement of the gingival tissue. It may occur as a result of inflammatory or fibrous lesions resulting from irritation or injury brought about by mechanical or chemical factors or systemic or localized pathologic processes. See also *fibromatosis gingivae* and *gingival hyperplasia.*

e. of heart cardiac e.

lumbar e., lumbosacral e. intumescentia lumbosacralis.

tympanic e. intumescentia tympanica.

En·lon (en′lon) trademark for a preparation of edrophonium chloride.

Enlon-Plus (en′lon plus′) trademark for a combination preparation of edrophonium chloride and atropine sulfate.

en·ni·a·tin (en-e-a′tin) a cyclic polypeptide antibiotic with a ring of 18 atoms, produced by a fungus of the genus *Fusarium.* It is active against certain gram-positive bacteria, functioning as an ionophore and altering membrane permeability.

enol (e′nol) [contraction from ethyl*ene* + alcoh*ol*] an organic compound in which one carbon of a double-bonded pair is also attached to a hydroxyl group; it is thus a tautomer of a ketone (see *keto-enol tautomerism* at *tautomerism*). The term is also used as a prefix or infix, often italicized.

eno·lase (e′no-lās) phosphopyruvate hydratase.

neuron-specific e. an isozyme of enolase that is found in normal neurons and in all the cells of the diffuse neuroendocrine system; it serves as a marker for neuroendocrine differentiation in tumors.

nonneuronal e. an isozyme of enolase found in normal astrocytes, ependymal cells, arachnoid cap cells, Schwann cells, and vascular endothelial cells; it serves as a marker for astrocytoma, ependymoma, meningioma, neurilemoma, and oligodendroglioma.

en·oph·thal·mos (en″of-thal′mos) [*en-* + Gr. *ophthalmos* eye] a backward displacement of the eyeball into the orbit.

en·oph·thal·mus (en″of-thal′məs) enophthalmos.

en·or·gan·ic (en″or-gan′ik) existing as a permanent quality of the organism.

en·os·to·sis (en″os-to′sis) [*en-* + *ostosis* (q.v.)] a morbid bony growth developed within the cavity of a bone or on the internal surface of the bone cortex.

enox·a·cin (ĕ-nok′sə-sin) a fluoroquinolone antibacterial effective against many gram-positive and gram-negative bacteria; administered orally in the treatment of gonorrhea and urinary tract infections due to susceptible organisms.

enox·a·par·in so·di·um (e-nok″sə-par′in) a low molecular weight heparin, prepared from porcine intestinal mucosa, that binds to and potentiates the action of antithrombin III, used to prevent pulmonary embolism and deep vein thrombosis following hip or knee replacement or high-risk abdominal surgery; administered subcutaneously. It is also used in conjunction with warfarin in the treatment of deep vein thrombosis, and in conjunction with aspirin in the prevention of coronary thrombosis associated with unstable angina or non–Q wave myocardial infarction.

enox·i·mone (ə-nok′sĭ-mōn) a phosphodiesterase inhibitor similar to inamrinone, having positive inotropic and vasodilator effects; used as a cardiotonic in the short-term management of congestive heart failure, administered intravenously.

enoyl CoA (e′no-əl ko-a′) enoyl coenzyme A.

enoyl-CoA hy·dra·tase (e′no-əl ko-a′ hi′drə-tās) [EC 4.2.1.17] an enzyme of the lyase class that catalyzes the stereospecific hydration of the double bond in enoyl coenzyme A, forming the L-hydroxy derivative of acyl coenzyme A from the *trans* isomer of enoyl coenzyme A. The reaction is a step in the beta oxidation of fatty acids.

enoyl CoA isom·er·ase (e′no-əl ko-a′ i-som′ə-rās) dodecenoyl-CoA Δ-isomerase.

enoyl co·en·zyme A (e′no-əl ko-en′zīm) dehydrogenated acyl coenzyme A; in the beta oxidation of fatty acids, the *trans* isomer of enoyl coenzyme A, with the double bond between carbons C-2 and C-3, is an intermediate.

en plaque (ahn-plak′) [Fr.] in the form of a plaque or plate.

en·rich·ment (ən-rich′mənt) the addition of nutrients, as to culture media; the medium resulting from such addition.

en·ro·flox·a·cin (en″ro-flok′sə-sin) a veterinary quinolone antibiotic with actions and uses similar to those of ciprofloxacin in humans.

En·roth sign (en′rot) [Emil Emanuel *Enroth,* Finnish physician, 1879–1953] see under *sign.*

en·si·form (en′sĭ-form) [L. *ensis* sword + *form*] xiphoid (def. 1).

en·sul·i·zole (en-sul′ĭ-zōl) [USP] a water soluble absorber of ultraviolet B radiation, used topically as a sunscreen. Called also *phenylbenzimidazole sulfonic acid.*

ENT ears, nose, and throat; see *otorhinolaryngology.*

en·tac·a·pone (en-tak′ə-pōn) a selective, reversible inhibitor of catechol *O*-methyltransferase, the enzyme mainly responsible for levodopa metabolism in the brain and periphery in the presence of carbidopa; used in conjunction with levodopa and carbidopa to enhance dopaminergic stimulation of the brain and the antiparkinsonian activity of levodopa in the treatment of idiopathic Parkinson disease, administered orally.

en·tac·tin (en-tak′tin) nidogen.

en·tad (en′tad) toward the center; inwardly.

en·tal (en′təl) [Gr. *entos* within] internal; inner; central.

ent·ame·bi·a·sis (en″tə-me-bi′ə-sis) amebiasis caused by *Entamoeba* species.

Ent·amoe·ba (en″tə-me′bə) [*ent-* + *ameba*] a genus of ramicristate amebae of the order Amoebida, parasitic in many different animals; the organism has a vesicular nucleus with a small central karyosome and numerous peripheral chromatin granules attached to the nuclear membrane.

E. bucca′lis *E. gingivalis.*

E. chatto′ni a species morphologically similar to *E. polecki,* found in the intestines of apes, monkeys, and occasionally humans.

E. co′li a common, nonpathogenic species found in the human intestine.

E. dis′par a species indistinguishable morphologically from *E. histolytica* but nonpathogenic.

E. gingiva′lis a species often found in the mouths of humans with periodontal disease; it has not been shown to be pathogenic.

E. hartman′ni a nonpathogenic species found in the human intestinal tract, almost identical to but smaller than *E. histolytica.*

E. histoly′tica the only species of *Entamoeba* that causes human amebiasis; it is transmitted through ingestion of cysts in contaminated food and water. Trophozoites may invade the tissue of the large intestine and may be spread to extraintestinal sites such as the liver, spleen, brain, lungs, and pericardium.

E. inva′dens a species that produces lesions of the gastrointestinal tract and liver in reptiles.

E. moshkov′kii a species indistinguishable morphologically from *E. histolytica* but nonpathogenic.

E. polec′ki a species found in the intestines of various different species of mammals.

en·tec·a·vir (en-tek′ə-vir) a guanosine nucleoside analogue that inhibits hepatitis B virus polymerase activity, used in the treatment of chronic hepatitis B; administered orally.

ent·epi·con·dyle (en-tep″ĭ-kon′dīl) the internal epicondyle of the humerus.

en·te·que (en-ta′ka) enzootic calcinosis.

en·ter·ad·e·ni·tis (en″tər-ad″ə-ni′tis) [*enter-* + *adenitis*] inflammation of the intestinal glands.

en·ter·al (en′tər-əl) enteric.

en·ter·al·gia (en″tər-al′jə) [*enter-* + *-algia*] pain or neuralgia of the intestine. Called also *enterodynia.*

en·ter·ec·to·my (en″tər-ek′tə-me) [*enter-* + *-ectomy*] excision of a part of the intestine; resection of the intestine.

En·te·reg (en′tə-reg) trademark for a preparation of alvimopan.

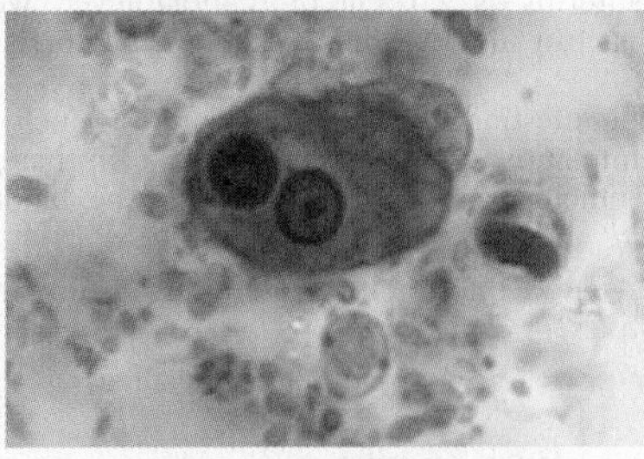

■ *Entamoeba histolytica* trophozoite with ingested erythrocyte. Nucleus has typical small centrally located karyosome and thin, uniform, peripheral chromatin (trichrome stain).

en·ter·ic (en-ter′ik) [Gr. *enterikos* intestinal] 1. intestinal. 2. within the small intestine. Called also *enteral.*

en·ter·ic-coat·ed (en-ter′ik-kōt′əd) a term designating a special coating applied to tablets or capsules which prevents release and absorption of their contents until they reach the intestines.

en·ter·i·tis (en″tər-i′tis) [*enter-* + *-itis*] inflammation of the intestine, usually referring only to the small intestine; see also *enterocolitis.*

bacterial e. enteritis caused by bacterial infection; the most common types in humans are *Campylobacter* enteritis, *Salmonella* enteritis, *Shigella* enteritis, and *Yersinia* enteritis.

***Campylobacter* e.** intestinal infection by a species of *Campylobacter;* characteristics include diarrhea that may be bloody, abdominal pain with cramps, and fever. The cause is usually ingestion of contaminated food or water. Called also *enteric campylobacteriosis.*

cat e. panleukopenia.

choleriform e. an acute, choleralike diarrheal disease with a high mortality rate, prevalent in epidemic and endemic form in the Western Pacific area since 1938, caused by the El Tor biovar of *Vibrio cholerae.*

chronic cicatrizing e. Crohn disease.

diphtheritic e. pseudomembranous enterocolitis.

duck virus e. duck plague.

feline e. panleukopenia.

granulomatous e. a type of enteritis seen in horses and dogs, with granuloma formation under the muscularis mucosa, especially in the jejunum and ileum; symptoms include hypoproteinemia, weight loss, edema, and diarrhea.

infectious feline e. panleukopenia.

lymphocytic-plasmacytic e. a type of enteritis seen in dogs, with infiltration of the walls of the stomach and intestines by lymphocytes and plasma cells, with malabsorption, protein-losing enteropathy, and diarrhea.

mink viral e. a highly contagious viral disease of mink resembling feline panleukopenia and caused by a closely related parvovirus.

necrotic e. 1. a type of porcine proliferative enteritis in which the intestinal walls become necrotic. 2. enterotoxemia in chickens, often with fatal hemorrhaging, due to infection by *Clostridium perfringens* type A or C.

e. necro′ticans a type of enteritis characterized by necrosis, caused by *Clostridium perfringens* type C.

phlegmonous e. a severe, acute type of enteritis that is usually secondary to other diseases, such as chronic intestinal obstruction, cirrhosis, strangulated hernia, or carcinoma.

e. polypo′sa enteritis marked by intestinal polyps.

porcine proliferative e. a disease of young pigs, caused by *Lawsonia intracellularis,* in which the walls of the intestines lose villi, immature epithelial cells proliferate, and the lamina propria becomes inflamed, resulting in diarrhea and anorexia. It is usually self-limiting, but it may develop into necrotic enteritis or proliferative hemorrhagic enteropathy that can be fatal.

pseudomembranous e. pseudomembranous enterocolitis.

radiation e., radiation-induced e. damage to the small intestine by ionizing radiation; symptoms include mucositis, edema in the crypts, increased motility with diarrhea, abdominal cramps, and nausea. Cf. *radiation colitis,* under *colitis.*

regional e. Crohn disease.

***Salmonella* e.** bacterial enteritis caused by species of *Salmonella;* see also *Salmonella gastroenteritis.*

segmental e. Crohn disease.

***Shigella* e.** bacterial enteritis caused by the *Shigella* infection of bacillary dysentery (see under *dysentery*).

streptococcus e. a type of bacterial enteritis caused by *Streptococcus pyogenes,* resembling phlegmonous enteritis.

terminal e. Crohn disease.

tuberculous e. enteritis secondary to advanced pulmonary tuberculosis, believed to be caused by the swallowing of large amounts of positive sputum; now rare due to antibiotic tuberculosis therapy.

typhoid e. enteritis as a result of typhoid fever, with hyperplastic Peyer patches that can ulcerate, and sometimes hemorrhage and perforation.

***Yersinia* e.** the intestinal symptoms of yersiniosis, including invasion of the mucosa, inflammation of the terminal ileum, pain that can be mistaken for that of appendicitis, and diarrhea that may be bloody. Called also *Yersinia enterocolitis* and *enteric* or *intestinal yersiniosis.*

enter(o)- [Gr. *enteron* intestine] a combining form denoting relationship to the intestines.

en·tero·ad·her·ent (en″tər-o-ad-hēr′ənt) adhering to the intestinal mucosa.

en·tero·ag·gre·ga·tive (en″tər-o-ag′rə-ga″tiv) adhering to, and forming colonies on, the intestinal mucosa.

en·tero·anas·to·mo·sis (en″tər-o-ə-nas″to-mo′sis) enteroenterostomy.

Enterobacteriaceae Associated with Infection

Cedecea	*Photorhabdus*
Citrobacter	*Plesiomonas*
Edwardsiella	*Proteus*
Enterobacter	*Providencia*
Escherichia	*Rahnella*
Ewingella	*Salmonella*
Hafnia	*Serratia*
Klebsiella	*Shigella*
Kluyvera	*Tatumella*
Morganella	*Yersinia*
Pantoea	

en·tero·ar·thric (en″tər-o-ahr′thrik) pertaining to or characterized by thallic-arthric conidiogenesis in which only the inner part of the cell wall forms the conidia.

En·tero·bac·ter (en″tər-o-bak′tər) [*entero-* + Gr. *baktron* a rod] a genus of gram-negative, facultatively anaerobic rod-shaped bacteria of the family Enterobacteriaceae, made up of motile, peritrichously flagellated cells, some being encapsulated. The organisms occur in the intestinal tracts of many different animals, and frequently cause nosocomial infections as a result of contaminated medical devices or personnel. The type species is *E. cloa′cae.*

E. aero′genes *Klebsiella mobilis.*

E. agglo′merans *Pantoea agglomerans.*

E. cloa′cae the most commonly occurring species, found in feces, soil, and water and, less commonly, in urine, pus, and pathological material; it can cause nosocomial pneumonia in debilitated patients (see Enterobacter *pneumonia,* under *pneumonia*).

E. gergo′viae a species that is lysine decarboxylase positive and can cause infections of the urinary tract, lung, or bloodstream.

E. sakaza′kii a species found in the environment and in foods; it sometimes contaminates infant formulas, so that babies contract septicemia or meningitis.

en·tero·bac·ter (en″tər-o-bak′tər) an organism of the genus *Enterobacter.*

En·tero·bac·te·ri·a·ceae (en″tər-o-bak-te″re-a′se-e) a large family of gram-negative, facultatively anaerobic, rod-shaped bacteria of the order Enterobacteriales, usually motile with peritrichous flagella, consisting of saprophytes and plant and animal parasites of worldwide distribution. In humans, disease results from both invasion and production of toxins. Members of this family are a common cause of nosocomial infection, and species not normally associated with disease may be opportunistic pathogens. See accompanying table.

En·tero·bac·te·ri·a·les (en″tər-o-bak-te″re-a′lēz) an order of bacteria of the class Gammaproteobacteria, phylum Proteobacteria, consisting of gram-negative, aerobic, motile or nonmotile, straight rods; it contains a single family, the Enterobacteriaceae.

en·tero·bi·a·sis (en″ter-o-bi′ə-sis) intestinal infection with nematodes of the genus *Enterobius,* especially *E. vermicularis.*

en·tero·bil·i·ary (en″tər-o-bil′e-ar-e) pertaining to or affecting both the small intestine and the biliary tract.

En·tero·bi·us (en″tər-o′be-əs) [*entero-* + Gr. *bios* life] a genus of intestinal nematodes of the family Oxyuridae.

E. vermicula′ris the most common species of parasitic intestinal oxyurid (pinworm or seatworm); it is small and white and inhabits the upper part of the large intestine, or occasionally the female genitals or bladder. Infection is frequent in children, sometimes causing itching. Formerly called *Ascaris vermicularis* and *Oxyuris vermicularis.*

en·tero·blas·tic (en″tər-o-blas′tik) pertaining to blastic conidiogenesis in which only the inner part of the cell wall is used to form the conidium.

en·tero·cele (en′tər-o-sēl″) [*entero-* + *-cele*[1]] 1. a hernia containing intestine; see entries under *hernia.* 2. hernia of intestine or a viscus into the posterior end of the labium majus; called also *posterior vaginal* or *vaginolabial hernia.*

pulsion e. see under *hernia.*

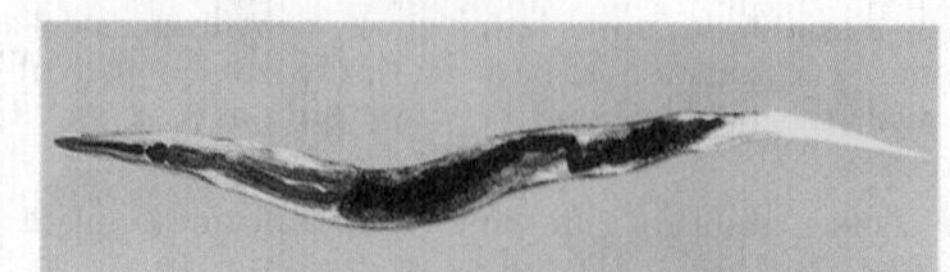

■ Adult female *Enterobius vermicularis.*

en·tero·cen·te·sis (en″tər-o-sen-te′sis) [*entero-* + *-centesis*] surgical puncture of the intestine.

en·tero·cho·le·cys·tost·o·my (en″tər-o-ko″lə-sis-tos′tə-me) cholecystoenterostomy.

en·tero·cho·le·cys·tot·o·my (en″tər-o-ko″lə-sis-tot′ə-me) [*entero-* + *cholecystotomy*] incision into the gallbladder and the intestine.

en·ter·o·chro·maf·fin (en″tər-o-kro′mə-fin) pertaining to cells in the gastrointestinal tract having granules that stain readily with silver and chromium salts; see *enterochromaffin cells,* under *cell.*

en·tero·clei·sis (en″tər-o-kli′sis) [*entero-* + Gr. *kleisis* closure] surgical closure of a wound in the intestine.

omental e. closure of an intestinal perforation by suturing the omentum over the defect.

en·ter·oc·ly·sis (en″tər-ok′lĭ-sis) [*entero-* + *clysis*] 1. the injection of a nutrient or medicinal liquid into the colon. 2. the introduction of barium into the small intestine through a nasogastric tube whose end is distal to the duodenojejunal junction, done for radiographic examination. Called also *small bowel enema.* **enteroclyt′ic** *adj*

En·tero·coc·ca·ceae (en″tər-o-kə-ka′se-e) a family of gram-positive, facultatively anaerobic to microaerophilic, nonmotile cocci of the order Lactobacillales, occurring singly or in pairs, tetrads, or short chains; medically important organisms are contained in the genus *Enterococcus.*

en·tero·coc·ce·mia (en″tər-o-kok-se′me-ə) enterococcal bacteremia.

En·tero·coc·cus (en″tər-o-kok′əs) [*entero-* + *coccus*] a large genus of gram-positive, facultatively anaerobic bacteria of the family Enterococcaceae. Organisms are round to ovoid, found in pairs or short chains, catalase-negative, non–spore-forming, and generally nonmotile. Members of this genus are common intestinal flora and sometimes cause opportunistic infections. The type species is *Enterococcus faeca′lis.*

E. a′vium a species found primarily in the feces of chickens; it is occasionally associated with appendicitis, otitis, and brain abscesses in humans.

E. faeca′lis a common species that is a normal inhabitant of the human intestinal tract but can also cause urinary tract infections, infective endocarditis, and bacteremia that is often fatal. Formerly called *Streptococcus faecalis.*

E. fae′cium a common species that is a normal inhabitant of the human intestinal tract but can also cause urinary tract infections, infective endocarditis, and bacteremia. Formerly called *Streptococcus faecium.*

en·tero·coc·cus (en″tər-o-kok′əs) pl. *enterococ′ci.* 1. An organism belonging to the genus *Enterococcus.* 2. name formerly given to any streptococcus normally found in the intestinal tracts of animals.

en·tero·coele (en″tər-o-se′le) [*entero-* + Gr. *koilia* belly] the body cavity formed by the outpouchings from the archenteron, typically found in echinoderms and chordates.

en·tero·coe·lom (en″tər-o-se′lom) enterocoele.

en·tero·coel·om·ate (en″tər-o-sēl′o-māt) 1. having an enterocoele. 2. any of a group of animals, such as echinoderms and chordates, having a body cavity (enterocoele) derived from the archenteron.

en·tero·co·lec·to·my (en″tər-o-ko-lek′tə-me) resection of portions of the intestines, including the ileum, cecum, and ascending colon.

en·tero·co·li·tis (en″tər-o-ko-li′tis) [*entero-* + *colitis*] inflammation involving both the small intestine and the colon; see also *enteritis* and *colitis.*

antibiotic-associated e. a type of pseudomembranous enterocolitis seen after treatment with antibiotics has altered intestinal flora, causing diarrhea and other changes. Called also *antibiotic-associated colitis.*

hemorrhagic e. enterocolitis characterized by hemorrhagic breakdown of the intestinal mucosa with inflammatory-cell infiltration; some cases have been linked to verotoxins produced by *Escherichia coli* 0157:H7.

necrotizing e., neutropenic e. a type of pseudomembranous enterocolitis around the ileocecal area; it was originally found in newborn infants, particularly premature ones, and later was found in adults with immunodeficiency or myelosuppression. Called also *neutropenic colitis* or *typhlitis.*

pseudomembranous e. an acute type with formation of pseudomembranous plaques that overlie superficial ulcerations and pass out in the feces; it may result from shock, ischemia, or aftereffects of antibiotic therapy (see *antibiotic-associated e.*). Called also *pseudomembranous colitis* or *enteritis.*

regional e. Crohn disease.

Yersinia **e.** see under *enteritis.*

en·tero·co·los·to·my (en″tər-o-kə-los′tə-me) [*entero-* + *colostomy*] 1. surgical formation of a communication between the small intestine and the colon. 2. the opening so constructed.

en·tero·cu·ta·ne·ous (en″tər-o-ku-ta′ne-əs) pertaining to or communicating between the intestine and the skin.

en·tero·cyst (en′tər-o-sist″) [*entero-* + *cyst*] enteric cyst.

en·tero·cys·to·cele (en″tər-o-sis′to-sēl) [*entero-* + *cysto-* + *-cele*[1]] hernia of intestine and a portion of the urinary bladder; called also *cystoenterocele.*

en·tero·cys·to·ma (en″tər-o-sis-to′mə) enteric cyst.

en·tero·cys·to·plas·ty (en″tər-o-sis′to-plas″te) the most common type of augmentation cystoplasty, in which an isolated segment of intestine is used for the added segment; types include cecocystoplasty, colocystoplasty, ileocystoplasty, ileocecocystoplasty, and sigmoid cystoplasty. Called also *intestinocystoplasty.* **enterocystoplas′tic** *adj*

en·tero·cyte (en′tər-o-sīt″) an epithelial cell of the intestinal wall.

En·tero·cy·to·zo·on (en″tər-o-si″to-zo′ən) a genus of protozoa of the order Microsporida. *E. bieneu′si* has been found in enterocytes of immunocompromised persons, causing microsporidiosis with diarrhea.

en·ter·odyn·ia (en″tər-o-din′e-ə) enteralgia.

en·er·o·en·do·crine (en″tər-o-en′do-krin) pertaining to endocrine activity in the intestine.

en·ter·o·en·ter·ic (en″tər-o-en-ter′ik) affecting or connecting two different parts of the intestine, as a fistula; cf. *intestinointestinal.*

en·tero·en·ter·os·to·my (en″tər-o-en″tər-os′tə-me) surgical anastomosis between two segments of the intestine. Called also *enteroanastomosis.*

en·tero·epip·lo·cele (en″tər-o-ə-pip′lo-sēl) [*entero-* + *epiplocele*] hernia of the small intestine and omentum.

en·tero·gas·tric (en″tər-o-gas′trik) 1. proceeding from the small intestine to the stomach. 2. gastrointestinal.

en·tero·gas·tri·tis (en″tər-o-gas-tri′tis) gastroenteritis.

en·tero·gas·trone (en″tər-o-gas′trōn) any of various hormones that mediate the humoral inhibition of gastric secretion and motility.

en·ter·o·gen·ic (en″tər-o-jen′ik) enterogenous.

en·ter·og·e·nous (en″tər-oj′ə-nəs) [*entero-* + *-genous*] 1. originating within the small intestine. 2. arising from the foregut. Called also *enterogenic.*

en·tero·glu·ca·gon (en″tər-o-gloo′kə-gon) [*entero-* + *glucagon*] any of several glucagonlike hyperglycemic polypeptides released by special cells of the mucosa of the upper intestine in response to the ingestion of food; the major ones are glicentin and oxyntomodulin. They are immunologically distinct from pancreatic glucagon but display some similar properties. Called also *gut glucagon* and *glucagonlike immunoreactivity.*

en·tero·gram (en′tər-o-gram″) 1. a radiograph of the intestines. 2. a tracing made by an instrument of the movements of the intestine.

en·ter·og·ra·phy (en″tər-og′rə-fe) radiographic examination of the intestines.

en·tero·hem·or·rha·gic (en″tər-o-hem″ə-raj′ik) causing bloody diarrhea, said of pathogenic microorganisms.

en·tero·he·pat·ic (en″tər-o-hə-pat′ik) pertaining to or connecting the liver and intestine; called also *hepatoenteric.*

en·tero·hep·a·ti·tis (en″tər-o-hep″ə-ti′tis) [*entero-* + *hepatitis*] 1. inflammation of the intestine and liver. 2. histomoniasis.

en·tero·hep·a·to·cele (en″tər-o-hep′ə-to-sēl″) an infantile umbilical hernia containing intestines and liver.

en·tero·hy·dro·cele (en″tər-o-hi′dro-sēl) [*entero-* + *hydrocele*] hernia with hydrocele.

en·tero·in·va·sive (en″tər-o-in-va′siv) capable of penetrating and spreading through the intestinal mucosal epithelium.

en·tero·ki·nase (en″tər-o-ki′nās) former name for *enteropeptidase.*

en·tero·ki·ne·sia (en″tər-o-kĭ-ne′zhə) peristalsis.

en·tero·ki·net·ic (en″tər-o-kĭ-net′ik) 1. peristaltic. 2. causing or stimulating peristalsis.

en·tero·lith (en′tər-o-lith″) [*entero-* + *-lith*] any concretion found in the intestine; called also *intestinal calculus.*

en·tero·li·thi·a·sis (en″ter-o-lĭ-thi′ah-sis) [*entero-* + *lithiasis*] the presence of calculi (enteroliths) in the intestine.

en·ter·ol·o·gy (en″tər-ol′ə-je) [*entero-* + *-logy*] the study of the intestines and the nature and treatment of their diseases.

en·ter·ol·y·sis (en″tər-ol′ə-sis) [*entero-* + *-lysis*] the operative division of adhesions between loops of intestine or between the intestine and abdominal wall.

en·tero·me·ga·lia (en″tər-o-mə-ga′le-ə) enteromegaly.

en·tero·meg·a·ly (en″tər-o-meg′ə-le) [*entero-* + *-megaly*] enlargement of the intestine.

en·tero·mere (en′tər-o-mēr″) [*entero-* + *-mere*] any segment of the embryonic alimentary tract.

en•tero•me•ro•cele (en″tər-o-me′ro-sēl) femoral hernia.

En•tero•mo•na•di•na (en″tər-o-mo″nə-di′nə) a suborder of parasitic protozoa of the order Diplomonadida, having one karyomastigont containing one to four flagella.

En•tero•mo•nas (en″tər-o-mo′nəs) [*entero-* + Gr. *monas* unit, from *monos* single] a genus of nonpathogenic, parasitic, intestinal protozoa of the order Diplomonadida, phylum Parabasalia, having four anterior flagella, one of which passes along the body and emerges and extends posteriorly.

en•tero•neu•ri•tis (en″tər-o-noo-ri′tis) inflammation of the nerves of the intestine.

en•tero•pan•cre•at•ic (en″ter-o-pan″kre-at′ik) pertaining to the intestine and pancreas; called also *pancreaticoenteric.*

en•tero•pa•re•sis (en″tər-o-pə-re′sis) [*entero-* + Gr. *paresis* relaxation] relaxation of the intestine resulting in dilatation.

en•ter•o•path•o•gen (en″tər-o-path′o-jən) a microorganism that causes intestinal disease.

en•tero•patho•gen•e•sis (en″tər-o-path″o-jen′ə-sis) the production of intestinal diseases or disorders.

en•ter•o•path•o•gen•ic (en″tər-o-path″o-jen′ik) pertaining to or producing intestinal disease.

en•ter•op•a•thy (en″tər-op′ə-the) [*entero-* + *-pathy*] any disease of the intestine.

AIDS e. HIV e.

gluten e., gluten-induced e., gluten sensitive e. celiac disease.

HIV e. gastrointestinal symptoms in immunocompromised persons infected with the human immunodeficiency virus. The most common is HIV-related diarrhea (see under *diarrhea*); less common symptoms include odynophagia, dysphagia, abdominal pain, jaundice, and anorectal disease.

nonsteroidal antiinflammatory drug e., NSAID e., NSAID-induced e. intestinal irritation caused by nonsteroidal antiinflammatory drugs, usually in long-term users; first there is increased permeability of the wall, and this may progress to perforations, ulcers, and strictures.

proliferative hemorrhagic e. a frequently fatal type of porcine proliferative enteritis characterized by anemia, diarrhea, and hemorrhagic intestinal lesions.

protein-losing e. a nonspecific term referring to conditions associated with excessive intestinal loss of plasma protein; these include extensive ulceration (such as inflammatory bowel disease), diffuse mucosal conditions involving rapid desquamation of mucosal epithelial cells (such as adult celiac disease), and obstruction of intestinal lymphatic vessels (intestinal lymphangiectasia).

radiation e. damage to the small intestine that is caused by ionizing radiation and is more chronic than that from radiation enteritis (q.v.); it may include mucosal atrophy, vascular sclerosis, intestinal stenosis, and eventually obstruction. In some patients it progresses to abscesses, ulceration, perforation, or fistula formation.

tropical e. changes in intestinal villus structure occurring in the tropics and subtropics, leading to decreased absorptive capacity and eventually a malabsorption syndrome. It may be caused by either subclinical intestinal infections or inadequate nutrition. See also *tropical sprue*, under *sprue.*

tufting e. a rare intestinal disorder, thought to be hereditary and autosomal recessive; infants have severe watery diarrhea with malabsorption of nutrients and will die unless put on total parenteral nutrition. Small tufts of enterocytes are visible in microscopic specimens, and the malabsorption is thought to be caused by abnormal interactions between the enterocytes and the mesenchymal cells.

en•tero•pep•ti•dase (en″tər-o-pep′tĭ-dās) [EC 3.4.21.9] a serine endopeptidase that catalyzes the cleavage of a specific peptide bond near the N-terminus of trypsinogen, converting it to the active form trypsin. The enzyme is secreted by the small intestine.

en•tero•pep•ti•dase de•fi•cien•cy (en″tər-o-pep′tĭ-dās) a rare autosomal recessive condition caused by mutation in the *PRSS7* gene (locus: 21q21), which encodes enteropeptidase, characterized by severe protein malabsorption, diarrhea, hypoproteinemic edema, and failure to thrive.

en•tero•pexy (en′tər-o-pek″se) [*entero-* + *-pexy*] surgical fixation of the intestine to the anterior or posterior abdominal wall, or occasionally of one segment to another.

en•tero•plas•ty (en′tər-o-plas″te) [*entero-* + *-plasty*] plastic surgery of the intestine, especially to enlarge the caliber of a constricted segment or area of bowel. Cf. *strictureplasty.* **enteroplas′tic** *adj*

en•ter•o•pli•ca•tion (en″tər-o-plĭ-ka′shən) surgical treatment of intussusception in cats and dogs by suturing loops of intestine to each other to maintain their relative positions.

en•tero•re•nal (en″tər-o-re′nəl) pertaining to or connecting the intestine and a kidney. Called also *renointestinal.*

en•ter•or•rha•gia (en″tər-o-ra′jə) [*entero-* + *-rrhagia*] hemorrhage from the intestine.

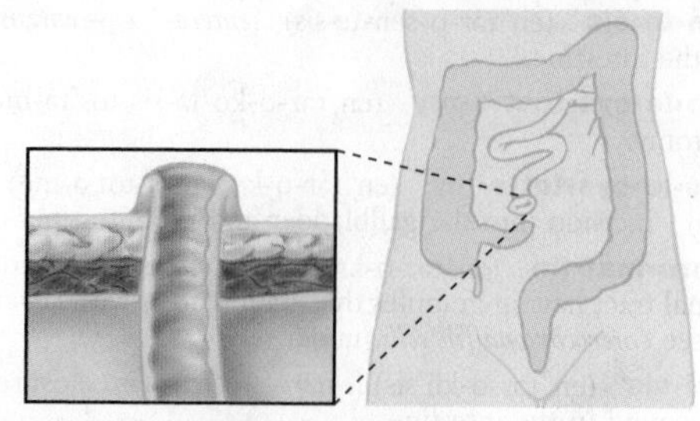

■ Ileostomy, a type of enterostomy, with inset showing in cross-section the protrusion of the everted ileal terminus through the abdominal wall, forming the stoma.

en•ter•or•rha•phy (en″tər-or′ə-fe) [*entero-* + *-rrhaphy*] repair or suture of the intestine.

en•ter•or•rhex•is (en″tər-o-rek′sis) [*entero-* + *-rrhexis*] rupture of the intestine.

en•tero•scope (en′tər-o-skōp) [*entero-* + *-scope*] an endoscope, usually fiberoptic, for examining the lumen of the intestine.

en•tero•scop•ic (en″tər-o-skop′ik) pertaining to enteroscopy or to an enteroscope.

en•ter•os•co•py (en″tər-os′kə-pe) examination of the intestine with an enteroscope.

capsule e. see under *endoscopy.*

double-balloon e. visualization and treatment of lesions along the entire length of the small intestine, using a flexible enteroscope with two balloons around its distal end; the balloons can be alternately inflated and deflated to allow advancement of the enteroscope.

push e. enteroscopy using a long, flexible endoscope that enters the small intestine and is pushed into the proximal jejunum.

sonde e. an older type of enteroscopy using a sonde that has a balloon on the tip so that it advances by peristalsis into the distal jejunum and the ileum; it visualizes while it is being slowly withdrawn.

en•tero•sep•sis (en″tər-o-sep′sis) [*entero-* + *sepsis*] intestinal sepsis due to putrefaction of the contents of the intestines.

en•tero•spasm (en′tər-o-spaz″əm) [*entero-* + *spasm*] a spasm of the intestine.

en•tero•sta•sis (en″tər-o-sta′sis) [*entero-* + *stasis*] intestinal stasis.

en•tero•ste•no•sis (en″tər-o-stə-no′sis) [*entero-* + *stenosis*] stenosis of the intestine; see also *ileus.*

en•tero•sto•mal (en″tər-o-sto′məl) relating to or having undergone enterostomy.

en•ter•os•to•my (en″tər-os′tə-me) [*entero-* + *-stomy*] 1. the formation of a permanent opening into the intestine through the abdominal wall, usually by surgical means. 2. the opening so created.

en•tero•tome (en′tər-ə-tōm″) [*entero-* + *-tome*] an instrument for cutting the intestine.

en•ter•ot•o•my (en″tər-ot′ə-me) [*entero-* + *-tomy*] incision into the intestine.

en•tero•tox•e•mia (en″tər-o-tok-se′me-ə) any of several usually fatal conditions in domestic animals characterized by presence in the blood of toxins or bacteria normally found in the intestines.

***Escherichia coli* e.** edema disease.

hemorrhagic e. struck.

infectious e. of sheep pulpy kidney disease in sheep.

en•ter•o•tox•i•gen•ic (en″tər-o-tok″sĭ-jen′ik) producing or containing an enterotoxin.

en•tero•tox•in (en′tər-o-tok″sin) [*entero-* + *toxin*] a toxin specifically affecting cells of the intestinal mucosa, causing vomiting and diarrhea, e.g., those elaborated by species of *Bacillus, Clostridium, Escherichia, Staphylococcus,* and *Vibrio.* See also *toxin.*

cholera e. see under *toxin.*

en•tero•tro•pic (en″tər-o-tro′pik) [*entero-* + *-tropic*] having a special affinity for or exerting its principal effect upon the intestines.

en•tero•vag•i•nal (en″tər-o-vaj′ĭ-nəl) pertaining to or communicating between the intestine and the vagina.

en•tero•ve•nous (en″tər-o-ve′nəs) communicating between the intestinal lumen and the lumen of a vein.

en•tero•ves•i•cal (en″tər-o-ves′ĭ-kəl) pertaining to or communicating between the urinary bladder and the intestine. Called also *vesicoenteric* and *vesicointestinal.*

En•tero•vi•rus (en′tər-o-vi″rəs) [*entero-* + *virus*] the enteroviruses, a genus of viruses of the family Picornaviridae that preferentially inhabit the intestinal tract. Infection is usually asymptomatic or mild but may result in a variety of disease syndromes. Human enteroviruses were originally classified as polioviruses, coxsackieviruses, or echoviruses and numbered sequentially within each group; because the boundaries between these groups have become indistinct, new enteroviruses are designated by a continuous numbering system, beginning with human enterovirus 68. The original groups continue to be used for previously discovered viruses. Enteroviruses also infect a wide range of animals and are grouped by host.

en·tero·vi·rus (en′tər-o-vi″rəs) any virus of the genus *Enterovirus.* **enterovi′ral** *adj*

bovine e. a species of the genus *Enterovirus,* separable into two serotypes, that have been associated with infertility and abortion in cattle.

human e. either of two species of the genus *Enterovirus* that infect humans; there are numerous different serogroups. Most strains cause only mild symptoms such as fever, but one causes acute hemorrhagic conjunctivitis and others cause aseptic meningitis, pericarditis, and pleurodynia.

porcine e. a species of the genus *Enterovirus,* separable into eleven serotypes, that are normal inhabitants of the intestinal tract of swine but may cause infectious porcine encephalomyelitis.

simian e. a species of the genus *Enterovirus,* separable into 18 serotypes, that causes usually asymptomatic infection in monkeys.

en·thal·py (en′thəl-pe) [*en-* + Gr. *thalpein* to warm] the heat content or chemical energy of a physical system; it is a thermodynamic function equal to the internal energy plus the product of the pressure and volume. Symbol *H.*

en·the·sis (en-the′sis) [Gr. "a putting in; insertion"] the site of attachment of a muscle or ligament to bone.

en·the·si·tis (en″thə-si′tis) inflammation of the muscular or tendinous attachment to bone.

en·the·sop·a·thy (en″thə-sop′ə-the) disorder of the muscular or tendinous attachment to bone.

en·theto·bio·sis (en-thet″o-bi-o′sis) [*enthesis* + *biosis*] dependency on a mechanical implant, as on an artificial cardiac pacemaker.

en·thla·sis (en′thlə-sis) [Gr. "a dent caused by pressure"] comminuted fracture of the skull, with depression of the bony fragments.

en·tire (en-tīr′) smooth and continuous with no projections or indentations; used to describe the border of a bacterial colony.

en·ti·ris (en-ti′ris) [*ent-* + *iris*] the posterior pigment layer of the iris.

en·ti·ty (en′tĭ-te) [L. *ens* being] an independently existing thing; a reality.

ent(o)- [Gr. *entos* inside] a prefix signifying within, or inner.

en·to·blast (en′to-blast) [*ento-* + *-blast*] endoderm.

en·to·chon·dros·to·sis (en″to-kon″dros-to′sis) [*ento-* + *chondro-* + *ostosis*] the development of bone taking place within cartilage.

en·toc·ne·mi·al (en″tok-ne′me-əl) on the inner side of the tibia.

en·to·cor·nea (en″to-kor′ne-ə) [*ento-* + *cornea*] lamina limitans posterior cornea.

En·to·cort (en′to-kort″) trademark for a preparation of budesonide.

en·to·cu·ne·i·form (en″to-ku-ne′ĭ-form) os cuneiforme mediale.

en·to·derm (en′to-dərm) [*ento-* + *-derm*] endoderm.

En·to·di·nio·mor·phi·da (en″to-di″ne-o-mor′fĭ-də) [*ento-* + Gr. *dinos* a whirling + *morphē* form] an order of ciliate protozoa (subclass Vestibuliferia, class Kinetofragminophorea) found as commensals in mammalian herbivores, including anthropoid apes. The somatic ciliature is reduced to unique tufts or bands and the oral ciliature is conspicuous, with the adoral zone being composed of membranelles that spiral toward the cytostome; the oral area is sometimes retractable, the pellicle is generally firm and may be drawn out into processes, and skeletal plates are present in many species.

en·to·ec·tad (en″to-ek′tad) [*ento-* + *ektad*] directed or proceeding from within outward.

en·to·mere (en′to-mēr) [*ento-* + *-mere*] a blastomere destined to become endoderm.

en·to·meso·derm (en″to-mes′o-dərm) endomesoderm.

en·to·mi·on (en-to′me-on) [Gr. *entomē* notch] the point at the tip of the mastoid angle of the parietal bone in the parietal notch of the temporal bone.

entom(o)- [Gr. *entomon* insect] a combining form denoting relationship to an insect, or to insects.

En·to·mo·brya (en″to-mo-bri′ə) a genus of insects, the spring tails, of the order Collembola, Australian species of which cause irritation by their bite.

en·to·mog·e·nous (en″to-moj′ə-nəs) [*entomo-* + *-genous*] 1. derived from insects, their bites, emanations, etc. 2. growing in the body of an insect.

en·to·mol·o·gist (en″to-mol′o-jist) a specialist in entomology.

en·to·mol·o·gy (en″tə-mol′ə-je) [*entomo-* + *-logy*] the branch of zoology that deals with the study of insects.

medical e. a branch of entomology concerned with insects that cause disease or serve as vectors of microorganisms causing disease in humans.

En·to·moph·tho·ra (en″to-mof′thə-rə) [*entomo-* + Gr. *phthora* destruction, death] a former genus of fungi of the family Entomophthoraceae, now divided into several separate genera. *E. corona′ta* is now called *Conidiobolus coronata.*

En·to·moph·tho·ra·ceae (en″to-mof″thə-ra′se-e) a family of fungi of the order Entomophthorales, found as saprobes and as parasites on higher fungi and insects. Pathogenic organisms are found in the genera *Basidiobolus* and *Conidiobolus.*

En·to·moph·tho·ra·les (en″to-mof″thə-ra′lēz) an order of perfect fungi of the phylum Zygomycota, class Zygomycetes, which are typically parasites of insects, although they can also infect humans (see *entomophthoromycosis*). Pathogenic organisms are found in the families Entomophthoraceae and Basidiobolaceae.

en·to·moph·tho·ra·my·co·sis (en″tə-mof″thə-rə-mi-ko′sis) entomophthoromycosis.

en·to·moph·tho·ro·my·co·sis (en″tə-mof″thə-ro-mi-ko′sis) 1. any disease caused by fungi of the order Entomophthorales; human infections are usually in apparently physiologically and immunologically normal individuals, although opportunistic infections also occur. See also *basidiobolomycosis* and *conidiobolomycosis.* 2. infection of the skin, oral mucosa, or nasal mucosa of horses by fungi of the order Entomophthorales, causing nodules or ulcerative granulomatous lesions. It is sometimes confused with cutaneous habronemiasis or pythiosis. See also *swamp cancer.*

e. basidio′bolae basidiobolomycosis.

e. conidio′bolae conidiobolomycosis.

en·toph·thal·mia (en″tof-thal′me-ə) endophthalmitis.

en·to·phyte (en′to-fīt) endophyte.

en·top·ic (en-top′ik) [*en-* + Gr. *topos* place] occurring in the proper place, as opposed to ectopic.

en·top·tic (en-top′tik) [*ent-* + *optic*] denoting visual phenomena which have their seat within the eye.

en·top·to·scope (en-top′to-skōp) an instrument for examining the media of the eyes, to ascertain their transparency.

en·top·tos·co·py (en″top-tos′ko-pe) [*ent-* + *opto-* + *-scopy*] the observation of the interior of the eye and its light and shadows.

en·to·ret·i·na (en″to-ret′ĭ-nə) [*ento-* + *retina*] the internal or nervous portion of the retina, disposed in five layers, which are named respectively outer plexiform, inner nuclear, inner plexiform, ganglion, and nerve fiber layers. See illustration at *retina.*

en·to·rhi·nal (en″to-ri′nəl) interior to the rhinal sulcus.

ent·os·to·sis (ent″os-to′sis) enostosis.

en·to·tym·pan·ic (en″to-tim-pan′ik) intratympanic.

en·to·zoa (en″to-zo′ə) [Gr.] plural of *entozoon.*

en·to·zo·al (en″to-zo′əl) pertaining to or caused by entozoa.

en·to·zo·on (en″to-zo′on) pl. *entozo′a* [*ento-* + Gr. *zōon* animal] a parasitic animal organism living within the body of its host.

en·train (en-trān′) to modulate the cardiac rhythm by gaining control of the rate of the pacemaker, cardiac or ectopic, with an external stimulus.

en·train·ment (en-trān′mənt) 1. a technique for identifying the slowest pacing necessary to terminate an arrhythmia, particularly atrial flutter; as the pacing rate is slowly increased incrementally, the electrocardiographic appearance of the flutter waves shifts incrementally away from a flutter morphology until the arrhythmia is terminated. 2. the synchronization and control of cardiac rhythm by an external stimulus.

en·trap·ment (en-trap′mənt) compression of a nerve or vessel by adjacent tissue, such as the walls of a fibrous or osseofibrous tunnel, muscle, tendon, or other tissue; see also *entrapment neuropathy.*

en·tro·pi·on (en-tro′pe-on) [*en-* + Gr. *tropein* to turn] 1. the turning inward (inversion) of an edge or margin. 2. specifically, the turning inward of the margin of the eyelid, with the tarsal cartilage turned inward toward the eyeball; called also *blepharelosis.*

cicatricial e. inversion of the margin of an eyelid caused by contraction of scar tissue in the palpebral conjunctiva or underlying tarsus.

spastic e. inversion of the eyelid caused by tonic spasm of the orbicularis oculi muscle.

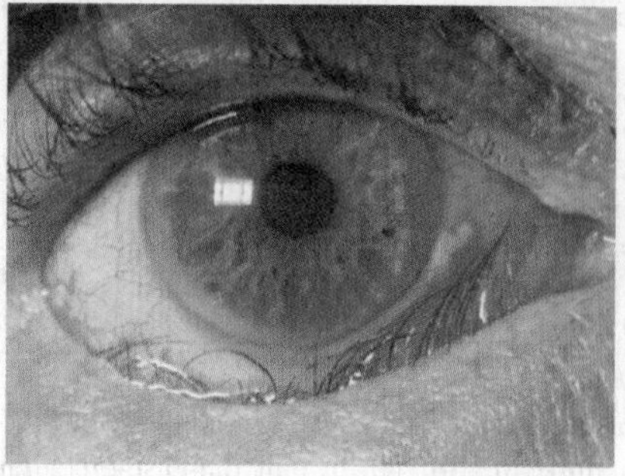

■ Entropion.

e. u'veae inversion of the margin of the pupil, usually the result of an iritis attended with exudate, and occurring rarely as a congenital condition.

en•tro•pi•um (en-tro'pe-əm) entropion.

en•tro•py (en'tro-pe) [Gr. *entropē* a turning inward] 1. the measure of that part of the heat or energy of a system which is not available to perform work; entropy increases in all natural (spontaneous and irreversible) processes. Symbol *S*. 2. the tendency of any system to move toward randomness or disorder. 3. diminished capacity for spontaneous change, as occurs in the psyche in aging.

ent•wick•lungs•me•cha•nik (ent″vik-loongs″mə-kahn'ik) [Ger. "developmental mechanics"] mechanisms of embryological development, as revealed by experimental study.

en•ty•py (en'tə-pe) [Gr. *entypē* pattern] a method of gastrulation in which the endoderm lies external to the amniotic ectoderm.

enu•cle•ate (e-noo'kle-āt) [L. *enucleare*] to remove whole and clean, as a tumor from its envelope or the eyeball; see *enucleation.*

enu•cle•at•ed (e-noo'kle-āt″əd) removed; said of an organ, tumor, or cell nucleus.

enu•cle•a•tion (e-noo″kle-a'shən) [L. *e* out + *nucleus* kernel] the removal of an organ, of a tumor, or of another body in such a way that it comes out clean and whole, like a nut from its shell. Used in connection with the eye, it denotes removal of the eyeball after the eye muscles and optic nerve have been severed.

en•ure•sis (en″u-re'sis) [Gr. *enourein* to void urine] urinary incontinence.

en•uret•ic (en″u-ret'ik) 1. pertaining to enuresis. 2. an agent that causes enuresis. 3. a person with enuresis.

en•ve•lope (en'və-lōp) [Old Fr. *enveloper* to wrap up] 1. an encompassing structure or membrane. 2. in virology, a lipoprotein bilayer surrounding the capsid of some viruses, acquired by budding through the cell membrane of the host cell; the lipids are derived from the host cell and the proteins are encoded by the virus. Called also *peplos.* 3. in bacteriology, the cell wall and the plasma membrane considered together.

cell e. the plasma membrane and the cell wall considered together.

egg e. see under *membrane.*

nuclear e. the structure enclosing the cell nucleus and separating it from the cytoplasm, consisting of two concentric lipid bilayers (the inner and outer membranes) separated by a 30-nm wide perinuclear space. The outer membrane is continuous with the rough endoplasmic reticulum, and nuclear pore complexes bridging both membranes provide communication between the nucleus and the cytoplasm. Called also *nuclear membrane.*

en•ven•om•a•tion (en-ven″o-ma'shən) poisoning by venom.

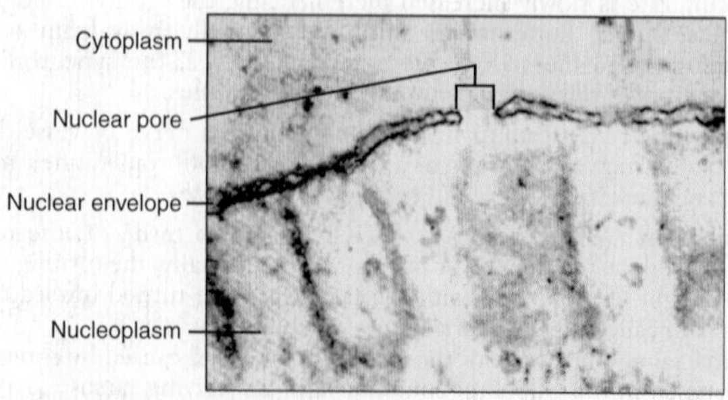

■ Nuclear envelope, showing the inner and outer membrane and a nuclear pore (electron micrograph).

en•vi•ron•ment (en-vi'ron-mənt) [Fr. *environner* to surround, to encircle] the sum total of all the conditions and elements making up the surroundings and influencing the development and actions of an individual.

protected e. an area maintained as free as possible from disease-causing agents, to be used by debilitated or immunocompromised patients. See also *isolation.*

en•vy (en've) a desire to have another's possessions or qualities for oneself.

penis e. in psychoanalysis, the concept that the female envies the male for his possession of a penis, first described by Freud as occurring during the phallic stage in little girls as they become aware of anatomical differences between the sexes; sometimes used to denote a woman's generalized envy of men or their characteristics.

en•za•cam•ene (en″zə-kam'ēn) [USP] an absorber of ultraviolet radiation, used topically as a sunscreen. Called also *methyl benzylidene camphor.*

En•zac•tin (en-zak'tin) trademark for preparations of triacetin.

en•zo•ot•ic (en″zo-ot'ik) [*en-* + *zootic*] 1. present in an animal community at all times, but occurring in only small numbers of cases. 2. a disease of low morbidity which is constantly present in an animal community. Cf. *epizootic.*

en•zy•got•ic (en″zi-got'ik) developed from the same zygote.

en•zy•mat•ic (en″zi-mat'ik) 1. pertaining to or of the nature of an enzyme. 2. caused by an enzyme.

en•zyme (en'zīm) [*en-* + Gr. *zymē* leaven] a protein molecule that catalyzes chemical reactions of other substances without itself being destroyed or altered upon completion of the reactions. Symbol E. Enzymes are classified according to the recommendations of the Nomenclature Committee of the International Union of Biochemistry. Each enzyme is assigned a recommended name and an Enzyme Commission (EC) number. They are divided into six main groups: oxidoreductases, transferases, hydrolases, lyases, isomerases, and ligases. For individual enzymes, see under the specific name, e.g., *glucose-6-phosphate dehydrogenase.*

adaptive e. induced e.

allosteric e. an enzyme whose catalytic activity is altered by binding of specific ligands at sites other than the substrate binding site.

brancher e., branching e. 1,4-α-glucan branching enzyme.

constitutive e. an enzyme that is produced constantly, irrespective of environmental conditions or demand.

cryptic e. in bacteriology, an enzyme that can attack added substrate in a cell lysate but not in intact cells, owing to selective action of a permeability barrier.

debrancher e., debranching e. 1. amylo-1,6-glucosidase. 2. a term used to describe any enzyme removing branches from macromolecules, usually polysaccharides, by cleaving at branch points.

extracellular e. exoenzyme.

fat-splitting e. lipase.

hydrolytic e. hydrolase.

induced e., inducible e. an enzyme whose production can be stimulated by another compound, often a substrate or a structurally related compound (inducer). The inducers studied first were substrates whose utilization thus became possible; hence these enzymes were known earlier as *adaptive enzymes.* Cf. *constitutive e.*

intracellular e. endoenzyme.

proteolytic e. peptidase.

receptor-destroying e. (RDE) an enzyme that renders red cells insusceptible to viral hemolysis by destroying its receptors.

redox e. oxidoreductase.

repressible e. an enzyme whose rate of formation is decreased by an increased concentration of one or more end products. The process serves as a control mechanism in certain bacterial and mammalian metabolic systems.

respiratory e. an enzyme that is part of an electron transport (respiratory) chain.

restriction e. restriction endonuclease.

stratum corneum chymotryptic e. [EC 3.4.21.117] a serine endopeptidase that is abundant in the stratum corneum and together with stratum corneum tryptic enzyme catalyzes degradation of the constituent proteins of corneodesmosomes, which is necessary for desquamation.

stratum corneum tryptic e. a serine endopeptidase that is abundant in the stratum corneum and together with stratum corneum chymotryptic enzyme catalyzes degradation of the constituent proteins of corneodesmosomes, which is necessary for desquamation. An excess of this enzyme together with an excess of cathelicidin results in the formation of an abnormal peptide that causes the lesions of rosacea.

yellow e's any of a number of enzymes having a flavin as a prosthetic group. Historically, NADPH dehydrogenase (occurring in plants and yeast) was called the *old yellow enzyme* to distinguish it from D-amino acid oxidase, known as the *new yellow enzyme.* See also *flavoprotein.*

en•zym•ic (en-zim'ik) enzymatic.

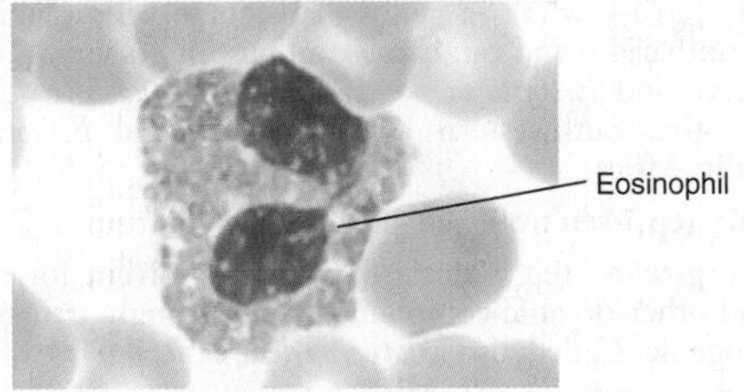

en·zy·mol·o·gy (en″zi-mol′ə-je) the study of enzymes and enzymatic action.

en·zy·mop·a·thy (en″zi-mop′ə-the) an inborn error of metabolism consisting of defective or absent enzymes, as in the glycogen storage diseases or the mucopolysaccharidoses.

lysosomal e. lysosomal storage disease.

EOG electro-olfactogram.

eo·sin (e′o-sin) [Gr. *ēōs* dawn] any of a group of related pink to red acid dyes that are halogenated derivatives of fluorescein, including eosins B and Y and ethyl eosin, as well as other related compounds. When used specifically, the term usually denotes eosin Y.

e. B, e. I bluish dibromodinitrofluorescein, a dye having staining properties similar to eosin Y, but having a bluish rather than yellow cast.

ethyl e. the ethyl ester of eosin Y, an alcohol soluble dye that can be used instead of eosin Y to counterstain hematoxylin in hematoxylin-eosin stain.

e. Y, e. yellowish, e. Y ws the sodium salt of tetrabromofluorescein, $C_{20}H_6Br_4Na_2O_5$, a water-soluble, red, anionic dye of the eosin group; widely used in bacteriologic and histologic staining.

eo·sin·o·cyte (e″o-sin′o-sīt) eosinophil.

eo·sin·o·pe·nia (e″o-sin-o-pe′ne-ə) [*eosinophil* + *-penia*] abnormal deficiency of eosinophils in the blood; called also *hypoeosinophilia*.

eo·sin·o·phil (e″o-sin′o-fil) [*eosin* + *-phil*] 1. a granular leukocyte with a nucleus that usually has two lobes connected by a slender thread of chromatin, and cytoplasm containing coarse, round granules that are uniform in size. Called also *eosinocyte* and *eosinophilic leukocyte*. 2. any structure, cell, or histologic element readily stained by eosin.

eo·sin·o·phile (e″o-sin′o-fil) 1. eosinophil. 2. eosinophilic.

eo·sin·o·phil·ia (e″o-sin″o-fil′e-ə) [*eosin* + *-philia*] 1. the formation and accumulation of an abnormally large number of eosinophils in the blood; see also *hypereosinophilia*. Called also *eosinophilic leukocytosis*. 2. the presence of eosinophils in a location where they are not normally found. 3. the condition of being readily stained with eosin.

Löffler e. see under *syndrome*.

pulmonary infiltration e. pulmonary infiltration with eosinophilia; see under *infiltration*.

simple pulmonary e. Löffler syndrome.

tissue e. the presence of eosinophils in tissues outside the bloodstream, usually seen as part of an inflammatory response.

tropical e., tropical pulmonary e. a subacute or chronic form of occult filariasis, usually involving *Brugia malayi*, *Wuchereria bancrofti*, or filariae that infect animals; it occurs in the tropics, especially in India, where some groups may have a genetic predisposition for the disease. It is characterized by episodic nocturnal wheezing and coughing, strikingly elevated eosinophilia, and diffuse reticulonodular infiltrations of the lung. Microfilariae are seldom detected in peripheral blood films since the parasites are confined primarily to the lungs. However, there is evidence of both humoral and cellular immunity to the filariae, and the illness often improves following antifilarial chemotherapy. Called also *filarial hypereosinophilia* and *Weingarten syndrome*.

eo·sin·o·phil·ic (e″o-sin″o-fil′ik) 1. readily stainable with eosin. 2. pertaining to eosinophils. 3. pertaining to or characterized by eosinophilia.

eo·sin·o·philo·poi·e·tin (e″o-sin″o-fil″o-poi′ə-tin) a peptide of low molecular weight that induces production of eosinophils.

eo·sin·o·phi·lo·sis (e″o-sin″o-fi-lo′sis) eosinophilia (def. 1).

eo·sin·oph·i·lous (e″o-sin-of′ĭ-ləs) eosinophilic.

eo·sin·o·phil·uria (e″o-sin″o-fil-u′re-ə) the presence of eosinophils in the urine, as in certain drug sensitivity conditions or disorders of the genitourinary tract.

eo·sin·o·tac·tic (e″o-sin″o-tak′tik) [*eosinophil* + *tactic*] exhibiting an influence on eosinophils, either repelling them *(negatively e.)* or attracting them *(positively e.)*.

EP evoked potential.

ep- see *epi-*.

EPA eicosapentaenoic acid; Environmental Protection Agency.

ep·ac·me (əp-ak′me) [Gr. *epakmazein* to come to its height] in evolution, the stage or period of development.

epac·tal (e-pak′təl) [Gr. *epaktos* brought in] 1. supernumerary. 2. os suturale.

ep·al·lo·bi·o·sis (əp-al″o-bi-o′sis) [*epi-* + *allo-* + *biosis*] dependency on an external life-support system, as on a heart-lung machine or hemodialyzer.

ep·ar·sal·gia (ep″ahr-sal′jə) [Gr. *epairein* to lift + *-algia*] any painful disorder due to overstrain of a part, including dilatation of the heart, hernia, enteroptosis, coughing, etc.

ep·ar·te·ri·al (ep″ahr-te′re-əl) [*epi-* + *arterial*] over an artery; applied especially to the first branch of the right primary bronchus which is so situated.

ep·ax·i·al (əp-ak′se-əl) [*epi-* + *axial*] situated upon or above an axis, such as the axis of a limb.

EPEC enteropathogenic *Escherichia coli*.

ep·en·dop·a·thy (ep″ən-dop′ə-the) ependymopathy.

epen·dy·ma (ə-pen′də-mə) [Gr. *ependyma* upper garment] [TA] the lining membrane of the ventricles of the brain and of the central canal of the spinal cord. **epen′dymal** *adj*

epen·dy·mi·tis (ə-pen″də-mi′təs) inflammation of the ependyma.

granular e. irritation of the ependyma on the floor of the fourth ventricle as a result of viral or bacterial infections such as neurosyphilis; granules appear, made up of neurological material and sometimes covered with ependyma. Obstruction of outflow of cerebrospinal fluid may cause hydrocephalus.

epen·dy·mo·blast (ə-pen′də-mo-blast) an embryonic ependymal cell; an ependymal spongioblast.

epen·dy·mo·blas·to·ma (ə-pen′də-mo-blas-to′mə) a rare malignant tumor composed of primitive ependymal cells. Some neuropathologists classify such tumors as malignant forms of ependymoma but some consider them a type of primitive neuroectodermal tumor.

epen·dy·mo·cyte (ə-pen′də-mo-sīt″) an ependymal cell.

epen·dy·mo·cy·to·ma (ə-pen″də-mo-si-to′mə) ependymoma.

epen·dy·mo·ma (ə-pen″də-mo′mə) a neoplasm composed of differentiated ependymal cells, occurring most often in the posterior cranial fossa in children and in the spinal cord in adults. Most are slow growing and benign, but a few are malignant.

epen·dy·mop·a·thy (ə-pen″də-mop′ə-the) disease of the ependyma.

Ep·eryth·ro·zo·on (ep″ə-rith″ro-zo′on) [*epi-* + *erythros-* + Gr. *zoon* animal] a genus of hematropic bacteria of the family Mycoplasmataceae that sometimes cause disease in rodents, cattle, sheep, and swine. The type species is *E. coccoi′des*.

ep·eryth·ro·zoo·no·sis (ep″ə-rith″ro-zo″o-no′sis) infection with rickettsiae of the genus *Eperythrozoon*.

ephapse (ə-faps′) [Gr. *ephapsis* a touching] electrical synapse.

ephap·tic (ə-fap′tik) pertaining to an electrical synapse (ephapse) or to conduction across it.

ep·har·mo·ny (ep-hahr′mo-ne) development in complete harmony with environment; harmonic relation between structure and environment.

ephe·bi·at·rics (ə-fe″be-at′riks) [Gr. *ephēbos* one arrived at puberty + *-iatrics*] a branch of medicine consisting of the diagnosis and treatment of diseases of youth (18–25 years).

Ephed·ra (ə-fed′rə) [Gr. *epi* upon + *hedra* seat] a genus of low, branching shrubs of the family Gnetaceae, indigenous to China and India. *E. equiseti′na* Bunge., *E. sini′ca* Stapf., *E. vulga′ris*, and other species (all called *ma huang* in China) are sources of ephedrine.

ephed·rine (ə-fed′rin, ef′ə-drin) [USP] an adrenergic obtained from *Ephedra* species or prepared synthetically. It stimulates both α- and β-adrenergic receptors and causes increased systolic and diastolic blood pressure and cardiac output by enhancing the release of endogenous norepinephrine from sympathetic neurons. It is also a central nervous system stimulant. It has been used as an ingredient in numerous supplements, with purported benefits including weight loss, increased energy, and enhanced athletic performance, but has been banned from nonprescription use in the United States by the Food and Drug Administration.

e. hydrochloride [USP] the hydrochloride salt of ephedrine, used as a bronchodilator and nasal decongestant in asthma and allergy; administered orally, parenterally, or intranasally.

e. sulfate [USP] the sulfate salt of ephedrine, used as a bronchodilator and nasal decongestant in asthma and allergy and to counteract hypotension secondary to spinal or infiltration anesthesia, sympathectomy, and overdose of adrenergic blocking agents, ganglionic blocking agents, or other drugs that lower blood pressure; administered orally, parenterally, or intranasally.

e. tannate the tannate salt of ephedrine, used as a bronchodilator and nasal decongestant; administered orally.

ephel·i·des (ə-fel′ĭ-dēz) [Gr.] plural of *ephelis*.

ephe·lis (ə-fe′lis) pl. *ephe′lides* [Gr. *ephēlis*] freckle.

ephem·era (ə-fem′ər-ə) [Gr. *ephēmeros* short-lived] a transitory condition or thing.

ephem·er·al (ə-fem′ər-əl) short-lived; transient.

Ephe·mer·i·da (e″fə-mer′i-də) a family of flies whose exuviae may cause sensitization and severe asthmatic paroxysms when inhaled.

Ephem·er·op·tera (e-fem″ər-op′tər-ə) [Gr. *ephemeros* short-lived + *pteron* wing] the mayflies, an order of elongated insects with net-veined paired wings, and two or three caudal filiform appendages; the adults have only vestigial mouth parts and starve to death soon after laying their eggs. See also *Hexagenia bilineata*.

Ephem·ero·vi·rus (e-fem′ər-o-vi″rəs) [Gr. *ephemeros* short-lived + *virus*] a genus of viruses of the family Rhabdoviridae that includes bovine ephemeral fever virus and related viruses.

epi- [Gr. *epi* on] a prefix meaning upon, above, or beside. In chemistry, it denotes a chemical compound or group that is related to another chemical compound or group. Also, *ep-*.

epi·al·lo·preg·nan·o·lone (ep″e-al″o-preg-nan′ə-lōn) a 21-carbon corticoid hormone present in pregnancy urine, thought to originate in the fetal adrenal cortex; probably a precursor of C19 androgens.

epi·an·dros·ter·one (ep″e-an-dros′tər-ōn) an anabolic-androgenic steroid, one of the urinary 17-ketosteroids, less active than androsterone and excreted in small amounts in normal human urine. Called also *isoandrosterone*.

epi·blast (ep′ĭ-blast) [*epi-* + *-blast*] 1. the upper layer of the bilaminar embryonic disc present during the second week; it gives rise to ectoderm. 2. ectoderm. 3. the ectoderm except for the neural plate.

epi·blas·tic (ep″ĭ-blas′tik) 1. pertaining to or arising from the epiblast. 2. ectodermal.

epi·bleph·a·ron (ep″ĭ-blef′ə-ron) [*epi-* + Gr. *blepharon* eyelid] a developmental anomaly in which a horizontal fold of skin stretches across the border of the eyelid, pressing the eyelashes inward against the eyelid.

epib·o·le (e-pib′o-le) epiboly.

epib·o·ly (e-pib′o-le) [Gr. *epibolē* cover] a process by which an outside cell layer spreads to envelop a yolk mass or deeper layer of cells, such as when the blastoderm spreads over the surface of a telolecithal egg in gastrulation.

epi·bul·bar (ep″ĭ-bul′bər) upon the eyeball.

epi·can·thal (ep″ĭ-kan′thəl) 1. pertaining to the epicanthus. 2. overlying the canthus.

epi·can·thic (ep″ĭ-kan′thik) epicanthal.

epi·can·thine (ep″ĭ-kan′thīn) epicanthal.

epi·can·thus (ep″ĭ-kan′thəs) [*epi-* + *canthus*] a vertical fold of skin on either side of the nose, sometimes covering the inner canthus. It is present as a normal characteristic in persons of certain races and as a congenital anomaly in others. Called also *epicanthal* or *palpebronasal fold*, and *plica palpebronasalis* [TA].

ep·i·car·cin·o·gen (ep″ĭ-kahr-sin′o-jən) epigenetic carcinogen.

epi·car·dia (ep″ĭ-kahr′de-ə) 1. plural of *epicardium*. 2. pars abdominalis oesophagi.

epi·car·di·ec·to·my (ep″ĭ-kahr″de-ek′tə-me) [*epicardium* + *-ectomy*] surgical removal of the epicardium, usually performed in constrictive pericarditis to permit greater diastolic filling of the heart.

epi·car·di·um (ep″ĭ-kahr′de-əm) [*epi-* + Gr. *kardia* heart] TA alternative for *lamina visceralis pericardii serosi*. **epicar′dial** *adj*

epi·cau·ma (ep″ĭ-kaw′mə) [*epi-* + Gr. *kauma* a burn] a superficial burn or ulcer on the eye.

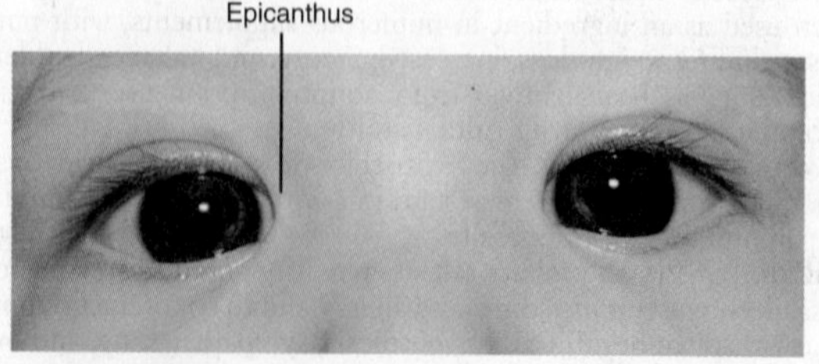

Ep·i·cau·ta (ep″ĭ-kaw′tə) a genus of blister beetles (family Meloidae) that secrete cantharidin and can cause cantharidin poisoning in ruminants. *E. pennsylva′nica* and *E. vitta′ta* are found in the eastern United States, *E. cine′rea* in the southwestern United States, and *E. tormento′sa* and *E. sapphiri′na* in Africa.

epi·cen·tral (ep″ĭ-sen′trəl) attached to the centrum of a vertebra.

epi·chlo·ro·hy·drin (ep″ə-klor″o-hi′drin) a solvent for resins, paints, varnishes, and other organic compounds; it is strongly irritant to the skin and is carcinogenic. Called also *chloropropylene oxide*.

epi·chor·dal (ep″ĭ-kor′dəl) situated dorsad of the notochord.

epi·cho·ri·on (ep″ĭ-kor′e-on) [*epi-* + *chorion*] the part of the uterine mucosa that encloses the implanted conceptus.

epi·coe·lo·ma (ep″ĭ-se-lo′mə) the portion of the coeloma nearest the notochord.

epic·o·mus (e-pik′o-məs) [*epi-* + Gr. *komē* hair] asymmetrical conjoined twins with the parasitic twin joined at the summit of the head of the larger twin.

epi·con·dy·lal·gia (ep″ĭ-kon″də-lal′jə) [*epicondyle* + *-algia*] pain in the muscles or tendons attached to the epicondyle of the humerus; see also *tennis elbow*, under *elbow*.

epi·con·dyle (ep″ĭ-kon′dīl) [*epi-* + *condyle*] epicondylus. **epicon′dylar, epicondylian, epicondylic** *adj*

external e. of femur epicondylus lateralis femoris.

external e. of humerus epicondylus lateralis humeri.

internal e. of femur epicondylus medialis femoris.

internal e. of humerus epicondylus medialis humeri.

lateral e. of femur epicondylus lateralis femoris.

lateral e. of humerus epicondylus lateralis humeri.

medial e. of femur epicondylus medialis femoris.

medial e. of humerus epicondylus medialis humeri.

epi·con·dy·li (ep″ĭ-kon′də-li) [L.] plural of *epicondylus*.

epi·con·dy·li·tis (ep″ĭ-kon″də-li′tis) inflammation of an epicondyle of the humerus or of the tissues adjoining it, usually from an overuse injury.

external humeral e., lateral e. an overuse injury of the lateral humeral epicondyle at the elbow, due to inflammation or irritation of the area where the extensor tendon attaches to it. Called also *radiohumeral e.* or *bursitis*, and popularly, *tennis elbow*.

medial e. an overuse injury with pain around the medial epicondyle of the humerus where the flexor muscles of the arm and hand attach; popularly called *golfer's elbow*.

radiohumeral e. lateral e.

epi·con·dy·lus (ep″ĭ-kon′də-ləs) pl. *epicon′dyli* [L.] [TA] epicondyle: an eminence on a bone above its condyle.

e. latera′lis fe′moris [TA] lateral epicondyle of femur: a projection from the distal end of the femur, above the lateral condyle, for the attachment of collateral ligaments of the knee. Called also *external epicondyle of femur*.

e. latera′lis hu′meri [TA] lateral epicondyle of humerus: a projection from the distal end of the humerus, giving attachment to a common tendon of origin of the extensor carpi radialis brevis, extensor digitorum communis, extensor digiti minimi, extensor carpi ulnaris, and supinator muscles. Called also *external epicondyle of humerus*.

e. media′lis fe′moris [TA] medial epicondyle of femur: a projection from the distal end of the femur, above the medial condyle, for the attachment of collateral ligaments of the knee; called also *internal epicondyle of femur*.

e. media′lis hu′meri [TA] medial epicondyle of humerus: a projection from the distal end of the humerus, giving attachment to the pronator teres above; a common tendon of origin of the flexor carpi radialis, palmaris longus, flexor digitorum superficialis, and flexor carpi ulnaris muscles in the middle, and the ulnar collateral ligament below. Called also *internal epicondyle of humerus*.

epi·cor·a·coid (ep″ĭ-kor′ə-koid) situated above the coracoid process.

epi·cor·nea·scle·ri·tis (ep″ĭ-kor″ne-ə-sklə-ri′tis) a chronic inflammatory condition affecting the cornea and sclera.

epi·cos·tal (ep″ĭ-kos′təl) [*epi-* + *costal*] situated upon a rib.

epi·cot·yl (ep″ĭ-kot′əl) the part of the stem of a plant embryo or seedling above the cotyledons and below the leaves.

epi·cra·ni·um (ep″ĭ-kra′ne-əm) [*epi-* + *cranium*] the integument, aponeurosis, and muscular expansions of the scalp.

epi·cra·ni·us (ep″ĭ-kra′ne-əs) [L.] pertaining to the epicranium; see under *musculus*.

epi·cri·sis (ep′ĭ-kri″sis) [*epi-* + *crisis*] 1. a second or supplementary crisis. 2. a critical analysis or discussion of a case of disease after its termination.

epi•crit•ic (ep″ĭ-krit′ik) [Gr. *epikrisis* determination] relating to or serving the purpose of accurate determination; applied to cutaneous nerve fibers that serve the purpose of perceiving fine variations of touch or temperature. See under *sensibility.*

ep•i•cu•ta•ne•ous (ep″ĭ-ku-ta′ne-əs) [*epi-* + L. *cutis* skin] upon the skin; pertaining to the surface of the skin.

epi•cu•ti•cle (ep″ĭ-ku′tĭ-kəl) [*epi-* + L. *cuticula*] the thin, flexible, colorless, outermost layer of the exoskeleton of certain crustaceans and arthropods, composed of wax and cuticulin.

epi•cys•ti•tis (ep″ĭ-sis-ti′tis) [*epi-* + *cystitis*] inflammation of structures adjacent to the bladder.

epi•cys•tot•o•my (ep″ĭ-sis-tot′ə-me) suprapubic cystotomy.

epi•cyte (ep′ĭ-sīt) [*epi-* + *cyte*] the cell membrane covering gregarine trophozoites.

ep•i•dem•ic (ep″ĭ-dem′ik) [Gr. *epidēmios* prevalent] occurring suddenly in numbers clearly in excess of normal expectancy; said especially of infectious diseases but applied also to any disease, injury, or other health-related event occurring in such outbreaks. Cf. *endemic* and *sporadic.*

ep•i•de•mic•i•ty (ep″ĭ-də-mis′ĭ-te) the state or quality of being epidemic.

ep•i•de•mi•og•ra•phy (ep″ĭ-de″me-og′rə-fe) [*epidemic* + *-graphy*] a treatise upon or an account of epidemics.

ep•i•de•mi•ol•o•gist (ep″ĭ-de″me-ol′ə-jist) a specialist in epidemiology.

ep•i•de•mi•ol•o•gy (ep″ĭ-de″me-ol′ə-je) [*epidemic* + *-logy*] the science concerned with the study of the factors determining and influencing the frequency and distribution of disease, injury, and other health-related events and their causes in a defined human population for the purpose of establishing programs to prevent and control their development and spread. Also, the sum of knowledge gained in such a study.

epi•derm (ep′ĭ-dərm) epidermis.

epi•der•mal (ep″ĭ-dur′məl) 1. pertaining to or resembling epidermis. Called also *epidermic.* 2. epidermoid (def. 1).

epi•der•mal•i•za•tion (ep″ĭ-dur″məl-ĭ-za′shən) squamous metaplasia.

epi•der•ma•ti•tis (ep″ĭ-dur″mə-ti′tis) epidermitis.

epi•der•ma•to•plas•ty (ep″ĭ-dər-mat′o-plas″te) [*epidermis* + *-plasty*] skin grafting done by transplanting pieces of epidermis to denuded areas. **epidermatoplas′tic** *adj*

epi•der•mic (ep″ĭ-dur′mik) epidermal (def. 1).

epi•der•mi•dal•iza•tion (ep″ĭ-dur″mĭ-dəl-ĭ-za′shən) squamous metaplasia.

epi•der•mis (ep″ĭ-dur′mis) pl. *epider′mides* [*epi-* + *dermis*] [TA] the outermost, nonvascular layer of the skin, derived from the embryonic ectoderm, varying in thickness from 0.07 to 0.12 mm, except on the palms and soles where it may be 0.8 to 1.4 mm. On the palms and soles it exhibits maximal cellular differentiation and layering, and comprises, from within outward, five layers: the stratum basale (basal layer); the stratum spinosum (prickle cell or spinous layer); the stratum granulosum (granular layer); the stratum lucidum (clear layer); and the stratum corneum (horny layer). In the thinner epidermis of the general body surface, the stratum basale, stratum spinosum, and stratum corneum are constantly present and the stratum granulosum is usually identifiable, but the stratum lucidum is usually absent.

epi•der•mi•tis (ep″ĭ-dər-mi′tis) a term sometimes used to denote dermatitis restricted to the epidermis; in actuality the inflammation also invariably affects the dermis. Called also *epidermatitis.*

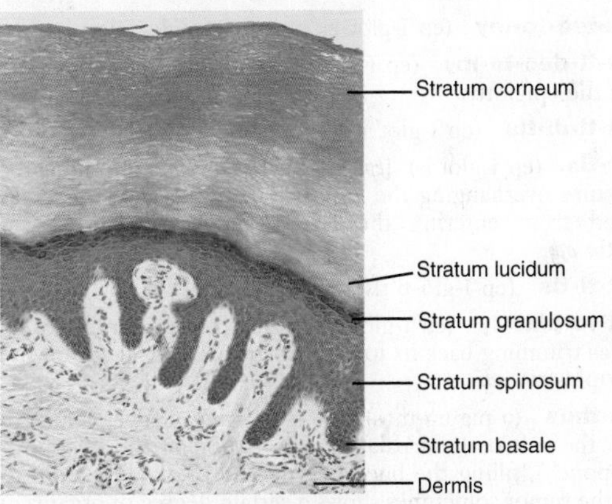

■ Section of epidermis.

exudative e. greasy pig disease.

epi•der•mi•za•tion (ep″ĭ-dur″mĭ-za′shən) the process of covering or of becoming covered with epidermis.

epi•der•mo•dys•pla•sia (ep″ĭ-dur″mo-dis-pla′zhə) faulty development of the epidermis.

e. verrucifor′mis a rare, autosomal recessive condition consisting of widespread and persistent dissemination, sometimes for many years, of verruca plana, caused by infection with human papillomavirus and with a tendency to malignant degeneration. It typically begins as isolated lesions in early childhood, which later increase in number and coalesce to form large plaques. Called also *Lewandowsky-Lutz disease.*

epi•der•moid (ep″ĭ-dur′moid) 1. resembling epidermis. Called also *epidermal.* 2. epidermal (def. 1). 3. epidermoid cyst (def. 2).

epi•der•moi•do•ma (ep″ĭ-dur″moi-do′mə) epidermoid cyst (def. 2).

epi•der•mol•y•sin (ep″ĭ-dər-mol′ə-sin) exfoliatin.

epi•der•mol•y•sis (ep″ĭ-dər-mol′ə-sis) [*epidermis* + *-lysis*] a loosened state of the epidermis, with formation of blebs and bullae, either spontaneously or following trauma. **epidermolyt′ic** *adj*

acquired e. bullosa epidermolysis bullosa that is not hereditary, usually seen in adulthood. It appears to be an autoimmune condition, with autoantibodies on the dermal side of the dermal-epidermal junction against type VII collagen, a major component of fibrils at the junction. The bullae and vesicles are often almost identical to those found in bullous pemphigoid, occurring most often on pressure areas of the hands and feet, although they may be anywhere on the body; they heal leaving atrophic scars and milia. Called also *e. bullosa acquisita* and *dermolytic pemphigoid.*

e. bullo′sa a heterogeneous group of chronic, mostly hereditary, mechanobullous skin diseases. Inherited types are divided into three major groups on the basis of the level at which blistering occurs in the basement membrane: *e. bullosa dystrophica, junctional e. bullosa,* and *e. bullosa simplex;* these are further divided into subtypes based on pattern of inheritance, morphology, and distribution of lesions.

e. bullo′sa acquisi′ta acquired epidermolysis bullosa.

e. bullo′sa dystro′phica epidermolysis bullosa caused by mutations in the *COL7A1* gene (locus: 3p21.3), which encodes type VII collagen, characterized by blistering beneath the lamina densa, with atrophy of previously blistered areas, severe scarring after healing, and dystrophy or absence of the nails. Inheritance may be autosomal dominant or recessive; see *dominant e. bullosa dystrophica* and *recessive e. bullosa dystrophica*. Called also *dystrophic e. bullosa*.

e. bullo′sa junctiona′lis junctional e. bullosa.

e. bullo′sa leta′lis the Herlitz type of junctional e. bullosa.

e. bullo′sa sim′plex any of a heterogeneous group of nonscarring forms of epidermolysis bullosa caused mainly by mutations in either of two genes that encode basal layer keratins: *KRT5* (locus: 12q13), which encodes keratin 5, or *KRT14* (locus: 17q12-q21), which encodes keratin 14; rarely, it may result from other mutations. It is characterized by blistering within the basal layer of the epidermis, or more uncommonly within the epidermis above the basal layer; age of onset is variable; and progressive improvement is common. Inheritance is mainly autosomal dominant, The *localized* or *Weber-Cockayne* type is the mildest form and appears in infancy or sometimes later and is characterized by blistering primarily on the hands and feet. In the *Koebner* type, the lesions are generalized and onset is at birth or in early infancy. The *Dowling-Meara* type is the most severe, with generalized lesions that often occur in clusters and onset at birth or in early infancy.

dominant e. bullosa dystrophica, dominant dystrophic e. bullosa a group of relatively mild autosomal dominant forms of epidermolysis bullosa dystrophica. There are two main variants: The more severe *Pasini* or *albopapuloid variant* is usually present at birth or in infancy, and is characterized by extensive blistering that heals to leave atrophic scarring and albopapuloid lesions, primarily on the skin over the joints and limbs but sometimes elsewhere; and frequent involvement of the mucous membranes, including the oral, esophageal, and pharyngeal mucosa. The less severe *Cockayne-Touraine (dysplastic* or *hyperplastic) variant* usually occurs in infancy or early childhood and is characterized by keratotic lesions that may show ichthyotic changes, generally confined to the extremities, which may heal with hypertrophic rather than atrophic scars. See also *Bart syndrome*, under *syndrome.*

dystrophic e. bullosa e. bullosa dystrophica.

junctional e. bullosa a genetically heterogeneous, autosomal recessive type of epidermolysis bullosa, caused by mutations in genes that encode the subunits of laminin 332. It is characterized by severe generalized blistering in the lamina lucida, affecting the head, trunk, or lower limbs. Extensive denudation may cause secondary infection and death from septicemia. The more severe *Herlitz* type *(e. bullosa letalis, Herlitz disease)* is caused by null mutations that result in a complete lack of laminin 332 in the skin; lesions are present at birth and death often occurs in infancy. The milder *non-Herlitz* type is caused by missense mutations and may also be caused by mutations in the *COL17A1* gene (locus: 10q24.3), which encodes type

XVII collagen; it is often present at birth but sometimes does not manifest until early adulthood. Called also *e. bullosa junctionalis.*

recessive e. bullosa dystrophica, recessive dystrophic e. bullosa the autosomal recessive forms of epidermolysis bullosa dystrophica; these tend to be more severe than the dominant forms. Most are characterized by extensive denuded hemorrhagic erosions and blisters on all body surfaces (including mucous membranes) at birth or in early infancy. Lesions in the esophagus heal to leave esophageal strictures that can impair feeding; other healed lesions can restrict mobility by causing syndactyly and sometimes flexion contractures. Called also *Hallopeau-Siemens syndrome.*

epi·der·mo·my·co·sis (ep″ĭ-dur″mo-mi-ko′sis) 1. dermatophytosis. 2. dermatomycosis.

epi·der·moph·y·tid (ep″ĭ-dər-mof′ə-tid) dermatophytid.

Epi·der·moph·y·ton (ep″ĭ-dər-mof′ĭ-ton) [*epidermis* + Gr. *phyton* plant] a genus of Fungi Imperfecti of the form-class Hyphomycetes, form-family Moniliaceae. *E. flocco′sum* is a species of dermatophytes that attacks skin and nails but not hair; it causes tinea cruris, tinea pedis, and onychomycosis.

epi·der·mo·phy·to·sis (ep″ĭ-dur″mo-fi-to′sis) 1. dermatophytosis. 2. infection by fungi of the genus *Epidermophyton.*

epi·did·y·mec·to·my (ep″ĭ-did″ə-mek′tə-me) [*epididymis* + *-ectomy*] surgical removal of the epididymis.

ep·i·did·y·mis (ep″ĭ-did′ə-mis) pl. *epididy′mides* [Gr., from *epi-* + *didymos* testis] [TA] the elongated cordlike structure along the posterior border of the testis, whose elongated coiled duct provides for storage, transit, and maturation of spermatozoa and is continuous with the ductus deferens. It consists of a head (caput epididymidis), body (corpus epididymidis), and tail (cauda epididymidis). Called also *parorchis.* **epidid′ymal** *adj*

epi·did·y·mi·tis (ep″ĭ-did″ə-mi′tis) inflammation of the epididymis.

spermatogenic e. an inflammatory reaction to spermatozoa that have escaped from the lumen of the epididymal tubules into the tissues of the epididymis.

tuberculous e. inflammation and swelling of the epididymis due to infection with *Mycobacterium tuberculosis,* such as from spread of renal tuberculosis.

epi·did·y·mo·def·er·en·tial (ep″ĭ-did″ə-mo-def″ər-en′shəl) pertaining to the epididymis and ductus deferens.

epi·did·y·mo·or·chi·dec·to·my (ep″ĭ-did″ə-mo-or-kĭ-dek′tə-me) epididymo-orchiectomy.

epi·did·y·mo·or·chi·ec·to·my (ep″ĭ-did″ə-mo-or-ke-ek′tə-me) surgical removal of an epididymis and a testis.

epi·did·y·mo·or·chi·tis (ep″ĭ-did″ə-mo-or-ki′tis) inflammation of the epididymis and testis; called also *orchiepididymitis.*

epi·did·y·mot·o·my (ep″ĭ-did″ə-mot′ə-me) [*epididymis* + *-tomy*] incision of the epididymis.

epi·did·y·mo·vas·os·to·my (ep″ĭ-did″ə-mo-və-sos′tə-me) [*epididymo-* + *vaso-* + *-stomy*] vasoepididymostomy.

epi·du·ral (ep″ĭ-doo′rəl) situated upon or outside the dura mater.

epi·du·rog·ra·phy (ep″ĭ-doo-rog′rə-fe) radiography of the spine after a radiopaque medium has been injected into the epidural space.

epi·du·ros·co·py (ep″ĭ-doo-ros′kə-pe) insertion of an endoscope into the epidural space, usually in the lumbar region, for administration of drugs or visualization.

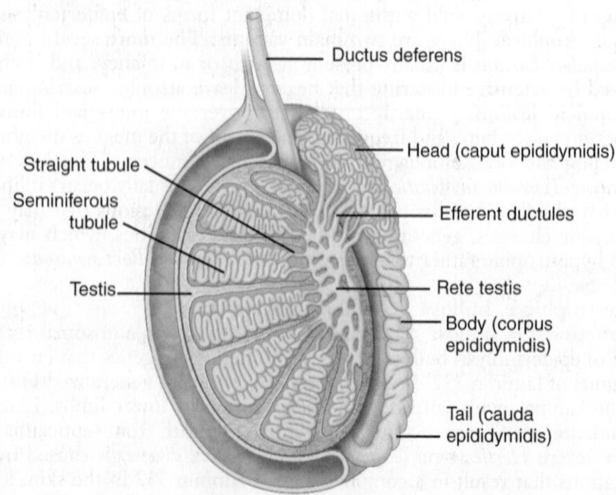

■ Epididymis in a cross section of the testis, showing its division into head, body, and tail.

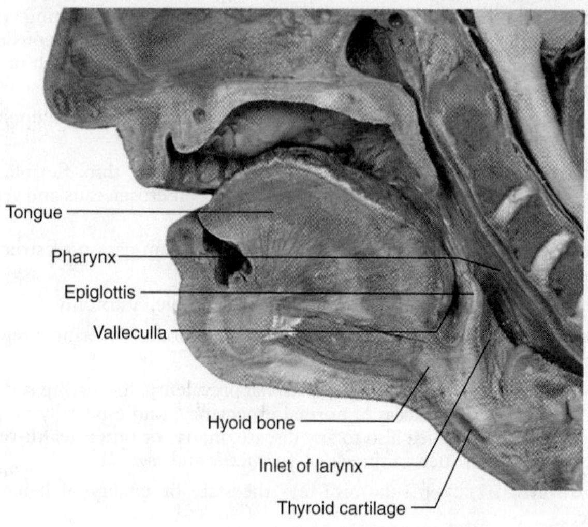

■ Epiglottis in a sagittal section of the head and neck.

epi·es·tri·ol (ep″e-es′tre-ol) any epimer of estriol found in the urine of pregnant women and originating in the fetoplacental unit.

epi·fas·cial (ep″ĭ-fash′əl) upon a fascia.

Epi·foam (ep′ĭ-fōm) trademark for a preparation of hydrocortisone acetate.

Epi·frin (ep′ĭ-frin) trademark for a preparation of epinephrine.

epi·gas·ter (ep″ĭ-gas′tər) [*epi-* + *gaster*] the hindgut: the embryonic structure from which the large intestine is formed.

epi·gas·tral·gia (ep″ĭ-gəs-tral′jə) [*epigastrium* + *-algia*] pain in the epigastrium.

epi·gas·tri·um (ep″ĭ-gas′tre-əm) [Gr. *epigastrion*] [TA] the upper middle region of the abdomen, located within the infrasternal angle; called also *antecardium, regio epigastrica* [TA alternative], *fossa epigastrica* [TA alternative], and *epigastric region* or *zone.* **epigas′tric** *adj*

epi·gas·tri·us (ep″ĭ-gas′tre-əs) [*epi-* + *gaster*] asymmetrical conjoined twins in which the parasitic twin forms a tumor on the epigastrium of the larger twin.

epi·gen·e·sis (ep″ĭ-jen′ə-sis) [*epi-* + *genesis*] the development of an organism from an undifferentiated cell, consisting in the successive formation and development of organs and parts that do not preexist in the zygote.

epi·ge·net·ic (ep″ĭ-jə-net′ik) 1. pertaining to epigenesis. 2. altering the activity of genes without changing their DNA sequence, or affecting the phenotype without changing the genotype.

epi·ge·net·ics (ep″ĭ-jə-net′iks) the study of heritable changes in the function of genes that occur without changes in the DNA sequence, occurring during development and cell proliferation and including mechanisms such as DNA methylation, histone modification, and RNA interference.

epi·ge·nome (ep″ĭ-je′nōm) the set of heritable modifications that interact with a genome to affect gene expression in a given differentiated cell without altering the nucleotide sequence.

epi·ge·no·type (ep″ĭ-je′no-tīp) the pattern of gene expression in a differentiated cell, being a function of the combination of the genotype and epigenetic mechanisms such as DNA methylation.

epi·glot·tec·to·my (ep″ĭ-glot-ek′tə-me) epiglottidectomy.

epi·glot·ti·dec·to·my (ep″ĭ-glot″ĭ-dek′tə-me) [*epiglottis* + *-ectomy*] excision of the epiglottis.

epi·glot·ti·di·tis (ep″ĭ-glot″ĭ-di′tis) supraglottitis.

epi·glot·tis (ep″ĭ-glot′is) [*epi-* + *glottis*] [TA] the lidlike cartilaginous structure overhanging the entrance to the larynx and serving to prevent food from entering the larynx and trachea while swallowing. **epiglot′tic** *adj*

epi·glot·ti·tis (ep″ĭ-glŏ-ti′tis) supraglottitis.

epi·glot·to·plas·ty (ep″ĭ-glot′o-plas″te) plastic surgery of the epiglottis, such as trimming back its folds to correct laryngeal stridor in infants. **epiglottoplas′tic** *adj*

epig·na·thus (ə-pig′nə-thəs) [*epi-* + Gr. *gnathos* jaw] a fetal tumor arising from the soft or hard palate in the region of the hypophysial pouch (Rathke pouch), filling the buccal cavity and protruding from the mouth. Because the tumor sometimes shows a certain degree of organization, it has been considered a parasitic fetus.

epig·o·nal (ə-pig'o-nəl) [*epi-* + *gon-* + *-al*[1]] situated on an embryonic gonad.

epi·hy·drin·al·de·hyde (ep″ĭ-hi″drin-al'də-hīd) a chemical compound, one of the substances that give rancid fats their disagreeable odor.

epi·hy·oid (ep″ĭ-hi'oid) situated upon the hyoid bone.

epi·ker·a·to·pha·kia (ep″ĭ-ker″ə-to-fa'ke-ə) [*epi-* + *kerato-* + *phak-* + *-ia*] a corneal operation in which a piece of donor cornea is implanted on the patient's own cornea to change its curvature in order to correct refractive error.

epi·ker·a·to·plas·ty (ep″ĭ-ker'ə-to-plas″te) epikeratophakia. **epikeratoplas'tic** *adj*

epi·la·mel·lar (ep″ĭ-lə-mel'ər) situated upon the basement membrane.

ep·i·late (ep'ĭ-lāt) depilate.

ep·i·la·tion (ep″ĭ-la'shən) depilation.

epil·a·to·ry (ə-pil'ə-tor″e) depilatory.

ep·i·lem·ma (ep″ĭ-lem'ə) [*epi-* + *-lemma*] the endoneurium. **epilem'mal** *adj*

ep·i·lep·sia (ep″ĭ-lep'se-ə) [L., from Gr. *epilēpsia*] epilepsy.

e. partia'lis conti'nua a form of status epilepticus with focal motor seizures, marked by continuous clonic movements of a limited part of the body. Called also *simple partial status*.

ep·i·lep·sy (ep'ĭ-lep″se) [Gr. *epilēpsia* seizure] any of a group of syndromes characterized by paroxysmal transient disturbances of the brain function that may be manifested as episodic impairment or loss of consciousness, abnormal motor phenomena, psychic or sensory disturbances, or perturbation of the autonomic nervous system. A single episode is called a *seizure* (q.v.). Many types of epilepsy are combinations of different kinds of seizures. Epilepsy is classified as either *symptomatic* or *idiopathic* according to whether the cause is known or unknown. Both of these types may be further subdivided into *partial* and *generalized* types depending on whether the seizures begin with localized, limited brain dysfunction or with widespread brain dysfunction.

abdominal e. paroxysmal abdominal pain, the expression of an abnormal neuronal discharge from the brain; called also *Moore syndrome*.

absence e. epilepsy characterized by absence seizures, usually having its onset in childhood or adolescence; called also *petit mal*, *petit mal e.*, *absence*, and *minor e.*

acquired e. symptomatic e.

activated e. epileptic seizures induced by electrical or drug stimulation for the purpose of observing the pattern of clinical and electroencephalographic response.

audiogenic e. reflex epilepsy caused by auditory stimuli.

Baltic myoclonic e. Unverricht-Lundborg disease.

benign e. with centrotemporal spikes, benign rolandic e., benign e. with rolandic spikes a self-limited childhood disorder consisting of partial seizures manifested by facial movements and grimaces, often followed by tonic-clonic seizures. The electroencephalogram from the primary somatomotor area (rolandic area) shows characteristic repetitive high-voltage spikes. Both autosomal dominant and complex patterns of inheritance have been observed. Called also *rolandic e.*

Bravais-jacksonian e. jacksonian e.

centralopathic e. benign rolandic e.

chronic focal e. epilepsia partialis continua.

cortical e. seizure phenomena originating in the cerebral cortex.

cryptogenic e. idiopathic e.

diurnal e. epileptic attacks occurring in the daytime or when the patient is awake.

essential e. idiopathic e.

focal e. epilepsy consisting of focal seizures.

gelastic e. temporal lobe epilepsy in which the automatisms consist of fits of uncontrollable mirthless laughter.

generalized e. epilepsy in which the seizures are generalized; they may have a focal onset or be generalized from the beginning.

generalized flexion e. hypsarrhythmia.

gestational e. epilepsy that first occurs during pregnancy; the cause is unknown. Cf. *eclampsia*.

grand mal e., haut mal e. a symptomatic form of epilepsy often preceded by an aura; characterized by loss of consciousness with generalized tonic-clonic seizures (q.v.). Called also *grand mal*, *major e.*, and *haut mal e.*

idiopathic e. epilepsy of unknown origin, possibly associated with some inherited predisposition for seizures; called also *cryptogenic e.* or *essential e.*

idiopathic generalized e's a group of epilepsies characterized by generalized seizures but no irregularities on the electroencephalogram; these are genetically determined and are not idiopathic in the usual sense of the word. Included are several types of absence epilepsy as well as juvenile myoclonic epilepsy.

jacksonian e. epilepsy characterized by focal motor seizures with unilateral clonic movements that start in one group of muscles and spread systematically to adjacent groups, reflecting the march of the epileptic activity through the motor cortex. The seizures are due to a discharging focus in the contralateral motor cortex; called also *Bravais-jacksonian e.*

juvenile myoclonic e. a syndrome of sudden myoclonic jerks, occurring particularly in the morning or under conditions of stress or fatigue; seen primarily in children and adolescents. Occasionally the jerks may progress to generalized tonic-clonic seizures, but there is no mental deterioration. Called also *Janz syndrome*.

Koshevnikoff (Koschewnikow, Kozhevnikov) e. epilepsia partialis continua.

Lafora myoclonic e. Lafora disease.

larval e. unerupted epileptic seizures, represented only by characteristic waves in the electroencephalogram; called also *latent e.*

late e. epilepsy beginning in middle age or later.

latent e. larval e.

localized e. focal e.

major e. grand mal e.

menstrual e. epileptic seizures associated with menstruation.

minor e. absence e.

minor focal e. simple partial seizures; see under *seizure*.

musicogenic e. reflex epilepsy occurring in response to a musical stimulus.

myoclonic e., myoclonus e. any of a group of disorders, of varying etiologies, in which seizures (epilepsy) are accompanied by muscle contractions (myoclonus); the group includes a benign idiopathic form, juvenile myoclonic epilepsy, as well as various progressive inherited disorders, including Unverricht-Lundborg disease, MERRF syndrome, and Lafora disease.

nocturnal e. epileptic attacks occurring at night or while the patient is asleep.

organic e. symptomatic e.

partial e. focal e.

petit mal e. absence e.

photic e., photogenic e. reflex epilepsy in which seizures are induced by a flickering light.

physiologic e. biologic or electrobiologic seizures based on physiologic and not on organic or structural abnormalities of the brain.

posttraumatic e. epileptic seizures that occur after head injury; called also *traumatic e.*

procursive e. temporal lobe epilepsy in which the automatisms consist of aimless running.

progressive myoclonic e. (EPM) any of the group of disorders causing progressive forms of myoclonic epilepsy (q.v.); Unverricht-Lundborg disease is progressive myoclonic epilepsy type 1 (EMP1), and Lafora disease is progressive myoclonic epilepsy type 2 (EMP2).

psychic e., psychomotor e. temporal lobe e.

reading e. reflex epilepsy that is triggered when the patient tries to read.

reflex e. epileptic seizures occurring in response to sensory (tactile, visual, auditory, or musical) stimuli; called also *sensory e.* See also *audiogenic e.*, *musicogenic e.*, *photogenic e.*, and *reading e.*

rolandic e. benign rolandic e.

rotatory e. temporal lobe epilepsy in which the automatisms consist of rotating body movements.

sensory e. 1. seizures manifested by paresthesias or hallucinations of sight, smell, or taste; see also *somatosensory e.*, *uncinate e.*, and *visual e.* 2. reflex e.

somatosensory e. sensory epilepsy with paresthesias such as tingling, numbness, or burning.

symptomatic e. acquired epileptic seizures caused by disease of the central nervous system itself; a generalized systemic disorder, such as hypoglycemia or uremia; or poisoning, as with lead or pentylenetetrazol; called also *organic e.*

tardy e. late e.

temporal lobe e. a form of epilepsy characterized by complex partial seizures; called also *psychomotor e.*

traumatic e. post-traumatic e.

uncinate e. temporal lobe epilepsy caused by a lesion in the uncinate region and therefore associated with hallucinations of smell and taste.

vertiginous e. focal seizures giving rise to a sensation of vertigo; occasionally these are auras of more general seizures. See also *vertiginous aura*.

visual e. sensory epilepsy in which there are visual hallucinations such as flashes of light or colors.

ep·i·lep·tic (ep″ĭ-lep'tik) [Gr. *epilēptikos*] 1. pertaining to or affected with epilepsy. 2. a person affected with epilepsy.

ep·i·lep·ti·form (ep″ĭ-lep'tĭ-form) [*epileptic* + *form*] 1. resembling epilepsy or its manifestations. 2. occurring in severe or sudden paroxysms. Called also *epileptoid*.

epi·lep·to·gen·e·sis (ep″ĭ-lep″to-jen′ə-sis) the production or development of epilepsy.

ep·i·lep·to·gen·ic (ep″ĭ-lep-to-jen′ik) [*epilepsy* + *-genic*] producing epileptic attacks.

ep·i·lep·tog·e·nous (ep″ĭ-lep-toj′ə-nəs) epileptogenic.

ep·i·lep·toid (ep″ĭ-lep′toid) epileptiform.

ep·i·lep·tol·o·gist (ep″ĭ-lep-tol′ə-jist) a specialist in epileptology.

ep·i·lep·tol·o·gy (ep″ĭ-lep-tol′ə-je) the study, diagnosis, and treatment of epilepsy.

ep·i·loia (ep″ĭ-loi′ə) tuberous sclerosis complex.

ep·i·lu·mi·nes·cence (ep″e-loo″mĭ-nes′əns) illumination of the surface of the skin through an oil immersion; see *epiluminescence microscopy*, under *microscopy*.

epi·man·dib·u·lar (ep″ĭ-man-dib′u-lər) [*epi-* + *mandibular*] situated upon the lower jaw.

epi·mas·ti·gote (ep″ĭ-mas′tĭ-gōt) [*epi-* + Gr. *mastix* whip] a morphologic stage in the life cycle of certain trypanosomatid protozoa; the kinetoplast and basal body are located anterior to the central vesicular nucleus of the slender elongate cell, and the flagellum passes anteriorly attached to the body by an undulating membrane, at the anterior end becoming free-flowing. Cf. *amastigote*, *choanomastigote*, *opisthomastigote*, *promastigote*, and *trypomastigote*.

ep·i·mer (ep′ĭ-mər) either of two diastereomers that differ in the configuration around one asymmetric carbon atom.

epim·er·ase (ə-pim′ə-rās) a term used in the names of some enzymes of the subclass racemases and epimerases [EC 5.1] to denote those that catalyze inversion of the configuration about an asymmetric carbon atom in a substrate having more than one center of asymmetry; thus epimers are interconverted.

ep·i·mere (ep′ĭ-mēr) [*epi-* + *-mere*] the dorsal portion of a somite, from which is formed muscles innervated by the dorsal ramus of a spinal nerve.

epim·er·iza·tion (ə-pim″ər-ĭ-za′shən) the changing of one epimeric form of a compound into another, as by enzymatic action.

epi·mes·trol (ep″ĭ-mes′trol) the 3-methyl ether of 17-epiestriol, an anterior pituitary activator used to stimulate ovulation.

epi·mor·pho·sis (ep″ĭ-mor-fo′sis) [*epi-* + *morphosis*] the regeneration of a part of an organism by proliferation at the cut surface. **epimor′phic** *adj*

Ep·i·mys (ep′ĭ-mis) [*epi-* + Gr. *mys* mouse] *Rattus*.

epi·mys·i·ot·omy (ep″ĭ-mis″e-ot′ə-me) [*epimysium* + *-tomy*] incision of the epimysium.

epi·mys·i·um (ep″ĭ-mis′e-əm) [*epi-* + Gr. *mys* muscle] [TA] the fibrous sheath about an entire muscle; called also *perimysium externum* or *external perimysium*.

Ep·i·nal (ep′ĭ-nəl) trademark for a preparation of epinephryl borate.

epi·neph·rine (ep″ĭ-nef′rin) 1. a catecholamine hormone secreted by the adrenal medulla and a neurotransmitter, released by certain neurons and active in the central nervous system. It is stored in the chromaffin granules and is released in response to hypoglycemia, stress, and other stimuli. It is a potent stimulator of the adrenergic receptors of the sympathetic nervous system and a powerful cardiac stimulant that accelerates the heart rate and increases cardiac output. It also promotes glycogenolysis and exerts other metabolic effects. 2. [USP] a synthetic preparation of the levorotatory form of epinephrine, used topically as a vasoconstricting adjunct to local or regional anesthesia, intravenously as a cardiac stimulant and vasopressor; subcutaneously, intramuscularly, or intravenously as a systemic antiallergic in the treatment of severe allergic reactions; subcutaneously, intramuscularly, intranasally, or by inhalation as a bronchodilator; and topically to the conjunctiva in the treatment of open-angle glaucoma. Called also *adrenaline* (Great Britain).

e. bitartrate [USP] the bitartrate salt of epinephrine, having the same actions as the base; applied topically to the conjunctiva to reduce intraocular pressure in the management of open-angle glaucoma and administered by inhalation as a bronchodilator.

epi·neph·rin·emia (ep″ĭ-nef″rĭ-ne′me-ə) the presence of epinephrine in the blood.

epi·neph·ryl bo·rate (ep″ĭ-nef′rəl) a compound containing epinephrine as a borate complex; applied topically to the conjunctiva in the treatment of open-angle glaucoma.

epi·neu·ral (ep″ĭ-noo′rəl) situated upon a neural arch.

epi·neu·ri·um (ep″ĭ-noor′e-um) [epi- + Gr. *neuron* nerve] [TA] the outermost layer of connective tissue of a peripheral nerve, surrounding the entire nerve and containing its supplying blood vessels and lymphatics. See also *perineurium* and *endoneurium*. **epineu′rial** *adj*

epi·ot·ic (ep″e-ot′ik) [*epi-* + *otic*] situated on or above the ear.

Epi·Pen (ep′e-pen) trademark for preparations of epinephrine.

epi·pha·ryn·ge·al (ep″ĭ-fə-rin′je-əl) nasopharyngeal.

epi·phar·yn·gi·tis (ep″ĭ-far″in-ji′tis) nasopharyngitis.

epi·phar·ynx (ep″ĭ-far′inks) pars nasalis pharyngis.

epi·phe·nom·e·non (ep″ĭ-fə-nom′ə-non) [*epi-* + *phenomenon*] an accessory, exceptional, or accidental occurrence in the course of an attack of any disease.

epiph·o·ra (ə-pif′ə-rə) [Gr. *epiphora* sudden burst] an abnormal overflow of tears down the cheek, mainly due to stricture of the lacrimal passages; called also *illacrimation*.

epi·phren·ic (ep″ĭ-fren′ik) next to the diaphragm.

epi·phys·e·od·e·sis (ep″ĭ-fiz″e-od′ə-sis) epiphysiodesis.

epiph·y·ses (ə-pif′ə-sēz) [Gr.] plural of *epiphysis*.

epi·phys·i·al (ep″ĭ-fiz′e-əl) epiphyseal.

epi·phys·i·od·e·sis (ep″ĭ-fiz″e-od′ə-sis) [*epiphysis* + *-desis*] the operation of premature fusion of an epiphysis to arrest growth.

epi·phys·i·oid (ep″ĭ-fiz′e-oid) resembling epiphyses; a term applied to carpal and tarsal bones which develop like epiphyses from centers of ossification.

epi·phys·i·ol·y·sis (ep″ĭ-fiz″e-ol′ə-sis) [*epiphysis* + *-lysis*] separation of an epiphysis from its bone; especially slipping of the upper femoral epiphysis.

epi·phys·i·om·e·ter (ep″ĭ-fiz″e-om′ə-tər) an instrument for measuring the epiphyses, used in the diagnosis of rickets.

epi·phys·i·op·a·thy (ep″ĭ-fiz″e-op′ə-the) [*epiphysis* + *-pathy*] 1. any disease of the pineal body. 2. any disease of an epiphysis of a bone.

epiph·y·sis (ə-pif′ə-sis) pl. *epi′physes* [Gr. "an ongrowth; excrescence"] [TA] the expanded articular end of a long bone, developed from a secondary ossification center, which during the period of growth is either entirely cartilaginous or is separated from the shaft by the epiphyseal cartilage. **epiphys′eal** *adj*

annular e., e. anula′ris [TA] a raised ring of compact bone at the periphery of the superior and inferior surfaces of the vertebral body, giving attachment to the anulus fibrosus and the longitudinal ligaments; generally considered to be a secondary ossification center. Called also *ring e.* and *annular* or *ring apophysis*.

capital e. the epiphysis at the head of a long bone.

e. ce′rebri glandula pinealis.

ring e. e. anularis.

slipped e. dislocation of the epiphysis of a bone, as of the epiphysis of the head of the femur.

stippled e's chondrodysplasia punctata.

epiph·y·si·tis (ə-pif″ə-si′tis) inflammation of an epiphysis or of the cartilage that separates it from the main bone.

e. juveni′lis Köhler bone disease (def.1).

vertebral e. osteochondrosis (q.v.) of the vertebra.

ep·i·phyte (ep′ĭ-fīt) [*epi-* + *-phyte*] 1. a plant organism growing upon another plant. 2. a plant ectoparasite.

ep·i·phyt·ic (ep″ĭ-fit′ik) 1. pertaining to epiphytes. 2. caused by epiphytes.

epi·pia (ep″ĭ-pi′ə) [*epi-* + *pia*] the part of the pia mater adjacent to the arachnoid mater, as distinguished from the pia-glia.

epi·pi·al (ep″ĭ-pi′əl) 1. situated on the pia mater. 2. pertaining to the epipia.

epi·pleu·ral (ep″ĭ-ploor′əl) situated on a pleural element, or pleurapophysis.

epipl(o)- [Gr. *epiploon* omentum] a combining form denoting relationship to the omentum.

epip·lo·cele (ə-pip′lo-sēl) omental hernia.

epip·lo·ec·to·my (ə-pip″lo-ek′tə-me) omentectomy.

epip·lo·itis (ə-pip″lo-i′tis) omentitis.

epip·lo·on (ə-pip′lo-on) [Gr.] omentum. **epiplo′ic** *adj*

greater e. omentum majus.

lesser e. omentum minus.

epip·lo·pexy (ə-pip′lo-pek″se) [*epiplo-* + *-pexy*] omentopexy.

epip·lo·plas·ty (ə-pip′lo-plas″te) [*epiplo-* + *-plasty*] omentoplasty. **epiploplas′tic** *adj*

epi·podo·phyl·lo·tox·in (ep″ĭ-pod″o-fil′o-tok″sin) [*epi-* + *podophyllotoxin*] a chemical derivative of podophyllotoxin from which the antineoplastic drugs etoposide and teniposide are derived.

epi·py·gus (ep″ĭ-pi′gəs) pygomelus.

epi·pyr·a·mis (ep″ĭ-pir′ə-mis) a small supernumerary carpal bone sometimes found between the triquetrum, lunate, hamate, and capitate bones; called also *epitriquetrum.*

epi·ret·i·nal (ep″ĭ-ret′ĭ-nəl) overlying the retina.

epi·ru·bi·cin (ep″ĭ-roo′bĭ-sin) an anthracycline antibiotic that is a stereoisomer of doxorubicin, having the same antineoplastic actions as but lower toxicity than doxorubicin; used in the treatment of carcinoma of the breast, ovary, stomach, colon, and rectum, leukemia, lymphoma, and multiple myeloma, administered intravenously. Available as *epirubicin hydrochloride.*

epi·scle·ra (ep″ĭ-skler′ə) the loose connective tissue forming the external surface of the sclera.

epi·scle·ral (ep″ĭ-skler′əl) 1. overlying the sclera. 2. of or pertaining to the episclera.

epi·scle·ri·tis (ep″ĭ-sklə-ri′tis) inflammation of the episclera and adjacent tissues; it may be confined to a sector or diffuse, and is usually idiopathic and self-limited. Visual acuity is usually normal. Cf. *scleritis.*

nodular e. episcleritis characterized by a tender, localized, injected nodule within the inflamed area; it can be moved over the sclera. Cf. *nodular scleritis.*

epi·scle·ro·ti·tis (ep″i-skler″o-ti′tis) episcleritis.

episi(o)- [Gr. *epision* pubic region] a combining form denoting relationship to the vulva.

epis·io·per·i·neo·plas·ty (ə-piz″e-o-per″ĭ-ne′o-plas″te) [*episio-* + *perineoplasty*] plastic repair of the vulva and perineum.

epis·io·per·i·ne·or·rha·phy (ə-piz″e-o-per″ĭ-ne-or′ə-fe) [*episio-* + *perineum* + *-rrhapy*] the suturing of the vulva and perineum.

epis·io·plas·ty (ə-piz′e-o-plas″te) [*episio-* + *-plasty*] plastic repair of the vulva. **episioplas′tic** *adj*

epis·i·or·rha·phy (ə-piz″e-or′ə-fe) [*episio-* + *-rrhaphy*] the suturing of the labia majora for repair of the vulva and perineum.

epis·io·ste·no·sis (ə-piz″e-o-stə-no′sis) [*episio-* + *stenosis*] the narrowing of the vulvar orifice.

epis·i·ot·o·my (ə-piz″e-ot′o-me) [*episio-* + *-tomy*] surgical incision into the perineum and vagina to prevent traumatic tearing during delivery.

ep·i·sode (ep′ĭ-sōd) a noteworthy happening or series of happenings occurring in the course of continuous events, as an episode of illness; a separate but not unrelated incident.

acute schizophrenic e. acute schizophrenia.

hypomanic e. [DSM-IV] a period during which there is elevated, expansive, or irritable mood, with symptoms resembling those of a manic episode but less severe and not including any psychotic features.

major depressive e. [DSM-IV] a period of two weeks or longer characterized by daily and day-long depressed mood or loss of interest or pleasure in virtually all activities; in children or adolescents the mood may be irritable. Also present is some combination of the following symptoms: altered appetite, weight, or sleep patterns, psychomotor agitation or retardation, diminished capacity for thinking, concentration, or decisiveness, lack of energy and fatigue, feelings of worthlessness, self-reproach, or inappropriate guilt, recurrent thoughts of death or suicide, and plans or attempts to commit suicide.

manic e. [DSM-IV] a period of predominantly elevated, expansive, or irritable mood accompanied by some of the following symptoms: inflated self-esteem or grandiosity, decreased need for sleep, talkativeness, flight of ideas, distractibility, hyperactivity or psychomotor agitation, hypersexuality, and reckless behavior.

mixed e. [DSM-IV] a period during which the criteria are met both for a major depressive episode and for a manic episode nearly every day, with rapidly alternating moods and with symptoms characteristic of each type of episode.

ep·i·some (ep′ĭ-sōm) in bacterial genetics, any accessory extrachromosomal replicating genetic element that can exist either autonomously or integrated with the chromosome, e.g., the F factor, colicinogens, and (drug) resistance transfer factor. See also *plasmid.*

epi·spa·dia (ep″ĭ-spa′de-ə) epispadias.

epi·spa·di·ac (ep″ĭ-spa′de-ak) 1. pertaining to or exhibiting epispadias; called also *epispadial.* 2. an individual with epispadias.

epi·spa·di·al (ep″ĭ-spa′de-əl) epispadiac (def. 1).

epi·spa·di·as (ep″ĭ-spa′de-əs) [*epi-* + Gr. *spadōn* a rent] a developmental anomaly consisting of absence of the upper wall of the urethra, with various degrees of severity; it occurs in both sexes but is more common in males, with the urethral opening somewhere on the dorsum of the penis, manifested as a groove or cleft without a covering.

balanic e., balanitic e. incomplete epispadias in a male with the urethral opening above and behind the glans; the dorsum of the penis is usually indented to its tip, but the opening may end at the corona or proximal to it. Called also *glandular e.*

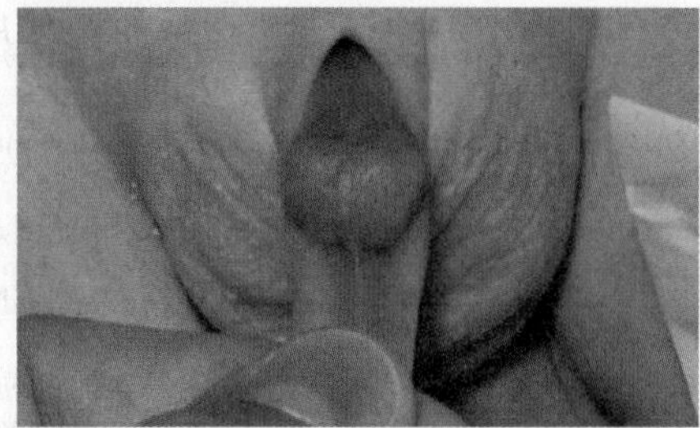

■ Penopubic epispadias.

clitoral e. incomplete epispadias in a female with the urethra opening superior to the clitoris or into it.

complete e. epispadias in which the urethra is entirely open to the bladder neck in males, and there may be complete failure of fusion of the anterior urethral wall in females; it is frequently associated with exstrophy of bladder.

glandular e. balanic e.

incomplete e. epispadias in which the bladder does not entirely open to the outside; designated according to the location of urethral opening in the male as either *balanic* or *penile,* and in the female as either *clitoral* or *subsymphyseal.*

penile e. incomplete epispadias in a male with the urethral orifice somewhere between the postglandular sulcus and the suspensory ligament, usually at the base of the penis.

penopubic e. complete epispadias in a male with the urethral opening at the junction of the penis and pubis; unless associated with bladder exstrophy, the urethral passage emerges between the corpora cavernosa under the pubic symphysis.

subsymphyseal e. incomplete epispadias in a female with the urethral opening beneath the symphysis pubis.

epi·spi·nal (ep″ĭ-spi′nəl) situated upon the spinal cord or the vertebral (spinal) column.

epi·sple·ni·tis (ep″ĭ-splə-ni′tis) [*epi-* + *splen-* + *-itis*] inflammation of the capsule of the spleen.

epis·ta·sis (ə-pis′tə-sis) [*epi-* + *stasis*] 1. suppression of a secretion or excretion, as of blood, menses, or lochia. 2. a scum on the surface of urine. 3. the interaction between genes at different loci that results in one gene masking the expression of the other. Cf. *dominance.*

epis·ta·sy (ə-pis′tə-se) epistasis.

epi·stat·ic (ep″ĭ-stat′ik) 1. pertaining to or characterized by epistasis. 2. superimposed.

ep·i·stax·is (ep″ĭ-stak′sis) [Gr.] hemorrhage from the nose; called also *nosebleed* and *nasal hemorrhage.*

anterior e. bleeding from the anterior part of the nasal cavity, more common in children than in older patients.

Gull renal e. essential hematuria.

posterior e. bleeding from the posterior part of the nasal cavity, more common in older patients than in children; mild cases may go undetected because the blood does not exit through the nares.

epis·te·mol·o·gy (ep″ĭ-stə-mol′ə-je) [Gr. *epistēmē* knowledge + *-logy*] the science of the methods and validity of knowledge.

epi·ster·nal (ep″ĭ-stur′nəl) 1. situated on or over the sternum. 2. pertaining to the episternum.

epi·ster·num (ep″ĭ-stur′nəm) [*epi-* + *sternum*] a bone present in reptiles and monotremes that may be represented as part of the manubrium, or first piece of the sternum.

epis·thot·o·nos (e″pis-thot′ə-nos) emprosthotonos.

epi·stro·phe·us (ep″ĭ-stro′fe-əs) [Gr. "the pivot"] axis (def. 3).

epi·tar·sus (ep″ĭ-tahr′səs) [*epi-* + *tarsus*] a congenital anomaly of the eye consisting of a fold of conjunctiva passing from the fornix to near the lid border; called also *congenital pterygium.*

epi·taxy (ep″ĭ-tak′se) the oriented growth and binding of a crystalline substance on a substrate of crystals of another compound, such as in formation of some renal calculi.

epi·te·la (ep″ĭ-te′lə) [*epi-* + *tela*] the delicate tissue of the rostral medullary velum.

epi·ten·din·e·um (ep″ĭ-tən-din′e-əm) 1. vagina tendinis. 2. epitenon.

epi·te·non (ep″ĭ-te′non) [*epi-* + Gr. *tenōn* tendon] the connective tissue covering a tendon inside the tendon sheath.

epi·tes·tos·te·rone (ep-e-tes-tos′tə-rōn) an epimer of testosterone, occurring in a ratio with testosterone that is specific for any given individual.

epi·tha·lam·ic (ep″ĭ-thə-lam′ik) 1. overlying the thalamus. 2. pertaining to the epithalamus.

epi·thal·a·mus (ep″ĭ-thal′ə-məs) [TA] the caudal part of the roof and the adjoining lateral walls of the third ventricle of the diencephalon, comprising the habenular nuclei and their commissure, pineal body, and commissure of the epithalamus.

epi·tha·lax·ia (ep″ĭ-thə-lak′se-ə) [*epithelium* + Gr. *allaxis* exchange] desquamation of the epithelium, especially of the intestinal mucosa.

ep·i·the·lia (ep″ĭ-the′le-ə) plural of *epithelium.*

ep·i·the·li·al·iza·tion (ep″ĭ-the″le-əl-ĭ-za′shən) healing by the growth of epithelium over a denuded surface.

ep·i·the·li·a·lize (ep″ĭ-the′le-əl-īz″) to cover with epithelium.

ep·i·the·li·itis (ep″ĭ-the″le-i′tis) inflammation of epithelium.

epitheli(o)- [L. *epithelium,* q.v.] a combining form denoting relationship to the epithelium.

ep·i·the·lio·chor·i·al (ep″ĭ-the″le-o-kor′e-əl) [*epithelio-* + *chorial*] denoting a type of placenta in which the chorion is apposed to the uterine epithelium but does not erode it.

ep·i·the·lio·fi·bril (ep″ĭ-the′le-o-fi″bril) one of the fibrils which run through the cytoplasm of epithelial cells.

epi·the·lio·gen·e·sis (ep″ĭ-the″le-o-jen′ə-sis) the forming of new epithelium.

e. imperfec′ta a condition in domestic animals similar to human aplasia cutis congenita; animals are born with patches of skin missing and the area covered by a thin membranelike covering.

e. imperfec′ta lin′guae bo′vis smooth tongue.

ep·i·the·lio·ge·net·ic (ep″ĭ-the″le-o-jə-net′ik) [*epithelio-* + *genetic*] due to epithelial proliferation.

ep·i·the·li·o·gen·ic (ep″ĭ-the″le-o-jen′ik) tending to produce epithelium.

ep·i·the·lio·glan·du·lar (ep″ĭ-the″le-o-glan′du-lər) pertaining to the epithelial cells of a gland.

ep·i·the·li·oid (ep″ĭ-the′le-oid) resembling epithelium.

ep·i·the·li·ol·y·sin (ep″ĭ-the″le-ol′ə-sin) a cytolysin formed in the serum of an animal when epithelial cells from an animal of a different species are injected. The epitheliolysin has the power of destroying epithelial cells of an animal of the same species as that from which the epithelial cells were originally taken.

ep·i·the·li·ol·y·sis (ep″ĭ-the″le-ol′ə-sis) [*epithelio-* + *-lysis*] destruction of epithelial cells.

ep·i·the·lio·lyt·ic (ep″ĭ-the″le-o-lit′ik) 1. pertaining to or characterized by epitheliolysis. 2. causing epitheliolysis.

ep·i·the·li·o·ma (ep″ĭ-the″le-o′mə) [*epithelio-* + *-oma*] 1. a neoplasm of epithelial origin; these range from benign (adenomas and papillomas) to malignant (carcinomas). 2. sometimes used loosely and incorrectly as a synonym for *carcinoma.*

e. adenoi′des cys′ticum multiple trichoepithelioma.

basal cell e. see under *carcinoma.*

benign calcified e., benign calcifying e. pilomatricoma.

Brooke e. multiple trichoepithelioma.

calcified e., calcifying e., calcifying e. of Malherbe pilomatricoma.

chorionic e. choriocarcinoma.

Ferguson Smith e. self-healing squamous e.

Malherbe calcifying e. pilomatricoma.

malignant e. carcinoma.

multiple self-healing squamous e. self-healing squamous e.

sebaceous e. see under *hyperplasia.*

self-healing squamous e. an autosomal dominant form of multiple keratoacanthoma, characterized by a succession of lesions resembling those of squamous cell carcinoma; they heal spontaneously with scarring and are most common on the face and limbs of male adolescents and young adults. Called also *Ferguson Smith e.*

ep·i·the·li·o·ma·to·sis (ep″ĭ-the″le-o-mə-to′sis) the state of being subject to or afflicted with epitheliomas.

ep·i·the·li·o·ma·tous (ep″ĭ-the″le-o′mə-təs) pertaining to or of the nature of epithelioma.

ep·i·the·lio·mus·cu·lar (ep″ĭ-the″le-o-mus′ku-lər) composed of epithelium and muscle.

ep·i·the·lio·tox·in (ep″ĭ-the′le-o-tok″sin) a cytotoxin which destroys epithelial cells.

ep·i·the·lite (ep″ĭ-the′līt) a lesion produced as a reaction to irradiation, in which the epithelium is replaced by a fibrous exudate.

ep·i·the·li·um (ep″ĭ-the′le-əm) pl. *epithe′lia* [*epi-* + Gr. *thēlē* nipple] the covering of internal and external surfaces of the body, including skin and the lining of vessels and other small cavities. It consists of cells joined by small amounts of cementing substances. Epithelium is classified into types on the basis of the number of layers deep and the shape of the superficial cells; see illustration. **epithel′ial** *adj*

e. ante′rius cor′neae [TA] anterior epithelium of cornea: the outer epithelial layer of the cornea, consisting of stratified squamous epithelium continuous with that of the conjunctiva; called also *e. corneae* or *corneal e.*

Barrett e. the metaplastic columnar epithelium of the esophagus seen in Barrett syndrome.

capsular e. parietal layer of glomerular capsule.

ciliated e. epithelium that has vibratile cilia on its free surface.

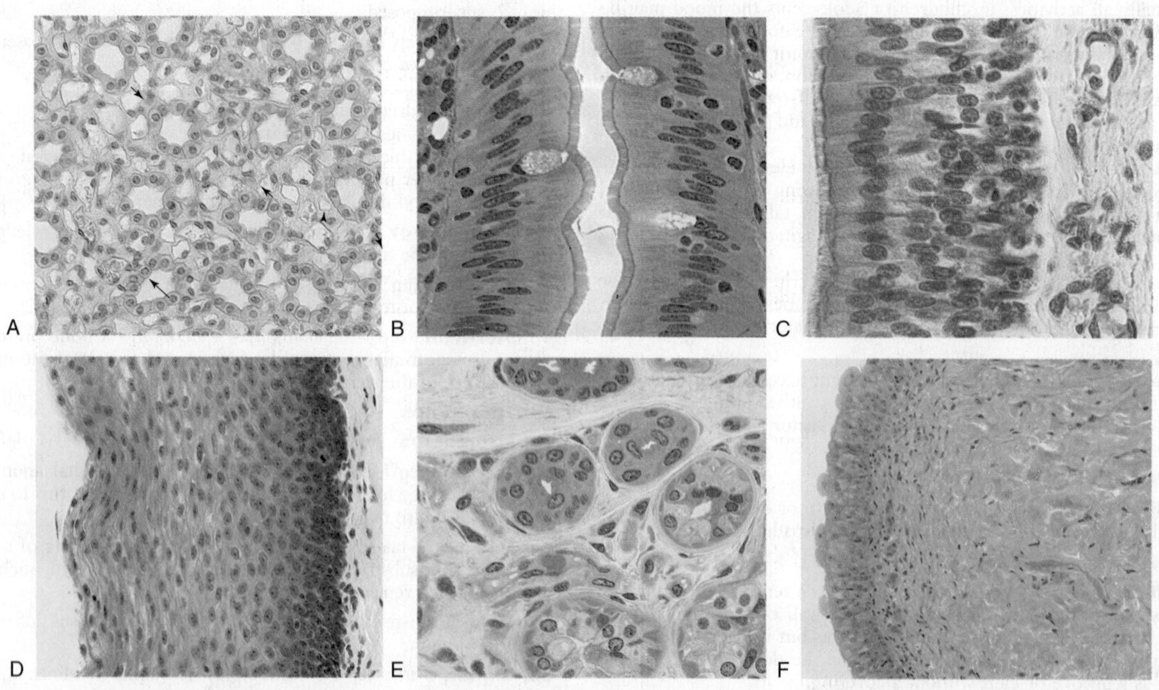

■ Epithelium of different types. *(A),* Simple squamous epithelium *(arrows)* and simple cuboidal epithelium *(arrowheads); (B),* simple columnar epithelium; *(C),* pseudostratified columnar epithelium; *(D),* stratified squamous (nonkeratinized) epithelium; *(E),* stratified cuboidal epithelium; *(F),* transitional epithelium.

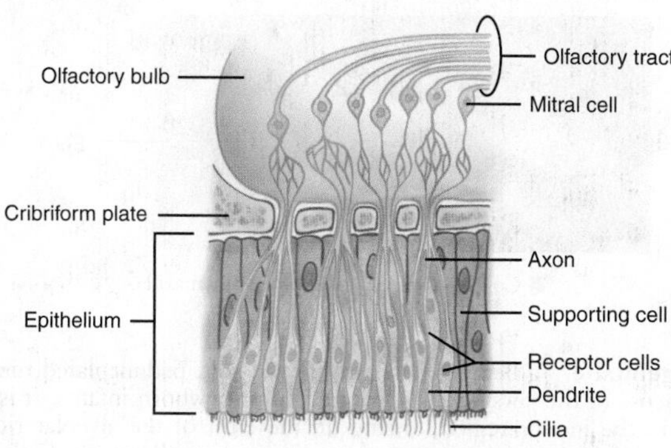

■ Schematic diagram of the receptors in the olfactory epithelium.

coelomic e. the epithelium of the coelom in an embryo or fetus; in children and adults it is seen primarily in tumors.
columnar e. epithelium that is composed of columnar cells.
e. cor′neae, corneal e. e. anterius corneae.
cubical e., cuboidal e. epithelium that is composed of cuboidal cells.
dome e. a type of epithelium in the embryo that forms sheets of epithelial cells to line or cover the body, body cavities, and other internal spaces.
e. duc′tus semicircula′ris the inner, simple epithelium lining the semicircular ducts.
enamel e. in the developing tooth, the inner or internal layer of cells (ameloblasts) of the enamel organ that deposit the organic matrix of enamel, plus the outer or external layer of cuboidal cells. The reduced enamel epithelium is the remains of both layers after enamel formation is complete.
false e. the lining of joint cavities.
germinal e. former term for the thickened coelomic epithelium covering the gonad from earliest development; misnamed because it was thought to give rise to the primordial germ cells.
gingival e. the stratified squamous epithelium covering the gingival tissues; it varies in architecture according to location, functional demands, and adaptation.
glandular e. epithelium made up of glandular or secreting cells.
glomerular e. visceral layer of glomerular capsule.
junctional e. a collarlike band of stratified squamous epithelium adhering on one side to the free gingiva and on the other to the crown of a tooth.
laminated e. stratified e.
e. len′tis [TA] epithelium of lens: the cuboidal epithelium on the front of the lens; called also *subcapsular e.*
mesenchymal e. the epithelium that lines the subdural and subarachnoid spaces, the perilymphatic spaces in the internal ear, and the chambers of the eye.
e. muco′sae, mucosal e. the epithelium that lines the tunica mucosa.
olfactory e. a type of pseudostratified epithelium that lines the olfactory region of the nasal cavity and contains olfactory receptors.
pavement e. simple squamous epithelium.
pigmentary e., pigmented e. epithelium containing granules of pigment.
pigmented e. of iris epithelium pigmentosum iridis.
pigmented e. of retina stratum pigmentosum retinae.
e. pigmento′sum i′ridis [TA] pigmented epithelium of iris: the anterior epithelium of the iris, situated just posterior to the stroma, that contains pigment cells.
e. poste′rius cor′neae [TA] endothelium of anterior chamber: the single layer of flattened squamous cells lining the posterior surface of the cornea and facing the anterior chamber of the eye. The cells have prominent interdigitations and tight junctions and gap junctions between them; they control fluid and solid transport across the posterior layer of the cornea and so control corneal hydration. Called also *corneal endothelium.*
pseudostratified e. a type of epithelium found in the large excretory ducts of the parotid and several other glands and in the male urethra. The nuclei are spaced at different levels and the cells are variable in shape, giving the appearance of stratified epithelium.
pyramidal e. columnar epithelium whose cells have been modified by pressure into truncated pyramids.
respiratory e. the pseudostratified epithelium that lines all but the finer divisions of the respiratory tract.
retinal pigment e. (RPE) stratum pigmentosum retinae.
rod e. epithelium whose cells are rod-shaped.
seminiferous e. a type of stratified epithelium that lines the seminiferous tubules.
sense e., sensory e. neuroepithelium (def. 1).
simple e. epithelium that is composed of a single layer of cells.
simple squamous e. squamous epithelium that has only one layer, such as in endothelium, mesothelium, and pulmonary alveoli. Called also *pavement* or *tessellated e.*
squamous e. epithelium composed of squamous cells; it may be either *simple* or *stratified.*
stratified e. epithelium in which the cells are arranged in several layers; called also *laminated e.*
stratified squamous e. epithelium such as that of typical skin, having a basal layer of cuboidal cells and overlying layers of squamous cells.
subcapsular e. 1. the epithelioid lining of the capsule of a ganglion; cf. *satellite cell.* 2. epithelium lentis.
sulcal e., sulcular e. the parakeratinized part of the gingival epithelium that covers the soft tissue wall of the gingival sulcus, extending from the gingival margin to the line of attachment of the epithelium to the tooth surface.
tessellated e. simple squamous epithelium.
transitional e. a type of epithelium formerly thought to represent a transitional form between stratified squamous and columnar epithelium, found characteristically in the mucous membrane of the excretory passages of the urinary system. In the contracted condition it consists of many cell layers, whereas in the stretched condition usually only two layers can be distinguished.

ep·i·the·li·za·tion (ep″ĭ-the″lĭ-za′shən) epithelialization.

ep·i·the·lize (ep″ĭ-the′līz) epithelialize.

epith·e·sis (ə-pith′ə-sis) [Gr. "a laying on"] 1. surgical correction of deformity, such as crooked limbs. 2. a splint or other appliance to be worn.

ep·i·ton·ic (ep″ĭ-ton′ik) [Gr. *epitonos* strained] abnormally tense or tonic; exhibiting an abnormal degree of tension or of tone.

ep·i·tope (ep′ĭ-tōp) antigenic determinant.

ep·i·trich·i·um (ep″ĭ-trik′e-əm) [*epi-* + Gr. *trichion* hair] periderm (def. 1).

epi·tri·que·trum (ep″ĭ-trĭ-kwe′trəm) epipyramis.

epi·troch·lea (ep″ĭ-trok′le-ə) [*epi-* + *trochlea*] the inner condyle of the humerus.

epi·troch·le·ar (ep″ĭ-trok′le-ər) 1. pertaining to the epitrochlea. 2. above a trochlea, such as the trochlea of the humerus.

epi·tu·ber·cu·lo·sis (ep″ĭ-too-bur″ku-lo′sis) a form of primary tuberculosis in children, producing mild symptoms despite large, usually lobar, consolidations, probably due to bronchial compression by enlarged hilar lymph nodes, with atelectasis.

epi·tym·pan·ic (ep″ĭ-tim-pan′ik) 1. situated upon or over the tympanum. 2. pertaining to the epitympanum (recessus epitympanicus [TA]).

epi·tym·pa·num (ep″ĭ-tim′pə-nəm) recessus epitympanicus.

ep·i·type (ep′ĭ-tīp) a group of related epitopes.

epi·vag (ep′ĭ-vag) [*epididymitis* + *vaginitis*] a venereal disease of cattle, probably of viral origin, in Kenya, southern Africa, and the United States, marked in cows by vaginal inflammation and discharge and by sterility. In bulls it is marked by epididymitis.

Epi·vir (ep′ĭ-vir″) trademark for preparations of lamivudine.

epi·zoa (ep″ĭ-zo′ə) [Gr.] plural of *epizoon.*

epi·zo·ic (ep″ĭ-zo′ik) 1. pertaining to epizoa. 2. caused by epizoa.

epi·zo·i·cide (ep″ĭ-zo′ĭ-sīd) [*epizoon* + *-cide*] an agent that destroys epizoa.

epi·zo·on (ep″ĭ-zo′on) pl. *epizo′a* [*epi-* + Gr. *zōon* animal] an animal ectoparasite.

epi·zo·ot·ic (ep″ĭ-zo-ot′ik) 1. attacking many animals in any region at the same time; widely diffused and rapidly spreading. 2. a disease of high morbidity which is only occasionally present in an animal community. Cf. *enzootic.*

epi·zo·ot·i·ol·o·gy (ep″ĭ-zo-ot″e-ol′ə-je) the study of the factors determining frequencies and distributions of infectious diseases among animals other than humans; animal epidemiology. See also *epizootic.*

epler·e·none (ĕ-pler′ə-nōn) an aldosterone antagonist used in treatment of hypertension and to improve survival in cardiac failure after acute myocardial infarction; administered orally.

éplu·chage (a″ploo-shahzh′) [Fr. "cleaning," "picking"] removal of contused and contaminated tissues from a wound. Cf. *débridement.*

EPM progressive myoclonic epilepsy.
EPM1 progressive myoclonic epilepsy type 1; see *Unverricht-Lundborg disease,* under *disease.*
EPM2 progressive myoclonic epilepsy type 2; see *Lafora disease,* under *disease.*

EPOCH a cancer chemotherapy regimen consisting of etoposide, prednisone, Oncovin (vincristine), cyclophosphamide, and hydroxydaunomycin (doxorubicin).

epo•e•tin (e-po′ə-tin) a 165–amino acid glycoprotein produced by recombinant DNA technology. It has the same amino acid sequence and mechanism of action as endogenous erythropoietin and is used in the treatment of anemia of various causes, including chronic renal failure, zidovudine therapy, and cancer chemotherapy and is also used prior to surgery in anemic patients to reduce the need for blood transfusion; administered intravenously or subcutaneously. It occurs in several forms, which have the same amino acid sequence but differ in glycosylation pattern; that used in the United States is *epoetin alfa*, while *epoetin beta* is often used in other countries. Called also *recombinant human erythropoietin (rHuEPO).*

Ep•o•gen (e′po-jən) trademark for a preparation of epoetin alfa.

Epon (e′pon) trademark for a plastic material in which specimens are imbedded for ultrastructural study.

epon•tic (ə-pon′tik) growing on any surface, plant, animal, or mineral.

ep•o•nych•i•um (ep″o-nik′e-əm) [*epi-* + *onyx*] 1. [TA] the narrow band of epidermis that extends from the nail wall onto the nail surface; called also *cuticle* and *perionychium*. 2. the horny fetal epidermis at the site of the future nail.

ep•oöph•o•ron (ep″o-of′ə-rən) [*epi-* + *oophoron*] [TA] a vestigial structure associated with the ovary, consisting of a more cranial group of mesonephric tubules and a corresponding portion of the mesonephric duct; called also *pampiniform body, parovarium,* and *Rosenmüller organ.* Spelled also *epoophoron*.

epo•pros•te•nol (e″po-pros′tə-nol) name given to prostacyclin when used pharmaceutically; it is used in the form of the sodium salt as an inhibitor of platelet aggregation when blood contacts nonbiological systems, as in renal dialysis, as a pulmonary antihypertensive, and as a vasodilator.

ep•or•ni•thol•o•gy (ep-or″nĭ-thol′ə-je) the scientific study of diseases of high morbidity that are only occasionally present in bird communities.

ep•or•nit•ic (ep″or-nit′ik) [*epi-* + Gr. *ornis* bird] 1. attacking many birds in a region at the same time. 2. a disease of high morbidity that is only occasionally present in a bird population.

epox•ide (ə-pok′sīd) an organic compound containing a reactive group resulting from the union of an oxygen atom with two other atoms, usually carbon, that are themselves joined together. Commonly referred to as *epoxy*. See also *epoxy resin*, under *resin*.

epoxy (ə-pok′se) 1. epoxide. 2. see under *resin*.

EPP erythropoietic protoporphyria.

Ep•py/N (ep′e) trademark for a preparation of epinephryl borate.

EPR electron paramagnetic resonance; electrophrenic respiration.

ep•ro•sar•tan mes•y•late (ep″ro-sahr′tan) an angiotensin II receptor antagonist, used as an antihypertensive; administered orally.

ep•si•lon (ep′si-lon) [E, ε] the fifth letter of the Greek alphabet. See also ε-.

Ep•si•lon•pro•teo•bac•te•ria (ep″sĭ-lon-pro″te-o-bak-tēr′e-ə) [*epsilon* the fifth letter of the Greek alphabet + *Proteobacteria*] a class of bacteria of the Proteobacteria, grouped together on the basis of 16S rRNA sequence analysis; organisms of medical interest are included in the order Campylobacterales.

EPSP excitatory postsynaptic potential.

Ep•stein disease, pearls (ep′stīn) [Alois *Epstein*, Czech pediatrician, 1849–1918] see *pseudodiphtheria*, and see under *pearl*.

Ep•stein syndrome (ep′stīn) [Albert Arthur *Epstein*, New York physician, 1880–1965] nephrotic syndrome; see under *syndrome*.

Ep•stein-Barr virus (ep′stīn bahr′) [Michael Anthony *Epstein*, British physician, born 1921; Yvonne M. *Barr*, British virologist, born 1932] see under *virus*.

ep•ta•tre•tin (ep″tə-tre′tin) a potent cardiostimulant obtained from the branchial heart of the Pacific hagfish *Eptatretus stouti* and reported to be a highly unstable aromatic amine. Its chemical structure has not been fully defined, but it is not a catecholamine or other commonly occurring biochemical.

ep•ti•fib•a•tide (ep″tə-fib′ə-tīd) an inhibitor of platelet aggregation, acting by reversibly binding to glycoprotein IIb/IIIa; used as an adjunct for the prevention of thrombosis in patients with acute coronary syndrome or undergoing balloon angioplasty or other percutaneous coronary procedures, administered intravenously.

epu•li•des (ə-pu′lĭ-dēz) [Gr.] plural of *epulis*.

epu•lis (ə-pu′lis) pl. *epu′lides* [Gr. *epoulis* gumboil] 1. a nonspecific term applied to tumors and tumor-like masses of the gingiva. 2. peripheral ossifying fibroma.

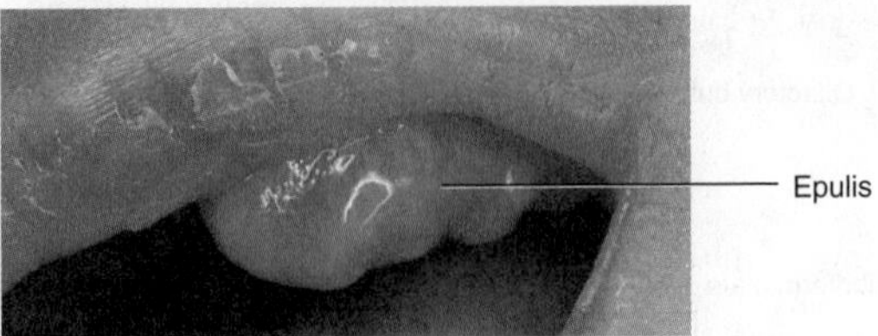

■ Congenital epulis of the anterior maxilla.

congenital e. a benign, nonencapsulated soft, pedunculated tumor of the mucosa of the jaws, usually the maxilla, of newborn infants. It is often found in the incisor region, arising on the crest of the alveolar ridge or process. Microscopically, it resembles a granular cell tumor. Called also *e. of newborn*.

e. fibromato′sa, fibromatous e. 1. a fibroma arising from the alveolar periosteum and the periodontal ligament. 2. a benign fibromatous tumor arising in periodontal stroma on the gum of a dog, usually an older animal. Some breeds are more susceptible than others, suggesting a genetic component. Called also *fibromatosis gingivae*.

e. fissura′ta fibrous inflammatory hyperplasia.

giant cell e., e. gigantocellula′ris a sessile or pedunculated lesion of the gingiva, or less often the mucous membrane covering edentulous ridges, which represents inflammatory reactions to injury or hemorrhage, and is not considered a true neoplasm. Histologically, it is composed of a spindle cell stroma punctuated by multinucleate giant cells. Called also *peripheral giant cell granuloma* and *peripheral giant cell reparative granuloma.*

e. granulomato′sa a pyogenic granuloma on the gingiva resulting from mechanical or other irritation.

e. of newborn congenital e.

ep•u•lo•fi•bro•ma (ep″u-lo″fi-bro′mə) a fibroma of the gingiva.

ep•u•loid (ep′u-loid) resembling an epulis.

ep•u•lo•sis (ep″u-lo′sis) [Gr. *epoulōsis*] cicatrization.

ep•u•lot•ic (ep″u-lot′ik) [Gr. *epoulōtikos*] cicatricial.

Equa•ge•sic (ek″wə-je′zik) trademark for a combination preparation of meprobamate and aspirin.

equate (e-kwāt′) to make equal or equivalent. In color vision, the physiologic faculty of combining two colors to match a third, as to combine red and green to make a homogeneous yellow.

equa•tion (e-kwa′zhən) [L. *aequatio*, from *aequare* to make equal] an expression made up of two members connected by the sign of equality, =.

Arrhenius e. an equation describing the temperature dependence of a reaction rate constant,

$$k = Ae^{-\Delta E_a}/RT,$$

where k is the rate constant, e is the base of natural logarithms, ΔE_a the activation energy, R the gas constant, T the absolute temperature, and A is a constant called the frequency factor, representing the frequency of encounters between reactant molecules.

chemical e. an equation that expresses a chemical reaction, the symbols on the left of the equation denoting the substances before, and those on the right those after, the reaction.

generalized estimation e. a method used to analyze correlated repeated measures; it must be robust to the correlation structure and computationally feasible.

Harden and Young e. an equation showing the chemical reaction in the fermentation of glucose to carbon dioxide, alcohol, and hexose diphosphate.

Henderson-Hasselbalch e. an equation giving the pH of a buffer system:

$$\mathrm{pH} = \mathrm{p}K_a + \log\frac{[\mathrm{A}^-]}{[\mathrm{HA}]}$$

where [HA] is the concentration of the free acid, $[A^-]$ is the concentration of the ionized form, and pK_a is the negative logarithm of the acid dissociation constant (K_a).

Hill e. an equation used in enzyme characterization, describing the fraction of the enzyme saturated by ligand as a function of the ligand concentration; it is used in determining the degree of cooperativity of the enzyme.

Lineweaver-Burk e. a rearrangement of the Michaelis-Menten equation of enzyme kinetics to give

$$\frac{1}{v} = \frac{K_M}{V_{max}[S]} + \frac{1}{V_{max}}$$

where v is the reaction velocity, [S] is the substrate concentration, V_{max} is the maximum velocity, and K_M is the Michaelis constant. If an enzyme reaction follows Michaelis-Menten kinetics, then a plot of $1/v$ against 1/[S] results in a straight line with defined slope and intercepts; see *Lineweaver-Burk plot*, under *plot*.

MDRD e. see under *formula*.

Michaelis-Menten e. a fundamental equation of enzyme kinetics:

$$v = \frac{V_{max}[S]}{K_M + [S]}$$

where v is the "initial velocity" of an enzyme-catalyzed reaction (the velocity when the product concentration is near zero); [S] is the substrate concentration; and V_{max} and K_M are two constants that characterize a specific enzyme: V_{max}, the maximum velocity, is the initial velocity seen when the enzyme is completely saturated with substrate, and K_M is the Michaelis constant, defined operationally as the substrate concentration at which $v = V_{max}/2$. The Michaelis-Menten equation does not apply to allosteric enzymes for which the binding of the substrate at the active site is altered by binding of the substrate at a second (allosteric) site. See also *Lineweaver-Burk e.*

Nernst e. an equation for the voltage produced by an electrochemical reaction:

$$E = E^\circ - \frac{RT}{zF}\ln Q$$

where E is the voltage produced, E° is the standard reduction potential for the reaction, R is the gas constant, T the absolute temperature, z the number of electrons transferred in the reaction, F Faraday constant, Q the reaction quotient (q.v.), and ln the natural logarithm. The same formula gives the membrane potential produced by a concentration of a diffusible ion across a membrane; in this case E° is zero, z is the ionic charge, and Q is the ratio of the concentrations on the two sides of the membrane.

Poiseuille e. see under *law*.

Ussing e. a method for determining active transport across a biologic membrane, by considering the unidirectional fluxes.

equa·tor (e-kwa′tər) [L. *aequator* equalizer] an imaginary line encircling a globe, equidistant from the poles. Used in anatomical nomenclature to designate such a line on a spherical organ, dividing the surface into two approximately equal parts. Called also *aequator*.

e. bul′bi o′culi [TA] equator of eyeball: an imaginary line encircling the eyeball equidistant from the anterior and the posterior poles, dividing the eye into anterior and posterior halves.

e. of cell the boundary of the plane of separation of a dividing cell.

e. of crystalline lens e. lentis.

e. of eyeball e. bulbi oculi.

e. len′tis [TA] equator of lens: the rounded peripheral margin of the lens at which the anterior and posterior surfaces meet.

equa·to·ri·al (e″kwə-tor′e-əl) 1. pertaining to an equator. 2. occurring at the same distance from each extremity of an axis.

equi·an·al·ge·sic (e″kwĭ-an″əl-je′sik) having the same analgesic effect as a given dose of another analgesic agent.

equi·ax·i·al (e″kwĭ-ak′se-əl) having axes of the same length.

equi·ca·lor·ic (e″kwĭ-kə-lor′ik) isocaloric.

Equi·dae (ek′wĭ-de) [L. *equus* horse] a family of perissodactylous mammals containing a single living genus, *Equus*, which includes horses, asses, zebras, and onagers.

equi·lat·er·al (e″kwĭ-lat′ər-əl) having sides that are equal or identical.

equi·li·bra·tion (e-kwil″ĭ-bra′shən) the achievement of a balance between opposing elements or forces.

mandibular e. 1. the act or acts performed to place the mandible in equilibrium. 2. a condition in which all of the forces acting upon the mandible are neutralized. 3. a term applied to adjustive grinding of an interfering tooth structure during the functional stroke.

occlusal e. see under *adjustment*.

equi·li·bra·tor (e-kwil″ĭ-bra′tər) an apparatus used to produce or maintain a state of balance between opposing forces.

equi·li·bri·um (e″kwĭ-lib′re-əm) [L. *aequus* equal + *libra* balance] 1. a condition in which opposing forces exactly counteract each other; called also *balance*. 2. postural balance of the body; see *sense of equilibrium*, under *sense*.

acid-base e. see under *balance*.

body e. physiologic e.

carbon e. the condition in which the total carbon of the excreta is balanced by the carbon of the food.

Donnan e. the conditions that exist at equilibrium when two solutions are separated by a membrane permeable to some but not all of the ions of the solutions. There is a complex distribution of the ions between the two solutions, an electrical potential develops between the two sides of the membrane, and the two solutions vary in osmotic pressure. Called also *Gibbs-Donnan e.* and *Donnan effect* or *e.*

dynamic e. the condition of balance between varying, shifting, and opposing forces which is characteristic of living processes.

fluid e. see under *balance*.

genetic e. the condition that exists when genotype frequencies in a population are constant in successive generations; i.e., the frequency of each allele in the population remains unchanged in successive generations. See also *Hardy-Weinberg law*, under *law*. Called also *Hardy-Weinberg e.*

Gibbs-Donnan e. Donnan e.

Hardy-Weinberg e. genetic e.

linkage e. in genetics, the situation in which the population frequency of each combination of alleles for two linked loci is equal to the product of their population frequencies at the individual loci.

nitrogen e., nitrogenous e. the condition in which the body is metabolizing and excreting as much nitrogen as it is receiving in the food, i.e. the nitrogen balance is neither positive nor negative. Called also *protein e.*

nutritive e., physiologic e. the condition in which the amount of material taken into the body exactly equals the amount discharged.

protein e. nitrogen e.

radioactive e. the fixed ratio between a radioactive element and one of its disintegration products that results after the lapse of a suitable time, owing to their half value periods. That of uranium and radium is 2,380,000:1.

water e. fluid balance.

equil·in (ek′wil-in) an estrogen, $C_{18}H_{20}O_2$, with both rings A and B aromatized, occurring in the urine of pregnant mares; a component of conjugated estrogens.

equi·mo·lar (e″kwĭ-mo′lər) containing the same number of moles, or having the same molarity.

equi·mo·lec·u·lar (e″kwĭ-mo-lek′u-lər) containing the same number of molecules; said of solutions.

equine (e′kwīn) [L. *equus* a horse] pertaining to, characteristic of, or derived from the horse.

equi·no·pho·bia (e-kwi″no-fo′be-ə) [L. *equinus* relating to horses + *phobia*] irrational fear of horses.

equi·no·val·gus (e-kwi″no-val′gəs) talipes equinovalgus.

equi·no·va·rus (e-kwi″no-va′rəs) talipes equinovarus.

equi·nus (e-kwi′nəs) talipes equinus.

equi·poise (e′kwĭ-poiz) a state of genuine uncertainty concerning the relative merits of a set of therapies or interventions; an ethical requirement for performing a randomized clinical trial.

equi·po·ten·tial (e″kwĭ-po-ten′shəl) [L. *aequus* equal + *potential*] possessed of similar and equal power; capable of developing in the same way and to the same extent.

equi·po·ten·ti·al·i·ty (e″kwĭ-po-ten″she-al′ĭ-te) the quality or state of having similar and equal power; the capacity for developing in the same way and to the same extent.

equi·se·to·sis (ek″wĭ-sə-to′sis) incoordination and cardiac irregularities due to thiamine deficiency in animals that consume hay contaminated with *Equisetum*.

Equi·se·tum (ek″wĭ-se′təm) the horsetails, a genus of plants of the family Equisetaceae. *E. arven′se* and *E. palus′tre* contain a thiamine antagonist that causes equisetosis in horses that eat them along with hay.

equiv·a·lence (e-kwiv′ə-ləns) 1. the condition of being equivalent; having equal valence. 2. in immunology, the ratio of antigen to antibody concentration at which maximal antigen-antibody combination takes place, yielding a precipitate or aggregate; see also *precipitin reaction*, under *reaction*.

equiv·a·lent (e-kwiv′ə-lent) [L. *aequivalens*, from *aequus* equal + *valere* to be worth] 1. having the same value; neutralizing or counterbalancing each other. 2. something that is essentially equal to another, or can take its place entirely. 3. equivalent weight; see under *weight*.

alpha-tocopherol e. the specific biological activity of 1.0 milligram of *d*-alpha-tocopherol. See also *international unit of vitamin E*.

aluminum e. the thickness of pure aluminum affording the same radiation attenuation, under specified conditions, as the material or materials being considered.

anxiety e. physical symptoms resulting from somatization of underlying anxiety.

combustion e. the heat value of a gram of fat or carbohydrate burned outside the body. It measures the amount of potential energy of the substance available, in the form of food, for the production of heat or the supply of energy.

concrete e. the thickness of concrete having a density of 2.35 g/cm^3 which would afford the same radiation attenuation, under specified conditions, as the material or materials being considered.

dose e. in radiation biology, the product of absorbed dose in rads and the modifying factors, namely the quality factor (QF), distribution factor (DF), and any other necessary factors. The unit of dose equivalent is the rem.

gold e. the amount of protective colloid, expressed in milligrams, which is just enough to prevent the precipitation of 10 mL of a 0.0055 per cent gold solution by 1 mL of a 10 per cent sodium chloride solution.

gram e. equivalent weight.

isodynamic e. the ratio, from a food-energy standpoint, between carbohydrate and fat. It is 9.3 to 4.1, or 2.3 to 1; that is, one part of fat is equivalent to 2.3 parts of sugar or starch.

Joule e. an expression of the relationship between mechanical energy and heat; numerically 4.186 joules = 1 calorie.

lead e. the thickness of pure lead which would afford the same radiation attenuation, under specified conditions, as the material or materials under consideration.

lethal e. a gene carried in the heterozygous state which, if homozygous, would be lethal, or any combination of genes which would be lethal to 100 percent of homozygotes; for example, a combination of two genes in the heterozygous state either of which in the homozygous state would have 50 per cent lethality.

migraine e. migraine aura without headache; see under *aura.*

neutralization e. the equivalent weight of an acid as determined by neutralization with a base regarded as a primary standard.

protein e. the protein content of a food plus the nonprotein content that can be converted into protein in the animal body.

psychic e. temporal lobe epilepsy.

retinol e. (RE) the specific biological activity of 1.0 microgram of all-*trans* retinol, 6.0 micrograms of β-carotene, or 12.0 micrograms of other provitamin A carotenoids; it is equivalent to 3.3 international units of vitamin A activity from retinol (10 from β-carotene).

skin e. a skin substitute created by tissue engineering from skin cells or a biomaterial, used as a dressing or replacement on a wound where skin has been damaged or destroyed. See also *tissue-engineered skin.*

starch e. a number (nearly 2.4) expressing the amount of oxygen which a given weight of fat will require for its complete combustion as compared with the amount required by the same weight of starch.

toxic e. the amount of poison per kilogram of body weight necessary to kill an animal.

ventilation e., ventilatory e. the ratio of the total volume of ventilation to the volume of oxygen absorbed by the lungs per unit of time.

water e. the product of the weight of an animal by its specific heat, it being also the number which represents the specific thermal capacity of an equal weight of water.

equu•lo•sis (ek″wə-lo′sis) [L. *equulus* a foal + *-osis*] actinobacillosis in horses and sometimes pigs, usually seen in the first few weeks of life, involving infection with *Actinobacillus equuli.* Symptoms in foals are purulent arthritis, synovitis, and enteritis, often with kidney abscesses and death; in piglets the symptoms are septicemia, fever, listlessness, and often death. When foals show extreme prostration, the condition is called *sleepy foal disease.*

Eq•uus (ek′wəs) the single living genus of the family Equidae, including horses, asses, and zebras.

Eq•va•lan (ek′və-lan) trademark for a preparation of ivermectin.

ER emergency room; endoplasmic reticulum; estrogen receptor.

Er erbium.

erab•u•tox•in (ə-rab′u-tok″sin) the active toxic principle of the venom of the sea snake *Laticauda semifasciata.*

Er•a•ty•rus (er″ə-ti′rəs) a genus of reduviid bugs that transmit Chagas disease.

Er•ax•is (ər-ak′sis) trademark for a preparation of anidulafungin.

Erb spastic paraplegia, etc. (erb) [Wilhelm Heinrich *Erb,* German neurologist, 1840–1921] see under *paraplegia* and *point,* see *primary lateral sclerosis* under *sclerosis,* and see *Duchenne muscular dystrophy,* under *dystrophy.*

Erb-Char•cot disease (erb′ shahr-ko′) [W.H. *Erb;* Jean Martin *Charcot,* French neurologist, 1825–1893] Erb spastic paraplegia.

Erb-Du•chenne paralysis (erb′ du-shen′) [W.H. *Erb;* Guillaume Benjamin Amand *Duchenne,* French neurologist, 1806–1875] see under *paralysis.*

Erb-Gold•flam disease (erb′ gōlt′flahm) [W.H. *Erb;* Samuel V. *Goldflam,* Polish neurologist, 1852–1932] myasthenia gravis.

Er•ben reflex (phenomenon, sign) (ur′bən) [Siegmund *Erben,* Austrian neurologist, late 19th century] see under *reflex.*

ERBF effective renal blood flow.

Er•bi•tux (ur′bĭ-tuks) trademark for a preparation of cetuximab.

er•bi•um (Er) (ur′be-əm) a rare metallic element, atomic number 68, atomic weight 167.26.

ERCP endoscopic retrograde cholangiopancreatography.

Erd•heim disease (cystic medial necrosis) (erd′hīm) [Jakob *Erdheim,* Austrian physician, 1874–1937] cystic medial necrosis.

erec•tile (ə-rek′tīl) capable of erection; see under *tissue.*

erec•tion (ə-rek′shən) [L. *erectio*] the condition of being made rigid and elevated, such as in erectile tissue when filled with blood.

erec•tor (ə-rek′tər) [L., from *erigere* to set up] something that erects, such as a muscle that raises or holds up a part. Cf. *arrector.*

er•e•ma•cau•sis (er″ə-mə-kaw′sis) [Gr. *ērema* gently + *kausis* burning] the slow oxidation, combustion, or decay of organic matter.

er•e•mo•pho•bia (er″ə-mo-fo′be-ə) [Gr. *erēmos* solitary + *-phobia*] irrational fear of being alone.

ere•thism (er′ə-thiz″əm) psychologic changes (memory loss, irritability, emotional lability, insomnia, and social withdrawal) caused by toxic damage to the central nervous system, seen especially in chronic mercury poisoning.

Ereth•ma•pod•i•tes (ə-reth″mə-pod′ĭ-tēs) a genus of mosquitoes, species of which transmit Rift Valley fever.

ERG electroretinogram.

erg (urg) [Gr. *ergon* work] a unit of work or energy, being the work performed when a force of 1 dyne moves its point of operation through a distance of 1 cm; equal to 10^{-7} joule.

Er•ga•mi•sol (ər-gam′ĭ-sol) trademark for a preparation of levamisole hydrochloride.

ERGIC endoplasmic reticulum–Golgi intermediate compartment

erg(o)- [Gr. *ergon* work] a combining form denoting relationship to work.

er•go•cal•cif•er•ol (ur″go-kal-sif′ər-ol) [USP] a sterol occurring naturally in fungi and some fish oils or synthesized from ergosterol; it is administered orally or added to food (e.g., milk) as a dietary source of vitamin D. It is also used in the treatment of hypocalcemia, hypophosphatemia, rickets, and osteodystrophy associated with a variety of disorders, such as chronic renal failure and hypoparathyroidism; administered orally, intravenously, or intramuscularly. The activity and metabolism of ergocalciferol are similar to those of cholecalciferol (q.v.). Called also *vitamin* D_2.

er•go•cor•nine (ur″go-kor′nēn) a toxic ergot alkaloid of the ergotoxine group.

er•go•cris•tine (ur″go-kris′tēn) a toxic ergot alkaloid of the ergotoxine group.

er•go•cryp•tine (ur″go-krip′tēn) a toxic ergot alkaloid of the ergotoxine group.

er•go•dy•namo•graph (ur″go-di-nam′o-graf) [*ergo-* + *dynamo-* + *-graph*] an apparatus for recording the force exhibited and the work done in muscular contraction.

er•go•es•the•sio•graph (ur″go-es-the′ze-o-graf) [*ergo-* + *esthesio-* + *-graph*] an apparatus for recording graphically muscular reactions to various stimuli.

er•go•gen•ic (ur″go-jen′ik) [*ergo-* + *-genic*] tending to increase work output.

er•go•gram (ur′go-gram) [*ergo-* + *-gram*] a tracing made by an ergograph.

er•go•graph (ur′go-graf) [*ergo-* + *-graph*] an instrument for recording work done in muscular exertion. **ergograph′ic** *adj*

Mosso e. an apparatus for recording the force and frequency of flexion of the fingers.

er•go•loid mes•y•lates (ur′go-loid) [USP] a mixture consisting of equal proportions by weight of the methanesulfonate (mesylate) salts of the hydrogenated ergot alkaloids dihydroergocristine, dihydroergocornine, and dihydroergocryptine; it has been administered orally in the treatment of mild to moderate dementia in the elderly.

Er•go•mar (ur′go-mahr) trademark for a preparation of ergotamine tartrate.

er•gom•e•ter (er-gom′ə-tər) [*ergo-* + *-meter*] dynamometer.

bicycle e. a bicyclelike apparatus for measuring the muscular, metabolic, and respiratory effects of exercise; used to determine cardiac status. See also *bicycle ergometer exercise test,* under *test.*

er•go•met•rine (ur″go-met′rin) INN and BAN for *ergonovine.*

er•go•nom•ics (ur″go-nom′iks) [*ergo-* + Gr. *nomos* law] the scientific study of humans and their work, including the anatomic, physiologic, psychologic, and mechanical principles affecting the efficient use of human energy.

er•gon•o•mist (ər-gon′ə-mist) an individual with professional credentials in ergonomics or a closely related field.

er•go•no•vine (ur″go-no′vin) a water-soluble alkaloid, from ergot or produced synthetically; an oxytocic and vasoconstrictor. Called also *ergometrine.*

e. maleate [USP] the bimaleate salt of ergonovine; used as an oxytocic in the prevention or treatment of postpartum or postabortion hemorrhage, administered orally, intramuscularly, or intravenously. It is also used intravenously as a provocative test in detection of variant angina due to coronary artery spasm.

er•go•stat (ur′go-stat) a machine to be worked for muscular exercise.

er•gos•te•rol (ər-gos′tə-rol″) a sterol occurring mainly in yeast and forming ergocalciferol (vitamin D_2) upon irradiation by ultraviolet rays or electronic bombardment. Called also *provitamin* D_2.

activated e., irradiated e. ergocalciferol.

er•got (ur′got) [Fr.; L. *ergota*] 1. the dried sclerotium of *Claviceps purpurea*, which is developed on rye plants *(Secale cereale);* it is the source of the ergot alkaloids (q.v.). 2. a small mass of horn in the tuft of hair at the flexion surface of the fetlock in horses.

er•got•amine (ər-got′ə-min) an alkaloid derived from ergot, consisting of lysergic acid, ammonia, proline, phenylalanine, and pyruvic acid combined in amide linkages; used in the treatment of migraine and cluster headaches.

e. tartrate [USP] the tartrate salt of ergotamine, administered orally, sublingually, by oral inhalation, or rectally in the treatment of migraine and cluster headaches.

er•go•tam•i•nine (ur″go-tam′ĭ-nēn) an isomer of ergotamine.

er•go•ther•a•py (ur″go-ther′ə-pe) [*ergo-* + *therapy*] treatment of disease by physical effort.

er•go•thi•o•ne•ine (ur″go-thi″o-ne′in) the trimethylbetaine of thiolhistidine, originally found in ergot and later isolated from human blood; it occurs in abnormal amounts in the urine of cancer patients; called also *erythrothioneine, thiazine,* and *thioneine.*

er•go•tism (ur′go-tiz-əm) poisoning from excessive or misdirected medicinal use of ergot, or from eating ergotized grain; it is marked by cerebrospinal symptoms, spasms, cramps, and sometimes a kind of dry gangrene. Called also *ergot poisoning* and *ergotoxicosis.*

er•got•ized (ur′got-īzd) diseased or otherwise affected by ergot.

er•go•tox•i•co•sis (ur″go-tok″sĭ-ko′sis) ergotism.

er•go•tox•ine (ur″go-tok′sēn) a mixture of three toxic ergot alkaloids, ergocornine, ergocristine, and ergocryptine, formerly used medicinally for its oxytocic and adrenergic blocking effects but no longer used because of the variability of these effects.

Er•go•trate (ur′go-trāt) trademark for preparations of ergonovine maleate.

Er•ich•sen sign (test) (er′ik-sən) [Sir John Eric *Erichsen*, English surgeon, 1818–1896] see under *sign.*

Er•i•o•dic•ty•on (er″e-o-dik′te-on) [Gr. *erion* wool + *diktyon* net] a genus of resinous shrubs of the family Hydrophyllaceae that grow in the southwestern United States and Mexico. The most important species is *E. califor′nicum*, the source of the flavoring called eriodictyon. Called also *mountain balm* and *yerba santa.*

er•i•o•dic•ty•on (er″e-o-dik′te-on) 1. any plant of the genus *Eriodictyon.* 2. the dried leaf of *E. californicum;* its fluidextract is used as a flavoring and its aromatic syrup as a vehicle for dispensing drugs. See under *fluidextract* and *syrup.*

er•i•o•nite (er′e-o-nīt) a common form of zeolite used as an absorbent and filtering material; excessive inhalation of its dust can cause pulmonary fibrosis or silicatosis.

er•is•i•phake (er-is′ĭ-fāk) erysiphake.

Er•is•ta•lis (er-is′tə-lis) a genus of flies, the hover flies, of the family Syrphidae. *E. te′nax* is the drone fly; it breeds in drains and its maggots (rat-tail maggots) occasionally cause intestinal or nasal myiasis.

Er•len•mey•er flask (er′lən-mi″ər) [Emil Richard August Carl *Erlenmeyer*, German chemist, 1825–1909] see under *flask.*

er•lo•ti•nib hy•dro•chlo•ride (er-lo′ti-nib) an inhibitor of protein tyrosine kinase and epidermal growth factor, used as an antineoplastic in treatment of non–small-cell lung cancer and pancreatic cancer; administered orally.

ERM ezrin, radixin, and moesin; see *ERM proteins*, under *protein.*

erode (e-rōd′) to wear away.

erog•e•nous (ə-roj′ə-nəs) erotogenic; arousing erotic feelings.

erose (ə-rōs′) [L. *erodere* to eat away] having an irregularly toothed edge.

ero•sio (ə-ro′se-o) [L., from *erodere* to eat away] erosion.

e. interdigita′lis blastomyce′tica intertigo of the skinfolds between the fingers, with an area of macerated white skin that sometimes extends to the sides of the fingers; caused by *Candida* and seen most often in persons whose hands are frequently immersed in water.

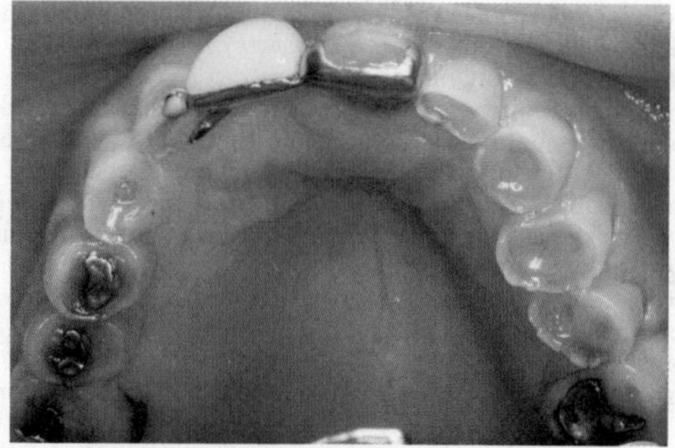

■ Erosion of the lingual surfaces of the maxillary teeth, showing concave depressions of the dentin surrounded by elevated rims of enamel.

ero•sion (ə-ro′zhən) [L. *erosio*, from *erodere* to eat out] 1. the wearing away or destruction of the surface of a tissue, material, or structure. 2. progressive loss of the hard substance of a tooth by chemical processes that do not involve bacterial action. See also *abrasion* and *attrition.* 3. a gradual breakdown or shallow ulceration of the skin, involving only the epidermis; it usually heals without scarring.

marginal e's areas of eroded cartilage near the edge of a joint, seen on a radiograph of a person with rheumatoid arthritis.

ero•sive (ə-ro′siv) 1. characterized by erosion. 2. causing or producing erosion. 3. an agent that produces erosion.

erot•ic (ə-rot′ik) [Gr. *erōtikos*] 1. charged with sexual feeling. 2. pertaining to sexual desire.

erot•i•cism (ə-rot′ĭ-siz-əm) a sexual instinct or desire; the expression of one's instinctual energy or drive, especially the sex drive. Called also *erotism.*

anal e. fixation of libido at (or regression to) the anal phase of infantile development, said in psychoanalytic theory to produce egotistic, dogmatic, stubborn, miserly character.

genital e. achievement and maintenance of libido at the genital phase of psychosexual development, said in psychoanalytic theory to permit acceptance of normal adult relationships and responsibilities.

oral e. 1. fixation of libido at (or regression to) the oral phase of infantile development, said in psychoanalytic theory to produce passive, insecure, sensitive character. 2. the pleasure derived from the use of the mouth for other than nutritional satisfactions.

erot•i•cize (ə-rot′ĭ-sīz) erotize.

er•o•tism (er′o-tiz″əm) eroticism.

er•o•tize (er′o-tīz) to endow with erotic or libidinous meaning or significance.

erot(o)- [Gr. *erōs*, gen. *erōtos* sexual desire] a combining form denoting relationship to sexual desire.

ero•to•gen•e•sis (ə-rot″o-jen′ə-sis) the formation or production of erotic feeling.

ero•to•gen•ic (ə-rot″o-jen′ik) erogenous.

ero•to•ma•nia (ə-rot″o-ma′ne-ə) [*eroto-* + *-mania*] 1. a type of delusional disorder in which the subject believes that a person, usually older and of higher social status, is deeply in love with him or her; failure of the object of the delusion to respond to the subject's advances are rationalized, and pursuit and harassment of that person may occur. 2. occasionally, hypersexuality.

ero•to•pho•bia (ə-rot″o-fo′be-ə) [*eroto-* + *-phobia*] fear of love, especially of sexual feelings and activity.

ERP endocardial resection procedure.

ERPF effective renal plasma flow.

er•rat•ic (ə-rat′ik) [L. *errare* to wander] 1. roving or wandering. 2. eccentric; deviating from an accepted course of thought or conduct.

er•rhine (er′īn) [Gr. *errhinon* a medicine that promotes nasal discharge] 1. promoting a nasal discharge. 2. a medicine that promotes nasal discharge or secretion.

er•ror (er′ər) a defect in structure or function; a deviation.

alpha e. Type I e.

beta e., false-negative e. Type II e.

false-positive e. Type I e.

inborn e. of metabolism a genetically determined biochemical disorder in which a specific enzyme defect produces a metabolic block that may have pathologic consequences at birth (e.g., phenylketonuria) or in later life (e.g., diabetes mellitus); called also *enzymopathy.*

nondifferential e. random e.

random e. indefiniteness or error in a measurement process that varies unsystematically or unpredictably from measurement to measurement; its magnitude may be quantifiable by statistical methods.

e. of refraction, refractive e. deviation from optimal focusing of light *(emmetropia)* by the lens of the eye onto the retina, such as myopia, hyperopia, astigmatism, or anisometropia.

standard e. in statistics, a measure of the variability that the calculated parameter estimate shows as repeated random samples are taken from the same population.

standard e. of the mean an indication of how well a sample mean estimates the population mean by measurement of the standard deviation of a sampling distribution of the means. It is approximately equal to

$$s/\sqrt{n},$$

where s is the sample estimate of the standard deviation and n is the sample size.

systematic e. reproducible inaccuracy; error in a measurement process that is predictable or in the same direction in all measurements; it may not be detectable by statistical methods. Called also *bias.*

Type I e. in a hypothesis test, the rejection of the null hypothesis when it is true; the probability of a Type I error (the significance level) is denoted by α.

Type II e. in a hypothesis test, failing to reject the null hypothesis when it is false; the probability of a Type II error is denoted by β.

er•ta•pen•em so•di•um (ər-tə-pen′em) an antibacterial that interferes with cell wall synthesis, effective against a wide variety of gram-positive and gram-negative, aerobic and anaerobic organisms; used in the treatment of complicated intra-abdominal, urinary tract, and skin infections, acute pelvic infections, community-acquired pneumonia, and diabetic foot infections; administered intramuscularly or intravenously.

Ertl procedure (amputation) (ur′təl) [Janos *Ertl*, Hungarian orthopedic surgeon, 1880–1951] see under *procedure.*

eru•cic ac•id (ə-roo′sik) [Lat. *eruca* caterpillar] a monounsaturated 22-carbon fatty acid occurring as a major constituent of most rapeseed and mustard oils. Because erucic acid has been linked to cardiac muscle damage, edible canola oil products are prepared from low erucic acid varieties of rapeseed plants. See also table accompanying *fatty acid.*

er•u•cism (er′u-siz″əm) caterpillar dermatitis.

eruc•ta•tion (ə-rək-ta′shən) [L. *eructatio*] the casting up of wind from the stomach through the mouth. Called also *belching.*

erup•tion (ĕ-rup′shən) [L. *eruptio* a breaking out] 1. a breaking out, appearing, or becoming visible. 2. any of various skin lesions due to disease; see also *exanthem* and *rash.* 3. tooth e.

active e. the continued eruption of the teeth after complete formation of their dentinal roots, consisting of movement of the teeth in the direction of the occlusal plane, and being coordinated with attrition.

continuous e. a concept that tooth eruption continues throughout life and does not cease when teeth meet their functional antagonists. See also *active e.* and *passive e.*

creeping e. 1. the development of migratory lesions corresponding to the movements of parasites beneath the skin of a human or other animal, such as occurs in cutaneous larva migrans and cutaneous myiasis. 2. cutaneous larva migrans.

delayed e. see under *dentition.*

drug e. an adverse cutaneous reaction produced by ingestion, parenteral use, or local application of a drug, which may produce various morphologic patterns and types of lesions. Called also *drug-induced dermatitis, dermatitis medicamentosa,* and *drug rash.*

fixed e. a circumscribed inflammatory skin lesion that recurs at the same site over a period of months or years; each attack lasts only a few days but leaves residual, cumulative pigmentation.

fixed drug e. a drug eruption that recurs at the same site (as a *fixed eruption*).

juvenile spring e. a type of polymorphic light eruption seen on the ears of young people, usually males.

Kaposi varicelliform e. a generalized and serious vesiculopustular, umbilicated eruption of viral origin, superimposed upon a preexisting atopic dermatitis; it may be caused by herpes simplex virus (eczema herpeticum), vaccinia virus (eczema vaccinatum), or a few other viruses.

passive e. the apparent eruption of a tooth that is actually the exposure of the crown of the tooth by separation of the epithelial attachment from the enamel and migration to the cementoenamel junction.

polymorphic light e. a common type of idiopathic photodermatosis in which lesions may be papular, papulovesicular, nodular, eczematoid, or plaquelike.

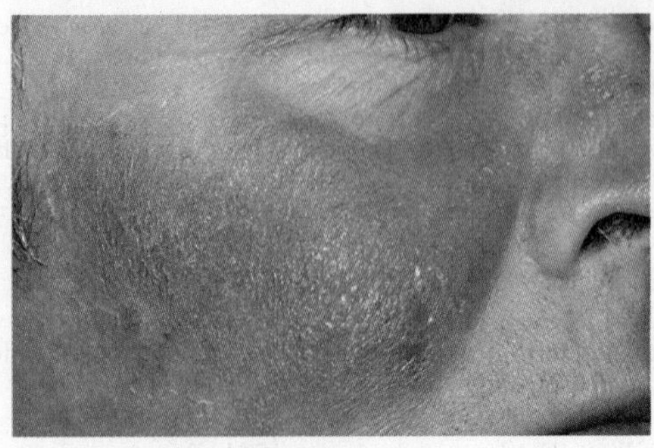

■ Erysipelas with characteristic sharply defined erythema and edema.

polymorphic e. of pregnancy pruritic urticarial papules and plaques of pregnancy; see under *plaque.*

pustular e., pustular drug e. acute generalized exanthematous pustulosis.

seabather's e. cercarial dermatitis.

serum e. an eruption or exanthem accompanying serum sickness.

surgical e. surgical removal of tissue blocking an unerupted tooth to permit eruption.

tooth e. the final stage of odontogenesis, in which a tooth breaks out from its crypt through surrounding tissue.

erup•tive (e-rup′tiv) pertaining to or characterized by eruption.

ERV expiratory reserve volume.

Er•win•ia (ər-win′e-ə) [*Erwin* F. Smith, American bacteriologist, 1854–1927] a genus of gram-negative, facultatively anaerobic, rod-shaped bacteria of the family Enterobacteriaceae, made up of plant pathogens, epiphytes, and saprophytes.

E. caroto′vora *Pectobacterium carotovora.*

E. herbi′cola a former species whose members are now included in *Pantoea agglomerans.*

Er•yc (er′ik) trademark for a preparation of erythromycin.

Ery•cette (er′ĭ-set) trademark for a preparation of erythromycin.

Ery•Derm (er′ĭ-dərm) trademark for a preparation of erythromycin.

Ery•gel (er′ĭ-jel) trademark for a preparation of erythromycin.

Ery•max (er′ĭ-maks) trademark for a preparation of erythromycin.

Ery•Ped (er′ə-ped) trademark for preparations of erythromycin ethylsuccinate.

er•y•sip•e•las (er″ə-sip′ə-ləs) [Gr. *erythros* red + *pella* skin] an acute superficial form of cellulitis involving the dermal lymphatics, usually caused by infection with group A streptococci. Characteristics include a peripherally spreading hot, bright red, edematous, brawny, infiltrated plaque with a circumscribed, raised, indurated border. Formerly called *St. Anthony fire.* **erysipel′atous** *adj*

coast e. (Sp. *erisipela de la costa*), a cutaneous manifestation of onchocerciasis seen in Central America, so called because of its resemblance to streptococcal erysipelas, characterized by an erythematous macular rash and edema of the face; in chronic cases the skin loses its elasticity, atrophies, becomes wrinkled, and causes leonine facies.

gangrenous e., necrotizing e. necrotizing fasciitis.

swine e. a contagious disease of swine caused by *Erysipelothrix rhusiopathiae.* It is of great economic importance around the world and occurs in four clinical forms: an *acute septicemic form,* marked by high fever, lesions of the internal organs and viscera, and a high mortality rate; an *urticarial form* (called also *diamonds* or *diamond skin disease*), the mildest form, rarely fatal, marked by sudden onset, high fever, general debility, red to purple blotches on the neck and body, and sometimes involvement of the viscera; a *chronic form,* sometimes fatal, marked by difficulty in breathing and vegetative endocarditis; and an *arthritic form,* not usually fatal, marked by stunting of growth; this form may occur alone or as a complication of other forms.

er•y•sip•e•loid (er″ə-sip′ə-loid) [*erysipelas* + *-oid*] 1. bacterial cellulitis due to infection with *Erysipelothrix rhusiopathiae,* usually occurring as an occupational disease associated with the handling of infected fish, shellfish, meat, or poultry. It presents in three forms: a *localized form,* usually self-limited and mild, manifested by an erythematous and painful swelling at the site of inoculation, which spreads peripherally with central clearing; a *generalized* or *diffuse form,* which may be accompanied by fever and arthritis symptoms and resolves spontaneously; and a rare *systemic form* associated with endocarditis that is sometimes fatal. 2. loosely, erysipelas-like.

Er•y•sip•e•lo•thrix (er″ə-sip′ə-lo-thriks″) [*erysipelas* + Gr. *thrix* hair] a genus of bacteria of the family Erysipelotrichaceae, consisting of gram-positive, asporogenous, rod-shaped organisms that form long filaments.

They occur as parasites in mammals, birds, and fish. The type species is *E. rhusiopa'thiae.*

E. rhusiopa'thiae a commonly seen species that causes swine erysipelas in pigs and erysipeloid in humans.

er•y•sip•e•lo•tox•in (er″ə-sip′ə-lo-tok″sin) the toxin produced by certain strains of *Streptococcus pyogenes* in bacterial erysipelas.

Ery•si•pe•lo•tri•cha•ceae (er″ə-sip″ə-lo-trĭ-ka′se-e) a family of bacteria incertae sedis of the class Mollicutes, consisting of gram-positive, straight or slightly curved, slender rods; organisms are nonmotile, aerobic to anaerobic, non–spore-forming, and chemo-organotrophic. It includes the genera *Erysipelothrix* and *Holdemania.*

Er•ys•i•pha•ceae (er-is″ĭ-fa′se-e) a family of fungi of the order Erysiphales, consisting of plant pathogens; it includes the genus *Erysiphe.*

er•ys•i•phake (er-is′ĭ-fāk) [Gr. *erysis* a drawing + *phakos* lentil] an instrument for removing a cataractous lens by suction. Cf. *phacoerysis.*

Er•ys•i•pha•les (er-is″ĭ-fa′lēz) the powdery mildews, an order of perfect fungi of the subphylum Ascomycotina, series Bitunicatae, which are parasitic on higher plants such as grapes and usually have closed ascocarps and large spherical stalked asci; it includes the family Erysiphaceae.

Er•ys•i•phe (er-is′ĭ-fe) a genus of powdery mildews, fungi of the family Erysiphaceae. *E. polygo'ni* attacks many species of fruits and vegetables. The imperfect (sexual) stage is *Oidium.*

Ery-Sol (er′ĭ-sol) trademark for a preparation of erythromycin.

Ery-Tab (er′ĭ-tab) trademark for a preparation of erythromycin.

er•y•the•ma (er″ə-the′mə) [Gr. *erythēma* flush upon the skin] redness of the skin produced by congestion of the capillaries. **erythem'atous** *adj*

acral e. erythema localized to the palms and soles, as in hand-foot syndrome.

e. annula're 1. gyrate erythema in which the lesions are ring shaped. 2. e. marginatum.

e. annula're centri'fugum an often mild but chronic and recurrent form of gyrate erythema characterized by ring-shaped, wheallike lesions with edematous, sometimes vesicular, borders and often a yellow central region with fine branny scaling; the lesions may coalesce. Called also *e. figuratum perstans* and *e. gyratum perstans.*

e. annula're rheuma'ticum e. marginatum.

e. area'ta mi'grans benign migratory glossitis.

e. arthri'ticum epide'micum Haverhill fever.

blanchable e. erythema that temporarily turns pale or white when pressure is applied; this is usually a normal reaction. Cf. *nonblanchable e.*

e. calo'ricum erythema caused by exposure to either heat *(e. ab igne)* or cold *(cold e.).*

e. chro'nicum mi'grans a deep form of gyrate erythema seen in Lyme disease. At the site of the tick bite a red papule develops and expands slowly, producing an annular lesion with central clearing.

chronic e. nodosum subacute nodular migratory panniculitis.

e. circina'tum, e. circina'tum rheuma'ticum e. marginatum.

cold e. a congenital hypersensitivity to cold seen in children, characterized by localized pain, widespread erythema, occasional muscle spasms, and vascular collapse on exposure to cold; some children cannot drink cold liquids without vomiting.

diaper e. see under *dermatitis.*

e. dyschro'micum per'stans an idiopathic dermatosis first identified in dark-skinned individuals in various countries in Latin America, but now seen elsewhere. Characteristics include single or multiple sharply demarcated gray macules of variable size and shape, which in their acute phase have a fine erythematous border. Some authorities consider it a variant of lichen planus. Called also *ashy dermatitis* and *ashy dermatosis of Ramirez.*

e. eleva'tum diu'tinum a benign cutaneous, small vessel vasculitis of unknown etiology characterized by pink or purple nodules and plaques, usually on the limbs and buttocks, sometimes with erosions or ulcers.

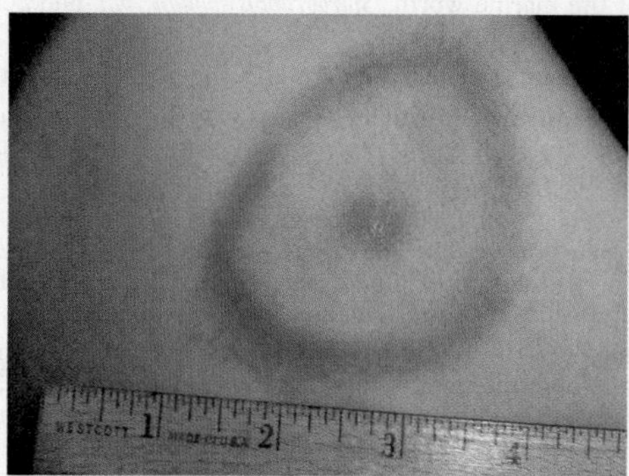

■ Erythema chronicum migrans.

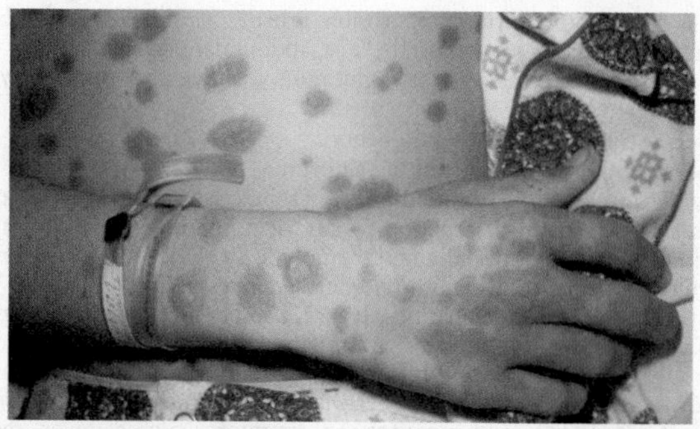

■ Erythema multiforme rash with discrete target lesions of the trunk and extremity, with confluence distally; dorsal wrist lesions have central bullae.

The lesions contain polymorphonuclear neutrophils and nuclear fragments that infiltrate vessel walls, which become fibrotic.

epidemic e. acrodynia.

epidemic arthritic e. Haverhill fever.

figurate e., e. figura'tum gyrate e.

e. figura'tum per'stans e. annulare centrifugum.

e. fu'gax erythema that comes and goes quickly.

gyrate e., e. gyra'tum erythema multiforme characterized by lesions of a variety of shapes, such as rings, arcs, or meshes, which tend to migrate and spread peripherally with central clearing. There are three basic types: *e. annulare centrifugum, e. chronicum migrans,* and *e. gyratum repens.* Called also *figurate e.* and *e. figuratum.*

e. gyra'tum per'stans e. annulare centrifugum.

e. gyra'tum re'pens a superficial form of gyrate erythema almost always associated with internal malignancy; it is characterized by migratory, elevated wavy bands having a scaly collarette and appearing over the entire body; it may be accompanied by pruritus.

e. ab ig'ne permanent erythema or a brown to red reticulated residual pigmentation produced by prolonged exposure to excessive radiant heat; it is seen most often on the lower limbs but under appropriate environmental circumstances can occur anywhere on the body.

indurated e., e. indura'tum 1. a type of predominantly lobular panniculitis of uncertain etiology, seen in young and middle-aged women, often seen in patients with cutaneous tuberculosis. It is initiated or exacerbated by cold weather and usually presents as recurrent erythrocyanotic nodules or plaques on the calves, with granulomas, vasculitis, and caseation; it sometimes progresses to form deep-seated indurations, ulcerations, and scars. 2. sometimes limited to those cases in which patients also have cutaneous tuberculosis, with nontubercular types being called *nodular vasculitis.* Called also *Bazin disease.*

e. infectio'sum a moderately contagious, often benign epidemic disease seen mainly in children and caused by B19 virus; the primary characteristic is a rash of abrupt onset that begins as redness of the cheeks, which appear to have been slapped; later there is a maculopapular rash on the trunk and limbs; when this fades,there may be central clearing that leaves a lacelike pattern. Immunocompromised patients may develop severe cases. Called also *fifth disease.*

e. i'ris target lesion (def. 3).

Jacquet e. diaper dermatitis.

e. margina'tum, e. margina'tum rheuma'ticum a superficial, often asymptomatic, form of gyrate erythema sometimes seen with rheumatic fever; it is characterized by transient eruption on the trunk and extensor surfaces of the limbs of multiple flat, indurated lesions. Called also *e. annulare, e. annulare rheumaticum, e. circinatum, e. circinatum rheumaticum,* and *e. marginatum.*

e. mi'grans 1. benign migratory glossitis. 2. e. chronicum migrans.

e. multifor'me either of two conditions characterized by sudden eruption of erythematous papules, some of which evolve into target lesions consisting of a central papule surrounded by a discolored ring or rings. Both represent reactions of the skin and mucous membranes to factors such as viral skin infections (especially herpes simplex); agents (including drugs) that are ingested or irritate the skin; malignancy; or pregnancy. The milder type is called *e. multiforme minus,* and the more severe type is called *Stevens-Johnson syndrome.*

e. multifor'me ma'jus Stevens-Johnson syndrome.

e. multifor'me mi'nus a mild self-limited mucocutaneous form of erythema multiforme that sometimes has a prodrome of fever, cough, and pharyngitis. In addition to the characteristic target lesions, there may be erythematous macules and papules, purpura, and occasional vesiculobullous lesions that burn or itch slightly. Called also *Hebra disease.*

necrolytic migratory e. a generalized, symmetrical, scaling, eczematous dermatitis with migratory necrolysis of the upper epidermis, liquefaction of the granular layer, and formation of clefts in the subcorneal region.

There is flaccid bulla formation, erosion, crusting, and healing with hyperpigmentation. It may be seen on the face, abdominal or groin area, or lower limbs. There is often an associated glucagonoma. See also *glucagonoma syndrome*, under *syndrome*.

e. necro′ticans Lucio phenomenon.

e. neonato′rum e. toxicum neonatorum.

e. nodo′sum a type of predominantly septal panniculitis usually occurring as a hypersensitivity reaction to any of numerous provoking agents, including infections (especially beta-hemolytic streptococcal infections and tuberculosis); drugs (especially oral contraceptives and sulfonamides); sarcoidosis; and certain enteropathies. It may also be idiopathic. It most often affects young women, with transient, inflammatory, nonulcerating nodules that are tender, multiple, and bilateral, usually on the shins. Lesions involute slowly, leaving bruiselike patches without scarring. The acute disease is often associated with mild constitutional symptoms such as fever, malaise, and arthralgias. A chronic variant sometimes occurs without serious associated systemic disease. See also *e. nodosum migrans.*

e. nodo′sum lepro′sum the type 1 kind of lepra reaction; it resembles an Arthus reaction, and usually occurs during chemotherapy for lepromatous or borderline lepromatous leprosy, although occasionally it appears spontaneously. It is usually characterized by vasculitis with small erythematous, tender cutaneous nodules or plaques widely distributed on the face and limbs, and it may be associated with severe systemic or visceral symptoms. Cf. *Lucio phenomenon.*

e. nodo′sum mi′grans subacute nodular migratory panniculitis.

nonblanchable e. erythema that persists when pressure is applied, seen in an early stage of pressure ulcer formation.

palmar e., e. palma′re persistent redness of the palms, which may be seen in pregnancy, liver disease, rheumatoid arthritis, regional ileitis, or skin diseases such as psoriasis, pityriasis rubra pilaris, and genodermatoses. One rare form is an autosomal dominant condition.

e. per′nio chilblain.

e. per′stans e. annula′re centri′fugum.

solar e., e. sola′re sunburn.

e. strepto′genes pityriasis alba.

toxic e. of chemotherapy erythema, usually the acral type, caused by a reaction to a chemotherapeutic agent.

e. tox′icum, e. tox′icum neonato′rum a common benign, idiopathic, generalized, transient eruption seen in infants during the first week of life, usually consisting of small papules or pustules that become sterile, light colored, firm vesicles surrounded by an erythematous halo and edema. Called also *e. neonatorum.*

er•y•them•a•to•edem•a•tous (er″ĭ-thēm″ə-to″ĕ-dem′ə-təs) pertaining to or affected by both erythema and edema.

er•y•the•mo•gen•ic (er″ĭ-the″mo-jen′ik) causing erythema.

er•y•thral•gia (er″ə-thral′jə) erythromelalgia.

er•y•thras•ma (er″ə-thraz′mə) a chronic, superficial bacterial infection of the skin involving the body folds and toe webs, sometimes becoming generalized, caused by *Corynebacterium minutissimum.* It is characterized by sharply demarcated, dry, brown, scaly, slowly spreading patches.

er•y•thre•mia (er″ə-thre′me-ə) [*erythro-* + *-emia*] polycythemia vera.

er•y•thre•mic (er″ə-thre′mik) pertaining to erythroid cells, particularly to those occurring in the blood in abnormal numbers or exhibiting abnormal development.

Er•y•thri•na (er″ə-thri′nə) a genus of tropical shrubs and trees of the family Leguminosae, long used in folk medicine; several species yield the alkaloids α-erythroidine and β-erythroidine.

eryth•rism (ə-rith′riz-əm) redness of the skin and hair of an animal; for humans this means having a ruddy complexion. **erythris′tic** *adj*

eryth•ri•tol (ə-rith′rĭ-tol) a four-carbon sugar formed from erythrose by reduction of the carbonyl group and occurring in algae, lichens, grasses, and several fungi; it is about twice as sweet as sucrose and is used as a low-calorie sweetener.

erythr(o)- [Gr. *erythros* red] a combining form denoting a relationship to red or to erythrocytes.

eryth•ro•blast (ə-rith′ro-blast) [*erythro-* + *-blast*] a term originally used to indicate any type of nucleated erythrocyte, but now usually limited to one of the nucleated precursors of an erythrocyte, i.e. one of the developmental stages in the erythrocytic series (q.v.), in contrast to a megaloblast. In this usage, it is called also *normoblast.* **erythroblas′tic** *adj*

acidophilic e. orthochromatic e.

basophilic e. see under *normoblast.*

definitive e's basophilic cells in the primordium of the liver that give rise to the mature non-nucleated erythrocytes; cf. *primordial e's.*

early e. basophilic normoblast.

eosinophilic e. orthochromatic e.

intermediate e. polychromatophilic e.

late e., orthochromatic e., oxyphilic e. the final stage of the nucleated, immature erythrocyte, before nuclear loss. Typically the cytoplasm is described as acidophilic, but it still shows a faint polychromatic tint. The nucleus is small and initially may still have coarse, clumped chromatin, as in its precursor, the polychromatophilic erythroblast, but ultimately it becomes pyknotic, and appears as a deeply staining, blue-black, homogeneous structureless mass. The nucleus is often eccentric and sometimes lobulated. Called also *acidophilic e., eosinophilic e.,* and *acidophilic, eosinophilic,* or *orthochromatic normoblast.*

polychromatic e., polychromatophilic e. a nucleated, immature erythrocyte in which the nucleus occupies a relatively smaller part of the cell than in its precursor, the basophilic erythroblast. The cytoplasm is beginning to acquire hemoglobin and thus is no longer a purely blue color, but takes on an acidophilic tint, which becomes progressively more marked as the cell matures. The chromatin of the nucleus is arranged in coarse, deeply staining clumps. Called also *intermediate e., intermediate, polychromatic,* or *polychromatophilic normoblast,* and *rubricyte.*

primitive e's, primordial e's cells arising from the blood islands of the yolk sac which are the precursors of the nucleated erythrocytes characteristic of the early embryo; cf. *definitive e's.*

eryth•ro•blas•te•mia (ə-rith″ro-blas-te′me-ə) erythroblastosis (def. 1).

eryth•ro•blas•to•ma (ə-rith″ro-blas-to′mə) a tumorlike mass composed of erythroblasts.

eryth•ro•blas•to•pe•nia (ə-rith″ro-blas″to-pe′ne-ə) abnormal deficiency of the erythroblasts, such as in an aplastic crisis.

transient e. of childhood temporary aplasia of erythropoietic tissue in young children, usually with anemia; the etiology is unknown, although there has often been a viral illness within the previous two months. The condition almost always resolves spontaneously without recurring.

eryth•ro•blas•to•sis (ə-rith″ro-blas-to′sis) 1. the presence in the peripheral blood of abnormally large numbers of erythroblasts (nucleated red cells); called also *erythroblastemia.* 2. one of the avian leukosis complex of diseases, a condition of fowl marked by increased erythroblasts in the circulating blood, with weakness, pallor, diarrhea, and spontaneous hemorrhages. Called also *erythroid leukosis* and *erythroleukosis.*

e. feta′lis, e. neonato′rum a type of hemolytic anemia of the fetus or newborn infant, caused by the transplacental transmission of maternally formed antibody, usually secondary to an incompatibility between the blood group of the mother and that of her offspring. The most common and frequently fatal type occurs when the baby or fetus is Rh positive and the mother is Rh negative. Another type is found in babies or fetuses of blood groups A and B whose mothers have type O blood; it is much milder than the Rh type because anti-A and anti-B antibodies only occasionally cross the placenta. Characteristics include accelerated destruction of erythrocytes, causing jaundice, increased red cell regeneration (nucleated red cells in the blood), and hepatosplenomegaly. In infants with severe jaundice, kernicterus may result. The most severe form is *hydrops fetalis.* Called also *congenital* or *hemolytic anemia of newborn* and *hemolytic disease of newborn.*

eryth•ro•blas•tot•ic (ə-rith″ro-blas-tot′ik) pertaining to or characterized by erythroblastosis.

eryth•ro•chro•mia (ə-rith″ro-kro′me-ə) [*erythro-* + *chrom-* + *-ia*] hemorrhagic pigmentation of the spinal fluid, giving it a red color.

Eryth•ro•cin (ə-rith′ro-sin) trademark for preparations of erythromycin.

er•y•throc•la•sis (er″ə-throk′lə-sis) [*erythro-* + Gr. *klasis* a breaking] fragmentation or splitting up of erythrocytes. Cf. *hemolysis.*

eryth•ro•clast (ə-rith′ro-klast) [*erythro-* + *-klast*] ghost cell.

eryth•ro•clas•tic (ə-rith″ro-klas′tik) 1. pertaining to or characterized by erythroclasis. 2. causing or producing erythroclasis.

eryth•ro•cru•o•rin (ə-rith″ro-kroo′ə-rin) a respiratory protein from the blood of the marine worm, *Spirographis spallanzanii,* and certain other worms.

eryth•ro•cu•prein (ə-rith″ro-koo′prēn) superoxide dismutase.

eryth•ro•cy•a•no•sis (ə-rith″ro-si″ə-no′sis) [*erythro-* + *cyanosis*] a slight swelling and a blue or pink tint to the skin of the lower limbs after prolonged exposure to cold; it is more common in girls and young women.

eryth•ro•cy•ta•phe•re•sis (ə-rith″ro-si″tə-fə-re′sis) [*erythrocyte* + *apheresis*] the withdrawal of blood, separation and retention of red blood cells, and retransfusion of the remainder into the donor.

eryth•ro•cyte (ə-rith′ro-sīt) [*erythro-* + *-cyte*] one of the elements found in peripheral blood; the normal mature form is a non-nucleated, yellowish, biconcave disk, adapted by virtue of its configuration and its hemoglobin content to the transport of oxygen. For immature forms, see *erythrocytic series,* under *series.* Called also *red blood cell* or *corpuscle* and *red cell* or *corpuscle.*

achromic e. achromocyte.

basophilic e. an abnormal erythrocyte that takes on basic stains; see *basophilia* (def. 1).

burr e., crenated e. burr cell.

hypochromic e. an erythrocyte with less than the normal concentration of hemoglobin, so that it appears paler than normal; it is usually also microcytic. Cf. *normochromic e.*

immature e. 1. normoblast. 2. erythroblast.

Mexican hat e. target cell.

normochromic e. an erythrocyte that has normal color and a normal concentration of hemoglobin, as opposed to a hypochromic erythrocyte. See also *orthochromatic erythroblast.*

nucleated e. 1. normoblast. 2. erythroblast.

polychromatic e., polychromatophilic e. an erythrocyte that, on staining, shows various shades of blue, combined with tinges of pink.

target e. see under *cell.*

eryth•ro•cy•the•mia (ə-rith″ro-si-the′me-ə) polycythemia.

eryth•ro•cyt•ic (ə-rith″ro-sit′ik) 1. pertaining to, characterized by, or of the nature of erythrocytes. 2. pertaining to the erythrocytic series; see under *series.*

eryth•ro•cy•to•blast (ə-rith″ro-si′to-blast) erythroblast.

eryth•ro•cy•tol•y•sin (ə-rith″ro-si-tol′ə-sin) hemolysin.

eryth•ro•cy•tol•y•sis (ə-rith″ro-si-tol′ə-sis) hemolysis.

eryth•ro•cy•tom•e•ter (ə-rith″ro-si-tom′ə-tər) [*erythrocyte* + *-meter*] a device for measuring or counting erythrocytes.

eryth•ro•cy•tom•e•try (ə-rith″ro-si-tom′ə-try) the measurement or counting of erythrocytes.

eryth•ro•cy•to•pe•nia (ə-rith″ro-si″to-pe′ne-ə) erythropenia.

eryth•ro•cy•toph•a•gy (ə-rith″ro-si-tof′ə-je) erythrophagocytosis. erythrocytoph′agous *adj*

eryth•ro•cy•to•poi•e•sis (ə-rith″ro-si″to-poi-e′sis) erythropoiesis.

eryth•ro•cy•tor•rhex•is (ə-rith″ro-si″to-rek′sis) [*erythrocyte* + *-rrhexis*] partial erythrocytoschisis with splitting off of particles and escape from the cells of round, shiny granules. Called also *erythrorrhexis.*

eryth•ro•cy•tos•chi•sis (ə-rith″ro-si-tos′kĭ-sis) [*erythrocyte* + *-schisis*] a morphological change in erythrocytes consisting of their degeneration into disklike bodies similar to platelets. See also *schistocytosis.*

eryth•ro•cy•to•sis (ə-rith″ro-si-to′sis) secondary polycythemia.

benign e., stress e. stress polycythemia.

eryth•ro•cy•tu•ria (ə-rith″ro-si-tu′re-ə) hematuria.

eryth•ro•de•gen•er•a•tive (ə-rith″ro-de-jen′ər-a″tiv) characterized by degeneration of erythrocytes; see also *hemolysis.*

eryth•ro•der•ma (ə-rith″ro-dur′mə) [*erythro-* + *derma*] 1. abnormal redness of the skin, usually meaning that it is over widespread areas of the body. 2. exfoliative dermatitis. Called also *erythrodermia.*

e. desquamati′vum Leiner disease.

exfoliative e. see under *dermatitis.*

nonbullous congenital ichthyosiform e. a genetically heterogeneous, autosomal recessive condition characterized by erythroderma and fine, white, semiadherent scales; other features include palmoplantar hyperkeratosis, nail dystrophy, and sparse hair. Most infants present as collodion babies.

psoriatic e., e. psoria′ticum erythrodermic psoriasis.

Sézary e. see under *syndrome.*

eryth•ro•der•mia (ə-rith″ro-dur′me-ə) erythroderma.

eryth•ro•dex•trin (ə-rith″ro-dek′strin) any of the class of water-soluble dextrins staining red with iodine and formed by partial hydrolysis of starch.

eryth•ro•don•tia (ə-rith″ro-don′shə) [*erythro-* + *odont-* + *-ia*] red to brown discoloration of the teeth.

eryth•ro•dys•es•the•sia (e-rith″ro-dis″es-the′zhə) erythema accompanied by dysesthesias of touch.

acral e., palmar-plantar e., palmoplantar e. hand-foot syndrome.

eryth•ro•gen (ə-rith′ro-jən) a fatty, crystalline compound from diseased bile.

eryth•ro•gen•e•sis (ə-rith″ro-jen′ə-sis) erythropoiesis.

e. imperfec′ta congenital hypoplastic anemia (def. 1).

eryth•ro•gen•ic (ə-rith″ro-jen′ik) [*erythro-* + *-genic*] 1. erythropoietic. 2. producing a sensation of red. 3. erythemogenic.

eryth•roid (ə-rith′roid, er′ĭ-throid″) 1. of a red color; reddish. 2. pertaining to any of the cells in the developmental series ending in erythrocytes; see *erythrocytic series,* under *series.*

eryth•ro•ker•a•to•der•ma (ə-rith″ro-ker″ə-to-dur′mə) erythrokeratodermia.

eryth•ro•ker•a•to•der•mia (ə-rith″ro-ker″ə-to-dur′me-ə) erythema with hyperkeratosis.

e. progressi′va symmet′rica, progressive symmetric e. a rare syndrome of aberrant keratinization, having variable inheritance; affected children develop verrucous plaques in symmetric distributions, especially over joints.

e. varia′bilis a rare autosomal dominant condition present at birth, characterized by both transient, migratory areas of erythroderma in various shapes and fixed plaques of hyperkeratosis. Called also *keratoderma palmoplantare transgrediens* and *keratosis palmoplantaris transgrediens.*

eryth•ro•ki•net•ics (ə-rith″ro-kĭ-net′iks) [*erythro-* + *kinetics*] the kinetics of erythrocytes, described by laboratory measurements of total red cell volume, rate of red cell production, and red cell life span (rate of destruction).

er•yth•rol (er′ith-rol) erythritol.

er•y•thro•lein (er″ə-thro′lēn) the ether-soluble fraction of the acid-precipitable part of the water-soluble pigments of litmus, occurring as a red oily substance.

eryth•ro•leu•ke•mia (ə-rith″ro-loo-ke′me-ə) a malignant blood dyscrasia, one of the myeloproliferative disorders, characterized by neoplastic proliferation of erythroblastic and myeloblastic elements, with atypical erythroblasts and myeloblasts in the peripheral blood. Symptoms are progressive anemia, myeloblastic erythroid hyperplasia, myeloid dysplasia, hepatosplenomegaly, and hemorrhagic phenomena. It may follow an acute or chronic course. Called also *Di Guglielmo syndrome* and *erythremic myelosis.*

acute e. a form of acute myelogenous leukemia representing erythroleukemia in which malignant precursors of leukocytes have proliferated and become predominant; called also *Di Guglielmo syndrome.*

eryth•ro•leu•ko•blas•to•sis (ə-rith″ro-loo″ko-blas-to′sis) icterus gravis neonatorum.

eryth•ro•leu•ko•sis (ə-rith″ro-loo-ko′sis) erythroblastosis (def. 2).

eryth•ro•lit•min (ə-rith″ro-lit′min) the alcohol-soluble fraction of the acid-precipitable part of the water-soluble pigments of litmus, occurring as a bright red powder.

er•y•throl•y•sin (er″ə-throl′ə-sin) hemolysin.

er•y•throl•y•sis (er″ə-throl′ə-sis) hemolysis.

eryth•ro•mel•al•gia (ə-rith″ro-məl-al′jə) [*erythro-* + *melalgia*] a disease affecting the feet and sometimes the hands, marked by paroxysmal, bilateral vasodilation with burning pain, increased skin temperature, and redness. Called also *acromelalgia* and *Gerhardt* or *Weir Mitchell disease.*

e. of the head cluster headache.

eryth•ro•mel•a•no•sis (ə-rith″ro-mel″ə-no′sis) erythrosis with melanosis.

e. follicula′ris fa′ciei a skin disorder seen most often in persons of East Asian ancestry, characterized by pinpoint papules over hair follicles on a red to red-brown patch of skin; some patients also have keratosis pilaris on their arms.

er•y•throm•e•ter (er″ə-throm′ə-tər) [*erythro-* + *-meter*] 1. an instrument or color scale for measuring degrees of redness. 2. erythrocytometer.

er•y•throm•e•try (er″ə-throm′ə-tre) 1. the measurement of the degree of redness. 2. erythrocytometry.

eryth•ro•my•cin (ə-rith″ro-mi′sin) [USP] a broad-spectrum macrolide antibiotic, produced by *Saccharopolyspora erythraea,* effective against most gram-positive and certain gram-negative bacteria, such as *Neisseria* species and *Haemophilus influenzae,* and against spirochetes, some rickettsias, and *Entamoeba;* it is also highly effective against *Mycoplasma pneumoniae.* It is used especially in patients allergic to penicillin and in those with penicillin-resistant infections and legionnaires' disease, and is also used in the prophylaxis of neonatal conjunctivitis and ophthalmia neonatorum, and in the treatment of acne vulgaris; administered orally as well as topically to the skin or to the conjunctiva.

e. estolate [USP] the lauryl sulfate ester of propionyl erythromycin, having the same actions as the base and administered orally as a systemic antibacterial and as an antiacne agent.

e. ethylsuccinate [USP] a salt of erythromycin having the same actions as the base; administered orally as a systemic antibacterial and as an antiacne agent. In combination with sulfisoxazole, it is used in the treatment of otitis media caused by *Haemophilus influenzae.*

e. gluceptate [USP] the glucoheptonate salt of erythromycin, having the same actions as the base; administered by intravenous infusion as a systemic antibacterial.

e. lactobionate [USP] a salt of erythromycin, having the same actions and uses as e. gluceptate.

e. stearate [USP] the stearate salt of erythromycin, having the same actions as the base; administered orally as a systemic antibacterial and an antiacne agent.

eryth·ro·my·elo·blas·to·sis (ə-rith″ro-mi″ə-lo-blas-to′sis) myeloblastosis (def. 2).

er·y·thron (er′ə-thron) [Gr. *erythros* red] the circulating erythrocytes in the blood, their precursors, and all the elements of the body concerned in their production. Cf. *leukon* and *thrombon.*

eryth·ro·neo·cy·to·sis (ə-rith″ro-ne″o-si-to′sis) [*erythro-* + *neo-* + *-cyte* + *-osis*] the presence of immature erythrocytes in the blood. Cf. *erythroblastosis.*

eryth·ro·par·a·site (ə-rith″ro-par′ə-sīt) a parasite of erythrocytes.

eryth·ro·pe·nia (ə-rith″ro-pe′ne-ə) [*erythro-* + *-penia*] deficiency in the number of erythrocytes; see also *anemia* and *pancytopenia.* Called also *erythrocytopenia.*

eryth·ro·phage (ə-rith′ro-fāj) [*erythro-* + *-phage*] a phagocyte that takes up erythrocytes and blood pigments.

eryth·ro·pha·gia (ə-rith″ro-fa′jə) erythrophagocytosis.

eryth·ro·phago·cy·to·sis (ə-rith″ro-fa″go-si-to′sis) [*erythro*cyte + *phagocytosis*] the engulfment or consumption of erythrocytes. Called also *erythrocytophagy* and *erythrophagia.* **erythrophagocyt′ic** *adj*

er·y·throph·a·gous (er″ĭ-throf′ə-gəs) erythrophagocytic.

eryth·ro·phil (ə-rith′ro-fil) [*erythro-* + *-phil*] 1. a cell or other element that is easily stained red. 2. erythrophilous.

er·y·throph·i·lous (er″ĭ-throf′ĭ-ləs) easily stained with red.

Eryth·ro·phloe·um (ə-rith″ro-fle′əm) [*erythro-* + Gr. *phloios* bark] a genus of trees of the family Leguminosae. *E. guineen′se* affords casca or Mancona bark, an African ordeal poison.

eryth·ro·pho·bia (ə-rith″ro-fo′be-ə) [*erythro-* + *-phobia*] 1. irrational fear of the color red, often accompanied by fear of blood (hematophobia). 2. fear of blushing; a distressing tendency to blush frequently.

eryth·ro·pho·bic (ə-rith″ro-fo′bik) having no affinity for red dye (acid fuchsin).

eryth·ro·phore (ə-rith′ro-for) [*erythro-* + *-phore*] a type of chromatophore containing granules of a red or brown alcohol-resistant pigment, found in the skin of many vertebrates.

eryth·ro·phose (ə-rith′ro-fōz) [*erythro-* + *phose*] any red phose.

eryth·ro·phyll (ə-rith′ro-fil″) [*erythro-* + Gr. *phyllon* leaf] a red coloring matter occurring in plants.

er·y·thro·pia (er″ə-thro′pe-ə) erythropsia.

eryth·ro·pla·kia (ə-rith″ro-pla′ke-ə) [*erythro-* + Gr. *plax* plate + *-ia*] a slow growing, erythematous, velvety red lesion with well-defined margins, occurring on a mucous membrane, most often in the oral cavity. It is usually associated with severe dysplasia or carcinoma, and occurs in middle-aged to older adults.

speckled e. a lesion in the oral cavity with characteristics of both erythroplakia and leukoplakia, yielding a speckled appearance. Called also *speckled leukoplakia.*

eryth·ro·pla·sia (ə-rith″ro-pla′zhə) a condition of the mucous membrane characterized by erythematous papular lesions.

e. of Queyrat penile intraepithelial neoplasia.

Zoon e. see under *balanitis.*

eryth·ro·plas·tid (ə-rith″ro-plas′tid) an erythrocyte that has no nucleus, such as the type normal in mammals.

eryth·ro·poi·e·sis (ə-rith″ro-poi-e′sis) [*erythro-* + *-poiesis*] the production of erythrocytes; in the fetus and neonate it takes place in the spleen and bone marrow, but in older individuals it is confined to the bone marrow. Called also *erythrocytopoiesis* and *erythrogenesis.*

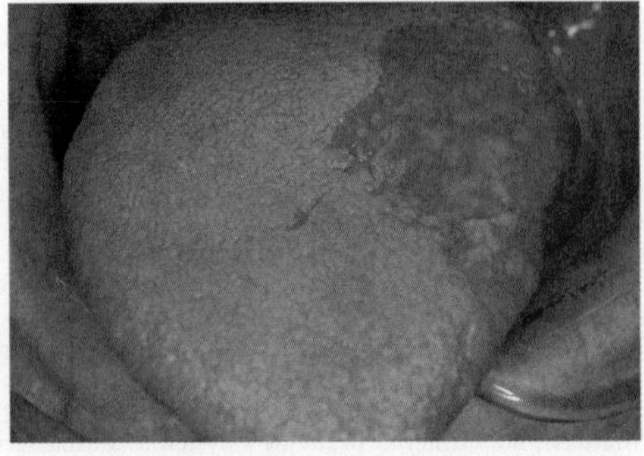

■ Erythroplakia of the tongue.

eryth·ro·poi·et·ic (ə-rith″ro-poi-et′ik) 1. pertaining to or characterized by erythropoiesis. 2. promoting erythropoiesis. Called also *erythrogenic.*

eryth·ro·poi·e·tin (ə-rith″ro-poi′ə-tin) a glycoprotein hormone secreted chiefly by the kidney in the adult and by the liver in the fetus, which acts on the bone marrow cells to stimulate erythropoiesis. Called also *hematopoietin* and *hemopoietin.*

recombinant human e. (r-HuEPO) epoetin.

eryth·ro·pros·o·pal·gia (ə-rith″ro-pros″o-pal′jə) [*erythro-* + *prosopalgia*] a disorder similar to erythromelalgia, but with the redness and pain in the face.

er·y·throp·sia (er″ə-throp′se-ə) [*erythro-* + *-opsia*] a chromatopsia in which all objects appear to have a red tinge, a symptom of aphakia.

er·y·throp·sin (er″ə-throp′sin) [*erythro-* + *opsin*] rhodopsin.

eryth·ro·pyk·no·sis (ə-rith″ro-pik-no′sis) pyknocytosis.

eryth·ror·rhex·is (ə-rith″ro-rek′sis) erythrocytorrhexis.

er·y·throse (ĕ-rith′rōs) an aldotetrose occurring in phosphorylated form (erythrose 4-phosphate) as an intermediate in the pentose phosphate pathway.

eryth·ro·sin (ə-rith′ro-sin) a red compound, used as a histologic stain.

eryth·ro·sine so·di·um (ə-rith′ro-sēn) a coloring agent used to disclose plaque on teeth; applied topically in solution, or tablets containing erythrosine sodium are chewed, after which the mouth is rinsed with water.

er·y·thro·sis (er″ə-thro′sis) a red to purple discoloration of the skin and mucous membranes, caused by capillary dilatation, such as in polycythemia vera.

eryth·ro·sta·sis (ə-rith″ro-sta′sis) the stoppage of erythrocytes in the capillaries, as in sickle cell anemia.

eryth·ro·thi·o·neine (ə-rith″ro-thi′ə-nēn) ergothioneine.

Eryth·ro·vi·rus (ə-rith′ro-vi″rəs) [*erythro-* + *virus*] a genus of viruses of the subfamily Parvovirinae (family Parvoviridae) containing viruses that infect erythrocyte progenitor cells; there is a single species, B19 virus.

Ery·throx·y·lon (er-ĭ-throk′sə-lon) a genus of South American trees and shrubs. *E. co′ca* is a shrub native to Andean regions whose leaves are a source of coca.

eryth·ru·lose (ə-rith′roo-lōs) the sole ketotetrose, an isomer of erythrose.

er·y·thru·ria (er″ĭ-throo′re-ə) [*erythr-* + *-uria*] chromaturia in which the urine is red.

Es einsteinium.

es·cape (əs-kāp′) the act of becoming free.

aldosterone e. a secondary response to the continuous presence of mineralocorticoids, in which the usual renal sodium-retaining effects of mineralocorticoids are time-limited, so that excessive retention of salt and water is limited.

atrioventricular junctional e. the occurrence of one or more escape beats in which the atrioventricular node acts as the cardiac pacemaker; see also under *beat* and *rhythm.*

nodal e. atrioventricular junctional e.

vagal e. the exhaustion of or adaptation to neural chemical mediators in the regulation of systemic arterial pressure.

ventricular e. the occurrence of one or more ectopic beats in which a ventricular pacemaker becomes effective before the pacemaker in the sinoatrial node. See also under *beat* and *rhythm.*

es·char (es′kahr) [Gr. *eschara* scab] 1. a slough produced by a thermal burn, by a corrosive application, or by gangrene. 2. the lesion seen in certain rickettsioses; see *tache noire.*

es·cha·rot·ic (es″kə-rot′ik) [Gr. *escharōtikos*] 1. corrosive to tissue. 2. an agent corrosive to tissue.

es·cha·rot·o·my (es″kə-rot′ə-me) surgical incision of the constricting eschar of a circumferentially burned limb in order to permit the cut edges to separate and restore blood flow to unburned tissue distal to the eschar.

Esch·e·rich bacillus (esh′ə-rik) [Theodor *Escherich*, German physician, 1857–1911] *Escherichia coli.*

Esch·e·rich·ia (esh″ə-rik′e-ə) [T. *Escherich*] a genus of gram-negative, facultatively anaerobic, rod-shaped bacteria of the family Enterobacteriaceae, found in the large intestines of many mammals and birds. Most species are nonpathogenic or opportunistic pathogens. This genus is a member of the "coliform" group of bacteria, their presence in water supplies being used as an indicator of fecal contamination. The type species is *E. cloa′cae.*

E. alber′tii a rare species that causes diarrhea in children.

E. co′li the principal species of the genus, a common facultative organism of the intestines of many different animals. The organisms are characteristically positive to indole and methyl red and negative to the

Voges-Proskauer and citrate tests; serovars are based on the distribution of heat-stable O antigens, envelope K antigens of varying heat stability, and flagellar H antigens that are heat labile. Most are nonpathogenic, but pathogenic strains producing fevers and diarrhea are common (see *colibacillosis*). The fever-causing strains are found in urinary tract infections, abscesses, conjunctivitis, and occasionally septicemic conditions such as *Winckel disease.* The enteropathogenic strains (EPEC) produce intestinal disease and diarrhea, especially in hospitalized infants and other baby animals. The enterotoxigenic strains (ETEC) cause diarrhea in piglets and calves and a choleralike disease in human infants and adults. Enteroinvasive serogroups (EIEC) related to *Shigella* invade the epithelial cells of the human colon, causing dysentery, sometimes associated with food poisoning. These often become the predominant bacteria in the flora of the mouth and throat during antibiotic therapy. Shiga toxin–producing groups (STEC, formerly called enterohemorrhagic, or EHEC) cause acute bloody diarrhea and hemolytic-uremic syndrome. A preparation of asparaginase derived from type EC-2 is used as an antineoplastic. Enteroadherent organisms (EAEC) are subdivided into enteroaggregative groups (EAggEC) (which adhere to the enteric mucosa to form colonies and can cause diarrhea in children), and diffusely adherent (DAEC) groups.

E. ferguso′nii a species isloated from human clinical specimens.

E. herma′nii a species that produces a yellow pigment, found in human clinical specimens.

E. vul′neris a species found in human clinical specimens.

Esch•scholt•zia (ə-shōlt′se-ə) a genus of plants of the family Papaveraceae. *E. califor′nica* Cham. is the California poppy, which is hypnotic and anodyne.

es•cin (es′kin) a strongly hemolytic saponin derived from the horse chestnut; it inhibits edema formation and reduces vascular fragility.

es•ci•tal•o•pram ox•a•late (es″i-tal′o-pram) a selective serotonin reuptake inhibitor (SSRI), the active *S*-isomer of citalopram, used as an antidepressant; administered orally.

Es•clim (es′klim) trademark for a preparation of estradiol.

Es•co•bar syndrome (es-ko-bahr′) [Victor *Escobar*, American dentist, 20th century] see under *syndrome.*

es•cu•lin (es′ku-lin) [L. *aesculus* horse-chestnut] a coumarin glycoside found in species of *Aesculus;* it has febrifuge properties but causes toxicity in livestock.

es•cutch•eon (es-kuch′ən) [L. *scutum* a shield] 1. a shield or something shaped like a shield. 2. the shieldlike pattern of distribution of the pubic hair.

esep•tate (e-sep′tāt) having no septa.

es•er•ine (es′ər-in) [*esere,* an African name of the Calabar bean] physostigmine.

ESF erythropoietic stimulating factor.

Es•gic (es′jik) trademark for combination preparations of butalbital, acetaminophen, and caffeine.

ESHAP a cancer chemotherapy regimen consisting of etoposide, methylprednisolone, ara-C (cytarabine), and Platinol (cisplatin).

Es•i•drix (es′ĭ-driks) trademark for a preparation of hydrochlorothiazide.

Es•i•mil (es′ĭ-mil) trademark for preparations of guanethidine monosulfate with hydrochlorothiazide.

-esis [Gr.] a word termination denoting action, process, or condition; see also *-sis.*

Es•ka•lith (es′kə-lith) trademark for preparations of lithium carbonate.

Es•march bandage (tourniquet) (es′mahrk) [Johann Friedrich August von *Esmarch*, German surgeon, 1823–1908] see under *bandage.*

es•march (es′mahrk) an Esmarch bandage.

ESMO European Society for Medical Oncology.

es•mo•lol hyd•ro•chlo•ride (es′mo-lol) a short-acting, cardioselective beta$_1$-blocker used as an antiarrhythmic in the short-term control of atrial fibrillation, atrial flutter, and noncompensatory sinus tachycardia; administered by intravenous infusion.

eso- [Gr. *esō* inward] a combining form meaning within.

eso•cata•pho•ria (es″o-kat″ə-for′e-ə) [*eso-* + *cataphoria*] a phoria in which the visual axes turn downward and inward.

eso•cine (es′o-sēn) a protamine from the sperm of the pike, *Esox lucius.*

eso•de•vi•a•tion (es″o-de″ve-a′shən) 1. esophoria. 2. esotropia.

es•o•mep•ra•zole mag•ne•si•um (es″o-mep′rə-zōl) a proton pump inhibitor used as a gastric acid secretion inhibitor in the treatment of symptomatic gastroesophageal reflux disease and in conjunction with antibiotics in the treatment of duodenal ulcer associated with *Helicobacter pylori* infection; administered orally.

esoph•a•gal•gia (ə-sof″ə-gal′ge-ə) [*esophag-* + *-algia*] pain in the esophagus; called also *esophagodynia.*

esoph•a•gec•to•my (ə-sof″ə-jek′tə-me) [*esophag-* + *-ectomy*] excision of part *(partial)* or all *(total)* of the esophagus.

Ivor Lewis e. transthoracic e.

transhiatal e. removal of the thoracic part of the esophagus by blunt dissection superiorly through a cervical incision and inferiorly with a transhiatal approach through an abdominal incision.

transthoracic e. removal of part or all of the thoracic part of the esophagus through abdominal and right thoracotomy incisions; called also *Ivor Lewis e.*

esoph•a•gism (ə-sof′ə-jiz-əm) diffuse esophageal spasm.

esoph•a•gis•mus (ə-sof″ə-jiz′məs) diffuse esophageal spasm.

esoph•a•gi•tis (ə-sof″ə-ji′tis) [*esophag-* + *-itis*] inflammation of the esophagus.

alkaline reflux e. inflammation of the esophagus resulting from repeated and prolonged contact with alkaline intestinal contents following gastrectomy.

***Candida* e., candidal e.** fungal esophagitis caused by *Candida* species.

caustic e. corrosive e.

chronic peptic e. reflux e.

corrosive e. esophagitis following ingestion of a caustic or corrosive substance, usually strongly alkaline or acid, such as when a child ingests a household cleaner. Injury may be limited to superficial mucosa or may extend deeper. Called also *caustic e.*

e. dis′secans superficia′lis infection of the esophagus, with sloughing of the squamous epithelial lining in the form of a tubular cast.

eosinophilic e. inflammation caused by eosinophilic infiltration of the esophageal mucosa; the etiology is unknown, although it sometimes accompanies gastroesophageal reflux disease and sometimes may be an allergic reaction.

fungal e. esophagitis caused by invasion of the epithelium by a fungus, usually a species of *Candida;* the incidence is increased among those with diabetes mellitus, hypoparathyroidism, adrenal insufficiency, or immunodeficiency.

herpes e., herpes simplex e., herpes simplex virus e., HSV e. viral esophagitis resulting from infection with herpes simplex virus, seen in both immunocompetent and immunocompromised persons; there are usually shallow ulcers and vesicles on the esophagus. Other symptoms include dysphagia, odynophagia, and sometimes nausea and vomiting.

peptic e. reflux e.

pill e. esophagitis resulting from irritation by pills that pass more slowly than expected through the esophagus.

radiation e. esophageal irritation caused by radiation therapy to the thorax, with retrosternal burning, difficulty swallowing, and slowed peristalsis; it usually clears up once the therapy is terminated.

reflux e. a serious and sometimes life-threatening form of gastroesophageal reflux disease that involves damage to the esophageal mucosa, often with erosion, ulceration, and infiltration by neutrophils or eosinophils. Stricture, scarring, and occasional perforation may occur in serious cases. Called also *peptic* or *chronic peptic e.*

viral e. esophagitis in which the infecting agent is a virus, usually herpes simplex virus, cytomegalovirus, or varicella zoster virus; the incidence is sharply increased among immunocompromised patients.

esophag(o)- [Gr. *oisophagos,* from *oisein* to carry + *phagēma* food] combining form denoting the esophagus.

esoph•a•go•bron•chi•al (ə-sof″ə-go-brong′ke-əl) bronchoesophageal.

esoph•a•go•car•dio•my•ot•o•my (ə-sof″ə-go-kahr″de-o-mi-ot′ə-me) incision of the muscular coats of the esophagus and cardiac part of the stomach for relief of esophageal achalasia. The original procedure involved

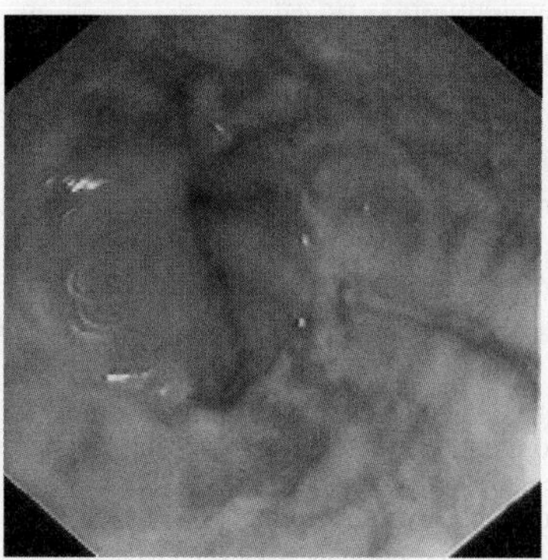

■ Linear streaks visible endoscopically in reflux esophagitis.

a myotomy on both anterior and posterior walls of the esophagus; in the later modification, only an extramucosal anterior myotomy is done. Called also *cardiomyotomy* and *Heller cardiomyotomy, esophagomyotomy, myotomy,* or *operation.*

esoph·a·go·cele (ə-sof′ə-go-sēl″) [*esophago-* + *-cele*[1]] herniation of the esophagus; protrusion of its mucous and submucous coats through a rupture in the muscular coat, producing a pouch or diverticulum.

esoph·a·go·co·lo·gas·tros·to·my (ə-sof″ə-go-ko″lo-gas-tros′tə-me) a formerly common type of esophagogastroplasty with interposition of a segment of colon between the esophagus and stomach.

esoph·a·go·co·lo·plas·ty (ə-sof″ə-go-ko′lo-plas″te) [*esophago-* + *colo-* + *-plasty*] excision of a portion of the esophagus and its replacement by a segment of the colon.

esoph·a·go·du·o·de·nos·to·my (ə-sof″ə-go-doo″o-de-nos′tə-me) [*esophago-* + *duodeno-* + *-stomy*] surgical anastomosis between the esophagus and the duodenum.

esoph·a·go·dyn·ia (ə-sof″ə-go-din′e-ə) esophagalgia.

esoph·a·go·en·ter·os·to·my (ə-sof″ə-go-en″tər-os′tə-me) [*esophago-* + *enterostomy*] surgical anastomosis between the esophagus and small intestine; see *esophagoduodenostomy* and *esophagojejunostomy.*

esoph·a·go·esoph·a·gos·to·my (ə-sof″ə-go-ə-sof″ə-gos′tə-me) anastomosis between two parts of the esophagus.

esoph·a·go·fun·do·pexy (ə-sof″ə-go-fun″do-pek′se) [*esophago-* + *fundo-* + *-pexy*] surgical fixation of the fundus of the stomach to the esophagus.

esoph·a·go·gas·trec·to·my (ə-sof″ə-go-gas-trek′tə-me) [*esophago-* + *gastrectomy*] excision of the esophagus and stomach, usually the distal portion of the esophagus and the proximal stomach.

esoph·a·go·gas·tric (ə-sof″ə-go-gas′trik) gastroesophageal (def. 1).

esoph·a·go·gas·tro·anas·to·mo·sis (ə-sof-ə-go-gas″tro-ə-nas″to-mo′sis) esophagogastrostomy.

esoph·a·go·gas·tro·du·o·de·nal (ə-sof″ə-go-gas″tro-doo″o-de′nəl) pertaining to the esophagus, stomach, and duodenum.

esoph·a·go·gas·tro·du·od·enos·co·py (EGD) (ə-sof″ə-go-gas″tro-doo″od-ə-nos′kə-pe) [*esophago-* + *gastro-* + *duodenoscopy*] endoscopic examination of the esophagus, stomach, and duodenum.

esoph·a·go·gas·tro·my·ot·o·my (ə-sof-ə-go-gas″tro-mi-ot′ə-me) esophagocardiomyotomy.

esoph·a·go·gas·tro·plas·ty (ə-sof″ə-go-gas′tro-plas″te) plastic repair of the esophagus and stomach; called also *cardioplasty.* **esophagogastroplas′tic** *adj*

esoph·a·go·gas·tros·co·py (ə-sof″ə-go-gas-tros′kə-pe) [*esophago-* + *gastro-* + *-scopy*] endoscopic examination of the esophagus and the stomach.

esoph·a·go·gas·tros·to·my (ə-sof″ə-go-gas-tros′tə-me) [*esophago-* + *gastro-* + *-stomy*] surgical creation of a new communication between the stomach and esophagus; called also *esophagogastroanastomosis* and *gastroesophagostomy.*

esoph·a·go·gram (ə-sof′ə-go-gram) a radiograph of the esophagus.

esoph·a·gog·ra·phy (ə-sof″ə-gog′rə-fe) [*esophago-* + *-graphy*] radiography of the esophagus.

esoph·a·go·je·ju·no·gas·tros·to·my (ə-sof″ə-go-jə-joo″no-gas-tros-tə-me) [*esophago-* + *jejuno-* + *gastrostomy*] surgical creation of a new connection between the esophagus and stomach, by interposition of a segment of jejunum.

esoph·a·go·je·ju·no·plas·ty (ə-sof″ə-go-jə-joo′no-plas″te) [*esophago-* + *jejuno-* + *-plasty*] replacement of the esophagus with a segment of jejunum. **esophagojejunoplas′tic** *adj*

esoph·a·go·je·ju·nos·to·my (ə-sof-ə-go-je″joo-nos′tə-me) [*esophago-* + *jejuno-* + *-stomy*] surgical anastomosis between the esophagus and the jejunum.

esoph·a·go·lar·yn·gec·to·my (ə-sof″ə-go-lar″in-jek′tə-me) [*esophago-* + *laryngectomy*] en bloc excision of the upper cervical esophagus and larynx.

esoph·a·gol·o·gy (ə-sof″ə-gol′ə-je) the study of the esophagus, including anatomy, physiology, and pathology.

esoph·a·go·ma·la·cia (ə-sof″ə-go-mə-la′shə) [*esophago-* + *-malacia*] softening of the walls of the esophagus.

esoph·a·go·my·ot·o·my (ə-sof″ə-go-mi-ot′ə-me) [*esophago-* + *myotomy*] incision through the muscular coat of the esophagus, usually in the distal part of the esophagus.
  Heller e. esophagocardiomyotomy.

esoph·a·go·plas·ty (ə-sof′ə-go-plas″te) [*esophago-* + *-plasty*] a plastic operation on the esophagus. **esophagoplas′tic** *adj*

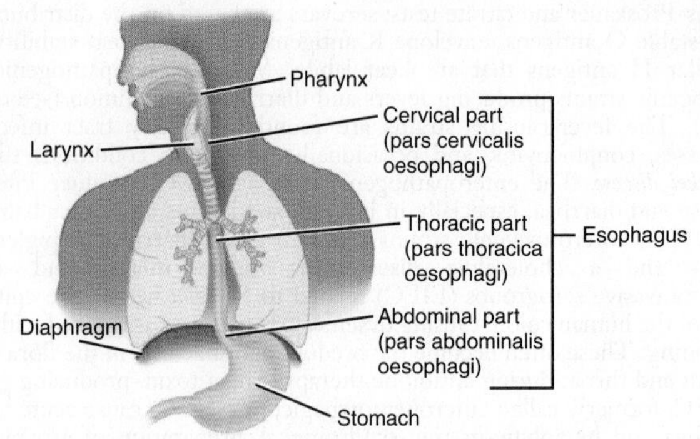

■ Esophagus, comprising cervical, thoracic, and abdominal parts.

esoph·a·go·pli·ca·tion (ə-sof″ə-go-plĭ-ka′shən) [*esophago-* + *plication*] the operation of narrowing the esophagus by folding in its wall.

esoph·a·gop·to·sis (ə-sof″ə-gop-to′sis, ə-sof″ə-go-to′sis) [*esophago-* + *-ptosis*] prolapse of the esophagus.

esoph·a·go·res·pi·ra·to·ry (ə-sof″ə-go-res′pĭ-rə-tor″e) pertaining to or communicating with the esophagus and respiratory tract (the trachea or a bronchus).

esoph·a·go·scope (ə-sof′ə-go-skōp) [*esophago-* + *-scope*] an endoscope for inspecting the lumen of the esophagus and carrying out diagnostic and therapeutic maneuvers such as taking biopsy specimens or removing foreign bodies.

esoph·a·gos·co·py (ə-sof″ə-gos′ko-pe) endoscopic examination of the esophagus.

esoph·a·go·spasm (ə-sof′ə-go-spaz″əm) diffuse esophageal spasm.

esoph·a·go·ste·no·sis (ə-sof″ə-go-stə-no′sis) [*esophago-* + *stenosis*] stricture or constriction of the esophagus.

esoph·a·gos·to·ma (e″sof-ə-gos′tə-mə) [*esophago-* + *stoma*] the external opening of an artificial opening leading into the esophagus.

esoph·a·go·sto·mi·a·sis (ə-sof″ə-go-sto-mi′ə-sis) oesophagostomiasis.

esoph·a·gos·to·my (ə-sof″ə-gos′tə-me) [*esophago-* + *-stomy*] the creation of an opening into the esophagus.

esoph·a·got·o·my (ə-sof″ə-got′ə-me) [*esophago-* + *-tomy*] incision of the esophagus.

esoph·a·go·tra·che·al (ə-sof″ə-go-tra′ke-əl) tracheoesophageal.

esoph·a·gram (ə-sof′ə-gram) esophagogram.

esoph·a·gus (ə-sof′ə-gəs) [Gr. *oisophagos,* from *oisein* to carry + *phagēma* food] the musculomembranous passage extending down from the pharynx and emptying into the stomach at the cardiac opening, passing through the diaphragm at the esophageal hiatus. It is divided anatomically into three parts; see *pars cervicalis oesophagi, pars thoracica oesophagi,* and *pars abdominalis oesophagi.* The official TA spelling is *oesophagus.* Called also *gullet.* **esoph′ageal** *adj*
  abdominal e. pars abdominalis oesophagi.
  Barrett e. see under *syndrome.*
  cervical e. pars cervicalis oesophagi.
  corkscrew e., curling e. the irregularly spiraling shape of the esophagus sometimes seen in diffuse esophageal spasm.
  nutcracker e. a motility disorder characterized by high-amplitude peristaltic contractions, often of prolonged duration, arising from the distal esophagus.
  thoracic e. pars thoracica oesophagi.

eso·pho·ria (es″o-fo′re-ə) [*eso-* + *phoria*] a form of heterophoria in which there is a deviation of the visual axis of an eye toward that of the other eye after the visual fusional stimuli have been eliminated; called also *esodeviation.* **esophor′ic** *adj*

eso·tro·pia (es″o-tro′pe-ə) [*eso-* + *tropia*] strabismus in which there is manifest deviation of the visual axis of an eye toward that of the other eye, resulting in diplopia. Called also *cross-eye* and *convergent* or *internal strabismus.* **esotrop′ic** *adj*

ESP extrasensory perception.

es·pun·dia (es-pōōn′jah) [Port. "sponge"] mucocutaneous leishmaniasis.

ESR erythrocyte sedimentation rate; electron spin resonance.

ESRD end-stage renal disease.

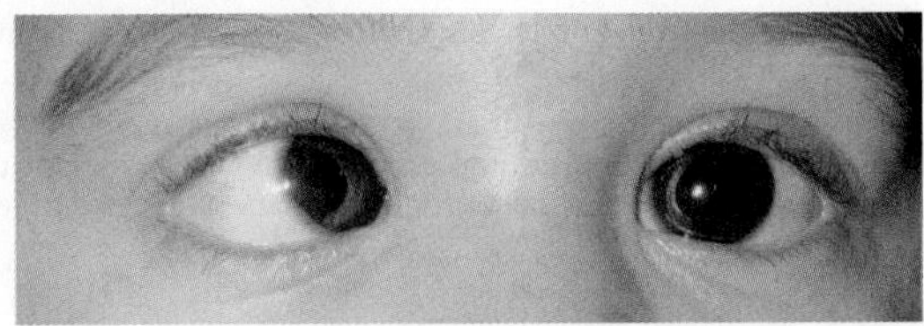

■ Esotropia.

es•sence (es′əns) [L. *essentia* quality or being] 1. that which is or necessarily exists as the cause of the properties of a body. 2. in traditional Chinese medicine, jing (q.v.). 3. a solution of a volatile oil in alcohol.

flower e's aqueous extracts of the fresh flowers of various plants chosen for their effects on specific mental or emotional symptoms, combined with brandy as a preservative; see also *Bach remedies*, under *remedy*.

e. of peppermint peppermint spirit.

es•sen•tial (ə-sen′shəl) [L. *essentialis*] 1. constituting the necessary or inherent part of a thing; giving a substance its peculiar and necessary qualities. 2. idiopathic; said of a disease. 3. indispensable; required in the diet, as essential fatty acids.

Es•ser graft, operation (es′ər) [Johannes Fredericus Samuel *Esser*, Dutch surgeon, 1877–1946] see under *graft*, and see *epithelial inlay*, under *inlay*.

es•si•ac (es′e-ak) [backward spelling of the last name of Rene M. *Caisse*, Canadian nurse, 1887–1978, who popularized the remedy] an herbal preparation, supposedly of Native American origin, used as a tea in the treatment of cancer; there are a number of variations on the original formula, which probably consisted of slippery elm bark, rhubarb root, burdock root, and sheep sorrel.

EST expressed sequence tag; electric shock (or electroshock) therapy; see *electroconvulsive therapy*, under *therapy*.

es•taz•o•lam (es-taz′o-lam) a benzodiazepine used as a sedative and hypnotic in the treatment of insomnia; administered orally.

es•ter (es′tər) a compound formed by removal of water from an acid and an alcohol, e.g., carboxylic acid esters, R—O—CO—R′, and phosphoric acid esters (organic phosphates), R—PO_4^{2-}; esters are named as if they were salts of the parent acid, e.g., methyl acetate, glucose 6-phosphate.

cholesteryl e. an ester formed from cholesterol and an acid; those in which the acid is a long chain fatty acid are major constituents of lipoproteins.

Cori e. glucose 1-phosphate.

Embden e. an equilibrium mixture of 75–80 per cent glucose 6-phosphate and 20–25 per cent fructose 6-phosphate.

Harden-Young e. fructose 1,6-bisphosphate.

Neuberg e. fructose 6-phosphate.

Robison e. glucose 6-phosphate.

es•ter•a•pe•nia (es″tər-ə-pe′ne-ə) [*esterase* + *-penia*] deficiency in the cholinesterase content of the blood.

es•ter•ase (es′tər-ās) 1. a term used in the recommended and trivial names of the hydrolases that act on ester bonds [EC 3.1] to produce an alcohol and an acid. 2. a general term used for any enzyme catalyzing this reaction.

C1 e. C1s; see under *complement*.

es•ter•i•fi•ca•tion (es-ter″ĭ-fĭ-ka′shən) the process of converting an acid into an ester.

es•ter•i•fy (es-ter′ĭ-fi) to combine with an alcohol with elimination of a molecule of water, forming an ester.

es•ter•ize (es′ter-īz) to convert, or be converted, into an ester.

es•ter•ol•y•sis (es″tər-ol′ə-sis) [*ester* + *-lysis*] the hydrolysis of an ester into its alcohol and acid.

es•tero•lyt•ic (es″tər-o-lit′ik) 1. pertaining to esterolysis. 2. causing esterolysis.

Es•tes operation (es′tēz) [William Lawrence *Estes*, Jr., American surgeon, 1885–1940] see under *operation*.

es•te•trol (es′tə-trol) 15α, 16α, 17β-estetrol, an estrogen produced in the fetoplacental unit by 15α-hydroxylation of estriol or estrogen precursors and found in the maternal serum, amniotic fluid, and urine.

es•the•sia (es-the′zhə) [*esthesi-* + *-ia*] perception, feeling, or sensation.

esthesi(o)- [Gr. *aisthēsis* perception, sensation] a combining form denoting relationship to feeling or to perception. Spelled also *aesthesi(o)-*.

es•the•sio•blast (es-the′ze-o-blast″) ganglioblast.

es•the•si•od•ic (es-the″ze-od′ik) esthesodic.

es•the•si•o•gen•ic (es-the″ze-o-jen′ik) producing sensation.

es•the•si•ol•o•gy (es-the″ze-ol′ə-je) [*esthesio-* + *-logy*] the science of sensation and the senses.

es•the•si•om•e•ter (es-the″ze-om′ə-tər) [*esthesio-* + *-meter*] an instrument for measuring tactile sensibility; called also *tactometer*.

es•the•sio•neu•ro•blas•to•ma (es-the″ze-o-noo″ro-blas-to′mə) olfactory neuroblastoma.

es•the•sio•phys•i•ol•o•gy (es-the″ze-o-fiz″e-ol′ə-je) the physiology of sensation and the sense organs.

es•the•sod•ic (es″thə-zod′ik) [*esthesio-* + Gr. *hodos* path] conducting or pertaining to the conduction of sensory impulses.

es•thet•ic (es-thet′ik) [Gr. *aisthēsis* sensation] pertaining to beauty, or the improvement of appearance. Also spelled *aesthetic*.

es•the•tics (es-thet′iks) in dentistry, a philosophy concerned especially with the appearance of a dental restoration, as achieved through its color and/or form. Also spelled *aesthetics*.

es•ti•mate[1] (es′tĭ-mət) [L. *aestimare* to value, to estimate] 1. a rough calculation or one based on incomplete data. 2. a statistic used to characterize the value of a population parameter. Called also *estimator*.

biased e. a point estimate that is not unbiased, i.e., a point estimate that for some reason should tend to be wrong in a given direction.

consistent e. a statistic that converges to the true value of the parameter being estimated (population parameter) as the sample size increases; i.e., the estimate value can be made as statistically close to the true value as desired by taking a large enough sample.

interval e. a statistical estimate that states with a specified degree of confidence that the parameter lies within a specified interval. Cf. *point e.*

maximum likelihood e. the estimate of a parameter describing a population distribution that makes the likelihood function take its maximum value; an estimate of the parameter that maximizes the probability of obtaining the sample values actually observed.

point e. a statistical estimate that specifies a value for the parameter. Cf. *interval e.*

product-limit e. Kaplan-Meier survival curve.

unbiased e. a point estimate having a sampling distribution with a mean equal to the parameter being estimated; i.e., the estimate will be greater than the true value as often as it is less than the true value.

es•ti•mate[2] (es′tĭ-māt) 1. to produce or use a rough calculation. 2. to measure or calculate a statistic for characterization of a population parameter.

es•ti•ma•tor (es′tĭ-ma″tər) estimate[1] (def. 2).

Es•ti•nyl (es′tĭ-nəl) trademark for a preparation of ethinyl estradiol.

es•ti•val (es′tĭ-vəl, ə-sti′vəl) [L. *aestivus*, from *aestas* summer] pertaining to or occurring in summer.

es•ti•va•tion (es″tĭ-va′shən) [L. *aestivus*, from *aestas* summer] the dormant state of decreased metabolism in which certain animal species, as some tropical amphibians, survive a hot, dry summer; summer dormancy. Cf. *hibernation*.

Est•lan•der operation (est′lahnd-ər) [Jakob August *Estlander*, Finnish surgeon, 1831–1881] see under *operation*.

es•to•late (es′to-lāt) USAN contraction for propionate lauryl sulfate.

Es•trace (es′trās) trademark for preparations of estradiol.

Es•tra•derm (es′trə-derm) trademark for a preparation of estradiol.

es•tra•di•ol (es″trə-di′ol, es-tra′de-ol) 1. the most potent naturally occurring ovarian and placental estrogen in mammals; it prepares the uterus for implantation of the fertilized oocyte and promotes the maturation and maintenance of the female accessory reproductive organs and secondary sex characters. It has also been produced semisynthetically. It exists in two isomeric forms: the active isomer is *estradiol-17*β and the inactive is *estradiol-17*α (formerly called β*-estradiol* and α*-estradiol* respectively). 2. [USP] a preparation of this hormone used in estrogen replacement therapy for conditions such as female hypogonadism, ovariectomy, or primary ovarian failure, and in treatment of abnormal uterine bleeding, vasomotor menopausal symptoms, postmenopausal osteoporosis, atrophic vaginitis or urethritis, vulvar squamous metaplasia, and certain advanced breast or prostatic carcinomas; administered orally, transdermally, intravaginally, or by intramuscular injection.

e. acetate an ester of estradiol used in the treatment of vasomotor symptoms of menopause; administered orally or intravaginally.

e. benzoate an ester of estradiol which has been injected intramuscularly in oil solution. It is also used as a feed additive to promote growth in cattle.

e. cypionate [USP] an ester of estradiol, having a longer duration of action than the base or other esters; used in the treatment of female hypogonadism and of vasomotor symptoms associated with menopause. Injected intramuscularly in oil solution.

ethinyl e. see under *ethinyl.*

e. valerate [USP] an ester of estradiol, having similar uses and more prolonged action than the base; injected intramuscularly in oil solution.

Es·tra-L (es′trə-el) trademark for preparations of estradiol valerate.

es·tra·mus·tine phos·phate (es″trə-mus′tēn) an antineoplastic agent consisting of estradiol joined to mechlorethamine (nitrogen mustard) by a carbamate link, phosphorylated to make it water soluble; administered orally for palliative treatment of metastatic or progressive carcinoma of the prostate. Available as *estramustine phosphate sodium.*

es·trane (es′trān) the 18-carbon tetracyclic hydrocarbon nucleus that is the parent structure of the estrogenic steroids; used for steroid hormone nomenclature.

Es·tra·tab (es′trə-tab) trademark for a preparation of esterified estrogens.

Es·tra·test (es′trə-test) trademark for combination preparations of esterified estrogens and methyltestosterone.

es·tri·a·sis (es-tri′ə-sis) oestriasis.

Es·tri·dae (es′trĭ-de) Oestridae.

es·trin (es′trin) estrogen.

Est·ring (est′ring) trademark for a preparation of estradiol.

es·trin·iza·tion (es″trin-ĭ-za′shən) production of the cellular changes in the vaginal epithelium characteristic of estrus.

es·tri·ol (es′tre-ol) an oxidation product of estradiol and estrone, having relatively weak estrogenic activity and detectable in high concentrations in the urine, especially human pregnancy urine.

Es·tro-Cyp (es′tro-sip″) trademark for a preparation of estradiol cypionate.

es·tro·gen (es′trə-jen) a generic term for any estrus-producing steroid. In humans estrogens are formed in the ovary, possibly the adrenal cortex, the testis, and the fetoplacental unit and have various functions in both sexes. They are responsible for the development of the female secondary sex characters, and during the menstrual cycle they act on the female genitalia to produce an environment suitable for the fertilization, implantation, and nutrition of the early embryo. Exogenous estrogens are used in oral contraceptives; in treatment of some kinds of advanced breast and prostate carcinoma; in replacement therapy for female hypogonadism, ovariectomy, primary ovarian failure, atrophic vaginitis, vasomotor menopausal symptoms, and vulvar squamous hyperplasia, treatment of atrophic urethritis and abnormal uterine bleeding, and prophylaxis of osteoporosis. Common naturally occurring estrogens include *estradiol* and *estrone.* Called also *estrin* and *female sex hormone.*

conjugated e's [USP] a mixture of the sodium salts of the sulfate esters of estrone and equilin, derived from pregnant mares' urine or prepared synthetically from estrone and equilin; the actions and uses are those of estrogens, administered orally, intravenously, intramuscularly, or intravaginally.

conjugated equine e's (CEE) conjugated estrogens that come from a mare.

esterified e's [USP] a mixture of the sodium salts of esters of estrogenic substances, principally estrone, having the actions and uses of estrogens; administered orally.

es·tro·gen·ic (es-tro-jen′ik) 1. producing estrus. 2. pertaining to, having the effects of, or similar to an estrogen. Called also *estrogenous.*

es·tro·ge·nic·i·ty (es″tro-jə-nis′ĭ-te) the quality of exerting or the ability to exert an estrus-producing or an estrogenic effect.

es·trog·e·nous (es-troj′ə-nəs) estrogenic.

es·trone (es′trōn) 1. an oxidation product of estradiol, the first of the estrogens isolated in pure form, found in human pregnancy urine, male human urine, human plasma, mare pregnancy urine, stallion urine, human ovarian follicular fluid and placenta, and palm kernel oil; also produced synthetically. It is less potent than estradiol but more so than estriol and is metabolically convertible to estradiol; it is secreted by the ovary but circulating estrone is for the most part derived from peripheral metabolism of estradiol and especially androstenedione. 2. [USP] a preparation of estrone; used in estrogen replacement therapy for hypogonadism, ovariectomy, primary ovarian failure, atrophic vaginitis, vasomotor menopausal symptoms, and vulvar atrophy, and in the treatment of dysfunctional uterine bleeding and advanced prostatic carcinoma; administered intramuscularly or intravaginally.

es·tro·phil·in (es″tro-fil′in) a cell protein that acts as a receptor for estrogen, found in estrogenic target tissue and in estrogen-dependent tumors and metastases.

es·tro·pi·pate (es′tro-pĭ-pāt) [USP] a compound of estrone sulfate and piperazine, having actions similar to those of other estrogen preparations and used in estrogen replacement therapy to treat estrogen deficiency of various causes, the vasomotor symptoms of menopause, and vulvar and vaginal atrophy, and also in the prophylaxis of osteoporosis. Administered orally or intravaginally.

Es·tro·step (es′tro-step) trademark for therapeutic regimens containing norethindrone acetate and ethinyl estradiol. When a week of placebo ferrous fumarate tablets are included, the trademark is Estrostep Fe.

es·tru·a·tion (es″troo-a′shən) estrus.

es·trum (es′trəm) estrus.

es·trus (es′trəs) [L. *oestrus* gadfly; Gr. *oistros* anything that drives mad, any vehement desire] the recurrent, restricted period of sexual receptivity in female mammals other than human females, marked by intense sexual urge. See also *estrous cycle,* under *cycle.* Called also *estruation, estrum, heat,* and *rut.* Also spelled *oestrus.* **es′trous, es′trual** *adj*

silent e. follicular development and ovulation occurring without the usual behavior of estrus.

esu electrostatic unit.

ESV end-systolic volume.

es·zo·pi·clone (es-zo′pĭ-klōn) a central nervous system depressant and hypnotic used in treatment of insomnia.

Et ethyl.

eta (a′tə) [H, η] the seventh letter of the Greek alphabet.

eta·fil·con A (a″tə-fil′kon) a hydrophilic contact lens material.

eta·ner·cept (e-tan′ər-sept) a soluble tumor necrosis factor receptor that inactivates tumor necrosis factor, used in the treatment of rheumatoid arthritis and juvenile idiopathic arthritis; administered subcutaneously.

état (a-tah′) [Fr. "state"] status.

é. criblé (krē-bla′) status cribalis.

é. mamelonné (mah-mel-un-a′) ["hillock-covered state"] hyperplasia of the mucous membrane of the stomach in chronic gastritis, resulting in the formation of small elevations.

é. marbré (mar-bra′) status marmoratus.

etch·ing (ech′ing) [Old High Ger. *ezzen* to eat] the cutting of a hard surface such as metal or glass by a corrosive chemical, usually an acid, in order to create a design.

acid e. etching of dental enamel with an acid in order to roughen the surface, increase retention of resin sealant, and promote mechanical retention.

ETEC enterotoxigenic *Escherichia coli.*

Eter·nod sinus (a-tər-no′) [Auguste François Charles *Eternod,* Swiss histologist, 1854–1932] see under *sinus.*

ETF electron transfer flavoprotein.

eth·a·cryn·ate so·di·um (eth″ə-krin′āt) [USP] the sodium salt of ethacrynic acid (q.v.), having the same actions as the base; administered intravenously when oral administration is impractical or onset of action must be rapid.

eth·a·cryn·ic ac·id (eth″ə-krin′ik) [USP] a loop diuretic used in the treatment of edema associated with congestive heart failure or hepatic or renal disease, of ascites due to malignancy, idiopathic edema, or lymphedema, or of hypertension, often in combination with other drugs, and as an adjunct in the treatment of acute pulmonary edema; administered orally.

etham·bu·tol hy·dro·chlo·ride (EMB) (ə-tham′bu-tol) [USP] an antibacterial, specifically effective against *Mycobacterium,* including *M. tuberculosis;* used in conjunction with one or more other antituberculous drugs in the treatment of pulmonary tuberculosis, administered orally.

etham·sy·late (ə-tham′sə-lāt) a hemostatic agent that acts by maintaining capillary wall stability, used for the prophylaxis and treatment of hemorrhage from small blood vessels; administered orally, intramuscularly, and intravenously.

eth·a·nal (eth′ə-nal) acetaldehyde.

eth·ane (eth′ān) a hydrocarbon of the methane series, C_2H_6, forming a constituent of natural gas, which occurs as a colorless, odorless, flammable gas.

eth·ane·di·al (eth″ān-di′al) glyoxal.

eth·ane·di·ni·trile (eth″ān-di-ni′tril) cyanogen (def. 2).

eth·a·no·ic ac·id (eth″ə-no′ik) systematic name for acetic acid.

eth·a·nol (eth′ə-nol) a primary alcohol existing as a transparent, colorless, volatile, flammable liquid, miscible with water, methanol, ether, chloroform and acetone; it is formed by microbial fermentation of carbohydrates or by synthesis from ethylene. Excessive ingestion results in acute intoxication, with psychological, gastrointestinal, neurological, and motor abnormalities; ingestion during pregnancy can harm the fetus. The official preparation is called *alcohol* [USP]. Called also *alcohol* and *ethyl* or *grain alcohol.*

eth•a•nol•amine (eth″ə-nol′ə-mēn) 1. monoethanolamine. 2. any of several related amine derivatives having one or more ethanol substituents.
 e. oleate the oleate salt of monoethanolamine, used as a sclerosing agent in the treatment of varicose veins and esophageal varices.

eth•a•nol•ism (eth′ə-nol″iz-əm) alcoholism.

eth•chlor•vy•nol (eth-klor′və-nol) [USP] a nonbarbiturate sedative and hypnotic, used for the short-term treatment of insomnia; administered orally.

eth•e•noid (eth′ə-noid) containing an ethylene linkage.

ether (e′thər) [L. *aether*, from Gr. *aithēr* "the upper and purer air"] 1. an organic compound having an oxygen atom bonded to two carbon atoms; general formula, R–O–R′. 2. [USP] a colorless, volatile, flammable liquid, $C_2H_5OC_2H_5$, with a characteristic odor; the first inhalational anesthetic used for surgical anesthesia (1846), now little used because of its flammability. Called also *diethyl e.* and *ethyl e.*
 anesthetic e. ether (def. 2); sometimes used more generally for any ether acting as an inhalational anesthetic.
 diethyl e. ether (def. 2).
 diethylene glycol monoethyl e. [NF] a condensation product of ethylene oxide and alcohol, used as a solvent in pharmaceutical preparations.
 ethyl e. ether (def. 2).
 petroleum e. see under *petroleum.*
 thio e. thioether.

ethe•re•al (ə-the′re-əl) 1. pertaining to, prepared with, containing, or resembling ether. 2. evanescent; delicate.

ether•i•fi•ca•tion (e″thər-ĭ-fĭ-ka′shən) the formation of an ether from alcohol.

ether•iza•tion (e″thər-ĭ-za′shən) the administration of ether by inhalation, and the consequent production of anesthesia.

ether•ize (e′thər-īz) to put under the anesthetic influence of ether.

eth•i•cal (eth′ĭ-kəl) 1. in accordance with the principles which govern right conduct. 2. pertaining to ethics in general or to the discipline of ethics.

eth•ics (eth′iks) [Gr. *ēthos* the manner and habits of man or of animals] 1. the rules or principles which govern right conduct. 2. the branch of philosophy that studies such principles.
 clinical e. the application of ethical analysis to decision making in the care of individual patients.
 medical e. the values and guidelines that should govern decisions in medicine.

ethid•i•um (ə-thid′e-əm) a fluorochrome that intercalates across double-stranded nucleic acids, particularly DNA. Its bromide salt is used to detect DNA after electrophoresis or in cytochemical preparations. In veterinary pharmacology, it is used as a trypanosomicide and is usually called *homidium.*

eth•i•nyl (eth′ĭ-nəl) the radical HC≡C—, derived from acetylene.
 e. estradiol [USP] a semisynthetic derivative of estradiol, one of the most potent estrogens. It is used in combination with a progestational agent in oral contraceptives and contraceptive patches, and administered orally in hormone replacement therapy and as an antineoplastic in treatment of advanced breast and prostate cancers.

Ethi•o•dol (ə-thi′o-dol) a trademark for a preparation of ethiodized oil.

ethio•fos (ĕ-thi″o-fos′) amifostine.

ethi•on•am•ide (ə-thi″ən-am′īd) [USP] an antibacterial, effective against *Mycobacterium tuberculosis;* used in conjunction with one or more other antituberculous drugs in the treatment of pulmonary tuberculosis, administered orally.

ethi•o•nine (ə-thi′ə-nēn) the ethyl homologue of methionine.

eth•mo•ceph•a•ly (eth″mo-sef′ə-le) [Gr. *ēthmos* sieve + *-cephaly*] a congenital anomaly in which a fetus has an imperfect head, more or less union of the eyes, and a rudimentary nose that may be displaced upward.

eth•mo•fron•tal (eth″mo-fron′təl) pertaining to the ethmoid and frontal bones.

eth•moid (eth′moid) [Gr. *ēthmos* sieve + *-oid*] 1. perforated like a sieve; see *os ethmoidale* . 2. ethmoidal.

eth•moi•dal (eth-moi′dəl) of or pertaining to the ethmoid bone; *ethmoid.*

eth•moid•ec•to•my (eth″moid-ek′tə-me) [*ethmoid* + *-ectomy*] excision of the ethmoid cells or of a portion of the ethmoid bone.

eth•moid•itis (eth″moi-di′tis) ethmoid sinusitis.

eth•moid•ot•o•my (eth″moi-dot′ə-me) surgical incision into the ethmoid sinus.

eth•mo•lac•ri•mal (eth″mo-lak′rĭ-məl) pertaining to the ethmoid and the lacrimal bones.

eth•mo•max•il•lary (eth″mo-mak′sĭ-lar-e) pertaining to the ethmoid and maxillary bones.

eth•mo•na•sal (eth″mo-na′zəl) pertaining to the ethmoid and nasal bones.

eth•mo•pal•a•tal (eth″mo-pal′ə-təl) pertaining to the ethmoid and palatine bones.

eth•mo•sphe•noid (eth″mo-sfe′noid) sphenoethmoid.

eth•mo•tur•bi•nal (eth″mo-tur′bĭ-nəl) pertaining to the superior and middle nasal conchae.

eth•mo•vo•mer•ine (eth″mo-vo′mər-ēn) pertaining to the ethmoid bone and the vomer.

Eth•mo•zine (eth′mo-zēn) trademark for a preparation of moricizine hydrochloride.

eth•nic (eth′nik) [Gr. *ethnikos* of a nation; national] pertaining to a social group who share cultural bonds (religious, national, etc.) or physical (racial) characteristics.

eth•nics (eth′niks) [Gr. *ethnikos* of a nation; national] ethnology.

eth•no•bi•ol•o•gy (eth″no-bi-ol′ə-je) the study of the interaction between cultural groups and the plant and animal life in their environment.

eth•no•bot•a•ny (eth″no-bot′ə-ne) the systematic study of the interactions between a culture and the plants in its environment, particularly the group's knowledge about and use of such plants.

eth•nog•ra•phy (eth-nog′rə-fe) [Gr. *ethnos* race + *-graphy*] a description of the ethnic groups of humanity. Cf. *anthropography.*

eth•nol•o•gy (eth-nol′ə-je) [Gr. *ethnos* race + *-logy*] the science that deals with the ethnic groups of humanity, their descent, relationship, and similar matters.

eth•no•med•i•cal (eth″no-med′ĭ-kəl) pertaining to systems of medicine specific to certain ethnic groups.

eth•no•med•i•cine (eth″no-med′ĭ-sin) medical systems based on the cultural beliefs and practices of specific ethnic groups, including alternative bodies of theory and practice such as traditional Chinese medicine, traditional therapies handed down from generation to generation, and various mystical or magical practices.

eth•no•phar•ma•col•o•gy (eth″no-fahr″mə-kol′ə-je) the systematic study of the use of medicinal plants by specific cultural groups.

ethol•o•gist (e-thol′ə-jist) a specialist in ethology.

ethol•o•gy (e-thol′ə-je) [Gr. *ēthos* manners and habits of humans or other animals + *-logy*] The scientific study of animal behavior, particularly in the natural state, the evolution of behavior, and its biologic significance. etholog′ical *adj*

etho•pab•ate (eth″o-pab′āt) [USP] an antiprotozoal agent used in veterinary practice for the control of coccidiosis.

etho•pro•pa•zine hy•dro•chlo•ride (eth″o-pro′pə-zēn) a phenothiazine derivative used as an antidyskinetic, believed to act by partially blocking central cholinergic receptors, so that cholinergic and dopaminergic activity in the basal ganglia is more balanced; used in the treatment of parkinsonism and for the control of drug-induced extrapyramidal reactions (except tardive dyskinesia); administered orally. Called also *profenamine hydrochloride.*

etho•sux•i•mide (eth″o-suk′sĭ-mīd) [USP] an anticonvulsant used in the treatment of seizures in absence epilepsy, administered orally.

etho•to•in (eth′o-to″in) an anticonvulsant used in the treatment of grand mal epilepsy and temporal lobe epilepsy; administered orally.

eth•ox•zol•a•mide (eth″oks-zol′ə-mīd) a carbonic anhydrase inhibitor used in treatment of glaucoma and edema.

Ēthrane (e′thrān) trademark for a preparation of enflurane.

eth•yl (eth′əl) [*ether* + *-yl*] the univalent alcohol radical, CH_3—CH_2—. Symbol Et.
 e. acetate [NF] a flavoring agent and solvent used in pharmaceutical preparations.
 e. aminobenzoate benzocaine.
 e. chloride [USP] a colorless, extremely volatile, flammable liquid, C_2H_5Cl, sprayed on skin to produce local anesthesia by superficial freezing caused by its rapid evaporation.
 e. ether ether (def. 2).
 e. mercaptan a thioalcohol which has a foul odor and contributes to the odor of feces.
 e. oleate [NF] a mobile, practically colorless liquid consisting of esters of ethyl alcohol and high-molecular-weight fatty acids, principally oleic acid; used as a vehicle for pharmaceutical preparations.

eth•yl•al•de•hyde (eth″əl-al′də-hīd) acetaldehyde.

eth•yl•ate (eth′əl-āt) any compound of ethyl alcohol in which the hydrogen of the hydroxyl is replaced by a base.

eth·yl·a·tion (eth″əl-a′shən) the act of combining or causing to combine with the ethyl radical.

eth·yl·cel·lu·lose (eth″əl-sel′u-lōs) [NF] a free-flowing, white to light tan powder, used as a tablet binder in pharmaceutical preparations.

eth·y·lene (eth′ə-lēn) $CH_2{=}CH_2$, a colorless, flammable gas with a sweet taste and odor, formerly used as an inhalational anesthetic.

e. dibromide a derivative of bromine and ethylene used as a fumigant and gasoline additive; it is irritating to the skin and mucous membranes and carcinogenic. Called also *1,2-dibromoethane.*

e. dichloride a colorless heavy liquid with a pungent odor, used as a solvent, gasoline additive, and intermediate; it is irritating to the eyes and respiratory tract and can cause central nervous system disturbances and renal and hepatic damage. Excessive exposure can be carcinogenic. Called also *1,2-dichloroethane.*

e. glycol a solvent with a sweetish, acrid taste, found in many industrial products such as antifreezes, drying agents, and inks. Ingestion or excessive skin exposure can be toxic; see *ethylene glycol poisoning,* under *poisoning.*

e. oxide a gas used in the manufacture of ethylene glycol, acrylonitrile, and other compounds and as a fumigant, fungicide, and sterilizing agent. It is highly irritating to the eyes and mucous membranes and is carcinogenic. Called also *oxirane.*

eth·y·lene·di·a·mine (eth″ə-lēn-di′ə-mēn) [USP] a clear, colorless or slightly yellow liquid with an ammonialike odor and a strong alkaline reaction; complexed with theophylline it forms aminophylline.

eth·y·lene·di·a·mine·tet·ra·ac·e·tate (eth″ə-lēn-di″ə-mēn-tet-rə-as′ə-tāt) a salt of ethylenediaminetetraacetic acid (EDTA). Called also *edetate.*

eth·y·lene·di·a·mine·tet·ra·a·ce·tic ac·id (EDTA) (eth″ə-lēn-di′ə-mēn-tet″rə-ə-se′tik) a chelating agent that binds calcium and heavy metal ions; used as an anticoagulant for blood specimens and also (see *edetate*) for treatment of lead poisoning and hypercalcemia.

eth·yl·ene·i·mine (eth″əl-ēn′ĭ-mēn) ethylenimine.

eth·yl·en·i·mine (eth″əl-en′ĭ-mēn) a toxic and carcinogenic compound, C_2H_5N, occurring as a colorless oily liquid with a strong odor of ammonia, used as an intermediate in a variety of industrial processes. Derivatives include alkylating agents used as antineoplastics. Spelled also *ethyleneimine.*

eth·yl·es·tre·nol (eth″əl-es′trə-nol) an anabolic-androgenic steroid; administered orally.

eth·yl·hy·dro·cu·pre·ine (eth″əl-hi-dro-ku′pre-ēn) optochin.

ethyl·ic (ə-thil′ik) pertaining to or derived from ethyl.

eth·yl·i·dene (eth′əl-ĭ-dēn) the bivalent radical, $CH_3CH{=}$.

e. chloride 1,1-dichloroethane; an oily liquid with a chloroformlike odor, used as a solvent and fumigant; it is irritating to the eyes and respiratory system and can cause central nervous system disturbances and renal and hepatic damage.

eth·yl·ism (eth′əl-iz-əm) poisoning or intoxication by ethyl alcohol.

eth·yl·ma·lon·ic-adip·ic·ac·id·uria (eth′əl-mə-lon′ik ə-dip″ik-as-ĭ-du′re-ə) glutaricaciduria, type II.

eth·yl·par·a·ben (eth″əl-par′ə-ben) [NF] an antifungal compound, closely related to butylparaben, methylparaben, and propylparaben; used as a preservative in pharmaceutic preparations.

ethy·no·di·ol di·ac·e·tate (ə-thi″no-di′ol) [USP] a progestational agent used in combination with an estrogen as an oral contraceptive.

eth·y·nyl (eth′ə-nəl) ethinyl.

Eth·y·ol (eth′e-ol) trademark for a preparation of amifostine.

eti·do·caine hy·dro·chlo·ride (ə-te′do-kān) a local anesthetic of the amide type used for percutaneous infiltration anesthesia, peripheral nerve block, retrobulbar block, and caudal or lumbar epidural block. It is also used for infiltration or nerve block in dental procedures.

eti·dro·nate (EHDP) (e-tĭ-dro′nāt) a diphosphonate compound that inhibits the resorption and deposition of hydroxyapatite crystals in bone and is used for treatment of various mineralization disorders of bone. Because of its affinity for sites of osteoid mineralization, it is also used as a complex with technetium 99m in bone scanning; see table at *technetium.*

e. disodium [USP] the disodium salt of etidronate; used to treat osteitis deformans, heterotopic ossification, and hypercalcemia of malignancy; administered orally or intravenously.

eti·dro·nic ac·id (e-tĭ-dro′nik) an acid used as a bone calcium regulator; see *etidronate.*

etio·cho·lan·o·lone (e″te-o-ko-lan′o-lōn) a degradation product of testosterone, androstenedione, and dehydroepiandrosterone excreted in the urine.

etio- [Gr. *aitia* cause] a combining form meaning cause. Spelled also *aetio-.*

eti·o·gen·ic (e″te-o-jen′ik) [*etio-* + *-genic*] causative.

eti·o·log·ic (e″te-o-loj′ik) pertaining to etiology, or to the causes of disease.

eti·o·log·i·cal (e″te-o-loj′ĭ-kəl) etiologic.

eti·ol·o·gy (e″te-ol′ə-je) [*etio-* + *-logy*] 1. the study or theory of the factors that cause disease and the method of their introduction to the host. 2. the causes or origin of a disease or disorder. Cf. *pathogenesis.*

etio·pa·thol·o·gy (e″te-o-pə-thol′ə-je) pathogenesis.

etio·por·phyr·in (e″te-o-por′fə-rin) a porphyrin (q.v.) in which each pyrrole ring has one methyl and one ethyl side chain.

eti·o·tro·pic (e″te-o-tro′pik) [*etio-* + *-tropic*] directed against the cause of a disease.

ET-NANB enterically transmitted non-A, non-B; see *hepatitis E,* under *hepatitis.*

eto·do·lac (e-to-do′lak) [USP] a nonsteroidal antiinflammatory drug used as an analgesic and antiinflammatory, especially to treat arthritis; administered orally. Called also *etodolic acid.*

eto·do·lic ac·id (e-to-do′lik) etodolac.

etom·i·date (ə-tom′ĭ-dāt) a short-acting sedative-hypnotic, administered intravenously for the induction and maintenance of general anesthesia and as a supplement to low-potency anesthetics for maintenance of anesthesia during short operative procedures.

eto·no·ges·trel (et-ə-no-jes′trel) the active metabolite of desogestrel, a synthetic progestin used as a contraceptive.

Eto·po·phos (e″to-po′fos) trademark for a preparation of etoposide phosphate.

eto·po·side (e″to-po′sīd) [USP] a semisynthetic derivative of podophyllotoxin used as an antineoplastic in the treatment of carcinoma of the testes, lung, and bladder, lymphoma, acute myelocytic leukemia, Ewing sarcoma, and AIDS-associated Kaposi sarcoma; administered orally or intravenously.

e. phosphate the phosphate salt of etoposide, having the same actions and uses as the base; administered intravenously.

etor·i·cox·ib (e-tor″ĭkok′sib) a nonsteroidal antiinflammatory drug of the COX-2 inhibitors group, used for symptomatic treatment of osteoarthritis and rheumatoid arthritis; administered orally.

etra·vir·ine (ĕ-trə-vir′ēn) a nonnucleoside reverse transcriptase inhibitor, used in combination with other antiretroviral agents in the treatment of human immunodeficiency virus type 1 (HIV-1) infection; administered orally.

ETS trademark for a preparation of erythromycin.

Eu europium.

eu- [Gr. *eu* well] a combining form meaning well, easily, or good; the opposite of *dys-.*

eu·adre·no·cor·ti·cism (u″ə-dre″no-kor′tĭ-siz-əm) the normal state of secretion by the adrenal cortex, as distinguished from hypoadrenocorticism and hyperadrenocorticism.

Eu·a·moe·bi·da (u″ə-me′bĭ-də) in newer systems of classification, an order of ramicristate amebae, protozoa of the class Lobosa, phylum Sarcomastigophora. The genera *Hartmannella* and *Paramoeba* are of medical significance.

Eu·bac·te·ria (u″bak-te′re-ə) [*eu-* + Gr. *baktērion* small rod] Bacteria.

eu·bac·te·ria (u″bak-te′re-ə) plural of *eubacterium.*

Eu·bac·te·ri·a·ceae (u″bak-tēr″e-a′se-e) a family of gram-positive, anaerobic, rod-shaped bacteria of the order Clostridiales; organisms of medical interest are contained in the genera *Eubacterium* and *Pseudoramibacter.*

Eu·bac·te·ri·um (u″bak-te′re-əm) [*eu-* + Gr. *baktērion* small rod] a genus of bacteria of the family Eubacteriaceae, consisting of nonsporulating, gram-positive, anaerobic rod-shaped organisms found as saprophytes in soil and water. They are normal inhabitants of the skin and cavities of mammals and occasionally cause infections of soft tissues.

E. alactoly′ticum *Pseudoramibacter alactolyticus.*

E. len′tum *Eggerthella lenta.*

E. limo′sum a species that synthesizes vitamin B_{12} and has been isolated from mud, feces, and infections.

eu·bac·te·ri·um (u″bak-te′re-əm) pl. *eubacte′ria.* 1. an organism of the genus *Eubacterium.* 2. formerly, an organism of the order Eubacteriales.

eu·bi·ot·ics (u″bi-ot′iks) [*eu-* + *biotics*] the science of healthy living.

eu·ca·lyp·tol (u″kə-lip′tol) [USP] a colorless liquid with a camphoraceous odor and a cooling, pungent taste, obtained from eucalyptus oil and other sources, used as a flavoring agent, expectorant, and local antiseptic. Called also *cajeputol* and *cineol.*

Eu•ca•lyp•tus (u″kə-lip′təs) [*eu-* + Gr. *kalyptos* covered] a genus of trees and shrubs of the family Myrtaceae, chiefly native to Australia. *E. glo′bulus* is the blue gum, source of eucalyptus oil.

eu•cap•nia (u-kap′ne-ə) [*eu-* + *capn-* + *-ia*] the condition in which the carbon dioxide tension of the blood is normal. Called also *normocapnia.* eucap′nic *adj*

Eu•carya (u-kar′e-ə) [*eu-* + Gr. *karyon* nucleus] in the three-domain system of classification, the division that includes all eukaryotic organisms: plants, animals, fungi, and protists. Spelled also *Eukarya.* Called also *Eukaryota.*

Eu•cary•o•tae (u-kar″e-o′te) [*eu-* + Gr. *karyon* nucleus] in some systems of classification, a proposed kingdom of organisms that would include everything except the Procaryotae (q.v.), i.e. all plants, animals, fungi, protozoa, and most algae, grouping together all the organisms that are made up of eukaryotic cells. Also written *Eukaryotae.*

eu•cary•ote (u-kar′e-ōt) eukaryote.

eu•cary•ot•ic (u″kar-e-ot′ik) eukaryotic.

eu•cat•ro•pine hy•dro•chlo•ride (u-kat′ro-pēn) [USP] an anticholinergic and antimuscarinic, used as a mydriatic, applied topically to the eye.

Eu•ces•to•da (u-səs-to′də) Cestoda.

Eu•cheu•ma (u-ku′mə) a genus of red algae that is a source of carrageenan.

eu•chlor•hy•dria (u″klor-hi′dre-ə) [*eu-* + *chlorhydric acid*] the presence of the normal proportion of free hydrochloric acid in the gastric juice.

eu•cho•lia (u-ko′le-ə) [*eu-* + *chol-* + *-ia*] normal condition of the bile.

eu•chro•ma•tin (u-kro′mə-tin) [*eu-* + *chromatin*] the form of chromatin that is genetically active and constitutes the majority of the chromosomes; it is relatively uncoiled and stains lightly during interphase and condenses and stains more darkly during nuclear division. Cf. *heterochromatin.* euchromat′ic *adj*

eu•chro•ma•top•sia (u-kro″mə-top′se-ə) normal color vision.

Eu•coc•ci•di•ida (u-kok″sĭ-di′ĭ-də) [*eu-* + Gr. *kokkos* berry] an order of parasitic protozoa (subclass Coccidia, class Sporozoea) found in the blood and epithelial cells of invertebrates and vertebrates, and having a life cycle involving merogony. Human pathogens are included in the suborders Eimeriina and Haemosporina.

Eu•coe•lo•ma•ta (u″se-lo-ma′tə) the major division of the higher invertebrates, including mollusks, annelids, arthropods, echinoderms, and chordates, which all have a separate mouth and anus, a true coelom, and a well-developed circulatory system. It is divided into two series, the Deuterostomia and the Protostomia.

eu•coe•lo•mate (u-se′lə-māt″) any member of the Eucoelomata; called also *coelomate.*

eu•col•loid (u-kol′oid) a colloid in which each dispersed particle consists of a single large molecule.

eu•cra•sia (u-kra′zhə) [*eu-* + *-crasia*] 1. a state of health; proper balance of different factors constituting a healthy state. 2. a state in which there is a decreased bodily reaction to ingested or injected drugs, proteins, etc.

eu•di•om•e•ter (u″de-om′ə-tər) [Gr. *eudia* fine weather + *-meter*] an instrument used in testing the purity of the air.

eu•dip•sia (u-dip′se-ə) [*eu-* + *-dipsia*] ordinary, mild thirst.

Eu•ge•nia (u-je′ne-ə) [Prince *Eugene* of Savoy, French-born Austrian general, 1663–1736] a genus of tropical trees and shrubs of the family Myrtaceae. *E. caryophyl′lus* is now called *Syzygium aromaticum.*

eu•gen•ic ac•id (u-jen′ik) eugenol.

eu•gen•ics (u-jen′iks) [*eu-* + *-genic*] the improvement of a population by selection of the individuals considered as its best specimens for breeding. Cf. *dysgenics.*

negative e. eugenics that concerns itself with prevention of reproduction (procreation) by individuals considered to possess inferior or undesirable traits.

positive e. eugenics that concerns itself with promotion of optimal reproduction of individuals considered to possess superior or desirable traits.

eu•gen•ol (u′jən-ol) [USP] a dental analgesic, obtained from clove oil or other natural sources; applied topically to dental cavities and also used as a component of dental protectives. Called also *allylguaiacol* and *eugenic acid.* See also *zinc oxide–eugenol cement.*

eu•gle•nid (u-gle′nid) a protozoan of the order Euglenida; called also *euglenoid.*

Eu•gle•ni•da (u-gle′nĭ-də) an order of plantlike, flagellate protozoa of the phylum Euglenozoa, order Euglenoidea. If there are chromatophores, they are green; there are usually one or two, rarely more, flagella protruding from an anterior invagination; and a small stigma is located anteriorly in colored forms. Species are usually found in fresh water, although some inhabit salt or brackish water, and a few are parasitic. See also *euglenoid movement,* under *movement.*

eu•gle•noid (u-gle′noid) pertaining to the order Euglenida; see also under *movement.*

Eu•gle•noi•dea (u″glə-noi′de-ə) in newer systems of classification, a class of protozoa of the phylum Euglenozoa, including the euglenids; it contains the order Euglenida.

Eu•gle•no•zoa (u″glə-no-zo′ə) in newer systems of classification, a phylum of protozoa that includes the euglenids and kinetoplastids; they usually have one or two flagella that arise from a pouchlike invagination.

eu•glob•u•lin (u-glob′u-lin) one of a class of globulins characterized by being insoluble in water but soluble in saline solutions; see *globulin.*

eu•gly•ce•mia (u″gli-se′me-ə) a blood glucose level that is within the normal range. Called also *normoglycemia.*

eu•gly•ce•mic (u″gli-se′mik) 1. pertaining to or characterized by euglycemia. 2. conducive to euglycemia. Called also *normoglycemic.*

eu•gna•thia (u-na′the-ə) [*eu-* + *gnath-* + *-ia*] an abnormality of the oral cavity which is limited to the teeth and their immediate alveolar supports and does not include the jaws. Cf. *dysgnathia.* eugnath′ic *adj*

eu•gno•sia (u-no′se-ə) [*eu-* + *gnosia*] ability to recognize and synthesize sensory stimuli into a normal perception. eugnos′tic *adj*

eu•gon•ic (u-gon′ik) [*eu-* + Gr. *gonē* seed] growing luxuriantly; said of bacterial cultures, especially of species of *Mycobacterium,* that produce heavy growth on culture media. Cf. *dysgonic.*

eu•hy•dra•tion (u-hi-dra′shən) a normal state of body water content; absence of absolute or relative hydration or of dehydration.

Eu•karya (u-kar′e-ə) Eucarya.

Eu•kary•o•ta (u-kar″e-o′tə) Eucarya.

Eu•kary•o•tae (u-kar″e-o′te) Eucaryotae.

eu•kary•ote (u-kar′e-ōt) [*eu-* + *karyon*] a member of the Eucarya; an organism whose cells have a true nucleus, i.e., one bounded by a nuclear membrane, within which lie the chromosomes and associated proteins and which exhibits mitosis; eukaryotic cells also contain membrane-bound compartments (organelles), in which cellular functions are performed, and have a cytoskeleton that provides mechanical support for the cell. The cells of plants, animals, fungi, and protists are eukaryotic. Cf. *prokaryote.* eukaryot′ic *adj*

eu•ker•a•tin (u-ker′ə-tin) a true keratin found in hair, nails, feathers, and horns.

eu•ki•ne•sia (u″kĭ-ne′zhə) [*eu-* + *kinesi-* + *-ia*] the state of possessing normal or proper motor function or activity; normal or proper mobility. eukinet′ic *adj*

eu•ki•ne•sis (u″kĭ-ne′sis) eukinesia.

eu•lam•i•nate (u-lam′ĭ-nāt) having the normal number of lamina, as certain areas of the cerebral cortex.

Eu•len•burg disease (oi′lən-bərg) [Albert *Eulenburg,* German neurologist, 1840–1917] paramyotonia congenita.

Eu•lex•in (u-lek′sin) trademark for a preparation of flutamide.

eu•mel•a•nin (u-mel′ə-nin) the most common type of melanin in humans, found in darkly colored skin and hair.

eu•men•or•rhea (u″mən-o-re′ə) [*eu-* + *menorrhea*] normal menstruation.

eu•me•tria (u-me′tre-ə) [Gr. "good measure," "good proportion"] a normal condition of nerve impulse, so that a voluntary movement just reaches the intended goal; the proper range of movement.

Eu•my•ce•tes (u″mi-se′tēz) Eumycota.

eu•my•ce•to•ma (u″mi-sə-to′mə) eumycotic mycetoma.

Eu•my•co•ta (u″mi-ko′tə) [*eu-* + Gr. *mykēs* fungus] the true fungi, a phylum in some systems of classification, consisting of fungi whose trophic phase is not motile but whose reproductive cells may be motile. Subphyla grouped under Eumycota are Ascomycotina, Basidiomycotina, Deuteromycotina, Mastigomycotina, and Zygomycotina.

eu•my•cot•ic (u″mi-kot′ik) pertaining to members of Eumycota (the true fungi).

eu•nuch (u′nək) [Gr. *eunouchos*] a man or boy deprived of the testes or the external genital organs, especially one castrated before puberty so that male secondary sex characters fail to develop.

fertile e. a person with fertile eunuch syndrome.

eu•nuch•ism (u′nək-iz-əm) [Gr. *eunouchismos* castration] 1. the condition of being a eunuch. 2. eunuchoidism.

eu•nuch•oid (u′nə-koid) [Gr. *eunouchoeidēs*] 1. resembling or having the characteristics of a eunuch. 2. a male with hypogonadism and deficient secondary sex characters.

eu•nuch•oid•ism (u′nə-koi″diz-əm) hypogonadism in a male, with deficiency of the testes or testicular secretions and secondary sex characters.

female e. a type of hypogonadism in females in which the ovaries fail to function at puberty, resulting in absence of secondary sex characters with infantile sexual organs and excessive growth of the long bones.

hypergonadotropic e. conditions caused by androgen deficiency that are associated with high levels of gonadotropins. See *hypergonadotropic hypogonadism*, under *hypogonadism.*

hypogonadotropic e. see under *hypogonadism.*

eu•os•mia (u-os′me-ə) [*eu-* + *osm-*[1] + *-ia*] 1. normosmia. 2. a pleasant odor.

eu•pan•cre•a•tism (u-pan′kre-ə-tiz″əm) normal pancreatic functioning.

Eu•pa•to•ri•um (u″pə-tor′e-əm) a genus of composite-flowered plants (family Compositae). *E. ayapa′na* (called also *Eupato′rium tripliner′ve*) is a Brazilian shrub whose leaves are used medicinally and called *ayapana* (q.v.). *E. rugo′sum* (called also *E. urticaefo′lium*) is the white snakeroot, which contains the toxic principle tremetol and causes trembles in cattle and sheep.

eu•pep•sia (u-pep′se-ə) [*eu-* + Gr. *pepsis* digestion + *-ia*] good digestion. Cf. *dyspepsia.*

eu•pep•tic (u-pep′tik) 1. pertaining to or characterized by eupepsia. 2. promoting eupepsia.

Eu•phor•bia (u-for′be-ə) the spurges, a large genus of trees, shrubs, and herbs of the family Euphorbiaceae, whose sap is emetic and cathartic and in some species poisonous.

eu•pho•ret•ic (u″fə-ret′ik) 1. producing euphoria. 2. euphoric. 3. an agent that produces euphoria.

eu•pho•ria (u-for′e-ə) [Gr. "the power of bearing easily"] an exaggerated feeling of physical and mental well-being, especially when not justified by external reality. Euphoria may be induced by drugs such as opioids, amphetamines, and alcohol and is also a feature of mania.

eu•pho•ri•ant (u-for′e-ənt) euphoretic.

eu•phor•ic (u-for′ik) characterized by euphoria. Called also *euphoretic.*

eu•phor•i•gen•ic (u-for″ĭ-jen′ik) euphoretic (def. 1).

eu•pho•ris•tic (u″fə-ris′tik) euphoretic (def. 1).

eu•plas•tic (u-plas′tik) [*eu-* + *plastic*] readily becoming organized; adapted to the formation of tissue, as in embryonic development or wound healing.

eu•ploid (u′ploid) [*eu-* + *-ploid*] having an exact multiple of the haploid number *(n)* of chromosomes.

eu•ploi•dy (u-ploi′de) the state of being euploid.

eup•nea (ūp-ne′ə) [*eu-* + *-pnea*] easy or normal respiration. **eupne′ic** *adj*

eu•prac•tic (u-prak′tic) 1. pertaining to or characterized by eupraxia. 2. promoting eupraxia.

eu•prax•ia (u-prak′se-ə) [*eu-* + Gr. *prassein* to do] intactness of reproduction of acquired, skilled movements.

eu•prax•ic (u-prak′sik) 1. concerned in the proper performance of a function. 2. eupractic.

Eu•proc•tis (u-prok′tis) a genus of moths. *E. chrysorrhoe′a* (called also *E. phaeorrhoe′a*) is the brown-tail moth, which causes brown-tail moth dermatitis.

eu•py•rene (u-pi′rēn) having a normal nucleus or chromatic material; said of certain spermatozoa.

eu•py•rex•ia (u″pĭ-rek′se-ə) a slight fever in the early stage of an infection, regarded as an attempt on the part of the individual to combat the infection.

eu•py•rous (u′pĭ-rəs) eupyrene.

Eu•rax (u′rəks) trademark for preparations of crotamiton.

Eu•re•sol (u′rə-sol) trademark for a preparation of resorcinol monoacetate.

eu•rhyth•mia (u-rith′me-ə) [Gr. "harmony"] harmonious relationships in body or organ development.

eu•ro•pi•um (Eu) (u-ro′pe-əm) a rare element, atomic number 63, atomic weight 151.965.

Eu•ro•ti•a•ceae (u-ro″she-a′se-e) Trichocomaceae.

Eu•ro•ti•a•les (u-ro″she-a′lēz) in some systems of classification, an order of mainly saprobic perfect fungi of the subphylum Ascomycotina, in which unitunicate asci are irregularly arranged within the primitive cleistothecium; it includes the family Trichocomaceae, which has human pathogens.

Eu•ro•ti•um (u-ro′she-əm) [Gr. *eurōs* mold] a genus of fungi or molds of the family Trichocomaceae; several species are perfect (sexual) stages of species of *Aspergillus. E. re′pens,* the sexual stage of *Aspergillus repens,* is sometimes found as a bread mold and occasionally infects human lungs.

eury- [Gr. *eurys* wide] a combining form meaning wide or broad.

eu•ry•ce•phal•ic (u″re-sə-fal′ik) [*eury-* + *cephalic*] brachycephalic.

eu•ry•cra•ni•al (u″re-kra′ne-əl) [*eury-* + *cranial*] brachycranic.

eu•ryg•na•thism (u-rig′nə-thiz-əm) [*eury-* + *gnatho-* + *-ism*] the state of having a wide jaw. **eurygnath′ic** *adj*

eu•ry•on (u′re-on) [Gr. *eurys* wide] the point on the right and left parietal bones marking the greatest transverse diameter of the skull or head.

Eu•ry•pel•ma (u″re-pel′mə) a genus of large spiders. *E. hent′zii* is the American tarantula.

eu•ry•ther•mal (u″re-thur′məl) [*eury-* + *thermal*] able to grow in a wide range of temperature, said of bacteria capable of good growth from 28°C to 50°C and above.

eu•ry•ther•mic (u″re-thur′mik) [*eury-* + *thermic*] eurythermal.

Eu•ry•tre•ma (u-re-tre′mə) a genus of trematodes of the family Dicrocoeliidae. *E. coeloma′ticum* and *E. pancrea′ticum* are found in the pancreatic ducts of sheep and cattle; humans can become infected by eating undercooked animal livers.

eu•ry•tre•mi•a•sis (u″re-trə-mi′ə-sis) infestation of the pancreatic ducts of a ruminant or occasionally a human by flukes of the genus *Eurytrema.*

Eu•scor•pi•us (u-skor′pe-əs) a genus of scorpions of the family Buthidae. *E. ita′licus* is the black scorpion of southern Europe and North Africa, which has a painful sting.

Eu•si•mu•li•um (u″sĭ-mu′le-əm) a genus of flies of the family Simuliidae; various species are common hosts of *Onchocerca volvulus,* a parasitic filarial worm.

eu•sper•mic (u-spur′mik) normospermic.

eu•splanch•nia (u-splank′ne-ə) [*eu-* + *splanchno-* + *-ia*] a normal condition of the internal organs.

eu•sple•nia (u-sple′ne-ə) normal splenic function.

eu•sta•chi•an (u-sta′ke-ən) named for Bartolommeo *Eustachio* (L. *Eustachius*), Italian anatomist, 1524–1574, as the *eustachian muscle, tube,* or *valve.*

eu•sta•chi•tis (u″stə-ki′tis) salpingitis (def. 2).

eu•sthen•ia (u-sthen′e-ə) [*eu-* + *stheno-* + *-ia*] a condition of normal strength and activity.

Eu•stron•gyl•i•des (u″stron-jil′ĭ-dēz) a genus of nematodes of the family Dioctophymidae. Larvae are parasitic in fish, and adults normally parasitize fish-eating birds; human infection also occurs after consumption of raw fish. Worms may reach 30 cm in length and penetrate the intestinal wall to invade the peritoneal cavity, causing peritonitis, abdominal pain, and fever.

eu•sys•to•le (u-sis′to-le) [*eu-* + *systole*] a normal state of the systole of the heart. **eusystol′ic** *adj*

Eu•tam•i•as (u-tam′e-əs) a genus of North American rodents, the western chipmunks, which can harbor the plague-infected flea *Monopsyllus eumolpi* and have sometimes been found infected with plague.

eu•tec•tic (u-tek′tik) [Gr. *eutēktos* easily melted or dissolved] 1. easily melted; used specifically of a mixture that melts at a lower temperature than any of its ingredients. 2. a solution or alloy of two or more components having the lowest possible melting temperature that could be obtained by manipulating the ratios of the components. 3. pertaining to such a solution, or to the lowest melting temperature so obtained.

eu•tha•na•sia (u″thə-na′zhə) [*eu-* + Gr. *thanatos* death] 1. an easy or painless death. 2. the deliberate ending of the life of a person suffering from an incurable and painful disease.

active e. the ending of life by the deliberate adminstration of drugs.

passive e. the ending of life by the deliberate withholding of drugs or other life-sustaining treatment.

Eu•the•ria (u-the′re-ə) [*eu-* + Gr. *thērion* beast, animal] in some systems of classification, a subclass of the Mammalia and in others an infraclass of the subclass Theria, including all the true placental mammals, and excluding the monotremes and marsupials.

eu•the•ri•an (u-the′re-ən) any member of the Eutheria.

eu•ther•mic (u-thur′mik) [Gr. *euthermos* very warm] 1. normothermic. 2. promoting warmth.

eu•thy•mia (u-thi′me-ə) [*eu-* + Gr. *thymos* mind] a state of mental tranquility and well-being; neither depressed nor manic.

eu•thy•mism (u-thi′miz-əm) a normal condition of thymus activity.

Eu•thy•neu•ra (u″thə-nu′rə) a subclass of gastropods, including snails and slugs found chiefly in fresh water or terrestrial habitats; many species are primary or intermediate hosts of trematodes and other pathogens. It includes the order Pulmonata.

eu•thy•roid (u-thi′roid) characterized by euthyroidism.

eu•thy•roid•ism (u-thi′roid-iz-əm) the condition of having normal thyroid function, as opposed to hyperthyroidism and hypothyroidism.

eu•to•cia (u-to′shə) [Gr. *eutokia*] normal labor, or childbirth.

eu•top•ic (u-top′ik) [*eu-* + *top-* + *-ic*] situated normally; arising from the normal site or tissue. Cf. *ectopic.*

Eu•tri•at•o•ma (u″tre-at′ə-mə) a genus of reduviid bugs, species of which transmit Chagas disease.

Eu•trom•bic•u•la (u″trom-bik′u-lə) a subgenus of the mite genus *Trombicula.*

E. alfreddugè′si a species whose larval form is the common chigger of the United States, a common cause of trombiculiasis. Called also *Trombicula alfreddugèsi* and *T. irritans.*

E. splen′dens a species whose larva (chigger) causes trombiculiasis in the southeastern United States; called also *Trombicula splendens.*

eu•tro•phia (u-tro′fe-ə) [*eu-* + *tropho-* + *-ia*] a state of normal (good) nutrition. eutroph′ic *adj*

eu•tro•phi•ca•tion (u″tro-fĭ-ka′shən) the promotion of excessive growth of an organism to the disadvantage of other organisms in the same ecosystem by oversupplying the former with nutrients; e.g., the stimulation of excessive growth of plants and algae in natural waters by an oversupply of inorganic nitrogen and phosphate compounds found in fertilizers.

eu•vo•le•mia (u-vo-le′me-ə) [*eu-* + *volume* + *-emia*] normovolemia. euvole′mic *adj*

eu•vo•lia (u-vo′le-ə) normal water content or volume of a given body compartment, e.g., extracellular euvolia.

eV electron volt.

evac•u•ant (e-vak′u-ənt) 1. emptying. 2. cathartic (defs. 1 and 2). 3. a remedy that empties any organ, such as a cathartic, emetic, or diuretic.

evac•u•a•tion (e-vak″u-a′shən) 1. an emptying. 2. emptying of the bowels, as by a medicine; called also *catharsis* and *purgation.*

evac•u•a•tor (e-vak′u-a-tər) an instrument for removing fluid or small particles from a body cavity or container.

evag•i•na•tion (e-vaj″ĭ-na′shən) obtrusion of a layer or part to form a pouch.

optic e. see under *vesicle.*

ev•a•nes•cent (ev″ə-nes′ənt) [L. *evanescere* to vanish away] vanishing; passing away quickly; unstable; unfixed.

Ev•ans syndrome (ev′ənz) [Robert Sherman *Evans*, American physician, 1912–1974] see under *syndrome.*

evap•o•ra•tion (e-vap″o-ra′shən) [L. *e* out + *vaporare* to steam] conversion of a liquid or solid into vapor.

eva•sion (e-va′zhən) in psychiatry, suppression of an idea that would come next in a thought sequence and substitution of a closely related idea; a form of paralogia.

even•tra•tion (e″ven-tra′shən) [L. *eventratio*] 1. herniation of intestines, such as in an abdominal hernia. 2. evisceration (def. 1).

diaphragmatic e. a congenital anomaly characterized by failure of muscular development of part or all of one (or occasionally both) hemidiaphragms, resulting in superior displacement of abdominal viscera and altered lung development.

umbilical e. omphalocele.

eve•ro•li•mus (ĕ-və-ro′lĭ-məs) a derivative of sirolimus, used as an immunosuppressant after transplant surgery.

Evers•busch operation (a′vərz-boosh″) [Oskar *Eversbusch*, German ophthalmologist, 1853–1912] see under *operation.*

ever•sion (e-vur′zhən) [L. *eversio*] 1. a turning inside out. Called also *ectropion.* 2. a turning outward, as of the sole of the foot or the eyelid.

cervical e. see under *ectropion.*

evert (e-vurt′) [L. *e* out + *vertere* to turn] 1. to turn inside out. 2. to turn outward, as the sole of the foot or the eyelid.

ever•tor (ə-vur′tər) a muscle that turns a part outward.

évide•ment (a-vēd-maw′) [Fr.] the operation of scooping out a cavity or diseased portion of an organ.

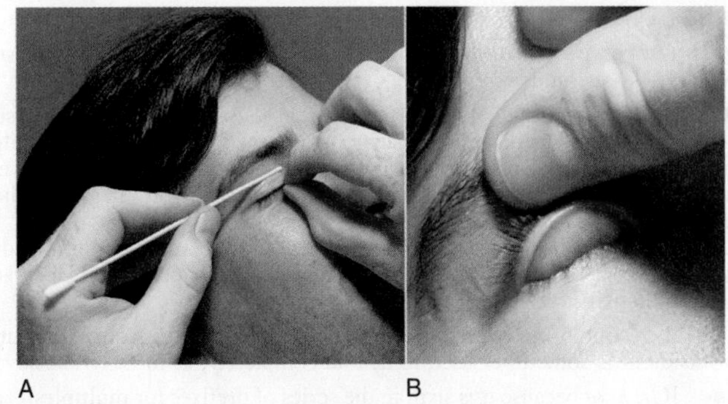

■ Eversion of the eyelid using a wooden applicator stick placed at the superior edge of the superior tarsal plate.

ev•i•dence-based (ev′ĭ-dəns-bāst) characterized by methods of diagnosis and treatment based on demonstrable evidence, i.e., whose effectiveness has been demonstrated by well-designed, peer-reviewed studies.

evil (e′vil) disease.

poll e. an abscess behind the ears of a horse, caused by a dual infection of the supra-atlantal bursa by *Brucella* and *Actinomyces;* this condition is virtually identical to fistulous withers.

quarter e. blackleg.

evi•ra•tion (e″vĭ-ra′shən) [L. *e* out + *vir* man] 1. male castration. 2. feminization. 3. a delusional belief of a man that he has become a woman.

evis•cer•a•tion (e-vis″ər-a′shən) [*e-* + *viscus*] 1. removal of viscera; called also *eventration.* 2. eventration (def. 1). 3. removal of the contents of the eyeball while leaving the sclera behind.

Evis•ta (e-vis′tə) trademark for a preparation of raloxifene hydrochloride.

evo•ca•tion (ev″o-ka′shən) [L. *e* out + *vocare* to call] the calling forth of morphogenetic potentialities through contact with organizer material.

evo•ca•tor (ev′o-ka″tər) a chemical substance emitted by an organizer region of an embryo that evokes a specific morphogenetic response from competent embryonic tissue in contact with it.

evo•lu•tion (ev″ə-loo′shən) [L. *evolutio*, from *e* out + *volvere* to roll] 1. an unrolling. 2. a process of development in which an organ or organism becomes more and more complex by the differentiation of its parts; a continuous and progressive change according to certain laws and by means of resident forces.

convergent e. the appearance of similar forms and/or functions in two or more lines not sufficiently related phylogenetically to account for the similarity.

emergent e. the assumption that each step in evolution produces something new and something that could not be predicted from its antecedents.

organic e. the origin and development of species; the theory that existing organisms are the result of descent with modification from those of past times.

parallel e. the independent evolution of similar structures in two or more rather closely related organisms.

saltatory e. evolution showing sudden changes; mutation or saltation.

Evo•xac (e′vo-zak″) trademark for a preparation of cevimeline hydrochloride.

evul•sion (e-vul′shən) [L. *evulsio*] forcible extraction; see *avulsion.*

Ew•art sign (u′ərt) [William *Ewart*, English physician, 1848–1929] see under *sign.*

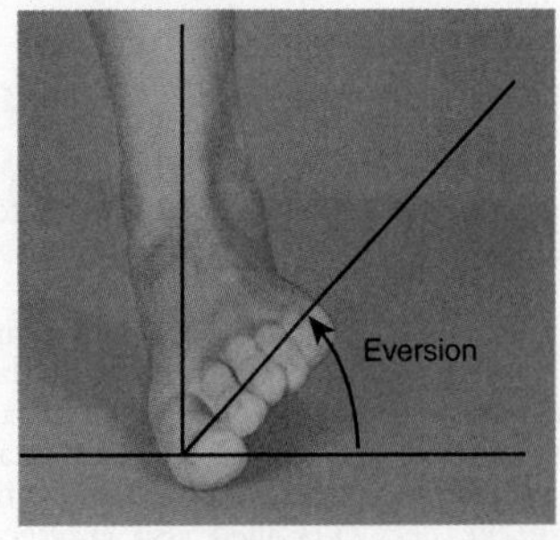

■ Eversion.

EWHO elbow-wrist-hand orthosis.

Ew•ing sarcoma (tumor) (u′ing) [James *Ewing*, American pathologist, 1866–1943] see under *sarcoma.*

Ew•ing•el•la (u″ing-el′ə) [William H. *Ewing*, American bacteriologist, 1914–1998] a genus of gram-negative, rod-shaped bacteria of the family Enterobacteriaceae, consisting of facultatively anaerobic, oxidase-negative, catalase-positive organisms that are motile by peritrichous flagella. The type species is *E. america′na.*

E. america′na a species that is a rare cause of human infection, including nosocomial bacteremia, peritonitis associated with peritoneal dialysis, and conjunctivitis.

ex- [L. *ex* out of, away from] a prefix meaning away from, without, or outside; it is sometimes used to denote completely, as in *exacerbation.*

exa- [Gr. *hexa* because it is sixth in the series of prefixes for multiples] a combining form used in naming units of measurement to indicate a quantity one quintillion (10^{18}) times the unit designated by the root with which it is combined. Symbol E.

ex•ac•er•ba•tion (eg-zas″ər-ba′shən) [*ex-* + L. *acerbus* harsh] increase in the severity of a disease or any of its symptoms.

ex•air•e•sis (ek-sār′ə-sis) [Gr. "a taking out"] exeresis.

ex•al•ta•tion (eg″zawl-ta′shən) a feeling of extreme elation, often associated with delusions of grandeur.

ex•a•meta•zime (eks″ə-met′ə-zēm) HMPAO; hexamethylpropyleneamine oxime, a neutral lipophilic compound that traverses the blood-brain barrier and localizes in the brain; complexed with technetium 99m it is used for imaging of cerebral regional blood flow in the detection of altered regional perfusion in stroke, identification of Alzheimer disease, evaluation of epilepsy, and diagnosis of brain death. The same complex can also be used to label autologous leukocytes for diagnostic studies of intra-abdominal inflammatory lesions and bowel disease. See table at *technetium.*

ex•am•i•na•tion (eg-zam″ĭ-na′shən) [L. *examinare*] inspection, palpation, auscultation, percussion, or other means of investigation, especially for diagnosing disease. See also *study, test,* and *trial.*

digital rectal e. (DRE) manual examination with the examiner's gloved hand of structures in and around the rectum, usually done as part of a general physical examination.

Mental Status E. (MSE) a component of the medical examination comprising the systematic evaluation of the mental status of the patient, including appearance, psychomotor behavior, speech, thinking and perception, emotional state including affect and mood, insight and judgment, intelligence, sensorium, attention and concentration, and memory.

Mini-Mental State E. (MMSE) trademark for a commonly-used written test of cognitive function and impairment, consisting of 30 questions assessing factors such as memory, orientation to space and time, and language ability.

physical e. examination of the bodily state of a patient by ordinary physical means, as inspection, palpation, percussion, and auscultation.

postmortem e. autopsy.

Present State E. a nondiagnostic semi-structured interview administered by a professional and measuring psychiatric symptoms in a variety of areas, concentrating on the one month interval preceding the interview.

ex•an•i•ma•tion (eg-zan″ĭ-ma′shən) unconsciousness; coma.

ex•an•them (eg-zan′thəm) [Gr. *exanthēma*] 1. a disease in which skin eruptions or rashes are a prominent manifestation. Classically, six exanthems of childhood were described that had similar rashes, and were numbered in the order in which they were reported: *first disease* was measles; *second disease* was scarlet fever; *third disease* was rubella; *fourth disease* was found to be a mild type of scarlet fever; *fifth disease* was erythema infectiosum; and *sixth disease* was exanthema subitum. Only the last two designations are still used. 2. rash.

Boston e. a mild febrile exanthematous illness caused by echovirus 16; an epidemic occurred in Boston, Massachusetts, in the 1970s, and sporadic cases continue to occur.

e. su′bitum exanthema subitum.

ex•an•the•ma (eg″zan-the′mə) pl. *exanthemas, exanthem′ata* [Gr. *exanthēma*] exanthem.

equine coital e. a benign venereal disease of horses, caused by a herpesvirus, characterized by vesicles and ulcers on the external genitalia, and occasionally on the lips, nares, and conjunctiva, that heal within a few weeks.

e. su′bitum an acute, short-lived disease of infants and young children, caused by human herpesvirus 6; after a high fever that lasta a few days, the temperature returns to normal; around this time, a macular or maculopapular rash appears on the trunk and spreads to other areas. The disease was given the ordinal designation *sixth disease* to differentiate it from other exanthems (see *exanthem,* def. 2). Called also *exanthem subitum, roseola,* and *roseola infantum.*

■ Exanthema subitum with rose-pink macules and papules.

ex•an•them•a•ta (eg″zan-them′ə-tə) [Gr.] plural of *exanthema.*

ex•an•them•a•tous (eg″zan-them′ə-təs) pertaining to, characterized by, or of the nature of an exanthem.

ex•an•thrope (ek′san-thrōp) [*ex-* + Gr. *anthrōpos* man] any source of disease not situated within the human body. **exanthrop′ic** *adj*

ex•ar•tic•u•la•tion (eks″ahr-tik″u-la′shən) disarticulation.

ex•ca•la•tion (eks″kə-la′shən) absence or exclusion of one member of a normal series, such as a vertebra.

ex•car•na•tion (eks″kahr-na′shən) [*ex-* + L. *caro, carnis* flesh] removal of superfluous fleshy tissue from a preparation.

ex•ca•va•tio (eks″kə-va′she-o) pl. *excavatio′nes* [L., from *ex* out + *cavus* hollow] excavation: a hollowed-out space, pouch, or cavity.

e. dis′ci [TA] depression of optic disk: the depression situated in the center of the optic disk; called also *optic* or *physiologic cup* and *excavation of optic disk.*

e. rectouteri′na [TA] rectouterine pouch: a sac or recess formed by a fold of the peritoneum dipping down between the rectum and the uterus; see also *e. rectovesicalis.* Called also *Douglas cul-de-sac, pouch,* or *space* and *rectovaginal pouch.*

e. rectovesica′lis [TA] rectovesical pouch: the space between the rectum and the bladder in the peritoneal cavity in the male; in females the corresponding cavity is divided by the uterus and broad ligament into the excavatio rectouterina and the excavatio vesicouterina.

e. vesicouteri′na [TA] vesicouterine pouch: the space between the bladder and the uterus in the female peritoneal cavity; see also *e. rectovesicalis.* Called also *uterovesical pouch.*

ex•ca•va•tion (eks″kə-va′shən) [L. *excavatio*] 1. the act of hollowing out. 2. a hollowed-out space, such as a pouch or cavity; see also *excavatio.*

dental e. removal of carious material from a tooth in preparation for restoration. See also *cavity preparation,* under *preparation,* and *prepared cavity,* under *cavity.*

e. of optic disk, physiologic e. excavatio disci.

rectouterine e. excavatio rectouterina.

rectovesical e. excavatio rectovesicalis.

vesicouterine e. excavatio vesicouterina.

ex•ca•va•ti•o•nes (eks″kə-va″she-o′nēz) [L.] plural of *excavatio.*

ex•ca•va•tor (eks′kə-va″tər) 1. an instrument for hollowing out something by removing the center or inner part, or for making a hole or cavity. 2. a scoop or gouge for surgical use.

dental e. a handcutting instrument designed for removing the carious dentin of a decayed tooth. See also *discoid* (def. 4).

hatchet e. hatchet.

spoon e. a dental excavator having a spoonlike blade with the entire margin tapered and sharpened to cut carious dentin out of tooth cavities. Called also *spoon.*

ex•cess (ek-ses′, ek′ses) the state of exceeding that which is normal, sufficient, or needed; superfluous.

antibody e. see *prozone.*

antigen e. see *precipitin reaction,* under *reaction.*

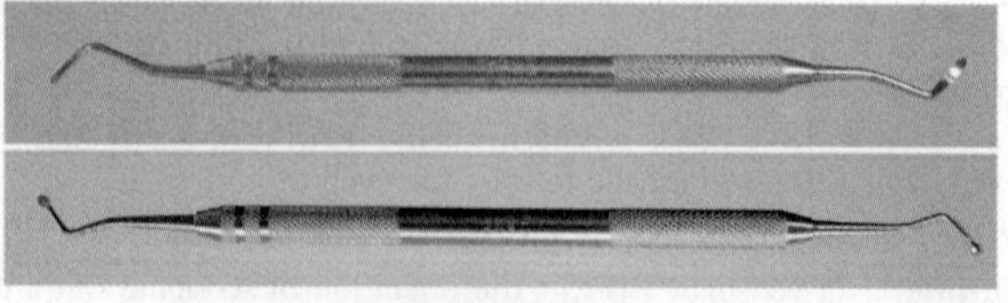

■ Dental excavators.

apparent mineralocorticoid e. (AME) a rare autosomal recessive enzyme deficiency syndrome caused by mutation in the *HSD11B2* gene (locus: 16q22), which encodes 11β-hydroxysteroid dehydrogenase type 2; it is characterized by accumulation of cortisol in the kidney in spite of normal plasma cortisol levels, with resulting hypertension, hypokalemia, metabolic alkalosis, and low plasma renin and aldosterone levels.

base e. the deviation from normal of the concentration of titratable base when blood or plasma is titrated to a plasma pH of 7.40 at a pCO_2 of 40 mm Hg at 37°C; it is 1.2 times the deviation of the standard bicarbonate from normal. Positive values indicate metabolic alkalosis; negative values, metabolic acidosis.

ex•change (eks-chānj′) 1. the substitution of one thing for another. 2. to substitute one thing for another.

plasma e. the removal of plasma from withdrawn blood, usually to a greater extent than in plasmapheresis, with retransfusion of the formed elements into the donor; done for removal of circulating antibodies or abnormal plasma constituents. The plasma removed is replaced by type-specific fresh frozen plasma or albumin.

alveolar gas e. the passage of oxygen and carbon dioxide in opposite directions across the alveolocapillary membrane.

sister chromatid e. the exchange of segments of DNA between sister chromatids, which is common in patients with Bloom syndrome.

ex•chang•er (eks-chānj′ər) an apparatus by which something may be exchanged.

heat e. a device placed in an extracorporeal circulation circuit to induce rapid cooling and rewarming of blood.

ex•cip•i•ent (ek-sip′e-ənt) [L. *excipiens*] any more or less inert substance added to a prescription in order to confer a suitable consistency or form to the drug; called also *vehicle*.

ex•cise (ek-sīz′) to cut out or off.

ex•ci•sion (ek-sizh′ən) [L. *excisio*, from *ex* out + *caedere* to cut] removal of a portion or all of an organ or other structure. Called also *resection* and *ectomy*.

intracapsular e. in surgery for soft tissue sarcoma, removal of the tumor alone by direct incision of the tumor capsule; of diagnostic value only since it leaves some gross tumor intact.

marginal e. surgical removal of an entire lesion, including only a very small margin of surrounding tissue.

radical e. in surgery for soft tissue sarcoma, removal of the entire anatomic compartment containing the tumor, as well as the origins and insertions of all muscles, bones, and joints contained in the compartment; frequently it involves the amputation of a limb.

total mesorectal e. (TME) a radical treatment for rectal cancer consisting of excision of the entire rectal mesentery, including that distal to the tumor.

wide e. in surgery for neoplasms, removal of both the tumor and a margin of apparently normal surrounding tissue; the limb, breast, or other body structure that is the site of the tumor is not amputated.

ex•ci•ta•bil•i•ty (ek-sīt″ə-bil′ĭ-te) 1. irritability. 2. the capacity of a cell to depolarize and form an action potential when in the presence of a stimulus stronger than a threshold value.

ex•ci•ta•ble (ek-sīt′ə-bəl) [L. *excitabilis*] irritable (def. 1).

ex•cit•ant (ek-sīt′ənt) stimulant.

ex•ci•ta•tion (ek″si-ta′shən) [L. *excitatio*, from *ex* out + *citare* to call] an act of irritation or stimulation or of responding to a stimulus; the addition of energy, as the excitation of a molecule by absorption of photons.

direct e. electrostimulation of a muscle by placing the electrode on the muscle itself.

indirect e. electrostimulation of a muscle by placing the electrode on its nerve.

reentrant e. reexcitation of cardiac tissue due to reentry; sometimes used synonymously with reentry.

ex•ci•ta•to•ry (ek-si′tə-tor″e) causing excitation.

ex•cite•ment (ek-sīt′ment) response to stimuli, often used specifically to denote excessive responsiveness to stimuli, particularly of an emotional nature, and often leading to impulsive activity.

catatonic e. periods of uncontrollable, unorganized, and apparently purposeless motor activity, without euphoria or other symptoms of mania; characteristic of catatonic schizophrenia.

psychomotor e. see under *acceleration*.

ex•ci•to•an•a•bol•ic (ek-si″to-an″ə-bol′ik) stimulating anabolism.

ex•ci•to•cat•a•bol•ic (ek-si″to-kat″ə-bol′ik) stimulating catabolism.

ex•ci•to•glan•du•lar (ek-si″to-glan′du-lər) causing glands to secrete.

ex•ci•to•met•a•bol•ic (ek-si″to-met″ə-bol′ik) producing metabolic changes.

ex•ci•to•mo•tor (ek-si″to-mo′tər) 1. tending to produce motion or motor function. 2. an agent that induces motion or functional activity.

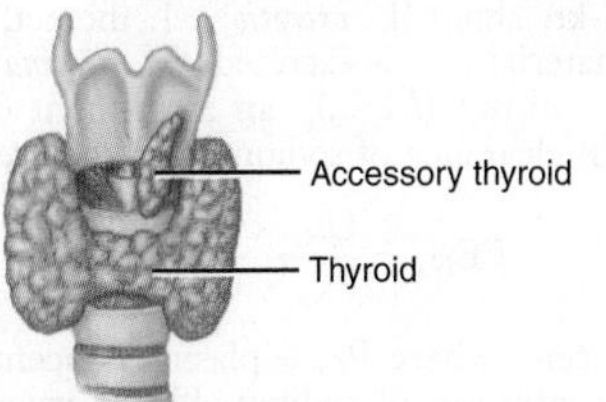

■ The accessory thyroid is an exclave of the thyroid.

ex•ci•to•mus•cu•lar (ek-si″to-mus′ku-lər) stimulating muscular activity.

ex•ci•tor (ek-si′tər) a nerve that when stimulated excites greater action in the part it supplies.

ex•ci•to•se•cre•to•ry (ek-si″to-sə-kre′tə-re) producing increased secretion.

ex•ci•to•tox•ic (ek-si′to-tok″sik) having a toxic excitatory effect on the nervous system; see *excitotoxin*.

ex•ci•to•tox•ic•i•ty (ek-si″to-tok-sis′ĭte) 1. the quality of being excitotoxic. 2. the degree to which a given substance has an excitotoxic effect on the nervous system.

ex•ci•to•tox•in (ek-si′to-tok″sin) any of a group of neurotoxic substances found in certain plants or made synthetically; they are analogous to glutamic acid and mimic its excitatory effects on neurons of the central nervous system as well as producing lesions on the perikarya; several of them are used experimentally to study the excitatory mechanisms of glutamate transmitters. They include ibotenic acid, kainic acid, quisqualic acid, and *N*-methyl-D-aspartate (NMDA).

ex•ci•to•vas•cu•lar (ek-si″to-vas′ku-lər) causing vascular changes.

ex•clave (eks′klāv) [*ex-* + L. *clavis* key, by analogy with *enclave*] a detached part of an organ, as of the pancreas, thyroid, or other gland.

ex•clu•sion (eks-kloo′zhən) [L. *exclusio*, from *ex* out + *claudere* to shut] 1. elimination, rejection, or extrusion. 2. an operation in which a portion of an organ is separated from the remainder but is not removed from the body.

allelic e. a mechanism that allows the expression of only one of a set of alleles, such as the expression of a single immunoglobulin by any one B lymphocyte or plasma cell or the expression of a single T cell receptor by any one T lymphocyte.

competitive e. the tendency for the better adapted species to exclude another related species from its particular ecological niche. See also *character displacement*, under *displacement*.

total vascular e. a technique used to limit hemorrhage during some stages of liver surgery, consisting of clamping of the inferior vena cava both above and below the liver as well as of the portal vein.

ex•coch•le•a•tion (eks-kok″le-a′shən) [*ex-* + L. *cochlea* spoon] the operation of curetting or scooping out a cavity.

ex•con•ju•gant (eks-kon′jŏŏ-gənt) [*ex-* + L. *conjugare* to join] either member of a pair of ciliate protozoa or bacteria (conjugants) after separation following conjugation.

ex•co•ri•ate (eks-ko′re-āt) scratch (def. 1).

ex•co•ri•a•tion (eks-ko″re-a′shən) scratch (def. 3).

neurotic e. a self-induced skin lesion, inflicted by the fingernails or other physical means.

ex•cre•ment (eks′krə-mənt) [L. *excrementum*, from *ex* out + *cernere* to sift, to separate] 1. feces. 2. any matter cast out as waste from the body; see also *discharge* (def. 3).

ex•cre•men•ti•tious (eks″krə-mən-tish′əs) 1. pertaining to excrement. 2. fecal.

ex•cres•cence (eks-kres′əns) [*ex-* + *-crescence*] any abnormal outgrowth; a projection of morbid origin.

fungating e., fungous e. a fungous growth in the umbilicus after separation of the umbilical cord; granuloma of the umbilicus.

Lambl e's small papillary projections on the cardiac valves, probably due to organized thrombi associated with the nodules of Arantius.

ex•cres•cent (eks-kres′ənt) resembling or of the nature of an excrescence.

ex•cre•ta (eks-kre′tə) [L., pl.] excretion (def. 2).

ex•crete (eks-krēt′) [L. *excernere*] to throw off or eliminate by a normal discharge, such as in defecation or urination. Called also *void*.

ex•cre•tin (eks-kre′tin) a crystalline compound, $C_{20}H_{36}O$, derivable from human feces.

ex•cre•tion (eks-kre′shən) [L. *excretio*] 1. the act, process, or function of excreting. 2. material that is excreted. Cf. *elimination.* **ex′cretory** *adj*

fractional e. of sodium (FE_{Na}) an assessment of acute renal failure comparing the renal clearance of sodium with the creatinine clearance:

$$FE_{Na} = \frac{U_{Na} \times P_{Cr}}{P_{Na} \times U_{Cr}} \times 100$$

expressed as a per cent, where P_{Cr} = plasma concentration of creatinine, P_{Na} = plasma concentration of sodium, U_{Cr} = urinary concentration of creatinine, and U_{Na} = urinary concentration of sodium. A value below 1.0 indicates that renal failure is due to prerenal azotemia, and a value above 2.0 suggests that it is due to acute tubular necrosis. Cf. *renal failure index*, under *index.*

pseudouridine e. increased excretion of pseudouridine in the urine of patients with gout; its significance remains to be established. A greater turnover of some forms of RNA has been suggested, possibly adding to the hyperuricemia of gout.

ex•cur•rent (eks-kur′ənt) excretory; efferent.

ex•cur•sion (eks-kur′zhən) [L. *excurrere* to run out from] movements occurring from a normal, or rest, position of a movable part in performance of a function, as those of the mandible to attain functional contact between the cusps of the mandibular and maxillary teeth in mastication, or of the chest wall in respiration. Called also *excursive movements.* **excur′sive** *adj*

lateral e. sideward movement of the mandible between the position of closure and that in which the tips of the cusps of opposing teeth are in vertical proximity.

protrusive e. movement of the mandible between the position of closure and that in which the incisal edges of the anterior teeth are in vertical approximation.

retrusive e. the slight backward and return movement of the mandible between the position of closure and one slightly posterior, more often present with mandibular overclosure.

ex•cy•clo•pho•ria (ek-si″klo-for′e-ə) [*ex-* + *cyclophoria*] cyclophoria in which the upper pole of the vertical axis of the eye deviates away from the midline of the face and toward the temple; called also *plus cyclophoria.* Cf. *incyclophoria.*

ex•cy•clo•tro•pia (ek-si″klo-tro′pe-ə) [*ex-* + *cyclotropia*] cyclotropia in which the upper pole of the vertical axis of the eye deviates away from the midline of the face, and toward the temple.

ex•cys•ta•tion (ek″sis-ta′shən) escape from a cyst or envelope; especially a stage in the life cycle of parasites occurring after the cystic form has been swallowed by the host.

Ex•el•derm (ek′sel-dərm″) trademark for a preparation of sulconazole nitrate.

Ex•e•lon (ek′sə-lon″) trademark for preparations of rivastigmine tartrate.

exe•mes•tane (ek″sə-mes′tān) an aromatase inhibitor structurally related to androstenedione; used as an antineoplastic in the treatment of advanced breast carcinoma in postmenopausal women, administered orally.

ex•e•mia (eg-se′me-ə) [*ex-* + *-emia*] loss of fluid from the blood vessels, with resultant hemoconcentration.

ex•en•a•tide (ek-sen′ə-tīd) a glucagon-like peptide 1 receptor agonist that stimulates insulin secretion, used in combination with metformin or a sulfonylurea in the treatment of type 2 diabetes mellitus; administered subcutaneously.

ex•en•ce•pha•lia (ek″sən-sə-fa′le-ə) exencephaly.

ex•en•ceph•a•lon (ek″sən-sef′ə-lon) exencephalus.

ex•en•ceph•a•lus (ek″sən-sef′ə-ləs) a fetus exhibiting exencephaly.

ex•en•ceph•a•ly (ek″sən-sef′ə-le) [*ex-* + Gr. *enkephalos* brain] a developmental anomaly characterized by acrania with the brain exposed. **exenceph′alous** *adj*

ex•en•din-4 (eks-en′din) exenatide.

ex•en•ter•a•tion (ek-sen″tər-a′shən) [*ex-* + Gr. *enteron* bowel] 1. a more extensive type of evisceration (removal of organs), usually radical excision of the contents of a body cavity, as of the pelvis. 2. in ophthalmology, removal of the entire contents of the orbit.

pelvic e. removal of the organs and adjacent structures of the pelvis; called also *Brunschwig operation.*

anterior pelvic e. excision en masse of the bladder, lower ureters, vagina, adnexa, pelvic lymph nodes, and pelvic peritoneum, with implantation of the ureters into the intact pelvic colon or an ileal conduit. See also *radical cystectomy*, under *cystectomy.*

posterior pelvic e. excision en masse of the pelvic colon, uterus, vagina, and adnexa, with or without pelvic lymph node excision, the lower urinary tract being undisturbed.

total pelvic e. excision en masse of the bladder, lower ureters, vagina, uterus, adnexa, and the pelvic and lower sigmoid colon, with excision of the pelvic lymph nodes, removal of all the pelvic peritoneum, and replantation of the ureters into an isolated ileal segment.

ex•en•ter•a•tive (ek-sen′tər-ə-tiv) 1. pertaining to exenteration. 2. requiring exenteration, as exenterative surgery.

ex•en•ter•itis (ek-sen″tər-i′tis) inflammation of the peritoneal covering of the intestine.

ex•er•cise (ek′sər-sīz) the performance of physical exertion for improvement of health or the correction of physical deformity.

active e. motion imparted to a part by voluntary contraction and relaxation of the muscles controlling the part. Called also *free e.*

active assisted e. motion imparted to a part of the body by voluntary contraction of muscles controlling the part, along with assistance from a therapist or some other means.

aerobic e. systematic exercise designed to increase oxygen consumption and improve the functioning of the respiratory and cardiovascular systems.

ballistic stretching e′s rapid, jerky movements whose purpose is to stretch muscles and connective tissue; they are much more strenuous than isometric exercises.

breathing e′s exercises to improve respiration, used both in primary respiratory disorders and in those due to musculoskeletal malformations, including relaxation techniques for slower, more efficient breathing patterns and techniques for better diaphragmatic, abdominal, and intercostal muscle coordination.

closed chain e′s, closed kinetic chain e′s exercises in which the kinetic chain of a limb is closed, i.e. the hand or foot cannot swing freely, such as when the foot is on the floor or some other surface.

corrective e. therapeutic e.

dynamic e. active e.

endurance e. any exercise that involves the use of several large groups of muscles and is thus dependent on the delivery of oxygen to the muscles by the cardiovascular system; used in both physical fitness programs and testing of cardiovascular and pulmonary function.

flexion back e′s an exercise regimen designed to decrease low back pain by flexing the lumbosacral spine and strengthening the muscles in the region.

free e. active e.

Frenkel e′s a series of movements of increasing difficulty and precision to be performed by ataxic patients for restoration of coordination.

functional e′s exercises designed to reinforce or improve performance of normal everyday activities.

isokinetic e. active exercise performed at a constant angular velocity; torque and tension remain constant while muscles shorten or lengthen.

isometric e. a type of exercise performed against stable resistance, without change in the length of the muscle. Called also *muscle-setting e.* and *static e.*

isotonic e. active exercise without appreciable change in the force of muscular contraction, with shortening of the muscle.

Kegel e′s exercises performed to strengthen the pubococcygeal muscle, for controlling or preventing stress incontinence, improving sexual response, and diminishing a variety of problems and discomfort in pregnancy.

muscle-setting e. isometric e.

open chain e′s, open kinetic chain e′s exercises in which the kinetic chain of a limb is open or free to move, i.e. the hand or foot can swing freely and is not pressed against the floor, a bar, or any other surface.

passive e. motion imparted to a segment of the body by another individual, machine, or other outside force, or produced by voluntary effort of another segment of the patient's own body.

plyometric e′s plyometrics.

progressive resistance e., progressive resistive e. a physical therapy method of strengthening debilitated muscles by increasing the amount of the resisting force at regular time intervals.

range of motion e. the putting of a joint through its full range of normal movements; it may be either active or passive.

relaxation e. any exercise designed to decrease muscle tension, whether due to psychogenic causes, excess of physical exertion, or an organic neurologic condition; it may involve breathing exercise or the rhythmic shaking of the affected part.

resistance e., resistive e. exercise performed by the patient against resistance supplied either by a weight or by the muscle power of the therapist.

sport-specific e. an exercise designed to improve performance in a particular sport.

static e. isometric e.

therapeutic e. the scientific use of bodily movement to restore normal function in diseased or injured tissues or to maintain a state of well being. Called also *corrective e.*

underwater e. exercise performed in a pool or a large tub of water. The buoyancy of the water allows much freer movement of weakened body

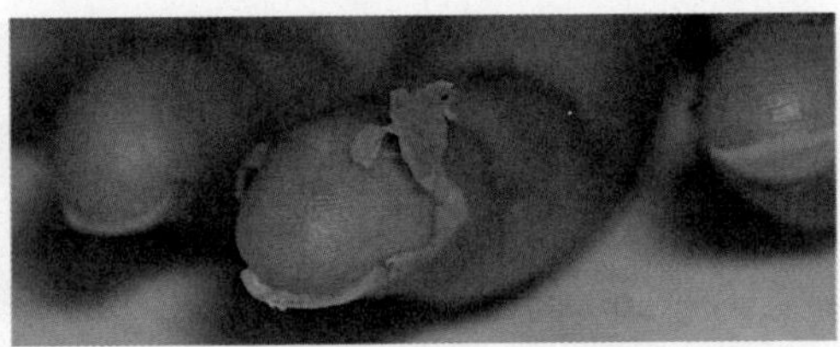

■ Exfoliation of fingertips in subacute phase of Kawasaki disease.

parts than is possible under normal atmospheric conditions; water temperature and water currents can be varied for different therapeutic effects. Cf. *Hubbard tank.*

Williams e's, Williams flexion e's widely used flexion back exercises involving flexion of the neck, trunk, pelvis, and lower limbs; designed to alleviate lower back pain by stretching the extensor muscles in the lower back and strengthening flexors such as the rectus abdominis and gluteus maximus.

ex•er•e•sis (ek-ser′ə-sis) [Gr. *exairesis* a taking out] surgical removal or excision.

ex•er•gon•ic (ek″sər-gon′ik) [*ex-* + Gr. *ergon* work] characterized or accompanied by the release of energy; said of reactions, particularly biochemical reactions, that release free energy, yielding products having a lower free energy than did the reactants. Opposed to *endergonic.*

ex•e•sion (eg-ze′zhən) [L. *exedere* to eat out] the gradual destruction of superficial parts of a tissue.

ex•flag•el•la•tion (eks-flaj″ə-la′shən) [*ex-* + L. *flagellum*] the rapid formation in the gut of the insect vector of microgametes from the microgamont in *Plasmodium* and certain other sporozoan protozoa.

ex•fo•li•a•tin (eks-fo″le-a′tin) [*ex-* + L. *folium* leaf] an erythrogenic, epidermolytic, heat-stabile, acid-labile exotoxin produced by certain strains of *Staphylococcus aureus* (phage group II), which causes intraepidermal separation by disturbing the adhesive forces between cells in the stratum granulosum to cause the clinical manifestations of staphylococcal scalded skin syndrome. Called also *epidermolysin.*

ex•fo•li•a•tio (eks″fo-le-a′she-o) [L., from *ex* away from + *folium* leaf] exfoliation.

e. area′ta lin′guae benign migratory glossitis.

ex•fo•li•a•tion (eks-fo″le-a′shən) [L. *exfoliatus*, past part. of *exfoliare* to strip of leaves] 1. a falling off in scales or layers, such as the stratum corneum of the skin or a superficial layer of bone. 2. the removal of scales or flakes from the surface of the skin. 3. the normal loss of deciduous teeth following loss of their root structure.

lamellar e. of the newborn the condition in a minority of collodion babies when shedding of the membrane leaves relatively normal skin. Called also *lamellar desquamation of the newborn.*

ex•fo•li•a•tive (eks-fo′le-ə-tiv″) pertaining to or characterized by exfoliation.

Ex•forge (ex′forj) trademark for a combination preparation of amlodipine besylate and valsartan.

ex•ha•la•tion (eks″hə-la′shən) [L. *exhalatio*, from *ex* out + *halare* to breathe] the act of breathing out; called also expiration.

ex•hale (eks′hāl) [*ex-* + L. *halare* to breathe] 1. to expel from the lungs by breathing. 2. to give off a watery or other vapor. Defs. 1 and 2 called also *expire.*

ex•haus•tion (eg-zaws′chən) [*ex-* + L. *haurire* to drain] 1. a state of extreme mental or physical fatigue. 2. the state of being drained, emptied, consumed, or used up.

combat e. former term for combat-related posttraumatic stress disorder; now used colloquially.

heat e. an effect of excessive exposure to heat, occurring among workers in hot places such as furnace rooms and foundries and sometimes in those under prolonged exposure to the sun's heat. It is marked by a core temperature that ranges from slightly subnormal to slightly elevated, with dizziness, headache, nausea, and sometimes delirium or collapse. Distinguished from *heat stroke* and *sunstroke*, in which the body temperature may be dangerously elevated. Called also *heat prostration.*

postactivation e., posttetanic e. changes at the cellular level, such as decreased neuromuscular transmission, seen when repetitive nerve stimulation is performed a few minutes after intense neuromuscular activity; see also *postactivation depression* and *postactivation facilitation.*

Exhib. [L.] exhibea′tur (let it be given).

ex•hi•bi•tion•ism (eg″zĭ-bish′ə-niz-əm) [DSM-IV] a paraphilia characterized by recurrent intense sexual urges and sexually arousing fantasies of exposing the genitals to an unsuspecting stranger. Exhibitionism occurs almost exclusively in males. **exhibi′tionist** *n*

ex•hu•ma•tion (eg″zu-ma′shən) [*ex-* + L. *humus* earth] disinterment; removal of the dead body from the earth after burial.

Ex•ner plexus (eks′nər) [Siegmund *Exner*, Austrian physiologist, 1846–1926] see under *plexus.*

exo- [Gr. *exō* outside] a prefix meaning outside, or outward.

exo•am•y•lase (ek″so-am′ə-lās) an amylase that catalyzes the cleavage of α-1,4-glucosidic bonds only at the nonreducing termini of polysaccharide chains. Cf. *endoamylase.*

exo•an•ti•gen (ek″so-an′tə-jən) ectoantigen.

exo•car•dia (ek″so-kahr′de-ə) ectocardia.

exo•carp (ek′so-kahrp) the outer layer of the pericarp of a flower.

exo•cata•pho•ria (ek″so-kat″ə-for′e-ə) [*exo-* + *cataphoria*] a phoria in which the visual axes turn downward and outward.

exo•cele (ek′so-sēl) extraembryonic coelom.

exo•cel•lu•lar (ek″so-sel′u-lər) external to the cell membrane, but still attached.

exo•cer•vix (ek″so-sur′viks) portio vaginalis cervicis.

exo•cho•ri•on (ek″so-kor′e-on) the part of the chorion derived from the ectoderm, as in those species in which extraembryonic membranes form by folding.

exo•coe•lom (ek″so-se′ləm) [*exo-* + *coelom*] extraembryonic coelom.

exo•coe•lo•ma (ek″so-se-lo′mə) extraembryonic coelom.

exo•crine (ek′so-krin) [*exo-* + Gr. *krinein* to separate] 1. secreting outwardly via a duct, as opposed to. *endocrine* (q.v.). 2. denoting such a gland or its secretion. See also under *gland.*

exo•cri•nol•o•gy (ek″so-krĭ-nol′ə-je) the study of substances secreted externally by individual organisms which effect integration of a group of organisms.

exo•cu•ti•cle (ek″so-ku′tĭ-kəl) [*exo-* + L. *cuticula*] the outer layer of the procuticle of certain crustaceans and arthropods, which contains cuticulin, chitin, and phenolic substances that are oxidized to produce the dark pigment of the cuticle.

exo•cyc•lic (ek″so-sik′lik, -si′klik) denoting one or more atoms attached to a ring structure but outside it.

exo•cy•to•sis (ek″so-si-to′sis) [Gk. *exo-* + *kutos* a hollow vessel] 1. the discharge of material from a cell by fusion of a membrane-bound vesicle with the plasma membrane and subsequent release of the vesicle's contents into the extracellular environment; cf. *endocytosis.* 2. the aggregation of migrating leukocytes in the epidermis as part of the inflammatory response.

exo•de•oxy•ri•bo•nu•cle•ase (ek″so-de-ok″se-ri″bo-noo′kle-ās) [EC 3.1.11] any of a sub-subclass of enzymes of the hydrolase class that catalyze the hydrolysis of terminal bonds of deoxyribonucleic acids, releasing mononucleotides.

exo•de•vi•a•tion (ek″so-de″ve-a′shən) 1. exophoria. 2. exotropia.

ex•odon•tia (ek″so-don′shə) exodontics.

ex•odon•tics (ek″so-don′tiks) the branch of dentistry that deals with extraction of the teeth. Called also *exodontia.*

ex•odon•tist (ek″so-don′tist) a dentist who practices exodontics.

exo•en•zyme (ek″so-en′zīm) an enzyme that acts outside of the cells in which it originates; called also *ectoenzyme* and *extracellular enzyme.* Cf. *endoenzyme.*

exo•er•gic (ek″so-ur′jik) 1. exergonic. 2. exothermic.

exo•eryth•ro•cyt•ic (ek″so-ə-rith″ro-sit′ik) outside the erythrocyte, said of stages in development of species of *Plasmodium.*

ex•og•a•mous (ek-sog′ə-məs) characterized by exogamy.

ex•og•a•my (ek-sog′ə-me) [*exo-* + Gr. *gamos* marriage] 1. fertilization by the union of cells not derived from the same parent cell. Cf. *autogamy* and *endogamy* (def. 1). 2. marriage outside a particular community, range, or other group.

exo•gas•tric (ek″so-gas′trik) extragastric.

exo•gas•tru•la (ek″so-gas′troo-lə) [*exo-* + *gastrula*] an abnormal gastrula in which invagination is hindered and the mesentoderm bulges outward.

exo•gas•tru•la•tion (ek″so-gas″troo-la′shən) the evagination to the exterior (or turning inside out) of the gut due to an interference with the normal processes of gastrulation, which can occur if the morula is cut transversely below the equator. It is usually followed by a migration of mesenchyme cells into the interior.

ex•o•gen (ek′so-jen) term used by some authorities for a fourth phase in the hair cycle during which the hair is shed.

ex•o•gen•ic (ek″so-jen′ik) exogenous.

ex•og•e•note (eks″oj′ə-nōt) in bacterial genetics, the extra piece of genetic information introduced by transduction into the recipient cell by the donor cell. Cf. *endogenote.*

ex•og•e•nous (ek-soj′ə-nəs) [*exo-* + *-genous*] 1. developed or originating outside the organism, such as a disease or infection. Called also *ectogenous* and *exogenic.* 2. growing by additions to the outside.

ex•og•na•thia (ek″sog-na′the-ə) prognathism.

ex•og•na•thi•on (ek″sog-na′the-on) [*exo-* + Gr. *gnathos* jaw] the maxilla exclusive of the premaxilla.

ex•om•pha•los (ek-som′fə-los) [*ex-* + Gr. *omphalos* navel] umbilical hernia.

e. ma′jor umbilical hernia in which the defect is at least 5 cm in diameter and contains liver and other viscera.

e. mi′nor umbilical hernia in which the defect is less than 5 cm in diameter and contains only bowel.

exo•mys•i•um (ek″so-mis′e-əm) perimysium.

ex•on (ek′son) [*ex*pressed (sequence) + *-on*] a coding sequence in a gene; see also *intron.*

exo•nu•cle•ase (ek″so-noo′kle-ās) [EC 3.1.11–16] any nuclease specifically catalyzing the hydrolysis of terminal bonds of deoxyribonucleotide or ribonucleotide chains, releasing mononucleotides. Cf. *endonuclease.*

exo•path•ic (ek″so-path′ik) of the nature of an exopathy; originating outside the body.

ex•op•a•thy (ek-sop′ə-the) [*exo-* + *-pathy*] a disease originating in some cause lying outside the organism; exogenous disease.

exo•pep•ti•dase (ek″so-pep′tĭ-dās) [EC 3.4.11–19] any peptidase that catalyzes the cleavage of the terminal or penultimate peptide bond, releasing a single amino acid or dipeptide from the peptide chain. Exopeptidases are classified as aminopeptidases, carboxypeptidases, dipeptidases, and omega peptidases.

Exo•phi•a•la (ek″so-fi′ə-lə) a widespread genus of saprobic Fungi Imperfecti of the form-class Hyphomycetes, form-family Dematiaceae. *E. jeansel′mei* (called also *Phialophora jeanselmei* and *Torula jeanselmei*) is commonly found in soil and sewage and causes eumycotic mycetoma and opportunistic infections in humans. *E. spini′fera* (called also *Phialophora spinifera*) occasionally causes phaeohyphomycosis of the skin. *E. wernec′kii* is now called *Hortaea werneckii.*

exo•pho•ria (ek-so-for′e-ə) [*exo-* + *phoria*] a form of heterophoria in which there is deviation of the visual axis of one eye away from that of the other eye in the absence of visual fusional stimuli. Called also *exodeviation.* **exopho′ric** *adj*

ex•oph•thal•mo•gen•ic (ek″sof-thal″mo-jen′ik) causing or producing exophthalmos.

ex•oph•thal•mom•e•ter (ek″sof-thəl-mom′ə-tər) an instrument for measuring the amount of exophthalmos; called also *ophthalmostatometer, orthometer, proptometer, protometer,* and *statometer.*

ex•oph•thal•mo•met•ric (ek″sof-thal″mo-met′rik) pertaining to exophthalmometry.

ex•oph•thal•mom•e•try (ek″sof-thəl-mom′ə-tre) [*exophthalmos* + *-metry*] measurement of the extent of protrusion of the eyeball in exophthalmos.

ex•oph•thal•mos (ek″sof-thal′mos) [*ex-* + Gr. *ophthalmos* eye] abnormal protrusion of the eyeball. Spelled also *exophthalmus;* called also *exorbitism* and *proptosis.* **exophthal′mic** *adj*

endocrine e. exophthalmos associated with disorder of an endocrine gland; the most common type is thyrotoxic exophthalmos.

malignant e. the severe exophthalmos of Graves orbitopathy, in which there is marked edema and infiltration of the orbital tissues and extraocular muscles, protrusion, and stare.

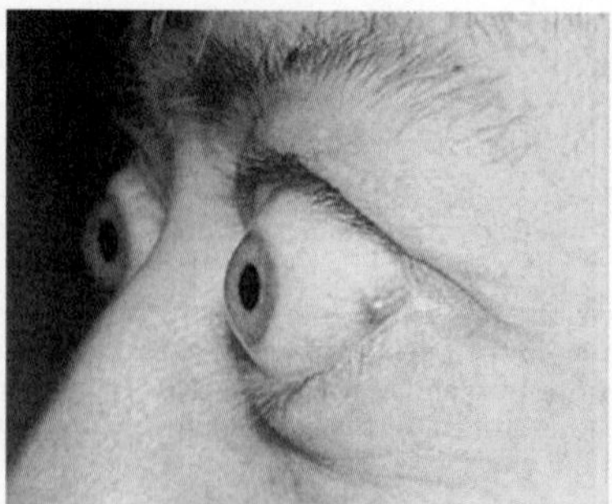

■ Exophthalmos and lid retraction associated with Graves disease.

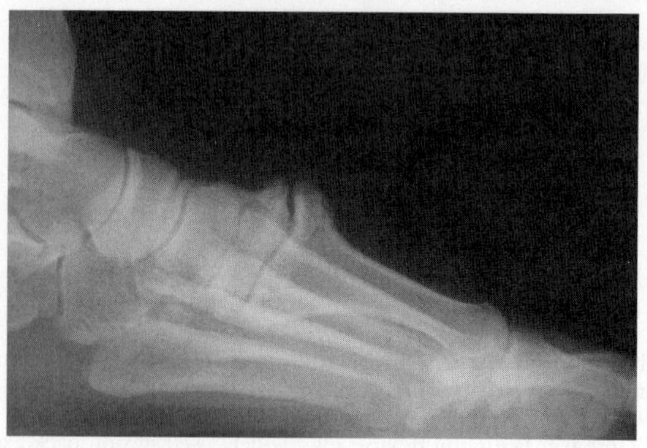

■ Exostosis at the metatarsocuneiform joint.

pulsating e. exophthalmos with pulsation and bruit, often due to aneurysm pushing the eye forward.

thyrotoxic e. exophthalmos due to thyrotoxicosis; see also *dysthyroid orbitopathy,* under *orbitopathy.*

ex•oph•thal•mus (ek″sof-thal′məs) exophthalmos.

exo•phyt•ic (ek″so-fit′ik) [*exo-* + *phyt-* + *-ic*] growing outward; in oncology, proliferating on the exterior or surface epithelium of an organ or other structure, in which the growth originated.

exo•plasm (ek′so-plaz″əm) ectoplasm.

exo•plas•mic (ek-so-plaz′mik) facing away from the cytoplasm.

ex•or•bi•tism (eg-sor′bĭ-tiz-əm) exophthalmos.

exo•ri•bo•nu•cle•ase (ek″so-ri-bo-noo′kle-ās) [EC 3.1.13–14] any member of two sub-subclasses of enzymes of the hydrolase class that catalyze the hydrolysis of terminal bonds of ribonucleotides, producing mononucleotides.

ex•or•phin (ek-sor′fin) any of various peptides that have opioid properties and are not normally found in humans; several are found in wheat gluten.

exo•se•ro•sis (ek″so-se-ro′sis) an oozing of serum or exudate, as in moist skin diseases and edema.

exo-α-si•al•i•dase (ek″so-si-al′ĭ-dās) [EC 3.2.1.18] EC nomenclature for *neuraminidase.*

exo•skel•e•tal (ek″so-skel′ə-təl) 1. pertaining to an exoskeleton. 2. resembling an exoskeleton.

exo•skel•e•ton (ek″so-skel′ə-ton) [*exo-* + *skeleton*] a hard structure developed on the outside of the body, as the shell of a crustacean. In vertebrates the term is applied to structures produced by the epidermis, as hair, nails, hoofs, teeth, etc.

ex•os•mose (ek′sos-mōs) to diffuse from within outward.

ex•os•mo•sis (ek″sos-mo′sis) [*ex-* + *osmosis*] diffusion or osmosis from within outward; movement outward through a diaphragm or through vessel walls. Cf. *endosmosis.*

exo•some (ek′so-sōm) 1. a large complex of exonucleases, present in both the nucleoplasm and the cytoplasm, that degrade RNA in a 3′ to 5′ direction, involved in a number of RNA processing and degradation pathways. 2. a small (10–30 nm) cytoplasmic vesicle, generated in many cell types by inward budding of the membrane of multivesicular bodies and containing a mixture of proteins and lipids; the vesicles are released into the extracellular environment and are involved in membrane remodeling and cell signaling.

exo•spore (ek′so-spor) conidium.

exo•spo•ri•um (ek″so-spor′e-əm) the external layer of the envelope of a spore.

ex•os•to•sec•to•my (ek-sos″to-sek′tə-me) excision of an exostosis.

ex•os•to•sis (ek″sos-to′sis) [*ex-* + *ostosis*] 1. a benign bony growth projecting outward from the surface of a bone. 2. osteochondroma.

e. bursa′ta an exostosis from the epiphyseal portion of a bone, consisting of bone and cartilaginous tissue covered by a connective-tissue capsule.

e. cartilagi′nea a variety of osteoma consisting of a layer of cartilage developing beneath the periosteum of a bone.

hereditary multiple e's multiple cartilaginous exostoses.

ivory e. compact osteoma.

multiple e's, multiple cartilaginous e's, multiple osteocartilaginous e's 1. an autosomal dominant disorder characterized by exostoses near the ends of diaphyses of long bones, which may be cartilaginous or osteocartilaginous growths; it is generally benign, although sarcomatous changes have occurred. Called also *diaphyseal aclasis* and *hereditary multiple e's.* 2. a bone

disease in dogs and sometimes cats, often hereditary, characterized by exostoses on bones such as ribs, long bones, or vertebrae. They may impinge on blood vessels, nerves, or the spinal cord; the latter case can cause paresis or paralysis.
osteocartilaginous e. osteochondroma.
subungual e. a cartilage-capped reactive bone spur on the distal phalanx, seen most often on the great toe in women.

ex•os•tot•ic (ek″sos-tot′ik) pertaining to or of the nature of exostosis.

Exo•surf Neo•na•tal (ek′so-sərf ne″o-na′təl) trademark for a combination preparation of colfosceril palmitate, cetyl alcohol, and tyloxapol.

exo•ter•ic (ek″so-ter′ik) [Gr. *exōterikos* outer] generated or developed outside the organism; exogenous.

exo•ther•mal (ek″so-thur′məl) exothermic.

exo•ther•mic (ek″so-thur′mik) [*exo-* + *thermic*] characterized or accompanied by the evolution of heat, as in a chemical reaction during and by which heat is released; liberating heat or energy from its potential forms. Cf. *endothermic.*

ex•ot•ic (eg-zot′ik) of foreign origin; not native.

exo•tox•ic (ek′so-tok″sik) [*exo-* + *toxic*] pertaining to or produced by an exotoxin.

exo•tox•in (ek′so-tok″sin) [*exo-* + *toxin*] a toxic substance that is formed by species of certain bacteria, such as *Bacillus, Bordetella, Clostridium, Corynebacterium, Escherichia, Pseudomonas, Salmonella, Shigella, Staphylococcus, Streptococcus, Vibrio,* and *Yersinia,* and is found either on the outside of the bacterial cell or free in the culture medium. Exotoxins are protein in nature and heat-labile; they are detoxified with retention of antigenicity by treatment with formaldehyde (formol toxoid), and are the most poisonous substances known to humans. The LD_{50} of crystalline botulinum type A toxin for the mouse is 4.5×10^{-9} mg.
streptococcal pyrogenic e. an exotoxin that is produced by *Streptococcus pyogenes* and exists in several antigenically distinct types; it causes fever, the rash of scarlet fever, organ damage, increased permeability of the blood-brain barrier, and alterations in immune response, including increased susceptibility to endotoxic shock and changes in T cell function. Formerly called *erythrogenic toxin.*

exo•tro•pia (ek″so-tro′pe-ə) [*exo-* + *tropia*] strabismus in which there is permanent deviation of the visual axis of one eye away from that of the other, resulting in diplopia; called also *divergent* or *external strabismus,* and *walleye.* **exotro′pic** *adj*

ex•pan•der (ek-span′dər) [L. *expandere* to spread out] extender.
plasma volume e. artificial plasma extender.
subperiosteal tissue e. (STE) a fillable tube inserted temporarily into the subperiosteal tissue prior to reconstruction of the alveolar ridge with hydroxylapatite granules; by progressively inflating the tube the periosteal mucosa can be expanded to create space for the granules.

ex•pan•sion (ek-span′shən) [L. *expandere* to spread out] 1. the process or state of being increased in extent, surface, or bulk. 2. a region or area of increased bulk or surface. 3. abnormal, excessive occurrence of a triplet repeat.
e. of the arch maxillary e.
clonal e. an immune response in which lymphocytes stimulated by antigen proliferate and amplify the population of relevant cells.
cubical e. increase in volume by an increase in all dimensions.
dorsal digital e., extensor e. a triangular aponeurotic extension of the digital extensor tendon on the dorsum of the proximal phalanx of each digit, to which the tendons of the lumbrical and interosseous muscles are also attached; it forms a movable hood around the metacarpophalangeal joint. Called also *extensor aponeurosis* or *hood.*
hygroscopic e. an increase in dimensions of a body or substance as a result of absorption of moisture.
maxillary e. an orthodontic method of correcting narrow or collapsed maxillary arches and functional posterior crossbite, whereby increased maxillary arch width is obtained with the use of various appliances that provide laterally expansive force resulting in orthopedic and orthodontic movements. Called also *e. of the arch.*

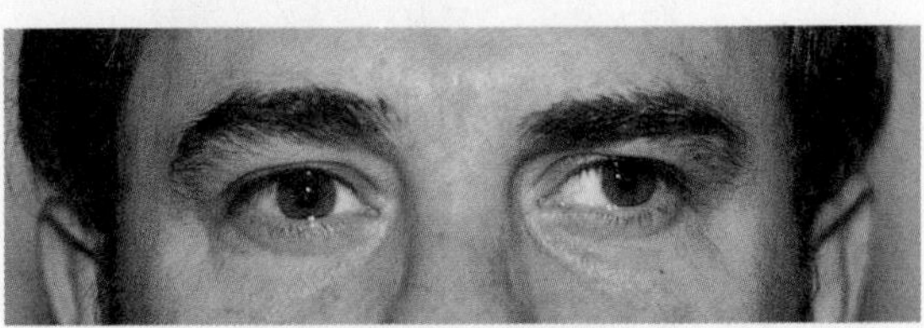

■ Exotropia.

setting e. the increase in dimensions of a material, such as plaster of Paris, which occurs concurrently with its hardening.
thermal e. an increase in dimensions of a body or substance as a result of an increase in its temperature; used in dentistry to enlarge an investment mold to compensate for shrinkage of the metal casting.
wax e. a type of thermal expansion consisting of an increase in the dimensions of a wax pattern for a dental restoration to compensate for shrinkage of the gold during the casting process.

ex•pan•sive•ness (ek-span′siv-nis) behavior marked by euphoria, loquacity, and grandiosity.

ex•pec•tan•cy (ek-spek′tən-se) the expected value or probability of occurrence for a specific event. Symbol *E.*
life e. 1. the number of years, based on statistical averages, that a given person of a specific age, class, or other demographic variable may be expected to continue living. 2. the average length of survival expected for an organism from a given point in its life cycle.

ex•pec•to•rant (ek-spek′tə-rənt) [*ex-* + L. *pectus* breast] 1. promoting the ejection, by spitting, of mucus or other fluids from the lungs and trachea. 2. an agent that promotes the ejection of mucus or exudate from the lungs, bronchi, and trachea; sometimes extended to all remedies that quiet cough (antitussives).
liquefying e. an expectorant that promotes the ejection of mucus from the respiratory tract by decreasing its viscosity.
stimulant e. an expectorant that stimulates secretion of mucus by the respiratory tract mucosa.

ex•pec•to•ra•tion (ek-spek″tə-ra′shən) 1. the act of coughing up and spitting out materials from the respiratory tract. 2. sputum.

ex•per•i•ment (ek-sper′ĭ-mənt) [L. *experimentum* proof from experience] a procedure done in order to discover or to demonstrate some fact or general truth.
check e. crucial e.
control e. an experiment that is made under standard conditions, to test the correctness of other observations; see also *control.*
crucial e. an experiment so designed and so prepared for by previous work that it will definitely settle some point.
Cyon e. the application of a stimulus to an intact anterior spinal nerve root, which induces a stronger contraction of muscle than the same stimulus to the peripheral end of a divided nerve root.
defect e. observation of an embryo, after destruction of a region or part, to ascertain the effect on development.
Küss e. injection of a solution of opium or belladonna into the bladder, which produces no symptoms of poisoning and thus proves the impermeability of the bladder epithelium to these substances.
Mariotte e. an experiment to demonstrate the blind spot of the eye: the eye is fixed on the center of a cross marked on a card on which is also marked a large spot; the card is moved to or from the face, and at a certain distance the image of the spot will disappear.
Müller e. see under *maneuver.*
Nussbaum e. ligation of the renal arteries of an animal in order to isolate the glomeruli of the kidneys from the circulation.
Scheiner e. an experiment in accommodation: one looks at an object through two pinholes closer together than pupil diameter in a card. If the object is in focus, only one image is observed; if it is not, two or more images are seen.
Stensen e. the experiment of cutting off the blood supply from the lumbar region of the spinal cord of an animal by compressing the abdominal aorta; it produces paralysis of the posterior parts of the body.
Toynbee e. see under *maneuver.*
Valsalva e. Valsalva maneuver (def. 1).

ex•pi•rate (eks′pĭ-rāt) exhalation (def. 3).
single e. the gas exhaled in a single breath.

ex•pi•ra•tion (ek″spĭ-ra′shən) [*ex-* + L. *spirare* to breathe] 1. exhalation (def. 1, 2, or 3). 2. termination, or death.

ex•pi•ra•to•ry (ek-spi′rə-tor″e) pertaining to exhalation (expiration).

ex•pire (ek-spīr′) 1. to exhale. 2. to die, or terminate.

ex•plant[1] (eks′plant) tissue taken from its original site and transferred to an artificial medium for growth.

ex•plant[2] (eks-plant′) 1. to remove an implant from the body. 2. to take tissue from the body and place in an artificial medium for growth.

ex•plan•ta•tion (eks″plan-ta′shən) 1. removal of an explant from the body. 2. the removal of an implant.

ex•plode (ek-splōd′) [L. *explodere,* from *ex* out +*plaudere* to clap the hands] 1. to undergo sudden and violent decomposition or combustion; see also *blast*[2]. 2. to burst; to spread rapidly, as an epidemic.

ex•plo•ra•tion (ek″splə-ra′shən) [L. *exploratio,* from *ex* out + *plorare* to cry out] investigation or examination, sometimes including surgery, for diagnostic purposes. **explor′atory** *adj*

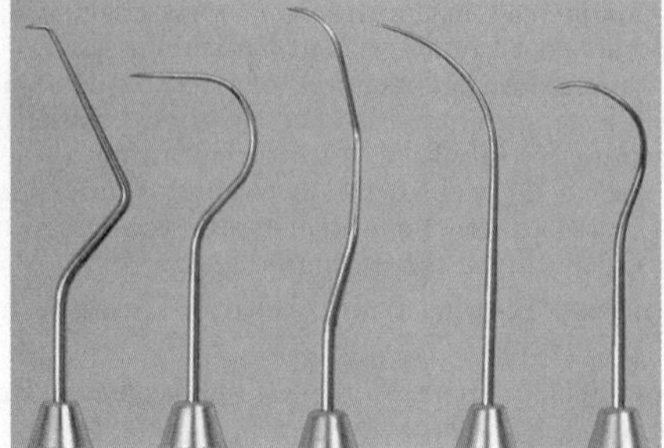
■ Typical explorers.

ex·plor·er (ek-splor′ər) 1. an instrument for use in exploration, particularly for foreign bodies. 2. an instrument with a flexible, sharp point, used to examine the crown of a tooth for defects or caries.

ex·plo·sion (ek-splo′zhən) [L. *explosio*] 1. the act of exploding. 2. a sudden and violent outbreak, as of emotion.

ex·plo·sive (ek-splo′siv) characterized by explosions.

ex·po·nent (ek-spo′nənt) a number or symbol placed above and to the right of another number or symbol indicating the number of times that that value is to be multiplied by itself; a negative exponent indicates the reciprocal of the quantity arrived at by multiplication. For example, $3^3 = 3 \times 3 \times 3 = 27$, and $x^{-2} = 1/(x \times x)$.

ex·po·nen·tial (ek″spə-nen′shəl) denoting a mathematical function in which the variable or variables appear in exponents, e.g., $y = a^x$, where a is a constant and x is a variable.

ex·po·sure (ek-spo′zhər) [L. *exponere* to put out] 1. the act of laying open, as surgical exposure. 2. the condition of being subjected to something that could have a harmful effect., such as an infectious agent or extremes of weather or radiation. 3. in radiology, a measure of the x-ray or gamma radiation at a certain place based on its ability to cause ionization. The unit of exposure is the roentgen. Symbol X. Called also *exposure dose.* 4. in radiology, the product of the intensity of x-rays and the time the film is exposed.

acute e. radiation exposure of short duration, usually referring to a heavy dose. See also *acute radiation syndrome*, under *syndrome.*

air e. the amount of exposure to ionizing radiation, measured in a small mass of air, excluding backscatter from irradiated objects, Called also *air dose.*

chronic e. a long-term radiation exposure, either continuous *(protraction exposure)* or intermittent *(fractionation exposure)*, usually referring to exposure to low-intensity radiation; effects may include accelerated aging, neoplastic disease, and genetic damage.

ex·pres·sate (ek-spres′āt) the material forced out by expression.

ex·pres·sion (ek-spresh′ən) [L. *expressio*] 1. the aspect or appearance of the face as determined by the physical or emotional state. 2. the act of squeezing or evacuating by pressure. 3. gene e.

gene e. 1. the flow of genetic information from gene to protein. 2. the process, or the regulation of the process, by which the effects of a gene are manifested. 3. the manifestation of a heritable trait in an individual carrying the gene or genes that determine it.

ex·pres·siv·i·ty (ek″sprĕ-siv′ĭ-te) in genetics, the level of phenotypic expression of an inherited trait in an individual.

variable e. expressivity that ranges in its manifestation under different conditions, being influenced by factors such as the environment and other genes.

ex·pul·sive (ek-spul′siv) [*ex-* + L. *pellere* to drive] driving or forcing out; tending to expel.

ex·san·gui·nate (ek-sang′wĭ-nāt) [*ex-* + L. *sanguis* blood] 1. to deprive of blood. 2. bloodless (def. 1).

ex·san·gui·na·tion (ek-sang″wĭ-na′shən) extensive loss of blood due to hemorrhage.

ex·san·guine (ek-sang′win) bloodless (def. 1).

ex·san·gui·no·trans·fu·sion (ek-sang″wĭ-no-trans-fu′zhən) exchange transfusion.

ex·sect (ek-sekt′) excise.

ex·sec·tion (ek-sek′shən) excision.

ex·sec·tor (ek-sek′tər) a cutting instrument for use in performing exsections (excisions).

Ex·sel (ek-sel′) trademark for a preparation of selenium sulfide.

Ex·se·ro·hi·lum (ek″sər-o-hi′ləm) a genus of Fungi Imperfecti of the form-class Hyphomycetes, form-family Dematiaceae, closely related to *Bipolaris* and *Drechslera. E. longirostra′tum, E. macgin′nisii,* and *E. rostra′tum* have been isolated from cases of sinusitis and meningitis.

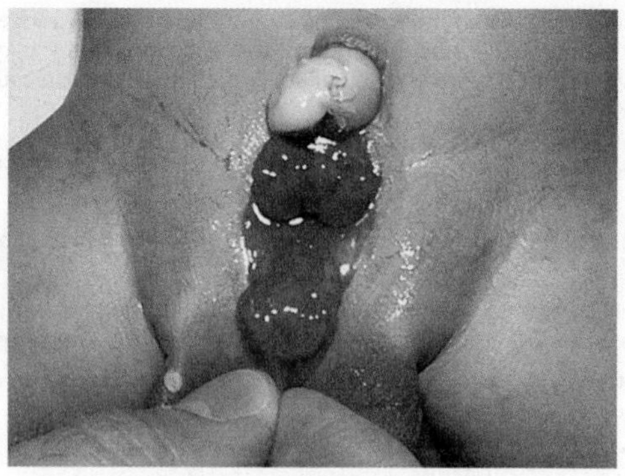
■ Exstrophy of the bladder in a male infant.

ex·sic·cant (ek-sik′ənt) desiccant.

ex·sic·cate (ek′sĭ-kāt) desiccate.

ex·sic·ca·tion (ek″sĭ-ka′shən) 1. desiccation. 2. xerosis. 3. in chemistry, the depriving of a crystalline substance of its water of crystallization.

ex·sic·co·sis (ek″sĭ-ko′sis) xerosis.

ex·sorp·tion (ek-sorp′shən) the movement of substances out of the blood, through the intestinal epithelial cells, and into the intestinal lumen.

ex·stro·phia (ek-stro′fe-ə) exstrophy.

ex·stro·phy (ek′stro-fe) [Gr. *ekstrephein* to turn inside out] the congenital eversion or turning inside out of an organ, such as the urinary bladder.

e. of bladder a developmental anomaly marked by absence of a portion of the lower anterior abdominal wall and the anterior bladder wall, with eversion of the posterior bladder wall through the defect and with an open pubic arch and widely separated ischia connected by a fibrous band. Called also *ectopia vesicae.*

e. of cloaca, cloacal e. a developmental anomaly in which two segments of bladder (hemibladders) are separated by an area of intestine with a mucosal surface, resembling a large red tumor in the midline of the lower abdomen. Called also *ectopia cloacae.*

ex·suf·fla·tion (ek″sə-fla′shən) [*ex-* + L. *sufflatio* a blowing up] the act of removing the air from a cavity by artificial or mechanical means, especially such action upon the lungs by means of an exsufflator.

ex·suf·fla·tor (ek″sə-fla′tər) an apparatus that produces sudden negative pressure in order to reproduce in the bronchial tree the effects of a natural, vigorous cough.

ext. extract.

ex·tend·ed-re·lease (ek-stend′əd-re-lēs′) allowing a twofold or greater reduction in frequency of administration of a drug in comparison with the frequency required by a conventional dosage form.

ex·ten·der (ek-sten′dər) [*ex-* + L. *tendere* to stretch] something that enlarges or prolongs; called also *expander.*

artificial plasma e. a substance that can be transfused to maintain fluid volume of the blood in an emergency, supplemental to the use of whole blood and plasma.

ex·ten·sion (ek-sten′shən) [L. *extensio*] 1. the movement that straightens or increases the angle between the bones or parts of the body. 2. the bringing of the members of a limb into or toward a straight relation. 3. enlargement or prolongation.

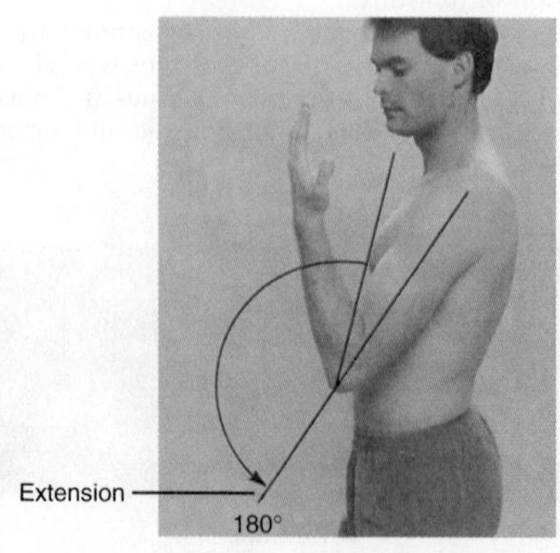

Buck e. the extension of a fractured lower limb by weights, the foot of the bed being raised so that the body makes counterextension.

nail e. extension exerted on the distal fragment of a fractured bone by means of a nail or pin driven into the fragment.

e. per contiguita'tem the spreading of a morbid process through one tissue or part into one adjacent to it.

e. per continuita'tem the spreading of a morbid process throughout a single tissue or part.

ridge e. an intraoral surgical operation for deepening the vestibular and oral sulci so as to increase the relative intraoral height of the alveolar ridge to facilitate denture retention.

ex•ten•sor (ek-sten'sor) [L.] 1. causing extension. 2. [TA] any muscle that extends a joint.

ex•te•ri•or (ek-stēr'e-ər) [L.] situated on or near the outside; outer.

ex•te•ri•or•ize (ek-stēr'e-ə-rīz") 1. to form a correct mental reference of the image of an object seen. 2. in psychiatry, to turn one's interest outward. 3. to transpose an internal organ to the exterior of the body.

ex•tern (ek'stərn) a medical student or graduate in medicine who assists in the care of patients in a hospital but does not reside in the hospital.

ex•ter•nal (ek-stur'nəl) [L. *externus* outside] situated or occurring on the outside; many anatomical structures formerly called external are now more correctly termed lateral.

ex•ter•nal•iza•tion (ek-stur"nəl-ĭ-za'shən) 1. the tendency to perceive in the external world and external objects components of one's own personality, including instinctual impulses, conflicts, moods, attitudes, and ways of thinking. 2. the process of learning the difference between self and non-self in childhood. 3. the process by which external rather than internal stimuli become capable of arousing a drive.

ex•terne (ek'stərn) extern.

ex•ter•nus (ek-stur'nəs) [TA] external: a term denoting a structure or an aspect farther from the center of a part or cavity.

ex•tero•cep•tion (ek"stər-o-sep'shən) the perception of stimuli originating outside or at a distance from the body.

ex•tero•cep•tive (ek"stər-o-sep'tiv) 1. pertaining to exteroceptors. 2. pertaining to exteroception.

ex•tero•cep•tor (ek"stər-o-sep'tər) a sensory nerve terminal that is stimulated by the immediate external environment, such as those in the skin and mucous membranes; cf. *interoceptor*, *proprioceptor*, and *receptor* (def. 2).

ex•tero•ges•tate (ek"stər-o-jes'tāt) 1. developing outside the uterus, but still requiring complete care to meet all physical needs. 2. an infant during the period of exterior gestation.

ex•ti•ma (ek'stĭ-mə) [L.] outermost.

ex•tinc•tion (ek-stink'shən) in psychology, the disappearance or reduction in frequency of a conditioned response as a result of nonreinforcement; also, the process by which the disappearance is accomplished.

ex•tin•guish (ek-sting'wish) [L. *extinguere*] to render extinct.

ex•tir•pa•tion (ek"stər-pa'shən) [L. *extirpare* to root out, from *ex* out + *stirps* root] complete removal or eradication of an organ or tissue; see also *excision* and *resection*.

dental pulp e. pulpectomy.

ex•tor•sion (ek-stor'shən) [*ex-* + *torsion*] outward rotation of the upper pole of the vertical meridian of each eye; called also *disclination*. Cf. *intorsion*.

ex•tor•tor (ek-stor'tər) [L. *extorquēre* to twist outward] 1. an outward rotator. 2. an extraocular muscle that produces extorsion, such as the inferior oblique or the inferior rectus muscle. Cf. *intortor*.

extra- [L. *extra* outside] a prefix meaning outside of, beyond, or in addition.

ex•tra•ab•dom•i•nal (eks"trə-ab-dom'ĭ-nəl) outside the abdomen.

ex•tra•adre•nal (eks"trə-ə-dre'nəl) situated or occurring outside the adrenal gland.

ex•tra•an•a•tom•ic (eks"trə-an"ə-tom'ik) not following the normal anatomic path; said of certain arterial bypass procedures.

ex•tra•an•throp•ic (eks"trə-an-throp'ik) exanthropic.

ex•tra•ar•tic•u•lar (eks"trə-ahr-tik'u-lər) [*extra-* + L. *articulus* joint] situated or occurring outside a joint.

ex•tra•bron•chi•al (eks"trə-brong'ke-əl) outside or independent of the bronchial tubes.

ex•tra•buc•cal (eks"trə-buk'əl) outside the mouth or cheek.

ex•tra•bul•bar (eks"trə-bul'bər) outside of or away from a bulb, as the medulla oblongata or the urethral bulb.

ex•tra•cap•su•lar (eks"trə-kap'su-lər) situated or occurring outside a capsule.

ex•tra•car•di•ac (eks"trə-kahr'de-ak) outside the heart.

ex•tra•car•di•al (eks"trə-kahr'de-əl) extracardiac.

ex•tra•car•pal (eks"trə-kahr'pəl) just outside the region of the wrist.

ex•tra•cel•lu•lar (eks"trə-sel'u-lər) outside a cell or cells.

ex•tra•cer•e•bral (eks"trə-ser'ə-brəl) situated or having its origin outside the cerebrum.

ex•tra•chro•mo•so•mal (eks"trə-kro"mo-so'məl) outside or not involving the chromosome, as in mitochondrial inheritance, which involves only mitochondrial DNA.

ex•tra•co•lon•ic (ek"strə-ko-lon'ik) outside the colon.

ex•tra•cor•o•nal (eks"trə-kor'ə-nəl) outside the crown of a tooth.

ex•tra•cor•po•ral (eks"trə-kor'pər-əl) extracorporeal.

ex•tra•cor•po•re•al (eks"trə-kor-por'e-əl) [*extra-* + *corporeal*] situated or occurring outside the body.

ex•tra•cor•pus•cu•lar (eks"trə-kor-pus'ku-lər) outside or on the exterior of the blood corpuscles.

ex•tra•cor•ti•co•spi•nal (eks"trə-kor"tĭ-ko-spi'nəl) outside the corticospinal tract; see under *tract*.

ex•tra•cra•ni•al (eks"trə-kra'ne-əl) outside the cranium.

ex•tract (ek'strakt) [L. *extractum*] a concentrated preparation of a vegetable or animal drug obtained by removing the active constituents therefrom with a suitable menstruum, evaporating all or nearly all the solvent, and adjusting the residual mass or powder to a prescribed standard. Extracts are prepared in three forms: semiliquid or of syrupy consistency, pilular or solid, and dry or powdered.

allergenic e. an extract of allergenic components from a crude preparation of an allergen, e.g., weed, grass, or tree pollen, molds, house dust, or animal dander, used for diagnostic skin testing or for immunotherapy (hyposensitization) of allergy.

belladonna e. [USP] a preparation containing, in each 100 g, between 1.15 and 1.35 g of alkaloids of belladonna leaf and having anticholinergic and antimuscarinic effects; it has been used as an antispasmodic in the gastrointestinal tract. Cf. *belladonna tincture*.

cell-free e. see under *system*.

compound e. an extract prepared from more than one drug.

dry e. powdered e.

liver e. a brownish, somewhat hygroscopic powder prepared from mammalian livers; used as a hematopoietic.

e. of male fern oil of male fern.

malt e. an extract of malt with dextrin, glucose, and small amounts of other carbohydrates and protein, used as an emulsifying and flavoring agent.

malt soup e. an extract of malt from barley grains, containing also a small amount of polymeric carbohydrates, proteins, electrolytes, and vitamins; administered orally as a bulk-forming laxative.

pilular e. an extract prepared as a plastic mass.

poison ivy e. an extract of the fresh leaves of poison ivy *(Rhus radicans)* used in desensitization for prevention of rhus dermatitis due to poison ivy.

poison oak e. an extract of the fresh leaves of poison oak *(Rhus diversiloba)*, used for desensitization in prevention of rhus dermatitis due to poison oak.

pollen e. a preparation of the pollen of certain plants, such as ragweed, used in the diagnosis and treatment of inhalant allergy.

powdered e. an extract prepared in a dry powdered form; called also *dry e.*

pyrethrum e. [USP] a mixture of pyrethrin I and pyrethrin II, used as a pediculicide.

semiliquid e. an extract evaporated to a syrupy consistency.

solid e. pilular e.

trichinella e. an aqueous extract of specially treated larvae of *Trichinella spiralis*, usually obtained from inoculated rodents; formerly widely used as a skin test for *Trichinella* infection.

yeast e. a powder prepared from a water-soluble, peptonelike derivative of yeast cells; see also *yeast extract agar*, under *culture medium*.

ex•trac•tion (ek-strak'shən) [*ex-* + *traction*] 1. the process or act of pulling or drawing out. 2. the preparation of an extract. 3. tooth e.

breech e. extraction of the infant from the uterus in breech presentation, i.e., when the buttocks of the fetus are presented in labor.

breech e., partial extraction of the remainder of the infant's body after it has been extruded from the uterus by natural forces as far as the umbilicus.

breech e., total extraction of the entire body of the infant from the uterus in cases of breech presentation.

cataract e. the surgical removal of a cataractous lens.

cataract e., extracapsular the surgical removal of the anterior capsule of a cataractous lens and of the lens contents (cortex and nucleus).

cataract e., intracapsular the surgical removal of a cataractous lens and its capsule.

first-pass e. clearance or biotransformation of a substance in the blood the first time it is carried through the organs of the body.

flap e. a cataract extraction by means of an incision that makes a flap of cornea.

progressive e. serial e.

selected e. serial e.

serial e. the selective extraction of deciduous teeth during the stage of mixed dentition in accordance with the shedding and eruption of the teeth; it is done over an extended period to allow autonomous adjustment to relieve crowding of the dental arches during the eruption of the lateral incisors, canines, and premolars, and may involve eventual extraction of the permanent first premolar teeth. Called also *selected e.* and *progressive e.*

testicular sperm e. (TESE) for men with obstructive azoospermia, extraction of spermatozoa directly from the testis.

tooth e. the surgical removal of a tooth; odontectomy.

ex•trac•tive (ek-strak′tiv) any substance present in an organized tissue, or in a mixture in a small quantity, and requiring to be extracted by a special method.

ex•trac•tor (ek-strak′tər) an instrument used for removing a calculus or foreign body.

basket e. a device for removal of calculi from the upper urinary tract, consisting of a network of filaments on a catheter that is passed into the ureter through a ureteroscope; the filaments surround the calculus and snare it so that it is withdrawn when the catheter is withdrawn.

vacuum e. a device to assist delivery consisting of a metal or plastic traction cup that is attached to the fetus' head; negative pressure is applied and traction is made.

ex•trac•tum (ek-strak′təm) gen. *extrac′ti*, pl. *extrac′ta* [L.] extract.

ex•tra•cys•tic (eks″trə-sis′tik) 1. outside a cyst. 2. extravesical.

ex•tra•du•ral (eks″trə-doo′rəl) situated or occurring outside the dura mater.

ex•tra•em•bry•on•ic (eks″trə-em″bre-on′ik) external to the embryo proper, as the extraembryonic coelom or extraembryonic membranes. Cf. *intraembryonic.*

ex•tra•epi•phys•e•al (eks″trə-ep″ĭ-fiz′ə-əl) away from, or unconnected with, an epiphysis.

ex•tra•esoph•a•ge•al (eks″trə-e-sof″ə-je′əl) outside the esophagus.

ex•tra•fu•sal (eks″trə-fu′zəl) [*extra-* + *fusus*] pertaining to striated muscle fibers outside the muscle spindle.

ex•tra•gas•tric (eks″trə-gas′trik) outside or on the outer surface of the stomach; called also *exogastric.*

ex•tra•gen•i•tal (eks″trə-jen′ĭ-təl) unrelated to, not originating in, or remote from the genital organs.

ex•tra•glo•mer•u•lar (eks″trə-glo-mer′u-lər) outside of or remote from a glomerulus.

ex•tra•he•pat•ic (eks″trə-hə-pat′ik) outside the liver.

ex•tra•im•mu•ni•za•tion (eks″trə-im″u-nĭ-za′shən) immunization using at least one dose of the vaccine in excess of the number recommended.

ex•tra•lig•a•men•tous (eks″trə-lig″ə-men′təs) occurring outside a ligament.

ex•tra•lu•mi•nal (ek″strə-loo′mĭ-nəl) outside the lumen of an organ.

ex•tra•lym•phat•ic (ek″strə-lim-fat′ik) situated or occurring outside the lymphatic system.

ex•tra•mal•le•o•lus (eks″trə-mə-le′o-ləs) the outer malleolus of the ankle joint.

ex•tra•mam•ma•ry (eks″trə-mam′ə-re) somewhere on the body other than around the breast.

ex•tra•mas•toi•di•tis (eks″trə-mas″toi-di′tis) inflammation of the outer surface of the mastoid process and nearby tissues.

ex•tra•med•ul•lary (eks″trə-med′u-lar″e) situated or occurring outside any medulla, especially the medulla oblongata.

ex•tra•me•nin•ge•al (eks″trə-mə-nin′jəl) occurring outside the meninges.

ex•tra•mu•ral (eks″trə-mu′rəl) [*extra-* + *mural*] situated or occurring outside the wall of an organ or structure.

ex•tra•ne•ous (ek-stra′ne-əs) [L. *extraneus* external] existing or belonging outside the organism.

ex•tra•nu•cle•ar (eks″trə-noo′kle-ər) situated or occurring outside a cell nucleus.

ex•tra•oc•u•lar (eks″trə-ok′u-lər) situated outside the eye.

ex•tra•os•se•ous (eks″trə-os′e-əs) occurring outside a bone or bones.

ex•tra•pan•cre•at•ic (ek″strə-pan″kre-at′ik) outside the pancreas.

ex•tra•pa•ren•chy•mal (eks″trə-pə-ren′kə-məl) occurring or formed outside the parenchyma.

ex•tra•pel•vic (eks″trə-pel′vik) unconnected with the pelvis.

ex•tra•peri•car•di•al (eks″trə-per″ĭ-kahr′de-əl) outside the pericardium.

ex•tra•per•i•ne•al (eks″trə-per″ĭ-ne′əl) away from, or not connected with, the perineum.

ex•tra•peri•os•te•al (eks″trə-per″e-os′te-əl) outside or independent of the periosteum.

ex•tra•peri•to•ne•al (eks″trə-per″ĭ-to-ne′əl) outside the peritoneal cavity.

ex•tra•pla•cen•tal (eks″trə-plə-sen′təl) outside of or independent of the placenta.

ex•tra•plan•tar (eks″trə-plan′tər) on the outside of the sole of the foot.

ex•tra•pleu•ral (eks″trə-ploor′əl) outside the pleural cavity.

ex•trap•o•la•tion (ek-strap″o-la′shən) inference of one or more unknown values on the basis of that which is known or has been observed; usually applied to estimation beyond the upper and lower ranges of observed data. Cf. *interpolation.*

ex•tra•pon•tine (eks″trə-pon′tēn) outside the pons.

ex•tra•pros•tat•ic (eks″trə-pros-tat′ik) outside of or not connected with the prostate.

ex•tra•psy•chic (eks″trə-si′kik) occurring outside the mind; taking place between the mind and the external environment.

ex•tra•pul•mo•nary (eks″trə-pool′mo-nar″e) not connected with the lungs.

ex•tra•py•ram•i•dal (eks″trə-pĭ-ram′ĭ-dəl) outside of the pyramidal tracts; see under *system.*

ex•tra•rec•tus (eks″trə-rek′təs) musculus rectus lateralis bulbi.

ex•tra•re•nal (eks″trə-re′nəl) outside the kidney.

ex•tra•se•rous (eks″trə-se′rəs) outside a serous cavity.

ex•tra•so•mat•ic (eks″trə-so-mat′ik) unconnected with the body.

ex•tra•stim•u•lus (ek″strə-stim′u-ləs) a premature stimulus delivered, singly or in a group of several stimuli, at precise intervals during a tachyarrhythmia in order to terminate it. Delivery of stimuli may be synchronous or asynchronous with the arrhythmia; if synchronous, delivery may be preprogrammed or adaptive to the tachycardia cycle length. Premature stimuli may also be delivered during cardiac electrophysiologic testing to initiate supraventricular or ventricular tachycardia.

ex•tra•su•pra•re•nal (eks″trə-soo″prə-re′nəl) extra-adrenal.

ex•tra•sys•to•le (eks″trə-sis′to-le) a premature contraction of the heart that is independent of the normal rhythm and arises in response to an impulse in some part of the heart other than the sinoatrial node; called also *premature beat* or *systole.*

atrial e. atrial premature complex.

atrioventricular (AV) e. atrioventricular junctional premature complex.

infranodal e. ventricular e.

interpolated e. see under *beat.*

junctional e. atrioventricular junctional premature complex.

nodal e. atrioventricular e.

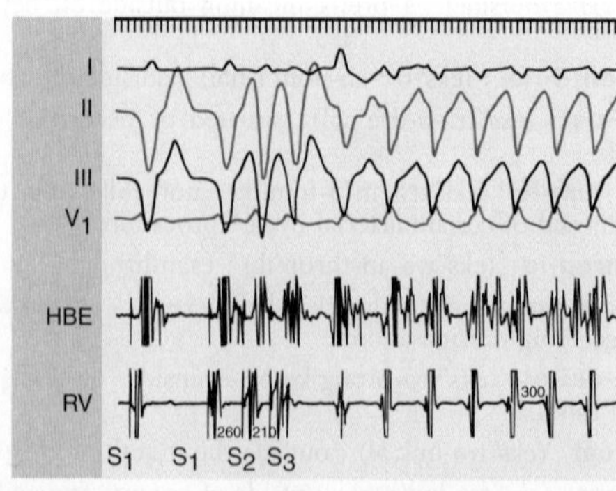

■ Programmed extrastimulus used to initiate ventricular tachycardia. The last two ventricular-paced beats at a cycle length of 600 milliseconds are shown. Two premature stimuli (S_1, S_2) initiate a sustained monomorphic tachycardia at a cycle length of 300 milliseconds.

retrograde e. a premature ventricular contraction followed by a premature atrial contraction, due to transmission of the stimulus backward, usually over the bundle of His.
ventricular e. ventricular premature complex.

ex·tra·ten·di·nous (eks″trə-ten′dĭ-nəs) outside a tendon.

ex·tra·tho·rac·ic (eks″trə-thə-ras′ik) outside the thorax.

ex·tra·thy·roi·dal (eks″trə-thi-roid′əl) outside or not involving the thyroid gland.

ex·tra·tra·che·al (eks″trə-tra′ke-əl) outside the trachea.

ex·tra·tu·bal (eks″trə-too′bəl) outside a tube.

ex·tra·tym·pan·ic (eks″trə-tim-pan′ik) outside the tympanum of the ear.

ex·tra·uter·ine (eks″trə-u′tər-in) outside the uterus.

ex·tra·vag·i·nal (eks″trə-vaj′ĭ-nəl) outside the vagina.

ex·trav·a·sa·tion (ek-strav″ə-sa′shən) [*extra-* + L. *vas* vessel] 1. a discharge or escape of blood or some other fluid normally found in a vessel or tube, into the surrounding tissues. 2. the process of being so discharged. 3. fluid that has been so discharged.
peripelvic e. extravasation of urine (see *urinoma*) into the area around the renal pelvis.
punctiform e. extravasation that causes a tissue to be covered with minute bloody points.

ex·tra·vas·cu·lar (eks″trə-vas′ku-lər) outside a vessel or vessels.

ex·tra·ven·tric·u·lar (eks″trə-vən-trik′u-lər) outside a ventricle.

ex·tra·ver·sion (eks″trə-vur′zhən) extroversion.

ex·tra·vert (eks′trə-vərt) extrovert.

ex·tra·ves·i·cal (eks″trə-ves′ĭ-kəl) outside the urinary bladder.

ex·trem·i·tal (ek-strem′ĭ-təl) pertaining to or situated at an extremity.

ex·trem·i·tas (ek-strem′ĭ-təs) pl. *extremita′tes* [L.] extremity: the distal or terminal portion of an elongated or pointed structure.
e. acromia′lis clavi′culae [TA] acromial end of clavicle: the lateral end of the clavicle, which articulates with the acromion of the scapula.
e. ante′rior sple′nis [TA] anterior extremity of spleen: the lower pole of the spleen, which is situated anterior to the upper pole.
e. infe′rior re′nis [TA] inferior extremity of kidney: the lower, smaller end of the kidney; called also *polus inferior renis* [TA alternative] and *inferior* or *lower pole of kidney* .
e. infe′rior tes′tis [TA] lower pole of testis: the inferior end of the testis, which is attached to the tail of the epididymis. Called also *polus inferior testis* [TA alternative] and *inferior pole of testis.*
e. poste′rior sple′nis [TA] posterior extremity of spleen: the uppermost pole of the spleen, situated somewhat posterior to the lower pole; called also *head of spleen.*
e. sterna′lis clavi′culae [TA] sternal end of clavicle: the medial end of the clavicle, which articulates with the sternum.
e. supe′rior re′nis [TA] superior extremity of kidney: the upper, larger end of the kidney; called also *polus superior renis* [TA alternative] and *superior* or *upper pole of kidney.*
e. supe′rior tes′tis [TA] upper pole of testis: the superior end of the testis, which is attached to the head of the epididymis. Called also *polus superior testis* [TA alternative] and *superior pole of testis*
e. tuba′ria ova′rii [TA] tubal extremity of ovary: the upper end of the ovary, related to the free end of the uterine tube.
e. uteri′na ova′rii [TA] uterine extremity of ovary: the lower end of the ovary, directed toward the uterus.

ex·trem·i·ta·tes (ek-strem″ĭ-ta′tēz) [L.] plural of *extremitas.*

ex·trem·i·ty (ek-strem′ĭ-te) 1. extremitas. 2. an upper or lower limb; see *membrum inferius* and *membrum superius.* 3. a hand or foot.
anterior e. of spleen extremitas anterior splenis.
inferior e. of kidney extremitas inferior renis.
lower e. membrum inferius.
posterior e. of spleen extremitas posterior splenis.
superior e. of kidney extremitas superior renis.
tubal e. of ovary extremitas tubaria ovarii.
upper e. membrum superius.
uterine e. of ovary extremitas uterina ovarii.

ex·trin·sic (ek-strin′zik) [L. *extrinsecus* situated on the outside] coming from or originating outside; having relation to parts outside the organ or limb in which found.

extro- [L. *extra* outside] a prefix meaning outward, outside.

ex·tro·gas·tru·la·tion (eks″tro-gas″troo-la′shən) malformation resulting from exogastrulation.

ex·tro·ver·sion (eks″tro-vur′zhən) [L. *extroversio,* from *extra* outside + *vertere* to turn] extraversion; 1. a turning inside out, as of an organ. 2. the turning outward to the external world of one's interest; cf. *introversion.* 3. in orthodontics, malocclusion in which the teeth or other maxillary structures are further from the median plane than normal, resulting in a wide dental arch. Cf. *intraversion.*

ex·tro·vert (eks′tro-vərt) 1. a person whose interest is turned outward to the external world. 2. to turn one's interest outward to the external world.

ex·trude (ek-strōōd′) 1. to force, thrust, or press out. 2. to force out, or to occupy a position mesial, distal, labial or buccal, or lingual or palatal to that normally occupied. 3. to occupy a position occlusal to that normally occupied, said of an overerupted tooth.

ex·tru·sion (ek-stroo′zhən) 1. thrusting or pushing out; expulsion by force. 2. the overeruption or movement of a tooth beyond its normal occlusal plane in the absence of opposing occlusal force. 3. an orthodontic technique for the elongation or elevation of a tooth. Cf. *intrusion.*
disk e. see *extruded disk,* under *disk.*

ex·tu·bate (eks-too′bāt) [*ex-* + L. *tuba* tube] to remove a tube from.

ex·tu·ba·tion (eks″too-ba′shən) the removal of a previously inserted tube; called also *detubation.* Cf. *decannulation.*

ex·u·ber·ant (eg-zoo′bər-ənt) [L. *exuberare* to be very fruitful] copious or excessive in production; showing excessive proliferation.

ex·u·date (eks′u-dāt) [L. *exsudare* to sweat out] material, such as fluid, cells, or cellular debris, which has escaped from blood vessels and has been deposited in tissues or on tissue surfaces, usually as a result of inflammation. An exudate, in contrast to a transudate, is characterized by a high content of protein, cells, or solid materials derived from cells.
cotton-wool e's see under *spot.*

ex·u·da·tion (eks″u-da′shən) 1. the escape of fluid, cells, and cellular debris from blood vessels and their deposition in or on the tissues, usually as the result of inflammation. 2. an exudate.

ex·u·da·tive (ek-soo′də-tiv) of or pertaining to a process of exudation.

ex·um·bil·i·ca·tion (eks″əm-bil″ĭ-ka′shən) [*ex-* + *umbilicus*] 1. marked protrusion of the navel. 2. umbilical hernia.

ex·u·vi·a·tion (eks-u″ve-a′shən) [L. *exuere* to divest oneself of] the shedding of any epithelial structure, as of the deciduous teeth.

ex vi·vo (eks ve′vo) [L.] outside the living body, such as removal of an organ for reparative surgery, after which it is returned to its original site.

eye (i) [L. *oculus;* Gr. *ophthalmos*] the organ of vision; called also *oculus* [TA]. In shape the eyeball (bulbus oculi [TA]) is a large sphere, with the segment of a smaller sphere, the cornea, in front. It is composed of three coats: the external tough *fibrous layer,* consisting of the white sclera over most of the eyeball and the cornea on the anterior surface; the middle *vascular layer* or *uvea,* consisting of the choroid, the ciliary body, and the iris; and the *inner layer,* which is neural and sensory and consists primarily of the retina. Within the three layers are the refracting media: the *aqueous humor,* the *crystalline lens,* and the *vitreous humor.* The lens is a double convex transparent body between the vitreous and aqueous humors; its convexity is altered by the ciliary muscle during accommodation. Posteriorly, fibers of the optic nerve enter the ganglionic layer and receive sensations from the visual cells of the retina (the *retinal rods* and *retinal cones*). The arteries of the eye are the short ciliary, the long ciliary, the anterior ciliary, and the central artery of the retina. The nerves are the optic and the long and short ciliary nerves. See Plate 15.
aphakic e. an eye lacking the crystalline lens; see also *aphakia.*
artificial e. a ready-made (stock) or custom-made prosthesis of glass or plastic shaped and colored to resemble the anterior portion of a normal eye and inserted for cosmetic reasons in the socket of an enucleated or eviscerated eye.
black e. ecchymosis of the eyelids and surrounding area.
cherry e. hypertrophy and prolapse of the gland of the nictitating membrane of a dog, with conjunctivitis and swelling in the form of a red mass.
compound e. the multifaceted eye of arthropods composed of units (ommatidia), each of which contains all of the structural and functional elements of the eye (including lens, retina, and photoreceptor cells).
crab's e. 1. *Abrus precatorius.* 2. jequirity bean.
crossed e's esotropia.
cystic e. a malformed eye consisting of a cystic structure.
dancing e's opsoclonus.
dark-adapted e. an eye that has undergone the changes produced by adequate exposure to darkness; it is more sensitive to very weak light.
deviating e. in strabismus, the nonfixating eye; called also *following e.*
dry e. keratoconjunctivitis sicca.
epiphyseal e. a modification of the parapineal organ of certain lower vertebrates to form an eyelike structure lying subepidermally on the median dorsal aspect of the head; it is a photoreceptor rather than an image forming eye, enabling the organism to respond to darkness or to light. Called also *parietal e., parietal body,* and *pineal e.*

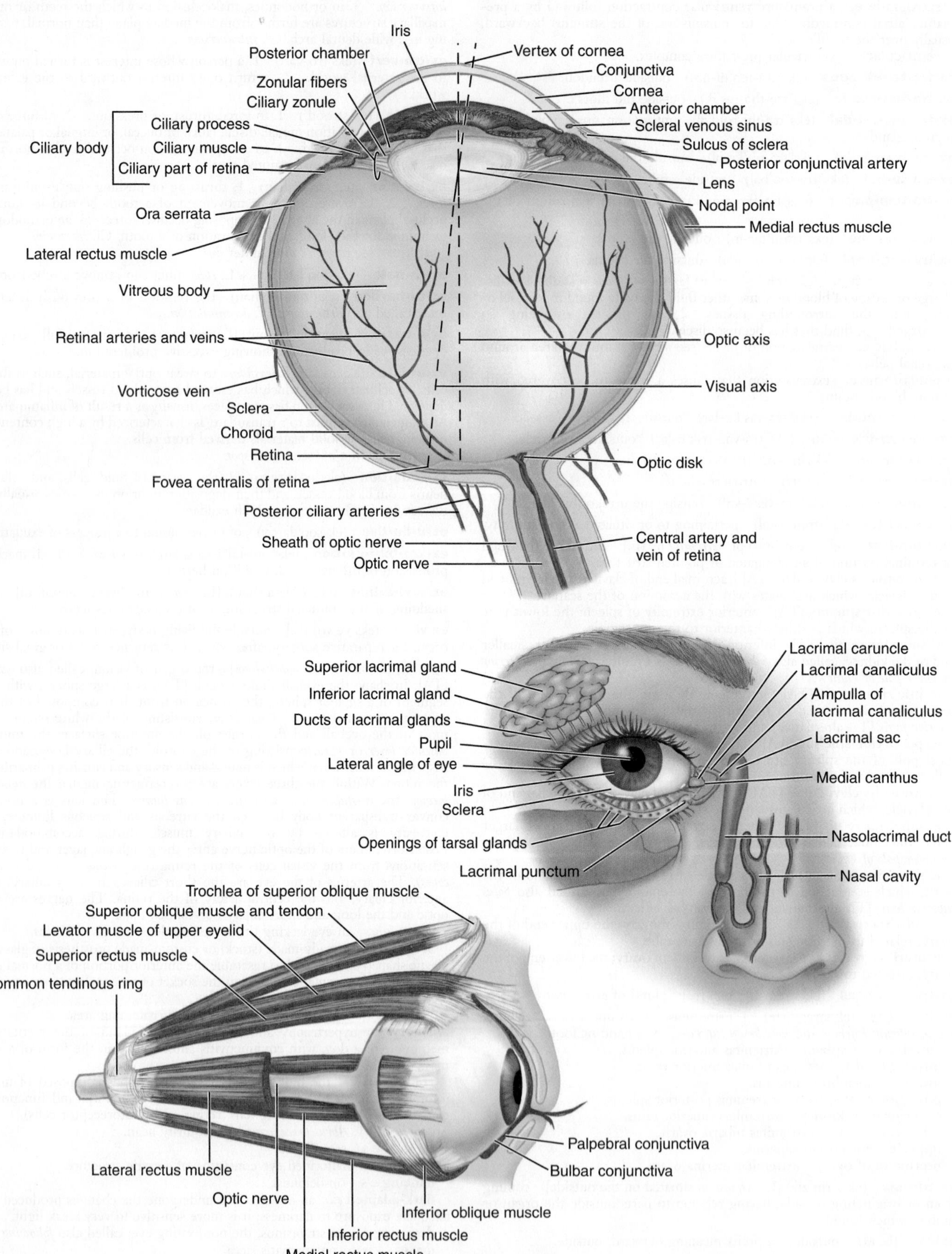

■ **PLATE 15—THE EYE AND RELATED STRUCTURES**

exciting e. the eye that is primarily injured and from which the influences start which involve the other eye in sympathetic ophthalmia; called also *primary e.*
fixating e. in strabismus, the eye directed toward the object of vision.
following e. deviating e.
hop e. conjunctivitis in hop pickers caused by irritation from the spine-like hairs of the hop plant.
light-adapted e. an eye that has undergone the changes produced by adequate exposure to rather strong light; it is less sensitive to weak light.
median e. an organ on the top of the head of many reptiles; it plays an important role in the response to light.
monochromatic e. an eye that can perceive only one color; see *monochromatic vision*, under *vision.*
parietal e. epiphyseal e.
pineal e. epiphyseal e.
pink e. 1. acute contagious conjunctivitis. 2. infectious keratoconjunctivitis.
primary e. exciting e.
pseudophakic e. an eye with an intraocular lens implant.
raccoon e's areas of ecchymosis around both eyes, most often indicating a basilar skull fracture; a similar finding is seen in AL amyloidosis. Called also *raccoon sign.*
reduced e. a mathematical model of the eye in which the optical systems are diagrammatically reduced to one refracting unit.
schematic e. 1. a diagrammatic illustration of the ideal normal eye, with constants for curvature, indices of refraction, and distances between the optical elements. 2. a model of the eye, usually simplified and enlarged, showing its anatomical and mechanical features.
secondary e. sympathizing e.
Snellen reform e. an artificial eye composed of two concavoconvex plates with an empty space between.
squinting e. in strabismus, the eye the visual axis of which deviates from the object of vision while the sound eye fixates.
sympathizing e. the uninjured eye that becomes secondarily involved in sympathetic ophthalmia; called also *secondary e.*
wall e. 1. leukoma of the cornea. 2. exotropia.

eye•ball (i′bawl) bulbus oculi.

eye•brow (i′brou) 1. the transverse elevation at the junction of the forehead and the upper eyelid, consisting of five layers: skin, subcutaneous tissue, a layer of interwoven fibers of the orbicularis oculi and occipitofrontalis muscles, a submuscular areolar layer, and pericranium; called also *supercilium* [TA]. 2. the hairs growing on this elevation; called also *supercilia* [TA].

eye•cup (i′kəp) 1. a small vessel for the application of cleansing or medicated solution to the exposed area of the eyeball. 2. optic cup (def. 2).

eye•glass•es (i′glas-əz) glasses.

eye•ground (i′ground) the fundus of the eye as revealed by ophthalmoscopic examination.

eye•lash (i′lash) one of the hairs growing at the edge of an eyelid; collectively called *cilia.*

eye•let (i′let) an orthodontic attachment, usually used with an edgewise appliance, welded or soldered for better rotational control.

eye•lid (i′lid) either of the two movable folds (upper and lower) that protect the anterior surface of the eyeball; called also *palpebra.*
third e. nictitating membrane.

eye-mind•ed (i′mīnd-əd) visile.

eye•piece (i′pēs) the lens or system of lenses in a microscope (or telescope) that is nearest to the eye of the user and that serves to further magnify the image produced by the objective.
comparison e. an eyepiece which presents, as though in juxtaposition, the images of separate objects being transmitted through two different objectives.
compensating e. an eyepiece especially designed to correct chromatic and spherical aberrations of the light rays produced by the objective.
demonstration e. a device consisting of two eyepieces which may be affixed to the eyepiece tube of a microscope, permitting two observers to see the same field simultaneously.
high-eyepoint e. an eyepiece whose eyepoint is higher than usual, for use by viewers wearing eyeglasses.
huygenian e. a negative eyepiece consisting of two planoconvex lenses, the convexities being directed toward the objective.
negative e. a combination of two lenses, one of which is below the plane in which the real image from the objective is formed.
positive e. a single lens combination, consisting of two planoconvex lenses or of an achromatic doublet or triplet, the combination being above the plane in which the real image from the objective is formed.
Ramsden e. a positive eyepiece consisting of two planoconvex lenses with the convexities turned toward each other.
widefield e. a positive eyepiece consisting of a doublet and a single element, giving a wider field of view than that afforded by other eyepieces.

eye•point (i′point) the point above a microscope eyepiece where the image is focused and where the eye should be positioned for viewing.

eye•spot (i′spot) 1. a light-sensitive pigmented spot with a visual function occurring in various invertebrates. See also *stigma* (def. 5) and *ocellus* (def. 1). 2. eye spot; see under *spot.*

eye•strain (i′strān) fatigue of the eye from overuse or from uncorrected defect in focus of the eye.

eye•worm (i′wərm) see under *worm.*

ezet•i•mibe (ĕ-zet′ĭ-mīb) an inhibitor of intestinal cholesterol absorption, used alone or in combination with an HMG-CoA reductase inhibitor in the treatment of primary hypercholesterolemia; administered orally.

ez•rin (ez′rin) an actin-binding protein, related to moesin and radixin; see *ERM proteins*, under *protein.*

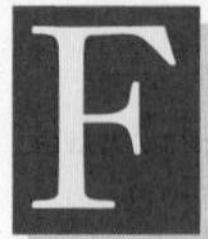

F Fahrenheit (see under *scale*); farad; fertility (see under *plasmid*); visual field; fluorine; formula; French (see under *scale*); phenylalanine.

F. [L.] fi'at (let there be made).

F coefficient of inbreeding; faraday; force.

F_1, F_2, F_3, etc. filial generation, with the generation specified by the subscript numeral.

°F degree Fahrenheit; see *Fahrenheit scale*, under *scale*.

f femto-; focal length.

f frequency (def. 2).

FA fatty acid; fluorescent antibody (see under *test*).

FAB French-American-British; see under *classification*.

Fab [*f*ragment, *a*ntigen-*b*inding] originally, either of two identical fragments, each containing an antigen combining site, obtained by papain cleavage of the IgG molecule; now generally used as an adjective, e.g., Fab region, segment, to refer to an "arm" of any immunoglobulin monomer, i.e., one light chain and the adjoining heavy chain V_H and C_H1 domains. Cf. *Fc*.

Crotalidae polyvalent immune Fab (ovine) an antivenin against the poison of snakes of the family Crotalidae (the pit vipers), consisting of immunoglobulin fragments from the blood of sheep that have been immunized against the venom of the snakes.

digoxin immune Fab (ovine) a preparation of antigen-binding fragments derived from specific antidigoxin antibodies produced in sheep that have been immunized with digoxin coupled as a hapten to human serum albumin, used as an antidote to life-threatening digoxin and digitoxin overdose; administered intravenously.

$F(ab')_2$ the fragment, containing both Fab regions and the hinge region connecting them by interchain disulfide bonds, obtained by pepsin cleavage of the IgG molecule; called also *$F(ab')_2$ fragment*.

fa·bel·la (fə-bel'ə) pl. *fabel'lae* [L. "little bean"] a sesamoid fibrocartilage occasionally found on the gastrocnemius muscle; it is visible radiographically as a small bony shadow behind the knee joint.

Fa·ber syndrome (fah'bər) [Knud Helge *Faber*, Danish physician, 1862–1956] hypochromic anemia.

fa·bism (fa'biz-əm) [L. *faba* bean] favism.

fab·ri·ca·tion (fab"rĭ-ka'shən) confabulation.

Fa·bri·ci·us bursa (fə-bris'e-əs) [H. *Fabricius*] see under *bursa*.

Fa·bry disease (fah'bre) [Johannes *Fabry*, German dermatologist, 1860–1930] see under *disease*.

fab·u·la·tion (fab"u-la'shən) confabulation.

Facb [*f*ragment, *a*ntigen-and-*c*omplement-*b*inding] the fragment, containing both light chains and the V_H and C_H2 domains of both heavy chains, obtained by plasmin cleavage of an IgG molecule.

FACD Fellow of the American College of Dentists.

face (fās) [L. *facies*] facies.

adenoid f. adenoid facies.

bovine f. facies bovina.

***cis* f. of Golgi complex** the surface of the Golgi complex nearest the endoplasmic reticulum, through which products from the endoplasmic reticulum are received.

cleft f. see *lateral facial cleft* and *oblique facial cleft*, under *cleft*.

cow f. facies bovina.

cytosolic f. the surface of a biomembrane directed toward the cytoplasm; in the plasma membrane, it faces the interior of the cell; in organelles it is the exterior face, away from the lumen. For structures having a double membrane, it is the surface directed away from the space between the membranes.

dish f., dished f. a facial deformity characterized by a prominence of the forehead, a recession of the midface and lower half of the nose, a lengthening of the upper lip, and a prognathic chin; called also *facies scaphoidea*.

exoplasmic f. the surface of a biomembrane directed away from the cytoplasm. In the plasma membrane it faces the extracellular environment; in organelles it faces the lumen. For structures having a double membrane, it is the surface facing the space between the membranes.

frog f. flatness of the face due to intranasal disease.

hippocratic f. see under *facies*.

moon f., moon-shaped f. moon facies.

***trans* f. of Golgi complex** the surface of the Golgi complex furthest from the endoplasmic reticulum, through which products of the Golgi complex are released to the *trans*-Golgi network.

face-bow (fās'bo) 1. a caliper-like device used in dentistry to record the positional relationship of the maxillary arch to the temporomandibular joints (or opening axis of the jaw) and to orient dental casts in this same relationship to the opening axis of the articulator. 2. an extraoral wire arch or bow used in orthodontics to connect an intraoral appliance to an extraoral anchorage.

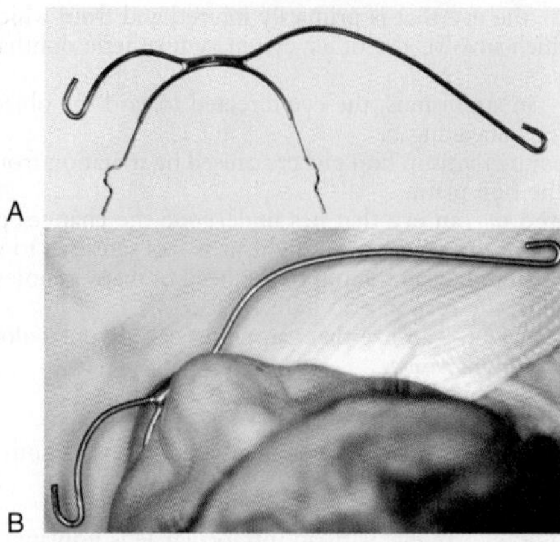

■ Asymmetric face-bow, used to regain bilateral but asymmetric space. The outer bow is shorter on the side that will need the smaller distal tooth movement *(A)*; when the appliance is in place, without the neck strap attached, the long side is farther from the cheek *(B)*.

adjustable axis f.-b. a face-bow with caliper ends that can be adjusted in such a way as to permit location of the hinge axis of rotation of the mandible. Called also *hinge-bow* and *kinematic f.-b.*

kinematic f.-b. adjustable axis f.-b.

face·lift (fās'lift) popular term for *rhytidectomy;* written also *face lift*.

face·om·e·ter (fās-om'ə-tər) an instrument for measuring the dimensions of the face.

fac·et (fas'ət, fə-set') [Fr. *facette*] a small plane surface on a hard body, as on a bone; see also *fovea*.

acromial f. of clavicle facies articularis acromialis claviculae.

anterior articular f. of dens of axis facies articularis anterior dentis.

anterior calcaneal f., anterior f. for calcaneus facies articularis calcanea anterior tali.

anterior talar f. of calcaneus facies articularis talaris anterior calcanei.

articular f. a small plane surface on a bone at the site where it articulates with another structure; see terms beginning *facies articularis*.

articular f. of head of fibula facies articularis capitis fibulae.

articular f. of head of radius fovea articularis capitis radii.

articular f. of head of rib facies articularis capitis costae.

articular f. of lateral malleolus facies articularis malleoli lateralis.

articular f. of medial malleolus facies articularis malleoli medialis.

articular f. of tubercle of rib facies articularis tuberculi costae.

f. for calcaneonavicular ligament facies articularis partis calcaneonavicularis ligamenti bifurcati.

clavicular f. incisura clavicularis sterni.

clavicular f. of acromion facies articularis clavicularis acromii.

f. for dens fovea dentis atlantis.

fibular articular f. on tibia facies articularis fibularis tibiae.

inferior articular f. of atlas facies articularis inferior atlantis.

inferior articular f. of vertebra facies articularis inferior vertebrae.

inferior costal f. fovea costalis inferior.

lateral malleolar f. of talus facies malleolaris lateralis tali.

locked f's of spine dislocation of articular processes of the spine.

medial malleolar f. of talus facies malleolaris medialis tali.

middle calcaneal f., middle f. for calcaneus facies articularis calcanea media tali.

middle talar f. of calcaneus facies articularis talaris media calcanei.

f. for plantar calcaneonavicular ligament facies articularis ligamenti calcaneonavicularis plantaris.

posterior articular f. of dens of axis facies articularis posterior dentis.

posterior calcaneal f., posterior calcaneal articular f. of talus facies articularis calcanea posterior tali.

posterior talar f. of calcaneus facies articularis talaris posterior calcanei.

squatting f. a smooth area observed on the anterior surface of the lower end of the tibia in persons who habitually squat for long periods.

sternal f. of clavicle facies articularis sternalis clavicularis.

superior articular f. of atlas facies articularis superior atlantis.

superior articular f. of vertebra facies articularis superior vertebrae.

superior costal f. fovea costalis superior.

superior f. of trochlea of talus facies superior trochleae tali.

transverse costal f., f. for tubercle of rib fovea costalis processus transversi.

fac•e•tec•to•my (fas″ə-tek′tə-me) [*facet* + *-ectomy*] excision of the articular facet of a vertebra.

fa•cette (fah-set′) [Fr.] facet.

fa•cial (fa′shəl) [L. *facialis*, from *facies* face] 1. pertaining to the face. 2. directed toward the face.

-facient [L. *faciens*, present participle of *facere* to do, to make] a word termination meaning making or causing to become.

fa•ci•es (fa′she-ēz) pl. *fa′cies* [L.] 1. a specific surface of a body structure, part, or organ. 2. [TA] face. the anterior, or ventral, aspect of the head, generally from the forehead to the chin, including the eyes, nose, mouth, cheeks, and chin but excluding the auricles. The forehead is excluded by some authorities. 3. the expression or appearance of the face; see *expression* (def. 1).

Facies

Descriptions of anatomic structures are given on TA terms, and include anglicized names of specific structures.

adenoid f. the dull expression, with open mouth, sometimes seen in children with hypertrophy of the pharyngeal tonsils ("adenoids").
f. ante′rior cor′dis TA alternative for *f. sternocostalis cordis.*
f. ante′rior cor′neae [TA] the anterior surface of the cornea.
f. ante′rior cor′poris maxil′lae [TA] anterior surface of maxilla: the surface of the body of the maxilla that is directed forward and somewhat laterally; it is bounded roughly by the infraorbital margin, root of the frontal process, nasal notch, alveolar process, and zygomatic process.
f. ante′rior glan′dulae suprarena′lis [TA] the anterior surface of the adrenal (suprarenal) gland, where the hilum is located.
f. ante′rior i′ridis [TA] the anterior surface of the iris, directed toward the anterior chamber of the eye.
f. ante′rior len′tis [TA] the surface of the lens directed toward the anterior surface of the eye.
f. ante′rior pal′pebrae [TA] anterior surface of eyelid: the exterior surface of the eyelid.
f. ante′rior par′tis petro′sae os′sis tempora′lis [TA] anterior surface of petrous part of temporal bone: the surface of the petrous part of the temporal bone that forms the posterior portion of the floor of the middle cranial fossa.
f. ante′rior patel′lae [TA] anterior surface of patella: the slightly convex, longitudinally striated front surface of the patella, which is perforated by small openings for the nutrient vessels.
f. ante′rior pro′statae [TA] anterior surface of prostate: the surface towards the pubic symphysis, separated from the symphysis by adipose tissue and the prostatic venous plexus.
f. ante′rior ra′dii [TA] anterior surface of radius; it gives attachment to the flexor pollicis longus and pronator quadratus muscles.
f. ante′rior re′nis [TA] anterior surface of kidney: the kidney surface that is directed toward the viscera and covered by peritoneum.
f. ante′rior sca′pulae TA alternative for *f. costalis scapulae.*
f. ante′rior ul′nae [TA] the anterior surface of the ulna.
f. ante′rior u′teri TA alternative for *f. vesicalis uteri.*
f. anteroinfe′rior cor′poris pancre′atis [TA] the anterior and inferior surface of the body of the pancreas.
f. anterolatera′lis cartila′ginis arytenoi′deae [TA] anterolateral surface of arytenoid cartilage: the external surface of the cartilage, which bears the triangular pit, the oblong pit, and the arcuate crest.

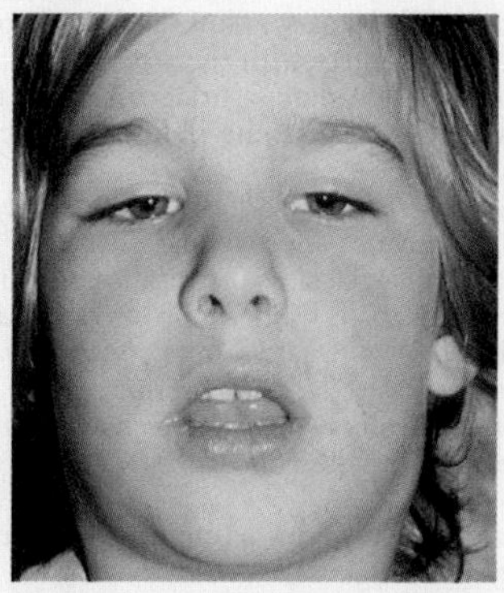

■ Adenoid facies in a child with marked enlargement of tonsils and adenoids necessitating mouth breathing and disrupting sleep and resultant signs of fatigue.

f. anterolatera′lis hu′meri [TA] anterolateral surface of humerus: the surface that provides attachment to the deltoid muscle and lateral part of the brachialis muscle.
f. anteromedia′lis hu′meri [TA] anteromedial surface of humerus: the surface of the humerus that begins above at the intertubercular groove and spreads out inferiorly to form the wide smooth area for origin of the brachialis muscle.
f. anterosupe′rior cor′poris pancre′atis [TA] the anterior and superior surface of the body of the pancreas.
f. approxima′lis den′tis [TA] approximal surface of tooth: the surface of a tooth facing an adjoining tooth in the same dental arch. The proximal surface facing toward the median line is known as the mesial surface (facies mesialis); the surface facing away from the median line is known as the distal surface (facies distalis). See also *area contingens dentis.*
f. articula′ris [TA] articular surface: a surface on bone or cartilage that forms a joint with another.
f. articula′ris acromia′lis clavi′culae [TA] acromial facet of clavicle: the smooth area on the lateral end of the clavicle for articulation with the acromion of the scapula.
f. articula′ris ante′rior den′tis [TA] anterior articular facet of dens of axis: an oval facet on the anterior surface of the dens of the axis, articulating with the fovea dentis of the atlas.
f. articula′ris arytenoi′dea cartila′ginis cricoi′deae [TA] arytenoid articular surface on cricoid cartilage: the surface that articulates with the arytenoid cartilage.
f. articula′ris calca′nea ante′rior ta′li [TA] anterior calcaneal facet: the small surface on the trochlea of the talus that rests upon the anterior talar articular surface of the calcaneus.
f. articula′ris calca′nea me′dia ta′li [TA] middle calcaneal facet: the convex part of the head of the talus that articulates with the sustentaculum tali of the calcaneus.
f. articula′ris calca′nea poste′rior ta′li [TA] posterior calcaneal facet: a transverse concavity on the inferior surface of the talus, articulating with the posterior talar articular surface of the calcaneus.
f. articula′ris ca′pitis cos′tae [TA] articular facet of head of rib: the surface on the head of a rib where it articulates with the body of a vertebra. Typically it is divided into two facets by a transverse crest, the lower facet articulating with the corresponding vertebra, and the upper facet with the superjacent vertebra. The articular surfaces of the heads of the first, tenth, eleventh, and twelfth ribs generally consist of only one facet.
f. articula′ris ca′pitis fi′bulae [TA] articular facet of head of fibula: the medial surface of the head of the fibula, which articulates with the lateral condyle of the tibia.
f. articula′ris carpa′lis ra′dii [TA] carpal articular surface of radius: the convex surface of the distal end of the radius, which articulates with the lunate and scaphoid bones.
f. articula′ris cartila′ginis arytenoi′dea [TA] articular surface of arytenoid cartilage: the surface that articulates with the cricoid cartilage.
f. articula′ris clavicula′ris acro′mii [TA] clavicular facet of acromion: a smooth oval area directed upwards and medially on the medial border of the acromion of the scapula for articulation with the lateral end of the clavicle.
f. articula′ris cuboi′dea calca′nei [TA] articular surface for cuboid: the saddle-shaped area on the anterior surface of the calcaneus where it articulates with the cuboid bone.
f. articula′ris fibula′ris ti′biae [TA] fibular articular facet on tibia: the surface on the posteroinferior aspect of the lateral condyle of the tibia that articulates with the head of the fibula.

Facies *Continued*

f. articula′ris fos′sae mandibula′ris [TA] articular surface of mandibular fossa: the articular surface found in the deep part of the mandibular fossa.
f. articula′ris infe′rior atlan′tis [TA] inferior articular surface of atlas: either of the two inferior articular surfaces found on the lateral masses of the atlas. Called also *inferior articular facet of atlas.*
f. articula′ris infe′rior ti′biae [TA] inferior articular surface of tibia: the surface on the distal end of the tibia where it articulates with the talus.
f. articula′ris infe′rior ver′tebrae [TA] inferior articular facet of vertebra: the articulating surface on the inferior articular process of a vertebra.
f. articula′ris ligamen′ti calcaneonavicula′ris planta′ris [TA] facet for plantar clacaneonavicular ligament: the lowest part of the articular surfaces of the head of the talus, which is in contact with the plantar calcaneonavicular ligament.
f. articula′ris malle′oli latera′lis [TA] articular facet of lateral malleolus: the anterosuperior surface of the lateral malleolus, which articulates with the lateral side of the talus.
f. articula′ris malle′oli media′lis [TA] articular facet of medial malleolus: the lateral aspect of the medial malleolus, which articulates with the talus.
f. articula′ris navicula′ris ta′li [TA] navicular articular surface of talus: the surface of the head of the talus that articulates with the navicular bone.
f. articula′ris par′tis calcaneonavicula′ris ligamen′ti bifurca′ti [TA] facet for calcaneonavicular ligament: a small facet on the talus, on the lateral edge of the navicular articular surface, serving as a point of attachment for the calcaneonavicular ligament.
f. articula′ris patel′lae [TA] articular surface of patella: the posterior surface of the patella, which is largely covered by a thick cartilaginous layer.
f. articula′ris poste′rior den′tis [TA] posterior articular facet of dens of axis: a smooth groove on the posterior surface of the dens, which lodges the transverse ligament of the atlas.
f. articula′ris sterna′lis clavi′culae [TA] sternal facet of clavicle: a triangular surface on the medial end of the clavicle for articulation with the sternum.
f. articula′ris supe′rior atlan′tis [TA] superior articular surface of atlas: the large oval facet on the superior aspect of either lateral mass of the atlas; called also *superior articular facet of atlas.*
f. articula′ris supe′rior ti′biae [TA] superior articular surface of tibia: the surface on the proximal end of the tibia that articulates with the condyles of the femur.
f. articula′ris supe′rior ver′tebrae [TA] superior articular facet of vertebra: the articulating surface on the superior articular process of a vertebra.
f. articula′ris tala′ris ante′rior calca′nei [TA] anterior talar articular surface of calcaneus: the small area on the superior surface of the calcaneus just anterior to the middle articular surface, which articulates with the talus. Called also *anterior talar facet of calcaneus.*
f. articula′ris tala′ris me′dia calca′nei [TA] middle talar articular surface of calcaneus: the area on the superior surface of the calcaneus just in front of the calcaneal sulcus, which articulates with the talus. Called also *middle talar facet of calcaneus.*
f. articula′ris tala′ris poste′rior calca′nei [TA] posterior talar articular surface of calcaneus: the area on the superior surface of the calcaneus just posterolateral to the calcaneal sulcus, which articulates with the talus. Called also *posterior talar facet of calcaneus.*
f. articula′ris thyroi′dea cartila′ginis cricoi′deae [TA] thyroid articular surface on cricoid cartilage: the surface that articulates with the thyroid cartilage.
f. articula′ris tuber′culi cos′tae [TA] articular facet of tubercle of rib: the convex facet on the costal tubercle that articulates with the transverse process of a vertebra.
f. auricula′ris os′sis i′lii [TA] auricular surface of ilium: a somewhat ear-shaped area on the sacropelvic surface of the ilium, which articulates with the auricular surface of the sacrum to form the sacroiliac joint.
f. auricula′ris os′sis sa′cri [TA] auricular surface of sacrum: the broad irregular surface on the superior half of the lateral aspect of the sacrum, which articulates with the ilium.
f. bovi′na [L. "cow face"] a term sometimes applied to the appearance of the face in craniofacial dysostosis; called also *bovine* or *cow face.*
f. bucca′lis den′tis [TA] buccal surface of tooth: the vestibular surface of the molars and premolars that faces the cheek. See also *f. vestibularis dentis.*
f. cerebra′lis a′lae majo′ris os′sis sphenoida′lis [TA] cerebral surface of greater wing of sphenoid bone: the smooth, concave part of the greater wing of the sphenoid bone that forms the anterior part of the floor of the middle cranial fossa, lying anterior to the petrous and squamous parts of the temporal bone.
f. cerebra′lis os′sis tempora′lis [TA] cerebral surface of temporal bone: the inner surface of the squamous part of the temporal bone forming the lateral wall of the middle cranial fossa.
f. co′lica sple′nis [TA] colic impression on spleen: the concave surface of the spleen in contact with the colon.
f. costa′lis pulmo′nis [TA] costal surface of lung: the convex surface of each lung in close adaptation to the curvatures of the ribs and the costal cartilages, which joins the mediastinal surface at the anterior and posterior borders and the diaphragmatic surface at the inferior border. It is related behind to the sides of the vertebral bodies *(pars vertebralis faciei costalis pulmonis).*
f. costa′lis sca′pulae [TA] costal surface of scapula: the anteromedially facing, concave surface of the scapula; called also *anterior* or *ventral surface of scapula,* and *f. anterior scapulae* [TA alternative].
f. diaphragma′tica cor′dis [TA] diaphragmatic surface of heart: the surface of the heart (within the pericardium) that rests on the diaphragm and is directed inferiorly and somewhat posteriorly; it is formed by the two ventricles, the left ventricle contributing a little more than the right; called also *f. inferior cordis* [TA alternative].
f. diaphragma′tica he′patis [TA] diaphragmatic surface of liver: the surface of the liver that is in contact with the diaphragm, divided anatomically into superior, anterior, right, and posterior parts (*pars superior, pars anterior, pars dexter,* and *pars posterior*).
f. diaphragma′tica pulmo′nis [TA] diaphragmatic surface of lung: the surface of each lung that is adjacent to the diaphragm.
f. diaphragma′tica sple′nis [TA] diaphragmatic surface of spleen: the convex posterolateral surface of the spleen, directed toward the diaphragm.
f. dista′lis den′tis [TA] distal surface of tooth: the proximal or contact surface of a tooth that is farthest from the midline of the dental arch.
f. doloro′sa the facial expression of a patient experiencing pain or severe sickness.
f. dorsa′les digito′rum ma′nus [TA] the posterior or dorsal surfaces of the fingers.
f. dorsa′les digito′rum pe′dis [TA] the dorsal or superior surfaces of the toes.
f. dorsa′lis os′sis sac′ri [TA] dorsal surface of sacrum: the markedly convex and rough posterior surface of the sacral bone, which gives origin to the sacrospinalis and multifidus muscles; called also *posterior surface of sacrum.*
elfin f. facial features including wide-set eyes, low-set ears, and hirsutism; seen in children with congenital conditions such as Donohue syndrome and Williams syndrome.
f. exter′na os′sis fronta′lis [TA] the external surface of the squama of the frontal bone; called also *outer table of frontal bone.*
f. exter′na os′sis parieta′lis [TA] the externally directed surface of the parietal bone.
f. gas′trica sple′nis [TA] gastric impression on spleen: the concave surface of the spleen in contact with the stomach.
f. glu′tea os′sis i′lii [TA] gluteal surface of ilium: the large external, or posterior, surface of the ala of the ilium, on which are located the three gluteal lines.
hippocratic f., f. hippocra′tica a drawn, pinched, and pale appearance of the face, indicative of approaching death.
Hutchinson f. a peculiar facial expression in persons having external ophthalmoplegia, with eyeballs fixed, eyebrows raised, and lids drooping.
f. infe′rior cor′dis TA alternative for *f. diaphragmatica cordis.*
f. infe′rior hemisphe′rii ce′rebri inferior surface of cerebral hemisphere: the part of the cerebral hemisphere that rests on the tentorium and in the anterior and middle cranial fossae. See *f. medialis et inferior hemispherii cerebri.*
f. infe′rior lin′guae [TA] inferior surface of tongue: the under surface of the body of the tongue.
f. infe′rior par′tis petro′sae os′sis tempora′lis [TA] inferior surface of petrous part of temporal bone: that surface of the petrous part of

the temporal bone which appears on the external surface of the base of the cranium.
f. inferolatera′lis pro′statae [TA] inferolateral surface of prostate: either of the surfaces on the convex end of the gland away from the base, separated from the superior fascia of the pelvic diaphragm by a venous plexus.
f. infratempora′lis a′lae majo′ris os′sis sphenoida′lis [TA] infratemporal surface of greater wing of sphenoid bone: the lower part of the lateral surface of the greater wing of the sphenoid bone, inferior to the infratemporal crest and to which attach the upper fibers of the lateral pterygoid plate. It forms part of the wall of the infratemporal fossa.
f. infratempora′lis cor′poris maxil′lae [TA] infratemporal surface of maxilla: the posterior convex surface of the body of the maxilla, bounded roughly by the inferior orbital fissure, the zygomatic process and associated ridge, maxillary tuberosity, and posterior margin of the nasal surface.
f. interloba′ris pulmo′nis [TA] interlobar surface of lung: the surface of each lung lying within the oblique and horizontal fissures.
f. inter′na os′sis fronta′lis [TA] internal surface of frontal bone: the vertically situated, concave cerebral surface of the frontal bone; in its midline the sagittal sulcus is seen superiorly and the frontal crest inferiorly. Called also *inner table of frontal bone.*
f. inter′na os′sis parieta′lis [TA] the internal surface of the parietal bone; it is concave and marked by cerebral gyri and grooves for vessels.
f. intervertebra′lis [TA] the surface of the vertebral body adjacent to the intervertebral disk, having an elevated rim (the annular apophysis) surrounding a rough center.
f. intestina′lis u′teri [TA] intestinal surface of uterus: the convex posterior surface of the uterus, adjacent to the intestine. Called also *f. posterior uteri* [TA alternative].
f. labia′lis den′tis [TA] labial surface of tooth: the vestibular surface of an incisor or canine tooth, which faces the lips. See also *f. vestibularis dentis.*
f. latera′lis fi′bulae [TA] lateral surface of fibula: the area between the anterior and posterior borders of the body of the fibula.
f. latera′lis os′sis zygoma′tici [TA] lateral surface of zygomatic bone: the more anterior surface, which is convex.
f. latera′lis ova′rii [TA] lateral surface of ovary: the surface of the ovary in contact with the lateral pelvic wall.
f. latera′lis ra′dii [TA] lateral surface of radius: the surface of the radius that gives attachment to the supinator and pronator teres muscles proximally, and underlies the tendons of the extensor carpi radialis longus and brevis muscles distally.
f. latera′lis tes′tis [TA] lateral surface of testis: the surface of the testis that is directed away from its fellow of the opposite side.
f. latera′lis ti′biae [TA] lateral surface of tibia: the surface of the body of the tibia between the interosseous and anterior borders.
leonine f., f. leonti′na ["lion's face"] a deeply furrowed, lionlike appearance of the face, seen in certain cases of advanced lepromatous leprosy and in other diseases associated with facial edema, such as coast erysipelas. Called also *leontiasis.*
f. lingua′lis den′tis [TA] lingual surface of tooth: the surface that faces inward toward the tongue (oral cavity), and opposite the vestibular (or facial) surface. Called also *oral surface of tooth.*
f. luna′ta aceta′buli [TA] lunate surface of acetabulum: the articular portion of the acetabulum.
f. malleola′ris latera′lis ta′li [TA] lateral malleolar facet of talus: the large triangular facet on the superior surface of the talus talus that articulates with the lateral malleolus of the fibula.
f. malleola′ris media′lis ta′li [TA] medial malleolar facet of talus: the narrow facet on the superior part of the talus, articulating with the medial malleolus of the tibia.
Marshall Hall f. the facies of hydrocephalus: a triangular face with a broad forehead and prominent frontal bones.
f. maxilla′ris a′lae majo′ris os′sis sphenoida′lis [TA] maxillary surface of greater wing of sphenoid bone: a small surface on the inferior part of the greater wing superior to the pterygoid processes; it is perforated by the foramen rotundum.
f. maxilla′ris la′minae perpendicula′ris os′sis palati′ni [TA] maxillary surface of perpendicular plate of palatine bone: the lateral surface of the perpendicular plate of the palatine bone, which is in relation to the maxilla. Posteriorly and inferiorly it contains the greater palatine sulcus, which forms the greater palatine canal with a corresponding groove on the maxilla.
f. media′lis cartila′ginis arytenoi′deae [TA] medial surface of arytenoid cartilage: the surface that faces medially toward the opposite arytenoid cartilage.
f. media′lis fi′bulae [TA] medial surface of fibula: the narrow area on the body of the fibula between the interosseous and anterior borders.
f. media′lis hemisphe′rii ce′rebri medial surface of cerebral hemisphere: the surface of the cerebral hemisphere parallel to and facing both the median plane and the corresponding surface of the opposite hemisphere. See *f. medialis et inferior hemispherii cerebri.*
f. media′lis et infe′rior hemisphe′rii ce′rebri [TA] the medial and inferior surfaces of the cerebral hemisphere considered as a unit.
f. media′lis ova′rii [TA] medial surface of ovary: the side of the ovary in contact with the fimbriated end of the uterine tube and the intestine.
f. media′lis tes′tis [TA] medial surface of testis: the surface of the testis that is directed toward its fellow of the opposite side.
f. media′lis ti′biae [TA] medial surface of tibia: the slightly convex surface of the body of the tibia between the anterior and medial borders.
f. media′lis ul′nae [TA] medial surface of ulna: the smooth, transversely convex surface of the ulna lying between the anterior and posterior borders.
f. mediastina′lis pulmo′nis [TA] mediastinal surface of lung: the surface of each lung lying medially to the vertebral column and mediastinum; it contains the cardiac impression.
f. mesia′lis den′tis [TA] mesial surface of tooth: the contact or proximal surface of a tooth that is closest to the midline of the dental arch.
mitral f., mitrotricuspid f. the appearance of the face of some patients with mitral stenosis of long duration, marked by rosy, flushed cheeks and dilated capillaries.
moon f. the peculiar rounded face observed in various conditions, such as Cushing syndrome, or following administration of corticosteroids.
myasthenic f. the characteristic facial expression in myasthenia gravis, caused by ptosis and weakness of the facial muscles.
myopathic f. the peculiar facial expression produced by relaxation of the facial muscles, as in Landouzy-Dejerine dystrophy.
f. nasa′lis cor′poris maxil′lae [TA] nasal surface of maxilla: the surface of the body of the maxilla that helps form the lateral wall of the nasal cavity; it is bounded roughly by the following: medial margin of the orbital surface, medial margin of the infratemporal surface, the palatine process, and the nasal notch.
f. nasa′lis la′minae horizonta′lis os′sis palati′ni [TA] nasal surface of horizontal plate of palatine bone: the superior surface of the horizontal plate, which forms the posterior part of the floor of the nasal cavity.
f. nasa′lis la′minae perpendicula′ris os′sis palati′ni [TA] nasal surface of perpendicular plate of palatine bone: the medial surface of the perpendicular plate; it articulates with the middle and inferior nasal conchae.

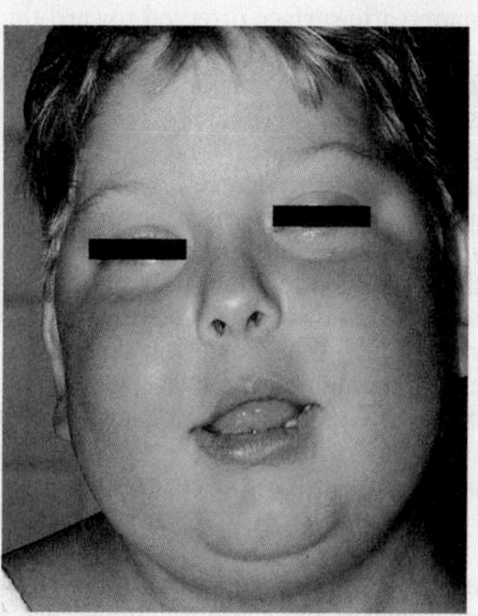

■ Moon facies associated with corticosteroid therapy for chronic asthma.

Facies *Continued*

f. occlusa′lis den′tis [TA] occlusal surface of tooth: the surface of the posterior or artificial teeth coming in contact with those of the opposite jaw during the act of occlusion. In natural teeth, restricted to the anatomic tooth surfaces of the posterior teeth limited mesially and distally by the marginal ridges and buccally and lingually by the buccal and lingual boundaries of the cusp eminences. By extension, the term *occlusal surface* is used to designate the incisal surface (q.v.) of the anterior teeth. Called also *masticatory surface*.
f. orbita′lis a′lae majo′ris os′sis sphenoida′lis [TA] orbital surface of greater wing of sphenoid bone: the quadrilateral surface on the greater wing of the sphenoid bone that forms the major part of the lateral wall of the orbit.
f. orbita′lis cor′poris maxil′lae [TA] orbital surface of maxilla: a triangular surface on the body of the maxilla that forms the greater part of the floor of the orbit.
f. orbita′lis os′sis fronta′lis [TA] orbital surface of frontal bone: the triangular plates of the frontal bone that form most of the roof of each orbit and the floor of the anterior cranial fossa; they are separated by the ethmoidal notch.
f. orbita′lis os′sis zygoma′tici [TA] orbital surface of zygomatic bone: the part of the zygomatic bone that helps form the lateral wall of the orbit.
f. palati′na la′minae horizonta′lis os′sis palati′ni [TA] palatine surface of horizontal plate of palatine bone: the inferior surface of the horizontal plate, forming the posterior part of the hard palate.
f. palatina′lis den′tis [TA] palatal surface of tooth: the lingual surface of a maxillary tooth.
f. palma′res digito′rum ma′nus [TA] the anterior or palmar surfaces of the fingers.
f. pancrea′tica sple′nis [TA] pancreatic impression on spleen: an inconstant concave surface of the spleen in contact with the pancreas; it is usually small when present and lies between the colic impression and the lateral part of the hilum.
Parkinson f., parkinsonian f. a stolid masklike expression of the face, with infrequent blinking, pathognomonic of parkinsonism.
f. patella′ris fe′moris [TA] patellar surface of femur: the smooth anterior continuation of the condyles that forms the surface of the femur articulating with the patella.
f. pel′vica os′sis sa′cri [TA] pelvic surface of sacrum: the smooth, concave, ventrocaudally directed surface of the sacrum that helps form the posterior wall of the pelvis; called also *anterior surface of sacrum*.
f. planta′res digito′rum pe′dis [TA] the plantar or inferior surfaces of the toes.
f. popli′tea fe′moris [TA] popliteal surface of femur: the triangular lower third of the posterior surface of the femur, between the medial and lateral supracondylar lines, which forms the superior part of the floor of the popliteal fossa.
f. poste′rior cartila′ginis arytenoi′deae [TA] posterior surface of arytenoid cartilage: the concave dorsal surface, to which various laryngeal muscles are attached.
f. poste′rior cor′neae [TA] the posterior surface of the cornea, which forms the anterior boundary of the anterior chamber.
f. poste′rior cor′poris pancre′atis [TA] posterior surface of body of pancreas: the pancreatic surface directed toward the posterior part of the body.
f. poste′rior fi′bulae [TA] posterior surface of fibula: the large area between the posterior and interosseous borders of the body of the fibula, presenting the medial crest.
f. poste′rior glan′dulae suprarena′lis [TA] the posterior surface of the adrenal (suprarenal) gland, which borders the peritoneum.
f. poste′rior hu′meri [TA] posterior surface of humerus: the surface of the humerus that is subdivided obliquely by the radial groove to give attachment to the lateral and medial heads of the triceps muscle.
f. poste′rior i′ridis [TA] the posterior surface of the iris, directed toward the posterior chamber of the eye.
f. poste′rior len′tis [TA] the posterior surface of the lens, directed toward the vitreous body of the eye.
f. poste′rior pal′pebrae [TA] posterior surface of eyelid: the inner surface of the eyelid, which is covered with conjunctiva and in contact with the eyeball.
f. poste′rior par′tis petro′sae os′sis tempora′lis [TA] the surface of the petrous part of the temporal bone that forms part of the anterior portion of the floor of the posterior cranial fossa.
f. poste′rior pro′statae [TA] posterior surface of prostate: the surface towards the anterior wall of the rectum, separated from it by fascia.
f. poste′rior ra′dii [TA] posterior surface of radius: a surface giving attachment to the supinator, abductor pollicis longus, and extensor pollicis brevis muscles.
f. poste′rior re′nis [TA] posterior surface of kidney: the kidney surface directed toward the posterior body wall, and not covered by peritoneum.
f. poste′rior sca′pulae [TA] posterior surface of scapula: the convex posterior surface of the scapula, which is divided into two unequal parts by the spine of the scapula. Called also *dorsal surface of scapula* and *dorsum of scapula*.
f. poste′rior ti′biae [TA] posterior surface of tibia: the surface of the body of the tibia between the medial and interosseous borders; in the proximal third it presents the soleal line.
f. poste′rior ul′nae [TA] posterior surface of ulna: the posterolaterally directed surface of the ulna.
f. poste′rior u′teri TA alternative for *f. intestinalis uteri*.
Potter f. the characteristic facial appearance seen with oligohydramnios sequence (see under *sequence*), consisting of a flattened nose, receding chin, wide interpupillary space, large low-set ears, and sometimes other anomalies.
f. pulmona′lis dex′tra/sinis′tra cor′dis [TA] right/left pulmonary surface of heart: the surface of the heart that faces either of the lungs.
f. rena′lis glan′dulae suprarena′lis [TA] renal surface of adrenal gland: the surface directed toward the kidney, being separated from it by a layer of fat.
f. rena′lis sple′nis [TA] renal impression on spleen: the concave surface of the spleen in contact with the left kidney.
f. sacropel′vica os′sis i′lii [TA] sacropelvic surface of ilium: an irregular area on the inner surface of the ala of the ilium, posterior to the iliac fossa; it contains the iliac tuberosity and the auricular surface.
f. scaphoi′dea dish face.
f. sternocosta′lis cor′dis [TA] sternocostal surface of heart: the convex surface of the heart, which in general is directed anteriorly and somewhat superiorly, being formed mainly by the right ventricle, and to a lesser degree by the left ventricle and the atria; called also *f. anterior cordis* [TA alternative].
f. supe′rior troch′leae ta′li [TA] superior facet of trochlea of talus: the smooth superior surface of the trochlea of the talus, articulating with the tibia.
f. superolatera′lis hemisphe′rii ce′rebri [TA] superolateral surface of cerebral hemisphere: the convex outer surface of the cerebrum, which faces the calvaria.
f. symphysia′lis os′sis pu′bis [TA] symphysial surface of pubic bone: the rough, ovoid, medial surface of the body of the pubic bone, by which it articulates at the pubic symphysis with its fellow of the opposite side.
f. tempora′lis a′lae majo′ris os′sis sphenoida′lis [TA] temporal surface of greater wing of sphenoid bone: the upper part of the lateral surface of the greater wing of the sphenoid bone, superior to the infratemporal crest; it forms a portion of the wall of the temporal fossa.
f. tempora′lis os′sis fronta′lis [TA] temporal surface of frontal bone: the slightly concave surface of the frontal bone that forms the superior part of the wall of the temporal fossa and gives attachment to the anterosuperior part of the temporalis muscle.
f. tempora′lis os′sis zygoma′tici [TA] temporal surface of zygomatic bone: the internal, concave surface of the bone, facing the temporal and infratemporal fossae.
f. tempora′lis par′tis squamo′sae os′sis tempora′lis [TA] temporal surface of squamous part of temporal bone: the external surface of the squamous part, the anterior part of which forms a portion of the temporal fossa.
f. urethra′lis pe′nis [TA] urethral surface of penis: the surface of the penis overlying the urethra, and opposite the dorsum penis.
f. vesica′lis u′teri [TA] vesical surface of uterus: the flat anterior surface of the uterus, adjacent to the urinary bladder. Called also *f. anterior uteri* [TA alternative].
f. vestibula′ris den′tis [TA] vestibular surface of tooth: the surface of a tooth that is directed outward toward the vestibule of the mouth, including the buccal and labial surfaces, and opposite the lingual (or oral) surface. Called also *facial surface of tooth*.

Facies *Continued*

f. viscera′lis he′patis [TA] visceral surface of liver: the posteroinferior surface of the liver, which is in contact with various abdominal viscera. Called also *inferior surface of liver.*

f. viscera′lis sple′nis [TA] visceral surface of spleen: the surface of the spleen that comes in contact with various other viscera, including the colon (facies colica), kidney (facies renalis), and stomach (facies gastrica).

fa•cil•i•ta•tion (fə-sil″ĭ-ta′shən) [L. *facilis* easy] 1. the promotion or hastening of any natural process; the reverse of inhibition. 2. in neurophysiology, the effect of a nerve impulse acting across a synapse, resulting in increased postsynaptic action potential of subsequent impulses in that nerve fiber or in other convergent nerve fibers.

postactivation f., posttetanic f. facilitation at the neuromuscular junction, consisting of a decreased decrementing response or increased amplitude of the M wave, when nerve stimulation is repeated a few seconds after a strong voluntary contraction or after tetanus has occurred. See also *postactivation depression* and *postactivation exhaustion.*

proprioceptive neuromuscular f. a system of therapeutic exercise for the inhibition of spasticity, with emphasis on the training of specific diagonal or spiral body movements against resistance in synergistic patterns; long repetition of involuntary reflex movements is aimed at the eventual development of greater voluntary motor control.

Wedensky f. facilitation across a block; when there is a complete block to nerve conduction the threshold of the nerve below the block to electric stimulation is lowered.

fa•cil•i•ta•tive (fə-sil′ĭ-ta″tiv) in pharmacology, denoting a reaction arising as an indirect result of drug action, as development of an infection after the normal microflora has been altered by an antibiotic.

fac•ing (fās′ing) a porcelain reproduction of the labial or buccal surface of a tooth; it may be constructed with or without pins and is soldered or cemented to a metal backing.

faci(o)- [L. *facies* face] a combining form denoting relationship to the face.

fa•cio•bra•chi•al (fa″she-o-bra′ke-əl) [*facio-* + *brachial*] pertaining to the face and upper limb.

fa•cio•ceph•a•lal•gia (fa″she-o-sef″ə-lal′jə) [*facio-* + *cephalalgia*] neuralgic pain in the face and neck attributed to disorders of the autonomic nervous system.

fa•cio•cer•vi•cal (fa″she-o-sur′vĭ-kəl) [*facio-* + *cervical*] pertaining to or affecting the face and neck.

fa•cio•dig•ito•gen•i•tal (fa″she-o-dij″ĭ-to-gen′ĭ-təl) [*facio-* + *digito-* + *genital*] pertaining to or affecting the face, digits, and genitalia

fa•cio•gen•i•tal (fa″she-o-gen′ĭ-təl) [*facio-* + *genital*] pertaining to or affecting the face and genitalia

fa•cio•lin•gual (fa″she-o-ling′wəl) [*facio-* + *lingual*] pertaining to the face and tongue.

fa•cio•plas•ty (fa′she-o-plas″te) [*facio-* + *-plasty*] plastic surgery of the face. **facioplas′tic** *adj*

fa•cio•ple•gia (fa″she-o-ple′jə) [*facio-* + *-plegia*] facial paralysis.

fa•cio•scap•u•lo•hu•mer•al (fa″she-o-skap″u-lo-hu′mər-əl) pertaining to the face, scapula, and upper limb.

fa•cio•ste•no•sis (fa″she-o-stə-no′sis) failure of the midface to grow.

FACOG Fellow of the American College of Obstetricians and Gynecologists.

FACP Fellow of the American College of Physicians.

FACR Fellow of the American College of Radiology.

FACS fluorescence-activated cell sorter; Fellow of the American College of Surgeons.

FACSM Fellow of the American College of Sports Medicine.

F-act•in see *actin.*

fac•ti•tial (fak-tish′əl) factitious.

fac•ti•tious (fak-tish′əs) artificially induced; not natural. Called also *factitial.*

Fac•tive (fak′tiv) trademark for a preparation of gemifloxacin mesylate.

fac•tor (fak′tər) [L. "maker"] 1. any of several substances or activities that are necessary to produce a result, e.g., a coagulation factor. Often, use of the term "factor" indicates that the chemical nature of the substance or its mechanism of action is unknown, as in endocrinology, where "factors" are renamed as "hormones" when their chemical nature is determined. 2. one of two or more quantities that multiplied together form a product. 3. a coefficient or conversion factor, a number by which a quantity is multiplied to produce a change of units of measurement.

Factor

f. I see under *coagulation f's.*
f. II see under *coagulation f's.*
f. III see under *coagulation f's.*
f. IV see under *coagulation f's.*
f. V see under *coagulation f's.*
f. VI see under *coagulation f's.*
f. VII see under *coagulation f's.*
f. VIII see under *coagulation f's.*
f. IX see under *coagulation f's.*
f. X see under *coagulation f's.*
f. XI see under *coagulation f's.*
f. XII see under *coagulation f's.*
f. XIII see under *coagulation f's.*
f. A former name for the alternative pathway complement factor *C3;* see under *complement.*
accelerator f. f. V; see under *coagulation f's.*
activation f. f. XII; see under *coagulation f's.*
angiogenesis f. a substance that causes the growth of new blood vessels, found in tissues with high metabolic requirements such as cancers and the retina; it is also released by hypoxic macrophages at the edges or outer surface of a wound and initiates revascularization in wound healing.
antigen-specific T-cell helper f. a soluble factor produced by helper T cells that activates other lymphocytes that are specific for the stimulating antigen; it may itself bind antigen.
antigen-specific T-cell suppressor f. a soluble factor produced by suppressor T cells following immunization; it produces antigen-specific suppression of the immune response and may itself bind antigen.
antihemophilic f. (AHF) 1. *f. VIII,* see under *coagulation f's.* 2. a preparation of factor VIII used in the treatment of hemophilia A, including preparations derived from human plasma (antihemophilic factor and cryoprecipitated antihemophilic factor) or porcine plasma (antihemophilic factor [porcine]) and those produced by recombinant technology (antihemophilic factor [recombinant]). 3. [USP] a sterile freeze-dried powder containing the factor VIII fraction prepared from human venous plasma; used to arrest hemorrhage or to prevent hemorrhage during surgery or other procedures in patients with hemophilia A and in the treatment of von Willebrand disease; administered intravenously.

Factor *Continued*

antihemophilic f. A f. VIII; see under *coagulation f's.*
antihemophilic f. B f. IX; see under *coagulation f's.*
antihemophilic f. C f. XI; see under *coagulation f's.*
antihemophilic f. (human) antihemophilic f. (def. 3).
antihemophilic f. (porcine) a highly purified sterile freeze-dried concentrate of porcine coagulation factor VIII obtained from porcine plasma; it is less antigenic than human factor VIII and is used in the treatment of hemophilia A in patients with circulatory antibodies to factor VIII and in patients with spontaneously acquired inhibitors to human factor VIII; administered by intravenous infusion.
antihemophilic f. (recombinant) a sterile, purified, concentrate produced by recombinant technology using cultured hamster cell lines that have been transfected with a gene for human coagulation factor VIII, and having biological activity comparable to that of plasma-derived coagulation factor VIII; used to prevent or arrest hemorrhage during surgery or other procedures in patients with hemophilia A; administered intravenously.
antinuclear f. (ANF) see under *antibody.*
antiperinuclear f. an antibody against perinuclear keratohyalin granules in cells of the buccal mucosa, found at increased levels in rheumatoid arthritis.
apoptotic protease activating f. 1 (Apaf-1) a cytoplasmic protein that is activated by cytochrome *c* (released from mitochondria) and deoxyadenosine triphosphate (dATP); it in turn binds to and activates caspase 9, initiating the apoptotic cascade.
atrial natriuretic f. (ANF) 1. atrial natriuretic peptide. 2. sometimes more specifically, the prohormone form of atrial natriuretic peptide.
autocrine growth f. a polypeptide, produced endogenously by a cell free from usual external growth controls, that may act on its producer cell to cause malignant transformation.
autocrine motility f. name given to glucose-6 isomerase in its identity as a stimulator of motility in cancer cells.
f. B a complement component that participates in the alternative pathway of complement activation (see *complement*), binding to C3b to form C3bB, which is a substrate for factor D.
basophil chemotactic f. (BCF) a lymphokine produced by activated lymphocytes that is chemotactic for basophils, possibly responsible for the influx of basophils into sites of inflammation (Jones-Mote reaction).
B cell differentiation f's (BCDF) factors derived from T cells that stimulate B cells to differentiate into antibody-secreting cells. Cf. *B lymphocyte stimulatory f's.*
B cell growth f's (BCGF) factors derived from T cells that stimulate B cells to proliferate in vitro but (unlike B cell differentiation factors) do not stimulate antibody secretion. Cf. *B lymphocyte stimulatory f's.*
blastogenic f. (BF) lymphocyte mitogenic f.
B lymphocyte stimulatory f's (BSF) a system of nomenclature for factors that stimulate B cells, replacing individual factor names (e.g., B cell differentiation factor). Each factor is designated by BSF and a number, BSF1, BSF2, etc., with the letter p prefixed to the number for factors that have not been purified or whose structure has not been identified. BSF1 is interleukin-4 and BSF2 is interleukin-6.
bone f. in periodontal disease, the systemic influence on alveolar bone loss in response to local inflammatory processes.
brain-derived neurotrophic f. (BDNF) a protein related to nerve growth factor, found in the brain and near peripheral nerves; it promotes growth and survival of neurons.
CAMP f. see under *test.*
Castle f., Castle intrinsic f. intrinsic f.
chemotactic f. a substance that induces chemotaxis. See *chemoattractant* and *chemorepellent.* Called also *chemotaxin.*
Christmas f. f. IX; see under *coagulation f's.*
citrovorum f. folinic acid.
clotting f's coagulation factors.
C3 nephritic f. (C3 NeF) an autoantibody that binds the alternative complement pathway C3 convertase C3b,Bb and prevents its inactivation by factor H, resulting in chronic fluid phase alternative pathway activation and complete consumption of plasma C3; found in the serum of many patients with type II membranoproliferative glomerulonephritis.
coagulation f's substances in the blood that are essential to the clotting process and hence, to the maintenance of normal hemostasis. They are designated by Roman numerals, to which the notation "a" is added to indicate the activated state. Platelet factors (q.v.) also play a role in coagulation.

f. I fibrinogen: a high-molecular-weight plasma protein, composed of three subunits (α, β, γ) encoded by separate genes, which is converted to fibrin through the action of thrombin. Deficiency of this factor results in afibrinogenemia or hypofibrinogenemia.

f. II prothrombin: a plasma protein that is converted to the active form thrombin (factor IIa) by cleavage by activated factor X (Xa) in the common pathway of coagulation; thrombin then cleaves fibrinogen to its active form fibrin. Deficiency of the factor leads to hypoprothrombinemia.

f. III tissue thromboplastin: a lipoprotein functioning in the extrinsic pathway of coagulation, activating factor X. Called also *tissue f.*

f. IV calcium: a factor required in many phases of blood coagulation.

f. V proaccelerin: a heat- and storage-labile material, present in plasma but not in serum, functioning in both the intrinsic and extrinsic pathways of coagulation, catalyzing the cleavage of prothrombin to the active thrombin. Deficiency of this factor, an autosomal recessive trait, leads to a rare hemorrhagic tendency called parahemophilia, with varying degrees of severity. Called also *accelerator globulin (AcG)* and *labile f.*

f. VI a factor (accelerin) previously thought to be an activated form of factor V. It no longer is considered in the scheme of hemostasis, and hence it is currently assigned neither a name nor a function.

f. VII proconvertin: a heat- and storage-stable factor participating in the extrinsic pathway of coagulation. It is activated by contact with calcium and in concert with factor III (tissue thromboplastin) activates factor X. Deficiency of this factor, which may be hereditary (autosomal recessive) or acquired (associated with vitamin K deficiency), results in a hemorrhagic tendency. Called also *serum prothrombin conversion accelerator (SPCA)* and *stable f.* The activated form is called also *convertin.*

f. VIII antihemophilic factor (AHF): a relatively storage-labile factor participating in the intrinsic pathway of coagulation, acting (in concert with von Willebrand factor) as a cofactor in the activation of factor X. Deficiency, an X-linked recessive trait, causes hemophilia A (classical hemophilia). Called also *antihemophilic globulin (AHG)* and *antihemophilic f. A.*

f. IX 1. plasma thromboplastin component (PTC): a relatively storage-stable substance involved in the intrinsic pathway of coagulation; upon activation, it activates factor X. Deficiency results in a hemorrhagic syndrome called hemophilia B, resembling hemophilia A. Called also *Christmas f.* and *antihemophilic f. B.* 2. any of several preparations of factor IX used therapeutically; see *factor IX complex,* under *complex, coagulation f. IX (human),* and *coagulation f. IX (recombinant).*

f. X Stuart factor: a storage-stable factor that participates in both the intrinsic and extrinsic pathways of coagulation, uniting them to begin the common pathway of coagulation. Once activated, it forms a complex with calcium, phospholipid, and factor V; the complex (prothrombinase) can cleave and activate prothrombin to thrombin. Deficiency of this factor may cause a systemic coagulation disorder. Called also *Prower factor* and *Stuart-Prower factor.* The activated form is called also *thrombokinase.*

f. XI plasma thromboplastin antecedent (PTA): a stable factor involved in the intrinsic pathway of coagulation; once activated, it activates factor IX. *Factor XI deficiency* (see under *deficiency*) results in a systemic blood-clotting defect that resembles hemophilia A. Called also *antihemophilic f. C.*

f. XII Hageman factor: a stable factor activated by contact with glass or other foreign surfaces, which initiates the intrinsic pathway of coagulation by activating factor XI and participates in activation of the kinin and fibrinolytic pathways. Deficiency of this factor results in a tendency toward thrombotic disorders, due to lack of activation of the fibrinolytic pathway. Called also *glass, contact,* or *activation f.*

f. XIII fibrin-stabilizing factor (FSF): a factor that polymerizes fibrin monomers so that they become stable and insoluble in urea, thus enabling fibrin to form a firm blood clot. Deficiency of this factor produces a clinical hemorrhagic diathesis. Called also *fibrinase, protransglutaminase,* and *Laki-Lorand f.* The activated form is also called *transglutaminase.*

coagulation f. IX (human) a purified, sterile, dried concentrate of factor IX derived from pooled human plasma; used in the prophylaxis and treatment of bleeding in patients with hemophilia B, administered intravenously. Cf. *coagulation f. IX (recombinant)* and *factor IX complex.*
coagulation f. IX (recombinant) a sterile, dried concentrate of factor IX prepared by recombinant means; used in the prophylaxis and treatment of bleeding in patients with hemophilia B, administered intravenously. Cf. *coagulation f. IX (human)* and *factor IX complex.*
colony-stimulating f's a group of glycoprotein lymphokine growth factors produced by blood monocytes, tissue macrophages, and stimulated lymphocytes; they are required for differentiation of stem cells into granulocyte and monocyte cell colonies, and were originally named according to their ability to stimulate the production of morphologically distinguishable myeloid cell colonies in vitro. In vivo, they

stimulate the production of granulocytes and macrophages and enhance the actions of mature cells. Colony-stimulating factors can be produced by recombinant DNA techniques and have been used experimentally as anticancer agents and for the restoration of hematopoietic function after myelosuppression in transplantation and cancer chemotherapy.
contact f. f. XII; see under *coagulation f's.*
cord f. a mycoside produced by those strains of *Mycobacterium tuberculosis* that characteristically grow in long serpentine cords.
cryoprecipitated antihemophilic f. [USP] a sterile, frozen concentrate of antihemophilic factor prepared from the coagulation factor VIII–rich cryoprotein fraction of human venous plasma; used for autologous replacement of factor VIII in patients with hemophilia A and for the treatment of von Willebrand disease, hypofibrinogenemia, and coagulation factor XIII deficiency, administered intravenously.
crystal-induced chemotactic f. (CCF) a glycoprotein produced by neutrophils upon ingestion of monosodium urate or calcium pyrophosphate crystals, which is directly chemotactic for neutrophils and is thought to be involved in the inflammatory process in gouty arthritis.
f. D a serine protease of the alternative complement pathway that cleaves factor B bound to C3b. The reaction releases Ba while leaving Bb bound to C3b to form the C3bBb that is the C3 convertase of the alternative pathway.
decay accelerating f. (DAF) a protein of most blood cells as well as endothelial and epithelial cells, CD55; it protects the cell membranes from attack by autologous complement, either by preventing assembly of convertase on the cell surface or by accelerating its decay once bound.
diabetogenic f. see under *hormone.*
diffusion f., Duran-Reynals f. hyaluronidase.
elongation f. one of two soluble proteins (EF-1 and EF-2) involved in the addition of each amino acid to the growing polypeptide chain in protein synthesis (see *translation).*
endothelial-derived relaxing f., endothelium-derived relaxing f. (EDRF) nitric oxide.
eosinophil chemotactic f. (ECF) 1. eosinophil chemotactic f. of anaphylaxis. 2. a lymphokine produced by activated lymphocytes that is chemotactic for eosinophils.
eosinophil chemotactic f. of anaphylaxis (ECF-A) eosinophil chemoattractants released by basophils and mast cells in immediate hypersensitivity reactions. ECF-A activity is associated with two acidic tetrapeptides (Ala-Gly-Ser-Glu and Val-Gly-Ser-Glu) and with less well characterized larger peptides, which are chemotactic for eosinophils and, to a lesser degree, for neutrophils. Some ECF-A activity is due to arachidonic acid metabolites (leukotriene B, 12-HETE, and 12-HHT). Called also *eosinophil chemotactic f. (ECF).*
epidermal growth f. (EGF) a mitogenic polypeptide originally extracted from the submandibular glands of male mice; it is produced by many cell types and is made in large amounts by some tumors. It promotes growth and differentiation, is essential in embryogenesis, and is also important in wound healing. It has been found to be part of a family of compounds that includes human epidermal growth factor, transforming growth factors, and amphiregulin.
epidermal growth f., human a mitogenic polypeptide found in humans that is 70 per cent homologous with the epidermal growth factor of mice; it promotes growth and differentiation, is essential in embryogenesis, and is important in wound healing. It is produced by many normal cell types and is made in large amounts by some tumors; the kidneys are the major source of the circulating factor. Called also *urogastrone.*
epithelial growth f. human epidermal growth f.
erythropoietic stimulating f. (ESF) erythropoietin.
extrinsic f. vitamin B_{12} (cyanocobalamin).
F f., fertility f. F plasmid.
fibrin-stabilizing f. (FSF) f. XIII; see under *coagulation f's.*
fibroblast growth f. see under *hormone.*
Fitzgerald f. high-molecular-weight kininogen.
Fletcher f. prekallikrein.
glass f. f. XII; see under *coagulation f's.*
glucose tolerance f. a biologically active complex of chromium and nicotinic acid that facilitates the reaction of insulin with receptor sites on tissues.
granulocyte colony-stimulating f. (G-CSF) a colony-stimulating factor, secreted by stimulated endothelial cells, fibroblasts, and macrophages, that stimulates the production of neutrophils from precursor cells. A recombinant form used therapeutically is called *filgrastim.*
granulocyte-macrophage colony-stimulating f. (GM-CSF) a colony-stimulating factor, secreted by activated T lymphocytes and macrophages and by stimulated endothelial cells, that binds to a specific receptor found on stem cells and most myelocytes and stimulates their differentiation into granulocytes and macrophages. GM-CSF also enhances the function of mature granulocytes and macrophages in vitro. A recombinant form used therapeutically is called *sargramostim.*
growth f. any of numerous substances that promote normal or pathological growth of cells or tissue, including the epidermal growth factors, insulin-like growth factors, nerve growth factors, platelet-derived growth factors, and transforming growth factors.
f. H a glycoprotein that binds to C3b (see under *complement*) and acts as an alternative pathway complement inhibitor by interfering with the binding of factor B to C3b; it also acts as a cofactor in the conversion of C3b to the inactive form iC3b by factor I.
Hageman f. (HF) f. XII; see under *coagulation f's.*
hematopoietic growth f's a group of substances with the ability to support hematopoietic colony formation in vitro, including erythropoietin, interleukin-3, and colony-stimulating factors. All except erythropoietin stimulate mature cells, have overlapping capabilities to affect progenitor cells of several blood cell lines, and also affect cells outside the hematopoietic system.
hepatocyte growth f. (HGF) a potent mitogen and inducer of hepatocyte proliferation, produced by nonparenchymal cells in the liver and by mesenchymal cells in many other organs. Called also *scatter f.*
hepatocyte nuclear f. (HNF) any of a group of transcription factors of liver-specific genes involved in a variety of functions, including carcinogenesis, atherosclerosis, hyperlipidemia, insulin resistance, and hypertension.
high-molecular-weight neutrophil chemotactic f. (HMW-NCF) neutrophil chemotactic f.
histamine-releasing f. (HRF) a lymphokine, believed to be produced by macrophages and B lymphocytes, that induces the release of histamine by IgE-bound basophils occurring in late phase allergic reaction in sensitive individuals.
homologous restriction f. (HRF) a regulatory protein that binds to the membrane attack complex factor C8 of autologous cells and by preventing C9 insertion into the membrane and subsequent polymerization so inhibits the final stages of complement activation.
hyperglycemic-glycogenolytic f. 1. former name for *glucagon.* 2. the hyperglycemic component of growth hormone extracts.
f. I a plasma enzyme that regulates both classical and alternative pathways of complement activation (see *complement*). In the classical pathway, it blocks the formation of C3 convertase by catabolizing C4b; in the alternative pathway, it inactivates C3b by cleaving it to form iC3b, requiring also a cofactor such as factor H, MCP (membrane cofactor protein), or CR1 (complement receptor 1).
immunoglobulin-binding f. (IBF) a lymphokine having the ability to bind IgG complexed with antigen and prevent complement activation, possibly Fc receptors shed from T cells.
inhibiting f's factors elaborated by one structure (such as the hypothalamus) that inhibit release of hormones by other structures (such as the adenohypophysis). The term is applied to substances of unknown chemical structure; those of established chemical identity are called *inhibiting hormones.*
initiation f. one of three soluble proteins (IF-1, IF-2, and IF-3) involved in the binding of mRNA and the first aminoacyl-tRNA to the small ribosomal subunit and the attachment of the small subunit to the large subunit at the beginning of protein synthesis (see *translation*).
insulinlike growth f's (IGF) serum peptides with insulin-like actions, formerly called *somatomedins* (q.v.). IGF-I (formerly *somatomedin C*) is an important growth hormone–dependent mediator of cell growth and replication. IGF-II (formerly *somatomedin A*) appears to be essential for normal embryonic development and may play special roles in the central nervous system. Both are similar in sequence and structure to proinsulin.
intestinal trefoil f. trefoil f. 3.
intrinsic f. a glycoprotein secreted by the parietal cells of the gastric glands, necessary for the absorption of vitamin B_{12} (cyanocobalamin). Lack of intrinsic factor, with consequent deficiency of vitamin B_{12}, results in pernicious anemia.
labile f. f. V; see under *coagulation f's.*
Laki-Lorand f. f. XIII; see under *coagulation f's.*

LE f. an antinuclear antibody present in the blood serum in systemic lupus erythematosus, having a sedimentation rate of 7S and reacting with leukocyte nuclei in the LE cell test.
leukocyte inhibitory f. (LIF) a lymphokine that inhibits the migration of polymorphonuclear leukocytes but not macrophages.
lymph node permeability f. (LNPF) a vasoactive factor, distinct from histamine, serotonin, bradykinin, and kallikrein, that is released without immunologic stimulus from many tissues, including lymph nodes, spleen, kidney, liver, and muscle.
lymphocyte-activating f. interleukin-1.
lymphocyte blastogenic f. (BF) lymphocyte mitogenic f.
lymphocyte mitogenic f. (LMF), lymphocyte-transforming f. (LTF) a nondialyzable heat-stable macromolecule, mol. wt. approximately 20,000–30,000, released by lymphocytes stimulated by specific antigen, that causes nonstimulated lymphocytes to undergo blast transformation and cell division.
macrophage-activating f. (MAF) interferon-γ.
macrophage chemotactic f. (MCF) a lymphokine produced by activated lymphocytes that is chemotactic for macrophages.
macrophage colony-stimulating f. (M-CSF) a colony-stimulating factor secreted by macrophages, stimulated endothelial cells, and most tissues, that stimulates the production of macrophages from precursor cells and maintains the viability of mature macrophages in vitro.
macrophage-derived growth f. a substance released by macrophages below the surface of a wound that induces the proliferation of fibroblasts, with consequent deposition of collagen, fibronectin, and glycosaminoglycan.
macrophage growth f. (MGF) any of various glycoproteins that permit macrophages harvested from peritoneal exudates to proliferate in liquid-suspension cultures and form colonies consisting solely of mononuclear phagocytes.
macrophage inhibition f., macrophage inhibitory f. migration inhibitory f.
migration inhibition f., migration inhibitory f. (MIF) a lymphokine that inhibits macrophage migration.
mitogenic f. lymphocyte mitogenic f.
müllerian duct inhibitory f., müllerian inhibiting f., müllerian regression f. antimüllerian hormone.
myocardial depressant f. (MDF) a peptide putatively formed in response to a fall in systemic blood pressure related to sepsis; it has a negatively inotropic effect on myocardial muscle fibers.
necrotizing f. necrotoxin.
nerve growth f. (NGF) a neurotrophin, secreted by a wide variety of cells, that regulates the proliferation, differentiation, and survival of sympathetic and sensory neurons; it is also involved in the initiation of pain and is a mediator of inflammation, particularly in the airways. It was originally discovered as a high-molecular-weight complex consisting of α, β, and γ subunits; the active form in humans is the β dimer.
neutrophil chemotactic f. (NCF) 1. a poorly characterized chemotactic factor, mol. wt. approximately 750,000, that attracts neutrophils but not eosinophils or monocytes and is released by basophils or mast cells in immediate hypersensitivity reactions. Called also *high-molecular-weight neutrophil chemotactic f. (HMW-NCF)*. 2. a lymphokine produced by activated lymphocytes that is chemotactic for neutrophils.
osteoclast-activating f. (OAF) a lymphokine that stimulates bone resorption; it is a small protein unrelated to parathyroid hormone and may be involved in the bone resorption associated with multiple myeloma and other hematologic neoplasms or inflammatory disorders such as rheumatoid arthritis and periodontal disease.
f. P properdin.
pellagra-preventive f. niacin.
platelet f's factors important in hemostasis, contained in or attached to the platelets; they act together with coagulation factors.

platelet f. 1 adsorbed factor V from the plasma.

platelet f. 2 an accelerator of the thrombin-fibrinogen reaction, attached to platelets.

platelet f. 3 a lipoprotein, extracted from platelets, that contributes to the interaction of activated plasma coagulation factors IX and VIII to produce activated factor X as well as of activated factors X and V to cleave and activate prothrombin.

platelet f. 4 an intracellular protein component of platelets, capable of neutralizing the antithrombic activity of heparin in the fibrinogen-fibrin reaction and the inhibitory effect of heparin in the thromboplastin generation test.

platelet-activating f. (PAF) a substance released by basophils and mast cells in immediate hypersensitivity reactions and macrophages and neutrophils in other inflammatory responses; it is an extremely potent mediator of bronchoconstriction and of the platelet aggregation and release reactions. It differs from other known biochemical mediators in being a phospholipid. Called also *PAF-acether* or *AGEPC* (acetyl glyceryl ether phosphoryl choline).
platelet-derived growth f. a substance found in the alpha granules of platelets, capable of inducing proliferation of vascular endothelial cells, vascular smooth muscle cells, fibroblasts, and glia cells; its action contributes to the repair of damaged vascular walls.
P.-P. f. niacin.
prolactin-inhibiting f. (PIF) see under *hormone.*
prolactin-releasing f. (PRF) see under *hormone.*
proteolysis-inducing f. a sulfated glycoprotein, mass 28 kD, isolated from certain types of tumors; it stimulates protein breakdown and causes cachexia.
Prower f. f. X; see under *coagulation f's.*
R f. R plasmid.
recruitment f. lymphocyte mitogenic f.
releasing f's 1. factors elaborated in one structure (such as the hypothalamus) that effect the release of hormones from another structure (such as the adenohypophysis). The term is applied to substances of unknown chemical structure; those of established chemical identity are called *releasing hormones* (see under *hormone*). 2. two soluble proteins (RF-1 and RF-2) involved in the release of the completed polypeptide chain from the ribosome when a termination codon is encountered during protein synthesis (see *translation*). RF-1 recognizes the termination codon UAA or UAG and RF-2 recognizes UAA or UGA.
resistance-inducing f. (RIF) see *Rubin test* (def. 2), under *test.*
resistance transfer f. (RTF) the portion of an R plasmid in a bacterial cell that contains the genes for conjugation and replication.
Rh f., Rhesus f. any of numerous antigens (agglutinogens) that may be present on the membrane of erythrocytes and that determine the Rh blood group system; the most common ones are called (in one system) Rh 1, Rh 3, Rh 4, Rh 5, and Rh 21. See *Rh blood group,* under *blood group.* Called also *Rh antigen.*
rheumatoid f. (RF) antibodies directed against antigenic determinants, i.e., Gm, in the Fc region of the IgG class of immunoglobulins; these are found in the serum of about 80 per cent of persons with classical or definite rheumatoid arthritis, but only about 20 per cent of those with juvenile rheumatoid arthritis. Rheumatoid factors may be of the IgM, IgG, or IgA classes of immunoglobulins, although serologic tests measure only IgM. Rheumatoid factors also occur in other connective tissue diseases and infectious diseases, such as Sjögren syndrome, systemic lupus erythematosus, sarcoidosis, subacute bacterial endocarditis, hepatitis A, and leprosy.
risk f. a clearly defined occurrence or characteristic that has been associated with the increased rate of a subsequently occurring disease; causality may or may not be implied.
scatter f. hepatocyte growth f.
sex f. F plasmid.
skeletal growth f. a protein that stimulates growth of osteocytes.
skin reactive f. (SRF) a lymphokine derived from antigen-stimulated lymphocytes that augments delayed hypersensitivity skin reaction, increasing capillary permeability and infiltration of monocytes; perhaps a mixture of other lymphokines.
somatotropin release–inhibiting f. (SRIF) somatostatin.
spreading f. hyaluronidase.
stable f. f. VII; see under *coagulation f's.*
steroidogenic f. 1 (SF-1) a zinc finger orphan nuclear receptor expressed in primary steroidogenic tissues and important for the development of the adrenal glands and for the regulation of several genes involved in reproduction, steroidogenesis, and male sexual differentiation; SF-1 disruption results in adrenal and gonadal agenesis, absence of pituitary gonadotrophs, ambiguous genitalia, and abnormalities of the hypothalamus.
Stuart f., Stuart-Prower f. f. X; see under *coagulation f's.*
sulfation f's former name for *insulin-like growth f's.*
sun protection f. (SPF), sun protective f. the ratio between the number of minimal erythema doses required to induce erythema through a film of sunscreen and that for unprotected skin.
T-cell growth f. former name for *interleukin-2.*

Factor *Continued*

tissue f. f. III; see under *coagulation f's.*

transcription f. a protein that regulates gene expression by binding to a DNA sequence adjacent to a sequence encoding a protein or RNA product, thus switching the gene on or off.

transfer f. (TF) 1. a dialyzable extract obtained from lysates of peripheral blood lymphocytes that is capable of transferring antigen-specific cell-mediated immunity (delayed-type hypersensitivity) from donor to recipient and also has nonspecific immunostimulatory activity; it appears to contain both protein and RNA but not DNA and to consist of small molecules (mol. wt. less than 10,000). TF is nonantigenic and does not transfer humoral immunity. It has been used in the treatment of a variety of immunodeficiency diseases. 2. elongation f.

transforming growth f. (TGF) either of two types of proteins secreted by transformed cells and stimulating growth of normal cells, although not causing transformation. *TGF-α* binds the epidermal growth factor receptor and also stimulates growth of microvascular endothelial cells. *TGF-β* comprises several proteins, which are found in hematopoietic tissue, stimulate wound healing, and in vitro are antagonists of lymphopoiesis and myelopoiesis. Similar proteins involved in inducing the change of undifferentiated tissues into specific types of tissues, including bone morphogenetic proteins, activins, and inhibins, are said to belong to the superfamily of TGF-β proteins.

trefoil f. (TFF) any of a family of protease-resistant peptides having a three-loop structure consisting of six cysteine residues and three disulfide bonds, expressed throughout the gastrointestinal tract. They promote epithelial cell migration and gastrointestinal wound healing, prevent apoptosis and anoikis, and contribute to mucosal protection; TFF1 is also a tumor suppressor. TFF1 is called also *pS2*; TFF2, *spasmolytic polypeptide* or *spasmolysin*; and TFF3, *intestinal trefoil f.*

tumor-angiogenesis f. a factor produced by cancer cells of solid tumors that stimulates the growth of blood vessels into the tumor.

tumor necrosis f. (TNF) either of two lymphokines that are capable of causing in vivo hemorrhagic necrosis of certain tumor cells, but not affecting normal cells; they have been used as experimental anticancer agents but can also induce shock when bacterial endotoxins cause their release. *Tumor necrosis factor α,* contains 157 amino acids and is produced by macrophages, eosinophils, and NK cells. *Tumor necrosis factor β* is lymphotoxin and contains 171 amino acids.

V f. an accessory substance required for the growth of certain species of *Haemophilus,* replaceable by nicotinamide-adenine dinucleotide (NAD) or nicotinamide-adenine dinucleotide phosphate (NADP) and present in red blood cells. Cf. *X f.*

vascular endothelial growth f. (VEGF), vascular permeability f. (VPF) a peptide factor, existing in four forms with different lengths (121, 165, 189, and 206 amino acids), that is mitogenic for vascular endothelial cells and promotes tissue vascularization; levels are elevated in hypoxia and it is important in tumor angiogenesis.

virulence f. a substance or environmental factor that increases the pathogenicity of a disease-causing microorganism.

von Willebrand f. (vWF) a glycoprotein synthesized in endothelial cells and megakaryocytes that circulates complexed to factor VIII (see under *coagulation f's*); it mediates adhesion of platelets to damaged epithelial surfaces and may participate in platelet aggregation. Deficiency results in the prolonged bleeding time seen in von Willebrand disease. NOTE: this factor was originally considered to be part of factor VIII, so that in older terminology the term factor VIII generally refers to the complex of the two factors.

X f. an accessory substance required for the aerobic growth of certain species of *Haemophilus* replaceable by hemin or other iron porphyrin compounds, and present in red blood cells. It is heat stable and is not destroyed by autoclaving. Cf. *V f.*

Fac·trel (fak′trəl) trademark for a preparation of gonadorelin hydrochloride.

fac·ul·ta·tive (fak′əl-ta″tiv) 1. not obligatory; capable of adaptation to different conditions. 2. in bacteriology, a bacterium that can grow either aerobically or anaerobically.

fac·ul·ty (fak′əl-te) [L. *facultas*] 1. any normal power or function, especially a mental one. 2. the corps of professors and instructors of a college or university.

fusion f. the power of blending into one the two images viewed by the two eyes.

FAD flavin adenine dinucleotide, sometimes used specifically for the oxidized form.

$FADH_2$ the reduced form of flavin adenine dinucleotide.

fad·ing (fād′ing) progressive weakness in puppies, so that suckling is impossible; it is usually accompanied by a falling body temperature, paddling movements, and death within a few days of birth. The cause may be a viral infection, a bacterial infection, or adverse environmental conditions.

fae- for words beginning thus, see those beginning *fe-*.

fag·op·y·rism (fəg-op′ĭ-riz-əm) [L. *fagopyrum* buckwheat] buckwheat allergy.

Fag·o·py·rum (fag″o-pi′rəm) a genus of herbs of the family Polygonaceae, native to temperate regions of Europe and Asia. *F. escu-len′tum* is buckwheat, a food and fodder crop that can cause fagopyrism if eaten in large quantities.

Fahr-Vol·hard disease (fahr′ fōl′hahrt) [Karl Theodor *Fahr,* German pathologist, 1877–1945; Franz *Volhard,* German physiologist, 1872–1950] malignant nephrosclerosis; see under *nephrosclerosis.*

Fah·rae·us-Lind·qvist effect (fah-re′əs lind′kvist) [Robert Sanno *Fahraeus,* Swedish pathologist, 1888–1968; Johan Törsten *Lindqvist,* Swedish physician, 20th century] see under *effect.*

Fahr·en·heit scale, thermometer (far′ən-hīt) [Gabriel Daniel *Fahrenheit,* German physicist, 1686–1736] see under *scale* and *thermometer.*

fail·ure (fāl′yər) inability to perform or to achieve a desired outcome; see also *insufficiency.*

acute congestive heart f. rapidly occurring deficiency in cardiac output marked by venocapillary congestion, hypertension, and edema, usually pulmonary edema.

acute hepatic f., acute liver f. sudden loss of hepatic cell function and metabolic functions of the liver, with coagulopathy and hepatic encephalopathy, seen most often in viral hepatitis or drug toxicity.

acute renal f. (ARF) renal failure of sudden onset, such as from physical trauma, infection, inflammation, or toxicity; symptoms include uremia and usually oliguria or anuria, with hyperkalemia and pulmonary edema. Three types are distinguished: *prerenal,* associated with poor systemic perfusion and decreased renal blood flow, such as with hypovolemic shock or congestive heart failure; *intrarenal,* associated with disease of the renal parenchyma, such as tubulointerstitial nephritis, acute interstitial nephritis, or nephrotoxicity; and *postrenal,* resulting from obstruction of urine flow out of the kidneys.

autonomic f. dysautonomia.

backward heart f. a concept of heart failure stating that imbalance of performance of the ventricles due to dysfunction of one results in a rise in pressure behind that ventricle, with backward transmission of the increased pressure and consequent rise in venous pressure and distention. Cf. *forward heart f.*

bone marrow f. failure of the hematopoietic function of the bone marrow; see also bone marrow suppression, under *suppression.*

cardiac f. heart f.

chronic renal f. (CRF) chronic kidney disease.

congestive heart f. (CHF) a clinical syndrome due to heart disease, characterized by breathlessness and abnormal sodium and water retention, often resulting in edema. The congestion may occur in the lungs or peripheral circulation or both, depending on whether the heart failure is right-sided or general.

diastolic heart f. heart failure due to a defect in ventricular filling caused by an abnormality in diastolic function.

end-stage renal f. see under *disease.*

fatigue f. slow failure of a body part, prosthesis, or appliance owing to repeated small stresses that would not cause failure individually.

forward heart f. a concept of heart failure that emphasizes the inadequacy of cardiac output relative to body needs; edema is attributed primarily to renal retention of sodium and water, and venous distention is considered a secondary feature.

heart f. inability of the heart to pump blood at an adequate rate to fill tissue metabolic requirements or the ability to do so only at an elevated filling pressure. It can be defined clinically as a syndrome of ventricular dysfunction accompanied by reduced exercise capacity and other characteristic hemodynamic, renal, neural, and hormonal responses.

high-output heart f. heart failure in which the cardiac output remains high enough to maintain a brisk circulation with warm extremities but is inadequate to meet demand; it is most often associated with hyperthyroidism, anemia, arteriovenous fistulas, beriberi, osteitis deformans, or sepsis.

idiopathic sudomotor f. a defect in cholinergic neural regulation of sweating, with anhidrosis, heat intolerance, tingling of the skin, nausea, and palpitation.

kidney f. renal f.

lactation f. in swine a variable syndrome in sows with agalactia occurring during the first two days after they have given birth; it may be accompanied by mastitis with fever, anorexia, and increased respiratory and heart rates, and occasionally by metritis with a vaginal discharge. Called also *farrowing fever* and *mastitis-metritis-agalactia.*

left-sided heart f., left ventricular f., left ventricular heart f. failure of adequate output by the left ventricle despite an increase in distending pressure and in end-diastolic volume, with dyspnea, orthopnea, and other signs and symptoms of pulmonary congestion and edema.

low-output heart f. heart failure in which cardiac output is decreased, as in most forms of heart disease, leading to clinical manifestations of impaired peripheral circulation and peripheral vasoconstriction (cold, pale extremities, cyanosis, narrowed pulse pressure).

pituitary f. severe to complete hypopituitarism; it may be congenital or acquired.

premature ovarian f. premature menopause.

primary autonomic f., pure autonomic f. Bradbury-Eggleston syndrome.

renal f. the inability of a kidney to excrete metabolites at normal plasma levels under conditions of normal loading, or the inability to retain electrolytes under conditions of normal intake, so that waste products and metabolites accumulate in the blood. It is often accompanied by oliguria. See *acute renal f.* and *chronic kidney disease.*

respiratory f. a condition resulting from respiratory insufficiency, in which there is persistent abnormally low arterial oxygen tension (Pa_{O_2}) or abnormally high carbon dioxide tension (Pa_{CO_2}). Called also *ventilatory f.*

right-sided heart f., right ventricular f., right ventricular heart f. failure of proper functioning of the right ventricle, with venous engorgement, hepatic enlargement, and subcutaneous edema; it is often combined with left-sided heart failure.

systolic heart f. heart failure due to a defect in expulsion of blood that is caused by an abnormality in systolic function.

f. to thrive physical and developmental retardation in infants and small children, seen in those with a physical illness or suffering psychosocial effects such as maternal deprivation. Characteristics include lack of physical growth and below normal achievement in fine and gross motor, social-adaptive, and language skills as assessed by psychometric testing.

ventilatory f. respiratory f.

virologic f. the failure of a given antiviral regimen.

faint (fānt) syncope.

Fa·jer·sztajn crossed sciatic sign (fah-zher-stīn′) [Jean *Fajersztajn,* French neurologist, early 20th century] see under *sign.*

fal·cate (fal′kāt) falciform.

fal·ces (fal′sēz) [L.] plural of *falx.*

fal·ci·form (fal′sĭ-form) [*falx* + *form*] shaped like a sickle.

fall·ing-out (fawl′ing out) a culture-specific syndrome occurring primarily in southern United States and Caribbean groups, characterized by an episode of sudden collapse, sometimes without forewarning, with temporary inability to speak, see, or move.

fal·lo·pi·an (fə-lo′pe-ən) named for Gabriele *Fallopio* (L. *Fallopius*), Italian anatomist, pupil of Vesalius, 1523–1562, as *fallopian aqueduct, fallopian artery, fallopian ligament,* and *fallopian tube.*

fal·lo·pos·co·py (fə-lo-pos′kə-pe) endoscopic visualization of the uterine tubes with a flexible hysteroscope, using a nonincisional transcervical approach to access the oviduct via the uterotubal ostium.

Fal·lot's pentalogy, tetralogy (tetrad), trilogy (fə-lōz′) [Étienne-Louis Arthur *Fallot,* French physician, 1850–1911] see under *pentalogy, tetralogy,* and *trilogy.*

false-neg·a·tive (fawls′ neg′ə-tiv) 1. denoting a test result that wrongly excludes an individual from a diagnostic or other category, e.g., one that labels a diseased person as healthy in screening for detection of that disease. 2. an individual so excluded. 3. an instance of a false-negative result.

false-pos·i·tive (fawls′ pos′ĭ-tiv) 1. denoting a test result that wrongly assigns an individual to a diagnostic or other category, e.g., one that labels a healthy person as diseased in screening for detection of that disease. 2. an individual so categorized. 3. an instance of a false-positive result.

biologic f.-p. (BFP) a false positive result on a serologic test. *Acute BFP* is usually associated with an infectious disease such as bacterial pneumonia, mycoplasma pneumonias, subacute bacterial endocarditis, varicella, infectious mononucleosis, or scarlet fever. *Chronic BFP* is usually associated with immune complex diseases, systemic lupus erythematosus, and leprosy.

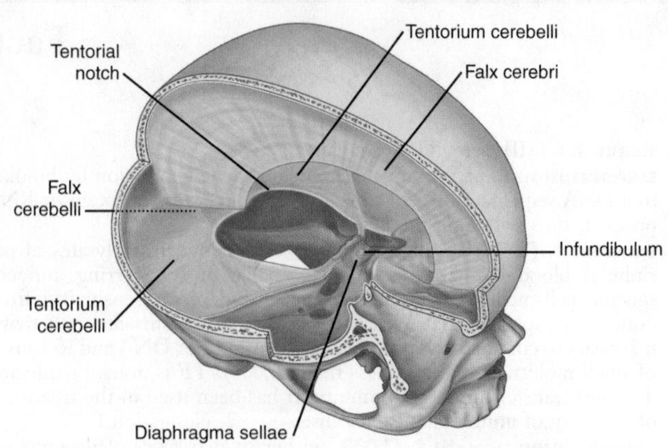

■ Falx cerebri, falx cerebelli, and other dural partitions.

fal·si·fi·ca·tion (fawl″sĭ-fĭ-ka′shən) an often deliberate misstatement or misrepresentation.

retrospective f. unconscious distortion of memories of past experiences to conform to present emotional needs.

falx (falks) pl. *fal′ces* [L. "sickle"] a general term in anatomical nomenclature for a sickle-shaped organ or structure. **fal′cial** *adj*

aponeurotic f., f. aponeuro′tica f. inguinalis.

f. cerebel′li [TA], **f. of cerebellum** cerebellar falx: the small fold of dura mater in the midline of the posterior cranial fossa, projecting forward toward the vermis of the cerebellum.

f. ce′rebri [TA], **f. of cerebrum** cerebral falx: the fold of dura mater, sickle-shaped when viewed in sagittal section, that extends downward in the longitudinal cerebral fissure and separates the two cerebral hemispheres.

inguinal f., f. inguina′lis [TA] the united tendons of the transverse and internal oblique muscles going to the linea alba and pectineal line of the pubic bone; called also *Henle ligament, tendo conjunctivus* [TA alternative] and *conjoined* or *conjoint tendon.*

ligamentous f., f. ligamento′sa processus falciformis ligamenti sacrotuberosi.

f. sep′ti valvula foraminis ovalis.

fam·ci·clo·vir (fam-si′klo-vir) a prodrug of penciclovir that is converted to the active drug by cellular kinases following administration, used in the treatment of herpes zoster and herpes genitalis and of mucocutaneous herpes simplex in immunocompromised patients; administered orally.

fa·mes (fa′mēz) [L.] hunger.

fa·mil·i·al (fə-mil′e-əl) [L. *familia* family] occurring in or affecting more members of a family than would be expected by chance. The term is often incorrectly equated with *genetic.*

fam·i·ly (fam′ĭ-le) 1. a group of individuals descended from a common ancestor. 2. a taxonomic subdivision subordinate to an order (or suborder) and superior to a tribe (or subfamily). 3. a group of related objects or individuals of any kind.

gene f., multigene f. a group of genes with a similar DNA sequence and evolved from a common ancestral gene by duplication and variation; they may cluster on a single chromosome.

secretin f. a group of peptides related to secretin, several of which are active in the alimentary tract; it includes secretin, glucagon, growth hormone–releasing hormone, glucose-dependent insulinotropic polypeptide, and vasoactive intestinal polypeptide.

systematic f. see *family* (def. 2).

tachykinin f. a family of hormones that are potent, rapidly acting secretagogues and cause smooth muscle contraction and vasodilation; it includes substance P and several less common peptides.

fam·o·ti·dine (fam-o′tĭ-dīn) [USP] a histamine H_2 receptor antagonist; it inhibits gastric acid secretion and is used in the prophylaxis and treatment of peptic ulcer, the relief of symptoms associated with hyperacidity, and the treatment of gastroesophageal reflux disease and of pathologic gastric hypersecretion, as that associated with Zollinger-Ellison syndrome; administered orally or intravenously.

Fam·vir (fam′vir) trademark for a preparation of famciclovir.

fan (fan) an area, figure, or structure in the shape of a sector of a circle containing less than a semicircle.

Fan•co•ni syndrome (anemia, pancytopenia, panmyelopathy) (fahn-ko′ne) [Guido *Fanconi*, Swiss pediatrician, 1892–1979] see under *syndrome*.

F and R force and rhythm (of pulse).

fang (fang) 1. a large canine tooth of a carnivore. 2. the envenomed tooth of a snake.

Fan•nia (fan′e-ə) a genus of flies of the family Muscidae whose larvae can cause intestinal and urinary myiasis in humans. This genus is sometimes calssified as part of the family Anthomyiidae.

F. canicula′ris the lesser housefly, a small gray species that lays its eggs on decaying vegetable matter or animal manure, from which the eggs or larvae may gain access to human hosts.

F. scala′ris the latrine flies, a species similar to but larger than *F. canicularis*, which usually deposits its eggs on feces only, not vegetable matter.

fan•ta•sy (fan′tə-se) [Gr. *phantasia* imagination; the power by which an object is made apparent to the mind] a consciously or unconsciously imagined situation or sequence of events, such as a daydream. Fantasy can serve as a realistic rehearsal of future events; it may also serve as an unconscious defense mechanism providing wish-fulfillment, gratification of repressed impulses, and resolution of unconscious conflicts.

autistic f. a defense mechanism characterized by excessive daydreaming as a solution for emotional conflict or stressors, substituting for human relationships or for more effective actions.

FAP familial adenomatous polyposis.

FAPHA Fellow of the American Public Health Association.

Far•a•beuf amputation, triangle (fahr″ə-boof′) [Louis Hubert *Farabeuf*, French surgeon, 1841–1910] see under *amputation* and *triangle*.

far•ad (F) (far′əd) [M. *Faraday*] the SI unit of electric capacitance; the capacitance of a condenser that charged with 1 coulomb gives a difference of potential of 1 volt. This unit is so large that one-millionth part of it has been adopted as a practical unit called a microfarad.

Far•a•day constant, law (far′ə-da) [Michael *Faraday*, English physicist, 1791–1867] see under *constant* and *law*.

far•a•day (*F*) (far′ə-da) [M. *Faraday*] the electric charge carried by one mole of electrons or one equivalent weight of ions, equal to 9.649×10^4 coulomb. Called also *Faraday constant*.

fa•rad•ic (fə-rad′ik) pertaining to faradism.

far•a•dim•e•ter (far″ə-dim′ə-tər) [*farad* + *-meter*] an instrument for measuring faradic electricity.

far•a•dism (far′ə-diz-əm) 1. induced current. 2. induced current in a rapidly alternating current. 3. faradization.

surging f. a faradic current of gradually increasing and decreasing amplitude; obtained by introducing a rhythmically varying series resistance into the circuit.

far•a•di•za•tion (far″ə-dĭ-za′shən) the therapeutic use of an interrupted current, derived from an induction coil; principally for the stimulation of muscles and nerves.

Far•ber disease (lipogranulomatosis, syndrome) (fahr′bər) [Sidney *Farber*, American pediatrician, 1903–1973] see under *disease*.

Far•ber-Uz•man syndrome (fahr′bər o͞oz′mən) [S. *Farber*; Lahut *Uzman*, American physician, 1923–1962] Farber disease.

far•cy (fahr′se) 1. the more chronic and constitutional lymphatic form of glanders, marked by thickening of the superficial lymph vessels. 2. any of several other animal diseases that resemble this condition.

bovine f. a benign type of nocardiosis in cattle, caused by infection with *Nocardia farcinica* and characterized by formation of nodules in subcutaneous tissues and organs. Called also *cattle f.*

button f. farcy in which there are small tubercular nodules *(farcy buds)* on the skin.

cattle f. bovine f.

Japanese f., Neapolitan f. lymphangitis epizootica.

far•cy pipes (fahr′se pīps) farcy cords; see under *cord*.

Far•es•ton (far′es-ton) trademark for a preparation of toremifine citrate.

Farr's law (fahrz) [William *Farr*, English medical statistician, 1807–1883] see under *law*.

Farre tubercles (fahr) [John Richard *Farre*, English physician, 1775–1862] see under *tubercle*.

Farre white line (fahr) [Arthur *Farre*, British obstetrician, 1811–1887] see under *line*.

far•sight•ed (fahr′sīt-əd) hyperopic.

far•sight•ed•ness (fahr′sīt-əd-nis) hyperopia.

fasc. [L.] fasci′culus (bundle).

fas•cia (fash′e-ə) gen. and pl. *fas′ciae* [L. "band"] a sheet or band of fibrous tissue such as lies deep to the skin or forms an investment for muscles and various other organs of the body. **fas′cial** *adj*

Fascia

Descriptions of anatomic structures are given on TA terms, and include anglicized names of specific fasciae.

abdominal f. f. abdominis.
abdominal f., internal f. transversalis.
abdominal f., parietal f. abdominis parietalis.
abdominal f., visceral f. abdominis visceralis.
f. abdo′minis [TA] abdominal fascia: an inclusive term for the fascia that forms part of the general layer lining the walls of the abdominal cavity and investing the abdominal organs; it is subdivided into *visceral abdominal fascia*, *parietal abdominal fascia*, and *extraperitoneal fascia*.
f. abdo′minis parieta′lis [TA] parietal abdominal fascia: the fascia lining the wall of the abdominal cavity.
f. abdo′minis viscera′lis [TA] the fascia that invests the abdominal viscera.
Abernethy f. f. iliopsoas.
f. adhe′rens an extensive adherens junction analogous to the zonula adherens but occurring in cardiac myocytes, primarily in the transverse portions of intercalated disks; it has multiple dense attachment plaques acting as sites of insertion of actin filaments into the sarcolemma and thus linking the cellular membrane and contractile apparatus with those of adjacent cells.
alar f. an ancillary layer of the deep cervical fascia, anterior to the prevertebral fascia and extending from the base of the skull to the level of the second thoracic vertebra, where it merges with the pretracheal fascia.
anal f. f. inferior diaphragmatis pelvis.
antebrachial f., f. antebra′chii [TA] the investing fascia of the forearm; called also *f. of forearm* and *deep f. of forearm*.
aponeurotic f. deep f.
f. axilla′ris [TA], **axillary f.** the investing fascia of the armpit which passes between the lateral borders of the pectoralis major and latissimus dorsi muscles.
bicipital f. aponeurosis musculi bicipitis brachii.
brachial f., f. bra′chii [TA] the investing fascia of the upper limb.
buccinator f., f. buccopharyn′gea [TA], **buccopharyngeal f.** a fibrous membrane forming the external covering of the constrictor muscles of the pharynx, and passing forward superiorly to the surface of the buccinator muscle.
Buck f. f. penis.
bulbar f. vagina bulbi.
Camper f. panniculus adiposus telae subcutaneae abdominis.
f. ca′pitis et col′li [TA] a collective term for the various layers of fascia found in the head and neck.
cervical f. f. cervicalis.
cervical f., deep deep layers of cervical fascia.
cervical f., superficial a thin layer of cervical fascia just beneath the skin, investing the platysma.
f. cervica′lis [TA] cervical fascia: the fascia of the neck, consisting of a thin superficial layer (superficial cervical fascia), three deep layers *(lamina superficialis*, *lamina pretrachealis*, and *lamina prevertebralis fasciae cervicalis)*, and the carotid sheath *(vagina carotica fasciae cervicalis)*.
clavipectoral f., f. clavipectora′lis [TA] a fascial sheet investing the subclavius muscle, attached to the clavicle above and continuing to the pectoralis minor muscle below; called also *coracoclavicular f.*
f. clito′ridis [TA], **f. of clitoris** the dense fibrous tissue that encloses the two corpora cavernosa of the clitoris.

Fascia *Continued*

Colles f. membrana perinei.
f. col′li TA alternative for *f. cervicalis.*
Cooper f. f. cremasterica.
coracoclavicular f. f. clavipectoralis.
cremasteric f., f. cremaste′rica [TA] the thin covering of the spermatic cord formed by the investing fascia of the cremaster muscle; it is adjacent to the external surface of the internal spermatic fascia. Called also *Cooper f.*
cribriform f., f. cribro′sa [TA] the part of the superficial fascia of the thigh that covers the saphenous opening; called also *Hesselbach f.*
crural f., f. cru′ris [TA] the investing fascia of the leg; it is continuous with the fascia lata.
Cruveilhier f. tela subcutanea perinei.
dartos f. tunica dartos.
deep f. a dense, firm, fibrous membrane investing the trunk and limbs, and giving off sheaths to the various muscles; formerly officially called *f. profunda* and now subdivided into fasciae of muscles (fasciae musculorum) and visceral fascia (fascia visceralis).
deep f. of arm f. brachii.
deep f. of back, deep dorsal f. f. thoracolumbalis.
deep f. of forearm f. antebrachii.
deep investing abdominal f. f. investiens profunda abdominis.
deep f. of leg f. cruris.
deep f. of thigh f. lata.
deltoid f., f. deltoi′dea [TA] the deep fascia covering the deltoid muscle of the shoulder.
Denonvilliers f. f. rectoprostatica.
diaphragmatic f., f. diaphragma′tica [TA] the fascia on the inferior surface of the diaphragm.
dorsal f. of foot f. dorsalis pedis.
dorsal f. of hand, f. dorsa′lis ma′nus [TA] the investing fascia of the back of the hand.
f. dorsa′lis pe′dis [TA] dorsal fascia of foot: the investing fascia on the dorsum of the foot.
Dupuytren f. aponeurosis palmaris.
endoabdominal f. 1. f. transversalis. 2. f. abdominis parietalis.
f. endoabdomina′lis TA alternative for *f. abdominis parietalis.*
endopelvic f. f. pelvis parietalis.
f. endopelvi′na TA alternative for *f. pelvis parietalis.*
endothoracic f., f. endothora′cica [TA] the extrapleural fascial sheet beneath the serous lining of the thoracic cavity; called also *parietal fascia of thorax* and *fascia parietalis thoracis* [TA alternative].
external intercostal f. f. thoracica.
extraperitoneal f., f. extraperitonea′lis [TA] the thin layer of areolar connective tissue separating the parietal peritoneum from the transversalis fascia in the abdomen and pelvis. It is currently considered synonymous with *tela subserosa peritonei* [TA]. Called also *extraperitoneal tissue.*
extraserosal f., f. extraserosa′lis [TA] a general term for any fascial layer of the trunk lying inside the fascia parietalis and outside the fascia visceralis.
femoral f. f. lata.
f. of forearm f. antebrachii.
fusion f. a double connective tissue band derived from the fusion of closely apposed surfaces of peritoneum as a result of degeneration of the lubricating serous layer between them; such fasciae are seen in the pelvic and abdominal cavities where crowding of organs occurs.

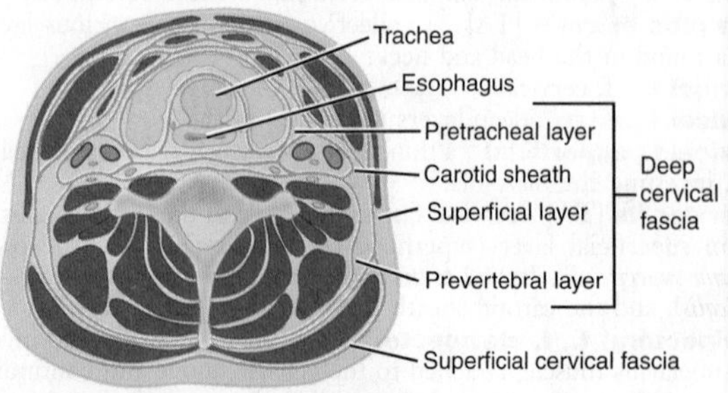

■ Fascia cervicalis (cervical fascia), showing both deep and superficial layers.

Gerota f. the anterior part of the renal fascia; sometimes used to denote the entire renal fascia.
f. of head and neck f. capitis et colli.
Hesselbach f. f. cribrosa.
iliac f. a term used variably to denote some or all of the fascia iliopsoas, either the fascia covering the ilacus musle in the abdomen (pars iliaca), that covering the iliacus muscle in the thigh (fascia iliaca), both of those collectively, or even sometimes the entire iliopsoas fascia.
f. ili′aca 1. [TA] iliac fascia: the fascia covering the iliacus muscle in the thigh, forming part of the iliopsoas fascia. 2. TA alternative for *f. iliopsoas.*
iliopectineal f. arcus iliopectineus.
f. iliopso′as [TA], **iliopsoas f.** a strong fascia covering the inner surface of the iliac and psoas muscles; it has both an iliac part *(pars iliaca)* and a psoas part *(pars psoatica)*. Called also *f. iliaca* [TA alternative].
f. of individual extraperitoneal abdominal organ f. propria organi extraperitonealis abdominis.
f. of individual extraperitoneal pelvic organ f. propria organi extraperitonealis pelvis.
f. of individual intraperitoneal abdominal organ f. propria organi intraperitonealis abdominis.
f. of individual intraperitoneal pelvic organ f. propria organi intraperitonealis pelvis.
f. of individual muscle f. propria musculi.
f. infe′rior diaphrag′matis pel′vis [TA], **inferior f. of pelvic diaphragm** the fascia that covers the lower surface of the coccygeus and levator ani muscles, forming the medial wall of the ischiorectal fossa; called also *ischiorectal f.* and *inferior layer of pelvic diaphragm.*
f. infraspina′ta [TA], **infraspinous f.** a thick, dense layer of deep fascia overlying the infraspinatus muscle on the posterior aspect of the scapula, attached to the margins of the infraspinous fossa; it is continuous with the deltoid fascia.
infundibuliform f. f. spermatica interna.
intermediate investing abdominal fasciae fasciae investientes intermediae abdominis.
f. inves′tiens [TA] investing layer: a layer of fascia that closely invests a muscle or ligament.
f. inves′tiens abdo′minis [TA] investing abdominal fascia: a collective term for the thin layers of deep fascia covering the external aspects of the muscle layers of the anterolateral abdominal wall and their aponeuroses; it is subdivided into superficial, intermediate, and deep layers.
fas′ciae investien′tes interme′diae abdo′minis [TA] intermediate investing abdominal fasciae: the deep fascia investing the middle layer of the anterolateral abdominal wall musculature, overlying the internal oblique muscle.
f. inves′tiens perine′i superficia′lis TA alternative for *f. perinei.*
f. inves′tiens profun′da abdo′minis [TA] deep investing abdominal fascia: the deep fascia investing the deepest of the three layers of musculature in the anterolateral abdominal wall; it overlies the transversus abdominis muscle.
f. inves′tiens superficia′lis abdo′minis [TA] superficial investing abdominal fascia: the deep fascia investing the most superficial of the three layers of musculature in the anterolateral abdominal wall; it overlies the external oblique muscle.
investing f. f. investiens.
investing abdominal f. f. investiens abdominis.
ischiorectal f. f. inferior diaphragmatis pelvis.
f. la′ta [TA] the investing fascia of the thigh; it is continuous with the fascia cruris.
lateroconal f. the lateral part of the renal fascia where its anterior and posterior parts join; this extends on either side posteriorly to the ascending and descending colon and is continuous with the parietal peritoneum.
f. of limbs f. membrorum.
lumbodorsal f. f. thoracolumbalis.
masseteric f., f. massete′rica [TA] a layer of fascia covering the masseter muscle.
f. membro′rum [TA] fascia of limbs: a collective term for the deep fascia of the upper and lower limbs. The term usually does not include the fascia forming an investing layer or surrounding individual muscles.
fasciae of muscles fasciae musculorum.

Fascia *Continued*

muscular fasciae of eye, fas'ciae muscula'res bul'bi [TA] the sheets of fascia investing the extraocular muscles, continuous with the vagina bulbi.
fas'ciae musculo'rum [TA] fasciae of muscles: a collective term for the fascia associated with specific muscles, including both the investing layer (fascia investiens) and the fascia associated with individual muscles (fascia propria musculi).
f. mus'culi pirifor'mis [TA] piriformis fascia: an extension of the parietal pelvic fascia that surrounds the piriformis muscle.
f. mus'culi quadra'ti lumbo'rum TA alternative for *lamina anterior fasciae thoracolumbalis.*
f. of nape f. nuchae.
f. of neck f. cervicalis.
f. nu'chae [TA], **nuchal f.** the fascia on the muscles in the dorsal region of the neck.
obturator f., f. obturato'ria [TA] the part of the parietal pelvic fascia that covers the obturator internus muscle.
orbital fasciae fibrous tissue surrounding the posterior part of the eyeball, supporting and binding together the structures within the orbit, including the periorbita, septum orbitale, vagina bulbi, spatium episclerale, corpus adiposum orbitae, and fasciae musculares bulbi.
palmar f. aponeurosis palmaris.
palpebral f. septum orbitale.
parietal f. f. parietalis.
parietal f. of pelvis f. pelvis parietalis.
parietal f. of thorax f. endothoracica.
f. parieta'lis [TA] parietal fascia: a general term for any fascia that lies outside the parietal layer of a serosa and lines the wall of a body cavity.
f. parieta'lis thora'cis TA alternative for *f. endothoracica.*
parotid f., f. parotide'a [TA] an extension of the deep cervical fascia that splits to enclose the parotid gland and sends extensions into the gland that become continuous with its stroma.
parotideomasseteric f. the fascia parotidea and fascia masseterica (qq.v.) considered as a unit.
pectineal f. the pubic portion of the fascia lata; called also *Cowper ligament.*
pectoral f., f. pectora'lis [TA] the sheet of fascia investing the pectoralis major muscle.
pelvic f. f. pelvis.
pelvic f., parietal f. pelvis parietalis.
pelvic f., visceral f. pelvis visceralis.
f. pel'vica TA alternative for *f. pelvis.*
f. pel'vis [TA] pelvic fascia: an inclusive term for the fascia that forms part of the general layer lining the walls of the pelvis and invests the pelvic organs; called also *f. pelvica* [TA alternative].
f. pel'vis parieta'lis [TA] parietal pelvic fascia: the fascia on the wall of the pelvis that covers the muscles passing from the interior of the pelvis to the thigh. Called also *f. endopelvina* [TA alternative] and *endopelvic f.*
f. pel'vis viscera'lis [TA] visceral pelvic fascia: the fascia that covers the organs and vessels of the pelvis.
penile f., penile f., deep f. penis.
penile f., superficial tela subcutanea penis.
f. pe'nis [TA], **f. of penis** the firm inner fascial layer that surrounds the corpora cavernosa and the corpus spongiosum of the penis collectively. Called also *deep penile fascia.*
perineal f., perineal f., deep f. perinei.
perineal f., superficial tela subcutanea perinei.
f. perine'i [TA] perineal fascia: fascia that invests the ischiocavernosus, bulbospongiosus, and superficial transverse perineal muscles; it is attached to the ischiopubic rami, perineal membrane, and perineal body, and anteriorly it is continuous with the suspensory ligament of the penis or clitoris. Called also *f. investiens perinei superficialis* [TA alternative], *superficial investing f. of perineum,* and *deep perineal f.*
perinephric f., perirenal f. f. renalis.
pharyngobasilar f., f. pharyngobasila'ris [TA] a strong fibrous membrane in the wall of the pharynx, lined internally with mucous membrane and incompletely covered on its outer surface by the overlapping constrictor muscles of the pharynx. It blends with the periosteum at the base of the skull. Called also *pharyngeal aponeurosis.*
phrenicopleural f., f. phrenicopleura'lis [TA] the fascial layer on the upper surface of the diaphragm, beneath the pleura.
piriformis f. f. musculi piriformis.
plantar f. aponeurosis plantaris.
f. precaecoco'lica [TA], **prececocolic f.** an extension sometimes found in the parietal abdominal fascia, crossing anterior to the cecum adjacent to the ascending colon.
presacral f., f. presacra'lis [TA] a layer of parietal pelvic fascia between the sacrum and the rectum; the superior and inferior hypogastric plexuses are imbedded in it.
pretracheal f. lamina pretrachealis fasciae cervicalis.
prevertebral f. lamina prevertebralis fasciae cervicalis.
f. profun'da see *deep f.*
f. pro'pria mus'culi [TA] fascia of individual muscle: the thin sheet of fascia that surrounds a single muscle, separating it from others. Called also *muscle sheath.*
f. pro'pria or'gani extraperitonea'lis abdo'minis [TA] fascia of individual extraperitoneal abdominal organ: the layer of fascia that surrounds each abdominal organ not covered by visceral peritoneum.
f. pro'pria or'gani extraperitonea'lis pel'vis [TA] fascia of individual extraperitoneal pelvic organ: the layer of fascia that surrounds each pelvic organ not covered by visceral peritoneum.
f. pro'pria or'gani intraperitonea'lis abdo'minis [TA] fascia of individual intraperitoneal abdominal organ: the layer of visceral fascia that surrounds individual organs within the abdomen.
f. pro'pria or'gani intraperitonea'lis pel'vis [TA] fascia of individual intraperitoneal pelvic organ: the layer of visceral fascia that surrounds individual organs within the pelvis.
quadratus lumborum f. lamina anterior fasciae thoracolumbalis.
rectoprostatic f., f. rectoprosta'tica [TA] a membranous partition separating the rectum from the prostate and urinary bladder; this structure in the male corresponds to the fascia rectovaginalis in the female. Called also *Denonvilliers* or *Tyrrell f.* and *septum rectovesicale* [TA alternative].
rectosacral f., f. rectosacra'lis [TA] the fusion of the inferior part of the presacral fascia with the visceral fascia on the posterior aspect of the rectum.
rectovaginal f., f. rectovagina'lis [TA] the membranous partition between the rectum and the vagina; this structure in the female corresponds to the fascia rectoprostatica in the male. Called also *septum rectovaginale* [TA alternative].
rectovesical f. f. rectoprostatica.
renal f., f. rena'lis [TA] a thin membranous sheath that encloses the kidney, perirenal fat, and adrenal gland, formed by condensation of fibroareolar tissue. Some authorities distinguish between *anterior renal fascia* and *posterior renal fascia,* which join laterally to form the *lateroconal fascia.* Called also *Gerota capsule* and *Gerota, perinephric,* or *perirenal f.*
Scarpa f. stratum membranosum telae subcutaneae abdominis.
semilunar f. aponeurosis musculi bicipitis brachii.
Sibson f. membrana suprapleuralis.
spermatic f., external f. spermatica externa.
spermatic f., internal f. spermatica interna.
f. sperma'tica exter'na [TA] external spermatic fascia: the thin outer covering of the spermatic cord, which is continuous with the investing fascia of the external oblique muscle.
f. sperma'tica inter'na [TA] internal spermatic fascia: the thin innermost covering of the spermatic cord, derived from the transversalis fascia of the abdominal wall.
subperitoneal f. f. extraperitonealis.
superficial f. tela subcutanea.
superficial investing abdominal f. f. investiens superficialis abdominis.
superficial investing f. of perineum f. perinei.
superficial f. of perineum tela subcutanea perinei.
superficial f. of scrotum tunica dartos.
f. superficia'lis former official nomenclature for the layer of connective tissue now considered to be tela subcutanea (q.v.).
f. supe'rior diaphrag'matis pel'vis [TA], **superior f. of pelvic diaphragm** the fascia on the upper surface of the levator ani and coccygeus muscles. Called also *superior layer of pelvic diaphragm.*
f. supraspina'ta [TA], **supraspinous f.** the deep fascia overlying the supraspinatus muscle, thick medially but thinner laterally, and attached to the posterior of the scapula around the boundaries of the attachment of the muscle.

Fascia *Continued*

temporal f., f. tempora′lis [TA] a strong fibrous sheet covering the temporalis muscle, consisting of deep and superficial layers *(lamina profunda* and *lamina superficialis)*, which attach inferiorly to the zygomatic arch. Called also *temporal aponeurosis.*
f. of Tenon vagina bulbi.
thoracic f., f. thora′cica [TA] the deep fascia that covers the outside of the thoracic cavity; called also *external intercostal f.*
f. thoracolumba′lis [TA], **thoracolumbar f.** the fascia of the back that attaches medially to the spinous processes of the vertebral column for its entire length and blends laterally with the aponeurosis of the transversus abdominis muscle; inferiorly it attaches to the iliac crest and the sacrum. Called also *lumbodorsal f.*
f. transversa′lis [TA], **transversalis f.** part of the inner investing layer of the abdominal wall, continuous with the fascia of the other side behind the rectus abdominis muscle and its sheath, as well as with the diaphragmatic fascia, iliopsoas fascia, and parietal pelvic fascia.
f. trun′ci [TA], **f. of trunk** the layers of fascia of the trunk, comprising the fascia parietalis, fascia extraserosalis, and fascia visceralis.
Tyrrell f. f. rectoprostatica.
umbilical f., f. umbilica′lis [TA] a thickening of the fascia transversalis extending along the median umbilical ligament downward from the umbilicus.
visceral f., f. viscera′lis [TA] a general term including the fascia lying immediately outside the visceral layer of the serosae together with the fascia immediately surrounding the viscera.
volar f. aponeurosis palmaris.
Waldeyer f. rectosacral f.
Zuckerkandl f. the posterior part of the renal fascia.

fas•ciae (fash′e-e) [L.] genitive and plural of *fascia.*

fas•cia•plas•ty (fash′e-ə-plas″te) [*fascia* + *-plasty*] a plastic operation on fascia; spelled also *fascioplasty.*

fas•ci•cle (fas′ĭ-kəl) fasciculus.

fas•cic•u•lar (fə-sik′u-lər) 1. pertaining to a fasciculus. 2. fasciculated.

fas•cic•u•lat•ed (fə-sik′u-lāt-əd) clustered together or occurring in bundles.

fas•cic•u•la•tion (fə-sik″u-la′shən) 1. the formation of fasciculi. 2. a small local contraction of muscles, visible through the skin, representing a spontaneous discharge of a number of fibers innervated by a single motor nerve filament.

contraction f′s brief, rhythmic twitching of a muscle during weak voluntary or postural contractions; seen in some elderly patients and those with neurogenic muscle atrophy.

fas•cic•u•li (fə-sik′u-li) [L.] genitive and plural of *fasciculus.*

fas•cic•u•lo•ven•tric•u•lar (fə-sic″u-lo-ven-trik′u-lər) [*fasciculus* + *ventricular*] connecting the bundle of His to the ventricle.

fas•cic•u•lus (fə-sik′u-ləs) gen. and pl. *fasci′culi* [L. dim. of *fascis* bundle] 1. a fascicle; a small bundle or cluster. 2. [TA] a small bundle of nerve, muscle, or tendon fibers. 3. a tract, bundle, or group of nerve fibers that are more or less associated functionally; see also under *bundle, lemniscus, tract,* and *tractus.*

Fasciculus

Descriptions of anatomic structures are given on TA terms, and include anglicized names of specific fasciculi.

alvear f. a bundle of fibers originating in the medial part of the entorhinal area and extending to the alveus of the hippocampus, where it has synapses with fibers that go to the dentate gyrus; called also *alvear path.*
anterior f. proprius of spinal cord f. proprius anterior medullae spinalis.
arcuate f. f. longitudinalis superior cerebri.
f. arcua′tus TA alternative for *f. longitudinalis superior cerebri.*
f. atrioventricula′ris [TA] bundle of His.
Burdach f. f. cuneatus medullae spinalis.
cuneate f. of medulla oblongata f. cuneatus medullae oblongatae.
cuneate f. of spinal cord f. cuneatus medullae spinalis.
f. cunea′tus medul′lae oblonga′tae [TA] cuneate fasciculus of medulla oblongata: the continuation into the medulla oblongata of the fasciculus cuneatus of the spinal cord.
f. cunea′tus medul′lae spina′lis [TA] cuneate fasciculus of spinal cord: the lateral portion of the posterior funiculus of the spinal cord, composed of ascending fibers that terminate in the nucleus cuneatus of the medulla oblongata; called also *Burdach f.*
dorsal f. proprius of spinal cord f. proprius posterior medullae spinalis.
dorsolateral f., f. dorsolatera′lis tractus posterolateralis.
f. exi′lis a cluster of muscle fibers connecting the flexor pollicis longus with the medial condyle of the humerus, or with the coronoid process of the ulna.
fibrous f. of biceps muscle aponeurosis musculi bicipitis brachii.
Foville f. stria terminalis.
fronto-occipital f. f. subcallosus.
Goll f. f. gracilis medullae spinalis.
Gowers f. tractus spinocerebellaris anterior.
gracile f. of medulla oblongata f. gracilis medullae oblongatae.
gracile f. of spinal cord f. gracilis medullae spinalis.
f. gra′cilis medul′lae oblonga′tae [TA] the continuation into the medulla oblongata of the fasciculus gracilis of the spinal cord; called also *posteromedian column of medulla oblongata.*
f. gra′cilis medul′lae spina′lis [TA] the median portion of the posterior funiculus of the spinal cord, composed of ascending fibers that terminate in the nucleus gracilis of the medulla oblongata; called also *Goll column.*

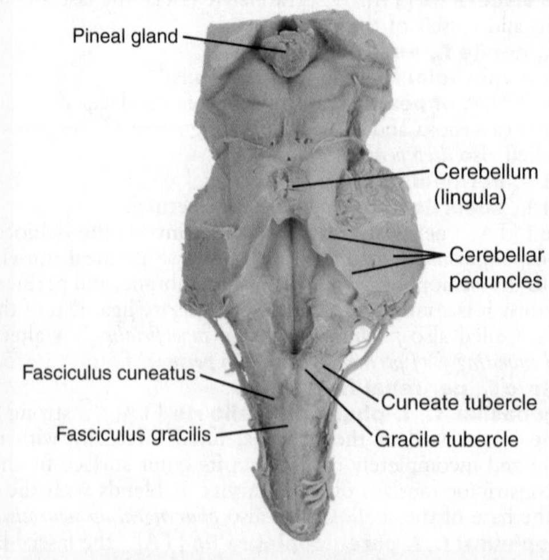

■ Fasciculus cuneatus and fasciculus gracilis on the dorsal surface of the brainstem.

Fasciculus *Continued*

f. interfascicula′ris [TA] interfascicular fasciculus: a collection of fibers situated between the fasciculus gracilis and the fasciculus cuneatus, containing some of the descending branches of the fibers of the medial division of the posterior roots of the spinal nerves; called also *comma tract of Schultze, f. semilunaris* [TA alternative], *Schultze tract*, and *semilunar f.* or *tract*.
intersegmental f. of spinal cord, anterior f. proprius anterior medullae spinalis.
intersegmental f. of spinal cord, dorsal f. proprius posterior medullae spinalis.
intersegmental f. of spinal cord, lateral f. proprius lateralis medullae spinalis.
intersegmental f. of spinal cord, posterior f. proprius posterior medullae spinalis.
intersegmental f. of spinal cord, ventral f. proprius anterior medullae spinalis.
lateral f. of brachial plexus, f. latera′lis plex′us brachia′lis [TA] lateral cord of brachial plexus: the lateral bundle of fibers of the brachial plexus, formed by the union of the anterior divisions of the superior and middle trunks, C5 through C7, and from which arise the lateral pectoral and musculocutaneous nerves and the lateral root of the median nerve.
lateral f. proprius of spinal cord f. proprius lateralis medullae spinalis.
f. lenticula′ris [TA] lenticular fasciculus: a bundle of pallidofugal nerve fibers arising from the dorsal surface of the globus pallidus; they pass through the internal capsule, traverse field H_2 of Forel, join and mingle with the fibers of the ansa lenticularis, and continue to the nuclei of the ventral thalamus as part of the thalamic fasciculus.
longitudinal f., dorsal f. longitudinalis posterior.
longitudinal f., medial f. longitudinalis medialis.
longitudinal f., posterior f. longitudinalis posterior.
longitudinal f. of cerebrum, inferior f. longitudinalis inferior cerebri.
longitudinal f. of cerebrum, superior f. longitudinalis superior cerebri.
longitudinal fasciculi of cruciform ligament fasciculi longitudinales ligamenti cruciformis atlantis.
longitudinal f. of medulla oblongata, medial f. longitudinalis medialis medullae oblongatae.
f. longitudina′lis dorsa′lis TA alternative for *f. longitudinalis posterior.*
f. longitudina′lis infe′rior ce′rebri [TA] inferior longitudinal fasciculus of cerebrum: a bundle of assumed association fibers interconnecting the cortex of the occipital and temporal lobes, extending through the occipital and temporal lobes of the cerebrum, and consisting chiefly of geniculocalcarine projection fibers.
fasci′culi longitudina′les ligamen′ti crucifor′mis atlan′tis [TA] longitudinal fasciculi of cruciform ligament: vertical midline longitudinal fibers that, together with the transverse ligament of the atlas, form the cruciform ligament of the atlas. The fibers arise in two groups from the root of the dens; one group extends cranially to the anterior margin of the foramen magnum and the other proceeds caudally to the body of the axis.
f. longitudina′lis media′lis [TA] medial longitudinal fasciculus: a fiber tract extending between the mesencephalon and the upper part of the spinal cord; it lies close to the median plane, just ventral to the central gray matter, and interconnects the vestibular nuclei with motor nuclei, chiefly those of the third, fourth, sixth, and eleventh cranial nerves.
f. longitudina′lis media′lis medul′lae oblonga′tae the portion of the fasciculus longitudinalis medialis within the medulla oblongata.
f. longitudina′lis media′lis pon′tis the portion of the fasciculus longitudinalis medialis within the pons.
f. longitudina′lis poste′rior [TA] posterior longitudinal fasciculus: a lightly myelinated fiber bundle that runs in the periventricular gray substance throughout the extent of the mesencephalon, near the medial longitudinal fasciculus; called also *Schütz bundle* or *tract, f. longitudinalis dorsalis* [TA alternative], and *dorsal longitudinal f.*
f. longitudina′lis supe′rior ce′rebri [TA] superior longitudinal fasciculus of cerebrum: a bundle of association fibers in the cerebrum, extending from the frontal lobe to the posterior end of the lateral sulcus, and interrelating the cortex of the frontal, temporal, parietal, and occipital lobes; called also *f. arcuatus* [TA alternative] and *arcuate f.*
maculary f. a system of nerve fibers originating in the macula lutea; some are uncrossed (on the temporal side) and others are crossed fibers (on the nasal side of the retina).
f. mammillotegmenta′lis [TA] mammillotegmental fasciculus: a bundle of fibers from the mammillary body to the tegmental nuclei of the reticular formation of the mesencephalon; called also *mammillotegmental tract.*
f. mammillothala′micus [TA] mammillothalamic fasciculus: a stout bundle of fibers from the mammillary body to the anterior nucleus of the thalamus; called also *mammillothalamic tract, thalamomammillary f.*, and *Vicq d'Azyr f.*
medial f. of brachial plexus f. medialis plexus brachialis.
medial prosencephalic f., medial telencephalic f. f. medialis telencephali.
f. media′lis plex′us brachia′lis [TA] medial cord of brachial plexus: the medial bundle of fibers of the brachial plexus, formed by the anterior division of the inferior trunk, C8 through T1, and from which arise the medial pectoral, medial brachial cutaneous, medial antebrachial cutaneous, and ulnar nerves, and the medial root of the median nerve.
f. media′lis telencepha′li [TA] medial forebrain bundle: a fiber system that is the main pathway for longitudinal connection in the hypothalamus; it runs through the lateral hypothalamic region, connecting the tegmentum of the mesencephalon and elements of the limbic system. Called also *f. prosencephalicus medialis, medial prosencephalic f.*, and *medial telencephalic f.*
Meynert f. tractus habenulointerpeduncularis.
f. of middle cerebellar peduncle, deep the most dorsal part of the transverse fibers of the pons, connecting pontine nuclei with the folia on the anterior superior surface of the cerebellum.
f. of middle cerebellar peduncle, inferior the most caudal portion of the transverse fibers of the pons, connecting pontine nuclei with the cerebellar folia near the vermis.
f. of middle cerebellar peduncle, superior the most rostral portion of the transverse fibers of the pons, connecting pontine nuclei with inferior lobules and posterior and lateral margins of the cerebellum.
Monakow f. tractus rubrospinalis.
occipitofrontal f., inferior f. occipitofrontalis inferior.
occipitofrontal f., superior f. occipitofrontalis superior.
f. occipitofronta′lis infe′rior [TA] inferior occipitofrontal fasciculus: a collection of association fibers in the inferior part of the extreme capsule near the uncinate fasciculus, connecting various inferior gyri of the temporal and frontal lobes.
f. occipitofronta′lis supe′rior [TA] superior occipitofrontal fasciculus: a collection of association fibers lying just internal to the intersection of the internal capsule and corpus callosum, interconnecting the cortex of the occipital and temporal lobes with that of the insula and frontal lobe, and probably comprising a significant part of the tapetum. Called also *f. subcallosus* [TA alternative] and *subcallosal f.*
olivocochlear f. tractus olivocochlearis.
f. parietooccipitoponti′nus a bundle of nerve fibers arising in the parietal and occipital lobes and passing through the retrolenticular part and caudal portions of the thalamolenticular part of the posterior limb of the internal capsule to end in the pontine nuclei.
perforating f. perforant pathway.
posterior f. of brachial plexus, f. poste′rior plex′us brachia′lis [TA] posterior cord of brachial plexus: the posterior bundle of fibers of the brachial plexus, formed by the union of the posterior divisions of the superior, middle, and inferior trunks, C5 through C8 and sometimes T1, and from which arise the subscapular, thoracodorsal, radial, and axillary nerves.
posterior f. proprius of spinal cord f. proprius posterior medullae spinalis.
f. pro′prius ante′rior medul′lae spina′lis [TA] anterior fasciculus proprius of spinal cord: any of the bundles of white substance in the anterior funiculus of the spinal cord at the gray–white matter interface, consisting of intersegmental fibers, some of which pass from the contralateral side, and probably also reticulospinal and descending autonomic fibers. Called also *anterior* or *ventral intersegmental f. of spinal cord, ventral f. proprius of spinal cord*, and *anterior* or *ventral intersegmental tract of spinal cord.*
f. pro′prius latera′lis medul′lae spin′alis [TA] lateral fasciculus proprius of spinal cord: any of the bundles of white substance in the

Fasciculus *Continued*

lateral funiculus of the spinal cord at the gray–white matter interface, consisting of intersegmental fibers, some of which have passed from the contralateral side, and probably reticulospinal and autonomic fibers; called also *lateral intersegmental f. of spinal cord* and *lateral intersegmental tract of spinal cord.*
f. pro′prius poste′rior medul′lae spina′lis [TA] posterior fasciculus proprius of spinal cord: any of the bundles of white substance in the deepest part of the posterior funiculus of the spinal cord at the gray–white matter interface, consisting chiefly of intersegmental fibers derived from the cells of the posterior gray column, which divide into ascending and descending association fibers that reenter the gray substance and ramify in it. Called also *dorsal* or *posterior intersegmental f. of spinal cord, dorsal f. proprius of spinal cord,* and *dorsal* or *posterior intersegmental tract of spinal cord.*
f. prosencepha′licus media′lis f. medialis telencephali.
pyramidal f. of medulla oblongata, f. pyramida′lis medul′lae oblonga′tae tractus pyramidalis (def. 1).
f. retroflex′us TA alternative for *tractus habenulo-interpeduncularis.*
Schütz f. f. longitudinalis posterior.
semilunar f. f. interfascicularis.
f. semiluna′ris TA alternative for *f. interfascicularis.*
septomarginal f., f. septomargina′lis [TA] a bundle of nerve fibers situated along the dorsal periphery of the dorsal funiculus of the spinal cord in the thoracic region and bordering the dorsal median septum in the lumbar region; called also *septomarginal tract.*
solitary f. tractus solitarius medullae oblongatae.
subcallosal f. f. occipitofrontalis superior.
f. subcallo′sus TA alternative for *f. occipitofrontalis superior.*
f. subthala′micus [TA] subthalamic fasciculus: a bundle of fibers that passes through the internal capsule and interconnects the subthalamic nucleus with the globus pallidus and putamen.
f. sulcomargina′lis [TA] sulcomarginal fasciculus: a layer of descending branches from the midbrain tectum situated in the ventral funiculus of the spinal cord, along the border of the ventral median fissure.
thalamic f., f. thala′micus [TA] a conjoined bundle of fibers beginning in field H of Forel, where the ansa lenticularis and lenticular fasciculus join and pass dorsal to the zona incerta to reach some of the ventral nuclei of the thalamus; it contains continuations of the ansa lenticularis and the fasciculus lenticularis and dentatothalamic, rubrothalamic, and thalamostriate fibers. See also *fields of Forel,* under *field.*
thalamomammillary f. f. mammillothalamicus.
fasci′culi transver′si aponeuro′sis palma′ris transverse fasciculi of palmar aponeurosis: the transverse fascial bands that support the webs between the fingers.
fasci′culi transver′si aponeuro′sis planta′ris [TA] transverse fasciculi of plantar aponeurosis: transverse bundles in the plantar aponeurosis near the toes.
Türck f. tractus corticospinalis anterior.
unciform f., uncinate f., f. uncina′tus [TA] a collection of association fibers interconnecting the cortex of the orbital surface of the frontal lobe with the parahippocampal gyrus and perhaps with the amygdala; other temporofrontal connections probably also exist.
ventral f. proprius of spinal cord f. proprius anterior medullae spinalis.
Vicq d'Azyr f. f. mammillothalamicus.

fas•ci•ec•to•my (fas″e-ek′tə-me) [*fasci-* + *-ectomy*] excision of fascia.

fas•ci•itis (fas″e-i′tis) pl. *fascii′tides.* inflammation of fascia.
eosinophilic f. inflammation of fasciae of the limbs, associated with eosinophilia, edema, and swelling; the etiology is unknown but frequently it occurs following strenuous exercise. Called also *Shulman syndrome.*
intravascular f. a variant form of nodular fasciitis occurring in small to medium sized arteries and veins, usually in infants or young children.
necrotizing f. a fulminating subcutaneous soft tissue infection beginning with extensive cellulitis that rapidly spreads to involve the superficial and often the deep fascia, producing thrombosis of subcutaneous vessels and gangrene of the underlying tissues. A cutaneous lesion often serves as a portal of entry for the infection. Although the infection is most closely linked to group A streptococci, it can be caused by other bacteria, either alone or in combination, and is categorized based on the infectious agents isolated. Polymicrobial infections with aerobic and anaerobic organisms are *type 1,* infection by group A streptococci is *type 2,* and gas gangrene is sometimes considered to be *type 3.* Called also *gangrenous* or *necrotizing cellulitis* and *gangrenous* or *necrotizing erysipelas.*
nodular f. a benign reactive proliferation of fibroblasts occurring as a rapidly growing nodular mass in the subcutaneous or deep somatic tissues, particularly of the upper limbs, usually in young adults or adults; histologically it closely resembles sarcoma. The term is sometimes used broadly to encompass variant forms such as proliferative fasciitis. Called also *pseudosarcomatous f.*
palmar f. fasciitis with nodules or whorls in the subcutaneous tissue of the hands, sometimes progressing to cause contractures; it is most often seen as part of a paraneoplastic condition (see *palmar fasciitis and polyarthritis syndrome,* under *syndrome*).
perirenal f. retroperitoneal fibrosis.
plantar f. inflammation of plantar fascia, owing to repetitive stretching or tearing of muscle fibers near their attachment to the calcaneal tuberosity; it is one of the most common causes of heel pain.
proliferative f. a benign reactive proliferation of fibroblasts in subcutaneous tissues, resembling nodular fasciitis (q.v.) but characterized also by basophilic giant cells resembling ganglion cells or rhabdomyoblasts; it usually occurs in the skeletal muscles in older adults.
pseudosarcomatous f. nodular f.

fas•cin (fas′in) any of a family of actin-binding proteins that participate in the formation of a variety of protrusions, such as filopodia and dendrites, and in the formation of cytoplasmic actin bundles. Fascins are expressed by the nervous system and by tissue derived from the mesenchyme; in epithelium, they are normally absent or expressed at low levels but are overexpressed in several types of carcinoma.

fasci(o)- [L. *fascia* band] a combining form denoting a relationship to a band or to fascia.

fas•ci•od•e•sis (fas″e-od′ə-sis) [*fascio-* + *-desis*] the operation of suturing a fascia to skeletal attachment.

Fas•ci•o•la (fə-si′o-lə) [L., dim. of *fascia*] a genus of flukes of the family Fasciolidae.
F. gigan′tica a large liver fluke that infects cattle, sheep, wild animals, and occasionally humans in Africa, Asia, and certain Pacific islands.
F. hepa′tica the common liver fluke that infests many herbivores and is occasionally found in the human liver, causing dangerous symptoms by obstructing the biliary passages or invading the liver parenchyma. Several snails of the genus *Lymnaea* act as invertebrate hosts.
F. hetero′phyes *Heterophyes heterophyes.*
F. mag′na *Fascioloides magna.*

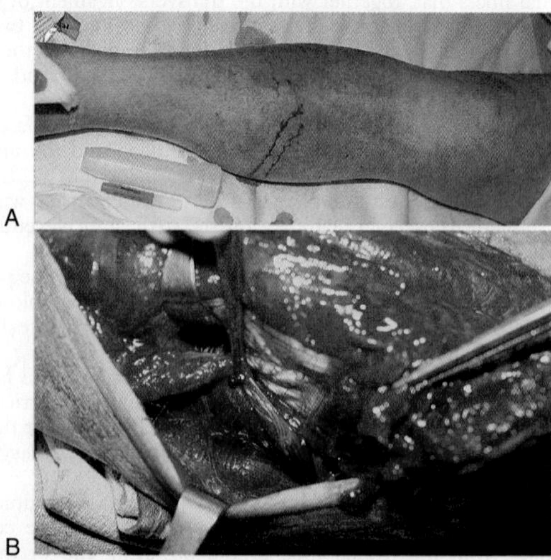

■ Necrotizing fasciitis caused by group A streptococci in a 60-year-old man with diabetes mellitus type 2. *(A),* The calf is swollen but the skin looks relatively normal except for two small purple bullae. *(B),* Surgical view shows extensive necrotizing fasciitis with myonecrosis beneath the fascia.

fas•ci•o•la (fə-si′o-lə) pl. *fasci′olae* [L., dim. of *fascia*] a small band or striplike structure. fasci′olar *adj*

f. cine′rea, f. cine′rea cin′guli gyrus fasciolaris.

fas•ci•o•lae (fə-si′o-le) [L.] genitive and plural of *fasciola.*

fas•cio•li•a•sis (fas″e-o-li′ə-sis) infection with either of the liver flukes *Fasciola hepatica* or *F. gigantica.*

fas•ci•o•li•cide (fas″e-o′lĭ-sīd) a substance lethal to flukes of the genus *Fasciola.*

Fas•ci•o•li•dae (fas″e-o′lĭ-de) a family of trematodes parasitic to mammals and birds; genera include *Fasciola, Fascioloides,* and *Fasciolopsis.*

Fas•ci•o•loi•des (fas″e-o-loi′dēz) a genus of flukes of the family Fasciolidae. *F. mag′na* is a large fluke found in the liver and lungs of herbivorous animals in North America.

fas•ci•o•lop•si•a•sis (fas″e-o-lop-si′ə-sis) infection with an intestinal fluke of the genus *Fasciolopsis.*

Fas•ci•o•lop•sis (fas″e-o-lop′sis) [*fasciola* + Gr. *opsis* appearance] a genus of trematodes of the family Fasciolidae.

F. bus′ki a trematode found in the small intestine of humans and pigs in many parts of Asia. It is the largest of the intestinal flukes, and may cause nausea, diarrhea, and a malabsorption syndrome if present in large numbers. The intermediate hosts are the snails *Planorbis coenosus* and various species of *Segmentina.*

fas•cio•plas•ty (fash′e-o-plas″te) fasciaplasty.

fas•ci•or•rha•phy (fash″e-or′ə-fe) [*fascio-* + *-rrhaphy*] suture of lacerated fascia.

fas•ci•ot•o•my (fash″e-ot′ə-me) [*fascio-* + *-tomy*] surgical incision or transection of fascia, often performed to release pressure in compartment syndrome.

fas•ci•tis (fə-si′tis) fasciitis.

Fas•lo•dex (fas′lo-deks) trademark for a preparation of fulvestrant.

fast (fast) [A.S. *faest* firm; *faestan* to abstain from food] 1. immovable, or unchangeable; resistant to the action of a specific agent, such as a stain or destaining agent (e.g., acid-fast). 2. abstention from food, or from food and liquid. 3. to abstain from food, or from food and liquid.

fas•tid•i•ous (fas-tid′e-əs) in bacteriology, a microorganism having complex nutritional or cultural requirements for growth.

fas•ti•ga•tum (fas″tĭ-ga′təm) [L.] pointed; sharpened to a point.

fas•tig•i•al (fas-tij′e-əl) of or pertaining to the fastigium or to the cerebellar fastigial nucleus.

fas•tig•i•um (fas-tij′e-əm) [L. "gable end"] 1. [TA] the highest point in the roof of the fourth ventricle of the brain, at the junction between the superior medullary velum and the nodulus. 2. the acme, or highest point, as of a fever.

fast•ing (fast′ing) abstinence from all food and drink except water for a prescribed period, performed for both spiritual and therapeutic purposes; among its uses is as a means of detoxification, def. 3 (q.v.).

fast•ness (fast′nis) the quality, in bacteria, of being resistant to the action of specific stains or inhibitors.

fat (fat) 1. a white or yellowish tissue which forms soft pads between various organs of the body, serves to smooth and round out bodily contours, and furnishes a reserve supply of energy. See also *adipose tissue,* under *tissue.* 2. an ester of glycerol with fatty acids, usually oleic acid, palmitic acid, or stearic acid; triglyceride; neutral fat.

bound f. masked f.

brown f. brown adipose tissue.

chyle f. fat in the form of an extremely fine emulsion taken into the chyle by the lymphatics of the intestine.

fetal f. a term sometimes used in pathology to refer to brown adipose tissue.

hydrous wool f. lanolin (def. 2).

masked f. fat that can be detected in a cell or tissue by chemical methods but is not revealed by staining methods; called also *bound f.*

milk f. the suspension in milk that can separate out as cream.

molecular f. fat occurring in fine specks within the cells.

neutral f. see *fat* (def. 2).

paranephric f., pararenal f. corpus adiposum pararenale.

perinephric f., perirenal f. capsula adiposa renis.

polyunsaturated f. a fat containing polyunsaturated fatty acids.

refined wool f. lanolin (def. 1).

retrobulbar f. corpus adiposum orbitae.

saturated f. a fat containing saturated fatty acids.

subcutaneous f. panniculus adiposus.

***trans* f's** see under *fatty acid.*

unsaturated f. a fat containing unsaturated fatty acids.

wool f. lanolin.

fa•tal (fa′təl) causing death; called also *mortal* and *lethal.*

fate (fāt) [L. *fatum* what is ordained by the gods] 1. the ultimate disposition or decreed outcome; see also *fate map,* under *map.* 2. in pharmacology, the intermediate and ultimate disposition of a drug in the body.

prospective f. the development normally achieved by any region of the zygote or early embryo when there is no interference.

fat•i•ga•bil•i•ty (fat″ĭ-gə-bil′ĭ-te) easy susceptibility to fatigue.

fa•tigue (fə-tēg′) [Fr.; L. *fatigatio*] 1. a state of increased discomfort and decreased efficiency resulting from prolonged or excessive exertion; loss of power or capacity to respond to stimulation. 2. the gradual fracturing of a material due to repetitive or cyclic stress.

battle f., combat f. former term for combat-related posttraumatic stress disorder; now used colloquially.

pseudocombat f. a term applied to psychiatric combat casualties whose functional impairment is attributed to preexisting personality disorder rather than to reaction to combat stress.

stimulation f. an increase in the threshold of a neural element due to repeated stimulation.

vocal f. phonasthenia.

fat•ty (fat′e) pertaining to or characterized by fat. Called also *adipose.*

fat•ty ac•id (fat′e) any straight chain monocarboxylic acid, especially those naturally occurring in fats. Fatty acids are classified as saturated or unsaturated; the latter are further classified as polyunsaturated or monounsaturated. The absolute and relative amounts of the various fatty acids consumed have been linked to plasma lipid levels, atherosclerosis, and coronary artery disease. See accompanying table and illustration.

essential f. a. (EFA) any fatty acid that cannot be synthesized by the human body and must be obtained from dietary sources, e.g., linoleic acid and linolenic acid.

free f. a's (FFA) nonesterified f. a's.

long-chain f. a's fatty acids with a chain length of 14–18 carbon atoms.

medium-chain f. a's (MCFA) fatty acids with a chain length of roughly 8 to 12 carbon atoms; they are absorbed directly into the portal blood, bypassing the lymphatic system.

monounsaturated f. a's unsaturated fatty acids containing a single double bond; they occur predominantly as oleic acid, in peanut, olive, and canola oils. Monounsaturated fatty acids have been shown to reduce low-density lipoprotein levels and thus the blood cholesterol level.

n-3 f. a's ω-3 f. a's.

nonesterified f. a's (NEFA) the fraction of plasma fatty acids that are not in the form of glycerol esters. Called also *free fatty a's* (a misnomer because they are transported complexed with albumin).

ω-3 f. a's, omega-3 f. a's unsaturated fatty acids in which the double bond closest to the methyl (omega) terminus of the molecule occurs at the third carbon from that end; they are present in marine animal fats and some vegetable oils. These fatty acids can modulate leukotriene composition, alter prostaglandin synthesis, inhibit platelet aggregation, and increase the ratio of high-density to low-density lipoproteins while lowering overall plasma lipid levels (particularly of triglycerides). There is evidence that they may inhibit some cancers. See accompanying table and illustration.

ω-6 f. a's, omega-6 f. a's unsaturated fatty acids in which the double bond closest to the methyl (omega) terminus of the molecule occurs at the sixth carbon from that end; they are present predominantly in vegetable and seed oils. Diets in which the ratio of omega-6 to omega-3 fatty acids is high have been linked to promotion of some cancers. See accompanying table and illustration.

ω-9 f. a's polyunsaturated fatty acids from animal and vegetable fats.

polyunsaturated f. a's (PUFA) unsaturated fatty acids (q.v.) containing two or more double bonds; they occur predominantly as linoleic, linolenic, and arachidonic acids, in vegetable and seed oils. Dietary polyunsaturated fatty acids can lower plasma lipid levels and thus lower serum cholesterol; however, they have been shown to lower both low-density and high-density lipoprotein levels, and excessive consumption of these fatty acids has also been linked to cancer.

saturated f. a's fatty acids without double bonds in their chains; they occur predominantly in animal fats and tropical oils and can be produced by hydrogenation of unsaturated fatty acids. Fats composed of saturated fatty acids increase serum low-density lipoproteins and blood cholesterol levels. See accompanying table and illustration.

short-chain f. a's (SCFA) fatty acids with a chain length of up to roughly 6 carbon atoms; they are produced by bacterial anaerobic fermentation, particularly of dietary carbohydrates, in the large intestine. They are readily absorbed and are metabolized in the liver and muscle tissues, producing energy.

***trans*–f. a's** stereoisomers of the naturally occurring *cis*–fatty acids, created by the partial hydrogenation of unsaturated fatty acids during the manufacture of margarine and shortening. Like saturated fatty acids, they raise the levels low-density lipoproteins and cholesterol. Called also *trans* fats.

Some Naturally Occurring Fatty Acids

Symbol*	Common Name	Systematic Name	Structural Formula
Saturated			
$C_{4:0}$	Butyric acid	Butanoic acid	$CH_3(CH_2)_2COOH$
$C_{6:0}$	Caproic acid	Hexanoic acid	$CH_3(CH_2)_4COOH$
$C_{8:0}$	Caprylic acid	Octanoic acid	$CH_3(CH_2)_6COOH$
$C_{10:0}$	Capric acid	Decanoic acid	$CH_3(CH_2)_8COOH$
$C_{12:0}$	Lauric acid	Dodecanoic acid	$CH_3(CH_2)_{10}COOH$
$C_{14:0}$	Myristic acid	Tetradecanoic acid	$CH_3(CH_2)_{12}COOH$
$C_{16:0}$	Palmitic acid	Hexadecanoic acid	$CH_3(CH_2)_{14}COOH$
$C_{18:0}$	Stearic acid	Octadecanoic acid	$CH_3(CH_2)_{16}COOH$
$C_{20:0}$	Arachidic acid	Eicosanoic acid	$CH_3(CH_2)_{18}COOH$
$C_{22:0}$	Behenic acid	Docosanoic acid	$CH_3(CH_2)_{20}COOH$
$C_{24:0}$	Lignoceric acid	Tetracosanoic acid	$CH_3(CH_2)_{22}COOH$
Unsaturated			
$C_{16:1\ \omega-7}$	Palmitoleic acid	*cis*-9-Hexadecenoic acid	$CH_3(CH_2)_5CH{=}CH(CH_2)_7COOH$
$C_{18:1\ \omega-9}$	Oleic acid	*cis*-9-Octadecenoic acid	$CH_3(CH_2)_7CH{=}CH(CH_2)_7COOH$
$C_{18:1\ \omega-7}$	Vaccenic acid	11-Octadecenoic acid	$CH_3(CH_2)_5CH{=}CH(CH_2)_9COOH$
$C_{18:2\ \omega-6}$	Linoleic acid	*cis,cis*-9,12-Octadecadienoic acid	$CH_3(CH_2)_4(CH{=}CHCH_2)_2(CH_2)_6COOH$
$C_{18:3\ \omega-3}$	Linolenic acid	all *cis*-9,12,15-Octadecatrienoic acid	$CH_3CH_2(CH{=}CHCH_2)_3(CH_2)_6COOH$
$C_{20:4\ \omega-6}$	Arachidonic acid	all *cis*-5,8,11,14-Eicosatetraenoic acid	$CH_3(CH_2)_4(CH{=}CHCH_2)_4(CH_2)_2COOH$
$C_{20:5\ \omega-3}$	—	all *cis*-5,8,11,14,17-Eicosapentaenoic acid	$CH_3(CH_2CH{=}CH)_5(CH_2)_3COOH$
$C_{22:1\ \omega-9}$	Erucic acid	*cis*-13-Docosenoic acid	$CH_3(CH_2)_7CH{=}CH(CH_2)_{11}COOH$
$C_{22:6\ \omega-3}$	—	all *cis*-4,7,10,13,16,19-Docosahexaenoic acid	$CH_3(CH_2CH{=}CH)_6(CH_2)_2COOH$
$C_{24:1\ \omega-9}$	Nervonic acid	*cis*-15-Tetracosenoic acid	$CH_3(CH_2)_7CH{=}CH(CH_2)_{13}COOH$

*Symbol subscripts denote *carbon chain length:number of double bonds*; in unsaturated fatty acids *position of the initial double relative to the ω-carbon* is also indicated.

unsaturated f. a's fatty acids containing one (monounsaturated) or multiple (polyunsaturated) double bonds; they predominate in most plant-derived fats. The number and position of each double bond can be specified, as in the systematic names, or the position of the double bond closest to the methyl (omega) terminus can be specified to denote functional subdivisions of the overall group, e.g., omega-3 fatty acids (see illustration). The numbers and positions of the double bonds have been linked to effects on plasma lipid, triglyceride, and cholesterol levels; see also *polyunsaturated f. a's*, *monounsaturated f. a's*, and accompanying table.

very-long-chain f. a's fatty acids with a chain length of over 18 carbon atoms; they are oxidized in the peroxisomes and accumulate in the tissues in disorders affecting peroxisome function.

fat·ty-ac·id syn·thase (fat′e as′id sin′thās) [EC 2.3.1.85] an enzyme complex that catalyzes the synthesis of long-chain fatty acids. Two-carbon units are successively added to the growing chain in a process similar to fatty acid oxidation in reverse, with each unit added via a series of condensation and decarboxylation, reduction, and dehydration reactions. The overall reaction is: acetyl CoA + n malonyl CoA + 2n NADPH = long-chain fatty acid anion + n CO_2 + 2n $NADP^+$ + (n + 1) CoA. Palmitate is the preferred product of the mammalian liver enzyme complex, which includes catalytic sites for the seven sequential reactions.

fat·ty ac·id thio·ki·nase (fat′e as′id thi″o-ki′nās) acyl CoA synthetase (def. 1).

fat-wrap·ping (fat rap′ing) excessive fat deposits around the exterior of the intestine as the result of mesenteric fat hypertrophy in Crohn disease. Spelled also *fat wrapping.*

fau·ces (faw′sēz) [L., pl. of *faux* "a gorge, narrow pass"] [TA] the passage from the mouth to the pharynx, including both the lumen and its boundaries; called also *throat.* fau′cial *adj*

Fau·chard disease (fo-shahr′) [Pierre *Fauchard*, French dentist, 1678–1761] marginal periodontitis.

fau·ci·tis (faw-si′tis) inflammation of the fauces; called also *sore throat.*

Saturated: (Palmitic acid, $C_{16:0}$)

```
16.......3  2  1
CH3(CH2)12CH2CH2COOH
ω          β  α
```

Unsaturated: (Palmitoleic acid, $C_{16:1\ \omega-7}$)

```
16......10   9.......2  1
CH3(CH2)5CH= CH(CH2)6CH2COOH
ω.....................α
ω-1.......ω-7 ω-8....ω-16
```

Palmitoleic acid is designated an ω-7 fatty acid, specifically *cis*-9-hexadecenoic acid.

■ Fatty acid numbering and nomenclature.

fau·na (faw′nə) [L. *Faunus* mythical deity of herdsmen] the animal life present in or characteristic of a given region or locality. It may be discernible with the unaided eye (macrofauna), or only with the aid of a microscope (microfauna).

fa·va (fa′və) *Vicia faba* L. (Leguminosae).

fa·ve·o·lar (fa-ve′o-lər) having small pits; cf. *foveolar.*

fa·ve·o·late (fa-ve′o-lāt) alveolate.

fa·vism (fa′vis-əm) [Italian *fava* bean] an acute hemolytic anemia caused by ingestion of fava beans or inhalation of the pollen of the plant *Vicia faba (fava)*, occurring in susceptible individuals usually as a result of a hereditary deficiency of glucose-6-phosphate dehydrogenase in erythrocytes; see *glucose-6-phosphate dehydrogenase deficiency.*

Fav·re-Du·rand-Nic·o·las disease (fahv′rə du-rah′ ne-ko-lah′) [Maurice Jules *Favre*, French physician, 1876–1954; J. *Durand*, French physician, 20th century; Joseph *Nicolas*, French physician, 1868–1960] lymphogranuloma venereum.

Fav·re-Ra·cou·chot syndrome (fahv′rə rah-koo-sho′) [M.J. *Favre;* Jean *Racouchot*, French physician, 1908–1994] see under *syndrome.*

fa·vus (fa′vəs) [L. "honeycomb"] a type of ringworm seen in many different animals, caused by species of *Trichophyton.* In humans the fungus is usually *T. schoenleinii* and is in the scalp *(tinea capitis)*, although it may also affect glabrous skin *(tinea corporis).* Yellow cup-shaped crusts form, called *scutula*, and may enlarge and coalesce to form honeycomblike masses; this may be associated with hair loss, cutaneous atrophy, and scarring. Called also *honeycomb ringworm* and *tinea favosa.*

f. of fowl a chronic dermatomycosis affecting the combs of fowls, usually males, caused by *Trichophyton gallinae;* called also *comb disease* and *honeycomb ringworm.*

f. herpetifor′mis, mouse f., f. mu′rium a skin disease in mice caused by infection with a strain of the fungus *Trichophyton mentagrophytes;* it can be transmitted to humans, causing ringworm.

Fay method (fa) [T. *Fay*, American physical therapist, 20th century] see under *method.*

Fa·zio-Londe atrophy, disease (fahz′e-o lōnd′) [E. *Fazio*, Italian physician, 1849–1902; P.F.L. *Londe*, French neurologist, 1864–1944] progressive bulbar palsy of childhood.

FBG fasting blood glucose.

5-FC flucytosine.

Fc [*f*ragment, *c*rystallizable] originally, the fragment, not containing antigen combining sites, obtained by papain cleavage of the IgG molecule; now generally used as an adjective, e.g., Fc region, segment, to refer to the part of any immunoglobulin monomer comprising the hinge region and C_H2, C_H3, and C_H4 domains of both heavy chains. The Fc region contains the allotypic markers and mediates all biologic activities including complement activation, binding to cell-surface receptors (Fc receptors, IgE receptors), and transplacental transport of IgG. Cf. *Fab.*

Fc´ a fragment produced in minute quantities by papain digestion of IgG molecules, a noncovalently bonded dimer containing most of the C_H3 domains of both heavy chains.

fCi femtocurie.

Fd the heavy chain portion of an Fab fragment.

FDA[1] [L.] fronto-dextra anterior (right frontoanterior, a position of the fetus; see *position*).

FDA[2] Food and Drug Administration.

FDH familial dysalbuminemic hyperthyroxinemia.

FDI [Fr.] Fédération Dentaire Internationale (International Dental Association).

FDP[1] [L.] fronto-dextra posterior (right frontoposterior, a position of the fetus; see *position*).

FDP[2] fibrin (or fibrinogen) degradation products.

FDT [L.] fronto-dextra transversa (right frontotransverse, a position of the fetus; see *position*).

F-duc·tion (ef-duk′shən) in bacterial genetics, the process whereby part of the bacterial chromosome is attached to the autonomous F factor (fertility factor) and thus is transferred with high frequency from the donor (male) bacterium to the recipient (female) bacterium. Called also *sexduction*.

F-dUMP 5-fluorodeoxyuridine monophosphate; see under *floxuridine*.

FE_{Na} fractional excretion of sodium.

FE_{Na} excreted fraction of filtered sodium; see under *test*.

Fe iron (L. *fer′rum*).

fear (fēr) the unpleasant emotional state consisting of psychological and psychophysiological responses to a real external threat or danger, including agitation, alertness, tension, and physiological mobilization of the alarm reaction. Cf. *anxiety*.
 ictal f. an aura, ranging from mild anxiety to intense fear, preceding temporal lobe seizures in some patients.

feb·an·tel (feb′ən-təl) a benzimidazole prodrug that is a precursor of fenbendazole; used as an anthelmintic in sheep, cattle, and horses.

Feb. dur. [L.] feb′re duran′te (while the fever lasts).

febr(i)- [L. *febris* fever] a combining form denoting relationship to fever.

fe·bric·i·ty (fə-bris′ĭ-te) feverishness.

fe·bric·u·la (fə-brik′u-lə) [L.] a slight or temporary attack of fever of indefinite origin or pathology.

feb·ri·fa·cient (feb″rĭ-fa′shənt) 1. pyrogenic. 2. pyrogen.

fe·brif·u·gal (fəb-rif′ə-gəl) [*febri-* + *-fugal*[1]] antipyretic (def. 1).

feb·ri·fuge (feb′rĭ-fūj) antipyretic (def. 2).

feb·rif·u·gine (fə-brif′u-jin) an antimalarial alkaloid from the plant *Dichroa febrifuga* (ch′ang shan).

feb·rile (feb′ril) [L. *febrilis*] pertaining to or characterized by fever. Called also *feverish* and *pyretic*.

fe·bris (fe′bris) [L.] fever.
 f. meliten′sis brucellosis.

fe·ca·lith (fe′kə-lith) [*fecal* + *-lith*] an intestinal concretion of fecal matter. Called also *coprolith* and *stercolith*.

fe·cal·oid (fe′kəl-oid) resembling feces.

fe·ca·lo·ma (fe′kə-lo′mə) [*feces* + *-oma*] an accumulation of feces forming a tumorlike mass in the rectum; called also *coproma*, *scatoma*, and *stercoroma*.

fe·cal·u·ria (fe″kəl-u′re-ə) [*feces* + *-uria*] the presence of fecal matter in the urine, such as with a fistula.

fe·ces (fe′sēz) [L. *faeces*, pl. of *faex* refuse] material discharged from the intestines, consisting of bacteria, cells exfoliated from the intestines, secretions, chiefly of the liver, and a small amount of food residue. Called also *excrement* and *stool*. fe′cal *adj*

fec·u·lent (fek′u-lənt) [L. *faeculentus*] 1. having dregs or a sediment. 2. fecal.

fe·cun·da·bil·i·ty (fə-kun″də-bil′ĭ-te) the probability that conception will occur in a given population of couples during a specific time period such as the length of one menstrual cycle.

fe·cun·date (fe′kən-dāt) fertilize.

fe·cun·da·tion (fe″kən-da′shən) [L. *fecundatio*] fertilization.
 artificial f. artificial insemination.

fe·cun·di·ty (fə-kun′dĭ-te) 1. in demography, the physiological ability to reproduce, as opposed to fertility. 2. ability to produce offspring rapidly and in large numbers.

feed·back (fēd′bak) the return of some of the output of a system as input so as to exert some control in the process; see also *endproduct inhibition*, under *inhibition*.
 alpha f. see under *biofeedback*.
 negative f. the condition of maintaining a constant output of a system by exertion of an inhibitory control on a key step in the system by a product of that system.
 positive f. a condition causing the output of a system to increase continually by exertion of a stimulatory effect on a key step in the system by a product of that system.
 tubuloglomerular f. a feedback mechanism in the juxtaglomerular apparatus of the kidney, so that changes in solute concentration at the macula densa link to control of the glomerular filtration rate and help ensure a relatively constant delivery of solutes to the distal tubule.

feed·for·ward (fēd-for′wərd) the anticipatory effect that one intermediate in a metabolic or endocrine control system exerts on another intermediate further along in the pathway; such effect may be stimulatory (positive f.) or inhibitory (negative f.).

feed·ing (fēd′ing) the taking or giving of food.
 artificial f. feeding of a baby with food other than mother's milk.
 breast f. breastfeeding.
 extrabuccal f. the administration of nutriment other than by mouth.
 Finkelstein f. feeding of infants based upon decrease in the milk sugar of the food.
 forced f., forcible f. the administration of food by force to those who cannot or will not receive it.
 sham f. 1. an experimental procedure that has been performed on dogs, in which food is chewed and swallowed but does not enter the stomach, because of diversion to the exterior by an esophageal fistula or other device. 2. sham feeding test; see under *test*.

Feer disease (fār) [Emil *Feer*, Swiss pediatrician, 1864–1955] acrodynia.

fee-split·ting (fe′split″ing) the division of moneys received by a specialist, such as a surgeon, between the specialist and the physician who referred the patient.

feet (fēt) plural of *foot*.

FEF forced expiratory flow.

Feh·ling solution (fa′ling) [Hermann Christian von *Fehling*, German chemist, 1812–1885] see under *solution*.

Fei·ba VH (fi′bə) trademark for a preparation of antiinhibitor coagulant complex.

fel·ba·mate (fel′bə-māt″) an anticonvulsant used in the treatment of partial seizures in adults with severe epilepsy and as an adjunct in the treatment of seizures associated with Lennox-Gastaut syndrome in children; administered orally.

Fel·ba·tol (fel′bə-tol) trademark for preparations of felbamate.

Fel·dene (fel′dēn) trademark for preparations of piroxicam.

Fel·den·krais meth·od (fel′den-krīs) [Moshe *Feldenkrais*, Israeli physicist, 1904–1984] see under *method*.

Fel·der·struk·tur (fel″dər-shtrook′tər) [Ger.] the term used to describe the pattern of organization of the myofilaments in cardiac and red skeletal muscles, in which the myofilaments are not associated in discrete myofibrils, but instead form a continuous field interrupted by mitochondria. Cf. *Fibrillenstruktur*.

Fel·i·co·la (fel-ĭ-ko′lə) a genus of parasitic biting lice of the order Mallophaga; *F. subros′trata* infests cats.

fe·line (fe′līn) [L. *feles* cat] pertaining to, characteristic of, or derived from a cat.

fel·la·tio (fə-la′she-o) [L. *fellare* to suck] oral stimulation or manipulation of the penis.

fe·lo·di·pine (fə-lo′dĭ-pēn) [USP] a calcium channel blocking agent used as a vasodilator in the treatment of hypertension; administered orally.

fel·on (fel′ən) whitlow.

Fel·ton phenomenon (fel′tən) [Lloyd D. *Felton*, American physician, 1885–1953] see under *phenomenon*.

felt·work (felt′wərk) a complex of closely interwoven fibers, as of nerve fibrils.
 Kaes f. Kaes-Bekhterev layer.

Fel·ty syndrome (fel′te) [Augustus Roi *Felty*, American physician, 1895–1963] see under *syndrome*.

fe·male (fe′māl) [L. *femella* young woman] 1. an individual organism of the sex that bears young or produces ova or eggs. 2. feminine.

Fem·a·ra (fem′ə-rə) trademark for a preparation of letrozole.

fem·hrt (fem′hahrt) trademark for a combination preparation of ethinyl estradiol and norethindrone acetate.

fem•i•nine (fem′ĭ-nin) 1. pertaining to the female sex. 2. having qualities normally associated with females.

fem•i•nin•i•ty (fem″ĭ-nin′ĭ-te) possession of normal feminine qualities by a girl or woman.

fem•i•ni•za•tion (fem″ĭ-nĭ-za′shən) 1. the normal development of primary and secondary sex characters in females. 2. the induction or development of female secondary sex characters in the male. Called also *effemination.*
 testicular f. complete androgen insensitivity syndrome.
 testicular f., incomplete partial androgen insensitivity syndrome.

fem•i•niz•ing (fem′ĭ-nīz″ing) causing feminization.

fem•i•no•nu•cle•us (fem″ĭ-no-noo′kle-əs) female pronucleus.

Fem. intern. [L.] femo′ribus inter′nus (at the inner side of the thighs).

fem•o•ra (fem′ə-rə) [L.] plural of *femur.*

fem•o•ral (fem′ə-rəl) [L. *femoralis*] pertaining to the femur, or to the thigh.

femor(o)- a combining form denoting relationship to the femur.

fem•o•ro•cele (fem′o-ro-sēl″) [*femoro-* + *-cele*[1]] femoral hernia.

fem•o•ro•fem•o•ral (fem″ə-ro-fem′ə-rəl) pertaining to both the right and left femoral arteries.

fem•o•ro•fem•o•ro•pop•lit•e•al (fem″ə-ro-fem″ə-ro-pop-lit′e-əl) pertaining to the left femoral, right femoral, and popliteal arteries.

fem•o•ro•il•i•ac (fem″o-ro-il′e-ak) pertaining to the femur and the ilium.

fem•o•ro•pop•lit•e•al (fem″ə-ro-pop-lit′e-əl) pertaining to the femoral and popliteal arteries.

fem•o•ro•tib•i•al (fem″o-ro-tib′e-əl) pertaining to the femur and tibia.

Fem•Patch (fem′pach) trademark for a preparation of estradiol.

Fem•ring (fem′ring) trademark for a preparation of estradiol acetate.

Fem•stat (fem′stat) trademark for a preparation of butoconazole nitrate.

femto- [Danish *femten* fifteen] a combining form used in naming units of measurement to indicate one quadrillionth (10^{-15}) of the unit designated by the root with which it is combined. Symbol f.

fem•to•cu•rie (fCi) (fem″to-ku′re) a unit of radioactivity, being one quadrillionth (10^{-15}) of a curie.

Fem•trace (fem′trās) trademark for a preparation of estradiol acetate.

fe•mur (fe′mər) pl. *fem′ora, femurs* [L.] 1. [TA] the bone that extends from the pelvis to the knee, being the longest and largest bone in the body; its head articulates with the acetabulum of the hip bone, and distally, the femur, along with the patella and tibia, forms the knee joint. Called also *os femoris* [TA alternative], and *thigh bone.* See also Plate 40. 2. official terminology for *thigh.*

fen•a•mate (fen′ə-māt) any of a class of analgesic and antiinflammatory agents derived from *N*-phenylanthranilic acid.

fen•ben•da•zole (fən-ben′də-zōl) [USP] a benzimidazole used as an anthelmintic.

fen•bu•fen (fən-bu′fən) a nonsteroidal antiinflammatory drug derived from propionic acid, used for the relief of pain in musculoskeletal and joint disorders; administered orally.

Head
Neck
Greater trochanter
Intertrochanteric crest
Lesser trochanter
Shaft
Popiteal surface
Adductor tubercle
Lateral epicondyle
Medial epicondyle
Lateral condyle
Medial condyle
Intercondylar fossa

■ Posterior view of right femur.

Fen•e•sin (fen′ə-sin) trademark for a preparation of guaifenesin.

fe•nes•tra (fə-nes′trə) gen. and pl. *fenes′trae* [L. "window"] 1. window (def. 1). 2. an opening in a bandage or cast. 3. an opening in the blade of a forceps.
 f. coch′leae [TA] fenestra or window of cochlea: a round opening in the inner wall of the middle ear inferior to and a little posterior to the fenestra vestibuli; it is covered by the secondary tympanic membrane. Called also *f. rotunda, cochlear window,* and *round window.*

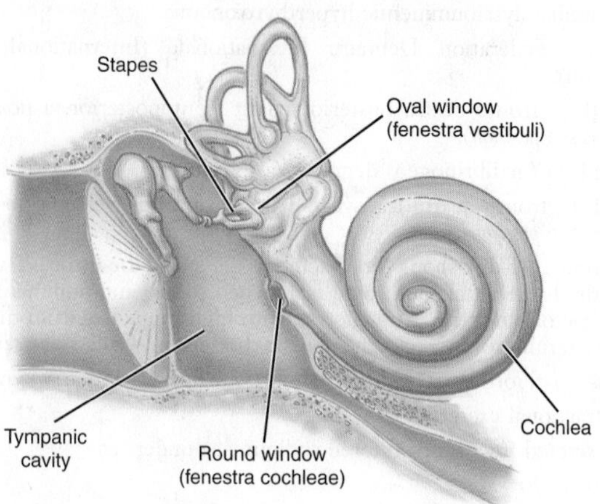

 f. nov-ova′lis a surgically created oval window in the lateral semicircular canal in the Lempert fenestration operation.
 f. ova′lis f. vestibuli.
 f. rotun′da f. cochleae.
 f. vesti′buli [TA] fenestra or window of vestibule: an oval opening in the internal ear, which is closed by the base of the stapes; called also *f. ovalis, oval window,* and *vestibular window.*

fe•nes•trae (fə-nes′tre) [L.] genitive and plural of *fenestra.*

fen•es•trate (fen′əs-trāt) to pierce with one or more openings.

fen•es•trat•ed (fen′əs-trāt″əd) [L. *fenestratus*] pierced with one or more openings.

fen•es•tra•tion (fen″əs-tra′shən) 1. the act of being perforated. 2. the presence of perforations or windows; see *fenestra.* 3. the surgical creation of a new opening in the labyrinth of the ear for the restoration of hearing in cases of otosclerosis; see *Lempert fenestration operation,* under *operation.*
 alveolar plate f. apical f.
 aorticopulmonary f. aortic septal defect.
 apical f. a condition seen in children, consisting of round or oval openings perforating the cortical plate of bone that overlies part of a pulpless primary tooth; it may involve all the primary teeth but usually affects only the upper primary incisors. Called also *alveolar plate f.*

feng shui (fung′ shwa′) [Mandarin Chinese "wind (and) water"] the Chinese art of positioning objects based on the premise that patterns of arrangement affect the balance of yin and yang and the flow of qi within an area. Such patterns are believed to have positive or negative effects, including effects on health.

fen•nel (fen′əl) 1. *Foeniculum vulgare.* 2. the edible seeds of *F. vulgare,* used as a flavoring agent and source of fennel oil.

fen•o•fi•bric ac•id (fen″o-fi′brik) the active form of fenofibrate, used in combination with statins to reduce elevated serum lipids; administered orally.

fen•o•fi•brate (fen″o-fi′brāt) [USP] a fibric acid derivative used to reduce elevated serum lipids, administered orally.

Feno•glide (fen′o-glīd) trademark for a preparation of fenofibrate.

fe•nol•do•pam mes•y•late (fe-nol′do-pam) a vasodilator with agonist effects on specific dopamine receptors; used for short-term, inpatient management of severe hypertension, administered intravenously.

fen•o•pro•fen cal•ci•um (fen″o-pro′fən) [USP] a nonsteroidal antiinflammatory drug derived from propionic acid; used in the treatment of rheumatoid arthritis, osteoarthritis, and other rheumatic and nonrheumatic inflammatory disorders, pain, dysmenorrhea, and vascular headaches; administered orally.

fen•o•ter•ol hy•dro•bro•mide (fen″o-ter′ol) a β-adrenergic agonist, selective for $β_2$-adrenergic receptors, used as a bronchodilator for the treatment of asthma-associated bronchospasm and the treatment and prophylaxis of reversible bronchospasm in obstructive airway disease; administered by inhalation.

fen•ta•nyl cit•rate (fen′tə-nəl) [USP] an opioid analgesic that interacts predominantly with opioid μ-receptors and is used mainly preoperatively, postoperatively, and during surgery; administered intravenously or intramuscularly. It may be used in combination with a neuroleptic agent such as droperidol to produce neuroleptanalgesia. It is also used to relieve chronic severe pain and administered transmucosally via the buccal cavity or transdermally.

Fen•to•ra (fen-to′rə) trademark for a preparation of fentanyl citrate.

fen•u•greek (fen′u-grēk) [L. *faenum graecum* Greek hay] 1. *Trigonella foenum-graecum.* 2. the seeds of *T. foenum-graecum,* used as a flavoring agent and used for loss of appetite and skin inflammations; it also has a variety of uses in traditional Chinese medicine and in Indian medicine. In veterinary medicine it is used to flavor powdered feed additives.

FEP free erythrocyte protoporphyrin.

fe•ral (fe′rəl) [L. *feralis*] savage; wild; living in the wild state, especially after having been domesticated.

fer-de-lance (fār-də-lahs′) [Fr. "lance head"] 1. *Bothrops lanceolatus,* a large venomous pit viper found in the West Indies. See table at *snake.* 2. name sometimes erroneously given to *Bothrops atrox,* the barba amarilla.

-ferent [L. *ferens* present part. of *ferre* to bear or carry] a word termination meaning bearing.

Fer•gu•son Smith epithelioma (fur′gə-sən″ smith) [John *Ferguson Smith,* British physician, 1888–1978] self-healing squamous epithelioma; see under *epithelioma.*

Fer•gus•son operation (incision) (fur′gə-sən) [Sir William *Fergusson,* British surgeon, 1808–1877] see under *operation.*

fer•ment (fər-ment′) [L. *fermentum* leaven] to undergo fermentation; the term is applied to decomposition of carbohydrates.

fer•men•ta•tion (fur″mən-ta′shən) the anaerobic enzymatic conversion of organic compounds, especially carbohydrates, to simpler compounds, especially to ethyl alcohol, resulting in energy in the form of adenosine triphosphate (ATP). It differs from *respiration* in that organic substances rather than molecular oxygen are used as electron acceptors. In the body this takes place in the large intestine, and the process is used commercially in the production of alcohol, bread, vinegar, and other food or industrial products. Fermentation occurs widely in bacteria and yeasts, the process usually being identified by the product formed; e.g., acetic, alcoholic, butyric, and lactic fermentation are those that result in the formation of acetic acid, alcohol, butyric acid, and lactic acid, respectively.

colonic f. fermentation of carbohydrates by the flora of the large intestine.

heterolactic f. fermentation that produces lactic acid and one or more additional products, such as ethanol, acetic acid, or carbon dioxide.

homolactic f. fermentation that produces only lactic acid as a product.

mixed acid f. fermentation carried out by most Enterobacteriaceae, in which acetic, lactic, succinic, and formic acids are formed in proportions varying by species and growth conditions.

stormy f. the rapid fermentation of milk produced by *Clostridium perfringens,* marked by rupture of the clotted milk by the pressure of the gas which develops.

fer•mi•um (Fm) (fur′me-əm) [Enrico *Fermi,* Italian physicist, 1901–1954; winner of the Nobel prize for physics in 1938] the chemical element number 100, atomic weight 253, originally discovered in debris from a thermonuclear explosion in 1952.

fern (fərn) any of a large number of flowerless, seedless plants that reproduce by spores; some are toxic.

bracken f. *Pteridium aquilinum;* see *bracken.*

jimmy f. *Cheilanthes sinnata.*

maidenhair f. any of several ferns of the genus *Adiantum,* including *A. pedatum,* which is used as an expectorant and demulcent.

male f., male shield f. *Dryopteris filix-mas.*

rock f. *Cheilanthes seiberi.*

Fer•nan•dez reaction (fār-nahn′dās) [J.M.M. *Fernandez,* Argentine physician, 20th century] see under *reaction.*

fern•ing (furn′ing) the appearance of a fernlike pattern in a dried specimen, due to the presence of sodium chloride and other electrolytes. In a specimen of cervical mucus this indicates the presence of estrogen that is not being counteracted by progesterone. In a specimen of vaginal fluid not contaminated by cervical mucus, it indicates the presence of amniotic fluid.

-ferous [L. *ferre* to bear] a word termination meaning bearing or producing.

fer•pen•te•tate (fər-pen′tə-tāt) a chelate of iron and ascorbate with pentetic acid; complexed with technetium 99m it is used in renal scanning.

fer•rat•ed (fer′āt-əd) charged with iron.

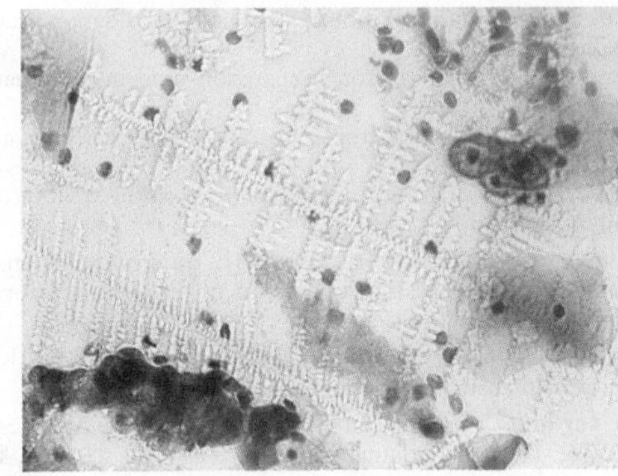

■ Ferning of postovulation cervical mucus.

fer•re•dox•in (fer″ə-dok′sin) a nonheme iron-containing protein, also having a high sulfide content and a very low redox potential; the ferredoxins participate in electron transport in photosynthesis, nitrogen fixation, and various other biological processes.

Fer•rein canal, ligament, etc. (fer-ă′) [Antoine *Ferrein,* French physician, 1693–1769] see under *ligament* and *tubule* and see *rivus lacrimalis* and *radii medullares* (under *radius*).

ferri- see *ferr(o)-.*

fer•ri•al•bu•min•ic (fer″e-al-bu-min′ik) [*ferri-* + *albumin* + *-ic*] containing iron and albumin.

fer•ric (fer′ik) [L. *ferrum*] containing iron in its plus-three oxidation state, Fe(III) (sometimes designated Fe^{3+}).

f. **chloride** orange-yellow or brownish yellow crystalline pieces, $FeCl_3 \cdot 6H_2O$; used as a reagent and as a diagnostic aid in phenylketonuria; it was formerly used as a hematinic in the treatment of iron deficiency anemias and as a topical astringent and styptic. Called also *iron chloride.*

f. **citrate** garnet-red scales or brown granules, $FeC_6H_5O_7 \cdot xH_2O$, used as a reagent; called also *iron citrate.*

f. **oxide** [NF] Fe_2O_3, a coloring agent used in pharmaceutical preparations.

fer•ri•heme (fer′e-hēm) hematin.

fer•ri•tin (fer′ĭ-tin) the iron-apoferritin complex, one of the chief forms in which iron is stored in the body; it occurs at least in the gastrointestinal mucosa, liver, spleen, bone marrow, and reticuloendothelial cells generally. See also *immunoferritin.*

Ferr•le•cit (fer′lə-sit) trademark for a preparation of sodium ferric gluconate.

ferr(o)- [L. *ferrum* iron] a combining form denoting a relationship to iron; a variant form is *ferri.*

fer•ro•che•la•tase (fer″o-ke′lə-tās) [EC 4.99.1.1] a mitochondrial enzyme of the lyase class that catalyzes the insertion of ferrous iron into protoporphyrin IX to form protoheme IX, the heme of hemoglobin. Inhibition of the enzyme in lead poisoning results in accumulation of protoporphyrin IX. Deficiency of the enzyme, an autosomal dominant trait, results in erythropoietic protoporphyria.

fer•ro•heme (fer′o-hēm) the Fe(II) chelate of heme; sometimes called simply *heme.*

fer•ro•ki•net•ics (fer″o-kĭ-net′iks) [*ferro-* + *kinetics*] the movement of iron in the body from plasma transferrin to red cell precursors in bone marrow to circulating red cells to macrophages in the reticuloendothelial system and back to plasma transferrin. Ferrokinetic studies, using the radioisotope iron-59 as a tracer, measure kinetic parameters helpful in evaluating certain anemias and in detecting abnormal iron storage or extramedullary hematopoiesis by external counting over the liver, spleen, and bone marrow. Studies include *plasma iron clearance half-time, plasma iron turnover, red cell utilization,* and *erythrocyte iron turnover.* **ferrokinet′ic** *adj*

fer•ro•por•tin (fer″o-por′tin) a protein that binds iron and transports it out of cells; it is normally kept in balance with hepcidin.

fer•ro•pro•tein (fer″o-pro′tēn) a protein combined with an iron-containing radical; the ferroproteins are respiratory carriers. Cf. *cytochrome* (def. 1).

fer•ro•so•fer•ric (fər-o″so-fer′ik) combining a ferrous with a ferric compound; containing iron in two different oxidation states, as in the oxide Fe_3O_4.

fer•ro•ther•a•py (fer″o-ther′ə-pe) [*ferro-* + *therapy*] therapeutic use of iron and iron compounds.

fer•rous (fer′əs) containing iron in its plus-two oxidation state, Fe(II) (sometimes designated Fe^{2+}).

f. fumarate [USP] an oral iron preparation used in the treatment of iron deficiency.

f. gluconate [USP] an oral iron preparation used in the treatment of iron deficiency.

f. sulfate [USP] an oral iron preparation used in the treatment of iron deficiency.

fer•rox•i•dase (fer-ok′sĭ-dās) [EC 1.16.3.1] an enzyme or enzyme activity that catalyzes the oxidation of ferrous to ferric ions prior to their transport in the blood by transferrins.

fer•ru•gi•nous (fə-roo′jĭ-nəs) [L. *ferruginosus; ferrugo* iron rust] 1. containing iron or iron rust. 2. of the color of iron rust.

Fer•ry-Por•ter law (fer′e por′tər) [Ervin Sidney *Ferry*, American physicist, 1868–1956; Thomas Cunningham *Porter*, English scientist, late 19th century] see under *law*.

fer•tile (fur′til) [L. *fertilis*] 1. fruitful; having the capacity to reproduce. 2. capable of developing into a new individual; said of a zygote.

fer•til•i•ty (fər-til′ĭ-te) 1. the capacity to conceive or induce conception. 2. see under *rate*.

fer•ti•li•za•tion (fur′tĭ-lĭ-za′shən) the act of rendering gametes fertile or capable of further development; it is a sequence of events that begins with contact between a spermatozoon and an oocyte, leading to their fusion, which stimulates the completion of oocyte maturation with release of the second polar body. Male and female pronuclei then form and merge; synapsis follows, which restores the diploid number of chromosomes and results in biparental inheritance and the determination of sex. The process of fertilization leads to the formation of a zygote and ends with the initiation of its cleavage. Called also *fecundation* and *impregnation*.

cross f. the fertilization of one flower by the pollen of another; allogamy.

external f. union of the gametes outside the bodies of the originating organisms, as in most fish.

internal f. union of the gametes inside the body of the female, the sperm having been transferred from the body of the male by an accessory sex organ or other means.

in vitro f. (IVF) removal of a secondary oocyte, fertilization of it in a culture medium in the laboratory, and placement of the dividing zygote into the uterus.

in vivo f. union of the sperm and oocyte within the reproductive tract of the female; usually referring to those types of artificial insemination in which the sperm is artificially introduced into the vagina, cervix, or uterine cavity.

fer•ti•lize (fur′tĭ-līz) to render a gamete fertile; see *fertilization*. Called also *fecundate* and *impregnate*.

fer•ti•li•zin (fur″tĭ-li′zin) a substance of the plasma membrane and gelatinous coat of the oocyte of some species, considered to possess the specific receptor groups that bind the sperm to the oocyte.

Fer•tin•ex (fer′tin-eks) trademark for a preparation of urofollitropin.

Fe•ru•la (fə-roo′lə) a genus of umbelliferous plants. *F. asafoe′tida* is a source of asafetida. *F. commu′nis* is a species found in Mediterranean regions that contains an anticoagulant and can cause fatal hemorrhaging in ruminants.

Ferv. [L.] fer′vens (boiling).

fer•ves•cence (fər-ves′əns) [L. *fervescere* to become hot] development of an increased body temperature, or fever.

FES fat embolism syndrome; functional electrical stimulation; functional endoscopic sinus surgery.

fes•cue (fes′ku) 1. any grass of the genus *Festuca*. 2. fescue foot.

fes•ter (fes′tər) to suppurate superficially.

fes•ti•nant (fes′tĭ-nənt) accelerating; characterized by festination.

fes•ti•na•tion (fes″tĭ-na′shən) [L. *festinatio*] an involuntary tendency to take short accelerating steps in walking; see *festinating gait*, under *gait*.

fes•toon (fes-to͞on′) a carving in the base material of a denture that simulates the contours of the natural tissues being replaced by the denture.

gingival f. the contour of the gingiva and oral mucosa over the roots of teeth with a thin alveolar process.

McCall f. a lifesaver-like enlargement of the marginal gingiva occurring on the vestibular surface, most commonly in the canine and premolar areas.

Fes•tu•ca (fes-too′kə) a genus of grasses (family Gramineae). *F. arundina′cea* is tall fescue, a species found in New Zealand, Australia, and the United States, sometimes host to the endophytic fungus *Acremonium coenophialum*, which causes fescue foot in cattle.

fe•tal (fe′təl) 1. of or pertaining to a fetus. 2. pertaining to in utero development after the embryonic period.

fe•tal•ism (fe′təl-iz-əm) fetalization.

fe•tal•iza•tion (fe″təl-ĭ-za′shən) the retention, into adult life, of bodily characters which at some earlier stage of evolutionary history were actually only infantile and were rapidly lost as the organism attained maturity.

fe•ta•tion (fe-ta′shən) 1. the development of a fetus within the uterus. 2. pregnancy.

fe•ti•cide (fe′tĭ-sīd) [*fetus* + *-cide*] the destruction of the fetus.

fet•id (fĕ′tid, fe′tid) [L. *foetidus*] having a rank or disagreeable smell.

fet•ish (fet′ish, fe′tish) [Fr. *fétiche*, from Port. *feitico* charm, sorcery] 1. a material object, such as an idol, charm, or talisman, believed to have supernatural powers. 2. an inanimate object used to obtain sexual gratification.

fet•ish•ism (fet′ish-iz-əm) [DSM-IV] a paraphilia characterized by recurrent, intense sexual urges and sexually arousing fantasies of the use of inanimate objects (fetishes), most commonly articles of feminine clothing such as shoes, earrings, or undergarments, as a preferred or necessary adjunct to sexual arousal or orgasm. **fet′ishist** *n*

transvestic f. [DSM-IV] a paraphilia of heterosexual males, characterized by recurrent, intense sexual urges, arousal, or orgasm associated with fantasized or actual cross-dressing. Called also *transvestism*.

fet•lock (fet′lok) the metacarpophalangeal and metatarsophalangeal regions in the horse.

fet(o)- [L. *fetus*, q.v.] a combining form denoting relationship to the fetus.

fe•tog•ra•phy (fe-tog′rə-fe) [*fetus* + *-graphy*] radiography of the fetus *in utero*.

fe•tol•o•gy (fe-tol′ə-je) maternal-fetal medicine.

fe•tom•e•try (fe-tom′ə-tre) [*fetus* + *-metry*] the measurement of the fetus, especially of the diameters of its head.

fe•top•a•thy (fe-top′ə-the) a disease or disorder seen in a fetus; cf. *embryopathy*.

fe•to•pla•cen•tal (fe″to-plə-sen′təl) pertaining to the fetus and placenta.

α-fe•to•pro•tein (fe″to-pro′tēn) see *alpha fetoprotein*.

fe•tor (fe′tor) [L.] an offensive odor.

f. ex o′re halitosis.

f. hepa′ticus a peculiar odor of the breath that often accompanies liver disease; called also *liver breath*.

f. o′ris halitosis.

fe•to•scope (fe′to-skōp) 1. a specially designed stethoscope for listening to the fetal heart. 2. an endoscope for viewing the fetus in utero.

DeLee-Hillis f. see under *stethoscope*.

fe•tos•co•py (fe-tos′kə-pe) viewing of the fetus in utero by means of the fetoscope. **fetoscop′ic** *adj*

fe•to•tox•ic (fe″to-tok′sik) characterized by or producing fetal toxicity.

fe•to•tox•ic•i•ty (fe″to-tok-sis′ĭ-te) fetal toxicity.

fe•tu•in (fe′tu-in) a low-molecular-weight globulin that constitutes nearly the total globulin in the blood of the fetus and newborn of ungulates.

fe•tus (fe′təs) [L.] the unborn offspring of any viviparous animal; specifically, the unborn offspring in the postembryonic period, after major structures have been outlined, in humans from nine weeks after fertilization until birth. Cf. *embryo*.

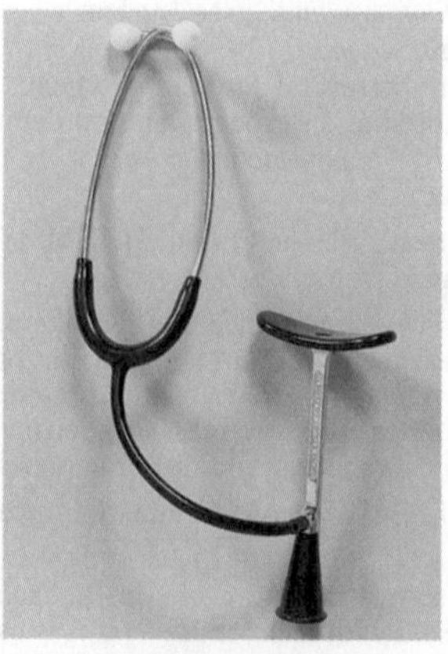

■ Fetoscope.

f. acardi′acus acardius.
f. amor′phus holoacardius amorphus.
calcified f. lithopedion.
f. compres′sus f. papyraceus.
f. in fe′tu a well-differentiated fetal teratoma having axial formation of limbs and organs. Cf. *endadelphos.*
harlequin f. a fetus covered with thick, horny armorlike plates as a result of an autosomal recessive keratinizing disorder; it may also be a severe form of collodion baby or it may represent the extreme form of lamellar ichthyosis. Babies born with this condition usually are stillborn or die within days after birth.
mummified f. a dried-up and shriveled fetus.
paper-doll f., papyraceous f. f. papyraceus.
f. papyra′ceus a dead fetus pressed flat by the growth of a living twin.
parasitic f. in asymmetrical conjoined twins, an incomplete minor fetus attached to the larger, more completely developed twin.
f. sanguinolen′tis a dead fetus that has undergone maceration.
sireniform f. sirenomelus.

Feu•er•stein-Mims syndrome (foi′ər-stīn mimz′) [Richard C. *Feuerstein,* American physician, 20th century; Leroy C. *Mims,* American physician, 20th century] sebaceous nevus syndrome.

Feul•gen reaction (foil′gən) [Robert *Feulgen,* German physiologic chemist, 1884–1955] see under *reaction.*

FEV forced expiratory volume.

fe•ver (fe′vər) [L. *febris*] 1. elevation of body temperature above the normal; it may be due to physiological stresses such as ovulation, excess thyroid hormone secretions, or vigorous exercise; to central nervous system lesions or infection by microorganisms; or to any of a host of noninfectious processes, such as inflammation or the release of certain materials, as in leukemia. Called also *pyrexia.* 2. any disease characterized by elevated body temperature.

Fever

African Coast f. East Coast f.
African swine f. a highly contagious, usually fatal disease of pigs in Africa, Southern Europe, and Brazil, transmitted by the African swine fever virus; symptoms closely resemble those of hog cholera. Transmission of the virus is by ticks of the genus *Ornithodoros,* by direct contact, by fomites, or by ingestion of infected meat. In Africa warthogs serve as a reservoir.
African tick f., African tick-bite f. 1. a type of spotted fever seen in southern Africa, caused by infection with *Rickettsia africae* and spread by the bites of ticks of species *Amblyomma hebraeum* and *A. variegatum;* symptoms are similar to those of boutonneuse fever. 2. a type of relapsing fever caused by *Borrelia duttonii.* 3. boutonneuse f.
aphthous f. foot-and-mouth disease.
Argentine hemorrhagic f., Argentinian hemorrhagic f. a hemorrhagic fever primarily affecting agricultural workers in northern Argentina, caused by the Junin virus and transmitted by contact with the excreta of infected rodents, especially *Calomys musculinus.* Characteristics include high fever, leukopenia, thrombocytopenia, generalized myalgia, hemorrhagic manifestations, exanthema, renal involvement, neurologic disturbances, and shock. Called also *Junin f.*
artificial f. pyretotherapy (def. 1).
aseptic f. fever associated with aseptic wounds, presumably due to the disintegration of leukocytes or to the absorption of avascular or traumatized but uninfected tissue.
Astrakhan f. a type of spotted fever observed in the summer in the Russian city of Astrakhan; it may be a variant of boutonneuse fever.
Australian Q f. Q f.
autumn f. mud f. (def. 1).
biliary f. of dogs canine babesiosis.
biliary f. of horses equine babesiosis.
black f. visceral leishmaniasis.
blackwater f. a severe complication of malaria characterized by intravascular hemolysis, hemoglobinuria, renal failure, and passage of dark brown or red urine, seen in association with intermittent quinine therapy, with *Plasmodium falciparum* infection in the nonimmune, or with interrupted exposure in the partially immune. The hemolysis is believed to be caused primarily by an autoimmune response to the infection. Called also *malarial hemoglobinuria.*
Bolivian hemorrhagic f. a hemorrhagic fever seen in tropical northeastern Bolivia, caused by the Machupo virus, whose natural reservoir is the mouse *Calomys callosus;* humans become infected by direct contact with mice or their excreta. Symptoms and epidemiology are similar to those of Argentine hemorrhagic fever.
boutonneuse f. an acute type of spotted fever caused by *Rickettsia conorii,* transmitted by the bites of ixodid ticks, with dogs and rodents being the chief hosts. There is a primary lesion (tache noire) at the site of the tick bite, as well as a maculopapular or petechial rash, headache, arthralgia, myalgia, chills, fever, and photophobia, usually without sequelae. It occurs from the Mediterranean and Black Seas across Central Asia, and variant forms occur in East Africa and on the Indian subcontinent. Called also *Marseilles f., Mediterranean spotted f.,* and *African, Indian, Israeli,* or *Kenyan tick f.*
bovine ephemeral f., bovine epizootic f. an acute viral disease of cattle in Africa, parts of Asia, and Australia, caused by a rhabdovirus transmitted by insect vectors; its symptoms resemble those of mild African horse sickness and include high fever lasting about three days, stiffness, and lameness. Called also *stiff sickness* and *three-day sickness.*
brassfounder's f. metal fume fever caused by fumes of any of several metals, most commonly zinc, copper, or magnesium.
Brazilian purpuric f. an acute illness in children characterized by fever, abdominal pain, vomiting, petechiae, purpura, and a recent history of conjunctivitis.
Brazilian spotted f. Rocky Mountain spotted f.
breakbone f. dengue.
Bwamba f. a mild, mosquito-borne febrile infection, caused by a bunyavirus, seen in many parts of sub-Saharan Africa.
cachectic f., cachexial f. visceral leishmaniasis.
camp f. epidemic typhus.
canicola f. Stuttgart disease.
cat-scratch f. see under *disease.*
central f. sustained fever resulting from damage to the thermoregulatory centers of the hypothalamus.
cerebrospinal f. meningococcal meningitis.
Charcot f., Charcot intermittent f. intermittent hepatic f.
chikungunya f. chikungunya.
childbed f. puerperal f.
Colombian tick f. Rocky Mountain spotted f.
Colorado tick f. an acute, benign febrile infection with a biphasic course, caused by an arenavirus transmitted by the bite of the wood tick, *Dermacentor andersoni,* occurring in the western United States and Canada. Characteristics include leukopenia with fever, chills, and pain in various parts of the body. Called also *mountain tick f.*
continued f., continuous f. persistently elevated body temperature, showing no or little variation and never falling to normal during any 24-hour period.
cotton-mill f. 1. mill f. (def. 1). 2. byssinosis.
Crimean-Congo hemorrhagic f. a hemorrhagic fever caused by the Crimean-Congo hemorrhagic fever virus, transmitted by ticks, especially those of the genus *Hyalomma,* and by contact with blood, secretions, or fluids from infected humans or domestic animals; it occurs in southern Russia, Central Asia, and sub-Saharan Africa.
dandy f. dengue.
deer fly f. tularemia.
dehydration f. 1. inanition f. 2. fever due to loss of body water or inadequate fluid intake, sometimes occurring as a postoperative complication.
dengue f. dengue.
dengue hemorrhagic f. hemorrhagic dengue.
desert f. primary coccidioidomycosis.
digestive f. a slight rise of temperature during the process of digestion.
drug f. a reaction marked by prolonged fever during administration of a drug, such as an antibiotic, antineoplastic, or vaccine.; it may be associated with vasculitis affecting small vessels, and usually disappears rapidly on discontinuance of the drug.
duck f. a type of hypersensitivity pneumonitis caused by sensitivity to duck proteins in duck feathers.
Dumdum f. visceral leishmaniasis.
Dutch type periodic f. hyperimmunoglobulinemia D syndrome.
Dutton relapsing f. a form of tick-borne relapsing fever seen in Central and Southern Africa, caused by *Borrelia duttonii.*

Fever *Continued*

East Coast f. a highly fatal form of theileriasis, seen in cattle from South Africa north to Kenya, caused by *Theileria parva* and transmitted by ticks of the genera *Rhipicephalus* and *Hyalomma.* Characteristics include high fever, dyspnea, emaciation, lymphadenopathy, and tarry feces. Called also *African Coast f.* and *bovine theileriasis.*
Ebola hemorrhagic f. Ebola virus disease.
elephantoid f. a recurrent acute febrile condition occurring with filariasis, sometimes associated with elephantiasis or lymphangitis.
Elokomin fluke f. a mild form of salmon poisoning (q.v.) in dogs, usually not fatal; the infective agent is an unidentified rickettsia. Characteristics include fever, anorexia, and diarrhea.
endemic relapsing f. tick-borne relapsing f.
enteric f. any of a group of febrile illnesses with enteric symptoms caused by species of *Salmonella;* the most common conditions are typhoid fever and paratyphoid fever. Cf. *salmonellosis.*
ephemeral f. a slight fever lasting for only one or two days.
ephemeral f. of cattle bovine ephemeral f.
epidemic hemorrhagic f. an acute type of hemorrhagic fever occurring in epidemics in northeastern Asia, and in a milder form in Russia, Central Asia, Eastern Europe, Scandinavia, and the southwestern United States. Symptoms include fever, prostration, vomiting, hemorrhagic phenomena, shock, and renal failure. It is caused by viruses of the genus *Hantavirus,* which are believed to be transmitted to humans by direct or indirect contact with the excreta of infected rodents. Called also *Far Eastern* or *Korean hemorrhagic f., hemorrhagic nephrosonephritis,* and *hemorrhagic f. with renal syndrome.*
epidemic relapsing f. louse-borne relapsing f.
equine biliary f. equine babesiosis.
eruptive f. any fever accompanied by a skin eruption or exanthem; called also *exanthematous f.*
essential f. fever for which no cause has been found.
exanthematous f. eruptive f.
familial Hibernian f. TNF-receptor–associated periodic syndrome.
familial Mediterranean f. an autoinflammatory disease (q.v.) of autosomal recessive inheritance, usually occurring in Armenians and Sephardic Jews, caused by mutation of the *MEFV* gene (locus: 16p13), which encodes pyrin. It is characterized by short recurrent attacks of fever with pain in the abdomen, chest, or joints and erythema resembling that seen in erysipelas; it is sometimes complicated by AA amyloidosis (q.v.). Called also *benign paroxysmal peritonitis, periodic peritonitis, familial recurrent polyserositis,* and *periodic* or *recurrent polyserositis.*
familial periodic f's autoinflammatory diseases.
Far Eastern hemorrhagic f. epidemic hemorrhagic f.
farrowing f. lactation failure in swine; see under *failure.*
fatigue f. a febrile attack due to overexercise and the absorption of waste products.
field f. 1. harvest f. 2. mud f.
filarial f. acute, recurrent fever with headache, malaise, and chills, occurring in filariasis; it subsides after 3 to 5 days and is usually accompanied by episodic adenolymphangitis or other manifestations of filariasis.
five-day f. trench f.
Flinders Island spotted f. an acute infection occurring during the summer months in Australia, caused by *Rickettsia honei* and transferred to humans by the reptile tick *Aponomma hydrosauri;* characteristics include fever, myalgia, headache, and an eschar and rash.
fog f. an often fatal acute adenomatoid reaction in the lungs of cattle, believed to be a response to chemicals generated in the rumen after being fed cut second-growth grass *(aftermath* or *fog).* Called also *acute bovine pulmonary emphysema, acute pulmonary emphysema of cattle, aftermath* or *lunger disease,* and *atypical interstitial pneumonia.*
Fort Bragg f. pretibial f.
foundryman's f. metal fume f.
glandular f. infectious mononucleosis.
grain f. a syndrome of malaise, fever, chills, and myalgia, occurring in grain elevator workers and others who have heavy exposure to grain dust; the cause is usually inhalation of endotoxins or contaminants such as mites. In some workers there is chronic asthma. See also *grain handler's lung,* under *lung.*
harvest f. a type of leptospirosis affecting harvest workers, characterized by fever, conjunctivitis, stupor, diarrhea, vomiting, and abdominal pains. Called also *field f.*
Haverhill f. a febrile disease caused by *Streptobacillus moniliformis,* resulting from ingestion of food or water contaminated by rat excrement and clinically resembling the bacillary form of rat-bite fever but with more severe vomiting and a higher incidence of pharyngitis. Called also *erythema arthriticum epidemicum* and *epidemic arthritic erythema.*
hay f. a type of allergic rhinitis that occurs at the same time every year, marked by acute conjunctivitis with lacrimation and itching, swelling of the nasal mucosa, sneezing, and often asthmatic symptoms. It is regarded as an anaphylactic or allergic condition excited by an allergen such as a pollen to which the individual is sensitized. Called also *pollen allergy, seasonal allergic rhinitis,* and *pollinosis.*
hay f., nonseasonal, hay f., perennial nonseasonal allergic rhinitis.
hectic f. a fever that recurs each day, with profound sweating, chills, and facial flushing.
hemoglobinuric f. malaria accompanied by hemoglobinuria; see *blackwater f.*
hemorrhagic f's a diverse group of severe epidemic viral infections, found in many parts of the world, mainly in tropical climates. Causative viruses are often geographically restricted, and they are usually transmitted to humans by arthropod bites or contact with virus-infected rodents. All the infections share certain features, such as fever, hemorrhagic manifestations, thrombocytopenia, shock, and neurologic disturbances. The group comprises Argentine hemorrhagic fever, Bolivian hemorrhagic fever, Crimean-Congo hemorrhagic fever, hemorrhagic dengue, Ebola virus disease, epidemic hemorrhagic fever, Kyasanur Forest disease, Lassa fever, Marburg virus disease, Omsk hemorrhagic fever, and yellow fever. Called also *viral hemorrhagic f's.*
hemorrhagic f. with renal syndrome epidemic hemorrhagic f.
hereditary periodic f's autoinflammatory diseases.
HIV-associated f. of unknown origin a fever of at least 38.3°C occurring on several occasions over a period of four weeks of outpatient care or three days of hospitalization in a patient with human immunodeficiency virus infection, and for which a cause cannot be determined after three days of investigation, including two days of incubation of cultures.
horse sickness f. a mild nonfatal form of African horse sickness, characterized by a slow onset of fever with only slight respiratory distress.
humidifier f. a syndrome of malaise, fever, cough, and myalgia, caused by inhalation of air that has been passed through humidifiers, dehumidifiers, or air conditioners contaminated by fungi, amebas, or thermophilic actinomycetes. See also *humidifier lung,* under *lung.*
inanition f. a transitory fever that frequently occurs in infants during the first few days of life; it is believed to be due to dehydration and is also called *dehydration f.*
intermittent f. an attack of malaria or other fever characterized by recurring paroxysms of elevated temperature separated by intervals during which the temperature is normal.
intermittent hepatic f. a fever occurring intermittently as the result of intermittent impaction of a calculus in the common bile duct with inflammation of the duct.
island f. scrub typhus.
Israeli spotted f. boutonneuse f.
jail f. epidemic typhus.
Japanese flood f., Japanese river f. scrub typhus.
Japanese spotted f. an acute infection occurring in Japan and caused by *Rickettsia japonica,* transmitted by ticks of the family Ixodidae; characterized by fever and headache and the appearance of an eschar and rash. Called also *Oriental spotted f.*
jungle yellow f. see *yellow f.*
Junin f. Argentine hemorrhagic f.
Katayama f. an acute type of schistosomiasis japonica, resembling serum sickness, characterized by fever, chills, nausea and vomiting, cough, headache, urticaria, hepatosplenomegaly, lymphadenopathy, marked eosinophilia, and usually increased levels of IgE and IgG.
Kew Gardens spotted f. rickettsialpox.
Korean hemorrhagic f. epidemic hemorrhagic f.
land f. a set of symptoms resembling seasickness sometimes experienced when, after an ocean voyage, the ship enters a relatively landlocked body of water.
Lassa f. an acute type of hemorrhagic fever caused by an arenavirus, endemic throughout West Africa but seen globally, usually transmitted via the multimammate mouse *(Mastomys natalensis)* or other *Mastomys* rodents but occasionally spread between persons. Most infections are subclinical or mild, although severe infection with multisystem involvement can be fatal. Clinical manifestations are variable, but may include

fever, headache, dry cough, back pain, vomiting, diarrhea, pharyngitis, and occasionally a rash; some patients develop deafness that can be permanent. Hypotension, peripheral vasoconstriction, facial and pulmonary edema, and hemorrhage from mucosal surfaces, usually occurring in the second week of infection, are all associated with fatal infection.
lechuguilla f. a disease of sheep and goats in western Texas, marked by toxic encephalitis, nephritis, photosensitization, listlessness, icterus, and a yellow discharge from the eyes and nostrils; it is caused by eating the plant *Agave lechuguilla.* Popularly known as *swellhead.*
louse-borne relapsing f. a type of relapsing fever caused by infection with *Borrelia recurrentis,* spread from person to person with a vector of the human body louse, *Pediculus humanus humanus,* which has humans as its reservoir. The condition occurs in epidemics when people are living in crowded or unsanitary conditions and can be spread either through louse bites or through contamination of a break in the skin by bodily secretions of lice. Called also *epidemic relapsing f.*
malignant catarrhal f. a highly fatal viral disease of cattle and other ungulates, characterized by exudative inflammation of mucous membranes, especially in the mouth, digestive tract, and respiratory tract, with corneal opacities, encephalitis, and enlargement of lymph nodes. The cause is thought to be a herpesvirus. Called also *bovine malignant catarrh* and *malignant catarrh of cattle.*
Malta f. brucellosis.
Marburg hemorrhagic f. Marburg disease.
Marseilles f. boutonneuse f.
marsh f. mud f. (def. 1).
Mediterranean f. 1. brucellosis. 2. boutonneuse f.
Mediterranean coast f. tropical theileriasis.
Mediterranean exanthematous f., Mediterranean spotted f. boutonneuse f.
metal fume f. an occupational disorder occurring in those engaged in welding and other metallic operations and due to inhalation of volatilized metals; it is characterized by sudden onset of thirst and a metallic taste in the mouth, followed by high fever, muscular aches and pains, shaking chills, headache, weakness, diaphoresis, and leukocytosis. Subtypes include *brassfounder's fever* and *spelter's fever.* A related condition is *polymer fume f.* Called also *foundryman's f.*
milk f. parturient paresis.
mill f. 1. fever and nausea in cotton mill workers, a rare manifestation of byssinosis. Called also *cotton-mill f.* 2. byssinosis.
mountain tick f. Colorado tick f.
mud f. 1. a type of leptospirosis seen in Germany and Russia, affecting workers in flooded fields or in swamps. Called also *autumn f., marsh f.,* and *swamp f.* 2. a disease of horses consisting of dermatophilosis, leptospirosis, and greasy heel.
Murchison-Pel-Ebstein f. Pel-Ebstein f.
nanukayami f. nanukayami.
neutropenic f. of unknown origin a fever of at least 38.3°C occurring on several occasions in a patient whose neutrophil level is lower than 500/mm^3 or is expected to fall below that level within one or two days, and for which a cause cannot be determined after three days of investigation, including two days of incubation of cultures.
nine-mile f. Q f.
nosocomial f. of unknown origin a fever of at least 38.3°C occurring on several occasions in a hospitalized patient in whom neither fever nor infection was present on admission, and for which a cause cannot be determined after three days of investigation, including two days of incubation of cultures.

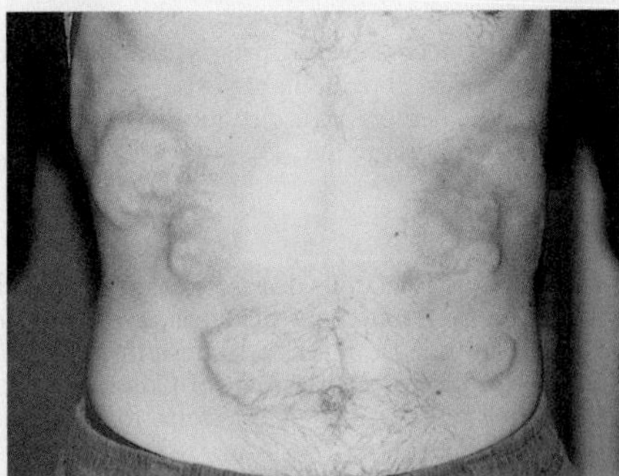
■ Urticaria associated with Katayama fever.

Omsk hemorrhagic f. a hemorrhagic fever similar in its clinical manifestations to Kyasanur Forest disease, endemic in a forested region of western Siberia, and caused by a flavivirus, transmitted to humans by the bites of infected ticks of the genus *Dermacentor* or by direct contact with infected muskrats, as by fur trappers.
o'nyong-nyong f. o'nyong-nyong.
Oriental spotted f. Japanese spotted f.
Oroya f. the first or acute stage of bartonellosis, marked by muscle pains, chills, fever, and severe hemolytic anemia that can be fatal. Called also Bartonella *anemia.*
Pahvant Valley f. tularemia.
papataci f., papatasi f., pappataci f. [It. *pappataci* silent sufferer] phlebotomus f.
paratyphoid f. a febrile illness clinically indistinguishable from but usually less severe than typhoid fever, caused by serovars of *Salmonella enterica* other than the one that causes typhoid fever. Occasionally paratyphoid fever may follow an attack of salmonella food poisoning. Called also *paratyphoid.*
parrot f. psittacosis.
parturient f. see under *paresis.*
Pel-Ebstein f. a cyclic fever occasionally seen in Hodgkin disease or certain other diseases, characterized by irregular episodes of pyrexia of several days' duration, with intervening afebrile periods lasting for days or weeks. Called also *Murchison-Pel-Ebstein f.*
pharyngoconjunctival f. a highly infectious febrile disease caused by an adenovirus, occurring in epidemic form, usually in schoolchildren, and characterized by fever, pharyngitis, rhinitis, conjunctivitis, and enlarged cervical lymph nodes.
Philippine hemorrhagic f. hemorrhagic dengue.
phlebotomus f. an acute, self-limited, febrile viral disease seen in warm weather from the Mediterranean Basin through the Middle East to Central Asia, as well as in Central and South America, and caused by any of several types of *Phlebovirus.* In Europe, North Africa, and Asia it is transmitted by the urban sandfly *Phlebotomus papatasi,* whereas in the Americas the vectors are sylvan sandflies (genus *Lutzomyia*). Called also *papataci, papatasi,* or *pappataci f.* and *sandfly f.*
pinta f. Mexican name for Rocky Mountain spotted fever.
polymer fume f. an occupational disorder due to exposure to the products of combustion of polymers, chiefly polytef (also known as Teflon); manifestations are similar to those of metal fume fever.
Pontiac f. an influenzalike disease caused by infection with any of various species of *Legionella;* characteristics include fever, chills, cough, muscle pain, headache, chest pain, and pleurisy.
Potomac horse f. equine monocytic ehrlichiosis.
pretibial f. a type of leptospirosis marked by a rash in the pretibial region accompanied by pain in the lumbar region and behind the eyes, with malaise, coryza, and fever. Called also *Fort Bragg f.*
prison f. epidemic typhus.
protein f. an increase in body temperature produced by the injection of protein material into the body.
puerperal f. an infectious, sometimes fatal, type of septicemia with fever, associated with childbirth; the focus of infection is the uterus, and the etiologic agent is frequently a streptococcus. Called also *childbed f.,* and *puerperal sepsis* or *septicemia.*
Q f. an acute, generally self-limited infection caused by *Coxiella burnetii,* characterized by fever, chills, headache, myalgia, malaise, and occasionally rash, and sometimes complicated by mild pneumonia (*Q fever pneumonia,* q.v.), hepatitis, and endocarditis. In humans, it is usually acquired by inhalation of airborne organisms in dust or aerosols contaminated by infected domestic animals, with no vector involved in transmission. Called also *Australian Q f.* and *nine-mile f.*
quartan f. a fever that occurs every fourth day, such as quartan malaria.
quintan f. trench f.
quotidian f. a fever that recurs every day, such as quotidian malaria.
rabbit f. tularemia.
rat-bite f. either of two clinically similar but etiologically distinct acute infectious diseases, transmitted by the bite of a rat or other small rodent: (1) the bacillary or streptobacillary form, seen mainly in North America, is caused by *Streptobacillus moniliformis* and has a latent

period of about a week, during which the initial wound heals without inflammation; the bite site later becomes inflamed and indurated, and this is followed by adenitis, chills, vomiting, headache, high fever, morbilliform eruption, especially on the hands and feet, and polyarthritis that is often severe. Cf. *Haverhill f.* (2) The spirillary form (called also *sodoku*), seen mainly in East Asia and nearby islands, is caused by *Spirillum minus* and has a latent period of usually more than ten days. Inflammation recurs at the primary wound site; the rash is less evident than in the bacillary form; arthritis is rare; and the fever is commonly of the relapsing type.

recurrent f. 1. a paroxysmal fever that recurs, seen in diseases such as malaria, meningococcemia, rat-bite fever, and tularemia. 2. relapsing f.

redwater f. bovine babesiosis.

relapsing f. either of two acute infectious, systemic, usually self-limited diseases, caused by infection with species of *Borrelia. Louse-borne relapsing fever* (q.v.) is spread by the human body louse, and *tick-borne relapsing fever* (q.v.) is spread by ticks of the genus *Ornithodoros.* Both types are characterized by alternating periods several days long with and without fever and spirochetemia. During the febrile periods, symptoms include chills, headache, fatigue, myalgia, arthralgia, anorexia, cough, abdominal pain, and sometimes coagulation disturbance, hepatosplenomegaly, psychic disturbances, petechial rash, and vomiting. Called also *recurrent*, or *spirillum f.*

remittent f. a fever in which the diurnal variation is 1°C or more, but in which the temperature never falls to a normal level; see *malaria.*

rheumatic f. a febrile disease occurring as a delayed sequela of infections with group A beta-hemolytic streptococci, characterized by multiple focal inflammatory lesions of connective tissue, especially of the heart (rheumatic heart disease), blood vessels, and joints (acute rheumatic arthritis); other manifestations include sudden fever, joint pain, abdominal pain, and Sydenham chorea. Aschoff bodies are typically present in the myocardium and skin. Atypical manifestations may also be seen, particularly in adults.

Rhodesian f., Rhodesian tick f. East Coast f.

rice field f. leptospirosis in workers in rice fields.

Rift Valley f. an acute febrile infection of sheep and cattle, zoonotic in humans, caused by a bunyavirus; it spreads to humans by the bites of mosquitoes of the genera *Aedes*, *Culex*, and *Anopheles* or by contact with tissues and secretions of infected animals. In humans it may be in a mild form with nonspecific influenzalike symptoms, or in a severe form with encephalitis, retinitis, or hemorrhagic fever. In other animals it is characterized by fever, listlessness, hepatitis, melena, bloodstained nasal discharge, and abortion in pregnant animals. First observed in the Rift Valley of Kenya, it is now seen throughout southern and eastern Africa as far north as Egypt.

Rocky Mountain spotted f. an acute, infectious, sometimes fatal disease caused by *Rickettsia rickettsii*, usually transmitted by the bite of an infected tick such as *Dermacentor andersoni* or *D. variabilis;* it occurs only in North and South America. It is characterized by sudden onset; chills; fever lasting 2 to 3 weeks; a cutaneous rash that appears early and spreads from the limbs upwards onto the trunk and face; myalgias; severe headache; and prostration. Called also *tick-borne typhus.* Several diseases observed in other places were found to be this, such as *Brazilian spotted fever*, *Colombian tick fever*, and *pinta fever*.

rose f. hay fever caused by grass pollens or rose pollen.

salt f. fever associated with excess of salt in the body, due to the retention by the salt of the water normally eliminated in perspiration.

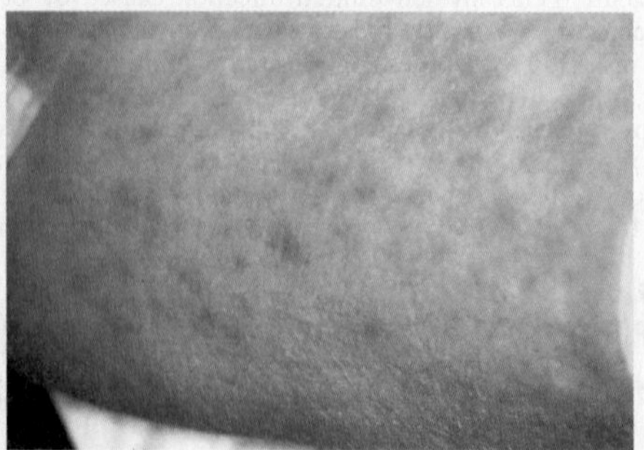

■ Petechial rash of Rocky Mountain spotted fever.

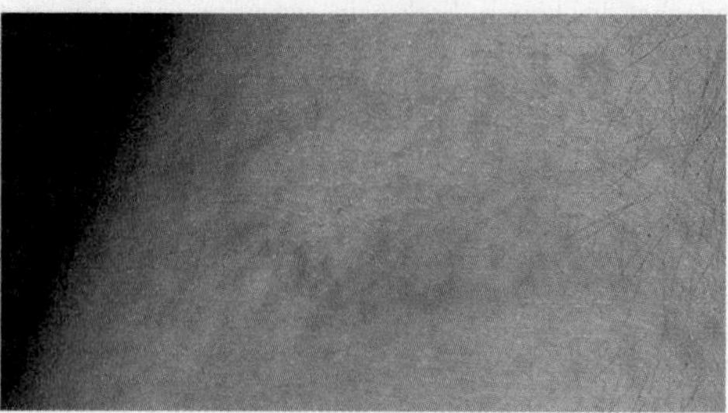

■ Rash of scarlet fever with characteristic Pastia lines.

sandfly f. phlebotomus f.

San Joaquin f., San Joaquin Valley f. primary coccidioidomycosis.

scarlet f. infection with group A β-hemolytic streptococci, now usually milder than in the past when septic complications were common, such as otitis media, mastoiditis, and lymphadenitis. It is characterized by pharyngitis, tonsillitis, and a rash produced by an exotoxin called streptococcal pyrogenic exotoxin, progressing from the trunk and neck to the limbs and face and sometimes followed by desquamation. Other symptoms include a red or white strawberry tongue and lines of hyperpigmentation in body creases (Pastia lines). Called also *scarlatina.*

sennetsu f. [Jap. *sennetsu* infectious mononucleosis, which it resembles] a febrile disease occurring in Japan and Malaysia and caused by *Neorickettsia sennetsu;* symptoms include headache, nausea or vomiting, lymphocytosis, and postauricular and posterior lymphadenopathy.

septic f. fever due to septicemia.

seven-day f. benign leptospirosis.

shin bone f. trench f.

shipping f. a disease of the respiratory tract of cattle caused by *Mannheimia haemolytica* in association with a virus; infection occurs when the resistance of the animal is lowered by stress. Characteristics include fever, pneumonialike symptoms, and sometimes death. Called also *stockyards f.* and *pneumonic pasteurellosis.*

Sindbis f. an epidemic-endemic febrile disease caused by infection with Sindbis virus, an alphavirus that has its normal reservoir in birds and is transmitted to humans by mosquitoes of the genus *Culex.* It has been observed in a belt from eastern Africa (South Africa to Egypt) across to Australia, as well as in Scandinavia. Symptoms include macular rash and arthritis.

South African tick-bite f. boutonneuse f.

South American hemorrhagic f's Argentine hemorrhagic fever, Bolivian hemorhagic fever, and Venezuelan hemorrhagic fever considered as a group.

spelter's f. metal fume fever caused by fumes in zinc smelters; called also *zinc fume f.*

spirillum f. relapsing f.

spotted f. any of a group of febrile diseases characterized by a skin eruption, especially several that are caused by tick-borne rickettsiae, such as boutonneuse fever, Rocky Mountain spotted fever, and others.

sthenic f. fever characterized by a full, strong pulse, hot and dry skin, high temperature, thirst, and active delirium.

stockyards f. shipping f.

swamp f. 1. mud f. (def. 1). 2. equine infectious anemia.

swine f. hog cholera.

tertian f. a fever that occurs every third day, such as tertian malaria.

Texas f., Texas cattle f. bovine babesiosis.

Thai hemorrhagic f. hemorrhagic dengue.

therapeutic f. pyretotherapy (def. 1).

thermic f. sunstroke.

three-day f. phlebotomus f.

threshing f. grain f.

tick f., tick-bite f. any infectious disease transmitted by the bite of a tick. The causative parasite may be a rickettsia, as in Rocky Mountain spotted fever and boutonneuse fever; a bacterium such as *Anaplasma*, *Babesia*, or *Borrelia;* or a virus, such as that of Colorado tick fever.

tick-borne f. 1. tick-bite f. 2. a general term for a condition spread by ticks.

tick-borne relapsing f. a type of relapsing fever that is caused by various species of *Borrelia*, spread to humans from animal reservoirs

Fever *Continued*

through tick vectors that are usually species of *Ornithodoros.* It is endemic in many parts of the world where the ticks and their hosts are found. Called also *endemic relapsing f.*
trench f. a self-limited rickettsial disease due to *Bartonella quintana*, transmitted by the body louse, *Pediculus humanus humanus*, characterized by intermittent fever, pain at various sites, especially the shins, chills, sweating, vertigo, malaise, typhuslike rash, and multiple relapses. It was first recognized during trench warfare in World War I, and was found to be endemic in Mexico, North Africa, Eastern Europe, and parts of Asia. Called also *quintan*, or *shin bone f.*
tsutsugamushi f. scrub typhus.
typhoid f. an acute, generalized, systemic febrile illness caused by *Salmonella enterica* subsp. *enterica* serovar Typhi; it is usually spread by ingestion of contaminated food or water. Characteristics include sustained bacteremia with invasion and multiplication inside the mononuclear phagocytes of the liver, spleen, lymph nodes, and ileal Peyer patches; prolonged hectic fever with malaise and later delirium; a characteristic transient skin rash known as *rose spots;* abdominal pain, splenomegaly, leukopenia, and bradycardia. Intestinal hemorrhages and perforation may be late complications. Called also *typhoid.*
typhus f. typhus.
undulant f. brucellosis.
f. of unknown origin (FUO) a febrile illness of at least three weeks' duration (some authorities permit a shorter duration), with a temperature of at least 38.3°C on at least three occasions and failure to establish a diagnosis in spite of intensive inpatient or outpatient evaluation (three outpatient visits or three days' hospitalization). Classic fever of unknown origin, as defined by the preceding criteria, is to be distinguished from neutropenic FUO, nosocomial FUO, and that associated with human immunodeficiency virus infection.
urban yellow f. see *yellow f.*
urethral f., urinary f. fever following the use of a urethral bougie, catheter, or sound.
uveoparotid f. Heerfordt syndrome.
valley f. primary coccidioidomycosis.
Venezuelan hemorrhagic f. a sometimes fatal hemorrhagic fever occurring in west central Venezuela, primarily in settlers moving into areas of cleared forest, caused by infection with the Guanarito virus, whose major reservoir is the cotton rat *Sigmodon alstoni.* Besides the fever and hemorrhaging, other characteristics include headache, myalgia, weakness, nausea, vomiting, and sometimes convulsions.
viral hemorrhagic f's hemorrhagic f's.
war f. epidemic typhus.
West Nile f. see under *encephalitis.*
Wolhynia f. trench f.
yellow f. an acute infectious disease caused by a flavivirus, now limited to tropical parts of Central and South America and Africa. It is considered one of the hemorrhagic fevers and is transmitted to humans by mosquitoes that have acquired the virus from either other humans (urban type) or animals (jungle type). In its severe form it is marked by fever, hemorrhage, renal damage, and jaundice from necrosis of the liver. It sometimes occurs as a mild or even inapparent febrile illness. *Urban yellow fever* affects chiefly persons living in close contact with one another, and is transmitted by *Aedes aegypti,* which usually breeds near human habitations. *Jungle yellow f.* most often affects those working in or living near forests; it has a variety of mosquito

fe•ver•few (fe′vər-fu″) [A.S. *feferfuge,* febrifuge, from L. *febrifugia*] [NF] the dried leaves of *Tanacetum parthenium,* used for migraine, arthritis, rheumatic diseases, and allergy; it has a wide variety of uses in folk medicine.

fe•ver•ish (fe′vər-ish) febrile.

Fèv•re-Langue•pin syndrome (fev′rə lahn-gə-pă′) [Marcel Paul Louis Edmond *Fèvre,* French physician, 1897–1978; Anne *Languepin,* French pediatrician, 20th century] see under *syndrome.*

fex•o•fen•a•dine hy•dro•chlo•ride (fek″so-fen′ə-dēn) [USP] an antihistamine (H_1-receptor antagonist) used in the treatment of seasonal allergic rhinitis (hay fever) and the skin manifestations of chronic idiopathic urticaria; administered orally.

FFA free fatty acids; see *nonesterified fatty acids,* under *fatty acid.*

FFT flicker fusion threshold; see *critical fusion frequency,* under *frequency.*

FG syndrome [initials of the last names of the first two children diagnosed with the condition] see under *syndrome.*

F.h. [L.] fi′at haus′tus (let a draft be made).

FIA fluorescence (or fluorescent) immunoassay (or fluoroimmunoassay).

FIAC Fellow of the International Academy of Cytology.

fi•at (fi′ət) pl. *fi′ant* [L.] let there be made. Abbreviated F.

fi•ber (fi′bər) 1. an elongated, threadlike structure; see also *fibra* [TA]. 2. neurofibra. 3. dietary f.

Fiber

For anatomic structures not listed here, see under *fibra* and see under the terms listed in def. 2 above.

A f's myelinated afferent or efferent fibers of the somatic nervous system having a diameter of 1 to 22 μm and a conduction velocity of 5 to 120 meters per second; they include the alpha, beta, delta, and gamma fibers.
accelerating f's, accelerator f's adrenergic fibers that transmit the impulses that accelerate the heartbeat; called also *augmentor* or *cardiac accelerator f's.*
accessory f's fibers of the zonule of Zinn that are perpendicular to the chief fibers and do not reach the lens of the eye, supporting and bracing the fibers running from the ciliary body to the chief fibers; they include the interciliary fibers and the orbiculociliary fibers. Called also *auxiliary f's.*
A delta f's a type of small myelinated afferent A fibers that respond to pressure, temperature, or chemical stimuli, conducting from the cutaneous tissues the initial stimulus perceived as the primary painful event. Their conducting velocity is slow, about the same as that of B fibers.
adrenergic f's nerve fibers, usually sympathetic, that release epinephrine or related substances as neurotransmitters.
afferent f's, afferent nerve f's 1. neurofibrae afferentes. 2. fibers or axons that are projecting toward a nucleus, using that nucleus as a reference point.
alpha f's motor and proprioceptive fibers of the A type having conduction velocities of 70 to 120 meters per second and ranging from 13 μm to 22 μm in diameter. See also under *motoneuron.*
alveolar f's fibers of the periodontal ligament extending from the cementum of the tooth root to the walls of the alveolus, distinguished as alveolar crest, horizontal, oblique, and apical fibers. Called also *cementoalveolar f's.*
alveolar crest f's fibers of the periodontal ligament extending from the cementum of the tooth root to the alveolar crest.
amianthoid f's asbestoslike crystalline fibers seen in some degenerated costal and laryngeal cartilage.
aminergic f's nerve fibers that liberate one of the biogenic amines at a synapse as a nerve impulse passes; nearly all nerve fibers are this type. Cf. *peptidergic f's.*
amygdalofugal f's the nerve fibers of the ventral amygdalofugal tract and the stria terminalis.

Fiber *Continued*

anastomosing f's, anastomotic f's fibers extending from one muscle bundle or nerve trunk to another.
apical f's fibers of the periodontal ligament extending from the cementum to the fundus of the alveolus.
arcuate f's association fibers that follow arc-shaped paths; see *fibrae arcuatae cerebri, fibrae arcuatae internae,* and *fibrae arcuatae externae posteriores* and *anteriores,* under *fibra.*
arcuate f's, anterior external fibrae arcuatae externae anteriores.
arcuate f's, dorsal external fibrae arcuatae externae posteriores.
arcuate f's, internal fibrae arcuatae internae.
arcuate f's, long long association f's.
arcuate f's, posterior external fibrae arcuatae externae posteriores.
arcuate f's, short short association f's.
arcuate f's, ventral external fibrae arcuatae externae anteriores.
arcuate f's of cerebrum fibrae arcuatae cerebri.
argyrophilic f's reticular f's; named for their staining properties with silver.
association f. fibra associationis.
association f's, long fibrae associationis longae.
association f's, short fibrae associationis breves.
association nerve f. fibra associationis.
association f's of telencephalon fibrae associationis telencephali.
augmentor f's accelerating f's.
autonomic f's neurofibrae autonomicae.
autonomic afferent f's see *neurofibrae autonomicae.*
autonomic efferent f's see *neurofibrae autonomicae.*
autonomic nerve f's neurofibrae autonomicae.
auxiliary f's accessory f's.
axial f. axon (def. 1).
B f's myelinated preganglionic autonomic axons having a fiber diameter ≤3 μm and a conduction velocity of 3 to 15 meters per second; these include only efferent fibers.
bag f. nuclear bag f.
basilar f's fibers that form the middle layer of the zona arcuata and the zona pectinata of the basilar membrane in the internal ear.
Bergmann f's processes which radiate from the molecular layer of the cerebellum and enter the pia.
beta f's motor and proprioceptive fibers of the A type having conduction velocities of 30 to 70 meters per second and ranging from 8 to 13 μm in diameter. See also *beta motoneurons.*
bone f's Sharpey f's (def. 1).
Brücke f's fibrae meridionales musculi ciliaris.
bulbospiral f's spiral muscle fibers that begin near the root of the aorta and spiral upward in bundles within the ventricles.
Burdach f's fasciculus cuneatus medullae spinalis.
C f's unmyelinated nerve fibers, having a smaller diameter (0.3 to 1.3 μm) and a slower conduction velocity (0.6 to 2.3 meters per second) than alpha fibers. They are found as postganglionic (efferent) fibers of the autonomic nervous system, and as afferent fibers at posterior roots, receiving impulses from free nerve endings that act as thermoreceptors, nociceptors, and interoceptors.
cardiac accelerator f's accelerating f's.
cardiac depressor f's vagal nerve fibers to the heart which when activated cause a decrease in cardiac output.
cardiac pressor f's sympathetic nerve fibers to the heart which when activated cause an increase in cardiac output.
cemental f's the fibers of the periodontal ligament extending from the cementum to the zone of the intermediate plexus, where their terminations are interspersed with the terminations of the alveolar group of periodontal fibers.
cementoalveolar f's alveolar f's.
cerebellovestibular f's nerve fibers in the fastigiobulbar tract that run from the cerebellar cortex to the vestibular nuclei.
cerebrospinal f's fibrae corticospinales.
chain f. nuclear chain f.
chief f's fibers of the zonule of Zinn that run from the ciliary body to the lens, including the orbiculoposterocapsular, the orbiculoanterocapsular, the cilioposterocapsular, and cilioequatorial fibers; called also *main* or *principal f's.*
cholinergic f's nerve fibers that liberate acetylcholine as a neurotransmitter.
chromatin f. the partially compacted chromatin structure formed by folding and condensation of the nucleosomes, having a diameter of 30 nm (and so sometimes called the 30-nm fiber). The exact arrangement of nucleosomes remains controversial; a classic model places them in a helical solenoid (q.v.).

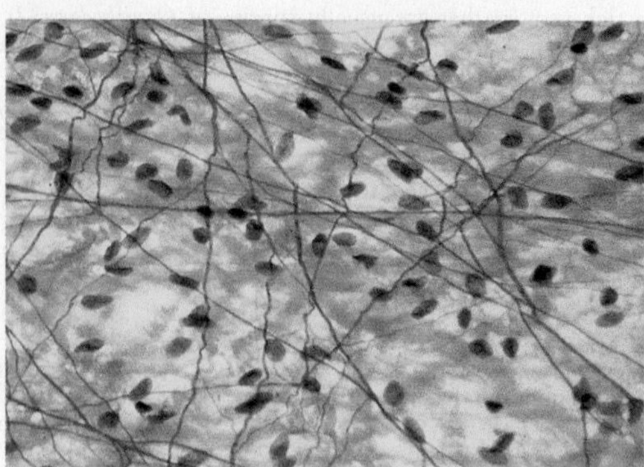

■ Loose connective tissue in the mesentery in a whole mount preparation, showing collagen fibers *(red)* and a network of thin elastin fibers *(black),* with interspersed oval gray nuclei, mainly of fibroblasts.

cilioequatorial f's chief fibers that pass from the summits of the ciliary processes to the equator of the lens.
cilioposterocapsular f's the most numerous of the chief fibers, arising from the tips and sides of the ciliary processes, passing posteriorly and crossing the anteriorly directed fibers, to insert into the posterior capsule anterior to the insertion of the orbiculoposterocapsular fibers.
circular f's 1. gingival fibers that pass through the connective tissue of the marginal and interdental gingivae and encircle the tooth in ringlike fashion. 2. fibrae circulares musculi ciliaris. 3. circular f's of eardrum.
circular f's of ciliary muscle fibrae circulares musculi ciliaris.
circular f's of eardrum the fibers in the stratum circulare membranae tympanicae.
climbing f's, clinging f's afferent fibers arising in part from the middle cerebellar peduncle and passing through the granular layer of the cerebellar cortex to terminate on Purkinje cell dendrites. Called also *tendril f's.* Cf. *mossy f's.*
collagen f's, collagenous f's the soft, flexible, white fibers that are the most characteristic constituent of all types of connective tissue. They consist of the protein collagen and are composed of bundles of fibrils that are in turn made up of smaller unit fibrils; see also *collagen fibrils,* under *fibril.* In describing the hierarchy of arrangement of collagen structure, the terms fiber and fibril are sometimes loosely interchanged.
commissural f. fibra commissuralis.
commissural f's of telencephalon fibrae commissurales telencephali.
cone f. a fiberlike extension of a retinal cone, running from the inner segment of the dendrite to the nucleus to the pedicle.
Corti f's pillar cells.
corticobulbar f's fibrae corticonucleares.
corticonuclear f's 1. fibrae corticonucleares. 2. Purkinje cells axons that connect to nuclei of the cerebellum.
corticopontine f's fibrae corticopontinae.
corticopontocerebellar f's the corticopontine fibers and pontocerebellar fibers considered together; see *fibrae corticopontinae* and *fibrae pontocerebellares.*
corticoreticular f's fibrae corticoreticulares.
corticorubral f's fibrae corticorubrales.
corticospinal f's fibrae corticospinales.
corticostriate f's afferent fibers originating in many parts of the cerebral cortex and descending to the caudate nucleus and putamen in the corpus striatum.
corticothalamic f's fibrae corticothalamicae.
crude f. dietary fiber that remains after food is digested with alkali and acid that have destroyed all of the soluble and some of the insoluble fiber; it comprises mainly lignin and cellulose.
dark f's muscle fibers rich in sarcoplasm and having a dark appearance.
decussating f's any set of interconnecting fibers.

dentatorubral f's fibrae dentatorubrales.
dentatothalamic f's nerve fibers in the cranial cerebellar peduncle that make up the dentatothalamic tract.
dentinal f. odontoblastic process.
dentinogenic f's Korff f's.
depressor f's 1. nerve fibers which, when stimulated reflexly, cause a diminished vasomotor tone and thereby a decrease in arterial pressure. 2. cardiac depressor f's.
dietary f. the part of whole grains, vegetables, fruits, and nuts that resists digestion in the gastrointestinal tract; it includes soluble fibers such as pectins, gums, mucilages, and some hemicelluloses and insoluble fibers such as cellulose, and other hemicelluloses.
Edinger f's fibers in the cerebrum of amphibia, forming part of the visual paths.
efferent f's, efferent nerve f's 1. neurofibrae efferentes. 2. fibers or axons that are projecting away from a nucleus, using that nucleus as a reference point.
elastic f's yellowish fibers of elastic quality, composed of a core of cross-linked elastin surrounded by fibrillin microfibrils, traversing the intercellular substance of connective tissue; called also *yellow f's.*
endogenous f's nerve fibers of the spinal cord which arise from cells the bodies of which are situated inside the cord.
exogenous f's fibers of the spinal cord which arise from cells the bodies of which are situated outside the cord.
extrafusal f's ordinary muscle fibers, as opposed to the intrafusal fibers of the muscle spindle.
fasciculoventricular f's Mahaim fibers that connect the bundle of His directly to the ventricular myocardium.
frontopontine f's fibrae frontopontinae.
fusimotor f's efferent A fibers that innervate the intrafusal fibers of the muscle spindle; see also *gamma f's.* Called also *fusimotor axons.*
gamma f's any A fibers that conduct at velocities of 15 to 40 meters per second and range from 3 to 7 μm in diameter; the only such fibers are the fusimotor fibers. See also under *loop* and *motoneuron.*
geniculostriate f's the fibers of the optic radiation; see *radiatio optica* under *radiatio.*
Gerdy f's the fibers of the superficial ligament connecting the clefts of the palmar surfaces of the fingers.
gingival f's the collagen fibers which make up the gingival corium and support the gingiva. They are attached and adapted to the tooth surface and act as a barrier to the apical migration of the epithelial attachment.
gingivodental f's gingival fibers of the vestibular, oral, and interproximal surfaces, embedded in the cementum just beneath the epithelium at the base of the gingival crevice.
Goll f's fasciculus gracilis medullae spinalis.
Gratiolet radiating f's radiatio optica.
gray f's unmyelinated nerve fibers, found largely, but not exclusively, in the sympathetic nerves.
hair f. a type of horny fiber containing the remains of a nucleus; a group of these makes up the main substance of each hair.
Henle f's the fibers of either of the elastic membranes of an artery.
heterodesmotic f's nerve fibers connecting dissimilar structures of the central nervous system. Cf. *homodesmotic f's.*
homodesmotic f's nerve fibers connecting similar structures of the central nervous system. Cf. *heterodesmotic f's.*
horizontal f's fibers of the periodontal ligament extending horizontally from the cementum of the tooth root to the walls of the alveolus.
impulse-conducting f's Purkinje f's.
insoluble f. dietary fiber that is not soluble in water, composed mainly of lignin, cellulose, and hemicelluloses and primarily found in the bran layers of cereal grains; its actions include increasing fecal bulk and decreasing free radicals in the gastrointestinal tract.
interciliary f's those accessory fibers that run between the ciliary processes.
intercolumnar f's, intercrural f's fibrae intercrurales.
internuncial f's nerve fibers connecting two or more neurons.
intersegmental f's see *fasciculus proprius posterior medullae spinalis, fasciculus proprius lateralis medullae spinalis,* and *fasciculus proprius anterior medullae spinalis.*
intrafusal f's modified muscle fibers which, surrounded by fluid and enclosed in a connective tissue envelope, compose the muscle spindle.
intrasegmental f's fibers in the white commissures of the spinal cord that link neurons to contralateral neurons at the same level.
intrathalamic f's fibrae intrathalamicae.
James f's in the heart, junctional tissue or a tract that bypasses the atrioventricular node and thus permits ventricular preexcitation.
kinetochore f's a component of the mitotic spindle, consisting of kinetochore microtubules (q.v.).
Korff f's collagen fibrils extending from fibroblasts (preodontoblasts), which project their processes toward the inner enamel epithelium (preameloblasts), whence they reach the area of aperiodic fibrils and basal lamina, where they form bundles and make up the matrix for dentin, particularly the mantle dentin.
f's of lens fibrae lentis.
light f's muscle fibers poor in sarcoplasm and therefore more transparent than dark fibers.
longitudinal f's of ciliary muscle fibrae meridionales musculi ciliaris.
longitudinal pontine f's fibrae pontis longitudinales.
Luschka f's fibers of the levator ani muscle that meet between the anus and the vagina in the perineal body.
macular f's the fibers of the maculary fasciculus.
Mahaim f's specialized tissue in the heart, connecting components of the conduction system directly to the ventricular septum; this is usually important functionally only when it is abundant. These fibers are often classified as either *fasciculoventricular f's* or *nodoventricular f's.*
main f's chief f's.
Mauthner f. an axon that extends from the metencephalon to the caudal end of the spinal cord of fishes and amphibians, and provides the final common path for impulses to the tail.
medullated f's, medullated nerve f's myelinated f's.
meridional f's of ciliary muscle fibrae meridionales musculi ciliaris.
Monakow f's tractus rubrospinalis.
moss f's, mossy f's thick afferent nerve fibers arising from the inferior cerebellar peduncle and passing into the cerebellar cortex to terminate in numerous branches or mosslike appendages around the cells of the granular layer. Cf. *climbing f's.*
motor f's neurofibrae efferentes.
Müller f's 1. fibrae circulares musculi ciliaris. 2. elongated neuroglial cells traversing all the layers of the retina and forming its most important supporting element; called also *sustentacular f's, cells of Müller, radial cells of Müller,* and *retinal gliocytes.*
muscle f. any of the cells of skeletal or cardiac muscle tissue. Skeletal muscle fibers are cylindrical multinucleate cells containing contracting myofibrils, across which run transverse striations, enclosed in a sarcolemma. Cardiac muscle fibers contain one or sometimes two nuclei and myofibrils and are separated from one another by an intercalated disk; although striated, cardiac muscle fibers branch to form an interlacing network. See also *muscle cell,* under *cell.*
muscle f's, fast twitch paler-colored muscle fibers of larger diameter than slow twitch fibers, and having less sarcoplasm and more prominent cross-striping; used for forceful and rapid contractions over short periods of time.
muscle f's, intermediate muscle fibers having characteristics intermediate between red and white muscle fibers.
muscle f's, red slow twitch muscle f's.
muscle f's, slow twitch small dark muscle fibers rich in mitochondria, myoglobin, and sarcoplasm and with only faint cross-striping; designed for slow but repetitive contractions over long periods of time.
muscle f's, type I slow twitch muscle f's.
muscle f's, type II fast twitch muscle f's.
muscle f's, white fast twitch muscle f's.
myelinated f's, myelinated nerve f's grayish white nerve fibers whose axons are encased in a myelin sheath, which may in turn be enclosed by a neurilemma; called also *medullated f's* and *medullated nerve f's.* Cf. *unmyelinated f's.*
nerve f. neurofibra.
neuroglial f. one of the fibrillar structures embedded in the cytoplasm and expansions of neuroglial cells, particularly fibrous astrocytes.
nigrostriatal f's the nerve fibers of the nigrostriatal tract.
nodoventricular f's Mahaim fibers that connect the atrioventricular node directly to the ventricle.
nonmedullated f's, nonmedullated nerve f's unmyelinated f's.
nuclear bag f. an intrafusal fiber that contains a nuclear bag; it is longer and thicker and contracts more slowly than a nuclear chain fiber.

nuclear chain f. an intrafusal fiber that contains a nuclear chain; it is shorter and thinner and contracts more rapidly than a nuclear bag fiber.
oblique f's the largest fibers of the periodontal ligament, extending from the cementum in a coronal direction obliquely to the apical two thirds of the alveolus; they suspend and anchor the tooth in its socket and resist surface tooth pressures.
oblique f's of ciliary muscle fibrae radiales musculi ciliaris.
oblique gastric f's, oblique f's of muscular coat, oblique f's of muscular layer, oblique f's of stomach fibrae obliquae tunicae mucosae.
occipitopontine f's see *fibrae corticopontinae*, under *fibra*.
odontogenic f's fibers of connective tissue (periodontium and pulp) contributing to the matrix of dentin and cementum.
olivocerebellar f's tractus olivocerebellaris.
orbiculoanterocapsular f's the chief fibers that have the most posterior and internal position, lying in close relation to the anterior boundary of the vitreous.
orbiculociliary f's those accessory fibers that pass from the pars orbicularis to the ciliary processes.
orbiculoposterocapsular f's the chief fibers that spring from the prolongation of the hyaloid membrane investing the ciliary ring.
osteocollagenous f's fibers gathered together into bundles and united by a special binding substance in the interstitial substance of bone.
osteogenetic f's, osteogenic f's precollagenous fibers formed by osteoclasts and becoming the fibrous component of bone matrix.
oxytalan f. 1. a connective tissue fiber, resistant to acid hydrolysis, found in structures subjected to mechanical stress, such as tendons, ligaments, adventitia, and connective tissue sheaths that surround the skin appendages. 2. oxytalan.
pallidofugal f's nerve fibers that conduct impulses from the globus pallidus across the internal capsule and fields of Forel to the thalamus and nearby areas; see also *ansa lenticularis* and *fasciculus lenticularis*.
parallel f's axons of granule cells in the cerebellum that cross the molecular layer at a right angle and synapse with gemmules of Purkinje cell dendrite; many thousands of parallel fibers may innervate a single Purkinje cell.
paraventricular f's fibrae paraventriculohypophysiales.
parietopontine f's fibrae parietopontinae.
parietotemporopontine f's fibrae parietotemporopontinae.
peptidergic f's nerve fibers that secrete neuropeptides as neurotransmitters. Cf. *aminergic f's*.
perforating f's Sharpey f's (def. 2).
periventricular f's fibrae periventriculares.
pilomotor f's unmyelinated nerve fibers going to the small muscles of the hair follicles.
pontocerebellar f's fibrae pontocerebellares.
postcommissural f's the nerve fibers of the commissure of the epithalamus that lie behind the pineal body.
postganglionic f's, postganglionic nerve f's neurofibrae postganglionicae.
precollagenous f's a name given reticular fibers on the supposition that they are immature collagenous fibers.
preganglionic f's, preganglionic nerve f's neurofibrae preganglionicae.
pressor f's 1. nerve fibers that, when stimulated reflexly, cause or increase vasomotor tone. 2. cardiac pressor f's.
principal f's 1. chief f's. 2. fibers of the periodontal ligament, which are collagen fibers arranged in bundles along the length of the root of a tooth that suspend and anchor the tooth to the alveolus. They include the transseptal, alveolar crest, horizontal, oblique, and apical fibers.
projection f., projection nerve f's fibra projectionis.
Prussak f's two short fibers from the end of the short process of the malleus to the notch of Rivinus.
Purkinje f's modified cardiac fibers composed of Purkinje cells, occurring as an interlaced network in the subendocardial tissue and constituting the terminal ramifications of the conducting system of the heart. The term is sometimes used loosely to denote the entire system of conducting fibers. See also *rami subendocardiales* and *systema conducens cordis*.
radial f's of ciliary muscle fibrae radiales musculi ciliaris.
radiating f's of anterior chondrosternal ligaments ligamenta sternocostalia radiata.

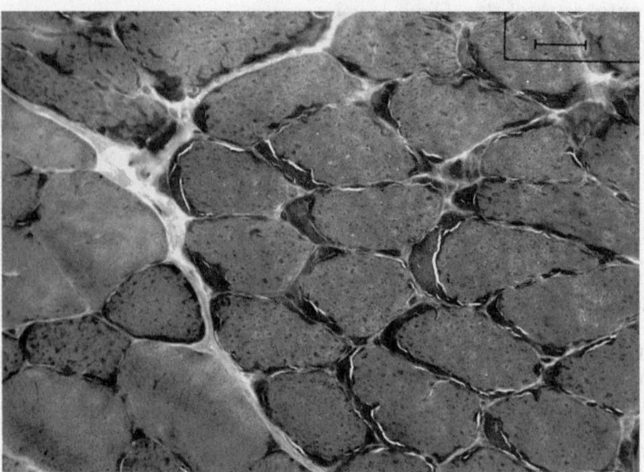

■ Ragged red fibers in mitochondrial myopathy (Gomori trichrome stain).

radiating f's of eardrum the fibers in the stratum radiatum membranae tympanicae.
radicular f's fibers in the roots of the spinal nerves.
ragged red f's muscle fibers characterized by large collections of structurally abnormal mitochondria below the sarcolemmal surface and within the fiber itself that stain red with Gomori trichrome stain; seen in mitochondrial myopathy and occasionally in other myopathic disorders.
Rasmussen nerve f's tractus olivocochlearis.
Reissner f. a highly refractive longitudinal nerve fiber in the central canal of the spinal cord.
reticular f's Type III collagen fibers, differing from most other type of collagen fibers in staining with silver; they form the reticular supporting meshwork of lymphoid and myeloid tissue and occur also in the interstitial tissue of glandular organs, the papillary layer of the skin, and other highly cellular tissues. Called also *argyrophilic f's* for their staining properties.
retinothalamic projection f's nerve fibers that connect the visual receptors of the retina with the thalamus and form part of the optic nerve and optic tract.
Retzius f's the stiff filaments of Deiters cells in the organ of Corti.
ring f. a band of circumferentially oriented myofibrils located beneath the sarcolemma of a muscle fiber and encircling the longitudinally oriented myofibrils within the fiber; seen in myotonic dystrophy.
Ritter f. a fiber in the axis of a retinal rod, probably a nerve fiber.
rod f. a fiberlike extension of a retinal rod, running from the inner segment of the dendrite to the nucleus to the spherule.
Rosenthal f's thick, elongated, irregular, eosinophilic structures that contain heat shock proteins and ubiquitin and occur within the processes of astrocytes. They are associated with long-standing gliosis and also are seen in certain astrocytomas and in Alexander disease.
Sappey f's smooth muscle fibers in the check ligaments of the eye near their orbital attachments.
sensory f's neurofibrae afferentes.
Sharpey f's 1. collagenous fibers that pass from the periosteum and are embedded in the outer circumferential and interstitial lamellae of bone; called also *bone f's*. 2. terminal portions of principal fibers that insert into the cementum of a tooth. Called also *perforating f's*.
sinospiral f's, sinuspiral f's spiral muscle fibers that begin near the posterior aspect of one or both atrioventricular fibrous rings and spiral upward in bundles within one or both ventricles.
soluble f. dietary fiber that has an affinity for water, either dissolving or swelling to form a gel; it includes gums, pectins, mucilages, and some hemicelluloses, and is primarily found in fruits, vegetables, oats, barley, legumes, and seaweed. It acts to decrease the rate of stomach emptying and increase transit time, and also binds bile acids, increasing their excretion.
somatic f's neurofibrae somaticae.
somatic afferent f's see *neurofibrae somaticae*.
somatic efferent f's see *neurofibrae somaticae*.
somatic nerve f's neurofibrae somaticae.

Fiber *Continued*

sphincter f's of ciliary muscle fibrae circulares musculi ciliaris.
spindle f's the microtubules radiating from the centrioles during mitosis and forming a spindle-shaped configuration. See *spindle* (def. 2).
spinohypothalamic f's fibrae spinohypothalamicae.
spinomesencephalic f's fibrae spinomesencephalicae.
spino-olivary f's fibrae spinoolivares.
spinoperiaqueductal f's fibrae spinoperiaqueductales.
spinoreticular f's fibrae spinoreticulares.
spinotectal f's fibrae spinotectales.
spinothalamic f's fibrae spinothalamicae.
Stilling f's nerve fibers in the reticular formation of the medulla oblongata.
f's of stria terminalis fibrae striae terminalis.
striatonigral f's the fibers of the strionigral tract.
sudomotor f's unmyelinated nerve fibers going to the sweat glands.
supraoptic f's fibrae supraopticohypophysiales.
sustentacular f's Müller f's.
T f. a nerve fiber that branches at right angles from the axon, as seen in pseudounipolar neurons.
tangential f's, tangential nerve f's neurofibrae tangentiales.
temporopontine f's fibrae temporopontinae.
tendril f's climbing f's.
terminal conducting f's of Purkinje Purkinje f's.
thalamocortical f's sensory nerve fibers that connect the dorsal thalamus to the cerebral cortex, which together form the peduncles of the thalamus; called also *thalamic radiations, radiations of thalamus,* and *thalamocortical projections.*
thalamoparietal f's fibrae thalamoparietales.
Tomes f. odontoblastic process.
transseptal f's fibers of the periodontal ligament extending interproximally over the alveolar crest and embedding in the cementum of adjacent teeth; they support the interproximal gingiva and secure the adjacent tooth.
transverse pontine f's fibrae pontis transversae.
trigeminothalamic f's nerve fibers that convey sensory information from the spinal tract and the nuclei of the trigeminal nerve to the sensory nuclei of the thalamus.
U f's fibrae arcuatae cerebri.
ultraterminal f. the thin unmyelinated twig that is the last ramification of the axon at the motor end plate.
unmyelinated f's, unmyelinated nerve f's nerve fibers (axons) that lack the myelin sheath but may be enclosed by a neurilemma. Called also *nonmedullated f's* and *nonmedullated nerve f's.* Cf. *myelinated f's.*
varicose f's certain myelinated fibers which have no neurilemma; after death a fluid accumulates between the myelin and the axon, giving the fibers a varicose appearance.
vasomotor f's unmyelinated nerve fibers going chiefly to arteriolar muscles.
visceral f's neurofibrae autonomicae.
visceral afferent f's autonomic afferent f's; see *neurofibrae autonomicae.*
visceral efferent f's autonomic efferent f's; see *neurofibrae autonomicae.*
visceral nerve f's neurofibrae autonomicae.
von Monakow f's tractus rubrospinalis.
Weissmann f's fibers within the muscle spindle.
white f's collagenous f's.
yellow f's elastic f's.
zonular f's fibrae zonulares.

fi·ber·co·lono·scope (fi″bər-ko-lon′o-skōp) fiberoptic colonoscope.

Fi·ber·Con (fi′bər-kon) trademark for a preparation of calcium polycarbophil.

fi·ber·gas·tro·scope (fi″bər-gas′tro-skōp) fiberoptic gastroscope.

fi·ber-il·lu·mi·nat·ed (fi′bər-ĭ-loo′mĭ-nāt″əd) transmitting light by means of bundles of glass or plastic fibers, utilizing a lens system to transmit the image; said of endoscopes of such design.

fi·ber·op·tic (fi″bər-op′tik) 1. pertaining to fiberoptics. 2. coated with glass or plastic fibers having special optical properties.

fi·ber·op·tics (fi″bər-op′tiks) 1. the transmission of an image along flexible bundles of coated parallel glass or plastic fibers that propagate light by internal reflections. 2. the branch of optics dealing with such transmission.

fi·ber·scope (fi′bər-skōp) a flexible endoscope that uses bundles of fibers with special optical properties (see *fiberoptics*) for the transmission of light and the collection of images; it also contains channels for insufflation and suction and for the introduction of a variety of accessories for diagnostic and therapeutic procedures. Called also *fiberoptic endoscope.*

fi·bra (fi′brə) gen. and pl. *fi′brae* [L.] [TA] fiber: a general term designating an elongated, threadlike structure. See also *neurofibra.*

fi′brae annula′res see *pars anularis vaginae fibrosae digitorum manus* and *pars anularis vaginae fibrosae digitorum pedis.*

fi′brae arcua′tae ce′rebri [TA] arcuate fibers of cerebrum: short association fibers within the cerebral cortex, having arc- or U-shaped paths that connect adjacent gyri. Called also *U fibers.*

fi′brae arcua′tae exter′nae anterio′res [TA] anterior external arcuate fibers: nerve fibers that arise from the arcuate nuclei, emerging from the anterior median fissure; they run laterally, backward, and upward over the medulla oblongata to reach the cerebellum by way of the inferior cerebellar peduncle.

fi′brae arcua′tae exter′nae posterio′res [TA] posterior external arcuate fibers: nerve fibers that arise from the accessory cuneate nucleus and enter the cerebellum by way of the ipsilateral inferior cerebellar peduncle.

fi′brae arcua′tae inter′nae [TA] internal arcuate fibers: nerve fibers that arise from the nucleus cuneatus and nucleus gracilis and pass ventromedially around the central gray substance of the medulla oblongata to form the decussation of the medial lemnisci.

f. associatio′nis [TA] association fiber: one of the nerve fibers connecting different cortical areas within one hemisphere. Called also *neurofibra associationis.* See also *fibrae associationis telencephali.*

fi′brae associatio′nis bre′ves [TA] short association fibers: association fibers that connect adjacent areas of the cerebral cortex; called also *short arcuate fibers.*

fi′brae associatio′nis lon′gae [TA] long association fibers: association fibers connecting areas of the cerebral cortex that are not adjacent; called also *long arcuate fibers.*

fi′brae associatio′nis telence′phali [TA] association fibers of telencephalon: nerve fibers that interconnect portions of the cerebral cortex within a hemisphere. See *fibrae associationis breves, fibrae associationis longae,* and *fibrae arcuatae cerebri.*

fi′brae circula′res mus′culi cilia′ris [TA] circular fibers of ciliary muscle: the most internal fibers of the ciliary muscle that form a discrete portion of the ciliary muscle and extend around the apex of the ciliary body close to the root of the iris. Called also *Müller fibers* or *muscle* and *sphincter fibers of ciliary muscle.*

f. commissura′lis [TA] commissural fiber: one of the nerve fibers that pass between the cortices of opposite hemispheres of the brain, or between two sides of the brainstem or spinal cord. Called also *neurofibra commissuralis.* See also *fibrae commissuralis telencephali.*

fi′brae commissura′les telence′phali [TA] commissural fibers of telencephalon: the nerve fibers that interconnect regions of the two hemispheres, crossing the median plane.

fi′brae corticonuclea′res corticonuclear fibers: longitudinal fibers of the pyramidal tract (see *tractus pyramidalis*) that arise in the cerebral cortex, descend in the internal capsule, and synapse in the various motor nuclei of the mesencephalon, pons, and medulla oblongata. Together they form the corticonuclear tract. Called also *corticobulbar fibers.*

fi′brae corticoponti′nae [TA] corticopontine fibers: nerve fibers that arise in the cerebral cortex of the frontal, temporal, parietal, and occipital lobes, descend in the internal capsule and cerebral peduncle, and terminate at different levels in the pontine nuclei where they are relayed chiefly to the opposite cerebellar hemisphere. Collectively called *corticopontine tract* or *tractus corticopontinus.*

fi′brae corticoreticula′res [TA] corticoreticular fibers: nerve fibers that arise chiefly in the sensorimotor areas of the cerebral cortex, descend with corticospinal fibers, and synapse with cells of the reticular formation, especially in the pons and medulla oblongata.

fi′brae corticorubra′les [TA] corticorubral fibers: nerve fibers that descend from the cortex of the frontal lobe through the posterior limb of the internal capsule to terminate in the red nucleus.

fi′brae corticospina′les [TA] corticospinal fibers: longitudinal fibers that arise in the cerebral cortex, descend in the internal capsule, mesencephalon, pons, and pyramids of the medulla oblongata, and which form, upon reaching the spinal cord, the lateral and ventral corticospinal tracts; see also *tractus pyramidalis.*

fi′brae corticothala′micae [TA] corticothalamic fibers: nerve fibers that project from the cerebral cortex through the centrum semiovale to terminate in the thalamus.

fi′brae dentatorubra′les dentatorubral fibers: afferent nerve fibers received by the red nucleus from the contralateral dentate nucleus.

fi′brae frontoponti′nae [TA] frontopontine fibers: nerve fibers that arise in the frontal lobe of the cerebral hemisphere and traverse the internal capsule and peduncle, ending in the pontine nuclei. Together they form the frontopontine tract (tractus frontopontinus).

fi′brae intercrura′les [TA] intercrural fibers: muscle fibers joining the medial and lateral crura of the superficial inguinal ring. Called also *intercolumnar fibers.*

fi′brae intrathala′micae [TA] intrathalamic fibers: neurons located within the thalamus whose axons project to other areas within the thalamus

fi′brae len′tis [TA] fibers of lens: long bands, derived from the epithelium, that make up the substance of the lens.

fi′brae longitudina′les mus′culi cilia′ris fibrae meridionales musculi ciliaris.

fi′brae meridiona′les mus′culi cilia′ris [TA] meridional fibers of ciliary muscle: the most external fibers of the ciliary muscle that run meridionally or longitudinally from the reticulum trabeculae toward the ciliary processes. Called also *Brücke fibers* and *longitudinal fibers of ciliary muscle.*

fi′brae obli′quae tu′nicae muscula′ris [TA], **fi′brae obli′quae ventri′culi** oblique fibers of muscular layer or coat: the inner obliquely coursing fibers of the muscular layer or coat of the stomach; called also *oblique fibers of stomach.*

fi′brae paraventricula′res, fi′brae paraventriculohypophysia′les [TA] paraventricular fibers: the efferent fiber components of the hypothalamicohypophysial tract that arise in the paraventricular nucleus and form the paraventriculohypophysial tract.

fi′brae parietoponti′nae [TA] parietopontine fibers: nerve fibers that arise in the cerebral cortex of the parietal lobe, descend in the sublentiform part of the posterior limb of the internal capsule to become constituent fibers of the basis pedunculi cerebri of the ventral part of the cerebral peduncle, and end in the pontine nuclei.

fi′brae parietotemporoponti′nae parietotemporopontine fibers: the fibrae parietopontinae and fibrae temporopontinae considered together.

fi′brae periventricula′res [TA] periventricular fibers: fibers that arise from the hypothalamus, then descend in the central gray matter through the tegmentum of the mesencephalon and the reticular formation of the pons and medulla oblongata; some are found in the dorsal longitudinal fasciculus.

fi′brae pon′tis longitudina′les [TA] longitudinal pontine fibers: a group of longitudinal nerve fibers that arise in the crus cerebri and run to the ventral part of the pons, where they become dispersed into smaller bundles, separated by the nuclei of the pons and the transverse fibers of the pons. The group includes the corticospinal, corticonuclear, corticoreticular, and corticopontine fibers.

fi′brae pon′tis profun′dae the more deeply situated of the fibrae pontis transversae.

fi′brae pon′tis superficia′les the more superficial of the fibrae pontis transversae.

fi′brae pon′tis transver′sae [TA] transverse pontine fibers: fibers within the ventral part of the pons which arise from the pontine nuclei and run laterally to form the middle cerebellar peduncles. Most of these fibers cross the midline. They are part of the frontopontocerebellar pathway.

fi′brae pontocerebella′res [TA] pontocerebellar fibers: longitudinal fibers in the ventral part of the pons that terminate in the vermis of the cerebellum.

f. projectio′nis [TA] projection fiber: one of the nerve fibers that connect the cerebral cortex with the subcortical centers, the brainstem, and the spinal cord; called also *neurofibra projectionis.*

fi′brae radia′les mus′culi cilia′ris [TA] radial fibers of ciliary muscle: the fibers of the ciliary muscle lying between the meridional (external) fibers and the circular (internal) fibers; they run in a radial or oblique direction from one to another and may form a fibrous network. Called also *oblique fibers of ciliary muscle.*

fi′brae spinohypothala′micae [TA] spinohypothalamic fibers: nerve fibers originating in the spinal cord and ascending as part of the anterolateral system to terminate in the hypothalamic areas and nuclei.

fi′brae spinomesencepha′licae [TA] spinomesencephalic fibers: nerve fibers originating in the spinal cord and ascending as part of the anterolateral system to terminate in the mesencephalon; they are subclassified as spinoperiaqueductal (fibrae spinoperiaqueductales) and spinotectal fibers (fibrae spinotectales).

fi′brae spinooliva′res [TA] spino-olivary fibers: nerve fibers originating in the spinal cord and ascending as part of the anterolateral system to terminate in the olivary nuclei.

fi′brae spinoperiaqueducta′les [TA] spinoperiaqueductal fibers: the subgroup of spinomesencephalic fibers of the anterolateral system that originate in the spinal cord and project to the periaqueductal gray substance.

fi′brae spinoreticula′res [TA] spinoreticular fibers: nerve fibers originating in the spinal cord and ascending as part of the anterolateral system to terminate in the reticular formation of the medulla, pons, and midbrain.

fi′brae spinotecta′les [TA] spinotectal fibers: the subgroup of spinomesencephalic fibers of the anterolateral system that originate in the spinal cord and project to the tectum.

fi′brae spinothala′micae [TA] spinothalamic fibers: nerve fibers originating in the spinal cord and ascending to terminate in the thalamus, most decussating in the anterior white commissure. They constitute one of the fiber populations of the anterolateral system.

fi′brae stri′ae termina′lis [TA] fibers of stria terminalis: the myelinated nerve fibers that make up the stria terminalis.

fi′brae supraop′ticae, fi′brae supraopticohypophysia′les [TA] supraoptic fibers: the efferent fiber components of the hypothalamicohypophysial tract that arise in the supraoptic nucleus and form the supraopticohypophysial tract.

fi′brae temporoponti′nae [TA] temporopontine fibers: nerve fibers that arise in the cerebral cortex of the temporal lobe, descend in the sublentiform part of the posterior limb of the internal capsule to become constituent fibers of the crus cerebri, and end in the pontine nuclei.

fi′brae thalamoparieta′les [TA] thalamoparietal fibers: nerve fibers that project from the parietal lobe through the posterior limb of the internal capsule to end in the thalamus.

fi′brae zonula′res [TA] zonular fibers: the fibers that anchor the lens capsule to the ciliary body and the retina; called also *aponeurosis of Zinn.*

fi•brae (fi′bre) [L.] genitive and plural of *fibra.*

fi•brates (fi′brāts) general term for fibric acid (q.v.) derivatives.

fi•bre (fi′bər) fiber.

fi•bric ac•id (fi′brik) any of a group of compounds structurally related to clofibrate that can reduce plasma levels of triglycerides and cholesterol; used to treat hypertriglyceridemia and hypercholesterolemia.

fi•bril (fi′bril) [L. *fibrilla*] a minute filament, such as a component of a fiber. **fi′brillar, fib′rillary** *adj*

anchoring f. a Type VII collagen fibril having a central cross-banded region and a fanlike group of filaments at each end that attach the dermis to the basement membrane by interweaving with collagen fibers in the dermis and lamina densa; these also occur in the gingiva, where they attach the epithelium to the lamina propria.

border f′s myoglia.

collagen f′s delicate fibrils of collagen in connective tissue, composed of molecules of tropocollagen in linear arrays. In Type I collagen, the most common type, the tropocollagen molecules are associated in periodic, staggered arrays that give the appearance of cross-banding, with a period of approximately 65 nm in the unit fibril; these unit fibrils are aggregated in bundles to form larger fibrils, with longitudinal striations, which may themselves be aggregated into fibers. Some other types of collagen also associate into fibrils (e.g., Types II, III, VI) but may not aggregate to show cross-banding or to form fibers. The terms fiber and fibril are sometimes interchanged loosely in descriptions of the hierarchy of collagen aggregation. See also under *fiber* and see illustration.

dentinal f′s component fibrils of the dentinal matrix.

fibroglia f′s see *fibroglia.*

muscle f., muscular f. myofibril.

nerve f. neurofibril.

perichromatin f′s fibrils, consisting of RNA polymerase II together with splicing factors and RNA packaging proteins, that occur on the surface

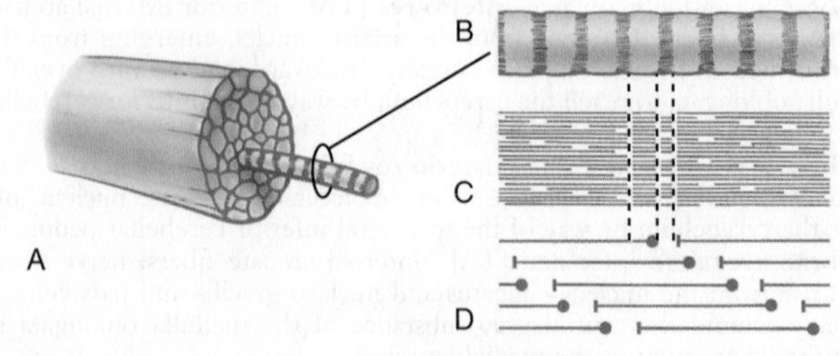

■ Type I collagen fibril *(A)*; it is composed of unit fibrils, here shown negatively stained *(B)*. The unit fibrils themselves comprise tropocollagen molecules in regular staggered arrays *(C, D)*.

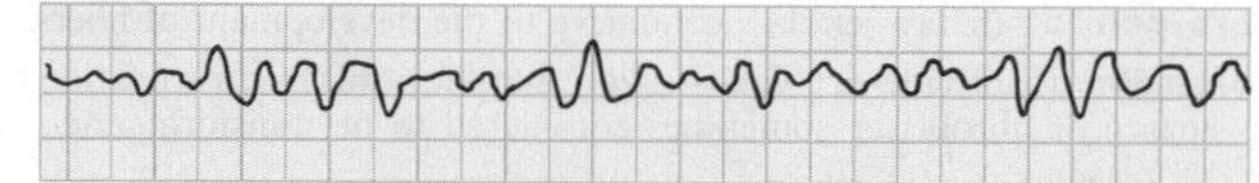

■ Ventricular fibrillation, characterized by an irregular undulating baseline.

of chromatin domains in the cell nucleus and are believed to be sites of RNA transcription and processing.

side f. of Golgi a twig that branches off at a right angle near the beginning of an axon of a ganglion cell.

Tomes f. odontoblastic process.

fi•bril•la (fi-bril′ə) gen. and pl. *fibril′lae* [L., dim. of *fibra*] a fibril.

fi•bril•lae (fi-bril′e) [L.] genitive and plural of *fibrilla.*

fi•bril•lat•ed (fi′brĭ-lāt″əd) made up of fibrils.

fi•bril•la•tion (fib″rĭ-la′shən) 1. the quality of being fibrillar. 2. a small, local, involuntary contraction of muscle, invisible under the skin, resulting from spontaneous activation of single muscle cells or muscle fibers whose nerve supply has been damaged or cut off. 3. the initial degenerative changes in osteoarthritis, characterized by softening of the articular cartilage and development of vertical clefts between groups of cartilage cells. 4. irregular, uncoordinated contraction of cardiac myocytes, either individually or in small groups; see *atrial f.* and *ventricular f.*

atrial f. (AF, AFib) an arrhythmia in which minute areas of the atrial myocardium are in various uncoordinated stages of depolarization and repolarization due to multiple reentry circuits within the atrial myocardium; instead of intermittently contracting, the atria quiver continuously in a chaotic pattern, causing a totally irregular, often rapid ventricular rate.

ventricular f. (VF, VFib) an arrhythmia characterized by fibrillary contractions of the ventricular muscle because of rapid repetitive excitation of myocardial fibers without coordinated contraction of the ventricle; it is an expression of randomized circus movement or of an ectopic focus with a very rapid cycle.

Fi•bril•len•struk•tur (fe-bril″en-shtrook′tər) [Ger.] the term used to describe the pattern of separate myofibrils that is typical of white skeletal muscles. Cf. *Felderstruktur.*

fi•bril•lin (fi-bril′in) a glycoprotein that is the main component of extracellular microfibrils and, with elastin, forms elastic fibers; in humans, there are two forms, designated fibrillin 1 and fibrillin 2. Abnormal fibrillin metabolism results in a variety of connective tissue disorders.

fi•bril•lo•blast (fi-bril′o-blast) odontoblast.

fi•bril•lo•gen•e•sis (fi-bril″o-jen′ə-sis) the formation of fibrils.

fi•bril•lol•y•sis (fi″brĭl-ol′ə-sis) destruction or dissolution of fibrils.

fi•bril•lo•lyt•ic (fi″bril-o-lit′ik) destructive to fibrils; causing fibrillolysis.

fi•brin (fi′brin) the insoluble protein formed from fibrinogen by the proteolytic action of thrombin during normal clotting of blood; it forms the essential portion of the blood clot. **fi′brinous** *adj*

stroma f. fibrin obtained from the stroma of blood cells.

fi•brin•ase (fi′brin-ās) factor XIII; see under *coagulation factors,* at *factor.*

fi•bri•no•cel•lu•lar (fi″brĭ-no-sel′u-lər) made up of fibrin and cells.

fi•brin•o•gen (fi-brin′o-jən) [*fibrin* + *-gen*] factor I; see under *coagulation factors,* at *factor.*

fi•brin•og•en•ase (fi″brin-oj′ə-nās) [*fibrinogen* + *-ase*] thrombin.

fi•brin•o•gen•emia (fi-brin″o-jə-ne′me-ə) hyperfibrinogenemia.

fi•bri•no•gen•e•sis (fi″brĭ-no-jen′ə-sis) the production or formation of fibrin.

fi•bri•no•gen•ic (fi″brĭ-no-jen′ik) producing or causing the formation of fibrin; called also *fibrinogenous.*

fi•bri•no•ge•nol•y•sis (fi″brĭ-no-jə-nol′ə-sis) [*fibrinogen* + *-lysis*] the dissolution or inactivation of fibrinogen in the blood.

fi•bri•no•geno•lyt•ic (fi″brĭ-no-jen″o-lit′ik) 1. pertaining to fibrinogenolysis. 2. inducing or causing fibrinogenolysis.

fi•brino•geno•pe•nia (fi-brin″o-jen″o-pe′ne-ə) hypofibrinogenemia.

fi•bri•nog•e•nous (fi″brĭ-noj′ə-nəs) 1. fibrinogenic. 2. caused by fibrin, or resulting from the formation of fibrin.

fi•brin•oid (fi′brin-oid) [*fibrin* + *-oid*] 1. resembling fibrin. 2. a homogeneous, eosinophilic, refractile, relatively acellular material with some of the tinctorial properties of fibrin.

fi•bri•nol•y•sin (fi″brĭ-nol′ə-sin) plasmin.

fi•bri•nol•y•sis (fi″brĭ-nol′ə-sis) the dissolution of fibrin by enzymatic action.

fi•bri•no•lyt•ic (fi″brĭ-no-lit′ik) 1. pertaining to or characterized by fibrinolysis. 2. causing fibrinolysis.

fi•bri•no•pep•tide (fi″brĭ-no-pep′tīd) either of two substances (*fibrinopeptide A* and *fibrinopeptide B*) split off from fibrinogen during coagulation, by the action of thrombin.

fi•bri•no•plate•let (fi″brĭ-no-plāt′lət) composed of fibrin and platelets, as a blood clot.

fi•bri•no•pu•ru•lent (fi″brĭ-no-pu′roo-lənt) characterized by the presence of both fibrin and pus.

fi•bri•nor•rhea (fi″brĭ-no-re′ə) a profuse discharge containing fibrin.

fi•bri•nos•co•py (fi-brĭ-nos′kə-pe) inoscopy.

fi•brin•uria (fi″brĭ-nu′re-ə) the presence of fibrin in the urine.

fibr(o)- [L. *fibra* fiber] a combining form denoting relationship to fibers.

fi•bro•ad•e•no•ma (fi″bro-ad″ə-no′mə) adenoma containing fibrous tissue. **fibroadeno′matous** *adj*

giant f. of breast phyllodes tumor.

intracanalicular f. a fibroadenoma of the breast with irregularly shaped clefts within a fibrous stroma that contains strands or cords of epithelial tissue; polypoid masses grow inward and compress the ducts.

pericanalicular f. a fibroadenoma of the breast with glandlike or cystlike spaces lined by epithelial cells in single or multiple layers.

fi•bro•ad•e•no•sis (fi″bro-ad″ə-no′sis) a nodular condition of the breast not due to neoplasm.

fi•bro•ad•i•pose (fi″bro-ad′ĭ-pōs) both fibrous and fatty.

fi•bro•an•gi•o•ma (fi″bro-an″je-o′mə) [*fibro-* + *angioma*] an angioma containing much fibrous tissue.

nasopharyngeal f. juvenile nasopharyngeal angiofibroma.

fi•bro•are•o•lar (fi″bro-ə-re′o-lər) [*fibro-* + *areolar*] both fibrous and areolar.

fi•bro•at•ro•phy (fi″bro-at′ro-fe) a combination of fibrosis and atrophy.

fi•bro•blast (fi′bro-blast) [*fibro-* + *-blast*] 1. a flat, elongated connective tissue cell with cytoplasmic processes at each end, capable of differentiating into a chondroblast, collagenoblast, or osteoblast, and forming fibrous tissues in the body such as tendons, aponeuroses, and other supporting and binding tissues. Called also *fibrocyte* and *desmocyte.* 2. collagenoblast.

pericryptal f′s flattened fibroblasts forming a sheath around the intestinal glands of the colon.

fi•bro•blas•tic (fi″bro-blas′tik) 1. pertaining to fibroblasts. 2. fibroplastic.

fi•bro•blas•to•ma (fi″bro-blas-to′mə) [*fibroblast* + *-oma*] a tumor arising from fibroblasts; types are divided into fibromas and fibrosarcomas.

perineural f. neurilemoma.

fi•bro•bron•chi•tis (fi″bro-brong-ki′tis) fibrinous bronchitis.

fi•bro•cal•cif•ic (fi″bro-kal-sif′ik) pertaining to or characterized by partially calcified fibrous tissue.

fi•bro•car•ci•no•ma (fi″bro-kahr″sĭ-no′mə) scirrhous carcinoma.

fi•bro•car•ti•lage (fi″bro-kahr′tĭ-ləj) a type of cartilage made up of typical cartilage cells (chondrocytes), with parallel thick, compact collagenous bundles forming the interstitial substances, separated by narrow clefts enclosing the encapsulated cells; called also *stratified cartilage.* For names of specific structures composed of such tissue, see under *fibrocartilago.* **fibrocartilag′inous** *adj*

basal f. fibrocartilago basalis.

circumferential f. fibrocartilage that forms a rim about a joint cavity.

connecting f. a disk of fibrocartilage that attaches opposing bones to each other by synchondrosis; called also *spongy f.*

cotyloid f. labrum acetabulare.

elastic f. fibrocartilage containing elastic fibers.

interarticular f. discus articularis.

semilunar f′s crescent-shaped structures resting on the articulating surfaces of the upper end of the tibia, increasing the concavity of the tibial condyles and acting as cushions or shock absorbers; the lateral and medial menisci.

spongy f. connecting f.

stratiform f. cartilage such as that lining the bony grooves lodging certain tendons.

white f. fibrocartilage in which strong bundles of white fibrous tissue predominate.

yellow f. fibrocartilage containing bundles of yellow elastic fibers but with little or no white fibrous tissue.

fi•bro•car•ti•lag•i•nes (fi″bro-kahr″tĭ-laj′ĭ-nēz) [L.] plural of *fibrocartilago.*

fi•bro•car•ti•la•go (fi″bro-kahr″tĭ-lah′go) pl. *fibrocartilag′ines* [L.] fibrocartilage.

f. basa′lis basal fibrocartilage: the cartilage that fills the foramen lacerum of the skull.

f. navicula′ris a fibrocartilaginous facet on the dorsal surface of the plantar calcaneonavicular ligament that helps form the articular cavity for the head of the talus.

fi•bro•ca•seous (fi″bro-ka′shəs) both fibrous and caseous.

fi•bro•cel•lu•lar (fi″bro-sel′u-lər) partly fibrous and partly cellular.

fi•bro•chon•dri•tis (fi″bro-kon-dri′tis) [*fibro-* + *chondritis*] inflammation of a fibrocartilage.

fi•bro•chon•dro•ma (fi″bro-kon-dro′mə) chondrofibroma.

fi•bro•col•lag•e•nous (fi″bro-ko-laj′ə-nəs) both fibrous and collagenous; pertaining to or composed of fibrous tissue mainly composed of collagen.

fi•bro•cys•tic (fi″bro-sis′tik) characterized by the development of cystic spaces, especially in relation to some duct or gland, accompanied by an overgrowth of fibrous tissue.

fi•bro•cyte (fi′bro-sīt) [*fibro-* + *-cyte*] fibroblast.

fi•bro•cy•to•gen•e•sis (fi′bro-si″to-jen′ə-sis) [*fibrocyte* + *-genesis*] the development of connective tissue fibrils.

fi•bro•dys•pla•sia (fi″bro-dis-pla′zhə) abnormality in development of fibrous connective tissue.

f. ossi′ficans progressi′va a rare, progressive, fatal, autosomal dominant disorder caused by mutation of the *ACVR1* gene (locus: 2q23-q24), which encodes a receptor that signals a specific transcriptional response related to growth and differentiation. It is characterized by extensive fibroblastic proliferation of various muscles and soft tissues followed by disabling ossification of skeletal muscles, tendons, fascia, and ligaments. Called also *myositis ossificans progressiva.*

fi•bro•elas•tic (fi″bro-e-las′tik) composed of fibrous and elastic tissue.

fi•bro•elas•to•ma (fi″bro-e-las-to′mə) a benign neoplasm consisting of fibroelastic elements.

papillary f. the most common heart valve tumor, composed of a characteristic cluster of hairlike projections consisting of collagen surrounded by elastic fibers and connective tissue and covered by endothelium, attached to a valve or to the papillary muscles, chordae tendineae, or endocardium.

fi•bro•elas•to•sis (fi″bro-e″las-to′sis) overgrowth of fibroelastic elements.

endocardial f. diffuse patchy thickening of the mural endocardium, particularly in the left ventricle, due to proliferation of collagenous and elastic tissue. It usually occurs in infants without other cardiac defects, but may occur in adolescents and adults, usually in association with congenital cardiac malformations. Thickening and incompetence of mitral and aortic valves is often associated. It is usually classified as *dilated* if the left ventricle is enlarged and hypertrophied or *contracted* if the left ventricle is of normal or reduced size.

primary endocardial f. a congenital form of endocardial fibroelastosis, manifest in infancy and occurring unassociated with other cardiac defects.

fi•bro•en•chon•dro•ma (fi″bro-en″kon-dro′mə) [*fibro-* + *enchondroma*] enchondroma containing fibrous elements.

fi•bro•ep•i•the•li•al (fi″bro-ep″ĭ-the′le-əl) having fibrous and epithelial elements.

fi•bro•ep•i•the•li•o•ma (fi″bro-ep″ĭ-the″le-o′mə) a tumor composed of fibrous and epithelial elements.

premalignant f. a rare, usually indolent variant of basal cell carcinoma, presenting as a firm sessile to pedunculated papule, usually on the lower trunk or lumbosacral area in middle-aged or older adults. Histologically it is characterized by prominent stromal fibrosis with long anastomosing cords of basal cells. Called also *premalignant fibroepithelial tumor* and *Pinkus tumor.*

fi•bro•fas•ci•tis (fi″bro-fə-si′tis) fibrositis.

fi•bro•fat•ty (fi″bro-fat′e) both fibrous and fatty.

fi•bro•fi•brous (fi″bro-fi′brəs) joining or connecting fibers.

fi•bro•fol•lic•u•lo•ma (fi″bro-fə-lik″u-lo′mə) [*fibro-* + *folliculus* + *-oma*] a type of benign adnexal tumor, a hamartoma of the perifollicular connective tissue, closely related to perifollicular fibroma and trichodiscoma, occurring as a yellow to white, smooth, dome-shaped papule, sometimes in groups. The usual location is on the face, and histologically it is characterized by proliferation of strands of follicular epithelium extending into the stroma. When there are multiple lesions, the patient may have *Birt-Hogg-Dube syndrome.*

fi•bro•gen•e•sis (fi″bro-jen′ə-sis) [*fibro-* + *genesis*] the development of fibers.

f. imperfec′ta os′sium a rare collagen disorder causing osteomalacia, with progressive skeletal pain and tenderness.

fi•bro•gen•ic (fi″bro-jen′ik) conducive to the development of fibers.

fi•brog•lia (fi-brog′le-ə) [*fibro-* + *-glia*] border fibrils in close relation to the surface of fibroblasts, sometimes considered to be transformations of the ectoplasm.

fi•bro•gly•can (fi″bro-gli′kan) syndecan-2; see *syndecan.*

fi•bro•hem•or•rhag•ic (fi″bro-hem″o-raj′ik) attended with hemorrhage and fibrin formation.

fi•bro•his•tio•cyt•ic (fi″bro-his″te-o-sit′ik) having fibrous and histiocytic elements.

fi•broid (fi′broid) [*fibr-* + *-oid*] 1. having a fibrous structure; resembling a fibroma. 2. fibroma. 3. leiomyoma. 4. *(in the pl.)* a colloquial term for *uterine leiomyoma.*

fi•broid•ec•to•my (fi″broid-ek′tə-me) [*fibroid* + *-ectomy*] uterine myomectomy.

fi•bro•in (fi-bro′in) a white albuminoid, $C_{15}H_{23}N_3O_6$, from spiders' webs and the cocoons of insects.

fi•bro•ker•a•to•ma (fi″bro-ker″ə-to′mə) a skin lesion with aspects of both fibroma and keratosis.

acquired digital f., acral f. a rare, benign growth on the skin consisting of a flesh-colored, keratotic papulonodule surrounded by a collarette; the usual location is on a finger, but it can also appear elsewhere.

fi•bro•la•mel•lar (fi″bro-lə-mel′ər) characterized by the formation of fibers of collagen arranged in layers.

fi•bro•li•po•ma (fi″bro-lĭ-po′mə) [*fibro-* + *-lipoma*] lipoma containing an excess of fibrous tissue. **fibrolipo′matous** *adj*

fi•bro•ma (fi-bro′mə) pl. *fibromas, fibro′mata* [*fibr-* + *-oma*] a tumor composed mainly of fibrous or fully developed connective tissue; called also *fibroid* and *fibroid tumor.* **fibro′matous** *adj*

ameloblastic f. an odontogenic tumor characterized by the simultaneous proliferation of both epithelial and mesenchymal tissue, without the formation of enamel or dentin.

aponeurotic f., calcifying aponeurotic f. a recurrent benign tumor usually seen on the hands of persons under 20 years of age, occurring as a firm, fixed nodule composed of fibroblastic tissue with finely stippled calcifications, not attached to the overlying skin and infiltrating into surrounding soft tissue. Called also *juvenile aponeurotic f.*

f. caverno′sum a cavernous hemangioma containing an excess of fibrous tissue.

cementifying f. a tumor usually occurring in the mandible of older persons and consisting of fibroblastic tissue containing masses of cementum-like tissue.

cemento-ossifying f. an ossifying fibroma, particularly when characterized by globular cementoid calcifications.

central odontogenic f. a rare, benign, unencapsulated, odontogenic tumor of the jaw, usually the mandible, characterized by islands of odontogenic epithelium within fibrous connective tissue and sometimes by calcifications.

chondromyxoid f. a rare, benign, slowly growing tumor of bone of chondroblastic origin, usually affecting the large long bones of the lower extremity; it is characterized by chondroid, myxoid, and fibrous areas in a lobular pattern and often has a deceptively malignant histologic appearance resembling chondrosarcoma.

cutaneous f. a fibroma of the skin; see also *dermatofibroma.*

cystic f. a fibroma that has undergone cystic degeneration.

desmoplastic f. a rare, benign, fibrous, osteolytic neoplasm usually occurring in the mandible, in long tubular bones, or in the hip bone; it is characterized by abundant collagen formation and an absence of significant cellularity or pleomorphism.

f. du′rum a fibroma composed of fibrous tissue with few cells; called also *hard f.*

follicular f. fibrofolliculoma.

hard f. f. durum.

infantile digital f. see under *fibromatosis.*

intracanalicular f. see under *fibroadenoma.*

juvenile aponeurotic f. aponeurotic f.

juvenile nasopharyngeal f. see under *angiofibroma.*

f. mol′le, f. mollus′cum acrochordon.

f. myxomato′des myxofibroma.

nonossifying f., nonosteogenic f. an osteolytic, proliferative, sometimes painful lesion comprising a focus of fibrous tissue in the metaphyseal region of long bones, particularly of the lower extremities, usually occurring in late childhood or adolescence; it is similar to fibrous cortical defect (q.v.) but is generally larger and actively growing. Called also *metaphyseal fibrous defect.*

odontogenic f. see *central odontogenic f.* and *peripheral odontogenic f.*

ossifying f., ossifying f. of bone a benign, relatively slow-growing, central bone tumor, usually of the jaws, especially the mandible, composed of fibrous connective tissue within which bone is formed.

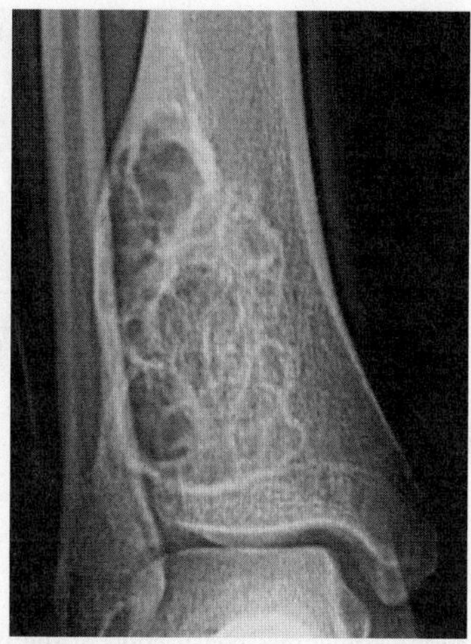

■ Nonossifying fibroma in the right distal tibia, with a characteristic scalloped border and bubblelike appearance.

parasitic f. see under *leiomyoma*.
f. pen′dulum acrochordon.
perifollicular f. a type of benign adnexal tumor consisting of a small, flesh-colored papule found on the head or neck near a hair follicle, often found in groups and probably a type of fibrofolliculoma.
peripheral odontogenic f. an extraosseous counterpart to a central odontogenic fibroma; it is a gingival mass of vascularized fibrous connective tissue with strands of odontogenic epithelium.
peripheral ossifying f. a fibroma, usually of the gingiva, showing areas of calcification or ossification. Called also *epulis*.
periungual f. a smooth, firm, protruding nodule on a nail fold; these are usually found in groups, are histologically angiofibromas, and are considered to be pathognomonic of tuberous sclerosis complex. Called also *Koenen tumor*.
pleomorphic f. a rare, benign, fibroblastic tumor of the skin or mucous membranes, characterized by pleomorphic hyperchromatic cells or giant cells in a collagenous stroma.
rabbit f. a benign viral disease of the wild cottontail rabbit, caused by a poxvirus, transmissible to laboratory rabbits, and marked by the development of fibromas that regress; called also *Shope f.*
recurrent digital f., recurring digital f. infantile digital fibromatosis.
Shope f. rabbit f.
f. sim′plex dermatofibroma.
soft f. acrochordon.
telangiectatic f. angiofibroma.
f. thecocellula′re xanthomato′des theca cell tumor.

fi•bro•ma•to•gen•ic (fi-bro″mə-to-jen′ik) producing or causing the formation of fibroma.

fi•bro•ma•toid (fi-bro′mə-toid) resembling fibroma; fibroma-like.

fi•bro•ma•to•sis (fi-bro″mə-to′sis) pl. *fibromatoses*. 1. a condition characterized by the formation of multiple fibromas. 2. the formation of a fibrous, tumorlike nodule arising from the deep fascia with a tendency to local recurrence, such as in a desmoid tumor.
aggressive f. desmoid tumor, particularly one that is extra-abdominal.
aggressive infantile f. an uncommon condition, present at birth or developing during infancy or childhood, characterized by fast-growing, firm, painless, single or multiple nodules involving subcutaneous tissue, muscle, fascia, and tendons and seen anywhere on the body; tumors are locally invasive but do not metastasize and have a high tendency to recur after excision.
f. col′li a firm, fusiform, fibrous mass in the midportion of the sternocleidomastoid muscle, usually occurring between two weeks and two months of age, and commonly disappearing in four to eight months; in some instances, torticollis may develop. It is believed by some to be a small hematoma due to injury to the muscle at birth.
congenital generalized f. a type of infantile myofibromatosis characterized by multiple small, firm, spherical or ovoid fibromas of subcutaneous tissue, muscle, viscera, and bone. Visceral involvement may be responsible for symptoms such as intestinal obstruction, diarrhea due to diffuse involvement of the intestines, and respiratory disturbances. Death frequently occurs during the neonatal period or early infancy.
desmoid f. see under *tumor*.
congenital multiple f. see *infantile myofibromatosis*, under *myofibromatosis*.
f. gin′givae, gingival f. 1. generalized or localized diffuse fibrous overgrowth of the gingival tissue, usually transmitted as an autosomal dominant trait, but some cases are idiopathic and others produced by drugs (see *Dilantin gingivitis*, under *gingivitis*). The enlarged gingiva is pink, firm, and leatherlike with a minutely pebbled surface and in severe cases the teeth are almost completely covered and the enlargement projects into the oral vestibule. Called also *elephantiasis gingivae*, *keloid of gums*, and *macrogingivae*. 2. fibromatous epulis (def. 2).
infantile digital f. a rare, often recurrent condition, usually seen in infants less than a year old, in which one or more small, smooth, dome-shaped, skin-colored to red nodules occur on the lateral or dorsal aspects of the fingers and toes; histologically, the lesions are composed of fibrous connective tissue and abundant collagen, and contain characteristic viruslike, black intracellular inclusions. Called also *infantile digital*, *recurrent digital*, or *recurring digital fibroma*.
juvenile hyaline f. a rare disorder, of autosomal recessive inheritance, characterized by multiple painless cutaneous papules containing spindle-shaped cells in an amorphous, acidophilic ground substance, occurring on the head, back, and extremities; lesions recur after removal and may continue to appear into adulthood.
palmar f. fibromatosis involving the palmar fascia, and resulting in Dupuytren contracture.
plantar f. fibromatosis involving the plantar fascia, manifested as single or multiple nodular swellings, sometimes accompanied by pain but usually unassociated with contractures.
subcutaneous pseudosarcomatous f. nodular fasciitis.

fi•bro•mec•to•my (fi″bro-mek′tə-me) [*fibroma* + *-ectomy*] 1. excision of a fibroma. 2. uterine myomectomy.

fi•bro•mem•bra•nous (fi″bro-mem′brə-nəs) composed of membrane containing much fibrous tissue.

fi•bro•mod•u•lin (fi″bro-mod′u-lin) a small (about 60 kD) leucine-rich repeat protein of the extracellular matrix, consisting of four keratan sulfate chains and associated oligosaccharides; it binds collagen I and II and may play a role in the assembly of the extracellular matrix.

fi•bro•mus•cu•lar (fi″bro-mus′ku-lər) composed of fibrous and muscular tissue.

fi•bro•my•al•gia (fi″bro-mi-al′jə) pain and stiffness in the muscles and joints that either is diffuse or has multiple trigger points.

fi•bro•my•itis (fi″bro-mi-i′tis) [*fibro-* + *myitis*] inflammation and fibrous degeneration of a muscle.

fi•bro•my•o•ma (fi″bro-mi-o′mə) [*fibro-* + *myoma*] leiomyoma.
f. u′teri leiomyoma uteri.

fi•bro•myo•mec•to•my (fi″bro-mi″o-mek′tə-me) uterine myomectomy.

fi•bro•myo•si•tis (fi″bro-mi″o-si′tis) [*fibro-* + *myositis*] inflammation of fibromuscular tissue.
nodular f. a disease marked by inflammation and the formation of nodules in the muscles.

fi•bro•myx•o•ma (fi″bro-mik-so′mə) myxofibroma.

fi•bro•myx•o•sar•co•ma (fi″bro-mik″so-sahr-ko′mə) [*fibro-* + *myxo-* + *sarcoma*] sarcoma containing fibromatous and myxomatous elements.

fi•bro•nec•tin (fi″bro-nek′tin) [*fibro-* + *nexus*] any of several related adhesive glycoproteins. One form circulates in plasma, acting as an opsonin; another is a cell-surface protein that mediates cellular adhesive interactions. Fibronectins are important in connective tissue, where they cross-link to collagen, and are also involved in aggregation of platelets.

fi•bro•neu•ro•ma (fi″bro-noŏ-ro′mə) neurofibroma.

fi•bro•nod•u•lar (fi″bro-nod′u-lər) consisting of nodules and fibrous tissue, often used to describe a pattern of nodules and linear opacities on a chest radiograph.

fi•bro•nu•cle•ar (fi″bro-noo′kle-ər) made up of nucleated fibers.

fi•bro-odon•to•ma (fi″bro-o″don-to′mə) [*fibro-* + *odont-* + *oma*] a tumor containing both fibrous and odontogenic elements.
ameloblastic f. a variant form of ameloblastic fibroma in which enamel and dentin are formed.

fi•bro-os•se•ous (fi″bro-os′e-əs) composed of both fibrous and bony tissue.

fi•bro-os•te•o•ma (fi″bro-os″te-o′mə) ossifying fibroma.

fi•bro•pap•il•lo•ma (fi″bro-pap″ĭ-lo′mə) fibroepithelial papilloma.

fi•bro•pi•tu•i•cyte (fi″bro-pĭ-too′ĭ-sīt) see *pituicyte*.

fi•bro•pla•sia (fi″bro-pla′zhə) the formation of fibrous tissue, as occurs normally in the healing of wounds and abnormally in some tissues.
adventitial f. perimedial f.
intimal f. a type of fibromuscular dysplasia that affects mainly children and young adult men, characterized by short localized areas of smooth stenosis of the tunica intima, either symmetrical or asymmetrical; sometimes it is secondary to trauma, surgery, or infection.

medial f. the most common type of fibromuscular dysplasia, seen mainly in adult women, characterized on an angiogram by the string of beads sign (areas of the artery wall having protruding aneurysms alternating with stenosis and thinning).

perimedial f. a rare type of fibromuscular dysplasia usually seen in women, characterized by stenotic fibrous tissue with dense collagen and a few aneurysms underlying an intact tunica media and tunica externa. Called also *adventitial* or *subadventitial f.*

retrolental f. (RLF) retinopathy of prematurity.

subadventitial f. perimedial f.

fi•bro•plas•tic (fi″bro-plas′tik) promoting or causing fibroplasia.

fi•bro•poly•cys•tic (fi″bro-pol″e-sis′tik) characterized by development of cystic spaces and an overgrowth of fibrous tissue.

fi•bro•pu•ru•lent (fi″bro-pu′roo-lənt) characterized by the presence of both fibers and pus.

fi•bro•re•tic•u•late (fi″bro-rə-tik′u-lāt) composed of a network of fibers.

fi•bro•sar•co•ma (fi″bro-sahr-ko′mə) [*fibro-* + *sarcoma*] a malignant tumor composed of cells and fibers derived from fibroblasts, which produce collagen but otherwise lack cellular differentiation; it is grossly grayish white and firm, invades locally, and metastasizes hematogenously. Several varieties occur: an aggressive *adult* form, a rarely metastasizing *infantile* or *congenital* form, an *inflammatory* form, and a *postirradiation* form.

ameloblastic f. an odontogenic tumor that is the malignant counterpart to an ameloblastic fibroma, within which it usually arises. Called also *ameloblastic sarcoma.*

odontogenic f. a malignant tumor of the jaws, originating from one of the mesenchymal components of the tooth or tooth germ, and histologically identical with other fibrosarcomas; the malignant counterpart of odontogenic fibroma.

fi•bro•scle•ro•sis (fi″bro-sklə-ro′sis) fibrosis associated with sclerosis.

multifocal f. any of a group of disorders of unknown etiology characterized by fibrosis, including mediastinal, hilar, and retroperitoneal fibrosis, Riedel struma, and sclerosing cholangitis.

fi•brose (fi′brōs) 1. to form fibrous tissue. 2. fibrous.

fi•bro•se•rous (fi″bro-se′rəs) composed of both fibrous and serous elements.

fi•bro•sis (fi-bro′sis) the formation of fibrous tissue, as in repair or replacement of parenchymatous elements. **fibrot′ic** *adj*

African endomyocardial f. endomyocardial f.

congenital hepatic f. a developmental disorder of the liver marked by formation of irregular broad bands of fibrous tissue containing multiple cysts formed by disordered terminal bile ducts, chiefly in the portal areas, resulting in vascular constriction, which leads to portal hypertension. It may be associated with polycystic renal disease.

cystic f., cystic f. of pancreas an autosomal recessive disorder of infants, children, and young adults in which there is widespread dysfunction of the exocrine glands, with signs of chronic pulmonary disease (due to excess mucus production in the respiratory tract), pancreatic insufficiency, abnormally high levels of electrolytes in the sweat, and occasionally biliary cirrhosis. Pathologically, the pancreas shows obstruction of its ducts by amorphous eosinophilic concretions, causing the insufficiency and resultant steatorrhea and azotorrhea. The degree of involvement of organs and glandular systems may vary greatly, with consequent variations in the clinical picture. It is caused by mutations in the *CFTR* gene, which encodes the cystic fibrosis transmembrane regulator (q.v.), a cAMP-regulated chloride channel that regulates other ion channels.

diatomite f. a form of silicosis caused by inhalation of the dust of diatomite (hard, dry infusorial earth).

diffuse interstitial pulmonary f. idiopathic pulmonary f.

endomyocardial f. idiopathic cardiomyopathy occurring endemically in various regions of Africa and rarely in other areas, characterized by cardiomegaly, marked thickening of the endocardium with dense, white fibrous tissue that frequently extends to involve the inner third or half of the myocardium, and congestive heart failure. Called also *African endomyocardial f.*

graphite f. see under *pneumoconiosis.*

idiopathic pulmonary f. chronic inflammation and progressive fibrosis of the pulmonary alveolar walls, with steadily progressive dyspnea, resulting finally in death from oxygen lack or right heart failure. Sometimes it is a component of bronchiolitis obliterans with organizing pneumonia (see under *bronchiolitis*).The acute, rapidly fatal form is called *acute interstitial pneumonia* or *Hamman-Rich syndrome.* Called also *chronic fibrous pneumonia, interstitial* or *usual interstitial pneumonia, diffuse interstitial pulmonary f., fibrosing alveolitis,* and *interstitial* or *interstitial pulmonary f.*

idiopathic retroperitoneal f. retroperitoneal f.

interstitial f., interstitial pulmonary f. idiopathic pulmonary f.

mediastinal f. development of hard white fibrous tissue in the upper mediastinum, causing compression, distortion, or obliteration of the superior vena cava, and sometimes constriction of the bronchi and large pulmonary vessels.

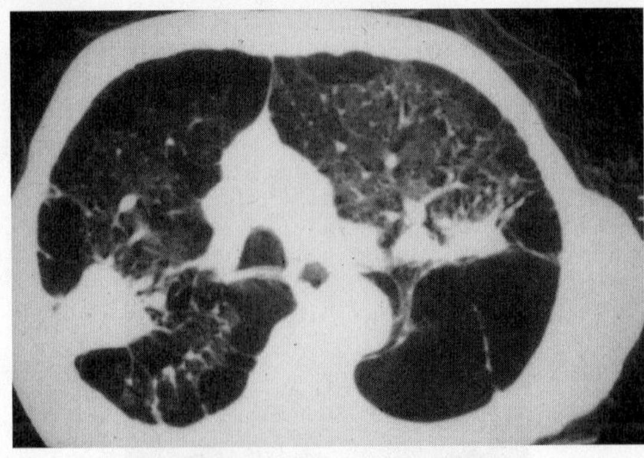

■ High resolution CT scan of progressive massive fibrosis, showing bilateral masses, with a background of nodules and bullous changes.

neoplastic f. proliferative f.

nephrogenic systemic f. nephrogenic fibrosing dermopathy.

nodular subepidermal f. 1. benign fibrous histiocytoma. 2. a subtype of benign fibrous histiocytoma characterized by multiple fibrous nodules beneath the epidermis resulting from inflammation. 3. dermatofibroma.

panmural f. of the bladder interstitial cystitis.

periureteral f., periureteric f. retroperitoneal f.

pipestem f. fibrosis around hepatic portal veins, seen as a complication of hepatic schistosomiasis. Called also *Symmers f.*

pleural f. fibrosis of the visceral pleura so that part or all of a lung becomes covered with a plaque or a thick layer of nonexpansible fibrous tissue. The more extensive form is called *fibrothorax.*

postfibrinous f. fibrosis occurring in tissues in which fibrin has been deposited.

progressive massive f. a complication of silicosis or coal workers' pneumoconiosis in which there is at least one dense lung lesion more than 1 cm in diameter; there are usually multiple lesions in the upper parts of the lungs, and they grow larger and more dense over time. The condition may be accompanied by emphysema or ischemia adjacent to the lesions.

proliferative f. fibrosis in which the fibrous elements continue to proliferate after the original causative factor has ceased to operate; called also *neoplastic f.*

pulmonary f. see *idiopathic pulmonary f.*

replacement f. the development of fibrous tissues to replace tissue that has been damaged.

retroperitoneal f. deposition of fibrous tissue in the retroperitoneal space; it may cause blockage of an intestinal loop or a ureter; in the latter case the result will be hydronephrosis, impaired renal function, and eventually renal failure. Called also *Ormond disease* and *perirenal fasciitis.*

root sleeve f. fibrosis and thickening of the dura mater resulting from prolonged nerve root pressure.

Symmers f. pipestem f.

fi•bro•si•tis (fi″bro-si′tis) [*fibro-* + *-itis*] inflammation especially of the muscle sheaths and fascial layers of the locomotor system; it is marked by pain and stiffness. Called also *fibrofascitis* and *muscular rheumatism.*

fi•bro•tho•rax (fi″bro-thor′aks) adhesion of the two layers of pleura, so that the lung is covered by a thick layer of nonexpansible fibrous tissue (see *dry pleurisy*). It is often a consequence of traumatic hemothorax or of pleural effusion.

fi•brous (fi′brəs) composed of or containing fibers.

fi•bro•vas•cu•lar (fi″bro-vas′ku-lər) both fibrous and vascular.

fi•bro•xan•tho•ma (fi″bro-zan-tho′mə) [*fibro-* + *xanthoma*] a type of xanthoma containing fibromatous elements; it is sometimes described as synonymous with or a subtype of either benign or malignant fibrous histiocytoma.

atypical f. (AFX) a small nodular cutaneous neoplasm usually occurring on sun-exposed areas of the face and neck in older white adults; it contains cells resembling histiocytes and fibroblasts and is sometimes considered to be related to or a subtype of either benign or malignant fibrous histiocytoma.

fi•bro•xan•tho•sar•co•ma (fi″bro-zan″tho-sahr-ko′mə) [*fibro-* + *xanthosarcoma*] malignant fibrous histiocytoma.

fib•u•la (fib′u-lə) [L. "buckle"] [TA] the outer and smaller of the two bones of the leg, which articulates proximally with the tibia and distally is joined to the tibia in a syndesmosis. See Plate 40.

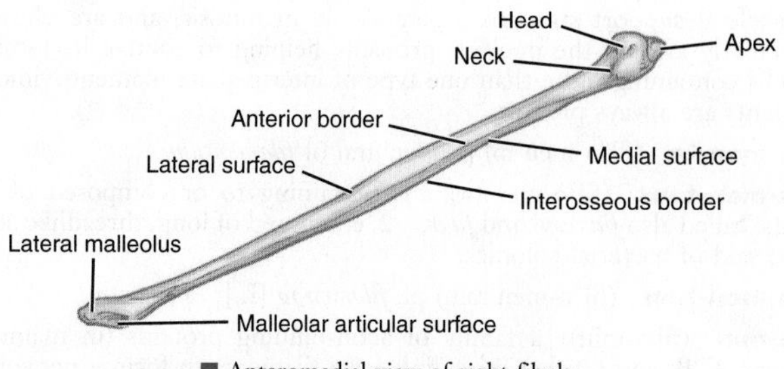

■ Anteromedial view of right fibula.

fib·u·lar (fib′u-lər) pertaining to the fibula or to the lateral aspect of the leg; peroneal. See also *fibularis.*

fib·u·la·ris (fib′u-lar′is) [L., from *fibula*] [TA] fibular; pertaining to the fibula. Called also *peroneal* and *peronealis* [TA alternative].

fib·u·lin (fib′u-lin) any of a family of calcium-binding glycoproteins, characterized by repeated epidermal growth factor–like domains and present in plasma and the extracellular matrix, that act as modulators of cell morphology, growth, adhesion, and motility.

fib·u·lo·cal·ca·ne·al (fib″u-lo-kal-ka′ne-əl) pertaining to the fibula and calcaneus.

fi·cain (fi′kān) [EC 3.4.22.3] an enzyme of the hydrolase class that catalyzes the cleavage of proteins on the carboxyl side of lysine, alanine, tyrosine, glycine, asparagine, leucine, and valine bonds. It is a cysteine endopeptidase derived from the sap of fig trees. Because it enhances the agglutination of red blood cells with IgG antibodies, it is used in the determination of the Rh factor; it is also used as a protein digestant in a variety of industrial applications.

FICD Fellow of the International College of Dentists.

fi·cin (fi′sin) ficain.

Fick's first law of diffusion, formula, etc. (fiks) [Adolf Eugen *Fick*, German physiologist, 1829–1901] see under *formula, law, method,* and *principle.*

FICS Fellow of the International College of Surgeons.

Fi·cus (fi′kəs) the figs, a genus of tropical shrubs and trees of the family Moraceae. *F. anthelmin′tica* Mart. is a wild species native to Central and South America whose sap, *leche de higuerón,* is medicinal. *F. bengalen′sis* is the banyan or banian, a species native to India and the East Indies whose branches send down auxiliary trunks that take root in the soil; its seeds and bark are tonic, antipyretic, and diuretic. *F. cari′ca* is the common fig tree. *F. elas′ticus* is the source of one kind of rubber.

Fied·ler disease, myocarditis (fēd′lər) [Carl Ludwig Alfred *Fiedler*, German physician, 1835–1921] see *Weil syndrome,* under *syndrome,* and see *acute isolated myocarditis,* under *myocarditis.*

field (fēld) 1. an area or open space, as an operative field or visual field. 2. a range of specialization in knowledge, study, or occupation. 3. in embryology, the developing region within a range of modifying factors.

auditory f. the space or range within which stimuli may be perceived as sound.

Cohnheim f's see under *area.*

cribriform f. of vision a field of vision over which a number of isolated scotomas lie dispersed.

dark-f. see under *microscope,* and see *ultramicroscope.*

electric f. a region of space in which an electric intensity exists at every point, causing charged bodies to be attracted to or repelled from each other; it is associated with an electromagnetic wave or a changing magnetic field.

electromagnetic f. a field of force resulting from electric charge in motion and having associated electric and magnetic components.

extended f. in radiotherapy, as for malignant lymphoma, an area of irradiation beyond the involved field.

eye f. see *frontal eye f.* and *occipital eye f.*

f. of fixation the region bounded by the utmost limits of central or clear vision, the eye being allowed to move, but the head being fixed.

Flechsig f. myelinogenetic f.

f's of Forel, Forel f's three areas in the ventral thalamus that are rich in nerve fibers and associated with cell groups. They are designated *fields H, H_1,* and *H_2.* Called also *areas of Forel.*

frontal eye f. an area in the precentral and frontal gyri (Brodmann areas 8, part of 6, and part of 9) concerned with the control of conjugate eye movements. Cf. *occipital eye f.*

gamma f. any area subjected to radiation from an unshielded or slightly shielded gamma radiation source.

f. H, f. H of Forel one of the fields of Forel, lying medial to the subthalamic nucleus, immediately rostral to the red nucleus; it is a large area in which pallidofugal, dentatothalamic, and rubrothalamic fibers and associated nuclei merge, uniting fields H_1 and H_2. Called also *prerubral f.* and *tegmental f.*

f. H_1, f. H_1 of Forel one of the fields of Forel; it is the area occupied by the thalamic fasciculus, although the term is sometimes used synonymously with thalamic fasciculus.

f. H_2, f. H_2 of Forel one of the fields of Forel; it is the area along the course of the lenticular fasciculus where the fibers of the fasciculus merge with the dorsal aspect of the subthalamic nucleus and the ventral aspect of the zona incerta.

high-power f. the area of a slide visible under the high magnification system of a microscope.

individuation f. a region in which an organizer influences adjacent tissue to become a part of a total embryo.

inverted Y f. in radiotherapy, as for malignant lymphoma, a circumscribed area of irradiation below the diaphragm, covering the spleen, extending down the midline, and branching inferiorly to form tails across the inguinal areas.

involved f. in radiotherapy, as for malignant lymphoma, the irradiated area when irradiation has been limited to sites of detectable macroscopic disease.

low-power f. the area of a slide visible under the low magnification system of a microscope.

magnetic f. that portion of space about a magnet in which its action is perceptible.

mantle f. in radiotherapy, as for malignant lymphoma, a circumscribed area of irradiation around the shoulders and chest, including the neck, clavicular regions, axillae, and mediastinum.

f. of a microscope the area that can be seen through a microscope at one time. The *high-power f.* is that area which is visible under the high-power objective; the *low-power f.* is that which is visible under low power.

morphogenetic f. an embryonic region, larger than its main derivatives, out of which definite structures normally develop.

myelinogenetic f. a collection of fibers in the neuraxis which at a definite stage of development receive myelin sheaths; called also *Flechsig's f.*

occipital eye f. any of several motor areas of the visual cortex that control voluntary or involuntary movements of the eye muscles. Cf. *frontal eye f.*

operating f., operative f. an isolated area where surgery is performed; it must be kept sterile by aseptic techniques (q.v.). Called also *surgical f.*

para-aortic f. in radiotherapy, as for malignant lymphoma, an area of irradiation below the diaphragm, covering the spleen and extending down the midline but ending before the pelvic area.

penumbra f. the region of free space which is irradiated by primary photons coming from only part of the radiation source.

prerubral f. f. H (of Forel).

primary nail f. a flat area on the terminal phalanx in the embryo where the nail is to develop.

spiral visual f. a visual field pattern, seen in functional visual loss, in which there is a continuous contraction of the visual field as it is plotted from meridian to meridian, so that the line connecting the limits of all of the meridians takes the form of a spiral.

sterile f. an operative field that is properly sterile according to aseptic techniques (q.v.).

surgical f. operative f.

surplus f. the portion of the field of vision in partial hemianopia which passes beyond the point of fixation.

tegmental f. f. H (of Forel).

tubular visual f. see *tunnel vision* (def. 1), under *vision.*

f. of vision visual f.

visual f. (F, vf) the area within which stimuli produce the sensation of sight with the eye in a straight-ahead position; also called *f. of vision.*

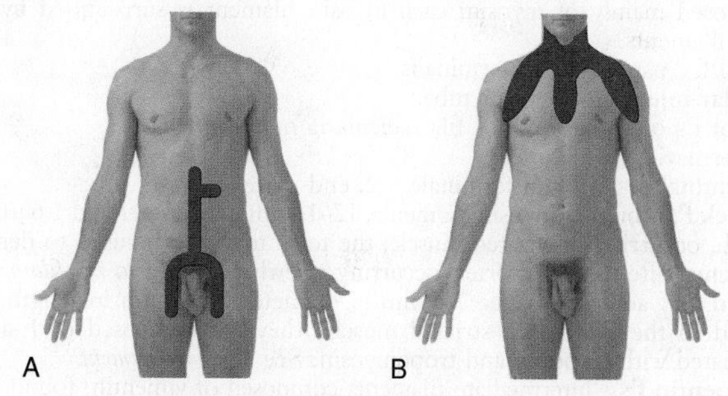

■ *(A),* Inverted Y field; *(B),* mantle field.

Wernicke f. see under *area*.

Fies·sing·er-Le·roy-Rei·ter syndrome (fe'sing-er lə-rwah' ri'tər) [Noël Armand *Fiessinger*, French physician, 1881–1946; Emile *Leroy*, French physician, early 20th century; Hans Conrad *Reiter*, German physician, 1881–1969] Reiter syndrome.

FIGLU formiminoglutamic acid.

FIGO [Fr.] Fédération Internationale de Gynécologie et d'Obstétrique (International Federation of Gynecology and Obstetrics); see under *classification*.

fig·u·ra·tum (fig″u-ra'təm) [L.] figured; said of skin lesions that have geometric patterns.

fig·ure (fig'yər) [L. *figura*, from *fingere* to shape or form] 1. an object of a particular form. 2. a number, or numeral.

flame f. a skin lesion seen with Wells syndrome, in which eosinophils and histiocytes surround collagenous masses and form small areas of necrosis.

fortification f's fortification spectrum; see under *spectrum*.

Lichtenberg f. a fernlike pattern of transient, erythematous skin lesions caused by a lightning strike.

Minkowski f. a numerical expression of the relation between glucose and nitrogen in the urine on a pure meat diet, and when fasting. It is 2.8:1.

mitotic f's stages of chromosome aggregation exhibiting a pattern characteristic of mitosis.

Purkinje f's patterns of shadows of retinal blood vessels cast onto the retina by obliquely projected light; called also *Purkinje shadows*.

Stifel f. a black disk having a white spot in the center, used for locating and measuring the blind spot in the eye.

Zöllner f's see under *line*.

fi·la (fi'lə) [L.] plural of *filum*.

fi·la·ceous (fi-la'shəs) filamentous (def. 1).

fil·ag·grin (fil-ag'rin) a protein that is synthesized in the granular layer of the epidermis and aggregates intermediate filaments of keratin by promoting formation of disulfide bonds.

fil·a·ment (fil'ə-mənt) [L. *filamentum*, from *filum* thread] a delicate fiber or thread.

actin f. one of the thin contractile myofilaments in a myofibril, composed mainly of actin; each actin filament is surrounded by three myosin filaments.

axial f. axoneme.

chromatin f. see under *fiber*.

desmin f's intermediate filaments composed of desmin, found in muscle cells; they provide a cytoskeletal framework to hold myofibrils in place and thus coordinate contraction of the cells.

glial f's intermediate filaments composed of glial fibrillary acidic protein, found in nonneuronal cells of the central nervous system, particularly astrocytes; they provide a framework for the cells and their cytoplasmic processes.

intermediate f's a class of cytoplasmic filaments, 8–11 nm in diameter, that predominantly act as structural components of the cytoskeleton and also allow various movements in cellular processes. Different types contain different, tissue-specific proteins; see also *desmin f's*, *glial filaments*, *keratin filaments*, *vimentin filaments*, *neurofilament*, and *lamin*.

keratin f's intermediate filaments composed of cytokeratins; they are usually heteropolymers formed from one acidic and one basic cytokeratin and are present in most epithelial cells. The cytokeratin composition varies in different types, states, and degrees of differentiation of the epithelia and has been used as an immunohistochemical marker. These filaments form a cytoskeletal framework, anchoring other elements and inserting into sites of cell-to-cell contact and are thus tonofilaments (q.v.).

lymphatic anchoring f's filaments that attach the endothelial cells of lymphatic capillaries to the connective tissue between surrounding tissue cells.

muscle f. myofilament.

myosin f. one of the thick contractile myofilaments in a myofibril, composed mainly of myosin; each myosin filament is surrounded by six actin filaments.

pial f. pars pialis fili terminalis.

polar injecting f. polar tube.

root f's of spinal nerve fila radicularia nervi spinalis.

spermatic f. end piece.

terminal f. 1. filum terminale. 2. end piece.

thick f's bipolar myosin filaments, 12–14 nm in diameter and 1.6 μm in length, occurring in striated muscle; the term may also be used to denote filaments, often much shorter, occurring elsewhere. See also *myofilament*.

thin f's actin filaments, 7–9 nm in diameter and 1 μm in length, attached to the Z-disks in striated muscle; they are composed of F-actin associated with troponin and tropomyosin. See also *myofilament*.

vimentin f's intermediate filaments composed of vimentin, found in a variety of cells derived from embryonic mesenchyme; they act as cytoskeletal support structures, play a role in mitosis, and are clustered particularly around the nucleus, probably helping to control its location. In cells containing more than one type of intermediate filament, vimentin filaments are always present.

fil·a·men·ta (fil″ə-men'tə) [L.] plural of *filamentum*.

fil·a·men·tous (fil″ə-men'təs) 1. pertaining to or composed of filaments; called also *filaceous* and *filar*. 2. composed of long, threadlike structures; said of bacterial colonies.

fil·a·men·tum (fil″ə-men'təm) pl. *filamen'ta* [L.] a filament.

fil·a·min (fil'ə-min) a family of actin-binding proteins (in mammals, filamins A, B, and C) that cross-link actin filaments to form a network in the cortex of many cells and regulate changes in cellular shape and motility; they also play a role in second messenger signaling.

fi·lar (fi'lər) filamentous (def. 1).

Fi·la·ria (fĭ-lar'e-ə) [L. *filum* thread] a name formerly used as a genus to include some members of the superfamily Filarioidea, now classified in a variety of genera.

fi·la·ria (fĭ-lar'e-ə) pl. *fila'riae* [L. *filum* thread] a nematode worm of the superfamily Filarioidea.

Bancroft f. *Wuchereria bancrofti*.

fi·la·riae (fĭ-lar'e-e) [L.] plural of *filaria*.

fi·la·ri·al (fĭ-lar'e-əl) 1. pertaining to filariae. 2. caused by filariae.

fil·a·ri·a·sis (fil″ə-ri'ə-sis) infestation by filariae.

bancroftian f. infection with the filarial worm *Wuchereria bancrofti*, adults of which live in the lymphatic system, producing recurrent lymphangitis with fibrosis and obstruction. In extensive obstruction, chronic edema may result, progressing to elephantiasis. Microfilariae circulate in the blood, where they are transmitted to feeding mosquitoes, the vector and intermittent host.

brugian f. infection with filarial worms of the species *Brugia malayi* and *B. timori*, the adult forms of which reside in the lymphatics, lymph nodes, and connective tissue; symptoms range from asymptomatic adenitis, to periodic attacks of fever and lymphangitis, to elephantiasis, especially of the lower limbs and feet. Microfilariae circulate in the blood, where they are transmitted to feeding mosquitoes, the vector and intermediate host.

lymphatic f. a general term comprising bancroftian and brugian filariasis.

Malayan f. brugian filariasis caused by *Brugia malayi*.

occult f. a condition in which microfilariae are present in the tissues but not in the blood; see *tropical pulmonary eosinophilia*, under *eosinophilia*.

Ozzard f. infection with *Mansonella ozzardi*.

perstans f. infection with *Mansonella perstans* (see also*mansonellosis*). Symptoms are usually mild and may include eosinophilia, abdominal and chest pain, edema, fever, and enlargement of the spleen and liver.

Timorian f. brugian filariasis caused by *Brugia timori*.

fi·lar·i·cid·al (fĭ-lar″ĭ-sīd'əl) [*filaria* + L. *caedere* to kill] destructive to filariae; cf. *antifilarial*.

fi·lar·i·cide (fĭ-lar'ĭ-sīd) an agent that destroys filariae.

fi·lar·i·form (fĭ-lar'ĭ-form) threadlike; resembling filariae; denoting that developmental stage in the life cycle of certain nematodes which is characterized by the possession of an esophagus of uniform diameter and which is often, as in hookworms, the infective stage.

Fi·lar·i·oi·dea (fĭ-lar″e-oi'de-ə) a superfamily or order of nematodes that are parasitic in many different animals. The adults are threadlike worms that invade the tissues and body cavities where the female deposits embryonated eggs (prelarvae) known as microfilariae. The microfilariae are then ingested by blood-sucking insects, in whom they pass their developmental stage, to be later returned to host animals when the insects bite them. Genera infecting humans include *Brugia*, *Loa*, *Mansonella*, *Onchocerca*, and *Wuchereria*. Those infecting domestic animals include *Dirofilaria*, *Parafilaria*, *Setaria*, and *Stephanofilaria*.

Fi·la·roi·des (fil″ə-roi'dēz) a genus of nematodes of the family Filaroididae. *F. hir'thi* and *F. os'leri* are lungworms that cause verminous bronchitis and occasionally verminous pneumonia in dogs.

Fil·a·roi·di·dae (fil″ə-roi'dĭ-de) a family of nematodes that infest the respiratory tract of mammals. It includes one genus of veterinary interest, *Filaroides*.

Fil·des enrichment agar (fil'dəz) [Sir Paul Gordon *Fildes*, English bacteriologist, 1882–1971] see under *culture medium*.

file (fil) a surgical or a dental instrument with a finely serrated surface, for reducing surplus hard substance such as bone or materials used in dental restorations, or for smoothing roughened surfaces.

endodontic f. root canal f.

root canal f. a file used in root canal therapy for cleaning and shaping the canal. Called also *endodontic f.*

fil·gras·tim (fil-gras′tim) a human granulocyte colony-stimulating factor (G-CSF) produced by recombinant DNA technology, used to stimulate neutrophil production, reduce the duration of neutropenia, and reduce the incidence of infection in patients receiving myelosuppressive chemotherapy for nonmyeloid malignancies or following induction or consolidation chemotherapy for acute myelogenous leukemia, to accelerate recovery and promote engraftment after bone marrow transplantation, to enhance peripheral progenitor cell yield in autologous hematopoietic stem cell transplantation, and to treat chronic, severe neutropenia; administered subcutaneously or intravenously.

fil·i·cin (fil′ĭ-cin) a compound found in oil of male fern.

fil·i·form (fil′ĭ-form, fi′lĭ-form) [*filum* + *form*] 1. thread-shaped. 2. an extremely slender bougie.

fil·io·pa·ren·tal (fil″e-o-pə-ren′təl) pertaining to the relationships between children and their parents.

fi·lix mas (fi′liks mas) [L. "male fern"] *Dryopteris filix-mas*, the male fern.

fil·let (fil′et) 1. a loop, as of cord or tape, for making traction on the fetus. 2. lemniscus.

fill·ing (fil′ing) 1. the material inserted into a prepared tooth cavity, usually gold, amalgam, cement, or a synthetic resin. 2. the process of inserting, condensing, shaping, and finishing this material in a prepared tooth cavity or root canal. Called also *restoration*.

complex f. a filling for a complex cavity.

composite f. a filling that consists of a composite resin.

compound f. a filling for a cavity that involves two surfaces of a tooth.

direct f. a filling that is formed and completed directly in the prepared tooth cavity.

direct resin f. a direct filling made from a synthetic resin.

ditched f. the marginal failure of an amalgam restoration due to fracture of either the material or the tooth structure itself in the affected area.

indirect f. a filling that is constructed on a die that has been made from an accurate impression of the tooth and that is then inserted into the tooth cavity.

permanent f. a filling intended to provide complete function while the tooth remains in the oral cavity.

retrograde f. in root canal therapy, an amalgam or other restoration placed in the apical portion of the canal to seal it after surgical removal of a periapical lesion; this is done through the apex, approached through the alveolar bone. Called also *retrograde amalgam*.

reverse f. retrofilling.

root canal f. 1. in root canal therapy, material(s) placed inside the canal to obturate or seal it. 2. canal obturation.

root-end f. retrofilling.

temporary f. a filling placed in a tooth cavity with the intention of removing it within a short period of time.

treatment f. a filling used to allay sensitive dentin prior to final preparation of the cavity.

film (film) 1. a thin layer or coating. 2. a thin transparent sheet of cellulose acetate or similar material coated on one or both sides with an emulsion that is sensitive to light or radiation.

absorbable gelatin f. [USP] a sterile, nonantigenic, absorbable, water-insoluble sheet of gelatin, used as an aid in surgical closure and repair of defects, as in the dura mater or pleura or after ocular surgery, and as a local hemostatic.

bite-wing f. radiographic film with a central protruding tab or wing to be held between the upper and lower teeth; used in dental radiography.

fixed blood f. a thin film of blood spread on a slide, dried quickly, and fixed.

lateral jaw f. a radiograph showing either the ramus or the body of the mandible.

occlusal f. a radiograph showing topographic and cross-sectional views of the maxillary or mandibular dental structure and adjacent tissue.

periapical f. film used in radiography of the root apex of a tooth and the surrounding structures.

plain f. a radiograph made without the use of a contrast medium.

spot f. a radiograph of a small anatomic area obtained either by rapid exposure during fluoroscopy to provide a permanent record of a transiently observed abnormality, or by limitation of radiation passing through the area to improve definition and detail of the image produced.

x-ray f. a film specially prepared for use in radiography; also, a radiograph.

film badge (film baj) a pack of radiographic film or films, usually worn on the body during potential exposure to radiation in order to detect and quantitate the dosage of exposure.

Fi·lo·ba·sid·i·el·la (fi″lo-bə-sid″e-el′ə) a genus of fungi classified in either order Ustilaginales or order Sporidiales.

F. bacillispo′ra *F. gattii.*

F. gat′tii the perfect (sexual) stage of *Cryptococcus gattii;* called also *F. bacillispora.*

F. neofor′mans the perfect (sexual) stage of *Cryptococcus neoformans.*

Fi·lo·ba·sid·i·um (fi″lo-bə-sid′e-əm) a genus of fungi classified in either order Ustilaginales or order Sporidiales. *F. florifor′me* is the perfect (sexual) stage of *Cryptococcus albidus.*

fi·lo·po·di·um (fi″lo-po′de-əm) pl. *filopo′dia* [*filum* + Gr. *pous* foot] a thin projection from a cell, supported by bundles of actin filaments and often associated with lamellipodium formation, thought to have an exploratory or sensory function.

fi·lo·var·i·co·sis (fi′lo-var″ĭ-ko′sis) the development of varicosities on the axon of a nerve fiber.

Fi·lo·vi·ri·dae (fi″lo-vir′ĭ-de) Marburg and Ebola viruses: a family of RNA viruses having enveloped filamentous virions, sometimes branching or U- or 6-shaped, 80 nm in diameter and varying greatly in length, with large peplomers, surrounding a helical nucleocapsid. The genome consists of a single molecule of negative-sense single-stranded RNA (MW 4.2×10^6, size 19.1 kb). Viruses contain seven major polypeptides and are sensitive to heat, ultraviolet and gamma radiation, beta-propiolactone, and formalin. Replication occurs in the cytoplasm and assembly is by budding through the plasma membrane. There is a single genus, *Filovirus.*

Fi·lo·vi·rus (fi′lo-vi″rəs) [L. *filum* thread + *virus*] the Marburg and Ebola viruses, a genus of viruses of the family Filoviridae that cause hemorrhagic fevers (Marburg virus disease, Ebola virus disease).

fi·lo·vi·rus (fi′lo-vi″rəs) any virus of the genus *Filovirus.* **filovi′ral** *adj*

fil·ter (fil′tər) [L. *filtrum*] 1. a membrane or other porous substance or device for the separation of impurities or particulate matter from liquid or gas. 2. to pass liquid or gas through such a device or material. 3. a device used to absorb electromagnetic radiation, particularly light, of specific wavelengths. 4. in radiology, a solid screen usually of varying thickness of metal (aluminum, copper, tin, lead, etc.) which when placed in the pathway of the radiation beam prevents transmission of beta particles and photons of longer wavelengths.

bird's nest f. an inferior vena cava filter consisting of four long, thin stainless steel wires with many bends, attached to struts that are fixed into place.

Greenfield f. an umbrella filter consisting of six stainless steel struts; small hooks on the ends of the struts anchor the filter in the vena cava when it is opened. Called also *Kimray-Greenfield f.*

inferior vena cava f. a filter used in transvenous vena caval interruption for the prevention of pulmonary embolism; the most common type is the umbrella filter. Called also *vena cava* or *vena caval f.*

Kimray-Greenfield f. Greenfield f.

membrane f. a filter made of a thin film of nylon, cellulose acetate, or other material, available in a range of defined pore sizes, usually in the range of 0.1–5 μm.

Millipore f. trademark for any of a variety of membrane filters.

Mobin-Uddin f. an umbrella filter consisting of six stainless steel spokes connected to a hub and covered by a perforated, heparin-impregnated Silastic membrane.

sintered glass f. a filter of sintered glass, available in various porosities, often designated from coarse to ultrafine.

umbrella f. the most common kind of vena cava filter for prevention of pulmonary embolism; it is inserted in a folded position and springs open like an umbrella to engage the caval wall. Common types are the Greenfield filter and Mobin-Uddin filter.

vena cava f., vena caval f. a filter used in transvenous vena caval interruption for the prevention of pulmonary embolism; the most common type is the umbrella filter. Called also *inferior vena cava f.*

Wood f. a filter of glass containing nickel oxide, which holds back all but a few violet rays of the visible spectrum and passes ultraviolet wavelengths of about 365 nm, used in Wood lamp. Called also *Wood glass.*

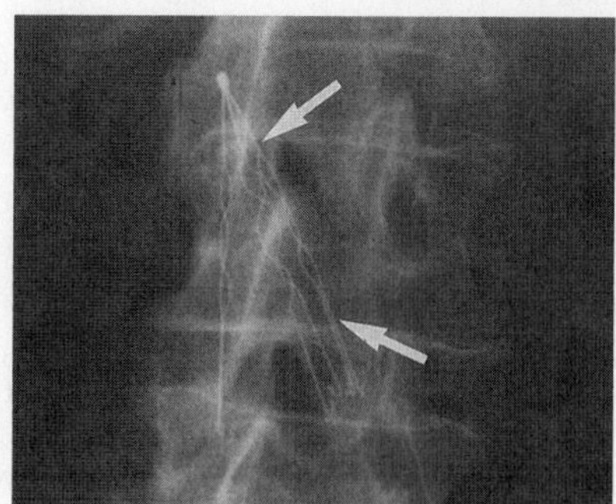

■ Vena cava filter. Expandable wire mesh basket *(arrows)* in the inferior vena cava.

fil·ter·a·ble (fil′tər-ə-bəl) capable of passing through the pores of a filter; usually referring to living infectious agents (i.e., viruses) able to pass through a filter that retains the usual pathogenic bacteria.

fil·tra·ble (fil′trə-bəl) filterable.

fil·trate (fil′trāt) a liquid or gas that has passed through a filter.
 glomerular f. the ultrafiltrate of plasma that passes across the membranes of the renal corpuscles into the urinary space.

fil·tra·tion (fil-tra′shən) 1. the passage of a liquid or gas through a filter. 2. in radiology, the use of a solid screen usually made of metal (aluminum, copper, tin, lead, etc.) to absorb beta particles and photons of longer wavelengths.
 gel f. a method for column chromatography in which high molecular weight substances are separated according to molecular size; see *gel-filtration chromatography.*
 reverse f. backfiltration.

fil·trum ven·tric·u·li (fil′trəm ven-trik′u-li) [L.] a depression between the two projections formed in the lateral wall of the vestibule of the larynx by the arytenoid and cuneiform cartilages.

fi·lum (fi′ləm) pl. *fi′la* [L.] a threadlike structure or part.
 f. corona′rium a tapering collagenous bundle that forms part of the fibrous annulus at each atrioventricular orifice; in the mitral valve one extends anteriorly and one posteriorly from the right fibrous trigone, partially encircling the orifice, and in the tricuspid valve they extend similarly from the left fibrous trigone.
 fi′la olfacto′ria [TA] olfactory nerves (1st cranial): the nerves of smell, consisting of about 20 bundles which arise in the olfactory epithelium and pass through the cribriform plate of the ethmoid bone to the olfactory bulb.
 fi′la radicula′ria ner′vi spina′lis [TA] rootlets of spinal nerve: the threadlike filaments by which the anterior and posterior roots of each spinal nerve are attached to the spinal cord. Called also *root filaments of spinal nerve.*
 f. termina′le [TA] terminal filum: a slender threadlike filament of connective tissue that descends from the conus medullaris to attach to the inner aspect of the dural sac and from there to the base of the coccyx; divided into a pial part *(pars pialis fili terminalis)* and a dural part *(pars duralis fili terminalis)*, the dividing line being the lower border of the second sacral vertebra.
 f. termina′le exter′num pars duralis fili terminalis.
 f. termina′le inter′num pars pialis fili terminalis.

fim·bria (fim′bre-ə) [L. *fimbriae* (pl.) a fringe] 1. a fringe, border, or edge. 2. pilus (def. 2).
 f. hippocam′pi [TA], **f. of hippocampus** the band of white matter along the medial edge of the ventricular surface of the hippocampus.
 ovarian f., f. ova′rica [TA] the longest of the processes that make up the fimbriae tubae uterinae, extending along the free border of the mesosalpinx; it is fused to the ovary, so that the ostium of the tube relates to the ovary.

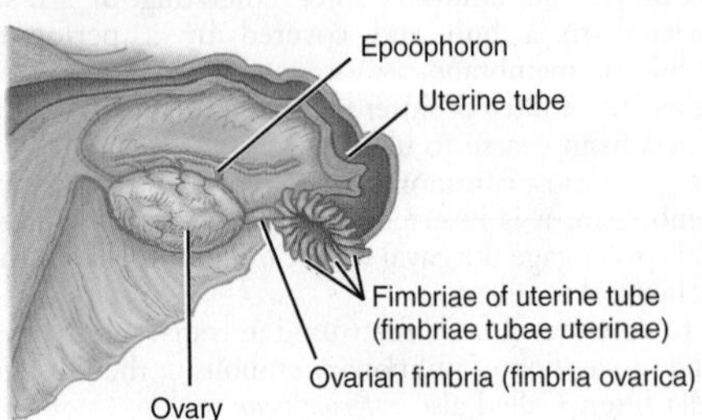

 fim′briae tu′bae uteri′nae [TA], **fimbriae of uterine tube** the numerous divergent fringelike processes on the distal part of the infundibulum of the uterine tube.

Fim·bri·a·ria (fim″bre-ar′e-ə) a genus of tapeworms of the family Hymenolepididae, which are parasites of anseriform birds. *F. fasciola′ris* infects wild and domestic fowl.

fim·bri·at·ed (fim′bre-āt″əd) fringed.

fim·bri·a·tion (fim″bre-a′shən) the formation of or the possession of fimbriae.

fim·bri·a·tum (fim″bre-a′təm) [L.] fringed.

fim·bri·ec·to·my (fim″bre-ek′tə-me) surgical removal of the fimbriae of the uterine tube along with tubal ligation as a method of female sterilization.

fim·brin (fim′brin) a 68-kD actin-binding protein that cross-links actin filaments to form tight, regular bundles in the epithelial brush border microvilli and the stereocilia of hair cells. Called also *plastin.*

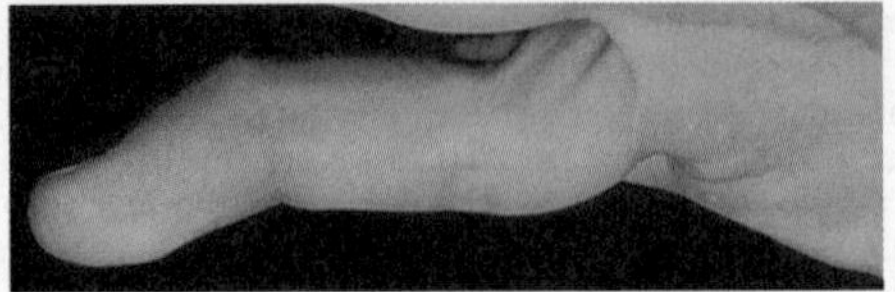
■ Mallet finger with secondary swan neck deformity.

fim·brio·cele (fim′bre-o-sēl″) [*fimbria* + *-cele*[1]] hernia containing fimbriae of the uterine tube.

fim·bri·o·plas·ty (fim′bre-o-plas″te) plastic surgery to the fimbriae of the uterine tube. **fimbrioplas′tic** *adj*

fin (fin) [A.S. *finn*] 1. a membranous appendage resembling a wing or paddle on the body of a fish or other aquatic animal; used for propulsion, guidance, or balance. 2. something resembling a fin in function or shape.
 nasal f. a thickened platelike ectodermal structure between the lateral and medial nasal prominences; it thins to form the oronasal membrane.

fi·nas·te·ride (fĭ-nas′tər-īd) [USP] an inhibitor of 5α-reductase, used in the treatment of benign prostatic hyperplasia and as a hair growth stimulant in the treatment of androgenetic alopecia; administered orally.

find·er (fīnd′ər) a device on a microscope to facilitate the finding of some object in the field.

find·ing (fīnd′ing) an observation; a condition discovered.

Fine·gol·dia (fīn-gol′de-ə) [Sydney M. *Finegold*, American microbiologist, born 1921] a genus of obligately anaerobic, gram-positive bacteria of the family Peptostreptococcaceae; organisms are non–spore-forming, nonmotile, pleomorphic cocci, occurring usually in masses and tetrads, but occasionally in pairs and short chains. The type species is *F. ma′gna.*
 F. mag′na a species that is part of the normal flora of the gastrointestinal and female genitourinary tracts and probably of the skin; it is a cause of septic arthritis and soft tissue infections. Formerly called *Peptostreptococcus magnus.*

Fine·vin (fin′vin) trademark for a preparation of azelaic acid.

fin·ger (fing′gər) any of the five digits of the hand. See *pollex, index, digitus medius, digitus anularis,* and *digitus minimus manus.*
 baseball f. mallet f.
 blubber f. seal f.
 clubbed f. a finger whose terminal phalanx is enlarged (cf. *clubbing*), sometimes having a coarse, curving nail called a hippocratic or watch crystal nail. Called also *drumstick* or *hippocratic f.*
 dead f. 1. a numb, mottled finger, as one seen in acrocyanosis. Called also *waxy* or *white f.* 2. hand-arm vibration syndrome.
 drop f. mallet f.
 drumstick f. clubbed f.
 fifth f. digitus minimus manus.
 first f. pollex.
 fourth f. digitus anularis.
 giant f. megalodactyly of the fingers.
 hammer f. mallet f.
 hippocratic f. clubbed f.
 index f. index (def. 1).
 little f. digitus minimus manus.
 lock f. a finger that is fixed in a flexed position, owing to the presence of a small fibrous growth in the sheath of the flexor tendon.
 Madonna f′s the thin, delicate fingers seen in acromicria.
 mallet f. partial permanent flexion of the terminal phalanx of a finger caused by a ball or other object striking the end or back of the finger, resulting in rupture of the attachment of the extensor tendon. Called also *baseball f., drop f.,* and *hammer f.*
 middle f. digitus medius manus.
 ring f. digitus anularis.
 seal f., sealer's f. a cellulitis of the hand, of unknown etiology and clinically resembling erysipeloid, occurring in handlers of seals and seal skins; called also *blubber f.*
 second f. index (def. 1).
 snapping f. trigger f.
 spider f. arachnodactyly.
 spring f. a condition in which flexion and extension of the finger beyond certain points are difficult.
 third f. digitus medius.
 trigger f. a finger liable to have a momentary spasmodic arrest of flexion or extension followed by a snapping into place, due either to stenosing tenosynovitis or to a nodule in the flexor tendon. See also *lock f.*
 tulip f′s a type of allergic contact dermatitis of the fingers in susceptible persons handling tulip bulbs.
 vibration white f. hand-arm vibration syndrome.
 waxy f. dead f. (def. 1).

webbed f's syndactyly of the fingers.
white f. dead f. (def. 1).
zinc f. see under *protein*.

fin·ger·ag·no·sia (fing″gər-ag-no′zhə) finger agnosia; see under *agnosia*.

fin·ger·nail (fing′gər-nāl) the nail of a finger; see *unguis* [TA].

fin·ger·print (fing′gər-print) 1. an impression of the cutaneous ridges of the fleshy distal portion of a finger; such records (as well as prints of hand or foot) are used as means of establishing identification. 2. the image obtained from fingerprinting (q.v.) of proteins or nucleic acids. 3. the infrared absorption spectrum of a molecule.
DNA f., genetic f. the image obtained by DNA fingerprinting (q.v.).

fin·ger·print·ing (fing′gər-print″ing) 1. originally, a technique for determining the structure of a protein in which the protein is enzymatically split into peptides and the fragments are separated in one direction by electrophoresis and at right angles by chromatography. After staining, the peptide fragments are seen to be in characteristic locations. The term has been extended to include related methods using other support media and other separation techniques. 2. DNA f.
DNA f. a technique for examining nucleic acids or nucleotides by digestion with a restriction enzyme and electrophoretic separation of the resulting fragements; the separated fragments are transferred to a nylon filter and hybridized with radioactive minisatellite probes. Because the number of repeats characterizing each specific minisatellite varies between individuals, the overall pattern obtained is unique to an individual genome; uses of the technique include identification of individuals and of lineage.

fin·ish (fin′ish) a desired surface texture given to something, such as a denture or an artificial crown.

Fin·kel·stein feeding (fing′kəl-shtīn) [Heinrich *Finkelstein*, German pediatrician, 1865–1942] see under *feeding*.

Fin·ney pyloroplasty (operation) (fin′e) [John Miller Turpin *Finney*, American surgeon, 1863–1942] see under *pyloroplasty*.

Fi·no·chi·et·to stirrup (fe-no″ke-et′o) [Enrique *Finochietto*, Argentine surgeon, 1881–1948] see under *stirrup*.

Fi·or·i·nal (fe-or′ĭ-nal) trademark for combination preparations of butalbital, aspirin, and caffeine.

Fi·or·tal (fe-or′təl) trademark for combination preparations of butalbital, aspirin, and caffeine.

fip·ro·nil (fip′ro-nil) a parasiticide used on cats and dogs to kill fleas and ticks; it acts by interfering with the insect's nervous system.

fire (fīr) fever; inflammation.
St. Anthony's f. 1. former name for *ergotism* (in humans). 2. former name for *erysipelas*.

fir·ing (fīr′ing) 1. the sintering of powder to produce porcelain, such as for a dental restoration. 2. the initiation of a nerve impulse.

Fir·mi·cu·tes (fər-mik′u-tēz, fur″mĭ-ku′tēz) [L. *firmus* strong + *cutis* skin] a phenotypically diverse phylum of mainly gram-positive bacteria; most have DNA that contains a lower percentage of guanine and cytosine in comparison with other bacteria and most have a cell wall that consists of a thick layer of peptidoglycan containing muramic acid. With Bacteroidetes, it is one of the two main constituents of the intestinal flora. There are three classes: Bacilli, Clostridia, and Mollicutes.

first aid (furst ād) emergency care and treatment of an injured or ill person before definitive medical and surgical management can be secured.

FISH fluorescence in situ hybridization.

Fish·berg concentration test (fish′bərg) [Arthur Maurice *Fishberg*, American physician, 1898–1992] see under *test*.

Fish·er exact test (fish′ər) [Sir Ronald Aylmer *Fisher*, British statistician, 1890–1962] see under *test*.

Fish·er syndrome (fish′er) [Charles Miller *Fisher*, Canadian neurologist, born 1913] see under *syndrome*.

fish·pox (fish′poks) a hyperplastic epidermal disease of viral origin occurring in fresh-water and marine fish.

fish (fish) any of various cold-blooded aquatic vertebrates, including some with bony skeletons and some with cartilaginous skeletons.
puffer f. any of several species of marine fish of the order Tetraodontidae, which when disturbed can inflate themselves to a spherical shape. Their flesh contains tetrodotoxin and can cause fatal poisoning. Called also *puffer*.
weever f. any of various fish of the family Trachinidae, found in the eastern Atlantic and the Mediterranean; their dorsal spines are venomous and cause severe pain in animals that get pricked.

fis·sile (fis′il) capable of being split; fissionable.

fis·sion (fish′ən) [L. *fissio*] 1. the act of splitting. 2. a form of asexual reproduction in which the cell divides into two or more daughter parts of equal size, each of which becomes a new, independent organism; it is seen chiefly in unicellular organisms such as bacteria. See also *binary f.* and *multiple f.*
binary f. fission of a cell in which the cell divides into two approximately equal daughter parts.
multiple f. fission of a cell in which the cell divides into a number of daughter cells.
nuclear f. the splitting of the nucleus of an atom, releasing a great quantity of kinetic energy.

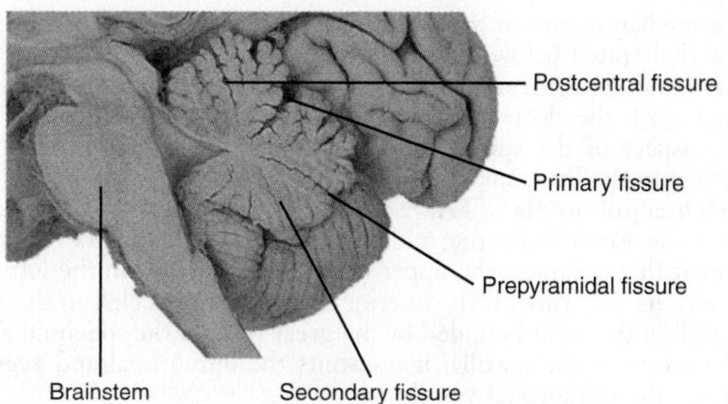

■ Fissurae cerebelli (cerebellar fissures).

fis·sion·a·ble (fish′ən-ə-bəl) capable of undergoing fission; fissile.

fis·sip·a·rous (fĭ-sip′ə-rəs) [L. *fissus* cleft + *-parous*] propagated by fission.

fis·su·la (fis′u-lə) [L., dim. of *fissura*] a little cleft.
f. an′te fenes′tram an irregular ribbon of connective tissue that extends through the bony otic capsule from the vestibule just anterior to the oval window, to the tympanic cavity near the processus cochleariformis.

fis·su·ra (fis-u′rə) gen. and pl. *fissu′rae* [L., from *findere* to split] fissure: a cleft or groove, especially a deep fold in the cerebral cortex that involves its entire thickness. Cf. *sulcus*.
f. in a′no anal fissure.
f. ansoparamedia′nis cerebel′li TA alternative for *f. lunogracilis cerebelli*.
f. ante′rior infe′rior cerebel′li TA alternative for *f. intrabiventralis*.
f. antitragohelici′na [TA] antitragohelicine fissure: a fissure in the auricular cartilage between the cauda helicis and the antitragus; called also *posterior fissure of auricle*.
fissu′rae cerebel′li [TA] cerebellar fissures: the numerous shallow grooves in the cortex of the cerebellum, on the surface and within the deep fissures, which divide the cortex into folia. See illustration.
f. choroi′dea ventri′culi latera′lis [TA] choroid fissure of lateral ventricle: the medially located line in the lateral ventricle along which the choroid plexus invaginates.
f. horizonta′lis cerebel′li [TA] horizontal fissure of cerebellum: the fissure that separates the superior from the inferior semilunar lobule of the cerebellum. Called also *f. intercruralis cerebelli* [TA alternative], *great horizontal fissure*, and *intercrural fissure*.
f. horizonta′lis pulmo′nis dex′tri [TA] horizontal fissure of right lung: the cleft that extends forward from the oblique fissure in the right lung, separating the upper and middle lobes.
f. intercrura′lis cerebel′li TA alternative for *f. horizontalis cerebelli*.
f. intrabiventra′lis [TA] intrabiventral fissure: a fissure occurring within the biventral lobule of the cerebellum and dividing it into lateral and medial parts. Called also *f. anterior inferior cerebel′li* [TA alternative] and *anterior inferior fissure*.
f. intraculmina′lis [TA] intraculminate fissure: a transverse cerebellar fissure dividing the culmen into anterior and posterior parts.
f. ligamen′ti te′retis [TA] fissure for ligamentum teres: the fissure or fossa on the visceral surface of the liver lodging the ligamentum teres in the adult; in the traditional anatomic conception, it forms part of the boundary between the right and left lobes of the liver. Called also *fissure of round ligament umbilical fissure* or *fossa (of liver)*, and *fossa of umbilical vein*.
f. ligamen′ti veno′si [TA] fissure for ligamentum venosum: a fossa on the posterior part of the diaphragmatic surface of the liver, lodging the ligamentum venosum in the adult.
f. longitudina′lis ce′rebri [TA] longitudinal fissure of cerebrum: the deep fissure between the cerebral hemispheres extending inferiorly to the corpus callosum.
f. lunogra′cilis cerebel′li [TA] lunogracile fissure; a fissure that separates the inferior semilunar lobule from the gracile lobule of the cerebellum. Called also *f. ansoparamedianis cerebelli* [TA alternative] and *ansoparamedian fissure*.
f. media′na ante′rior medul′lae oblonga′tae [TA] anterior median fissure of medulla oblongata: the longitudinal fissure in the median plane of the anterior aspect of the medulla oblongata, continuous with the

anterior median fissure of the spinal cord; it separates the pyramids and is partially obliterated below by their decussation.

f. media'na ante'rior medul'lae spina'lis [TA] anterior median fissure of spinal cord: the deep longitudinal fissure in the median plane of the anterior aspect of the spinal cord; it contains the anterior spinal artery ensheathed in the linea splendens.

f. obli'qua pulmo'nis [TA] oblique fissure of lung: 1. the cleft that separates the lower from the middle and upper lobes in the right lung. 2. the cleft that separates the upper from the lower lobe in the left lung.

f. orbita'lis infe'rior [TA] inferior orbital fissure: a cleft in the inferolateral wall of the orbit bounded by the great wing of the sphenoid and the orbital process of the maxilla; it transmits the infraorbital and zygomatic nerves and the infraorbital vessels.

f. orbita'lis supe'rior [TA] superior orbital fissure: an elongated cleft between the small and great wings of the sphenoid bone, which transmits various nerves and vessels.

f. petrooccipita'lis [TA] petrooccipital fissure: a fissure extending posteriorly from the foramen lacerum to the jugular foramen, between the basioccipital area and the posterior and inner border of the petrous portion of the temporal bone; called also *petrobasilar fissure.*

f. petrosquamo'sa [TA] petrosquamous fissure: a slight fissure of varying distinctness in the floor of the middle cranial fossa, marking the line of fusion between the squamous and petrous portions of the temporal bone.

f. petrotympa'nica [TA] petrotympanic fissure: a narrow transversely running slit just posterior to the articular surface of the mandibular fossa of the temporal bone; an arteriole and the chorda tympani nerve pass through it, and it lodges a portion of the malleus. Called also *glaserian fissure.*

f. porta'lis dex'tra [TA] right portal fissure: a plane across the right liver, separating the right lateral division from the right medial division; the right hepatic vein forms part of it.

f. porta'lis principa'lis [TA] main portal fissure: a plane through the liver, dividing the left liver from the right liver; it is approximately demarcated by the Cantlie line, and the middle hepatic vein is a prominent part of it.

f. postcentra'lis cerebel'li TA alternative for *f. preculminalis cerebelli.*

f. postcliva'lis cerebel'li TA alternative for *f. posterior superior cerebelli.*

f. poste'rior supe'rior cerebel'li [TA] posterior superior fissure: a fissure of the cerebellum between the simple lobule and the folium vermis. Called also *f. postclivalis cerebelli* [TA alternative], *postclival fissure,* and *postlunate fissure.*

f. posterolatera'lis cerebel'li [TA] posterolateral fissure: the fissure separating the nodulus from the uvula of the vermis and the flocculus from the tonsilla of the cerebellar hemisphere; called also *dorsolateral fissure.*

f. postlingua'lis cerebel'li TA alternative for *f. precentralis cerebelli.*

f. postpyramida'lis TA alternative for *f. secunda cerebelli.*

f. prebiventra'lis cerebel'li [TA] prebiventral fissure: a fissure of the cerebellum separating the tuber vermis from the pyramid. Called also *f. prepyramidalis cerebelli* [TA alternative] and *prepyramidal fissure.*

f. precentra'lis cerebel'li [TA] precentral fissure of cerebellum: a fissure in the anterior part of the superior vermis of the cerebellum, separating the lingula from the central lobule. Called also *f. postlingualis cerebelli* [TA alternative] and *postlingual fissure.*

f. precliva'lis cerebel'li TA alternative for *f. prima cerebelli.*

f. preculmina'lis cerebel'li [TA] preculminate fissure: a fissure separating the central lobule of the cerebellum with its alae from the more dorsal culmen and quadrangular lobules. Called also *f. postcentralis cerebellaris* [TA alternative] and *postcentral fissure of cerebellum.*

f. prepyramida'lis cerebel'li TA alternative for *f. prebiventralis cerebelli.*

f. pri'ma cerebel'li [TA] primary fissure of cerebellum: the fissure that separates the anterior from the posterior lobe in the cerebellum; it lies between the culmen and declive of the vermis, and between the anterior quadrangular lobule and simple lobule in the hemisphere of the cerebellum. Called also *f. preclivalis cerebelli* [TA alternative] and *preclival fissure.* See illustration.

f. pterygomaxilla'ris [TA] pterygomaxillary fissure: a cleft just posterior to the inferior orbital fissure between the lateral pterygoid plate and the maxilla; called also *pterygopalatine fissure.*

f. secun'da cerebel'li [TA] secondary fissure of cerebellum: a fissure that lies between the uvula of the cerebellum and the pyramid; called also *f. postpyramidalis* [TA alternative] and *postpyramidal fissure.* See illustration.

f. spheno-occipita'lis sphenooccipital fissure: the fissure between the basilar part of the occipital bone and the body of the sphenoid bone; called also *basilar* or *occipitosphenoidal fissure.*

f. sphenopetro'sa [TA] sphenopetrosal fissure: a fissure in the floor of the middle cranial fossa between the posterior edge of the greater wing of the sphenoid bone and the petrous part of the temporal bone; called also *angular* or *petrosphenoidal fissure.*

f. transver'sa ce'rebri [TA] transverse fissure of cerebrum: the fissure between the dorsal surface of the diencephalon and the ventral surface of the cerebral hemispheres, produced by the folding back of the hemispheres during their development; called also *great* or *great transverse fissure of cerebrum* and *fissure of Bichat.*

f. tympanomastoi'dea [TA] tympanomastoid fissure: an external fissure on the inferior and lateral aspect of the skull between the tympanic portion and the mastoid process of the temporal bone; the auricular branch of the vagus nerve often passes through it. Called also *petromastoid fissure.*

f. tympanosquamo'sa [TA] tympanosquamous fissure: a line seen on the posterior wall of the external acoustic meatus at the junction between the tympanic and squamous parts of the temporal bone. Called also *squamotympanic fissure.*

fis•su•rae (fĭ-su'reː) [L.] genitive and plural of *fissura.*

fis•su•ral (fish'u-rəl) pertaining to a fissure.

fis•sure (fish'ər) [L. *fissura,* q.v.] 1. fissura. 2. any cleft, groove, or sulcus, normal or otherwise. 3. a deep cleft in the tooth surface, usually due to imperfect fusion of the enamel of the adjoining dental lobes. Cf. *pit.* Considered as belonging to Class I in the Black classification (see table at *caries*). Called also *enamel f.*

Fissure

For descriptions of specific anatomic structures not listed here, see under *fissura.*

abdominal f. a congenital cleft in the abdominal wall. See also *gastroschisis* and *thoracogastroschisis.* Called also *celoschisis.*

accessory f. any of various inconstant fissures on the lung surface; the most common one is the azygos fissure.

adoccipital f. an inconstant sulcus which crosses the caudal part of the precuneus and joins the occipital fissure.

Ammon f. a pear-shaped aperture in the sclera at an early fetal period.

amygdaline f. a slight groove inconstantly present near the extremity of the temporal lobe.

anal f., f. in ano a painful linear ulcer at the margin of the anus.

angular f. fissura sphenopetrosa.

ansoparamedian f. fissura lunogracilis cerebelli.

anterior inferior f. fissura intrabiventralis.

antitragohelicine f. fissura antitragohelicina.

auricular f. of temporal bone fissura tympanomastoidea.

azygos f. an inconstant fissure at the apex of the right lung, produced when the azygos vein arches over the superior part of the lung instead of near the hilum; it sets off the azygos lobe.

basilar f. fissura sphenooccipitalis.

basisylvian f. the part of the lateral sulcus between the temporal lobe and the orbital surface of the frontal bone.

f. of Bichat fissura transversa cerebri.

branchial f's 1. branchial clefts (def. 1). 2. pharyngeal grooves.

Broca f. a term loosely applied to the anterior and ascending rami of the cerebral lateral sulcus which invade the left inferior frontal gyrus.

Burdach f. the groove between the lateral surface of the insula and the inner surface of the operculum.

calcarine f. sulcus calcarinus.

callosal f. sulcus corporis callosi.

callosomarginal f. sulcus cinguli.

central f. sulcus centralis cerebri.

cerebellar f's fissurae cerebelli.

cerebral f's 1. sulci cerebri. 2. see *fissura longitudinalis cerebri* and *fissura transversa cerebri.*

choroid f. 1. fissura choroidea ventriculi lateralis. 2. retinal f.

choroid f. of lateral ventricle fissura choroidea ventriculi lateralis.

collateral f. sulcus collateralis.

Fissure *Continued*

corneal f. the cleft or groove in the scleral margin into which the limbus corneae fits; called also *corneal cleft.*
craniofacial f. a vertical fissure separating the mesethmoid bone into two parts.
dentate f. sulcus hippocampalis.
dorsolateral f. fissura posterolateralis cerebelli.
f. of ductus venosus fossa ductus venosi.
enamel f. fissure (def. 2).
entorbital f. a sulcus occasionally seen between the orbital and olfactory sulci.
glaserian f. fissura petrotympanica.
f. of glottis rima glottidis.
great f. of cerebrum, great transverse f. of cerebrum fissura transversa cerebri.
great horizontal f. fissura horizontalis cerebelli.
hippocampal f. sulcus hippocampalis.
horizontal f. of cerebellum fissura horizontalis cerebelli.
horizontal f. of right lung fissura horizontalis pulmonis dextri.
intercrural f. fissura horizontalis cerebelli.
intrabiventral f. fissura intrabiventralis.
intraculminate f. fissura intraculminalis.
lateral cerebral f. sulcus lateralis cerebri.
f. for ligamentum teres fissura ligamenti teretis.
f. for ligamentum venosum fissura ligamenti venosi.
longitudinal f. of cerebellum vallecula cerebelli.
longitudinal f. of cerebrum fissura longitudinalis cerebri.
lunogracile f. fissura lunogracilis cerebelli.
mandibular f's the two lowest facial fissures of the embryo.
median f. of medulla oblongata, anterior fissura mediana anterior medullae oblongatae.
median f. of medulla oblongata, dorsal, median f. of medulla oblongata, posterior sulcus medianus posterior medullae oblongatae.
median f. of medulla oblongata, ventral fissura mediana anterior medullae oblongatae.
median f. of spinal cord, anterior fissura mediana anterior medullae spinalis.
median f. of spinal cord, dorsal, median f. of spinal cord, posterior sulcus medianus posterior medullae spinalis.
median f. of spinal cord, ventral fissura mediana anterior medullae spinalis.
oblique f. of lung fissura obliqua pulmonis.
occipitosphenoidal f. fissura sphenooccipitalis.
optic f. retinal f.
oral f. rima oris.
orbital f., inferior fissura orbitalis inferior.
orbital f., superior fissura orbitalis superior.
f. of palpebrae, palpebral f. rima palpebrarum.
parieto-occipital f. sulcus parietooccipitalis.
petrobasilar f. fissura petrooccipitalis.
petromastoid f. fissura tympanomastoidea.
petrooccipital f. fissura petrooccipitalis.
petrosphenoidal f. fissura sphenopetrosa.
petrosquamosal f., petrosquamous f. fissura petrosquamosa.
petrotympanic f. fissura petrotympanica.
portal f. porta hepatis.
portal f., main fissura portalis principalis.
portal f., right fissura portalis dextra.
postcentral f. of cerebellum fissura preculminalis cerebelli.
postcentral f. of cerebrum sulcus postcentralis cerebri.
postclival f. fissura posterior superior cerebelli.
posterior f. of auricle fissura antitragohelicina.
posterior superior f. fissura posterior superior cerebelli.
posterolateral f. fissura posterolateralis cerebelli.
postlingual f. fissura precentralis cerebelli.
postlunate f. fissura posterior superior cerebelli.
postpyramidal f. fissura secunda cerebelli.
prebiventral f. fissura prebiventralis.
precentral f. of cerebellum fissura precentralis cerebelli.
precentral f. of cerebrum sulcus precentralis cerebri.
preclival f. fissura prima cerebelli.
preculminate f. fissura preculminalis cerebelli.
precuneal f. a sulcus in the precuneus.
prepyramidal f. fissura prebiventralis.
presylvian f. the anterior branch of the lateral cerebral sulcus.
primary f. of cerebellum fissura prima cerebelli.
pterygoid f. incisura pterygoidea.
pterygomaxillary f. fissura pterygomaxillaris.
pterygopalatine f. fissura pterygomaxillaris.
retinal f. a ventral groove formed by invagination of the optic cup and its stalk by vascular mesenchyme from which the hyaloid vessels develop; called also *choroid* or *optic f.*
retrocuticular f. a fissure in the oral epithelium made by a tooth at the time of eruption.
retrotonsillar f. either of a pair of curving fissures in the inferior cerebellum, lateral continuations of the sulcus valleculae, between the tonsils and the biventral lobes.
f. of Rolando sulcus centralis cerebri.
f. for round ligament fissura ligamenti teretis.
Santorini f's the two notches in the cartilage of the acoustic meatus; see *incisura cartilaginis meatus acustici.*
Schwalbe f. fissura choroidea ventriculi lateralis.
secondary f. of cerebellum fissura secunda cerebelli.
spheno-occipital f. fissura sphenooccipitalis.
sphenopetrosal f. fissura sphenopetrosa.
squamotympanic f. fissura tympanosquamosa.
subtemporal f. an occasional fissure in the inferior and middle temporal convolutions.
sylvian f., Sylvius f. sulcus lateralis cerebri.
transverse f. porta hepatis.
transverse f. of cerebrum fissura transversa cerebri.
tympanic f. fissura petrotympanica.
tympanomastoid f. fissura tympanomastoidea.
tympanosquamous f. fissura tympanosquamosa.
umbilical f. fissura ligamenti teretis.
f. of venous ligament fossa ductus venosi.
f. of the vestibule rima vestibuli.
zygal f. a cerebral fissure that consists of two portions united by a short perpendicular third portion.

Fis·su·rel·la (fis″ə-rel′ə) the keyhole limpets, a genus of snaillike marine gastropods of the subclass Streptoneura, order Aspidobranchiae. See *keyhole-limpet hemocyanin,* under *hemocyanin.*

fis·tu·la (fis′tu-lə) pl. *fistulas, fis′tulae* [L. "pipe"] an abnormal passage or communication, usually between two internal organs, or leading from an organ to the surface of the body; see illustration. Such passages may also be created surgically for arteriovenous access or experimentally to obtain body secretions for physiologic study. **fis′tulous** *adj*

abdominal f. a fistula between a hollow abdominal organ and the surface of the abdomen.

amphibolic f. an opening made into the gallbladder of an animal in order to obtain bile for study, with the common bile duct left intact so that the bile may flow through it when the fistula is closed.

anal f., f. in a′no a cutaneous fistula opening on the body surface near the anus; it may or may not communicate with the rectum. See illustration.

anorectal f. an anal fistula that communicates with the rectum.

aortocaval f. a fistula between the abdominal aorta and inferior vena cava caused by erosion of an aortic aneurysm into the vena cava.

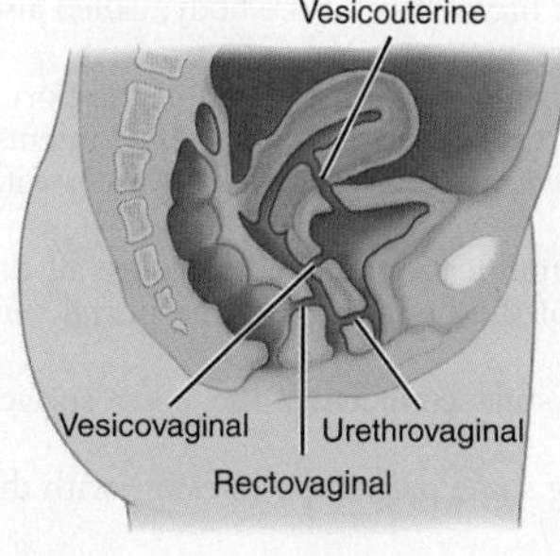

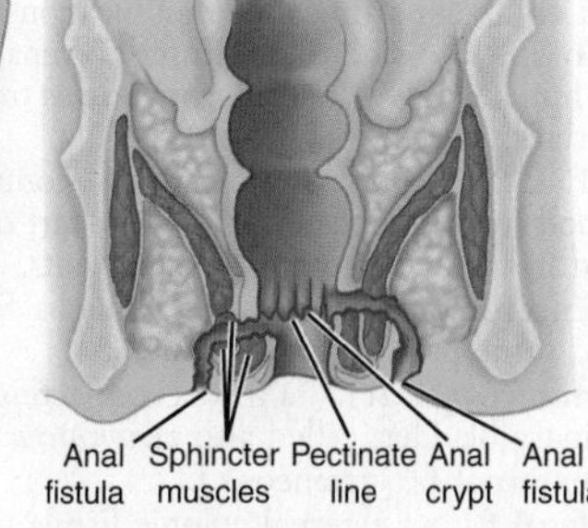

■ Various types of fistulae, designated according to site or to the organs with which they communicate. *(A),* Genitourinary fistulae; *(B),* anal fistulae.

aortoenteric f. a fistula between the aorta and intestine caused by erosion of an abdominal aortic aneurysm into the duodenum; it may be primary or it may be a late complication of prosthetic reconstruction of the aorta and the iliac arteries.

arteriovenous f. 1. a communication, sometimes congenital but often traumatic, between an artery and a nearby vein, so that blood flows directly into the vein *(aneurysmal varix)* or else is carried into the vein by a connecting sac *(varicose aneurysm)*. 2. a surgically created arteriovenous connection that provides a site for vascular access.

f. au′ris conge′nita congenital preauricular f.

biliary f. a fistula communicating between the biliary tract and some other organ or part.

f. bimuco′sa a complete fistula of the anus, with both ends opening on the mucous surface of the anal canal.

blind f. a fistula that is open at one end only; it may open only on the surface of the body *(external blind f.)* or on an internal mucous surface *(internal blind f.)*. Called also *incomplete f.*

brachiocephalic f. an arteriovenous fistula for hemodialysis, located in the wrist and connecting the brachial artery with the cephalic vein.

branchial f. a cutaneous fistula running between the side of the neck and the pharynx, resulting from failure of closure of the second pharyngeal (branchial) groove and second pharyngeal pouch; called also *cervical f.*

Brescia-Cimino f. an arteriovenous fistula for hemodialysis, located in the elbow region, consisting of a side-to-side anastomosis of the cephalic vein and radial artery. Called also *radiocephalic f.*

bronchobiliary f. a fistula between a bronchus and a bile duct, often with leakage of bile into the respiratory system.

bronchocavitary f. a fistula connecting a bronchus and a cavity within the lung.

bronchopleural f. a fistula between a bronchus and the pleural cavity, sometimes seen after lung surgery or as a complication of empyema, fibrosis, or pneumonia.

carotid-cavernous f., carotid–cavernous sinus f. a fistula between an injured internal carotid artery and the cavernous sinus; the adjacent orbital veins may swell and press against various ocular nerves, causing visual symptoms.

cerebrospinal fluid f. a fistula between the subarachnoid space and a body cavity, with leakage of cerebrospinal fluid, usually in the form of rhinorrhea or otorrhea; causes include head trauma and bone erosion caused by a mass or other pathologic process.

cervical f. 1. branchial f. 2. a fistula communicating with the canal of the cervix uteri.

f. col′li conge′nita branchial f.

colonic f. a fistula communicating between the colon and the surface of the body *(external colonic f.)*, or between the colon and another hollow organ *(internal colonic f.)*.

colovesical f. a fistula connecting the colon and the urinary bladder; called also *vesicocolonic f.*

complete f. a fistula in which each end opens on a mucous surface or on the exterior surface of the body.

congenital preauricular f. an epidermis-lined tract communicating with an ear pit (q.v.) on the skin; it results from imperfect fusion of the first and second branchial arches in formation of the auricle; see also *congenital preauricular cyst.* Called also *f. auris congenita.*

f. cor′neae a fistula remaining after failure of a corneal ulcer to heal.

coronary arteriovenous f., coronary artery f. a congenital fistula between a coronary artery and a cardiac chamber, pulmonary trunk or vein, coronary sinus, or vena cava, particularly between the right artery and the right heart.

craniosinus f. a fistula between the intracranial space and a paranasal sinus, permitting escape of cerebrospinal fluid into the nose.

cutaneous f. a fistula that opens on the surface of the body; called also *external f.*

Eck f. an artificial communication made between the end of the portal vein and the side of the inferior vena cava; used in animal experiments. In humans this was formerly done as treatment for esophageal varices with portal hypertension.

Eck f. in reverse an artificial communication created to route all the blood from the posterior (lower) part of the body through the portal vein and liver; used in animal experiments.

enterocutaneous f. a cutaneous fistula connecting the body surface and some part of the intestine.

enterovesical f. a fistula connecting some part of the intestine with the urinary bladder; called also *vesicoenteric f.*

external f. cutaneous f.

fecal f. an external colonic fistula that discharges feces.

gastric f. 1. a fistula communicating between the stomach and another organ or the surface of the body. 2. gastrostomy (def. 2).

gastrocolic f. a fistula connecting the stomach and the colon.

gastropericardial f. a fistula connecting the stomach with the pericardium, usually a complication after gastroesophageal surgery.

genitourinary f. a fistula between two organs of the urogenital system or between one of those organs and some other system. See illustration.

hepatic f. a fistula between the liver and another body part or organ.

horseshoe f. a cutaneous fistula near the anus running in a semicircular tract, with both openings on the body surface.

incomplete f. blind f.

internal f. a fistula between two internal organs.

intestinal f. 1. enterocutaneous f. 2. enterostomy (def. 2).

labyrinthine f. circumscribed labyrinthitis.

lacrimal f. a fistula communicating with the lacrimal sac or duct.

lymphatic f., f. lympha′tica a fistula communicating with a lymphatic vessel.

Mann-Bollman f. an artificial opening into an isolated segment of intestine, having its proximal end sutured to the abdominal wall and its distal end attached by end-to-side anastomosis to the duodenum or other part of the small intestine; used in animal experiments.

omphalomesenteric f. an abnormal passageway between the umbilicus and the terminal ileum, formed by persistence of the intraembryonic part of the yolk stalk.

oroantral f. a fistula connecting the oral cavity and the maxillary antrum, usually as a result of extraction of a molar during which a small piece of bone is accidentally also extracted.

pancreatic f. a fistula between the pancreas and another organ or structure.

pancreaticocutaneous f. external pancreatic f.

pancreaticoenteric f. a fistula connecting the pancreas with some part of the intestine.

pancreaticopleural f. a fistula connecting the pancreas with the pleural cavity.

parietal f. cutaneous f.

perianal f. anal f.

perilymph f., perilymphatic f. rupture of the round window with leakage of perilymph into the middle ear, causing sensorineural hearing loss; it usually results from trauma such as barotrauma or from an erosive disease process.

perineal f. a congenital malformation of the anus and rectum, consisting of an imperforate anus and a fistula that exits via a tiny hole in the perineum.

pharyngeal f. a fistula communicating with the pharynx. Cf. *branchial f.*

pilonidal f. see under *sinus.*

pulmonary f. a fistula communicating with the lung.

pulmonary arteriovenous f. a congenital fistula between the pulmonary arterial and venous systems, allowing unoxygenated blood to enter the systemic circulation.

radiocephalic f. Brescia-Cimino f.

rectovaginal f. a fistula between the rectum and vagina. See illustration.

rectovesical f. a fistula between the rectum and urinary bladder.

rectovestibular f. a congenital malformation of the anus and rectum of females, consisting of an imperforate anus and a fistula exiting via a hole in the vestibule of the vagina. Called also *vestibular f.*

salivary f. a fistula between a salivary duct or gland and the body surface, or into the oral cavity through other than a normal pathway.

saphenous loop f. an arteriovenous fistula for hemodialysis, connecting the saphenous vein and the side of the femoral artery.

spermatic f. a fistula communicating with any of the seminal ducts.

spinal dural arteriovenous f. a common type of malformation of the vasculature in the spinal dura mater, with an artery developing a fistulous connection to a vein, resulting in venous congestion and hypoperfusion of that area of the cord. Many are idiopathic, and others are the result of trauma.

stercoral f. fecal f.

submental f. a salivary fistula opening below the chin.

Thiry f. an artificial opening into an isolated segment of intestine, with its proximal end sutured to the abdominal wall and its distal end closed; used in animal experiments.

Thiry-Vella f. an artificial opening into an internal closed loop of intestine, which communicates with the abdominal wall through an intestinal segment interposed between the surface and the loop; used in animal experiments.

thoracic f. a fistula communicating with the thoracic cavity.

tracheal f. a fistula communicating with the trachea.

tracheocutaneous f. a cutaneous fistula between the trachea and the surface of the neck, due to epithelialization of a tracheotomy opening.

tracheoesophageal f. a fistula between the trachea and the esophagus; it may be either pathological (the result of trauma or a congenital anomaly) or surgically created (see *tracheoesophageal puncture*).

umbilical f. a fistula communicating with the intestine or urachus at the umbilicus.

urachal f. a fistula resulting from a patent urachus communicating with the umbilicus and urinary bladder.

ureteroarterial f. a rare, life-threatening fistula that communicates between a ureter and a nearby artery, usually seen as a complication of a surgical procedure of the ureter.

urethrocutaneous f. a cutaneous fistula between the urethra and the skin, such as after repair of hypospadias or exstrophy of bladder.

urethrovaginal f. a fistula between the urethra and vagina. See illustration.

urinary f. a fistula between the urinary tract and another organ or the surface of the body.

Vella f. an artificial opening into an isolated segment of intestine, with both open ends sutured to the abdominal wall; used in animal experiments.

vesical f. a fistula communicating with the urinary bladder.

vesicocolonic f. colovesical f.

vesicoenteric f. enterovesical f.

vesicorectal f. rectovesical f.

vesicouterine f. a fistula between the urinary bladder and uterus. See illustration.

vesicovaginal f. a fistula from the bladder to the vagina. See illustration.

vestibular f. rectovestibular f.

fis•tu•lae (fis'tu-le) [L.] genitive and plural of *fistula.*

fis•tu•la•gram (fis'tu-lə-gram) fistulogram.

fis•tu•la•tome (fis'tu-lə-tōm) [*fistula* + *-tome*] an instrument for incising a fistula; called also *syringotome.*

fis•tu•lec•to•my (fis″tu-lek'tə-me) [*fistula* + *-ectomy*] excision of a fistulous tract.

fis•tu•li•za•tion (fis″tu-lĭ-za'shən) 1. the process of becoming fistulous. 2. the creation of a communication between two structures which were not previously connected. 3. the surgical creation of an opening into a hollow organ, cavity, or abscess.

fis•tu•lo•en•ter•os•to•my (fis″tu-lo-en″tər-os'tə-me) the operation of making a fistula empty permanently into the intestine.

fis•tu•lo•gram (fis'tu-lo-gram) the radiograph taken during fistulography; called also *fistulagram.*

fis•tu•log•ra•phy (fis″tu-log'rə-fe) angiographic examination of a fistula, such as to assess a pathological one or check on patency of an arteriovenous fistula used for hemodialysis access.

fis•tu•lot•o•my (fis″tu-lot'ə-me) incision of a fistula.

fit (fit) 1. seizure (def. 2). 2. the adaptation of one structure into another, as the adaptation of any dental restoration to its site in the mouth.

FITC fluorescein isothiocyanate.

fit•ness (fit'nis) 1. in genetics, the probability of transmitting one's genotype to the next generation relative to the average probability for the population. 2. physical f.

aerobic f., cardiorespiratory f. the capacity of the cardiovascular and respiratory systems of an individual to supply oxygen and energy during sustained physical activity.

physical f. the capacity of an individual to perform physical activities requiring cardiorespiratory exertion, muscular endurance, strength, or flexibility.

Fitz-Hugh–Cur•tis syndrome (fitz'hu kur'tis) [Thomas *Fitz-Hugh* Jr., American physician, 1894–1963; Arthur H. *Curtis*, American gynecologist, 1881–1955] see under *syndrome.*

Fitz•pat•rick scale, skin type (fitz-pat'rik) [Thomas B. *Fitzpatrick*, American dermatologist, 1919–2003] see under *scale* and *type.*

FIV feline immunodeficiency virus.

fix (fiks) to fasten or hold firm; see *fixation.*

fix•a•tion (fik-sa'shən) [L. *fixatio*] 1. the act or operation of holding, suturing, or fastening in a fixed position. 2. the condition of being held in a fixed position. 3. in psychiatry, a term with two related meanings: *(a)* arrest of development at a particular stage, which if temporary is a normal reaction to difficulties but if continued is a cause of emotional problems; and *(b)* a close and suffocating attachment to another person, especially a childhood figure, such as a parent. Both meanings are derived from psychoanalytic theory and refer to "fixation" of libidinal energy either in a specific erogenous zone, hence fixation at the oral, anal, or phallic stage, or in a specific object, hence mother or father fixation. 4. the use of a fixative (q.v.) to preserve histological or cytological specimens. 5. in chemistry, the process whereby a substance is removed from the gaseous or solution phase and localized, as in carbon dioxide fixation or nitrogen fixation. 6. in ophthalmology, direction of the gaze so that the visual image of the object falls on the fovea centralis. 7. in film processing, the chemical removal of all undeveloped salts of the film emulsion, leaving only the developed silver to form a permanent image.

autotrophic f. the cyclic mechanism whereby carbon dioxide is fixed into organic linkage by autotrophic organisms, e.g., plants and autotrophic bacteria.

bifoveal f., binocular f. training both eyes on the same object as in ordinary vision.

Bovin f. an acetic fixation which destroys the mitochondria of the cell.

carbon dioxide f. conversion of atmospheric carbon dioxide to organic carbon compounds, as in photosynthesis.

complement f., f. of complement the consumption of complement upon reaction with immune complexes containing complement-fixing antibodies; this is the basis of complement fixation tests, two-stage procedures in which heat-inactivated antiserum (or antigen) is reacted with the test material in the presence of a known amount of complement. If the homologous antigen (or antibody) is present in the test material, complement is fixed. Then sheep red blood cells and antisheep erythrocyte antibody are added; lack of hemolysis indicates complement fixation, i.e., a positive test result. Quantitative results are obtained by determining the highest dilution of antiserum or test material that gives a positive reaction. Called also *Bordet-Gengou phenomenon* or *reaction.*

elastic band f. the stabilization of fractured segments of the jaws by means of intermaxillary elastic bands applied to splints or appliances.

external pin f. in oral surgery, a method for stabilizing fractures by means of pins drilled into the bony parts through the overlying skin and connected by metal bars.

external pin f., biphase external pin fixation in which the rigid metal bar connector is replaced with an acrylic bar adapted at the time of the reduction.

intermaxillary f. maxillomandibular f.

internal f., intraosseous f. the open reduction and stabilization of fractured bony parts by direct fixation to one another with surgical wires, screws, pins, and plates.

maxillomandibular f. the fixation of fractures of the maxilla or mandible in a functional relationship with the opposing dental arch, through the use of elastics, wire ligatures, arch bars, or other splints. Called also *intermaxillary f.*

nasomandibular f. mandibular immobilization, especially for edentulous jaws, using maxillomandibular splints; a circummandibular wire is connected with an intraoral interosseous wire passed through a hole drilled into the anterior nasal spine of the maxilla.

nitrogen f. the union of the free atmospheric nitrogen with other elements to form chemical compounds, such as ammonia and nitrates or amino groups. This occurs primarily through the action of soil bacteria of the genus *Rhizobium* or *Bradyrhizobium* in symbiosis with leguminous plants. Nonbiological nitrogen fixation processes include electrical methods and chemical catalysis (Haber process).

ossicular f. the fixing of one or more of the auditory ossicles by fibrous adhesion, tympanosclerosis, or bony fixation; it may be congenital or secondary to infection or trauma.

skeletal f. immobilization of the ends of a fractured bone by metal wires or plates applied directly to the bone *(internal skeletal fixation)* or on the body surface *(external skeletal fixation).*

fix•a•tive (fik'sə-tiv) a fluid, often a mixture of several reactive chemicals, into which histological or cytological specimens are placed so that, by processes such as denaturation and cross-linking of proteins, autolysis is prevented, the specimen is hardened to withstand further processing, and the specimen is preserved in a close facsimile of the living state in regard to both cellular morphology and the location of subcellular constituents.

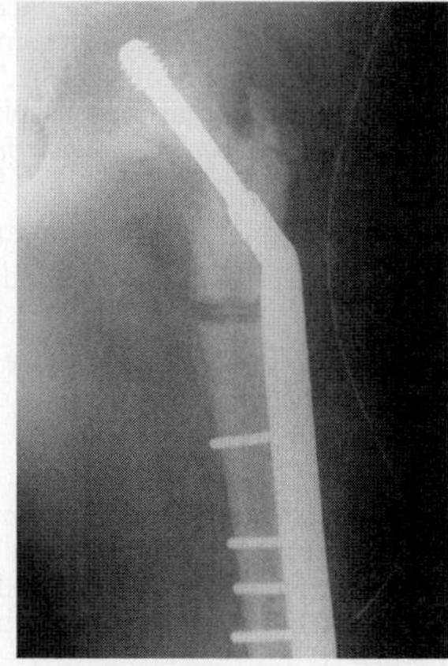

■ Internal fixation of hip fracture using side plate and bone graft after subtrochanteric valgus osteotomy.

glutaraldehyde f. a fixative used in specimen preparation for electron microscopy that does not simultaneously stain the tissue.
Carnoy f. see under *fluid.*
Maximow f. a fixing solution similar to Helly fluid but containing twice as much formaldehyde solution; used in preserving animal tissue.
Zenker f. a fixative solution consisting of mercury bichloride, potassium dichromate, glacial acetic acid, and water.
Zenker-formol f. a solution similar to Zenker fixative but containing also formaldehyde solution; see *Helly fluid,* under *fluid.*

fix·a·tor (fik′sa-tər) see under *muscle.*

Fl. fluid.

FLA [L.] fronto-laeva anterior (left frontoanterior, a position of the fetus; see *position*).

F.l.a. [L.] fi′at le′ge ar′tis (let it be done according to rule).

Flab·el·li·na (flab″ə-li′nə) [L. *flabellum* fan] in older classifications, a suborder of ameboid protozoa of the order Amoebida, having a flattened, broad, sometimes discoid body with an extensive hyaline zone but no obvious pellicle-like layer.

flac·cid (flak′sid, flas′id) [L. *flaccidus*] 1. weak or soft. 2. atonic.

fla·che·rie (flă-shre′) [Fr. "flaccidity"] a fatal disease of silkworms occurring in two forms: an infectious form due to a small nonoccluded virus and a noninfectious form due to environmental changes, such as a sudden increase in temperature and humidity. It is marked by diarrhea, weakness, flaccidity, and death, after which the body quickly turns dark and the tissues liquefy. See also *gattine.*

Flack node, test (flak) [Martin William *Flack,* British physiologist, 1882–1931] see *nodus sinuatrialis* and see under *test.*

fla·gel·la (flə-jel′ə) [L.] plural of *flagellum.*

flag·el·lan·tism (flaj′ə-lən-tiz″əm) a type of sadomasochism characterized by the practice of whipping or being whipped for sexual arousal or gratification.

Flag·el·la·ta (flaj″ə-la′tə) former name for Mastigophora.

flag·el·late[1] (flaj′ə-lāt) 1. any microorganism having flagella as organs of locomotion. 2. mastigophoran. 3. to practice flagellation.
animallike f. zooflagellate.
plantlike f. phytoflagellate.

flag·el·late[2] (flaj′ə-lit, -lāt, flə-jel′it) flagellated.

flag·el·lat·ed (flaj′ə-lāt″ed) having a flagellum or flagella.

flag·el·la·tion (flaj″ə-la′shən) 1. the act or instance of whipping or beating, particularly as a sexual excitant. 2. the formation of flagella. 3. the arrangement of flagella on an organism or surface.

fla·gel·li·form (flə-jel′ĭ-form) [*flagellum* + *form*] shaped like a flagellum.

fla·gel·lin (flə-jel′in) a protein (mol. wt. approximately 40,000) occurring in the flagella of bacteria, which is composed of subunits arranged in several-stranded helix formation somewhat resembling myosin in structure, and sometimes containing ε-N-methyl lysine. Its composition varies with the species; thus flagellin antibodies are species-specific.

flag·el·lo·sis (flaj″ə-lo′sis) infection with flagellate protozoa.

fla·gel·lo·spore (flə-jel′o-spor) zoospore.

fla·gel·lum (flə-jel′əm) pl. *flagel′la* [L. "whip"] a long, mobile, whiplike projection from the free surface of a cell, serving as a locomotor organelle. In eukaryotes, it is composed of nine pairs of microtubules arrayed around a central pair. Arising from basal bodies, flagella are common to all mastigophoran protozoa and occur in such specialized cells as spermatozoa. Bacterial flagella are thinner and simpler, being composed of strands of flagellin tightly woven in a helical filament, attached to a basal body in the cell wall. Based on the configuration of their flagella, bacteria are characterized as either *monotrichous, lophotrichous, amphitrichous,* or *peritrichous.* See also *cilia* (def. 3). **flagel′lar** *adj*

Flag·yl (flag′əl) trademark for preparations of metronidazole.

flail (flāl) exhibiting abnormal or paradoxical mobility, as flail joint, flail chest, or flail valve.

flame (flām) 1. the luminous, irregular appearance usually accompanying combustion caused by the light emitted from energetically excited chemical species, or an appearance resembling it. 2. to render an object sterile by exposure to a flame.

flange (flanj) the part of the denture base that extends from the cervical ends of the teeth to the border of the denture. Called also *denture f.*
buccal f. the portion of the flange of a denture that occupies the buccal vestibule of the mouth and extends distally from the buccal notch.
denture f. flange.
labial f. the portion of the flange of a denture that occupies the labial vestibule of the mouth.
lingual f. the portion of the flange of a mandibular denture which occupies the space adjacent to the residual ridge and next to the tongue.

flank (flank) the side of the body inferior to the ribs and superior to the ilium; called also *latus* [TA].

flap (flap) 1. a mass of tissue for grafting, usually including skin, only partially removed from one part of the body so that it retains its own blood supply during its transfer to a new location; used to repair defects in an adjacent or distant part of the body. 2. an uncontrolled movement.
Abbe f. a triangular flap from the median portion of the lower lip, used to fill a defect in the upper lip.
advancement f. a local flap carried forward to its new position by a sliding technique to close the defect; called also *sliding f.*
arterialized f. a flap whose blood supply in the new site is maintained by a vein that is grafted to an artery.
axial pattern f. a flap whose blood supply is derived from an artery contained in its long axis. Cf. *random pattern f.*
bilobed f. a transposition flap consisting of two lobes: a large lobe that is transposed into the primary defect and a second, smaller lobe that is transposed to fill the defect left by mobilization of the large one.
bipedicle f. a pedicle flap with two vascular attachments.
Boari f. in a ureteroneocystostomy, a flap of bladder wall that is fashioned into a tube and attached to a remnant ureter to replace a missing ureteral segment.
bone f. craniotomy involving elevation of a section of skull; used to correct skull abnormalities or to allow surgical access to a relatively large area of the brain.
cross-arm f. a flap cut from one arm and attached to the other to repair a defect.
cross-leg f. a surgical flap cut from one leg and attached to the other to repair a defect.
delayed transfer f. a flap partially raised from the donor bed and then replaced; done to permit development of collateral circulation through the pedicle.
deltopectoral f. an axial pattern flap whose blood supply is the internal mammary artery and its branches; tissue is transferred from the deltoid and pectoral regions to the neck.
direct transfer f. immediate transfer f.
distant f. a pedicle flap brought from a distant area and transplanted by bringing the donor area and the recipient site into close approximation; called also *Italian f.*
double pedicle f. bipedicle f.
Eloesser f. a flap of skin created over the ribs for open drainage of chronic empyema.
endorectal advancement f. an advancement flap consisting of of rectal mucosa and internal anal sphincter, used to cover the defect created by excision of an anal fistula tract.
envelope f. a mucoperiosteal flap retracted from a horizontal linear incision (as along the free gingival margin) with no vertical component of that incision.
Estlander f. a triangular flap from the side of the lower lip used to fill a defect on the same side of the upper lip.
free f. an island flap detached from the body and reattached at the distant recipient site by microvascular anastomosis.
French f. advancement f.
gauntlet f. pedicle f.
Gillies f. tube f.
immediate transfer f. a skin flap applied to the recipient site immediately after being elevated from its bed; called also *direct transfer f.*
Indian f. interpolated f.
interpolated f. a local pedicle flap that is twisted or rotated on its base and placed into a contiguous area; called also *Indian f.*
island f. an advancement flap consisting of the skin and subcutaneous tissue with a pedicle composed only of subcutaneous tissue, which constitutes the sole vascular supply.
Italian f. distant f.
jump f. a skin flap cut from the abdomen and attached to the forearm; the flap is transferred later to some other part of the body to fill a defect there.

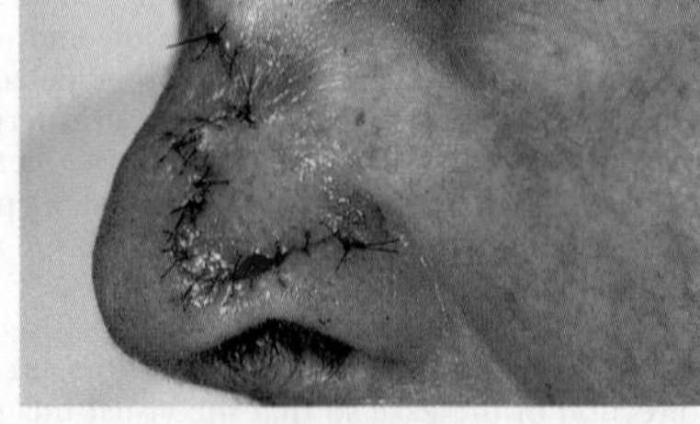
■ Bilobed flap.

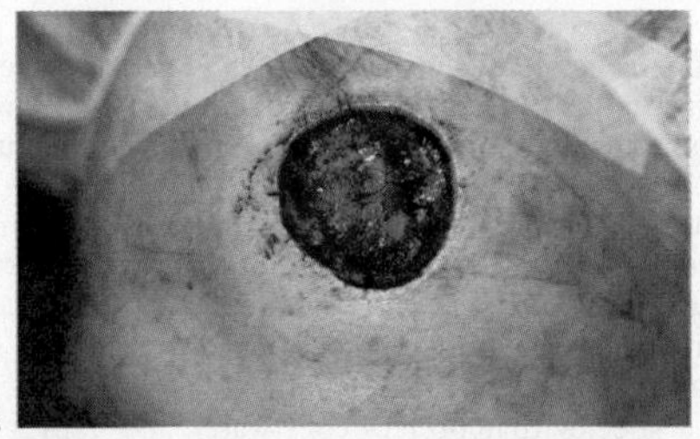

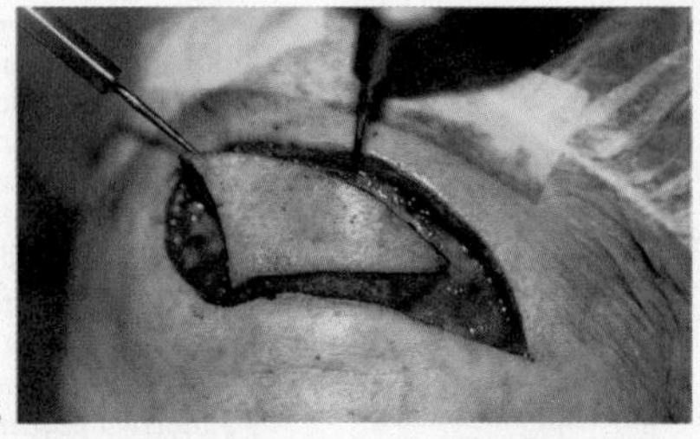

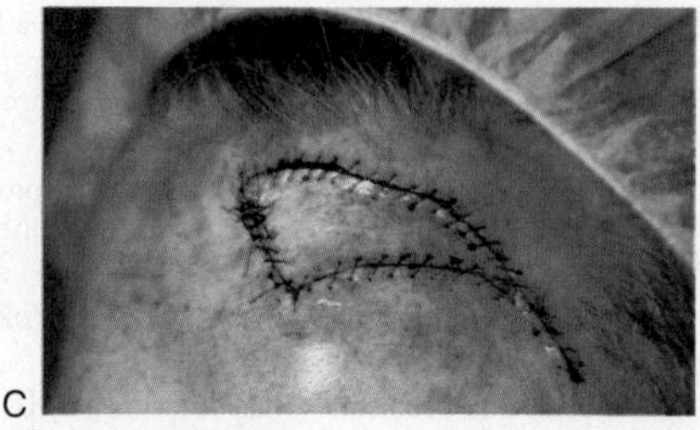

■ Island flap. *(A)*, Large forehead defect. *(B)*, Island flap with a single pedicle that is based inferior to the flap on the blood supply of the supratrochlear and supraorbital arteries. *(C)*, After advancement of the flap and closure.

Karydakis f. a flap technique for repair of pilonidal sinuses.

Limberg f. a rhomboid skin flap, originally used in plastic surgery of the face but now used almost exclusively for repair of pilonidal sinuses.

lingual tongue f. a combination type used to repair fistulae of the hard palate: a flap of palatal tissue forms the floor of the nose, and one taken from the back or edge of the tongue replaces the palatal surface.

liver f. asterixis.

local f. a flap cut from tissue neighboring the defect, such as an advancement flap or some kinds of pedicle flaps.

modified Widman f. see *surgical curettage*, under *curettage*.

mucoperiosteal f. a flap of mucosal tissue, including the periosteum, reflected from bone.

musculocutaneous f., myocutaneous f. a combination of skin and muscle with vascularity adequate for the necessary amount of tissue to be transferred to the recipient site.

pedicle f. a flap consisting of the full thickness of the skin and subcutaneous tissue, attached by tissue through which it receives its blood supply. See also *local f.* and *distant f.*

random pattern f. a flap whose blood supply is derived from multiple vessels of the dermal and subdermal vascular plexuses rather than from a specific artery. Cf. *axial pattern f.*

rope f. tube f.

rotation f. a local pedicle flap whose width is increased by having the edge distal to the defect form a curved line; the flap is then rotated and a counterincision is made at the base of the curved line, which increases the mobility of the flap.

Rubens f. a flap consisting of tissue from above the iliac crest, used in breast reconstruction after mastectomy in patients who have had a previous abdominoplasty and have few other tissues available for an autologous graft; so called from the fullness above the iliac crest appearing in female figures in paintings by Rubens.

skin f. a full-thickness mass or flap of tissue containing epidermis, dermis, and subcutaneous tissue.

sliding f. advancement f.

TRAM f. an autogenous myocutaneous flap that uses transverse rectus abdominis muscle to carry lower abdominal skin and fat to the breast for reconstruction.

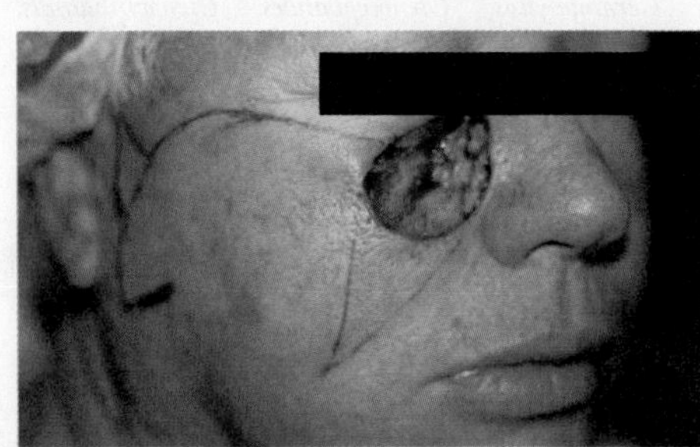

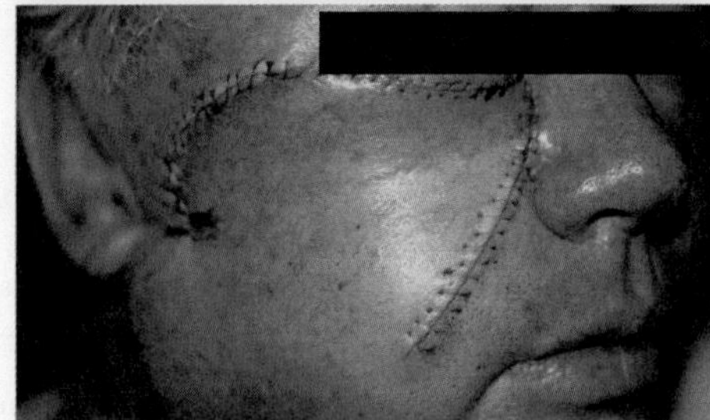

■ Rotation flap.

transposition f. a flap that is carried over intervening skin to a recipient site.

tube f., tubed pedicle f. a type of bipedicle flap made by elevating a long strip of tissue from its bed except at the two ends, the cut edges then being sutured together to form a tube; it has largely been replaced by the free flap. Called also *rope f.*, *tunnel f.*, and *Gillies f.*

tunnel f. tube f.

tympanomeatal f. a flap made by an incision of the inferior part of the external auditory meatus, including the tympanum and part of the meatus, created surgically for access to the middle ear.

von Langenbeck bipedicle mucoperiosteal f. a bipedicle flap of the conjoined mucoperiosteal tissues, used for closure of a cleft palate.

V-Y f. a procedure in which an incision is made in the shape of a V and is sutured in the shape of a Y so as to lengthen an area of tissue; or conversely the incision is Y-shaped and the closure V-shaped to shorten an area of tissue.

Z-f. Z-plasty.

Zimany bilobed f. bilobed f.

flare (flār) 1. the red outermost zone of the wheal and flare reaction, a manifestation of immediate, as opposed to delayed, allergy or hypersensitivity. 2. a spreading flush or area of redness on the skin, spreading out around an infective lesion or extending beyond the main point of reaction to an irritant. 3. sudden exacerbation of a disease.

flash (flash) excess material extruded from a mold, as in the packing of a denture by the compression technique.

flash•lamp (flash′lamp) a lamp that produces an intense light in pulses with alternate on and off phases of a few microseconds each; used with pulsed dye lasers.

flask (flask) 1. a container, such as a narrow-necked vessel of glass for containing liquid. 2. a metal case in which the materials used in the creation of artificial dentures are placed for processing. 3. to place a denture in a flask for processing.

casting f. refractory f.

crown f. denture f.

denture f. a sectional, boxlike metal, ceramic, or polymer case that can be tightly closed, and with which sectional molds of plaster of Paris or dental stone are used to compress and form a resinous denture base or crown material during curing. Called also *crown f.*

Erlenmeyer f. a glass flask with a conical body, broad base, and narrow neck.

refractory f. a metal tube in which a refractory mold is made for casting metal dental restorations or appliances; called also *casting f.*

volumetric f. a narrow-necked vessel of glass calibrated to contain or deliver an exact volume at a given temperature.

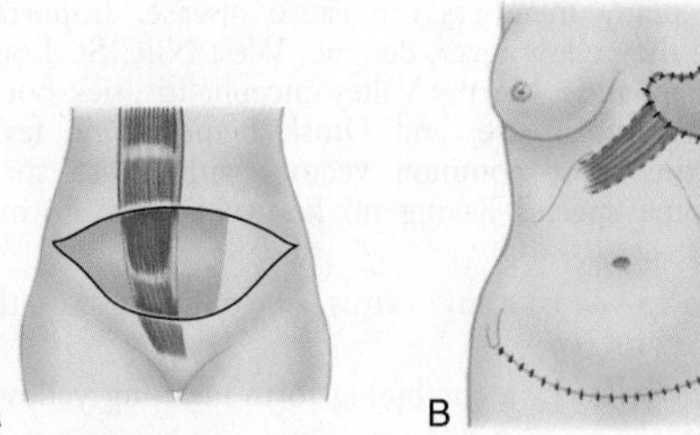

■ TRAM flap. *(A)*, Rectus abdominis muscle and the attached skin and subcutaneous tissue *(brown shading)*, which will be used to form the flap. *(B)*, The skin and tissue on the muscle pedicle have been transferred to the contralateral chest wall via a subcutaneous tunnel in the abdomen and chest, then sculpted and sutured to reconstruct the breast.

flask·ing (flask′ing) 1. the act of investing in a flask. 2. the process of investing the cast and a wax denture in a flask preparatory to molding the denture base material into the form of the denture.

flat (flat) 1. lying in one plane; having an even surface. 2. having little or no resonance. 3. slightly below the normal pitch of a musical tone.

optical f. a glass plate so perfectly flat that only an interferometer can measure its unevenness.

Fla·tau's law (flah′touz) [Edward *Flatau*, Polish neurologist, 1869–1932] see under *law*.

Fla·tau-Schil·der disease (flah′tou shil′dər) [E. *Flatau;* Paul Ferdinand *Schilder*, German-born American psychiatrist, 1886–1940] see *Schilder disease*, under *disease*.

flat·foot (flat′foot) a condition in which one or more of the arches of the foot have been lowered and flattened out; called also *pes planovalgus*, *pes planus*, and *pes valgus*.

rocker-bottom f. see under *foot*.

spastic f. a painful form of flatfoot due to spasm of the peroneal muscles.

flat·ness (flat′nis) a peculiar sound lacking resonance, heard on percussing a part that is abnormally solid.

flat·ten·ing (flat′ə-ning) making flat; diminishing.

f. of affect see under *affect*.

flat·u·lence (flat′u-ləns) [L. *flatulentia*] the presence of excessive amounts of air or gas in the stomach or intestine, leading to distention of the organs. **flat′ulent** *adj*

fla·tus (fla′təs) [L. "a blowing"] 1. gas or air in the gastrointestinal tract. 2. gas or air expelled through the anus.

f. vagina′lis noisy expulsion of gas from the vagina.

flat·worm (flat′wərm) platyhelminth.

fla·vec·to·my (fla-vek′tə-me) [*flavo-* + *-ectomy*] excision of the ligamentum flavum.

fla·ves·cent (flə-ves′ənt) yellowish.

fla·vin (fla′vin) [L. *flavus* yellow] any one of a group of compounds containing the isoalloxazine nucleus, especially riboflavin. Flavin compounds are characterized by a yellow color and intense green fluorescence in the oxidized form; the reduced form is colorless.

f. adenine dinucleotide (FAD) a coenzyme composed of riboflavin 5′-phosphate (FMN) and adenosine 5′-phosphate linked by a pyrophosphate bond; it forms the prosthetic group of many flavoprotein enzymes, including D-amino acid oxidase and xanthine oxidase, serving as an electron carrier by being alternately oxidized (FAD) and reduced ($FADH_2$). It is important in electron transport in mitochondria and the endoplasmic reticulum.

f. mononucleotide (FMN) riboflavin 5′-phosphate; it acts as a coenzyme for a number of oxidative enzymes, including NADH dehydrogenase, serving as an electron carrier by being alternately oxidized (FMN) and reduced ($FMNH_2$).

fla·vin mono·oxy·ge·nase (fla′vin mon″o-ok′sə-jən-ās) unspecific monooxygenase.

Fla·vi·vi·ri·dae (fla″vĭ-vir′ĭ-de) the flaviviruses: a family of RNA viruses having a virion 40–60 nm in diameter consisting of a lipid envelope, with fine peplomers, surrounding a spherical nucleocapsid. The genome consists of a single molecule of positive-sense single-stranded RNA (MW 4×10^6, size 9.5–12.5 kb). Viruses contain two or three major structural polypeptides and are sensitive to lipid solvents, detergents, ultraviolet radiation, and heat. Replication occurs in the cytoplasm and assembly is by budding through the plasma membrane. It includes the genera *Flavivirus*, *Hepacivirus*, and *Pestivirus*.

Fla·vi·vi·rus (fla′vĭ-vi″rəs) [*flavo-* + *virus*] a genus of viruses of the family Flaviviridae of worldwide distribution, containing about 75 species in 9 serogroups; many members can cause disease. Important human pathogens include the yellow fever, dengue, West Nile, St. Louis encephalitis, Japanese encephalitis, Murray Valley encephalitis, tick-borne encephalitis, Kyasanur Forest disease, and Omsk hemorrhagic fever viruses. Mosquitoes are the most common vector, with some species being tick-borne and some species having no known vector. Formerly called group B arboviruses.

fla·vi·vi·rus (fla′və-vi″rəs) any virus belonging to the family *Flaviviridae*. **flavivi′ral** *adj*

flav(o)- [L. *flavus* yellow] a combining form meaning yellow.

Fla·vo·bac·te·ri·a·ceae (fla″vo-bak-tēr″e-a′se-e) a family of bacteria of the phylum Bacteroidetes, consisting of gram-negative, aerobic or anaerobic, non–spore-forming, short to moderately long rods; flagella are generally absent and organisms are nonmotile or move by gliding. Most are soil or water saprophytes; some are pathogenic. Genera of medical interest are *Capnocytophaga*, *Flavobacterium*, and *Riemerella*.

Fla·vo·bac·te·ri·um (fla″vo-bak-tēr′e-əm) [*flavo-* + *bacterium*] a genus of gram-negative, aerobic or facultatively anaerobic, rod-shaped bacteria of the family Flavobacteriaceae, characterized by production of a yellow pigment. The organisms occur widely in soil and water, and are opportunistic pathogens in humans.

F. columna′re a species that prefers warm water and causes columnaris disease in fish. Called also *Cytophaga columnaris* and *Flexibacter columnaris*.

F. meningosep′ticum *Elizabethkingia meningoseptica*.

F. odora′tum a former species whose members are now classified in the *Myroides odoratimimus* and *M. odoratus*.

F. psychro′philum a species that prefers cold water and causes cold-water disease in fish. Called also *Cytophaga psychrophila* and *Flexibacter psychrophilus*.

fla·vo·en·zyme (fla″vo-en′zīm) any enzyme that is a flavoprotein.

fla·vo·noid (fla′və-noid) any of a group of compounds containing a characteristic aromatic trimeric heterocyclic nucleus, usually occurring in glycosidic form and widely distributed in plants, often as a pigment. A subgroup with biological activity in mammals is termed the bioflavonoids (q.v.).

fla·vo·pro·tein (fla″vo-pro′tēn) a protein containing a flavin nucleotide (FAD or FMN) as a prosthetic group. Most flavoproteins are enzymes; many are found in complexes containing metal ions and an iron-sulfur complex or a heme. They catalyze a wide variety of oxidation-reduction reactions.

electron transfer f. (ETF) a component of a side chain of redox reactions by which electrons are funneled to ubiquinone and thus the electron transport chain; electrons from acyl CoA thioesters and choline are transferred via the flavin of acyl CoA dehydrogenases, dimethylglycine dehydrogenase, and sarcosine dehydrogenase to the FAD prosthetic group of ETF, which is then oxidized via reduction of electron transfer flavoprotein: ubiquinone oxidoreductase (q.v.). Deficiency of ETF results in glutaricaciduria, type II.

fla·vor (fla′vər) 1. that quality of any substance which affects the taste. 2. a pharmaceutical or other preparation for improving the taste of a food or medicine.

fla·vo·xan·thin (fla″vo-zan′thin) a minor, yellow, carotenoid pigment from the petals of ranunculaceous plants, structurally related to vitamin A but having no vitamin A activity.

fla·vox·ate hy·dro·chlo·ride (fla-voks′āt) a smooth muscle relaxant used as an antispasmodic for the urinary system, administered orally to treat the symptoms of urologic disorders and irritative voiding.

flax (flak) any of various plants of the genus *Linum*, especially *L. usitatis′simum*.

Flax·e·dil (flak′sə-dil) trademark for a preparation of gallamine triethiodide.

flax·seed (flak′sēd) linseed.

fld fluid.

fl dr fluid dram.

flea (fle) any insect of the order *Siphonaptera;* many are parasitic and may act as carriers of disease. Genera of medical importance include *Cediopsylla*, *Ceratophyllus*, *Ctenocephalides*, *Ctenophthalmus*, *Diamanus*, *Echidnophaga*, *Hoplopsyllus*, *Leptopsylla*, *Monopsyllus*, *Neopsylla*, *Nosopsyllus*, *Oropsylla*, *Pulex*, *Rhopalopsyllus*, *Tunga*, and *Xenopsylla*.

Asiatic rat f. *Xenopsylla cheopis*.

burrowing f. chigoe.

cat f. *Ctenocephalides felis*.

cavy f. *Rhopalopsyllus cavicola*.

chigoe f. chigoe.

common human f. *Pulex irritans*.

dog f. *Ctenocephalides canis*.

European mouse f. *Ctenophthalmus agrytes*.

European rat f. *Nosopsyllus fasciatus*.

human f. *Pulex irritans*.

Indian rat f. *Xenopsylla astia*.

jigger f. chigoe.

mouse f. *Leptopsylla segnis*.

rat f. any of various species of *Nosopsyllus* and *Xenopsylla*.

sand f. chigoe.

squirrel f. *Hoplopsyllus anomalus*.

sticktight f. *Echidnophaga gallinacea*.

suslik f. any of several species of fleas that infest the suslik (Russian ground squirrel) and are vectors of plague.

tropical rat f. *Xenopsylla cheopis*.

fle·cai·nide ace·tate (flə-ka′nīd) [USP] a sodium channel blocker that decreases the rate of cardiac conduction and increases the ventricular refractory period; used in the treatment of life-threatening arrhythmias.

Flech•sig field, tract, zone (flek′sig) [Paul Emil *Flechsig*, German neurologist, 1847–1929] see under *zone* and see *myelinogenetic field* under *field* and *tractus spinocerebellaris posterior.*

fleck (flek) a flake, particle, speckle, or spot.
 tobacco f's Gamna nodules.

fleck•milz (flek′milts) [Ger.] a condition of the spleen in myeloid leukemia and other leukemic or lymphomatous diseases characterized by multiple pale ischemic infarcts.

Flec•tor (flek′tor) trademark for a skin patch preparation of diclofenac epolamine.

fleece (flēs) 1. the thick, woolly or hairy coat of a sheep or other animal. 2. a network of interlacing fibers; see *neuropil.*
 f. of Stilling the lacework of myelinated fibers surrounding the dentate nucleus.

Fle•gel disease (fla′gəl) [Heinz *Flegel,* German physician, born 1923] hyperkeratosis lenticularis perstans.

Fleisch•ner disease (flīsh′nər) [Felix *Fleischner,* Austrian-born American radiologist, 1893–1969] see under *disease.*

Flem•ming center, solution (fixing fluid) (flem′ing) [Walther *Flemming,* German anatomist, 1843–1905] see *germinal center,* under *center,* and see under *solution.*

fler•ox•a•cin (flə-rok′sə-sin) a fluoroquinolone antibiotic having actions and uses similar to those of ciprofloxacin; administered orally or by intravenous infusion.

flesh (flesh) [A.S. *flaesc*] 1. muscular tissue. 2. skin.
 goose f. cutis anserina.
 proud f. exuberant amounts of soft, edematous, granulation tissue that may develop during the healing of large surface wounds.

fleshy (flesh′e) 1. pertaining to or resembling flesh. 2. characterized by abundant flesh.

fleur•ette (floor-et′) [Fr. "small flower"] a type of cell found in clusters in retinoblastomas and retinocytomas, representing differentiation of tumor cells into photoreceptors; eosinophilic processes project through the cell membrane so that the cell resembles a flower with petals.

flex (fleks) [L. *flexus* bent] to bend or put in a state of flexion.

Flex•er•il (flek′sə-ril) trademark for a preparation of cyclobenzaprine hydrochloride.

Flexi•bac•ter (flek′sĭ-bak″tər) a genus of gram-negative, rod-shaped, aerobic or facultatively aerobic bacteria.
 F. columna′ris *Flavobacterium columnare.*
 F. psychro′philus *Flavobacterium psychrophilum.*

flex•i•bil•i•tas (flek″sĭ-bil′ĭ-təs) [L.] flexibility.
 ce′rea f. waxy flexibility.

flex•i•bil•i•ty (flek″sĭ-bil′ĭ-te) [L. *flexibilitas*] the quality of being flexible.
 waxy f. the rigidity of the body seen in some severe cases of catatonic schizophrenia, in which the patient maintains whatever body position they are placed in, the limbs having a heavy waxy malleability.

flex•i•ble (flek′sĭ-bəl) [L. *flexibilis, flexilis*] readily bent without tendency to break.

flex•ile (fleks′īl) flexible.

flex•ion (flek′shən) [L. *flexio*] 1. the act of bending or condition of being bent. 2. in gynecology, a displacement of the uterus in which the organ is bent so far anteriorly or posteriorly that an acute angle forms between the fundus and the cervix. See *version* (def. 3). 3. in obstetrics, the normal bending forward of the head of the fetus in the uterus or the birth canal.

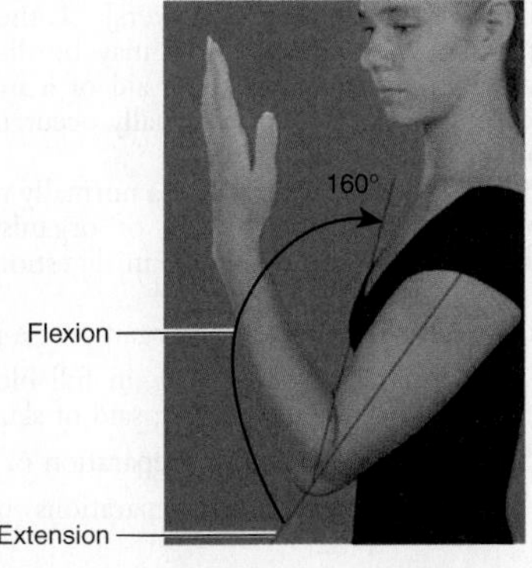

■ Flexion and extension of the elbow.

 fixed f. loss of ability to extend a joint, so that it remains permanently flexed. Cf. *flexion contracture,* under *contracture.*
 plantar f. bending of the toes or foot downward toward the sole.

flex•I•ther•a•py (flek″se-ther′ə-pe) combination chemotherapy in which two regimens thought to be not cross-resistant are alternated and new drugs may be added at given intervals in a flexible pattern that depends on the patient's individual rate of tumor response.

Flex•ner bacillus, dysentery (fleks′nər) [Simon *Flexner,* American pathologist, 1863–1946] see *Shigella flexneri,* and see *bacillary dysentery,* under *dysentery.*

Flex•ner-Win•ter•stei•ner rosette (fleks′nər vin′tər-shti″nər) [S. *Flexner;* Hugo *Wintersteiner,* Austrian ophthalmologist, 1865–1918] see under *rosette.*

flex•or (flek′sor) [L.] 1. [TA] causing flexion. 2. any muscle that flexes a joint; see under *musculus.*
 f. retina′culum see *retinaculum musculorum flexorum manus* and *retinaculum musculorum flexorum pedis.*

flex•or•plas•ty (flek′sor-plas″te) plastic surgery of flexor muscles.

flex•u•ose (flek′su-ōs) winding or wavy.

flex•u•ra (flek-shoo′rə) gen. and pl. *flexu′rae* [L.] flexure: an anatomical bend, such as a bent portion of a structure or organ.
 f. anorecta′lis [TA] anorectal flexure: the bend at the caudal end of the rectum, where it deviates caudally and posteriorly. Called also *f. perinealis* [TA alternative] and *perineal flexure.*
 f. co′li dex′tra [TA] right colic flexure: the bend in the large intestine at which the ascending colon becomes the transverse colon; called also *f. coli hepatica* [TA alternative], *f. hepatica coli,* and *right* or *hepatic flexure of colon.*
 f. co′li hepa′tica TA alternative for *f. coli dextra.*
 f. co′li sinis′tra [TA] left colic flexure: the bend in the large intestine at which the transverse colon becomes the descending colon; called also *f. coli splenica* and *left* or *splenic flexure of colon.*
 f. co′li sple′nica TA alternative for *f. coli sinistra.*
 f. duode′ni infe′rior [TA] inferior duodenal flexure: the bend where the descending part of the duodenum ends and the horizontal part begins.
 f. duode′ni supe′rior [TA] superior duodenal flexure: the bend where the superior part of the duodenum ends and the descending part begins.
 f. duodenojejuna′lis [TA] duodenojejunal flexure: the bend in the small intestine at the junction between the duodenum and jejunum; the suspensory muscle of the duodenum attaches to this point.
 f. hepa′tica co′li f. coli dextra.
 f. infe′rior latera′lis rec′ti TA alternative for *f. inferodextra lateralis recti.*
 f. inferodex′tra latera′lis rec′ti [TA] inferior right lateral flexure of rectum: the fourth bend of the rectum, where it deviates laterally to the right. Called also *inferior lateral flexure of rectum* and *f. inferior lateralis recti* [TA alternative].
 f. interme′dia latera′lis rec′ti TA alternative for *f. intermediosinistra lateralis recti.*
 f. intermediosinis′tra latera′lis rec′ti [TA] intermediate left lateral flexure of rectum: the third bend of the rectum, where it deviates laterally to the left. Called also *intermediate lateral flexure of rectum* and *f. intermedia lateralis recti* [TA alternative].
 flexu′rae latera′les rec′ti [TA] lateral flexures of rectum: the three lateral bends in the rectum; see *f. inferodextra lateralis recti, f. intermediosinistra lateralis recti,* and *f. superodextra lateralis recti.*
 f. liena′lis co′li f. coli sinistra.
 f. perinea′lis TA alternative for *f. anorectalis.*
 f. sacra′lis rec′ti [TA] sacral flexure of rectum: the first bend in the rectum, where it deviates posteriorly.
 f. supe′rior latera′lis rec′ti TA alternative for *f. superodextra lateralis recti.*
 f. superodex′tra latera′lis rec′ti [TA] superior right lateral flexure of rectum: the second bend in the rectum, where it deviates laterally to the right. Called also *superior lateral flexure of rectum* and *f. superior lateralis recti* [TA alternative].

flex•u•rae (flek-shoo′re) [L.] genitive and plural of *flexura.*

flex•ure (flek′shər) a bend; a bent portion of a structure or organ; see *flexura.* **flex′ural** *adj*
 anorectal f. flexura anorectalis.
 basicranial f. pontine f.
 caudal f. the bend at the aboral (caudal) end of the embryo; called also *sacral f.*
 cephalic f. the curve in the midbrain (mesencephalon) of the neural tube; called also *cranial f.* and *mesencephalic f.*
 cerebral f., cervical f. a bend in the neural tube of the embryo at the junction of the brain and spinal cord; called also *head bend, neck bend,* and *nuchal f.*
 colic f., left flexura coli sinistra.
 colic f., right flexura coli dextra.

cranial f. cephalic f.
dorsal f. one of the flexures of the embryo in the mid-dorsal region.
duodenal f., inferior flexura duodeni inferior.
duodenal f., superior flexura duodeni superior.
duodenojejunal f. flexura duodenojejunalis.
hepatic f. of colon flexura coli dextra.
inferior f. of duodenum flexura duodeni inferior.
lateral f's of rectum flexurae laterales recti.
lateral f. of rectum, inferior, lateral f. of rectum, inferior right flexura inferodextra lateralis recti.
lateral f. of rectum, intermediate, lateral f. of rectum, intermediate left flexura intermediosinistra lateralis recti.
lateral f. of rectum, superior, lateral f. of rectum, superior right flexura superodextra lateralis recti.
left f. of colon flexura coli sinistra.
lumbar f. the ventral curvature of the back in the lumbar region.
mesencephalic f. cephalic f.
nuchal f. cervical f.
perineal f. flexura anorectalis.
pontine f. a flexure in the hindbrain of the embryo; called also *basicranial f.*
right f. of colon flexura coli dextra.
sacral f. 1. caudal f. 2. flexura sacralis recti.
sacral f. of rectum flexura sacralis recti.
sigmoid f. colon sigmoideum.
splenic f. of colon flexura coli sinistra.
superior f. of duodenum flexura duodeni superior.

flick•er (flik'ər) [A.S. *flicorian* to flutter] the visual sensation produced by regular flashes of light; the flashes may appear to flutter or to be steady according to the rate of interruption; called also *flicker phenomenon*. See also *critical fusion frequency*, under *frequency*.

flight of ideas (flīt of i-de'əz) a nearly continuous flow of rapid speech that jumps from topic to topic, usually based on discernible associations, distractions, or plays on words, but in severe cases so rapid as to be disorganized and incoherent. It is most commonly seen in manic episodes but may also occur in other mental disorders such as in manic phases of schizophrenia.

Flin•ders Is•land spotted fever (flin'dərz i'lənd) [*Flinders Island*, northeast of Tasmania, Australia] see under *fever*.

Flint arcade, law (flint) [Austin *Flint*, Jr., American physiologist, 1836–1915] see under *arcade* and *law*.

Flint murmur (flint) [Austin *Flint*, American physician, 1812–1886] see under *murmur*.

float•ers (flo'tərz) "spots before the eyes"; deposits in the vitreous of the eye, usually moving about and probably representing fine aggregates of vitreous protein occurring as a benign degenerative change. Called also *vitreous f's* and *muscae volitantes*.

floc•cil•la•tion (flok"sĭ-la'shən) [L. *floccilatio*] the aimless picking at bedclothes by a patient with delirium, dementia, fever, or exhaustion; called also *carphology*, *crocidismus*, and *tilmus*.

floc•cose (flok'ōs) [L. *floccosus* full of flocks of wool] woolly; said of a bacterial growth which is composed of short, curved chains variously oriented.

floc•cu•lar (flok'u-lər) pertaining to the flocculus.

floc•cu•la•tion (flok"u-la'shən) 1. the formation of lumpy or fluffy masses. 2. a colloid phenomenon in which the disperse phase separates in discrete, usually visible, fleecy particles rather than in a continuous mass, as in coagulation.

floc•cule (flok'ūl) flocculus.
toxoid-antitoxin f. a suspension of the precipitate formed when toxoid and antitoxin are mixed.

floc•cu•lent (flok'u-lənt) containing downy or flaky masses.

floc•cu•lus (flok'u-ləs) pl. *floc'culi* [L. "tuft"] 1. a small tuft, as of wool or similar material, or a small mass of other fibrous material such as one of the flakes of a flocculent solution. 2. [TA] (HX); one of a pair of small lateral lobules of the cerebellum, continuous by a small stalk of nerve fibers with the nodulus vermis, and separated from the cerebellar uvula and tonsillae by the posterolateral fissure; it is part of the flocculonodular lobe.
accessory f. paraflocculus.

floc•ta•fen•ine (flok"tə-fen'ēn) a nonsteroidal antiinflammatory drug derived from anthranilic acid, used for the short-term relief of pain, including that associated with vascular headaches, and the treatment of attacks of gout or calcium pyrophosphate deposition disease; administered orally.

Flo•lan (flo'lan) trademark for a preparation of epoprostenol sodium.

Flo•max (flo'maks) trademark for a preparation of tamsulosin hydrochloride.

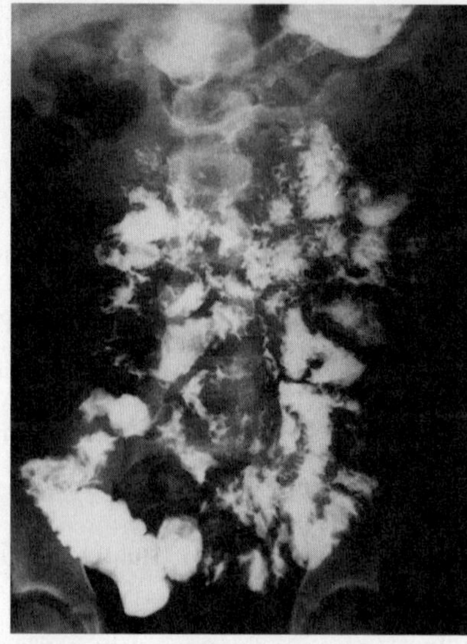

■ Flocculation and segmentation of barium with mild dilatation of the bowel in a small bowel series in a child with celiac disease.

Flo•nase (flo'nāz) trademark for a preparation of fluticasone propionate.

Flood ligament (flud) [Valentine *Flood*, Irish surgeon, 1800–1847] see under *ligament*.

flood•ing (flud'ing) in behavior therapy, a form of desensitization for the treatment of phobias and related disorders in which the patient is repeatedly exposed to highly distressing stimuli without being able to escape but without danger, until the lack of reinforcement of the anxiety response causes its extinction. In general, the term is used for actual exposure to the stimuli, with *implosion* used for imagined exposure, but the two terms are sometimes used synonymously to describe either or both types of exposure. Cf. *systematic desensitization*.

floor (flor) [A.S. *flōr*] the inferior inner surface of a hollow organ or other space.
cavity f. f. of prepared cavity.
f. of fourth ventricle fossa rhomboidea.
inguinal f., f. of inguinal canal the posterior wall of the inguinal canal, formed by the fascia transversalis and the aponeurosis of the transversus abdominis muscle.
f. of lateral ventricle the inferior interior surface of the lateral ventricle, formed by the caudate nucleus, the stria terminalis, the thalamostriate veins, the collateral eminence, and the superior surfaces of the thalamus, the rostrum of the corpus callosum, and the hippocampus.
f. of nasal cavity the inferior surface of the cavity, formed by the palatine process of the maxilla and the horizontal plate of the palatine bone.
f. of orbit, orbital f. paries inferior orbitae.
pelvic f., f. of pelvis the layer of tissue just below the outlet of the pelvis, formed by the coccygeal and levator ani muscles and the perineal fascia. See also *diaphragma pelvis*.
f. of prepared cavity the bottom or enclosing base wall of a prepared cavity, which the restoration material rests on.
f. of third ventricle the inferior interior surface of the third ventricle, formed by the optic chiasm, the tuber cinereum, the infundibulum, the mammillary bodies, and the posterior perforated substance.
f. of tympanic cavity paries jugularis cavitatis tympani.

flo•ra (flor'ə) [L. *Flora*, the goddess of flowers] 1. the plant life present in or characteristic of a special location; it may be discernible with the unaided eye (macroflora), or only with the aid of a microscope (microflora). 2. the bacteria and fungi, both normally occurring and pathological, found in or on an organ.
enteric f., gut f., intestinal f. the bacteria normally residing within the lumen of the intestine, consisting mainly of organisms of the phyla Bacteroidetes and Firmicutes; some are aids in digestion and food breakdown.
resident f. flora occurring in or on an organ over a protracted period.

flor•id (flor'id) [L. *floridus* blossoming] 1. in full bloom; occurring in fully developed form. 2. having a red color; said of skin.

Flor•i•din (flor'ĭ-din) trademark for a preparation of fuller's earth.

Flor•i•nef (flor'ĭ-nef) trademark for preparations of fludrocortisone acetate.

Flor•one (flor'ōn) trademark for preparations of diflorasone diacetate.

Flo•vent (flo′vent) trademark for preparations of fluticasone propionate.

flow (flo) 1. the movement of a liquid or gas. 2. the rate at which a fluid passes through an organ or part, expressed as volume per unit of time. Called also *flow rate.*

blood f. 1. circulation (def. 2). 2. circulation rate.

effective renal blood f. (ERBF) that portion of the total blood flow through the kidneys that perfuses functional renal tissue such as the glomeruli.

effective renal plasma f. (ERPF) the amount of plasma that perfuses the renal tubules per unit time, generally measured by the *p*-aminohippurate clearance.

estimated hepatic blood f. (EHBF) an estimate of the rate of blood flow through the liver in a liver function test, such as by calculating indocyanine green clearance.

forced expiratory f. (FEF) the rate of airflow recorded in measurements of forced vital capacity, usually calculated as an average flow over a given portion of the expiratory curve; the portion between 25 and 75 per cent of forced vital capacity is called the *maximal* or *maximum midexpiratory f.*

gene f. the movement of genes between populations due to migration and interbreeding.

laminar f. the movement of corresponding parts of a fluid along parallel and relatively smooth paths; it has a lower Reynolds number than turbulent flow. See also *axial current,* under *current.*

maximal expiratory f. maximum expiratory f.

maximal midexpiratory f. maximum midexpiratory f.

maximum expiratory f. the rate of airflow during a forced vital capacity maneuver, often specified at a given volume; see also *forced expiratory f.* Called also *maximal expiratory f.*

maximum midexpiratory f. the average rate of airflow measured between exhaled volumes of 25 and 75 per cent of the vital capacity during a forced exhalation. See also *forced expiratory f.* Called also *maximal midexpiratory f.* and *maximal* or *maximum midexpiratory flow rate.*

mean inspiratory f. tidal volume divided by the duration of inhalation.

peak expiratory f. (PEF) the greatest rate of airflow that can be achieved during forced exhalation, beginning with the lungs fully inflated. Called also *peak expiratory flow rate.*

peak inspiratory f. (PIF) the greatest rate of airflow that can be achieved during forced inhalation, beginning with the lungs maximally deflated. Called also *peak inpiratory flow rate.*

regional cerebral blood f. (rCBF) the rate of blood flow to a specific region of the brain, assessed in the monitoring of danger of cerebral infarction and other conditions.

renal plasma f. (RPF) the total amount of plasma that perfuses the kidneys per unit time, approximately 10 per cent greater than the effective renal plasma flow.

turbulent f. the movement of corresponding parts of a fluid through chaotic, nonparallel paths; it has a higher Reynolds number than laminar flow.

flower (flou′ər) [Old Fr. *flor,* from L. *flos,* gen. *floris*] the blossom of a plant; preparations of the flowers of some plants are used medicinally.

balloon f. 1. *Platycodon grandiflorum.* 2. a preparation of the roots of *P. grandiflorum,* used in traditional Chinese medicine as an expectorant.

passion f. 1. any plant of the genus *Passiflora.* 2. a preparation of the aerial parts of *P. incarnata,* having anxiolytic and sedative properties and used for anxiety and insomnia; it is also used in homeopathy.

Flow•er index (flou′ər) [Sir William Henry *Flower,* British zoologist, 1831–1899] dental index; see under *index.*

flow•ers (flou′ərz) a sublimed drug.

f. of benzoin benzoic acid.

f. of sulfur sublimed sulfur.

flow•me•ter (flo′me-tər) an apparatus for measuring the rate of flow of liquids or gases; written also *flow meter.* See also *velocimetry.*

blood f. an apparatus that measures the rate of blood flow in the arteries or veins.

Doppler ultrasonic f., Doppler ultrasound f. a flowmeter that is sensitive to the Doppler effect, such as measuring blood flow by noting the Doppler effect in ultrasonic waves reflected off moving red blood cells. Called also *ultrasonic* or *ultrasound Doppler f.*

electromagnetic f. an apparatus that measures flow of a conductive fluid through a tube (such as blood through a vessel) in a magnetic field, and analysis of the resultant voltage; the voltage is perpendicular to the direction of movement and to the magnetic field and is proportional to the velocity of movement.

laser Doppler f. an apparatus that examines flow of a fluid such as blood using a laser beam; the light is shifted by moving objects in the fluid, in accordance with the Doppler effect, and the scattered light is detected with a photodetector.

transit time f., transit time ultrasonic f., transit time ultrasound f. a type of ultrasonic flowmeter that compares the ultrasound transit time in both directions between two transducers and from the difference is able to calculate velocity and direction of flow of the fluid in question.

ultrasonic f. ultrasound f.

ultrasonic Doppler f. Doppler ultrasonic flowmeter.

ultrasound f. any of various types of flowmeters that use ultrasound techniques to measure flow of fluids.

ultrasound Doppler f. Doppler ultrasonic f.

flow•me•try (flo′met-re) measurement of the rate of flow of gases or liquids using a flowmeter.

flox•a•cil•lin (flok″sə-sil′in) a penicillinase-resistant, semisynthetic isoxazolyl penicillin which has been used primarily in the treatment of infections due to benzylpenicillin-resistant staphylococci. Called also *flucloxacillin.*

Flox•in (flok′sin) trademark for preparations of ofloxacin.

flox•uri•dine (floks-ūr′ĭ-dēn) [USP] a fluoropyrimidine that is metabolically activated to the monophosphate nucleotide (F-dUMP), the metabolite of 5-fluorouracil (q.v.) that blocks DNA synthesis; FUDR is also metabolized to 5-fluorouracil; it is used as an antineoplastic by intra-arterial administration for treatment of liver metastases from gastrointestinal malignancies.

fl oz fluid ounce.

FLP [L.] fronto-laeva posterior (left frontoposterior, a position of the fetus; see *position*).

FLT [L.] fronto-laeva transversa (left frontotransverse, a position of the fetus; see *position*).

flu (floo) popular name for *influenza.*

trimellitic anhydride (TMA) f. influenzalike symptoms in workers inhaling excessive amounts of trimellitic anhydride fumes. See also *trimellitic anhydride pneumonitis.*

Flu•a•rix (floo′ə-riks) trademark for a preparation of influenza virus vaccine.

flu•ben•da•zole (floo-ben′də-zōl) a benzimidazole anthelmintic used to treat roundworm infestations of pigs.

flu•clox•a•cil•lin (floo-klok″sə-sil′in) BAN and INN for floxacillin.

flu•con•a•zole (floo-kon′ə-zōl) a triazole antifungal used in the systemic treatment of candidiasis and cryptococcal meningitis; administered orally or intravenously.

Flu•cort (floo′kort) trademark for preparations of flumethasone.

fluc•tu•ant (fluk′choo-ənt) 1. showing varying levels. 2. conveying the sensation of or exhibiting wavelike motion on palpation, owing to a liquid content.

fluc•tu•a•tion (fluk″choo-a′shən) [L. *fluctuatio*] 1. a variation, as about a fixed value or mass. 2. a wavelike motion, as of a fluid in a cavity of the body after succussion.

flu•cy•to•sine (floo-si′to-sēn″) [USP] an antifungal used in the treatment of serious infections, such as septicemia, endocarditis, and urinary tract infections, due to *Candida* and *Cryptococcus* species; administered orally.

Flu•da•ra (floo-dar′ə) trademark for a preparation of fludarabine phosphate.

flu•dar•a•bine phos•phate (floo-dar′ə-bēn) an adenine analogue and purine antimetabolite that inhibits DNA synthesis, used as an antineoplastic in the treatment of chronic lymphocytic leukemia; administered intravenously.

flu•de•oxy•glu•cose F 18 (floo″de-ok″se-gloo′kōs) [USP] 2-deoxy-D-glucose labeled with ^{18}F; used in positron emission tomography in the diagnosis of brain disorders, cardiac disease, and tumors of various organs. Called also *fluorodeoxyglucose.*

flu•dro•cor•ti•sone ac•e•tate (floo″dro-kor′tĭ-sōn) [USP] the acetate salt of a synthetic steroid with potent mineralocorticoid and high glucocorticoid activity, used in replacement therapy for primary or secondary adrenocortical insufficiency in Addison disease and for the treatment of salt-losing adrenogenital syndrome; administered orally.

flu•ent (floo′ənt) [L. *fluens* flowing] flowing effortlessly; said of speech.

flu•id (floo′id) [L. *fluidus*] 1. a liquid or a gas. 2. composed of elements or particles which freely change their relative positions without separating. See also *humor, liquid, liquor,* and *solution.*

allantoic f. the fluid contained in the allantois.

Altmann f. a histologic fixing fluid composed of equal parts of 2 per cent osmic acid solution and a 5 per cent potassium dichromate solution.

amniotic f. fluid within the amniotic cavity produced by the amnion during the early embryonic period, and later by the lungs and kidneys; at first crystal clear, it later becomes cloudy. It protects the embryo and fetus from injury. The amount at term normally varies from 500 to 1500 mL. Called also *liquor amnii* and, popularly, *waters.*

antral f. follicular f.

ascitic f. the serous fluid found in the peritoneal cavity in ascites.

bleaching f. a fluid prepared by passing chlorine gas into an emulsion of calcium hydrate.

Bouin f. a histologic fixing fluid consisting of formaldehyde solution, glacial acetic acid, and saturated solution of trinitrophenol.

bursal f. synovia.

Callison f. a solution of distilled water, Löffler methylene blue, formaldehyde solution, glycerin, ammonium oxalate, and sodium chloride; used as a diluent in counting erythrocytes.

Carnoy f. see under *solution.*

Carrel-Dakin f. Dakin solution.

cerebrospinal f. (CSF) liquor cerebrospinalis.

chorionic f. fluid in the chorionic sac; it is resorbed as the amniotic sac enlarges and fuses with the chorionic sac.

Condy f. a disinfecting solution of sodium and potassium permanganates.

crevicular f. gingival f.

decalcifying f. a fluid that removes the calcium from samples or equipment, as from tissues before sectioning.

extracellular f. (ECF) a general term for all the body fluids outside the cells, such as interstitial fluid, plasma, lymph, and cerebrospinal fluid. Extracellular fluid consists of ultrafiltrates of the blood plasma and transcellular fluid (fluid produced by active cellular secretion). It provides a constant external environment for the cells.

Flemming fixing f. Flemming solution.

follicular f. an albuminous fluid in the follicular antrum of a vesicular ovarian follicle. Called also *antral f.* and *liquor folliculi.*

formol-Müller f. Müller fluid to which formaldehyde solution has been added.

gingival f. interstitial fluid and plasma that seeps in minute amounts into the gingival sulcus through its well. Called also *crevicular f.* and *sulcular f.*

Helly f. a histologic fixative consisting of Zenker fixative in which the glacial acetic acid is replaced by formaldehyde solution; the most widely used formula consists of 9 parts Zenker stock solution and 1 part neutral formalin (Zenker-Helly-Maximow) and is usually called *Zenker-formol fixative.*

interstitial f. the extracellular fluid that bathes the cells of most tissues but which is not within the confines of the blood or lymph vessels and is not a transcellular fluid; it is formed by filtration through the blood capillaries and is drained away as lymph. It is the extracellular fluid volume minus the lymph volume, the plasma volume, and the transcellular fluid volume.

intracellular f. (ICF) the portion of the total body water and its dissolved solutes that is within the cell membranes.

labyrinthine f. perilympha.

Locke f. see under *solution.*

Müller f. a hardening solution consisting of potassium dichromate, sodium sulfate, and water.

Parker f. a hardening fluid composed of formaldehyde solution and alcohol.

pericardial f. a fluid found in small amounts in the potential space between the parietal and visceral laminae of the serous pericardium.

Piazza f. a blood-coagulating fluid composed of sodium chloride and ferric chloride in water.

prostatic f. the secretion of the prostate gland, which contributes to formation of the semen.

Scarpa f. endolympha.

Schaudinn f. a hardening fluid consisting of mercury bichloride, dehydrated alcohol, and distilled water.

seminal f. semen (def. 1).

serous f. normal lymph of a serous cavity.

spinal f. the fluid within the spinal canal.

sulcular f. gingival f.

synovial f. synovia.

Thoma f. a decalcifying fluid for histologic work, consisting of alcohol and nitric acid.

tissue f. interstitial f.

Toison f. see under *solution.*

transcellular f. the portion of the extracellular fluid produced by active cellular secretion.

ventricular f. the portion of the cerebrospinal fluid contained in the cerebral ventricles.

Wickersheimer f. a fluid composed of arsenic trioxide, sodium chloride, and the sulfate, carbonate, and nitrate of potassium in a mixture of water, alcohol, and glycerin; used for preserving anatomical specimens.

Zenker f. see under *fixative.*

flu•id•ex•tract (floo″id-ek′strakt) a liquid preparation of a vegetable drug, containing alcohol as a solvent or as a preservative, or both, of such strength that each milliliter contains the therapeutic constituents of 1 g of the standard drug which it represents.

aromatic cascara f. [USP] a preparation of cascara sagrada, magnesium oxide, suitable sweetening agents, essential oils, flavoring agents, and alcohol; used as a cathartic.

eriodictyon f. a fluidextract prepared from eriodictyon; used as a pharmaceutical flavoring agent and in the preparation of aromatic eriodictyon syrup.

licorice f. [NF] a fluidextract prepared from ground licorice, used as a pharmaceutical flavoring agent.

senna f. [USP] a fluidextract prepared from senna; used as a laxative and in the preparation of senna syrup.

flu•id•ounce (floo-id-ouns′) fluid ounce; see under *ounce.*

flu•i•dram (floo″ĭ-dram′) fluid dram; see under *dram.*

fluke (flo͞ok) trematode.

blood f. *Schistosoma.*

conical f. paramphistome.

intestinal f. a fluke that inhabits the intestine, usually a species of family Fasciolidae, Heterophyidae, or Paramphistomatidae.

lancet f. *Dicrocoelium dendriticum.*

liver f. a fluke found in the liver, such as species of *Clonorchis, Dicrocoelium, Fasciola, Fascioloides,* or *Opisthorchis.*

lung f. *Paragonimus westermani.*

rumen f., ruminal f. the usual type of paramphistome, found in the rumen of a ruminant.

Flu•La•val (floo′lə-val) trademark for a preparation of influenza virus vaccine.

flu•like (floo′līk) 1. resembling influenza. 2. characterized by symptoms resembling those of influenza.

Flu•ma•dine (floo′mə-dīn) trademark for preparations of rimantadine hydrochloride.

flu•ma•ze•nil (floo′ma-zə-nil″) [USP] a specific agonist to benzodiazepines that binds competitively to central nervous system benzodiazepine receptors, used to reverse the effects of benzodiazepines following sedation, general anesthesia, or overdose; administered intravenously.

flu•men (floo′mən) pl. *flu′mina* [L.] a stream.

flu′mina pilo′rum [TA] hair streams: continuous lines formed by the pattern of hair growth on various parts of the body, with the hairs lying in the same direction.

flu•me•quine (floo′mə-kwin) a quinolone antibacterial with actions and uses similar to those of nalidixic acid; administered orally.

flu•meth•a•sone (floo-meth′ə-sōn″) a low potency synthetic corticosteroid used in veterinary medicine as an antiinflammatory for a variety of corticosteroid-responsive conditions; administered intramuscularly, intravenously, intra-arterially, and orally.

f. pivalate [USP] the pivalate salt of flumethasone, used topically for the relief of inflammation and pruritus in corticosteroid-responsive dermatoses.

flu•mi•na (floo′mĭ-nə) [L.] plural of *flumen.*

Flu•Mist (floo′mist) trademark for a preparation of influenza virus vaccine for intranasal administration.

flu•nar•i•zine hy•dro•chlo•ride (floo-nar′ĭ-zēn) a calcium channel blocking agent with antihistaminic activity, derived from cinnarizine, used for the prophylaxis of migraine; administered orally.

flu•nis•o•lide (floo-nis′o-līd″) [USP] a synthetic glucocorticoid administered by inhalation for treatment of bronchial asthma and intranasally for treatment of allergic rhinitis and other inflammatory nasal conditions.

flu•ni•traz•e•pam (floo″nĭ-traz′ə-pam) a short-acting benzodiazepine with properties similar to those of diazepam, administered orally as a hypnotic and intramuscularly as an induction agent in anesthesia. It is not used legally in the United States.

flu•nix•in (floo-nik′sin) an antiinflammatory and analgesic.

f. meglumine [USP] the meglumine salt of flunixin, used as a veterinary antiinflammatory and analgesic.

flu•o•cin•o•lone acet•o•nide (floo″ə-sin′ə-lōn) [USP] a synthetic corticosteroid used topically for the relief of inflammation and pruritus in corticosteroid-responsive dermatoses.

flu•o•cin•o•nide (floo″ə-sin′ə-nīd) [USP] a high potency synthetic corticosteroid, derived from fluocinolone acetonide; used topically for the relief of inflammation and pruritus in corticosteroid-responsive dermatoses.

Flu•o•nid (floo′ə-nid) trademark for preparations of fluocinolone acetonide.

flu•or•ane (floor′ān) the parent compound of fluorescein and related dyes; 9-hydroxy-9-xanthene-*o*-benzoic acid lactone.

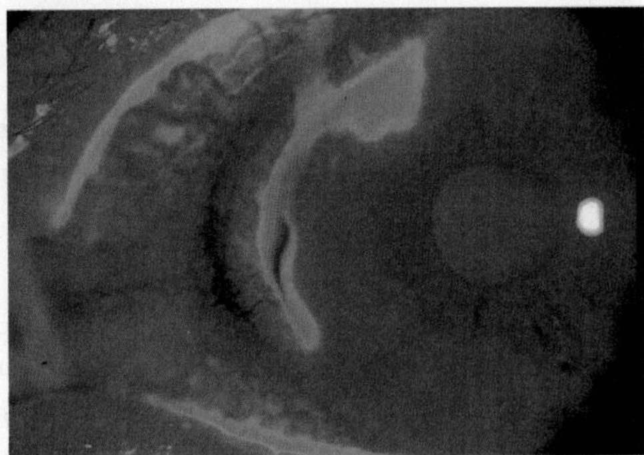

■ Fluorescein staining of an area of ulceration in progressive circumferential peripheral corneal ulceration.

flu•o•res•ce•in (floo͝-res′ēn) [USP] the simplest of the fluorane dyes and the parent compound of eosin; used as a diagnostic indicator in assessing corneal trauma and fitting contact lenses.

f. isothiocyanate (FITC) a fluorescein derivative that can be conjugated to proteins, particularly antibodies, and is used as a fluorescent label in various assays.

f. dilaurate an ester of fluorescein with two molecules of laurate, used in the pancreolauryl test of pancreatic function.

f. sodium [USP] an odorless, water-soluble, orange-red powder used in dilute solution to reveal corneal trauma, in contact lens fitting, and in retinal angiography. Called also *uranin*.

soluble f. f. sodium.

flu•o•res•ce•in•uria (floo͝-res″e-nu′re-ə) the presence of fluorescein in the urine.

flu•o•res•cence (floo͝-res′əns) [first observed in *fluorspar*] the property of emitting light while exposed to light, the wavelength of the emitted light being only slightly longer than that of the light absorbed. Cf. *phosphorescence*.

secondary f. fluorescence in tissues which is induced by staining with fluorescent dyes *(fluorochromes)*. Cf. *autofluorescence*.

flu•o•res•cent (floo͝-res′ənt) exhibiting fluorescence.

flu•o•ri•da•tion (floor″ĭ-da′shən) treatment with fluorides; specifically, the addition of fluoride to the public water supply as part of the public health program to prevent or reduce the incidence of dental caries.

flu•o•ride (floor′īd) a binary compound of fluorine. See also *stannous fluoride*, under *stannous*.

flu•o•rim•e•ter (floo͝-rim′ə-tər) fluorometer.

flu•o•rim•e•try (floo͝-rim′ə-tre) fluorometry.

flu•o•rine (F) (floor′ēn) [L. *fluor* any of a group of minerals, including fluorite (calcium fluoride), used as metallurgical fluxes, from *fluere* to flow] a nonmetallic, gaseous element, belonging to the halogen group; atomic number 9, atomic weight 18.998. Fluorine, in the form of fluoride, is incorporated into the structure of bone and teeth and provides protection against dental caries; an excess of fluorine may result in fluorosis.

f. 18 a radioactive isotope of fluorine, atomic mass 18, having a half-life of 1.8925 hours; it decays primarily by positron emission, with energy 0.635 MeV and has been used as a tracer in positron emission tomography.

flu•o•ro•ac•e•tate (floor″o-as′ə-tāt) a salt of fluoroacetic acid; the sodium salt and others are used in rodenticides and are toxic to many mammalian species. See *fluoroacetate poisoning*, under *poisoning*.

flu•o•ro•ace•tic ac•id (floor″o-ə-se′tik) a toxin from a South African tree, used as a rodenticide; see *sodium fluoroacetate*.

flu•o•ro•car•bon (floor′o-kahr″bən) any of the class of organic compounds consisting of carbon and fluorine only; fluorocarbons are analogous to hydrocarbons but with the hydrogen atoms replaced by fluorine. Fluorocarbon emulsions dissolve oxygen and carbon dioxide and can be used in place of red blood cell preparations in the prevention and treatment of ischemia.

flu•o•ro•chrome (floor′o-krōm) any fluorescent dye used as a stain or label, e.g., fluorescein isothiocyanate attached to an antibody. Called also *fluorophore*.

flu•o•ro•cyte (floor′o-sīt) a reticulocyte showing red fluorescence.

flu•o•ro•de•oxy•glu•cose (floor″o-de-ok″se-gloo′kōs) fludeoxyglucose F 18.

flu•o•ro•do•pa F 18 (floor″o-do′pə) [USP] a compound containing fluorine and levodopa, in which some of the molecules are labeled with ^{18}F; used for positron emission tomography of the cerebrum.

flu•o•rog•ra•phy (floo͝-rog′rə-fe) photofluorography.

flu•o•ro•im•mu•no•as•say (FIA) (floor″o-im″u-no-as′a) fluorescence immunoassay.

flu•o•rom•e•ter (floo͝-rom′ə-tər) the instrument used in fluorometry, consisting of an energy source (e.g., a mercury arc lamp or xenon lamp) to induce fluorescence, filters or monochromators for selection of the wavelength, and a detector; called also *fluorimeter*.

flu•o•ro•meth•o•lone (floor″o-meth′ə-lōn) [USP] a synthetic glucocorticoid used topically in the treatment of corticosteroid-responsive allergic and inflammatory conditions of the eye.

flu•o•rom•e•try (floo͝-rom′ə-tre) an analytical technique for identifying and characterizing minute amounts of a substance by excitation of the substance with a beam of ultraviolet light and detection and measurement of the characteristic wavelength of fluorescent light emitted. Called also *fluorimetry*.

flu•o•ro•naph•thy•ri•done (floor″o-naf-thi′rĭ-dōn) any of a group of antibiotics structurally related to the fluoroquinolones and including alatrofloxacin and trovafloxacin.

flu•o•ro•neph•e•lom•e•ter (floor″o-nef″ə-lom′ə-tər) an instrument for analysis of a solution by measuring the light scattered or emitted by it. Called also *nefluorophotometer*.

flu•o•ro•phore (floor′o-for) fluorochrome.

Fluor-Op (floor′op) trademark for a preparation of fluorometholone.

***p*-flu•o•ro•phen•yl•al•a•nine** (floor″o-fen″əl-al′ə-nēn) a modified molecule of phenylalanine that binds to enzymes but is incapable of performing the functions of the natural molecule and thus acts as an antagonist.

flu•o•ro•phos•phate (floor″o-fos′fāt) a salt or ester containing fluorine and phosphorus.

diisopropyl f. see under *D*.

flu•o•ro•pho•tom•e•try (floor″o-fo-tom′ə-tre) fluorometry.

vitreous f. the measurement of light given off by intravenously injected fluorescein that has leaked through the retinal vessels into the vitreous; done to detect the breakdown of the blood-retinal barrier, an early ocular change in diabetes mellitus.

Flu•or•o•plex (floor′o-pleks″) trademark for preparations of fluorouracil.

flu•o•ro•py•rim•i•dine (flo͞or″o-pə-rim′ĭ-dēn) any of a group of uracil analogues having fluorine substitutions at the 5 position and demonstrating antineoplastic activity, including fluorouracil and floxuridine.

flu•o•ro•quin•o•lone (floor″o-kwin′o-lōn) any of a subgroup of quinolones that have a piperazinyl group and a fluorine atom at position 6 and a broader spectrum of activity than nalidixic acid, including ciprofloxacin, norfloxacin, and ofloxacin. Called also fluorinated 4-quinolone.

flu•o•ro•ra•di•og•ra•phy (floor″o-ra″de-og′rə-fe) photofluorography.

flu•o•ro•scope (floor′o-skōp) a device used for examining deep structures by means of x-rays; it consists of a screen *(fluorescent screen)* covered with crystals of calcium tungstate on which are projected the shadows of x-rays passing through the body placed between the screen and the source of irradiation.

biplane f. a fluoroscope by which examinations can be made in two planes, horizontal and vertical.

flu•o•ros•co•py (floo͝-ros′kə-pe) examination by means of the fluoroscope. **fluoroscop′ic** *adj*

flu•o•ro•sil•i•cate (floor″o-sil′ĭ-kāt) a compound of silicon and some other base with fluorine, such as sodium silicofluoride; fluorosilicates are sometimes used as insecticides, and are very toxic when ingested. Called also *silicofluoride*.

flu•o•ro•sis (floo͝-ro′sis) 1. a condition caused by ingestion of excessive amounts of fluorine or its compounds, such as by from accidental ingestion of an insecticide or rodenticide, chronic inhalation of industrial dusts or gases, or prolonged ingestion of water that contains large amounts of fluorides. Symptoms include skeletal changes such as osteofluorosis, and mottled enamel if the exposure occurs during enamel formation. 2. a condition in

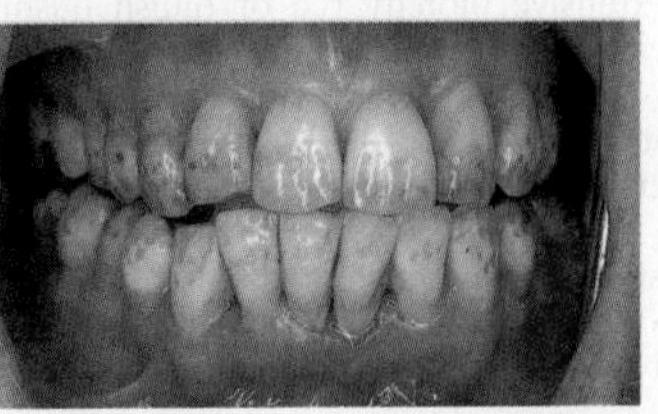

■ Fluorosis resulting from excessive levels of fluoride in drinking water.

livestock that is similar to human fluorosis and may be due to the same factors, to ingestion of feed containing toxic levels of fluorides, or grazing on pastures contaminated from industrial dusts or gases. Called also *chronic endemic f.* and *chronic fluoride* or *fluorine poisoning*.

chronic endemic f. fluorosis.

dental f. mottled enamel.

skeletal f. skeletal changes due to long term ingestion of excessive fluoride; they may include hyperostosis, osteopetrosis, and osteoporosis.

flu•o•ro•ura•cil (floor″o-ūr′ə-sil″) [USP] 5-fluorouracil (5-FU); a fluoropyrimidine metabolically activated like uracil; used intravenously as an antineoplastic for the treatment of solid tumors, especially palliative treatment of carcinomas of the breast and gastrointestinal tract. It is also used topically for the treatment of actinic keratoses and other precancerous skin conditions and for superficial basal cell carcinomas.

Flu•o•sol (floo′o-sol) trademark name for a frozen perfluorochemical used as a temporary carrier of oxygen in the blood.

Flu•o•thane (floo′o-thān) trademark for a preparation of halothane.

flu•ox•e•tine (floo-ok′sə-tēn) a selective serotonin uptake inhibitor used as the hydrochloride salt.

f. hydrochloride [USP] the hydrochloride salt of fluoxetine, used in the treatment of depression, obsessive-compulsive disorder, bulimia nervosa, and premenstrual dysphoric disorder; administered orally.

flu•ox•y•mes•ter•one (floo-ok″se-mes′tər-ōn) [USP] an anabolic-androgenic steroid used in treatment of primary and secondary male hypogonadism and delayed male puberty and in palliation of metastatic breast carcinoma in postmenopausal women; administered orally.

flu•pen•thix•ol (floo″pen-thik′sol) a thioxanthene antipsychotic agent with actions similar to those of chlorpromazine.

flu•pen•tix•ol (floo″pen-tik′sol) INN for *flupenthixol*.

flu•phen•a•zine (floo-fen′ə-zēn) the 2-trifluromethyl derivative of perphenazine, the most potent of the phenothiazine antipsychotic agents.

f. decanoate [USP] the decanoate ester of fluphenazine, having the same actions as the hydrochloride salt, but of longer duration; administered subcutaneously or intramuscularly in maintenance therapy for psychotic disorders.

f. enanthate [USP] the enanthate ester of fluphenazine, having the same uses as the hydrochloride salt, but of longer duration; administered intramuscularly and subcutaneously.

f. hydrochloride [USP] the dihydrochloride salt of fluphenazine, used as an antipsychotic; administered orally and intramuscularly.

flu•pros•te•nol so•di•um (floo-pros′tə-nol) a prostaglandin of the F series used in the treatment of infertility.

flur•an•dren•o•lide (floor″ən-dren′ə-līd) [USP] a synthetic corticosteroid used topically for the relief of inflammation and pruritus in corticosteroid-responsive dermatoses.

flu•raz•e•pam hy•dro•chlo•ride (flo͞o-raz′ə-pam) [USP] a benzodiazepine used as a sedative and hypnotic in the treatment of insomnia; administered orally.

flur•bi•pro•fen (floor-bi′pro-fen) a nonsteroidal antiinflammatory drug derived from propionic acid and structurally related to ibuprofen; administered orally in the treatment of rheumatoid arthritis, osteoarthritis, ankylosing spondylitis, bursitis, tendinitis, soft tissue injuries, and dysmenorrhea.

f. sodium the sodium salt of flurbiprofen, applied topically to the conjunctiva to inhibit miosis during, and as an antiinflammatory following, ophthalmic surgery.

Flur•ess (flo͞o-res′) trademark for a preparation of benoxinate hydrochloride and fluorescein sodium.

flush (flush) 1. transient, episodic redness of the face and neck; it occurs normally in situations of heat, physical exertion, or certain emotions, and pathologically after ingestion of some drugs or other substances and in certain diseases. See also *erythema*. 2. to wash out with fluid.

atropine f. flushing and dryness of the skin of the face and neck from overdosage with atropine.

breast f. a condition sometimes occurring in late pregnancy, consisting of a tense and flushed state of the breasts with prominent veins.

carcinoid f. extensive blotchy red or bluish flushing on the face or trunk, often associated with diarrhea and abdominal pain and sometimes bronchospasm; it is possibly due to vasoactive kinins or other peptides associated with carcinoid tumor.

hectic f. a persistent or chronic flush associated with a hectic fever (q.v.).

histamine f. sudden symmetric erythema of the face and upper trunk, usually associated with throbbing headache, bounding pulse, and histaminuria. Seen in a type of urticaria pigmentosa and also in scombroid poisoning.

malar f. flushing, such as a hectic flush, at the malar eminence.

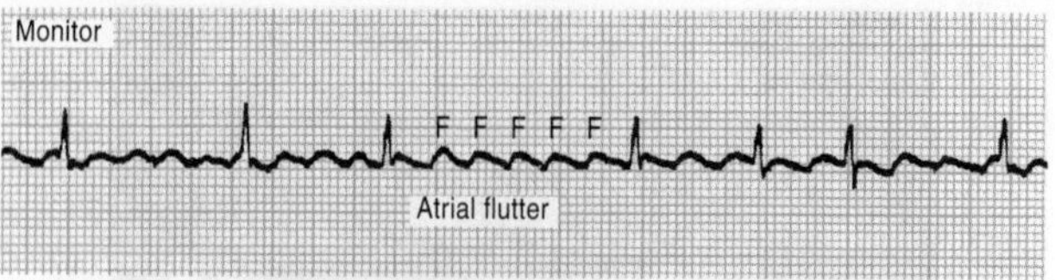

■ Atrial flutter with characteristic sawtooth waves *(F)*.

flu•spir•i•lene (floo-spēr′ĭ-lēn) a diphenylbutylpiperidine antipsychotic, used for the treatment of schizophrenia; administered intramuscularly.

flu•ta•mide (floo′tə-mīd) [USP] a nonsteroidal antiandrogen, administered orally in the treatment of metastatic prostatic carcinoma.

flu•ti•a•zin (floo-ti′ə-zin) a veterinary antiinflammatory agent.

flu•tic•a•sone pro•pi•o•nate (floo-tik′ə-sōn″) [USP] a synthetic corticosteroid used topically as an antiinflammatory and antipruritic in treatment of corticosteroid-responsive dermatoses, intranasally in treatment of allergic rhinitis, other inflammatory nasal conditions, and nasal polyps, and by inhalation in maintenance treatment of asthma.

flut•ter (flut′ər) a rapid vibration or pulsation.

atrial f. a condition of cardiac arrhythmia in which the atrial contractions are rapid (250 to 350 per minute), but regular. In many instances, a circus movement caused by reentry is probably present. The ventricles are unable to respond to each atrial impulse, so that at least a partial atrioventricular block must develop and the ventricular rate is usually approximately 150 beats per minute.

diaphragmatic f. peculiar, wavelike fibrillations of the diaphragm of unknown cause; the condition may be paroxysmal or persist indefinitely.

impure f. an arrhythmia in which the electrocardiogram shows alternating periods of atrial flutter and fibrillation or periods not clearly distinguishable as one versus the other.

mediastinal f. a condition of abnormal motility of the mediastinum during respiratory movements.

ocular f. short bursts of rapid horizontal oscillations of the eye.

pure f. atrial f.

ventricular f. (VFl) a ventricular tachyarrhythmia characterized electrocardiographically by smooth undulating waves with QRS complexes merged with T waves and a rate of approximately 250 per minute. If untreated it usually progresses to ventricular fibrillation.

flut•ter-fib•ril•la•tion (flut′ər-fib″rĭ-la′shən) a type of impure flutter that varies from moment to moment in resemblance to flutter or fibrillation.

flu•va•stat•in so•di•um (floo′və-stat″in) [USP] an inhibitor of HMG-CoA reductase, which can lower plasma levels of cholesterol and raise the plasma level of high-density lipoprotein C (HDL-C); used in the treatment of hypercholesterolemia and other forms of dyslipidemia and to slow the progression of atherosclerosis in patients with coronary heart disease; administered orally.

Flu•vi•rin (floo-vi′rin) trademark for a preparation of influenza virus vaccine.

flu•vox•amine (floo-vok′sə-mēn) a selective serotonin uptake inhibitor used as the maleate salt.

f. maleate [USP] the maleate salt of fluvoxamine, used to relieve the symptoms of obsessive-compulsive and depressive disorders; administered orally.

flux (fluks) [L. *fluxus*] 1. the rate of the flow of some quantity (or magnetic field) per unit area. 2. a substance that maintains the cleanliness of metals to be united and facilitates the easy flow and attachment of solder.

ceramic f. a type of flux used in manufacturing of powdered silicate and porcelain for dental materials.

ionic f. the number of mols per second passing through an area of 1 cm oriented perpendicularly to the direction of flow of the substance.

luminous f. the rate of flow of radiant energy, specifically that of the visible spectrum; its SI unit is the lumen.

magnetic f. (Φ) a quantitative measure of a magnetic field, equal to the integral over a specified surface of the magnetic flux density perpendicular to the surface.

neutral f. a fusible material, usually an inorganic salt, which does not unite with the combined oxygen in the metal but merely dissolves the metal oxide (barium chloride, sodium chloride).

oxidizing f. a material which, when heated, gives up oxygen that may unite with base metals and form oxides (as potassium nitrate, potassium chlorate).

reducing f. a material that unites with the oxygen of metallic oxides and frees the metal from such combinations.

flux•ion (fluk′shən) a flowing; especially an abnormal or excessive flow of fluid to a part.

Flu•zone (floo′zōn) trademark for preparations of influenza virus vaccine.

fly (fli) general term for any of numerous two-winged insects of the order Diptera. Called also *musca*.
black f. any of various insects of the family Simuliidae.
blackbottle f. see *Phormia*.
bloodsucking f's see *Chrysops* and *Tabanus*.
blow f. 1. any member of the genus *Calliphora*. 2. any member of the family Calliphoridae that lays its eggs on injured or decayed animal flesh and causes cutaneous myiasis; this includes most species of *Calliphora* and *Phaenicia* and some of *Cochliomyia* and *Phormia*.
bluebottle f. *Calliphora vomitoria*.
bot f. botfly.
caddis f. a fly of the order Trichoptera; hairs and scales from these flies are a cause of allergic symptoms in susceptible persons.
cheese f. see *Piophila*.
deer f. *Chrysops discalis*.
drone f. *Eristalis tenax*.
dung f. *Sepsis violacea*.
eye f. any fly that attacks the eye, such as species of *Hippelates* and *Siphunculina funicola*.
face f. *Musca autumnalis*.
filth f. *Musca domestica*.
flesh f. any member of the family Sarcophagidae.
fruit f. see *Drosophila*.
gad f. tabanid.
greenbottle f. see *Phaenicia*.
head f. *Hydrotaea irritans*.
heel f. any fly of the genus *Hypoderma*.
horn f. *Haematobia irritans*.
horse f. tabanid.
house f. *Musca domestica*.
hover f's flies of the family Syrphidae.
lake f. *Hexagenia bilineata*.
latrine f. *Fannia scalaris*.
Lund f. *Cordylobia rodhaini*.
mango f., mangrove f. *Chrysops dimidiata*.
moth f. a fly of the family Psychodidae.
nose f., nostril f. *Oestrus ovis*.
owl f. any member of the family Psychodidae.
ox-warble f. any fly of the genus *Hypoderma*.
phlebotomus f. see *Phlebotomus*.
pomace f. *Drosophila*.
Russian f. *Lytta*.
sand f. see *sandfly*.
screw-worm f. *Cochliomyia hominivorax*.
Seroot f. *Tabanus gratus*.
sheep maggot f. a fly whose larvae are sheep maggots.
snipe f. a fly of the family *Rhagionidae*.
soldier f. *Hermetia illucens*.
Spanish f. 1. *Lytta vesicatoria*. 2. cantharides.
stable f. *Stomoxys calcitrans*.
tabanid f. tabanid.
tick f. see *Hippobosca*.
tsetse f. any member of the genus *Glossina*.
tumbu f. *Cordylobia anthropophaga*.
warble f. any fly of the genus *Hypoderma*.

Flynn-Aird syndrome (flin′ ārd′) [P. *Flynn*, American physician, 20th century; Robert Burns *Aird*, American neurologist, 1903–2000] see under *syndrome*.

F.M. [L.] fi′at mistu′ra (make a mixture).

Fm fermium.

FML trademark for preparations of fluorometholone.

FMN flavin mononucleotide, sometimes used specifically for the oxidized form.

FMN ad•e•nyl•yl•trans•fer•ase (ad″ə-nəl″əl-trans′fər-ās) [EC 2.7.7.2] an enzyme of the transferase class that catalyzes the formation of flavin adenine dinucleotide (FAD) by transferring AMP from ATP to flavin mononucleotide (FMN).

FMNH$_2$ the reduced form of flavin mononucleotide.

FMTC familial medullary thyroid carcinoma.

FNH focal nodular hyperplasia.

FNS functional neuromuscular stimulation.

FNTC fine needle transhepatic cholangiography.

foam (fōm) [A.S. *fām*] 1. a dispersion of gas in a liquid or solid, e.g., whipped cream or pumice. 2. frothy saliva, produced particularly on exertion or pathologically. 3. the frothy sweat of an equine. 4. to produce or cause production of such a substance.

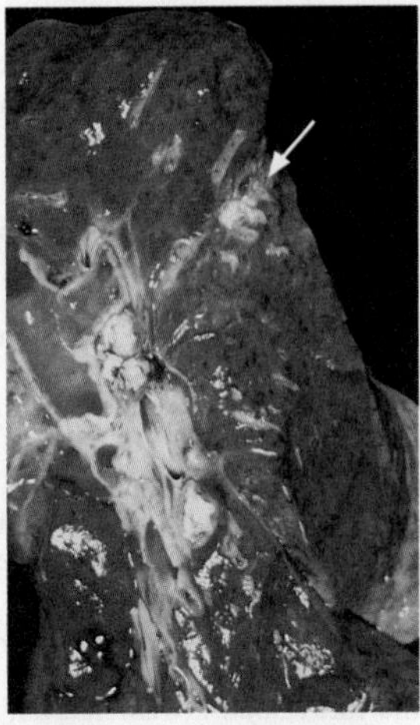

■ Ghon focus *(arrow)* in pulmonary tuberculosis.

fo•cal (fo′kəl) pertaining to or occupying a focus.

Fo•ca•lin (fo′kə-lin) trademark for preparations of dexmethylphenidate hydrochloride.

fo•ci (fo′si) [L.] genitive and plural of *focus*.

fo•cim•e•ter (fo-sim′ə-tər) [*focus* + *-meter*] an apparatus for finding the focus of a lens.

fo•cus (fo′kəs) pl. *fo′ci* [L. "fire-place"] 1. the point of convergence of light rays or of the waves of sound. 2. the chief center of a morbid process. 3. cardiac pacemaker.
aplanatic f. the focus or point from which diverging rays pass the lens without spherical aberration.
Assmann f. the early exudative lesion of pulmonary tuberculosis, occurring most frequently in the subapical region; called also *Assmann tuberculous infiltrate*.
conjugate f. the point at which rays that come from some definite point are brought together.
dysplastic f. a collection of dysplastic hepatocytes less than 1 mm in diameter, occurring as a precancerous condition in the liver. Cf. *dysplastic nodule*, under *nodule*.
ectopic f. see under *pacemaker*.
epileptogenic f. the area of the cerebral cortex responsible for causing epileptic seizures.
epileptogenic f., secondary a second focus that develops in a different part of the brain because of a spread of the pathologic process outward from the original epileptogenic focus; it may develop into a new, independent focus that continues to operate after the original one has been treated.
Ghon f. the primary parenchymal lesion of primary pulmonary tuberculosis; when associated with a corresponding lymph node focus, it is known as the *primary* or *Ghon complex*. Called also *Ghon primary lesion* and *Ghon tubercle*.
mirror f. a type of secondary epileptogenic focus that develops in the opposite hemisphere as an approximate mirror image of the original focus.
principal foci points of convergence of rays parallel with the principal axis of a lens, or system: in the eye (approx.) 18 mm from the anterior nodal point, and 24 mm from the posterior nodal point, and holding the ratio of the indices of air and vitreum.
real f. the point at which convergent rays intersect.
Simon foci hematogenous areas in the apices of the lungs of children regarded as precursors of apical tuberculosis in later life.
virtual f. the point at which divergent rays would intersect if prolonged backward.

fo•cus•ing (fo′kəs-ing) the act of converging at a point.
isoelectric f. electrophoresis in which the protein mixture is subjected to an electric field in a gel medium in which a pH gradient has been established; each protein then migrates until it reaches the site (or focus) at which the pH is equal to its isoelectric point. Called also *electrofocusing*.

fo•drin (fo′drin) an isoform of spectrin found in cells of the brain and intestinal microvilli; it helps form and dismantle microfilaments, thus aiding or inhibiting cell movements.

foe- for words beginning thus, see those beginning *fe-*.

Foe•nic•u•lum (fe-nik′u-ləm) a genus of flowering herbs of the family Umbelliferae, native to Europe and Asia. *F. vulga′re* is fennel, the source of fennel oil.

Foer•ster see *Förster.*

fog (fog) 1. a colloid system in which the dispersion medium is a gas and the disperse particles are liquid, e.g., a cloudlike mass of water droplets dispersed in air. 2. an artifact seen on a radiograph caused by unintentional exposure to reducing contrast. 3. aftermath.

mental f. clouding of consciousness.

Fo•gar•ty catheter (fo′gər-te) [Thomas J. *Fogarty,* American thoracic surgeon, born 1934] see under *catheter.*

fog•ging (fog′ing) in ophthalmology, a method employed in determining the refractive error, the patient being first made artificially myopic by means of plus spheres, in order to relax all accommodation before using cylinders.

fo•go (faw′goo) [Port. "fire"] a skin condition in South America.

f. selva′gem (sāl-vah′zha) [Port. "wild fire"] a progressive, sometimes fatal variant of pemphigus foliaceus endemic in certain areas of South America, characterized by a burning sensation with blisters that rupture to form erosions with peripheral rolls of epidermis. Called also *Brazilian, South American,* or *wildfire pemphigus.*

foil (foil) metal in the form of an extremely thin, pliable sheet.

gold f. pure gold beaten and/or rolled into thin sheets, used as a direct filling material in dental restorations; gold foil used in direct restorations has a thickness of 0.5 μm or less. Occasionally used loosely to refer to mat gold and powdered gold.

gold f., cohesive gold foil that has been rendered cohesive by the process of annealing or degassing; pieces of cold gold foil are welded together into a desired shape or thinness. Called also *cohesive gold.*

mat f. foil produced by sandwiching mat gold (see under *gold*) between two sheets of cohesive gold foil; used as a direct filling dental material.

platinum f. a very thin foil of pure platinum, suitable for use as a matrix to provide internal forms for porcelain restorations during their fabrication.

tin f. a thin sheet rolled from tin, used as a protective wrapping; also used as a separating material between the cast and denture base material during flasking and curing. Written also *tinfoil.*

Foix syndrome (fwah) [Charles *Foix,* French neurologist, 1882–1927] cavernous sinus syndrome.

Foix-Ala•jou•a•nine syndrome (fwah′ ah-lah-zhoo-ah-nēn′) [C. *Foix;* Théophile *Alajouanine,* French neurologist, 1890–1980] see under *syndrome.*

Foix-Cha•va•ny-Ma•rie syndrome (fwah′ shah-vah-ne′ mah-re′) [C. *Foix;* Jean Alfred Emile *Chavany,* French neurologist, 1892–1959; Julien *Marie,* French pediatrician, 1899–1987] anterior opercular syndrome.

fo•la•cin (fo′lə-sin) folic acid or derivatives with similar vitamin activity.

fo•late (fo′lāt) 1. the anionic form of folic acid. 2. more generally, any of the pteroylglutamate derivatives having various levels of reduction of the bicyclic pteridine portion, substitutions of this structure, and numbers of glutamate residues.

f. polyglutamate pteroylpolyglutamate.

fold (fōld) a thin, recurved margin, or doubling over; called also *plica.*

Fold

For descriptions of specific anatomic structures not found here, see under *plica.*

alar f's plicae alares.
amniotic f. the folded edge of the amniotic membrane where it rises over and finally encloses the embryo.
anal f's slight elevations flanking the anal membrane and derived from the cloacal folds; they form the margin of the anus.
anterior f. of malleus plica mallearis anterior tunicae mucosae cavitatis tympanicae.
aryepiglottic f. plica aryepiglottica.
axillary f., anterior a shallow skin furrow in the axilla consisting of a fold of skin and muscle, produced by the lower border of the pectoralis major muscle, forming the anterior boundary of the axillary fossa. Called also *plica axillaris anterior.*
axillary f., posterior a shallow skin furrow consisting of skin and muscle produced by the latissimus dorsi and teres major muscles, forming the posterior boundary of the axillary fossa. Called also *plica axillaris posterior.*
Brachet mesolateral f. mesolateral f.
bulboventricular f. a fold between the bulbus cordis and the ventricle that disappears as the bulbus cordis is absorbed into the right ventricle.
caval f. a ridge that contains the superior segment of the embryonic inferior vena cava.
cecal f's plicae caecales.
cholecystoduodenocolic f. an occasionally present fold of peritoneum sometimes uniting the colon, duodenum, and gallbladder.
ciliary f's plicae ciliares.
circular f's, circular f's of Kerckring plicae circulares.
cloacal f's slight elevations located just lateral to the cloacal membrane early in the fifth week of embryonic development, later dividing into urogenital folds and anal folds.
conjunctival f. the cul-de-sac formed where the conjunctiva is reflected from the eyeball to the upper or lower eyelid; called also *palpebral f.* and *retrotarsal f.*
Dennie-Morgan f. Morgan f.
Douglas f. 1. plica rectouterina. 2. linea arcuata vaginae musculi recti abdominis.
Duncan f's the loose folds of peritoneum which cover the uterus immediately following delivery.
duodenal f., inferior plica duodenalis inferior.
duodenal f., superior plica duodenalis superior.
duodenojejunal f. plica duodenalis superior.
duodenomesocolic f. plica duodenalis inferior.
epicanthal f., epicanthine f. epicanthus.
epigastric f. plica umbilicalis lateralis.
fimbriated f. plica fimbriata.
gastric f's plicae gastricae.
gastropancreatic f., left plica gastropancreatica.
gastropancreatic f., right plica hepatopancreatica.
genital f. gonadal ridge.
glossoepiglottic f., lateral plica glosso-epiglottica lateralis.
glossoepiglottic f., median plica glosso-epiglottica mediana.
gluteal f. sulcus glutealis.
Guérin f. valvula fossae navicularis.
Hasner f. plica lacrimalis.
head f. a crescentic, ventral fold of the embryonic disc at the future head end of the embryo.
Heister f. plica spiralis.
hepatopancreatic f. plica hepatopancreatica.
horizontal f's of rectum plicae transversae recti.
ileocecal f. plica ileocaecalis.
incudal f., f. of incus plica incudialis.
inframammary f. (IMF) the angle of deflection where the breast tissue meets the chest wall below the breast.
interarticular f. of hip ligamentum capitis femoris.
interarytenoid f. plica interarytenoidea.
interdigital f. see under *web.*
interureteric f. plica interureterica.
iridial f's plicae iridis.
Jonnesco f., Juvara f. parietoperitoneal f.
Kerckring f's, Kerkring f's plicae circulares.
Kohlrausch f's plicae transversae recti.
labioscrotal f's see under *swelling.*
lacrimal f. plica lacrimalis.
longitudinal f. of duodenum plica longitudinalis duodeni.
malleolar f. of mucous membrane of tympanic cavity, anterior plica mallearis anterior tunicae mucosae cavitatis tympanicae.
malleolar f. of mucous membrane of tympanic cavity, posterior plica mallearis posterior tunicae mucosae cavitatis tympanicae.
malleolar f. of tympanic membrane, anterior plica mallearis anterior membranae tympanicae.
malleolar f. of tympanic membrane, posterior plica mallearis posterior membranae tympanicae.
mammary f. inframammary f.
Marshall f. plica venae cavae sinistrae.
medullary f. neural f.
mesolateral f. the right lamella of the primordial mesentery running to the right liver; called also *Brachet mesolateral f.*

Fold *Continued*

mesonephric f. see under *ridge*.
mesouterine f. a fold of peritoneum supporting the uterus.
Morgan f. a secondary crease in the lower eyelids in atopic dermatitis; called also *Dennie-Morgan f.* or *line* and *Morgan line*.
mucobuccal f. the cul-de-sac formed where the mucous membrane is reflected from the upper or lower jaw to the cheek.
mucolabial f. the line of flexure of the oral mucous membrane as it passes from the mandible or maxilla to the lip.
mucosal f. a fold of mucous membrane; called also *mucous f.*
mucosal f's of gallbladder plicae mucosae vesicae biliaris.
mucosobuccal f. mucobuccal f.
mucous f. mucosal f.
mucous f's of rectum columnae anales.
nail f. vallum unguis.
nasopharyngeal f. plica salpingopalatina.
Nélaton f. one of the transverse folds of the rectum, marking the junction of its lower and middle thirds.
neural f. one of the paired folds of the neural plate, lying one on either side of the neural groove, that fuse to form the neural tube; called also *medullary f.*
opercular f. a fold of tissue constituting an adhesion between the tonsil and the anterior pillar of the fauces.
palatine f's, palatine f's, transverse plicae palatinae transversae.
palmate f's plicae palmatae.
palpebral f. conjunctival f.
palpebronasal f. epicanthus.
paraduodenal f. plica paraduodenalis.
parietoperitoneal f. a fold of peritoneum in the fetus, arising at the left side of the ascending colon and attached to the parietal peritoneum at the right of the ascending colon; called also *Jonnesco* or *Juvara f.*
pharyngoepiglottic f. plica glosso-epiglottica lateralis.
pleuropericardial f's a pair of small ridges that originate along the lateral body walls in the fifth week of embryonic development and project into the cranial ends of the pericardioperitoneal canals to divide the pleural cavities from the pericardial cavity; they later develop into the pleuropericardial membranes.
pleuroperitoneal f's a pair of crescent-shaped ridges that originate along the lateral body walls of in the fifth week of embryonic development and project into the caudal ends of the pericardioperitoneal canals to divide the pleural cavities from the peritoneal cavity; they later develop into the pleuroperitoneal membranes.
posterior f. of malleus plica mallearis posterior.
primitive f. one of the two ridges flanking the primitive groove in the primitive streak, one on either side.
Rathke f's two fetal folds of mesoderm which unite at the median line to form the Douglas septum and to render the rectum a complete canal.
rectal f's plicae transversae recti.
rectouterine f. plica rectouterina.
rectovaginal f. a fold of peritoneum interposed between the rectum and vagina.
rectovesical f. plica rectouterina.
retrotarsal f. conjunctival f.
Rindfleisch f's folds in the serous surface of the pericardium around the beginning of the aorta.
sacrogenital f. plica rectouterina.
salpingopalatine f. plica salpingopalatina.
salpingopharyngeal f. plica salpingopharyngea.
Schultze f. a sickle-shaped fold of the amnion extending from the point of insertion of the cord into the placenta to the remains of the umbilical vesicle.
semilunar f's of colon plicae semilunares coli.
semilunar f. of conjunctiva plica semilunaris conjunctivae.
semilunar f. of fauces plica semilunaris faucium.
semilunar f. of fascia transversalis ligamentum interfoveolare.
serosal f., serous f. a fold of serous membrane.
sigmoid f's of colon plicae semilunares coli.
skin f. 1. skinfold. 2. a skin furrow deeper than a groove.
spiral f., spiral f. of cystic duct plica spiralis.
stapedial f., f. of stapedius plica stapedialis.
sublingual f. plica sublingualis.
synovial f. plica synovialis.
synovial f., infrapatellar plica synovialis infrapatellaris.
synovial f., mediopatellar plica synovialis mediopatellaris.
synovial f., patellar plica synovialis infrapatellaris.
synovial f., suprapatellar plica synovialis suprapatellaris.
synovial f. of hip ligamentum capitis femoris.
tail f. a crescentic, ventral fold of the embryonic disc at the future caudal end of the embryo.
tracheoesophageal f's longitudinal folds in the embryonic respiratory diverticulum that fuse to form the tracheoesophageal septum.
transverse f's of rectum plicae transversae recti.
Treves f. plica ileocaecalis.
triangular f. plica triangularis.
tubal f's of uterine tube plicae tubariae tubae uterinae.
f's of tunica mucosa of gallbladder plicae mucosae vesicae biliaris.
umbilical f., lateral plica umbilicalis lateralis.
umbilical f., medial plica umbilicalis medialis.
umbilical f., median, umbilical f., middle plica umbilicalis mediana.
urachal f. plica umbilicalis mediana.
urethral f's, urogenital f's a pair of folds derived from the cloacal folds; in male embryos they close over the urethral plate and fuse to form the spongy urethra and ventral aspect of the penis, and in female embryos they fuse only anterior to the anus and form the labia minora.
urorectal f. see under *septum*.
vaginal f's rugae vaginales.
vascular cecal f. plica caecalis vascularis.
Vater f. a fold in the mucous membrane of the duodenum superior to the hepatopancreatic ampulla.
ventricular f. plica vestibularis.
vesical f., transverse plica vesicalis transversa.
vestibular f. plica vestibularis.
vestigial f. of Marshall plica venae cavae sinistrae.
villous f's of stomach plicae villosae gastricae.
vocal f. plica vocalis.
vocal f., false plica vestibularis.

Fo•lex (fo′leks) trademark for preparations of methotrexate sodium.

Fo•ley catheter, Y-V pyeloplasty (ureteropelvioplasty) (fo′le) [Frederic Eugene Basil *Foley*, American urologist, 1891–1966] see under *catheter* and *pyeloplasty*.

FOLFOX a cancer chemotherapy regimen consisting of folinic acid, fluorouracil, and oxaliplatin.

fo•lia (fo′le-ə) plural of *folium*.

fo•li•a•ceous (fo″le-a′shəs) foliate.

fo•li•an (fo′le-ən) named for Caecilius *Folius*, as *folian process*.

fo•li•ate (fo′le-ət) [L. *folia* leaves] 1. having, pertaining to, or resembling leaves. 2. consisting of thin, leaflike layers.

fo•lic ac•id (fo′lik) 1. a water-soluble vitamin of the B complex composed of pteroic acid linked to L-glutamic acid (pteroylglutamic acid); more generally, any derivatives having various levels of reduction of the bicyclic pteridine portion, substitutions at this structure, and number of glutamate residues. Folic acid is necessary for hematopoiesis and is found in liver, green vegetables, and yeast. After absorption, it is successively reduced to dihydrofolic acid and then tetrahydrofolic acid (q.v.), the parent compound of the derivatives that act as coenzyme carriers of one-carbon groups in various metabolic reactions. Deficiency of folic acid results in anemia (see *folic acid deficiency anemia*, under *anemia*). 2. [USP] a preparation of folic acid administered orally or parenterally in the prophylaxis and treatment of folic acid deficiency states, including megaloblastic anemia.

fo•lie (fo-le′) [Fr.] psychosis; insanity.

f. **à deux** (ah doo̅) ["madness between two"] mental disorder affecting two persons who share the same delusions; classified as *shared psychotic disorder* (q.v.) by DSM-IV.

f. **du pourquoi** (doo poor-kwah′) ["madness of why"] psychopathologic constant questioning.

f. **gémellaire** (zha″mĕ-lăr′) ["madness of twins"] psychosis occurring simultaneously in twins.

Fol•in method (fol′in) [Otto Knut Olof *Folin*, American physiologic chemist, 1867–1934] see under *method*.

fo•lin•ic ac•id (fo-lin′ik) the 5-formyl derivative of tetrahydrofolic acid; it can act as a coenzyme carrier in certain folate-mediated reactions but does not require dihydrofolate reductase activity and thus it is used, as the calcium salt leucovorin calcium, in treating some disorders of folic acid deficiency. Called also *leucovorin* and *citrovorum factor.*

fo•li•um (fo′le-əm) pl. *fo′lia* [L. "leaf"] a leaflike structure, especially one of the leaflike subdivisions of the cerebellar cortex.

fo′lia cerebel′li [TA] folia of cerebellum: the numerous long narrow folds of the cerebellar cortex, separated by fissures and supported by white laminae; they are aggregated into the various subdivisions of the cerebellum. Called also *gyri cerebelli.*

lingual folia papillae foliatae.

f. ver′mis [TA] folium of vermis (VII A): a lobule of the vermis of the cerebellum, in the posterior superior region, between the declive and the tuber vermis and continuous with the superior semilunar lobule on each side.

Fo•li•us muscle, process (fo′le-əs) [Caecilius *Folius,* Italian anatomist, 1615–1660] see *ligamentum mallei laterale* and *processus anterior mallei.*

fol•li•cle (fol′ĭ-kəl) 1. a sac or pouchlike depression or cavity; see also *folliculus.* 2. lymphoid nodule.

antral f′s folliculi ovarici vesiculosi.

atretic ovarian f. an ovarian follicle that began to mature but did not become the dominant follicle and has involuted.

dental f. tooth f.

dominant ovarian f. the growing ovarian follicle in a given menstrual cycle that matures completely and forms the corpus luteum.

Fleischmann f. an occasional follicle in the mucosa of the floor of the mouth, near the anterior border of the genioglossus muscle.

gastric f′s fundic glands.

graafian f′s folliculi ovarici vesiculosi.

growing ovarian f. a follicle that has undergone recruitment and is either a primary or a vesicular ovarian follicle.

hair f. folliculus pili.

intestinal f′s glandulae intestinales.

Lieberkühn f′s glandulae intestinales.

lingual f′s noduli lymphoidei tonsillae lingualis.

lymphatic f., lymphoid f. lymphoid nodule.

Montgomery f′s Naboth f′s.

Naboth f′s, nabothian f′s cystlike formations caused by occlusion of the lumina of glands in the mucosa of the uterine cervix, causing them to be distended with retained secretion; called also *Montgomery f′s* and *Naboth cysts* or *glands.*

ovarian f. the oocyte and its encasing cells, at any stage of its development.

pilosebaceous f. see under *unit.*

primary lymphoid f. see under *nodule.*

primary ovarian f′s growing ovarian follicles that are partially mature, each comprising an immature oocyte and the specialized epithelial cells (follicle cells) that surround it.

primordial ovarian f. an immature ovarian follicle that has not undergone recruitment and consists of an oocyte enclosed by a single layer of cells. Called also *unilaminar ovarian f.*

sebaceous f. glandula sebacea.

secondary lymphoid f. see under *nodule.*

secondary ovarian f′s folliculi ovarici vesiculosi.

solitary f′s, solitary lymphatic f′s, solitary lymphoid f′s noduli lymphoidei solitarii; see under *nodulus.*

f. of Stannius a lymphoid unit in chicks, resembling the thymus and developing from nodules formed by proliferation of points of the epithelium of the bursa of Fabricius.

thyroid f′s, f′s of thyroid gland discrete, cystlike units of the thyroid gland that are lined with cuboidal epithelium and are filled with a colloid substance; there are about 30 to each lobule. Called also *thyroid acini.*

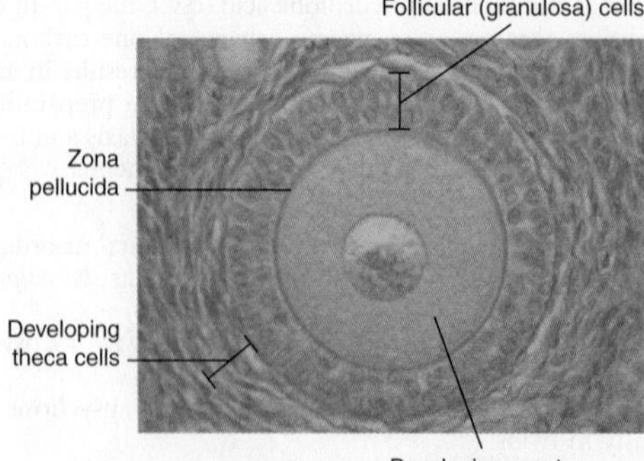

■ Ovarian follicle in early stage of oocyte development.

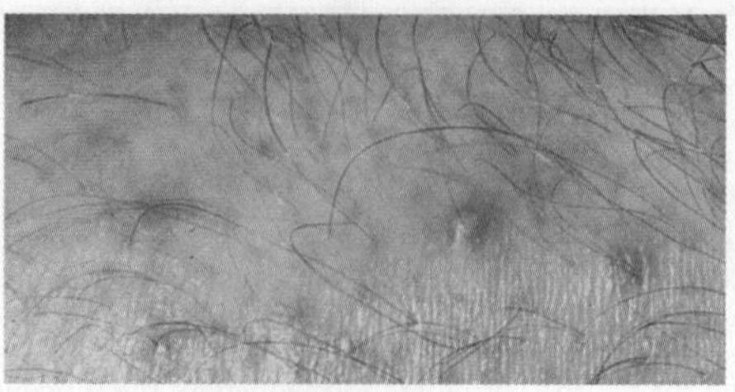

■ Folliculitis.

f′s of tongue noduli lymphoidei tonsillae lingualis.

tooth f. the structure within the developing alveolar bone of the jaws enclosing the tooth germ. Called also *dental f.*

unilaminar ovarian f. primordial ovarian f.

vesicular ovarian f′s folliculi ovarici vesiculosi.

fol•lic•u•lar (fə-lik′u-lər) [L. *follicularis*] of or pertaining to a follicle or follicles.

fol•lic•u•li (fə-lik′u-li) [L.] genitive and plural of *folliculus.*

fol•lic•u•li•tis (fə-lik″u-li′tis) inflammation of a follicle or follicles; usually referring to hair follicles, but sometimes to follicles of other kinds.

f. absce′dens et suffo′diens perifolliculitis capitis abscedens et suffodiens.

agminate f. inflammation of a number of follicles in one area.

f. bar′bae see under *pseudofolliculitis.*

f. decal′vans a rare, localized, spreading, suppurative folliculitis of unknown cause, leading to scarring, with permanent hair loss.

dissecting f. perifolliculitis capitis abscedens et suffodiens.

eosinophilic pustular f. a rare dermatosis characterized by pruritic sterile pustules on the face, trunk, and limbs, coalescing to form plaques that tend toward central clearing with hyperpigmentation and have spontaneous exacerbation and remission. There is spongiosis of the follicular epithelium and leukocytic infiltration of the hair follicle root sheath and nearby dermis, which results in destruction of the follicle and sometimes formation of abscesses. Called also *Ofuji disease.*

gram-negative f. a superinfection complicating long-term systemic antibiotic treatment of acne vulgaris, particularly with tetracyclines, usually caused by species of *Enterobacter, Klebsiella,* or *Proteus.* Infection with the first two species is manifested by a superficial pustular eruption, often around the nares; *Proteus* infections are characterized by deep nodular cysts, usually on the back.

hot tub f. *Pseudomonas* f.

keloidal f., f. keloida′lis acne keloidalis.

f. keloida′lis nu′chae see under *acne.*

f. na′res per′forans inflammation of a hair follicle in the nose, with pustulation and destruction of the follicle, leading to extension of the process through the tissues to the external surface.

perforating f. a type of acquired perforating dermatosis in which hair follicles are associated with small, discrete, erythematous papules with a keratotic plug. It occurs most often on the upper arms, buttocks, and thighs of young adults and in diabetics receiving hemodialysis; lesions have a central hair or a central umbilication containing keratinous material, and the Koebner phenomenon may occur.

***Pseudomonas* f.** a pruritic skin rash with follicular papules, vesicles, and pustules, seen after exposure to water contaminated with *Pseudomonas aeruginosa.* Called also *hot tub f.* or *whirlpool f.*

tufted hair f. an inflammatory, exudative scalp condition of unknown etiology, possibly related to folliculitis decalvans, in which multiple hairs emerge from single follicles in a localized area, often resulting in scarring and alopecia (cicatricial alopecia).

f. ulerythemato′sa reticula′ta a type of atrophoderma vermiculatum that is usually confined to the cheek but sometimes spreads to the ears, forehead, and scalp.

f. variolifor′mis see under *acne.*

whirlpool f. *Pseudomonas* f.

fol•lic•u•lo•cen•tric (fə-lik″u-lo-sen′trik) centered around the hair follicles; said of adnexal tumors.

fol•lic•u•lo•gen•e•sis (fə-lik″u-lo-jen′ə-sis) the formation of ovarian follicles. **folliculogen′ic** *adj*

fol•lic•u•lo•ma (fə-lik″u-lo′mə) [*folliculus* + *-oma*] 1. a benign adnexal tumor of a hair follicle; see *fibrofolliculoma* and *trichofolliculoma.* 2. granulosa–theca cell tumor; see under *tumor.*

f. lipidique a granulosa-theca cell tumor in which streamers or trabeculae of tall, columnar, lipid-laden cells are interspersed among the more characteristic collections of granulosa cells.

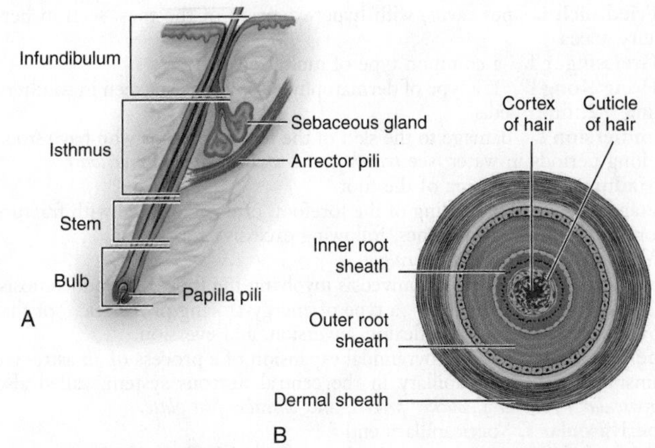

■ Folliculus pili (hair follicle). *(A)*, Longitudinal section, comprising the infundibulum, isthmus, stem, and bulb; *(B)*, transverse section of follicle, showing the hair shaft and surrounding follicular sheaths.

fol·lic·u·lo·sis (fə-lik″u-lo′sis) a disease characterized by excessive development of lymph follicles.

fol·lic·u·lo·stat·in (fə-lik″u-lo-stat′in) [*follicle*-stimulating hormone + *-statin*] follistatin.

fol·lic·u·lo·trop·ic (fə-lik″u-lo-trop′ik) spreading into hair follicle structures; said of adnexal tumors.

fol·lic·u·lus (fə-lik′u-ləs) gen. and pl. *folli′culi* [L., dim. of *follis* a leather bag] follicle: a very small excretory or secretory sac or gland.

folli′culi ova′rici vesiculo′si [TA] vesicular ovarian follicles: growing ovarian follicles that are nearing maturity and among whose cells fluid has begun to accumulate, leading to formation of a single cavity called the follicular antrum. The oocyte is eccentrically located in the cumulus oophorus, a hillock of follicle cells. Called also *antral follicles* and *graafian follicles.*

f. pi′li [TA] hair follicle: one of the tubular invaginations of the epidermis that enclose the hairs, and from which they grow. It is divided into upper and lower segments: the upper comprises the follicular infundibulum (extending from the free surface to the sebaceous gland) and the isthmus (extending from the sebaceous gland to the arrector pili muscle); the lower comprises the hair bulb and the part sometimes referred to as the stem. In the lower part, the hair cuticle is surrounded by the inner and outer root sheaths, enclosed within a dermal sheath.

fol·li·stat·in (fol′ĭ-stat″in) [*follicle*-stimulating hormone + *-statin*] a peptide that suppresses the secretion of follicle-stimulating hormone; called also *folliculostatin.*

Fol·lis·tim (fol′is-tim) trademark for a preparation of follitropin beta.

fol·li·tro·pin (fol′ĭ-tro″pin) follicle-stimulating hormone.

f. alfa, f. beta two synthetic isoforms of follicle-stimulating hormone derived from genetically modified Chinese hamster ovary cells, differing in method of manufacture; used to stimulate the development of ovarian follicles in the treatment of female infertility and to induce ovulation in women undergoing an assisted reproductive technology procedure; administered subcutaneously or intramuscularly. Follitropin alfa is also used to induce spermatogenesis in men with primary and secondary hypogonadotropic hypogonadism.

fol·low·ing (fol′o-ing) an effect seen on an electroencephalogram, in which brain waves change their frequencies in response to certain repetitive sensory stimuli. Cf. *driving.*

fol·low-through (fol′o throo′) a barium study done over time.

small bowel f.-t. (SBFT) a type of barium study in which contrast medium is administered orally and monitored on a series of radiographs as it travels through the small intestine.

Foltz valve (fōlts) [Jean Charles Eugène *Foltz,* French ophthalmologist, 1822–1876] see under *valve.*

Fol·vite (fol′vīt) trademark for preparations of folic acid.

fo·men·ta·tion (fo″mən-ta′shən) [L. *fomentatio; fomentum,* a poultice] treatment by warm and moist applications; also the substance thus applied.

fo·mep·i·zole (fo-mep′ĭ-zōl) an alcohol dehydrogenase inhibitor, used as an antidote to poisoning by methanol or ethylene glycol. Called also *4-methyl-1H-pyrazole.*

fo·mes (fo′mēz) pl. *fo′mites* [L. "tinder"] fomite.

fo·mite (fo′mīt) [back-formation from Latin plural *fomites*] an object, such as a book, wooden object, or an article of clothing, that is not in itself harmful, but is able to harbor pathogenic microorganisms and thus may serve as an agent of transmission of an infection. Called also *fomes.*

fom·i·tes (fo′mĭ-tēz) plural of *fomes.*

fo·mi·vir·sen so·di·um (fo-miv′ər-sən) an antiviral agent, administered by intravitreal injection in the treatment of cytomegalovirus retinitis associated with AIDS.

fon·da·par·i·nux so·d·ium (fon″də-par′ĭ-nuks) an antithrombotic compound that inhibits factor Xa by selectively binding antithrombin III, used in the treatment of deep vein thrombosis; administered subcutaneously.

Fon·se·caea (fon-se-se′ə) [O. da *Fonseca,* Brazilian scientist, early 20th century] a genus of Fungi Imperfecti of the form-class Hyphomycetes, form-family Dematiaceae; some species were formerly included in the genera *Hormodendrum* and *Cladosporium. F. compac′tum* and *F. pedro′soi* are etiologic agents of chromoblastomycosis.

Fon·tan procedure (fawn-tah′) [François Maurice *Fontan,* French heart surgeon, born 1929] see under *procedure.*

Fon·ta·na spaces (fōn-tah′nah) [Felice *Fontana,* Italian naturalist and physiologist, 1730–1805] spatia anguli iridocornealis; see under *spatium.*

fon·ta·nel (fon″tə-nel′) fontanelle.

fon·ta·nelle (fon″tə-nel′) [Fr., dim. of *fontaine* spring, filter] fonticulus; see *fonticuli cranii.*

anterior f. fonticulus anterior.
anterolateral f. fonticulus sphenoidalis.
bregmatic f. fonticulus anterior.
Casser f., casserian f., Casserio f. fonticulus mastoideus.
cranial f's fonticuli cranii.
frontal f. fonticulus anterior.
Gerdy f. a fontanelle occasionally occurring in the sagittal suture; called also *sagittal f.*
mastoid f. fonticulus mastoideus.
occipital f., posterior f. fonticulus posterior.
posterolateral f., posterotemporal f. fonticulus mastoideus.
quadrangular f. fonticulus anterior.
sagittal f. Gerdy f.
sphenoidal f. fonticulus sphenoidalis.
triangular f. fonticulus posterior.

fon·tic·u·li (fon-tik′u-li) [L.] genitive and plural of *fonticulus.*

fon·tic·u·lus (fon-tik′u-ləs) pl. *fontic′uli* [L., dim. of *fons* fountain] fontanelle: one of the fonticuli cranii (q.v.).

f. ante′rior [TA] anterior fontanelle: the unossified area of the skull situated at the junction of the frontal, coronal, and sagittal sutures; called also *f. frontalis [major]* and *frontal fontanelle.*

f. anterolatera′lis TA alternative for *f. sphenoidalis.*

fontic′uli cra′nii [TA] fontanelles: the membrane-covered spaces, or soft spots, remaining at the incomplete angles of the parietal and adjacent bones, until ossification of the skull is completed. Popularly called *soft spots.*

f. ma′jor f. anterior.

f. mastoi′deus [TA] mastoid fontanelle: the unossified area of the skull at the junction of the lambdoidal, parietomastoid, and occipitomastoid sutures. Called also *posterolateral fontanelle, f. posterolateralis* [TA alternative], and *posterotemporal fontanelle.*

f. mi′nor f. posterior.

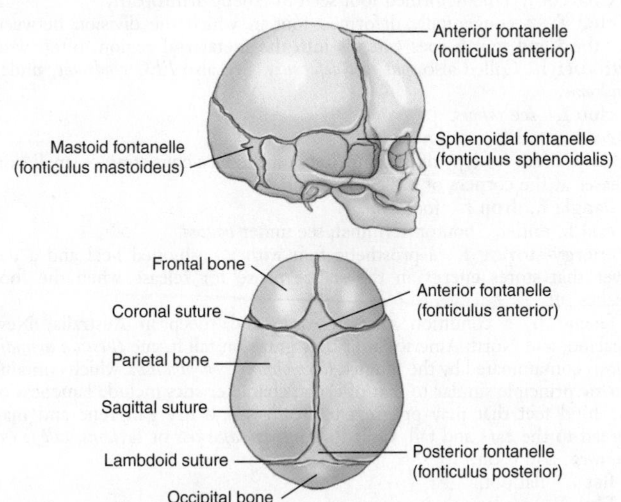

■ Neonatal skull showing the four fonticuli cranii (cranial fontanelles): the anterior, mastoid, posterior, and sphenoidal.

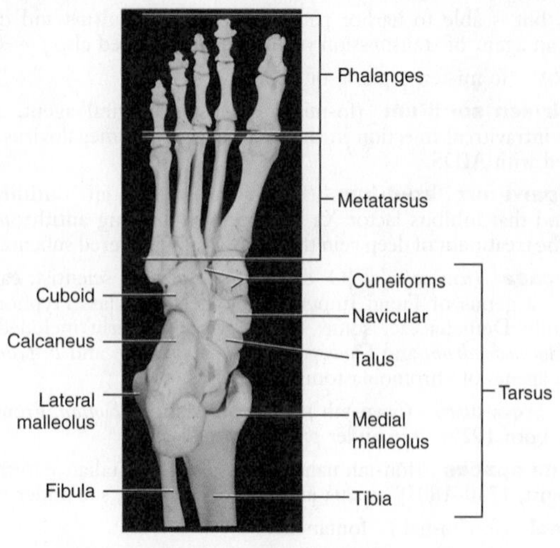

■ Inferior view of right foot.

f. occipita′lis, f. poste′rior [TA] posterior fontanelle: the unossified area of the skull at the junction of the sagittal and lambdoidal sutures; called also *f. minor*, and *occipital* or *triangular fontanelle*.

f. posterolatera′lis TA alternative for *f. mastoideus*.

f. sphenoida′lis [TA] sphenoidal fontanelle: the unossified area at the junction of the parietal and frontal bones, the greater wing of the sphenoidal, and the squamous part of the temporal bones. Called also *anterolateral fontanelle* and *f. anterolateralis* [TA alternative].

food (fo͞od) anything which, when taken into the body, serves to nourish or build up the tissues or to supply body heat; aliment; nutriment.

functional f's foods and food supplements marketed for presumed health benefits, such as vitamin supplements and certain herbs; called also *nutraceuticals*.

isodynamic f's foods that generate equal amounts of energy in heat units.

foot (foot) [A.S. *fōt*] 1. the distal portion of the lower limb, upon which an individual stands and walks. In humans it consists of the tarsus, metatarsus, and phalanges and the tissues encompassing them; other animals may use only part of the analogous structures for walking. Called also *pes* [TA]. 2. something resembling this structure. 3. a unit of linear measure, 12 inches, being the equivalent of 0.3048 meter. Abbreviated ft.

athlete's f. tinea pedis.

broad f. metatarsus latus.

burning feet 1. burning sensations in the soles of the feet; there are many causes such as the hyperalgesia of diabetes, alcoholism, or toxicity. 2. Gopalan syndrome.

buttress f. periostitis or ostitis in the region of the pyramidal process of the coffin bone of the horse, with fracture of the process, deformity of the hoof, and alteration of the normal angle of the joint. Called also *extensor process disease*, *pyramidal disease*, and *low ring-bone*.

cavus f. talipes cavus.

Charcot f. the deformed foot seen in tabetic arthropathy.

cleft f. a congenitally deformed foot in which the division between the third and fourth toes extends into the metatarsal region, often with ectrodactyly. Called also *split-foot deformity*. See also *EEC syndrome*, under *syndrome*.

club f. see *talipes*.

contracted f. see under *hoof*.

crow's feet a type of dynamic lines on the face consisting of small skin creases at the corners of the eyes.

dangle f., drop f. footdrop.

end f., end-f. bouton terminal; see under *bouton*.

energy-storing f. a prosthetic foot with a cushioned heel and a toe lever that stores energy in the stance phase for release when the foot pushes off.

fescue f. a condition seen in cattle and sheep in Australia, New Zealand, and North America after they graze on tall fescue *(Festuca arundinacea)* contaminated by the fungus *Acremonium coenophialum*, which contains a toxic principle similar to that of ergot; characteristics include lameness of the hind feet that may progress to necrosis and dry gangrene and may spread to the ears and tail. Called also *fescue lameness* or *toxicosis*, *tall fescue lameness*, and *fescue*.

flat f. flatfoot.

Flex-F. trademark for a type of energy-storing foot.

forced f. a painful swelling of the feet of soldiers after forced marches, due to fracture of a metatarsal bone.

Friedreich f. pes cavus, with hyperextension of the toes; seen in hereditary ataxia.

Greissinger f. a common type of multiaxial foot.

Hong Kong f. 1. a type of dermatophytosis of the foot seen in southern China. 2. tinea pedis.

immersion f. damage to the skin of the feet of persons who have stood for long periods in water; see *trench f.* and *warm water immersion f.*

Madura f. mycetoma of the foot.

march f. painful swelling of the forefoot, often associated with fracture of one of the metatarsal bones, following excessive foot strain.

Morton f. see under *neuralgia*.

mossy f. 1. chromoblastomycosis involving the foot. 2. podoconiosis.

multiaxial f., multiaxis f. a type of energy-storing prosthetic foot that allows plantar flexion, dorsiflexion, inversion, and eversion.

pericapillary end f. a pyramidal expansion of a process of an astrocyte against the wall of a capillary in the central nervous system; called also *perivascular f.*, *sucker f.*, *sucker process*, and *vascular foot plate*.

perivascular f. pericapillary end f.

pricked f. a condition in the horse in which the soft tissue of the foot has been punctured either by a horseshoe nail or by a nail or other object the animal has stepped on, causing pain and lameness. A nail that is near, but not into, the soft tissue may cause *nail bind*. Called also *nail prick*.

red f. redfoot.

reel f. talipes.

rocker-bottom f. 1. congenital convex pes valgus, due to primary dislocation of the talonavicular joint; it may occur as an isolated primary deformity or be associated with autosomal trisomy, including trisomy 13–15 and trisomy 18; called also *rocker-bottom flatfoot*. 2. talipes equinovarus in which the foot is shaped like a rocker of a rocking chair, occurring as a result of a transverse break in the midtarsal area; called also *rocker-bottom deformity*.

SACH f. (*s*olid *a*nkle *c*ushion *h*eel) a common type of multiaxial foot.

SAFE f. (*s*tationary *a*ttachment *f*lexible *e*ndoskeleton) a type of endoskeletal prosthetic foot.

sag f. sagging of the arch of the foot.

Seattle f. a type of energy-storing prosthetic foot that allows flexion, extension, inversion, and eversion; it is made of plastic and resembles a normal human foot.

spatula f. a foot in which several toes are fused together.

spread f. metatarsus latus.

sucker f. pericapillary end f.

tabetic f. the flat, distorted foot seen in tabes dorsalis, due to disease of the tarsus.

taut f. a shortening and contraction of the calf muscles and plantar flexors of the foot, due to high-heeled shoes.

trench f. a type of immersion foot resembling frostbite, caused by prolonged action of cold water on the skin combined with circulatory disturbance due to cold and inaction.

tropical immersion f., warm water immersion f. a type of immersion foot caused by standing in warm water, characterized by maceration, blanching, and wrinkling of the skin and swelling of the soles with ridging of the surface.

weak f. an early stage of flatfoot.

foot•board (foot′bord) a device placed at the foot of the bed in such a way that the feet rest firmly against it and are at right angles to the legs, used to relieve the weight of bedclothes, to maintain proper positioning of the feet while the patient is confined to bed, and to prevent development of footdrop.

foot•drop (foot′drop) dropping of the foot from a peroneal or tibial nerve lesion that causes paralysis of the anterior muscles of the leg; see also *steppage gait*. Called also *dangle foot* and *drop foot*.

foot•plate (foot′plāt) basis stapedis.

floating f. abnormal mobilization of the stapedial footplate.

stapedial f. basis stapedis.

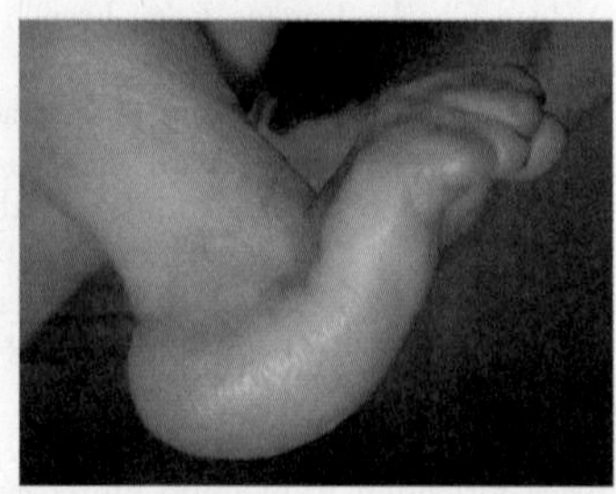
■ Rocker-bottom foot.

foot•print•ing (foot′print-ing) a technique for determining the location of binding between a protein and a DNA molecule; the two are bound, enzymes or chemicals are used to hydrolyze unbound, unprotected DNA, and the resulting protected DNA fragments can be identified electrophoretically.

For•a•dil (for′ə-dil) trademark for a preparation of formoterol fumarate.

fo•ra•men (fo-ra′mən) pl. *fora′mina* [L.] a natural opening or passage, especially one into or through a bone.

Foramen

Descriptions of anatomic structures are given on TA terms, and include anglicized names of specific foramina.

alveolar foramina of maxilla, fora′mina alveola′ria cor′poris maxil′lae [TA] the openings of the alveolar canals at the deepest portion of the tooth sockets in the maxilla.
aortic f. hiatus aorticus.
apical f. of tooth, f. a′picis den′tis [TA] a minute aperture usually at or near the apex of a root of a tooth but on occasion located on a side of a root, which gives passage to the vascular, lymphatic, and neural structures supplying the pulp; the main foramen sometimes branches near the apex to form two or more apical ramifications. Called also *pulpal f.* and *root f.*
f. of Bochdalek hiatus pleuroperitonealis.
Botallo f. f. ovale cordis.
f. cae′cum lin′guae [TA] foramen cecum of tongue: a depression on the dorsum of the tongue at the end of the median sulcus, representing the remains of the superior end of the thyroglossal duct of the embryo.
f. cae′cum medul′lae oblonga′tae [TA] a small triangular expansion at the lower border of the pons, formed by the termination of the anterior median fissure of the medulla oblongata; called also *f. of Vicq d'Azyr.*
f. cae′cum os′sis fronta′lis [TA] foramen cecum of frontal bone: a blind opening formed between the frontal crest and the crista galli, which sometimes transmits a vein from the nasal cavity to the superior sagittal sinus.
caroticoclinoid f. the foramen between the anterior and middle clinoid processes in the minority of sphenoid bones where those processes meet at their outer ends.
carotid f. the inferior aperture of the carotid canal, giving passage to the carotid vessels.
caval f. foramen venae cavae.
cecal f., f. cecum an apparent foramen that ends as a blind sac; see terms beginning *f. caecum.*
f. cecum of frontal bone f. caecum ossis frontalis.
f. cecum of medulla oblongata foramen caecum medullae oblongatae.
f. cecum of tongue f. caecum linguae.
condyloid f., anterior canalis nervi hypoglossi.
condyloid f., posterior canalis condylaris.
conjugate f. a foramen formed by a notch in each of two opposed bones.
f. costotransversa′rium [TA], **costotransverse f.** the narrow space between the posterior surface of the neck of a rib and the anterior surface of the transverse process of the corresponding vertebra.
cribriform foramina, fora′mina cribro′sa os′sis ethmoida′lis [TA] the openings in the cribriform plate of the ethmoid bone for passage of the olfactory nerves. Called also *olfactory foramina.*
emissary f. any foramen in a cranial bone that gives passage to an emissary vein.
epiploic f. *f. omentale.*
f. epiplo′icum TA alternative for *f. omentale.*
esophageal f. hiatus oesophageus.
ethmoidal f., anterior f. ethmoidale anterius.
ethmoidal f., posterior f. ethmoidale posterius.
f. ethmoida′le ante′rius [TA] anterior ethmoidal foramen: the anterior of two small grooves found as a pair crossing the superior surface on both sides of the ethmoid labyrinth, at its junction with the roof of each orbit; it transmits the nasal branch of the ophthalmic nerve and the anterior ethmoid artery and vein. Called also *anterior ethmoidal canal.*
f. ethmoida′le poste′rius [TA] posterior ethmoidal foramen: the posterior of two small grooves found as a pair crossing the superior surface on both sides of the ethmoid labyrinth, at its junction with the roof of each orbit; it transmits the posterior ethmoid artery and vein. Called also *posterior ethmoidal canal.*
external auditory f. meatus acusticus externus.
frontal f., f. fronta′le [TA] the frontal notch when it is bridged by osseous tissue; see *incisura frontalis.*
greater ischiadic f. f. ischiadicum majus.
greater palatine f. f. palatinum majus.
greater sacrosciatic f., greater sciatic f. f. ischiadicum majus.
Huschke f. a passage formed by union of the tubercles of the tympanic ring; it normally becomes ossified and disappears during childhood. Called also *Huschke canal.*
fora′mina incisi′va [TA] incisive foramina: the openings in the incisive fossa of the hard palate that transmit the nasopalatine nerves. Called also *foramina of Stensen.* See also *canales incisivi.*
infraorbital f., f. infraorbita′le [TA] the opening of the infraorbital canal on the anterior surface of the maxilla giving passage to the infraorbital nerve and vessels.
infrapiriform f. an opening below the piriformis muscle through which the inferior gluteal vessels and nerve pass out of the pelvis.
interatrial f. primum ostium primum.
interatrial f. secundum ostium secundum.
internal auditory f. porus acusticus internus.
interventricular f., f. interventricula′re [TA] a passage through which the lateral and third ventricles communicate.
intervertebral f., f. intervertebra′le [TA] the passage formed by the inferior and superior notches on the pedicles of adjacent vertebrae; it transmits a spinal nerve and vessels.
intervertebral foramina of sacrum, fora′mina intervertebra′lia os′sis sa′cri [TA] the four short, forked tunnels in each lateral wall of the sacral canal, connecting it with the pelvic and posterior sacral foramina.
f. ischia′dicum ma′jus [TA] greater sciatic foramen: a hole converted from the major sciatic notch by the sacrotuberal and sacrospinal ligaments; called also *greater ischiadic* or *greater sacrosciatic f.*
f. ischia′dicum mi′nus [TA] lesser sciatic foramen: a hole converted from the minor sciatic notch by the sacrotuberal and sacrospinal ligaments; called also *lesser ischiadic* or *lesser sacrosciatic f.*
jugular f., f. jugula′re [TA] the opening formed by the jugular notches on the temporal and occipital bones, for the transmission of various veins, arteries, and nerves.
f. of Key and Retzius apertura lateralis ventriculi quarti.
lacerate f., anterior fissura orbitalis superior.
lacerate f., middle f. lacerum.
lacerate f., posterior f. jugulare.
f. la′cerum [TA] an irregular gap formed at the junction of the base of the greater wing of the sphenoid bone, the tip of the petrous part of the temporal bone, and the basilar part of the occipital bone; in life, it does not exist, being occupied by an unossified part of the petrous part of the temporal bone.
lesser ischiadic f. f. ischiadicum minus.
lesser palatine foramina foramina palatina minora.
lesser sacrosciatic f., lesser sciatic f. f. ischiadicum minus.
f. of Luschka apertura lateralis ventriculi quarti.
f. of Magendie apertura mediana ventriculi quarti.
f. mag′num [TA] the large opening in the anterior and inferior part of the occipital bone, interconnecting the vertebral canal and the cranial cavity.
f. mandi′bulae [TA] mandibular foramen: the opening on the medial surface of the ramus of the mandible, leading into the mandibular canal.
mastoid f., f. mastoi′deum [TA] a prominent opening in the temporal bone posterior to the mastoid process and near its occipital articulation; an artery and vein usually pass through it.
median incisor f. Scarpa f.
medullary f. f. vertebrale.
mental f., f. menta′le [TA] an opening on the lateral part of the body of the mandible, opposite the second bicuspid tooth, for passage of the mental nerve and vessels.

Foramen *Continued*

f. of Monro f. interventriculare.
Morgagni f. 1. a small defect on either side, between the sternal and costal portions of the diaphragm, allowing passage of the superior epigastric blood vessels and a few lymphatic vessels; called also *pleuroperitoneal f.* 2. f. caecum linguae. 3. f. singulare.
nasal foramina, fora′mina nasa′lia [TA] openings on the outer surface of each nasal bone for the transmission of blood vessels.
fora′mina nervo′sa [TA] numerous small openings in the labium limbi tympanicum for the passage of the cochlear nerves; called also *habenulae perforatae.*
neural f. f. intervertebrale.
f. nutri′cium [TA], **nutrient f.** any one of the passages that admit the nutrient vessels to the medullary cavity of a bone.
obturator f., f. obtura′tum [TA] the large opening between the os pubis and the ischium.
olfactory foramina foramina cribrosa ossis ethmoidalis.
omental f., f. omenta′le [TA] the opening connecting the greater and lesser peritoneal sacs, situated below and behind the porta hepatis. Called also *epiploic f., f. epiploicum* [TA alternative], and *foramen of Winslow.*
optic f., f. op′ticum canalis opticus.
oval f. of heart f. ovale cordis.
oval f. of sphenoid bone foramen ovale ossis sphenoidalis.
f. ova′le cor′dis [TA], **f. ovale of heart** the aperture in the septum secundum of the fetal heart that provides a communication between the atria. Called also *oval foramen of heart.*
f. ova′le os′sis sphenoida′lis [TA], **f. ovale of sphenoid** an opening in the greater wing of the sphenoid bone, on the posterior part of the medial portion; it transmits the mandibular branch of the trigeminal nerve and some vessels.
f. palati′num ma′jus [TA] greater palatine foramen: the inferior opening of the great palatine canal, found laterally on the horizontal plate of each palatine bone opposite the root of each third molar tooth; it transmits a palatine nerve and artery.
fora′mina palati′na mino′ra [TA] lesser palatine foramina: the openings of the lesser palatine canals behind the palatine crest and the greater palatine foramina.
fora′mina papilla′ria rena′lis [TA], **papillary foramina of kidney** minute openings in the summit of each renal papilla, the orifices of the collecting tubules. Called also *openings of papillary ducts.*
parietal f., f. parieta′le [TA] an opening on the posterior part of the superior portion of the parietal bone near the sagittal suture, for the passage of a vein and arteriole.
patent f. ovale (PFO) a type of septal defect consisting of abnormal persistence of the fetal foramen ovale cordis after birth, often resulting in a left-to-right or right-to-left shunt.
f. petro′sum [TA] petrosal foramen: a small opening sometimes present posterior to the oval foramen for transmission of the lesser petrosal nerve; called also *canaliculus innominatus* and *innominate canaliculus.*
pleuroperitoneal f. 1. hiatus pleuroperitonealis. 2. Morgagni f. (def. 1).
pterygopalatine f. f. sphenopalatinum.
pulpal f. f. apicis dentis.
Retzius f. apertura lateralis ventriculi quarti.
root f. f. apicis dentis.

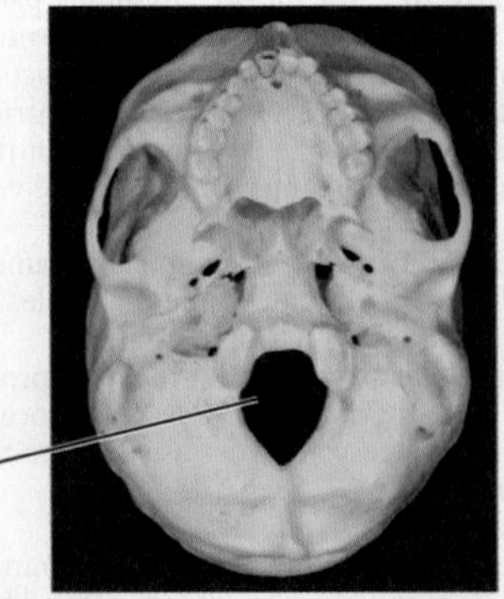

■ Inferior view of the base of the skull, showing the foramen magnum.

f. rotun′dum os′sis sphenoida′lis [TA] round foramen of sphenoid: a round opening in the medial part of the greater wing of the sphenoid bone that transmits the maxillary branch of the trigeminal nerve.
sacral foramina, anterior foramina sacralia anteriora.
sacral foramina, dorsal, sacral foramina, posterior foramina sacralia posteriora.
sacral foramina, ventral foramina sacralia anteriora.
fora′mina sacra′lia anterio′ra [TA] anterior sacral foramina: the eight openings (four on each side) on the pelvic surface of the sacrum for the anterior rami of the sacral nerves.
fora′mina sacra′lia posterio′ra [TA] posterior sacral foramina: the eight openings (four on each side) on the posterior surface of the sacrum for the posterior rami of the sacral nerves.
Scarpa f. one of the two foramina, one behind either upper medial incisor, for transmission of the nasopalatine nerves; called also *median incisor f.*
f. singula′re [TA] singular foramen: the opening in the inferior vestibular area of the fundus of the internal acoustic meatus that gives passage to the nerves of the ampulla of the posterior semicircular duct; called also *Morgagni f.* and *singular canal.*
foramina of smallest cardiac veins foramina venarum minimarum.
sphenoidal emissary f. f. venosum.
sphenopalatine f., f. sphenopalati′num [TA] an opening on the medial wall of the pterygopalatine fossa, interconnecting this fossa with the nasal cavity, and transmitting the sphenopalatine artery and nasal nerves. Called also *pterygopalatine f.*
spinal f. f. vertebrale.
f. spino′sum [TA] spinous foramen: an opening in the greater wing of the sphenoid bone, near its posterior angle, for the middle meningeal artery.
Spöndel f. a small transient foramen in the cartilaginous base of the developing cranium between the ethmoid bone and the lesser wings of the sphenoid.
foramina of Stensen foramina incisiva.
stylomastoid f., f. stylomastoi′deum [TA] a foramen on the inferior part of the temporal bone between the styloid and mastoid processes, for the facial nerve and the stylomastoid artery.
supraorbital f., f. supraorbita′le [TA] a passage in the frontal bone for the supraorbital vessels and nerve, representing a supraorbital notch whose open side of fibrous tissue has changed to bone.
suprapiriform f. an opening above the piriformis muscle through which the gluteal vessels and superior gluteal nerve pass out of the pelvis.
thebesian foramina foramina venarum minimarum.
thyroid f., f. thyroi′deum [TA] an inconstantly present opening in the upper part of the lamina of the thyroid cartilage, resulting from incomplete union of the fourth and fifth branchial cartilages.
f. transversa′rium [TA] the passage in either process of a cervical vertebra that, in the upper six vertebrae, transmits the vertebral vessels; it is small or may be absent in the seventh.
transverse f. f. transversarium.
f. ve′nae ca′vae [TA] caval opening: the opening in the diaphragm that transmits the inferior vena cava and some branches of the right vagus nerve. Called also *caval f.*
fora′mina vena′rum minima′rum [TA] foramina of smallest cardiac veins: minute openings in the walls of the heart through which small veins, the venae cardiacae minimae, empty their blood directly into the heart; they are most numerous in the right atrium and ventricle, occasional in the left atrium, and rare in the left ventricle. Called also *thebesian* or *Vieussens foramina.*
f. veno′sum [TA] sphenoidal emissary foramen: an opening occasionally found medial to the foramen ovale of the sphenoid for the passage of a vein from the cavernous sinus; called also *f. of Vesalius.*
venous f. 1. f. venae cavae. 2. f. venosum.
f. vertebra′le [TA] vertebral foramen: the large opening in a vertebra formed by its body and arch; called also *medullary f.,* and *spinal f.*
vertebroarterial f. f. transversarium.
f. of Vesalius f. venosum.
f. of Vicq d'Azyr f. caecum medullae oblongatae.
Vieussens foramina foramina venarum minimarum.
Weitbrecht f. an opening in the capsule of the shoulder joint through which passes the synovial membrane to the bursa that lines the under surface of the subscapularis muscle.

Foramen *Continued*

f. of Winslow f. omentale.
zygomaticofacial f., f. zygomaticofacia′le [TA] the opening on the anterior surface of the zygomatic bone for the zygomaticofacial nerves and vessels.
zygomatico-orbital f., f. zygomaticoorbita′le [TA] either of the two openings on the orbital surface of each zygomatic bone, which transmit branches of the zygomatic branch of the trigeminal nerve and branches of the lacrimal artery.
zygomaticotemporal f., f. zygomaticotempora′le [TA] the opening on the temporal surface of the zygomatic bone for passage of the zygomaticotemporal nerve.

fo•ram•i•na (fo-ram′ĭ-nə) [L.] plural of *foramen*.

fo•ram•i•not•o•my (fo-ram″ĭ-not′ə-me) [*foramina* + *-tomy*] the operation of removing the roof of intervertebral foramina, done for the relief of nerve root compression.

For•ane (for′ān) trademark for a preparation of isoflurane.

Forbes disease (forbz) [Gilbert Burnett *Forbes*, American pediatrician, 1915–2003] glycogen storage disease, type III; see under *disease*.

For•bes-Al•bright syndrome (forbz′ awl′brīt) [Anne Poppenheimer *Forbes*, American physician, 1911–1992; Fuller *Albright*, American physician, 1900–1969] see under *syndrome*.

force (fors) [L. *fortis* strong] any influence that acts to change the motion of an object, either accelerating or decelerating it, including changes in direction of motion. Symbol *F*.
bite f. masticatory f.
catabolic f. energy derived from the metabolism of food.
chewing f. masticatory f.
electromotive f. the force which, by reason of differences in potential, causes a flow of electricity from one place to another, giving rise to an electric current; it is measured in volts. Abbreviated EMF. Symbol *E*.
extraoral f. force applied by orthodontic anchorage units (calvarial, occipital, or cervical) outside the oral cavity.
field f's hypothetical forces that have a part in the individuation processes of the early embryo.
G f., g f. the unit of force exerted on a resting body that is equal to the force on it due to gravity. An accelerating body experiences multiple units of this force, symbolized *G* or *g* following the number of units.
masticatory f. the degree of force applied against the occlusal surfaces of the teeth by the muscles of mastication during the chewing of food. Called also *chewing f.*
occlusal f. the force exerted on opposing teeth when the jaws are brought into approximation.
reciprocal f. a force applied by an orthodontic anchorage in which the resistance of one or more dental units is utilized to move one or more opposing dental units. Cf. *reciprocal anchorage*.
reserve f. energy above that required for normal functioning; in the heart it is the power which will take care of the additional circulatory burden imposed by bodily exertion.
rest f. the power of the heart necessary to maintain the circulation when the patient is at rest.
van der Waals f's the relatively weak, short-range forces of attraction existing between atoms and molecules and arising from brief shifts of orbital electrons on one side of the atom or molecule and the corresponding electron shifts in adjacent molecules; it results in the attraction of nonpolar organic compounds to each other.
vital f. the energy that characterizes a living organism. Most systems of complementary medicine seek to affect or to use this energy. Called also *vital energy*.

force•plate (fors′plāt) force platform.

for•ceps (for′seps) [L.] 1. an instrument with two blades and a handle for compressing or grasping tissues in surgical operations, and for handling sterile dressings and other surgical supplies. See accompanying table. 2. an organ or part shaped like the surgical instrument, particularly the terminal fibers of the corpus callosum.
alligator f. a long, sharply angled forceps with a jawlike mechanism at the tip.
Adson f. a small thumb forceps having a fine tip, with or without teeth.
Adson-Brown f. a thumb forceps similar to the Adson forceps, having fine teeth at the tip, used for grasping delicate tissue; called also *Brown-Adson f.*
Allis f. a grasping forceps with opposing serrated edges with short teeth, used for grasping fascia or exerting traction on subcutaneous tissue.
artery f. forceps for grasping and compressing an artery.
Asch f. forceps used for reduction and fixation of nasal fractures.
axis-traction f. specially jointed obstetrical forceps so constructed that traction may be applied in the line of the pelvic axis.
Bailey-Williamson f. a form of obstetrical forceps.
Barton f. an obstetrical forceps with a hinge in one blade, which can be applied correctly to the fetal head without disturbing its relationship to the pelvic axis; used mainly for deep transverse arrests in a flat pelvis.
bayonet f. a forceps whose blades are offset from the axis of the handle.
bone-cutting f. a forceps with heavy jaws for cutting bone.
Brown-Adson f. Adson-Brown f.
bulldog f. spring forceps for seizing an artery to arrest or prevent hemorrhage; the jaws are usually covered with rubber tubing to prevent injury to the vascular wall.
bullet f. a forceps for extracting bullets.
capsule f. forceps for removing the lens capsule in membranous cataract.
chalazion f. a thumb forceps with a flattened plate at the end of one arm and a matching ring on the other; it is an ophthalmologic instrument, also used for isolation of lip and cheek lesions to facilitate removal.
Chamberlen f. the original form of obstetrical forceps, invented by Peter Chamberlen (1560–1631), and disclosed by Hugh Chamberlen (1664–1728).
clamp f. 1. a forceps with an automatic lock, used for compressing arteries, the pedicle of a tumor, etc.; called also *pedicle clamp*. 2. rubber dam f.
clip f. 1. a double-action forceps for applying wound clips. 2. a McKenzie forceps for applying brain clips.
Cornet f. a forceps for holding a coverglass.
DeBakey f. atraumatic tissue forceps used to grasp fine tissue.
DeLee f. a modified Simpson forceps.
dental f. forceps for the extraction of teeth. Called also *extracting f.*
disk f. a forceps for grasping the scleral disk in trephining the eyeball.
dressing f. a thumb forceps with a blunt end and serrated teeth, used to apply and remove dressings and to handle items in surgical wounds.
ear f. delicate forceps for ear surgery or extraction of foreign bodies from the ear.
Elliot f. a form of obstetrical forceps used in vaginal delivery and breech presentations with aftercoming head.
epilating f., epilation f. forceps for use in plucking out hairs.
extracting f. dental f.
fixation f. forceps for holding a part during an operation.

Selected Surgical Forceps

Adair-Allis forceps	Johns Hopkins forceps
Adson-Brown forceps	Judd-DeMartel forceps
Babcock forceps	Kahler forceps
Barraquer forceps	Kelly-Murphy forceps
Bishop-Harmon forceps	Kelman forceps
Blake forceps	Kelman-McPherson forceps
Blakesley-Weil forceps	Kerrison forceps
Bozeman forceps	Kocher forceps
Castroviejo forceps	Lahey forceps
Castroviejo-Arruga forceps	Lewkowitz forceps
Colibri forceps	Mixter forceps
Dandy forceps	Moynihan forceps
Desjardins forceps	Ochsner forceps
Doyen forceps	Potts-Smith forceps
Duval-Allis forceps	Rampley forceps
Elliot forceps	Randall forceps
Fenger forceps	Rochester-Ochsner forceps
Frankfeldt forceps	Rochester-Péan forceps
Gavin-Miller forceps	Schnidt forceps
Gaylor forceps	Somers forceps
Heaney forceps	Struyken forceps
Jacobs forceps	Takahashi forceps
Jameson forceps	Varco forceps
Jansen forceps	

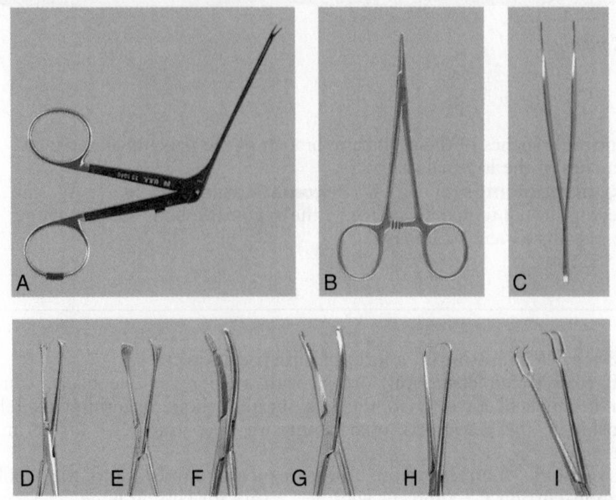

■ Some types of forceps. *(A)*, Alligator forceps (straight); *(B)*, Halsted mosquito hemostatic forceps (straight); *(C)*, Adson tissue forceps (teeth); *(D)*, Allis tissue forceps; *(E)*, Allis-Adair tissue forceps; *(F)*, Heaney hysterectomy forceps (single tooth, curved); *(G)*, Heaney-Ballentine hysterectomy forceps (single tooth, curved); *(H)*, Schroeder uterine tenaculum forceps (single tooth); *(I)*, Schroeder uterine vulsellum forceps (double tooth, straight).

frontal f. f. minor.
f. fronta'lis TA alternative for *f. minor.*
Garrison f. an obstetrical forceps with unfenestrated blades; called also *Luikart f.*
grasping f. any forceps for grasping tissue and exerting traction, having finger rings and a locking mechanism.
Haig Ferguson f. a form of obstetrical forceps.
Hawks-Dennen f. a form of obstetrical forceps.
hemostatic f. a locking forceps for compressing a blood vessel to control hemorrhage.
high f. see *forceps delivery, high,* under *delivery.*
jeweler's f. a thumb forceps with fine, pointed tips, used for microvascular and ophthalmic procedures.
Kazanjian f. cutting forceps used for resection of the nasal dorsal hump.
Kielland (Kjelland) f. obstetrical forceps having no pelvic curve, a marked cephalic curve, and an articulation permitting a gliding movement of one blade over the other, thus allowing the blades to adapt to the sides of the fetal head when the head lies with its long diameter in the transverse diameter of the pelvis.
Kocher f. a strong forceps with sharp points at the tips and transverse serrations along the full length for holding tissues during operation or for compressing bleeding tissue.
Laufe f. a form of obstetrical forceps.
Levret f. modified Chamberlen forceps, curved to correspond with the curve of the parturient canal.
lithotomy f. forceps for removing a vesical calculus in lithotomy.
low f. see *forceps delivery, low,* under *delivery.*
Löwenberg f. forceps for removing adenoid growths.
Luikart f. Garrison f.
McKenzie f. a forceps for applying silver clips.
Magill f. angled forceps used to guide a tracheal tube into the larynx or a nasogastric into the esophagus under direct vision; also used to place pharyngeal packs and remove foreign bodies.
f. ma'jor [TA] major forceps: the terminal fibers of the corpus callosum that pass from the splenium into the occipital lobes; called also *f. occipitalis* [TA alternative], and *occipital f.*
mid f. see *midforceps delivery,* under *delivery.*
f. mi'nor [TA] minor forceps: the terminal fibers of the corpus callosum that pass from the genu into the frontal lobes; called also *frontal f.,* and *f. frontalis* [TA alternative].
mosquito f. see under *clamp.*
mouse-tooth f. forceps with one or more fine teeth at the tip of each blade.
obstetrical f. an instrument designed to extract the fetus by the head from the maternal passages without injury to it or to the mother.
occipital f. f. major.
f. occipita'lis TA alternative for *f. major.*
Péan f. see under *clamp.*
Piper f. a special obstetrical forceps for an aftercoming head.
point f. forceps used in root canal therapy to securely hold the cones or points during placement.
rongeur f. a forceps designed for use in cutting bone.
rubber dam f., rubber dam clamp f. a forceps for placing rubber dam clamps in position. Called also *clamp f.*
sequestrum f. forceps with small but strong serrated jaws for removing the portions of bone forming a sequestrum.
Simpson f. a form of obstetrical forceps.
speculum f. long slender forceps for use through a speculum.
suture f. forceps used to hold the needle in passing a suture; a needle holder.
Tarnier f. a form of axis-traction forceps.
tenaculum f. forceps having a sharp hook at the end of each jaw.
thumb f. 1. a forceps consisting of two strips of metal joined at one end and designed to be used between the thumb and the index and middle fingers. 2. tissue f.
tissue f. forceps with one or more fine teeth at the tip of each blade, designed for handling tissues with minimal trauma during surgery; called also *thumb f.*
torsion f. forceps for making torsion on an artery to arrest hemorrhage.
Tucker-McLane f. a long obstetrical forceps with a solid blade.
tying f. a thumb forceps with fine, smooth tips for tying sutures in ophthalmologic surgery.
volsella f., vulsellum f. a forceps with teeth for grasping tissues and applying traction.
Walsham f. forceps used for reduction and fixation of nasal fractures.

for·ci·pate (for'sĭ-pāt) shaped like forceps.

For·ci·po·my·ia (for"sĭ-po-mi'yə) a genus of midges, family Chironomidae. *F. townsen'di* and *F. u'tae* were once thought to transmit mucocutaneous leishmaniasis.

for·ci·pres·sure (for'sĭ-presh"ər) pressure with forceps, chiefly for the arrest of hemorrhage.

For·dyce disease, granule (spot) (for'dīs) [John Addison *Fordyce,* American dermatologist, 1858–1925] see *Fox-Fordyce disease,* under *disease,* and see under *granule.*

fore·arm (for'ahrm) 1. the part of the upper limb of the body between the elbow and the wrist; called also *antebrachium* [TA]. 2. the corresponding part of the foreleg in horses and certain other quadrupeds.

fore·brain (for'brān) prosencephalon.

fore·con·scious (for'kon-shəs) preconscious.

fore·fin·ger (for'fing-gər) index (def. 1).

fore·foot (for'foot) 1. the foot on the foreleg of a quadruped. 2. the fore part of the foot.

fore·gut (for'gət) 1. the endodermal canal of the embryo cephalic to the junction of the yolk stalk; it gives rise to the pharynx, lung, esophagus, stomach, liver, and part of the duodenum. 2. the anterior, chitin-lined, ectodermal portion of the alimentary tract of invertebrates, such as arthropods; it usually comprises a pharynx, crop, and proventriculus.

fore·head (for'hed) the anterior aspect of the head superior to the superciliary arches and extending up to the hairline; some authorities consider it to be the upper part of the face while others exclude it from the face. In official terminology, called *frons* when considered as part of the skull, and *sinciput* when considered as part of the body. Called also *brow.*

for·eign (for'ən) in immunology, pertaining to substances not recognized as "self" and capable of inducing an immune response.

fore·kid·ney (for-kid'ne) pronephros.

Fo·rel decussation, fields (areas) (fo-rel') [Auguste Henri *Forel,* Swiss psychiatrist, 1848–1931] see *decussationes tegmentales,* under *decussatio,* and see under *field.*

fore·leg (for'leg) the front leg (thoracic limb) of a quadruped. Cf. *hind leg,* under *leg.*

fore·limb (for'lim) a foreleg or a wing.

fore·lock (for'lok) 1. the hair just above the forehead. 2. the anterior portion of the mane of a horse, covering the forehead. Called also *foretop.*
white f. lack of melanin in the forelock, as seen in piebaldism.

fo·ren·sic (fə-ren'zik) [L. *forēnsis* relating to a market place or forum] pertaining to or applied in legal proceedings.

fore·play (for'pla) the sexually stimulating, usually pleasurable activity preceding intercourse.

fore·pleas·ure (for'plezh-ər) sexual pleasure that precedes orgasm. Cf. *end-pleasure.*

fore·skin (for'skin) preputium penis.
hooded f. absence of the ventral foreskin, usually associated with hypospadias.

Fo·res·tier disease (fo"res-tya') [Jacques *Forestier,* French neurologist, 1890–1978] diffuse idiopathic skeletal hyperostosis; see under *hyperostosis.*

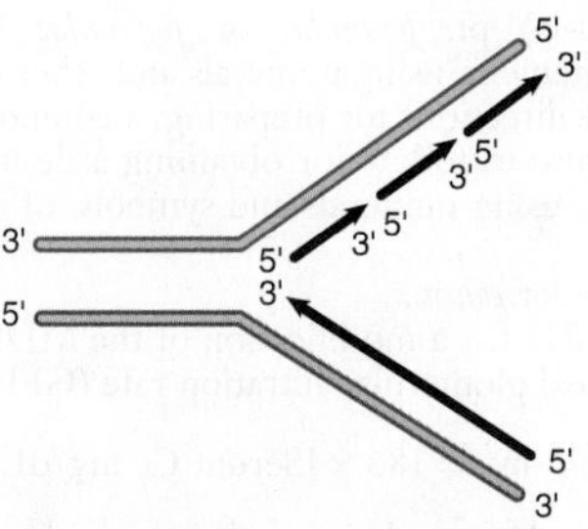

■ Replication fork, showing simultaneous synthesis of both strands; since synthesis occurs in the 5′ to 3′ direction, one strand, the leading strand, can be synthesized continuously while the other, the lagging strand, must be synthesized discontinuously in short fragments (Okazaki fragments) which are later joined.

fore·stom·ach (for′stum-ək) any of the first three stomachs of a ruminant, i.e., the rumen, reticulum, or omasum.

fore·top (for′top) forelock.

fore·wa·ters (for′waw-tərz) the amniotic fluid that presents at the cervix uteri.

fork (fork) 1. an instrument with prongs. 2. something resembling such an instrument.

replication f. a site on a DNA molecule at which unwinding of the helices and synthesis of daughter molecules are both occurring.

tuning f. a fork-shaped metal instrument with two tines, which produces harmonic vibration when the tines are struck; used to test hearing by air and bone conduction. See also *tuning fork tests*, under *test*.

form (form) [L. *forma*] 1. the characteristic of a structure or entity generally determined by its shape and size, or other external or visible feature. 2. in taxonomy, a prefix indicating that the taxon to which it is affixed is composed of organisms whose sexual phase is nonexistent or unknown; used in the classification of the *Deuteromycota* (Fungi Imperfecti).

accolé f. (ak″o-la′) appliqué f.

appliqué f. (ap″le-ka′) a term used to describe the early trophozoite of *Plasmodium falciparum* that does not assume a ring form but lies spread out along the periphery of the infected cell where it appears to have been "applied." Called also *accolé f.*

arch f. the shape and contour of a dental arch.

band f. see under *cell*.

involution f. an abnormally shaped bacterial cell that occurs in an old culture or one that has been exposed to unfavorable conditions.

juvenile f. metamyelocyte.

L-f. L-phase variant; see under *variant*.

racemic f. racemate.

retention f. adaptation of the form of a tooth cavity in such a way as to help maintain the filling material in the cavity.

ring f. the early trophozoite in the erythrocytic stage of the life cycle of hemosporian protozoa, which after Romanovsky staining has blue cytoplasm surrounding a clear zone with a red nucleus at one side, giving the cell the appearance of a signet ring. Called also *ring stage* and *signet ring*.

spherical f. of occlusion see under *occlusion*.

tooth f. the characteristic contour of a tooth, with its curves, lines, and angles, which permits the tooth to be differentiated from other teeth and its identity to be established.

young f. metamyelocyte.

-form [L. *forma*] a word termination meaning shape.

for·mal·de·hyde (for-mal′də-hīd) a gas formerly used as a strong disinfectant; an aqueous solution called *formaldehyde solution* (see under *solution*) is used as a disinfectant and as a preservative and fixative for pathologic specimens. The gas is toxic if inhaled or absorbed through the skin and is carcinogenic. Called also *methanal* and *formic aldehyde*.

for·mal·de·hyde de·hy·dro·gen·ase (glu·ta·thi·one) (for-mal′də-hīd de-hi′dro-jən-ās gloo″tə-thi′ōn) former name for *S-(hydroxymethyl) glutathione dehydrogenase*.

for·mal·de·hyd·o·gen·ic (for-mal″də-hīd″o-jen′ik) producing formaldehyde; pertaining to the production of formaldehyde by certain compounds when subjected to chemical reactions (i.e., steroids with α-ketol grouping in the C-17 position which on treatment with periodic acid liberate formaldehyde).

for·ma·lin (for′mə-lin) formaldehyde solution.

for·ma·lin·ize (for′mə-lin-īz) to treat with formaldehyde.

For·ma·lyde-10 (for′mə-līd) trademark for a preparation of dilute formaldehyde in solution.

for·mam·i·dase (for-mam′ĭ-dās) 1. [EC 3.5.1.49] an enzyme of the hydrolase class that catalyzes the deamination of formamide to produce formate. The enzyme also acts on similar amides. 2. arylformamidase.

for·ma·mide (for′mə-mīd) the simplest amide, $HCONH_2$, derived from formic acid.

for·mam·i·dox·im (for-mam′ĭ-dok″sim) isouretin.

form·ant (for′mənt) a combination of tones produced in the articulation of a vowel sound.

for·mate (for′māt) any salt of formic acid.

for·mate de·hy·dro·gen·ase (for′māt de-hi′dro-jən-ās) [EC 1.2.1.2] an enzyme of the oxidoreductase class that catalyzes the oxidation of formate to CO_2, using NAD^+ as an electron acceptor. The reaction occurs in bacteria but not in mammals. The fact that bacteria containing the enzyme (e.g., *Escherichia coli*) produce gas in mixed acid fermentations, and those that do not form the enzyme (e.g., *Shigella*) produce acid but no gas, is the basis for a test for the identification of Enterobacteriaceae.

for·mate–tet·ra·hy·dro·fo·late li·gase (for′māt tet″rə-hi″dro-fo′lāt li′gās) [EC 6.3.4.3] an enzyme activity of the ligase class that catalyzes the ATP-dependent synthesis of 10-formyltetrahydrofolate from formate and tetrahydrofolate, a step in the system of folate-mediated one-carbon transfer reactions. The enzyme activity is part of a trifunctional enzyme that also includes methenyltetrahydrofolate cyclohydrolase (q.v.) and methylenetetrahydrofolate dehydrogenase ($NADP^+$) activities.

for·ma·tio (for-ma′she-o) pl. *formatio′nes* [L.] formation: an anatomical structure of definite shape.

f. reticula′ris [TA] reticular formation: any of several diffuse networks of cells and fibers in the spinal cord and brainstem; generally subdivided into the reticular formations of the spinal cord, medulla oblongata, mesencephalon, and pons.

f. reticula′ris medul′lae oblonga′tae reticular formation of medulla oblongata: the phylogenetically old part of the medulla oblongata which has a reticular structure, i.e., which is composed of diffuse aggregations of nerve cells in the midst of a wealth of nerve fibers and, with certain exceptions, lacks circumscribed cell groups; it fills the spaces between the major nuclei and fiber tracts.

f. reticula′ris spina′lis [TA] spinal reticular formation: numerous small islets of gray matter and intersecting myelinated fibers located lateral to the posterior horn of the spinal cord at the interface of gray and white matter, especially at cervical levels; in the thoracic cord, the formation occurs immediately dorsal to the lateral horn. Called also *reticular formation of spinal cord*.

f. reticula′ris tegmen′ti mesence′phali [TA] reticular formation of mesencephalon: the part of the mesencephalon that has a reticular structure like that of the medulla oblongata; it lies between the substantia nigra and the central gray matter.

f. reticula′ris tegmen′ti pon′tis [TA] reticular formation of pons: the part of the pars dorsalis pontis, anterior to the central gray matter, that has a structure similar to that of the reticular formation of the medulla oblongata.

for·ma·tion (for-ma′shən) 1. the process of giving shape or form; the creation of an entity or of a structure of definite shape. 2. a structure of definite shape; see *formatio*.

coffin f. the surrounding of dead nerve cells by satellite cells in neuronophagia.

compromise f. in psychoanalysis, a disguised idea or act representing and permitting partial expression of a repressed conflict.

Gothic arch f. Henning sign.

hippocampal f. a term used to denote the hippocampus in its entirety, including the hippocampus proper, dentate gyrus, and subiculum; used particularly when hippocampus is used to denote the hippocampus proper.

palisade f. arrangement of cells in a palisade; see *palisade*.

pedestal f. in an intestinal infection by enteropathogenic *Escherichia coli*, the destruction of microvilli to form little pedestals for attachment of bacteria.

reaction f. a defense mechanism in which a person adopts conscious attitudes, interests, or feelings that are the opposites of his unconscious feelings, impulses, or wishes.

reticular f. formatio reticularis.

reticular f. of brainstem see *formatio reticularis medullae oblongatae*, *formatio reticularis tegmenti pontis*, and *formatio reticularis tegmenti mesencephali*.

reticular f. of medulla oblongata formatio reticularis medullae oblongatae.

reticular f. of mesencephalon formatio reticularis tegmenti mesencephali.

reticular f. of pons formatio reticularis tegmenti pontis.

reticular f. of spinal cord formatio reticularis spinalis.

rouleau f., f. of rouleaux the aggregation of erythrocytes in structures resembling piles of coins, caused by adhesion of their flat surfaces. Called also *impilation*, *pseudoagglutination*, and *pseudohemagglutination*.

spinal reticular f. formatio reticularis spinalis.

for·ma·ti·o·nes (for-ma-she-o′nēz) [L.] plural of *formatio.*

for·ma·tive (for′mə-tiv) concerned in the origination and development of an organism, part, or tissue.

for·ma·zan (for′mə-zan) reduced nitroblue tetrazolium that is dark blue and water-insoluble; the reduction process is the basis of the nitroblue tetrazolium test (see under *test*).

form·board (form′bord) a board containing variously shaped cutouts into which blocks corresponding to the cutouts are to be fitted; used as a test in mental retardation.

form-class (form′klas″) an artificial taxonomic category comparable to a class, to which organisms are provisionally assigned, as are imperfect fungi until their perfect (sexual) stages are identified. Form-classes are subdivided into form-orders, form-families, and so on.

forme (form) pl. *formes* [Fr.] form.

f. fruste (froost) pl. *formes frustes* ["defaced form"] an atypical, especially a mild or incomplete, form, as of a disease or anomaly.

f. tardive (tahr-dēv′) ["late form"] a late-occurring form of a disease that usually makes its appearance at an earlier age.

form-fam·i·ly (form′fam′ĭ-le) see *form-class.*

For·mi·ca (for-mi′kə) a genus of ants (family Formicidae), including most of those that are household pests.

for·mic ac·id (for′mik) HCO_2H, an acid from the distillation of ants and derivable from oxalic acid, glycerin, and the oxidation of formaldehyde. Formic acid resembles acetic acid in its actions but is far more irritating and pungent and is dangerously caustic to skin. The acid and its sodium and calcium salts are used as food preservatives.

for·mi·ca·tion (for″mĭ-ka′shən) [L. *formica* ant] a tactile hallucination in which there is a sensation of tiny insects crawling over the skin; most commonly seen in cocaine or amphetamine intoxication. Called also *Magnan sign.*

for·mi·ci·a·sis (for″mĭ-si′ə-sis) [L. *formica* ant] poisoning resulting from ant bites.

For·mic·i·dae (for-mis′ĭ-de) the ants, a family of usually crawling insects of the order Hymenoptera, having a complex social organization with castes; some females become temporarily winged. Some varieties are human pests or reservoirs for disease, and others have venomous bites. Genera include *Formica* and *Solenopsis.*

For·mi·coi·dea (for″mĭ-koi-de′ə) a superfamily of the order Hymenoptera, containing a single family, Formicidae; the ants.

for·mim·i·no (for-mim′ĭ-no) the group —CH═NH.

for·mim·i·no·glu·ta·mate (for-mim″ĭ-no-gloo′tə-māt) the anionic form of formiminoglutamic acid.

for·mim·i·no·glu·tam·ic ac·id (for-mim″ĭ-no-gloo-tam′ik) an intermediate in the catabolic pathway from histidine to glutamate. It may be excreted in the urine in liver disease, in vitamin B_{12} or folic acid deficiency, or in glutamate formiminotransferase deficiency. Abbreviated FIGLU.

5-for·mim·i·no·tet·ra·hy·dro·fo·late (for-mim″ĭ-no-tet″rə-hi″dro-fo′lāt) a substituted derivative of tetrahydrofolate, carrying a formimino group; it is an intermediate in the degradation of histidine.

for·mim·i·no·tet·ra·hy·dro·fo·late cy·clo·de·am·i·nase (for-mim″ĭ-no-tet″rə-hi″dro-fo′lāt si″klo-de-am′ĭ-nās) [EC 4.3.1.4] an enzyme of the lyase class that catalyzes the deamination of 5-formiminotetrahydrofolate to form 5,10-methenyltetrahydrofolate, a step in the degradation of histidine. The enzyme activity occurs in a bifunctional enzyme, along with glutamate formiminotransferase (q.v.) activity.

for·mim·i·no·trans·fer·ase (for-mim″ĭ-no-trans′fər-ās) any enzyme that transfers a formimino group; usually used to refer to glutamate formiminotransferase.

for·mim·i·no·trans·fer·ase de·fi·cien·cy (for-mim″ĭ-no-trans′fər-ās) deficiency of glutamate formiminotransferase.

for·min (for′min) any of a class of large, multidomain proteins that regulate the dynamic remodeling of the cytoskeleton by acting on the actin and microtubule networks; it is important in meiosis and mitosis, the maintenance of cell polarity, transport of lipids and proteins between organelles, signaling to the nucleus, and embryonic development.

for·mol (for′mol) formaldehyde solution.

form-ord·er (form′or′dər) see *form-class.*

for·mot·er·ol fu·ma·rate (for-mot′ə-rol) a long-acting β_2-adrenergic receptor agonist, used as a bronchodilator for maintenance treatment of asthma; administered by oral inhalation.

for·mu·la (for′mu-lə) pl. *formulas* or *for′mulae* [L., dim. of *forma* form] a specific statement, using numerals and other symbols, of the composition of, or of the directions for preparing, a compound, such as a medicine, or of a procedure to follow for obtaining a desired value or result; a simplified statement, using numerals and symbols, of a single concept. See also *chemical f.*

Arneth f. see under *count.*

abbreviated MDRD f. a modification of the MDRD formula for estimating a person's ideal glomerular filtration rate (GFR) in mL per minute:

$$\text{GFR mL/min/1.73 m}^2 = 186 \times [\text{Serum Cr mg/dL}]^{-1.154} \times \text{age}^{-0.203}.$$

For persons of black African descent, the result should be multiplied by 1.210, and for women it should be multiplied by 0.742.

Arrhenius f. $\log x = \theta c$, in which x is the viscosity of the solution relative to that of the medium of suspension, c the percentage of volume occupied by the suspended particles, and θ a constant.

Bazett f. a formula correcting the Q–T interval for heart rate by dividing the duration of the Q–T interval by the square root of the duration from the R wave to the one preceding: $Q\text{–}Tc = (Q\text{–}T)/\sqrt{R-R}$.

Beckmann f. a formula used in cryoscopy, $\Delta T = K \times m$, in which ΔT is the difference in freezing points of the pure solvent and the solution containing a solute at molality m, and K is a constant characteristic of the particular solvent.

Berkow f. an adaptation of the rule of nines to burned children, taking into account the difference in proportional size of body parts between children and adults.

chemical f. a combination of symbols used to express the chemical constitution of a substance; in practice, different types of formulas, of varying complexity, are employed. See *empirical f., molecular f., spatial f.,* and *structural f.*

Cockcroft-Gault f. a formula for estimating a person's ideal creatinine clearance in mL per minute; for males:

$$\frac{(140 - \text{age}) \times \text{weight in kg}}{\text{serum creatinine (mg/dL)} \times 72}$$

for females:

$$\frac{0.85(140 - \text{age}) \times \text{weight in kg}}{\text{serum creatinine (mg./dL)} \times 72}.$$

configurational f. spatial f.

constitutional f. structural f.

dental f. an expression in symbols of the number and arrangement of teeth in the jaws. Letters represent the various types of teeth: I, *incisor;* C, *canine;* P, *premolar;* M, *molar.* Each letter is followed by a horizontal line. Numbers above the line represent maxillary teeth; those below, mandibular teeth. The human dental formula is $I\frac{2}{2}C\frac{1}{1}M\frac{2}{2} = 10$ (one side only) for deciduous teeth, and $I\frac{2}{2}C\frac{1}{1}P\frac{2}{2}M\frac{3}{3} = 16$ (one side only) for permanent teeth.

digital f. a formula expressing the relative lengths of the digits, usually $3 > 4 > 2 > 5 > 1$, or $3 > 2 > 4 > 5 > 1$, for the fingers, and $1 > 2 > 3 > 4 > 5$, or $2 > 1 > 3 > 4 > 5$, for the toes.

Einthoven f. see under *law.*

empirical f. a chemical formula that expresses the proportions of the elements present in a substance. For substances composed of discrete molecules, it expresses the relative numbers of atoms present in a molecule of the substance in the smallest whole numbers. For example, the empirical formula for ethane is written CH_3, whereas its actual *molecular formula* is C_2H_6.

Fick f. the equation used to determine cardiac output in the Fick method.

Fischer projection f. a type of projection formula used to depict chirality, particularly for monosaccharides; in reference to the plane of symmetry defined by the central carbon chain, horizontal lines are drawn to depict substituents falling in front of the plane, or toward the viewer, while vertical lines depict substituents falling behind the plane, or away from the viewer.

D-glucose	L-glucose
CHO	CHO
H–C–OH	HO–C–H
HO–C–H	H–C–OH
H–C–OH	HO–C–H
H–C–OH	HO–C–H
CH_2OH	CH_2OH

■ Fischer projection formula depicting the enantiomers D- and L-glucose.

Gompertz f. see under *law*.

Gorlin f. a formula yielding an estimated area of the opening of a cardiac valve by calculating flow through the opening and pressure gradient across the valve.

graphic f. a term occasionally used to describe a "complete" structural formula, i.e., one in which every individual atom and bond is represented in the formula. The distinction is made because structural formulas are frequently written in a simplified or shortened form. See *structural f.*

Hamilton-Stewart f. a formula for measuring cardiac output following the rapid intravenous injection of an indicator dye: $F = i/ct$, in which F represents the blood flow in liters per minute; i, the injected substance in milligrams; c>, the average dye concentration of the primary curve; and t, the duration of the primary curve in seconds, i.e., the time from appearance to disappearance of the dye at a fixed site if there were no recirculation of the dye.

MDRD f. [*M*odification of *D*iet in *R*enal *D*isease] a formula for calculating a person's ideal glomerular filtration rate, drawn up by a study of the effect of restricting protein intake in dialysis patients. It has now been replaced by the abbreviated MDRD formula. Called also *MDRD equation.*

Modification of Diet in Renal Disease Study f. MDRD f.

molecular f. a chemical formula giving the number of atoms of each element present in a molecule of a substance, without indicating how they are linked.

official f. a formula officially established by a pharmacopeia or other recognized authority.

projection f. a planar, and therefore simplified, representation of a spatial formula.

rational f. structural f.

spatial f. a chemical formula giving the numbers of atoms of each element present in a molecule of a substance, which atom is linked to which, the types of linkages involved, and the relative positions of the atoms in space.

stereochemical f. spatial f.

structural f. a chemical formula telling how many atoms of each element are present in a molecule of a substance, which atom is linked to which, and the type of linkages involved; for convenience, abbreviated structural formulas are sometimes used. Called also *constitutional f.*, *graphic f.*, and *rational f.*

```
  H  H
  |  |
H—C—C—O—H        CH3CH2OH
  |  |              or
  H  H            C2H5OH

 Complete       Abbreviated
```

■ Structural formulas for ethanol.

Van Slyke f. the urinary coefficient of various substances is equal to $D/(Bl \times \sqrt{Wt} \times V)$, in which D is the daily output in grams of the substance in the urine; Bl, the grams of the same substance per liter of blood; Wt, the weight of the patient in kilograms; and V, the total volume of urine in 24 hours.

vertebral f. an expression in symbols of the number of vertebrae in each region of the vertebral column; for humans it is C7 T12 L5 S5 Cd4 = 33.

for·mu·lary (for′mu-lar″e) a collection of recipes, formulas, and prescriptions.

National F. see under *N.*

for·mu·late (for′mu-lāt) 1. to state in the form of a formula. 2. to prepare in accordance with a prescribed or specified method.

for·mu·la·tion (for″mu-la′shən) the act or product of formulating.

American Law Institute F. a section of the American Law Institute Model Penal Code: "A person is not responsible for criminal conduct if at the time of such conduct as a result of mental disease or defect he lacks substantial capacity either to appreciate the criminality [wrongfulness] of his conduct or to conform his conduct to the requirements of the law ... the terms 'mental disease or defect' do not include an abnormality manifested only by repeated criminal or otherwise antisocial conduct [antisocial personality]." This test of criminal responsibility or closely related rules have been adopted by many state and federal jurisdictions.

Working F. of Non-Hodkgin Lymphomas for Clinical Usage a classification of non-Hodgkin lymphomas that updated the Lukes-Collins classification and others; it grouped lymphomas by pathologic classification, then assigned them to one of three clinical prognostic groups (low, intermediate, and high grade). It has been superseded by the Revised European-American Lymphoma (REAL) Classification.

for·myl (for′məl) [L. *formic* +Gr. *hylē* matter] the radical, HCO—, of formic acid.

for·myl·ase (form′əl-ās) arylformamidase.

for·myl·ky·nu·re·nine (for″məl-kīn′u-rə-nēn″) the intermediate formed in tryptophan catabolism by oxidative cleavage of the indole ring of tryptophan.

for·myl·tet·ra·hy·dro·fo·late (for″məl-tet″rə-hi″dro-fo′lāt) any derivative of tetrahydrofolate that carries a formyl group substitution. The 5-formyl derivative is folinic acid (q.v.); the 10-formyl derivative is important in purine synthesis and in the liver-mediated release of excess one-carbon units.

5-for·myl·tet·ra·hy·dro·fo·late cy·clo·li·gase (form″əl-tet″rə-hi″dro-fo′lāt si″klo-li′gās) [EC 6.3.3.2] an enzyme of the ligase class that catalyzes the ATP-dependent formation of 5,10-methenyltetrahydrofolate from 5-formyltetrahydrofolate (folinic acid). The reaction provides a means of utilization of folinic acid in the absence of dihydrofolate reductase activity. Called also *5,10-methenyltetrahydrofolate synthetase.*

for·myl·tet·ra·hy·dro·fo·late de·hy·dro·gen·ase (form″əl-tet″rə-hi″dro-fo′lāt de-hi′dro-jən-ās) [EC 1.5.1.6] an enzyme of the oxidoreductase class that catalyzes the oxidative decarboxylation of 10-formyltetrahydrofolate to produce tetrahydrofolate, using $NADP^+$as an electron acceptor. The reaction occurs in liver to release excess active one-carbon fragments and maintain sufficient tetrahydrofolate for metabolism.

for·myl·trans·fer·ase (for″məl-trans′fər-ās) a term used in the names of some of the enzymes of the sub-subclass hydroxymethyl-, formyl-, and related transferases [EC 2.1.2] to denote those that catalyze the transfer of a formyl group from a donor to an acceptor compound. Cf. *hydroxymethyltransferase.*

for·ni·cal (for′nĭ-kəl) [L. *fornix*, arch] pertaining to a fornix.

for·ni·cate (for′nĭ-kāt) [L. *fornicatus* arched] shaped like an arch.

for·nic·e·al (for-nis′e-əl) fornical.

for·nix (for′niks) pl. *for′nices* [L. "arch"] 1. an archlike anatomical structure or the vaultlike space created by such a structure. 2. [TA] fornix of brain: the efferent pathway of the hippocampus, projecting chiefly to the mammillary bodies and habenular nuclei; each fornix of the pathway is an arched tract that is united under the corpus callosum with the other fornix, so that together they comprise two columns, a body, and two crura.

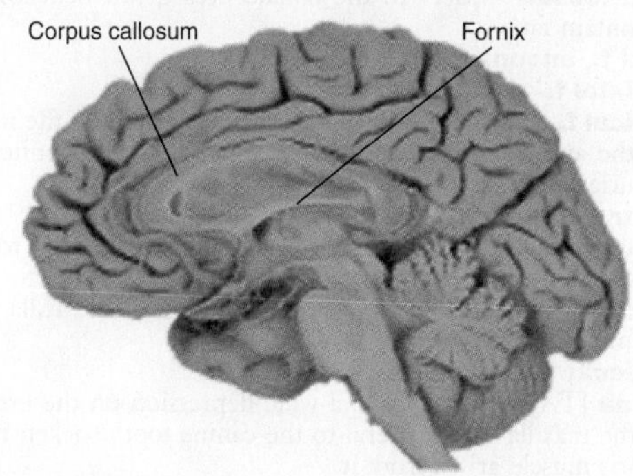

anterior f. pars anterior fornicis vaginae.

f. of brain fornix (def. 2).

caliceal f., calyceal f. the inner border of a renal calyx where it touches one or more papillae.

f. conjuncti′vae infe′rior [TA] inferior conjunctival fornix: the inferior line of reflection of the conjunctiva from the eyelid to the eyeball.

f. conjuncti′vae supe′rior [TA] superior conjunctival fornix: the superior line of reflection of the conjunctiva from the eyelid to the eyeball; it receives the openings of the lacrimal duct.

gastric f., f. gas′tricus [TA] a term used in radiographic anatomy to refer to the arch of the fundus of the stomach. Called also *f. of stomach, f. ventricularis,* and *f. ventriculi.*

lateral f. pars lateralis fornicis vaginae.

f. pharyn′gis [TA] pharyngeal fornix: the archlike roof of the nasopharynx; called also *nasopharyngeal roof* and *roof of nasopharynx.*

posterior f. pars posterior fornicis vaginae.

f. sac′ci lacrima′lis [TA] fornix of lacrimal sac: the upper, blind extremity of the lacrimal sac.

f. of stomach f. gastricus.

f. vagi′nae [TA] the recess formed between the vaginal wall and the vaginal part of the cervix; sometimes subdivided into anterior *(pars anterior fornicis vaginae)*, posterior *(pars posterior fornicis vaginae)*, and lateral *(pars lateralis fornicis vaginae)* fornices, depending on the relation of the recess to the wall of the vagina. Called also *vaginal vault.*

f. ventricula′ris, f. ventri′culi f. gastricus.

Forns index (fornz) [Xavier *Forns*, Spanish hepatologist, 21st century] see under *index.*

For•o•blique (for″o-blek′) trademark for an obliquely forward visual telescopic system used in panendoscopes.

For•res•ter classification (for′əs-tər) [James S. *Forrester*, American cardiologist, 20th century] see under *classification.*

For•si•us-Eriks•son syndrome (for′se-əs er′ik-sən) [Henrik *Forsius*, Finnish physician, born 1921; Aldur W. *Eriksson*, Finnish geneticist, 20th century] see under *syndrome.*

Fors•sell sinus (for′səl) [Gösta *Forssell*, Swedish radiologist, 1876–1950] see under *sinus.*

Forss•man antibody, antigen (fors′mən) [John *Forssman*, Swedish pathologist, 1868–1947] see under *antibody* and *antigen.*

För•ster choroiditis (disease), photometer (fur′stər) [Carl Friedrich Richard *Förster*, German ophthalmologist, 1825–1902] see *areolar choroiditis*, under *choroiditis*, and see *photoptometer.*

För•ster diplegia (syndrome, atonic-astatic syndrome) (fur′stər) [Otfrid *Förster*, German neurosurgeon, 1873–1941] atonic-astatic diplegia.

For•taz (for′taz) trademark for a preparation of ceftazidime.

Fort Bragg fever (fört′ brag′) [*Fort Bragg*, North Carolina, USA, where cases were observed] pretibial fever; see under *fever.*

For•teo (for-ta′o) trademark for a preparation of teriparatide.

For•to•vase (for′to-vās) trademark for a preparation of saquinavir.

Fo•sa•max (fos′ə-maks) trademark for a preparation of alendronate sodium.

fos•am•pren•a•vir cal•ci•um (fos″am-pren′ə-vir) a prodrug of amprenavir (q.v.), to which it is converted by cellular proteases; used in the treatment of human immunodeficiency virus infections, administered orally.

fosa•prep•i•tant di•meg•lu•mine (fos-ə-prep′ĭ-tənt) a prodrug of aprepitant that rapidly converts to aprepitant in the body; administered intravenously as an antiemetic.

fos•car•net so•di•um (fos-kahr′net) a virostatic agent used in the treatment of cytomegalovirus retinitis and acyclovir-resistant herpes simplex in immunocompromised patients.

Fos•ca•vir (fos′kə-vir) trademark for a preparation of foscarnet sodium.

fos•fo•my•cin tro•meth•amine (fos-fo-mi′sin) an antibacterial agent derived from phosphonic acid, active against a wide range of gram-positive and gram-negative bacteria, used in the treatment of urinary tract infection; administered orally.

fo•sin•o•pril so•di•um (fo-sin′o-pril) an angiotensin-converting enzyme inhibitor used in the treatment of hypertension; also used as a vasodilator in the treatment of congestive heart failure. Administered orally.

fos•phen•y•to•in so•di•um (fos′fen-ĭ-toin″) [USP] a prodrug of phenytoin used as an anticonvulsant in the treatment of epilepsy, excluding petit mal epilepsy; administered intravenously or intramuscularly.

fos•pi•rate (fos′pĭ-rāt) a veterinary anthelmintic.

fos•sa (fos′ə) gen. and pl. *fos′sae* [L.] [TA] a trench, channel, or hollow place.

Fossa

Descriptions are given on TA terms, and include anglicized names of specific fossae.

acetabular f., f. aceta′buli [TA] a rough nonarticular area in the floor of the acetabulum above the acetabular notch.

adipose fossae spaces in the female breast, just beneath the skin, which contain fat.

anconal f., anconeal f. f. olecrani.

antecubital f. f. cubitalis.

antihelical f., f. antihe′lica [TA] the depression on the medial surface of the auricle of the ear that corresponds to the antihelix on the lateral surface.

articular f. 1. f. articularis. 2. f. mandibularis.

f. articula′ris [TA] articular fossa: a general term used to denote a fossa associated with a synovial joint.

f. axilla′ris [TA], **axillary f.** the small hollow at the axilla where the upper limb joins the body at the shoulder.

Biesiadecki f. iliacosubfascial f.

f. cani′na [TA] canine fossa: a wide depression on the external surface of the maxilla superolateral to the canine tooth socket; the levator anguli oris muscle arises from it.

f. cerebella′ris [TA] cerebellar fossa: either of a pair of depressions in the internal surface of the occipital bone posterior to the foramen magnum, separated from one another by the internal occipital crest, that lodge the hemispheres of the cerebellum.

cerebral f. f. cerebralis.

cerebral f., lateral f. lateralis cerebri.

f. cerebra′lis [TA] cerebral fossa: either of a pair of depressions in the internal surface of the occipital bone, immediately superior to the cerebellar fossae, that house the occipital lobes of the cerebrum.

f. condyla′ris [TA] condylar fossa: either of two pits on the lateral portions of the occipital bone, one on either side of the foramen magnum, posterior to the occipital condyle. Called also *condyloid f.*

condyloid f. f. condylaris.

f. coronoi′dea hu′meri [TA] coronoid fossa of humerus: the cavity in the humerus that receives the coronoid process of the ulna when the elbow is flexed. Called also *ulnar f.*

cranial f., anterior f. cranii anterior.

cranial f., middle f. cranii media.

cranial f., posterior f. cranii posterior.

f. cra′nii ante′rior [TA] anterior cranial fossa: the anterior subdivision of the floor of the cranial cavity, supporting the frontal lobes of the brain, and composed of portions of three bones: the ethmoid, frontal, and sphenoid.

f. cra′nii me′dia [TA] middle cranial fossa: the middle subdivision of the floor of the cranial cavity, supporting the temporal lobes of the brain and the pituitary gland; it is composed of the body and greater wings of the sphenoid bone and the squamous and petrous portions of the temporal bone.

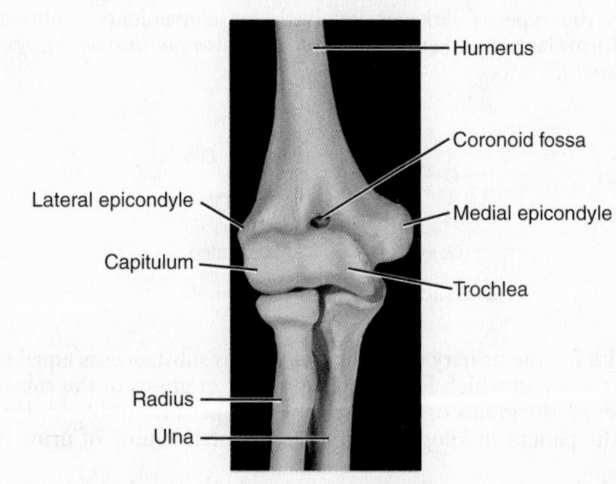

■ Fossa coronoidea humeri (coronoid fossa) in an anterior view of the right elbow joint.

f. cra′nii poste′rior [TA] posterior cranial fossa: the posterior subdivision of the floor of the cranial cavity, lodging the cerebellum, pons, and medulla oblongata; it is formed by portions of the sphenoid, temporal, parietal, and occipital bones.

crural f. femoral f.

cubital f. f. cubitalis.

f. cubita′lis [TA] cubital fossa: the depression in the anterior region of the elbow.

digastric f. f. digastrica.

f. digas′trica [TA] digastric fossa: a depression on the internal surface of the body of the mandible on each side of the symphysis to which is attached the anterior belly of the digastric muscle.

digital f. f. trochanterica.

f. duc′tus veno′si fossa of ductus venosus: an impression on the posterior part of the diaphragmatic surface of the liver in the fetus, lodging the ductus venosus.

duodenal f., inferior recessus duodenalis inferior.

duodenal f., superior, duodenojejunal f. recessus duodenalis superior.

epigastric f. epigastrium.

f. epigas′trica TA alternative for *epigastrium.*
ethmoid f. a groove situated in the cribriform plate of the ethmoid bone; it lodges the olfactory bulb of the brain. Called also *olfactory groove.*
femoral f. a small depression on the peritoneum of the lower anterior abdominal wall, inferomedial to the lateral inguinal fossa; it overlies the femoral ring (anulus femoralis).
floccular f. f. subarcuata ossis temporalis.
f. for gallbladder f. vesicae biliaris.
f. glan′dulae lacrima′lis [TA] fossa for lacrimal gland: a shallow depression in the lateral part of the roof of the orbit, lodging the lacrimal gland; called also *lacrimal f.*
glenoid f. of scapula cavitas glenoidalis.
glenoid f. of temporal bone f. mandibularis.
f. he′licis scapha.
f. hyaloi′dea [TA] hyaloid fossa: a depression on the anterior surface of the vitreous body, in which the lens is lodged; called also *lenticular f.* and *patellar f.*
f. hypophysia′lis [TA] hypophysial fossa: a deep depression in the middle of the sella turcica of the sphenoid bone, lodging the pituitary gland; called also *pituitary f.* and *sellar f.*
ileocecal f., inferior recessus ileocaecalis inferior.
ileocecal f., superior recessus ileocaecalis superior.
ileocolic f. recessus ileocaecalis superior.
f. ili′aca [TA] iliac fossa: a large, smooth concave area occupying much of the inner surface of the ala of the ilium, especially anteriorly; from it arises the iliacus muscle.
iliacosubfascial f. an inconstant depression on the inner surface of the abdomen between the psoas muscle and the crest of the ilium; called also *Biesiadecki f.*
f. iliopecti′nea iliopectineal fossa: a depression between the iliopsoas and pectineus muscles in the center of the femoral triangle; called also *lesser f. of Scarpa.*
implantation f. a shallow depression at the site where the tail of a spermatozoon attaches to the head.
f. inci′siva [TA] incisive fossa: a depression in the midline of the bony palate, immediately posterior to the central incisors, into which the incisive canals open.
incisive f. 1. f. incisiva. 2. a shallow depression on the anterior surface of the maxilla above the incisor teeth, to which the depressor septi nasi muscle is attached; called also *prenasal f.* 3. a shallow depression on the body of the mandible, immediately posterior to the symphysis and above the mental protuberance, situated below the alveolar border of the central and lateral incisors.
incudal f., f. incu′dis [TA] fossa for incus: a groove in the posterior wall of the tympanic cavity, lodging the short limb of the incus and the posterior ligament of the incus.
f. infraclavicula′ris [TA] infraclavicular fossa: the triangular region of the thorax or chest just inferior to the clavicle, between the deltoid and pectoralis major muscles; called also *infraclavicular triangle* and *Mohrenheim f.* or *triangle.*
infraduodenal f. recessus retroduodenalis.
f. infraspina′ta [TA], **infraspinous f.** the large, slightly concave area below the spinous process on the dorsal surface of the scapula; it is the site of origin of the infraspinatus muscle.
f. infratempora′lis [TA] infratemporal fossa: the area on the side of the cranium limited superiorly by the infratemporal crest, posteriorly by the mandibular fossa, anteriorly by the infratemporal surface of the maxilla, and laterally by the zygomatic arch and part of the ramus of the mandible; called also *zygomatic f.*.
inguinal f., external f. inguinalis lateralis.
inguinal f., internal f. inguinalis medialis.
inguinal f., lateral f. inguinalis lateralis.
inguinal f., medial, inguinal f., middle f. inguinalis medialis.
f. inguina′lis latera′lis [TA] lateral inguinal fossa: the depression on the inside of the anterior abdominal wall lateral to the lateral umbilical fold; called also *external inguinal f.*
f. inguina′lis media′lis [TA] medial inguinal fossa: the depression on the inside of the anterior abdominal wall between the medial and lateral umbilical folds; called also *internal inguinal f.*
intercondylar f. of femur f. intercondylaris femoris.
intercondylar f. of tibia, anterior area intercondylaris anterior tibiae.
intercondylar f. of tibia, posterior area intercondylaris posterior tibiae.
f. intercondyla′ris fe′moris [TA] intercondylar fossa of femur: the posterior depression between the condyles of the femur; called also *intercondylar notch of femur* and *popliteal notch.*
intercondyloid f. 1. f. intercondylaris femoris. 2. either of the intercondylar areas of the tibia; see *area intercondylaris anterior tibiae* and *area intercondylaris posterior tibiae.*
f. interpeduncula′ris [TA] interpeduncular fossa: a depression between the two cerebral peduncles, the floor of which is the posterior perforated substance.
intersigmoid f. recessus intersigmoideus.
f. ischioana′lis [TA] ischioanal fossa: the potential space between the pelvic diaphragm and the skin inferior to it; an anterior recess extends a variable distance, sometimes reaching the retropubic space. Called also *ischiorectal f.* and *perineal f.*
ischiorectal f. f. ischioanalis.
Jobert f. the fossa in the popliteal region bounded above by the adductor magnus and below by the gracilis and sartorius, best seen when the knee is bent and the thigh strongly rotated outward.
f. of Jonnesco the duodenojejunal fossa between the superior and inferior duodenal folds.
jugular f., f. jugula′ris [TA] a prominent depression on the inferior surface of the petrous part of the temporal bone, forming the major part of the jugular notch; it forms the anterior and lateral wall of the jugular foramen and lodges the superior bulb of the internal jugular vein.
lacrimal f., f. for lacrimal gland f. glandulae lacrimalis.
f. for lacrimal sac f. sacci lacrimalis.
Landzert f. recessus paraduodenalis.
f. of lateral malleolus f. malleoli lateralis.
f. latera′lis ce′rebri [TA] lateral cerebral fossa: a depression, in fetal life, on the lateral surface of each cerebral hemisphere at the bottom of which lies the insula; later it is closed over by the operculum, the edges of which form the lateral sulcus. Called also *sylvian f.,* and *f. of Sylvius.*
lenticular f. f. hyaloidea.
lesser f. of Scarpa f. iliopectinea.
Malgaigne f. trigonum caroticum.
malleolar f., f. malle′oli latera′lis [TA] a depression on the medial aspect of the lateral malleolus behind its articular surface.
f. mandibula′ris [TA] mandibular fossa: a prominent depression in the inferior surface of the squamous part of the temporal bone at the base of the zygomatic process, in which the condyloid process of the mandible rests. Called also *glenoid f. of temporal bone.*
mastoid f. foveola suprameatica.
mesentericoparietal f. parajejunal f.
Mohrenheim f. f. infraclavicularis.
f. of Morgagni f. navicularis urethrae.
nasal f. the portion of the nasal cavity anterior to the middle meatus.
navicular f. of Cruveilhier f. scaphoidea ossis sphenoidalis.
navicular f. of male urethra f. navicularis urethrae.
navicular f. of sphenoid bone f. scaphoidea ossis sphenoidalis.
f. navicula′ris ure′thrae [TA] navicular fossa of urethra: the lateral expansion of the urethra in the glans penis. Called also *fossa of Morgagni.*
occlusal f., f. occlusa′lis [TA] a depression between cusps on the occlusal surface of a tooth.

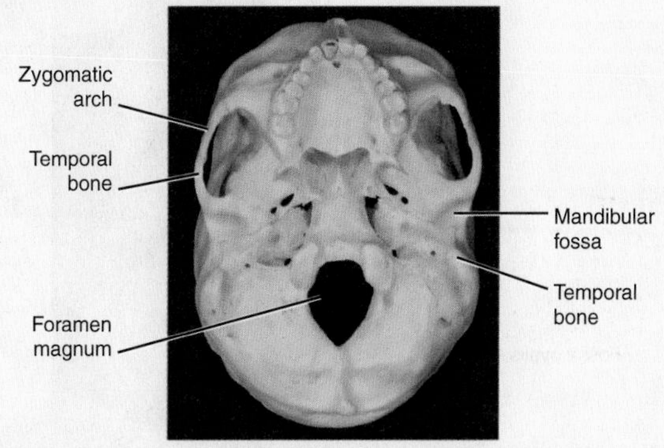

■ Fossa mandibularis (mandibular fossa), in an inferior view of the base of the skull.

Fossa *Continued*

f. ole′crani [TA], **olecranon f.** a depression on the posterior surface of the humerus, above the trochlea, for lodging the olecranon of the ulna when the elbow is extended.
oral f. stomodeum.
oval f. 1. f. ovalis (def. 1). 2. hiatus saphenus.
f. ova′lis 1. [TA] an oval depression in the right atrium on the lower part of the interatrial septum, within a triangular area bounded by the openings of the two venae cavae and the coronary sinus. It represents the remains of the fetal foramen ovale, its floor composed of the fetal septum primum. 2. hiatus saphenus.
f. ova′rica [TA] ovarian fossa: a shallow pouch on the posterior surface of the broad ligament, in which the ovary is located.
paraduodenal f. recessus paraduodenalis.
parajejunal f. a pouch of peritoneum sometimes seen below the lower end of the first part of the jejunum.
pararectal f., f. pararecta′lis [TA] either of two cavities formed by folds of peritoneum, one on either side of the rectum, varying in size according to distention of the rectum; in males this is continuous with the rectovesical pouch and in females it is continuous with the rectouterine pouch. Called also *pararectal pouch*.
paravesical f., f. paravesica′lis [TA] the fossa formed by the peritoneum on each side of the urinary bladder, into which the obturator canal opens; in females it is the lateral part of the vesicouterine pouch.
parietal f. the deepest portion of the inner surface of the parietal bone.
patellar f. f. hyaloidea.
perineal f. f. ischioanalis.
petrosal f. fossula petrosa.
piriform f. recessus piriformis.
pituitary f. f. hypophysialis.
f. popli′tea [TA], **popliteal f.** the depression in the posterior region of the knee; called also *popliteal cavity*.
prenasal f. incisive f. (def. 2).
prescapular f., prespinous f. a depression in the anterior surface of the spine of the scapula.
f. pterygoi′dea [TA] pterygoid fossa: the posteriorly facing fossa which is formed by the divergence of the medial and lateral pterygoid plates of the sphenoid bone, and lodges the origins of the internal pterygoid muscle and tensor veli palatini muscle.
pterygomaxillary f. f. pterygopalatina.
f. pterygopalati′na [TA] pterygopalatine fossa: a small space between the anterior aspect of the root of the pterygoid process of the sphenoid bone and the posterior aspect of the maxilla.
f. radia′lis hu′meri [TA] radial fossa of humerus: a depression on the anterior surface of the humerus just above the capitulum.
retrocecal f. recessus retrocaecalis.
retroduodenal f. recessus retroduodenalis.
f. retromandibula′ris retromandibular fossa: the depression posterior to the angle of the mandible, on either side, inferior to the auricle.
retromolar f., f. retromola′ris [TA] a shallow fossa posterior to the last molar, bounded by the lowest portion of the temporal crest and the external oblique ridge.
f. rhomboi′dea [TA] rhomboid fossa: the floor of the fourth ventricle of the brain, made up of the dorsal surfaces of the medulla oblongata and pons. It is divided into superior, intermediate, and inferior parts.

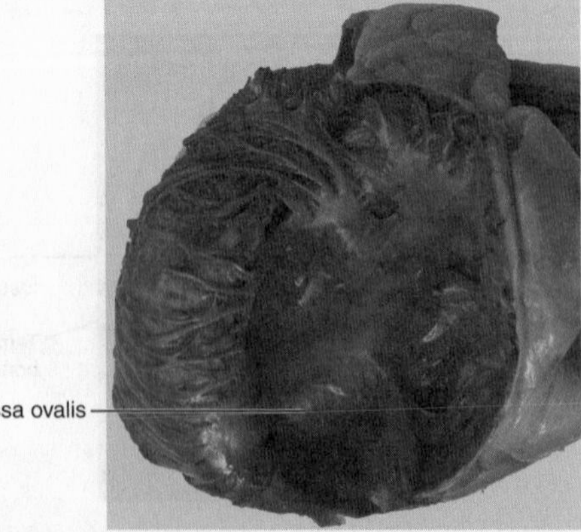

■ Fossa ovalis, in the right atrium, from the front and right.

Rosenmüller f. recessus pharyngeus.
f. sac′ci lacrima′lis [TA] fossa for lacrimal sac: the fossa that lodges the lacrimal sac, formed by the lacrimal sulcus of the lacrimal bone and the frontal process of the maxilla.
scaphoid f. 1. f. scaphoidea ossis sphenoidalis. 2. scapha.
f. scaphoi′dea os′sis sphenoida′lis [TA] scaphoid fossa of sphenoid bone: a depression on the superior part of the posterior portion of the medial plate of the pterygoid process of the sphenoid bone, giving attachment to the tensor veli palatini muscle. Called also *navicular f. of Cruveilhier* or *of sphenoid bone*.
sellar f. f. hypophysialis.
f. subarcua′ta [TA] subarcuate fossa: a small fossa on the internal surface of the petrous part of the temporal bone just inferior to the arcuate eminence, most prominent in the fetus. In the adult it lodges a piece of dura and transmits a small vein.
sublingual f. fovea sublingualis.
submandibular f., submaxillary f. fovea submandibularis.
f. subscapula′ris [TA] subscapular fossa: the shallow concavity covering most of the costal surface of the body of the scapula.
supraclavicular f., greater fossa supraclavicularis major.
supraclavicular f., lesser fossa supraclavicularis minor.
f. supraclavicula′ris ma′jor [TA] greater supraclavicular fossa: a depression on the surface of the body, located superior and posterior to the clavicle, lateral to the tendon of the sternocleidomastoid muscle. See also *trigonum omoclaviculare*.
f. supraclavicula′ris mi′nor [TA] lesser supraclavicular fossa: the region of the neck in the depression posterior to the clavicle, about the interval between the two tendons of the sternocleidomastoid muscle.
supramastoid f. foveola suprameatica.
f. supraspina′ta [TA], **supraspinous f.** the deeply concave area above the spinous process on the dorsal surface of the scapula from which the supraspinous muscle takes origin.
f. supratonsilla′ris [TA] supratonsillar fossa: the triangular space between the palatoglossal and palatopharyngeal arches superior to the tonsil.
f. supravesica′lis [TA] supravesical fossa: the depression on the inside of the anterior abdominal wall between the median and the medial umbilical fold.
sylvian f., f. of Sylvius 1. f. lateralis cerebri. 2. sulcus lateralis cerebri.
temporal f., f. tempora′lis [TA] the area on the side of the cranium outlined posteriorly and superiorly by the temporal lines, anteriorly by the frontal and zygomatic bones, laterally by the zygomatic arch, and inferiorly by the infratemporal crest.
f. tonsilla′ris [TA] tonsillar fossa: the depression between the palatoglossal and palatopharyngeal arches in which the palatine tonsil is located; called also *tonsillar sinus*.
transverse intermesocolic f. a recess of the peritoneum in a similar position to that of the recessus duodenalis superior, but extending transversely.
Treitz f. recessus duodenalis superior.
f. triangula′ris auri′culae [TA] triangular fossa of auricle: the cavity just above the concha of the ear between the crura of the anthelix.
f. trochante′rica [TA] trochanteric fossa: a deep depression on the medial surface of the greater trochanter that receives the insertion of the tendon of the obturator externus muscle.
trochlear f. fovea trochlearis.
ulnar f. f. coronoidea humeri.
umbilical f. of liver, f. of umbilical vein fissura ligamenti teretis.
vermian f. a small fossa sometimes present on the interior surface of the occipital bone at the inferior end of the internal occipital crest; it houses part or all of the inferior cerebellar vermis.
f. vesi′cae bilia′ris [TA] fossa for gallbladder: the fossa on the visceral surface of the liver that lodges the gallbladder and helps to separate the right and left lobes. Called also *f. vesicae felleae* [TA alternative].
f. vesi′cae fel′leae TA alternative for *f. vesicae biliaris*.
vestibular f., f. vesti′buli vagi′nae [TA] fossa of vestibule of vagina: the part of the vestibule between the orifice of the vagina and the frenulum of the pudendal labia.
Waldeyer f. the recessus duodenalis inferior and recessus duodenalis superior considered as one space.
zygomatic f. f. infratemporalis.

fos•sae (fos′e) [L.] genitive and plural of *fossa*.

fos•sette (fos-et′) [Fr.] 1. a small depression. 2. a small and deep corneal ulcer.

fos•su•la (fos′u-lə) gen. and pl *fos′sulae* [L., dim. of *fossa*] a small fossa; a slight depression in the surface of a structure or organ.

f. fenes′trae coch′leae [TA] fossula of cochlear window: a depression on the medial wall of the tympanic cavity, at the bottom of which is the fenestra cochleae; called also *f. of round window* and *niche of round window*.

f. fenes′trae vesti′buli [TA] fossula of vestibular window: a depression on the medial wall of the tympanic cavity, at the bottom of which is the fenestra vestibuli; called also *f. of oval window*.

f. of oval window f. fenestrae vestibuli.

f. petro′sa [TA], **f. of petrous ganglion** petrosal fossula: a small depression on the inferior surface of the petrous portion of the temporal bone, on a small ridge separating the jugular fossa from the external carotid foramen.

f. post fenes′tram a connective tissue tract just behind the oval window, resembling the fissula ante fenestram, but smaller and less constant.

f. of round window f. fenestrae cochleae.

fos′sulae tonsilla′res [TA] tonsillar pits: the mouths of the tonsillar crypts of the pharyngeal tonsils and palatine tonsils.

f. of vestibular window f. fenestrae vestibuli.

fos•su•lae (fos′u-le) [L.] genitive and plural of *fossula*.

fos•su•late (fos′u-lāt) marked by a small fossa; hollowed or grooved.

Fos•ter Ken•ne•dy see *Kennedy*.

Foth•er•gill operation (foth′ər-gil) [William Edward *Fothergill*, Manchester gynecologist, 1865–1926] Manchester operation; see under *operation*.

Fou•chet test (foo-sha′) [André *Fouchet*, French chemist, 20th century] see under *test*.

foul•brood (foul′brood) a contagious disease of honeybees in which larvae are abnormal; the two kinds are *American foulbrood*, caused by *Bacillus larvae*, and *European foulbrood*, caused by *B. alvei*.

foul in the foot foot rot of cattle.

foun•da•tion (foun-da′shən) the structure or basis on which something is built.

denture f. denture-bearing area.

found•er (foun′dər) laminitis (def. 2).

grain f. laminitis in the horse with indigestion or an overloaded stomach, probably due to overeating that results in metabolic disturbance.

four•chette (foor-shet′) [Fr. "a fork-shaped object"] frenulum labiorum pudendi.

Four•neau 309 (foor′no) trademark for a preparation of suramin hexasodium.

Four•nier gangrene (disease), test (foor-nya′) [Jean Alfred *Fournier*, French dermatologist, 1832–1914] see under *gangrene* and *test*.

fo•vea (fo′ve-ə) gen. and pl. *fo′veae* [L. "a pit"] 1. a small pit or depression in the surface of a structure or organ. 2. f. centralis retinae.

f. articula′ris ca′pitis ra′dii [TA] articular facet of head of radius: a depression on the proximal surface of the head of the radius for articulation with the capitulum of the humerus.

f. ca′pitis fe′moris [TA] fovea of head of femur: a depression in the head of the femur where the ligament of head of femur is attached.

f. centra′lis re′tinae [TA] central fovea of retina: a tiny pit, about 1 degree wide, in the center of the macula lutea, which in turn presents an extremely small depression (foveola) containing rodlike elongated cones; it is the area of most acute vision, because here the layers of the retina are spread aside, permitting light to fall directly on the cones.

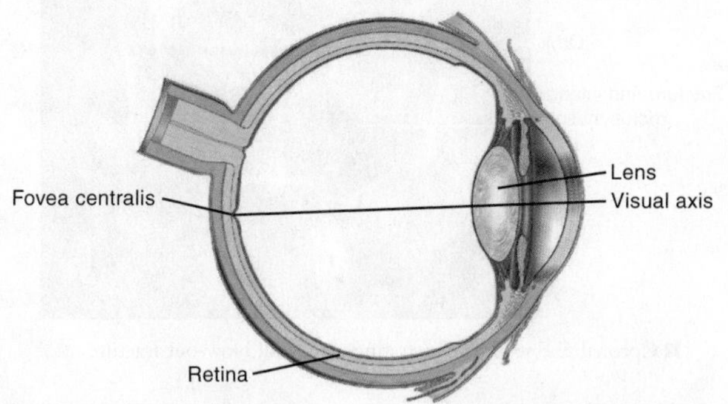

f. costa′lis infe′rior [TA] inferior costal facet: a small facet, really a demifacet, on the lower edge of the body of a vertebra, articulating with the head of a rib.

f. costa′lis proces′sus transver′si [TA] transverse costal facet: a facet on the transverse process of a vertebra for articulation with the tubercle of a rib.

f. costa′lis supe′rior [TA] superior costal facet: a small facet, really a demifacet, on the upper edge of the body of a vertebra, articulating with the head of a rib.

f. den′tis atlan′tis [TA] facet for dens: the facet on the inner surface of the anterior arch of the atlas for the articulation of the dens of the axis.

f. dista′lis den′tis [TA], **distal f. of tooth** a minute depression located at the point of intersection of developmental grooves on the distal aspect of the occlusal surface of bicuspid and molar teeth. Called also *distal pit*.

f. of head of femur f. capitis femoris.

f. infe′rior [TA] inferior fovea: a slight depression in the inferior part of the floor of the fourth ventricle, at the upper end of the vagal trigone, marking the position of the sulcus limitans.

f. lim′bica a sulcus marking the lateral border of the lateral area olfactoria and gyrus hippocampi in lower mammals.

f. mesia′lis den′tis [TA], **mesial f. of tooth** a minute depression located at the point of intersection of developmental grooves on the mesial aspect of the occlusal surface of bicuspid and molar teeth. Called also *mesial pit*.

f. oblon′ga cartila′ginis arytenoi′deae [TA] oblong fovea of arytenoid cartilage: a depression on the anterolateral surface of the arytenoid cartilage, separated from the triangular pit above by the arcuate crest; called also *oblong pit of arytenoid cartilage*.

f. palati′na, palatine f. either of a pair of small pits, situated at or near the junction between the hard and soft palate, just lateral to the midline; it is an orifice through which some of the ducts of the minor mucus glands of the palate empty and plays a role in the gag reflex.

f. pterygoi′dea [TA] pterygoid fovea: a depression on the inner side of the neck of the condyloid process of the mandible, for attachment of the external pterygoid muscle; called also *pterygoid depression* or *pit*.

f. sublingua′lis [TA] sublingual fossa: a depression on the inner surface of the body of the mandible, lodging a portion of the sublingual gland.

f. submandibula′ris [TA] submandibular fossa: a depression on the medial aspect of the body of the mandible, lodging a small portion of the submandibular gland.

f. supe′rior [TA] superior fovea: an angular depression in the floor of the fourth ventricle produced by widening of the sulcus limitans immediately lateral to the facial colliculus.

f. triangula′ris cartila′ginis arytenoi′deae [TA] triangular fovea of arytenoid cartilage: a depression on the anterolateral surface of the arytenoid cartilage, separated from the oblong pit below by the arcuate crest.

f. trochlea′ris [TA] trochlear fovea: a depression on the anteromedial part of the orbital surface of the frontal bone for the attachment of the trochlea of the superior oblique muscle; it is often replaced by the trochlear spine.

fo•ve•ae (fo′ve-e) genitive and plural of *fovea*.

fo•ve•ate (fo′ve-āt) [L. *foveatus*] pitted.

fo•ve•a•tion (fo″ve-a′shən) 1. the formation of pits or foveae. 2. a pitted condition.

fo•ve•o•la (fo-ve′o-lə) gen. and pl. *fove′olae* [L., dim. of *fovea*] a small pit or depression. **foveo′lar** *adj*

f. coccy′gea [TA], **coccygeal f.** a small pit in the skin near the tip of the coccyx, indicative of the site of attachment of the embryonic neural tube to the skin; called also *postanal dimple* or *pit*.

fove′olae gas′tricae [TA] gastric pits: the numerous pits in the gastric mucosa marking the openings of the gastric glands.

granular foveolae, fove′olae granula′res [TA] small pits on the internal surface of the cranial bones on either side of the sagittal sulcus; they are occupied by the arachnoidal granulations.

f. re′tinae [TA] foveola of retina: an extremely small depression in the floor of the fovea centralis, which is devoid of rod cells but contains rodlike elongated cones.

f. suprameata′lis TA alternative for *f. suprameatica*.

f. supramea′tica [TA] suprameatal pit: a small triangular depression at the junction of the posterior and superior borders of the external acoustic meatus, posterior to the suprameatal spine; called also *f. suprameatalis* [TA alternative], *mastoid* or *supramastoid fossa*, and *Macewen* or *suprameatal triangle*.

fo•ve•o•lae (fo-ve′o-le) [L.] genitive and plural of *foveola*.

fo•ve•o•late (fo-ve′o-lāt) pitted.

Fo•ville syndrome (fo-vēl′) [Achille Louis François *Foville*, French neurologist, 1799–1878] see under *syndrome*.

Fow•ler position (fou′lər) [George Ryerson *Fowler*, American surgeon, 1848–1906] see under *position*.

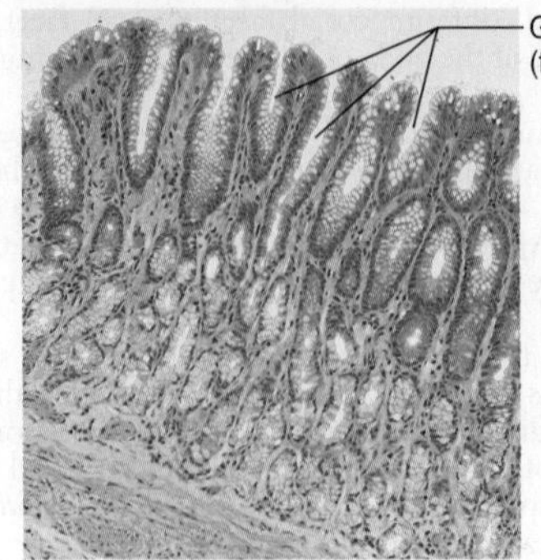

■ Foveolae gastricae (gastric pits) in the pyloric stomach.

fowl·pox (foul′poks) a contagious disease of domestic poultry and birds due to a poxvirus; characteristics include epithelial nodules on unfeathered areas of skin, especially the wattles, comb, and legs, sometimes with membranous lesions in the respiratory passages.

Fox-For·dyce disease (foks′ for′dīs) [G.H. *Fox*, American dermatologist, 1846–1937; John Addison *Fordyce*, American dermatologist, 1858–1925] see under *disease*.

fox·glove (foks′glov) see *digitalis*.
 purple f. digitalis.

F.p. [L.] fi′at po′tio (let a potion be made).

fp freezing point.

FPG fasting plasma glucose.

F.pil. [L.] fi′ant pil′ulae (let pills be made).

Fr francium.

Fract. dos. [L.] frac′ta do′si (in divided doses).

frac·tion (frak′shən) 1. a portion of something larger; see also *fractionation* and *fractional dose*, under *dose*. 2. in chemistry, one of the separable constituents of a substance.
 attributable f. see under *risk*.
 ejection f. the proportion of the volume of blood in the ventricles at the end of diastole that is ejected during systole; it is the stroke volume divided by the end-diastolic volume, often expressed as a percentage. It is normally 65 ± 8 per cent; lower values indicate ventricular dysfunction.
 filtration f. the portion of the plasma that is filtered through the renal glomerular capillary membrane, calculated as the fraction of total glomerular filtration rate divided by total renal blood flow.
 growth f. a fraction whose numerator is the number of cells in a population that are actively passing through the cell cycle and whose denominator is the total number in the population.
 human plasma protein f. plasma protein f.
 mole f. in a system, the ratio of the mass in moles of a component to the mass in moles of all components.
 plasma f's the various components separated from the blood plasma by electrophoresis or by other means.
 plasma protein f. [USP] a sterile preparation of serum albumin and globulin obtained by fractionating material (source blood, plasma, or serum) from healthy human donors; used as a blood volume supporter.
 population attributable f. see under *risk*.
 recombination f. see under *frequency*.
 regurgitant f. the percentage of the stroke volume of blood ejected from a ventricle that returns by regurgitation.
 survival f. after exposure to a cytotoxic substance or irradiation, the ratio between surviving exposed cells per unit of volume and unexposed control cells per unit.

frac·tion·al (frak′shən-əl) [L. *fractio* a breaking] pertaining to a fraction; see also *fractional dose*, under *dose*.

frac·tion·ate (frak′shən-āt) to break up into smaller, generally equal, parts, such as in a fractionated dose of chemotherapy or radiotherapy.

frac·tion·a·tion (frak″shən-a′shən) 1. in radiotherapy, division of the total dose of radiation into small doses administered at intervals, which usually causes less biological damage than the same total dose given at one time; see also *hyperfractionation*. Called also *dose fractionation*. 2. division of the total dosage of a drug into smaller doses *(fractional doses)* administered at frequent intervals. Called also *dose f.* 3. in chemistry, separation of a substance into components, as by distillation or crystallization. 4. in histology, isolation of components of living cells by differential centrifugation.
 dose f. see *fractionation* (defs. 1 and 2).
 plasma f. separation and removal of plasma fractions, using membrane filtration, specific sorption, or other physicochemical methods.

frac·tog·ra·phy (frak-tog′rə-fe) [*fracture* + *-graphy*] a technique of photography which permits observation of jagged surfaces at high magnification.

frac·ture (frak′chər) [L. *fractura*, from *frangere* to break] 1. the breaking of a part, especially a bone. 2. a break or rupture in a bone.

Fracture

agenetic f. spontaneous fracture due to imperfect osteogenesis.
apophyseal f. a fracture in which a small fragment or a bony prominence is torn from the bone.
articular f. a fracture of the joint surface of a bone; called also *joint f.*
atrophic f. a spontaneous fracture resulting from atrophy of the bone.
avulsion f. an indirect fracture caused by avulsion or pull of a ligament.
axial compression f. fracture of a vertebra by excessive vertical force, so that pieces of it move out in horizontal directions, often injuring the spinal cord; it usually occurs in the thoracic or lumbar region as a result of flexion. Called also *burst f.*
Barton f. fracture of the distal end of the radius into the wrist joint.
basal neck f. fracture of the neck of the femur at its junction with the trochanteric region.
bending f. an indirect fracture caused by bending of the limb.
Bennett f. a fracture of the base of the first metacarpal bone running into the carpometacarpal joint and complicated by subluxation.
blow-out f. fracture of the orbital floor caused by a sudden increase of intraorbital pressure due to traumatic force; the orbital contents herniate into the maxillary sinus so that the inferior rectus or inferior oblique muscle may become incarcerated in the fracture site, producing diplopia on looking up. In the pure type there is disruption of the orbital floor without involvement of the orbital rim; the impure type involves the rim, i.e., there is concomitant midfacial fracture.
boxer's f. fracture of the metacarpal neck with volar displacement of the metacarpal head caused by striking a hard object with the closed fist.
bucket-handle f. a tear in the semilunar cartilage, along the middle portion, leaving a loop of cartilage lying in the intercondylar notch.
bumper f. fracture of one or both lower limbs immediately below the knee caused by an automobile bumper, often involving the tibial plateau.

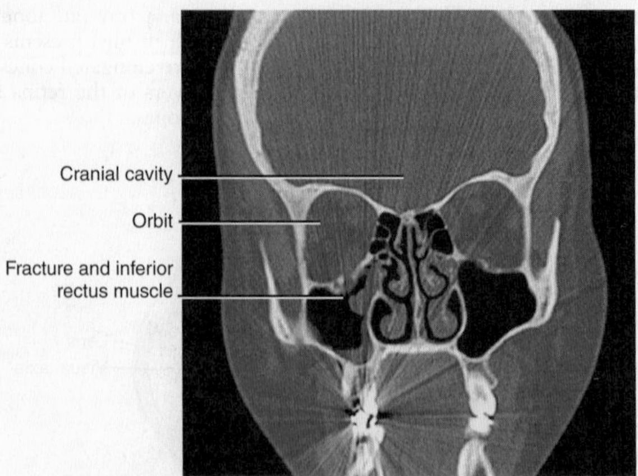

■ Coronal CT scan demonstrating an orbital blow-out fracture.

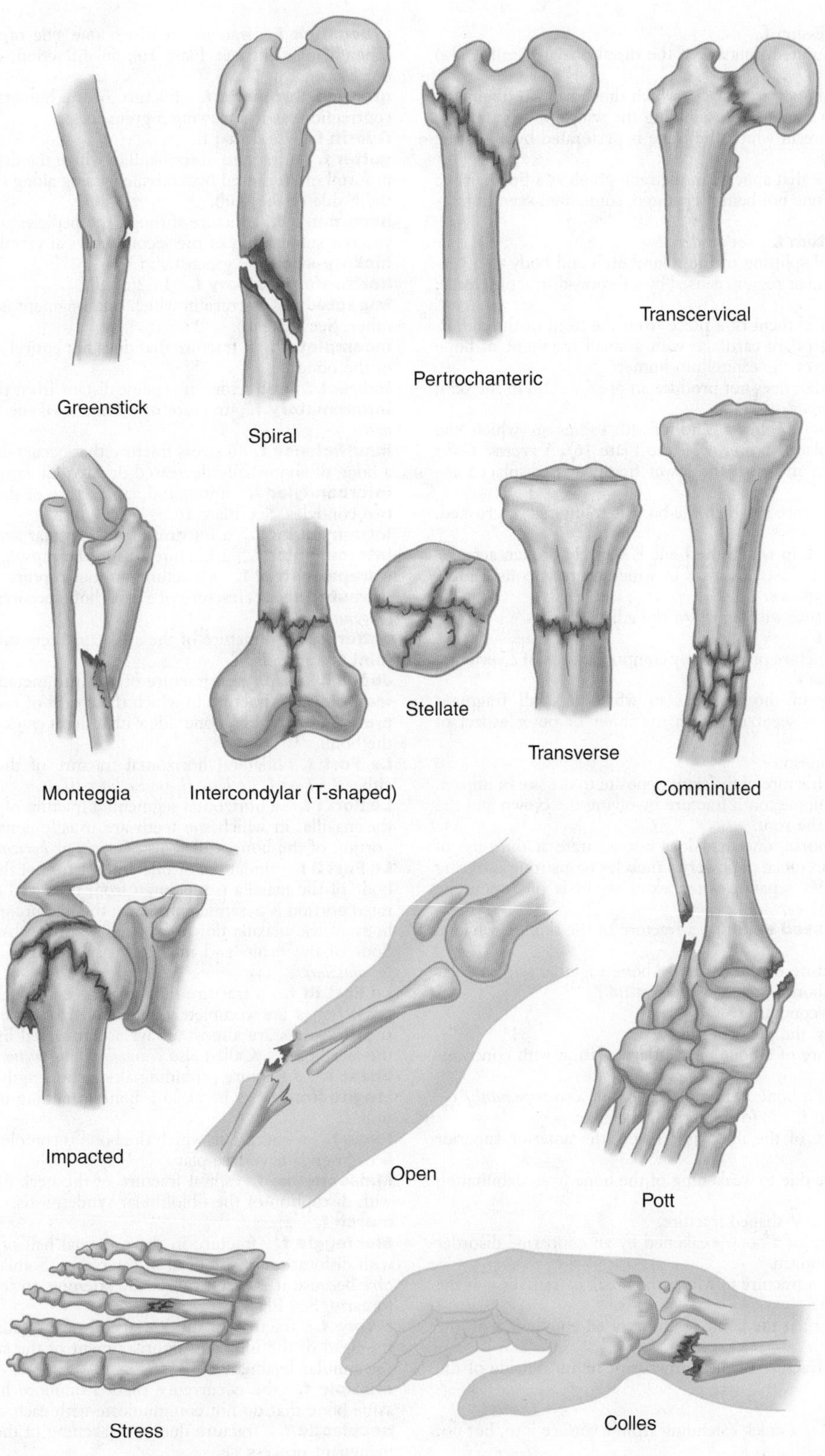

■ **PLATE 16—VARIOUS TYPES OF FRACTURES**

Fracture *Continued*

burst f. axial compression f.
bursting f. a comminuted fracture of the distal phalanx; called also *tuft f.*
butterfly f. a comminuted fracture in which there are two fragments on each side of a main fragment, resembling the wings of a butterfly.
buttonhole f. fracture in which the bone is perforated by a missile; called also *perforating f.*
capillary f. a fracture that appears in the radiograph as a fine hairlike line, the segments of bone not being separated; sometimes seen in fractures of the skull.
cemental f., cementum f. see under *tear.*
Chance f. horizontal splitting of the neural arch and body of a vertebra, usually in the lumbar region, caused by a flexion-distraction force; called also *seat belt f.*
chisel f. oblique detachment of a piece from the head of the radius.
cleavage f. shelling off of cartilage with a small fragment of bone from the upper surface of the capitellum humeri.
closed f. a fracture that does not produce an open wound in the skin; cf. *open f.* Called also *simple f.*
Colles f. fracture of the lower end of the radius in which the lower fragment is displaced posteriorly (see Plate 16). A *reverse Colles* or *Smith fracture* is one in which the lower fragment is displaced anteriorly.
comminuted f. a fracture in which the bone is splintered or crushed. See Plate 16.
complete f. a fracture in which the bone is entirely broken across.
complex simple f. a closed fracture in which there is considerable injury to adjacent soft tissues.
complicated f. fracture with injury of the adjacent parts.
compound f. open f.
compression f. a fracture produced by compression, as of a vertebra; see also *axial compression f.*
condylar f. fracture of the humerus in which a small fragment including the condyle is separated from the inner or outer aspect of the bone.
congenital f. intrauterine f.
f. by contrecoup a fracture of the skull opposite to the site of impact.
crown-root f. an oblique tooth fracture involving the crown and the adjacent distal part of the root.
deferred f. in the horse, one that does not separate at the time of injury because of the presence of powerful muscles or a strong covering of periosteum, but does separate when extra strain is put upon the injured part.
depressed f., depressed skull f. a fracture of the skull in which a fragment is depressed.
de Quervain f. fracture of the navicular bone together with a volar luxation of the lunate bone. Called also *Quervain f.*
diacondylar f. transcondylar f.
direct f. a fracture at the point of injury.
dislocation f. fracture of a bone near an articulation with concomitant dislocation of that joint.
double f. fracture of a bone in two places; called also *segmental f.*
Dupuytren f. 1. Pott f. 2. (of forearm) Galeazzi f.
Duverney f. fracture of the ilium just below the anterior superior spine.
dyscrasic f. fracture due to weakening of the bone from debilitating disease.
f. en coin (ah kwă′) a V-shaped fracture.
endocrine f. fracture of a bone weakened by an endocrine disorder such as hyperparathyroidism.
f. en rave (ah rahv′) a fracture in which the break is transverse at the surface, but not within.
epiphyseal f. fracture at the point of union of an epiphysis with the shaft of a bone.
extracapsular f. a fracture of the humerus or femur outside of the capsule.
fatigue f. stress f.
fissure f., fissured f. a crack extending from a surface into, but not through, a long bone.
freeze f. see *freeze-fracturing.*
Galeazzi f. fracture of the radius above the wrist combined with dislocation of the distal end of the ulna; called also *Dupuytren f.*
Gosselin f. a V-shaped fracture of the distal end of the tibia, extending into the ankle joint.
greenstick f. fracture in which one side of a bone is broken, the other being bent (see Plate 16); an infraction; called also *hickory-stick* or *willow f.*
grenade-thrower's f. fracture of the humerus caused by muscular contraction, as in throwing a grenade.
Guérin f. Le Fort I f.
gutter f. a fracture of the skull in which the depression is long elliptic in form; often caused by a missile passing along the outside or grooving the inside of the skull.
hangman's f. fracture through the pedicles of the axis (C2) with or without subluxation of the second cervical vertebra on the third.
hickory-stick f. greenstick f.
horizontal maxillary f. Le Fort I f.
impacted f. fracture in which one fragment is firmly driven into the other. See Plate 16.
incomplete f. a fracture that does not entirely destroy the continuity of the bone.
indirect f. a fracture at a point distant from the site of injury.
inflammatory f. fracture of a bone weakened by inflammatory disease.
insufficiency f. a stress fracture that occurs during normal stress on a bone of abnormally decreased density. Cf. *osteoporosis.*
intercondylar f. a longitudinal fracture of the humerus between its two condyles. See Plate 16.
intraarticular f. a fracture of the articular surface of a bone.
intracapsular f. a fracture within the capsule of a joint.
intraperiosteal f. a fracture without rupture of the periosteum.
intrauterine f. fracture of a fetal bone occurring *in utero;* called also *congenital f.*
Jefferson f. fracture of the atlas (first cervical vertebra).
joint f. articular f.
Jones f. diaphyseal fracture of the fifth metatarsal.
lead pipe f. fracture in which the cortex of the bone is slightly compressed and bulges on one side with a slight crack on the opposite side of the bone.
Le Fort f. bilateral horizontal fracture of the maxilla, classified as either *Le Fort I, Le Fort II,* or *Le Fort III.*
Le Fort I f. a horizontal segmented fracture of the alveolar process of the maxilla, in which the teeth are usually contained in the detached portion of the bone; called also *Guérin* or *horizontal maxillary f.*
Le Fort II f. unilateral or bilateral fracture of the maxilla, in which the body of the maxilla is separated from the facial skeleton and the separated portion is pyramidal in shape; the fracture may extend through the body of the maxilla down the midline of the hard palate, through the floor of the orbit, and into the nasal cavity. Called also *pyramidal f. (of maxilla).*
Le Fort III f. a fracture in which the entire maxilla and one or more facial bones are completely separated from the craniofacial skeleton; such fractures are almost always accompanied by multiple fractures of the facial bones. Called also *craniofacial disjunction* and *transverse facial f.*
linear f. a fracture extending along the length of a bone.
longitudinal f. a break in a bone extending in a longitudinal direction.
loose f. a fracture in which the bone is completely broken so that the broken ends have free play.
Maisonneuve f. spiral fracture of the neck of the fibula, associated with disruption of the tibiofibular syndesmosis.
march f. stress f.
Monteggia f. fracture in the proximal half of the shaft of the ulna, with dislocation of the head of the radius. Sometimes called *parry fracture* because it is often caused by attempts to fend off blows with the forearm. See Plate 16.
Moore f. fracture of the lower end of the radius with dislocation of the head of the ulna and imprisonment of the styloid process beneath the annular ligaments.
multiple f. the occurrence of two or more lines of fracture in the same bone that do not communicate with each other.
neoplastic f. fracture due to weakening of the bone as a result of a malignant process.
neurogenic f. fracture due to weakening of the bone as a result of a neurological condition such as tabes dorsalis or paresis.
oblique f. fracture in which the break is in an oblique direction.
open f. a fracture in which there is an external wound leading to the break in the bone; cf. *closed f.* Called also *compound f.* See Plate 16.

Fracture *Continued*

paratrooper f. fracture of the posterior articular margin of the tibia and/or of the internal or external malleolus.
parry f. Monteggia f.
pathologic f. a fracture due to weakening of the bone structure by pathologic processes, such as neoplasia, osteomalacia, osteomyelitis, and other diseases. Called also *secondary f.* and *spontaneous f.*
perforating f. buttonhole f.
periarticular f. a fracture extending close to, but not into, a joint.
pertrochanteric f. fracture of the femur passing through the greater trochanter. See Plate 16.
pillion f. a fracture of the lower end of the femur occurring when the knee of a person riding pillion on a motorcycle is struck in a collision; it is a T-shaped fracture with displacement of the condyles behind the femoral shaft.
pilon f. comminuted fracture of the inferior articular surface of the tibia and the malleoli, caused by axial compression of the ankle joint.
ping-pong f., pond f. a type of depressed skull fracture usually seen in young children, resembling the indentation that can be produced with the finger in a ping-pong ball; when elevated it resumes and retains its normal position.
Pott f. fracture of the lower part of the fibula, with serious injury of the lower tibial articulation, usually a chipping off of a portion of the medial malleolus, or rupture of the medial ligament; called also *Dupuytren f.* See Plate 16.
pressure f. a fracture caused by pressure on the bone from an adjoining tumor.
pyramidal f., pyramidal f. of maxilla Le Fort II f.
Quervain f. de Quervain f.
resecting f. a fracture in which a piece of the bone is removed by violence, as by a bullet.
sagittal slice f. fracture of a vertebra breaking it in an oblique direction; the vertebral column above is displaced horizontally, usually causing paraplegia.
Salter-Harris f. an epiphyseal fracture in children that involves the epiphyseal disk.
seat belt f. Chance f.
secondary f. pathologic f.
segmental f. double f.
Segond f. avulsion fracture of the tibial attachment of the iliotibial band.
Shepherd f. fracture of the astragalus, with detachment of the outer protecting edge.

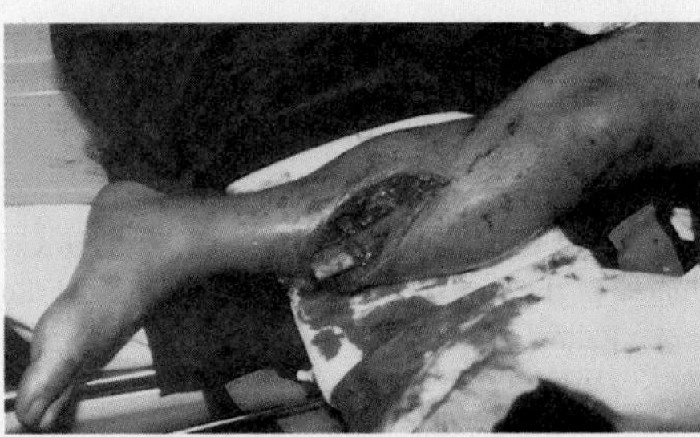
■ Open fracture of the lower leg.

silver fork f. a name sometimes given to Colles fracture because of the shape of the deformity that it causes.
simple f. closed f.
Skillern f. complete fracture of the lower third of the radius with greenstick fracture of the lower third of the ulna.
Smith f. a fracture of the lower end of the radius near its articular surface with forward displacement of the lower fragment; sometimes called *reverse Colles fracture.*
spiral f. a fracture in which the bone has been twisted apart; called also *torsion f.* See Plate 16.
splintered f. a type of comminuted fracture in which the bone is splintered into thin, sharp fragments.
spontaneous f. pathologic f.
sprain f. the separation of a tendon or ligament from its insertion, taking with it a piece of bone.
sprinter's f. fracture of the anterior superior or of the anterior inferior spine of the ilium, a fragment of the bone being pulled off by muscular violence, as at the start of a sprint.
stellate f. a fracture that has a central point of injury from which numerous fissures radiate out. See Plate 16.
Stieda f. fracture of the internal condyle of the femur.
stress f. a fracture caused by unusual or repeated stress on a bone, such as with soldiers or athletes. Called also *fatigue* or *march f.* See Plate 16.
subcapital f. fracture of a bone just below its head, especially an intracapsular fracture of the neck of the femur at the junction of the head and neck.
subcutaneous f. closed f.
subperiosteal f. a crack through a bone without alteration in its alignment or contour, the supposition being that the periosteum is not broken.
supracondylar f. fracture of the humerus in which the line of fracture is through the lower end of the shaft of the humerus.
Tillaux f. vertical fracture of the distal lateral margin of the tibia.
torsion f. spiral f.
torus f. a fracture in which there is a localized expansion or torus of the cortex, with little or no displacement of the lower end of the bone.
transcervical f. fracture through the neck of the femur. See Plate 16.
transcondylar f. fracture of the humerus in which the line of fracture is at the level of the condyles, traverses the fossae, and is in part within the capsule of the joint; called also *diacondylar f.*
transverse f. a fracture at right angles to the axis of the bone. See Plate 16.
transverse facial f. Le Fort III f.
transverse maxillary f. Le Fort I f.
trimalleolar f. fracture of the medial and lateral malleoli and the posterior tip of the tibia.
triplane f. fracture of the distal lateral tibia occurring in three planes: sagittally through the epiphysis, horizontally through the physis, and coronally through the metaphysis.
T-shaped f. an intercondylar fracture that has both longitudinal and transverse portions in the form of a T.
tuft f. bursting f.
Wagstaffe f. separation of the internal malleolus.
wedge-compression f. compression fracture of only the anterior part of a vertebra, leaving a wedge-shaped vertebra.
willow f. greenstick f.

frac·ture-dis·lo·ca·tion (frak′chər-dis″lo-ka′shən) a fracture of a bone near a joint, also involving dislocation.

Fraenk·el see *Fränkel.*

frag·i·form (fraj′ĭ-form) [L. *fraga* strawberry + *form*] shaped like a strawberry.

fra·gil·i·tas (frə-jil′ĭ-təs) [L., from *frangere* to break] fragility.
 f. cri′nium fragility of the hair; see *trichorrhexis.*
 f. un′guium brittleness of the nails; see *onychorrhexis.*

fra·gil·i·ty (frə-jil′ĭ-te) susceptibility, or lack of resistance, to factors capable of causing disruption of continuity or integrity.
 capillary f. unusual susceptibility of capillaries under stress to disruption with extravasation, usually with spots visible on the skin, such as ecchymoses, petechiae, or telangiectasias.
 erythrocyte f. susceptibility of erythrocytes to hemolysis under conditions such as decreased osmotic pressure or when subjected to mechanical trauma.
 osmotic f. susceptibility of erythrocytes to rupture when subjected to increasingly hypotonic saline solutions; seen in some forms of hemolytic anemia and spherocytosis. See also *osmotic fragility test,* under *test.*

fra·gilo·cyte (frə-jil′o-sīt) an erythrocyte characterized by osmotic fragility.

fra·gilo·cy·to·sis (frə-jil″o-si-to′sis) the presence of fragilocytes in the blood, as seen in some types of hemolytic anemia and spherocytosis.

frag·ment (frag′mənt) one of the small pieces into which a larger entity has been broken.
 Fab f. see *Fab.*
 $F(ab')_2$ f. see $F(ab')_2$.

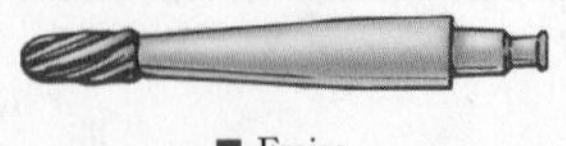

■ Fraise.

Fc f. see *Fc.*

Okazaki f's the short fragments of DNA, each consisting of an RNA primer and a short DNA chain and ranging in length from 100–200 nucleotides in eukaryotes to 1000–2000 nucleotides in prokaryotes, formed in synthesis of the lagging strand during DNA replication; later the primers are replaced by DNA and the fragments are joined by DNA ligase to form a continuous strand. See illustration at *replication fork,* under *fork.*

restriction f. a DNA fragment produced by a restriction endonuclease.

frag•men•ta•tion (frag″mən-ta′shən) 1. a division into fragments. 2. a form of reproduction seen in certain organisms, such as flatworms, in which the body of the parent may break into several pieces, each piece then regenerating the missing parts and developing into a whole animal.

f. of myocardium transverse rupture of the muscle fibers of the heart.

Frag•min (frag′min) trademark for a preparation of dalteparin sodium.

fraise (frāz) [Fr. "strawberry"] a conical or hemispherical bur for cutting osteoplastic flaps or enlarging trephine openings.

Fra•ley syndrome (fra′le) [Elwin E. *Fraley,* American urologist, born 1934] see under *syndrome.*

fram•be•sia (fram-be′zhə) [Fr. *framboise* raspberry] yaws.

f. tro′pica yaws.

fram•be•si•o•ma (fram-be″ze-o′mə) mother yaw; see under *yaw.*

fram•boe•sia (fram-be′zhə) yaws.

fram•boe•si•o•ma (fram-be″ze-o′mə) mother yaw; see under *yaw.*

frame (frām) a structure, usually rigid, designed for giving support to or for immobilizing a part.

Balkan f. a rectangular frame attached to and overhanging a bed; particularly useful in allowing bedridden patients to move more effectively and for attachment of splints. Called also *Balkan splint.*

Bradford f. a rectangular frame of pipe with a sheet of heavy canvas attached, used as a bed frame for patients who must remain immobile.

Deiters terminal f. plates in the lamina reticularis that unite Deiters phalanges with Hensen cells.

Foster f. a device similar to the Stryker frame.

occluding f. dental articulator.

open reading f. (ORF) see *reading f.*

quadriplegic standing f. standing f.

reading f. one of the three possible ways of reading a nucleotide sequence as a series of triplets. An open reading frame contains no termination codons and is thus potentially translatable into protein.

standing f. a device for supporting in the upright position a patient whose four limbs are paralyzed.

Stryker f. trademark for an apparatus constructed of canvas stretched over pipes, which allows the patient to be rotated to lie in the prone or supine position; used in the treatment of persons with injuries to the spinal column or cord and those with severe burns.

trial f. a frame specially devised to permit easy insertion of different lenses used in correcting refractive errors of vision.

Whitman f. a bed frame similar to the Bradford frame except that it is curved.

frame•work (frām′wərk) 1. the basic structure about which something is formulated or built. 2. the metallic skeletal portion of a dental prosthesis to which are attached the resin flange and base components of the partial denture and the artificial teeth.

central f. middle ring.

implant f. see under *substructure.*

scleral f. the larger and coarser part of the angle of the iris which is adjacent to the sclera.

uveal f. ligamentum pectinatum anguli iridocornealis.

fra•my•cet•in sul•fate (frə-mi′sə-tin) a broad-spectrum aminoglycoside antibiotic administered topically to the conjunctiva in the treatment of ocular infection caused by pyogenic bacteria.

Fran•ce•schet•ti syndrome (frahn″chĕ-sket′e) [Adolphe *Franceschetti,* Swiss ophthalmologist, 1896–1968] see under *syndrome.*

Fran•ce•schet•ti-Jad•as•sohn syndrome (frahn″chĕ-sket′e yah′dahsōn) [A. *Franceschetti;* Josef *Jadassohn,* German dermatologist, 1863–1936] see under *syndrome.*

Fran•cis disease (fran′sis) [Edward *Francis,* American bacteriologist, 1872–1957] tularemia.

Fran•ci•sel•la (fran-sĭ-sel′ə) [E. *Francis*] a genus of gram-negative bacteria of the familyFrancisellaceae, consisting of small, pleomorphic, rod-shaped or coccoid cells. Organisms are aerobic and nonmotile, do not produce endospores, and are pathogenic in various animals, particularly lagomorphs. The type species is *F. tularen′sis.*

F. philomira′gia a species that is an opportunistic pathogen and causes septicemia and pneumonia in immunocompromised persons.

F. tularen′sis the etiologic agent of tularemia in humans; it is divided into several subspecies, all of which cause disease. Its natural reservoir is various wild animals, such as rabbits, squirrels, and muskrats, and it is transmitted to humans by contact with infected animals or their products, by inhalation of aerosolized bacteria, or by being bitten by blood-sucking insect carriers.

Fran•ci•sel•la•ceae (fran″sis-el-a′se-e) a family of gram-negative bacteria of the order Thiotrichales, consisting of short rod-shaped or coccoid cells; organisms are aerobic, nonmotile, non–spore-forming and weakly catalase positive. It contains the genus *Francisella.*

fran•ci•um (Fr) (fran′se-əm) the chemical element of atomic number 87, atomic weight 223, all isotopes of which are radioactive.

Fran•çois syndrome (frahn-swah′) [Jules *François,* Belgian ophthalmologist, 1907–1984] oculomandibulofacial syndrome.

frange (frahnzh) [Fr. "brush"] a fringe or band of cilia in the oral area of certain ciliate protozoa, made up of kinetofragments. Called also *hypostomial frange.* Cf. *pseudomembranelle.*

Frank-Star•ling curve (frahngk′ stahr′ling) [Otto *Frank,* German physiologist, 1865–1944; Ernest Henry *Starling,* English physiologist, 1866–1927] see under *curve.*

Fran•kel classification (frang′kəl) [Hans Ludwig *Frankel,* British physician, born 1932] see under *classification.*

Frän•kel sign (freng′kel) [Albert *Fränkel,* German physician, 1848–1916] see under *sign.*

Frank•en•häu•ser ganglion (frahngk′en-hoi″zər) [Ferdinand *Frankenhäuser,* German gynecologist, 1832–1894] see under *ganglion.*

Frantz tumor (frants) [Virginia Kneeland *Frantz,* American surgical pathologist, 1896–1967] solid pseudopapillary tumor of pancreas.

Fra•ser syndrome (fra′zer) [George Robert *Fraser,* Czechoslovakian-born American geneticist, born 1932] cryptophthalmos syndrome.

fra•tax•in (frə-tak′sin) a mitochondrial protein involved in iron metabolism and normally present in the nervous system, heart, and pancreas; levels in these tissues are severely reduced in patients with Friedreich ataxia (q.v.).

fra•ter•nal (frə-tur′nəl) [L. *frater* brother] 1. of or pertaining to brothers. 2. derived from two zygotes; said of twins.

***F*-ratio, test** [Sir Ronald Aylmer *Fisher,* British statistician, 1890–1962] see under *ratio* and *test.*

Frax•i•nus (frak-si′nəs) the ashes, a genus of deciduous trees of the family Oleaceae. *F. or′nus* and other species are sources of mannitol, and the bark of many species is astringent and antiperiodic.

Fra•zier-Spil•ler operation (fra′zhər spil′ər) [Charles Harrison *Frazier,* American surgeon, 1870–1936; William Gibson *Spiller,* American neurologist, 1863–1940] see under *operation.*

FRC functional residual capacity.

FRCP Fellow of the Royal College of Physicians.

FRCP(C) Fellow of the Royal College of Physicians of Canada.

FRCPE Fellow of the Royal College of Physicians of Edinburgh.

FRCP(Glasg) Fellow of the Royal College of Physicians and Surgeons of Glasgow *qua* Physician.

FRCPI Fellow of the Royal College of Physicians in Ireland.

FRCS Fellow of the Royal College of Surgeons.

FRCS(C) Fellow of the Royal College of Surgeons of Canada.

FRCSEd Fellow of the Royal College of Surgeons of Edinburgh.

FRCS(Glasg) Fellow of the Royal College of Physicians and Surgeons of Glasgow *qua* Surgeon.

FRCSI Fellow of the Royal College of Surgeons in Ireland.

FRCVS Fellow of the Royal College of Veterinary Surgeons.

Fre•Am•ine II (fre-am′ēn) trademark for a crystalline amino acid solution for intravenous administration, containing a mixture of essential and nonessential amino acids but no peptides.

freck•le (frek′əl) [Middle English *frakel, frekel*] 1. a benign, small, tan to brown macule occurring on sun-exposed skin; these are most common in children and tend to fade in adult life. Freckles resemble lentigines, but differ in not darkening after exposure to sunlight; also, freckles do not have increased numbers of melanocytes the way lentigines do. Called also *ephelis.* 2. to develop these macules on the skin.

Hutchinson f., melanotic f. of Hutchinson lentigo maligna.

freck•ling (frek′ling) the occurrence of freckles.
axillary f. Crowe sign.

Fre•det-Ram•stedt operation (frĕ-da′ rahm′shtet) [Pierre *Fredet*, French surgeon, 1870–1946; Conrad *Ramstedt*, German surgeon, 1867–1963] see under *operation.*

Free•man-Shel•don syndrome (fre′mən shel′dən) [Ernest Arthur *Freeman*, British orthopedic surgeon, 1900–1975; Joseph Harold *Sheldon*, British physician, 1920–1964] see under *syndrome.*

free•mar•tin (fre′mahr-tin) a sexually maldeveloped female calf born as a twin to a normal male calf; it is commonly sterile and intersexual as the result of male hormone reaching it through anastomosed placental vessels.

freeze-cleav•ing (frēz-clēv′ing) freeze-etching.

freeze-dry•ing (frēz′dri″ing) a method of tissue preparation in which the tissue specimen is frozen and then dehydrated at low temperature in a high vacuum. See also *lyophilization.*

freeze-etch•ing (frēz′ech″ing) a method used to study unfixed cells by electron microscopy, in which the object to be studied is placed in 20 per cent glycerol, frozen at −100°C, and then mounted on a chilled holder.

freeze-frac•tur•ing (frēz′frak″chər-ing) a method of preparing cells for electron-microscopical examination: a tissue specimen is frozen at −150°C, inserted into a vacuum chamber, and fractured by a microtome; a platinum carbon replica of the exposed surfaces is made, freed of the underlying specimen, and then examined.

freeze-sub•sti•tu•tion (frēz′sub″stĭ-too′shən) a modification of freeze-drying in which the ice within the frozen tissue is replaced by alcohol or other solvents at a very low temperature.

Frei•berg infraction (disease) (fri′bərg) [Albert Henry *Freiberg*, American surgeon, 1868–1940] Köhler bone disease (def. 2); see under *disease.*

Frej•ka pillow (pillow splint) (frāj′kah) [Bedrich *Frejka*, Czechoslovakian orthopedic surgeon, 1890–1972] see under *pillow.*

frem•i•tus (frem′ĭ-təs) [L.] a vibration perceptible on palpation; cf. *thrill.*
bronchial f. rhonchal f.
friction f. rub.
pectoral f. vocal f.
pericardial f. a thrill of the chest wall due to the friction of the surfaces of the pericardium over each other.
pleural f. a palpable vibration of the wall of the thorax due to a friction rub between the opposing surfaces of the pleura.
rhonchal f. palpable vibrations produced by the passage of air through a large bronchial tube filled with mucus; see also *rhonchus.* Called also *bronchial f.*
subjective f. vibration felt by the patient on humming with the mouth closed.
tactile f. a strong vocal fremitus that can be felt by a hand on the thorax.
tussive f. vibration felt on the chest when the patient coughs.
vocal f. (VF) a thrill caused by speaking, perceived by the ear of the auscultator applied to the chest; called also *pectoral f.*

fre•na (fre′nə) [L.] plural of *frenum.*

fre•nal (fre′nəl) pertaining to a frenum or frenulum.

French (french) see *French scale*, under *scale.*

fre•nec•to•my (fre-nek′tə-me) [*frenum* + *-ectomy*] excision of a frenum (frenulum).

Fren•kel movements (treatment) (freng′kəl) [Heinrich S. *Frenkel*, Swiss neurologist in Germany, 1860–1931] see under *movement.*

fre•no•plas•ty (fre′no-plas″te) the correction of an abnormally attached frenum by surgically repositioning it. **frenoplas′tic** *adj*

fre•not•o•my (fre-not′ə-me) [L. *frenum* + *-tomy*] cutting the frenum (frenulum), especially for release of ankyloglossia (tongue-tie).
lingual f. incision of the lingual frenum; ankylotomy.

fren•u•la (fren′u-lə) [L.] plural of *frenulum.*

fren•u•lec•to•my (fren″u-lek′tə-me) frenectomy.

fren•u•lo•plas•ty (fren′u-lo-plas″te) frenoplasty. **frenuloplas′tic** *adj*

fren•u•lum (fren′u-ləm) pl. *fren′ula* [L., dim. of *frenum* bridle] a small fold of integument or mucous membrane that checks, curbs, or limits the movements of an organ or part; see also *frenum.*
f. clito′ridis [TA] the tissue fold on the under surface of the clitoris formed by union of the two medial parts of the labia minora.
f. of cranial medullary velum f. veli medullaris superioris.
f. of ileal orifice, f. of ileocecal valve f. ostii ilealis.
labial f. the frenulum of either lip; see *f. labii superioris* and *f. labii inferioris.*

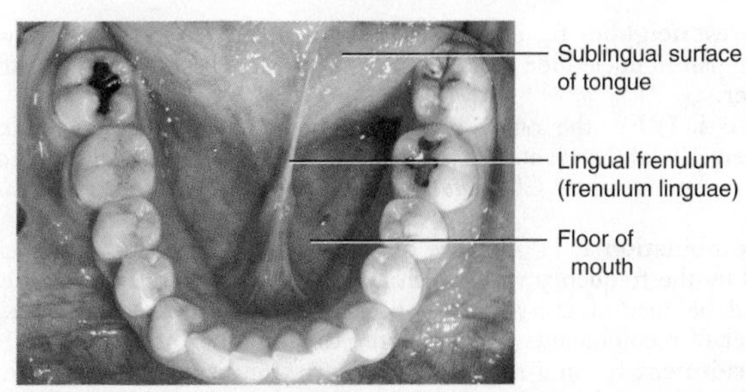

■ Frenulum linguae (lingual frenulum) in a view of the floor of the mouth from above.

f. la′bii inferio′ris [TA] frenulum of lower lip: the fold of mucous membrane on the inside of the middle of the lower lip, connecting the lip with the gums.
f. la′bii superio′ris [TA] frenulum of upper lip: the fold of mucous membrane on the inside of the middle of the upper lip, connecting the lip with the gums.
f. labio′rum puden′di [TA] frenulum of labia minora: the posterior union of the labia minora, anterior to the posterior commissure; called also *fourchette* and *frenum of labia.*
f. lin′guae [TA], **lingual f.** frenulum of tongue: the vertical fold of mucous membrane inferior to the tongue, attaching it to the floor of the mouth; called also *frenum of tongue.*
f. os′tii ilea′lis [TA] frenulum of ileal orifice: a fold formed by the joined extremities of the ileal orifice, extending partly around the lumen of the colon; it was called *frenulum of ileocecal valve* before it was discovered that the valve was found only in cadavers.
f. prepu′tii pe′nis [TA] frenulum of prepuce of penis: the fold on the lower surface of the glans penis that connects it with the prepuce.
f. of pudendal labia f. labiorum pudendi.
f. of rostral medullary velum f. veli medullaris superioris.
f. of superior lip f. labii superioris.
f. of superior medullary velum f. veli medullaris superioris.
f. of tongue f. linguae.
f. val′vae ilea′lis, f. val′vae ileocaeca′lis former names for the frenulum ostii ilealis.
f. ve′li medulla′ris crania′lis, f. ve′li medulla′ris rostra′lis f. veli medullaris superioris.
f. ve′li medulla′ris superio′ris [TA] frenulum of superior medullary velum: a median ridge that descends upon the rostral medullary velum from between the inferior colliculi; called also *f. of cranial medullary velum, f. of rostral medullary velum, f. veli medullaris cranialis*, and *f. veli medullaris rostralis.*

fre•num (fre′nəm) pl. *fre′na* [L. "bridle"] a restraining structure or part; see *frenulum.*
buccal f. a fold of mucous membrane connecting the alveolar ridge to the cheek and separating the labial vestibule from the buccal vestibule.
f. of labia frenulum labiorum pudendi.
lingual f. frenulum linguae.
Macdowel f. a group of fibers attached to the tendon of the pectoralis muscle and strengthening the intermuscular septum.
f. of tongue frenulum linguae.

fre•quen•cy (fre′kwən-se) 1. the number of occurrences of a periodic or recurrent process per unit time. 2. the number of occurrences of a particular event or the number of members of a population or statistical sample falling in a particular class. Symbol *f.* 3. relative f.
audio f. any frequency corresponding to a normally audible sound wave. See also *audibility limits*, under *limit.*
class f. in statistics, the number of variables contained in a class.
critical flicker f., critical fusion f. the number of flashes per second at which a flickering light just appears to be continuous; see also *flicker.*
fusion f. critical fusion frequency.
gene f. the proportion of loci at which a given allele is found in a given population.
high f. 1. said of any periodic event or process that recurs at a rate greater than a specified norm. 2. an alternating current where frequency in cycles per second is high in reference to a certain standard. 3. a frequency of sound waves that is above a certain standard such as middle C. 4. the rate of oscillation in an alternating current exceeding the rate at which muscular contraction ceases, approximately 10,000 per second.
infrasonic f. any frequency below the audio frequency range.
low f. 1. said of any periodic event or process that recurs at a rate below a specified norm. 2. an alternating current where frequency in cycles per second is low in reference to a certain standard. 3. a frequency of sound waves that is below a certain standard such as middle C.

nearest neighbor f. in a nucleic acid, the relative frequency with which a given pair of nucleotide bases, of the four possible bases, occur next to one another.

radio f. (RF) the range of frequencies of electromagnetic radiation between 10 kilohertz and 100 gigahertz, which are the ones used for radio communication. Cf. *radio waves,* under *wave.* Written also *radiofrequency.*

recombination f. a measure of the distance separating two loci, assessed by the frequency with which new combinations of linked genes are formed because of crossing over occurring between their loci, i.e., the number of recombinants divided by the total number of progeny.

recruitment f. in a recruitment pattern, the firing rate of one motor unit action potential at the time that a different potential first appears; cf. *recruitment interval.*

relative f. the ratio of the number of occurrences of a specified phenomenon in a population to the total size of the population.

subsonic f. infrasonic f.

supersonic f. ultrasonic f.

ultrasonic f. any frequency above the audio frequency range; see *ultrasonics.*

urinary f. urination at short intervals without increase in daily volume of urinary output, due to reduced bladder capacity. Called also *pollakisuria* and *pollakiuria.*

Fres•nel lens (fra-nel′) [Augustin Jean *Fresnel,* French physicist and engineer, 1788–1827] see under *lens.*

fress•re•flex (fres′re-fleks) [Ger. "eating reflex"] rhythmic sucking, chewing, and swallowing movements elicited by stroking of the lips and cheeks.

FRET fluorescence resonance energy transfer.

fre•ta (fre′tə) [L.] plural of *fretum.*

fre•tum (fre′təm) pl. *fre′ta* [L.] a constriction or isthmus.

Freud (froid) Sigmund, 1856–1939. German-born psychiatrist in Austria; the founder of psychoanalysis. He developed such fundamental concepts as the unconscious, infantile sexuality, repression, sublimation, and superego, ego, and id formation and their applications to all human behavior.

freud•i•an (froi′de-ən) 1. pertaining to Sigmund Freud or his psychological theories and method of psychotherapy (psychoanalysis). 2. an adherent or user of freudian theory or methods.

Freund adjuvant (froind) [Jules Thomas *Freund,* Hungarian-born bacteriologist in the United States, 1890–1960] see under *adjuvant.*

Freund anomaly (froind) [Wilhelm Alexander *Freund,* German surgeon, 1833–1918] see under *anomaly.*

Frey hairs (fri) [Max Rupert Franz von *Frey,* Austrian physiologist, 1852–1932] see under *hair.*

Frey procedure (fri) [Charles F. *Frey,* American surgeon, late 20th century] see under *procedure.*

Frey syndrome (fri) [Lucja *Frey,* Polish neurologist, 1889–1944] auriculotemporal syndrome; see under *syndrome.*

FRFPSG Fellow of the Royal Faculty of Physicians and Surgeons of Glasgow.

fri•a•ble (fri′ə-bəl) [L. *friabilis*] easily pulverized or crumbled.

Fri•berg test (fri′bərg) [J. *Friberg,* American physician, 20th century] tray agglutination test; see under *test.*

fric•a•tive (frik′ə-tiv) a speech sound produced by forcing an air stream through a narrow opening, such as *f* or *s.*

fric•tion (frik′shən) [L. *frictio*] 1. the act of rubbing; attrition. 2. massage using a circular or back-and-forth rubbing movement, used especially for massage of deep tissues.

Frid•er•ich•sen-Wa•ter•house syndrome (frid′rik-sən waw′tər-hous) [Carl *Friderichsen,* Danish pediatrician, 20th century; Rupert *Waterhouse,* British physician, 1873–1958] Waterhouse-Friderichsen syndrome.

Fried•län•der disease (frēd′len-dər) [Karl *Friedländer,* German pathologist, 1847–1887] see *endarteritis obliterans.*

Fried•reich ataxia, etc. (frēd′rīk) [Nikolaus *Friedreich,* German physician, 1825–1882] see under *ataxia, foot,* and *sign,* and see *paramyoclonus multiplex.*

fri•gid•i•ty (frĭ-jid′ĭ-te) 1. coldness. 2. former name for *female sexual arousal disorder.*

frigo•la•bile (frig″o-la′bəl, -la′bīl) [L. *frigor* cold + *labile*] easily affected or destroyed by cold.

frigo•rif•ic (frig″o-rif′ik) [L. *frigorificus*] producing coldness.

frigo•sta•bile (frig″o-sta′bəl, -sta′bīl) frigostable.

frigo•sta•ble (frig″o-sta′bəl) [L. *frigor* cold + *stable*] resistant to cold or low temperature.

frit (frit) a fused mass produced by firing a mixture of quartz, kaolin, pigments, opacifiers, a suitable flux, and other substances, which is ground to form a fine powder for use in fabricating dental porcelain restorations and artificial teeth.

frog (frog) 1. any of various tailless leaping amphibians of the order Anura, with a smooth skin and fully webbed feet, often used in laboratory experiments. Cf. *toad.* 2. the band of horny substance in the middle of the sole of a horse's foot, dividing into two branches and running toward the heel in the form of a fork.

clawed f. *Xenopus laevis.*

Fröh•lich syndrome (frur′lik) [Alfred *Fröhlich,* Austrian pharmacologist in the United States, 1871–1953] adiposogenital dystrophy.

Fröh•se arcade (frer′zə) [Fritz *Fröhse,* German anatomist, 1871–1916] see under *arcade.*

Froin syndrome (frwah) [Georges *Froin,* French physician, 1874–1932] see under *syndrome.*

frole•ment (frōl-maw′) [Fr.] a rustling sound often heard in auscultation in disease of the pericardium.

Fro•ment paper sign (fro-maw′) [Jules *Froment,* French physician, 1878–1946] see under *sign.*

From•mann lines (from′ən) [Carl *Frommann,* German anatomist, 1831–1892] see under *line.*

From•mel disease (from′əl) [Richard Julius Ernst *Frommel,* German gynecologist, 1854–1912] Chiari-Frommel syndrome; see under *syndrome.*

From•mel-Chi•a•ri syndrome (from′əl ke-ah′re) [R.J.E. *Frommel;* Johann Baptist *Chiari,* German obstetrician 1817–1854] Chiari-Frommel syndrome; see under *syndrome.*

fron•dose (fron′dōs) [L. *frondosus* leafy] bearing fronds, or villi, as the chorion frondosum.

frons (fronz) [L. "the front, forepart"] [TA] official name for *forehead,* considered as part of the skull; cf. *sinciput.*

fron•tad (frun′tad) toward a frontal aspect.

fron•tal (frun′təl) [L. *frontalis*] 1. pertaining to the forehead. 2. denoting a longitudinal plane of the body at right angles to the sagittal plane; see under *plane.*

fron•ta•lis (frən-tal′is) [L., from *frons,* forehead] [TA] frontal: a general term denoting a relationship to the frontal or coronal planes.

fron•tip•e•tal (frən-tip′ə-təl) [*frontalis* + *-petal*] directed to the front; moving in a frontal direction.

fron•to•ma•lar (frun″to-ma′lər) pertaining to the frontal and zygomatic (malar) bones; zygomaticofrontal.

fron•to•max•il•lary (frun″to-mak′sĭ-lar″e) pertaining to the frontal bone and the maxilla.

fron•to•na•sal (frun″to-na′zəl) nasofrontal.

fron•to•oc•cip•i•tal (frun″to-ok-sip′ĭ-təl) pertaining to the forehead and the occiput.

fron•to•pa•ri•e•tal (frun″to-pə-ri′ə-təl) pertaining to the frontal and parietal bones.

fron•to•tem•por•al (frun″to-tem′por-əl) pertaining to the frontal and temporal bones.

fron•to•zy•go•mat•ic (frun″to-zi″go-mat′ik) zygomaticofrontal.

Fro•riep ganglion (fro′rēp) [August von *Froriep,* German anatomist, 1849–1917] see under *ganglion.*

frost (frost) 1. frozen dew or vapor. 2. a deposit resembling this.

urea f., uremic f. crystals of uric acid carried in the sweat and deposited on the skin of patients with uremia, such as in end stage renal disease. Called also *urhidrosis crystallina.*

frost•bite (frost′bīt) damage to tissues as the result of exposure to low environmental temperatures; called also *congelation.*

deep f. frostbite extending through the skin and subcutaneous tissue to deeper tissue, often causing gangrene. See *third degree f.* and *fourth degree f.*

first-degree f. a superficial frostbite characterized by erythema, edema, and epidermal anesthesia of the part; there is usually full recovery. Called also *frostnip.*

fourth-degree f. severe deep frostbite extending through a part that subsequently develops gangrene and must be amputated.

second-degree f. a superficial frostbite that includes hyperemia, edema, and blistering with clear fluid; the part heals, but sometimes there is long-term neuropathy.

superficial f. frostbite involving only the epidermis and upper dermis; see *first degree f.* and *second degree f.*

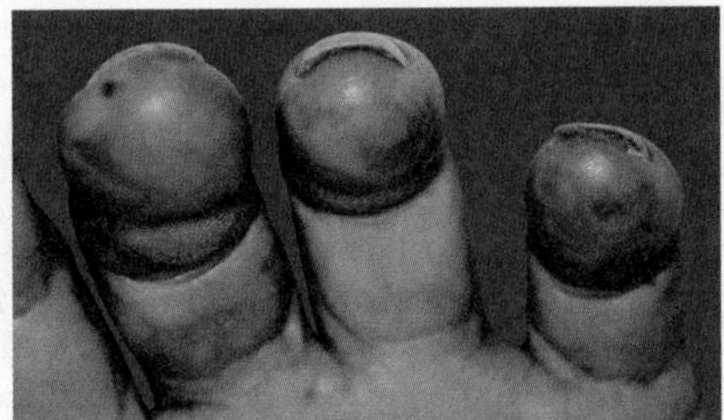

■ First degree frostbite.

third-degree f. a deep frostbite extending through the entire skin and into the subcutaneous tissue. Severe edema develops and can last for a month, and there may be blisters containing blood. In some cases the skin becomes dry and sloughs off.

frost•nip (frost′nip) first degree frostbite.

frot•tage (fro-tahzh′) [Fr. "rubbing"] frotteurism.

frot•teur (fro-toor′) an individual who achieves sexual gratification by practicing frotteurism.

frot•teur•ism (fro-toor′iz-əm) [DSM-IV] a paraphilia in which sexual arousal or orgasm is achieved by rubbing up against another person, usually in a crowded place with an unsuspecting victim, or by fantasies of such actions. Sexual arousal achieved by real or fantasized touching or fondling may also be included or may be classified separately as *toucherism.* Called also *frottage.*

Fro•va (fro′və) trademark for a preparation of frovatriptan succinate.

fro•va•trip•tan suc•ci•nate (fro″və-trip′tən) a selective serotonin receptor agonist used in the acute treatment of migraine; administered orally.

fro•zen (fro′zən) 1. turned into, covered by, or surrounded by ice. 2. very cold. 3. stiff or immobile, or rendered immobile.

FRS Fellow of the Royal Society.

fruc•tan (frook′tan) fructosan.

fruc•ti•fi•ca•tion (frook″tĭ-fĭ-ka′shən) 1. the production of fruit. 2. a fruiting body. 3. a spore-bearing structure.

fruc•tiv•o•rous (frook-tiv′ə-rəs) [L. *fructus* fruit + *vorare* to eat] subsisting on or eating fruits.

fruc•to•fu•ra•nose (frook″to-fu′rə-nōs) fructose occurring in the cyclic furanose configuration; it is the more reactive form of fructose.

fruc•to•ki•nase (frook″to-ki′nās) an enzyme of the transferase class that catalyzes the ATP-dependent phosphorylation of fructose to form fructose 1-phosphate as an initial step in the utilization of fructose. The enzyme is present in the liver, intestine, and kidney cortex. Deficiency of the enzyme, an autosomal recessive trait, causes essential fructosuria. In official nomenclature, called *ketohexokinase* [EC 2.7.1.3].

fruc•to•py•ra•nose (frook″to-pi′rə-nōs) fructose occurring in the cyclic pyranose configuration; it is the more common form in solution.

fruc•to•sa•mine (frook-tōs′ə-mēn) a glycosated protein formed by the attachment of fructose to an amine, as when glucose forms a bond with the amino group of a protein. Levels of fructosamine in the serum can be used to monitor glycemic control in diabetes, measuring blood glucose levels over a period of several weeks prior to the test; see *frutosamine test*, under *test.*

fruc•to•san (frook′to-san) any polymer composed solely or mainly of fructose residues; e.g., inulin.

fruc•to•sa•zone (frook-tōs′ə-zōn) the osazone formed from fructose by reaction with phenylhydrazine; it is identical to glucosazone.

fruc•tose (frook′tōs) [L. *fructus* fruit] 1. chemical name: D-fructose. A ketohexose found in honey and many sweet fruits and as a component of many di- and polysaccharides; it is obtainable by inversion of aqueous solutions of sucrose and subsequent separation of fructose from glucose. Called also *fructopyranose*, *fruit sugar*, and *levulose.* 2. [USP] an official preparation of fructose, administered intravenously in solution as a fluid and nutrient replenisher.

f. 1,6-bisphosphate a key intermediate in the Embden-Meyerhof pathway (q.v.) and in gluconeogenesis.

f. 2,6-bisphosphate an effector synthesized in small amounts in the liver to activate phosphofructokinase and inhibit fructose-1,6-bisphosphatase. Its formation is inhibited by catecholamines or glucagon, which thereby promote gluconeogenesis and diminish conversion of glucose to fatty acids.

f. 1,6-diphosphate f. 1,6-bisphosphate.

f. 1-phosphate an intermediate in fructose metabolism.

f. 6-phosphate an intermediate in the Embden-Meyerhof pathway (q.v.) of glucose metabolism.

fruc•tose-bis•phos•pha•tase (frook′tōs bis-fos′fə-tās″) [EC 3.1.3.11] EC nomenclature for *fructose-1,6-bisphosphatase.*

fruc•tose-1,6-bis•phos•pha•tase (frook′tōs bis-fos′fə-tās″) an enzyme of the hydrolase class that catalyzes the hydrolysis of fructose 1,6-bisphosphate to form fructose 6-phosphate. The reaction is part of the route of gluconeogenesis in the liver and kidneys. In EC nomenclature, called *fructose-bisphosphatase.*

fruc•tose-1,6-bis•phos•pha•tase de•fi•cien•cy (frook′tōs bis-fos′fə-tās″) an autosomal recessive disorder caused by mutations in the *FBP1* gene (locus: 9q22.2-q22.3), which encodes hepatic fructose-1,6-bisphosphatase. It is marked by apnea, hyperventilation, hypoglycemia, ketosis, and lactic acidosis resulting from impaired gluconeogenesis due to deficiency of the enzyme; it may be fatal to untreated newborns but once past early childhood, patients develop normally.

fruc•tose-2,6-bis•phos•pha•tase (frook′tōs bis-fos′fə-tās) fructose-2,6-bisphosphate 2-phosphatase.

fruc•tose-bis•phos•phate al•do•lase (frook′tōs bis-fos′fāt al′do-lās) [EC 4.1.2.13] an enzyme of the lyase class that catalyzes the cleavage of fructose 1,6-bisphosphate to form dihydroxyacetone phosphate and glyceraldehyde 3-phosphate, a reaction of the Embden-Meyerhof pathway (see illustration under *pathway*). The enzyme also catalyzes the conversion of fructose 1-phosphate to dihydroxyacetone phosphate and glyceraldehyde. Three isozymes are recognized: A (occurring primarily in skeletal muscle), B (in liver, kidney, small intestine, and leukocytes), and C (in brain). Isozyme B, often referred to as fructose 1-phosphate aldolase, has greater affinity for fructose 1-phosphate. Deficiency of the latter activity, an autosomal recessive trait, results in hereditary fructose intolerance. Called also *aldolase.*

fruc•tose-2,6-bis•phos•phate 2-phos•pha•tase (frook′tōs bis-fos′fāt fos′fə-tās) [EC 3.1.3.46] an enzyme activity that catalyzes the hydrolysis of fructose 2,6-bisphosphate to form fructose 6-phosphate; it occurs on the same polypeptide as the enzyme activity 6-phosphofructo-2-kinase (q.v.); in liver, the two activities form part of a mechanism for regulating carbohydrate metabolism. The liver enzyme activity is activated via phosphorylation by cyclic-AMP–dependent protein kinase, thus increasing the rate of removal of fructose 2,6-bisphosphate and slowing glycolysis. Called also *fructose-2,6-bisphosphatase.*

fruc•tose 1,6-di•phos•pha•tase (frook′tōs di-fos′fə-tās″) former name for *fructose-1,6-bisphosphatase.*

fruc•to•se•mia (frook″to-se′me-ə) the presence of fructose in the blood, as occurs in hereditary fructose intolerance and essential fructosuria.

fruc•tose 1-phos•phate al•do•lase (frook′tōs fos′fāt al′do-lās) fructose-bisphosphate aldolase, isozyme B.

fruc•to•side (frook′to-sīd) a glycoside of fructose.

fruc•to•su•ria (frook″to-su′re-ə) the presence of fructose in the urine, as occurs in hereditary fructose intolerance and essential fructosuria (q.v.).

essential f. a benign, asymptomatic, autosomal recessive disorder of carbohydrate metabolism due to deficiency of hepatic fructokinase resulting from mutations in the *KHK* gene (locus: 2p23.3-23.2); the only manifestations are fructosemia and fructosuria. See also *hereditary fructose intolerance*, under *intolerance.*

fruc•to•syl (frook′to-səl) a radical of fructose.

fruc•to•veg•e•ta•tive (frook″to-vej′ə-ta″tiv) composed of or pertaining to fruits and vegetables.

fru•giv•o•rous (froo-jiv′ə-rəs) fructivorous.

fruit (frōōt) [L. *fructus*] the developed ovary of a plant, including the seed and its envelopes.

fruit•ar•i•an (froo-tar′e-ən) one who practices fruitarianism.

fruit•ar•i•an•ism (froo-tar′e-ən-izm) restriction of the diet to fruits, nuts, honey, and olive oil.

fruit bro•me•lain (frōōt bro′mə-lān) [EC 3.4.22.33] see *bromelain.*

frus•e•mide (frus′ə-mīd) furosemide.

Frust. [L.] frustilla′tim (in small pieces).

frus•tra•tion (frəs-tra′shən) 1. the blocking or thwarting of purposes, desires, actions, or impulses. 2. a feeling of tension arising when such thwarting occurs.

F.s.a. [L.] fi′at secun′dum ar′tem (let it be made skillfully).

FSF fibrin-stabilizing factor (factor XIII; see *coagulation factors*, under *factor*).

FSG focal segmental glomerulosclerosis.

FSGS focal segmental glomerulosclerosis.

FSH follicle-stimulating hormone.

FSH/LH-RH follicle-stimulating hormone and luteinizing hormone–releasing hormone; see *gonadotropin-releasing hormone*, under *hormone*.

FSH-RH follicle-stimulating hormone–releasing hormone; see *gonadotropin-releasing hormone*, under *hormone*.

Ft. [L.] fi′at, fi′ant (let there be made).

ft foot.

Ft. mas. div. in pil. [L.] fi′at mas′sa dividen′da in pil′ulae (let a mass be made and divided into pills).

Ftor·a·fur (ftor′ə-fur) trademark for preparations of tegafur.

Ft. pulv. [L.] fi′at pul′vis (let a powder be made).

5-FU 5-fluorouracil; see *fluorouracil.*

Fuchs coloboma, etc. (fŭks) [Ernst *Fuchs*, Austrian ophthalmologist, 1851–1930] see under *coloboma, dimple, dystrophy,* and *syndrome.*

fuch·sin (fūk′sin) [from the pink, red, or purple flower *fuchsia*, after Leonard *Fuchs*, German botanist, 1501–1566] any of several red to purple triphenylmethane dyes, sometimes specifically basic fuchsin.

acid f. a mixture of sulfonated fuchsins used in Andrade indicator and in various complex stains; called also *acid magenta.*

basic f. [USP] a triphenylmethane dye, a mixture of rosaniline and pararosaniline hydrochlorides and magenta II, used in the form of carbolfuchsin in various stains for acid-fast bacteria, as an antifungal agent in carbolfuchsin topical solution, as a germicide, and as a histologic stain. Called also *basic magenta.*

new f. a basic dye with staining properties much like those of basic fuchsin; it is a tricyclic compound, trimethyl fuchsin.

fuch·sin·o·phil (fūk-sin′o-fil) [*fuchsin* + *-phil*] 1. any cell or other element readily stained with fuchsin. 2. fuchsinophilic.

fuch·sin·o·phil·ia (fūk″sin-o-fil′e-ə) the property of staining readily with fuchsin dyes; especially the affinity of infarcted areas of the heart for acid fuchsin. **fuchsinophil′ic, fuchsinoph′ilous** *adj*

fu·co·san (fu′ko-san) any of a group of pentosans composed of L-fucose residues; they are constituents of the cell walls of many seaweeds and occur in human milk.

fu·cose (fu′kōs) a methylpentose structurally derived from galactose (6-deoxygalactose); the L-isomer occurs naturally in various oligo- and polysaccharides (fucosans) and fucosides and in the carbohydrate portion of some mucopolysaccharides and glycoproteins, including the A, B, and O blood group antigens.

α-L-fu·co·si·dase (fu-ko′sĭ-dās) [EC 3.2.1.51] an enzyme of the hydrolase class that catalyzes cleavage of terminal α-linked L-fucose residues from fucosides. The reaction is important in the degradation of fucose-containing oligosaccharides and glycoproteins. Deficiency of the enzyme, an autosomal recessive trait, results in fucosidosis.

fu·co·side (fu′ko-sīd) a glycoside of fucose.

fu·co·si·do·sis (fu″ko-sĭ-do′sis) a lysosomal storage disease caused by defective α-L-fucosidase and accumulation of fucose-containing glycoconjugates. It results from mutations in the *FUCA1* gene (locus: 1p34). Clinical symptoms include angiokeratoma, psychomotor deterioration, coarse facies, growth retardation, hepatosplenomegaly, cardiomegaly, and seizures. There are two clinical types based on age of onset: *Type I*, the fatal infantile type, has age of onset by 18 months and causes death before six years of age. Marked increase of sodium chloride in sweat is an additional feature. *Type II*, the juvenile form, has age of onset by four years of age and slower psychomotor and neurologic deterioration; patients survive to their twenties.

fu·co·xan·thin (fu″ko-zan′thin) [L. *fucus* rock lichen + *xanthin*] the brown carotenoid found in diatoms, brown algae, and dinoflagellates.

FUDR 1. abbreviation for floxuridine (5-fluorouracil deoxyribonucleoside). 2. trademark for a preparation of floxuridine.

FUdR 5-fluorouracil deoxyribonucleoside; see *floxuridine.*

fu·gac·i·ty (fu-gas′ĭ-te) [L. *fugacitas*, from *fugere* to flee] a measure of the escaping tendency of a substance from one phase to another phase, or from one part of a phase to another part of the same phase. The logarithm of the fugacity is proportional to the chemical potential, measured by the correction for the deviation of the behavior of a gas from ideal.

-fugal[1] [L., *fugare* to put to flight] a word termination implying banishing, or driving away, affixed to a stem designating the object of banishment, as *vermifugal*, expelling parasitic worms, or *febrifugal*, relieving or dispelling fever.

-fugal[2] [L. *fugere* to flee from] a word termination implying traveling away from, affixed to a stem designating the object from which flight is made, as *centrifugal*, traveling away from a center, or *corticifugal*, directed away from the cortex.

-fuge [L. *fugare* to put to flight] a word termination denoting an agent that drives away or banishes, as *febrifuge*, that which drives away fever.

fu·gi·tive (fu′jĭ-tiv) [L. *fugitivus*] 1. wandering. 2. transient.

Fugl-Mey·er assessment (foo′gəl-mi′ər) [Axel R. *Fugl-Meyer*, Swedish neurologist, 20th century] see under *assessment.*

Fu·gu (foo′goo) [Japanese] a genus of Japanese marine puffer fish of the family Tetraodontidae. Their gonads and viscera contain tetrodotoxin, and when they are eaten without special cooking, fatal tetrodotoxism may result.

fu·gu (foo′goo) [Japanese] 1. a puffer fish of the genus *Fugu.* 2. the flesh of such fish, which contains tetrodotoxin.

fugue (fūg) [L. *fuga* a flight] a pathological state of altered consciousness in which an individual may act and wander around as though conscious but with behavior not directed by the complete, normal personality; the behavior is not remembered after the fugue ends. The term is often used to denote *dissociative f.* specifically.

dissociative f. [DSM-IV] a dissociative disorder characterized by an episode of sudden, unexpected travel away from home or business, with amnesia for the past and partial to total confusion about identity or assumption of a new identity; the disorder is usually related to emotional conflicts due to some traumatic, stressful, or overwhelming event, remits spontaneously, and rarely recurs.

epileptic f. a fuguelike state of running or wandering that occasionally occurs as an ictal or postictal phenomenon in psychomotor (temporal lobe) epilepsy.

psychogenic f. dissociative f.

fu·gu·ism (foo′goo-iz-əm) [*fugu* + *-ism*] tetrodotoxism (def. 1).

fu·gu·tox·in (foo′goo-tok″sin) tetrodotoxin.

Fu·ku·ya·ma type congenital muscular dystrophy (syndrome) (foo″koo-yah′mah) [Yukio *Fukuyama*, Japanese neurologist, born 1928] see under *dystrophy.*

ful·gu·rant (ful′gu-rənt) [L. *fulgurans*, from *fulgur* lightning] coming and going like a flash of lightning.

ful·gu·rate (ful′gu-rāt) 1. to come and go like a flash of lightning. 2. to destroy by fulguration.

ful·gu·ra·tion (ful″gu-ra′shən) [L. *fulgur* lightning] destruction of living tissue by electric sparks generated by a high frequency current. See *electrocautery.*

direct f. fulguration in which an insulated electrode with a metal point is connected to the uniterminal and an electric spark is allowed to impinge on the area being treated.

indirect f. fulguration in which the patient is connected directly by a metal handle to the uniterminal and the operator uses an active electrode to complete an arc from the patient.

fu·lig·i·nous (ful-lij′ĭ-nəs) [L. *fuligo* soot] sooty in color or appearance.

Fül·le·born method (fēl′ə-born) [Friedrich *Fülleborn*, German parasitologist, 1866–1933] see under *method.*

ful·mi·nant (ful′mĭ-nənt) [L. *fulminare* to flare up] sudden, severe; occurring suddenly and with great intensity.

ful·mi·nate (ful′mĭ-nāt) [L. *fulminare*] to occur suddenly with great intensity.

ful·ves·trant (ful-ves′trənt) an antiestrogen administered by intramuscular injection in treatment of breast cancer.

Ful·vi·cin (ful′vĭ-sin) trademark for preparations of griseofulvin.

fu·ma·rase (fu′mə-rās) fumarate hydratase.

fu·ma·rate (fu′mə-rāt) a salt or anionic form of fumaric acid.

fu·ma·rate hy·dra·tase (fu′mə-rāt hi′drə-tās) [EC 4.2.1.2] an enzyme of the lyase class that catalyzes the hydration of fumarate to form L-malate in a reaction of the tricarboxylic acid cycle (see illustration under *cycle*). Deficiency causes mental retardation and failure to thrive. Called also *fumarase.*

fu·mar·ic ac·id (fu-mar′ik) *trans*-butanedioic acid, the trans isomer of maleic acid, an intermediate in the tricarboxylic acid cycle (q.v.).

fu·mar·ic·ac·id·uria (fu-mar″ik-as″ĭ-du′re-ə) excretion of fumaric acid in the urine, as seen in children with fumarate hydratase deficiency.

fu·ma·ryl·ace·to·ac·e·tase (fu″mə-ril″ə-se″to-as′ə-tās) [EC 3.7.1.2] an enzyme of the hydrolase class that catalyzes the cleavage of fumarylacetoacetate to form acetoacetate and fumarate; the reaction is a step in the tyrosine catabolic pathway. Deficiency of the enzyme, an autosomal recessive trait, causes tyrosinemia, type I.

fu·ma·ryl·ace·to·ac·e·tate (fu″mə-ril″ə-se″to-as′ə-tāt) a compound composed of fumarate linked to acetoacetate; it is an intermediate in the degradation of tyrosine and phenylalanine.

fu·ma·ryl·ace·to·ac·e·tate hy·dro·lase (fu″mə-ril″ə-se″to-as′ə-tāt hi′dro-lās) fumarylacetoacetase.

fu·mi·gant (fu′mĭ-gənt) a substance used in fumigation.

fu·mi·ga·tion (fu″mĭ-ga′shən) [L. *fumus* smoke, steam, vapor] exposure of an area or object to disinfecting fumes.

fum·ing (fūm′ing) [L. *fumus* smoke] smoking; emitting a visible vapor.

fu·mon·i·sin (fu-mon′ĭ-sin) any of a group of mycotoxins produced by *Fusarium moniliforme*, which contaminates corn; they cause moldy corn poisoning in livestock and are carcinogenic.

func·tio (funk′she-o) [L.] function.

f. lae′sa loss of function, one of the cardinal signs of inflammation.

func·tion (funk′shən) [L. *functio*, from *fungi* to do] 1. the special, normal, or proper physiologic activity of an organ or part. 2. to perform such activity. 3. in chemistry, a characteristic behavior of a chemical compound due to the presence of a specific functional group (q.v.) 4. in mathematics, a rule that assigns to each member of one set (the domain) a value in another set (the range).

cumulative distribution f. (cdf) a mathematical function that defines the probability distribution of a random variable by giving for each random variable X the probability of observing a value less than or equal to a specified value x.

density f. probability density f.

distribution f. cumulative distribution f.

fine motor f. the ability to perform precise, coordinated movements such as writing, visual tracking, sewing, or cutting; called also *fine motor skills.*

gross motor f. the ability to use large muscle groups for activities or functions such as maintaining balance, walking, and running; called also *gross motor skills.*

likelihood f. see *likelihood.*

probability density f. in statistics, a mathematical function that describes the distribution of measurements for a population; a curve that describes a population. Its integral is the cumulative distribution function, so the probability that an individual measurement will fall between two numbers a and b is equal to the proportion of the area under the curve between points a and b, with the entire area under the function being 1.

ventricular f. ventricular performance (q.v.) as related to end-diastolic volume, dimension, or pressure; Starling curves (ventricular function curves) are used in the assessment of loading conditions and of cardiac contractility.

func·tion·al (funk′shən-əl) 1. of or pertaining to a function. 2. affecting the function but not the structure; see under *disorder.*

func·ti·o·na·lis (funk″she-o-na′lis) [L.] 1. functional. 2. stratum functionale.

func·tion·ing (funk′shən-ing) carrying out an activity.

borderline intellectual f. [DSM-IV] a classification of mental ability covering persons with I.Q. scores in the range of 71 to 84, with only slight impairments in adaptive behavior. Called also *borderline mental retardation.*

fun·dal (fun′dəl) pertaining to a fundus.

fun·da·ment (fun′də-mənt) [L. *fundamentum*] 1. a base or foundation, such as the breech or rump. 2. the anus and parts adjacent to it.

fun·da·men·tal (fun″də-men′təl) pertaining to a base or foundation.

fun·dec·to·my (fun-dek′tə-me) fundusectomy.

fun·di (fun′di) [L.] genitive and plural of *fundus.*

fun·dic (fun′dik) pertaining to a fundus.

fun·di·form (fun′dĭ-form) [L. *funda* sling + *form*] shaped like a sling.

fun·do·pli·ca·tion (fun″do-plĭ-ka′shən) [*fundus* + *plication*] plication of the fundus of the stomach around the lower end of the esophagus, done as treatment for reflux esophagitis that may be associated with disorders such as hiatal hernia. Called also *fundic wrapping.*

Belsey Mark IV f. see under *operation.*

Nissen f. a procedure in which the fundus is wrapped completely around the distal esophagus. Called also *Nissen operation.*

Thal f. fundoplication of less than the entire circumference of the lower esophagus to correct a benign stricture or treat gastroesophageal reflux. Called also *Thal procedure.*

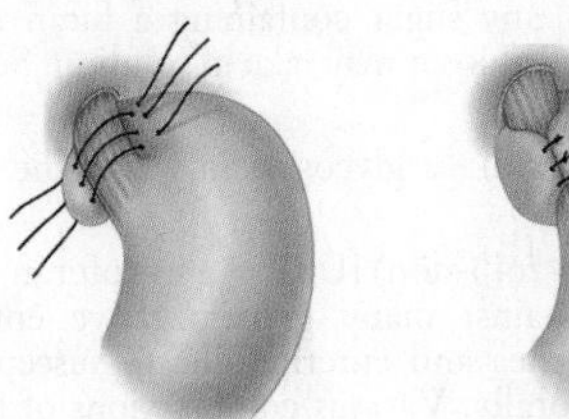

■ Nissen fundoplication for control of gastroesophageal reflux.

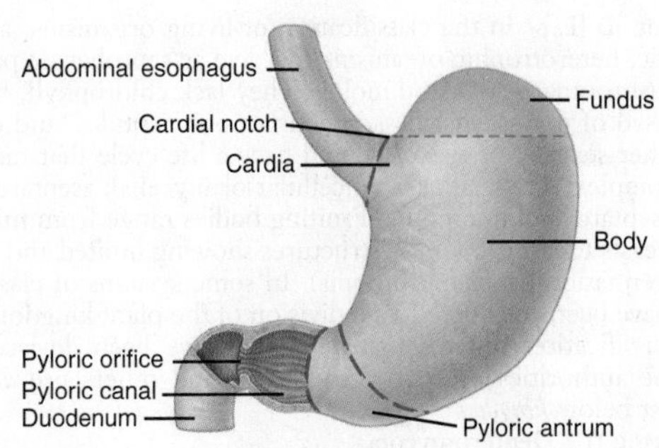

■ Fundus gastricus (gastric fundus).

Toupet f. a procedure in which the fundus is wrapped 180° to 200° around the distal esophagus; done for patients with poor esophageal clearance and asymmetrical extrinsic pressure. Called also *Toupet operation.*

Fun·du·lus (fun′du-ləs) the killifish, a genus of the order Cyprinodontidae. *F. heterocli′tus* is the common or green killifish, a species much used in biological research.

fun·dus (fun′dəs) gen. and pl. *fun′dus* [L.] 1. the bottom or base of something. 2. the bottom or base of an organ, or the part of a hollow organ farthest from its mouth.

albinotic f. a fundus of the eye which permits clear visualization of the choroidal vasculature, owing to lack of pigment in the pigment epithelium and choroid.

f. albipuncta′tus a disorder in which gray or white mottling of the fundus of the eye is associated with night blindness; called also *Lauber disease.*

f. of bladder f. vesicae urinariae.

f. diabe′ticus a fundus of the eye having dilated veins, a prodrome of diabetic retinopathy.

f. of eye f. oculi.

f. flavimacula′tus a condition characterized by the presence of yellow to white atrophic lesions in the midperiphery or perimacular region of the fundus of the eye.

f. of gallbladder f. vesicae biliaris.

gastric f., f. gas′tricus [TA] the part of the stomach to the left and above the level of the entrance of the esophagus; called also *f. of stomach, f. ventricularis,* and *f. ventriculi.*

f. of internal acoustic meatus f. mea′tus acus′tici inter′ni.

leopard f. the mottled fundus of the eye seen in tapetoretinal degeneration; called also *leopard retina.*

f. mea′tus acus′tici inter′ni [TA] fundus of internal acoustic meatus: the laterally placed end or bottom of the internal acoustic meatus.

ocular f., f. o′culi fundus of eye: the back portion of the interior of the eyeball, as seen by means of the ophthalmoscope.

salt and pepper f. a fundus of the eye that is dusted with fine blue pigmented and orange depigmented spots, characteristic of hereditary syphilis; also seen in other disorders, e.g., rubella.

f. of stomach f. gastricus.

tessellated f., f. ti′gre, tigroid f. a normal, nonpathological fundus of the eye with marked exposure of the choroidal vessels due to scanty pigmentation; called also *tessellated* or *tigroid retina.*

f. tym′pani paries jugularis cavi tympani.

f. of urinary bladder f. vesicae urinariae.

f. u′teri [TA] fundus of uterus: the part of the uterus above the orifices of the uterine tubes.

f. ventricula′ris, f. ventri′culi f. gastricus.

f. vesi′cae bilia′ris [TA] fundus of gallbladder: the inferior dilated portion of the gallbladder; called also *f. vesicae felleae* [TA alternative].

f. vesi′cae fel′leae TA alternative for *f. vesicae biliaris.*

f. vesi′cae urina′riae [TA] fundus of urinary bladder: an area formed by the posterior surface of the bladder and containing the lowest section (trigone of bladder) where urine empties out through the internal urethral orifice. Called also *f. of bladder, base of bladder,* and *infundibulum of urinary bladder.*

fun·du·scope (fun′də-skōp) ophthalmoscope.

fun·dus·co·py (fən-dus′kə-pe) ophthalmoscopy.

fun·du·sec·to·my (fun″də-sek′tə-me) [*fundus* + *-ectomy*] excision of the fundus of an organ, as of the fundus of the stomach or uterus; called also *fundectomy.*

fun·gate (fung′gāt) 1. to produce funguslike growths. 2. to grow rapidly, like a fungus.

fun·ge·mia (fən-je′me-ə) the presence of fungi in the bloodstream.

Fun·gi (fun′ji) [L.] in the classification of living organisms, a kingdom of eukaryotic, heterotrophic organisms that live as saprobes or parasites; it includes mushrooms, yeasts, and molds. They lack chlorophyll, have a cell wall composed of polysaccharides, sometimes polypeptides, and chitin, reproduce either sexually or asexually, and have a life cycle that ranges from simple to complex. The thallus is unicellular or mycelial; aseptate, partially septate, or septate; and nonmotile. Fruiting bodies range from microscopic hyphae in yeasts to large, complex structures showing limited and reversible tissue differentiation (as in mushrooms). In some systems of classification, the Fungi have been considered a subdivision of the plant kingdom. Several different classification systems for the Fungi have been devised; for example, some authorities use the term *phylum* and others use *division* for the level just below *kingdom*.

F. Imperfec′ti Deuteromycota.

fun·gi (fun′ji) [L.] plural of *fungus*.

fun·gi·ci·dal (fun″jĭ-si′dəl) [*fungus* + L. *caedere* to kill] destroying fungi; cf. *antifungal*.

fun·gi·cide (fun′jĭ-sīd) an agent that destroys fungi.

fun·gi·ci·din (fun″jĭ-si′din) nystatin.

fun·gi·form (fun′jĭ-form) shaped like a fungus; see also *fungoid*.

fun·gi·sta·sis (fun-jĭ-sta′sis) [*fungus* + *-stasis*] inhibition of growth of fungi.

fun·gi·stat (fun′jĭ-stat) an antifungal agent that inhibits growth of fungi.

fun·gi·stat·ic (fun″jĭ-stat′ik) inhibiting growth of fungi; cf. *antifungal*.

fun·gis·ter·ol (fən-jis′tər-ol) a sterol, $C_{25}H_{44}O$, found in ergot and other fungi.

fun·gi·tox·ic (fun′jĭ-tok″sik) deleterious to fungi; cf. *antifungal*.

fun·gi·tox·ic·i·ty (fun″jĭ-tok-sis′ĭ-te) the quality of being toxic to fungi.

Fun·gi·zone (fun′jĭ-zōn) trademark for preparations of amphotericin B.

Fun·goid (fun′goid) trademark for a preparation of clotrimazole.

fun·goid (fung′goid) [*fungus* + *-oid*] resembling a fungus; see also *fungiform*.

fun·go·ma (fəng-go′mə) [*fungus* + *-oma*] fungus ball.

fun·gous (fung′gəs) [L. *fungosus*] 1. fungal. 2. fungoid.

fun·gu·ria (fung-gu′re-ə) the presence of fungi in the urine.

fun·gus (fung′gəs) pl. *fun′gi* [L.] an organism belonging to the Fungi. See also *mycosis* and *mycotoxicosis*. **fun′gal** *adj*

club fungi Basidiomycotina.

conidial fungi mitosporic fungi.

dimorphic f. a fungus that can live as either a yeast or a mold, depending on environmental conditions.

imperfect f. a fungus whose perfect (sexual) stage is unknown; all such fungi are classified in the phylum Deuteromycota.

mitosporic fungi fungi that have asexual reproduction by mitosis without meiosis; called also *conidial fungi*.

mosaic f. a mycelium-like intercellular deposit of cholesterol sometimes seen in scrapings from lesions thought to be fungal in origin.

perfect f. a fungus for which both sexual and asexual types of spore formation are known; these fungi are classified in the subphyla Ascomycotina and Basidiomycotina, and the phylum Zygomycota.

proper fungi Eumycota.

ray f. *Actinomyces*.

sac fungi Ascomycotina.

slime f. see under *mold*.

true fungi Eumycota.

fu·nic (fu′nik) 1. pertaining to a funis. 2. funicular.

fu·ni·cle (fu′nĭ-kəl) funiculus.

fu·nic·u·li (fu-nik′u-li) genitive and plural of *funiculus*.

fu·nic·u·li·tis (fu-nik″u-li′tis) 1. inflammation of the spermatic cord. 2. inflammation of the portion of a spinal nerve root lying within the intervertebral canal.

endemic f., filarial f. secondary involvement of the spermatic cord in lymphatic filariasis.

fu·nic·u·lo·ep·i·did·y·mi·tis (fu-nik″u-lo-ep″ĭ-did″ĭ-mi′tis) inflammation of the spermatic cord and the epididymis.

fu·nic·u·lus (fu-nik′u-ləs) pl. *funic′uli* [L.] [TA] cord: anatomic terminology for a cordlike structure or part. **funic′ular** *adj*

f. am′nii a cord of tissue by which the amnion and chorion are temporarily united in certain ruminant animals.

f. ante′rior medul′lae spina′lis [TA], **anterior f. of spinal cord** the white substance of the spinal cord lying on either side between the anterior median fissure and the anterior roots of the spinal nerves; called also *ventral f. of spinal cord*.

cuneate f. fasciculus cuneatus medullae spinalis.

dorsal f. of spinal cord f. posterior medullae spinalis.

lateral f. of medulla oblongata f. lateralis medullae oblongatae.

lateral f. of spinal cord f. lateralis medullae spinalis.

f. latera′lis medul′lae oblonga′tae [TA] lateral funiculus of medulla oblongata: the continuation into the medulla oblongata of all the fiber tracts of the lateral funiculus of the spinal cord, with the exception of the lateral corticospinal tract.

f. latera′lis medul′lae spina′lis [TA] lateral funiculus of spinal cord: the white substance of the spinal cord that lies on either side between the dorsal and ventral roots of the spinal nerves.

funi′culi medul′lae spina′lis [TA] funiculi of spinal cord: the large bundles of fiber tracts that make up the white substance of the spinal cord.

f. poste′rior medul′lae spina′lis [TA], **posterior f. of spinal cord** the white substance of the spinal cord lying on either side between the posterior median sulcus and the posterior roots of the spinal nerves; called also *dorsal f. of spinal cord*.

f. se′parans [TA] a narrow translucent ridge of thickened ependyma in the floor of the fourth ventricle that runs across the lower part of the trigone of the vagus nerve and separates it from the area postrema; the blood-brain barrier may be modified in this area. See also *circumventricular organs*, under *organ*.

f. sperma′ticus [TA] spermatic cord: a structure that extends from the abdominal inguinal ring to the testis, comprising the ductus deferens and associated structures including the testicular artery, pampiniform plexus, and nerves, as well as various other vessels and loose connective tissue.

funiculi of spinal cord funiculi medullae spinalis.

ventral f. of spinal cord f. anterior medullae spinalis.

fu·ni·form (fu′nĭ-form) [*funis* + *form*] resembling a rope or cord.

fu·ni·punc·ture (fu′nĭ-pungk″chər) cordocentesis.

fu·nis (fu′nis) [L. "cord"] 1. any cordlike structure; see *chorda* and *funiculus*. 2. umbilical cord.

f. hippoc′ratis tendo calcaneus.

fu·ni·si·tis (fu″nĭ-si′tis) inflammation of the umbilical cord.

necrotizing f. inflammation of the umbilical cord resulting from infection with organisms that cause sexually transmitted diseases or with normal lower genital tract flora and characterized by yellowish-white chalky stripes that parallel the umbilical vessels and an inflammatory cell infiltrate extending from the vascular intima to Wharton jelly.

fun·nel (fun′əl) 1. a hollow conical structure with a narrow opening at the apex, such as the vessels used in chemistry and pharmacy for filtering and other purposes. 2. infundibulum.

mitral f. the cone-shaped mitral valve seen in mitral stenosis, the orifice being at the apex of the cone.

muscular f. the funnel-shaped space bounded by the four rectus muscles of the eye.

pial f. a sheath of adventitia, extended from the pia mater, loosely surrounding blood vessels as they enter the brain or spinal cord; see also *Virchow-Robin spaces*, under *space*.

vascular f. the light-colored depression at the center of the disk of the retina.

FUO fever of unknown origin.

Fu·ra·cin (fu′rə-sin) trademark for preparations of nitrofurazone.

Fur·a·dan·tin (fūr″ə-dan′tin) trademark for preparations of nitrofurantoin.

fu·ral·ta·done (fu-ral′tə-dōn) a nitrofuran antibacterial and antiprotozoal used in poultry.

fu·ran (fu′ran) a heterocyclic compound,

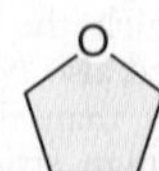

the ring structure that is the basis of the furanoses and furfural.

fu·ra·nose (fu′rə-nōs) any sugar containing a furan ring structure, a cyclic form that ketoses and aldoses may take in solution. See also individual sugars, e.g., *fructofuranose*.

fu·ran·o·side (fu-ran′o-sīd) a glycoside in which the sugar is in furanose configuration.

fu·ra·zol·i·done (fu″rə-zol′ĭ-dōn) [USP] a nitrofuran antibacterial and antiprotozoal, effective against many gram-negative enteric organisms, used in treatment of diarrhea and enteritis due to susceptible organisms, and usually administered orally. Various combinations of furazolidone and nifuroxime are administered intravaginally in treatment of bacterial, candidal, and trichomonal vaginitis.

fur·ca (fur′kə) gen. and pl. *fur′cae* [L. "fork"] furcation.

fur·cal (fur′kəl) [L. *furca* fork] shaped like a fork; forked.

fur·ca·tion (fər-ka′shən) the area where the roots divide on a multi-rooted tooth. See also *bifurcation* and *trifurcation.*

fur·co·cer·cous (fur″ko-sur′kəs) [*furca* + *cerc-* + *-ous*] having a forked tail.

fur·cu·la (fur′ku-lə) [L. "little fork"] a horseshoe-shaped ridge in the embryonic larynx, bounding the pharyngeal aperture ventrally and laterally.

fur·fu·ra·ceous (fur″fu-ra′shəs) [L. *furfur* bran] fine and loose; said of scales resembling bran or dandruff.

fur·fu·ral (fur′fu-rəl) furan carrying a carbonyl substituent, an intermediate formed from pentosans of cereal straws and brans and used in a variety of industrial processes; it irritates mucous membranes and causes photosensitivity and headaches.

fur·fu·ran (fur′fu-rən) furan.

fur·i·fos·min (fu″rĭ-foz′min) a phosphine which when labeled with technetium 99m is used in myocardial perfusion imaging; see table at *technetium.*

fu·ro·cou·ma·rin (fu″ro-koo′mə-rin) any of a group of antifungal substances produced by certain species of plants to ward off fungi; when they come in contact with human skin, they can cause photosensitization. Common plants containing furocoumarins include celery, fig, and parsley.

fu·ror (fu′ror) [L.] fury; rage.

fu·ro·sem·ide (fu-ro′sə-mīd) [USP] a loop diuretic used in the treatment of edema associated with congestive heart failure or hepatic or renal disease, as an adjunct in the treatment of acute pulmonary edema, and in the treatment of hypertension, usually in combination with other drugs; administered orally, intramuscularly, or intravenously.

Fu·rox·one (fūr-ok′sōn) trademark for preparations of furazolidone.

fur·row (fur′o) sulcus.

cleavage f. a deepening constriction of the plasma membrane at the equator of a dividing cell, formed by the pinching in of the membrane as the diameter of the contractile ring decreases.

genital f. a groove that appears on the genital tubercle of the fetus at the end of the second month.

gluteal f. 1. crena analis. 2. sulcus glutealis.

Jadelot f's see under *line.*

mentolabial f. see under *sulcus.*

nympholabial f. a groove separating the labium majus and labium minus on either side.

primitive f., primordial f. see under *groove.*

scleral f. sulcus sclerae.

Sibson f. the inferior border of the pectoralis major muscle.

skin f's sulci cutis.

fu·run·cle (fu′rung-kəl) [L. *furunculus*] a painful nodule formed in the skin by circumscribed inflammation of the dermis and subcutaneous tissue after staphylococci enter through the hair follicles; its formation may be favored by digestive disorders, local irritation, or more general systemic disorders including immunodeficiency. Called also *boil.* **furun′cular** *adj*

fu·run·cu·loid (fu-rung′ku-loid) resembling a furuncle.

fu·run·cu·lo·sis (fu-rung″ku-lo′sis) 1. the persistent sequential occurrence of furuncles over a period of weeks or months. 2. the simultaneous occurrence of a number of furuncles.

aural f. a type of circumscribed otitis externa in which a furuncle forms in the external auditory canal, caused by infection of a hair follicle or sebaceous gland.

fu·run·cu·lus (fu-rung′ku-ləs) pl. *furun′culi* [L.] furuncle.

FUS feline urological syndrome.

fu·sar·io·tox·i·co·sis (fu-sar″e-o-tok″sĭ-ko′sis) any of numerous types of mycotoxicosis caused by fungi of the genus *Fusarium.*

fu·sar·i·o·sis (fu-sar″e-o′sis) fungal infection with a species of *Fusarium,* seen most often as an opportunistic infection in an immunocompromised patient. It may be manifested as a skin lesion or may invade the bloodstream with a fatal outcome.

Fu·sar·i·um (fu-sar′e-əm) a genus of Fungi Imperfecti of the form-class Hyphomycetes, form-family Moniliaceae (sometimes classified in the small form-family Tuberculariaceae). Perfect stages of many species are included in the order Hypocreales. Some species are important pathogens of plants, and some cause opportunistic infections in animals. Certain species produce trichothecene mycotoxins, and others have been isolated from otomycosis and keratomycosis. See also *fusariotoxicosis.*

F. graminea′rum *F. roseum.*

F. monilifor′me a species that contains fumonisins and sometimes contaminates corn, causing moldy corn poisoning in domestic animals.

F. oxyspo′rum a species causing banana wilt, and occasionally human eumycotic mycetoma.

F. po′ae a species that contaminates grain and contains T-2 toxin, causing fusariotoxicosis in farm animals and alimentary toxic aleukia in humans.

F. ro′seum a species that contaminates grain and produces the estrogenic mycotoxin zearalenone; farm animals that eat contaminated grain or flour products may develop fertility problems or vulvovaginitis. Called also *F. graminearum.*

F. so′lani a species causing potato wilt and occasionally human eumycotic mycetoma or mycotic keratitis.

F. sporotrichiel′la a species believed to be the etiologic agent of Kashin-Bek disease.

F. sporotrichioi′des a species that sometimes contaminates grain and contains T-2 toxin, causing fusariotoxicosis in livestock and alimentary toxic aleukia in humans.

F. tricinc′tum a species that sometimes contaminates corn and contains T-2 toxin, causing fusariotoxicosis in livestock and alimentary toxic aleukia in humans.

fu·sa·ri·um (fu-sar′e-əm) pl. *fusa′ria.* Any fungus of the genus *Fusarium.*

fus·cin (fu′sin) [L. *fuscus* brown] a yellow to brown pigment of the retinal epithelium.

fuse (fūz) 1. a bar, strip, or wire of easily fusible metal inserted for safety in an electric circuit; when the current increases beyond a safe strength the metal melts, thus breaking the circuit and thereby saving an apparatus from overload. 2. to join together, as the abnormal coherence of adjacent body structures.

fu·seau (fu-zo′) pl. *fuseaux′* [Fr.] a macroaleuriospore or macroconidium.

fu·si (fu′si) [L.] plural of *fusus.*

fu·si·ble (fu′zĭ-bəl) susceptible of being melted or fused.

fu·si·cel·lu·lar (fu″sĭ-sel′u-lər) fusocellular.

fu·si·date (fu′si-dāt) a salt of fusidic acid.

fu·sid·ic ac·id (fu-sid′ik) a fermentation product of the fungus *Fusidium coccineum* used as an antibiotic.

fu·si·form (fu′zĭ-form) [*fus-* + *form*] shaped like a spindle; tapered at each end.

fu·si·gen·ic (fu-zi-jen′ik) fusogenic.

fu·si·mo·tor (fu″sĭ-mo′tər) [*fus-* + *motor*] innervating intrafusal fibers of the muscle spindle; said of motor nerve fibers of gamma motoneurons.

fu·sion (fu′zhən) [L. *fusio*] 1. the act, process, or result of melting. 2. merging or coherence of adjacent parts or bodies. 3. coordination of separate images of the same object in the two eyes into one. 4. operative formation of an ankylosis or arthrodesis; called also *f. of joint.*

anterior interbody f. spinal fusion using an anterior approach, with immobilization by bone grafts on the anterior and lateral surfaces, used in the cervical region to treat degenerative disk disease and herniated nucleus pulposus, and in the lumbar region primarily for patients in whom other types of fusion have failed.

binocular f. see *fusion* (def. 3).

cell f. the production of a hybrid cell by merging the contents of two previously separate cells; it may occur naturally, as in the formation of skeletal muscle, or may be induced artificially. Cf. *heterokaryon.*

centric f. robertsonian translocation.

cervical spinal f. spinal fusion in the cervical region to correct instability when traumatic vertebral fractures do not heal with other techniques.

diaphyseal-epiphyseal f. operative establishment of bony union between the diaphysis and epiphysis, to arrest growth in the length of a bone.

f. of joint fusion (def. 4).

midline f. the process of symmetrical union along the midline that forms the neural tube in the embryo; cf. *dysraphism.*

penoscrotal f. a developmental anomaly in which the penis is fused to the scrotum; see also *penoscrotal transposition,* under *transposition.*

renal f. fused kidney.

spinal f. operative immobilization or ankylosis of two or more vertebrae, often with diskectomy or laminectomy; types are named for the surface immobilized, such as *anterior spinal f., lateral spinal f., posterior spinal f.,* and *posterolateral spinal f.* Called also *spondylosyndesis.*

fu·sion·al (fu′zhən-əl) marked by fusion.

fus(o)- [L. *fusus* spindle] a combining form denoting relationship to a spindle.

Fu·so·bac·te·ria (fu″zo-bak-tēr′e-ə) 1. a phenotypically homogeneous phylum of gram-negative bacteria, consisting of anaerobic, chemo-organotrophic, non–spore-forming, rod-shaped organisms. 2. the sole class of this phylum, containing a single order, the Fusobacteriales.

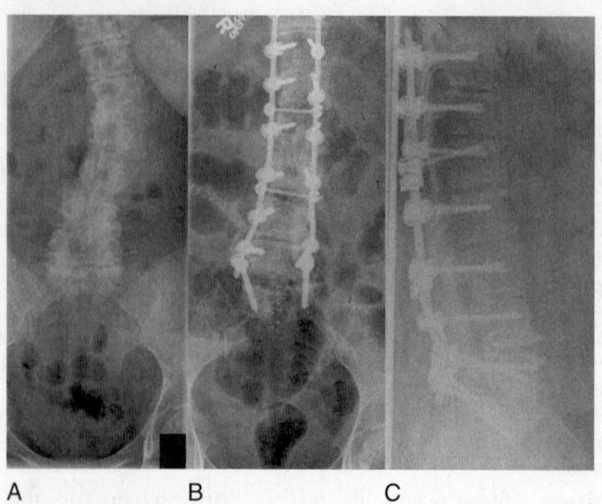

■ Spinal fusion. *(A)*, Posteroanterior (PA) radiograph of degenerative scoliotic deformity of the thoracolumbar spine. Postoperative PA *(B)* and lateral *(C)* views showing spinal fusion with rod and long pedicle screws from T11 to S1.

Fu•so•bac•te•ri•a•ceae (fu″zo-bak-tēr″e-a′se-e) a family of gram-negative, rod-shaped bacteria of the order Fusobacteriales; medically important organisms are contained in the genera *Fusobacterium*, *Leptotrichia*, and *Streptobacillus*.

Fu•so•bac•te•ri•a•les (fu″zo-bak-tēr″e-a′lēz) an order of bacteria of the class Fusobacteria; it contains the family Fusobacteriaceae.

Fu•so•bac•te•ri•um (fu″zo-bak-tēr′e-əm) [L. *fusus* spindle + *bacterium*] a genus of gram-negative, anaerobic, nonsporulating bacteria of the family Fusobacteriaceae, consisting of slender cells with tapered ends. Some species are normal inhabitants of the body cavities of animals, and others are pathogenic. The type species is *Fusobacterium nuclea′tum*.

F. gonidiafor′mans a species isolated from human infections of the respiratory, urogenital, and gastrointestinal tracts.

F. morti′ferum a species isolated from normal sources and from abscesses, septicemia, pleurisy, and urinary tract infections.

F. navifor′me a species isolated from human abscesses and other clinical specimens, and from the intestines of rats.

F. necro′phorum a pleomorphic species, divided into several subspecies, that is the cause of foot rot in cattle, sheep, and pigs; interdigital dermatitis in sheep; calf diphtheria; and Schmorl disease.

F. nuclea′tum a species, divided into several subspecies, isolated from the normal mouth, the upper respiratory, genital, and gastrointestinal tracts, and infections of the mouth, lungs, and brain. It is the organism most commonly found, in association with spirochetes *(Treponema vincentii)*, in acute necrotizing ulcerative gingivitis.

F. rus′sii a species isolated from perianal abscesses and feces.

F. va′rium a species isolated from intestinal cavities and purulent infections.

fu•so•bac•te•ri•um (fu″zo-bak-tēr′e-əm) pl. *fusobacte′ria*. 1. a rod-shaped bacterium in which the cell is thicker in the center and tapers toward the ends. 2. an organism of the genus *Fusobacterium*.

fu•so•cel•lu•lar (fu″so-sel′u-lər) [*fuso-* + *cellular*] having spindle-shaped cells.

fu•so•gen•ic (fu-zo-jen′ik) inducing or enabling fusion.

fu•so•spi•ril•lary (fu″so-spi′rĭ-lar″e) pertaining to or caused by fusobacteria and spirilla, as in necrotizing ulcerative gingivitis.

fu•so•spi•ril•lo•sis (fu″so-spi″rĭ-lo′sis) necrotizing ulcerative gingivitis.

fu•so•spi•ro•che•tal (fu″so-spi″ro-ke′təl) pertaining to or caused by fusobacteria and spirochetes.

fu•so•spi•ro•che•to•sis (fu″so-spi″ro-ke-to′sis) infection with fusobacteria and spirochetes, as in acute necrotizing ulcerative gingivitis.

fu•sus (fu′səs) pl. *fu′si* [L.] a spindle-shaped object.

cortical fusi tiny air spaces that appear among the cells of the cortex of a hair shaft as it grows, produced by evaporation of the fluid that originally filled the spaces in the living portion of the root of the hair.

Fut•cher line (fuch′ər) [Palmer Howard *Futcher*, American physician, 1910–2004] Voigt line; see under *line*.

Fu•ze•on (fu′ze-on) trademark for a preparation of enfuvirtide.

FVC forced vital capacity.

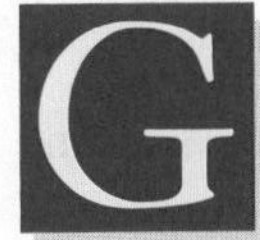

G gauss; giga-; glycine; gravida; guanine or guanosine.

G conductance; gravitational constant; Gibbs free energy; G force.

g gram.

g standard gravity.

γ gamma, the third letter of the Greek alphabet; symbol for the heavy chain of IgG (see *immunoglobulin*) and the γ chains of fetal hemoglobin.

γ- a prefix designating (1) the third carbon atom along a chain starting with that adjacent to the principal functional group, e.g., γ-aminobutyric acid (see α-); (2) a plasma protein migrating with the γ band in protein electrophoresis, a gamma globulin; (3) one in a series of related entities or chemical compounds, e.g., γ-carotene or γ-ray. For terms prefixed with the symbol γ-, see the unprefixed form.

Ga gallium.

GABA γ-aminobutyric acid.

GABA·er·gic (gab″ə-ur′jik) transmitting or secreting γ-aminobutyric acid; said of nerve fibers, synapses, and other neural structures.

gab·a·pen·tin (gab″ə-pen′tin) [USP] an anticonvulsant that is a structural analogue of γ-aminobutyric acid (GABA), used as adjunctive therapy in the treatment of partial seizures; administered orally.

GABA trans·am·i·nase (gab″ə-trans-am′ĭ-nās) 1. 4-aminobutyrate transaminase. 2. a renal transaminase that catalyzes the transfer of an amino group from γ-aminobutyrate (GABA) to pyruvate, forming alanine and succinate semialdehyde; the reaction may play a role in chloride permeability in the nephron.

Gab·i·tril (gab′ĭ-tril) trademark for a preparation of tiagabine hydrochloride.

G-ac·tin see *actin*.

GAD generalized anxiety disorder; glutamic acid decarboxylase (see *glutamate decarboxylase*).

gad·fly (gad′fli) tabanid.

gad·o·di·a·mide (gad″o-di′ə-mīd) a complex of gadolinium with diethylenetriamine pentetic acid bismethylamide; used as a paramagnetic contrast medium in magnetic resonance imaging.

gad·o·lin·i·um (Gd) (gad″o-lin′e-əm) a rare element of atomic number 64, atomic weight 157.25; chelated gadolinium is used as a paramagnetic contrast medium in magnetic resonance imaging.

g. 153 an artificial isotope of gadolinium used in dual photon absorptiometry; it has a half-life of 241.6 days and decays by electron capture and emission of 0.070, 0.097, and 0.103 MeV gamma rays.

gad·o·lin·i·um-pen·tet·ic ac·id (gad″o-lin′e-əm) a paramagnetic contrast medium used in magnetic resonance imaging.

gad·o·pen·te·tate di·meg·lu·mine (gad″o-pen′tə-tāt) [USP] the dimeglumine salt of the gadolinium complex of pentetic acid; a paramagnetic contrast medium used in magnetic resonance imaging of intracranial lesions and lesions of the spine and associated tissues, administered intravenously.

gado·ver·set·a·mide (gad″o-vər-set′ə-mīd) a nonionic chelate of gadolinium, used as a paramagnetic contrast medium in magnetic resonance imaging of intracranial lesions, lesions of the spine and associated tissues, and lesions of the liver; administered intravenously.

Ga·dus (ga′dəs) [L., from Gr. *gados* a kind of fish] a genus of marine fishes of the family Gadidae. *G. mor′rhua* is the common cod, source of cod liver oil.

Gaens·len sign (test) (genz′lən) [Frederick Julius *Gaenslen*, American surgeon, 1877–1937] see under *sign*.

Gaff·ky scale (gahf′ke) [Georg Theodor August *Gaffky*, German bacteriologist, 1850–1918] see under *scale*.

GAG glycosaminoglycan.

gag (gag) 1. a surgical device for holding the mouth open. 2. to prevent from speaking. 3. retch.

gage (gāj) gauge.

Gai·ge·ria (ga-je′re-ə) a genus of hookworms of the family Ancylostomatidae. *G. pachysce′lis* infests the intestines of sheep in India, Indonesia, Africa, and South America; it is a voracious blood sucker and often kills its host.

Gail·lard-Arlt suture (ga-yahr′ ahrlt′) [François Lucien *Gaillard*, French physician, 1805–1869; Carl Ferdinand Ritter von *Arlt*, Austrian ophthalmologist, 1812–1887] see under *suture*.

gain (gān) 1. an increase in amount or value; a benefit or advantage. 2. the increase achieved by amplification of a signal. 3. to acquire, obtain, or increase.

antigen g. the acquisition by cells of new antigenic determinants not normally present or not normally accessible in the parent tissue.

primary g. the direct alleviation of anxiety by a defense mechanism; the relief from emotional conflict or tension provided by neurotic symptoms or illness.

secondary g. external and incidental advantage derived from an illness, such as rest, gifts, personal attention, release from responsibility, and disability benefits.

Gais·böck disease (gīs′bərk) [Felix *Gaisböck*, German physician, 1868–1955] stress polycythemia.

gait (gāt) the manner or style of walking. See also *gait cycle*, under *cycle*.

antalgic g. a limp adopted so as to avoid pain on weight-bearing structures (as in hip injuries), characterized by a very short stance phase.

ataxic g. an unsteady, uncoordinated walk, with a wide base and the feet thrown out, due to some form of ataxia; see *cerebellar g.*, *Charcot g.*, and *tabetic g.*

calcaneus g. the gait resulting when the gastrocnemius-soleus muscles are paralyzed, with lack of push-off and shift of the tibia posteriorly over the talus at the end of the stance phase.

cerebellar g. a staggering ataxic gait, sometimes with a tendency to fall to one side, indicative of cerebellar lesions.

Charcot g. the peculiar gait seen in Friedreich ataxia.

circumduction g. hemiplegic g.

compensated gluteus medius g. Trendelenburg g.

double-step g. a gait in which the length and/or timing of alternate steps is noticeably different; see also *intermittent double-step g.*

drag-to g. a gait in which the feet are dragged (rather than lifted) toward the crutches.

drop-foot g. steppage g.

dystrophic g. myopathic g.

equine g. steppage g.

festinating g. a gait in which the patient involuntarily moves with short, accelerating steps, often on tiptoe, as seen in parkinsonism and certain other neurologic disorders; called also *propulsive g.* See also *festination.*

four-point g. a gait in forward motion: first one crutch and then the opposite leg, followed by the other crutch and then the other leg, and so on.

gluteal g. Trendelenburg g.

gluteus medius g. see *Trendelenburg g.* and *uncompensated gluteus medius g.*

heel-toe g. the normal, nonpathologic gait in which the heel touches down first and the toes last.

helicopod g. a gait in which the feet describe half circles, as in some cases of conversion disorder.

hemiplegic g. a gait involving flexion of the hip because of footdrop and circumduction of the leg. Called also *circumduction g.*

hip extensor g. an abnormal gait due to weakness or paralysis of the gluteus maximus and other hip extensor muscles; with each step on the affected side, after the heel strikes the floor the hip is thrown forward and the trunk and pelvis are thrown back.

hysterical g. a bizarre gait pattern not due to a physical cause, such as *helicopod g.* or *stuttering g.*

intermittent double-step g. a hemiplegic gait in which there is a pause after the short step of the normal foot, or in some cases after the step of the affected foot.

maximus g. hip extensor g.

myopathic g. exaggerated alternation of lateral trunk movements with an exaggerated elevation of the hip, suggesting the gait of a duck or penguin; characteristic of muscle diseases such as progressive muscular dystrophy, spinal muscular atrophy, and sometimes Guillain-Barré syndrome.

paraplegic spastic g. a walk in which the legs are held together and move in a stiff manner, the toes seeming to drag and catch; caused by lesions of the central nervous system.

point g. any of several gaits in which at least one foot and one crutch are on the ground at any given time; see *two-point g.*, *three-point g.*, and *four-point g.*

propulsive g. festinating g.

quadriceps g. a gait seen when the quadriceps muscle is paralyzed or absent; with each step of the affected leg, the knee goes into hyperextension and the trunk tends to lurch forward.

scissors g. a gait in which one foot is passed in front of the other, producing a cross-legged progression.

spastic g. paraplegic spastic g.

staggering g. a reeling, tottering, and tipping gait in which the individual appears as if they may fall backward or lose balance; it is associated with alcohol or barbiturate intoxication.

steppage g. the gait in footdrop in which the advancing leg is lifted high in order that the toes may clear the ground. It is due to paralysis of the anterior tibial and peroneal muscles and is seen in lesions of lower motoneurons, such as multiple neuritis, lesions of the anterior motor horn cells, and lesions of the cauda equina. Called also *drop-foot g.* and *equine g.*

stuttering g. a walking disorder characterized by hesitancy that resembles stuttering; seen in some hysterical or schizophrenic patients as well as in patients with neurologic damage.

swaying g. cerebellar g.
swing g. a gait in which the lower body is swung between the crutches at each step; see *swing-through g.* and *swing-to g.*
swing-through g. a gait in which the crutches are advanced and then the legs are swung past them.
swing-to g. a gait in which the crutches are advanced and the legs are swung to the same point.
tabetic g. an ataxic gait that accompanies tabes dorsalis.
tandem g. a gait used in neurologic assessments; the patient is told to walk in a straight line and at the end of each step to touch the heel of the foot in front to the toe of the foot behind.
three-point g. a gait in which both crutches and the affected leg are advanced together and then the normal leg is moved forward.
Trendelenburg g. the gait characteristic of paralysis of the gluteus medius muscle, marked by a listing of the trunk toward the affected side at each step. See also *Trendelenburg test* (def. 2), under *test.* Called also *compensated gluteus medius g.* and *gluteal g.*
two-point g. a gait in which the right foot and left crutch (or cane) are advanced together, and then the left foot and right crutch.
uncompensated gluteus medius g. a gait that occurs with moderate weakness of the gluteus medius muscle; with each step of the affected leg, the pelvis on the opposite side dips, causing protrusion of the stationary affected hip. Cf. *Trendelenburg g.*
waddling g. myopathic g.

ga•lac•ta•cra•sia (gə-lak″tə-kra′zhə) [*galact-* + *a-*[1] + *-crasia*] abnormal condition of the breast milk.

ga•lac•ta•gogue (gə-lak′tə-gog) [*galact-* + *-agogue*] 1. promoting the flow of milk. 2. an agent that promotes the flow of milk.

ga•lac•tan (gə-lak′tən) any polymer composed of galactose residues and occurring in plants, e.g., agar.

gal•ac•te•mia (gal″ak-te′me-ə) [*galact-* + *-emia*] the presence of milk in the blood.

ga•lac•tic (gə-lak′tik) 1. lactic. 2. galactagogue.

gal•ac•tis•chia (gal″ak-tis′ke-ə) [*galact-* + *isch-* + *-ia*] suppression of lactation.

ga•lac•ti•tol (gə-lak′tĭ-tol) the alcohol obtained on reduction of galactose, occurring naturally in manna and other plant products. Galactitol is formed in excess in the lens of the eye in galactosemia caused by deficiency of galactokinase; the result is cataracts in infancy.

galact(o)- [Gr. *gala*, gen. *galaktos* milk] a combining form denoting relationship to milk.

ga•lac•to•cele (gə-lak′to-sēl) [*galacto-* + *-cele*[1]] a cystic enlargement of the mammary gland containing milk; called also *lactocele.*

ga•lac•to•ce•re•bro•side (gə-lak″to-sə-re′bro-sīd″) any of the cerebrosides in which the monosaccharide head group is galactose; they are abundant in the cell membranes of nervous tissue, particularly the myelin sheath, and in the kidney, and they accumulate abnormally in Krabbe disease.

ga•lac•to•cer•e•bro•side β-ga•lac•to•si•dase (gə-lak″to-sə-re′bro-sīd″ gə-lak″to-si′dās) galactosylceramidase.

ga•lac•to•cra•sia (gə-lak″to-kra′zhə) galactacrasia.

gal•ac•tog•e•nous (gal″ak-toj′ə-nəs) [*galacto-* + *-genous*] favoring the production of milk.

ga•lac•to•gogue (gə-lak′to-gog) galactagogue.

gal•ac•tog•ra•phy (gal″ak-tog′rə-fe) [*galacto-* + *-graphy*] radiography of the mammary ducts after injection of a radiopaque medium into the duct system.

ga•lac•to•ki•nase (gə-lak″to-ki′nās) [EC 2.7.1.6] an enzyme of the transferase class that catalyzes the reaction ATP + galactose = ADP + galactose 1-phosphate; the initial step of galactose utilization. Absence of enzyme activity, an autosomal recessive trait, results in galactokinase deficiency galactosemia.

ga•lac•to•ki•nase de•fi•cien•cy (gə-lak″to-ki′nās) a form of galactosemia caused by mutations in the galactokinase gene (*GALK1*, locus: 17q24); deficiency of the enzyme results in accumulation of galactose in blood and tissues and of galactitol in the lens of the eye and causes cataracts in infants and children.

gal•ac•tom•e•ter (gal″ak-tom′ə-tər) [*galacto-* + *-meter*] an instrument for measuring the specific gravity of milk.

ga•lac•to•pex•ic (gə-lak″to-pek′sik) fixing or holding galactose.

ga•lac•to•pexy (gə-lak′to-pek″se) [*galacto-* + *-pexy*] the fixation of galactose by the liver.

gal•ac•toph•a•gous (gal″ak-tof′ə-gəs) lactivorous.

ga•lac•to•phle•bi•tis (gə-lak″to-flə-bi′tis) phlegmasia alba dolens.

ga•lac•to•phore (gə-lak′to-for) 1. galactophorous. 2. a milk duct; see *ductus lactiferi.*

ga•lac•to•pho•ri•tis (gə-lak″to-for-i′tis) [*galacto-* + Gr. *pherein* to carry + *-itis*] inflammation of the lactiferous ducts.

gal•ac•toph•o•rous (gal″ak-tof′o-rəs) lactiferous.

ga•lac•to•poi•e•sis (gə-lak″to-poi-e′sis) [*galacto-* + *-poiesis*] the production of milk by the mammary glands; called also *lactogenesis.*

ga•lac•to•poi•et•ic (gə-lak″to-poi-et′ik) 1. pertaining to, characterized by, or promoting the production of milk. 2. an agent that promotes the secretion of milk. Called also *lactogenic.*

ga•lac•to•py•ra•nose (gə-lak″to-pir′ə-nōs) galactose occurring in the cyclic pyranose configuration.

ga•lac•tor•rhea (gə-lak″to-re′ə) [*galacto-* + *-rrhea*] excessive or spontaneous flow of milk irrespective of nursing; it is sometimes associated with hyperprolactinemia (q.v.).

gal•ac•to•sa•mine (gal″ak-to′sə-mēn) the amino sugar derivative of galactose, substituted at the 2 position; it occurs in a variety of glycosaminoglycans and complex polysaccharides, such as blood group substances, and is generally acetylated.

gal•ac•to•sa•mine-6-sul•fa•tase (gal″ak-to′sə-mēn sul′fə-tās) *N*-acetylgalactosamine-6-sulfatase.

ga•lac•to•san (gə-lak′to-san) galactan.

gal•ac•to•sa•zone (gal″ak-to′sə-zōn) the osazone formed from galactose by reaction with phenylhydrazine; it has been used to identify galactose.

ga•lac•tose (gə-lak′tōs) [Gr. *gala*, gen. *galaktos* milk] an aldohexose epimeric with glucose at the 4 carbon but less soluble and less sweet, occurring naturally in both D- and L- forms (the latter in plants); it is a component of lactose and other oligosaccharides, cerebrosides and gangliosides, and various glycolipids and glycoproteins.
g. 1-phosphate galactose containing a phosphate substitution, an intermediate in carbohydrate metabolism.

ga•lac•tos•e•mia (gə-lak″to-se′me-ə) [*galactose* + *-emia*] a general term encompassing three autosomal recessive disorders resulting from defective galactose metabolism. *Classic galactosemia*, which is often fatal to neonates, is caused by mutations in the *GALT* gene (locus: 9p13), which encodes UDP-glucose–hexose-1-phosphate uridylyltransferase. Enzyme deficiency results in accumulation of galactose 1-phosphate and galactose, with cataracts, cirrhosis, hepatomegaly, vomiting, diarrhea, jaundice, poor weight gain, and malnutrition in infancy, and mental retardation in survivors. The other two disorders are *galactokinase deficiency* and *UDP-glucose 4-epimerase deficiency* (qq.v.).

ga•lac•tose 1-phos•phate u•ri•dyl•trans•fer•ase (gə-lak″tōs fos′fāt u″rĭ-dəl-trans′fər-ās) UDP-glucose–hexose-1-phosphate uridylyltransferase.

ga•lac•tose 1-phos•phate uri•dyl•yl•trans•fer•ase (gə-lak′tōs fos′fāt u″rĭ-dil″əl-trans′fər-ās) UTP–hexose-1-phosphate uridylyltransferase.

ga•lac•to•si•al•i•do•sis (gə-lak″to-si-al″ĭ-do′sis) an autosomal recessive lysosomal storage disease caused by mutations in the *CTSA* gene (locus: 20q13.1), which encodes cathepsin A, resulting in deficiency of both neuraminidase (sialidase) and β-galactosidase. It is clinically almost indistinguishable from sialidosis type II. Three phenotypic variants occur, of increasing severity with decreasing age of onset: early infantile, characterized by fetal hydrops, ascites, visceromegaly, and early death; late infantile, characterized by cardiac involvement, hepatosplenomegaly, and growth retardation; and juvenile, characterized by progressive neurological deterioration without visceromegaly.

α-ga•lac•to•si•dase (gə-lak″to-si′dās) 1. [EC 3.2.1.22] an enzyme of the hydrolase class that catalyzes the cleavage of terminal, nonreducing, α-linked galactose residues from galactosides. 2. α-g. A.

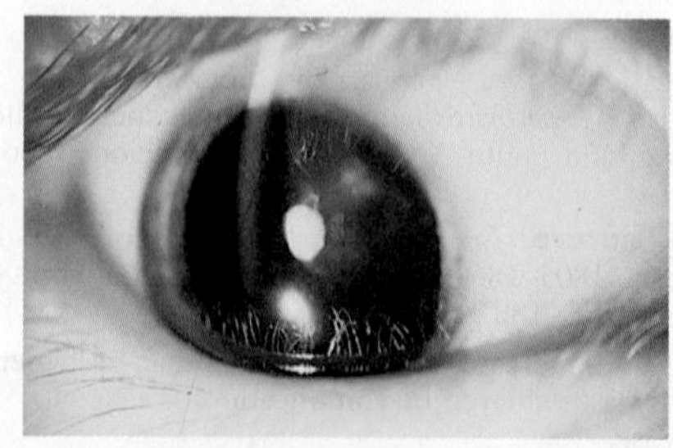

■ Cataract associated with galactosemia, the opacity of the lens having an oil-droplet appearance.

α-g. A a lysosomal enzyme that catalyzes the cleavage of terminal galactose residues from glycosphingolipids, particularly ceramide trihexosides. Deficiency of the enzyme, an X-linked trait, causes accumulation of ceramide trihexosides and other glycosphingolipids in plasma and tissues and results in Fabry disease. Called also *ceramide trihexosidase* and *α-g*.

α-g. B α-*N*-acetylgalactosaminidase.

β-ga•lac•to•si•dase (gə-lak″to-si′dās) [EC 3.2.1.23] any of a group of enzymes of the hydrolase class that catalyze the cleavage of terminal, β-linked, nonreducing galactose residues from a variety of substrates, including ganglioside GM_1, lactosylceramides, lactose, and various glycoproteins and oligosaccharides. See also *lactase*. The lysosomal (acid) isozyme catalyzes the hydrolysis of β-galactosides in gangliosides and keratan sulfate, and its catalytic activity with these substrates is differentially impaired in several autosomal recessive disorders caused by allelic mutations. In GM_1 gangliosidosis, activity toward ganglioside GM_1 is particularly decreased or absent, while in Morquio syndrome, type B, this activity is normal but activity toward keratan sulfate is decreased.

ga•lac•to•side (gə-lak′to-sīd) a glycoside containing galactose.

gal•ac•to•sis (gal″ak-to′sis) the formation of milk by the lacteal glands.

ga•lac•to•sta•sia (gə-lak″to-sta′shə) galactostasis.

gal•ac•tos•ta•sis (gal″ak-tos′tə-sis) [*galacto-* + *-stasis*] 1. cessation of lactation. 2. an abnormal collection of milk in the mammary glands.

ga•lac•tos•uria (gə-lak″to-su′re-ə) presence of galactose in the urine owing to deficiency of enzymes that normally would convert it to glucose.

ga•lac•to•syl (gə-lak′to-səl) a radical of galactose.

ga•lac•to•syl•ce•ram•i•dase (gə-lak″to-səl-sə-ram′ĭ-dās) [EC 3.2.1.46] an enzyme of the hydrolase class that catalyzes the hydrolytic cleavage of galactose from galactocerebrosides to form ceramides, a reaction occurring in the lysosomal degradation of sphingolipids. Deficiency of the enzyme, an autosomal recessive trait, causes Krabbe disease. Called also *galactocerebroside β-galactosidase*.

ga•lac•to•syl•cer•a•mide (gə-lak″to-səl-ser′ə-mīd) galactocerebroside.

ga•lac•to•syl•cer•a•mide β-ga•lac•to•si•dase (gə-lak″to-səl-ser′ə-mīd gə-lak″to-si′dās) galactosylceramidase.

ga•lac•to•syl•hy•droxy•ly•syl glu•co•syl•trans•fer•ase (gə-lak″to-səl-hi-drok″se-li′səl gloo″ko-səl-trans′fər-ās) procollagen glucosyltransferase.

ga•lac•to•syl•trans•fer•ase (gə-lak″to-səl-trans′fər-ās) a term used in the trivial and recommended names of some hexosyltransferases [EC 2.4.1] that catalyze the transfer of a galactosyl group from a donor to an acceptor compound.

ga•lac•to•tox•in (gə-lak′to-tok″sin) [*galacto-* + *toxin*] a basic substance formed in milk.

ga•lac•to•tox•ism (gə-lak′to-tok″siz-əm) poisoning by milk.

gal•ac•tox•ism (gal″ak-tok′siz-əm) galactotoxism.

ga•lac•tu•ron•ic ac•id (gə-lak″tu-ron′ik) the uronic acid formed by the oxidation of C-6 of galactose to a carboxy group; it occurs in pectins.

gala•nin (gal′ə-nin) a hormone expressed in the central and peripheral nervous systems and in neural structures of various organs. It is released in a variety of stimulus and stress situations and may have functions including regulation of food intake, memory and cognition, antinociception, and regulation of certain neuroendocrine processes.

ga•lan•ta•mine hy•dro•bro•mide (gə-lan′tə-mēn) the hydrobromide salt of an alkaloid obtained from the daffodil *Narcissus pseudonarcissus*; it is a reversible competitive inhibitor of acetylcholinesterase and is administered orally in the treatment of mild to moderate Alzheimer disease. It is believed to act by increasing the concentration of acetylcholine and so enhancing cholinergic function.

ga•lea (ga′le-ə) [L. "helmet"] a helmetlike structure or part.

g. aponeuro′tica [TA] the aponeurotic structure of the scalp, connecting the frontal and occipital bellies of the occipitofrontalis muscle. Called also *aponeurosis epicranialis* [TA alternative] and *epicranial aponeurosis*.

Ga•le•a•ti glands (gah-la-ah′te) [Domenico Gusmano *Galeati*, Italian physician, 1686–1775] glandulae duodenales.

ga•le•at•o•my (gal″e-at′ə-me) galeotomy.

gal•e•a•tus (gal″e-a′təs) [L., from *galea* helmet] born with a caul.

Ga•le•az•zi fracture, sign (gah-la-aht′se) [Riccardo *Galeazzi*, Italian orthopedic surgeon, 1866–1952] see under *fracture* and *sign*.

Ga•len (ga′lən) a Greek physician and teacher, c. 129– c. 200, born in Pergamum (Asia Minor); author of 500 books on philosophy, philology, and medicine (83 medical books survive). He was court physician to Marcus Aurelius, a surgeon to gladiators, and a practicing anatomist. Galen was the great compiler and systemizer of Greco-Roman medicine, physiology, and anatomy. By experiment he showed that arteries carried blood, believed the brain to be the seat of intelligence, and understood the diagnostic value of the pulse. His work was superseded by that of Vesalius in anatomy and of Harvey in physiology.

Ga•len nerve (anastomosis), etc. (ga′lən) [*Galen*] see *ramus communicans nervi laryngei superioris cum nervo laryngeo inferiore, venae internae cerebri, vena magna cerebri*, and *ventriculus laryngis*.

ga•len•ic (gə-len′ik) pertaining to the ancient system of medicine taught and practiced by Galen.

ga•len•i•ca (gə-len′ĭ-kə) galenicals.

ga•len•i•cals (gə-len′ĭ-kəlz) medicines prepared according to the formulas of Galen; the term is now used to denote standard preparations containing one or several organic ingredients, as contrasted with pure chemical substances.

ga•len•ics (gə-len′iks) galenicals.

ga•leo•pho•bia (ga″le-o-fo′be-ə) [Gr. *galeē* weasel, cat + *-phobia*] ailurophobia.

ga•le•ot•o•my (gal″e-ot′ə-me) incision of the galea aponeurotica; called also *galeatomy*.

Gal•er•i•na (gal-ə-ri′nə) a genus of mushrooms of the family Cortinariaceae. They contain amatoxins but cause mushroom poisoning less frequently than *Amanita* species because of being considerably smaller in size.

gal•er•o•pia (gal″ər-o′pe-ə) [Gr. *galeros* cheerful + *-opia, -opsia*] abnormal clearness of vision due to a pathologic condition.

gal•er•op•sia (gal″ər-op′se-ə) galeropia.

gall (gawl) [L. *galla*] 1. bile. 2. nutgall. 3. a localized swelling or skin sore caused by friction.

Aleppo g. nutgall.

collar g. a wound or pressure ulcer on a horse caused by repeated trauma from an ill-fitting harness or collar.

saddle g. a wound or pressure ulcer on a horse caused by repeated trauma from an ill-fitting saddle. Called also *saddle sore*.

wind g. windgall.

gal•la•mine tri•eth•io•dide (gal′ə-mēn tri″ə-thi′o-dīd) [USP] a quaternary ammonium compound used to induce skeletal muscle relaxation during surgery and other procedures, such as endoscopy or intubation, administered intravenously.

gal•late (gal′āt) any salt or ester of gallic acid.

Gal•la•var•din phenomenon (gahl-ə-var-dă′) [Louis *Gallavardin*, French cardiologist, 1875–1957] see under *phenomenon*.

gall•blad•der (gawl′blad″ər) vesica biliaris.

Courvoisier g. a distended gallbladder resulting from biliary tract obstruction, sometimes in premalignant conditions.

floating g. wandering g.

folded fundus g. phrygian cap.

hourglass g. a gallbladder divided into a wide upper and a narrower lower compartment by an annular constriction; the anomaly may be congenital or acquired.

mobile g. wandering g.

porcelain g. diffuse or focal calcification of the gallbladder wall, arising in chronic cholecystitis and frequently associated with the development of carcinoma.

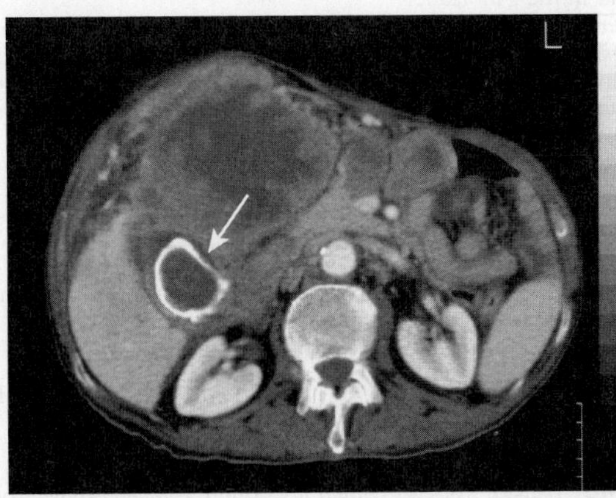

■ Porcelain gallbladder with concentric calcification of the gallbladder wall *(arrow)*. A large gallbladder cancer is also present.

sandpaper g. a rough state of the mucous membrane of the gallbladder caused by the presence of cholesterol gallstones.

strawberry g. a strawberrylike appearance of the gallbladder due to fine grains of cholesterol-fat material embedded in the mucosa, seen in cholesterolosis with inflammation.

wandering g. abnormal mobility of the gallbladder; called also *floating* or *mobile g.*

gal·le·in (gal′e-in) an aniline dye indicator that is changed in color by an alkali to red and by an acid to yellow.

gal·lic ac·id (gal′ik) 3,4,5-trihydroxybenzoic acid, obtained from nutgalls and formerly used as an astringent. Its alkyl esters are antioxidants and are used as preservatives in pharmaceuticals, foods, and cosmetics.

gal·lid (gal′id) [L. *gallus* cock] pertaining to fowl. Cf. *avian.*

Gal·lie transplant (gal′e) [William Edward *Gallie*, Canadian surgeon, 1882–1959] see under *transplant.*

gal·li·um (Ga) (gal′e-əm) [L., from *Gallia* Gaul] a rare metal liquid at room temperature; atomic number 31, atomic weight 69.72; some of its compounds are poisonous.

g. 67 a radioisotope of gallium, atomic mass 67, having a half-life of 3.26 days and decaying by electron capture and emission of 0.093, 0.184, 0.300, and 0.393 MeV gamma rays; used primarily chelated with citrate; see *g. Ga 67 citrate.*

g. Ga 67 citrate a radiopharmaceutical imaging agent, the citrate salt of ^{67}Ga; it binds initially to plasma proteins, then localizes primarily in the liver, spleen, bone marrow, and skeleton. It is used to image neoplasms, particularly of soft tissues, and sites of inflammation and abscess.

g. nitrate a hydrated nitrate salt of gallium, a potent inhibitor of bone calcium resorption; administered intravenously to treat cancer-related hypercalcemia.

gall·nut (gawl′nət) nutgall.

gal·lon (gal′on) [A.S. "a liquid measure"] a measure of liquid volume, four quarts. In the United States it is equivalent to 3.785 liters *(standard gallon);* in Great Britain it is equivalent to 4.546 liters *(imperial gallon).*

gal·lop (gal′op) a disordered rhythm of the heart; see under *rhythm.*

atrial g. S_4 g.

diastolic g. S_3 g.

fourth heart sound g. S_4 g.

presystolic g. S_4 g.

protodiastolic g. an older term for *S_3 g.*

S_3 g. an accentuated third heart sound detected in patients with cardiac disease characterized by pathologic alterations in ventricular filling in early diastole.

S_4 g. an accentuated, audible fourth heart sound usually associated with cardiac disease, often that characterized by altered ventricular compliance.

summation g. a gallop rhythm in which the third and fourth sounds are superimposed, appearing as one loud sound; it may occur in some patients with tachycardia but is usually associated with cardiac disease.

third heart sound g. S_3 g.

ventricular g. S_3 g.

gal·lo·tan·nic ac·id (gal″o-tan′ik) tannic acid.

gall·sick·ness (gawl′sik-nis) anaplasmosis.

gall·stone (gawl′stōn) a concretion formed in the gallbladder or bile duct; the usual composition is cholesterol, a blood pigment liberated by hemolysis, or a calcium salt. Called also *biliary calculus* and *cholelith.* See also *cholelithiasis.*

cholesterol g. a gallstone whose main component is cholesterol, usually found in the gallbladder.

pigment g. a gallstone whose major component is a bile pigment. Black stones, usually found in the gallbladder, are composed of calcium bilirubinate or pigment polymers, with or without calcium carbonate, calcium phosphate, and mucin; they are hard and often have spicules on the surface. Brown stones, usually found in the common bile duct, are not as hard as black ones, and are composed of calcium bilirubinate and calcium salts of fatty acids, as well as more cholesterol than black ones have.

GalNAc *N*-acetylgalactosamine.

gal·sul·fase (gal-sul′fās) a recombinant form of the enzyme *N*-acetylgalactosamine 4-sulfatase, used in treatment of Maroteaux-Lamy syndrome; administered by intravenous infusion.

GALT gut-associated lymphoid tissue.

Gal·ton's law of regression (gawl′tənz) [Sir Francis *Galton*, English anthropologist and biologist, 1822–1911] see under *law.*

Galv. galvanic.

gal·van·ic (gal-van′ik) 1. named for Luigi *Galvani*, Italian physicist and physiologist, 1737–1798, as *galvanic current.* 2. pertaining to galvanism.

gal·va·nism (gal′və-niz-əm) [Luigi *Galvani*] 1. galvanic current. 2. the therapeutic use of this current, particularly for stimulation of nerves and muscle.

dental g. production of galvanic current in the oral cavity due to the presence of two or more dissimilar metals in dental restorations that are bathed in saliva, or a single metal restoration and two electrolytes, saliva and pulp tissue fluid, thus producing an electrolytic cell and an electric current. When such restorations touch each other, the current may be high enough to irritate the dental pulp and cause sharp pain. The anodic restoration or areas of a restoration are subject to electrolytic corrosion.

gal·va·ni·za·tion (gal″və-nĭ-za′shən) treatment by galvanic current.

gal·va·no·con·trac·til·i·ty (gal″və-no-kon″trak-til′ĭ-te) contractility in response to a galvanic stimulus.

gal·va·no·gus·tom·e·ter (gal″və-no-gəs-tom′ə-tər) an apparatus for the clinical determination of taste thresholds by the use of a galvanic current.

gal·va·nom·e·ter (gal″və-nom′ə-tər) [*galvanism* + *-meter*] an instrument for measuring current by electromagnetic action.

Einthoven g., string g. the original type of electrocardiograph, which consisted of a delicate thread of silvered quartz or platinum stretched between the poles of a strong magnet; the thread is displaced by an electric current flowing through it in proportion to the strength of the current.

gal·va·no·pal·pa·tion (gal″və-no-pal-pa′shən) a method of testing the sensory and vasomotor nerves of the skin by applying a sharp-pointed anode electrode to the part of the skin to be tested, the cathode being applied to some other part of the body.

gal·va·no·tax·is (gal″və-no-tak′sis) the tendency of an organism to arrange itself in a medium so that its axis bears a certain relation to the direction of the current in the medium.

gal·va·no·ther·a·py (gal″və-no-ther′ə-pe) the therapeutic use of galvanic current.

gal·va·not·rop·ism (gal″və-not′ro-piz-əm) [*galvanism* + *-tropism*] the tendency of an organism to turn or move under the action of an electric current.

Gam·a·stan (gam′ə-stan″) trademark for a preparation of immune human serum globulin.

Gam·bi·an horse sickness, trypanosomiasis (sleeping sickness) (gam′be-ən) [*Gambia*, West Africa] see under *sickness* and *trypanosomiasis.*

Gam·bi·er·dis·cus (gam″be-ər-dis′kəs) a genus of plantlike marine protozoa of the order Gonyaulacales, phylum Dinoflagellata, sometimes the cause of red tide.

G. tox′icus a species that produces a pretoxin that is biotransformed to the active toxin ciguatoxin (q.v.) upon ingestion by certain marine fish.

gam·bir (gam′bēr) the dried aqueous, astringent extract from the leaves and twigs of the shrub *Uncaria gambier;* its main constituents are catechin, catechutannic acid, and quercetin. Formerly used as an antidiarrheal and as a gargle for sore throat. Called also *catechu* or *pale catechu.*

gam·bling (gam′bling) betting money or other valuables on the outcome of a game or event.

pathological g. [DSM-IV] an impulse control disorder consisting of persistent failure to resist the urge to gamble, to such an extent that personal, family, and vocational life are seriously disrupted.

Gam·bu·sia (gam-boo′se-ə) a genus of fish effective in destroying mosquito larvae.

G. affi′nis a top minnow that has been introduced into every major malarious region in the world; it feeds upon the larvae of *Anopheles* mosquitoes along the surface of the water.

gam·e·tan·gi·um (gam″ə-tan′je-əm) pl. *gametan′gia* [*gamet-* + Gr. *angeion* vessel] the structure in which zygospores are developed. See also *zygophore.*

gam·ete (gam′ēt) [Gr. *gametē* wife, *gametēs* husband] 1. one of two haploid reproductive cells, male *(spermatozoon)* and female *(oocyte)*, whose union is necessary in sexual reproduction to initiate the development of a new individual. 2. the malarial parasite in its sexual form in the gut of the mosquito vector, either male *(microgamete)* or female *(macrogamete);* the latter fertilizes the former to form a zygote, which develops into an ookinete.

ga·met·ic (gə-met′ik) pertaining to gametes or to primordial sexual elements.

gamet(o)- [Gr. *gametē* wife, *gametēs* husband] a combining form denoting relationship to a gamete.

ga·me·to·ci·dal (gə-me″to-si′dəl) capable of destroying gametes or gametocytes.

ga·me·to·cide (gə-me′to-sīd) [*gameto-* + *-cide*] an agent that destroys gametes or gametocytes.

ga•me•to•cyte (gə-me′to-sīt) [*gameto-* + *cyte*] 1. a cell capable of dividing to form gametes; an oocyte or spermatocyte. 2. gamont.

ga•me•to•cy•te•mia (gə-me″to-si-te′me-ə) the presence of malarial gametocytes in the blood.

gam•e•to•gen•e•sis (gə-me″to-jen′ə-sis) [*gameto-* + *-genesis*] the development of the male and female sex cells, or gametes.

gam•e•to•gen•ic (gə-me″to-jen′ik) producing or favoring gametogenesis.

gam•e•tog•o•ny (gam″ə-tog′ə-ne) 1. in malarial plasmodia and other sporozoa, the development of merozoites into male and female gametes, which later fuse to form a zygote. Called also *gamogony*. 2. reproduction by means of gametes.

gam•e•toid (gam′ə-toid) resembling gametes.

gam•e•to•ki•net•ic (gam″ə-to-kĭ-net′ik) [*gameto-* + *kinetic*] stimulating gamete action.

gam•e•to•pha•gia (gam″ə-to-fa′jə) gamophagia.

gam•e•to•phyte (gam′ə-to-fīt″) [*gameto-* + *-phyte*] the haploid or sexual stage in organisms having alternation of generations (metagenesis); it may be female (megagametophyte) or male (microgametophyte).

Gam•gee tissue (gam′je) [Joseph Sampson *Gamgee*, British surgeon, 1828–1886] see under *tissue*.

gam•ic (gam′ik) of or requiring fertilization to reproduce.

Gam•i•mune N (gam′ĭ-mūn) trademark for preparations of immune globulin intravenous (human).

gam•ma (gam′ə) [Γ, γ] the third letter of the Greek alphabet. See also γ-.

gam•ma-ami•no•bu•tyr•ic ac•id (gam′ə-ə-me″no-bu-tir′ik) γ-aminobutyric acid; see under *A*.

gam•ma ben•zene hex•a•chlo•ride (gam′ə ben′zēn hek″sə-klor′īd) lindane.

gam•ma•cism (gam′ə-siz-əm) [*gamma* + *-ism*] a speech disorder involving deficient pronunciation of velar speech sounds such as *g* and *k*. Called also *paragammacism*.

Gam•ma•gard (gam′ə-gahrd) trademark for preparations of immune globulin intravenous (human).

gam•ma glob•u•lin (gam′ə glob′u-lin) see under *globulin*.

gam•ma•glob•u•li•nop•a•thy (gam″ə-glob″u-lin-op′ə-the) gammopathy.

gam•ma•gram (gam′ə-gram) a graphic record of the gamma rays emitted by an object or substance.

Gam•ma•her•pes•vi•ri•nae (gam″ə-hur″pēz-vir-I′ne) a subfamily of the Herpesviridae, members of which are specific for either B or T lymphocytes. Genera *Lymphocryptovirus* and *Rhadinovirus* infect humans, and there are a number of unassigned species.

gam•ma-lac•tone (gam″ə-lak′tōn) a compound having a five-membered ring structure formed by internal reaction of a carboxylic acid group with a hydroxyl group on the gamma carbon of a carbon chain.

Gam•ma•pap•il•lo•ma•vi•rus (gam″ə-pap″ĭ-lo′mə-vi″rəs) a genus of viruses of the family Papillomaviridae that contains several of the human papillomaviruses.

Gam•ma•pro•teo•bac•te•ria (gam″ə-pro″te-o-bak-tēr′e-ə) [*gamma* the third letter of the Greek alphabet + *Proteobacteria*] a class of bacteria of the Proteobacteria, grouped together on the basis of 16S rRNA sequence analysis; organisms of medical interest are included in the orders Aeromonadales, Cardiobacteriales, Enterobacteriales, Legionellales, Pasteurellales, Pseudomonadales, Thiotrichales, Vibrionales, and Xanthomonadales.

Gam•ma•ret•ro•vi•rus (gam″mə-ret′ro-vi″rəs) a genus of the family Retroviridae, characterized by a dense, spherical, symmetrically located inner core. These can cause leukemia and other cancers in various animals but not humans; species include feline leukemia virus and murine leukemia virus. **gammaretrovi′ral** *adj*

Gam•mar-P (gam′ahr) trademark for a preparation of immune globulin intravenous (human).

gam•mop•a•thy (gam-op′ə-the) [*gamma* globulin + *-pathy*] a condition marked by disturbed immunoglobulin synthesis.

benign monoclonal g. the presence of a serum M component without signs or symptoms of multiple myeloma, Waldenström macroglobulinemia, or other plasma cell neoplasms; it occurs in about 3 per cent of the population over age 70. A few patients eventually develop a malignant plasma cell dyscrasia. Called also *monoclonal g. of undetermined significance*.

monoclonal g′s plasma cell dyscrasias.

monoclonal g. of undetermined significance (MGUS) benign monoclonal g.

Gam•na disease (gahm′nə) [Carlo *Gamna*, Italian physician, 1896–1950] see under *disease*.

gam(o)- [Gr. *gamos* marriage] a combining form denoting relationship to marriage or sexual union.

gamo•gen•e•sis (gam″o-jen′ə-sis) sexual reproduction. **gamogenet′ic** *adj*

gam•og•o•ny (gam-og′ə-ne) gametogony (def. 1).

gam•one (gam′ōn) 1. a sex hormone released by certain plants. 2. a biological agent released by a gamete to act on gametes of the opposite sex and facilitate fusion and fertilization.

gam•ont (gam′ont) [*gam-* + Gr. *ōn* being] the sexual (gametic) stage in the sporozoan life cycle, produced by gamogony from a trophozoite or a merozoite. Called also *gametocyte*.

gamo•pha•gia (gam″o-fa′jə) [*gamo-* + *-phagia*] the disappearance of the male or female element in the conjugation of unicellular organisms.

gamp•so•dac•ty•ly (gamp″so-dak′tə-le) [Gr. *gampsos* crooked + *daktylos* digit] deformity of the toes marked by hyperextension of the first phalanx on the metatarsal and flexion of the other two phalanges; called also *clawfoot*.

Gam•storp disease (gahm′storp) [Ingrid *Gamstorp*, Swedish pediatrician, born 1924] hyperkalemic periodic paralysis; see under *paralysis*.

Gam•u•lin Rh (gam′u-lin) trademark for a preparation of Rh_0(D) immune globulin.

Gam•u•nex (gam′u-neks) trademark for a preparation of immune globulin intravenous (human).

gan•ci•clo•vir (gan-si′klo-vir) a derivative of acyclovir that inhibits replication of herpesviruses. When used for the treatment of cytomegalovirus infections, ganciclovir is preferentially phosphorylated in infected cells, with the phosphorylated form inhibiting viral DNA synthesis. Administered orally and by intravitreal implant. Called also *DHPG*.

g. sodium the monosodium salt of ganciclovir, used for the treatment of cytomegalovirus retinitis in immunocompromised patients; administered intravenously or by intravitreal injection.

gan•glia (gang′gle-ə) [Gr.] plural of *ganglion*.

gan•gli•al (gang′gle-əl) ganglionic.

gan•gli•at•ed (gang′gle-āt″əd) ganglionated.

gan•gli•ec•to•my (gang″gle-ek′tə-me) ganglionectomy.

gan•gli•form (gang′glĭ-form) having the form of a ganglion.

gan•gli•itis (gang″gle-i′tis) ganglionitis.

gangli(o)- [Gr. *ganglion*, q.v.] a combining form denoting relationship to a ganglion.

gan•glio•blast (gang′gle-o-blast″) [*ganglio-* + *-blast*] an embryonic cell of the cerebrospinal ganglia.

gan•glio•cyte (gang′gle-o-sīt″) [*ganglio-* + *-cyte*] ganglion cell (def. 1).

gan•glio•cy•to•ma (gang″gle-o-si-to′mə) ganglioneuroma.

gan•glio•form (gang′gle-o-form″) gangliform.

gan•glio•gli•o•ma (gang″gle-o-gli-o′mə) a ganglioneuroma in the central nervous system; called also *ganglioglioneuroma* and *neuroglioma ganglionare*.

gan•glio•glio•neu•ro•ma (gang″gle-o-gli″o-nōō-ro′mə) ganglioneuroma.

gan•glio•lyt•ic (gang″gle-o-lit′ik) ganglioplegic.

gan•gli•o•ma (gang″gle-o′mə) [*gangli-* + *-oma*] ganglioneuroma.

gan•gli•on (gang′gle-on) pl. *gang′lia* or *ganglions* [Gr. "knot"] 1. a knot, or knotlike mass. 2. [TA] anatomical terminology for a group of nerve cell bodies located outside the central nervous system; occasionally applied to certain nuclear groups within the brain. 3. a benign cystic tumor occurring on an aponeurosis or tendon, as in the wrist or dorsum of the foot; it consists of a thin fibrous capsule enclosing a clear mucinous fluid.

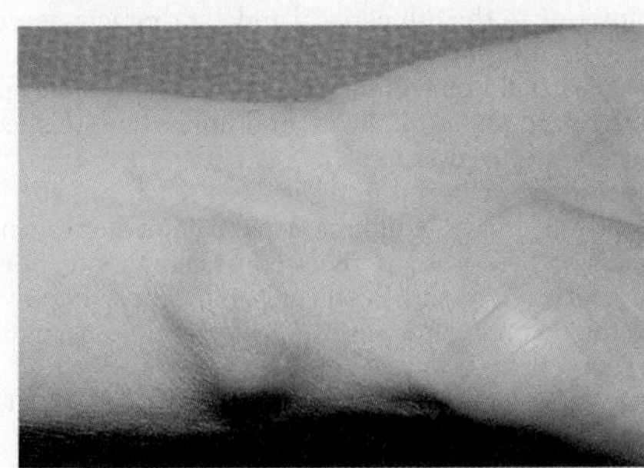

■ Ganglion overlying the wrist joint and flexor tendons.

Ganglion

Descriptions of specific anatomic structures are given on TA terms, and include anglicized names of specific ganglia.

aberrant g. a small ganglion sometimes found on a dorsal cervical nerve root between the spinal ganglia and the spinal cord.
accessory ganglia ganglia intermedia.
acousticofacial g. a ganglion of early embryonic life, a portion of which persists as the geniculate ganglion.
Acrel g. a cystic tumor on an extensor tendon of the wrist.
Andersch g. g. caudalis nervi glossopharyngei.
ganglia aorticorena′lia [TA] aorticorenal ganglia: a more or less detached inferolateral extension of the celiac ganglion.
auditory g. 1. g. cochleare. 2. *(in the pl.)* nuclei cochleares.
Auerbach g. any of the small ganglia of Auerbach plexus.
g. autono′micum [TA] autonomic ganglion: the ganglia found along the sympathetic trunks, on the peripheral plexuses, and within the walls of organs supplied by the autonomic nervous system; they are divided into two structurally similar groups, the sympathetic ganglia and the parasympathetic ganglia. Called also *visceral g.* and *g. viscerale.*
ganglia of autonomic plexuses ganglia plexuum autonomicorum.
basal ganglia see under *nucleus.*
Bezold g. a series of ganglion cells in the interatrial septum.
Bidder ganglia ganglia on the cardiac nerves, situated at the lower end of the atrial septum. Called also *ventricular ganglia.*
Blandin g. g. submandibulare.
Bochdalek g. plexus dentalis superior.
Bock g. carotid g.
gan′glia cardi′aca [TA] cardiac ganglia: ganglia of the cardiac plexus near the arterial ligament; called also *Wrisberg ganglia.*
carotid g. a ganglion of the internal carotid plexus in the cavernous sinus; called also *Bock g.*
caudal g. of glossopharyngeal nerve g. inferius nervi glossopharyngei.
caudal g. of vagus nerve g. inferius nervi vagi.
g. cauda′lis ner′vi glossopharyn′gei g. inferius nervi glossopharyngei.
g. cauda′lis ner′vi va′gi g. inferius nervi vagi.
celiac ganglia, gan′glia celi′aca ganglia coeliaca.
cerebrospinal ganglia the ganglia associated with the cranial and spinal nerves.
cervical g., inferior ganglion cervicale inferioris.
cervical g., middle g. cervicale medium.
cervical g., superior g. cervicale superius.
cervical g. of uterus a ganglion situated near the cervix uteri; called also *Lee g.* and *Frankenhäuser g.*
g. cervica′le inferio′ris [TA] inferior cervical ganglion: an inconstant ganglion formed in place of the usual cervicothoracic ganglion by fusion of the lower two cervical ganglia in instances where the first thoracic ganglion remains separate.
g. cervica′le me′dium [TA] middle cervical ganglion: a variable ganglion, often fused with the vertebral ganglion, on the sympathetic trunk at about the level of the cricoid cartilage; its postganglionic fibers are distributed mainly to the heart, cervical region, and upper limb.
g. cervica′le supe′rius [TA] superior cervical ganglion: the uppermost ganglion on the sympathetic trunk, lying behind the internal carotid artery and in front of the second and third cervical vertebrae; it gives rise to postganglionic fibers to the heart via cervical cardiac nerves, to the pharyngeal plexus and thence to the larynx and pharynx, and to the head via the external and internal carotid plexuses.
g. cervicothora′cicum [TA] cervicothoracic ganglion: a ganglion on the sympathetic trunk at the level of the 7th cervical and 1st thoracic vertebrae, anterior to the 8th cervical and 1st thoracic nerves; it has two components, the inferior cervical and first thoracic ganglia, which are usually fused, partially or completely. Its postganglionic fibers are distributed to the head and neck, heart, and upper limb. Called also *stellate g.* and *g. stellatum* [TA alternative].
cervicouterine g. cervical g. of uterus.
g. cilia′re [TA] ciliary ganglion: a parasympathetic ganglion in the posterior part of the orbit; it receives preganglionic fibers from the oculomotor nerve, and its postganglionic fibers supply the ciliary muscle and the sphincter pupillae. Sensory and postganglionic sympathetic fibers pass through the ganglion.
Cloquet g. an enlargement of the nasopalatine nerve in the anterior palatine canal.
g. cochlea′re [TA] cochlear ganglion: the sensory ganglion located within the spiral canal of the modiolus. It consists of bipolar cells that send fibers peripherally through the foramina nervosa to the spiral organ and centrally through the internal acoustic meatus to the cochlear nuclei of the brainstem. Called also *g. spirale cochleae* [TA alternative], *Corti* or *spiral g.,* and *spiral g. of cochlea.*
gan′glia coelia′ca [TA] celiac ganglia: two irregularly shaped ganglia, one on each crus of the diaphragm, within the celiac plexus; each contains sympathetic nerve cells and preganglionic sympathetic fibers from the greater and lesser splanchnic nerves: preganglionic parasympathetic and sensory fibers pass through the ganglia. Called also *ganglia celiaca.*
collateral ganglia prevertebral ganglia.
compound g. a cystic tumor of a tendon sheath that has been compressed into two parts by a ligament.
Corti g. g. cochleare.
cranial sensory g. g. sensorium nervi cranialis.
g. craniospina′le senso′rium [TA] craniospinal sensory ganglion: the ganglia sensoria nervorum spinalium and the ganglia sensoria nervorum cranialium considered together.
diffuse g. a swelling of several adjoining tendon sheaths due to inflammatory effusion.
dorsal root g. g. sensorium nervi spinalis.
Ehrenritter g. g. superius nervi glossopharyngei.
gan′glia encepha′lica g. sensorium nervi cranialis.
encephalospinal g., g. encephalospina′le g. craniospinale sensorium.
false g. an enlargement on a nerve that does not have a true ganglionic structure.
first thoracic g. a portion of the ganglion cervicothoracicum, present sometimes as a separate ganglion.
Frankenhäuser g. cervical g. of uterus.
Froriep g. the ganglion of the lowest occipital segment in the human embryo.
Gasser g., gasserian g. g. trigeminale.
geniculate g. g. geniculi nervi facialis.
g. genicula′tum ner′vi facia′lis TA alternative for *g. geniculi nervi facialis.*
g. geni′culi ner′vi facia′lis [TA] the sensory ganglion of the facial nerve, situated on the geniculum of the facial nerve. Called also *geniculate g.* and *g. geniculatum nervi facialis* [TA alternative].
glossopharyngeal ganglia, ganglia of glossopharyngeal nerve see *g. inferius nervi glossopharyngei* and *g. superius nervi glossopharyngei.*
hepatic g. a ganglion situated near the hepatic artery.
hypogastric ganglia ganglia pelvica.
hypoglossal g. a ganglion of the hypoglossal nerve; rarely found in humans except in the embryo.
g. im′par [TA] the ganglion commonly found in front of the coccyx, where the sympathetic trunks of the two sides unite.
inferior g. of glossopharyngeal nerve g. inferius nervi glossopharyngei.
inferior g. of vagus nerve g. inferius nervi vagi.
g. infe′rius ner′vi glossopharyn′gei [TA] inferior ganglion of glossopharyngeal nerve: the lower of two ganglia on the glossopharyngeal nerve as it passes through the jugular foramen; it contains cell bodies for some of the afferent fibers of the nerve. See also *g. superius nervi glossopharyngei.* Called also *g. caudalis nervi glossopharyngei, caudal g. of glossopharyngeal nerve, inferior petrosal g., petrosal g.,* and *petrous g.*
g. infe′rius ner′vi va′gi [TA] inferior ganglion of vagus nerve: a ganglion of the vagus nerve just below the jugular foramen, in front of the transverse processes of the first and second cervical vertebrae; it contains cell bodies for some of the afferent fibers of the nerve. Called also *caudal g. of vagus nerve, g. caudalis nervi vagi,* and *nodose g.* See also *g. superius nervi vagi.*
inhibitory g. any ganglion performing an inhibitory function.
gan′glia interme′dia [TA] intermediate ganglia: small groups of sympathetic nerve cells present on spinal nerves and on rami communicantes, especially in the cervical, lower thoracic, and upper lumbar regions; called also *accessory ganglia.*

Ganglion *Continued*

jugular g. of glossopharyngeal nerve g. superius nervi glossopharyngei.
jugular g. of vagus nerve g. superius nervi vagi.
Langley g. a collection of nerve cells in the hilus of the submaxillary gland in some animals.
Laumonier g. carotid g.
Lee g. cervical g. of uterus.
lesser g. of Meckel g. submandibulare.
Lobstein g. g. thoracicus splanchnicum.
lower g. of glossopharyngeal nerve g. inferius nervi glossopharyngei.
Ludwig g. a ganglion connected with the cardiac plexus and situated near the right atrium of the heart.
gan′glia lumba′lia [TA] lumbar ganglia: the ganglia on the lumbar part of the sympathetic trunk, usually four or five on either side. Called also *ganglia lumbaria* [TA alternative].
gan′glia lumba′ria TA alternative for *ganglia lumbalia.*
Meckel g. g. pterygopalatinum.
Meissner g. one of the small groups of nerve cells in the submucosal (Meissner) plexus.
mesenteric g., inferior g. mesentericum inferius.
mesenteric g., superior g. mesentericum superius.
g. mesente′ricum infe′rius [TA] inferior mesenteric ganglion: a sympathetic ganglion in the inferior mesenteric plexus near the beginning of the inferior mesenteric artery.
g. mesente′ricum supe′rius [TA] superior mesenteric ganglion: one or more sympathetic ganglia at the sides of, or just below, the superior mesenteric artery; commonly fused with the celiac ganglia.
g. of Müller g. superius nervi glossopharyngei.
nerve g. ganglion (def. 2).
g. ner′vi splanch′nici g. thoracicum splanchnicum.
neural g. ganglion (def. 2).
nodose g. g. inferius nervi vagi.
olfactory g. a mass of tissue in the embryo that develops into the olfactory nerves.
g. o′ticum [TA] otic ganglion: a parasympathetic ganglion in the infratemporal fossa, medial to the mandibular nerve and just inferior to the foramen ovale: its preganglionic fibers are derived from the glossopharyngeal nerve via the lesser petrosal nerve, and its postganglionic fibers supply the parotid gland. Sensory and postganglionic sympathetic fibers pass through the ganglion.
parasympathetic g., g. parasympathe′ticum g. parasympathicum.
g. parasympa′thicum [TA] parasympathetic ganglion: one of the aggregations of cell bodies of primarily cholinergic neurons of the parasympathetic nervous system, located near, on, or within the wall of the organs being innervated; see also *cholinergic.*
gan′glia pel′vica [TA] pelvic ganglia: small sympathetic and parasympathetic ganglia located within the pelvic plexus.
gan′glia pelvi′na ganglia pelvica.
petrosal g., petrosal g., inferior, petrous g. g. inferius nervi glossopharyngei.
gan′glia phre′nica [TA] phrenic ganglia: any of various small sympathetic ganglia often found within the phrenic plexus at its junction with the celiac plexus.
gan′glia plex′uum autonomico′rum ganglia of autonomic plexuses: groups of nerve cell bodies found in the autonomic plexuses, composed primarily of sympathetic postganglionic neurons; called also *ganglia of visceral plexuses.*
gan′glia plex′uum viscera′lium ganglia plexuum autonomicorum.
posterior root g. g. sensorium nervi spinalis.
prevertebral ganglia sympathetic ganglia (other than those of the sympathetic trunk) in the prevertebral plexuses of the thorax and abdomen.
primary g. a ganglion on a tendon or aponeurosis that does not follow a local inflammation.
g. pterygopalati′num [TA] pterygopalatine ganglion: a parasympathetic ganglion in the pterygopalatine fossa; its preganglionic fibers are derived from the facial nerve via the greater petrosal nerve and the nerve of the pterygopalatine canal. Its postganglionic fibers supply the lacrimal, nasal, and palatine glands; sensory and sympathetic fibers pass through the ganglion. Called also *Meckel, sphenomaxillary,* or *sphenopalatine g.*
Remak g. 1. a sympathetic ganglion in the heart wall near the superior vena cava; called also *sinoatrial g.* 2. one of the sympathetic ganglia in the diaphragmatic opening for the inferior vena cava. 3. one of the ganglia in the gastric plexus.
gan′glia rena′lia [TA] renal ganglia: small sympathetic ganglia within the renal plexus.
Ribes g. a small ganglion sometimes seen in the termination of the internal carotid plexus around the anterior communicating artery of the brain.
rostral g. of glossopharyngeal nerve g. superius nervi glossopharyngei.
rostral g. of vagus nerve g. superius nervi vagi.
g. rostra′lis ner′vi glossopharyn′gei g. superius nervi glossopharyngei.
g. rostra′lis ner′vi va′gi g. superius nervi vagi.
gan′glia sacra′lia [TA] sacral ganglia: the ganglia of the sacral part of the sympathetic trunk, usually three or four on either side.
Scarpa g. g. vestibulare.
Schmiedel g. carotid g.
semilunar g. 1. ganglion trigeminale. 2. *(in the pl.)* ganglia coeliaca.
g. sensoria′le sensory g.; see *g. craniospinale sensorium, g. sensorium nervi cranialis,* and *g. sensorium nervi spinalis.*
g. senso′rium ner′vi crania′lis [TA] sensory ganglion of cranial nerve: the ganglion found on the root of each cranial nerve, containing the cell bodies of afferent (sensory) neurons. Called also *cranial sensory g.*
g. senso′rium ner′vi spina′lis [TA] spinal ganglion: the ganglion found on the posterior root of each spinal nerve, composed of the unipolar nerve cell bodies of the sensory neurons of the nerve. Called also *g. spinale* and *dorsal* or *posterior root g.*
sensory g. see *g. craniospinale sensorium, g. sensorium nervi cranialis,* and *g. sensorium nervi spinalis.*
sensory g. of cranial nerve, sensory g. of encephalic nerve g. sensorium nervi cranialis.
simple g. a cystic tumor in a tendon sheath.
sinoatrial g. Remak g. (def. 1).
sinus g. a group of nerve cells around the junction of the coronary sinus and the right atrium of the heart.
sphenomaxillary g., sphenopalatine g. g. pterygopalatinum.
spinal g., g. spina′le g. sensorium nervi spinalis.
spiral g., spiral g. of cochlea, spiral g. of cochlear nerve g. cochleare.
g. spira′le coch′leae TA alternative for *g. cochleare.*
splanchnic g., splanchnic thoracic g., g. splanch′nicum g. thoracicum splanchnicum.
stellate g. g. cervicothoracicum.
g. stella′tum TA alternative for *g. cervicothoracicum.*
g. sublingua′le [TA] sublingual ganglion: a ganglion of nerve cells sometimes found on the fibers passing distally from the submandibular ganglion to the lingual nerve.
g. submandibula′re [TA] submandibular ganglion: a parasympathetic ganglion located superior to the deep part of the submandibular gland, on the lateral surface of the hyoglossus muscle; its preganglionic fibers are derived from the facial nerve by way of the chorda tympani and lingual nerve, and its postganglionic fibers supply the

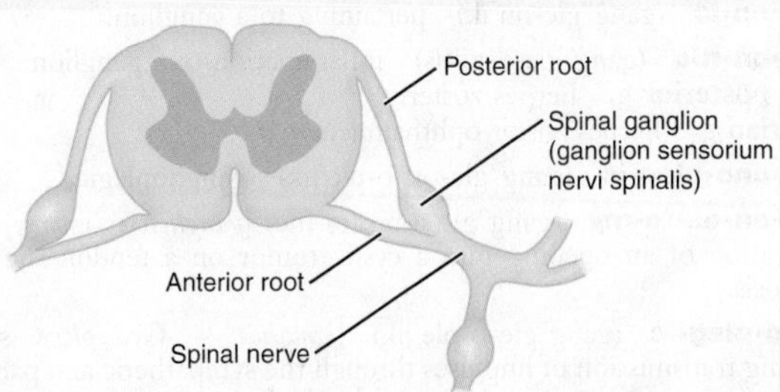

■ Ganglion sensorium nervi spinalis (spinal ganglion), seen in a cross-section of the spinal cord.

Ganglion *Continued*

submandibular and sublingual glands; sensory and postganglionic sympathetic fibers pass through the ganglion.

superior g. of glossopharyngeal nerve g. superius nervi glossopharyngei.

superior g. of vagus nerve g. superius nervi vagi.

g. supe′rius ner′vi glossopharyn′gei [TA] superior ganglion of glossopharyngeal nerve: the upper of two ganglia on the glossopharyngeal nerve as it passes through the jugular foramen; it contains cell bodies for some of the afferent fibers of the nerve. Called also *jugular g. of glossopharyngeal nerve, rostral g. of glossopharyngeal nerve,* and *g. rostralis nervi glossopharyngei.* See also *g. inferius nervi glossopharyngei.*

g. supe′rius ner′vi va′gi [TA] superior ganglion of vagus nerve: a small ganglion on the vagus nerve in the jugular foramen, giving off a meningeal and an auricular branch and containing cell bodies for some of the afferent fibers of the nerve. Called also *rostral g. of vagus nerve, g. rostralis nervi vagi,* and *jugular g. of vagus nerve.* See also *g. inferius nervi vagi.*

suprarenal g. a small sympathetic ganglion in the suprarenal plexus.

ganglia of sympathetic trunk ganglia trunci sympathetici.

g. sympathe′ticum, g. sympa′thicum [TA] sympathetic ganglion: any of the aggregations of cell bodies of primarily adrenergic neurons of the sympathetic nervous system, including the ganglia of the sympathetic trunks, the intermediate ganglia, the prevertebral ganglia, and some ganglionic cells in the autonomic plexuses. See also *adrenergic.*

synovial g. digital mucous cyst.

g. termina′le [TA] terminal ganglion: a group of nerve cells found along the terminal nerves, medial to the olfactory bulb.

gan′glia thoraca′lia ganglia thoracica.

gan′glia thora′cica [TA] thoracic ganglia: the ganglia on the thoracic portion of the sympathetic trunk, about eleven or twelve on either side.

g. thora′cicum splanch′nicum [TA] splanchnic thoracic ganglion: a small ganglion formed on the greater thoracic splanchnic nerve near the twelfth thoracic vertebra; called also *ganglion splanchnicum* and *splanchnic g.*

g. of trigeminal nerve, g. trigemina′le [TA] trigeminal ganglion: one on the sensory root of the fifth cranial nerve, situated in a cleft within the dura mater (trigeminal cave) on the anterior surface of the petrous portion of the temporal bone. It gives off the ophthalmic and maxillary nerves and part of the mandibular nerve, and contains the cells of origin of most of the sensory fibers of the trigeminal nerve. Called also *Gasser g., gasserian g.,* and *semilunar g.*

Troisier g. signal node.

gan′glia trun′ci sympathe′tici, gan′glia trun′ci sympa′thici [TA] ganglia of sympathetic trunk: sympathetic ganglia that are arranged in a chainlike fashion along each sympathetic trunk, about twenty to twenty-three on either side.

tympanic g. intumescentia tympanica.

tympanic g. of Valentin 1. a ganglion on a superior dental nerve. 2. intumescentia tympanica.

g. tympa′nicum TA alternative for *intumescentia tympanica.*

vagal g., inferior g. inferius nervi vagi.

vagal g., superior g. superius nervi vagi.

Valentin g. 1. intumescentia tympanica. 2. a ganglion on a superior dental nerve.

ventricular ganglia Bidder ganglia.

g. vertebra′le [TA] vertebral ganglion: a small ganglion almost always present between the middle and inferior sympathetic ganglia, usually anterior to the vertebral artery; it contributes to the ansa subclavia and sends postganglionic fibers to the vertebral nerve and plexus and to the brachial plexus.

g. vestibula′re [TA] vestibular ganglion: the sensory ganglion located in the upper part of the lateral end of the internal acoustic meatus, the bipolar nerve cells of which give rise to the fibers of the vestibular nerve.

visceral g., g. viscera′le g. autonomicum.

ganglia of visceral plexuses ganglia plexuum autonomicorum.

Wrisberg ganglia ganglia cardiaca.

wrist g. cystic enlargement of a tendon sheath on the back of the wrist.

---

gan·gli·on·at·ed (gang′gle-ə-nāt″əd) provided with ganglia. Called also *gangliated.*

gan·gli·on·ec·to·my (gang″gle-ə-nek′tə-me) [*ganglion* + *-ectomy*] excision of a ganglion. Called also *gangliectomy.*

gan·glio·neu·ro·blas·to·ma (gang″gle-o-noor″o-blas-to′mə) a tumor with elements of both ganglioneuroma and neuroblastoma; regarded as a partially differentiated neuroblastoma.

gan·glio·neu·ro·fi·bro·ma (gang″gle-o-noor″o-fi-bro′mə) a ganglioneuroma outside of the central nervous system.

gan·glio·neu·ro·ma (gang″gle-o-noo̅-ro′mə) a benign neoplasm composed of nerve fibers and mature ganglion cells; regarded by many as a fully differentiated neuroblastoma. Called also *gangliocytoma, ganglioma, neurocytoma,* and *ganglionar, ganglionated,* or *ganglionic neuroma.* See also *ganglioglioma* and *ganglioneurofibroma.*

gan·glio·neu·ro·ma·to·sis (gang″gle-o-noo̅-ro″mə-to′sis) overgrowth of nerve tissue in the walls of the upper gastrointestinal tract, seen in some patients with neurofibromatosis I or multiple endocrine neoplasia type III.

gan·gli·on·ic (gang″gle-on′ik) pertaining to a ganglion.

gan·gli·on·itis (gang″gle-ə-ni′tis) inflammation of a ganglion.

acute posterior g. herpes zoster.

gasserian g. herpes zoster ophthalmicus.

gan·gli·ono·pleg·ic (gang″gle-on″o-ple′jik) ganglioplegic.

gan·gli·on·os·to·my (gang″gle-ə-nos′tə-me) [*ganglion* + *-ostomy*] surgical creation of an opening into a cystic tumor on a tendon sheath or aponeurosis.

gan·glio·pleg·ic (gang″gle-o-ple′jik) [*ganglio-* + Gr. *plēgē* stroke] 1. blocking transmission of impulses through the sympathetic and parasympathetic ganglia. 2. an agent with ganglioplegic activity.

gan·glio·side (gang′gle-o-sīd″) any of a group of glycosphingolipids in which the polar head group on ceramide is a sialic acid–containing oligosaccharide linked via a glucose residue; they occur predominantly in tissues of the central nervous system. The most basic core structure is ceramide-glucose-galactose-*N*-acetylneuraminic acid.

g. G_{M1} a ganglioside structurally similar to ganglioside GM_2 but with an additional galactose residue linked to the *N*-acetylgalactosamine residue of GM_2; it accumulates abnormally in tissues in GM_1 gangliosidoses.

g. G_{M2} a ganglioside containing an *N*-acetylgalactosamine residue linked to the galactose of the core structure; it accumulates abnormally in tissues in GM_2 gangliosidoses.

gan·gli·o·si·do·sis (gang″gle-o-si-do′sis) pl. *gangliosido′ses.* Any of a group of lysosomal storage diseases generally characterized by abnormal accumulation of ganglioside GM_1 or GM_2 and related glycoconjugates due to a deficiency of specific lysosomal hydrolases, and by progressive psychomotor deterioration usually beginning in infancy or childhood and usually fatal. Two subgroups exist (GM_1 and GM_2), each having several forms of varying severity.

generalized g. GM_1 g., usually specifically the infantile form.

GM_1 g. an autosomal recessive disorder due to a deficiency of lysosomal β-galactosidase activity as a result of mutation in the *GLB1* gene (locus: 21.33), with accumulation of ganglioside GM_1, glycoproteins, and keratan sulfate. It occurs as several forms, decreasing in severity with increasing age of onset. The *infantile,* or *type I,* form is characterized by onset at birth, severe retardation of mental and motor development, cerebral degeneration, dysostosis multiplex, hepatosplenomegaly, early blindness, coarse facies, edema, seizures, hypotonia, hyperacusis, dysarthria, and sometimes cherry-red macular spot; death occurs by the age of 2. The *juvenile,* or *type II,* form is characterized by onset between 6 and 20 months, accumulation of ganglioside GM_1 in brain but not viscera, seizures, late blindness, spasticity, and ataxia; death occurs between 3 and 10 years of age. The *adult,* or *type III,* form is characterized by onset in the teens, spasticity, and dysarthria, with little intellectual impairment and survival into the third decade.

GM_2 g. any of a group of lysosomal storage diseases characterized by abnormal accumulation of ganglioside GM_2 and related glycoconjugates, due to deficiency of activity of one or more hexosaminidase isozymes or of an activator protein necessary for enzyme activity.

GM_2 g., type I Tay-Sachs disease; often specifically the classic infantile form.

GM_2 g., type II Sandhoff disease.

GM_2 g., type III the juvenile form of Tay-Sachs disease.

GM_2 g., 0 variant Sandhoff disease.

GM_2 g., AB variant a GM_2 gangliosidosis caused by mutation in the *GM2A*gene (locus: 5q31.3-q33.1), which encodes GM_2 activator protein, a sphingolipid activator protein necessary for hexosaminidase A activity; this variant is clinically identical to infantile Tay-Sachs disease.

GM_2 g., B variant Tay-Sachs disease.

gan•glio•spore (gang′gle-o-spor″) [*ganglion* + *spore*] a type of aleuriospore developed from the swollen tip of a hypha.

gan•glio•sym•pa•thec•to•my (gang″le-o-sim″pə-thek′tə-me) excision of a sympathetic ganglion.

gan•grene (gang′grēn) [L. *gangraena;* Gr. *gangraina* an eating sore] death of tissue, usually in considerable mass and generally associated with loss of vascular (nutritive) supply; it can be followed by bacterial invasion and putrefaction (wet gangrene). Cf. *necrosis* and *necrobiosis.* **gang′renous** *adj*

atherosclerotic g. dry gangrene caused by vascular sclerosis.

circumscribed g. gangrene that is clearly separated from normal tissue by a zone of inflammatory reaction.

cold g. gangrene that is not preceded by inflammation.

diabetic g. moist gangrene, usually of the feet, in persons with diabetes mellitus, due to neuropathy, angiopathy, and other complications. Cf. *diabetic ulcer.*

dry g. necrosis occurring without subsequent bacterial decomposition, the tissues becoming dry and shriveled.

embolic g. gangrene following the blocking of the blood supply by an embolism.

emphysematous g. gas g.

Fournier g. an acute gangrenous type of necrotizing fasciitis of the scrotum, penis, or perineum involving gram-positive organisms, enteric bacilli, or anaerobes; it may occur following local trauma, operative procedures, an underlying urinary tract disease, or a distant acute inflammatory process. Called also *Fournier disease.*

gas g., gaseous g. 1. an acute, severe, painful condition, often resulting from dirty, lacerated wounds, with muscles and subcutaneous tissues becoming filled with gas and a serosanguineous exudate. The condition is due to infection by anaerobic bacteria, among which are *Clostridium perfringens, C. novyi, C. septicum, C. sporogenes,* and other species of *Clostridium.* Called also *clostridial myonecrosis.* 2. a similar condition in domestic animals, such as occurs with malignant edema, blackleg, and braxy.

hot g. gangrene that follows an inflammation.

humid g. moist g.

inflammatory g. gangrene due to acute inflammation.

Meleney g. see under *ulcer.*

Meleney synergistic g. progressive synergistic g.

moist g. wet g.

pressure g. gangrene due to pressure, as in decubitus ulcer.

primary g. gangrene without preceding inflammation of the part.

progressive g. gangrene in which an effective limiting zone of inflammatory reaction does not form.

progressive bacterial synergistic g., progressive synergistic g., progressive synergistic bacterial g. gangrene of the skin due to synergistic infection by bacteria such as aerobic hemolytic *Staphylococcus aureus,* microaerophilic nonhemolytic streptococci, or gram-negative rods; it occurs most often as a complication of abdominal surgery, thoracic surgery, or a traumatic wound. The characteristic lesion is a wide area of cellulitis that later ulcerates and enlarges to form a plaque with central granulation surrounded by gangrenous skin having an undermined, rolled, darker border. See also *Meleney ulcer* (def. 1). Called also *burrowing phagedenic ulcer, Meleney ulcer, Meleney synergistic g.,* and *undermining burrowing ulcer.*

pulp g. gangrenous pulp necrosis.

Raynaud g. Raynaud disease (def. 1).

secondary g. gangrene following local inflammation.

senile g. dry gangrene affecting the extremities of the elderly.

static g. gangrene that results from stasis of blood in a part.

■ Extensive gas gangrene due to *Clostridium perfringens* that has developed in an untreated knife wound.

symmetric g. gangrene of corresponding digits on both sides, due to vasomotor disturbances.

sympathetic g. gangrene that results from some primary condition.

thrombotic g. gangrene from thrombosis of an artery.

traumatic g. gangrene caused by accidental injury.

venous g. static g.

wet g. necrosis of tissues, with proteolytic decomposition resulting from bacterial action; called also *moist g.*

gan•gre•no•sis (gang″rə-no′sis) the development of gangrene.

gan•i•re•lix ac•e•tate (gan″ĭ-rel′iks) a synthetic decapeptide derived from, and an antagonist to, gonadotropin-releasing hormone; used to inhibit premature luteinizing hormone surges in women undergoing ovarian hyperstimulation in treatment of female factor infertility, administered subcutaneously.

Gan•ite (gan′īt) trademark for a preparation of gallium nitrate.

gan•o•blast (gan′o-blast) ameloblast.

Gan•ser commissure, syndrome (gahn′sər) [Sigbert Joseph Maria *Ganser,* German psychiatrist, 1853–1931] see under *syndrome,* and see *supraoptic commissures,* under *commissure.*

Gan•ta•nol (gan′tə-nol) trademark for a preparation of sulfamethoxazole.

Gan•tri•sin (gan′trĭ-sin) trademark for preparations of sulfisoxazole.

gap (gap) 1. hiatus. 2. an unoccupied interval in time.

air-bone g. the lag between the audiographic curves for air- and bone-conducted stimuli, as an indication of a conductive hearing loss.

anion g. the concentration of plasma anions not routinely measured by laboratory screening, accounting for the difference between the routinely measured anions and cations and equal to the plasma sodium − (chloride + bicarbonate); used in the evaluation of acid-base disorders.

auscultatory g. time in which sound is not heard in the auscultatory method of sphygmomanometry, occurring particularly in hypertension and in aortic stenosis.

Bochdalek g. hiatus pleuroperitonealis.

excitable g. in cardiology, the area of repolarized, excitable tissue that can exist between the head of an approaching depolarizing wavefront and the tail of that preceding.

interocclusal g. see under *distance.*

silent g. auscultatory g.

urinary anion g. the amount of urinary anion not routinely measured by laboratory screening, which accounts for the difference between the routinely measured anion and cation, equal to sodium + potassium − chloride. It is an indirect measure of ammonium excretion and is used in the evaluation of hyperchloremic acidosis.

GAPD glyceraldehyde-3-phosphate dehydrogenase.

gapes (gāps) infestation of the trachea of birds by the gapeworm *Syngamus trachea,* which causes gasping and choking.

gape•worm (gāp′wərm) *Syngamus trachea.*

Ga•ra•my•cin (gar″ə-mi′sin) trademark for preparations of gentamicin sulfate.

gar•ban•zo (gahr-bahn′zo) [Sp.] chickpea.

Gar•cin syndrome (gahr-să′) [Raymond *Garcin,* French physician, 1897–1971] see under *syndrome.*

Gar•da•sil (gahr′də-sil) trademark for a preparation of human papillomavirus quadrivalent vaccine, recombinant.

Gard•ner syndrome (gahrd′nər) [Eldon John *Gardner,* American geneticist, 1909–1989] see under *syndrome.*

Gard•ner-Dia•mond syndrome (gahrd′nər di′ah-mənd) [Frank H. *Gardner,* American physician, born 1919; Louis Klein *Diamond,* American pediatrician, 1902–1999] painful bruising syndrome.

Gard•ner•el•la (gahrd″nər-el′ə) [H.L. *Gardner,* American bacteriologist] a genus of small, pleomorphic, gram-negative, rod-shaped bacteria of the family Bifidobacteriaceae, found in the normal female genital tract and also as a major cause of bacterial vaginitis. It comprises a single species, *G. vagina′lis.* Formerly called *Haemophilus vaginalis.*

Garg. [L.] gargaris′ma (gargle).

gar•gal•an•es•the•sia (gahr″gəl-an″es-the′zhə) absence or loss of gargalesthesia.

gar•gal•es•the•sia (gahr″gəl-es-the′zhə) [Gr. *gargalos* itching + *esthesia*] the perception of tickling (q.v.). **gargalesthet′ic** *adj*

gar•get (gahr′gət) bovine mastitis.

gar•gle (gahr′gəl) [L. *gargarisma*] 1. to agitate a solution in the throat by forcing air through it so as to rinse or medicate the mucous membranes. 2. a solution used for rinsing or medicating the mouth and throat.

gar•goyl•ism (gahr′goil-iz-əm) Hurler syndrome.

Gar•land triangle (gahr′lənd) [George Minot *Garland,* American physician, 1848–1926] see under *triangle.*

gar•lic (gahr′lik) 1. *Allium sativum,* a flowering plant with a bulbous stem base. 2. [NF] the bulbous stem base of *A. sativum,* containing the antibacterial sulfur ester derivative allicin; preparations of the dried or fresh bulbs are used for hyperlipidemia, hypertension, and arteriosclerosis. It is also commonly used in folk medicine as an antitussive, antiseptic, rubefacient, diaphoretic, toothache and earache remedy, vermifuge, and aid in nervous conditions.

gar•ment (gahr′mənt) an article of clothing.

pneumatic antishock g. an inflatable garment used to combat shock, stabilize fractures, promote hemostasis, increase peripheral vascular resistance, and permit autotransfusion of small amounts of blood.

pressure g. a garment that applies continual pressure over large areas of healing skin after burns, trauma, and surgical intervention; worn continually for several months to a year, it limits the hypertrophy and contraction of scar tissue.

gar•net (gahr′nət) a silicate of any combination of aluminum, cobalt, magnesium, iron, and manganese. Garnet particles are one of the abrasives commonly used on dental disks.

Gar•ré osteomyelitis (disease, osteitis) (gah-ra′) [Karl *Garré,* Swiss surgeon, 1857–1928] sclerosing nonsuppurative osteomyelitis; see under *osteomyelitis.*

Gart•ner cyst, duct (canal) (gahrt′nər) [Hermann Treschow *Gartner,* Danish surgeon and anatomist, 1785–1827] see under *cyst,* and see *ductus longitudinalis epoöphori.*

Gärt•ner tonometer (gert′nər) [Gustav *Gärtner,* Austrian pathologist, 1855–1937] see under *tonometer.*

gas (gas) any elastic aeriform fluid in which the molecules are separated from one another and so have free paths.

alveolar g. (A) the gas in the alveoli of the lungs, where gaseous exchange with the capillary blood takes place; called also *alveolar air.*

blood g's the partial pressures of oxygen and carbon dioxide in blood; see under *analysis.*

expired g. gas exhaled from the lungs, especially a mixture of gas from the dead space and alveolar gas.

hemolytic g. arsine.

inert g. a gas that does not react chemically with the other constituents of a system, especially in reference to the noble gases, such as helium and argon.

lacrimator g. tear g.

laughing g. nitrous oxide.

mustard g. dichlorodiethyl sulfide.

noble g. the gas elements of group VIII of the periodic table, i.e., helium, neon, argon, krypton, xenon, and radon.

pepper g. a powdered form of capsicum, used as a tear gas; as a liquid aerosol it is called *pepper spray.*

sneezing g. diphenylchlorarsine.

suffocating g. any of several war gases, such as phosgene, causing intense irritation of the bronchial tubes and lungs that results in pulmonary edema.

tear g. a gas that produces severe lacrimation by irritating the conjunctivae.

vesicating g. dichlorodiethyl sulfide.

war g. any noxious gas manufactured for possible use in warfare.

gas•e•ous (gash′əs) of the nature of a gas.

gas•e•ous•ness (gas′e-əs-nis, gash′əs-nis) burbulence.

gas•i•form (gas′ĭ-form) gaseous.

gas•kin (gas′kin) the part of the upper leg of the horse between the stifle joint and the hock, equivalent to the human calf.

gas•o•gen•ic (gas-o-jen′ik) producing gas.

gas•om•e•ter (gas-om′ə-tər) a calibrated container for measuring the volume of gases.

gas•om•e•try (gas-om′ə-tre) [*gas* + *-metry*] the determination of the amounts of various gases present in a mixture. **gasomet′ric** *adj*

Gas•ser ganglion (gahs′ər) [Johann Laurentius *Gasser,* Austrian professor, 1725–1765] ganglion trigeminale.

Gas•ser syndrome (gahs′ər) [Konrad Joseph *Gasser,* Swiss pediatrician, 20th century] hemolytic uremic syndrome; see under *syndrome.*

gas•se•ri•an (gə-se′re-ən) named for Johann Laurentius *Gasser.*

gas•ter (gas′tər) [Gr. *gastēr* the stomach] [TA] stomach: the musculomembranous expansion of the alimentary tract between the esophagus and the duodenum. The proximal portion is the *cardia;* the portion above the entrance of the esophagus is the *fundus;* the distal portion is the *pyloric part;* and the *body* is between the fundus and the pyloric part. The upper concave surface or edge is the *lesser curvature,* and the lower convex edge is the *greater curvature.* The stomach wall has four coats or layers: an outer, peritoneal, or *serous coat (tunica serosa gastrica);* a *muscular coat (tunica muscularis gastrica),* made up of longitudinal, oblique, and circular fibers; a *submucosa (tela submucosa gastrica);* and the *mucosa tunica mucosa gastrica* that forms the inner lining. Gastric glands, found in the mucosa, secrete gastric juice into the cavity of the stomach; it contains hydrochloric acid, pepsin, and various other digestive enzymes. Food mixed with this juice forms a semifluid substance called chyme that is suitable for further digestion by the intestine. Called also *ventriculus.*

Gas•tero•my•ce•tes (gas″tər-o-mi-se′tēz) [*gaster* + Gr. *mykēs* fungus] in some systems of classification, a class of perfect fungi of the subphylum Basidiomycotina; it includes the order Lycoperdales. In other classifications its members are placed in the class Holobasidiomycetes.

Gas•ter•oph•i•lus (gas″tər-of′ĭ-ləs) [*gaster* + Gr. *philein* to love] a genus of botflies of the family Oestridae; the adults do not eat and die soon after laying their eggs on the hairs of the host. The eggs hatch into larvae that migrate through the skin and internal organs of the host.

G. haemorrhoida′lis the nose botfly, a species with red orange terminal segments whose larvae usually infest the facial skin and pharynx of horses and migrate to the stomach; they sometimes attack humans.

G. intestina′lis the most common species of *Gasterophilus;* its larvae usually infest the legs of horses. On their occasional human hosts, migration of their larvae beneath the skin causes larva migrans.

G. nasa′lis the throat botfly, a species whose larvae infest horses and migrate from the mouth down to the duodenum.

gas•trad•e•ni•tis (gas″trad-ə-ni′tis) [*gastr-* + *adenitis*] inflammation of the stomach glands; called also *gastroadenitis.*

gas•tral•gia (gas-tral′jə) [*gastr-* + *-algia*] pain in the stomach; called also *gastrodynia.*

gas•tral•go•ke•no•sis (gas-tral″go-kə-no′sis) [*gastr-* + *algo-* + *keno-* + *-sis*] paroxysmal gastric pain when the stomach is empty, which is easily relieved by taking food.

gas•trec•to•my (gas-trek′tə-me) [*gastr-* + *-ectomy*] excision of all *(total g.)* or part *(subtotal* or *partial g.)* of the stomach. Called also *gastric resection.*

Billroth g. Billroth operation.

sleeve g. a surgical procedure for morbid obesity consisting of removal of the inferior part of the stomach so that the remainder is shaped like a banana or sleeve.

gas•tric (gas′trik) [L. *gastricus;* Gr. *gastēr* stomach] 1. pertaining to or affecting the stomach. 2. originating in the stomach.

gas•tric ac•id (gas′trik) the hydrochloric acid that is secreted by glands in the stomach wall and forms part of the gastric juice.

gas•tric•sin (gas-trik′sin) [EC 3.4.23.3] EC nomenclature for *pepsin C.*

gas•trin (gas′trin) any of several polypeptide hormones released from peptidergic fibers in the vagus nerve and from G cells in the pyloric glands of the gastric antrum. Forms include *little gastrins* (G_{17}, chain lengths of 17 amino acids), *big gastrins* (G_{34}, chain lengths of 34), and *minigastrins* (G_{14}, chain lengths of 14). Gastrin stimulates secretion of gastric acid, causing contraction of the lower esophageal sphincter and modifying gastric and esophageal motility; increases growth of acid-secreting mucosa cells; and weakly stimulates secretion of pancreatic enzymes and gallbladder contraction.

fasting serum g. measurement of the levels of gastrin in blood serum after the patient has fasted for 12 hours, so that presence of food is not a factor; it is markedly increased in conditions such as Zollinger-Ellison syndrome and G cell hyperplasia.

gas•tri•no•ma (gas″trĭ-no′mə) a tumor that secretes gastrin. Most are islet cell tumors of cells other than the beta cells; some are found at sites such as the antrum of the stomach, the hilum of the spleen, or regional lymph nodes. This is the usual cause of Zollinger-Ellison syndrome.

gas•tri•tis (gas-tri′tis) [*gastr-* + *-itis*] inflammation of the stomach. **gastrit′ic** *adj*

acute g. acute inflammation of the gastric mucosa with edema, hyperemia, and infiltration by polymorphonuclear leukocytes; it may be transient or it may develop into acute erosive gastritis.

acute erosive g., acute hemorrhagic g. acute gastritis involving erosions of the full thickness of the stomach mucosa, usually with some degree of hemorrhaging; it may be either localized or diffuse.

alkaline reflux g. chronic gastritis caused by reflux of alkaline intestinal contents after partial gastrectomy.

antral g., antrum g. the usual type of type B gastritis, found in the antrum of the stomach.

atrophic g. a type of chronic nonerosive gastritis characterized by infiltration of the lamina propria by inflammatory cells, similar to superficial gastritis but involving the entire mucosa. The amount of chief cells and parietal cells decreases, lymphoid nodules may be present, the total thickness of the mucosa decreases, and intestinal metaplasia may develop.

atrophic-hyperplastic g. a variant of atrophic gastritis in which the mucosa is of normal or even increased thickness.

autoimmune g. a rare type of chronic gastritis due to an autoimmune condition of the stomach, resulting from the presence of circulating autoantibodies against the parietal cells. Characteristics include inflammation and atrophy of the mucosa of the body of the stomach, with replacement of normal mucosa by antral, pseudopyloric, and intestinal metaplasia. Destruction of the mucosal glands results in achlorhydria and a decrease in production of intrinsic factor, in severe cases leading to failure of vitamin B_{12} absorption and pernicious anemia. Called also *diffuse atrophic g.*, *diffuse corporal atrophic g.*, and *type A g.*

bile g., bile reflux g. alkaline reflux g.

chemical g. acute gastritis caused by ingestion of a corrosive substance; complete mucosal destruction may cause death. Called also *corrosive g.*

chronic g. chronic inflammatory changes of the gastric mucosa, usually with atrophy; it may be either erosive or nonerosive (see *chronic erosive g.* and *chronic nonerosive g.*).

chronic cystic g. a type of chronic gastritis in which the gastric and pyloric glands are dilated and lined by flattened epithelium, suggestive of a degenerative rather than an inflammatory condition.

chronic erosive g. a type of chronic gastritis with mild symptoms, characterized by multiple punctate or aphthous ulcers, found by endoscopy; some patients have nausea and vomiting but others are symptom free. The cause may be a reaction to nonsteroidal antiinflammatory drugs, a complication of Crohn disease or a viral infection, or an unknown factor. Called also *varioliform g.*

chronic follicular g. a type of atrophic gastritis in which the size and number of lymphoid follicles in the mucosa and submucosa are greatly increased, with heavy infiltration of the entire mucosa by lymphocytes.

chronic nonerosive g. any type of chronic gastritis that does not involve deep penetration of the gastric mucosa.

collagenous g. a rare type of gastritis characterized by subepithelial fibrosis in the stomach. Children have pain and other symptoms of gastritis; in adults it may be related to collagenous sprue or celiac disease, and symptoms include anemia, abdominal pain, diarrhea, and sometimes blood in the feces.

corrosive g. chemical g.

g. cys′tica profun′da a type of gastritis in which there are cysts in the submucosa of the stomach, consisting of abnormal extensions of gastric glands; it is most often a late complication of partial gastrectomy and may be due to ischemia or inflammation at the suture site.

diffuse atrophic g., diffuse corporal atrophic g. autoimmune g.

emphysematous g. infectious gastritis in which the infectious agents are gas-producing bacteria; radiologically it resembles gastric emphysema but is much more serious, even life-threatening.

eosinophilic g. a rare type of chronic gastritis in which there is considerable edema with heavy infiltration of all coats of the wall of the pyloric antrum by eosinophils. The cause is unknown; in some patients it may be linked to an allergic condition, while others may have parasites in the stomach.

erosive g., exfoliative g. gastritis in which the surface epithelium is eroded, manifesting as a patchy or a diffuse lesion. See *acute erosive g.* and *chronic erosive g.*

follicular g. see *chronic follicular g.*

fundal g., fundic g. gastritis whose focus is in the gastric fundus.

giant hypertrophic g. hypertrophic g.

granulomatous g. chronic gastritis with granulomas of the stomach mucosa, seen with Crohn disease, sarcoidosis, or certain other conditions.

***Helicobacter pylori* g.** gastritis caused by the presence of *Helicobacter pylori* in the stomach mucosa; *H. pylori* may be present for many years as chronic gastritis before finally causing an attack of acute gastritis.

hemorrhagic g. acute hemorrhagic g.

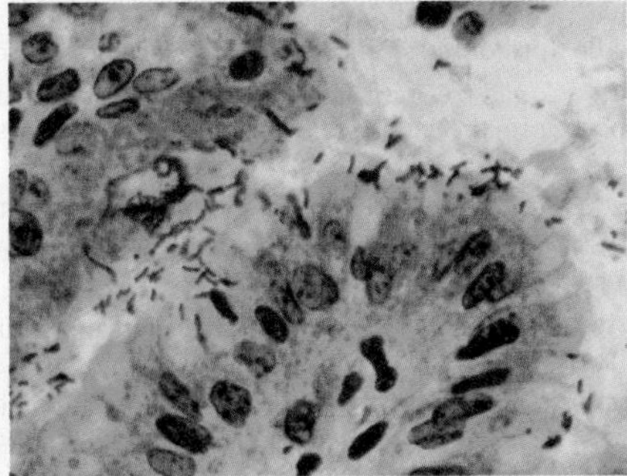

■ *Helicobacter pylori* gastritis; spiral-shaped bacteria are abundant within surface mucus.

hypertrophic g. chronic gastritis with excessive proliferation of the mucosa and diffuse thickening of the stomach wall; inflammatory changes may be associated. Called also *giant hypertrophic g.* and *Ménétrier disease.*

infectious g. any type of gastritis, usually chronic, caused by a bacterial infection in the stomach; the most common type is *Helicobacter pylori* gastritis. In immunocompromised patients, gastritis may occur as a complication of tuberculosis, syphilis, or other conditions.

lymphocytic g. chronic gastritis with large numbers of T lymphocytes in the epithelium of the stomach; sometimes it is associated with celiac disease or *Helicobacter pylori* infection.

phlegmonous g. infectious gastritis with abscesses in the stomach walls; the most common infectious agents implicated are hemolytic streptococci.

radiation g. acute gastritis resulting from radiation injury.

reactive g. gastritis caused by a harmful substance in the stomach, such as a nonsteroidal antiinflammatory drug, bile refluxing from the duodenum, or a toxic chemical *(chemical g.).* It may be either acute or chronic.

stress g. changes in the gastric mucosa, often with bleeding, owing to stress; a serious type is acute hemorrhagic gastritis. See also *stress ulcer*, under *ulcer.*

superficial g. chronic gastritis with inflammation limited to the outer third of the mucosa in the foveolar area and infiltration of the lamina propria by neutrophils, lymphocytes, plasma cells, and a few eosinophils. Columnar cells of the surface epithelium are often morphologically abnormal. Cf. *atrophic g.*

toxic g. chemical gastritis caused by the action of a poison or a corrosive agent.

type A g. autoimmune g.

type B g. any type of chronic gastritis not having circulating autoantibodies, as opposed to autoimmune gastritis; most types are found in the gastric antrum.

varioliform g. chronic erosive g.

zonal g. acute gastritis in the vicinity of a gastric lesion, such as that associated with peptic ulcer or gastric carcinoma.

gastr(o)- [Gr. *gastēr* stomach] a combining form denoting relationship to the stomach.

gas·tro·aceph·a·lus (gas″tro-ə-sef′ə-ləs) [*gastro-* + *acephalus*] asymmetrical conjoined twins in which the larger twin bears the smaller one as a headless parasite on its abdomen.

gas·tro·ad·e·ni·tis (gas″tro-ad″ə-ni′tis) gastradenitis.

gas·tro·amor·phus (gas″tro-a-mor′fəs) [*gastro-* + *amorphus*] asymmetrical conjoined twins in which the larger one has fetal parts of the smaller one concealed within its abdomen.

gas·tro·anas·to·mo·sis (gas″tro-ə-nas″to-mo′sis) gastrogastrostomy.

gas·tro·cam·era (gas″tro-kam′ə-rə) a small camera that can be swallowed or passed down the esophagus on an appropriate instrument to photograph the inside of the stomach.

gas·tro·car·di·ac (gas″tro-kahr′de-ak) pertaining to the stomach and heart.

gas·tro·cele (gas′tro-sēl) [*gastro-* + *-cele*[1]] hernial protrusion of the stomach or of a gastric pouch.

gas·troc·ne·mi·us (gas″trok-ne′me-əs, gas″tro-) [*gastro-* + Gr. *knēmē* leg] see under *musculus.*

gas·tro·coele (gas′tro-sēl) [*gastro-* + *-coele*] archenteron.

gas·tro·col·ic (gas″tro-kol′ik) 1. pertaining to or communicating between the stomach and colon. 2. proceeding from the stomach to the colon.

gas·tro·co·li·tis (gas″tro-ko-li′tis) [*gastro-* + *colitis*] inflammation of the stomach and colon.

gas·tro·co·los·to·my (gas″tro-kə-los′tə-me) [*gastro-* + *colostomy*] 1. surgical creation of an opening between the stomach and the colon. 2. the opening so created.

gas·tro·co·lot·o·my (gas″tro-ko-lot′ə-me) incision into the stomach and colon.

Gas·tro·crom (gas′tro-crom) trademark for preparations of cromolyn sodium.

gas·tro·cu·ta·ne·ous (gas″tro-ku-ta′ne-əs) pertaining to or communicating between the stomach and skin.

gas·tro·cys·to·plas·ty (gas″tro-sis′to-plas″te) [*gastro-* + *cystoplasty*] augmentation cystoplasty using a portion of the stomach for the added segment.

gas·tro·der·mis (gas″tro-dur′mis) [*gastro-* + Gr. *derma* skin] the tissue lining the gut cavity of an invertebrate, which is responsible for digestion and absorption.

gas·tro·did·y·mus (gas″tro-did′ə-məs) [*gastro-* + *-didymus*] symmetrical conjoined twins joined in the abdominal region.

gas·tro·dis·ci·a·sis (gas″tro-dis-ki′ə-sis) intestinal infection caused by *Gastrodiscoides hominis.*

Gas·tro·dis·coi·des (gas″tro-dis-koi′dēz) [*gastro-* + Gr. *diskos* disk + *eidos* form] a genus of trematodes of the family Paramphistomatidae; many are parasitic in the intestinal tract, causing paramphistomiasis. Called also *Gastrodiscus. G. ho′minis* is found in the cecum and colon of pigs and occasionally humans in India, Indochina, and Malaysia.

Gas·tro·dis·cus (gas″tro-dis′kəs) *Gastrodiscoides.*

gas·tro·du·o·de·nal (gas″tro-doo″o-de′nəl) 1. pertaining to or communicating between the stomach and duodenum. 2. proceeding from the stomach to the duodenum.

gas·tro·du·o·de·nec·to·my (gas″tro-doo″o-də-nek′tə-me) surgical removal of the stomach and duodenum.

gas·tro·du·o·de·ni·tis (gas″tro-doo″o-də-ni′tis) [*gastro-* + *duodenitis*] an inflammation of the stomach and duodenum.

gas·tro·du·o·de·nos·co·py (gas″tro-doo″o-də-nos′kə-pe) [*gastro-* + *duodeno-* + *-scopy*] examination of the stomach and duodenum, through a gastroscope passed through the mouth and esophagus.

gas·tro·du·o·de·nos·to·my (gas″tro-doo″o-də-nos′tə-me) [*gastro-* + *duodeno-* + *-stomy*] 1. gastroenterostomy between the stomach and the duodenum. 2. the opening so created.

gas·tro·dyn·ia (gas″tro-din′e-ə) gastralgia.

gas·tro·en·ter·ic (gas″tro-ən-ter′ik) gastrointestinal.

gas·tro·en·ter·i·tis (gas″tro-en″tər-i′tis) [*gastro-* + *enteritis*] inflammation of the lining of the stomach and intestines, characterized by anorexia, nausea, diarrhea, abdominal pain, and weakness. Causes include food poisoning (see *bacterial g.*); viral infections (see *viral g.*); consumption of irritating food or drink; and sometimes psychological factors such as anger, stress, or fear. Called also *enterogastritis.*

acute infectious g. bacterial or viral gastroenteritis that has an acute onset.

bacterial g. gastroenteritis caused by bacteria or bacterial toxins (such as in food poisoning);

***Campylobacter* g.** bacterial gastroenteritis caused by infection with species of *Campylobacter*, characterized by diarrhea that may be bloody, abdominal pain with cramps, and fever. The cause is usually ingestion of contaminated food or water.

canine coronaviral g. vomiting and diarrhea in dogs and other canines infected with coronaviruses; it has a sudden onset and can be fatal in puppies.

canine hemorrhagic g. a syndrome of intestinal hemorrhage in dogs, of unknown etiology; characteristics include sudden onset, bloody diarrhea, dehydration, and hemoconcentration, often followed by collapse and death. Smaller dogs are most often affected.

coliform g. a diarrheal disease of baby pigs caused by enterotoxigenic strains of *Escherichia coli*, marked by profuse, watery diarrhea, dehydration, and acidosis, frequently leading to death; see also *edema disease*, under *disease.* Called also *enteric* or *enterotoxigenic colibacillosis.*

eosinophilic g. a rare condition marked by infiltration of the mucosa of the small intestine and sometimes the stomach by eosinophils, with edema but without vasculitis, and usually with eosinophilia of the peripheral blood. Symptoms depend on the site and extent of disease, and include abdominal pain, diarrhea, nausea, fever, and malabsorption. The disorder is commonly associated with intolerance to specific foods. See also *eosinophilic granuloma* (def. 2), under *granuloma.* Called also *eosinophilic gastroenteropathy.*

epidemic nonbacterial g., epidemic viral g. former names for *Norwalk virus g.*

nonbacterial g. viral g.

Norwalk g., Norwalk virus g. viral gastroenteritis due to infection with a Norwalk virus, one of the most common causes of diarrhea in the United States; the virus is usually ingested in contaminated food or water, although person-to-person infection also occurs. This type is most common in older children and adults. Symptoms include vomiting, diarrhea, abdominal cramps, and sometimes fever.

rotavirus g. viral gastroenteritis due to a rotavirus infection, one of the most common causes of diarrhea in the United States; the virus is usually ingested in contaminated food or water. Young children are particularly susceptible and can suffer severe dehydration or even death.

***Salmonella* g.** gastroenteritis caused by serovars of *Salmonella enterica*, which usually enter the body in contaminated food. Symptoms include inflammation of the mucosa, nausea, vomiting, abdominal pain, and bloody diarrhea. A more virulent form can occur in immunocompromised patients, sometimes resulting in septicemia.

***Shigella* g.** bacterial gastroenteritis caused by the *Shigella* infection of bacillary dysentery (see under *dysentery*).

transmissible g. of swine a viral disease of swine caused by the porcine transmissible gastroenteritis virus, occurring chiefly during the winter and characterized by severe diarrhea and acute inflammation of the gastric mucosa, which may lead to ulceration and hemorrhage. The mortality rate among piglets is very high.

viral g. gastroenteritis caused by a virus; the most common types are rotavirus gastroenteritis and Norwalk virus gastroenteritis. Adenoviruses, astroviruses, and Norwalk-like viruses also commonly cause symptoms.

gas·tro·en·tero·anas·to·mo·sis (gas″tro-en″tər-o-ə-nas″to-mo′sis) gastroenterostomy.

gas·tro·en·tero·co·li·tis (gas″tro-en″tər-o-ko-li′tis) inflammation of the stomach, small intestine, and colon.

gas·tro·en·tero·co·los·to·my (gas″tro-en″tər-o-kə-los′tə-me) [*gastro-* + *entero-* + *colostomy*] 1. surgical creation of an opening between the stomach, intestine, and colon. 2. an opening surgically created between the stomach, intestine, and colon.

gas·tro·ent·er·ol·o·gist (gas″tro-en″tər-ol′ə-jist) a specialist in gastroenterology.

gas·tro·en·ter·ol·o·gy (gas″tro-en″tər-ol′ə-je) [*gastro-* + *entero-* + *-logy*] the study of the stomach and intestines and the nature and treatment of their diseases.

gas·tro·en·tero·pan·cre·at·ic (gas″tro-en″tər-o-pan″kre-at′ik) pertaining to the stomach, intestine, and pancreas.

gas·tro·en·ter·op·a·thy (gas″tro-en″tər-op′ə-the) any disease of the stomach and intestines; see also *gastroenteritis.*

allergic g. eosinophilic gastritis in children with food allergies, particularly to cows' milk; signs of the disease include edema, malabsorption, eosinophilia, iron deficiency anemia, elevated levels of serum IgE, and protein-losing enteropathy.

diabetic g. gastrointestinal changes seen with diabetes mellitus, especially those caused by gastroparesis and delayed gastric emptying; some persons have rapid gastric emptying of fluids.

eosinophilic g. eosinophilic gastroenteritis.

protein-losing g. gastrointestinal disease accompanied by leakage of serum proteins from blood vessels into the gastrointestinal tract, causing hypoproteinemia and other symptoms. The numerous conditions accompanied by this symptom have been grouped into mucosal damage without erosion or ulceration, mucosal damage with erosion or ulceration, obstructive conditions of the intestinal lymphatics, and those in which the mechanism of protein loss is not known.

gas·tro·en·tero·plas·ty (gas″tro-en′tər-o-plas″te) a plastic operation on the stomach and small intestine.

gas·tro·en·ter·os·to·my (gas″tro-en″tər-os′tə-me) [*gastro-* + *enter-* + *ostomy*] 1. surgical creation of an anastomosis between the stomach and the small intestine; the most common type is the gastrojejunostomy. 2. the opening so created.

Billroth g. see under *operation.*

gas·tro·en·ter·ot·o·my (gas″tro-en″tər-ot′ə-me) [*gastro-* + *entero-* + *-tomy*] surgical incision into the stomach and intestine.

gas·tro·ep·i·plo·ic (gas″tro-ep″ĭ-plo′ik) [*gastro-* + *epiploic*] pertaining to the stomach and epiploon (omentum).

gas·tro·esoph·a·ge·al (gas″tro-ə-sof″ə-je′əl) 1. pertaining to the stomach and esophagus. 2. proceeding from the stomach to the esophagus.

gas·tro·esoph·a·gi·tis (gas″tro-ə-sof″ə-ji′tis) inflammation of the stomach and esophagus.

gas·tro·esoph·a·gos·to·my (gas″tro-ə-sof″ə-gos′tə-me) esophagogastrostomy.

gas·tro·fi·ber·scope (gas″tro-fi′bər-skōp) fiberoptic gastroscope.

gas·tro·gas·tros·to·my (gas″tro-gas-tros′tə-me) [*gastro-* + *gastro-* + *-stomy*] surgical creation of an anastomosis between the pyloric and cardiac ends of the stomach, usually performed because of hourglass contraction of the middle third of the stomach; also, the anastomosis so established.

gas·tro·ga·vage (gas″tro-gə-vahzh′) [*gastro-* + *gavage*] the introduction of nutriment into the stomach by means of a tube passed through the esophagus.

gas·tro·gen·ic (gas″tro-jen′ik) formed or originating in the stomach.

Gas·tro·graf·in (gas″tro-graf′in) trademark for a preparation of meglumine diatrizoate.

gas·tro·graph (gas′tro-graf) [*gastro-* + *-graph*] an apparatus for recording the motions of the stomach.

gas·trog·ra·phy (gas-trog′rə-fe) radiographic examination of the stomach.

gas·tro·he·pat·ic (gas″tro-hə-pat′ik) [*gastro-* + *hepatic*] pertaining to the stomach and liver.

gas•tro•hep•a•ti•tis (gas″tro-hep-ə-ti′tis) inflammation of the stomach and liver.

gas•tro•il•e•ac (gas″tro-il′e-ak) gastroileal.

gas•tro•il•e•al (gas″tro-il′e-əl) pertaining to the stomach and ileum.

gas•tro•il•e•itis (gas″tro-il-e-i′tis) inflammation of the stomach and ileum.

gas•tro•il•e•os•to•my (gas″tro-il″e-os′tə-me) 1. a gastroenterostomy in which the anastomosis is between the stomach and ileum. 2. the opening so created.

gas•tro•in•tes•ti•nal (gas″tro-in-tes′tĭ-nəl) [*gastro-* + *intestinal*] pertaining to or communicating with the stomach and intestine. Called also *enterogastric* and *gastroenteric.*

gas•tro•je•ju•no•col•ic (gas″tro-jə-joo″no-kol′ik) pertaining to or communicating between the stomach, jejunum, and colon.

gas•tro•je•ju•nos•to•my (gas″tro-jə-joo-nos′tə-me) [*gastro-* + *jejunostomy*] 1. a gastroenterostomy between the stomach and the jejunum. 2. the anastomosis so created.

gas•tro•ki•neso•graph (gas″tro-kĭ-nes′o-graf) gastrograph.

gas•tro•li•e•nal (gas″tro-li′ən-əl) [*gastro-* + *lienal*] gastrosplenic.

gas•tro•lith (gas′tro-lith) [*gastro-* + *-lith*] a concretion in the stomach; called also *gastric calculus.*

gas•tro•li•thi•a•sis (gas″tro-lĭ-thi′ə-sis) [*gastro-* + *lithiasis*] the presence or formation of gastroliths.

Gas•tro•lo•bi•um (gas″tro-lo′be-um) a genus of leguminous plants found in Australia; most species contain fluoroacetate and can cause fatal fluoroacetate poisoning in ruminants.

gas•trol•o•gist (gas-trol′ə-jist) a specialist in gastrology.

gas•trol•o•gy (gas-trol′ə-je) [*gastro-* + *-logy*] the study of the stomach and the nature and treatment of its diseases.

gas•trol•y•sis (gas-trol′ə-sis) [*gastro-* + *-lysis*] surgical division of perigastric adhesions in order to mobilize the stomach.

gas•tro•ma•la•cia (gas″tro-mə-la′shə) [*gastro-* + *malacia*] abnormal softening of the wall of the stomach.

gas•tro•meg•a•ly (gas″tro-meg′ə-le) [*gastro-* + *-megaly*] enlargement of the stomach; called also *megalogastria.*

gas•trom•e•lus (gas-trom′ə-ləs) [*gastro-* + Gr. *melos* limb] a fetus with a supernumerary lower limb attached to the abdomen.

gas•tro•my•ot•o•my (gas″tro-mi-ot′ə-me) [*gastro-* + *myotomy*] incision through the muscular coats of the stomach down to the mucosa.

gas•trone (gas′trōn) a reputed hormonal inhibitor of gastric acid secretion, extracted from gastric mucosa.

gas•tro•pan•cre•a•ti•tis (gas″tro-pan″kre-ə-ti′tis) inflammation of the stomach and pancreas.

gas•tro•pa•ral•y•sis (gas″tro-pə-ral′ə-sis) gastroparesis.

gas•tro•pa•re•sis (gas″tro-pə-re′sis) [*gastro-* + *paresis*] paralysis of the stomach, usually from damage to its nerve supply, so that food empties out much more slowly, if at all. Symptoms include early satiety, nausea, and vomiting. Called also *gastroparalysis* and *gastroplegia.*

diabetic g., g. diabetico′rum gastroparesis due to changes caused by diabetes mellitus, usually because of damage to the vagus nerve. Symptoms include postprandial bloating and vomiting, and often hypoglycemia because of food not moving properly into the duodenum.

gas•tro•pa•ri•e•tal (gas″tro-pə-ri′ə-təl) pertaining to the stomach wall.

gas•tro•path•ic (gas″tro-path′ik) pertaining to or characterized by gastropathy.

gas•trop•a•thy (gas-trop′ə-the) [*gastro-* + *-pathy*] any disease of the stomach; see also *gastritis* and *gastroenteropathy.*

congestive g. multiple ectasias of the blood vessels of the stomach, and sometimes the duodenum and colon, often associated with cirrhosis and appearing as discrete red spots or as a pattern of red patches outlined in white; bleeding may be acute or may result in occult blood loss and anemia.

hypertrophic g. see under *gastritis.*

nonsteroidal antiinflammatory drug g., NSAID g., NSAID-induced g. damage to the gastric mucosa resulting from use of nonsteroidal antiinflammatory drugs; the most common changes are mucosal erosions and small hemorrhages, especially in the fundus and body of the stomach.

portal hypertensive g. changes in the gastric mucosa accompanying portal hypertension, sometimes with varices, telangiectasias, and bleeding.

reactive g. damage to the gastric mucosa with epithelial change but no inflammation, commonly seen in areas near an ulcer; some authorities put alkaline reflux gastritis and similar conditions in this category because they do not show true inflammation.

gas•tro•peri•car•di•al (gas″tro-per″ĭ-kahr′de-əl) pertaining to the stomach and pericardium.

gas•tro•peri•to•ni•tis (gas″tro-per″ĭ-to-ni′tis) inflammation of the stomach and peritoneum.

gas•tro•pexy (gas′tro-pek″se) [*gastro-* + *-pexy*] surgical fixation of the stomach to prevent displacement.

Hill posterior g. an operation for gastroesophageal reflux in which the reduced gastroesophageal junction is anchored by sutures between the proximal lesser curvature and the preaortic fascia, and sutures are placed in the crura to narrow the hiatus.

Gas•troph•i•lus (gas-trof′ĭ-ləs) *Gasterophilus.*

gas•tro•pho•tog•ra•phy (gas″tro-fo-tog′rə-fe) photography of the interior of the stomach with a gastrocamera.

gas•tro•phren•ic (gas″tro-fren′ik) [*gastro-* + *phrenic*] phrenogastric.

gas•tro•phthis•is (gas″tro-this′is) [*gastro-* + *phthisis* (def. 1)] 1. hyperplasia of the gastric mucosa and submucosa, leading to thickening of the stomach walls and diminution of its cavity. 2. emaciation due to abdominal disease.

gas•tro•plas•ty (gas′tro-plas″te) [*gastro-* + *-plasty*] a plastic operation on the stomach. **gastroplas′tic** *adj*

ring g. a type of vertical banded gastroplasty in which the band is a plastic ring.

vertical banded g. (VBG) a surgical treatment for morbid obesity consisting of the construction of a small pouch in the stomach that empties through a narrow stoma into the distal stomach and duodenum.

gas•tro•ple•gia (gas″tro-ple′jə) gastroparesis.

gas•tro•pli•ca•tion (gas″tro-plĭ-ka′shən) [*gastro-* + *plication*] the surgical treatment of gastric dilatation by stitching a fold in the stomach.

gas•tro•pod (gas′tro-pod) a mollusk of the class Gastropoda.

Gas•trop•o•da (gas-trop′ə-də) [*gastro-* + Gr. *pous* foot] a class of mollusks embracing the snails, slugs, whelks, abalones, and others, including many species that serve as primary and intermediate hosts of pathogens.

gas•tro•pro•tec•tive (gas″tro-pro-tek′tiv) reducing the risk of damage to the stomach or the upper gastrointestinal tract.

gas•trop•to•sis (gas″trop-to′sis, gas″tro-to′sis) [*gastro-* + *-ptosis*] downward displacement of the stomach; a term based on the outmoded concept that variation in position of abdominal organs is pathologic.

gas•tro•pul•mo•nary (gas″tro-pool′mo-nar-e) pneumogastric.

gas•tro•py•lo•rec•to•my (gas″tro-pi″lə-rek′tə-me) [*gastro-* + *pylorectomy*] excision of the pyloric portion of the stomach.

gas•tro•py•lor•ic (gas″tro-pi-lor′ik) pertaining to the stomach in its entirety and to the pylorus.

gas•tro•re•nal (gas″tro-re′nəl) pertaining to or communicating between the stomach and kidney. Called also *renogastric.*

gas•tror•rha•gia (gas″tro-ra′jə) [*gastro-* + *-rrhagia*] hemorrhage from the stomach.

gas•tror•rha•phy (gas-tror′ə-fe) [*gastro-* + *-rrhaphy*] suture of a wound of the stomach.

gas•tror•rhea (gas″tro-re′ə) [*gastro-* + *-rrhea*] excessive secretion by the stomach of gastric juice *(hyperchlorhydria)* or mucus.

gas•tror•rhex•is (gas″tro-rek′sis) [*gastro-* + *-rrhexis*] rupture of the stomach.

gas•tros•chi•sis (gas-tros′kĭ-sis) [*gastro-* + *-schisis*] a congenital fissure of the anterior abdominal wall not involving the site of insertion of the umbilical cord, and usually accompanied by protrusion of the small intestine and part of the large intestine.

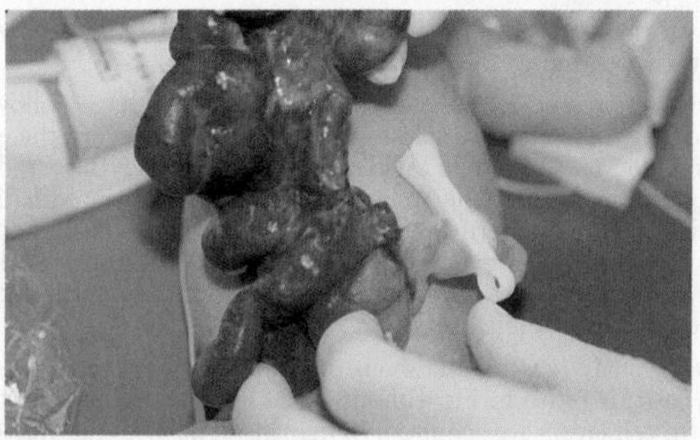

■ Gastroschisis. The abdominal defect lies to the right of an intact umbilical cord without a sac, and the intestines have been exposed to the amniotic fluid, resulting in an inflammatory response.

gas•tro•scope (gas′tro-skōp) [*gastro-* + *-scope*] an endoscope for inspecting the interior of the stomach.

fiberoptic g. a gastroscope that uses fiberoptic technology. Called also *fibergastroscope* and *gastrofiberscope.*

gas•tros•co•py (gas-tros′kə-pe) [*gastro-* + *-scopy*] inspection of the interior of the stomach by means of the gastroscope. **gastroscop′ic** *adj*

gas•tro•se•lec•tive (gas″tro-sə-lek′tiv) having an affinity for receptors involved in regulation of gastric activities.

gas•tro•spasm (gas′tro-spaz″əm) [*gastro-* + *spasm*] spasm of the stomach.

gas•tro•splen•ic (gas″tro-splen′ik) pertaining to the stomach and spleen.

gas•tro•stax•is (gas″tro-stak′sis) [*gastro-* + *staxis*] oozing of blood from the mucous membrane of the stomach, as in hemorrhagic gastritis.

gas•tro•ste•no•sis (gas″tro-stə-no′sis) [*gastro-* + *stenosis*] contraction or shrinkage of the stomach.

gas•tros•to•ga•vage (gas-tros″to-gə-vahzh′) gavage (def. 1).

gas•tros•to•la•vage (gas-tros″to-lə-vahzh′) irrigation of the stomach through a gastric fistula.

gas•tros•to•ma (gas-tros′to-mə) 1. gastric fistula (def. 1). 2. gastrostomy (def. 2).

gas•tros•to•my (gas-tros′tə-me) [*gastro-* + *-stomy*] 1. surgical creation of an artificial opening into the stomach. 2. the opening so established; called also *gastric fistula.*

Janeway g. surgical creation of a permanent gastric fistula via a tube between the anterior gastric wall to the surface of the abdominal wall.

percutaneous endoscopic g. (PEG) a method used for long-term tube feeding, in which a tube is inserted through the chest wall into the stomach under endoscopic guidance.

Stamm g. surgical placement of a tube through an incision in the abdominal wall into the gastric lumen; the stomach is sutured to the peritoneum at the exit site.

Witzel g. insertion of a tube into the gastric lumen, the tube being implanted so as to create a serosal tunnel of stomach as it enters the gastric lumen. Called also *Witzel operation.*

gas•tro•tho•ra•cop•a•gus (gas″tro-thor″ə-kop′ə-gəs) [*gastro-* + *thoracopagus*] conjoined twins joined at the abdomen and thorax.

g. dipy′gus asymmetrical conjoined twins in which there is a parasitic twin consisting of only the pelvis and lower limbs attached to the abdomen of the larger twin. Called also *dipygus parasiticus.*

gas•tro•tho•rax (gas″tro-thor′aks) a severe type of hiatal hernia in which the entire stomach is above the diaphragm in the thoracic cavity.

tension g. gastrothorax that increases the pressure within the thoracic cavity similarly to a tension pneumothorax.

gas•trot•o•my (gas-trot′ə-me) [*gastro-* + *-tomy*] incision into the stomach.

gas•tro•to•nom•e•ter (gas″tro-to-nom′ə-tər) [*gastro-* + *tono-* + *-meter*] an instrument for measuring intragastric pressure.

gas•tro•to•nom•e•try (gas″tro-to-nom′ə-tre) the measurement of intragastric pressure.

gas•tro•tox•in (gas′tro-tok″sin) a substance that exerts a toxic effect on the stomach.

Gas•tro•tricha (gas″tro-trik′ə) [*gastro-* + Gr. *trichos* hair] a class of very small aquatic animals of the phylum Aschelminthes, which have cilia on the ventral surface and a triradiate esophagus. In some systems of classification, they are considered to be a separate phylum.

gas•tro•tro•pic (gas″tro-tro′pik) [*gastro-* + *-tropic*] having an affinity for or exerting a special effect upon the stomach.

gas•tro•tym•pa•ni•tes (gas″tro-tim″pə-ni′tēz) [*gastro-* + *tympanites*] tympanitic distention of the stomach.

gas•tru•la (gas′troo-lə) the early embryo in the stage following the blastula or blastocyst. The simplest type consists of two layers, the ectoderm and the endoderm, and of two cavities, one lying between the ectoderm and the endoderm; the other (the archenteron) is formed by invagination so as to lie within the endoderm and having an opening (the blastopore). In human embryos the gastrula stage occurs during the third week, as the embryonic disc becomes trilaminar, establishing the ectoderm, mesoderm, and endoderm from the epiblast.

gas•tru•la•tion (gas″troo-la′shən) the process by which a blastula becomes a gastrula or, in forms without a true blastula, the process by which three germ cell layers are acquired. In humans, it denotes the conversion of the bilaminar embryonic disc into a trilaminar embryonic disc as cells from the epiblast migrate through the primitive streak to become ectoderm, mesoderm, and endoderm.

Gatch bed (gach) [Willis Dew *Gatch*, American surgeon, 1878–1954] see under *bed.*

gate (gāt) 1. an electronic circuit that passes a pulse only when a signal (the gate pulse) is present at a second input; called also *gate circuit.* 2. a mechanism for opening or closing a channel in a cell membrane, regulated by a signal such as increased concentration of a neurotransmitter, change in electrical potential, or physical binding of a ligand molecule to the channel protein to cause a conformational change in the protein molecule. 3. to open and close selectively and function as a gate.

gat•i•flox•a•cin (gat″ĭ-flok′sə-sin) a fluoroquinolone antibacterial effective against many gram-positive and gram-negative bacteria; administered orally and intravenously as the sesquihydrate in the treatment of bacterial exacerbation of chronic bronchitis, acute sinusitis, community-acquired pneumonia, gonorrhea, pyelonephritis, and urinary tract infections due to susceptible organisms.

gat•ing (gāt′ing) 1. controlling access or passage through gates or channels. 2. selection of electrical signals by a gate, which passes signals only when a control signal, the gate pulse, is present, or which passes only signals with certain characteristics, such as a pulse height. 3. substrate-binding– or ligand-binding–induced opening and closing of a biologic membrane channel, believed to be due to conformational changes in proteins lining the channels. 4. sensory g.

cardiac g. selective acquisition of cardiac function information at specific points in the cardiac cycle by using information from the electrocardiographic signal to time the cardiac cycle and control image sampling. It has been used in digital subtraction angiography, computed tomography, nuclear cardiology, and magnetic resonance imaging.

sensory g. inhibition or blocking of incoming sensory stimuli or channels when attention is occupied by another channel or stimulus.

ga•to•pho•bia (gat″o-fo′be-ə) [Sp. *gato*, from L. *catus* cat + *-phobia*] ailurophobia.

gat•tine (gat′ēn) [Fr.] a form of flacherie in which the cephalic end of a silkworm larva becomes swollen and almost translucent; thought to be caused by a mixed infection with an unidentified virus and an enterococcus related to *Streptococcus faecalis.*

Gau•cher cells, disease (go-sha′) [Phillippe Charles Ernest *Gaucher*, French physician, 1854–1918] see under *cell* and *disease.*

gauge (gāj) an instrument for determining physical properties of anything, including caliber, dimensions, or pressure.

Boley g. a watchmaker's gauge used in dentistry for accurate measurement of arch, tooth, and facial dimensions.

catheter g. a plate with graduated perforations for measuring the outside diameter of catheters.

Gaul•the•ria (gawl-the′re-ə) [Jean-François *Gaultier*, Canadian physician and botanist, 1708–1756] a genus of plants of the family Ericaceae. *G. procum′bens* is wintergreen, a North American species whose leaves contain methyl salicylate (see under *salicylate*).

gaunt•let (gawnt′lət) [Fr. *gant* glove] gauntlet bandage.

Gauss sign (gous) [Karl Johann *Gauss*, German obstetrician, 1875–1957] see under *sign.*

gauss (gous) [Karl Friedrich *Gauss*, German mathematician and physicist, 1777–1855] a unit of magnetic flux density, equal to 10^{-4} tesla.

gauss•i•an (gou′se-ən) named for Karl Friedrich *Gauss.*

gauze (gawz) a light, open-meshed fabric of muslin or similar material used in bandages, dressings, and surgical sponges. Before use in surgery, it is usually sterilized and frequently impregnated with various antiseptics.

absorbable g. gauze made from oxidized cellulose.

absorbent g. [USP] a plain woven cloth of cotton or of a mixture of cotton and rayon; it is classified as Type I (the heaviest) to Type VIII (the lightest) on the basis of thread count and weight. It is supplied in various lengths and widths in the form of rolls and folds.

absorbent g., sterile absorbent gauze that has been sterilized and subsequently protected from contamination.

petrolatum g. [USP] absorbent gauze saturated with white petrolatum; used as a protective covering for wounds.

zinc gelatin–impregnated g. absorbent gauze impregnated with zinc gelatin that may contain a small amount of ferric oxide as coloring matter; see also *Unna boot*, under *boot.*

ga•vage (gə-vahzh′) [Fr. "cramming"] 1. forced feeding, especially through a tube passed into the stomach. 2. the therapeutic use of a very full diet; superalimentation.

Ga•vard muscle (gah-vahr′) [Hyacinthe *Gavard*, French anatomist, 1753–1802] see under *muscle.*

GAVE gastric antral vascular ectasia.

Gav•is•con (gav′is-kon) trademark for preparations of aluminum hydroxide and magnesium carbonate.

Gay glands (ga) [Alexander Heinrich *Gay*, Russian anatomist, 1842–1907] circumanal glands.

Gay-Lus•sac's law (ga′-lu-sahks′) [Joseph Louis *Gay-Lussac*, French naturalist, 1778–1850] see under *law*.

gaze (gāz) 1. to look steadily in one direction. 2. the act of looking steadily at something.

conjugate g. the normal movement of the two eyes simultaneously in the same direction to bring something into view.

GBG glycine-rich β glycoprotein, former name for *factor B*.

GBM glomerular basement membrane.

GBS Guillain-Barré syndrome.

GC gas chromatography.

g-cal. gram calorie; see *small calorie*, under *calorie*.

GCS Glasgow Coma Scale.

G-CSF granulocyte colony-stimulating factor.

Gd gadolinium.

GDM gestational diabetes mellitus.

GDP guanosine diphosphate.

Ge germanium.

gear (gēr) equipment.

cervical g. an extraoral appliance by means of which the back of the neck is used for anchorage or as a base of traction in effecting tooth movement.

head g. headgear.

Gee disease (ge) [Samuel Jones *Gee*, English physician, 1839–1911] the infantile form of celiac disease.

Gee-Her•ter disease (ge′ hur′tər) [S.J. *Gee;* Christian Archibald *Herter*, American physician, 1865–1910] the infantile form of celiac disease.

Gee-Her•ter-Heub•ner disease (ge′ hur′tər hoib′nər) [S.J. *Gee;* C.A. *Herter;* Johann Otto Leonard *Heubner*, German pediatrician, 1843–1926] the infantile form of celiac disease.

Gee-Thay•sen disease (ge′ ti′sən) [S.J. *Gee;* Thorwald Einar Hess *Thaysen*, Danish physician, 1883–1936] the adult form of celiac disease.

ge•fit•i•nib (gĕ-fit′ĭ-nib) a tyrosine kinase inhibitor, used in treatment of non–small-cell lung cancer; administered orally.

Ge•gen•baur cell (ga′gən-bou″ər) [Carl *Gegenbaur*, German anatomist, 1826–1903] osteoblast.

ge•gen•hal•ten (ga″gən-hahlt′ən) [Ger., from *gegen* against + *halten* to hold] involuntary resistance to passive movement, as may occur in cerebral cortical disorders. Called also *paratonia*.

Gei•gel reflex (gi′gəl) [Richard *Geigel*, German physician, 1859–1930] see under *reflex*.

Gei•ger counter (gi′gər) [Hans Wilhelm *Geiger*, German physicist, 1882–1945] see under *counter*.

Gei•ger-Mül•ler counter (gi′gər mu′ler) [H.W. *Geiger;* Walther Müller, German physicist, 20th century] see under *counter*.

Geis•so•spe•rum (gi″so-spe′rəm) a genus of plants of the family Apocyanaceae. *G. lae′ve* and *G. vello′sii* Allem. are poisonous species that contain vellosine.

gel (jel) 1. a colloid in which the solid disperse phase forms a network in combination with the fluid continuous phase to produce a viscous semirigid sol. 2. to form such a compound or any similar semi-solid material.

acidulated phosphate fluoride g. sodium fluoride and phosphoric acid g.

aluminum hydroxide g. [USP] a suspension of amorphous aluminum hydroxide in which there is partial substitution of carbonate for hydroxide; used as a gastric antacid, especially in treatment of peptic ulcer, and as a phosphate binder in treatment of hyperphosphatemia and phosphate nephrolithiasis. Called also *colloidal aluminum hydroxide*.

aluminum phosphate g. [USP] an aqueous suspension of aluminum phosphate, used as an antacid and to reduce excretion of phosphates in the feces.

APF g. sodium fluoride and phosphoric acid g.

basic aluminum carbonate g. an aqueous suspension of a complex of aluminum hydroxide and aluminum carbonate, used as an antacid, for the treatment of hyperphosphatemia in renal insufficiency, and to prevent the formation of phosphate urinary calculi.

corticotropin g. repository corticotropin injection.

dried aluminum hydroxide g. [USP] an amorphous form of aluminum hydroxide in which there is partial substitution of carbonate for hydroxide, prepared by drying aluminum hydroxide gel at low temperature; used as an antacid and phosphate binder.

silica g. a purified form of silica (silicon dioxide) obtained by the reaction of sodium silicate with a mineral acid; used as a dispersing and suspending agent in pharmaceutical preparations.

sodium fluoride and phosphoric acid g. [USP] a fluoride-containing preparation, consisting of sodium fluoride, hydrofluoric acid, and phosphoric acid, with concentrations of 1.23 per cent fluoride ion and 0.98 per cent phosphoric acid, pH of 3.0 to 3.5, and flavoring, coloring, sweetening, and thickening agents; applied topically to the teeth as a dental caries prophylactic.

ge•las•mus (jə-las′məs) [G. *gelasma* a laugh] hysterical laughter. **gelas′tic** *adj*

gel•ate (jel′āt) to form a gel.

ge•lat•i•fi•ca•tion (jə-lat″ĭ-fĭ-ka′shən) conversion into gelatin.

gel•a•tig•e•nous (jel″ə-tij′ə-nəs) producing or forming gelatin.

gel•a•tin (jel′ə-tin) [L. *gelatina*, from *gelare* to congeal] [NF] a product obtained by partial hydrolysis of collagen derived from the skin, white connective tissue, and bones of animals; used as a suspending agent. It is also used pharmaceutically in the manufacture of capsules and suppositories, has been suggested for intravenous use as a plasma substitute, and has been used as an adjuvant protein food.

silk g. sericin.

g. of Wharton Wharton jelly.

zinc g. a preparation of zinc oxide, gelatin, glycerin, and purified water, used as a topical skin protectant. See also *Unna boot*, under *boot*.

ge•lat•i•nase (jə-lat′ĭ-nās) a nonspecific extracellular proteolytic enzyme, produced by certain microorganisms, that hydrolyzes gelatin.

gel•a•ti•nif•er•ous (jel″ə-tĭ-nif′ər-əs) [*gelatin* + *-ferous*] producing gelatin.

ge•lat•i•nize (jə-lat′ĭ-nīz) 1. to convert into gelatin. 2. to become converted into gelatin.

ge•lat•i•noid (jə-lat′ĭ-noid) resembling gelatin.

gel•a•ti•no•lyt•ic (jel″ə-tin-o-lit′ik) [*gelatin* + *-lytic*] dissolving or splitting up gelatin.

gel•a•ti•no•sa (jel″ə-tĭ-no′sə) [L.] gelatinous; see entries beginning with *substantia gelatinosa*, under *substantia*.

ge•lat•i•nous (jə-lat′ĭ-nəs) [L. *gelatinosus*] like jelly or softened gelatin.

ge•la•tion (jə-la′shən) the conversion of a sol into a gel.

ge•la•tum (jə-la′təm) [L., from *gelare* to congeal] jelly, or gel.

geld (geld) to castrate a male animal, especially a horse.

geld•ing (gel′ding) a castrated male animal, especially a horse.

gel•eo•phys•ic (jel″e-o-fiz′ik) [Gr. *gelan* to laugh + *physis* nature] appearing to have a happy nature; used of the characteristic happy facies of geleophysic dysplasia.

Gel•film (jel′film) trademark for absorbable gelatin film.

Gel•foam (jel′fōm) trademark for an absorbable gelatin sponge.

Gé•li•neau syndrome (zha-le-no′) [Jean Baptiste Edouard *Gélineau*, French neurologist, 1859–1906] narcolepsy.

Gell and Coombs classification (jel′ ko͞omz′) [Philip George Howthern *Gell*, British immunologist, 1914–2001; Robert Royston Amos *Coombs*, British immunologist, 1921–2006] see under *classification*.

gel•om•e•ter (jel-om′ə-tər) a device for determining the time required for a solution to gel.

Gel. quav. gelati′na qua′vis (in any kind of jelly).

gel•se•mine (jel′sə-mēn) a toxic alkaloid found in the roots and rhizomes of *Gelsemium sempervirens;* it acts as a central nervous system stimulant and also causes double vision, muscular weakness, and sometimes respiratory arrest.

Gel•se•mi•um (gel-sem′e-um) a genus of woody vines of the family Loganaceae, native to Asia and the southeastern United States. *G. semper-vi′rens* (L.) Alt. is the yellow jessamine, a flowering plant of North America that contains gelsemine and other toxic alkaloids and can cause neurologic symptoms in animals that eat it.

gel•sol•in (jel-sol′in) any of a family of actin-binding proteins that sever and cap actin filaments at high calcium concentrations, thus controlling the length of actin filaments and lowering the viscosity of cytoplasm in processes such the formation of filopodia. They also bind to phosphatidylinositol bisphosphate, linking actin organization and signal transduction. See also *profilin*.

Gé•ly suture (zha-le′) [Jules Aristide *Gély*, French surgeon, 1806–1861] see under *suture*.

ge•mäs•te•te (gə-mes′tə-tə) [Ger.] swollen or bloated: a term applied to enlarged astrocytes in the region of a degenerated area.

gem·cit·a·bine hy·dro·chlo·ride (jem-sit′ə-bēn) [USP] a pyrimidine analogue, which acts as an antineoplastic by preventing DNA chain elongation; used in chemotherapy for pancreatic adenocarcinoma and non–small cell lung carcinoma; administered intravenously.

Ge·mel·la (jə-mel′ə) [L., dim. of *gemellus* a twin] a genus of gram-positive, aerobic or facultatively anaerobic cocci of the family Staphylococcaceae, occurring singly or in pairs, tetrads, or short chains, with adjacent sides flattened. Organisms are part of the normal oropharyngeal, gastrointestinal, and urogenital flora of many different animals but can also cause infectious illnesses, particularly in immunocompromised persons. The type species is *G. haemoly′sans.*

G. haemoly′sans a species that is a part of the normal flora of the upper respiratory tract; it is an opportunistic pathogen, causing endocarditis, septic shock, meningitis, arthritis, and pneumonia.

G. morbillo′rum a species that is a part of the normal flora of the oropharyngeal, gastrointestinal, and urogenital tracts and causes opportunistic infections in immunocompromised persons.

gem·el·lary (jem′ə-lar″e) pertaining to twins.

gem·el·lip·a·ra (jem′ə-lip′ə-rə) [L. *gemelli* twins + *para*] a woman who has given birth to twins.

gem·el·lol·o·gy (jem″əl-ol′ə-je) [L. *gemellus* twin + *-logy*] the scientific study of twins and twinning.

gem·fib·ro·zil (jem-fib′ro-zil) [USP] a fibric acid derivative used in the treatment of very high serum triglyceride levels that are not responsive to diet, administered orally.

gemi·flox·a·cin mes·y·late (jem-ĭ-flok′sə-sin) a broad-spectrum fluoroquinolone antibacterial agent used in the treatment of infection by susceptible organisms, including bronchitis and community-acquired pneumonia; administered orally.

gem·i·nate (jem′ĭ-nāt) [L. *geminatus*] paired; occurring in pairs.

gem·i·na·tion (jem″ĭ-na′shən) a doubling; a form of fusion of two teeth that results in the formation of two teeth or of a double crown formed on a single root with a single pulp canal. The term is usually applied to fusion of two supernumerary teeth or union of one supernumerary with a regular tooth.

gem·i·ni (jem′ĭ-ni) [L.] plural of *geminus.*

gem·i·nous (jem′ĭ-nəs) geminate.

gem·i·nus (jem′ĭ-nəs) pl. *ge′mini* [L.] twin.

ge·mis·to·cyte (jə-mis′to-sīt″) [Gr. *gemistos* laden, full + *-cyte*] a pathologic astrocyte in which the cell body swells considerably, the nucleus assumes an eccentric position, and the cytoplasm is clearly visible; seen particularly in demyelinating and neoplastic conditions. Called also *gemistocytic astrocyte.*

ge·mis·to·cyt·ic (jə-mis″to-sĭ′tik) composed of gemistocytes stuffed with fatty debris; said of a type of astrocytoma.

gem·ma (jem′ə) [L. "bud"] a budlike body or structure.

g. gustato′ria TA alternative for *caliculus gustatorius.*

gem·ma·tion (jə-ma′shən) [L. *gemmare* to bud] budding (def. 1).

gem·mule (jem′ūl) [L. *gemmula*, dim. of *gemma* bud] 1. a reproductive bud; the immediate product of gemmation (budding). 2. any of numerous small excrescences on the dendrites of a neuron; they are particularly common on Purkinje cells and pyramidal cells. Called also *dendritic spine.*

gem·tu·zu·mab ozo·ga·mi·cin (gem-too′zoo-mab″ o″zo-gə-mi′sin) a recombinant DNA–derived monoclonal antibody conjugated with a cytotoxic antitumor antibiotic, calicheamicin, isolated from the bacterium *Micromonospora echinospora* sp. *calichensis*. It is used as an antineoplastic in the treatment of relapsed CD33-positive acute myelogenous leukemia, administered intravenously.

Gem·zar (jem′zahr) trademark for a preparation of gemcitabine hydrochloride.

-gen [Gr. *-genēs* born, with an alteration in meaning to "producing"] a word termination denoting an agent productive of the object or state indicated by the word stem to which it is affixed, as allergen (allergy), cryogen (cold), and pathogen (disease).

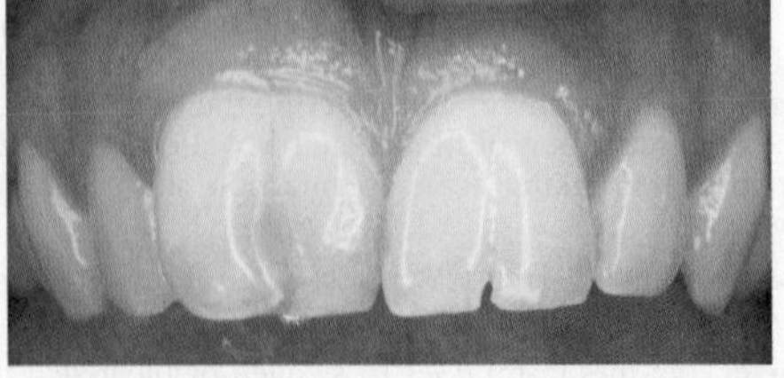

■ Gemination of both upper central incisors.

ge·nal (je′nəl) buccal.

gen·der (jen′dər) 1. sex (def. 1). 2. see *gender identity*, under *identity.*

gene (jēn) [Gr. *gennan* to produce] a segment of a DNA molecule (RNA in certain viruses) that contains all the information required for synthesis of a product (polypeptide chain or RNA molecule), including both coding and noncoding sequences where the latter occur. It is the biologic unit of inheritance, self-reproducing, and transmitted from parent to progeny. Each gene has a specific position (locus) in the genome.

allelic g. allele.

autosomal g. a gene located on a chromosome that is not a sex chromosome.

BRCA g. [*br*east *ca*ncer] either of two tumor suppressor genes, *BRCA1* and *BRCA2*, that encode ubiquitously expressed nuclear proteins involved in regulation of DNA repair, transcriptional activation, and the cell cycle; germline mutations of either gene are associated with inherited predisposition to ovarian and female breast cancers. *BRCA1* mutations also confer an increased risk for prostate and colon cancers and *BRCA2* for prostate, pancreatic, bile duct, gallbladder, and male breast cancers.

candidate g. a DNA sequence that because of its biochemical product, chromosomal location, or other property is considered as a gene of interest; used particularly for a gene considered as potentially causing a particular genetic disorder.

caretaker g. any of those involved in maintenance of the stability of the genome, as one involved in the function of DNA repair or replication enzymes; inactivation can result in increased levels of mutations and cancer. Cf. *gatekeeper g.*

cell interaction g's genes of the major histocompatibility complex that control cell-cell interactions between B cells, T cells, and macrophages and between cytotoxic T cells and target cells. Called also *CI g's.*

chimeric g. an artificial gene constructed by juxtaposition of fragments of unrelated genes or other DNA, which may themselves have been altered in sequence.

CI g's cell interaction g's.

codominant g. see under *allele.*

complementary g's two or more nonallelic genes that act together to produce a phenotype that is produced by neither individually; called also *reciprocal g's.*

DCC g. [*d*eleted in *c*olorectal *c*arcinoma] a gene normally expressed in the mucosa of the colon but reduced or absent in many patients with colorectal cancer.

derepressed g. a gene that is freed from its usual inhibition of expression, resulting in increased synthesis of the gene product; cf. *repressed g.*

DMPK g. [*d*ystrophia *m*yotonica *p*rotein *k*inase] a protein kinase gene on chromosome 19 that is associated with myotonic dystrophy (q.v.).

dominant g. see under *allele.*

FMR1 g. [*f*ragile X *m*ental *r*etardation *1*] a gene expressed in human brain and testes cells and associated with fragile X syndrome (q.v.).

gatekeeper g. any of those involved in regulation of cellular proliferation and the maintenance of a constant cell number; inactivation may be the genetic threshold beyond which ensues unrestrained cell growth and cancer. Cf. *caretaker g.*

H g., histocompatibility g. a gene that determines a histocompatibility antigen.

holandric g. a gene that is located on the Y chromosome and thus appears only in males.

homeobox g's a large, diverse group of genes that contain homeobox (q.v.) sequences; many play important roles in the development of embryonic organ morphogenesis and cell fate.

homeotic g's a family of genes, first observed in *Drosophila*, that orchestrate the development of individual embryonic segments into specific body parts; they occur in one or more clusters, are expressed in specific patterns at particular stages in embryogenesis, and are highly conserved across many species, all of them containing conserved homeobox (q.v.) sequences. They encode transcription factors, and mutations often have pleiotropic effects, particularly developmental defects or cancer.

housekeeping g. a gene that encodes a protein needed for basic cell function and so is expressed in all cells. Cf. *luxury g.*

HOX g's [*ho*meobo*x*-containing] name for homeotic genes (q.v.) of vertebrates; they occur in four clusters of approximately 11 genes each, and are expressed along the dorsal axis from the hindbrain to the tail region. By convention, written *Hox g's* for nonhuman animals.

immune response g's genes that govern the immune response to certain antigens. Animals carrying the gene are responders; those lacking the gene are nonresponders. In all species studied, these are autosomal dominant genes that map with those for class II major histocompatibility antigens; thus the HLA-D/DR genes are probably immune response genes in humans.

immune suppressor g's genes governing the ability of suppressor T cells to respond to certain antigens.

immunoglobulin g's the genes coding for immunoglobulin heavy and light chains, which are organized in three loci coding for κ light chains, λ light chains, and heavy chains found on human chromosomes 2, 22, and 14, respectively. These genes undergo several DNA rearrangements during the differentiation of stem cells into B cells and plasma cells, permitting synthesis of the various immunoglobulin classes.
imprinted g. a gene whose expression has been affected by genomic imprinting so that only a single allele functions, the other being turned off by epigenetic mechanisms during embryonic development.
Ir g's immune response g's.
Is g's immune suppressor g's.
lethal g. a gene the expression of which brings about the death of the organism; see also *lethal equivalent.*
luxury g. a gene that encodes a specialized function, which is generally needed, and therefore synthesized, at a high level only in a particular cell type; e.g., the hemoglobin gene, expressed only in erythrocytes. Cf. *housekeeping g.*
mismatch repair g. any of various genes involved in mismatch repair of DNA, correcting errors introduced during replication; defects lead to slow accumulation of errors and increased frequency of recombination and mutation, and are associated with microsatellite instability and tumorigenesis.
MITF g. [*mi*crophthalmia-associated *t*ranscription *f*actor] a gene expressed in the developing eye; it encodes a transcription factor that converts fibroblasts into melanocyte-like cells by transactivation of a tyrosinase gene; inactivation causes hypopigmentation.
modifier g. a gene that alters the expression of another gene at a separate locus.
mutant g. a gene that has undergone a detectable mutation.
operator g. operator.
orthologous g's genes in different species that are similar in DNA sequence and encode proteins having the same function; they originate from a single ancestral gene that diverged after speciation, e.g., the genes encoding β-globin chains in different species. Cf. *paralogous g's.*
p53 g. a tumor suppressor gene that encodes the DNA-binding p53 protein (q.v.). Mutations have been associated with malignant transformation of cells, including germline mutations in Li-Fraumeni syndrome and sporadic somatic mutations.
paired box g's PAX genes.
paralogous g's genes in a single species that have similar DNA sequences and encode proteins with similar or related functions; they are likely to have originated from a single ancestral gene, diverging after duplication, e.g., the genes encoding α- and β-globin chains. Cf. *orthologous g's.*
PAX g's [*pa*ired bo*x*; named for a conserved protein domain] a family of genes involved in developmental control, regulating tissue development and cellular differentiation in embryos. They encode transcription factors and are highly conserved across vertebrate and invertebrate species; all encode a DNA-binding paired domain, and some also encode a homeodomain and other conserved sequences. In humans, mutations in different *PAX* genes have been associated with a variety of birth defects and with cancer. By convention, written *Pax g's* for nonhuman animals.
pleiotropic g. a gene that produces many apparently unrelated effects in the phenotype.
presenilin g. either of two genes, *PSEN1* (locus: 14q24.3) and *PSEN2* (locus: 1q31-q42), encoding similar polypeptides found in many cell types both within and outside the brain and involved in cellular lipid metabolism; mutations are associated with early-onset autosomal dominant Alzheimer disease (q.v.).
recessive g. see under *allele.*
reciprocal g's complementary g's.
regulator g., regulatory g. a gene whose product controls the activity of other, distant genes; the term was originally used specifically to denote a gene that synthesizes a repressor, and is still sometimes so used.
repressed g. a gene that under normal conditions is inhibited from synthesizing the maximum possible amount of gene product; cf. *derepressed g.*
repressor g. a gene that synthesizes a repressor.
sex-linked g. a gene carried on a sex chromosome (X or Y); the term has been used synonymously with X-linked gene (q.v.), because the human Y chromosome carries so few genes other than those determining maleness, but is now little used to avoid ambiguity.
SHH g. [*S*onic *H*edge*h*og; from the animated character] a human gene homologous to the *Drosophila* hedgehog gene, which is required for embryonic segmentation; it encodes a dosage-sensitive signaling molecule that induces and organizes development of cells and tissues, including the brain and spinal cord and the limb buds. Mutations have been associated with holoprosencephaly.
silent g. a mutant gene having no detectable phenotypic effect or producing no product.
SOX g's [*S*RY (sex-determining region Y)-b*ox*] a family of genes encoding transcription factors that contain a DNA-binding sequence similar to the HMG box of the SRY gene; they are important in the formation of tissues and organs during embryonic development, and also maintain the normal function of certain cells after birth. By convention, written *Sox g's* for nonhuman animals.
split g. a gene containing multiple exons and at least one intron.
SRY g. [*s*ex-determining *r*egion *Y*] a mammalian gene, locus Yp11.3, responsible for testis determination; it encodes a transcription factor containing a highly conserved DNA-binding region called an HMG box. It is the only Y chromosome gene needed for sex determination, and mutations are associated with primary sex reversal.
structural g. 1. a gene that is transcribed into messenger RNA (mRNA) and thus encodes the amino acid sequence of a polypeptide chain. 2. more generally, a gene that encodes an mRNA, ribosomal RNA (rRNA), or transfer RNA (tRNA) product. Cf. *regulatory g.*
suicide g. a protein-coding sequence that produces an enzyme capable of converting a nontoxic prodrug to a cytotoxic compound; it is coupled to a promoter from a tumor-associated marker gene and introduced into tumor cells by a virus vector.
suppressor g. a gene that by its presence can reverse the effects of a specific mutation in another gene; see *suppression* (def. 3).
syntenic g's genes located on the same chromosome.
T-box g's, Tbx g's a highly conserved family of transcription factors having a common DNA-binding sequence (the T-box), which are important in the regulation of a wide variety of developmental processes in animals.
TP53 g. p53 g.
tumor suppressor g. a gene whose function is to limit cell proliferation and loss of whose function leads to cell transformation and tumor growth; called also *antioncogene.*
wild-type g. the allele commonly found in nature and designated as the normal; sometimes symbolized by +.
XIST g. [*X-i*nactivation–*s*pecific *t*ranscript] a gene, expressed only by the inactive X chromosome (see *lyonization*), that is responsible for the inactivation of genes on that chromosome. It does not encode a protein and is believed to function via binding of its RNA transcription product to the same X chromosome.
X-linked g. a gene carried on the X chromosome; it shows patterns of inheritance that differ between the sexes. See also under *inheritance.*
Y-linked g. a gene carried on the Y chromosome; it shows patterns of inheritance that differ between the sexes. Other than the genes that determine maleness, few human Y-linked genes have been identified. See also under *inheritance.*

gen•era (jen′ər-ə) [L.] plural of *genus.*

gen•er•al (jen′ər-əl) [L. *generalis*] affecting many parts or all parts of the organism; not local.

gen•er•al•iza•tion (jen″ər-əl-ĭ-za′shən) 1. act or process of generalizing. 2. a general principle or idea.
stimulus g. exhibition of a conditioned response to stimuli similar but not identical to the conditioned stimulus.

gen•er•al•ize (jen′ər-əl-īz) 1. to spread throughout the body, as when local disease becomes systemic. 2. to form a general principle; to reason inductively.

gen•er•a•tion (jen″ər-a′shən) [L. *generatio*] 1. reproduction (def. 1). 2. a class composed of all individuals removed by the same number of successive ancestors from a common predecessor, or occupying positions on the same level in a pedigree chart. 3. in pharmacology, a subgroup of a larger class of agents that share a certain characteristic and usually were developed around the same time as each other.
alternate g. reproduction by alternate asexual and sexual means in an animal or plant species.
asexual g. see under *reproduction.*
direct g. asexual g.
filial g. the offspring produced by the mating of the individuals of a given generation, with the offspring of the parental generation constituting the *first filial generation* (F_1), and their offspring constituting the *second filial generation* (F_2), and so on. See illustration.

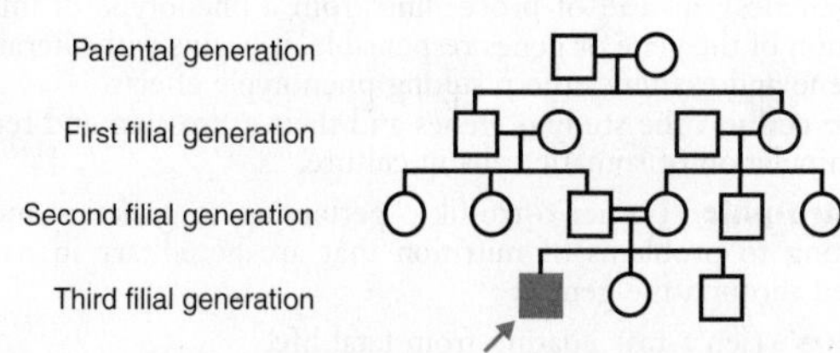

■ Pedigree in which consanguinity in the second filial generation suggests autosomal recessive inheritance (proband in third filial generation) *(arrow).*

nonsexual g. asexual g.

parental g. (P_1) the generation with which a particular genetic study is begun. See illustration.

sexual g. see under *reproduction.*

spontaneous g. the discredited concept of the development of living organisms from nonliving matter.

gen·er·a·tive (jen′ər-ə-tiv″) reproductive.

gen·er·a·tor (jen′ər-a″tər) 1. something that produces or causes to exist. 2. a machine that converts mechanical to electrical energy.

pattern g. a network of neurons, in vertebrates most often located in the central nervous system, that produces a stereotyped form of complex movement, such as ambulation or chewing, that is almost invariable from one performance to the next.

pulse g. 1. a physiologic mechanism that yields regular pulses of a hormone or other substance within the body. 2. an apparatus that delivers regular pulses of electricity for therapeutic purposes. 3. the power source for an artificial cardiac pacemaker system, usually fueled by lithium, supplying impulses to the implanted electrodes, either at a fixed rate or in some programmed pattern.

ge·ner·ic (jə-ner′ik) [L. *genus, generis* kind] 1. pertaining to a genus. 2. nonproprietary; denoting a drug name not protected by a trademark, usually descriptive of its chemical structure; such a name is sometimes called a *public name.*

ge·ne·si·al (jə-ne′ze-əl) pertaining to generation or to origin.

ge·nes·ic (jə-nes′ik) genesial.

ge·ne·si·ol·o·gy (jə-ne″ze-ol′ə-je) [*genesis* + *-logy*] the scientific study of reproduction.

gen·e·sis (jən′ə-sis) [Gr. "production," "generation"] the coming into being of anything; the process of originating.

-genesis a word termination used to denote the production, formation, or development of the object or state indicated by the word stem to which it is affixed, as *gametogenesis,* and *pathogenesis.*

gen·e·sis·ta·sis (jen″ə-sis′tə-sis) [*genesis* + *-stasis*] interruption of the reproduction of organisms by chemotherapy so as to permit the body cells or fluids to dispose of them.

gen·e·sta·tic (jen″ə-stat′ik) tending to prevent sporulation.

ge·net·ic (jə-net′ik) 1. pertaining to or determined by genes. 2. pertaining to reproduction or to birth or origin.

ge·net·i·cist (jə-net′ĭ-sist) a specialist in genetics.

ge·net·ics (jə-net′iks) [Gr. *gennan* to produce] the study of genes and their heredity.

bacterial g. the study of mechanisms of heredity in bacteria.

biochemical g. the branch of genetics concerned with the chemical and physical nature of genes and the mechanisms by which they function at the molecular level, specifically the roles of genes in controlling steps in metabolic pathways.

clinical g. the application of genetics to the diagnosis of genetic disorders and patient care, including counseling and management of the disorder.

developmental g. the branch of genetics concerned with how development is controlled by specific genes.

forward g. see *reverse g.*

mathematical g. the statistical analysis of probabilities of genetic transmission, genes in populations, and hypothesis testing.

molecular g. the branch of genetics concerned with the molecular structure and functioning of genes, including the replication of DNA, its transcription into RNA, and the translation of RNA to form proteins.

population g. the study of the distribution of genes in populations and of how genes and genotype frequencies are maintained or changed. See also *Hardy-Weinberg law,* under *law.*

reproductive g. the use of a combination of clinical genetics, dysmorphology, maternal-fetal medicine, and assisted reproductive technologies for detection, understanding, and prevention of reproductive abnormalities.

reverse g. a branch of molecular genetics that proceeds in the opposite direction from traditional molecular genetics (sometimes in contrast called forward genetics); instead of proceeding from a phenotype of interest to identification of the gene or genes responsible, it begins with alteration of a specific gene and examines the resulting phenotypic effects.

somatic cell g. the study of genes and their expression and regulation using manipulation of somatic cells in culture.

ge·neto·tro·phic (jə-net″o-tro′fik) pertaining to genetics and nutrition; relating to problems of nutrition that are hereditary in nature, or transmitted through the genes.

gen·e·tous (jen′ə-təs) dating from fetal life.

Ge·ne·va Con·ven·tion (jə-ne′və) an international agreement of 1864 whereby, among other pledges, the signatory nations pledged themselves to treat the wounded and the military medical and nursing staffs as neutrals on the field of battle.

Gen·gou phenomenon (zhaw-goo′) [Octave *Gengou,* Belgian bacteriologist, 1875–1957] complement fixation.

Gen·graf (jen′graf) trademark for preparations of cyclosporine.

ge·ni·al (jə-ni′əl) [*geni-* + *-al*[1]] mental[2].

ge·ni·an (je′ne-ən) mental[2].

gen·ic (jen′ik) genetic (def. 1).

-genic [Gr. *gennan* to produce] a word termination meaning producing, or productive of.

ge·nic·u·la (jə-nik′u-lə) [L.] plural of *geniculum.*

ge·nic·u·lar (jə-nik′u-lər) pertaining to the knee.

ge·nic·u·late (jə-nik′u-lāt) [L. *geniculatus*] bent, like a knee.

ge·nic·u·lo·cal·car·ine (jə-nik″u-lo-kal′kə-rīn) [*geniculum* + *calcarine*] pertaining to, or connecting, one of the geniculate bodies and the calcar avis or calcarine sulcus.

ge·nic·u·lo·stri·ate (jə-nik″u-lo-stri′āt) connecting one of the geniculate nuclei with the striate cortex.

ge·nic·u·lum (jə-nik′u-ləm) pl. *genic′ula* [L., dim. of *genu*] [TA] a general term designating a sharp, kneelike bend in a small structure or organ, such as a nerve.

g. cana′lis facia′lis, g. cana′lis ner′vi facia′lis [TA], **g. of facial canal** the bend in the facial canal lodging the geniculum nervi facialis; called also *genu of facial canal.*

g. of facial nerve, g. ner′vi facia′lis [TA] the part of the facial nerve at the lateral end of the internal acoustic meatus, where the fibers turn sharply posteroinferiorly, and where the geniculate ganglion is found; called also *external genu of facial nerve.*

gen·in (jen′in) aglycon.

geni(o)- [Gr. *geneion* chin] a combining form denoting relationship to the chin. See also words beginning *ment(o)-.*

ge·nio·chei·lo·plas·ty (je″ne-o-ki′lo-plas″te) [*genio-* + *cheilo-* + *-plasty*] plastic surgery of the chin and lip.

ge·nio·glos·sus (je″ne-o-glos′əs) see under *musculus.*

ge·nio·hyo·glos·sus (je″ne-o-hi″o-glos′əs) musculus genioglossus.

ge·nio·hy·oid (je″ne-o-hi′oid) pertaining to the chin and hyoid bone.

ge·nio·hy·oi·de·us (je″ne-o-hi-oi′de-əs) see under *musculus.*

ge·nio·plas·ty (je′ne-o-plas″te) [*genio-* + *-plasty*] plastic surgery of the chin. **genioplas′tic** *adj*

gen·i·tal (jen′ĭ-təl) [L. *genitalis* belonging to birth] 1. reproductive. 2. pertaining to the organs of reproduction; see terms beginning *organa genitalia.*

gen·i·ta·lia (jen″ĭ-ta′le-ə) [L., pl.] the organs of reproduction, particularly those external to the body; see entries beginning *organa genitalia,* under *organum.*

ambiguous g. genital organs with characteristics typical of both male and female, as seen in hermaphroditism and some types of pseudohermaphroditism.

female external g. organa genitalia feminina externa.

female internal g. organa genitalia feminina interna.

indifferent g. the reproductive organs of the embryo prior to the establishment of definitive sex. In human embryos this stage occurs during the fourth to seventh weeks.

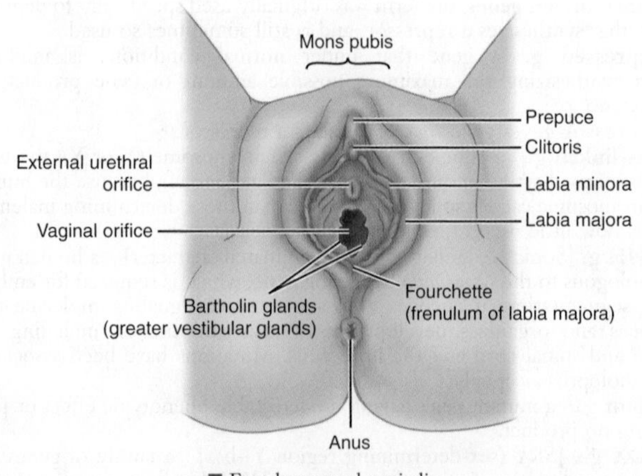

■ Female external genitalia.

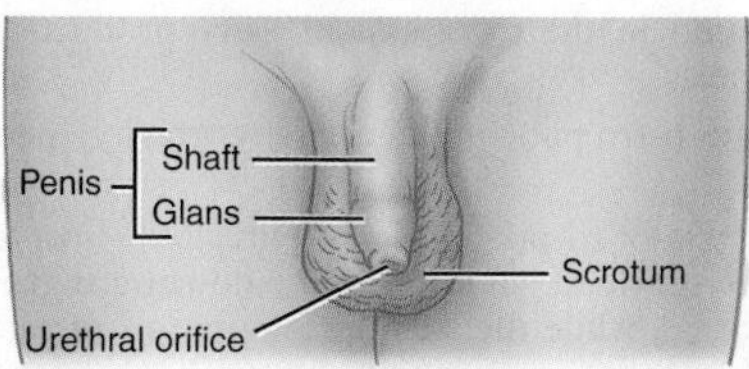

■ Male external genitalia.

male external g. organa genitalia masculina externa.
male internal g. organa genitalia masculina interna.

gen·i·tal·oid (jen′ĭ-tal-oid) [*genitalia* + *-oid*] pertaining to the primordial germ cells, before future sexuality is distinguishable.

gen·i·tals (jen′ĭ-təlz) [L. *genitalia*] genitalia.

genit(o)- [*genital*, q.v.] a combining form denoting relationship to the organs of reproduction.

gen·i·to·cru·ral (jen″ĭ-to-kroo′rəl) [*genital* + *crural*] pertaining to the genitalia and lower limb.

gen·i·to·fem·o·ral (jen″ĭ-to-fem′or-əl) genitocrural.

gen·i·tog·ra·phy (jen″ĭ-tog′rə-fe) radiography of the urogenital sinus and internal duct structures after injection of a contrast medium through the opening of the sinus.

gen·i·to·plas·ty (jen′ĭ-to-plas″te) [*genital* + *-plasty*] plastic surgery on the genital organs. **genitoplas′tic** *adj*

gen·i·to·uri·nary (jen″ĭ-to-u′rĭ-nar-e) pertaining to the genital and urinary systems; called also *urinogenital* and *urogenital.*

ge·nius (jēn′yəs) 1. distinctive character or peculiar nature. 2. superlative aptitude or ability. 3. a person with superlative aptitude or ability.

Gen·na·ri line (band, stria, stripe) (jĕ-nah′re) [Francesco *Gennari*, Italian anatomist, 1750–1796] see under *line.*

gen(o)- [Gr. *genos* offspring, race, kind] a combining form denoting relationship to (1) reproduction, (2) sex, (3) race or kind, or (4) a gene or genes.

ge·no·blast (je′no-blast) [*geno-* + *-blast*[1]] the nucleus of the fertilized oocyte.

ge·no·copy (je′no-kop″e) a phenotype that appears identical to another phenotype but that is caused by a different genetic mechanism. See also *phenocopy.*

ge·no·der·ma·tol·o·gy (je″no-dur″mə-tol′ə-je) the branch of dermatology that treats hereditary skin diseases.

ge·no·der·ma·to·sis (je″no-dur″mə-to′sis) [*geno-* + *dermatosis*] a genetically determined disorder of the skin, usually generalized; if circumscribed, it is usually called a *nevus.*

ge·nome (je′nōm) [*gene* + chromoso*me*] the entirety of the genetic information encoded by the nucleotide sequence of an organism, cell, organelle, or virus; it is DNA in eukaryotes and prokaryotes, and DNA or RNA in viruses. In a human being, the genome size is approximately 3 billion base pairs of DNA and approximately 25,000 genes. **genom′ic** *adj*

mitochondrial g. a circular double-stranded DNA molecule present in 5 to 10 copies within each mitochondrion, and thus in thousands of copies per cell, with a slightly different genetic code and a higher rate of mutation than those of the nuclear genome. Because the mitochondria are cytoplasmic, the genome is transmitted by maternal inheritance (q.v.). In humans, it is 16.6 kb in size and contains 37 genes; 13 encode polypeptides that function in the electron transport system and oxidative phosphorylation, 22 encode types of tRNA, and two encode types of rRNA, with other components of the protein-synthesizing apparatus and other mitochondrial proteins encoded in the nucleus.

ge·no·mics (je-no′miks) the study of the structure and function of the genome, including information about sequence, mapping, and expression, and how genes and their products work in organisms.

cancer g. the study of genome structure in cancer cells to enhance understanding of the molecular mechanisms involved, in order to improve disease prevention, detection, diagnosis, and treatment. Called also *oncogenomics.*

functional g. the study of the roles of DNA and RNA in the progression from genetic information to the production of a given protein.

Gen·op·tic (jen-op′tik) trademark for preparations of gentamicin sulfate.

ge·no·spe·cies (je′no-spe″shēz) a group of bacterial strains capable of genetic transfer and recombination.

ge·no·tox·ic (je′no-tok″sik) damaging to DNA: pertaining to agents (radiation or chemical substances) known to damage DNA, thereby causing mutations, which can result in cancer.

Geno·tro·pin (jen-o′tro-pin) trademark for a preparation of somatropin.

ge·no·type (je′no-tīp) [*geno-* + *type*] 1. the entire genetic constitution of an individual. 2. the alleles present at one or more specific loci. Cf. *phenotype.*

ge·no·typ·ic (je″no-ti′pik) pertaining to or expressive of the genotype.

-genous [Gr. *-genēs* born] a word termination with two opposite meanings: (1) arising or resulting from, or produced by (endogenous, pyogenous); (2) producing (androgenous).

Gen·ta·ci·din (jen″tə-si′din) trademark for preparations of gentamicin sulfate.

Gen·tak (jen′tak) trademark for preparations of gentamicin sulfate.

gen·ta·mi·cin (jen″tə-mi′sin) an aminoglycoside antibiotic complex derived from *Micromonospora echinospora*, consisting of components designated A, B, C, etc. The form in clinical use is a mixture of three fractions of the C component (C_1, C_{1A}, C_2); it is effective against a wide range of aerobic gram-negative bacilli, especially the Enterobacteriaceae and *Pseudomonas*, and some gram-positive bacteria.

g. sulfate [USP] the sulfate salt of gentamicin, applied topically to the skin, ear canal, or conjunctiva or administered intramuscularly or intravenously in the treatment of a wide variety of infections caused by susceptible gram-negative organisms.

gen·tian (jen′shən) the dried rhizome and roots of *Gentiana lutea* L. (Gentianaceae); used as a bitter tonic. It contains gentiin, gentiamarin, gentisin, gentisic acid, gentiopicrin, gentianose, and pectin. Also known as *yellow* or *pale gentian.*

g. violet [USP] a dye occurring as a dark green powder or greenish glistening pieces having a metallic luster, with antibacterial, antifungal, and anthelmintic properties, applied topically in the treatment of infections of the skin and mucous membranes associated with gram-positive bacteria and molds, and also used to kill trypanosomes in blood collected in blood banks in areas endemic for Chagas disease. Called also *crystal violet* and *methyl violet.*

gen·tian·o·phil (jen′shən-o-fil) 1. an element staining readily with gentian violet. 2. gentianophilic.

gen·tian·o·phil·ic (jen′shən-o-fil′ik) [*gentian* + *-philic*] staining readily with gentian violet.

gen·tian·o·pho·bic (jen″shən-o-fo′bik) not staining readily with gentian violet.

Gen·tran (jen′tran) trademark for a preparation of dextran.

ge·nu (je′nu) gen. *ge′nus* pl. *ge′nua* [L.] [TA] 1. the knee; the site of articulation between the thigh (femur) and leg. 2. a general term used to designate any anatomic structure bent like the knee.

g. cap′sulae inter′nae [TA] genu of internal capsule: the blunt angle formed by the union of the two limbs of the internal capsule, situated posterior to the caudate nucleus, anterior to the thalamus, and medial to the lentiform nucleus; called also *knee of internal capsule.*

g. cor′poris callo′si [TA] genu of corpus callosum: the sharp ventral curve at the anterior end of the trunk of the corpus callosum.

external g. of facial nerve geniculum nervi facialis.

g. extror′sum g. varum.

g. of facial canal geniculum canalis facialis.

g. of facial nerve 1. genu nervi facialis. 2. geniculum nervi facialis.

g. impres′sum a flattening and bending of the knee joint to one side, with consequent displacement of the patella up and to the same side.

g. of internal capsule g. capsulae internae.

internal g. of facial nerve g. nervi facialis.

g. intror′sum g. valgum.

g. ner′vi facia′lis [TA] genu of facial nerve: the bend in the fibers arising from the nucleus of the facial nerve, which with the abducens nucleus produces the facial colliculus in the floor of the fourth ventricle; fibers of this genu loop from caudal to rostral around the abducens nucleus.

g. recurva′tum hyperextension of the knee; called also *back knee.*

g. val′gum a deformity in which the knees are abnormally close together and the space between the ankles is increased; known also as *knock knee.*

g. va′rum a deformity in which the knees are abnormally separated and the lower extremities are bowed inwardly; the deformity may be in the thigh or leg, or both. Known also as *bowleg.*

gen·ua (jen′u-ə) [L.] plural of *genu.*

gen·u·al (jen′u-əl) 1. relating to a genu or knee. 2. resembling a genu or knee.

genu·cu·bi·tal (jen″u-ku′bĭ-təl) [*genu* + *cubital*] pertaining to the knees and elbows; see under *position.*

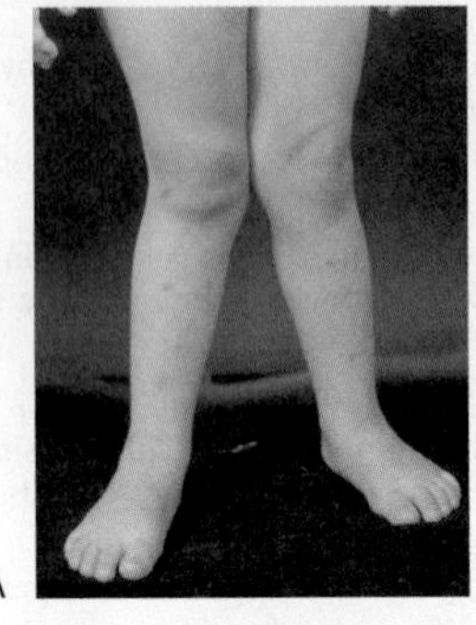

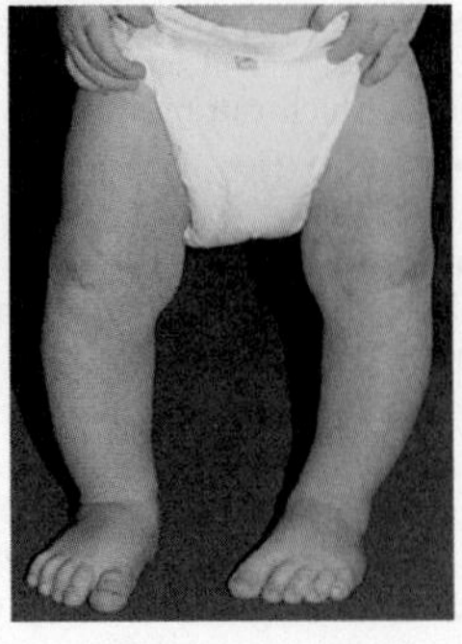

■ *(A)*, Genu valgum; *(B)*, genu varum.

genu·fa·cial (jen″u-fa′shəl) [*genu* + *facial*] pertaining to the knees and face; see under *position*.

genu·pec·to·ral (jen″u-pek′tər-əl) [*genu* + *pectoral*] pertaining to the knees and chest; see under *position*.

ge·nus (je′nəs) pl. *gen′era* [L.] a taxonomic category subordinate to a tribe (or subtribe) and superior to a species (or subgenus).

-geny [Gr. *-geneia*, from *-genēs* born] a word termination denoting generation or origin.

ge(o)- [Gr. *gē* earth] a combining form denoting relationship to the earth, or to soil.

Geo·ba·cil·lus (je″o-bə-sil′əs) a genus of bacteria of the family Bacillaceae, consisting of thermophilic, gram-positive, motile or nonmotile, spore-producing rods, occurring singly or in short chains; organisms are chemoorganotrophic and aerobic or facultatively anaerobic. Many species were formerly classified in the genus *Bacillus*.

G. stearothermo′philus a thermophilic species that produces very resistant spores and is capable of growth at 65°C. It is used to test for autoclave quality control. Formerly called *Bacillus stearothermophilus*.

geo·bi·ol·o·gy (je″o-bi-ol′ə-je) [*geo-* + *biology*] the biology of terrestrial life.

geo·chem·is·try (je″o-kem′is-tre) [*geo-* + *chemistry*] the science concerned with study of the elements in the earth's crust and the chemical changes that occur therein.

Ge·o·cil·lin (je′o-sil″in) trademark for a preparation of carbenicillin indanyl sodium.

ge·ode (je′ōd) [Gr. *geōdes* earthlike: so called from a fancied resemblance to a mineral geode] a dilated lymph space.

Ge·o·don (je′o-don″) trademark for a preparation of ziprasidone hydrochloride.

ge·o·gen (je′o-jən) an aspect of the geography or geochemistry of an area that affects organisms in it, particularly with reference to disease.

geo·graph·ic (je″o-graf′ik) a term used in pathology referring to a pattern that is well demarcated, resembling the outline of a land mass against water on a map.

geo·med·i·cine (je″o-med′ĭ-sin) [*geo-* + *medicine*] the branch of medicine dealing with the influence of geographic factors, such as climate and environmental conditions, on health and disease. Called also *nosogeography* and *geographic medicine*. See also *geographic pathology*, under *pathology*.

geo·pa·thol·o·gy (je″o-pə-thol′ə-je) [*geo-* + *pathology*] the study of the peculiarities of disease in relation to topography, climate, food habits, etc., of various regions of the earth.

Ge·o·pen (je′o-pen) trademark for a preparation of carbenicillin disodium.

geo·pha·gia (je-o-fa′jə) [*geo-* + *-phagia*] the habit of eating clay or earth, a form of pica.

ge·oph·a·gism (je-of′ə-jiz-əm) geophagia.

ge·oph·a·gy (je-of′ə-je) geophagia.

geo·phil·ic (je″o-fil′ik) [*geo-* + *-philic*] characterized by an affinity for soil; said of parasitic organisms that have this quality and infect only animals that are weak or immunocompromised. Cf. *anthropophilic* and *zoophilic*.

geo·tax·is (je″o-tak′sis) [*geo-* + *taxis*] taxis of an animal in response to gravitational force. **geotac′tic** *adj*

geo·tri·cho·sis (je″o-trĭ-ko′sis) infection by *Geotrichum candidum*, which may attack the bronchi, lungs, mouth, or intestinal tract; its manifestations resemble those of candidiasis.

Ge·ot·ri·chum (je-ot′rĭ-kəm) a genus of yeastlike imperfect fungi of the form-family Cryptococcaceae, closely related to *Trichosporon*. *G. can′didum*, found in the feces and in dairy products, is the etiologic agent of geotrichosis.

ge·o·tro·pic (je″o-tro′pik) influenced by gravity; pertaining to geotropism.

ge·ot·ro·pism (je-ot′ro-piz-əm) [*geo-* + *tropism*] tropism in an organism in response to gravitational force, as the downward growth of the roots of a plant *(positive g.)*, while the stem grows upward *(negative g.)*.

ge·phyr·in (jə-fir′in) a peripheral membrane protein associated with the cytoplasmic domain of neuronal glycine receptors; it binds microtubules and is necessary for the clustering of glycine receptors.

ge·ra·ni·ol (jə-ra′ne-ol) 1. a 10-carbon branched-chain alcohol occurring widely in essential oils of plants. 2. a pheromone of certain species of bees, being secreted by worker bees to signal the location of food.

ge·rat·ic (jə-rat′ik) [Gr. *gēras* old age] pertaining to old age.

ger·a·tol·o·gy (jer″ə-tol′ə-je) gerontology.

Ger·bich blood group (gur′bich) [*Gerbich*, surname of the American propositus first observed in 1960] see under *blood group*.

ger·bil (jur′bəl) any of several species of small burrowing rodents of genus *Gerbillus* and related genera, native to arid parts of Africa and southwestern Asia. Some species serve as reservoirs for bubonic plague and others as reservoirs for Old World cutaneous leishmaniasis.

great g. *Rhombomys opimus*.

Ger·bil·lus (jər-bil′əs) a genus of rodents of the family Muridae, including most types of gerbils.

GERD gastroesophageal reflux disease.

Ger·dy fibers, etc. (zher-de′) [Pierre Nicholas *Gerdy*, French surgeon, 1797–1856] see under *fiber*, *fontanelle*, *loop*, *ligament*, and *tubercle*.

Ge·ref (je′ref) trademark for a preparation of sermorelin acetate.

Ger·hardt disease, triangle (dullness) (ger′hahrt) [Carl Adolf Christian Jacob *Gerhardt*, German physician, 1833–1902] see under *triangle* and see *erythromelalgia*.

Ger·hardt-Se·mon law (ger′harht se′mon) [C.A.C.J. *Gerhardt;* Sir Felix *Semon*, German-born English laryngologist, 1849–1921] see under *law*.

ger·i·at·ric (jer″e-at′rik) 1. pertaining to elderly persons or to the aging process. 2. pertaining to geriatrics.

ger·i·atri·cian (jer″e-ə-trish′ən) a specialist in geriatrics.

ger·i·at·rics (jer″e-at′riks) [*ger-* + *-iatrics*] the branch of medicine that treats problems peculiar to old age and the aging, including the clinical problems of senescence and senility.

dental g. gerodontics.

Ger·i·mal (jer′ĭ-mal) trademark for preparations of ergoloid mesylates.

geri·odon·tics (jer″e-o-don′tiks) gerodontics.

geri·odon·tist (jer″e-o-don′tist) gerodontist.

Ger·lach valve (ger′lahk) [Joseph von *Gerlach*, German anatomist, 1820–1896] valve of vermiform appendix.

Ger·lier disease (zher-le-a′) [Felix *Gerlier*, Swiss physician, 1840–1914] see under *disease*.

germ (jurm) [L. *germen*] 1. a pathogenic microorganism. 2. living substance capable of developing into an organ, part, or organism as a whole; a primordium.

dental g. tooth g.

enamel g. the epithelial rudiment of the enamel organ.

hair g. an ectodermal concentration in the basal layer of the embryonic epidermis, the precursor of a hair follicle and related structures.

tooth g. a budlike thickening of the dental lamina that is the primordium of a tooth, and in which the enamel knot develops; the collective structures from which a tooth is formed, including the dental follicle, enamel organ, and dental papilla. Called also *dental g.* See also *tooth bud*, under *bud*.

Ger·ma·nin (jur′mə-nin) trademark for a preparation of suramin hexasodium.

ger·ma·ni·um (Ge) (jər-ma′ne-əm) a rare element, having the appearance of a bluish gray metalloid, atomic number 32, atomic weight 72.59.

ger·mer·ine (jur′mər-ēn) a crystalline alkaloid, $C_{36}H_{57}O_{11}N$, from *Veratrum senecio*.

ger·mi·ci·dal (jur″mĭ-si′dəl) [L. *germen* germ + *caedere* to kill] lethal to pathogenic microorganisms.

ger·mi·cide (jur′mĭ-sīd) an agent that kills pathogenic microorganisms; see also *antibiotic* and *antimicrobial*.

ger·mi·nal (jur′mĭ-nəl) [L. *germinalis*] pertaining to or of the nature of a gamete (germ cell) or the primordial stage of development.

ger·mi·na·tion (jur″mĭ-na′shən) [L. *germinatio*] the sprouting of a seed, spore, or plant embryo.

ger·mi·na·tive (jur′mĭ-na″tiv) 1. pertaining to germination. 2. causing germination.

ger·mi·no·ma (jur″mĭ-no′mə) a type of germ cell tumor consisting of large round cells with vesicular nuclei, usually found in the ovary, undescended testis, anterior mediastinum, or pineal gland; in males these are called *seminomas* and in females *dysgerminomas*.

pineal g. a common type of pineal tumor, consisting of nests of large spherical germ cells that are surrounded by a network of reticular connective tissue and are histologically identical to the germ cells of the testes or ovaries. Symptoms include obstructive hydrocephalus, headache, papilledema, nausea, vomiting, diplopia, and lethargy.

suprasellar g. a germinoma located superior to the sella turcica, causing symptoms including hypopituitarism, diabetes insipidus, and visual disturbances.

germ·line (jərm′līn) the sequence of cells in the line of direct descent from zygote to gamete, as opposed to somatic cells (all other body cells). Mutations in germline cells are transmitted to progeny; those in somatic cells are not. Written also *germ line.*

ger(o)- [Gr. *gēras* old age] a combining form denoting relationship to old age or to the aged.

gero·der·ma (jer″o-dur′mə) [*gero-* + *derma*] dystrophy of the skin and genitals, producing the appearance of old age.

g. osteodysplas′ticum an autosomal recessive disorder caused by mutation in the *SCYL1BP1* gene (locus: 1q24.2), which encodes a protein which has been identified as a golgin. It is characterized by geroderma associated with osseous changes, including osteoporosis, lines in the bones that resemble growth rings of a tree, and dwarfism. Called also *Walt Disney dwarfism.*

gero·der·mia (jer″o-dur′me-ə) geroderma.

ger·odon·tia (jer″o-don′shə) gerodontics.

ger·odon·tic (jer″o-don′tik) [*gero-* + *odontic*] 1. pertaining to changes in the dental tissues with age. 2. pertaining to the practice of gerodontics.

ger·odon·tics (jer″o-don′tiks) [*gero-* + *odontic*] the delivery of dental care to aging persons; the diagnosis, prevention, and treatment of problems peculiar to advanced age. Called also *dental geriatrics* and *gerodontia.*

ger·odon·tist (jer″o-don′tist) a dentist who practices gerodontics.

ger·odon·tol·o·gy (jer″o-don-tol′ə-je) the study of the dentition and dental problems in the aged or aging.

gero·mor·phism (jer″o-mor′fiz-əm) [*gero-* + *morph-* + *-ism*] premature aging of a body part.

cutaneous g. geroderma.

ger·on·tal (jer-on′təl) senile.

ger·on·tic (jə-ron′tik) senile.

geront(o)- [Gr. *gerōn*, gen. *gerontos* old man] a combining form denoting relationship to old age or to the aged.

ger·on·tol·o·gist (jer″on-tol′ə-jist) a specialist in gerontology.

ger·on·tol·o·gy (jer″on-tol′ə-je) [*geronto-* + *-logy*] the scientific study of aging and its problems in all their aspects—clinical, biologic, historical, and sociologic.

ger·on·to·phil·ia (jer″on-to-fil′e-ə) [*geronto-* + *-philia*] sexual attraction to old people.

ger·on·to·ther·a·peu·tics (jer-on″to-ther″ə-pu′tiks) [*geronto-* + *therapeutics*] therapeutic management of aging persons designed to retard and prevent the development of many of the aspects of senescence.

ger·on·to·ther·a·py (jer-on″to-ther′ə-pe) gerontotherapeutics.

ger·on·to·tox·on (jer-on″to-tok′son) arcus corneae.

g. len′tis equatorial couching of the lens in the aged; no longer done.

ger·on·tox·on (jer″on-tok′son) gerontotoxon.

gero·psy·chi·a·try (jer″o-si-ki′ə-tre) a subspecialty of psychiatry dealing with mental illness in the elderly.

Ge·ro·ta fascia (capsule), method (ga-ro′tah) [Dumitru *Gerota*, Romanian anatomist, 1867–1939] see under *method* and see *fascia renalis* under *fascia.*

Gerst·mann syndrome (gerst′mahn) [Josef *Gerstmann*, Austrian neurologist, 1887–1969] see under *syndrome.*

Gerst·mann-Sträus·sler syndrome (gerst′mahn shtrois′lər) [J. *Gerstmann;* E. *Sträussler*, Austrian physician, 20th century] Gerstmann-Strässler-Scheinker syndrome.

Gerst·mann-Sträus·sler-Schein·ker syndrome (gerst′mahn shtrois′lər shīn′kər) [J. *Gerstmann;* E. *Sträussler;* I. *Scheinker*, Austrian physician, 20th century] see under *syndrome.*

ge·rüst·mark (gĕ-rūst′mahrk) [Ger., from *Gerüst* scaffolding + *Mark* marrow] a unique, collagen-poor zone of connective tissue lying across the bone marrow adjoining the growing ends of bones; observed in scurvy.

GES gastric electrical stimulation.

Ge·sell developmental schedule (gə-zel′) [Arnold Lucius *Gesell*, American pediatrician and psychologist, 1880–1961] see under *schedule.*

ges·ta·gen (jes′tə-jen) progestational agent.

ge·stalt (gə-stawlt′, gə-shtawlt′) [Ger.] form, shape; a whole perceptual configuration. See *gestaltism.*

ge·stal·tism (gə-stawl′tiz-əm, gə-shtawl′tiz-əm) [*gestalt* + *-ism*] a theory in psychology that claims that objects of the mind, as immediately presented to direct experience, come as complete, unanalyzable wholes or forms (Gestalten) that cannot be split up into parts; called also *gestalt theory.*

ges·ta·tion (jes-ta′shən) [L. *gestatio*] pregnancy. **gesta′tional** *adj*

multiple g. see under *pregnancy.*

geste (zhest) [Fr.] gesture.

g. antagoniste′ (ahn-tag-o-nēst′) ["antagonistic gesture"] a sensory trick, such as lightly touching the eyelid in blepharospasm, that temporarily alleviates dystonic movements.

ges·to·sis (jes-to′sis) pl. *gesto′ses* [L. *gestare* to bear] any manifestation of preeclampsia in pregnancy.

ges·tri·none (jes′trĭ-nōn) a synthetic steroid hormone with androgenic, antiestrogenic, and antiprogestogenic properties, used in the treatment of endometriosis; administered orally.

GeV gigaelectron volt; one billion electron volts.

GFAP glial fibrillary acidic protein.

GFR glomerular filtration rate.

GGR global genome repair.

GGT γ-glutamyltransferase.

GH growth hormone.

GHA glucoheptonate (gluceptate).

GHB γ-hydroxybutyric acid.

Ghon complex, focus (primary lesion, tubercle) (gon) [Anton *Ghon*, Austrian-born pathologist in Czechoslovakia, 1866–1936] see *primary complex*, and see under *focus.*

Ghon-Sachs bacillus (gon′ sahks′) [A. *Ghon;* Anton *Sachs*, Austrian physician, 19th century] *Clostridium septicum.*

ghost (gōst) a faint or shadowy figure, lacking the customary substance of reality.

red cell g. ghost cell (def. 2).

ghrel·in (grel′in) [Indo-European root *ghrē-* to grow] a peptide hormone related to motilin, expressed primarily by the stomach and secondarily by the small intestine and colon and possibly other tissues. It is a growth hormone secretagogue; stimulates the sensation of hunger and regulates energy balance and glucose homeostasis; and has regulatory functions in the gastrointestinal, cardiovascular, and immune systems.

GH-RH growth hormone–releasing hormone.

GI gastrointestinal.

Gia·co·mi·ni band (jah-ko-me′ne) [Carlo *Giacomini*, Italian anatomist, 1841–1898] see under *band.*

Gia·nel·li sign (jah-nel′e) [Giuseppe *Gianelli*, Italian physician, 1799–1871] Tournay sign.

Gian·nuz·zi crescents (bodies, cells, demilunes) (jah-nōōt′se) [Guiseppe *Giannuzzi*, Italian anatomist, 1839–1876] see under *crescent.*

Gia·not·ti-Cros·ti syndrome (jah-not′e kros′te) [Fernando *Gianotti*, Italian dermatologist, 1920–1984; Agostino *Crosti*, Italian dermatologist, 20th century] see under *syndrome.*

gi·ant (ji′ənt) [Gr. *gigas*] a person or organism of very great size; see *gigantism.*

gi·ant·ism (ji′ənt-iz-əm) gigantism.

Gian·tur·co coil (jahn-tōōr′ko) [Cesare *Gianturco*, Italian-born American radiologist, 1905–1995] see under *coil.*

Gi·ar·dia (je-ahr′de-ə) [Alfred *Giard*, French biologist, 1846–1908] a genus of usually nonpathogenic, flagellate intestinal protozoa of the order Diplomonadida, phylum Parabasalia, parasitic in vertebrates. A large sucking disk on the organism's ventral body surface enables it to adhere to microvilli in the host's intestinal epithelium; there are two anterior nuclei and eight flagella in four pairs.

G. intestina′lis a species that is the usual cause of giardiasis in humans; it may also infect domestic animals.

G. lamb′lia former name for *G. intestinalis.*

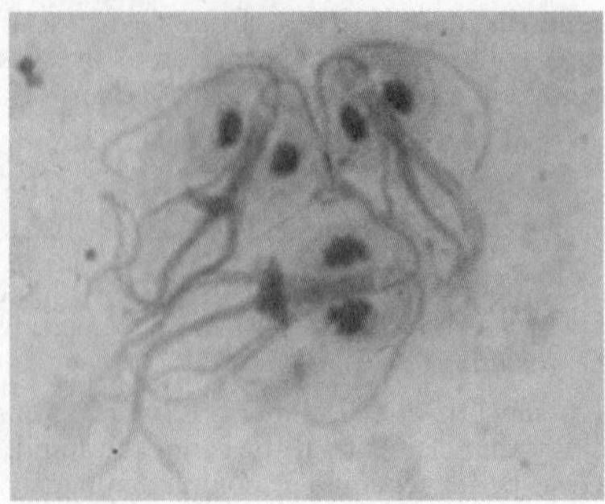

■ *Giardia intestinalis* trophozoites from duodenal mucosa biopsy, each with two large nuclei and flagella (Giemsa stain).

gi·ar·di·a·sis (je″ahr-di′ə-sis) 1. a common infection of the human small intestine with the protozoan *Giardia lamblia*, spread via contaminated food or water or by direct person-to-person contact. Most patients are asymptomatic, but a few have symptoms ranging from nonspecific gastrointestinal discomfort to mild or profuse diarrhea, nausea, lassitude, anorexia, and weight loss. 2. infection of a dog or cat with *Giardia lamblia*, characterized by copious diarrhea and anorexia; it may be persistent or self-limiting.

gib·bos·i·ty (gĭ-bos′ĭ-te) [L. *gibbosus* crooked] the condition of being humped; kyphosis.

gib·bous (gib′əs) [L. *gibbosus*] convex; humped; protuberant; humpbacked.

Gibbs free energy, theorem (gibz) [Josiah Willard *Gibbs*, American physicist, 1839–1903] see under *theorem.*

Gibbs-Don·nan equilibrium (effect) (gibz′ don′ən) [J.W. *Gibbs;* Frederick George *Donnan*, English chemist, 1870–1956] Donnan equilibrium.

gib·bus (gib′əs) [L.] hump.

Gib·ney bandage (strapping), boot, perispondylitis (disease) (gib′ne) [Virgil Pendleton *Gibney*, American surgeon, 1847–1927] see under *bandage* and *perispondylitis.*

Gib·son murmur (gib′sən) [George Alexander *Gibson*, Scottish physician, 1854–1913] see under *murmur.*

gid (gid) a disease of the brain and spinal cord of ruminants caused by the presence of *Coenurus cerebralis* (the larva of *Taenia multiceps*), and marked by unsteadiness of gait, which if untreated can progress to paralysis and blindness. Called also *coenurosis, coenuriasis, staggers, sturdy*, and *turnsickness.*

Giem·sa stain (gēm′sə) [Gustav *Giemsa*, German chemist and bacteriologist, 1867–1948] see *Stains and Staining Methods*, under *stain.*

Gier·ke corpuscles (gēr′kə) [Hans Paul Bernhard *Gierke*, German anatomist, 1847–1886] see under *corpuscle.*

Gie·son see *van Gieson.*

Gif·ford operation, reflex (gif′ərd) [Harold *Gifford*, American oculist, 1858–1929] see under *operation* and see *orbicularis pupillary reflex*, under *reflex.*

GIFT gamete intrafallopian transfer.

giga- [Gr. *gigas* giant] a prefix designating gigantic size; used in naming units of measurement to indicate a quantity one billion (10^9) times the unit designated by the root with which it is combined. Symbol G.

gi·gan·ti·form (ji-gan′tĭ-form) very large.

gi·gan·tism (ji-gan′tiz-əm, ji′gan-tiz-əm) [*gigant-* + *-ism*] abnormal overgrowth; excessive size and stature. Called also *giantism, hypersomia*, and *somatomegaly.*

acromegalic g. pituitary gigantism in which the body also has the changes in the short and flat bones and in the distal parts that are characteristic of acromegaly.

cerebral g. gigantism in the absence of increased levels of growth hormone, attributed to a cerebral defect; infants are large, and accelerated growth continues for the first four or five years, the rate being normal thereafter. The hands and feet are large, the head large and dolichocephalic, the medial portion of the palpebral fissure is higher than the temporal portion, and there is hypertelorism. The child is clumsy, and mental retardation of varying degrees is usually present. Called also *Sotos syndrome.*

eunuchoid g. gigantism in which the body has eunuchoid features and hypogonadism.

fetal g. see under *macrosomia.*

hyperpituitary g. pituitary g.

normal g. gigantism in which the body proportions and sexual development are normal.

pituitary g. gigantism due to excessive pituitary secretion of growth hormone, occurring before puberty and before the epiphyses close; it is most often caused by eosinophilic cell hyperplasia or an eosinophilic adenoma, but sometimes results from a chromophobe adenoma. Called also *hyperpituitary g.* and *Launois syndrome.*

gigant(o)- [Gr. *gigas*, gen. *gigantos* giant] a combining form meaning huge.

gi·gan·to·cel·lu·lar (ji-gan″to-sel′u-lər) pertaining to giant cells.

gi·gan·to·mas·tia (ji-gan″to-mas′te-ə) extreme macromastia.

Gi·gar·ti·na (ji″gahr-ti′nə) a genus of red algae. *G. mammillo′sa* (Goodenough & Woodward) J. Aghardt. is a source of carrageenan and chondrus.

gi·gan·to·so·ma (ji-gan″to-so′mə) gigantism.

Gi·gli wire saw (jēl′ye) [Leonardo *Gigli*, Italian gynecologist, 1863–1908] see under *saw.*

Gil·bert syndrome (cholemia) (zhēl-bār′) [Nicolas Augustin *Gilbert*, French physician, 1858–1927] see under *syndrome.*

Gil·christ disease (gil′krist) [Thomas Caspar *Gilchrist*, American dermatologist, 1862–1927] North American blastomycosis.

gil·da·ble (gil′də-bəl) susceptible of being colored with gold stains.

gill (gil) 1. the respiratory organ of aquatic animals, such as fish, mollusks, and many arthropods, usually a thin-walled projection from the body surface or from some part of the digestive tract whose surface is increased by filaments, lamellae, or other folds. 2. one of the thin perpendicular plates found on the underside of a mushroom cap and along which the basidia are produced. Called also *lamella.*

Gilles de la Tou·rette syndrome (zhēl-də-lah-too-ret′) [Georges Edouard Albert Brutus *Gilles de la Tourette*, French physician, 1857–1904] see under *syndrome.*

Gil·les·pie syndrome (gĭ-les′pe) [Frank David *Gillespie*, American ophthalmologist, born 1927] see under *syndrome.*

Gil·li·am operation (gil′e-əm) [David Tod *Gilliam*, American gynecologist, 1844–1923] see under *operation.*

Gil·lies flap, operation (gil′ēz) [Sir Harold Delf *Gillies*, British plastic surgeon, 1882–1960] see *tube flap*, under *flap*, and see under *operation.*

Gil·mer splint, wiring (gil′mər) [Thomas Lewis *Gilmer*, American oral surgeon, 1849–1931] see under *splint* and *wiring.*

gilt (gilt) a female pig that is intended for breeding but has not yet given birth.

Gil-Ver·net technique (jēl′-ver-net′) [Josep María *Gil-Vernet*, Spanish urologist, 20th century] see under *technique.*

Gim·ber·nat ligament, reflex ligament (hēm-bār-naht′) [Antonio de *Gimbernat*, Spanish surgeon and anatomist, 1734–1817] see *ligamentum lacunare* and *ligamentum inguinale reflexum.*

gin·ger (jin′jər) [L. *zingiber;* Gr. *zingiberis*] 1. *Zingiber officinale.* 2. [NF] the dried rhizome of *Z. officinale*, used primarily as a flavoring agent. It is also used for the treatment of loss of appetite, flatulence, and colic and to prevent motion sickness in humans, and as a stimulant, carminative, and anticolic medication for horses.

gin·gi·va (jin′jĭ-və, jin-ji′və) pl. *gin′givae* [L. "gum of the mouth"] [TA] gum: that part of the oral mucosa overlying the crowns of unerupted

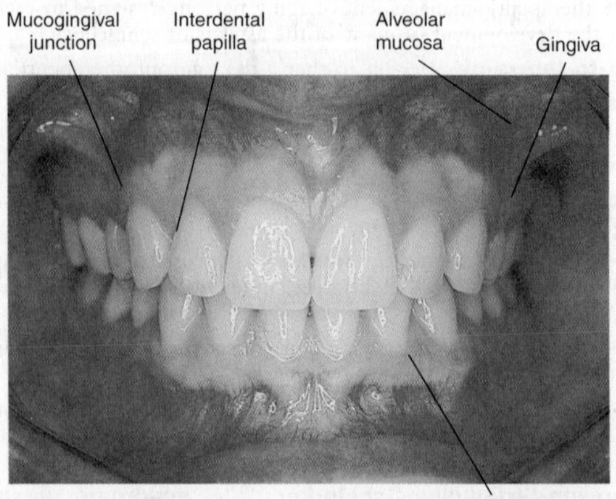

■ Gingiva and alveolar mucosa.

teeth and encircling the necks of those that have erupted, serving as the supporting structure for subjacent tissues. It is formed by pale pink tissue immovably attached to the bone and the teeth, which joins the alveolar mucosa at the mucogingival junction. **gin′gival** *adj*

alveolar g. periodontium protectionis.

areolar g. the oral mucous membrane lying beyond the keratinized mucosa over the alveolar process, being continuous with the buccal and labial mucosa.

attached g. periodontium protectionis.

buccal g. the portion of the gingiva located on the buccal aspect of the teeth.

cemental g. the portion of the attached gingiva adherent to the cementum.

free g. periodontium insertionis.

interdental g., interproximal g. the portion of the gingiva occupying the interproximal space beneath the area of tooth contact, consisting of two papillae and a depression (col) that connects the papillae and conforms to the shape of the interproximal contact area; called also *papillary g.* and *septal g.*

labial g. the portion of the gingiva found on the labial aspect of the teeth.

lingual g. the portion of the gingiva found on the lingual aspect of the teeth.

marginal g. margo gingivalis.

papillary g. interdental g.

septal g. interdental g.

unattached g. periodontium insertionis.

gin•gi•vae (jin′jĭ-ve, jin-ji′ve) [L., plural of *gingiva*] the gums; see under *gingiva.*

gin•gi•val•gia (jin″jĭ-val′jə) [*gingivo-* + *-algia*] pain in the gingivae.

gin•gi•val•ly (jin′jĭ-vəl″e) toward the gingivae.

gin•gi•vec•to•my (jin″jĭ-vek′tə-me) [*gingiv-* + *ectomy*] surgical excision of the gingiva at the level of its attachment, thus creating new marginal gingiva; used to eliminate gingival or periodontal pockets or to provide an approach for extensive surgical interventions, and to gain access necessary to remove calculus within the pocket.

gin•gi•vi•tis (jin″jĭ-vi′tis) [*gingiv-* + *-itis*] inflammation of the gingivae; when it is associated with bony changes, the condition is referred to as *periodontitis.*

acute necrotizing ulcerative g. (ANUG), acute ulcerative g. necrotizing ulcerative g.

atrophic senile g. inflammation of the gingiva and oral mucosa in menopausal and postmenopausal women, characterized microscopically by atrophy of the germinal and prickle cell layers of the gingival epithelium and sometimes by areas of ulceration; considered to be caused by altered estrogen metabolism.

bismuth g. see under *stomatitis.*

catarrhal g. transitory gingivitis, sometimes associated with stomatitis, accompanied by erythema, swelling, and occasionally epithelial desquamation; believed to be caused by the oral bacterial flora.

cotton roll g. secondary infection of denuded areas of gingivae caused by adherence of epithelium to cotton rolls placed in the mouth during dental procedures.

desquamative g. an inflammatory condition characterized by tendency of the surface epithelium of the gingivae to desquamate. Chronic desquamative gingivitis is called also *gingivosis.*

Dilantin g. generalized hyperplasia of the gingivae, and occasionally other areas of the oral mucosa, resulting from overgrowth of the fibrous tissue following anticonvulsant therapy with Dilantin (phenytoin). Called also *Dilantin hyperplasia.*

eruptive g. gingivitis occurring at the time of tooth eruption, particularly the permanent teeth; food impaction and debris accumulation may be associated.

fusospirochetal g. necrotizing ulcerative g.

g. gravida′rum pregnancy g.

hemorrhagic g. gingivitis characterized by profuse bleeding, as in ascorbic acid deficiency (see *scurvy*).

herpetic g. gingivitis due to herpesvirus infection. See also under *gingivostomatitis.*

hormonal g. gingivitis associated with endocrine imbalance.

hyperplastic g. gingivitis associated with proliferation of the gingival cells. See *gingival enlargement*, under *enlargement*, and *gingival hyperplasia*, under *hyperplasia.*

marginal g. inflammation of the marginal gingivae.

marginal g., generalized inflammation of the marginal gingivae in all the teeth, frequently extending to the interdental papillae.

marginal g., simple hyperemia of the gingivae with edema of the margins and gingival papillae, resulting from slight trauma or neglected dental hygiene.

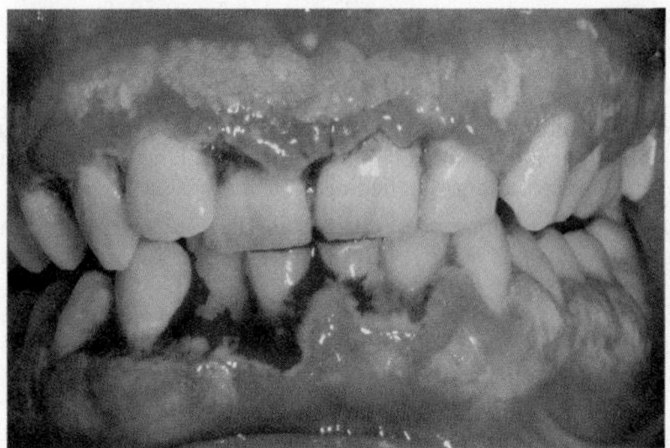

■ Necrotizing ulcerative gingivitis.

marginal g., suppurative, g. margina′lis suppurati′va inflammation of the gingival margins, with formation of a purulent discharge.

necrotizing ulcerative g. a progressive painful infection, also seen in subacute and recurrent forms, marked by crateriform lesions of interdental papillae with pseudomembranous slough circumscribed by linear erythema; fetid breath; increased salivation; and spontaneous gingival hemorrhage. The etiology is uncertain, but fusiform bacilli, spirochetes, and other microorganisms are present in the lesions; many postulate an etiology of a bacterial complex in the presence of predisposing factors such as gingival disease or nutritional deficiency. Although it often occurs in an epidemic pattern, it has not been shown to be contagious. Called also *fusospirillosis, fusospirochetal g., acute necrotizing ulcerative g., phagedenic g., trench mouth*, and *Vincent g.* or *stomatitis.* When it spreads to nearby structures, it may be called *necrotizing ulcerative gingivostomatitis* or *Vincent angina.*

papillary g. inflammation of the interdental papillae.

phagedenic g. necrotizing ulcerative g.

pregnancy g. any of various gingival changes during pregnancy, ranging from gingivitis to the so-called pregnancy tumor; called also *g. gravidarum.*

scorbutic g. gingivitis associated with scurvy; see also *hemorrhagic g.*

streptococcal g. inflammation of the gingival margins caused by streptococcal infection.

tuberculous g. tuberculous infection of the gingiva, characterized by diffuse, hyperemic, nodular or papillary proliferation of the gingival tissue. See also *oral tuberculosis*, under *tuberculosis.*

Vincent g. necrotizing ulcerative g.

gingiv(o)- [L. *gingiva* gum] a combining form denoting relationship to the gingivae.

gin•gi•vo•buc•co•ax•i•al (jin″jĭ-vo-buk″o-ak′se-əl) pertaining to or formed by the gingival, buccal, and axial walls of a tooth cavity preparation.

gin•gi•vo•glos•si•tis (jin″jĭ-vo-glos-i′tis) [*gingivo-* + *gloss-* + *-itis*] inflammation of gingivae and tongue.

gin•gi•vo•la•bi•al (jin″jĭ-vo-la′be-əl) pertaining to the gingivae and lips.

gin•gi•vo•lin•guo•ax•i•al (jin″jĭ-vo-ling″wo-ak′se-əl) pertaining to or formed by the gingival, lingual, and axial walls of a tooth cavity preparation.

gin•gi•vo•peri•odon•ti•tis (jin″jĭ-vo-per″e-o-don-ti′tis) inflammation involving the gingivae and periodontium.

necrotizing ulcerative g. a severe form of periodontitis occurring after prolonged repeated bouts of necrotizing ulcerative gingivitis, manifested by generalized or localized destruction of interdental bone, and characterized by periods of exacerbation in which a gray pseudomembrane may be present in affected areas and by necrotic odor.

gin•gi•vo•plas•ty (jin′jĭ-vo-plas″te) [*gingivo-* + *-plasty*] surgical reshaping of the gingivae and papillae for correction of deformities (particularly enlargements) and to provide the gingivae with a normal and functional form, the incision creating an external bevel. **gingivoplas′tic** *adj*

gin•gi•vo•sis (jin″jĭ-vo′sis) chronic desquamative gingivitis.

gin•gi•vo•sto•ma•ti•tis (jin″jĭ-vo-sto″mə-ti′tis) inflammation involving both the gingivae and the oral mucosa.

herpetic g. an infection of the oral mucosa (including the gingivae) by the herpes simplex virus, characterized by redness of oral tissues, formation of multiple vesicles and painful ulcers, and fever.

necrotizing ulcerative g. gingivostomatitis caused by extension to the oral mucosa of necrotizing ulcerative gingivitis, characterized by ulceration, pseudomembrane, and odor, with lesions involving the palate or pharynx as well as the oral mucosa. Called also *fusospirochetal stomatitis* and *pseudomembranous angina.*

gin•gly•form (jin′glĭ-form) ginglymoid.

gin·gly·mo·ar·thro·di·al (jin″glə-mo-ahr-thro′de-əl) partly ginglymoid and partly arthrodial.

gin·gly·moid (jin′glə-moid) [*ginglymus* + *-oid*] resembling a ginglymus.

gin·gly·mus (jin′glĭ-məs) [L., from Gr. *ginglymos* hinge] [TA] a type of synovial joint that allows movement in but one plane, forward and backward, as the hinge of a door; called also *ginglymoid* or *hinge joint.*

Gink·go (ging′ko) a genus of deciduous, diecious trees with fan-shaped leaves and malodorous fleshy yellow fruit native to China, Japan, and Korea.

G. bilo′ba the sole species of the genus. The leaves and seeds are used medicinally; see *ginkgo* (def. 2). The foul-smelling pulp around the seeds contains urushiol and can cause urushiol dermatitis in susceptible individuals.

gink·go (ging′ko) 1. a tree of the genus *Ginkgo.* 2. [NF] the dried leaves of *Ginkgo biloba,* used for symptomatic relief of brain dysfunction, for intermittent claudication, and for tinnitus and vertigo of vascular origin. It is also used in traditional Chinese medicine for asthma, tinnitus, hypertonia, and angina pectoris, and in homeopathy for tonsillitis and headache.

gin·seng (jin′seng) [Chinese *jin-tsan* life of man] 1. any herb of the genus *Panax,* especially *P. ginseng* (Chinese ginseng) and *P. quinquefolius* (American ginseng). 2. the root of Chinese or American ginseng, used as a tonic and stimulant in fatigue and during convalescence.

Asian g. [NF] the dried roots of *Panax ginseng* (Chinese ginseng). Formerly called *oriental ginseng.*

eleuthero g. Siberian g.

oriental g. Asian g.

Siberian g. 1. *Eleutherococcus senticosus.* 2. a preparation of the root of *E. senticosus,* used internally to improve general well-being and used for a variety of indications in traditional Chinese medicine. Called also *eleuthero* and *eleuthero ginseng.*

GIP gastric inhibitory polypeptide.

Gi·ral·dés organ (zhe-rahl-dāz′) [Joachim Albin Cardozo Cazado *Giraldés,* Portuguese surgeon in Paris, 1808–1875] paradidymis.

Gi·rar·di·nus (jĭ-rar′dĭ-nus) *Poecilia.*

G. poeciloi′des *Poecilia reticulata.*

gir·dle (gur′dəl) 1. an encircling structure or part. 2. cingulum.

limbus g. a benign type of corneal degeneration in the form of an opaque line concentric with the limbus; called also *white limbal g. of Vogt.*

g. of lower limb cingulum pelvicum.

pectoral g. cingulum pectorale.

pelvic g. cingulum pelvicum.

shoulder g., thoracic g., g. of upper limb cingulum pectorale.

white limbal g. of Vogt limbus g.

Gir·dle·stone resection (operation) (ger′dəl-stōn) [Gathorne Robert *Girdlestone,* British orthopedic surgeon, 1881–1950] see under *resection.*

GIST gastrointestinal stromal tumor.

git·a·lin (jit′ə-lin) a mixture of the digitalis glycosides gitoxin, gitaloxin, and digitoxin, having the same actions and uses as for digitalis; administered orally. Called also *amorphous g.*

git·a·lox·in (jit″ə-lok′sin) a cardiac glycoside from *Digitalis purpurea;* a component of gitalin.

Git·el·man syndrome (git′əl-mən) [Hillel Jonathan *Gitelman,* American nephrologist, born 1932] see under *syndrome.*

gith·a·gism (gith′ə-jiz-əm) poisoning from seeds of *Agrostemma githago* that contaminate human or animal food; called also *corn cockle poisoning.*

gi·tox·i·gen·in (jĭ-tok′sĭ-jən-in) the steroid nucleus that is the aglycon of gitoxin.

gi·tox·in (jĭ-tok′sin) a cardiac glycoside, principally from *Digitalis purpurea* but also a constituent of *D. lanata,* consisting of gitoxigenin linked to three digitoxose molecules; a component of gitalin.

Giuf·fri·da-Rug·gi·eri stigma (joo-fre″də-roo″je-er′e) [Vincenzo *Giuffrida-Ruggieri,* Italian anthropologist, 1872–1922] see under *stigma.*

giz·zard (giz′ərd) [L. *gigeria* cooked entrails of poultry] 1. the highly modified posterior portion of the stomach in birds, characterized by muscular walls and glands that secrete a horny lining, in which food passed from the proventriculus is ground with the aid of ingested gravel. 2. a similar organ in the alimentary tract of certain invertebrates, such as insects.

Gjes·sing syndrome (yes′ing) [Rolv *Gjessing,* Norwegian psychiatrist, 1887–1959] see under *syndrome.*

GL greatest length.

gl. [L.] glan′dula (gland).

gla·bel·la (glə-bel′ə) [L. *glabellus* smooth, dim. of *glaber*] 1. [TA] a craniometric landmark, being the most prominent point in the median plane between the superciliary arches. 2. more broadly, the smooth area on the frontal bone between the superciliary arches.

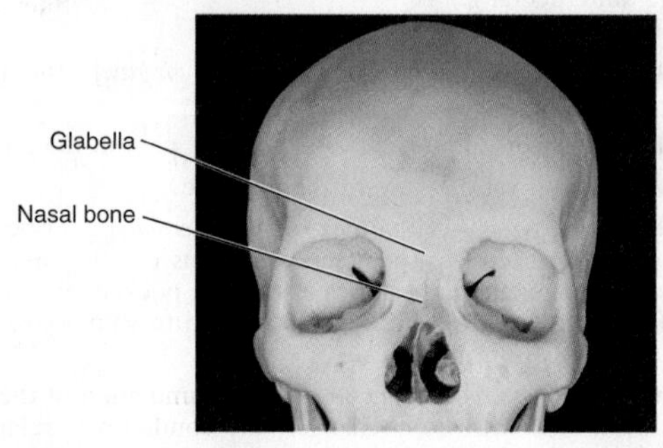

gla·bel·lad (glə-bel′əd) [*glabella* + *-ad*[1]] toward the glabella.

gla·brous (gla′brəs) [L. *glaber* smooth] smooth and bare.

gla·cial (gla′shəl) [L. *glacialis*] 1. resembling ice; vitreous; solid. 2. designating a highly pure state of certain acids, e.g., acetic or phosphoric acid, so called because the freezing point is only slightly below room temperature.

gla·di·ate (gla′de-āt) [L. *gladius* sword] xiphoid (def. 1).

gla·di·o·lus (glə-di′o-ləs) [L., dim. of *gladius* sword] corpus sterni.

gla·dio·ma·nu·bri·al (glad″e-o-mə-noo′bre-əl) pertaining to gladiolus (corpus sterni) and manubrium.

glair·in (glār′in) [L. *clarus* clear] a gelatinous substance of bacterial origin found on the surface of certain thermal and sulfur waters.

glairy (glār′e) resembling the white of an egg.

gland (gland) [L. *glans* acorn] glandula.

Gland

For descriptions of specific glands not listed here, see under *glandula.*

accessory g. a minor mass of glandular tissue situated near or at some distance from a gland of similar structure.

accessory adrenal g's glandulae suprarenales accessoriae.

accessory lacrimal g's glandulae lacrimales accessoriae.

accessory mammary g. mamma accessoria.

accessory parotid g. glandula parotidea accessoria.

accessory suprarenal g's glandulae suprarenales accessoriae.

accessory thyroid g's glandulae thyroideae accessoriae.

acid g's fundic g's.

acinar g. acinous g.

acinotubular g. tubuloacinar g.

acinous g. a gland made up of one or more acini.

admaxillary g. glandula parotidea accessoria.

adrenal g. glandula suprarenalis.

aggregate g's, aggregated g's aggregated lymphoid nodules; see terms beginning *noduli lymphoidei aggregati,* under *nodulus.*

Albarrán g. a term sometimes used for that part of the median lobe of the prostate underneath the uvula vesicae.

alveolar g. acinous g.

anal g's circumanal g's.

apical g's of tongue anterior lingual g's.

apocrine g. a gland whose discharged secretion contains part of the secreting cells. Cf. *holocrine g.* and *merocrine g.* NOTE: the term is often used to denote the apocrine sweat glands specifically.

Gland *Continued*

apocrine sweat g. a type of large, branched, specialized sweat gland that empties into the upper portion of a hair follicle instead of directly onto the skin surface; found only on certain areas of the body, such as around the anus and in the axilla; after puberty they produce a viscous secretion that is acted on by bacteria to produce a characteristic acrid odor.
areolar g's glandulae areolares.
arteriococcygeal g. glomus coccygeum.
arytenoid g's mucous glands in the posterior part of the larynx, near the aryepiglottic fold and the arytenoid cartilages; called also *posterior laryngeal g's.*
Aselli g's see under *pancreas.*
axillary g's nodi lymphoidei axillares.
Bartholin g. glandula vestibularis major.
Bauhin g's anterior lingual g's.
g's of bile duct, biliary g's, g's of biliary mucosa glandulae ductus choledochi.
Blandin g's, Blandin and Nuhn g's anterior lingual g's.
Bowman g's glandulae olfactoriae.
bronchial g's glandulae bronchiales.
Bruch g's the lymph follicles of the conjunctiva of the lower lid.
Brunner g's glandulae duodenales.
buccal g's glandulae buccales.
bulbocavernous g., bulbourethral g. glandula bulbourethralis.
cardiac g's, cardial g's mucous glands in the lower end of the esophagus and the cardiac end of the stomach surrounding the cardiac opening.
carotid g. glomus caroticum.
celiac g's lymph nodes anterior to the abdominal aorta.
ceruminous g's glands in the skin of the external auditory canal that secrete cerumen.
cervical g's of uterus glandulae cervicales uteri.
cheek g's glandulae buccales.
Ciaccio g's glandulae lacrimales accessoriae.
ciliary g's, ciliary g's of conjunctiva glandulae ciliares.
circumanal g's specialized sweat and sebaceous glands situated in an annular zone around the anus; called also *anal* or *Gay glands.*
Cloquet g. nodus lymphoideus ingunalis profundus proximalis.
coccygeal g. glomus coccygeum.
compound g. a gland made up of a number of smaller units whose excretory ducts combine to form ducts of progressively higher order.
conjunctival g's glandulae conjunctivales.
Cowper g. glandula bulbourethralis.
cutaneous g's glandulae cutis.
ductless g's endocrine g's.
duodenal g's glandulae duodenales.
Ebner g's serous secreting glands in the posterior part of the tongue near the vallate papillae; called also *gustatory g's.*
eccrine g., eccrine sweat g. an ordinary, or simple, sweat gland *(glandula sudorifera)*; they are of the merocrine type, unbranched, coiled, tubular glands that are distributed over almost all of the body surface, and promote cooling by evaporation of their secretion.
endocrine g's ductless organs that secrete specific substances *(hormones)* that are released directly into the circulatory system and influence metabolism and other body processes. The endocrine glands include the hypothalamus, pituitary, thyroid, parathyroid, and adrenal glands, the pancreatic islets, the pineal body, and the gonads. See also under *system*, and see Plate 17. Called also *glandulae endocrinae* [TA] and *ductless g's.*
endoepithelial g. intraepithelial g.
esophageal g's glandulae oesophageae.
excretory g. any gland that excretes waste products from the system.
exocrine g. a gland that discharges its secretion through a duct opening on an internal or external surface of the body, as a lacrimal gland. Cf. *endocrine g's.*
extraparotid lymph g's lymph nodes overlying the parotid gland, between the superficial and deep fasciae.
fundic g's, fundus g's numerous nearly straight tubular glands in the mucosa of the fundus and body of the stomach; they contain the cells that produce gastric acid and pepsin.
Galeati g's glandulae duodenales.
gastric g's glandulae gastricae.
gastric g's proper fundic g's.
Gay g's circumanal g's.
genal g's glandulae buccales.
genital g. gonad.
gingival g's glandlike infoldings of epithelium at the junction of gingiva and tooth.
glossopalatine g's mucous glands at the posterior end of the smaller sublingual glands.
greater vestibular g. glandula vestibularis major.
gustatory g's Ebner g's.
Harder g's, harderian g's accessory lacrimal glands at the inner corner of the eye in animals that possess nictitating membranes; they excrete an unctuous fluid that facilitates the movement of the third eyelid. They are rudimentary in humans.
haversian g's villi synoviales.
hedonic g's glands in certain animals that function during the season of sexual activity. See also *scent g.*
hemal g's, hemal lymph g's hemal nodes.
hemolymph g's 1. hemal nodes. 2. hemolymph nodes (def. 2).
Henle g's tubular glands in the conjunctiva of the eyelids.
heterocrine g. mixed g. (def. 2).
holocrine g. a gland whose discharged secretion contains entire secreting cells.
intercarotid g. glomus caroticum.
intermediate g's in some classifications, a fourth type of gastric gland, which is found in a narrow region between the fundic and pyloric glands.
interstitial g. the interstitial cells of the ovary, collectively; so called because of their epithelioid appearance and presumed secretory function.
intestinal g's glandulae intestinales.
intraepithelial g. a gland situated in an epithelial layer.
intramuscular g's of tongue anterior lingual g's.
jugular g. a lymph node behind the clavicular insertion of the sternomastoid muscle.
Krause g's glandulae conjunctivales.
labial g's of mouth glandulae labiales.
lacrimal g. glandula lacrimalis.
lactiferous g. glandula mammaria.
g's of large intestine see *glandulae intestinales.*
laryngeal g's glandulae laryngeales.
laryngeal g's, anterior mucous glands in the anterior part of the larynx.
laryngeal g's, middle mucous glands located in the arytenoepiglottic fold.
laryngeal g's, posterior arytenoid g's.
lesser vestibular g's glandulae vestibulares minores.
g's of Lieberkühn glandulae intestinales.
lingual g's glandulae linguales.
lingual g's, anterior deeply placed mucoserous glands near the apex of the tongue.
Littre g's 1. glandulae preputiales. 2. glandulae urethrales urethrae masculinae.
Luschka g. glomus coccygeum.
lymph g., lymphatic g. see under *node.*
major salivary g's glandulae salivariae majores.
malar g's glandulae buccales.
mammary g. glandula mammaria.
mandibular g. glandula submandibularis.
Mehlis g. gland cells surrounding the ootype of trematodes.
meibomian g's glandulae tarsales.
merocrine g. a gland in which the secretory cells maintain their integrity throughout the secretory cycle.
minor salivary g's glandulae salivariae minores.
mixed g. 1. a gland having both endocrine and exocrine portions. 2. a gland composed of both mucous and serous secreting cells, such as the labial glands. Called also *heterocrine g.* and *seromucous g.*
molar g's glandulae molares.
Moll g's glandulae ciliares.
monoptychial g. a gland in which the tubules or alveoli are lined with a single layer of secreting cells.
Montgomery g's glandulae areolares.

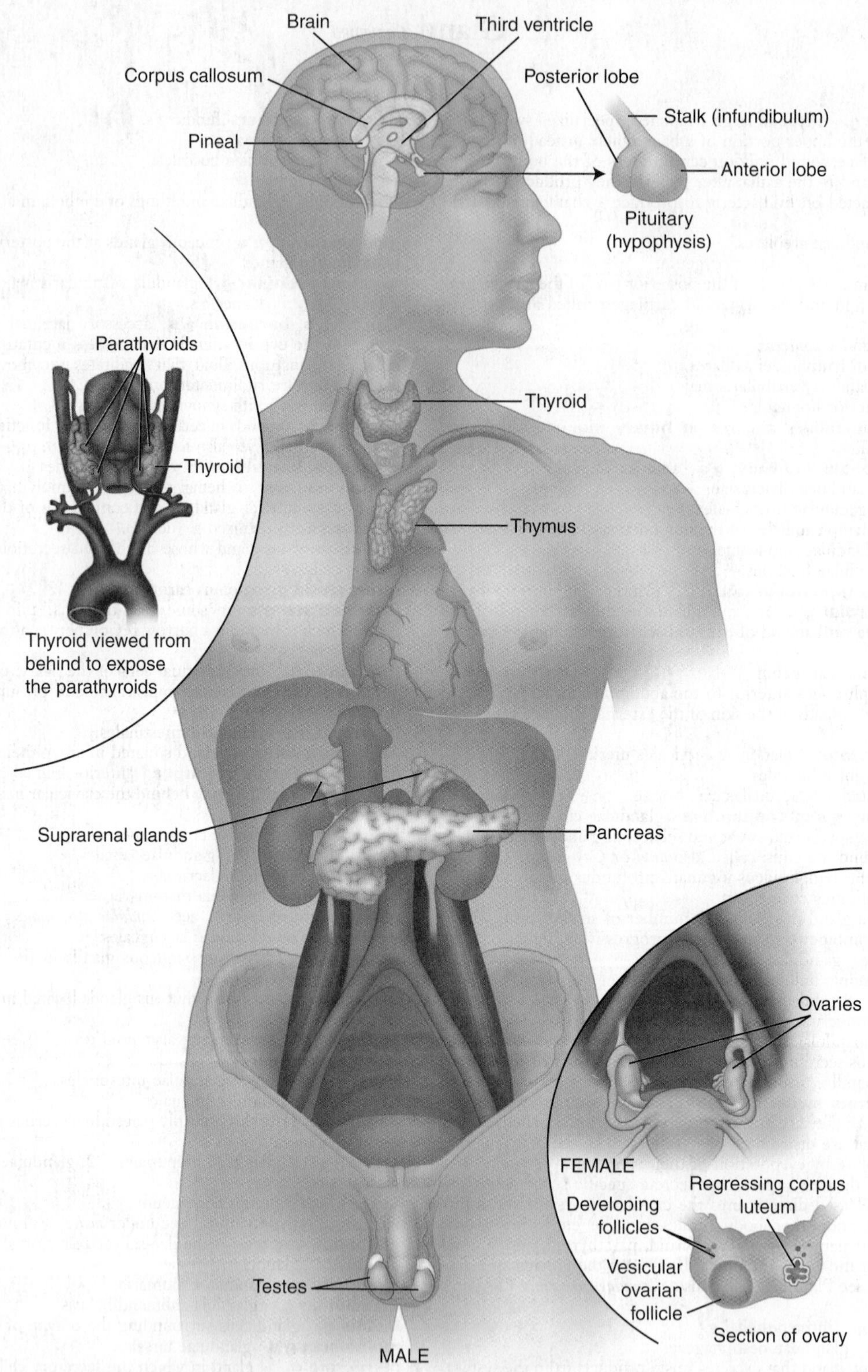

■ **PLATE 17—THE ENDOCRINE GLANDS**

Gland *Continued*

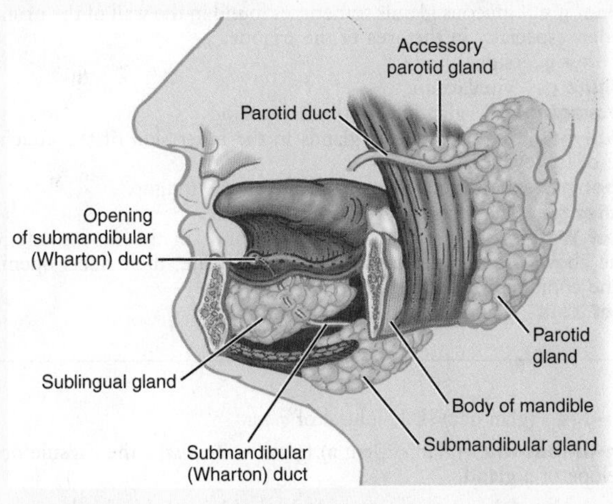

■ Salivary glands.

Morgagni g's glandulae urethrales urethrae masculinae.
g's of mouth glandulae oris.
mucilaginous g's villi synoviales.
muciparous g., mucous g. a gland that secretes mucus or a similar chemically inert slimy material.
mucous g's of auditory tube glandulae tubariae.
mucous g's of duodenum glandulae duodenales.
mucous g's of eustachian tube glandulae tubariae.
multicellular g. a gland in which many cells cooperate to produce a gland complex, represented in its simplest form by a secretory sheet (q.v.) of epithelial cells.
Naboth g's, nabothian g's see under *follicle.*
nasal g's glandulae nasales.
Nuhn g's anterior lingual g's.
odoriferous g's of prepuce glandulae preputiales.
oil g. glandula sebacea.
olfactory g's glandulae olfactoriae.
oxyntic g's fundic g's.
palatine g's glandulae palatinae.
palpebral g's glandulae tarsales.
parathyroid g's small bodies apposed to the posterior surface of the thyroid gland, developed from the endoderm of the branchial clefts, occurring in a variable number of pairs, commonly two (*glandula parathyroidea inferior* and *glandula parathyroidea superior* [TA]) (see inset on Plate 17). The parenchyma comprises masses and cords of epithelial cells, which have been divided into two main types: chief cells and oxyphil cells, but intermediate forms exist. The chief cells secrete parathyroid hormone, a major regulator of calcium and phosphorus metabolism. Called also *parathyroids* and *parathyroid bodies.*
paraurethral g's a group of urethral glands of the female urethra that are drained by the paraurethral ducts. Called also *Skene glands* and *female prostate.*
parotid g. glandula parotidea.
peptic g's fundic g's.
Peyer g's noduli lymphoidei aggregati intestini tenuis.
pharyngeal g's glandulae pharyngeales.
pilosebaceous g. the sebaceous gland next to a hair follicle in a pilosebaceous unit.
pineal g. glandula pinealis.
pituitary g. hypophysis.
Poirier g's lymph nodes on the conoid ligament at the upper border of the isthmus of the thyroid.
polyptychic g. a gland whose tubules or alveoli are lined with more than one layer of secreting cells.
preen g. a large compound alveolar structure on the back of birds, above the base of the tail, which secretes an oily waterproof material that the bird applies to its feathers and skin by preening. Called also *uropygial g.*
pregnancy g's the glands containing female genital hormone, that is, the ovarian follicle, corpus luteum, and placenta.
prehyoid g's glandulae thyroidea accessoriae.
preputial g's glandulae preputiales.
prostate g. prostate.
pyloric g's mucous glands found in the pyloric part of the stomach.
racemose g's glands composed of acini arranged like grapes on a stem.
retromolar g's glandulae molares.
Rivinus g. glandula sublingualis.
Rosenmüller g. 1. pars palpebralis glandulae lacrimalis. 2. nodus lymphoideus ingunalis profundus proximalis.
saccular g. a gland consisting of a sac or sacs, lined with glandular epithelium.
salivary g's the glands of the oral cavity whose combined secretion constitutes the saliva; see *glandulae salivariae majores* and *glandulae salivariae minores.*
salivary g., external glandula parotidea.
salivary g., internal the glandula sublingualis and glandula submandibularis regarded as a unit.
scent g. any gland that secretes a pheromone, such as occurs in many animal species during mating season.
sebaceous g. glandula sebacea.
sebaceous g's of conjunctiva, sebaceous g's of eyelids glandulae sebaceae palpebrarum.
seminal g. glandula vesiculosa.
sentinel g. an enlarged lymph node, considered to be indicative of a pathological condition elsewhere in the body.
seromucous g. mixed g. (def. 2).
serous g. a gland that secretes a watery albuminous material, commonly but not always containing enzymes.
Serres g's Epstein pearls.
sex g., sexual g. gonad.
simple g. a gland with a nonbranching duct.
Skene g's paraurethral g's.
g's of small intestine see *glandulae intestinales.*
Stahr g. lymph node situated on the facial artery.
sublingual g. glandula sublingualis.
submandibular g., submaxillary g. glandula submandibularis.
sudoriferous g., sudoriparous g. glandula sudorifera.
suprarenal g. glandula suprarenalis
Suzanne g. a mucous gland of the mouth, beneath the alveololingual groove.
sweat g. glandula sudorifera.
synovial g's villi synoviales.
target g. a gland such as the thyroid, adrenal, or a gonad that is specifically affected by the secretory product of another gland; see also *releasing hormones* and *inhibiting hormones,* under *hormone.*
tarsal g's, tarsoconjunctival g's glandulae tarsales.
thymus g. thymus.
thyroid g. glandula thyroidea.
g's of tongue glandulae linguales.
tracheal g's glandulae tracheales.
trachoma g's lymphoid follicles of the conjunctiva, found chiefly near the inner canthus of the eye.
tubal g's glandulae tubariae.
tubular g. any gland made up of or containing a tubule or a number of tubules.

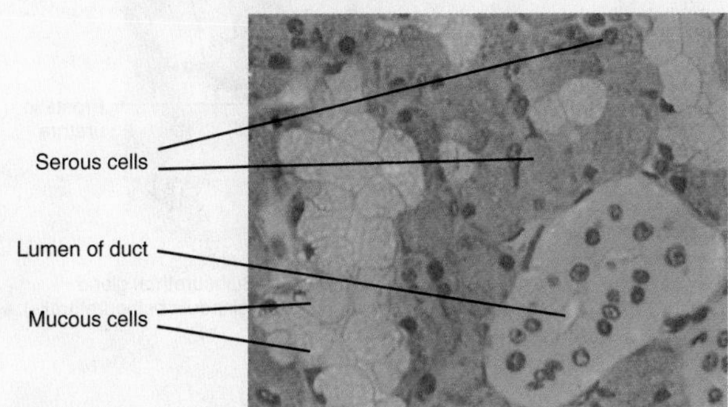

■ Detail of submandibular salivary gland, showing mucus-secreting mucous cells and enzyme-secreting serous cells; duct cross sections are also visible.

Gland *Continued*

tubuloacinar g. a gland that is both tubular and acinous.
Tyson g's glandulae preputiales.
ultimobranchial g's see under *body.*
unicellular g. a single cell that functions as a gland, e.g., a goblet cell.
urethral g's of female urethra glandulae urethrales urethrae femininae.
urethral g's of male urethra glandulae urethrales urethrae masculinae.
uropygial g. preen g.
uterine g's glandulae uterinae.
vaginal g. a type of mucus-secreting gland found in the vaginal mucous membrane.
vascular g. a hemal node.
vesical g's mucous glands sometimes found in the wall of the urinary bladder, especially in the area of the trigone.
Virchow g. signal node.
vitelline g. vitellarium.
vulvovaginal g. glandula vestibularis major.
Waldeyer g's acinotubular glands in the inner skin of the attached edge of the eyelid.
Weber g's the tubular mucous glands of the tongue.
Wölfler g's glandulae thyroideae accessoriae.
g's of Wolfring small tubuloalveolar glands in the subconjunctival tissue above the upper border of the tarsal plate, their ducts opening on the conjunctival surface.
g's of Zeis glandulae sebaceae palpebrarum.

glan•ders (glan′dərz) a contagious disease of horses, communicable to humans, caused by *Burkholderia mallei.* The acute form, which may be fatal, is marked by a purulent inflammation of mucous membranes and an eruption on the skin of nodules that coalesce and break down, forming deep ulcers that may end in necrosis of cartilages and bones. A chronic form known as *farcy* involves the lymphatic system. Called also *malleus.* glan′derous *adj*
African g., Japanese g. lymphangitis epizootica.

glan•des (glan′dēz) [L.] plural of *glans.*

glan•di•lem•ma (glan″dĭ-lem′ə) [*gland* + *-lemma*] the capsule or outer envelope of a gland.

glan•du•la (glan′du-lə) gen. and pl. *glan′dulae* [L.] gland: an aggregation of cells, specialized to secrete or excrete materials not related to their ordinary metabolic needs.

Glandula

Descriptions of glands are given on TA terms, and include anglicized names of specific glands.

glan′dulae areola′res [TA] areolar glands: sebaceous glands of the mammary areola; called also *Montgomery glands.*
glan′dulae bronchia′les [TA] bronchial glands: seromucous glands in the mucosa and submucosa of the bronchial walls.
glan′dulae bucca′les [TA] buccal glands: the serous and mucous glands on the inner surface of the cheeks.
g. bulbourethra′lis [TA] bulbourethral gland: either of two glands embedded in the substance of the external sphincter of the male urethra, just posterior to the membranous part of the urethra; they are homologues of the greater vestibular glands in the female. Called also *Cowper gland.*
glan′dulae cervica′les u′teri [TA] cervical glands of uterus: mucus-secreting glands located in clefts in the wall of the uterine cervix.
glan′dulae cilia′res [TA] ciliary glands: sweat glands that have become arrested in their development, situated obliquely in contact with and parallel to the bulbs of the eyelashes; called also *Moll glands.*
glan′dulae conjunctiva′les [TA] conjunctival glands: accessory lacrimal glands situated deep in the subconjunctival connective tissue, mainly in the upper fornix; called also *Krause glands.*

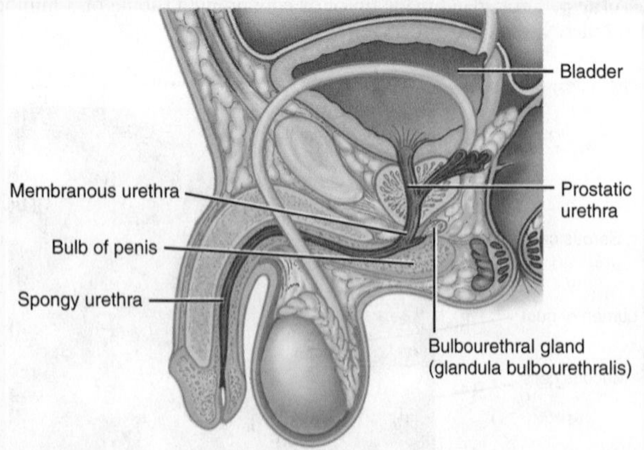

■ Glandula bulbourethralis (bulbourethral gland) in relation to other genitourinary structures.

glan′dulae cu′tis [TA] cutaneous glands: the glands of the skin, including the sweat glands (see *glandula sudorifera*), sebaceous glands (see *glandula sebacea*), and the ceruminous glands.
glan′dulae duc′tus bilia′ris TA alternative for *glandulae ductus choledochi.*
glan′dulae duc′tus chole′dochi [TA] glands of bile duct: tubuloacinar glands in the mucosa of the bile ducts and the neck of the gallbladder; called also *glandulae ductus biliaris* [TA alternative] and *biliary glands.*
glan′dulae duodena′les [TA] duodenal glands: tubuloacinar glands in the submucous layer of the duodenum that open into the crypts of Lieberkühn; they secrete urogastrone. Called also *Brunner glands.*
glan′dulae endocri′nae [TA] the endocrine glands (q.v.), including the thyroid, parathyroid, pituitary, and adrenal glands, and the gonads.
glan′dulae esopha′geae glandulae oesophageae.
glan′dulae gas′tricae [TA] gastric glands: the secreting glands of the stomach, including the fundic, cardiac, and pyloric glands; sometimes used specifically to denote the fundic glands.
g. incisi′va a small intraoral gland in the median line of the upper jaw near the incisors.
glan′dulae intestina′les [TA] intestinal glands: simple tubular glands in the mucous membrane of either the small intestine *(glandulae intestinales intestini tenuis),* opening between the bases of the villi and containing argentaffin cells; or the large intestine *(glandulae intestinales intestini crassi).* Called also *crypts* or *glands of Lieberkühn,* and *Lieberkühn* or *intestinal follicles.*
glan′dulae labia′les [TA] labial glands of the mouth: the serous and mucous glands on the inner part of the lips.
g. lacrima′lis [TA] lacrimal gland: either of a pair of glands, one at the upper outer angle of each orbit, secreting the tears; they are divided into two portions, the orbital and palpebral, by the orbital fascia.
glan′dulae lacrima′les accesso′riae [TA] accessory lacrimal glands: portions of the lacrimal gland sometimes found near the superior fornix of the conjunctiva.
glan′dulae laryngea′les [TA] laryngeal glands: the mucous glands in the mucosa of the larynx.
glan′dulae lingua′les [TA] lingual glands: the mucous and serous glands on the surface of the tongue.
g. mamma′ria [TA] mammary gland: the specialized accessory gland of the skin of female mammals that secretes milk. In the human female, it is a compound tubuloalveolar gland composed of 15 to 25 lobes

arranged radially about the nipple and separated by connective and adipose tissue, each lobe having its own excretory (lactiferous) duct opening on the nipple. The lobes are subdivided into lobules, with the alveolar ducts and alveoli being the secretory portion of the gland. Called also *lactiferous gland*.

glan′dulae mola′res [TA] molar glands: the glands on the external aspect of the buccinator muscle, their ducts piercing it to open on the internal aspect of the cheek; called also *retromolar glands*.

glan′dulae nasa′les [TA] nasal glands: numerous large mucous and serous glands in the respiratory part of the nasal cavity.

glan′dulae oesopha′geae [TA] esophageal glands: the mucous glands in the submucous layer of the esophagus. Written also *glandulae esophageae*.

glan′dulae olfacto′riae [TA] olfactory glands: small mucous glands in the olfactory mucosa; called also *Bowman glands*.

glan′dulae o′ris [TA] the glands of the mouth; see *glandulae salivariae majores* and *glandulae salivariae minores*.

glan′dulae palati′nae [TA] palatine glands: the mucous glands on the soft palate and the posteromedial part of the hard palate.

g. parathyroi′dea infe′rior [TA] inferior parathyroid gland; see *parathyroid glands*, under *gland*.

g. parathyroi′dea supe′rior [TA] superior parathyroid gland; see *parathyroid glands*, under *gland*.

g. paroti′dea [TA] parotid gland: the largest of the three glands occurring in pairs, which together with numerous small glands in the mouth constitute the salivary glands; it is located below the zygomatic arch, below and in front of the external acoustic meatus.

g. paroti′dea accesso′ria [TA] accessory parotid gland: a frequently present, more or less detached portion of the parotid gland.

glan′dulae pharyngea′les [TA] pharyngeal glands: mucous glands beneath the tunica mucosa of the pharynx.

g. pinea′lis [TA] pineal gland: a small flattened cone-shaped body in the epithalamus, lying in the midline above the superior colliculi and below the splenium of the corpus callosum. Its hormonal function in human physiology is not firmly established; in response to norepinephrine it synthesizes and releases melatonin, whose rate of release declines when light activates retinal photoreceptors. Called also *epiphysis cerebri*, *corpus pineale* [TA alternative], and *pineal body*.

g. pituita′ria TA alternative for *hypophysis*.

glan′dulae preputia′les [TA] preputial glands: small sebaceous glands of the corona of the penis and the inner surface of the prepuce, which secrete smegma; called also *Littre* or *Tyson glands*.

glan′dulae saliva′riae majo′res [TA] major salivary glands: the larger exocrine glands of the oral cavity, which together with the smaller salivary glands *(glandulae salivariae minores)* secrete saliva; the group includes the sublingual, submandibular, and parotid glands.

glan′dulae saliva′riae mino′res [TA] minor salivary glands: the smaller exocrine glands of the oral cavity, which together with the larger salivary glands *(glandulae salivariae majores)* secrete saliva; the group includes the labial, buccal, molar, palatine, and lingual glands, and the anterior lingual gland.

g. seba′cea [TA] sebaceous gland: one of the holocrine glands of the skin that are are located in the dermis and secrete sebum. Called also *oil gland*.

glan′dulae seba′ceae la′bii majo′ris pudenda′lis sebaceous glands in the skin of the labia majora.

glan′dulae seba′ceae palpebra′rum [TA] sebaceous glands of eyelids: modified rudimentary sebaceous glands attached directly to the follicles of the eyelashes; called also *glands of Zeis*.

g. semina′lis TA alternative for *glandula vesiculosa*.

g. sublingua′lis [TA] sublingual gland: the smallest of the three salivary glands, occurring in pairs, predominantly mucous in type, and draining into the oral cavity through 10 to 30 sublingual ducts; called also *Rivinus gland*.

g. submandibula′ris [TA], **g. submaxilla′ris** submandibular gland: one of the three chief, paired salivary glands, predominantly serous, lying partly above and partly below the posterior half of the base of the mandible.

g. sudori′fera [TA] sudoriferous or sweat gland: one of the glands that secrete sweat, located in the dermis or subcutaneous tissue, and opening by a duct on the surface of the body. There are two types: the ordinary or *eccrine sweat glands* and the *apocrine sweat glands*.

g. suprarena′lis [TA] suprarenal or adrenal gland: a flattened body found in the retroperitoneal tissues at the cranial pole of the kidney. In humans it consists of two components of different embryologic origin, the cortex and medulla. The adrenal cortex, under control of the pituitary hormone corticotropin, elaborates steroid hormones. The adrenal

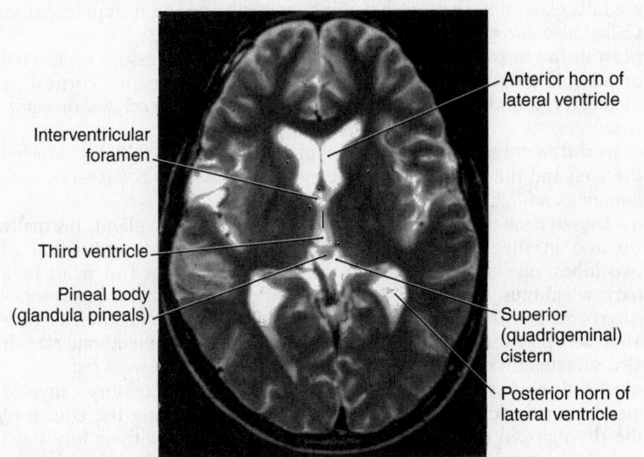

■ Glandula pinealis (pineal body) and adjacent structures in an axial MRI scan.

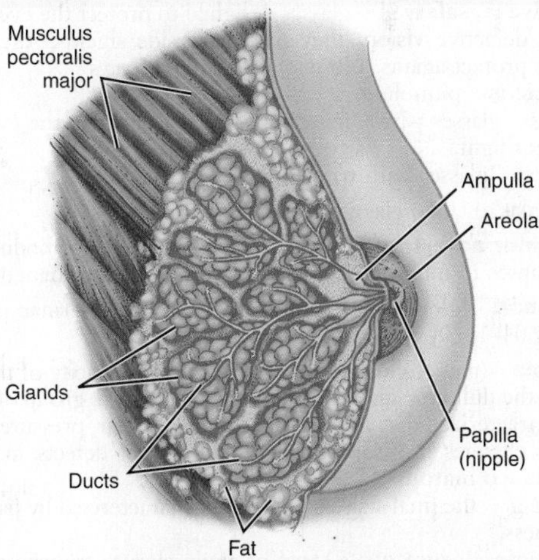

■ Glandula mammaria (mammary gland).

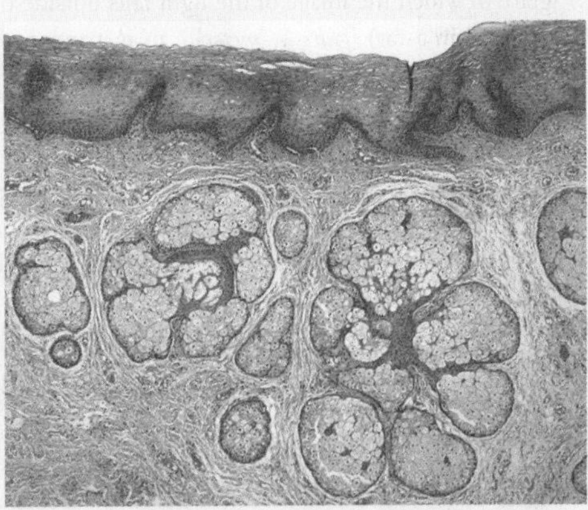

■ Cross section of multiple sebaceous glands (glandulae sebaceae) in the superficial lamina propria.

Glandula *Continued*

medulla elaborates the catecholamines epinephrine and norepinephrine. Called also *adrenal* or *suprarenal body.*

glan′dulae suprarena′les accesso′riae [TA] accessory suprarenal or adrenal glands: adrenal glandular tissue, usually either cortical or medullary, found in the abdomen or pelvis. Called also *adrenal* or *suprarenal rests.*

glan′dulae tarsa′les [TA] tarsal glands: sebaceous follicles between the tarsi and the conjunctiva of the eyelids; called also *palpebral* or *meibomian glands.*

g. thyroi′dea [TA] thyroid gland: an endocrine gland normally situated in the lower part of the front of the neck, consisting of two lobes, one on either side of the trachea and joined in front by a narrow isthmus. It secretes, stores, and liberates the thyroid hormones (thyroxine and triiodothyronine), which require iodine for their elaboration and play major endocrine roles in regulating the metabolic rate. It also secretes thyrocalcitonin. Called also *thyroid* and *thyroid body.*

glan′dulae thyroi′deae accesso′riae [TA] accessory thyroid glands: small exclaves of the thyroid gland, found along the course of the thyroglossal duct and elsewhere; types (named for their locations) include *intrathoracic thyroid, lingual thyroid, suprahyoid thyroid,* and *retrosternal thyroid.* Called also *aberrant thyroids* and *prehyoid glands.*

glan′dulae trachea′les [TA] tracheal glands: mucous glands in the elastic submucous coat between the cartilaginous rings and on the posterior wall of the trachea.

glan′dulae tuba′riae [TA] tubal glands: mucous glands within the mucosa of the auditory tube, especially near its nasopharyngeal end; called also *mucous glands of auditory* or *eustachian tube.*

glan′dulae urethra′les ure′thrae femini′nae [TA] urethral glands of female urethra: numerous small mucous glands in the mucosa of the female urethra. See also *paraurethral glands,* under *gland.*

glan′dulae urethra′les ure′thrae masculi′nae [TA] urethral glands of male urethra: mucous glands in the wall of the male urethra; called also *Littre glands.*

glan′dulae uteri′nae [TA] uterine glands: simple tubular glands throughout the entire thickness and extent of the endometrium, which become enlarged during the premenstrual period.

g. vesiculo′sa [TA] seminal gland: either of the paired, sacculated pouches attached to the posterior part of the urinary bladder; the duct of each joins the ipsilateral ductus deferens to form the ejaculatory duct. Called also *seminal vesicle, vesicula seminalis* [TA alternative], and *g. seminalis* [TA alternative].

g. vestibula′ris ma′jor [TA] greater vestibular gland: either of two small reddish yellow bodies in the vestibulovaginal bulbs, one on each side of the vaginal orifice; they are homologues of the bulbourethral glands in the male. Called also *Bartholin gland.*

glan′dulae vestibula′res mino′res [TA] lesser vestibular glands: small mucous glands opening upon the vestibular mucous membrane between the urethral and the vaginal orifice.

---

glan·du·lae (glan′du-le) [L.] genitive and plural of *glandula.*

glan·du·lar (glan′du-lər) 1. pertaining to or of the nature of a gland. Called also *adenic* and *adenous.* 2. glanular.

glan·dule (glan′dūl) a small gland.

glan·du·lous (glan′du-ləs) glandular (def. 1).

glans (glanz) pl. *glan′des* [L. "acorn"] a small rounded mass or glandlike body.

g. clito′ridis [TA] glans of clitoris: erectile tissue at the end of the clitoris, which is continuous with the intermediate part of the vestibulovaginal bulbs.

g. pe′nis [TA] the cap-shaped expansion of the corpus spongiosum at the end of the penis; called also *balanus.*

glan·u·lar (glan′u-lər) pertaining to the glans penis or glans clitoridis.

glan·u·lo·plas·ty (glan′u-lo-plas″te) plastic surgery on a glans, such as the glans penis to correct hypospadias. **glanuloplas′tic** *adj*

Glanz·mann thrombasthenia (disease) (glahnts′mən) [Eduard *Glanzmann,* Swiss pediatrician, 1887–1959] see *thrombasthenia.*

glare (glār) [Middle English *glaren*] a condition of discomfort in the eye and of depression of central vision produced when a bright light enters the field of vision, especially when the eye is adapted to dark. The amount of glare is directly proportional to the candle power of the light and inversely proportional to the square of the distance of the light from the eye and to its angular distance from the visual axis.

direct g. glare in which the image of the light falls on the fovea.

indirect g. glare in which the image of the light falls outside the fovea.

glar·om·e·ter (glār-om′ə-tər) [*glare* + *-meter*] an instrument for measuring a person's resistance to glare from the lights of an approaching automobile.

gla·se·ri·an (gla-se′re-ən) named for Johann Heinrich *Glaser* (Glaserius), Swiss anatomist, 1629–1675, as *glaserian fissure.*

Glas·gow Coma Scale, Outcome Scale (glas′go) [*Glasgow,* Scotland, where the scales were developed] see under *scale.*

Glas·gow sign (glas′go) [William Carr *Glasgow,* American physician, 1845–1907] see under *sign.*

glass (glas) [L. *vitrum*] 1. a hard, brittle, and often transparent material, usually consisting of the fused amorphous silicates of potassium or sodium, and of calcium, with silica in excess. 2. a container, usually cylindrical, made from glass.

cover g. a thin glass plate used to cover an object for microscopic examination. Written also *coverglass.*

crown g. a glass of low refractive index (achieved by incorporating a considerable percentage of phosphorus pentoxide); used in combination with flint glass in multielement lenses.

cupping g. a small vessel from which the air has been or can be exhausted, applied to the body in the practice of cupping (q.v.).

flint g. a highly refractive glass in which calcium has been replaced in large part by lead; used for lenses and prisms and in the manufacture of cut glass.

object g. see *objective.*

optical g. glass of high quality and controlled composition, used for lenses.

quartz g. pure fused silica, used for prisms, lenses, and chemical vessels because its index of thermal expansion is so small that it does not crack when heated or cooled and because it transmits more ultraviolet radiation than does ordinary glass.

test g. a small glass vessel, resembling a beaker, used in a chemical laboratory.

Wood g. see under *filter.*

glass·es (glas′əz) spectacles; a pair of lenses arranged in a frame holding them in the proper position before the eyes, as an aid to vision. See also entries under *lens* and *spectacles.*

bifocal g. glasses with bifocal lenses.

crutch g. glasses that will elevate and support the upper lids of patients with ptosis.

Hallauer g. glasses with grayish-green lenses which prevent the passage of blue light and ultraviolet rays.

industrial g. safety glasses.

pinhole g. glasses that have opaque disks in place of lenses, with only small central apertures. Called also *stenopeic g.*

protective g., safety g. glasses designed to protect the eyes rather than to correct defective vision; they may have side shields, safety lenses, or lenses that protect against ultraviolet or infrared rays

stenopeic g. pinhole g.

tinted g. glasses whose lenses are tinted to protect the eyes from certain kinds of light.

trifocal g. glasses with trifocal lenses.

glassy (glas′e) like glass; hyaline or vitreous.

gla·tir·a·mer ac·e·tate (glə-tir′ə-mər) an immunomodulator used to reduce relapses in multiple sclerosis; administered subcutaneously.

Glau·ber salt (glou′ber) [Johann Rudolf *Glauber,* German physician and chemist, 1604–1670] sodium sulfate.

glau·co·ma (glaw-, glou-ko′mə) [Gr. *glaukōma* opacity of the crystalline lens (from the dull gray gleam of the affected eye)] a group of eye diseases usually characterized by an increase in intraocular pressure that causes pathologic changes in the optic disk and typical defects in the field of vision. **glauco′matous** *adj*

absolute g. the final stage of glaucoma characterized by pain in the eye and blindness.

acute angle-closure g. a stage of angle-closure glaucoma that can be intensely painful, with intraocular pressure rising, although the obstruction of the trabecular meshwork is still reversible.

acute congestive g. angle-closure g.

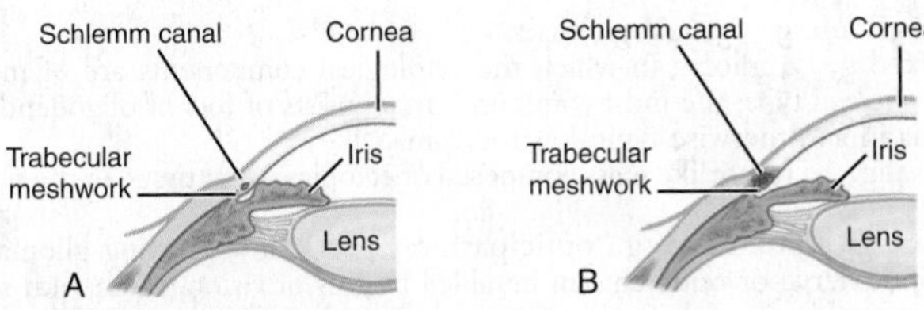

■ Glaucoma. Impairment of outflow of aqueous humor is caused by closure of the anterior angle, with apposition of the iris and trabecular meshwork, in angle-closure glaucoma *(A)*, and by other obstruction in open-angle glaucoma *(B)*.

air-block g. a form of postoperative glaucoma, resulting from blockage of the flow of aqueous humor by air injected behind the iris.

angle-closure g. glaucoma caused by closure of the anterior angle by contact between the iris and the inner surface of the trabecular meshwork; called also *closed-angle g.*, *narrow-angle g.*, and *pupillary block g.*

angle-recession g. glaucoma secondary to contusion injury of the eye, in which the anterior chamber is deep and the angle recedes, with exposure of the ciliary body, as seen gonioscopically, with blocking of the trabecular spaces; called also *contusion g.*

aphakic g. a general term referring to glaucoma in an eye from which the lens has been removed; the glaucoma may be related to the cataract extraction or to its sequelae, or it may have existed prior to the cataract extraction.

apoplectic g. hemorrhagic g.

auricular g. glaucoma associated with increased pressure in the labyrinth of the ear.

capsular g., g. capsula're open-angle glaucoma associated with the exfoliation syndrome, and with particles of iris pigment scattered in the anterior angle.

chronic g. open-angle g.

chronic angle-closure g. the final stage of angle-closure glaucoma, in which there is an irreversible increase in intraocular pressure resulting from progressive damage to the angle structures and from permanent, at least partial closure of the anterior angle by synechiae.

closed-angle g. angle-closure g.

congenital g. a form of glaucoma that may be fully developed at birth or may develop later, up to two or three years of age; characteristics are enlargement and hazing of the corneas, resulting from inability of the cornea and sclera to withstand the increased intraocular pressure. Called also *infantile g.*, *buphthalmos*, and *hydrophthalmos*. Cf. *juvenile g.*

congestive g. angle-closure g.

g. consumma'tum absolute g.

contusion g. angle-recession g.

exfoliation g. g. capsulare.

ghost cell g. a type of open-angle glaucoma caused by erythroclasts that obstruct outflow of aqueous humor; it may occur after vitreous hemorrhage caused by trauma, after retinal neovascularization, or after cataract extraction.

hemolytic g. a type of open-angle glaucoma caused by blood clots that fill the anterior angle or by erythrocytes that infiltrate the trabecular meshwork.

hemorrhagic g. glaucoma caused by pressure from retinal hemorrhage.

infantile g. congenital g.

inflammatory g. a type of glaucoma attended with ciliary congestion, corneal opacity, and blindness, recurring in paroxysmal attacks.

intermittent angle-closure g. an intermediate stage of angle-closure glaucoma, usually lasting for several months, and characterized by intermittent, transient attacks of glaucoma with rapidly rising intraocular pressure, edematous cornea, and dull or throbbing pain in or around the eye.

juvenile g. a type of glaucoma similar to congenital glaucoma but differing in that it occurs in older children and young adults up to 30 years of age, and does not involve gross enlargement of the eyeball.

latent angle-closure g. the earliest stage of angle-closure glaucoma; patients may be free of symptoms or have minor attacks of varying severity, duration, and frequency for months or years before a crisis. Gonioscopy reveals narrow angles capable of closure. Called also *prodromal g.*

lenticular g. glaucoma occurring in association with congenital or traumatic dislocation of the lens, or with swelling of the lens, usually due to mechanical obstruction at the peripheral angle of the anterior chamber.

low-tension g. open-angle glaucoma without increased intraocular pressure.

malignant g. glaucoma that grows rapidly worse in spite of iridectomy.

melanomalytic g. glaucoma caused by mechanical blockage of the anterior angle by macrophages in the eye with necrotic malignant melanoma.

narrow-angle g. angle-closure g.

neovascular g. a form of secondary glaucoma caused by neovascularization in the chamber angle.

noncongestive g. open-angle g.

obstructive g. angle-closure g.

open-angle g. any glaucoma in which the angle of the anterior chamber remains open, but filtration is gradually diminished because of the tissues of the angle; called also *chronic*, *simple*, or *wide-angle g.*

phacogenic g., phacolytic g. open-angle glaucoma secondary to leakage of lens protein into the aqueous humor from a mature or hypermature cataract with subsequent ingestion of the protein by macrophages, which swell and block the trabecular spaces.

pigmentary g. a form of open-angle glaucoma associated with an abnormal amount of pigment dispersion in the anterior segment of the eyeball.

primary g. increased intraocular pressure occurring in an eye without previous disease; see *angle-closure g.* and *open-angle g.*

prodromal g. latent angle-closure g.

pupillary block g. angle-closure g.

secondary g. increased intraocular pressure resulting from a preexisting disease or injury.

simple g. primary open-angle g.

steroid g. a secondary open-angle glaucoma due to chronic use of topical or systemic corticosteroids.

traumatic g. an increase in intraocular pressure due to a nonperforating injury of the globe, resulting in vascular congestion.

vitreous-block g. postoperative glaucoma in which the vitreous body plugs the pupil, so that the aqueous humor, which is unable to move to the anterior chamber, forces the vitreous body and iris forward, producing occlusion of the chamber angle and eventually peripheral anterior synechiae.

wide-angle g. open-angle g.

Glau·con (glou'kon) trademark for a preparation of epinephrine.

glau·kom·fleck·en (glou'kom-flek″ən) [Ger. "glaucoma spots"] glaucomatous cataract.

glaze (glāz) 1. to cover with a glossy, smooth surface or coating. 2. a ceramic veneer added to a dental porcelain restoration after it has been fired, to give a completely nonporous, glossy or semiglossy surface. 3. the final firing (in air) of dental porcelain, when formation of a thin, vitreous, glossy surface takes place.

GLC gas-liquid chromatography.

GlcNAc *N*-acetylglucosamine.

Glea·son grade (score) (gle'sən) [Donald F. *Gleason*, American pathologist, born 1920] see under *grade*.

gleet (glēt) old popular term for a purulent urethral discharge, such as that seen in gonorrhea.

vent g. cloacitis in domestic fowl.

Glee·vec (gle'vek) trademark for a preparation of imatinib mesylate.

Glenn operation (anastomosis, shunt) (glen) [William Wallace Lumpkin *Glenn*, American surgeon, 1914–2003] see under *operation*.

Glenn-An·der·son technique (glen' an'dər-sən) [James Francis *Glenn*, American urologist, born 1928; E.E. *Anderson*, American urologist, 20th century] see under *technique*.

gle·no·hu·mer·al (gle″no-hu'mər-əl) pertaining to the glenoid cavity and the humerus.

gle·noid (gle'noid, glen'oid) [Gr. *glēnē* socket + *-oid*] resembling a pit or socket; see *cavitas glenoidalis*.

GLI glucagon-like immunoreactivity; see *enteroglucagon*.

glia (gli'ə) [Gr. "glue"] neuroglia. **gli'al** *adj*

ameboid g. degenerated neuroglial cells that are rich in pale protoplasm, possess few processes, and have densely staining nuclei.

Bergmann g. see under *cell*.

cytoplasmic g. enlarged neuroglial cells, rich in cytoplasm, containing vacuoles and supplied with fibrils; seen in degeneration of the spinal cord.

g. of Fañanás see under *cell*.

fibrillary g. degenerated neuroglial cells containing an abundance of fibrils.

radial g. a special type of glia in the developing central nervous system, whose cells have radial processes extending through the entire thickness from the ventricular surface to the exterior cortical surface; neurons formed on the ventricular surface are thought to migrate along these processes to their final positions in other parts of the cortex.

-glia [Gr. *glia* glue] a word termination denoting the neuroglia.

glia·cyte (gli'ə-sīt) neuroglia cell.

Gli·a·del (gli'ə-del) trademark for a preparation of polifeprosan 20 with a carmustine implant.

gli•a•din (gli′ə-din) [Gr. *glia* glue] a protein of the prolamin group, found in wheat and occurring in various forms (α-, β-, γ-, and ω-gliadins); it contains the toxic factor associated with celiac disease.

gli•ben•cla•mide (gli-ben′klə-mīd) INN and BAN for *glyburide.*

gli•born•ur•ide (gli-born′ūr-īd) a sulfonylurea compound used as a hypoglycemic in the treatment of type 2 diabetes mellitus; administered orally.

gli•cen•tin (gli-sen′tin) a common enteroglucagon, secreted in the intestinal tract and having glycogenolytic activity.

glic•la•zide (glik′lə-zīd) a sulfonylurea compound used as a hypoglycemic in the treatment of type 2 diabetes mellitus; administered orally.

glide (glīd) 1. a smooth continuous movement. 2. a speech sound that is transitional between a vowel and a consonant.
mandibular g. the side-to-side, protrusive, and intermediate movement of the mandible occurring when the teeth or other occluding surfaces are in contact.
occlusal g. the movement induced by deflective tooth contact that diverts the mandible from a normal path of closure to a centric jaw relation.

gli•mep•i•ride (gli-mep′ĭ-rīd) [USP] a sulfonylurea compound used as a hypoglycemic in the treatment of type 2 diabetes mellitus; administered orally.

gli(o)- [Gr. *glia* glue] a combining form denoting relationship to a gluey substance or, specifically, to the neuroglia.

glio•bac•te•ria (gli″o-bak-tēr′e-ə) [*glio-* + *bacteria*] bacteria that are surrounded by a gelatinous matrix.

glio•blast (gli′o-blast) spongioblast (def. 1).

glio•blas•to•ma (gli″o-blas-to′mə) [*glio-* + *blastoma*] the most malignant type of astrocytoma, classified as Grade IV, one of the most common primary tumors of the brain; it also occurs in the brainstem in children and occasionally in the spinal cord of an adult or child. It grows rapidly, is usually found in the cerebral hemispheres, and is composed of a mixture of spongioblasts, astroblasts, and astrocytes. Called also *glioblastoma multifor′me* and *spongioblastoma multiforme.* **glioblastom′atous** *adj*

glio•coc•cus (gli″o-kok′əs) [*glio-* + *coccus*] a micrococcus that forms gelatinous matter.

glio•cyte (gli′o-sīt) neuroglial cell.
retinal g's Müller fibers.

glio•fi•bril•lary (gli″o-fi′brĭ-lar-e) pertaining to fibrils of the neuroglia.

gli•o•ma (gli-o′mə) [*gli-* + *-oma*] originally, a tumor composed of tissue representing neuroglia in any of its stages of development; the term has been extended to include all the primary intrinsic neoplasms of the brain and spinal cord, including astrocytomas, ependymomas, medulloblastomas, medulloepitheliomas, and others. Called also *neurogliocytoma, neuroglioma,* and *neurospongioma.* **glio′matous** *adj*
astrocytic g. astrocytoma.
brainstem g. a heterogeneous group that includes gliomas anywhere in the brainstem; they are seen mainly in children and cause neuropathy with motor symptoms and problems of gait, speech, and swallowing. The *diffuse, intrinsic type* is difficult to treat and usually fatal within two years. The *dorsal, exophytic type* is focal, arises in the floor of the fourth ventricle, grows slowly, and may be amenable to resection.
g. endo′phytum endophytic retinoblastoma.
ependymal g. ependymoma.
g. exo′phytum exophytic retinoblastoma.

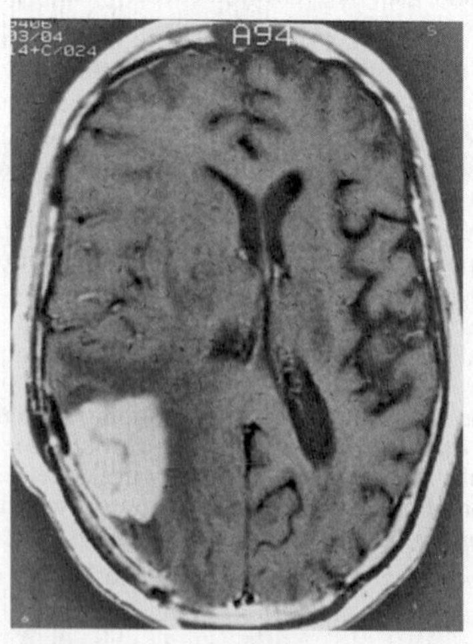

■ Glioblastoma. MRI demonstrates a large contrast-enhancing left temporal lesion with an irregular border as well as a central lucency suggesting an area of necrosis.

ganglionic g. ganglioglioma.
mixed g. a glioma in which the cytological components are of more than one cell type; the most common form consists of foci of oligodendroglioma in an otherwise typical astrocytoma.
nasal g. a tumorlike mass composed of ectopic neural tissue in the nasal cavity.
optic g., optic nerve g., optic pathway g. a slow-growing glioma of the optic nerve or optic chiasm heralded by loss of vision, often with secondary strabismus, followed by proptosis and loss of eye movement.
peripheral g. schwannoma.
g. re′tinae retinoblastoma.

gli•o•ma•to•sis (gli″o-mə-to′sis) diffuse formation of gliomas; called also *neurogliosis.*
cerebral g., g. ce′rebri a rare variant of glioblastoma in which one hemisphere or the entire brain is infiltrated diffusely with anaplastic astrocytes.
peritoneal g., g. perito′nei the metastatic implantation of immature neuroectodermal tumor tissue on peritoneal surfaces.

glio•neu•ro•ma (gli″o-noo̅-ro′mə) ganglioglioma.

glio•pha•gia (gli″o-fa′jə) [*glio-* + *-phagia*] phagocytosis of neuroglial cells.

glio•pil (gli′o-pil) [*glio-* + Gr. *pilos* felt] a dense feltwork of glial processes, as in the subependymal tissue around the ventricles.

glio•sar•co•ma (gli″o-sahr-ko′mə) [*glio-* + *sarcoma*] a glioma, usually a glioblastoma, that has sarcomatous components.

gli•o•sis (gli-o′sis) an excess of astroglia in damaged areas of the central nervous system; see also *astrocytosis.* Called also *astrogliosis.*
diffuse g. gliosis affecting the whole of the cerebral tissue, or widely scattered through it.
g. endome′trii g. uteri.
hemispheric g. gliosis affecting one of the cerebral hemispheres.
hypertrophic nodular g. a form of gliosis in which the brain is symmetrically enlarged because of hyperplasia of the neuroglial tissue.
isomorphic g. gliosis in which there is a regular and parallel arrangement of glial fibers.
perivascular g. a form of arteriosclerosis of the cerebral vessels, marked by an increase of neuroglia.
unilateral g. hemispheric g.
g. u′teri proliferation of neural tissue in the endometrium or endocervix.

glio•some (gli′o-sōm) [*glio-* + *-some*] one of the small cytoplasmic granules seen in neuroglial cells.

glio•tox•in (gli′o-tok″sin) an antibiotic obtained from several unrelated species of fungi, including species of *Trichoderma, Aspergillus,* and *Penicillium;* it is a neutral, nitrogen- and sulfur-containing compound.

glip•i•zide (glip′ĭ-zīd) [USP] a sulfonylurea compound used as a hypoglycemic in the treatment of type 2 diabetes mellitus; administered orally.

Gli•ric•o•la (gli-rik′o-lə) a genus of biting lice of the order Mallophaga; *G. porcel′li* infests guinea pigs.

glis•sade (glĭ-sād′) [Fr. "sliding"] a gliding involuntary movement of the eye in changing the point of fixation; it is a slower, smoother movement than is a saccade. **glissad′ic** *adj*

Glis•son capsule, sling, sphincter (glis′ən) [Francis *Glisson,* English physician and anatomist, 1597–1677] see *capsula fibrosa perivascularis hepatis* and *musculus sphincter ampullae hepatopancreaticae,* and see under *sling.*

glis•so•ni•tis (glis″o-ni′tis) [F. *Glisson*] inflammation of the Glisson capsule (capsula fibrosa perivascularis hepatis).

gli•ta•zone (glĭ-ta′zōn) [from the ending *-glitazone* that occurs in the names of drugs of this class] thiazolinedione.

Gln glutamine.

globe (glōb) 1. sphere. 2. bulbus oculi.

glo•bi (glo′bi) [L.] genitive and plural of *globus.*

Glo•bid•i•um (glo-bid′e-əm) former name for *Besnoitia.*

glo•bin (glo′bin) 1. the protein constituent of hemoglobin; see also *globin chain,* under *chain.* 2. any member of a group of proteins similar to the typical globin.

Glo•bo•ceph•a•lus (glo″bo-sef′ə-lus) a genus of blood-sucking nematodes of the family Ancylostomatidae. *G. urosubula′tus* and other species infest the intestines of pigs, causing anemia.

glo•boid (glo′boid) spheroid.

glo•bose (glo′bōs) spherical.

glob•o•side (glob′o-sīd) a glycosphingolipid containing acetylated amino sugars and simple hexoses of the general composition N-acetylgalactosamine-galactose-galactose-glucose-ceramide; it accumulates in tissues in Sandhoff disease, but not in Tay-Sachs disease.

glo·bo·tri·a·o·syl·cer·a·mide (glo″bo-tri-a″o-səl-ser′ə-mīd) ceramide trihexoside.

glob·u·lar (glob′u-lər) 1. like a globe. 2. like a globule. 3. composed of globules.

Glo·bu·la·ria (glob″u-lar′e-ə) a genus of shrubs of the family Globulariaceae. *G. aly′pum* L. is a perennial herb indigenous to the Mediterranean region used as a cathartic and for intermittent fevers.

glob·ule (glob′ūl) [L. *globulus*] 1. a small spherical mass or body. 2. a small spherical drop of fluid or semifluid substance, e.g., a fat droplet in milk or a drop of water. 3. a little globe or pellet, as of medicine.

dentin g's small spherical bodies in the peripheral dentin, created by beginning calcification of the matrix about discrete foci.

Dobie g. a minute stainable mass in the middle of the transparent disk of a muscle fibril.

Marchi g's fragments and particles of broken-up myelin that stain by Marchi method, seen in degeneration of the spinal cord.

Morgagni g's round fragments of cells in the cortex of the lens; they are a sign of mature cataract.

polar g's polar bodies (def. 1).

glo·bu·li (glob′u-li) genitive and plural of *globulus.*

glob·u·lin (glob′u-lin) [L. *globulus* globule] any member of a class of proteins, most of which are insoluble in water but soluble in saline solutions *(euglobulins)*, but some of which *(pseudoglobulins)* are water soluble proteins whose other physical properties closely resemble those of the true globulins. See also *serum g's.*

α-g's the serum globulins with the most rapid electrophoretic migration, further subdivided into the faster $α_1$-globulins and the slower $α_2$-globulins. Written also *alpha g's.*

AC g., accelerator g. factor V; see under *coagulation factors,* at *factor.*

alpha g's α-g's.

antihemophilic g. (AHG) factor VIII; see under *coagulation factors,* at *factor.*

anti–human g. serum [USP] monospecific or broad spectrum antiserum produced by immunizing a rabbit or other animal with human plasma proteins; used in the antiglobulin test (Coombs test) and immunoelectrophoresis.

antilymphocyte g. (ALG) the gamma globulin fraction of antilymphocyte serum (q.v.), used as an immunosuppressant in organ transplantation. The term is sometimes used interchangeably with *antithymocyte globulin.*

antithymocyte g. (ATG) the gamma globulin fraction of antiserum derived from animals that have been immunized against human thymocytes; an immunosuppressive agent that causes specific destruction of T lymphocytes and is used in treatment of allograft rejection. The term is sometimes used interchangeably with *antilymphocyte globulin.*

antithymocyte g. (rabbit) a purified gamma globulin obtained from rabbits immunized with human thymocytes; administered intravenously in the treatment of acute rejection occurring after renal transplantation and experimentally in the treatment of rejection occurring after various other transplant procedures.

β-g's globulins of plasma that have an electrophoretic mobility in neutral or alkaline solutions intermediate between that of the alpha and the gamma globulins.

bacterial polysaccharide immune g. (BPIG) a human hyperimmune globulin derived from the blood plasma of adult human donors immunized with *Haemophilus influenzae* type b, pneumococcal, and meningococcal polysaccharide vaccines; used for passive immunization of infants under 18 months of age.

beta g's β-g's.

corticosteroid-binding g., cortisol-binding g. (CBG) transcortin.

cytomegalovirus immune g. a purified immunoglobulin derived from pooled adult human plasma selected for high titers of antibody against cytomegalovirus (CMV); administered intravenously for the treatment and prophylaxis of cytomegalovirus disease in transplant recipients.

γ-g's, gamma g's serum globulins having the least rapid electrophoretic migration. Since the gamma globulin fraction is composed almost entirely of immunoglobulin, gamma globulin came to be used as a synonym for "immunoglobulin" or "immune globulin." Because some immunoglobulins have α or β electrophoretic mobility, this usage is imprecise and is in decline.

hepatitis B immune g. [USP] a specific immune globulin derived from plasma of human donors with high titers of antibodies against hepatitis B surface antigen (HB_sAg); used for postexposure prophylaxis following contact with HB_sAg-positive materials, also administered to infants of HB_sAg-positive mothers.

hyperimmune g. any of various immunoglobulin preparations that are especially high in antibodies against certain specific diseases.

immune g. 1. immunoglobulin. 2. [USP] a concentrated preparation containing mostly gamma globulins, predominantly IgG, from a large pool of human donors; used for passive immunization against measles, hepatitis A, and varicella and for treatment of hypogammaglobulinemia or agammaglobulinemia in immunodeficient patients, administered intramuscularly. See also *immune g. intravenous (human).*

immune human serum g. immune g. (def. 2).

immune g. intravenous (human) (IGIV) a preparation of immune globulin (q.v.) suitable for intravenous administration; used in the treatment of primary immunodeficiency disorders and idiopathic thrombocytopenic purpura, and as an adjunct in the treatment of Kawasaki disease and the prevention of infections associated with chronic lymphocytic leukemia, bone marrow transplantation, and pediatric human immunodeficiency virus infection.

immune serum g. immune g. (def. 2).

lymphocyte immune g. antilymphocyte g.

pertussis immune g. [USP] a specific immune globulin derived from human donors immunized with pertussis vaccine; used for prophylaxis and treatment of pertussis. Formerly called *pertussis immune human g.*

rabies immune g. [USP] a specific immune globulin derived from plasma of human donors hyperimmunized with rabies vaccine; administered in conjunction with rabies vaccine in cases of bite or scratch exposure to animals known or suspected to be rabid.

respiratory syncytial virus immune g. intravenous a preparation of immunoglobulin G (IgG) from pooled adult human plasma selected for high titers of antibodies against respiratory syncytial virus; used for passive immunization of infants and children less than 24 months of age, administered by intravenous infusion.

Rh_0(D) immune g. [USP] a specific immune globulin derived from plasma of human donors immunized to produce high levels of antibodies against the Rh_0 antigen (D antigen); used to prevent Rh-sensitization of Rh-negative females and thus prevent erythroblastosis fetalis in subsequent pregnancies; administered within 72 hours after exposure to Rh-positive blood resulting from delivery of an Rh-positive child, abortion or miscarriage of an Rh-positive fetus, or transfusion of Rh-positive blood. It is also used as a platelet count stimulator in the treatment of idiopathic thrombocytopenic purpura. Formerly called *Rh_0(D) immune human g.*

serum g's all plasma proteins except albumin, which is not a globulin, and fibrinogen, which is not in the serum. The serum globulins are subdivided into α-, β-, and γ-globulins on the basis of their relative electrophoretic mobilities.

sex hormone–binding g. (SHBG), sex steroid–binding g. a β-globulin in plasma that binds to and transports testosterone, and to a lesser degree estrogens; it is formed in the liver. Called also *testosterone-estradiol–binding g.* and *testosterone-estrogen–binding g.*

specific immune g. a preparation of immune globulin derived from a donor pool preselected for high antibody titer against a specific antigen, such as hepatitis B immune globulin.

testosterone-estradiol–binding g. (TEBG), testosterone-estrogen–binding g. sex hormone–binding g.

tetanus immune g. [USP] a specific immune globulin derived from blood of human donors hyperimmunized with tetanus toxoid; used for prophylaxis and treatment of tetanus. Formerly called *tetanus immune human g.*

thyroxine-binding g. (TBG) a 54-kD acidic glycoprotein that is the main transport protein in the blood for thyroxine (and less firmly, triiodothyronine); it is a serum globulin synthesized by the liver and has electrophoretic mobility intermediate between that of the $α_1$- and $α_2$-globulins.

vaccinia immune g. (VIG) [USP] a specific immune globulin derived from blood of human donors immunized with vaccinia virus smallpox vaccine; used for prophylaxis and treatment of vaccinia or smallpox. Formerly called *vaccinia immune human g.*

varicella-zoster immune g. (VZIG) a specific immune globulin derived from plasma of human donors with high titers of varicella-zoster antibodies; used for prevention or amelioration of varicella in immunodeficient or immunosuppressed patients exposed to the disease and in neonates whose mothers develop varicella in the perinatal period.

glob·u·lin·uria (glob″u-lĭ-nu′re-ə) proteinuria in which globulin is excreted in the urine.

glob·u·lose (glob′u-lōs) a proteose produced by action of pepsin on the globulins; several varieties have been described.

glo·bu·lus (glob′u-ləs) gen. and pl. *glo′buli* [L.] globule.

glo′buli os′sei intrachondrial bone.

glo·bus (glo′bəs) gen. and pl. *glo′bi* [L. "sphere"] 1. a sphere or spherical structure. 2. bulbus oculi. 3. one of the encapsulated globular masses containing bacilli, seen in smears of lepromatous leprosy lesions.

g. of the heel the portion of the wall of a horse's hoof that curves around the heel to form the bar.

g. hyste′ricus globus pharyngeus resulting from a conversion disorder.

g. pal′lidus the smaller and more medial part of the lentiform nucleus of the brain, separated from the putamen by the lateral medullary lamina. In official anatomic terminology, it is divided by the medial medullary lamina into two parts, lateral and medial (see *g. pallidus lateralis* and *g. pallidus medialis*), both of which have extensive connections with the corpus

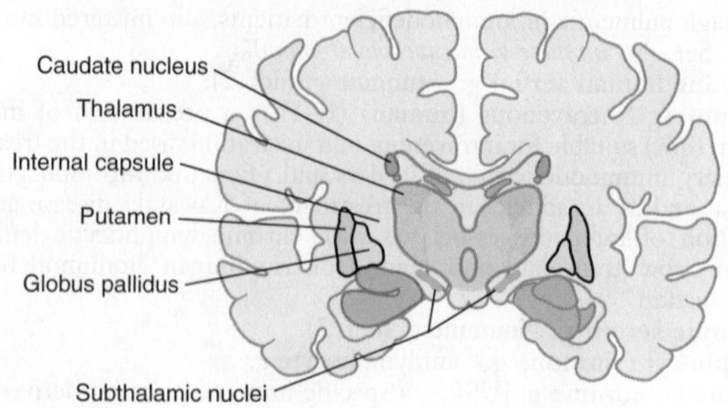

■ Globus pallidus in relation to other components of the basal ganglia and closely associated brain regions; coronal section.

striatum, thalamus, and mesencephalon. Called also *pallidum.* See also *paleostriatum.*

g. pal′lidus exter′na g. pallidus lateralis.

g. pal′lidus inter′na g. pallidus medialis.

g. pal′lidus latera′lis [TA] globus pallidus lateral segment: the larger, lateral (or external) part of the globus pallidus, separated from the putamen by the lateral medullary lamina and from the smaller, medial part of the globus pallidus by the medial medullary lamina; called also *globus pallidus external segment* and *pallidum I.* See also *g. pallidus.*

g. pal′lidus media′lis [TA] globus pallidus medial segment: the smaller, medial (or internal) part of the globus pallidus, separated from the larger, lateral part by the medial medullary lamina; called also *globus pallidus internal segment* and *pallidum II.* See also *g. pallidus.*

g. pharyn′geus an uncomfortable feeling of having a lump in the throat when none is there; it may be psychogenic *(globus hystericus)* or due to some disorder of the esophagus or nearby cervical structures.

glo·chid (glo′kid) a small barbed hair or bristle found on certain species of cactus, such as the prickly pears (species *Opuntia*), a common cause of mechanical irritant dermatitis.

Gloe·o·trich·ia (gle″o-trik′e-ə) a genus of cyanobacteria that sometimes contaminate water and can cause cyanobacteria poisoning.

Glo·fil (glo′fil) trademark for a preparation of iothalamate I 125 sodium.

glo·man·gi·o·ma (glo-man″je-o′mə) [*glomus* + *angioma*] glomus tumor (def. 1).

glo·mec·to·my (glo-mek′tə-me) excision of a glomus, especially one containing a glomus tumor.

glom·era (glom′ər-ə) [L.] plural of *glomus.*

glom·er·ate (glom′ər-āt) [L. *glomeratus* wound into a ball] crowded together into a ball.

glo·mer·u·lar (glo-mer′u-lər) pertaining to or of the nature of a glomerulus.

glo·mer·u·li (glo-mer′u-li) [L.] genitive and plural of *glomerulus.*

glo·mer·u·li·tis (glo-mer″u-li′tis) inflammation of renal glomeruli, such as in glomerulonephritis.

glomerul(o)- [L. *glomerulus,* q.v.] a combining form denoting relationship to the renal glomeruli.

glo·mer·u·loid (glo-mer′u-loid) resembling a glomerulus.

glo·mer·u·lo·meg·a·ly (glo-mer″u-lo-meg′ə-le) excessive size of the renal glomeruli, such as in glomerulosclerosis.

glo·mer·u·lo·ne·phri·tis (glo-mer″u-lo-nə-fri′tis) [*glomerulo-* + *nephritis*] nephritis accompanied by inflammation of the capillary loops in the renal glomeruli. It occurs in acute, subacute, and chronic forms and may be secondary to hemolytic streptococcal infection. Evidence also supports possible immune or autoimmune mechanisms. Called also *glomerular nephritis.*

acute g. glomerulonephritis characterized by proteinuria, edema, hematuria, renal failure, and hypertension; it may be preceded by tonsillitis or febrile pharyngitis.

anti-GBM g., anti–GBM antibody g., anti–glomerular basement membrane g. see under *nephritis.*

chronic g. slowly progressive glomerulonephritis that generally leads to end-stage renal disease; it may be a primary disease, follow acute glomerulonephritis, or be secondary to systemic disease. Symptoms and course vary widely.

chronic hypocomplementemic g. membranoproliferative g.

crescentic g. 1. any glomerulonephritis in which epithelial crescents are present, such as types of diffuse glomerulonephritis and rapidly progressive glomerulonephritis. 2. rapidly progressive glomerulonephritis when crescents are present.

diffuse g., diffuse proliferative g. a severe form in which there are proliferative changes in more than half the glomeruli, frequently with epithelial crescent formation and necrosis; it is often seen in cases of advanced systemic lupus erythematosus.

fibrillary g. a rare form of glomerulonephritis characterized by infiltration of the glomeruli with fibrils slightly larger than amyloid fibrils that do not stain with Congo red. Immunotactoid glomerulopathy is a variety having particularly large fibrils. Called also *microtubular glomerulopathy.*

focal g. glomerulonephritis in which some glomeruli show inflammatory changes but others appear normal.

focal embolic g. focal glomerulonephritis associated with bacterial endocarditis; see *Löhlein-Baehr lesion,* under *lesion.*

IgA g. see under *nephropathy.*

immune complex g. glomerulonephritis due to formation of circulating immune complexes and their deposition in tissue, a type III hypersensitivity reaction, which causes activation of complement and an inflammatory response, leading to activation of leukocytes and damage to the glomerular basement membrane layer.

immunotactoid g. see under *glomerulopathy.*

lobular g., lobulonodular g. membranoproliferative g.

lupus g. see under *nephritis.*

malignant g. rapidly progressive g.

membranoproliferative g. a chronic glomerulonephritis characterized by mesangial cell proliferation and irregular thickening of the glomerular capillary wall. There are two subtypes: *Type I* is marked by subendothelial electron-dense deposits and classical complement pathway activation, and *Type II* (called also *dense deposit disease*) is marked by heavy electron-dense deposits in the glomerular basement membrane and alternative complement pathway activation involving C3 nephritic factor. Both types occur in older children and young adults and follow a slowly progressive course with irregular remissions ultimately resulting in renal failure. Called also *chronic hypocomplementemic g., lobular* or *lobulonodular g.,* and *mesangiocapillary g.*

membranous g. glomerulonephritis characterized histologically by proteinaceous deposits on the glomerular basement membrane or by thickening of the membrane, with circulating antigen-antibody complexes indicating immune complex disease. It may be secondary to a number of other conditions, and clinical features are those of chronic glomerulonephritis. In some cases it may develop into the nephrotic syndrome. Called also *membranous glomerulopathy* or *nephropathy.*

mesangial proliferative g. glomerulonephritis characterized by diffuse glomerular proliferation of mesangial and endocapillary cells and mesangial matrix, seen in patients with the nephrotic syndrome; IgM deposits and complement 3 are often found in the mesangium. Called also *IgM nephropathy.*

mesangiocapillary g., nodular g. membranoproliferative g.

pauci-immune crescentic g., pauci-immune rapidly progressive g. a type of rapidly progressive glomerulonephritis in which there are epithelial crescents and antineutrophil cytoplasmic antibodies, but few, if any, immune deposits.

postinfectious g. glomerulonephritis following infection, usually by group A streptococci, seen mainly in children, adolescents, and young adults; characteristics include onset 10 days or more after the infection, oliguria, and hematuria, often with edema, hypertension, and circulatory congestion that can be resolved by diuresis. Serious cases sometimes lead to renal failure.

poststreptococcal g. the most common type of postinfectious glomerulonephritis, which follows infection by group A streptococci *(Streptococcus pyogenes).*

proliferative g. any of various types accompanied by proliferation of endothelial or mesangial cells in the glomeruli, including acute, diffuse, membranoproliferative, mesangial proliferative, and rapidly progressive glomerulonephritis.

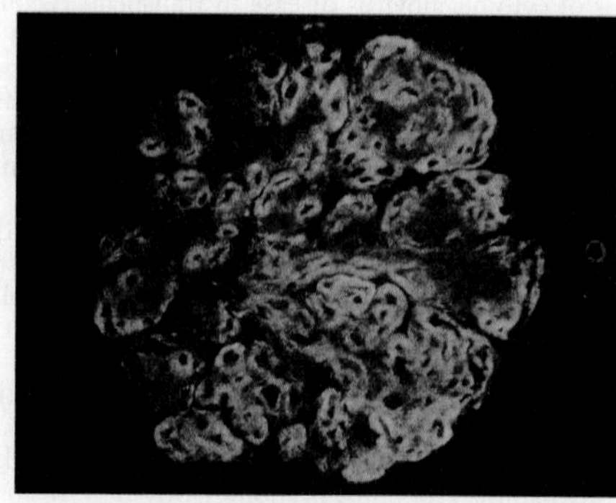

■ Type I membranoproliferative glomerulonephritis; immunofluorescence demonstrates immunoreactivity for C3 along capillary loops.

rapidly progressive g. acute glomerulonephritis marked by a rapid progression to end-stage renal disease and, histologically, by profuse epithelial proliferation, often with epithelial crescents; principal signs are anuria, proteinuria, hematuria, and anemia. Called also *crescentic g.*

segmental g. focal glomerulonephritis in which only limited segments of affected glomeruli are diseased.

subacute g. persistence of acute glomerulonephritis, with or without periods of remission, which may develop into lobular or malignant glomerulonephritis.

glo•mer•u•lo•ne•phrop•a•thy (glo-mer″u-lo-nə-frop′ə-the) glomerulopathy.

glo•mer•u•lop•a•thy (glo-mer″u-lop′ə-the) any disease of the renal glomeruli.

collapsing g. focal segmental glomerulosclerosis with extensive collapse of glomerular capillaries and heavy proteinuria, usually progressing to end-stage renal disease within two years.

diabetic g. intercapillary glomerulosclerosis.

immunotactoid g. a type of fibrillary glomerulonephritis having particularly large fibrils (immunotactoids). Called also *immunotactoid glomerulonephritis.*

membranous g. see under *glomerulonephritis.*

microtubular g. fibrillary glomerulonephritis.

minimal change g. see under *disease.*

glo•mer•u•lo•scle•ro•sis (glo-mer″u-lo-sklə-ro′sis) fibrosis and scarring with senescence of the renal glomeruli.

diabetic g. intercapillary g.

focal g., focal segmental g. the occurrence of focal sclerosing lesions of the renal glomeruli, marked by proteinuria, hematuria, hypertension, and the nephrotic syndrome; it may be idiopathic or secondary to another disease, such as heroin-abuse nephropathy, chronic interstitial nephritis, or a malignancy. Exacerbations and remissions may occur, most often in children; progression to renal failure occurs at a variable and unpredictable rate. Called also *focal glomerular sclerosis.*

intercapillary g. a degenerative complication of diabetes mellitus in which there is glomerular mesangial expansion with either diffuse or nodular lesions; the nodular lesions are known as *Kimmelstiel-Wilson lesions.* Symptoms include albuminuria, nephrotic edema, hypertension, renal insufficiency, and retinopathy. Called also *diabetic g.* The type with nodular lesions is also called *Kimmelstiel-Wilson syndrome.*

glo•mer•u•lose (glo-mer′u-lōs) glomerular.

glo•mer•u•lo•tu•bu•lar (glo-mer″u-lo-too′bu-lər) pertaining to the renal tubules and glomeruli; called also *tubuloglomerular.*

glo•mer•u•lus (glo-mer′u-ləs) pl. *glomer′uli* [L., dim. of *glomus* ball] 1. a tuft or cluster; used in anatomic nomenclature as a general term to designate such a structure, as one composed of blood vessels or nerve fibers. 2. g. renis.

glome′ruli arterio′si coch′leae an arterial network surrounding the cochlea.

juxtamedullary g. a renal glomerulus located particularly close to the corticomedullary border.

g. of kidney, malpighian g. glomerulus renis.

nonencapsulated nerve g. a type of free nerve ending in the connective tissue of various organs, with the terminal branches of the nerve forming spherical or elongated structures resembling glomeruli.

olfactory g. one of the small globular masses of dense neuropil in the olfactory bulb; it contains the first synapse in the olfactory pathway and the axons of olfactory cells synapse here with dendrites primarily of mitral cells and tufted cells.

renal g., g. re′nis a globular tuft formed by capillaries in the kidney, the site of the filtration barrier between the blood and the kidney; it projects into the expanded end of a renal tubule, and together with its surrounding capsule (*glomerular capsule*) it constitutes a renal corpuscle. Called also *malpighian g.* See Plate 20.

synaptic g. a glomerulus formed by the coming together of a number of end-feet around a central dendrite, all enclosed by a layer of neuroglial cells; found in the sensory nuclei of the thalamus, in the olfactory bulbs, and in a few other locations in the brain. See also *olfactory g.*

glo•mic (glo′mik) 1. pertaining to a glomus. 2. affecting a glomus.

glo•moid (glo′moid) resembling a glomus.

glo•mus (glo′məs) pl. *glom′era* [L. "a ball"] 1. a small, histologically recognizable body, composed of fine arterioles connecting directly with veins, and possessing a rich nerve supply. 2. glomus body.

glo′mera aor′tica corpora paraaortica.

g. caro′ticum [TA] carotid body: a small neurovascular structure lying in the bifurcation of the right and left carotid arteries, made up of richly innervated epithelioid glomus cells (type I) surrounded by type II cells. It functions as an arterial chemoreceptor (although which component is responsible is uncertain), with stimulation by hypoxia, hypercapnia, or elevated hydrogen ion concentration resulting in increases in blood pressure,

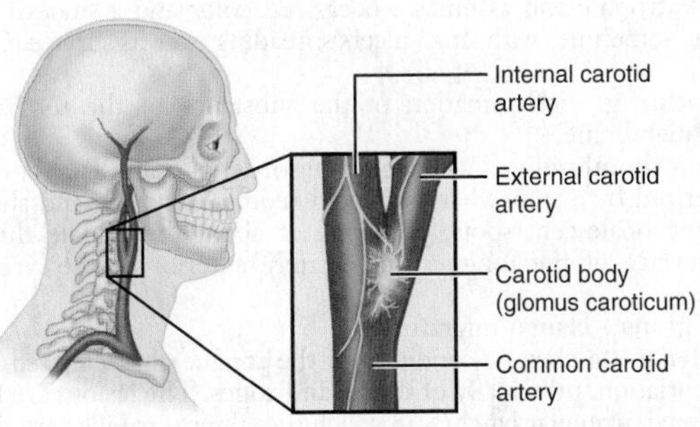

■ Glomus caroticum (carotid body), located deep to the carotid bifurcation and innervated by a plexus of glossopharyngeal, vagal, and sympathetic components.

cardiac rate, and respiratory movements. Another function may be as an endocrine gland.

g. choroi′deum [TA] choroidal enlargement: an enlargement of the choroid plexus in the atrium of the lateral ventricle, where the body, temporal horn, and posterior horn of the lateral ventricle converge.

g. coccy′geum [TA] coccygeal body: an oval structure consisting of irregular masses of spherical or polyhedral epithelioid cells grouped around a dilated, sinusoidal capillary vessel, occurring anterior to, or immediately inferior to, the apex of the coccyx, at the termination of the median sacral vessels. Called also *coccygeal gland, corpus coccygeum,* and *Luschka body* or *gland.*

jugular g., g. jugula′re tympanic body.

g. tympa′nicum a tympanic body located adjacent to the middle ear. See also *g. tympanicum tumor,* under *tumor.*

g. vaga′le a glomus along the vagus nerve. See also *glomus vagale tumor,* under *tumor.*

glos•sa (glos′ə) [Gr. *glōssa*] the tongue (lingua [TA]). **glos′sal** *adj*

glos•sa•gra (glos-ag′rə) [*gloss-* + *-agra*] gouty pain of the tongue.

glos•sal•gia (glos-al′jə) [*gloss-* + *-algia*] pain in the tongue; called also *glossodynia.*

glos•san•thrax (glos-an′thraks) [*gloss-* + *anthrax*] carbuncle of the tongue.

glos•sec•to•my (glos-ek′tə-me) [*gloss-* + *-ectomy*] partial or total surgical excision of the tongue.

Glos•si•na (glŏ-si′nə) the tsetse flies, a genus of biting flies of the family Muscidae. It is divided into three subgenera, *Nemorhina* (*palpalis* or riverine group), *Glossina* (*morsitans* or savannah group), and *Austenina* (*fusca* or forest group). The groups transmit pathogenic trypanosomes by their bites. The *palpalis* group transmits mainly *Trypanosoma brucei gambiense,* causing West African trypanosomiasis; the *morsitans* group transmits mainly *T. brucei rhodesiense,* causing East African trypanosomiasis; and the *fusca* group transmits trypanosomes pathogenic to livestock.

G. fus′cipes a species in the *palpalis* group; its subspecies transmit both West African and East African trypanosomiasis.

G. mor′sitans a South African species that transmits *Trypanosoma brucei,* the cause of nagana in domestic animals, and *T. rhodesiense,* the cause of East African trypanosomiasis in humans.

G. palli′dipes a species that transmits *Trypanosoma brucei,* the cause of nagana in domestic animals.

G. palpa′lis a Central African species that transmits *Trypanosoma gambiense* to cause West African trypanosomiasis.

G. swynnerto′ni a species in the *morsitans* group that transmits East African trypanosomiasis.

G. tachinoi′des a species in the *palpalis* group that transmits both West African and East African trypanosomiasis.

glos•si•tis (glos-i′tis) [*gloss-* + *-itis*] inflammation of the tongue.

g. area′ta exfoliati′va benign migratory g.

atrophic g. Hunter g.

benign migratory g. a condition of the tongue, of unknown etiology, characterized by annular areas of desquamation of the filiform papillae on the dorsal surface of the tongue, usually presenting pinkish-red central lesions outlined by thin, yellowish lines or bands that change patterns and shift location every few days. Called also *g. areata exfoliativa, g. migrans, erythema areata migrans, erythema migrans,* and *geographic tongue.*

herpetic geometric g. painful longitudinal, crossed, or branched fissures on the dorsum of the tongue, occurring as a manifestation of herpes simplex virus type 1 infection in immunocompromised patients.

Hunter g. a chronic condition of the tongue seen in pernicious anemia, characterized by glossitis, glossodynia, glossopyrosis, and altered sense of taste; the pain and burning sensation are usually confined to the tongue but may also extend to other parts of the oral mucosa. Ultimately, the tongue becomes atrophic and assumes a beefy red color and a smooth shiny appearance, sometimes with small ulcers spreading over its surface. Called also *atrophic g.*

idiopathic g. inflammation of the substance of the tongue and its mucous membrane.

median rhomboid g. a congenital disorder of noninflammatory origin, characterized by a somewhat rhomboid reddish, smooth, and shiny lesion with some opalescent spots, occurring at about the middle third of the dorsal surface of the tongue, immediately anterior to the circumvallate papillae.

g. mi′grans benign migratory g.

Moeller g. a chronic condition of the tongue characterized by superficial excoriation, principally of the tip and edges. The lesions are beefy red, well-defined, irregular patches, in which the filiform papillae are thinned or absent and the fungiform papillae are swollen. Called also *bald tongue* and *glossodynia exfoliativa.*

g. rhomboi′dea media′na median rhomboid g.

gloss(o)- [Gr. *glōssa* tongue] a combining form denoting relationship to the tongue.

glos·so·cele (glos′o-sēl) [*glosso-* + *-cele*[1]] swelling and protrusion of the tongue.

glos·so·cin·es·thet·ic (glos″o-sin-əs-thet′ik) glossokinesthetic.

glos·soc·o·ma (glos-ok′o-mə) retraction of the tongue.

glos·so·dy·na·mom·e·ter (glos″o-di″nə-mom′ə-tər) [*glosso-* + *dynamometer*] an instrument for recording the power of the tongue to resist pressure.

glos·so·dyn·ia (glos″o-din′e-ə) [*glosso-* + *-odynia*] glossalgia.

g. exfoliati′va Moeller glossitis.

psychogenic g. glossopyrosis.

glos·so·epi·glot·tic (glos″o-ep-ĭ-glot′ik) glossoepiglottidean.

glos·so·epi·glot·tid·e·an (glos″o-ep-ĭ-glŏ-tid′e-ən) pertaining to the tongue and epiglottis.

glos·so·graph (glos′o-graf) [*glosso-* + *-graph*] an apparatus for recording the tongue movements in speech.

glos·so·hy·al (glos″o-hi′əl) [*glosso-* + *hyoid*] pertaining to the tongue and hyoid bone.

glos·so·kin·es·thet·ic (glos″o-kin″əs-thet′ik) [*glosso-* + *kinesthetic*] pertaining to the subjective perception of the movements of the tongue in speech.

glos·so·la·lia (glos″o-la′le-ə) [*glosso-* + *lal-* + *-ia*] speech in unknown or imaginary language, simulating coherent speech, seen in some types of schizophrenia.

glos·sol·o·gy (glos-ol′ə-je) [*glosso-* + *-logy*] the sum of knowledge regarding the tongue.

glos·so·man·tia (glos″o-man-ti′ə) [*glosso-* + Gr. *manteia* divination] prognosis based on the appearance of the tongue.

glos·son·cus (glos-ong′kəs) [*glosso-* + Gr. *onkos* mass] a swelling of the tongue.

glos·so·pal·a·tine (glos″o-pal′ə-tīn) palatoglossal.

glos·so·pal·a·ti·nus (glos″o-pal″ə-ti′nəs) musculus palatoglossus.

glos·sop·a·thy (glos-op′ə-the) [*glosso-* + *-pathy*] any disease of the tongue.

glos·so·pexy (glos″o-pek′se) lip-tongue adhesion.

glos·so·pha·ryn·ge·al (glos″o-fə-rin′je-əl) [*glosso-* + *pharynx*] pertaining to the tongue and pharynx.

glos·so·pha·ryn·ge·us (glos″o-fə-rin′je-əs) [L.] 1. pertaining to the tongue and pharynx. 2. musculus glossopharyngeus; see *pars glossopharyngea musculi constrictoris pharyngis superioris.*

glos·so·pho·bia (glos″o-fo′be-ə) [*glosso-* + *-phobia*] lalophobia.

glos·so·phyt·ia (glos″o-fit′e-ə) black hairy tongue.

glos·so·plas·ty (glos′o-plas″te) [*glosso-* + *-plasty*] plastic surgery of the tongue. **glossoplas′tic** *adj*

glos·sop·to·sis (glos″op-to′sis, glos″o-to′sis) [*glosso-* + *-ptosis*] downward displacement or retraction of the tongue.

glos·so·py·ro·sis (glos″o-pi-ro′sis) [*glosso-* + Gr. *pyrōsis* burning] a form of paresthesia characterized by pain, burning, itching, and stinging of the mucous membranes of the tongue without apparent lesions of the affected areas. Called also *burning tongue.*

glos·sor·rha·phy (glos-or′ə-fe) [*glosso-* + *-rrhaphy*] suture of the tongue.

glos·sos·co·py (glos-os′kə-pe) [*glosso-* + *-scopy*] examination of the tongue.

glos·so·spasm (glos′o-spaz″əm) [*glosso-* + *spasm*] spasm of the tongue muscles.

glos·so·ster·e·sis (glos″o-stə-re′sis) glossectomy.

glos·sot·o·my (glos-ot′ə-me) [*glosso-* + *-tomy*] incision of the tongue.

glos·so·trich·ia (glos″o-trik′e-ə) [*glosso-* + *trich-* + *-ia*] hairy tongue.

glot·tis (glot′is) pl. *glot′tides* [Gr. *glōttis*] [TA] the vocal apparatus of the larynx, consisting of the true vocal cords (plicae vocales) and the opening between them (rima glottidis). **glot′tal, glot′tic** *adj*

false g. rima vestibuli.

intercartilaginous g., g. respirato′rius, respiratory g. pars intercartilaginea rimae glottidis.

true g. rima glottidis.

g. voca′lis pars intermembranacea rimae glottidis.

glot·tog·ra·phy (glŏ-tog′rə-fe) the recording of the movements of the vocal cords during respiration and phonation, usually measured as electrical potentials generated with movement.

glot·tol·o·gy (glot-ol′ə-je) glossology.

glox·a·zone (glok′sə-zōn) an anaplasmodastat used in cattle.

GLP glucagon-like peptide.

Glu glutamic acid.

Glu·ca·Gen (gloo′kə-jən) trademark for a preparation of glucagon (recombinant).

glu·ca·gon (gloo′kə-gon) 1. a polypeptide hormone secreted by the alpha cells of the islets of Langerhans in response to hypoglycemia or the presence of acetylcholine, certain amino acids, or growth hormone. It stimulates glycogenolysis in the liver by activating liver phosphorylase, promotes gluconeogenesis and ketogenesis, and stimulates the release of insulin by the pancreatic islets. Formerly called *hyperglycemic-glycogenolytic factor.* 2. [USP] a preparation of this hormone obtained from the organs of slaughtered food animals; used in the treatment of severe hypoglycemia, administered intramuscularly, intravenously, or subcutaneously. Because it decreases gastrointestinal motility, it is also used as an adjunct in gastrointestinal radiography. 3. g. (recombinant).

gut g. enteroglucagon.

g. (recombinant) a form of recombinant DNA origin, having the same actions and uses as that of animal origin.

glu·ca·gon·o·ma (gloo″kə-gon-o′mə) a type of islet cell tumor of the alpha cells that secretes glucagon; some are malignant. See also *glucagonoma syndrome,* under *syndrome.*

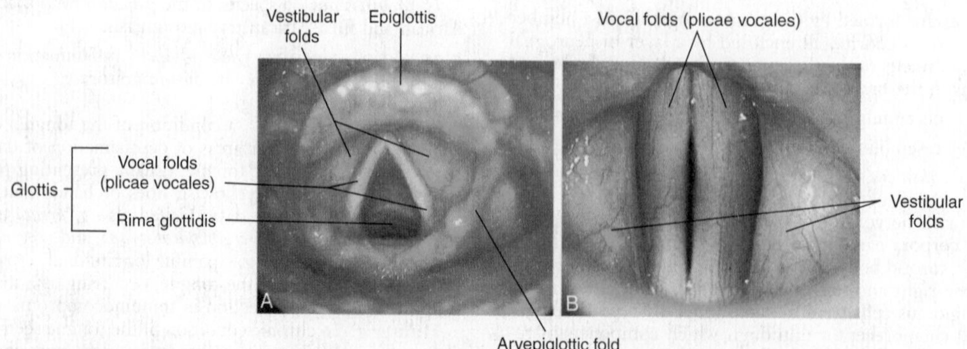

■ Glottis, comprising the vocal folds (cords) and rima glottidis, seen in a laryngoscopic view of the larynx. *(A),* Open during inspiration; *(B),* closed during expiration.

glu•cal (gloo′kal) a glycal of glucose.

glu•can (gloo′kan) any polysaccharide (e.g., glycogen, starch, and cellulose) composed only of recurring units of glucose; a homopolymer of glucose.

1,4-α-glu•can branch•ing en•zyme (gloo′kan branch′ing en′zīm) [EC 2.4.1.18] an enzyme of the transferase class that catalyzes the cleavage of internal α-1,4-glucoside linkages in glycogen (or, in plants, amylopectin) and transfer of the fragments into α-1,6 linkages, thus creating branches in the glycogen molecule. Deficiency of the enzyme, an autosomal recessive trait, results in glycogen storage disease, type IV. Called also *brancher* or *branching enzyme.*

glu•can 1,4-α-glu•co•si•dase (gloo′kan gloo-ko′sĭ-dās) [EC 3.2.1.3] a lysosomal enzyme of the hydrolase class that catalyzes the cleavage of glucose residues from polyglucoside chains by hydrolyzing terminal α-1,4 or α-1,6 bonds; the enzyme degrades glycogen to glucose in the lysosomes. Deficiency or absence of enzyme activity, an autosomal recessive trait, results in glycogen storage disease, type II. Called also *acid maltase* and *lysosomal α-glucosidase.*

glu•can trans•fer•ase (gloo′kan trans′fər-ās) an enzyme transferring glucosyl chains in glucans from one site to another, usually with specific conformations of donor and acceptor sites; see *oligo-1,4,-1,4-glucantransferase* and *1,4-α-glucan branching enzyme.*

glu•car•ic ac•id (gloo-kar′ik) the aldaric acid resulting from oxidation of glucose.

glu•cep•tate (gloo-sep′tāt) USAN contraction for *glucoheptonate.* See also table at *technetium.*

glu•ci•tol (gloo′sĭ-tol) sorbitol.

gluc(o)- [Gr. *glykys* sweet] a combining form denoting relationship to sweetness, or to glucose. Cf. *glyc(o)-.*

glu•co•am•y•lase (gloo″ko-am′ə-lās) glucan 1,4-α-glucosidase.

glu•co•ascor•bic ac•id (gloo″ko-ə-skor′bik) a seven-carbon homologue of ascorbic acid having no vitamin C activity.

Glu•co•bay (gloo′ko-ba) trademark for a preparation of acarbose.

glu•co•cer•e•bro•si•dase (gloo″ko-sə-re″bro-si′dās) glucosylceramidase.

glu•co•cer•e•bro•side (gloo″ko-sə-re′bro-sīd″) any of the cerebrosides whose monosaccharide head group is glucose; they occur mostly in nonneuronal tissue and accumulate abnormally in Gaucher disease. Called also *glucosylceramide.*

glu•co•cin•in (gloo″ko-sin′in) glucokinin.

glu•co•cor•ti•coid (gloo″ko-kor′tĭ-koid) 1. any of the corticosteroids (steroids produced by the adrenal cortex) that regulate carbohydrate, lipid, and protein metabolism and inhibit the release of corticotropin. They also affect muscle tone and the microcirculation, participate in the maintenance of arterial blood pressure, increase gastric secretion, alter connective tissue response to injury, impede cartilage production, inhibit inflammatory, allergic, and immune responses, invoke shrinkage of lymphatic tissue, reduce the number of circulating lymphocytes, and affect the functions of the central nervous system. Some exert varying degrees of mineralocorticoid activity. In humans the most important ones are cortisol, cortisone, and corticosterone. Cf. *mineralocorticoid.* 2. of, pertaining to, having the properties or effects of, or resembling one of these substances.

glu•co•fu•ra•nose (gloo″ko-fu′rə-nōs) glucose occurring in the cyclic furanose configuration; it is a minor constituent of glucose solutions.

glu•co•gen•e•sis (gloo″ko-jen′ə-sis) [*gluco-* + *-genesis*] the formation of glucose from any of the products of glycolysis.

glu•co•gen•ic (gloo″ko-jen′ik) [*gluco-* + *-genic*] giving rise to or producing glucose.

glu•co•hep•to•nate (GHA) (gloo″ko-hep′tə-nāt) a seven-carbon carbohydrate derivative; complexed with technetium 99m, it is used in renal and brain imaging and in dynamic renal and cerebral perfusion studies. See table at *technetium.* Called also *gluceptate* (USAN contraction).

glu•co•ki•nase (gloo″ko-ki′nās) 1. [EC 2.7.1.2] an enzyme of the transferase class that catalyzes the phosphorylation of D-glucose at the 6 carbon. The enzyme is found in invertebrates and microorganisms and is highly specific for glucose. 2. hexokinase, type IV (liver).

glu•co•ki•net•ic (gloo″ko-kĭ-net′ik) activating sugar so as to maintain the sugar level of the blood.

glu•co•kin•in (gloo″ko-kin′in) [*gluco-* + Gr. *kinein* to move] a hormonelike substance obtained from vegetable tissues and yeast, subcutaneous injection of which produces hypoglycemia in animals and acts on depancreatized dogs in a manner similar to that of insulin.

glu•col•y•sis (gloo-kol′ə-sis) glycolysis.

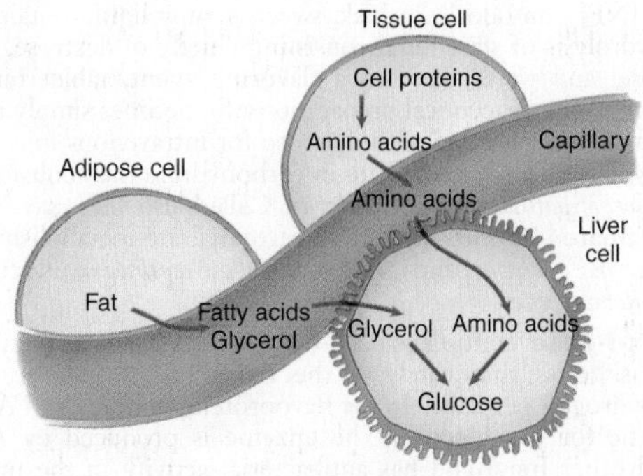

■ Gluconeogenesis.

glu•co•nate (gloo′ko-nāt) a salt, ester, or anionic form of gluconic acid.

glu•co•neo•gen•e•sis (gloo″ko-ne″o-jen′ə-sis) [*gluco-* + *neo-* + *-genesis*] the formation of glucose from molecules that are not themselves carbohydrates, as from amino acids, lactate, and the glycerol portion of fats. Called also *glyconeogenesis.* **gluconeogenet′ic** *adj*

glu•con•ic ac•id (gloo-kon′ik) the hexonic acid derived from glucose by oxidation of the aldehyde group at C-1 to a carboxyl group.

glu•co•no•lac•tone (gloo″kon-o-lak′tōn) [USP] glucono delta-lactone; a chelating agent produced by the oxidation of glucose, used as a moisturizer in preparations applied topically to the skin.

glu•co•pe•nia (gloo-ko-pe′ne-ə) deficiency of sugar in the tissues; called also *glycopenia.* **glucope′nic** *adj*

Glu•co•phage (gloo′ko-fāj″) trademark for preparations of metformin hydrochloride.

glu•co•phore (gloo′ko-for) [*gluco-* + *phore*] the group of atoms in a molecule of a compound that is responsible for its sweet taste.

glu•co•priv•ic (gloo″ko-priv′ik) glucopenic.

glu•co•pro•tein (gloo″ko-pro′tēn) glycoprotein.

glu•co•py•ra•nose (gloo″ko-pir′ə-nōs) glucose occurring in the cyclic pyranose configuration; it is the major form in glucose solutions, polysaccharides, and glucosides.

glu•co•reg•u•la•tion (gloo″ko-reg″u-la′shən) regulation of glucose metabolism.

glu•co•sa•mine (gloo-kōs′ə-mēn) the amino sugar derivative of glucose, substituted at the 2 position, occurring in glycosaminoglycans and a variety of complex polysaccharides such as blood group substances. It is generally acetylated (*N*-acetylglucosamine).

g. sulfate the sulfate salt of glucosamine, prepared artificially as a nutritional supplement and as a popular remedy for osteoarthritis.

glu•co•sa•mine-phos•phate *N*-ac•e•tyl•trans•fer•ase (gloo-kōs′ə-mēn fos′fāt as″ə-tēl-trans′fər-ās) [EC 2.3.1.4] an enzyme of the transferase class that catalyzes the transfer of an acetyl group from acetyl coenzyme A to glucosamine 6-phosphate to form *N*-acetylglucosamine 6-phosphate, a step in the synthesis of UDP-*N*-acetylglucosamine.

glu•co•san (gloo′ko-san) glucan.

glu•co•sa•zone (gloo-ko′sə-zōn) the osazone formed from glucose by reaction with phenylhydrazine; it is a yellow crystalline substance that has been used to identify glucose. It is chemically identical to fructosazone and mannosazone.

Glu•co•scan (gloo′ko-skan″) trademark for a kit for the preparation of technetium Tc 99m gluceptate.

glu•cose (gloo′kōs) [Gr. *gleukos* sweetness] 1. an aldohexose, $C_6H_{12}O_6$, occurring naturally as the D- form and found as a free monosaccharide in fruits and other plants and in the normal blood of all animals; it also is combined in glucosides and di-, oligo-, and polysaccharides. It is the end product of carbohydrate metabolism and is the chief source of energy for living organisms, its utilization being controlled by insulin. Excess glucose is converted to glycogen and stored in the liver and muscles for use as needed and, beyond that, is converted to fat and stored as adipose tissue. See also *hyperglycemia* and *hypoglycemia.* In pharmaceuticals it is called *dextrose.* 2. liquid g.

Brun g. a histologic clearing solution composed of glucose, distilled water, camphor, and glycerin.

fasting blood g. (FBG), fasting plasma g. (FPG) a measurement of the concentration of glucose in the plasma after the patient has not eaten for at least 8 hours; see also *oral glucose tolerance test.* Called also *fasting blood sugar.*

liquid g. [NF] an odorless, thick, sweet, syrupy liquid obtained by incomplete hydrolysis of starch and consisting chiefly of dextrose, with dextrins, maltose, and water; used as a flavoring agent, tablet binder, and coating agent in pharmaceutical preparations. Sometimes simply called *glucose.* It is not interchangeable with dextrose for intravenous injection.

g. 1-phosphate an intermediate in carbohydrate metabolism. See also *Embden-Meyerhof pathway,* under *pathway.* Called also *Cori ester.*

g. 6-phosphate an intermediate in carbohydrate metabolism. See also *Embden-Meyerhof pathway* and *pentose phosphate pathway,* under *pathway.* Called also *Robison ester.*

glu•cose ox•i•dase (gloo′kōs ok′sĭ-dās) [EC 1.1.3.4] an enzyme of the oxidoreductase class that catalyzes the oxidation of glucose, reducing oxygen to hydrogen peroxide. It is a flavoprotein, containing FAD, and is highly specific for β-D-glucose. The enzyme is produced by *Penicillium notatum* and other fungi and has antibacterial activity in the presence of glucose and oxygen because of the hydrogen peroxide produced. It is used to estimate glucose concentration in blood or urine samples through the formation of colored dyes by the hydrogen peroxide.

glu•cose-6-phos•pha•tase (gloo″kōs fos′fə-tās″) [EC 3.1.3.9] an enzyme of the hydrolase class that catalyzes the dephosphorylation of glucose 6-phosphate. It occurs in the endoplasmic reticulum of liver, kidney, and intestinal mucosa, but not of muscle, and its reaction is the principal route for hepatic gluconeogenesis, controlling blood glucose concentrations. Deficiency of the enzyme, an autosomal recessive trait, results in glycogen storage disease, type I.

glu•cose-6-phos•phate de•hy•dro•gen•ase (G6PD) (gloo′kōs fos′fāt de-hi′dro-jən-ās) [EC 1.1.1.49] an enzyme of the oxidoreductase class that catalyzes the oxidation of glucose-6-phosphate to a lactone, reducing $NADP^+$ to NADPH. The reaction is the first step in the pentose phosphate pathway of glucose metabolism. Genetic deficiency of the enzyme causes severe hemolytic crises in affected individuals. In EC nomenclature, called *glucose-6-phosphate 1-dehydrogenase.*

glu•cose-6-phos•phate de•hy•dro•gen•ase de•fi•cien•cy (gloo′kōs fos′fāt de-hi′dro-jən-ās) the most common inborn error of metabolism, an X-linked enzyme deficiency causing varying degrees of hemolytic anemia in many millions of people around the world. It can cause favism, some drug-induced hemolytic anemias, or chronic nonspherocytic hemolytic anemia. The G6PD gene is highly polymorphic, with about 400 variants known.

glu•cose-6-phos•phate isom•er•ase (gloo′kos fos′fāt i-som′ər-ās) [EC 5.3.1.9] an enzyme of the isomerase class that catalyzes the interconversion glucose 6-phosphate = fructose 6-phosphate. The forward reaction is a step in the Embden-Meyerhof pathway (see illustration under *pathway*), and the reverse is a step in gluconeogenesis. Deficiency of the enzyme, an autosomal recessive trait, results in hemolytic anemia. Called also *phosphoglucose isomerase.* The enzyme also has the effect of promoting motility and metastasis in cancer cells, and is increased in certain types of cancer; in that case it has been called *autocrine motility factor.*

glu•cose 6-phos•phate trans•lo•case (gloo′kōs fos′fāt trans-lo′kās) a transport system occurring in the endoplasmic reticulum of liver, kidney, and intestinal mucosa cells; it transports glucose 6-phosphate into the endoplasmic reticulum, where glucose-6-phosphatase is located. Deficiency of this system results in glycogen storage disease, type IB.

α-glu•co•si•dase (gloo-ko′sĭ-dās) [EC 3.2.1.20] any of a group of enzymes that catalyzes the hydrolysis of terminal, nonreducing 1,4-linked α-D-glucose residues, primarily in oligosaccharides but also in polysaccharides, with release of α-D-glucose. Called also *maltase.*

lysosomal α-g. glucan 1,4-α-glucosidase.

α-1,4-glu•co•si•dase (gloo-ko′sĭ-dās) 1. glucan 1,4-α-glucosidase. 2. more generally, any enzyme able to cleave α-1,4-glucosidic linkages (e.g., α-glucosidase).

α-1,4-glu•co•si•dase de•fi•cien•cy (gloo-ko′sĭ-dās) glycogen storage disease, type II.

β-glu•co•si•dase (gloo-ko′sĭ-dās) [EC 3.2.1.21] any of a group of enzymes of the hydrolase class that catalyze the hydrolysis of terminal, nonreducing, β-linked glucose residues from glycosides.

glu•co•side (gloo′ko-sīd) a glycoside in which the sugar constituent is glucose; originally the term glucoside was given to any of a variety of natural plant products containing a sugar, but it is now generally restricted to those in which the sugar is glucose. See *glycoside.*

glu•co•si•do•lyt•ic (gloo″ko-si″do-lit′ik) causing the splitting up of glucosides.

glu•cos•u•ria (gloo″ko-su′re-ə) glycosuria.

glu•co•syl (gloo′ko-səl) a glucose radical.

glu•co•syl•cer•am•i•dase (gloo″ko-səl-sə-ram′ĭ-dās) [EC 3.2.1.45] an enzyme of the hydrolase class that catalyzes the hydrolytic cleavage of glucose from glucocerebrosides to form ceramides, a reaction occurring in the lysosomal degradation of sphingolipids. Deficiency of enzyme activity, an autosomal recessive trait, results in Gaucher disease. Called also *glucocerebrosidase.*

glu•co•syl•cer•a•mide (gloo-kos″əl-ser′ə-mīd) glucocerebroside.

glu•co•syl•trans•fer•ase (gloo″ko-səl-trans′fər-as) a term used in the trivial and recommended names of some hexosyltransferases [EC 2.4.1] that catalyze the transfer of a glucosyl group from a donor to an acceptor compound. Called also *transglucosylase.*

glu•co•tox•ic•i•ty (gloo″ko-tok-sis′ĭ-te) the toxic effects of long-term hyperglycemia, as in diabetes mellitus (q.v.). Called also *glucose toxicity.*

Glu•co•trol (gloo′ko-trōl″) trademark for preparations of glipizide.

Glu•co•vance (gloo′ko-vans″) trademark for a combination preparation of glyburide and metformin hydrochloride.

glu•cu•ro•nate (gloo-ku′ro-nāt) a salt, ester, or anionic form of glucuronic acid.

glu•cu•ron•ic ac•id (gloo″ku-ron′ik) the uronic acid derived from glucose; it is a constituent of several glycosaminoglycans and also forms conjugates (glucuronides) with drugs and toxins in their biotransformation.

β-glu•cu•ron•i•dase (gloo″ku-ron′ĭ-dās) [EC 3.2.1.31] a lysosomal enzyme of the hydrolase class that catalyzes cleavage of terminal glucuronic acid residues from a variety of β-glucuronides. It is important for the degradation of a variety of glycosaminoglycans, including dermatan sulfate, heparan sulfate, and the chondroitin sulfates. Deficiency of the enzyme, an autosomal recessive trait, results in Sly syndrome (mucopolysaccharidosis VII).

glu•cu•ron•ide (gloo″ku-ron′īd) a glycoside of glucuronic acid; glucuronides are common soluble conjugates formed as a step in the metabolism and excretion of many toxins and drugs, such as phenols and alcohols.

glu•cu•ron•o•syl•trans•fer•ase (gloo″ku-ron″o-səl-trans′fər-ās) [EC 2.4.1.17] an enzyme of the transferase class that catalyzes the transfer of a glucuronate moiety from UDP-glucuronate to an acceptor to form a glucuronide conjugate. The reaction occurs with a wide range of substrates and is important in the conversion of bilirubin to its more soluble glucuronide conjugates, which are then secreted into the bile. Deficiency of the enzyme, an autosomal recessive trait, results in Crigler-Najjar syndrome.

glu•cu•ron•yl trans•fer•ase (gloo″ku′ron-əl trans′fər-ās) a less accurate term for *glucuronosyltransferase.*

glue (gloo) a preparation used to adhere or bond substances together.

fibrin g. a mixture of fibrin, factor XIII, and other clotting components, used to bring about hemostasis in a wound during surgery. Called also *fibrin sealant.*

tissue g. glue used instead of sutures or staples to repair dissected tissue.

Glu•gea (gloo′je-ə) a genus of intracellular protozoa (suborder Apansporoblastina, order Microsporida) parasitic in fishes.

glu•ta•mate (gloo′tə-māt) a salt, ester, or anionic form of glutamic acid; glutamate is the principal excitatory neurotransmitter in the central nervous system.

g.-γ-semialdehyde glutamic-γ-semialdehyde.

glu•ta•mate–am•mo•nia li•gase (gloo′tə-māt ə-mōn′yə li′gās) [EC 6.3.1.2] an enzyme of the ligase class that catalyzes the ATP-dependent amination of glutamate by ammonium ions to form glutamine. Called also *glutamine synthetase.*

glu•ta•mate–cys•te•ine li•gase (gloo′tə-māt sis′te-ēn li′gās) [EC 6.3.2.2] an enzyme of the ligase class that catalyzes the ATP-dependent formation of a peptide bond between the γ-carboxyl group of glutamate and the amino group of cysteine to form γ-glutamylcysteine as a step in the synthesis of glutathione.

glu•ta•mate de•car•box•y•lase (gloo′tə-māt de-kahr-bok′sə-lās) [EC 4.1.1.15] an enzyme of the lyase class that catalyzes the decarboxylation of glutamate to form γ-aminobutyrate (GABA). The enzyme is a pyridoxal phosphate protein, and the reaction occurs within the mitochondria in kidney, and outside the mitochondria in brain. Deficiency of the brain enzyme may be the cause of convulsions that begin in infancy and are responsive to pyridoxine therapy. Called also *glutamic acid decarboxylase.*

glu•ta•mate de•hy•dro•gen•ase [NAD(P)⁺] (gloo′tə-māt de-hi′dro-jən-ās) [EC 1.4.1.3] an enzyme of the oxidoreductase class that catalyzes the oxidative deamination of glutamate to form α-ketoglutarate, using either NAD^+ or $NADP^+$ as an electron acceptor. The reversible reaction has a major function in both synthesis and degradation of glutamic acid and, via transaminases, other amino acids as well.

glu•ta•ma•ter•gic (gloo″tə-ma-tur′jik) 1. activated or transmitted by glutamate. 2. pertaining to neurons that release glutamate.

glu•ta•mate for•mim•i•no•trans•fer•ase (gloo′tə-māt for-mim″ĭ-no-trans′fər-ās) [EC 2.1.2.5] an enzyme of the transferase class that catalyzes the transfer of a formimino group from formiminoglutamate to tetrahydrofolate, forming 5-formiminotetrahydrofolate. The reaction is a step in the degradation of histidine. The enzyme is bifunctional; it also contains a catalytic site with formiminotetrahydrofolate cyclodeaminase (q.v.) activity. Urinary excretion of formiminoglutamate and mental retardation have been associated with decreased enzyme activity, resulting from either a genetic disorder or a deficiency of tetrahydrofolate. Called also *formiminotransferase.*

glu·tam·ic ac·id (gloo-tam′ik) a nonessential amino acid, α-aminoglutaric acid, occurring in proteins. It also serves as an excitatory neurotransmitter in all regions of the central nervous system. Symbols Glu and E. See also table at *amino acid.*

g. a. hydrochloride a compound used as a gastric acidifier in replacement therapy for achlorhydria and hypochlorhydria.

glu·tam·ic ac·id de·car·box·y·lase (GAD) (gloo-tam′ik as′id de-kahr-bok′sĭ-lās) glutamate decarboxylase.

glu·tam·ic-ox·a·lo·ace·tic trans·am·i·nase (GOT) (gloo-tam′ik oks″ə-lo-ə-se′tik trans-am′ĭ-nās) aspartate transaminase.

glu·tam·ic-py·ru·vic trans·am·i·nase (GPT) (gloo-tam′ik pi-roo′vik trans-am′ĭ-nās) alanine transaminase.

glu·tam·i·nase (gloo-tam′ĭ-nās) [EC 3.5.1.2] an enzyme of the hydrolase class that catalyzes the deamination of glutamine to form glutamate and ammonium ions; most of the latter are converted to urea via the urea cycle.

glu·ta·mine (gloo′tə-mēn) [USP] the monoamide of glutamic acid, a nonessential amino acid occurring in the juices of many plants and in some animal tissues; it is an important carrier of urinary ammonia and is broken down in the kidney by the enzyme glutaminase. Symbols Gln and Q. See also table at *amino acid.*

glu·ta·mine syn·the·tase (gloo′tə-mēn sin′thə-tās) glutamate–ammonia ligase.

glu·tam·i·nyl (gloo-tam′ĭ-nəl) the acyl radical of glutamine.

glu·ta·myl (gloo′tə-məl) the acyl radical of glutamic acid.

γ-glu·ta·myl·cy·clo·trans·fer·ase (gloo″tə-məl-si″klo-trans′fər-ās) [EC 2.3.2.4] an enzyme of the transferase class that catalyzes the hydrolytic cyclization of glutamyl–amino acid to form 5-oxoproline and a free amino acid. The reaction is part of the γ-glutamyl cycle for transporting amino acids across the plasma membrane.

γ-glu·ta·myl·cys·te·ine (gloo″tə-məl-sis′te-ēn) glutamate linked via its γ-carboxyl group to the amino group of cysteine; it is an intermediate in the synthesis of glutathione.

γ-glu·ta·myl·cys·te·ine syn·the·tase (gloo″tə-məl-sis′te-ēn sin′thə-tās) glutamate-cysteine ligase.

γ-glu·ta·myl·cys·te·ine syn·the·tase de·fi·cien·cy (gloo″tə-məl-sis′te-ēn sin′thə-tās) an autosomal recessive aminoacidopathy of glutathione synthesis caused by mutation in the *GCLC* gene (locus: 6p12), which encodes glutamate-cysteine ligase (γ-glutamylcysteine synthetase), characterized by hemolytic anemia, spinocerebellar degeneration, peripheral neuropathy, myopathy, and aminoaciduria.

γ-glu·ta·myl·trans·fer·ase (GGT) (gloo″tə-məl-trans′fər-ās) [EC 2.3.2.2] an enzyme of the transferase class that catalyzes the transfer of the γ-glutamyl group from glutathione to an amino acid to form a glutamyl–amino acid and the dipeptide cysteinyl-glycine. The enzyme occurs on the outside of the plasma membrane, primarily in cells of the kidney and other sites involved in transport; the glutamyl–amino acids formed can cross the membrane and enter the cell as part of the glutamyl cycle. Deficiency of the enzyme, an autosomal recessive trait, results in γ-glutamyl transpeptidase deficiency.

γ-glu·ta·myl trans·pep·ti·dase (gloo′tə-məl trans-pep′tĭ-dās) γ-glutamyltransferase.

γ-glu·ta·myl trans·pep·ti·dase de·fi·cien·cy (gloo′tə-məl trans-pep′tĭ-dās) an autosomal recessive aminoacidopathy of glutathione synthesis, caused by mutation in the *GGT1* gene (locus: 22q11.2), a member of the gamma-glutamyltransferase gene family. It is characterized by mental retardation, behavioral disorders, glutathionemia, and urinary excretion of glutathione, γ-glutamylcysteine, and cysteine. Called also *glutathionuria.*

glu·ta·ral (gloo′tə-rəl) glutaraldehyde.

g. concentrate [USP] a solution of glutaraldehyde in purified water, used as a disinfectant.

glu·ta·ral·de·hyde (gloo″tə-ral′də-hīd) a disinfectant, $C_5H_8O_2$, effective against vegetative gram-positive, gram-negative, and acid-fast bacteria, bacterial spores, some fungi, and viruses; used in an aqueous solution for sterilization of endoscopic equipment, thermometers, and plastic, rubber, or other non–heat-resistant equipment. Glutaraldehyde is also used as a tissue fixative for light and electron microscopy because of its preservation of fine structural detail and localization of enzyme activity. Called also *glutaral.*

glu·tar·ic ac·id (gloo-tar′ik) a dicarboxylic acid occurring at high levels in the blood and urine in glutaricaciduria.

glu·tar·ic·ac·i·de·mia (gloo-tar″ik-as″ĭ-de′me-ə) 1. glutaricaciduria (def. 1). 2. an excess of glutaric acid in the blood.

glu·tar·ic·ac·id·uria (gloo-tar″ik-as″ĭ-du′re-ə) 1. a genetically and clinically heterogeneous, autosomal recessive aminoacidopathy characterized by accumulation and excretion of glutaric acid in the urine. 2. excretion of glutaric acid in the urine.

g. type I a disorder caused by mutation in the *GCDH* gene (locus: 19p13.2), resulting in a deficiency of glutaryl-CoA dehydrogenase; 3-hydroxyglutaric acid is excreted in addition to glutaric acid, and there are progressive dystonia and dyskinesia, hypoglycemia, mild ketosis and acidosis, opisthotonus, choreoathetosis, seizures, motor delay, hypotonia, and death within the first decade of life.

g. type II a genetically heterogeneous disorder due to deficiencies in the electron transport system, characterized by accumulation and excretion of glutaric and 2-hydroxyglutaric acids as well as multiple organic acids normally oxidized by mitochondrial flavin-containing acyl-CoA dehydrogenases, which require both proteins for activity. It is caused by defects in any of three proteins: the α- or the β- subunit of electron transfer flavoprotein or electron transfer flavoprotein:ubiquinone oxidoreductase. There are three subtypes, designated A, B, and C, based on the genetic defect involved. Additional manifestations include hypoglycemia without ketosis, metabolic acidosis, and a spectrum of phenotypic manifestations varying in severity, which is inversely correlated with increasing age of onset. When of neonatal onset it may be accompanied by congenital anomalies and is rapidly fatal. Called also *multiple acyl CoA dehydrogenation deficiency.*

g. type III a rare, generally benign metabolic abnormality caused by mutation in the *C7ORF10* gene (locus: 7p14), characterized by urinary excretion of glutaric acid, with no consistent clinical phenotype; it may result from impaired peroxisomal metabolism.

glu·ta·ryl (gloo′tə-rəl) the divalent radical of glutaric acid; as glutaryl CoA, a thioester formed with coenzyme A, it is an intermediate in the catabolism of lysine, hydroxylysine, and tryptophan.

glu·ta·ryl-CoA de·hy·dro·gen·ase (gloo′tə-rəl ko-a′ de-hi′dro-jən-ās) [EC 1.3.99.7] an enzyme of the oxidoreductase class that catalyzes the oxidative decarboxylation of glutaryl CoA, with sequential reduction of FAD and then electron transfer flavoprotein; the reaction is a step in the degradation of lysine, hydroxylysine, and tryptophan. Deficiency of the enzyme, an autosomal recessive trait, causes glutaricaciduria, type I.

glu·ta·thi·one (gloo″tə-thi′ōn) a tripeptide, γ-glutamyl-cysteinyl-glycine, that is widely distributed in animal and plant tissues; it exists in both the reduced thiol form (GSH) and the oxidized disulfide form (GSSG). It functions in various redox reactions, such as the destruction of peroxides and free radicals, the detoxification of harmful compounds, and activity as a cofactor for enzymes. In erythrocytes, these reactions prevent oxidative damage by reduction of methemoglobin and peroxides. Glutathione is also involved in the formation and maintenance of disulfide bonds in proteins and in transport of amino acids across cell membranes.

glu·ta·thi·one-di·sul·fide re·duc·tase (gloo″tə-thi′ōn di-sul′fīd re-duk′tās) [EC 1.6.4.2] an enzyme of the oxidoreductase class that catalyzes the reduction of glutathione via oxidation of NADPH. It is a flavoprotein (FAD), occurring in erythrocytes, and is involved in many redox reactions. Deficiency of enzyme activity in erythrocytes usually results from nutritional or metabolic inadequacy of FAD and, except when severe, has not been linked to hemolysis. Diminished enzyme activity does decrease protection of cells from oxidative damage.

glu·ta·thi·on·emia (gloo″tə-thi″o-ne′me-ə) the presence of glutathione in the blood.

glu·ta·thi·one per·ox·i·dase (gloo″tə-thi′ōn pə-rok′sĭ-dās) [EC 1.11.1.9] an enzyme of the oxidoreductase class that catalyzes the detoxifying reduction of hydrogen peroxide and organic peroxides via oxidation of glutathione. The enzyme requires selenium at the active site; deficiency of enzyme activity may be linked to jaundice and hemolytic anemia in neonates.

glu·ta·thi·one re·duc·tase (NADPH) (gloo″tə-thi′ōn re-duk′tās) glutathione-disulfide reductase.

glu·ta·thi·one syn·thase (gloo″tə-thi′ōn sin′thās) [EC 6.3.2.3] official nomenclature for *glutathione synthetase.*

glu·ta·thi·one syn·the·tase (gloo″tə-thi′ōn sin′thə-tās) an enzyme of the ligase class that catalyzes the ATP-dependent formation of glutathione from glycine and γ-glutamylcysteine. In EC nomenclature, called *glutathione synthase.*

glu·ta·thi·one syn·the·tase de·fi·cien·cy (gloo″tə-thi′ōn sin′thə-tās) an autosomal recessive aminoacidopathy due to mutation in the *GSS* gene (locus: 20q11.2), which encodes glutathione synthetase, resulting in decreased levels of glutathione and altering the γ-glutamyl cycle; γ-glutamylcysteine synthesized futilely is converted to excess 5-oxoproline and cysteine. It occurs in two forms. Deficiency of glutathione synthetase confined to the erythrocytes results in a well-compensated hemolytic anemia; generalized deficiency of the enzyme causes high levels of 5-oxoproline in plasma and urine, metabolic acidosis, and often neurologic dysfunction, along with hemolytic anemia.

glu•ta•thi•on•uria (gloo″tə-thi″on-u′re-ə) 1. the excretion of excessive amounts of glutathione in the urine. 2. γ-glutamyl transpeptidase deficiency.

glu•te•al (gloo′te-əl) [Gr. *gloutos* buttock] pertaining to the buttocks. Called also *natal* and *pygal.*

glu•ten (gloo′tən) [L. "glue"] the protein of wheat and other grains that gives to the dough its tough elastic character.

glu•teo•fem•o•ral (gloo″te-o-fem′or-əl) [*gluteal* + *femoral*] pertaining to the buttock and thigh.

glu•teo•in•gui•nal (gloo″te-o-in′gwĭ-nəl) pertaining to the buttock and groin.

glu•teth•i•mide (gloo-teth′ĭ-mīd) a nonbarbiturate structurally related to phenobarbital, used as a sedative and hypnotic. It is no longer sold legally in the United States, but has been found as a drug of abuse.

glu•ti•nous (gloo′tĭ-nəs) [L. *glutinosus*] sticky; adhesive; gluey; viscid.

glu•ti•tis (gloo-ti′tis) [Gr. *gloutos* buttock + *-itis*] inflammation of the buttock.

Glu•tose (gloo′tōs) trademark for preparations of glucose.

Gly glycine.

gly•bur•ide (gli′būr-īd) [USP] a sulfonylurea compound used as a hypoglycemic in the treatment of type 2 diabetes mellitus; administered orally. Called also *glibenclamide.*

gly•cal (gli′kal) an unsaturated derivative of a monosaccharide, in which a double bond between carbons 1 and 2 replaces their hydroxyl groups.

gly•can (gli′kan) polysaccharide.

gly•cate (gli′kāt) the product of glycation.

gly•ca•tion (gli-ka′shən) a nonenzymatic form of glycosylation in which glucose is incorporated into a protein when the environment has a high concentration of glucose.

gly•ce•mia (gli-se′me-ə) [*glyc-* + *-emia*] the presence of glucose in the blood; see also *hyperglycemia.* Called also *glycosemia.*

gly•ce•mic (gli-se′mik) pertaining to glycemia.

gly•cen•tin (gli-sen′tin) glicentin.

Glyc•e•ra (glis′ə-rə) a family of parasitic nematodes native to temperate regions of North America. *G. dibranchia′ta* has venom-containing fangs, and its bite produces painful swelling with erythema.

glyc•er•al•de•hyde (glis″ər-al′də-hīd) an aldose, the aldehyde form of the triose derived by oxidation of glycerol; it is isomeric with dihydroxyacetone.

g. **3-phosphate** an intermediate in the metabolism of glucose, both in the Embden-Meyerhof pathway (see illustration under *pathway*) and in the pentose phosphate pathway.

glyc•er•al•de•hyde-3-phos•phate de•hy•dro•gen•ase (phos•phor•y•lat•ing) (glis″ər-al′də-hīd fos′fāt de-hi′dro-jən-ās fos-for′ə-lāt′ing) [EC 1.2.1.12] an enzyme of the oxidoreductase class that catalyzes the phosphorylation of glyceraldehyde 3-phosphate, one of two reactions by which high-energy phosphate is generated in the Embden-Meyerhof pathway. Abbreviated GAPD. (See illustration under *pathway.*) Called also *triosephosphate dehydrogenase.*

glyc•er•ate (glis′ər-āt) a salt or ester of glyceric acid.

glyc•er•ate de•hy•dro•gen•ase (glis′ər-āt de-hi′dro-jən-ās) [EC 1.1.1.29] an enzyme of the oxidoreductase class that catalyzes the reduction of hydroxypyruvate to form D-glycerate, using NADH as an electron donor. Deficiency of the enzyme is believed to be a cause of primary hyperoxaluria, type II, and of D-glycericacidemia.

gly•cer•ic ac•id (gli-sēr′ik) a hydroxy acid derived by oxidation of C1 of glycerol or glyceraldehyde to a carboxyl group; various phosphorylated derivatives are important intermediates in glucose metabolism. See also *1,3-* and *2,3-bisphosphoglycerate* and *phosphoglycerate.*

D-gly•cer•ic•ac•i•de•mia (gli-ser″ik-as″ĭ-de′me-ə) an autosomal recessive disorder characterized by an increased concentration of D-glyceric acid in the blood, believed to be due to a defect in glycerate dehydrogenase and characterized by hyperglycinemia without ketosis or acidosis, delayed psychomotor development, mental retardation, and seizures.

L-gly•cer•ic•ac•id•uria (gli-ser″ik-as″ĭd-u′re-ə) primary hyperoxaluria, type II.

glyc•er•i•dase (glis′ər-ĭ-dās) any enzyme that catalyzes the cleavage of a glyceride, such as a lipase.

glyc•er•ide (glis′ər-īd) glycerol esterified with one or more organic acids, particularly with long chain fatty acids. Glycerides are classified as mono-, di-, or triglycerides as a function of the number of such substituents. Called also *acylglycerol.*

glyc•er•in (glis′ər-in) [L. *glycerinum*] [USP] a clear, colorless, syrupy liquid, $C_3H_8O_3$; administered rectally as a laxative, orally as a diuretic to reduce intraocular pressure, and orally as a demulcent in cough preparations. It is also used as a solvent, humectant, and vehicle in various pharmaceutical preparations. See also *glycerol.*

glyc•er•in•at•ed (glis′ər-in-āt″əd) treated with or preserved in glycerin.

glyc•ero•gel (glis′ər-o-jel) a gel in which glycerin is the dispersed medium.

glyc•er•ol (glis′ər-ol) a trihydroxy sugar alcohol that is the backbone of many lipids and an important intermediate in carbohydrate and lipid metabolism. Pharmaceutical preparations are called glycerin (q.v.).

g. **phosphate,** (L-)g. **3-phosphate** an intermediate in the glycerol phosphate shuttle, in the utilization of glycerol, and in the biosynthesis of lipids.

glyc•er•ol•ize (glis′ər-ol-īz″) to treat with or preserve in glycerol, as in the treatment of red blood cells with a glycerol solution before they are frozen for preservation.

glyc•er•ol ki•nase (glis″ər-ol-ki′nās) [EC 2.7.1.30] an enzyme of the transferase class that catalyzes the phosphorylation of glycerol to form glycerol 3-phosphate. Deficiency of the enzyme, an X-linked trait, causes hyperglycerolemia.

glyc•er•ol-3-phos•phate O-ac•yl•trans•fer•ase (glis′ər-ol fos′fāt a″səl-trans′fər-ās) [EC 2.3.1.15] an enzyme of the transferase class that catalyzes the transfer of an acyl group to glycerol 3-phosphate from an acyl CoA with a chain longer than ten carbons, yielding a lysophosphatidate. The reaction is a step in the synthesis of triglycerides and phosphatidates, and the enzyme also catalyzes the addition of a second acyl group to the lysophosphatidate to form a phosphatidate.

glyc•er•ol-3-phos•phate de•hy•dro•gen•ase (glis′ər-ol fos′fāt de-hi′dro-jə-nās) [EC 1.1.99.5] an enzyme of the oxidoreductase class that catalyzes the oxidation of glycerol 3-phosphate to dihydroxyacetone phosphate. In mitochondria of striated muscle and of nervous tissue, the enzyme contains iron and the acceptor is FAD. The dihydroxyacetone phosphate formed can cross into the cytosol, where glycerol-3-phosphate dehydrogenase (NAD^+) catalyzes its reduction via electrons from NADH, regenerating glycerol 3-phosphate. See also *glycerol phosphate shuttle,* under *shuttle.*

glyc•er•ol-3-phos•phate de•hy•dro•gen•ase (NAD^+) (glis′ər-ol fos′fāt de-hi′dro-jən-ās) [EC 1.1.1.8] a cytosolic enzyme of the oxidoreductase class that catalyzes the oxidation of glycerol 3-phosphate to dihydroxyacetone phosphate, with NAD^+ as the electron acceptor. NADH formed from NAD^+ by other reactions displaces the equilibrium, producing glycerol 3-phosphate and the oxidized nucleotide NAD^+. The glycerol phosphate produced can cross into the mitochondria, where it is reoxidized by glycerol-3-phosphate dehydrogenase, regenerating dihydroxyacetone phosphate and donating electrons to FAD. See also *glycerol phosphate shuttle,* under *shuttle.*

glyc•er•ol•uria (glis″ər-ol-u′re-ə) excretion of glycerol in the urine, such as in hyperglycerolemia.

glyc•er•one (glis′ər-ōn) [*glycer*ol + ket*one*] formal, seldom used, term for *dihydroxyacetone.*

glyc•er•yl (glis′ər-əl) the mono-, di-, or trivalent radical formed by removal of a hydrogen from one, two, or three of the hydroxy groups of glycerol.

g. **guaiacolate** guaifenesin.

g. **monostearate** [NF] a compound prepared from glycerin and stearic acid, occurring as a white, waxlike solid, or white, waxlike beads or flakes with a slight, pleasant, fatty odor and taste; used as an emulsifying agent.

g. **triacetate** triacetin.

g. **trinitrate** nitroglycerin.

g. **trioleate** olein.

g. **tripalmitate** palmitin.

gly•cin•a•mide ri•bo•nu•cleo•tide (gli-sin′ə-mīd ri″bo-noo′kle-o-tīd) an intermediate of purine biosynthesis in which glycine is linked to the amino group of phosphoribosylamine.

gly•cin•ate (gli′sin-āt) any salt of glycine (aminoacetic acid).

gly•cine (G, Gly) (gli′sēn) 1. the smallest of the amino acids, a nonessential amino acid occurring as a constituent of many proteins. It is glycogenic, participates in a variety of synthetic reactions such as purine formation, and is an inhibitory neurotransmitter in the central nervous system. See table at *amino acid.* 2. [USP] an official preparation used as a dietary supplement and gastric antacid, and as a bladder irrigation in surgery, particularly in transurethral prostatectomy. Called also *aminoacetic acid.*

gly·cine am·i·di·no·trans·fer·ase (gli′sēn am″ĭ-dēn″o-trans′fər-ās) [EC 2.1.4.1] an enzyme of the transferase class that catalyzes the transfer of an amidino group from arginine to glycine to form guanidinoacetate and ornithine. The reaction is a step in the synthesis of creatine.

gly·cine hy·droxy·meth·yl·trans·fer·ase (gli′sēn hi-drok″se-meth″əl-trans′fər-ās) [EC 2.1.2.1] an enzyme of the transferase class that catalyzes the reversible transfer of a methylene group from serine to tetrahydrofolate to form 5,10-methylenetetrahydrofolate and glycine. The enzyme is a pyridoxal phosphate protein. The reaction occurs in mitochondria and is a major source of one-carbon units for folate-mediated transfer reactions. Called also *serine hydroxymethyltransferase.*

gly·cine trans·a·mid·in·ase (gli′sēn trans″ə-mid′in-ās) glycine amidinotransferase.

gly·cin·emia (gli″sin-e′me-ə) hyperglycinemia.

glyc·i·nin (glis′ĭ-nin) a globulin which constitutes 90 to 95 per cent of the protein content of soybean.

Gly·ciph·a·gus (gli-sif′ə-gəs) *Glycyphagus.*

glyc(o)- [Gr. *glykys* sweet] a combining form denoting relationship to *(a)* sweetness, *(b)* sugar, sometimes specifically glucose, *(c)* glycerine, or *(d)* glycogen. Cf. *gluc(o)-.*

gly·co·al·de·hyde (gli″ko-al′də-hīd) glycolaldehyde.

gly·co·bi·ol·o·gy (gli″ko-bi-ol′ə-je) research examining the biological functions of glycoconjugates, including glycoproteins, glycolipids, and proteoglycans, as well as free oligosaccharides, and the proteins that specifically interact with them, including lectins, glycosyltransferases, and glycosidases.

gly·co·cal·yx (gli″ko-kal′iks) the glycoprotein and polysaccharide covering that surrounds many cells; in bacterial cells the glycocalyx forms masses of fibers that extend from the cell and by means of which the cell adheres to surfaces; it also protects the cell form injury and functions in cell-cell recognition.

gly·co·che·no·de·oxy·cho·late (gli″ko-ke″no-de-ok″se-ko′lāt) chenodeoxycholylglycine.

gly·co·che·no·de·oxy·cho·lic ac·id (gli″ko-ke″no-de-ok″se-ko′lik) chenodeoxycholylglycine.

gly·co·cho·late (gli″ko-ko′lāt) cholylglycine.

gly·co·cho·lic ac·id (gli″ko-ko′lik) cholylglycine.

gly·co·con·ju·gate (gli″ko-kon′jə-gət) any of the complex molecules containing glycosidic linkages, such as glycolipids, glycopeptides, oligosaccharides, or glycosaminoglycans.

gly·co·cy·amine (gl″ko-si′ə-mēn) guanidinoacetic acid.

gly·co·gel·a·tin (gli″ko-jel′ə-tin) an ointment base containing glycerin and gelatin.

gly·co·gen (gli′ko-jən) [*glyco-* + *-gen*] a large polysaccharide similar to amylopectin but more highly branched, consisting of chains of glucose residues in α-(1,4) linkage with branches created by α-(1,6) linkages. It constitutes the major carbohydrate reserve of animals, stored primarily in liver and muscle, and is synthesized and degraded for energy as demanded.

hepatic g. glycogen stored in the liver.

tissue g. glycogen stored in tissues other than the liver, especially in muscle.

gly·co·gen·e·sis (gli″ko-jen′ə-sis) [*glyco-* + *-genesis*] the formation or synthesis of glycogen.

gly·co·ge·net·ic (gli″ko-jə-net′ik) 1. pertaining to or characterized by glycogenesis. 2. promoting glycogenesis.

gly·co·gen·ic (gli″ko-jen′ik) [*glyco-* + *-genic*] 1. glycogenetic. 2. pertaining to or involving glycogen.

gly·co·ge·nol·y·sis (gli″ko-jə-nol′ə-sis) [*glycogen* + *-lysis*] the breakdown of glycogen to glucose by hydrolysis (as in digestion or within lysosomes) or phosphorolysis (as in mobilization of glycogen as a fuel).

gly·co·geno·lyt·ic (gli″ko-jen″o-lit′ik) 1. pertaining to or characterized by glycogenolysis. 2. promoting glycogenolysis.

gly·co·ge·no·sis (gli″ko-jə-no′sis) glycogen storage disease.

brancher deficiency g. glycogen storage disease, type IV.

generalized g. glycogen storage disease, type II.

hepatophosphorylase deficiency g. glycogen storage disease, type VI.

hepatorenal g. glycogen storage disease, type I.

myophosphorylase deficiency g. glycogen storage disease, type V.

gly·cog·e·nous (gli-koj′ə-nəs) glycogenetic.

gly·co·gen phos·phor·y·lase (gli′ko-jən fos-for′ə-lās) [EC 2.4.1.1] an enzyme of the transferase class that catalyzes the phosphorolysis of a terminal α-1,4-glycosidic bond at the non-reducing end of a glycogen molecule, releasing a glucose 1-phosphate residue. The inactive form of the enzyme (phosphorylase *b*) is converted to the active, phosphorylated form (phosphorylase *a*) by phosphorylase kinase, and phosphorylase *a* is deactivated by phosphorylase phosphatase; phosphorylase *b* can also be activated by AMP without being phosphorylated. Two isozymes exist: the liver isozyme replenishes blood glucose, while the muscle isozyme mobilizes glycogen as fuel. Deficiency of glycogen phosphorylase, an autosomal recessive trait, causes glycogen storage disease. The muscle isozyme is absent in glycogen storage disease, type V; the liver isozyme is deficient in type VI. Called also *phosphorylase.*

gly·co·gen phos·phor·y·lase ki·nase (gli′ko-jən fos-for′ə-lās ki′nās) phosphorylase kinase.

gly·co·gen (starch) syn·thase (gli′ko-jən stahrch sin′thās) [EC 2.4.1.11] official nomenclature for *glycogen synthase.*

gly·co·gen syn·thase (gli′ko-jən sin′thās) an enzyme of the transferase class that catalyzes the synthesis of glycogen by forming an α-1,4-glucoside linkage between the terminal hydroxyl group of glycogen chain and a glucosyl group donated by UDP-glucose. The reaction is highly regulated by allosteric effectors, by kinases and phosphatases, and by insulin. There are liver and muscle isoforms, each encoded by a separate gene; deficiency of either isoform, particularly the former, causes glycogen storage disease, type 0. In official nomenclature, called *glycogen (starch) synthase.*

[gly·co·gen-syn·thase-D] phos·pha·tase (gli′ko-jən sin′thās fos′fə-tās) [EC 3.1.3.42] an enzyme of the hydrolase class that catalyzes the cleavage of a phosphoryl group from (inactive) glycogen synthase *b* to form (active) glycogen synthase *a;* the reaction is part of the mechanism of regulation of glycogen metabolism. This enzyme is considered to be an activity of the more general enzyme protein phosphatase 1 (q.v.).

gly·co·geu·sia (gli″ko-goo′zhə) [*glyco-* + Gr. *geusis* taste] a condition in which there is a sweet taste in the mouth.

gly·co·he·mo·glo·bin (gli″ko-he″mo-glo′bin) glycated hemoglobin.

gly·col (gli′kol) any of a group of aliphatic dihydric alcohols having marked hygroscopic properties and useful as solvents and plasticizers.

polyethylene g. see under *P.*

gly·col·al·de·hyde (gli″kol-al′də-hīd) a two-carbon aldehyde moiety that is the activated intermediate transferred to aldoses by transketolase and is the precursor of glycolic acid. Called also *glycoaldehyde.*

gly·co·late (gli′ko-lāt) a salt, anion, or ester of glycolic acid.

gly·col·ic ac·id (gli-kol′ik) hydroxyacetic acid, an intermediate in the conversion of serine to glycine; it is accumulated and excreted in primary hyperoxaluria, type I.

gly·col·ic·ac·id·uria (gli-kol″ik-as″ĭ-du′re-ə) primary hyperoxaluria, type I.

gly·co·lip·id (gli″ko-lip′id) a lipid containing carbohydrate groups, usually galactose but also glucose, inositol, or others. While it can describe those lipids derived from either glycerol or sphingosine, with or without phosphate groups, the term is used almost exclusively to denote the sphingosine derivatives lacking phosphate groups (glycosphingolipids).

gly·co·lyl (gli′ko-ləl) the acyl radical of glycolic acid.

gly·col·y·sis (gli-kol′ə-sis) [*glyco-* + *-lysis*] the anaerobic enzymatic conversion of glucose to the simpler compounds lactate and pyruvate, resulting in energy stored in the form of adenosine triphosphate (ATP), as occurs in muscle; it differs from *respiration* in that organic substances, rather than molecular oxygen, are used as electron acceptors. See *Embden-Meyerhof pathway,* under *pathway.*

gly·co·lyt·ic (gli″ko-lit′ik) 1. pertaining to or characterized by glycolysis. 2. promoting glycolysis.

gly·come (gli′kōm) [*glyc-* + *-ome*] the entire set of carbohydrates, free and conjugated, in a particular cell or organism under certain conditions.

gly·co·mics (gli-ko′miks) the study of the interaction of the polysaccharides and proteins of a cell, and the resulting effects on cellular phenotype, as in cell–cell communication.

gly·cone (gli′kōn) the sugar portion of a glycoside. Cf. *aglycon.*

gly·co·neo·gen·e·sis (gli″ko-ne″o-jen′ə-sis) gluconeogenesis.

gly·co·nu·cleo·pro·tein (gli″ko-noo″kle-o-pro′tēn) a nucleoprotein bearing carbohydrate groups.

gly·co·pe·nia (gli″ko-pe′ne-ə) glucopenia. **glycope′nic** *adj*

gly·co·pep·tide (gli″ko-pep′tīd) any of a class of peptides that contain carbohydrates, including some containing amino sugars.

gly·co·pex·ic (gli″ko-pek′sik) 1. pertaining to or characterized by glycopexis. 2. promoting glycopexis.

gly·co·pex·is (gli″ko-pek′sis) [*glyco-* + *pexis*] the fixation or storing of sugar or glycogen.

Gly·coph·a·gus (gli-kof′ə-gəs) *Glycyphagus.*

gly·co·phil·ia (gli″ko-fil′e-ə) [*glyco-* + *-philia*] a condition in which a very small amount of glucose produces hyperglycemia.

gly·co·phor·in (gli″ko-for′in) any of a group of transmembrane glycoproteins of erythrocytes, attaching to oligosaccharides at the outer cell membrane surface and to contractile proteins (spectrin and actin) at the cytoplasmic surface; some carry blood group antigens. Defects of glycophorin C lead to in elliptocytosis, spherocytosis, and pyropoikilocytosis.

gly·co·poly·uria (gli″ko-pol″e-u′re-ə) [*glyco-* + *poly-* + *-uria*] polyuria due to glycosuria.

gly·co·pri·val (gli″ko-pri′vəl) glucopenic.

gly·co·pro·tein (gli″ko-pro′tēn) a conjugated protein containing one or more covalently linked carbohydrate residues. While technically describing conjugates in which the carbohydrate is less than 4 per cent by weight, the term is often used generically to include the mucoproteins (q.v.) and proteoglycans (q.v.).

g. IIb/IIIa a transmembrane protein of platelets; it is an integrin that binds fibrinogen, von Willebrand factor, and other adhesive ligands and plays a role in platelet aggregation and thrombus formation.

α1-acid g. an acute phase protein found in blood plasma, an indicator of tissue necrosis and inflammation. Called also orosomucoid.

glycine-rich β g. (GBG) former name for *factor B.*

human cartilage g.-39 a 42-kilodalton glycoprotein produced by chondrocytes, synovial cells, macrophages, and neutrophils, thought to play a role in tissue remodeling; serum levels are increased in rheumatoid arthritis and certain inflammatory conditions.

g. Mac-1 a β_2 integrin (CD11b/CD18) expressed on monocytes, macrophages, neutrophils, and NK cells that mediates leukocyte adhesion and serves as a receptor for inactivated complement fragment C3b (iC3b) and for some carbohydrates of certain bacteria and yeasts; it also plays a role in antibody-dependent cellular cytotoxicity. It comprises an α and a β chain; the latter is common also to CR4. Called also *Mac-1* and *complement receptor 3 (CR3).*

P-g. (Pgp) a 170-kilodalton cell-surface protein occurring normally in the colon, small intestine, adrenal glands, kidney, and liver, and also expressed by tumor cells. It is a modulator of multidrug resistance, mediating the transport of antineoplastic agents out of tumor cells.

g. p150,95 complement receptor CR4; see under *complement receptor*, at *receptor.*

variable surface g. (VSG) any of an array of glycoproteins that forms the antigenic protein coating of *Trypanosoma brucei.* The organisms contain numerous genes encoding hundreds of such glycoproteins and, by expressing individual ones successively, evade the immune system of the host.

gly·co·pro·tein 4-β-ga·lac·to·syl·trans·fer·ase (gli″ko-pro′tēn gə-lak″to-səl-trans′fər-ās) an enzyme of the transferase class that catalyzes the attachment of galactose moieties derived from UDP-galactose to *N*-acetylglucosamine residues of glycoproteins. The enzyme is present in many tissues; in secreting mammary gland cells it complexes with α-lactalbumin to form lactose synthase. In EC nomenclature, called *β-N-acetylglucosaminyl-glycopeptide β-1,4-galactosyltransferase.*

gly·co·pty·al·ism (gli″ko-ti′əl-iz-əm) [*glyco-* + *ptyal-* + *-ism*] glycosialia.

gly·co·pyr·ro·late (gli″ko-pir′o-lāt) [USP] a synthetic quaternary anticholinergic used as an antispasmodic to help treat peptic ulcer and other gastrointestinal disorders, a preanesthetic antisialagogue to decrease salivation and respiratory secretions, and an antiarrhythmic to counteract vagal inhibitory reflexes during induction of anesthesia and surgery; administered orally, intramuscularly, or intravenously. Called also *glycopyrronium bromide.*

gly·co·pyr·ro·ni·um bro·mide (gli″ko-pir-o′ne-əm) INN for *glycopyrrolate.*

gly·cor·rha·chia (gli″ko-ra′ke-ə) [*glyco-* + *rhachi-* + *-ia*] presence of glucose in the cerebrospinal fluid.

gly·cor·rhea (gli″ko-re′ə) [*glyco-* + *-rrhea*] a sugary discharge, as with glycosuria.

gly·co·sam·ine (gli-ko′sə-mēn) an amino sugar, usually glucosamine.

gly·cos·ami·no·gly·can (gli″kōs-ə-me″no-gli′kan) any of several high-molecular-weight linear heteropolysaccharides having disaccharide repeating units containing an *N*-acetylhexosamine and a hexose or hexuronic acid; either or both residues may be sulfated. This class of compounds includes the chondroitin sulfates, dermatan sulfates, heparan sulfate and heparin, keratan sulfates, and hyaluron. All except heparin occur in proteoglycans. One or more glycosaminoglycans are accumulated abnormally in the various mucopolysaccharidoses. Abbreviated GAG. Formerly called *mucopolysaccharide.*

gly·co·se·cre·to·ry (gli″ko-se-kre′to-re) causing or concerned in the deposition of glycogen.

gly·co·se·mia (gli″ko-se′me-ə) glycemia.

gly·co·si·a·lia (gli″ko-si-a′le-ə) [*glyco-* + *sial-* + *-ia*] presence of glucose in the saliva.

gly·co·si·a·lor·rhea (gli″ko-si″ə-lo-re′ə) [*glyco-* + *sialo-* + *-rrhea*] excessive flow of saliva containing glucose.

gly·co·si·dase (gli-ko′sĭ-dās) glycosylase; sometimes restricted to those catalyzing the hydrolytic cleavage of *O*-, or *S*-linked glycosyl compounds specifically [EC 3.2.1].

β-g. 1. a glycosidase specifically cleaving β-linked sugar residues from glycosides. 2. see under *complex.*

gly·co·side (gli′ko-sīd) any compound that contains a carbohydrate molecule (sugar), particularly any such natural product in plants, convertible, by hydrolytic cleavage, into sugar and a nonsugar component (aglycon), and named specifically for the sugar contained, as glucoside (glucose), pentoside (pentose), fructoside (fructose), etc.

cardiac g. any of a group of glycosides characterized by an aglycone consisting of a steroid nucleus with an α,β-unsaturated lactone ring attached at the C-17 position, occurring in certain plants (e.g., *Digitalis, Strophanthus, Urginea*). Cardiac glycosides increase the force of contraction of cardiac muscle and some are used as cardiotonics and antiarrhythmics.

digitalis g. any of a number of cardiotonic and antiarrhythmic glycosides derived from *Digitalis purpurea* and *D. lanata*, consisting of a steroid nucleus with an α, β-unsaturated lactone ring attached at the C-17 position and a digitoxose moiety attached at C-3. The term is often used to denote any drug chemically and pharmacologically related to these glycosides, although not all are derived from *Digitalis* (e.g., ouabain); in this case it is equivalent to *cardiac g.*

gly·co·some (gli′ko-sōm) a microbody (q.v.) containing glycolytic enzymes, occurring in protozoa of the order Kinetoplastida.

gly·co·sphingo·lip·id (gli″ko-sfing″o-lip′id) any sphingolipid in which the head group is a mono- or oligosaccharide unit; included are the cerebrosides, sulfatides, and gangliosides. See also *glycolipid.*

gly·co·sphing·o·lip·i·do·sis (gli″ko-sfing″o-lip″ĭ-do′sis) [*glyco-* + *sphingolipid* + *-osis*] Fabry disease.

gly·co·stat·ic (gli″ko-stat′ik) [*glyco-* + *static*] tending to maintain a constant sugar level.

gly·cos·uria (gli″ko-su′re-ə) [*glycose*, older variant of *glucose* + *-uria*] the presence of glucose in the urine, especially excretion of an abnormally large amount in the urine, such as more than 1 g in 24 hours. Called also *dextrosuria* and *glucosuria.*

alimentary g. digestive g.

benign g. renal g.

digestive g. normal glycosuria following the ingestion of sugar; called also *alimentary g.*

emotional g. glycosuria induced by violent emotion.

epinephrine g. glycosuria following the injection of epinephrine.

hyperglycemic g. glycosuria associated with hyperglycemia.

magnesium g. glycosuria due to high concentration of magnesium in the blood.

nondiabetic g., nonhyperglycemic g., normoglycemic g., orthoglycemic g. renal g.

pathologic g. appearance of large amounts of sugar in the urine for a considerable period of time.

phlorhizin g. glycosuria following the experimental administration of phlorhizin.

renal g. glycosuria occurring when there is only the normal amount of sugar in the blood, due to inability of the renal tubules to reabsorb glucose completely. Called also *nondiabetic* or *normoglycemic g.* and *renal diabetes.*

toxic g. glycosuria produced by poisons.

gly·co·syl (gli′ko-sil″) the radical formed from a saccharide by removal of the anomeric hydroxyl group.

gly·co·syl·ase (gli-ko′səl-ās) [EC 3.2] any of a large subclass of enzymes of the hydrolase class that catalyze the hydrolytic cleavage of *O*-, *N*-, or *S*-linked glycosyl compounds; most are of broad specificity.

gly·co·syl·at·ed (gli-ko′sə-lāt″əd) having formed a linkage with a glycosyl group.

gly·co·syl·a·tion (gli-ko″sə-la′shən) the formation of linkages with glycosyl groups.

***N*-linked g.** the addition of an *N*-linked oligosaccharide to a protein, a cotranslational process occurring in the endoplasmic reticulum; the oligosaccharide is added as a preformed precursor that is modified by later processing.

nonenzymatic g. glycation.

***O*-linked g.** the addition of an *O*-linked oligosaccharide to a protein, a process that occurs in the Golgi complex; the oligosaccharide is synthesized by sequential addition of individual sugars.

gly·co·syl·cer·am·i·dase (gli″ko-sil″sə-ram′ĭ-dās) [EC 3.2.1.62] an enzyme of the hydrolase class that catalyzes the cleavage of a β-linked sugar residue from β-glycosides with large hydrophobic aglycons, such as galactosyl- and glycosylceramides and phlorizin. Such enzyme activity occurs as part of the β-glycosidase complex (q.v.), along with lactase, in the intestinal brush border membrane, where it is frequently referred to as *phlorhizin hydrolase*. In this context, it is sometimes described as a composite of glucosylceramidase [EC 3.2.1.45] and galactosylceramidase [EC 3.2.1.46] activities and denoted *glycosylceramidase* [EC 3.2.1.45–6].

gly·co·syl·trans·fer·ase (gli″ko-səl-trans′fər-ās) [EC 2.4] any enzyme that catalyzes the transfer of glycosyl groups from one molecule to another; the glycosyltransferases include the hexosyltransferases (EC 2.4.1), the pentosyltransferases (EC 2.4.2), and those transferring other glycosyl groups (EC 2.4.99). Called also *transglycosylase*.

gly·co·tax·is (gli″ko-tak′sis) [*glyco-* + *-taxis*] the metabolic distribution of glucose to the body tissues.

gly·co·tro·pic (gli″ko-tro′pik) [*glyco-* + *-tropic*] having an affinity for or attracting sugar; antagonizing the effects of insulin, causing hyperglycemia.

gly·cu·re·sis (gli″ku-re′sis) [*glyc-* + *-uresis*] glycosuria.

gly·cu·ron·ic ac·id (gli″ku-ron′ik) uronic acid.

gly·cu·ro·nide (gli″ku-rōn′īd) a glycoside of a glycuronic (uronic) acid, often specifically a glucuronide.

gly·cyl (gli′səl) the acyl radical of glycine.

gly·cyl·cy·cline (gli″səl-si′klēn) any member of a class of antibiotics derived from the tetracyclines for treatment of bacterial infections that are tetracycline-resistant.

gly·cyl·gly·cine (gli″səl-gli′sēn) the simplest dipeptide, $CH_2(NH_2)$•CO•NH•CH_2•CO_2•H.

Gly·cyph·ag·i·dae (gli″sĭ-faj′ĭ-de) a family of mites similar to Acaridae, free-living mites often found on organic material. The one genus of medical interest is *Glycyphagus*.

Gly·cyph·a·gus (gli-sif′ə-gəs) [Gr. *glykys* sweet + *phagein* to eat] a genus of free-living mites of the family Glycyphagidae. *G. domes′ticus* is the food mite, a cause of grocer's itch. Spelled also *Glyciphagus*.

Glyc·yr·rhi·za (glis″ə-ri′zə) [Gr. *glykys* sweet + *rhiza* root] a widely distributed genus of perennial herbs of the family Leguminosae. *G. glab′ra* is licorice.

glyc·yr·rhi·za (glis″ə-ri′zə) licorice (def. 2).

Gly·nase (gli′nās) trademark for a preparation of glyburide.

gly·ox·al (gli-ok′səl) a yellow crystalline compound prepared by the oxidation of acetaldehyde and used in organic synthesis, glues, and biocides; called also *biformyl*, *ethanedial*, and *oxalaldehyde*.

gly·ox·a·lase (gli-ok′sə-lās) a term used to describe the enzyme activity that converts methylglyoxal to lactic acid. It is composed of two enzymes: *lactoylglutathione lyase* (glyoxalase I) and *hydroxyacylglutathione hydrolase* (glyoxalase II).

gly·ox·a·lin (gli-ok′sə-lin) imidazole.

gly·ox·y·late (gli-ok′sə-lāt) a salt, anion, or ester of glyoxylic acid.

gly·ox·yl·ic ac·id (gli″ok-sil′ik) an α-keto acid occurring as an intermediate in the conversion of glycolic acid to glycine; it is also the primary precursor of oxalic acid and is excreted in primary hyperoxaluria, type I. See also *glyoxylate cycle*, under *cycle*.

gly·ox·y·some (gli-ok′sĭ-sōm) any of the microbodies present in certain plants and microorganisms, resembling the peroxisomes of vertebrate animal cells, but having, in addition to catalase and oxidase enzymes, the enzymes of the glyoxylate cycle, a metabolic pathway involved in the conversion of fat to carbohydrate. Glyoxosomes, in association with chloroplasts, also participate in the process of photorespiration. Spelled also *glyoxisome* and *glyoxosome*. See also *microbody*.

gly·pi·can (gli′pĭ-kan) any of a family of integral membrane proteoglycans, consisting of a 62-kD core and four heparan sulfate chains, and expressed by lung, skin, epithelial, endothelial, and smooth muscle cells; the extracellular domain binds to a number of proteins of the extracellular matrix and mediates cell adhesion.

Glyp·to·cra·ni·um (glip″to-kra′ne-əm) *Mastophora*.

Gly·set (gli′set) trademark for a preparation of miglitol.

Gm See under *allotype*.

gm gram.

GMC General Medical Council (British).

GM-CSF granulocyte-macrophage colony-stimulating factor.

GMK a preparation of green monkey kidney cells used as culture system for growing viruses, e.g., for recovering the rubella virus.

GMO genetically modified organism.

GMP guanosine monophosphate.
 3′,5′-GMP, cyclic GMP cyclic guanosine monophosphate.

GMS Gomori methenamine silver; see *methenamine silver stain*, under *stain*.

gnat (nat) a small dipterous insect; see also *Diptera*. In England the term includes mosquitoes, but in North America it includes only members of *Diptera* smaller than mosquitoes.
 buffalo g. any of various insects of the family Simuliidae.
 eye g. *Hippelates pusio*.
 turkey g. any of various insects of the family Simuliidae.

gnath·al·gia (nath-al′jə) [*gnath-* + *-algia*] pain in the jaw.

gnath·ic (nath′ik) pertaining to the jaw or cheek.

gnath·i·on (nath′e-on) a craniometric landmark indicating the lowest median point on the inferior border of the mandible; it is a derived point midway between the most anterior (pogonion) and inferior (menton), established by bisecting the angle between the nasion–pogonion and mandibular planes.

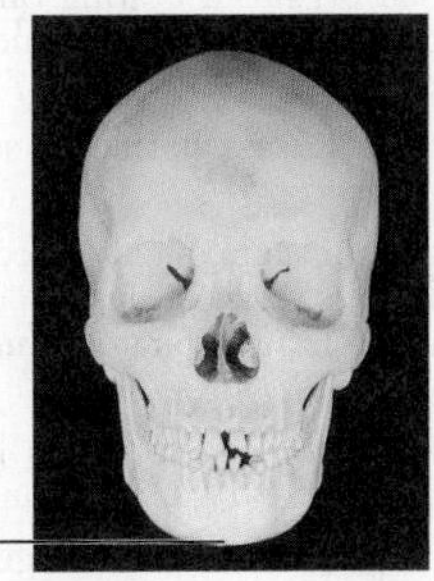

gnath·itis (nath-i′tis) [*gnath-* + *-itis*] inflammation of the jaw.

gnath(o)- [Gr. *gnathos* jaw] a combining form denoting relationship to the jaw.

Gnath·ob·del·li·dae (nath″ob-del′ĭ-de) a family of leeches (class Hirudinea); it includes the genera *Dinobdella*, *Haemadipsa*, *Haemopis*, *Hirudinaria*, *Hirudo*, *Limnatis*, *Macrobdella*, and *Theromyzon*.

gnatho·ceph·a·lus (nath″o-sef′ə-ləs) [*gnatho-* + *-cephalus*] a fetus with no head except the jaws.

gnatho·dy·nam·ics (nath″o-di-nam′iks) [*gnatho-* + *dynamics*] the study of the physical forces used in mastication.

gnatho·dy·na·mom·e·ter (nath″o-di″nə-mom′ə-tər) [*gnatho-* + *dynamometer*] an instrument for measuring the force exerted in closing the jaws; called also *occlusometer*.
 bimeter g. a gnathodynamometer equipped with a central-bearing point of adjustable height.

gnath·odyn·ia (nath″o-din′e-ə) [*gnatho-* + *-odynia*] gnathalgia.

gnath·og·ra·phy (nath-og′rə-fe) [*gnatho-* + *-graphy*] the recording of the strength of a patient's bite by a tracing of the changes in the flow of an electric current through a bite gauge.

gnath·ol·o·gy (nath-ol′ə-je) [*gnatho-* + *-logy*] the science that deals with the anatomy, histology, physiology, and pathology of the jaws and the masticatory system as a whole, including the applicable diagnostic, therapeutic, and rehabilitative procedures. **gnatholog′ic** *adj*

gnatho·plas·ty (nath′o-plas″te) [*gnatho-* + *-plasty*] plastic surgery of the jaw. **gnathoplas′tic** *adj*

gnath·os·chi·sis (nath-os′kĭ-sis) [*gnatho-* + *-schisis*] cleft jaw.

gnatho·so·ma (nath″o-so′mə) [*gnatho-* + *soma*] the capitulum of an acarine.

gnatho·stat (nath′o-stat) a jaw-positioning device used in dental radiology, facial photography, cephalometry, and other procedures requiring exact positioning of the jaws. See also *cephalostat*.

gnatho·stat·ics (nath″o-stat′iks) [*gnatho-* + *-static*] a method of prosthodontic and orthodontic diagnosis based on determination of the basal and osteometric relationships between the teeth and their supporting structures.

Gnath·os·to·ma (nath-os′to-mə) [*gnatho-* + *stoma*] a genus of nematodes of the family Gnathostomatidae, which are parasitic in various mammals. *G. spini′gerum* causes gnathostomiasis in cats, dogs, and humans.

Gnatho·sto·mat·i·dae (nath″o-sto-mat′ĭ-de) a family of nematodes parasitic in mammals, part of the superfamily Spiruroidea; it includes the genus *Gnathostoma*.

gnatho·sto·mi·a·sis (nath″o-sto-mi′ə-sis) infection with the nematode *Gnathostoma spinigerum*, occurring in animals that eat raw or undercooked fish harboring the larvae. Usually the larvae migrate in subcutaneous tissue and cause cutaneous larva migrans. Occasionally they migrate to deeper tissues to cause abscesses, or to the central nervous system to cause eosinophilic myeloencephalitis.

gno•sia (no′se-ə) [Gr. *gnosis* knowledge] the faculty of perceiving and recognizing.

gno•to•bi•ol•o•gy (no″to-bi-ol′ə-je) gnotobiotics.

gno•to•bio•ta (no″to-bi-o′tə) the specifically and entirely known microfauna and microflora of a specially reared laboratory animal.

gno•to•bi•ote (no″to-bi′ōt) a specially reared laboratory animal the microfauna and microflora of which are specifically known in their entirety.

gno•to•bi•ot•ic (no″to-bi-ot′ik) pertaining to a gnotobiote or to gnotobiotics. Cf. *axenic.*

gno•to•bi•ot•ics (no″to-bi-ot′iks) [Gr. *gnotos* known + *biota* the fauna and flora of a region] the science of raising laboratory animals whose microfauna and microflora are specifically known in their entirety.

gno•to•phor•e•sis (no″to-fə-re′sis) [Gr. *gnotos* known + *-phoresis*] the state of existence of an organism bearing one or more known species in intimate contact with it and no other demonstrable viable microorganisms. **gnotophor′ic** *adj*

Gn-RH gonadotropin-releasing hormone; see *luteinizing hormone–releasing hormone*, under *hormone.*

goat•pox (gōt′poks) an acute, highly infectious disease of goats, caused by a poxvirus and less severe than sheep-pox; characteristics include vesicular eruption with catarrh of the respiratory mucous membranes. Called also *variola caprina.*

Goeck•er•man treatment (go′kər-mən) [William Henry *Goeckerman*, American dermatologist, 1884–1954] see under *treatment.*

Gog•gia sign (go′jah) [Carlo Paolo *Goggia*, Italian physician, 1871–1948] see under *sign.*

goi•ter (goi′tər) [L. *guttur* throat] an enlargement of the thyroid gland, causing a swelling in the front part of the neck. Called also *struma.* **goi′trous** *adj*

aberrant g. enlargement of an ectopic or supernumerary thyroid gland.

adenomatous g. goiter caused by hyperplasia of thyroid follicular cells or by multiple colloid nodules. See also *follicular adenoma*, under *adenoma.*

Basedow g. a colloid goiter that becomes hyperfunctional after administration of iodine.

colloid g. a large soft goiter in which the thyroid follicular cells are greatly distended with colloid.

congenital g. goiter present at birth, resulting from congenital absence of enzymes required for production of thyroxine and consequent overstimulation of the thyroid by thyrotropin.

cystic g. a goiter containing cysts formed by mucoid or colloid degeneration.

diffuse g. a goiter in which the gland is diffusely enlarged, as in Graves disease.

diffuse toxic g. 1. exophthalmic goiter. 2. Graves disease.

diving g. a movable goiter located sometimes above and sometimes below the sternal notch. Called also *plunging g.* and *wandering g.*

dyshormonogenetic g. hypothyroidism caused by defective production of hormones by the thyroid gland, usually because of an inborn error of metabolism.

endemic g. goiter that is endemic to a region, usually because the soil and hence the diet has a low iodide content; seen in mountainous areas around the world and various other regions.

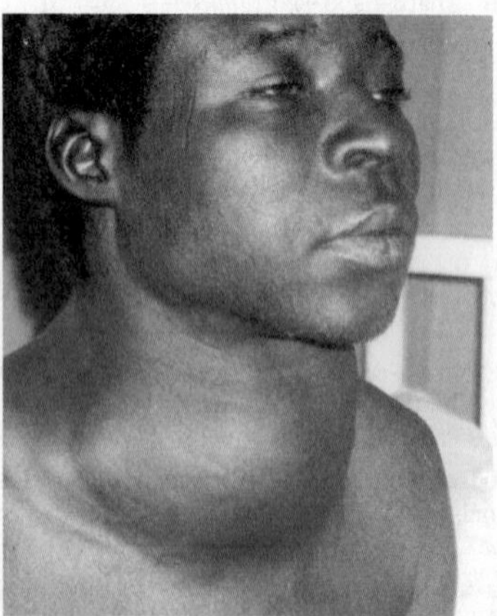

■ Goiter secondary to iodine deficiency.

exophthalmic g. goiter accompanied by protrusion of the eyeballs, as in Graves orbitopathy. Called also *diffuse toxic g.*

fibrous g. goiter caused by hyperplasia of the capsule and stroma.

follicular g. parenchymatous g.

intrathoracic g. goiter in which a portion is in the thoracic cavity.

iodide g. a goiter that occurs in response to high concentrations of exogenous iodides, which inhibits iodide oxidation and incorporation into thyroglobulin *(Wolff-Chaikoff effect).*

lingual g. an enlargement of the upper end of the original thyroglossal duct, forming a tumor at the posterior part of the dorsum of the tongue.

lymphadenoid g. Hashimoto disease.

multinodular g. a goiter containing circumscribed nodules within its substance.

nodular g. multinodular g.

nontoxic g. goiter occurring sporadically and not associated with hyperthyroidism.

parenchymatous g. goiter marked by enlarged thyroid follicular cells and increased numbers of follicles.

perivascular g. a goiter that surrounds a large blood vessel.

plunging g. diving g.

retrovascular g. a goiter with a portion behind a large blood vessel.

simple g. simple hyperplasia of the thyroid gland.

substernal g. a goiter in which a portion is beneath the sternum.

suffocative g. a goiter that causes dyspnea by pressure on the trachea.

toxic multinodular g. hyperthyroidism arising in a multinodular goiter, usually of long standing. Called also *toxic adenoma* and *Parry* or *Plummer disease.*

vascular g. goiter due chiefly to dilatation of the blood vessels.

wandering g. diving g.

goi•tre (goi′tər) [Fr.] goiter.

goi•trin (goi′trin) a goitrogenic substance isolated from rutabagas and turnips.

goi•tro•gen (goi′tro-jən) a goiter-producing compound.

goi•tro•gen•ic (goi-tro-jen′ik) producing goiter; called also *goitrogenous.*

goi•tro•ge•nic•i•ty (goi″tro-jə-nis′ĭ-te) the tendency to produce goiter.

goi•trog•e•nous (goi-troj′ə-nəs) goitrogenic.

gold (Au) (gōld) a yellow metallic element, atomic number 79, atomic weight 196.967, specific gravity 19.32. When alloyed, in carats, pure gold has 24 parts (or carats). Gold compounds are used in medicine, chiefly in arthritis (see *chrysotherapy*). However, all the compounds are poisonous; see also *chrysiasis* and *chrysoderma.*

g. Au 198 the most common radioactive isotope of gold, atomic mass 198, used in solid form (seed) or colloidal solution. It has a half-life of 2.69 days and emits gamma (0.412 MeV) and beta particles (1.371, 0.962 MeV); it has been used by intracavitary or interstitial injection or implantation in the treatment of certain types of cancer and has also been used, in colloidal form, as a scintiscanning agent.

cohesive g. cohesive gold foil.

colloidal g. a purplish suspension of minute particles of metallic gold, used in medicine since alchemical times. The radioactive form, made by exposure to neutrons, has been used by intracavitary or interstitial injection in the treatment of certain types of cancer and also has been used as a scintiscanning agent.

mat g. spongy strips of pure gold produced by the process of electroplating, which can be formed into ropes and cylinders and used in the base of dental restorations and as a direct filling material. See also under *foil.*

g. sodium thiomalate [USP] a monovalent gold salt used as a disease-modifying antirheumatic drug in treatment of early active rheumatoid arthritis not controlled by nonsteroidal antiinflammatory drugs, rest, and physical therapy; administered intramuscularly. Called also *sodium aurothiomalate.*

g. thioglucose aurothioglucose.

Gold•berg syndrome (gōld′bərg) [Morton Falk *Goldberg*, American physician, born 1937] see under *syndrome.*

Gold•blatt clamp, hypertension (phenomenon), kidney (gōld′blat) [Harry *Goldblatt*, American physician, 1891–1977] see under *clamp, hypertension*, and *kidney.*

Gold•en S sign (gōl′dən) [Ross *Golden*, American radiologist, 1889–1975] see under *sign.*

Gol•den•har syndrome (gōl′dən-hahr) [Maurice *Goldenhar*, Swiss physician, 20th century] oculoauriculovertebral dysplasia; see under *dysplasia.*

gol•den•rod (gōl′dən-rod) any plant of the genus *Solidago.*

gol•den•seal (gōl′dən-sēl″) 1. *Hydrastis canadensis.* 2. a preparation of the dried rhizome of *H. canadensis*, widely used in folk medicine and used in homeopathy for irregular menstruation, digestive problems, and bronchitis.

Gold•flam disease (gōlt′flahm) [Samuel Vulfovich *Goldflam,* Polish neurologist, 1852–1932] myasthenia gravis.

Gold•flam-Erb disease (gōlt′flahm erb′) [S.V. *Goldflam;* Wilhelm Heinrich *Erb,* German neurologist, 1840–1921] myasthenia gravis.

Gold•schei•der percussion, test (gōlt′shi-dər) [Johannes Karl August Eugen Alfred *Goldscheider,* German physician, 1858–1935] see *threshold percussion,* under *percussion,* see *orthopercussion;* and see under *tests.*

Gold•stein disease, sign (gōld′stīn) [Hyman Isaac *Goldstein,* American physician, 1887–1954] see under *disease* and *sign.*

Gold•thwait brace, sign (gōld′thwāt) [Joel Ernest *Goldthwait,* American orthopedic surgeon, 1866–1961] see under *brace* and *sign.*

Gol•gi complex, etc. (gol′je) [Camillo *Golgi,* Italian neurologist, histologist, and Nobel prize winner, 1843–1926] see under *complex, neuron,* and *organ,* and at *Stains and Staining Methods,* under *stain.*

gol•gin (gol′jin) any of a large family of proteins associated with the Golgi complex, having a number of transport and maintenance functions, including tethering vesicles to target membranes prior to fusion and biogenesis of membranes of the Golgi stack.

Goll fasciculus (column, fibers, tract), nucleus (gol) [Friedrich *Goll,* Swiss anatomist, 1829–1903] see *fasciculus gracilis medullae spinalis* and *nucleus gracilis.*

Goltz syndrome (gōlts) [Robert William *Goltz,* American dermatologist, born 1923] focal dermal hypoplasia; see under *hypoplasia.*

Go-LYTELY (go-līt′le) trademark for combination preparations of polyethylene glycol 3350 and electrolytes (sodium sulfate, sodium bicarbonate, sodium chloride, and potassium chloride).

Gom•bault-Phi•lippe triangle (gom-bo′ fe-lēp′) [François Alexis Albert *Gombault,* French neurologist, 1844– 1904; Claudien *Philippe,* French pathologist, 1866–1903] see under *triangle.*

go•mit•o•li (go-mit′o-li) [It. plural of *gomitolo* coil] a network of capillaries in the upper infundibular stem (of the hypothalamus) that surround terminal arterioles of the superior hypophysial arteries and that lead into portal veins to the adenohypophysis.

Go•mo•ri stains (go-mo′re) [George *Gomori,* Hungarian histochemist in the United States, 1904–1957] see *Stains and Staining Methods,* under *stain.*

Gom•pertz' law (formula) (gom′pərts) [Benjamin *Gompertz,* British actuary, 1779–1865] see under *law.*

gom•pho•sis (gom-fo′sis) [Gr. *gomphōsis* a bolting together] 1. [TA] a type of fibrous joint in which a conical process is inserted into a socketlike portion, such as the styloid process in the temporal bone, or the teeth in the dental alveoli. Called also *socket.* 2. TA alternative for *syndesmosis dentoalveolaris.*

go•nad (go′nad) [L. *gonas,* from Gr. *gonos* procreation] a gamete-producing gland; an ovary, testis, or ovotestis. Called also *genital gland* and *sex gland.* **gonad′al** *adj*

indifferent g. the sexually undifferentiated gonad of the early embryo. In human embryos this stage occurs during the fifth to seventh weeks.

streak g's undeveloped gonadal structures found in the broad ligament below the fallopian tube, composed of whorled connective-tissue stroma with no germinal or secretory cells; seen most often in Turner syndrome.

go•nad•ar•che (go″nə-dahr′ke) the onset of gonadal functioning.

go•nad•ec•to•mize (go″nə-dek′tə-mīz) to surgically remove one or both of the gonads; see also *castrate.*

go•nad•ec•to•my (go″nə-dek′tə-me) [*gonad-* + *-ectomy*] surgical removal of an ovary or testis. See also *castration.*

gonad(o)- [L. *gonas,* gen. *gonadis* gonad, from Gr. *gonos* procreation] a combining form denoting relationship to the gonads.

go•na•do•blas•to•ma (go″nə-do-blas-to′mə) a rare benign type of germ cell tumor, usually arising in dysgenetic gonads, often bilaterally. It contains all gonadal elements, including germ cells, sex cord derivatives, and stromal derivatives and is frequently associated with an abnormal chromosomal karyotype. It may give rise to development of a dysgerminoma or other more malignant germ cell tumor.

go•na•do•gen•e•sis (go″nə-do-jen′ə-sis) [*gonado-* + *-genesis*] the development of the gonads in the embryo.

go•na•do•in•hib•i•to•ry (go″nə-do-in-hib′ĭ-tor-e) inhibiting or preventing gonadal activity.

go•na•do•ki•net•ic (go″nə-do-kĭ-net′ik) gonadotropic.

go•na•do•lib•er•in (go″nə-do-lib′ər-in) [*gonado*tropin + *-liberin*] luteinizing hormone–releasing hormone.

go•na•do•mi•met•ic (go″nə-do-mĭ-met′ik) imitating the effects of the sex hormones; said of drugs.

gon•a•dop•a•thy (gon″ə-dop′ə-the) [*gonado-* + *-pathy*] any disease of the gonads.

go•na•do•rel•in (gə-nad″o-rel′in) synthetic luteinizing hormone–releasing hormone, structurally identical to the natural hormone.

g. acetate the acetate ester of gonadorelin, having the same actions and uses as the hydrochloride salt; also used in the treatment of delayed puberty, female infertility, and amenorrhea; administered subcutaneously or intravenously.

g. hydrochloride [USP] the dihydrochloride salt of gonadorelin, used in the evaluation of the functional capacity and response of the anterior pituitary gonadotrophs in hypogonadism; administered subcutaneously or intravenously.

go•na•do•tox•ic (gə-nad′o-tok″sik) having a deleterious effect on the gonads, such as radiation or a chemotherapeutic agent.

go•na•do•tox•ic•i•ty (go″nə-do-tok-sis′ĭ-te) 1. the quality of being gonadotoxic. 2. the extent to which something damages the gonads.

go•na•do•tox•in (go′nə-do-tok″sin) a substance having a deleterious effect on the gonads.

go•nado•trope (go-nad′o-trōp) gonadotroph.

go•nado•troph (go-nad′o-trōf) 1. a basophil of the adenohypophysis whose granules secrete follicle-stimulating hormone and luteinizing hormone. Called also *delta basophil, delta cell,* and *gonadotrope* or *gonadotropic cell.* 2. a substance that stimulates the gonads.

go•na•do•tro•phic (go″nə-do-tro′fik) gonadotropic.

go•na•do•tro•phin (go′nə-do-tro″fin) gonadotropin.

go•nado•tro•pic (go″nə-do-tro′pik) [*gonado-* + *-tropic*] stimulating the gonads; applied to hormones of the anterior pituitary.

go•nado•tro•pin (go″nə-do-tro′pin) any hormone that stimulates the gonads, especially follicle-stimulating hormone and luteinizing hormone. See also *chorionic g.* Called also *gonadotropic hormone.*

chorionic g., human chorionic g. (HCG, hCG) 1. a two-subunit glycopeptide hormone produced by syncytiotrophoblasts of the fetal placenta that maintains the function of the corpus luteum during the first few weeks of pregnancy, and is thought to promote steroidogenesis in the fetoplacental unit and to stimulate fetal testicular secretion of testosterone. The α subunit is identical to that of luteinizing hormone, follicle-stimulating hormone, and thyrotropin; the β subunit shares homology with luteinizing hormone but is antigenically unique, containing an additional glycopeptide sequence. Chorionic gonadotropin can be detected by immunoassay in the maternal urine within days after fertilization and thus provides the basis for the most commonly used pregnancy tests. 2. [USP] the same principle obtained from the urine of pregnant women, used to treat certain cases of cryptorchidism and male hypogonadism, to induce ovulation and pregnancy in anovulatory women in whom the anovulation is secondary and not due to ovarian failure, and to increase the numbers of oocytes for patients attempting conception using assisted reproductive technologies such as gamete intrafallopian transfer (GIFT) or in vitro fertilization; administered intramuscularly. Called also *choriogonadotropin.* See also *choriogonadotropin alfa.*

human menopausal g. (hMG) menotropins.

gon•a•do•tro•pi•no•ma (gon″ə-do-tro″pĭ-no′mə) gonadotroph adenoma.

gon•a•duct (gon′ə-dəkt) the duct of a gonad; a uterine tube or seminal duct.

Gon•al-F (gon′əl) trademark for a preparation of follitropin alfa.

go•nal•gia (go-nal′jə) [Gr. *gony* knee + *-algia*] pain in the knee.

go•nane (go′nān) a 17-carbon tetracyclic hydrocarbon nucleus that is the parent structure of some steroid hormones and bile acids.

gon•ar•thri•tis (gon″ahr-thri′tis) [Gr. *gony* knee + *arthritis*] inflammation of a knee or knee joint.

gon•ar•thro•men•in•gi•tis (gon-ahr″thro-men″in-ji′tis) [Gr. *gony* knee + *arthro-* + *mening-* + *-itis*] inflammation of the synovial membrane of the knee joint.

gon•ar•thro•sis (gon″ahr-thro′sis) arthropathy of the knee joint.

gon•e•cyst (gon′ə-sist) [*gon-* + *cystis*] glandula vesiculosa. **gonecys′tic** *adj*

Gon•gy•lo•ne•ma (gon″jĭ-lo-ne′mə) [Gr. *gongylos* round + *nema*] a genus of nematodes of the superfamily Spiruroidea; infections cause only mild symptoms if any at all, but the meat of slaughtered animals must be discarded. *G. ingluvi′cola* infects chickens. *G. neoplas′ticum* infects rats and other laboratory rodents. *G. pul′chrum* (called also *G. scuta′tum*) infects the esophageal and oral mucous membranes of sheep, goats, cattle, pigs, and sometimes humans.

gon•gy•lo•ne•mi•a•sis (gon″jĭ-lo-ne-mi′ə-sis) infection with the nematode *Gongylonema.*

go•nia (go′ne-ə) [Gr.] plural of *gonion.*

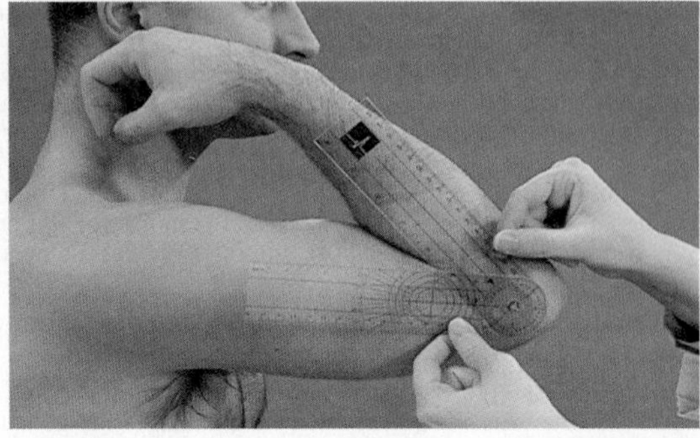

■ Goniometer being used to measure range of motion of a joint.

gon·id·an·gi·um (gon″id-an′je-əm) a cell within which gonidia are formed.

go·nid·i·um (go-nid′e-əm) pl. *gonid′ia* [Gr. *gonē* seed] the algal cell part of the thallus of a lichen.

goni(o)- [Gr. *gōnia* angle] a combining form denoting relationship to an angle, especially the angle of the anterior chamber of the eye.

Go·nio·ba·sis (go″ne-o-ba′sis) a genus of small fresh water snails of the family Pleuroceridae. *G. sili′cula* is a species found in the northwestern United States that acts as a host for the fluke *Troglotrema salmincola.*

go·nio·dys·gen·e·sis (go″ne-o-dis-jen′ə-sis) [*gonio-* + *dysgenesis*] defective development of the anterior segment of the eyeball.

go·ni·om·e·ter (go″ne-om′ə-tər) [*gonio-* + *-meter*] 1. an instrument for measuring angles; used clinically to measure angles of joint motion. Called also *arthrometer.* 2. a plank, one end of which may be tilted to any height, used in testing for labyrinthine disease.

finger g. an apparatus for measuring the limits of flexion and extension of the interphalangeal joints of the fingers.

universal g. a goniometer consisting of a metal or plastic protractor in a full circle or half circle with two indicating arms that are several inches to a foot (10 to 30 cm) in length; the arms are held in place by a tight pivot at the center of the circle so that the instrument can be picked up and read; used to measure range of motion of a joint.

go·ni·om·e·try (go″ne-om′ə-tre) the measurement of angles, particularly those of range of motion of a joint.

go·ni·on (go′ne-on) pl. *go′nia* [Gr. *gōnia* angle] [TA] a craniometric landmark located at the most inferior, posterior, and lateral point on the external angle of the mandible, being the apex of the maximum curvature of the mandible, where the ascending ramus becomes confluent with the corpus. **go′nial** *adj*

Go·nio·ne·mus (go″ne-o-ne′məs) a genus of invertebrates of the phylum Cnidaria, class Hydrozoa, resembling small jellyfish. *G. ver′tens* is a common species found in oceans and seas in temperate climates and has a painful sting that causes a painful skin lesion and sometimes a systemic reaction.

go·nio·pho·tog·ra·phy (go″ne-o-fo-tog′rə-fe) photography of the angle of the anterior chamber of the eye.

Gon·i·ops (gon′e-ops) a genus of biting flies of the family Tabanidae.

go·nio·punc·ture (go″ne-o-punk′chər) [*gonio-* + *puncture*] an infrequently used filtering operation for glaucoma, done by inserting a knife blade through clear cornea just within the limbus, across the anterior chamber, and through the opposite corneoscleral wall.

go·nio·scope (go′ne-o-skōp″) [*gonio-* + *-scope*] an optical instrument for examining the angle of the anterior chamber and for demonstrating ocular motility and rotation.

go·ni·os·co·py (go″ne-os′kə-pe) examination of the angle of the anterior chamber of the eye with the gonioscope.

go·nio·syn·ech·ia (go′ne-o-sə-nek′e-ə) adhesion of the iris to the cornea at the angle of the anterior chamber of the eye.

go·ni·ot·o·my (go″ne-ot′ə-me) [*gonio-* + *-tomy*] an operation for types of glaucoma characterized by an open angle and normal depth of the anterior chamber; it consists of the opening of Schlemm canal under direct vision secured by a contact glass.

go·ni·tis (go-ni′tis) [*gon-* + *-itis*] 1. inflammation of the knee. 2. inflammation of the stifle joint in a horse.

fungous g. inflammation of the knee joint in which the capsule is diffusely thickened.

g. tuberculo′sa tuberculosis of the knee joint.

gon(o)-[1] [Gr. *gonē* offspring, seed, genitalia] a combining form meaning sexual or generative, or denoting relationship to semen or seed, or to the reproductive organs.

gon(o)-[2] [Gr. *gony* knee] a combining form denoting relationship to the knee.

gono·blen·nor·rhea (gon″o-blen″o-re′ə) gonococcal conjunctivitis.

gono·camp·sis (gon″o-kamp′sis) [*gono-*[2] + Gr. *kamptos* bent] permanent flexion of the knee.

gon·och·o·rism (gon-ok′ə-riz-əm) [*gono-*[1] + Gr. *chōrizein* to separate] differentiation of the gonads with normal development of the reproductive organs appropriate to the sex; cf. *hermaphroditism.*

gono·coc·ce·mia (gon″o-kok-se′me-ə) [L. *gonococci* + *-emia*] the presence of gonococci in the blood.

gono·coc·ci (gon″o-kok′si) [L.] plural of *gonococcus.*

gono·coc·cide (gon″o-kok′sīd) [*gonococcus* + *-cide*] an agent that kills gonococci.

gono·coc·co·cide (gon″o-kok′o-sīd) [*gonococcus* + *-cide*] gonococcide.

gono·coc·cus (gon″o-kok′əs) pl. *gonococ′ci* [*gono-*[1] + *coccus*] an individual microorganism of the species *Neisseria gonorrhoeae*, the organism causing gonorrhea. **gonococ′cal, gonococ′cic** *adj*

gono·cyte (gon′o-sīt) [*gono-*[1] + *-cyte*] primordial germ cell.

gono·neph·ro·tome (gon″o-nef′rə-tōm) [*gono-*[1] + *nephrotome*] that part of the mesoderm which develops into the reproductive and excretory organs of the embryo.

gono·phage (gon′o-fāj) a bacteriophage having the gonococcus as its natural host.

gono·phore (gon′o-for) [*gono-*[1] + *-phore*] an accessory generative organ, such as the uterine tube and uterus in the female, or spermiduct and seminal vesicle in the male.

gon·or·rhea (gon″o-re′ə) [*gono-*[1] + *-rrhea*] infection due to *Neisseria gonorrhoeae*, usually a sexually transmitted disease; children in households with infected persons may become infected, and health care workers having contact with infected exudates may contract it. In males it is marked by urethritis with pain and purulent discharge, but in females it is commonly asymptomatic, although it may extend to produce suppurative salpingitis, oophoritis, tubo-ovarian abscess, and peritonitis. Bacteremia occurs in both sexes, resulting in cutaneous lesions, arthritis, and occasionally meningitis or endocarditis. **gonorrhe′al** *adj*

gono·tome (gon′o-tōm) [*gono-*[1] + *-tome*] that part of the mesoderm which develops into the reproductive organs of the embryo.

gon·y·au·la·ca·les (gon″e-aw-lə-ka′lēz) an order of plantlike marine protozoa of the phylum Dinoflagellata.

Gony·au·lax (gon″e-aw′laks) [*gony-* + Gr. *aulakos* a furrow] a genus of plantlike marine protozoa of the order Gonyaulacales, phylum Dinoflagellata, having mainly brown to yellow chromatophores. Like other dinoflagellates, they can produce red tide when present in vast numbers. Certain species have been associated with a form of shellfish poisoning (q.v.). Representative species include *G. acatenella, G. catenella, G. polyedra,* and *G. tamarensis.*

Gon·za·lez diet (gon-zah′lez) [Nicholas J. *Gonzalez*, American physician, late 20th century] see under *diet.*

Good syndrome (good) [Robert Alan *Good*, American pediatrician, born 1922] immunodeficiency with thymoma.

Goo·dell sign (law) (go͝o-del′) [William *Goodell*, American gynecologist, 1829–1894] see under *sign.*

Good·man syndrome (good′mən) [Richard M. *Goodman*, Israeli physician, 1932–1989] see under *syndrome.*

Good·pas·ture stain, syndrome (good′pas-chər) [Ernest William *Goodpasture*, American pathologist, 1886–1960] see *Stains and Staining Methods*, under *stain*, and see under *syndrome.*

Good·sall rule (good′sawl) [David H. *Goodsall*, British surgeon, 1843–1906] see under *rule.*

Goor·magh·tigh apparatus (cells) (go͞or′mah-ti) [Norbert *Goormaghtigh*, Belgian physician, 1890–1960] juxtaglomerular cells.

Go·pa·lan syndrome (go′pah-lahn) [Coluthur *Gopalan*, Indian biochemist, born 1918] see under *syndrome.*

Gor·di·a·cea (gor″de-a′se-ə) Nematomorpha.

Gor·di·us (gor′de-əs) [Gordian knot] a genus of worms of the class Nematomorpha, the hair snakes or horsehair worms.

G. aqua′ticus a species occasionally found as a pseudoparasite of the intestinal tract of a person who has accidentally eaten infected insects.

G. robus'tus a species that is generally found as a pseudoparasite similarly to *G. aquaticus*, but has also been found in periorbital tissues of a few persons.

Gor•don reflex, sign (gor'dən) [Alfred *Gordon*, American neurologist, 1874–1953] see *flexor reflex, paradoxical,* under *reflex*, and *finger phenomenon* (def. 1), under *phenomenon*.

Gor•don syndrome (gor'dən) [Richard D. *Gordon*, Australian physician, 20th century] see under *syndrome*.

Gor•do•nia (gor-do'ne-ə) [Ruth E. *Gordon*, American bacteriologist, 20th century] a genus of nocardioform actinomycetes of the family Gordoniaceae, occurring widely in soil and water; organisms are gram-positive to gram-variable, aerobic, catalase-positive, nonmotile, non-spore-forming short rods and cocci that occur singly or in pairs, V-shaped arrangements, or short chains. Some species have rarely been associated with human infections, chiefly in immunocompromised patients. The type species is *G. bronchia'lis*. Formerly called (incorrectly) *Gordona*.

G. bronchia'lis the species that most commonly causes human infection, most often associated with sternal wounds resulting from surgery. Formerly called *Rhodococcus bronchialis*.

Gor•do•ni•a•ceae (gor-do″ne-a'se-e) a family of aerobic, nonmotile, gram-positive to gram-variable soil and water bacteria of the suborder Corynebacterineae, order Actinomycetales; medically important organisms are contained in the genus *Gordonia*.

gor•get (gor'jet) a wide-grooved lithotome director.

Gor•ham disease (gor'əm) [Lemuel Whittington *Gorham*, American physician, 1885–1968] disappearing bone disease.

Gor•ham-Stout disease (gor'əm stout) [L. W. *Gorham;* Arthur Purdy *Stout*, American pathologist, mid-20th century] disappearing bone disease.

Gor•lin formula (gor'lin) [Richard *Gorlin*, American cardiologist, born 1926] see under *formula*.

Gor•lin cyst, sign, syndrome (gor'lin) [Robert James *Gorlin*, American oral pathologist and geneticist, born 1923] see *calcifying odontogenic cyst*, under *cyst*, see under *sign*, and see *nevoid basal cell carcinoma syndrome*, under *syndrome*.

Gor•lin-Goltz syndrome (gor'lin gōltz') [R.J. *Gorlin;* Robert William *Goltz*, American physician, born 1923] nevoid basal cell carcinoma syndrome.

go•se•rel•in (go'sə-rel″in) a synthetic gonadotropin-releasing hormone analogue; upon administration it initially stimulates release of follicle-stimulating hormone and luteinizing hormone and on prolonged administration later suppresses them.

g. acetate the acetate salt of goserelin, used to treat breast and prostate carcinomas and endometriosis, and to thin the endometrium prior to endometrial ablation; administered by subcutaneous implant.

Gos•lee tooth (goz'le) [Hart John *Goslee*, American dentist, 1871–1930] see under *tooth*.

Gos•se•lin fracture (gos-ə-lă') [Léon Athanase *Gosselin*, French surgeon, 1815–1887] see under *fracture*.

Gos•syp•i•um (gŏ-sip'e-əm) [L.] cotton; a genus of tropical and subtropical plants of the family Malvaceae. Three species, *G. barbaden'se*, *G. herba'ceum*, and *G. hirsu'tum*, yield most of the commercial cotton and are also sources of cottonseed and cottonseed oil.

gos•sy•pol (gos'ə-pol) [*Gossypium* + *-ol*] a poisonous yellow pigment, found in cottonseed and detoxified by heating; it has male antifertility properties, apparently having its effects in the seminiferous tubules. Gossypol poisoning (q.v.) occurs when cottonseed cakes containing excessive gossypol are fed to pigs.

GOT glutamic-oxaloacetic transaminase; see *aspartate transaminase*.

Gott•lieb's epithelial attachment (got'lēbz) [Bernhard *Gottlieb*, Austrian dentist, 1885–1950] see under *attachment*.

Gott•ron papules, sign (got'ron) [Heinrich Adolf *Gottron*, German dermatologist, 1890–1974] see under *papule* and *sign*.

go•tu ko•la (go'too ko'lə) 1. *Centella asiatica*. 2. a preparation of the leaves and stems of *C. asiatica*, used externally to promote wound healing and to treat the lesions of leprosy; it is also widely used in ayurveda, traditional Chinese medicine, and Asian folk medicine

gouge (gouj) a hollow chisel used in cutting and removing bone.

Kelley g. an instrument for removing cartilage grafts.

Gou•ger•ot-Blum syndrome (goo-zher-o' bloom') [Henri *Gougerot*, French physician, 1881–1955; Paul *Blum*, French physician, 1878–1933] pigmented purpuric lichenoid dermatitis.

Gou•ger•ot-Car•teaud syndrome (goo-zher-o' kahr-to') [H. *Gougerot;* Alexandre *Carteaud*, French physician, 20th century] confluent and reticulate papillomatosis.

Gou•ley catheter (goo'le) [John Williams Severin *Gouley*, American surgeon, 1832–1920] see under *catheter*.

goun•dou (gōōn-doo') [West African] a late sequel of yaws and endemic syphilis manifested by massive periostitis of the nasal processes of the maxillae, characterized by the formation of bony hornlike exostoses at the sides of the nose, leading to distortion of the facial features and destruction of the nose and orbit. Called also *anakhré*.

gou•siek•te (goo-sēk'te) [Afrikaans "rapid disease"] a condition in sheep and cattle marked by myocarditis, dilatation, and heart failure, caused by eating any of several poisonous plants including species of *Pavetta* and the shrub *Vangueria pygmora*.

gout (gout) [L. *gutta* a drop, because of the ancient belief that the disease was due to a "noxa" falling drop by drop into the joint] a group of disorders of purine metabolism, manifested by various combinations of (1) hyperuricemia and uric acid calculi; (2) recurrent acute inflammatory arthritis induced by crystals of monosodium urate monohydrate; and (3) tophaceous deposits of these crystals in and around the joints of the extremities, sometimes causing crippling destruction of the joints. **gout'y** *adj*

articular g. gout affecting the joints.

chalky g. tophaceous g.

idiopathic g. a gout of uncertain classification; see *primary g.* and *secondary g.*

lead g. gout occurring as a complication of lead poisoning.

oxalic g. oxalate poisoning.

polyarticular g. a rare type of gout that attacks many joints.

primary g. gout that seems to be innate, not a consequence of an acquired disorder or condition such as use of thiazide diuretics, and not secondary to an inborn error of metabolism such as glycogen storage disease, type I; it afflicts almost entirely men from the fourth to sixth decades, as well as a few postmenopausal women.

regular g. articular g.

saturnine g. lead g.

secondary g. gout resulting from an acquired disorder such as polycythemia vera or chronic myelogenous leukemia, or from an inborn error of metabolism.

tophaceous g. gout in which there are tophi or chalky deposits of sodium urate.

visceral g. a disease of birds characterized by the deposition of sodium urates on the viscera.

Gow•ers tract (column, fasciculus), etc. (gou'ərz) [Sir William Richard *Gowers*, English neurologist, 1845–1915] see under *sign* and *solution*, see *tractus spinocerebellaris anterior*, and see *vasovagal syncope*, under *syncope*.

GP general paresis; general practitioner.

GPCR G protein–coupled receptor.

G6PD glucose-6-phosphate dehydrogenase.

GPT glutamic-pyruvic transaminase; see *alanine transaminase*.

gr grain (def. 2).

graaf•i•an (grah'fe-ən) named for Reijnier (Regner) de *Graaf*, Dutch physician and anatomist, 1641–1673, as *graafian follicles*.

Grac•i•la•ria (gras″ĭ-lar'e-ə) a genus of seaweeds. *G. lichenoi'des* (L.) Harv. is Ceylon moss, used as food, as a source of agar, and in China as an antidysenteric.

grac•ile (gras'il) [L. *gracilis*] slender or delicate.

grac•il•o•plas•ty (gras'il-o-plas″te) plastic surgery on the gracilis muscle. **graciloplas'tic** *adj*

dynamic g. a surgical technique sometimes used for treatment of anal incontinence, consisting of detaching the distal end of the gracilis muscle from the thigh and wrapping it around the anal canal to make a neosphincter.

Grad. grada'tim (by degrees).

gra•da•tim (gra-da'tim) [L.] gradually; by degrees.

grade (grād) score.

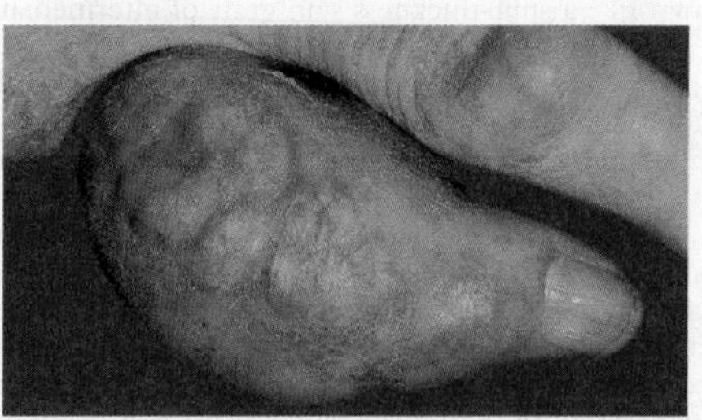

■ Tophaceous gout.

Gleason g. a rating of localized cancer of the prostate that assigns scores of 1 to 5 for degree of primary and secondary growth, with undifferentiated and destructive types having higher scores. Called also *Gleason score*.

-grade [L. *gradi* to walk or take steps] a word termination meaning progression.

Gra•de•ni•go syndrome (grah-də-ne′go) [Giuseppe *Gradenigo*, Italian physician, 1859–1926] see under *syndrome*.

gra•di•ent (gra′de-ənt) 1. the increase or decrease of one variable expressed as a function of a second. 2. the graphic representation of such a change.

alveolar-arterial oxygen g. the difference between the predicted alveolar oxygen tension (PA_{O2}) and the measured arterial oxygen tension (P_{O2}); it is elevated in pulmonary conditions in which there is impaired gas exchange.

concentration g. variation in the concentration of a solute over a distance or on two sides of a permeable barrier.

density g. progressive variation in density over a distance; used particularly for that of a solute along the height or width of a confined solution; see also under *centrifugation*.

electrochemical g. the difference in ion concentration and electrical potential from one point to another, so that ions tend to move passively along it.

hepatic vein pressure g., hepatic venous pressure g. the difference between the wedged hepatic venous pressure and the free hepatic venous pressure, used to assess portal hypertension.

magnetic field g. in magnetic resonance imaging, the change in the magnetic field in a given direction.

mitral g. the difference in pressure between the left atrium and the left ventricle in diastole.

serum-ascites albumin g. (SAAG) a method for categorizing ascites: the albumin concentration of serum and ascitic fluid specimens is measured, and the value of the ascitic fluid specimen is subtracted from the value of the serum specimen. A difference equal to or greater than 1.1 g/dL indicates the presence of portal hypertension.

systolic g. the pressure difference between two communicating cardiac chambers or across a semilunar valve during systole.

ventricular g. the net differences in ventricular electrical activity of varying duration, as determined by the algebraic sum of the electrocardiographic vectors representing the QRS and T-wave areas; as an index of duration of the excited state of the ventricles, it represents the local rate of repolarization.

grad•u•ate (graj′oo-ət) [L. *graduatus*] 1. a person who has received a degree from a university or college. 2. a measuring vessel marked by a series of lines.

grad•u•at•ed (graj′oo-āt″əd) [L. *gradus* step] marked by a succession of lines, steps, or degrees.

Grae•fe knife, operation, sign (gra′fə) [Albrecht Friedrich Wilhelm Ernst von *Graefe*, German ophthalmologist, 1828–1870] see under *knife*, *operation*, and *sign*.

graft (graft) 1. any tissue or organ for implantation or transplantation. 2. to implant or transplant such tissues. This term is preferred over *transplant* in the case of skin grafts. See also *implant*.

accordion g. mesh g.

activated g. a graft in which the nerves and blood supply have grown to nourish it, after a period of denervation and tenuous vascularity.

allogeneic g. allograft.

arteriovenous g. a means of arteriovenous access consisting of a venous autograft or xenograft or a synthetic tube, often made of polytef, grafted onto the artery and vein.

autochthonous g. autograft.

autodermic g., autoepidermic g. a skin graft taken from the patient's own body.

autogenous g., autologous g., autoplastic g. autograft.

avascular g. a graft of tissue in which not even transient vascularization is achieved.

Blair-Brown g. a split-thickness skin graft of intermediate depth.

bone g. bone transplanted from one site to another.

brephoplastic g. the transplantation of tissue from an embryo or newborn to an adult animal.

bypass g. an autograft consisting of a segment of vein or artery grafted into place in a bypass.

cable g. a nerve graft made up of several sections of nerve in the manner of a cable.

chorioallantoic g. the placing of cells, tissues, or parts on the chorioallantoic membrane of the embryonic chick.

composite g. a graft that has more than one component, such as a bypass graft consisting of both a vein and a prosthesis or an autograft containing more than one tissue.

coronary artery bypass g. (CABG) see under *bypass*.

cutis g. dermal g.

Davis g. pinch g.

delayed g. a skin graft that is sutured back into its bed and subsequently shifted to a new recipient bed.

dermal g., dermic g. skin from which epidermis and subcutaneous fat have been removed; used instead of fascia in various plastic procedures. Called also *cutis g.*

diced cartilage g's numerous small segments of cartilage that can be packed or molded into any desired contour like wet grains of sand; used to repair faulty cartilage or bone structure.

dowel g. a cylindrical plug of bone used to immobilize adjacent vertebrae in anterior spinal fusion.

epidermal g. a skin graft in which a piece of epidermis is implanted on a raw surface.

Esser g. inlay g.

fascia g. a graft taken from the fascia lata or from the lumbar fascia.

fascicular g. a nerve graft in which the bundles of nerve fibers are approximated and sutured separately.

fat g. a graft of fat completely freed from its bed; used in filling depressions.

filler g. a graft used for the filling of defects, as the filling of depressions with fatty tissue or of a bony cyst cavity with bone chips or dried cartilage.

free g. a graft of tissue completely freed from its bed, in contrast to a flap.

full-thickness g. a skin graft consisting of the epidermis and the full depth of the dermis.

heterodermic g. a skin graft taken from a donor of another species.

heterologous g., heteroplastic g. xenograft.

heterotopic g. a graft transplanted into a site or position that it does not normally occupy.

homologous g., homoplastic g. allograft.

human umbilical vein g. a specially prepared umbilical vein used as an allograft.

hyperplastic g. a skin graft that is in a state of active repair.

inlay g. a skin or mucosal graft applied by spreading the graft over a stent and suturing the graft and mold into a prepared pocket; called also *Esser g.* and *Stent g.*

interposition g. a graft consisting of a part, such as a section of a tubular organ, that is surgically removed from its normal location and reattached to aid functioning of a different part. Called also *interposition*.

island g. see under *flap*.

isogeneic g., isologous g., isoplastic g. syngraft.

jump g. see under *flap*.

Kimura cartilage g. a split-thickness costal cartilage graft used in the management of tracheal stenosis.

Krause-Wolfe g. a full-thickness skin graft.

lamellar g. replacement of the superficial layers of an opaque cornea by a thin layer of clear cornea from a donor eye.

mesh g. a thin split-thickness skin graft in which many tiny slits have been made to allow the graft to expand and be stretched to cover a large area.

mucosal g. a graft of mucosal tissue, usually comprising the entire thickness of the mucosa.

nerve g. a nerve segment used to repair an area of defective nerve.

nonvascularized g. a graft in which the blood supply to the grafted tissue is not maintained.

Ollier-Thiersch g. a very thin skin graft consisting of epidermis and a thin layer of dermis, often cut in long, broad strips.

omental g. a free or attached segment of omentum used for reparative surgery in the chest, such as covering suture lines after gastrointestinal surgery or repairing weak structures.

onlay bone g. bone used as a graft that is laid on or over cortical bone of the recipient site(s).

osseous g. bone g.

outlay g. a modification of an inlay graft, used in ectropion of the eyelid.

patch g. a graft of living tissue or prosthetic material used to repair a vascular incision in order to enlarge the lumen of the vessel.

pedicle g. see under *flap*.

penetrating g. a full-thickness corneal transplant.

periosteal g. a piece of periosteum applied to a denuded area of a bone.

Phemister g. a bone graft of cortical bone with cancellous bone chips to enhance callus formation.

pinch g. a small free skin graft obtained by lifting the skin with a needle to form a cone, which is cut across the base resulting in a graft 2–4 mm in diameter with a full thickness of skin at the center; a number of them are placed at intervals on an open wound.

porcine g. a split-thickness graft of skin from a pig, applied to a denuded area on a human as a temporary dressing for treatment of a severe burn.
Reverdin g. pinch g.
sieve g. a skin graft from which very small circular islands of skin are removed so that a larger denuded area can be covered, the sievelike portion being placed over one area, and the individual islands over surrounding or other denuded areas.
skin g. skin transplanted to replace a lost portion of the body skin surface; it may be a full-thickness or split-thickness graft.
sleeve g. a graft for repairing traumatic gaps in nerves by a sleevelike extension from the distal stump which is sutured to the central stump.
Smith-Robinson g. a horseshoe-shaped bone graft obtained from the iliac crest, used to immobilize adjacent vertebrae in anterior spinal fusion.
split-skin g., split-thickness g. a skin graft consisting of the epidermis and a portion of dermis, or a mucosal graft consisting of only a partial thickness of mucosa.
Stent g. inlay g.
syngeneic g. syngraft.
tendon g. a free graft of tendon used to replace a damaged tendon segment.
thick-split g. a skin graft consisting of the epidermis and about two thirds of the dermis.
Thiersch g. Ollier-Thiersch g.
thin-split g. Ollier-Thiersch g.
tube g., tunnel g. tube flap.
vascularized g. a graft in which the blood supply to the grafted tissue is maintained, as with a pedicle flap.
vein g. a bypass graft using a segment of vein, often the saphenous vein.
white g. avascular g.
Wolfe g., Wolfe-Krause g. Krause-Wolfe g.
xenogeneic g. xenograft.

graf·tec·to·my (graf-tek′tə-me) surgical removal of a previously transplanted organ or tissue.

graft·ing (graft′ing) transplantation; see also *graft*.
skin g. implantation of patches of healthy skin on a denuded area to provide epithelial covering.

graft·skin (graft′skin) an artificial skin product produced through biomedical engineering, containing both epidermis and dermis, used in skin grafts.

Gra·ham's law (gra′əmz) [Thomas *Graham*, British chemist, 1805–1869] see under *law*.

Gra·ham test (gra′əm) [Evarts Ambrose *Graham*, American surgeon, 1883–1957] see under *test*.

Gra·ham Lit·tle syndrome (gra′əm lit′əl) [Sir Ernest Gordon *Graham Little*, British physician, 1867–1950] see under *syndrome*.

Gra·ham Steell murmur (gra′əm stēl) [*Graham Steell*, British physician, 1851–1942] see under *murmur*.

grain (grān) [L. *granum*] 1. a seed, especially of a cereal plant. 2. the smallest unit of weight in the apothecaries' and avoirdupois systems, equivalent to 64.8 mg; in the apothecaries' system there are 20 grains to the scruple, with 480 grains in 1 ounce; in the avoirdupos system, there are 27.34 grains to the dram, with 437.5 grains in 1 ounce. Abbreviated gr. 3. an individual crystal of a metal or other crystalline structure.

Gram method, stain, solution (gram) [Hans Christian Joachim *Gram*, Danish physician, 1853–1938] see *Stains and Staining Methods*, under *stain*, and see *gram-negative* and *gram-positive*.

gram (g) (gram) [Gr. *gramma* a small weight] a unit of mass in the SI system; it is one thousandth of a kilogram (q.v.).

-gram [Gr. *gramma* something drawn or written] a word termination meaning that which is drawn, written, or recorded.

gram·i·ci·din (gram″ĭ-si′din) [USP] an antibiotic produced by *Bacillus brevis* which acts by damaging bacterial cell membranes, applied topically in pyodermic, ocular, and other localized infections due to susceptible gram-positive organisms. It is also one of the two major components of tyrothricin, the other being tyrocidine.

gram·ine (gram′ēn) a crystalline indole alkaloid found in barley; called also *donaxine*.

Gra·min·eae (grə-min′e-e) the grass family, a large family of plants that have hollow stems and slender leaves. Besides the plants popularly called *grass*, it includes food plants such as many grains and sugar cane.

gram·i·niv·o·rous (gram″ĭ-niv′ə-rəs) feeding or subsisting on grass or cereal grains.

gram-neg·a·tive (gram-neg′ə-tiv) losing the stain or decolorized by alcohol in the Gram method of staining, a primary characteristic of bacteria having a cell wall composed of a thin layer of peptidoglycan covered by an outer membrane of lipoprotein and lipopolysaccharide. Cf. *gram-positive*.

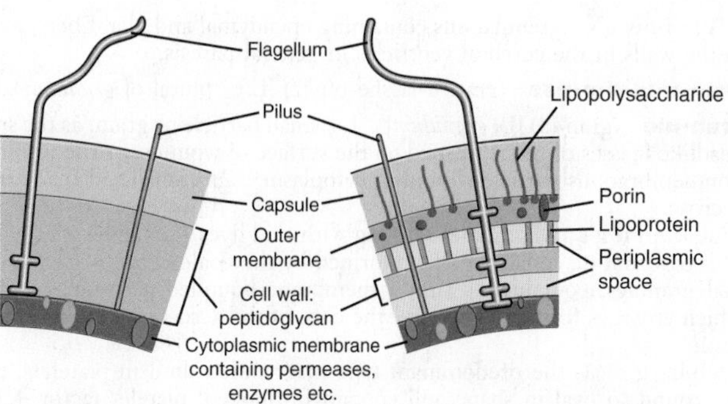

■ Characteristic cell wall structures of gram-positive *(left)* and gram-negative *(right)* bacteria.

gram-pos·i·tive (gram-poz′ĭ-tiv) retaining the stain or resisting decolorization by alcohol in the Gram method of staining, a primary characteristic of bacteria whose cell wall is composed of a thick layer of peptidoglycan with attached teichoic acids. Cf. *gram-negative*.

gram-var·i·a·ble (gram-var′e-ə-bəl) appearing to be a mixture of gram-positive and gram-negative organisms, said of gram-positive bacteria that lose the stain easily, so that some bacteria in a sample are decolorized and others retain the stain.

gra·na (gra′nə) [pl. of L. *granum* grain] dense green, chlorophyll-containing bodies in chloroplasts consisting of numerous, closely packed lamellae which make them appear to be suspended in a matrix.

gran·di·ose (gran′de-ōs″) in psychiatry, pertaining to exaggerated beliefs or claims of one's importance or identity, often manifested by delusions of great wealth, power, or fame.

gran·di·os·i·ty (gran″de-os′ĭ-te) the condition of being grandiose; an exaggerated belief of one's importance or identity.

grand mal (grahn mahl) [Fr.] see under *epilepsy*.

Gran·ger line, sign (grān′jər) [Amedee *Granger*, American radiologist, 1879–1939] see under *line* and *sign*.

gran·is·e·tron hy·dro·chlo·ride (grā-nis′ə-tron) an antiemetic used in conjunction with cancer chemotherapy or radiotherapy; administered orally or intravenously.

Gra·nit loop (grah′nēt) [Ragnar Arthur *Granit*, Finnish-born physiologist in Sweden and Nobel prize winner, 1900–1991] gamma loop; see under *loop*.

gran·u·la (gran′u-lə) pl. *gran′ulae* [L.] 1. a small particle or grain. 2. granule (def. 2).
g. iri′dica a black or brown outgrowth from the edge of the iris in cattle and horses; called also *nigroid body*.

gran·u·lar (gran′u-lər) [L. *granularis*] made up of or marked by presence of granules or grains.

gran·u·la·tio (gran″u-la′she-o) pl. *granulatio′nes* [L.] a general term denoting a granule, or granular mass.
granulatio′nes arachnoi′deae [TA], **granulatio′nes arachnoidea′les** arachnoid granulations: small elevations, visible to the naked eye, thought by some to be enlargements of arachnoid villi, which project into the superior sagittal sinus and associated venous lacunae and create slight depressions on the inner surface of the cranium; these granulations are the structures through which cerebrospinal fluid is reabsorbed into the blood in the venous system. Called also *arachnoidal granulations* or *villi*, *cerebral granulations*, *meningeal granules*, and *pacchionian bodies*, *corpuscles*, or *granulations*.
granulatio′nes cerebra′les granulationes arachnoideae.

gran·u·la·tion (gran″u-la′shən) [L. *granulatio*] 1. the process of forming granulation tissue. 2. the process of forming cytoplasmic granules. 3. granule (def. 1). 4. any granular material on the surface of a tissue, membrane, or organ. 5. the rendering of hard or metallic substances into granules or grains.
arachnoid g's, arachnoidal g's granulationes arachnoideae.
cerebral g's granulationes arachnoideae.
exuberant g's excessive proliferation of granulation tissue in healing wounds.
pacchionian g's granulationes arachnoideae.
pyroninophilic g's structures seen in liver and other cells, which stain red with methyl green–pyronine by Pappenheim stain; they are one of the early effects of carbon tetrachloride poisoning.
Reilly g's large azurophilic granules in the cytoplasm of polymorphonuclear leukocytes and lymphocytes, occurring in Hurler syndrome.

Virchow g's granulations containing ependymal and glial fibers, found in the walls of the cerebral ventricles in general paresis.

gran·u·la·ti·o·nes (gran″u-la″she-o′nēz) [L.] plural of *granulatio.*

gran·ule (gran′ūl) [L. *granulum*] 1. a small particle or grain, as the small beadlike masses of tissue formed on the surface of wounds, or the insoluble nonmembranous particles found in cytoplasm. 2. a small pill made from sucrose.

acidophil g's 1. granules staining with acid dyes. 2. alpha g's (def. 3).

acrosomal g. a large globule formed by the coalescence of proacrosomal granules, contained within a membrane-bounded acrosomal vesicle, which enlarges further to become the core of the acrosome of a spermatozoon.

alpha g's 1. the predominant type of granule found in platelets; they are round to oval in shape and contain fibrinogen, platelet factor 4, and various other proteins. 2. large granules in the alpha cells of the islets of Langerhans, which are insoluble in alcohol and contain glucagon. 3. the granules found in the acidophils (alpha cells) of the adenohypophysis. Called also *acidophil g's.*

amphophil g's granules that stain with either acid or basic dyes.

argentaffin g's granules that stain with silver.

atrial g's specific atrial g's.

azurophil g. 1. any granule that stains easily with azure dyes. See also *azurophilia.* 2. a specific type of azurophilic granule found in the promyelocyte; it contains numerous compounds that are antimicrobial, including myeloperoxidase. Called also *primary g.*

basal g. basal body.

basophil g. 1. any granule staining with basic dyes. 2. one of the coarse bluish-black granules found in basophils (def. 2). 3. *(in the pl.)* beta g's (def. 2).

beta g's 1. the granules in the beta cells of the islets of Langerhans, which contain insulin. 2. granules found in the basophils (beta cells) of the adenohypophysis; called also *basophil g's.*

Birbeck g's membrane-bound, rod- or tennis racquet–shaped inclusions with a central linear, longitudinally striated nucleus, found in the cytoplasm of Langerhans cells. Called also *Langerhans g's.*

bull's eye g. dense body (def. 2).

chromaffin g's organelles found in the chromaffin cells of the adrenal medulla, where epinephrine and norepinephrine are synthesized, stored, and released when needed.

chromatic g's, chromophilic g's Nissl bodies.

cone g's the nuclei of the visual cells of the retina in its outer nuclear layer which are connected with the cones.

cortical g's special structures in the cortex of the ovum of many animals, including humans; they break up during fertilization and supply the material for the development of the fertilization membrane.

cytoplasmic g. general term for a condensed area of cellular material.

delta g. dense body.

dense g. dense body (def. 2).

Ehrlich g's, Ehrlich-Heinz g's cell granules that stain with Ehrlich triacid stain.

elementary g's hemoconia.

eosinophil g. one of the coarse round granules that stain with eosin and are found in eosinophils.

fuchsinophil g's granules staining with fuchsin.

Fordyce g's ectopic sebaceous glands found on the lips and gums and in the mucosa of the cheeks, which present as yellowish white milia. Called also *Fordyce disease* or *spots.*

gamma g's a name applied to basophilic granules found in the blood, marrow, and in the tissues.

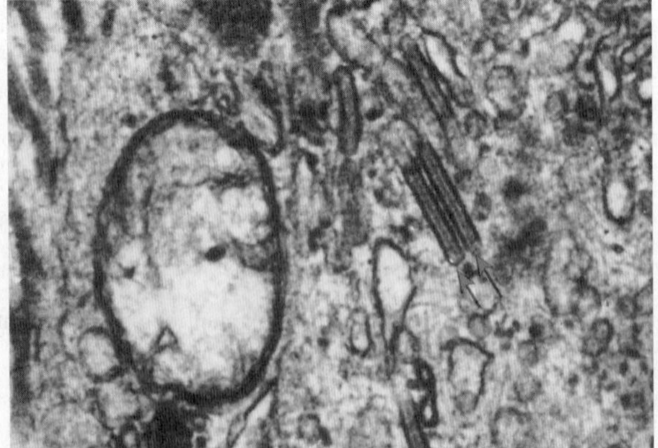

■ Birbeck granules *(arrows)* in the cytoplasm of a Langerhans cell (electron micrograph).

gelatinase g. a type of neutrophil granule found primarily in mature cells and seen sedimenting out with specific granules in some fractionation techniques. Called also *tertiary g.*

Heinz g's Heinz-Ehrlich bodies.

interchromatin g's particles 20–25 nm in diameter, consisting of small nuclear ribonucleoproteins and other protein factors involved in RNA processing, that occur in clusters in the interchromosomal domain of the cell nucleus.

iodophil g's granules staining brown with iodine, seen in polymorphonuclear leukocytes in various acute infectious diseases.

juxtaglomerular g's stainable osmophilic secretory granules present in the juxtaglomerular cells, closely resembling zymogen granules.

kappa g. azurophil g. (def. 2).

keratohyalin g's irregularly shaped granular deposits of keratohyalin, found on tonofibrils in the granular cells of the stratum granulosum of the epidermis; they stain with some acid dyes and some basic dyes.

Kölliker interstitial g's granules of various sizes seen in the sarcoplasm of muscle fibers.

lamellar g. see under *body.*

Langerhans g's Birbeck g's.

Langley g's granules seen in secreting serous glands.

membrane-coating g. lamellar body.

meningeal g's granulationes arachnoideae.

metachromatic g. 1. a granular cell inclusion that stains a color different from that of the dye used. 2. in certain bacteria, yeasts, yeastlike fungi, and protozoa, granules that appear red when stained with a blue dye, composed of complex polyphosphate, lipid, and volutin; they serve as an intracellular phosphate reserve.

monocytic g. one of the fine red azurophilic granules of a monocyte.

Much g's gram-positive, nonacid-fast granules and rods found in tuberculous sputum and thought to be modified tubercle bacilli.

neutrophil g. any of the granules found in the cytoplasm of neutrophils; those in immature cells are called *primary* or *azurophil granules* and those in mature cells are called *secondary* or *specific granules.*

Nissl g's Nissl bodies.

oxyphil g's acidophil g's.

perichromatin g's granules occurring in the perichromatin region of the cell nucleus and containing heterogeneous nuclear ribonucleoproteins (hnRNPs); they are involved in the storage of various RNAs and in messenger RNA transport.

pigment g's small masses of coloring matter occurring in pigment cells.

polar g's polar bodies (def. 2).

primary g. azurophil g. (def. 2).

proacrosomal g. any of the small, dense bodies found inside one of the vacuoles of the Golgi body, which fuse to form an acrosomal granule.

protein g's microscopically observable particles of various proteins, some anabolic and others catabolic.

rod g's the nuclei of rod visual cells in the outer nuclear layer of the retina that are connected with the rods.

secondary g. specific g.

secretory g's membrane-bound vesicles derived from the trans-Golgi network that contain secretory products for delivery to the plasma membrane and subsequent release from the cell. Called also *secretory vesicles.*

seminal g's small granular bodies found in semen.

specific g. a type of neutrophil granule found primarily in mature cells; most are released into the extracellular fluid. They contain lactoferrin, plasminogen activator, leukocyte alkaline activator, and collagenase, as well as membrane-bound molecules that they release onto the cell surface. Called also *secondary g.*

specific atrial g's membrane-bound spherical granules with a dense homogeneous interior that are concentrated in the core of sarcoplasm of the atrial cardiac muscle, extending in either direction from the poles of the nucleus, usually near the Golgi complex; they also may be found in limited numbers in other regions of the cell. They are the storage site of atrial natriuretic peptide.

sphere g. a large granular cell or corpuscle seen in serous exudation.

sulfur g's granular bodies found in lesions and discharges of actinomycosis, so called because they are usually a yellow color that resembles sulfur, although they are sometimes other colors.

tertiary g. gelatinase g.

toxic g's dark-staining basophilic granules observed in neutrophils in infections and other toxic states; they are probably phagosomes or autophagic vacuoles.

vermiform g's Birbeck g's.

volutin g's see *volutin.*

zymogen g's secretory granules in certain cells, containing the precursors of enzymes that become active after they have left the cell.

Gran·u·lex (gran′u-leks) trademark for a combination preparation of crystallized trypsin and balsam of Peru.

Gran•u•lic•a•tel•la (gran″u-lik″ə-tel′ə) a genus of gram-positive bacteria of the family Carnobacteriaceae, found growing in satellite colonies around other bacteria, especially *Streptococcus aureus;* many are penicillin-resistant. They are found as normal flora in the upper respiratory, urogenital, and gastrointestinal tracts, and have been implicated in some cases of bacterial endocarditis. The type species is *G. adiacens.*

G. adia′cens a species isolated from cases of bacteremia and endocarditis; formerly called *Abiotrophia adiacens* and *Streptococcus adjacens.*

G. e′legans a species isolated from cases of infective endocarditis and occasionally other infections.

gran•u•li•form (gran′u-lĭ-form″) in the form of, or resembling, small grains.

granul(o)- [L. *granulum,* dim. of *granum* grain] a combining form denoting relationship to granules.

gran•u•lo•ad•i•pose (gran″u-lo-ad′ĭ-pōs) [*granulo-* + *adipose*] showing fatty degeneration which contains granules of fat.

gran•u•lo•cyte (gran′u-lo-sīt″) [*granulo-* + *-cyte*] 1. any cell containing granules. 2. granular leukocyte.

band-form g. band cell.

segmented g. see under *cell.*

gran•u•lo•cyt•ic (gran″u-lo-sit′ik) 1. pertaining to, characterized by, or of the nature of granulocytes. 2. pertaining to the granulocytic series; see under *series.*

gran•u•lo•cy•top•a•thy (gran″u-lo-si-top′ə-the) [*granulocyte* + *-pathy*] any disorder of the granular leukocytes (granulocytes).

gran•u•lo•cy•to•pe•nia (gran″u-lo-si″to-pe′ne-ə) [*granulocyte* + *-penia*] reduction in the number of granular leukocytes in the blood. Cf. *agranulocytosis.* Called also *granulopenia* and *hypogranulocytosis.*

gran•u•lo•cy•to•poi•e•sis (gran″u-lo-si″to-poi-e′sis) granulopoiesis. **granulocytopoiet′ic** *adj*

gran•u•lo•cy•to•sis (gran″u-lo-si-to′sis) an abnormally large number of granulocytes in the blood.

gran•u•lo•fat•ty (gran″u-lo-fat′e) granuloadipose.

gran•u•lo•ma (gran″u-lo′mə) pl. *granulomas, granulo′mata* [*granul-* + *-oma*] an imprecise term applied to either a small, nodular, delimited aggregation of mononuclear inflammatory cells, or a similar collection of epithelioid cells; it is usually surrounded by a rim of lymphocytes and often includes multinucleated giant cells. Some granulomas contain eosinophils and plasma cells, and many are accompanied by fibrosis. Granuloma formation represents a chronic inflammatory response that can be initiated by infectious or noninfectious agents. See also *granulomatosis.*

acral lick g. see under *dermatitis.*

actinic g. annular elastolytic giant cell g.

amebic g. granulomatous lesions of the colon sometimes seen in amebiasis.

annular elastolytic giant cell g. a variant of granuloma annulare seen on skin chronically exposed to the sun. The border is raised and contains many histiocytes and giant cells; many of the normal elastic fibers are gathered near the giant cells or phagocytized by them. Called also *Miescher g.* and *actinic g.*

g. annula′re a group of benign, usually self-limited granulomatous diseases of unknown etiology with both localized and disseminated varieties, most often seen in children and young adults. The lesions chiefly involve the dermis and are perforating papules or subcutaneous nodules grouped in rings. Histopathologic findings include palisading macrophages surrounding foci of necrobiosis of the dermis.

apical g. periapical g.

aquarium g. swimming pool g.

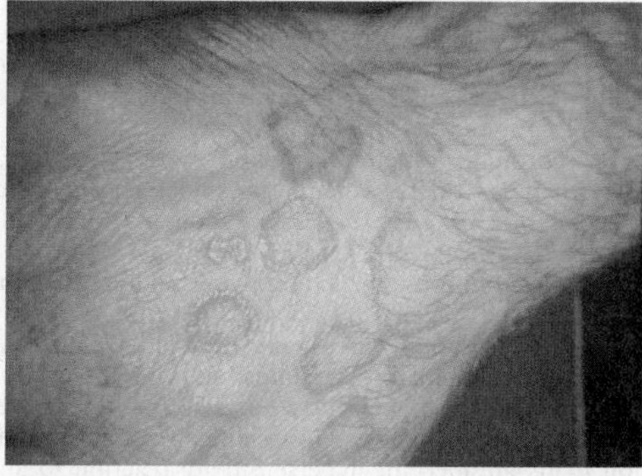

■ Granuloma annulare of the dorsum of the hand.

beryllium g. a complication of chronic berylliosis, consisting of a chronic, local, noncaseating, sarcoidlike granulomatous reaction, usually in the lungs; it often progresses to fibrosis and hyalinization.

***Candida* g., candidal g.** a rare response to invasive candidiasis of the skin, usually seen in immunocompromised children, with granulomatous lesions on the skin of the face, scalp, and less often other parts of the body. There are primary vascularized papules covered with a thick, adherent crust, and they sometimes develop into horns or protrusions.

canine venereal g. canine transmissible venereal tumor.

central giant cell g., central giant cell reparative g. a lesion of the jaws, considered by some authorities to be a type of giant cell tumor, and by others to be a form of osteogenic sarcoma; lesions vary in degree of malignancy. It seems to be a central lesion of the bone of the jaws, representing an inflammatory reaction to injury or hemorrhage, and not a true neoplasm. It is composed of a spindle cell stroma punctuated by multinucleate giant cells.

cholesterol g. a granulomatous lesion in which crystals of cholesterol esters are surrounded by foreign-body giant cells in a mass of fibrotic granulation tissue. The mass may grow and press against nearby structures, with symptoms depending on the location in the body.

Churg-Strauss g. cutaneous extravascular necrotizing g.

coccidioidal g. secondary coccidioidomycosis.

collagenolytic g. equine nodular necrobiosis.

contact g. a benign lesion on the posterior part of a vocal fold, consisting of a pale to red mass on the medial aspect of the vocal process of the arytenoid cartilage; the cause may be voice overuse, irritation from a gastric or esophageal tube, or gastroesophageal reflux. Called also *contact ulcer.*

cutaneous extravascular necrotizing g. an umbilicated granuloma surrounded by palisading histiocytes; it is similar in appearance to a rheumatoid papule and may be a variant. Called also *Churg-Strauss* or *Winkelmann g.*

dental g. periapical g.

eosinophilic g. 1. the mildest form of Langerhans cell histiocytosis, affecting primarily children, adolescents, and young adults. There may a single cranial lesion or a few foci, most often in the skull, spine, pelvis, ribs, or mandible and less commonly in the long bones, with localized pain and tenderness and sometimes pathologic fracture. 2. a disorder similar to eosinophilic gastroenteritis, characterized by localized nodular or pedunculated lesions of the submucosa and muscle walls, usually in the pyloric area of the stomach, but sometimes involving the small intestine. The cause is infiltration by eosinophils, but it does not involve peripheral eosinophilia or allergic symptoms. 3. anisakiasis in humans. 4. see *eosinophilic granuloma complex,* under *complex.*

epithelioid g., epithelioid cell g. any granuloma characterized by epithelioid cells.

g. facia′le a rare, chronic, benign skin disorder in which papules, nodules, or plaques appear on the face and occasionally elsewhere; the etiology is unknown, but in some patients sun exposed areas are more vulnerable. In the dermis there is an infiltrate of neutrophils, eosinophils, and plasma cells.

fish tank g. swimming pool g.

g. fissura′tum 1. a circumscribed, firm, reddish, fissured, fibrotic granuloma of the gum and buccal mucosa, occurring on an edentulous alveolar ridge and in the fold between the ridge and cheek; it is caused by an ill-fitting denture. 2. acanthoma fissuratum.

foreign body g. a localized reaction in the skin or a mucous membrane to the presence of a foreign body such as starch, talc, or oil; it is usually a firm nodule with infiltration of macrophages.

g. fungoi′des mycosis fungoides.

g. gangraenes′cens lethal midline g.

giant cell g., giant cell reparative g. a type of lesion of the jaws characterized by a proliferation of vascular connective tissue and multinucleate giant cells. The etiology is unknown, but a possible link to earlier trauma has made some authorities use the word *reparative* with these lesions. Two types are distinguished: the *central giant cell granuloma* and the *peripheral giant cell granuloma* or *giant cell epulis.*

g. glutea′le infan′tum a type of dermatosis seen in the diaper area or buttocks of infants, characterized clinically by oval nodules resembling hemangiomas or hematomas, and histologically by hyperkeratosis, acanthosis, and an infiltrate of polymorphonuclear leukocytes mixed with plasma cells and macrophages throughout the dermis. Recovery is usually spontaneous. Called also *infantile gluteal g.*

g. gravida′rum pregnancy tumor.

Hodgkin g. see under *disease.*

infantile gluteal g. g. gluteale infantum.

infectious g. a granulomatous lesion due to an infectious agent, such as a bacterium or fungus.

g. inguina′le a chronic, slowly progressive, ulcerative granulomatous disease, spread by uncleanliness and sometimes by sexual transmission, seen in the tropics and subtropics. It is caused by *Klebsiella granulomatis* and primarily involves the skin and lymphatics of the anogenital region;

sometimes it spreads to the adjacent perineal or inguinal regions. Called also *donovanosis*, *g. pudendi*, *g. venereum*, and *pudendal ulcer*.

laryngeal g. a firm nodule on the larynx due to trauma, particularly from endotracheal intubation or from excessive use of the voice.

lethal midline g. a progressive, localized, destructive process of the face, occurring chiefly in males; it involves predominantly the nose, paranasal sinuses, and palate, with erosion through contiguous structures such as the orbit and face and destruction of soft tissue, bone, and cartilage. There is also associated nonspecific acute and chronic inflammation, as well as necrosis with or without granuloma formation. Called also *g. gangraenescens* and *midline g.*

linear g. a skin lesion of young cats, consisting of circumscribed raised discolored linear plaques, usually on the posterior thigh but sometimes on the lips or in the mouth. It is part of the eosinophilic granuloma complex.

lipoid g. xanthoma.

lipophagic g. a granuloma resulting from loss or breakdown of subcutaneous fat, such as in panniculitis and certain other conditions.

Majocchi g. trichophytic g.

malarial g. a granulomatous lesion sometimes seen in the brain in fatal cases of cerebral malaria.

midline g. lethal midline g.

Miescher g. annular elastolytic giant cell g.

g. multifor′me a rare type of granuloma seen most often in women in Central Africa and other tropical areas, thought to be an atypical form of granuloma annulare, characterized by multiple round, papulonodular lesions with plaques and nodules.

oil g. a granuloma formed around an abnormal collection of oil in the body; some are due to repeated inhalation of oil droplets by workers in certain occupations, and others are the result of injection under the skin of oily substances.

paracoccidioidal g. paracoccidioidomycosis.

periapical g. a slowly expanding, spherical, granulomatous lesion adjacent to the root apex of a tooth, usually occurring as a complication of pulpitis. It consists of a proliferating mass of chronic inflammatory tissue enclosed within a fibrous capsule that is an extension of the periodontal ligament. Called also *apical g.*, *dental g.*, and *chronic apical periodontitis*.

peripheral giant cell g., peripheral giant cell reparative g. giant cell epulis.

plasma cell g. inflammatory pseudotumor.

pseudopyogenic g. a superficial variant of angiolymphoid hyperplasia with eosinophilia; see under *hyperplasia*.

g. puden′di g. inguinale.

pyogenic g., g. pyoge′nicum a usually solitary polypoid type of capillary hemangioma (which is neither pyogenic nor a true granuloma). The usual location is on the skin or oral mucous membranes; it is often associated with trauma or local irritation, representing a vasoproliferative inflammatory response. It presents as a small papule that enlarges, may pedunculate, and may become infected and ulcerate to release blood or exudate. Called also *g. telangiectaticum*. See also *angiogranuloma*.

reparative giant cell g. giant cell g.

reticulohistiocytic g. a solitary reticulohistiocytoma, seen mainly in men; in contrast to multicentric reticulocytosis, this type of reticulohistiocytoma is not associated with systemic involvement.

rheumatic g′s nodules found in various parts of the body in rheumatic fever.

sarcoid g., sarcoidal g. the granuloma seen with sarcoidosis, consisting of multinucleated giant cells surrounded by macrophages and epithelioid cells. The appearance is nonspecific; similar granulomas may be seen in other conditions.

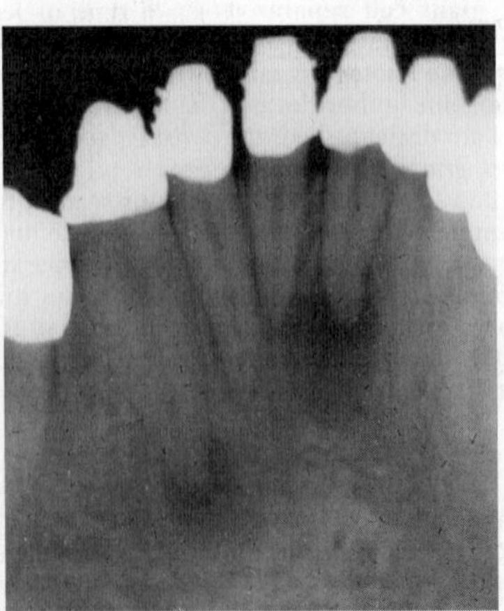

■ Periapical granulomas associated with nonvital teeth.

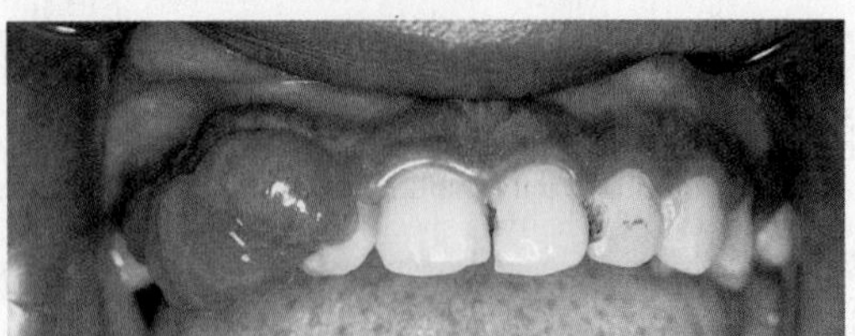

■ Pyogenic granuloma.

schistosomal g., schistosome g. a granuloma formed around deposited eggs of the parasites in schistosomiasis; the location depends on the species of parasite, but the intestines and liver are most common.

sea urchin g. a type of foreign body granuloma in the skin around the spine of a sea urchin.

silicotic g. a granuloma induced by silica particles; see *silicosis*.

stitch g. a foreign-body granuloma occurring around a buried nonabsorbable suture.

swimming pool g. a chronic granulomatous bacterial infection caused by contamination of an abrasion by *Mycobacterium marinum* from a swimming pool, aquarium, or similar enclosed tank of water that does not circulate enough. The most common sites of abrasions are on the elbows, fingers, backs of the hands, and knees. There is a papule or pustule at the site of inoculation that enlarges and may break down and become covered by a brownish crust; if there is no reinfection, the lesion heals spontaneously over several months. Called also *aquarium* or *fish tank g.*

g. telangiecta′ticum pyogenic g.

trichophytic g., g. trichophy′ticum a rare form of tinea corporis of the lower legs, also infecting the hair shafts, caused by *Trichophyton rubrum*. It is characterized by elevated, circumscribed, red to blue granulomas, either disseminated or in chains. After several months, lesions either are absorbed slowly or undergo necrosis and leave depressed scars. Called also *Majocchi g.* and *tinea profunda*.

tuberculoid g. a granuloma characterized by the grouping of macrophages into follicles that resemble tubercles, often with central necrosis; seen most often in the lungs in any of various inflammatory conditions.

umbilical g. granulation tissue on the stem of the umbilical cord in newborn infants.

g. vene′reum g. inguinale.

Winkelmann g. cutaneous extravascular necrotizing g.

xanthomatous g. eosinophilic g.

zirconium g. a papular granulomatous eruption consisting of shiny, red or brown lesions, representing an allergic reaction to zirconium ions or salts that may be components of antiperspirants, deodorants, or lotions used to treat poison ivy.

gran·u·lo·ma·to·sis (gran″u-lo″mə-to′sis) any condition characterized by formation of granulomas.

allergic g. Churg-Strauss syndrome.

bronchocentric g. a rare disorder consisting of necrosis of the walls of the lower airways, filling of the lumen with granular necrotic material, and eventually areas of lung consolidation; many cases are due to a hypersensitivity reaction to infection by fungi, such as with allergic bronchopulmonary aspergillosis.

eosinophilic g. eosinophilic granuloma.

intestinal lipophagic g. Whipple disease.

Langerhans cell g. see under *histiocytosis*.

lymphomatoid g. an immunoproliferative disorder that is angiogenic and characterized by tissue infiltration and nodular granulomatous inflammation with atypical lymphocytes and plasmacytoid cells; the organs involved are usually the lungs, skin, central nervous system, or kidneys. Presenting symptoms include cough, shortness of breath, and chest pain; extrapulmonary manifestations are common, such as skin nodules.

necrotizing sarcoid g., necrotizing sarcoidal g. a rare lung condition characterized by focal areas of vasculitis with necrosis and confluent granulomas; it resembles sarcoidosis and usually has a benign course.

orofacial g. chronic, nontender swelling of the lips, face, and oral cavity. In some patients this is a manifestation of Crohn disease and in others it is an allergic response to certain foods or food additives. See also *cheilitis granulomatosa*.

g. sidero′tica a condition in which brownish nodules (Gamna nodules) are seen in the enlarged spleen.

Wegener g. a multisystem disease chiefly affecting males, characterized by necrotizing granulomatous vasculitis involving the upper and lower respiratory tracts, glomerulonephritis, and variable degrees of the ANCA-associated type of small vessel vasculitis. Most authorities consider this condition to be an aberrant hypersensitivity reaction to an unknown antigen.

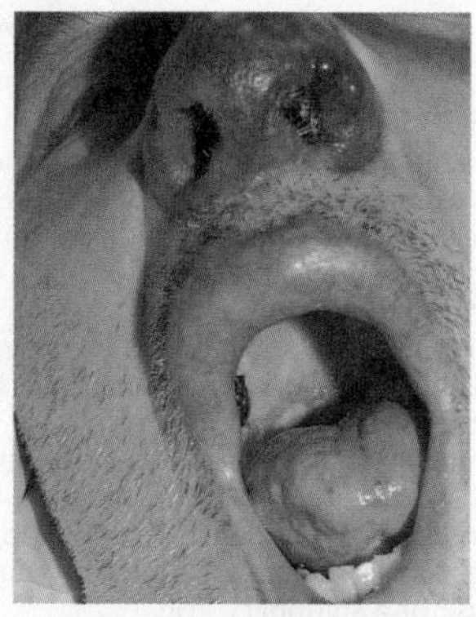

■ Wegener granulomatosis, with necrotic lesions of the nose and ulcerations in the mouth due to vasculitis of larger vessels.

gran·u·lom·a·tous (gran″u-lom′ə-təs) containing granulomas.

gran·u·lo·mere (gran′u-lo-mēr″) the center portion of a platelet, which in a dry, stained blood smear appears to be filled with fine purplish granules; it is surrounded by the hyalomere.

gran·u·lo·pe·nia (gran″u-lo-pe′ne-ə) granulocytopenia.

gran·u·lo·plas·tic (gran″u-lo-plas′tik) [*granulo-* + *plastic*] forming granules.

gran·u·lo·poi·e·sis (gran″u-lo-poi-e′sis) [*granulocyte* + *-poiesis*] the production or formation of granulocytes; see also *granulocytic series*, under *series*. Called also *granulocytopoiesis*. **granulopoiet′ic** *adj*

gran·u·lo·poi·e·tin (gran″u-lo-poi′ə-tin) a hypothesized substance, probably a colony-stimulating factor, that serves as the humoral regulator of granulopoiesis. Called also *leukopoietin*.

Gran·u·lo·re·tic·u·lo·sea (gran″u-lo-rə-tik″u-lo′se-ə) [*granulo-* + *reticular*] a class of ameboid protozoa (superclass Rhizopoda, subphylum Sarcodina), the organisms of which have delicate, finely granular or hyaline reticulopodia or, rarely, finely pointed, granular but nonanastomosing pseudopodia. It includes three orders: Athalamida, Monothalamida, and Foraminiferida.

gran·u·lo·sa (gran″u-lo′sə) pertaining to the cells of the cumulus oophorus; see also under *cell*.

gran·u·lose (gran′u-lōs) 1. a bacterial polysaccharide resembling amylopectin, occurring as cytoplasmic granules and staining red violet with iodine. 2. having a granular appearance.

gran·u·lo·sis (gran″u-lo′sis) the formation of a mass of granules.

g. ru′bra na′si a rare autosomal dominant condition of the skin of the face, consisting of hyperhidrosis of the nose, adjacent areas of the face, and sometimes the chin, accompanied by red papules and sometimes many small vesicles. It is usually seen in children, clearing up at puberty, although in some individuals it persists into adulthood.

gran·u·los·i·ty (gran″u-los′ĭ-te) a mass of granulations.

gran·u·lo·vac·u·o·lar (gran″u-lo-vak″u-o′lər) [*granulo-* + *vacuole*] characterized by granules and vacuoles.

gra·num (gra′nəm) pl. *gra′na* [L. "grain"] see *grana*.

grapes (grāps) bovine tuberculosis.

grape·seed (grāp′sēd) see under *seed*.

graph (graf) [Gr. *graphein* to write, or record] a diagram or curve representing varying relationships between sets of data.

graph·an·es·the·sia (graf-an″es-the′zhə) agraphesthesia.

-graph a word termination denoting an instrument for writing or recording; also, the record made by such an instrument.

graph·es·the·sia (graf″es-the′zhə) [*graph-* + *esthesia*] the ability to recognize figures or numbers written on the skin with a dull-pointed object.

graph·ic (graf′ik) [*graph-* + *-ic*] written or drawn; pertaining to representation by diagrams.

graph·ite (graf′īt) [L. *graphites*, from Gr. *graphis* a writing instrument] a form of native mineralized carbon; inhalation of its dust causes a form of pneumoconiosis. Called also *plumbago*.

graph·i·to·sis (graf″ĭ-to′sis) graphite pneumoconiosis.

Graph·i·um (graf′e-əm) a genus of imperfect fungi of the form-class Hyphomycetes that produce several cultural spore types; inhalation of sawdust containing the spores causes sequoiosis.

graph(o)- [Gr. *graphein* to write] a combining form denoting relationship to writing or to a record.

grapho·anal·y·sis (graf″o-ə-nal′ə-sis) analysis of personality based on handwriting.

gra·phol·o·gy (graf-ol′ə-je) [*grapho-* + *-logy*] the study of handwriting, applied to personal identification or psychological study of the writer.

grapho·mo·tor (graf″o-mo′tər) [*grapho-* + *motor*] pertaining to, or affecting, the movements required in writing.

graph·or·rhea (graf″o-re′ə) [*grapho-* + *-rrhea*] the writing of a long succession of meaningless and unconnected words.

grapho·spasm (graf′o-spaz″əm) writers' cramp.

-graphy [Gr. *-graphia*, from *graphein* to write] a word termination meaning the process of writing or recording, or a method of recording.

Gra·ser diverticulum (grah′zər) [Ernst *Graser*, German surgeon, 1860–1929] see under *diverticulum*.

grass (gras) any plant of the family Gramineae; many are commonly used as fodder for cattle and horses, and the family also includes food plants such as grains and sugar cane. Grasses whose pollen is important as a cause of hay fever include Bermuda grass *(Cynodon dactylon);* Kentucky bluegrass or June grass *(Poa pratensis);* Johnson grass *(Sorghum halepense);* orchard grass *(Dactylis glomerata);* redtop grass *(Agrostis alba);* sweet vernal grass *(Anthoxanthum odoratum);* and timothy or timothy grass *(Phleum pratense)*. Johnson grass, Sudan grass, and arrow grass (*Triglochin* species) contain cyanogenetic compounds; timothy sometimes contains the mold *Claviceps purpurea;* and sweet vernal grass contains dicumarol. Any of these, when eaten in large quantities, can be fatal to livestock.

canary g. any of various species of grasses of the genus *Phalaris*. See also *Phalaris staggers*, under *staggers*.

couch g. the perennial grass *Agropyrum repens;* its long roots are diuretic, demulcent, and antitussive and have been used to treat cystitis.

panic g. any of several members of the genus *Panicum*.

scurvy g. *Cochlearia officinalis*.

Gras·set phenomenon (sign) (grah-sa′) [Joseph *Grasset*, French physician, 1849–1918] see under *phenomenon*.

Gras·set-By·chow·ski sign (grah-sa′ be-kof′ske) [J. *Grasset;* Zygmunt *Bychowski*, Polish neurologist, 1860–1935] Grasset phenomenon; see under *phenomenon*.

Gras·set-Gaus·sel phenomenon (grah-sa′ go-sel′) [J. *Grasset;* Amans *Gaussel*, French physician, 1871–1937] Grasset phenomenon; see under *phenomenon*.

Gras·set-Gaus·sel-Hoo·ver sign (grah-sa′ go-sel′ hoo′vər) [J. *Grasset;* A. *Gaussel;* Charles Franklin *Hoover*, American physician, 1865–1927] Hoover sign (def. 1); see under *sign*.

grat·ing (gra′ting) a grill or grid, or something resembling such a structure.

diffraction g. a surface, usually glass or polished metal, that is ruled closely with fine parallel lines, grooves, or slits; used to separate the wavelengths of light in a spectroscope.

Gra·ti·o·la (grə-ti′o-lə) a genus of small herbs of the family Scrophulaceae. *G. officina′lis* is the hedge hyssop, a European species used as a cathartic, emetic, and diuretic.

Gra·ti·o·let radiating fibers, radiation (grah-te″o-la′) [Louis Pierre *Gratiolet*, French anatomist, 1815–1865] see under *fiber*, and see *radiatio optica*.

grat·tage (grah-tahzh′) [Fr.] the removal of granulations (as in trachoma) by scraping or by friction with a stiff brush.

grave (grāv) [L. *gravis*] severe or serious.

grav·el (grav′əl) fairly coarse concretions of mineral salts, as from the kidneys or bladder, of smaller size than the usual calculi.

Graves dermopathy, disease, orbitopathy (ophthalmopathy) (grāvz) [Robert James *Graves*, Irish physician, 1796–1853] see *pretibial myxedema*, under *myxedema*, and see under *disease* and *orbitopathy*.

gravi- [L. *gravis* heavy] a combining form denoting relationship to weight or pregnancy.

grav·id (grav′id) [L. *gravida* heavy, pregnant] pregnant.

grav·i·da (grav′ĭ-də) [L.] a pregnant woman. Called *gravida I* or *primigravida* during the first pregnancy, *gravida II* or *secundigravida* during the second pregnancy, *gravida III* or *tertigravida* during the third pregnancy, and so on. Symbol G. Cf. *para*.

gra·vid·ic (grə-vid′ik) occurring in pregnancy.

gra·vid·i·tas (grə-vid′ĭ-təs) [L.] pregnancy.

g. examnia′lis pregnancy in which the amnion has burst and is retracted around the insertion of the umbilical cord, but the chorion is intact.

g. exochoria′lis pregnancy in which the membranes have burst and shrunk, leaving the fetus in the uterus but outside of the chorion.

gra•vid•i•ty (grah-vid′ĭ-te) [L. *graviditas*] 1. pregnancy. 2. the condition of being pregnant, without regard to the outcome. Cf. *parity.*

grav•i•do•car•di•ac (grav″ĭ-do-kahr′de-ak) [*gravida* + *cardiac*] pertaining to heart disease of pregnancy.

grav•i•do•pu•er•per•al (grav″ĭ-do-pu-ur′pər-əl) [*gravida* + *puerperal*] pertaining to pregnancy and the puerperium.

gra•vim•e•ter (grə-vim′ə-tər) [L. *gravis* heavy + *-meter*] an instrument for determining specific gravities.

grav•i•met•ric (grav″ĭ-met′rik) pertaining to measurement by weight; performed by weight, as a gravimetric method of drug assay.

grav•i•ta•tion (grav″ĭ-ta′shən) the phenomenon of attraction between massive bodies; see *law of gravitation.*

grav•i•tom•e•ter (grav″ĭ-tom′ə-tər) a balance for measuring specific gravity.

grav•i•ty (grav′ĭ-te) [L. *gravitas*] 1. the phenomenon by which two bodies having mass are attracted to each other. 2. the gravitational attraction near a large body having mass, particularly near or on the surface of a planet or star.

specific g. (sp gr) the ratio of the density of a substance to that of a reference substance at a specific temperature.

standard g. (g) the acceleration due to gravity at mean sea level on earth, 9.80616 meters per second squared. Called also *acceleration of gravity.*

Gra•witz tumor (grah′vits) [Paul Albert *Grawitz*, German pathologist, 1850–1932] see under *tumor.*

gray (gra) 1. of a hue between white and black. 2. a unit of absorbed radiation dose equal to 100 rads. Abbreviated Gy.

silver g., steel g. nigrosin.

gray•a•no•tox•in (gra′ə-no-tok″sin) andromedotoxin.

grease (grēs) greasy heel.

grease-heel (grēs-hēl′) greasy heel.

Gre•be chondrodysplasia (gra′bə) [Hans *Grebe*, German internist and geneticist, 1913–1999] see under *chondrodysplasia.*

green (grēn) 1. a color between yellow and blue, produced by energy with wavelengths between 490 and 570 nm. 2. a dye or stain with this color.

acid g. any of several green acid dyes, generally light g. SF.

bromcresol g. an indicator, tetrabromo-*m*-cresolsulfonphthalein, used in the determination of hydrogen ion concentration, being yellow at pH 4.0 and blue at pH 5.4. Written also *bromocresol g.*

diazin g. S Janus g. B.

fast g. FCF a green acid dye used as a histologic stain for plasma and collagen.

fast acid g. N light g. SF yellowish.

Hoffman g. iodine g.

indocyanine g. [USP] a dye occurring as an olive-brown, dark green, dark blue, or black powder; used intravenously as a diagnostic aid in determination of plasma volume and of blood flow in organs such as the eyes, kidneys, and lungs; in measurement of cardiac output; and in liver function tests.

iodine g. a triphenylmethane dye used as a chromatin stain.

Janus g. B an azo dye used supravitally for the demonstration of mitochondria.

light g., 2 G or 2 GN light g. SF yellowish.

light g. SF see *acid g.*

light g. SF yellowish an acid dye used as a plasma stain.

malachite g. a triphenylmethane dye used as a biologic stain.

methyl g. a green basic triphenylmethane dye used as a histologic counterstain and as the DNA-staining component of methyl green–pyronin stain.

methylene g. a dye formed by nitrating methylene blue, interesting for its dark green metachromasia; it is a component of polychrome methylene blue.

Paris g. copper acetoarsenite.

Schweinfurt g. copper acetoarsenite.

Victoria g. malachite g.

Green•field filter (grēn′fēld) [Lazar J. *Greenfield*, American surgeon, 20th century] see under *filter.*

greg•a•loid (greg′ə-loid) [L. *grex* flock + *-oid*] said of a type of loose colony of protozoa; see under *colony.*

Greig syndrome (greg) [David Middleton *Greig*, Scottish physician, 1864–1936] ocular hypertelorism; see under *hypertelorism.*

Grei•ther disease (keratosis) (gri′ter) [Aloys *Greither*, German dermatologist, 1914–1986] see under *disease.*

grenz (grents) [Ger. *Grenze* border] the abnormal type of histopathological border seen in a grenz zone.

Grey Tur•ner sign (gra′ tur′nər) [George *Grey Turner*, British surgeon, 1877–1951] Turner sign; see under *sign.*

GRH growth hormone–releasing hormone.

grid (grid) 1. an arrangement of thin lead strips separated by a radiolucent medium; used to reduce the amount of scattered radiation reaching the x-ray film. 2. a chart with horizontal and perpendicular lines for plotting curves.

Amsler g. the grid on an Amsler chart.

baby g. a direct reading control chart on infant growth.

crossed g. two parallel grids arranged so that the lead strips of one are at right angles to the lead strips of the other.

focused g. a parallel grid in which the lead strips are angled so that they all point toward a focus at a specified distance.

moving g. a parallel grid that is moved continuously or oscillated throughout the making of a radiograph; used to eliminate the grid lines that occur with the use of a stationary grid.

parallel g. in radiography, one in which the lead strips are oriented parallel to each other; rather than angled as in a focused grid.

Potter-Bucky g. a type of parallel grid that is an integral part of the x-ray table, located below the table top and above a cassette tray. It decreases the amount of secondary radiation reaching the film, thus increasing detail and contrast, and moves during exposure so that no grid lines appear in the radiograph.

stationary g. a parallel grid placed in apposition to a radiographic film for its accentuation of detail; the grid lines will be visible on the resultant radiographs.

Wetzel g. a direct reading chart for evaluating physical fitness in terms of body build, developmental level, and basal metabolism.

grief (grēf) the normal emotional response to an external and consciously recognized loss; it involves a period of mourning and generally is self-limited, gradually subsiding within a reasonable time. See also *mourning.*

Grie•sin•ger disease, sign (gre′zing-ər) [Wilhelm *Griesinger*, German neurologist, 1817–1868] see *hookworm disease*, under *disease*, and see under *sign.*

Griess test (grēs) [Johann Peter *Griess*, German-born chemist in England, 1829–1888] see under *test.*

Grif•fith sign (grif′ith) [J. *Griffith*, English ophthalmologist, late 19th century] see under *sign.*

Grig•nard reagent (compound) (grēn-yahr′) [François Auguste Victor *Grignard*, French chemist, 1871–1935] see under *reagent.*

Gri•ful•vin (grĭ-ful′vin) trademark for preparations of griseofulvin.

grind•ing (grīnd′ing) 1. rubbing together with force; wearing away or polishing by rubbing. 2. crushing of food by the posterior teeth in mastication, especially by molars. 3. bruxism. 4. shaping of a tooth contour through the use of abrasive tools. See also *occlusal adjustment*, under *adjustment.*

selective g. modification of the occlusal forms of teeth by grinding at select places.

spot g. elimination of high places or occlusal interferences on natural dentitions or dentures by grinding.

grind•ing-in (grīnd′ing-in) the process of correcting errors in the centric and eccentric occlusions of natural or artificial teeth. See also *milling-in.*

grip[1] (grip) [A.S. *gripe*, grasp] a grasping or seizing.

devil's g. epidemic pleurodynia.

hook g. a functional posture of the hand, as that usually assumed when grasping handles or straps or suspending or pulling upon an object: the fingers are flexed toward the palm, to a degree depending on the size of the grasped object.

power g. a functional posture of the hand, as that usually assumed when holding a hammer or piece of rope: the fingers are flexed around an object, with counter pressure from the thumb, which is positioned to bring either its pad or its medial border firmly against the held object.

precision g. a functional posture of the hand, as that usually assumed when holding a pen or pencil: the object is grasped between the tips of the thumb and fingers (most often the index, with the middle often involved).

grip[2] (grip) [Fr. *grippe*] influenza.

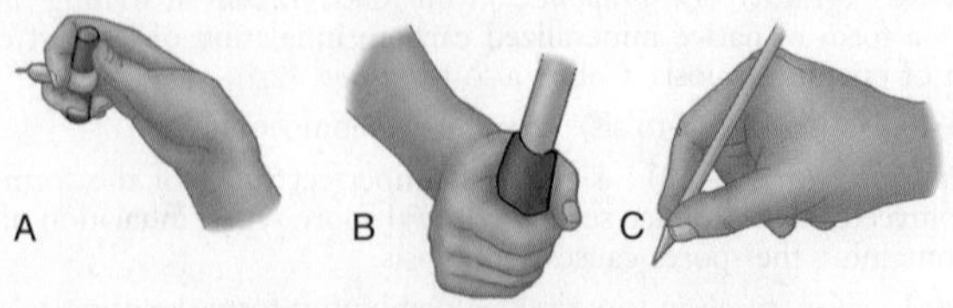

■ *(A)*, Hook grip; *(B)*, power grip; *(C)*, precision grip.

gastric g. a groove or canal through the reticulum, omasum, and abomasum of a ruminant, analogous to the gastric canal of humans. It is subdivided into the *reticular*, *omasal*, and *abomasal grooves*.
genital g. urethral g.
gingival g. sulcus gingivalis.
greater palatine g. of maxilla sulcus palatinus major maxillae.
greater palatine g. of palatine bone sulcus palatinus major ossis palatini.
greater petrosal g., g. for greater petrosal nerve sulcus nervi petrosi majoris.
Harrison g. a horizontal depression along the lower border of the thorax, corresponding to the costal insertion of the diaphragm; seen in advanced rickets in children.
hyopharyngeal g. second pharyngeal g.
inferior interventricular g. sulcus interventricularis posterior.
g. for inferior petrosal sinus sulcus sinus petrosi inferioris.
infraorbital g. sulcus infraorbitalis.
interatrial g. a slight depression on the external surface of the heart, marking the separation of the atria.
interdental g. a linear, vertical depression on the surface of the interdental papillae; it functions as a sluiceway for the egress of food from the interproximal areas.
intersphincteric g. sulcus intersphinctericus analis.
intertubercular g. of humerus sulcus intertubercularis humeri.
interventricular g. of heart interventricular sulcus of heart.
labial g. an embryonic groove produced by degeneration of the central cells of the labial lamina, which later becomes the vestibule of the oral cavity.
lacrimal g. sulcus lacrimalis.
lacrimal g. in lacrimal bone sulcus lacrimalis ossis lacrimalis.
lacrimal g. in maxilla sulcus lacrimalis maxillae.
laryngotracheal g. a furrow at the caudal end of the floor of the embryonic pharynx that develops into the respiratory tract.
lateral bicipital g. sulcus bicipitalis lateralis.
lateral g. of mesencephalon sulcus lateralis mesencephali.
lateral nail g. the groove where the nail plate meets a lateral nail wall.
g. for lesser petrosal nerve sulcus nervi petrosi minoris.
lingual g., lingual developmental g. a developmental groove on the lingual surface of a posterior tooth.
major g. in DNA, the larger groove occurring between successive turns of the two antiparallel chains around the helical axis. See illustration at *deoxyribonucleic acid.* Cf. *minor g.*
malleolar g. of fibula sulcus malleolaris fibulae.
malleolar g. of tibia sulcus malleolaris tibiae.
g. for marginal sinus sulcus sinus marginalis.
medial bicipital g. sulcus bicipitalis medialis.
medullary g. neural g.
mesiobuccal g., mesiobuccal developmental g. the mesial of the two buccal grooves ordinarily found on the mandibular first molar.
mesiolingual g., mesiolingual developmental g. a groove marking the junction of the fifth cusp with the palatal surface on an upper molar tooth.
g. for middle meningeal artery sulcus arteriae meningeae mediae.
g. for middle temporal artery sulcus arteriae temporalis mediae.
minor g. in DNA, the smaller groove occurring between the two antiparallel chains as they wind around the helical axis. See illustration at *deoxyribonucleic acid.* Cf. *major g.*
musculospiral g. sulcus nervi radialis.
mylohyoid g. sulcus mylohyoideus mandibulae.
nail g. 1. a pathologic groove in a nail, such as a Beau line (see under *line*). 2. see *lateral nail g.* and *proximal nail g.*
g. of nail matrix the cutaneous fold in which the proximal edge of the nail is embedded; called also *sulcus matricis unguis.*
nasolacrimal g. an epithelial ingrowth parallel with but medial to the nasomaxillary groove of the embryo, which marks the site of later development of the nasolacrimal duct.
nasomaxillary g. a furrow located between the maxillary and the lateral nasal prominences of the same side in the embryo.
nasopalatine g. a furrow on the lateral surface of the vomer for the nasopalatine nerve and vessels.
nasopharyngeal g. a faint line between the nasal cavity and the nasopharynx.
neural g. the groove produced by the invagination of the neural plate of the embryo during the process of formation of the neural tube; called also *medullary g.*
obturator g. sulcus obturatorius.
occipital g. sulcus arteriae occipitalis.
g. for occipital sinus sulcus sinus occipitalis.
occlusal g. one of the developmental grooves on the occlusal surface of a posterior tooth.

olfactory g. 1. sulcus olfactorius nasi. 2. ethmoid fossa. 3. sulcus olfactorius lobi frontalis.
omasal g. the part of the gastric groove of a ruminant that is located in the omentum.
optic g. sulcus prechiasmaticus.
palatine g's of maxilla sulci palatinae maxillae.
palatovaginal g. sulcus palatovaginalis.
pharyngeal g's the embryonic ectodermal clefts between successive pharyngeal arches; each one is named for the pharyngeal arch just in front of it. Called also *branchial g's* or *clefts*.
g. for popliteus sulcus popliteus femoris.
posterior auricular g. sulcus posterior auriculae.
posterior interventricular g. sulcus interventricularis posterior.
posterolateral g. of medulla oblongata sulcus posterolateralis medullae oblongatae.
posterolateral g. of spinal cord sulcus posterolateralis medullae spinalis.
preauricular g. of ilium see under *sulcus*.
primitive g. a lengthwise median furrow in the primitive streak of the embryo; in human embryos it is clearly visible during the third week. Called also *primordial g.* or *furrow*.
primitive dental g. a groove in the border of the jaws of the embryo.
primordial g. primitive g.
g. of promontory of tympanic cavity sulcus promontorii tympani.
proximal nail g. the groove next to a cuticle where the nail plate meets the proximal nail wall.
g. of pterygoid hamulus sulcus hamuli pterygoidei.
pulmonary g. sulcus pulmonalis.
radial g., g. for radial nerve sulcus nervi radialis.
reticular g. the part of the gastric groove of a ruminant that is located in the reticulum.
retro-olivary g. sulcus retroolivaris.
sagittal g. sulcus sinus sagittalis superioris.
Sibson g. a furrow sometimes seen at the lower border of the pectoralis major muscle.
sigmoid g., g. for sigmoid sinus sulcus sinus sigmoidei.
skin g's sulci cutis.
g. for spinal nerve sulcus nervi spinalis.
spiral g. sulcus nervi radialis.
subclavian g. 1. sulcus arteriae subclaviae. 2. sulcus musculi subclavii. 3. sulcus venae subclaviae. 4. g. for subclavian artery (def. 2).
g. for subclavian artery 1. sulcus arteriae subclaviae. 2. a broad, shallow, transverse groove across the top of each lung, lodging the subclavian artery.
g. for subclavian vein sulcus venae subclaviae.
g. for subclavius sulcus musculi subclavii.
subcostal g. sulcus costae.
g. for superior petrosal sinus sulcus sinus petrosi superioris.
g. for superior sagittal sinus sulcus sinus sagittalis superioris.
supplemental g's grooves on the surface of a tooth that do not mark (as do the developmental grooves) the junction of the primary lobes of the tooth.
supra-acetabular g. sulcus supraacetabularis.
g. for tendon of fibularis longus, g. for tendon of peroneus longus sulcus tendinis musculi fibularis longi.
g. for tendon of flexor hallucis longus sulcus tendinis musculi flexoris hallucis longi.
g. for tibialis posterior sulcus malleolaris tibiae.
g. for transverse sinus sulcus sinus transversi.
trigeminal g. the embryonic structure that develops into the trigeminal (gasserian) ganglion.
ulnar g., g. for ulnar nerve sulcus nervi ulnaris.
urethral g. the embryonic groove that becomes the penile urethra as the urogenital folds on each side fuse.
g. for vena cava sulcus venae cavae.
venous g's sulci venosi.
Verga lacrimal g. a groove running downward from the lower orifice of the nasal duct.
vertebral g. the depression on each side of the spine between the spinous processes, laminae, and transverse processes; it lodges the deep back muscles.
g. for vertebral artery sulcus arteriae vertebralis atlantis.
vomerine g. sulcus vomeris.
vomerovaginal g. sulcus vomerovaginalis.

Gross disease (grōs) [Samuel David *Gross*, American surgeon, 1805–1884] see under *disease*.

gross (grōs) [L. *grossus* rough] 1. coarse or large. 2. visible to the naked eye without the use of magnification; called also *macroscopic*.

ground (ground) 1. a path of conduction from an electrical circuit to the earth. 2. to connect an electrical circuit or electrical equipment to the earth.

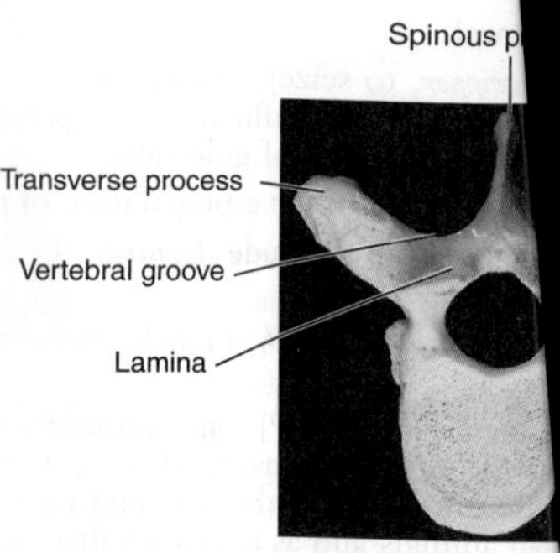

■ Vertebral groove, shown in a superior view of the se

ground-glass (ground-glas) having a filmy, h radiographs of a lung containing excess fluid.

ground•hog (ground′hog) woodchuck.

group (gro͞op) 1. an assemblage of objects or ind qualities in common; see also *population*. 2. a numb recognizable and usually a transferable portion of a
alcohol g. a combination of carbon, hydrogen, a molecule, which is characteristic of a chemical com alcohol. There are three: —CH_2OH, the primary; = ary; and ≡COH, the tertiary alcohol group.
amide g. the monovalent radical —$CONH_2$, der the replacement of the OH of the carboxyl group wit
azo g. a bivalent chemical group composed of —N=N—.
blood g. see *blood group*, under *B*.
CMN g. a group of bacteria composed of the *Mycobacterium*, and *Nocardia*, characterized by common mycolic acid constituents in the cell walls. Organisms o used as adjuvants in experimental immunization.
coli-aerogenes g. coliform bacteria.
colon-typhoid-dysentery g. a collective term refer the genera *Escherichia*, *Salmonella*, and *Shigella*.
control g. see *control* (def. 3).
coryneform g. see under *bacterium*.
Diagnosis-Related G's (DRG) groupings of diag used as a basis for hospital payment schedules by Me third-party payment plans.
dorsal respiratory g. part of the medullary respirator the length of the medulla oblongata, largely within the nu tary tract; its main function is to control the basic rhythm o *ventral respiratory g.*
encounter g. a sensitivity group in which the membe emotional rather than intellectual insight with emphasis o of interpersonal feelings in the group situation.
functional g. a part of a molecule that gives it charact properties, e.g., an aldehyde, alcohol, amine, carboxylic acid, ketone group.
glucophore g. see *glucophore*.
HACEK g. *Haemophilus aphrophilus*, *Actinobacillus acti tans*, *Cardiobacterium hominis*, *Eikenella corrodens*, and vari *Kingella*, species of gram-negative, capnophilic bacilli that a likely to infect heart valves or cause endocarditis.
hemorrhagic-septicemia g. a group of bacteria of whi *multocida* is the type organism.
Lancefield g. one of the groups of hemolytic strepto Lancefield classification.
methyl g. a monovalent chemical group, —CH_3.
osmophore g. see *osmophore*.
paratyphoid-enteritidis g. a group of organisms of *Salmonella* that cause food poisoning and other diseases.
peptide g. the bivalent radical, —CO•NH—, formed by tween the NH_2 and COOH groups of adjacent amino acids, a linkage building up compounds known as dipeptides, tripeptide tides, etc., depending on the number of amino acids making u ecule.
platelet g. a subset of platelets expressing a particular plate antigen, such as Pl(A1) antigen.
prosthetic g. a low-molecular-weight, nonprotein comp binds with a protein component (apoprotein, specifically apoe form a protein (e.g., holoenzyme) with biologic activity.
Runyon g. one of four divisions of nontuberculous mycobact sified according to pigmentation and rate of growth. See *nont mycobacteria*, under *mycobacterium*.

sapophore g. see *sapophore.*

sensitivity g., sensitivity training g. a nonclinical group not intended for persons with mental illnesses or substantial emotional problems, which, in an effort to develop the assets of leadership, management, counseling, or other roles, focuses on self-awareness and understanding and on interpersonal interactions. Called also *training g. (T-g.).*

sulfonic g. a monovalent radical, —SO_2OH.

T-g. sensitivity g.

training g. sensitivity g.

ventral respiratory g. part of the medullary respiratory center running the length of the medulla oblongata within and next to the nucleus ambiguus; these neurons mainly function during strong, active respiration, moving voluntary muscles in the control of inhalation and exhalation or modifying the behavior of other respiratory motoneurons. Cf. *dorsal respiratory g.*

group·er (gro͞op′ər) any of various large, carnivorous, marine fish of the genera *Epinepherus* and *Mycteroperca,* found in tropical waters; they are often eaten, but may contain ciguatoxin and cause ciguatera.

group·ing (gro͞op′ing) the classification of individual entities according to certain common characteristics.

blood g. the classification of blood according to blood group, done to determine its suitability for transfusion in a given recipient, to settle cases of disputed paternity, and to trace substances in certain criminal cases. See *blood group,* under *B.*

haptenic g. hapten.

group-spe·cif·ic (gro͞op″spə-sif′ik) specific for a given group; as a blood group or certain microorganisms; said of agglutinins.

group-trans·fer (gro͞op″trans′fər) denoting a chemical reaction, excluding oxidation and reduction, in which molecules exchange functional groups, a process catalyzed by enzymes called transferases.

Gro·ver disease (gro′vər) [R.W. *Grover,* American dermatologist, 20th century] transient acantholytic dermatosis; see under *dermatosis.*

growth (grōth) 1. a normal process of increase in size of an organism as a result of accretion of tissue similar to that originally present. Cf. *differentiation.* 2. an abnormal formation, such as a tumor. 3. the proliferation of cells, as in a bacterial culture.

absolute g. an expression of the actual increase in size of an individual, or of a particular organ or part.

accretionary g. increase in size resulting from increase in number of special cells by mitotic division, other more differentiated cells which perform various physiologic functions having lost the ability to proliferate.

allometric g. the growth of different organs or parts of an organism at different rates.

appositional g. growth by addition at the periphery of a particular structure or part. Cf. *interstitial g.*

auxetic g. auxesis.

condylar g. the growth of the condyle of the temporomandibular joint, usually reflected in a downward and forward positioning of the mandible and teeth.

differential g. an expression of the comparison of the increases in size of dissimilar organisms, organs, or parts.

heterogonous g. growth of such a nature that, when it is plotted logarithmically, it gives a straight line.

histiotypic g. uncontrolled growth of cells as occurs in tissue cultures.

interstitial g. growth occurring in the interior of parts or structures already formed. Cf. *appositional g.*

intussusceptive g. auxesis.

isometric g. the growth of different organs or parts of an organism at the same rate.

multiplicative g. increase in the size of an organism, organ, or part, resulting from increase in the number of cells brought about by their mitotic division, the average size of the cells remaining about the same.

new g. a neoplasm, or tumor.

organotypic g. controlled growth of cells as occurs normally in the production of organs and parts.

relative g. an expression of the comparison of the increases in size of similar organisms, organs, or parts.

grü·bel·sucht (gre′bel-sookt) [Ger. *grübeln* to brood, ponder + *sucht* illness] the drawing of overly fine distinctions (hair-splitting); worrying over trifles. Seen particularly in obsessive-compulsive personalities.

Gru·ber syndrome (groo′ber) [Georg Benito Otto *Gruber,* German pathologist, 1884–1977] Meckel syndrome.

Gruen·tzig balloon catheter (grēn′tsig) [Andreas Roland *Gruentzig,* German radiologist, 1939–1985] see under *catheter.*

gru·mose (groo′mōs) grumous.

gru·mous (groo′məs) [L. *grumus* heap] clotted or lumpy.

Gryn·feltt hernia, triangle (grā-felt′) [Joseph Casimir *Grynfeltt,* French surgeon, 1840–1913] see under *hernia,* and see *Lesshaft triangle,* under *triangle.*

Gryn·feltt-Less·haft triangle (grā-felt′ les′hahft) [J.C. *Grynfeltt;* Peter Frantsevich *Lesshaft,* Russian physician, 1837–1909] Lesshaft triangle.

gryo·chrome (gri′o-krōm) [Gr. *gry* morsel + *-chrome*] a nerve cell in which the stainable matter of the cell body appears as fine granules.

gry·pho·sis (grĭ-fo′sis) gryposis.

gry·po·sis (grĭ-po′sis) [Gr. *grypōsis* a crooking, hooking] abnormal curvature, as of the nails; called also *gryphosis.*

GSC gas-solid chromatography.

GSH reduced glutathione.

GSS Gerstmann-Sträussler-Scheinker syndrome.

GSSG oxidized glutathione.

gt. [L.] gut′ta (drop).

GTH gonadotropic hormone; see *gonadotropin.*

GTN gestational trophoblastic neoplasia.

GTP guanosine triphosphate.

GTPase (je-te-pe′ās) enzyme activity that catalyzes the hydrolysis of guanosine triphosphate to guanosine diphosphate and orthophosphate. GTPase converts GTP-binding proteins (q.v.) from the active to the inactive form.

GTP cy·clo·hy·dro·lase I (si′klo-hi′dro-lās) [EC 3.5.4.16] an enzyme of the hydrolase class that catalyzes the first step in the biosynthesis of tetrahydrobiopterin from guanosine triphosphate. Deficiency of the enzyme, an autosomal recessive trait caused by mutation of the *GCH1* gene encoding the enzyme, is a form of tetrahydrobiopterin deficiency (q.v.) with hyperphenylalaninemia; an autosomal dominant disorder with sex-influenced reduced penetrance caused by mutation of same gene manifests as a dopa-responsive dystonia without hyperphenylalaninemia, with reduced rate of tetrahydrobiopterin synthesis.

GTT glucose tolerance test.

gtt. [L.] gut′tae (drops).

GU genitourinary.

gua·co (gwah′ko) [Spanish American] any of several plants, especially *Mikania guaco,* used in South America to treat asthma, dyspepsia, gout, rheumatism, skin diseases, and snakebite.

guai·ac (gwi′ək) a resin from the wood of the tropical trees *Guaiacum officinale* and *G. sanctum,* used as a reagent in tests for occult blood and formerly in the treatment of rheumatism.

Guai·a·cum (gwi′ə-kəm) a genus of trees and shrubs of the family Zygophyllaceae, native to tropical regions of the Americas. *G. officina′le* L. and *G. sanc′tum* L. are trees found in Haiti and the Dominican Republic whose wood yields the resin guaiac.

guai·fen·e·sin (gwi-fen′ə-sin) [USP] an expectorant believed to act by reducing sputum viscosity, administered orally. Called also *glyceryl guaiacolate.*

gua·na·benz (gwah′nə-benz) an α_2-adrenergic agonist that stimulates the α_2-adrenergic receptors of the central nervous system, resulting in a reduction of sympathetic outflow to the heart and peripheral vascular system; used as an antihypertensive.

g. acetate [USP] an antihypertensive agent having the same actions as the base, administered orally.

gua·na·drel sul·fate (gwah′nə-drel) [USP] an adrenergic neuron blocking agent, used in the treatment of hypertension; administered orally.

gua·nase (gwah′nās) guanine deaminase.

guan·eth·i·dine mo·no·sul·fate (gwahn-eth′ĭ-dēn) [USP] an adrenergic neuron blocking agent used as an antihypertensive; administered orally.

guan·fa·cine hy·dro·chlo·ride (gwahn′fə-sēn) [USP] an α_2-adrenergic agonist that stimulates the α_2-adrenergic receptors of the central nervous system, resulting in a reduction of sympathetic outflow to the heart and peripheral vascular system, used as an antihypertensive; administered orally.

gua·ni·dine (gwah′nĭ-dēn) the compound $NH{=}C(NH_2)_2$, a strong base found in the urine as a normal product of protein metabolism. It is used in laboratory research as a protein denaturant.

g. phosphate a less correct term for *phosphoguanidine.*

gua·ni·dine-acet·ic ac·id (gwah′nĭ-dēn-ə-se′tik) guanidinoacetic acid.

gua·ni·din·emia (gwah″nĭ-dĭ-ne′me-ə) the presence of guanidine in the blood.

gua·ni·din·i·um (gwah″nĭ-din′e-əm) the radical derived from guanidine; the guanidinium group is an important component of arginine and creatine.

gua·ni·di·no (gwah″nĭ-de′no) guanidinium.

gua·ni·di·no·ac·e·tate (gwah″nĭ-de″no-as′ə-tāt) a salt or anionic form of guanidinoacetic acid.

gua·ni·di·no·ac·e·tate *N*-meth·yl·trans·fer·ase (gwah″nĭ-de″no-as′ə-tāt meth″əl-trans′fər-ās) [EC 2.1.1.2] a cytosolic enzyme of the transferase class that catalyzes the methylation of guanidinoacetate to form creatine, the final step in the biosynthesis of creatine. The methyl donor is *S*-adenosylmethionine, and the enzyme is concentrated in the kidney and pancreas.

gua·ni·di·no·a·ce·tic ac·id (gwah″nĭ-de″no-ə-se′tik) a nitrogenous compound formed enzymatically in the liver, pancreas, and kidney by a reaction transfering an amidino group between arginine and glycine, and *N*-methylated in the liver by *S*-adenosylmethionine to form creatine. Called also *glycocyamine, guanidine-acetic acid,* and *guanido-acetic acid.*

gua·ni·do (gwah′nĭ-do) guanidinium.

gua·ni·do-ace·tic ac·id (gwah″nĭ-do-ə-se′tik) guanidinoacetic acid.

gua·nine (gwah′nēn) a purine base, in animal and plant cells usually occurring condensed with ribose or deoxyribose to form the nucleosides guanosine and deoxyguanosine; these nucleosides are components of nucleic acids and of free nucleotides important in metabolism. Symbol G. See also illustration of *purine and pyrimidine bases,* under *base.*

g. nucleotide guanylic acid.

gua·nine de·am·i·nase (gwah′nēn de-am′ĭ-nās) [EC 3.5.4.3] an enzyme of the hydrolase class that catalyzes the deamination of guanine to form xanthine. The reaction is a step in the degradation of guanine to uric acid. The enzyme is present in liver, kidney, spleen, and other tissues. Called also *guanase.*

gua·no·phore (gwah′no-for″) [*guanine* + *phore*] a cell filled with guanine crystals that produce interference in the light and thus give the cell a silvery or golden appearance; found in the skin of some cold-blooded vertebrates such as fishes.

gua·no·sine (gwah′no-sēn) a purine nucleoside, guanine linked by its N9 nitrogen to the C1 carbon of ribose. It is a component of ribonucleic acid and its nucleotides play important roles in metabolism. Symbol G.

cyclic g. monophosphate a cyclic nucleotide, guanosine 3′,5′-cyclic monophosphate, an intracellular "second messenger" similar in action to cyclic adenosine monophosphate (q.v.); the two cyclic nucleotides activate different protein kinases and usually produce opposite effects on cell function. Abbreviated 3′,5′-GMP, cGMP, and cyclic GMP.

g. diphosphate (GDP) a nucleotide, the 5′-pyrophosphate of guanosine, which serves as a carrier for mannose residues in glycoprotein synthesis and as a substrate for a phosphorylation reaction of the tricarboxylic acid cycle.

g. monophosphate (GMP) a nucleotide, the 5′-phosphate of guanosine; it is a constituent of ribonucleic acid and a regulator of pyrimidine nucleotide biosynthesis.

g. triphosphate (GTP) a nucleotide, the 5′-triphosphate of guanosine; it is an activated precursor in the synthesis of ribonucleic acid and is also involved in energy metabolism, being produced from GDP by substrate level phosphorylation in the tricarboxylic acid (Krebs) cycle and serving as a source of free energy to drive protein synthesis. The ratio of GTP to ATP is maintained by the reversible transfer of phosphate catalyzed by GDP kinase.

gua·nyl·ate (gwah′nə-lāt) a dissociated form of guanylic acid.

gua·nyl·ate cy·clase (gwah′nə-lāt si′klās) [EC 4.6.1.2] an enzyme of the lyase class that catalyzes the cyclization of guanosine triphosphate to form cyclic guanosine monophosphate and pyrophosphate.

gua·nyl·ate ki·nase (gwah′nə-lāt ki′nās) [EC 2.7.4.8] an enzyme of the transferase class that catalyzes the phosphorylation of GMP or dGMP to form the corresponding phosphate compound.

gua·nyl·ic ac·id (gwah-nil′ik) guanosine monophosphate.

gua·nyl·yl (gwah-nil′əl) the radical formed by removal of OH from the phosphate group of guanosine monophosphate.

gua·ra·na (gwə-rah′nə) [Tupi-Guarani] 1. *Paullinia cupana.* 2. a dried paste prepared from the seeds of *P. cupana,* a woody vine of Brazil; used as a stimulant and tonic in folk medicine and for the treatment of headache in homeopathy.

gua·ra·nine (gwə-rah′nēn) caffeine.

guard (gahrd) a protective device.

bite g. occlusal splint.

mouth g. a removable, soft plastic intraoral appliance that covers all occlusal surfaces and the palate and extends to the border of the attached gingiva on the vestibular surface of the teeth; used to protect the teeth, lips, and cheeks during contact sports.

night g., occlusal g. occlusal splint.

Gua·rea (gwa′re-ə) a genus of tropical American trees and shrubs of the family Meliaceae. *G. rus′byi* (Britt.) has bark that is dried to yield the medicinal substance cocillana.

Guar·ni·eri bodies (gwahr″ne-er′e) [Giuseppi *Guarnieri,* Italian physician, 1856–1918] see under *body.*

gua sha (wah shaw) [Chinese *gua* to scrape + *sha* petechiae] coin rubbing.

gu·ber·nac·u·lum (goo″bər-nak′u-ləm) pl. *guberna′cula* [L. "helm, rudder"] a structure that guides. **gubernac′ular** *adj*

chorda g. a portion of the gubernaculum testis and round ligament that develops in the body wall of the embryo.

Hunter g. g. testis.

g. tes′tis the fetal ligament attached to the inferior end of the epididymis and testis and, at its other end, to the bottom of the scrotum; it is present during, and is thought to guide, the descent of the testis into the scrotum and then atrophies. Called also *Hunter g.*

Gub·ler hemiplegia (goo-bla′) [Adolphe Marie *Gubler,* French physician, 1821–1879] Millard-Gubler syndrome; see under *syndrome.*

Gud·den's commissure, law (good′enz) [Bernhard Alloys von *Gudden,* German psychiatrist, 1824–1886] see *supraoptic commissures,* under *commissure,* and see under *law.*

Guenz see *Günz.*

Gué·rin fold, fracture, etc. (ga-ră′) [Alphonse François Marie *Guérin,* French surgeon, 1817–1895] see *lacuna magna* and *valvula fossae navicularis;* and see *Le Fort I fracture* under *fracture.*

Gue·rrei·ro-Ma·cha·do test (ga-ra′roo mah-shah′doo) [Cesar *Guerreiro,* Brazilian medical researcher, 1885–1949; Astrogildo *Machado,* Brazilian medical researcher, 1885–1945] Machado-Guerreiro test.

guid·ance (gi′dəns) 1. a guide. 2. an act of guiding.

condylar g. the path that the horizontal rotation axis of the condyles travels during normal mandibular opening, measured in degrees as related to the Frankfort horizontal plane. It also influences mandibular movements from the temporomandibular joint, articular guidance, or condylar elements. Called also *condylar guide.* See also under *inclination.*

incisal g. the influence on mandibular movements by the contacting surfaces of the mandibular and maxillary anterior teeth.

guide (gīd) a device by which another object is led in its proper course, such as a grooved sound or filiform bougie over which a tunneled sound is passed, as in stricture of the urethra.

adjustable anterior g. an anterior guide whose superior surface may be varied to provide desired separation of dental casts in various eccentric relationships.

anterior g. the part of a dental articulator on which the anterior guide pin rests to maintain the vertical dimension of occlusion; it influences the degree of separation of the casts in eccentric relationships.

condylar g. see under *guidance.*

incisal g. the part of a dental articulator that maintains the incisal guide angle.

guide·line (gīd′līn) any line used as a marker or indicator.

clasp g. survey line (def. 3).

guide·wire (gīd′wīr″) a thin, usually flexible wire that can be inserted into a confined or tortuous space to act as a guide for subsequent insertion of a stiffer or bulkier instrument, such as a catheter.

Gui·di canal (gwe′de) [Guido *Guidi* (L. *Vidius*), Italian physician and anatomist, 1500–1567] canalis pterygoideus.

Guil·lain-Bar·ré syndrome (polyneuritis) (ge-yă′ bə-ra′) [Georges Charles *Guillain,* French neurologist, 1876–1961; Jean Alexander *Barré,* French neurologist, 1880–1967] see under *syndrome.*

Guil·lain-Mol·la·ret triangle (ge-yă′ mol-ah-ra′) [G.C. *Guillain;* Pierre *Mollaret,* French neurologist, 1898–1987] see under *triangle.*

guil·lo·tine (ge′o-tēn) [Fr.] an instrument for excising a tonsil or the uvula.

guin·ea pig (gin′e pig) [possibly a corruption of *Guiana,* South America + fancied resemblance to the domestic pig] *Cavia cobaya,* a rodent native to South America, much used in laboratory experiments.

Gui·non disease (ge-naw′) [Georges *Guinon,* French physician, 1859–1929] Gilles de la Tourette syndrome.

Gull disease (gul) [Sir William Withey *Gull,* English physician, 1816–1890] see under *disease.*

gul·let (gul′ət) 1. the esophagus. 2. the pharynx and the esophagus together.

Gull•strand's slit lamp, law (gool'strahndz) [Allvar *Gullstrand*, Swedish ophthalmologist and Nobel prize winner, 1862–1930] see *slit lamp* under *lamp*, and see under *law*.

gu•lon•ic ac•id (gu-lon'ik) the hexonic acid derived from glucose and formed by the reduction of the aldehyde group of glucuronic acid to an alcohol; it is an intermediate in the synthesis of ascorbic acid by many mammals.

L-gu•lo•no•lac•tone (gu"lo-no-lak'tōn) the immediate precursor of ascorbic acid in plants and in those animals capable of its biosynthesis; gulonolactone is itself formed from L-gulonic acid.

gu•lose (gu'lōs) an aldohexose isomeric with glucose but nonfermentable.

gum (gum) [L. *gummi*] 1. a mucilaginous excretion from various plants; on hydrolysis gums yield hexoses, pentoses, and uronic acids. 2. gingiva.

g. arabic acacia (def. 2).

g. benjamin, g. benzoin benzoin (def. 1).

blue g. 1. *Eucalyptus globulus*, source of eucalyptus oil. 2. the bluish discoloration of the gums seen in lead poisoning.

British g. dextrin, particularly that prepared by dry heating of starch in the absence of acid.

g. camphor camphor.

free g. periodontium insertionis.

ghatti g. a gum from *Anogeissus latifolia*, the dhava tree of India; used like acacia.

guar g. [NF] a gum obtained from the ground endosperms of the leguminous tree *Cyamopsis tetragonolobus;* used as a tablet binder and disintegrant in pharmaceutical preparations. It can also be used as a source of soluble dietary fiber.

karaya g. the dried gummy exudation from *Sterculia urens* or other species of *Sterculia*, which becomes gelatinous when moisture is added; used as a bulk laxative. Because of its adhesive properties, products containing karaya gum are used as dental adhesives and as skin adhesives and protective skin barriers in the fitting and care of colostomy appliances and in other conditions involving an artificial stoma. Called also *sterculia g.*

Kordofan g. a superior type of acacia (gum arabic) from trees found in the Sudan.

sterculia g. karaya g.

g. tragacanth tragacanth.

xanthan g. [NF] a dried, purified, high-molecular-weight polysaccharide gum produced by pure-culture fermentation of a carbohydrate with the bacterium *Xanthomonas campestris;* it contains D-glucose and D-mannose, along with D-glucuronic acid. It is used as the sodium, potassium, and calcium salts as a suspending agent in pharmaceutical preparations.

gum•boil (gum'boil) parulis.

Gum•boro disease (gum'bər-o) [*Gumboro*, Delaware, where the disease was first identified] see *infectious bursal disease*, under *disease*.

gum•ma (gum'ə) pl. *gummas, gum'mata* [L. *gummi* gum] 1. a chronic focal area of inflammatory destruction in tertiary syphilis from localization of *Treponema pallidum* in a tissue. The lesion is indolent and has a center of rubbery, gray-white coagulation necrosis surrounded by epithelioid cells, fibroblastic cells, and sometimes giant cells. Gummata vary in size from microscopic to large and tumorlike; they may be single or multiple and may involve any organ or tissue, although most commonly they affect mucocutaneous tissues, the liver, bones, or testes. Called also *syphiloma.* 2. late benign syphilis.

tuberculous g. a variant of scrofuloderma consisting of a subcutaneous nodule that becomes fluctuant and drains, with undermined ulceration and sinus formation; it is caused by hematogenous spread of tubercle bacilli from a primary focus of infection owing to lowered resistance or immunodeficiency, especially in children. Called also *metastatic tuberculous abscess.*

gum•ma•ta (gum'ə-tə) [L.] plural of *gumma.*

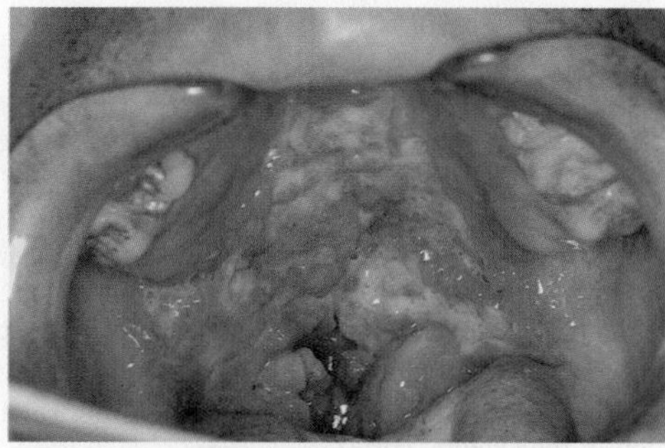

■ Gumma of the palate.

gum•ma•tous (gum'ə-təs) pertaining to or characterized by a gumma.

gum•mi (gum'i) [L., from Gr. *kommi*] gum (def. 1).

gum•my (gum'e) 1. pertaining to gum. 2. soft and mucilaginous, like gum (def. 1).

gum•res•in (gum"rez'in) a dried exudation from various trees, consisting of a principle soluble in water and insoluble in alcohol, combined with a volatile oil or resin soluble in alcohol, but not in water, and including myrrh and scammony.

soluble g.-r. pyroxylin.

gu•na (goo'nah) [Sanskrit] according to ayurveda, any of the three attributes of the universe and self that compose mind and body: sattva (equilibrium), rajas (activity), and tamas (inertia).

gun•cot•ton (gun-kot'ən) pyroxylin.

Gunn crossing sign, dots, pupil, etc. (gun) [Robert Marcus *Gunn*, British ophthalmologist, 1850–1909] see under *dot, sign*, and *syndrome;* see *Marcus Gunn pupil*, under *pupil;* and see *Marcus Gunn pupillary phenomenon*, under *phenomenon.*

Gun•ning splint (gun'ing) [Thomas Brian *Gunning*, American dentist, 1813–1889] see under *splint.*

Gün•ther disease (gēn'ter) [Hans *Günther*, German physician, 1884–1956] see *congenital erythropoietic porphyria*, under *porphyria.*

Günz ligament (gēnts) [Justus Gottfried *Günz*, German anatomist, 1714–1754] see under *ligament.*

gur•ney (gur'ne) a wheeled cot used in hospitals.

Gus•sen•bau•er suture (goo'sən-bou"ər) [Karl *Gussenbauer*, Austrian surgeon, 1842–1903] see under *suture.*

gus•ta•tion (gəs-ta'shən) taste.

colored g. a pseudogeusia in which tastes are associated with colors; called also *color taste.*

gus•ta•tism (gus'tə-tiz-əm) pseudogeusia.

gus•tin (gus'tin) a polypeptide (molecular weight, 27,000) present in saliva and containing two zinc atoms; it is apparently necessary for normal development of the taste buds.

gus•tom•e•ter (gəs-tom'ə-tər) [L. *gustare* to taste + *-meter*] an apparatus used in the quantitative determination of taste thresholds; see also *electrogustometer.*

gus•tom•e•try (gəs-tom'ə-tre) the clinical determination of thresholds of the sense of taste.

gut (gut) 1. intestinum. 2. the primordial digestive tube, consisting of the foregut, midgut, and hindgut. 3. surgical g.

blind g. caecum (def. 2).

chromic g., chromicized g. surgical gut treated with a chromic salt to increase its resistance to absorption in tissues.

postanal g. a temporary extension of the embryonic hindgut caudal to the cloaca.

preoral g. Seessel pouch.

primitive g., primordial g. archenteron.

ribbon g. an absorbable ribbon of the intestinal tissue of animals used for suturing where broad support is to be secured.

surgical g. an absorbable sterile strand obtained from collagen derived from healthy mammals, originally prepared from the submucous layer of the intestines of sheep; used as a surgical ligature. See also *absorbable suture*, under *suture.* Called also *catgut.*

tail g. postanal g.

Guth•rie muscle (guth're) [George James *Guthrie*, English surgeon, 1785–1856] see *musculus sphincter urethrae externus urethrae femininae* and *musculus sphincter urethrae externus urethrae masculinae.*

Guth•rie test (guth're) [Robert *Guthrie*, American microbiologist, 1916–1995] see under *test.*

Gu•ti•er•re•zia (goo"te-ə-re'ze-ə) the broomweeds or snakeweeds, a genus of herbs that have yellow flowers; several species, such as *G. diversifo'lia* and *G. saro'thrae*, may cause selenium poisoning in livestock when growing in selenium-rich soil. *G. microce'phala* causes abortion in pregnant female animals.

gut•ta (gut'ə) pl. *gut'tae* [L.] drop.

gut•tae (gut'e) [L.] plural of *gutta.*

gut•ta-per•cha (gut"ə-pur'chə) [Malay *getah perca* sap of the percha tree] [USP] the coagulated, dried, and purified latex of trees of the genera *Palaquium* and *Payena*, particularly *Palaquium gutta;* used in orthopedics for fracture splints, in dental surgery for temporary sealing of cavities, and in dentistry in the form of cones for filling the root canal and in the form of sticks for sealing cavities over treatment.

Guttat. [L.] gutta'tim (drop by drop).

gut•tate (gut'āt) characterized by lesions that are drop-shaped.

gut·ta·tim (gə-ta′tim) [L.] drop by drop.

gut·ter (gut′ər) a deep sulcus.
 paracolic g's sulci paracolici.

gut·tie (gut′ti) 1. a hernia in cattle in which a loop of intestine passes through a tear in the peritoneum and is held there, producing obstruction of the bowels. 2. a twisting of the intestine in domestic animals.

Gutt. quibusd. [L.] gut′tis quibus′dam (with a few drops).

gut·tur (gut′ər) [L.] fauces.

gut·tur·al (gut′ər-əl) 1. pertaining to the throat; see also *pharyngeal.* Called also *faucial.* 2. velar (def. 2).

gut·tur·oph·o·ny (gut″ər-of′ə-ne) [*guttur* + Gr. *phōnē* voice] a throaty quality of the voice.

gut·turo·tet·a·ny (gut″ər-o-tet′ə-ne) [*guttur* + *tetany*] a guttural spasm, resulting in a kind of stutter.

Guy·on amputation (operation), canal (ge-yaw′) [Felix Jean Casimir *Guyon*, French surgeon, 1831–1920] see under *amputation* and *canal.*

GVH graft-versus-host; see under *disease.*

GVHD graft-versus-host disease.

GXT graded exercise test; see *exercise test,* under *test.*

Gy gray (def. 2).

gym·na·moe·bae (jim″nə-me′be) ramicristate amebae.

Gym·na·moe·bia (jim″nə-me′be-ə) [*gymn-* + *ameba*] the ramicristate amebae when they are considered a subclass; see under *ameba.*

gym·nas·tics (jim-nas′tiks) [Gr. *gymnastikos* pertaining to athletics] systematic muscular exercise.
 ocular g. systematic exercise of the eye muscles in order to secure proper movement, accommodation, or fixation.
 Swedish g. a system of exercise including carefully chosen free, active, deliberate movement, using little equipment and stressing correct posture.

Gym·ne·ma (jim-ne′mə) a genus of trees of the family Asclepiadaceae. *G. sylves′tre* R. Bv. is an African species whose leaves are used as a flavoring agent for medicines.

gymn(o)- [Gr. *gymnos* naked] a combining form meaning naked or denoting relationship to nakedness.

Gym·no·as·ca·ceae (jim″no-as-ka′se-e) a family of keratinophilic fungi of the order Onygenales in which the reproductive organs are in the form of naked asci. It includes the genera *Ajellomyces, Arthroderma,* and *Gymnoascus.*

Gym·no·as·cus (jim″no-as′kəs) a genus of fungi of the family Gymnoascaceae, some species of which are pathogenic.

gym·no·car·pous (jim″no-kahr′pəs) [*gymno-* + Gr. *karpos* fruit] of certain fungi, having the hymenium, or fertile layer, exposed during spore formation.

Gym·no·din·i·um (jim″no-din′e-əm) [*gymno-* + Gr. *dinein* to whirl] a genus of plantlike marine and freshwater protozoa of the phylum Dinoflagellata; most species have many colored (yellow, brown, green, or blue) chromatophores. Like other dinoflagellates, they produce red tide when present in vast numbers. *G. breve* has been renamed *Karenia brevis.*

Gym·no·phal·loi·des (jim″no-fə-loi′dēz) a genus of minute trematodes. The species *G. seo′I* is usually found in shore birds, but has been found as an intestinal parasite in humans in Korea.

gym·no·sperm (jim′no-spərm) [*gymno-* + *sperma*] a plant in which the seeds are not enclosed in an ovary.

gym·no·spore (jim′no-spor) a spore without any protective envelope.

gym·no·the·ci·um (jim″no-the′se-əm) a type of fruiting body (ascocarp) composed of a loose network of mycelia through which ascospores filter and are released at maturity; its reproductive organs are in the form of naked asci. Seen in fungi of the family Gymnoascaceae.

gynaec(o)- for words beginning thus, see those beginning *gynec(o)-.*

gy·nan·der (gi-, jə-nan′dər) [*gyn-* + Gr. *anēr, andros* man] 1. female pseudohermaphrodite. 2. hermaphrodite. 3. any female exhibiting masculinization.

gy·nan·dria (gi-, jə-nan′dre-ə) 1. female pseudohermaphroditism. 2. hermaphroditism. 3. masculinization in a female.

gy·nan·drism (gi-, jə-nan′driz-əm) 1. female pseudohermaphroditism. 2. hermaphroditism. 3. masculinization in a female.

gy·nan·dro·blas·to·ma (gi-, jə-nan″dro-blas-to′mə) [*gyn-* + *andro-* + *blastoma*] a rare ovarian tumor containing histologic features of both arrhenoblastoma and granulosa cell tumor.

gy·nan·droid (gi-, jə-nan′droid) [*gyn-* + *andr-* + *-oid*] 1. like a gynander. 2. hermaphrodite. 3. hermaphroditic.

gy·nan·dro·mor·phism (gi-, jə-nan″dro-mor′fiz-əm) [*gyn-* + *andro-* + *morph-* + *-ism*] the condition of having both male and female characteristics; properly used to denote the presence of chromosomes of both sexes in different tissues of the body in insects, resulting from cell-specific X chromosome inactivation.

gy·nan·dry (gi′-, ji′nan-dre) 1. female pseudohermaphroditism. 2. hermaphroditism. 3. masculinization in a female.

gyn·atre·sia (gi″nə-, jin″ə-tre′zhə) [*gyn-* + *atresia*] occlusion of some part of the female genital tract, especially of the vagina.

Gy·na·zole-1 (gi′nə-zōl) trademark for a preparation of butoconazole nitrate.

gyne- see *gynec(o)-.*

gy·nec·ic (gi-, jə-nes′ik) feminine.

gy·ne·ci·um (jə-ne′se-əm) [*gyn-* + Gr. *oikos* house] the female part of a flower; called also *pistil.*

gynec(o)- [Gr. *gynē*, gen. *gynaikos* woman] a combining form meaning female or denoting relationship to women or to the female reproductive organs. Also, *gynaec(o)-, gyne-,* and *gyn(o)-.*

gy·ne·co·gen·ic (gi″nə-, jin″ə-ko-jen′ik) feminizing.

gy·ne·cog·ra·phy (gi″nə-, jin″ə-kog′rə-fe) radiography of the female reproductive tract.

gy·ne·coid (gi′nə, jin′ə-koid) [*gynec-* + *oid*] womanlike; see also *feminine.*

gy·ne·co·log·ic (gi″nə-, jin″ə-kə-loj′ik) pertaining to the female reproductive tract or to gynecology.

gy·ne·co·log·i·cal (gi″nə-, jin″ə-kə-loj′ĭ-kəl) gynecologic.

gy·ne·col·o·gist (gi″nə-, jin″ə-kol′ə-jist) a specialist in gynecology.

gy·ne·col·o·gy (gi″nə-, jin″ə-kol′ə-je) [*gyneco-* + *-logy*] the branch of medicine that deals with female health and disease, particularly the diagnosis and treatment of diseases of the female reproductive system, including the breasts.

gy·ne·co·ma·nia (gi″nə-, jin″ə-ko-ma′ne-ə) hypersexuality in a male.

gy·ne·co·mas·tia (gi″nə-, jin″ə-ko-mas′te-ə) [*gyneco-* + *mast-* + *-ia*] excessive growth of the male mammary glands, in some cases including development to the stage at which milk is produced, usually associated with metabolic derangements that lead to estrogen accumulation, testosterone deficiency, and hyperprolactinemia. A mild form may develop transiently during normal puberty. Cf. *pseudogynecomastia.*
 nutritional g., refeeding g., rehabilitation g. transitory enlargement of the male breast developing during rehabilitation and recovery from a state of malnutrition or starvation.

gy·ne·co·mas·tism (gi″nə-, jin″ə-ko-mas′tiz-əm) gynecomastia.

gy·ne·co·mas·ty (gi′nə-, jin′ə-ko-mas″te) gynecomastia.

gy·ne·cop·a·thy (gi″nə-, jin″ə-kop′ə-the) [*gyneco-* + *-pathy*] a disease peculiar to women.

gy·ne·coph·o·ral (gi″nə-, jin″ə-kof′ə-rəl) see under *canal.*

Gyne-Lo·tri·min (gi″nə-lo′trĭ-min) trademark for a preparation of clotrimazole.

gy·ne·pho·bia (gi″nə-, jin″ə-fo′be-ə) [*gyne-* + *-phobia*] irrational fear of or aversion to women.

gy·ne·plas·ty (gi′nə-, jin′ə-plas″te) gynoplasty.

gyn·e·sin (jin′ə-sin) trigonelline.

gyn(o)- see *gynec(o)-.*

Gy·no·di·ol (gi″no-di′ol) trademark for preparations of estradiol.

gyno·gen·e·sis (gi″no-, jin″o-jen′ə-sis) [*gyno-* + *-genesis*] development of an egg that is stimulated by a spermatozoon in the absence of any participation of the spermatozoon nucleus.

gy·noid (gi′-, ji′noid) [*gyn-* + *-oid*] gynecoid.

gyno·pho·bia (gi″no-, jin″o-fo′be-ə) gynephobia.

gyno·plas·tics (gi″no-, jin″o-plas′tiks) gynoplasty.

gyno·plas·ty (gi′no-, jin′o-plas″te) plastic or reconstructive surgery of the female reproductive organs. Called also *gyneplasty* and *gynoplastics.* gynoplas′tic *adj*

Gy·no·rest (gi′no-rest) trademark for a preparation of dydrogesterone.

gyp·sum (jip′səm) [L., from Gr. *gypsos* chalk] native calcium sulfate dihydrate (see *calcium sulfate;*); when calcined, it becomes *plaster of Paris.*

gy·rate (ji′rāt) [L. *gyratus* turned round] twisted in a ring or spiral shape.

gy·ra·tion (ji-ra′shən) revolution in a circle or in circles.

gy·rec·to·my (ji-rek′tə-me) excision or resection of a cerebral gyrus, or of a portion of the cerebral cortex.
 frontal g. topectomy.

gy•ren•ce•phal•ic (ji″rən-sə-fal′ik) having cerebral hemispheres marked by convolutions, such as normally occurs in humans and some other animals. Cf. *lissencephalic.*

gy•ri (ji′ri) [L.] genitive and plural of *gyrus.*

gyr(o)- [Gr. *gyros* circle] a combining form meaning round or denoting relationship to a gyrus.

Gy•ro•dac•ty•lus (ji″ro-dak′tĭ-lus) a genus of trematodes that infect the skin and gills of aquarium fish, causing hyperactivity and breathing difficulty that can be fatal.

gy•rom•e•ter (ji-rom′ə-tər) [*gyro-* + *-meter*] an instrument for measuring the cerebral gyri.

Gy•ro•mi•tra (ji″ro-mi′trə) a genus of mushrooms of the family Helvellaceae, found in North America and Europe; many species contain the toxin monomethylhydrazine.

Gy•ro•pus (gi′ro-pəs) a genus of biting lice of the order Mallophaga; *G. ova′lis* is found on guinea pigs.

gy•rose (ji′rōs) marked by curved lines or circles.

gy•ro•spasm (ji′ro-spaz″əm) [*gyro-* + *spasm*] rotatory spasm of the head.

gy•rous (ji′rəs) gyrose.

gy•rus (ji′rəs) gen. and pl. *gy′ri* [L., from Gr. *gyros* circle] one of the convolutions of the surface of the cerebral hemispheres caused by infolding of the cortex; see *gyri cerebri.*

Gyrus

Descriptions of gyri are given on TA terms, and include anglicized names of specific gyri.

g. angula′ris [TA] angular gyrus: a convolution of the inferior parietal lobule, arching over the posterior end of the superior temporal sulcus and continuous with the middle temporal gyrus.
annectant gyri, annectent gyri, gy′ri annecten′tes gyri transitivi cerebri.
anterior paracentral g. g. paracentralis anterior.
ascending parietal g. g. postcentralis.
gy′ri bre′ves in′sulae [TA] short gyri of insula: the short, rostrally placed gyri on the surface of the insula; called also *preinsular gyri.*
Broca g. see under *convolution.*
callosal g., g. callo′sus g. cinguli.
central g., anterior g. precentralis.
central g., posterior g. postcentralis.
gy′ri cerebel′li folia cerebelli.
cerebral gyri, gy′ri ce′rebri [TA] the tortuous convolutions of the surface of the cerebral hemispheres, caused by infolding of the cortex and separated by sulci. Many are constant enough that they have been given special names.
cingulate g., g. cingula′tus g. cinguli.
g. cin′guli [TA] cingulate gyrus: an arch-shaped convolution closely related to the surface of the corpus callosum, from which it is separated by the callosal sulcus; called also *callosal g., g. callosus,* and *g. cingulatus.*
dentate g., g. denta′tus [TA] a serrated strip of gray matter under the medial border of the hippocampus and in its depths; it is an archaeocortex which develops along the edge of the hippocampal fissure and which consists of molecular, granular, and multiform layers.
g. fasciola′ris [TA] fasciolar gyrus: a posterior and upward extension of the dentate gyrus, forming a transitional area between the dentate gyrus and the indusium griseum; called also *fasciola cinerea.*
g. fornica′tus the marginal portion of the cerebral cortex on the medial aspect of the hemisphere, including the gyrus cinguli, gyrus parahippocampalis, isthmus, and uncus; it forms a major part of the limbic system.
frontal g., ascending g. precentralis.
frontal g., inferior g. frontalis inferior.
frontal g., medial g. frontalis medialis.

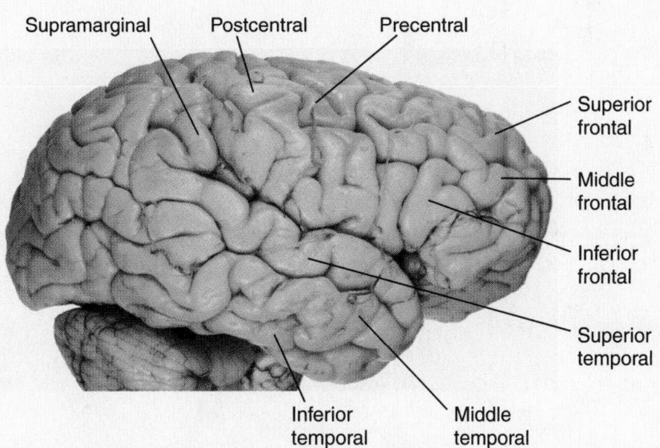

■ Gyri cerebri (cerebral gyri) in a lateral view of the right hemisphere.

frontal g., middle g. frontalis medius.
frontal g., superior g. frontalis superior.
g. fronta′lis infe′rior [TA] inferior frontal gyrus: a convolution of the frontal lobe below the inferior frontal sulcus; it is divided by the anterior and ascending branches of the lateral sulcus into orbital, triangular, and opercular parts. Cf. *Broca convolution.*
g. fronta′lis media′lis [TA] medial frontal gyrus: the medial surface of the frontal lobe, separated from the cingulate gyrus by the cingulate sulcus, and continuous with the superior frontal gyrus above and the gyrus rectus below.
g. fronta′lis me′dius [TA] middle frontal gyrus: a convolution of the frontal lobe between the superior and inferior frontal sulci, extending anteriorly from the precentral gyrus; a longitudinal sulcus may be present, dividing the gyrus into superior and inferior parts.
g. fronta′lis supe′rior [TA] superior frontal gyrus: a convolution of the frontal lobe above the superior frontal sulcus, extending anteriorly from the precentral gyrus.
g. fusifor′mis fusiform gyrus: a gyrus of the temporal lobe on the inferior surface of the hemisphere between the inferior temporal gyrus and the parahippocampal gyrus. It consists of a lateral and a medial part, called *g. occipitotemporalis lateralis* [TA] and *g. occipitotemporalis medialis* [TA].
g. geni′culi a vestigial gyrus at the anterior end of the corpus callosum.
Heschl gyri gyri temporales transversi.
hippocampal g., g. hippocam′pi g. parahippocampalis.
infracalcarine g. g. lingualis.
gy′ri in′sulae [TA] insular gyri: the gyri that are found on the surface of the insula, including the *gyrus longus insulae* and the *gyri breves insulae.*
interlocking gyri small gyri in the opposing walls of the central sulcus which interlock with each other like gears.
intralimbic g. the posterior part of the inferior surface of the uncus, separated from the uncinate gyrus by the Giacomini band.
g. lingua′lis [TA] lingual gyrus: a gyrus of the occipital lobe on the inferior surface of the hemisphere, forming the inferior lip of the calcarine sulcus and, with the cuneus, the visual cortex; it is continuous anteriorly with the parahippocampal gyrus.
g. lon′gus in′sulae [TA] long gyrus of insula: the long, occipitally directed gyrus on the surface of the insula.
marginal g. g. frontalis medialis.
occipital g., inferior the lower of the two gyri separated by the lateral occipital sulcus on the lateral aspect of the occipital lobe.
occipital gyri, lateral see *occipital g., inferior* and *occipital g., superior.*
occipital g., superior the upper of the two gyri separated by the occipital lateral sulcus on the lateral aspect of the occipital lobe.
occipitotemporal g., lateral g. occipitotemporalis lateralis.
occipitotemporal g., medial g. occipitotemporalis medialis.
g. occipitotempora′lis latera′lis [TA] lateral occipitotemporal gyrus: the lateral portion of the gyrus fusiformis on the inferior surface of the cerebral hemisphere, separated from the medial portion by the occipitotemporal sulcus, and continuous laterally with the inferior temporal gyrus.
g. occipitotempora′lis media′lis [TA] medial occipitotemporal gyrus: the medial portion of the gyrus fusiformis on the inferior surface of the cerebral hemisphere, separated from the lateral portion by the occipitotemporal sulcus, and from the parahippocampal gyrus by the collateral sulcus.

Gyrus *Continued*

g. olfacto′rius latera′lis [TA] lateral olfactory gyrus: the layer of gray substance covering the lateral olfactory stria.
g. olfacto′rius media′lis [TA] medial olfactory gyrus: the layer of gray substance covering the medial olfactory stria.
olfactory g., lateral g. olfactorius lateralis.
olfactory g., medial g. olfactorius medialis.
gy′ri orbita′les [TA] orbital gyri: the various irregular convolutions lateral to the olfactory sulcus on the orbital surface of the frontal lobe.
paracentral g. lobulus paracentralis.
g. paracentra′lis ante′rior [TA] anterior paracentral gyrus: the anterior portion of the paracentral lobule, medial to and continuous with the precentral gyrus; it is the primary somatomotor cortex for the lower extremities and genitalia.
g. paracentra′lis poste′rior [TA] posterior paracentral gyrus: the posterior portion of the paracentral lobule, medial to and continuous with the postcentral gyrus; it is the primary somatosensory cortex for the lower extremities and genitalia.
parahippocampal g., g. parahippocampa′lis [TA] a convolution on the inferior surface of each cerebral hemisphere, lying between the hippocampal and collateral sulci; called also *hippocampal g.* and *g. hippocampi.*
g. paratermina′lis [TA] paraterminal gyrus: a thin sheet of gray substance in front of the lamina terminalis and ventral to the genu of the corpus callosum; see also *septum precommissurale.*
parietal g. any one of the convolutions into which the surface of the parietal lobe is divided.
g. postcentra′lis [TA] postcentral gyrus: the convolution of the parietal lobe lying between the central and postcentral sulci; the primary sensory area of the cerebral cortex for the face, upper extremity, trunk, and hip. Called also *posterior central g.* and *ascending parietal g.*
posterior paracentral g. g. paracentralis posterior.
g. precentra′lis [TA] precentral gyrus: the convolution of the frontal lobe lying between the precentral and central sulci; the primary motor area of the cerebral cortex for the face, upper extremity, trunk and hip. Called also *anterior central g.*
preinsular gyri gyri breves insulae.
g. rec′tus [TA] straight gyrus: a convolution on the orbital surface of the frontal lobe, medial to the olfactory sulcus and continuous with the medial frontal gyrus on the medial surface.
short gyri of insula gyri breves insulae.
splenial g. g. fasciolaris.
straight g. g. rectus.
subcallosal g. area subcallosa.
supracallosal g. indusium griseum.
g. supramargina′lis [TA] supramarginal gyrus: the convolution of the inferior parietal lobe that curves around the upper end of the posterior branch of the lateral fissure and is continuous behind it with the superior temporal gyrus.
temporal g., anterior transverse g. temporalis transversus anterior.
temporal g., inferior g. temporalis inferior.
temporal g., middle g. temporalis medius.
temporal g., posterior transverse g. temporalis transversus posterior.
temporal g., superior g. temporalis superior.
temporal gyri, transverse gyri temporales transversi.
g. tempora′lis infe′rior [TA] inferior temporal gyrus: the convolution of the temporal lobe lying between the inferior temporal sulcus and the lateral occipitotemporal gyrus, the two gyri being continuous at the inferolateral margin of the temporal lobe.
g. tempora′lis me′dius [TA] middle temporal gyrus: the convolution of the temporal lobe lying between the superior and the inferior temporal sulci; it is continuous posteriorly with the angular gyrus.
g. tempora′lis supe′rior [TA] superior temporal gyrus: the convolution of the temporal lobe lying between the superior temporal sulcus and the lateral sulcus, continuous posteriorly with the supramarginal gyrus.
gy′ri tempora′les transver′si [TA] transverse temporal gyri: the transverse convolutions marking the posterior extremity of the superior temporal gyrus and lying mostly in the lateral sulcus; usually two, anterior and posterior, but sometimes single on one or both sides. Called also *Heschl gyri* or *convolutions.*
g. tempora′lis transver′sus ante′rior [TA] anterior transverse temporal gyrus: the anterior, more marked, of the two transverse temporal gyri, where two exist; it represents the cortical center for hearing. See *gyri temporales transversi.*
g. tempora′lis transver′sus poste′rior [TA] posterior transverse temporal gyrus: the posterior of the two transverse temporal gyri, where two exist; it represents the cortical area for hearing. See *gyri temporales transversi.*
gy′ri transiti′vi ce′rebri various small folds on the cerebral surface that are too inconstant to bear special names; called also *annectant* or *annectent gyri.*
uncinate g. the anterior part of the inferior surface of the uncus, separated from the intralimbic gyrus by the Giacomini band.

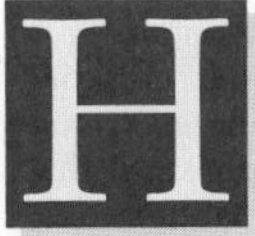

H Hauch; henry; histidine; Hounsfield unit; hydrogen; hyperopia.

H enthalpy.

H_0 null hypothesis.

H_1 alternative hypothesis.

H_a alternative hypothesis.

h hecto-; hour.

h. [L.] ho′ra (hour).

h Planck constant; height.

HA hemadsorbent; hemagglutinin; hepatitis A.

Ha element 105 (hahnium); see table at *element*.

HAA hepatitis-associated antigen; see *hepatitis B surface antigen*, under *antigen*.

Haab reflex (hahb) [Otto *Haab*, Swiss ophthalmologist, 1850–1931] see under *reflex*.

HAART highly active antiretroviral therapy.

ha•be•na (hə-be′nə) pl. *habe′nae* [L. "rein"] any straplike anatomic structure; cf. *habenula*.

ha•ben•u•la (hə-ben′u-lə) gen. and pl. *haben′ulae* [L., dim. of *habena*, q.v.] 1. a frenulum, or reinlike structure, such as one of a set of such structures in the cochlea. 2. [TA] a component of the epithalamus, being the small eminence on the dorsomedial surface of the thalamus, just in front of the posterior commissure on the lateral edge of the habenular trigone; called also *pineal peduncle*.

h. cona′rii habenula (def. 2).

habe′nulae perfora′tae foramina nervosa; see under *foramen*.

h. urethra′lis either of two whitish lines extending from the urinary meatus to the clitoris in girls and young women.

ha•ben•u•lae (hə-ben′u-le) [L.] genitive and plural of *habenula*.

ha•ben•u•lar (hə-ben′u-lər) pertaining to a habenula.

Ha•ber•mann disease (hah′ber-mahn) [Rudolf *Habermann*, German dermatologist, 1884–1941] pityriasis lichenoides et varioliformis acuta.

hab•it (hab′it) [L. *habitus*, from *habere* to hold] 1. a fixed or constant practice established by frequent repetition. 2. predisposition or bodily temperament; see also *type*.

clamping h., clenching h. centric bruxism.

glaucomatous h. shallowness of the anterior chamber of the eye with dilated pupil; seen in persons who have a predisposition to glaucoma.

oral h. a habit that causes changes in occlusal relationships, e.g., finger, thumb, and lip sucking, tongue thrusting, and the like. See also *habit-breaking appliance*, under *appliance*.

hab•i•tat (hab′ĭ-tat) the natural abode or home of an animal or plant species.

ha•bit•u•al (hə-bich′u-əl) 1. according to or of the nature of a habit. 2. established through long use or frequent repetition.

ha•bit•u•a•tion (hə-bich″u-a′shən) 1. the gradual adaptation to a stimulus or to the environment. 2. extinction or decrease of a conditioned reflex over time by repetition of the conditioned stimulus. 3. an older term used in describing habitual drug use, used sometimes to denote drug tolerance (see under *tolerance*) and other times to denote psychological but not physical dependence on a drug as a consequence of repeated consumption, with a desire to continue its use but with little or no tendency to increase the dose.

hab•i•tus (hab′ĭ-təs) [L. "habit"] 1. posture or position of the body. 2. physique; body build and constitution. See also entries under *type*.

Hab•ro•ne•ma (hab″ro-ne′mə) [Gr. *habros* graceful + *nema*] a genus of nematodes of the family Habronematidae. The larval forms are taken up from the feces of horses by flies and the flies, when swallowed along with the feed by the same or a different horse, can then transmit the larvae back into the horse's stomach. Larvae may also be transmitted to the skin of horses to produce cutaneous habronemiasis.

H. ma′jus *H. microstoma.*

H. megasto′ma *Draschia megastoma.*

H. microsto′ma a species that causes habronemiasis in horses; called also *H. majus.*

H. mus′cae a species that causes habronemiasis in horses.

Hab•ro•ne•mat•i•dae (hab″ro-ne-mat′ĭ-de) a family of nematodes that includes the genera *Draschia* and *Habronema* and cause habronemiasis in horses.

hab•ro•ne•mi•a•sis (hab″ro-ne-mi′ə-sis) infection of a horse with a nematode of the family Habronematidae. *Habronema muscae* and *H. microstoma* in the stomach can cause a mild catarrhal type of gastritis. *Draschia megastoma* causes gastric habronemiasis. Any of these species can also cause cutaneous habronemiasis.

cutaneous h. infection of the skin of a horse with larvae of *Habronema* or *Draschia* species; cutaneous granulomas grow in size until the skin around them is destroyed, leaving a large raw surface. Because of the clinical similarity between cutaneous habronemiasis and pythiosis, the disorders are often confused. See also *swamp cancer*, under *cancer*. Called also *bursati, bursautee*, and *summer sores*.

gastric h. infestation of the stomach wall of a horse with larvae of *Draschia megastoma*, which form large nodules filled with worms and necrotic material. Many affected horses do not show clinical signs, but they may die if the stomach wall is perforated.

ha•bu (hah′boo) [native name in Ryukyu Islands] 1. *Trimeresurus flavoviridis*, an extremely venomous pit viper inhabiting the warmer parts of East Asia, especially the Ryukyu Islands. 2. *Trimeresurus mucrosquamatus* (also called the *Chinese habu*), a venomous pit viper found in Taiwan, southern China, and Southeast Asia.

Had•field-Clarke syndrome (had′fēld klahrk′) [Geoffrey *Hadfield*, British physician, 1889–1968; Cecil *Clarke*, British physician, 20th century] Clarke-Hadfield syndrome.

hae- for words beginning thus, see also those beginning *he-*.

Haeck•el's law (hek′əlz) [Ernst Heinrich Philipp August *Haeckel*, German naturalist, 1834–1919] see *recapitulation theory*, under *theory*.

haem (hēm) heme.

hae•ma (he′mə) [Gr. *haima, haimatos* blood] [TA] the blood (q.v.). Spelled also *hema*. Called also *sanguis* [TA alternative].

haema- see *hem(o)-*; for words beginning thus, see also those beginning *hema-*.

Hae•mac•cel (he′mak-sel″) trademark for a preparation of polygeline.

Hae•ma•dip•sa (he′mə-dip′sə) [*haema-* + *dipsia*] the land leeches, a genus of the family Gnathobdellidae.

H. ceylo′nica a species common in Sri Lanka that has a painful bite.

H. chilia′ni a species that attacks horses and cattle in South America.

H. japo′nica a species found in Japan.

H. zeylan′dica a species that attacks mammals in the tropical jungles of Asia.

Hae•ma•gog•us (hem″ə-gog′əs) [*haem-* + Gr. *agōgos* leading] a genus of mosquitoes of the tribe Aedini, family Culicinae, some of which transmit jungle yellow fever in tropical Central and South America.

Hae•ma•phys•a•lis (he″mə-fis′ə-lis) [*haema-* + *physallis* bubble] a large genus of ticks of the family Ixodidae.

H. concin′na a species of northern Europe and Asia that attacks mammals and is a vector of Siberian tick typhus and tularemia.

H. humero′sa the bandicoot tick, an Australian species that is a vector of *Coxiella burnetii*, which causes Q fever.

H. lea′chi the common dog tick of South Africa, a vector for the protozoa causing canine babesiosis.

H. leporispalus′tris the rabbit tick, a North American species that usually parasitizes wild animals and is a vector for Rocky Mountain spotted fever and tularemia.

H. longicor′nis a species of eastern Asia and nearby islands from Japan to Australia, which infests mammals and is a vector for species of *Theileria* and *Babesia, Coxiella burnetii*, and Russian spring-summer encephalitis virus.

H. puncta′ta a species that infests mammals and birds from Central Asia across much of Europe and is a vector for diseases such as babesiosis, tularemia, Q fever, and tick paralysis.

H. spinige′ra a species that attacks rodents and a few other mammals in the tropical forests of India and is a vector of the virus causing Kyasanur Forest disease in forest workers.

haemat(o)- see *hemat(o)-*.

Hae•ma•to•bia (he″mə-to′be-ə) a genus of flies of the family Muscidae. *H. ir′ritans* is the horn fly, a small species that is very troublesome to cattle.

Hae•ma•to•pi•nus (he″mə-to-pi′nəs) [*haemato-* + Gr. *pinein* to drink] a genus of sucking lice (order Anoplura). *H. asi′ni* infests horses; *H. eurys-ter′ni*, the short-nosed cattle louse, infests cattle; *H. quadrister′ni* infests cattle; and *H. su′is* is the most common louse of pigs.

Hae•ma•top•o•ta (he″mə-top′ə-tə) a genus of horseflies (family Tabanidae), large biting bloodsuckers that attack horses, cattle, and other mammals and cause anemia, mastitis, anthrax, anaplasmosis, and trypanosomiasis.

Hae•ma•to•si•phon (he″mə-to-si′fon) a genus of insects closely related to the genus *Cimex*, but having longer legs and a very long beak. *H. in′dorus*, a species of the southwestern United States and Mexico, may be a serious pest of poultry and sometimes attacks humans.

Hae•ma•tox•y•lon (he″mə-tok′sə-lon) [*haemato-* + Gr. *xylon* wood] a genus of trees of the family Leguminosae, native to Mexico, Central America, and the West Indies. *H. campechia′num* L. is campechy or logwood, whose heartwood contains tannin, hematoxylin, and resin, and yields a purplish-red dye.

Hae•men•te•ria (he″mən-tēr′e-ə) a genus of leeches. *H. officina′lis* is used for medicinal purposes in Mexico and elsewhere in Latin America.

haem(o)- see *hem(o)-*.

Hae•mo•bar•to•nel•la (he″mo-bahr″to-nel′ə) [*haemo-* + *Bartonella*] in former systems of classification, a genus of bacteria of the family Mycoplasmataceae; members are now classified in the genus *Mycoplasma*.

H. ca′nis *Mycoplasma haemocanis*.

H. fe′lis *Mycoplasma haemofelis*.

H. mu′ris *Mycoplasma haemomuris*.

hae•mo•bar•to•nel•lo•sis (he″mo-bahr″tə-nə-lo′sis) feline infectious anemia.

Hae•mo•dip•sus (he″mo-dip′səs) a genus of lice. *H. ventrico′sus* is the common sucking louse of the rabbit and transmits the infective agent of tularemia from rabbit to rabbit.

Hae•mo•greg•a•ri•na (he″mo-greg″ə-ri′nə) [*hemo-* + L. *gregarius* crowding together] a genus of coccidian protozoa (suborder Adeleina, order Eucoccidiida) in which the life cycle involves two hosts, the vertebrate circulatory system (e.g., reptiles, amphibians, birds, certain mammals) and the invertebrate digestive system (e.g., blood-sucking invertebrates such as an insect or leech).

hae•mon•cho•sis (hēm″ong-ko′sis) infection of a ruminant with nematodes of the genus *Haemonchus*, especially *H. contortus*, characterized by weakness and anemia that can be fatal.

Hae•mon•chus (he-mon′kəs) a genus of parasitic nematodes of the family Trichostrongylidae. *H. contor′tus* is the wireworm or barber's pole worm, a stomach worm that parasitizes the abomasum of ruminants, causing haemonchosis.

Hae•moph•i•lus (he-mof′ĭ-ləs) [*hemo-* + Gr. *philein* to love] a genus of gram-negative, aerobic or facultatively anaerobic, rod-shaped or coccobacillary bacteria of the family Pasteurellaceae, consisting of cells that sometimes form threads and filaments. The organisms require one or both growth factors (X factor, which can be replaced by hematin, or V factor, which can be replaced by nicotinamide adenine dinucleoside) present in blood. They are normal inhabitants of the upper respiratory tract but may become primary or secondary pathogens.

H. aegyp′tius a biovar of *H. influenzae* that causes infectious conjunctivitis, especially in hot climates; it was formerly classified as a separate species.

H. aphro′philus a species that is part of the normal oral microflora and is occasionally found as a cause of endocarditis.

H. ducre′yi a species that causes soft genital chancres and chancroids. Called also *Ducrey bacillus*.

H. equigenita′lis *Taylorella equigenitalis*.

H. haemoly′ticus a nonpathogenic species found as a normal inhabitant of the upper respiratory tract.

H. influen′zae a species once thought to be the cause of epidemic influenza. Noncapsulated strains are normal inhabitants of the human nasopharynx (biovars II and III). In children, capsulated strains of biovar I are the major cause of bacterial meningitis, and may also cause potentially fatal acute epiglottitis. In both children and immunocompromised patients it can cause pneumonia (see *Haemophilus influenzae pneumonia*).

H. paragallina′rum a species that causes infectious avian coryza in chickens.

H. parainfluen′zae a species that is part of the normal oral flora and is occasionally associated with bacterial endocarditis.

H. paraphro′philus a species that is part of the normal oral microflora, has been associated with endocarditis, and has been found in abscessed internal organs.

H. parasu′is a species that is a normal inhabitant of the upper respiratory tract of swine, but is also a potential pathogen and may cause respiratory tract infections and polyserositis. See also *Glasser disease*.

H. som′nus *Histophilus somni*.

H. vagina′lis *Gardnerella vaginalis*.

Hae•mo•pho•ruc•tus (he″mo-fə-ruk′təs) a genus of blood-sucking flies of the family Heleidae.

Hae•mo•pis (he-mo′pis) a genus of leeches of the family Gnathobdellidae. *H. palu′dum* infests the nose and throat of horses in Sri Lanka. *H. sanguisu′ga* infests the nasal passages of horses in Europe and North Africa.

Hae•mo•pro•te•us (he″mo-pro′te-əs) [*haemo-* + *Proteus*] a genus of coccidian protozoa (suborder Haemosporina, order Eucoccidiida) in which the vectors are blood-sucking insects other than mosquitoes and the vertebrate hosts are mammals, reptiles, and wild and domestic birds including ducks, pigeons, and turkeys. In these organisms merogony takes place not in erythrocytes but in the vascular endothelial cells, and the gametocytes are found only in the circulating erythrocytes.

Hae•mo•spo•ri•na (he″mo-spor-i′nə) [*hemo-* + *spore*] a suborder of heteroxenous protozoa (subclass Coccidia, class Sporozoea) in which merogony takes place in a vertebrate, usually in the blood, and sporogony in the alimentary canal of a blood-sucking insect. Hemosporians are characterized by the independent development of macrogamete and microgamont; the absence of syzygy; the usual absence of a conoid; the production by the microgamont of eight flagellated microgametes; and the formation of a motile zygote (ookinete). Representative genera include *Haemoproteus*, *Hepatocystis*, *Leucocytozoon*, and *Plasmodium*.

hae•mo•zo•in (he″mo-zo′in) hemozoin.

Haff disease (hahf) [Ger. *Haff*, bay; named for Königsberg (or Frisches) *Haff*, a bay connected with the Baltic Sea, where epidemics occurred in 1924–5, 1932–3, and 1940] see under *disease*.

Haf•nia (haf′ne-ə) [L. *Hafnia* the old name for Copenhagen] a genus of gram-negative facultatively anaerobic bacteria of the family Enterobacteriaceae, made up of motile, peritrichously flagellated, non-encapsulated straight rods. The type species is *H. alvei*.

H. al′vei a species found in soil, water, sewage, and dairy products and as part of the normal intestinal flora of many animals; it can cause infection and diarrhea in debilitated persons.

haf•ni•um (Hf) (haf′ne-əm) [L. *Hafnia* Copenhagen] a chemical element of atomic number 72 and atomic weight 178.49. Discovered in a zircon, in 1923, by Coster and Hevesy of Copenhagen.

Ha•ge•dorn needles (hah′gə-dorn) [Werner *Hagedorn*, German surgeon, 1831–1894] see under *needle*.

Hag•lund deformity, disease (hahg′loond) [Sims Emil Patrik *Haglund*, Swedish orthopedist, 1870–1937] retrocalcaneal bursitis.

Hag•ner disease (hahg′nər) [*Hagner*, surname of the original propositus studied in the 19th century] hypertrophic pulmonary osteoarthropathy; see under *osteoarthropathy*.

Hahn sign (hahn) [Eugen Heinrich *Hahn*, German physician, 1841–1902] see under *sign*.

hah•ne•man•ni•an (hahn″ə-mah′ne-ən) pertaining to Christian Friedrich Samuel *Hahnemann*, German physician, 1755–1843, founder of homeopathy.

hah•ne•man•nism (hahn′ə-mən″iz-əm) homeopathy.

HAI hemagglutination inhibition; see under *test*.

Hai•ding•er brushes (hi′ding-ər) [Wilhelm von *Haidinger*, Austrian mineralogist, 1795–1871] see under *brush*.

Hai•ley-Hai•ley disease (ha′le ha′le) [Hugh Edward *Hailey*, American dermatologist, 1909–1964; William Howard *Hailey*, American dermatologist, 1898–1967] benign familial pemphigus; see under *pemphigus*.

hair (hār) [L. *pilus*; Gr. *thrix*] 1. a long, slender filament. 2. in most mammals, one of the filamentous appendages growing out of the skin, consisting primarily of keratin, and comprising a cylindrical shaft and a root, which is contained in a follicle. The base of the root expands to form the hair bulb, which rests upon and encloses the hair papilla. The three phases from production of a hair to its final shedding are called the *hair cycle* (q.v.). In anatomical terminology, hairs in different locations are given specific names, e.g., pili, capilli, tragi, vibrissae, pubes, hirci.

axillary h's hirci.

bamboo h. trichorrhexis invaginata.

beaded h. hair marked with alternate swellings and constrictions, as in monilethrix. Called also *moniliform h.*

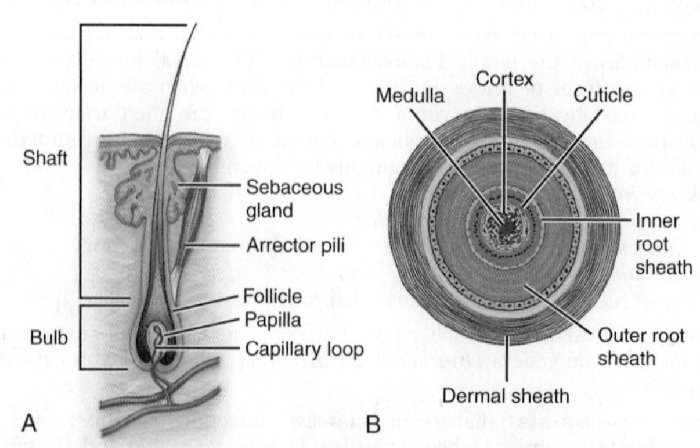

■ Hair in longitudinal section *(A)*, and in cross section *(B)*, showing the surrounding root and dermal sheaths.

club h. a hair whose root is surrounded by a bulbous enlargement composed of keratinized cells, usually just before normal loss of the hair from the follicle; see *telogen.*

downy h. lanugo.

exclamation point h. a hair that when pulled out shows atrophy and attenuation of its bulb; this is characteristic of alopecia areata.

Frey h's stiff hairs of varying diameters, individually mounted in a handle; used for testing the sensitiveness of the pressure points of the skin.

gustatory h's taste h's.

ingrown h. a hair that emerges from the skin but curves and reenters it, exciting a foreign body papule that may become infected. See also *pili incarnati*, under *pilus.*

kinky h. twisted h.

knotted h. trichonodosis.

lanugo h. lanugo.

moniliform h. beaded h.

olfactory h's modified cilia that are extremely long and nonmotile, project from the olfactory vesicle, and function as sensory receptors. Called also *olfactory cilia.*

primary h. lanugo.

pubic h. pubes (def. 1).

resting h. hair during the resting phase of growth; see *telogen.*

ringed h. a peculiar ringed type of hair seen in pili annulati (see under *pilus*).

sensory h's hairlike projections on the cells of sensory epithelium; see also *olfactory h's* and *taste h's.*

spun glass h. uncombable h.

steely h. twisted h.

stellate h. a hair split at the end in a starlike form.

tactile h's hairs that are sensitive to touch, such as the vibrissae of certain animals.

taste h's clumps of microvilli that form short hairlike processes projecting into the lumen of a taste pore from the peripheral ends of the taste cells.

terminal h. the coarse hair growing on various areas of the body during adult years.

twisted h. a hair that at spaced intervals, twisted through an axis of 180 degrees, and abnormally flattened, as in Menkes disease. See also *pili torti*, under *pilus.*

uncombable h. the peculiar triangular hair seen in the uncombable hair syndrome; called also *spun glass h.*

vellus h. vellus (def. 1).

hair·ball (hār′bawl) trichobezoar.

hair·worm (hār′wərm) threadworm.

hairy (hār′e) 1. pertaining to or characterized by hair; called also *pilar.* 2. hirsute.

Ha·kim syndrome (hah-kēm′) [S. *Hakim*, American neurologist, 20th century] normal-pressure hydrocephalus; see under *hydrocephalus.*

Ha·kim-Ad·ams syndrome (hah-kēm′ ad′əmz) [S. *Hakim;* R.D. *Adams*, American physician, 20th century] normal-pressure hydrocephalus; see under *hydrocephalus.*

Hal·a·rach·ni·dae (hal″ə-rak′nĭ-de) a family of mites that parasitize monkeys and dogs; it includes the genera *Pneumonyssoides* and *Pneumonyssus.*

hal·a·tion (hal-a′shən) [Gr. *halōs* halo] indistinctness or blurring of the visual image by strong illumination coming from the same direction as the viewed object.

hal·az·e·pam (hal-az′ə-pam) a benzodiazepine used as an antianxiety agent in the treatment of anxiety disorders and for short-term relief of anxiety symptoms; administered orally.

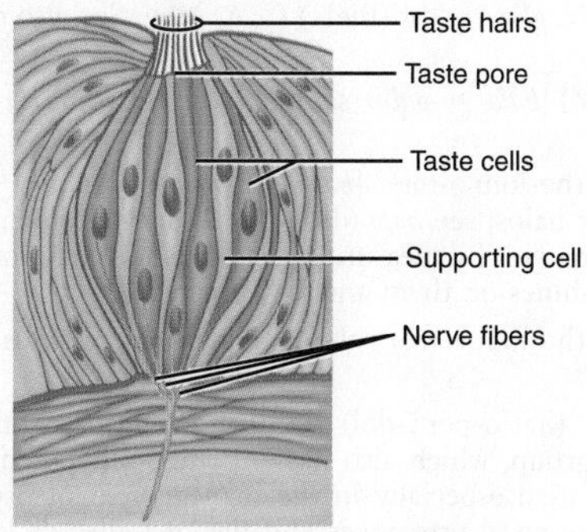

■ Taste hairs protruding from the pore of a taste bud.

hal·a·zone (hal′ə-zōn) [USP] a white, crystalline powder, $C_7H_5Cl_2NO_4S$, having a chlorine-like odor; used as a disinfectant for water supplies.

hal·cin·o·nide (hal-sin′ə-nīd) [USP] a high potency synthetic corticosteroid used topically for the relief of inflammation and pruritus in corticosteroid-responsive dermatoses.

Hal·ci·on (hal′se-ən) trademark for a preparation of triazolam.

Hal·dane effect (hawl′dān) [John Scott *Haldane*, Scottish physiologist, 1860–1936] see under *effect.*

Hal·dol (hal′dol) trademark for preparations of haloperidol.

Hal·drone (hal′drōn) trademark for a preparation of paramethasone acetate.

Hales piesimeter (hālz) [Stephen *Hales*, English physiologist, 1677–1761] see under *piesimeter.*

Hal·fan (hal′fan) trademark for a preparation of halofantrine hydrochloride.

half-ax·i·al (haf-ak′se-əl) hemiaxial.

half-life (haf′līf″) 1. the time required for the decay of half of a sample of particles of a radionuclide or elementary particle, equal to 0.693 divided by the decay constant; symbol $t_{1/2}$ or $T_{1/2}$. 2. half-time.

antibody h.-l. a measure of the mean survival time of antibody molecules following their formation, usually expressed as the time required to eliminate 50 percent of a known quantity of immunoglobulin from the animal body. Half-life varies from one immunoglobulin class to another.

biological h.-l. the time required for a living tissue, organ, or organism to eliminate one half of a radioactive substance which has been introduced into it.

drug h.-l. the time required for the plasma level of a drug to fall to half of a certain measured level.

effective h.-l. the time required for the radioactivity of a radioactive nuclide to be diminished 50 per cent through the combined action of radioactive decay and biological elimination.

half-time ($T_{1/2}$, $t_{1/2}$) (haf′tīm) the time required for one half of a quantity of a substance to be eliminated from a system when the substance is eliminated at a rate proportional to its concentration (i.e., exhibits first-order kinetics).

plasma iron clearance h.-t. the time required for half of the iron in the blood plasma at a given time to be removed, determined by administering radioactive iron-59 bound to the patient's own transferrin and calculating the slope of the best-fit line to a semilogarithmic plot of the amount of plasma radioactive iron over time.

half-val·ue (haf″val′u) see under *layer.*

half·way house (haf′wa hous′) a residence for patients, such as mental patients, drug addicts, and alcoholics, who do not require complete hospitalization but who need an intermediate degree of care until they have again become established in the community.

Hal·i·ceph·a·lo·bus (hal″ĭ-sef″ə-lo′bus) a genus of phasmid parasites of the order Rhabditoidea. *H. dele′trix* is a species that usually inhabits decaying organic matter and manure but sometimes infests horses, such as in nasal sinuses and the central nervous system. Called also *Micronema.*

hal·ide (hal′īd) 1. haloid. 2. a binary compound of one of the halogens (fluorine, chlorine, bromine, or iodine).

ha·lis·te·re·sis (hə-lis″tə-re′sis) [*hal-* + Gr. *sterēsis* privation] osteomalacia. **halisteret′ic** *adj*

h. ce′rea waxy softening of the bones.

hal·i·to·sis (hal″ĭ-to′sis) [L. *halitus* exhalation] offensive-smelling breath; called also *fetor ex ore, fetor oris,* and *stomatodysodia.*

Hall sign (hawl) [Josiah Newhall *Hall*, American physician, 1859–1939] see under *sign.*

hall·a·chrome (hal′ə-krōm) a compound formed from dihydroxyphenylalanine by tyrosinase.

Hal·lau·er glasses (hahl′ou-ər) [Otto *Hallauer*, Swiss ophthalmologist, late 19th century] see under *glasses.*

Hall·berg effect (hawl′bərg) [Josef Hendrik *Hallberg*, American electrician, 20th century] see under *effect.*

Hallé point (ah-la′) [Adrien Joseph Marie Noël *Hallé*, French physician, 1859–1947] see under *point.*

Hal·ler arch, circle, etc. (hahl′er) [Albrecht von *Haller*, Swiss physiologist, 1708–1777] see *circulus vasculosus nervi optici, ductulus aberrans inferior, lamina vasculosa choroideae, ligamentum arcuatum laterale, ligamentum arcuatum mediale, rete testis,* and *truncus coeliacus.*

Hal·ler·mann-Streiff syndrome (hah′lər-mahn shtrīf′) [Wilhelm *Hallermann*, German ophthalmologist, 1901–1976; Enrico Bernardo *Streiff*, Swiss ophthalmologist, 20th century] oculomandibulofacial syndrome.

Hal•ler•mann-Streiff-Fran•çois syndrome (hah′lər-mahn shtrīf′ frahn-swah′) [W. *Hallermann;* E.B. *Streiff;* Jules *François,* Belgian ophthalmologist, 1907–1984] oculomandibulofacial syndrome.

Hal•ler•vor•den-Spatz disease (hah′lər-for″dən shpahts′) [Julius *Hallervorden,* German (Nazi) neurologist, 1882–1965; Hugo *Spatz,* German (Nazi) neurologist and psychiatrist, 1888–1969] see under *disease.*

hal•lex (hal′əks) pl. *hal′lices.* hallux.

Hal•lo•peau acrodermatitis (ah-lo-po′) [François Henri *Hallopeau,* French dermatologist, 1842–1919] acrodermatitis continua.

Hal•lo•peau-Sie•mens syndrome (ah-lo-po′ se′mənz) [F.H. *Hallopeau;* Hermann Werner *Siemens,* German dermatologist, 1891–1969] recessive epidermolysis bullosa dystrophica; see under *epidermolysis.*

Hall•pike maneuver (hawl′pīk) [Charles Skinner *Hallpike,* British otologist, 1900–1979] Dix-Hallpike maneuver; see under *maneuver.*

hal•lu•ces (hal′ə-sēz, hal′u-sēz) [L.] plural of *hallux.*

hal•lu•ci•na•tion (hə-loo″sĭ-na′shən) [L. *hallucinatio;* Gr. *alyein* to wander in the mind] a sense perception without a source in the external world; a perception of an external stimulus object in the absence of such an object.

auditory h. a hallucination involving the sense of hearing. Called also *paracusia* and *paracusis.*

gustatory h. a hallucination involving the sense of taste.

haptic h. tactile h.

hypnagogic h. a vivid dreamlike hallucination occurring at sleep onset.

hypnopompic h. a vivid dreamlike hallucination occurring on awakening.

kinesthetic h. a hallucination involving the sense of bodily movement.

lilliputian h. a visual hallucination in which the imagined objects, usually people or animals, seem smaller than they would be in reality. Cf. *micropsia.*

olfactory h. a hallucination involving the sense of smell.

somatic h. a hallucination involving the perception of a physical experience occurring with the body.

tactile h. a hallucination involving the sense of touch.

visual h. a hallucination involving the sense of sight.

hal•lu•ci•na•tive (hə-loo′sĭ-nə-tiv) pertaining to or characterized by hallucinations; called also *hallucinatory.*

hal•lu•ci•na•to•ry (hə-loo′sĭ-nə-tor″e) hallucinative.

hal•lu•ci•no•gen (hə-loo′sĭ-no-jen″) [*hallucin*ation + *-gen*] an agent that induces hallucinations.

hal•lu•ci•no•gen•e•sis (hə-loo″sĭ-no-jen′ə-sis) the production of hallucinations.

hal•lu•ci•no•ge•net•ic (hə-loo″sĭ-no-jə-net′ik) hallucinogenic.

hal•lu•ci•no•gen•ic (hə-loo″sĭ-no-jen′ik) producing hallucinations.

hal•lu•ci•no•sis (hə-loo″sĭ-no′sis) a state characterized by the presence of hallucinations without other impairment of consciousness. hallucinot′ic *adj*

alcoholic h. hallucinations occurring in a clear sensorium in alcoholics with a long history of dependence and heavy intake, usually following a bout of unusually heavy drinking.

organic h. a term used in a former system of classification, denoting an organic mental syndrome characterized by the presence of hallucinations caused by a specific organic factor and not associated with delirium. Such disorders are now mainly classified as *substance-induced psychotic disorders* and *psychotic disorders due to general medical condition.*

hal•lux (hal′əks) gen. *hal′lucis* pl. *hal′luces* [L.] [TA] the great toe, or first digit of the foot; called also *digitus primus (I) pedis* [TA alternative]. hal′lucal *adj*

h. doloro′sus a painful condition of the great toe usually associated with flatfoot.

h. flex′us h. rigidus.

h. mal′leus hammer toe of the hallux.

h. ri′gidus painful flexion deformity of the great toe in which there is limitation of motion at the metatarsophalangeal joint.

h. val′gus angulation of the great toe away from the midline of the body, or toward the other toes; the great toe may ride under or over the other toes.

h. va′rus angulation of the great toe toward the midline of the body, or away from the other toes.

Hall•wachs effect (hahl′vahks) [Wilhelm Ludwig Franz *Hallwachs,* German physiologist, 1859–1922] photoelectric effect; see under *effect.*

ha•lo (ha′lo) [L., from Gr. *halōs* disk of the sun or moon] 1. a luminous or colored circle, such as the colored circle seen around a light in glaucoma. 2. a ring seen around the macula luteae in ophthalmoscopical examination. 3. the imprint of the ciliary processes upon the vitreous body.

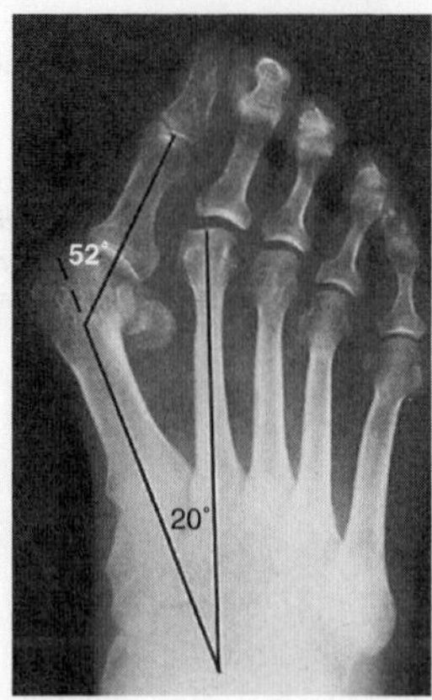

■ Hallux valgus, showing the increased intermetatarsal angle, lateral dislocation of sesamoids, subluxation of first metatarsophalangeal joint, and pronation of great toe.

4. a metal or plastic band that encircles the head or neck, providing support and stability as part of a halo device.

Fick h. a colored circle appearing around a light, caused by the wearing of contact lenses; see also *Fick phenomenon.*

h. glaucomato′sus, glaucomatous h. peripapillary atrophy seen in severe or chronic glaucoma.

h. saturni′nus lead line.

senile h. a zone of variable width surrounding the optic papilla, caused by exposure of various elements of the choroid as a result of senile atrophy of the pigmented epithelium.

hal(o)- [Gr. *hals,* gen. *halos* salt] a combining form denoting relationship to a salt.

hal•o•be•ta•sol pro•pi•o•nate (hal″o-ba′tə-sol) a very high potency synthetic corticosteroid used topically for the relief of inflammation and pruritus in corticosteroid-responsive dermatoses.

halo•der•mia (hal″o-dur′me-ə) halogenoderma.

Hal•o•drin (hal′o-drin) trademark for a combination preparation of fluoxymesterone and ethinyl estradiol.

halo•du•ric (hal″o-du′rik) [*halo-* + L. *durare* to endure] capable of existing in a medium containing a high concentration of salt.

hal•o•fan•trine hy•dro•chlor•ide (hal″o-fan′trēn) an antimalarial chemically related to quinine and mefloquine, effective against the asexual forms of *Plasmodium* in the blood stream; used in the treatment of acute falciparum and vivax malaria.

Hal•og (hal′og) trademark for preparations of halcinonide.

hal•o•gen (hal′ə-jən, ha′lə-jən) [*halo-* + *-gen*] an element of a closely related chemical family, all of which form similar (saltlike) compounds in combination with sodium and most other metals. The halogens are bromine, chlorine, fluorine, iodine, and astatine.

hal•o•gen•a•tion (hal″o-jə-na′shən) incorporation of a halogen into a chemical compound.

hal•o•gen•o•der•ma (hal″ə-jən-o-dur′mə) dermatosis caused by ingestion of a halogen or halide, such as in a medication. See *bromoderma* and *iododerma.*

Hal•o•ge•ton (hal-ə-ge′tən) a genus of small plants of the family Polygonaceae, which were introduced into the southwestern United States; they contain soluble oxalates that can be highly poisonous to grazing animals, causing respiratory difficulty, hemorrhage, and hypocalcemia. The major species is *H. glomera′tus* (Bieb.) C. A. Mey. See also *oxalate poisoning,* under *poisoning.*

hal•oid (hal′oid) [*halo-* + *-oid*] saltlike; derived from or resembling a halogen.

ha•lom•e•ter (hə-lom′ə-tər) [*halo* + *-meter*] 1. an instrument for measuring ocular halos; see *halo* (def. 1). 2. an instrument for estimating the size of erythrocytes by measuring the halos formed around them when a beam of light shines on them and is diffracted.

ha•lom•e•try (hə-lom′ə-tre) the measurement of halos with a halometer.

hal•o•peri•dol (hal″o-per′ĭ-dol) [USP] an antipsychotic agent of the butyrophenone group, which also has antiemetic, hypotensive, and hypothermic actions; used especially in the management of psychoses and for the control of the vocal utterances and tics of Gilles de la Tourette syndrome; administered orally and intramuscularly.

h. decanoate the decanoate ester of haloperidol, having the same actions as the base but of longer duration; administered intramuscularly in maintenance therapy for psychotic disorders.

hal·o·phil (hal′o-fil) a microorganism that requires a high concentration of salt for optimal growth.

hal·o·phile (hal′o-fīl) 1. halophil. 2. halophilic.

hal·o·phil·ic (hal″o-fil′ik) [*halo-* + *-philic*] pertaining to or characterized by an affinity for salt; applied to microorganisms which require a high concentration of salt for optimal growth.

hal·o·pro·gin (hal″o-pro′jin) a synthetic topical antifungal used in the treatment of various forms of tinea.

Hal·o·tes·tin (hal″o-tes′tin) trademark for a preparation of fluoxymesterone.

Hal·o·tex (hal′o-teks) trademark for a preparation of haloprogin.

hal·o·thane (hal′o-thān) [USP] a potent inhalational anesthetic, widely used for induction and maintenance of general anesthesia; it is nonflammable, induction and recovery are smooth and rapid, and the depth of anesthesia is rapidly altered.

hal·quin·ol (hal′kwin-ol) BAN for *halquinols*.

hal·quin·ols (hal′kwin-ols) a topical anti-infective compound, consisting of a mixture of 5,7-dichloro-8-quinolinol, 5-chloro-8-quinolinol, and 7-chloro-8-quinolinol in proportions resulting naturally from chlorination of 8-quinolinol; it has antiamebic, antifungal, and antibacterial actions.

Hal·sted mastectomy (operation), suture (hal′sted) [William Stewart *Halsted*, American surgeon, 1852–1922] see under *suture* and see *radical mastectomy*, under *mastectomy*.

Hal·tia-San·ta·vu·ori disease (hahl′te-ah sahn″tah-vwo′re) [M. *Haltia*, Finnish physician, 20th century; Pirkko *Santavuori*, Finnish physician, 20th century] see under *disease*.

hal·zoun (hal′zən) [Ar. *halzun* snail] 1. a pharyngeal form of fascioliasis occurring in the Middle East, caused by eating raw animal livers infected with *Fasciola;* young adult worms attach to the pharyngeal mucosa and produce pain, bleeding, and facial and neck edema. 2. a similar condition caused by ingestion of pentastomes from the livers or visceral lymph nodes of sheep or goats, which were eaten without being adequately cooked. Called also *halzoun syndrome*.

Ham test (ham) [Thomas Hale *Ham*, American physician, 1905–1987] acidified serum test.

Ham·a·me·lis (ham″ə-me′lis) [Gr. *hama* together + *mēlon* apple] a genus of trees and shrubs of the family Hamamelidaceae. *H. virginia′na* is witch hazel; an extract of its twigs is made into the astringent liquid also called witch hazel.

ham·a·me·lis (ham″ə-me′lis) the dried leaves of *Hamamelis virginiana*, which have been used as an astringent; see also *witch hazel* (def. 2).

ham·ar·tia (ham-ahr′shə) [Gr. "defect"] a defect in tissue combination during development. **hamar′tial** *adj*

hamart(o)- [Gr. *hamartia* fault] a combining form denoting relationship to a defect or to a hamartoma.

ham·ar·to·blas·to·ma (ham-ahr″to-blas-to′mə) [*hamarto-* + *blastoma*] a tumor developing from a hamartoma.

ham·ar·to·ma (ham″ahr-to′mə) [*hamart-* + *-oma*] a benign tumorlike nodule composed of an overgrowth of mature cells and tissues that normally occur in the affected part, but with disorganization and often with one element predominating.

bile duct h., biliary h. a generally benign hepatic lesion resulting from an embryonic ductal plate defect, consisting of well-defined nodules containing bile ducts surrounded by a fibrous stroma; malignant transformation rarely occurs.

fibrous h. of infancy a benign, nonencapsulated tumor, present at birth or appearing in the first few months of life, usually on the shoulder, axilla, or upper arm. It is a firm, painless, skin-colored nodule composed of well-defined fibrous trabeculae, immature mesenchymal tissue, and mature adipose cells, and often invades surrounding subcutaneous tissue.

hepatic mesenchymal h. a rare type of benign tumor of the liver, usually seen in young children and thought to be a developmental anomaly of portal connective tissue; it is characterized by overgrowth of mesenchymal stroma and may be solid or cystic.

pulmonary h. a benign tumor, usually a circumscribed nodule or coin lesion in peripheral lung parenchyma or in a bronchus; tissue types and degree of calcification vary.

sclerosing epithelial h. desmoplastic trichoepithelioma.

smooth muscle h. a rare type of hamartoma consisting of smooth muscle bundles forming skin-colored or hyperpigmented plaques on the skin of the trunk or the proximal part of a limb; it may be congenital or acquired.

sweat gland h. hidradenoma.

ham·ar·to·ma·to·sis (ham″ahr-to-mə-to′sis) the development of multiple hamartomas.

ham·ar·to·ma·tous (ham″ahr-to′mə-təs) pertaining to a disturbance in growth of a tissue in which the cells of a circumscribed area outstrip those of the surrounding areas.

ham·ate (ham′āt) shaped like a hook (hamulus). Cf. *uncinate*.

ha·ma·tum (hə-ma′təm) [L. "hooked"] 1. hamate. 2. os hamatum.

Ham·man disease, syndrome, sign (ham′ən) [Louis *Hamman*, American physician, 1877–1946] see *pneumomediastinum*, and see under *sign*.

Ham·man-Rich syndrome (ham′ən rich′) [L. *Hamman;* Arnold Rice *Rich*, American pathologist, 1893–1968] idiopathic pulmonary fibrosis.

ham·mer (ham′ər) 1. an instrument with a head designed for striking blows. 2. malleus.

percussion h. a small hammer, usually with a rubber head, for performing percussion.

reflex h. a type of percussion hammer used to tap tendons, nerves, or muscles to test various reflexes, such as the patellar reflex.

Ham·mond disease (ham′ənd) [William Alexander *Hammond*, American neurologist, 1828–1900] athetosis.

Hamp·ton hump (hamp′tən) [Aubrey Otis *Hampton*, American radiologist, 1900–1955] see under *hump*.

ham·ster (ham′stər) any member of four genera of the rodent family Muridae; genera used as laboratory animals are *Cricetulus*, *Cricetus*, and *Mesocricetus*.

Chinese h. *Cricetulus griseus*, a species that was formerly a common laboratory animal and is the source of the Chinese hamster ovary (CHO) cell line.

European h. *Cricetus cricetus*, a species native to Europe and the Middle East, commonly used as a laboratory animal.

golden h. *Mesocricetus auratus*, a species widely used as a laboratory animal and pet. Called also *Syrian h.*

Syrian h. golden h.

Syrian cardiomyopathic h. an inbred strain of Syrian hamster used as an animal model of hypertrophic cardiomyopathy.

ham·string (ham′string) 1. one of the tendons that border the popliteal fossa laterally and medially. 2. pertaining to or related to these tendons; see under *muscle*.

inner h's the tendons of the gracilis, sartorius, and two other muscles.

outer h. the tendon of the biceps flexor femoris.

ham·u·lar (ham′u-lər) shaped like a hook.

ham·u·lus (ham′u-ləs) pl. *ham′uli* [L. "little hook"] hook; a long, thin, curved structure.

h. of hamate bone h. ossis hamati.

h. lacrima′lis [TA] lacrimal hamulus: the hooklike process on the anterior part of the inferolateral border of the lacrimal bone, articulating with the maxilla.

h. la′minae spira′lis [TA] hamulus of spiral lamina: the hooklike upper end of the osseous spiral lamina.

h. os′sis hama′ti [TA] hook of hamate bone: a hooklike process on the volar surface of the hamate bone, to which numerous structures are attached. Called also *hamulus of hamate bone*.

h. pterygoi′deus [TA] pterygoid hamulus: a hooklike process on the inferior extremity of the medial pterygoid plate of the sphenoid bone, around which the tendon of the tensor veli palatini muscle passes.

h. of spiral lamina h. laminae spiralis.

Han·cock amputation (operation) (han′kok) [Henry *Hancock*, English surgeon, 1809–1880] see under *amputation*.

Hand disease (hand) [Alfred *Hand*, Jr., American pediatrician, 1868–1949] Hand-Schüller-Christian disease; see under *disease*.

Hand-Schül·ler-Chris·tian disease (hand′ she′lər kris′chən) [A. *Hand*, Jr.; Arthur *Schüller*, Austrian neurologist, 1874–1958; Henry Asbury *Christian*, American physician, 1876–1951] see under *disease*.

hand (hand) the distal region of the upper limb, including the carpus, metacarpus, and digits. In official terminology, called *manus*.

ape h. a hand with the thumb permanently extended.

benediction h. a hand in which the ring and little fingers are flexed; there is weakness of abduction and adduction of the index and middle fingers but they can be extended normally, and the thumb remains normal; seen in ulnar paralysis and syringomyelia.

claw h. clawhand.

cleft h. a congenital anomaly of the hand in which the division between the fingers extends into the metacarpus; often there are just two large digits, one on either side of the cleft. Called also *lobster-claw h.* or *deformity*, *split h.*, *split-hand deformity*, and *main fourchée*. See also *EEC syndrome*, under *syndrome*.

club h. clubhand.

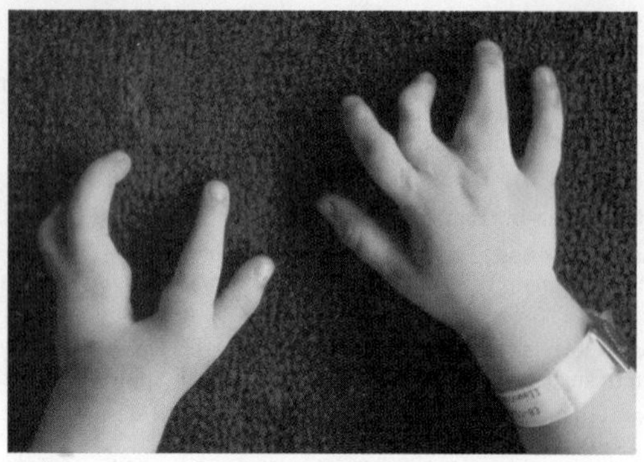

■ Cleft hands.

dead h. an occupational disorder seen sometimes in those who use vibratory tools, and apparently caused by the multitude of concussions. The hands are painful and dark blue in color, but blanch on exposure to cold.

drop h. wristdrop.

flat h. manus plana.

frozen h. stiffness of the hand resulting from edema accompanying trauma.

lobster-claw h. cleft h.

Marinesco succulent h. a soft, swollen, cyanotic, and cold hand caused by thickening and edema of the subcutaneous tissues; seen in syringomyelia. Called also *main succulente* and *Marinesco sign.* See also *Morvan syndrome* (def. 2), under *syndrome.*

mechanic's h's hands with chronic, eczematous skin that is fissured and scaly, seen in various systemic connective tissue disorders.

mirror h's an anomaly in which there are two crude hands growing from a common wrist.

mitten h. mitten deformity (q.v.) of the hand.

monkey h. adduction and extension of the thumb, which cannot be opposed to touch the tips of the other fingers because of thenar muscle weakness, usually because of a lesion of the median nerve. Called also *main en singe* and *monkey paw.*

myelopathy h. dysfunction of the hand associated with cervical myelopathy, characterized by loss of the ability to adduct and extend the fourth and fifth, and sometimes the middle, fingers (finger-escape sign) and inability to grip and release rapidly with these fingers.

obstetrician's h. the contraction of the hand in tetany, flexed at the wrist with fingers at the metacarpophalangeal joints but extended at the interphalangeal joints, the thumb being strongly flexed into the palm; so called because of a dubious resemblance to the position assumed by the hand of the obstetrician when examining the vagina.

opera-glass h. a pawlike hand marked by telescoping of the fingers caused by absorption of the phalanges, seen in chronic arthritis.

phantom h. a paresthetic feeling as if the hand were still present after amputation.

preacher's h. benediction h.

skeleton h. a hand markedly atrophied and held in a position of extension: seen in progressive muscular atrophy; called also *main en squelette.*

spade h. the thick square hand of myxedema and acromegaly.

split h. cleft h.

trench h. contracture or other incapacity of the hand from frostbite; so called from its occurrence in the trenches during World War I.

trident h. the characteristic hand of achondroplasia: the fingers are relatively of the same length, and there is a peculiar separation of the second and third fingers at the second phalangeal joint, causing the fingers to spread out.

writing h. a peculiar position of the hand in which it appears poised for writing; seen in Parkinson disease.

H and E hematoxylin-eosin; see *Stains and Staining Methods,* under *stain.*

hand•ed•ness (hand′əd-nis) the preferential use in voluntary motor acts of the hand of one side; see *dextrality* and *sinistrality.*

left h. the preferential use in voluntary motor acts of the left hand.

right h. the preferential use in voluntary motor acts of the right hand.

hand•i•cap (han′dĭ-kap) any physical or mental characteristic or defect, congenital or acquired, that prevents or restricts a person from participating in normal life or limits the capacity to work; see also *disability* and *impairment.*

han•dle (han′dəl) a part of a larger object enabling it to be grasped with the hand; see also *manubrium.*

h. of malleus manubrium mallei.

hand•piece (hand′pēs″) a hand-held device that engages rotary instruments used for removing tooth structures, cleaning teeth, and polishing dental restorations, connected to the dental engine by an adjustable arm in the case of a belt-driven instrument or by flexible tubing if air driven.

contra-angle h. a handpiece in which two or more angles or bends are used to set the shaft at a desired angle in order to access hard-to-reach areas of the oral cavity.

HANE hereditary angioneurotic edema; see *hereditary angioedema,* under *angioedema.*

hang•nail (hang′nāl) a shred of eponychium on a proximal or lateral nail fold.

Han•hart syndrome (hahn′hahrt) [Ernst *Hanhart,* Swiss physician, 1891–1973] see under *syndrome.*

Han•no•ver canal (hahn′o-vər) [Adolph *Hannover,* Danish anatomist, 1814–1894] see under *canal.*

Ha•not-Chauf•fard syndrome (ahn-o′ sho-fahr′) [Victor Charles *Hanot,* French physician, 1844–1896; Anatole Marie Emile *Chauffard,* French physician, 1855–1932] see under *syndrome.*

Han•se•mann macrophages (hahn′sə-mahn) [David Paul von *Hansemann,* German pathologist, 1858–1920] von Hansemann cells.

Han•sen bacillus, disease (hahn′sən) [Gerhard Henrik Armauer *Hansen,* Norwegian physician, 1841–1912] see *Mycobacterium leprae* and *leprosy.*

han•se•ni•a•sis (han″sə-ni′ə-sis) leprosy.

Han•sen•u•la (hən-sen′u-lə) a genus of yeasts of the family Saccharomycetaceae. *H. ano′mala* is a species commonly found in soil and as normal flora in the human respiratory and intestinal tracts.

Han•ta•vi•rus (han′tə-vi″rəs) [*Hantaan* River, Korea] a genus of viruses of the family Bunyaviridae that cause epidemic hemorrhagic fever and respiratory tract infections (see *hantavirus pulmonary syndrome,* under *syndrome*). There are at least 20 species included in one serogroup, and several unclassified species. Each species of virus appears to have a single rodent species as a host; transmission to humans is believed to be by contact, direct or indirect, with the excreta of infected rodents.

han•ta•vi•rus (han′tə-vi″rəs) any virus of the genus *Hantavirus.* hantavi′ral *adj*

Hap•a•lo•chlae•na (hap″ə-lo-kle′nə) [Gr. *hapalos* soft + *chlaina* cloak] a genus of octopus. *H. maculo′sa* is the venomous blue-ringed octopus (q.v.).

hap•a•lo•nych•ia (hap″ə-lo-nik′e-ə) onychomalacia.

HAPE high-altitude pulmonary edema.

haph•al•ge•sia (haf″al-je′ze-ə) [Gr. *haphē* touch + *algesia*] a type of tactile hyperesthesia in which normally painless touch sensations cause pain, as in Pitres sign (def. 1) or certain mental disorders.

haphe•pho•bia (haf″e-fo′be-ə) [Gr. *haphē* touch + *-phobia*] irrational fear of being touched.

hapl(o)- [Gr. *haploos* simple, single] a combining form meaning simple or single.

Hap•lo•chi•lus (hap″lo-ki′ləs) a genus of small fish. *H. pan′chax,* called *ikan kapala timah* in Malay, is a species placed in fishponds in Indonesia to eat the larvae of *Anopheles* mosquitoes.

hap•lo•dip•loi•dy (hap″lo-dip′loi-de) [*haplo-* + *diploidy*] the state in which males develop from unfertilized eggs and are haploid, and females develop from fertilized eggs and are diploid, as in honeybees.

hap•lo•dont (hap′lo-dont) [*haplo-* + Gr. *odous* tooth] having molar teeth without cusps or ridges.

hap•loid (hap′loid) [*hapl-* + *-oid*] having a single set of chromosomes, representing the normal complement of the species, as found in prokaryotes and in eukaryotic gametes. In humans, the haploid number, *n,* is 23. Cf. *diploid.*

hap•lo•iden•ti•cal (hap″lo-i-den′tĭ-kəl) sharing a haplotype; having the same alleles at a set of closely linked genes on one chromosome.

hap•lo•iden•ti•ty (hap″lo-i-den′tĭ-te) the condition of being haploidentical.

hap•loi•dy (hap′loi-de) the state of being haploid.

hap•lo•in•suf•fi•cien•cy (hap″lo-in″sə-fish′ən-se) the situation in which the contribution from a single copy of a normal allele, as in an individual carrying a heterozygous mutation or hemizygous at a particular locus, is inadequate to provide normal function.

hap•lo•my•co•sis (hap″lo-mi-ko′sis) adiaspiromycosis.

hap•lont (hap′lont) [Gr. *haploun* to make single] an individual having haploid somatic cells or nuclei, as many algae and fungi.

Hap•lo•pap•pus (hap-lo-pap′əs) a genus of composite-flowered plants (family Compositae). Several species, such as *H. hetero′phyllus,* the rayless goldenrod, contain the toxin tremetol and cause trembles in cattle and sheep.

hap•lop•a•thy (hap-lop′ə-the) [*haplo-* + *-pathy*] an uncomplicated disease.

hap•lo•pia (hap-lo′pe-ə) [*hapl-* + *-opia*] single vision; the condition in which an object looked at is seen single and not double.

Hap•lor•chis (hap-lor′kis) a genus of minute trematodes found in tropical areas; they are intestinal parasites of numerous types of vertebrates. *H. tai′chui* infects birds and mammals.

hap•lo•scope (hap′lo-skōp) [*haplo-* + *-scope*] an instrument that presents two separate views to the two eyes so that the views may be seen as one integrated view; it is used to measure, test, or stimulate various binocular functions. **haploscop′ic** *adj*

mirror h. a haploscope that uses mirrors to separate or displace the fields of vision of the two eyes.

hap•lo•spo•ran•gin (hap″lo-spor-an′jin) an antigen derived from the fungus *Emmonsia parva.*

Hap•lo•spo•ran•gi•um (hap″lo-spor-an′je-əm) *Emmonsia.*

hap•lo•type (hap′lo-tīp) [from *haplo*id geno*type*] 1. a set of alleles of a group of closely linked related genes on one chromosome of an individual, usually inherited as a unit; used particularly of the combination of alleles of the HLA complex. 2. the genetic constitution of an individual at such a set of closely linked genes.

Haps•burg jaw, lip, disease (haps′bərg) [*Hapsburg*, a German-Austrian royal family, including rulers of several European states, such as Austria (1278–1918) and Spain (1504–1700)] see under *jaw* and *lip*, and see *hemophilia.*

hap•ten (hap′tən) [Ger., from Gr. *haptein* to fasten] a small molecule, not antigenic by itself, that can react with antibodies of appropriate specificity and elicit the formation of such antibodies when conjugated to a larger antigenic molecule, usually a protein, called in this context the carrier or schlepper. Antibody production involves activation of B lymphocytes by the hapten and helper T lymphocytes by the carrier.

hap•tene (hap′tēn) hapten.

hap•ten•ic (hap-ten′ik) 1. pertaining to haptens. 2. caused by haptens.

hap•te•pho•bia (hap″te-fo′be-ə) [*hapt-* + *-phobia*] haphephobia.

hap•tic (hap′tik) [Gr. *haptikos* able to lay hold of] tactile.

hap•tics (hap′tiks) the study of the sense of touch; see *touch.*

hapt(o)- [Gr. *haptein* to fasten, grasp, touch] a combining form denoting relationship to touch or to binding.

hap•to•cor•rin (hap″to-kor′in) R protein.

hap•to•glo•bin (hap″to-glo′bin) a 100,000-dalton plasma glycoprotein with alpha electrophoretic mobility that irreversibly binds free hemoglobin to form a hemoglobin-haptoglobin complex, which is promptly removed by the liver; this prevents loss of free hemoglobin in the urine. Haptoglobin levels are decreased by hemolysis and increased by increased synthesis in conditions resulting in extensive tissue damage and necrosis. Haptoglobin has two major genetic variants, designated Hp 1 and Hp 2.

hap•tom•e•ter (hap-tom′ə-tər) [*hapto-* + *-meter*] an instrument for measuring sensitivity to touch.

Ha•ra•da syndrome (hah-rah′dah) [Einosuke *Harada*, Japanese ophthalmologist, 1892–1947] Vogt-Koyanagi-Harada syndrome; see under *syndrome.*

ha•rara (hə-rar′ə) [Ar. *al harara* heat] 1. an allergic skin reaction caused by bites of the sand fly *Phlebotomus papatasi* in the Middle East; characteristics include urticarial and inflammatory papules and blisters. After the initial exposure, most persons develop immunity in time. Called also *urticaria multiformis endemica.* 2. popular name for any of various other skin eruptions.

Har•den-Young ester (hahr′dən yung′) [Sir Arthur *Harden*, English biochemist, 1865–1940; William John *Young*, Australian biochemist, 20th century] fructose 1,6-bisphosphate.

hard•en•ing (hahr′dən-ing) 1. induration (def. 2). 2. sclerosis. 3. the procedure of rendering tissue firm, so that it may be more readily cut for purposes of microscopic examination.

h. of arteries popular term for *arteriosclerosis.*

Har•der glands (hahr′dər) [Johann Jacob *Harder*, Swiss physician, 1656–1711] see under *gland.*

hard•er•i•an (hahr′dər-e-ən) named for Johann Jacob *Harder*, as *harderian glands.*

hard•ero•por•phy•ria (hahr″dər-o-por-fīr′e-ə) a severe variant of hereditary coproporphyria differing in having earlier onset of attacks, excretion of harderoporphyrin in the feces, and virtual absence of coproporphyrinogen oxidase activity.

hard•ero•por•phy•rin (hahr″dər-o-por′fə-rin) an intermediate in heme biosynthesis, formed in the conversion of coproporphyrinogen to protoporphyrinogen and excreted excessively in the feces in harderoporphyria.

hard•ness (hahrd′nis) 1. a quality of water produced by soluble salts of calcium and magnesium or other substances which form an insoluble curd with soap and thus interfere with its cleansing power. 2. the quality of firmness produced by cohesion of the particles composing a substance, as evidenced by its inflexibility or resistance to indentation, distortion, or scratching. See also *hardness number*, under *number.* 3. the quality of x-rays that determines their penetrating power; hardness depends on wavelength: the shorter the wavelength, the harder the rays and the greater their penetrating power. 4. the degree of refraction of the residual gas in a glass tube: the higher the vacuum, the shorter the wavelength of the resulting x-rays.

diamond pyramid h. Vickers hardness number.

permanent h. hardness of water not removed by boiling; it is usually due to sulfates and chlorides.

temporary h. hardness of water removed by boiling; it is due to soluble bicarbonates, which lose CO_2 on boiling and precipitate as normal carbonates.

Har•dy-Wein•berg equilibrium, law (principle, rule) (hahr′de vīn′bərg) [Godfrey Harold *Hardy*, British mathematician, 1877–1947; Wilhelm *Weinberg*, German physician, 1862–1937] see under *law*, and see *genetic equilibrium*, under *equilibrium.*

Hare syndrome (hār) [Edward Selleck *Hare*, British surgeon, 1812–1838] Pancoast syndrome (def. 1).

hare•lip (hār′lip) former name for *cleft lip.*

har•le•quin (hahr′lə-kwin) [It. *arlecchino* a conventional stock character in European comedies who wore colorful checkered clothing] 1. having a pattern of diamond shapes, particularly in bright colors. 2. coral snake.

har•ma•line (hahr′mə-lēn) an alkaloid that has hallucinogenic properties, found in the seeds of African rue *(Peganum harmala)* and the South American vine *Banisteria caapi.*

har•mine (hahr′mēn) an alkaloid that has hallucinogenic properties, found in the seeds of African rue *(Peganum harmala)* and the South American vine *Banisteria caapi.* Called also *banisterine.*

har•mo•nia (hahr-mo′ne-ə) [L.] sutura plana.

har•mo•ny (hahr′mo-ne) the state of working together smoothly.

occlusal h. proper occlusion of the teeth occurring in various positions of the mandible.

occlusal h., functional such occlusion of the teeth in all positions of the mandible during mastication as will provide the greatest masticatory efficiency without imposing undue strain or trauma on the supporting tissues.

Har•mo•nyl (hahr′mo-nəl) trademark for preparations of deserpidine.

har•ness (hahr′nis) the combination of straps, bands, and other pieces that forms the working gear of a draft animal, or a device resembling such gear.

Pavlik h. a type of hip abduction orthosis consisting of a set of straps that hold the hips in flexion and abduction to correct hip dislocations in infants with developmental dysplasia of the hip.

Har•pa•go•phy•tum (hahr″pə-gof′ĭ-təm) [L. *harpago* grappling hook + Gr. *phyton* plant] a genus of herbs native to southern Africa, including *H. procum′bens*, the devil's claw, which is used medicinally.

Har•pi•rhyn•chus (hahr″pe-ring′kəs) [Gr. *harpē* bird of prey + Gr. *rhynchos* snout] a genus of mites parasitic on birds.

har•poon (hahr-po͞on′) [Gr. *harpazein* to seize] an instrument for removing small pieces of living tissue for diagnostic examination.

Har•ring•ton instrumentation, rod (har′ing-tən) [Paul Randall *Harrington*, American orthopedic surgeon, 1911–1980] see under *instrumentation* and *rod.*

Har•ris hematoxylin stain (har′is) [Downey Lamar *Harris*, American pathologist, 1875–1956] see *Stains and Staining Methods*, under *stain.*

Har•ris lines (har′is) [Henry Albert *Harris*, Welsh anatomist, 1886–1968] see under *line.*

Har•ris syndrome (har′is) [Seale *Harris*, American physician, 1870–1957] see under *syndrome.*

Har•ri•son groove (curve, sulcus) (har′ĭ-sən) [Edward *Harrison*, English physician, 1766–1838] see under *groove.*

Har•tel treatment (hahr′təl) [Fritz *Hartel*, German surgeon, 20th century] see under *treatment.*

Hart•ley-Krause operation (hahrt′le krou′zə) [Frank *Hartley*, American surgeon, 1857–1913; Fedor *Krause*, German surgeon, 1857–1937] see under *operation*.

Hart•mann curet (hahrt′mahn) [Arthur *Hartmann*, German laryngologist, 1849–1931] see under *curet*.

Hart•mann pouch, procedure (operation, colostomy) (hahrt′mahn) [Henri *Hartmann*, French surgeon, 1860–1952] see under *pouch* and *procedure*.

Hart•man•nel•la (hahrt″mən-el′ə) a genus of free-living ramicristate amebae, protozoa of the order Euamoebida, found in fresh water and soil. *H. vermifor′mis* and a few other species can cause opportunistic infections in immunocompromised persons, usually primary amebic meningoencephalitis and sometimes other conditions such as amebic keratitis.

hart•man•nel•li•a•sis (hahrt″mə-nel-i′ə-sis) opportunistic infection with *Hartmannella*, such as primary amebic meningoencephalitis or amebic keratitis.

Hart•nup disease (hahrt′nəp) [*Hartnup*, surname of the British propositus] see under *disease*.

harts•horn (hahrts′horn) ammonium carbonate.

har•vest (hahr′vəst) to remove tissues or cells from a donor and preserve for transplantation.

Har•vey (hahr′ve) William, 1578–1657. English physician; he practiced in London and was physician to James I and Charles I. In his *Exercitatio anatomica de motu cordis et sanguinis* (1628), Harvey demonstrated that (1) contraction of the heart muscle coincides with the pulse as the ventricles pump blood into the aorta and pulmonary artery; (2) the pulse is produced by the arteries' filling with blood; (3) the septum is impervious; (4) venous and arterial blood are the same; and (5) the blood in the right ventricle goes through the arteries to the lungs and thence through the pulmonary veins to the left ventricle and thence through the arteries to the body whence it returns along the smaller veins to the venae cavae and then into the right ventricle—a complete circulation of the blood.

Ha•shi•mo•to disease (thyroiditis, struma), encephalopathy (hah″-she-mo′to) [Hakaru *Hashimoto*, Japanese surgeon, 1881–1934] see under *disease* and *encephalopathy*.

hash•ish (hă-shēsh′) [Ar. "herb"] a preparation of the unadulterated resin scraped from the flowering tops of cultivated female hemp plants, *Cannabis sativa* L. (Cannabaceae), which is smoked or chewed for its intoxicating effects. It is far more potent than marijuana. See *cannabis*.

hash•i•tox•i•co•sis (hash″ĭ-tok″sĭ-ko′sis) [*Hashi*moto disease + *toxicosis*] hyperthyroidism in patients with Hashimoto disease. Cf. *painless thyroiditis*, under *thyroiditis*.

Has•ner fold, valve (hahs′nər) [Joseph Ritter von Artha *Hasner*, Czech ophthalmologist, 1819–1892] see *plica lacrimalis*.

Has•sall corpuscles (bodies) (has′əl) [Arthur Hill *Hassall*, English chemist and physician, 1817–1894] see under *corpuscle*.

HAT hypoxanthine-aminopterin-thymidine (medium); see under *culture medium*.

hatch•et (hach′ət) a bibeveled or single beveled cutting dental instrument having its cutting edge in line with the axis of its blade; used for breaking down tooth structures undermined by caries, for smoothing cavity walls, and for sharpening line and point angles. Called also *hatchet excavator*.

enamel h. a hatchet in which the broad side of the blade is parallel with the angle of the shank; used with a chipping or a lateral scraping stroke in developing an internal cavity form.

hatch•ing (hach′ing) emergence from an egg.

assisted embryo h., embryo h. treatment of infertility caused by an abnormally thick covering to the egg; using micromanipulation techniques, the fertilized egg is helped to emerge from the covering and implant in the endometrium.

H$^+$-ATP•ase (a-te-pe′ās) H$^+$-transporting ATP synthase.

Hauch (H) (houk) [Ger. "breath" (because motile bacteria form a spreading film around colonies resembling that produced by breathing on glass)] used to describe certain bacterial colonies; see *H antigen* under *antigen* and *H colony* under *colony*.

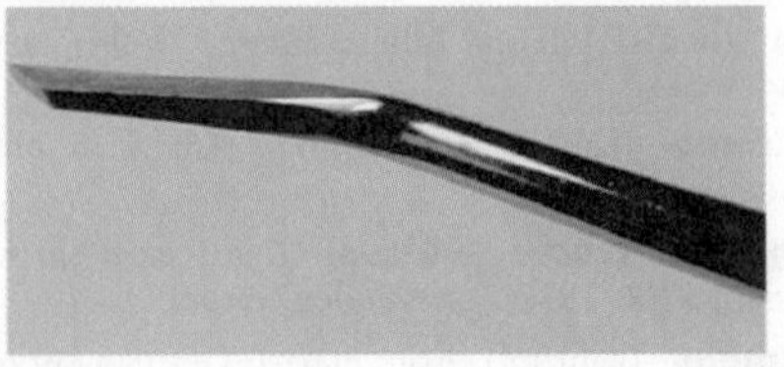

■ Hatchet.

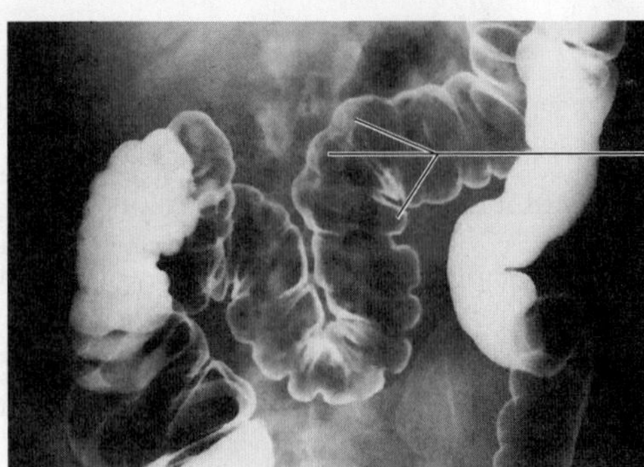

■ Haustra coli in a double-contrast radiograph after barium enema (anteroposterior view).

Hau•dek sign (niche) (hou′dek) [Martin *Haudek*, Austrian radiologist, 1880–1931] see under *sign*.

haunch (hawnch) the hip and buttock.

Haust. haus′tus (a draft).

haus•tel•lum (haw-stel′əm) pl. *haustel′la* [L., from *haustus* draw up] a mouthpart of certain ectoparasites, such as bedbugs and lice, modified for piercing and sucking, consisting of a hollow tube with an eversible set of five stylets, by which the organism attaches itself to the host and through which the blood is drawn up.

haus•tor•i•um (haws-tor′e-əm) pl. *hausto′ria* [L., from *haustus* a drawing in] a structure of certain parasites adapted specially to penetrate the host's tissues and absorb nutrients and water.

haus•tra (haws′trə) [L.] plural of *haustrum*.

haus•tral (haws′trəl) pertaining to the haustra of the colon.

haus•tra•tion (haws-tra′shən) 1. the formation of a haustrum. 2. a haustrum.

haus•trum (haws′trəm) pl. *haus′tra* [L. *haustor* drawer] a recess or sacculation.

haus′tra co′li [TA], **haustra of colon** sacculations in the wall of the colon produced by adaptation of its length to that of the taeniae coli, or by the arrangement of the circular muscle fibers.

haut-mal (o-mahl′) [Fr.] grand mal; see under *epilepsy*.

Haut•mann neobladder (hout′mahn) [Richard E. *Hautmann*, German urologist, late 20th century] see under *neobladder*.

HAV hepatitis A virus.

Ha•ver•hill fever (ha′vər-il) [*Haverhill*, Massachusetts, where an epidemic occurred in 1925] see under *fever*.

ha•ver•sian (ha-vur′zhən) named for Clopton *Havers*, English physician and anatomist, 1650–1702, as *haversian lamella* and *haversian system*.

Hav•rix (hav′riks) trademark for a preparation of hepatitis A vaccine inactivated.

haw (haw) 1. popular term for *nictitating membrane*. 2. haw syndrome.

haw•kin•sin (haw′kin-sin) a cyclic amino acid metabolite of tyrosine excreted in hawkinsinuria, a rare aminoacidopathy. It is formed from an intermediate of the 4-hydroxyphenylpyruvate dioxygenase reaction combined with glutathione.

haw•kin•sin•u•ria (haw″kin-sin-u′re-ə) a rare autosomal dominant disorder caused by heterozygous mutation in the *HPD* gene (locus: 12q24-qter), which encodes 4-hydroxyphenylpyruvate dioxygenase, an enzyme important in tyrosine catabolism. It is characterized by excretion of hawkinsin in urine, metabolic acidosis, and failure to thrive in infancy; hypertyrosinemia is absent or minimal. Cf. *tyrosinemia type III*.

Haw•ley retainer (appliance) (haw′le) [C.A. *Hawley*, American dentist, early 20th century] see under *retainer*.

haw•thorn (haw′thorn″) [A.S. *hagathorn*, from *haga* hedge + *thorn*] 1. a shrub or tree of the genus *Crataegus*. 2. a preparation of the flowers, fruit, and leaves of certain species of *Crataegus*, having a mechanism of action similar to that of digitalis, used to decrease output in congestive heart failure (New York Heart Association (NYHA) classification stages I and II and possibly III); also used in traditional Chinese medicine and homeopathy, and for a wide variety of indications in folk medicine.

Hay-Wells syndrome (ha′ welz′) [R.J. *Hay*, British dermatologist, 20th century; Robert Stuart *Wells*, British dermatologist, 20th century] see under *syndrome*.

Ha·yem solution (ah-yahn′) [Georges *Hayem*, French physician, 1841–1933] see under *solution.*

Ha·yem-Wi·dal syndrome (ah-yah′ ve-dahl′) [G. *Hayem;* Georges Fernand Isidore *Widal*, French physician, 1862–1929] hemolytic anemia.

Hay·flick limit (ha′flik) [Leonard *Hayflick*, American microbiologist, born 1928] see under *limit.*

HB hepatitis B.

Hb hemoglobin.

HBc hepatitis B core (antigen).

HBcAg hepatitis B core antigen.

HbCV *Haemophilus* b conjugate vaccine.

HBE His bundle electrogram.

HBe hepatitis B e (antigen).

HBeAg hepatitis B e antigen.

HbO_2 oxyhemoglobin.

HBs hepatitis B surface (antigen).

HBsAg hepatitis B surface antigen.

HBV hepatitis B virus.

HC Hospital Corps.

HCFA Health Care Financing Administration, part of the Department of Health and Human Services.

HCG, hCG human chorionic gonadotropin.

HCM hypertrophic cardiomyopathy.

HCP hereditary coproporphyria.

Hct hematocrit.

HCV hepatitis C virus.

HD Huntington disease; hemodialysis.

H.d. ho′ra decu′bitus (at bedtime).

HDCV human diploid cell (rabies) vaccine.

HDL high-density lipoprotein.

HDL_1 Lp(a) lipoprotein.

HDL_2 see *high-density lipoprotein*, under *lipoprotein.*

HDL_3 see *high-density lipoprotein*, under *lipoprotein.*

HDL-C high-density-lipoprotein cholesterol.

HDN hemolytic disease of newborn; see *erythroblastosis fetalis.*

HDP oxidronate (hydroxymethylene diphosphonate).

HDV hepatitis D virus.

H & E hematoxylin-eosin; see *Stains and Staining Methods*, under *stain.*

He helium.

he- for words beginning thus, see also those beginning *hae-*.

Head zones (hed) [Sir Henry *Head*, British neurologist, 1861–1940] see under *zone.*

head (hed) [A.S. *hēafod*] 1. caput (def. 1). 2. the upper, anterior, or proximal extremity of a structure or body. See also *caput.*

anterior h. of rectus femoris muscle caput rectum musculi recti femoris.

articular h. an eminence on a bone by which it articulates with another bone.

h. of astragalus caput tali.

big h. bighead.

h. of caudate nucleus caput nuclei caudati.

h. of condyloid process of mandible caput mandibulae.

coronoid h. of pronator teres muscle caput ulnare musculi pronatoris teretis.

deep h. of flexor pollicis brevis muscle caput profundum musculi flexoris pollicis brevis.

deep h. of triceps brachii muscle caput mediale musculi tricipitis brachii.

deep h. of triceps extensor cubiti muscle caput mediale musculi tricipitis brachii.

drum h. membrana tympanica.

engaged h. the position of the fetal head when the biparietal plane has passed the pelvic inlet.

h. of epididymis caput epididymidis.

femoral h., h. of femur caput femoris.

h. of fibula caput fibulae.

first h. of triceps brachii muscle caput longum musculi tricipitis brachii.

first h. of triceps extensor cubiti muscle caput longum musculi tricipitis brachii.

floating h. the head of the fetus when it is freely movable above the inlet of the birth canal.

great h. of adductor hallucis muscle caput obliquum musculi adductoris hallucis.

great h. of triceps brachii muscle caput laterale musculi tricipitis brachii.

great h. of triceps extensor cubiti muscle caput laterale musculi tricipitis brachii.

great h. of triceps femoris muscle musculus adductor magnus.

hot cross bun h. former name for caput quadratum.

hourglass h. a head in which the coronal suture is depressed.

humeral h. of extensor carpi ulnaris muscle caput humerale musculi extensoris carpi ulnaris.

humeral h. of flexor carpi ulnaris muscle caput humerale musculi flexoris carpi ulnaris.

humeral h. of pronator teres muscle caput humerale musculi pronatoris teretis.

humeroulnar h. of flexor digitorum superficialis muscle caput humero-ulnare musculi flexoris digitorum superficialis.

h. of humerus caput humeri.

inferior h. of lateral pterygoid muscle caput inferius musculi pterygoidei lateralis.

lateral h. of flexor hallucis brevis muscle caput laterale musculi flexoris hallucis brevis.

lateral h. of gastrocnemius muscle caput laterale musculi gastrocnemii.

lateral h. of triceps brachii muscle caput laterale musculi tricipitis brachii.

lateral h. of triceps extensor cubiti muscle caput laterale musculi tricipitis brachii.

little h. of humerus capitulum humeri.

long h. of adductor hallucis muscle caput obliquum musculus adductoris hallucis.

long h. of adductor triceps muscle musculus adductor longus.

long h. of biceps brachii muscle caput longum musculi bicipitis brachii.

long h. of biceps femoris muscle caput longum musculi bicipitis femoris.

long h. of biceps flexor cruris muscle caput longum musculi bicipitis femoris.

long h. of biceps flexor cubiti muscle caput longum musculi bicipitis brachii.

long h. of triceps brachii muscle caput longum musculi tricipitis brachii.

long h. of triceps extensor cubiti muscle caput longum musculi tricipitis brachii.

long h. of triceps femoris muscle musculus adductor longus.

lower h. of lateral pterygoid muscle caput inferius musculi pterygoidei lateralis.

h. of malleus caput mallei.

h. of mandible caput mandibulae.

medial h. of biceps brachii muscle caput breve musculi bicipitis brachii.

medial h. of biceps flexor cubiti muscle caput breve musculi bicipitis brachii.

medial h. of flexor hallucis brevis muscle caput mediale musculi flexoris hallucis brevis.

medial h. of gastrocnemius muscle caput mediale musculi gastrocnemii.

medial h. of triceps brachii muscle caput mediale musculi tricipitis brachii.

medial h. of triceps extensor cubiti muscle caput mediale musculi tricipitis brachii.

medusa h. caput medusae.

h. of metacarpal caput ossis metacarpi.

h. of metatarsal caput ossis metatarsi.

middle h. of triceps brachii muscle caput longum musculi tricipitis brachii.

middle h. of triceps extensor cubiti muscle caput longum musculi tricipitis brachii.

h. of muscle the end of a muscle at the site of its attachment (origin) to a bone or other fixed structure; called also *caput musculi.*

nasal h. of levator labii superioris alaeque nasi muscle musculus levator labii superioris alaeque nasi.

oblique h. of adductor hallucis muscle caput obliquum musculus adductoris hallucis.

oblique h. of adductor pollicis muscle caput obliquum musculi adductoris pollicis.

h. of pancreas caput pancreatis.

h. of penis glans penis.

h. of phalanx of hand caput phalangis manus.

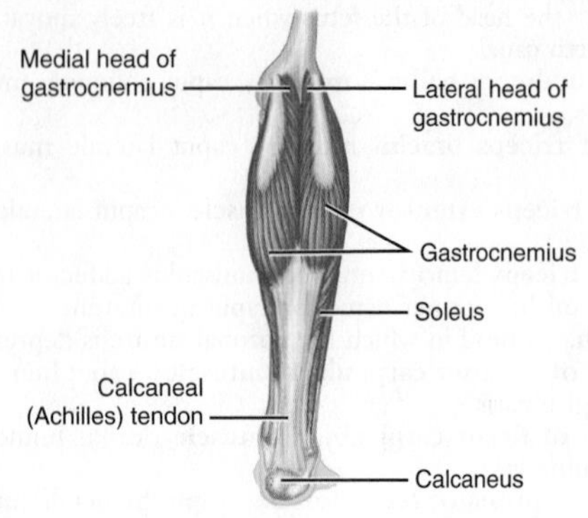

■ Lateral and medial heads of the gastrocnemius muscle.

h. of phalanx of foot caput phalangis pedis.
plantar h. of flexor digitorum pedis longus muscle musculus quadratus plantae.
h. of posterior horn of spinal cord caput cornus posterioris medullae spinalis.
posterior h. of rectus femoris muscle caput reflexum musculi recti femoris.
quadrate h. of flexor digitorum pedis longus muscle musculus quadratus plantae.
radial h. of flexor digitorum sublimis muscle caput radiale musculi flexoris digitorum superficialis.
radial h. of flexor digitorum superficialis muscle caput radiale musculi flexoris digitorum superficialis.
radial h. of humerus capitulum humeri.
h. of radius caput radii.
reflected h. of rectus femoris muscle caput reflexum musculi recti femoris.
h. of rib caput costae.
saddle h. a head with a sunken crown.
scapular h. of triceps brachii muscle caput longum musculi tricipitis brachii.
scapular h. of triceps extensor cubiti muscle caput longum musculi tricipitis brachii.
second h. of triceps brachii muscle caput laterale musculi tricipitis brachii.
short h. of biceps brachii muscle caput breve musculi bicipitis brachii.
short h. of biceps femoris muscle caput breve musculi bicipitis femoris.
short h. of biceps flexor cruris muscle caput breve musculi bicipitis femoris.
short h. of biceps flexor cubiti muscle caput breve musculi bicipitis brachii.
short h. of triceps brachii muscle caput mediale musculi tricipitis brachii.
short h. of triceps extensor cubiti muscle caput mediale musculi tricipitis brachii.
short h. of triceps femoris muscle musculus adductor brevis.
sperm h., h. of spermatozoon the oval anterior end of a spermatozoon, which contains the male pronucleus and is surrounded by the acrosome. See illustration at *spermatozoon.*
h. of spleen extremitas posterior splenis.
h. of stapes caput stapedis.
steeple h. oxycephaly.
straight h. of rectus femoris muscle caput rectum musculi recti femoris.
superficial h. of flexor pollicis brevis muscle caput superficiale musculi flexoris pollicis brevis.
superior h. of lateral pterygoid muscle caput superius musculi pterygoidei lateralis.
swelled h. bighead (def. 2).
h. of talus caput tali.
tower h. oxycephaly.
transverse h. of adductor hallucis muscle caput transversum musculi adductoris hallucis.
transverse h. of adductor pollicis muscle caput transversum musculi adductoris pollicis.
h. of ulna caput ulnae.
ulnar h. of extensor carpi ulnaris muscle caput ulnare musculi extensoris carpi ulnaris.
ulnar h. of flexor carpi ulnaris muscle caput ulnare musculi flexoris carpi ulnaris.
ulnar h. of pronator teres muscle caput ulnare musculi pronatoris teretis.
upper h. of lateral pterygoid muscle caput superius musculi pterygoidei lateralis.
zygomatic h. of quadratus labii superioris muscle musculus zygomaticus minor.

head•ache (hed′āk″) pain in the head; called also *cephalalgia, cephalgia,* and *cephalodynia.*
benign cough h. primary cough headache.
chronic tension h. see *tension h.*
cluster h. a primary headache characterized by attacks of unilateral excruciating pain over the eye and forehead, with temperature elevation, lacrimation, and rhinorrhea; attacks last from 15 minutes to about an hour and tend to occur in clusters, sometimes a few times a day for two to eight weeks followed by months or years without occurrence. Because attacks identical to the spontaneous attacks may be induced in sufferers by subcutaneous injection of histamine phosphate, it is also known as *histamine cephalalgia* or *h.* See also *chronic paroxysmal hemicrania,* under *hemicrania.* Called also *Horton disease* and *vasomotor h.*
cough h. severe, stabbing, bilateral head pain brought on by coughing or some other Valsalva maneuver; it may be due to a structural lesion such as a Chiari malformation, or it may be without an underlying cause *(primary cough h.).*
dynamite h. a severe headache occurring in persons handling high explosives.
episodic tension h. see *tension h.*
exertional h. a headache that follows physical exercise; many are of short duration. Cf. *cough h.* and *postcoital h.*
functional h. a headache caused by tension or other emotional upset.
helmet h. pain involving the upper half of the head.
histamine h., Horton h. cluster h.
hypnic h. a rare primary headache, occurring mainly in individuals over 50 years of age, that wakes the person from sleep, often at about the same time each night. Pain is dull, diffuse, and often bilateral and throbbing and lasts 15 minutes or longer.
lumbar puncture h. headache occurring a few hours after lumbar puncture, due to lowering of intracranial pressure after leakage of cerebrospinal fluid; see also post–lumbar puncture syndrome. Called also *post–dural puncture, post–lumbar puncture, postspinal,* or *post–spinal puncture h.,* and *spinal h.*
migraine h. migraine.
occipital h. see under *neuralgia.*
organic h. a headache due to intracranial disease or other organic disease.
postcoital h. exertional headache occurring during or after sexual activity, usually in males; one subtype lasts for hours.
post–dural puncture h., post–lumbar puncture h. lumbar puncture headache.
postspinal h., post–spinal puncture h. lumbar puncture h.
posttraumatic h. a headache occurring after trauma to the head or neck; it may be either physical or psychogenic in origin and may resemble either a cluster or a tension headache. Physical causes include subdural hematoma, stretching or tearing of ligaments and muscles in the neck, and injury to cervical soft tissues.
primary h. one of the two broad categories of headache, comprising headaches that occur without a discernible underlying cause; it includes cluster headache, tension headache, and migraine. Cf. *secondary h.*
primary cough h. severe bilateral head pain of sudden onset following coughing or some other Valsalva maneuver, without any underlying pathologic cause. Called also *benign cough h.*
puncture h. lumbar puncture h.
rhinogenous h. head pain caused by nasal disease or pathology.
secondary h. one of the two broad categories of headache, comprising headaches caused by an underlying pathologic condition, such as a neoplastic or vascular disorder, an adverse drug reaction, or a psychiatric disorder. Cf *primary h.*
sick h. migraine.
spinal h. lumbar puncture h.
tension h., tension-type h. a primary headache brought on by prolonged overwork or emotional strain, or both, affecting especially the occipital region; it is usually continuous for weeks or months. Some individuals are particularly susceptible, possibly because of a defect in neurologic pathways controlling pain. A distinction is made between *episodic tension headaches,* which abate within a few weeks to six months, and *chronic tension headaches,* which persist uninterrupted for six months or longer.
thunderclap h. a severe headache of rapid onset, reaching maximum intensity in less than a minute and lasting from an hour to several days. It is most often associated with intracranial vascular disorders; in rare instances it may be a primary headache.
toxic h. headache caused by systemic poisoning or certain illnesses.

vacuum h. headache caused by obstruction of the outlet of the frontal sinus.

vascular h. a classification for certain types of headaches, based on a proposed etiology involving abnormal functioning of the blood vessels or vascular system of the brain; included are migraine, cluster headache, toxic headache, and headache caused by chronic or episodic increases in blood pressure.

vasomotor h. cluster h.

head·cap (hed′kap) headgear.

head·gear (hed′gēr) a harnesslike device fitting over the top and back of the head, serving as a source of resistance for extraoral anchorage for an orthodontic appliance. Called also *headcap.*

head·grit (hed′grit) yellows (def. 2).

head·gut (hed′gət) foregut.

heal (hēl) 1. to restore wounded parts or to make healthy. 2. to become well or healthy.

heal·ing (hēl′ing) 1. a process of cure. 2. the restoration of integrity to injured tissue.

h. by first intention healing in which union or restoration of continuity occurs directly without the intervention of granulations.

h. by granulation h. by second intention.

h. by primary intention h. by first intention.

h. by second intention union by closure of a wound with granulations which form from the base and both sides toward the surface of the wound.

spiritual h. the use of spiritual practices, such as prayer, for the purpose of effecting a cure of or an improvement in an illness.

h. by third intention a method of closing a grossly contaminated wound: the wound is left open until contamination has been markedly reduced and inflammation has subsided and then is closed by first intention. Called also *delayed primary closure.*

Heal·on (hēl′on) trademark for a preparation of hyaluronan.

health (helth) a state of optimal physical, mental, and social well-being; the popular idea that it is merely an absence of disease and infirmity is not complete.

allied h. any of diverse health care professions, including clinical laboratory personnel, physical therapy, occupational therapy, dietetic services, medical records personnel, radiology services, speech-language pathology and audiology, and respiratory therapy. It does not include physicians, nurses, dentists, or podiatrists.

holistic h. a system of preventive medicine that takes into account the whole individual, his own responsibility for his well-being and the total influences—social, psychological, environmental—that affect health, including nutrition, exercise, and mental relaxation.

public h. the field of medicine concerned with safeguarding and improving the health of the community as a whole.

healthy (hel′the) 1. pertaining to or characterized by health. 2. promoting health.

hear·ing (hēr′ing) [L. *auditus*] the sense by which sounds are perceived; capacity to perceive sound. Called also *audition.*

color h. a form of chromesthesia in which sounds cause sensations of color.

double disharmonic h. diplacusis.

monaural h. hearing with one ear.

visual h. lip reading.

hear·ing loss (hēr′ing los′) deafness; partial or complete loss of the sense of hearing.

acoustic trauma h. l. noise-induced hearing loss caused by a single loud noise such as blast injury.

Alexander h. l. see under *deafness.*

central h. l. hearing loss due to causes in the auditory pathways or in the auditory cortex of the brain.

cochlear h. l. sensorineural hearing loss due to a defect in the receptor or transducing mechanisms of the cochlea.

conduction h. l., conductive h. l. hearing loss due to a defect of the sound conducting apparatus, i.e., of the external auditory canal or middle ear. Called also *transmission h. l.*

functional h. l. hearing loss that lacks any organic lesion. Called also *nonorganic h. l.*

high-frequency h. l., high-tone h. l. sensorineural hearing loss of tones at high frequencies, most commonly seen with noise-induced hearing loss.

low-frequency h. l., low-tone h. l. sensorineural hearing loss of tones at low frequencies.

mixed h. l. hearing loss that is both conductive and sensorineural in nature.

neural h. l. sensorineural hearing loss caused primarily by a lesion of the vestibulocochlear nerve or the central neural pathways.

noise-induced h. l. sensorineural hearing loss caused either by a single very loud noise (acoustic trauma hearing loss) or by prolonged exposure to high levels of noise (socioacusis).

nonorganic h. l. functional h. l.

organic h. l. hearing loss due to defect in the ear or auditory apparatus.

ototoxic h. l. hearing loss caused by ingestion of toxic substances; called also *toxic h. l.*

pagetoid h. l. see under *deafness.*

paradoxic h. l. hearing loss in which the hearing is better during loud noise. Called also *paracusis of Willis.*

perceptive h. l. sensorineural h. l.

postlingual h. l. hearing loss that occurs after the person has learned to speak.

prelingual h. l. hearing loss that occurs before the person has learned to speak.

retrocochlear h. l. sensorineural hearing loss in which the lesion is proximal to the cochlea, in the vestibulocochlear nerve or one of the auditory areas of the brain.

sensorineural h. l. hearing loss due to a lesion in either the cochlea (sensory mechanism of the ear), the vestibulocochlear nerve, the central neural pathways, or a combination of these structures. It is sometimes subdivided into *cochlear h. l.* and *retrocochlear h. l.*

sensory h. l. sensorineural hearing loss caused primarily by damage to the sensory mechanisms in the internal ear.

toxic h. l. ototoxic h. l.

transmission h. l. conductive h. l.

heart (hahrt) [L. *cor;* Gr. *kardia*] the viscus of cardiac muscle that maintains the circulation of the blood. Called also *cor* [TA]. It is divided into four cavities—two atria and two ventricles. The left atrium receives oxygenated blood from the lungs. From there the blood passes to the left ventricle, which forces it via the aorta through the arteries to supply the tissues of the body. The right atrium receives the blood after it has passed through the tissues and given up much of its oxygen. The blood then passes to the right ventricle, and then to the lungs, to be oxygenated. The major valves are four in number: the *left atrioventricular valve (mitral),* between the left atrium and ventricle; the *right atrioventricular valve (tricuspid),* between the right atrium and ventricle; the *aortic valve,* at the orifice of the aorta; and the *pulmonary valve,* at the orifice of the pulmonary trunk. The heart tissue itself is nourished by the blood in the coronary arteries. See Plate 18.

armored h. a condition marked by calcareous deposits in the pericardium.

artificial h. a pumping mechanism that duplicates the output, rate, and blood pressure of the natural heart. It may replace the function of the entire heart or a portion of it, and may be permanent or temporary, intracorporeal or extracorporeal.

athletic h. hypertrophy or dilation of the heart with no disease of the valves or other disorder of the circulation, sometimes seen in athletes.

beer h. beer-drinkers' cardiomyopathy.

beriberi h. heart failure from thiamine deficiency.

boat-shaped h. the radiologic appearance of the heart in aortic regurgitation, due to dilatation and hypertrophy of the left ventricle.

booster h. auxiliary ventricle.

bovine h. cor bovinum.

chaotic h. a heart which exhibits frequent extrasystoles.

dynamite h. a condition seen in workers exposed to nitroglycerin, in which blood vessels become dilated during exposure, and when exposure is discontinued they contract and reduce the blood supply to the heart.

encased h. a heart affected with chronic constrictive pericarditis.

extracorporeal h. an artificial heart located outside the body and usually performing a pumping and an oxygenating function.

fat h., fatty h. 1. a heart affected with fatty degeneration. 2. a condition in which there is an excessive layer of fat deposited about and in the heart muscle. Called also *cor adiposum.*

fibroid h. a heart in which fibrous tissue replaces portions of the myocardium, such as sometimes occurs in chronic myocarditis.

flask-shaped h. the x-ray appearance of the heart in pericarditis with effusion.

hairy h. shaggy pericardium.

horizontal h. a counterclockwise rotation of the electrical axis (deviation to the left) of the heart; a moderate deviation (0° to −20°) is normally observed in asthenic persons with a transversely situated heart, in the obese, and in pregnant women.

hyperthyroid h. the heart in thyrotoxic heart disease.

hypoplastic h. a heart of small size.

intracorporeal h. an artificial heart implanted in the body.

irritable h. neurocirculatory asthenia.

Jarvik-7 artificial h. original name for an air-driven artificial heart consisting of two smooth-surfaced, sac-like polyurethane pumps that replaced the ventricles, and two pneumatic power units that regulated blood flow by pulsing air through tubing drive lines; it is still used as a bridge to transplantation.

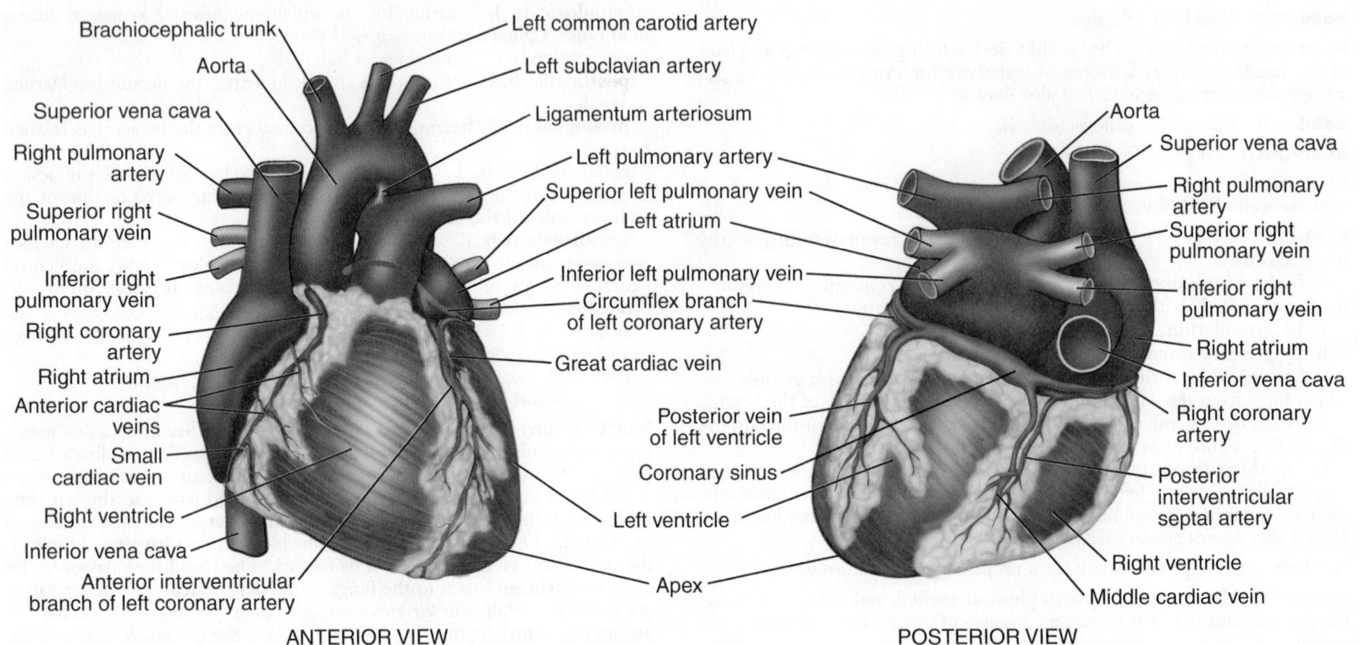

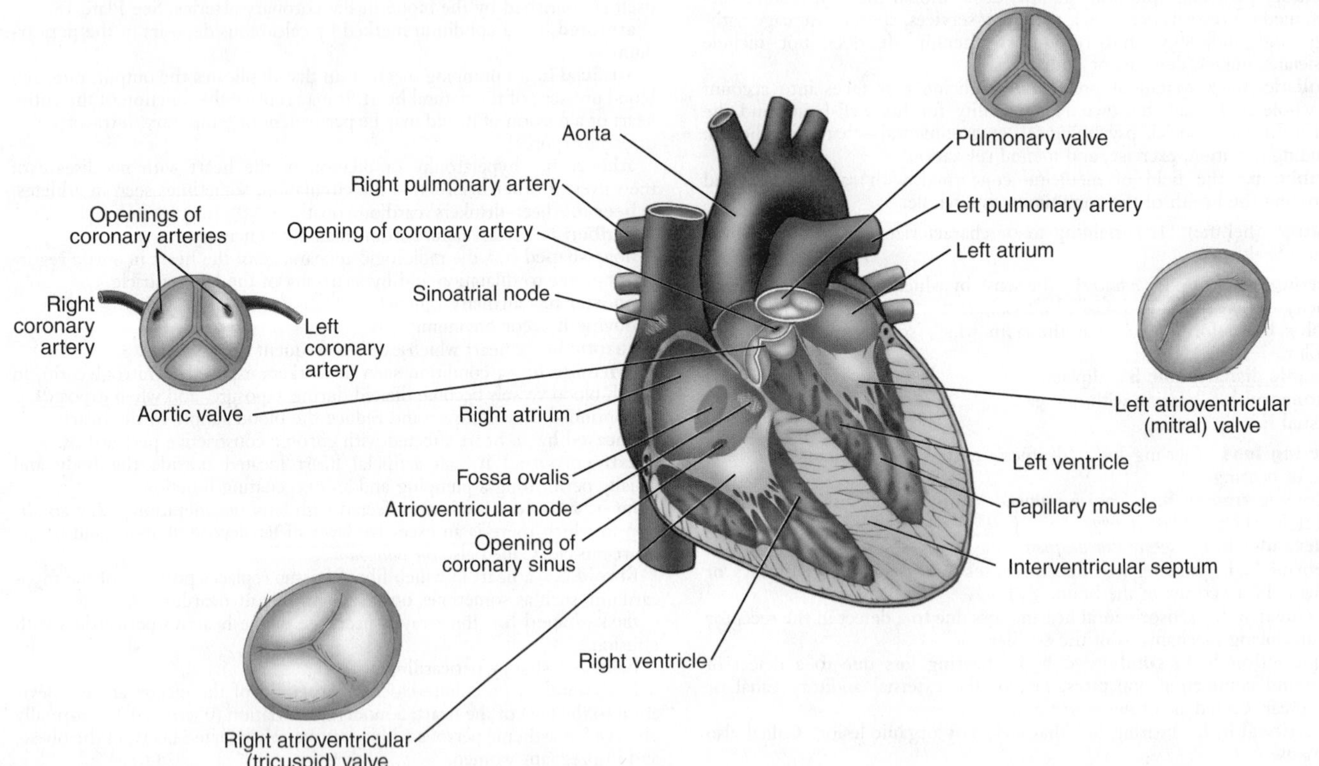

■ **PLATE 18**—STRUCTURES OF THE HEART

left h. the left atrium and ventricle; that portion of the heart which propels the blood in systemic circulation.

lymph h. an organ in frogs and fishes concerned in the distribution of lymph.

mechanical h. artificial h.

myxedema h. an enlarged heart associated with hypothyroidism.

ox h. cor bovinum.

parchment h. the appearance of the right ventricle in Uhl anomaly.

pulmonary h. right h.

right h. the right atrium and ventricle; that portion of the heart which propels the blood in the pulmonary circulation.

sabot h. coeur en sabot.

soldier's h. neurocirculatory asthenia.

stone h. massive contraction band necrosis in an irreversibly noncompliant hypertrophied heart, occurring as a complication of cardiac surgery; it is believed due to a combination of low levels of adenosine triphosphate and calcium overload.

systemic h. left h.

tabby cat h. a condition of the heart in which the inner surface of the ventricular wall and the papillary muscles are streaked and spotted; seen in marked cases of fatty degeneration. Called also *thrush breast h.*, *tiger h.*, and *tiger lily h.*

three-chambered h. a developmental anomaly in which the heart is missing the interventricular septum (common ventricle) or the interatrial septum (common atrium) and so has only three compartments. Called also *cor triloculare* or *trilocular h.*

thrush breast h., tiger h., tiger lily h. tabby cat h.

triatrial h. cor triatriatum.

trilocular h. three-chambered h.

vertical h. a clockwise rotation of the electrical axis (deviation to the right) of the heart; a moderate deviation (90° to 100°) is normally observed in asthenic persons with a vertically situated heart and in early infancy.

water-bottle h. a radiographic sign of pericardial effusion: the cardiopericardial silhouette is enlarged and assumes the shape of a flask or water bottle, with blurring of the left cardiac border and obscuring of the hilar vessels.

heart•beat (hahrt′bēt) a complete cardiac cycle, during which the electrical impulse is conducted and mechanical contraction occurs.

heart block (hahrt blok) impairment of conduction of an impulse in heart excitation; often applied specifically to atrioventricular block. For specific types of heart block, see under *block*.

heart•burn (hahrt′bərn) a feeling of burning or warmth that begins in the lower esophagus, tends to rise upward toward the neck, and occurs in waves. It is often associated with gastroesophageal reflux and may be accompanied by a reflux of fluid into the mouth (water brash). Called also *pyrosis*.

heart•wa•ter (hahrt′waw-tər) a fatal rickettsial disease of cattle, sheep, and goats in sub-Saharan Africa and on certain islands in the Indian Ocean, marked by fluid accumulation in the pleura, pericardium, and pleural cavity. It is caused by *Ehrlichia ruminantium*, which is transmitted by the ticks *Amblyomma hebraeum* and *A. variegata*. Called also *cowdriosis*, *veld* or *veldt disease*, and *veld* or *veldt sickness*.

heart•worm (hahrt′wərm) *Dirofilaria immitis*.

heat (hēt) [L. *calor*] 1. the sensation of an increase in temperature. 2. the energy which produces the sensation of heat. It exists in the form of molecular or atomic vibration (thermal agitation) and may be transferred, as a consequence of a gradient in temperature, by conduction through a substance, by convection by a substance, and by radiation as electromagnetic waves. Symbol Q or q. 3. estrus. 4. to become, or to cause to become, warm or hot.

atomic h. the product of the atomic weight of an element and its specific heat.

conductive h. heat transmitted to the body by contact with a heated object, such as a hot water bag.

convective h. heat conveyed to the surface of the body from warm currents of water or air.

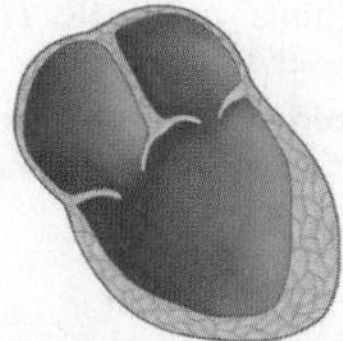

■ Three-chambered heart in which the interventricular septum is absent (common ventricle).

conversive h. heat developed in the tissues by the resistance of the tissues to the passage of high-frequency electromagnetic radiation through them; used in various kinds of diathermy.

dry h. heat that is not moist; usually produced by heated dry air that rapidly absorbs from the skin the moisture of perspiration.

h. of fusion the enthalpy change at constant temperature and pressure in converting a unit amount of a substance from the solid to the liquid state, usually specified in cal/g or cal/mol. Called also *latent h. of fusion*.

latent h. the amount of heat absorbed or given off by a body without changing temperature, as when it undergoes a change of state.

latent h. of fusion h. of fusion.

latent h. of sublimation h. of sublimation.

latent h. of vaporization h. of vaporization.

molecular h. the product of the molecular weight of a substance multiplied by its specific heat.

prickly h. miliaria rubra.

radiant h. heat applied to the surface of the body by rays from a source of infrared radiation, such as a heat lamp.

specific h. the ratio of the heat capacity of a substance to the heat capacity of water at constant volume or pressure; it is equivalent to the amount of heat required to raise the temperature of one gram of the substance by one degree Celsius, since the corresponding value for water is defined as 1.0.

h. of sublimation the enthalpy change at constant temperature and pressure in converting a unit amount of a substance from the solid to the gas state, usually specified in cal/g or cal/mol. Called also *latent h. of sublimation*.

h. of vaporization the enthalpy change at constant temperature and pressure in converting a unit amount of a substance from the liquid to the gas state, usually specified in cal/g or cal/mol. Called also *latent h. of vaporization*.

heat•stroke (hēt′strōk″) see under *stroke*.

heaves (hēvz) 1. chronic obstructive pulmonary disease in equines, resulting from reduced elasticity and rupture of the elastic network of the respiratory bronchioles and pulmonary alveoli; characteristics include coughing, bronchitis, and labored respiration. 2. retching.

dry h. retching.

heb•dom•a•dal (heb-dom′ə-dəl) [L. *hebdomada* a week] pertaining to the first week of life.

Heb•e•lo•ma (heb″ə-lo′mə) a genus of fungi of the family Cortinariaceae. Certain species are called *asetake* in Japan and are gastrointestinal poisons.

he•be•phre•nia (he″bə-fre′ne-ə) [Gr. *hēbē* youth + *phren* + *-ia*] disorganized schizophrenia.

he•be•phren•ic (he″bə-fren′ik) 1. pertaining to hebephrenia (disorganized schizophrenia). 2. a person with disorganized schizophrenia.

He•ber•den disease, nodes (sign) (he′bər-dən) [William *Heberden*, English physician, 1710–1801] see under *disease* and *node*.

he•bet•ic (hə-bet′ik) [Gr. *hēbētikos* youthful] pubertal.

heb•e•tude (heb′ə-tōōd) [L. *hebetudo*, from *hebes* dull] apathy or dullness from any cause; in psychiatry, emotional dullness, a characteristic of schizophrenia.

He•bra disease, prurigo (ha′brah) [Ferdinand Ritter von *Hebra*, Austrian dermatologist, 1816–1880] see *erythema multiforme minus*, and see under *prurigo*.

hec•a•tom•er•al (hek″ə-tom′ər-əl) hecatomeric.

hec•a•to•mer•ic (hek″ə-to-mer′ik) [Gr. *hekateron* each of two + *meros* part] having processes which divide into two, one going to each side of the spinal cord; said of certain neurons.

Hecht syndrome (hekt) [Frederick *Hecht*, American physician, born 1930] trismus-pseudocamptodactyly syndrome.

Hecht-Beals syndrome (hekt′ bēlz′) [F. *Hecht;* Rodney K. *Beals*, American orthopedic surgeon, 20th century] trismus-pseudocamptodactyly syndrome.

Hecht-Beals-Wil•son syndrome (hekt′ bēlz′ wil′sən) [F. *Hecht;* R.K. *Beals;* Ralph V. *Wilson*, American orthopedic surgeon, born 1938] trismus-pseudocamptodactyly syndrome.

Heck disease (hek) [John W. *Heck*, American dentist, born 1923] focal epithelial hyperplasia; see under *hyperplasia*.

Heck•a•thorn disease (hek′ə-thorn) [*Heckathorn*, surname of the propositus first observed in the 1970s] see under *disease*.

hec•tic (hek′tik) [L. *hecticus;* Gr. *hektikos* consumptive] fluctuating each day; see under *fever*.

hect(o)- [Fr., from Gr. *hekaton* one hundred] a combining form designating one hundred; used in naming units of measurement to indicate a quantity 100 (10^2) times the unit designated by the root with which it is combined. Symbol h.

hec•to•gram (hek′to-gram) a unit of mass of the metric system, being 10^2 grams.

Hec•to•rol (hek′tə-rol) trademark for preparations of doxercalciferol.

HED [Ger.] Haut-Einheits-Dosis (unit skin dose), a unit of x-ray dosage established by Seitz and Wintz.

hedge•hog (hej′hog) any of a family of proteins, or the homologous genes encoding them, related to the *hedgehog* gene of *Drosophila*. The original gene was named for its ability to alter the direction of epidermal bristles, and other genes in the family also encode developmental morphogens.

Sonic H. a human homolog of *Drosophila hedgehog;* see *SHH gene*, under *gene*.

he•don•ic (he-don′ik) pertaining to pleasure or to hedonism.

he•do•nism (he′don-iz-əm) [Gr. *hēdonē* pleasure] 1. pleasure-seeking behavior. 2. the ethical doctrine that regards pleasure and happiness as the highest good. 3. in psychology, the theory that the attainment of pleasure and the avoidance of pain are the prime motivators of human behavior.

heel (hēl) 1. calx (def. 2). 2. the posterior part of the wall of a horse's hoof.

anterior h. a triangular-shaped piece of leather fastened obliquely across the ball of the shoe just behind the heads of the metatarsal bones, the object being to support the heads, equalize the pressure, and support the anterior arch.

basketball h. black heel (q.v.) in basketball players.

black h. a benign condition characterized by sudden appearance of minute, blood-filled, punctate black macules on the bottom of the heel and sometimes the ends of toes; it is due to the shearing stress of athletic activities such as basketball, volleyball, tennis, or lacrosse. Called also *calcaneal petechiae* and *talon noir*.

contracted h. see under *hoof*.

Elso h. inherited spastic paresis.

gonorrheal h. the development of exostoses on the heel, attributed to gonorrheal infection.

greasy h. swelling and seborrheic dermatitis in the region of the fetlock and pastern on the back of a horse's leg, with formation of cracks in the skin and excretion of oily matter, usually due to prolonged standing in wet or unsanitary quarters. A similar condition occurs in cattle. Called also *grease*, *grease-heel*, and *scratches*.

painful h. the causing of pain by pressure on the heel.

prominent h. a swelling on the back of the heel due to thickening of the periosteum of the os calcis.

Thomas h. a shoe correction consisting of a heel about 0.5 inch (1 cm) longer and slightly higher on the inside, used to bring the heel of the foot into varus and to prevent depression in the region of the head of the talus.

Heer•fordt syndrome (hār′fort) [Christian Frederik *Heerfordt*, Danish oculist, 1872–1953] see under *syndrome*.

he•fil•con (hə-fil′kon) either of two hydrophilic contact lens materials, designated A or B.

He•gar dilator, sign (ha′gahr) [Alfred *Hegar*, German gynecologist, 1830–1914] see under *dilator* and *sign*.

hEGF human epidermal growth factor.

Hei•den•hain's demilunes, law, iron hematoxylin stain (hi′dən-hīn) [Rudolf Peter *Heidenhain*, German physiologist, 1834–1897] see *Giannuzzi crescents*, under *crescent*, and see under *law* and *stain*.

Hei•den•hain syndrome (hi′dən-hīn) [Adolf *Heidenhain*, German neurologist, 20th century] see under *syndrome*.

height (hīt) the vertical measurement of an object or body.

h. of contour the line encircling a tooth at its greatest bulge with reference to a predetermined path of insertion for a removable partial denture.

h. of contour, surveyed a line scribed or marked on a cast that designates the greatest bulge or diameter with respect to a selected path of denture placement or removal.

cusp h. 1. the shortest distance between the tip of a cusp of a tooth and its base plane. 2. the shortest distance between the deepest part of the central fossa of a posterior tooth and a line connecting the points of the cusps of the tooth.

facial h. the linear measurement of portions of the face, in the midline, using specified reference points; see *anterior*, *upper*, *lower*, and *posterior facial heights*, and see illustration.

facial h., anterior the linear distance from the nasion to the bottom of the chin, the precise point variously specified as the pogonion, gnathion, or menton. It is subdivided into *upper* and *lower facial h.* See illustration.

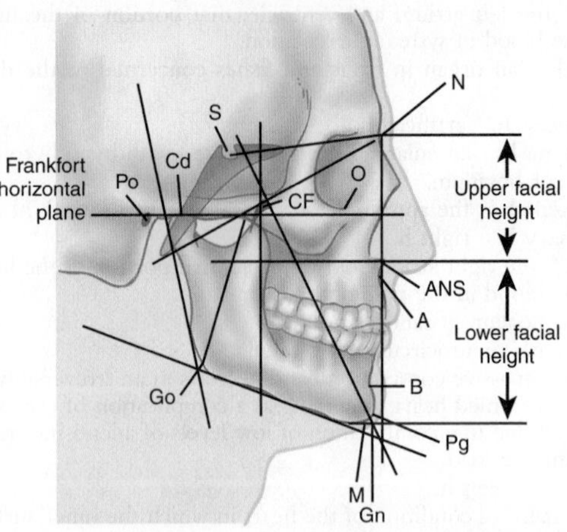

■ Facial height. Anterior facial height is the sum of upper and lower facial heights, the lower limit of the latter variously defined as the pogonion, gnathion, or menton. Posterior facial height is often measured from the gonion to the condylare, sella, or center of face point. *A*, subspinale; *ANS*, anterior nasal spine; *B*, supramentale; *Cd*, condylare; *CF*, center of face; *Gn*, gnathion; *Go*, gonion; *M*, menton; *N*, nasion; *O*, orbitale; *Pg*, pogonion; *Po*, porion; *S*, sella.

facial h., lower the linear distance between the chin, specified as either the menton, gnathion, or pogonion, and the region of the teeth, usually the anterior nasal spine or the interdentale inferius. See illustration.

facial h., posterior a quite variable measure of the linear height of the face in the region of the ear. The most common measure is between a point on the inferior border of the mandible, generally the gonion, and the condylare, sella, or a point defined as the center facial point. Other measurements of height exist, some involving lines of intersection drawn between major facial planes. See illustration.

facial h., upper the linear distance between the nasion and a point in the region of the maxillary teeth, usually the anterior nasal spine but sometimes the interdentale superius or prosthion. See illustration.

sitting h. sitting vertex h.

sitting suprasternal h. the distance from the middle of the anterior-superior border of the manubrium sterni to the surface on which the subject is seated.

sitting vertex h. the distance from the highest point of the head in the sagittal plane to the surface on which the subject is seated; commonly called *sitting h.* Cf. *crown-rump length*.

standing h. the distance from the highest point of the head in the sagittal plane to the surface on which the individual is standing, measured when the subject is not wearing shoes. Cf. *crown-heel length*.

Heil•bron•ner thigh (sign) (hīl′bron-ər) [Karl *Heilbronner*, Dutch physician, 1869–1914] see under *thigh*.

Heim-Krey•sig sign (hīm′ kri′sig) [Ernst Ludwig *Heim*, German physician, 1747–1834; Friedrich Ludwig *Kreysig*, German physician, 1770–1839] see under *sign*.

Heim•lich maneuver (hīm′lik) [Henry Jay *Heimlich*, American surgeon, born 1920] see under *maneuver*.

Hei•ne-Med•in disease (hi′nĕ ma′din) [Jacob von *Heine*, German physician, 1800–1879; Karl Oskar *Medin*, Swedish physician, 1847–1927] see *poliomyelitis*.

Hei•ne•ke-Mik•u•licz pyloroplasty (operation) (hi′nĕ-ke me′koo-lich) [Walter Hermann *Heineke*, German surgeon, 1834–1901; Johann von *Mikulicz*-Radecki, Romanian-born surgeon in Germany, 1850–1905] see under *pyloroplasty*.

Hei•nig projection (hi′nig) [C.F. *Heinig*, American radiologist, 20th century] see under *projection*.

Heinz bodies (granules) (hīnts) [Robert *Heinz*, German pathologist, 1865–1924] Heinz-Ehrlich bodies; see under *body*.

Heinz-Ehr•lich bodies (hīnts′ er′lik) [R. *Heinz;* Paul *Ehrlich*, German bacteriologist, 1854–1915] see under *body*.

Heis•ter diverticulum, fold, valve (hīs′tər) [Lorenz *Heister*, German anatomist, 1683–1758] see *bulbus superior venae jugularis* and *plica spiralis*.

HEK human embryo kidney (cell culture).

HEL human embryo lung (cell culture).

HeLa cells (he′lə) [*H*enrietta *La*cks, the patient from whose carcinoma of the cervix uteri the parent carcinoma cells were isolated in 1951] see under *cell*.

Hel•bing sign (hel′bing) [Carl Ernst *Helbing*, German physician, 1842–1914] see under *sign*.

hel•coid (hel′koid) [Gr. *helkos* ulcer + *-oid*] resembling an ulcer.

hel•col•o•gy (hel-kol′ə-je) [Gr. *helkos* ulcer + *-logy*] the scientific study of ulcers.

hel•co•ma (hel-ko′mə) [Gr.] corneal ulcer.

hel•co•sis (hel-ko′sis) [Gr. *helkōsis*] ulceration.

Held end-bulb (held) [Hans *Held*, German anatomist, 1866–1942] see under *end-bulb*.

He•le•i•dae (hə-le′ĭ-de) a family of flies of the suborder Nematocerca, order Diptera, containing, among others, the four genera *Culicoides, Haemophoructus, Lasiohelea*, and *Leptoconops*, various species of which suck blood and may serve as vectors of disease. Called also *Ceratopogonidae*.

He•le•ni•um (hə-le′ne-um) sneezeweed, a genus of composite plants found in North America that cause vomiting and neurological symptoms in sheep.

he•li•an•thin (he-le-an′thin) methyl orange; see under *orange*.

hel•i•cal (hel′ĭ-kəl) spiral (def. 2).

hel•i•case (he′lĭ-kās) any of a diverse group of enzymes that use energy from ATP hydrolysis to unwind nucleic acid helixes. Some unwind the DNA helix at the replication fork so that the individual strands can be copied; others unwind RNA and participate in processes such as RNA splicing and messenger RNA translation.

He•li•cel•la (he″lĭ-sel′ə) a genus of snails of the family Helicellidae; they serve as hosts of the liver fluke *Dicrocoelium dentriticum* in Europe.

He•li•cel•li•dae (he″lĭ-sel′ĭ-de) a family of snails of the suborder Stylommatophora that serve as hosts of trematodes.

He•lic•i•dae (he-lis′ĭ-de) a family of terrestrial and fresh water snails of the order Pulmonata, suborder Stylommatophora. It includes the genera *Alocinma* and *Helix*.

hel•i•cine (hel′ĭ-sēn) spiral (def. 2).

helic(o)- [Gr. *helix* coil, gen. *helikos*] a combining form denoting relationship to a coil.

He•li•co•bac•ter (hel′ĭ-ko-bak′tər) [*helico-* + *-bacter*] a genus of gram-negative, microaerophilic bacteria of the family Helicobacteraceae, consisting of motile, spiral organisms with multiple sheathed flagella; formerly classified in the genus *Campylobacter*.

H. cinae′di a species found in cases of proctitis and colitis in homosexual men; it has also been implicated in septicemia in immunocompromised patients and as a cause of neonatal septicemia and meningitis. Formerly called *Campylobacter cinaedi*.

H. fennel′liae a species associated with proctitis and proctocolitis in homosexual men and isolated from blood and feces of children with diarrhea. Formerly called *Campylobacter fennelliae*.

H. pylo′ri a species that causes gastritis and pyloric ulcers and is also associated with stomach cancer. Formerly called *Campylobacter pylori*.

He•li•co•bac•ter•a•ceae (hel″ĭ-ko-bak″tər-a′se-e) a morphologically, metabolically, and ecologically diverse family of bacteria of the order Campylobacterales, grouped together on the basis of 16S rRNA sequence analysis; pathogenic organisms are included in the genus *Helicobacter*.

he•li•co•bac•te•ri•o•sis (hel″ĭ-ko-bak-te-re-o′sis) infection with *Helicobacter pylori*, a cause of gastric and duodenal ulcers.

hel•i•coid (hel′ĭ-koid) [*helico-* + *-oid*] resembling a coil or helix; cf. *spiroid*.

hel•i•co•pod (hel′ĭ-ko-pod″) denoting a peculiar dragging gait; see under *gait*.

hel•i•co•tre•ma (hel″ĭ-ko-tre′mə) [*helico-* + Gr. *trēma* hole] [TA] the passage of the ear that connects the scala tympani and scala vestibuli at the apex of the cochlea.

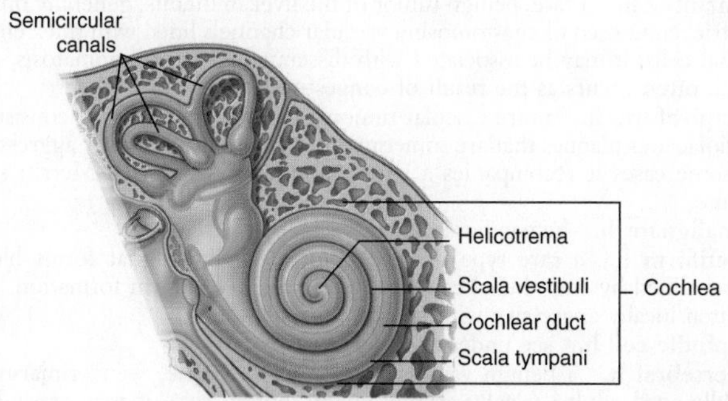

■ Helicotrema, shown in the right bony labyrinth.

Heli•dac (hel′ĭ-dak) trademark for a prepackaged oral therapeutic regimen of bismuth subsalicylate, metronidazole, and tetracycline hydrochloride.

heli(o)- [Gr. *hēlios* sun] a combining form denoting relationship to the sun.

he•lio•sin (he″le-o′sin) a compound containing keratin and various inorganic salts.

he•li•o•sis (he″le-o′sis) [*helio-* + *-osis*] sunstroke.

he•lio•tax•is (he″le-o-tak′sis) [*helio-* + *taxis*] the movement of cells and microorganisms in response to either or both light and heat from the sun. The response may be toward *(positive h.)* or away *(negative h.)* from the source of stimulus. Cf. *heliotropism, phototaxis*, and *thermotaxis*.

he•lio•ther•a•py (he″le-o-ther′ə-pe) [*helio-* + *therapy*] the treatment of disease by exposing the body to the sun's rays; the therapeutic use of the sun bath.

he•li•ot•ro•pism (he″le-ot′ro-piz-əm) [*helio-* + *tropism*] the turning of an organism, especially a plant, toward *(positive h.)* or away from *(negative h.)* the sun. Cf. *heliotaxis*.

he•li•ox (he′le-oks) a low-density mixture of helium and oxygen that reduces resistance to flow within the airways, used in the treatment of asthma, bronchiolitis, and other conditions characterized by increased airway resistance.

he•li•um (He) (he′le-əm) [Gr. *hēlios* sun] a colorless, odorless, tasteless gas, which is not combustible and does not support combustion. It is one of the inert gaseous elements, which was first detected in the sun and is now obtained from natural gas. Atomic number, 2; atomic weight, 4.003. Used in medicine [USP] as a diluent for other gases, being especially useful with oxygen in the treatment of certain cases of respiratory obstruction, and as a vehicle for general anesthetics.

He•lix (he′liks) a genus of snails of the family Helicidae, including some of the common garden snails.

he•lix (he′liks) pl. *helixes* or *he′lices* [Gr. "snail," "coil"] 1. a winding structure. See also *coil* and *spiral*. 2. [TA] the superior and posterior free margin of the pinna of the ear.

α-h., alpha h. a secondary structure occurring in many proteins; it is a right-handed helix with 3.6 amino acid residues per turn stabilized by hydrogen bonds between the imino hydrogen of each peptide bond and the carbonyl oxygen of the peptide bond four residues further along the polypeptide chain.

double h., Watson-Crick h. the usual configuration of double-stranded DNA in vivo, being two complementary antiparallel polynucleotide chains coiled into a helix, with the sugar-phosphate backbone on the outside and the two chains held together by hydrogen bonds between pairs of bases. The most common form is the classical right-handed helical B-DNA (q.v.), but alternative forms also exist, such as A-DNA and Z-DNA (qq.v.). See illustration at *deoxyribonucleic acid*.

He•lix•ate (he′lik-sāt) trademark for a preparation of antihemophilic factor (recombinant).

hel•le•bore (hel′ə-bor) [L. helleborus; Gr. helleboros] 1. any plant of the genus *Helleborus*, perennial herbs that were formerly used medicinally. See *black h.* 2. any of various plants of the genus *Veratrum*, used medicinally but sometimes toxic to livestock.

American h. *Veratrum viride*.

black h. 1. *Helleborus niger*. 2. a preparation of the rhizome, with or without the roots, of *H. niger*, used for a variety of indications in folk medicine and homeopathy.

European h. *Veratrum album*.

green h. *Veratrum viride*.

white h. 1. *Veratrum album*. 2. a highly toxic preparation of the rhizome and roots of *V. album*, having a wide variety of uses in folk medicine and homeopathy.

Hel•le•bo•rus (hel″ə-bo′rəs) a genus of plants of the family Ranunculaceae, native to Europe and Asia. *H. ni′ger* is the black hellebore, a perennial herb whose root (also called *black hellebore*) contains a cardiac glycoside and is used in folk medicine and homeopathy.

Hel•ler esophagomyotomy (myotomy, operation) (hel′ər) [Ernst *Heller*, German surgeon, 1877–1964] esophagocardiomyotomy.

Hel•ler plexus (hel′ər) [Arnold Ludwig Gotthilf *Heller*, German pathologist, 1840–1913] see under *plexus*.

Hel•ler•work (hel′ər-wərk) [Joseph *Heller*, Polish-born American bodyworker, born 1940] a bodywork system derived from Rolfing that uses deep massage, movement reeducation, and dialogue to improve body alignment, establish less stressful movement patterns, and promote awareness of the mind-body relationship; used for musculoskeletal pain, improvement of posture, and enhancement of well-being.

Hel•lin's law (hel'inz) [Dyonizy *Hellin*, Polish pathologist, 1867–1935] see under *law*.

Helm•holtz ligament, theory (helm'holtz) [Hermann Ludwig Ferdinand von *Helmholtz*, German physiologist, inventor of the ophthalmoscope, 1821–1894] see under *ligament* and *theory*.

hel•minth (hel'minth) [Gr. *helmins* worm] a parasitic worm. **helmin'thic, helmin'thous** *adj*

hel•min•tha•gogue (hel-min'thə-gog) anthelmintic (def. 2).

hel•min•them•e•sis (hel"min-them'ə-sis) [*helminth* + *emesis*] the vomiting of worms.

hel•min•thi•a•sis (hel"min-thi'ə-sis) infection with worms; called also *vermination*.

hel•min•thi•cide (hel-min'thĭ-sīd) [*helminth* + *-cide*] anthelmintic (def. 2).

hel•min•thoid (hel-min'thoid) resembling a parasitic worm.

hel•min•thol•o•gy (hel"min-thol'ə-je) [*helminth* + *-logy*] the scientific study of parasitic worms.

hel•min•tho•ma (hel"min-tho'mə) [*helminth* + *-oma*] a tumor caused by a parasitic worm.

hel(o)- [Gr. *hēlos* nail, corn, callus] a combining form denoting relationship to a nail, or to a wart or callus.

He•lo•der•ma (he"lo-dur'mə) [*helo-* + *derma*] a genus of venomous lizards of the southwestern United States and Mexico. *H. hor'ridum* is the beaded lizard and *H. suspec'tum* is the Gila monster.

he•lo•ma (he-lo'mə) corn (def. 1).
 h. du'rum hard corn.
 h. mol'le soft corn.

He•loph•i•lus (hə-lof'ĭ-ləs) a genus of hover flies of the family Syrphidae, whose larvae (rat-tail maggots) may cause nasal and intestinal myiasis.

He•lo•ti•a•les (he"lo-she-a'lēz) an order of fungi of the subphylum Ascomycotina, series Unitunicatae, having inoperculate asci; some species are saprobes and others are parasites of plants. It includes the genus *Sclerotinia*.

Hel•vel•la (hel-vel'ə) the saddle fungi, a genus of the family Helvellaceae. Some species contain a heat-stable hemolysin. *H. esculen'ta* and other species cause mycetismus sanguinarius, a form of mushroom poisoning.

Hel•vel•la•ceae (hel"vəl-a'se-e) a family of fungi of the order Pezizales; some species are edible and others are poisonous. It includes the genera *Gyromitra* and *Helvella*.

Hel•weg tract (hel'veg) [Hans Kristian Saxtorph *Helweg*, Danish physician, 1847–1901] olivospinal tract; see under *tract*.

Hel•weg-Lar•sen syndrome (hel'veg-lahr'sən) [Hans Frederik *Helweg-Larsen*, Danish dermatologist and geneticist, 1917–1969] see under *syndrome*.

he•ma (he'mə) [Gr. *haima, haimatos* blood] haema; see also *blood*.

hema- see *hem(o)-*.

He•ma•bate (he'mə-bāt) trademark for a preparation of carboprost tromethamine.

he•ma•chro•ma•to•sis (he"mə-kro"mə-to'sis) hemochromatosis.

he•ma•chrome (he'mə-krōm) an oxygen-carrying blood pigment, e.g., hemoglobin or hemocyanin.

he•ma•cyte (he'mə-sīt) blood cell.

he•ma•cy•tom•e•ter (he"mə-si-tom'ə-tər) a device used in manual blood counts, consisting of a microscopic slide with a depression whose base is marked in grids, and into which a measured volume of a sample of blood or bacterial culture is placed and covered with a cover glass. The number of cells and formed blood elements in the squares is counted under a microscope and used as a representative sample for calculating the unit volume. Called also *counting cell, counting chamber*, and *hemocytometer*.

he•ma•cy•tom•e•try (he"mə-si-tom'ə-tre) the counting of blood cells using a hemacytometer; called also *hemocytometry*.

he•ma•do•ste•no•sis (he"mə-do-, hem-ə-do-stə-no'sis) stenosis of a blood vessel; see also *angiostenosis*.

he•mad•sor•bent (he"mad-zor'bənt) 1. characterized by hemadsorption. 2. inducing or causing hemadsorption.

he•mad•sorp•tion (he"mad-zorp'shən) the adherence of red cells to other cells, particles, or surfaces; see *hemadsorption test*, under *test*.

he•ma•dy•na•mom•e•try (he"mə-di"nə-mom'ə-tre) measurement of blood pressure.

he•ma•fa•cient (he"mə-fa'shənt) hematopoietic.

he•mag•glu•ti•na•tion (he"mə-gloo"tĭ-na'shən) agglutination of erythrocytes, which may be caused by antibodies such as hemagglutinins, by viruses such as those of influenza and mumps, or by other substances such as lectins.
 indirect h., passive h. agglutination of erythrocytes due to the reaction of specific antibody with antigen passively adsorbed on the surface or chemically coupled to the cells; the basis of many serologic tests.
 viral h. the agglutination of erythrocytes by viruses, either by intact virions or by viral products; the basis of hemagglutination or hemagglutination inhibition methods for viral titration.

he•mag•glu•ti•na•tive (he"mə-gloo'tĭ-nə"tiv) 1. pertaining to or characterized by hemagglutination. 2. causing hemagglutination.

he•mag•glu•ti•nin (HA) (he"mə-gloo'tĭ-nin) [*hem-* + *agglutinin*] an agglutinin, e.g., an antibody or lectin, that agglutinates erythrocytes.
 cold h. a cold agglutinin (q.v.) that agglutinates red cells.
 warm h. a warm agglutinin (q.v.) that agglutinates red cells.

he•mal (he'məl) 1. ventral to the spinal axis, where the heart and great vessels are located, as, e.g., the hemal arches. Cf. *neural*. 2. hemic. 3. pertaining to the blood vessels; see *vascular*.

hem•al•um (he'mə-ləm) a mixture of hematoxylin and alum introduced by Mayer, widely used as a nuclear stain, especially in combination with eosin as a general oversight method. Also, any alum and hematoxylin stain. Called also *alum hematoxylin*.

hem•a•nal•y•sis (he"mə-nal'ə-sis) [*hem-* + *analysis*] analysis or examination of the blood.

he•man•gi•ec•ta•sia (he-man"je-ek-ta'shə) angiectasis.

he•man•gi•ec•ta•sis (he-man"je-ek'tə-sis) angiectasis.

hemangi(o)- [Gr. *haima* blood + *angeion* vessel] a combining form denoting relationship to the blood vessels.

he•man•gio•amelo•blas•to•ma (he-man"je-o-ə-mel"o-blas-to'mə) [*hemangio-* + *ameloblastoma*] a highly vascular ameloblastoma.

he•man•gio•blast (he-man'je-o-blast) [*hemangio-* + *-blast*] a mesodermal cell that gives rise to both vascular endothelium and hemocytoblasts.

he•man•gio•blas•to•ma (he-man"je-o-blas-to'mə) [*hem-* + *angioblast* + *-oma*] a benign blood vessel tumor of the cerebellum, spinal cord, or retina, consisting of proliferated blood vessel cells and angioblasts. Called also *angioblastoma* and *Lindau tumor*.
 cerebellar h. hemangioblastoma of the cerebellum, often cystic; an autosomal dominant form is associated with von Hippel-Lindau disease.
 retinal h. von Hippel disease.
 spinal h. a hemangioblastoma of the spinal cord, usually small and encapsulated and in an intramedullary location.

he•man•gio•blas•to•ma•to•sis (he-man"je-o-blas"to-mə-to'sis) multiple or widespread hemangioblastomas.

he•man•gio•en•do•the•li•al (he-man"je-o-en"do-the'le-əl) pertaining to the vascular endothelium.

he•man•gio•en•do•the•lio•blas•to•ma (he-man"je-o-en"do-the"le-o-blas-to'mə) [*hemangioendothelioma* + *blastoma*] a hemangioendothelioma with embryonic elements of mesenchymal origin.

he•man•gio•en•do•the•lio•ma (he-man"je-o-en"do-the"le-o'mə) [*hemangioma* + *endothelioma*] a true neoplasm of vascular origin, characterized by proliferation of endothelial cells in and about the vascular lumen; it is usually considered to be intermediate in grade between hemangioma and hemangiosarcoma but sometimes is used to denote the latter.
 benign h. a benign neoplasm of blood-vessel endothelium; the term is usually used to denote an infantile hemangioendothelioma.
 epithelioid h. a rare vascular neoplasm occurring in the medium to large veins of the distal extremities of adults, particularly young males; it may be benign or malignant and is characterized by proliferation of epithelioid or histiocytoid endothelial cells lining dilated vascular channels.
 infantile h. a rare, benign tumor of the liver in infants, generally multicentric, composed of anastomosing vascular channels lined with thick endothelial cells; it may be associated with disseminated hemangiomatosis, and death often occurs as the result of congestive heart failure.
 kaposiform h. a rare vascular tumor, usually seen in infants, consisting of violaceous plaques that are sometimes deep-seated and locally aggressive. In some cases it accompanies a lymphangioma or Kasabach-Merritt syndrome.
 malignant h. hemangiosarcoma.
 retiform h. a rare type of hemangioendothelioma that forms blood vessels lined by endothelial cells, has a treelike or retiform formation, and is often locally aggressive without metastases.
 spindle cell h. see under *hemangioma*.
 vertebral h. a benign vascular tumor of the spine, seen primarily in middle-aged adults; usually asymptomatic, but in time it may expand or hemorrhage and compress the spinal canal and cord.

he•man•gio•en•do•the•lio•sar•co•ma (he-man″je-o-en″do-the″le-o-sahr-ko′mə) hemangiosarcoma.

he•man•gio•fi•bro•ma (he-man″je-o-fi-bro′mə) [*hemangio-* + *fibroma*] a hemangioma containing fibrous tissue.

he•man•gi•o•ma (he-man″je-o′mə) [*hem-* + *angioma*] 1. a common type of vascular malformation, usually seen in infancy and childhood, consisting of newly formed blood vessels that result from malformation of angioblastic tissue of fetal life. There are two main types: capillary hemangiomas and cavernous hemangiomas. 2. a general term denoting a benign or malignant vascular malformation that resembles the classic type of hemangioma but occurs at any age. Cf. *angioma* and *lymphangioma*.

ameloblastic h. hemangioameloblastoma.

capillary h. 1. the most common type of hemangioma; most are composed of closely packed aggregations of capillaries that are separated by scant connective stroma and conform to the caliber of normal capillaries. According to one classification, *strawberry h.*, *nevus flammeus*, *cherry angioma*, and *pyogenic granuloma* are all types of capillary hemangiomas. 2. strawberry h.

cavernous h. a vascular tumor composed mainly of large dilated blood vessels that often contain large amounts of blood; the usual location is in the skin, subcutaneous tissue, or both, although it may also be found in viscera such as the liver, spleen, pancreas, or brain. Most present in early life but usually not at birth. The typical superficial lesions are bright to dark red in color; deep lesions have a blue color. Called also *cavernoma*, *cavernous angioma*, and *strawberry mark* or *nevus*.

hobnail h. targetoid hemosiderotic h.

sclerosing h. 1. a type of benign fibrous histiocytoma characterized not only by histiocytic and fibroblastic elements but also by numerous blood vessels and hemosiderin deposits. 2. dermatofibroma.

h. sim′plex strawberry h.

spindle cell h. a rare type of vascular tumor usually seen in children or young adults on the distal part of a limb, characterized by dark blue, firm nodules with vascular cavities containing fascicles of spindle cells. Called also *spindle cell hemangioendothelioma*.

strawberry h. a firm, red, dome-shaped hemangioma, sharply demarcated from surrounding skin, usually found on the head or neck; it grows rapidly and generally undergoes regression and involution without scarring. It is caused by proliferation of immature capillary vessels in active stroma, and is usually present at birth or within the first 2 or 3 months of life. See also *capillary h.* and *vascular nevus*. Called also *h. simplex*, *strawberry mark*, and *strawberry nevus*.

targetoid hemosiderotic h. a benign vascular malformation presenting as a solitary papule on a limb or the trunk of a young or middle-aged person; it can mimic disorders such as angiosarcoma, melanoma, and Kaposi sarcoma. Some authorities believe it is a reactive condition, and others believe it to be caused by trauma. Called also *hobnail h.*

venous h. a type of cavernous hemangioma in which the dilated vessels have thick, fibrous walls.

he•man•gio•ma•to•sis (he-man″je-o-mə-to′sis) a condition in which multiple hemangiomas are developed.

disseminated h. the presence of multiple hemangiomas on the skin, frequently with others on internal organs such as the liver, gastrointestinal tract, lungs, or central nervous system; death may result from high-output heart failure, respiratory obstruction, or central nervous system compression.

he•man•gio•peri•cyte (he-man″je-o-per′ĭ-sīt) pericyte.

he•man•gio•peri•cy•to•ma (he-man″je-o-per″ĭ-si-to′mə) [*hemangiopericyte* + *-oma*] a tumor composed of spindle cells with a rich vascular network, which apparently arises from pericytes. It may be benign or malignant and usually occurs in the lower extremities or retroperitoneum.

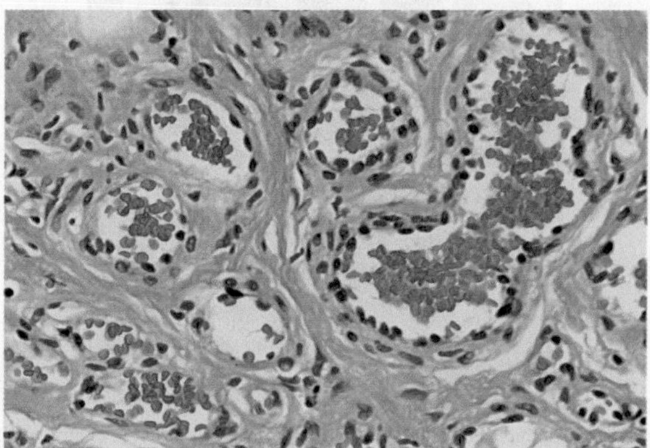

■ Capillary hemangioma demonstrating well-formed capillary-sized vessels.

h. of kidney juxtaglomerular cell tumor.

he•man•gio•sar•co•ma (he-man″je-o-sahr-ko′mə) [*hemangio-* + *sarcoma*] a rare malignant tumor of vascular origin, formed by proliferation of endothelial tissue lining irregular vascular channels; it usually occurs in the skin, soft tissues, breast, or liver. Called also *angiosarcoma* and *malignant hemangioendothelioma*. See also *lymphangiosarcoma*.

he•ma•phe•ic (he″mə-fe′ik) pertaining to or characterized by hemaphein.

he•ma•phe•in (he′mə-fēn″) [*hema-* + Gr. *phaios* dusky, gray] a brown coloring matter of the blood and urine.

he•ma•phe•ism (he″mə-fe′iz-əm) the presence of hemaphein in the urine.

he•ma•phe•re•sis (he″mə-fə-re′sis) apheresis.

he•ma•poi•e•sis (he″mə-poi-e′sis) hematopoiesis. **hemapoiet′ic** *adj*

he•ma•poph•y•sis (he″mə-pof′ə-sis) [*hem-* + *apophysis*] a costal cartilage regarded as an apophysis of the hemal spine.

he•mar•thros (he-mahr′thros) hemarthrosis.

he•mar•thro•sis (he″mahr-thro′sis) [*hem-* + *arthrosis*] extravasation of blood into a joint or its synovial cavity.

he•ma•stron•ti•um (he″mə-stron′she-əm) a tissue stain prepared by adding strontium chloride to a solution of hematein and aluminum chloride in alcohol and citric acid.

he•ma•tal (he′mə-təl) hemic.

he•mat•apos•te•ma (he″mat-ap″os-te′mə) [*hemat-* + Gr. *apostēma* abscess] an abscess containing effused blood.

he•ma•te•in (he′mə-tēn) a brownish-red, crystalline substance derived from hematoxylin by oxidation; used as an indicator and stain.

he•ma•tem•e•sis (he″mə-tem′ə-sis) [*hemat-* + *emesis*] the vomiting of blood.

he•mat•en•ceph•a•lon (he″mat-, hem″at-en-sef′ə-lon) cerebral hemorrhage.

he•ma•ther•a•py (he″mə-ther′ə-pe) hemotherapy.

he•ma•ther•mal (he″mə-thur′məl) homeothermic.

he•ma•ther•mous (he″mə-thur′məs) homeothermic.

he•ma•tho•rax (he″mə-thor′aks) hemothorax.

he•mat•ic (he-mat′ik) 1. hemic. 2. hematinic.

he•ma•ti•dro•sis (he″mə-, hem″ə-tĭ-dro′sis) [*hemat-* + Gr. *hidrōsis* sweating] the excretion of bloody sweat. Called also *hematohidrosis*.

he•ma•tim•e•ter (he″mə-, hem″ə-tim′ə-tər) hemacytometer.

he•ma•tin (he′mə-tin) 1. a porphyrin chelate of iron (III) formed by the oxidation of free heme; the hydroxide of heme. It stimulates the synthesis of globin and inhibits the synthesis of porphyrin by inactivation of 5-aminolevulinate synthase and is a component of the cytochromes and peroxidases. Hematin derived synthetically from hemin is used as a reagent. 2. hemin (def. 1).

he•ma•tin•emia (he″mə-, hem″ə-tĭ-ne′me-ə) the presence of hematin (heme) in the blood.

he•ma•tin•ic (he″mə-tin′ik) 1. pertaining to hematin. 2. an agent that increases the hemoglobin level and the number of erythrocytes in the blood.

he•ma•tin•uria (he″mə-tĭ-nu′re-ə) the presence of hematin in the urine, seen in hemoglobinuria.

he•ma•tite (he′mə-tīt) a mineral made up of ferric oxide with a small amount of silica; inhalation of its dust can cause hematite pneumoconiosis.

hemat(o)- [Gr. *haima*, gen. *haimatos* blood] a combining form denoting relationship to the blood. Also, *haemat(o)-*.

he•ma•to•bil•ia (he″mə-to-, hem″ə-to-bil′e-ə) hemobilia.

he•ma•to•blast (he′mə-to-, he-mat′o-blast″) blast cell (def. 2).

he•ma•to•cele (he′mə-to-, hem′ə-to-sēl″) [*hemato-* + *-cele*[1]] an effusion of blood into a cavity, such as in the tunica vaginalis testis.

parametric h., pelvic h., retrouterine h. swelling caused by effusion of blood into the pouch of Douglas.

scrotal h. effusion of blood into the tissues of the scrotum.

he•ma•to•ceph•a•lus (he″mə-to-, hem″ə-to-sef′ə-ləs) [*hemato-* + *-cephalus*] a fetus born with its head distended with blood.

he•ma•to•che•zia (he″mə-to-, hem″ə-to-ke′zhə) [*hemato-* + Gr. *chezein* to defecate] presence of blood in the feces.

he•ma•to•chro•ma•to•sis (he″mə-to-, hem″ə-to-kro″mə-to′sis) [*hemato-* + *chromato-* + *-sis*] 1. staining of tissues with blood pigment. 2. hemochromatosis.

he•ma•to•chy•lu•ria (he″mə-to-, hem″ə-to-ki-lu′re-ə) [*hemato-* + *chyluria*] the discharge of blood and chyle with the urine, a symptom of filariasis.

he•ma•to•coe•lia (he″mə-to-, hem″ə-to-se′le-ə) hemoperitoneum.

he•ma•to•col•po•me•tra (he″mə-to-, hem″ə-to-kol″po-me′trə) [*hemato-* + *colpo-* + *metra*] accumulation of menstrual blood in the vagina and uterus.

he•ma•to•col•pos (he″mə-to-, hem″ə-to-kol′pəs) [*hemato-* + Gr. *kolpos* vagina] an accumulation of menstrual blood in the vagina.

he•mat•o•crit (Hct) (he-mat′ə-krit) [*hemato-* + Gr. *krinein* to separate] the proportion of the volume of a blood sample that is red blood cells (packed red blood cells), measured in mL per dL of whole blood or as a per cent.

large vessel h. the hematocrit of blood from a large vessel, usually a vein; cf. *total body h.*

total body h., whole body h. the average hematocrit of the whole body, as determined by tracer dilution methods; it is normally about 0.92 times the large vessel hematocrit.

he•ma•toc•ry•al (he″mə-, hem″ə-tok′re-əl) poikilothermic.

he•ma•to•cy•a•nin (he″mə-to-, hem″ə-to-si′ə-nin) [*hemato-* + Gr. *kyanos* blue] hemocyanin.

he•ma•to•cyst (he′mə-to-, he-mat′o-sist″) [*hemato-* + *cyst*] an effusion of blood into the bladder or into a cyst.

he•ma•to•cys•tis (he″mə-to-, hem″ə-to-sis′tis) hematocyst.

he•ma•to•cyte (he′mə-to-, he-mat′o-sīt″) blood cell.

he•ma•to•cy•to•blast (he″mə-to-, hem″ə-to-si′to-blast) blast cell (def. 2).

he•ma•to•cy•tol•y•sis (he″mə-to-, hem″ə-to-si-tol′ĭ-sis) hemolysis.

he•ma•to•cy•tom•e•ter (he″mə-to-, hem″ə-to-si-tom′ə-tər) hemacytometer.

he•ma•to•cy•to•pe•nia (he″mə-to-, hem″ə-to-si″to-pe′ne-ə) cytopenia.

he•ma•to•cy•tu•ria (he″mə-to-, hem″ə-to-si-tu′re-ə) hematuria.

he•ma•to•en•ce•phal•ic (he″mə-to-, hem″ə-to-en″sə-fal′ik) [*hemato-* + *encephalic*] pertaining to the blood and the brain.

he•ma•to•gen•e•sis (he″mə-to-, hem″ə-to-jen′ə-sis) hematopoiesis.

he•ma•to•gen•ic (he″mə-to-, he-mat″o-jen′ik) 1. hematopoietic. 2. hematogenous.

he•ma•tog•e•nous (he″mə-toj′ə-nəs) 1. produced by or derived from the blood. 2. disseminated by the circulation or through the bloodstream.

he•ma•to•hi•dro•sis (he′mə-to-, hem″ə-to-hĭ-dro′sis) hematidrosis.

he•ma•to•hy•a•loid (he″mə-to-, hem″ə-to-hi′ə-loid) [*hemato-* + *hyaloid*] pertaining to a thrombus that has undergone hyaline degeneration.

he•ma•toid (he′mə-toid) [*hemato-* + *-oid*] resembling blood.

he•ma•toid•in (he-mə-toid′in) a yellow-brown or red pigment, apparently chemically identical with bilirubin but with a different site of origin, formed locally in the tissues from hemoglobin, particularly under conditions of reduced oxygen tension.

he•ma•to•kol•pos (he″mə-to-, hem″ə-to-kol′pəs) hematocolpos.

he•ma•tol•o•gist (he″mə-tol′ə-jist) a specialist in hematology.

he•ma•tol•o•gy (he″mə-tol′ə-je) [*hemato-* + *-logy*] the branch of medical science that deals with the blood and blood-forming tissues.

he•ma•to•lymph•an•gi•o•ma (he″mə-to-, hem″ə-to-lim″fan-je-o′mə) [*hemato-* + *lymph-* + *angioma*] a benign tumor composed of blood vessels and lymph vessels. Called also *hemolymphangioma.*

he•ma•tol•y•sis (he″mə-tol′ə-sis) hemolysis. **hematolyt′ic** *adj*

he•ma•to•ma (he″mə-to′mə) [*hemato-* + *-oma*] a localized collection of blood, usually clotted, in an organ, space, or tissue, usually due to a break in the wall of a blood vessel.

aneurysmal h. false aneurysm.

auricular h., h. au′ris hematoma of the perichondrium of the auricle, a common precursor of cauliflower ear.

dissecting h. dissecting aneurysm.

epidural h. accumulation of blood in the epidural space, due to damage to and leakage of blood from the middle meningeal artery, producing compression of the dura mater and thus compression of the brain. Unless evacuated, it may result in herniation through the tentorium, and death.

parenchymatous h. a mass of blood within the brain tissue itself, usually from rupture of an artery or vein within the brain.

pelvic h. a collection of blood in the pelvic soft tissue.

perianal h. a painful hematoma under the perianal skin, caused by rupture of a subcutaneous vessel.

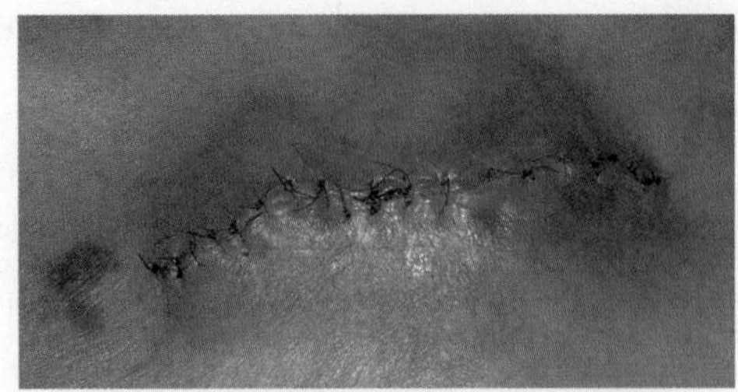

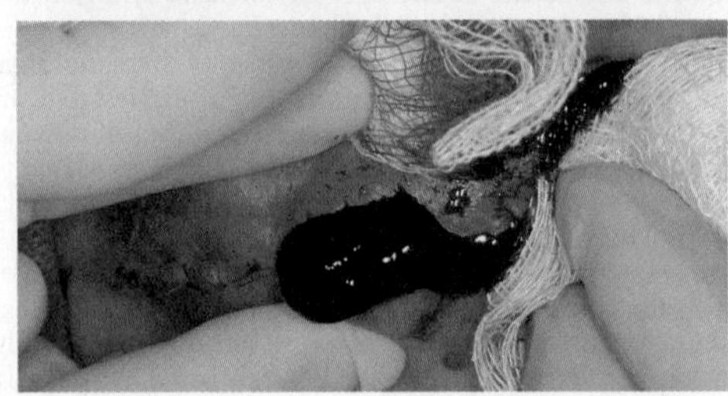

■ Hematoma. Postoperative formation *(A)* and evacuation *(B)*.

perinephric h., perirenal h. a hematoma resulting from hemorrhage into the perirenal space.

pulsating h. pseudoaneurysm.

retroperitoneal h. a hematoma resulting from a hemorrhage into the retroperitoneal space.

retrouterine h. an effusion of blood into the retrouterine connective tissue.

subdural h. accumulation of blood between the dura mater and the arachnoid, resulting in the creation of an abnormal space (*subdural space,* q.v.). In the severe *acute* form, both blood and cerebrospinal fluid enter the space as a result of laceration of the brain and a tear in the arachnoid, adding subdural compression to the direct injury to the brain. In the *chronic* form, only blood effuses into the subdural space as a result of rupture of the bridging veins, usually due to closed head injury. The effusion is a gradual process resulting, weeks after the injury, in headache and progressive focal signs that reflect the location of the mass.

subungual h. an accumulation of blood under the nail plate.

he•ma•to•ma•nom•e•ter (he″mə-to-, hem″ə-to-mə-nom′ə-tər) sphygmomanometer.

he•ma•to•me•di•as•ti•num (he″mə-to-, hem″ə-to-me″de-əs-ti′nəm) [*hemato-* + *mediastinum*] hemomediastinum.

he•ma•to•me•tra (he″mə-to-, hem″ə-to-me′trə) [*hemato-* + *metra*] an accumulation of blood in the uterus.

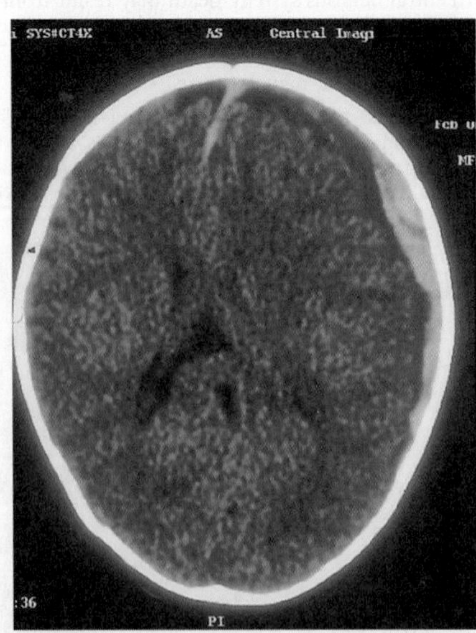

■ Acute focal subdural hematoma of the left frontal area of a six-month-old infant. The layering of subdural blood is due to rapid collection and consists of newly clotted blood and fresh hemorrhage.

he•ma•tom•e•try (he″mə-tom′ə-tre) [*hemato-* + *-metry*] measurement of various parameters of the blood, such as the complete blood count (see under *count*).

he•ma•to•my•elia (he″mə-to-, hem″ə-to-mi-e′le-ə) [*hemato-* + *myel-* + *-ia*] hemorrhage into the spinal cord, usually confined to the gray substance, most often due to trauma but also seen in arteriovenous malformations; marked by the sudden onset of flaccid paralysis with sensory disturbances.

he•ma•to•my•eli•tis (he″mə-to-, hem″ə-to-mi″ə-li′tis) [*hemato-* + *myelitis*] acute myelitis with bloody effusion within the spinal cord.

he•ma•to•my•elo•pore (he″mə-to-, hem″ə-to-mi′əl-o-por″) [*hemato-* + *myelo-* + *pore*] a disease marked by the formation of canals in the spinal cord, due to hemorrhage.

he•ma•to•pa•thol•o•gy (he″mə-to-, hem″ə-to-pə-thol′ə-je) hemopathology.

he•ma•to•pe•nia (he″mə-to-, hem″ə-to-pe′ne-ə) [*hemato-* + *-penia*] deficiency of blood; see also *anemia*.

he•ma•to•peri•car•di•um (he″mə-to-, hem″ə-to-per″ĭ-kahr′de-əm) hemopericardium.

he•ma•to•peri•to•ne•um (he″mə-to-, hem″ə-to-per″ĭ-to-ne′əm) hemoperitoneum.

he•ma•to•phage (he′mə-to-, he-mat′o-fāj) hemophagocyte.

he•ma•to•pha•gia (he″mə-to-, hem″ə-to-fa′jə) 1. blood drinking. 2. subsisting on the blood of another animal.

he•ma•to•phago•cyte (he″mə-to-, hem″ə-to-fa′go-sīt) hemophagocyte.

he•ma•toph•a•gous (he″mə-, hem″ə-tof′ə-gəs) [*hemato-* + *phag-* + *-ous*] characterized by hematophagia.

he•ma•toph•a•gy (he″mə-, hem″ə-tof′ə-je) hematophagia.

he•ma•to•pho•bia (he″mə-to-, hem″ə-to-fo′be-ə) hemophobia.

he•ma•to•plas•tic (he″mə-to-, hem″ə-to-plas′tik) hematopoietic.

he•ma•to•poi•e•sis (he″mə-to-, hem″ə-to-poi-e′sis) [*hemato-* + *-poiesis*] the formation and development of blood cells. In the embryo and fetus it takes place in a variety of sites including the liver, spleen, thymus, lymph nodes, and bone marrow; from birth throughout the rest of life it is mainly in the bone marrow with a small amount occurring in lymph nodes. See also *erythropoiesis*, *leukopoiesis*, and *thrombocytopoiesis*. Called also *hematogenesis*, *hemogenesis*, and *hemopoiesis*.

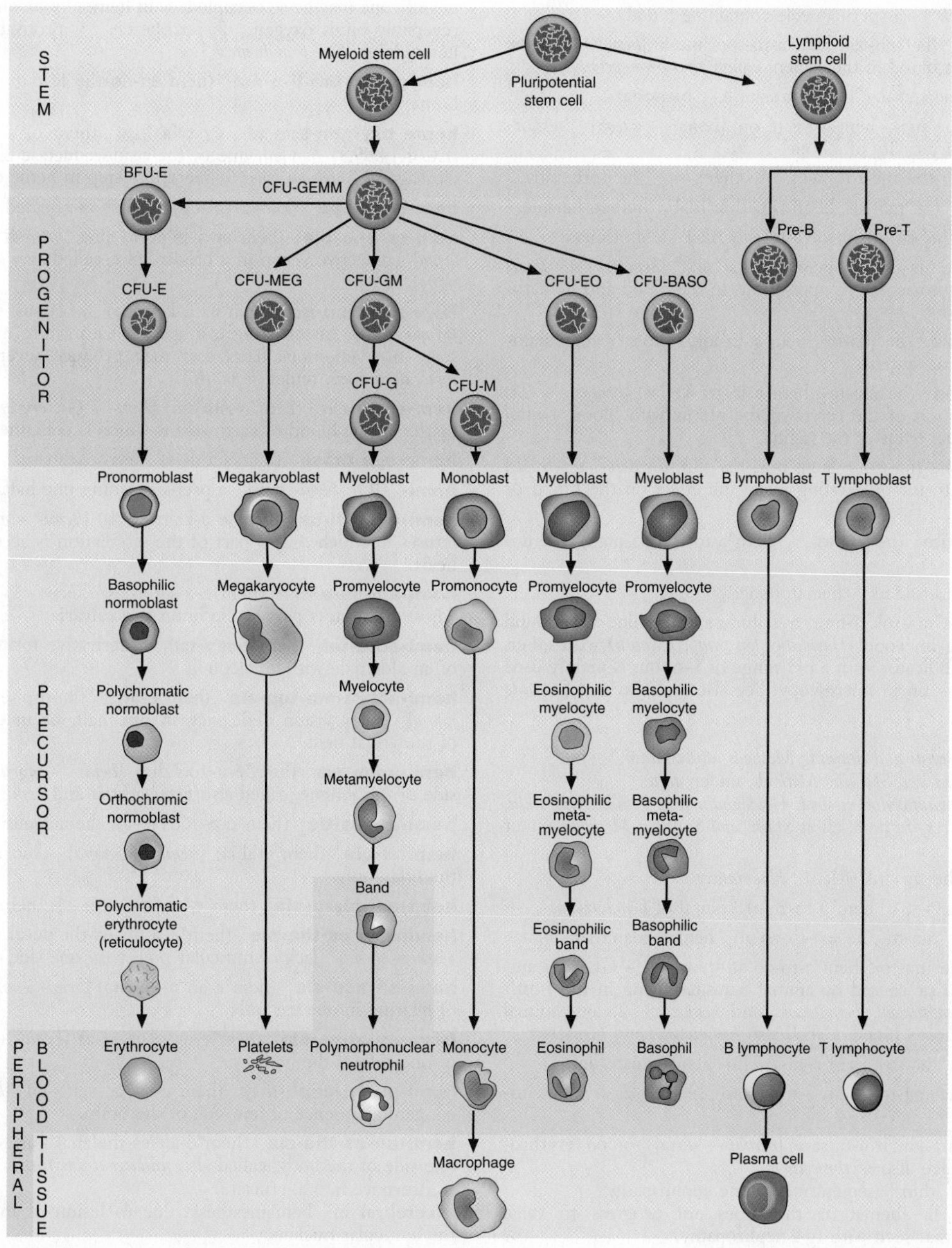

■ Hematopoiesis. *CFU-GEMM*, colony-forming unit–granulocyte, erythrocyte, monocyte, megakaryocyte. *BFU-E*, burst-forming unit–erythroid. *CFU-E*, colony-forming unit–erythroid. *CFU-MEG*, colony-forming unit–megakaryocytic. *CFU-GM*, colony-forming unit–granulocyte-macrophage. *CFU-EO*, colony-forming unit–eosinophilic. *CFU-BASO*, colony-forming unit–basophilic. *CFU-G*, colony-forming unit–granulocytic. *CFU-M*, colony-forming unit–macrophage.

cyclic h. see under *neutropenia.*
extramedullary h. the formation and development of blood cells outside the bone marrow; it is normal in the fetus but rare in later life.

he•ma•to•poi•et•ic (he″mə-to-, hem″ə-to-poi-et′ik) 1. pertaining to or effecting hematopoiesis; called also *hemapoietic, hematogenic, hematoplastic, hemogenic,* and *hemopoietic.* 2. an agent that promotes hematopoiesis.

he•ma•to•poi•e•tin (he″mə-to-, hem″ə-to-poi′ə-tin) erythropoietin.

he•ma•to•por•phy•rin (he″mə-to-, hem″ə-to-por′fə-rin) a dark red to purple pigment, a porphyrin (q.v.) in which two pyrrole rings have one methyl and one propionate side chain and the other two pyrrole rings have one methyl and one 1-hydroxyethyl side chain.

He•ma•top•o•ta (he″mə-, hem″ə-top′o-tə) *Haematopota.*

he•ma•tor•rha•chis (he″mə-, hem″ə-tor′ə-kis) hematomyelia.

he•ma•to•sal•pinx (he″mə-to-, hem″ə-to-sal′pinks) an accumulation of blood in the uterine tube.

he•ma•to•spec•tro•scope (he″mə-to-, hem″ə-to-spek′tro-skōp) [*hemato-* + *spectroscope*] a spectroscope for examining thin layers of blood.

he•ma•to•spec•tros•co•py (he″mə-to-, hem″ə-to-spek-tros′ko-pe) [*hemato-* + *spectroscopy*] spectroscopic examination of the blood.

he•ma•to•sper•mato•cele (he″mə-to-, hem″ə-to-spər-mat′o-sēl) [*hemato-* + *spermato-* + *-cele*[1]] a spermatocele containing blood.

he•ma•to•sper•mia (he″mə-to-, hem″ə-to-spur′me-ə) [*hemato-* + *sperm* + *-ia*] the presence of blood in the semen; called also *hemospermia.*

he•ma•to•stat•ic (he″mə-to-, hem″ə-to-stat′ik) hemostatic.

he•ma•tos•te•on (he″mə-, hem″ə-tos′te-on) [*hemat-* + *osteon*] hemorrhage into the medullary cavity of a bone.

he•ma•to•ther•a•py (he″mə-to-, hem″ə-to-ther′ə-pe) hemotherapy.

he•ma•to•ther•mal (he″mə-to-, hem″ə-to-thur′məl) homeothermic.

he•ma•to•tho•rax (he″mə-to-, hem″ə-to-thor′aks) hemothorax.

he•ma•to•tox•ic (he′mə-to-, hem′ə-to-tok″sik) [*hemato-* + *toxic*] 1. pertaining to hematotoxicosis. 2. poisonous to the blood and hematopoietic system.

he•ma•to•tox•i•co•sis (he″mə-to-, hem″ə-to-tok″sĭ-ko′sis) toxic damage to the hematopoietic system.

he•ma•to•tra•che•los (he″mə-to-, hem″ə-to-trə-ke′ləs) [*hemato-* + Gr. *trachēlos* neck] distention of the cervix of the uterus with blood, owing to atresia of the external os or of the vagina.

he•ma•to•tro•pic (he″mə-to-, hem″ə-to-tro′pik) [*hemato-* + *-tropic*] having a special affinity for or exerting a specific effect on the blood or blood cells.

he•ma•to•tym•pa•num (he″mə-to-, hem″ə-to-tim′pə-nəm) hemotympanum.

he•ma•tox•ic (he′mə-tok″sik) hematotoxic.

he•ma•tox•y•lin (he″mə-tok′sĭ-lin) a colorless crystalline compound obtained by extracting logwood *(Haematoxylon campechianum)* with ether. It may be used as an indicator with a pH range of 5–6, but is mainly used in oxidized form as a stain in microscopy. See also at *Stains and Staining Methods,* under *stain.*
alum h. hemalum.
Delafield h. see *Stains and Staining Methods,* under *stain.*
Harris h. see *Stains and Staining Methods,* under *stain.*
iron h. see *iron hematoxylin method, Heidenhain iron hematoxylin stain,* and *Weigert iron hematoxylin stain,* all at *Stains and Staining Methods,* under *stain.*

He•ma•tox•y•lon (he″mə-tok′sĭ-lən) *Haematoxylon.*

he•ma•to•zoa (he″mə-to-, hem″ə-to-zo′ə) plural of *hematozoon.*

he•ma•to•zo•al (he″mə-to-, he″mə-to-zo′əl) hematozoan (def. 1).

he•ma•to•zo•an (he″mə-to-, hem″ə-to-zo′ən) [*hemato-* + Gr. *zōon* animal] 1. pertaining to or caused by animal parasites living in the host's blood. Called also *hematozoal, hematozoic,* and *hemozoic.* 2. any animal parasite living in the host's blood. Called also *hematozoon* and *hemozoon.*

he•ma•to•zo•ic (he″mə-to-, hem″ə-to-zo′ik) hematozoan (def. 1).

he•ma•to•zo•on (he″mə-to-, hem″ə-to-zo′ən) pl. *hematozo′a.* hematozoan (def. 2).

he•ma•tu•ria (he″mə-, hem″ə-tu′re-ə) [*hemat-* + *-uria*] blood (erythrocytes) in the urine; called also *erythrocyturia.*
benign familial h. thin basement membrane nephropathy.
benign recurrent h. hematuria that does not progress to renal insufficiency, such as that seen with IgA nephropathy.
endemic h. urinary schistosomiasis.
enzootic bovine h. a disease of cattle marked by passing of blood in the urine, anemia, and debilitation; it is usually due to bracken poisoning.
essential h. hematuria for which no cause has been determined; called also *primary h.* and *functional h.*
false h. pseudohematuria.
functional h. essential h.
gross h. hematuria in which redness of the urine can be seen by the naked eye; called also *macroscopic h.*
macroscopic h. gross h.
microscopic h. blood in the urine visible only with a microscope, defined as at least two or three red blood cells per high power field. Called also *microhematuria.*
persistent h. hematuria present in every specimen.
primary h. essential h.
renal h. hematuria in which the blood comes from the kidney.
urethral h. hematuria in which the blood comes from the urethra.
vesical h. hematuria in which the blood comes from the bladder.

heme (hēm) 1. any quadridentate chelate of iron with the four pyrrole groups of a porphyrin, further distinguished as ferroheme or ferriheme referring to the chelates of Fe(II) and Fe(III) respectively. The four porphyrin ligands form a square-planar complex; the fifth and sixth coordination positions of the iron atom are perpendicular to the plane of the porphyrin and both may be occupied by strong field ligands, such as a nitrogen atom of a histidine residue of a protein, as in cytochromes, or only one may be so occupied, as in hemoglobin where the sixth position reversibly binds oxygen. 2. ferroheme. 3. protoheme IX, the heme of hemoglobin. See *protoheme.*

hem•en•do•the•li•o•ma (hēm″en-do-the″le-o′mə) hemangioendothelioma.

heme oxy•gen•ase (de•cy•cliz•ing) (hēm ok′sĭ-jən-ās de-si′kli-zing) [EC 1.14.99.3] an enzyme of the oxidoreductase class that catalyzes the cleavage of heme to form biliverdin, a step in heme catabolism.

hem•er•al•ope (hem′ər-əl-ōp) a person affected with hemeralopia.

hem•er•a•lo•pia (hem″ər-ə-lo′pe-ə) [Gr. *hēmera* day + *alaos* blind + *-opia*] defective vision in a bright light; called also *day blindness* and *night sight.*

Hem•ero•cam•pa (hem″ər-o-kam′pə) a genus of moths. *H. leukostig′ma* is the tussock moth, a species with white markings whose larval stage has venomous hairs that may produce severe urticaria. See also *insect dermatitis,* under *dermatitis.*

hem•eryth•rin (hēm″ə-rith′rin) [*hem-* + Gr. *erythros* red] the coloring matter of the blood of earthworms which is contained in the plasma.

heme syn•thase (hēm sin′thās) ferrochelatase.

hemi- [Gr. *hēmi-* half] a prefix meaning one half.

hemi•acar•di•us (hem″e-ə-kahr′de-əs) [*hemi-* + *acardius*] one of twin fetuses in which only a part of the circulation is accomplished by its own heart.

hemi•aceph•a•lus (hem″e-ə-sef′ə-ləs) [*hemi-* + *acephalus*] a fetus whose head lacks part of the brain and calvaria.

hemi•ac•e•tal (hem″e-as′ə-tal) a derivative formed by a combination of an aldehyde with an alcohol.

hemi•achro•ma•top•sia (hem″e-ə-kro″mə-top′se-ə) [*hemi-* + *achromatopsia*] color vision deficiency in one half, or in corresponding halves, of the visual field.

hemi•ageu•sia (hem″e-ə-goo′zhə) [*hemi-* + *ageusia*] ageusia on one side of the tongue; called also *hemiageustia* and *hemigeusia.*

hemi•ageus•tia (hem″e-ə-gōōs′te-ə) hemiageusia.

hemi•al•gia (hem″e-al′jə) [*hemi-* + *-algia*] pain affecting one side of the body only.

hemi•am•bly•o•pia (hem″e-am″ble-o′pe-ə) hemianopia.

hemi•amy•os•the•nia (hem″e-ə-mi″os-the′ne-ə) [*hemi-* + *a-*[1] + *myo-* + *sthen-* + *-ia*] lack of muscular power on one side of the body.

hemi•an•acu•sia (hem″e-an″ə-ku′zhə) [*hemi-* + *an-*[1] + *acou-* + *-ia*] loss of hearing in one ear only.

hemi•an•al•ge•sia (hem″e-an″əl-je′ze-ə) [*hemi-* + *analgesia*] analgesia of one side of the body.

hemi•an•en•ceph•a•ly (hem″e-an″ən-sef′ə-le) [*hemi-* + *anencephaly*] congenital absence of one side of the brain.

hemi•an•es•the•sia (hem″e-an″es-the′zhə) anesthesia affecting only one side of the body; called also *unilateral anesthesia.*
alternate h. h. cruciata.
cerebral h. hemianesthesia due to lesion of the internal capsule of the lenticular nucleus.
crossed h. h. cruciata.
h. crucia′ta loss of sensation on one side of the face with contralateral loss of pain and temperature sense on the body, resulting from a lateral

lesion in the pons or medulla, affecting both the sensory root of the trigeminal nerve and the spinothalamic tract.

mesocephalic h., pontile h. hemianesthesia due to disease of the pons.

spinal h. hemianesthesia due to a lesion of the spinal cord.

hemi•an•o•pia (hem″e-ə-no′pe-ə) [*hemi-* + *an-*[1] + *-opia*] defective vision or blindness in half of the visual field of one or both eyes; loosely, scotoma in less than half of the visual field of one or both eyes. **hemianop′ic** *adj*

absolute h. blindness to light, color, and form, in half of the visual field.

altitudinal h. hemianopia in the upper or lower half of the visual field.

bilateral h. hemianopia affecting both eyes.

binasal h. heteronymous hemianopia in which the defects are in the nasal half of the field of vision in each eye.

binocular h. bilateral h.

bitemporal h. heteronymous hemianopia in which the defects are in the temporal half of the field of vision in each eye.

complete h. hemianopia affecting an entire half of the visual field of each eye.

congruous h. homonymous hemianopia in which the defects in the field of vision in each eye are symmetrical in position, shape, size, and degree.

crossed h. altitudinal hemianopia affecting the upper field of one eye and the lower field of the other.

heteronymous h. hemianopia affecting the nasal or the temporal half of the field of vision of each eye.

homonymous h. hemianopia affecting the right halves or the left halves of the visual fields of the two eyes.

horizontal h. altitudinal h.

incomplete h. hemianopia affecting less than an entire half of the visual field.

incongruous h. homonymous hemianopia in which the defects in the field of vision in the two eyes differ in one or more respects, as in extent or intensity.

lateral h. homonymous h.

nasal h. hemianopia in the nasal halves of the visual fields.

quadrant h., quadrantic h. quadrantanopia.

relative h. defective vision of or blindness to form or color in half of the visual field, the perception of light being retained.

temporal h. hemianopia in the temporal halves of the visual fields.

unilateral h. hemianopia in one eye only.

hemi•an•op•sia (hem″e-ə-nop′se-ə) hemianopia. **hemianop′tic** *adj*

hemi•an•os•mia (hem″e-ə-noz′me-ə) [*hemi-* + *anosmia*] anosmia in one of the nostrils.

hemi•aprax•ia (hem″e-ə-prak′se-ə) [*hemi-* + *apraxia*] apraxia affecting one side of the body only.

hemi•ar•thro•plas•ty (hem″e-ahr′thro-plas″te) arthroplasty in which just one joint surface is replaced. **hemiarthroplas′tic** *adj*

hemi•ar•thro•sis (hem″e-ahr-thro′sis) [*hemi-* + *arthrosis*] a spurious synchondrosis.

hemi•aso•ma•tog•no•sia (hem″e-ə-so″mə-tog-no′zhə) defective or lack of awareness of the condition of one side of one's body.

hemi•asyn•er•gia (hem″e-as″ə-nur′jə) [*hemi-* + *asynergia*] asynergia affecting one side of the body only.

hemi•atax•ia (hem″e-ə-tak′se-ə) [*hemi-* + *ataxia*] ataxia affecting one side of the body only.

hemi•ataxy (hem″e-ə-tak′se) hemiataxia.

hemi•ath•e•to•sis (hem″e-ath″ə-to′sis) [*hemi-* + *athetosis*] athetosis affecting one side of the body only.

hemi•at•ro•phy (hem″e-at′ro-fe) [*hemi-* + *atrophy*] atrophy of one side of the body or of one half of an organ or part.

facial h. a condition of unknown etiology, characterized by progressive atrophy of the tissues of one side of the face, frequently with pigmentation disorders and alopecia, jacksonian epilepsy, and trigeminal neuralgia. Sometimes it spreads to involve both sides of the face or the ipsilateral trunk, viscera, or limbs. Called also *hemifacial atrophy, Romberg disease, facial trophoneurosis,* and *Parry-Romberg syndrome.*

progressive lingual h. progressive atrophy of one lateral half of the tongue.

hemi•ax•i•al (hem″e-ak′se-əl) at any oblique angle to the long axis of the body or a part.

hemi•bal•lism (hem″e-bal′iz-əm) hemiballismus.

hemi•bal•lis•mus (hem″e-bə-liz′məs) [*hemi-* + *ballismus*] a violent form of dyskinesia involving only one side of the body and being most marked in the upper extremity, resulting from a destructive lesion of the nucleus subthalamicus (Luys body). Cf. *hemichorea.* Called also *body of Luys syndrome.*

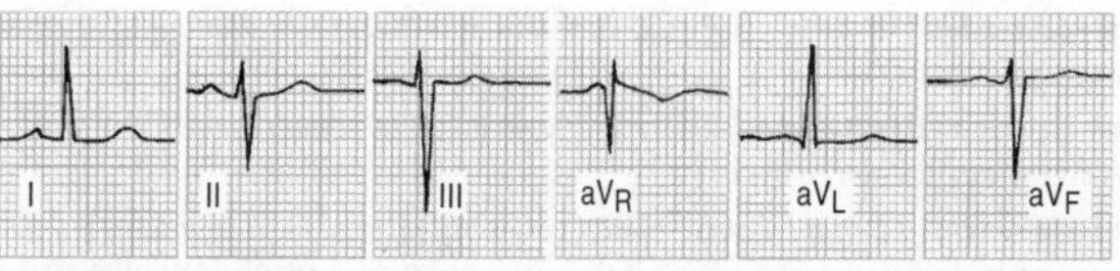

■ Left anterior hemiblock showing marked left axis deviation without significant widening of the QRS duration.

hemi•blad•der (hem′e-blad″ər) a half bladder, as seen in exstrophy of the cloaca; the urinary bladder is formed as two physically separated parts, each with its own ureter.

hemi•block (hem′e-blok) failure in conduction of the cardiac impulse in either of the two main divisions of the left ventricular conducting system (bundle of His); it is called *left anterior hemiblock* when the anterior-superior division is interrupted and *left posterior hemiblock* when the posterior division is interrupted.

he•mic (he′mik, hem′ik) [Gr. *haima* blood] pertaining to the blood; called also *hemal, hematal,* and *hematic.*

hemi•ca•nit•i•es (hem″e-kə-nish′e-ēz) grayness of the hair on one side of the body.

hemi•car•dia (hem″e-kahr′de-ə) [*hemi-* + *cardia*] 1. a congenital anomaly characterized by the presence of only half of a four-chambered heart. 2. either lateral half of a normal heart.

hemi•car•di•us (hem″e-kahr′de-əs) a free twin fetus whose development is greatly reduced but whose body form and various parts are still recognizable.

hemi•cel•lu•lose (hem″e-sel′u-lōs) a general name for a group of high molecular weight polysaccharides, found in plant cell walls, similar to cellulose but smaller, alkali-soluble, and composed of various sugars, including aldopentoses, aldohexoses, and uronic acids; the most ubiquitous are the xylans.

hemi•cen•trum (hem″e-sen′trəm) [*hemi-* + *centrum*] either lateral half of a vertebral centrum.

hemi•ce•pha•lia (hem″e-sə-fa′le-ə) [*hemi-* + *cephal-* + *-ia*] congenital absence of the cerebrum.

hemi•ceph•a•lus (hem″e-sef′ə-ləs) a fetus whose brain is rudimentary and lacks a cerebrum; see *hemicephalia.*

hemi•cer•e•brum (hem″e-sə-re′brəm, -ser′ə-brəm) hemispherium cerebri.

hemi•cho•rea (hem″e-kə-re′ə) [*hemi-* + *chorea*] chorea which affects only one side; called also *hemilateral chorea.* Cf. *hemiballismus.*

hemi•chro•ma•top•sia (hem″e-kro″mə-top′se-ə) hemiachromatopsia.

he•mi•chrome (he′mĭ-krōm) an oxidized derivative of methemoglobin in which a functional group of globin has replaced the normal water substituent of the heme; it precipitates readily, aggregating to form Heinz bodies and ultimately causing cell lysis.

hemi•co•lec•to•my (hem″e-ko-lek′tə-me) [*hemi-* + *colectomy*] excision of approximately half of the colon.

left h. surgical removal of the left colon.

right h. surgical removal of the right colon.

hemi•cor•por•ec•to•my (hem″e-kor-por-ek′tə-me) [*hemi-* + *corpus* + *-ectomy*] surgical removal of the lower part of the body through the lumbar region, including the entire lower limbs, bony pelvis, genitalia, and pelvic contents such as the anus and lower rectum.

hemi•cor•ti•cec•to•my (hem″e-kor″tĭ-sek′tə-me) excision of a cerebral hemisphere leaving the basal ganglia intact; done in intractable epilepsy.

hemi•cra•nia (hem″e-kra′ne-ə) [*hemi-* + Gr. *kranion* skull] 1. unilateral headache. 2. incomplete anencephaly or meroanencephaly.

chronic paroxysmal h. one-sided headache resembling a cluster headache but occurring in paroxysms of half an hour or less, several times a day, sometimes daily for years; it is accompanied by conjunctival hyperemia, rhinorrhea and occasionally Horner's syndrome.

h. conti′nua continual, generally mild to moderate, one-sided headache that responds to indomethacin, with periodic exacerbations accompanied by conjunctival injection, lacrimation, nasal congestion, rhinorrhea, ptosis, or eyelid edema.

hemi•cra•ni•ec•to•my (hem″ĭ-kra″ne-ek′tə-me) [*hemi-* + *craniectomy*] exposure of half of the brain by sectioning the vault of the skull from front to back near the median line and forcing the entire side outward.

hemi•cra•ni•o•sis (hem″e-kra″ne-o′sis) a condition marked by hyperostosis on one half of the cranium or face, with cerebral involvement. The condition is believed to be due to endothelioma of the dura.

hemi·cra·ni·ot·o·my (hem″e-kra″ne-ot′ə-me) [*hemi-* + *craniotomy*] hemicraniectomy.

hemi·de·cor·ti·ca·tion (hem″e-de-kor″tĭ-ka′shən) removal of one half of the cerebral cortex.

hemi·des·mo·some (hem″e-des′mo-sōm) [*hemi-* + *desmosome*] a structure, morphologically similar to half a desmosome but chemically and functionally distinct, found on the basal surface of some epithelial cells and forming the site of attachment between the basal surface of the cell and the basement membrane; the transmembrane linking proteins are integrins.

hemi·dia·pho·re·sis (hem″e-di″ə-fə-re′sis) hemihyperhidrosis.

hemi·dia·phragm (hem″e-di′ə-fram) one half of the diaphragm.

hemi·dys·er·gia (hem″e-dis-ur′je-ə) dysergia affecting one side of the body.

hemi·dys·es·the·sia (hem″e-dis″es-the′zhə) [*hemi-* + *dysesthesia*] a dysesthesia affecting one side of the body only.

hemi·dys·to·nia (hem″e-dis-to′ne-ə) dystonia affecting just one side of the body.

hemi·dys·tro·phy (hem″e-dis′trə-fe) unequal development of the two sides of the body.

hemi·ec·tro·me·lia (hem″e-ek-tro-me′le-ə) a developmental anomaly characterized by imperfect development of the limbs of one side of the body.

hemi·elas·tin (hem″e-ə-las′tin) a substance formed by the digestion or hydrolysis of elastin.

hemi·en·ceph·a·lus (hem″e-ən-sef′ə-ləs) [*hemi-* + Gr. *enkephalos* brain] a fetus that lacks one cerebral hemisphere.

hemi·epi·lep·sy (hem″e-ep′ĭ-lep-se) [*hemi-* + *epilepsy*] epilepsy affecting one side of the body only.

hemi·fa·cial (hem″e-fa′shəl) pertaining to or affecting one half of the face.

hemi·gas·trec·to·my (hem″e-gas-trek′tə-me) excision of half of the stomach.

hemi·geu·sia (hem″e-goo′zhə) hemiageusia.

hemi·ghost (hem′e-gōst) an abnormal erythrocyte seen in anemia.

hemi·gi·gan·tism (hem″e-ji-gan′tiz-əm) overgrowth of one side of the entire body or of a portion of one side, as of the face.

hemi·glos·sal (hem″e-glos′əl) hemilingual.

hemi·glos·sec·to·my (hem″e-glos-ek′tə-me) [*hemi-* + *glossectomy*] resection of one side of the tongue.

hemi·glos·si·tis (hem″e-glos-i′tis) [*hemi-* + *glossitis*] inflammation involving only one side of the tongue.

hemi·gna·thia (hem″e-na′the-ə) [*hemi-* + *gnath-* + *-ia*] a developmental anomaly characterized by partial to complete absence of the lower jaw on one side.

hemi·hep·a·tec·to·my (hem″e-hep″ə-tek′tə-me) excision of half of the liver.

hemi·hi·dro·sis (hem″e-hĭ-dro′sis) [*hemi-* + *hidr-* + *-osis*] sweating on one side of the body only.

hemi·hy·pal·ge·sia (hem″e-hi″pəl-je′ze-ə) [*hemi-* + *hypalgesia*] hypalgesia on one side of the body.

hemi·hy·per·es·the·sia (hem″e-hi″pər-es-the′zhə) [*hemi-* + *hyperesthesia*] hyperesthesia on one side of the body.

hemi·hy·per·hi·dro·sis (hem″e-hi″pər-hĭ-dro′sis) [*hemi-* + *hyperhidrosis*] excessive sweating on one side of the body only; called also *hemidiaphoresis.*

hemi·hy·per·me·tria (hem″e-hi″pər-me′tre-ə) hypermetria affecting one side of the body.

hemi·hy·per·pla·sia (hem″e-hi″pər-pla′zhə) overdevelopment of one side of the body, or of one half of an organ or part, as of the cranium.

hemi·hy·per·to·nia (hem″e-hi″pər-to′ne-ə) [*hemi-* + *hypertonia*] increased tone of the muscles of one side, which may result in contractures; sometimes seen after a stroke. Called also *hemitonia.*

hemi·hy·per·tro·phy (hem″e-hi-pur′trə-fe) [*hemi-* + *hypertrophy*] 1. overgrowth of one half of the body or unilateral hypertrophy of a part. 2. Curtius syndrome.

facial h. overgrowth of one side of the face. Called also *hemifacial hypertrophy.*

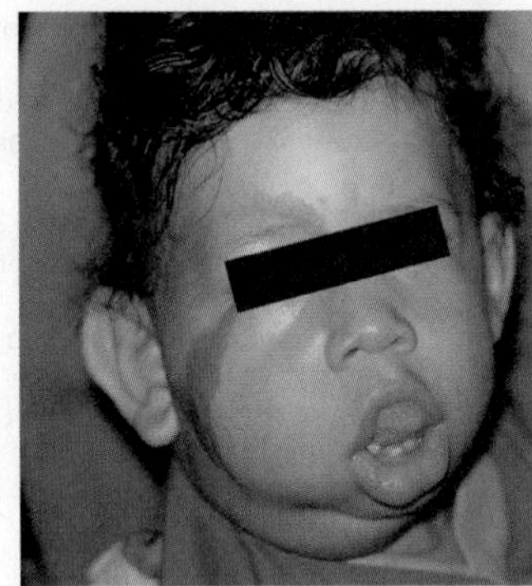

■ Facial hemihypertrophy as part of epidermal nevus syndrome.

hemi·hy·pes·the·sia (hem″e-hi″pes-the′zhə) hypoesthesia on one side of the body; called also *hemihypoesthesia.*

hemi·hy·po·es·the·sia (hem″e-hi″po-es-the′zhə) hemihypesthesia.

hemi·hy·po·me·tria (hem″e-hi″po-me′tre-ə) hypometria affecting one side of the body.

hemi·hy·po·pla·sia (hem″e-hi″po-pla′zhə) underdevelopment of one side of the body, or of one half of a part or organ, as of the brain.

hemi·hy·po·to·nia (hem″e-hi″po-to′ne-ə) [*hemi-* + *hypotonia*] reduced muscle tone of one side of the body.

hemi-in·at·ten·tion (hem″e-in-ə-ten′shən) unilateral neglect.

hemi·ke·tal (hem″ĭ-ke′təl) a derivative formed by a combination of a ketone group with an alcohol.

hemi·lam·i·nec·to·my (hem″e-lam″ĭ-nek′tə-me) surgical removal of one side of the vertebral lamina.

hemi·lar·yn·gec·to·my (hem″e-lar″in-jek′tə-me) excision of one lateral half of the larynx.

hemi·lat·er·al (hem″e-lat′ər-əl) affecting one lateral half.

hemi·lin·gual (hem″ĭ-ling′gwəl) [*hemi-* + *lingual*] affecting one side of the tongue; called also *hemiglossal.*

hemi·liv·er (hem″e-liv′ər) either the right liver or the left liver; see *pars hepatis dextra* and *pars hepatis sinistra.*

hemi·ma·cro·glos·sia (hem″ĭ-mak″ro-glos′e-ə) enlargement of one side of the tongue.

hemi·man·dib·u·lec·to·my (hem″ĭ-man-dib″u-lek′tə-me) surgical excision of half of the mandible.

hemi·max·il·lec·to·my (hem″i-mak″sil-ek′tə-me) [*hemi-* + *maxillectomy*] surgical excision of half or part of the maxilla.

hemi·me·lia (hem″e-me′le-ə) [*hemi-* + *-melia*] a developmental anomaly characterized by absence of all or part of the forearm or the lower leg.

fibular h. hemimelia of the lower limb in which the fibula is primarily affected, ranging in severity from mild shortening to total absence of the fibula. It results in leg-length discrepancy with deformity of the foot (usually equinovalgus), flexion contracture of the knee, and instability of the knee and ankle.

radial h. hemimelia of the upper limb in which the radius is primarily affected; see *radial clubhand,* under *hand.*

tibial h. hemimelia of the lower limb in which the tibia is primarily affected, ranging in severity from mild hypoplasia to total absence of the tibia. The proximal fibular head may be displaced, and the knee is flexed and may lack extension. It may occur as an isolated anomaly or as part of a larger syndrome. Most cases are sporadic but autosomal dominant and recessive patterns of inheritance have been reported.

ulnar h. hemimelia of the upper limb in which the ulna is primarily affected; see *ulnar clubhand,* under *hand.*

hem·im·e·lus (hem-im′ə-ləs) an individual exhibiting hemimelia.

hemi·meth·yl·a·tion (hem″e-meth″əl-a′shən) the presence of methylated nucleotides in only one strand of a double-stranded DNA molecule, as a result of semiconservative replication. The unmethylated strand is then methylated by specific DNA methyltransferases, using the methylated strand as a template.

he·min (he′min) 1. a porphyrin chelate of iron (III), derived from red blood cells; the chloride of heme. It is used to ameliorate the symptoms of acute intermittent porphyria, porphyria variegata, and hereditary coproporphyria; administered intravenously. 2. hematin (def. 1).

hemi·ne·glect (hem″e-nə-glekt′) unilateral neglect.

hemi·ne·phrec·to·my (hem″e-nə-frek′tə-me) excision of a portion of a kidney.

hemi·neph·ro·ure·ter·ec·to·my (hem″e-nef″ro-u-re″tər-ek′tə-me) excision of a portion of a kidney and ureter.

hemi·obe·si·ty (hem″e-o-bēs′ĭ-te) [*hemi-* + *obesity*] obesity of one side of the body only.

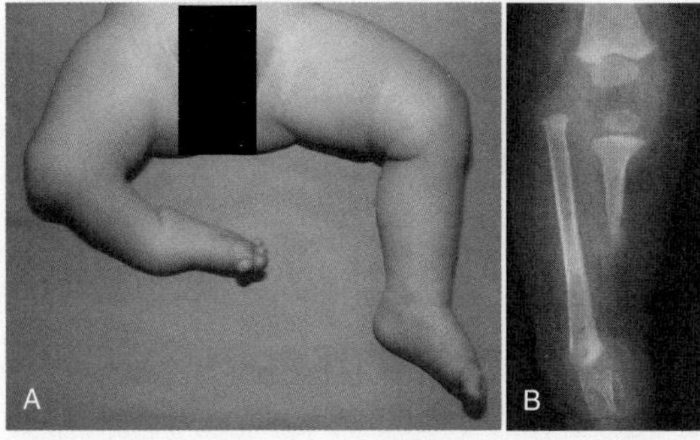

■ Congenital tibial hemimelia with proximal dislocation of fibula and radiographically visible proximal tibia with normal-appearing knee joint; clinical *(A)* and radiographic *(B)* appearance.

hemi·op·al·gia (hem″e-op-al′jə) [*hemi-* + *opalgia*] pain in one side of the head and in one eye.

hemi·opia (hem″e-o′pe-ə) hemianopia. **hemiop′ic** *adj*

hem·ip·a·gus (hem-ip′ə-gəs) [*hemi-* + *-pagus*] conjoined twins united laterally at the thorax.

hemi·pa·ral·y·sis (hem″e-pə-ral′ə-sis) hemiplegia.

hemi·par·a·ple·gia (hem″e-par″ə-ple′jə) [*hemi-* + *paraplegia*] paralysis of the lower half of one side of the body.

hemi·pa·re·sis (hem″e-pə-re′sis) [*hemi-* + *paresis*] muscular weakness or partial paralysis affecting one side of the body.

ataxic h. a type of lacunar stroke characterized by weakness and ataxia in a lower limb and sometimes the upper limb on the same side.

pure motor h. a type of lacunar stroke characterized by paralysis without sensory deficits on one side of the body, usually involving the face, upper limb, and lower limb.

hemi·par·es·the·sia (hem″e-par″es-the′zhə) [*hemi-* + *paresthesia*] perverted sensation on one side of the body.

hemi·pa·ret·ic (hem″e-pə-ret′ik) 1. pertaining to hemiparesis. 2. an individual with hemiparesis.

hemi·par·kin·son·ism (hem″ĭ-pahr′kin-son-iz-əm) parkinsonism affecting only one side of the body.

hemi·pel·vec·to·my (hem″ĭ-pel-vek′tə-me) amputation of a lower limb through the sacroiliac joint. Called also *hindquarter*, *interilioabdominal*, or *interpelviabdominal amputation* and *Jaboulay amputation* or *operation*.

hemi·phal·an·gec·to·my (hem″ĭ-fal″ən-jek′tə-me) the excision of part of a digital phalanx.

hemi·pla·cen·ta (hem″e-plə-sen′tə) [*hemi-* + *placenta*] an organ, composed of the chorion, yolk sac, and, usually, allantois, that puts marsupial embryos into temporary relation with the maternal uterus.

hemi·ple·gia (hem″e-ple′jə) [*hemi-* + *-plegia*] paralysis of one side of the body. **hemiple′gic** *adj*

h. al′ternans hypoglos′sica hemiplegia due to lesion of the hypoglossal nerve on the side opposite the paralyzed part.

alternate h. hemiplegia that affects a part on one side of the body and another part on the opposite side.

alternating oculomotor h. Weber syndrome.

ascending h. ascending paralysis of one lateral half of the body.

capsular h. hemiplegia due to lesion of the internal capsule.

cerebral h. hemiplegia which is due to a lesion of the brain.

contralateral h. hemiplegia on the side of the body opposite the site of the brain lesion causing it.

crossed h., h. crucia′ta alternate h.

facial h. paralysis of one side of the face, the body being unaffected.

faciobrachial h. paralysis of one half of the face and of the upper limb on the same side.

faciolingual h. paralysis of one side of the face and tongue.

flaccid h. hemiplegia with loss of tone of the muscles of the paralyzed part and absence of tendon reflexes. Cf. *spastic h.*

Gubler h. Millard-Gubler syndrome.

infantile h. hemiplegia due to cerebral thrombosis or hemorrhage at delivery or occurring before birth.

laryngeal h. paralysis of one side of the larynx of a horse, which produces roaring (q.v.).

spastic h. hemiplegia marked by spasticity of the muscles of the paralyzed part and increased tendon reflexes. Cf. *flaccid h.*

spinal h. hemiplegia due to a lesion of the spinal cord.

Wernicke-Mann h. partial hemiplegia of the extremities.

He·mip·tera (he-mip′tər-ə) [*hemi-* + Gr. *pteron* wing] an order of insects that may be winged or wingless and have mouth parts adapted to piercing or sucking; it includes ticks and lice. The families Cimicidae and Reduviidae (suborder Heteroptera) contain species of considerable medical importance. See also *bug*.

he·mip·ter·ous (he-mip′tər-əs) of or pertaining to insects of the order Hemiptera.

hemi·py·lor·ec·to·my (hem″ĭ-pi″lor-ek′tə-me) excision of half of the pylorus.

hemi·pyo·ne·phro·sis (hem″ĭ-pi″o-nə-fro′sis) pyonephrosis in a portion of a kidney or in half of a double kidney.

hemi·ra·chis·chi·sis (hem″e-rə-kis′kĭ-sis) rachischisis without prolapse of the spinal cord.

hemi·sa·cral·iza·tion (hem″e-sa″krəl-ĭ-za′shən) fusion of the fifth lumbar vertebra to the first segment of the sacrum on only one side.

Hemi·scor·pi·i·dae (hem″e-skor-pi′ĭ-de) a family of scorpions (order Scorpionida), containing the single genus *Hemiscorpius*.

Hemi·scor·pi·us (hem″e-skor′pe-əs) a genus of scorpions of the family Hemiscorpiidae, found in southwestern Asia from the Arabian Peninsula to Pakistan. *H. leptu′rus* has a venomous bite that causes serious skin wounds.

hemi·sco·to·sis (hem″e-sko-to′sis) hemianopia.

hemi·sec·tion (hem″e-sek′shən) 1. division into two equal parts. 2. surgical division of a multiple rooted tooth from the crown to the furcation with removal of a root and part of the crown.

hemi·sec·to·my (hem″e-sek′tə-me) [*hemi-* + *-ectomy*] amputation of one root of a two-rooted mandibular tooth. Cf. *apicoectomy*.

hemi·sep·tum (hem″e-sep′təm) either half of a septum, especially the lamina of the septum pellucidum of the brain.

h. ce′rebri the lateral half of the septum pellucidum of the brain.

hemi·so·mus (hem″e-so′məs) [*hemi-* + Gr. *sōma* body] an imperfectly developed fetus.

hem·iso·ton·ic (hem″i-so-ton′ik) [*hem-* + *isotonic*] having the same osmotic pressure as the blood.

hemi·spasm (hem′e-spaz″əm) spasm affecting one side only.

hemi·sphere (hem′ĭ-sfēr) [*hemi-* + *sphere*] half of a spherical or roughly spherical structure; see also *hemispherium*.

animal h. the half of the mass of cells formed by cleavage of a zygote that is nearest the animal pole.

cerebellar h. hemispherium cerebelli.

cerebral h. hemispherium cerebri.

dominant h. the cerebral hemisphere that is more concerned than the other in the integration of sensations and the control of many functions, such as speech and language and the preferential use of one or the other of paired organs in voluntary movements. The hemisphere opposite to the handedness of the individual, i.e., the left cerebral hemisphere in right-handed persons, and vice versa, is the dominant one for many functions, but the left hemisphere is usually dominant for speech and language functions regardless of handedness.

nondominant h. the hemisphere opposite to the dominant one; it plays a far smaller role in speech and language but may play a far larger role in mediating spatial responses and emotional responses.

vegetal h. the half of the mass of cells formed by cleavage of a zygote that is nearest the vegetal pole.

hemi·spher·ec·to·my (hem″ĭ-sfēr-ek′tə-me) [*hemisphere* + *-ectomy*] resection of a cerebral hemisphere.

hemi·sphe·ri·um (hem″ĭ-sfēr′e-əm) pl. *hemisphe′ria* [L.] hemisphere.

h. cerebel′li [TA] cerebellar hemisphere: the part of the cerebellum lateral to the vermis. Each hemisphere is subdivided into lobules designated HII–X, which correspond to the lobules of the vermis (I–X); there is no HI in humans to correspond to I (lingula). See also *cerebellum*.

h. ce′rebri [TA] cerebral hemisphere: either of the pair of structures, formed by evagination of the embryonic telencephalon, lying on either side of the midline, partly separated by the longitudinal cerebral fissure, containing a central cavity, the lateral ventricle, and covered by a layer of gray substance, the cerebral cortex; together they constitute the largest part of the human brain.

hemi·sphyg·mia (hem″ĭ-sfig′me-ə) [*hemi-* + *sphygm-* + *-ia*] a condition in which there appear to be twice as many pulse beats as heart beats, such as pulsus bisferiens.

hemi·spore (hem′ĭ-spor) a spore formed by the differentiation and division of the terminal portion of a hypha.

hemi·syn·drome (hem″e-sin′drom) a syndrome that affects just one side of the body.

hemi·ter·a·ta (hem″e-ter′ə-tə) [*hemi-* + *teras*] a grouping of congenitally deformed individuals whose anomalies are less severe than teratisms.

hemi·ter·at·ic (hem″e-tər-at′ik) congenitally deformed, but not exhibiting teratism.

hemi·tet·a·ny (hem″e-tet′ə-ne) tetany limited to one side of the body.

hemi·ther·mo·an·es·the·sia (hem″e-thur″mo-an″es-the′zhə) thermanesthesia on one side of the body.

hemi·tho·rax (hem″e-thor′aks) [*hemi-* + *thorax*] one side of the chest.
  frozen h. prevention of a mediastinal shift away from the affected lung in diffuse pleural mesothelioma, caused by encasement of the lung by nodular thickening of the pleura.

hemi·thy·roi·dec·to·my (hem″e-thi″roid-ek′tə-me) excision of one lobe of the thyroid gland.

hemi·to·nia (hem″e-to′ne-ə) [*hemi-* + *ton-* + *-ia*] hemihypertonia.

hemi·tox·in (hem′e-tok″sin) a toxin whose toxicity has been reduced by one half.

hemi·tre·mor (hem″e-trĕ′mər) tremor of one side of the body.

hemi·tri·gone (hem″e-tri′gōn) 1. half a trigone. 2. congenital absence of half of a bladder trigone, sometimes with absence of one ureter.

hemi·va·got·o·ny (hem″e-və-got′o-ne) vagotonia on one side.

hemi·ver·te·bra (hem″e-vur′tə-brə) 1. a developmental anomaly characterized by incomplete development of one half of a vertebra. 2. a vertebra which is incompletely developed on one side.

hemi·zo·na (hem″e-zo′nə) half of a zone, such as the zona pellucida.

hemi·zy·gos·i·ty (hem″e-zi-gos′ĭ-te) [*hemi-* + *-zygosity*] possession of only one of a pair of alleles; refers particularly to the state of the male for X-linked genes, and also to abnormal conditions in which a segment of DNA has been deleted from one member of a chromosome pair, so that the individual is *hemizygous* for the genes lost with that segment. **hemizy′gous** *adj*

hemi·zy·gote (hem″e-zi′gōt) an individual or cell exhibiting hemizygosity.

hem·lock (hem′lok) 1. any fir tree of the genus *Tsuga*. 2. any of the plants of the genera *Cicuta* and *Conium*. 3. poison h.
  poison h. *Conium maculatum*, a large herb that contains the poisonous alkaloid coniine; animals that eat it develop nausea and vomiting, followed by muscle paralysis and respiratory failure that can be fatal. The dried, fully grown, but unripe fruit has sedative, anodyne, and antispasmodic properties. Called also *hemlock*.
  water h. any tree of the genus *Cicuta*.

hem(o)- [Gr. *haima* blood] a combining form denoting relationship to the blood; variant forms are *haema-*, *haem(o)-*, and *hema-*.

he·mo·ac·cess (he″mo-ak′səs) vascular access.

he·mo·ag·glu·ti·na·tion (he″mo-ə-gloo″tĭ-na′shən) hemagglutination.

he·mo·ag·glu·ti·nin (he″mo-ə-gloo′tĭ-nin) hemagglutinin.

he·mo·bil·ia (he″mo-bil′e-ə) bleeding into the biliary passages.

he·mo·blast (he′mo-blast) blast cell (def. 2).
  lymphoid h. of Pappenheim pronormoblast.

he·mo·ca·ther·e·sis (he″mo-kə-ther′ə-sis) hemolysis.

He·moc·cult (he′mo-kəlt) trademark for a modification of the guaiac test for occult blood, in which guaiac-impregnated filter paper is used; the test is positive if the specimen turns blue.

he·mo·cele (he′mo-sēl) hemocoelom.

he·mo·ce·lom (he″mo-se′lom) hemocoelom.

he·mo·cho·le·cyst (he″mo-ko′lə-sist) nontraumatic hemorrhage of the gallbladder.

he·mo·cho·le·cys·ti·tis (he″mo-ko-lə-sis-ti′tis) hemorrhagic cholecystitis.

he·mo·cho·ri·al (he″mo-kor′e-əl) [*hemo-* + *chorion*] denoting a type of placenta in which maternal blood comes in direct contact with the chorion, as in humans.

he·mo·chro·ma·to·sis (he″mo-kro″mə-to′sis) [*hemo-* + *chromatosis*] a syndrome of organ damage resulting from accumulation of iron in the tissues, causing damage and dysfunction of the liver, pancreas, heart, joints, and endocrine organs, and leading to organ failure. Classic clinical signs include bronze pigmentation of skin, arthropathy, diabetes mellitus, cirrhosis, hepatosplenomegaly, hypogonadism, and loss of body hair. Full development of the condition among women is restricted by menstruation and pregnancy. Cf. *hemosiderosis* and *siderosis*. **hemochromatot′ic** *adj*
  acquired h. hemochromatosis resulting from blood transfusions or excessive dietary iron, or secondary to other disease, e.g., thalassemia or sideroblastic anemia; called also *secondary h.*
  exogenous h. acquired h.

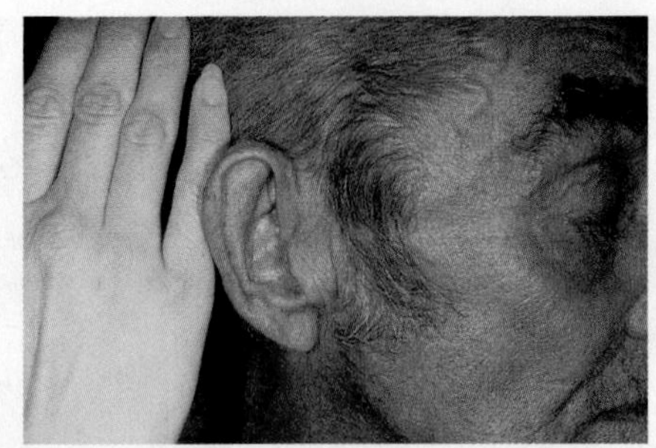

■ Hemochromatosis.

  genetic h., hereditary h. a genetically heterogeneous group of inherited disorders of iron metabolism characterized by failure to prevent excessive amounts of iron from entering the circulatory pool and accumulating in the tissues. It comprises most cases of hemachromatosis; four types have been identified.
    type 1 the most common hereditary hemochromatosis, an autosomal recessive disorder caused by mutation in the *HFE* gene (locus: 6p21.3), which encodes a transferrin-binding transmembrane protein the occurs in the villi of the small intestine. Transferrin iron saturation, serum ferritin levels, and liver iron content are all elevated. Iron accumulation is lifelong, with symptoms appearing usually in the fifth or sixth decades of life.
    type 2 juvenile h.
    type 3 an autosomal recessive form, clinically resembling type 1 but with normal transferrin iron saturation and serum ferritin levels, caused by mutation in the *TFR2* gene (locus: 7q22), which encodes transferrin receptor-2.
    type 4 a rare autosomal dominant form caused by mutation in the *SLC40A1* gene (locus: 2q32), which encodes ferroportin, characterized by hepatic iron deposition mainly in reticuloendothelial cells, elevated serum ferritin, and transferrin iron saturation that is frequently normal.
  idiopathic h. hereditary h.
  juvenile h. either of two autosomal recessive iron overload disorders that clinically resemble hereditary hemochromatosis type 1 but have their onset in childhood and lead to death by age 30. The most common of these is caused by mutation in the *HJV* gene (locus: 1q21), which encodes hemojuvelin; the other is caused by mutation in the *HAMP* gene (locus: 19q13), which encodes hepcidin. Called also *hereditary h. type 2*.
  neonatal h., perinatal h. a rare fulminant disease of the liver, of unknown cause, characterized by massive deposition of iron in the liver, pancreas, heart, and endocrine glands; symptoms are those of neonatal hepatitis and appear in utero or within the first week of life, with death usually occurring by 4 months of age.
  primary h. hereditary h.
  secondary h. acquired h.

he·mo·chrome (he′mo-krōm) [*hemo-* + *-chrome*] a heme compound in which the fifth and sixth coordination positions of the central iron atom are occupied by strong field ligands, usually nitrogen atoms, as in cytochromes; originally a complex of 2 moles of a nitrogenous base per mole of heme. Called also *hemochromogen*.

he·mo·chro·mo·gen (he″mo-kro′mo-jən) hemochrome.

he·mo·cla·sis (he-mok′lə-sis) hemolysis. **hemoclas′tic** *adj*

he·mo·clip (he′mo-klip) a metal clip used to ligate blood vessels.

he·mo·co·ag·u·lin (he″mo-ko-ag′u-lin) a constituent of the venom of certain snakes which causes coagulation of the blood.

he·mo·coe·lom (he″mo-se′lom) [*hemo-* + *coelom*] 1. the part of the coelom in which the heart is developed. 2. collectively, the spaces between the cells and tissues of many invertebrates, such as most mollusks, arthropods, and tunicates, through which a bloodlike fluid (hemolymph) circulates. Sometimes spelled *hemocele* or *hemocoel*.

he·mo·coe·lo·ma (he″mo-se-lo′mə) hemocoelom.

he·mo·con·cen·tra·tion (he″mo-kon″sən-tra′shən) decrease of the fluid content of the blood, with resulting increase in its concentration. Cf. *exemia*.

he·mo·co·nia (he″mo-ko′ne-ə) [*hemo-* + *coni-* + *-ia*] small, round, or dumbbell-shaped particles demonstrating brownian movement, observed in platelets in a wet film of blood under darkfield microscopy. Called also *blood dust*.

he·mo·co·ni·o·sis (he″mo-ko″ne-o′sis) the presence in the blood of abnormal amounts of hemoconia.

he·mo·cry·os·co·py (he″mo-kri-os′kə-pe) [*hemo-* + *cryoscopy*] cryoscopy of the blood; the ascertaining of the freezing point of the blood.

he•mo•cul•ture (he″mo-kul′chər) [*hemo-* + *culture*] blood culture.

he•mo•cu•pre•in (he″mo-ku′pre-in) superoxide dismutase.

he•mo•cy•a•nin (he″mo-si′ə-nin) a nonheme blue respiratory pigment that is found in the blood plasma of many mollusks and arthropods and is composed of monomers each of which contains two atoms of Cu^+ and can bind one molecule of O_2.

keyhole-limpet h. (KLH) a hemocyanin from the keyhole limpet; it is a commonly used antigen in laboratory immunology.

he•mo•cyte (he′mo-sīt) blood cell.

he•mo•cy•to•blast (he″mo-si′to-blast) blast cell (def. 2).

he•mo•cy•to•ma (he′mo-si-to′mə) acute undifferentiated leukemia.

he•mo•cy•tom•e•ter (he″mo-si-tom′ə-tər) hemacytometer.

he•mo•cy•tom•e•try (he″mo-si-tom′ə-tre) hemacytometry.

he•mo•cy•to•pe•nia (he″mo-si″to-pe′ne-ə) cytopenia.

he•mo•cy•to•pha•gia (he″mo-si″to-fa′jə) hemophagocytosis.

he•mo•cy•to•phag•ic (he″mo-si″to-faj′ik) hemophagocytic.

he•mo•cy•to•poi•e•sis (he″mo-si″to-poi-e′sis) hematopoiesis.

he•mo•cy•to•trip•sis (he″mo-si″to-trip′sis) [*hemocyte* + *tripsis*] disintegration of the blood corpuscles by pressure.

he•mo•di•a•fil•tra•tion (he″mo-di″ə-fil-tra′shən) hemofiltration with a dialytic component added; blood flow is accelerated to twice that of conventional dialysis. Called also *high flux hemodiafiltration.*

he•mo•di•ag•no•sis (he″mo-di″əg-no′sis) [*hemo-* + *diagnosis*] diagnosis by examination of the blood.

he•mo•di•al•y•sis (he″mo-di-al′ə-sis) the removal of certain elements from the blood by virtue of the difference in the rates of their diffusion through a semipermeable membrane (see *hemodialyzer*). Two distinct physical processes are involved, diffusion and ultrafiltration (qq.v.). See also *clearance.* Called also *dialysis, kidney dialysis,* and *renal dialysis.*

high efficiency h. hemodialysis using a membrane with a high diffusive clearance so that solutes with large molecules can be efficiently cleared; it filters slightly less rapidly than high flux hemodialysis.

high flux h. hemodialysis using a high flux membrane so that solutes composed of large molecules can be cleared rapidly; it filters slightly more rapidly than high efficiency hemodialysis.

he•mo•di•a•lyt•ic (he″mo-di-ə-lit′ik) 1. pertaining to hemodialysis. 2. undergoing hemodialysis.

he•mo•di•a•lyz•er (he″mo-di′ə-līz″ər) an apparatus by which hemodialysis may be performed; blood is brought in contact with a semipermeable membrane on whose other side is a dialysate solution of such composition as to secure diffusion of certain elements out of the blood.

he•mo•di•a•pe•de•sis (he″mo-di″ə-pə-de′sis) [*hemo-* + *diapedesis*] the extravasation of blood through the skin.

he•mo•di•lu•tion (he″mo-di-loo′shən) increase of the fluid content of the blood with resulting decrease in concentration of its erythrocytes. See also *hypervolemia.*

he•mo•dy•nam•ic (he″mo-di-nam′ik) pertaining to the movements involved in the circulation of the blood.

he•mo•dy•nam•ics (he″mo-di-nam′iks) the study of the movements of the blood and of the forces concerned therein.

he•mo•dy•na•mom•e•try (he″mo-di″nə-mom′ə-tre) measurement of blood pressure.

he•mo•dys•tro•phy (he″mo-dis′trə-fe) [*hemo-* + *dystrophy*] any blood disease due to faulty blood nutrition.

he•mo•en•do•the•li•al (he″mo-en-do-the′le-əl) [*hemo-* + *endothelium*] denoting a type of placenta in which maternal blood comes in contact with the endothelium of chorionic vessels, as in rabbits.

He•mo•fil (he′mo-fil) trademark for a preparation of antihemophilic factor (human).

he•mo•fil•ter (he′mo-fil″tər) a filter used in hemofiltration.

he•mo•fil•tra•tion (he″mo-fil-tra′shən) the removal of waste products from the blood by passing the blood through extracorporeal filters. Cf. *hemoperfusion.*

continuous arteriovenous h. an uncommon form of continuous renal replacement therapy, similar to continuous venovenous hemofiltration but with vascular access in an arteriovenous fistula, powered by the patient's own arterial pressure without need for a mechanical pump.

continuous venovenous h. a form of continuous renal replacement therapy consisting of hemofiltration with venovenous access, small-volume, low-resistance hemofilters, and a mechanical pump; used as an alternative to conventional hemodialysis ultrafiltration.

high-volume h. a type of continuous venovenous hemofiltration in which the average ultrafiltration rate is above 75 liters per day; it is used primarily with critically ill patients, such as those with septic shock, and requires large hemofilters and high flux membranes.

he•mo•flag•el•late (he″mo-flaj′ə-lāt) [*hemo-* + *flagellate*] any flagellate microorganism parasitic in the blood, especially protozoa of the suborder Trypanosomatina.

he•mo•fus•cin (he″mo-fūs′in) [*hemo-* + *fuscus*] a brownish-yellow pigment that results from the decomposition of hemoglobin; it is sometimes seen in the urine.

he•mo•gen•e•sis (he″mo-jen′ə-sis) hematopoiesis.

he•mo•gen•ic (he″mo-jen′ik) 1. hematopoietic. 2. hematogenous.

he•mo•glo•bin (Hb) (he′mo-glo″bin) the red oxygen-carrying pigment of erythrocytes, formed by developing erythrocytes in bone marrow. It is a type of hemoprotein that contains four heme groups and globin and has the property of reversible oxygenation. A molecule of hemoglobin contains four polypeptide globin chains, composed of between 141 and 146 amino acids; those most often found are α and β chains, with γ and δ chains seen somewhat less often. Different types of hemoglobins are determined by different combinations of chains, with the number of chains of each type in the molecule being indicated by a subscript. For example, *hemoglobin F (fetal h.),* the predominant type in the newborn, may be written $\alpha_2{}^A\gamma_2{}^F$, and *hemoglobin A (adult h.),* which is normally predominant in the adult, may be written $\alpha_2{}^A\beta_2{}^A$ or $\alpha_2\beta_2$. Another hemoglobin, *hemoglobin A_2* (designated $\alpha_2{}^A\delta_2{}^{A2}$ or $\alpha_2{}^A\delta_2$), is usually present in limited minor concentrations. Hundreds of hemoglobins with differing electrophoretic mobilities and characteristics have been reported; the first ones were given capital letters, such as S, C, D, E, G, H, I, J, K, L, M, N, and Q. As refined biochemical techniques led to the discovery of many additional hemoglobins, newer standards for nomenclature were devised: those with electrophoretic mobility equal to one of the lettered hemoglobins could be named with that letter using the place of discovery as a subscript, such as hemoglobin $M_{Saskatoon}$ or hemoglobin $M_{Milwaukee}$. New hemoglobins with unique electrophoretic mobilities are now often named simply for the laboratory, hospital, or town where they were discovered, such as hemoglobin Chesapeake or hemoglobin Gun Hill. When known, the number of each amino acid substituting in each polypeptide in the molecule should be indicated by the appropriate superscript numeral. Symbol *Hb.*

h. A normal adult hemoglobin, composed of two α and two β chains, $\alpha_2{}^A\beta_2{}^A$.

h. A_{1c} a type of glycated hemoglobin A, having a hexose attached to the N terminal of its β chain; its levels are increased in persons with poorly controlled diabetes mellitus.

h. A_2 $\alpha_2{}^A\delta_2$, a type of normal adult hemoglobin present in small amounts, in which δ chains replace the β chains.

h. anti-Lepore an abnormal crossover hemoglobin similar to hemoglobin Lepore but whose non-α chains have fusion in the opposite configuration from those of hemoglobin Lepore (β chain portions at the N terminus and δ chain portions at the C terminus); most individuals with this hemoglobin have predominantly normal hemoglobin and do not suffer from anemia or thalassemia.

h. Bart's an abnormal hemoglobin composed of four γ chains having high oxygen affinity, seen in Southeast Asians and a few other groups; infants born with only this type of hemoglobin have hydrops fetalis and usually die within a few hours. Hemoglobin Bart's is often found mixed with hemoglobin H, resulting in α-thalassemia.

h. C a common abnormal hemoglobin in which lysine replaces glutamic acid at position six of the β chains; it was one of the earliest hemoglobins to have its molecular abnormality defined. The homozygous state manifests as the anemic condition called *hemoglobin C disease,* and the asymptomatic heterozygous state is called *hemoglobin C trait.*

h. carbamate carbaminohemoglobin.

h. Chesapeake an abnormal hemoglobin in which leucine is substituted for arginine in the α chain, resulting in high oxygen affinity so that the individual has polycythemia.

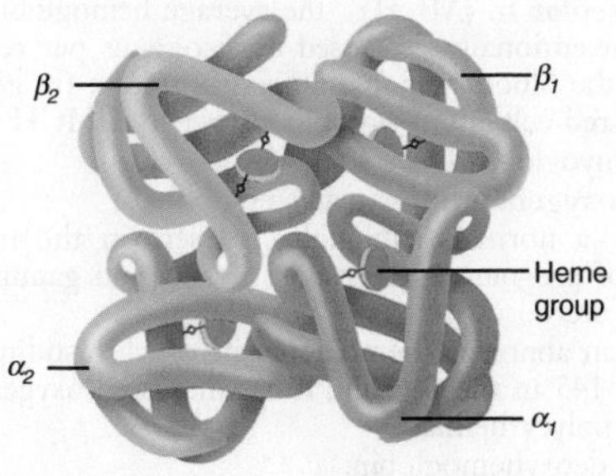

■ Hemoglobin, comprising four globin chains, each with a heme group.

h. Constant Spring an abnormal hemoglobin seen in Southeast Asians, characterized by 31 extra amino acid residues at the C terminus of the α chain, resulting in a form of α-thalassemia.

crossover h. an abnormal hemoglobin that has a globin chain formed from parts of two chains that have undergone crossover, such as hemoglobin Lepore, h. anti-Lepore, and h. Kenya.

h. D any of several abnormal hemoglobins, all characterized by electrophoretic mobility equal to that of hemoglobin S on paper or cellulose acetate but unequal on acid agar gel. The most common one is *h. D Los Angeles* (also known as *h. D Punjab*), which has glycine substituted for glutamic acid at position 121 of the β chain. In the homozygous state, hemoglobin D manifests as the anemic state called hemoglobin D disease; the heterozygous state is clinically silent.

deoxygenated h. deoxyhemoglobin.

h. E an abnormal hemoglobin with lysine substituted for glutamic acid at position 26 of the β chain, seen most often in Southeast Asia, especially Thailand. The homozygous state may be asymptomatic or may be manifested as the anemic state called hemoglobin E disease, while the heterozygous state is clinically silent.

h. F fetal h.

fast h's hemoglobins with greater mobility on electrophoresis (in an alkaline buffer) than normal hemoglobin A, such as hemoglobin K, J, or N.

fetal h. the hemoglobin normally comprising more than half of that in the fetus, composed of two alpha and two gamma polypeptides ($\alpha_2{}^{A}\gamma_2{}^{F}$); it has higher affinity for oxygen under physiologic conditions than does hemoglobin A. It is present in minimal amounts in adulthood and is abnormally elevated in aplastic anemia, leukemia, and certain types of thalassemia. Called also *h. F.*

h. G any of various abnormal hemoglobins with an amino acid substitution on the α chain; the most common one is *h. G Philadelphia*, which causes α-thalassemia.

glycated h., glycosylated h. any of various hemoglobins to which glucose is bound by glycation; the most common one is hemoglobin A_{1c}.

Gower h., h. Gower a normal hemoglobin present in early embryonic life and disappearing before birth; it occasionally consists entirely of epsilon chains (ε_4), but the usual forms are *h. Gower-1*, consisting of two zeta and two epsilon chains ($\zeta_2\varepsilon_2$) and *h. Gower-2*, consisting of two alpha and two epsilon chains ($\alpha_2\varepsilon_2$).

h. Gun Hill an unstable hemoglobin with a segmental deletion of amino acids in the β chain that causes inability to bind heme and mild hemolytic anemia.

h. H a rapidly migrating abnormal hemoglobin composed of four β chains, having a high oxygen affinity, found mainly in Southeast Asians, natives of the Mediterranean region, and a few other ethnic groups. Infants may be born with a mixture of hemoglobin H and hemoglobin Bart's. See *hemoglobin H disease*, under *disease*.

h. I an abnormal hemoglobin resulting from an amino acid substitution in the α chain, causing α-thalassemia.

h. Kansas an abnormal hemoglobin with threonine substituted for asparagine at position 102 of the β chain, resulting in decreased oxygen affinity and cyanosis.

h. Kenya an abnormal type of crossover hemoglobin in which the non-α chain has a γ chain portion at the N terminus and a β chain portion at the C terminus, resulting in β-thalassemia.

h. Köln an unstable hemoglobin that has methionine substituted for valine at position 95 of the β chain, usually resulting in Heinz body anemia.

h. Lepore any of several abnormal crossover hemoglobins having two normal α chains and two globin chains that have portions of a δ chain at the N terminus and portions of a β chain at the C terminus. Homozygous individuals have about 90 per cent hemoglobin F, 10 per cent hemoglobin Lepore, and no hemoglobin A or A_2, which results in thalassemia major; heterozygotes have varying amounts of hemoglobin Lepore and hemoglobin A and may have mild anemia.

h. M any of several abnormal hemoglobins having amino acid substitutions in the α or β chains and all associated with methemoglobinemia.

mean corpuscular h. (MCH) the average hemoglobin content of an erythrocyte, conventionally expressed in picograms per red cell, obtained by multiplying the blood hemoglobin concentration (in g/dL) by ten and dividing by the red cell count (in millions per μL): MCH = Hb/RBC.

muscle h. myoglobin.

oxidized h., oxygenated h. oxyhemoglobin.

h. Portland a normal hemoglobin present in the fetus late in the first trimester of pregnancy, consisting of zeta and gamma chains ($\zeta_2\gamma_2$); it disappears in utero.

h. Rainier an abnormal hemoglobin in which histidine replaces tyrosine at position 145 in the β chain; it has increased oxygen affinity and is associated with polycythemia.

reduced h. deoxyhemoglobin.

h. S the most common abnormal hemoglobin, having valine substituted for glutamic acid at position 6 of the β chain; the homozygous state results in sickle cell anemia, and the asymptomatic heterozygous state is called *sickle cell trait.*

h. Seattle an abnormal hemoglobin in which glutamic acid is substituted for alanine at position 76 of the β chain; it has decreased oxygen affinity.

slow h's hemoglobins that are less mobile on electrophoresis (in an alkaline buffer) than normal hemoglobin A, such as hemoglobin S or D.

unstable h's abnormal hemoglobins whose molecule is unstable, usually owing to substitution or deletion of at least one amino acid. Many have increased oxygen affinity and some have Heinz bodies; affected individuals often have Heinz body anemia or some other type of hemolytic anemia.

h. Yakima an abnormal hemoglobin in which histidine is substituted for aspartic acid at position 99 of the β chain; it has increased oxygen affinity and is associated with polycythemia.

he•mo•glo•bin•at•ed (he″mo-glo′bin-āt-əd) containing hemoglobin.

he•mo•glo•bin•emia (he″mo-glo″bin-e′me-ə) the presence of free hemoglobin in the blood plasma, an indication of significant intravascular hemolysis.

he•mo•glo•bino•cho•lia (he″mo-glo″bin-o-ko′le-ə) [*hemoglobin* + *chol-* + *-ia*] the occurrence of hemoglobin in the bile.

he•mo•glo•bin•ol•y•sis (he″mo-glo″bin-ol′ə-sis) [*hemoglobin* + *-lysis*] splitting up of hemoglobin.

he•mo•glo•bin•om•e•ter (he″mo-glo″bin-om′ə-tər) [*hemoglobin* + *-meter*] an instrument for measuring the hemoglobin of the blood.

he•mo•glo•bin•om•e•try (he″mo-glo″bin-om′ə-tre) the measurement of the hemoglobin of the blood.

he•mo•glo•bin•op•a•thy (he″mo-glo″bin-op′ə-the) [*hemoglobin* + *-pathy*] 1. any inherited disorder caused by abnormalities of hemoglobin, resulting in conditions such as sickle cell anemia, hemolytic anemia, or thalassemia. 2. sometimes more specifically, a hemoglobin disorder involving a variation or variations of a globin chain such as changes or substitutions in the amino acid sequences, or moving of a chain from its usual place in the molecule. (In this case hemoglobinopathies are distinguished from thalassemias, which involve reduced or absent synthesis of normal polypeptide chains.) When the site of an aberration is known, the abnormality of the peptide chain, the number of the altered amino acid, and the nature of the replacement are indicated. For example, hemoglobin S is expressed as $\alpha_2{}^{A}\beta_2{}^{S}$, or $\alpha_2{}^{A}\beta_2{}^{6\ \text{valine}}$, and hemoglobin $G_{\text{Philadelphia}}$ is expressed as $\alpha_2{}^{G}\beta_2{}^{A}$, or $\alpha_2{}^{6\ \text{lysine}}\beta_2{}^{A}$. If more than one hemoglobin is present, the phenotype is designated by listing them in order of decreasing concentrations; for example, the phenotype for sickle cell trait is expressed as AS, for sickle cell anemia as SS, and for sickle cell–hemoglobin C disease as SC.

he•mo•glo•bi•nous (he″mo-glo′bĭ-nəs) hemoglobinated.

he•mo•glo•bin•uria (he″mo-glo″bĭ-nu′re-ə) the presence of free hemoglobin in the urine. **hemoglobinu′ric** *adj*

bacillary h. an infectious, often fatal toxemic disease of cattle and sometimes sheep, caused by *Clostridium haemolyticum;* it is marked by anorexia, fever, bloody diarrhea, dark red urine, anemia, and hemoglobinuria. Called also *bovine h.* and *redwater disease.*

bovine h. 1. Texas fever. 2. bacillary h.

malarial h. blackwater fever.

march h. hemolysis caused by repeated uncushioned shocks to some body part, such as in soldiers on long marches, in marathon runners, or in karate practitioners.

paroxysmal cold h. an autoimmune or postviral disease marked by episodes of hemoglobinemia and hemoglobinuria after exposure to cold, caused by complement-dependent hemolysis due to IgG antibody (Donath-Landsteiner antibody) directed against the P blood group antigen; it is detected by the Donath-Landsteiner test.

paroxysmal nocturnal h. (PNH) a chronic acquired blood cell dysplasia with proliferation of a clone of stem cells producing erythrocytes, platelets, and granulocytes that are abnormally susceptible to lysis by complement; it is marked by episodes of intravascular hemolysis, causing hemolytic anemia, particularly following infections, and by venous thromboses, especially of the hepatic veins. Diagnosis is based on the acidified serum test (Ham test) or the sucrose lysis test. Called also *Marchiafava-Micheli syndrome.*

toxic h. hemoglobinuria caused by ingestion of a poison.

he•mo•gram (he′mo-gram) [*hemo-* + *-gram*] a written record or graphic representation of a detailed blood assessment such as the complete blood count or differential leukocyte count.

he•mo•ju•ve•lin (he-mo-joo′və-lin) a peptide hormone, expressed in the liver, heart, and skeletal muscle, that is a coreceptor for bone morphogenetic proteins and plays a role in the regulation of hepcidin release.

he•mo•ki•ne•sis (he″mo-kĭ-ne′sis) [*hemo-* + *-kinesis*] circulation. **hemokinet′ic** *adj*

he•mol•o•gy (he-mol′ə-je) hematology.

he•mo•lymph (he′mo-limf″) [*hemo-* + *lymph*] 1. the blood and lymph. 2. the bloodlike fluid moving through the hemocoelom of those invertebrates (e.g., mollusks, arthropods, and tunicates) with open circulatory systems, which combines the properties of blood and lymphlike interstitial fluid.

he•mo•lymph•an•gi•o•ma (he″mo-lim-fan″je-o′mə) hematolymphangioma.

he•mol•y•sate (he-mol′ə-sāt) the product of hemolysis.

he•mol•y•sin (he-mol′ə-sin) [*hemo-* + *lysin*] a substance that causes hemolysis; called also *erythrocytolysin* and *erythrolysin.*

alpha h. 1. a hemolysin producing alpha hemolysis. 2. the hemolysin of the alpha toxin of *Staphylococcus aureus,* which hemolyzes rabbit, sheep, cow, and goat but not human erythrocytes. See also *staphylococcal toxin,* under *toxin.*

bacterial h. a toxic hemolysin produced by bacteria.

beta h. 1. a hemolysin that produces beta hemolysis. 2. the hemolysin of the beta toxin of *Staphylococcus aureus;* it is a sphingomyelinase that lyses human and sheep erythrocytes in the cold following a warm incubation. See also *staphylococcal toxin,* under *toxin.*

heterophile h. a hemolysin that has affinity for erythrocytes of animal species in addition to the one for which it is specific.

hot-cold h. a hemolysin that lyses erythrocytes in the cold following preliminary warm incubation, such as the beta hemolysin of *Staphylococcus aureus.*

immune h. a hemolysin produced by deliberate immunization of an animal with blood or blood cells foreign to it, such as the rabbit anti-sheep red blood cell serum (hemolysin) that is used in complement fixation tests.

he•mol•y•sis (he-mol′ə-sis) [*hemo-* + *-lysis*] disruption of the integrity of the erythrocyte membrane causing release of hemoglobin; it may be caused by bacterial hemolysins, by antibodies that cause complement-dependent lysis, by placing erythrocytes in a hypotonic solution, or by defects in the cell membrane. Called also *erythrocytolysis, erythrolysis,* and *hematolysis.*

alpha h. the production of a zone of greenish discoloration surrounding a bacterial colony on blood-agar medium, caused by partial decomposition of the hemoglobin of the erythrocytes; it is characteristic of pneumococci and certain streptococci.

beta h. the production of a clear zone immediately surrounding a bacterial colony on blood-agar medium, which is characteristic of certain pathogenic bacteria.

colloid osmotic h. hemolysis due to swelling of the erythrocyte when defective membrane permeability allows excessive sodium to enter followed by excessive water.

contact h. the hastened hemolysis of erythrocytes in contact with a surface.

gamma h. a term used to indicate absence of hemolysis around a bacterial colony on blood agar, which indicates that the bacteria is nonhemolytic.

immune h. the lysis by complement of erythrocytes sensitized as a consequence of interaction with specific antibody to the erythrocytes.

passive h. the lysis of erythrocytes on which antigen has been adsorbed in the presence of complement and antiserum to that antigen.

venom h. hemolysis produced by snake venom.

he•mo•lyt•ic (he″mo-lit′ik) 1. pertaining to or characterized by hemolysis. 2. causing or producing hemolysis.

he•mo•lyz•a•ble (he″mo-li′zə-bəl) capable of undergoing hemolysis.

he•mo•ly•za•tion (he″mo-li-za′shən) the production of hemolysis.

he•mo•lyze (he′mo-līz) 1. to subject to hemolysis. 2. to undergo hemolysis.

he•mo•ma•nom•e•ter (he″mo-mə-nom′ə-tər) a manometer for determining blood pressure.

he•mo•me•di•as•ti•num (he″mo-me″di-əs-ti′nəm) an effusion of blood in the mediastinum.

he•mo•me•tra (he″mo-me′trə) hematometra.

he•mom•e•try (he-mom′ə-tre) hematometry.

he•mo•ne•phro•sis (he″mo-nə-fro′sis) presence of blood in the renal pelvis.

he•mo•pa•thol•o•gy (he″mo-pə-thol′ə-je) [*hemo-* + *pathology*] the study of diseases of the blood; called also *hematopathology.*

he•mop•a•thy (he-mop′ə-the) [*hemo-* + *-pathy*] any disease of the blood. **hemopath′ic** *adj*

he•mo•per•fu•sion (he″mo-pər-fu′zhən) the passing of large volumes of blood over an extracorporeal adsorbent substance in order to remove toxic substances. Cf. *hemofiltration.*

he•mo•peri•car•di•um (he″mo-per″ĭ-kahr′de-əm) [*hemo-* + *pericardium*] an effusion of blood within the pericardium.

he•mo•peri•to•ne•um (he″mo-per″ĭ-to-ne′əm) [*hemo-* + *peritoneum*] an effusion of blood in the peritoneal cavity.

he•mo•pex•in (he″mo-pek′sin) a plasma glycoprotein, mol. wt. 57,000, in the β_1-globulin band; it is produced by hepatocytes and its function is the binding of free heme in plasma; it has one binding site for hematin forming a tight complex that is taken up and degraded by hepatocytes.

he•mo•phage (he′mo-fāj) hemophagocyte.

he•mo•phago•cyte (he″mo-fa′go-sīt) [*hemo-* + *phagocyte*] a macrophage that destroys blood cells. Called also *hemophage* and *hematophage.*

he•mo•phag•o•cyt•ic (he″mo-fa″go-sit′ik) 1. pertaining to hemophagocytes. 2. pertaining to or characterized by hemophagocytosis; called also *hemocytophagic.*

he•mo•phago•cy•to•sis (he″mo-fa″go-si-to′sis) [*hemo-* + *phagocytosis*] the ingestion and destruction of blood cells by macrophages. Called also *hemocytophagia.*

he•mo•phane (he′mo-fān) a membranous substance made of regenerated cellulose, used in low-flux hemodialyzer membranes.

he•mo•phil (he′mo-fil) [*hemo-* + *-phil*] 1. an organism thriving on blood. 2. a microorganism which grows best in media containing hemoglobin.

he•mo•phil•ia (he″mo-fil′e-ə) [*hemo-* + *-philia*] a hemorrhagic diathesis occurring in two main forms, designated *hemophilia A* and *hemophilia B.* Both are determined by a mutant gene near the telomere of the long arm of the X chromosome, but at different loci, and are characterized by subcutaneous and intramuscular hemorrhages; bleeding from the mouth, gums, lips, and tongue; hematuria; and hemarthroses.

h. A the most common type of hemophilia, an X-linked recessive condition caused by mutation in the coagulation factor VIII gene (*F8,* locus: Xq28) that results in deficiency of the factor. Called also *classical h.*

h. B an X-linked recessive condition, clinically indistinguishable from hemophilia A, caused by mutation in the coagulation factor IX gene (*F9,* locus: Xq27.1-q27.2) that results in deficiency of the factor. Called also *Christmas disease.*

h. B Leyden a transient condition in which there is a deficiency of coagulation factor IX, the bleeding tendency abating after puberty, caused by point mutations in the promoter region of the *F9* gene.

h. C factor XI deficiency.

classical h. h. A.

vascular h. von Willebrand disease.

he•mo•phil•i•ac (he″mo-fil′e-ak) an individual exhibiting hemophilia.

he•mo•phil•ic (he-mo-fil′ik) 1. having an affinity for blood; living in blood. In bacteriology, growing especially well in culture media containing blood or having a nutritional affinity for constituents of fresh blood; said of bacteria of the genera *Haemophilus* and *Bordetella.* 2. pertaining to or characterized by hemophilia.

he•mo•phil•i•oid (he″mo-fil′e-oid) [*hemophilia* + *-oid*] resembling hemophilia but not due solely to a deficiency of factor VIII, such as any of the hemorrhagic disorders due to deficiencies of other coagulation factors.

he•moph•i•lus (he-mof′ĭ-ləs) any bacterium of the genus *Haemophilus.*

he•mo•pho•bia (he″mo-fo′be-ə) [*hemo-* + *-phobia*] irrational fear of blood.

he•moph•thal•mia (he″mof-thal′me-ə) hemophthalmos.

he•moph•thal•mos (he″mof-thal′mos) [*hemo-* + Gr. *ophthalmos* eye] an extravasation of blood within the eye.

he•moph•thal•mus (he″mof-thal′məs) hemophthalmos.

he•mo•pi•ezom•e•ter (he″mo-pi″ə-zom′ə-tər) [*hemo-* + Gr. *piesis* pressure + *meter*] any apparatus for measuring blood pressure.

he•mo•plas•tic (he″mo-plas′tik) hematopoietic.

he•mo•pleu•ra (he″mo-ploor′ə) hemothorax.

he•mo•pneu•mo•peri•car•di•um (he″mo-noo″mo-per″ĭ-kahr′de-əm) pneumohemopericardium.

he•mo•pneu•mo•tho•rax (he″mo-noo″mo-thor′aks) pneumothorax with hemorrhagic effusion; called also *pneumohemothorax.*

he•mo•poi•e•sis (he″mo-poi-e′sis) hematopoiesis.

he•mo•poi•et•ic (he″mo-poi-et′ik) hematopoietic.

he•mo•poi•e•tin (he″mo-poi-e′tin) erythropoietin.

he•mo•po•sia (he″mo-po′zhə) hematophagia.

he•mo•pre•cip•i•tin (he″mo-pre-sip′ĭ-tin) a precipitin that precipitates leukoantigens.

he•mo•proc•tia (he″mo-prok′shə) [*hemo-* + *proct-* + *-ia*] hemorrhage from the rectum.

he•mo•pro•tein (he′mo-pro″tēn) a conjugated protein containing heme as the prosthetic group; examples include catalase, cytochrome, hemoglobin, and myoglobin.

he•mop•so•nin (he″mop-so′nin) [*hemo-* + *opsonin*] an opsonin that renders red blood cells more liable to phagocytosis.

he•mop•to•ic (he-mop-to′ik) hemoptysic.

he•mop•ty•sis (he-mop′tĭ-sis) [*hemo-* + Gr. *ptyein* to spit] the expectoration of blood or of blood-stained sputum. **hemopty′sic** *adj*

cardiac h. hemoptysis due to heart disease and related pulmonary hypertension, as in mitral stenosis or Eisenmenger syndrome.

endemic h. parasitic h.

Goldstein h. hemoptysis due to bleeding telangiectases in the tracheobronchial tree.

Manson h. parasitic h.

parasitic h. a type of paragonimiasis, usually infestation with *Paragonimus westermani;* symptoms include coughing, spitting of blood, and gradual deterioration of health. Called also *endemic h.*

vicarious h. hemoptysis occurring at the time of normal menstruation; see *vicarious menstruation.*

he•mo•rhe•ol•o•gy (he″mo-re-ol′ə-je) [*hemo-* + *rheology*] the scientific study of the deformation and flow properties of cellular and plasmatic components of blood in macroscopic, microscopic, and submicroscopic dimensions, and the rheological properties of vessel structure with which the blood comes in direct contact. Also spelled *hemorrheology.*

he•mor•rha•chis (he-mor′ə-kis) hematomyelia.

hem•or•rhage (hem′ə-rəj) [*hemo-* + *-rrhage*] the escape of blood from the vessels; bleeding. Small hemorrhages are classified according to size as petechiae (very small), purpura (up to 1 cm), and ecchymoses (larger). A large accumulation of blood within a tissue is called a hematoma. See also *bleeding.* **hemorrhag′ic** *adj*

alveolar h. hemorrhage from a dental alveolus.

arterial h. the escape of blood from an artery, e.g., ruptured aneurysm.

brain h. cerebral h.

capillary h. the oozing of blood from a capillary.

capsuloganglionic h. hemorrhage into the basal ganglia and internal and external capsule of the brain.

cerebral h. hemorrhage into the cerebrum, an often fatal type of stroke syndrome. Called also *intracerebral, intraparenchymal,* or *parenchymatous h.*

choroidal h. expulsive h.

concealed h. internal h.

Duret h's small, linear hemorrhages in the midline of the brainstem and upper pons caused by traumatic downward displacement of the brainstem.

expulsive h., expulsive choroidal h. hemorrhage of the eye, breaking through both the choroid and the retina and extruding the contents of the eye; it usually occurs during the course of an intraocular surgical procedure.

external h. hemorrhage in which blood escapes from the body.

extradural h. intracranial hemorrhage into the epidural space; it is often caused by external trauma to the skull.

fetomaternal h. the leakage of fetal red blood cells into the maternal circulation.

fibrinolytic h. hemorrhage due to abnormalities of fibrinolysis rather than hypofibrinogenemia.

flame-shaped h's large hemorrhagic spots in the eyeground; called also *flame spots.*

internal h. hemorrhage in which the extravasated blood remains within the body.

intracerebral h. cerebral h.

intracranial h. bleeding within the cranium, which may be extradural, subdural, subarachnoid, or cerebral (parenchymatous); all types can cause brain damage because of increased intracranial pressure. See also *stroke syndrome,* under *syndrome.*

intramedullary h. hematomyelia.

intraparenchymal h. cerebral h.

intrapartum h. hemorrhage occurring during parturition.

intraventricular h. cerebral hemorrhage into the ventricles.

massive h. loss of blood so rapid and profuse that shock supervenes unless appropriate replacement is instituted promptly.

nasal h. epistaxis.

parenchymatous h. 1. hemorrhage into the parenchyma of an organ. 2. cerebral h.

perinephric h., perirenal h. hemorrhage from the kidney into the perirenal space. Cf. *retroperitoneal h.*

h. per rhexin hemorrhage from rupture of a blood vessel.

petechial h. the tiny capillary hemorrhage that causes a petechia; called also *punctate h.*

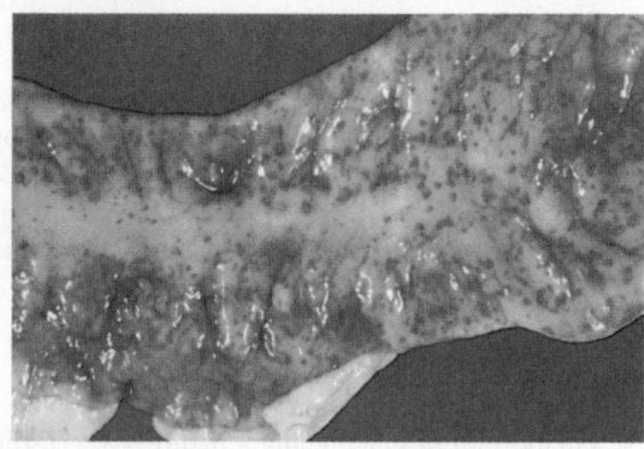

■ Petechial hemorrhage of the colonic mucosa in thrombocytopenia.

postpartum h. hemorrhage which occurs soon after labor or childbirth.

preretinal h. hemorrhage from retinal vessels into the space between the retina and the vitreous body. Called also *subhyaloid h.*

pulmonary h. hemorrhage from the lungs; called also *pneumorrhagia.*

punctate h. petechial h.

renal h. hemorrhage from the kidney; it may be either internal or into the perirenal space. Called also *nephrorrhagia.*

retroperitoneal h. hemorrhage from the kidney into the retroperitoneal space. Cf. *perirenal h.*

splinter h. a linear hemorrhage beneath a nail; most are benign, but when located near the base of the nail it may signify subacute bacterial endocarditis.

spontaneous h. bleeding occurring without overt provocation.

subarachnoid h. intracranial hemorrhage into the subarachnoid space; the most common cause is rupture of an aneurysm.

subdural h. cerebral hemorrhage into the subdural space; see also *subdural hematoma,* under *hematoma,* and *stroke syndrome,* under *syndrome.*

subhyaloid h. preretinal h.

venous h. the escape of blood from a vein.

vitreous h. bleeding into the vitreous body, resulting from any of numerous causes including diabetic retinopathy, spread of hemorrhage from a subarachnoid or choroid hemorrhage, and Terson syndrome.

hem•or•rha•gen•ic (hem″o-rə-jen′ik) [*hemorrhage* + *-genic*] causing hemorrhage.

hem•or•rha•gin (hem″ə-ra′jin) a cytolysin existing in certain venoms and poisons, such as snake venom and ricin, which is destructive to endothelial cells and blood vessels. Cf. *endotheliotoxin.*

he•mor•rhe•ol•o•gy (he″mo-re-ol′ə-je) hemorheology.

hem•or•rhoid (hem′ə-roid) [Gr. *haimorrhois*] prolapse of an anal cushion, resulting in bleeding and painful swelling in the anal canal.

combined h. mixed h.

external h. a hemorrhoid distal to the pectinate line, covered with modified anal skin.

internal h. a hemorrhoid originating above the pectinate line, covered by mucous membrane.

mixed h., mucocutaneous h. prolapse of an anal cushion on both sides of the pectinate line, forming an external and an internal hemorrhoid in continuity.

prolapsed h. an internal hemorrhoid that has descended below the pectinate line and protruded outside the anal sphincter.

strangulated h. a prolapsed hemorrhoid whose blood supply has become occluded by the constricting action of the anal sphincter.

thrombosed h. a hemorrhoid containing clotted blood.

hem•or•rhoi•dal (hem″ə-roi′dəl) 1. pertaining to, or of the nature of, hemorrhoids. 2. a term formerly used for blood vessels now described as *rectal.*

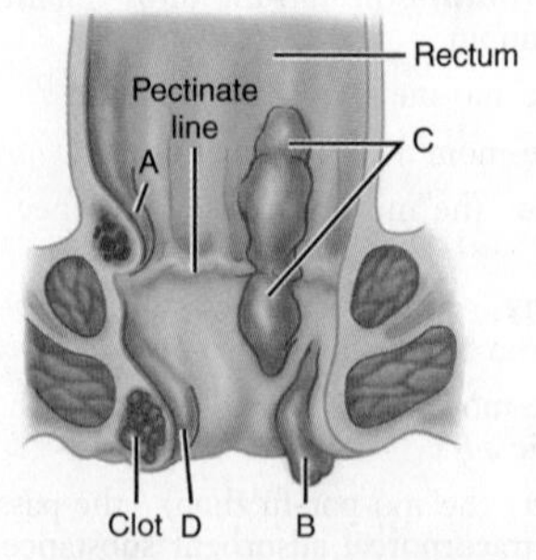

■ Hemorrhoids: *(A),* internal; *(B),* external; *(C),* mixed; *(D),* thrombosed.

hem•or•rhoid•ec•to•my (hem″ə-roid-ek′tə-me) excision of hemorrhoids.

hem•or•rhoid•o•pexy (hem″ə-roi′do-pek″se) surgical fixation of hemorrhoids.

stapled h. a method of treating hemorrhoids by excising a band of prolapsed tissue with a special circular stapling device into which excess tissue is pulled while the remaining tissue is stapled, so that the hemorrhoidal tissue is restored to its original anatomical position. Called also *circumferential mucosectomy.*

he•mo•sal•pinx (he″mo-sal′pinks) [*hemo-* + *salpinx*] hematosalpinx.

he•mo•sid•er•in (he″mo-sid′ər-in) [*hemo-* + Gr. *sidēros* iron] an intracellular storage form of iron, found in the form of pigmented yellow to brown granules consisting of a complex of ferric hydroxides, polysaccharides, and proteins with an iron content of about 33 per cent by weight.

he•mo•sid•er•in•uria (he″mo-sid″ər-ĭ-nu′re-ə) the presence of hemosiderin in the urine, such as in hemochromatosis. Called also *urinary siderosis.*

he•mo•sid•er•o•sis (he″mo-sid″ər-o′sis) a focal or general increase in tissue iron stores without associated tissue damage; called also *siderosis.* Cf. *hemochromatosis.*

hepatic h. the deposit of an abnormal quantity of hemosiderin in the liver, usually in Kupffer cells, when this is not associated with cirrhosis, as hemochromatosis is. Called also *hepatic siderosis.*

pulmonary h. the deposition of abnormal amounts of hemosiderin in the lungs, due to bleeding into the lung. The hemosiderin is found mainly in macrophages in the air spaces, but also in the interstitium. It is seen in any condition, such as severe congestive heart failure, in which repeated hemorrhages into the lungs occur.

he•mo•sper•mia (he″mo-spur′me-ə) hematospermia.

he•mo•spo•ri•an (he″mo-spor′e-ən) 1. any protozoan of the suborder Haemosporina. 2. pertaining to protozoa of the suborder Haemosporina. Called also *hemosporidian.*

he•mo•spo•rid•i•an (he″mo-spor-id′e-ən) hemosporian.

he•mo•sta•sia (he″mo-sta′zhə) hemostasis.

he•mo•sta•sis (he″mo-sta′sis, he-mos′tə-sis) [*hemo-* + *stasis*] 1. arrest of bleeding, either by the physiological properties of vasoconstriction and coagulation or by surgical means. 2. interruption of blood flow through a vessel or to a part.

he•mo•stat (he′mo-stat) 1. a small surgical clamp for constricting a blood vessel. 2. an agent that checks hemorrhage when properly applied to a bleeding point.

he•mo•stat•ic (he″mo-stat′ik) [*hemo-* + *-static*] 1. causing hemostasis. 2. an agent that arrests the flow of blood. 3. due to or characterized by stasis of the blood; called also *hematostatic.*

capillary h. an agent that reduces capillary bleeding time by increasing the contractility and resistance and decreasing the permeability of the capillary wall.

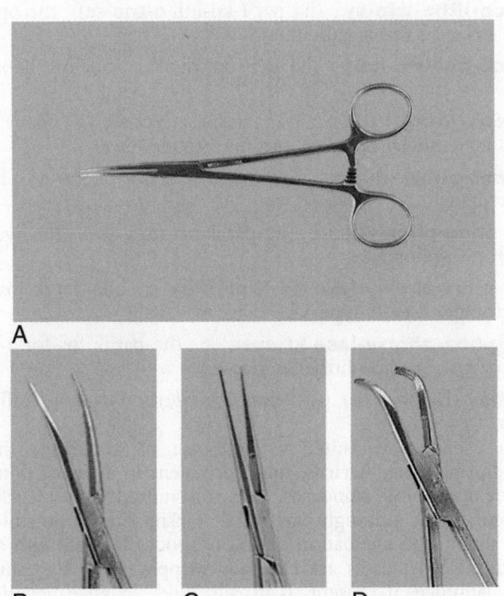

■ Hemostats. *(A),* Crile hemostat; *(B),* tip of Crile hemostat; *(C),* tip of Halsted hemostat; *(D),* tip of Westphal hemostat.

he•mo•styp•tic (he″mo-stip′tik) hemostatic.

he•mo•suc•cus pan•cre•at•i•cus (he″mo-suk′əs pan-kre-at′ĭ-kəs) [L., from *hemo-* + *succus* sap, juice; L. "pancreatic"] bleeding through the pancreatic duct into the intestine, usually after a pancreatic pseudocyst has eroded into an artery.

he•mo•ther•a•peu•tics (he″mo-ther″ə-pu′tiks) hemotherapy.

he•mo•ther•a•py (he″mo-ther′ə-pe) [*hemo-* + *therapy*] treatment of disease by the administration of blood or blood products, such as blood plasma. Called also *hematherapy* and *hematotherapy.*

he•mo•tho•rax (he″mo-thor′aks) [*hemo-* + *thorax*] a pleural effusion containing blood. Cf. *hemorrhagic pleurisy.* Called also *hemathorax, hematothorax,* and *hemopleura.*

he•mo•tox•ic (he′mo-tok″sik) hematotoxic.

he•mo•tox•in (he′mo-tok″sin) an exotoxin that causes hemolysis; see also *hemolysin.*

cobra h. the constituent of cobra venom that can lyse red blood cells without the presence of blood serum.

he•mo•troph (he′mo-trōf) [*hemo-* + Gr. *trophē* nourishment] the totality of the nutritive substances supplied to the embryo from the maternal blood during gestation. Cf. *embryotroph* and *histotroph.*

he•mo•tro•phic (he″mo-tro′fik) pertaining to or derived through hemotroph.

he•mo•tro•pic (he″mo-tro′pik) hematotropic.

he•mo•tym•pa•num (he″mo-tim′pə-nəm) a hemorrhagic exudation into the middle ear; called also *hematotympanum.*

he•mo•zo•ic (he″mo-zo′ik) hematozoan (def. 1).

he•mo•zo•in (he″mo-zo′in) [*hemo-* + Gr. *zōon* animal] a pigment produced from the hemoglobin in the host's erythrocytes by malarial parasites and enabling the parasites to sequester in benign form. In chronic cases of malaria, hemozoin collects in tissues, e.g., the spleen, giving the organ a grayish to dark brown or black color. Also written *haemozoin.* Called also *malarial pigment.*

he•mo•zo•on (he″mo-zo′on) hematozoan (def. 2).

hem•pa (hem′pə) a colorless liquid with an ammonia-like odor, used as a de-icing additive in jet fuel, as a solvent, and as a chemosterilant for insect pests; it is carcinogenic. Called also *hexamethylphosphoramide* and abbreviated *HMPA.*

HEM•PAS (hem′pəs) [*h*ereditary *e*rythroblastic *m*ultinuclearity with *p*ositive *a*cidified *s*erum] the most common type of congenital dyserythropoietic anemia.

hen•bane (hen′bān) 1. *Hyoscyamus niger.* 2. hyoscyamus.

Hench-Ro•sen•berg syndrome (hench′ ro′zən-bərg) [P.S. *Hench;* Edward Frank *Rosenberg,* American physician, 1908–1982] palindromic rheumatism; see under *rheumatism.*

Hen•der•son-Has•sel•balch equation (hen′dər-sən has′əl-bahlk) [Lawrence Joseph *Henderson,* American chemist, 1878–1942; Karl A. *Hasselbalch,* Danish biochemist, 1874–1962] see under *equation.*

Hen•der•son-Jones disease (hen′dər-sən jōnz′) [Melvin Starkey *Henderson,* American orthopedic surgeon, 1883–1954; Hugh T. *Jones,* American orthopedic surgeon, 20th century] see under *disease.*

Hen•der•son-Pat•er•son bodies (hen′dər-sən pat′ər-sən) [William *Henderson,* Scottish pathologist, 1810–1872; Robert *Paterson,* Scottish physician, 1814–1889] molluscum bodies.

Hen•der•son•u•la (hen″dər-son′u-lə) a genus of Fungi Imperfecti of the form-class Coelomycetes. *H. toruloi′dea* has been isolated from numerous cases of dermatomycosis and phaeohyphomycosis; it is a synanamorph of *Scytalidium hyalinum.*

Hen•i•pa•vi•rus (hen′ĭ-pə-vi″rəs) a genus of viruses of the family Paramyxoviridae, subfamily Paramyxovirinae. Species causing human disease include Hendra virus and Nipah virus.

Hen•ke space, triangle (trigone) (heng′kə) [Philipp Jakob Wilhelm *Henke,* German anatomist, 1834–1896] see under *space* and *triangle.*

Hen•le ampulla, loop, etc. (hen′le) [Friedrich Gustav Jakob *Henle,* German anatomist, 1809–1885] see under *fiber, gland, layer, membrane,* and *reaction,* and see *ampulla ductus deferentis, ansa nephroni, falx inguinalis,* and *spina suprameatica.*

Henne•bert sign (en″ə-bār′) [Camille *Hennebert,* Belgian otologist, 1867–1958] see under *sign.*

Hen•nings sign (hen′ingz) [Wilhelm *Hennings,* German physician, 1716–1794] see under *sign.*

Hen•och purpura (hen′ok) [Edouard Heinrich *Henoch,* German pediatrist, 1820–1910] see under *purpura.*

Hen·och-Schön·lein purpura (syndrome) (hen′ok shərn′līn) [E.H. *Henoch;* Johann Lukas *Schönlein,* German physician, 1793–1864] see under *purpura.*

heno·gen·e·sis (hen″o-jen′ə-sis) ontogeny.

Hen·ry's law (hen′rēz) [William *Henry,* English chemist, 1774–1836] see under *law.*

hen·ry (H) (hen′re) [Joseph *Henry,* American physicist, 1797–1878] the SI unit of electric inductance, equivalent to 1 weber per ampere.

Hen·sen body, etc. (hen′sən) [Victor *Hensen,* German anatomist and physiologist, 1835–1924] see under *body* and *cell;* see *H band* and *M band,* under *band;* see *primitive node,* under *node;* and see *ductus reuniens.*

HEP hepatoerythropoietic porphyria.

Hep·aci·vi·rus (hep-as′ĭ-vi″rəs) [*hepatitis C* + *virus*] the hepatitis C–like viruses: a genus of viruses of the family Flaviviridae consisting of hepatitis C virus and related viruses.

Hep·ad·na·vi·ri·dae (hep-ad″nə-vir′ĭ-de) [*hepat-* + *DNA* + *virus*] the hepatitis B–like viruses: a family of DNA viruses having a virion 42 nm in diameter consisting of a lipid-containing envelope (containing hepatitis B surface antigen, HBsAg) surrounding an icosahedral nucleocapsid (containing hepatitis B core antigen, HBcAg). The genome consists of a single circular molecule of DNA that contains a large single-stranded gap (size of fully double-stranded molecule 3.2 kbp). Viruses contain two major polypeptides comprising HBsAg, one comprising HBcAg, and a number of others comprising the e antigen (HBeAg); they are resistant to heat and organic solvents. Replication occurs in the nuclei of hepatocytes. HBsAg occurs in the cytoplasm and shedding of 22-nm HBsAg particles into the bloodstream produces antigenemia. Persistent infection is common and is associated with chronic disease and neoplasia. There are two genera, one *(Orthohepadnavirus)* containing species infecting mammals and the other *(Avihepadnavirus)* containing species infecting birds.

Hep·ad·na·vi·rus (hep-ad′nə-vi″rəs) a former genus of the Hepadnaviridae; see *Avihepadnavirus* and *Orthohepadnavirus.*

hep·ad·na·vi·rus (hep-ad′nə-vi″rəs) any virus belonging to the family Hepadnaviridae. **hepadnavi′ral** *adj*

he·par (he′pahr) [Gr. *hēpar* liver] 1. [TA] the liver (q.v.), a large gland in the upper abdomen. 2. the liver of certain animals, used in pharmaceutical preparations.

h. adipo′sum fatty liver.

h. loba′tum a liver divided into numerous lobes by deep fissures produced by syphilis.

hep·a·ran-α-glu·co·sam·i·nide *N*-ac·e·tyl·trans·fer·ase (hep′ə-ran gloo″ko-sam′ĭ-nīd as″ə-tēl-trans′fər-ās) [EC 2.3.1.78] a lysosomal enzyme of the transferase class that catalyzes the acetylation of the amino groups of terminal desulfated glucosamine residues in heparan sulfate chains, a step in the degradation of heparan sulfate. Acetyl coenzyme A is the acetyl donor. Deficiency of the enzyme, an autosomal recessive trait, results in Sanfilippo syndrome, type C. Called also *acetyl CoA:α-glucosaminide* N-*acetyltransferase.*

hep·a·ran *N*-sul·fa·tase (hep′ə-ran sul′fə-tās) a lysosomal enzyme of the hydrolase class that catalyzes the removal of sulfate from terminal *N*-sulfated glucosamine residues of heparan sulfate chains. Deficiency of the enzyme, an autosomal recessive trait, causes Sanfilippo syndrome, type A. See also N-*sulfoglucosamine sulfohydrolase.*

hep·a·ran sul·fate (hep′ə-ran) a glycosaminoglycan occurring in the cell membrane of most cells. It consists of repeating disaccharide units in specific linkage, each composed of a glucosamine residue linked to a uronic acid, either glucuronic acid or L-iduronic acid, which may be sulfated. The glucosamine residues frequently contain acetyl or sulfate group substituents. It is an accumulation product in several mucopolysaccharidoses.

hep·a·ran sul·fate sul·fam·i·dase (hep′ə-ran sul′fāt səl-fam′ĭ-dās) heparan *N*-sulfatase.

hep·a·rin (hep′ə-rin) [Gr. *hēpar* liver] a sulfated glycosaminoglycan of mixed polysaccharide nature varying in molecular weights and composed of polymers of alternating derivatives of D-glycosamine and L-iduronic acid or D-glucuronic acid; it is released by mast cells and by basophils of the blood and is present in many tissues, especially the liver and lungs. Heparin is a mixture of active principles, some of which have potent anticoagulant properties that result from binding to and greatly enhancing the activity of antithrombin III and from inhibition of a number of coagulation factors, particularly activated factor X (factor Xa). Heparin also has lipotrophic properties, promoting transfer of fat from the blood to the fat depots by activation of lipoprotein lipase.

h. calcium [USP] the calcium salt of the mixture of active principles that compose heparin, usually obtained from the intestinal mucosa or other suitable tissues of domestic food animals; used in the prophylaxis and treatment of disorders in which there is undesirable or excessive clotting, such as deep venous thrombosis, thromboembolism, and disseminated intravascular coagulation and to prevent clotting during extracorporeal circulation, blood transfusion, and blood sampling. Administered intravenously or subcutaneously.

h. sodium [USP] the sodium salt of the mixture of active principles that compose heparin, usually obtained from the intestinal mucosa or other suitable tissues of domestic food animals, and having the same indications, uses, and routes of administration as the calcium salt.

hep·a·rin·ate (hep′ə-rin-āt) any salt of heparin.

hep·a·rin·emia (hep″ə-rĭ-ne′me-ə) the presence of heparin in the blood.

hep·a·ri·nize (hep′ə-rĭ-nīz″) to treat with heparin in order to increase the clotting time of the blood.

hep·a·rin·oid (hep′ə-rin-oid) a substance with anticoagulant activity similar to that of heparin.

hep·a·ri·tin sul·fate (hep′ə-rĭ-tin) heparan sulfate.

hep·a·tal·gia (hep″ə-tal′jə) [*hepat-* + *-algia*] pain in the liver; called also *hepatodynia.*

hep·a·ta·tro·phia (hep″ə-tə-tro′fe-ə) [*hepat-* + *atrophia*] atrophy of the liver.

hep·a·tat·ro·phy (hep″ə-tat′rə-fe) hepatatrophia.

hep·a·tec·to·mize (hep″ə-tek′tə-mīz) to surgically remove all or part of the liver.

hep·a·tec·to·my (hep″ə-tek′tə-me) [*hepat-* + *-ectomy*] excision of all *(total h.)* or part *(partial* or *subtotal h.)* of the liver.

he·pat·ic (hə-pat′ik) [L. *hepaticus;* Gr. *hēpatikos*] pertaining to the liver.

hepatic(o)- [Gr. *hēpatikos* of the liver] a combining form denoting relationship to a hepatic duct, or, sometimes, to the liver.

he·pat·ic li·pase (hə-pat′ik li′pās) see under *lipase.*

he·pat·i·co·cho·led·o·chos·to·my (hə-pat′ĭ-ko-ko-led″o-kos′tə-me) surgical anastomosis of the common hepatic duct and common bile duct.

he·pat·i·co·do·chot·o·my (hə-pat″ĭ-ko-do-kot′ə-me) surgical incision of the hepatic duct and the common bile duct.

he·pat·i·co·du·o·de·nos·to·my (hə-pat″ĭ-ko-doo″o-də-nos′tə-me) a type of hepaticoenterostomy in which the hepatic duct empties into the duodenum.

he·pat·i·co·en·ter·os·to·my (hə-pat″ĭ-ko-en″tər-os′tə-me) [*hepatico-* + *enterostomy*] surgical creation of a communication between the hepatic duct and part of the intestine.

he·pat·i·co·gas·tros·to·my (hə-pat″ĭ-ko-gas-tros′tə-me) [*hepatico-* + *gastrostomy*] surgical creation of a communication between the hepatic duct and the stomach.

he·pat·i·co·je·ju·nos·to·my (hə-pat″ĭ-ko-jə-joo-nos′tə-me) [*hepatico-* + *jejunostomy*] a type of hepaticoenterostomy in which the hepatic duct empties into the jejunum.

he·pat·i·co·li·thot·o·my (hə-pat″ĭ-ko-lĭ-thot′ə-me) incision of the hepatic duct and removal of one or more calculi.

he·pat·i·co·litho·trip·sy (hə-pat″ĭ-ko-lith′o-trip-se) the operation of crushing a stone in the hepatic duct.

he·pat·i·co·pul·mo·nary (hə-pat″ĭ-ko-pool′mo-nar″e) hepatopulmonary.

he·pat·i·cos·to·my (hə-pat″ĭ-kos′tə-me) [*hepatico-* + *-stomy*] surgical creation of an artificial opening into the hepatic duct.

he·pat·i·cot·o·my (hə-pat″ĭ-kot′ə-me) [*hepatico-* + *-tomy*] incision of the hepatic duct.

he·pat·ic phos·phor·y·lase (hə-pat′ik fos-for′ə-lās) the liver isozyme of glycogen phosphorylase.

he·pat·ic phos·phor·y·lase de·fi·cien·cy (hə-pat′ik fos-for′ə-lās) glycogen storage disease, type VI.

he·pat·ic phos·phor·y·lase ki·nase (hə-pat′ik fos-for′ə-lās ki′nās) the liver isozyme of phosphorylase kinase.

hep·a·ti·tis (hep″ə-ti′tis) pl. *hepati′tides* [*hepat-* + *-itis*] inflammation of the liver.

h. A a usually self-limited viral disease of worldwide distribution caused by the hepatitis A virus, more prevalent in areas of poor hygiene and low socioeconomic standards. It is transmitted almost exclusively by the fecal-oral route, although parenteral transmission is possible; there is no carrier state. The incubation period is about 30 days, with a range of 15 to 50 days. Most cases are clinically inapparent or have mild flulike symptoms; jaundice, if present, is usually mild. Massive hepatic necrosis (fulminant hepatitis) does occur, but much less commonly than with hepatitis B or C. Formerly called *epidemic* or *infectious h.*

acute parenchymatous h. former name for massive hepatic necrosis.

alcoholic h. liver inflammation resulting from alcoholism, often a precursor of cirrhosis.

amebic h. hepatic amebiasis.

anicteric h. viral hepatitis without jaundice.

autoimmune h. 1. an autoimmune disease of the liver, occurring more often in females, characterized by circulating autoantibodies and hypergammaglobulinemia; it is associated with extrahepatic complaints such as malaise, fever, and arthralgia. *Type 1* is characterized by antinuclear and anti–smooth muscle antibodies; *type 2* is less common and is characterized by antibodies against the microsomal antigen of liver and kidney. 2. chronic active h.

avian infectious h., avian vibrionic h. avian campylobacteriosis.

h. B a viral disease caused by the hepatitis B virus; it is endemic worldwide, with the areas of highest endemicity being China, Southeast Asia, sub-Saharan Africa, most Pacific islands, and the Amazon basin. The virus is shed in all body fluids by individuals with acute or chronic infections and by asymptomatic carriers, and is transmitted primarily by parenteral routes, such as by blood transfusion or by sharing of needles among drug users. Oral transmission can occur but has low efficiency; the disease can also be spread by intimate contact (such as sexual contact), as well as by vertical transmission from mother to neonate. The incubation period is about 90 days (range, 40 to 180 days), and the clinical course is more variable than that of hepatitis A. In the prodromal phase there may be fever, malaise, anorexia, nausea, and vomiting (which decline with the onset of clinical jaundice), as well as urticaria, angioedema, arthritis, and occasionally glomerulonephritis or a serum sickness–like syndrome. Most patients recover completely and become HB_SAg-negative in 3 to 4 months, but some remain chronic carriers or develop chronic active hepatitis or chronic persistent hepatitis. Massive hepatic necrosis (fulminant hepatitis) is a rare complication. In areas of high endemicity a relationship has been shown between hepatitis and virus infection, cirrhosis, and hepatocellular carcinoma. Formerly called *inoculation* or *serum h.* See also under *antigen.*

h. C a viral disease caused by the hepatitis C virus, the most common form of posttransfusion hepatitis; it can also follow parenteral drug abuse or other intimate personal contact with an infected person. This is a common acute sporadic form of hepatitis, and approximately 50 per cent of acutely infected persons develop chronic hepatitis. Although the chronic infection is usually mild and asymptomatic, cirrhosis may occur. See also *chronic active h.* and *non-A, non-B h.*

canine virus h. infectious canine h.

cholangiolitic h., cholangitic h. cholestatic h. (def. 1).

cholestatic h. 1. a rare form of viral hepatitis in which there is cholestasis with obstructive jaundice, pruritus, dark urine, light-colored feces, and elevated levels of alkaline phosphatase and conjugated bilirubin; the course is prolonged compared to that of other forms of hepatitis. Called also *cholangitic h.* and *cholangiolitic h.* 2. hepatic inflammation and cholestasis resulting from reaction to drugs; numerous ones have been implicated. It often resembles primary biliary cirrhosis, with the difference that it eventually resolves.

chronic active h., chronic aggressive h. chronic inflammation of the liver occurring as a sequel to hepatitis B or certain other types of hepatitis, in congenital or acquired hypogammaglobulinemia, or following administration of certain drugs; in some cases an autoimmune mechanism is suspected. It is characterized by infiltration of portal areas by plasma cells and macrophages, piecemeal necrosis from destruction of liver cells, and fibrosis. It runs a variable course; there may be long asymptomatic periods with periods of symptomatic hepatitis and jaundice; there may be a variety of extrahepatic manifestations; or the disease may progress to cirrhosis and liver failure. Called also *autoimmune, lupoid, plasma cell,* or *subacute h.* and *acute juvenile cirrhosis.*

chronic persistent h., chronic persisting h. a chronic, nonprogressive inflammatory process affecting primarily the portal areas without producing fibrosis, necrosis, or cirrhosis, an uncommon sequel of one of the forms of viral hepatitis. It may be asymptomatic or may produce symptoms of mild hepatitis; it does not progress to cirrhosis or liver failure but may persist for years.

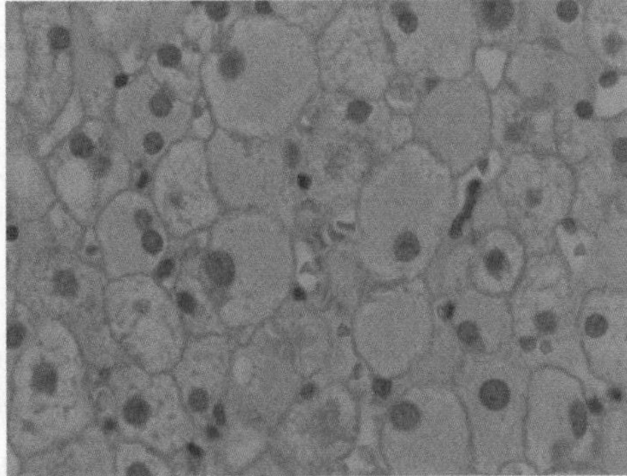

■ Chronic active hepatitis caused by hepatitis B virus, with characteristic ground-glass cells.

h. contagio′sa ca′nis infectious canine h.

h. D, delta h. infection with the hepatitis D virus, requiring antecedent or simultaneous infection with hepatitis B virus; manifestations are similar to those of hepatitis B, whose severity it may increase.

duck virus h. a highly fatal, rapidly spreading disease of waterfowl ducklings, caused by a virus of the genus *Avihepadnavirus,* characterized primarily by hepatitis marked by an enlarged, mottled, hemorrhagic liver.

h. E a type of viral hepatitis caused by exposure to hepatitis E virus, transmitted by the fecal-oral route, usually via contaminated water. It is endemic in many tropical regions and in India and China. The incubation period is 15 to 60 days, and there is a prodromal phase. Chronic infection does not occur, but acute hepatitis may be fatal in pregnant women. Called also *enterically transmitted non-A, non-B h.* and *ET-NANB h.*

enterically transmitted non-A, non-B h. h. E.

epidemic h. former name for hepatitis A.

ET-NANB h. h. E.

familial h. Wilson disease.

fatty liver h. nonalcoholic steatohepatitis.

fibrosing cholestatic h. a rapidly progressive form of hepatitis B or C with fibrosis and cholestasis, seen in rare cases following immunosuppression to prevent transplant rejection.

fulminant h. massive hepatic necrosis (q.v.) resulting from viral hepatitis, usually hepatitis B, C, or E.

h. G a posttransfusion disease caused by the hepatitis G virus, ranging in severity from asymptomatic infection to fulminant hepatitis.

giant cell h. neonatal h.

granulomatous h. a rare, nonviral type of hepatitis characterized by granulomas in the liver; it can have any of numerous different causes, including systemic infections, sarcoidosis, autoimmune conditions, and reactions to certain drugs.

halothane h. a rare complication of halothane anesthesia, consisting of transient jaundice or massive hepatic necrosis.

homologous serum h. h. B.

hypoxic h. hepatic ischemia.

inclusion body h. a viral disease of young chickens, caused by an adenovirus and characterized by hemorrhage, jaundice, and anemia; hepatocytes have eosinophilic inclusion bodies. Mortality in a flock may reach 25 per cent.

infectious h. former name for hepatitis A.

infectious canine h. a highly contagious type of hepatitis in canines, caused by an adenovirus; symptoms may be mild to severe and range from fever, vomiting, and abdominal pain to convulsions, hemorrhage, and death. Called also *canine virus h., h. contagiosa canis,* and *Rubarth disease.*

infectious necrotic h. a usually fatal infectious disease of sheep, and occasionally cattle, pigs, and horses, caused by multiplication of *Clostridium novyi* in areas of hepatic necrosis from liver flukes, with resultant septicemia. Called also *black disease.*

inoculation h. 1. any type of viral hepatitis spread by inoculations or injections, most commonly hepatitis B or hepatitis C. 2. former name for hepatitis B.

interface h. destruction of liver cells at the interface between liver parenchyma and portal triads, usually associated with lymphocytic infiltration; it is characteristic of severe chronic active hepatitis and primary biliary cirrhosis. Called also *piecemeal necrosis.*

ischemic h. hepatic ischemia.

Labrea h. a fulminant type of viral hepatitis seen in the western Amazon basin in Brazil, thought to be related to hepatitis B or D.

lupoid h. chronic active h.

neonatal h., neonatal giant cell h. hepatitis of unknown etiology with onset in the first few weeks of life; some cases are associated with viral or bacterial infection; a few are familial. It is characterized by the transformation of hepatocytes into multinucleated giant cells and by conjugated hyperbilirubinemia with jaundice. Most children recover completely, but some develop chronic disease or fatal cirrhosis. Cf. *neonatal hemochromatosis.* Called also *giant cell h.*

non-A–E h. viral hepatitis occurring without the serotypic markers of hepatitis viruses A, B, C, D, or E.

non-A, non-B h. former name for types of acute viral hepatitis that lacked the serologic markers of hepatitis A or B, now identified as hepatitis C and hepatitis E.

plasma cell h. chronic active h.

posttransfusion h. viral hepatitis transmitted via transfusion of blood or blood products, especially multiple pooled donor products such as clotting factor concentrates. The first cases were all hepatitis B, but now most are hepatitis C. Called also *transfusion h.*

pseudoalcoholic h. nonalcoholic steatohepatitis.

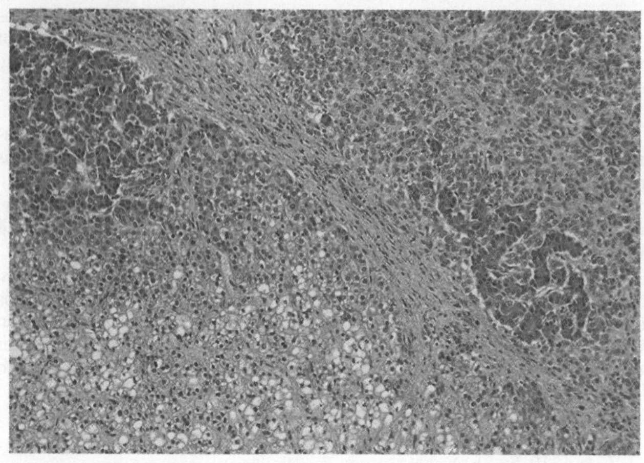

■ Hepatoblastoma, composed of cuboidal cells that resemble fetal hepatocytes embedded in a mesenchymal matrix.

relapsing h. hepatitis A that returns weeks to months after apparent resolution of the first attack.
serum h. h. B.
subacute h. chronic active h.
syncytial giant cell h. h. G.
toxic h. see under *hepatopathy*.
transfusion h. posttransfusion h.
vibrionic h. avian campylobacteriosis.
viral h. hepatitis caused by a viral infection; see *h. A*, *h. B*, *h. C*, *h. D*, and *h. E*.

hep·a·ti·za·tion (hep″ə-tĭ-za′shən) consolidation of tissue into a liver-like mass, especially as seen in the lung in pneumococcal pneumonia.
gray h. a usually late stage of hepatization in which the affected lung tissue is grayish.
red h. a usually early stage of hepatization in which the solidified lung tissue is red from excess of blood.
yellow h. hepatization in which lung tissue is yellowish from a purulent exudate.

hep·a·tized (hep′ə-tīzd) changed into a liverlike substance.

hepat(o)- [Gr. *hēpar*, gen. *hēpatos* liver] a combining form denoting relationship to the liver.

hep·a·to·bil·i·ary (hep″ə-to-bil′e-ar″e) pertaining to the liver and the bile or the bile ducts.

hep·a·to·blas·to·ma (hep″ə-to-blas-to′mə) a malignant intrahepatic tumor occurring in infants and young children and consisting chiefly of embryonic hepatic tissue.

hep·a·to·bron·chi·al (hep″ə-to-brong′ke-əl) pertaining to or communicating between the liver and a bronchus.

hep·a·to·car·ci·no·gen·e·sis (hep″ə-to-kahr″sĭ-no-jen′ə-sis) the production of carcinoma of the liver.

hep·a·to·car·cin·o·gen·ic (hep″ə-to-kahr″sĭ-no-jen′ik) causing carcinoma of the liver.

hep·a·to·car·ci·no·ma (hep″ə-to-kahr″sĭ-no′mə) hepatocellular carcinoma.

hep·a·to·cele (hə-pat′o-sēl) [*hepato-* + *-cele*[1]] hernial protrusion of a part of the liver.

hep·a·to·cel·lu·lar (hep″ə-to-sel′u-lər) pertaining to or affecting hepatic cells.

hep·a·to·cho·lan·ge·itis (hep″ə-to-ko-lan″je-i′tis) hepatocholangitis.

hep·a·to·cho·lan·gio·car·ci·no·ma (hep″ə-to-ko-lan″je-o-kahr″sĭ-no′mə) cholangiohepatoma.

hep·a·to·cho·lan·gi·os·to·my (hep″ə-to-ko-lan″je-os′tə-me) the operation of establishing drainage of the hepatic duct either through the abdominal wall *(external h.)* or into some part of the gastrointestinal tract *(internal h.)*.

hep·a·to·cho·lan·gi·tis (hep″ə-to-ko″lan-ji′tis) inflammation of the liver and bile ducts.

hep·a·to·cir·rho·sis (hep″ə-to-sĭ-ro′sis) [*hepato-* + *cirrhosis*] former name for cirrhosis.

hep·a·to·col·ic (hep″ə-to-kol′ik) pertaining to the liver and the colon.

hep·a·to·cu·prein (hep″ə-to-koo′prēn) a soluble, bluish-green copper protein present in liver tissue; it contains about 0.34 per cent copper.

hep·a·to·cys·tic (hep″ə-to-sis′tik) pertaining to the liver and gallbladder.

Hep·a·to·cys·tis (hep″ə-to-sis′tis) [*hepato-* + *cyst*] a genus of coccidian protozoa (suborder Haemosporina, subclass Sporozoea) comprising parasites of Old World lower monkeys, fruit bats, and squirrels, in which merogony takes place in the hepatocytes, resulting in large glistening schizonts (merocysts) on the surface of the liver, from which merozoites are released to invade erythrocytes and develop into gametocytes.

hep·a·to·cyte (hep′ə-to-sīt) a hepatic cell. **hepatocyt′ic** *adj*
ground-glass h. see under *cell*.

hep·a·to·di·a·phrag·mat·ic (hep″ə-to-di″ə-frag-mat′ik) pertaining to or connecting the liver and diaphragm; called also *hepatophrenic*.

hep·a·to·du·o·de·nal (hep″ə-to-doo″o-de′nəl) pertaining to or connecting the liver and the duodenum.

hep·a·to·du·o·de·nos·to·my (hep″ə-to-doo″o-də-nos′tə-me) [*hepato-* + *duodenostomy*] the surgical creation of a communication between the liver and the duodenum.

hep·a·to·dyn·ia (hep″ə-to-din′e-ə) [*hepat-* + *-odynia*] hepatalgia.

hep·a·to·en·ter·ic (hep″ə-to-ən-ter′ik) enterohepatic.

hep·a·to·en·ter·os·to·my (hep″ə-to-en″tər-os′tə-me) surgical creation of a communication between the liver and the intestine.

hep·a·tof·u·gal (hep″ə-tof′u-gəl) [*hepato-* + *-fugal*[2]] directed or flowing away from the liver.

hep·a·to·gas·tric (hep″ə-to-gas′trik) gastrohepatic.

hep·a·to·gen·ic (hep″ə-to-jen′ik) 1. giving rise to or forming liver tissue. 2. produced in or originating in the liver; called also *hepatogenous*.

hep·a·tog·e·nous (hep″ə-toj′ə-nəs) hepatogenic.

hep·a·to·gram (hep′ə-to-gram) a radiograph of the liver.

hep·a·tog·ra·phy (hep″ə-tog′rə-fe) [*hepato-* + *-graphy*] the making of a radiograph of the liver.

hep·a·toid (hep′ə-toid) [*hepat-* + *-oid*] resembling the liver in structure.

hep·a·to·jug·u·lar (hep″ə-to-jug′u-lər) pertaining to the liver and jugular vein; see under *reflux*.

hep·a·to·len·tic·u·lar (hep″ə-to-lən-tik′u-lər) pertaining to the liver and the lenticular nucleus.

hep·a·to·li·e·nal (hep″ə-to-li-e′nəl) pertaining to the liver and spleen.

hep·a·to·li·e·nog·ra·phy (hep″ə-to-li″ə-nog′rə-fe) hepatosplenography.

hep·a·to·li·e·no·meg·a·ly (hep″ə-to-li″ə-no-meg′ə-le) hepatosplenomegaly.

He·pat·o·lite (hə-pat′o-līt″) trademark for a kit for the preparation of technetium Tc 99m disofenin.

hep·a·to·lith (hep′ə-to-lith″) [*hepato-* + *-lith*] a gallstone within the liver, usually in the intrahepatic bile ducts. Called also *hepatic calculus*.

hep·a·to·li·thec·to·my (hep″ə-to-lĭ-thek′tə-me) [*hepato-* + *lithectomy*] removal of a calculus from the liver.

hep·a·to·li·thi·a·sis (hep″ə-to-lĭ-thi′ə-sis) [*hepato-* + *lithiasis*] the formation or presence of calculi in the liver.

hep·a·tol·o·gist (hep″ə-tol′ə-jist) a specialist in hepatology.

hep·a·tol·o·gy (hep″ə-tol′ə-je) [*hepato-* + *-logy*] the study of the liver and the nature and treatment of its diseases.

hep·a·tol·y·sin (hep″ə-tol′ĭ-sin) a cytolysin destructive to liver cells.

hep·a·tol·y·sis (hep″ə-tol′ĭ-sis) [*hepato-* + *-lysis*] destruction of liver cells.

hep·a·to·lyt·ic (hep″ə-to-lit′ik) 1. pertaining to or characterized by hepatolysis. 2. causing hepatolysis.

hep·a·to·ma (hep″ə-to′mə) 1. a tumor of the liver. 2. hepatocellular carcinoma.
fibrolamellar h. see under *carcinoma*.
malignant h. hepatocellular carcinoma.

hep·a·to·ma·la·cia (hep″ə-to-mə-la′shə) [*hepato-* + *-malacia*] softening of the liver.

hep·a·to·me·ga·lia (hep″ə-to-mə-ga′le-ə) hepatomegaly.

hep·a·to·meg·a·ly (hep″ə-to-meg′ə-le) [*hepato-* + *-megaly*] enlargement of the liver.

hep·a·to·mel·a·no·sis (hep″ə-to-mel″ə-no′sis) melanosis of the liver.

hep·a·tom·e·try (hep″ə-tom′ə-tre) determination of the size of the liver.

hep·a·tom·pha·lo·cele (hep″ə-tom′fə-lo-sēl) hepatomphalos.

hep·a·tom·pha·los (hep″ə-tom′fə-los) [*hepat-* + Gr. *omphalos* navel] an omphalocele with part of the liver in the sac. Called also *hepatomphalocele*.

hep·a·to·neph·ric (hep″ə-to-nef′rik) pertaining to the liver and kidney.

hep·a·to·ne·phri·tis (hep″ə-to-nə-fri′tis) [*hepato-* + *nephritis*] a form of severe jaundice due to simultaneous inflammation of the liver and kidneys from the same cause, e.g., leptospiral infection. **hepatonephrit′ic** *adj*

hep·a·to·neph·ro·meg·a·ly (hep″ə-to-nef″ro-meg′ə-le) [*hepato-* + *nephro-* + *-megaly*] enlargement of the liver and kidney.

hep·a·to·pan·cre·as (hep″ə-to-pang′kre-əs) any of certain digestive glands of invertebrates, as the so-called liver of certain crustaceans, which secretes a fluid acting on both fats and proteins.

hep·a·to·pan·cre·at·ic (hep″ə-to-pan″kre-at′ik) pertaining to or connecting the liver and pancreas.

hep·a·top·a·thy (hep″ə-top′ə-the) [*hepato-* + *-pathy*] any disease of the liver, such as cirrhosis or hepatitis.

alcoholic h. liver disease resulting from alcoholism, progressing in time to fibrosis and cirrhosis.

cardiac h. see under *cirrhosis.*

congestive h. see under *cirrhosis.*

sickle cell h. the liver damage that accompanies sickle cell disease, owing especially to vascular occlusion and ischemia, sequestration, and cholestasis.

toxic h. liver disease produced by a hepatotoxin such as *Amanita phalloides* toxin, carbon tetrachloride, or any of various drugs. It can range in severity from subclinical abnormalities to jaundice to fulminant liver failure.

hep·a·to·peri·to·ni·tis (hep″ə-to-per″ĭ-to-ni′tis) [*hepato-* + *peritonitis*] inflammation of the peritoneum covering the liver.

hep·a·top·e·tal (hep″ə-top′ə-təl) [*hepato-* + *-petal*] directed or flowing toward the liver.

hep·a·to·pexy (hep″ə-to-pek′se) [*hepato-* + *-pexy*] surgical fixation of the displaced liver.

hep·a·to·phle·bi·tis (hep″ə-to-flə-bi′tis) inflammation of the veins of the liver.

hep·a·to·phle·bog·ra·phy (hep″ə-to-flə-bog′rə-fe) radiologic visualization of the outflow of the venous network of the liver performed through retrograde injection of a radiopaque solution.

hep·a·to·phren·ic (hep″ə-to-fren′ik) hepatodiaphragmatic.

hep·a·to·pleu·ral (hep″ə-to-ploor′əl) pertaining to or communicating between the liver and the pleura.

hep·a·to·pneu·mon·ic (hep″ə-to-noo-mon′ik) hepatopulmonary.

hep·a·to·poi·e·tin A (HPTA) (hep″ə-to-poi′ə-tin) hepatocyte growth factor.

hep·a·to·por·tal (hep″ə-to-por′təl) 1. pertaining to the hepatic portal circulation. 2. connecting a hepatic artery with a portal vein, such as a fistula.

hep·a·to·por·to·en·ter·os·to·my (hep″ə-to-por″to-en″tər-os′tə-me) portoenterostomy.

hep·a·top·to·sis (hep″ə-top-to′sis, hep″ə-to-to′sis) [*hepato-* + *-ptosis*] 1. downward displacement of the liver, such as from laxness of suspensory ligaments, diminished tone of abdominal muscles, emphysema, right pleural effusion or empyema, subphrenic abscess, or spinal deformity. 2. Chilaiditi sign.

hep·a·to·pul·mo·nary (hep″ə-to-pool′mo-nar-e) pertaining to, affecting, or communicating with the liver and lungs; called also *hepatopneumonic.*

hep·a·to·re·nal (hep″ə-to-re′nəl) pertaining to the liver and kidneys.

hep·a·tor·rha·gia (hep″ə-to-ra′jə) [*hepato-* + *-rrhagia*] hemorrhage from the liver.

hep·a·tor·rha·phy (hep″ə-tor′ə-fe) [*hepato-* + *-rrhaphy*] operative repair of the liver.

hep·a·tor·rhex·is (hep″ə-to-rek′sis) [*hepato-* + *-rrhexis*] rupture of the liver.

hep·a·to·scan (hep′ə-to-skan) a surface scintiscan of the liver.

hep·a·tos·co·py (hep″ə-tos′kə-pe) [*hepato-* + *-scopy*] examination of the liver.

hep·a·to·sis (hep″ə-to′sis) hepatopathy.

h. diete′tica a form of vitamin E–selenium deficiency syndrome (q.v.) in pigs, characterized by necrosis of the liver, edema, and often sudden death. Called also *dietary hepatic necrosis.*

serous h. veno-occlusive disease of the liver; see under *disease.*

toxic h. see under *hepatopathy.*

hep·a·to·sple·ni·tis (hep″ə-to-splə-ni′tis) inflammation of the liver and spleen.

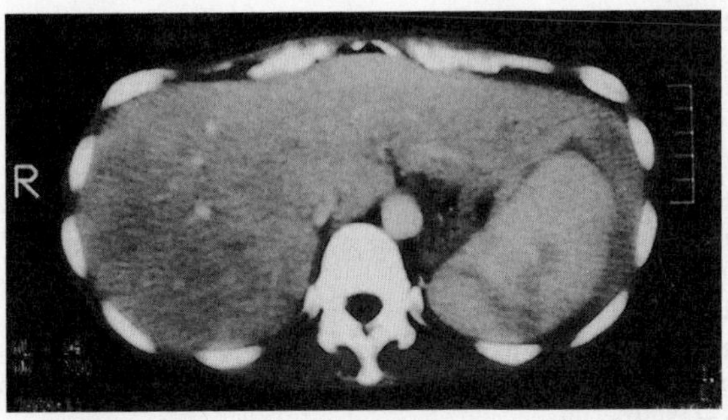

■ Massive hepatosplenomegaly demonstrated by CT scan in a patient with severe malarial anemia due to *Plasmodium falciparum* infection.

hep·a·to·sple·nog·ra·phy (hep″ə-to-splə-nog′rə-fe) radiography of the liver and spleen.

hep·a·to·sple·no·me·ga·lia (hep″ə-to-sple″no-mə-ga′le-ə) hepatosplenomegaly.

hep·a·to·sple·no·meg·a·ly (hep″ə-to-sple″no-meg′ə-le) [*hepato-* + *spleno-* + *-megaly*] enlargement of the liver and spleen; called also *splenohepatomegaly.*

hep·a·to·sple·nop·a·thy (hep″ə-to-splə-nop′ə-the) any combined disorder of the liver and spleen.

hep·a·tos·to·my (hep″ə-tos′tə-me) [*hepato-* + *-stomy*] surgical creation of an opening into the liver.

hep·a·to·ther·a·py (hep″ə-to-ther′ə-pe) [*hepato-* + *therapy*] treatment of disease by the administration of liver or liver extract.

hep·a·tot·o·my (hep″ə-tot′ə-me) [*hepato-* + *-tomy*] surgical incision of the liver.

hep·a·to·tox·ic (hep′ə-to-tok″sik) toxic to liver cells.

hep·a·to·tox·ic·i·ty (hep″ə-to-tok-sis′ĭ-te) the quality or property of exerting a destructive or poisonous effect upon liver cells.

hep·a·to·tox·in (hep′ə-to-tok″sin) [*hepato-* + *toxin*] a toxin that destroys liver cells.

hep·a·tot·ro·pism (hep″ə-tot′ro-piz-əm) [*hepato-* + *-tropism*] special affinity for or attraction to the liver; said of chemical compounds or pathogenic agents such as the hepatitis viruses. **hepatotrop′ic** *adj*

Hep·a·to·vi·rus (hep′ə-to-vi″rəs) [*hepato-* + *virus*] a genus of viruses of the family Picornaviridae that contains just one species, hepatitis A virus. **hepatovi′ral** *adj*

hep·a·tox·ic (hep′ə-tok″sik) hepatotoxic.

Hep·a·to·zo·on (hep″ə-to-zo′on) [*hepato-* + Gr. *zōon* animal] a genus of coccidian protozoa (suborder Adeleina, order Eucoccidiida) found in the red blood cells of birds and mammals such as dogs, foxes, and rats. *H. ca′nis* is transmitted to canines by the tick *Rhipicephalus sanguineus* (see *hepatozoonosis*). *H. muris,* found in the liver cells of rats, and *H. perniciosum,* found in dogs, are transmitted by the mite *Echinolaelaps echidninus.*

hep·a·to·zoo·no·sis (hep″ə-to-zo″o-no′sis) an infectious, sometimes fatal disease of dogs caused by *Hepatozoon canis,* and characterized by intermittent fever, emaciation, mild anemia, muscular hyperesthesia, especially affecting the back, purulent ocular and nasal discharge, and sometimes diarrhea.

hep·ci·din (hep′si-din) [*hep*atocyte bacteri*cid*al prote*in*] a peptide hormone, expressed in the liver, that regulates iron homeostasis by inhibiting iron uptake in the duodenum and inhibiting release of iron from macrophages by interfering with the activity of ferroportin. Overexpression results in iron deficiency anemia and deficiency results in hemochromatosis.

Hep·e·vi·rus (hep-e′vi-rəs) a genus of viruses that includes hepatitis E virus; it has not yet been assigned to a family.

Hep·sera (hep-sēr′ə) trademark for a preparation of adefovir dipivoxil.

hept(a)- [Gr. *hepta* seven] a combining form meaning seven.

hep·ta·chro·mic (hep″tə-kro′mik) [*hepta-* + *chrom-* + *-ic*] 1. pertaining to or exhibiting seven colors. 2. able to distinguish all seven colors of the spectrum; possessing full color vision.

hep·tad (hep′təd) any element having a valency of seven.

hep·ta·dac·tyl·ia (hep″tə-dak-til′e-ə) heptadactyly.

hep·ta·dac·ty·lism (hep″tə-dak′tə-liz-əm) heptadactyly.

hep·ta·dac·ty·ly (hep″tə-dak′tə-le) [*hepta-* + Gr. *daktylos* finger] the occurrence of seven digits on one hand or foot.

hep·ta·ene (hep′tə-ēn) a chemical compound in which there are seven conjugated double bonds.

-hep·ta·ene suffix denoting a chemical compound in which there are seven conjugated double bonds.

hep·ta·no·ate (hep″tə-no′āt) enanthate.

hep·ta·no·ic ac·id (hep″tə-no′ik) systematic name for *enanthic acid.*

hep·ta·pep·tide (hep″tə-pep′tīd) a polypeptide containing seven amino acids.

hep·ta·tom·ic (hep″tə-tom′ik) septivalent.

hep·ta·va·lent (hep′tə-va″lənt) [*hepta-* + L. *valere* to be able] 1. effective against seven different entities, as diseases or strains of a pathogen. 2. septivalent.

hep·to·glo·bin (hep″to-glo′bin) a protein that is one of the fractions of blood plasma and may be increased in infections, malignancy, and certain endocrine disorders.

hep·tose (hep′tōs) [*hept-* + *-ose*] a monosaccharide containing seven carbon atoms in a molecule.

hep·tos·uria (hep″to-su′re-ə) presence of a heptose in the urine.

herb (urb, hurb) [L. *herba*] any leafy plant without a woody stem, especially one used medicinally or as a flavoring.
 death's h. belladonna (def. 1).

her·ba·ceous (ər-, hər-ba′shəs) having the characters of an herb.

her·bal (ur′-, hur′bəl) 1. pertaining to herbs. 2. a book on herbs.

her·bal·ism (ur′-, hur′bəl-iz-əm) the medical use of preparations containing only plant material.

her·bal·ist (ur′-, hur′bəl-ist) a person versed in the use of herbs, especially medicinal herbs.

Her·bert pits (hur′bərt) [Major Herbert *Herbert,* English ophthalmic surgeon in India, 1865–1942] see under *pit.*

her·bi·cide (ur′-, hur′bĭ-sīd) [*herb* + *-cide*] an agent that is destructive to weeds or causes an alteration in their normal growth.

her·bi·vore (ur′-, hur′bĭ-vor) a herbivorous animal.

her·biv·o·rous (ər-, hər-biv′ə-rəs) [L. *herba* herb + *vorare* to eat] subsisting upon plants.

Herb. recent. herba′rium recen′tium (of fresh herbs).

Herbst corpuscles (hərbst) [Ernst Friedrich Gustav *Herbst,* German physician, 1803–1893] see under *corpuscle.*

Her·cep·tin (hər-sep′tin) trademark for a preparation of trastuzumab.

he·red·i·tary (hə-red′ĭ-tar-e) [L. *hereditarius*] genetically transmitted from parent to offspring.

he·red·i·ty (hə-red′ĭ-te) [L. *hereditas*] 1. the genetic transmission of a particular quality or trait from parent to offspring. 2. the genetic constitution of an individual.
 autosomal h. the transmission of a quality or trait by a gene located on an autosome.
 X-linked h. transmission of a quality or trait by a gene located on the X chromosome.
 Y-linked h. transmission of a quality or trait by a gene located on the Y chromosome.

hered(o)- [L. *heres,* gen. *heredis* heir] a combining form denoting relationship to heredity.

her·e·do·atax·ia (her″ə-do-ə-tak′se-ə) any hereditary type of ataxia, such as Friedreich ataxia.

her·e·do·di·ath·e·sis (her″ə-do-di-ath′ə-sis) [L. *heres* heir + *diathesis*] hereditary diathesis or predisposition.

her·e·do·fa·mil·i·al (her″ə-do-fə-mil′e-əl) pertaining to an inherited trait or condition occurring in multiple members of a family. The term has generally been replaced by *familial, hereditary,* or *genetic,* whichever is more appropriate.

her·e·do·in·fec·tion (her″ə-do-in-fek′shən) germinal infection.

her·e·do·path·ia (her″ə-do-path′e-ə) a hereditary disease.
 h. atac′tica polyneuritifor′mis Refsum disease.

He·relle see *d'Herelle.*

Her·ing law, test, theory (her′ing) [Karl Ewald Constantin *Hering,* German physiologist, 1834–1918] see under *law, test,* and *theory.*

Her·ing nerve (her′ing) [Heinrich Ewald *Hering,* German physiologist, 1866–1948] see *ramus sinus carotici nervi glossopharyngei.*

Her·ing-Breu·er reflex (her′ing broi′ər) [H.E. *Hering;* Josef Robert *Breuer,* Austrian physician, 1842–1925] see under *reflex.*

her·i·ta·bil·i·ty (her″ĭ-tə-bil′ĭ-te) 1. the quality of being heritable. 2. a measure of the extent to which a phenotype is influenced by the genotype.

her·i·ta·ble (her′ĭ-tə-bəl) capable of being inherited, as a genetic trait.

Her·litz disease (her′lits) [Carl Gillis *Herlitz,* Swedish pediatrician, 20th century] see *junctional epidermolysis bullosa,* under *epidermolysis.*

Her·man·sky-Pud·lak syndrome (hər-mahn′ske pood′lahk) [Frantisek *Hermansky,* Czech physician, 1916–1980; P. *Pudlak,* Czech physician, 20th century] see under *syndrome.*

her·maph·ro·dism (hər-maf′ro-diz-əm) hermaphroditism.

her·maph·ro·dite (hər-maf′ro-dīt) [Gr. *hermaphroditos*] an individual having hermaphroditism.
 pseudo-h. see *pseudohermaphrodite.*
 true h. an individual with true hermaphroditism, having both testicular and ovarian tissue. Called also *true intersex.*

her·maph·ro·di·tism (hər-maf′rə-dĭ-tiz″əm) [Gr. *hermaphroditos* hermaphrodite] the presence of both male and female gonadal tissue in the same individual. *True hermaphroditism* (q.v.) is distinguished from *male pseudohermaphroditism* and *female pseudohermaphroditism.* Called also *gynandrism, hermaphrodism,* and *intersexuality.* **hermaphrodit′ic** *adj*
 bilateral h. hermaphroditism in which gonadal tissue typical of both sexes occurs on each side of the body.
 false h. pseudohermaphroditism.
 lateral h. presence of gonadal tissue typical of one sex on one side of the body and tissue typical of the other sex on the opposite side.
 spurious h. pseudohermaphroditism.
 transverse h. a condition in which the external genital organs are characteristic of one sex and the gonads are typical of the other.
 true h. coexistence, in the same individual, of both ovarian and testicular tissue, caused by anomalous differentiation of the gonads; secondary sex characters of both genders may be present.
 unilateral h. presence of gonadal tissue typical of both sexes on one side and of an ovary or testis on the other.

Her·me·tia il·lu·cens (hər-me′sh-e-ə il-u′sənz) the soldier fly, a species whose larvae may cause intestinal myiasis or pseudomyiasis.

her·met·ic (hər-met′ik) [L. *hermeticus*] impervious to air; airtight.

her·nia (hur′ne-ə) [L.] the protrusion of a loop or knuckle of an organ or tissue through an abnormal opening. See also *herniation.* **her′nial** *adj*

Hernia

abdominal h. herniation of omentum, intestine, or some other internal body structure through the abdominal wall; it may be congenital or found as a complication of pregnancy or a surgical incision. Called also *ventral h.* and *laparocele.*

acquired h. a hernia brought on by lifting or by a strain or other injury.

axial hiatal h. sliding hiatal h.

Barth h. hernia of intestine between the serosa of the abdominal wall and that of a persistent vitelline duct.

Béclard h. femoral hernia through the saphenous opening.

Birkett h. synovial h.

Bochdalek h. a congenital diaphragmatic hernia due to failure of closure of the pleuroperitoneal hiatus (foramen of Bochdalek). Called also *foramen of Bochdalek h., parasternal h.,* and *retrosternal h.* See illustration.

cecal h. a hernia of intestine including all or part of the cecum.

cerebral h., h. ce′rebri protrusion of brain substance through the cranium, through either a cranium bifidum, the foramen magnum, or the tentorial notch. See *encephalocele* and see *tonsillar herniation* and *transtentorial herniation,* under *herniation.*

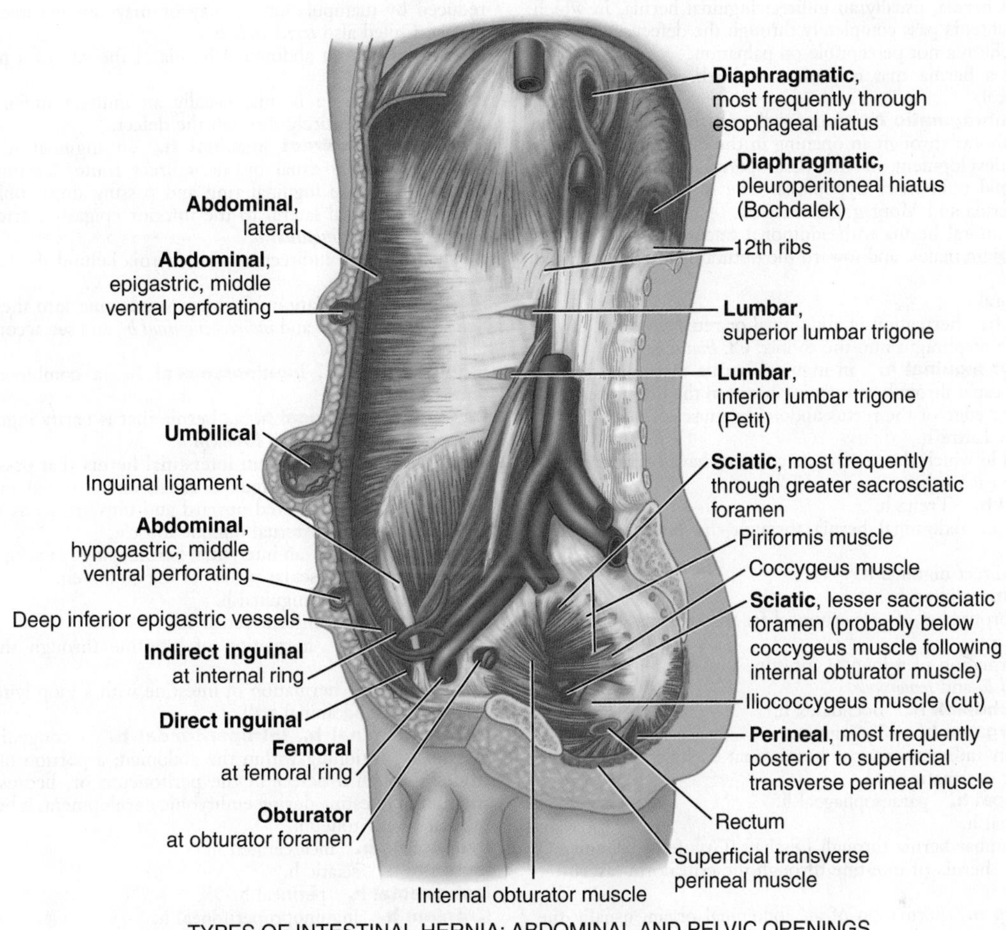

TYPES OF INTESTINAL HERNIA: ABDOMINAL AND PELVIC OPENINGS

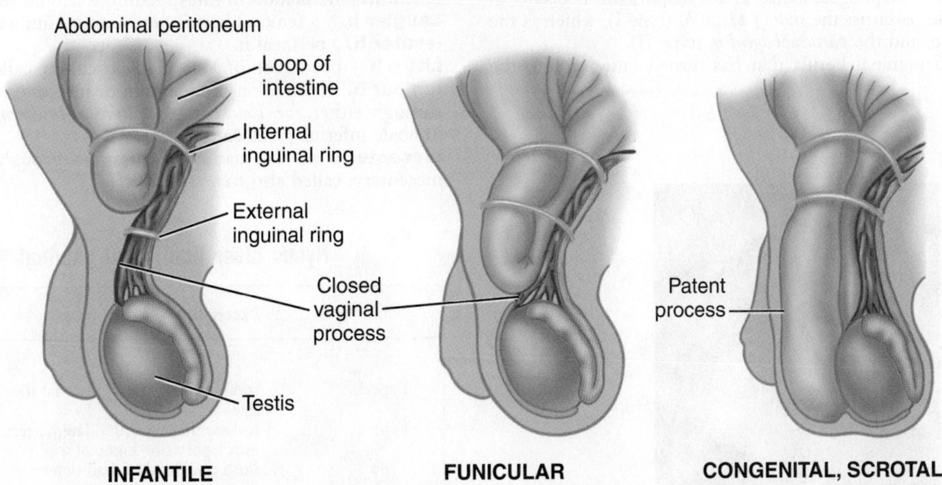

TYPES OF INDIRECT INGUINAL HERNIA

■ **PLATE 19—INTESTINAL AND INGUINAL HERNIAS**

Cloquet h. pectineal h.
complete h. a hernia, usually an indirect inguinal hernia, in which the sac and its contents pass completely through the defect.
concealed h. hernia not perceptible on palpation.
congenital h. a hernia that is present at birth, most commonly scrotal or umbilical.
congenital diaphragmatic h. congenital protrusion of abdominal viscera into the thorax through an opening in the diaphragm resulting from defective development of the pleuroperitoneal membrane; it often leads to fatal pulmonary hypoplasia. The most common types are Bochdalek hernia and Morgagni hernia.
Cooper h. a femoral hernia with additional tracts into the scrotum or toward the labium majus, and toward the obturator foramen. Called also *Hey h.*
crural h. femoral h.
diaphragmatic h. herniation of abdominal or retroperitoneal structures through the diaphragm into the thorax. Cf. *hiatal h.*
direct h., direct inguinal h. an inguinal hernia that goes directly into the inguinal canal through an opening between the inferior epigastric artery and the edge of the rectus abdominis muscle.
diverticular h. Littre h.
dry h. a hernia in which the sac and its contents have become intimately adherent to each other.
duodenojejunal h. Treitz h.
epigastric h. an abdominal hernia through the linea alba above the navel.
external h. indirect inguinal h.
extrasaccular h. sliding h.
fat h. hernial protrusion of preperitoneal fat through the abdominal wall.
femoral h. herniation of a loop of intestine into the femoral canal. Called also *crural h.* and *femorocele.*
foramen of Bochdalek h. Bochdalek h.
foramen of Morgagni h. Morgagni h.
funicular h. an indirect inguinal hernia that includes part of the umbilical cord or spermatic cord.
gastroesophageal h. paraesophageal h.
groin h. inguinal h.
Grynfeltt h. lumbar hernia through Lesshaft (Grynfeltt) triangle.
Hesselbach h. hernia of intestine through the cribriform fascia.
Hey h. Cooper h.
hiatal h., hiatus h. herniation of an abdominal organ, usually the stomach, through the esophageal hiatus of the diaphragm. It occurs in two major anatomic patterns: the *sliding hiatal h.* (type I), which is the more common type, and the *paraesophageal h.* (type II).
Holthouse h. an inguinal hernia that has turned outward into the groin.

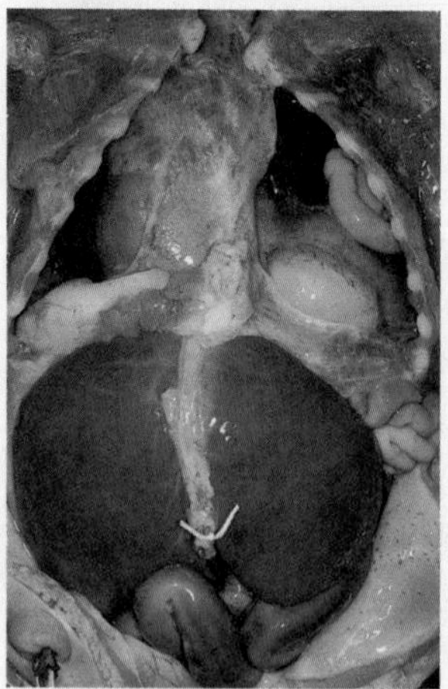

■ Bochdalek hernia in an infant, with right lung compression, cardiomediastinal shift, left lung hypoplasia, and visceral herniation through the diaphragmatic defect.

incarcerated h. hernia of intestine that cannot be returned or reduced by manipulation; it may or may not become a strangulated hernia. Called also *irreducible h.*
incisional h. an abdominal hernia at the site of a previously made incision.
incomplete h. a hernia, usually an indirect inguinal hernia, that has not passed entirely through the defect.
indirect h., indirect inguinal h. an inguinal hernia that goes into the inguinal canal by an indirect route, leaving the abdomen through the deep inguinal ring and passing down obliquely through the inguinal canal lateral to the inferior epigastric artery. Called also *oblique* or *oblique inguinal h.*
infantile h. an indirect inguinal hernia behind the funicular process of the peritoneum.
inguinal h. herniation of a loop of intestine into the inguinal canal. See *direct inguinal h.* and *indirect inguinal h.*, and see accompanying table. Called also *groin h.*
inguinocrural h., inguinofemoral h. a combined inguinal and femoral hernia.
inguinoproperitoneal h. a hernia that is partly inguinal and partly properitoneal; called also *Krönlein h.*
inguinosuperficial h. an interstitial hernia that passes through the internal inguinal ring, inguinal canal, and external inguinal ring, at which point it is deflected upward and outward so as to lie upon the aponeurosis of the external oblique muscle.
intermuscular h. an interstitial hernia lying between one or another of the fascial or muscular planes of the abdomen.
internal h. direct inguinal h.
interparietal h. intermuscular h.
intersigmoid h. herniation of intestine through the intersigmoid fossa.
interstitial h. herniation of intestine with a loop lying between two layers of the abdominal wall.
intra-abdominal h., intraperitoneal h. a congenital anomaly of intestinal positioning within the abdomen; a portion of intestine protrudes through a defect in the peritoneum or, because of abnormal rotation of intestine during embryonic development, it becomes trapped in a sac of peritoneum.
irreducible h. incarcerated h.
ischiatic h. sciatic h.
ischiorectal h. perineal h.
Krönlein h. inguinoproperitoneal h.
labial h. herniation of intestine into a labium majus.
Laugier h. a femoral hernia perforating Gimbernat ligament.
levator h. perineal h.
Littre h. protrusion of Meckel diverticulum; called also *diverticular h.*
lumbar h. herniation of omentum or intestine in the lumbar region, through either the Lesshaft space *(Grynfeltt hernia)* or the trigonum lumbale inferius *(Petit hernia).*
mesenteric h. herniation of intestine through an opening in the mesentery; called also *transmesenteric h.*

Nyhus Classification of Inguinal Hernias

Hernia Type	Description
Type 1	Indirect hernia with internal inguinal ring of normal size
Type 2	Indirect hernia with dilated internal inguinal ring but intact posterior inguinal wall
Type 3	Posterior inguinal wall defect
Type 3A	Direct inguinal hernia
Type 3B	Indirect hernias with a large, dilated internal inguinal ring that encroaches on the posterior inguinal wall; includes pantaloon, scrotal, and sliding hernias
Type 3C	Femoral hernia
Type 4	Recurrent hernias
Type 4A	Direct
Type 4B	Indirect
Type 4C	Femoral
Type 4D	Combined

Hernia *Continued*

mesentericoparietal h., mesocolic h. paraduodenal h.
Morgagni h. a congenital diaphragmatic hernia with extrusion of tissue into the thorax through the foramen of Morgagni; called also *foramen of Morgagni h.* and *pleuroperitoneal h.*
oblique h., oblique inguinal h. indirect inguinal h.
obturator h. herniation of intestine or other abdominal organs through the obturator foramen.
omental h. an abdominal hernia containing omentum.
ovarian h. hernial protrusion of an ovary.
pantaloon h. inguinal hernia in which there are both direct and indirect hernial sacs.
paraduodenal h. an intra-abdominal hernia in which the small intestine rotates incompletely during development and becomes trapped within the mesentery of the colon. Called also *mesentericoparietal* or *mesocolic h.*
paraesophageal h., parahiatal h. hiatal hernia in which part or almost all of the stomach protrudes through the hiatus into the thorax to the left of the esophagus, with the gastroesophageal junction remaining in place. Called also *type II hiatal hernia.*
paraperitoneal h. a vesical hernia in which only part of the protruded bladder is covered by the peritoneum of the sac.
parasaccular h. sliding h.
parasternal h. Bochdalek h.
parastomal h. an incisional hernia in the abdominal wall adjacent to a stoma.
parietal h. Richter h.
pectineal h. a type of femoral hernia that enters the femoral canal and then perforates the aponeurosis of the pectineus muscle; called also *Cloquet h.*
perineal h. herniation of intestine into the perineum through a fissure in the levator muscle and its fascia; called also *levator h.* and *pudendal h.*
Petit h. lumbar hernia through the trigonum lumbale inferius (Petit triangle).
pleuroperitoneal h. Morgagni h.
posterior labial h. enterocele (def. 2).
posterior vaginal h. 1. downward protrusion of the pouch of Douglas, with its intestinal contents, between the posterior vaginal wall and the rectum. 2. enterocele.
preperitoneal h. an interstitial hernia located between the parietal peritoneum and the transversalis fascia.
prevascular femoral h. a femoral hernia in the femoral sheath anterior to the femoral vessels. Called also *Velpeau h.*
properitoneal h. preperitoneal h.
pudendal h. 1. labial h. 2. perineal h.

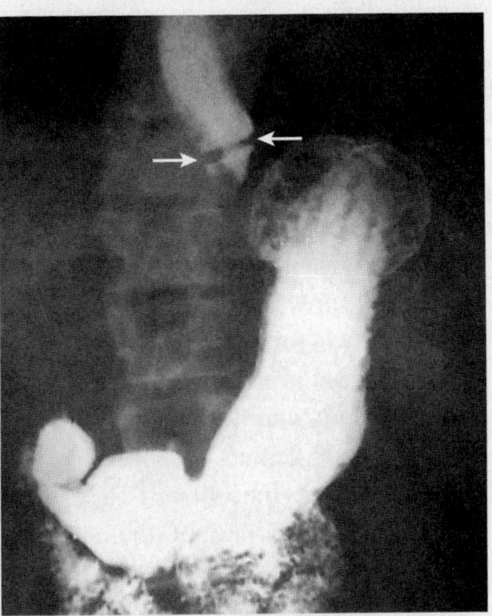

■ Sliding hiatal hernia with esophageal ring *(arrows).*

pulsion h. a hernia produced by sudden increase of intra-abdominal pressure.
rectovaginal h. rectocele.
reducible h. a hernia that can be returned to its proper place by manipulation.
retrograde h. herniation of two loops of intestine, with the part between them lying inside the abdominal cavity. Called also W *h.*
retroperitoneal h. Treitz h.
retrosternal h. Bochdalek h.
retrovascular h. a femoral hernia that passes within the femoral sheath but exits posterior to the femoral vessels.
Richter h. an incarcerated or strangulated hernia in which only a portion of the circumference of the bowel wall is involved; called also *parietal h.*
Rokitansky h. protrusion of a sac of mucous membrane or of the peritoneum through separated muscular fibers of the intestine.
rolling h. paraesophageal h.
sciatic h. herniation of intestine through the greater or lesser sciatic foramen. Called also *ischiatic h.* and *ischiocele.*
scrotal h. an inguinal hernia that has descended into the scrotum.
sliding h. hernia of the cecum (on the right) or the sigmoid colon (on the left) in which the intestinal wall forms a portion of the hernial sac, the remainder of the sac being formed by the parietal peritoneum. Called also *extrasaccular, slip,* or *slipped h.*
sliding hiatal h. hiatal hernia in which the upper stomach and the cardioesophageal junction protrude upward into the posterior mediastinum; the protrusion, which may be fixed or intermittent, is partially covered by a peritoneal sac. Called also *axial hiatal h.* and *type I hiatal h.*
slip h., slipped h. sliding h.
spigelian h. an abdominal hernia through the linea semilunaris (spigelian line).
strangulated h. an incarcerated hernia that is so tightly constricted as to compromise the blood supply of the contents of the hernial sac, leading to gangrene.
synovial h. protrusion of the inner lining membrane through the fibrous membrane of an articular capsule; called also *Birkett h.*
tonsillar h. tonsillar herniation.
transmesenteric h. mesenteric h.
Treitz h. herniation of intestine through the superior duodenal recess (Treitz fossa); called also *duodenojejunal h.* and *retroperitoneal h.*
umbilical h. a type of abdominal hernia in which part of the intestine protrudes at the umbilicus and is covered with skin and subcutaneous tissue; it may occur as a congenital anomaly or as a complication of pregnancy or a surgical incision. Cf. *omphalocele.* Called also *exomphalos* and *exumbilication.*
h. u′teri inguina′lis a common type of persistent müllerian duct syndrome.
uterine h. hernial protrusion of the uterus.
vaginal h. herniation of intestine or a viscus into the vagina. Called also *colpocele* and *vaginocele.*
vaginolabial h. enterocele (def. 2).
Velpeau h. prevascular femoral h.
ventral h. abdominal h.
vesical h. herniation of the urinary bladder; see *cystocele* and *exstrophy of bladder.*
W **h.** retrograde h.

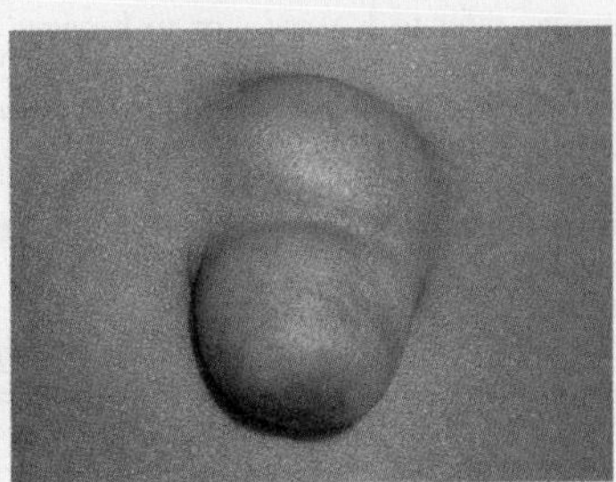

■ Umbilical hernia.

her•ni•at•ed (hur′ne-āt″əd) protruding like a hernia; enclosed in a hernia.

her•ni•a•tion (hur″ne-a′shən) the abnormal protrusion of an organ or other body structure through a defect or natural opening in a covering, membrane, muscle, or bone. See also *hernia.*

ascending transtentorial h. a rare kind of transtentorial herniation in which part of the cerebellum protrudes upward through the tentorial notch. Symptoms may include nausea, vomiting, and eventually coma.

caudal transtentorial h. descending transtentorial h.

central h. descending transtentorial herniation with downward shift of the brainstem and diencephalon, causing Cheyne-Stokes respirations with pinpoint nonreactive pupils.

cingulate h. subfalcial h.

descending transtentorial h. the most common kind of transtentorial herniation, with downward displacement of the most medially-placed cerebral structures through the tentorial notch, compressing parts of the cerebrum and structures beneath the notch; it is caused by a supratentorial mass. Symptoms depend on which structures are compressed and may include ocular changes or hemiparesis. Called also *caudal transtentorial h.*

disk h., h. of intervertebral disk protrusion of the nucleus pulposus or anulus fibrosus of an intervertebral disk, which may impinge on nerve roots; this occurs most often in lumbar vertebrae, and sometimes in cervical vertebrae. The herniated disk may be either *contained* or *noncontained* (see under *disk*). Called also *herniated, protruded,* or *ruptured disk.*

h. of nucleus pulposus see *h. of intervertebral disk.*

painful fat h. piezogenic papules.

rostral transtentorial h. ascending transtentorial h.

subfalcial h. a shift of the cingulate gyrus to below the falx cerebri; called also cingulate herniation.

tentorial h. transtentorial h.

tonsillar h. protrusion of the cerebellar tonsils through the foramen magnum, exerting pressure on the medulla oblongata. Called also *tonsillar hernia.*

transtentorial h. protrusion of brain structures through the tentorial notch; the two types are *descending transtentorial h.* and *ascending transtentorial h.* Called also *tentorial h.*

uncal h. descending transtentorial herniation in which the uncus protrudes through the notch.

her•ni•oid (hur′ne-oid) resembling a hernia.

her•nio•lap•a•rot•o•my (hur″ne-o-lap″ə-rot′ə-me) laparotomy for treatment of hernia.

her•nio•plas•ty (hur′ne-o-plas″te) surgical repair of a hernia; sometimes used specifically to denote repair using a mesh patch or plug to reinforce the area of the defect. Cf. *herniorrhaphy.* **hernioplas′tic** *adj*

tension-free h. hernia repair using a mesh sheet or plug to reinforce the defect, thus avoiding the tension caused by suturing together structures not normally in apposition.

her•ni•or•rha•phy (hur″ne-or′ə-fe) [*hernia* + *-rrhaphy*] surgical repair of a hernia; sometimes used specifically to denote a simple apposition and suturing of the defect. Cf. *hernioplasty.*

her•ni•ot•o•my (hə-r″ne-ot′ə-me) [*hernia* + *-tomy*] incision of an inguinal hernia, usually preceding herniorrhaphy.

her•o•in (her′o-in) diacetylmorphine.

herp•an•gi•na (hur″pən-ji′nə) [*herpes* + *angina*] an acute infectious disease caused by either group A or group B coxsackievirus or by echoviruses, chiefly affecting young children in the summer; characteristics include vesiculoulcerative lesions on the mucous membranes of the throat, dysphagia, vomiting, and fever. Called also *aphthous pharyngitis, vesicular pharyngitis,* and *herpes angina.*

her•pes (hur′pēz) [L., from Gr. *herpēs* a spreading cutaneous eruption, from *herpein* to creep] any inflammatory skin disease caused by a herpesvirus and characterized by the formation of clusters of small vesicles. When used alone, the term may refer to *h. simplex* or to *h. zoster.*

h. blat′tae a rare type of allergic contact dermatitis that resembles a herpes lesion and is caused by a cockroach of the genus *Blatta* crawling on the skin of a susceptible person.

h. cor′neae herpetic keratitis.

cutaneous h., cutaneous h. simplex herpes simplex of the skin, characterized by a vesicular eruption.

h. digita′lis herpes simplex of the fingers.

h. facia′lis herpes febrilis of the face; called also *h. simplex facialis.*

h. febri′lis herpes simplex caused mainly by human herpesvirus 1 but also by human herpesvirus 2, and primarily spread by oral secretions; it usually occurs as a concomitant of fever, but may develop in the absence of fever or prior illness, and commonly involves the facial region, especially the vermilion border of the lips *(h. labialis)* and the nares; the vesicular lesions are self-limited. Called also *cold sore* and *fever blister.*

genital h., h. genita′lis, genital h. simplex herpes simplex in the genital region, seen in both males and females; it is caused mainly by human herpesvirus 2, but also may be caused by human herpesvirus 1, and is transmitted primarily sexually via genital secretions, and contact with viroids. Although symptoms in the female are more severe than in the male, the vesicular lesions are self-limited. Genital herpes at term in the pregnant female may lead to infection of the neonate that can progress from localized to disseminated disease that often results in death of the baby. Called also *progenital h.* and *h. progenitalis.*

h. gestatio′nis a rare, self-limited blistering skin disorder seen in pregnant women during the second and third trimesters, resembling cutaneous herpes but not due to a herpesvirus; it may be an autoimmune disease. It usually begins on the abdomen and spreads to other sites and is an intensely pruritic polymorphous eruption that may recur with subsequent pregnancies. Called also *gestational pemphigoid* and *pemphigoid gestationis.*

h. gladiato′rum cutaneous herpes acquired by direct exogenous infection of traumatized skin, such as in wrestlers, usually associated with localization of lesions to the area of trauma and regional lymphadenopathy and often with symptoms of systemic illness such as fever and malaise. Called also *traumatic h.*

h. labia′lis herpes simplex on the vermilion border of the lips; called also *h. simplex labialis.*

neonatal h., neonatal h. simplex, h. neonato′rum herpes simplex in a neonate, usually contracted while passing through the birth canal of a mother with active genital herpes. It may be localized with skin eruptions or generalized, affecting the liver, adrenal glands, and lungs. In a minority of cases, virus from the mother crosses the placenta and the fetus is infected in utero; these neonates may have brain involvement such as microcephaly and seizures.

ocular h. herpes simplex of the eye and its adnexa; see *herpetic keratitis.*

h. ophthal′micus h. zoster ophthalmicus.

progenital h., h. progenita′lis genital h.

h. sim′plex a group of acute infections caused by human herpesviruses 1 and 2, characterized by small fluid-filled vesicles on the skin or a mucous membrane with a raised erythematous base; it may be a primary infection or recurrent because of reactivation of a latent infection. Type 1 herpesvirus infections usually involve nongenital regions of the body, whereas type 2 infections are primarily on the genitals and surrounding areas, although there is overlap between the two types. Precipitating factors include fever, exposure to cold temperature or ultraviolet rays, sunburn, cutaneous or mucosal abrasions, emotional stress, and nerve injury.

h. sim′plex facia′lis h. facialis.

h. sim′plex genita′lis genital h.

h. sim′plex labia′lis h. labialis.

traumatic h., wrestler's h. h. gladiatorum.

h. zos′ter an acute, infectious, usually self-limited disease believed to represent activation of latent human herpesvirus 3 in those who have become partially immune after an attack of chickenpox. It involves the sensory ganglia and their areas of innervation, and is characterized by severe neuralgic pain along the distribution of the affected nerve with crops of clustered vesicles over the area of the corresponding dermatome; it is usually unilateral and confined to one dermatome or adjacent ones. Postherpetic neuralgia may be a complication. In immunocompromised patients it may disseminate and be fatal. Called also *acute posterior ganglionitis, shingles, zona,* and *zoster.*

h. zos′ter auricula′ris Ramsay Hunt syndrome (def. 1).

h. zos′ter ophthal′micus herpes zoster involving the ophthalmic division of the trigeminal nerve, characterized by a cutaneous vesicular rash on an erythematous base along the nerve path, preceded by lancinating pain, usually accompanied by conjunctivitis and sometimes by keratitis, scleritis, iridocyclitis, extraocular muscle palsies, ptosis, and mydriasis. In some patients it can lead to glaucoma and blindness. Called also *gasserian ganglionitis, h. ophthalmicus,* and *ophthalmic zoster.*

h. zos′ter o′ticus Ramsay Hunt syndrome (def. 1).

Her•pes•vi•ri•dae (hur″pēz-vi′rĭ-de) the herpesviruses: a family of DNA viruses having a virion 102–200 nm in diameter consisting of four components: a lipid bilayer envelope with surface projections, a tegument

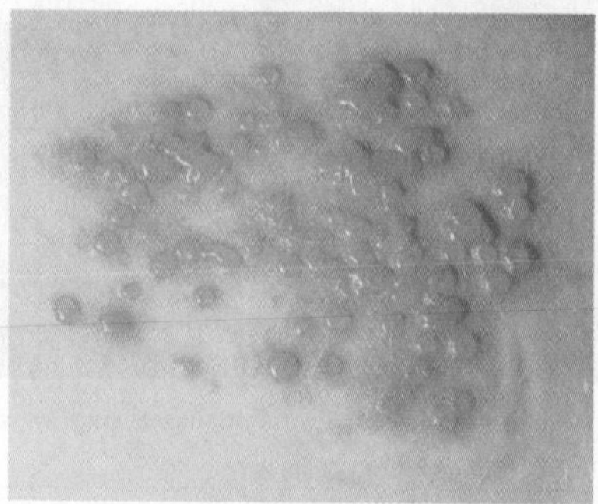

■ Herpes simplex, characterized by grouped epidermal vesicles and dermal erythema.

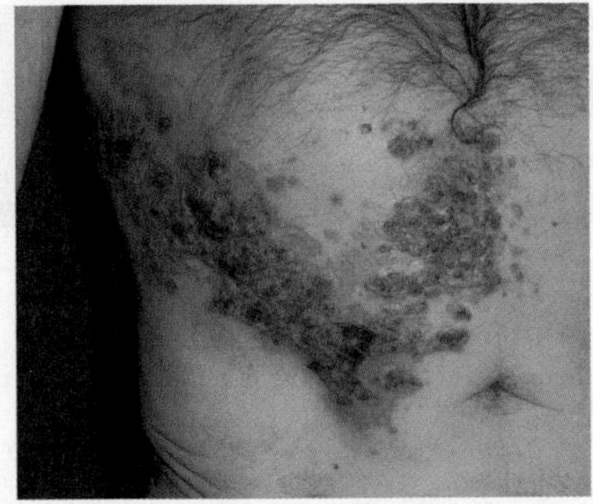

■ Herpes zoster, with diffuse involvement of a dermatome.

of amorphous material, an icosahedral nucleocapsid with 162 prismatic capsomers, and a protein spool on which the DNA is wrapped. The genome consists of a single molecule of linear double-stranded DNA (MW 70–150 × 10^6, size 124–235 kbp). Viruses contain at least 20 structural polypeptides and are sensitive to lipid solvents, heat, and extremes of pH. Replication occurs in the nucleus and the envelope is acquired by budding through the inner lamella of the nuclear membrane; virions are released by transport via the endoplasmic reticulum to the cell membrane. Persistence for the lifetime of the host is common and some herpesviruses induce neoplasia. There are three subfamilies: Alphaherpesvirinae, Betaherpesvirinae, and Gammaherpesvirinae. A large number of herpesviruses have not yet been assigned to a subfamily or genus.

her•pes•vi•rus (hur′pēz-vi″rəs) [*herpes* + *virus*] any virus belonging to the family Herpesviridae. **herpesvi′ral** *adj*

h. B a virus of the genus *Simplexvirus* that infects Asiatic macaques. Human infection, usually fatal, can result from monkey bites and may cause ascending myelopathy or acute meningitis. Called also *B virus* and *cercopithecine herpesvirus 1.*

bovine h. 1 a virus of the genus *Varicellovirus* that is the etiologic agent of infectious bovine rhinotracheitis. Called also *infectious bovine rhinotracheitis virus.*

bovine h. 2 a virus of the genus *Simplexvirus* that is the etiologic agent of bovine ulcerative mammillitis.

cercopithecine h. 1 h. B.

equid h. 1 a virus of the genus *Varicellovirus* that is an etiologic agent of equine viral rhinopneumonitis; see also *equid h. 4.* Called also *equine h. 1.*

equid h. 3 a virus of the subfamily Alphaherpesvirinae that is the etiologic agent of equine coital exanthema.

equid h. 4 a virus of the genus *Varicellovirus*, closely related to equid herpesvirus 1, that is an etiologic agent of equine viral rhinopneumonitis. Called also *equine h. 4.*

equine h. 1 equid h. 1.

equine h. 3 equid h. 3.

equine h. 4 equid h. 4.

felid h. 1, feline h. 1 a virus in the subfamily Alphaherpesvirinae (family Herpesviridae) that is the main cause of disease in the feline respiratory disease complex. See also *feline rhinotracheitis.* Called also *feline rhinotracheitis virus.*

gallid h. 1 a species of the genus *Iltovirus* that causes infectious laryngotracheitis in poultry. Called also *infectious laryngotracheitis virus.*

gallid h. 2 a species of the genus *Mardivirus*, family Herpesviridae that is an etiologic agent of Marek disease. Called also *Marek disease h. 1.*

gallid h. 3 a species of the genus *Mardivirus*, family Herpesviridae that is an etiologic agent of Marek disease. Called also *Marek disease h. 2.*

human h. 1 a virus of the genus *Simplexvirus* that is an etiologic agent of herpes simplex and causes predominantly non-genital infections. Primary infection usually occurs in early childhood and is often asymptomatic, although gingivostomatitis and pharyngitis may occur. The virus can pass along nerves and remain latent in ganglia, from which it may be reactivated. Called also herpes simplex virus 1. See Plate 49.

human h. 2 a virus of the genus *Simplexvirus* that is an etiologic agent of herpes simplex, is transmitted venereally, and causes primarily genital infections. Called also *herpes simplex virus 2.* See Plate 49.

human h. 3 a virus of the genus *Varicellovirus* that is the etiologic agent of chickenpox and herpes zoster. Called also *varicella-zoster virus.*

human h. 4 Epstein-Barr virus.

human h. 5 the sole species of the genus *Cytomegalovirus*, the cause of cytomegalic inclusion disease.

human h. 6 a species of the genus *Roseolovirus* that is the etiologic agent of exanthema subitum. Most healthy adults carry the virus and are asymptomatic; infection results in lifelong persistence.

human h. 7 a species closely related to human herpesvirus 6 but not known to be associated with any disease.

human h. 8 a virus in the family Herpesviridae that has been implicated as the etiologic agent of Kaposi sarcoma, primary effusion lymphoma, and multicentric plasma cell–type Castleman disease. Called also *Kaposi sarcoma h.* and *Kaposi sarcoma–associated h.*

Kaposi sarcoma h., Kaposi sarcoma–associated h. human h. 8.

Marek disease h. 1 gallid h. 2.

Marek disease h. 2 gallid h. 3.

suid h. 1 pseudorabies virus.

her•pet•ic (hər-pet′ik) [L. *herpeticus*] 1. pertaining to or of the nature of herpes. 2. pertaining to or caused by herpesviruses.

her•pet•i•form (hər-pet′ĭ-form) [*herpet-* + *form*] resembling herpes; having grouped vesicles.

herpet(o)- [Gr. *herpeton* creeping thing, crawler, reptile, from *herpein* to creep] a combining form denoting a relationship to (1) herpes or (2) a snake or other reptile.

her•pe•tol•o•gist (hur″pə-tol′o-jist) a specialist in herpetology.

her•pe•tol•o•gy (hur″pə-tol′ə-je) [*herpeto-* + *-logy*] the branch of zoology that specializes in the study of reptiles and amphibians.

her•peto•pho•bia (hər-pet″o-fo′be-ə) irrational fear of reptiles or amphibians.

Her•pe•to•so•ma (hər-pet″o-so′mə) [*herpeto-* + *soma*] in some systems of classification, a subgenus of *Trypanosoma* that includes *T. lewisi* and various nonpathogenic species.

Her•plex (hur′pleks) trademark for a preparation of idoxuridine.

Her•ring bodies (her′ing) [Percy Theodore *Herring*, English physiologist, 1872–1967] see under *body.*

Herr•mann syndrome (hur′mən) [Christian *Herrmann*, Jr., American physician, born 1921] see under *syndrome.*

Hers disease (ārz) [Henri-Géry *Hers*, Belgian physiologist and biochemist, 20th century] glycogen storage disease, type VI; see under *disease.*

her•sage (ār-sahzh′) [Fr. "combing"] surgical dissociation of the fibers in a scarred area of a peripheral nerve by splitting the sheath and separating the nerve into a ribbon of fine free fibers. Called also *endoneurolysis.*

Her•ter disease (hur′tər) [Christian Archibald *Herter*, American physician, 1865–1910] the infantile form of celiac disease (q.v.).

Her•ter-Heub•ner disease (hur′tər hoib′nər) [C.A. *Herter*; Johann Otto Leonhard *Heubner*, German pediatrician, 1843–1926] the infantile form of celiac disease (q.v.).

Her•tig-Rock ova (hur′tig rok) [Arthur Tremain *Hertig*, American pathologist, 1904–1990; John *Rock*, American gynecologist, 1890–1984] see under *ovum.*

Hert•wig sheath (hert′vik) [Richard Carl Wilhelm Theodor von *Hertwig*, German zoologist, 1850–1937] root sheath (def. 1).

Hert•wig-Ma•gen•die phenomenon (hert′vik mah-zhahn-de′) [R.C.W.T. von *Hertwig*; François *Magendie*, French physiologist, 1783–1855] skew deviation.

hertz (Hz) (hurts) the SI unit of frequency, equal to 1 cycle per second.

HERV human endogenous retroviruses.

Herx•heim•er reaction (hərks′hi-mər) [Karl *Herxheimer*, German dermatologist, 1861–1944] Jarisch-Herxheimer reaction; see under *reaction.*

herz•tod (herts′tōt) [Ger. "cardiac death"] porcine stress syndrome.

Heschl gyri (convolutions) (hesh′əl) [Richard L. *Heschl*, Austrian pathologist, 1824–1881] see *gyri temporales transversi*, under *gyrus.*

Hes•pan (hes′pan) trademark for a preparation of hetastarch.

hes•per•i•din (hes-per′ĭ-din) a bioflavonoid predominant in lemons and oranges.

Hess capillary test (hes) [Alfred Fabian *Hess*, American physician, 1875–1933] tourniquet test (def. 1); see under *test.*

Hes•sel•bach fascia, hernia, ligament, triangle (hes′əl-bahk) [Franz Kaspar *Hesselbach*, German surgeon, 1759–1816] see under *hernia*, and see *fascia cribrosa*, *ligamentum interfoveolare*, and *trigonum inguinale.*

het•a•cil•lin (het″ə-sil′in) a semisynthetic penicillin which itself has no antibacterial activity, but is converted in the body to ampicillin and has actions and uses similar to those of ampicillin (q.v.); administered orally.

h. potassium the potassium salt of hetacillin, having antibacterial actions and uses similar to those of ampicillin; administered intravenously and intramuscularly.

het·a·starch (het′ə-stahrch) a starch containing not more than 90 per cent of amylopectin, and that has been etherified so that an average of 7 to 8 of the OH groups in every 10-D-glucopyranose units of starch polymer have been converted into OCH_2CH_2OH groups; used as a plasma volume expander, administered by infusion.

HETE hydroxyeicosatetraenoic acid.

het·er·a·del·phus (het″ər-ə-del′fəs) [*heter-* + *-adelphus*] asymmetrical conjoined twins; see under *twin.*

Het·er·ak·i·dae (het″ər-ak′ĭ-de) a family of nematodes some of which parasitize birds; it includes the genus *Heterakis.*

Het·er·a·kis (het″ər-a′kis) [*heter-* + Gr. *akis* pointed object] a genus of nonpathogenic nematodes of the family Heterakidae, parasitic in the ceca of chickens, turkeys, and other birds. *H. galli′nae* serves as a paratenic host for *Histomonas meleagridis,* the etiologic agent of histomoniasis.

het·er·aux·e·sis (het″ər-awk-ze′sis) [*heter-* + *auxesis*] disproportionate growth of a part in relation to another part.

het·er·ax·i·al (het″ər-ak′se-əl) [*heter-* + *axial*] having axes of unequal length.

het·er·e·cious (het″ər-e′shəs) heteroecious.

het·er·e·cism (het″ər-e′siz-əm) the state of being heteroecious.

het·er·er·gic (het″ər-ur′jik) [*heter-* + Gr. *ergon* work] having different effects; said of two drugs one of which produces a particular effect and the other does not.

het·er·es·the·sia (het″ər-es-the′zhə) [*heter-* + *esthesia*] variation in the degree of cutaneous sensibility on adjoining areas of the body surface.

heter(o)- [Gr. *heteros* other, different] a combining form meaning other, different, or abnormal, or denoting relationship to another.

het·ero·ag·glu·ti·na·tion (het″ər-o-ə-gloo″tĭ-na′shən) agglutination of particulate antigens (on cells or adsorbed on inert carrier particles) of one species by agglutinins derived from organisms of another species.

het·ero·ag·glu·ti·nin (het″ər-o-ə-gloo′tĭ-nin) an agglutinin with reactive specificity for particulate antigen(s) in one or more species other than the species in which it originates.

het·ero·an·ti·body (het″ər-o-an″tĭ-bod′e) an antibody specific for antigens originating in a species other than that of the antibody producer.

het·ero·an·ti·gen (het″ər-o-an′tĭ-jən) an antigen originating in a species different from, and therefore foreign to, the antibody producer.

het·er·o·at·om (het″ər-o-at′om) any atom in an organic compound other than carbon or hydrogen.

Het·ero·bil·har·zia (het″ər-o-bil-hahr′zhə) a genus of trematodes of the family Schistosomatidae that parasitize mammals. *H. america′na* has cercariae that can cause visceral schistosomiasis and cercarial dermatitis.

het·ero·blas·tic (het″ər-o-blas′tik) [*hetero-* + *blast-* + *-ic*] having origin in different kinds of tissue.

het·ero·cel·lu·lar (het″ər-o-sel′u-lər) composed of cells of different kinds.

het·ero·cen·tric (het″ər-o-sen′trik) [*hetero-* + *centric*] 1. made up of rays of light that neither are parallel nor meet in one point. 2. allocentric.

het·ero·chi·ral (het″ər-o-ki′rəl) [*hetero-* + *chiral*] reversed as regards right and left, but otherwise the same in form and size, as the hands.

het·ero·chro·ma·tin (het″ər-o-kro′mə-tin) [*hetero-* + *chromatin*] the form of chromatin that is darkly staining and tightly coiled in interphase; it is composed of repetitive DNA, is late to replicate, and is transcriptionally inactive. Cf. *euchromatin.*

constitutive h. the chromatin in regions of the chromosomes that are invariably heterochromatic, located mainly to both sides of the centromeres and to the telomeres; it contains highly repetitive sequences of DNA that are genetically inactive, and may serve as a structural element of the chromosome. See also *C banding,* under *banding.*

facultative h. the chromatin in regions of the chromosomes that become heterochromatic in certain cells and tissues; e.g., it makes up the inactive X chromosome in female somatic cells.

pericentric h. constitutive heterochromatin located in the region of the centromere.

telomeric h. constitutive heterochromatin located near the end of a chromosome.

het·ero·chro·ma·tin·iza·tion (het″ər-o-kro″mə-tin-ĭ-za′shən) the condensation of euchromatin into heterochromatin.

het·ero·chro·ma·ti·za·tion (het″ər-o-kro″mə-tĭ-za′shən) heterochromatinization.

het·ero·chro·ma·to·sis (het″ər-o-kro″mə-to′sis) heterochromia.

het·ero·chro·mia (het″ər-o-kro′me-ə) [*hetero-* + *chrom-* + *-ia*] diversity of color in a part or parts that should normally be of one color. heterochro′mic *adj*

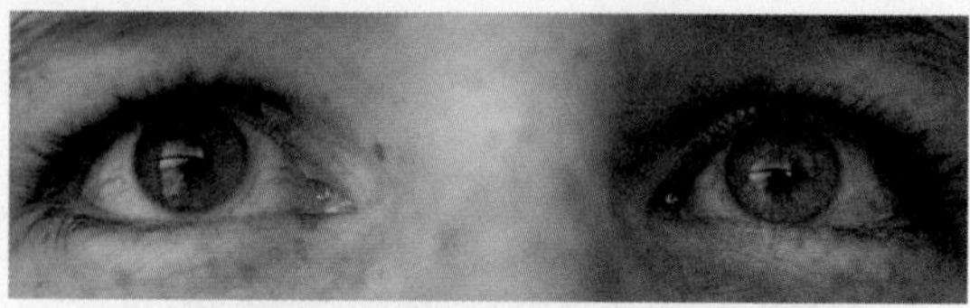

■ Heterochromia iridum.

binocular h. h. iridum.

h. i′ridis the presence of two colors in different areas of the same iris; called also *uniocular h.* and *iris bicolor.*

h. i′ridum difference of color of the two irides; called also *binocular h.*

uniocular h. h. iridis.

het·ero·chro·nia (het″ər-o-kro′ne-ə) heterochrony.

het·ero·chron·ic (het″ər-o-kron′ik) 1. pertaining to or characterized by heterochrony. 2. denoting different ages or stages of development, as between the excised organ and the implanted organ in transplantation procedures.

het·er·och·ro·nous (het″ər-ok′ro-nəs) heterochronic.

het·er·och·ro·ny (het″ər-ok′rə-ne) [*hetero-* + *chron-*] 1. the formation of parts or tissues, or the occurrence of a phenomenon, at an unusual time. Cf. *synchronia* (def. 2). 2. a difference in the rate or time of occurrence between two processes. Called also *heterochronia.*

het·ero·clad·ic (het″ər-o-klad′ik) [*hetero-* + Gr. *klados* branch] pertaining to or characterized by an anastomosis between terminal branches from different arteries.

het·ero·clit·ic (het″ər-o-klit′ik) [Gr. *heteroklitos* irregularly inflected (a grammatical term)] irregular; said of a kind of antibody (see under *antibody*).

het·ero·crine (het′ər-o-krin) [*hetero-* + Gr. *krinein* to separate] secreting more than one kind of matter.

het·ero·cyc·lic (het″ər-o-sik′lik, -si′klik) having or pertaining to a closed chain or ring formation which includes atoms of different elements.

het·ero·cy·to·tro·pic (het″ər-o-si″to-tro′pik) [*hetero-* + *cyto-* + *-tropic*] having an affinity for cells of different species; see under *antibody.*

Het·er·od·era rad·i·cic·o·la (het″ər-od′ə-ra rad″ĭ-sik′o-lə) a nematode parasitic on the common root vegetables, such as radishes, carrots, turnips, potatoes, etc., as well as on celery. When infested vegetables are eaten, ova of the parasite may appear in the stools and must be distinguished from those of true parasites.

het·ero·der·mic (het″ər-o-dur′mik) [*hetero-* + *dermic*] denoting a skin graft taken from a member of another species. See *dermatoheteroplasty.*

het·ero·des·mot·ic (het″ər-o-des-mot′ik) [*hetero-* + *desmo-* + *-ic*] joining dissimilar parts of the central nervous system; see under *fiber.*

het·ero·did·y·mus (het″ər-o-did′ə-məs) heterodymus.

het·ero·di·mer (het″ər-o-di′mər) a dimer consisting of unlike subunits.

het·ero·dont (het′ər-o-dont) [*heter-* + Gr. *odous* tooth] having teeth of different types, such as incisors and molars.

Het·ero·dox·us (het″ər-o-dok′səs) a genus of parasitic biting lice (order Mallophaga). *H. longitar′sus* is parasitic on kangaroos, wallabies, and sometimes dogs in Australia. *H. spi′niger* is parasitic on coyotes, wolves, and sometimes dogs in North and South America.

het·er·od·ro·mous (het″ər-od′ro-məs) [*hetero-* + *drom-* + *-ous*] moving, acting, or arranged in the opposite direction.

het·er·od·y·mus (het″ər-od′ə-məs) [*hetero-* + *-didymus*] asymmetrical conjoined twins in which one fetus has a second head, neck, and thorax attached to its thorax.

het·er·oe·cious (het″ər-e′shəs) [*heter-* + Gr. *oikos* house] requiring two or more hosts to complete the life cycle; said of certain fungi and insects, as opposed to *autoecious.*

het·ero·erot·ic (het″er-o-ĕ-rot′ik) 1. pertaining to or characterized by heteroeroticism. 2. alloerotic.

het·ero·erot·i·cism (het″ər-o-ə-rot′ĭ-siz-əm) 1. sexual feeling directed toward someone of the opposite sex. 2. alloeroticism (def. 1). 3. a stage in the development of object relationships in which the erotic energy is directed toward objects other than oneself, specifically to those of the opposite sex. Cf. *alloeroticism, autoeroticism.*

het·ero·fer·men·ta·tion (het″ər-o-fur″mən-ta′shən) fermentation producing more than one major product; the term is often used as a synonym of heterolactic fermentation (q.v.).

het·ero·fer·ment·er (het″ər-o-fər-men′tər) a microorganism that exhibits heterofermentation.

het·ero·gam·ete (het″ər-o-gam′ēt) a gamete of different size and structure from the one with which it unites.

het·ero·ga·met·ic (het″ər-o-gə-met′ik) pertaining to production of gametes containing more than one kind of sex chromosome, as in human males (XY).

het·ero·gam·e·ty (het″ər-o-gam′ə-te) the production of unlike gametes by an individual of one sex, such as the production of X- and Y-bearing gametes by the human male.

het·er·og·a·mous (het″ər-og′ə-məs) pertaining to heterogamy.

het·er·og·a·my (het″ər-og′ə-me) [*hetero-* + Gr. *gamos* marriage] 1. reproduction resulting from the union of two dissimilar gametes, particularly in higher organisms. See also *anisogamy* and *oogamy*. 2. alternation of generations in which the two types of sexual reproduction alternate, as bisexual and parthenogenetic.

het·ero·gan·gli·on·ic (het″ər-o-gang″le-on′ik) interganglionic.

het·ero·ge·ne·i·ty (het″ər-o-jə-ne′ĭ-te) the state or quality of being heterogeneous.

allelic h. see *genetic h.*

genetic h. the production of identical or similar phenotypes by more than one genetic mutation; either by different mutant alleles at the same locus *(allelic h.)* or by mutations at two or more loci *(locus h.)*.

locus h. see *genetic h.*

het·ero·ge·ne·ous (het″ər-o-je′ne-əs) [*hetero-* + Gr. *genos* kind] 1. consisting of or composed of dissimilar elements or ingredients; not having a uniform quality throughout. 2. in genetics, pertaining to a phenotype that can be produced by different mutations.

het·ero·gen·e·sis (het″ər-o-gen′ə-sis) [*hetero-* + *-genesis*] alternation of generations.

het·ero·ge·net·ic (het″ər-o-jə-net′ik) 1. pertaining to heterogenesis. 2. not arising within the organism.

het·er·o·gen·ic (het′ər-o-jen′ik) xenogeneic.

het·ero·ge·nic·i·ty (het″ər-o-jə-nis′ĭ-te) heterogeneity.

het·ero·ge·note (het′ər-o-je″nōt) [*hetero-* + *gene* (analogy with zygote)] in bacterial genetics, a merozygote in which the corresponding alleles at a specific locus of the diploid region of the genome are different. See also *homogenote* and *merozygote*.

het·er·og·e·nous (het″ər-oj′ə-nəs) 1. xenogeneic. 2. heterogeneous.

het·ero·geu·sia (het″ər-o-goo′zhə) [*hetero-* + Gr. *geusis* taste + *-ia*] any parageusia in which all gustatory stimuli are distorted in a similar way. Cf. *cacogeusia*.

het·er·og·o·ny (het″ər-og′ə-ne) [*hetero-* + Gr. *gonos* procreation] alternation of generations; used particularly to denote alternation of parthenogenetic and sexual reproductive cycles or alternation of parasitic and free-living forms.

het·ero·graft (het′ər-o-graft″) xenograft.

het·ero·he·mag·glu·ti·na·tion (het″ər-o-he″mə-gloo″tĭ-na′shən) agglutination of erythrocytes of one species by hemagglutinins derived from an individual of a different species.

het·ero·he·mag·glu·ti·nin (het″ər-o-he″mə-gloo′tĭ-nin) a hemagglutinin derived from one species that agglutinates erythrocytes of organisms of one or more other species.

het·ero·he·mol·y·sin (het″ər-o-he-mol′ə-sin) 1. a hemolysin occurring spontaneously in the blood of an untreated animal that will hemolyze the blood cells of an animal of another species. 2. hemolysin established in one species by deliberate immunization with blood cells of an animal of another species.

het·ero·hex·o·san (het″ər-o-hek′so-san) any of a class of heterosaccharides in which the sugar components are hexoses.

Het·er·o·hy·rax (het″ə-ro-hi′raks) a genus of rock hyraxes. *H. bru′cei* is a species found in hilly regions of Ethiopia that is a common reservoir for *Leishmania aethiopica*.

het·ero·im·mune (het″ər-o-ĭ-mūn′) pertaining to or characterized by heteroimmunity.

het·ero·im·mu·ni·ty (het″ə-ro-ĭ-mu′nĭ-te) 1. an immune state that results from the immunization of an animal of one species with cells of one of a different species. 2. a state in which the immune response by the body to exogenous antigens (including drugs and infectious agents) results in immunopathological changes.

het·ero·kary·on (het″ər-o-kar′e-on) [*hetero-* + *karyon*] a multinucleate cell in which the nuclei are from genetically different sources, as commonly occurs in fungal hyphae. It may also be produced artificially for the study of nuclear processes. Cf. *homokaryon*.

het·ero·kary·o·sis (het″ər-o-kar″e-o′sis) [*heterokaryon* + *-osis*] 1. the formation of heterokaryons. 2. the state of containing heterokaryons.

het·ero·ker·a·to·plas·ty (het″ər-o-ker′ə-to-plas″te) [*hetero-* + *keratoplasty*] corneal transplantation in which tissue is grafted from an animal of one species into one of a different species.

het·ero·lac·tic (het″ər-o-lak′tik) producing large quantities of lactic acid along with acetic acid, ethanol, and carbon dioxide; said of bacterial fermentation.

het·ero·la·lia (het″ər-o-la′le-ə) the uttering of words other than those intended by the speaker; called also *heterophasia*.

het·ero·lat·er·al (het″ər-o-lat′ər-əl) contralateral.

het·ero·lit·er·al (het″ər-o-lit′ər-əl) marked by the substitution of one letter for another in pronouncing words.

het·er·ol·o·gous (het″ər-ol′ə-gəs) [*hetero-* + Gr. *logos* due relation, proportion] 1. made up of tissue not normal to the part. 2. xenogeneic. 3. pertaining to antigen and antibody that are not homologous, i.e., the antigen is not the one that elicited the production of the antibody.

het·er·ol·o·gy (het″ər-ol′ə-je) 1. abnormality in structure, arrangement, or manner of formation. 2. in chemistry, the relationship between substances of partial identity of structure but of different properties.

het·er·ol·y·sin (het″ər-ol′ĭ-sin) a lysin that dissolves cells of species other than the one in which it is formed, by leading to interruption of the integrity of the cell membranes; a lysin formed on the introduction of antigen from a different species.

het·er·ol·y·sis (het″ər-ol′ĭ-sis) [*hetero-* + *-lysis*] lysis of the cells of one species by lysin from a different species.

het·ero·lyt·ic (het″ər-o-lit′ik) pertaining to or caused by heterolysis or a heterolysin.

het·er·om·er·al (het″ər-om′ər-əl) heteromeric.

het·ero·mer·ic (het″ər-o-mer′ik) [*hetero-* + *mer-*[1] + *-ic*] sending processes through one of the commissures to the white matter of the other side of the spinal cord; said of spinal nerves.

het·er·om·er·ous (het″ər-om′ər-əs) heteromeric.

het·ero·meta·pla·sia (het″ər-o-met″ə-pla′zhə) [*hetero-* + *metaplasia*] development of tissue into a variety foreign to the part where it is produced.

het·ero·met·ric (het″ər-o-met′rik) involving or dependent on a change in size; cf. *homeometric*.

het·ero·me·tro·pia (het″ər-o-mə-tro′pe-ə) [Gr. *heterometros* of different measure + *-opia*] the state in which there are differences in degree of refraction in the two eyes.

het·ero·mor·phic (het″ər-o-mor′fik) [*hetero-* + *-morph* + *-ic*] 1. of abnormal shape or structure. 2. morphologically dissimilar.

het·ero·mor·phism (het″ər-o-mor′fiz-əm) the state of being heteromorphic.

het·ero·mor·pho·sis (het″ər-o-mor-fo′sis) [*hetero-* + *morphosis*] the development, particularly through regeneration, of an organ or structure inappropriate to the location.

het·ero·mor·phous (het′ər-o-mor′fəs) heteromorphic.

het·er·on·o·mous (het″ər-on′ə-məs) [*hetero-* + *nom-* + *-ous*] in biology, subject to different laws of growth; specialized along different lines.

het·er·on·y·mous (het″ər-on′ĭ-məs) [*heter-* + Gr. *onyma* name] in ophthalmology, pertaining to the noncorresponding vertical halves of the visual fields of both eyes, i.e., the nasal half of the left eye and the nasal of the right, or the temporal half of the left eye and the temporal of the right.

het·ero·os·teo·plas·ty (het″ər-o-os′te-o-plas″te) [*hetero-* + *osteoplasty*] osteoplasty in which bone from an individual of one species is grafted to one of a different species.

het·ero·ov·u·lar (het″ər-o-ov′u-lər) dizygotic.

het·er·op·a·gus (het″ər-op′ə-gəs) [*hetero-* + *-pagus*] asymmetrical conjoined twins; see under *twin*.

het·er·op·a·thy (het″ər-op′ə-the) [*hetero-* + *-pathy*] 1. hyperesthesia. 2. allopathy.

het·ero·pen·to·san (het″ər-o-pen′to-san) any of a class of heterosaccharides in which the sugar components are pentoses, including gums, mucilages, and pectins.

het·er·oph·a·gy (het″ər-of′ə-je) [*hetero-* + *-phagy*] the taking into a cell of exogenous material by phagocytosis or pinocytosis, and digestion of the ingested material after fusion of the newly formed vacuole with a lysosome. Cf. *autophagy*.

het·er·oph·a·ny (het″ər-of′ə-ne) [*hetero-* + Gr. *phainein* to appear] a difference in the manifestations of the same condition.

het·ero·pha·sia (het″ər-o-fa′zhə) heterolalia.

het•ero•phil (het′ər-o-fil″) [*hetero-* + *-philic*] 1. a type of granular leukocyte represented in humans by the neutrophil and in other mammals by cells whose granules have variable sizes and staining characteristics. Called also *heterophilic leukocyte*. 2. heterophile.

het•ero•phile (het′ər-o-fīl″) pertaining to a group of cross-reacting antigens found in several species and having a species distribution that does not correspond to phylogenetic relationships, or to antibody directed against such antigens. Called also *heterophil.*

het•ero•phil•ic (het″ər-o-fil′ik) 1. pertaining to or having heterophils. 2. staining with a type of stain other than the usual one. 3. heterophile. 4. of cell adhesion molecules, binding to a nonidentical cell adhesion molecule in an adjacent cell.

het•ero•pho•ral•gia (het″ər-o-fo-ral′jə) [*hetero-* + Gr. *phoros* bearing + *-algia*] heterophoria associated with pain.

het•ero•pho•ria (het″ər-o-for′e-ə) [*hetero-* + Gr. *phora* movement, range] failure of the visual axes to remain parallel after the visual fusional stimuli have been eliminated. Types are named using the suffix *phoria* with a prefix indicating the direction of deviation. See *cyclophoria*, *esophoria*, *exophoria*, *hyperphoria*, and *hypophoria*. Called also *latent deviation*.

het•ero•phor•ic (het″ər-o-for′ik) pertaining to or characterized by heterophoria.

het•er•oph•thal•mia (het″ər-of-thal′me-ə) [*hetero-* + *ophthalm-* + *-ia*] difference in the direction of the axes, or in the color, of the two eyes.

het•er•oph•thal•mos (het″ər-of-thal′mos) heterophthalmia.

het•ero•phy•di•a•sis (het″ər-o-fə-di′ə-sis) heterophyiasis.

Het•er•oph•y•es (het″ər-of′e-ēz) [*hetero-* + Gr. *phyē* stature] a genus of minute trematodes of the family Heterophyidae, found in the middle third of the small intestine of fish-eating mammals. *H. heteroph′yes* is found in the Middle East and elsewhere in Asia. *H. katsura′dai* and *H. brevicae′ca* have been found in Japan and the Philippines.

het•ero•phy•i•a•sis (het″ər-o-fi-i′ə-sis) intestinal infection with trematodes of the genus *Heterophyes;* it is generally asymptomatic.

Het•ero•phy•i•dae (het″ər-o-fi′ĭ-de) a family of trematodes that includes the genera *Heterophyes* and *Metagonimus.*

het•ero•pla•sia (het″ər-o-pla′zhə) [*hetero-* + *-plasia*] the replacement of normal by abnormal tissue; malposition of normal cells.

progressive osseous h. osteoma cutis.

het•ero•plasm (het′ər-o-plaz″əm) any heterologous tissue.

het•ero•plas•my (het′ər-o-plaz″me) [*hetero-* + *-plasm*] the presence of multiple types of mitochondrial or chloroplast DNA within a single cell or individual.

het•ero•plas•tic (het′ər-o-plas″tik) 1. pertaining to heteroplasia. 2. xenogeneic.

het•ero•ploid (het′ər-o-ploid″) 1. pertaining to or characterized by heteroploidy. 2. an individual or cell with an abnormal number of chromosomes; cf. *aneuploid.*

het•ero•ploi•dy (het′ər-o-ploi″de) the state of having an abnormal number of chromosomes; cf. *aneuploidy.*

Het•er•op•o•da (het″ər-op′o-də) a genus of large spiders sometimes confused with tarantulas.

H. venato′ria a large spider found in shipments of tropical fruit, particularly bananas; its bite is painful, but not serious.

het•er•op•o•dal (het″ər-op′o-dəl) [*hetero-* + *pod-* + *-al*[1]] having branches or processes of different kinds; said of neurons.

het•ero•poly•mer•ic (het″ər-o-pol″e-mer′ik) [*hetero-* + *poly-* + Gr. *meros* a part] composed of dissimilar constituent building units; said of a macromolecule such as a protein.

het•ero•poly•sac•cha•ride (het″ər-o-pol″e-sak′ə-rīd) any polysaccharide macromolecule containing two or more different sugars, its function varying with the nature of its residues.

het•ero•pro•so•pus (het″ər-o-pro′so-pəs) [*hetero-* + Gr. *prosōpon* face] janiceps.

het•ero•pro•te•ose (het″ər-o-pro′te-ōs) a primary proteose that is insoluble in water but soluble in dilute salt solution.

het•er•op•sia (het″ər-op′se-ə) [*hetero-* + *-opsia*] unequal vision in the two eyes.

Het•er•op•tera (het″ər-op′tər-ə) [*hetero-* + Gr. *pteron* wing] a suborder of Hemiptera characterized by the possession of two pairs of wings, one horny, the other membranous; it includes the medically important families Cimicidae and Reduviidae.

het•er•op•tics (het″ər-op′tiks) [*hetero-* + *optics*] false or perverted vision; visual perception of objects not in the field of vision or misinterpretation of visual images.

het•ero•pyk•no•sis (het″ər-o-pik-no′sis) [*hetero-* + *pyknosis*] 1. the quality of showing variations in density throughout. 2. a state of differential condensation observed in comparison of different chromosomes, or of different regions of the same chromosome; it may be attenuated *(negative h.)* or accentuated *(positive h.).*

het•ero•pyk•not•ic (het″ər-o-pik-not′ik) pertaining to or characterized by heteropyknosis.

het•ero•re•sis•tant (het″ər-o-re-zis′tənt) having variable degrees of resistance, usually referring to a population of bacteria in which some are susceptible and some are resistant to a given drug.

het•ero•sac•cha•ride (het″ər-o-sak′ə-rīd) a polysaccharide containing a carbohydrate and a noncarbohydrate unit. Cf. *holosaccharide.*

het•ero•sce•das•tic•i•ty (het″ər-o-skə-das-tis′ĭ-te) [*hetero-* + Gr. *skedastikos* tending to scatter] the property of having unequal variances.

het•ero•scope (het′ər-o-skōp) [*heterophoria* + *-scope*] a pair of tubes so mounted as to allow observation of the progress of cases of heterophoria; called also *fusion tubes.*

het•er•os•co•py (het′ər-os′kə-pe) 1. inequality of vision in the two eyes. 2. examination with a heteroscope.

het•ero•sex•u•al (het″ər-o-sek′shoo-əl) 1. pertaining to the opposite sex; directed toward a person of the opposite sex, as opposed to *homosexual.* 2. one who is sexually attracted to persons of the opposite sex. 3. contrasexual (def. 2).

het•ero•sex•u•al•i•ty (het″ər-o-sek″shoo-al′ĭ-te) [*hetero-* + *sexuality*] sexual orientation to or activity with those of the opposite sex, as distinguished from *homosexuality.*

het•er•o•sis (het″ər-o′sis) [Gr. *heterōsis* alteration] the condition in which a first generation hybrid shows more vigor, as measured by growth, survival, or fertility, than either of the parent strains, usually a reflection of increased heterozygosity. Called also *hybrid vigor.*

het•er•os•mia (het″ər-os′me-ə) [*heter-* + *osm-*[1] + *-ia*] any parosmia in which all olfactory stimuli are distorted in a similar way; cf. *cacosmia.*

het•er•os•po•rous (het″ər-os′pə-rəs) having spores of two kinds (such as megaspores and microspores), which reproduce asexually.

het•ero•sug•ges•tion (het″ər-o-səg-jes′chən) [*hetero-* + *suggestion*] suggestion received from another person; opposed to *autosuggestion.*

het•ero•tax•ia (het″ər-o-tak′se-ə) [*hetero-* + Gr. *taxis* arrangement] anomalous placement or transposition of viscera or parts; called also *situs ambiguus.* See also *heterotaxy syndrome*, under *syndrome.*

het•ero•tax•ic (het″ər-o-tak′sik) affected with heterotaxia.

het•ero•tax•is (het″ər-o-tak′sis) heterotaxia.

het•ero•taxy (het′ə-ro-tak″se) heterotaxia.

het•ero•thal•lism (het″ər-o-thal′iz-əm) a form of sexual reproduction in which the isogamete must fuse with a gamete formed by a cell of a different mating type, as in various algae and fungi. **heterothal′lic** *adj*

het•ero•therm (het′ər-o-thərm″) an animal that exhibits heterothermy.

het•ero•ther•my (het′ər-o-thur″me) [*hetero-* + Gr. *thermē* heat] the exhibition of widely different body temperatures at different times or under different conditions, as certain species of birds, marsupials, or hibernating species. **heterother′mic** *adj*

het•ero•to•nia (het″ər-o-to′ne-ə) [*hetero-* + *ton-* + *-ia*] a state characterized by variations in tension or tone. **heteroton′ic** *adj*

het•ero•to•pia (het″ər-o-to′pe-ə) [*hetero-* + *top-* + *-ia*] 1. malposition. 2. ectopia. 3. choristoma.

band h., laminar h. an anomaly of the cerebral cortex in which a heterotopic band of gray matter is found between the lateral ventricles and the cortex; affected patients may have mental retardation or epilepsy.

periventricular nodular h. a genetically heterogeneous anomaly of the cerebral cortex in which nodular masses of gray matter line the walls of the ventricles and protrude into the lumen. Many persons with this condition develop absence epilepsy around the second decade of life.

het•ero•top•ic (het″ər-o-top′ik) 1. ectopic. 2. transplanted into a site or position that an organ or tissue does not normally occupy; said of a graft or transplant.

het•er•ot•o•py (het″ər-ot′ə-pe) 1. malposition. 2. ectopia.

het•ero•trans•plant (het″ər-o-trans′plant) xenograft.

het•ero•trans•plan•ta•tion (het″ər-o-trans″plan-ta′shən) xenogeneic transplantation.

het•ero•tri•cho•sis (het″ər-o-trĭ-ko′sis) [*hetero-* + *trichosis*] growth of hair of different colors on the body.

het•ero•tri•mer (het″ər-o-tri′mər) a trimer having at least one subunit that differs from the others.

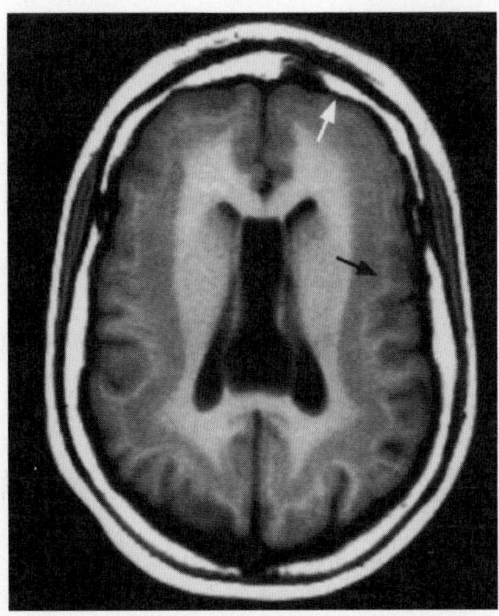

■ Band heterotopia in a T1 weighted MRI scan. A thin layer of white matter *(black arrow)* lies between the band of heterotopic gray matter and the cortical surface. Failure of cortical organization with lissencephaly is present in both frontal lobes *(white arrow)*.

het·ero·troph (het′ər-o-trōf″) an individual or organism suffering from heterotrophia.

het·ero·tro·phia (het″ər-o-tro′fe-ə) [*hetero-* + *troph-* + *-ia*] 1. any disorder or fault of nutrition. 2. a type of nutrition in which organisms derive energy from the oxidation of organic compounds by either consumption or absorption of other organisms.

het·ero·tro·phic (het″ər-o-tro′fik) 1. pertaining to or characterized by heterotrophia. 2. not self-sustaining; see *heterotrophia* (def. 2). Called also *organotrophic.* Cf. *autotrophic.*

het·er·ot·ro·phy (het″ər-ot′rə-fe) heterotrophia.

het·ero·tro·pia (het″ər-o-tro′pe-ə) strabismus.

het·ero·tro·pic (het′ər-o-tro″pik) [*hetero-* + *-tropic*] pertaining to an allosteric enzyme that is stimulated or inhibited by one or more effector molecules other than its substrate. Cf. *homotropic.*

het·er·ot·ro·py (het″ər-ot′rə-pe) strabismus.

het·ero·typ·ic (het″ə-ro-tip′ik) pertaining to, characteristic of, or belonging to a different type.

het·ero·typ·i·cal (het″ər-o-tip′ĭ-kəl) of a type differing from that usually or normally encountered; having characteristics peculiar to a different type; sometimes applied to the first meiotic division of the germ cells.

het·er·ox·e·nous (het″ər-ok′sə-nəs) [*hetero-* + Gr. *xenos* host] requiring more than one host in the life cycle; said of certain parasites. Called also digenetic.

het·er·ox·e·ny (het″ər-ok′sə-ne) the state of being heteroxenous.

het·ero·zo·ic (het″ər-o-zo′ik) [*hetero-* + *zoic*] pertaining to another animal or species of animal.

het·ero·zy·go·sis (het″ər-o-zi-go′sis) formation of a zygote by union of gametes of unlike genetic constitution.

het·ero·zy·gos·i·ty (het″ər-o-zi-gos′ĭ-te) [*hetero-* + *-zygosity*] the state of possessing pairs of different alleles at one or more loci. Cf. *homozygosity.* heterozy′gous *adj*

het·ero·zy·gote (het″ər-o-zi′gōt) [*hetero-* + *zygote*] an individual exhibiting heterozygosity.

compound h. an individual possessing two different mutant alleles at the same locus, one on each homologous chromosome.

double h. an individual possessing two different mutant alleles at each of two separate loci.

manifesting h. a female heterozygous for an X-linked disorder in whom, because of unfavorable X inactivation, the trait is expressed clinically with the same severity as in hemizygous affected males.

obligate h. see under *carrier.*

Heub·lein method (hoib′līn) [Arthur Carl *Heublein*, American radiologist, 1879–1932] see under *method.*

Heub·ner disease (endarteritis) (hoib′nər) [Johann Otto Leonhard *Heubner*, German pediatrician, 1843–1926] see under *disease.*

Heub·ner-Her·ter disease (hoib′nər hur′tər) [J.O.L. *Heubner;* Christian Archibald *Herter*, American physician, 1865–1910] the infantile form of celiac disease (q.v.).

heu·ris·tic (hu-ris′tik) [Gr. *heuriskein* to find out, discover] encouraging or promoting investigation; conducive to discovery.

Heu·ser membrane (hoi′zər) [Chester *Heuser*, American embryologist, 1885–1965] see *exocoelomic membrane*, under *membrane.*

HEV hepatitis E virus.

He·vea (he′ve-ə) the rubber trees, a genus of tropical trees of the family Euphorbiaceae, whose latex is the source of one kind of rubber. The most important species is *H. brasilien′sis.*

HEW Department of Health, Education, and Welfare; succeeded by the Department of Health and Human Services (HHS).

hex(a)- [Gr. *hex* six] a combining form meaning six.

hexa·ba·sic (hek″sə-ba′sik) [*hexa-* + *basic*] having six atoms replaceable by a base.

hexa·canth (hek″sə-kant′) having six hooks, such as an oncosphere.

hexa·chlo·ro·ben·zene (hek″sə-klor″o-ben′zēn) a compound used in organic synthesis and as a fungicide; it is toxic, causing cutaneous porphyria and liver disease, and may be carcinogenic. Since it does not break down easily, when used to preserve livestock feeds it may build up in the tissues of the animals.

hexa·chlo·ro·cy·clo·hex·ane (hek″sə-klor″o-si″klo-hek′sān) benzene hexachloride.

hexa·chlo·ro·eth·ane (hek″sə-klor″o-eth′ān) a crystalline anthelmintic used to treat fascioliasis in cattle and sheep.

hexa·chlo·ro·phene (hek″sə-klor′o-fēn) [USP] an antibacterial effective against gram-positive organisms; used as a topical anti-infective and detergent, mainly in soaps and dermatological preparations, and in veterinary medicine to combat flukes in poultry and ruminants.

hex·a·co·sane (hek″sə-ko′sān) [*hexa-* + Gr. *eikosi* twenty] an aliphatic hydrocarbon extracted from plant waxes.

hex·ad (hek′sad) 1. a group or combination of six similar or related entities. 2. any element having a valence of six.

hexa·dac·tyl·ia (hek″sə-dak-til′e-ə) hexadactyly.

hexa·dac·ty·lism (hek″sə-dak′tə-liz-əm) hexadactyly.

hexa·dac·ty·ly (hek″sə-dak′tə-le) [*hexa-* + *daktyl-* + *-ia*] the occurrence of six digits on one hand or foot.

hexa·dec·a·no·ate (hek″sə-dek″ə-no′āt) palmitate.

hexa·dec·a·no·ic ac·id (hek″sə-dek″ə-no′ik) systematic name for *palmitic acid;* see table at *fatty acid.*

Hex·a·drol (hek′sə-drol) trademark for preparations of dexamethasone.

hex·a·ene (hek′sə-ēn) a chemical compound in which there are six conjugated double bonds.

-hex·a·ene (hek′sə-ēn) a suffix denoting a chemical compound in which there are six conjugated double bonds.

Hex·a·ge·nia (hek″sə-je′ne-ə) a genus of mayflies (order Ephemeroptera). *H. bilinea′ta* is the lake fly, a species found on the shores of Lake Erie whose cast skins may cause asthma.

hexa·hy·dric (hek″sə-hi′drik) containing six atoms of hydrogen.

Hex·a·len (hek′sə-len) trademark for a preparation of altretamine.

hex·a·mer (hek′sə-mər) 1. a polymer molecule composed of six monomers. 2. a capsomer having six structural subunits.

hexa·meth·y·lat·ed (hek″sə-məth′ə-lāt-əd) containing six methyl groups.

hexa·meth·yl·en·amine (hek″sə-meth″əl-ēn-am′ēn) methenamine.

hexa·meth·yl·mel·amine (HMM) (hek″sə-meth″əl-mel′ə-mēn) altretamine.

hexa·meth·yl·phos·phor·a·mide (hek″sə-meth″əl-fos-for′ə-mīd) hempa.

hex·a·mine (hek″sə-mēn) methenamine.

Hex·am·i·ta (hek-sam′ĭ-tə) [*hexa-* + Gr. *mitos* thread] a genus of flagellate protozoa of the order Diplomonadida, phylum Parabasalia, having two anterior nuclei, six anterior flagella, and two posterior flagella. It comprises free-living species as well as intestinal parasites. *H. melea′gridis* causes enteritis in wild and domestic fowl; *H. mu′ris* is found in rats, mice, hamsters, and various wild rodents; *H. salmo′nis* is found in trout and salmon; and *H. colum′bae* is found in pigeons.

hex·am·i·ti·a·sis (heks-am″ĭ-ti′ə-sis) infection of birds, rodents, or fish with protozoa of the genus *Hexamita;* the most economically significant disease is an often fatal enteritis in turkeys caused by *H. meleagridis.*

hex·ane (hek′sān) n-hexane; an aliphatic hydrocarbon of the methane series, C_6H_{14}, obtained by distillation from petroleum, occurring as a colorless, volatile, highly flammable liquid with a characteristic odor; it is a constituent of petroleum benzin, and is used as a solvent and in spectrophotometry. Prolonged exposure can result in sensorimotor polyneuropathy.

hex·a·no·ate (hek″sə-no′āt) caproate.

hex·a·no·ic ac·id (hek″sə-no′ik) systematic name for *caproic acid.*

Hex·ap·o·da (hek-sap′o-də) [*hexa-* + Gr. *pous* foot] Insecta.

hex·atom·ic (hek″sə-tom′ik) containing six atoms of an element, or six replaceable univalent atoms.

hexa·va·lent (hek″sə-va′lənt) having a valence of six.

hex·en·milch (hek′sən-milk) [Ger. "witches' milk"] a milklike secretion from the breast of a newborn infant; called also *witch's milk.*

hex·et·i·dine (hek-set′ĭ-dēn) an antifungal, antiprotozoal, and antibacterial agent used mainly as a topical antiinfective in the treatment of vaginitis.

hex·hy·dric (heks-hi′drik) containing six atoms of replaceable hydrogen.

hexo·bar·bi·tal (hek″so-bahr′bĭ-təl) a short-acting barbiturate used as a sedative and hypnotic; administered orally.

hexo·bar·bi·tone (hek″so-bahr′bĭ-tōn) hexobarbital.

hexo·ben·dine (hek″so-ben′dēn) a vasodilator which has been used in the treatment of coronary insufficiency and stable angina.

hexo·ki·nase (hek″so-ki′nās) [EC 2.7.1.1] an enzyme of the transferase class that catalyzes the phosphorylation of hexose at the 6 carbon, the initial step in the cellular utilization of free hexoses. The enzyme occurs in all tissues and exists as various isozymes. Those in brain and muscles are relatively nonspecific; glucose, fructose, and mannose are effective substrates at low concentrations. The liver isozyme, often designated type IV, is called also *glucokinase* because it is more specific for glucose.

hex·on·ic ac·id (hek-son′ik) an aldonic acid formed specifically from an aldohexose, e.g., gluconic acid.

hex·o·pren·a·line sul·fate (hek″so-pren′ə-līn) a β_2-adrenergic receptor agonist used as a bronchodilator and sometimes as a tocolytic agent.

hex·os·amine (hek-sōs′ə-mēn) any of a class of amino sugars derived from hexoses.

hex·os·amin·i·dase (hek″sōs-ə-min′ĭ-dās) 1. any of the enzymes that cleave hexosamine or *N*-acetylhexosamine residues from gangliosides or other glycosides. Specific enzymes are named for the specific amino sugar and linkage that are potential substrates (e.g., α-*N*-acetylglucosaminidase). 2. β-*N*-acetylhexosaminidase.

h. A β-*N*-acetylhexosaminidase, isozyme A.

h. B β-*N*-acetylhexosaminidase, isozyme B.

hex·o·san (hek′so-san) any of the class of polysaccharides composed of hexose residues; included are fructosans, galactans, glucans, and mannans.

hex·o·sa·zone (hek-sōs′ə-zōn) any osazone formed from a hexose.

hex·ose (hek′sōs) a monosaccharide such as glucose or fructose that contains six carbon atoms in each molecule.

h. monophosphate a general term used to describe any or all of the phosphorylated hexoses involved in carbohydrate metabolism.

hex·ose 1-phos·phate uri·dyl·yl·trans·fer·ase (hek″sōs fos′fāt u″rĭ-dil″əl-trans′fər-ās) UDP-glucose–hexose-1-phosphate uridylyltransferase.

hex·o·side (hek′so-sīd) any glycoside in which the sugar component is a hexose.

hex·o·syl·trans·fer·ase (hek″so-səl-trans′fər-ās) [EC 2.4.1] one of a sub-subclass of enzymes of the transferase class that catalyze the transfer of a hexose group from one compound to another.

hex·u·lose (hek′su-lōs) ketohexose.

hex·uron·ic ac·id (hek″su-ron′ik) any uronic acid formed by oxidation of a hexose.

hex·yl (hek′səl) [*hex-* + *-yl*] a hydrocarbon, C_6H_{13}, in many isomeric forms.

hex·yl·re·sor·ci·nol (hek″səl-rə-sor′sĭ-nol) [USP] a substituted phenol with bactericidal properties used as an antiseptic in mouthwashes and skin wound cleansers.

Hey amputation (operation), hernia, ligament (ha) [William *Hey*, English surgeon, 1736–1819] see under *amputation;* see *Cooper hernia*, under *hernia;* and see *margo falciformis hiatus saphenus.*

Hey·mann nephritis (ha′mahn) [Walter *Heymann*, Belgian-born American physician, 1901–1985] see under *nephritis.*

HF Hageman factor (factor XII; see *coagulation factors*, under *factor*); high frequency.

Hf hafnium.

Hfr high frequency of recombination; see under *cell.*

Hg mercury (L. *hydrargyrum*).

HGA human granulocytic anaplasmosis.

Hgb hemoglobin.

HGBV hepatitis GB virus.

HGE human granulocytic ehrlichiosis; see *human granulocytic anaplasmosis*, under *anaplasmosis.*

HGF hepatocyte growth factor.

HGG human gamma globulin.

HGH, hGH human growth hormone.

hGHr human growth hormone recombinant; see *somatropin.*

HGPRT hypoxanthine-guanine phosphoribosyltransferase, a common name for hypoxanthine phosphoribosyltransferase (HPRT).

HGV hepatitis G virus.

HHS Department of Health and Human Services (formerly Department of Health, Education, and Welfare), a department of the United States Government.

HHT hydroxyheptadecatrienoic acid.

HI hemagglutination inhibition; see under *test.*

5-HIAA 5-hydroxyindoleacetic acid.

hi·a·tion (hi-a′shən) yawning.

hi·a·tus (hi-a′təs) gen. and pl. *hia′tus* [L.] a gap, cleft, or opening. hia′tal *adj*

h. adducto′rius [TA] adductor hiatus: the opening between the long tendon of the adductor magnus and the femur, marking the distal end of the adductor canal; called also *h. tendineus.*

h. aor′ticus [TA] aortic hiatus: the opening in the diaphragm through which the aorta and thoracic duct pass.

h. cana′lis ner′vi petro′si majo′ris [TA] hiatus for greater petrosal nerve: an opening in the petrous part of the temporal bone in the floor of the middle cranial fossa that transmits the greater petrosal nerve and a branch of the middle meningeal artery.

h. cana′lis ner′vi petro′si mino′ris [TA] hiatus for lesser petrosal nerve: the small, laterally placed opening on the anterior surface of the pyramid of the temporal bone that transmits the lesser petrosal nerve.

esophageal h. h. oesophageus.

h. of facial canal h. canalis nervi petrosi majoris.

h. for greater petrosal nerve h. canalis nervi petrosi majoris.

h. for lesser petrosal nerve h. canalis nervi petrosi minoris.

leukemic h., h. leuke′micus a condition observed in acute myelogenous leukemia in which there are numerous myeloblasts and a number of mature neutrophils in the peripheral blood, with few or no intermediate forms.

h. maxilla′ris [TA], **maxillary h.** a small round or oval opening connecting the maxillary sinus and the middle nasal meatus; it is often indented so that the opening appears tubular. Called also *maxillary ostium* and *maxillary sinus ostium.*

h. oesopha′geus [TA] esophageal hiatus: the opening in the diaphragm for the passage of the esophagus and the vagus nerves.

pleuroperitoneal h., h. pleuroperitonea′lis a posterolateral opening in the fetal diaphragm; its failure to close leaves a congenital posterolateral defect that may become a site for a congenital diaphragmatic hernia. Called also *foramen of Bochdalek.*

h. sacra′lis [TA] sacral hiatus: the opening at the inferior end of the sacral canal formed by failure of the laminae of the fifth and sometimes the fourth sacral vertebrae to meet in the midline.

h. saphe′nus [TA] saphenous opening: the depression in the fascia lata that is bridged by the cribriform fascia and perforated by the great saphenous vein.

h. semiluna′ris [TA] semilunar hiatus: the deep semilunar groove anterior and inferior to the bulla of the ethmoid bone; the anterior

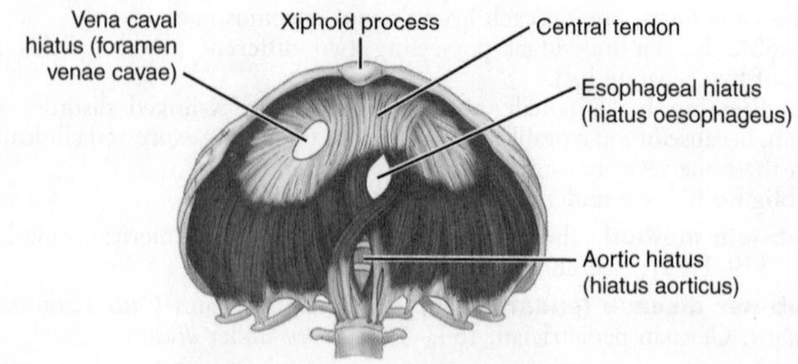

■ Inferior view of the diaphragm, showing the openings through which the aorta, esophagus, and vena cava pass.

ethmoidal (air) cells, the maxillary sinus, and sometimes the frontonasal duct drain through it via the ethmoid infundibulum.

h. tendi′neus h. adductorius.

tentorial h. incisura tentorii cerebelli.

urogenital h., h. urogenita′lis [TA] an opening in the pelvic floor between the medial borders of the levator ani muscles of each side, which gives passage to the urethra and, in females, the vagina.

vena caval h. foramen venae cavae.

Hibbs operation (hibz) [Russell Aubra *Hibbs*, New York surgeon, 1869–1932] see under *operation.*

hi•ber•na•tion (hi″bər-na′shən) [L. *hibernare* to spend the winter] 1. the dormant state in which certain animal species pass the winter; it is characterized by narcosis and by sharp reduction in body temperature and metabolic activity. Cf. *estivation.* 2. an analogous temporary reduction in function, such as of an organ.

artificial h. a dormant state that mimics a natural state of hibernation but is artificially induced in animals in captivity that would normally hibernate in the wild.

myocardial h. chronic but potentially reversible cardiac dysfunction caused by chronic myocardial ischemia, persisting at least until blood flow is restored. Cf. *myocardial stunning.*

hi•ber•no•ma (hi″bər-no′mə) [L. *hibernus* pertaining to the winter + *-oma*] a rare, benign, encapsulated lipoma arising from vestiges of brown fat resembling that in certain hibernating animals; it is a small, lobulated, nontender, tan to dark lesion occurring usually on the mediastinum or intrascapular region of female adults.

Hi•bic•lens (hi′bik-lens) trademark for a preparation of chlorhexidine gluconate.

HibTITER (hib′ti-ter) trademark for a preparation of *Haemophilus* b conjugate vaccine.

hic•cough (hik′əp) hiccup.

hic•cup (hik′əp) an involuntary spasmodic contraction of the diaphragm, causing a beginning inhalation that is suddenly checked by closure of the glottis, causing a characteristic sound; called also *hiccough* and *singultus.*

epidemic h's persistent hiccups sometimes seen with certain kinds of encephalitis.

Hick•man catheter (hik′mən) [R.O. *Hickman*, American surgeon, 20th century] see under *catheter.*

Hicks version (hiks) [John Braxton *Hicks*, English gynecologist, 1825–1897] see *Braxton Hicks version*, under *version.*

HIDA hepatobiliary iminodiacetic acid.

hide•bound (hīd′bound) bound down tightly to the subcutaneous tissues, said of the skin in scleroderma.

hi•drad•e•ni•tis (hi″drad-ə-ni′tis) [*hidraden-* + *-itis*] inflammation of a sweat gland, usually of the apocrine type. Called also *hydradenitis.*

h. axilla′ris h. suppurativa.

neutrophilic eccrine h. a skin eruption seen most often in cancer patients undergoing chemotherapy, consisting of edematous macules, papules, or plaques, usually on the trunk or limbs, with pathological changes in the eccrine sweat glands and an inflammatory neutrophilic infiltrate.

h. suppurati′va a chronic suppurative disease of skin that bears apocrine sweat glands, chiefly in the axillae or anogenital region, caused by occlusion of pores with secondary bacterial infection of the glands. Tender red abscesses develop, enlarge, and eventually break through the skin, yielding purulent or seropurulent drainage. When lesions heal, fibrosis remains, and recurrences lead to sinus tract formation and scarring. Called also *acne inversa* and *apocrinitis.*

hidraden(o)- a combining form denoting relationship to a sweat gland.

hi•drad•e•no•car•ci•no•ma (hi-drad″ə-no-kahr″sĭ-no′mə) [*hidradeno-* + *carcinoma*] a type of adnexal carcinoma arising in a sweat gland; called also *sweat gland carcinoma, syringadenocarcinoma,* and *syringocystadenocarcinoma.*

clear cell h. a very rare tumor occurring as an erythematous, sometimes ulcerated, nodule on the face or scalp; histologically, it resembles a clear cell hidradenoma but displays cellular atypia and frequently deep invasion.

hi•drad•e•noid (hi-drad′ə-noid) resembling a sweat gland; having components resembling elements of a sweat gland.

hi•drad•e•no•ma (hi-drad″ə-no′mə) [*hidraden-* + *-oma*] an adnexal adenoma originating in sweat gland epithelial cells; subtypes are variously designated according to histologic pattern and specific component from which the tumor appears to be derived.

clear cell h. a usually solitary, well circumscribed, nodular, solid or cystic adenoma originating in the eccrine sweat glands in middle-aged or older women; it is characterized histologically by large, glycogen-rich clear cells. Called also *eccrine acrospiroma, nodular h.,* and *solid-cystic h.*

eruptive h., h. erupti′vum see under *syringoma.*

nodular h. clear cell h.

papillary h., h. papilli′ferum a usually solitary, firm, nodular, and well circumscribed adenoma originating in the apocrine sweat glands and occurring in the vulva or anal region in adult women; it is characterized by a central cystic space into which papilliferous projections extend.

solid-cystic h. clear cell h.

hidr(o)- [Gr. *hidrōs* sweat] a combining form denoting relationship to sweat or to a sweat gland.

hi•dro•ac•an•tho•ma (hi″dro-ak″an-tho′mə) [*hidro-* + *acanthoma*] a type of eccrine adenoma.

h. sim′plex a keratotic lesion thought to be the intraepidermal counterpart of an eccrine poroma.

hi•dro•ad•e•no•ma (hi″dro-ad″ə-no′mə) hidradenoma.

hi•dro•cys•to•ma (hi″dro-sis-to′mə) [*hidro-* + *cystoma*] 1. a retention cyst of a sweat gland. 2. syringocystadenoma.

apocrine h. a type of benign adnexal tumor that is smooth, bluish, dome-shaped, and translucent; it is usually found as a solitary lesion on the face and is an adenomatous cystic proliferation of the apocrine sweat glands. Called also *apocrine cystadenoma.*

eccrine h. a type of small, cystic adnexal tumor thought to develop from secretions of eccrine sweat glands. It may occur singly or in groups, most often on the faces of older adults, and is often exacerbated by hot weather and perspiration.

hi•dro•poi•e•sis (hi″dro-poi-e′sis) [*hidro-* + *-poiesis*] the formation and secretion of sweat. **hidropoiet′ic** *adj*

hi•dros•ad•e•ni•tis (hi″dros-ad″ə-ni′tis) hidradenitis.

hi•dros•che•sis (hi-dros′kə-sis) anhidrosis.

hi•dro•sis (hi-dro′sis) sweating.

hi•drot•ic (hi-drot′ik, hĭ-drot′ik) 1. diaphoretic. 2. sudoriparous.

HIDS hyperimmunoglobulinemia D syndrome.

hi•e•mal (hi′ə-məl) [L. *hiemalis*, from *hiems* winter] pertaining to or occurring in winter.

hi•e•ma•lis (hi″ĕ-ma′lis) [L.] hiemal.

HIES hyper-immunoglobulin E syndrome.

high-grade (hi′grād′) occurring near the high end of a range, as of a malignancy.

High•more antrum, body (hi′mor) [Nathaniel *Highmore*, English anatomist, 1613–1685] see *sinus maxillaris* and *mediastinum testis.*

hi•la (hi′lə) [L.] plural of *hilum.*

hi•li (hi′li) [L.] plural of *hilus.*

Hill posterior gastropexy (hil) [Lucius D. *Hill*, American surgeon, born 1921] see under *gastropexy.*

Hill sign (hil) [Sir Leonard Erskine *Hill*, English physiologist, 1866–1952] see under *sign.*

Hill-Sachs lesion (hill′ saks′) [Harold Arthur *Hill*, American radiologist, 1901–1973; Maurice D. *Sachs*, American radiologist, 1909–1987] see under *lesion.*

hill•ock (hil′ək) a small prominence or elevation.

auricular h's embryonic tubercles adjoining the first pharyngeal groove; they give rise to the auricle of the ear and adjacent structures. Called also *h's of His.*

axon h. the conical expansion of an axon at its point of attachment to the body of the nerve cell.

h's of His auricular h's.

seminal h. colliculus seminalis.

Hil•ton muscle, sac, white line (hil′tən) [John *Hilton*, English surgeon, 1804–1878] see under *line* and see *musculus aryepiglotticus* and *sacculus laryngis.*

hi•lum (hi′ləm) pl. *hi′la* [L. "a small thing, a trifle"] a depression or pit at the part of an organ where vessels and nerves enter. Formerly called *hilus.* **hi′lar** *adj*

h. of adrenal gland h. glandulae suprarenalis.

h. of caudal olivary nucleus h. nuclei olivaris inferioris.

h. of dentate nucleus h. nuclei dentati.

h. glan′dulae suprare′nalis [TA] hilum of adrenal or suprarenal gland: the depression on the anterior surface of the gland where the suprarenal vein enters it.

h. of inferior olivary nucleus h. nuclei olivaris inferioris.

h. of kidney h. renale.

h. liena′le TA alternative for *h. splenicum.*

h. of liver porta hepatis.

h. of lung h. pulmonis.

h. of lymph node, h. lymphoglan′dulae h. nodi lymphoidei.

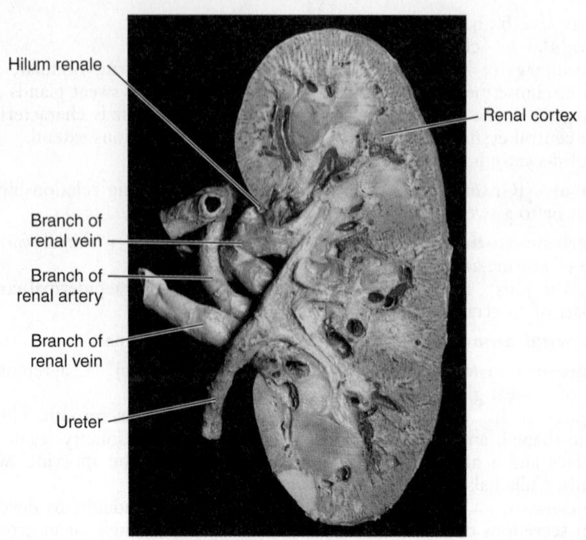

■ Longitudinal section through the kidney, showing the hilum renale.

h. no′di lympha′tici, h. no′di lymphoi′dei [TA] hilum of lymph node: the indentation on a lymph node where the arteries enter and the veins and efferent lymphatic vessels leave.

h. nu′clei denta′ti [TA] hilum of dentate nucleus: the white core of the dentate nucleus of the cerebellum.

h. nu′clei oliva′ris cauda′lis h. nuclei olivaris inferioris.

h. nu′clei oliva′ris inferio′ris [TA] hilum of inferior olivary nucleus: the white core of the inferior olivary nucleus of the medulla oblongata, most prominent medially. Called also *h. of caudal olivary nucleus* and *h. nuclei olivaris caudalis.*

h. ova′rii [TA] hilum of ovary: the point on the mesovarial border of the ovary where the vessels and nerves enter.

h. pulmo′nis [TA] hilum of lung: the depression on the mediastinal surface of the lung where the bronchus and the blood vessels and nerves enter.

h. rena′le [TA] hilum of kidney: the indented area on the medial margin of the kidney where the vessels, nerves, and ureter enter.

h. sple′nicum [TA] hilum of spleen: the fissure on the gastric surface of the spleen where the vessels and nerves enter; called also *h. lienale* [TA alternative].

h. of suprarenal gland h. glandulae suprarenalis.

hi•lus (hi′ləs) pl. *hi′li.* hilum.

hi•man•to•sis (hi″mən-to′sis) [Gr. *himantōsis,* from *himas* strap] elongation of the uvula.

hind•brain (hīnd′brān″) rhombencephalon.

hind•foot (hīnd′foot″) the posterior portion of the foot, comprising the region of the talus and calcaneus.

hind•gut (hīnd′gut″) 1. the embryonic structure from which chiefly the colon is formed. 2. the posterior ectodermal portion of the alimentary tract of invertebrates, such as arthropods; it comprises an intestine and a rectum.

hind-kid•ney (hīnd-kid′ne) metanephros.

hind•quar•ter (hīnd′kwor-tər) in a quadruped, the hind limb with the adjacent loin, pelvis, and musculature.

Hines-Ban•nick syndrome (hīnz′ ban′ik) [Edgar Alphonso *Hines,* Jr., American physician, 1905–1978; Edwin *Bannick,* American physician, 20th century] see under *syndrome.*

Hines-Brown test (hīnz′ broun′) [E.A. *Hines,* Jr.; George Elgie *Brown,* American physician, 1885–1935] see under *test.*

hinge-bow (hinj′bo) adjustable axis face-bow.

Hin•man syndrome (hin′mən) [Frank *Hinman* Jr., American urologist, born 1915] see under *syndrome.*

hip (hip) 1. the area of the body lateral to and including the hip joint; in official terminology called *coxa.* 2. loosely, the hip joint (*articulatio coxae* [TA]).

irritable h. term used for a group of inflammatory conditions of the hip, including coxitis, septic arthritis, and transient synovitis.

snapping h. a condition characterized by an audible or palpable snapping sensation that occurs during hip movement associated with exercise or normal daily activities, often accompanied by pain. It is classified as *external,* caused by sudden displacement of a thickened iliotibial band or gluteus maximus muscle over the greater trochanter; *internal,* caused by snapping of the iliopsoas tendon over the iliopectineal eminence; or *intra-articular,* caused by mechanical abnormalities within the joint.

HIPAA Health Insurance Portability and Accountability Act.

Hip•pel see *von Hippel.*

Hip•pe•la•tes (hip″ə-la′tēz) a genus of small flies of the family Chloropidae. *H. fla′vipes* and *H. pal′lipes* may be mechanical vectors of yaws in Haiti and Jamaica. *H. pu′sio* is the eye gnat, a mechanical vector of epidemic conjunctivitis across the entire southern part of the United States.

Hip•peu•tis (hi-pu′tis) a genus of fresh water snails of the family Planorbidae. *H. canto′ri* is a species found in eastern China that is one of the principal intermediate hosts of the trematode *Fasciolopsis buski.*

hipp(o)- [Gr. *hippos* horse] a combining form denoting relationship to a horse.

Hip•po•bos•ca (hip″o-bos′kə) [*hippo-* + Gr. *boskein* to feed] the typical genus of the family Hippoboscidae; the winged tick flies. They are pupiparous, dipterous, and parasitic to various mammals. *H. ru′fipes* is a South American species whose bite transmits *Trypanosoma theileri.*

hip•po•bos•cid (hip″o-bos′kid) 1. pertaining to the family Hippoboscidae. 2. any fly of the family Hippoboscidae.

Hip•po•bos•ci•dae (hip″o-bos′kĭ-de) a family of parasitic flies found on birds and mammals; some have wings, others are wingless. It includes the genera *Hippobosca, Melophagus,* and *Pseudolynchia.*

hip•po•cam•pus (hip″o-kam′pəs) [Gr. *hippokampos* sea horse] [TA] a convoluted elevation of gray matter extending the entire length of the floor of the temporal horn of the lateral ventricle; it is part of the limbic system and plays major roles in short term memory and spatial navigation. Official anatomical terminology and many authorities use the term to denote the entire structure including the hippocampus proper, the dentate gyrus, and the subicular complex (presubiculum, parasubiculum, and subiculum), but it can also be used more restrictively, most often denoting the hippocampus proper, in which case the entire structure may be called the *hippocampal formation.* **hippocam′pal** *adj*

h. proper, h. pro′prius [TA] the tightly curved region of the hippocampus between the dentate gyrus and the subiculum. Called also *cornu ammonis* [TA alternative] and *Ammon's horn.* The term is often used more broadly to denote the entire hippocampus (q.v.).

hip•po•co•pros•ter•ol (hip″o-ko-pros′tər-ol) [*hippo-* + *copro-* + *sterol*] a sterol found in the feces of herbivorous animals and derived from the phytosterol of grass and other food plants; possibly related to coprostanol.

Hip•poc•ra•tes of Cos (hĭ-pok′rə-tēz) the Father of Medicine, c. 460–c. 375 B.C., a student and teacher at the medical school on Cos. Of the many writings in the Hippocratic corpus, none can be surely ascribed to him. Hippocrates' anatomy was vague: he knew only bones in detail, not being sure of the organs, muscles, nerves, tendons, or blood vessels. His physiology was based on humoralism, diagnosis was directed toward general pathology, and prognosis predicted the stages, duration, and end of disease. Hippocrates' therapy was to restore the humoral equilibrium by ridding the body of excess humors and replacing the deficient humors. He relied on the healing power of nature and recommended diet and moderate exercise, but rejected drugs.

hip•po•crat•ic (hip″o-krat′ik) pertaining to or described by Hippocrates of Cos, or pertaining to his school of medicine.

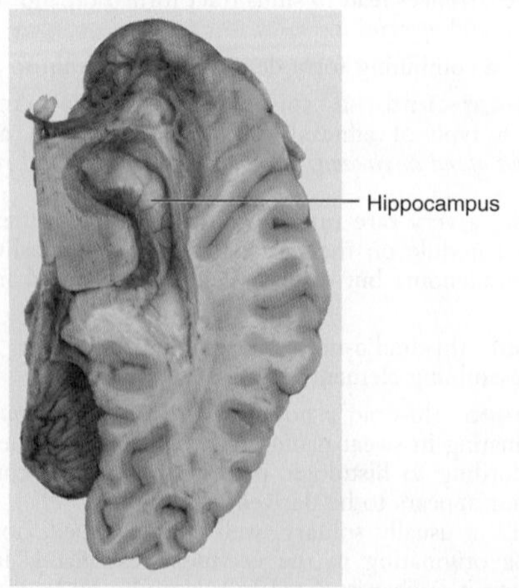

■ Hippocampus in a dissection of the right lateral ventricle.

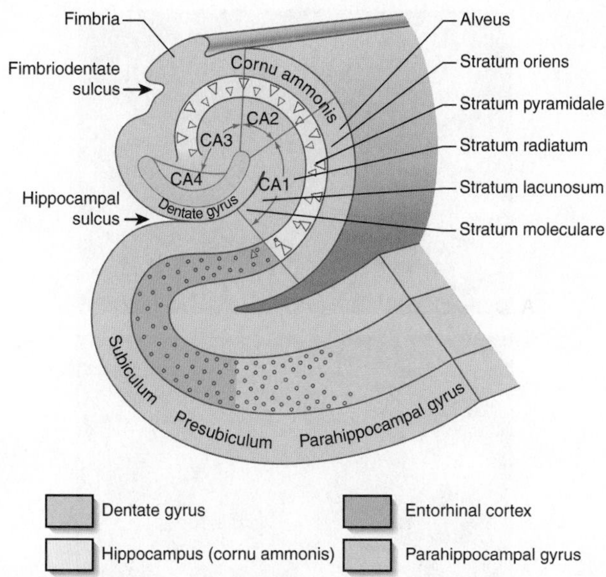

■ Schematic diagram of the hippocampal formation showing the disposition of the various cell fields. *CA1–4* denotes a classification scheme for subdividing the cornu region into a series of radially disposed fields.

Hip•po•crat•ic Oath (hip″o-krat′ik ōth) an oath of professional behavior sworn by physicians as they embark upon their medical careers; it is attributed to Hippocrates: "I swear by Apollo the physician, by Aesculapius, Hygeia, and Panacea, and I take to witness all the gods, all the goddesses, to keep according to my ability and my judgment the following Oath: To consider dear to me as my parents him who taught me this art; to live in common with him and if necessary to share my goods with him; to look upon his children as my own brothers, to teach them this art if they so desire without fee or written promise; to impart to my sons and the sons of the master who taught me and the disciples who have enrolled themselves and have agreed to the rules of the profession, but to these alone, the precepts and the instruction. I will prescribe regimen for the good of my patients according to my ability and my judgment and never do harm to anyone. To please no one will I prescribe a deadly drug, nor give advice which may cause his death. Nor will I give a woman a pessary to procure abortion. But I will preserve the purity of my life and my art. I will not cut for stone, even for patients in whom the disease is manifest; I will leave this operation to be performed by practitioners (specialists in this art). In every house where I come I will enter only for the good of my patients, keeping myself far from all intentional ill-doing and all seduction, and especially from the pleasures of love with women or with men, be they free or slaves. All that may come to my knowledge in the exercise of my profession or outside of my profession or in daily commerce with men, which ought not to be spread abroad, I will keep secret and will never reveal. If I keep this oath faithfully, may I enjoy my life and practice my art, respected by all men and in all times; but if I swerve from it or violate it, may the reverse be my lot."

Hip•pom•a•ne (hĭ-pom′ə-ne) a genus of tropical American trees of the family Euphorbiaceae. *H. mancinel′la* is the manchineel, a species with poisonous sap.

hip•pom•a•ne (hĭ-pom′ə-ne) small, rounded, flat, amber bodies found in the allantoic fluid of various animals, especially the ungulates and ruminants.

hip•pu•rate (hip′u-rāt) any salt of hippuric acid.

hip•pu•ric ac•id (hĭ-pūr′ik) a crystallizable acid from the urine of domestic animals, occasionally found in human urine. Called also *benzoylglycine* and *urobenzoic acid.*

hip•pu•ri•case (hip-ūr′i-kās) aminoacylase.

hip•pus (hip′əs) [Gr. *hippos*] abnormally exaggerated rhythmic contraction and dilation of the pupil, independent of changes in illumination or in fixation of the eyes; called also *pupillary athetosis.*

Hi•prex (hi′preks) trademark for a preparation of methenamine hippurate.

hir•ci (hur′si) (sing. *hir′cus*) [L.] [TA] axillary hairs: the hairs growing in the axilla.

hir•cis•mus (hir-siz′məs) [L. *hircus* goat] the strong odor of the axillae caused by bacterial decomposition of apocrine sweat.

hir•cus (hur′kəs) pl. *hir′ci* [L. "a goat"] see *hirci.*

Hirsch•berg method (hirsh′bərg) [Julius *Hirschberg,* German ophthalmologist, 1843–1925] see under *method.*

Hirsch•berg sign (hərsh′bərg) [Leonard Keene *Hirschberg,* American physician, early 20th century] see under *sign.*

Hirsch•feld canals (hərsh′feld) [Isador *Hirschfeld,* American dentist 1881–1965] interdental canals.

Hirsch•sprung disease (hirsh′sproong) [Harald *Hirschsprung,* Danish physician, 1830–1916] congenital megacolon.

hir•sute (hur′soot) [L. *hirsutus*] having abundant or excessive hair; see also *hirsutism.*

hir•su•ti•es (hir-soo′she-ēz) hirsutism.

hir•sut•ism (hur′soot-iz-əm) abnormal hairiness, especially an adult male pattern of hair distribution in women. Cf. *hypertrichosis.*

hi•ru•di•ci•dal (hĭ-roo″dĭ-si′dəl) destructive to leeches.

hi•ru•di•cide (hĭ-roo′dĭ-sīd) an agent that is destructive to leeches.

hi•ru•din (hĭ-roo′din) [L. *hirudo* leech] the active principle of the secretion of the buccal glands of leeches, which prevents coagulation of the blood by acting as an antithrombin; hirudin prepared by recombinant technology is a direct thrombin inhibitor that is used as an anticoagulant.

Hi•ru•di•na•ria (hir″oo-dĭ-nar′e-ə) a genus of leeches of the family Gnathobdellidae.

Hir•u•din•ea (hir″oo-din′e-ə) the leeches, a class of the phylum Annelida; it includes the genera *Haemadipsa, Haementeria, Haemopis, Hirudinaria, Hirudo, Limnatis,* and *Macrobdella.* See also *leech.*

hir•u•di•ni•a•sis (hir″oo-dĭ-ni′ə-sis) infection or infestation by leeches, such as in the nose, mouth, pharynx, or larynx or on the skin.

hir•u•di•ni•za•tion (hĭ-roo″dĭ-nĭ-za′shən) [L. *hirudo* leech] 1. the process of rendering the blood noncoagulable by the injection of hirudin. 2. leeching.

hi•ru•di•nize (hĭ-roo′dĭ-nīz) to render the blood noncoagulable by the injection of hirudin.

Hi•ru•do (hĭ-roo′do) [L. "leech"] a genus of leeches of the family Gnathobdellidae. *H. japo′nica* and *H. medicina′lis* have been used medicinally (see *leeching*). Other species include *H. java′nica* of Indonesia and Burma, *H. quinquestria′ta* of Australia, and *H. trocti′na* of Europe. *H. aegypti′aca* has been renamed *Limnatis nilotica.*

His histidine.

His bundle (band), disease, spindle (his) [Wilhelm *His,* Jr., Swiss physician, 1863–1934] see under *bundle,* and see *trench fever,* under *fever,* and *aortic spindle* under *spindle.*

His bursa, space, zones (his) [Wilhelm *His,* Swiss anatomist and embryologist in Germany, 1831–1904] see under *bursa, space,* and *zone.*

His-Pur•kin•je system (his′ pər-kin′je) [W. *His,* Jr.; Johannes Evangelista *Purkinje,* Czech physiologist, 1787–1869] see under *system.*

His-Wer•ner disease (his′ ver′ner) [W. *His,* Jr.; Heinrich *Werner,* German physician, 1874–1946] trench fever.

Hiss capsule stain (his) [Philip Hanson *Hiss,* Jr., American bacteriologist, 1868–1913] see *Stains and Staining Methods,* under *stain.*

his•tam•i•nase (his-tam′ĭ-nās) amine oxidase (copper-containing).

his•ta•mine (his′tə-mēn) chemical name: 1*H*-imidazole-4-ethanamine. A decarboxylation product of histidine, $C_5H_9N_3$, found in all body tissues, particularly in the mast cells and their related blood basophils, the highest concentration being in the lungs. It is also present in ergot and other plants and may be synthesized outside the body from histidine or citric acid. It has several functions, including (1) dilation of capillaries, which increases capillary permeability and results in a drop of blood pressure, (2) contraction of most smooth muscle tissue, including bronchial smooth muscle of

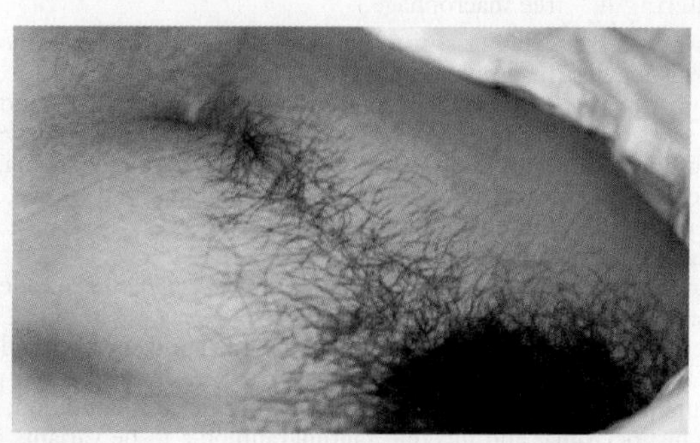

■ Hirsutism of the abdomen in a woman.

the lung, (3) induction of increased gastric secretion, and (4) acceleration of the heart rate. It is also responsible for the triple response, and is implicated as a mediator of immediate hypersensitivity. Cellular receptors of histamine include three types: the H_1 receptors mediate the contraction of smooth muscle and the effects on capillaries; the H_2 receptors mediate the acceleration of heart rate and the promotion of gastric acid secretion. Both H_1 and H_2 receptors mediate the contraction of vascular smooth muscle. H_3 receptors occur in a number of systems including the central nervous system and peripheral nerves, and are believed to play a role in regulation of the release of histamine and other neurotransmitters from neurons.

h.$_1$ the cellular receptor site for histamine responsible for the dilation of blood vessels and the contraction of smooth muscle; abbreviated H_1.

h.$_2$ the cellular receptor site for histamine responsible for the stimulation of heart rate and gastric secretion; abbreviated H_2.

h. phosphate [USP] the phosphate salt of histamine, having the same actions as the base; used in testing airway hyperresponsiveness in the diagnosis of asthma, administered by inhalation, and as a positive control in skin testing for allergy, administered subcutaneously.

his•tam•i•ne•mia (his-tam″ĭ-ne′me-ə) the presence of histamine in the blood.

his•ta•min•er•gic (his″tə-min-ur′jik) denoting those responses by histamine receptors to histamine that are blocked by histamine antagonists (e.g., cimetidine).

his•tan•ox•ia (his″tan-ok′se-ə) [*hist-* + *anoxia*] oxygen deprivation of the tissues due to a lessening of the blood supply.

His•ta•span (his′tə-span) trademark for preparations containing chlorpheniramine maleate.

his•tic (his′tik) pertaining to or of the nature of tissue.

his•ti•dase (his′tĭ-dās) histidine ammonia-lyase.

his•ti•dine (his′tĭ-dēn) an essential amino acid, α-amino-1H-imidazole-4-propanoic acid, first found as a decomposition product of the protamine of sturgeon testes; it is obtainable from many proteins by the action of sulfuric acid and water. The decarboxylation of histidine results in the formation of histamine. Symbols His and H. See table at *amino acid.*

his•ti•dine am•mo•nia-ly•ase (his′tĭ-dēn ə-mo′ne-ə li′ās) [EC 4.3.1.3] an enzyme of the lyase class that catalyzes the deamination of histidine to urocanate, the initial step of histidine catabolism. Deficiency of the enzyme, an autosomal recessive trait, causes histidinemia. Called also *histidase.*

his•ti•din•emia (his″tĭ-dĭ-ne′me-ə) an autosomal recessive aminoacidopathy caused by mutation in the histidine ammonia-lyase gene (*HAL*, locus: 12q22-q23), resulting in deficiency of the enzyme; it is characterized by accumulation of histidine in serum and urinary excretion of histidine and metabolites, but is usually benign. In some cases it may cause mild central nervous system dysfunction.

his•ti•din•uria (his″tĭ-dĭ-nu′re-ə) an aminoaciduria consisting of excessive histidine in the urine, usually in either histidinemia or during pregnancy.

his•ti•dyl (his′tĭ-dəl) the acyl radical of histidine.

histi(o)- [Gr. *histion* web] a combining form denoting relationship to tissue.

his•tio•blast (his′te-o-blast″) a local histiocyte (macrophage).

his•tio•cyte (his′te-o-sīt″) [*histio-* + *-cyte*] macrophage. **histiocyt′ic** *adj*

cardiac h. Anichkov cell.

palisaded h's, palisading h's histiocytes in a palisaded formation around a skin lesion of degenerated collagen, seen in rheumatoid neutrophilic dermatitis.

sea-blue h. an abnormal foamy, granulated histiocyte, sea-blue in color, containing ceroid material; seen in the sea-blue histiocyte syndrome, adult varieties of Niemann-Pick disease, and some forms of hemolytic anemia.

wandering h. free macrophage.

his•tio•cy•to•ma (his″te-o-si-to′mə) [*histiocyte* + *-oma*] a tumor containing histiocytes (macrophages).

benign fibrous h. any of a group of benign skin tumors found in the dermis and containing macrophages and fibroblasts. This term is variable; some authorities broadly include neoplasms such as dermatofibroma, nodular subepidermal fibrosis, and sclerosing hemangioma, but others limit it to cover only one of the conditions.

h. cu′tis dermatofibroma.

fibrous h. 1. see *benign fibrous h.* and *malignant fibrous h.* 2. dermatofibroma.

generalized eruptive h. a rare, self-limited skin disorder usually seen on the face, trunk, or proximal limbs, characterized by discolored papules that contain macrophages; some authorities consider this condition, benign fibrous histiocytoma, and juvenile xanthogranuloma to be variants of each other.

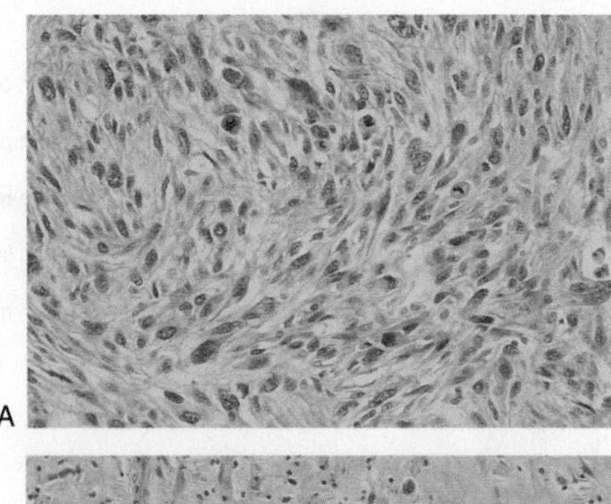

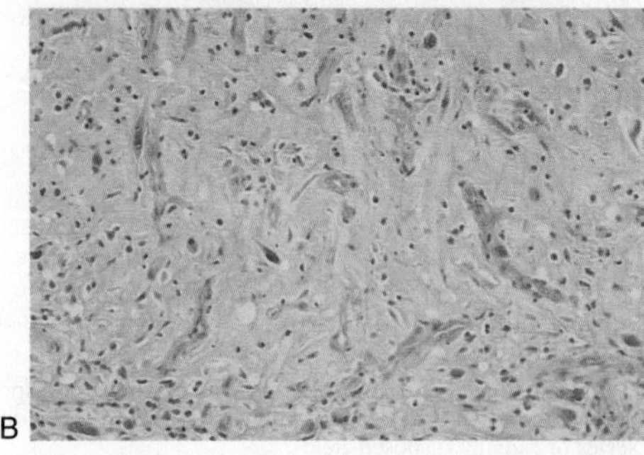

■ Malignant fibrous histiocytoma (MFH). *(A)*, Storiform-pleomorphic MFH, characterized by spindle-shaped and larger pleomorphic cells; *(B)*, myxoid MFH, characterized by myxoid tissue surrounding prominent blood vessels.

lipoid h. fibroxanthoma.

malignant fibrous h. any of a group of malignant neoplasms found mainly in soft tissues in middle-aged adults; depending on the tumor location and the classification system, the term is sometimes used synonymously with or as a general term including similar lesions such as atypical fibroxanthoma and dermatofibrosarcoma protuberans. The group is usually divided into five histological subtypes: *angiomatoid, giant cell, inflammatory, myxoid,* and *storiform-pleomorphic malignant fibrous histiocytomas.*

his•tio•cy•to•ma•to•sis (his″te-o-si″to-mə-to′sis) any generalized disorder of the reticuloendothelial system, such as xanthomatosis, Gaucher disease, Niemann-Pick disease, or lymphogranulomatosis.

his•tio•cy•to•sis (his″te-o-si-to′sis) any of a variety of proliferative disorders of macrophages (histiocytes), marked by the abnormal appearance of macrophages in the blood, or by abnormally elevated numbers of macrophages in lymphoid tissue.

benign cephalic h. a rare, self-limited skin disorder usually seen on the faces of young children, characterized by comma-shaped, discolored macules and papules that contain macrophages. Some authorities consider this condition, benign fibrous histiocytoma, and juvenile xanthogranuloma to be variants of each other.

crystal-storing h. the presence in bone marrow and other organs of macrophages that contain immunoglobulins, a rare finding in multiple myeloma and lymphoproliferative disorders.

generalized eruptive h. see under *histiocytoma.*

Langerhans cell h. any of a group of disorders characterized by proliferation of Langerhans cells, affecting children more often than adults. Lesions may be unifocal or multifocal and may involve the bone marrow, endocrine system, or lungs (the last being more common in adults than in children). Although the cause is uncertain, these disorders are believed to arise from disturbances in regulation of the immune system. Called *Langerhans cell granulomatosis.* Formerly called *h. X.*

Langerhans cell h., acute disseminated Letterer-Siwe disease.

Langerhans cell h., multifocal Langerhans cell histiocytosis occurring as erosive accumulations of proliferating Langerhans cells, commonly within the medullary cavities of bones, but also affecting the skin, gingiva, lungs, and stomach. It most commonly affects children and is accompanied by seborrheic eruptions, fever, frequent occurrences of otitis media, mastoiditis, and upper respiratory tract infection, often with lymphadenopathy and splenomegaly. When the triad of calvarial bone defects, exophthalmos, and diabetes insipidus is present, it is referred to as *Hand-Schüller-Christian disease.*

Langerhans cell h., unifocal Langerhans cell histiocytosis occurring as a single osteolytic lesion, usually in a long or flat bone; it may be asymptomatic or may produce bone pain, tenderness, and swelling and, sometimes, pathologic fracture.

malignant h. a rare type of histiocytosis found accompanying malignancies such as acute myelogenous leukemia; it may be a malignant transformation of stem cells of the monocyte series. It usually affects children or young adults and has a poor prognosis.

sea-blue h. sea-blue histiocyte syndrome.

sinus h. a disorder of the lymph nodes in which the distended sinuses are completely, or nearly completely, filled by histiocytes, as a result of active multiplication of the littoral cells.

sinus h. with massive lymphadenopathy (SHML) Rosai-Dorfman disease.

h. X Langerhans cell h.

his·ti·o·gen·ic (his″te-o-jen′ik) histogenous.

his·ti·oid (his′te-oid) histoid.

hist(o)- [Gr. *histos* web] a combining form denoting relationship to tissue.

his·to·blast (his′to-blast) [*histo-* + *-blast*] a tissue-forming cell.

his·to·chem·i·cal (his″to-kem′ĭ-kəl) pertaining to histochemistry or to the chemical components or activities of cells or tissues.

his·to·chem·is·try (his″to-kem′is-tre) the branch of histology which deals with the identification of chemical components in cells and tissues.

his·to·clas·tic (his″to-klas′tik) [*histo-* + *clastic*] breaking down tissue; said of certain cells.

his·to·clin·i·cal (his″to-klin′ĭ-kəl) combining histological and clinical evaluation.

his·to·com·pa·ti·bil·i·ty (his″to-kəm-pat″ĭ-bil′ĭ-te) 1. the quality or state of being histocompatible. 2. the degree to which two individuals are histocompatible.

his·to·com·pat·i·ble (his″to-kəm-pat′ĭ-bəl) pertaining to a donor and recipient who share a sufficient number of histocompatibility antigens (q.v.) so that a graft is accepted and remains functional.

his·to·cyte (his′to-sīt) macrophage.

his·to·di·ag·no·sis (his″to-di″əg-no′sis) [*histo-* + *diagnosis*] diagnosis by microscopic examination of the tissues.

his·to·dif·fer·en·ti·a·tion (his″to-dif″ər-en″she-a′shən) the acquisition of tissue characteristics by cell groups.

his·to·flu·o·res·cence (his″to-flo͞o″res′əns) fluorescence produced in the body by exposure to x-rays following the administration of a fluorescing drug.

his·to·gen·e·sis (his″to-jen′ə-sis) [*histo-* + *-genesis*] the formation or development of tissues from the undifferentiated cells of the germ layers of the embryo. histogenet′ic *adj*

his·tog·e·nous (his-toj′ə-nəs) [*histo-* + *-genous*] formed by the tissues.

his·tog·e·ny (his-toj′ə-ne) histogenesis.

his·to·gram (his′to-gram) [Gr. *histos* mast + *-gram*] a graphic display of a frequency distribution, represented by a series of rectangles dividing the data into classes, the height of a rectangle indicating the number of values that are contained in that class (class frequency) and the width of each base being the size of the intervals into which the classes have been divided.

his·tog·ra·phy (his-tog′rə-fe) [*histo-* + *-graphy*] description of the tissues.

his·to·hem·a·tog·e·nous (his″to-hem″ə-toj′ə-nəs) [*histo-* + *hemato-* + *-genous*] formed from both the tissues and the blood.

his·to·hy·dria (his″to-hi′dre-ə) the presence of an excessive amount of water in body tissue.

his·to·hy·pox·ia (his″to-hi-pok′se-ə) an abnormally diminished concentration of oxygen in the tissues.

his·toid (his′toid) [*hist-* + *-oid*] 1. weblike. 2. developed from but one kind of tissue. 3. like one of the tissues of the body.

his·to·in·com·pat·i·bil·i·ty (his″to-in″kəm-pat″ĭ-bil′ĭ-te) the quality or state of being histoincompatible.

his·to·in·com·pat·i·ble (his″to-in″kəm-pat′ĭ-bəl) pertaining to a donor and recipient who have sufficient differences in histocompatibility antigens to cause rejection of grafts.

his·to·ki·ne·sis (his″to-kĭ-ne′sis) [*histo-* + *-kinesis*] movement in the tissues of the body.

his·to·log·ic (his″to-loj′ik) pertaining to histology.

his·to·log·i·cal (his″to-loj′ĭ-kəl) histologic.

his·tol·o·gist (his-tol′ə-jist) a specialist in histology.

his·tol·o·gy (his-tol′ə-je) [*histo-* + *-logy*] that department of anatomy which deals with the minute structure, composition, and function of the tissues; called also *microscopic anatomy.*

normal h. the histology of normal tissues.

pathologic h. the histology of diseased tissues; called also *histopathology.*

his·tol·y·sate (his-tol′ə-zāt) a substance formed by histolysis.

his·tol·y·sis (his-tol′ə-sis) [*histo-* + *-lysis*] the dissolution or the breaking down of tissues.

his·to·lyt·ic (his″to-lit′ik) 1. pertaining to or characterized by histolysis. 2. causing histolysis.

his·to·meta·plas·tic (his″to-met″ə-plas′tik) pertaining to, characterized by, or stimulating metaplasia of tissue.

his·tom·e·try (his-tom′ə-tre) the measurement of changes in cells, such as in laboratory animals administered a given substance.

His·to·mo·nas (his″to-mo′nəs) [*histo-* + Gr. *monas* unit, from *monos* single] a genus of ameboflagellate protozoa of the order Trichomonadida, parasitic in the cecum and liver of turkeys, chickens, pheasants, guinea fowl, and other wild and domestic fowl. *H. melea′gridis* is the only pathogenic species, being the etiologic agent of histomoniasis, which is especially severe in turkeys. It is usually transmitted in the eggs of the nematode coparasite *Heterakis gallinae.*

his·to·mo·ni·a·sis (his″to-mo-ni′ə-sis) an infectious protozoal disease caused by *Histomonas meleagridis,* which is especially lethal to turkeys although chickens and other fowl may also be affected. It is characterized by ulcerative and necrotic lesions of the cecum and liver, and the head may be cyanotic. Called also *blackhead* and *enterohepatitis.*

h. of turkeys the lethal type of histomoniasis seen in turkeys; there are lesions of the intestine and liver and a dark discoloration of the comb.

his·to·mor·phol·o·gy (his″to-mor-fol′ə-je) histology.

his·to·mor·phom·e·try (his″to-mor-fom′ə-tre) [*histo-* + *morpho-* + *-metry*] computerized characterization of tissue comparing physical measurements and other qualities of different tissue areas. histomorphomet′ric *adj*

his·tone (his′tōn) any of various simple proteins containing many basic groups, soluble in water and insoluble in dilute ammonia; the globin of hemoglobin is a histone. Combined with nucleic acids they form nucleohistone, and are associated with DNA in chromatin. Some are poisonous and contain a great deal of phosphorus. Blood treated with histone is altered and has lower coagulability. Cf. *protamine.*

h. nucleinate a compound of nucleic acid and histone, the characteristic constituent of lymph glands, spleen, and thymus.

his·tone ace·tyl·trans·fer·ase (his′tōn ə-se″til-trans′fər-ās) [EC 2.3.1.48] any of a group of enzymes that add an acetyl group to histone, resulting in release of the restricted access to DNA that histone usually imposes.

his·tone de·ace·tyl·ase (his′tōn de″ə-se′til-ās) [EC 3.5.1.48] any of a group of enzymes that remove an acetyl group from histone and thus allow it to bind DNA and inhibit transcription.

his·tone meth·yl·trans·fer·ase (his′tōn meth″il-trans′fər-ās) any of several enzymes that add methyl groups to histones, causing them to retract into chromosomes to block further transcription.

his·ton·o·my (his-ton′ə-me) [*histo-* + Gr. *nomos* law] the scientific study of tissues based on the translation, into biological terms, of quantitative laws derived from histological measurement.

his·ton·uria (his-to-nu′re-ə) [*histone* + *-uria*] the presence of histone in the urine, seen in some types of leukemia and febrile illnesses.

his·to·pa·thol·o·gy (his″to-pə-thol′ə-je) [*histo-* + *pathology*] pathologic histology.

his·toph·a·gous (his-tof′ə-gəs) [*histo-* + *phag-* + *-ous*] eating or subsisting on tissues; applied to certain protozoa, especially those ciliates ectoparasitic on or endoparasitic in nonvital tissues of their hosts.

his·to·phi·lo·sis (his″to-fĭ-lo′sis) septicemic infection of cattle with *Histophilus somni*; the most serious form is fatal thromboembolic meningoencephalitis, but it may also take the form of bronchopneumonia, fibrinous pleuritis, myocarditis, or mastitis.

His·toph·i·lus (his-tof′ĭ-ləs) a genus of gram-negative, facultatively anaerobic bacteria of the family Pasteurellaceae.

H. somni a species that causes thromboembolic meningoencephalitis and histophilosis in cattle. Formerly called *Haemophilus somnus.*

his·to·phys·i·ol·o·gy (his″to-fiz″e-ol′ə-je) [*histo-* + *physiology*] the correlation of function with the microscopic structure of cells and tissues.

His·to·plas·ma (his″to-plaz′mə) a genus of Fungi Imperfecti of the form-class Hyphomycetes, form-family Moniliaceae.

H. capsula′tum the etiologic agent of classic histoplasmosis, occurring as small, oval, yeastlike cells which in tissue seem to be encapsulated but are not. It grows as a mycelial fungus in the soil and as a yeast at 37° C on agar or in tissue. Its perfect (sexual) stage is *Ajellomyces capsulatus.*

H. capsula′tum var. *duboi′sii* a variant form larger than other variants, the cause of the African form of histoplasmosis.

H. capsula′tum var. *farcimino′sum* the etiologic agent of lymphangitis epizootica, differing from the other variants in having smooth macroaleuriospores in the saprobic stage. Called also *H. farciminosum.*

H. farcimino′sum *H. capsulatum* var. *farciminosum.*

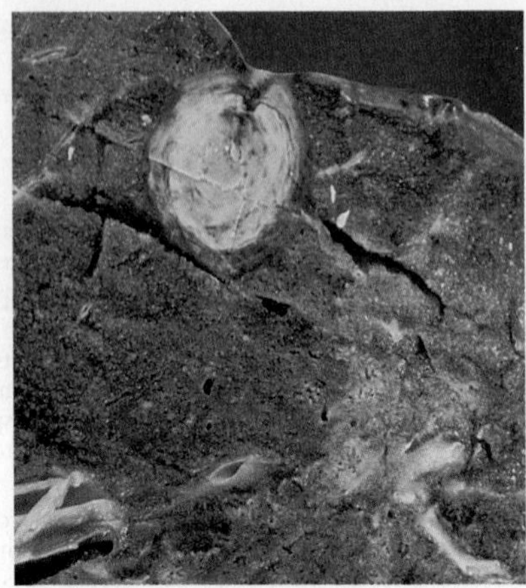

■ *Histoplasma* causing laminated granuloma of lung.

his·to·plas·min (his″to-plaz′min) [USP] a skin test antigen prepared from mycelial phase *Histoplasma capsulatum* organisms. Because positive skin tests are common in endemic areas and indicate only previous exposure, not necessarily active disease, histoplasmin is not useful in diagnosis of histoplasmosis. It is used primarily in epidemiologic surveys and in testing for cutaneous anergy in diagnosis of immunodeficiency.

his·to·plas·mo·ma (his″to-plaz-mo′mə) [*Histoplasma* + *-oma*] a rounded granuloma of the lung caused by infection with *Histoplasma capsulatum*, seen radiographically as a coin-shaped lesion.

his·to·plas·mo·sis (his″to-plaz-mo′sis) infection resulting from inhalation, or sometimes ingestion, of spores of *Histoplasma capsulatum*. It is usually asymptomatic, but in a few cases it may cause acute pneumonia, disseminated reticuloendothelial hyperplasia with hepatosplenomegaly and anemia, or an influenzalike illness with joint effusion and erythema nodosum. Reactivated infection, such as in immunocompromised patients, involves the lungs, meninges, heart, peritoneum, and adrenals, in that order of frequency. Called also *Darling disease*.

African h. a variant form of histoplasmosis seen across tropical parts of Africa, differentiated from the classic form by large yeast forms of *Histoplasma capsulatum* var. *duboisii* in the tissues.

h. capsula′tum incorrect term used for histoplasmosis caused by *H. capsulatum*.

h. duboi′sii African h.

equine h. epizootic lymphangitis.

ocular h. a disseminated type of choroiditis thought to be caused by *Histoplasma capsulatum*, resulting in scars in the periphery of the fundus near the optic nerve and characteristic disciform macular lesions.

progressive disseminated h. a condition, seen primarily in infants and in immunocompromised adults, caused by dissemination of *Histoplasma capsulatum* from the lungs to other areas of the body; in the oral, pharyngeal, and gastrointestinal tracts it may cause ulceration, bleeding, or obstruction and in the central nervous system it may present as focal cerebritis or diffuse meningitis.

his·to·ra·di·og·ra·phy (his″to-ra″de-og′rə-fe) [*histo-* + *radiography*] radiography of microscopic sections of tissue.

his·to·re·ten·tion (his″to-re-ten′shən) retention of matter by the tissues.

his·to·tel·i·o·sis (his″to-tel″e-o′sis) [*histo-* + Gr. *tēle* + *-osis*] the final differentiation of cells whose fate has already been determined irreversibly.

his·to·ther·a·py (his″to-ther′ə-pe) [*histo-* + *therapy*] the treatment of disease by the administration of animal tissues.

his·to·throm·bin (his″to-throm′bin) thrombin from connective tissue.

his·to·tome (his′to-tōm) [*histo-* + *-tome*] microtome.

his·tot·o·my (his-tot′ə-me) [*histo-* + *-tomy*] the dissection of the tissues; microtomy.

his·to·tox·ic (his′to-tok″sik) [*histo-* + *toxic*] poisonous to tissue or tissues.

his·to·troph (his′to-trōf) [*histo-* + Gr. *trophē* nourishment] in viviparous animals such as mammals, the totality of nutritive substances supplied to the embryo from sources other than the mother's blood. Cf. *embryotroph* and *hemotroph*.

his·to·tro·phic (his″to-tro′fik) 1. encouraging the formation of tissue. 2. pertaining to histotroph; with reference to nutrition through histotroph.

his·to·tro·pic (his″to-tro′pik) [*histo-* + *-tropic*] having special affinity for tissue cells.

his·to·zo·ic (his″to-zo′ik) [*histo-* + Gr. *zōē* life] living on or within the tissues; said of parasites.

his·trel·in ace·tate (his-trel′in) a synthetic preparation of gonadotropin-releasing hormone, used in treatment of central precocious puberty; administered by injection.

his·tri·on·ic (his″tre-on′ik) excessively dramatic or emotional; of or relating to the behavioral characteristics of histrionic personality disorder (q.v.).

hitch (hich) a device that fastens one thing to another.

psoas h. a type of ureteroneocystostomy in which the urinary bladder is raised within the abdominal cavity and sutured to the psoas minor muscle or tendon, in order for a ureter with a gap at the inferior end to be reimplanted.

Hit·torf number (hit′orf) [Johann Wilhelm *Hittorf*, German physicist, 1824–1914] see under *number*.

HIV human immunodeficiency virus.

hive (hīv) wheal.

hives (hīvz) urticaria.

Hiv·id (hiv′id) trademark for a preparation of zalcitabine.

HKAFO hip-knee-ankle-foot orthosis.

H⁺,K⁺-ATP·ase (a-te-pe′ās) a membrane-bound enzyme occurring on the secretory surfaces of parietal cells; it uses the energy derived from the hydrolysis of ATP to drive the exchange of ions across the cell membrane, secreting acid into the gastric lumen. Protons and chloride ions are pumped against gradients across the apical membranes of activated parietal cells into the gastric lumen, in exchange for potassium ions. In EC nomenclature, called *H^+/K^+-exchanging ATPase*. See also *adenosinetriphosphatase*.

H^+/K^+-ex·chang·ing ATP·ase (eks-chānj′ing a-te-pe′ās) [EC 3.6.3.10] EC nomenclature for *H^+,K^+-ATPase*.

H^+/K^+-trans·port·ing ATP·ase (trans-port′ing a-te-pe′ās) H^+,K^+-ATPase.

Hl latent hyperopia.

HLA human leukocyte antigens.

HLHS hypoplastic left heart syndrome.

Hm manifest hyperopia.

HMDP oxidronate (hydroxymethylene diphosphonate).

HMG 3-hydroxy-3-methylglutaryl.

hMG human menopausal gonadotropin; see *menotropins*.

HMM hexamethylmelamine.

HMO health maintenance organization.

HMPA hexamethylphosphoramide; see *hempa*.

HMPAO hexamethylpropyleneamine oxime; see *exametazime*.

HMS trademark for a preparation of medrysone.

HMSN hereditary motor and sensory neuropathy.

HMWK high-molecular-weight kininogen.

HMW-NCF high-molecular-weight neutrophil chemotactic factor.

HN2 mechlorethamine; see *mechlorethamine hydrochloride*.

HNF hepatocyte nuclear factor.

HNPCC hereditary nonpolyposis colorectal cancer.

hnRNA heterogeneous nuclear RNA.

hnRNP heterogeneous nuclear ribonucleoprotein.

HO hand orthosis; hip orthosis.

Ho holmium.

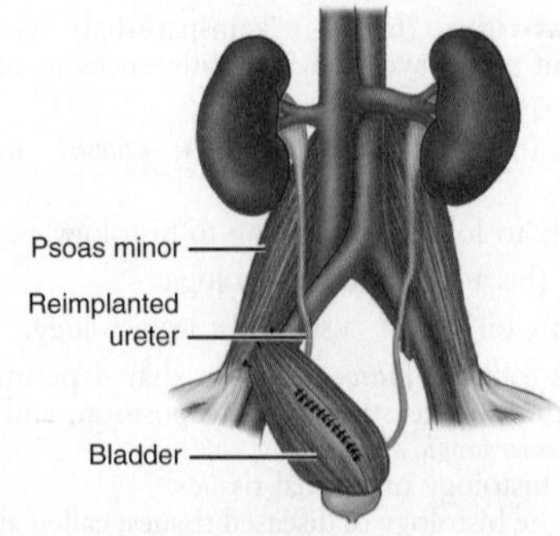

■ Psoas hitch in which the bladder has been opened by anterior cystotomy.

hoarse•ness (hors′nis) a rough or noisy quality of voice. Called also *trachyphonia.*

Ho•bo•ken nodules, valves (ho′bo-kən) [Nicolas van *Hoboken,* Dutch anatomist and physician, 1632–1678] see under *nodule* and *valve.*

hock (hok) the tarsal joint or region of the tarsus in the hind leg of a quadruped. Called also *ankle* and *hock joint.*
capped h. a hygromalike cyst or a thickening of the skin over the point of the calcaneus in the horse. Cf. *capped elbow.*
curby h. a hock affected with curb.
spring h. stringhalt.

HOCM hypertrophic obstructive cardiomyopathy.

Hodge pessary, plane (hoj) [Hugh Lenox *Hodge,* American gynecologist, 1796–1873] see under *pessary* and *plane.*

Hodg•en splint (hoj′ən) [John Thompson *Hodgen,* American surgeon, 1826–1882] see under *splint.*

Hodg•kin cells, disease (granuloma), sarcoma (hoj′kin) [Thomas *Hodgkin,* English physician, 1798–1866] see *Reed-Sternberg cells,* under *cell,* and see under *disease* and *sarcoma.*

Hodg•kin cycle (hoj′kin) [Alan Lloyd *Hodgkin,* British physiologist and Nobel prize winner, 1914–1998] see under *cycle.*

Hodg•son disease (hoj′son) [Joseph *Hodgson,* English physician, 1788–1869] see under *disease.*

ho•do•neu•ro•mere (ho″do-noor′o-mēr) [Gr. *hodos* path + *neuro-* + *-mere*] a segment of the embryonic trunk with its pair of nerves and their branches.

hoe (ho) a cutting dental instrument having its cutting edge at a right angle to the axis of its blade and no constriction at the junction of its shank and blade; used for breaking down tooth structure undermined by caries, smoothing cavity walls, and sharpening line and point angles.

Hoeh•ne sign (her′nə) [Ottomar *Hoehne,* German gynecologist, 1871–1932] see under *sign.*

Hof•bau•er cells (hawf′bou-ər) [J. Isfred Isidore *Hofbauer,* American gynecologist, 1878–1961] see under *cell.*

Hoff see *van't Hoff.*

Hof•fa disease, operation (haw′fə) [Albert *Hoffa,* German surgeon, 1859–1907] see under *disease,* and see *Lorenz operation,* under *operation.*

Hof•fa-Lo•renz operation (haw′fə lo′rənts) [A. *Hoffa;* Adolf *Lorenz,* Austrian surgeon, 1854–1946] Lorenz operation.

Hoff•mann phenomenon, sign (reflex) (hawf′mahn) [Johann *Hoffmann,* German neurologist, 1857–1919] see under *phenomenon* and *sign.*

Hoff•mann-Werd•nig syndrome (hawf′mahn vərd′nig) [J. *Hoffmann;* Guido *Werdnig,* Austrian neurologist, 1844–1919] Werdnig-Hoffmann disease.

Hof•mann bacillus (hawf′mahn) [Georg von *Hofmann*-Wellenhof, Austrian bacteriologist, 1843–1890] *Corynebacterium pseudodiphtheriticum.*

Hof•mann violet (hawf′mahn) [August Wilhelm von *Hofmann,* German chemist, 1818–1892] dahlia.

Hog•ness box (hog′nəs) [David S. *Hogness,* American molecular biologist, born 1925] TATA box.

hol•an•dric (hol-an′drik) [*hol-* + *andr-* + *-ic*] inherited exclusively through the male descent; transmitted through genes located on the Y chromosome.

Hol•de•ma•nia (hol″də-man′e-ə) [Lillian V. *Holdeman* Moore, American microbiologist, 20th century] a genus of bacteria of the family Erysipelotrichaceae, consisting of gram-positive, anaerobic, short rods that occur in pairs and short chains, isolated from human feces. The type species is *H. filifor′mis.*

Hol•den line (hōl′dən) [Luther *Holden,* English surgeon, 1815–1905] see under *line.*

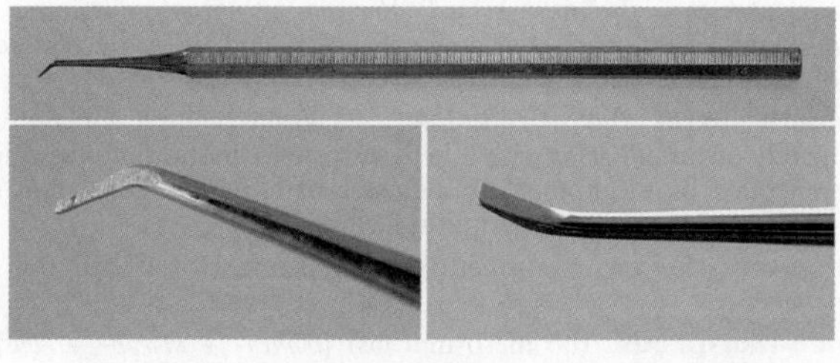

■ Hoes.

hold•fast (hōld′fast) a mass of material secreted by a cell or organism by which it is attached to a substrate or surface; called also *holdfast organ* or *organelle.*

hole (hōl) an opening or perforation.
bur h. one of a series of holes in the skull made with a bur in craniotomy.
macular h. loss of part or all of the thickness of an area of the macula lutea owing to trauma or degeneration, visible ophthalmoscopically as a round red spot with sharply defined edges.

Hol•ger Niel•sen method (hōl′gər nēl′sen) [*Holger Nielsen,* Danish army officer, 1866–1955] see under *method.*

hol•ism (hōl′iz-əm) [*hol-* + *-ism*] the theory that the determining factors in nature are organisms, which are wholes and not mechanisms and are irreducible, autonomous, and functionally greater than the sums of their parts.

ho•lis•tic (ho-lis′tik) considering the person as a functioning whole, or relating to the conception of a human being as a functioning whole; see also under *health.*

Hol•len•horst plaques (hol′ən-horst) [Robert W. *Hollenhorst,* American ophthalmologist, 1913–2008] see under *plaque.*

hol•low (hol′o) 1. a depressed area or concavity. 2. enclosing an empty space or cavity.
Sebileau h. a depressed area beneath the tongue, formed by the oral mucosa and the sublingual glands.

hol•low-back (hol′o-bak) see *lordosis.*

Holmes degeneration, phenomenon (sign) (hōmz) [Sir Gordon Morgan *Holmes,* Irish neurologist, 1876–1965] see under *degeneration,* and see *rebound phenomenon,* under *phenomenon.*

Holmes-Adie syndrome (hōmz′ a′de) [Sir G.M. *Holmes;* William John *Adie,* Australian neurologist in England, 1886–1935] Adie syndrome.

hol•mi•um (Ho) (hōl′me-əm) one of the rare earth elements, atomic number 67, atomic weight 164.930.

hol(o)- [Gr. *holos* entire] a combining form meaning entire, or denoting relationship to the whole.

holo•acar•di•us (hōl″o-ə-kahr′de-əs) [*holo-* + *acardius*] a separate, monozygotic twin represented by a more or less shapeless and unidentifiable mass; the vascular systems of the two fetuses are connected, and the circulation is accomplished solely by the heart of the well-developed twin.
h. ace′phalus an imperfectly formed free twin fetus lacking the cranial part of the body.
h. acor′mus an imperfectly formed free twin fetus lacking the caudal part of the body.
h. amor′phus an imperfectly formed free twin fetus entirely without form and recognizable parts.

holo•an•ti•gen (hōl″o-an′tĭ-jən) complete antigen, as opposed to hapten.

holo•ar•thric (hōl″o-ahr′thrik) pertaining to thallic-arthric conidiogenesis in which both of the cell walls form the conidia.

Holo•ba•sid•io•my•ce•tes (ho″lo-bə-sid″e-o-mi-se′tēz) [*holo-* + *basidium* + Gr. *mykēs* fungus] a class of perfect fungi of the subphylum Basidiomycotina, characterized by having an aseptate basidium; its orders include Agaricales, Aphyllophorales, Lycoperdales, and Phallales.

Holo•ba•sid•io•my•ce•ti•dae (ho″lo-bə-sid″e-o-mi-set′ĭ-de) name given to Holobasidiomycetes in some systems of classification, considering it a subclass.

holo•blas•tic (hōl″o-blas′tik) [*holo-* + *blast-* + *-ic*] 1. dividing completely; undergoing cleavage in which the entire zygote participates; see under *cleavage.* 2. pertaining to blastic conidiogenesis in which all of the cell wall is used to form the conidium.

holo•car•boxy•lase syn•the•tase (hōl″o-kahr-bok′sə-lās sin′thə-tās) an enzyme catalyzing the ATP-dependent biotinylation of the apoenzyme forms of the carboxylases acetyl-CoA carboxylase, methylcrotonoyl-CoA carboxylase, propionyl-CoA carboxylase, and pyruvate carboxylase, forming the active holoenzymes.

holo•car•boxy•lase syn•the•tase de•fi•cien•cy (hōl″o-kahr-bok′sə-lās sin′thə-tās) a biotin-responsive, autosomal recessive aminoacidopathy caused by mutations in the *HLCS* gene (locus: 21q22.1), which encodes holocarboxylase synthetase, leading to deficiency of activity of the biotin-containing carboxylases. It appears during the neonatal period or in infancy; features include metabolic ketoacidosis, organic aciduria, hyperammonemia, breathing difficulties, alopecia, skin rash, developmental delay, hypotonia, seizures, ataxia, and coma. Urine contains organic acids characteristic of each individual carboxylase deficiency. Called also *early-onset, neonatal,* or *infantile multiple carboxylase deficiency.*

holo•ce•phal•ic (hōl″o-sə-fal′ik) [*holo-* + *cephalic*] having a complete head but deficiencies in other parts of the body; said of a fetus.

holo•crine (ho′lo-krin) [*holo-* + Gr. *krinein* to separate] wholly secretory: denoting that type of glandular secretion in which the entire secreting cell, along with its accumulated secretion, forms the secreted matter of the gland, as in the sebaceous glands. Cf. *merocrine* and *apocrine.*

holo•di•a•stol•ic (hōl″o-di″ə-stol′ik) [*holo-* + *diastole*] pertaining to the entire diastole.

holo•en•dem•ic (hōl″o-en-dem′ik) [*holo-* + *endemic*] endemic at a high level early in life in a population and leading to a state of equilibrium such that the adult population shows evidence of the disease less often than do the children. Cf. *hyperendemic.*

holo•en•zyme (hōl″o-en′zīm) the functional compound formed by the combination of an apoenzyme and its appropriate coenzyme.

ho•log•a•my (ho-log′ə-me) [*holo-* + Gr. *gamos* marriage] the condition in which the gametes are of the same size and structural type as the somatic cells.

holo•gas•tros•chi•sis (hōl″o-gas-tros′kĭ-sis) [*holo-* + *gastro-* + *-schisis*] a developmental anomaly characterized by a fissure extending the entire length of the abdomen.

holo•gen•e•sis (hōl″o-jen′ə-sis) [*holo-* + *-genesis*] the theory that humans originated everywhere on earth, instead of in a certain special region or regions.

holo•gram (hōl′o-gram″) a three-dimensional image produced by holography.

hol•og•ra•phy (hōl-og′rə-fe) the recording of images in three-dimensional form on photographic film by exposing it to a laser beam reflected from the object under study.

acoustical h. holography in which sound waves reflected from an object under study are converted into light waves, which act on the emulsion of the film. The film is then exposed to a laser beam to give a three-dimensional effect.

holo•morph (hōl′o-morf″) [*holo-* + *-morph*] a whole fungus in all of its forms and stages; a *perfect fungus* includes a *teleomorph* (sexual stage) and one or more *anamorphs* (asexual stages), whereas an *imperfect fungus* includes an anamorph only.

holo•mor•pho•sis (hōl″o-mor-fo′sis) [*holo-* + *morphosis*] the complete regeneration of a lost part.

holo•phyt•ic (hōl″o-fit′ik) [*holo-* + *phyt-* + *-ic*] having a type of nutrition or feeding resembling that of a plant; said of certain photosynthesizing protozoa. Cf. *holozoic.*

holo•pros•en•ceph•a•ly (hōl″o-pros″ən-sef′ə-le) [*holo-* + *prosencephalon*] failure of cleavage of the prosencephalon resulting in incomplete or absent cortical separation and deficits in midline facial development; usually subdivided into alobar, semilobar, and lobar forms on the basis of degree of lobar separation. Facial dysmorphisms may include cyclopia, micro- or macrocephaly, micro- or anophthalmia, hypo- or hypertelorism, single nostril, and cleft lip or palate. It has a variety of causes, including chromosomal and single-gene disorders and environmental factors, and may occur alone or associated with various syndromes. Nonsyndromic familial forms show genetic heterogeneity, variable expressivity, and variable penetrance; mutations in the *Sonic Hedgehog (SHH)* gene are a major cause of the nonsyndromic autosomal dominant form.

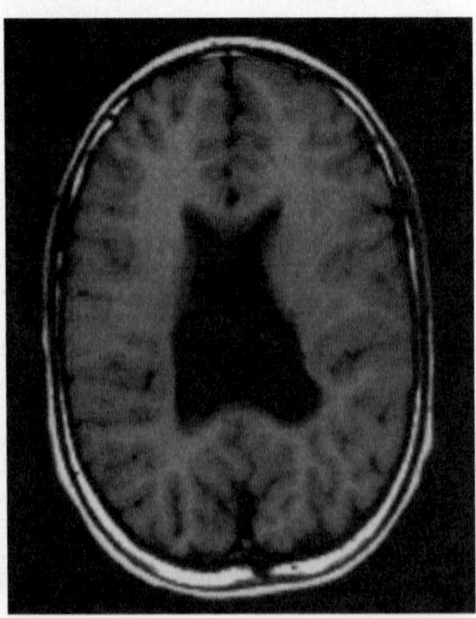

■ Lobar holoprosencephaly. MRI scan demonstrates failure of separation of the hemispheres and a persistent fused ventricle.

holo•ra•chis•chi•sis (hōl″o-rə-kis′kĭ-sis) [*holo-* + *rhachischisis*] rachischisis totalis.

holo•sac•cha•ride (hōl″o-sak′ə-rīd) a polysaccharide composed of sugar units only. Cf. *heterosaccharide.*

holo•sys•tol•ic (hōl″o-sis-tol′ik) [*holo-* + *systole*] pertaining to the entire systole.

holo•thal•lic (hōl″o-thal′ik) pertaining to or characterized by thallic conidiogenesis in which just one part of the parent cell disarticulates to form the conidium.

Hol•o•thu•ria (hōl″o-thu′re-ə) the most common genus of sea cucumbers; several species contain toxic holothurin.

holo•thu•rin (hōl″o-thoo′rin) a hemotoxic mixture of steroid glycosides obtained from sea cucumbers of the genus *Holothuria.*

Holo•thy•rus (hōl″o-thi′rəs) a genus of mites. *H. coccinel′la*, is a poisonous species found in Mauritius that can cause fatal poisoning in birds and painful swelling of the tongue and throat in humans.

ho•lot•o•py (ho-lot′ə-pe) [*holo-* + Gr. *topos* place] the position of an organ in relation to the whole body.

ho•lot•ri•chous (ho-lot′rĭ-kəs) [*holo-* + *trich-* + *-ous*] covered uniformly with cilia.

holo•type (hōl′o-tīp) the type culture of a species or subspecies of microorganisms, either because it was so designated in the original description or because the original description was based on only one strain.

holo•xen•ic (hōl″o-zen′ik) [*holo-* + *xen-* + *-ic*] raised under usual circumstances; said of an animal not raised under special laboratory conditions, as opposed to one raised in a germ-free environment. See also *axenic* and *gnotobiotic.*

holo•zo•ic (hōl″o-zo′ik) [*holo-* + *zoic*] having a type of nutrition or feeding resembling that of an animal, such as ingestion of whole organisms or relatively large particles. Called also *phagotrophic.* Cf. *holophytic* and *saprozoic.*

Holt-Oram syndrome (hōlt′ or′əm) [Mary Clayton *Holt*, British cardiologist, born 1924; Samuel *Oram*, British cardiologist, 1913–1991] see under *syndrome.*

Hol•ter monitor (hōl′tər) [Norman Jefferis *Holter*, American biophysicist, 1914–1983] see under *monitor.*

Holt•house hernia (hōlt′hous) [Carsten *Holthouse*, English surgeon, 1810–1901] see under *hernia.*

Holz•knecht space (holts′knekt) [Guido *Holzknecht*, Austrian radiologist, 1872–1931] see under *space.*

Ho•mans operation, sign (ho′mənz) [John *Homans*, American surgeon, 1877–1954] see under *operation* and *sign.*

Ho•ma•pin (ho′mə-pin) trademark for preparations of homatropine methylbromide.

hom•a•rine (hom′ə-rēn) an organic nitrogen compound which is found in lobster muscle and tissues of other marine animals. It is the methyl betaine of picolinic acid, $C_5H_4N^+(CH_3)CO_2^-$.

ho•mat•ro•pine (ho-mat′ro-pēn) a belladonna alkaloid having anticholinergic and antispasmodic actions.

h. hydrobromide [USP] the hydrobromide salt of homatropine, used in ophthalmology as a cycloplegic and mydriatic, applied topically to the conjunctiva.

h. methylbromide [USP] the 8-methyl derivative of homatropine hydrobromide, used as an antispasmodic and inhibitor of secretions, especially in gastrointestinal disorders, administered orally.

ho•max•i•al (ho-mak′se-əl) having axes of the same length.

home(o)- [Gr. *homoios* like, resembling] a combining form denoting sameness or similarity.

ho•meo•box (ho′me-o-boks″) any of a class of highly conserved DNA sequences, approximately 180 base pairs long, encoding a protein domain involved in binding to DNA; named for its initial discovery as a *Drosophila* locus important in homeotic mutation, but it also occurs in many other species, including humans, and is usually found in genes that control development.

ho•meo•chrome (ho′me-o-krōm″) [*homeo-* + *-chrome*] staining with mucin stains after formol-bichromate fixation; applied to certain serous cells of the salivary glands. Cf. *tropochrome.*

ho•meo•do•main (ho′me-o-do-mān″) a DNA-binding domain of approximately 60 amino acids with a helix-turn-helix motif, first identified as being encoded by the homeobox sequence of homeotic genes, but since then also found in other transcription factors.

ho•meo•met•ric (ho″me-o-met′rik) independent of a change in size; cf. *heterometric.*

ho•meo•mor•phous (ho″me-o-mor′fəs) [*homeo-* + *morph-* + *-ous*] of like form and structure.

ho•meo•os•teo•plas•ty (ho″me-o-os′te-o-plas″te) [*homeo-* + *osteo-* + *-plasty*] the grafting of bone from one individual to another within the same species.

ho•meo•path (ho′me-o-path) homeopathist.

ho•me•op•a•thist (ho″me-op′ə-thist) a specialist in homeopathy.

ho•me•op•a•thy (ho″me-op′ə-the) [*homeo-* + *-pathy*] a system of therapeutics founded by Samuel Hahnemann (1755–1843), in which diseases are treated by drugs which are capable of producing in healthy persons symptoms like those of the disease to be treated, the drug being administered in minute doses. Cf. *allopathy*. **homeopath′ic** *adj*

ho•meo•pla•sia (ho″me-o-pla′zhə) [*homeo-* + *-plasia*] the formation of new tissue like that adjacent to it and normal to the part.

ho•meo•plas•tic (ho″me-o-plas′tik) 1. resembling in structure the adjacent parts. 2. pertaining to, characterized by, or stimulating homeoplasia.

ho•me•or•rhe•sis (ho″me-o-re′sis) [*homeo-* + Gr. *rhein* to flow] the tendency to maintain a biological process, as a growth process, along a particular pathway despite the operation of factors tending to divert it.

ho•me•o•sis (ho″me-o′sis) [Gr. *homoiōsis* likeness, resemblance] the formation of a body part having the characteristics normally found in a related part at a different body site.

ho•meo•sta•sis (ho″me-o-sta′sis) [*homeo-* + *-stasis*] a tendency to stability in the normal body states (internal environment) of the organism. It is achieved by a system of control mechanisms activated by negative feedback; e.g., a high level of carbon dioxide in extracellular fluid triggers increased pulmonary ventilation, which in turn causes a decrease in carbon dioxide concentration. See also *equilibrium* (def. 1). **homeostat′ic** *adj*

ho•meo•ther•a•py (ho″me-o-ther′ə-pe) [*homeo-* + *therapy*] treatment or prevention of disease with a substance similar to but not the same as the causative agent of the disease.

ho•meo•therm (ho′me-o-thurm″) [*homeo-* + Gr. *thermē* heat] an animal that exhibits homeothermy; a so-called warm-blooded animal, as opposed to a poikilotherm.

ho•meo•ther•mism (ho″me-o-thur′miz-əm) homeothermy.

ho•meo•ther•my (ho′me-o-thur″me) the maintenance of a constant body temperature despite changes in the environmental temperature. Cf. *poikilothermy* (defs. 1, 2). **homeother′mal, homeother′mic** *adj*

ho•meo•typ•ic (ho″me-o-tip′ik) [*homeo-* + Gr. *typos* type] resembling the normal or usual type.

ho•meo•typ•i•cal (ho″me-o-tip′ĭ-kəl) homeotypic.

hom•er•gic (hōm-ur′jik) [*hom-* + Gr. *ergon* work] having the same effect; said of two drugs each of which produces the same overt effect.

Ho•mer Wright rosette (ho′mər rīt′) [James *Homer Wright*, American pathologist, 1871–1928] see under *rosette*.

hom•i•cide (hom′ĭ-sīd) [L. "murderer," from *homo* man + *caedere* to kill] the taking of the life of one person by another.

ho•mid•i•um (ho-mid′e-əm) a trypanosomicide used as the bromide and chloride salts in the treatment of infections with *Trypanosoma congolense* and *T. vivax* in cattle and horses. Its bromide salt is used in molecular genetics as a fluorochrome in the detection of double-stranded nucleic acids; in that context it is usually called *ethidium*.

hom•i•nal (hom′i-nəl) [L. *homo* man] 1. pertaining to human beings. 2. pertaining to male human beings.

hom•ing (ho′ming) any mechanism seen in cells causing them to migrate to a specific tissue, organ, or other location, such as that causing organ-specific metastasis or that mediating binding of particular lymphocytes to specific vascular endothelium.

hom•i•nid (hom′ĭ-nid) 1. pertaining to the family of humans (Hominidae). 2. a living or extinct human or humanlike type.

Ho•min•i•dae (ho-min′ĭ-de) [L. *homo* man + Gr. *eidos* resemblance] a family of primates (superfamily Hominoidea, suborder Anthropoidea), including both modern humans *(Homo sapiens)* and fossil hominids.

hom•i•noid (hom′ĭ-noid) 1. pertaining to the Hominoidea. 2. a member of the Hominoidea.

Hom•i•noi•dea (hom″ĭ-noi′de-ə) [L. *homo* man + Gr. *oeidos* likeness] a superfamily of primates, including the families Pongidae and Hominidae. Cf. *Anthropoidea*.

homme (um) [Fr.] man.

h. rouge (rōōzh) ["red man"] 1. a stage in mycosis fungoides in which the red plaques become infiltrated and coalesce over a wide area of the body. 2. the severe erythroderma seen in some cases of mycosis fungoides.

Ho•mo (ho′mo) [L. *man*] a genus of primates of the family Hominidae, including humans *(H. sa′piens)* and fossil hominids.

hom(o)- [Gr. *homos* same] 1. a combining form meaning the same. 2. a prefix in chemical names indicating the addition of one CH_2 group to the main compound.

ho•mo•ar•te•re•nol hy•dro•chlo•ride (ho″mo-ahr″tə-re′nol) nordefrin hydrochloride.

ho•mo•bio•tin (ho″mo-bi′o-tin) a homologue of biotin having an additional CH_2 group in the side chain and acting as a biotin antagonist.

ho•mo•body (ho′mo-bod″e) an antibody with an idiotypic determinant that is stereochemically similar to the epitope on the antigen against which the antibody was originally directed; it is therefore able to mimic the behavior of the antigen.

ho•mo•car•no•sin•ase (ho″mo-kahr′no-sĭ-nās) former name for an enzyme activity now believed to be part of the serum isozyme of X-His dipeptidase (carnosinase).

ho•mo•car•no•sine (ho″mo-kahr′no-sēn) a dipeptide consisting of γ-aminobutyric acid and histidine, found in the brain.

ho•mo•car•no•sin•o•sis (ho″mo-kahr″no-sĭ-no′sis) an autosomal recessive aminoacidopathy characterized by accumulation of homocarnosine in cerebrospinal fluid and the brain but not in plasma or urine, accompanied by carnosinuria. Progressive spastic paraplegia, mental deterioration, and retinal pigmentation may be sequelae. The disorder is due to deficiency of the serum isozyme of X-His dipeptidase, but its relationship to serum carnosinase deficiency (q.v.) has not been elucidated.

ho•mo•cen•tric (ho″mo-sen′trik) [*homo-* + *centric*] having the same center or focus.

ho•mo•chron•ic (ho″mo-kron′ik) homochronous.

ho•moch•ro•nous (ho-mok′ro-nəs) [*homo-* + *chron-* + *-ous*] 1. occurring at the same age or life stage in successive generations. 2. denoting the same age or stage of development, as tissue from one organism transplanted into another of the developmental stage.

ho•mo•cit•rul•line (ho″mo-sit′roo-lēn) an unusual amino acid formed by carbamoylation of the epsilon amino group of lysine; it is not normally present in urine but is excreted in hyperornithinemia-hyperammonemia-homocitrullinuria syndrome (q.v.).

ho•mo•cit•rul•lin•uria (ho″mo-sit″roo-lĭ-nu′re-ə) excess of homocitrulline in the urine; see *hyperornithinemia-hyperammonemia-homocitrullinuria syndrome*, under *syndrome*.

ho•mo•clad•ic (ho″mo-klad′ik) [*homo-* + Gr. *klados* branch] formed between small branches of the same artery; said of such an anastomosis.

ho•mo•cyc•lic (ho″mo-sik′lik, -si′klik) having or pertaining to a closed chain or ring formation which includes only atoms of the same element.

ho•mo•cys•te•ine (ho″mo-sis′te-ēn) a sulfur-containing amino acid homologous with cysteine and produced by demethylation of methionine. It can serve as an intermediate in the biosynthesis of cysteine from methionine via cystathionine or can be remethylated to methionine.

ho•mo•cys•te•in•emia (ho″mo-sis″te-in-e′me-ə) hyperhomocysteinemia.

ho•mo•cys•te•ine–tet•ra•hy•dro•fo•late meth•yl•trans•fer•ase (ho″mo-sis′teēn tet″rə-hi″dro-fo′lāt meth″əl-trans′fər-ās) methionine synthase.

ho•mo•cys•tine (ho″mo-sis′tēn) a disulfide homologous with cystine, formed by oxidation and subsequent condensation of two molecules of homocysteine; it is a source of sulfur in the body.

ho•mo•cys•tin•emia (ho″mo-sis″tin-e′me-ə) an excess of homocystine in the blood; see *homocystinuria*.

ho•mo•cys•tin•uria (ho″mo-sis″tin-u′re-ə) excretion of excess homocystine in the urine, a biochemical abnormality with a variety of autosomal recessive genetic as well as nongenetic causes, characterized by developmental delay, failure to thrive, and neurologic abnormalities, with other features such as hematologic abnormalities varying with specific causes. Principal causes include deficiency of activity of cystathionine β-synthase, any of several genetic disorders causing deficiency of activity of methionine synthase, and nutritional vitamin B_{12} or folate deficiency; certain drugs can also elevate urinary homocystine. In older literature, the term usually denotes the disorder caused by deficiency of cystathionine β-synthase activity.

ho•mo•cy•to•tro•pic (ho″mo-si″to-tro′pik) [*homo-* + *cyto-* + *-tropic*] having an affinity for cells from the same species; see under *antibody*.

ho•mo•des•mot•ic (ho″mo-dəs-mot′ik) [*homo-* + Gr. *desmos* bond] joining similar parts of the central nervous system; see under *fiber*.

ho•mo•di•mer (ho″mo-di′mər) a dimer consisting of identical subunits.

ho•mo•dont (ho′mo-dont) [*hom-* + Gr. *odous* tooth] having teeth of only one type.

ho•mod•ro•mous (ho-mod′ro-məs) [*homo-* + *dromo-* + *-ous*] moving or acting in the same direction.

homoe(o)- see *home(o)-*.

ho•moe•o•sis (ho″me-o′sis) homeosis.

ho•mo•erot•ic (ho″mo-ə-rot′ik) pertaining to or characterized by homoeroticism.

ho•mo•erot•i•cism (ho″mo-ə-rot′ĭ-siz-əm) 1. sexual feeling directed toward a person of the same sex. 2. a stage in the development of object relationships characterized by suppression of libidinal energies and occurring between the Oedipal stage and adolescence; see also *latency stage*, under *stage*.

ho•mo•fer•men•ta•tion (ho″mo-fur″mən-ta′shən) fermentation that produces one major product; the term is often used as a synonym of homolactic fermentation (q.v.).

ho•mo•fer•ment•er (ho″mo-fər-ment′ər) a microorganism that exhibits homofermentation.

ho•mo•gam•ete (ho″mo-gam′ēt) one of two gametes of the same size and structure, as the X chromosome in the human female.

ho•mo•ga•met•ic (ho″mo-gə-met′ik) pertaining to production of gametes containing only one kind of sex chromosome, as in the human female.

ho•mog•a•mous (ho-mog′ə-məs) characterized by or pertaining to homogamy.

ho•mog•a•my (ho-mog′ə-me) [*homo-* + Gr. *gamos* marriage] 1. inbreeding. 2. maturation of the male (stamens) and female (pistils) gametes of a flower at the same time. 3. the mating of like with like.

ho•mog•e•nate (ho-moj′ə-nāt) material subjected to homogenization, as tissue that is finely shredded and mixed.

ho•mo•ge•ne•i•ty (ho″mo-jə-ne′ĭ-te) 1. the state or quality of being homogeneous. 2. in magnetic resonance imaging, evenness of magnetic field strength across the entire field.

ho•mo•ge•ne•iza•tion (ho″mo-je″ne″ĭ-za′shən) homogenization.

ho•mo•ge•ne•ous (ho″mo-je′ne-əs) [*homo-* + Gr. *genos* kind] consisting of or composed of similar elements or ingredients; of a uniform quality throughout.

ho•mo•gen•e•sis (ho″mo-jen′ə-sis) [*homo-* + *-genesis*] reproduction by the same process in each generation. **homogenet′ic** *adj*

ho•mo•gen•ic (ho″mo-jen′ik) homozygous.

ho•mo•ge•nic•i•ty (ho″mo-jə-nis′ĭ-te) homogeneity.

ho•mog•e•ni•za•tion (ho-moj″ə-nĭ-za′shən) the act or process of rendering homogeneous.

ho•mog•e•nize (ho-moj′ə-nīz) to render homogeneous, or of uniform quality or consistency throughout.

ho•mo•ge•note (ho″mo-je′nōt) in bacterial genetics, a merozygote in which the corresponding alleles at a specific locus of the diploid region of the genome are identical.

ho•mog•e•nous (ho-moj′ə-nəs) 1. having a similarity of structure because of descent from a common ancestor. 2. homogeneous.

ho•mo•gen•tis•ate (ho″mo-jən-tis′āt) the anionic form of homogentisic acid.

ho•mo•gen•tis•ate 1,2-di•oxy•gen•ase (ho″mo-jən-tis′āt di-ok′sə-jən-ās) [EC 1.13.11.5] an enzyme of the oxidoreductase class that catalyzes the oxidation of homogentisate to form 4-methylacetoacetate as a step in the degradation of tyrosine and phenylalanine. Deficiency of the enzyme, an autosomal recessive trait, causes alkaptonuria.

ho•mo•gen•tis•ic ac•id (ho″mo-jen-tis′ik) an aromatic hydrocarbon formed as an intermediate in the catabolism of tyrosine and phenylalanine. It is accumulated abnormally and excreted in the urine in alkaptonuria.

ho•mo•gen•tis•ic ac•id ox•i•dase (ho″mo-jen-tis′ik as′id ok′sĭ-dās) homogentisate 1,2-dioxygenase.

ho•mo•gen•tis•ic ac•id ox•i•dase de•fi•cien•cy (ho″mo-jen-tis′ik as′id ok′sĭ-dās) alkaptonuria.

ho•mo•gen•ti•su•ria (ho″mo-jen″tĭ-su′re-ə) excretion of homogentisic acid in the urine, as occurs in alkaptonuria.

ho•mo•glan•du•lar (ho″mo-glan′du-lər) pertaining to the same gland.

ho•mo•graft (ho′mo-graft) allograft.

homoi(o)- see *home(o)-*.

ho•moi•op•o•dal (ho″moi-op′o-dəl) [*homoio-* + Gr. *pous* foot] having processes of one kind only; said of nerve cells.

ho•mo•kary•on (ho″mo-kar′e-on) [*homo-* + *karyon*] a multinucleate cell in which the nuclei are genetically identical. Cf. *heterokaryon*.

ho•mo•ker•a•to•plas•ty (ho″mo-ker′ə-to-plas″te) [*homo-* + *keratoplasty*] corneal transplantation with tissue derived from another individual of the same species.

ho•mo•lac•tic (ho″mo-lak′tik) producing lactic acid by way of the Embden-Meyerhof pathway; said of bacterial fermentation.

ho•mo•lat•er•al (ho″mo-lat′ər-əl) situated on, pertaining to, or affecting the same side; ipsilateral.

ho•mol•o•gen (ho-mol′o-jən) homologue (def. 2).

ho•mo•log•ic (ho″mə-loj′ik) homologous.

ho•mol•o•gous (ho-mol′ə-gəs) [Gr. *homologos* agreeing, correspondent] 1. corresponding in structure, position, origin, etc., as *(a)* the feathers of a bird and the scales of a fish, *(b)* antigen and its specific antibody, *(c)* allelic chromosomes. Cf. *analogous*. 2. allogeneic. 3. pertaining to an antibody and the antigen that elicited its production.

ho•mo•logue (ho′mo-log) 1. any homologous organ or part; an organ similar in structure, position, and origin to another organ, as the front flippers of a seal and human hands. See *analogue*. 2. in chemistry, one of a series of compounds, each of which is formed from the one before it by the addition of a constant element or a constant group of elements, as in the homologous series CH_4, C_2H_6, C_3H_8, etc.; called also *homologen*.

Propane Butane Pentane

■ Homologues.

ho•mol•o•gy (ho-mol′ə-je) [Gr. *homologia* agreement] the quality of being homologous; the morphological identity of corresponding parts; structural similarity due to descent from a common form.

ho•mol•y•sin (ho-mol′ə-sin) a lysin (e.g., isohemolysin) produced by injection into the body of antigen derived from an individual of the same species.

ho•mol•y•sis (ho-mol′ə-sis) [*homo-* + *-lysis*] lysis of a cell by extracts of the same type of tissue.

ho•mo•mor•phic (ho-mo-mor′fik) [*homo-* + *morph-* + *-ic*] morphologically similar.

ho•mo•mor•pho•sis (ho″mo-mor-fo′sis) [*homo-* + *morphosis*] regenerative replacement of a lost part by a similar part.

ho•mon•o•mous (ho-mon′ə-məs) [*homo-* + Gr. *nomos* law] designating homologous serial parts, such as somites.

ho•mon•y•mous (ho-mon′ĭ-məs) [*hom-* + Gr. *onoma* name] 1. having the same or corresponding sound or name. 2. in ophthalmology, pertaining to the corresponding vertical halves of the visual fields of both eyes, i.e., the right visual field (the nasal half of the left eye, the temporal of the right) and the left visual field (the temporal half of the left eye, the nasal of the right).

ho•mo•phil (ho′mo-fil) pertaining to antibody that reacts only with its homologous antigen.

ho•mo•phil•ic (ho″mo-fil′ik) [*homo-* + *-philic*] 1. having affinity for or reacting with a specific antigen; said of an antibody. 2. of cell adhesion molecules, binding to an identical cell adhesion molecule in an adjacent cell.

ho•mo•plas•my (ho′mo-plaz″me) [*homo-* + *-plasm*] the presence of only a single type of mitochondrial or chloroplast DNA within a cell or individual.

ho•mo•plas•tic (ho″mo-plas′tik) [*homo-* + *plastic*] 1. allogeneic. 2. denoting organs or parts, as the wings of birds and insects, that resemble one another in structure and function but not in origin or development.

ho•mo•plas•ty (ho′mo-plas″te) 1. allogeneic transplantation. 2. similarity between organs or parts not due to common ancestry.

ho•mo•poly•mer (ho″mo-pol′ĭ-mər) [*homo-* + *polymer*] a polymer containing the same repeating units of one amino acid in a molecule.

ho•mo•poly•sac•cha•ride (ho″mo-pol″e-sak′ə-rīd) a polysaccharide consisting of a single recurring monosaccharide unit, as glycogen is a polymer of glucose.

hom•or•gan•ic (hom″or-gan′ik) [*homo-* + *organic*] produced by the same or by homologous organs.

ho•mo•sal•ate (ho″mo-sal′āt) [USP] a salicylate compound used as a sunscreen, effective against ultraviolet B; applied topically to the skin.

ho•mo•sce•das•tic•i•ty (ho″mo-skə-das-tis′ĭ-te) [*homo-* + Gr. *skedastikos* tending to scatter] the property of having equal variances.

ho•mo•sex•u•al (ho″mo-sek′shoo-əl) 1. pertaining to the same sex; directed toward a person of the same sex; the opposite of heterosexual. 2. one who is sexually attracted to persons of the same sex.

ho•mo•sex•u•al•i•ty (ho″mo-sek″shoo-al′ĭ-te) [*homo-* + *sexuality*] sexual orientation toward or activity with those of the same sex, as distinguished from heterosexuality.

ho•mo•spore (ho′mo-spor) a homosporous organism.

ho•mos•po•rous (ho-mos′pə-rəs) [*homo-* + *spor-* + *-ous*] having spores of only one kind, which reproduce asexually.

ho•mo•thal•lism (ho″mo-thal′iz-əm) a form of sexual reproduction in which the isogamete produced by one cell can fuse with another isogamete produced by the same cell, as in various algae and fungi. Cf. *heterothallism.* **homothal′lic** *adj*

ho•mo•therm (ho′mo-thərm) homeotherm.

ho•mo•ther•mal (ho″mo-thur′məl) homeothermic.

ho•mo•ther•mic (ho″mo-thur′mik) homeothermic.

ho•mo•top•ic (ho″mo-top′ik) [*homo-* + *top-* + *-ic*] occurring at the same place upon the body.

ho•mo•trans•plant (ho″mo-trans′plant) allograft.

ho•mo•tro•pic (ho′mo-tro″pik) [*homo-* + *-tropic*] pertaining to an allosteric enzyme that is modulated by its usual substrate. Cf. *heterotropic.*

ho•mo•type (ho′mo-tīp″) [*homo-* + Gr. *typos* type] a part that has a reversed symmetry with its fellow of the opposite side of the body, as the hand. **homotyp′ic** *adj*

ho•mo•va•nil•lic ac•id (ho″mo-və-nil′ik) a product of catecholamine metabolism; elevated urinary levels occur in patients with pheochromocytoma or other catecholamine-secreting tumors. Abbreviated HVA.

ho•mox•e•nous (ho-mok′sə-nəs) [*homo-* + Gr. *xenos* host] requiring only one host in the life cycle; said of certain parasites. Called also *monoxenous.*

ho•mo•zo•ic (ho″mo-zo′ik) [*homo-* + *zoic*] pertaining to the same animal or the same species.

ho•mo•zy•go•sis (ho″mo-zi-go′sis) the formation of a zygote by the union of gametes that possess identical alleles at one or more loci.

ho•mo•zy•gos•i•ty (ho″mo-zi-gos′ĭ-te) [*homo-* + *-zygosity*] the state of possessing a pair of identical alleles at a given locus. Cf. *heterozygosity.* **homozy′gous** *adj*

ho•mo•zy•gote (ho″mo-zi′gōt) [*homo-* + *zygote*] an individual exhibiting homozygosity.

ho•mun•cu•lus (ho-munk′u-ləs) [L. "little man"] a grotesque drawing or model of a human figure that maps the motor and sensory regions of the body to the motor and primary somatosensory areas of the cerebral cortex; the representation of each body part is proportionate in size to its distribution in the cortex.

hon•ey (hun′e) a sweet-tasting substance deposited by the honeybee, which contains between 62 and 83 per cent glucose and fructose, and small amounts of sucrose, dextrin, and malic and acetic acids; its pH is 3.8 to 4.3.

hon•ey•comb (hun′e-kōm) 1. a network of hexagonal cells, made out of beeswax by honeybees. 2. something resembling this structure, such as a honeycomb lung. 3. reticulum (def. 3).

hon•ey•comb•ing (hun′e-kōm-ing) see *honeycomb lung*, under *lung.*

Hong Kong foot, influenza (hong′ kong″) [*Hong Kong*, China, where the conditions were first observed] see under *foot* and *influenza.*

hood (hood) a flexible covering.

extensor h. see under *expansion.*

tooth h. dental operculum.

hoof (hoof) [L. *ungula*] the hard, horny casing of the end of certain digits of a group of mammals that are, because of this feature, known as the *ungulates.* Called also *ungula.*

contracted h. a condition in a horse's hoof in which it becomes dried out and reduced in size, which causes inadequate pressure on the frog and lameness. Called also *contracted foot* and *contracted heel.*

ribbed h., ringed h. a condition in which the wall of a horse's hoof is marked by ridges running parallel with the coronary margin.

hook (hook) 1. a curved instrument, usually with a sharp point, designed for holding, elevating, or exerting traction on a tissue. 2. something with a long, thin, curved shape resembling that of this instrument; see *hamulus* and *uncus.*

h. of hamate bone hamulus ossis hamati.

muscle h. a hook for securing and isolating an extraocular muscle; called also *squint h.*

palate h. a hook for raising the palate in posterior rhinoscopy.

skin h. a forcepslike surgical instrument for retracting skin from an incision site.

squint h. muscle h.

Tyrrell h. a slender hook used in eye surgery.

hook-up (hook′əp) the method of arranging circuits, appliances, and electrodes for a particular diagnostic or therapeutic procedure.

hook•worm (hook′wurm″) any nematode of the family Ancylostomatidae. See also *hookworm disease*, under *disease.*

American h. *Necator americanus.*

dog h. any type that infests dogs, such as *Ancylostoma braziliense* or *A. caninum.*

European h. *Ancylostoma duodenale.*

New World h. *Necator americanus.*

Old World h. *Ancylostoma duodenale.*

rat h. *Nippostrongylus brasiliensis.*

h. of ruminants *Bunostomum.*

hoose (hōōz) verminous bronchitis in sheep, cattle, goats, and swine, caused by the presence of nematodes of genera *Dictyocaulus*, *Metastrongylus*, *Muellerius*, and *Protostrongylus* in the bronchial tubes or lungs; it is marked by cough, dyspnea, anorexia, and constipation. Called also *husk.*

Hoo•ver sign (hoo′vər) [Charles Franklin *Hoover*, American physician, 1865–1927] see under *sign.*

HOP a cancer chemotherapy regimen consisting of hydroxydaunomycin (doxorubicin), Oncovin (vincristine), and prednisone.

Hope sign (hōp) [James *Hope*, English physician, 1801–1841] see under *sign.*

Hop•lop•syl•lus anom•a•lus (hop″lo-sil′əs ə-nom′ə-ləs) a species of flea found in the ground squirrels of western United States and transmitting plague.

Hop•pe-Sey•ler test (hawp′ə-si′lər) [Ernst Felix Immanuel *Hoppe-Seyler*, German physiologic chemist, 1825–1895] see under *test.*

hops (hops) the dried flowers and cones of *Humulus lupulus*, the hop plant, used in brewing and medicinally for nervousness and insomnia.

Hor. decub. [L.] ho′ra decu′bitus (at bedtime).

hor•de•o•lum (hor-de′o-ləm) [L. "barleycorn"] a localized, purulent, inflammatory staphylococcal infection of one or more sebaceous glands (meibomian or zeisian) of the eyelids; called also *stye.*

external h. a hordeolum that occurs on the surface of the skin at the edge of the lid.

internal h. a hordeolum that is marked by swelling on the conjunctival surface of the lid.

hore•hound (hor′hound) 1. *Marrubium vulgare.* 2. the leaves and tops of *M. vulgare*, which have been used as an expectorant, bitter tonic, vermifuge, and laxative.

Hor. interm. [L.] ho′ris interme′diis (at the intermediate hours).

ho•ri•zons (hə-ri′zənz) numbered stages of human embryonic development defined by anatomical characteristics in order to circumvent individual uncertainties of age and variations of dimension from both natural and technical causes. Streeter outlined 23 horizons, each spanning 2 or 3 days, covering the 7-week period beginning with fertilization; they have been revised to the currently used Carnegie stages (q.v.).

Streeter h. see *horizons.*

hor•i•zon•tal (hor″ĭ-zon′təl) 1. parallel to the plane of the horizon; see also *horizontalis.* 2. occupying or confined to a single level in a hierarchy; see under *transmission.*

hor•i•zon•ta•lis (hor″ĭ-zon-ta′lis) [TA] horizontal: a term denoting relationship to this orientation when the body is in the anatomical, i.e., the upright, position.

hor•me•sis (hor-me′sis) [Gr. *hormēsis* rapid motion] the stimulating or beneficial effect of small doses of a toxic substance that at higher doses has an inhibitory or adverse effect.

hor•mi•on (hor′me-on) [Gr. *hormos* a wreath] the median anterior point of the spheno-occipital bones.

Hor•mo•car•di•ol (hor″mo-kahr′de-ol) [*hormone* + Gr. *kardia* heart] a commercial preparation of an extract from the sinus of the frog's heart that

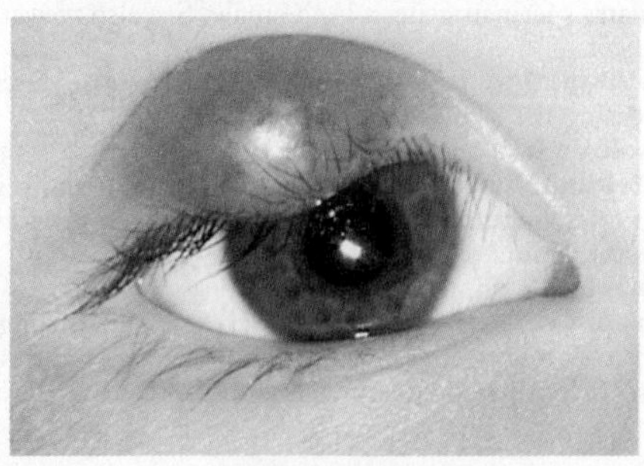

■ Hordeolum.

stimulates the contraction of the frog's ventricle; used as a coronary vasodilator.

Hor•mo•den•drum (hor″mo-den′drəm) a former genus of Fungi Imperfecti; many saprobic species have been placed in the genus *Cladosporium*, and human pathogens in *Fonsecaea*.

hor•mon•a•gogue (hor-mōn′ə-gog) [*hormone* + *-agogue*] an agent that stimulates the production of hormones.

hor•mone (hor′mōn) [Gr. *hormaein* to set in motion, spur on, from *hormē* impulse] a chemical substance produced in the body by an organ, cells of an organ, or scattered cells, having a specific regulatory effect on the activity of an organ or organs. The term was originally applied to substances secreted by endocrine glands and transported in the bloodstream to distant target organs, but later it was applied to various substances having similar actions but not produced by special glands. See also *endocrine system*, under *system*. **hormo′nal, hormon′ic** *adj*

Hormone

adaptive h. a hormone secreted during the organism's adaptation to unusual circumstances, which contributes to the ability to cope; e.g., corticosteroids and corticotropin.
adenohypophysial h's anterior pituitary h's.
adipokinetic h. 1. former name for β-lipotropin. 2. *(in the pl.)* lipolytic h's.
adrenocortical h. 1. any of the corticosteroids elaborated by the adrenal cortex; besides the glucocorticoids and mineralocorticoids, this classification also includes some androgens, progesterone, and perhaps estrogens. See also *corticosteroid.* 2. corticosteroid.
adrenocorticotropic h. (ACTH) corticotropin.
adrenomedullary h's substances secreted by the adrenal medulla, such as epinephrine and norepinephrine.
androgenic h. androgen.
anterior pituitary h's the hormones secreted by the adenohypophysis (anterior pituitary), including growth hormone, thyrotropin, prolactin, follicle-stimulating hormone, luteinizing hormone, β-lipotropin, and corticotropin. Called also *adenohypophysial h's.*
antidiuretic h. vasopressin.
antimüllerian h. a glycoprotein produced by Sertoli cells of the fetal testis that acts ipsilaterally in the male to suppress the paramesonephric (müllerian) ducts, consequently preventing development of the uterus and uterine tubes, thus influencing control of the formation of the male phenotype. Called also *müllerian inhibiting factor* or *substance*, *müllerian duct inhibitory factor*, and *müllerian regression factor.*
chromaffin h. a hormone released from chromaffin cells; epinephrine is a major type.
corpus luteum h. progesterone.
cortical h. corticosteroid.
corticotropin-releasing h. (CRH) a neuropeptide elaborated by the median eminence of the hypothalamus, the pancreas, and the brain; it binds to specific receptors on the corticotrophs of the adenohypophysis and stimulates production of corticotropin.
diabetogenic h. a hormone such as cortisol that causes gluconeogenesis. Called also *diabetogenic factor.*
ectopic h. a hormone released from a neoplasm or cells outside the usual source of the hormone. Such hormones may be useful as tumor markers. Cf. *eutopic h.*
estrogenic h. estrogen.
eutopic h. a peptide hormone released from its usual site or from a neoplasm of that tissue; cf. *ectopic h.*
fat-mobilizing h's lipolytic h's.
female sex h. estrogen.
fibroblast growth h. a peptide hormone secreted by the adenohypophysis, affecting many of the same cell types as platelet-derived growth factor; it is a potent mitogen of vascular endothelial cells and is a regulator of tissue vascularization.
follicle-stimulating h. (FSH) an anterior pituitary hormone that is a gonadotropic hormone, a glycopeptide of about 30,000 daltons that stimulates the growth and maturation of ovarian follicles, stimulates estrogen secretion, promotes the endometrial changes characteristic of the first portion (proliferative phase) of the mammalian menstrual cycle, and stimulates spermatogenesis in the male. See also *menotropins.* Called also *follitropin.*
follicle-stimulating h.–releasing h. (FSH-RH) luteinizing hormone–releasing h.
galactopoietic h. prolactin.
gastrointestinal h's hormones that originate in and regulate motor and secretory activity of the digestive organs, such as gastrin, secretin, and cholecystokinin.
gonadotropic h. gonadotropin.
gonadotropin-releasing h. (Gn-RH) 1. luteinizing hormone–releasing h. 2. more generally, any hypothalamic factor that stimulates the release of both follicle-stimulating hormone and luteinizing hormone.
growth h. (GH) 1. any of several related anterior pituitary hormones secreted episodically by the adenohypophysis that affect protein, carbohydrate, and lipid metabolism and control the rate of skeletal and visceral growth; their secretion is in part controlled by the hypothalamus. The major form of human growth hormone (hGH) is a single chain of 191 amino acids (about 21,500 daltons). Called also *somatotrophin*, *somatotropin*, and *somatotrophic* or *somatotropic h.* 2. a preparation of human growth hormone for pharmaceutical use; see *somatropin* and *somatrem.* 3. any substance that stimulates growth, such as a growth factor (q.v.).
growth h. release–inhibiting h. somatostatin.
growth h.–releasing h. (GH-RH) a neuropeptide elaborated in the hypothalamus that binds to specific receptors on the somatotrophs of the adenohypophysis and stimulates the secretion of growth hormone. Called also *somatocrinin*, *somatoliberin*, and *somatotropin-releasing h.*
human growth h. (hGH) see *growth h.*
hypophysiotropic h's hormones produced by the hypothalamus, usually releasing hormones, which maintain the endocrine functions of cells of the adenohypophysis.
inhibiting h's hormones elaborated by one structure that inhibit release of hormones from another structure, such as those from the hypothalamus that act on the adenohypophysis. Examples include follistatin, prolactin-inhibiting hormone (prolactostatin), and somatostatin. The term is applied to substances of established chemical identity; substances of unknown chemical structure are called *inhibiting factors* (see under *factor*).
interstitial cell–stimulating h. luteinizing h.
intestinal h's hormones that are active in the intestines, including both those produced by the enteroendocrine cells and those produced elsewhere that aid in digestion or other intestinal processes. Cf. *gastrointestinal h's.*
juvenile h. the secretion of the corpora allata which prevents metamorphosis, keeping the insect in the larval state and ensuring that the larva will molt several times and reach large size before pupating.
lactation h., lactogenic h. prolactin.
lipolytic h's hormones that promote the degradation of triacylglycerols to diacylglycerols, monoacylglycerols, glycerols, and fatty acids; they include the catecholamines, glucagon, growth hormone, and (in high levels only) corticotropin and thyroid-stimulating hormone. Called also *fat-mobilizing h's.*
lipotropic h. (LPH) lipotropin.
local h. a substance with hormonelike properties that acts at an anatomically restricted site; most are rapidly degraded. Examples are histamine, serotonin, angiotensin, and the prostaglandins. Called also *autacoid* and *autocoid.*
luteal h. progesterone.
luteinizing h. (LH) a glycoprotein anterior pituitary hormone that is a gonadotropin (28,000 daltons) and acts with follicle-stimulating hormone to promote ovulation as well as secretion of androgens and progesterone. It instigates and maintains the second (secretory) portion of the mammalian estrus and menstrual cycle. In females it is concerned with corpus luteum formation and in males it stimulates the development and functional activity of testicular Leydig cells. Called also *interstitial cell–stimulating h.* and *lutropin.*
luteinizing h.–releasing h. 1. a decapeptide hormone elaborated by the median eminence of the hypothalamus that binds to specific receptor sites on gonadotrophs of the adenohypophysis and stimulates the release of follicle-stimulating hormone and luteinizing hormone. High levels continuously maintained desensitize gonadotrophs and terminate gonadotropin release. Long-acting analogs are used to inhibit gonadal steroid secretion in individuals with prostate cancer and some other hormone-responsive cancers. Called also *follicle-stimulating hormone–releasing h.*, *gonadotropin-releasing h.*, *gonadoliberin*, and *luliberin.* 2. a preparation of the acetate and hydrochloride salts of this hormone obtained from the brains of certain food animals, used in the differential diagnosis of hypothalamic, pituitary, and gonadal dysfunction and

Hormone *Continued*

sometimes in treatment of types of male or female infertility or hypogonadism.

luteotropic h. prolactin.

male sex h. androgen.

melanin-concentrating h. a hormone expressed in the lateral hypothalamus that regulates food intake and sleep similarly to the orexins.

melanocyte-stimulating h., melanophore-stimulating h. (MSH) a melanotropic peptide that is an anterior pituitary hormone derived from pro-opiomelanocortin. Types are designated α, β, and γ_1 to γ_3. The acylated forms cause dispersion of pigment granules of melanocytes, producing a rapid change in skin coloration, while the non-acylated forms are neurotransmitters. α-MSH is identical to the N-terminal 13 residues of corticotropin, and β-MSH to the C-terminal 18 residues of γ-lipotropin. Immunoreactive "β-MSH" in humans consists of β- and γ-lipotropin. Administration of α-MSH or elevation of corticotropin in humans causes a slight increase in melanization. Called also *intermedin* and *melanotropin.*

neurohypophysial h's posterior pituitary h's.

ovarian h's the hormones secreted by the ovary, such as estrogens and progestational agents.

parathyroid h. a polypeptide hormone (84 amino acid residues) secreted by the parathyroid glands. It promotes release of calcium from bone to extracellular fluid by activating osteoclasts and inhibiting osteoblasts, indirectly promotes increased intestinal absorption of calcium, promotes renal tubular reabsorption of calcium and increased renal excretion of phosphates, and is a major regulator of bone metabolism. Secretion of parathyroid hormone increases when the level of calcium in the extracellular fluid is low. Its action is opposed by that of calcitonin. Called also *parathormone* and *parathyrin.*

pituitary h's see *anterior pituitary h's* and *posterior pituitary h's.*

placental h's the hormones produced by the placenta during pregnancy, including chorionic gonadotropin and certain other substances having estrogenic, progestational, or adrenocorticoid activity.

placental growth h. human placental lactogen.

posterior pituitary h's the hormones released from the neurohypophysis (posterior pituitary), which are formed in the neuronal cells of the hypothalamic nuclei and stored in nerve cell endings in the neurohypophysis. The principal ones are vasopressin and oxytocin. Called also *neurohypophysial h's.*

progestational h. 1. progesterone. 2. see under *agent.*

prolactin-inhibiting h. a hormone released by the hypothalamus that inhibits secretion of prolactin by the adenohypophysis. Called also *prolactin-inhibiting factor* and *prolactostatin.*

prolactin-releasing h. any of various hormones elaborated by the hypothalamus that stimulate the release of prolactin by the adenohypophysis. Most such activity is exerted by vasoactive intestinal peptide, although in humans thyrotropin-releasing h. can also have this action. Called also *prolactin-releasing factor* and *prolactoliberin.*

proparathyroid h. an inactive biosynthetic precursor of parathyroid hormone; it is of larger molecular size than the active hormone.

prothoracicotropic h. in the development of insects, the hormone that controls secretion of ecdysone by the prothoracic glands. It is secreted by a gland in the brain.

releasing h's hormones elaborated in one structure that cause the release of hormones from another structure, such as those from the hypothalamus that act on the adenohypophysis. The term is applied to substances of established chemical identity, whereas substances of unknown chemical structure are called *releasing factors* (see under *factor*).

sex h's the estrogens and androgens considered together.

somatotrophic h., somatotropic h. growth h.

somatotropin release–inhibiting h. somatostatin.

somatotropin-releasing h. (SRH) growth hormone–releasing h.

steroid h's hormones that are biologically active steroids; they are secreted by the adrenal cortex, testis, ovary, and placenta and include the progestogens, glucocorticoids, mineralocorticoids, androgens, and estrogens. They act by binding to specific receptors to form complexes, which then enhance or inhibit the expression of specific genes.

thyroid h's the hormones produced by the thyroid gland: thyroxine, triiodothyronine, and calcitonin.

thyroid-stimulating h. (TSH), thyrotropic h. thyrotropin.

thyrotropin-releasing h. (TRH) a tripeptide hormone, elaborated by the median eminence of the hypothalamus, which stimulates release of thyrotropin from the adenohypophysis. In human subjects, it can also promote a prolactin-releasing factor. It is used in diagnosis of mild hyperthyroidism and Graves disease, and in differentiating among primary, secondary, and tertiary hypothyroidism. Called also *thyroliberin.* A synthetic preparation is called *protirelin.*

hor•mo•no•gen•e•sis (hor-mo″no-jen′ə-sis) the production of hormones; called also *hormonopoiesis.*

hor•mo•no•gen•ic (hor-mo″no-jen′ik) pertaining to, characterized by, or stimulating hormonogenesis; called also *hormonopoietic.*

hor•mo•nol•o•gy (hor″mo-nol′ə-je) the study of hormones; see endocrinology.

hor•mo•no•poi•e•sis (hor-mo″no-poi-e′sis) hormonogenesis. **hormonopoiet′ic** *adj*

hor•mo•no•priv•ia (hor-mo″no-priv′e-ə) [*hormone* + L. *privus* deprived of] a hormone deficiency.

hor•mo•no•sis (hor-mo-no′sis) a condition caused by excessive quantities of one or more hormones; cf. *endocrinopathy.*

exogenous h. hormonosis caused by administration of pharmacologic amounts of a hormone as in cortisone therapy.

hor•mo•no•ther•a•py (hor-mo″no-ther′ə-pe) endocrine therapy.

horn (horn) [L. *cornu*] 1. a pointed projection, often paired, found on the heads of various animals. 2. cornu (def. 2). 3. an excrescence or projection resembling the horn of an animal.

Ammon's h. hippocampus proprius.

anterior h. of lateral ventricle cornu frontale ventriculi lateralis.

anterior h. of spinal cord cornu anterius medullae spinalis.

■ Cutaneous horn arising from an actinic keratosis.

cicatricial h. a hard, dry outgrowth from a scar, usually scaly but occasionally osseous.

coccygeal h. cornu coccygeum.

cutaneous h. a horny excrescence of the skin, usually on the scalp or face; these sometimes overlie premalignant keratoses or squamous or basal cell carcinoma.

dorsal h. of spinal cord cornu posterius medullae spinalis.

frontal h. of lateral ventricle cornu frontale ventriculi lateralis.

gray h's of spinal cord see *columnae griseae.*

greater h. of hyoid bone cornu majus ossis hyoidei.

inferior h. of falciform margin cornu inferius marginis falciformis.

inferior h. of lateral ventricle cornu temporale ventriculi lateralis.

inferior h. of thyroid cartilage cornu inferius cartilaginis thyroideae.

lateral h. of spinal cord cornu laterale medullae spinalis.

lesser h. of hyoid bone cornu minus ossis hyoidei.

occipital h. of lateral ventricle, posterior h. of lateral ventricle cornu occipitale ventriculi lateralis.

posterior h. of spinal cord cornu posterius medullae spinalis.

h. of pulp an extension of the pulp into an accentuation of the roof of the pulp chamber directly under a cusp or lobe of the tooth.

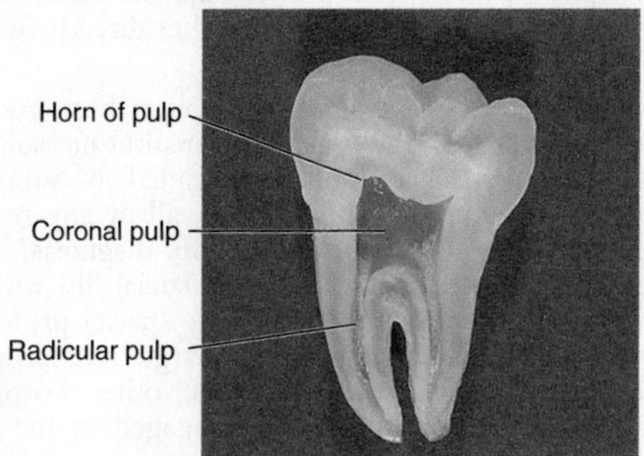

sacral h. cornu sacrale.
sebaceous h. a hard outgrowth of the contents of a sebaceous cyst.
superior h. of falciform margin cornu superius marginis falciformis.
superior h. of thyroid cartilage cornu superius cartilaginis thyroideae.
temporal h. of lateral ventricle cornu temporale ventriculi lateralis.
h. of uterus cornu uteri.
ventral h. of spinal cord cornu anterius medullae spinalis.

Hor·ner muscle (hor′nər) [William Edmonds *Horner*, American anatomist, 1793–1853] pars profunda partis palpebralis musculi orbicularis oculi.

Hor·ner ptosis, syndrome (hor′nər) [Johann Friedrich *Horner*, Swiss ophthalmologist, 1831–1886] see under *ptosis* and *syndrome.*

Horn·er sign (hor′nər) [David Alfred *Horner*, American obstetrician and gynecologist, 20th century] Spalding sign; see under *sign.*

hor·net (hor′nət) any of various wasps of the genera *Vespa* and *Vespula* that build papery nests.

horn·i·fi·ca·tion (hor″nĭ-fĭ-ka′shən) cornification (def. 1).

hor·ny (hor′ne) having the nature and appearance of horn; called also *corneous, keratic,* and *keratinous.*

ho·rop·ter (ho-rop′tər) [Gr. *horos* limit + *optēr* observer] the sum of all the spatial points whose images at a given distance fall on corresponding points of the retina. If the point of fixation is 2 meters, the horopter is a straight line across the observer's front (the *apparent frontoparallel plane h.*); if the point of fixation is less than 2 meters, the horopter is a curve concave to the observer *(concave h.);* and if the point of fixation is more than 2 meters, the horopter is a curve convex to the observer *(convex h.).* **horopter′ic** *adj*

Vieth-Müller h. a circle which joins the fixation point with the nodal points of the two eyes; called also *Vieth-Müller circle.*

hor·rip·i·la·tion (hor″ĭ-pĭ-la′shən) [L. *horrere* to bristle, to stand on end + *pilus* hair] erection of the fine hairs of the skin, as in cutis anserina; called also *piloerection.*

horse·fly (hors′fli) tabanid.

horse·pox (hors′poks) a mild form of poxvirus infection in horses, marked by a pustular eruption of the skin and sometimes of the oral and nasal mucosa.

Canadian h. contagious acne of horses.

horse·rad·ish (hors′rad-ish) 1. *Armoracia lapathifolia.* 2. any of several other plants of the family Cruciferae resembling *A. lapathifolia.* 3. the pungent root of one of these plants, used as a condiment and appetite stimulant; in the past it was used as a rubefacient and plaster like mustard, because it contains sinigrin.

horse·rad·ish per·ox·i·dase (HRP) (hors′rad-ish pər-ok′sĭ-dās″) peroxidase [EC 1.11.1.7] (q.v.) isolated from horseradish *(Armoracia lapathifolia);* used as a reagent in biochemical assays.

Hors·ley operation, sign (hors′le) [Sir Victor Alexander Haden *Horsley*, English surgeon, 1857–1916] see under *operation* and *sign.*

Hor·taea (hor-te′ə) a genus of Fungi Imperfecti of the family Dothioraceae. Its only species is *H. wernec′kii* (formerly called *Exophiala werneckii* and *Phaeoannellomyces werneckii*), a halophilic, dematiaceous yeast that inhabits the soil, particularly in tropical and subtropical climates, and is the cause of tinea nigra.

Hor·te·ga cell, method (or-ta′gə) [Pío del Río *Hortega*, Spanish histologist in Argentina, 1882–1945] see *microglia* and see *Stains and Staining Methods*, under *stain.*

Hor·ton arteritis (syndrome), headache (disease) (hor′tən) [Bayard Taylor *Horton*, American physician, 1895–1980] see *giant cell arteritis*, under *arteritis*, and see *cluster headache* under *headache.*

Hor. un. spatio [L.] ho′rae uni′us spa′tio (at the end of one hour).

Ho·sack·ia (ho-sak′e-ə) [David *Hosack*, American biologist, 19th century] a genus of herbaceous plants found in the western United States, one of the groups called *locoweed.*

hos·pice (hos′pis) a facility that provides palliative and supportive care for terminally ill patients and their families, either directly or on a consulting basis.

hos·pi·tal (hos′pĭ-təl) [L. *hospitalium*, from *hospes*, host, guest] an institution for the treatment of the sick. "An institution suitably located, constructed, organized, managed and personneled, to supply, scientifically, economically, efficiently and unhindered, all or any recognized part of the complex requirements for the prevention, diagnosis, and treatment of physical, mental, and the medical aspect of social ills; with functioning facilities for training new workers in the many special professional, technical and economic fields essential to the discharge of its proper functions; and with adequate contacts with physicians, other hospitals, medical schools and all accredited health agencies engaged in the better health program."—Council on Medical Education.

base h. a hospital unit within the line of communication of a branch of the armed forces, usually in a permanent building, designed for the reception of wounded and other patients received via field hospitals from the battle front, and for cases originating within the line of communication itself.

camp h. an immobile military unit organized and equipped for the care of the sick and wounded in camp in order to allow continued mobility of field hospitals or other mobile sanitary organizations.

closed h., closed staff h. a hospital in which only members of the staff are permitted to treat patients.

cottage h. a hospital consisting of a number of detached buildings.

day h. see *partial hospitalization*, under *hospitalization.*

evacuation h. a mobile advance hospital unit within the line of communication, designed to take over the functions of field hospitals when they move away with their divisions and to supplement base hospitals in their functions.

field h. a portable military hospital, manned by noncommissioned officers and men, located beyond the zone of conflict, 3–4 miles beyond the dressing stations, designed to shelter and care for wounded brought in by ambulance companies until they can be transported to the line of communications.

lying-in h., maternity h. an institution for the care of obstetric patients.

night h. see *partial hospitalization*, under *hospitalization.*

surgical h. a hospital specializing in surgical procedures.

teaching h. a hospital that allocates a substantial part of its resources to conduct, in its own name or in association with a college or university, formal educational programs or courses of instruction that lead to granting of recognized certificates, diplomas, degrees, or other documents required for professional certification or licensure.

voluntary h. a private, not-for-profit hospital; one of the major purposes of voluntary hospitals is the provision of uncompensated care to the poor.

weekend h. see *partial hospitalization*, under *hospitalization.*

hos·pi·tal·ist (hos′pĭ-təl-ist) a physician specializing in hospital inpatient care; called also *hospital-based* or *inpatient physician.*

hos·pi·tal·iza·tion (hos″pĭ-təl-ĭ-za′shən) the confinement of a patient in a hospital, or the period of such confinement.

partial h. a psychiatric treatment program for patients who do not need full-time hospitalization, involving a special facility or an arrangement within a hospital setting to which the patient may come for treatment during the day and return home at night *(day hospital);* or return at night after a day in the community to receive treatment during the evening and to remain all night *(night hospital);* or return at the end of the week to receive treatment and remain all weekend, resuming his normal activities during the week *(weekend hospital).*

hos·pi·tal·ize (hos′pĭ-təl-īz) to place a patient in a hospital.

host (hōst) [L. *hospes*] 1. an animal or plant that harbors or nourishes another organism (parasite). 2. the recipient of an organ or tissue transplanted from another organism (the donor).

accidental h. a host that harbors an organism that is not ordinarily parasitic in the particular species.

amplifying h. a host in which the level of a pathogen can become high enough that a vector such as a mosquito that feeds on it will probably become infectious.

compromised h. a person with an impaired ability to resist infection; the defect can be acquired or congenital.

dead end h. incidental h.

definitive h., final h. a host in which a parasite either attains sexual maturity (helminths) or undergoes sexual stages of development (protozoa). Called also *primary h.*

incidental h. a host that harbors a pathogenic organism but cannot pass it on to another host; called also *dead end h.*

intermediate h. a host in which a parasite passes through one or more of its asexual stages (protozoa) or larval stages (helminths); if there is more than one, the stages may be designated first, second, and so on.

paratenic h. a potential or substitute intermediate host that serves until the appropriate definitive host is reached, and in which no development of the parasite occurs; it may or may not be necessary to the completion of the parasite's life cycle. Called also *transfer* or *transport h.*

h. of predilection the host preferred by a parasite.
primary h. definitive h.
reservoir h. reservoir (def. 3).
secondary h. intermediate h.
transfer h., transport h. paratenic h.

hot (hot) 1. characterized by high temperature. 2. radioactive; particularly used to denote the presence of significantly or dangerously high levels of radioactivity.

hot line (hot līn) telephone assistance for those in need of crisis intervention (q.v.), as in suicide prevention, usually available 24 hours a day, seven days a week, and staffed by nonprofessionals with mental health professionals serving as advisors or in a back-up capacity.

Houns•field unit (hounz′fēld) [Sir Godfrey Newbold *Hounsfield*, British electronics engineer and Nobel prize winner, 1919–2004] see under *unit.*

Hous•say animal, phenomenon (o-si′) [Bernardo Alberto *Houssay*, Argentine physiologist and Nobel prize winner, 1887–1971] see under *animal* and *phenomenon.*

Hous•ton muscle, valve (hu′ston) [John *Houston*, Irish surgeon, 1802–1845] see under *muscle* and see *plicae transversae recti*, under *plica.*

ho•ven (ho′vən) tympany of the stomach.

Ho•vi•us canal, circle, plexus (ho′ve-əs) [Jacobus *Hovius*, Dutch ophthalmologist, 1710–1786] see under *canal*, *circle*, and *plexus.*

How•el-Ev•ans syndrome (hou′əl-ev′ənz) [William *Howel-Evans*, British physician, 1925–1997] see under *syndrome.*

How•ell bodies (hou′əl) [William Henry *Howell*, American physiologist, 1860–1945] see under *body.*

How•ell-Jol•ly bodies (hou′əl zho-le′) [W.H. *Howell;* Justin Marie Jules *Jolly*, French histologist, 1870–1953] see under *body.*

How•ship lacuna (hou′ship) [John *Howship*, English surgeon, 1781–1841] see *absorption lacuna*, under *lacuna.*

How•ship-Rom•berg sign (hou′ship rom′berg) [J. *Howship;* Moritz Heinrich von *Romberg*, German neurologist, 1795–1873] see under *sign.*

HP house physician.

Hp haptoglobin.

HPA hyperphenylalaninemia.

H. P. Ac•thar Gel (ak′thahr) trademark for a preparation of repository corticotropin injection.

HPETE hydroperoxyeicosatetraenoic acid.

HPF high-power field.

HPL, hPL human placental lactogen.

HPLC high-performance liquid chromatography.

HPRT hypoxanthine phosphoribosyltransferase.

HPTA hepatopoietin A.

HPV human papillomavirus.

HRA high right atrial; see under *electrogram.*

HRCT high-resolution computed tomography.

HRF histamine-releasing factor; homologous restriction factor.

HRP horseradish peroxidase.

HRSA Health Resources and Services Administration, an agency of the United States Public Health Service.

HRT hormone replacement therapy.

HS house surgeon.

h.s. [L.] ho′ra som′ni (at bedtime).

HSA human serum albumin.

HSAN hereditary sensory and autonomic neuropathy.

HSC hepatic stellate cell.

hs-CRP high-sensitivity C-reactive protein; see under *test.*

HSR homogeneously staining regions.

HSV herpes simplex virus.

5-HT 5-hydroxytryptamine; see *serotonin.*

Ht total hyperopia.

HTACS human thyroid adenylate cyclase stimulators.

HTC homozygous typing cells.

^{3}H-TdR tritium-labeled thymidine.

HTLV-1 human T-lymphotropic virus 1.

HTLV-2 human T-lymphotropic virus 2.

HTLV-III human T-cell lymphotropic virus type III; see *human immunodeficiency virus*, under *virus.*

H^+-trans•port•ing ATP syn•thase (trans-port′ing sin′thās) [EC 3.6.3.14] an enzyme complex of the mitochondrial membrane that catalyzes the phosphorylation of ADP to form ATP. The energy for the synthesis of ATP is produced at three sites in the electron transport chain (see illustration under *chain*) and oxidative phosphorylation and electron transport are coupled via translocation of protons across the mitochondrial membrane. When removed from the membrane, the enzyme acts as an ATPase. Called also *ATP synthase*, *H^+-ATPase*, and *mitochondrial ATPase.* In official nomenclature, the preferred name is now *H^+-transporting two-sector ATPase.*

Hua (hu′ə) a genus of fresh water snails of the family Thiaridae.

H. ningpoen′sis a species of central and southern China that ingests eggs of the liver fluke *Opisthorchis sinensis*, which then hatch in its body.

H. touchea′na a first intermediate host of the lung fluke *Paragonimus westermani.*

huang-qi (hwang che) preparations of *Astragalus* root used in traditional Chinese medicine.

Hub•bard tank (hub′ərd) [Carl *Hubbard*, American engineer, 20th century] see under *tank.*

Hu•chard disease (u-shahr′) [Henri *Huchard*, French physician, 1844–1910] see under *disease.*

Hud•son line (hud′sən) [Arthur Cyril *Hudson*, British ophthalmologist, 1875–1962] see under *line.*

Hud•son-Stäh•li line (hud′sən sta′le) [A. C. *Hudson;* Jean *Stähli*, Swiss ophthalmologist, 20th century] see under *line.*

Hueck ligament (hēk) [Alexander Friedrich *Hueck*, German anatomist, 1802–1842] reticulum trabeculare.

Hue•ter line, maneuver, sign (he′tər) [Karl *Hueter*, German surgeon, 1838–1882] see under *line*, *maneuver*, and *sign.*

Hughes reflex (hūz) [Charles Hamilton *Hughes*, American neurologist, 1839–1916] virile reflex (def. 2).

Hughes-Sto•vin syndrome (hūz sto′vin) [John Patterson *Hughes*, British physician, 20th century; Peter George Ingle *Stovin*, British physician, 20th century] see under *syndrome.*

Hugh•ston projection (hu′stən) [J.C. *Hughston*, American radiologist, 20th century] see under *projection.*

Hu•guier canal, circle, sinus (u-gya′) [Pierre Charles *Huguier*, French surgeon, 1804–1873] see under *circle* and *sinus* and see *anterior canaliculus for chorda tympani.*

Huh•ner test (hu′nər) [Max *Huhner*, American urologist, 1873–1947] postcoital test.

HuIFN human interferon.

hum (hum) an indistinct, low, prolonged sound.

venous h. a continuous blowing, singing, or humming murmur heard on auscultation over the right jugular vein in the sitting or erect position; it is an innocent sign that is obliterated on assumption of the recumbent position or on exerting pressure over the vein. Called also *bruit de diable* and *humming-top murmur.*

Hu•ma•log (hu′mə-log) trademark for preparations of insulin lispro.

Hu•mate-P (hu′māt) trademark for a combination preparation of antihemophilic factor (human) and von Willebrand factor.

Hu•ma•tin (hu′mə-tin) trademark for preparations of paromomycin sulfate.

Hu•ma•trope (hu′mə-trōp) trademark for a preparation of somatropin.

hu•mec•tant (hu-mek′tənt) [L. *humectus*, from *humectare* to be moist] 1. moistening. 2. a moistening or diluent substance.

hu•mec•ta•tion (hu″mək-ta′shən) the act of moistening.

Hu•me•gon (hu′mə-gon) trademark for a preparation of menotropins.

hu•meri (hu′mər-i) [L.] genitive and plural of *humerus.*

hu•mero•ra•di•al (hu″mər-o-ra′de-əl) pertaining to the humerus and the radius.

hu•mero•scap•u•lar (hu″mər-o-skap′u-lər) pertaining to the humerus and the scapula.

hu•mero•ul•nar (hu″mər-o-ul′nər) pertaining to the humerus and the ulna.

hu•mer•us (hu′mər-əs) gen. and pl. *hu′meri* [L.] [TA] the bone that extends from the shoulder to the elbow articulating proximally with the scapula and distally with the radius and ulna; see illustration and Plate 40. **hu′meral** *adj*

h. va′rus a bent humerus.

Hu•mi•bid (hu′mĭ-bid) trademark for a preparation of guaifenesin.

hu•mid•i•fi•er (hu-mid′ĭ-fi″ər) an apparatus for controlling humidity by adding moisture to the air of a room.

hu•mid•i•ty (hu-mid′ĭ-te) [L. *humiditas*] 1. the degree of moisture, especially of that in the air. 2. relative h.

absolute h. the actual amount of vapor in the atmosphere expressed in weight per unit volume.

relative h. the percentage of moisture in the air as compared to the amount necessary to cause saturation, which is taken as 100.

Hu•mi•ra (hu-mi′rə) trademark for a preparation of adalimumab.

hu•mor (hu′mər) pl. *humors*, *humo′res* [L. "a liquid"] 1. a fluid or semifluid substance; used in anatomical nomenclature to designate certain fluid

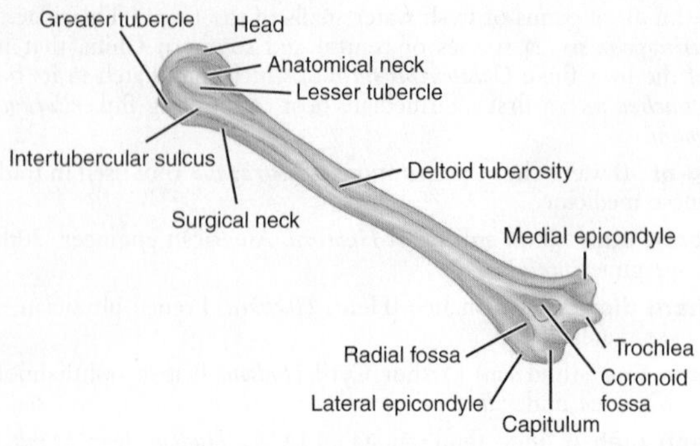

■ Anterior view of right humerus.

materials in the body. 2. one of the four hypothetical fluids of humoralism.

aqueous h., h. aquo′sus [TA] the fluid produced in the eye, occupying the anterior and posterior chambers, and diffusing out of the eye into the blood via the canal of Schlemm. It supplies nutrients to the cornea and lens and maintains the intraocular pressure. Called also *aqueous*.

crystalline h. see under *lens*.

ocular h. one of the humors of the eye; see *aqueous h.* and *vitreous h.*

plasmoid h. aqueous or vitreous humor containing an abnormally high amount of protein; formed after trauma or inflammation, it has a cloudy appearance and the proteins tend to coalesce.

vitreous h., h. vi′treus [TA] the watery substance, resembling aqueous humor, contained within the interstices of the stroma in the vitreous body.

hu•mor•al (hu′mər-əl) 1. pertaining to elements dissolved in the blood or body fluids, e.g., humoral immunity from antibodies in the blood as opposed to cellular immunity. 2. pertaining to one of the humors of the body or to humoralism.

hu•mor•al•ism (hu′mər-əl-iz″əm) the ancient theory that health and illness result from a balance or imbalance of bodily liquids ("humors"). The theory is especially associated with Hippocratic writers, but it long antedates Hippocrates. The four humors and associated qualities are phlegm (cold and moist), blood (hot and moist), black bile or gall (secreted from the kidneys and spleen, cold and dry), and yellow bile or choler (secreted from the liver, hot and dry). Elements of humoralism may be seen in traditional systems such as curanderismo.

Hu•mor•sol (hu′mor-sol) trademark for a solution of demecarium bromide.

hump (hump) a rounded eminence; called also *gibbus*.

buffalo h. obesity confined to the neck, head, and trunk; seen in Cushing syndrome.

dowager's h. popular name for dorsal kyphosis caused by multiple wedge fractures of the thoracic vertebrae seen in osteoporosis.

dromedary h. a bulge on the lateral surface of a kidney (usually the left), resembling the hump of a dromedary camel, seen in persons whose spleen or liver presses down.

Hampton h. a homogeneous wedge-shaped density in the peripheral region of the lung, with a convex apex toward the hilum; seen on the radiograph after pulmonary infarction.

hump•back (hump′bak) kyphosis.

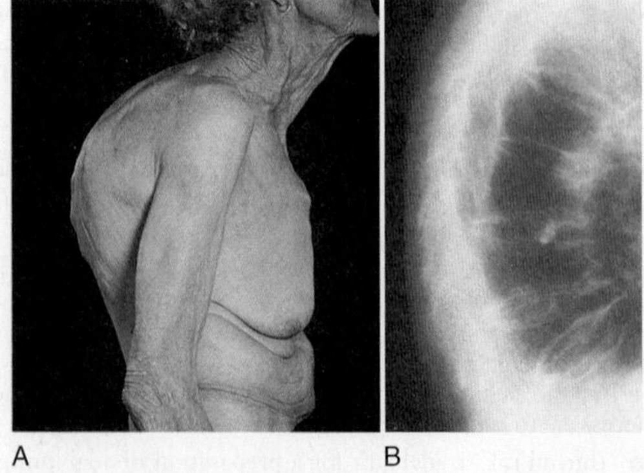

■ Dowager's hump. Marked thoracic kyphosis due to multiple osteoporotic fractures *(A)* and corresponding radiograph. *(B)*.

Hum•phry ligament (hum′fre) [Sir George Murray *Humphry*, English anatomist, 1820–1896] ligamentum meniscofemorale anterius.

Hu•mu•lin (hu′mu-lin) trademark for preparations of insulin human produced by recombinant DNA technology; different forms are identified by letters following the trademark, e.g., Humulin U denotes extended insulin human zinc suspension, or by numerals, e.g., Humulin 70/30 denotes a preparation of isophane insulin human suspension and buffered insulin human in a 7:3 ratio.

Hu•mu•lus (hu′mu-ləs) [L.] a genus of herbaceous vines of the family Urticaceae, including *H. lu′pulus*, the hop (see *hops*), which is used medicinally.

hun•ger (hung′gər) a craving, as for food.

air h. Kussmaul respiration.

calcium h. a condition due to calcium deficit, marked by severe headache, usually occurring during and after menstruation. See also *calcipenia*.

Hun•ner ulcer (hun′ər) [Guy LeRoy *Hunner*, American surgeon, 1868–1957] see under *ulcer*.

Hunt atrophy, phenomenon, syndrome (neuralgia) (hunt) [James Ramsay *Hunt*, American neurologist, 1872–1937] see under *atrophy* and *phenomenon*, and see *Ramsay Hunt syndrome*, under *syndrome*.

Hun•ter canal, gubernaculum (hun′tər) [John *Hunter*, Scottish anatomist and surgeon, 1728–1793] see *canalis adductorius* and *gubernaculum testis*.

Hun•ter glossitis (hun′tər) [William *Hunter*, English physician, 1861–1937] see under *glossitis*.

Hun•ter ligament, line (hun′tər) [William *Hunter*, Scottish anatomist, 1718–1783] see *ligamentum teres uteri* and *linea alba*.

Hun•ter syndrome (hun′tər) [Charles H. *Hunter*, Canadian physician, 1873–1955] see under *syndrome*.

Hun•ter-Thomp•son acromesomelic dysplasia (hun′tər tomp′sən) [Alasdair G. W. *Hunter*, Canadian pediatrician and geneticist, 20th century; Margaret W. *Thompson*, Canadian geneticist, born 1920] see under *dysplasia*.

hun•ting•tin (hun′ting-tin) a protein encoded by a gene located on 4p16.3 and altered in structure and function in Huntington disease. Mutation causes increased and unstable numbers of CAG triplet repeats in the gene and thus increased numbers of glutamine residues in the protein; above a threshold of 40 glutamine repeats, clinical disease is apparent, with age of onset inversely correlated with the number of repeats. The altered proteins tend to form tangled aggregates.

Hun•ting•ton disease (chorea), sign (hun′ting-tən) [George Sumner *Huntington*, American physician, 1850–1916] see under *disease* and *sign*.

Hur•ler syndrome (disease) (hur′lər) [Gertrud *Hurler*, Austrian pediatrician, 1889–1965] see under *syndrome*.

Hur•ler-Scheie syndrome (hur′lər sha′) [G. *Hurler*; Harold G. *Scheie*, American ophthalmologist, 1909–1990] see under *syndrome*.

Hürth•le cells, cell tumor (hērt′lə) [Karl *Hürthle*, German histologist, 1860–1945] see *Askanazy cells*, under *cell*, and see under *tumor*.

Husch•ke foramen (canal), etc. (hoosh′kə) [Emil *Huschke*, German anatomist, 1797–1858] see under *foramen* and see *dentes acustici* and *plica lacrimalis*.

husk (husk) 1. an outer covering or shell, as of some fruits and seeds. 2. hoose.

psyllium h. [USP] the cleaned, dried seed coat from the seeds of *Plantago ovata*, *P. psyllium*, or *P. indica;* used as a bulk-forming laxative, and as a dietary adjunct in the treatment of hypercholesterolemia. It also has a wide variety of uses in ayurveda and folk medicine.

Hutch diverticulum (huch) [J.A. *Hutch*, American urologist, mid-20th century] see under *diverticulum*.

Hutch•in•son facies, mask, etc. (huch′in-sən) [Sir Jonathan *Hutchinson*, English surgeon, 1828–1913] see under *facies*, *mask*, *pupil*, *sign*, *tooth*, and *triad;* see *angioma serpiginosum* and *lentigo maligna;* and see *salmon patch* (def. 1), under *patch*.

Hutch•in•son-Gil•ford syndrome (huch′in-sən gil′fərd) [Sir J. *Hutchinson;* Hastings *Gilford*, English physician, 1861–1941] progeria.

hutch•in•so•ni•an (huch″in-so′ne-ən) named for or described by Sir Jonathan *Hutchinson*.

Hutch•i•son syndrome (huch′ĭ-sən) [Sir Robert *Hutchison*, English pediatrician, 1871–1960] see under *syndrome*.

Hu•ti•nel disease (u-te-nel′) [Victor Henri *Hutinel*, French pediatrician, 1849–1933] see under *disease*.

HUVS hypocomplementemic urticarial vasculitis syndrome.

Hux•ley layer (huks′le) [Thomas Henry *Huxley*, English physiologist and naturalist, 1825–1895] see under *layer*.

huy•gen•i•an (hi-jen′e-ən) named for Christiaan *Huygens* (or Huyghens), Dutch physicist, 1629–1695.

HVA homovanillic acid.

HVL half-value layer.

hy•al (hi′əl) hyoid.

Hy•al•gan (hi′al-gan) trademark for a preparation of hyaluronan.

hy•a•lin (hi′ə-lin) [Gr. *hyalos* glass] 1. a translucent albuminoid substance, one of the products of amyloid degeneration. 2. a substance composing the walls of hydatid cysts.

hy•a•line (hi′ə-lēn) [Gr. *hyalos* glass] glassy and transparent or nearly so; called also *hyaloid.*

hy•a•lin•iza•tion (hi″ə-lin″ĭ-za′shən) conversion into a substance resembling glass.

Crooke h. degeneration of pituitary gland corticotrophs, with loss of specific granulation and progressive hyalinization, seen in the presence of elevated plasma corticosteroid levels of any cause. Called also *Crooke* or *Crooke-Russell changes* and *Crooke hyaline degeneration.*

hy•a•li•no•sis (hi″ə-lin-o′sis) hyaline degeneration.

h. cu′tis et muco′sae lipoid proteinosis.

hy•a•lin•u•ria (hi″ə-lĭ-nu′re-ə) the discharge of hyalin in the urine, usually in the form of casts composed of protein in an acid pH.

hy•a•li•tis (hi″ə-li′tis) [*hyal-* + *-itis*] inflammation of the hyaloid membrane of the eye or of the vitreous body. Called also *hyaloiditis* and *vitreitis.*

asteroid h. see under *hyalosis.*

h. puncta′ta, punctate h. inflammation of the vitreous body with formation of small opacities.

h. suppurati′va, suppurative h. a purulent inflammation of the vitreous body.

hyal(o)- [Gr. *hyalos* glass] a combining form denoting a relationship to glass or to the vitreous body or vitreous humor, or denoting a resemblance to glass.

hy•al•o•gen (hi-al′o-jən) [*hyalo-* + *-gen*] an albuminous substance occurring in cartilage, the vitreous body, etc., and convertible into hyalin.

hy•a•lo•hy•pho•my•co•sis (hi″ə-lo-hi″fo-mi-ko′sis) [*hyalo-* + *hyphomycosis*] a hyphomycosis caused by mycelial fungi with colorless walls; most are opportunistic.

hy•a•loid (hi′ə-loid) [*hyal-* + *-oid*] hyaline.

hy•a•loid•itis (hi″ə-loi-di′tis) hyalitis.

hy•a•lo•mere (hi′ə-lo-mēr″) [*hyalo-* + *-mere*] a zone of homogeneous or finely fibrillar pale blue cytoplasm surrounding the central granulomere of a platelet in a dry, stained blood smear.

Hy•a•lom•ma (hi″ə-lom′ə) [*hyal-* + Gr. *omma* eye] a genus of ticks of the family Ixodidae, found primarily in hot and dry regions of the world.

H. anato′licum a species found in arid regions from North Africa and southeastern Europe across Central Asia to Bangladesh, with several subspecies that attack large domestic animals with economic consequences. It is a vector for animal diseases such as babesiosis, theileriasis, and hemorrhagic fevers, as well as for Crimean-Congo hemorrhagic fever in humans.

H. margina′tum a species with subspecies found in various parts of Africa, Central Asia, Saudi Arabia, and the Indian subcontinent, attacking primarily birds and herbivores; it is a vector for various animal diseases and for Crimean-Congo hemorrhagic fever in humans.

H. plum′beum a species found on livestock in Eastern Europe and parts of Asia, a vector for canine and equine babesiosis.

H. trunca′tum a species that attacks cattle and sheep in dry regions of eastern Africa and is a vector for diseases such as Crimean-Congo hemorrhagic fever, Q fever, sweating sickness, tick paralysis, and tick typhus.

hy•a•lo•mu•coid (hi″ə-lo-mu′koid) [*hyalo-* + *mucoid* (def. 1)] the mucoid of the vitreous body.

hy•a•lo•nyx•is (hi″ə-lo-nik′sis) [*hyalo-* + *nyxis*] surgical puncturing of the vitreous body.

hy•a•lo•pha•gia (hi″ə-lo-fa′je-ə) [*hyalo-* + *-phagia*] the eating of glass, a form of pica.

hy•a•loph•a•gy (hi″ə-lof′ə-je) hyalophagia.

hy•a•lo•plasm (hi′ə-lo-plaz″əm) [*hyalo-* + *-plasm*] cytosol.

hy•a•lo•se•ro•si•tis (hi″ə-lo-se″ro-si′tis) [*hyalo-* + *serositis*] inflammation of serous membranes marked by hyalinization of the serous exudate into a pearly investment of the organ concerned.

progressive multiple h. Concato disease.

hy•a•lo•sis (hi″ə-lo′sis) [*hyal-* + *-osis*] degenerative changes in the vitreous body.

asteroid h. a condition of the eye, usually unilateral and in older men, characterized by spherical or star-shaped, calcium-containing opacities in the vitreous body that appear to sparkle when illuminated under an examining light. Vision is usually unaffected. Called also *asteroid hyalitis* and *Benson disease.*

hy•a•lu•ron•an (hi″ə-loo͝-ron′an) a glycosaminoglycan found in lubricating proteoglycans of synovial fluid, vitreous humor, cartilage, blood vessels, skin, and the umbilical cord. It is a linear chain of about 2500 repeating disaccharide units in specific linkage, each composed of an *N*-acetylglucosamine residue linked to one of glucuronic acid. A preparation extracted from chicken combs is used for the treatment of pain in osteoarthritis, administered by intra-articular injection. It is also used as an adjunct, injected into the anterior or posterior chamber during surgical procedures on the eye to maintain the shape of the eye, to manipulate and separate tissues by hydraulic pressure, and to protect intraocular structures from trauma. Called also *hyaluronate* and *hyaluronic acid.* See also *hylan.*

hy•a•lu•ro•nate (hi″ə-loo′rə-nāt) hyaluronan.

hy•a•lu•ro•nate ly•ase (hi″ə-loo′rə-nāt li′ās) [EC 4.2.2.1] an enzyme of the lyase class that catalyzes the fragmentation of hyaluronan via an elimination reaction in which the bond from *N*-acetylglucosamine to glucuronate is broken and a double bond introduced into the latter. It is one of the enzymes called hyaluronidases; see also *hyaluronoglucosaminidase* and *hyaluronoglucuronidase.*

hy•a•lu•ron•ic ac•id (hi″ə-loo͝-ron′ik) hyaluronan.

hy•a•lu•ron•i•dase (hi″ə-loo͝-ron′ĭ-dās) 1. any of three enzymes (hyaluronate lyase, hyaluronoglucosaminidase, and hyaluronoglucuronidase) that catalyze the breakdown of hyaluronan. These enzymes are found in mammalian testicular and spleen tissue, in bee and snake venoms, and in certain species of *Clostridium, Staphylococcus,* and *Streptococcus.* Called also *Duran-Reynals factor, invasin,* and *diffusion* or *spreading factor.* 2. [USP] a preparation derived from mammalian testes and capable of hydrolyzing hyaluronan and similar glycosaminoglycans, used to aid absorption and dispersion of other injected drugs and fluids, for hypodermoclysis, and for improving resorption of radiopaque media; administered intramuscularly or subcutaneously.

hy•a•lu•rono•glu•co•sa•min•i•dase (hi″ə-loo͝-ron″o-gloo″kōs-ə-min′ĭ-dās) [EC 3.2.1.35] an enzyme of the hydrolase class that catalyzes the hydrolysis of random β-1,4 linkages between *N*-acetylglucosamine and D-glucuronic acid residues in hyaluronan. It also hydrolyzes chondroitin, chondroitin 4- and 6-sulfates, and dermatan sulfate. It is one of the enzymes called hyaluronidases; see also *hyaluronate lyase* and *hyaluronoglucuronidase.*

hy•a•lu•rono•glu•cu•ron•i•dase (hi″ə-loo͝-ron″o-gloo″ku-ron′ĭ-dās) [EC 3.2.1.36] an enzyme of the hydrolase class that catalyzes the hydrolysis of β-1,3 linkages between glucuronic acid and *N*-acetylglucosamine residues in hyaluronan. It is one of the enzymes called hyaluronidases; see also *hyaluronate lyase* and *hyaluronoglucosaminidase.*

Hy•ate:C (hi′āt-se″) trademark for a preparation of antihemophilic factor (porcine).

hy•bar•ox•ia (hi″bar-ok′se-ə) inhalation therapy using hyperbaric oxygen, i.e., oxygen at pressures greater than 1 atmosphere.

hy•ben•zate (hi-ben′zāt) USAN contraction for *o*-(4-hydroxybenzoyl)-benzoate.

Hy•bo•lin (hi′bə-lin) trademark for preparations of nandrolone.

Hy•bo•mi•tra (hi″bo-mi′trə) a genus of biting horseflies of North America (family Tabanidae) that are vectors for anaplasmosis, anthrax, equine infectious anemia, and tularemia.

hy•brid (hi′brid) [L. *hybrida* mongrel] 1. an offspring produced by genetically different parents, particularly those of different species. 2. something of mixed origin or composition.

false h. an individual produced by a form of gynogenesis in which the foreign spermatozoon enters the egg and activates it to cell division, but does not fuse with the egg nucleus.

somatic cell h. the heterokaryon produced by somatic cell hybridization.

hy•brid•ism (hi′brid-iz-əm) the state of being a hybrid.

hy•brid•i•ty (hi-brid′ĭ-te) the state of being a hybrid.

hy•brid•iza•tion (hi″brid-ĭ-za′shən) 1. the act or process of producing hybrids. 2. nucleic acid h. 3. in chemistry, a procedure whereby orbitals of intermediate energy and desired directional character are constructed by taking an appropriate linear combination of atomic orbitals; e.g., sp^3 hybrid orbitals are formed from one s and three p orbitals.

allele-specific oligonucleotide h., ASO h. a procedure for detection of alleles of known composition, by measuring hybridization of a labeled DNA sample with oligonucleotide probes of known sequence, differing from each other by a single nucleotide, under conditions stringent enough that only perfectly matched sequences hybridize.

colony h. a screening method for detecting the occurrence of a specific nucleic acid sequence in a heterogeneous population of bacterial colonies: a replica of a plate of colonies is prepared and all colonies are lysed with preservation of their relative positions and their DNA denatured; hybridization to the nucleic acid sequence of interest reveals the colonies carrying this sequence, and they can be retrieved from the master plate.

comparative genomic h. (CGH) a cytogenetic technique in which genomic DNA preparations from two sources, reference DNA and the DNA to be studied, as from a tumor, are labeled with two different fluorochromes and then hybridized to a metaphase chromosome spread; copy number changes can be mapped as alterations in the ratio of colors observed.

differential h. subtractive h.

dot blot h. see *dot blot*, under *blot*.

filter h. any of various methods, e.g., Southern blotting, dot blotting, for detection of a specific nucleic acid sequence by immobilizing a population of single-stranded nucleic acids on a filter, exposing it to a specific labeled single-stranded nucleic acid probe, then washing off the unbound probe to reveal the location on the filter of hybrid double-stranded molecules.

fluorescence in situ h. (FISH) in situ hybridization in which DNA probes are labeled with fluorescent tags and hybridized to metaphase or nondividing (interphase) chromosome spreads to identify and localize specific sequences. See also *chromosome painting*, under *painting*.

in situ h. nucleic acid hybridization in which a labeled, single-stranded nucleic acid probe is applied to prepared cells or histologic sections and annealing occurs in situ; performed to analyze the intracellular or intrachromosomal distribution, transcription, or other characteristics of the nucleic acid.

liquid h. solution h.

molecular h. nucleic acid h.

Northern blot h. see *Northern blot*, under *blot*.

nucleic acid h. formation of a partially or wholly complementary DNA-RNA, DNA-DNA, or RNA-RNA duplex by association of single-stranded nucleic acids, sometimes specifically from different sources; used as the basis of a wide variety of techniques for analysis of nucleic acids and detection and isolation of specific sequences.

reverse Southern h. a variation on a Southern blot (q.v.) for detection of specific DNA sequences, in which DNA sequences in solution are first hybridized to a labeled probe and then separated electrophoretically.

saturation h. an in vitro nucleic acid hybridization reaction in which one nucleic acid component is in vast excess, ensuring that all complementary sequences in the other nucleic acid form duplexes.

slot blot h. a variation on a dot blot hybridization with substitution of a slotted template for the usual one with circular holes; it increases sample capacity and maintains precision.

solution h. the formation of double-stranded nucleic acid molecules from complementary single-stranded nucleic acids in solution.

somatic cell h. formation of a heterokaryon by fusion of two somatic cells, usually of different species.

Southern blot h. see *Southern blot*, under *blot*.

subtractive h. a technique for isolating sequences expressed in one cell type but not in another; when a cDNA population prepared from the mRNA of one cell type is hybridized to the mRNA population of the second, and the cDNA:mRNA hybrids removed, the remaining single-stranded cDNA molecules represent the mRNA sequences expressed only in the first cell type.

Western blot h. see *Western blot*, under *blot*.

hy•brid•o•ma (hi″brid-o′mə) [*hybrid* + *-oma*] a somatic cell hybrid formed by fusion of normal lymphocytes and tumor cells; the resulting hybridoma cells will produce the same secretion as the normal parent cells and proliferate indefinitely in culture like the parent tumor cells.

B cell h. a hybridoma formed by the fusion of antibody-secreting B lymphocytes and nonsecretory myeloma cells; used in the production of monoclonal antibodies.

T cell h. a hybridoma formed by the fusion of T lymphocytes and myeloma cells, used particularly in the production of T lymphocyte–derived lymphokines.

Hy•cam•tin (hi-kam′tin) trademark for a preparation of topotecan hydrochloride.

hy•clate (hi′klāt) USAN contraction for monohydrochloride hemiethanolate hemihydrate.

Hy•co•dan (hi′ko-dan) trademark for preparations of hydrocodone bitartrate.

Hy•co•mine (hi′ko-mēn″) trademark for a combination preparation of hydrocodone bitartrate, chlorpheniramine maleate, phenylephrine hydrochloride, acetaminophen, and caffeine.

Hy•co•tuss (hi′ko-tus″) trademark for a combination preparation of hydrocodone bitartrate and guaifenesin.

hy•dan•to•in (hi-dan′to-in) 1. a crystalline base derivable from allantoin:

2. any of a group of anticonvulsants, including phenytoin, ethotoin, and methyphenytoin, containing such a ring structure.

hy•dan•to•in•ate (hi″dan-to′in-āt) any salt of hydantoin.

hy•da•tid (hi′də-tid) [Gr. *hydatis*, water] 1. hydatid cyst. 2. any cystlike structure; see under *mole*.

h. of Morgagni 1. appendix testis. 2. *(in the pl.)* appendices vesiculosae epoophori.

sessile h. appendix testis.

hy•da•tid•i•form (hi″də-tid′ĭ-form) resembling a hydatid cyst; see under *mole*.

hy•da•tid•o•sis (hi″də-tĭ-do′sis) hydatid disease.

hy•da•tid•os•to•my (hi″də-tĭ-dos′tə-me) [*hydatid* + *-stomy*] incision and drainage of a hydatid cyst.

hy•da•tid•uria (hi″də-tĭ-du′re-ə) excretion in the urine of material from hydatid cysts involving the urinary tract.

Hy•da•tig•ena (hi″də-tij′ə-nə) *Taenia*.

hy•da•toid (hi′də-toid) [Gr. *hydōr* water + *-oid*] 1. aqueous humor. 2. pertaining to the aqueous humor. 3. the hyaloid membrane (membrana vitrea).

Hy•del•tra•sol (hi-del′trə-sol″) trademark for a preparation of prednisolone sodium phosphate.

Hy•der•gine (hi′dər-jēn) trademark for preparations of ergoloid mesylates.

hy•drad•e•ni•tis (hi″drad-ə-ni′tis) hidradenitis.

hy•drad•e•no•ma (hi″drad-ə-no′mə) hidradenoma.

hy•dra•gogue (hi′drə-gog) [*hydr-* + *-agogue*] 1. producing watery discharge, especially from the intestines. 2. a cathartic that has this action.

hy•dral•a•zine (hy-dral′ə-zēn) a peripheral vasodilator used as an antihypertensive.

h. hydrochloride [USP] the monohydrochloride salt of hydralazine, used as an antihypertensive; administered orally, intramuscularly, or intravenously. It is also used in combination with nitrates, diuretics, or digitalis glycosides, or a combination of these, in the treatment of congestive heart failure.

hy•dra•mine (hi′drə-mēn) an amine derived from a glycol in which one hydroxyl is replaced by an amino group.

hy•dram•ni•on (hi-dram′ne-on) polyhydramnios.

hy•dram•ni•os (hi-dram′ne-os) polyhydramnios.

hy•dran•en•ceph•a•ly (hi″dran-ən-sef′ə-le) complete or almost complete absence of the cerebral hemispheres, the space they normally occupy being filled with cerebrospinal fluid.

hy•drar•thro•sis (hi″drahr-thro′sis) [*hydr-* + *arthro-* + *-osis*] an accumulation of watery fluid in the cavity of a joint. **hydrarthro′dial** *adj*

intermittent h. serous effusion into a joint occurring periodically.

Hy•dras•tis (hi-dras′tis) a genus of North American herbs of the family Ranunculaceae. *H. canaden′sis* L. is goldenseal, whose dried root contains berberine and is used as a folk remedy and in homeopathy.

hy•dra•tase (hi′drə-tās) [EC 4.2.1] a term used in the recommended or trivial names of some enzymes of the sub-subclass hydro-lyase when the reaction equilibrium lies toward hydration.

hy•drate (hi′drāt) [L. *hydras*] 1. any compound of a radical with H_2O. 2. any salt or other compound that contains water of crystallization.

hy•drat•ed (hi′drāt-əd) [L. *hydratus*] combined with water; forming a hydrate or a hydroxide.

hy•dra•tion (hi-dra′shən) 1. the act of combining or causing to combine with water. 2. the condition of being combined with water.

hy•drau•lics (hi-draw′liks) [*hydr-* + Gr. *aulos* pipe] the branch of physics which treats of the action of liquids under physical laws.

Hy•dra-Zide (hy′drə-zīd) trademark for combination preparations of hydralazine hydrochloride and hydrochlorothiazide.

hy•dra•zine (hi′drə-zēn) a toxic, irritant, carcinogenic, colorless, gaseous diamine, $H_2N{\bullet}NH_2$; also any member of a group of its substitution derivatives.

hy•dra•zin•ol•y•sis (hi″drə-zin-ol′ə-sis) cleavage of the peptide bonds of a peptide by hydrazine, with the C-terminal residue appearing as a free amino acid.

hy•dra•zone (hi′drə-zōn) a compound containing the group —NH•N:C—, formed from an aldehyde or ketone by the action of phenylhydrazine or other hydrazine.

Hy•drea (hi-dre′ə) trademark for a preparation of hydroxyurea.

hy•dre•mia (hi-dre′me-ə) [*hydr-* + Gr. *haima* blood] excessive dilution of the blood, so that the proportion of serum to corpuscles is excessive; seen in splenomegaly and other conditions. Cf. *hypo-osmolality.* Called also *dilution anemia.*

hy•dren•ceph•a•lo•cele (hi″dren-sef′ə-lo-sēl″) hydroencephalocele.

hy•dren•ceph•a•lo•me•nin•go•cele (hi″drən-sef″ə-lo-mə-ning′o-sēl) hydroencephalocele.

hy•dren•ceph•a•lus (hi″drən-sef′ə-ləs) hydrocephalus.

hy•dren•ceph•a•ly (hi″drən-sef′ə-le) hydrocephalus.

hy•drepi•gas•tri•um (hi″drep-ĭ-gas′tre-əm) [*hydr-* + *epigastrium*] a collection of watery fluid between the peritoneum and the abdominal wall.

hy•dric (hi′drik) pertaining to or combined with hydrogen; containing replaceable hydrogen.

hy•dride (hi′drīd) [Gr. *hydōr* water] any compound of hydrogen with an element or radical.

hy•dri•od•ic ac•id (hi″dri-o′dik) a term applied to aqueous solutions of hydrogen iodide, HI, a strong mineral acid.

hy•dri•on (hi-dri′on) hydrogen ion.

hydr(o)- [Gr. *hydōr* water] a combining form denoting *(a)* relationship to water, *(b)* the accumulation of fluid in a body part, or *(c)* the presence of hydrogen in a chemical compound.

hy•droa (hi-dro′ə) [*hydro-* + Gr. *ōon* egg] a vesicular or bullous eruption.
h. estiva′le h. vacciniforme.
h. vaccinifor′me a type of vesicular and bullous eruption on sun-exposed areas of the skin, sometimes preceded by pruritus and a burning sensation; it is usually seen in children and tends to recur each summer. The lesion dries up and leaves a brown, adherent crust surrounded by an erythematous zone, with the appearance of a vaccination vesicle. Called also *h. estivale.*

hy•dro•adip•sia (hi″dro-ə-dip′se-ə) [*hydro-* + *a-*[1] + *dipsa*] absence of thirst for water.

hy•dro•al•co•hol•ic (hi″dro-al″kə-hol′ik) pertaining to or containing both water and alcohol.

hy•dro•ap•pen•dix (hi″dro-ə-pen′diks) distention of the vermiform appendix with a watery fluid.

Hy•dro•bi•i•dae (hi″dro-be′ĭ-de) a family of snails of the order Mesogastropoda, including the subfamilies Hydrobiinae and Buliminae, which are intermediate hosts of various species of parasitic flukes.

Hy•dro•bi•i•nae (hi″dro-be′ĭ-ne) a subfamily of snails (family Hydrobiidae, order Mesogastropoda) that includes the genus *Oncomelania,* the intermediate host of *Schistosoma japonicum.*

hy•dro•bleph•a•ron (hi″dro-blef′ə-ron) [*hydro-* + Gr. *blepharon* eyelid] edema of the eyelids.

hy•dro•bro•mic ac•id (hi-dro-bro′mik) a term applied to aqueous solutions of hydrogen bromide, HBr, a strong mineral acid.

hy•dro•bro•mide (hi″dro-bro′mīd) an addition salt of hydrobromic acid. Cf. *hydrochloride.*

hy•dro•ca•ly•co•sis (hi″dro-ka″lĭ-ko′sis) cystic dilatation of a major renal calyx, lined by transitional epithelium and due to obstruction of the infundibulum; it may be asymptomatic or may be accompanied by inflammation and pain. Called also *hydrocalyx.*

hy•dro•ca•lyx (hi″dro-ka′liks) hydrocalycosis.

hy•dro•car•bon (hi′dro-kahr″bən) an organic compound that contains carbon and hydrogen only. The hydrocarbons are divided into *alicyclic, aliphatic,* and *aromatic* hydrocarbons, according to the arrangement of the atoms and the chemical properties of the compounds.
alicyclic h. a hydrocarbon that has cyclic structure and aliphatic properties.
aliphatic h. a hydrocarbon in which no carbon atoms are joined to form a ring.
aromatic h. a hydrocarbon that has cyclic structure and a closed conjugated system of double bonds that gives it the characteristic chemical properties of the parent aromatic hydrocarbon, benzene (C_6H_6); other typical aromatic hydrocarbons are toluene (C_7H_8), naphthalene ($C_{10}H_8$), anthracene ($C_{14}H_{10}$), and phenanthrene ($C_{14}H_{10}$).
chlorinated h. any of a group of hydrocarbons with chlorine substitution, which accumulate in body fat and can build up to toxic levels. They are used mainly as refrigerants, industrial solvents, insecticides, and dry cleaning fluids, and some have been used as anesthetics. See table at *organochlorine.* Called also *chlorohydrocarbon.*

■ Hydrocarbons. *(A),* Benzene, C_6H_6, an aromatic hydrocarbon; *(B),* cyclohexane, C_6H_{12}, an alicyclic hydrocarbon; *(C), n*-hexane, C_6H_{14}, an aliphatic hydrocarbon.

cyclic h. one of a series of hydrocarbons having the general formula C_nH_{2n}, the carbon atoms being thought of as having a closed ring structure.
saturated h. a hydrocarbon that has the maximum number of hydrogen atoms for a given carbon structure, such as methane, ethane, propane, cyclopropane, and the butanes.
unsaturated h. any hydrocarbon that has at least one double or triple bond between a pair of carbon atoms and thus has less than the maximum number of hydrogen atoms for a given structure.

hy•dro•car•bon•ism (hi″dro-kahr′bon-iz-əm) poisoning by hydrocarbons.

hy•dro•cele (hi′dro-sēl) [*hydro-* + *-cele*[1]] a circumscribed collection of fluid, especially a collection of fluid in the tunica vaginalis testis or along the spermatic cord.

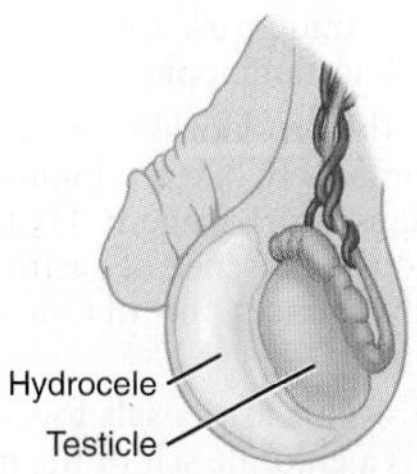

cervical h., h. col′li a serous dilatation of a persistent cervical duct, or sometimes of a deep cervical lymph space; called also *Maunoir h.*
communicating h. hydrocele in which the processus vaginalis testis is patent.
congenital h. hydrocele in the unobliterated canal between the peritoneal cavity and that of the tunica vaginalis testis.
h. of the cord funicular h.
Dupuytren h. a bilocular hydrocele that is partly in the tunica vaginalis testis and partly in the abdominal cavity.
h. fe′minae a collection of fluid in the round ligament of a female that resembles the ordinary hydrocele of a male.
funicular h. hydrocele of the spermatic cord and tunica vaginalis testis in a space closed toward the testis and open toward the peritoneal cavity. Called also *h. of the cord.*
Maunoir h., h. of neck cervical h.
h. rena′lis urinoma.
scrotal h. a circumscribed collection of fluid in the scrotum.
h. spina′lis spina bifida.

hy•dro•ce•lec•to•my (hi″dro-se-lek′tə-me) [*hydrocele* + *-ectomy*] excision of a hydrocele.

hy•dro•ceph•a•lo•cele (hi″dro-sef′ə-lo-sēl″) hydroencephalocele.

hy•dro•ceph•a•loid (hi″dro-sef′ə-loid) 1. resembling hydrocephalus. 2. see under *disease.*

hy•dro•ceph•a•lus (hi″dro-sef′ə-ləs) [*hydro-* + *-cephalus*] a condition marked by dilatation of the cerebral ventricles, most often occurring secondary to obstruction of the cerebrospinal fluid pathways (see *ventricular block,* under *block*), and accompanied by an accumulation of cerebrospinal fluid within the skull; the fluid is usually under increased pressure, but occasionally may be normal or nearly so. In children it may occur prior to closure of the skull sutures and is typically characterized by enlargement of the head, prominence of the forehead, brain atrophy, mental deterioration, and convulsions. In adults the syndrome includes incontinence, imbalance, and dementia. It may be congenital or acquired and may be of sudden onset *(acute h.)* or be slowly progressive *(chronic* or *primary h.).* Called also *hydrocephaly, hydrencephaly,* and *hydrencephalus.* **hydrocephal′ic** *adj*
acquired h. hydrocephalus resulting from a disease process, such as meningitis, or from trauma. Called also *secondary h.*

communicating h. hydrocephalus in which there is no obstruction in the ventricular system, and cerebrospinal fluid passes readily out of the brain into the spinal canal, but is not absorbed. Cf. *obstructive h. (noncommunicating h.)*.

congenital h. hydrocephalus resulting from a developmental obstruction of the cerebrospinal fluid pathways, called also *primary h.*

noncommunicating h. obstructive h.

normal-pressure h., normal-pressure occult h. dementia, ataxia, and urinary incontinence with hydrocephalus, i.e., with enlarged ventricles associated with inadequacy of the subarachnoid spaces, occurring in middle-aged and older persons. The cerebrospinal and spinal fluid pressures are at the upper end of normal, but with the excess spinal fluid volume, that pressure is actually abnormally high. Called also *occult normal-pressure h.*

obstructive h. hydrocephalus due to ventricular block (q.v.); called also *noncommunicating h.* Cf. *communicating h.*

occult normal-pressure h. normal-pressure h.

otitic h. acute hydrocephalus caused by spread of the inflammation of otitis media to the cranial cavity.

posthemorrhagic h. hydrocephalus in an infant following intracranial hemorrhage that has distended the ventricles and obstructed normal pathways for cerebrospinal fluid; in some infants it resolves spontaneously, but in others it leads to permanent neurodevelopmental deficits.

primary h. 1. congenital h. 2. chronic h.; see *hydrocephalus.*

secondary h. acquired h.

tension h. obstructive h.

h. ex va′cuo a compensatory replacement by cerebrospinal fluid of the volume of tissue lost in atrophy of the brain.

hy•dro•ceph•a•ly (hi″dro-sef′ə-le) hydrocephalus.

Hy•dro•cet (hi′dro-set″) trademark for a combination preparation of hydrocodone bitartrate and acetaminophen.

hy•dro•chlo•ric ac•id (hi″dro-klor′ik) a term applied to aqueous solutions of hydrogen chloride (HCl); it is a highly corrosive strong mineral acid commonly used as a laboratory reagent. HCl is secreted by the gastric parietal cells in response to the presence of gastrin or histamine or to vagal stimulation. This normally reduces the pH of the stomach contents to below 2.0.

hy•dro•chlo•ride (hi″dro-klor′īd) a salt formed by addition of hydrochloric acid; chemically it is a chloride salt of the moiety formed by protonation of a neutral organic compound. The term *hydrochloride* is used primarily in drug names.

hy•dro•chlo•ro•thi•a•zide (hi″dro-klor″o-thi′ə-zīd) [USP] a thiazide diuretic, used for treatment of hypertension and edema; administered orally. It is often used in combination with a potassium-sparing diuretic.

hy•dro•cho•le•cys•tis (hi″dro-ko″lə-sis′tis) [*hydro-* + *cholecystis*] distention of the gallbladder with watery fluid.

hy•dro•cho•le•re•sis (hi″dro-ko″lə-re′sis) [*hydro-* + *choleresis*] choleresis with excretion of watery bile (low in specific gravity, viscosity, and total solid content).

hy•dro•cho•le•ret•ic (hi″dro-ko″lər-et′ic) 1. pertaining to or characterized by hydrocholeresis. 2. causing or producing hydrocholeresis.

hy•dro•cho•les•ter•ol (hi″dro-kə-les′tər-ol) a reduced form of cholesterol.

hy•dro•co•done (hi″dro-ko′dōn) a semisynthetic opioid analgesic derived from codeine but having more powerful sedative and analgesic effects.

h. bitartrate [USP] the bitartrate salt of hydrocodone, used as an analgesic and antitussive; administered orally.

h. polistirex sulfonated styrene-divinylbenzene copolymer complex with hydrocodone, administered orally as an extended-release antitussive.

hy•dro•col•loid (hi″dro-kol′oid) [*hydro-* + *colloid*] a colloid system in which water is the dispersion medium.

irreversible h. a hydrocolloid that can be converted from the sol to the gel condition but cannot be reverted to a sol by any simple means. Common examples are the soluble alginates (see *alginate*).

reversible h. a hydrocolloid that can be reverted from the gel to the sol condition by increase in temperature; a common example is agar.

hy•dro•col•pos (hi″dro-kol′pos) [*hydro-* + Gr. *kolpos* vagina] a collection of watery fluid in the vagina.

hy•dro•co•ni•on (hi″dro-ko′ne-on) [*hydro-* + Gr. *konis* dust] an atomizer or vaporizer for throwing liquids in a fine spray.

hy•dro•cor•ta•mate hy•dro•chlo•ride (hi″dro-kor′tə-māt) a synthetic glucocorticoid, used topically as an antiinflammatory in the treatment of steroid-responsive dermatoses.

hy•dro•cor•ti•sone (hi″dro-kor′tĭ-sōn) [USP] the name given to cortisol when used as a pharmaceutical, applied to both the natural hormone and the same substance produced synthetically; it has life-maintaining and blood pressure–sustaining properties and also has limited mineralocorticoid activity. The official preparation and its salts are used primarily for their antiinflammatory and immunosuppressant properties, in the treatment of a wide variety of disorders, including allergic disorders, dermatologic disorders, adrenocortical insufficiency and other endocrine disorders, gastrointestinal disorders, hematologic disorders, musculoskeletal disorders, ophthalmologic disorders, respiratory disorders, rheumatic disorders, neoplasms, and shock. The base is administered orally, rectally, or topically.

h. acetate [USP] an ester of hydrocortisone, having actions and uses similar to those of the base; administered by intra-articular, intralesional, or soft-tissue injection, rectally, or applied topically to the skin, external acoustic canal, or conjunctiva. It is also applied topically to the oral mucosa to treat nonherpetic lesions and to the conjunctiva to treat inflammatory ophthalmic disorders.

h. butyrate [USP] an ester of hydrocortisone used topically for the relief of inflammation and pruritus in corticosteroid-responsive dermatoses.

h. hemisuccinate [USP] an ester of hydrocortisone, having actions and uses similar to those of the base.

h. probutate an ester of hydrocortisone used topically for the relief of inflammation and pruritus in corticosteroid-responsive dermatoses.

h. sodium phosphate [USP] a water-soluble ester of hydrocortisone having actions and uses similar to those of the base; administered intramuscularly, intravenously, or subcutaneously.

h. sodium succinate [USP] a water-soluble ester of hydrocortisone havng actions and uses similar to those of the base; administered intramuscularly or intravenously.

h. valerate [USP] an ester of hydrocortisone used topically for the relief of inflammation and pruritus in corticosteroid-responsive dermatoses.

Hy•dro•cor•tone (hi″dro-kor′tōn) trademark for preparations of hydrocortisone.

hy•dro•cy•an•ic ac•id (hi″dro-si-an′ik) hydrogen cyanide.

hy•dro•cy•an•ism (hi″dro-si′ən-iz-əm) cyanide poisoning (q.v.) caused by hydrogen cyanide.

hy•dro•cyst (hi′dro-sist) a cyst with watery contents.

hy•dro•cy•to•sis (hi″dro-si-to′sis) stomatocytosis.

hy•dro•de•lin•e•a•tion (hi″dro-de-lin″e-a′shən) the injection of fluid between the layers of the nucleus of the lens, using a blunt needle; done to delineate the nuclear zones during cataract surgery.

hy•dro•dif•fu•sion (hi″dro-dĭ-fu′zhən) diffusion in an aqueous medium.

hy•dro•dip•so•ma•nia (hi″dro-dip″so-ma′ne-ə) an epileptic condition characterized by attacks of insatiable thirst.

hy•dro•dis•sec•tion (hi″dro-dĭ-sek′shən) [*hydro-* + *dissection*] injection of a small amount of fluid, usually an isotonic salt solution, into the capsule of the lens in order to dissect its anterior part from the cortex of the lens and allow maneuverability of the nucleus of the lens during extracapsular or phacoemulsification surgery.

hy•dro•di•ure•sis (hi″dro-di″u-re′sis) [*hydro-* + *diuresis*] diuresis with hydruria.

Hy•dro•DI•U•RIL (hi″dro-di′u-ril) trademark for a preparation of hydrochlorothiazide.

hy•dro•dy•nam•ics (hi″dro-di-nam′iks) [*hydro-* + *dynamics*] the branch of the science of mechanics that studies the movement of fluids and of solids contained in fluids.

hy•dro•elec•tric (hi″dro-e-lek′trik) pertaining to water and electricity.

hy•dro•en•ceph•a•lo•cele (hi″dro-en-sef′ə-lo-sēl) encephalocele into a distended sac containing cerebrospinal fluid; called also *encephalocystocele*, *hydrencephalocele*, and *hydrocephalocele*.

hy•dro•flu•me•thi•a•zide (hi″dro-floo″mə-thi′ə-zīd) [USP] a thiazide diuretic, used for treatment of hypertension and edema; administered orally.

hy•dro•flu•o•ric ac•id (hi″dro-floor′ik) a term applied to aqueous solutions of hydrogen fluoride, an organic acid used in dilute solutions for cleaning and etching. It is extremely poisonous, as well as corrosive to the skin.

hy•dro•gel (hi′dro-jel″) a gel that has water as its dispersion medium.

hy•dro•gen (H) (hi′dro-jən) [*hydro-* + Gr. *gennan* to produce] the lightest element, an odorless, tasteless, colorless gas that is inflammable and explosive when mixed with air. It is found in water and in almost all organic compounds. Its ion is the active constituent of all acids in the water system. Atomic number 1, atomic weight 1.00797, specific gravity 0.069. Hydrogen exists in three isotopes: ordinary, or light, hydrogen is the mass 1 isotope, also called *protium;* heavy hydrogen is the mass 2 isotope, also called *deuterium;* the mass 3 isotope is *tritium.*

arseniuretted h. see *arsine.*

h. chloride a corrosive inorganic acid, HCl; see *hydrochloric acid.*

h. cyanide an extremely poisonous colorless liquid or gas, HCN, a decomposition product of various naturally occurring glycosides and a common cause of cyanide poisoning. Inhalation of the gas can cause death within a minute. Called also *hydrocyanic acid* and *prussic acid.*

h. disulfide an ill-smelling liquid, H_2S_2.

h. fluoride a corrosive inorganic acid, HF; see *hydrofluoric acid.*

heavy h. see *hydrogen.*

light h. see *hydrogen.*

ordinary h. see *hydrogen.*

h. peroxide a strongly disinfectant cleansing and bleaching liquid, H_2O_2, used in dilute solution in water, mainly as a wash or spray.

h. selenide a poisonous gas, H_2Se; its inhalation causes an obstinate coryza and destroys the sense of smell.

h. sulfide H_2S, a poisonous gas with an offensive smell, released from decaying organic material, natural gas, petroleum, and sulfur deposits, and sometimes used as a chemical reagent.

sulfuretted h. h. sulfide.

hy•dro•gen•ate (hi′dro-jən-at″) to cause to combine with hydrogen; to reduce with hydrogen.

hy•dro•gen•ize (hi′dro-jən-īz) hydrogenate.

hy•drog•e•noid (hi-droj′ə-noid) a homeopathic term denoting a constitution or temperament that will not tolerate much moisture.

hy•dro•gym•nas•tic (hi″dro-jim-nas′tik) pertaining to exercises performed in the water.

hy•dro•gym•nas•tics (hi″dro-jim-nas′tiks) therapeutic exercise performed in water.

hy•dro•hy•men•itis (hi″dro-hi″mən-i′tis) [*hydro-* + *hymen-* + *-itis*] inflammation of a serous membrane.

hy•dro•ki•net•ic (hi″dro-kĭ-net′ik) relating to the movement of water or other fluid, as in a whirlpool bath.

hy•dro•ki•net•ics (hi″dro-kĭ-net′iks) [*hydro-* + *kinet-* + *-ic*] the branch of mechanics that studies fluids in motion.

hy•dro•la•bile (hi″dro-la′bəl, -la′bīl) having a tendency to lose weight under carbohydrate or salt restriction or following infections or gastrointestinal disease. Cf. *hydrostabile.*

hy•dro•la•bil•i•ty (hi″dro-lə-bil′ĭ-te) [*hydro-* + *lability*] a condition in which tissue fluids tend to vary in quantity.

hy•dro•lase (hi′dro-lās) [EC 3] any member of the class of enzymes that catalyze the cleavage of a chemical bond with the addition of water, e.g., esterases, glycosidases, lipases, nucleotidases, peptidases, and phosphatases.

hy•drol•o•gy (hi-drol′ə-je) [*hydro-* + *-logy*] the sum of knowledge regarding water and its uses.

hy•dro•ly•ase (hi″dro-li′ās) [EC 4.2.1] a sub-subclass of enzymes of the lyase class. These enzymes catalyze the removal of water from a substrate by breakage of a carbon-oxygen bond, leading to formation of a double bond. The recommended name is usually dehydratase. The term synthase or hydratase is used when the reverse aspect of the reaction is dominant.

hy•dro•lymph (hi′dro-limf) [*hydro-* + *lymph*] the thin, watery nutritive fluid of certain animals other than humans.

hy•drol•y•sate (hi-drol′ə-zāt) a compound produced by hydrolysis.

protein h. a mixture of amino acids prepared by splitting a protein with acid, alkali, or enzyme. Such preparations provide the nutritive equivalent of the original material (casein, lactalbumin, fibrin, etc.) in the form of its constituent amino acids; used as a fluid and nutrient replenisher.

hy•drol•y•sis (hi-drol′ə-sis) pl. *hydrol′yses* [*hydro-* + *-lysis*] the splitting of a compound into fragments by the addition of water, the hydroxyl group being incorporated in one fragment, and the hydrogen atom in the other.

hy•dro•lyst (hi′dro-list) an agent that promotes hydrolysis.

hy•dro•lyte (hi′dro-līt) a substance undergoing hydrolysis.

hy•dro•lyt•ic (hi-dro-lit′ik) 1. pertaining to or characterized by hydrolysis. 2. promoting hydrolysis.

hy•dro•lyze (hi′dro-līz) to subject to hydrolysis.

hy•dro•ma (hi-dro′mə) hygroma.

hy•dro•mas•sage (hi″dro-mə-sahzh′) massage by means of moving water.

hy•dro•men•in•gi•tis (hi″dro-men″in-ji′tis) [*hydro-* + *meningitis*] meningitis with serous effusion.

hy•dro•me•nin•go•cele (hi″dro-mə-ning′go-sēl) [*hydro-* + *meningocele*] a meningocele forming a sac containing cerebrospinal fluid but no brain or spinal cord substance, in contrast to a myelomeningocele or an encephalocele.

hy•drom•e•ter (hi-drom′ə-tər) [*hydro-* + *-meter*] an instrument for determining the specific gravity of a fluid.

hy•dro•me•tra (hi″dro-me′trə) [*hydro-* + *metra*] a collection of watery fluid in the uterus.

hy•dro•me•tro•col•pos (hi″dro-me″tro-kol′pos) [*hydro-* + *metro-* + *kolpos* vagina] a collection of watery fluid in the uterus and vagina.

hy•drom•e•try (hi-drom′ə-tre) the measurement of the specific gravity of a fluid by means of the hydrometer. **hydromet′ric** *adj*

hy•dro•mi•cro•ceph•a•ly (hi″dro-mi″kro-sef′ə-le) microcephaly with an abnormal amount of cerebrospinal fluid.

hy•dro•mor•phone (hi″dro-mor′fōn) a morphine alkaloid, having opioid analgesic effects similar to but greater and of shorter duration than those of morphine.

h. hydrochloride [USP] the hydrochloride salt of hydromorphone, having the same actions as the base; administered orally, subcutaneously, intramuscularly, intravenously, or rectally for the relief of moderate to severe pain, as an antitussive, and as an adjunct to anesthesia.

Hy•dro•mox (hi′dro-moks) trademark for preparations of quinethazone.

hy•drom•pha•lus (hi-drom′fə-ləs) [*hydro-* + *omphalus*] a cystic accumulation of watery fluid at the umbilicus.

hy•dro•my•elia (hi″dro-mi-e′le-ə) [*hydro-* + *myel-* + *-ia*] a pathological condition in which there is dilation of the central canal of the spinal cord with increased fluid accumulation. Cf. *syringobulbia* and *syringomyelia.*

hy•dro•my•elo•cele (hi″dro-mi′ə-lo-sēl) hydromyelomeningocele.

hy•dro•my•elo•me•nin•go•cele (hi″dro-mi″ə-lo-mə-ning′go-sēl) [*hydro-* + *myelomeningocele*] a myelomeningocele that contains both cerebrospinal fluid and spinal cord tissue; cf. *hydromeningocele.*

hy•dro•my•o•ma (hi″dro-mi-o′mə) [*hydro-* + *myoma*] uterine leiomyoma with cystic degeneration.

hy•dro•ne•phro•sis (hi″dro-nə-fro′sis) [*hydro-* + *nephro-* + *-osis*] distention of the pelvis and calices of the kidney with urine, as a result of obstruction of the ureter. **hydronephrot′ic** *adj*

closed h. a permanent condition, resulting from complete obstruction of the ureter.

infected h. hydronephrosis that has become complicated by bacterial infection; see also *pyonephrosis.*

open h. an intermittent condition, resulting from sporadic or incomplete obstruction of the ureter.

h. of pregnancy hydronephrosis due to pressure against the ureter by the pregnant uterus.

ureterovascular h. hydronephrosis caused by crossed vessels next to the kidney that compress or deform the renal pelvis.

hy•dro•ni•um (hi-dro′ne-əm) the hydrated proton, H_3O^+; it is the form in which the proton (hydrogen ion, H^+) exists in aqueous solution, a combination of H^+ and H_2O.

Hy•dro•pane (hi′dro-pān) trademark for a combination preparation of hydrocodone bitartrate and homatropine methylbromide.

hy•dro•par•o•ti•tis (hi″dro-par″o-ti′tis) distention of the parotid gland with watery fluid.

hy•dro•pe•nia (hi″dro-pe′ne-ə) [*hydro-* + *-penia*] 1. water deprivation. 2. deficiency of water in the body.

hy•dro•pe•nic (hi″dro-pe′nik) relating to hydropenia.

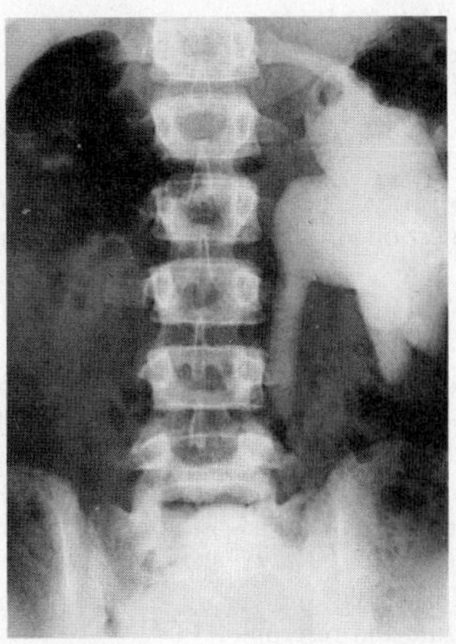

■ Hydronephrosis demonstrated in a percutaneous anterograde pyelogram.

hy·dro·peri·car·di·tis (hi″dro-per″ĭ-kahr-di′tis) [*hydro-* + *pericarditis*] pericarditis associated with a watery effusion in the pericardial sac.

hy·dro·peri·car·di·um (hi″dro-per″ĭ-kahr′de-əm) [*hydro-* + *pericardium*] abnormal accumulation of serous fluid in the pericardial cavity.

hy·dro·per·i·on (hi″dro-per′e-on) [*hydro-* + *peri-* + *ōon* egg] the fluid between the capsular and parietal decidua.

hy·dro·peri·to·ne·um (hi″dro-per″ĭ-to-ne′əm) ascites.

hy·dro·peri·to·nia (hi″dro-per″ĭ-to′ne-ə) ascites.

hy·dro·per·ox·ide (hi″dro-pər-ok′sīd) an organic peroxide in which one of the groups attached to the —O—O— is a hydrogen group; i.e., R—O—O—H.

hy·dro·per·oxy·ei·co·sa·tet·ra·eno·ic ac·id (HPETE) (hi″dro-pər-ok″se-i-ko″sə-tet″rə-e-no′ik) any of several arachidonic acid metabolites produced by the actions of lipoxygenases. 5-HPETE (5-hydroperoxy-6,8,11,14-eicosatetraenoic acid) is the precursor of the leukotrienes. 12-HPETE (12-hydroperoxy-5,8,10,14-eicosatetraenoic acid) is the precursor of 12-HETE, which is chemotactic for neutrophils and eosinophils. 15-HPETE is the precursor of 15-HETE and of lipoxins.

hy·dro·pex·ia (hi″dro-pek′se-ə) hydropexis.

hy·dro·pex·is (hi″dro-pek′sis) the fixation or holding of water. **hydropex′ic** *adj*

hy·dro·phago·cy·to·sis (hi″dro-fa″go-si-to′sis) [*hydro-* + *phagocytosis*] absorption by macrophages of plasma surrounding them.

Hy·dro·phi·idae (hi″dro-fi′ĭ-de) the sea snakes, a family of venomous snakes adapted for living in the ocean, found in the Indian and Pacific Oceans and characterized by an oarlike tail and immovable hollow fangs. Genera include *Enhydrina*, *Kerilia*, and *Pelamis*. See table at *snake*.

hy·dro·phil (hi′dro-fil) hydrophilic.

hy·dro·phil·ia (hi-dro-fil′e-ə) [*hydro-* + *-philia*] the property of absorbing water.

hy·dro·phil·ic (hi″dro-fil′ik) readily absorbing moisture; hygroscopic; having strongly polar groups that readily interact with water.

hy·droph·i·lism (hi-drof′ĭ-liz-əm) hydrophilia.

hy·droph·i·lous (hi-drof′ĭ-ləs) hydrophilic.

hy·dro·pho·bia (hi″dro-fo′be-ə) [*hydro-* + *-phobia*] 1. irrational fear of water. 2. choking, gagging, and fear on attempts to drink, a symptom of the paralytic phase of rabies. 3. former term for rabies.

hy·dro·pho·bic (hi″dro-fo′bik) 1. pertaining to or affected with hydrophobia (rabies). 2. not readily absorbing water; adversely affected by water. 3. lacking polar groups and, therefore, insoluble in water.

hy·droph·thal·mia (hi″drof-thal′me-ə) 1. hydrophthalmos. 2. congenital glaucoma.

hy·droph·thal·mos (hi″drof-thal′mos) [*hydro-* + Gr. *ophthalmos* eye] 1. a form of glaucoma characterized by marked enlargement and distention of the fibrous coats of the eye; called also *buphthalmia*, *buphthalmos*, *hydrophthalmia*, and *hydrophthalmus*. 2. congenital glaucoma.

h. ante′rior hydrophthalmos that affects only the anterior portion of the eyeball.

h. poste′rior hydrophthalmos that affects only the posterior part of the eyeball.

h. tota′lis hydrophthalmos that affects the entire eyeball.

hy·droph·thal·mus (hi″drof-thal′məs) 1. hydrophthalmos. 2. congenital glaucoma.

hy·dro·phy·so·me·tra (hi″dro-fi″so-me′trə) physohydrometra.

hy·dro·phyte (hi′dro-fit) [*hydro-* + *-phyte*] a plant adapted to grow in a very wet environment, either completely aquatic or rooted in water or mud but with stems and leaves above the water.

hy·dro·pneu·ma·to·sis (hi″dro-noo″mə-to′sis) [*hydro-* + *pneumatosis*] a collection of fluid and gas within the tissues.

hy·dro·pneu·mo·go·ny (hi″dro-noo-mo′gə-ne) [*hydro-* + *pneumo-* + Gr. *gony* knee] the injection of air into a joint to detect effusion or other abnormality.

hy·dro·pneu·mo·peri·car·di·um (hi″dro-noo″mo-per″ĭ-kahr′de-əm) pneumohydropericardium.

hy·dro·pneu·mo·peri·to·ne·um (hi″dro-noo″mo-per″ĭ-to-ne′əm) [*hydro-* + *pneumo-* + *peritoneum*] a collection of watery fluid and gas in the peritoneal cavity.

hy·dro·pneu·mo·tho·rax (hi″dro-noo″mo-thor′aks) [*hydro-* + *pneumothorax*] a collection of fluid and gas within the pleural cavity. Called also *pneumohydrothorax*, *pneumoserothorax*, and *seropneumothorax*.

Hy·dro·pres (hi′dro-pres) trademark for a combination preparation of hydrochlorothiazide and reserpine.

hy·drops (hi′drops) [L., from Gr. *hydrōps*] edema. **hydrop′ic** *adj*

h. arti′culi hydrarthrosis.

endolymphatic h. Meniere disease.

fetal h., h. feta′lis gross edema of the entire body of a fetus or newborn infant, associated with severe anemia, occurring in erythroblastosis fetalis.

h. fetalis, immune hydrops fetalis caused by maternal sensitization to a fetal blood group antigen; see *erythroblastosis fetalis*.

h. fetalis, nonimmune hydrops fetalis caused by any of a variety of nonimmunologic disorders, particularly cardiac defects.

h. folli′culi abnormal accumulation of fluid in the graafian follicle, forming a large solitary follicular cyst.

h. labyrin′thi, labyrinthine h. Meniere disease.

h. spu′rius pseudomyxoma peritonei.

h. tu′bae hydrosalpinx.

h. tu′bae pro′fluens a condition in which the abdominal opening of the uterine tube becomes closed, and the tube may reach enormous proportions as it fills with serum; peristaltic action of the tube causes colicky pain, until the fluid escapes through the uterine opening. Called also *intermittent hydrosalpinx*.

hy·dro·pyo·ne·phro·sis (hi″dro-pi″o-nə-fro′sis) [*hydro-* + *pyo-* + *nephro-* + *-osis*] accumulation of urine and pus in the renal pelvis, as seen in pyonephrosis.

hy·dro·quin·one (hi″dro-kwĭ-nōn′) [USP] the reduced form of quinone, containing two hydroxyl groups; applied topically to bleach hyperpigmented skin.

hy·dro·ra·chis (hi″dro-ra′kis) hydromyelia.

hy·dror·rhea (hi″dro-re′ə) [*hydro-* + *-rrhea*] a copious watery discharge.

h. gravida′rum a periodic or intermittent discharge of clear, yellowish, or bloody fluid from the uterus, caused by escape of amniotic fluid or resulting from decidual metritis.

hy·dro·sal·pinx (hi″dro-sal′pinks) [*hydro-* + *salpinx*] a collection of watery fluid in a uterine tube, occurring as the end stage of pyosalpinx.

h. follicula′ris hydrosalpinx in which there is no central cystic cavity, the lumen being broken up into compartments as the result of fusion of the tubal plicae.

intermittent h. hydrops tubae profluens.

h. sim′plex hydrosalpinx characterized by excessive distention and thinning of the wall of the uterine tube, the plicae being few and widely separated.

hy·dro·sol (hi′dro-sol) a sol in which the dispersion medium is water.

hy·dro·sol·u·ble (hi″dro-sol′u-bəl) soluble in water.

hy·dro·sphyg·mo·graph (hi″dro-sfig′mo-graf) [*hydro-* + *sphygmograph*] a sphygmograph with water for an index.

hy·dro·sta·bile (hi″dro-sta′bəl, -sta′bīl) preserving a stable weight under diet restrictions or gastrointestinal disease. Cf. *hydrolabile*.

hy·dro·stat (hi′dro-stat) [*hydro-* + *-stat*] a device by which the height of fluid in a container (column or reservoir) is regulated.

hy·dro·stat·ic (hi″dro-stat′ik) [*hydro-* + *-static*] pertaining to a liquid in a state of equilibrium; see under *pressure*.

hy·dro·stat·ics (hi″dro-stat′iks) the science of liquids in a state of rest or equilibrium and of the pressures they exert.

Hy·dro·stat IR (hi′dro-stat″) trademark for a preparation of hydromorphone hydrochloride.

hy·dro·syn·the·sis (hi″dro-sin′thə-sis) a chemical reaction in which water is formed.

hy·dro·sy·rin·go·my·elia (hi″dro-sĭ-ring″go-mi-e′le-ə) syringomyelia.

Hy·dro·taea (hi″dro-te′ə) a genus of flies of the family Muscidae that do not bite but often cause irritation by landing in large numbers on animals. *H. ir′ritans* is the head fly, a common species of northern Europe that is attracted to any surface of an animal's body where there are secretions such as sweat, blood, saliva, or tears. *H. meteo′rica* is a species that gathers around the eyes and nostrils.

hy·dro·tax·is (hi″dro-tak′sis) [*hydro-* + *-taxis*] an orientation movement of motile organisms or cells in response to stimulation by water or moisture.

hy·dro·ther·a·py (hi″dro-ther′ə-pe) [*hydro-* + *therapy*] the application of water in any form, but usually externally, in the treatment of disease.

colon h. an extension of the enema, used as a cleansing and detoxification procedure, in which the entire colon is irrigated by means of water, which may contain enzymes or herbs, introduced through the rectum and circulated through the colon. Called also *colonic*.

hy·dro·ther·mal (hi-dro-thur′məl) relating to the temperature effects of water, as in hot baths.

hy·dro·ther·mic (hi″dro-thur′mik) hydrothermal.

hy·dro·thio·ne·mia (hi″dro-thi″o-ne′me-ə) [*hydro-* + Gr. *theion* sulfur + *-emia*] the presence of hydrogen sulfide in the blood; see hydrogen sulfide poisoning, under *poisoning*.

hy·dro·thi·on·uria (hi″dro-thi″o-nu′re-ə) [*hydro-* + Gr. *theion* sulfur + *-uria*] the presence of hydrogen sulfide in the urine; see *hydrogen sulfide poisoning*, under *poisoning*.

hy·dro·tho·rax (hi″dro-thor′aks) [*hydro-* + *thorax*] a pleural effusion containing serous fluid. See also *pleurisy with effusion*.

chylous h. chylothorax.

hepatic h. pleural effusion that accompanies cirrhosis and portal hypertension without significant heart or lung disease.

hy·drot·o·my (hi-drot′ə-me) [*hydro-* + *-tomy*] the dissection or separation of parts by the forcible injection of water.

hy·drot·ro·pism (hi-drot′ro-piz-əm) [*hydro-* + *tropism*] a growth response of a nonmotile organism elicited by the presence of water or moisture.

hy·dro·tu·ba·tion (hi″dro-too-ba′shən) introduction of saline solution into the uterine tube; solution containing dye may be used to determine patency of the tube.

hy·dro·ure·ter (hi″dro-u-re′tər) abnormal distention of the ureter with urine or with a watery fluid, due to obstruction from any cause; cf. *megaureter*.

hy·dro·ure·tero·neph·ro·sis (hi″dro-u-re″tər-o-nə-fro′sis) [*hydro-* + *uretero-* + *nephr-* + *-osis*] distention of both the ureter and the renal pelvis and calices with urine because of obstruction of the ureter. Called also *ureterohydronephrosis*.

hy·dro·ure·ter·o·sis (hi″dro-u-re″tər-o′sis) hydroureter.

hy·dro·uria (hi″dro-u′re-ə) [*hydro-* + *-uria*] hydruria.

hy·drous (hi′drəs) containing water.

hy·dro·va·ri·um (hi″dro-var′e-əm) [*hydro-* + *ovarium*] a collection of serous fluid in an ovary.

hy·drox·ide (hi-drok′sīd) any compound of hydroxyl radical (OH), or of hydroxide ion, OH^-, with another radical or atom.

hy·droxo·co·bal·a·min (hi-drok″so-ko-bal′ə-min) [USP] a cobalamin derivative in which the substituent is a hydroxyl group; it is the naturally occurring form of vitamin B_{12} (see *cyanocobalamin*) and is sometimes used as a source of that vitamin. Abbreviated OH-Cbl.

hydroxy- a chemical prefix indicating presence of the univalent radical OH.

hy·droxy·ac·yl CoA (hi-drok″se-a′səl ko-a′) hydroxyacyl coenzyme A.

3-hy·droxy·ac·yl-CoA de·hy·dro·gen·ase (hi-drok″se-a′səl ko-a′ de-hi′dro-jən-ās) [EC 1.1.1.35] an enzyme of the oxidoreductase class that catalyzes the oxidation at the C-3 of L-hydroxyacyl coenzyme A to form ketoacyl coenzyme A, using NAD^+ as an electron acceptor. The reaction is one of the steps in fatty acid oxidation.

3-hy·droxy·ac·yl-CoA epim·er·ase (hi-drok″se-a′səl ko-a′ ə-pim′ər-ās) 3-hydroxybutyryl-CoA epimerase.

hy·droxy·ac·yl co·en·zyme A (hi-drok″se-a′səl ko-en′zīm) a hydroxy derivative of acyl coenzyme A; the L- stereoisomer hydroxylated at C-3 is an intermediate in fatty acid oxidation.

hy·droxy·ac·yl·glu·ta·thi·one hy·dro·lase (hi-drok″se-a″səl-gloo″tə-thi′ōn hi′dro-lās) [EC 3.1.2.6] an enzyme of the hydrolase class that catalyzes the cleavage of a hydroxyacylglutathione compound to the corresponding hydroxy acid and glutathione, specifically converting lactoylglutathione to lactic acid as the last step in the conversion of methylglyoxal to lactic acid. The enzyme is found in red cells and other animal tissues. See also *glyoxalase*.

hy·droxy·am·phet·amine hy·dro·bro·mide (hi-drok″se-am-fet′ə-mēn) [USP] an adrenergic used as a mydriatic, applied topically to the conjunctiva. It is also used topically as a nasal decongestant and orally as a pressor agent in the treatment of heart block, carotid sinus syndrome, and postural hypotension.

hy·droxy·an·thra·nil·ic ac·id (hi-drok″se-an″thrə-nil′ik) a cyclic aromatic compound formed in the catabolism of tryptophan.

hy·droxy·ap·a·tite (hi-drok″se-ap′ə-tīt) an inorganic compound found in bone matrix and teeth, giving them rigidity. Compounds having this approximate chemical formula are synthesized for use as calcium supplements (see *tribasic calcium phosphate*, def. 2) and prosthetic aids (see *durapatite*). Called also *hydroxylapatite*.

hy·droxy·ben·zene (hi-drok″se-ben′zēn) phenol (def. 1).

hy·droxy·bu·ty·rate (hi-drok″se-bu′tĭ-rāt) a salt or anionic form of hydroxybutyric acid.

3-hy·droxy·bu·ty·rate de·hy·dro·gen·ase (hi-drok″se-bu′tə-rāt de-hi′dro-jən-ās) [EC 1.1.1.30] an enzyme of the oxidoreductase class that catalyzes the oxidation of D-3-hydroxybutyrate to form acetoacetate, using NAD^+ as an electron acceptor. The enzyme functions in nervous tissues and muscles, enabling use of circulating hydroxybutyrate as a fuel. In the liver mitochondrial matrix, the enzyme can also catalyze the reverse reaction, a step in ketogenesis. Written also *β-hydroxybutyrate dehydrogenase*.

hy·droxy·bu·tyr·ic ac·id (hi-drok″se-bu′tə-rik) any of several hydroxy derivatives of butyric acid; they are intermediates occurring at elevated levels in some metabolic disorders. Called also *oxybutyric acid*.

3-h. a. β-h. a.

4-h. a. γ-h. a.

β-h. a. butyric acid substituted at the β, or 3, position, one of the ketone bodies produced in the liver and occurring at high levels in the blood and urine in ketosis. Called also *3-h. a.*

γ-h. a. (GHB) butyric acid substituted at the γ, or 4, position; it is an intermediate in the metabolism of γ-aminobutyric acid (GABA) and with GABA occurs at elevated levels in some body fluids in succinate semialdehyde dehydrogenase deficiency (q.v.). Because of its sedative and central nervous system depressant properties, this substance has become a drug of abuse; when taken with ethanol it causes respiratory depression and coma that can be fatal. Called also *4-h. a.* and *succinate semialdehyde*.

4-hy·droxy·bu·tyr·ic·ac·id·uria (hi-drok″se-bu-tir″ik-as″ĭ-du′re-ə) succinic semialdehyde dehydrogenase deficiency.

γ-hy·droxy·bu·tyr·ic·ac·id·uria (hi-drok″se-bu-tir″ik-as″ĭ-du′re-ə) succinic semialdehyde dehydrogenase deficiency.

hy·droxy·bu·ty·ryl (hi-drok″se-bu′tə-rəl) the acyl radical of hydroxybutyric acid.

3-hy·droxy·bu·ty·ryl-CoA epim·er·ase (hi-drok″se-bu′tə-rəl ko-a′ ə-pim′ə-rās) [EC 5.1.2.3] an enzyme of the isomerase class that catalyzes the epimerization around C-3 of a D-3-hydroxyacyl coenzyme A to form the L isomer, a substrate for beta oxidation. The reaction is necessary for metabolism of some unsaturated fatty acids. Called also *3-hydroxyacyl-CoA epimerase*.

hy·droxy·car·ba·mide (hi-drok″se-kahr′bə-mīd) hydroxyurea.

hy·droxy·chlo·ro·quine sul·fate (hi-drok″se-klor′o-kwin) [USP] a 4-aminoquinoline compound with antiprotozoal and antiinflammatory properties, used for suppression and treatment of malaria, for suppression of lupus erythematosus, and as an antiinflammatory disease-modifying antirheumatic drug in treatment of rheumatoid arthritis; administered orally.

25-hy·droxy·cho·le·cal·cif·e·rol (hi-drok″se-ko″lə-kal-sif′ə-rol) the major metabolite synthesized from cholecalciferol (vitamin D_3) in the liver and occurring in the serum; it is the precursor of 1,25-dihydroxycholecalciferol. See also table at *cholecalciferol*. Called also *calcifediol*, *calcidiol*, and *25-hydroxyvitamin D_3*.

hy·droxy·cho·les·ter·ol (hi-drok″se-kə-les′tə-rol) any of several hydroxylated derivatives of cholesterol. 7-α-Hydroxycholesterol is an intermediate in the metabolism of cholesterol to bile acids.

hy·droxy·cor·ti·co·ste·roid (hi-drok″se-kor″tĭ-ko-ster′oid) a corticosteroid bearing a hydroxyl group on a designated carbon atom.

17-h. (17-OHCS) any steroid hydroxylated at carbon 17; some are intermediates in the biosynthesis of steroid hormones and are accumulated and excreted abnormally in various disorders of steroidogenesis. Those with dihydroxyacetone side chains *(Porter-Silber chromogens)* react positively in the Porter-Silber reaction.

17β-hy·droxy·cor·ti·co·ster·one (hi-drok″se-kor″tĭ-kos′tər-ōn) cortisol.

hy·droxy·dau·no·my·cin (hi-drok″se-daw-no-mi′sin) doxorubicin.

hy·droxy·ei·co·sa·tet·ra·eno·ic ac·id (HETE) (hi-drok″se-i-ko″sə-tet″rə-e-no′ik) any of several arachidonic acid metabolites produced by lipoxygenases from hydroperoxyeicosatetraenoic acid. 5-HETE is a byproduct of leukotriene metabolism. 12-HETE and 5,12-HETE are chemotactic for neutrophils and eosinophils and 12-HETE and 15-HETE may inhibit leukotriene production.

2-hy·droxy·eth·ane·sul·fo·nate (hi-drok″se-eth″ān-sul′fə-nāt) any salt of 2-hydroxyethanesulfonic acid; see also *isethionate*.

2-hy·droxy·eth·ane·sul·fon·ic ac·id (hi-drok″se-eth″ān-sul-fon′ik) see *isethionic acid*.

hy·droxy·eth·yl cel·lu·lose (hi-drok″se-eth′əl sel′u-lōs) [NF] a partially substituted, nonionic, water-soluble cellulose ether available in several grades that vary in viscosity and degree of substitution and some of which are modified to improve their dispersion in water; it may contain suitable anticaking agents. Used as a pharmaceutic aid (suspending agent and viscosity-increasing agent).

hy·droxy·for·mo·ben·zo·yl·ic ac·id (hi-drok″se-for″mo-ben″zo-il′ik) a crystalline compound sometimes occurring in the urine in acute yellow atrophy of the liver.

hy·droxy·glu·tar·ic ac·id (hi-drok″se-gloo-tar′ik) any of several hydroxylated derivatives of glutaric acid; 2-hydroxyglutaric acid is accumulated and excreted in glutaricaciduria, type II, and 3-hydroxyglutaric acid in glutaricaciduria, type I.

hy·droxy·hep·ta·deca·tri·eno·ic ac·id (HHT) (hi-drok″se-hep″tə-dek″ə-tri″e-no′ik) a prostaglandin metabolite that is a chemoattractant for neutrophils and eosinophils.

5-hy·droxy·in·dole·ace·tic ac·id (5-HIAA) (hi-drok″se-in″dōl-ə-se′tik) a product of serotonin metabolism excreted in large amounts by patients with carcinoid tumors.

3-hy·droxy·iso·bu·ty·ryl (hi-drok″se-i″so-bu′tə-rəl) the acyl radical of an isomer of 3-hydroxybutyric acid; the thioester formed with coenzyme A, 3-hydroxyisobutyryl CoA, is an intermediate in the catabolism of valine.

3-hy·droxy·iso·bu·ty·ryl-CoA hy·dro·lase (hi-drok″se-i″so-bu′tə-rəl ko-a′ hi′dro-lās) [EC 3.1.2.4] an enzyme of the hydrolase class that catalyzes the cleavage of the coenzyme A (CoA) moiety from 3-hydroxyisobutyryl CoA as a step in the use of valine as a fuel. Deficiency results in toxic tissue accumulation of the CoA thioester of methacrylic acid and its cysteine compound conjugates.

3-hy·droxy·iso·va·ler·ic ac·id (hi-drok″se-i″so-və-ler′ik) a methylated form of isovaleric acid accumulating abnormally and excreted in the urine in several disorders of leucine catabolism.

hy·droxy·kyn·ure·nine (hi-drok″se-kīn′u-rə-nēn″) a hydroxylated derivative of kynurenine, formed from kynurenine in the catabolism of tryptophan.

hy·drox·yl (hi-drok′səl) the univalent radical OH.

hy·drox·yl·amine (hi″drok-sil′ə-mēn) an unstable inorganic compound, NH_2OH, used as a reducing agent and in organic synthesis.

hy·drox·yl·ap·a·tite (hi-drok″səl-ap′ə-tīt) hydroxyapatite.

hy·drox·y·lase (hi-drok′sə-lās) a general term used to denote enzymes of the oxidoreductase class that catalyze the formation of a hydroxyl group on a substrate by incorporation of oxygen from O_2 [EC 1.13, 1.14]. Most are monooxygenases incorporating one atom of oxygen; more rarely the term is applied to a dioxygenase hydroxylating two substrates.
11β-h. steroid 11β-monooxygenase.
17α-h. steroid 17α-monooxygenase.
18-h. corticosterone 18-monooxygenase; sometimes specifically the enzyme activity catalyzing the first (hydroxylation) reaction.
21-h. steroid 21-monooxygenase.
26-h. former name for *cholestanetriol 26-monooxygenase.*
27-h. cholestanetriol 26-monooxygenase.

11β-hy·drox·y·lase de·fi·cien·cy (hi-drok′sə-lās) an autosomal recessive disorder of steroidogenesis caused by a mutation in the *CYP11B1* gene (locus: 8q21), which encodes steroid 11β-monooxygenase; the resulting enzyme deficiency causes classic and nonclassic forms of one type of congenital adrenal hyperplasia (type IV). In the classic *(hypertensive)* form, the enzyme deficiency results in increased levels of cortisol precursors such as 11-deoxycortisol and the salt-retaining hormone 11-deoxycorticosterone, and decreased cortisol and aldosterone synthesis. Clinical manifestations include hypertension and, due to increased androgens, female pseudohermaphroditism and postnatal virilization of both sexes. The nonclassic *(late onset)* form is milder, and patients are frequently normotensive. See table at *hyperplasia.*

17α-hy·drox·y·lase de·fi·cien·cy (hi-drok′sə-lās) an autosomal recessive disorder of steroidogenesis caused by mutation in the *CYP17A1* gene (locus: 10q24.3), which encodes steroid 17α-monooxygenase; the resulting enzyme deficiency causes one type of congenital adrenal hyperplasia (type V). The disorder is characterized by decreased cortisol, androgens, estrogens, and aldosterone production and increases in 17-deoxysteroids such as corticosterone and deoxycorticosterone, resulting in hypertension, hypokalemia, and hypogonadism. Severe deficiency during fetal life can cause male pseudohermaphroditism; postnatally, it can impair sexual development in both males and females. See table at *hyperplasia* and see also *17,20 lyase deficiency.*

21-hy·drox·y·lase de·fi·cien·cy (hi-drok′sə-lās) an autosomal recessive disorder of steroidogenesis caused by mutation in the *CYP21* gene (locus: 6p21.3) , which encodes steroid 21-monooxygenase, and the adjacent pseudogene *CYP21P*; the resulting enzyme deficiency impairs the ability to produce all glucocorticoids. It is lethal if severe and untreated. It causes several forms of the most common type of congenital adrenal hyperplasia (type III): the more severe *classic forms* present at birth (*salt-wasting* and *simple virilizing*), and the less severe *nonclassic forms* of later onset (*late-onset*, or *attenuated*, and *cryptic*). The *simple virilizing* form is characterized clinically by female pseudohermaphroditism and postnatal virilization with advanced somatic development and biochemically by elevated androgens and decreased corticoids. The *salt-wasting* form is additionally characterized by aldosterone deficiency and salt wasting. Patients with nonclassic forms display variable expression of androgen excess later in life, ranging from hirsutism and infertility *(late onset)* to absence of clinical signs *(cryptic)*. See also table at *hyperplasia.*

hy·droxy·ly·sine (hi-drok″se-li′sēn) a hydroxylated derivative of the amino acid lysine; it is a component of collagen, where its residues participate in the formation of crosslinks and also act as attachment sites for disaccharide groups; it also occurs in complement C1q.

hy·droxy·ly·syl ga·lac·to·syl·trans·fer·ase (hi-drok″se-li′səl gal″ak-tōs″əl-trans′fər-ās) procollagen galactosyltransferase.

hy·droxy·meth·yl (hi-drok″se-meth′əl) the univalent radical $HOCH_2$— derived from methanol.

hy·droxy·meth·yl·bil·ane syn·thase (hi-drok″se-meth″əl-bil′ān sin′thās) [EC 2.5.1.61] an enzyme of the transferase class that catalyzes the deamination and condensation of four molecules of porphobilinogen to form a linear tetrapyrrole intermediate, hydroxymethylbilane, which cyclizes to form uroporphyrinogen. Alone, the enzyme produces uroporphyrinogen I; in the presence of uroporphyrinogen synthase it produces uroporphyrinogen III, the physiologically important isomer. Deficiency of the enzyme, an autosomal dominant trait, results in acute intermittent porphyria. Called also *porphobilinogen deaminase* and *uroporphyrinogen I synthase.*

3-hy·droxy-3-meth·yl·glu·tar·ic ac·id (hi-drok″sĭ-meth″əl-gloo-tar′ik) a dicarboxylic acid occurring at elevated levels in the urine in 3-hydroxy-3-methylglutaricaciduria.

3-hy·droxy-3-meth·yl·glu·tar·ic·ac·id·uria (hi-drok″sĭ-meth″əl-gloo-tar″ik-as″ə-du′re-ə) an autosomal recessive aminoacidopathy caused by mutation in the *HMGCL* gene (locus: 1pter-p33), which encodes hydroxymethylglutaryl-CoA lyase. The resulting enzyme deficiency is characterized by excessive urinary excretion of 3-hydroxy-3-methylglutaric, 3-methylglutaconic, and related organic acids. Onset is in the neonatal or infantile period. It resembles Reye syndrome clinically, with vomiting, lethargy, hypotonia, coma, nonketotic acidosis, hypoglycemia, and hyperammonemia.

3-hy·droxy-3-meth·yl·glu·ta·ryl (hi-drok″se-meth″əl-gloo′tə-rəl) a radical of 3-hydroxy-3-methylglutaric acid; the thioester it forms with coenzyme A, 3-hydroxy-3-methylglutaryl CoA, is an intermediate in the catabolism of leucine and in the synthesis of ketone bodies and cholesterol. Written also *β-hydroxy-β-methylglutaryl.*

hy·droxy·meth·yl·glu·ta·ryl-CoA ly·ase (hi-drok″se-meth″əl-gloo′tə-rəl ko-a′ li′ās) [EC 4.1.3.4] an enzyme of the lyase class that catalyzes the cleavage of 3-hydroxy-3-methylglutaryl CoA to form acetyl coenzyme A and acetoacetate. The reaction is a step in ketogenesis and in the catabolism of leucine. Deficiency of the enzyme, an autosomal recessive trait, causes 3-hydroxy-3-methylglutaricaciduria.

hy·droxy·meth·yl·glu·ta·ryl-CoA re·duc·tase (NADPH) (hi-drok″se-meth″əl-gloo′tə-rəl ko-a′ re-duk′tās) [EC 1.1.1.34] an enzyme of the oxidoreductase class that catalyzes the reduction of 3-hydroxy-3-methylglutaryl CoA to mevalonate, using NADPH as an electron donor. The reaction is a key rate-limiting step in the biosynthesis of cholesterol and the enzyme is inactivated by a specific kinase and reactivated by a specific phosphorylase.

hy·droxy·meth·yl·glu·ta·ryl-CoA syn·thase (hi-drok″se-meth″əl-gloo′tə-rəl ko-a′ sin′thās) [EC 2.3.3.10] an enzyme of the transferase class that catalyzes the condensation of acetyl coenzyme A and acetoacetyl coenzyme A to form 3-hydroxy-3-methylglutaryl CoA. A liver and kidney mitochondrial enzyme catalyzes the reaction as a step in ketogenesis; a cytosolic enzyme acts in the synthesis of cholesterol and other isoprenoids.

S-(hy·droxy·meth·yl)·glu·ta·thi·one de·hy·dro·gen·ase (hi-drok″se-meth″əl-gloo″tə-thi′ōn de-hi′dro-jən-ās) [EC 1.1.1.284] an enzyme of the oxidoreductase class that catalyzes the conversion of *S*-(hydroxymethyl)glutathione, a complex formed spontaneously from formaldehyde and glutathione, to *S*-formylglutathione, using NAD^+ or $NADP^+$ as an electron acceptor. The human enzyme belongs to the family of zinc-dependent alcohol dehydrogenases, and the reaction is part of the pathway that detoxifies formaldehyde. Formerly called *formaldehyde dehydrogenase (glutathione).*

hy·droxy·meth·yl·trans·fer·ase (hi″drok″se-meth″əl-trans′fər-ās) a term used in the names of some of the enzymes of the sub-subclass hydroxymethyl-, formyl-, and related transferases [EC 2.1.2] to denote those that catalyze the transfer of a hydroxymethyl group from a donor to an acceptor compound. Cf. *formyltransferase.*

4-hy·droxy-2-oxo·glu·ta·rate al·do·lase (hi-drok″se-ok″so-gloo′tə-rāt al′do-lās) [EC 4.1.3.16] an enzyme of the lyase class that catalyzes the cleavage of 4-hydroxy-α-ketoglutarate to form pyruvate and glyoxylate. The reaction is a step in the degradation of free hydroxyproline.

hy·droxy·phen·yl·eth·yl·amine (hi-drok″se-fen″əl-eth′əl-ə-mēn″) tyramine.

p-hy·droxy·phen·yl·py·ru·vate (hi-drok″se-fen″əl-pi′roo-vāt) the anionic form of *p*-hydroxyphenylpyruvic acid. Written also *4-hydroxyphenylpyruvate.*

4-hy·droxy·phen·yl·py·ru·vate di·oxy·gen·ase (hi-drok″se-fen″əl-pi′roo-vāt di-ok′sə-jən-ās) [EC 1.13.11.27] an enzyme of the oxidoreductase class that catalyzes the oxidation of *p*-hydroxyphenylpyruvate to homogentisate as a step in the use of tyrosine and phenylalanine as fuels. Deficiency of the enzyme due to heterozygous mutation in the gene encoding it causes hawkinsinuria; that due to homozygous mutation causes tyrosinemia type III.

p-hy·droxy·phen·yl·py·ru·vate ox·i·dase (hi-drok″se-fen″əl-pi′roo-vāt ok′sĭ-dās) 4-hydroxyphenylpyruvate dioxygenase.

p-hy·droxy·phen·yl·py·ru·vic ac·id (hi-drok″se-fen″əl-pi-roo′vik) the keto acid formed by transamination of tyrosine in the catabolism of tyrosine and phenylalanine; it occurs at elevated levels in the urine of patients with defects in tyrosine catabolism. Abbreviated PHPPA. Written also *4-hydroxyphenylpyruvic acid.*

hy·droxy·preg·nen·o·lone (hi-drok″se-preg-nēn′ə-lōn) pregnenolone bearing a hydroxyl; it is an intermediate in the biosynthesis of steroid hormones and is accumulated and excreted abnormally in some disorders of steroidogenesis.

hy·droxy·pro·ges·ter·one (hi-drok″se-pro-jes′tər-ōn) 17α-hydroxyprogesterone; an intermediate formed in the conversion of cholesterol to cortisol, androgens, and estrogens.

h. caproate [USP] a synthetic progestin used in the treatment of dysfunctional uterine bleeding and abnormalities of the menstrual cycle, and in the diagnosis of endogenous estrogen production; administered intramuscularly.

17α-hy·droxy·pro·ges·ter·one al·do·lase (hi-drok″se-pro-jes′tə-rōn al′do-lās) [EC 4.1.2.30] an enzyme of the lyase class that catalyzes the cleavage of the bond between carbons 17 and 20 in 17α-hydroxyprogesterone to form Δ^4-androstenedione, an androgen. It also catalyzes the conversion of 17α-hydroxypregnenolone to dehydroepiandrosterone. The enzyme activity is part of the enzyme steroid 17α-monooxygenase. Deficiency of enzyme activity is called 17,20-lyase deficiency. Called also *17,20-lyase* and *17,20-desmolase.*

hy·droxy·pro·line (hi-drok″se-pro′lēn) a hydroxylated form of the imino acid proline; it occurs in connective tissue proteins, particularly collagen. The majority is 4-hydroxyproline, but some of the 3-hydroxy form is also present.

hy·droxy·pro·lin·e·mia (hi-drok″se-pro″lĭ-ne′me-ə) 1. excess of hydroxyproline in the blood. 2. an autosomal recessive aminoacidopathy characterized by an excess of free hydroxyproline in the plasma and urine, due to a defect in the enzyme hydroxyproline oxidase; it may be associated with mental retardation. Called also *hyperhydroxyprolinemia.*

hy·droxy·pro·line ox·i·dase (hi-drok″se-pro′lēn ok′sĭ-dās) an enzyme of the oxidoreductase class that catalyzes the oxidation of 4-hydroxyproline to form the 3-hydroxy analog of Δ^1-pyrroline 5-carboxylate as part of the pathway of degradation of free hydroxyproline. Deficiency of the enzyme, an autosomal recessive trait, results in hydroxyprolinemia.

hy·droxy·pro·pyl cel·lu·lose (hi-drok″se-pro′pəl sel′u-lōs) [NF] a partially substituted, water-soluble cellulose ether, which may contain suitable anticaking agents; used as a pharmaceutic aid (emulsifying, thickening, and suspending agent, and tablet excipient, binder, and coating agent) and as an ophthalmic protectant and lubricant in the treatment of dry eye, applied topically.

hy·droxy·pro·pyl meth·yl·cel·lu·lose (hi-drok″se-pro′pəl meth″əl-sel′u-lōs) hypromellose.

hy·droxy·py·ru·vate (hi-drok″se-pi′roo-vāt) a carboxylic acid formed by the transamination of serine, serving as the primary source of D- and L-glyceric acid in plants and animals.

8-hy·droxy·quin·o·line (hi-drok″se-kwin′o-lēn) oxyquinoline.

hy·droxy·ste·roid (hi-drok″se-ster′oid) a steroid carrying a hydroxyl group, with the position and sometimes conformation of the group specified in the name of the compound.

17-h. a steroid hydroxylated at the 17 carbon; usually used to denote a 17-hydroxycorticosteroid.

3β-hy·droxy-Δ^5-ste·roid de·hy·dro·gen·ase (hi-drok″se-ster′oid de-hi′dro-jən-ās) [EC 1.1.1.145] an enzyme of the oxidoreductase class that catalyzes the dehydrogenation and isomerization of 3β-hydroxysteroids (e.g., pregnenolone) to 3-ketosteroids (e.g., progesterone), a step occurring in the biosynthetic pathways of all classes of corticosteroids.

3β-hy·droxy·ste·roid de·hy·dro·gen·ase de·fi·cien·cy (hi-drok″se-ster′oid de-hi′dro-jən-ās) an autosomal recessive disorder of steroidogenesis caused by mutation in the *HSD3B2* gene (locus: 1p13.1), which encodes 3β-hydroxysteroid dehydrogenase, resulting in several forms of one type of congenital adrenal hyperplasia (type II): the classic forms are *salt-wasting* and the milder *non–salt-wasting,* and the nonclassic form is *late onset.* The enzyme deficiency is present in adrenals and gonads; pathways to cortisol, sex steroids, and aldosterone are blocked; and pregnenolone, 17α-hydroxypregnenolone, and dehydroepiandrosterone are elevated in plasma. Males affected during fetal life are pseudohermaphroditic; both sexes have slight postnatal virilization. Most common is the mildest form (late onset) but of the classic forms, salt-wasting is predominant. See also table at *hyperplasia.*

11β-hy·droxy·ste·roid de·hy·dro·gen·ase (hi-drok″se-ster′oid de-hi′dro-jən-ās) [EC 1.1.1.146] an enzyme of the oxidoreductase class that catalyzes the reversible hydrogenation-dehydrogenation reaction between cortisone and cortisol. There are two isoforms: *type 1,* which is found in a wide range of tissues, catalyzes the conversion of cortisone to cortisol; *type 2,* found mainly in the kidney, colon, salivary glands, and placenta, catalyzes the inactivation of cortisol to cortisone.

11β-hy·droxy·ster·oid de·hy·dro·gen·ase de·fi·cien·cy (hi-drok″se-ster′oid de-hi′dro-jən-ās) deficiency of activity of either of the isoforms of 11β-hydroxysteroid dehydrogenase. Deficiency of the type 1 isozyme is caused by mutations involving two genes and three alleles and gives rise to a phenotype resembling polycystic ovary syndrome. Deficiency of the type 2 isozyme results in apparent mineralocorticoid excess (q.v.).

17β-hy·droxy·ste·roid de·hy·dro·gen·ase (hi-drok″se-ster′oid de-hi′dro-jən-ās) a large family of enzymes that modulate the potency of androgens and estrogens by catalyzing the interconversion of active 17-hydroxysteroids and inactive 17-ketosteroids. Members of this family are encoded by nonhomologous genes, have different substrate and cofactor specificities, subcellular locations, and tissue-specific patterns of expression. Deficiencies of types 3, 4 (D-bifunctional protein, q.v.), and 10 cause disease.

17β-hy·droxy·ste·roid de·hy·dro·gen·ase de·fi·cien·cy (hi-drok″se-ster′oid de-hi′dro-jən-ās) any of several disorders due to deficiency of one of the 17β-hydroxysteroid dehydrogenases.

17β-h. d. type 3 d. an autosomal recessive disorder of sexual development caused by mutation in the *HSD17B3* gene (locus: 9q22), which encodes the type 3 enzyme, characterized by male pseudohermaphroditism with variable gynecomastia.

17β-h. d. type 4 d. an autosomal recessive syndrome clinically similar to cerebrohepatorenal syndrome, caused by mutation in the *HSD17B4* gene (locus: 5q2), which encodes D-bifunctional protein (17β-hydroxysteroid dehydrogenase type 4), resulting in deficiency of either or both of the enzyme activities; it is classified into three types on the basis of the missing activity. Called also *D-bifunctional protein deficiency.*

17β-h. d. type 10 d. an X-linked dominant condition in which mutation in the *HSD17B10* gene (locus: Xp11.2) results in deficiency of the type 10 enzyme, a multifunctional mitochondrial enzyme that is involved in maintaining synaptic function; it is characterized by a number of neurologic abnormalities, including mental retardation, delayed psychomotor development, choreoathetosis, progressive neurodegeneration, and seizures.

18-hy·droxy·ste·roid de·hy·dro·gen·ase (hi-drok″se-ster′oid de-hi′dro-jən-ās) the enzyme activity of corticosterone 18-monooxygenase specifically catalyzing the second (oxidation) reaction. Deficiency of this enzyme activity is called corticosterone methyl oxidase deficiency, type II.

4a-hy·droxy·tet·ra·hy·dro·bi·op·ter·in de·hy·dra·tase (hi-drok″se-tet″rə-hi″dro-bi-op′tər-in de-hi′drə-tās) [EC 4.2.1.96] an enzyme of the lyase class that catalyzes the dehydration of 4α-hydroxytetrahydrobiopterin, a step in the regeneration of the cofactor tetrahydrobiopterin. It is encoded by the *PCDB* gene (locus 10q22), mutation of which, an autosomal recessive trait, causes a transient form of hyperphenylalaninemia with associated primapterinuria. Called also *pterin-4α-carbinolamine dehydratase (PCD).* Written also *4α-hydroxytetrahydrobiopterin dehydratase.*

5-hy·droxy·tryp·ta·mine (5-HT) (hi-drok″se-trip′tə-mēn) serotonin.

3-hy·droxy·ty·ra·mine (hi-drok″se-ti′rə-mēn) dopamine.

hy·droxy·urea (hi-drok″se-u-re′ə) [USP] an inhibitor of the enzyme ribonucleoside diphosphate reductase, which catalyzes the conversion of ribonucleotides to deoxyribonucleotides, an essential step in DNA synthesis. It is used as an antineoplastic agent primarily for treatment of busulfan-resistant chronic granulocytic leukemia, and also for the treatment of carcinoma of the head and neck, ovary, and cervix, malignant melanoma, and polycythemia vera; administered orally. It is also used orally in sickle cell disease to reduce the frequency of painful crises and to reduce the need for blood transfusions.

hy·droxy·val·ine (hi-drok″se-val′in) an amino acid obtained by protein hydrolysis.

25-hy·droxy·vi·ta·min D (hi-drok″se-vi′tə-min) either 25-hydroxycholecalciferol, the corresponding hydroxy- derivative of ergocalciferol, or both; assays evaluating stores of vitamin D by measuring serum levels of 25-hydroxyvitamin D usually reflect the total level of both compounds.

25-hy·droxy·vi·ta·min D_3 (hi-drok″se-vi′tə-min) 25-hydroxycholecalciferol.

hy·droxy·zine (hi-drok′sə-zēn) a piperazine derivative with central nervous system depressant, antispasmodic, antihistaminic, and antifibrillatory actions.

h. hydrochloride [USP] the dihydrochloride salt of hydroxyzine, used as an antianxiety agent and antiemetic, in urticaria and other manifestations of allergic dermatoses, and as an adjunct to preoperative and postoperative medications. Administered orally or intramuscularly.

h. pamoate [USP] the pamoate salt of hydroxyzine, having the actions and uses of the hydrochloride salt; administered orally.

Hy·dro·zoa (hi″drə-zo′ə) [Gr. *Hydra* a mythical nine-headed monster + *zoon* animal] a class of invertebrates of the phylum Cnidaria, usually possessing colonial branching polyps and small medusa-like bodies. It includes the poisonous genera *Gonionemus*, *Millepora*, and *Physalia*.

hy·dro·zo·an (hi″dro-zo′ən) an individual of the class Hydrozoa.

hy·dru·ria (hi-droo′re-ə) [*hydr-* + *-uria*] excessive dilution of the urine, so that it has a low osmolality or specific gravity. Cf. *hypo-osmolality*. **hydrur′ic** *adj*

Hy·ae·nan·che (hi-ə-nang′ke) a genus of trees of the family Euphorbiaceae, native to southern Africa. *H. globo′sa* has poisonous fruit that contains the alkaloid hyenanchin.

hy·e·nan·chin (hi″ə-nan′kin) a poisonous alkaloid from the outer envelope of the fruit of *Hyaenanche globosa;* it somewhat resembles strychnine in its action.

hy·giene (hi′jēn) [Gr. *hygieia* health] the science of health and of its preservation.

dental h. oral h.

industrial h. the branch of preventive medicine concerned with the protection of health of the industrial population.

mouth h. oral h.

oral h. the personal maintenance of cleanliness and hygiene of the teeth and oral structures by toothbrushing, tissue stimulation, gum massage, hydrotherapy, and other procedures recommended by the dentist or dental hygienist for the preservation of dental and oral health. Called also *dental h.* and *mouth h.*

radiation h. the science of practices involved in human protection from radiation injury.

hy·gien·ic (hi-jen′ik) 1. pertaining to hygiene. 2. conducive to health.

hy·gien·ics (hi-jen′iks) a system of principles for promoting health; hygiene.

hy·gien·ist (hi-jen′ist, hi-je′nist) a specialist in hygiene.

dental h. a dental auxiliary specially trained in dental prophylaxis, who meets certain prescribed standards of education and clinical competence. Dental hygienists work under the direct supervision of the dentist; their functions include scaling and polishing the teeth, dental radiography, and teaching oral hygiene. Some states permit them to apply fluoride solution to the teeth.

hy·gien·iza·tion (hi-jen″ĭ-za′shən) the establishment of hygienic conditions.

hy·gie·ol·o·gy (hi″je-ol′ə-je) [Gr. *hygieia* health + *-logy*] the complete science upon which the arts of hygiene and sanitation are based.

hy·gio·gen·e·sis (hi″je-o-jen′ə-sis) [Gr. *hygiēs* healthy + *-genesis*] the mechanism of the processes which lead to maintenance of health.

hy·gi·ol·o·gy (hi″je-ol′ə-je) hygieology.

hy·gre·che·ma (hi″grə-ke′mə) an auscultation sound caused by the presence of water.

hy·gric (hi′grik) [*hygr-* + *-ic*] pertaining or relating to moisture.

hygr(o)- [Gr. *hygros* moist] a combining form meaning moist or denoting relationship to moisture.

hy·gro·ble·phar·ic (hi″gro-blə-far′ik) [*hygro-* + *blephar-* + *-ic*] 1. denoting an excessive watery condition of the eyelids. 2. pertaining to any gland bringing moisture to the eyelids.

hy·gro·ma (hi-gro′mə) pl. *hygromas, hygro′mata* [*hygro-* + *-oma*] a sac, cyst, or bursa distended with a fluid. **hygrom′atous** *adj*

h. col′li a watery tumor of the neck.

cystic h., h. cys′ticum a lymphangioma, usually in the neck area, composed of large, multilocular, thin-walled cysts. It may become large and exert pressure on adjacent structures. Called also *cavernous* or *cystic lymphangioma*.

subdural h. a collection of fluid in the subdural space resulting from liquefaction of a subdural hematoma; see under *hematoma*.

hy·grom·e·ter (hi-grom′ə-tər) [*hygro-* + *-meter*] an instrument for measuring the moisture of the atmosphere.

hair h., Saussure h. a hygrometer whose action is determined by the elongation and contraction of a hair under the influence of moisture.

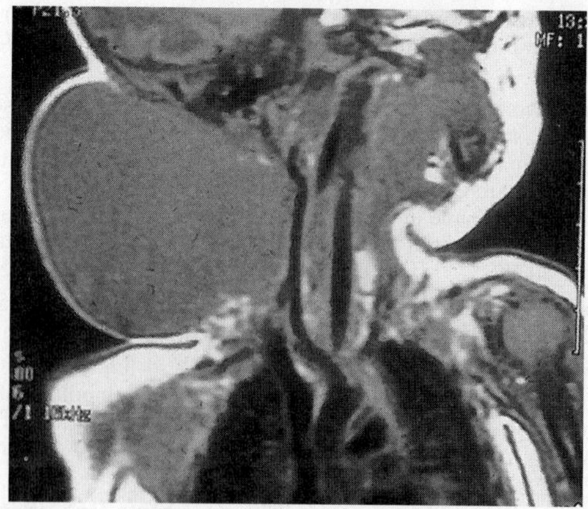

■ Large cervical cystic hygroma in an MRI scan.

hy·grom·e·try (hi-grom′ə-tre) [*hygro-* + *-metry*] the measurement of the proportion of moisture in the air. **hygromet′ric** *adj*

hy·gro·scop·ic (hi″gro-skop′ik) taking up and retaining moisture readily.

Hy·gro·ton (hi′gro-ton) trademark for a preparation of chlorthalidone.

Hy·la·form (hi′lə-form) trademark for a preparation of hylan B used as a tissue filler.

hy·lan (hi′lan) any of a family of viscoelastic cross-linked derivatives of hyaluronan, used in pharmaceutical preparations for the treatment of pain in osteoarthritis; administered by intra-articular injection. A preparation of hylan B is used as a tissue filler, injected subcutaneously.

hyle- see *hyl(o)-*.

Hy·le·my·ia (hi″lə-mi′ə) a genus of flies whose larvae infest vegetables and may be swallowed if the latter are eaten raw. *H. anti′qua* is the onion root maggot. *H. bras′sicae* is the cabbage root maggot.

Hy·le·sia (hi-le′zhə) a genus of moths native to Venezuela and nearby countries; they have venomous barbed spines on their abdomens that are often shed and can cause severe caterpillar dermatitis.

hyl(o)- [Gr. *hylē* matter] a combining form denoting relationship to matter, material, or substance. Also *hyle-*.

Hy·lo·rel (hi′lo-rel″) trademark for a preparation of guanadrel sulfate.

hy·lot·ro·py (hi-lot′rə-pe) [*hylo-* + *-tropy*] the ability of a substance to change from one physical form to another (e.g., solid to liquid, liquid to gas) without change in chemical composition; change of phase. **hylotrop′ic** *adj*

hy·men (hi′mən) [Gr. *hymēn* membrane] [TA] the membranous fold that partially or wholly occludes the external orifice of the vagina. **hy′menal** *adj*

annular h. circular h.

h. bifenestra′tus, h. bifo′ris a hymen having two openings side by side, separated by a broad septum.

circular h. a hymen having a circular opening.

cribriform h. a hymen pierced by many small perforations.

denticular h. a hymen having an opening with serrated edges.

falciform h. a sickle-shaped hymen.

fenestrated h. cribriform h.

imperforate h. a hymen that completely closes the vaginal orifice.

lunar h. a moon-shaped hymen.

persistent h. white heifer disease.

septate h. a hymen whose opening is divided by a narrow septum.

subseptate h. a hymen whose opening is partially filled by a septum that extends out of one wall but does not reach the other.

hy·men·ec·to·my (hi″mən-ek′tə-me) [*hymen-* + *-ectomy*] excision of the hymen.

hy·men·itis (hi″mən-i′tis) [*hymen-* + *-itis*] inflammation of the hymen.

hy·me·ni·um (hi-me′ne-əm) [dim. of Gr. *hymēn* membrane] the fertile, or spore-forming, surface of a fungus, which is composed of hyphae lining the fruiting body.

hymen(o)- [Gr. *hymēn* membrane] a combining form denoting a relationship to a membrane or a membranous structure, or to the hymen.

hy·me·no·lep·i·a·sis (hi″mə-no-lep-i′ə-sis) infection with *Hymenolepis;* in humans it is usually intestinal infestation by *H. nana.* Infected persons are usually asymptomatic, but in massive infection there may be dizziness, abdominal pain, diarrhea, insomnia, convulsions, and other symptoms.

Hy·me·no·lep·i·di·dae (hi″mən-o-lep′ĭ-di-de) a family of small to medium-sized tapeworms of the order Cyclophyllidea, subclass Cestoda,

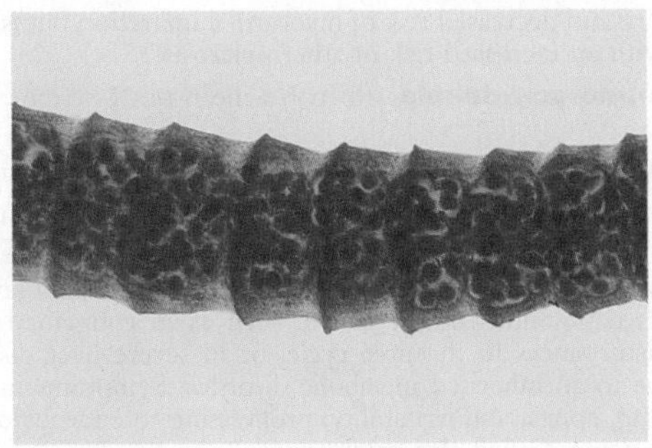

■ *Hymenolepis nana,* gravid proglottids (acetocarmine stain).

which parasitizes birds and mammals. *Hymenolepis* is the genus of medical importance.

Hy·me·nol·e·pis (hi″mə-nol′ə-pis) [Gr. *hymēn* membrane + *lepis* rind] a genus of tapeworms of the family Hymenolepididae.

H. diminu′ta a tapeworm of rats and mice, occasionally found in humans.

H. frater′na the rodent form of *H. nana;* often called *H. nana* var. *fraterna.*

H. lanceola′ta a species that infects ducks, geese, and occasionally humans.

H. na′na the dwarf tapeworm, a species from 70 to 80 mm long that is parasitic in the intestines of rats, mice, and humans, especially children, causing hymenolepiasis.

H. na′na var. *frater′na* *H. fraterna.*

hy·men·ol·o·gy (hi″mən-ol′ə-je) [*hymen-* + *-ology*] the sum of what is known regarding the membranes of the body.

Hy·me·no·my·ce·tes (hi″mə-no-mi-se′tēz) [*hymeno-* + Gr. *mykēs* fungus] in some classification systems, a category of perfect fungi at around the class level that would include the subclasses Phragmobasidiomycetidae and Holobasidiomycetidae.

hy·men·o·plas·ty (hi′mə-no-plas″te) restoration of the integrity of a ruptured hymen through plastic surgery; called also *hymenorrhaphy* and *hymen repair.* **hymenoplas′tic** *adj*

Hy·men·op·tera (hi″mən-op′tər-ə) [*hymeno-* + Gr. *pteron* wing] an order of insects usually having two pairs of well-developed membranous wings. It includes the families Apidae (bees), Formicidae (ants), and Vespidae (wasps).

hy·men·op·ter·an (hi″mən-op′tər-ən) any insect of the order Hymenoptera.

hy·men·op·ter·ism (hi″mən-op′tər-iz-əm) poisoning by the stings or bites of insects of the order Hymenoptera, as of a bee or wasp.

hy·men·or·rha·phy (hi″mən-or′ə-fe) hymenoplasty.

Hy·me·no·sto·ma·tia (hi″mə-no-sto-ma′she-ə) [*hymeno-* + Gr. *stoma* mouth] a subclass of chiefly freshwater, ciliate protozoa (class Oligohymenophorea, phylum Ciliophora) with uniform, heavy body ciliature and a ventral buccal cavity when one is present; if kinetodesmata are present, they are usually conspicuous. It comprises three orders: Hymenostomatida, Scuticociliatida, and Astomatida.

Hy·me·no·sto·ma·ti·da (hi″mə-no-sto-ma′tĭ-də) an order of ciliate protozoa (subclass Hymenostomatia, class Oligohymenophorea) characterized by the presence of a well-defined buccal cavity containing membranelles or peniculi with infraciliary bases typically three to four rows of kinetosomes wide; and by a ventral oral area, usually in the anterior half of the body. It comprises three suborders: Tetrahymenina, Ophryoglenina, and Peniculina.

hy·men·ot·o·my (hi″mən-ot′ə-me) [*hymeno-* + *-tomy*] surgical incision of the hymen.

hy·me·no·vin (hi″mə-no′vin) a toxic lactone that is the active principle in species of *Hymenoxys* and causes gastroenteritis in cattle and sheep.

Hy·men·ox·ys (hi″mə-nok′sis) a genus of herbs found in North America; some species contain the lactone hymenovin, which causes gastroenteritis and vomiting in cattle and sheep. Two common poisonous species are *H. odora′ta,* the bitterweed, and *H. richardso′nii,* the pingue or rubberweed.

hyo·epi·glot·tic (hi″o-ep″ĭ-glot′ik) pertaining to the hyoid bone and the epiglottis.

hyo·epi·glot·tid·e·an (hi″o-ep″ĭ-glŏ-tid′e-ən) hyoepiglottic.

hyo·glos·sal (hi″o-glos′əl) [hyoid bone + *glossal*] pertaining to the hyoid bone and the tongue or to the hyoglossal muscle.

hy·oid (hi′oid) [Gr. *hyoeides* shaped like the Greek letter upsilon (υ)] 1. shaped like the lower case Greek letter upsilon (υ). Cf. *hypsiloid.* 2. shaped like a U. 3. pertaining to the hyoid bone.

hyo·scine (hi′o-sēn) [L. *hyoscina*] scopolamine.

hyo·scy·amine (hi″o-si′ə-mēn) [USP] an anticholinergic and antimuscarinic alkaloid derived from *Hyoscyamus niger, Atropa belladonna,* and other solanaceous plants. It is the levorotatory component of racemic atropine; since the dextrorotatory component has little activity, hyoscyamine has approximately twice the potency of atropine. It is used primarily as an antispasmodic for gastrointestinal or urinary tract disorders; administered orally.

h. hydrobromide [USP] a salt of hyoscyamine, having actions and uses similar to those of the base.

h. sulfate [USP] a salt of hyoscyamine, having actions similar to those of the base, administered orally or parenterally as an antispasmodic in gastrointestinal disorders and orally in the treatment of hypermotility in cystitis or other urinary tract disorders.

Hyo·scy·a·mus (hi″o-si′ə-məs) [L., from Gr. *hys* swine + *kyamos* bean] a genus of annual or biennial plants of the family Solanaceae. *H. ni′ger* L. is henbane, whose leaves, seeds, flowers, and tops contain the anticholinergic alkaloids hyoscyamine and scopolamine and cause neurotoxicity in livestock. See also *hyoscyamus.*

hyo·scy·a·mus (hi″o-si′ə-məs) the dried leaf of *Hyoscyamus niger,* with or without its stem and top, which contains the anticholinergic alkaloids hyoscyamine and scopolamine; formerly used as a smooth muscle relaxant and to produce parasympathetic blockade. Called also *henbane* and *black henbane.*

Hyo·stron·gy·lus (hi″o-stron′jə-ləs) a genus of nematodes of the family Trichostrongylidae. *H. ru′bidus* is found in the stomachs of pigs.

hyo·thy·roid (hi″o-thi′roid) pertaining to the hyoid bone and the thyroid cartilage.

hyp·acu·sia (hi″pə-ku′zhə) hypoacusis.

hyp·acu·sis (hi″pə-koo′sis) hypoacusis.

hyp·al·bu·min·emia (hi″pəl-bu″mĭn-e′me-ə) hypoalbuminemia.

hyp·al·ge·sia (hi″pal-je′ze-ə) [*hyp-* + *algesia*] decreased nociception (pain sense); called also *hypalgia* and *hypoalgesia.*

hyp·al·ge·sic (hi″pəl-je′sik) 1. pertaining to or characterized by hypalgesia. 2. causing or producing hypalgesia.

hyp·al·get·ic (hi″pəl-jet′ik) hypalgesic.

hyp·al·gia (hi-pal′jə) hypalgesia.

hyp·am·ni·on (hi-pam′ne-on) oligohydramnios.

hyp·am·ni·os (hi-pam′ne-os) [*hypo* + *amnion*] oligohydramnios.

hyp·ana·ki·ne·sia (hi-pan″ə-kĭ-ne′zhə) hypokinesia.

hyp·ana·ki·ne·sis (hi-pan″ə-kĭ-ne′sis) hypokinesia.

hy·paph·o·rine (hi-paf′o-rin) a crystalline alkaloid that is poisonous and convulsive, obtained from *Erythrina americana* Mill., and other members of Leguminosae.

Hy·paque (hi′pāk) trademark for preparations of diatrizoate meglumine and diatrizoate sodium.

hyp·ar·te·ri·al (hi″pahr-tēr′e-əl) [*hypo* + *arterial*] beneath an artery, applied especially to the bronchi which are so situated.

hyp·ax·i·al (hi-pak′se-əl) ventral to the long axis of the body.

hyp·azo·tu·ria (hĭ-paz″o-tu′re-ə) hypoazoturia.

hyp·en·chyme (hi′pən-kīm) the primitive embryonic tissue formed in the cavity of the archenteron.

hyper- [Gr. *hyper* above] a prefix meaning above, beyond, more than normal, or excessive.

hy·per·ab·sorp·tion (hi″pər-ab-sorp′shən) increased intestinal absorption of a substance.

hy·per·ac·an·tho·sis (hi″pər-ak″ən-tho′sis) acanthosis.

hy·per·ac·id (hi″pər-as′id) abnormally or excessively acid.

hy·per·ac·id·i·ty (hi″pər-ə-sid′ĭ-te) excessive acidity, particularly in the stomach.

gastric h. hyperchlorhydria.

hy·per·acou·sia (hi″pər-ə-koo′zhə) hyperacusis.

hy·per·ac·ti·va·tion (hi″pər-ak″tĭ-va′shən) a stage of sperm motility after capacitation, in which the sperm moves extremely fast. If the sperm head is attached to the zona pellucida, only the tail will be moving; if it is not attached, the entire sperm will move rapidly and randomly.

hy·per·ac·tive (hi″pər-ak′tiv) pertaining to or characterized by hyperactivity; called also *hyperkinetic.*

hy•per•ac•tiv•i•ty (hi″pər-ak-tiv′ĭ-te) 1. excessive or abnormally increased muscular function or activity. 2. former name for, but now one of the signs of, *attention-deficit/hyperactivity disorder.*

autonomic h. pathologic overactivity of the autonomic nervous system, with symptoms such as tachycardia, sweating, and hypertension; this occurs in conditions such as alcohol withdrawal delirium and serotonin syndrome.

detrusor h. see under *overactivity.*

sympathetic h. autonomic hyperactivity expressed primarily in the sympathetic nervous system.

hy•per•acu•sia (hi″pər-ə-ku′zhə) hyperacusis.

hy•per•acu•sis (hi″pər-ə-koo′sis) [*hyper-* + *acou-* + *-sis*] exceptionally acute hearing, the hearing threshold being unusually low. It may or may not be accompanied by pain. Called also *hyperacousia, hyperacusia, hyperakusis,* and *acoustic* or *auditory hyperesthesia.*

hy•per•acute (hi″pər-ə-kūt′) extremely acute.

hy•per•ad•e•no•sis (hi″pər-ad″ə-no′sis) [*hyper-* + *adenosis*] a condition characterized by enlargement of the glands.

hy•per•ad•i•po•sis (hi″pər-ad″ĭ-po′sis) morbid obesity.

hy•per•ad•i•pos•i•ty (hi″pər-ad″ĭ-pos′ĭ-te) morbid obesity.

hy•per•adre•nal•ism (hi″pər-ə-dre′nəl-iz-əm) abnormally increased secretion of adrenal hormones; see *adrenocortical hormone* and *adrenomedullary hormones.*

hy•per•ad•ren•er•gic (hi″pər-ad″ren-ur′jik) excessive activity of adrenergic nerve fibers with an increase in the effects of adrenergic receptors (q.v.).

hy•per•adre•no•cor•ti•cism (hi″pər-ə-dre″no-kor′tĭ-siz-əm) abnormally increased secretion of adrenocortical hormones, as in *Cushing syndrome.* Called also *hypercorticalism* and *hypercorticism.*

hy•per•aer•a•tion (hi″pər-ār-a′shən) overexpansion of the lungs so that they contain an abnormal amount of air.

hy•per•aku•sis (hi″pər-ə-koo′sis) hyperacusis.

hy•per-β-al•a•nin•emia (hi″pər-ba″tə-al″ə-nĭ-ne′me-ə) a rare disorder of β-alanine metabolism, possibly an autosomal recessive trait, due to deficiency of β-alanine–α-ketoglutarate transaminase activity; β-alanine, β-aminoisobutyric acid, taurine, and γ-aminobutyric acid are accumulated and excreted at elevated levels and the disorder is characterized by lethargy, somnolence, and grand mal seizures. Called also *β-alaninemia.*

hy•per•al•bu•min•emia (hi″pər-al-bu″mĭ-ne′me-ə) an abnormally high albumin content of the blood.

hy•per•al•bu•min•o•sis (hi″pər-al-bu″mĭ-no′sis) a condition characterized by excessive albuminoids.

hy•per•al•dos•ter•on•emia (hi″pər-al-dos″tə-ro-ne′me-ə) abnormally increased aldosterone in the blood.

hy•per•al•dos•ter•on•ism (hi″pər-al-dos′tə-ro-niz″əm) aldosteronism.

hy•per•al•dos•ter•on•uria (hi″pər-al-dos″tə-ro-nu′re-ə) excessive aldosterone in the urine; called also *aldosteronuria.*

hy•per•al•ge•sia (hi″pər-al-je′ze-ə) [*hyper-* + Gr. *algesia*] abnormally increased nociception (pain sense); called also *hyperalgia.* **hyperalge′sic, hyperalget′ic** *adj*

auditory h. the condition in which slight noises cause pain.

muscular h. the condition in which slight exertion causes great pain.

primary h. hyperalgesia at a site where there has been an injury such as a burn.

secondary h. hyperalgesia in healthy tissue adjacent to the site where there has been an injury, usually owing to central nervous system mechanisms that have caused increased sensitivity.

hy•per•al•gia (hi-pər-al′jə) hyperalgesia.

hy•per•al•i•men•ta•tion (hi″pər-al″ĭ-men-ta′shən) 1. ingestion of excessive quantities; see also *bulimia* and *binge eating.* Called also *hypernutrition* and *overnutrition.* 2. administration of a greater than optimal amount of nutrients.

parenteral h. see *total parenteral alimentation,* under *alimentation.*

hy•per•al•i•men•to•sis (hi″pər-al″ĭ-men-to′sis) disease due to hyperalimentation (q.v.).

hy•per•al•ka•les•cence (hi″pər-al″kə-les′əns) hyperalkalinity.

hy•per•al•ka•lin•i•ty (hi″pər-al″kə-lin′ĭ-te) excessive alkalinity.

hy•per•al•lan•to•in•uria (hi″pər-ə-lan″to-ĭ-nu′re-ə) excretion of excessive allantoin in the urine; see *allantoinuria.*

hy•per•al•pha•lipo•pro•tein•emia (hi″pər-al″fə-lip″o-pro″te-ne′me-ə) the presence of abnormally high levels of high-density lipoproteins in the blood.

familial h. an autosomal dominant condition characterized by elevation of high-density–lipoprotein cholesterol (HDL-C), resulting from any of several mutations that affect HDL metabolism. It is frequently associated with longevity and decreased risk of myocardial infarction but is sometimes associated with an increased risk of atherosclerosis.

hy•per•am•i•no•ac•i•de•mia (hi″pər-ə-me″no-as″ĭ-de′me-ə) aminoacidemia.

hy•per•ami•no•ac•id•uria (hi″pər-ə-me″no-as″ĭ-du′re-ə) aminoaciduria.

hy•per-β-ami•no•iso•bu•tyr•ic•ac•id•uria (hi″pər-ə-me″no-i″so-bu-tir″ik-as″ĭ-du′re-ə) β-aminoisobutyricaciduria.

hy•per•am•mo•ne•mia (hi″pər-am″o-ne′me-ə) elevated levels of ammonia or its compounds in the blood, such as in congenital conditions including disturbances in the urea cycle, or in severe liver disease; some cases are due to an inherited metabolic disorder. Symptoms include lethargy, vomiting, apnea, and irritability, progressing to encephalopathy with seizures and coma. Called also *ammonemia.*

cerebroatrophic h. Rett syndrome.

hy•per•am•mo•nu•ria (hi″pər-am″o-nu′re-ə) increased excretion of ammonia in the urine, as with hyperammonemia; called also *ammoniuria.*

hy•per•am•y•las•emia (hi″pər-am″ə-la-se′me-ə) abnormally high elevation of amylase in the blood.

hy•per•an•dro•gen•ism (hi″pər-an′dro-jən-iz-əm) the state of having excessive secretion of androgens, as seen in congenital adrenal hyperplasia, some types of precocious puberty, and other conditions.

hy•per•aphia (hi″pər-a′fe-ə) tactile hyperesthesia. **hyperaph′ic** *adj*

hy•per•ar•gin•in•emia (hi″pər-ahr″jĭ-nĭ-ne′me-ə) 1. arginase deficiency. 2. excess of arginine in the blood.

hy•per•arou•sal (hi″pər-ə-rou′səl) a state of increased psychological and physiological tension marked by such effects as reduced tolerance to pain, anxiety, exaggerated startle responses, insomnia, fatigue, and accentuation of personality traits.

hy•per•azo•te•mia (hi″pər-az″o-te′me-ə) an excess of nitrogenous matter, usually urea, in the blood.

hy•per•azo•tu•ria (hi″pər-az″o-tu′re-ə) azoturia (def. 1).

hy•per•bar•ic (hi″pər-bar′ik) [*hyper-* + *bar-* + *-ic*] having greater than normal pressure or weight; applied to gases under greater than atmospheric pressure, or to a solution of greater specific gravity than another taken as a standard of reference.

hy•per•bar•ism (hi″pər-bar′iz-əm) the condition resulting from exposure to ambient gas pressure or atmospheric pressures that exceed the pressure within body tissues, fluids, and cavities.

hy•per•baso•phil•ic (hi″pər-ba″so-fil′ik) staining intensely with basic dyes.

hy•per•be•ta•lipo•pro•tein•emia (hi″pər-ba″tə-lip″o-pro″te-ne′me-ə) increased accumulation of low-density lipoproteins in the blood.

familial h. familial hypercholesterolemia.

hy•per•bi•car•bo•nat•emia (hi″pər-bi-kahr″bə-na-te′me-ə) excessive bicarbonates in the blood; see also *alkalosis.*

hy•per•bil•i•ru•bin•emia (hi″pər-bil″ĭ-roo″bĭ-ne′me-ə) excessive bilirubin in the blood, which may lead to jaundice; the hyperbilirubinemias are classified as either *conjugated* or *unconjugated,* according to the predominant form of bilirubin involved.

h. I Gilbert syndrome.

h. II Dubin-Johnson syndrome.

congenital h. Crigler-Najjar syndrome.

conjugated h. hyperbilirubinemia due to defective excretion of conjugated bilirubin by the liver cells or to anatomic obstruction to bile flow within the liver or in the extrahepatic bile duct system; conditions showing this include Dubin-Johnson syndrome and Rotor syndrome.

constitutional h. Gilbert syndrome.

neonatal h., newborn h. a type of mild, transient unconjugated hyperbilirubinemia seen in the normal neonate; a transient familial form also occurs, in which jaundice occurs within four days after birth and may lead to kernicterus.

unconjugated h. hyperbilirubinemia due to excessive bilirubin production (hemolysis), to defective clearance of bilirubin from the blood by the liver, or to defective conjugation by the liver; it includes hemolytic states, Crigler-Najjar syndrome, Gilbert syndrome, and neonatal hyperbilirubinemia.

hy•per•brachy•ce•phal•ic (hi″pər-brak″e-sə-fal′ik) pertaining to or characterized by hyperbrachycephaly.

hy•per•brachy•ceph•a•ly (hi″pər-brak″e-sef′ə-le) the condition of having a cephalic index of 85.5 or more.

hy•per•brady•ki•nin•emia (hi″pər-brad″e-ki″nĭ-ne′me-ə) elevated levels of bradykinin in the blood, marked by a warm feeling, flushing, wheezing, and sometimes nausea.

hy•per•brady•ki•nin•ism (hi″pər-brad″e-ki′nĭ-niz-əm) a syndrome characterized by high plasma levels of bradykinin, in which standing produces a fall in systolic blood pressure, an increase in diastolic blood pressure and heart rate, and purplish discoloration of the lower limbs with ecchymoses.

hy·per·cal·ce·mia (hi″pər-kal-se′me-ə) [*hyper-* + *calci-* + *-emia*] an excess of calcium in the blood; manifestations include fatigability, muscle weakness, depression, anorexia, nausea, and constipation. Called also *calcemia* and *hypercalcinemia.*

familial benign h., familial hypocalciuric h. a generally benign, usually asymptomatic, autosomal dominant condition characterized by hypercalcemia resulting from loss of function of the calcium-sensing receptor, so that higher than normal levels of blood calcium are needed to suppress parathyroid hormone secretion. Other characteristics include mild hypermagnesemia, normal or slightly elevated parathyroid hormone levels, and low urine levels of calcium. Homozygous individuals present with severe hyperparathyroidism at birth. Most cases are caused by mutation in the calcium-sensing receptor gene (*CASR*, locus: 3q13.3-q21); a few cases are caused by mutation at 19q13.

idiopathic h. a condition of infants, associated with vitamin D intoxication, and characterized by elevated serum calcium levels and increased density of the skeleton, with mental deterioration progressing to severe retardation, and nephrocalcinosis causing chronic uremia.

humoral h. of malignancy hypercalcemia of malignancy caused by bone resorption mediated by circulating osteoclast-activating factors released from distant tumor cells.

h. of malignancy, osteolytic h. abnormal elevation of serum calcium associated with malignant tumors, resulting from osteolysis caused by bone metastases or by the action of circulating osteoclast-activating factors released from tumor cells.

hy·per·cal·ci·ne·mia (hi″pər-kal″sĭ-ne′me-ə) hypercalcemia.

hy·per·cal·ci·nu·ria (hi″pər-kal″sĭ-nu′re-ə) hypercalciuria.

hy·per·cal·ci·pexy (hi″pər-kal′sĭ-pek″se) excessive fixation of calcium.

hy·per·cal·ci·to·nin·emia (hi″pər-kal″sĭ-to″nĭ-ne′me-ə) excessive calcitonin in the blood.

hy·per·cal·ci·uria (hi″pər-kal″se-u′re-ə) excess of calcium in the urine, such as in hypercalcemic conditions or in defective renal tubular reabsorption of calcium; some types predispose the patient to formation of renal calculi.

absorptive h. hypercalciuria due to hyperabsorption of calcium, with formation of calcium oxalate or calcium phosphate renal calculi.

idiopathic h. any type whose cause is unknown, often with formation of renal calculi. Some patients have increased turnover of bone calcium and in some there may be a genetic predisposition.

renal h. hypercalciuria due to primary renal wasting of calcium, which stimulates production of parathyroid hormone to increase calcium resorption in the intestine. This type is not linked to formation of renal calculi.

hy·per·ca·lor·ic (hi″pər-kə-lor′ik) high in calories.

hy·per·cap·il·lar·i·za·tion (hi″pər-kap″ĭ-lər-ĭ-za′shən) an abnormally increased number of capillaries in a tissue or organ.

hy·per·cap·nia (hi″pər-kap′ne-ə) [*hyper-* + *capn-* + *-ia*] excess of carbon dioxide in the blood. Called also *hypercarbia.* **hypercap′nic** *adj*

permissive h. artificially induced hypercapnia in patients with acute respiratory distress syndrome or respiratory failure, done to lower the inspiratory pressure and tidal volume and thus the possibility of lung injury.

hy·per·car·bia (hi″pər-kahr′be-ə) hypercapnia.

hy·per·car·o·ten·emia (hi″pər-kar″ə-tə-ne′me-ə) an elevated level of carotene in the blood, resulting from excessive ingestion of carotenoids or from decreased ability to convert carotenoids to vitamin A; it is often characterized by yellowing of the skin (see *carotenosis*). Called also *carotenemia.*

hy·per·cat·a·bol·ic (hi″pər-kat″ə-bol′ik) 1. pertaining to or characterized by hypercatabolism. 2. causing hypercatabolism.

hy·per·ca·tab·o·lism (hi″pər-kə-tab′o-liz-əm) abnormally increased catabolism.

hy·per·ca·thar·sis (hi″pər-kə-thahr′sis) excessive evacuation of feces. **hypercathar′tic** *adj*

hy·per·cel·lu·lar (hi″pər-sel′u-lər) pertaining to or characterized by hypercellularity.

hy·per·cel·lu·lar·i·ty (hi″pər-sel″u-lar′ĭ-te) a state characterized by an abnormal increase in the number of cells present, as in bone marrow.

hy·per·ce·men·to·sis (hi″pər-se″mən-to′sis) a regressive change of teeth characterized by excessive development of secondary cementum on the tooth surface; it may occur on any part of the root, but the apical two thirds is the part most often affected. Called also *cementosis* and *cementum hyperplasia.*

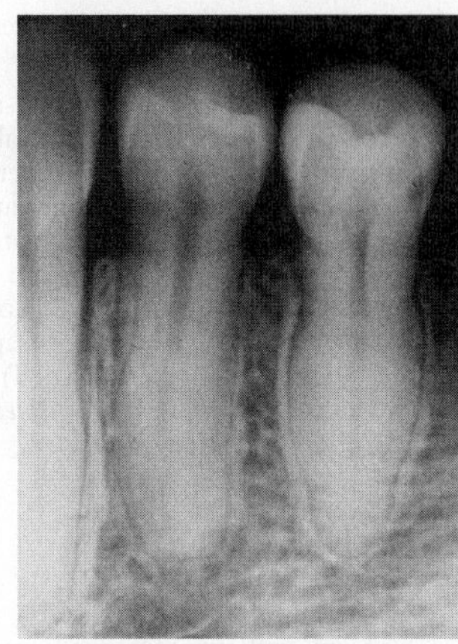

■ Hypercementosis, showing thickening and blunting of the roots of the mandibular bicuspids.

hy·per·chlor·emia (hi″pər-klor-e′me-ə) an excess of chloride in the blood. **hyperchlore′mic** *adj*

hy·per·chlor·hy·dria (hi″pər-klor-hi′dre-ə) excessive secretion of hydrochloric acid by the stomach cells. Called also *chlorhydria* and *hyperhydrochloria.*

hy·per·chlo·ri·du·ria (hi″pər-klo″rĭ-du′re-ə) chloruresis.

hy·per·cho·les·ter·emia (hi″pər-kə-les″tər-e′me-ə) hypercholesterolemia.

hy·per·cho·les·ter·ol·emia (hi″pər-kə-les″tər-ol-e′me-ə) excessive cholesterol in the blood.

autosomal dominant h. a genetically heterogeneous, autosomal domininant disorder of lipoprotein metabolism characterized by elevated LDL cholesterol, with development of tendinous xanthomas, corneal arcus, and coronary artery disease. The most common type is *familial h.*

familial h. an inherited disorder of lipoprotein metabolism resulting from defects in the cellular receptor for plasma low-density lipoprotein (LDL), inherited as an autosomal dominant trait with gene dosage effect. Defects in the receptor are caused by mutation in the *LDLR* gene (locus: p13.2); over 1000 different mutations have been described. It is characterized by cutaneous and tendinous xanthomas, corneal arcus, and premature coronary atherosclerosis. The biochemical phenotype, elevated plasma LDL and cholesterol, is that of a type II-a hyperlipoproteinemia; rarely, plasma very-low-density lipoproteins and triglycerides may also be elevated, a type II-b phenotype. See table at *hyperlipoproteinemia.*

polygenic h. any of a diverse group of disorders in which some combination of genetic, and frequently also environmental, factors interact to cause elevated plasma cholesterol (i.e., a hyperlipoproteinemia type II-a or II-b phenotype; see table at *hyperlipoproteinemia*). It is distinguished from familial hypercholesterolemia and familial combined hyperlipidemia.

hy·per·cho·les·ter·ol·emic (hi″pər-kə-les″tər-ol-e′mik) 1. pertaining to or characterized by hypercholesterolemia. 2. tending to produce hypercholesterolemia.

hy·per·cho·les·ter·ol·ia (hi″pər-kə-les″tər-ol′e-ə) abnormally high cholesterol in the bile.

hy·per·cho·lia (hi″pər-ko′le-ə) [*hyper-* + *chol-* + *-ia*] excessive secretion of bile.

hy·per·chon·dro·pla·sia (hi″pər-kon″dro-pla′shə) excessive development of cartilage.

hy·per·chro·maf·fin·ism (hi″pər-kro-maf′ĭ-niz-əm) a condition caused by excessive release of biogenic amines from chromaffin cells, as in pheochromocytoma; the major symptom is arterial hypertension.

hy·per·chro·ma·sia (hi″pər-kro-ma′zhə) hyperchromatism.

hy·per·chro·mat·ic (hi″pər-kro-mat′ik) 1. staining more intensely than is normal. 2. pertaining to or marked by hyperchromatism.

hy·per·chro·ma·tin (hi″pər-kro′mə-tin) the darkly staining chromatin seen in hyperchromatism.

hy·per·chro·ma·tism (hi″pər-kro′mə-tiz-əm) [*hyper-* + *chromato-* + *-ism*] excessive pigmentation in the form of a darkly staining cell nucleus, the consequence of an excess of chromatin. Called also *hyperchromasia, hyperchromatosis,* and *hyperchromia.*

hy·per·chro·ma·to·sis (hi″pər-kro″mə-to′sis) 1. increased staining capacity. 2. hyperchromatism.

hy·per·chro·mia (hi″pər-kro′me-ə) hyperchromatism.

hy·per·chro·mic (hi″pər-kro′mik) highly or excessively stained or colored.

hy·per·chy·lo·mi·cron·emia (hi″pər-ki″lo-mi″kro-ne′me-ə) the presence in the blood of an excess of chylomicrons. Called also *chylomicronemia.*

familial h. an inherited disorder of lipoprotein metabolism characterized by elevated plasma chylomicrons and triglycerides and manifested clinically by episodic abdominal pain and pancreatitis, cutaneous xanthomas, lipemia retinalis, and hepatosplenomegaly. It is due to deficiency of lipoprotein lipase, caused by mutation in the *LPL* gene (locus: 8p22) and resulting in a type I hyperlipoproteinemia, or its cofactor apolipoprotein C-II, caused by mutation in the *APOA5* gene (locus: 11q23) and resulting in a type V hyperlipoproteinemia. See table at *hyperlipoproteinemia.*

familial h. with hyperprebetalipoproteinemia see *familial h.*

hy·per·ci·ne·sia (hi″pər-sĭ-ne′zhə) hyperkinesia.

hy·per·cit·rul·lin·emia (hi″pər-sit-rul″in-e′me-ə) an excess of citrulline in the blood.

hyp·er·CK·emia (hi″pər-ce″ka″e′me-ə) persistent elevated levels of serum creatine kinase; a form without accompanying muscle weakness has been associated with mutation in the gene encoding caveolin-3.

hy·per·co·ag·u·la·bil·i·ty (hi″pər-ko-ag″u-lə-bil′ĭ-te) the state of being more readily coagulated than normal. **hypercoag′ulable** *adj*

hy·per·co·ria (hi″pər-kor′e-ə) hyperkoria.

hy·per·cor·ti·cal·ism (hi″pər-kor′tĭ-kəl-iz-əm) hyperadrenocorticism.

hy·per·cor·ti·cism (hi″pər-kor′tĭ-siz-əm) hyperadrenocorticism.

hy·per·cor·ti·sol·ism (hi″pər-kor′tĭ-sol″iz-əm) hyperadrenocorticism.

hy·per·cre·a·tin·emia (hi″pər-kre″ə-tĭ-ne′me-ə) an abnormality of creatine metabolism in skeletal muscle, a common feature of thyrotoxicosis.

hy·per·cry·al·ge·sia (hi″pər-kri″al-je′ze-ə) hypercryesthesia.

hy·per·cry·es·the·sia (hi″pər-kri″es-the′zhə) [*hyper-* + *cryesthesia*] particularly severe cryesthesia; called also *hypercryalgesia.*

hy·per·cu·pre·mia (hi″pər-ku-pre′me-ə) [*hyper-* + L. *cuprum* copper + *-emia*] an excess of copper in the blood. See also *copper poisoning,* under *poisoning.*

hy·per·cu·pri·uria (hi″pər-ku-pre-u′re-ə) [*hyper-* + L. *cuprum* copper + *-uria*] excretion of excessive copper in the urine, as seen in copper poisoning, Wilson disease, and similar conditions. Called also *cupriuria* and *cupruresis.*

hy·per·cy·a·not·ic (hi″pər-si″ə-not′ik) extremely cyanotic.

hy·per·cy·e·sis (hi″pər-si-e′sis) superfetation.

hy·per·cy·the·mia (hi″pər-si-the′me-ə) polycythemia.

hy·per·cy·to·chro·mia (hi″pər-si″to-kro′me-ə) [*hyper-* + *cyto-* + *chrom-* + *-ia*] increased staining capacity of a blood cell.

hy·per·dac·tyl·ia (hi″pər-dak-til′e-ə) polydactyly.

hy·per·dac·ty·ly (hi″pər-dak′tə-le) polydactyly.

hy·per·dense (hi′pər-dens″) being denser than other similar objects, such as an object or area that is denser than others on a radiograph.

hy·per·di·cro·tism (hi″pər-dik′rə-tiz-əm) [*hyper-* + *dicrotism*] a condition in which the pulse is extremely dicrotic. **hyperdicrot′ic** *adj*

hy·per·dip·loid (hi″pər-dip′loid) [*hyper-* + *diploid*] aneuploid with more than the diploid number of chromosomes (usually only a few more).

hy·per·dip·sia (hi″pər-dip′se-ə) [*hyper-* + *dipsia*] intense thirst of relatively brief duration.

hy·per·dis·ten·tion (hi″pər-dis-ten′shən) excessive distention.

hy·per·di·ure·sis (hi″pər-di″u-re′sis) extreme diuresis.

hy·per·don·tia (hi″pər-don′shə) [*hyper-* + *odont-* + *-ia*] an anomaly in which there are supernumerary teeth; called also *polyodontia.*

hy·per·dy·na·mia (hi″pər-di-na′me-ə) hyperactivity (def. 1). **hyperdynam′ic** *adj*

h. u′teri excessive uterine contractions in labor.

hy·per·ec·cris·ia (hi″pər-ə-kris′e-ə) [*hyper-* + *eccrisis* + *-ia*] abnormally increased excretion. **hypereccrit′ic** *adj*

hy·per·ec·cri·sis (hi″pər-ək′rĭ-sis) hypereccrisia.

hy·per·echo·gen·ic (hi″pər-ek″o-jen′ik) hyperechoic.

hy·per·echo·ic (hi″pər-ə-ko′ik) in ultrasonography, giving off many echoes; said of tissues or structures that reflect relatively many of the ultrasound waves directed at them. Called also *hyperechogenic.*

hy·per·ek·plex·ia (hi″pər-ek-plek′se-ə) [*hyper-* + Gr. *eklēxia* panic] a congenital condition of exaggerated startle reactions. In infants it has been observed in a syndrome accompanied by hypertonia, hypokinesia, and brisk cerebral bulbar reflexes, and in adults it is similar to jumping disease. Called also *startle disease* and *hyperexplexia.*

hy·per·elas·tic (hi″per-e-las′tik) excessively elastic; characterized by hyperelasticity.

hy·per·elas·tic·i·ty (hi″per-e-las-tis′ĭ-te) excessive elasticity, such as of the skin in cutis laxa and Ehlers-Danlos syndrome.

hy·per·elec·tro·ly·te·mia (hi″pər-e-lek″tro-li-te′me-ə) an abnormally high concentration of electrolytes in the blood.

hy·per·em·e·sis (hi″pər-em′ə-sis) [*hyper-* + *-emesis*] excessive vomiting. **hyperemet′ic** *adj*

h. gravida′rum severe, pernicious morning sickness.

h. lacten′tium excessive vomiting of nursing babies.

hy·per·emia (hi″pər-e′me-ə) [*hyper-* + *-emia*] an increase of blood in a part; cf. *congestion.* Called also *engorgement.* **hypere′mic** *adj*

active h. increased blood in a part due to local or general relaxation of the arterioles. Called also *arterial h.* and *fluxionary h.*

arterial h. active h.

collateral h. increased flow of blood through collateral vessels when the flow through the main artery is arrested.

exercise h. vasodilation of the capillaries in muscles in response to the onset of exercise; it is proportionate to the force of the muscular contractions.

fluxionary h. active h.

passive h. increased blood in a part resulting from obstruction to its outflow from the area. Called also *venous h.*

reactive h. an excess of blood in a part following restoration of its temporarily arrested flow.

venous h. passive h.

hy·per·emi·za·tion (hi″pər-e″mĭ-za′shən) the production of hyperemia, especially when done for therapeutic purposes.

hy·per·en·dem·ic (hi″pər-ən-dem′ik) [*hyper-* + *endemic*] equally endemic, at a high level, in all age groups of a population. Cf. *holoendemic.*

hy·per·eo·sin·o·phil·ia (hi″pər-e″o-sin″o-fil′e-ə) extreme eosinophilia.

filarial h. tropical pulmonary eosinophilia.

hy·per·epi·neph·rin·emia (hi″pər-ep″ĭ-nef″rĭ-ne′me-ə) an excess of epinephrine in the blood, as in pheochromocytoma.

hy·per·equi·lib·ri·um (hi″pər-e′kwĭ-lib′re-əm) an excessive tendency to vertigo; see also *sense of equilibrium,* under *sense.*

hy·per·er·gia (hi″pər-ur′jə) increased sensitivity in allergy.

hy·per·eryth·ro·cy·the·mia (hi″pər-ə-rith″ro-si-the′me-ə) polycythemia.

hy·per·eso·pho·ria (hi″pər-es″o-for′e-ə) [*hyper-* + *esophoria*] a tendency of the visual axis to deviate upward and inward.

hy·per·es·the·sia (hi″pər-es-the′zhə) [*hyper-* + *esthesia*] a dysesthesia consisting of increased sensitivity, particularly a painful sensation from a normally painless touch stimulus. Cf. *hyperalgesia.* **hyperesthet′ic** *adj*

acoustic h., auditory h. hyperacusis.

cerebral h. hyperesthesia due to a cerebral lesion.

gustatory h. hypergeusia.

muscular h. muscular oversensitivity to pain or fatigue.

olfactory h. hyperosmia.

oneiric h. increase of sensitivity or of pain during sleep and dreams.

optic h. abnormal sensitivity of the eye to light.

tactile h. a paraphia consisting of excessive sensitivity of the sense of touch; called also *hyperaphia.*

hy·per·es·tro·gen·emia (hi″pər-es″tro-jə-ne′me-ə) excessively high blood estrogen levels; in men it may cause gynecomastia and similar changes.

hy·per·es·tro·gen·ism (hi″pər-es′tro-jən-iz-əm) excessive amounts of estrogens in the body.

hy·per·es·tro·gen·o·sis (hi″pər-es″tro-jə-no′sis) hyperestrogenism.

hy·per·evol·u·tism (hi″pər-e-vol′u-tiz-əm) accelerated development.

hy·per·ex·ci·ta·bil·i·ty (hi″pər-ek-sīt″ə-bil′ĭ-te) hyperirritability.

peripheral nerve h. excessive irritability of peripheral nerves, with symptoms in the muscles they innervate, such as cramps, stiffness, and neuromyotonia.

hy·per·ex·cre·to·ry (hi″pər-eks′krə-tor-e) marked by excessive secretion or excretion.

hy·per·exo·pho·ria (hi″pər-ek″so-for′e-ə) [*hyper-* + *exophoria*] a tendency of the visual axis to deviate upward and outward.

hy·per·ex·plex·ia (hi″pər-eks-plek′se-ə) hyperekplexia.

hy·per·ex·pres·sion (hi″pər-eks-presh′ən) elaboration of more than a normal amount of a product such as a hormone or a gene product.

hy·per·ex·tend (hi″pər-ək-stend′) to extend beyond the normal.

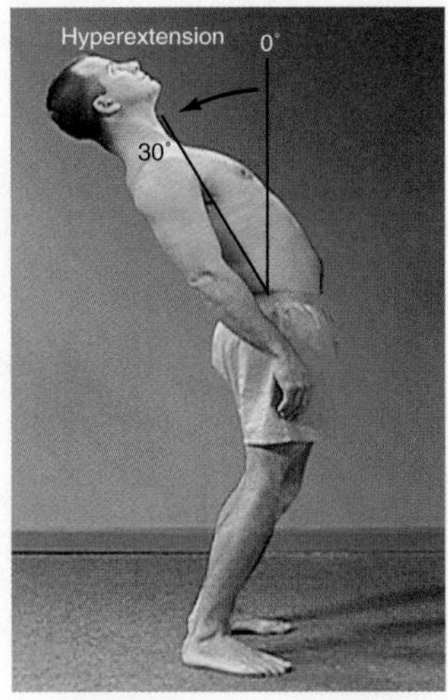

■ Hyperextension of the spine.

hy·per·ex·ten·sion (hi″pər-ək-sten′shən) extreme or excessive extension of a limb or part.

hy·per·fer·re·mia (hi″pər-fer-e′me-ə) [*hyper-* + *ferr-* + *-emia*] an excess of iron in the blood; see also *iron poisoning,* under *poisoning.* Called also *hyperferricemia* and *siderosis.* **hyperferre′mic** *adj*

hy·per·fer·ri·ce·mia (hi″pər-fer″ĭ-se′me-ə) hyperferremia.

hy·per·fi·bri·no·ge·ne·mia (hi″pər-fi-brin″o-jə-ne′me-ə) an excess of fibrinogen in the blood; called also *fibrinogenemia.*

hy·per·fil·tra·tion (hi″pər-fil-tra′shən) an increase in the glomerular filtration rate, often a sign of early type 1 diabetes mellitus.

hy·per·flex·ion (hi″pər-flek′shən) forcible excessive flexion of a limb or part.

hy·per·frac·tion·a·tion (hi″pər-frak″shən-a′shən) the subdivision of a radiotherapy schedule with reduction of dose per exposure but no decrease in overall treatment span; done to decrease side effects while delivering an equivalent or greater total dose. Called also *hyperfractionated radiotherapy.*

hy·per·func·tion (hi″pər-funk′shən) excessive functioning of an organ.

hy·per·ga·lac·tia (hi″pər-gə-lak′she-ə) [*hyper-* + *galact-* + *-ia*] excessive lactation.

hy·per·gal·ac·to·sis (hi″pər-gal″ak-to′sis) hypergalactia.

hy·per·ga·lac·tous (hi″pər-gə-lak′təs) 1. pertaining to or characterized by hypergalactia. 2. characterized by or causing hypergalactia.

hy·per·gam·ma·glob·u·lin·emia (hi″pər-gam″ə-glob″u-lĭ-ne′me-ə) an excess of gamma globulins in the blood, seen frequently in chronic infectious diseases.
monoclonal h's plasma cell dyscrasias.
polyclonal h. hypergammaglobulinemia due to increased quantity of all immunoglobulin classes, rather than only one.

hy·per·gas·trin·emia (hi″pər-gas′trĭ-ne′me-ə) excessively high blood gastrin levels, such as in Zollinger-Ellison syndrome. **hypergastrine′mic** *adj*

hy·per·gen·e·sis (hi″pər-jen′ə-sis) [*hyper-* + *-genesis*] excessive development, hypertrophy, or redundancy. **hypergenet′ic** *adj*

hy·per·gen·i·tal·ism (hi″pər-jen′ĭ-təl-iz-əm) hypergonadism.

hy·per·geus·es·the·sia (hi″pər-goos″es-the′zhə) hypergeusia.

hy·per·geu·sia (hi″pər-goo′zhə) [*hyper-* + Gr. *geusis* taste] a parageusia involving increased sensitivity of taste; called also *hypergeusesthesia* and *gustatory hyperesthesia.*

hy·per·glan·du·lar (hi″pər-glan′du-lər) marked by abnormally increased activity of any gland.

hy·per·glob·u·lin·emia (hi″pər-glob″u-lĭ-ne′me-ə) abnormally high content of any globulin in the blood; see also *hypergammaglobulinemia.*

hy·per·glu·ca·gon·emia (hi″pər-gloo″kə-gon-e′me-ə) abnormally high levels of glucagon in the blood.

hy·per·gly·ce·mia (hi″pər-gli-se′me-ə) [*hyper-* + *glyc-* + *emia*] abnormally increased glucose in the blood, such as in diabetes mellitus.
rebound h. Somogyi phenomenon.

hy·per·gly·ce·mic (hi″pər-gli-se′mik) 1. pertaining to, characterized by, or causing hyperglycemia. 2. an agent that causes increased levels of glucose in the blood.

hy·per·glyc·er·i·de·mia (hi″pər-glis″ər-i-de′me-ə) an excess of glycerides, usually triglycerides, in the blood.

hy·per·glyc·er·i·de·mic (hi″pər-glis′ər-i-de″mik) 1. pertaining to or characterized by hyperglyceridemia. 2. producing hyperglyceridemia.

hy·per·glyc·er·ol·emia (hi″pər-glis″ər-ol-e′me-ə) 1. accumulation and excretion of glycerol caused by deficiency of glycerol kinase activity, an X-linked trait caused by mutation in the glycerol kinase gene (*GK,* locus: Xp21.3-p21.2). The *infantile* or *microdeletion* form is caused by a chromosomal deletion that usually also involves one or both of the loci for Duchenne muscular dystrophy and congenital adrenal hypoplasia; resultant phenotypes include features characteristic to the defective locus or loci. The *juvenile* form is characterized by episodes of vomiting, metabolic acidosis, stupor, and coma and is caused by deficiency of glycerol kinase only, as is the *adult* form, which is generally symptomless. 2. excess of glycerol in the blood.

hy·per·gly·cin·e·mia (hi″pər-gli″sĭ-ne′me-ə) excess of glycine in the blood or other body fluids. Called also *glycinemia.*
ketotic h. 1. the elevated accumulation and excretion of glycine accompanied by ketosis that is secondary to propionicacidemia, methylmalonicacidemia, and other organic acidemias, as distinguished from nonketotic hyperglycinemia. 2. propionicacidemia (def. 1).
nonketotic h. glycine encephalopathy.

hy·per·gly·cin·uria (hi″pər-gli″sĭ-nu′re-ə) an aminoaciduria consisting of excessive glycine in the urine; see *hyperglycinemia.*

hy·per·gly·co·gen·ol·y·sis (hi″pər-gli″ko-jən-ol′ə-sis) excessive splitting up of glycogen, resulting in an excess of glucose in the body.

hy·per·gly·cor·rha·chia (hi″pər-gli″ko-ra′ke-ə) [*hyper-* + *glyco-* + *rhachi-* + *-ia*] the presence of greater than normal glucose in the cerebrospinal fluid.

hy·per·gly·co·se·mia (hi″pər-gli″ko-se′me-ə) hyperglycemia.

hy·per·gly·cos·uria (hi″pər-gli″ko-su′re-ə) extreme glycosuria.

hy·per·gno·sis (hi″pər-no′sis) [*hyper-* + Gr. *gnōsis* knowledge] an exaggerated perception, e.g., expansion of an isolated idea into a complex philosophical system; seen in paranoia.

hy·per·go·nad·ism (hi″pər-go′nad-iz-əm) a condition caused by excessive secretion of gonadal (sex) hormones; manifestations include accelerated and precocious sexual development. See also *hyperovarianism.*

hy·per·go·nado·tro·pic (hi″pər-gon″ə-do-tro′pik) relating to or caused by excessive amounts of gonadotropins.

hy·per·guan·i·din·emia (hi″pər-gwan″ĭ-dĭ-ne′me-ə) excessive guanidine in the blood.

hy·per·he·mo·glo·bin·emia (hi″pər-he″mo-glo″bĭ-ne′me-ə) excessive hemoglobin in the blood.

hy·per·hep·a·rin·emia (hi″pər-hep″ə-rĭ-ne′me-ə) excessive heparin in the blood, usually leading to increased clotting time and tendency to hemorrhage.

hy·per·hi·dro·sis (hi″pər-hĭ-dro′sis) [*hyper-* + Gr. *hidrōsis* sweating] excessive sweating. Called also *hyperidrosis* and *polyhidrosis.*
axillary h. a common type of emotional hyperhidrosis, occurring in the axillae.
compensatory h. excessive sweating on one part of the body to compensate for damage and inactivity of nearby sweat glands.
emotional h. 1. excessive sweating due primarily to emotional causes. 2. an autosomal dominant disorder of the eccrine sweat glands, most often of the palms, soles, and axillae, in which emotional stimuli (e.g., anxiety) and sometimes mental or sensory stimuli elicit axillary or volar sweating (usually not both in the same individual); eccrine sweat glands in other areas of the body are affected less often and are less sensitive to such stimuli.
gustatory h. 1. hyperhidrosis after certain kinds of taste sensations; called also *gustatory sweating.* 2. auriculotemporal syndrome.
palmar h. emotional hyperhidrosis of the palms only.
palmoplantar h. emotional hyperhidrosis of the palms and soles.
plantar h. emotional hyperhidrosis of the soles of the feet.
unilateral h., h. unilatera′lis excessive sweating on one side of the body only.
volar h. palmoplantar h.

hy·per·hi·drot·ic (hi″pər-hĭ-drot′ik) 1. pertaining to or characterized by hyperhidrosis. 2. causing hyperhidrosis.

hy·per·ho·mo·cys·te·in·emia (hi″pər-ho″mo-sis′te-in-e′me-ə) the presence of excessive homocysteine in the blood, a condition closely related to homocystinuria. Called also *homocysteinemia.*

hy•per•hy•dra•tion (hi″pər-hi-dra′shən) a state of excess fluids in the body; called also *overhydration.*

hy•per•hy•dro•chlo•ria (hi″pər-hi″dro-klor′e-ə) hyperchlorhydria.

hy•per•hy•dro•chlo•rid•ia (hi″pər-hi″dro-klor-id′e-ə) hyperchlorhydria.

hy•per•hy•droxy•pro•lin•e•mia (hi″pər-hi-drok″se-pro″lĭ-ne′me-ə) hydroxyprolinemia.

Hy•per•i•cum (hi-per′ĭ-kum) a genus of herbs with yellow flowers, including several types of St. John's wort; sheep and cattle that consume it suffer dermatitis and hepatogenous photosensitization.

H. perfora′tum the species of St. John's wort whose above-ground parts are used medicinally.

hy•per•idro•sis (hi″pər-ĭ-dro′sis) hyperhidrosis.

hy•per•im•ido•di•pep•tid•uria (hi″pər-im″ĭ-do-di-pep″tĭ-du′re-ə) 1. prolidase deficiency. 2. imidodipeptiduria.

hy•per•im•mune (hi″pər-ĭ-mūn′) having large quantities of specific antibodies in the serum.

hy•per•im•mu•ni•ty (hi″pər-ĭ-mu′nĭ-te) the high levels of specific antibodies produced by hyperimmunization.

hy•per•im•mu•ni•za•tion (hi″pər-im″u-nĭ-za′shən) any process of immunization that produces very high levels of circulating antibodies, especially immunization of an animal or human donor with repeated doses of antigen for the production of therapeutic antisera or immune globulins.

hy•per•im•mu•no•glob•u•lin•emia (hi″pər-im″u-no-glob″u-lĭ-ne′me-ə) abnormally high levels of immunoglobulins in the serum.

h. D an abnormal elevation of immunoglobulin D in the serum; see *hyperimmunoglobulinemia D syndrome*, under *syndrome.*

h. E extremely high levels of immunoglobulin E in the serum, associated with cutaneous anergy and deficient antibody response; see *hyperimmunoglobulinemia E syndrome*, under *syndrome.*

hy•per•in•fec•tion (hi″pər-in-fek′shən) infection by exceptionally high numbers of organisms in immunocompromised individuals, used especially of infection by high numbers of helminths as a result of autoinfection.

hy•per•in•fla•tion (hi″pər-in-fla′shən) excessive inflation or expansion, as of the lungs; called also *overinflation.*

hy•per•in•ges•tion (hi″pər-in-jes′chən) ingestion of a greater than optimal amount of nutrients.

hy•per•in•su•lin•ar (hi″pər-in′sə-lin-ər) pertaining to or characterized by excessive secretion of insulin.

hy•per•in•su•lin•emia (hi″pər-in″sə-lĭ-ne′me-ə) excessively high blood insulin levels. **hyperinsuline′mic** *adj*

hy•per•in•su•lin•ism (hi″pər-in′sə-lin-iz″əm) 1. excessive secretion of insulin by the pancreatic islets, resulting in hypoglycemia. 2. insulin shock. 3. hyperinsulinemia.

hy•per•in•tense (hi″pər-in-tens′) having a greater intensity than something else, such as strength of signals or imagery.

hy•per•in•vo•lu•tion (hi″pər-in″vo-loo′shən) superinvolution.

hy•per•io•de•mia (hi″pər-i″o-de′me-ə) excessive iodine in the blood; see also *iodism.*

hy•per•ir•ri•ta•bil•i•ty (hi″pər-ir″ĭ-tə-bil′ĭ-te) excessive irritability.

hy•per•iso•to•nia (hi″pər-i″so-to′ne-ə) [*hyper-* + *isotonia*] marked equality of tone or tonicity.

hy•per•iso•ton•ic (hi″pər-i″so-ton′ik) hypertonic.

hy•per•ka•le•mia (hi″pər-kə-le′me-ə) [*hyper-* + L. *kalium* potassium + *-emia*] abnormally high potassium concentration in the blood, most often due to defective renal excretion. It is characterized clinically by electrocardiographic abnormalities (elevated T waves, depressed P waves, and wide QRS complexes, eventually with atrial asystole). In severe cases, weakness and flaccid paralysis may occur. Called also *potassemia* and *hyperpotassemia.* **hyperkale′mic** *adj*

hy•per•kal•i•emia (hi″pər-kal″e-e′me-ə) hyperkalemia.

hy•per•ker•a•tin•iza•tion (hi″pər-ker″ə-tin″ĭ-za′shən) [*hyper-* + *keratinization*] the excessive development or retention of keratin by the epidermis.

hy•per•ker•a•to•sis (hi″pər-ker″ə-to′sis) [*hyper-* + *keratosis*] 1. hypertrophy of the stratum corneum of the skin; see also *callus* and *keratosis.* 2. a skin disease of cattle marked by inflammation and thickening of the stratum corneum, and caused by the ingestion of feed containing chlorinated naphthalenes. It was once thought to be caused by a virus and was called *x disease.*

epidermolytic h. an autosomal dominant disorder of keratinization caused by mutation in the keratin genes *KRT1* (locus: 12q13) and *KRT10* (locus: 17q21-q22), resulting in structural defects in tonofibrils. It is present at birth and characterized by generalized erythroderma and severe hyperkeratosis. There are small, hard, verrucous scales over the entire body, especially in flexural areas, including the creases on the palms and soles. Recurrent bullae, primarily on the lower limbs, are characteristic in infancy and childhood. See also *ichthyosis hystrix.*

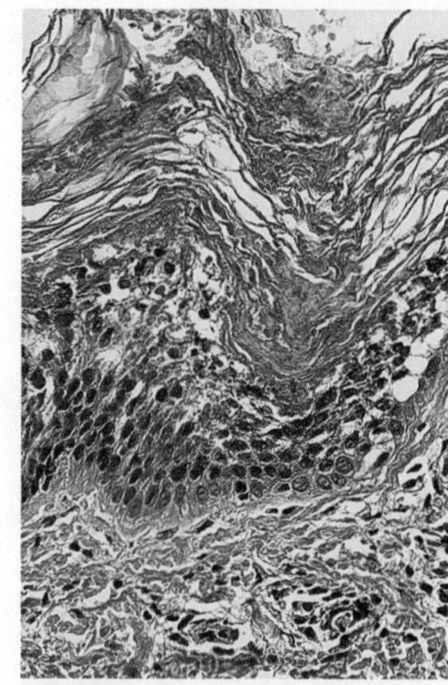

■ Epidermolytic hyperkeratosis. Compact orthokeratosis overlies an epidermis showing granular and vacuolar changes in its upper layers.

focal acral h. a rare skin condition consisting of hard papules on the hands and feet, similar to those of acrokeratoelastoidosis but without elastoidosis.

follicular h. a skin condition characterized by hyperkeratosis of hair follicles, resulting in rough, cone-shaped, elevated papules whose openings are often closed with a white plug of sebum. Deficiencies of vitamins A and E, B complex vitamins, and essential fatty acids have all been implicated in the etiology. Called also *phrynoderma* and *toad skin.*

h. follicula′ris in cu′tem pe′netrans, h. follicula′ris et parafollicula′ris in cu′tem pe′netrans Kyrle disease.

h. lacuna′ris keratosis pharyngea.

h. lenticula′ris per′stans a rare, possibly autosomal dominant skin disorder, usually seen in the third or fourth decade of life, characterized by discolored, hyperkeratotic, scaly papules on the lower limb and sometimes the trunk, thigh, or upper limb. It is usually associated with punctate keratoses on the palms and soles. Histologically there is a lack of keratinosomes, with reduction of keratohyalin granules in the epidermis underlying the lesions. Called also *Flegel disease.*

h. palma′ris et planta′ris, palmoplantar h., h. palmoplanta′ris, h. of palms and soles see under *keratoderma.*

h. pe′netrans Kyrle disease.

progressive dystrophic h. Vohwinkel syndrome.

subungual h., h. subungua′lis hyperkeratosis affecting the nail beds.

hy•per•ke•ton•emia (hi″pər-ke″to-ne′me-ə) ketonemia.

hy•per•ke•ton•uria (hi″pər-ke″to-nu′re-ə) ketonuria.

hy•per•ke•to•sis (hi″pər-ke-to′sis) ketosis.

hy•per•ki•ne•mia (hi″pər-kĭ-ne′me-ə) [*hyper-* + *kin-* + *-emia*] abnormally high cardiac output; increased rate of blood flow through the circulatory system.

hy•per•ki•ne•mic (hi″pər-kĭ-ne′mik) 1. increasing blood flow through a tissue. 2. an agent that increases blood flow through a tissue area.

hy•per•ki•ne•sia (hi″pər-kĭ-ne′zhə) hyperactivity. **hyperkinet′ic** *adj*

hy•per•ki•ne•sis (hi″pər-kĭ-ne′sis) hyperactivity.

hy•per•ko•ria (hi″pər-kor′e-ə) [*hyper-* + Gr. *koros* satiety + *-ia*] an early sense of satiety.

hy•per•lact•ac•i•de•mia (hi″pər-lak″tas-ĭ-de′me-ə) excessive lactic acid in the blood.

hy•per•lac•ta•te•mia (hi″pər-lak″ta-te′me-ə) increased level of lactate in the blood.

hy•per•lac•ta•tion (hi″pər-lak-ta′shən) lactation in greater than normal amount or for a longer than usual period.

hy•per•lec•i•thin•emia (hi″pər-les″ĭ-thĭ-ne′me-ə) excess of lecithin in the blood.

hy•per•lep•tin•emia (hi″pər-lep″tĭ-ne′me-ə) excess of leptins in the blood.

hy•per•le•thal (hi″pər-le′thəl) superlethal.

hy•per•leu•cin•emia (hi″pər-loo″sĭ-ne′me-ə) excessive amounts of leucine in the blood, as in some forms of maple syrup urine disease, tyrosinemia, and other conditions. See also *leucinuria.*

hy•per•leu•ko•cy•to•sis (hi″pər-loo″ko-si-to′sis) [*hyper-* + *leukocyte* + *-osis*] extreme leukocytosis, as seen in certain forms of leukemia.

hy•per•lip•ac•i•de•mia (hi″pər-lip″as-ĭ-de′me-ə) lipacidemia.

hy•per•lip•as•emia (hi″pər-lip″ās-e′me-ah) excessive lipases in the blood, as seen in pancreatitis, Crohn disease, and other conditions; called also *lipasemia.*

hy•per•li•pe•mia (hi″pər-lĭ-pe′me-ə) hyperlipidemia.

carbohydrate-induced h. elevated blood lipids, particularly triglycerides, after carbohydrate ingestion; it is characteristic of disorders with type IV or type V hyperlipoproteinemia phenotypes and is sometimes used as a synonym for these phenotypes or for the genetic disorders causing them.

combined fat- and carbohydrate-induced h. persistently elevated blood levels of very-low-density lipoproteins and chylomicrons after ingestion of fat or carbohydrates; it is characteristic of disorders with a type V hyperlipoproteinemia phenotype and is sometimes used as a synonym for this phenotype or for genetic disorders causing it.

endogenous h. elevated plasma lipids derived from body stores rather than dietary sources (i.e., very-low-density lipoproteins); used as a generic descriptor of the type IV hyperlipoproteinemia phenotype. See table of hyperlipoproteinemias.

essential familial h. a term used to describe an inherited disorder causing a type I hyperlipoproteinemia phenotype or the phenotype itself.

exogenous h. elevated plasma levels of lipoproteins derived from dietary sources (i.e., chylomicrons); used as a generic descriptor of the type I hyperlipoproteinemia phenotype. See table of hyperlipoproteinemias.

familial fat-induced h. persistently elevated blood chylomicrons after ingestion of fat; it is characteristic of disorders with a type I hyperlipoproteinemia phenotype and is sometimes used as a synonym for this phenotype or genetic disorders causing it.

mixed h. generic designation for a hyperlipoproteinemia in which several classes of lipoproteins are elevated; usually used to denote a type V phenotype but sometimes used for a type II-b phenotype. See table of hyperlipoproteinemias. Called also *mixed dyslipidemia.*

hy•per•lip•id•emia (hi″pər-lip″ĭ-de′me-ə) a general term for elevated concentrations of any or all of the lipids in the plasma, such as hypertriglyceridemia, hypercholesterolemia, and so on. See also table of hyperlipoproteinemias. Called also *hyperlipemia, lipemia,* and *lipidemia.* **hyperlipide′mic** *adj*

combined h. a generic designation for a hyperlipidemia in which several classes of lipids are elevated; usually used to denote the phenotype of a type II-b hyperlipoproteinemia. See table of hyperlipoproteinemias.

familial combined h. a genetically heterogeneous, autosomal dominant disorder of lipoprotein metabolism manifest in adulthood as either hypercholesterolemia (type II-a hyperlipoproteinemia phenotype), hypertriglyceridemia (type IV hyperlipoproteinemia phenotype), or a combination (type II-b hyperlipoproteinemia phenotype); different phenotypes may succeed each other in a single individual. The disorder is characterized by greatly elevated plasma apolipoprotein B and premature coronary atherosclerosis, but only occasionally xanthomas. Called also *multiple lipoprotein–type h.* See also table of hyperlipoproteinemias.

mixed h. see under *hyperlipemia.*

multiple lipoprotein–type h. familial combined h.

remnant h. a hyperlipoproteinemia in which the accumulated lipoproteins are normally transient intermediates, chylomicron remnants, and intermediate density lipoproteins. See table of hyperlipoproteinemias.

hy•per•lipo•pro•tein•emia (hi″pər-lip″o-pro″te-ne′me-ə) an excess of lipoproteins in the blood, due to a disorder of lipoprotein metabolism; it may be an acquired or familial condition or some combination. The disorder has been subdivided on the basis of biochemical phenotype, and each type has since been shown to have a variety of causes. See accompanying table for individual phenotypes as well as some primary genetic disorders that cause them. See also *familial h., hyperlipemia,* and *hyperlipidemia.*

acquired h. hyperlipoproteinemia occurring secondarily to some other disorder, such as hypothyroidism, nephrotic syndrome, or hypoadrenocorticism, or as a result of environmental factors, including diet.

familial h. an inherited hyperlipoproteinemia, classified on the basis of the type I–V phenotypes described in the accompanying table. For any given phenotype, the term is frequently used loosely to denote either the phenotype or any or all of the genetic disorders causing the phenotype. However, the latter usage is frequently imprecise or inaccurate because a single phenotype may have multiple causes and a single genetic disorder may result in multiple phenotypes.

Lp(a) h. greatly elevated levels of Lp(a) lipoprotein in plasma, an autosomal dominant trait caused by mutation in the *LPA* gene (locus: 6q27) and characterized by increased incidence of severe arteriosclerosis of coronary and carotid vessels, atherogenesis, and cutaneous and tendinous xanthomas.

hy•per•li•po•sis (hi″pər-lĭ-po′sis) an excess of fat in the blood *(hyperlipidemia)* or tissues.

hy•per•li•the•mia (hi″pər-lĭ-the′me-ə) excessive lithium in the blood.

hy•per•lo•gia (hi″pər-lo′jə) logorrhea.

hy•per•lor•do•sis (hi″pər-lor-do′sis) extremely marked lordosis.

hy•per•lu•cen•cy (hi″pər-loo′sən-se) increased radiolucency.

hy•per•lu•te•in•iza•tion (hi″pər-loo″te-in-ĭ-za′shən) excessive luteinization of cystic ovarian follicles.

hy•per•ly•sin•emia (hi″pər-li″se-ne′me-ə) 1. excess of lysine in the blood. 2. an autosomal recessive aminoacidopathy due to mutation in the *AASS* gene (locus: 7q31.3), which encodes α-aminoadipic semialdehyde synthase, causing deficiency of both of its enzyme activities (lysine-ketoglutarate dehydrogenase and saccharopine dehydrogenase); it is characterized by excess of lysine and, to a lesser degree, saccharopine, in the blood and urine. Cf. *saccharopinuria.*

hy•per•ly•sin•uria (hi″pər-li″sin-u′re-ə) lysinuria.

hy•per•mag•ne•se•mia (hi″pər-mag″nə-se′me-ə) an abnormally high magnesium content of the blood; manifestations include lethargy, weakness, electrocardiographic abnormalities and, as levels increase, loss of deep tendon reflexes, somnolence, and coma. Called also *magnesemia.*

hy•per•mag•ne•su•ria (hi″pər-mag″nə-soo′re-ə) abnormally high levels of magnesium in the urine, seen with hypermagnesemia and hypercalcemia; called also *magnesuria.*

hy•per•ma•nia (hi″pər-ma′ne-ə) intense mania with overwhelming tensions, marked disorientation, and incoherence.

Hyperlipoproteinemias

Phenotype	Generic Designation	Elevated Lipoprotein Class	Elevated Lipid Class	Primary Genetic Disorders
I	Exogenous hyperlipemia	Chylomicrons	Triglycerides	Familial lipoprotein lipase deficiency Familial apolipoprotein C-II deficiency Unclassified
II-a	Hypercholesterolemia	LDL	Cholesterol	Familial hypercholesterolemia Familial combined hyperlipidemia Polygenic hypercholesterolemia
II-b	Combined hyperlipidemia	LDL, VLDL	Cholesterol, Triglycerides	Familial combined hyperlipidemia Unclassified
III	Remnant hyperlipidemia	β-VLDL	Triglycerides, Cholesterol	Familial dysbetalipoproteinemia Unclassified
IV	Endogenous hyperlipemia	VLDL	Triglycerides	Familial hypertriglyceridemia (mild) Familial combined hyperlipidemia Sporadic hypertriglyceridemia Tangier disease
V	Mixed hyperlipemia	VLDL, Chylomicrons	Triglycerides, Cholesterol	Familial hypertriglyceridemia (severe) Familial lipoprotein lipase deficiency Familial apolipoprotein C-II deficiency

LDL, Low-density lipoproteins; VLDL, very-low-density lipoproteins; β-VLDL, a class of abnormal VLDL.

hy·per·mas·tia (hi″pər-mas′te-ə) [*hyper-* + *mast-* + *-ia*] 1. the presence of one or more supernumerary mammary glands. 2. macromastia.

hy·per·ma·ture (hi″pər-mə-choor′) past the stage of maturity.

hy·per·mel·a·no·sis (hi″pər-mel″ə-no′sis) melanosis. **hypermelanot′ic** *adj*

hy·per·men·or·rhea (hi″pər-men″o-re′ə) [*hyper-* + *menorrhea*] menstruation with an excessive flow but at regular intervals and of usual duration. Called also *menorrhagia.*

hy·per·met·a·bol·ic (hi″pər-met″ə-bol′ik) exhibiting an increased rate of metabolism.

hy·per·me·tab·o·lism (hi″pər-mə-tab′o-liz-əm) increased metabolism; abnormally increased utilization of oxygen, nutrients, and other materials by the body.

extrathyroidal h. abnormally elevated basal metabolism unassociated with thyroid disease.

hy·per·meta·mor·pho·sis (hi″pər-met″ə-mor′fə-sis) excessive attentiveness and reaction to visual stimuli, as in the Klüver-Bucy syndrome.

hy·per·meta·pla·sia (hi″pər-met″ə-pla′zhə) increased metaplasia.

hy·per·me·thi·o·nin·emia (hi″pər-mə-thi″o-nĭ-ne′me-ə) excess of methionine in the blood.

hy·per·me·tria (hi″pər-me′tre-ə) [Gr. "a passing all measure, overflow"] a condition in which voluntary muscular movement overreaches the intended goal.

hy·per·met·rope (hi″pər-me′trōp) hyperope.

hy·per·me·tro·pia (hi″pər-me-tro′pe-ə) hyperopia.

hy·per·mim·ia (hi″pər-mim′e-ə) [*hyper-* + Gr. *mimos* actor, mime + *-ia*] excessive use of gestures when speaking.

hy·per·min·er·al·iza·tion (hi″pər-min″ər-əl-ĭ-za′shən) the presence of an excess of mineral elements in the body.

hy·perm·ne·sia (hi″pərm-ne′zhə) [*hyper-* + Gr. *mnēmē* memory] extreme retentiveness or unusual clarity of memory. **hypermne′sic** *adj*

hy·per·mo·bil·i·ty (hi″pər-mo-bil′ĭ-te) greater than normal range of motion in a joint, which may occur naturally in otherwise normal persons or may be a sign of joint instability. Cf. *laxity.*

hy·per·mo·dal (hi″pər-mo′dəl) in statistics, relating to the values or items falling above the mode of the frequency distribution.

hy·per·morph (hi′pər-morf) [*hyper-* + *-morph*] a mutant gene characterized by an increase in the activity it influences. Cf. *hypomorph.*

hy·per·mo·til·i·ty (hi″pər-mo-til′ĭ-te) excessive or abnormally increased motility, as of the gastrointestinal tract.

hy·per·mu·ta·tion (hi″pər-mu-ta′shən) occurrence of mutations at a higher than normal frequency.

somatic h. extremely high-frequency point mutations that occur in the genes coding immunoglobulin heavy and light chain V regions during B lymphocyte maturation, leading to the increased affinity of antibodies for antigen seen in the secondary immune response.

hy·per·myo·to·nia (hi″pər-mi″o-to′ne-ə) hypertonia.

hy·per·my·ot·ro·phy (hi″pər-mi-ot′rə-fe) [*hyper-* + *myotrophy*] excessive development of the muscular tissue.

hy·per·na·sal·i·ty (hi″pər-na-zal′ĭ-te) an excessively nasal quality of voice, which may result in unintelligible speech; the cause is velopharyngeal insufficiency with emission of too much air through the nose. Called also *rhinolalia aperta* and *open rhinolalia.*

hy·per·na·tre·mia (hi″pər-nə-tre′me-ə) [*hyper-* + L. *natrium* sodium + *-emia*] excessive sodium in the blood.

hypodipsic h. an uncommon syndrome of chronic or recurrent episodes of severe hypernatremia with dehydration and lack of thirst, seen in persons with various congenital or acquired diseases of the brain.

hy·per·na·tre·mic (hi″pər-nə-tre′mik) 1. pertaining to or characterized by hypernatremia. 2. causing hypernatremia. 3. caused by hypernatremia.

hy·per·neo·cy·to·sis (hi″pər-ne″o-si-to′sis) [*hyper-* + *neocytosis*] hyperleukocytosis in which excessive immature leukocytes are present.

hy·per·neph·roid (hi″pər-nef′roid) resembling the adrenal gland.

hy·per·ne·phro·ma (hi″pər-nə-fro′mə) renal cell carcinoma.

hy·per·ni·tre·mia (hi″pər-ni-tre′me-ə) [*hyper-* + *nitrogen* + *-emia*] excessive nitrogen in the blood.

hy·per·nom·ic (hi″pər-nom′ik) [*hyper-* + *nom-* + *-ic*] above the law; unrestrained; excessive.

hy·per·nor·mal (hi″pər-nor′məl) in excess of what is normal.

hy·per·nu·tri·tion (hi″pər-noo-trish′ən) hyperalimentation (def. 1).

hy·per·onych·ia (hi″pər-o-nik′e-ə) onychauxis.

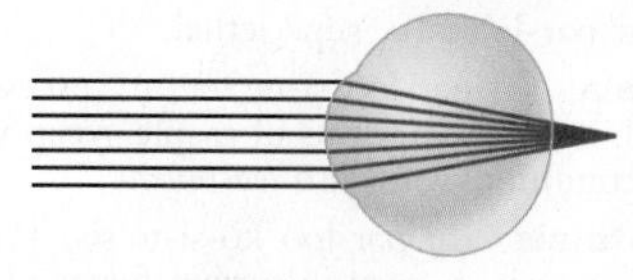

■ Hyperopia.

hy·per·ope (hi′pər-ōp) a person with hyperopia.

hy·per·opia (hi″pər-o′pe-ə) [*hyper-* + *-opia*] an error of refraction in which rays of light entering the eye parallel to the optic axis are brought to a focus behind the retina, as a result of the eyeball being too short from front to back. Symbol H. Called also *farsightedness* (because the near point is more distant than it is in emmetropia with an equal amplitude of accommodation) and *hypermetropia.* **hypero′pic** *adj*

absolute h. that amount of hyperopia which cannot be corrected by accommodation.

axial h. hyperopia which is due to shortness of the anteroposterior axis of the eye.

curvature h. hyperopia due to insufficient convexity of the refracting surfaces.

facultative h. that amount of hyperopia which can be entirely corrected by the ciliary muscle, i.e., by the effort of accommodation.

index h. hyperopia caused by deficient refractive power in the media of the eye.

latent h. that part of the total hyperopia corrected by the physiologic tone of the ciliary muscle and revealed only when that muscle is paralyzed by the use of a drug, such as atropine.

manifest h. that part of the total hyperopia not corrected by the physiologic tone of the ciliary muscle nor revealed with cycloplegic examination.

relative h. facultative hyperopia allowing clear vision, but causing excessive convergence or convergent strabismus.

total h. the sum of manifest and latent hyperopia; it can be determined only with mydriasis.

hy·per·o·ral·i·ty (hi″pər-o-ral′ĭ-te) excessive placing of inedible objects into the mouth; this is normal behavior in babies but in older persons it may signify mental illness or dementia.

hy·per·orex·ia (hi″pər-o-rek′se-ə) [*hyper-* + Gr. *orexis* appetite + *-ia*] an abnormally increased appetite. See also *hyperalimentation* (def. 1) and *bulimia.*

hy·per·or·ni·thin·emia (hi″pər-or″nĭ-thĭ-ne′me-ə) excessive ornithine in the plasma, such as occurs in the genetic disorders gyrate atrophy of choroid and retina and hyperornithinemia-hyperammonemia-homocitrullinemia syndrome.

hy·per·or·tho·cy·to·sis (hi″pər-or″tho-si-to′sis) [*hyper-* + *orthocytosis*] hyperleukocytosis in which the proportion of the various forms of leukocytes is normal.

hy·per·os·mia (hi″pər-oz′me-ə) [*hyper-* + *osm-*[1] + *-ia*] a parosmia involving increased sensitivity of smell; called also *olfactory hyperesthesia.*

hy·per·os·mo·lal·i·ty (hi″pər-oz″mo-lal′ĭ-te) an increase in the osmolality of the body fluids.

hy·per·os·mo·lar·i·ty (hi″pər-oz″mo-lar′ĭ-te) abnormally increased osmolar concentration.

hy·per·os·mot·ic (hi″pər-oz-mot′ik) 1. producing or caused by abnormally rapid osmosis. 2. containing a higher concentration of osmotically active components than a standard solution.

hy·per·os·te·og·e·ny (hi″pər-os″te-oj′ə-ne) [*hyper-* + *osteo-* + *-geny*] excessive development of bone.

hy·per·os·to·sis (hi″pər-os-to′sis) [*hyper-* + *osteo-* + *-osis*] hypertrophy of bone; cf. *exostosis.* **hyperostot′ic** *adj*

h. cortica′lis defor′mans juveni′lis an autosomal recessive disorder beginning in childhood and marked by multiple fractures and bowing of all extremities, by thickening of the frontal, parietal, and occipital bones, by osteoporosis, and by elevated concentrations of serum alkaline phosphatase and of urinary hydroxyproline. Called also *juvenile Paget disease, chronic congenital idiopathic hyperphosphatasemia,* and *familial osteoectasia.*

h. cortica′lis generalisa′ta an autosomal recessive disorder, characterized principally by osteosclerosis of the skull, mandible, clavicles, ribs, and diaphyses of long bones, associated with elevated blood alkaline phosphatase; beginning during puberty, it sometimes leads to optic atrophy and perceptive deafness due to nerve pressure exerted by thickening of the base of the skull. Called also *hyperphosphatasemia tarda* and *van Buchem syndrome.*

h. cra′nii hyperostosis involving the cranial bones.

diffuse idiopathic skeletal h. (DISH) a rheumatologic disorder characterized by hyperostosis, most prominently the anterior longitudinal ligament and other structures anterior to the vertebral column; it is seen most often in the elderly. Severe cases may resemble ankylosing spondylitis. Called also *Forestier disease* and *senile ankylosing h.*

flowing h. melorheostosis.

h. fronta'lis inter'na, frontal internal h. thickening of the inner table of the frontal bone, which may be associated with hypertrichosis and obesity; it most commonly affects women near menopause. Called also *Morel syndrome.*

infantile cortical h. a disease of young infants characterized by soft tissue swellings over the affected bones, fever, and irritability, and marked by periods of remission and exacerbation; called also *Caffey disease.*

senile ankylosing h. diffuse idiopathic skeletal h.

hy•per•ova•ri•an•ism (hi″pər-o-var′e-ən-iz-əm) [*hyper-* + *ovarian* + *-ism*] precocious puberty in girls due to excessive and untimely ovarian secretion.

hy•per•ova•rism (hi″pər-o′və-riz-əm) hyperovarianism.

hy•per•ox•al•uria (hi″pər-ok″sə-lu′re-ə) the excretion of an excessive amount of oxalates in the urine; high concentrations of oxalates may lead to formation of urinary calculi. Called also *oxaluria.*

enteric h. hyperoxaluria occurring after extensive resection or disease of the ileum and resulting from excessive absorption of oxalate from the colon, with formation of calcium oxalate calculi in the urinary tract.

primary h. an autosomal recessive disorder of glyoxylate metabolism, characterized by urinary excretion of large amounts of oxalate and deposition of calcium oxalate in the tissues, especially the kidney, with nephrolithiasis, nephrocalcinosis, and renal failure; there are two types, caused by different mutations.

type I primary hyperoxaluria due to deficiency of alanine–glyoxylate transaminase as the result of mutation in the *AGXT* gene (locus: 2q36-q37).

type II primary hyperoxaluria, milder than type I, caused by mutation in the *GRHPR* gene (locus: 9cen), resulting in a defect in an enzyme complex involved in the metabolism of hydroxypyruvate to D-glycerate.

hy•per•ox•emia (hi″pər-ok-se′me-ə) [*hyper-* + *ox-* + *-emia*] excessive acidity of the blood.

hy•per•ox•ia (hi″pər-ok′se-ə) excessive oxygen in the system, resulting from exposure to high oxygen concentrations, especially to hyperbaric pressures of oxygen. See *oxygen toxicity*, under *toxicity.* **hyperox′ic** *adj*

hy•per•ox•i•da•tion (hi″pər-ok″sĭ-da′shən) excessive oxidation.

hy•per•pal•les•the•sia (hi″pər-pal″es-the′zhə) [*hyper-* + *pallesthesia*] abnormally increased sensitivity of the vibration sense (pallesthesia).

hy•per•par•a•site (hi″pər-par′ə-sīt) [*hyper-* + *parasite*] a parasite that preys on another parasite.

second degree h. a parasite that preys on a hyperparasite.

hy•per•par•a•si•te•mia (hi″pər-par″ə-si-te′me-ə) excessive parasitemia.

hy•per•par•a•sit•ic (hi″pər-par″ə-sit′ik) pertaining to a hyperparasite. Called also biparasitic.

hy•per•par•a•sit•ism (hi″pər-par′ə-si″tiz-əm) infestation with a hyperparasite.

hy•per•para•thy•roid•ism (hi″pər-par″ə-thi′roid-iz-əm) a condition caused by excessive amounts of parathyroid hormone, which causes hypercalcemia and hypophosphatemia and affects the functions of many cell types. Manifestations include calcium deposits in the renal tubules; generalized decalcification of bone (osteoporosis) that results in pain and tenderness of bones and spontaneous fractures or in localized bone cysts; hypercalcemia that leads to muscular weakness, gastrointestinal symptoms such as anorexia, nausea, vomiting, and abdominal pains; and drowsiness or obtusion.

familial isolated h., familial isolated primary h. hypoparathyroidism inherited as an autosomal dominant trait in the absence of other inherited endocrinopathies; it is a genetically heterogeneous condition.

nutritional secondary h. secondary hyperparathyroidism in domestic animals due to an unbalanced diet; there may be insufficient calcium, excessive phosphorus that competes with calcium, or (in ruminants) oxalates that bind to calcium and form insoluble calcium oxalate crystals. The most prominent symptoms are swelling of the mandible and maxilla, loosening of the teeth, and lameness. Called also *bran disease*, *miller's disease*, and *bighead.*

primary h. hyperparathyroidism due to excessive production of parathyroid hormone, either from hyperplasia of the parathyroid gland or from a neoplasm.

secondary h. hyperparathyroidism occurring when the serum calcium falls below normal levels, such as in chronic disease or vitamin D deficiency.

tertiary h. hyperparathyroidism in which parathyroid adenomas arise from secondary hyperplasia caused by chronic renal failure.

hy•per•path•ia (hi″pər-path′e-ə) abnormally exaggerated subjective response to painful stimuli; see also *hyperesthesia* and *hyperalgesia.*

hy•per•pep•sia (hi″pər-pep′se-ə) [*hyper-* + Gr. *pepsis* digestion] impairment of digestion, due to hyperchlorhydria.

hy•per•peri•stal•sis (hi″pər-per″ĭ-stawl′sis) excessively active peristalsis.

hy•per•per•me•a•bil•i•ty (hi″pər-pur″me-ə-bil′ĭ-te) undue or abnormal permeability, as of a cell membrane or a vessel wall.

hy•per•pex•ia (hi″pər-pek′se-ə) [*hyper-* + *pexia*] fixation of an excessive amount of a substance by a tissue.

hy•per•pexy (hi″pər-pek′se) hyperpexia.

hy•per•pha•gia (hi″pər-fa′jə) polyphagia. **hyperpha′gic** *adj*

hy•per•pha•lan•gia (hi″pər-fə-lan′jə) hyperphalangism.

hy•per•pha•lan•gism (hi″pər-fə-lan′jiz-əm) greater than normal number of phalanges of a finger or toe.

hy•per•phen•yl•al•a•nin•emia (HPA) (hi″pər-fen″əl-al″ə-nĭ-ne′me-ə) 1. any of several autosomal recessive defects in the hydroxylation of phenylalanine resulting in accumulation and excretion of dietary phenylalanine. Most commonly the defect is in the enzyme phenylalanine hydroxylase (PAH); the most severe manifestation of this is phenylketonuria (q.v.), but less severe defects in the enzyme cause non-PKU hyperphenylalaninemia or variant phenylketonuria (qq.v.). Less commonly, the defect is in one of various enzymes involved in synthesis or regeneration of the cofactor tetrahydrobiopterin; see *tetrahydrobiopterin deficiency*, under *deficiency.* 2. excess of phenylalanine in the blood.

non-PKU h. an autosomal recessive condition caused by mutation in the *PAH* (locus: 12q24.1), which encodes phenylalanine hydroxylase; the resulting enzyme defect does not abolish enzyme activity; enough activity remains to keep plasma phenylalanine concentrations below 1mM without dietary restriction, and the clinical phenotype is normal.

hy•per•pho•ne•sis (hi″pər-fo-ne′sis) [*hyper-* + *phon-* + *-esis*] an increase in intensity of the vocal sound in auscultation, or of the percussion note.

hy•per•pho•nia (hi″pər-fo′ne-ə) [*hyper-* + *phon-* + *-ia*] a dysphonia with excessively energetic phonation, as in stuttering. Called also *superenergetic phonation.*

hy•per•pho•ria (hi′pər-for′e-ə) [*hyper-* + *phoria*] a form of heterophoria in which there is permanent upward deviation of the visual axis of an eye after the visual fusional stimulus has been eliminated.

hy•per•phos•pha•ta•se•mia (hi″pər-fos″fə-ta-se′me-ə) high levels of alkaline phosphatase in the blood.

chronic congenital idiopathic h. hyperostosis corticalis deformans juvenilis.

h. tar′da hyperostosis corticalis generalisata.

hy•per•phos•pha•ta•sia (hi″pər-fos″fə-ta′zhə) hyperphosphatasemia.

hy•per•phos•pha•te•mia (hi″pər-fos″fə-te′me-ə) excessive phosphates in the blood; it is usually asymptomatic.

hy•per•phos•pha•tu•ria (hi″pər-fos″fə-tu′re-ə) an excessive amount of phosphates in the urine, such as in hyperparathyroidism, rickets, or inability of renal tubules to reabsorb phosphorus.

hy•per•phos•pho•re•mia (hi″pər-fos″fə-re′me-ə) excessive phosphorus compounds in the blood.

hy•per•phra•sia (hi″pər-fra′zhə) logorrhea.

hy•per•phre•nia (hi″pər-fre′ne-ə) [*hyper-* + *phren-* + *-ia*] excessive mental activity.

hy•per•pig•men•ta•tion (hi″pər-pig″mən-ta′shən) abnormally increased pigmentation, such as of the skin or a mucous membrane.

photodistributed h. hyperpigmentation of sun-exposed areas of photosensitized skin.

reticular h., reticulate h., reticulated h. hyperpigmentation in a netlike pattern over the skin; called also *reticular*, *reticulate*, or *reticulated pigmentation.*

hy•per•pi•ne•al•ism (hi″pər-pin′e-əl-iz-əm) a presumed abnormal increase in secretion by the pineal body.

hy•per•pip•e•co•la•te•mia (hi″pər-pip″ə-kol″ə-te′me-ə) excess of pipecolic acid in the blood, usually associated with cerebrohepatorenal syndrome but also a consequence of hyperlysinemia.

hy•per•pi•tu•i•ta•rism (hi″pər-pĭ-too′ĭ-tə-riz″əm) a condition due to excessive secretion of pituitary hormones. Adenomas producing growth hormone can cause acromegaly and pituitary gigantism; those producing corticotropin can cause Cushing disease; and those producing prolactin can cause galactorrhea-amenorrhea syndrome.

hy•per•pla•sia (hi″pər-pla′zhə) [*hyper-* + *-plasia*] abnormal multiplication or increase in the number of normal cells in normal arrangement in a tissue. See also *hypertrophy* and *proliferation.* **hyperplas′tic** *adj*

adenomatous h. dysplastic nodule.

adrenal cortical h., adrenocortical h. hyperplasia of adrenal cortical cells, as in adrenogenital syndrome and Cushing syndrome.

angiolymphoid h. with eosinophilia a type of erythematous dermal or subcutaneous nodule, usually on the head or neck of a young adult, found singly or in groups, sometimes with lymphadenopathy, and characterized histologically by lymphoid hyperplasia, angioid proliferation, and tissue eosinophilia. The more superficial, usually larger, lesions have been called *pseudopyogenic granuloma*. See also *Kimura disease*, under *disease*.

antral G cell h. G cell h.

benign prostatic h. (BPH) age-associated enlargement of the prostate resulting from proliferation of both glandular and stromal elements, beginning generally in the fifth decade of life; it may cause urethral compression and obstruction. Called also *benign prostatic hypertrophy* and *nodular hyperplasia of the prostate*.

C-cell h. a premalignant stage in the development of the familial forms of medullary thyroid carcinoma, characterized by multicentric patches of parafollicular cells (C cells).

cementum h. hypercementosis.

chronic perforating pulp h. internal tooth resorption (def. 1).

congenital adrenal h. (CAH) a group of inherited disorders in which deficiencies of enzymes that catalyze the biosynthesis of cortisol result in compensatory hypersecretion of corticotropin and subsequent adrenal hyperplasia as well as excessive androgen production. There are several different forms, numbered in order of increasing severity, of which the most common type is type III, or 21-hydroxylase deficiency (see accompanying table). They range from "classic" forms present at birth with severe salt wasting or hypertension and pseudohermaphroditism to less severe "nonclassic" forms of later onset. See also deficiency conditions at names of specific enzymes.

cutaneous lymphoid h. an ill-defined, benign skin condition characterized by skin lesions ranging from a solitary plaque or nodule to several in a group or more widespread lesions; they are usually found on the face, ears, limbs, or areolae of the breasts. When multiple, they may resemble malignant lymphoma, although some may regress, sometimes with recurrences. Sometimes it is a reaction to an allergy hyposensitization injection, insect bite, light, trauma, or tattoo pigment. Called also *cutaneous lymphoplasia*, *lymphadenosis benigna cutis*, *lymphocytoma cutis*, and *Spiegler-Fendt pseudolymphoma* or *sarcoid*.

cystic prostatic h. a usually benign type of hyperplasia of the prostate in dogs, with fluid-filled cysts, often due to obstruction of excretory ducts.

diffuse nodular h. nodular regenerative h.

Dilantin h. see under *gingivitis*.

endometrial h., h. endome'trii abnormal overgrowth of the endometrium.

fibromuscular h. see under *dysplasia*.

fibrous inflammatory h. masses of collagenized, fibrous connective tissue along the borders of ill-fitting dentures or in other areas where chronic irritation exists. Called also *epulis fissurata*.

focal epithelial h. hyperplasia of oral mucous membranes, especially on the lower lip, with sessile papules, caused by infection with a human papillomavirus, seen most often in children and adolescents. Called also *Heck disease*.

focal nodular h. (FNH) presence of a single benign regenerative nodule in the liver, usually asymptomatic and chiefly in women; it is a firm, highly vascular mass resembling cirrhosis, usually with a stellate fibrous core containing numerous small bile ducts, and having vessels lined by Kupffer cells.

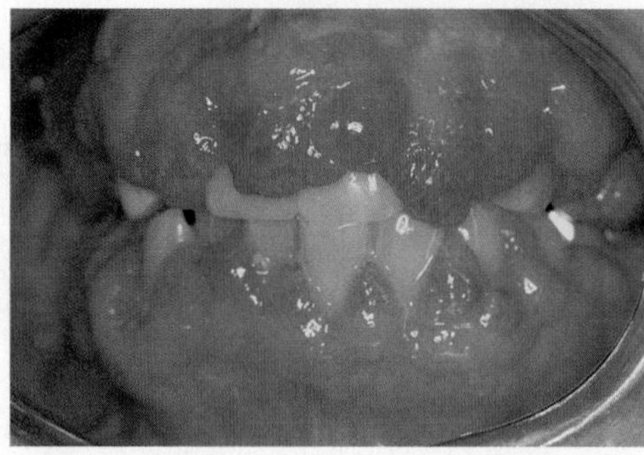

■ Generalized gingival hyperplasia associated with chronic monocytic leukemia.

follicular h. a form of chronic lymphadenitis, characterized by expansion of the germinal centers, which contain large numbers of rapidly proliferating lymphocytes in various stages of differentiation and histiocytes containing phagocytized debris; morphologically, it can resemble follicular lymphoma.

G cell h. increased numbers of G cells in the gastric mucosa, which causes marked hypergastrinemia resembling that seen in the Zollinger-Ellison syndrome.

giant follicular h. a disorder of the lymph nodes, generally confined to the cervical lymph nodes, which may simulate follicular lymphoma, but cytologically the follicles contain both macrophages and lymphoblasts.

giant lymph node h. Castleman disease.

gingival h. noninflammatory enlargement of the gingivae produced by factors other than local irritation. See also under *enlargement*.

hepatic nodular h. nodular h. of the liver.

inflammatory h. hyperplasia brought about by inflammation.

intimal h. thickening of the intima of a blood vessel as a complication of a reconstruction procedure or endarterectomy.

intravascular papillary endothelial h. a benign vascular tumor usually occurring as a solitary nodule of the head, neck, or finger; it is characterized by papillary lobules of proliferating endothelial cells with an underlying fibrous stroma, and often resembles angiosarcoma. Called also *Masson tumor*.

juxtaglomerular cell h. Bartter syndrome.

lipoid h. increased formation of lipoid-containing cells.

lipoid adrenal h., lipoid congenital adrenal h. the most severe type of congenital adrenal hyperplasia, caused by mutation in either of two genes (*STAR*, locus: 8p11.2, or *CYP11A*, locus: 15q23-q24) that encode proteins involved in steroidogenesis. It is characterized by accumulation of lipids and cholesterol in the adrenal cortex, decreased or absent steroid hormones, severe salt wasting, sexual infantilism, and male pseudohermaphroditism; the adrenal insufficiency is usually lethal. See table at *congenital adrenal hyperplasia*.

lymphoid h. a form of chronic lymphadenitis occurring as an immunologic response, often induced by drugs, and characterized by transformation of T cells to lymphoblasts, endothelial cell hypertrophy, and the presence of a mixed leukocyte infiltrate. Called also *reactive* or *reactive lymphoid h.*

macronodular adrenal h., macronodular adrenocortical h. nodular adrenal h.

Congenital Adrenal Hyperplasia

Type	Deficiency	Form	Ambiguous Genitalia	Postnatal Virilization	Salt Metabolism	Elevated Steroids	Decreased Steroids
I	Cholesterol desmolase	Lipoid hyperplasia	Males	No	Salt wasting	None	All
II	3*β*-Hydroxysteroid dehydrogenase	Classic					
		Salt-wasting	Males	Yes	Salt wasting	DHEA, 17-OH-Pregnenolone	Aldo, T, Cort, Estradiol
		Non–salt-wasting	Males	Yes	Normal	DHEA, 17-OH-Pregnenolone	Aldo, T, Cort, Estradiol
		Nonclassic	No	Yes	Normal	DHEA, 17-OH-Pregnenolone	—
III	21-Hydroxylase	Classic					
		Salt-wasting	Females	Yes	Salt wasting	17-OHP, Δ^4-A	Aldo, Cort
		Simple virilizing	Females	Yes	Normal	17-OHP, Δ^4-A	Cort
		Nonclassic	No	Yes	Normal	17-OHP, Δ^4-A	—
IV	11*β*-Hydroxylase	Classic	Females	Yes	Hypertension	DOC, 11-Deoxycortisol	Cort, Aldo
		Nonclassic	No	Yes	Normal	11-Deoxycortisol, DOC	—
V	17*α*-Hydroxylase	—	Males	No	Hypertension	DOC, Corticosterone	Aldo, Andro, Cort, Estro
	17,20-Lyase	—	Males	No	Normal	—	DHEA, T, Δ^4-A

Aldo = Aldosterone; T = Testosterone; Andro = Androgens; Δ^4-A = Δ^4-Androstenedione; Cort = Cortisol; DHEA = Dehydroepiandrosterone; DOC = (11-)Deoxycorticosterone; Estro = Estrogens; 17-OHP = 17*α*-Hydroxyprogesterone.

myofiber h. a hereditary condition of cattle characterized by increased muscle mass because of greater than average numbers of fibers in the muscles, with decreased fat and connective tissue. Called also *culard*, *doppellender*, and *double muscle*.

neoplastic h. hyperplasia brought about by a new growth.

nodular adrenal h., nodular adrenocortical h., nodular cortical h. uneven adrenocortical hyperplasia with small nests or masses of nodules resembling adenomas between the columns of cortical cells. Called also *macronodular adrenal* or *macronodular adrenocortical h*.

nodular h. of the liver the presence of a regenerative nodule or nodules in the liver; see *focal nodular h.* and *nodular regenerative h.*

nodular lymphoid h. a proliferation of small nodules of lymphoid tissue, seen in the terminal ileum and colon of children, in the small intestine and sometimes colon and stomach of adults with primary immunodeficiency disease, and, rarely, in adults with malignant lymphoma.

nodular h. of the prostate benign prostatic hyperplasia.

nodular regenerative h. a rare liver condition characterized by presence of regenerative nodules in the parenchyma that do not cause fibrosis or other major alterations in lobular architecture. Called also *nodular transformation of the liver*.

ovarian stromal h. thecomatosis.

polar h. excessive development at either extremity of the embryo, producing a fetus with either two heads or three or more lower limbs.

pseudoepitheliomatous h. a benign proliferative epithelial hyperplasia whose cytoarchitectural features are suggestive of squamous cell carcinoma, seen in conditions such as granulomatous inflammatory reactions, ulcerations, and granular cell tumors.

psoriasiform h., psoriasiform epidermal h. epidermal hyperplasia with acanthosis and lesions resembling those of psoriasis.

reactive h., reactive lymphoid h. lymphoid h.

sebaceous h., senile sebaceous h. single or multiple pale, round lesions, consisting of enlarged, malformed sebaceous glands; the most common location is on the face of an older adult. Called also *sebaceous adenoma* or *epithelioma*.

squamous h., squamous cell h. thickening of vulval tissue, often owing to chronic irritation such as from a chemical agent, allergic condition, or physical irritation; it may also be secondary to a vulval condition such as lichen sclerosus. Called also *hyperplastic dystrophy*.

verrucous h. a superficial, typically white, hyperplastic lesion of the oral mucosa, usually occurring in older males; it is believed to be a precursor to verrucous carcinoma.

hy•per•plas•mia (hi″pər-plaz′me-ə) hypervolemia.

hy•per•ploid (hi′pər-ploid) [*hyper-* + *-ploid*] 1. having more than the typical number of chromosomes in unbalanced sets, as in Down syndrome. 2. an individual or cell having more than the typical number of chromosomes in unbalanced sets.

hy•per•ploi•dy (hi″pər-ploi′de) the state of being hyperploid. Cf. *aneuploidy*.

hy•per•pnea (hi″pər-ne′ə, hi″pərp-ne′ə) [*hyper-* + *-pnea*] abnormal increase in the depth and rate of breathing; see also *hyperventilation* (def. 1) and *tachypnea*. Called also *polypnea*. **hyperpne′ic** *adj*

hy•per•po•lar•iza•tion (hi″pər-po″lər-ĭ-za′shən) any increase in the amount of electrical charge separated by the cell membrane and hence in the strength of the transmembrane potential; thus it is a negative shift in the resting potential of the cell.

hy•per•poly•pep•tid•emia (hi″pər-pol″e-pep″tĭ-de′me-ə) excessive polypeptides in the blood.

hy•per•po•ne•sis (hi″pər-po-ne′sis) [*hyper-* + *pon-* + *-esis*] dysponesis in which there is excessive output of action potentials from the motor and premotor areas of the cerebral cortex. **hyperponet′ic** *adj*

hy•per•po•sia (hi″pər-po′zhə) [*hyper-* + *posia*] abnormally increased ingestion of fluids for relatively brief periods. Cf. *polyposia*.

hy•per•po•tas•se•mia (hi″pər-po″tə-se′me-ə) hyperkalemia.

hy•per•pra•gia (hi″pər-pra′je-ə) excessive mental activity.

hy•per•prax•ia (hi″pər-prak′se-ə) [*hyper-* + *praxis*] excessive activity; restlessness.

hy•per•pre•be•ta•lipo•pro•tein•emia (hi″pər-pre-ba″tə-lip″o-pro″te-ne′me-ə) an excess of very-low-density lipoproteins (pre-beta lipoproteins) in the blood.

familial h. see under *hypertriglyceridemia*.

hy•per•pres•by•opia (hi″pər-pres″be-o′pe-ə) excessive presbyopia.

hy•per•pro•in•su•lin•emia (hi″pər-pro-in″sə-lĭ-ne′me-ə) elevated levels of proinsulin or proinsulin-like material in the blood.

hy•per•pro•lac•tin•emia (hi″pər-pro-lak″tĭ-ne′me-ə) increased levels of prolactin in the blood; in women it is associated with amenorrhea and galactorrhea, and in men it has been reported to cause hypogonadism, impotence, and in some cases gynecomastia. It is often associated with microadenoma of the adenohypophysis. **hyperprolactine′mic** *adj*

hy•per•pro•lin•emia (hi″pər-pro″lĭ-ne′me-ə) 1. an autosomal recessive aminoacidopathy characterized by excessive proline in the body fluids; it is considered to be relatively benign, although neurologic abnormalities have been reported in some patients. There are two types, caused by different enzyme deficiencies: *type I* results from mutation in the proline oxidase gene (*PRODH*, locus: 22q11.2); *type II* results from mutation in the 1-pyrroline-5-carboxylate dehydrogenase gene (*P5CDH*, locus: 1p36). 2. excess of proline in the blood; called also *prolinemia*.

hy•per•pro•sex•ia (hi″pər-pro-sek′se-ə) [*hyper-* + Gr. *prosechein* to heed] a condition in which the mind is occupied by one idea to the exclusion of others.

hy•per•pros•o•dy (hi″pər-pros′ə-de) dysprosody marked by exaggerated variations in stress, pitch, or rhythm.

hy•per•pro•tein•emia (hi″pər-pro″te-ne′me-ə) [*hyper-* + *protein* + *-emia*] abnormally high levels of protein in the blood; see also *hyperlipoproteinemia*.

hy•per•pro•te•o•sis (hi″pər-pro″te-o′sis) a condition caused by an excess of protein in the diet.

hy•per•pty•al•ism (hi″pər-ti′əl-iz″əm) ptyalism.

hy•per•py•re•mia (hi″pər-pi-re′me-ə) [*hyper-* + Gr. *pyreia* fuel + *-emia*] excess of unoxidized carbonaceous matter in the blood.

hy•per•py•ret•ic (hi″pər-pi-ret′ik) 1. hyperthermic. 2. causing hyperthermia.

hy•per•py•rex•ia (hi″pər-pi-rek′se-ə) hyperthermia. **hyperpyrex′ial** *adj*

malignant h. see under *hyperthermia*.

hy•per•re•ac•tio lu•te•in•a•lis (hi″pər-re-ak′she-o loo″te-ĭ-na′lis) bilateral ovarian enlargement during pregnancy due to the presence of numerous theca-lutein cysts, usually associated with abnormally high levels of human chorionic gonadotropin such as with hydatidiform moles, choriocarcinoma, fetal hydrops, or multiple gestations.

hy•per•re•ac•tive (hi″pər-re-ak′tiv) pertaining to or characterized by a greater than normal response to a stimulus or irritant. Cf. *irritability* and *reaction*.

hy•per•re•ac•tiv•i•ty (hi″pər-re-ak-tiv′ĭ-te) the quality of being hyperreactive. Cf. *irritability*. Called also *hyperresponsiveness*.

hy•per•re•flex•ia (hi″pər-re-flek′se-ə) [*hyper-* + *reflex* + *-ia*] dysreflexia characterized by exaggeration of reflexes.

autonomic h. paroxysmal hypertension, bradycardia, sweating of the forehead, severe headache, and gooseflesh due to distention of the bladder and rectum; it is associated with lesions above the outflow of the splanchnic nerves.

detrusor h. increased contractile activity of the detrusor urinae muscle, resulting in urge incontinence, seen in spinal neural disease, supraspinal neural or vascular disease, parkinsonism, and some forms of dementia. Cf. *detrusor instability*.

hy•per•re•nin•emia (hi″pər-re″nĭ-ne′me-ə) a condition of elevated levels of renin in the blood, which may lead to aldosteronism. See also *reninism*. **hyperrenine′mic** *adj*

hy•per•res•o•nance (hi″pər-rez′o-nəns) an exaggerated resonance.

hy•per•re•spon•sive (hi″pər-rə-spon′siv) hyperreactive.

hy•per•re•spon•sive•ness (hi″pər-rə-spon′siv-nis) hyperreactivity.

airway h. an abnormality of the airways in which there is an exaggerated bronchoconstrictor response to any of various physical or chemical stimuli; seen in conditions such as asthma and sometimes chronic obstructive pulmonary disease.

hy•per•sa•line (hi″pər-sa′lēn) excessively saline, a term applied to treatment by administration of large doses of sodium chloride.

hy•per•sal•i•va•tion (hi″pər-sal″ĭ-va′shən) ptyalism.

hy•per•sar•co•sin•e•mia (hi″pər-sahr″ko-sĭ-ne′me-ə) elevated plasma concentration of sarcosine; see *sarcosinemia*.

hy•per•se•cre•tion (hi″pər-se-kre′shən) excessive secretion.

gastric h. hyperchlorhydria.

hy•per•seg•men•ta•tion (hi″pər-seg″mən-ta′shən) a condition of having more segments or lobes than usual.

hereditary h. of neutrophils a hereditary condition in which the neutrophils are multilobed; called also *Undritz anomaly*.

hy•per•sen•si•bil•i•ty (hi″pər-sen″sĭ-bil′ĭ-te) excessive sensibility.

hy•per•sen•si•tive (hi″pər-sen′sĭ-tiv) 1. having abnormally increased sensitivity. 2. reacting with characteristic signs and symptoms to the application of or contact with certain substances (allergens) in amounts that are innocuous to nonsensitized individuals. See *hypersensitivity*.

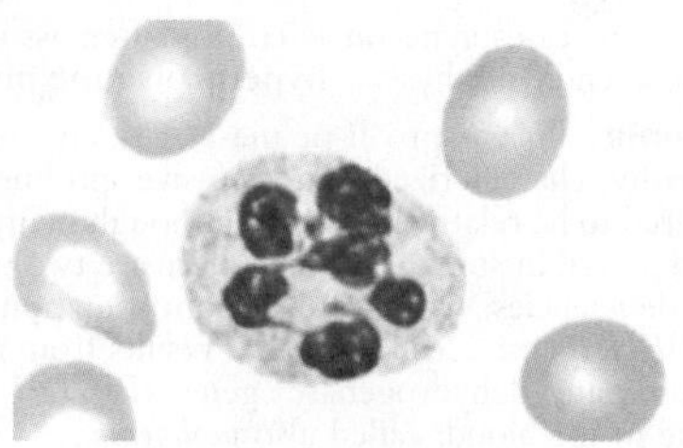

■ Neutrophil hypersegmentation.

hy·per·sen·si·tiv·i·ty (hi″pər-sen″sĭ-tiv′ĭ-te) a state of altered reactivity in which the body reacts with an exaggerated or inappropriate immune response to what is perceived to be a foreign substance. The resulting hypersensitivity reactions are usually subclassified as types I–IV on the basis of the Gell and Coombs classification of immune responses; see individual types under *hypersensitivity reaction* at *reaction.*

anaphylactic h. the most severe form of type I hypersensitivity, manifest as anaphylaxis. The term is sometimes used more loosely to describe any form of type I hypersensitivity, when contrasting this group with other types of hypersensitivity (e.g., types II–IV).

antibody-mediated h. 1. type II h. 2. occasionally, any form of hypersensitivity in which antibodies are the primary mediators, as contrasted with that mediated by T lymphocytes; included are *types I, II,* and *III h.*

antibody-mediated cytotoxic h. type II h.

cell-mediated h. type IV h.

contact h. type IV hypersensitivity produced by contact of the skin with a chemical substance having the properties of an antigen or hapten, the resulting skin condition being allergic contact dermatitis.

***Culicoides* h.** allergic dermatitis in horses as a reaction to the bites of various species of *Culicoides* flies, characterized by severe pruritus in the mane and tail region, alopecia or broken hairs from scratching, and a serous effusion with crusting. Called also *Queensland itch* and *sweet itch.*

cutaneous basophil h. Jones-Mote reaction.

cytotoxic h. type II h.

delayed h. (DH), delayed-type h. (DTH) a type of hypersensitivity that (in contrast to *immediate h.*) takes 24 to 72 hours to develop and is mediated by T lymphocytes rather than by antibodies; the term is usually used to denote the subset of type IV hypersensitivity involving cytokine release and macrophage activation, as opposed to direct cytolysis, but can be used more broadly, even sometimes being used synonymously with *type IV h.* (q.v.).

immediate h. 1. type I h. 2. occasionally, any form of hypersensitivity mediated by antibodies and developing rapidly, generally in minutes to hours (i.e., *type I, II,* or *III h.*), as distinguished from that mediated by T lymphocytes and macrophages and generally requiring 24 to 72 hours to develop (*type IV h.*, sometimes called *delayed h.).*

immune complex–mediated h. type III h.

T cell–mediated h. type IV h.

tuberculin-type h. delayed h.

type I h. hypersensitivity that occurs rapidly (within several minutes) upon reexposure to an antigen, due to interaction of IgE and the antigen; see *type I hypersensitivity reaction*, under *hypersensitivity reaction*, at *reaction.*

type II h. hypersensitivity resulting from antibody-antigen interactions on cell surfaces; see *type II hypersensitivity reaction*, under *hypersensitivity reaction*, at *reaction.* Called also *antibody-mediated h.*

type III h. hypersensitivity due to formation of circulating antigen-antibody complexes and their deposition in tissues; see *type III hypersensitivity reaction*, under *hypersensitivity reaction*, at *reaction.* Called also *immune complex–mediated h.*

type IV h. hypersensitivity initiated by antigen-specific T lymphocytes; unlike forms mediated by antibodies, it takes one or more days to develop and can be transferred by lymphocytes but not by serum. The term is often equated with *delayed hypersensitivity*, although the latter is sometimes restricted to hypersensitivity involving cytokine-mediated reactions (as contrasted with direct cytolysis). See *type IV hypersensitivity reaction*, under *hypersensitivity reaction*, at *reaction.* Called also *cell-* or *T cell–mediated h.*

hy·per·sen·si·ti·za·tion (hi″pər-sen″sĭ-tĭ-za′shən) the process of rendering, or the condition of being, abnormally sensitive. See *hypersensitivity.*

hy·per·sero·to·ne·mia (hi″pər-se″ro-to-ne′me-ə) excessive serotonin in the blood or serum; symptoms may include mental status changes and hyperactivity of the autonomic nervous system; see *serotonin syndrome*, under *syndrome.*

hy·per·sero·to·nin·e·mia (hi″pər-ser″o-to-nin-e′me-ə) hyperserotonemia.

hy·per·sex·u·al·i·ty (hi″pər-sek″shoo-al′ĭ-te) abnormally increased sexual desire or activity; see *nymphomania* and *satyriasis.*

hy·per·si·a·lor·rhea (hi″pər-si″ə-lo-re′ə) ptyalism.

hy·per·so·mato·trop·ism (hi″pər-so-mat″o-trop′iz-əm) excessive secretion of growth hormone, as seen in acromegaly and gigantism.

hy·per·so·mia (hi″pər-so′me-ə) gigantism.

hy·per·som·nia (hi″pər-som′ne-ə) [*hyper-* + *somn-* + *-ia*] excessive sleeping or sleepiness, as in any of a group of sleep disorders with a variety of physical and psychogenic causes.

primary h. [DSM-IV] a dyssomnia consisting of persistent excessive sleepiness and sleeping, with prolonged sleep episodes or regularly occurring voluntary or involuntary napping, and not due to any other psychological or physical condition.

hy·per·som·no·lence (hi″pər-som′no-lens) hypersomnia.

hy·per·sphyx·ia (hi″pər-sfik′se-ə) [*hyper-* + Gr. *sphyxis* pulse + *-ia*] increased activity of the circulation with increased blood pressure.

hy·per·sple·nia (hi″pər-sple′ne-ə) hypersplenism.

hy·per·splen·ism (hi″pər-splen′iz-əm) a condition characterized by exaggeration of the suggested inhibitory or destructive functions of the spleen, resulting in deficiency of the peripheral blood elements, singly or in combination, hypercellularity of the bone marrow, and usually, but not always, splenomegaly.

hy·per·spon·gi·o·sis (hi″pər-spon″je-o′sis) proliferation of spongy bone (substantia spongiosa ossium).

hy·per·ste·a·to·sis (hi″pər-ste-ə-to′sis) seborrhea.

hy·per·ster·eo·ra·di·og·ra·phy (hi″pər-ste″re-o-ra″di-og′rə-fe) stereoradiography with great distance between the homologous points.

hy·per·sthe·nia (hi″pər-sthe′ne-ə) great strength or tonicity. **hypersthen′ic** *adj*

hy·per·sthen·uria (hi″pər-sthə-nu′re-ə) [*hyper-* + *sthen-* + *-uria*] increased osmolality of the urine.

hy·per·stim·u·la·tion (hi″pər-stim″u-la′shən) excessive stimulation of an organ or part.

controlled ovarian h. a method of assisted reproductive technology consisting of carefully monitored administration of agents designed to induce ovulation by a greater number of ovarian follicles and thus increase the probability of an oocyte being fertilized. Called also *controlled ovarian stimulation.*

ovarian h. ovarian enlargement with exudation of fluid and protein; see *ovarian hyperstimulation syndrome*, under *syndrome.*

hy·per·sus·cep·ti·bil·i·ty (hi″pər-sə-sep″tĭ-bil′ĭ-te) a condition of abnormally increased susceptibility to poisons, infective agents, or agents to which the normal individual is less susceptible.

hy·per·ta·rach·ia (hi″pər-tə-rak′e-ə) [*hyper-* + Gr. *tarachē* confusion + *-ia*] extreme irritability of the nervous system. See *nervous irritability* (def. 2), under *irritability.*

hy·per·tau·ro·don·tism (hi″pər-taw″ro-don′tiz-əm) [*hyper-* + *taurodontism*] taurodontism in which the tooth roots do not branch.

hy·per·telo·rism (hi″pər-te′lor-iz-əm) [*hyper-* + Gr. *tēlouros* distant] 1. abnormally increased distance between two organs or parts. 2. ocular h.

ocular h., orbital h. a condition characterized by abnormal increase in the interorbital distance, often associated with cleidocranial or craniofacial dysostosis, and occasionally accompanied by mental deficiency.

hy·per·ten·sion (hi″pər-ten′shən) [*hyper-* + *tension*] high arterial blood pressure; various criteria for its threshold have been suggested, ranging from 140 mm Hg systolic and 90 mm Hg diastolic to as high as 200 mm Hg systolic and 110 mm Hg diastolic. Hypertension may have no known cause (*essential* or *idiopathic h.)* or be associated with other primary diseases (*secondary h.).*

accelerated h. progressive hypertension marked by the funduscopic vascular changes of malignant hypertension but without papilledema.

adrenal h. hypertension caused by an adrenal tumor that secretes mineralocorticoids, such as in hyperaldosteronism; in many cases it may be associated with excessive production of other adrenocortical hormones normally made in minute amounts.

benign intracranial h. pseudotumor cerebri.

borderline h. prehypertension.

chronic thromboembolic pulmonary h. persistent pulmonary hypertension due to obstruction of a major pulmonary artery by an unresolved embolus.

endocrine h. secondary hypertension caused by an endocrine disorder, such as adrenal hypertension.

essential h. hypertension occurring without discoverable organic cause; called also *primary h.* and *idiopathic h.*

gestational h. pregnancy-induced h.

Goldblatt h. hypertension experimentally induced with clamping that causes a Goldblatt kidney; called also *Goldblatt phenomenon.*

idiopathic h. essential h.

idiopathic intracranial h. pseudotumor cerebri.
intracranial h. increased intracranial pressure; if symmetrically distributed it may have few neurologic symptoms (see *pseudotumor cerebri*), but if it is asymmetrical, as with hydrocephalus, neurologic symptoms are often severe.
labile h. prehypertension.
low-renin h. essential hypertension associated with low levels of plasma renin concentration or low renin activity.
malignant h. a severe hypertensive state with poor prognosis; it is characterized by papilledema of the ocular fundus with vascular exudative and hemorrhagic lesions, medial thickening of small arteries and arterioles, and left ventricular hypertrophy. Diastolic pressures as high as 130 mm Hg or more are commonly present.
masked h. hypertension that is detectable on home monitoring devices but disappears when the patient is in a clinician's office. Cf. *white coat h.*
ocular h. persistently elevated intraocular pressure in the absence of any other signs of glaucoma; it may or may not progress to open-angle glaucoma.
office h. white coat h.
persistent pulmonary h. of the newborn a condition in newborns in which blood continues to flow through the foramen ovale and a patent ductus arteriosus, bypassing the lungs and resulting in hypoxemia. Called also persistent fetal circulation.
portal h. abnormally increased blood pressure in the portal venous system, a frequent complication of cirrhosis.
portopulmonary h. pulmonary hypertension in combination with portal hypertension.
h. of pregnancy, pregnancy-induced h. the spectrum of preeclampsia and eclampsia.
primary h. essential h.
pulmonary h., pulmonary arterial h. increased pressure (above 30 mm Hg systolic and 12 mm Hg diastolic) within the pulmonary arterial circulation.
renal h. hypertension due to or associated with renal disease with a factor of parenchymal ischemia.
renovascular h. hypertension due to occlusive disease of the renal arteries such as renal artery stenosis or fibromuscular dysplasia.
secondary h. hypertension due to or associated with a variety of primary diseases, such as renal disorders, disorders of the central nervous system, endocrine diseases, and vascular diseases.
splenoportal h. obstruction of the splenic venous system resulting in enlargement of the liver and manifestation of ascites and other evidence of portal cirrhosis.
symptomatic h. hypertension accompanied by symptoms such as dizziness or headache.
systemic venous h. elevation of systemic venous pressure, usually detected by inspection of the jugular veins.
vascular h. hypertension.
white coat h. hypertension detected when monitored in a clinician's office but not in other settings such as the patient's home; cf. *masked h.* Called also *office h.*

hy·per·ten·sive (hi″pər-ten′siv) 1. characterized by increased tension or pressure. 2. an agent that causes hypertension; called also *arteriopressor*. 3. a person with hypertension.

hy·per·ten·sor (hi″pər-ten′sər) pressor.

hy·per·the·co·sis (hi″pər-the-ko′sis) hyperplasia with excessive luteinization of the theca interna of the ovary; it may be associated with hirsutism and amenorrhea and is seen in most cases of polycystic ovary syndrome.

hy·per·the·lia (hi″pər-the′le-ə) polythelia.

hy·per·ther·mal·ge·sia (hi″pər-thur″məl-je′ze-ə) [*hyper-* + *thermalgesia*] abnormally increased sensitivity to heat (thermalgesia). Called also *hyperthermesthesia.*

hy·per·ther·mes·the·sia (hi″pər-thur″mes-the′zhə) hyperthermalgesia.

hy·per·ther·mia (hi″pər-thur′me-ə) [*hyper-* + *therm-* + *-ia*] 1. elevation of core body temperature to above 37.2°C (99°F). 2. the raising of body temperature to between 42°C (107.6°F) and 45° C (113.0°F) for therapeutic purposes. Cf. *thermotherapy.* **hyperther′mal, hyperther′mic** *adj*
h. of anesthesia malignant h.
malignant h. 1. a sudden, rapid rise in body temperature in patients undergoing general anesthesia, associated with signs of increased muscle metabolism, such as tachycardia, tachypnea, sweating, cyanosis, increased carbon dioxide production, and usually muscle rigidity. Susceptibility to this disorder is inherited as an autosomal dominant trait and can be caused by mutation in any of several genes. Called also *h. of anesthesia* and *malignant hyperpyrexia.* 2. a similar condition in pigs, a type of porcine stress syndrome in reaction to drugs such as halothane or succinylcholine chloride.

hy·per·ther·my (hi″pər-thur′me) hyperthermia.

hy·per·throm·bin·emia (hi″pər-throm″bĭ-ne′me-ə) abnormally high thrombin content of the blood.

hy·per·thy·mia (hi″pər-thi′me-ə) [*hyper-* + *thymo-* + *-ia*] 1. excessive emotionalism. 2. excessive activity, verging on hypomania.

hy·per·thy·mic (hi″pər-thi′mik) marked by hyperthymia.

hy·per·thy·mism (hi″pər-thi′miz-əm) a condition attributed to excessive activity of the thymus gland.

hy·per·thy·roid (hi″pər-thi′roid) marked by or due to hyperthyroidism.

hy·per·thy·roid·ism (hi″pər-thi′roid-iz-əm) a condition caused by excessive production of iodinated thyroid hormones; characteristics include goiter, tachycardia or atrial fibrillation, widened pulse pressure, palpitations, fatigability, nervousness and tremor, heat intolerance and excessive sweating, warm, smooth, moist skin, weight loss, muscular weakness, excessive defecation, emotional lability, and ocular signs such as stare, slowing of eyelid movements, photophobia, and sometimes exophthalmos. Called also *hyperthyroidosis.* See also *Graves disease* and *thyrotoxicosis.*
iodine-induced h. hyperthyroidism following administration of iodine or iodide, either as a dietary supplement or as contrast medium. Called also *jodbasedow.*
masked h. hyperactivity of the thyroid gland in which the classic signs and symptoms are subtle, and predominance of cardiovascular symptoms leads to suspicion of heart disease rather than thyroid disease; it occurs chiefly in middle-aged or elderly persons.

hy·per·thy·roid·osis (hi″pər-thi″roid-o′sis) hyperthyroidism.

hy·per·thy·rox·in·emia (hi″pər-thi-rok″sĭ-ne′me-ə) excessively high blood levels of thyroxine.
euthyroid h. a condition characterized by increased levels of thyroxine in the blood but a normal level of thyroid-stimulating hormone and normal thyroid function.
familial dysalbuminemic h. (FDH) an autosomal dominant disorder in which an elevation in total serum thyroxine suggests hyperthyroidism, but the patient is euthyroid by clinical evaluation and other tests because an excess of T_4-binding serum albumin results in normal free thyroxine concentration and triiodothyronine resin uptake.

hy·per·to·nia (hi″pər-to′ne-ə) [*hyper-* + *ton-* + *-ia*] excessive tone of the skeletal muscles, so that they have increased resistance to passive stretching and reflexes are often exaggerated; this usually indicates upper motor neuron injury.
h. polycythae′mica increased blood pressure associated with polycythemia.

hy·per·ton·ic (hi″pər-ton′ik) 1. denoting a solution which when bathing body cells causes a net flow of water across the semipermeable cell membrane out of the cell. 2. denoting a solution having a greater tonicity than another solution, e.g., the blood, with which it is compared. 3. exhibiting hypertonia.

hy·per·to·nic·i·ty (hi″pər-to-nis′ĭ-te) the state or quality of being hypertonic.

hy·per·to·nus (hi″pər-to′nəs) hypertonia.

hy·per·tox·ic (hi′pər-tok″sik) excessively toxic.

hy·per·tox·ic·i·ty (hi″pər-tok-sis′ĭ-te) the state or quality of being excessively toxic.

hy·per·trans·fu·sion (hi″pər-trans-fu′zhən) a regimen of regular transfusions, usually given to children with chronic conditions such as β-thalassemia or sickle cell disease to prevent anemia.

hy·per·tri·cho·sis (hi″pər-trĭ-ko′sis) [*hyper-* + *trich-* + *-osis*] excessive growth of the hair. Called also *polytrichia* and *polytrichosis.* Cf. *hirsutism.*
congenital universal h. universal h.
h. cu′biti localized hypertrichosis around the elbows, transmitted as an autosomal dominant trait.
generalized h. universal h.
h. lanugino′sa persistent or acquired production of lanugo. One form is a rare autosomal dominant disorder in which there is excessive hair over the entire body throughout life, sometimes in association with other congenital anomalies. This type is also called *generalized* or *universal h.* An acquired form occasionally accompanies certain types of internal carcinoma; it is usually on the face, with the degree of hairiness being variable.
localized h. acquired hypertrichosis in a circumscribed area; causes include repeated trauma, friction, irritation, and inflammation.
nevoid h. hypertrichosis associated with a nevus, such as a Becker nevus or melanocytic nevus.
h. pin′nae au′ris hypertrichosis in which the pinnae of the ears have hairs 7 cm long or longer; it may be a Y-linked or an autosomal dominant trait. Called also *hairy ears* and *hairy pinnae.*
universal h., h. universa′lis the congenital form of hypertrichosis lanuginosa; called also *generalized h.*
vellus h. 1. hypertrichosis with vellus hair. 2. h. lanuginosa.

hy·per·tri·glyc·er·i·de·mia (hi″pər-tri-glis′ə-ri-de′me-ə) excessive triglycerides in the blood.

familial h. a genetically heterogenous, autosomal dominant disorder of lipoprotein metabolism characterized by mildly elevated triglycerides and very-low-density lipoproteins, thus having a type IV hyperlipoproteinemia phenotype but lacking other biochemical or clinical features. The disorder can interact with secondary factors to cause more severe elevation of triglycerides with hyperchylomicronemia, a type V phenotype; see *familial hyperchylomicronemia* and see also table at *hyperlipoproteinemia.*

sporadic h. hypertriglyceridemia that appears to be identical to an inherited form but in which inheritance cannot be documented; used in classifying disorders of lipoprotein metabolism.

hy•per•tro•phia (hi″pər-tro′fe-ə) hypertrophy.

hy•per•tro•phy (hi-pur′trə-fe) [*hyper-* + *-trophy*] the enlargement or overgrowth of an organ or part due to an increase in size of its constituent cells. See also *hyperplasia* and *proliferation.* **hypertro′phic** *adj*

adaptive h. increase in size in response to changed conditions, as, for example, increased thickness of the walls of a hollow organ when the outflow is obstructed.

asymmetrical septal h. (ASH) 1. hypertrophic cardiomyopathy. 2. the term is sometimes limited to cases of hypertrophic cardiomyopathy in which the hypertrophy is localized to the interventricular septum. Cf. *hypertrophic obstructive cardiomyopathy.*

benign prostatic h. see under *hyperplasia.*

Bertin column h. congenital enlargement of renal columns (Bertin columns), a benign condition sometimes mistaken for a renal tumor. Called also *renal column h.*

cardiac h. enlargement of myocardial cells and hyperplasia of nonmuscular cardiac components due to pressure and volume overload and sometimes to neurohumoral factors.

compensatory h. hypertrophy that results from an increased workload due to some physical defect, such as occurs in one kidney when the other is absent or nonfunctional.

complementary h. increase in size of the remaining part of an organ to take the place of a portion which has been lost.

concentric h. hypertrophy of a hollow organ in which there is increased thickness of the walls with no enlargement in external size, with diminished capacity.

eccentric h. hypertrophy of a hollow organ in which there is dilatation of its cavity and enlargement of its external size.

false h. enlargement due to an increase in only one constituent element of an organ or part, commonly the stroma.

functional h. hypertrophy of an organ or part caused by its increased activity.

hemifacial h. facial hemihypertrophy.

Marie h. enlargement of the soft parts of the joints resulting from periostitis.

physiologic h. temporary increase in the size of an organ produced by physiologic activity, as in the female breast during pregnancy and lactation.

pseudomuscular h. pseudohypertrophic muscular dystrophy.

renal column h. Bertin column h.

simple h. hypertrophy that is due to a simple increase of the number of structural elements.

true h. enlargement due to an increase of all the component elements of an organ or part.

unilateral h. overgrowth of one side of the entire body or of a portion of one side, as of the face.

ventricular h. hypertrophy of the myocardium of a ventricle of the heart, due to chronic pressure overload; it is manifest electrocardiographically by increased QRS complex voltage, frequently accompanied by repolarization changes.

vicarious h. hypertrophy of an organ in consequence of the failure of another organ of allied function. Cf. *compensatory h.*

hy•per•tro•pia (hi″pər-tro′pe-ə) [*hyper-* + *trop-* + *-ia*] vertical strabismus in which there is permanent upward deviation of the visual axis of an eye.

Hy•per•tus•sis (hi″pər-tus′is) trademark for a preparation of pertussis immune globulin.

hy•per•ty•ro•sin•emia (hi″pər-ti″ro-sĭ-ne′me-ə) 1. excessive levels of tyrosine in the blood, as occurs in a variety of disorders of tyrosine catabolism. See also *tyrosinemia.* 2. tyrosinemia.

hy•per•ura•tu•ria (hi″pər-u″ra-tu′re-ə) hyperuricosuria.

hy•per•u•ric•ac•i•de•mia (hi″pər-u″rik-as″ĭ-de′me-ə) hyperuricemia.

hy•per•u•ric•ac•i•du•ria (hi″pər-u″rik-as″ĭ-du′re-ə) hyperuricosuria.

hy•per•uri•ce•mia (hi″pər-u″rĭ-se′me-ə) excess of uric acid or urates in the blood; it is a prerequisite for the development of gout and may lead to renal disease. Called also *hyperuricacidemia, uricacidemia,* and *uricemia.* **hyperurice′mic** *adj*

hy•per•uri•co•su•ria (hi″pər-u″rĭ-ko-su′re-ə) excess of uric acid or urates in the urine, such as with a high purine diet or in renal failure,

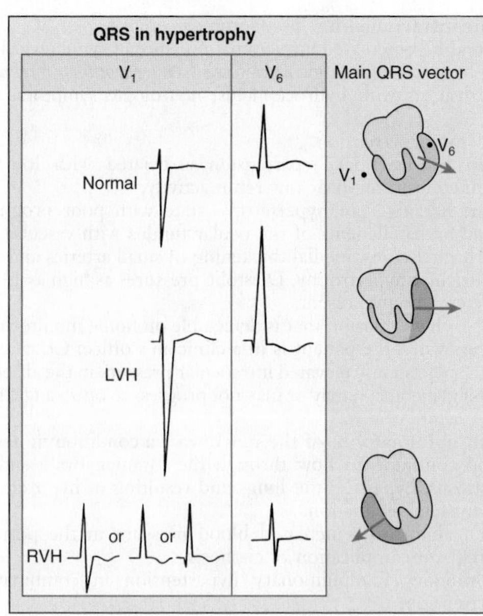

■ Ventricular hypertrophy. Diagram contrasting the effects of left *(LVH)* and right *(RVH)* ventricular hypertrophy on the QRS vector. LVH exaggerates the normal pattern, causing deeper right precordial S waves and taller left precordial R waves. RVH shifts the QRS vector to the right, causing increased right precordial R waves.

ketoacidosis, or a disorder of purine metabolism such as gout. Called also *hyperuricaciduria, hyperuricuria,* and *uricaciduria.*

hy•per•u•ric•uria (hi″pər-u″rĭ-ku′re-ə) hyperuricosuria.

hy•per•vac•ci•na•tion (hi″pər-vak″sĭ-na′shən) the subsequent inoculation (one or more times) of a previously immunized animal with enough vaccine to enable it to produce a serum protective to other animals.

hy•per•val•i•ne•mia (hi″pər-val″ĭ-ne′me-ə) 1. an autosomal recessive aminoacidopathy, due to a defect in valine transaminase, characterized by elevated levels of valine in the plasma and urine with failure to thrive. 2. elevated levels of valine in the plasma. Called also *valinemia.*

hy•per•vas•cu•lar (hi″pər-vas′ku-lər) extremely vascular.

hy•per•ven•ti•la•tion (hi″pər-ven″tĭ-la′shən) 1. a state in which there is an increased amount of air entering the pulmonary alveoli (increased *alveolar ventilation*; see under *ventilation*). This results in reduction of carbon dioxide tension, eventually leading to alkalosis. See also *hyperpnea, tachypnea,* and *hyperventilation syndrome.* 2. abnormally prolonged, rapid, and deep breathing (polypnea), frequently used as a test procedure in epilepsy and tetany.

hy•per•vig•i•lance (hi″pər-vij′ĭ-ləns) abnormally increased arousal, responsiveness to stimuli, and scanning of the environment for threats; it is often associated with delusional or paranoid states and with posttraumatic stress disorder.

hy•per•vis•cos•i•ty (hi″pər-vis-kos′ĭ-te) excessive viscosity, as of the blood; see also *hyperviscosity syndrome,* under *syndrome.*

hy•per•vi•ta•min•o•sis (hi″pər-vi″tə-mĭ-no′sis) a condition due to ingestion of an excess of one or more vitamins; called also *supervitaminosis.* **hypervitaminot′ic** *adj*

h. A a symptom complex resulting from ingestion of excessive amounts of vitamin A, with hair loss, skin disorders, headache, bone and joint pain, anorexia, fatigue, irritability, hyperostosis, hepatosplenomegaly, papilledema, and pseudotumor cerebri.

h. D a symptom complex resulting from ingestion of excessive amounts of vitamin D, with weakness, fatigue, loss of weight, and other symptoms.

hy•per•vo•le•mia (hi″pər-vo-le′me-ə) [*hyper-* + *volume* + *-emia*] abnormal increase in the volume of circulating blood plasma; see also *hemodilution.* **hypervole′mic** *adj*

hy•per•vo•lia (hi″pər-vo′le-ə) augmented water content or volume of a given compartment, such as a cell.

hyp•es•the•sia (hīp″es-the′zhə) hypoesthesia.

hy•pha (hi′fə) pl. *hy′phae* [L., from Gr. *hyphe* web] 1. one of the filaments or threads composing the mycelium of a fungus. 2. branching filamentous outgrowths produced by certain bacteria (e.g., *Actinomyces, Hyphomicrobium*), sometimes forming a mycelium.

aerial h. a hypha produced above the surface of a culture medium.

dematiaceous h. a hypha that is dark-colored owing to the presence of melanin.

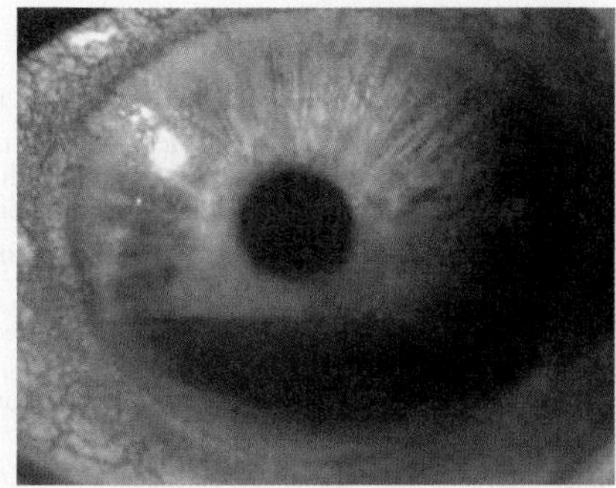

■ Thirty percent hyphema.

hyaline h. a hypha that is transparent, either completely clear or with a color.

racket h. a type of hypha composed of racket cells, found in various kinds of dermatophytes.

hy·phal (hi′fəl) pertaining to a hypha.

hyp·he·do·nia (hīp″hə-do′ne-ə) [*hypo-* + Gr. *hēdonē* pleasure + *-ia*] pathologic diminution of the feeling of pleasure in acts that normally give pleasure.

hy·phe·ma (hi-fe′mə) [Gr. *hyphaimos* suffused with blood, bloodshot; especially of the eyes] hemorrhage within the anterior chamber of the eye. Called also *hyphemia.*

hy·phe·mia (hi-fe′me-ə) hyphema.

hyp·hi·dro·sis (hīp″hĭ-dro′sis) hypohidrosis.

Hy·pho·my·ce·ta·les (hi″fo-mi″se-ta′lēz) name used for the form-order Moniales in some classifications of fungi.

hy·pho·my·cete (hi″fo-mi′sēt) any individual organism of the class Hyphomycetes. **hyphomyce′tous** *adj*

Hy·pho·my·ce·tes (hi″fo-mi-se′tēz) [pl., Gr. *hyphē* web + Gr. *mykēs* fungus] a form-class of Fungi Imperfecti (subphylum Deuteromycotina), consisting of the mycelial (hyphal) fungi, i.e., molds. It usually is considered to include the form-families Dematiaceae and Moniliaceae, and sometimes Cryptococcaceae.

hy·pho·my·co·sis (hi″fo-mi-ko′sis) any infection caused by an imperfect fungus of the form-class *Hyphomycetes*; the group has been divided into *hyalohyphomycosis* and *phaeohyphomycosis* based on the color of the mycelium and wall of the fungus.

h. de′struens e′qui pythiosis.

hyp·na·gog·ic (hip″nə-goj′ik) 1. hypnotic (defs. 1 and 2). 2. occurring just before sleep; applied to hallucinations occurring at sleep onset.

hyp·nal·gia (hip-nal′jə) [*hypn-* + *-algia*] pain that occurs during sleep.

hyp·nic (hip′nik) [Gr. *hypnikos*] hypnotic (def. 1).

hypn(o)- [Gr. *hypnos* sleep] a combining form denoting relationship to sleep or to hypnosis.

hyp·no·anal·y·sis (hip″no-ə-nal′ə-sis) [*hypno-* + *analysis*] a method of psychotherapy in which psychoanalysis is employed in conjunction with hypnosis.

hyp·no·an·es·the·sia (hip″no-an″es-the′zhə) induction of the anesthetic state by hypnosis.

hyp·no·cyst (hip′no-sist) [*hypno-* + *cyst*] a quiescent parasitic cyst; see *cyst* (def. 2).

hyp·no·don·tia (hip″no-don′shə) hypnodontics.

hyp·no·don·tics (hip″no-don′tiks) [*hypno-* + *odont-* + *-ic*] the application of controlled suggestion and hypnosis in the practice of dentistry.

hyp·no·gen·e·sis (hip″no-jen′ĕ-sis) [*hypno-* + *-genesis*] the causing or entering a state of hypnosis or of sleep.

hyp·no·ge·net·ic (hip″no-jə-net′ik) hypnotic (def. 1).

hyp·no·gen·ic (hip″no-jen′ik) hypnotic (def. 1).

hyp·nog·e·nous (hip-noj′ə-nəs) hypnotic (def. 1).

hyp·noid (hip′noid) pertaining to or resembling hypnosis, the hypnotic state, or sleep.

hyp·noi·dal (hip-noi′dəl) hypnoid.

hyp·nol·o·gy (hip-nol′ə-je) somnology.

hyp·no·pe·dia (hip″no-pe′de-ə) [*hypno-* + *paideia* education] sleep learning; learning during sleep, as by listening to recordings.

hyp·no·pom·pic (hip″no-pom′pik) [*hypno-* + Gr. *pompē* a sending away, a sending home] persisting after sleep; applied to hallucinations occurring on awakening.

hyp·no·sis (hip-no′sis) [Gr. *hypnos* sleep] a state of altered consciousness, usually artificially induced, characterized by focusing of attention, heightened responsiveness to suggestions and commands, suspension of disbelief with lowering of critical judgment, the potential of alteration in perceptions, motor control, or memory in response to suggestions, and the subjective experience of responding involuntarily.

hyp·no·ther·a·py (hip″no-ther′ə-pe) [*hypno-* + *therapy*] the use of hypnosis in the treatment of disease.

hyp·not·ic (hip-not′ik) 1. inducing sleep. 2. an agent that induces sleep. 3. pertaining to or of the nature of hypnosis or hypnotism.

hyp·no·tism (hip′no-tiz-əm) the study of or the method or practice of inducing hypnosis.

hyp·no·tist (hip′no-tist) an individual who induces hypnosis.

hyp·no·ti·za·tion (hip″no-tĭ-za′shən) the induction of hypnosis.

hyp·no·tize (hip′no-tīz) to induce a state of hypnosis.

hyp·no·tox·in (hip′no-tok″sin) a toxic substance derived from the tentacles of *Physalia*, the Portuguese man-of-war, characteristically causing a central nervous system depression, affecting both motor and sensory elements.

hyp·no·zo·ite (hip″no-zo′īt) [*hypno-* + Gr. *zōon* animal] the round or oval, uninucleate, dormant form of *Plasmodium* seen inside hepatic cells during the intrahepatic stage of the parasite's life; it is believed to be the true latent stage associated with relapse in malaria.

hy·po (hi′po) 1. popular designation for a hypodermic inoculation or syringe. 2. a contraction for sodium thiosulfate used as a photographic fixing agent.

hyp(o)- [Gr. *hypo* under] a prefix signifying beneath, under, below normal, or deficient. Cf. *sub-*. In chemistry, it denotes a compound, usually an acid or a salt, containing the lowest proportion of oxygen in a series of similar compounds, e.g., hypochlorous acid (HClO) or sodium hypochlorite (NaClO).

hy·po·ac·id·i·ty (hi″po-ə-sid′ĭ-te) deficiency of acid; lack of normal acidity.

hy·po·ac·tive (hi″po-ak′tiv) pertaining to or characterized by hypoactivity.

hy·po·ac·tiv·i·ty (hi″po-ak-tiv′ĭ-te) 1. abnormally diminished activity, as of peristalsis. 2. abnormally decreased motor and cognitive activity, with slowing of thought, speech, and movement.

hy·po·acu·sis (hi″po-ə-ku′sis) [*hypo-* + *acou-* + *-sis*] slightly diminished auditory sensitivity, with hearing threshold levels above the normal limit so that the impairment is measurable in decibels. Called also *hypacusia, hypacusis,* and *acoustic* or *auditory hypoesthesia.*

hy·po·ad·i·po·nec·tin·emia (hi″po-ad″ĭ-po-nek″tĭ-ne′me-ə) an abnormally low level of adiponectin in the blood.

hy·po·adren·a·lism (hi″po-ə-dre′nəl-iz-əm) adrenal insufficiency (def. 1).

hy·po·adre·no·cor·ti·cism (hi″po-ə-dre″no-kor′tĭ-siz-əm) adrenocortical insufficiency.

hy·po·al·bu·min·emia (hi″po-al-bu″min-e′me-ə) an abnormally low albumin content of the blood; called also *hypalbuminemia.*

hy·po·al·bu·min·o·sis (hi″po-al-bu″mĭ-no′sis) hypoalbuminemia.

hy·po·al·dos·ter·on·emia (hi″po-al-dos″tər-o-ne′me-ə) an abnormally low level of aldosterone in the blood.

hy·po·al·dos·ter·on·ism (hi″po-al-dos′tə-ro-niz″əm) aldosterone deficiency, usually associated with hypoadrenalism, and characterized by hypotension, dehydration, and a tendency to excrete excessive amounts of sodium.

hyporeninemic h. the most common type of isolated hypoaldosteronism, caused by decreased renin production by the kidney.

isolated h. a rare endocrine disorder characterized by aldosterone deficiency, with normal production of cortisol and all other adrenocortical steroids.

hy·po·al·dos·ter·on·uria (hi″po-al-dos″tə-ro-nu′re-ə) abnormally low levels of aldosterone in the urine.

hy·po·al·ge·sia (hi″po-al-je′ze-ə) hypalgesia.

hy·po·al·i·men·ta·tion (hi″po-al″ĭ-mən-ta′shən) insufficient nourishment.

hy·po·al·ka·line (hi″po-al′kə-līn, -lin) less alkaline than normal.

hy·po·al·ka·lin·i·ty (hi″po-al″kə-lin′ĭ-te) the state of being less alkaline than normal.

hy·po·al·pha·lipo·pro·tein·emia (hi″po-al″fə-lip″o-pro″te-ne′me-ə) 1. deficiency of high-density lipoproteins (alpha lipoproteins) in the blood. 2. Tangier disease.

hy·po·am·i·no·ac·i·de·mia (hi″po-ə-me″no-as″ĭ-de′me-ə) lower than normal levels of amino acids in the blood.

hy·po·an·dro·gen·ism (hi″po-an-dro′jən-iz-əm) a state characterized or caused by deficiency of androgens.

hy·po·azo·tu·ria (hi″po-az″o-tu′re-ə) [*hypo-* + *azote* + *-uria*] diminished excretion of nitrogenous material in the urine.

hy·po·bar·ic (hi″po-bar′ik) [*hypo-* + *bar-* + *-ic*] characterized by less than normal pressure or weight; applied to gases under less than atmospheric pressure or to a solution of lower specific gravity than another taken as a standard of reference. See under *solution.*

hy·po·bar·ism (hi″po-bar′iz-əm) the condition resulting from exposure to ambient gas pressure or atmospheric pressures that are below those within body tissues, fluids, cavities.

hy·po·bar·op·a·thy (hi″po-bar-op′ə-the) [*hypo-* + *baro-* + *-pathy*] 1. the disturbances experienced in high altitudes due to reduced air pressure; see *high-altitude sickness* and *mountain sickness,* under *sickness.* 2. hypobarism.

hy·po·be·ta·lipo·pro·tein·emia (hi″po-ba″tə-lip″o-pro″te-ne′me-ə) abnormally low levels of low-density lipoproteins (beta lipoproteins) in the serum, as in debilitating diseases and malabsorption syndromes.

familial h. a disorder of lipid metabolism clinically similar to abetalipoproteinemia, but of codominant inheritance and usually milder; the genetic basis is in most cases uncertain.

hy·po·bi·car·bo·nat·emia (hi″po-bi-kahr″bə-na-te′me-ə) an abnormally low level of bicarbonate in the blood; see *bicarbonate buffer,* under *buffer.*

hy·po·bil·i·ru·bin·emia (hi″po-bil″ĭ-roo″bĭ-ne′me-ə) abnormal diminution of bilirubin in the blood.

hy·po·blast (hi′po-blast) [*hypo-* + *-blast*] the lower layer of the bilaminar embryonic disc in a human embryo, present during the second week; it gives rise to the endoderm. **hypoblas′tic** *adj*

hy·po·bran·chi·al (hi″po-brang′ke-əl) [*hypo-* + *branchial*] located beneath the branchial (or pharyngeal) arches.

hy·po·bro·mite (hi″po-bro′mīt) any salt of hypobromous acid.

hy·po·bro·mous ac·id (hi″po-bro′məs) an unstable acid, HBrO; used as a disinfectant and bleaching agent and in testing for urea.

hy·po·cal·ce·mia (hi″po-kal-se′me-ə) [*hypo-* + *calci-* + *-emia*] reduction of the blood calcium below normal; manifestations include hyperactive deep tendon reflexes, Chvostek sign, muscle and abdominal cramps, and carpopedal spasm. **hypocalce′mic** *adj*

hy·po·cal·cia (hi″po-kal′se-ə) calcipenia.

hy·po·cal·ci·fi·ca·tion (hi″po-kal″sĭ-fĭ-ka′shən) diminished calcification.

enamel h. an autosomal dominant form of amelogenesis imperfecta due to faulty mineralization of enamel, characterized by a tooth crown that appears normal at eruption but soon assumes a white chalky appearance and gradually undergoes brown discoloration; the affected teeth are soft and rough.

hy·po·cal·ci·pexy (hi″po-kal′sĭ-pek″se) deficient calcium fixation. **hypocalcipec′tic** *adj*

hy·po·cal·ci·uria (hi″po-kal″se-u′re-ə) abnormally low levels of calcium in the urine.

hy·po·ca·lor·ic (hi″po-kə-lor′ik) low in calories.

hy·po·cap·nia (hi″po-kap′ne-ə) [*hypo-* + *capn-* + *-ia*] deficiency of carbon dioxide in the blood, resulting from hyperventilation and eventually leading to alkalosis. Called also *hypocarbia.* **hypocap′nic** *adj*

hy·po·car·bia (hi″po-kahr′be-ə) hypocapnia.

hy·po·cat·a·la·sia (hi″po-kat″ə-la′zhə) an asymptomatic variant of acatalasia in which some catalase activity is present; it occurs in some heterozygotes.

hy·po·cel·lu·lar (hi″po-sel′u-lər) pertaining to or characterized by hypocellularity.

hy·po·cel·lu·lar·i·ty (hi″po-sel″u-lar′ĭ-te) a state of abnormal decrease in the number of cells present, as in bone marrow.

hy·po·ce·lom (hi″po-se′lom) hypocoelom.

hy·po·chlor·emia (hi″po-klor-e′me-ə) abnormally low levels of chloride in the blood. **hypochlore′mic** *adj*

hy·po·chlor·hy·dria (hi″po-klor-hi′dre-ə) [*hypo-* + *chloro-* + *hydr-* + *-ia*] deficiency of hydrochloric acid in the gastric juice. Cf. *achlorhydria.*

hy·po·chlo·ri·da·tion (hi″po-klor″ĭ-da′shən) deficiency of chloride in the system.

hy·po·chlo·rid·emia (hi″po-klor″i-de′me-ə) hypochloremia.

hy·po·chlo·rite (hi″po-klor′īt) [*hypo-* + *chlorite*] any salt of hypochlorous acid; used as a medicinal agent, particularly as a diluted solution of sodium hypochlorite. See *sodium hypochlorite solution,* under *solution.*

hy·po·chlo·ri·za·tion (hi″po-klor″ĭ-za′shən) reduction of the amount of sodium chloride in the diet; see *low salt diet,* under *diet.*

hy·po·chlo·rous ac·id (hi″po-klor′əs) an unstable compound, HClO, a disinfectant and bleaching agent; its salts (hypochlorites) are used as medicinal agents, particularly as diluted sodium hypochlorite solution; see *sodium hypochlorite solution,* under *solution.*

hy·po·chlor·uria (hi″po-klor-u′re-ə) [*hypo-* + *chlor-* + *-uria*] deficiency of chlorides in the urine.

hy·po·cho·les·te·re·mia (hi″po-kə-les″tə-re′me-ə) hypocholesterolemia. **hypocholestere′mic** *adj*

hy·po·cho·les·ter·ol·emia (hi″po-kə-les″tər-ol-e′me-ə) abnormally low levels of cholesterol in the blood. **hypocholesterole′mic** *adj*

hy·po·chol·uria (hi″po-ko-lu′re-ə) abnormal reduction in the amount of bile in the urine.

hy·po·chon·dria (hi″po-kon′dre-ə) 1. plural of *hypochondrium.* 2. hypochondriasis.

hy·po·chon·dri·ac (hi″po-kon′dre-ak) 1. pertaining to the hypochondrium. 2. pertaining to hypochondriasis. 3. a person affected with hypochondriasis.

hy·po·chon·dri·a·cal (hi″po-kon-dri′ə-kəl) 1. pertaining to the hypochondrium. 2. pertaining to or affected with hypochondriasis.

hy·po·chon·dri·a·sis (hi″po-kon-dri′ə-sis) [so called because it was supposed by the ancients to be due to disturbed function of the organs of the upper abdomen; see also *regio hypochondriaca*] [DSM-IV] a somatoform disorder characterized by a preoccupation with bodily functions and the interpretation of normal sensations (such as heart beats, sweating, peristaltic action, and bowel movements) or minor abnormalities (such as a runny nose, minor aches and pains, or slightly swollen lymph nodes) as indications of serious problems needing medical attention. Negative results of diagnostic evaluations and reassurance by physicians only increase the patient's anxious concern about his health, although the concern is not of delusional intensity. Called also *hypochondriacal neurosis.*

hy·po·chon·dri·um (hi″po-kon′dre-əm) pl. *hypochon′dria* [*hypo-* + Gr. *chondros* cartilage] [TA] either of the superolateral regions of the abdomen, lateral to the epigastric region, overlying the costal cartilages. Called also *regio hypochondriaca* [TA alternative].

hy·po·chon·dro·pla·sia (hi″po-kon″dro-pla′zhə) a common autosomal dominant chondrodystrophy resembling achondroplasia but with milder clinical features, which include short stature with a long trunk and short limbs, broad and short fingers, and a normal face. It is genetically heterogeneous, with most cases being caused by mutation in the fibroblast growth factor receptor 3 *(FGFR3)* gene (locus: 4p16.3).

hy·po·chor·dal (hi″po-kor′dəl) beneath the notochord; called also *subchordal* and *subnotochordal.*

hy·po·chro·ma·sia (hi″po-kro-ma′zhə) [*hypo-* + Gr. *chrōma* color] 1. the condition of staining less intensely than normal. 2. hypochromia (def. 1).

hy·po·chro·mat·ic (hi″po-kro-mat′ik) 1. containing an abnormally small number of chromosomes; marked by hypochromatism. 2. characterized by hypochromatism.

hy·po·chro·ma·tism (hi″po-kro′mə-tiz-əm) [*hypo-* + *chromat-* + *-ism*] 1. abnormally deficient pigmentation, especially deficiency of the chromatin in a cell nucleus. 2. hypochromia (def. 1).

hy·po·chro·mia (hi″po-kro′me-ə) [*hypo-* + *chrom-* + *-ia*] 1. abnormal decrease in the hemoglobin content of the erythrocytes. Called also *hypochromasia* and *hypochromatism.* 2. hypochromatism (def. 1).

hy·po·chro·mic (hi″po-kro′mik) pertaining to or marked by hypochromia.

hy·po·chro·mo·trich·ia (hi″po-kro″mo-trik′e-ə) achromotrichia.

hy·po·ci·ne·sia (hi″po-sĭ-ne′zhə) hypokinesia.

hy·po·cit·ra·tu·ria (hi″po-sĭ-tra-tu′re-ə) excretion of urine containing an abnormally small amount of citrate, such as in persons forming renal calculi. Cf. *hypocitruria.*

hy·po·ci·tre·mia (hi″po-sĭ-tre′me-ə) [*hypo-* + *citric* acid + *-emia*] abnormally low content of citric acid in the blood.

hy·po·ci·tru·ria (hi″po-sĭ-troo′re-ə) [*hypo-* + *citric* acid + *-uria*] excretion of urine containing an abnormally small amount of citric acid, such as in persons forming renal calculi. Cf. *hypocitraturia.*

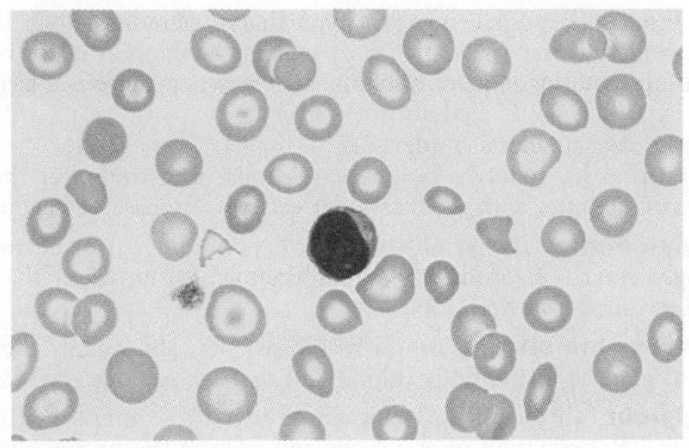

■ Hypochromia in a peripheral smear in hypochromic microcytic anemia.

hy•po•co•ag•u•la•bil•i•ty (hi″po-ko-ag″u-lə-bil′ĭ-te) the state of having less coagulability than normal.

hy•po•co•ag•u•la•ble (hi″po-ko-ag′u-lə-bəl) having abnormally decreased coagulability.

hy•po•coe•lom (hi″po-se′lom) [*hypo-* + *coelom*] the ventral portion of the coelom of the embryo of a vertebrate.

hy•po•com•ple•men•te•mia (hi″po-kom″plə-men-te′me-ə) abnormally low levels of complement in the blood. **hypocomplemente′mic** *adj*

hy•po•con•dy•lar (hi″po-kon′də-lər) inferior to a condyle.

hy•po•cone (hi′po-kōn) [*hypo-* + Gr. *kōnos* cone] the distolingual cusp of an upper molar tooth.

hy•po•con•id (hi″po-ko′nid) [*hypo-* + *con(o)-* + *-id*] the distobuccal cusp of a lower molar tooth.

hy•po•con•u•lid (hi″po-kon′u-lid) the distal, or fifth, cusp of a lower molar tooth; usually found on the mandibular first molar.

hy•po•cor•ti•cal•ism (hi″po-kor′tĭ-kəl-iz-əm) adrenocortical insufficiency.

hy•po•cor•ti•cism (hi″po-kor′ti-siz-əm) adrenocortical insufficiency.

hy•po•cot•yl (hi″po-kot′əl) [*hypo-* + *kotyle* hollow] the part of the axis of a plant embryo or seedling below the point of attachment of the cotyledon and from which the radicle, or primary root, grows.

Hy•po•crea (hi″po-kre′ə) a genus of fungi of the family Hypocreaceae, including the perfect (sexual) stage of some species of *Trichoderma.*

Hy•po•cre•a•ceae (hi″po-kre-a′se-e) a family of fungi of the order Hypocreales. It includes the genera *Hypocrea*, *Nectria*, and *Podostroma*, which contain the perfect (sexual) stages of several species of *Acremonium*, *Fusarium*, and *Trichoderma* and the etiologic agents of numerous types of plant wilt.

Hy•po•cre•a•les (hi″po-kre-a′ləs) an order of perfect fungi of the subphylum Ascomycotina, series Unitunicatae, characterized by inoperculate asci; it includes the family Hypocreaceae.

hy•po•cre•tin (hi-po-kre′tin) orexin.

hy•po•cu•pre•mia (hi″po-ku-pre′me-ə) [*hypo-* + L. *cuprum* copper + *-emia*] abnormally low levels of copper in the blood.

hy•po•cy•clo•sis (hi″po-si-klo′sis) [*hypo-* + *cycl-* + *-osis*] insufficiency of accommodation due either to undue rigidity of the crystalline lens *(lenticular h.)* or to weakness of the ciliary muscle *(ciliary h.)*.

hy•po•cy•the•mia (hi″po-si-the′me-ə) erythropenia.

hy•po•cy•to•sis (hi″po-si-to′sis) cytopenia.

hy•po•dac•ty•ly (hi″po-dak′tə-le) oligodactyly.

hy•po•dense (hi′po-dens″) being less dense than other similar objects, such as an object or area that is less dense than others on a radiograph.

hy•po•derm (hi′po-dərm) tela subcutanea.

Hy•po•der•ma (hi″po-dur′mə) [*hypo-* + Gr. *derma* skin] the ox-warble flies or heel flies, a genus of insects of the family Oestridae whose larvae cause larva migrans in humans and warbles in cattle.

H. bo′vis a species whose larvae cause warbles in cattle and larva migrans in humans; in cattle they prefer to migrate to the area near the spinal canal.

H. linea′tum a species that infests mainly cattle and prefers to migrate to the area near the esophagus.

hy•po•der•mi•a•sis (hi″po-dər-mi′ə-sis) infection by *Hypoderma*, particularly their larvae, which migrate through the host's body; see *larva migrans* and *warbles.*

hy•po•der•mic (hi″po-dur′mik) beneath the skin; called also *subcutaneous.*

hy•po•der•mis (hi″po-dur′mis) [*hypo-* + *dermis*] 1. TA alternative for tela subcutanea. 2. the outer cellular layer of the body of invertebrates, which secretes the cuticular exoskeleton.

hy•po•der•mi•tis (hi″po-dər-mi′tis) inflammation of the subcutaneous tissue (hypodermis); cf. *cellulitis* and *panniculitis.*

h. sclerodermifor′mis lipodermatosclerosis.

hy•po•der•moc•ly•sis (hi″po-dər-mok′lĭ-sis) [*hypoderm* + *clysis*] infusion of fluid, usually physiologic saline solution, into the subcutaneous tissue; called also *subcutaneous infusion.*

hy•po•der•mo•sis (hi″po-dər-mo′sis) hypodermiasis.

hy•po•di•a•phrag•mat•ic (hi″po-di″ə-frag-mat′ik) subphrenic.

hy•po•dip•loid (hi″po-dip′loid) 1. pertaining to or characterized by hypodiploidy. 2. an individual or cell with less than the diploid number of chromosomes (<2n).

hy•po•dip•loi•dy (hi″po-dip′loi-de) the state of being hypodiploid.

hy•po•dip•sia (hi″po-dip′se-ə) [*hypo-* + *dipsia*] abnormally diminished thirst. Cf. *subliminal thirst*, under *thirst.* **hypodip′sic** *adj*

hy•po•don•tia (hi″po-don′shə) [*hypo-* + *odont-* + *-ia*] partial absence of the teeth, a relatively common congenital condition characterized by absence of a tooth or teeth because of absence of the anlage; it is seldom associated with other anomalies. Called also *partial anodontia.*

hy•po•dy•na•mia (hi″po-di-na′me-ə) [*hypo-* + *dynam-* + *-ia*] diminished power.

h. cor′dis diminished cardiac power.

hy•po•dy•nam•ic (hi″po-di-nam′ik) marked by or exhibiting diminished power or strength; used particularly to describe poor ventricular contractility.

hy•po•echo•ic (hi″po-ə-ko′ik) in ultrasonography, giving off few echoes; said of tissues or structures that reflect relatively few of the ultrasound waves directed at them.

hy•po•elec•tro•ly•te•mia (hi″po-e-lek″tro-li-te′me-ə) abnormally decreased electrolyte content of the blood.

hy•po•eo•sin•o•phil•ia (hi″po-e″o-sin″o-fil′e-ə) eosinopenia.

hy•po•ep•i•neph•rin•emia (hi″po-ep″ĭ-nef″rĭ-ne′me-ə) an abnormally low level of epinephrine in the blood.

hy•po•equi•lib•ri•um (hi″po-e″kwĭ-lib′re-əm) decreased or absent reactions to changes in position; see also *sense of equilibrium*, under *sense.*

hy•po•er•gia (hi″po-ur′jə) hyposensitivity to allergens.

hy•po•er•gic (hi″po-ur′jik) 1. less energetic than normal. 2. pertaining to or characterized by hypoergia.

hy•po•er•gy (hi″po-ur′je) hypoergia.

hy•po•eso•pho•ria (hi″po-es″o-for′e-ə) a tendency of the visual axis to deviate downward and medially when fusion is prevented.

hy•po•es•the•sia (hi″po-es-the′zhə) [*hypo-* + *esthesia*] a dysesthesia consisting of abnormally decreased sensitivity, particularly to touch. Called also *hypesthesia.* **hypoesthet′ic** *adj*

acoustic h., auditory h. hypoacusis.

gustatory h. hypogeusia.

olfactory h. hyposmia.

tactile h. a paraphia consisting of diminution or dullness of the sense of touch.

hy•po•es•tro•gen•emia (hi″po-es″tro-jə-ne′me-ə) decreased levels of estrogen in the blood, such as after menopause.

hy•po•evol•u•tism (hi″po-e-vol′u-tiz-əm) retarded development.

hy•po•exo•pho•ria (hi″po-ek″so-for′e-ə) a tendency of the visual axis to deviate downward and laterally when fusion is prevented.

hy•po•fer•re•mia (hi″po-fer-e′me-ə) [*hypo-* + *ferr-* + *-emia*] deficiency of iron in the blood; see also *iron deficiency*, under *deficiency.*

hy•po•fer•rism (hi″po-fer′iz-əm) iron deficiency.

hy•po•fer•tile (hi″po-fur′til) subfertile.

hy•po•fer•til•i•ty (hi″po-fər-til′ĭ-te) subfertility.

hy•po•fi•brin•o•gen•emia (hi″po-fi-brin″o-jə-ne′me-ə) abnormally low levels of fibrinogen in the blood; called also *fibrinogenopenia.*

hy•po•func•tion (hi″po-funk′shən) diminished function.

hy•po•ga•lac•tia (hi″po-gə-lak′she-ə) deficiency of lactation. **hypogalac′tous** *adj*

hy•po•gam•ma•glob•u•lin•emia (hi″po-gam″ə-glob″u-lĭ-ne′me-ə) abnormally low levels of all classes of immunoglobulins in the blood; see also *agammaglobulinemia*, *dysglobulinemia*, and *immunodeficiency.*

acquired h. common variable immunodeficiency.

common variable h. see under *immunodeficiency.*

physiologic h. a normal period of hypogammaglobulinemia seen in all infants at about 5–6 months of age as the level of transplacentally acquired maternal immunoglobulins declines before endogenous immunoglobulin synthesis rises to normal levels.

transient h. of infancy prolongation of the normal physiologic hypogammaglobulinemia of infancy caused by delayed development of endogenous immunoglobulin production and associated with increased susceptibility to infections.

X-linked h., X-linked infantile h. see under *agammaglobulinemia.*

hy•po•gan•gli•o•no•sis (hi″po-gang″gle-ə-no′sis) deficiency in the number of myenteric ganglion cells in the distal segment of the large intestine, resulting in constipation; it is a variant of congenital megacolon.

hy•po•gas•tric (hi″po-gas′trik) [L. *hypogastricus*] 1. inferior to the stomach. 2. pertaining to the hypogastrium. 3. pertaining to the internal iliac artery.

hy•po•gas•tri•um (hi″po-gas′tre-əm) [*hypo-* + Gr. *gastēr* stomach] [TA] pubic region: the middle portion of the most inferior region of the abdomen, located inferior to the umbilical region and between the two inguinal regions. Called also *hypogastric region* and *regio pubica* [TA alternative].

hy•po•gas•trop•a•gus (hi″po-gəs-trop′ə-gəs) [*hypo-* + *gastro-* + *-pagus*] conjoined twins united at the hypogastric region.

hy•po•gas•tros•chi•sis (hi″po-gas-tros′kĭ-sis) [*hypo-* + *gastro-* + *-schisis*] a developmental anomaly in which an abdominal fissure is restricted to the hypogastric region.

hy•po•gen•e•sis (hi″po-jen′ə-sis) [*hypo-* + *-genesis*] defective embryonic growth or development. **hypogenet′ic** *adj*

polar h. defective development at either extremity of the embryo, resulting in deformity.

hy•po•gen•i•tal•ism (hi″po-jen′ĭ-təl-iz″əm) hypogonadism.

hy•po•geus•es•the•sia (hi″po-gōōs″es-the′zhə) hypogeusia.

hy•po•geu•sia (hi″po-goo′zhə) [*hypo-* + Gr. *geusis* taste] a parageusia involving diminished sensitivity of taste. Called also *amblygeustia, hypogeusesthesia,* and *gustatory hypoesthesia.*

hy•po•glan•du•lar (hi″po-glan′du-lər) marked by abnormally decreased glandular activity.

hy•po•glos•sal (hi″po-glos′əl) sublingual.

hy•po•glu•ca•gon•emia (hi″po-gloo″kə-gon-e′me-ə) abnormally reduced levels of glucagon in the blood.

hy•po•gly•ce•mia (hi″po-gli-se′me-ə) [*hypo-* + *glyc-* + *-emia*] an abnormally diminished concentration of glucose in the blood, which may lead to tremulousness, cold sweat, piloerection, hypothermia, and headache; when chronic and severe it may cause central nervous system manifestations that in rare cases can even be fatal (see *neuroglycopenia*).

alimentary h. a type of reactive hypoglycemia seen in patients who have had surgical modification of the digestive tract so that ingested food moves too quickly past the stomach into the duodenum.

autoimmune h. hypoglycemia caused by autoantibodies to insulin or occasionally by autoantibodies to insulin receptors; see *insulin autoimmune syndrome,* under *syndrome.*

factitial h., factitious h. hypoglycemia that appears spontaneous but actually is not, such as in a diabetic or nondiabetic after surreptitious injection of insulin.

fasting h. hypoglycemia occurring in the fasting state, i.e., after the glucose contents of the intestine have been absorbed; it occurs in such conditions as insulinoma, glycogen storage disease, severe hepatic failure, starvation, malabsorption, hypopituitarism, and adrenocortical insufficiency.

hyperinsulinemic h., insulin-induced h. hypoglycemia caused by inappropriately high levels of insulin in the plasma, usually referring to that from an endogenous source such as an insulinoma or injection of insulin (see *factitious hypoglycemia*).

ketotic h. the most common form of childhood hypoglycemia, characterized by episodic hypoglycemia, ketonuria, convulsions, and vomiting occurring in the early morning after carbohydrate deprivation; it generally begins between 18 months and 5 years and resolves spontaneously by 9 years of age.

leucine-induced h. an autosomal recessive type of neonatal hypoglycemia caused by mutation in the *SUR1* gene (locus: 11p15.1), which encodes a large membrane protein that modulates insulin release. Hypoglycemia is induced by ingestion of leucine-containing protein, which causes an exaggerated release of insulin in susceptible persons.

mixed h. hypoglycemia occurring both during the fasting state and following the ingestion of carbohydrate; it occurs in hypoglycemia of infancy, anterior pituitary and adrenocortical insufficiency, and insulin-secreting tumors of the islet cells of the pancreas.

neonatal h. 1. fasting hypoglycemia in a neonate; those most at risk have diabetic mothers or are premature or small for gestational age. Leucine-induced hypoglycemia is a type that is hereditary. 2. hypoglycemia during the first week of life of piglets, a common cause of death; it may result from inadequate nursing, such as when there is a large litter, or from hypothermia. Called also *h. of piglets.*

h. of piglets neonatal h. (def. 2).

postprandial h., reactive h. hypoglycemia occurring after the ingestion of carbohydrate, with a consequent excessive release of insulin.

hy•po•gly•ce•mic (hi″po-gli-se′mik) 1. pertaining to or characterized by hypoglycemia. 2. producing hypoglycemia. 3. an agent that lowers the level of glucose in the blood.

hy•po•gly•ce•mo•sis (hi″po-gli″sə-mo′sis) an abnormally diminished content of glucose in the body (blood and tissues); see *hypoglycemia.*

hy•po•gly•cin (hi″po-gli′sin) either of two toxic amino acids, designated A and B, occurring in the seeds and arils of the unripe akee (q.v.); they induce hypoglycemia by inhibiting cofactors responsible for hepatic gluconeogenesis. Hypoglycin A, the more potent of the two, is sometimes referred to simply as hypoglycin.

hy•po•gly•co•gen•ol•y•sis (hi″po-gli″ko-jən-ol′ə-sis) depressed glycogenolysis.

hy•po•gly•cor•rha•chia (hi″po-gli″ko-ra′ke-ə) [*hypo-* + *glyco-* + *rhachi-* + *-ia*] the presence of less than the normal amount of glucose in the cerebrospinal fluid; usually indicative of meningeal infection.

hy•pog•na•thous (hi-pog′nə-thəs) 1. having a protruding lower jaw. 2. of the nature of a hypognathus.

hy•pog•na•thus (hi-pog′nə-thəs) [*hypo-* + Gr. *gnathos* jaw] a parasitic twin attached to the lower jaw of the larger twin in asymmetrical conjoined twins. See also *polygnathus.*

hy•po•go•nad•ism (hi″po-go′nad-iz-əm) a condition resulting from abnormally decreased gonadal function, with retardation of growth, sexual development, and secondary sex characters; see *hypo-orchidism, hypo-ovarianism,* and *eunuchoidism.* Called also *hypogenitalism.*

eugonadotropic h. hypogonadism associated with normal levels of pituitary gonadotropins.

hypergonadotropic h. hypogonadism due to defective development or function of the gonads, with elevated levels of pituitary gonadotropins; usually there is some type of androgen insensitivity syndrome with steroid hormone receptor defects. Klinefelter syndrome is one type. Called also *primary h.*

hypogonadotropic h. hypogonadism due to lack of gonadotropin secretion; either luteinizing hormone or follicle-stimulating hormone or both may be deficient; it may also be caused by lack of secretion of gonadotropin-releasing hormone, as in Kallmann syndrome. Called also *secondary h.* and *hypogonadotropic eunuchoidism.*

hypothalamic h. hypogonadism caused by failure of the hypothalamus to secrete enough luteinizing hormone–releasing hormone.

primary h. hypergonadotropic h.

secondary h. hypogonadotropic h.

hy•po•go•nado•trop•ism (hi″po-go″nə-do-tro′piz-əm) deficiency in the amount of gonadotropins in the body, such as in hypogonadotropic hypogonadism. **hypogonadotro′pic** *adj*

hy•po•gran•u•lo•cy•to•sis (hi″po-gran″u-lo-si-to′sis) granulocytopenia.

hy•po•hi•dro•sis (hi″po-hĭ-dro′sis) [*hypo-* + Gr. *hidrōsis* sweating] abnormally diminished sweating; see also *anhidrosis.*

hy•po•hi•drot•ic (hi″po-hĭ-drot′ik) 1. pertaining to or characterized by hypohidrosis. 2. causing hypohidrosis.

hy•po•hy•dro•chlo•ria (hi″po-hi″dro-klor′e-ə) hypochlorhydria.

hy•po•hyp•not•ic (hi″po-hip-not′ik) marked by light sleep.

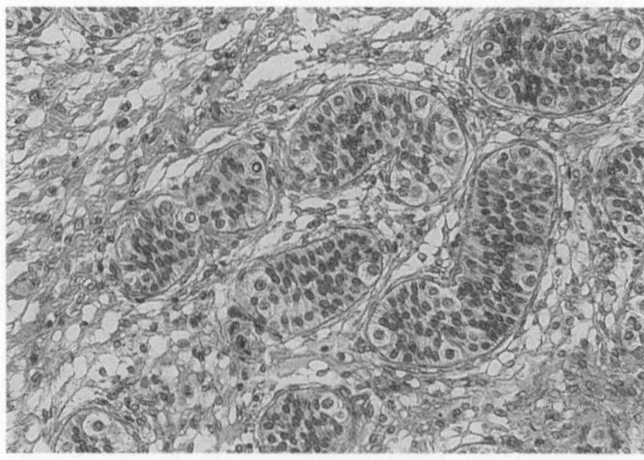

■ Hypogonadotropic hypogonadism. The small seminiferous tubules contain immature Sertoli cells and a few spermatogonia.

hy•po•idro•sis (hi″po-ĭ-dro′sis) hypohidrosis.

hy•po•in•su•lin•emia (hi″po-in″sə-lĭ-ne′me-ə) abnormally low insulin blood levels.

hy•po•in•su•lin•ism (hi″po-in′su-lin-iz″əm) insulinopenia.

hy•po•in•tense (hi″po-in-tens′) having a lower intensity than something else, such as strength of signals or imagery.

hy•po•io•di•dism (hi″po-i-o′dĭ-diz-əm) [*hypo-* + *iodide* + *-ism*] deficiency of iodide in the body.

hy•po•iso•ton•ic (hi″po-i″so-ton′ik) less than isotonic; said of a solution having a lesser osmotic power than another.

hy•po•ka•le•mia (hi″po-kə-le′me-ə) [*hypo-* + L. *kalium* potassium + *-emia*] abnormally low potassium concentration in the blood; it may result from excessive potassium loss by the renal or the gastrointestinal route, from decreased intake, or from transcellular shifts. It may be manifested clinically by neuromuscular disorders ranging from weakness to paralysis, by electrocardiographic abnormalities (depression of the T wave and elevation of the U wave), by renal disease, and by gastrointestinal disorders.

hy•po•ka•le•mic (hi″po-kə-le′mik) 1. pertaining to or characterized by hypokalemia. 2. an agent that acts to lower the potassium content of the blood.

hy•po•kali•emia (hi″po-kal″e-e′me-ə) hypokalemia.

hy•po•ke•to•sis (hi″po-ke-to′sis) an abnormally low plasma concentration of ketone bodies owing to their underproduction in the liver. **hypoketot′ic** *adj*

hy•po•ki•ne•mia (hi″po-kĭ-ne′me-ə) [*hypo-* + *kin-* + *-emia*] subnormal cardiac output; decreased rate of blood flow through the circulatory system.

hy•po•ki•ne•sia (hi″po-kĭ-ne′zhə) [*hypo-* + *kinesi-* + *-ia*] abnormally decreased mobility; abnormally decreased motor function or activity. Cf. *dyskinesia.* Called also *hypanakinesia, hypanakinesis, hypocinesia,* and *hypokinesis.* **hypokinet′ic** *adj*

hy•po•ki•ne•sis (hi″po-kĭ-ne′sis) hypokinesia.

hy•po•lac•ta•sia (hi″po-lak-ta′zhə) deficiency of lactase activity in the intestines; see *lactase deficiency.*

hy•po•lar•ynx (hi″po-lar′inks) cavitas infraglottica.

hy•po•lem•mal (hi″po-lem′əl) [*hypo-* + Gr. *lemma* sheath] located beneath a sheath, such as the end plates of motor nerves under the sarcolemma of muscle.

hy•po•le•thal (hi″po-le′thəl) not sufficient to cause death.

hy•po•ley•dig•ism (hi″po-li′dig-iz-əm) abnormally diminished functional activity of Leydig cells; resulting in hypoandrogenism.

hy•po•li•pe•mia (hi″po-lĭ-pe′me-ə) hypolipidemia.

hy•po•lip•i•de•mia (hi″po-lip″ĭ-de′me-ə) an abnormally decreased amount of fat in the blood; called also *hypolipemia.*

hy•po•lip•id•emic (hi″po-lip″ĭ-de′mik) 1. pertaining to or characterized by hypolipidemia. 2. promoting hypolipidemia.

hy•po•lipo•pro•tein•emia (hi″po-lip″o-pro″te-ne′me-ə) the presence of abnormally low levels of lipoproteins in the serum, as in hypobetalipoproteinemia and Tangier disease.

hy•po•li•po•sis (hi″po-lĭ-po′sis) a deficiency of lipids in the blood or tissues; lipids are transported in the blood as lipoproteins. See *hypolipoproteinemia.*

hy•po•lym•phe•mia (hi″po-lim-fe′me-ə) lymphocytopenia.

hy•po•mag•ne•se•mia (hi″po-mag″nə-se′me-ə) an abnormally low magnesium content of the blood plasma, usually the result of malabsorption, dehydration, alcoholism, or renal disease; the chief manifestation is neuromuscular irritability.

hy•po•ma•nia (hi″po-ma′ne-ə) [*hypo-* + *-mania*] an abnormality of mood resembling mania (persistent elevated or expansive mood, hyperactivity, inflated self-esteem, etc.) but of lesser intensity. **hypoman′ic** *adj*

hy•po•mas•tia (hi″po-mas′te-ə) micromastia.

hy•po•mel•a•no•sis (hi″po-mel″ə-no′sis) [*hypo-* + *melanosis*] a deficiency of melanin in the tissues, especially in the skin.

idiopathic guttate h. a common, benign condition of unknown etiology manifested by small, sharply demarcated, irregular hypopigmented spots primarily on sun-exposed areas of the limbs in persons over age 30.

h. of Ito a congenital neurocutaneous syndrome, not present at birth but appearing in early life, characterized by whorled, linear, and splatterlike patterns of hypopigmentation, often associated with other abnormalities such as hair loss and ocular, musculoskeletal, and mental disturbances. Called also *incontinentia pigmenti achromians.*

hy•po•men•or•rhea (hi″po-men″o-re′ə) [*hypo-* + *meno-* + *-rrhea*] menstruation in which the flow is less than the normal amount but at regular intervals, with the period of flow lasting the same or less time than average.

hy•po•mere (hi′po-mēr) 1. the ventrolateral portion of a myotome, innervated by an anterior ramus of a spinal nerve. 2. the lateral plate of mesoderm that develops into the walls of the body cavities.

hy•po•me•tab•o•lism (hi″po-mə-tab′o-liz-əm) [*hypo-* + *metabolism*] abnormally decreased utilization of any substance by the body in metabolism; low basal metabolic rate. **hypometabol′ic** *adj*

hy•po•me•thi•o•nin•emia (hi″po-mə-thi″o-nĭ-ne′me-ə) decreased concentration of methionine in the blood.

hy•po•meth•yl•a•tion (hi″po-meth″əl-a′shən) 1. presence of fewer methylated nucleotides in DNA than is usual for that DNA; it may be localized or global, and is related to DNA expression. Hypomethylation of specific regions has been linked to tumorigenesis, among other epigenetic mechanisms. 2. the formation of fewer methylated groups than usual on a compound, such as a DNA molecule; cf. *demethylation.*

hy•po•me•tria (hi″po-me′tre-ə) ["a deficiency"; by analogy with Gr. *eumetria, hypermetria*] dysmetria in which voluntary muscular movement falls short of reaching the intended goal.

hy•po•mim•ia (hi″po-mim′e-ə) [*hypo-* + Gr. *mimos* actor, mime + *-ia*] lack of facial expression with reduced blinking. **hypomimet′ic, hypomim′ic** *adj*

hy•po•min•er•al•iza•tion (hi″po-min″ər-əl-ĭ-za′shən) deficiency of mineral elements in the body.

hy•po•mo•dal (hi″po-mo′dəl) in statistics, relating to the values or items falling below the mode of the frequency distribution.

hy•po•morph (hi′po-morf″) [*hypo-* + *-morph*] hypomorphic allele.

hy•po•mo•til•i•ty (hi″po-mo-til′ĭ-te) deficient motility of a part.

hy•po•my•e•lin•a•tion (hi″po-mi″ə-lin-a′shən) disappearance, or inadequate formation, of myelin sheaths on nerves.

hy•po•myx•ia (hi″po-mik′se-ə) [*hypo-* + *myx-* + *-ia*] decreased secretion of mucus.

hy•po•na•sal•i•ty (hi″po-na-zal′ĭ-te) a quality of voice in which there is a complete lack of nasal emission of air and nasal resonance, so that speakers sound as if they have a cold. Called also *denasality* and *rhinolalia clausa.*

hy•po•na•tre•mia (hi″po-nə-tre′me-ə) [*hypo-* + L. *natrium* sodium + *-emia*] deficiency of sodium in the blood.

depletional h. euvolemic h.

dilutional h. low plasma concentration of sodium resulting from loss of sodium from the body with nonosmotic retention of water, such as that induced by vasopressin; there may also be hypovolemia.

euvolemic h. low plasma concentration of sodium associated with low total body sodium and normal blood volume; called also *depletional h.*

hy•po•na•tre•mic (hi″po-nə-tre′mik) 1. pertaining to or characterized by hyponatremia. 2. caused by hyponatremia.

hy•po•na•tru•ria (hi″po-nə-troo′re-ə) [*hypo-* + L. *natrium* sodium + *-uria*] an abnormally low level of sodium in the urine.

hy•po•neo•cy•to•sis (hi″po-ne″o-si-to′sis) [*hypo-* + *neocytosis*] leukopenia with immature forms of leukocytes present in the blood.

hy•po•ni•tre•mia (hi″po-ni-tre′me-ə) a low level of nitrogen in the blood, sometimes associated with protein malnutrition or overhydration.

hy•po•noia (hi″po-noi′ə) [*hypo-* + Gr. *noein* to think] sluggish mental activity.

hy•po•nych•i•al (hi″po-nik′e-əl) subungual.

hy•po•nych•i•um (hi″po-nik′e-əm) [*hypo-* + Gr. *onyx* nail] [TA] the thickened epidermis underneath the free distal end of the nail.

hy•pon•y•chon (hi-pon′ĭ-kon) [*hypo-* + Gr. *onyx* nail] ecchymosis beneath the nail.

hy•po•or•chi•dism (hi″po-or′kĭ-diz-əm) defective endocrine activity of the testes; see also *hypoandrogenism.*

hy•po•or•tho•cy•to•sis (hi″po-or″tho-si-to′sis) [*hypo-* + *orthocytosis*] leukopenia in which the proportion of the various forms of leukocytes is normal.

hy•po•os•mo•lal•i•ty (hi″po-oz″mo-lal′ĭ-te) a decrease in the osmolality of the body fluids. Body fluid volume increases and solute volumes usually decrease; the predominant symptoms are those of hyponatremia such as cerebral edema with neurologic manifestations including disorientation, focal deficits, and seizures.

hy•po•os•mot•ic (hi″po-oz-mot′ik) containing a lower concentration of osmotically active components than a standard solution.

hy•po•ova•ri•an•ism (hi″po-o-var′e-ən-iz-əm) deficient endocrine activity of the ovaries; see also *hypoestrogenemia.*

hy•po•pal•les•the•sia (hi″po-pal″es-the′zhə) [*hypo-* + *pallesthesia*] abnormally decreased sensitivity of vibration sense (pallesthesia).

hy•po•pan•cre•a•tism (hi″po-pan′kre-ə-tiz″əm) pancreatic insufficiency; diminished pancreatic activity.

hy•po•para•thy•roid (hi″po-par″ə-thi′roid) pertaining to or characterized by reduced function of the parathyroid glands; called also *parathyroprival.*

hy•po•para•thy•roid•ism (hi″po-par″ə-thi′roid-iz-əm) the condition produced by greatly reduced function of the parathyroid glands; it may be due to autoimmune disease, genetic factors, or the removal of the glands. Lack of parathyroid hormone leads to a fall in plasma calcium level (hypocalcemia), which may result in increased neuromuscular excitability and ultimately tetany, as well as a rise in plasma phosphate level. Bone turnover is reduced; there may also be dermatologic, ophthalmologic (cataracts), psychiatric, and dental symptoms, and associated primary failure of other endocrine glands such as the adrenal cortex. See also *pseudohypoparathyroidism.* Called also *parathyroid insufficiency.*

hy•po•pep•sia (hi″po-pep′se-ə) [*hypo-* + Gr. *pepsis* digestion + *-ia*] impairment of digestion, due to hypochlorhydria.

hy•po•per•fu•sion (hi″po-pər-fu′zhən) decreased perfusion of blood through an organ, as in hypovolemic shock; if prolonged it may result in permanent cellular dysfunction and death.

hy•po•peri•stal•sis (hi″po-per″ĭ-stawl′sis) abnormally sluggish peristalsis.

hy•po•pex•ia (hi″po-pek′se-ə) [*hypo-* + *pexia*] the fixation by a tissue of a deficient amount of a substance.

hy•po•pexy (hi′po-pek″se) hypopexia.

hy•po•pha•gia (hi″po-fa′jə) anorexia.

hy•po•pha•lan•gism (hi″po-fə-lan′jiz-əm) less than the usual number of phalanges of a finger or toe.

hy•po•pha•ryn•ge•al (hi″po-fə-rin′je-əl) pertaining to the hypopharynx.

hy•po•pha•ryn•go•scope (hi″po-fə-ring′go-skōp) an instrument for inspecting the hypopharynx.

hy•po•pha•ryn•gos•co•py (hi″po-far″in-gos′kə-pe) examination of the hypopharynx.

hy•po•phar•ynx (hi″po-far′inks) pars laryngea pharyngis.

hy•po•pho•ne•sis (hi″po-fo-ne′sis) [*hypo-* + *phon-* + *-esis*] diminished intensity of the sound in auscultation or percussion.

hy•po•pho•nia (hi″po-fo′ne-ə) [*hypo-* + *phon-* + *-ia*] a dysphonia in which there is decreased phonation, resulting in whispering. Called also *leptophonia, microphonia,* and *subenergetic phonation.*

hy•po•pho•ria (hi″po-for′e-ə) [*hypo-* + *phoria*] a type of heterophoria in which there is downward deviation of the visual axis of an eye when visual fusional stimuli are eliminated. When both eyes are affected, it is called *cataphoria.*

hy•po•phos•pha•ta•sia (hi″po-fos″fə-ta′zhə) [*hypo-* + *phosphatase* + *-ia*] an inherited metabolic disorder caused by mutation in the *ALPL* gene (locus: 1p36.1-p34), which encodes alkaline phosphatase; the resulting serum and bone enzyme deficiency leads to hypercalcemia, ethanolamine phosphatemia, and ethanolamine phosphaturia. Clinical manifestations include severe skeletal defects resembling vitamin D–resistant rickets, failure of the calvaria to calcify, dyspnea, cyanosis, vomiting, constipation, renal calcinosis, failure to thrive, movement disorders, beading where the ribs meet their cartilages, and rachitic bone changes (bowleg). There are three clinical types based upon age of onset and severity of symptoms. Two are autosomal recessive: the *infantile* type is the most severe, lethal in over half the cases; and the *childhood* type usually has as its first symptom spontaneous loss of deciduous teeth. The *adult* type is the mildest and is autosomal dominant. See also *pseudohypophosphatasia.*

hy•po•phos•pha•te•mia (hi″po-fos″fə-te′me-ə) [*hypo-* + *phosphate* + *-emia*] an abnormally decreased amount of phosphates in the blood; manifestations include hemolysis, lassitude, weakness, and convulsions. It may be found in hyperparathyroidism, rickets, osteomalacia, and several renal tubular abnormalities, including the Fanconi syndrome. **hypophosphate′mic** *adj*

familial h. familial hypophosphatemic rickets; the term is sometimes used specifically for X-linked hypophosphatemia.

X-linked h. a form of familial hypophosphatemic rickets, with X-linked dominant inheritance and caused by mutation at locus Xp22.2-p22.1; the bone disease is due to defects in the resorption of phosphate by the proximal renal tubule and in the regulation of renal 25-hydroxyvitamin D activation, and to decreased intestinal absorption of calcium with resulting hyperparathyroidism. Called also *X-linked hypophosphatemic rickets.*

hy•po•phos•pha•tu•ria (hi″po-fos″fə-tu′re-ə) an abnormally decreased amount of phosphate in the urine.

hy•po•phos•phite (hi″po-fos′fīt) any salt of hypophosphorous acid.

hy•po•phos•pho•re•mia (hi″po-fos″fə-re′me-ə) hypophosphatemia.

hy•po•phos•phor•ous ac•id (hi″po-fos-for′əs) a strong monobasic acid, H_3PO_2, used as a reducing agent.

hy•po•phren•ic (hi″po-fren′ik) [*hypo-* + *phrenic*] subphrenic.

hy•po•phre•ni•um (hi″po-fre′ne-əm) a peritoneal space between the diaphragm and the transverse colon.

hy•po•phys•e•al (hi″po-fiz′e-əl) hypophysial.

hy•po•phys•ec•to•mize (hi″po-fəz-ek′to-mīz) to remove the hypophysis (pituitary gland).

hy•po•phys•ec•to•my (hi-pof″ə-sek′tə-me) [*hypophysis* + *-ectomy*] surgical removal or destruction of the hypophysis (pituitary gland). Called also *pituitectomy.*

hy•po•phys•eo•por•tal (hi″po-fiz″e-o-por′təl) hypophysioportal.

hy•po•phys•eo•priv•ic (hi″po-fiz″e-o-priv′ik) hypophysioprivic.

hy•po•phys•eo•tro•pic (hi″po-fiz″e-o-tro′pik) hypophysiotropic.

hy•po•phys•io•por•tal (hi″po-fiz″e-o-por′təl) pertaining to the venules and capillaries that connect the hypothalamus and the adenohypophysis. Also spelled *hypophyseoportal.*

hy•po•phys•io•priv•ic (hi″po-fiz″e-o-priv′ik) pertaining to deficiency of hormone secretion by the hypophysis (pituitary gland); see *hypopituitarism.*

hy•po•phys•io•tro•pic (hi″po-fiz″e-o-tro′pik) acting on the pituitary gland (hypophysis), as certain hormones.

hy•poph•y•sis (hi-pof′ə-sis) [*hypo-* + Gr. *phyein* to grow] [TA] pituitary gland: an epithelial body located at the base of the brain in the sella turcica, attached by a stalk to the hypothalamus, from which it receives an important neural and vascular outflow. It consists of two lobes of differing embryonic origin, the anterior lobe (adenohypophysis), which secretes most of the hormones, and the posterior lobe (neurohypophysis), which stores and releases neurohormones that it receives from the hypothalamus. Called also *glandula pituitaria* [TA alternative] and *pituitary body.* **hypophys′ial** *adj*

h. ce′rebri hypophysis.

pharyngeal h., h. pharyngea′lis [TA] a small median residual collection of adenohypophysial glandular tissue in the mucoperiosteum of the roof of the nasopharynx; it develops from the Rathke pouch in the embryo. Called also *pharyngeal pituitary.*

hy•poph•y•si•tis (hi-pof″ə-si′tis) inflammation of the hypophysis (pituitary gland).

granulomatous h. a rare chronic inflammatory disorder of the hypophysis, characterized histologically by diffuse collections of histiocytes and multinucleated giant cells surrounded by lymphocytes and plasma cells. Headache is the most common manifestation; nausea, vomiting, meningitis, hyperprolactinemia, and occasionally diabetes mellitus also occur.

lymphocytic h. destruction of the normal parenchyma of the pituitary gland by infiltrating lymphocytes and plasma cells, with resultant hypopituitarism, usually seen during pregnancy and thought to be an autoimmune reaction.

xanthomatous h. an extremely rare inflammatory disorder of the hypophysis characterized by the presence of cysts filled with yellowish fluid and infiltrated by foamy histiocytes and small lymphocytes.

hy•po•pig•men•ta•tion (hi″po-pig″mən-ta′shən) [*hypo-* + *pigmentation*] abnormally diminished pigmentation. In the skin this is from decreased melanin production *(amelanosis* or *hypomelanosis).* See also *depigmentation.*

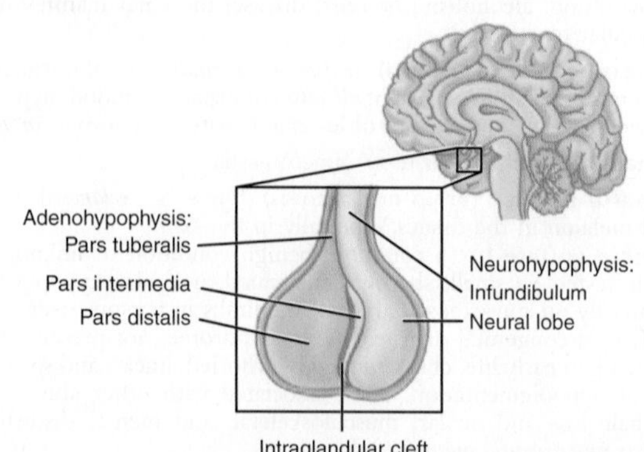

■ Hypophysis, subdivided into its two lobes, the adenohypophysis and neurohypophysis.

postinflammatory h. loss of color in the skin after healing of an inflammatory dermatosis, infection, burn, or wound; it is also sometimes seen after dermabrasion or intralesional steroid injections.

hy•po•pig•men•ter (hi″po-pig-men′tər) an agent that reduces pigmentation of the skin; a bleach.

hy•po•pin•e•al•ism (hi″po-pin′e-ə-liz″əm) a presumed decrease in normal secretory activity of the pineal body.

hy•po•pi•tu•i•ta•rism (hi″po-pĭ-too′ĭ-tə-riz″əm) diminution or cessation of function of the adenohypophysis due to surgical removal, to ablation by irradiation, or to spontaneous causes, as in chromophobe adenoma or postpartum necrosis (Sheehan syndrome). There is variable deficiency of hormones, including: gonadotropins (causing *secondary hypogonadism*); somatotropin (causing *pituitary dwarfism* in children); thyrotropin (causing secondary *hypothyroidism*); and corticotropin (causing secondary *adrenocortical insufficiency*).

hy•po•pla•sia (hi″po-pla′zhə) [*hypo-* + *-plasia*] incomplete development or underdevelopment of an organ or tissue; it is less severe in degree than aplasia. **hypoplas′tic** *adj*

cartilage-hair h. an autosomal recessive bone dysplasia caused by mutation in the *RMRP* gene (locus: 9p21-p12), which encodes an enzyme complex involved in processing mitochondrial RNA. It is characterized by short-limbed dwarfism with flaring of the lower rib cage and a prominent sternum; fine, sparse, light-colored hair; neutropenia with defective cell-mediated immunity; malabsorption; celiac disease; Hirschsprung disease; and increased susceptibility to malignancy.

congenital adrenal h. a rare hereditary condition in which the adrenal glands lack the usual adult cortical zone, resulting in adrenocortical insufficiency. The usual form is X-linked (locus: Xp21.3-p21.2) and seen in boys, who have sexual infantilism and skeletal abnormalities. An autosomal recessive condition has also been observed.

enamel h. a form of amelogenesis imperfecta characterized by incomplete formation of the dental enamel. It may be transmitted as an X-linked or autosomal dominant trait, or be associated with vitamin A, C, or D deficiency, measles, chickenpox, scarlet fever, congenital syphilis (Hutchinson teeth), prematurity, birth injuries, Rh incompatibility, trauma, local infection, or Morquio disease. Small grooves, pits, and fissures on the enamel surface may be seen in mild cases, deep horizontal rows of pits in severe cases; or absence of enamel in extreme cases; associated with yellow, reddish, or brown discoloration of the teeth. Called also *hypoplastic emphysema*.

focal dermal h. an X-linked dominant disorder caused by mutation in the *PORCN* gene (locus: Xp11.23), which encodes an endoplasmic reticulum transmembrane protein involved in processing of Wnt proteins. It is found almost exclusively in females, being lethal to males in utero, and is characterized by anomalies of the skin, digits, and eyes, and sometimes mental retardation. Called also *Goltz syndrome*.

myofibrillar h. a congenital condition of piglets in which leg muscles are weak, usually in the rear legs, and the legs spread apart. Affected animals have difficulty moving and may starve or be crushed by their mothers. It can have many causes, including in utero poisoning or infection or perinatal injury. Called also *splayleg, splay legs*, and *spraddle legs*.

oligomeganephronic renal h. oligomeganephronia.

renal h. a congenital anomaly of the renal parenchyma in which there are fewer than the usual number of nephrons; see also *oligomeganephronia*.

h. of right ventricle parchment heart.

segmental renal h. Ask-Upmark kidney.

thymic h. DiGeorge syndrome.

Turner h. see under *tooth*.

hy•po•plas•ty (hi′po-plas″te) hypoplasia.

hy•po•ploid (hi′po-ploid) [*hypo-* + *-ploid*] the aneuploid, almost always fatal condition in which there is less than the normal diploid number of chromosomes, such as 45 chromosomes in a human (the 2n − 1 state).

hy•pop•nea (hi-pop′ne-ə) [*hypo-* + *-pnea*] abnormal decrease in the depth and rate of breathing. Cf. *bradypnea* and *hypoventilation*. **hypopne′ic** *adj*

hy•po•po•ne•sis (hi″po-po-ne′sis) [*hypo-* + *pon-* + *-esis*] dysponesis in which there is insufficient action-potential output from the motor and premotor areas of the cerebral cortex.

hy•po•po•ro•sis (hi″po-po-ro′sis) [*hypo-* + *por-*[2] + *-osis*] deficient formation of callus after a fracture.

hy•po•po•sia (hi″po-po′zhə) [*hypo-* + Gr. *posis* drinking + *-ia*] abnormally diminished ingestion of fluids.

hy•po•po•tas•se•mia (hi″po-po″tə-se′me-ə) hypokalemia.

hy•po•po•ten•tia (hi″po-po-ten′shə) [*hypo-* + *potentia*] a condition of diminished power, especially of diminished electrical activity of the cerebral cortex.

hy•po•prax•ia (hi″po-prak′se-ə) abnormally diminished activity.

hy•po•pros•o•dy (hi″po-pros′o-de) dysprosody marked by diminution of the normal variation of stress, pitch, and rhythm of speech.

hy•po•pro•tein•emia (hi″po-pro″te-ne′me-ə) abnormally decreased levels of protein in the blood, sometimes resulting in edema and fluid accumulation in serous cavities. **hypoproteine′mic** *adj*

prehepatic h. hypoproteinemia occurring as a result of prolonged ingestion of faulty low or incomplete protein diet.

hy•po•pro•tein•o•sis (hi″po-pro″tēn-o′sis) deficiency of proteins or protein foods.

hy•po•pro•throm•bin•emia (hi″po-pro-throm″bĭ-ne′me-ə) deficiency of prothrombin (coagulation factor II) in the blood; called also *prothrombinopenia*.

hy•pop•sel•a•phe•sia (hi″pop-sel″ə-fe′zhə) tactile hypoesthesia.

hy•po•pty•al•ism (hi″po-ti′əl-iz″əm) [*hypo-* + *ptyal-* + *-ism*] abnormally decreased salivation, as in xerostomia. Called also *hyposalivation* and *hyposialosis*.

hy•po•pus (hi-po′pəs) a stage in the development of certain mites (family Acaridae), occurring between the first and the second nymph stages.

hy•po•py•on (hi-po′pe-on) [*hypo-* + Gr. *pyon* pus] an accumulation of pus in the anterior chamber of the eye.

hy•po•re•ac•tive (hi″po-re-ak′tiv) pertaining to or characterized by a less than normal response to stimuli. Cf. *irritability* and *reaction*.

hy•po•re•flex•ia (hi″po-re-flek′se-ə) dysreflexia characterized by weakening of the reflexes.

detrusor h. abnormal weakness of response of the detrusor urinae muscle to stimuli; see *detrusor areflexia*, under *areflexia*.

hy•po•re•nin•emia (hi″po-re″nĭ-ne′me-ə) low levels of renin in the blood.

hy•po•re•nin•emic (hi″po-re″nĭ-ne′mik) producing or characterized by hyporeninemia.

hy•po•re•spond•er (hi″po-re-spon′dər) a person or animal who after vaccination against a given virus shows very little immune response when challenged with the virus.

hy•po•sal•i•va•tion (hi″po-sal″ĭ-va′shən) hypoptyalism.

hy•po•sar•ca (hi″po-sahr′kə) anasarca.

hy•po•scle•ral (hi″po-skler′əl) under the sclera.

hy•po•se•cre•tion (hi″po-se-kre′shən) diminished secretion, as of a gland.

hy•po•sen•si•tive (hi″po-sen′sĭ-tiv) 1. exhibiting abnormally decreased sensitivity. 2. having the specific or general reaction to a given allergen reduced by repeated and gradually increasing doses of the offending substance.

hy•po•sen•si•tiv•i•ty (hi″po-sen″sĭ-tiv′ĭ-te) the condition of being hyposensitive.

hy•po•sen•si•ti•za•tion (hi″po-sen″sĭ-tĭ-za′shən) desensitization.

hy•po•sex•u•al•i•ty (hi″po-sek″shoo-al′ĭ-te) abnormally decreased sexual desire; see also *sexual arousal disorders*, under *disorder*.

hy•po•si•a•lo•sis (hi″po-si″ə-lo′sis) hypoptyalism.

hy•pos•mia (hi-poz′me-ə) [*hypo-* + *osm-*[1] + *-ia*] a parosmia involving diminished sensitivity of smell; called also *olfactory hypoesthesia*.

hy•pos•mo•lar•i•ty (hi-poz″mo-lar′i-te) abnormally decreased osmolar concentration.

hy•pos•mo•sis (hi″pos-mo′sis) decreased speed of osmosis.

hy•po•so•mato•tro•pism (hi″po-so-mat″o-tro′piz-əm) growth hormone deficiency; in children this causes pituitary dwarfism.

hy•po•so•mia (hi″po-so′me-ə) [*hypo-* + *-somia*] inadequate bodily development; see also *dwarfism*.

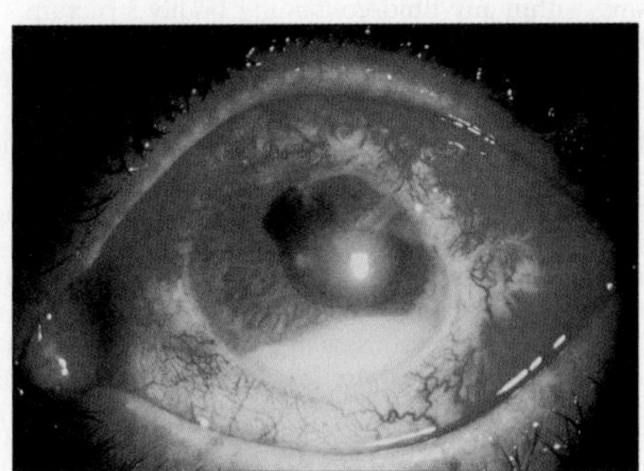

■ Hypopyon following cataract extraction; there is neovascularization of the iris.

hy•po•som•nia (hi″po-som′ne-ə) reduced time of sleep; cf. *insomnia.*

hy•po•spa•dia (hi″po-spa′de-ə) hypospadias.

hy•po•spa•di•ac (hi″po-spa′de-ak) 1. pertaining to or exhibiting hypospadias. 2. a person with hypospadias.

hy•po•spa•di•al (hi″po-spa′de-əl) hypospadiac (def. 1).

hy•po•spa•di•as (hi″po-spa′de-əs) [*hypo-* + Gr. *spadōn* a cleft or rent] a developmental anomaly in which the urethra opens inferior to its usual location; usually seen in males with the opening on the underside of the penis or on the perineum. See also *female h.*

balanic h., balanitic h. glandular h.

female h. a developmental anomaly in the female in which the urethra opens into the vagina.

glandular h., glanular h. the most common type of hypospadias in the male; the urethral orifice opens at the site of the frenum, which may be rudimentary or absent. The normal site of the urinary meatus is represented on the glans penis as a blind pit.

penile h. hypospadias in the male with the urethral opening lying somewhere between the glans and the junction of the penis and scrotum.

penoscrotal h. hypospadias in the male with the urethral orifice at the junction of the penis and scrotum, sometimes associated with congenital chordee.

perineal h. hypospadias in the male with anomalous development of the genitalia, the rudimentary penis often being engulfed by an overlying bifid scrotum; seen in 5α-reductase deficiency and other disorders. An extreme form is called *pseudovaginal h.*

pseudovaginal h. see *perineal h.*

hy•po•sper•ma•to•gen•e•sis (hi″po-spur″mə-to-jen′ə-sis) abnormally decreased production of spermatozoa; cf. *aspermatogenesis.*

hy•po•splen•ism (hi″po-splen′iz-əm) diminished functioning of the spleen.

hy•pos•ta•sis (hi-pos′tə-sis) [*hypo-* + *stasis*] poor or stagnant circulation of the blood in a dependent part of the body or organ, as in venous insufficiency.

hy•po•stat•ic (hi″po-stat′ik) 1. pertaining to, caused by, or associated with hypostasis. 2. pertaining to certain inherited traits that are particularly liable to be suppressed by other traits; see *epistasis.*

hy•pos•the•nia (hi″pos-the′ne-ə) weakness. **hyposthen′ic** *adj*

hy•pos•the•ni•ant (hi″pos-the′ne-ənt) reducing the strength.

hy•pos•then•uria (hi″pos-thə-nu′re-ə) inability to form urine of high osmolality.

tubular h. hyposthenuria occurring as a result of injury to the epithelial cells of the renal tubules.

hy•po•stome (hi′po-stōm) [*hypo-* + *stoma*] any of several structures, parts, or organs found in association with the mouth in various organisms; e.g., the rodlike piercing mouth part, sometimes with spines or teeth, used by certain ticks and mites to thrust into and hold firmly onto the tissues of a prey or host.

hy•po•sto•mia (hi″po-sto′me-ə) [*hypo-* + *stom-* + *-ia*] a developmental anomaly characterized by abnormal smallness of the mouth, the slit being vertical instead of horizontal.

hyp•os•to•sis (hip″os-to′sis) [*hypo-* + *osteo-* + *-osis*] deficient development of bone.

hy•po•sul•fite (hi″po-sul′fīt) thiosulfate.

hy•po•syn•er•gia (hi″po-sĭ-nur′jə) dyssynergia.

hy•po•telo•rism (hi″po-tel′ə-riz-əm) [*hypo-* + *tele-* + *-ism*] abnormally decreased distance between two organs or parts.

ocular h., orbital h. a condition characterized by abnormal decrease in the interorbital distance, consistently present in trigonocephaly.

hy•po•ten•sion (hi″po-ten′shən) 1. abnormally low blood pressure; seen in shock but not necessarily indicative of it. 2. abnormally low tension or pressure within any fluid-containing bodily structure.

chronic idiopathic orthostatic h., chronic orthostatic h., idiopathic orthostatic h. 1. Shy-Drager syndrome. 2. Bradbury-Eggleston syndrome.

intracranial h. abnormally low intracranial pressure, such as from leakage of cerebrospinal fluid or after lumbar puncture.

intradialytic h. hypotension sometimes seen as a complication of hemodialysis.

orthostatic h., postural h. a fall in blood pressure associated with dizziness, blurred vision, and sometimes syncope, occurring upon standing or when standing motionless in a fixed position; it can be acquired or idiopathic, transient or chronic, and may occur alone or secondary to a disorder of the central nervous system such as the Shy-Drager syndrome.

supine h. see under *syndrome.*

vascular h. severe hypotension from dilatation of the blood vessels.

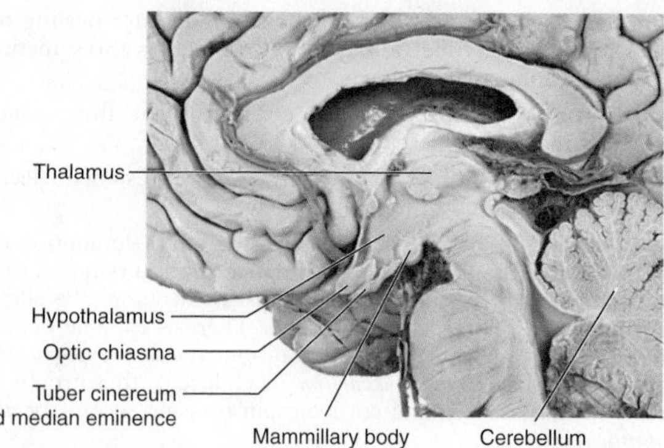

■ Hypothalamus as seen on the medial surface of a hemisection of the diencephalon and part of the brainstem and cerebellum.

hy•po•ten•sive (hi″po-ten′siv) 1. characterized by or causing diminished tension or pressure, as abnormally low blood pressure. 2. a person with abnormally low blood pressure.

hy•po•ten•sor (hi″po-ten′sər) a substance that lowers blood pressure; a hypotensive agent.

hy•po•thal•a•mot•o•my (hi″po-thal″ə-mot′ə-me) [*hypothalamus* + *-tomy*] production of lesions in the posterolateral part of the hypothalamus; performed in the treatment of psychotic disorders.

hy•po•thal•a•mus (hi″po-thal′ə-məs) [*hypo-* + *thalamus*] [TA] the ventral part of the diencephalon, forming the floor and part of the lateral wall of the third ventricle. Anatomically, it includes the preoptic area, optic tract, optic chiasm, mammillary bodies, tuber cinereum, infundibulum, and neurohypophysis, but for physiological purposes the neurohypophysis is considered a distinct structure. The hypothalamus may be divided into five regions or areas *(area hypothalamica rostralis, area hypothalamica dorsalis, area hypothalamica intermedia, area hypothalamica lateralis,* and *area hypothalamica posterior)* or into three longitudinal zones *(periventricular zone, medial zone,* and *lateral zone).* The hypothalamic nuclei constitute that part of the corticodiencephalic apparatus that activates, controls, and integrates the peripheral autonomic mechanisms, endocrine activity, and many somatic functions, such as general regulation of water balance, body temperature, sleep, and food intake, as well as development of secondary sex characters. The hypothalamus secretes vasopressin and oxytocin, which are stored in the pituitary, as well as many releasing factors (hypophysiotropic hormones), by means of which it exerts control over functions of the adenohypophysis. **hypothalam′ic** *adj*

hy•poth•e•nar (hi-poth′ə-nər, hi″po-the′nahr) [*hypo-* + *thenar*] 1. [TA] the fleshy eminence on the palm along the ulnar margin; called also *eminentia hypothenaris* [TA alternative] and *hypothenar eminence.* 2. relating to this eminence.

hy•po•ther•mal (hi″po-thur′məl) hypothermic.

hy•po•ther•mia (hi″po-thur′me-ə) [*hypo-* + *therm-* + *-ia*] 1. a reduction of core body temperature to 35°C or lower, usually due either to coldness of the environment or artificial inducement (see *induced h.*). 2. a state of low temperature induced in an excised organ being preserved for transplantation.

accidental h. unintentional reduction of the core body temperature, as in a cold environment, without primary disturbance of the thermoregulatory center.

endogenous h. abnormally reduced body temperature resulting from physiologic causes, due to hypofunction of the central nervous system (diencephalon) or of the endocrine system, e.g., the thyroid gland.

environmental h. accidental hypothermia due to heat loss due to a combination of convection, conduction, and radiation to the surrounding ambient air.

induced h. deliberate reduction of the temperature of all or part of the body as a means of decreasing metabolism of tissues and thereby the need for oxygen; sometimes used as an adjunct to anesthesia in surgical procedures involving a limb, and as a protective measure in cardiac and neurologic surgery.

mild h. a reduction in core body temperature to between 33° and 35°C.

moderate h. a reduction in core body temperature to between 28° and 33°C.

regional h. temperature reduction in a limb or organ resulting from application of external cold or perfusion with a cold solution.

severe h. reduction in core body temperature to between 9° and 28°C.

hy•po•ther•mic (hi″po-thur′mik) pertaining to or exhibiting hypothermia.

hy•po•ther•my (hi″po-thur′me) hypothermia.

hy·poth·e·sis (hi-poth′ə-sis) a supposition that appears to explain a group of phenomena and is advanced as a basis for further investigation; a proposition that is subject to proof or to an experimental or statistical test. See also *theory*.

alternative h. the hypothesis that is compared with the null hypothesis in a statistical test. Symbol H_1 or H_a.

biogenic amine h. the hypothesis that depression is associated with deficiency of biogenic amines (catecholamines and serotonin), especially norepinephrine, at functionally important receptor sites in the brain and that elation is associated with excess of such amines.

Dreyer and Bennett h. see *recombinational germline theory*, under *theory*.

gate h. gate theory.

insular h. the hypothesis that diabetes mellitus is due to disordered function of the pancreatic islets.

jelly roll h. a theory explaining the formation of nerve myelin, which states that it consists of successive layers of the plasma membrane of a Schwann cell wrapped spirally around the axon in a jelly roll fashion.

lattice h. a theory of the nature of the antigen-antibody reaction which postulates reaction between multivalent antigen and divalent antibody to give an antigen-antibody complex of a lattice-like structure.

Lyon h. in mammalian somatic cells, all X chromosomes in excess of one are inactivated (in the form of sex chromatin) on a random basis at an early stage of embryogenesis, around the time of implantation. Thus the normal human female is in effect a mosaic for heterozygous X-linked genes, since the paternal X chromosome is inactivated in some cells and the maternal one in the others, and females heterozygous for an X-linked disorder often exhibit some stigmata for the condition. See also *lyonization*.

Makeham h. the assumption that death is due to two co-existing causes: (1) chance, which is constant; (2) inability to withstand destruction, which progresses geometrically.

null h. the particular hypothesis under investigation; termed null because it frequently asserts a lack of effect or of difference. Symbol H_0. Cf. *alternative h.*

one gene–one enzyme h. the hypothesis that each gene is responsible for making a single enzyme; modified to the one gene–one polypeptide chain hypothesis when enzymes composed of multiple heterogeneous polymers were discovered.

one gene–one polypeptide chain h. the hypothesis that each gene codes for the production of a single polypeptide chain; there are exceptions, e.g., antibody genes, in which separate genes for variable and constant regions are rearranged to code for a single polypeptide.

response-to-injury h. a hypothesis explaining atherogenesis as initiating with some injury to the endothelial cells lining the artery walls, which causes a variety of forms of endothelial dysfunction and leads to abnormal cellular interactions and initiation and progression of atherogenesis.

sliding filament h. see under *mechanism*.

Starling h. the direction and rate of fluid transfer between blood plasma in the capillary and fluid in the tissue spaces depend on the hydrostatic pressure on each side of the capillary wall, on the osmotic pressure of protein in plasma and in tissue fluid, and on the properties of the capillary wall as a filtering membrane.

unitarian h. the theory that antibody is a single species of modified serum globulin regardless of the overt consequences of its reaction with homologous antigen, e.g., agglutination, precipitation, complement fixation, etc.

wobble h. the third base of a tRNA anticodon does not have to pair with a complementary codon (as do the first two bases) but can form base pairs with any of several mRNA codons, explaining how a specific transfer RNA (tRNA) molecule can translate different codons in a messenger RNA (mRNA) template.

hy·po·throm·bin·emia (hi″po-throm″bĭ-ne′me-ə) a deficiency of thrombin in the blood.

hy·po·thy·mia (hi″po-thi′me-ə) [*hypo-* + *thymo-*[2] + *-ia*] abnormal diminution of emotional tone, as in depression. **hypothy′mic** *adj*

hy·po·thy·mism (hi″po-thi′miz-əm) abnormally deficient activity of the thymus.

hy·po·thy·roid (hi″po-thi′roid) marked by or due to hypothyroidism. Called also *athyrotic*, *thyroprival*, and *thyroprivic*.

hy·po·thy·roid·ism (hi″po-thi′roid-iz-əm) deficiency of thyroid activity, characterized by decrease in basal metabolic rate, fatigue, and lethargy; if untreated, it progresses to myxedema. In adults it is more common in women than men, and in infants it can lead to cretinism. Called also *athyria*, *athyroidism*, *athyroidosis*, *hypothyrosis*, *thyroprivia*, and *thyroid insufficiency*.

central h. secondary h.

consumptive h. a rare type of hypothyroidism in which there are vascular tumors in the liver and excessive deiodination of thyroxine; it is usually seen in infants, but a few cases have occurred in older persons.

hypothalamic h. secondary hypothyroidism caused by a defect or lesion of the hypothalamus that interferes with its production of thyrotropin-releasing hormone. Called also *tertiary h.*

infantile h. hypothyroidism that is first seen in infancy; when severe, it leads to cretinism.

juvenile h. hypothyroidism that is first seen in childhood, with manifestations intermediate between those of the infantile and adult types, including slowed bone and dental growth and delayed sexual development; in children under age three it may cause mental retardation.

juvenile acquired h. hypothyroidism with an insidious onset in childhood, caused by thyrotropin deficiency; it is marked by slowing and cessation of growth, thickening and yellowing of the skin, coarse facies, delayed pubertal development, and short stature at maturity.

pituitary h. secondary hypothyroidism caused by a defect or lesion of the pituitary gland (usually a tumor) that interferes with production of thyrotropin.

primary h. hypothyroidism due to a disease or lesion of the thyroid gland itself, usually accompanied by increased levels of thyrotropin.

secondary h. hypothyroidism resulting from inadequate secretion of thyrotropin by the pituitary gland; see *hypothalamic h.* and *pituitary h.* Called also *central h.*

tertiary h. hypothalamic h.

hy·po·thy·ro·sis (hi″po-thi-ro′sis) hypothyroidism.

hy·po·thy·rox·in·emia (hi″po-thi-rok″sĭ-ne′me-ə) abnormally low blood levels of thyroxine.

hy·po·to·nia (hi″po-to′ne-ə) [*hypo-* + *ton-* + *-ia*] a condition of diminished tone of the skeletal muscles, so that they have diminished resistance to passive stretching and are flaccid; this usually means the nerve supply is compromised. See also *atony*.

benign congenital h. a condition marked by signs of weakness and floppiness in babies, due to nonprogressive weakness of skeletal muscles from birth.

h. o′culi low intraocular pressure.

hy·po·ton·ic (hi-po-ton′ik) 1. denoting a solution which, when bathing body cells, causes a net flow of water across the semipermeable cell membrane into the cell. 2. denoting a solution having less tonicity than another solution, e.g., the blood, with which it is compared. 3. exhibiting hypotonia.

hy·po·to·nic·i·ty (hi″po-to-nis′ĭ-te) the state or quality of being hypotonic.

hy·pot·o·nus (hi-pot′ə-nəs) hypotonia.

hy·po·tox·ic·i·ty (hi″po-tok-sis′ĭ-te) [*hypo-* + *toxicity*] the state or quality of having mitigated or diminished toxicity.

hy·po·trans·fer·rin·emia (hi″po-trans-fer″ĭ-ne′me-ah) deficiency of transferrin in the blood.

hy·po·tri·chi·a·sis (hi″po-trĭ-ki′ə-sis) 1. congenital alopecia. 2. hypotrichosis.

hy·po·tri·cho·sis (hi″po-trĭ-ko′sis) [*hypo-* + *trich-* + *-osis*] presence of less than the normal amount of hair; cf. *alopecia*.

Marie Unna h. a rare autosomal dominant disorder caused by mutation in the *HR* gene (locus: 8p21.2), which is the human analogue of the mouse "hairless" gene. Children are born with sparse, twisted hair that progresses to widespread alopecia; called also *hereditary trichodysplasia*.

hy·pot·ro·phy (hi-pot′rə-fe) [*hypo-* + *-trophy*] abiotrophy.

hy·po·tro·pia (hi″po-tro′pe-ə) [*hypo-* + *trop-* + *-ia*] vertical strabismus in which there is permanent downward deviation of the visual axis of an eye.

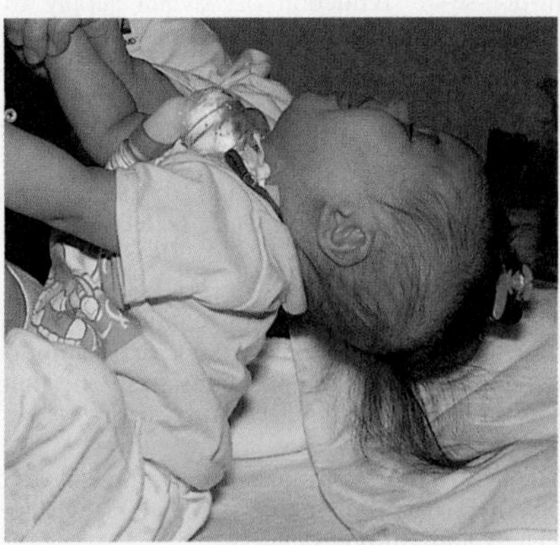

■ Hypotonia with severe head lag and failure of limbs to flex to counter the upward traction.

hy·po·tryp·to·phan·ic (hi″po-trip-to-fan′ik) caused by deficiency of tryptophan in the diet.

hy·po·tym·pan·ic (hi″po-tim-pan′ik) inferior to the sulcus tympanicus of the temporal bone.

hy·po·tym·pa·not·o·my (hi″po-tim″pə-not′ə-me) surgical opening of the hypotympanum.

hy·po·tym·pa·num (hi″po-tim′pə-nəm) a space in the middle ear, below the lower edge of the sulcus tympanicus of the temporal bone.

hy·po·ure·mia (hi″po-u-re′me-ə) abnormally low levels of urea in the blood.

hy·po·ure·sis (hi″po-u-re′sis) oliguria.

hy·po·uri·ce·mia (hi″po-u″rĭ-se′me-ə) deficiency of uric acid in the blood, seen along with xanthinuria, due to deficiency of xanthine oxidase, the enzyme required for conversion of hypoxanthine to xanthine and of xanthine to uric acid.

hy·po·uri·co·su·ria (hi″po-u″rĭ-ko-su′re-ə) deficiency of uric acid in the urine; called also *hypouricuria.*

hy·po·uri·cu·ria (hi″po-u″rĭ-ku′re-ə) hypouricosuria.

hyp·ovar·i·an·ism (hi″po-var′e-ən-iz-əm) hypo-ovarianism.

hy·po·ve·nos·i·ty (hi″po-ve-nos′ĭ-te) incomplete development of the venous system in any area.

hy·po·ven·ti·la·tion (hi″po-ven″tĭ-la′shən) a state in which there is a reduced amount of air entering the pulmonary alveoli (decreased *alveolar ventilation;* see under *ventilation*), resulting in increased carbon dioxide tension. Cf. *hypopnea* and *bradypnea.*

controlled h. permissive hypercapnia.

primary alveolar h. impairment of automatic control of respiration, usually due to a spinal cord or brainstem lesion; voluntary control remains intact but apnea occurs during sleep. Called also *Ondine curse.*

hy·po·vi·ta·min·o·sis (hi″po-vi″tə-min-o′sis) deficiency of one or more essential vitamins; see specific vitamins.

hy·po·vo·le·mia (hi″po-vo-le′me-ə) [*hypo-* + *volume* + *-emia*] abnormally decreased volume of circulating blood in the body; the most common cause is hemorrhage. **hypovole′mic** *adj*

hy·po·vo·lia (hi″po-vo′le-ə) diminished water content or volume, as of extracellular fluid.

hy·po·xan·thine (hi″po-zan′thēn) 6-oxypurine, a purine base formed as an intermediate in the degradation of purines and purine nucleosides to uric acid and in the salvage of free purines. It is found in some transfer RNA molecules and occurs complexed with ribose as the nucleoside inosine.

hy·po·xan·thine-guan·ine phos·pho·ri·bo·syl·trans·fer·ase (HGPRT) (hi″po-zan′thēn-gwahn′ēn fos″fo-ri″bo-səl-trans′fər-ās) hypoxanthine phosphoribosyltransferase.

hy·po·xan·thine phos·pho·ri·bo·syl·trans·fer·ase (HPRT) (hi″po-zan′thēn fos″fo-ri″bo-səl-trans′fər-ās) [EC 2.4.2.8] an enzyme of the transferase class that catalyzes the phosphorylation of hypoxanthine or guanine to its corresponding nucleoside monophosphate, a salvage mechanism for recovery of preformed purines, especially in the central nervous system. Absence of enzyme activity, an X-linked trait, results in Lesch-Nyhan syndrome; partially decreased enzyme activity results in hyperuricemia and severe gouty arthritis without the neurologic sequelae of Lesch-Nyhan syndrome. Called also *hypoxanthine-guanine phosphoribosyltransferase.*

hy·pox·emia (hi″pok-se′me-ə) [*hyp-* + *ox-* + *-emia*] deficient oxygenation of the blood; cf. *hypoxia.*

hy·pox·ia (hi-pok′se-ə) reduction of oxygen supply to tissue below physiological levels despite adequate perfusion of the tissue by blood. Cf. *anoxia.* **hypox′ic** *adj*

anemic h. hypoxia due to reduction of the oxygen-carrying capacity of the blood as a result of a decrease in the total hemoglobin or an alteration of the hemoglobin constituents. Cf. *anemic anoxia.*

affinity h. hypoxia resulting from failure of the hemoglobin to release oxygen to the tissues, as may occur with a left-shifted oxyhemoglobin dissociation curve.

circulatory h. stagnant h.

fetal h. hypoxia in utero, caused by conditions such as inadequate placental function (often abruptio placentae), preeclamptic toxicity, prolapse of the umbilical cord, or complications from anesthetic administration. See also *fetal asphyxia* under *asphyxia* and *hypoxic-ischemic encephalopathy* under *encephalopathy.*

histotoxic h. hypoxia due to impaired utilization of oxygen by tissues.

hypobaric h. hypoxia occurring in hypobaric environments, such as occurs in airsickness and altitude sickness.

hypoxemic h., hypoxic h. hypoxia due to insufficient oxygen reaching the blood. Cf. *anoxic anoxia.*

stagnant h. hypoxia resulting from failure to transport sufficient oxygen because of inadequate blood flow.

hy·pox·ia-is·che·mia (hi-pok′se-ə-is-ke′me-ə) the changes occurring in tissues when the blood supply is cut off, particularly in a fetus or infant with asphyxia; see also *hypoxic-ischemic encephalopathy* under *encephalopathy.*

hy·pox·i·do·sis (hi-pok″sĭ-do′sis) impaired cell function due to reduced supply of oxygen.

hyp·oxy·phi·lia (hi-pok″se-fil′e-ə) [*hyp-* + *oxy-* + *-philia*] a paraphilia in which sexual arousal or activity depends on oxygen deprivation.

hy·pro·mel·lose (hi-pro′mə-lōs) [USP] a propylene glycol ether of methylcellulose, supplied in differing degrees of viscosity; used as a suspending and viscosity-increasing agent and tablet binder, coating, and excipient in pharmaceutical preparations, and applied topically to the conjunctiva to protect and lubricate the cornea. Called also *hydroxypropyl methylcellulose.*

h. phthalate [NF] a phthalic acid ester of hydroxypropyl methylcellulose, used as a coating agent for tablets and granules.

Hyp·Rho-D (hi′pro-de) trademark for preparations of $Rh_0(D)$ immune globulin.

hyp·sa·rhyth·mia (hip″sə-rith′me-ə) see *hypsarrhythmia.*

hyp·sar·rhyth·mia (hip″sə-rith′me-ə) [*hyps-* + *arrhythmia*] an electroencephalographic abnormality sometimes observed in infants, with random, high-voltage slow waves and spikes that arise from multiple foci and spread to all cortical areas. It is seen most commonly in cases of jackknife seizures.

hypsi- [Gr. *hypsi* aloft] a combining form meaning high.

hyp·si·brachy·ce·phal·ic (hip″sĭ-brak″e-sə-fal′ik) [*hypsi-* + *brachycephalic*] having the head broad and high.

hyp·si·ceph·a·ly (hip″sĭ-sef′ə-le) oxycephaly. **hypsicephal′ic** *adj*

hyp·si·con·chous (hip″sĭ-kong′kəs) [*hypsi-* + *concha* + *-ous*] having an orbital index over 85.

hyp·si·loid (hip′sĭ-loid) [Gr. *hypsiloeidēs*] shaped like a capital Greek letter upsilon (Y). Cf. *hyoid.*

hyp·si·sta·phyl·ia (hip″sĭ-stə-fil′e-ə) [*hypsi-* + *staphyl-* + *-ia*] a condition characterized by an unusually high-arched, narrow palate.

hyp·si·steno·ce·phal·ic (hip″sĭ-sten″o-sə-fal′ik) [*hypsi-* + *steno-* + *cephalic*] having a high, curved vertex, prominent cheek bones, and prognathic jaws.

hyps(o)- [Gr. *hypsos* height] a combining form denoting relationship to height.

hyp·so·ceph·a·lous (hip″so-sef′ə-ləs) oxycephalic.

hyp·so·chrome (hip′so-krōm) [*hypso-* + *-chrome*] an atom or group whose introduction into a compound shifts the compound's absorption maximum to a shorter wavelength; cf. *bathochrome.*

hyp·so·chro·my (hip″so-kro′me) a shift of the absorption band toward higher frequencies (shorter wavelengths), with lightening of color.

hyp·so·dont (hip′so-dont) [*hypso-* + Gr. *odous* tooth] having prism-shaped teeth with high crowns, as in many herbivorous mammals.

hyp·so·ki·ne·sis (hip″so-kĭ-ne′sis) [*hypso-* + *kin-* + *-esis*] a backward swaying, retropulsion, or falling when in erect posture, seen in Parkinson disease, Wilson disease, and similar conditions.

hy·rax (hi′raks) any of several species of rabbit-sized ungulates of the genera *Procavia, Dendrohyrax,* and *Heterohyrax,* found in Africa and the Middle East; they have fat furry bodies, short legs, small ears, and short tails. Some are reservoirs for *Leishmania aethiopica.* Called also *coney.*

rock h. any of several ground-dwelling species of the genera *Procavia* and *Heterohyrax,* often reservoirs for *Leishmania aethiopica;* called also *dassie.*

tree h. any of several tree-dwelling species of the genus *Dendrohyrax,* often reservoirs for *Leishmania aethiopica.*

Hyrtl loop (anastomosis), recess, sphincter (hur′təl) [Jozsef *Hyrtl,* Hungarian anatomist in Austria, 1810–1894] see under *loop* and *sphincter,* and see *recessus epitympanicus.*

hys·sop (his′əp) a woody, evergreen Eurasian plant, *Hyssopus officinalis,* having small blue flowers and fragrant leaves, used in perfumery and as an expectorant and circulatory stimulant.

Hys·so·pus (his′ə-pəs) [L., from Gr. *hyssōpos,* probably of Semitic origin] a genus of Eurasian herbs and shrubs, including *H. officina′lis,* which is used medicinally.

hys·ter·al·gia (his″tər-al′jə) [*hyster-* + *-algia*] pain in the uterus; called also *hysterodynia* and *uteralgia.*

hys·ter·atre·sia (his″tər-ə-tre′zhə) atresia of the opening into the uterus.

hys·ter·ec·to·my (his″tər-ek′tə-me) [*hystero-* + *-ectomy*] the operation of excising the entire uterus, performed either through the abdominal wall (*abdominal h.*) or through the vagina (*vaginal h.*).

abdominal h. excision of the uterus through an incision in the abdominal wall.

cesarean h. cesarean section followed by removal of the uterus.

complete h. total h.

laparoscopically assisted vaginal h. (LAVH) hysterectomy in which the ligamentous attachments of the uterus are severed using laparoscopic instruments and the uterus is then removed through the vagina.

partial h. subtotal h.

radical h. hysterectomy with pelvic lymphadenectomy and wide lateral excision of parametrial and paravaginal supporting structures; called also *Wertheim operation* or, when done by the vaginal route, *Schauta operation.*

subtotal h., supracervical h., supravaginal h. hysterectomy in which the cervix is left in place.

total h. hysterectomy in which the uterus and cervix are completely excised; called also *panhysterectomy.*

vaginal h. excision of the uterus through the vagina.

hys·te·re·sis (his″tə-re′sis) [Gr. *hysterēsis* a lagging behind] 1. a time lag in the occurrence of two associated phenomena, as between cause and effect. 2. in cardiac pacemaker terminology, the number of pulses per minute below the programmed pacing rate that the heart must drop in order to cause initiation of pacing.

hys·ter·ia (his-ter′e-ə) [Gr. *hystera* womb, from the antiquated belief that wandering of the uterus caused mental disturbances] a now somewhat nebulous term formerly used widely in psychiatry. Its meanings have included (1) classic hysteria (now *somatization disorder*); (2) hysterical neurosis (now divided into *conversion disorder* and *dissociative disorders*); (3) anxiety hysteria; and (4) hysterical personality (now *histrionic personality disorder*).

anxiety h. Freud's term for phobias, reflecting his view that the same defense mechanisms, repression and displacement, and the same unconscious conflicts involving infantile sexuality are involved in both hysteria and phobias.

conversion h. former name for a subtype of hysterical neurosis (see *hysteria*); currently classified as conversion disorder.

dissociative h. former name for a subtype of hysterical neurosis (see *hysteria*); the current classification is *dissociative disorders.*

farrowing h. a psychological abnormality seen in sows that have just given birth, usually for the first time, in which they attack their offspring when the piglets attempt to nurse; sometimes the piglets may die of their injuries.

fixation h. a form of conversion disorder in which the symptoms are based on an existing or previous organic disease or injury, as the persistence of a nervous cough after pertussis.

hys·ter·ic (his-ter′ik) pertaining to or characterized by hysteria.

hys·ter·i·cal (his-ter′i-kəl) characterized by hysteria.

hys·ter·ics (his-ter′iks) popular term for an uncontrollable emotional outburst.

hys·ter·i·form (his-ter′ĭ-form) having the appearance of hysteria.

hyster(o)- [Gr. *hystera* uterus] a combining form denoting relationship to the uterus, or to hysteria; see also *metr(o)-*.

hys·tero·cele (his′tər-o-sēl″) uterine hernia.

hys·tero·col·pec·to·my (his″tər-o-kol-pek′tə-me) [*hystero-* + *colpo-* + *-ectomy*] surgical removal of the uterus and vagina.

hys·ter·odyn·ia (his″tər-o-din′e-ə) hysteralgia.

hys·tero·gram (his′tər-o-gram″) a radiograph of the uterus.

hys·tero·graph (his′tər-o-graf″) [*hystero-* + *-graph*] an apparatus for measuring the strength of uterine contractions in labor.

hys·ter·og·ra·phy (his″tər-og′rə-fe) [*hystero-* + *-graphy*] 1. graphic recording of the strength of uterine contractions in labor. 2. radiography of the uterus after instillation of a contrast medium; see also *hysterosalpingography.* Called also *metrography* and *uterography.*

hys·ter·oid (his′tər-oid) [*hyster-* + *-oid*] resembling hysteria.

hys·ter·ol·y·sis (his″tər-ol′ə-sis) [*hystero-* + *-lysis*] the operation of loosening the uterus from its attachments or adhesions.

hys·te·rom·e·try (his″tə-rom′ə-tre) [*hystero-* + *-metry*] the measurement of the dimensions of the uterus.

hys·tero·myo·ma (his″tər-o-mi-o′mə) uterine leiomyoma.

hys·tero·myo·mec·to·my (his″tər-o-mi″o-mek′tə-me) uterine myomectomy.

hys·tero·my·ot·o·my (his″tər-o-mi-ot′ə-me) [*hystero-* + *myotomy*] incision of the uterus.

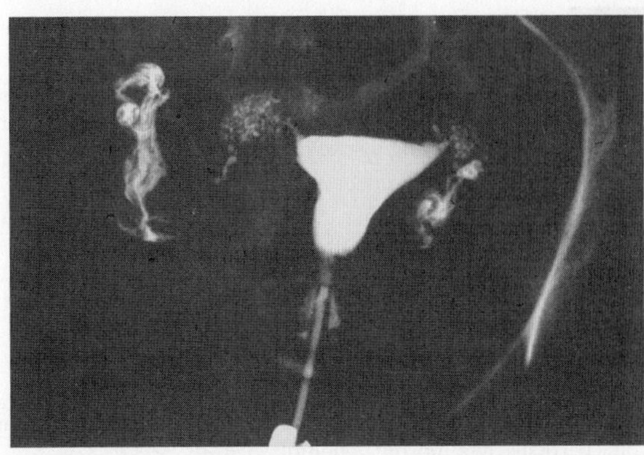

■ Hysterosalpingography showing characteristic honeycomb appearance in the proximal segment of the uterine tube in salpingitis isthmica nodosa as a result of penetration of contrast medium within the tubal wall.

hys·te·rop·a·thy (his″tə-rop′ə-the) [*hystero-* + *-pathy*] any uterine disease or disorder.

hys·tero·pexy (his′tər-o-pek″se) [*hystero-* + *-pexy*] surgical fixation of a displaced uterus, which may be done by ventrofixation, shortening of the round ligaments, shortening of the sacrouterine ligaments, or shortening of the endopelvic fascia. It is called *abdominal* or *vaginal,* depending on whether the uterus is fastened to the abdominal wall or to the vagina.

hys·ter·op·to·sis (his″tər-op-to′sis, his″tər-o-to′sis) uterine prolapse.

hys·ter·or·rha·phy (his″tər-or′ə-fe) [*hystero-* + *-rrhaphy*] 1. hysteropexy. 2. the operation of suturing of the lacerated uterus.

hys·ter·or·rhex·is (his″tər-o-rek′sis) metrorrhexis.

hys·tero·sal·pin·gec·to·my (his″tər-o-sal″pin-jek′tə-me) [*hystero-* + *salpingectomy*] excision of the uterus and uterine tubes.

hys·tero·sal·pin·gog·ra·phy (his″tər-o-sal″ping-gog′rə-fe) [*hystero-* + *salpingography*] radiography of the uterus and uterine tubes after the injection of opaque material. Called also *uterosalpingography.*

hys·tero·sal·pin·go-ooph·o·rec·to·my (his″tər-o-sal-ping″go-o-of″ə-rek′tə-me) excision of the uterus, uterine tubes, and ovaries.

hys·tero·sal·pin·gos·to·my (his″tər-o-sal″ping-gos′tə-me) [*hystero-* + *salpingostomy*] surgical creation of an anastomosis between the uterus and a fallopian tube after excision of a strictured or obstructed portion of the tube.

hys·tero·scope (his′tər-o-skōp″) [*hystero-* + *-scope*] an endoscope used in direct visual examination of the canal of the uterine cervix and the cavity of the uterus.

hys·ter·os·co·py (his″tər-os′kə-pe) inspection of the interior of the uterus with an endoscope.

hys·tero·spasm (his′tər-o-spaz″əm) spasm of the uterus.

hys·tero·stat (his′tər-o-stat) [*hystero-* + *-stat*] a mechanical intrauterine device for holding sealed sources of ionizing radiation (radium, cesium-137, etc.) in order to give planned patterns of irradiation.

hys·tero·ther·mom·e·try (his″tər-o-thər-mom′ə-tre) uterothermometry.

hys·tero·tome (his′tər-o-tōm″) [*hystero-* + *-tome*] an instrument for incising the uterus.

hys·ter·ot·o·my (his″tər-ot′ə-me) [*hystero-* + *-tomy*] incision of the uterus, usually for delivery of a fetus.

abdominal h. incision of the uterus through the wall of the abdomen. Called also *abdominohysterotomy, abdominouterotomy,* and *laparohysterotomy.*

vaginal h. incision of the uterus through the vagina.

Hy·tak·er·ol (hi-tak′ər-ol) trademark for preparations of dihydrotachysterol.

Hy·tone (hi′tōn) trademark for preparations of hydrocortisone.

Hy·trin (hi′trin) trademark for a preparation of terazosin hydrochloride.

Hy·zaar (hi′zahr) trademark for a combination preparation of losartan potassium and hydrochlorothiazide.

Hyz·yd (hiz′id) trademark for a preparation of isoniazid.

Hz hertz.

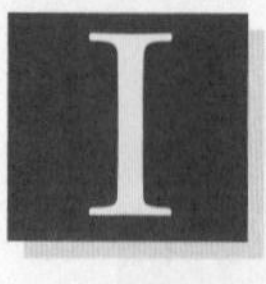

I incisor; iodine; inosine (in nucleotides); isoleucine.

I electric current; intensity (of radiant energy); ionic strength.

-ia [L. and Gr. noun-forming suffix] a word termination denoting a state or condition.

IAB intra-aortic balloon; see under *counterpulsation.*

IABP intra-aortic balloon pump.

IADL instrumental activities of daily living.

IAEA International Atomic Energy Agency.

IAHA immune adherence hemagglutination assay.

IAP inhibitor of apoptosis protein.

IAPP islet amyloid polypeptide; see *amylin.*

-iasis a word termination meaning a process or the condition resulting therefrom, particularly a morbid condition. See *-sis.*

iat•ric (i-at′rik) [Gr. *iatrikos*] pertaining to medicine or to a physician.

-iatric [Gr. *iatrikos* pertaining to a physician, from *iatros* physician] a combining form denoting relationship to medical treatment.

-iatrics [*-iatric*] a combining form denoting medical treatment.

iatr(o)- [Gr. *iatros* physician] a combining form denoting relationship to a physician or to medicine.

iat•ro•ep•i•dem•ic (i-at″ro-ep-ĭ-dem′ik) a trend in medical thought or procedure that becomes popular but causes harm or death in excess of its benefits.

iat•ro•gen•e•sis (i-at″ro-jen′ə-sis) [*iatro-* + *-genesis*] the creation of additional problems or complications resulting from treatment by a physician or surgeon.

iat•ro•gen•ic (i-at″ro-jen′ik) [*iatro-* + *-genic*] resulting from the activity of physicians.

iat•ro•phys•ics (i-at″ro-fiz′iks) [*iatro-* + *physics*] the physics of medicine or of medical and surgical treatment.

-iatry [Gr. *iatreia* healing, from *iatros* physician] a word termination denoting medical treatment.

IB inclusion body.

iban•dro•nate so•di•um (i-ban′drə-nāt) a bisphosphonate calcium-regulating agent used to inhibit the resorption of bone in the prevention and treatment of postmenopausal osteoporosis; administered orally.

IBC iron-binding capacity.

IBD inflammatory bowel disease.

IBF immunoglobulin-binding factor.

ibo•ga•ine (i-bo′gə-ēn) an alkaloid from the root of *Tabernanthe iboga* Baill. (Apocynaceae) that has antidepressant and euphoric properties; it has been used investigationally as an aid to withdrawal symptoms in the treatment of drug addiction.

ibo•ten•ic ac•id (i″bo-ten′ik) an excitotoxin found in the mushroom *Amanita muscaria;* it is 3 to 10 times as potent as glutamic acid and is used to study the excitatory mechanisms of glutamate transmitters.

ib•ri•tu•mo•mab (ib″rĭ-too′mo-mab) a monoclonal antibody directed against the CD20 surface antigen of B lymphocytes.

i. tiuxetan an immunoconjugate of ibritumomab and the linker-chelator tiuxetan, used as part of a regimen for non-Hodgkin lymphoma in conjunction with the monoclonal antibody rituximab and the radiopharmaceuticals indium 111 and yttrium 90.

IBS irritable bowel syndrome.

IBU trademark for preparations of ibuprofen.

ibu•pro•fen (i″bu-pro′fən) [USP] a nonsteroidal antiinflammatory drug derived from propionic acid and having also analgesic and antipyretic actions; administered orally in the treatment of pain, fever, dysmenorrhea, osteoarthritis, rheumatoid arthritis, and other rheumatic and nonrheumatic inflammatory disorders, and in the treatment and prophylaxis of vascular headaches.

ibu•ti•lide fu•ma•rate (ĭ-bu′tĭ-līd) a cardiac depressant used as an antiarrhythmic agent in the treatment of atrial arrhythmias; administered by intravenous infusion.

IC inspiratory capacity; irritable colon.

-ic [L. *-icus,* from Gr. *-ikos*] 1. a suffix meaning pertaining to or characteristic of, e.g., acidic. 2. in chemistry, a suffix used to indicate an ion or acid exhibiting the higher of two oxidation states, the other being indicated by the suffix *-ous.*

ICAM-1 intercellular adhesion molecule 1.

ICAM-2 intercellular adhesion molecule 2.

ICCs interstitial cells of Cajal.

ICC_{IM}, ICC_{MY}, ICC_{SM} functional types of interstitial cells of Cajal (q.v.).

ICD International Classification of Diseases (of the World Health Organization); intrauterine contraceptive device; implantable cardioverter-defibrillator.

ICE a cancer chemotherapy regimen consisting of ifosfamide, carboplatin, and etoposide.

ice (īs) the solid state of water occurring at or below 0°C and 1 atmosphere.

dry i. carbon dioxide snow.

Ice•land disease (īs′lənd) [*Iceland,* island country in the North Atlantic, where an epidemic occurred in 1948] chronic fatigue syndrome.

ICF intracellular fluid.

ich (ik) white spot disease (def. 3).

ich•tham•mol (ik′thəm-ol) [USP] a reddish brown to brownish black viscous fluid, with a strong, characteristic odor, obtained by the destructive distillation of certain bituminous schists, sulfonation of the distillate, and neutralization of the product with ammonia; used as a local skin anti-infective.

ich•thy•ism (ik′the-iz-əm) ichthyotoxism.

ichthy(o)- [Gr. *ichthys* fish] a combining form denoting relationship to fish.

ich•thyo•acan•tho•tox•in (ik′the-o-ə-kan′tho-tok″sin) [*ichthyo-* + *acantho-* + *toxin*] the venom secreted by venomous fishes, in connection with stings, spines, or "teeth."

ich•thyo•acan•tho•tox•ism (ik″the-o-ə-kan″tho-tok′siz-əm) intoxication resulting from injuries produced by the stings, spines, or "teeth" of venomous fishes.

ich•thyo•col•la (ik″the-o-kol′ə) [*ichthyo-* + Gr. *kolla* glue] isinglass.

ich•thyo•he•mo•tox•in (ik″the-o-he′mo-tok″sin) [*ichthyo-* + *hemo-* + *toxin*] a toxic substance found in the blood of certain fish.

ich•thyo•he•mo•tox•ism (ik″the-o-he″mo-tok′siz-əm) intoxication caused by the ingestion of ichthyohemotoxin, characterized by gastrointestinal and neurological disturbances.

ich•thy•oid (ik′the-oid) [*ichthyo-* + *-oid*] resembling a fish; shaped like a fish.

ich•thy•ol•o•gy (ik″the-ol′ə-je) the branch of zoology that specializes in the study of fishes.

ich•thy•oo•tox•in (ik″the-o′o-tok″sin) [*ichthyo-* + *oo-* + *toxin*] a toxic substance derived from the roe of certain fish; see also *ichthyootoxism.*

ich•thy•oo•tox•ism (ik″the-o″o-tok′siz-əm) intoxication caused by the ingestion of toxic fish roe, characterized by gastrointestinal and neurological disturbances.

ich•thyo•pha•gia (ik″the-o-fa′jə) [*ichthyo-* + *-phagia*] the practice of subsisting on fish.

ich•thy•oph•a•gous (ik″the-of′ə-gəs) eating or subsisting on fish.

ich•thy•oph•thi•ri•a•sis (ik″the-o-thi′re-ə-sis) [*Ichthyophthirius* + *-iasis*] white spot disease (def. 3).

Ich•thy•oph•thi•ri•us (ik″the-o-thi′re-əs) [*ichthyo-* + Gr. *phtheir* louse] a genus of histophagous protozoa of the order Hymenostomatida, suborder Ophryoglenina. *I. multifi′liis* causes white spot disease in marine and freshwater fishes.

ich•thyo•sar•co•tox•in (ik″the-o-sahr′ko-tok″sin) [*ichthyo-* + *sarco-* + *toxin*] the poison found in the flesh of poisonous fishes, excluding toxins which may result from bacterial contamination.

ich•thyo•sar•co•tox•ism (ik″the-o-sahr″ko-tok′siz-əm) intoxication characterized by various gastrointestinal and neurological disturbances, resulting from the ingestion of the flesh of poisonous fishes; the term excludes ordinary bacterial food poisoning. Some types are *elasmobranch, Gymnothorax, fugu* or *puffer fish,* and *scombroid poisoning* and *ciguatera.* Called also *fish poisoning.*

ich•thyo•si•form (ik″the-o′sĭ-form) resembling ichthyosis.

ich•thy•o•sis (ik″the-o′sis) [*ichthy-* + *-osis*] 1. any in a group of cutaneous disorders characterized by increased or aberrant keratinization, resulting in noninflammatory scaling of the skin. Metaphors sometimes used to describe the appearance or texture of the skin in various types or stages of ichthyosis include alligator, collodion, crocodile, fish, and porcupine skin. Most ichthyoses are genetically determined, but a few types may be acquired, usually developing in association with systemic diseases or genetic syndromes. 2. i. vulgaris. **ichthyot′ic** *adj*

acquired i. ichthyosis occurring secondary to systemic disease, such as Hodgkin disease, leprosy, or sarcoidosis, or occasionally as an adverse drug reaction.

i. bullosa of Siemens an autosomal dominant condition caused by mutation in the *KRT2* gene (locus: 12q11-q13), which encodes keratin 2e, characterized by mild blistering in infancy on skin surfaces that bump objects; the blisters shed to leave small areas denuded of stratum corneum. When this subsides, the child has hyperkeratosis of elbows, knees, and other joints.

bullous i. 1. ichthyosis bullosa of Siemens. 2. epidermolytic hyperkeratosis.

i. conge'nita, congenital i. 1. in humans, any type of ichthyosis that is present at birth. See also *collodion baby*, under *baby*, and *harlequin fetus*, under *fetus*. 2. in cattle, a lethal autosomal recessive condition in which calves are born with most hair lacking and the entire body covered with thick horny plaques.

i. exfoliati'va, exfoliative i. i. bullosa of Siemens.

i. feta'lis the ichthyosis affecting a harlequin fetus.

follicular i. a rare type of ichthyosis usually seen on the head, neck, or extensor surfaces of limbs of infant boys, with follicular plugging similar to that of Darier disease.

harlequin i. i. fetalis.

i. hys'trix [L. *hys'trix* porcupine] any of several rare autosomal dominant skin disorders in which large areas of the skin have wartlike growths that are sometimes pointed to resemble porcupine quills; some types are severe forms of epidermolytic hyperkeratosis.

lamellar i., i. lamella'ris a genetically and clinically heterogeneous, autosomal recessive form of ichthyosis, in which the affected infant is born encased in a collodionlike membrane (see *collodion baby*, under *baby*). The membrane is soon shed, and the skin becomes covered with large, coarse scales, including on all the flexures, the palms, and the soles. Universal erythroderma and pruritus are characteristic, and ectropion of variable degree is usually present.

i. linea'ris circumflex'a an autosomal recessive congenital disorder characterized by generalized erythroderma and scaling associated with migratory, polycyclic lesions with a peripheral double-edged scale and hyperkeratosis of the flexural areas, and palmoplantar hyperhidrosis. It is the form of ichthyosis characteristic of Netherton syndrome.

i. palma'ris et planta'ris palmoplantar keratoderma.

i. sim'plex i. vulgaris.

i. u'teri a condition marked by transformation of the columnar epithelium of the endometrium into stratified squamous epithelium.

i. vulga'ris the most common form of ichthyosis, an autosomal dominant disorder caused by mutation in the *FLG* gene (locus: 1q21), which encodes filaggrin. Onset is after the first year of life, often near puberty. It is characterized by prominent fine scaling, mainly on the extensor surfaces of the limbs and back, with flexures, the abdomen, and the face usually being spared; there is accentuated marking with creases on the palms and soles, and sometimes atopy. Called also *i. simplex*.

X-linked i. a chronic, X-linked ichthyosis caused by deficiency of the microsomal enzyme steryl-sulfatase as a result of mutation in the *STS* gene (locus: Xp22.32); it may be present at birth or appear in early infancy. It is characterized by prominent, adherent scales, often brown, especially on the neck, limbs, trunk, and buttocks. Corneal opacities that do not interfere with vision are often found; they may occur in minor form in heterozygotic female carriers.

ich•thyo•tox•ic (ik'the-o-tok"sik) caused by the toxic principle of fish.

ich•thyo•tox•i•col•o•gy (ik"the-o-tok"sĭ-kol'ə-je) [*ichthyo-* + *toxico-* + *-logy*] the science of poisons derived from certain fish, their cause, detection, and effects, and the treatment of conditions produced by them.

ich•thyo•tox•in (ik'the-o-tok"sin) [*ichthyo-* + *toxin*] a general term applied to any type of toxic substance derived from fish.

ich•thyo•tox•ism (ik"the-o-tok'siz-əm) [*ichthyo-* + *toxin* + *-ism*] a general term applied to intoxication caused by any toxic substance derived from fish.

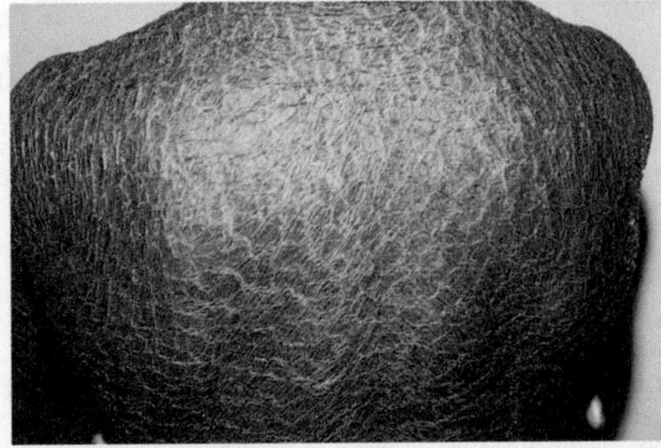

■ Lamellar ichthyosis, with thick, brown scales covering the entire skin surface.

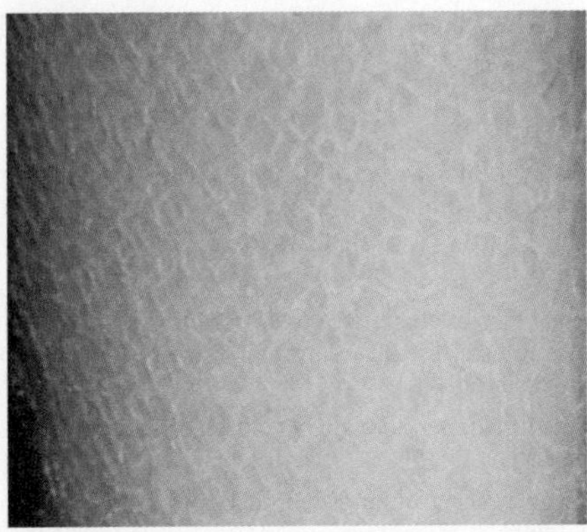

■ Ichthyosis vulgaris with typical fishlike scales.

ick (ik) white spot disease (def. 3).

ICN International Council of Nurses.

icon (i'kon) [Gr. *eikōn* likeness, image] 1. an image, model, or representation. 2. a brief sensory image in the mind, often pictorial, which may or may not become part of short-term memory.

ico•sa•he•dral (i"ko-sə-he'drəl) [Gr. *eikosi* twenty + *hedra* seat] pertaining to an icosahedron, a solid having 20 faces and 12 vertices.

ico•sa•no•ic ac•id (i"ko-sə-no'ik) arachidic acid.

ICP intracranial pressure.

ICRP International Commission on Radiological Protection.

ICRU International Commission on Radiological Units and Measurements.

ICS International College of Surgeons.

ICSH interstitial cell–stimulating hormone (luteinizing hormone).

ICSI intracytoplasmic sperm injection.

icter(o)- [L. *icterus*, q.v.] a combining form meaning affected with or pertaining to jaundice.

ic•tero•ane•mia (ik"tər-o-ə-ne'me-ə) anemia with jaundice.

ic•tero•gen•ic (ik"tər-o-jen'ik) [*ictero-* + *-genic*] causing jaundice.

ic•tero•ge•nic•i•ty (ik"tər-o-jə-nis'ĭ-te) ability to cause jaundice.

ic•tero•hem•a•tu•ria (ik"tər-o-hem"ə-tu're-ə) jaundice associated with hematuria. **icterohematu'ric** *adj*

ic•tero•he•mo•glob•in•uria (ik"tər-o-he"mo-glo"bĭ-nu're-ə) combined jaundice and hemoglobinuria.

ic•tero•hep•a•ti•tis (ik"tər-o-hep"ə-ti'tis) jaundice with hepatitis.

ic•ter•oid (ik'tər-oid) [*ictero-* + *-oid*] resembling jaundice.

ic•ter•us (ik'tər-əs) [L., from Gr. *ikteros*] jaundice. **icter'ic** *adj*

i. gra'vis neonato'rum a severe type of neonatal jaundice, usually a form of isoimmunization with Rh factor; it sometimes progresses to kernicterus. Called also *erythroleukoblastosis*.

neonatal i., i. neonato'rum see under *jaundice*.

nuclear i. kernicterus.

i. prae'cox a mild type of neonatal jaundice that sometimes develops in the first 24 hours of life and is due to incompatibility of the ABO blood group system between mother and infant; it usually clears spontaneously.

scleral i. a yellow discoloration of the sclerae owing to hyperbilirubinemia.

ic•tus (ik'təs) pl. *ic'tus* [L. "stroke"] a seizure, stroke, blow, or sudden attack. **ic'tal** *adj*

i. epilep'ticus seizure (def. 2).

i. paraly'ticus paralytic stroke.

i. san'guinis stroke syndrome.

i. so'lis sunstroke.

ICU intensive care unit.

ID intradermal; inside diameter; infective dose.

ID_{50} median infective dose.

Id. i'dem (the same).

id (id) [L. *id*, Ger. *es* it] in psychoanalytic theory, the innate, totally unconscious, primitive aspect of the personality dominated by the pleasure principle and harboring instinctive impulses that seek immediate personal pleasure, gratification, or satisfaction. Cf. *ego* and *superego*.

-id [Gr. *eidos* form, shape] a word termination denoting (1) having the shape of, or resembling or (2) an id reaction associated with the disorder specified by the root word.

IDA iminodiacetic acid.

-idae [Gr. *-idai*, pl. of *-ides* patronymic ending] in zoology, a word termination denoting a family.

Ida·my·cin (i″də-mi′sin) trademark for a preparation of idarubicin hydrochloride.

ida·ru·bi·cin hy·dro·chlo·ride (i″də-roo′bĭ-sin) [USP] an anthracycline antineoplastic used in the treatment of acute myelogenous leukemia; administered intravenously.

IDD, IDDM insulin-dependent diabetes mellitus; see *type 1 diabetes mellitus*, under *diabetes*.

-ide a suffix signifying a binary chemical compound, such as a chloride, sulfide, or carbide.

idea (i-de′ə) [Gr. "form"] an impression, thought, or conception resulting from mental activity.

autochthonous i. a persistent idea originating within the mind, usually from the unconscious, but seeming to have come from an outside source and often therefore felt to be of malevolent origin.

dominant i. an idea that controls or colors every action and thought.

fixed i. a morbid impression or belief which stays in the mind and cannot be changed by reason.

overvalued i. a false or exaggerated belief sustained beyond reason or logic but with less rigidity than a delusion, also often being less patently unbelievable.

i. of reference, referential i. the assumption by a patient that the words and actions of others refer to himself or the projection of the causes of his own imaginary difficulties upon someone else; if frequent or intense, or if organized and systematized, called *delusion of reference*.

ide·al (i-de′əl) 1. having some relation to ideas, impressions, or imaginations. 2. a standard of perfection.

ego i. the component of the superego comprising the internalized image of what one desires to become and toward the attainment of which the ego strives, formed through conscious or unconscious identification with or emulation of one who plays a significant role or has a place of esteem in the life of the developing child.

ide·al·iza·tion (i-de″əl-ĭ-za′shən) a conscious or unconscious mental mechanism in which the individual overestimates an admired aspect or attribute of another person.

ide·a·tion (i″de-a′shən) the formation of a mental concept, image, or thought. **idea′tional** *adj*

paranoid i. the persistent idea, not of delusional intensity, that one is being persecuted, harassed, or otherwise unfairly treated.

idée (e-da′) [Fr.] idea.

i. fixe (fēks) fixed idea.

iden·ti·fi·ca·tion (i-den″tĭ-fĭ-ka′shən) a largely unconscious process by which a person patterns himself or herself after one or more other people, associating closely with them and assuming their viewpoints; in some people this can be a type of defense mechanism.

cosmic i. identification of one's self with the universe, as in schizophrenic delusions of omnipotence.

projective i. a type of defense mechanism in which unacceptable aspects of the self are falsely attributed to others; it differs from projection in that the target is transformed, unconsciously identifying and responding, and the aspects that are projected are not completely disavowed but rather are perceived as justifiable reactions to the other person's induced responses.

iden·ti·ty (i-den′tĭ-te) the aggregate of characteristics by which individuals are recognized by themselves and others.

core gender i. gender i.

ego i. a sense of unity and continuity of oneself.

gender i. a person's self-conception as male and masculine or female and feminine, or ambivalent; usually based on physical characteristics, parental attitudes and expectations, and psychological and social pressures. It is the private experience of gender role. Cf. *gender role*.

ideo·ge·net·ic (i″de-o-jə-net′ik) related to mental processes in which images of sense impressions are used, rather than ideas that are ready for verbal expression.

ideo·ki·net·ic (i-de″o-ki-net′ik) ideomotor.

ide·ol·o·gy (i″de-ol′ə-je, id″e-ol′ə-je) [Gr. *idea* + *-logy*] 1. the science of the development of ideas. 2. the body of ideas characteristic of an individual or of a social unit.

ideo·mo·tion (i″de-o-mo′shən) motion or muscular action which is neither reflex nor volitional, but is induced by some dominant idea.

ideo·mo·tor (i″de-o-mo′tər) aroused by an idea or thought; said of involuntary motion so aroused.

IDET intradiscal electrothermal therapy.

idi(o)- [Gr. *idios* one's own, separate] a combining form meaning one's own, separate, or self-produced.

id·io·ag·glu·ti·nin (id″e-o-ə-gloo′tĭ-nin) [*idio-* + *agglutinin*] an agglutinin that originates independently of any transfer or artificial means in the animal in which it is formed.

id·io·gen·e·sis (id″e-o-jen′ə-sis) [*idio-* + *-genesis*] the origin of disease without a known cause, as in an idiopathic disease.

id·io·glos·sia (id″e-o-glos′e-ə) [*idio-* + *gloss-* + *-ia*] extremely defective imperfect articulation, with the utterance of vocal sounds that are virtually unintelligible. Called also *idiolalia*. **idioglot′tic** *adj*

id·io·gram (id′e-o-gram″) [*idio-* + *-gram*] a diagrammatic representation of a karyotype (q.v.).

id·io·het·ero·ag·glu·ti·nin (id″e-o-het″ər-o-ə-gloo′tĭ-nin) [*idio-* + *heteroagglutinin*] a heteroagglutinin normally present in the blood.

id·io·het·er·ol·y·sin (id″e-o-het″ər-ol′ə-sin) a heterolysin normally present in the blood.

id·io·hyp·no·tism (id″e-o-hip′no-tiz-əm) [*idio-* + *hypnotism*] spontaneous or self-induced hypnotism.

id·io·iso·ag·glu·ti·nin (id″e-o-i″so-ə-gloo′tĭ-nin) an isoagglutinin normally present in the blood, and not produced by artificial means.

id·io·isol·y·sin (id″e-o-i-sol′ə-sin) a lysin normally present which lyses the cells of other members of the same species as the animal in which it is formed.

id·io·la·lia (id″e-o-la′le-ə) idioglossia.

id·i·ol·y·sin (id″e-ol′ə-sin) [*idio-* + *lysin*] a lysin, normally present in the blood and not produced by artificial means, that lyses the cells of the animal in which it is formed.

id·io·mus·cu·lar (id″e-o-mus′ku-lər) [*idio-* + *muscular*] pertaining to the muscular tissue apart from any nerve stimulus; a term applied to certain muscular contractions which occur in degenerated muscles only.

id·io·path·ic (id″e-o-path′ik) of unknown cause or spontaneous origin; of the nature of an idiopathy. Called also *agnogenic*.

id·i·op·a·thy (id″e-op′ə-the) [*idio-* + *-pathy*] a pathologic condition of unknown cause or spontaneous origin.

id·io·re·flex (id″e-o-re′fleks) [*idio-* + *reflex*] a reflex brought about by a cause within the same organ.

id·io·ret·i·nal (id″e-o-ret′ĭ-nəl) pertaining to the retina alone; a term applied to a visual sensation occurring without any visual stimulus.

id·io·some (id′e-o-sōm″) [*idio-* + *-some*] the centrosome of a spermatocyte, together with surrounding Golgi apparatus and mitochondria.

id·io·spasm (id′e-o-spaz″əm) a spasm of a limited area or region.

id·io·syn·cra·sy (id″e-o-sin′krə-se) [*idio-* + Gr. *synkrasis* mixture] 1. a habit or quality of body or mind peculiar to any individual. 2. an abnormal susceptibility to some drug, protein, or other agent which is peculiar to the individual. **idiosyncrat′ic** *adj*

id·i·ot sa·vant (id′e-ət sə-vahnt′, e-dyo′ sah-vahn′) [Fr. "learned idiot"] a person who is severely mentally retarded in some respects, yet has a particular mental faculty that is developed to an unusually high degree, as memory, mathematics, or music.

id·io·tope (id′ĭ-o-tōp″) idiotypic determinant; an antigenic determinant on a variable domain of an immunoglobulin molecule. Cf. *allotope*.

id·io·topy (id′e-o-top″e) [*idio-* + Gr. *topos* place] the position and relation of the parts of an organ among themselves.

id·io·tro·phic (id″e-o-tro′fik) [*idio-* + *-trophic*] capable of selecting its own nourishment.

id·i·o·tro·pic (id″e-o-tro′pik) [*idio-* + *-tropic*] introspective; egocentric.

id·io·type (id′e-o-tīp′) a set of one or more idiotopes that distinguish a clone of immunoglobulin-producing cells from other clones. Idiotypes occur in the variable domains of immunoglobulin molecules and may be within, near to, or outside of the antigen-binding site; antibodies to idiotypes located within or near to the antigen-binding site will prevent the immunoglobulin from combining with antigen. **idiotyp′ic** *adj*

id·io·ven·tric·u·lar (id″e-o-vən-trik′u-lər) relating to or affecting the cardiac ventricles alone, as idioventricular rhythm.

idi·tol (i′dĭ-tol) the alcohol formed by reduction of the aldehyde group of idose.

L-idi·tol 2-de·hy·dro·ge·nase (i′dĭ-tol de-hi′dro-jən-ās) [EC 1.1.1.14] an enzyme of the oxidoreductase class that catalyzes the oxidation of L-iditol to L-fructose, using NAD^+ as an electron acceptor; the enzyme also acts on some other sugar alcohols. The enzyme occurs in significant quantities only in the liver; increased activity in serum is used as an indicator of parenchymal liver damage. Called also *sorbitol dehydrogenase*.

IDL intermediate-density lipoprotein.

idose (i'dōs) an aldohexose; structurally, L-idose is an epimer of D-glucose.

idox·ur·i·dine (IDU) (i-doks-ūr'ĭ-dēn) [USP] an analog of pyrimidine which inhibits viral DNA synthesis; used as an antiviral agent in the treatment of herpes simplex keratitis, applied topically to the conjunctiva.

IDU idoxuridine.

idu·ron·ate (i″du-ron'āt) a salt, ester, or anionic form of iduronic acid.

idu·ron·ate-2-sul·fa·tase (i″du-ron'āt sul'fə-tās) [EC 3.1.6.13] a lysosomal enzyme of the hydrolase class that catalyzes the cleavage of sulfate groups from the L-iduronate residues of dermatan sulfate and heparan sulfate, a step in the degradation of these glycosaminoglycans. Deficiency of the enzyme, an X-linked recessive trait, results in Hunter syndrome (mucopolysaccharidosis II).

idu·ron·ic ac·id (i″du-ron'ik) the uronic acid derived from idose; L-iduronic acid is an epimer of glucuronic acid and a constituent of dermatan sulfate, heparan sulfate, and heparin.

L-idu·ron·i·dase (i″du-ron'ĭ-dās) [EC 3.2.1.76] an enzyme of the hydrolase class that catalyzes the hydrolysis of terminal desulfated α-L-iduronic acid residues of dermatan sulfate and heparan sulfate, a step in the degradation of these glycosaminoglycans. Deficiency of the enzyme, an autosomal recessive trait, leads to mucopolysaccharidosis I.

IEP immunoelectrophoresis.

IF intrinsic factor.

IFA immunofluorescence assay; see *fluorescence immunoassay*, under *immunoassay*.

Ifex (i'feks) trademark for a preparation of sterile ifosfamide.

IFN interferon.

ifos·fa·mide (i-fos'fə-mīd) [USP] a cytotoxic alkylating agent of the nitrogen mustard group, a structural analogue of and similar in action to cyclophosphamide; it is itself pharmacologically inert and must be activated by the microsomal enzyme system of the liver. Used in the treatment of solid tumors of the testis, ovary, and lung as well as sarcomas; administered intravenously.

Ig immunoglobulin. The five classes are designated IgM, IgG, IgA, IgD, IgE. Subclasses are designated by numerical suffixes, e.g., IgG1.

IgA immunoglobulin A; see *immunoglobulin*.

IgD immunoglobulin D; see *immunoglobulin*.

IgE immunoglobulin E; see *immunoglobulin*.

IGF insulinlike growth factor.

IgG immunoglobulin G; see *immunoglobulin*.

IGIV immune globulin intravenous (human).

IgM immunoglobulin M; see *immunoglobulin*.

ig·na·tia (ig-na'she-ə) [L.] the poisonous dried ripe seed of *Strychnos ignatii;* it contains several alkaloids, the principal ones being strychnine and brucine, and has been used as a bitter tonic.

ig·ni·punc·ture (ig'nĭ-punk″chər) [*ignis* + *puncture*] therapeutic puncture with hot needles.

ig·nis (ig'nis) [L.] fire.
 i. inferna'lis [L. "infernal fire"] ergotism.

ig·ni·sa·tion (ig″nĭ-za'shən) [L. *ignis* fire] hyperthermia produced by exposure to artificial sources of heat.

ig·no·tine (ig'no-tēn) carnosine.

IGT impaired glucose tolerance.

IHD ischemic heart disease.

IHS Indian Health Service, an agency of the United States Department of Health and Human Services.

IHSS idiopathic hypertrophic subaortic stenosis.

IL interleukin; usually followed by a numeral designating a specific interleukin, e.g., IL-2.

il- see *in-*.

ILA International Leprosy Association.

Ile isoleucine.

il·e·ac (il'e-ak) 1. of the nature of ileus. 2. ileal.

ile·adel·phus (il″e-ə-del'fəs) iliopagus.

ile·ec·to·my (il″e-ek'tə-me) [*ile-* + *-ectomy*] surgical removal of the ileum.

il·e·itis (il″e-i'tis) inflammation of the ileum.
 distal i., regional i., terminal i. Crohn disease affecting the ileum.

ile(o)- [L. *ileum*] a combining form denoting relationship to the ileum.

il·eo·a·nal (il″e-o-a'nəl) pertaining to or connecting the ileum and the anus.

il·eo·ce·cal (il″e-o-se'kəl) pertaining to the ileum and cecum.

il·eo·ce·co·cys·to·plas·ty (il″e-o-se″ko-sis'to-plas″te) augmentation cystoplasty using a segment of ileum and cecum for the reconstruction.

il·eo·ce·cos·to·my (il″e-o-se-kos'tə-me) 1. surgical creation of a new opening between the ileum and the cecum. 2. the opening so created.

il·eo·ce·cum (il″e-o-se'kəm) the ileum and cecum considered as one organ.

il·eo·col·ic (il″e-o-kol'ik) pertaining to the ileum and colon.

il·eo·co·li·tis (il″e-o-ko-li'tis) inflammation of the ileum and colon.
 tuberculous i. tuberculous inflammation of the ileum and colon.

il·eo·co·lon·ic (il″e-o-ko-lon'ik) ileocolic.

il·eo·co·lon·os·co·py (il″e-o-ko″lən-os'kə-pe) examination of the colon and distal ileum through a colonoscope.

il·eo·co·los·to·my (il″e-o-kə-los'tə-me) [*ileo-* + *colo-* + *-stomy*] 1. surgical creation of an opening between the ileum and colon. 2. the opening so created.

il·eo·co·lot·o·my (il″e-o-ko-lot'ə-me) [*ileo-* + *colo-* + *-tomy*] surgical incision of the ileum and colon.

il·eo·cys·to·plas·ty (il″e-o-sis'to-plas″te) [*ileo-* + *cystoplasty*] augmentation cystoplasty using an isolated loop of the ileum for the added segment. ileocystoplas'tic *adj*

il·eo·cys·tos·to·my (il″e-o-sis-tos'tə-me) ileovesicostomy.

il·eo·gas·tros·to·my (il″e-o-gas-tros'tə-me) gastroileostomy.

il·eo·il·e·al (il″e-o-il'e-əl) pertaining to or connecting two different parts of the ileum.

il·eo·ile·os·to·my (il″e-o-il″e-os'tə-me) [*ileo-* + *ileo-* + *-stomy*] 1. surgical creation of an opening between two different parts of the ileum. 2. the opening so created.

il·eo·proc·tos·to·my (il″e-o-prok-tos'tə-me) [*ileo-* + *procto-* + *-stomy*] 1. surgical creation of an opening between the ileum and rectum; called also *ileorectostomy*. 2. the opening so created.

il·eo·rec·tal (il″e-o-rek'təl) pertaining to or communicating between the ileum and the rectum.

il·eo·rec·tos·to·my (il″e-o-rek-tos'tə-me) ileoproctostomy.

il·e·or·rha·phy (il″e-or'ə-fe) [*ileo-* + *-rrhaphy*] operative repair of the ileum.

il·eo·sig·moid (il″e-o-sig'moid) pertaining to or connecting the ileum and the sigmoid.

il·eo·sig·moi·dos·to·my (il″e-o-sig″moi-dos'tə-me) [*ileo-* + *sigmoidostomy*] 1. surgical creation of an opening between the ileum and the sigmoid colon. 2. the opening so created.

il·e·os·to·my (il″e-os'tə-me) [*ileo-* + *-stomy*] surgical creation of an opening into the ileum, usually by establishing an ileal stoma on the abdominal wall.
 Brooke i. the simplest conventional type of ileostomy, in which the intestinal mucosal surface is everted and sutured to the skin to form the stoma, so that the serosal surface is not exposed to the air.
 continent i. an ileostomy that maintains continence of feces, usually through construction of a continent ileal reservoir; now largely replaced by ileoanal anastomosis procedures.
 defunctioning i., diverting i., diverting loop i. an initial stage in colectomies or pouch creation in which the future anastomosis is not yet created and a loop of ileum is attached to a stoma; this allows healing of the distal structure that has been altered, with the expectation that later the ileum will be anastomosed to the altered colon or rectum.
 loop i. diverting i.

il·e·ot·o·my (il″e-ot'ə-me) [*ileo-* + *-tomy*] incision of the ileum.

il·eo·trans·verse (il″e-o-trans-vərs') pertaining to or connecting the ileum and the transverse colon.

il·eo·trans·vers·os·to·my (il″e-o-trans″vərs-os'tə-me) surgical creation of an opening between the ileum and the transverse colon.

il·eo·ure·ter·al (il″e-o-u-re'tər-əl) ureteroileal.

il·eo·ure·thral (il″e-o-u-re'thrəl) pertaining to or communicating between the ileum and the urethra. Called also *urethroileal*.

il·eo·ves·i·cal (il″e-o-ves'ĭ-kəl) pertaining to or communicating between the ileum and the urinary bladder. Called also *vesicoileal*.

il·eo·ves·i·cos·to·my (il″e-o-ves″ĭ-kos'tə-me) a type of urinary diversion consisting of creation of a channel made from a section of ileum, leading from the urinary bladder upwards to the abdominal surface; called also *ileocystostomy.*

Il·e·tin (il′ə-tin) trademark for preparations of insulin.
  Lente I. trademark for preparations of insulin zinc suspension.
  NPH I. trademark for preparations of insulin isophane suspension.
  Regular I. trademark for preparations of insulin (def. 3).

il·e·um (il′e-əm) [L.] [TA] the distal and longest portion of the small intestine, extending from the jejunum to the cecum. **il′eal** *adj*
  duplex i. congenital duplication of the ileum.
  terminal i. pars terminalis ilei.

il·e·us (il′e-əs) [L., from Gr. *eileos,* from *eilein* to roll up] 1. intestinal obstruction that is due to a nonmechanical cause, such as paralysis and failure of peristalsis. 2. formerly, any intestinal obstruction.
  adynamic i. ileus caused by inhibition of intestinal motility; it may be produced by any of numerous causes, most frequently by peritonitis.
  dynamic i. spastic i.
  gallstone i. a rare type of intestinal obstruction caused by impaction of a large gallstone in the intestine; seen mainly in elderly patients.
  hyperdynamic i. spastic i.
  mechanical i. term formerly used for intestinal obstructions from mechanical causes, such as hernias, adhesions, or volvulus.
  meconium i. ileus in the newborn due to blocking of the intestine with thick meconium, often associated with cystic fibrosis.
  occlusive i. mechanical i.
  paralytic i. adynamic i.
  spastic i. ileus due to persistent contracture of an intestinal segment, such as in Ogilvie syndrome. Called also *dynamic* or *hyperdynamic i.*

Ilex (i′leks) the hollies, a genus of small trees and shrubs of the family Aquifoliaceae. *I. paraguayen′sis* St. Hil. is a South American species whose leaves are the herb maté (q.v.). *I. verticilla′ta* L. Gray, the black alder or winterberry, has a tonic and astringent bark.

Il·he·us encephalitis, virus (ēl-ya′o͞os) [*Ilheus,* Brazil, where the disease was first observed in 1944] see under *encephalitis* and *virus.*

il·ia (il′e-ə) [L.] plural of *ilium.*

il·i·ac (il′e-ak) [L. *iliacus*] pertaining to the os ilium.

ili·adel·phus (il″e-ə-del′fəs) iliopagus.

ili(o)- [L. *ilium*] a combining form denoting relationship to the ilium or iliac region.

il·io·coc·cyg·e·al (il″e-o-kok-sij′e-əl) pertaining to the ilium and coccyx.

ilio·coc·cy·ge·us (il″e-o-kok-sij′e-us) [L., from *ilio-* + *coccygeus*] iliococcygeal; see under *musculus.*

il·io·cos·tal (il″e-o-kos′təl) [*ilio-* + *costal*] connecting or pertaining to the ilium and ribs.

il·io·fem·or·al (il″e-o-fem′or-əl) 1. pertaining to the ilium and femur. 2. pertaining to or connecting the iliac and femoral arteries.

il·io·hy·po·gas·tric (il″e-o-hi″po-gas′trik) pertaining to the ilium and hypogastrium.

il·io·in·gui·nal (il″e-o-in′gwĭ-nəl) pertaining to the iliac and inguinal regions.

il·io·lum·bar (il″e-o-lum′bər, -bahr) pertaining to the iliac and lumbar regions, or to the flank and loin.

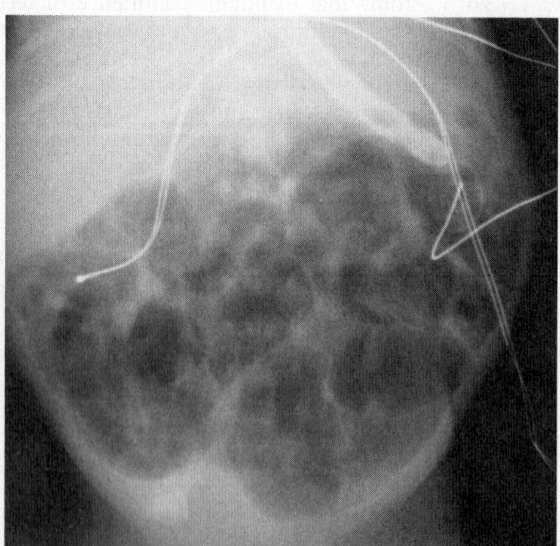

■ Meconium ileus in an anteroposterior view of the abdomen. The bowel is dilated and no gas is seen in the rectum.

il·io·lum·bo·cos·to·ab·dom·i·nal (il″e-o-lum″bo-kos″to-ab-dom′ĭ-nəl) pertaining to the iliac, lumbar, costal, and abdominal regions.

il·i·op·a·gus (il″e-op′ə-gəs) [*ilio-* + *-pagus*] symmetrical conjoined twins united in the iliac region.

il·io·pec·tin·e·al (il″e-o-pek-tin′e-al) pertaining to the ilium and pubic bone.

il·io·pel·vic (il″e-o-pel′vik) pertaining to the iliac region or muscle and to the pelvis.

il·io·pso·as (il″e-o-so′əs) see under *musculus.*

il·io·pu·bic (il″e-o-pu′bik) iliopectineal.

il·io·sa·cral (il″e-o-sa′krəl) pertaining to the ilium and the sacrum.

il·io·sci·at·ic (il″e-o-si-at′ik) pertaining to the ilium and the ischium.

il·io·spi·nal (il″e-o-spi′nəl) pertaining to the ilium and the vertebral (spinal) column.

il·io·tho·ra·cop·a·gus (il″e-o-thor″ə-kop′ə-gəs) [*ilio-* + *thoraco-* + *-pagus*] symmetrical conjoined twins fused from the pelvis to the thorax.

il·io·tib·i·al (il″e-o-tib′e-əl) pertaining to or extending between the ilium and tibia.

il·io·tro·chan·ter·ic (il″e-o-tro-kan-ter′ik) pertaining to the ilium and a trochanter.

il·io·xi·phop·a·gus (il″e-o-zi-fop′ə-gəs) symmetrical conjoined twins fused from the pelvis to the xiphoid process.

il·i·um (il′e-əm) pl. *il′ia* [L.] TA alternative for *os ilium.*

ill (il) 1. not well; sick. 2. a disease or disorder.
  föhn i. headache, weariness, and depression felt during the föhn (a wind from the south in Central Europe).
  joint i. navel i.
  louping i. a type of encephalomyelitis usually seen in sheep in Great Britain and Ireland, caused by a flavivirus transmitted by the tick, *Ixodes ricinus;* the sheep have tremors and sometimes jumping movements ("louping"), sometimes followed by paralysis.
  navel i. a generalized, often fatal septicemia seen in foals, lambs, and calves, usually characterized by omphalophlebitis with abscesses in the joints resulting in polyarthritis; it is due to infection through the open navel by organisms such as species of *Staphylococcus, Streptococcus, Shigella, Escherichia,* and *Pasteurella.* Called also *joint i.*
  quarter i. blackleg.

il·lac·ri·ma·tion (ĭ-lak″rĭ-ma′shən) epiphora.

Il·lic·i·um (ĭ-lis′e-əm) [L.] a genus of trees and shrubs of the family Magnoliaceae. *I. ve′rum* is an Asian tree whose fruit is Chinese or star anise (see under *anise*). *I. religio′sum* is the Japanese star anise or sikimi, a Japanese species whose leaves are poisonous.

il·li·ni·tion (il″ĭ-nish′ən) [L. *illinire* to smear] the application of an ointment or liniment with rubbing.

ill·ness (il′nis) disease.
  compressed-air i. decompression sickness.
  emotional i. a colloquialism roughly equivalent to "mental disorder," but not usually applied to those with a specific organic etiology or to mental retardation.
  influenzalike i. nonspecific respiratory illness whose symptoms resemble those of influenza; most cases are caused not by influenza virus infection but by other viruses or by bacteria.
  mental i. see under *disorder.*
  psychosomatic i. see under *disorder.*
  radiation i. see under *sickness.*

ill thrift (il thrift) unthriftiness.

il·lu·mi·na·tion (ĭ-loo″mĭ-na′shən) [L. *illuminatio*] 1. the lighting up of a part, cavity, organ, or object for inspection. 2. the luminous flux per unit area of a given surface; its SI unit is the lux. Symbol *E.*
  axial i. the transmission or reflection of light along the axis of a microscope.
  central i. axial i.
  contact i. illumination of the eye by means of an instrument which is pressed directly to the cornea and conjunctiva.
  critical i. the focusing of light precisely upon an object inspected.
  darkfield i., dark-ground i. the throwing of peripheral rays of light upon a microscopical object from the side, the center rays being blocked out: the object appears bright upon a dark background. See under *microscope,* and see *ultramicroscope.*
  direct i. the throwing of light upon a microscopical object from above or from the direction of observation.
  focal i. 1. the throwing of light upon the focus of a lens or mirror. 2. illumination of an object by focusing a source of light on it through an optical system.

Köhler i. an improved method of illumination by adjustment of the substage Abbe condenser, for obtaining the best image detail in microscopical work.
lateral i., oblique i. illumination in which the object is illuminated by oblique light.
through i. the transmission of light through an object, or from the direction opposite to that of observation.

il•lu•mi•na•tor (ĭ-loo″mĭ-na′tər) the source of light for viewing an object.
Abbe i. see under *condenser.*

il•lu•min•ism (ĭ-loo′min-iz-əm) a hallucinatory state characterized by conversations with imaginary, usually supernatural, beings.

il•lu•sion (ĭ-loo′zhən) [L. *illusio*] a false or misinterpreted sensory impression; a false interpretation of a real sensory image. Cf. *delusion.* **illu′sional** *adj*

Il•o•pan (il′o-pan) trademark for a preparation of dexpanthenol.

ilo•prost (i′lo-prost) a synthetic analogue of prostacyclin that is a systemic and pulmonary arterial dilator, used in the treatment of primary pulmonary hypertension; administered by inhalation.

Il•o•sone (il′o-sōn) trademark for a preparation of erythromycin estolate.

Ilo•ty•cin (i″lo-ti′sin) trademark for preparations of erythromycin.

Il•o•zyme (il′o-zīm) trademark for a preparation of pancrelipase.

ILT infectious laryngotracheitis.

Ili•to•vi•rus (il′ĭ-to-vi″rəs) [*i*nfectious *l*aryngo*t*racheitis + *virus*] a genus of viruses of the subfamily Alphaherpesvirinae, family Herpesviridae; the species gallid herpesvirus 1 causes infectious laryngotracheitis in poultry.

ILVEN inflammatory linear verrucous epidermal nevus.

IM intramuscular; see under *injection.*

im-[1] see *in-.*

im-[2] a prefix in chemical names indicating the bivalent group =NH.

ima (i′mə) [L.] lowest.

im•age (im′əj) [L. *imago*] a picture or conception with more or less likeness to an objective reality. See also *imaging.*
accidental i. afterimage.
body i. a three-dimensional concept of one's self, recorded in the cortex by the perception of ever-changing postures of the body and constantly changing with them.
direct i. virtual i.
eidetic i. an unusually vivid, elaborate, and exact mental image of objects previously seen or imagined.
erect i. virtual i.
false i. the one formed by the deviating eye in strabismus.
heteronymous i. the two images seen when the eyes are focused on a point beyond the object; cf. *crossed diplopia.*
homonymous i. the two images seen when the eyes are focused on a point nearer than the object; cf. *direct diplopia.*
incidental i. the impression of an image which remains on the retina after the object has been removed.
inverted i. real i.
memory i. a sensation or sense perception as it is pictured in the memory.
mental i. any concept corresponding to an object appreciated by the senses.
mirror i. 1. the image of light made visible by the reflecting surface of the cornea and lens when illuminated through the slit lamp. 2. an identical reproduction of an object except for transposition of right and left relations, as appears in the reflection of an object in a mirror.
motor i. the organized cerebral model of the possible movements of the body.
negative i. afterimage.
optical i. an image formed by the reflection of refraction of rays of light.
Purkinje-Sanson mirror i's reflected images formed on the anterior surface of the cornea and the anterior and posterior surfaces of the crystalline lens. The images on the two anterior surfaces are virtual and noninverted, and the image on the posterior surface is real and inverted. Useful in the study of the movement of the lens surfaces in accommodation and, formerly, in the evaluation of cataract.
radioisotope i. a quasi-pictorial representation of the distribution of radioactive materials in the body.
real i. an image formed where the emanating rays are collected, in which the object is pictured as being inverted.
retinal i. the representation formed upon the retina of an object seen.
Sanson i's Purkinje-Sanson mirror i's.
sensory i. a representation formed by means of one or more of the sense organs.

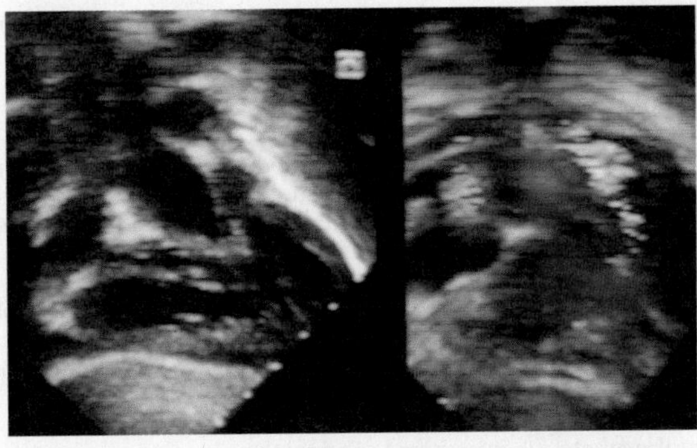

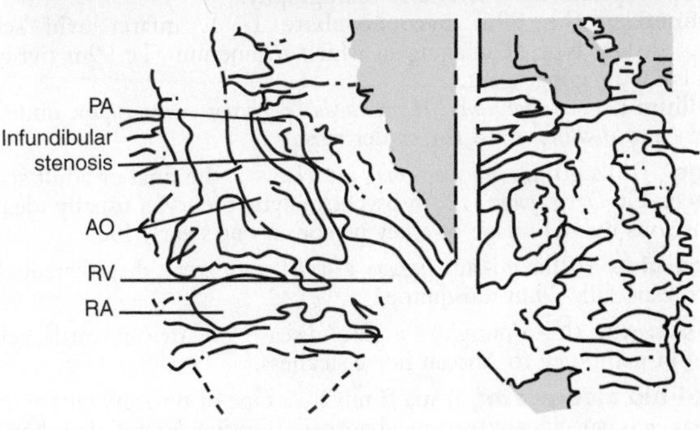

■ Color flow Doppler imaging *(right)* confirms turbulent flow across the stenotic area in tetralogy of Fallot; subcostal view *(left)* shows both valvular pulmonic and infundibular stenosis. *AO,* aorta; *PA,* pulmonary artery; *RA,* right atrium; *RV,* right ventricle.

specular i. mirror i. (def. 1).
virtual i. a picture from projected light rays that are intercepted before focusing, as by a plane mirror; it cannot be received on a screen, and it has the same orientation as the object. Called also *direct* or *erect i.*

im•age•ry (im′əj-re) 1. the formation of a mental representation of something perceived by the senses, often used synonymously with *visualization* (def. 2). 2. any of a number of therapeutic techniques that use the formation of such representations to elicit changes in attitudes, behaviors, or physiologic reactions.
guided i. a therapeutic technique in which the patient enters a relaxed state and focuses on an image related to the issue being confronted, which the therapist uses as the basis of an interactive dialogue in order to help the person resolve the issue; used for a wide variety of indications, including relaxation and stress management, behavior modification, pain management, and the treatment of life-threatening and terminal illness.

Im•a•gent GI (im′a-jənt) trademark for a preparation of perflubron.

imag•i•nes (ĭ-maj′ĭ-nēz) [L.] plural of *imago.*

imag•ing (im′ə-jing) the production of clarity, contrast, and detail in images, especially in radiological and ultrasound images.
color flow Doppler i. a method for visualizing direction and velocity of movement, as of blood flow within the cardiac chambers or blood vessels: color-coded flow direction and velocity information gathered by Doppler ultrasonography at multiple sites across the imaging field are superimposed onto a black and white cross-sectional image. Direction and velocity are coded as colors and shades, respectively, and used to produce color maps depicting blood flow.
echo planar i. a technique of magnetic resonance imaging in which the image is obtained in less than 50 msec; a single radiofrequency pulse is recalled several times in a series of echoes that are each encoded differently and from which the image can be reconstructed.
electrostatic i. a method of visualizing deep structures of the body, in which an electron beam, rather than x-rays, is passed through the patient and the emerging beam (unabsorbed electrons) strikes an electrostatically charged vacuum-packed plate, dissipating the charge according to the strength of the beam. A record (e.g., a film) is then made from the plate.
functional i. the use of imaging techniques such as magnetic resonance imaging and computed tomography to provide quantitative data about physiologic function.
gated cardiac blood pool i. equilibrium radionuclide angiocardiography.
gated magnetic resonance i. a method of magnetic resonance imaging in which motion and other artifacts are minimized by gating signal

acquisition, such as by linking sampling to electrocardiographic information in cardiac studies.

gray-scale i. see under *ultrasonography*.

hot spot i. infarct avid scintigraphy.

infarct avid i. see under *scintigraphy*.

magnetic resonance i. (MRI) a method of visualizing soft tissues of the body by applying an external magnetic field that makes it possible to distinguish between hydrogen atoms in different environments. This is an application of the principle of nuclear magnetic resonance (q.v.).

myocardial perfusion i. see under *scintigraphy*.

narrow band i. an endoscopic technique that creates a high-resolution image by means of filters that remove visible light except for a narrow bandwidth in the blue and green spectrum in order to increase the contrast between the epithelial surface and underlying blood vessels.

nuclear i., nuclear medicine i. radionuclide scanning.

pyrophosphate i. infarct avid scintigraphy.

technetium Tc 99m pyrophosphate i. 1. infarct avid scintigraphy. 2. any type of imaging in which technetium Tc 99m pyrophosphate is the imaging agent.

thallium i. see *thallium-201 myocardial perfusion scintigraphy*, under *scintigraphy* and *thallium stress test*, under *tests*.

ima•go (ĭ-ma′go) pl. *imagoes*, *imag′ines* [L.] 1. the final or adult stage of an insect. Cf. *larva*, *pupa*. 2. in psychoanalytic theory, a usually idealized, unconscious mental image of a key person in one's early life.

ima•go•cide (ĭ-ma′go-sīd) [*imago* + *-cide*] an agent that destroys adult insects, especially adult mosquitoes.

im•a•pun•ga (im-ə-pung′ə) a rare disease of African cattle, closely related in pathology to African horse sickness.

im•at•i•nib mes•y•late (ĭ-mă′tĭ-nib″) a type of tyrosine kinase inhibitor that acts specifically on an abnormal tyrosine kinase that has been created by the Philadelphia chromosome abnormality and is constitutively present in chronic myeloid leukemia. It is used in the treatment of chronic myeloid leukemia during blast crisis, accelerated phase, or chronic phase after failure of interferon-α therapy, administered orally.

im•bal•ance (im-bal′əns) 1. dysequilibrium (def. 2). 2. inability to stand upright; lack of balance between muscles.

autonomic i. 1. ataxia caused by a problem in the autonomic nervous system. 2. any disturbance of the autonomic nervous system.

binocular i. inequality in some aspect of binocular vision, such as aniseikonia, anisometropia, heterophoria, or strabismus.

vasomotor i. autonomic i.

im•bed (im-bed′) embed; see *embedding*.

im•bi•bi•tion (im″bĭ-bish′ən) [L. *imbibere* to drink] 1. the absorption of a liquid. 2. insudation.

im•bri•cat•ed (im′brĭ-kāt″əd) [L. *imbricatus*, from *imbrex* tile] overlapping like tiles or shingles.

im•bri•ca•tion (im″brĭ-ka′shən) the overlapping of apposing surfaces, like shingles on a roof.

ImD_{50} median immunizing dose.

Im•dur (im′dər) trademark for a preparation of isosorbide mononitrate.

Imers•lund syndrome (e′mər-slund) [Olga *Imerslund*, Norwegian physician, 20th century] see under *syndrome*.

Imers•lund-Graes•beck syndrome (e′mər-slund grās′bek) [O. *Imerslund;* Ralph Gustav *Graesbeck*, Finnish biochemist, born 1930] see under *syndrome*.

IMF inframammary fold.

im•id•a•clo•prid (im″id-ə-klo′prid) an insecticide used against pests of food crops and ectoparasites of domestic animals.

im•id•az•ole (im″id-az′ōl) 1. a five-membered heterocyclic organic compound containing two nitrogen atoms in the ring:

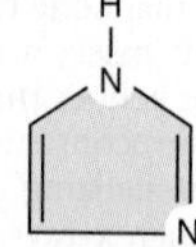

It is a type of azole, and is an antimetabolite and inhibitor of histamine and is used as an insecticide. 2. any of a class of fungistatic compounds containing such a ring, a subset of the class of azole antifungals, effective against a wide range of fungi; they alter cell membrane functions and permeability by inhibiting the biosynthesis of ergosterol.

im•i•daz•o•lone (im″id-az′ə-lōn) an advanced glycation end product seen in increased amounts in end-stage renal disease, diabetic nephropathy, and arthritis.

im•id•azo•lyl•eth•yl•amine (im″id-az″o-ləl-eth″əl-am′in) histamine.

im•ide (im′īd) any compound containing the bivalent group =NH, to which are attached only acid radicals.

imido- a prefix denoting the presence in a compound of the bivalent group =NH attached to two acid radicals.

imid•o•carb hy•dro•chlo•ride (im′ĭ-do-kahrb) a veterinary antiprotozoal used against *Babesia*.

imi•do•di•pep•tide (im″ĭ-do-di-pep′tīd) a dipeptide in which the C-terminal amino acid is an imino acid. Cf. *iminodipeptide*.

imi•do•di•pep•ti•du•ria (im″ĭ-do-di-pep″tĭ-du′re-ə) excretion of imidodipeptides in the urine, as in prolidase deficiency.

imi•do•gen (ĭ-mid′o-jən) the bivalent radical =NH.

im•i•glu•cer•ase (im″ĭ-gloo′sər-ās) an analogue of glucosylceramidase produced by recombinant DNA technology, used as an enzyme replenisher to replace glucosylceramidase (glucocerebrosidase) in type 1 Gaucher disease; administered by intravenous infusion.

im•in•az•ole (im″in-az′ōl) imidazole.

imine (ĭ-mēn′) an organic compound containing an imino group; in a *substituted imine*, a nonacyl group replaces the imino hydrogen.

imino- a prefix used to denote the presence of the bivalent group =NH attached to nonacid radicals.

im•i•no ac•id (im′ĭ-no) an organic acid containing the bivalent group =NH, such as proline or hydroxyproline.

imi•no•di•ace•tic ac•id (IDA) (im″ĭ-no-di″ə-se′tik) a simple dicarboxylic acid containing an imino group; radiolabeled (^{99m}Tc) analogues of iminodiacetic acid are used in hepatobiliary imaging.

hepatobiliary i. a. (HIDA) a term traditionally used as a synonym for lidofenin (q.v.), but sometimes used more broadly for the class of radiolabeled (^{99m}Tc), substituted analogues of iminodiacetic acid used in hepatobiliary imaging, including disofenin, lidofenin, and mebrofenin.

im•i•no•di•pep•tide (im″ĭ-no-di-pep′tīd) a dipeptide in which the N-terminal amino acid is an imino acid. Cf. *imidodipeptide*.

im•i•no•gly•cin•uria (im″ĭ-no-gli″sin-u′re-ə) a benign, polygenic, autosomal recessive disorder of renal tubular reabsorption of glycine and the imino acids proline and hydroxyproline, marked by excessive levels of all three substances in the urine without clinical symptoms.

im•i•no•stil•bene (im″ĭ-no-stil′bēn) a tricyclic tertiary amine similar in ring structure to the tricyclic antidepressants; the term is used to describe a class of anticonvulsants with such a structure that are employed in the treatment of epilepsy, e.g., carbamazepine.

imi•no•urea (im″ĭ-no-u′re-ə) guanidine.

im•i•pen•em (im″ĭ-pen′əm) [USP] a broad-spectrum antibiotic of the carbapenem group, having activity against a wide range of gram-positive and gram-negative organisms. Because it is hydrolyzed by a dipeptidase occurring in the proximal renal tubule, it is administered with the dipeptidase inhibitor cilastatin sodium.

imip•ra•mine (ĭ-mip′rə-mēn) a tricyclic antidepressant of the dibenzazepine class, the first of the tricyclic antidepressants to be used.

i. hydrochloride [USP] the monohydrochloride salt of imipramine, used especially in endogenous depression; used also in the treatment of childhood enuresis, panic disorder, chronic pain, attention-deficit/hyperactivity disorder, cataplexy associated with narcolepsy, urinary incontinence, and bulimia nervosa. Administered orally or intramuscularly.

i. pamoate a tricyclic antidepressant with uses similar to those of imipramine hydrochloride, except that it is not used to treat enuresis.

im•i•quim•od (im″ĭ-kwim′od) a biologic response modifier used topically in the treatment of condyloma acuminatum of the external genitalia and perianal region.

Im•i•trex (im-′ĭ-treks″) trademark for a preparation of sumatriptan succinate.

im•ma•ture (im″ə-chōōr′) [*in-*[2] + *mature*] unripe or not fully developed.

im•me•di•ate (ĭ-me′de-ət) [*in-*[2] + *mediate*] direct; with nothing intervening; occurring without delay.

im•mer•sion (ĭ-mur′zhən) [L. *immersio*] 1. the placing or plunging of a body into a liquid. 2. the use of the microscope with the object and object glass both covered with a liquid.

homogeneous i. the employment in microscopy of a liquid of nearly the same refractive power as the cover glass.

oil i. the covering of the microscopical objective and the object with oil.

water i. the covering of the microscopical objective and the object with water.

im•mis•ci•ble (ĭ-mis′ĭ-bəl) not susceptible to being mixed.

im•mit•tance (ĭ-mit′əns) [*im*pedance + ad*mittance*] a term coined to express the effect of both admittance and impedance.

acoustic i. measurement of energy flow through the middle ear by assessing acoustic admittance, acoustic impedance, or both.

im•mo•bil•i•ty (ĭ″mo-bil′ĭ-te) the state of being immovable.

im•mo•bil•iza•tion (ĭ-mo″bĭ-lĭ-za′shən) the act of rendering immovable, as by a cast or splint.

im•mo•bi•lize (ĭ-mo′bĭ-līz) [*in-*[2] + *mobilis* movable] to render incapable of being moved, as by a cast or splint.

im•mo•bi•liz•er (ĭ-mo′bĭ-li″zər) something that immobilizes.

sternal-occipital-mandibular i. (SOMI) any of a variety of cervical orthoses that have two or three posts running between head plates and a jacket or corset; called also *SOMI orthosis.*

im•mor•tal•i•za•tion (ĭ-mor″təl-ĭ-za′shən) acquisition of immunity to normal limitations on growth or life span, sometimes achieved by animal cells in vitro or by tumor cells; causes may be spontaneous mutation, exposure to chemical carcinogens, or viral infection.

im•mune (ĭ-mūn′) [L. *immunis* free, exempt] 1. protected against infectious disease by either specific or nonspecific mechanisms. 2. pertaining to the immune system and immune responses.

im•mu•ni•ty (ĭ-mu′nĭ-te) [L. *immunitas*] the condition of being immune; the protection against infectious disease conferred either by the immune response generated by immunization or previous infection or by other nonimmunologic factors.

acquired i. immunity involving the functioning of the immune system acquired by natural infection or vaccination (active immunity) or transfer of antibody or lymphocytes from an immune donor (passive immunity). Cf. *innate i.*

active i. acquired immunity that develops in response to antigenic stimulus. Cf. *passive i.*

adoptive i. passive immunity of the cell-mediated type conferred by the administration of sensitized lymphocytes from an immune donor.

antibacterial i. immunity against the action of bacteria, i.e., the ability to resist infection by bacteria.

antitoxic i. immunity against toxins, attributable to the presence of specific antitoxin(s) in the immune individual.

antiviral i. immunity against viruses.

artificial i. acquired immunity produced by deliberate exposure to an antigen *(active immunity),* as in vaccination, or by the transfer of immunoglobulins from an immune individual to a nonimmune one *(passive immunity).*

cell-mediated i. (CMI), cellular i. immunity mediated by T lymphocytes either through release of lymphokines or through exertion of direct cytotoxicity, transmissible by transfer of lymphocytes but not serum; it includes type IV hypersensitivity reactions, such as contact dermatitis, granulomatous disease, allograft rejection, graft-versus-host disease, and systemic responses to viral or microbial infections or to tumor cells. Called also *T cell–mediated i.* Cf. *humoral i.*

community i. herd i.

concomitant i. infection i.

cross i. immunity produced by inoculation with an agent (e.g., a bacterium or virus) that is different from, but closely related to, the agent causing the disease.

familial i. innate i.

genetic i. innate i.

herd i. the resistance of a group to attack by a disease because of the immunity of a large proportion of the members and the consequent lessening of the likelihood of an affected individual coming into contact with a susceptible individual.

humoral i. immunity mediated by antibodies. Cf. *cell-mediated i.*

infection i. the development of resistance to reinfection even though the original infection persists, an apparent paradox. Called also *concomitant i.*

inherent i. innate i.

inherited i. innate i.

innate i. immunity based on the genetic constitution of the individual, e.g., immunity of humans to canine distemper. Called also *familial i., genetic i., inherent i., inherited i.,* and *native i.*

intrauterine i. passive immunity acquired by the fetus as a consequence of the passage of maternal IgG antibodies from an immune mother through the placenta into the fetal circulation.

local i. immunity confined to a particular tissue or organ.

maternal i. passively transferred humoral immunity from the mother to the offspring, across the placenta before birth in primates, from the colostrum via the intestines in ungulates, and from the egg yolk in birds.

native i. innate i.

natural i. immunity mediated by cells capable of immune activity without being stimulated by immunization and without antigen specificity, e.g., the activity of NK cells against virus infection and tumor cells.

nonspecific i. immunity that does not involve the recognition of antigen by lymphocytes and the mounting of a specific immune response; e.g., the protection afforded by lysozyme, interferon, the cells involved in natural immunity, and anatomical barriers to infection.

passive i. acquired immunity that a person receives by transfer of antibody or lymphocytes from an immune donor. Cf. *active i.*

species i. resistance of members of a particular species to a disease; immunity enjoyed by members of a particular species and determined by their genetic constitution.

specific i. immunity against a particular disease, e.g., scarlet fever, or against a particular antigen.

T cell–mediated i. (TCMI) cell-mediated i.

tissue i. local i.

im•mu•ni•za•tion (im″u-nĭ-za′shən) the induction of immunity; see *active i.* and *passive i.*

active i. stimulation of the immune system to confer protection against disease, e.g., by administration of a vaccine or toxoid.

adoptive i. passive immunization by transfer of sensitized lymphocytes from an immune donor to a previously nonimmune recipient.

passive i. the conferring of specific immune reactivity on previously nonimmune individuals by the administration of sensitized lymphoid cells or serum from immune individuals.

im•mu•nize (im′u-nīz) to render immune.

im•mu•no•ab•la•tion (im″u-no-ab-la′shən) an immunotherapy technique involving severe or complete immunosuppression with ablation of a cell population, such as in the ablative step preceding bone marrow transplantation. **immunoab′lative** *adj*

im•mu•no•ad•ju•vant (im″u-no-aj′ə-vənt) a nonspecific stimulator of the immune response, e.g., BCG vaccine or Freund's complete and incomplete adjuvants.

im•mu•no•ad•sor•bent (im″u-no-ad-sor′bənt) a preparation of antigen or antibody in an insoluble form used to bind homologous antibody or antigen, respectively, and remove it from a mixture of substances.

im•mu•no•ad•sorp•tion (im″u-no-ad-sorp′shən) the use of an immunoadsorbent to effect a chemical separation of antigen or antibody, as in immunoassays or in affinity chromatography.

im•mu•no•as•say (im″u-no-as′a) any of several methods for the quantitative determination of chemical substances that utilize the highly specific binding between an antigen or hapten and homologous antibodies, including radioimmunoassay, enzyme immunoassay, and fluorescence immunoassay.

enzyme i. (EIA) any of several immunoassay methods that use an enzyme covalently linked to an antigen or antibody as a label, the two most common being ELISA (enzyme-linked immunosorbent assay) and EMIT (enzyme multiplied immunoassay technique).

fluorescence i., fluorescent i. (FIA) any immunoassay using fluorochrome-labeled antibody or antigen; classified as either *heterogeneous* or *homogeneous.* Called also *fluoroimmunoassay,* and *immunofluorescence assay.*

heterogeneous fluorescence i. a fluorescence immunoassay that has more than one phase, requiring separation of the bound label (antigen-antibody complex) from the free labeled immunoreactant by physiochemical methods.

homogeneous fluorescence i. a fluorescence immunoassay that is single-phase and uses a change in fluorescence (such as quenching or increased polarization) accompanying antigen-antibody binding to measure the amount of bound label without separation.

im•mu•no•bead (im′u-no-bēd″) a minute plastic bead coated with antigen or antibody so that it aggregates or agglutinates in the presence of the corresponding antibody or antigen; used in the immunobead assay.

im•mu•no•bio•log•i•cal (im″u-no-bi″o-loj′ĭ-kəl) an antigenic or antibody-containing preparation derived from a pool of human or animal donors, including vaccines, toxoids, immune globulins, and antitoxins; used for immunization and immune therapy.

im•mu•no•bi•ol•o•gy (im″u-no-bi-ol′ə-je) the branch of biology dealing with immunologic effects on such phenomena as infectious disease, growth and development, recognition phenomena, hypersensitivity, heredity, aging, cancer, and transplantation.

im•mu•no•blast (im′u-no-blast″) lymphoblast. **immunoblas′tic** *adj*

im•mu•no•blot (im′u-no-blot″) to transfer proteins onto a membrane or other immobilizing matrix, analyzing or identifying them via antigen-antibody specific reactions, or the blot resulting from this process, as in a Western blot or dot blot. The term is sometimes used synonymously with Western blot.

im•mu•no•chem•i•cal (im″u-no-kem′ĭ-kəl) pertaining to immunochemistry.

im•mu•no•chem•is•try (im″u-no-kem′is-tre) 1. the study of the chemical basis of immunologic phenomena. 2. the application of antibodies as chemical reagents.

im·mu·no·che·mo·ther·a·py (im″u-no-ke″mo-ther′ə-pe) a combination of immunotherapy and chemotherapy.

im·mu·no·chro·ma·tog·ra·phy (im″mu-no-kro″mə-tog′rə-fe) the separating out of components of a mixture by chromatographic and immunoassay methods.

im·mu·no·com·pe·tence (im″u-no-kom′pə-təns) the ability or capacity to develop an immune response (i.e., antibody production and/or cell-mediated immunity) following exposure to antigen; called also *immunoresponsiveness* and *immunologic competence*. **immunocom′petent** *adj*

im·mu·no·com·plex (im″u-no-kom′pləks) antigen-antibody complex.

im·mu·no·com·pro·mised (im″u-no-kom′prə-mīzd) having the immune response attenuated by administration of immunosuppressive drugs, by irradiation, by malnutrition, or by some disease processes (e.g., cancer or the acquired immune deficiency syndrome).

im·mu·no·con·glu·ti·nin (im″u-no-kən-gloo′tĭ-nin) an autoantibody, usually of the immunoglobulin M class, that is specific for activated C3 and C4 components of complement. It is found in low titer in most normal sera and in increased levels in certain infectious diseases, in autoimmune disease, and after immunization with many antigens. Not to be confused with *conglutinin*. Called also *immune conglutinin*.

im·mu·no·con·ju·gate (im″u-no-kon′jo͝o-gāt) a conjugate comprising an immune substance such as an antibody and a diagnostic or therapeutic substance such as a cytotoxic compound or a radioisotope, used especially to target specific cells in cancer therapy.

im·mu·no·cyte (im′u-no-sīt″) a cell of the lymphoid series that can react with antigen to produce antibody or to become active in cell-mediated immunity or delayed hypersensitivity reactions; called also *immunologically competent cell*.

im·mu·no·cy·to·ad·her·ence (im″u-no-si″to-ad-hēr′əns) the formation of rosettes by the binding of red cells bearing a homologous antigen to lymphocytes bearing surface immunoglobulin (B cells); used to identify B cells.

im·mu·no·cy·to·chem·is·try (im″u-no-si″to-kem′is-tre) a technique for detecting an antigen expressed by cells, using antibody specific for the antigen coupled to a label that is visible by light microscopy. Sometimes used interchangeably with *immunohistochemistry*. **immunocytochem′ical** *adj*

im·mu·no·cy·to·ma (im″u-no-si-to′mə) lymphoplasmacytic lymphoma.

cutaneous i. marginal zone lymphoma.

im·mu·no·de·fi·cien·cy (im″u-no-də-fish′ən-se) a deficiency of immune response or a disorder characterized by deficient immune response; classified as *antibody* (B cell), *cellular* (T cell), or *combined immunodeficiency*, or *phagocytic dysfunction disorders*. See accompanying table. See also *acquired immunodeficiency syndrome*, under *syndrome*. **immunodefi′cient** *adj*

antibody i. deficiency in immunity mediated by B lymphocytes, marked by hypo- or dysgammaglobulinemia and recurrent bacterial otitis media and sinopulmonary infections. For a list of disorders of this type, see table.

cellular i. deficiency in cellular immunity (q.v.), marked by recurrent infections with low-grade or opportunistic pathogens, by graft-versus-host reactions following blood transfusions, and by severe disease following immunization with live vaccines. For a list of disorders of this type, see table.

combined i. deficiency of lymphoid cells that mediate both humoral immunity (B lymphocytes) and cellular immunity (T lymphocytes). See table. Called also *combined immunodeficiency disease*.

common variable i. (CVID), common variable unclassifiable i. a heterogeneous group of disorders characterized by hypogammaglobulinemia, decreased antibody production in response to antigenic challenge, and recurrent pyogenic infections, and often associated with hematologic and autoimmune disorders. Most patients have normal numbers of circulating B lymphocytes, which can identify antigens and proliferate, but lack plasma cells and appear to have an intrinsic defect of B cell differentiation. However, two other forms are also recognized: that due to a disorder of T lymphocyte regulation and that due to production of autoantibodies against T and B lymphocytes. Called also *common variable agammaglobulinemia* or *hypogammaglobulinemia*.

i. with elevated IgM, i. with hyper-IgM a rare syndrome characterized by elevated immunoglobulin M levels and decreased levels of G and A immunoglobulins, associated with recurrent pyogenic infections, and possibly caused by failure of IgM-producing cells to switch to production of IgC and IgA. Most cases appear to exhibit X-linked recessive inheritance.

severe combined i. (SCID) a group of rare congenital disorders characterized by gross impairment of both humoral and cell-mediated immunity and absence of T lymphocytes; some forms are also characterized by a lack of B lymphocytes. In most cases all classes of immunoglobulins are nearly or completely absent, and there is marked lymphocytopenia. Persistent diarrhea, chronic mucocutaneous candidiasis, and failure to thrive occur in infancy. Blood transfusions can result in graft-versus-host disease and routine vaccinations in fatal infection. Unless immune function is restored by a histocompatible bone marrow or fetal tissue transplant or the patient is kept in gnotobiotic isolation, death from opportunistic infection usually occurs before the first birthday. In approximately 50 per cent of cases, the disorder is X-linked and due to a defect in the γ chain of the receptor for IL-2 and other interleukins. B lymphocyte numbers are usually normal. The remaining 50 per cent of cases are of autosomal recessive inheritance and have varying etiologies, including defects in activity of adenosine deaminase, purine-nucleoside phosphorylase, or Janus kinase 3 (JAK3). A rare type of the autosomal recessive form is called *reticular dysgenesis*.

i. with short-limbed dwarfism short-limbed dwarfism marked by short, pudgy hands, redundant skin, and hyperextensible joints of the hands and feet associated with immunodeficiency, which may be either antibody or cellular or combined.

i. with thymoma an immunodeficiency disorder in which thymoma, usually of the benign spindle-cell type, is associated with hypogammaglobulinemia; deficiencies of cell-mediated immunity, such as eosinopenia, hypoplastic or aplastic anemia, or autoimmune diseases, may occur also. Removal of the thymoma does not cure the immunodeficiency, and patients suffer from recurrent severe infections.

im·mu·no·de·pres·sion (im″u-no-də-presh′ən) immunosuppression.

Primary Immunodeficiency Disorders, Diseases, and Syndromes

Antibody (B-Cell) Deficiency Disorders
- X-linked agammaglobulinemia (Bruton disease)
- Common variable immunodeficiency
- Transient hypogammaglobulinemia of infancy
- Selective IgA deficiency
- Immunodeficiency with hyper-IgM
- Selective IgM deficiency
- Selective deficiency of IgG subclasses
- Kappa light chain deficiency
- Secretory component deficiency
- Specific antibody deficiency with normal immunoglobulins
- X-linked lymphoproliferative syndrome (Duncan syndrome)

Cellular (T-Cell) Deficiency Disorders
- Thymic hypoplasia (DiGeorge syndrome)
- Chronic mucocutaneous candidiasis
- Acquired immunodeficiency syndrome (AIDS)

Combined (B-Cell and T-Cell) Deficiency Disorders
- Severe combined immunodeficiency (SCID)*
  - Autosomal recessive SCID
  - SCID with adenosine deaminase deficiency
  - SCID with purine nucleoside phosphorylase deficiency
  - X-linked recessive SCID
  - Reticular dysgenesis
- Cellular immunodeficiency with immunoglobulins (Nezlof syndrome)
- Immunodeficiency with thrombocytopenia and eczema (Wiskott-Aldrich syndrome)
- Ataxia-telangiectasia
- Immunodeficiency with short-limbed dwarfism
- Immunodeficiency with thymoma
- Transcobalamin II deficiency
- Episodic lymphopenia with lymphotoxin

Phagocytic Dysfunction Disorders
- Chédiak-Higashi syndrome
- Chronic granulomatous disease
- Job syndrome
- Lazy leukocyte syndrome
- Deficiency disorders
  - Alkaline phosphatase deficiency
  - Glucose-6-phosphate dehydrogenase deficiency
  - Myeloperoxidase deficiency
  - Tuftsin deficiency
- Elevated IgE with defective chemotaxis, eczema, and recurrent infection
- Leukocyte movement disorders

*Some forms of SCID, although deficient in both antibody and cellular immunity, actually have normal numbers of B cells.

im•mu•no•de•pres•sive (im″u-no-də-pres′iv) immunosuppressive.

im•mu•no•der•ma•tol•o•gy (im″u-no-dur″mə-tol′ə-je) the study of immunologic phenomena as they affect skin disorders and their treatment or prophylaxis.

im•mu•no•de•tec•tion (im″u-no-de-tek′shən) detection of a substance or reaction by means of the specific interaction of antibody with antigen.

im•mu•no•de•vi•a•tion (im″u-no-de″ve-a′shən) split tolerance (def. 2).

im•mu•no•di•ag•no•sis (im″u-no-di″əg-no′sis) diagnosis based on blood serum reactions to antigens; serodiagnosis.

im•mu•no•dif•fu•sion (im″u-no-dĭ-fu′zhən) any technique involving diffusion of antigen or antibody through a semisolid medium, usually agar or agarose gel, resulting in a precipitin reaction. Precipitin lines or bands form where the concentrations of antigen and antibody are serologically equivalent.
radial i. (RID) a quantitative immunodiffusion technique in which the antigen solutions are placed in wells cut in an agar plate containing antiserum; the area or diameter of the precipitin ring around an unknown solution is compared with the rings of a serial dilution of a standard antigen solution to determine the amount of antigen present in the unknown. Called also *single radial diffusion.*

im•mu•no•dom•i•nance (im″u-no-dom′ĭ-nəns) the degree to which a subunit of an antigenic determinant is involved in binding or reacting with specific antibody.

im•mu•no•dom•i•nant (im″u-no-dom′ĭ-nənt) denoting the subunits of the antigenic determinant group that most influence the specificity of the induced antibodies.

im•mu•no•dot (im′u-no-dot″) dot blot.

im•mu•no•elec•tro•pho•re•sis (im″u-no-e-lek″tro-fə-re′sis) a technique combining protein electrophoresis and double immunodiffusion; proteins are separated by agarose gel electrophoresis; then specific antisera are placed in a trough cut parallel to the protein track, and the proteins and antibodies are allowed to diffuse through the gel, the proteins diffusing radially from their electrophoretic placement and the antibodies diffusing perpendicularly from the trough, resulting in a distinct elliptical precipitin arc for each protein detectable by the antisera. Abbreviated IEP.
counter i. counterimmunoelectrophoresis.
countercurrent i. counterimmunoelectrophoresis.
crossed i. a combination of protein electrophoresis and rocket immunoelectrophoresis; protein antigens are separated by agarose gel electrophoresis; then a strip containing the separated antigens is cut out and placed in a trough in a gel containing antiserum, and an electric field perpendicular to the trough is applied, producing a "rocket" precipitin pattern for each antigen.
rocket i. one-dimensional single electroimmunodiffusion; a technique in which antigen is placed in a row of wells in an agar plate containing antiserum and an electric field perpendicular to the line of wells is applied; this drives the antigen through the gel, forming a spike or "rocket" precipitin pattern trailing away from each well. The length of the rocket is proportional to the amount of antigen placed in the well. Called also *Laurell technique.*

im•mu•no•en•do•crine (im″u-no-en′do-krin) pertaining to the immune and endocrine systems or the interactions between them.

im•mu•no•en•do•cri•nop•a•thy (im″u-no-en″do-krĭ-nop′ə-the) a disease or condition that affects both endocrine glands and the immune system, such as Addison disease or the polyglandular autoimmune syndromes.

im•mu•no•fer•ri•tin (im″u-no-fer′ĭ-tin) an antibody labeled with ferritin; when combined with antigen, the antigenic determinant sites are visible under the electron microscope.

im•mu•no•fil•tra•tion (im″u-no-fil-tra′shən) the purification of antigen or antibody using an immunoadsorbent.

im•mu•no•flu•o•res•cence (im″u-no-floo̅-res′əns) any immunohistochemical method that uses antibody labeled with a fluorescent dye.
direct i. immunofluorescence involving a specific antibody or antiserum that is conjugated with a fluorochrome and is used as a specific fluorescent stain.
indirect i. immunofluorescence that involves a fluorochrome attached to an antiglobulin, with a tissue constituent that is stained using an unlabeled specific antibody and the labeled antiglobulin, which binds the unlabeled antibody.

im•mu•no•gen (im′u-no-jən) a substance capable of inducing an immune response, in most contexts synonymous with antigen; in some contexts immunogen is used to draw a distinction with substances capable of reacting only with antibody (antigens or haptens) or to denote a form of an antigen that induces an immune response as opposed to a tolerogen, a form that induces tolerance.

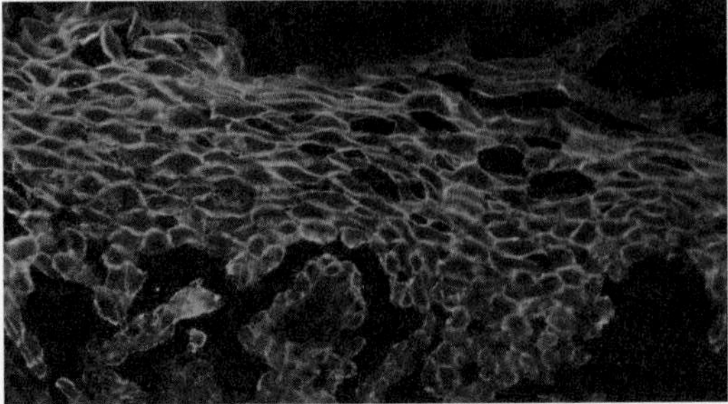

■ Immunofluorescence *(green)* used to detect pemphigus vulgaris.

im•mu•no•ge•net•ic (im″u-no-jə-net′ik) pertaining to immunology and genetics.

im•mu•no•ge•net•ics (im″u-no-jə-net′iks) [*immuno-* + *genetics*] the study of the genetics of the immune response, such as the study of immune response genes, or the association of human leukocyte antigens with disease susceptibility, or the generation of antibody diversity.

im•mu•no•gen•ic (im″u-no-jen′ik) producing immunity; evoking an immune response.

im•mu•no•ge•nic•i•ty (im″u-no-jə-nis′ĭ-te) the property that endows a substance with the capacity to provoke an immune response, or the degree to which a substance possesses this property.

im•mu•no•glob•u•lin (im″u-no-glob′u-lin) any of the structurally related glycoproteins that function as antibodies, divided into five classes (IgM, IgG, IgA, IgD, and IgE) on the basis of structure and biologic activity. The basic structural unit of the immunoglobulin molecule, referred to as a monomer, is a Y-shaped molecule composed of two heavy (H) chains and two light (L) chains (see illustration). IgD, IgG, and IgE occur only as monomers; IgM and IgA may occur as monomers or polymers. The polymeric forms contain an additional polypeptide called the J chain, and secretory IgA contains another structure called the secretory component (SC). Each chain consists of a variable region (V_H or V_L) and a constant region (C_H or C_L), which are coded for by different genes. Parts of the V_H and V_L regions make up the antigen-binding site, one on each "arm" (Fab region) of the monomer. An individual can make about 10^4 different V_H regions and 10^3 V_L regions, which combine to make about 10^7 different antigen-binding sites, each with a distinct antigenic specificity. Parts of the C_H regions make up the "body" (Fc region) of the monomer, which contains various sites responsible for the biological activity of the molecule. In any one immunoglobulin molecule, all of the H chains are identical, as are the L chains. The C_H region determines both the heavy chain class to which the H chain belongs and the immunoglobulin class to which the molecule belongs. The H chain classes are denoted by the Greek letters (μ, δ, γ, ε, and α) corresponding to the Latin letters of the immunoglobulin classes, e.g., μ to IgM. There are two types of light chains (denoted κ and λ), either of which may combine with any of the heavy chains and thus occur in any of the immunoglobulin classes. In human immunoglobulins, three of the classes (IgM, IgG, and IgA) have subclasses; i.e., there are several similar but distinct C_H region genes in these classes. In addition, the λ light chain type has subtypes. The subclasses (subtypes) are denoted by numerical suffixes, e.g., IgG1 and γ1 subclasses and λ2 subtype. Immunoglobulins (monomeric IgM and IgD) first appear on the surface of B cells as antigen receptors. When a cell is activated by contact with antigen and differentiates into a plasma cell, the cell continues to produce the same L chain and V_H region of the H chain, but gene rearrangement may occur to attach this V_H region to a different C_H region (class switching). Thus the secreted immunoglobulin may be of any class but has the same antigenic specificity as the antigen receptors of the parent B cell. In addition to the effects produced solely by the binding of antigen by antibody, e.g., viral neutralization or the inability of some bacteria to invade mucosal surfaces when coated by antibody, certain classes of antibodies can trigger other processes when bound to antigen: IgM and IgG activate the classic complement pathway, IgA and IgG activate the alternative pathway, and IgM, IgG1, and IgG3 act as opsonins, triggering phagocytosis of the bound antigens by macrophages and neutrophils. IgE has the unique function of mediating immediate hypersensitivity (q.v.) reactions; it binds to specific receptors on basophils and mast cells and triggers the release of mediators on contact with antigen. IgG is the only class transferred across the placenta, providing the fetus and neonate with protection against infection. See also *immunoglobulin genes,* under *gene, homology region,* under *region,* and *allotype, idiotype,* and *isotype.*
antilymphocyte i. see under *globulin.*
monoclonal i. see *M component.*
secretory i. A secretory IgA; the predominant immunoglobulin in secretions (oral, nasal, bronchial, urogenital, and intestinal mucous secretions

The Human Immunoglobulins

	Polypeptide Chains								
	H Chains					L Chains		Other	
	μ	γ	α	δ	ε	κ	λ	J	SC*
Immunoglobulin classes	IgM	IgG	IgA	IgD	IgE	all	all	IgM, IgA	IgA
Subclasses or subtypes	—	1–4	1,2	—	—	—	1–4	—	—
Allotypes	—	Gm (1–25)	Am (1–2)	—	—	Km (1–3)	—	—	—
Mol. wt. (kDa)	70	50	55	62	70	23	23	15	70
Carbohydrate (%)	15	4	10	18	18	—	—	8	16

	Immunoglobulins					
	Serum					Secretory
	IgM	IgG	IgA	IgD	IgE	IgA
Molecular formula	$(\mu_2L_2)_5J$	γ_2L_2	α_2L_2 or $(\alpha_2L_2)_nJ^{\dagger}$	δ_2L_2	ε_2L_2	$(\alpha_2L_2)_2J$, SC
Mol. wt (kDa)	900	150	153; 325; 580	180	190	400
Sedimentation coefficient (S)	19	7	7; 10; 14	7	8	—
Electrophoretic mobility	fast γ to β	γ	fast γ to β	fast γ	fast γ	—
Serum concentration (mg/dL)	25–200	700–1500	40–350	1–40	<0.06	—
Serum half-life (days)	5	23	6	3	2	—

*Secretory component.
†n = 2 or 3.

and tears, saliva, and milk), a dimer containing the J chain and the secretory component (SC).

thyroid-binding inhibitory i's (TBII) thyrotropin-binding inhibitory i's.

thyroid-stimulating i's (TSI) circulating IgG antibodies with the ability to mimic thyrotropin by binding to receptors for it on thyroid cells and activating adenylate cyclase, thus causing an increase in the level of the intracellular second messenger cyclic AMP, which results in the release of thyroid hormones; thought to be responsible for most cases of Graves disease. Called also *human thyroid adenylate cyclase stimulators* (HTACS). Formerly called *long-acting thyroid stimulator*.

thyrotropin-binding inhibitory i's (TBII), TSH-binding inhibitory i's proteins present in the serum of patients with Graves disease that inhibit the binding of thyrotropin to its receptors in human thyroid tissues. Called also *TSH-displacing antibody*.

im·mu·no·glob·u·lin·op·a·thy (im″u-no-glob″u-lin-op′ə-the) gammopathy.

monoclonal i's plasma cell dyscrasias.

im·mu·no·hem·a·tol·o·gy (im″u-no-hēm″ə-tol′ə-je) the branch of hematology that studies antigen-antibody reactions and analogous phenomena as they relate to the pathogenesis and clinical manifestations of blood disorders.

im·mu·no·his·to·chem·is·try (im″u-no-his″to-kem′is-tre) a technique for detecting an antigen in tissue by means of antibody that is specific for the antigen and is coupled to a label that is visible by light microscopy. Sometimes used interchangeably with *immunocytochemistry*. **immunohistochem′ical** *adj*

im·mu·no·his·to·flu·o·res·cence (im″u-no-his-to-floo″o-res′əns) histofluorescence accomplished by injection of antibody labeled with fluorochrome.

im·mu·no·in·com·pe·tent (im″u-no-in-kom′pə-tent) lacking the ability or capacity to develop an immune response to antigenic challenge. See also *immunodeficiency*.

im·mu·no·log·ic (im″u-no-loj′ik) 1. pertaining to immunology. 2. pertaining to the immune response or other immune mechanisms.

im·mu·no·log·i·cal (im″u-no-loj′ĭ-kəl) immunologic.

im·mu·no·lipo·some (im″mu-no-lip′o-sōm) a liposome conjugated with or containing specific antigen, as for targeted delivery of a drug to tumor cells.

im·mu·nol·o·gist (im″u-nol′ə-jist) a specialist in immunology.

im·mu·nol·o·gy (im″u-nol′ə-je) the branch of biomedical science concerned with the response of the organism to antigenic challenge, the recognition of self and not self, and all the biological (in vivo), serological (in vitro), and physical chemical aspects of immune phenomena. It encompasses the study of the structure and function of the immune system (basic immunology); immunization, organ transplantation, blood banking, and immunopathology (clinical immunology); laboratory testing of cellular and humoral immune function (laboratory immunology); and the use of antigen-antibody reactions in other laboratory tests (serology and immunochemistry).

im·mu·no·lym·pho·scin·tig·ra·phy (im″u-no-lim″fo-sin-tig′rə-fe) scintigraphic detection of metastatic tumor in lymph nodes using radiolabeled monoclonal antibodies or antibody fragments specific for tumor-associated antigens.

im·mu·no·mod·u·la·tion (im″u-no-mod″u-la′shən) adjustment of the immune response to a desired level.

im·mu·no·mod·u·la·tor (im″u-no-mod′u-la″tər) an agent that specifically or nonspecifically augments or diminishes immune responses, i.e., an adjuvant, immunostimulant, or immunosuppressant.

im·mu·no·neph·e·lom·e·try (im″mu-no-nef″ə-lom′ə-tre) immunoturbidimetry.

im·mu·no·par·a·si·tol·o·gy (im″u-no-par″ə-si-tol′ə-je) immunology as applied to the interaction of animal parasites and their hosts.

im·mu·no·patho·gen·e·sis (im″u-no-path″o-jen′ə-sis) a process in which the course of a disease is altered or affected by an immune response (either the cellular [T-cell] or humoral [B-cell] response) or by the products of an immune reaction, such as the antigen-antibody-complement complexes deposited in renal glomeruli.

im·mu·no·patho·log·ic (im″u-no-path″o-loj′ik) pertaining to immunopathology.

im·mu·no·pa·thol·o·gy (im″u-no-pə-thol′ə-je) 1. the branch of biomedical science concerned with immune responses to disease, with immunodeficiency diseases, and with diseases with an immunologic etiology or pathogenesis. 2. the structural and functional manifestations associated with immune responses to disease or with diseases having an immunologic etiology.

im·mu·no·per·ox·i·dase (im″u-no-pər-ok′sĭ-das) pertaining to immunocytochemical methods using antibody coupled to the enzyme peroxidase to stain tissue constituents; frequently used to identify tissue antigens to aid diagnosis in surgical pathology.

im·mu·no·phe·no·type (im″mu-no-fe′no-tīp) 1. the characterization of a set of cells according to the antigens expressed. 2. a phenotype of cells of hematopoietic neoplasms defined according to their resemblance to normal T cells and B cells of the immune system. See also listings under *leukemia* and *lymphoma*.

im·mu·no·phe·no·typ·ing (im″u-no-fe′no-tīp-ing) analysis of the antigens expressed by cells, as by flow cytometry.

im·mu·no·phys·i·ol·o·gy (im″u-no-fiz″e-ol′ə-je) the physiology of immunologic processes.

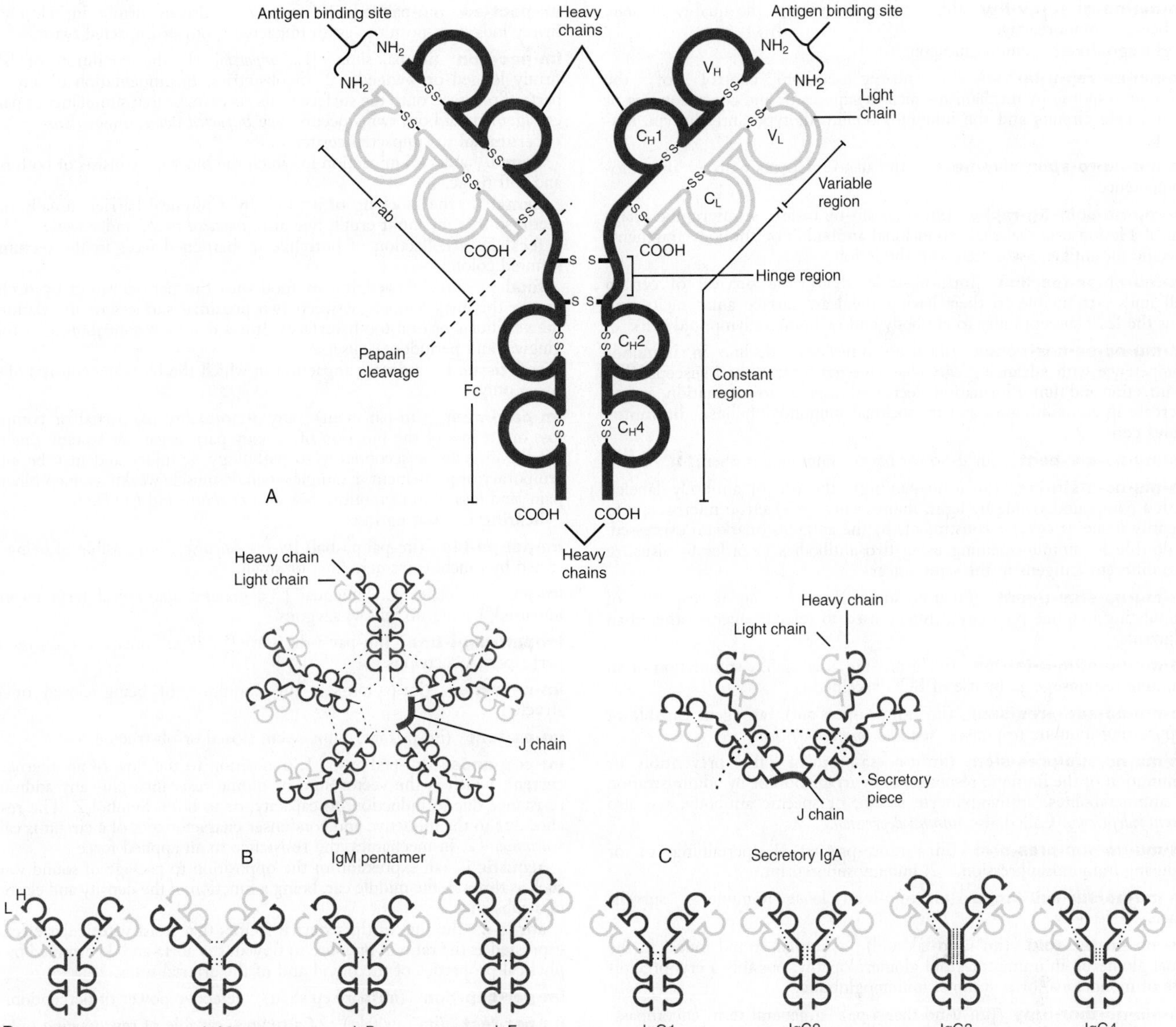

■ Molecular structure of the five classes of immunoglobulins. *(A)*, Schematic representation, using an IgG1 molecule, of the basic arrangement of heavy and light chains into the four-polypeptide chain unit, the antigen binding sites, the variable, constant, and hinge regions, and the site of papain cleavage generating the Fab and Fc fragments. Both intra- and interchain disulfide bonds are depicted (—SS—). *(B)*, IgM pentamer showing the arrangement of five four-chain monomers, interchain disulfide bonds *(dotted lines)*, and the J chain. *(C)*, Secretory IgA, here composed of IgA1 monomers, showing the position of the interchain disulfide bonds *(dotted lines)*, J chain, and secretory piece. *(D)*, Structure of IgA, IgD, IgE, and IgG subclasses, showing the interchain disulfide bonds *(dotted lines)*.

im•mu•no•po•ten•cy (im″u-no-po′tən-se) the immunogenic capacity of an individual antigenic determinant on an antigen molecule to initiate antibody synthesis.

im•mu•no•po•ten•ti•a•tion (im″u-no-po-ten″she-a′shən) enhancement of the immune response by use of an adjuvant or immunostimulant.

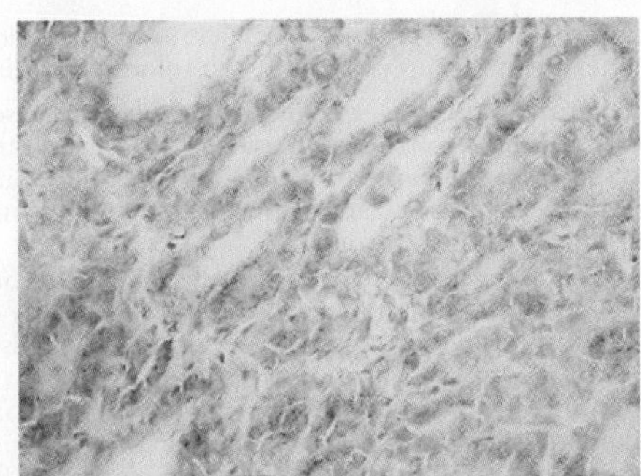

■ Immunoperoxidase used to stain thyroid tissue for HLA class II (DR) antigen in the diagnosis of Graves disease. DR antigen is markedly expressed in thyroid glands from patients with autoimmune thyroid disease, but not in normal thyroid epithelial cells; its expression causes cells to stain brown with immunoperoxidase.

im•mu•no•po•ten•ti•a•tor (im″u-no-po-ten′she-a-tər) an agent that specifically or nonspecifically enhances or augments the immune response, such as an adjuvant, BCG vaccine, or transfer factor.

im•mu•no•pre•cip•i•ta•tion (im″u-no-pre-sip″ĭ-ta′shən) precipitation resulting from interaction of specific antibody and antigen. See *precipitin reaction*, under *reaction*.

im•mu•no•pro•lif•er•a•tive (im″u-no-pro-lif′ər-ə-tiv) characterized by the uncontrolled proliferation of lymphoid cells.

im•mu•no•pro•phy•lax•is (im″u-no-pro″fə-lak′sis) the prevention of disease by the use of vaccines or therapeutic antisera.

im•mu•no•ra•dio•met•ric (im″u-no-ra″de-o-met′rik) pertaining to immunoradiometry or to immunoradiometric assay.

im•mu•no•ra•di•om•e•try (im″u-no-ra″de-om′ə-tre) the use of radiolabeled antibody (in the place of radiolabeled antigen) in radioimmunoassay techniques.

im•mu•no•re•ac•tant (im″u-no-re-ak′tənt) a substance that participates in an immune reaction, e.g., an antigen or antibody.

glucagon i. enteroglucagon.

im•mu•no•re•ac•tion (im″u-no-re-ak′shən) the reaction that takes place between an antigen and its antibody or between an antigen and an immunocyte sensitized to it.

im•mu•no•re•ac•tive (im″u-no-re-ak′tiv) exhibiting immunoreaction.

im•mu•no•re•ac•tiv•i•ty (im″u-no-re″ak-tiv′ĭ-te) the quality or state of being immunoreactive.

glucagonlike i. enteroglucagon.

im•mu•no•reg•u•la•tion (im″u-no-reg″u-la′shən) control of the immune response by mechanisms such as suppressor and contrasuppressor lymphocyte circuits and the immunoglobulin idiotype–anti-idiotype network.

im•mu•no•re•spon•sive•ness (im″u-no-re-spon′siv-nis) immunocompetence.

im•mu•no•scin•tig•raphy (im″u-no-sin-tig′rə-fe) scintigraphic imaging of a lesion using labeled monoclonal antibodies or antibody fragments specific for antigen associated with the lesion.

im•mu•no•se•lec•tion (im″u-no-sə-lek′shən) the survival of certain cell lines attributable to their having the least surface antigenicity and thus the least susceptibility to antibody and/or immune lymphoid cells.

im•mu•no•se•nes•cence (im″u-no-sə-nes′əns) decline in immunocompetence with advancing age, characterized by increased susceptibility to infection and tumor formation, decreased response to vaccination, and an increase in autoantibodies and monoclonal immunoglobulins. **immunosenes′cent** *adj*

im•mu•no•sor•bent (im″u-no-sor′bənt) immunoadsorbent.

im•mu•no•stain•ing (im″u-no-stān′ing) the use of antibody labeled with a compound visible by light, fluorescence, or electron microscopy to identify tissue or cellular constituents by the antigens (markers) expressed.

double i. immunostaining using two antibodies in order to visualize two different antigens in the same smear.

im•mu•no•stim•u•lant (im″u-no-stim′u-lənt) an agent capable of stimulating immune responses, usually used to refer to agents other than adjuvants.

im•mu•no•stim•u•la•tion (im″u-no-stim″u-la′shən) stimulation of an immune response, e.g., by use of BCG vaccine.

im•mu•no•sup•pres•sant (im″u-no-sə-pres′ənt) an agent capable of suppressing immune responses. See also *immunodeficiency.*

im•mu•no•sup•pres•sion (im″u-no-sə-presh′ən) the prevention or diminution of the immune response, as by irradiation or by administration of antimetabolites, antilymphocyte serum, or specific antibody; see also *immunodeficiency.* Called also *immunodepression.*

im•mu•no•sup•pres•sive (im″u-no-sə-pres′iv) 1. pertaining to or inducing immunosuppression. 2. immunosuppressant.

im•mu•no•sur•veil•lance (im″u-no-sər-va′ləns) immune surveillance.

im•mu•no•tac•toid (im″u-no-tak′toid) a fibrillar strand found in the renal glomeruli in immunotactoid glomerulopathy, possibly a cryoprecipitate of monoclonal or polyclonal immunoglobulin.

im•mu•no•ther•a•py (im″u-no-ther′ə-pe) a general term encompassing active and passive immunization, treatment with immunopotentiators and immunosuppressants, hyposensitization for allergic disorders, bone marrow transplantation, and thymus implantation.

adoptive i., adoptive cellular i. the treatment of cancer by transferring cultured lymphocytes having antitumor activity into the tumor-bearing host.

im•mu•no•tox•in (im′u-no-tok″sin) a hybrid molecule formed by coupling an entire toxin or the A chain of a toxin to an antibody or antigen molecule; the resulting molecule has the specificity of the antibody or antigen and the toxicity of the toxin.

im•mu•no•trans•fu•sion (im″u-no-trans-fu′zhən) transfusion of blood from donors previously immunized by the bacteria infecting the patient, or from the specific infection or of blood from persons recently recovered from the specific infection.

im•mu•no•tur•bi•dim•e•try (im″u-no-tər-bĭ-dim′ə-tre) a type of nephelometry that tests for a given antigenic substance (such as albumin or apolipoprotein) by immunologic techniques. A sample is diluted, mixed with antibody to the substance under investigation, and incubated; then a beam of light is passed through the solution and the reduction in light transmission by antigen-antibody complexes is measured by spectrophotometry. Called also *immunonephelometry.*

Imo•di•um (ĭ-mo′de-əm) trademark for preparations of loperamide hydrochloride.

Im•o•gam (im′o-gam″) trademark for preparations of rabies immune globulin.

Im•o•vax (im′o-vaks) trademark for a preparation of rabies vaccine (human diploid cell vaccine).

IMPA incisal mandibular plane angle.

im•pact (im′pakt) [L. *impactus*] a sudden and forcible collision.

im•pact•ed (im-pak′təd) [L. *impactus*] driven firmly in; closely or firmly lodged in position, as an impacted tooth or impacted twins.

im•pac•tion (im-pak′shən) [L. *impactio*] 1. the condition of being firmly lodged or wedged. 2. in obstetrics, the indentation of any fetal parts of one twin onto the surface of its co-twin, so that simultaneous partial engagement of both twins occurs. See *impacted twins,* under *twin.*

ceruminal i. impacted cerumen.

bony i. a dental impaction in which the blockage consists of both bone and soft tissue.

dental i. the blocking of a tooth by a physical barrier, usually other teeth, so that it cannot erupt. See also *impacted tooth,* under *tooth.*

fecal i. a collection of puttylike or hardened feces in the rectum or sigmoid colon.

food i. forceful wedging of food into the periodontium by occlusal forces; this may happen between two proximal surfaces or in relation to the vestibular or oral tooth surfaces. It is a common contributing factor in gingival and periodontal disease.

soft tissue i. a dental impaction in which the blockage consists of soft tissue only.

im•pair•ment (im-pār′mənt) any abnormality of, partial or complete loss of, or loss of the function of, a body part, organ, or system; this may be due directly or secondarily to pathology or injury and may be either temporary or permanent. Examples include muscle weakness, incontinence, pain, and loss of joint motion. See also *disability* and *handicap.*

hearing i. hearing loss.

im•pal•pa•ble (im-pal′pə-bəl) [*in-*[2] + *palpable*] impossible of being detected by touch; extremely fine, or small.

im•par (im′pahr) [L. "unequal"] a general anatomical term meaning unpaired; having no fellow; azygous.

im•pari•dig•i•tate (im-par″ĭ-dij′ĭ-tāt) [L. *impar* unequal + *digitus* finger] perissodactylous.

im•pa•ten•cy (im-pa′tən-se) the condition of being closed or obstructed.

im•pa•tent (im-pa′tənt) not open; closed or obstructed.

im•ped•ance (im-pēd′əns) 1. opposition to the flow of an alternating current, which is the vector sum of ohmic resistance plus any additional resistance due to induction, to capacity, or to both. Symbol Z. The resistance due to the inductive and condenser characteristics of a circuit is called *reactance.* 2. In mechanics, the resistance to an applied force.

acoustic i. an expression of the opposition to passage of sound waves, such as through the middle ear, being a function of the density and elasticity of a substance.

aortic i. the sum of the external factors that resist ventricular ejection, expressed as the ratio of pressure to flow in the aorta and determined by the physical properties of the blood and of the arterial walls.

im•per•cep•tion (im″pər-sep′shən) defective power of perception.

im•per•fect (im-pur′fəkt) of a fungus, capable of reproducing only by means of conidia (asexual spores). Cf. *perfect.*

im•per•fo•rate (im-pur′fə-rāt) [L. *imperforatus*] not open; abnormally closed, as imperforate anus.

im•per•fo•ra•tion (im-pur″fə-ra′shən) the state of being abnormally closed; see also *atresia.*

im•pe•ri•al•ine (im-pe′re-al″in) a toxic crystalline alkaloid, from the bulbs of the liliaceous plant *Fritillaria imperialis.*

im•per•me•a•ble (im-pur′me-ə-bəl) [*in-*[2] + *per-* + *meare* to move] not permitting passage, as of fluid.

im•per•vi•ous (im-pur′ve-əs) [L. *impervius*] impenetrable; not affording a passage.

im•pe•tig•i•ni•za•tion (im″pə-tij″ĭ-nĭ-za′shən) the development of impetigo upon an area previously affected with some other skin disease.

im•pe•ti•go (im″pə-ti′go) [L.] a contagious pyoderma, caused by direct inoculation of *Staphylococcus aureus* or occasionally a group A streptococcus into superficial cutaneous abrasions or compromised skin, usually on the face or a limb. Two main types are distinguished, bullous impetigo and nonbullous impetigo. **impetig′inous** *adj*

Bockhart i. a superficial folliculitis, usually caused by *Staphylococcus aureus,* characterized by small purulent pustules at the orifices of the pilosebaceous glands, especially on the scalp and limbs. Called also *superficial pustular perifolliculitis.*

i. bullo′sa, bullous i. impetigo caused by infection with *Staphylococcus aureus,* seen most often in newborns but sometimes in older children or adults. Skin eruptions begin as small vesicles that enlarge to form flaccid bullae, sometimes up to 5 cm in diameter, with erythematous rims; the lesions later rupture and form a thin, varnishlike crust. Called also *i. contagiosa bullosa* and *i. neonatorum.*

i. contagio′sa impetigo.

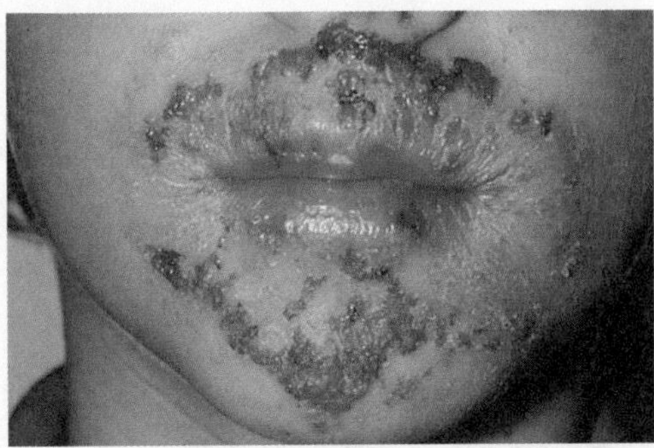

■ Nonbullous impetigo.

i. contagio'sa bullo'sa i. bullosa.

i. herpetifor'mis a rare, acute skin condition seen in late pregnancy, resembling generalized pustular psoriasis; if not treated promptly, it can be fatal to the mother or the unborn fetus. Characteristics include pruritic sterile pustules that resolve with desquamation; patients have hypocalcemia and hypoalbuminemia with fever, lethargy, and potentially fatal tetany.

i. neonato'rum i. bullosa.

nonbullous i. the most common kind of impetigo, caused by infection at sites of minor trauma such as scrapes, cuts, or insect bites; the infecting organism is usually *Staphylococcus aureus* and less often a group A streptococcus. The characteristic lesions are discrete fragile vesicles that have erythematous borders and later become pustular, rupture, and discharge a thin yellow seropurulent fluid that dries and forms a thick crust. The pustules may spread peripherally with central healing, evolving into annular, circinate, or gyrate patterns. Called also *i. vulgaris.*

staphylococcal i. former name for *bullous i.*

streptococcal i. former name for *nonbullous i.*

udder i. a staphylococcal infection of the udders of cows, with pustules near the teats that sometimes extend into boils. Cf. *staphylococcal mastitis.*

i. vulga'ris nonbullous i.

im·pi·la·tion (im″pĭ-la'shən) rouleau formation; see under *formation.*

im·pinge·ment (im-pinj'mənt) advancement of one thing out of its expected place to where it may collide with something else; see *impingement syndrome,* under *syndrome.*

femoroacetabular i. impingement of the femoral head onto the acetabular labrum, owing to hypermobility of the hip joint, with eventual delamination or ulceration of the articular cartilage.

Im·plan·on (im-plan'on) trademark for an implantable preparation of etonogestrel.

im·plant[1] (im-plant') to insert or graft an object or material, such as an alloplastic or radioactive material, a drug capsule, or tissue, into the body of a recipient.

im·plant[2] (im'plant) an object or material, such as an alloplastic or radioactive material or tissue, partially or totally inserted or grafted into the body for prosthetic, therapeutic, diagnostic, or experimental purposes. See also *graft* and *insert*[2].

Bosker i. a common type of transmandibular implant.

Brånemark i. a type of osseointegrated implant consisting of a two-stage system of titanium screws.

cochlear i. a device consisting of a microphone, signal processor, external transmitter, and implanted receiver; the receiver is surgically implanted under the skin near the mastoid process above and behind the ear. It is an alternative to total deafness, although it does not actually restore hearing.

dental i. a prosthetic device of alloplastic material implanted into the oral tissues beneath the mucosal or periosteal layer or within the bone to provide support and retention to a partial or complete denture.

endodontic i. a metallic implant extending through the root canal of a tooth into the periapical bone structure, thereby lengthening the root of a pulpless tooth.

endometrial i's fragments of endometrial mucosa transferred through the uterine tubes and implanted on the uterus, ovaries, or pelvic peritoneum.

endosseous i., endosteal i. a dental implant made of metal or sometimes ceramic or polymeric material, consisting of a blade, screw, pin, or vent, inserted into the jaw bone through the alveolar or basal bone, with a post protruding through the mucoperiosteum into the oral cavity to serve as an abutment for dentures or orthodontic appliances, or to serve in fracture fixation.

magnet i. denture magnet.

osseointegrated i. an endosseous implant containing pores into which osteoblasts and supporting connective tissue can migrate. Metallic, ceramic, and polymeric materials have been used.

penile i. see under *prosthesis.*

subdermal contraceptive i. a contraceptive that can be implanted subdermally for long-term use.

subperiosteal i. a dental implant consisting of a metal frame implanted under the periosteum and firmly bound by the mucoperiosteum, resting on the jaw bone, with a post protruding into the oral cavity.

transmandibular i. (TMI) a dental implant inserted via submandibular incision and fixed to the symphyseal border of the mandible; it traverses the mandible, bears the denture directly, and is designed for patients with severe mandibular alveolar atrophy.

transosteal i. a dental implant consisting of a bolt that crosses the mandible and is secured in place by a nut; a post protrudes into the oral cavity and serves as an abutment for dentures or orthodontic appliances.

im·plan·ta·tion (im″plan-ta'shən) [*in-*[1] + *plantation*] 1. attachment of the blastocyst to the epithelial lining of the uterus, its penetration through the epithelium, and its embedding in the compact layer of the endometrium, beginning six or seven days after fertilization of the oocyte. 2. the insertion of an organ or tissue, such as skin, nerve, or tendon, in a new site in the body. 3. the insertion or grafting into the body of biological, living, inert, or radioactive material.

central i., circumferential i. superficial i.

eccentric i. embedding of the blastocyst within a recess of the uterine cavity.

hypodermic i. the placing of a medicine in the subcutaneous tissue.

interstitial i. complete embedding of a blastocyst within the endometrium, as in humans.

LeDuc i. see under *technique.*

nerve i. the operation of inserting and attaching a nerve into the sheath of another nerve.

periosteal i. surgical insertion of a normal tendon into the periosteum of a bone at the insertion of a paralyzed tendon, to take its place.

superficial i. embedding of the blastocyst so that the blastocyst, and later the chorionic sac, come to occupy the uterine cavity. Called also *central* or *circumferential i.*

teratic i. the partial blending of an imperfect with a nearly perfect fetus.

im·plan·to·don·tics (im-plan″to-don'tiks) the branch of dentistry dealing with the implantation of artificial devices and materials into the oral hard and soft tissues for prosthetic, therapeutic, or diagnostic purposes. Called also *dental* or *oral implantology* and *implantodontology.*

im·plan·to·don·tist (im-plan″to-don'tist) a dentist who specializes in the practice of implantodontics; called also *implantologist.*

im·plan·to·don·tol·o·gy (im-plan″to-don'tol'ə-je) implantodontics.

im·plan·tol·o·gist (im″plan-tol'ə-jist) 1. a specialist in implantology. 2. implantodontist.

im·plan·tol·o·gy (im″plan-tol'ə-je) the science dealing with the study and practice of inserting implants into the body.

dental i., oral i. implantodontics.

im·plo·sion (im-plo'zhən) see *flooding.*

im·po·tence (im'pə-təns) [*in-*[2] + *potentia*] 1. lack of power. 2. specifically, lack of copulative power in the male due to inability to initiate an erection or to maintain an erection until ejaculation; usually classified as either *psychogenic i.* or *organic i.* Called also *erectile dysfunction.*

arteriogenic i. vasculogenic impotence due to a disorder in the arteries supplying the penis, such as atherosclerosis or stenosis.

diabetic i. impotence that commonly occurs in men with diabetes mellitus, resulting from a variety of organic effects of the disease.

endocrinologic i. organic impotence resulting from an endocrine disorder, usually of either the gonads or the hypothalamus and pituitary gland.

functional i. psychogenic i.

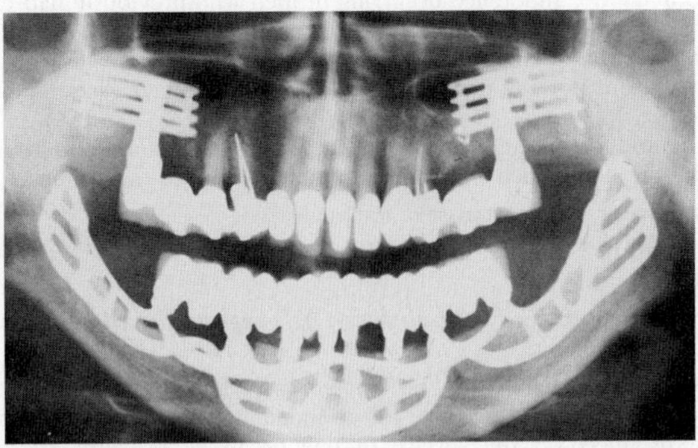

■ Panoramic radiograph of subperiosteal implant.

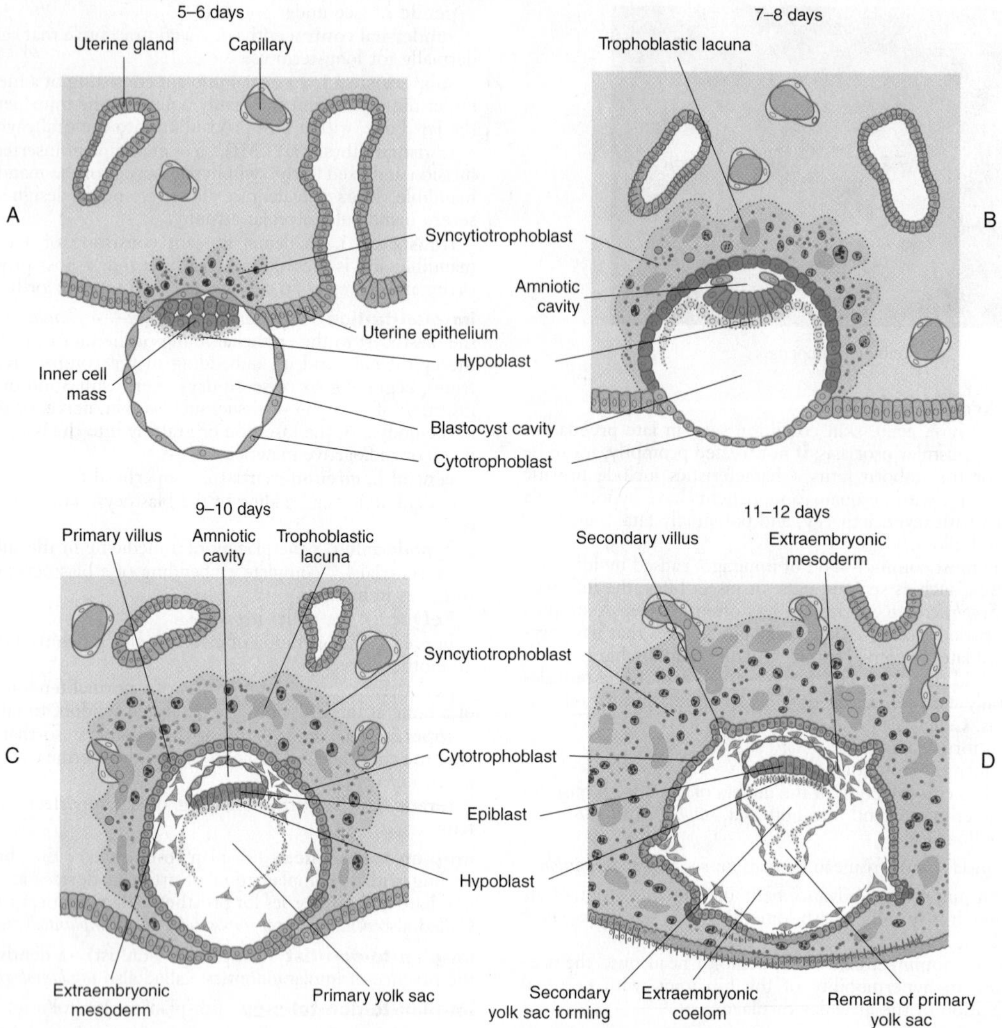

■ Major stages in implantation of a human embryo. *(A)*, The syncytiotrophoblast is just beginning to invade the endometrial stroma. *(B)*, Most of the embryo is embedded in the endometrium; there is early formation of the trophoblastic lacunae. The amniotic cavity and yolk sac are beginning to form. *(C)*, Implantation is almost complete; primary villi are forming, and the extraembryonic mesoderm is appearing. *(D)*, Implantation is complete; secondary villi are forming.

neurogenic i. organic impotence resulting from a lesion in the nervous system, either in the central nervous system or along peripheral nerves such as the nervi erigentes.

organic i. impotence caused by some physical disorder that affects the sexual apparatus, usually classified as either vasculogenic, neurogenic, or endocrinologic. It is sometimes caused by accidental or iatrogenic trauma or it may occur as a side effect of certain drugs. Cf. *psychogenic i.*

primary i. impotence that is persistent throughout the patient's life; formerly thought to be entirely psychogenic, it is now known sometimes to have physical causes such as trauma at a young age or organic disorders.

psychic i., psychogenic i., psychological i. impotence caused by some underlying psychological condition; in DSM-IV, called *male erectile disorder* (q.v.). Cf. *organic i.*

secondary i. impotence occurring in men who previously had experienced normal penile function.

vasculogenic i. organic impotence resulting from some disorder (usually insufficient flow) of penile arteries or veins; see *arteriogenic i.* and *venogenic i.*

venogenic i. vasculogenic impotence due to a disorder in the veins draining the penis, such as a failure to maintain venous occlusion.

im·po·ten·cy (im′pə-tən-se) impotence.

im·preg·nate (im-preg′nāt) [L. *impregnare*] 1. fertilize. 2. to saturate or charge with.

im·preg·na·tion (im″prəg-na′shən) [L. *impregnatio*] 1. fertilization. 2. saturation (def. 1).

im·pres·sio (im-pres′e-o) pl. *impressio′nes* [L.] impression: a term used in anatomic nomenclature for an indentation or concavity, especially one produced in the surface of one organ by pressure exerted by another.

i. cardi′aca he′patis [TA] cardiac impression on liver: a depression on the superior part of the diaphragmatic surface of the liver, corresponding to the position of the heart.

i. cardi′aca pulmo′nis [TA] cardiac impression on lung: the indentation on the medial surface of either lung produced by the heart and pericardium.

i. co′lica he′patis [TA] colic impression on liver: a variable concavity in the right liver, where it is in contact with the right flexure of the colon.

i.′nes digita′tae TA alternative for *impressiones gyrorum.*

i. duodena′lis he′patis [TA] duodenal impression on liver: a concavity on the right liver where it is in contact with the descending part of the duodenum.

i. esopha′gea he′patis i. oesophagea hepatis.

i. gas′trica he′patis [TA] gastric impression on liver: a large concavity in the left liver where it is in contact with the anterior wall of the stomach.

i.′nes gyro′rum [TA] impressions of cerebral gyri: poorly defined depressions on the inner surface of the cranium, corresponding to the gyri of the brain. Called also *digital* or *digitate impressions, gyrate impressions, impressiones digitatae* [TA alternative] and *juga cerebralia* [TA alternative].

i. ligamen′ti costoclavicula′ris [TA] impression for costoclavicular ligament: the point on the inferior surface of the clavicle where the costoclavicular ligament is attached; called also *costal tuberosity of clavicle.*

i. oesopha′gea he′patis [TA] esophageal impression on liver: a concavity on the left liver corresponding to the position of the abdominal part of the esophagus.

i. rena′lis he′patis [TA] renal impression on liver: the concavity on the right liver where it is in contact with the right kidney.

i. suprarena′lis he′patis [TA] suprarenal impression on liver: a small concavity on the right liver, superior to the renal impression, caused by contact with the right adrenal (suprarenal) gland.

i. trigemina'lis [TA] trigeminal impression: the shallow impression in the floor of the middle cranial fossa on the petrous part of the temporal bone, lodging the semilunar ganglion of the trigeminal nerve.

im•pres•sion (im-presh'ən) [L. *impressio*] 1. a slight indentation or depression; see *impressio.* 2. a negative copy or the impressed reverse of the surface of an object. 3. an effect produced upon the mind, body, or senses by some external stimulus or agent. 4. dental i.

anatomic i. an impression of the form of a dental arch or portion thereof that records the structures in a passive or unstrained form, making possible a static relationship of a prosthesis produced from such an impression.

basilar i. 1. platybasia. 2. basilar invagination.

bridge i. an impression made for the purpose of constructing or assembling a fixed restoration, fixed partial denture, or bridge.

cardiac i. on liver impressio cardiaca hepatis.

cardiac i. on lung impressio cardiaca pulmonis.

i's of cerebral gyri impressiones gyrorum.

cleft palate i. an impression of the upper jaw made in patients with cleft palate, to be used in the prosthetic repair of the defect.

colic i. on liver impressio colica hepatis.

colic i. on spleen facies colica splenis.

complete denture i. 1. an impression made of the entire edentulous arch of the maxilla or mandible, for the purpose of construction of a complete denture. 2. a negative registration of the entire denture-bearing area of the maxilla or mandible. 3. a negative registration of the entire denture-bearing and border seal areas of the edentulous mouth.

i. for costoclavicular ligament impressio ligamenti costoclavicularis.

dental i., denture i. an imprint or negative likeness of the teeth and edentulous areas, made in plastic material that becomes hardened or set while in contact with the tissue; it is later filled with plaster of Paris or artificial stone to produce a facsimile of the oral structures present.

digital i's, digitate i's impressiones gyrorum.

direct bone i. an impression of denuded bone used in the construction of dental implants.

duodenal i. on liver impressio duodenalis hepatis.

esophageal i. on liver impressio oesophagea hepatis.

final i. secondary i.

gastric i. on liver impressio gastrica hepatis.

gastric i. on spleen facies gastrica splenis.

gyrate i's impressiones gyrorum.

hydrocolloid i. a denture impression made of a hydrocolloid material.

lower i., mandibular i. an impression of the mandibular jaw and related tissues and dental structures.

maxillary i. an impression of the maxillary jaw and related tissues and dental structures; called also *upper i.*

pancreatic i. on spleen facies pancreatica splenis.

partial denture i. a negative copy of the partially edentulous dental arch or its section made for the purpose of constructing a partial denture.

preliminary i. primary i.

primary i. an impression of the edentulous mouth that usually lacks fine details of the tissue and is often used for construction of a secondary impression. Called also *preliminary i.*

renal i. on liver impressio renalis hepatis.

renal i. on spleen facies renalis splenis.

secondary i. an impression made by using an impression material in a tray, produced by the primary impression method for the reproduction of fine details of an edentulous mouth. Called also *final i.*

sectional i. a dental impression that is made in sections.

suprarenal i. on liver impressio suprarenalis hepatis.

trigeminal i. impressio trigeminalis.

upper i. maxillary i.

im•pres•sio•nes (im-pres″e-o'nēz) [L.] plural of *impressio.*

im•print (im'print) [L. *imprimere* to impress] a mark created on a surface by pressure.

touch i. a method of preparing specimens for cytopathologic examination: the freshly cut surface of a block of tissue is touched lightly to a slide several times to make a series of imprints, which are air-dried, fixed, and stained.

im•print•ing (im-print'ing) rapid learning of species-specific behavior patterns that occurs with exposure to the proper stimulus at a sensitive period of early life.

genomic i. differential expression of a gene or genes as a function of inheritance from the male versus the female parent, e.g., a deletion on chromosome 15 that causes Prader-Willi syndrome if inherited from the father causes instead Angelman syndrome if inherited from the mother. Imprinting appears to be controlled by DNA methylation patterns that are not erased during gametogenesis.

im•pulse (im'pəls) 1. a sudden pushing force. 2. a sudden uncontrollable determination to act. 3. nerve i.

apex i., apical i. see under *beat.*

cardiac i. the palpable or recorded movement of the chest wall caused by the heartbeat.

ectopic i. 1. the impulse that causes an ectopic beat. 2. a pathologic nerve impulse that begins in the middle of an axon and proceeds simultaneously towards the cell body and the periphery; it may be connected to a paresthesia or some other disorder of transmission.

irresistible i. an impulse to commit a criminal act that cannot be resisted because mental disease has destroyed the person's freedom of will and power to choose between right and wrong. The "irresistible impulse test" that a person is not criminally responsible if the act was due to an irresistible impulse is still used in some states.

left parasternal i's cardiac impulses categorized according to their location along the upper, mid, or lower left sternal border. An *upper left parasternal impulse* is usually caused by a systolic expansion of a dilated pulmonary artery; a *mid* to *lower left parasternal impulse* usually occurs as a result of a right ventricular contraction, and is characterized by an outward movement beginning synchronously with the first heart sound, but is sometimes caused by mitral incompetence.

nerve i., neural i. the electrochemical process propagated along nerve fibers.

right parasternal i's cardiac impulses categorized according to their location along the upper, mid, or lower right sternal border.

im•pul•sion (im-pul'shən) blind obedience to internal drives, without regard for acceptance by others or pressure from the superego; seen in children and in adults with weak defensive organization.

im•pu•ta•tion (im″pu-ta'shən) the use of statistical methods to estimate missing values from available values when data are missing, e.g., due to lack of response to a survey.

Im•u•ran (im'u-ran) trademark for preparations of azathioprine.

IMV intermittent mandatory ventilation.

IMViC, imvic a mnemonic indicating the tests used in classifying coliform bacteria, namely indole, methyl red, Voges-Proskauer, and citrate. See under *test.*

In indium.

in inch.

in-[1] [L. *in* in, into] a prefix meaning in or into; occurs as *il-* before *l*, *im-* before *b*, *m*, or *p*, and *ir-* before *r*.

in-[2] [L. *in-* not] a prefix meaning not; occurs as *il-* before *l*, *im-* before *b*, *m*, or *p*, and *ir-* before *r*.

INA International Neurological Association.

in•acid•i•ty (in″ə-sid'ĭ-te) anacidity.

in•ac•ti•vate (in-ak'tĭ-vāt) to render inactive; to destroy the activity of.

in•ac•ti•va•tion (in-ak″tĭ-va'shən) the destruction of biological activity, as of a virus or enzyme, by the action of heat or other physical or chemical means.

complement i. any method of destroying the complement activity of serum, such as heat inactivation or treatment with hydrazine.

heat i. any destruction of biological activity by heating, such as the destruction of complement activity in serum by heating to 56°C for 30 minutes.

X-chromosome i., X-i. lyonization.

in•ac•ti•va•tor (in-ak'tĭ-va″tər) an agent that renders another inactive.

anaphylatoxin i. (AI) a serum carboxypeptidase that destroys the anaphylatoxin activity of C3a, C4a, and C5a by removing C-terminal arginyl or lysyl residues.

C3b i. (C3b INA) former name for complement *factor I.*

electrocerebral i. (ECI) see under *silence.*

in•ac•tiv•i•ty (in″ak-tiv'ĭ-ty) lack of activity, especially in electroencephalography or electromyography.

electrocerebral i. see under *silence.*

in•ad•e•qua•cy (in-ad'ə-kwə-se) [*in-*[2] + *adaequare* to make equal] inability to perform an allotted function; insufficiency; incompetence.

in•al•i•men•tal (in″al-ĭ-men'təl) [*in-*[2] + *aliment* + *-al*[1]] not nutritious; not serviceable as food.

in•am•ri•none (in-am'rĭ-nōn) [USP] a phosphodiesterase inhibitor that prevents enzymatic breakdown of cyclic AMP by phosphodiesterase, having positive inotropic and vasodilator effects; used as a cardiotonic. Called also *amrinone.*

i. lactate the lactate salt of inamrinone, used for the short-term management of congestive heart failure in patients unresponsive to digitalis, diuretics, or vasodilators; administered intravenously.

in•an•i•mate (in-an'ĭ-mət) [*in-*[2] + *animatus* alive] 1. without life. 2. lacking in animation.

in•a•ni•tion (in″ə-nish'ən) [L. *inanis* empty] marked weakness, extreme weight loss, and decreased metabolism due to prolonged severe insufficiency of food (starvation).

in·ap·pe·tence (in-ap′ə-təns) [*in-*[2] + *appetere* to desire] lack of desire or appetite.

In·ap·sine (in-ap′sēn) trademark for a preparation of droperidol.

in·ar·tic·u·late (in″ahr-tik′u-lət) [*in-*[2] + *articulate*[2]] not having joints; disjointed; not uttered like articulate speech.

in ar·tic·u·lo mor·tis (in ahr-tik′u-lo mor′tis) [L.] at the very point of death.

in·as·sim·i·la·ble (in″ə-sim′ĭ-lə-bəl) [*in-*[2] + *assimilable*] not susceptible of being utilized as nutriment.

in·at·ten·tion (in″ə-ten′shən) [*in-*[2] + *attention*] lack of attention.
 selective i. 1. unilateral neglect. 2. the ignoring or otherwise screening out of stimuli that are threatening, anxiety-producing, or felt to be unimportant.

in·born (in′born) 1. genetically determined, and present at birth; see also *inborn error of metabolism,* under *error.* 2. congenital.

in·bred (in′bred) produced by inbreeding.

in·breed·ing (in′brēd-ing) the breeding of closely related individuals, or of individuals having closely similar genetic constitutions.

in·can·des·cent (in″cən-des′ənt) [L. *incandescens* glowing] glowing with heat and light; emitting light on being heated.

in·car·cer·at·ed (in-kahr′sər-āt″əd) [L. *incarceratus* imprisoned] imprisoned; constricted; subjected to incarceration.

in·car·cer·a·tion (in-kahr″sər-a′shən) [L. *in* in + *carcer* prison] unnatural retention or confinement of a part, as may occur in hernia.

in·car·na·tio (in″kahr-na′she-o) [L., from *in* in + *caro,* gen. *carnis* flesh] ingrowth.
 i. un′guis ingrown toenail.

in·car·na·tive (in-kahr′nə-tiv) [L. *incarnare* to invest in flesh] 1. promoting the formation of granulations. 2. an agent that promotes granulations.

in·cer·tae se·dis (in-ser′te se′dis) [L.] of uncertain position; said of taxa that are of uncertain classification.

in·cest (in′sest) [L. *incestus* impure] sexual intercourse or other sexual activity between persons so closely related that marriage between them is legally or culturally prohibited.

inch (in) (inch) a unit of linear measure, one twelfth of a foot, being the equivalent of 2.54 cm.

in·ci·dence (in′sĭ-dəns) [L. *incidere* to occur, to happen] 1. the rate at which a certain event occurs, e.g., the number of new cases of a specific disease occurring during a certain period in a population at risk (see *incidence rate,* under *rate*). Cf. *prevalence.* 2. the arrival of radiant energy at a surface.
 cumulative i. cumulative incidence rate.

in·ci·dent (in′sĭ-dənt) [L. *incidere* to fall upon] 1. an unusual or noteworthy occurrence. 2. falling or striking upon, as incident radiation.

in·ci·den·ta·lo·ma (in″sĭ-den″tə-lo′mə) an asymptomatic tumor, usually of an adrenal gland, discovered during a diagnostic imaging procedure performed for some other reason.

in·cin·e·ra·tion (in-sin″ə-ra′shən) [*in-*[1] + *cineres* ashes] the act of burning to ashes; cremation.

in·cip·i·ent (in-sip′e-ənt) beginning to exist; coming into existence.

in·ci·sal (in-si′zəl) 1. cutting. 2. pertaining to the cutting edge of an anterior tooth.

in·cised (in-sīzd′) [L. *incisus*] cut; made by cutting.

in·ci·sion (in-sizh′ən) [L. *incidere* to cut open, to cut through] 1. a cut, or a wound produced by cutting with a sharp instrument. 2. the act of cutting.
 Battle i., Battle-Jalaguier-Kammerer i. Kammerer-Battle i.
 Bevan i. an incision along the outer border of the rectus muscle, for operations in the upper abdominal quadrants.
 celiotomy i. an incision made through the abdominal wall to give access to the peritoneal cavity.
 Cherney i. an abdominal incision in the surgical approach to the female reproductive organs.
 clear corneal i. a tiny incision off to the side in the clear part of the cornea for cataract extraction.
 Deaver i. incision through the anterior sheath of the right rectus muscle, the muscle then being retracted medially.
 Dührssen i's incisions made in the cervix uteri to facilitate delivery.
 epigastric i. see illustration.
 Fergusson i. see under *operation.*
 gridiron i. McBurney i.
 Kammerer-Battle i. a vertical abdominal incision through the skin and superficial fascia, vertical division of the anterior layer of the rectus sheath, with retraction of the rectus muscle medialward, and vertical division of the posterior layer of the sheath nearer the median line, together with the subserous areolar tissue and peritoneum.

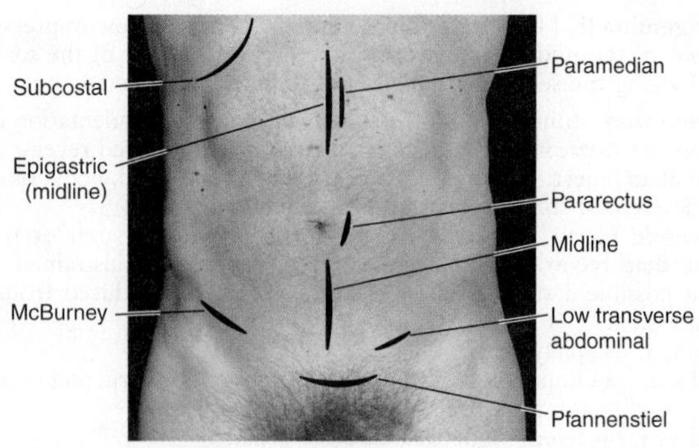

■ Various abdominal incisions.

 Kocher i. a subcostal incision that, when made on the right, provides exposure of the gallbladder and common bile duct and, when made on the left, provides exposure for splenectomy or splenorenal venous anastomosis.
 low transverse abdominal i. see illustration.
 Lynch i. the incision used in the Lynch operation, running midway between the medial canthus and nasion and extending into the inferior aspect of the brow.
 McBurney i. an abdominal incision parallel to the fibers of the external oblique muscle, about one-third the distance along a line from the anterior superior iliac spine to the umbilicus, half the incision being above and the remainder below this point. The skin and subcutaneous fat are incised down to the external oblique muscle, the fibers of which are split; the underlying internal oblique and transversus abdominalis are then split and separated.
 Maylard i. an abdominal incision in the surgical approach to the female reproductive organs.
 midline i. see illustration.
 Munro Kerr i. a transverse incision of the lower uterine segment for cesarean section.
 paramedian i. see illustration.
 pararectus i. see illustration.
 paravaginal i. incision of the vagina and perineum in order to secure enlargement of the vulvovaginal outlet, and thereby permit easy access to the vagina in cancer operations and, rarely, to facilitate childbirth; called also *Schuchardt i.* and *vaginoperineotomy.*
 Pfannenstiel i. a curved abdominal incision, the convexity being directed downward, just above the symphysis, passing through skin, superficial fascia, and aponeurosis, exposing the pyramidalis and rectus muscles, which are separated from each other in the midline, the peritoneum then being opened vertically. See illustration.
 relief i. an incision made to relieve tension in tissue.
 Rockey-Davis i. an incision similar to the McBurney incision, except that the skin incision is transverse rather than vertical.
 Schuchardt i. paravaginal i.
 scleral tunnel i. an incision used for cataract extraction, making a minute tunnel through the sclera for insertion of a keratome.
 subcostal i. see illustration.
 transurethral i. of prostate (TUIP) endoscopic bilateral incision from just distal to the ureteral orifice through the bladder neck up to the verumontanum, in order to relieve bladder outlet obstruction in the treatment of benign prostatic hyperplasia.
 Warren i. an incision following the thoracomammary fold, permitting access to any part of the breast.

in·ci·sive (in-si′siv) [L. *incisivus*] 1. having the power or quality of cutting. 2. pertaining to the incisor teeth.

in·ci·so·la·bi·al (in-si″zo-la′be-əl) denoting the incisal and labial surfaces of an anterior tooth.

in·ci·so·lin·gual (in-si″zo-ling′gwəl) denoting the incisal and lingual surfaces of an anterior tooth.

in·ci·so·prox·i·mal (in-si″zo-prok′sĭ-məl) denoting the incisal and proximal surfaces of an anterior tooth.

in·ci·sor (I) (in-si′zər) [L. *incidere* to cut into] 1. adapted for cutting. 2. incisor tooth.
 central i., first i. the two incisor teeth in each jaw that are located closer to the midline of the body.
 hawk-bill i's shovel-shaped i's.
 Hutchinson i's see under *tooth.*
 lateral i. the second incisor tooth on either side of the midline of each jaw, lateral to the central incisor and mesial to the canine tooth.
 medial i. central i.

second i. lateral i.

shovel-shaped i's large upper medial incisor teeth that are concave on the lingual side; called also *hawk-bill i's.*

winged i. a rotation deformity of a maxillary incisor tooth in which the distal edge of the tooth protrudes labially.

in•ci•su•ra (in-si-su'rə) gen. and pl. *incisu'rae* [L., from *incidere* to cut into] [TA] notch: an indentation or depression, usually on the side of a bone or other structure.

in•ci•su•rae (in″si-su′re) [L.] genitive and plural of *incisura.*

in•ci•sure (in-si′zhər) notch.

angular i. incisura angularis.

i's of Lanterman, Lanterman-Schmidt i's Schmidt-Lanterman i's.

Schmidt-Lanterman i's channels of cytoplasm in the myelin sheath of neurons that lead back to the Schwann cell body; they appear as oblique lines or slashes in the sheath. See Plate 39.

Incisura

Descriptions of anatomic structures are given on TA terms and include anglicized names of specific incisurae.

i. aceta′buli [TA] acetabular notch: a notch in the inferior portion of the lunate surface of the acetabulum.

i. angula′ris [TA] angular incisure: the lowest point on the lesser curvature of the stomach, marking the junction of the cranial two thirds and caudal one third of the stomach. Called also *angular* or *gastric notch.*

i. ante′rior auri′culae [TA] anterior notch of auricle: a depression between the crus of the helix and the tragus; called also *auricular notch.*

i. a′picis cor′dis [TA] notch of cardiac apex: a slight notch found at the site where the anterior and posterior interventricular sulci become continuous and cross the right margin of the heart.

i. cardi′aca pulmo′nis sinis′tri [TA] cardiac notch of left lung: a notch in the anterior border of the left lung.

i. cardia′lis [TA] cardial or cardiac notch of stomach: a notch at the junction of the esophagus and the greater curvature of the stomach.

i. cartila′ginis mea′tus acus′tici [TA] notch in cartilage of acoustic meatus: two vertical fissures in the anterior part of the cartilage of the external acoustic meatus.

i. clavicula′ris ster′ni [TA] clavicular notch of sternum: either of two oval surfaces, one on each side of the superior border of the manubrium of the sternum, where it articulates with the clavicle.

incisu′rae costa′les ster′ni [TA] costal notches of sternum: the facets on the sternum, seven on each lateral edge, for articulation with the costal cartilages.

i. ethmoida′lis os′sis fronta′lis [TA] ethmoidal notch of frontal bone: a space between the orbital parts of the frontal bone, in which the ethmoid bone is lodged.

i. fibula′ris ti′biae [TA] fibular notch of tibia: a depression on the lateral surface of the lower end of the tibia, which articulates with the lower end of the fibula.

i. fronta′lis [TA] frontal notch: a notch located in the supraorbital margin of the frontal bone medial to the supraorbital notch or foramen, for transmission of branches of the supraorbital nerve and vessels; frequently converted into a foramen *(foramen frontale)* by a bridge of osseous tissue.

i. interarytenoi′dea [TA] interarytenoid notch: the posterior portion of the aditus laryngis between the two arytenoid cartilages.

i. intertra′gica [TA] intertragic notch: the notch at the lower part of the pinna of the ear between the tragus and the antitragus.

i. ischia′dica ma′jor [TA] greater sciatic notch: the large notch on the posterior border of the hip bone, where the posterior borders of the ilium and the ischium become continuous.

i. ischia′dica mi′nor [TA] lesser sciatic notch: the notch on the posterior border of the ischium just inferior to the ischiadic spine.

i. jugula′ris os′sis occipita′lis [TA] jugular notch of occipital bone: a notch on the anterior surface of the jugular process of the occipital bone, forming the posterior wall of the jugular foramen.

i. jugula′ris os′sis tempora′lis [TA] jugular notch of temporal bone: a prominent depression on the inferior surface of the petrous part of the temporal bone. It forms the anterior and lateral wall of the jugular foramen and lodges the superior bulb of the internal jugular vein in its lateral part and the glossopharyngeal, vagus, and accessory nerves in its medial part.

i. jugula′ris ster′ni [TA] jugular notch of sternum: the notch on the upper border of the sternum between the incisurae claviculares (clavicular notches); called also *presternal, sternal,* or *suprasternal notch.*

i. lacrima′lis maxil′lae [TA] lacrimal notch of maxilla: an indentation on the posterior border of the frontal process of the maxilla, that lodges the lacrimal sac.

i. ligamen′ti te′retis [TA] notch for ligamentum teres: a notch in the inferior border of the liver, occupied by the ligamentum teres in the adult.

i. mandi′bulae [TA] mandibular notch: a deep notch on the upper edge of the ramus of the mandible between the condyle and the coronoid process. Called also *sigmoid notch.*

i. mastoi′dea os′sis tempora′lis [TA] mastoid notch: a deep groove on the medial surface of the mastoid process of the temporal bone, which gives origin to the posterior belly of the digastric muscle.

i. nasa′lis maxil′lae [TA] nasal notch of maxilla: the large notch in the anterior border of the maxilla that forms the lateral and inferior margins of the anterior nasal aperture.

i. pancre′atis [TA] pancreatic notch: a notch at the junction of the left half of the head of the pancreas and the neck of the pancreas.

i. parieta′lis os′sis tempora′lis [TA] parietal notch of temporal bone: the notch found on the upper margin of the temporal bone where the squamous and parietomastoid sutures meet.

i. preoccipita′lis [TA] preoccipital notch: a notch near the posterior end of the inferolateral border of the cerebral hemisphere. A line joining it to the parietooccipital sulcus serves to delineate the parietal and temporal lobes from the occipital lobe.

i. pterygoi′dea [TA] pterygoid notch: a notch on the inferior portion of the pterygoid processes of the sphenoid bone, where the pyramidal process of the palatine bone is inserted between the diverging medial and lateral pterygoid plates; called also *pterygoid fissure.*

i. radia′lis ul′nae [TA] radial notch of ulna: the cavity on the outer side of the coronoid process, articulating with the rim of the head of the radius.

i. sca′pulae [TA] suprascapular notch: a notch, converted into a foramen by a ligament, on the upper border of the scapula at the base of the coracoid process; called also *scapular notch.*

i. sphenopalati′na os′sis palati′ni [TA] sphenopalatine notch of palatine bone: a notch between the orbital and sphenoid processes of the palatine bone; it is converted into a foramen by the inferior surface of the sphenoid bone.

i. supraorbita′lis [TA] supraorbital notch: a palpable notch in the frontal bone at the junction of the medial one-third and lateral two-thirds of the supraorbital margin, for transmission of the supraorbital nerve and vessels to the forehead. In life it is bridged by fibrous tissue, which is sometimes ossified, forming a bony aperture *(foramen supraorbitale).*

i. tento′rii cerebel′li [TA], **i. of tentorium of cerebellum** tentorial notch: an opening at the anterior part of the cerebellum, formed

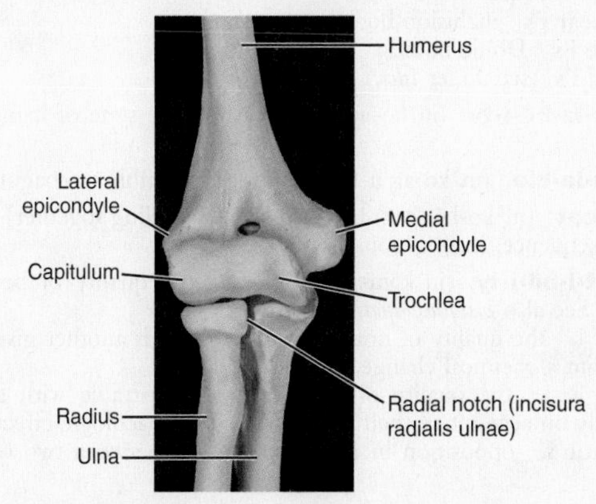

■ Incisura radialis ulnae (radial notch of ulna), in an anterior view of the right arm.

Incisura *Continued*

by the free, internal border of the tentorium cerebelli and the dorsum sellae of the sphenoid, and occupied chiefly by the mesencephalon.

i. termina′lis auricula′ris [TA] terminal notch of auricle: a deep notch separating the lamina tragi and cartilage of the external acoustic meatus from the main auricular cartilage.

i. thyroi′dea infe′rior [TA] inferior thyroid notch: a notch at the lower part of the anterior border of the thyroid cartilage.

i. thyroi′dea supe′rior [TA] superior thyroid notch: a deep notch in the upper portion of the anterior border of the thyroid cartilage.

i. trochlea′ris ul′nae [TA] trochlear notch: a large concavity on the anterior surface at the proximal end of the ulna, formed by the olecranon and coronoid processes, for articulation with the trochlea of the humerus. Called also *semilunar notch of ulna.*

i. tympa′nica [TA] tympanic notch: a defect in the upper portion of the tympanic part of the temporal bone, between the greater and lesser tympanic spines; it is filled in by the pars flaccida of the tympanic membrane. Called also *rivinian* or *Rivinus notch.*

i. ulna′ris ra′dii [TA] ulnar notch of radius: a concavity on the medial side of the distal extremity of the radius, articulating with the head of the ulna.

i. vertebra′lis infe′rior [TA] inferior vertebral notch: the indentation found below each pedicle of a vertebra which, with the indentation located above the pedicle of the vertebra below, forms the intervertebral foramen.

i. vertebra′lis supe′rior [TA] superior vertebral notch: the indentation found above each pedicle of a vertebra which, with the indentation located below the corresponding pedicle of the vertebra above, forms the intervertebral foramen.

temporal i. a slight fissure between the uncus of the parahippocampal gyrus and the apex of the temporal lobe.

in•cli•na•tio (in″klĭ-na′she-o) pl. *inclinatio′nes* [L., from *inclinare* to lean] inclination.

i. pel′vis [TA] pelvic inclination: the angle between the plane of the superior aperture of the minor pelvis and the horizontal plane, when the body is in the erect position; called also *pelvic incline.*

in•cli•na•tion (in″klĭ-na′shən) [L. *inclinare* to lean] 1. a deviation from the horizontal or vertical; a sloping or leaning. 2. deviation of the long axis of a tooth from the perpendicular line. 3. deviation of a portion of the surface of a tooth from the general plane of that surface. 4. description of the angles with the surface of a tooth at which the walls of a cavity may be cut, or of the relation of the opposing walls to each other, as *outward inclination, inward inclination,* etc. 5. inclination of enamel rods from a line perpendicular to the surface of a tooth.

condylar guidance i., condylar guide i. the angle of inclination of the condylar guidance to an accepted horizontal plane.

lateral condylar i. the direction of the lateral condyle path.

lingual i. deviation of a tooth from the vertical, in the direction of the tongue.

pelvic i., i. of pelvis inclinatio pelvis.

in•cli•na•ti•o•nes (in″klĭ-na″she-o′nēz) [L.] plural of *inclinatio.*

in•cline (in′klīn) inclination.

pelvic i., i. of pelvis inclinatio pelvis.

in•cli•nom•e•ter (in″klĭ-nom′ə-tər) [*inclination* + *-meter*] an instrument for determining ocular inclinations, angles, and directions of the visual axes.

in•clu•sion (in-kloo′zhən) [L. *inclusio*] 1. the act of enclosing or condition of being enclosed. 2. anything that is enclosed; often used alone to refer to cell inclusions.

cell i. a usually lifeless, often temporary, constituent of the cytoplasm of a cell, such as an accumulation of proteins, fats, carbohydrates, pigments, secretory granules, crystals, or other insoluble components.

dental i. 1. a tooth so surrounded with bony material that it is unable to erupt. 2. a cyst of oral soft tissue or bone.

fetal i. endadelphos.

intranuclear i's inclusion bodies.

leukocyte i's Döhle bodies.

Walthard i's see under *islet.*

in•co•ag•u•la•bil•i•ty (in″ko-ag″u-lə-bil′ĭ-te) the state of being incoagulable.

in•co•ag•u•la•ble (in″ko-ag′u-lə-bəl) not susceptible to coagulation.

in•co•her•ent (in″ko-hēr′ənt) [*in-*[2] + *cohaerere* to cling together] without proper sequence; incongruous.

in•com•pat•i•bil•i•ty (in″kəm-pat″ĭ-bil′ĭ-te) the quality of being incompatible. See also *histoincompatibility.*

chemical i. the quality of not being miscible with another given substance without a chemical change.

physiologic i. the quality of not being administrable with another given remedy on account of their antagonistic pharmacologic effects.

therapeutic i. opposition in therapeutic effect between two or more medicines.

in•com•pat•i•ble (in″kəm-pat′ĭ-bəl) [L. *incompatibilis*] not suitable for combination or simultaneous administration; mutually repellent. See also *histoincompatible.*

in•com•pe•tence (in-kom′pə-təns) [L. *in* not + *competens* sufficient] 1. insufficiency. 2. mental inadequacy. 3. the legal status of a person determined by the court to be unable to manage his own affairs.

aortic i. see under *insufficiency.*

atrial chronotropic i. inability to increase the heart rate to levels capable of satisfying the needs of the body.

congenital palatopharyngeal i. (CPI) a congenital variety of velopharyngeal insufficiency.

mitral i. see under *insufficiency.*

primary valvular i. venous insufficiency.

pulmonary i. see under *insufficiency.*

tricuspid i. see under *insufficiency.*

valvular i. see under *insufficiency.*

velopharyngeal i. see under *insufficiency.*

in•com•pe•ten•cy (in-kom′pə-tən″se) incompetence.

in•com•pe•tent (in-kom′pə-tənt) 1. lacking competence; unable to perform the required functions. 2. an individual who is unable to perform the required functions of everyday living. 3. a person determined by the court to be unable to manage his own affairs.

in•com•pres•si•ble (in″kəm-pres′ĭ-bəl) not susceptible of being squeezed together.

in•con•ti•nence (in-kon′tĭ-nəns) [L. *incontinentia*] 1. inability to control excretory functions, such as defecation (fecal i.) or urination (urinary i.). 2. immoderation or excess.

active i. urinary or fecal incontinence in which the bowel or bladder is emptied involuntarily, but at regular intervals and in the normal way.

anal i. fecal i.

anatomic i. urinary incontinence associated with instability or excessive mobility of the bladder neck and adjacent urethra.

bowel i. fecal i.

emotional i. pseudobulbar affect.

fecal i., i. of the feces failure of control of the anal sphincters, with involuntary passage of feces and flatus; it may be either psychogenic or organic in origin. Called also *encopresis* and *anal,bowel,* or *rectal i.*

melanin i., melanin pigment i. release of melanin from lysed keratinocytes with uptake by melanophages of the superficial epidermis, producing a slate-colored discoloration of the skin.

overflow i., paradoxical i. urinary incontinence due to pressure of retained urine in the bladder after the bladder has contracted to its limits, with dribbling of urine.

passive i. 1. urinary incontinence in which the bladder is full and cannot be emptied in the normal way, but the urine dribbles away from mere pressure. 2. fecal incontinence in which defecation does not occur in the normal way but can be induced by pressure.

pigment i., i. of pigment incontinentia pigmenti.

rectal i. fecal i.

reflex i. the urinary incontinence that accompanies detrusor hyperreflexia (see under *hyperreflexia*).

stress i. urinary incontinence due to anatomic displacement that exerts an opening pull on the bladder orifice, as in straining or coughing.

urge i., urgency i. urinary or fecal incontinence preceded by a sudden, uncontrollable impulse to evacuate. See also *urgency.*

urinary i., i. of urine failure of voluntary control of the vesical and urethral sphincters, with constant or frequent involuntary urination. Called also *enuresis.*

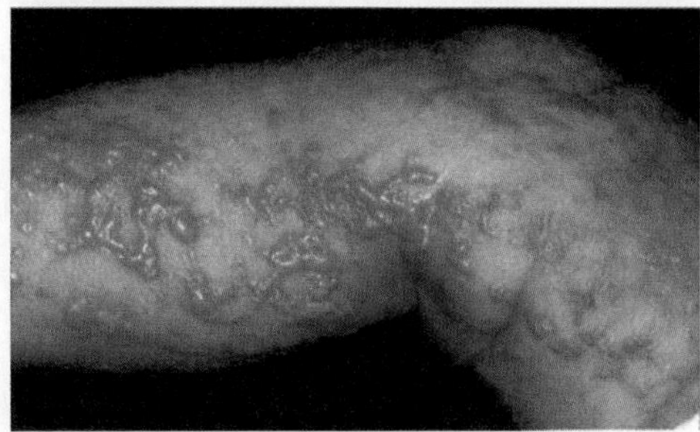

■ Whorled pattern of vesicles in incontinentia pigmenti.

in•con•ti•nent (in-kon′tĭ-nənt) 1. unable to control excretory functions; see *incontinence.* 2. immoderate.

in•con•ti•nen•tia (in-kon″tĭ-nen′shə) [L.] incontinence.
 i. al′vi fecal incontinence.
 Bloch-Sulzberger i. pigmen′ti i. pigmenti.
 i. pigmen′ti an X-linked dominant syndrome, usually lethal in utero to males, caused by mutation in the *IKBKG* gene (locus: Xq28), resulting in a mosaic pattern in which cells expressing the mutant chromosome die and are replaced by cells expressing the normal chromosome. In surviving infants, onset is at birth or shortly thereafter and proceeds through four phases, which may overlap. The first is characterized by erythematous linear streaks and vesiculation; in the second phase, the vesicles become dry and hyperkeratotic and form verrucous plaques. The third phase is characterized by hyperpigmented cutaneous lesions such as brown or gray-brown bands, whorls, swirls, or splatterlike patterns, which generally disappear by age 20. The fourth phase is marked by the appearance of hairless, anhidrotic, hypopigmented patches or streaks. It is often associated with developmental anomalies involving other structures such as the hair, eyes, skeletal system, and central nervous system. Called also *Bloch-Sulzberger i. pigmenti* and *Bloch-Sulzberger syndrome.*
 i. pigmen′ti achro′mians hypomelanosis of Ito.
 i. uri′nae urinary incontinence.

in•co•or•di•na•tion (in″ko-or″dĭ-na′shən) [*in-*[2] + *coordination*] 1. ataxia. 2. failure of organs to work harmoniously.

in•cor•po•ra•tion (in-kor″por-a′shən) [L. *in* into + *corpus* body] 1. the union of one substance with another, or with others, in a composite mass. 2. in psychoanalytic theory, a primitive unconscious defense mechanism in which aspects of another person are assimilated into the self through a figurative process of symbolic oral ingestion; it is the earliest mechanism of identification and is a form of introjection.

in•co•sta•pe•di•al (ing″ko-stə-pe′de-əl) incudostapedial.

in•cre•ment (in′krə-mənt) [L. *incrementum*] addition, or increase; the amount by which a given quantity or value is increased.

in•cre•tin (in-kre′tin) any of various gastrointestinal hormones and factors that act as potent stimulators of insulin secretion, such as gastric inhibitory polypeptide.

in•cre•tion (in-kre′shən) internal secretion.

in•cross (in′kros) [*in-*[1] + *cross* (def. 2)] the mating of individuals of the same genotype, particularly those of the same inbred strain; cf. *intercross.*

in•crus•ta•tion (in″krəs-ta′shən) [L. *in* on + *crusta* crust] 1. the formation of a crust. 2. a crust, scale, or scab.

in•cu•bate (in′ku-bāt) [L. *incubare* to lie in or on; to watch over jealously] 1. to place in an optimal situation for development, as by provision of the proper temperature and humidity for the growth of living cells, such as ova, microorganisms, or tissue cells. 2. to maintain a culture or a reaction mixture at a fixed temperature. 3. material which has been incubated.

in•cu•ba•tion (in″ku-ba′shən) [L. *incubatio*] 1. the development of the embryo in the eggs of oviparous animals. 2. the maintenance of an environment with controlled temperature, humidity, and oxygen for the development of an infant, especially of a premature one. 3. the development of an infectious disease from the entrance of the pathogen to the appearance of clinical symptoms. See also *incubation period,* under *period.* 4. the development of microorganisms or other cells in an appropriate medium under controlled environmental conditions, especially of temperature, to permit optimum growth. 5. the process of maintaining reaction mixtures at a given temperature for specified time periods for the development of chemical or enzymatic reactions.

in•cu•ba•tor (in′ku-ba″tər) 1. an apparatus for maintaining a premature infant in an environment of proper temperature and humidity. 2. an apparatus for maintaining a constant and suitable temperature for the development of eggs, cultures of microorganisms, or other living cells.

in•cu•dec•to•my (ing″ku-dek′tə-me) [*incus* + *-ectomy*] surgical removal of the incus.

in•cu•di•form (ing-ku′dĭ-form) anvil-shaped.

in•cu•do•mal•le•al (ing″ku-do-mal′e-əl) incudomalleolar.

in•cu•do•mal•le•ar (ing″ku-do-mal′e-ər) incudomalleolar.

in•cu•do•mal•le•o•lar (ing″ku-do-mal″e-o′lər) pertaining to the incus and the malleus, particularly to the articulation between them. Called also *incudomalleal* and *incudomallear.*

in•cu•do•sta•pe•di•al (ing″ku-do-stə-pe′de-əl) pertaining to the incus and stapes, particularly to the articulation between them.

in•cur•a•ble (in-kūr′ə-bəl) not susceptible of being cured.

in•cur•va•tion (in″kər-va′shən) [L. *incurvare* to bend in] a condition of being bent in.

in•cus (ing′kəs) gen. *incu′dis* [L. "anvil"] [TA] the middle of the three ossicles of the ear, which, with the stapes and malleus, serves to conduct vibrations from the tympanic membrane to the internal ear. Called also *anvil.* See illustration at *ossicula auditus,* under *ossiculum.* **in′cudal** *adj*

in•cy•clo•pho•ria (in-si″klo-for′e-ə) [L. *in* toward + *cyclophoria*] cyclophoria in which the upper pole of the vertical axis of the eye deviates toward the midline of the face, or toward the nose; called also *minus cyclophoria.* Cf. *excyclophoria.*

in•cy•clo•tro•pia (in-si″klo-tro′pe-ə) [L. *in* toward + *cyclotropia*] cyclotropia in which the upper pole of the vertical axis of the eye deviates toward the midline of the face, or toward the nose.

in d. [L.] in di′es (daily).

in•dane•di•one (in″dān-di′ōn) any of a group of synthetic anticoagulants derived from 1,3-indanedione; they are chemically different from the coumarin (q.v.) drugs but similar to them in structure and actions, i.e., they impair the hepatic synthesis of the vitamin K–dependent coagulation factors (prothrombin, factors VII, IX, and X).

in•dap•a•mide (in-dap′ə-mīd) [USP] an antihypertensive and diuretic with actions and uses similar to those of chlorothiazide; administered orally either alone or in combination with other antihypertensive agents.

In•de•cid•ua (in″də-sid′u-ə) a division of the class Mammalia, comprising the mammals without a decidua, including whales and ungulates.

in•den•iza•tion (in-den″ĭ-za′shən) innidiation.

in•den•ta•tion (in″dən-ta′shən) [L. *in* + *dens*] 1. a condition of being notched; a notch, pit, or depression. 2. the act of indenting, as with the finger.

In•der•al (in′dər-awl) trademark for preparations of propranolol hydrochloride.

In•der•ide (in′der-īd) trademark for preparations of propranolol hydrochloride with hydrochlorothiazide.

in•dex (in′deks) pl. *indexes* or *indices* [L. "that which points out," from *indicare*] 1. [TA] the second digit of the hand, the finger adjacent to the thumb; called also *forefinger, index finger,* and *digitus secundus (II) manus* [TA alternative]. 2. a unitless quantity, usually a ratio of two measurable quantities having the same dimensions, or such a ratio multiplied by 100. 3. a core or mold used in dentistry to record or maintain the relative position of a tooth or teeth to one another and/or to a cast, to ensure reproduction in the dental prosthesis of their original position. 4. a directory, in particular an alphabetized list of terms, each term accompanied by page numbers or other notations telling where it appears in a given work or set of works. 5. a subscript, as in x_i, used to indicate that there is a collection of objects, one corresponding to each value of the subscript, with the sequence indexed by i. For example, the sequence $x_1, x_2, x_3, \ldots$ can be written x_i, $i = 1, 2, 3, \ldots$.

Index

absorbancy i. absorptivity.
acetabular i. acetabular angle.
ACH i. an index for nutritional condition of children based on measurements of arm girth, chest depth, and hip width.

Index *Continued*

Addiction Severity I. (ASI) a scale used in assessing alcoholism and substance abuse by measuring the severity of problems in six areas, comprising drug and alcohol abuse, medical, psychological, legal, family and social, and employment and support.
altitudinal i. the relation of the cranial height to the cranial length; called also *height i.* and *length-height i.*
alveolar i. gnathic i.
ankle-brachial i. (ABI) the ratio of the resting systolic pressure in the arteries of the ankle to that of the brachial artery; an ABI of less than 0.9 indicates peripheral artery disease of the lower limb.
Arneth i. a calculation formerly much used in reference to the Arneth count of lobes of neutrophil nuclei; in a normal population the percentages with one or two lobes plus half the percentage with three lobes should total 60 per cent.
AST to platelet ratio i. (APRI) the ratio between aspartate transaminase and platelets in the blood, a noninvasive test for assessing liver fibrosis in conditions such as hepatitis B and C.
auricular i. the relation of the width to the height of the auricle of the ear.
auriculoparietal i. the ratio of the breadth of the skull between the auricular points to its greatest breadth.
auriculovertical i. the ratio of the height of the skull superior to the auricular point to its greatest height.
baric i. 100 times the body weight in grams divided by the cube of the height in centimeters.
Barthel i. a common method used for functional assessment (q.v.), using standardized classifications to measure skills such as activities of daily living and mobility.
basilar i. the ratio of the distance between the basion and the alveolar point to the total length of the skull.
Becker-Lennhoff i. Lennhoff i.
body build i. body weight in grams divided by the square of the height in centimeters.
body mass i. (BMI) the weight in kilograms divided by the square of the height in meters, a measure of body fat that gives an indication of nutritional status.
brachial i. 100 times the length of the upper limb from the head of the radius to the styloid process divided by the length of the limb from the acromion to the head of the radius.
Broders i. an index of malignancy based on the fact that the more undifferentiated or embryonic the cells of a tumor, the more malignant the tumor. Grade 1 contains one fourth undifferentiated cells; grade 2, one half undifferentiated cells; grade 3, three fourths undifferentiated cells; grade 4, all cells undifferentiated.
Brugsch i. 100 times the chest circumference divided by body length.
calcium i. the relative amount of calcium in the blood compared with that in a 1:6000 solution of calcium oxide.
cardiac i. (CI) cardiac output per unit time divided by body surface area; normally calculated in liters per minute per square meter.
cardiothoracic i. see under *ratio.*
I.-Catalogue Index-Catalogue of the Library of the Surgeon General's Office, published from 1880 to 1950; replaced by Current List of Medical Literature published to 1959; in 1960 replaced by Index Medicus.
centromeric i. the ratio of the length of the shorter arm of a mitotic chromosome to the total length of the chromosome.
cephalic i. 100 times the maximal head breadth divided by the maximal head length.
cephalorachidian i., cephalorhachidian i. cerebrospinal i.
cephalospinal i. the ratio of the area of the foramen magnum in square meters and the cranial capacity in cubic centimeters.
cerebral i. the ratio of the greatest transverse to the greatest anteroposterior diameter of the cranial cavity.
cerebrospinal i. the figure obtained by multiplying the final cerebrospinal pressure by the quantity of fluid withdrawn in spinal puncture and then dividing by the initial pressure.
chemotherapeutic i. therapeutic i.
Colour I. a publication of the Society of Dyers and Colourists and the American Association of Textile Chemists and Colorists containing an extensive list of dyes and dye intermediates. Each chemically distinct compound is identified by a specific number, the CI number, avoiding the confusion of trivial names used for dyes in the dye industry.
coronofrontal i. the ratio of the greatest frontal to the greatest coronal breadth of the head.
cranial i. 100 times the maximal breadth of the skull divided by its length.
Cumulated I. Medicus an annual publication of the National Library of Medicine, comprising the twelve monthly issues of the Index Medicus.
dental i. a craniometric index obtained by multiplying the dental length by 100 and dividing the product by the basinasal length. Called also *Flower i.*
digital i. a measure of the extent of clubbing: for each of the ten fingers, circumferences are measured for the nail bed (NB) and distal interphalangeal joint (DIP) and the ratio NB/DIP is calculated. The sum of the ten ratios is calculated; if it exceeds 10.0, clubbing is present.
dyspnea i. the ratio of peak exercise ventilation to maximal voluntary ventilation.
effective temperature i. an index indicating the warmth due to air temperature, air movement, and humidity.
endemic i. the percentage of persons in any locality affected with an endemic disease.
erythrocyte indices the mean corpuscular volume, mean corpuscular hemoglobin, and mean corpuscular hemoglobin concentration. Called also *red blood cell indices* and *red cell indices.*
facial i. the relation of the length of the face to its width, obtained by multiplying by 100 the bizygomatic width and dividing the product by the distance from the ophryon to the alveolar point.
fatigue i. the ratio between the muscle tension after a period of intermittent tetanic stimulation and the tension present before stimulation was applied.
femorohumeral i. 100 times the length of the humerus divided by the length of the femur.
Flower i. dental i.
forearm-hand i. 100 times the length of the hand divided by the length of the forearm.
Forns i. a noninvasive formula for assessing liver fibrosis in conditions such as hepatitis B and C, calculating patient age, platelet count, serum cholesterol, and serum γ-glutamyl transferase.
free T_3 i. free triiodothyronine i.
free T_4 i. free thyroxine i.
free thyroxine i. an estimate of the physiologically active free thyroxine in serum, obtained by multiplying the total serum thyroxine concentration by the thyroxine uptake. Called also *free T_4 i.*
free triiodothyronine i. an estimate of the physiologically active free triiodothyronine in serum, obtained by multiplying the total serum triiodothyronine concentration by the triiodothyronine uptake. Called also *free T_3 i.*
gnathic i. the degree of prominence of the upper jaw, expressed as a percentage of the distance from basion to nasion. Called also *alveolar i.*
habitus i. 100 times the sum of the chest girth and the abdominal girth divided by the stature.
hair i. the figure obtained by dividing the least diameter of the cross section of a hair by its greatest diameter and multiplying by 100; a high index indicates an approximately round shape; a low index indicates an ovoid cross section.
hand i. 100 times the breadth of the hand divided by its length.
height i. altitudinal i.
intermembral i. 100 times the length of the humerus plus radius divided by the length of the femur plus tibia.
length-breadth i. the breadth of the skull expressed as a percentage of its length.
length-height i. the height of the skull expressed as a percentage of its length.
Lennhoff i. 100 times the distance from the sternal notch to the symphysis pubis divided by the greatest circumference of the abdomen.
lower leg–foot i. 100 times the length of the foot divided by the length of the lower leg.
maturation i. the ratio between three different types of cells shed from the vaginal squamous epithelium, done from a random sample. The cell types are parabasal cells, intermediate cells, and superficial cells, and the ratio between them varies at different times in the normal menstrual cycle or in a woman's life (such as before and after menopause). A predominance of parabasal cells indicates absence of estrogen stimulation, and a predominance of superficial cells indicates presence of estrogen stimulation.
maxilloalveolar i. the distance between the two most lateral points on the external surface of the upper alveolar margin, usually opposite

Index *Continued*

the middle of the second permanent molar teeth, divided by the maxilloalveolar length.
I. Medicus a monthly publication of the National Library of Medicine in which the world's leading biomedical literature is indexed by author and subject; see also *Cumulated I. Medicus.*
metacarpal i. the average of the figures obtained by dividing the lengths of the right second, third, fourth, and fifth metacarpal bones by their respective breadths at the exact midpoint; stated to range normally between 5.4 and 7.9. A value above 8.4 is diagnostic of arachnodactyly.
mitotic i. an expression of the number of cells in a population undergoing mitosis, either as the number of cells in a given area of a sample (e.g., per 10 high-power fields) or as a percentage of the total number of cells.
morphologic face i. 100 times the distance from the nasion to the gnathion divided by the bizygomatic breadth.
morphological i. the volume of the trunk divided by the length of the limbs.
nasal i. 100 times the maximal breadth of the nasal aperture divided by the nasion-nasospinale height.
nucleoplasmic i. the relation of the size of the nucleus of a cell to that of the cytoplasm, expressed numerically by the quotient of the nuclear volume divided by the difference between the volume of the cell and the nuclear volume.
obesity i. body weight divided by body volume.
opsonic i. a measure of opsonic activity determined by the ratio of the number of microorganisms phagocytized by normal leukocytes in the presence of serum from an individual infected by the microorganism, to the number phagocytized in serum from a normal individual.
orbital i. 100 times the height of the opening of the orbit, divided by its width.
oxygenation i. (OI) a measure of the efficiency or impairment of oxygenation of the blood, expressed by the formula

$$\frac{(F_IO_2 \times 100)(MAP)}{P_{O_2}}$$

where F_IO_2 = functional concentration of oxygen; MAP = mean arterial pressure; and P_{O_2} = the partial pressure of oxygen. Values above 40 are life-threatening.
palatal i., palatine i., palatomaxillary i. a numerical expression of the ratio of various proportions of the palate obtained by multiplying the palatal breadth by 100 and dividing the product by the palatal length. See also *brachystaphyline* and *leptostaphyline.*
parasite i. the percentage of individuals in a population whose blood smears show the presence of parasites.
penile brachial i. the ratio of the penile systolic pressure to the radial systolic pressure in the arm; a ratio of less than 0.6 indicates organic impotence resulting from vascular incompetence.
peripheral vascular resistance i. a measure of the total vascular resistance, normalized for body surface area.
phagocytic i. any arbitrary measure of the ability of neutrophils to ingest native or opsonized particles determined by various assays; it reflects either the average number of particles ingested or the rate at which particles are cleared from the blood or culture medium.
physiognomonic upper face i. 100 times the distance from the nasion to the stomion divided by the bizygomatic breadth.
Pirquet i. (of nutritional status), multiply the weight in grams by 10, divide this product by the sitting height in centimeters and extract the cube root of this quotient. A result lower than 0.945 indicates faulty nutrition.
ponderal i. an index of body mass equal to 100 times the weight in grams divided by the square of the height (or of the crown-heel length in newborns) in centimeters.
radiohumeral i. 100 times the maximal length of the radius divided by the maximal length of the humerus.
rapid shallow breathing i. the ratio of respiratory rate to tidal volume during spontaneous breathing; a higher value means less effective spontaneous breathing and greater likelihood of need for assisted ventilation.
red blood cell indices, red cell indices erythrocyte indices.
refractive i. the refractive power of a medium compared with that of air, which is assumed to be 1. Symbol n, *n*, or n_D.
renal failure i. (RFI) an assessment of acute renal failure comparing the sodium clearance with the creatinine clearance:

$$RFI = \frac{U_{Na}}{U_{Cr}/P_{Cr}}$$

where P_{Cr} = plasma concentration of creatinine, U_{Cr} = urinary concentration of creatinine, and U_{Na} = urinary concentration of sodium. A value below 1.0 indicates renal failure due to prerenal azotemia and a value above 2.0 suggests that it is due to acute tubular necrosis. Cf. *fractional excretion of sodium,* under *excretion.*
Ritchie i. assessment of several different joints of a person with rheumatoid arthritis, measuring the degree of tenderness when pressure is applied, with numerical scores from 0 (no tenderness) to 3 (very tender).
sacral i. 100 times the breadth of the sacrum divided by the length.
short increment sensitivity i. (SISI) tones of 1- to 5-decibel increments in intensity and lasting 0.5 second are superimposed on a continuous (carrier) tone of the same frequency at random intervals, the carrier tone being 20 decibels above the speech reception threshold; only patients with cochlear damage can detect these increments.
spleen i., splenic i. the percentage of individuals in the population having enlarged spleens; used in malaria surveys.
stimulation i. (SI) see *lymphocyte proliferation test,* under *test.*
stroke i., stroke volume i. the stroke volume per heartbeat corrected for body surface area; usually expressed in mL per beat per square meter.
sulcus bleeding i. any of various methods of assessing bleeding in the gingival sulcus before or after treatment.
therapeutic i. originally, the ratio of the maximum tolerated dose to the minimum curative dose; now defined, so as to account for variability of individual response, as the ratio of the median lethal dose (LD_{50}) to the median effective dose (ED_{50}). It is used in assessing the safety of a drug. Called also *chemotherapeutic i.*
thoracic i. the ratio of the anteroposterior diameter of the thorax to the transverse diameter.
tibiofemoral i. 100 times the length of the tibia divided by the length of the femur.
tibioradial i. 100 times the length of the radius divided by the length of the tibia.
trunk i. 100 times the bi-acromial breadth divided by the sitting suprasternal height.
uricolytic i. the percentage of uric acid oxidized to allantoin before being secreted.
venous filling i. a measure of the rate of refilling of the veins, usually in the legs, expressed in milliliters per second; calculated by dividing 0.9 of the functional venous volume by the time needed to go from minimum volume (after patient has been supine with legs elevated) to 0.9 of the venous volume (with patient standing up).
vertical i. 100 times the height of the skull divided by the length of the skull.
zygomaticoauricular i. the ratio between the zygomatic and auricular diameters of the skull.

in·di·can (in′dĭ-kən) 1. a yellow indoxyl glycoside from plants that yield indigo. On hydrolysis it yields glucose and indoxyl. 2. potassium indoxyl sulfate, formed by decomposition of tryptophan in the intestines, absorbed, conjugated, and excreted in the urine.

in·di·can·emia (in″dĭ-kə-ne′me-ə) the presence of indican in the blood.

in·di·can·me·ter (in″dĭ-kən-me′tər) an instrument for estimating the amount of indican in the urine.

in·di·cano·ra·chia (in″dĭ-kan-o-ra′ke-ə) the presence of indican in the spinal fluid.

in·di·cant (in′dĭ-kənt) 1. indicating. 2. a symptom which indicates the true diagnosis or treatment.

in·di·can·uria (in″dĭ-kə-nu′re-ə) the presence of excessive indican in the urine.

in·di·car·mine (in″dĭ-kahr′mēn) indigotindisulfonate sodium.

in·di·ca·tion (in″dĭ-ka′shən) [L. *indicatio*] a sign or circumstance that points to or shows the cause, pathology, treatment, or issue of an attack of disease; something that points out, or serves as a guide or warning.

in·di·ca·tor (in′dĭ-ka″tər) [L.] 1. the index finger (index [TA]). 2. the extensor muscle of the index finger (musculus extensor indicis [TA]). 3. a substance, usually a dye or intermediate, that shows the concentration of a substance, the completion of a reaction, or the attainment of a particular pH range by a change in color or other visible sign.
anaerobic i. a dilute solution of methylene blue is decolorized in the absence of oxygen.
biological i. a viable culture of specific microorganisms resistant to a given sterilization process, used to develop sterilization processes or monitor sterilization cycles; it may consist of spores added to a paper, glass, or plastic carrier or of spores added to representative units of the lot to be sterilized (or to similar units).
radioactive i. see under *tracer*.
redox i. a pigment which indicates by a change of color a change in the oxidation potential.
Schneider i. an index designed to reflect cardiovascular fitness, based mainly on heart rate during and after mild exercise.

in·di·co·phose (in′dĭ-ko″fōz) an indigo-colored phose.

in·dif·fer·ence (in-dif′ər-əns) lack of appropriate feeling or emotion or of response to a stimulus; apathy. **indif′ferent** *adj*
congenital i. to pain analgesia or hypoalgesia owing to a congenital condition, usually an autosomal recessive condition; it may occur with few other abnormalities or as part of a syndrome such as familial dysautonomia.

in·dif·fé·rence (ă-de″fa-rahns′) [Fr.] indifference.
la belle i. [Fr. "beautiful indifference"] an inappropriately complacent attitude toward their condition and symptoms shown by individuals with conversion disorder.

in·dig·e·nous (in-dij′ə-nəs) [L. *indigenus*] native, or not exotic; native to a particular place or country.

in·di·gest·i·ble (in″di-jes′tĭ-bəl) [*in-*[2] + *digestible*] not susceptible of being digested.

in·di·ges·tion (in″dĭ-jes′chən) lack or failure of digestion; commonly used to denote vague abdominal discomfort after meals.
acid i. hyperchlorhydria.
fat i. steatorrhea.
gastric i. indigestion taking place in the stomach, or due to a disorder of the stomach.
intestinal i. inadequacy of digestive function of the intestine.
sugar i. defective ability to digest sugar, resulting in fermentative diarrhea.
vagus i. a condition in cattle and sometimes sheep caused by damage to the vagus nerve, such as after traumatic reticuloperitonitis; characteristics include impaired motility through the stomachs and intestines, abdominal distention, chronic constipation, and anorexia.

in·dig·i·ta·tion (in-dij″ĭ-ta′shən) [L. *in* into + *digitus* finger] intussusception (def. 1).

in·di·go (in′dĭ-go) [Gr. *Indikon* Indian dye] 1. any of various plants of the genus *Indigofera*. 2. a blue dyeing material, the aglycon of indican, found in *I. tinctoria* and other plants, or made synthetically. It is sometimes found in the sweat and the urine, where it is derived from urinary indican (indoxyl sulfate). 3. a color between blue and violet, produced by energy of wavelengths between 420 and 450 nm.

In·di·gof·e·ra (in″dĭ-gof′ə-rə) a genus of leguminous herbs. *I. do′minii* (formerly called *I. ennea′phylla*) causes Birdsville disease among horses in Australia. *I. spica′ta* causes liver damage in horses. *I. tincto′ria* is a source of indigo.

in·di·go·gen (in′dĭ-go-jən) a crystalline principle from indigo.

in·di·go·pur·pu·rine (in″dĭ-go-pur′pu-rin) a purple pigment occasionally found in the urine.

in·dig·o·tin (in″dĭ-go′tin) a neutral, tasteless, dark blue powder, the principal ingredient of commercial indigo; called also *indigo blue*.

in·di·go·tin·di·sul·fon·ate so·di·um (in″dĭ-go″tin-di-sul′fo-nāt) [USP] a dye, occurring as a dusky, purplish blue powder or blue granules; used as a diagnostic aid in cystoscopy and other studies of the urinary tract; administered intravenously. Called also *indigo carmine*, *indicarmine*, and *soluble indigo blue*.

in·din·a·vir sul·fate (in-din′ə-vir) [USP] an HIV protease inhibitor that causes formation of immature, noninfectious viral particles; used in the treatment of human immunodeficiency virus infection and acquired immunodeficiency syndrome; administered orally.

in·di·rect (in″di-rekt′) [L. *indirectus*] 1. not immediate or straight. 2. acting through an intermediary agent.

in·di·ru·bin (in″di-roo′bin) a red pigment occasionally found in the urine.

in·di·ru·bin·uria (in″di-roo″bĭ-nu′re-ə) the presence of indirubin in the urine.

in·dis·crim·i·nate (in″dis-krim′ĭ-nət) [L. *in* not + *discrimen* distinction] affecting various parts without distinction.

in·dis·po·si·tion (in″dis-pə-zish′ən) the condition of being slightly ill; a slight illness.

in·di·um (In) (in′de-əm) [L. *indicum* indigo] a metallic element, atomic number 49, atomic weight 114.82; named from its blue line in the spectrum.
i. 111 an artificial radioactive isotope of indium, having a half-life of 2.81 days; it decays by electron capture, emitting 0.172 and 0.247 MeV gamma rays, and is used as a tracer in nuclear medicine.
i. 113m a radioactive isotope having a half-life of 1.66 hours, decaying by isomeric transition and emitting gamma rays of energy 0.393 MeV; used as a radioactive tracer in nuclear medicine.
i. In 111 chloride [USP] a solution of ^{111}In in dilute hydrochloric acid, used for the radiolabeling of proteins such as monoclonal antibodies.
i. In 111 DTPA i. In 111 pentetate.
i. In 111 ibritumomab tiuxetan [USP] a chelate of ^{111}In and the immunoconjugate ibritumomab tiuxetan, used in the treatment of non-Hodgkin lymphoma; administered intravenously
i. In 111 oxine i. In 111 oxyquinoline.
i. In 111 oxyquinoline [USP] a chelate of ^{111}In with oxyquinoline, used to label platelets and leukocytes; labeled leukocytes are used for the diagnosis and localization of inflammatory lesions, as in abscesses, infections, or inflammatory bowel diseases, and labeled platelets are used in the detection of thrombi and studies of platelet survival.
i. In 111 pentetate [USP] a chelate of ^{111}In with pentetic acid, administered intrathecally, intracisternally, or intraventricularly in radionuclide cisternography to evaluate disorders of the flow of cerebrospinal fluid.
i. In 111 pentetreotide [USP] a chelate of ^{111}In with the somatostatin analogue pentetreotide, used in the imaging of neuroendocrine tumors with somatostatin receptors; administered intravenously.
i. In 111 satumomab pentetide an ^{111}In–labeled monoclonal antibody used as a diagnostic imaging agent to determine the location and extent of extrahepatic malignant lesions in patients with colorectal or ovarian cancer.

in·di·vid·u·a·tion (in″dĭ-vid″u-a′shən) 1. the process of developing individual characteristics. 2. differential regional activity in the embryo occurring in response to organizer influence.

In·do·cin (in′do-sin) trademark for preparations of indomethacin.

in·dol·amine (in-dol′ə-mēn) an amine-substituted derivative of indole, such as serotonin or melatonin.

in·dole (in′dōl) 1. a heterocyclic compound, obtained from coal tar and also produced by the decomposition of tryptophan in the intestine; it is partly responsible for the peculiar odor of the feces. 2. any of numerous compounds containing the ring structure of this compound.

in·do·lent (in′do-lənt) [L. *in* not + *dolens* painful] 1. causing little pain, as an indolent lesion. 2. slow growing, as an indolent tumor.

in·do·log·e·nous (in″do-loj′ə-nəs) causing the formation of indole.

in·dol·uria (in″dōl-u′re-ə) the presence of an indole in the urine.

in·do·meth·a·cin (in″do-meth′ə-sin) [USP] a nonsteroidal antiinflammatory drug; used in the treatment of rheumatoid arthritis, osteoarthritis, ankylosing spondylitis, acute gouty arthritis, other rheumatic and nonrheumatic inflammatory conditions, and dysmenorrhea, and the treatment and prophylaxis of vascular headaches; administered orally or rectally. It is also applied topically to the conjunctiva to prevent miosis during cataract surgery and to reduce the severity and occurrence of postoperative cystoid macular edema.
i. sodium [USP] the trihydrated sodium salt of indomethacin, used to induce closure of a hemodynamically significant patent ductus arteriosus in premature infants weighing between 500 and 1750 g who do not respond to conservative treatment; administered intravenously.

in·do·phe·nol (in″do-fe′nol) any one of a series of dyes which are nitrogen derivatives of quinone.

in·dor·a·min (in-dor′ə-min) a selective antagonist of α_1-adrenergic receptors, used as an antihypertensive; administered orally.

in·dox·yl (in-dok′səl) [*indigo* + *ox-* + *-yl*] an oxidation product of indole, formed by decomposition from tryptophan and excreted in the urine as indican (potassium indoxyl sulfate).

in·dox·yl·emia (in-dok″sə-le′me-ə) the presence of indoxyl in the blood.

in·dox·yl·uria (in-dok″sə-lu′re-ə) the presence of an excess of indoxyl in the urine.

in·duced (in-dōōst′) [L. *inducere* to lead in] 1. produced artificially. 2. produced by induction.

in·duc·er (in-dōōs′ər) in molecular genetics, a molecule that causes a cell or organism to accelerate synthesis of an enzyme or sequence of enzymes in response to an environmental signal. The inducer often acts by antagonizing the action of a corresponding repressor, and may be a substrate of the enzyme or may be some other molecule, such as a hormone.

in•du•ci•ble (in-doo'sĭ-bəl) produced because of stimulation by an inducer; cf. *constitutive.*

in•duc•tance (in-duk'təns) that property of a circuit whereby changing current generates an electromotive force (EMF) in the same or a neighboring circuit; the EMF is proportional to the rate of change of the current and inductance is quantitated as the ratio of these two, in SI units expressed as the henry. It is sometimes used to denote mutual inductance specifically. See also *self-inductance.*

mutual i. (*M*) inductance generated in a neighboring circuit. Called also *inductance.*

in•duc•tion (in-duk'shən) [L. *inductio*] 1. the act or process of inducing or causing to occur. See also under *chemotherapy.* 2. the production of a specific morphogenetic effect in the developing embryo through the influence of evocators or organizers. 3. the production of anesthesia or unconsciousness by use of appropriate agents. 4. the generation of an electric current or of magnetic properties in a body because of the presence of another electric current or magnetic field nearby.

autonomous i. induction in which the inductor forms no part of the portion produced.

complementary i. induction in which the inductor forms a part of the portion produced.

enzyme i. increased synthesis of an enzyme in response to an inducer or other stimulus.

magnetic i. magnetic flux density.

ovulation i. treatment of infertility in the female by administration of hormones that stimulate the ovaries.

Spemann i. the stimulating and directing effect shown by certain tissues on neighboring tissues or parts in early development of the embryo.

spinal i. the process by which one reflex lowers the threshold of another reflex which otherwise cannot be penetrated.

in•duc•tor (in-duk'tər) a tissue elaborating a chemical substance which acts to determine the growth and differentiation of embryonic parts. Cf. *activator* (def. 2) and *organizer.*

in•duc•to•therm (in-duk'to-thərm) an apparatus for producing high body temperature by electric induction.

in•duc•to•ther•my (in-duk'to-thur"me) the production of artificial fever by electric induction.

in•du•lin (in'du-lĭn) a coal tar dye, used as a histologic stain.

in•du•lin•o•phil (in"du-lin'o-fil) 1. an element easily stainable with indulin. 2. indulinophilic.

in•du•lin•o•phil•ic (in"du-lin-o-fil'ik) [*indulin* + *-philic*] stainable with indulin.

in•du•rat•ed (in'du-rāt"əd) [L. *indurare* to harden] hardened; rendered hard. Called also *sclerous.*

in•du•ra•tion (in"du-ra'shən) [L. *induratio*] 1. the quality of being hard. 2. the process of becoming hard; called also *hardening* and *sclerosis.* 3. an abnormally hard spot or place. **indur'ative** *adj*

black i. the hardening and pigmentation of lung tissue seen in coal workers' pneumoconiosis.

brawny i. inflammatory hardening and thickening of tissues.

brown i. 1. a deposit of altered blood pigment in the lung. 2. marked increase of the connective tissue of the lung and excessive pigmentation, due to long-continued congestion from heart disease. Cf. *gray i.*

cyanotic i. a hard, dense, purple state of an organ due to congestion.

fibrous i. fibrous hardening of tissue induced by diffuse scarring.

gray i. an induration of lung tissue in or after pneumonia, without the pigmentation seen in brown induration.

penile i. Peyronie disease.

plastic i. sclerosis of the corpora cavernosa of the penis.

red i. red, congested lung tissue seen in idiopathic pulmonary fibrosis.

in•du•si•um gris•e•um (in-doo'ze-əm gris'e-əm) [L.] [TA] a thin layer of gray substance on the dorsal aspect of the corpus callosum; called also *supracallosal gyrus.*

in•dwell•ing (in'dwel-ing) pertaining to a catheter or other tube left within an organ or body passage for drainage, maintenance of patency, or administration of drugs or nutrients.

-ine a suffix indicating an alkaloid, an organic base, or a halogen.

in•e•bri•ant (in-e'bre-ənt) [L. *inebriare* to make drunk] 1. causing inebriation. 2. an agent that causes inebriation.

in•e•bri•ate (in-e'bre-āt) to intoxicate with alcohol. See also *alcoholism.*

in•e•bri•a•tion (in-e"bre-a'shən) [L. *inebriare* to make drunk] 1. intoxication with alcohol; see also *alcoholism.* 2. a state resembling alcoholic intoxication. Called also *drunkenness.*

in•e•bri•e•ty (in"ə-bri'ə-te) inebriation.

in•elas•tic (in"e-las'tik) lacking elasticity.

In•er•mi•cap•si•fer (in-ur"mĭ-kap'sĭ-fər) a genus of tapeworms of the family Linstowiidae, usually parasitic in hyraxes and rodents in Africa. *I. arvican'thidis* has been found in humans in Cuba and Central America.

in•ert (in-urt') having no action; not reacting with other elements, as inert gases.

in•er•tia (in-ur'shə) [L.] inactivity; inability to move spontaneously.

colonic i. weak muscular activity of the colon, leading to distention of the organ and constipation.

immunologic i. specific depression of immunity in a mother toward the histocompatibility antigens of a fetus, or in a fetus toward those of the mother; it does not include immunologic tolerance.

i. u'teri insufficiently strong or poorly coordinated uterine contractions during labor.

in ex•tre•mis (in ek-stre'mis) [L. "at the end"] at the point of death.

Inf. [L.] infun'de (pour in).

in•fan•cy (in'fən-se) the early period of life; see *infant.*

In•fan•rix (in'fan-riks) trademark for a preparation of diphtheria and tetanus toxoids and acellular pertussis vaccine.

in•fant (in'fənt) a young child; considered to designate the human young from birth (see *neonate*) to 12 months.

dysmature i. postmature i.

extremely low birthweight (ELBW) i. an infant weighing less than 1000 grams at birth. See also *low birth weight i.*

floppy i. see under *syndrome.*

immature i. an infant usually weighing less than 2500 grams at birth and not physiologically fully developed.

large-for-gestational-age (LGA) i. a preterm, term, or postterm infant who is above the 90th percentile for gestational age in head circumference, body weight, or length.

low birth weight (LBW) i. an infant weighing less than 2500 grams at birth.

mature i. an infant weighing 2500 grams or more at birth, usually at or near full term, physiologically fully developed, and having an optimum chance of survival.

moderately low birth weight (MLBW) i. an infant weighing at least 1500 but less than 2500 grams at birth. See also *low birth weight i.*

newborn i. the human young during the first four weeks after birth; called also *newborn* and *neonate.*

postmature i. 1. an infant with postmaturity syndrome. Called also *dysmature i.* 2. postterm i.

postterm i. an infant born at or after the forty-second completed week (294 days) of gestation.

premature i. 1. an infant usually born after the twentieth completed week and before full term, arbitrarily defined as one weighing 500 to 2499 grams at birth, having poor to good chance of survival, depending on the weight. In countries where adults are smaller than in the United States, the upper limit may be lower. Other criteria such as crown-heel length (less than 47 cm) and occipitofrontal diameter (less than 11.5 cm) have also been used. 2. preterm i.

preterm i. an infant born before the thirty-seventh completed week (259 days) of gestation.

small-for-gestational-age (SGA) i. a preterm, term, or postterm infant who is below the 10th percentile for gestational age in head circumference, body weight, or length.

term i. an infant born in the interval from the thirty-seventh completed week to the forty-second completed week of gestation; 259 days to 293 days, inclusive.

very low birth weight (VLBW) i. an infant weighing less than 1000 grams at birth. See also *low birth weight i.*

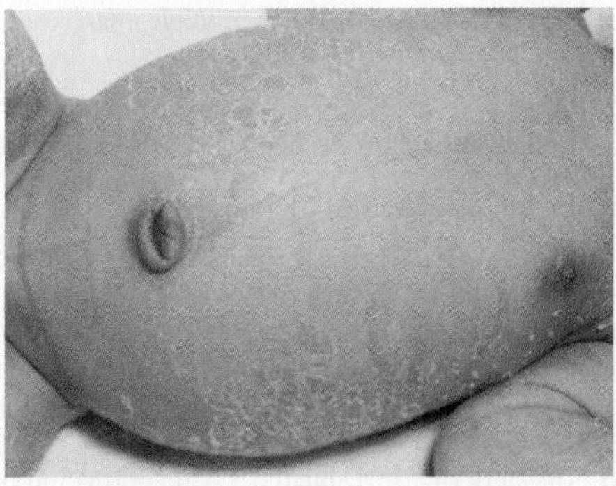

■ Postmature infant with characteristic skin changes; the skin is dry, cracking, and desquamating.

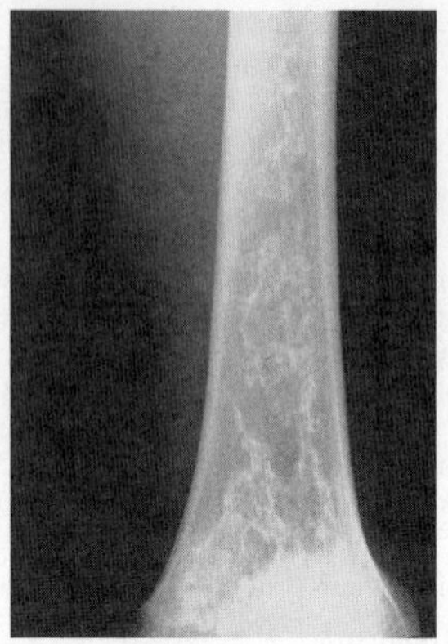

■ Bone infarcts seen as areas of diffuse and amorphous calcification within the medullary space of the distal femur.

in·fan·ti·cide (in-fan′tĭ-sīd) [*infant* + *-cide*] the taking of the life of an infant.

in·fan·tile (in′fən-tīl) pertaining to an infant or to infancy.

in·fan·ti·lism (in′fən-tĭ-liz″əm, in-fan′tĭ-liz″əm) persistence of the characteristics of childhood into adult life; it is marked by mental retardation, underdevelopment of the sexual organs, and often, but not always, dwarfism. Cf. *progeria.*

celiac i. infantilism accompanying the infantile form of celiac disease.

hypophysial i. old name for *pituitary dwarfism.*

pancreatic i. infantilism caused by inadequate secretion of pancreatic islet hormones, especially insulin. See also *Clarke-Hadfield syndrome,* under *syndrome.*

partial i. arrested development of a single part or tissue.

pituitary i. old name for *pituitary dwarfism.*

regressive i. reversion to an infantile state after body growth has been completed.

sexual i. retardation of sexual development, as in adiposogenital dystrophy and some types of pituitary dwarfism.

universal i. short stature with undeveloped secondary sex characters, as in some types of pituitary dwarfism.

in·farct (in′fahrkt) [L. *infarctus*] an area of coagulation necrosis in a tissue due to local ischemia resulting from obstruction of circulation to the area, most commonly by a thrombus or embolus. Called also *infarction.*

anemic i. an infarct in a tissue produced by sudden arrest of circulation in a vessel; called also *pale i.* and *white i.*

bilirubin i's masses of crystals of bilirubin in the pyramids of the kidneys, especially in the newborn.

bland i. an uninfected infarct.

bone i. an area of bone tissue that has become necrotic as a result of loss of its arterial blood supply.

Brewer i's dark-red, wedge-shaped areas, resembling infarcts, seen on section of a kidney in pyelonephritis.

calcareous i. a deposit of calcium salt in infarcted tissues.

cystic i. an infarct in which dead tissue is enclosed in a membrane.

embolic i. an infarct caused by an embolus.

hemorrhagic i. an infarct that is red in color owing to the oozing of red corpuscles into the dead area; seen most often in the brain or lung. Called also *red i.*

lacunar i. a small (less than 1.5 cm) infarct in the brain, found most often in the basal ganglia, internal capsule, pons, or white matter and usually in older hypertensive patients or diabetics. Depending on their location, these may be asymptomatic or may cause significant impairment; those with symptoms are called *lacunar strokes.* When multiple infarcts are present, the condition is called *status lacunaris.* Called also *lacune.*

pale i. anemic i.

red i. hemorrhagic i.

septic i. an infarct in which the tissues have been invaded by pathogenic organisms.

thrombotic i. an infarct caused by a thrombus.

uric acid i. a deposit of uric acid crystals in the renal tubules of the newborn.

white i. anemic i.

i. of Zahn an area of reddish blue discoloration in the liver, with stasis and hepatocellular atrophy, seen following occlusion of an intrahepatic branch of the portal vein; not a true infarct, because there is no necrosis.

in·farc·tec·to·my (in″fahrk-tek′tə-me) surgical removal of an infarct.

in·farc·tion (in-fahrk′shən) 1. infarct. 2. the formation of an infarct.

acute myocardial i. (AMI) myocardial infarction occurring during the period when circulation to a region of the heart is obstructed and necrosis is occurring; it is usually characterized by severe pain, frequently associated with pallor, perspiration, nausea, dyspnea, and dizziness; electrographic abnormalities may include Q wave, ST segment, and T wave alterations.

anterior myocardial i. myocardial infarction localized to the left ventricular free wall between the interventricular groove and the lateral margin of the anterior papillary muscle.

anteroinferior myocardial i. myocardial infarction involving features of both the anterior and inferior types; on the EKG there are abnormal Q waves in leads II, III, and aV_L and in one or more of leads V_1 to V_4.

anterolateral myocardial i. myocardial infarction involving features of both the anterior and lateral types; on the EKG there are abnormal Q waves in leads I, aV_L, and V_3 to V_6.

anteroseptal myocardial i. myocardial infarction involving features of both the anterior and septal types; on the EKG there are abnormal Q waves in leads V_1 to V_4.

apical myocardial i. anteroinferior myocardial I.

atrial i. the formation of an infarct in a cardiac atrium, which may be due to coronary artery occlusion, periarteritis nodosa, obliterating endarteritis of the small branches of coronary arteries, or other conditions.

cardiac i. myocardial I.

cerebral i. an ischemic condition of the brain, producing local tissue death and usually a persistent focal neurological deficit in the area of distribution of one of the cerebral arteries. See also *stroke syndrome,* under *syndrome, reversible ischemic neurologic deficit,* under *deficit,* and *transient ischemic attack,* under *attack.* Called also *cerebral ischemia.*

cortical i. a focal type of cerebral infarction limited to the cortex.

diaphragmatic myocardial i. inferior myocardial I.

extensive anterior myocardial i. myocardial infarction in the anterior region of the heart, with a more diffuse distribution than anterior myocardial infarction; on the EKG there are abnormal Q waves in leads I, aV_L, and V_1 to V_6.

high lateral myocardial i. myocardial infarction localized to the upper portion of the lateral region; on the EKG there are abnormal Q waves in leads I and aV_L.

inferior myocardial i. myocardial infarction localized in the region between the lateral border of the posterior papillary muscle and the posterior septum; on the EKG there are abnormal Q waves in leads II, III, and aV_F.

inferolateral myocardial i. myocardial infarction involving features of both the inferior and lateral types; on the EKG there are abnormal Q waves in leads II, III, aV_F, V_5, and V_6.

intestinal i. occlusion of an artery or arteriole in the wall of the intestine, resulting in the formation of an area of coagulation necrosis.

lacunar i. see under *infarct.*

lateral myocardial i. myocardial infarction in the region between the lateral margin of the anterior papillary muscle and the lateral margin of the posterior papillary muscle; on the EKG there are abnormal Q waves in leads I, aV_L, V_5, and V_6.

maternal floor i. a disorder of the placenta resulting from decreased maternal blood flow and characterized by the deposition of fibrin in the decidua basalis with induration of the maternal surface of the placenta.

mesenteric i. coagulation necrosis of the intestines due to a decrease in blood flow in the mesenteric vasculature (see also *mesenteric ischemia,* under *ischemia*). Two types are distinguished, *occlusive* and *nonocclusive mesenteric I.*

migrainous i. a focal neurologic deficit that constituted part of a migrainous aura but that has persisted for a long period and may be permanent. Called also *complicated migraine.*

myocardial i. (MI) gross necrosis of the myocardium as a result of interruption of the blood supply to the area; it is almost always caused by atherosclerosis of the coronary arteries, upon which coronary thrombosis is usually superimposed.

non–Q wave i., non–Q wave myocardial i. myocardial infarction in which the Q waves are not abnormal. Cf. *Q wave I.*

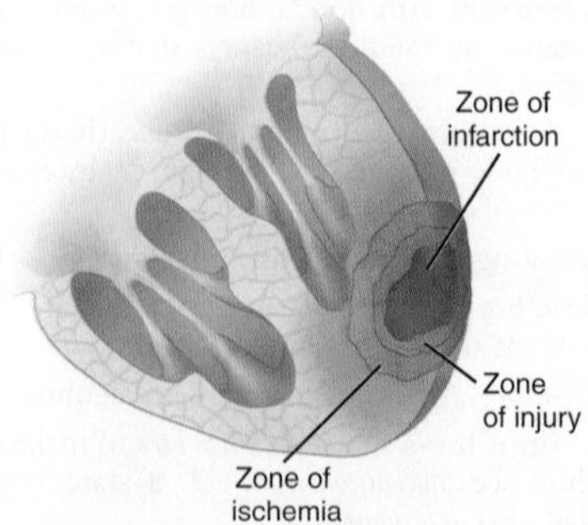

■ Myocardial infarction shown in cross-section of heart (ventricles only).

nonocclusive mesenteric i. mesenteric infarction having a nonocclusive cause, such as arteritis, a cardiogenic abnormality, or hypovolemia.

nontransmural myocardial i. a myocardial infarction that involves less than the full thickness of the myocardial wall; sometimes used synonymously with *subendocardial myocardial infarction.*

occlusive mesenteric i. mesenteric infarction due to occlusion of one of the mesenteric arteries, such as by a thrombus or by mechanical compression.

posterior myocardial i. myocardial infarction localized in the basal third of the posteroinferior heart wall; on the EKG there are abnormally large R waves in leads V_1 or V_2.

pulmonary i. localized necrosis of lung tissue caused by obstruction of the arterial blood supply, most often due to pulmonary embolism. Clinical manifestations range from the subclinical to pleuritic chest pain, dyspnea, hemoptysis, and tachycardia.

Q wave i., Q wave myocardial i. any type of myocardial infarction in which Q waves are abnormal in character or number or both. Cf. *transmural myocardial I.*

right ventricular myocardial i. myocardial infarction localized to the free wall of the right ventricle, usually associated with inferior myocardial infarctions of the left ventricle; on the EKG there are ST segment elevation in one or more right precordial leads.

septal myocardial i. myocardial infarction localized to the interventricular septum; on the EKG there are abnormal Q waves in leads V_1 and V_2.

silent myocardial i. myocardial infarction without pain or other symptoms; it may be recognized by electrographic or postmortem examination.

ST elevation myocardial i. (STEMI), ST segment elevation myocardial i. any type of myocardial infarction in which the ST segment is elevated in one lead or several leads.

subendocardial myocardial i. myocardial infarction localized to the inner one third to one half of the myocardial wall; sometimes described as *nontransmural myocardial infarction.*

transmural myocardial i. myocardial infarction involving the entire thickness of the heart wall. The term is sometimes incorrectly used as a synonym for *Q wave I.*

watershed i. cerebral infarction in a watershed area (q.v.) during a time of prolonged systemic hypotension.

In•fa•surf (in′fə-sərf) trademark for a preparation of calfactant.

in•fect (in-fekt′) [L. *inficere* to stain, infect] 1. to invade and produce infection in. 2. to transmit a pathogen or disease to.

in•fec•ti•ble (in-fek′tĭ-bəl) capable of being infected.

in•fec•tion (in-fek′shən) 1. invasion and multiplication of microorganisms or parasites in body tissues; it may be clinically inapparent (subclinical infection) or remain localized with cellular injury due to competitive metabolism, toxins, intracellular replication, or antigen-antibody reaction. Infections remain localized, subclinical, and temporary if the body's defense mechanisms are effective. However, they may persist, become symptomatic, and spread by extension to become acute, subacute, or chronic disease states. A local infection may also become systemic when the microorganisms gain access to the lymphatic system or the bloodstream. 2. infectious disease.

airborne i. an infection contracted by inhalation of microorganisms or spores suspended in air on water droplets *(droplet i.)* or dust particles *(dust-borne i.).* Microorganisms are often rendered airborne as a result of a sneeze or cough.

apical i. an infection at the apex of the root of a tooth.

ascending i. infection of the fetus by microorganisms that gain access to the uterus from the vagina, usually following rupture of membranes but sometimes acquired in utero while the membranes are intact; called also *transcervical i.*

asymptomatic i. subclinical i.

chronic Epstein-Barr virus i. chronic fatigue syndrome.

colonization i. an infection that follows colonization of tissue by the infecting agent.

cross i. infection transmitted from one individual to another.

disseminated gonococcal i. spread of gonorrhea beyond the initial site of infection via the bloodstream, seen more often in women because gonorrhea has fewer symptoms in women than in men. The most common presentation is gonococcal arthritis.

droplet i. airborne infection due to inhalation of droplet nuclei.

dust-borne i. airborne infection by pathogens that have become attached to particles of dust.

endogenous i. an infection caused by reactivation of organisms present in a dormant focus.

exit site i. infection in the area where an artificial tube exits from the body.

exogenous i. an infection caused by organisms that are not normally present in the body but have gained entrance from the environment.

germinal i. transmission of infection to the fetus or child by means of the oocyte or sperm of the parent.

hematogenous i. transplacental i.

HIV i. human immunodeficiency virus infection.

horizontal i. an infection spread by horizontal transmission.

human immunodeficiency virus i. an epidemic, transmissible retroviral disease due to infection with human immunodeficiency virus (HIV), which attacks the subset of T lymphocytes known as the CD4 cells. The primary method of transmission is transfer from one person to another of bodily fluids that contain the virus, most commonly semen during sexual intercourse or blood or blood products during transfusions or intravenous injection with a contaminated needle. In its most severe manifestation, meeting specific clinical criteria, it is classified as AIDS (acquired immunodeficiency syndrome; see under *syndrome*).

iatrogenic i. infection acquired by the patient during the course of treatment by a health care professional. Cf. *nosocomial i.*

inapparent i. subclinical i.

latent i. 1. a phase during the course of some established infections during which the pathogenic microorganisms are dormant and manifestations of disease that may have been recognizable earlier are no longer detectable, as in latent syphilis. 2. subclinical i.

mass i. infection produced by a large number of pathogenic organisms in the circulation.

mixed i. infection of an organ or tissue by more than one microorganism, such as in wound infections, abscesses, or pneumonia. Mixtures of every type occur, e.g., bacterial and viral, bacterial and fungal, and protozoan and viral. Called also *polyinfection.*

nosocomial i. an infection not present or incubating prior to admittance to a hospital, but occurring a few days after admittance; the term is usually used to refer to patient disease, but hospital personnel may also acquire nosocomial infection. Cf. *iatrogenic i.*

opportunistic i. infection by an organism that does not ordinarily cause disease but that becomes pathogenic under certain circumstances, such as with immunodeficiency disorders.

perinatal i. infection in the newborn acquired shortly before or during delivery, due to ascending infection following rupture of the membranes or contact with microorganisms in the birth canal during delivery.

pyogenic i. an infection caused by pus-producing microorganisms, such as pyogenic bacteria.

secondary i. infection by a second pathogen after that by a previous pathogen.

sexually transmitted i. see under *disease.*

subclinical i. infection in which symptoms and signs are not detectable by clinical examination or laboratory tests; this may be in an early stage of the infection, with symptoms and signs becoming manifest later, or the symptoms and signs may never become apparent. Called also *asymptomatic* or *inapparent i.*

TORCH i. see under *syndrome.*

transcervical i. ascending i.

transplacental i. infection acquired by the fetus in utero by the hematogenous spread of a maternal infection across the placenta via the chorionic villi; called also *hematogenous i.*

tunnel i. subcutaneous infection of an artificial passage into the body that has been kept patent for continuous or repeated entry of a catheter or other tube.

vector-borne i. an infection caused by microorganisms transmitted from one host to another by a carrier such as a biting insect.

vertical i. an infection spread by vertical transmission.

water-borne i. an infection caused by microorganisms transmitted through water and acquired through ingestion, bathing, or other means.

in•fec•ti•os•i•ty (in-fek″she-os′ĭ-te) infectivity.

in•fec•tious (in-fek′shəs) 1. caused by or capable of being communicated by infection, as an infectious disease. Cf. *communicable* and *contagious.* 2. infective (def. 1).

in•fec•tious•ness (in-fek′shəs-nis) infectivity.

in•fec•tive (in-fek′tiv) 1. capable of producing infection. 2. infectious (def. 1).

in•fec•tiv•i•ty (in″fek-tiv′ĭ-te) 1. the state or quality of being infectious; called also *infectiousness.* 2. virulence.

in•fe•cun•di•ty (in″fe-kun′dĭ-te) [L. *infecunditas*] infertility.

InFeD (in′fed) trademark for a preparation of iron dextran.

in•fer•ent (in′fər-ənt) afferent.

In•fer•gen (in′fər-jen) trademark for a preparation of interferon alfacon-1.

in•fe•ri•or (in-fēr′e-ər) [L. "lower"] 1. situated below, or directed downward. 2. [TA] a term used in reference to the lower surface of an organ or other structure, or to the lower of two (or more) similar structures.

in•fe•ro•lat•er•al (in″fər-o-lat′ər-əl) situated inferiorly and to one side.

in•fe•ro•me•di•an (in″fər-o-me′de-ən) situated in the middle of the inferior side.

in•fe•ro•na•sal (in″fər-o-na′zəl) in ophthalmology, that quadrant of the eye or of the visual field inferior to the horizontal meridian of the eye and medial to the vertical meridian.

in•fe•ro•pos•te•ri•or (in″fər-o-pos-tēr′e-ər) situated inferiorly and posteriorly.

in•fe•ro•tem•po•ral (in″fər-o-tem′pər-əl) in ophthalmology, that quadrant of the eye or of the visual field inferior to the horizontal meridian of the eye and lateral to the vertical meridian.

in•fer•tile (in-fur′til) not fertile; exhibiting infertility.

in•fer•til•i•ty (in″fər-til′ĭ-te) [*in-*[2] + *fertility*] diminished or absent capacity to produce offspring; the term does not denote complete inability to produce offspring as does *sterility.* Called also *relative sterility.*

cervical i., cervical factor i. female factor infertility caused by abnormal interaction between the sperm and the cervical mucus.

female factor i. infertility of a couple due to a problem in the female's reproductive system; types include cervical factor infertility and tubal factor infertility.

immunologic i. any of several types of female factor infertility believed to be caused by presence of antibodies that interfere with functioning of the sperm, such as antisperm antibody.

male factor i. infertility of a couple due to a problem in the male's reproductive system, such as anejaculation, aspermatogenesis, or azoospermia.

primary i. infertility in a patient who has never conceived.

secondary i. infertility in a patient who has previously conceived.

tubal factor i. female factor infertility caused by an abnormality of the uterine tubes, such as scarring or obstruction following a urinary tract infection.

in•fes•ta•tion (in-fes-ta′shən) parasitic attack or subsistence on the skin and its appendages by ectoparasites such as insects, mites, or ticks.

in•fib•u•la•tion (in-fib″u-la′shən) [L. *infibulare* to buckle together] 1. the act of buckling, or fastening as if with buckles. 2. a practice done in extreme types of female circumcision in certain cultures; after excision of the clitoris and the labia minora, the vaginal orifice is largely closed up with stitches or clasps. This has been declared harmful by the World Health Organization.

in•fil•trate (in-fil′trāt) 1. to penetrate the interstices of a tissue or substance. 2. the material or solution so deposited; called also *infiltration.*

Assmann tuberculous i. see under *focus.*

in•fil•tra•tion (in″fil-tra′shən) [*in-*[1] + *filtration*] 1. the pathological accumulation in tissue or cells of substances not normal to it or in amounts in excess of the normal. 2. infiltrate (def. 2). 3. the deposition of a solution directly into tissue; see under *anesthesia.*

adipose i. fatty i.; see *fatty change,* under *change.*

calcareous i. a deposit of lime and magnesium salts in the tissues.

calcium i. a deposit of calcium salts within the tissues of the body.

cellular i. the migration and accumulation of cells within the tissues.

fatty i. 1. a deposit of fat in the tissues, especially between the cells; the term describes an older concept now included in *fatty change* (see under *change*). 2. the presence of fat vacuoles in the cytoplasm of cells, as occurs in fatty change in the liver, myocardium, and kidneys.

gelatinous i. gray i.

glycogen i. abnormal accumulations of glycogen within the cytoplasm of cells, as occurs in diabetes mellitus and the glycogen storage diseases.

gray i. a condition of the lungs in acute pulmonary tuberculosis in which they have large amounts of semisolid grayish exudate; seen primarily at autopsy. Called also *gelatinous i.*

inflammatory i. penetration of the interstices of a tissue by an inflammatory exudation.

Jessner lymphocytic i., lymphocytic i. of skin a variable skin condition seen most often in middle-aged persons, characterized by asymptomatic, single or multiple, firm, reddish papules or plaques that expand peripherally to form annular lesions, sometimes with central clearing; it may be induced or aggravated by light exposure. Some authorities consider this a variant of cutaneous lymphoid hyperplasia or lupus erythematosus tumidus, while others consider it premalignant, an early stage of cutaneous T-cell lymphoma.

paraneural i., perineural i. perineural anesthesia.

pulmonary i. with eosinophilia infiltration of the pulmonary parenchyma by eosinophils; see *PIE syndrome,* under *syndrome.*

sanguineous i. infiltration with extravasated blood.

serous i. the abnormal presence of lymph in a tissue.

tuberculous i. the formation of a collection of tuberculous cells and bacilli in a tissue.

in•fil•tra•tive (in′fil-tra″tiv) pertaining to or characterized by infiltration.

in•firm (in-firm′) weak; feeble, as from disease or old age.

in•fir•ma•ry (in-fur′mə-re) [L. *infirmarium*] a hospital or place where sick or infirm persons are maintained or treated; commonly used to denote a space or a building set aside for the care of members of a group or community; a dispensary.

in•fir•mi•ty (in-fur′mĭ-te) [L. *infirmitas*] 1. a feeble or weak state of the body or mind. 2. a disease or condition producing weakness.

In•fla•mase (in′flə-mās″) trademark for preparations of prednisolone sodium phosphate.

in•flam•ma•gen (in-flam′ə-jən) an irritant that elicits both edema and the cellular response of inflammation. Cf. *edemagen.*

in•flam•ma•some (in-flam′ə-sōm) a complex of cryopyrin, caspase-1, and other proteins, found in phagocytic cells and related to the body's system of innate immunity; they are necessary for activation of cytokine and caspase-1 during the inflammatory response.

in•flam•ma•tion (in″flə-ma′shən) [L. *inflammare* to set on fire] a localized protective response elicited by injury or destruction of tissues, which serves to destroy, dilute, or wall off (sequester) both the injurious agent and the injured tissue. It is characterized in the acute form by the classical signs of pain (dolor), heat (calor), redness (rubor), swelling (tumor), and loss of function (functio laesa). Histologically, it involves a complex series of events, including dilatation of arterioles, capillaries, and venules, with increased permeability and blood flow; exudation of fluids, including plasma proteins; and leukocytic migration into the inflammatory focus.

acute i. inflammation, usually of sudden onset, characterized by the classical signs (see *inflammation*), with predominance of the vascular and exudative processes.

adhesive i. inflammation that promotes adhesion of contiguous surfaces.

atrophic i. inflammation that results in atrophy and deformity.

catarrhal i. inflammation affecting primarily a mucous surface, marked by a copious discharge of mucus and epithelial debris.

chronic i. inflammation of slow progress and marked chiefly by the formation of new connective tissue; it may be a continuation of an acute form or a prolonged low-grade form, and usually causes permanent tissue damage.

cirrhotic i. atrophic i.

diffuse i. inflammation that is both interstitial and parenchymatous or is spread over a large area.

disseminated i. inflammation that has a number of distinct foci.

exudative i. inflammation in which the prominent feature is an exudate.

fibrinous i. inflammation characterized by an exudate of coagulated fibrin.

fibrosing i. atrophic i.

focal i. inflammation confined to a single spot or to a few limited spots.

granulomatous i. inflammation, usually chronic, characterized by formation of granulomas (q.v.).

hyperplastic i. inflammation that leads to formation of new connective tissue fibers. Called also *productive* or *proliferative i.*

hypertrophic i. inflammation marked by increase in size of the elements composing the affected tissue.

interstitial i. inflammation that primarily affects the stroma of an organ.

metastatic i. inflammation reproduced in a distant part by conveyance of infectious material through blood vessels and lymph organs.

necrotic i., necrotizing i. necroinflammation.

obliterative i. inflammation of the lining membrane of a cavity or vessel, producing adhesions between the surfaces and consequent obliteration of the lumen.

parenchymatous i. inflammation primarily affecting essential tissue elements of an organ.

plastic i., productive i., proliferative i. hyperplastic i.

pseudomembranous i. an acute inflammatory response to a powerful necrotizing toxin, such as the diphtheria toxin, characterized by the formation on a mucosal surface, most often in the pharynx, larynx, respiratory passages, and intestinal tract, of a false membrane composed of precipitated fibrin, necrotic epithelium, and inflammatory leukocytes.

purulent i. suppurative i.

sclerosing i. atrophic i.

seroplastic i. inflammation with both serous and plastic exudation.

serous i. inflammation producing an exudation of serum.

simple i. inflammation with no flow of pus or other inflammatory products.

specific i. inflammation due to a particular microorganism.

subacute i. a condition intermediate between chronic and acute inflammation, exhibiting some of the characteristics of each.

suppurative i. inflammation with formation of pus.

toxic i. inflammation that is caused by a poison, such as a bacterial product.

traumatic i. inflammation caused by an injury.

ulcerative i. inflammation in which necrosis on or near the surface leads to loss of tissue and creation of a local defect (ulcer).

in•flam•ma•to•ry (in-flam′ə-tor″e) pertaining to or characterized by inflammation.

in•fla•tion (in-fla′shən) [L. *in-*[1] + *flare* to blow] 1. distention with air, gas, or fluid. 2. the act of distending with air, gas, or fluid.

in•fla•tor (in-fla′tər) an instrument for inflating any organ for therapeutic or diagnostic purposes.

in•flec•tion (in-flek′shən) [L. *inflexio*] the act of bending inward or the state of being bent inward, as of a limb.

in•flex•ion (in-flek′shən) inflection.

in•flix•i•mab (in-flik′sĭ-mab) a chimeric human-murine immunoglobulin that acts as an anti–tumor necrosis factor antibody; administered intravenously in treatment of Crohn disease and rheumatoid arthritis.

in•flo•res•cence (in″flo-res′əns) the structure or arrangement of the flowers of a plant.

in•flu•en•za (in″floo-en′zə) [Ital., from L. *influentia* influence, from the belief that the stars influenced epidemics] an acute viral infection of the respiratory tract that may occur in isolated cases, in epidemics, or in pandemics; causative viruses are classified in genera Influenzavirus A, Influenzavirus B, and Influenzavirus C. Influenza usually has a 3-day incubation period and lasts for 3 to 10 days. It is marked by inflammation of the nasal mucosa, pharynx, and conjunctiva; headache; myalgia; often fever, chills, and prostration; and occasionally involvement of the myocardium or central nervous system. Necrotizing bronchitis and interstitial pneumonia may occur in severe cases, opening the way for secondary bacterial pneumonia due to *Streptococcus pneumoniae*, *Haemophilus influenzae*, or *Staphylococcus aureus*. Called also *flu* and *grippe*. **influen′zal** *adj*

i. A the most common variety of influenza, caused by Influenzavirus A; epidemics occur at two- to three-year intervals. The causative strain has wide variations in antigenic type (see *antigenic shift*, under *shift*). Outbreaks caused by various antigenic types have been given the names *Asian i.*, *Spanish i.*, *Russian i.*, and others.

Asian i. a pandemic of influenza A that occurred in 1957 and was first observed in China.

avian i. a highly contagious disease of wild and domesticated birds caused by *avian influenza virus*, a subspecies of Influenzavirus A; it occurs in both mild and severe, fulminating, highly fatal forms. It may be transmitted to humans through contact with bird droppings or surfaces contaminated by them or through intermediate hosts such as pigs; person-to-person transmission appears to be rare. Symptoms in humans range from typical influenzalike symptoms to eye infections, pneumonia, acute respiratory distress, and other severe and life-threatening complications.

i. B influenza caused by Influenzavirus B and occurring in epidemics at four- to five-year intervals.

i. C influenza caused by Influenzavirus C and occurring sporadically.

endemic i. infection with influenza virus occurring continuously within a population, i.e., between epidemics, either sporadically and not recognized as influenza or as a subclinical infection.

equine i. a highly contagious febrile respiratory disease of horses caused by two immunologically distinct strains of Influenzavirus A. Called also *equine infectious bronchitis*.

feline i. feline respiratory disease complex.

goose i. 1. infectious avian serositis in geese. 2. a type of serositis in geese, caused by a parvovirus.

Hong Kong i. a type of influenza A that occurred in a pandemic in 1968 and was first observed in Hong Kong.

Russian i. a type of influenza A that occurred in a pandemic in 1978 and was first observed in Russia.

Spanish i. a virulent type of influenza A that occurred in a pandemic in 1918 and 1919, with more than 20 million deaths around the world.

swine i. an acute, highly contagious, respiratory disease of hogs caused by a species of Influenzavirus A.

In•flu•en•za•vi•rus (in″floo-en′zə-vi″rəs) [*influenza* + *virus*] a former genus of the Orthomyxoviridae that comprised *Influenzavirus A* and *Influenzavirus B*, which are now considered to be separate genera.

I. A influenza A virus; a genus of viruses of the family Orthomyxoviridae containing the agent of influenza A. See *influenza virus*, under *virus*.

I. B influenza B virus; a genus of viruses of the family Orthomyxoviridae containing the agent of influenza B. See *influenza virus*, under *virus*.

I. C influenza C virus; a genus of viruses of the family Orthomyxoviridae containing the agent of influenza C. See *influenza virus*, under *virus*.

in•fold•ing (in-fōld′ing) 1. the folding inward of a layer of tissue, as in the formation of the neural tube in the embryo. 2. the enclosing of redundant tissue by suturing together the walls of the organ on either side of it.

infra- [L. *infra* beneath] a prefix meaning inferior to, below, or beneath.

in•fra-ax•il•lary (in″frə-ak′sĭ-lar″e) subaxillary.

in•fra•bulge (in′frə-bəlj) the surfaces of a tooth gingival to the height of contour, or sloping cervically; the surface of the crown of a tooth cervical to the clasp guideline or surveyed height of contour, being the retention area of a tooth. Cf. *suprabulge*.

in•fra•cal•ca•rine (in″frə-kal′kə-rīn) inferior to the calcarine sulcus.

in•fra•cil•i•a•ture (in″frə-sil′e-ə-chər) [*infra-* + *cilium*] the basal bodies and kinetodesmata of ciliate protozoa considered collectively.

in•fra•class (in′frə-klas) a taxonomic category sometimes established, subordinate to a subclass and superior to an order.

in•fra•cla•vic•u•lar (in″frə-klə-vik′u-lər) subclavian.

in•fra•clu•sion (in″frə-kloo′zhən) malocclusion in which a tooth has failed to erupt fully and reach the line of occlusion and is out of contact with the opposing tooth. Called also *infraversion*.

in•fra•col•ic (in″frə-kol′ik) [*infra-* + *colon*] inferior to the colon.

in•fra•con•stric•tor (in″frə-kən-strik′tər) musculus constrictor pharyngis inferior.

in•fra•cor•ti•cal (in″frə-kor′tĭ-kəl) subcortical.

in•fra•cos•tal (in″frə-kos′təl) subcostal.

in•fra•cot•y•loid (in″frə-kot′ə-loid) inferior to the acetabulum (cotyloid cavity).

in•frac•tion (in-frak′shən) [L. *in* into + *fractio* break] incomplete fracture of a bone without displacement of the fragments.

Freiberg i. Köhler bone disease (def. 2).

in•fra•den•ta•le (in″frə-dən-ta′le) an osteometric landmark, being the highest anterior point on the gingiva between the mandibular central incisors.

in•fra•di•an (in″frə-de′ən) [*infra-* + L. *dies* day] pertaining to the rhythmic repetition of certain phenomena in living organisms occurring in cycles of less frequency than circadian, that is, less frequently than once a day. Cf. *circadian* and *ultradian*.

in•fra•di•a•phrag•mat•ic (in″frə-di″ə-frag-mat′ik) subphrenic.

in•fra•duc•tion (in″frə-duk′shən) [*infra-* + *duction*] 1. the downward rotation of an eye around its horizontal axis. 2. the downward rotation of one eye independent of the other by a base-up prism in testing for vertical divergence. See also *infravergence* and *infraversion*. Called also *deorsumduction* and *subduction*.

in•fra•gle•noid (in″frə-gle′noid) subglenoid.

in•fra•glot•tic (in″frə-glot′ik) subglottic.

in•fra•hy•oid (in″frə-hi′oid) subhyoid.

in•fra•in•gui•nal (in″frə-ing′gwə-nəl) inferior to the inguinal ligament.

in•fra•le•va•tor (in″frə-lĕ-va′tər) beneath a levator muscle.

in•fra•mal•le•o•lar (in″frə-mal-e-o′lər) inferior to one or both of the malleoli.

in•fra•mam•ma•ry (in″frə-mam′ə-re) submammary.

in•fra•mam•mil•lary (in″frə-mam′ĭ-lar″e) inferior to the nipple.

in•fra•man•dib•u•lar (in″frə-man-dib′u-lər) submandibular.

in•fra•mar•gin•al (in″frə-mahr′jĭ-nəl) submarginal.

in•fra•max•il•lary (in″frə-mak′sĭ-lar″e) submaxillary.

in•fra•no•dal (in″frə-no′dəl) below a node.

in•fra•nu•cle•ar (in″frə-noo′kle-ər) inferior to a nucleus in the nervous system.

in•fra•or•bi•tal (in″frə-or′bĭ-təl) lying under, or on the inferior surface of, the orbit. Called also *suborbital*.

in•fra•pa•tel•lar (in″frə-pə-tel′ər) inferior to the patella; called also *subpatellar*.

in•fra•pop•lit•e•al (in″frə-pop-lit′e-əl) inferior to the posterior surface of the knee or fossa poplitea.

in•fra•psy•chic (in″frə-si′kik) below the conscious level; subconscious or automatic.

in•fra•red (in-frə-red′) denoting thermal radiation of wavelength greater than that of the red end of the visible spectrum, between the red waves and the radio waves, having wavelengths between 0.75 and 1000 μm. Infrared rays emanating from tissues are the basis of thermography.

far i., long-wave i. infrared radiation of the longest wavelength, i.e., furthest from the visible spectrum (wavelength about 3.0 to 1000 μm).

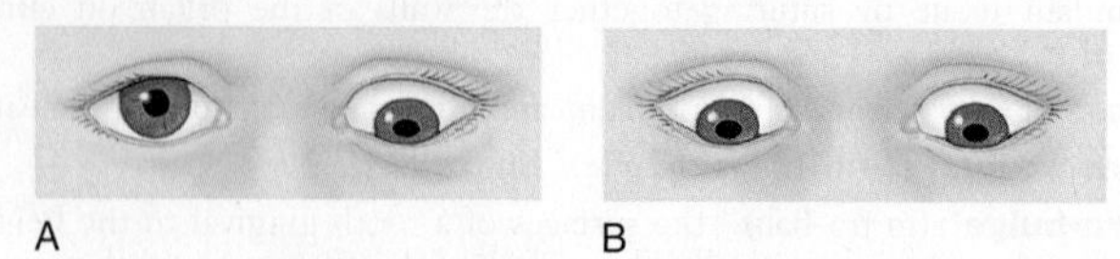

■ Infraversion of one *(A)* or both *(B)* eyes.

near i., short-wave i. infrared radiation of the shortest wavelength, i.e., closest to the visible spectrum (wavelength about 0.75 to 3.0 μm).

in·fra·scap·u·lar (in″frə-skap′u-lər) subscapular.

in·fra·son·ic (in″frə-son′ik) below the frequency range of the waves normally perceived as sound by the human ear.

in·fra·spi·nous (in″frə-spi′nəs) inferior to the spine of the scapula.

in·fra·ster·nal (in″frə-stur′nəl) substernal.

in·fra·struc·ture (in″frə-struk′chər) substructure (def. 2).
implant i. see under *substructure.*

in·fra·tem·po·ral (in″frə-tem′pə-rəl) inferior to the temple or temporal fossa; called also *subtemporal.*

in·fra·ten·to·ri·al (in″frə-ten-tor′e-əl) subtentorial.

in·fra·ton·sil·lar (in″frə-ton′sĭ-lər) inferior to the palatine tonsil.

in·fra·tra·che·al (in″frə-tra′ke-əl) inferior to the trachea.

in·fra·troch·le·ar (in″frə-trok′le-ər) subtrochlear.

in·fra·tu·bal (in″frə-too′bəl) inferior to a tube.

in·fra·tym·pan·ic (in″frə-tym-pan′ik) inferior to the tympanic membrane; called also *subtympanic.*

in·fra·um·bil·i·cal (in″frə-əm-bil′ĭ-kəl) subumbilical.

in·fra·ver·gence (in″frə-vur′jəns) [*infra-* + *vergence*] disjunctive reciprocal movement of the eyes in which one eye rotates downward while the other one remains still; called also *deorsumvergence.*

in·fra·ver·sion (in″frə-vur′zhən) [*infra-* + *version*] 1. infraclusion. 2. the downward deviation of one eye. 3. conjugate downward rotation of both eyes; called also *deorsumversion.*

in·fra·ves·i·cal (in″frə-ves′ĭ-kəl) [*infra-* + *vesical*] inferior to the urinary bladder.

in·fric·tion (in-frik′shən) [L. *in* on + *friction*] the rubbing of medicaments upon the skin.

In·fu·morph (in′fu-morf″) trademark for a preparation of morphine sulfate.

in·fun·dib·u·la (in″fən-dib′u-lə) [L.] plural of *infundibulum.*

in·fun·dib·u·lar (in″fən-dib′u-lər) 1. pertaining to an infundibulum; called also *choanal.* 2. funnel-shaped; called also *infundibuliform* and *choanoid.*

in·fun·dib·u·lec·to·my (in″fən-dib″u-lek′tə-me) excision of the infundibulum of the heart.
Brock i. transventricular closed valvotomy.

in·fun·dib·u·li·form (in″fən-dib′u-lĭ-form) [*infundibulum* + *form*] infundibular (def. 2).

in·fun·dib·u·lo·fol·lic·u·li·tis (in″fun-dib″u-lo-fə-lik″u-li′tis) inflammation of the follicular infundibulum.
disseminate and recurrent i. a rare skin condition seen primarily in persons of black African descent, characterized by widespread tiny pruritic papules on hair follicles, usually on the neck, face, or trunk; it resembles keratosis pilaris but is less keratotic and on a different part of the body.

in·fun·dib·u·lo·ma (in″fən-dib″u-lo′mə) a tumor of the infundibulum hypothalami.

in·fun·dib·u·lo·neu·ro·hy·poph·y·si·tis (in″fun-dib″u-lo-noor″o-hi-pof″ə-si′tis) inflammation of the infundibulum of the neurohypophysis.
lymphocytic i. autoimmune inflammation of the infundibulum, a rare neuroendocrine condition that interferes with pituitary function and causes central diabetes insipidus.

in·fun·dib·u·lo·pel·vic (in″fən-dib″u-lo-pel′vik) pertaining to an infundibulum and a pelvis, as of the kidney.

in·fun·dib·u·lum (in″fən-dib′u-ləm) pl. *infundi′bula* [L. "funnel"] 1. a general anatomical term for a funnel-shaped structure; called also *choana.* 2. i. neurohypophyseos. 3. a downgrowth from the neuroectoderm of the embryonic diencephalon that gives rise to the neurohypophysis. 4. conus arteriosus. 5. the deep, often tubular or funnel-shaped part of the buccal cavity seen in certain protozoa, especially peritrichous ciliates.
crural i., i. crura′le canalis femoralis.
ethmoidal i. of cavity of nose i. ethmoidale cavitatis nasi.
ethmoidal i. of ethmoid bone i. ethmoidale ossis ethmoidalis.
i. ethmoida′le cavita′tis na′si [TA] ethmoidal infundibulum of nasal cavity: a passage connecting the cavity of the nose with the anterior ethmoidal cells and the frontal sinus.
i. ethmoida′le os′sis ethmoida′lis [TA] ethmoidal infundibulum of ethmoid bone: a variable sinuous passage extending upward from the middle nasal meatus through the ethmoidal labyrinth, communicating with the anterior ethmoidal cells and often with the frontal sinus.
i. of fallopian tube i. tubae uterinae.
follicular i. the portion of a hair follicle between the isthmus and the skin surface; called also *pilary canal.*
i. of gallbladder i. vesicae biliaris.
i. of heart conus arteriosus.
i. of hypophysis, i. hypotha′lami, i. of hypothalamus i. neurohypophyseos.
infundibula of kidney calices renales minores.
i. lo′bi posterio′ris hypophy′seos TA alternative for *i. neurohypophyseos.*
i. na′si, i. of nose 1. i. ethmoidale cavi nasi. 2. i. ethmoidale ossis ethmoidalis.
i. neurohypophy′seos [TA] infundibulum of neurohypophysis: a hollow, funnel-shaped mass in front of the tuber cinereum, which extends to the neurohypophysis. Called also *i. of hypophysis* or *of hypothalamus, i. hypothalami, i. lobi posterioris hypophyseos* [TA alternative], and *hypophysial, infundibular, neural,* or *pituitary stalk.*
i. tu′bae uteri′nae [TA] infundibulum of uterine tube: the funnel-like dilation at the distal end of the uterine tube.
i. of urinary bladder fundus vesicae.
i. of uterine tube i. tubae uterinae.
i. vesi′cae bilia′ris [TA] infundibulum of gallbladder: the tapering part of the gallbladder, ending at the neck. Called also *i. vesicae felleae* [TA alternative].
i. vesi′cae fel′leae TA alternative for *i. vesicae biliaris.*

in·fu·si·ble (in-fu′zĭ-bəl) incapable of being melted.

in·fu·sion (in-fu′zhən) [L. *infusio*] 1. the steeping of a substance in water to obtain its medicinal principles. 2. the product of the process of steeping a drug for the extraction of its medicinal principles. 3. the therapeutic introduction of a fluid other than blood, as saline solution, into a vein. NOTE: An *infusion* flows in by gravity, an *injection* is forced in by a syringe, an *instillation* is dropped in, and an *insufflation* is blown in.
cold i. the product of steeping a drug in cold water.
continuous subcutaneous insulin i. (CSII) insulin pump.
donor leukocyte i. a treatment for a viral infection or relapse of cancer after a bone marrow transplant, consisting of infusion with leukocytes from the same donor; see also *leukocytotherapy.*
meat i. (for bacteriological use), fresh lean meat free from fat is ground and extracted with water; the mixture is infused overnight in the refrigerator, gradually raised to the boiling point, and filtered.
saline i. administration, either subcutaneously or intravenously, of saline solution.
subcutaneous i. hypodermoclysis.

in·fu·so·de·coc·tion (in-fu″so-de-kok′shən) a mixture of the infusion and the decoction of a substance.

in·ges·ta (in-jes′tə) [L. pl., *in* into + *gerere* to carry] food and drink taken into the stomach.

in·ges·tant (in-jes′tənt) a substance that is or may be taken into the body by way of the mouth, or through the digestive system.

in·ges·tion (in-jes′chən) the act of taking food, medicines, etc., into the body, by mouth. **inges′tive** *adj*

in·glu·vi·es (in-gloo′ve-ēz) [L.] 1. crop (def. 1). 2. rumen.

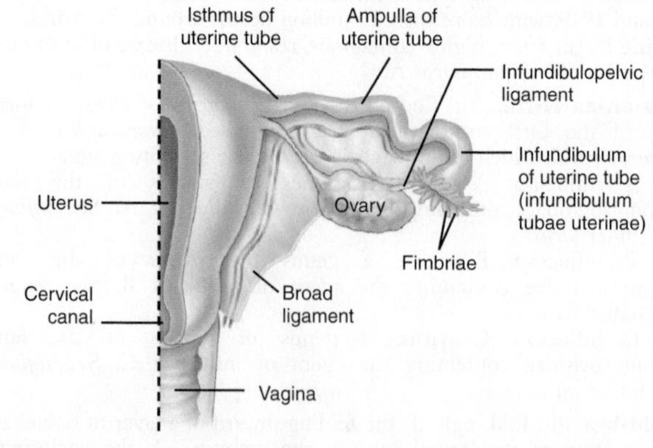

in·gras·sia process (wing) (in-grah′se-ah) [Giovanni Filippo *Ingrassia*, Italian anatomist, 1510–1580] ala minor ossis sphenoidalis.

in·gra·ves·cent (in″grə-ves′ənt) [L. *in* upon + *gravesci* to grow heavy] gradually increasing in severity.

in·grown (in′grōn) having grown inward, into the flesh.

in·growth (in′grōth) an inward growth; something that grows inward or into.

epithelial i. a complication of intraocular surgery, most often cataract extraction, or of penetrating wounds of the cornea where wound healing is poor, in which epithelium proliferates through the wound into the anterior chamber, causing obstruction of the trabecula, and sometimes pupillary block, resulting in glaucoma.

stromal fatty i. the replacement of connective tissue stroma by adipose tissue, most often occurring in the pancreas and heart, usually without any alteration in the organ's function.

in·guen (ing′gwən) pl. *in′guina* [L.] [TA] groin: the junctional region between the abdomen and thigh. Called also *regio inguinalis* [TA alternative] and *iliac* or *inguinal region.* **in′guinal** *adj*

in·gui·na (ing′gwĭ-nə) [L.] plural of *inguen.*

in·gui·no·ab·dom·i·nal (ing″gwĭ-no-ab-dom′ĭ-nəl) pertaining to the groin and the abdomen.

in·gui·no·cru·ral (ing″gwĭ-no-kroo′rəl) pertaining to the groin and the thigh.

in·gui·no·dyn·ia (ing″gwĭ-no-din′e-ə) pain in the groin.

in·gui·no·la·bi·al (ing″gwĭ-no-la′be-əl) pertaining to the groin and labium.

in·gui·no·scro·tal (ing″gwĭ-no-skro′təl) pertaining to the groin and the scrotum.

INH isoniazid (isonicotine hydrazine).

in·hal·ant (in-ha′lənt) 1. something meant to be inhaled; see *inhalation* (def. 3). 2. a class of psychoactive substances whose volatile vapors are subject to abuse; see *substance abuse*, under *abuse.*

antifoaming i. an agent inhaled as a vapor to prevent the formation of foam in the respiratory passages of a patient with pulmonary edema.

in·ha·la·tion (in″hə-la′shən) [L. *inhalatio*] 1. the drawing of air into the lungs; called also *inspiration.* 2. the drawing of an aerosolized drug into the lungs with the breath. 3. something inhaled, such as a drug or solution of drugs administered (as by a nebulizer or aerosol) by the nasal or oral respiratory route for local or systemic effect.

in·hale (in-hāl′) [L. *inhalare*] to take into the lungs by breathing; called also *inspire.*

in·hal·er (in-hāl′ər) 1. an apparatus for administering vapor or volatilized medications by inhalation. 2. ventilator (def. 2).

dry powder i. an inhaler that disperses a cloud of dry powdered medication; most types are breath-activated.

metered dose i. an inhaler used to deliver aerosolized medications in fixed doses to patients with respiratory disease.

in·her·ent (in-her′ənt) [L. *inhaerens* sticking fast] implanted by nature; intrinsic; innate.

in·her·i·tance (in-her′ĭ-təns) [L. *inhereditare* to appoint an heir] 1. the acquisition of characters or qualities by transmission from parent to offspring. 2. a character or quality that is transmitted from parent to offspring. See also entries under *character, trait,* and *gene.*

codominant i. inheritance characterized by full expression of both alleles in heterozygotes.

complex i. multifactorial i.

cytoplasmic i. inheritance of traits carried by genes not located on chromosomes of the nucleus, e.g., those of mitochondria or chloroplasts. Called also *extrachromosomal i.*

dominant i. the inheritance of a trait that is expressed in both heterozygotes and homozygotes.

extrachromosomal i. cytoplasmic i.

holandric i. Y-linked i.

maternal i. transmission of characters only from the maternal parent, as is characteristic of genes carried on the mitochondrial genome or other cytoplasmic organelle.

mendelian i. that which follows Mendel's laws (q.v.).

mitochondrial i. the inheritance of traits controlled by genes on the DNA of mitochondria in the ooplasm; the genes are thus inherited entirely from the mother (maternal inheritance). Inheritance is nonmendelian, since mitochondria are randomly distributed to the daughter cells at meiosis or mitosis. Mutations of the mitochondrial DNA cause a number of maternally inherited disorders; phenotypic expression of these disorders is variable and depends on the proportions of normal and mutant DNA.

monofactorial i. transmission of a character determined by a single gene.

multifactorial i. inheritance determined by multiple factors, genetic and possibly nongenetic (environmental), each with only a partial effect. See also *polygenic i.*

polygenic i., quantitative i. inheritance determined by many genes at different loci, with small additive effects. See also *multifactorial i.*

pseudoautosomal i. inheritance of traits controlled by genes located in the pseudoautosomal regions of the sex chromosomes and mimicking the patterns of inheritance seen with autosomal genes.

quasidominant i. inheritance characterized by an apparently dominant pattern, but actually resulting from the mating of a carrier of a recessive gene with an individual homozygous for the recessive allele.

recessive i. the inheritance of a trait that is only expressed in homozygotes, not in a heterozygote also possessing a dominant allele for that locus.

sex-influenced i. the inheritance of a trait expressed differently in males and females; see under *trait.*

sex-limited i. the inheritance of a trait expressed in one sex only; see under *trait.*

sex-linked i. the pattern of inheritance shown by genes carried on a sex (X or Y) chromosome, differing for males and females. See also under *gene* and *trait.*

X-linked i. the pattern of inheritance shown by genes carried on the X chromosome (X-linked genes); affected males, having only one X chromosome, always express the phenotype, and they transmit the gene to all their daughters but none of their sons. Heterozygous affected females do not express the phenotype if the trait is recessive, and they transmit the gene equally to their sons and daughters.

Y-linked i. the pattern of inheritance shown by genes carried on the Y chromosome (Y-linked genes); only males can be affected, and they always express the phenotype and transmit the gene to all of their sons.

in·hib·in (in-hib′in) either of two glycoproteins, A and B, each composed of a common alpha subunit and one of two beta subunits; they are secreted by the gonads and found in seminal plasma and follicular fluid, and inhibit pituitary production of follicle-stimulating hormone. They also contribute to the control of gametogenesis, embryonic and fetal development, and hematopoiesis. They are members of the transforming growth factor-β superfamily of proteins, and their actions are opposed by activins, which share the same beta subunits.

in·hib·it (in-hib′it) [L. *inhibēre*] to retard, arrest, or restrain.

in·hi·bi·tion (in″hĭ-bish′ən) 1. restraint or termination of a process. 2. in psychoanalytic theory, the conscious or unconscious restraining of an impulse or desire.

allogenic i. injury to cells in vitro as a consequence of contact with lymphocytes that are of a different genotype.

allosteric i. inhibition of an enzyme by binding of an inhibitor at an allosteric site that causes at the catalytic site either reduced binding affinity of the enzyme for the substrate or decreased rate of catalytic turnover.

competitive i. inhibition of enzyme activity in which the inhibitor (substrate analogue) reversibly combines with catalytic sites, thus competing with the substrate for binding on the enzyme. The inhibition is reversible since it can be overcome by increasing the substrate concentration. Similarly, the reversible binding of a physiologic antagonist to a receptor site for a hormone or neurotransmitter.

contact i. the inhibition of cell division and motility in normal cells when in close contact with each other, as in the formation of differentiated tissues; loss of inhibition of cell division is a step in carcinogenesis.

endproduct i. feedback i.

enzyme i. inhibition of enzyme activity, as in competitive or endproduct inhibition.

feedback i. inhibition of the initial steps of a process by an endproduct of the reaction.

hemagglutination i. (HI, HAI) see under *test.*

mixed i. inhibition of enzyme activity in a manner that has features of both competitive and noncompetitive inhibition, both substrate binding and rate of turnover of the enzyme being affected.

noncompetitive i. inhibition of enzyme activity by a substance that combines with the enzyme at a site other than that utilized by the substrate, causing a change in enzyme configuration and a decrease in activity. Similarly, the inhibition of a hormone or neurotransmitter by binding of a physiologic antagonist to a receptor at a site other than the active center.

proactive i. the interference of earlier learning in the retention of new learning; cf. *retroactive i.*

reciprocal i. the inhibition of one group of muscles on excitation of their antagonists, a phenomenon resulting from reciprocal innervation (q.v.).

retroactive i. the interference of new learning in the recall of earlier learning; cf. *proactive i.*

uncompetitive i. inhibition of an enzyme by a substance that binds reversibly to the enzyme-substrate complex. The enzyme-substrate-inhibitor complex cannot yield the normal product until the inhibitor is released.

Wedensky i. a partial block to conduction in a nerve may transmit impulses at low frequencies but not at higher frequencies.

in·hib·i·tive (in-hib′ĭ-tiv) inhibitory.

in·hib·i·tor (in-hib′ĭ-tər) 1. any substance that interferes with a chemical reaction, growth, or other biological activity. 2. a chemical substance that inhibits an enzyme reaction. See also *inhibition.*

ACE i's angiotensin-converting enzyme i's.

alpha$_1$-protease i., alpha$_1$-proteinase i. 1. alpha$_1$-antitrypsin. 2. alpha$_1$-proteinase inhibitor (human).

alpha$_1$-proteinase i. (human) a sterile, stable, lyophilized preparation of human alpha$_1$-proteinase inhibitor (alpha$_1$-antitrypsin) obtained from the pooled plasma of normal human donors; used in the treatment of congenital alpha$_1$-antitrypsin deficiency.

angiogenesis i. any of a group of drugs that prevent neovascularization of solid tumors.

angiotensin-converting enzyme i's competitive inhibitors of peptidyl-dipeptidase A (angiotensin-converting enzyme), used for treatment of hypertension, usually in conjunction with a diuretic. They are effective in both renovascular and essential low-renin hypertension. They are also used as vasodilators in the treatment of congestive heart failure. Called also *ACE i's.*

aromatase i's a class of drugs that inhibit aromatase activity and thus block production of estrogens; used to treat breast cancer and endometriosis.

C1 i. (C1 INH) an α_2-globulin of the serpin family that inhibits the complement component C1 (see under *complement*), binding the complex of C1r and C1s, removing it from C1q and preventing activation of the classical complement pathway. It also inhibits plasmin, thrombin, and kallikrein. Deficiency of or defect in the protein causes hereditary angioedema.

calcineurin i. any of a group of compounds that inhibit the action of calcineurin and are used as immunosuppressants.

carbonic anhydrase i. any of a group of agents that inhibit activity of carbonic anhydrase (carbonate dehydratase). In the kidney this decreases hydrogen ion concentration in the renal tubule, resulting in increased excretion of bicarbonate, sodium, potassium, and water; in the eye it depresses production of aqueous humor and lowers intraocular pressure. These were originally used as diuretics but were replaced by other agents because their diuretic effect is self-limiting; now they are used chiefly for treatment of glaucoma, and also for epilepsy, familial periodic paralysis, acute mountain sickness, and uric acid calculi.

CDK i. cyclin-dependent kinase i.

C1 esterase i. C1 i.

cholesterol i. an agent that suppresses the production of cholesterol or decreases its level in the blood.

cholinesterase i. a compound that prevents the hydrolysis of acetylcholine by acetylcholinesterase, permitting high levels of acetylcholine to accumulate at reactive sites. Some are used as drugs, some are insecticides, and certain potent ones are nerve gases that can be deadly to humans or other animals. Called also *anticholinesterase.*

coagulation i. anticoagulant.

COX-2 i., cyclooxygenase-2 i. any of a group of nonsteroidal antiinflammatory drugs (NSAIDs) that act by inhibiting cyclooxygenase-2 (COX-2) activity; they have fewer gastrointestinal side effects than other NSAIDs. Called also *coxib.*

cyclin-dependent kinase i., cyclin kinase i. any of a group of substances that inhibit or suppress the activity of cyclin-dependent kinase; some show antineoplastic activity. Called also *CDK inhibitor.*

direct thrombin i. any of a group of agents that bind to the thrombin active site and inhibit various thrombin-catalyzed reactions.

fusion i. any of a group of antiretroviral drugs active against the human immunodeficiency virus; they prevent the virus from replicating by blocking its fusion with the inside of a cell.

gastric acid pump i. proton pump i.

α-glucosidase i. any of a group of oral antihyperglycemic agents that act by competitive inhibition of α-glucosidase, delaying intestinal carbohydrate absorption and lessening postprandial increases in glucose levels.

HIV protease i. any of a group of antiretroviral drugs active against the human immunodeficiency virus; they prevent protease-mediated cleavage of viral polyproteins, causing production of immature viral particles that are noninfective.

HMG-CoA reductase i's a group of drugs that competitively inhibit the enzyme hydroxymethylglutaryl-CoA reductase, which catalyzes the rate-limiting step in cholesterol biosynthesis; used to lower plasma lipoprotein levels in treatment of hyperlipoproteinemia. Called also *statins.*

lupus i. see under *anticoagulant.*

MAO i. monoamine oxidase inhibitor.

membrane attack complex i. former name for *S protein;* see *vitronectin.*

membrane i. of reactive lysis (MIRL) protectin.

microtubule i's a large group of substances that interfere with the growth of microtubules on target cells, especially tumor cells, so that many are useful as antineoplastics. Taxanes and vinca alkaloids are important examples.

mitotic i. a substance such as colchicine that slows or arrests the process of mitosis.

monoamine oxidase i. (MAOI) any of a group of antidepressant drugs that have the ability to block the oxidative deamination of monoamines. It is thought that by inhibiting monoamine oxidase activity the inhibitors increase the level of catecholamines in the central nervous system, which would have been otherwise neutralized by the enzyme, and that these increased concentrations are responsible for their antidepressant effects. They are also used in the prophylaxis of migraine.

non-nucleoside reverse transcriptase i. (NNRTI) see *reverse transcriptase i.*

pancreatic secretory trypsin i. (PSTI) a peptide that is expressed inside the pancreas and inhibits intrapancreatic activation of trypsin so that trypsin does not digest the pancreas itself; lack of this peptide leads to acute or chronic pancreatitis.

phosphodiesterase i. any of a class of drugs that inhibit the activity of phosphodiesterases, each agent having a different effect because of differing affinities for the various phosphodiesterase fractions; the class includes amrinone, dipyridamole, enoximone, milrinone, papaverine, and theophylline.

α_2-plasmin i. α_2-antiplasmin.

plasminogen activator i. (PAI) any of several members of the serpin group, regulators of fibrinolysis that act by binding to and inhibiting free plasminogen activator. The concentration in plasma of the inhibitors is normally low, but is altered in some disturbances of the hemostatic system. *PAI-1* is an important fast-reacting inhibitor of t-PA and u-PA; its synthesis, activity, and release are highly regulated, and elevated levels of it have been described in a number of disease states. *PAI-2* is a normally minor inhibitor that greatly increases in concentration during pregnancy and in certain disorders. *PAI-3* is another name for *protein C inhibitor.*

platelet i. any of a group of agents that inhibit the clotting activity of platelets. See also *antiplatelet therapy,* under *therapy.*

protease i. (PI) 1. a substance that blocks activity of endopeptidase (protease), such as in a virus. 2. HIV protease i.

proteasome i's a class of antineoplastic agents that disrupt the ubiquitin-proteasome system of cells, thereby interfering with growth and other cellular processes.

protein C i. the primary inhibitor of activated anticoagulant protein C; it is a glycoprotein, M_r 57,000, of the serpin superfamily of proteinase inhibitors and also inhibits several other proteins involved in coagulation and urokinase. Called also *plasminogen activator inhibitor 3.*

proton pump i. (PPI) an agent that inhibits the proton pump in the stomach, thus limiting gastric acid secretion; it works by blocking the action of H^+,K^+-ATPase at the secretory surface of gastric parietal cells; called also *gastric acid pump i.*

reverse transcriptase i. a substance that blocks activity of the reverse transcriptase of a retrovirus and is used as an antiretroviral agent. Some are nucleosides or nucleoside analogues, and those that are not are therefore often called *non-nucleoside reverse transcriptase inhibitors.*

selective norepinephrine reuptake i. (NRI) any of a group of compounds that elevate the extracellular level of norepinephrine in the central nervous system by inhibiting its reuptake into the synapse via the presynaptic norepinephrine transporter, but that have only weak or no effects on neuronal uptake of serotonin and dopamine; used to treat attention-deficit/hyperactivity disorder and depression. NOTE: SNRI is sometimes used as an abbreviation, but is confusing since it also is used for *serotonin-norepinephrine reuptake inhibitor.*

selective serotonin reuptake i. (SSRI) any of a group of compounds that inhibit the inactivation of serotonin by blocking its absorption in the central nervous system, but that have only weak or no effects on neuronal uptake of norepinephrine and dopamine; used to treat depressive, obsessive-compulsive, and panic disorders.

serine protease i., serine proteinase i. serpin.

serotonin-norepinephrine reuptake i. (SNRI) any of a group of compounds that limit the reabsorption of serotonin and norepinephrine by blocking their transporter proteins, acting also weakly on dopamine, and thereby potentiating neurotransmitter activity in the central nervous system; used in the treatment of depression and other affective disorders, as well as anxiety disorders, obsessive-compulsive disorder, attention-deficit/hyperactivity disorder, and chronic neuropathic pain. See also note at *selective norepinephrine reuptake i.*

topoisomerase i. any of a group of antineoplastic agents that interfere with the arrangement of DNA in cells.

tyrosine kinase i. any of a class of antineoplastic agents that inhibit protein-tyrosine kinase and interfere with the action of epidermal growth factor in cancer cells.

in·hib·i·to·ry (in-hib′ĭ-tor″e) restraining or arresting any process; effecting a stay or arrest, partial or complete.

in·ho·mo·ge·ne·i·ty (in-ho″mo-jə-ne′ĭ-te) lack of normal homogeneity.

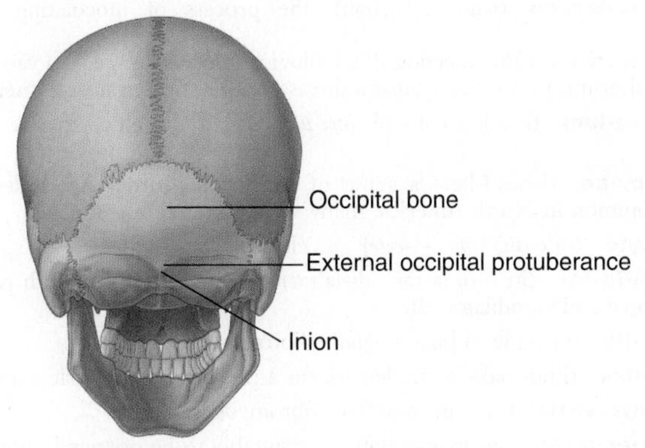

in·ho·mo·ge·neous (in-ho″mo-je′ne-əs) lacking homogeneity.

in·i·ad (in′e-əd) toward the inion.

in·i·en·ceph·a·lus (in″e-ən-sef′ə-ləs) a fetus exhibiting iniencephaly.

in·i·en·ceph·a·ly (in″e-ən-sef′ə-le) [*ini-* + Gr. *enkephalos* brain] a developmental anomaly characterized by enlargement of the foramen magnum and absence of the laminae and spinous processes of the cervical, dorsal, and sometimes lumbar vertebrae, with vertebrae reduced in number and irregularly fused, the brain and much of the spinal cord occupying a single cavity.

ini(o)- [Gr. *inion* occiput] a combining form denoting relationship to the occiput.

in·i·od·y·mus (in″e-od′ĭ-məs) iniopagus.

in·i·on (in′e-on) [Gr. "the back of the head"] [TA] the most prominent point of the external occipital protuberance. **in′iac, in′ial** *adj*

in·i·op·a·gus (in″e-op′ə-gəs) [*inio-* + *-pagus*] symmetrical conjoined twins fused at the occiput.

in·i·ops (in′e-ops) [*inio-* + Gr. *ōps* eye] a double-faced fetus with the posterior face incomplete.

ini·tial (ĭ-nish′əl) [L. *initialis*, from *initium* beginning] pertaining to the very first stage of any process.

ini·ti·a·tion (ĭ-nĭ″she-a′shən) in toxicology, the creation of a small alteration in the genetic makeup of a cell by a low level of exposure to a carcinogen; the cell may later become neoplastic upon repeated exposure to the same carcinogen or exposure to a promoter.

ini·ti·a·tor (ĭ-nish′e-a″tər) an agent that initiates polymerization of a resin when mixed with the resin.

in·ject·a·ble (in-jek′tə-bəl) 1. capable of being injected. 2. a substance that may be injected.

in·ject·ed (in-jek′təd) 1. introduced by injection. 2. congested.

in·jec·tion (in-jek′shən) [L. *injectio*, from *inicere* to throw into] 1. the act of forcing a liquid into a part, as into the subcutaneous tissues, the vascular tree, or an organ. Cf. *infusion* (def. 3). 2. a substance so forced or administered. Officially, in pharmacy, a solution of a medicament suitable for injection. See also under specific substances. 3. congestion.

aminophylline i. [USP] a sterile solution of aminophylline in water for injection, or of theophylline in water for injection prepared with the aid of ethylenediamine; used as a bronchodilator in the treatment and prophylaxis of asthma and the treatment of chronic obstructive pulmonary disease and of dipyridamole toxicity.

anatomical i. an injection into the vessels or organs of the cadaver, designed to facilitate dissection or demonstration.

circumcorneal i. dilatation of the ciliary and conjunctival blood vessels close to the limbus, and diminishing toward the periphery.

coarse i. an anatomical injection that fills only the larger vessels.

cytarabine liposome i. liposomal cytarabine.

depot i. injection of a medication that stays in a local area (a *depot*) and is distributed slowly into the body; absorption is often kept slow by mixing the medication with a suitable excipient.

endermic i. intradermal i.

fine i. an anatomical injection that fills even the smallest vessels.

gaseous i. injection of gas or air for therapeutic purposes as in collapse therapy; for diagnostic purposes, as in ventriculography; or for facilitating anatomical demonstrations.

gelatin i. a preservative injection of which gelatin is the base.

hypodermic i. subcutaneous i.

intracutaneous i. intradermal i.

intracytoplasmic sperm i. (ICSI) a micromanipulation technique, in which a single spermatocyte is inserted into an oocyte by micropuncture.

intradermal i., intradermic i. an injection made into the dermis or substance of the skin.

intramuscular i. an injection into the substance of a muscle.

intrathecal i. injection of a substance through the theca of the spinal cord into the subarachnoid space.

intravascular i. an injection made into a vessel.

intravenous i. an injection made into a vein.

invert sugar i. [USP] a sterile aqueous solution prepared by mixing equal amounts of dextrose and fructose or by hydrolysis of an equivalent amount of sucrose; used as a fluid and nutrient replenisher.

iodinated I 131 albumin aggregated i. [USP] a sterile aqueous suspension of albumin human iodinated with ^{131}I and denatured to produce aggregates of controlled particle size; each mL contains 300 μg to 3.0 mg of aggregated albumin with specific activity of 200 microcuries to 1.2 millicuries per mg.

jet i. injection of a drug in solution through the intact skin by an extremely fine jet of the solution under high pressure.

lactated Ringer i. [USP] a sterile solution of calcium chloride, potassium chloride, sodium chloride, and sodium lactate in water for injection, given as a fluid and electrolyte replenisher by intravenous infusion; called also *lactated Ringer solution.*

multiple electrolytes i. a sterile solution of electrolytes in water for injection to provide various combinations of ions; official preparations [USP] contain different combinations of salts and may also include carbohydrates (see table at *electrolyte*).

opacifying i. the injection of a radiopaque medium into the vessels or into some body cavity for diagnostic radiological study.

parenchymatous i. an injection made into the substance of an organ.

preservative i. an injection that serves to protect a cadaver or specimen from decay.

protein hydrolysate i. [USP] a sterile solution of amino acids and short-chain peptides, representing the approximate nutritive equivalent of the protein from which it is derived; used as a fluid and nutrient replenisher.

repository corticotropin i. [USP] corticotropin in a solution of partially hydrolyzed gelatin, a gel form having prolonged effects; administered subcutaneously or intramuscularly as an anticonvulsant for treating infantile spasms.

Ringer i. [USP] a sterile solution of sodium chloride, potassium chloride, and calcium chloride in water for injection, given as a fluid and electrolyte replenisher by intravenous infusion.

sclerosing i. sclerotherapy.

sodium chloride i. [USP] a sterile isotonic solution of sodium chloride in water for injection, used as a fluid and electrolyte replenisher and as an irrigating solution. It is also used as a vehicle for the injection of medications.

subcutaneous i. an injection made into the subcutaneous tissues; called also *hypodermic i.*

subzonal i. of sperm subzonal insemination.

Z-track i. a technique for intramuscular injection of a substance that may be irritating, or that requires strict deposition and absorption. The tissue to be injected is pulled downward in the direction of the body's midline and held during and after injection. When the tissue is released, the usually straight needle track becomes a broken line shaped like a Z, which holds the medication deep in the muscle.

in·jec·tor (in-jek′tər) an instrument used in making injections.

in·ju·ry (in′jə-re) [L. *injuria*] harm or hurt; usually applied to damage inflicted on the body by an external force. Called also *trauma* and *wound.*

acute kidney i. acute renal failure.

birth i. see under *trauma.*

blast i. the injuries caused by an explosion (see *blast*[2]), most commonly blast chest (q.v.), laceration of other thoracic and abdominal viscera, ruptured ear drums, and minor effects on the central nervous system.

cold i. any tissue damage caused by hypothermia. *Freezing cold injury* occurs when environmental temperature is at or below 0°C and involves the more severe forms of frostbite and often gangrene. *Nonfreezing cold injury* occurs at warmer temperatures and causes conditions such as superficial frostbite and immersion foot. Called also *hypothermic i.*

deceleration i. an injury sustained by sudden deceleration in the movement of the body, as in a motor vehicle accident; the brain is especially liable to such trauma.

diffuse axonal i. diffuse damage to the white matter of the brain caused by stretching or shearing in head injury, resulting in a coma that may last a few hours or days or may be permanent.

hypothermic i. cold i.

overuse i. injury to a part, such as a muscle, nerve, or bone, caused by repetitive motion, such as in certain occupations or sports. See also *entrapment neuropathy*, under *neuropathy*. Called also *overuse syndrome* and *repetitive strain i.*

reperfusion i. adverse effects of the restoration of blood flow following an ischemic episode, including cellular swelling and necrosis, edema, hemorrhage, the no-reflow phenomenon, and tissue damage by free oxygen radicals.

repetitive strain i. overuse i.

steering wheel i. injury to the chest and sometimes contusion of the heart in motorists, caused by being thrown forward against the steering wheel.

straddle i. injury to the distal urethra by falling astride a blunt object such as bicycle handlebars or the top of a fence or railing.

transfusion-related acute lung i. (TRALI) a syndrome seen in persons receiving transfusions, characterized by pulmonary edema, dyspnea, hypoxemia, hypotension, and fever; it is thought to be a reaction to antibodies or other components of the donor blood product. Patients need oxygen support, and in some cases the syndrome can be fatal.

unintentional i. in public health, the cause of death when the death occurs under accidental circumstances.

whiplash i. a popular nonspecific term applied to injury to the spine and spinal cord at the junction of the fourth and fifth cervical vertebrae, occurring as the result of rapid acceleration or deceleration of the body. Because of their greater mobility, the four upper vertebrae act as the lash, and the lower three act as the handle of the whip.

in·lay (in′la) 1. material, such as bone or skin, inserted into a tissue defect. 2. a dental restoration made outside of a tooth to correspond with the form of a prepared cavity and then cemented into the tooth.

epithelial i. a method of securing epithelialization of an unhealed deep wound. A mold of the wound cavity is taken and covered with a Thiersch graft of epidermis, the whole being inserted into the wound cavity, and the edges then approximated with sutures. The mold is removed after ten days, leaving the cavity completely epithelialized. Called also *Esser operation.* See also under *onlay.*

in·let (in′lət) a means or route of entrance.

esophageal i. constrictio pharyngooesophagealis.

laryngeal i. aditus laryngis.

pelvic i. apertura pelvis superior.

thoracic i. apertura thoracis superior.

INN International Nonproprietary Name.

in·nate (ĭ-nāt′) [L. *in* in + *nasci* to be born] inborn.

in·ner·va·tion (in″ər-va′shən) [*in-*[1] + *nervus*] 1. the distribution or supply of nerves to a part. 2. the supply of nervous energy or of nerve stimulus sent to a part.

double i. innervation of a structure by two kinds of nerve fibers, e.g., sympathetic and parasympathetic.

reciprocal i. the innervation of muscles around the joints, where the motor centers are so connected in pairs that when one is excited the center of the corresponding antagonist is inhibited.

in·nid·i·a·tion (ĭ-nid″e-a′shən) [*in-*[1] + *nidus*] the development of cells in a part to which they have been carried by metastasis; called also *colonization* and *indenization.*

in·no·cent (in′o-sənt) [L. *innocens; in* not +*nocere* to harm] not malignant; benign; not tending of its own nature to a fatal issue. See *innocent bystander,* under *bystander.*

in·noc·u·ous (ĭ-nok′u-əs) harmless.

In·no·hep (in′o-hep″) trademark for a preparation of tinzaparin sodium.

in·nom·i·na·tal (ĭ-nom″ĭ-na′təl) pertaining to the innominate (brachiocephalic) artery or to the innominate (hip) bone.

in·nom·i·nate (ĭ-nom′ĭ-nāt) [L. *innominatus* nameless; *in* not + *nomen* name] not having a name; nameless. The term has been applied to certain structures better identified by their descriptive names, as the innominate (brachiocephalic) artery and the innominate (hip) bone.

In·no·var (in′o-vahr) a trademark for a preparation of droperidol and fentanyl citrate in a 50:1 ratio; used as a neuroleptanalgesic.

in·nox·ious (ĭ-nok′shəs) [*in-*[2] + *noxius*] not injurious; not hurtful.

in(o)- [Gr. *is,* gen. *inos* fiber] a combining form denoting relationship to a fiber, or fibrous material.

ino·chon·dri·tis (in″o-kon-dri′tis) [*ino-* + *chondr-* + *-itis*] inflammation of a fibrocartilage.

In·o·cor (in′o-kor) trademark for a preparation of inamrinone lactate.

in·oc·u·la (ĭ-nok′u-lə) [L.] plural of *inoculum.*

in·oc·u·la·ble (ĭ-nok′u-lə-bəl) 1. susceptible to being inoculated. 2. transmissible by inoculation.

in·oc·u·late (ĭ-nok′u-lāt) [L. *inoculare*] 1. to implant microbes or other infective materials in or on culture media. 2. to introduce immune serum, vaccines of various kinds, or some other antigenic material into a healthy individual to produce a mild form of the disease followed by immunity. 3. to spread a disease by inserting its etiologic agent.

in·oc·u·la·tion (ĭ-nok″u-la′shən) the process of inoculating something.

protective i. the injection of a biological preparation, e.g., a vaccine or an antiserum, to protect against a disease; vaccination against a disease.

in·oc·u·lum (ĭ-nok′u-ləm) pl. *inoc′ula* [L.] a substance that is inoculated.

I·no·cy·be (i-nos′ĭ-be) a genus of mushrooms (order Agaricales) that are common in North America; many species contain muscarine.

ino·cyte (in′o-sīt) [*ino-* + *-cyte*] a cell of fibrous tissue.

ino·di·la·tor (in″o-di′la-tər, -di-la′tər) an agent that has both positive inotropic and vasodilator effects.

in·og·lia (in-og′le-ə) [*ino-* + *-glia*] fibroglia.

INO·max (i′no-maks″) trademark for a preparation of nitric oxide.

ino·myo·si·tis (in″o-mi″o-si′tis) fibromyositis.

in·op·er·a·ble (in-op′ər-ə-bəl) not suitable to be operated upon.

in·o·per·cu·late (in″o-pur′ku-lāt) not having an operculum; said of an ascus.

ino·phrag·ma (in″o-frag′mə) [*ino-* + Gr. *phragmos* a fencing in] ground membrane; a name given to the Z band and M band (q.q.v.) because they continue uninterruptedly as transverse membranes through all the adjoining fibrils of a muscle fiber. See *mesophragma* and *telophragma.*

in·or·gan·ic (in″or-gan′ik) [*in-*[2] + *organic*] 1. having no organs. 2. not of organic origin. 3. pertaining to substances not of organic origin. 4. in chemistry, denoting substances not derived from hydrocarbons.

in·or·gan·ic py·ro·phos·pha·tase (in″or-gan′ik pi″ro-fos′fə-tās) [EC 3.6.1.1] an enzyme of the hydrolase class that catalyzes the cleavage of pyrophosphate into two phosphate molecules. The enzyme is present in all cells and regulates the concentration of endogenous pyrophosphate. Specificity varies with the source and with the activating metal ion. The enzyme from some sources may be identical with alkaline phosphatase or with glucose-6-phosphatase. In official nomenclature, the preferred name is now *inorganic diphosphatase.*

ino·scle·ro·sis (in″o-sklə-ro′sis) [*ino-* + *sclerosis*] sclerosis or induration by increase of fibrous tissue.

in·os·co·py (in-os′ko-pe) [*ino-* + *-scopy*] the diagnosis of disease by artificial digestion and examination of the fibers or fibrinous matter of the sputum, blood, effusions, etc.

in·os·cu·late (in-os′ku-lāt) [*in-*[1] + *osculum*] to unite or communicate by means of small openings or anastomoses.

in·os·cu·la·tion (in-os″ku-la′shən) the establishment of communication by means of small openings or anastomoses; especially, establishment of such communication between blood vessels or other tubular structures that come in contact.

in·ose (in′ōs) inositol.

in·o·se·mia (in″o-se′me-ə) 1. the presence of inose (inositol) in the blood. 2. an excess of fibrin in the blood.

in·o·si·nate (in-o′sĭ-nāt) a salt, anion, or ester of inosinic acid (inosine monophosphate).

in·o·sine (I) (in′o-sēn) a purine nucleoside, hypoxanthine linked by its N9 nitrogen to the C1 carbon of ribose. It is an intermediate in the degradation of purines and purine nucleosides to uric acid and in pathways of purine salvage. It also occurs in the anticodon of certain transfer RNA molecules.

i. monophosphate (IMP) a nucleotide, the 5′-phosphate of inosine, formed by deamination of adenosine monophosphate (AMP); it is the precursor of AMP and GMP (guanosine monophosphate) in purine biosynthesis and an intermediate in the salvage of purines and the degradation of purines to uric acid.

i. triphosphate (ITP) a nucleotide, the 5′-triphosphate of inosine; it acts as a phosphate donor in certain carboxylation reactions.

in·o·sin·ic ac·id (in″o-sin′ik) inosine monophosphate.

in·o·site (in′o-sīt) inositol.

ino·sit·ide (in-o′sĭ-tīd) a compound containing inositol, particularly phosphatidylinositol and related lipids.

in·o·si·tis (in″o-si′tis) [*ino-* + *-itis*] inflammation of fibrous tissue.

ino·si·tol (ĭ-no′sĭ-tol) a cyclic sugar alcohol, the fully hydroxylated derivative of cyclohexane, occurring naturally in a variety of stereoisomers, particularly the *myo*-isomer. Used alone, the term usually denotes this isomer.

***myo*-i.** a stereoisomer of inositol occurring in a variety of plant and animal tissues and microorganisms; it is often phosphorylated and is a component of phosphatidylinositols. It often classified as a member of the vitamin B complex and can be obtained from vegetables, citrus fruits, cereal grains, and organ and other meats.

i. 1,4,5-triphosphate ($InsP_3$, IP_3) a second messenger generated by cleavage of phosphatidylinositol 4,5-bisphosphate in calcium-mediated hormonal responses; it causes the release of calcium from certain intracellular organelles.

ino•si•tol-phos•phate phos•pha•tase (in-o′sĭ-tol fos′fāt fos′fə-tās) [EC 3.1.3.25] an enzyme of the hydrolase class that catalyzes the dephosphorylation of *myo*-inositol phosphate to form *myo*-inositol, acting on five of the six monophosphate isomers of *myo*-inositol phosphate (all except *myo*-inositol 2-phosphate). Inhibition of this reaction by lithium breaks the hormonally dependent cycle of degradation and regeneration of phosphoinositides. Formerly officially called *myo-inositol-1 (or 4)-monophosphatase.*

in•o•si•tol•uria (in″o-sĭ″tol-u′re-ə) inosituria.

in•o•si•tu•ria (in″o-sĭ-tu′re-ə) the occurrence of inositol in the urine; called also *inosuria.*

in•os•to•sis (in″os-to′sis) the re-formation of bony tissue to replace bone that has been destroyed.

in•os•uria (in″o-su′re-ə) 1. fibrinuria. 2. inosituria.

ino•tag•ma (in″o-tag′mə) [*ino-* + Gr. *tagma* arrangement] a linear arrangement of the contractile structural elements of a muscle cell.

ino•trope (in′o-trōp) an agent that affects the force or energy of muscle contractions.

in•o•tro•pic (in″o-tro′pik) [*ino-* + *-tropic*] affecting the force or energy of muscular contractions.

negatively i. weakening the force of muscular contraction.

positively i. increasing the force of muscular contraction.

in•ot•ro•pism (in-ot′rə-piz-əm) the quality of influencing the contractility of muscle fibers.

in ovo (in o′vo) [L.] in the egg; referring specifically to various experimental procedures involving the use of chick embryos.

in•pa•tient (in′pa-shənt) a patient who comes to a hospital or other health care facility for diagnosis or treatment that requires an overnight stay.

in•quest (in′kwest) [L. *in* into + *quaerere* to seek] a legal inquiry before a coroner or medical examiner, and usually a jury, into the manner of a death.

in•qui•line (in′kwĭ-līn) [L. *inquilinus* a lodger] an organism that lives within the body of another, but does not derive its nourishment from the host.

in•sal•i•va•tion (in″sal-ĭ-va′shən) [*in-*[1] + *salivation*] the saturation of the food with saliva in mastication.

In•sall-Sal•va•ti ratio (in′səl sahl-vah′te) [John N. *Insall*, American orthopedist, 1930–2000; E. *Salvati*, American orthopedist, 20th century] see under *ratio.*

in•sa•lu•bri•ous (in″sə-loo′bre-əs) not salubrious; not conducive to health.

in•san•i•tary (in-san′ĭ-tar-e) not in a good sanitary condition; not conducive to good health; unclean.

in•san•i•ty (in-san′ĭ-te) [L. *insanitas*, from *in* not + *sanus* sound] mental derangement or disorder, a legal rather than a medical term denoting a condition due to which a person lacks criminal responsibility for a crime and therefore cannot be convicted of it. **insane′** *adj*

in•scrip•tio (in-skrip′she-o) pl. *inscriptio′nes* [L., from *inscribere* to write on] 1. inscription. 2. intersectio.

i. tendi′nea intersectio tendinea.

i.′nes tendin′eae mus′culi rec′ti abdom′inis intersectiones tendineae musculi recti abdominis.

in•scrip•tion (in-skrip′shən) [L. *inscriptio*] 1. a mark, or line. 2. that part of a prescription which contains the names and amounts of the ingredients.

tendinous i. intersectio tendinea.

tendinous i's of rectus abdominis muscle intersectiones tendineae musculi recti abdominis.

in•scrip•ti•o•nes (in-skrip″she-o′nēz) [L.] plural of *inscriptio.*

in•sect (in′sekt) any individual of the class Insecta.

In•sec•ta (in-sek′tə) [L., from *in* + *sectum* cut] a class of the Arthropoda whose members are characterized by division of the body into three parts: head, thorax, and abdomen; there are three orders of medical interest, Diptera, Hemiptera, and Siphonaptera.

in•sec•ta•ri•um (in″sek-tar′e-əm) a place for breeding and raising insects.

in•sec•ti•cide (in-sek′tĭ-sīd) [*insect* + *-cide*] any substance selectively poisonous to insects.

in•sec•ti•fuge (in-sek′tĭ-fūj) [*insect* + *-fuge*] a preparation that repels insects.

In•sec•tiv•o•ra (in″sek-tiv′o-rə) [*insect* + L. *vorare* to devour] an order of small, terrestrial mammals, including the moles and shrews, which feed primarily on insects and other invertebrates.

in•sec•ti•vore (in-sek′tĭ-vor) an individual of the order Insectivora.

in•sec•tiv•o•rous (in″sek-tiv′ə-rəs) subsisting on insects.

in•sem•i•na•tion (in-sem″ĭ-na′shən) [L. *inseminatus* sown] the deposit of semen or seminal fluid within the vagina or cervix, as during sexual intercourse.

artificial i. (AI) introduction of semen into the vagina or cervix by artificial means; the sperm may be from the woman's husband *(artificial i. by husband)* or from a donor known or unknown to the woman *(donor i.).* Called also *therapeutic i.*

artificial i. by donor (AID) donor i.

artificial i. by husband (AIH) artificial insemination in which the semen used is from the woman's mate; called also *homologous i.*

direct intraperitoneal i. a method of assisted reproductive technology in which semen is injected into the pouch of Douglas.

donor i., heterologous i. artificial insemination in which the semen used is that of a man other than the woman's mate. Called also *artificial i. by donor (AID).*

homologous i. artificial i. by husband.

intrafallopian i. intratubal i.

intrafollicular i. a method of assisted reproductive technology in which semen is injected into an ovarian follicle.

intraperitoneal i. injection of semen into the peritoneal cavity; see *direct intraperitoneal i.*

intratubal i. a method of assisted reproductive technology in which washed semen is injected into the fallopian tube; called also *intrafallopian i.*

intrauterine i. (IUI) artificial insemination in which specially washed sperm is injected through the cervix directly into the uterus.

subzonal i. (SUZI) a micromanipulation technique used in cases of male factor infertility; spermatozoa are inserted into the perivitelline space after breaching of the zona pellucida by mechanical or chemical means. Called also *subzonal injection* or *insertion of sperm.*

therapeutic i. artificial i.

therapeutic i. by donor, therapeutic donor i. donor i.

in•se•nes•cence (in″sə-nes′əns) the process of growing old.

in•sen•si•ble (in-sen′sĭ-bəl) [*in-*[2] + *sensible*] 1. not appreciable by or perceptible to the senses. 2. devoid of consciousness or of sensibility.

in•sen•si•tiv•i•ty (in-sen″sĭ-tiv′ĭ-te) lack of the expected response to a stimulus or chemical.

androgen i. lack of response to stimulation by androgens: see *androgen insensitivity syndrome*, under *syndrome.* Called also *androgen resistance.*

in•sert[1] (in-sərt′) [L. *inserere* to graft, insert] to put in, introduce, or implant something into another thing.

in•sert[2] (in′sərt) something that is put in or introduced; cf. *implant*[2].

intramucosal i., mucosal i. a nonreactive metal stud, consisting of a base, cervix, and head, attached to a prosthesis inserted into a pocket of oral mucosa just before fitting of a denture; most commonly used for added retention of complete upper dentures.

in•ser•tio (in-sur′she-o) [L.] [TA] insertion.

i. velamento′sa velamentous insertion.

in•ser•tion (in-sur′shən) [L. *inserere* to join to] 1. the putting of one thing into something else or among other things. 2. a place of attachment, as of a muscle to the bone it moves. 3. in genetics, a rare nonreciprocal type of translocation involving three breaks in which a segment is removed from one chromosome and then inserted into a broken region of a nonhomologous chromosome. See illustration at *aberration.*.

parasol i. a type of attachment of the umbilical cord to the placenta in which the vessels of the cord separate before they join the placenta and resemble the ribs of a parasol.

subzonal i. of sperm subzonal insemination.

velamentous i. a type of attachment of the umbilical cord to the membranes (amnion and chorion) in which the vessels course for a long or short distance between the amnion and the smooth chorion before reaching the placenta.

in•sheathed (in-shēthd′) enclosed within a sheath.

in•sid•i•ous (in-sid′e-əs) [L. *insidiosus* deceitful, treacherous] coming on in a stealthy manner; of gradual and subtle development.

in•sight (in′sīt) 1. in psychiatry, the patient's awareness and understanding of the origins and meaning of his attitudes, feelings, and behavior and of his disturbing symptoms; self-understanding. 2. in problem solving, the sudden perception of the appropriate relationships of things that results in a solution.

intellectual i. understanding of the objective reality of a situation without the ability to apply that knowledge in the future or without true feeling.

true i. understanding of the objective reality of a situation coupled to true feeling and to the motivation and capability to use the understanding in the future.

in si•tu (in si′tu) [L.] in the natural or normal place; confined to the site of origin without invasion of neighboring tissues.

in•so•la•tion (in″so-la′shən) 1. heliotherapy. 2. sunstroke.

asphyxial i. sunstroke with low temperature, cold skin, and feeble pulse.

hyperpyrexial i. thermic fever with very high temperature, coma, and congested skin.

in•sol•u•ble (in-sol′u-bəl) not susceptible of being dissolved.

in•som•nia (in-som′ne-ə) [*in-*[2] + *somn-* + *-ia*] inability to sleep; abnormal wakefulness.

fatal familial i. an autosomal dominant prion disease caused by mutation in the prion protein gene (*PRNP*, locus: 20pter-p12), affecting primarily the ventral and dorsomedial nuclei of the thalamus and characterized by progressive insomnia, hallucinations, stupor, and coma ending in death within 6 months to 3 years of onset; autonomic and motor disturbances are also present.

initial i. insomnia characterized by difficulty falling asleep, often due to anxiety, tension, or depression.

middle i. insomnia characterized by awakening during the sleep period, with difficulty in falling back to sleep.

primary i. [DSM-IV] a dyssomnia characterized by persistent difficulty initiating or maintaining sleep or by persistently nonrestorative sleep; it is not due to another sleep disorder or mental disorder or to a general medical condition or substance use.

terminal i. insomnia characterized by early awakening with difficulty in falling back to sleep, often occurring in depression, bereavement, chronic anxiety, and cerebral arteriosclerosis.

in•som•ni•ac (in-som′ne-ak) 1. pertaining to insomnia. 2. an individual exhibiting insomnia.

in•som•nic (in-som′nik) insomniac.

in•so•nate (in-so′nāt) to expose to ultrasound waves.

in•sorp•tion (in-sorp′shən) the movement of a substance into the blood, such as intestinal absorption of the contents of the gastrointestinal tract.

$InsP_3$ inositol 1,4,5-triphosphate.

in•sper•sion (in-spur′zhən) the act of sprinkling, as with a powder.

in•spi•ra•tion (in″spĭ-ra′shən) inhalation (def. 1). **inspi′ratory** *adj*

in•spire (in-spīr′) [L. *inspirare*] inhale.

in•spi•rom•e•ter (in″spi-rom′ə-tər) [*inspire* + *-meter*] an apparatus for measuring the amount of air inhaled.

in•spis•sat•ed (in-spis′āt-əd) being thickened, dried, or rendered less fluid.

in•spis•sa•tion (in″spis-a′shən) [L. *inspissatio*] 1. the act or process of rendering dry or thick by the evaporation of readily vaporizable parts. 2. the condition of being rendered less thin by evaporation.

in•spis•sa•tor (in-spis′a-tər) an apparatus for inspissating fluids, such as blood serum.

In•spra (in′sprə) trademark for a preparation of eplerenone.

in•sta•bil•i•ty (in-stə-bil′ĭ-te) lack of steadiness or stability.

detrusor i. involuntary contraction of the detrusor muscle of the bladder caused by nonneurological problems such as bladder outlet obstruction. Cf. *detrusor hyperreflexia.*

functional i. inability of a joint to maintain support during use.

glenohumeral i. slippage or subluxation of the humeral head out of the glenoid fossa; it may or may not be traumatic in origin. The traumatic type is seen particularly in athletes who throw.

microsatellite i. (MSI) the presence of unusual microsatellite lengths in an individual, caused by defects in the DNA mismatch repair genes; it has been identified as a marker for a variety of cancers, both hereditary, such as hereditary nonpolyposis colorectal cancer, and sporadic. The phenotype is sometimes referred to as *replication error–positive.*

in•star (in′stahr) [L. "a form"] any stage of an arthropod between molts.

in•step (in′step) the dorsal part of the arch of the foot.

in•stil•la•tion (in″stĭ-la′shən) administration of a liquid drop by drop.

in•stil•la•tor (in′stĭ-la″tər) an instrument for performing instillations.

in•stinct (in′stinkt) a complex of unlearned responses that is characteristic of a species.

aggressive i. death i.

death i. Freud's concept of an unconscious drive toward dissolution and death, in opposition to the life instinct.

ego i. one of the nonsexual, self-preservative instincts originally postulated by Freud; they were later subsumed under the life instinct.

herd i. the instinct or urge to be one of a group and to conform to the standards of that group in conduct and opinion.

life i. Freud's concept of all the constructive tendencies of the organism aimed at maintenance and perpetuation of the individual and species, in opposition to the death instinct.

mother i. the complex behavior in a mother which accomplishes the care of the young; whether such an instinct exists in human females is questioned.

sexual i. life i.

in•stinc•tive (in-stink′tiv) of the nature of, related to, or prompted by instinct; performed spontaneously, without thinking.

in•sti•tu•tion•al•iza•tion (in-stĭ-too″shən-əl-ĭ-za′shən) 1. commitment of a patient to a health care facility for treatment, often psychiatric. 2. in patients hospitalized for a long period, the development of excessive dependency on the institution and its routines, with diminishing of the will to function independently.

in•stru•ment (in′strə-mənt) [L. *instrumentum*] any tool, appliance, or apparatus.

in•stru•men•tal (in″strə-men′təl) 1. pertaining to or performed by instruments. 2. serving as a means to a particular result.

in•stru•men•tar•i•um (in″strə-mən-tar′e-əm) the instruments or equipment required for any particular operation or purpose; the physical adjuncts with which a physician combats disease.

in•stru•men•ta•tion (in″strə-mən-ta′shən) 1. the use of instruments; work performed with instruments. 2. a group of instruments used for a specific purpose.

Cotrel-Dubousset i. a system of rods, hooks, and screws used to treat scoliosis in the thoracic and lumbar regions with spinal fusion and also to set vertebral fractures.

Dwyer i. a method to correct scoliosis by using rods, screws, and staples for anterior spinal fusion in the lumbar region.

Harrington i. a system of metal hooks and rods inserted surgically in the posterior elements of the spine to provide distraction and compression in treatment of scoliosis and other deformities.

Knodt i. a system of rods and hooks used in spinal stabilization of limited areas of the lumbar spine to correct scoliosis.

Luque i. a method to correct scoliosis by using rigid (Luque) rods and sublaminar wiring for spinal fusion in the lumbar region.

Zielke i. a method to correct scoliosis by using rods and screws for anterior spinal fusion in the lumbar region.

in•suc•ca•tion (in″sə-ka′shən) [L. *insuccare* to soak in] the thorough soaking of a drug before preparing an extract from it.

in•su•date (in-soo′dāt) the substance accumulated in insudation.

in•su•da•tion (in″soo-da′shən) [*in-* + L. *sudare* to sweat] the accumulation, as in the kidney or the arterial (intimal) wall, of substances derived from the blood.

in•suf•fi•cien•cy (in″sə-fish′ən-se) the condition of being insufficient or inadequate to the performance of the allotted function; see also *failure.* Called also *incompetence.*

active i. the inability of a muscle to act owing to the abnormal (or other) approximation of its insertion to its origin.

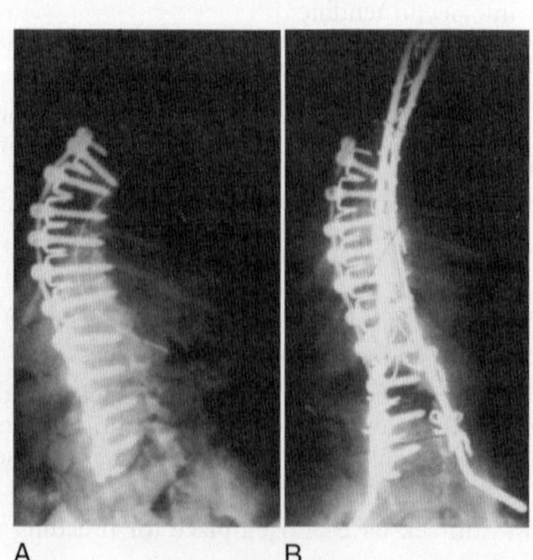

■ Anterior fusion with Dwyer instrumentation for correction of severe scoliosis *(A)*, followed by posterior fusion with rods *(B)*.

adrenal i. 1. abnormally diminished activity of the adrenal gland; see also *adrenocortical i. Primary adrenal i.* is another name for *Addison disease.* Called also *hypoadrenalism.* 2. adrenocortical i.

adrenocortical i. abnormally diminished secretion of corticosteroids by the adrenal cortex. *Acute adrenocortical i.* is another name for addisonian crisis and *primary* or *chronic adrenocortical i.* is another name for Addison disease. *Secondary adrenocortical* (or *adrenal*) *insufficiency* is any type caused by dysfunction of the pituitary or hypothalamus, with low plasma levels of cortisol and often of corticotropin. Called also *hypoadrenocorticism, hypocorticalism,* and *hypocorticism.*

aortic i., aortic valve i. defective functioning of the aortic valve, with incomplete closure resulting in aortic regurgitation.

basilar i. vertebrobasilar i.

cardiac i. insufficiency of the heart muscle or function; see also *heart failure.*

coronary i. decrease in flow of blood through the coronary blood vessels.

i. of the externi insufficient power in the externi muscles of the eye, so that they are overbalanced by the interni, producing esophoria.

i. of the eyelids a condition in which the eyes are closed only by a conscious effort.

gastric i., gastromotor i. inability of the stomach to empty itself.

hepatic i. inability of the liver to perform its usual functions properly.

i. of the interni insufficient power in the interni muscles of the eye, so that they are overbalanced by the externi, producing exophoria.

mitral i., mitral valve i. defective functioning of the mitral valve, with incomplete closure causing mitral regurgitation.

muscular i. the inability of a muscle to do its normal work by a normal contraction.

myocardial i. functional insufficiency of the heart muscle; see also *heart failure.*

pancreatic i. diminished secreting activity of the pancreas, either endocrine or exocrine or both, with resultant excess of undigested food elements in the urine and feces; affected individuals may have steatorrhea, azotorrhea, or diabetes mellitus.

parathyroid i. hypoparathyroidism.

pituitary i. hypopituitarism.

placental i. dysfunction of the placenta, with reduction in the area of exchange of nutrients; it often leads to fetal growth retardation.

primary adrenal i., primary adrenocortical i. Addison disease.

pulmonary i. 1. respiratory i. 2. pulmonary valve i.

pulmonary valve i. defective functioning of the pulmonary valve, with incomplete closure resulting in pulmonic regurgitation.

renal i. a state of disordered function of the kidneys verifiable by quantitative tests; it may progress to renal failure (see under *failure*).

respiratory i. inability of the lungs to provide adequate oxygen intake or carbon dioxide expulsion as needed by the body and its cells; if not managed successfully, it can progress to respiratory failure (see under *failure*).

thyroid i. hypothyroidism.

tricuspid i., tricuspid valve i. incomplete closure of the tricuspid valve, resulting in tricuspid regurgitation; it is usually secondary to systolic overload in the right ventricle.

uterine i. weakness of the contractile power of the uterus.

i. of the valves, valvular i. 1. dysfunction of one of the cardiac valves, with incomplete valve closure resulting in valvular regurgitation; see *aortic i., mitral i., pulmonary i.,* and *tricuspid i.* 2. venous i.

velopharyngeal i. inability to achieve velopharyngeal closure, due to muscular dysfunction, deficiency of the soft palate or superior constrictor muscle, cleft palate, or some other disorder; it often results in a speech disorder. Called also *velopharyngeal incompetence.*

venous i. inadequacy of the venous valves and impairment of venous return from the lower limbs (venous stasis), usually characterized by edema, warmth, and erythema, particularly of the lower third of the extremity; chronic insufficiency leads to stasis ulcers of the ankle or over the medial malleolus. Called also *primary valvular incompetence* and *valvular incompetence.*

vertebrobasilar i. transient or intermittent ischemia of the brainstem and cerebellum due to stenosis, thrombosis, or other obstruction of the vertebral or basilar artery; this results in symptoms such as vertigo, diplopia, nystagmus, muscle weakness, and dysarthria. A similar but more severe syndrome consists of paralysis, coma, and death. Cf. *subclavian steal.* Called also *basilar i., basilar artery syndrome,* and *vertebrobasilar ischemia* or *syndrome.*

in•suf•fla•tion (in″sə-fla′shən) [L. *in* into + *sufflatio* a blowing up] 1. the act of blowing a powder, vapor, gas, or air into a body cavity. Cf. *infusion* (def. 3). 2. finely powdered or liquid drugs carried into the respiratory passages by such devices as aerosols.

cranial i. the forcing of air into the subdural space and the cerebral ventricles.

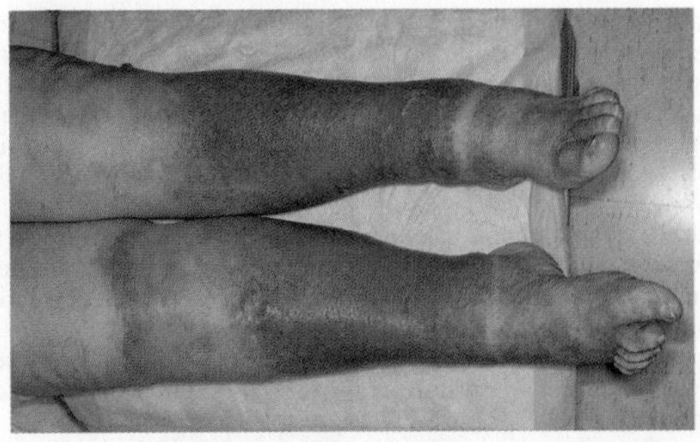

■ Chronic venous insufficiency.

i. of the lungs the act of blowing air into the lungs for the purpose of artificial respiration.

perirenal i. the injection of air around the kidneys for the purpose of radiographic visualization of the adrenal glands.

presacral i. the injection of gas, usually carbon dioxide, around the kidneys through a needle inserted into the retrorectal space for the purpose of radiographic visualization of the entire retroperitoneal space, with delineation of renal and adrenal areas.

tubal i. Rubin test (def. 1); see under *test.*

in•suf•fla•tor (in′sə-fla″tər) an instrument used in performing insufflation.

in•su•la (in′sə-lə) gen. and pl. *in′sulae* [L. "island"] 1. an islandlike structure. 2. [TA] a portion of the cerebral cortex lying deep in the lateral sulcus, almost surrounded by the circular sulcus; it is covered over and hidden from view by juxtaposition of the opercula. Called also *lobus insularis* [TA alternative], *insular lobe* or *>cortex* and *insula of Reil.*

in′sulae pancrea′ticae [TA] islets of Langerhans.

i. of Reil insula (def. 2).

in•su•lar (in′sə-lər) pertaining to an island, especially to the insula or to the pancreatic islets.

in•su•la•tion (in″sə-la′shən) [L. *insulare* to make an island of] 1. the surrounding of a space or body with material designed to prevent the entrance or escape of radiant or electrical energy. 2. the material so used.

in•su•la•tor (in′sə-la″tər) any substance or appliance of such nonconducting properties that it can be used to secure insulation.

in•su•lin (in′sə-lin) [L. *insula* island + *-in*] 1. a protein hormone secreted by the beta cells of the pancreatic islets, serving as a hormonal signal of the fed state; it is secreted in response to elevated blood levels of glucose and amino acids and promotes efficient storage and use of these fuel molecules by controlling transport of metabolites and ions across cell membranes and regulating intracellular biosynthetic pathways. It promotes entry of glucose, fatty acids, and amino acids into cells; promotes glycogen, protein, and lipid synthesis; and inhibits gluconeogenesis, glycogen degradation, protein degradation, and lipolysis. Its secretion is also influenced by gastrointestinal hormones and by autonomic nervous activity. It is formed from a single polypeptide chain *(proinsulin)* that is cleaved by proteases at two points; the end pieces *(A* and *B chains),* held together by disulfide bridges, make up insulin; the connecting *C peptide* is also secreted but has no physiologic activity. Relative insulin deficiency is the cause of most cases of diabetes mellitus. 2. a preparation of the hormone, used in the treatment of diabetes mellitus; it may be bovine or porcine in origin or a recombinant human type, although insulin preparations of bovine origin are no longer available in the United States. Types vary in rapidity of onset,

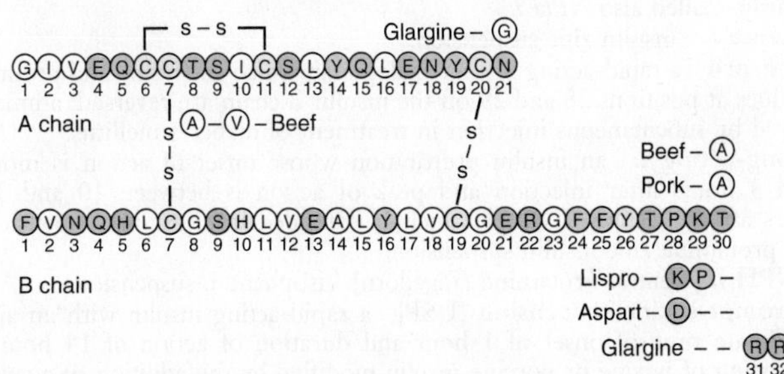

■ Primary structure of insulin. The amino acid sequences of the A and B chains of human insulin are shown and the inter- and intrachain disulfide bridges are indicated. Residues in beef and pork insulin and in several modified insulins that differ from those of unmodified human insulin are shown above or below the A and B chains. For the key to the letter codes for individual amino acids, see the illustration at *amino acid.*

duration of action, and degree of purification (most containing some proinsulin and other antigenic components). 3. [USP] a rapid-acting, unmodified form of the hormone with an approximate time of onset of 30 minutes to 1 hour and duration of action of 6 to 8 hours, prepared from crystalline bovine or porcine insulin, or both. Administered subcutaneously, intramuscularly, intravenously, or by continuous infusion pump. Called also *regular i.*

i. aspart a rapid-acting insulin analogue in which an aspartate residue has been substituted for the usual proline at position 28 on the insulin B chain; administered by subcutaneous injection in treatment of diabetes mellitus.

buffered i. human insulin human buffered with phosphate; used particularly in continuous infusion pumps, but also administered subcutaneously, intramuscularly, or intravenously.

i. detemir a long-acting insulin analogue in which the threonine at position 30 of the B insulin chain is omitted, and a 14-carbon fatty acid chain is attached to the amino acid at position B29; administered subcutaneously in the treatment of diabetes mellitus.

extended i. human zinc suspension [USP] a long-acting insulin consisting of insulin human reacted with a zinc salt to produce zinc-insulin crystals. Administered subcutaneously.

extended i. zinc suspension [USP] a long-acting insulin with time of onset about 4 to 6 hours after injection and duration of action of 36 hours, consisting of bovine or porcine insulin modified by addition of a suitable zinc salt such that the solid phase of the suspension is predominantly crystalline. Administered subcutaneously.

i. glargine an insulin analogue that differs from human insulin in that the asparagine at position A21 is replaced by glycine and two arginines are added to the C-terminus of the B-chain; administered subcutaneously for once-daily insulin replacement therapy.

i. glulisine an insulin analogue having a more rapid onset and shorter duration of action than regular human insulin, administered subcutaneously at mealtimes for the control of hyperglycemia; it is used in combination with a longer-acting insulin or insulin analogue.

i. human 1. [USP] a protein corresponding to insulin elaborated in the human pancreas, derived from pork insulin by enzymatic action that changes its amino acid sequence or produced synthetically by recombinant DNA techniques. The term may be used specifically to denote a preparation of regular insulin having the sequence of that in humans, or may be used generally to denote any insulin preparation with this sequence, including slow, intermediate, and fast-acting preparations. 2. [USP] a preparation of regular insulin in which the insulin has the same sequence as that occurring in humans. Administered subcutaneously, intramuscularly, intravenously, or by continuous infusion pump. 3. any insulin preparation with this sequence, including slow, intermediate, and fast-acting preparations.

i. human zinc suspension [USP] an intermediate-acting insulin consisting of a sterile suspension of insulin human in buffered water for injection with the addition of a suitable zinc salt such that the solid phase of the suspension contains a 7:3 ratio of crystalline to amorphous insulin. Administered subcutaneously.

intermediate-acting i. an insulin preparation whose onset of action is from 1.5 to 3.0 hours after injection and peak of action is between about 6 and 12 hours after injection. Examples include isophane insulin suspension and insulin zinc suspension.

isophane i. human suspension [USP] an intermediate-acting insulin consisting of insulin human reacted with zinc chloride and protamine sulfate such that the solid phase of the suspension consists of crystals composed of insulin, protamine, and zinc. Administered subcutaneously.

isophane i. suspension [USP] an intermediate-acting insulin with time of onset about 2 hours after injection and duration of action of 24 hours, consisting of bovine or porcine insulin reacted with zinc chloride and protamine sulfate such that the solid phase of the suspension consists of crystals composed of insulin, protamine, and zinc. Administered subcutaneously. Called also *NPH i.*

Lente i. insulin zinc suspension.

i. lispro a rapid-acting insulin analogue in which the lysine and proline residues at positions 28 and 29 on the insulin B chain are reversed; administered by subcutaneous injection in treatment of diabetes mellitus.

long-acting i. an insulin preparation whose onset of action is more than 3 hours after injection and peak of action is between 10 and 30 hours after injection. Examples include extended insulin zinc suspension and protamine zinc insulin suspension.

NPH i. [*N*eutral *P*rotamine *H*agedorn] isophane i. suspension.

prompt i. zinc suspension [USP] a rapid-acting insulin with an approximate time of onset of 1 hour and duration of action of 14 hours, consisting of bovine or porcine insulin modified by the addition of a suitable zinc salt to produce a suspension of amorphous insulin. Administered subcutaneously.

protamine zinc i. suspension a long-acting insulin with time of onset about 7 hours after injection and duration of action of 36 hours, consisting of bovine or porcine insulin reacted with zinc chloride and protamine to form a protein complex from which insulin is slowly released. It is unpredictable and is no longer used in the United States.

rapid-acting i. an insulin preparation whose onset of action is from 0.5 to 1.5 hours after injection and peak of action is about 2 to 4 hours after injection. Examples include insulin (def. 3) and prompt insulin zinc suspension. Called also *short-acting i.*

regular i. insulin (def. 3).

regular i. human insulin human (def. 2).

Semilente i. prompt insulin zinc suspension.

short-acting i. rapid-acting i.

Ultralente i. extended insulin zinc suspension.

i. zinc suspension [USP] an intermediate-acting insulin with an approximate time of onset of 2 hours and duration of action of 24 hours, consisting of a sterile suspension of insulin in buffered water for injection with the addition of a suitable zinc salt such that the solid phase of the suspension contains a 7:3 ratio of crystalline to amorphous insulin. Administered subcutaneously.

in•su•lin•emia (in″sə-lĭ-ne′me-ə) [*insulin* + *-emia*] 1. the presence of insulin in the blood. 2. hyperinsulinemia.

in•su•lin•li•po•dys•tro•phy (in″sə-lin-li″po-dis′trə-fe) the local disappearance of fat at the sites of injection in diabetic patients on insulin treatment.

in•su•lin•o•gen•e•sis (in″sə-lin-o-jen′ə-sis) the formation and release of insulin by the islets of Langerhans.

in•su•lin•o•gen•ic (in″sə-lin″o-jen′ik) 1. pertaining to or characterized by insulinogenesis. 2. promoting insulinogenesis.

in•su•lin•oid (in′sə-lin-oid″) 1. resembling insulin. 2. any substance with hypoglycemic properties like those of insulin.

in•su•li•no•ma (in″sə-lin-o′mə) an islet cell tumor of the beta cells; although usually benign, such tumors secrete excessive amounts of insulin and are among the most important causes of hypoglycemia. Called also *insuloma.*

in•su•lin•op•a•thy (in″sə-lin-op′ə-the) any defect in the genetically determined molecular structure of insulin, usually manifested as hyperinsulinemia and a mild syndrome similar to type 2 diabetes mellitus.

in•su•lino•pe•nia (in″sə-lin″o-pe′ne-ə) deficient secretion of insulin by the pancreas, resulting in hyperglycemia. Called also *hypoinsulinism.* **insulinope′nic** *adj*

in•su•li•tis (in″sə-li′tis) lymphocytic infiltration of the islets of Langerhans, suggesting an inflammatory or immunologic reaction.

in•su•lo•gen•ic (in″sə-lo-jen′ik) insulinogenic.

in•su•lo•ma (in″sə-lo′mə) insulinoma.

in•sult (in′səlt) [L. *insultus* attack] 1. injury. 2. attack.

in•sus•cep•ti•bil•i•ty (in″sə-sep″tĭ-bil′ĭ-te) the quality of not being susceptible; immunity.

in•take (in′tāk) the substances, or the quantities thereof, taken in and utilized by the body.

caloric i. the food ingested or otherwise taken into the body.

fluid i. the fluid taken into the body by drinking or parenterally.

In•tal (in′tal) trademark for a preparation of cromolyn sodium.

In•teg•ra (in-teg′rə) trademark for a type of synthetic semipermeable membrane consisting of a collagen matrix on a silicone sheet, used as a covering for burns.

in•te•gra•tion (in″tə-gra′shən) 1. coordination. 2. assimilation (def. 1). 3. anabolism. 4. the covalent insertion of one segment of DNA into another, such as the incorporation of viral or prophage DNA or a transposable element into genomic DNA.

biological i. the acquisition of functional coordination during embryonic development through humoral and nervous influences.

functional i. see *Feldenkrais method*, under *method.*

structural i. general term for systems of bodywork, derived from Rolfing, that use soft tissue manipulation to correct dysfunctional structural relationships within the body; see *Hellerwork* and *Rolfing.*

in•te•gra•tor (in′tə-gra′tər) an instrument for measuring body surfaces.

In•teg•ri•lin (in-teg′rĭ-lin) trademark for a preparation of eptifibatide.

in•teg•rin (in-teg′rin) any of a family of heterodimeric cell adhesion molecules, consisting of two noncovalently linked polypeptide chains, designated α and β, that mediate cell-to-cell and cell-to–extracellular matrix interactions.

β_1 i. any integrin containing a β_1 chain; members of this group are variously expressed on leukocytes, platelets, and some non-blood cells and mediate cell-matrix adhesion. Heterodimers of this class were first identified on T cells 2 to 4 weeks after activation in vitro and were called very late activation (VLA) antigens; the designation VLA has been continued for other proteins of this group, with numbers designating individual members.

β_2 i. any integrin containing a β_2 chain; members of this group (LFA-1, Mac-1, and p150,95) are expressed on leukocytes and mediate leukocyte adhesion and act as complement receptors; called also *leukocyte adhesion protein*.

β_3 i. any integrin containing a β_3 chain; members of this group are expressed on nonlymphoid cells and serve as receptors for fibrinogen, fibronectin, thrombospondin, von Willebrand factor, and vitronectin.

in•teg•u•ment (in-teg′u-mənt) [L. *integumentum*] 1. a covering or investment. 2. integumentum commune.

common i. integumentum commune.

in•teg•u•men•ta•ry (in-teg-u-men′tə-re) 1. pertaining to or composed of an integument such as skin. 2. serving as a covering, like the skin.

in•teg•u•men•tum (in-teg″u-men′təm) [L., from *in* on + *tegere* to cover] 1. integument; a covering or investment. 2. i. commune.

i. commu′ne [TA] common integument: the covering of the body; the skin with its various layers and appendages, including the epidermis, dermis, subcutaneous tissue, hair, nails, cutaneous glands, the breast, and mammary glands. Called also *integument, integumentum,* and *dermal* or *integumentary system*.

in te•la (in te′lə) [L.] in tissue; relating especially to stained histological preparations.

In•tel•ence (in-tel′ens) trademark for a preparation of etravirine.

in•tel•lect (in′tə-lekt) the mind, thinking faculty, or understanding.

in•tel•lec•tu•al•iza•tion (in″tə-lek″choo-əl-ĭ-za′shən) a type of defense mechanism in which reasoning is used to avoid confronting an objectionable impulse, emotional conflict, or other stressor and thus to defend against anxiety.

in•tel•li•gence (in-tel′ĭ-jəns) [L. *intelligere* to understand] the ability to acquire knowledge and use it effectively; see also under *quotient*.

artificial i. a branch of computer science in which machines are made to perform functions similar to the intellectual functions of the human mind, such as learning and reasoning.

in•tem•per•ance (in-tem′pər-əns) [L. *in* not + *temperare* to moderate] excess or lack of self-control in respect of food and drink, particularly in the use of alcoholic drinks.

in•ten•si•fi•ca•tion (in-ten″sĭ-fĭ-ka′shən) [L. *intensus* intense + *facere* to make] 1. the act of adding intensity to something. 2. the process of becoming intense.

in•ten•sio•nom•e•ter (in-ten″se-o-nom′ə-tər) an ionometric instrument for measuring the intensity of x-rays. Two series of plates, separated by an air gap that serves as the dielectric, are connected to opposite terminals in a closed chamber. An electric circuit is completed when the air becomes ionized by the x-rays, and the difference in electric potential is registered by deflection of a galvanometer needle.

in•ten•si•ty (in-ten′sĭ-te) [L. *intensus* intense] the condition or quality of having a high degree of tension, activity, or energy.

electric i. the force exerted on a unit charge at a point in an electric field. Symbol *E*. Called also *electric field strength*.

luminous i. the light-giving power of a source of light. Cf. *candle power*.

i. of x-rays the x-ray energy passing per unit time through unit area normal to the direction of propagation.

in•ten•sive (in-ten′siv) of great force or intensity; see also *intensive care unit*, under *unit*.

in•ten•siv•ist (in-ten′sĭ-vist) a physician who specializes in the provision of care in the intensive care unit.

in•ten•tion (in-ten′shən) [L. *intentio*] 1. a manner of healing; see under *healing*. 2. a goal or desired end; a term used to refer to neurogenic abnormalities that arise when a goal is consciously sought.

paradoxical i. the hypothesis that struggling against one's mental symptoms only exacerbates them whereas invoking them deliberately may do the opposite; used as a form of psychotherapy in which the behavior or feelings to be avoided are commanded to be performed or felt.

inter- [L. *inter* between] a prefix meaning between or among.

in•ter•ac•ces•so•ry (in″tər-ak-ses′ər-e) connecting the accessory processes of the vertebrae.

in•ter•ac•i•nar (in″tər-as′ĭ-nər) situated between acini.

in•ter•ac•i•nous (in″tər-as′ĭ-nəs) interacinar.

in•ter•ac•tion (in″tər-ak′shən) the quality, state, or process of (two or more things) acting on each other.

drug i. alteration of the effects of a drug by reaction with another drug or drugs, with foods or beverages, or with a preexisting medical condition.

in•ter•ac•tome (in″tər-ak′tōm) [*interaction* + *-ome*] the totality of protein–protein interactions in a cell or organism.

in•ter•al•ve•o•lar (in″tər-al-ve′ə-lər) between alveoli.

in•ter•an•gu•lar (in″tər-ang′u-lər) situated or occurring between two or more angles.

in•ter•an•nu•lar (in″tər-an′u-lər) [*inter-* + *annular*] situated between two rings or constrictions.

in•ter•ar•tic•u•lar (in″tər-ahr-tik′u-lər) [*inter-* + *articular*] situated between articular surfaces.

in•ter•ar•y•te•noid (in″tər-ar″e-te′noid) between the arytenoid cartilages.

in•ter•atri•al (in″tər-a′tre-əl) situated between the atria of the heart.

in•ter•au•ric•u•lar (in″tər-aw-rik′u-lər) 1. interatrial. 2. situated between the auricles or pinnae. 3. situated between the auricles of the heart.

in•ter•brain (in′tər-brān″) diencephalon.

in•ter•ca•lary (in-tur′kə-lar″e) intercalated.

in•ter•ca•late (in-tur′kə-lāt) [L. *intercalare*] to insert between.

in•ter•ca•lat•ed (in-tur′kə-lāt″əd) inserted or placed between; interposed.

in•ter•can•a•lic•u•lar (in″tər-kan″ə-lik′u-lər) between canaliculi.

in•ter•cap•il•lary (in″tər-kap′ĭ-lar-e) among or between capillaries.

in•ter•ca•pit•u•lar (in′tər-kə-pit′u-lər) passing between small heads; see under *vein*.

in•ter•ca•rot•ic (in″tər-kə-rot′ik) between the carotid arteries.

in•ter•ca•rot•id (in″tər-kə-rot′id) intercarotic.

in•ter•car•pal (in″tər-kahr′pəl) between the carpal bones.

in•ter•car•ti•lag•i•nous (in″tər-kahr″tĭ-laj′ĭ-nəs) connecting or situated between two or more cartilages.

in•ter•cav•er•nous (in″tər-kav′ər-nəs) between two cavities.

in•ter•cel•lu•lar (in″tər-sel′u-lər) between or among cells.

in•ter•cen•tral (in″tər-sen′trəl) situated between or connecting two or more nerve centers.

in•ter•cer•e•bral (in″tər-ser′ə-brəl) connecting or situated between the two cerebral hemispheres.

in•ter•change (in′tər-chānj″) 1. translocation (def. 3). 2. an exchange or trading.

in•ter•chon•dral (in″tər-kon′drəl) intercartilaginous.

in•ter•chro•mo•so•mal (in″tər-kro″mə-so′məl) between chromosomes.

in•ter•chro•ma•tin (in″tər-kro′mə-tin) interchromosomal.

in•ter•cil•i•um (in″tər-sil′e-əm) [*inter-* + *cilium*] the space between the eyebrows.

in•ter•cla•vic•u•lar (in″tər-klə-vik′u-lər) [*inter-* + *clavicular*] situated between the clavicles.

in•ter•cli•noid (in″tər-kli′noid) pertaining to or passing between the clinoid processes.

in•ter•coc•cyg•e•al (in″tər-kok-sij′e-əl) situated between the segments of the coccyx.

in•ter•co•lum•nar (in″tər-kə-lum′nər) [*inter-* + *column*] situated between columns or pillars.

in•ter•con•dy•lar (in″tər-kon′də-lər) between two condyles.

in•ter•con•dy•loid (in″tər-kon′də-loid) intercondylar.

in•ter•con•dy•lous (in″tər-kon′də-ləs) intercondylar.

in•ter•cos•tal (in″tər-kos′təl) [*inter-* + *costal*] situated between the ribs.

in•ter•cos•to•hu•mer•al (in″tər-kos-to-hu′mər-əl) pertaining to an intercostal space and the humerus.

in•ter•course (in′tər-kors) [L. *intercursus* running between] 1. mutual exchange. 2. sexual i.

sexual i. 1. coitus. 2. any physical contact between two individuals involving stimulation of the genital organs of at least one.

in•ter•cri•co•thy•rot•o•my (in″tər-kri″ko-thi-rot′o-me) cricothyrotomy.

in•ter•cris•tal (in″tər-kris′təl) between two crests.

in•ter•crit•i•cal (in″tər-krit′ĭ-kəl) denoting the period between attacks, as of gout.

in•ter•cross (in′tər-kros) [*inter-* + *cross* (def. 2)] the mating of heterozygotes; cf. *incross*.

in•ter•cru•ral (in″tər-kroo′rəl) between two crura.

in•ter•cur•rent (in″tər-kur′ənt) breaking into and modifying the course of an already existing disease.

in·ter·cus·pa·tion (in″tər-kəs-pa′shən) the fitting together of cusps of opposing teeth in occlusion; the cusp-to-fossa relationship of the upper and lower posterior teeth to each other.

in·ter·cusp·ing (in″tər-kusp′ing) the occlusion of the cusps of the teeth of one jaw with the depressions in the teeth of the other jaw.

in·ter·def·er·en·tial (in″tər-def″ər-en′shəl) between the two ductus deferentes.

in·ter·den·tal (in″tər-den′təl) [*inter-* + *dental*] situated between the proximal surfaces of adjacent teeth in the same dental arch. See also *interocclusal* and *interproximal.*

in·ter·den·ta·le (in″tər-dən-ta′le) a craniometric landmark located between the right and left central incisors, in the midline on the tip of the alveolar septum.

in·ter·den·ti·um (in″tər-den′she-əm) the interproximal space; see under *space.*

in·ter·dia·lyt·ic (in″tər-di″ə-lit′ik) pertaining to the time between hemodialysis treatments.

in·ter·di·ges·tive (in″tər-di-jes′tiv) between two times of digestion.

in·ter·dig·it (in″tər-dij′it) the space between two contiguous fingers or toes.

in·ter·dig·i·tal (in″tər-dij′ĭ-təl) [*inter-* + *digital*] between two fingers or toes.

in·ter·dig·i·tate (in″tər-dij′ĭ-tāt) [*inter-* + *digitate*] to interlock and interrelate, as the fingers of clasped hands.

in·ter·dig·i·ta·tion (in″tər-dij″ĭ-ta′shən) [*inter-* + *digitation*] 1. an interlocking of parts by fingerlike processes. 2. any one of a set of fingerlike processes.

in·ter·do·mal (in″tər-do′məl) between the nasal domes over the two major alar cartilages.

in·ter·face (in′tər-fās″) in chemistry, the surface of separation or boundary between two phases of a heterogeneous system. **interfa′cial** *adj*

dineric i. the interface between two immiscible liquids.

in·ter·fas·cic·u·lar (in″tər-fə-sik′u-lər) [*inter-* + *fascicular*] situated between fasciculi.

in·ter·fem·o·ral (in″tər-fem′o-rəl) between the thighs.

in·ter·fer·ence (in″tər-fēr′əns) [*inter-* + L. *ferire* to strike] 1. opposition to or hampering of an action or procedure. 2. the process in which two or more light, sound, or electromagnetic waves of the same frequency combine to reinforce or cancel each other, the amplitude of the resulting wave being equal to the sum of the amplitudes of the combining waves. 3. impairment of cardiac impulse conduction due to refractoriness of the tissue where the refractoriness is a physiological response to passage of a preceding impulse. See also *interference dissociation*, under *dissociation.* 4. any premature contact point along the occlusal surface of the teeth that prevents maximum contact, function, and proper alignment in full occlusion. See also *deflective occlusal contact*, under *contact.*

cuspal i. deflective occlusal contact.

occlusal i's areas of interference on teeth that hamper smooth, gliding, harmonious jaw movements with the teeth maintaining contact.

proactive i. see under *inhibition.*

retroactive i. see under *inhibition.*

RNA i. (RNAi) a mechanism of posttranscriptional gene silencing in which RNA-induced silencing complexes bind to complementary messenger RNA sequences and induce degradation.

in·ter·fer·ing (in″tər-fēr′ing) the striking or rubbing of the fetlock of a horse by the opposite foot during locomotion.

in·ter·fe·rom·e·ter (in″tər-fēr-om′ə-tər) an instrument for measuring lengths or movements by means of the phenomena caused by the interference of two rays of light, or of sound (acoustic i.).

in·ter·fe·rom·e·try (in″tər-fēr-om′ə-tre) the use of the interferometer for measuring distances or movements.

in·ter·fer·on (in″tər-fēr′on) any of a family of glycoproteins that exert virus-nonspecific but host-specific antiviral activity by inducing the transcription of cellular genes coding for antiviral proteins that selectively inhibit the synthesis of viral RNA and proteins. Interferons also have immunoregulatory functions (inhibition of B cell activation and antibody production enhancement of T cell activity, and enhancement of NK cell cytotoxic activity) and can inhibit the growth of nonviral intracellular parasites. Production of interferon can be stimulated by viral infection, especially by the presence of double-stranded RNA, by intracellular parasites (chlamydiae, rickettsiae), by protozoa *(Toxoplasma)*, and by bacteria (streptococci, staphylococci) and bacterial products (endotoxins). Interferons have been divided into three distinct types (α, β, and γ) associated with specific producer cells and functions, but all animal cells are able to produce interferons, and certain producer cells (leukocytes and fibroblasts) produce more than one type (both interferon-α and interferon-β). Abbreviated IFN.

i.-α (IFN-α) the major interferon produced by virus-induced leukocyte cultures; the primary producer cells are null lymphocytes, and the major activities are antiviral activity and activation of NK cells. It is used in the experimental treatment of hairy cell leukemia and other selected neoplasias. Called also *leukocyte i.*

i.-alfa i.-α.

i. alfa-2a a synthetic form of interferon-α produced by recombinant technology that acts as a biological response modifier, used as an antineoplastic in the treatment of hairy cell leukemia and AIDS-related Kaposi sarcoma; administered intramuscularly or subcutaneously.

i. alfa-2b a synthetic form of interferon-α produced by recombinant technology that acts as a biologic response modifier, used in the treatment of condylomata acuminata, hepatitis B, and chronic hepatitis C and as an antineoplastic in the treatment of hairy cell leukemia, AIDS-related Kaposi sarcoma, and other neoplasms; administered intramuscularly, subcutaneously, or intralesionally.

i. alfacon-1 a synthetic interferon produced by recombinant DNA technology, consisting of 166 amino acids whose sequence was derived by comparing the sequences of several naturally occurring interferon subtypes and assigning the most commonly occurring amino acid at each position, with changes in four amino acids being made to facilitate construction of the molecule; used in the treatment of chronic hepatitis C virus infection, administered subcutaneously.

i. alfa-n3 a highly purified mixture of natural human interferon proteins, manufactured from pooled human leukocytes that have been induced to produce interferon alfa-n3, that acts as a biologic response modifier; used in the treatment of condylomata acuminata, administered intralesionally.

i.-β (IFN-β) the major interferon produced by double-stranded RNA–induced fibroblast cultures; the primary producer cells are fibroblasts, epithelial cells, and macrophages, and the major activity is antiviral activity. Called also *epithelial, fibroblast,* or *fibroepithelial i.*

i. beta-1a a synthetic form of interferon-β produced by recombinant DNA techniques that acts as a biologic response modifier; used in the treatment of relapsing forms of multiple sclerosis; administered intramuscularly.

i. beta-1b a synthetic modified form of interferon-β produced by recombinant DNA techniques, having 165 amino acids, substituting serine for cysteine at position 17, and lacking the carbohydrate side chains of the natural form. It has both antiviral and immunoregulatory properties and is used as a biologic response modifier in the treatment of relapsing forms of multiple sclerosis; administered subcutaneously.

i. beta-2 former name for *interleukin-6.*

consensus i. i. alfacon-1.

epithelial i., fibroblast i., fibroepithelial i. i.-β.

i.-γ (IFN-γ) the major interferon produced by lymphocyte cultures immunologically stimulated by mitogens or antigens; the primary producer cells are T lymphocytes, and the major activity is immunoregulation. IFN-γ has been implicated in aberrant expression of class II histocompatibility antigens by tissue cells (such as thyroid cells) that do not normally express them, leading to autoimmune disease. Called also *immune i.*

i. gamma-1b a synthetic form of interferon-γ produced by recombinant technology that acts as a biologic response modifier; used to enhance phagocytic function in order to reduce the frequency and severity of serious infections associated with chronic granulomatous disease, administered subcutaneously. Also used in the treatment of renal cell carcinoma and severe congenital osteopetrosis.

immune i. i.-γ.

leukocyte i. i.-α.

type I i. i.-α and i.-β.

type II i. i.-γ.

in·ter·fi·bril·lar (in″tər-fi′bril-ər) between or among fibrils.

in·ter·fi·bril·lary (in″tər-fi′brĭ-lar″e) interfibrillar.

in·ter·fi·brous (in″tər-fi′brəs) between fibers.

in·ter·fil·a·men·tous (in″tər-fil″ə-men′təs) between filaments.

in·ter·fi·lar (in″tər-fi′lər) [*inter-* + *filar*] between or among the fibrils of a reticulum.

in·ter·fron·tal (in″tər-fron′təl) between the halves of the frontal bone.

in·ter·fur·ca (in″tər-fur′kə) pl. *interfur′cae* [*inter-* + L. *furca* fork] the area lying between and at the base of divided tooth roots.

in·ter·fur·cae (in″tər-fur′se) [L.] plural of *interfurca.*

in·ter·gan·gli·on·ic (in″tər-gang″gle-on′ik) between ganglia.

in·ter·gem·mal (in″tər-jem′əl) between taste buds or other buds.

in·ter·glob·u·lar (in″tər-glob′u-lər) [*inter-* + *globular*] between or among globules, as of the dentin.

in·ter·glu·te·al (in″tər-gloo′te-əl) between the buttocks. Called also *internatal.*

in·ter·go·ni·al (in″tər-go′ne-əl) between the tips of the two angles of the mandible.

in·ter·gran·u·lar (in″tər-gran′u-lər) between the granule cells of the brain.

in·ter·gy·ral (in″tər-ji′rəl) between cerebral gyri or convolutions.

in·ter·hemi·cer·e·bral (in″tər-hem″e-ser′ə-brəl) intercerebral.

in·ter·hemi·sphe·ric (in″tər-hem″ĭ-sfēr′ik) intercerebral.

in·ter·ic·tal (in″tər-ik′təl) occurring between attacks or paroxysms; called also *interparoxysmal.*

in·te·ri·or (in-tēr′e-ər) [L. "inner"; neut. *interius*] 1. situated inside; inward. 2. an inner part or cavity.

in·ter·is·chi·ad·ic (in″tər-is″ke-ad′ik) between the two ischia.

in·ter·ki·ne·sis (in″tər-kĭ-ne′sis) [*inter-* + Gr. *kinēsis* motion] a period intervening between meiosis I and meiosis II, similar to interphase in mitosis but without DNA replication.

in·ter·la·bi·al (in″tər-la′be-əl) [*inter-* + *labial*] between the lips, or between any two labia.

in·ter·la·mel·lar (in″tər-lə-mel′ər) between lamellae.

in·ter·leu·kin (in′tər-loo″kin) [*inter-* + *leukocyte*] a generic term for a group of multifunctional cytokines that are produced by a variety of lymphoid and nonlymphoid cells and have effects at least partly within the lymphopoietic system; originally believed to be produced chiefly by and to act chiefly upon leukocytes.

i.-1 (IL-1) a predominately macrophage-produced interleukin that mediates the host inflammatory response in innate immunity; two principal forms exist, designated α and β, with apparently identical biological activity. At low concentrations, IL-1 principally acts to mediate local inflammation, causing mononuclear phagocytes and endothelial cells to synthesize leukocyte-activating chemokines; at high concentrations IL-1 enters the blood stream and acts as an endocrine hormone, in some actions resembling tumor necrosis factor by its ability to cause fever, initiate hepatic synthesis of acute phase proteins, and induce cachexia.

i.-2 (IL-2) an interleukin produced by T cells in response to antigenic or mitogenic stimulation, acting to regulate the immune response. It stimulates the proliferation of T cells and the synthesis of other T cell–derived cytokines, stimulates the growth and cytolytic function of NK cells to produce lymphokine-activated killer cells, is a growth factor for and stimulates antibody synthesis in B cells, and may promote apoptosis in antigen-activated T cells. IL-2 is used as an anticancer drug in the treatment of a wide variety of solid malignant tumors. Formerly called *T-cell growth factor.*

i.-3 (IL-3) a lymphokine produced by antigen- or mitogen-activated T lymphocytes, which stimulates proliferation of hematopoietic as well as lymphoid stem cells; a colony-stimulating factor for all bone marrow progenitor cells. IL-3 supports the growth and differentiation of early hematopoietic and lymphoid stem cells as well as that of more mature hematopoietic cells, including granulocytes, macrophages, and mast cells.

i.-4 (IL-4) a lymphokine produced by antigen- or mitogen-activated T cells; its principal role is regulation of IgE- and eosinophil-mediated immune reactions. It stimulates switching of B cells for production of IgE, is a growth and differentiation factor for T cells, particularly T_H2 cells, is a growth factor for mast cells, and stimulates the expression of some adhesion molecules on endothelial cells. Formerly called *B lymphocyte stimulatory factor 1.*

i.-5 (IL-5) a lymphokine produced by antigen- or mitogen-activated T cells and by activated mast cells that stimulates the growth and differentiation of eosinophils and activates mature eosinophils to kill helminths. It may act as a cofactor in the growth and differentiation of B cells and may also be involved in increasing synthesis of IgA by mature B cells.

i.-6 (IL-6) a lymphokine produced by antigen- or mitogen-activated T cells, fibroblasts, macrophages, and adipose and other cells that serves as a differentiation factor for B cells and thymocytes and stimulates immunoglobulin production by B cells; it also induces hepatocytes to synthesize various plasma proteins involved in the acute phase response and is a cofactor in initiation of the cell cycle in primitive hematopoietic cells in vitro.

i.-7 (IL-7) an interleukin produced by epithelial and mesangial stromal cells that serves as a differentiation factor for B cells in the early stages of their development and also supports the growth of some thymocytes and T lymphocytes.

i.-8 (IL-8) a chemokine produced by monocytes, endothelial cells, and other cells that acts as a chemotactic and activator for neutrophils and may play a role in the extravasation of neutrophils in inflammation.

i.-9 (IL-9) a cytokine produced by T cells and macrophages that acts as a growth factor for some T cell populations and bone marrow–mast cell progenitors.

i.-10 (IL-10) a cytokine produced by activated macrophages, certain lymphocytes, and other cells that decreases both innate and T cell–mediated immune inflammation; it inhibits the production of cytokines by activated T cells, plays a role in B cell activation, inhibits production of interferon-γ, and blocks antigen presentation and macrophage formation of IL-1, IL-6, and tumor necrosis factor.

i.-11 (IL-11) a cytokine produced by bone marrow stromal cells that stimulates megakaryocyte proliferation and B cell differentiation.

i.-12 (IL-12) a heterodimeric cytokine produced by phagocytic cells, B cells, and other antigen-presenting cell types; it is a potent inducer of cytokine production, causes T and NK cells to secrete interferon-γ, is a growth factor for preactivated T and NK cells, and enhances cytotoxic activity in $CD8^+$ T cells and NK cells. It also has a role in the generation of T-helper type 1 cells and in the differentiation of cytotoxic T lymphocytes.

i.-13 (IL-13) a cytokine produced by activated T lymphocytes that has structural and functional similarities to IL-4; it inhibits inflammatory cytokine production by lipopolysaccharide in human peripheral blood monocytes and may be involved in promoting B cell division.

i.-14 (IL-14) a cytokine produced by T lymphocytes and malignant B lymphocytes that induces B cell proliferation and inhibits immunoglobulin secretion.

i.-15 (IL-15) a cytokine released by mononuclear phagocytes and some tissue cells in response to events triggering innate immunity, such as viral infection; its primary function appears to be promotion of NK cell proliferation.

in·ter·lig·a·men·ta·ry (in″tər-lig″ə-men′tə-re) between or among ligaments.

in·ter·lig·a·men·tous (in″tər-lig″ə-men′təs) interligamentary.

in·ter·lo·bar (in″tər-lo′bər) [*inter-* + *lobar*] situated or occurring between lobes.

in·ter·lo·bi·tis (in″tər-lo-bi′tis) interlobular pleurisy.

in·ter·lob·u·lar (in″tər-lob′u-lər) [*inter-* + *lobular*] situated or occurring between lobules.

in·ter·lock·ing (in″tər-lok′ing) 1. closely joined, as by hooks or dovetails; locking into one another. 2. a complication of labor in twin births in which the inferior surface of the chin of one twin is hooked to that of its co-twin above or below the pelvic inlet. When this condition occurs in the true pelvis, it is called *compaction.*

in·ter·mal·le·o·lar (in″tər-mə-le′o-lər) between the malleoli.

in·ter·mam·ma·ry (in″tər-mam′ə-re) between the breasts.

in·ter·mam·mil·lary (in″tər-mam′ĭ-lar″e) between the nipples.

in·ter·mar·riage (in″tər-mar′əj) [*inter-* + L. *maritare* to wed] the marriage of persons related by blood or consanguinity.

in·ter·max·il·lary (in″tər-mak′sĭ-lar″e) situated between the two maxillae.

in·ter·me·di·ary (in″tər-me′de-ar″e) [*inter-* + L. *medius* middle] 1. performed or occurring in a median stage; neither early nor late; intermediate. 2. an intermediate stage.

in·ter·me·di·ate (in″tər-me′de-ət) [*inter-* + L. *medius* middle] 1. placed between; see *medial* and *median.* 2. resembling, in part, each of two extremes. 3. a substance formed in a chemical process that is essential to the formation of the end product of the process.

in·ter·me·din (in″tər-me′din) melanocyte-stimulating hormone.

in·ter·me·dio·lat·er·al (in″tər-me″de-o-lat′ər-əl) both intermediate and lateral.

in·ter·me·di·us (in″tər-me′de-əs) [TA] intermediate: a term denoting the middle of three structures, one of which is situated closer to and the other farther from the median plane of the body or part.

in·ter·mem·bra·nous (in″tər-mem′brə-nəs) situated or occurring between membranes.

in·ter·me·nin·ge·al (in″tər-mə-nin′je-əl) situated or occurring between the meninges.

in·ter·men·stru·al (in″tər-men′stroo-əl) [*inter-* + *menstrual*] occurring between the menstrual periods.

in·ter·men·stru·um (in″tər-men′stroo-əm) the interval between two menstrual periods.

in·ter·meta·car·pal (in″tər-met″ə-kahr′pəl) [*inter-* + *metacarpal*] situated between the metacarpal bones.

in·ter·meta·mer·ic (in″tər-met″ə-mer′ik) between two metameres.

in·ter·meta·tar·sal (in″tər-met″ə-tahr′səl) situated or occurring between the metatarsal bones.

in·ter·mis·sion (in″tər-mish′ən) [L. *intermissio*] an interval; a period of temporary cessation, as between two occurrences or paroxysms.

in·ter·mi·tot·ic (in″tər-mi-tot′ik) pertaining to or occurring during the interval between successive mitoses.

in·ter·mit·tent (in″tər-mit′ənt) [L. *intermittens*] occurring at separated intervals; having periods of cessation of activity.

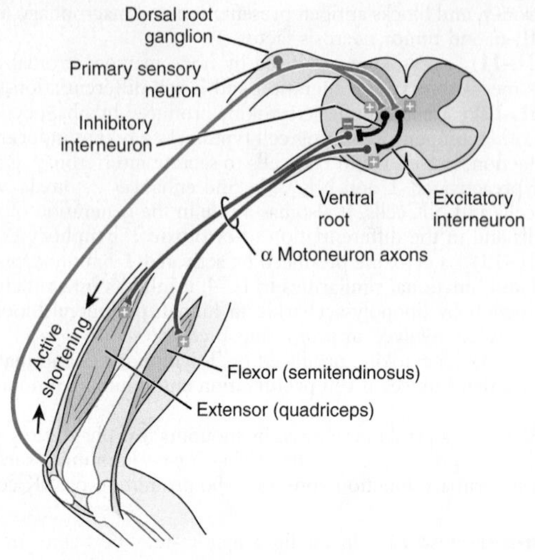

■ Excitatory and inhibitory interneurons in three-neuron reflex arcs of the quadriceps and semitendinosus muscles of the thigh.

in•ter•mo•lec•u•lar (in″tər-mo-lek′u-lər) between molecules.

in•ter•mu•ral (in-tər-mu′rəl) between the walls of organs.

in•ter•mus•cu•lar (in″tər-mus′ku-lər) situated between muscles.

in•tern[1] (in′tərn) [Fr. *interne*, internal] a graduate of a medical or dental school serving in a hospital preparatory to being licensed to practice medicine or dentistry. Cf. *resident.*

in•tern[2] (in-turn′) to confine within certain geographical or physical boundaries.

in•ter•nal (in-tur′nəl) [L. *internus*] situated or occurring within or on the inside; many anatomical structures formerly called internal are now correctly termed medial.

in•ter•nal•iza•tion (in-tur″nəl-ĭ-za′shən) the mental process whereby certain attributes, attitudes, or standards of others are unconsciously taken as one's own.

in•ter•nar•i•al (in″tər-nar′e-əl) between the nostrils.

in•ter•na•sal (in″tər-na′zəl) situated between the nasal bones.

in•ter•na•tal (in″tər-na′təl) intergluteal.

In•ter•na•tion•al Non•pro•pri•e•tary Name see *INN.*

in•terne (ă-tern′) [Fr.] intern.

in•ter•neu•ron (in″tər-noor′on) 1. any neuron in a chain of neurons that is situated between a primary sensory neuron and the final motoneuron. 2. any neuron whose processes are entirely confined within a specific area, as within the olfactory lobe, and which synapse with neurons extending into that area. Called also *intercalary, intercalated,* or *internuncial neuron.*

in•tern•ist (in-tur′nist) a physician who specializes in the diagnosis and medical, as opposed to surgical and obstetrical, treatment of diseases of adults.

in•ter•no•dal (in″tər-no′dəl) between two nodes.

in•ter•node (in′tər-nōd) [*inter-* + *node*] internodal segment.
 i. of Ranvier internodal segment.

in•ter•nod•u•lar (in″tər-nod′u-lər) between two nodules.

in•tern•ship (in′tərn-ship) the position or term of service of an intern in a hospital.

in•ter•nu•cle•ar (in″tər-noo′kle-ər) 1. pertaining to or affecting structures between nuclei, as internuclear ophthalmoplegia. 2. between the nuclear layers of the retina.

in•ter•nun•ci•al (in″tər-nun′she-əl) [L. *internuncius* a go-between] serving as a medium of communication between nerve cell bodies or neurons; see *interneuron.*

in•ter•nus (in-tur′nəs) [TA] internal: anatomical terminology denoting something situated nearer to the center of an organ or a cavity.

in•ter•oc•clu•sal (in″tər-o-kloo′zəl) situated between the occlusal surfaces of opposing teeth of the mandibular and maxillary arches. See also *interdental* and *interproximal.*

in•tero•cep•tion (in″tər-o-sep′shən) the perceiving of stimuli within the viscera by interoceptors.

in•tero•cep•tive (in″tər-o-sep′tiv) 1. pertaining to interoceptors. 2. pertaining to interoception.

in•tero•cep•tor (in″tər-o-sep′tər) any of the sensory nerve terminals that are located in and transmit impulses from the viscera; see *receptor* (def. 3), *exteroceptor,* and *proprioceptor.*

in•ter•oc•u•lar (in″tər-ok′u-lər) between the eyes.

in•tero•in•fe•ri•or•ly (in″tər-o-in-fēr′e-ər-le) inwardly and in a downward position or direction.

in•ter•ol•i•vary (in″tər-ol′ĭ-var″e) situated between the olivary bodies of the brain.

in•ter•or•bi•tal (in″tər-or′bĭ-təl) between the orbits.

in•ter•os•se•al (in″tər-os′e-əl) [*inter-* + *osse-* + *-al*[1]] 1. interosseous. 2. pertaining to the interossei muscles.

in•ter•os•se•ous (in″tər-os′e-əs) [L. *interosseus; inter* between + *os* bone] between bones; called also *interosseal.*

in•ter•pal•pe•bral (in″tər-pal′pə-brəl) between the eyelids.

in•ter•pa•ri•e•tal (in″tər-pə-ri′ə-təl) [*inter-* + *parietal*] 1. intermural. 2. situated between the parietal bones.

in•ter•par•ox•ys•mal (in″tər-par″ok-siz′məl) interictal.

in•ter•pe•dic•u•late (in″tər-pə-dik′u-lāt) between the pedicles of a vertebra, as interpediculate distance.

in•ter•pe•dun•cu•lar (in″tər-pə-dunk′u-lər) [*inter-* + *peduncular*] situated between two peduncles, as between two cerebellar peduncles.

in•ter•pha•lan•ge•al (in″tər-fə-lan′je-əl) [*inter-* + *phalangeal*] situated between two contiguous phalanges.

in•ter•phase (in′tər-fāz) the portion of the cell cycle between two successive cell divisions, during which normal cellular metabolism occurs and DNA is synthesized; chromosomes are not individually distinguishable but occupy chromosomal territories. It is divided into three phases: G_1, S, and G_2.

in•ter•pi•al (in″tər-pi′əl) situated between the two layers of the pia mater.

in•ter•plant (in′tər-plant) [*inter-* + L. *plantare* to set] an embryonic part isolated by transference to an indifferent environment provided by another embryo.

in•ter•pleu•ral (in″tər-ploor′əl) between two layers of the pleura.

in•ter•po•lar (in″tər-po′lər) [*inter-* + *polar*] situated between two poles.

in•ter•po•lat•ed (in-tur′po-la″təd) inserted between other elements or parts.

in•ter•po•la•tion (in-tur″po-la′shən) the determination of intermediate values in a series on the basis of observed values.

in•ter•po•si•tion (in″tər-pə-zish′ən) 1. the act of placing between; the condition of being interposed. 2. interposition graft.
 colonic i. an interposition graft of a section of colon to replace a section of esophagus that has been removed in cancer surgery.
 free jejunal i. an interposition graft of a section of jejunum to replace a section of esophagus that has been removed in cancer surgery.

in•ter•pos•i•tum (in″tər-poz′ĭ-təm) [L.] interposed; see under *velum.*

in•ter•pre•ta•tion (in-tur″prə-ta′shən) in psychotherapy, the therapist's explanation of the latent or hidden meanings of what the patient says, does, or experiences, in terms which are understandable to him.

in•ter•pro•to•met•a•mere (in″tər-pro″to-met′ə-mēr) [*inter-* + *proto* + *meta-* + *-mere*] the structure between the primary segments of the embryo.

in•ter•prox•i•mal (in″tər-prok′sĭ-məl) between adjoining surfaces, as the space between adjacent teeth. See also *interdental* and *interocclusal.*

in•ter•pu•bic (in″tər-pu′bik) [*inter-* + *pubic*] between the pubic bones.

in•ter•pu•pil•lary (in″tər-pu′pĭ-lar″e) between the pupils.

in•ter•ra•di•al (in″tə-ra′de-əl) situated between rays.

in•ter•ra•dic•u•lar (in″tər-rə-dik′u-lər) between or among roots or radicles.

in•ter•re•nal (in″tər-re′nəl) [*inter-* + *renal*] between the kidneys.

in•ter•re•nic•u•lar (in″tə-rə-nik′u-lər) interrenuncular.

in•ter•re•nunc•u•lar (in″tə-rə-nung′ku-lər) between two renal lobes.

in•ter•rupt•ed (in″tə-rup′təd) [L. *interruptus*] not continuous; marked by intermissions or breaches of continuity.

in•ter•rup•tion (in″tər-rup′shən) an interference or blocking.
 vena caval i. interference with free flow of blood through the inferior vena cava by means of a filter to trap emboli and prevent pulmonary embolism; see also *vena cava filter,* under *filter.*

in•ter•scap•u•lar (in″tər-skap′u lər) between the scapulae.

in·ter·scap·u·lum (in″tər-skap′u-ləm) the space between the scapulae.

in·ter·sci·at·ic (in″tər-si-at′ik) between the two ischia.

in·ter·sec·tio (in″tər-sek′she-o) pl. *intersectio′nes* [L., from *inter* between + *secare* to cut] 1. a cutting across or between. 2. a site at which one structure cuts across another.

i. tendi′nea [TA] tendinous intersection: a fibrous band that crosses the belly of a muscle and more or less completely divides it into two parts; called also *inscriptio tendinea.*

i.′nes tendi′neae mus′culi rec′ti abdo′minis [TA] tendinous intersections of rectus abdominis muscle: three or more fibrous bands that cross the front of the rectus abdominis muscle, fusing with the anterior layer of its sheath; called also *inscriptiones tendineae musculi recti abdominis.*

in·ter·sec·tion (in″tər-sek′shən) a site at which one structure cuts across another.

tendinous i. intersectio tendinea.

in·ter·sec·ti·o·nes (in″tər-sek″she-o′nēz) [L.] plural of *intersectio.*

in·ter·seg·ment (in″tər-seg′mənt) 1. any one of a series of segments, like the angiotomes, etc. 2. a metamere.

in·ter·seg·men·tal (in″tər-seg-men′təl) between segments.

in·ter·sep·tal (in″tər-sep′təl) between two septa.

in·ter·sep·tum (in″tər-sep′təm) [L.] the diaphragm.

in·ter·sex (in′tər-seks) 1. hermaphrodite. 2. pseudohermaphrodite. 3. androgyne.

female i. female pseudohermaphrodite.

male i. male pseudohermaphrodite.

true i. true hermaphrodite.

in·ter·sex·u·al (in″tər-sek′shoo-əl) 1. hermaphroditic. 2. androgynous.

in·ter·sex·u·al·i·ty (in″tər-sek″shoo-al′ĭ-te) 1. hermaphroditism. 2. pseudohermaphroditism. 3. androgyny.

in·ter·space (in′tər-spās) a space between two similar structures.

dineric i. the surface between two liquid phases.

in·ter·sphinc·ter·ic (in″tər-sfingk-ter′ik) between the internal and external anal sphincters.

in·ter·spi·nal (in″tər-spi′nəl) between two spinous processes.

in·ter·spi·nous (in″tər-spi′nəs) interspinal.

in·ter·ster·nal (in″tər-stur′nəl) between parts of the sternum.

in·ter·stice (in-tur′stis) [L. *interstitium*] a small interval, space, or gap in a tissue or structure.

in·ter·sti·tial (in″tər-stish′əl) pertaining to or situated between parts or in the interstices of a tissue.

in·ter·sti·ti·um (in″tər-stish′e-əm) [L.] 1. interstice. 2. stroma.

in·ter·tar·sal (in″tər-tahr′səl) situated between the tarsal bones.

in·ter·tha·lam·ic (in″tər-thə-lam′ik) between thalami, particularly the optic thalami.

in·ter·trans·verse (in″tər-trans-vərs′) [*inter-* + *transverse*] situated between or connecting the transverse processes of the vertebrae.

in·ter·tri·go (in″tər-tri′go) [*inter-* + L. *terere* to rub] a superficial dermatitis occurring on apposed skin surfaces, such as in the axillae or groin, beneath pendulous breasts, or in skin furrows. It is caused by moisture, friction, warmth, and sweat retention, and obesity is a predisposing factor. Characteristics include erythema, maceration, burning, itching, and sometimes erosions, fissures, exudations, and secondary infections. Called also *eczema intertrigo.* **intertrig′inous** *adj*

i. labia′lis perlèche.

in·ter·tro·chan·ter·ic (in″tər-tro″kan-ter′ik) [*inter-* + *trochanter*] situated in or pertaining to the space between the greater and the lesser trochanter.

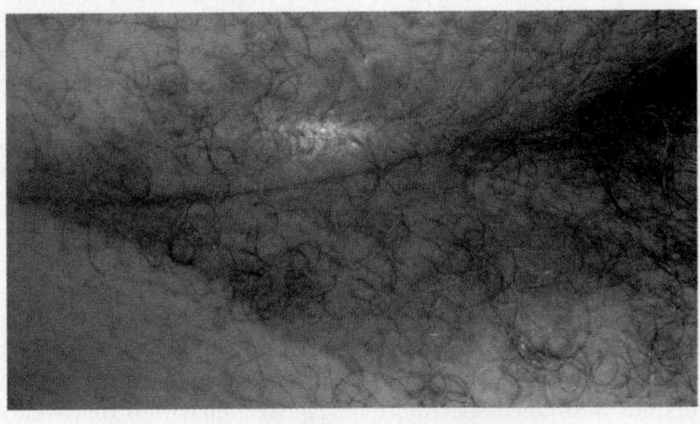

■ Intertrigo.

in·ter·tu·ber·cu·lar (in″tər-too-bur′ku-lər) between tubercles.

in·ter·tu·bu·lar (in″tər-too′bu-lər) between or among tubules.

in·ter·ure·ter·al (in″tər-u-re′tər-əl) interureteric.

in·ter·ure·ter·ic (in″tər-u″rə-ter′ik) between the ureters.

in·ter·vag·i·nal (in″tər-vaj′ĭ-nəl) situated between sheaths.

in·ter·val (in′tər-vəl) [*inter-* + L. *vallum* rampart] the space between two objects or parts; the lapse of time between two recurrences or paroxysms.

A–H i. the period between the onset of depolarization of the lower right atrium, measured as the A wave, and that of the bundle of His, measured as the His bundle deflection; approximates the time for impulse conduction across the atrioventricular node.

atrioventricular i., AV i. the time between the start of atrial and the start of ventricular systole; it is equivalent to the P–R interval of electrocardiography. Called also *atrioventricular delay.*

cardioarterial i. the time between the apex beat and arterial pulsation; it measures the rate of propagation of the pulse wave.

confidence i. a type of statistical interval estimate for an unknown parameter: a range of values believed to contain the parameter, with a predetermined degree of confidence. Its endpoints are the *confidence limits* and it has a stated probability (the *confidence coefficient*) of containing the parameter.

conservative confidence i. a confidence interval having a confidence coefficient at least as great as a stated nominal value.

coupling i. the length of time between an ectopic beat and the sinus beat preceding it; in an arrhythmia characterized by such beats, the intervals may be constant *(fixed coupling intervals)* or inconstant *(variable coupling intervals).*

escape i. the interval between an escape beat and the normal beat preceding it.

focal i. the distance from the anterior to the posterior focal point; called also *Sturm i.*

H–V i. the period between the onset of depolarization of the bundle of His, the H deflection in a His bundle electrogram, and the onset of ventricular activity, measured by surface or intracardiac leads; it approximates the time for conduction through the His-Purkinje system.

interdischarge i. the time between two discharges of the action potential of a single muscle fiber.

interpotential i. the length of time between discharges of action potentials of two different fibers from the same motor unit.

lucid i. 1. a brief period of remission of symptoms in a psychosis. 2. a brief return to consciousness after loss of consciousness in head injury.

P–A i. the period from the onset of atrial activity, measured as the P wave in an electrocardiogram, and the onset of activity of the lower right atrial septum, measured as the A wave in a His bundle electrogram; it approximates the time for intra-atrial impulse conduction.

pacemaker escape i. the period between the last sensed spontaneous cardiac activity and the first beat stimulated by the pacemaker.

P–P i. in electrocardiography, the time from the beginning of one P wave to that of the next P wave; it is the length of the cardiac cycle. See also illustration at *electrocardiogram.*

PQ i. P–R i.

P–R i. the portion of the electrocardiogram between the onset of the P wave (atrial depolarization) and the onset of the QRS complex (ventricular depolarization), lasting approximately 0.12 to 0.20 second in the adult. It is the time taken for an impulse to traverse the atrioventricular node, bundle of His, and bundle branches. See also illustration at *electrocardiogram.*

QRS i. in electrocardiography, the interval from the beginning of the Q wave to the termination of the S wave, representing the time for ventricular depolarization. See also illustration at *electrocardiogram.*

QRST i., Q–T i. in electrocardiography, the time from the beginning of the Q wave to the end of the T wave; it represents the duration of ventricular electrical activity. See also illustration at *electrocardiogram.*

Q–Tc i. the Q–T interval corrected for heart rate; see *Bazett formula,* under *formula.*

recruitment i. the inverse of the recruitment frequency; in a recruitment pattern, the length of time between two consecutive discharges of a given motor unit when an additional motor unit is recruited.

reference i. see under *value.*

ST i. the portion of the electrocardiogram from the end of the S wave to the end of the T wave, comprising the ST segment and the T wave.

Sturm i. focal i.

systolic time i's (STI) any of several intervals measured for assessing left ventricular performance, particularly left ventricular ejection time (LVET), electromechanical systole (QS_2), and preejection period (PEP); electrocardiography, phonocardiography, and carotid pulse tracings are used to determine LVET and QS_2, and from them, PEP. See also individual intervals.

V–A i. the time between a ventricular stimulus and the atrial stimulus following it.

in·ter·val·vu·lar (in″tər-val′vu-lər) between valves.

in·ter·vas·cu·lar (in″tər-vas′ku-lər) between blood vessels.

in·ter·ve·nous (in″tər-ve′nəs) between veins.

in·ter·ven·tion (in″tər-ven′shən) [L. *intervenire* to come between] 1. the act or fact of interfering so as to modify. 2. specifically, any measure whose purpose is to improve health or to alter the course of a disease.

crisis i. 1. an immediate, short-term, psychotherapeutic approach, the goal of which is to help resolve a personal crisis within the individual's immediate environment. 2. the procedures involved in responding to an emergency.

percutaneous coronary i. (PCI) the management of coronary artery occlusion (q.v.) by any of various catheter-based techniques, such as percutaneous transluminal coronary angioplasty, rotational atherectomy, directional atherectomy, transluminal endarterectomy, angioplasty using the excimer laser, or implantation of coronary stents or similar devices.

in·ter·ven·tric·u·lar (in″tər-vən-trik′u-lər) between ventricles.

in·ter·ver·te·bral (in″tər-vur′tə-brəl) between two contiguous vertebrae.

in·ter·vil·lous (in″tər-vil′əs) between or among villi.

in·tes·ti·nal·iza·tion (in-tes″tĭ-nəl-ĭ-za′shən) replacement of the normal mucosa of the body of the stomach by mucosa resembling that of the large intestine, occurring in certain cancers and in autoimmune gastritis.

in·tes·tine (in-tes′tin) intestinum. **intes′tinal** *adj*

iced i. peritonitis chronica fibrosa encapsulans.

large i. intestinum crassum.

mesenterial i. the portion of the small intestine that has a mesentery, comprising the jejunum and ileum.

small i. intestinum tenue.

in·tes·ti·no·cys·to·plas·ty (in-tes″tĭ-no-sis′to-plas″te) enterocystoplasty.

in·tes·ti·no·in·tes·ti·nal (in-tes″tĭ-no-in-tes′tĭ-nəl) in anatomy or physiology, pertaining to or affecting two different parts of the intestine. Cf. *enteroenteric*.

in·tes·ti·num (in″tes-ti′nəm) pl. *intesti′na* [L., from *intestinus* inward, internal] intestine: the portion of the alimentary canal extending from the pyloric opening of the stomach to the anus; it is a membranous tube, comprising the intestinum tenue (small intestine) and intestinum crassum (large intestine). Its function is to complete the processes of digestion; to provide the body (through absorption) with water, electrolytes, and nutrients; and to move along and store fecal wastes until they are expelled. Called also *bowel* and *gut*.

i. cras′sum [TA] large intestine: the distal portion of the intestine, about 1.5 meters (5 feet) long, extending from its junction with the small intestine to the anus; it comprises the cecum, colon, rectum, and anal canal.

i. te′nue [TA] small intestine: the proximal portion of the intestine, smaller in caliber than the large intestine, and about 6 meters (20 feet) long, extending from the pylorus to the cecum; it comprises the duodenum, jejunum, and ileum.

in·ti·ma (in′tĭ-mə) [L. "innermost"] 1. innermost. 2. tunica intima vasorum.

in·ti·mal (in′tĭ-məl) pertaining to the inner layer of the blood vessels (tunica intima vasorum).

in·ti·mi·tis (in″tĭ-mi′tis) endangiitis.

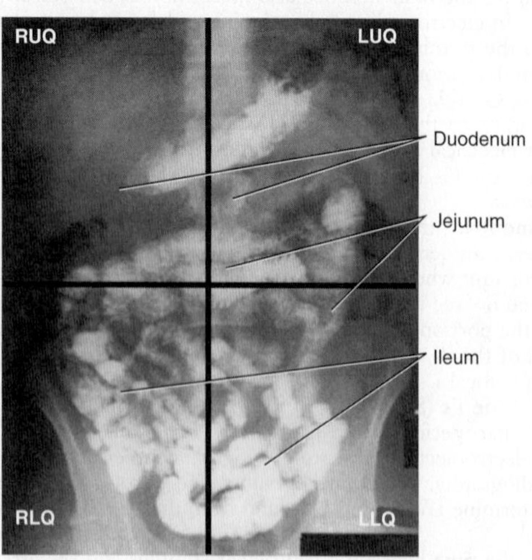

■ Barium-filled intestinum tenue and stomach.

in·toe·ing (in′to-ing) pigeon toe.

in·tol·er·ance (in-tol′ər-əns) [*in-*[2] + *tolerance*] inability to withstand; sensitivity, as to a drug.

carbohydrate i. inability to properly metabolize one or more carbohydrates, as in glucose intolerance, hereditary fructose intolerance, and the various types of disaccharide intolerance.

congenital lactose i. lactose intolerance present at birth, due to deficiency of lactase activity; see *lactase deficiency*.

congenital sucrose i. a disaccharide intolerance specific for sucrose, usually due to a congenital defect in the sucrase-isomaltase enzyme complex; see *sucrase-isomaltase deficiency*, under *deficiency*.

disaccharide i. a symptom complex occurring after ingestion of normal quantities of dietary carbohydrates, characterized by abdominal symptoms including diarrhea, flatulence, borborygmus, distention, and pain; it is usually due to deficiency of one or more disaccharidases but may have other causes such as impaired absorption. See also *lactose i.* and *α,α-trehalase*, and see *sucrase-isomaltase deficiency* and *disaccharidase deficiency*, under *deficiency*.

drug i. 1. inability to continue taking, or difficulty in continuing to take, a medication because of an adverse side effect that is not immunity-mediated. 2. the state of reacting to the normal pharmacologic doses of a drug with the symptoms of overdosage.

exercise i. limitation of ability to perform work or exercise at normally accepted levels; cf. *exercise tests*, under *test*.

fructose i. inability to metabolize fructose, as in fructose-1,6-bisphosphatase deficiency.

glucose i. inability to properly metabolize glucose, a type of carbohydrate intolerance; see also *impaired glucose tolerance*, under *tolerance*, and *diabetes mellitus*.

hereditary fructose i. an autosomal recessive carbohydrate intolerance with onset in infancy, caused by mutation in the *ALDOB* gene (locus: 9q22.3), which encodes fructose-bisphosphate aldolase, isozyme B; the resulting enzyme deficiency is characterized by hypoglycemia, with variable manifestations of fructosuria, fructosemia, anorexia, vomiting, failure to thrive, jaundice, splenomegaly, and an aversion to fructose-containing foods. If untreated, it may be fatal. See also *essential fructosuria*, under *fructosuria*.

lactose i. a disaccharide intolerance specific for lactose, usually due to an inherited deficiency of lactase activity in the intestinal mucosa; see also *lactase deficiency*.

lysinuric protein i. a rare autosomal recessive disorder of metabolism caused by mutation in the *SLC7A7* gene (locus: 14q11.2), which encodes a subunit of a cationic amino acid transport, resulting in a defect in transport of lysine, ornithine, and arginine in the kidneys and intestine. It is characterized by episodic hyperammonemia, aversion to protein-rich food, vomiting, and mild diarrhea, which may result in failure to thrive, wasting, and hypotonia, and is treated by citrulline supplementation.

orthostatic i. an abnormal response to standing upright that results from decreased blood pressure and inadequate blood flow to the brain, characterized by a variety of symptoms including lightheadedness, palpitations, tremulousness, visual disturbances, and syncope. It occurs in both acute and chronic forms and is frequently seen as a transient condition in space travelers returning from microgravity. The etiology is unknown but may be related to abnormalities in the autonomic regulation of cardiovascular function.

in·tor·sion (in-tor′shən) [L. *in* toward + *torsio* twisting] inward rotation of the upper pole of the vertical meridian of each eye; called also *adtorsion* and *conclination*. Cf. *extorsion*.

in·tort·or (in′tor-tər) [L. *intorquēre* to twist] 1. an internal rotator. 2. an extraocular muscle that produces intorsion, such as the superior oblique or the superior rectus muscle. Cf. *extortor*.

in·tox·i·ca·tion (in-tok″sĭ-ka′shən) [L. *in* intensive + Gr. *toxikon* poison] 1. stimulation, excitement, or stupefaction produced by a chemical substance, or as if by one. 2. substance i., particularly that in which the substance is alcohol (see *alcohol i.*). 3. poisoning.

alcohol i. [DSM-IV] a type of substance intoxication seen during or shortly after ingestion of alcohol, characterized by maladaptive psychological or behavioral changes combined with physiologic responses such as slurred speech, incoordination, impaired memory or attention, and unsteady gait, progressing eventually to stupor or coma.

alcohol idiosyncratic i. a term previously used for maladaptive behavioral change, usually belligerence, produced by ingestion of amounts of alcohol insufficient to cause intoxication in most persons. It is no longer considered to be separate from alcohol intoxication because evidence for a distinction is lacking.

bongkrek i. see under *poisoning*.

pathological i. alcohol idiosyncratic i.

roentgen i. radiation sickness.

substance i. [DSM-IV] a type of substance-induced disorder comprising reversible, substance-specific, maladaptive behavioral or psychological changes directly resulting from the physiologic effects on the central nervous system of recent ingestion of or exposure to a psychoactive substance. Specific cases are named on the basis of etiology, e.g., alcohol intoxication. DSM-IV recognizes specific syndromes for these drugs: alcohol, amphetamines or related substances, caffeine, cannabis, cocaine, hallucinogens, inhalants, opioids, PCP or related substances, and sedatives, hypnotics, or anxiolytics.

water i. a condition resulting from undue retention of water with decrease in sodium concentration, marked by lethargy, nausea, vomiting, and mild mental aberrations; in severe cases there may be convulsions and coma.

intra- [L. *intra* within] a prefix meaning within, into, or during.

in·tra·ab·dom·i·nal (in″trə-ab-dom′ĭ-nəl) within the abdomen.

in·tra·ac·i·nous (in″trə-as′ĭ-nəs) within an acinus.

in·tra·aor·tic (in″trə-a-or′tik) within the aorta.

in·tra·ap·pen·dic·u·lar (in″trə-ap′ən-dik′u-lər) within the appendix.

in·tra·arach·noid (in″trə-ə-rak′noid) within or underneath the arachnoid.

in·tra·ar·te·ri·al (in″trə-ahr-tēr′e-əl) within an artery or arteries; called also *endarterial.*

in·tra·ar·tic·u·lar (in″trə-ahr-tik′u-lər) within a joint.

in·tra·atri·al (in″trə-a′tre-əl) within one or both atria of the heart.

in·tra·au·ral (in″trə-aw′rəl) within the ear; called also *endaural.*

in·tra·au·ric·u·lar (in″trə-aw-rik′u-lər) within an auricle of the ear.

in·tra·bron·chi·al (in″trə-brong′ke-əl) situated or occurring within a bronchus.

in·tra·buc·cal (in″trə-buk′əl) within the mouth or within the cheek.

in·tra·can·a·lic·u·lar (in″trə-kan″ə-lik′u-lər) within a canaliculus or canaliculi.

in·tra·cap·su·lar (in″trə-kap′su-lər) within a capsule.

in·tra·car·di·ac (in″trə-kahr′de-ak) within the heart.

in·tra·car·pal (in″trə-kahr′pəl) within the wrist.

in·tra·car·ti·lag·i·nous (in″trə-kahr″tĭ-laj′ĭ-nəs) within a cartilage; endochondral.

in·tra·cav·er·no·sal (in″trə-kav″ər-no′səl) within the corpus cavernosum.

in·tra·cav·i·tary (in″trə-kav′ĭ-tar″e) within a cavity, as that of the cervix or of the uterus.

in·tra·ce·li·al (in″trə-se′le-əl) within one of the body cavities.

in·tra·cel·lu·lar (in″trə-sel′u-lər) within a cell.

in·tra·ce·phal·ic (in″trə-sə-fal′ik) within the brain.

in·tra·cer·e·bel·lar (in″trə-ser″ə-bel′ər) situated within the cerebellum.

in·tra·cer·e·bral (in″trə-ser′ə-brəl) situated within the cerebrum.

in·tra·cer·e·bro·ven·tric·u·lar (in-trə-ser″əbro-ven-trik′u-lər) within the ventricles of the brain.

in·tra·cer·vi·cal (in″trə-sur′vĭ-kəl) situated within the canal of the cervix uteri.

in·tra·chon·dral (in″trə-kon′drəl) endochondral.

in·tra·chon·dri·al (in″trə-kon′dre-əl) endochondral.

in·tra·chor·dal (in″trə-kor′dəl) within the notochord.

in·tra·cis·ter·nal (in″trə-sis-tur′nəl) within a cistern, especially the cisterna cerebellomedullaris.

in·tra·col·ic (in″trə-kol′ik) intracolonic.

in·tra·co·lon·ic (in″trə-ko-lon′ik) within the colon.

in·tra·cor·po·ral (in″trə-kor′por-əl) intracorporeal.

in·tra·cor·po·re·al (in″trə-kor-por′e-əl) situated or occurring within the body.

in·tra·cor·pus·cu·lar (in″trə-kor-pus′ku-lər) within a blood corpuscle. Called also *endocorpuscular*, *endoglobular*, and *intraglobular*.

in·tra·cos·tal (in″trə-kos′təl) on the inner surface of the rib.

in·tra·cra·ni·al (in″trə-kra′ne-əl) within the cranium.

in·tra·crine (in′trə-krin) denoting a type of hormone function in which a regulatory factor acts within the cell that synthesizes it by binding to intracellular receptors.

in·tra·cri·nol·o·gy (in″trə-krĭ-nol′ə-je) the study of the processes of intracrine hormones.

in·tra·cru·re·us (in″trə-kroo′re-əs) the internal part of the musculus vastus intermedius.

in·trac·ta·ble (in-trak′tə-bəl) resistant to cure, relief, or control.

in·tra·cu·ta·ne·ous (in″trə-ku-ta′ne-əs) within the skin; called also *intradermal.*

in·tra·cys·tic (in″trə-sis′tik) within a cyst.

in·tra·cy·to·plas·mic (in″trə-si″to-plaz′mik) within the cytoplasm of a cell.

in·trad (in′trad) [*intra-* + *-ad*[1]] inward in direction.

in·tra·der·mal (in″trə-dur′məl) 1. within the dermis. 2. intracutaneous.

in·tra·di·a·lyt·ic (in″trə-di″ə-lit′ik) taking place during hemodialysis.

in·tra·dip·lo·ic (in″trə-dip-lo′ik) within the diploë.

in·tra·dis·cal (in″trə-dis′kəl) within an intervertebral disk.

in·tra·duc·tal (in″trə-duk′təl) situated or occurring within the duct of a gland.

in·tra·du·o·de·nal (in″trə-doo″o-de′nəl) within the duodenum.

in·tra·du·ral (in″trə-doo′rəl) within or beneath the dura.

in·tra·em·bry·on·ic (in″trə-em″bre-on′ik) within the body of the embryo. Cf. *extraembryonic.*

in·tra·epi·der·mal (in″trə-ep″ĭ-dur′məl) within the epidermis.

in·tra·ep·i·phys·e·al (in″trə-ep″ĭ-fiz′e-əl) within an epiphysis.

in·tra·ep·i·the·li·al (in″trə-ep″ĭ-the′le-əl) situated among the cells of the epithelium.

in·tra·eryth·ro·cyt·ic (in″trə-ə-rith″ro-sit′ik) within an erythrocyte.

in·tra·fal·lo·pi·an (in″trə-fə-lo′pe-ən) within the uterine (fallopian) tube.

in·tra·fas·cic·u·lar (in″trə-fə-sik′u-lər) within a fascicle.

in·tra·fat (in″trə-fat′) situated in or introduced into fatty tissue, as the subcutaneous tissue.

in·tra·fe·ta·tion (in″trə-fe-ta′shən) the development of a fetus within another fetus; see *endadelphos.*

in·tra·fi·lar (in″trə-fi′lər) within a reticulum.

in·tra·fis·su·ral (in″trə-fish′ə-rəl) within a cerebral fissure.

in·tra·fis·tu·lar (in″trə-fis′tu-lər) within a fistula.

in·tra·fol·lic·u·lar (in″trə-fo-lik′u-lər) within a follicle.

in·tra·fu·sal (in″trə-fu′zəl) [*intra-* + *fusus*] pertaining to the striated fibers within a muscle spindle.

in·tra·gas·tric (in″trə-gas′trik) situated or occurring within the stomach; called also *endogastric.*

in·tra·gem·mal (in″trə-jem′əl) within a bud, such as a taste bud.

in·tra·gen·ic (in″trə-jen′ik) within a gene.

in·tra·glan·du·lar (in″trə-glan′du-lər) within a gland.

in·tra·glob·u·lar (in″trə-glob′u-lər) 1. within a globe or globule. 2. intracorpuscular.

in·tra·gy·ral (in″trə-ji′rəl) within a cerebral gyrus.

in·tra·he·pat·ic (in″trə-hə-pat′ik) within the liver.

in·tra·hy·oid (in″trə-hi′oid) within the hyoid bone.

in·tra·ic·tal (in″trə-ik′təl) occurring during an attack or seizure.

in·tra·in·tes·ti·nal (in″trə-in-tes′tĭ-nəl) within the intestine.

in·tra·jug·u·lar (in″trə-jug′u-lər) within the jugular foramen, process, or vein.

in·tra·la·mel·lar (in″trə-lə-mel′ər) within lamellae.

in·tra·la·ryn·ge·al (in″trə-lə-rin′je-əl) endolaryngeal.

in·tra·le·sion·al (in″trə-le′zhən-əl) occurring in or introduced directly into a localized lesion.

in·tra·leu·ko·cyt·ic (in″trə-lu″ko-sit′ik) within a leukocyte.

in·tra·lig·a·men·ta·ry (in″trə-lig″ə-men′tə-re) intraligamentous.

in·tra·lig·a·men·tous (in″trə-lig″ə-men′təs) within a ligament.

in·tra·lin·gual (in″trə-ling′gwəl) within the tongue.

in·tra·lo·bar (in″trə-lo′bər) within a lobe.

in·tra·lob·u·lar (in″trə-lob′u-lər) within a lobule.

in·tra·loc·u·lar (in″trə-lok′u-lər) within the loculi of a structure.

in·tra·lu·mi·nal (in″trə-loo′mĭ-nəl) within the lumen of a tube, as of a blood vessel; endoluminal.

in·tra·ly·so·so·mal (in-trə-li″so-so′məl) within a lysosome.

in·tra·mam·ma·ry (in″trə-mam′ə-re) within the breast.

in·tra·mar·gin·al (in″trə-mahr′jĭ-nəl) within a margin.

in·tra·mat·ri·cal (in″trə-mat′rĭ-kəl) within a matrix.

in·tra·med·ul·lary (in″trə-med′u-lar″e) 1. within the spinal cord. 2. within the medulla oblongata. 3. within the marrow cavity of a bone.

in·tra·mem·bra·nous (in″trə-mem′brə-nəs) within a membrane.

in·tra·me·nin·ge·al (in″trə-mə-nin′je-əl) within the meninges.

in·tra·me·nis·cal (in″trə-mə-nis′kəl) within a meniscus.

in·tra·mo·lec·u·lar (in″trə-mo-lek′u-lər) within the molecule.

in·tra·mu·ral (in″trə-mu′rəl) within the wall of an organ.

in·tra·mus·cu·lar (in″trə-mus′ku-lər) within the substance of a muscle.

in·tra·my·eli·nic (in-trə-mi″ə-lin′ik) within white matter or a myelin sheath.

in·tra·myo·car·di·al (in″trə-mi″o-kahr′de-əl) within the myocardium.

in·tra·nar·i·al (in″trə-nar′e-əl) within the nares.

in·tra·na·sal (in″trə-na′zəl) within the nose. Called also *endonasal.*

in·tra·na·tal (in″trə-na′təl) occurring during birth.

in·tra·neu·ral (in″trə-nōōr′əl) endoneural.

in·tra·nu·cle·ar (in″trə-noo′kle-ər) within a nucleus, as a cell nucleus.

in·tra·oc·u·lar (in″trə-ok′u-lər) within the eye.

in·tra·op·er·a·tive (in″trə-op′ər-ə-tiv) occurring during the course of a surgical operation.

in·tra·oral (in″trə-or′əl) within the mouth.

in·tra·or·bi·tal (in″trə-or′bĭ-təl) within the orbit.

in·tra·os·se·ous (in″trə-os′e-əs) within a bone.

in·tra·os·te·al (in″trə-os′te-əl) intraosseous.

in·tra·ovar·i·an (in″trə-o-var′e-ən) within the ovary.

in·tra·ov·u·lar (in″trə-ov′u-lər) within an oocyte or ovum.

in·tra·pan·cre·at·ic (in″trə-pan″kre-at′ik) within the pancreas.

in·tra·par·en·chym·a·tous (in″trə-par″ən-kim′ə-təs) within the parenchyma of an organ.

in·tra·pa·ri·e·tal (in″trə-pə-ri′ə-təl) [*intra-* + *parietal*] 1. intramural. 2. situated in the parietal region of the brain.

in·tra·par·tal (in″trə-pahr′təl) intrapartum.

in·tra·par·tum (in″trə-pahr′təm) occurring during childbirth, or during delivery.

in·tra·pel·vic (in″trə-pel′vik) within the pelvis.

in·tra·peri·car·di·al (in″trə-per″ĭ-kahr′de-əl) within the pericardium.

in·tra·per·i·ne·al (in″trə-per″ĭ-ne′əl) within the tissues of the perineum.

in·tra·peri·to·ne·al (in″trə-per″ĭ-to-ne′əl) within the peritoneal cavity; called also *endoperitoneal.*

in·tra·pet·rous (in″trə-pet′rəs) within the petrous part of the temporal bone.

in·tra·pi·al (in″trə-pe′əl) within or beneath the pia mater.

in·tra·pi·tu·i·tary (in″trə-pĭ-too′ĭ-tar″e) within the pituitary gland.

in·tra·pla·cen·tal (in″trə-plə-sen′təl) within the placenta.

in·tra·pleu·ral (in″trə-ploor′əl) within the pleura.

in·tra·pon·tine (in″trə-pon′tin) [*intra-* + *pontine*] within the substance of the pons.

in·tra·pros·tat·ic (in″trə-pros-tat′ik) within the prostate gland.

in·tra·pro·to·plas·mic (in″trə-pro″to-plaz′mik) within the protoplasm.

in·tra·psy·chic (in″trə-si′kik) arising, occurring, or situated within the mind.

in·tra·pul·mo·nary (in″trə-pool′mo-nar″e) within a lung.

in·tra·py·ret·ic (in″trə-pi-ret′ik) during the stage of fever.

in·tra·ra·chid·i·an (in″trə-rə-kid′e-ən) intraspinal.

in·tra·rec·tal (in″trə-rek′təl) within the rectum.

in·tra·re·nal (in″trə-re′nəl) within the kidney.

in·tra·ret·i·nal (in″trə-ret′ĭ-nəl) within the retina.

in·tra·scle·ral (in″trə-skler′əl) within the sclera.

in·tra·scro·tal (in″trə-skro′təl) within the scrotum.

in·tra·seg·men·tal (in″trə-seg-men′təl) within a single segment, such as a bronchopulmonary segment or spinal segment.

in·tra·sel·lar (in″trə-sel′ər) within the sella turcica.

in·tra·spi·nal (in″trə-spi′nəl) within the vertebral column.

in·tra·sple·nic (in″trə-sple′nik) within the spleen.

in·tra·ster·nal (in″trə-stur′nəl) within the sternum.

in·tra·sti·tial (in″trə-stish′əl) within the cells or fibers of a tissue.

in·tra·stro·mal (in″trə-stro′məl) within the stroma of an organ.

in·tra·syno·vi·al (in″trə-sĭ-no′ve-əl) within the synovial membrane or fluid of a joint.

in·tra·tar·sal (in″trə-tahr′səl) within or on the inner side of the tarsus.

in·tra·ten·di·nous (in″trə-ten′dĭ-nəs) within a tendon.

in·tra·tes·tic·u·lar (in″trə-tes-tik′u-lər) within the testis.

in·tra·the·cal (in″trə-the′kəl) within a sheath; see also under *injection.*

in·tra·the·nar (in″trə-the′nər) situated between the thenar and hypothenar eminences.

in·tra·tho·rac·ic (in″trə-thə-ras′ik) endothoracic.

in·tra·ton·sil·lar (in″trə-ton′sĭ-lər) within a tonsil.

in·tra·tra·bec·u·lar (in″trə-trə-bek′u-lər) within a trabecula.

in·tra·tra·che·al (in″trə-tra′ke-əl) endotracheal.

in·tra·tu·bal (in″trə-too′bəl) situated or occurring within a tube, especially within a uterine tube.

in·tra·tu·bu·lar (in″trə-too′bu-lər) within the tubules of an organ.

in·tra·tym·pan·ic (in″trə-tim-pan′ik) within the tympanic cavity.

in·tra·ure·ter·al (in″trə-u-re′tər-əl) within the ureter.

in·tra·ure·ter·ic (in″trə-u″rə-ter′ik) intraureteral.

in·tra·ure·thral (in″trə-u-re′thrəl) within the urethra; called also *endourethral.*

in·tra·uter·ine (in″trə-u′tər-in) within the uterus; called also *endouterine.*

in·tra·vag·i·nal (in″trə-vaj′ĭ-nəl) within the vagina.

in·trav·a·sa·tion (in-trav″ə-sa′shən) the entrance of foreign material into a blood vessel.

in·tra·vas·cu·lar (in″trə-vas′ku-lər) within a vessel.

in·tra·ve·na·tion (in″trə-ve-na′shən) the entrance or injection of foreign matter into a vein.

in·tra·ve·nous (in″trə-ve′nəs) within a vein or veins.

in·tra·ven·tric·u·lar (in″trə-ven-trik′u-lər) within a ventricle.

in·tra·ver·sion (in″trə-vur′zhən) in orthodontics, malocclusion in which the teeth or other maxillary structures are too near the median plane. Cf. *extroversion* (def. 3).

in·tra·ver·te·bral (in″trə-vur′tə-brəl) intraspinal.

in·tra·ves·i·cal (in″trə-ves′ĭ-kəl) within the urinary bladder; called also *endovesical.*

in·tra·vil·lous (in″trə-vil′əs) situated within a villus.

in·tra·vi·tal (in″trə-vi′təl) occurring during life.

in·tra vi·tam (in′trə vi′təm) [L.] during life.

in·tra·vi·tel·line (in″trə-vi-tel′in) within the yolk.

in·tra·vit·re·al (in-trə-vit′re-əl) into or within the vitreous.

in·tra·vit·re·ous (in″trə-vit′re-əs) intravitreal.

in·trin·sic (in-trin′sik) [L. *intrinsecus* situated on the inside] situated entirely within or pertaining exclusively to a part.

intro- [L. *intro* within] a prefix meaning into or within.

in·tro·duc·er (in″trə-doo′sər) an intubator.

in·tro·fi·er (in′tro-fi″ər) a liquid which has the property of lowering the interfacial tension of emulsions.

in·tro·flex·ion (in″tro-flek′shən) a bending inward.

in·tro·gas·tric (in″tro-gas′trik) [*intro-* + *gastric*] conveyed or leading into the stomach.

in·tro·gres·sion (in″tro-gresh′ən) [*intro-* + L. *gressus* course] the incorporation of a gene or genes of one species into the gene pool of another species.

in·troi·tus (in-tro′ĭ-təs) pl. *intro′itus* [L.] an entrance or opening.
- **i. pel′vis** apertura pelvis superior.
- **vaginal i.** ostium vaginae.

in·tro·jec·tion (in″tro-jek′shən) [*intro-* + L. *jacēre* to throw] an immature, unconscious defense mechanism in which loved or hated external objects are absorbed into the self; anxiety is diminished by reducing the possibility of loss in the case of a loved object, or by internally controlling aggression on the part of a hated object.

in·tro·mis·sion (in″tro-mish′ən) [*intro-* + L. *mittere* to send] the insertion of one part into another, as of the penis into the vagina.

in•tron (in′tron) [*inter*vening (sequence) + *-on*] in eukaryotic genes, a noncoding DNA sequence separating two coding sequences (exons); it is initially transcribed into heterogeneous nuclear RNA (hnRNA) as part of the primary transcript, but is spliced out in the generation of mature messenger RNA (mRNA), prior to translation. By extension, the term also denotes the same sequences in the primary RNA transcript. Called also *intervening sequence*.

In•tron A (in′tron) trademark for a preparation of interferon alfa-2b.

In•tro•pin (in′tro-pin) trademark for a preparation of dopamine hydrochloride.

in•tro•spec•tion (in″tro-spek′shən) [*intro-* + L. *spicere* to look] the contemplation or observation of one's own thoughts and feelings; self-analysis.

in•tro•sus•cep•tion (in″tro-sə-sep′shən) intussusception.

in•tro•ver•sion (in″tro-vur′zhən) [*intro-* + *version*] 1. the turning outside in, more or less completely, of an organ, or the resulting condition. 2. the turning inward to the self of one's interest, with lack of interest in the external world. 3. intraversion.

in•tro•vert (in′tro-vərt) 1. a person whose interest is turned inward to the self. 2. to turn one's interest inward to the self. 3. a structure that can be turned or drawn inwards. 4. to turn a part or organ inward upon itself.

in•tru•sion (in-troo′zhən) in orthodontic therapy, a technique of depressing a tooth back into the occlusal plane or an effort to prevent its eruption or elongation during the correction of an excessive overbite. Called also *tooth depression*. Cf. *extrusion* (def. 3).

in•tu•bate (in′too-bāt) to treat by intubation.

in•tu•ba•tion (in″too-ba′shən) [L. *in* into + *tuba* tube] the insertion of a tube into a body canal or cavity; see also *cannulation* and *catheterization*.

endotracheal i. insertion of an endotracheal tube; see under *tube*.

nasal i. insertion of a tube through the nose, such as a nasogastric or endotracheal tube.

nasotracheal i. insertion of a nasotracheal tube.

oral i. insertion of a tube through the mouth.

orotracheal i. insertion of an orotracheal tube.

in•tu•ba•tion•ist (in-too-ba′shən-ist) an individual who performs intubations.

in•tu•ba•tor (in′too-ba-tər) an instrument used in intubation.

in•tu•mesce (in-too-mes′) to swell up.

in•tu•mes•cence (in-too-mes′əns) [L. *intumescentia*] 1. a swelling, normal or abnormal. 2. the process of swelling.

in•tu•mes•cent (in-too-mes′ənt) [L. *intumescens*] swelling or becoming swollen.

in•tu•mes•cen•tia (in-too-mə-sen′she-ə) pl. *intumescen′tiae* [L.] an enlargement or swelling.

i. cervica′lis [TA] cervical enlargement: the enlargement of the cervical spinal cord at the level of attachment of the nerves to the upper limbs, generally extending from the third cervical to the second thoracic vertebra.

i. lumbosacra′lis [TA] lumbosacral enlargement: the enlargement of the lumbar spinal cord at the level of attachment of the nerves to the lower limbs, generally extending from the first lumbar to the third sacral vertebra.

i. tympa′nica [TA] tympanic enlargement: a pseudoganglion on the tympanic branch (nerve) of the glossopharyngeal nerve; called also *ganglion tympanicum* [TA alternative], *tympanic ganglion, tympanic ganglion of Valentin*, and *Valentin pseudoganglion*.

in•tus•sus•cep•tion (in″tə-sə-sep′shən) [L. *intus* within + *suscipere* to receive] 1. a receiving within. 2. prolapse of one part of the intestine into the lumen of an immediately adjoining part. It is most common in infants, and in adults it is often associated with a neoplasm. Symptoms include partial obstruction, a palpable abdominal mass, and abdominal pain with cramping.

appendiceal i. invagination of one part of the vermiform appendix into an adjoining part, ranging in severity from invagination of the tip into the distal appendix to prolapse of the entire appendix into the cecum.

colic i., colonic i. intussusception involving two segments of the colon.

double i. the enveloping of one intussusception by an even larger one.

enteric i. intussusception involving two segments of the small intestine.

ileal i. intussusception involving two segments of the ileum.

ileocecal i. intussusception at the ileocecal junction, with the cecum being drawn back into the ileum. Cf. *ileocolic i.*

ileocolic i. intussusception at the ileocecal junction, with the distal ileum being drawn forward into the colon. Cf. *ileocecal i.*

jejunogastric i. a complication sometimes seen after gastrojejunostomy, with the anastomosed jejunum prolapsing into the stomach.

retrograde i. invagination of a distal part of the intestine into a proximal part.

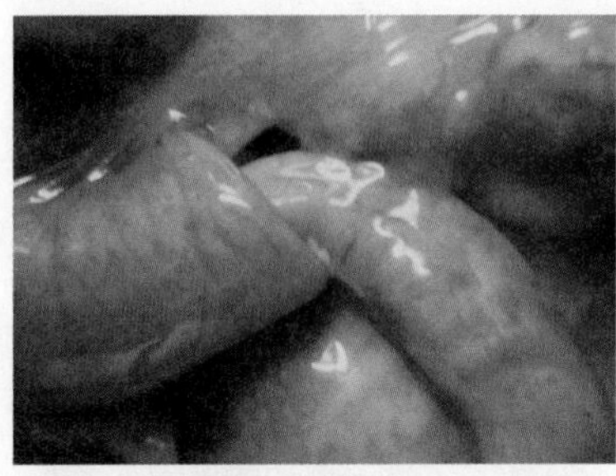

■ Enteric intussusception.

in•tus•sus•cep•tum (in″tə-sə-sep′təm) [L.] in intussusception, the portion of intestine that has been invaginated within another part.

in•tus•sus•cip•i•ens (in″tə-sə-sip′e-əns) [L.] in intussusception, the portion of intestine into which another portion has invaginated.

In•u•la (in′u-lə) [L.] a genus of composite-flowered plants (family Compositae), whose rhizomes contain inulin. The root has numerous uses in folk medicine.

in•u•lase (in′u-lās) inulinase.

in•u•lin (in′u-lin) an indigestible polysaccharide vegetable starch found in the rhizome of certain plants (Compositae). It is a polymer of fructofuranose, yields fructose on hydrolysis, and is used in a test for determining glomerular filtration rate. See *inulin clearance*, under *clearance*.

in•u•lin•ase (in′u-lin-ās) [EC 3.2.1.7] an enzyme of the hydrolase class that catalyzes the cleavage of specific linkages between fructose residues in inulin, releasing fructose. The enzyme occurs in a variety of fungi and in higher plants.

in•unc•tion (in-ungk′shən) [*in-*[1] + *unction*] the act of anointing or of applying an ointment with rubbing.

in utero (in u′tər-o) [L.] inside the uterus.

Inv [from the name of the propositus] see *Km allotypes*, under *allotype*.

in vac•uo (in vak′u-o) [L.] in a vacuum.

in•vag•i•nate (in-vaj′ĭ-nāt) to infold one portion of a structure within another portion.

in•vag•i•na•tion (in-vaj″ĭ-na′shən) [L. *invaginatio*, from *in* within + *vagina* sheath] 1. the state of being or the process of becoming invaginated. 2. in embryology, a process by which *(a)* one region of a hollow, single-walled, spherical blastula caves in to form and line a new cavity in the now cup-shaped, double-walled gastrula, or *(b)* an ever-deepening pit develops into a diverticulum or tube from the surface into the tissues below. 3. intussusception.

basilar i. a developmental deformity of the occipital bone and upper end of the cervical spine in which the latter appears to have pushed the floor of the occipital bone upward; see also *platybasia*. Called also *basilar impression*.

in•va•lid (in′və-lid) [L. *invalidus; in* not + *validus* strong] 1. not well and strong. 2. a person who is disabled by illness or infirmity.

In•vanz (in′vanz) trademark for a preparation of ertapenem sodium.

in•va•sin (in-va′zin) hyaluronidase.

in•va•sion (in-va′zhən) [L. *invasio*, from *in* into + *vadere* to go] 1. the attack or onset of a disease. 2. the infiltration and active destruction of surrounding tissue by a malignant tumor.

in•va•sive (in-va′siv) 1. pertaining to or characterized by invasion. 2. involving puncture or incision of the skin or insertion of an instrument or foreign material into the body; said of diagnostic techniques.

in•va•sive•ness (in-va′siv-nis) 1. the ability of a pathogenic microorganism to enter and spread throughout the body. 2. the ability of a malignant tumor to be invasive.

in•ven•to•ry (in′vən-tor″e) a comprehensive list of personality traits, aptitudes, and interests.

Beck Depression I. a self-report questionnaire for measuring the symptoms of depression, focusing on the cognitive symptoms.

California Personality I. (CPI) a self-report, true-false test designed to measure aspects of personality style; generally used in counseling situations or for less than severe psychopathology.

Millon Clinical Multiaxial I. (MCMI) a self-report inventory designed to produce a profile of the personality style and structure underlying mental disorders.

Minnesota Multiphasic Personality I. (MMPI) a self-report, true-false test designed to evaluate personality and particularly to assess psychopathology.

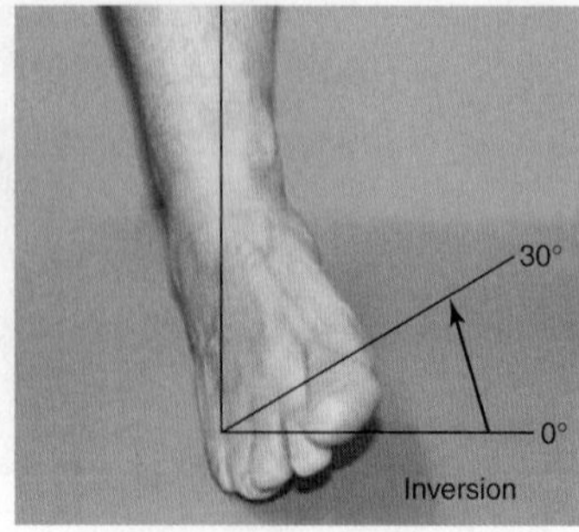

■ Inversion and eversion of the foot.

in•ver•mi•na•tion (in-vur″mĭ-na′shən) 1. vermination (def. 1). 2. helminthiasis.

in•verse (in′vərs) 1. reversed in order, effect, or nature. 2. the reciprocal of a particular quantity.

In•ver•sine (in-vur′sēn) trademark for a preparation of mecamylamine hydrochloride.

in•ver•sion (in-vur′zhən) [L. *inversio; in* into +*vertere* to turn] 1. a turning inward, inside out, upside down, or other reversal of the normal relation of a part. 2. in genetics, a chromosomal aberration caused by the inverted reunion of a chromosome segment after breakage of a chromosome at two points, resulting in a change in sequence of genes or nucleotides; e.g., the sequence *abcdefg* may be inverted to *abfedcg.* See illustration at *aberration.*

carbohydrate i. hydrolysis of disaccharides or polysaccharides to monosaccharides.

paracentric i. inversion in which the inverted chromosome segment is on one side of the centromere, i.e., both breaks occur in one arm. See illustration at *aberration.*

pericentric i. inversion in which the inverted chromosome segment includes the centromere.

thermic i. the state in which the body temperature is highest in the morning.

i. of uterus a turning of the uterus inside out, whereby the fundus is forced through the cervix and protrudes into or outside of the vagina.

visceral i. the more or less complete right and left transposition of the viscera; see *situs inversus.*

in•ver•sus (in-vur′səs) [L., past part. of *invertere* to invert] opposite to, or inverted from, the normal; see *situs inversus.*

in•ver•te•brate (in-vur′tə-brāt) 1. any animal that has no vertebral column; a nonvertebrate animal. 2. having no vertebral column.

in•ver•tor (in-vur′tər) a muscle that turns a part inward.

in•vest (in-vest′) 1. to envelop in or cover another tissue or part (as fascia). 2. to surround, envelop, or embed in an investment material.

in•vest•ing (in-vest′ing) 1. the act or process of covering or enveloping wholly or in part an object, such as a denture, tooth, wax form, or crown with a refractory investment material before curing, soldering, or casting. 2. the covering or enveloping of a tissue or part by another tissue, such as a fascia.

i. the pattern surrounding the wax pattern with an investment material, such as a mix of a plaster, for low temperature casting, or a mix consisting of dental stone and a silica refractory for high temperature casting; the investment hardens to form a mold into which casting materials are poured.

vacuum i. subjecting the water-investment mixture to a vacuum during the investing procedure in order to remove air bubbles from the mixture.

in•vest•ment (in-vest′mənt) 1. any tissue, such as fascia, that envelops or covers other tissues or parts. 2. a material applied as a soft paste to a pattern that hardens to form a mold for casting.

gypsum-bonded i. an investment bonded by gypsum or one of its derivatives, used with metals or alloys that have low fusion temperatures.

phosphate-bonded i. an investment bonded by phosphate and a metallic oxide, used with metals or alloys that have high fusion temperatures.

silica-bonded i. an investment bonded by silica, used with metals or alloys that have high fusion temperatures.

in•vet•er•ate (in-vet′ər-ət) [L. *inverteratus*] chronic and confirmed; long established and of difficult cure.

In•vi•rase (in′vĭ-rās) trademark for a preparation of saquinavir mesylate.

in•vis•ca•tion (in″vis-ka′shən) [L. *in* among + *viscum* slime] the mixing of the food with the mucous secretion of the mouth in mastication.

in vi•tro (in ve′tro) [L.] within a glass; observable in a test tube; in an artificial environment.

in vi•vo (in ve′vo) [L.] within the living body.

in•vo•lu•cre (in′vo-loo″kər) an involucrum.

in•vo•lu•crum (in″vo-loo′krəm) pl. *involu′cra* [L.; *in* in + *volvere* to wrap] a covering or sheath, such as contains the sequestrum of a necrosed bone.

in•vol•un•tary (in-vol′ən-tar″e) [L. *involuntarius; in* against + *voluntas* will] 1. independent of the will. 2. contrary to the will.

in•vo•lute (in′vo-lo͞ot) [L. *in* into + *volvere* to roll] 1. to return to normal size after enlargement. 2. to regress; to change to an earlier or to a more primitive condition. See *involution.*

in•vo•lu•tion (in″vo-loo′shən) [L. *involutio; in* into + *volvere* to roll] 1. a rolling or turning inward. 2. a retrograde change of the entire body or in a particular organ, as the retrograde changes in the female genital organs that result in normal size after delivery. 3. the progressive degeneration occurring naturally with advancing age, resulting in a reduction in size or function of organs or tissues.

senile i. involution (def. 3).

in•vo•lu•tion•al (in″vo-loo′shən-əl) pertaining to, due to, or occurring in involution.

io•ben•guane (i″o-ben′gwān) *m*-iodobenzylguanidine (mIBG), an analogue of norepinephrine with affinity for the sympathetic nervous system and related tumors; it is believed to share the same transport pathway with norepinephrine and displace norepinephrine from intraneuronal storage granules in adrenergic nerves.

i. I 123 iobenguane in which a portion of the molecules are labeled with ^{123}I, used as a radioactive tracer for diagnostic imaging of neuroendocrine tumors and disorders of the adrenal medulla; administered intravenously as the sulfate salt.

i. I 131 iobenguane in which a portion of the molecules are labeled with ^{131}I, used as a radioactive tracer for diagnostic imaging of neuroendocrine tumors and disorders of the adrenal medulla. It is also used for local radiation therapy in the treatment of carcinoid syndrome, pheochromocytoma, and neuroblastoma.

io•da•mide (i-o′də-mīd) a water-soluble iodinated radiopaque medium, used for intravenous excretory urography and computed tomography of the brain.

Io•da•moe•ba (i-o″də-me′bə) [*iod-* + *ameba*] a genus of ramicristate amebae of the order Amoebida, parasitic in mammals; they have a vesicular nucleus with a large chromatin-rich endosome surrounded by a layer of globules, and achromatic strands between the endosome and membrane. Their cysts are usually uninucleate with a large glycogenous vacuole that readily stains brown with iodine.

I. bütsch′lii a generally nonpathogenic species found in the intestines of primates and pigs; it is characterized by trophozoites and cysts. Rare cases of disease caused by this organism are clinically similar to those caused by *Entamoeba histolytica.*

io•date (i′o-dāt) any salt of iodic acid; the IO_3^- anion.

iod-Bas•e•dow (i″ōd baz′ə-do) iodine-induced hyperthyroidism.

io•de•mia (i″o-de′me-ə) [*iodine* + *-emia*] the presence of iodides in the blood.

iod•ic ac•id (i-o′dik) a strong inorganic acid, HIO_3, which is a highly corrosive oxidizing agent.

io•dide (i′o-dīd) any binary compound of iodine; the I^- anion. Dietary iodine is reduced to iodide, absorbed in the intestines, and later taken up from the bloodstream by the thyroid gland for incorporation into thyroid hormones.

io•dide per•ox•i•dase (i′o-dīd pər-ok′sĭ-dās) [EC 1.11.1.8] an enzyme of the oxidoreductase class that catalyzes a series of reactions occurring in the synthesis of thyroxine; it catalyzes the oxidation of iodide to iodine, the iodination of tyrosyl residues of thyroglobulins, and the intramolecular condensation of such iodinated residues to form iodothyronines. Deficiency of the enzyme, an autosomal recessive disorder, results in congenital goiter. Called also *thyroid peroxidase* and *thyroperoxidase.*

io•dim•e•try (i″o-dim′ə-tre) [*iodine* + *-metry*] 1. the estimation of the quantity of iodine in a mixture or compound. 2. in quantitative analysis, the procedure used to determine an oxidizing agent consisting of the quantitative oxidation of potassium iodide to free iodine, and then titration with sodium thiosulfate.

io•di•nate (i-o′dĭ-nāt) to combine or compound with iodine.

io•din•a•tion (i″o-din-a′shən) the incorporation or addition of iodine in a compound.

io•dine (I) (i′o-dīn) [Gr. *ioeides* violetlike, from the color of its vapor] 1. a halogen element of a peculiar odor and acrid taste; atomic number, 53; atomic weight, 126.904. It is a nonmetallic element, occurring in heavy, grayish black plates or granules. Iodine is essential in nutrition, being especially necessary for the synthesis of thyroid hormones (thyroxine and triiodothyronine), which regulate the metabolic rate in all cells. 2. [USP] a preparation of iodine used as a topical antiinfective (see also under *solution*). Iodine, usually in the form of iodides, is used in the treatment of hyperthyroidism.

i. 123 a radioactive isotope of iodine, atomic mass 123, having a half-life of 13.2 hours; it decays by electron capture, emitting gamma rays (0.159 MeV) and x-rays. It is used as a tracer in diagnostic imaging and as a radiation source in radiation therapy.

i. 125 a radioisotope of iodine, atomic mass 125, having a half-life of 60.14 days and emitting gamma rays (0.035 MeV); used as a radioactive tracer, particularly as a label in radioimmunoassays and other in vitro tests, and also for thyroid imaging.

i. 131 a radioactive isotope of iodine, atomic mass 131, having a half-life of 8.04 days; it emits beta particles (0.607, 0.81, 0.336 MeV) and gamma rays (0.080, 0.284, 0.364, 0.637, 0.723 MeV) and is used as a tracer in diagnostic imaging and as a radiation source in radiation therapy.

Lugol i. strong iodine solution.

povidone-i. see *povidone-iodine* at *P.*

protein-bound i. (PBI) iodine bound to protein in the blood serum, measured in the protein-bound iodine test.

radioactive i. radioiodine.

io·din·o·phil (i″o-din′o-fil) [*iodine* + *-phil*] 1. any cell or other element readily stainable with iodine. 2. iodinophilous.

io·din·oph·i·lous (i″o-din-of′ĭ-ləs) readily stainable with iodine.

io·dip·a·mide (i″o-dip′ə-mīd) [USP] a water-soluble iodinated contrast medium used for intravenous cholangiography and cholecystography.

i. meglumine [USP], **i. methylglucamine** the meglumine salt of iodipamide, used as a radiopaque medium in cholangiography and cholecystography, administered intravenously.

i. sodium the sodium salt of iodipamide, used as a radiopaque medium in cholangiography and cholecystography, administered intravenously.

io·dism (i′o-diz-əm) chronic poisoning by iodine or iodine compounds; it is marked by coryza, ptyalism, frontal headache, emaciation, weakness, and skin eruptions (iododerma). Called also *iodine poisoning.*

io·dix·a·nol (i″o-dik′sə-nol) a nonionic contrast medium used in angiography, computed tomography, and excretory urography.

io·dize (i′o-dīz) to impregnate with iodine or to incorporate iodine or one of its compounds.

iod(o)- [Fr. *iode* iodine] word element denoting a relationship to iodine.

io·do·ace·tic ac·id (i-o″do-ə-se′tik) a compound, used in biochemical studies; it alkylates free thiol groups but not disulfide bridges.

***m*-io·do·ben·zyl·gua·ni·dine** (i-o″do-ben″zəl-gwah′nĭ-dēn) iobenguane.

io·do·chlor·hy·drox·y·quin (i-o″do-klor″hi-drok′sə-kwin) clioquinol.

io·do·cho·les·ter·ol I 131 (i-o″do-kə-les′tər-ol) a radiopharmaceutical, cholesterol iodinated with ^{131}I, which has been used in radionuclide imaging of the adrenal cortex; now largely replaced by iodomethylnorcholesterol.

io·do·der·ma (i-o″do-dur′mə) [*iodo-* + *derma*] a halogenoderma resulting from ingestion of iodine or its compounds; see also *iodism.*

io·do·form (i-o′do-form) [*iodo-* + *formyl*] [USP] chemical name: triiodomethane. A greenish yellow powder or crystals, CHI_3, having a strong, penetrating odor, containing about 96 per cent iodine, and soluble in chloroform and ether and somewhat in alcohol and water: used as a topical antiinfective, applied to the skin, and used for packing cavities in oral and otorhinologic surgery.

io·do·form·ism (i-o″do-form′iz-əm) poisoning by iodoform.

io·do·gen·ic (i-o″do-jen′ik) [*iodine* + *genic*] yielding or producing iodine.

io·do·glob·u·lin (i-o″do-glob′u-lin) an iodine-containing globulin.

io·do·gor·gor·ic ac·id (i-o″do-gor′gər-ik) diiodotyrosine.

io·do·hip·pu·rate so·di·um (i-o″do-hip′u-rāt) an iodine-containing compound that has been used as a radiopaque medium in pyelography.

i. s. I 123 [USP] iodohippurate sodium in which a portion of the molecules are labeled with ^{123}I; administered intravenously in renography to determine renal function, urinary obstruction, and effective renal plasma flow and also in renal imaging.

i. s. I 131 [USP] iodohippurate sodium in which a portion of the molecules are labeled with ^{131}I; administered intravenously in renography to determine renal function, urinary obstruction, and effective renal plasma flow and also in renal imaging.

io·do·log·ra·phy (i-o″do-log′rə-fe) radiographic visualization of an organ or part after the injection into it of iodized oil.

io·do·meth·ane (i-o″do-meth′ān) methyl iodide.

io·do·meth·yl·nor·cho·les·ter·ol (i-o″do-meth″əl-nor″kə-les′tər-ol) norcholesterol, a cholesterol analogue, iodinated with ^{131}I, used in radionuclide imaging of the adrenal cortex. Called also *NP-59.*

io·dom·e·try (i″o-dom′ə-tre) [*iodo-* + *-metry*] estimation of the quantity of a chemical by titration with iodine. **iodomet′ric** *adj*

io·do·pa·no·ic ac·id (i-o″do-pə-no′ik) iopanoic acid.

io·do·phil (i-o′do-fil) iodinophil.

io·do·phil·ia (i-o″do-fil′e-ə) [*iodo-* + *-philia*] the reaction shown by leukocytes in certain conditions when treated with iodine or iodides. Normal leukocytes are colored bright yellow, but in certain pathologic conditions, such as toxemia and severe anemia, the polymorphonuclear leukocytes show diffuse brownish coloration. When the staining affects the leukocytes themselves, it is termed *intracellular;* when only the particles around the leukocytes are affected, it is *extracellular.*

io·do·phor (i-o′do-for) any of various compounds of iodine with carriers such as polyvinylpyrrolidone; used as surgical scrubs, surface disinfectants, and veterinary medicine skin disinfectants.

io·do·phthal·ein so·di·um (i-o″do-thal′ēn) the disodium salt of tetraiodophenolphthalein; used as a radiopaque medium in cholecystography.

io·dop·sin (i″o-dop′sin) [Gr. *iōdēs* violet colored + *opsis* vision] a photosensitive violet retinal pigment found in the retinal cones of some animals and important for color vision.

io·do·pyr·a·cet (i-o″do-pi′rə-set) a radiopaque medium, used especially in urography; administered intravenously or intramuscularly.

io·do·quin·ol (i-o″do-kwin′ol) [USP] an amebicide used in the treatment of amebic dysentery, administered orally. It has also been used topically in fungal and bacterial skin infections and in seborrheic dermatitis, usually in conjunction with a corticosteroid. Called also *diiodohydroxyquin.*

io·do·sul·fate (i-o″do-sul′fāt) a combination of a base with iodine and sulfuric acid.

io·do·ther·a·py (i-o″do-ther′ə-pe) [*iodo-* + *therapy*] treatment, usually of a goiter, with iodine or iodides.

io·do·thy·ro·glob·u·lin (i-o″do-thi″ro-glob′u-lin) iodinated thyroglobulin.

io·do·thy·ro·nine (i-o″do-thi′ro-nēn) an iodinated thyronine, such as the thyroid hormones triiodothyronine and tetraiodothyronine (thyroxine).

io·do·ty·ro·sine (i-o″do-ti′ro-sēn) any iodinated derivative of tyrosine.

io·do·ty·ro·sine de·hal·o·gen·ase (i-o″do-ti′ro-sēn de-hal′o-jən-ās) iodotyrosine deiodinase.

io·do·ty·ro·sine de·io·din·ase (i″o-do-ti′ro-sēn de-i′o-dĭ-nās) an enzyme that catalyzes the removal of iodine from monoiodotyrosine and diiodotyrosine. The reaction is a step in the conservation of iodine by the thyroid. Congenital deficiency of the enzyme results in severe loss of iodine, resulting in hypothyroidism and goiter. Called also *iodotyrosine dehalogenase.*

io·do·ven·tric·u·log·ra·phy (i-o″do-vən-trik″u-log′rə-fe) ventriculography with iodine contrast medium.

io·do·vol·a·til·iza·tion (i-o″do-vol″ə-til-ĭ-za′shən) the liberation of free iodine by living epidermal cells in the iodogenic layer of certain brown algae or kelp. It accumulates in the algae as potassium iodide and has been used as a commercial source of iodine.

io·dox·am·ic ac·id (i-o″dok-sam′ik) an ionic, dimeric radiopaque medium used in cholecystography.

io·du·ria (i″o-du′re-ə) the presence of iodine or iodides in the urine.

io·fet·amine hy·dro·chlo·ride I 123 (i″o-fet′ə-mēn) an aromatic hydrocarbon iodinated with ^{123}I; it is used as a brain imaging agent in the localization and evaluation of certain kinds of stroke.

io·gly·cam·ic ac·id (i″o-gli-kam″ik) an acid whose meglumine and sodium salts are used as radiopaque media in cholecystography.

io·hex·ol (i″o-hek′sol) [USP] a nonionic, water-soluble, low-osmolality radiopaque medium, administered by intrathecal or intravascular injection.

IOL intraocular lens.

ion (i′on) [Gr. *iōn* going] an atom or radical having a charge of positive (cation) or negative (anion) electricity owing to the loss or gain of one or more electrons. Substances that form ions are called electrolytes. See *ionic theory*, under *theory.* **ion′ic** *adj*

dipolar i. zwitterion.

hydrogen i. the nucleus of the hydrogen atom or a hydrogen atom that has lost its electron, H^+; it bears a positive charge equivalent to the negative charge of the electron and is called a proton.

hydronium i. the hydrated form, H_3O^+, in which the proton (hydrogen ion, H^+) exists in aqueous solution; a combination of H^+ and H_2O.

Io•na•min (i-on′ə-min) trademark for a preparation of phentermine.

ion•iza•tion (i″on-ĭ-za′shən) 1. any process by which a neutral atom or molecule gains or loses electrons, thus acquiring a net charge, as the dissociation of a substance in solution into ions or ion production by the passage of radioactive particles. 2. iontophoresis.

avalanche i. the multiplicative process in which a single charged particle, accelerated by a strong electric field, produces additional charged particles through collision with neutral gas molecules; called also *Townsend i.*

Townsend i. avalanche i.

ion•ize (i′on-īz) to separate into ions.

ion•o•col•or•im•e•ter (i″ŏ-no-kul″ər-im′ə-tər) an apparatus for measuring the ionic acidity of a solution.

ion•o•gen•ic (i-on″o-jen′ik) forming or supplying ions.

ion•o•mer (i-on′ə-mər) a polymer having covalent bonds within the long-chain molecules and ionic bonds between the chains; see also *glass ionomer cement*, under *cement*, and *ionomer resin*, under *resin*.

ion•om•e•ter (i″ŏ-nom′ə-tər) an instrument for the measurement of the intensity or quantity of radiation from an ionizing radiation source.

ion•o•phore (i-on′ə-for″) any molecule, as of a drug, that increases the permeability of cell membranes to a specific ion.

ion•o•phose (i′ŏ-no-fōz″) [Gr. *ion* violet + *phose*] a violet phose.

ion•o•scope (i-on′o-skōp) an instrument for detecting alkaline or acid impurity in nitrous oxide.

ion•o•ther•a•py[1] (i″o-no-ther′ə-pe) [*ion* + *therapy*] iontophoresis.

ion•o•ther•a•py[2] (i″o-no-ther′ə-pe) [Gr. *ion* violet + *therapy*] radiotherapy.

ion-pro•tein (i-on-pro′tēn) a protein molecule combined with an inorganic ion.

ion•ther•a•py (i″on-ther′ə-pe) iontophoresis.

ion•to•pho•re•sis (i-on″to-fə-re′sis) the introduction by means of the electric current, of ions of soluble salts into the tissues of the body, often for therapeutic purposes; a form of electro-osmosis. Called also *iontherapy.*

ion•to•pho•ret•ic (i-on″to-fə-ret′ik) pertaining to iontophoresis.

IOP intraocular pressure.

io•pam•i•dol (i″o-pam′ĭ-dol) a nonionic, water-soluble, low-osmolality radiopaque medium used in myelography; administered intravenously or orally.

io•pa•no•ic ac•id (i″o-pə-no′ik) [USP] an iodinated contrast medium that after oral administration is absorbed from the duodenum, conjugated with glucuronic acid in the liver, and secreted in the bile; it is used for oral cholecystography and cholangiography.

io•phen•dy•late (i″o-fen′də-lāt) [USP] a radiopaque medium used in myelography, administered intrathecally or by special injection.

io•phen•ox•ic ac•id (i″o-fən-ok′sik) a radiopaque medium used in cholecystography. Called also *triiodoethionic acid.*

Io•pi•dine (i-o′pĭ-dēn) trademark for a preparation of apraclonidine hydrochloride.

io•pro•mide (i″o-pro′mīd) [USP] a nonionic, low-osmolality radiopaque medium used for imaging of the cardiovascular system, for excretory urology, and for contrast enhancement in computed tomography; administered intra-arterially or intravenously.

IORT intraoperative radiotherapy.

io•ser•ic ac•id (i″o-ser′ik) a compound used as a radiopaque medium.

io•sul•a•mide meg•lu•mine (i″o-sul′ə-mīd) a compound used as a radiopaque medium.

io•ta (i-o′tə) [I, ι] the ninth letter of the Greek alphabet.

io•thal•a•mate (i″o-thal′ə-māt) a water-soluble iodinated contrast medium used for a wide variety of radiographic procedures, including angiography, angiocardiography, arthrography, cholangiography, urography, and contrast enhancement of computed tomographic images.

i. meglumine [USP] a radiopaque medium consisting of iothalamic acid in water for injection, prepared with the aid of meglumine. Alone, it is used intravascularly in angiography, arteriography, venography, computed tomographic brain or body imaging, and excretory urography; intraductally in cholangiography and cholangiopancreatography; intrasynovially in arthrography; and intravesically or intraureterally in cystography, cystourethrography, and pyelography. It is also often used in combination with iothalamate sodium.

i. sodium [USP] a radiopaque medium consisting of iothalamic acid in water for injection, prepared with the aid of sodium hydroxide. Alone, it is used intravascularly in angiocardiography, renal arteriography, aortography, computed tomographic brain or body imaging, and excretory urography. It is also often used in combination with iothalamate meglumine.

i. I 125 sodium [USP] sodium iothalamate in which a portion of the molecules have been iodinated with ^{125}I; used in determination of the glomerular filtration rate.

io•tha•lam•ic ac•id (i″o-thal′ə-mik) [USP] the free acid of iothalamate, used in the preparation of certain radiopaque media.

io•ver•sol (i″o-vur′sol) [USP] a nonionic contrast medium used in angiography and urography and for contrast enhancement in computed tomography.

iox•ag•late (i″ok-sag′lāt) a salt or ester of ioxaglic acid.

i. meglumine [USP] a salt of ioxaglic acid used as a low-osmolality radiopaque medium.

i. sodium [USP] a salt of ioxaglic acid used as a low-osmolality radiopaque medium.

iox•ag•lic ac•id (i″ok-sag′lik) [USP] a low-osmolality radiopaque medium.

iox•i•lan (i-ok′sĭ-lan) [USP] a low-viscosity, low-osmolality, nonionic contrast medium used in arteriography, excretory urography, and computed tomography.

IP intraperitoneal; isoelectric point.

IP$_3$ inositol 1,4,5-triphosphate.

IPAA International Psychoanalytical Association.

IPD intermittent peritoneal dialysis.

ip•e•cac (ip′ə-kak) [USP] the dried rhizome and roots of *Cephaelis ipecacuanha* (Brotero) Rich. (Rubiaceae) (Rio or Brazilian i.) or of *C. acuminata* Karsten (Cartagena, Nicaragua, or Panama i.). Originally introduced as a remedy for dysentery, it has been replaced by its alkaloid emetine for that purpose, and is now used in syrup as an emetic, particularly in cases of poisoning. It also has expectorant properties.

ipo•date (i′po-dāt) a contrast medium usually given as the calcium or sodium salt.

i. calcium the calcium salt of ipodate, used as a radiopaque medium in cholecystography, administered orally.

i. sodium [USP] the sodium salt of ipodate, used as a radiopaque medium in cholecystography, administered orally.

Ipol (i′pōl) trademark for a preparation of poliovirus vaccine inactivated.

ipo•mea (i″po-me′ə) the dried root of *Ipomoea orizabensis*, used as a cathartic; called also *Mexican scammony* and *orizaba jalap root.*

Ipo•moea (i″po-me′ə) a large genus of herbs and shrubs of the family Convolvulaceae, including morning glories and sweet potatoes. Some species, such as *I. orizaben′sis*, contain cathartic resins; others, such as some morning glories, contain toxic psychotomimetic indole alkaloids such as lysergic acid amide.

I. calo′bra the weir plant, an Australian weed that is poisonous to ruminants and can cause neurotoxic effects and blindness.

I. muelle′ri the most common species of morning glory; it contains toxic psychotomimetic alkaloids and can cause fatal neurological disease in ruminants.

***I. orizaben′sis* Ledenois** a Mexican species that is the source of the cathartic ipomea.

***I. viola′cea* L.** a species of morning glory that contains the toxic psychotomimetic alkaloid lysergic acid amide.

IPPB intermittent positive pressure breathing.

ipra•tro•pi•um bro•mide (ip″rə-tro′pe-əm) a synthetic congener of atropine with anticholinergic and antimuscarinic effects; it is administered by oral inhalation as a bronchodilator in the maintenance treatment of chronic bronchitis, pulmonary emphysema, and other forms of chronic obstructive pulmonary disease, and intranasally for the relief of rhinorrhea associated with rhinitis or the common cold.

iprin•dole (ĭ-prin′dōl) a tricyclic antidepressant with actions similar to those of amitriptyline; administered orally.

ipro•nid•a•zole (i-pro-nīd′ə-zōl) an antiprotozoal effective against *Histomonas.*

ipro•pla•tin (i′pro-plat″in) an antineoplastic analogue of cisplatin, administered intravenously; its actions are similar to those of cisplatin, but its toxicities are different and usually milder.

ipsi- [L. *ipse* self] a combining form meaning the same.

IPSID immunoproliferative small intestine disease.

ip•si•lat•er•al (ip″sĭ-lat′ər-əl) [*ipsi-* + *lateral*] situated on, pertaining to, or affecting the same side, as opposed to contralateral.

IPSP inhibitory postsynaptic potential.

IPSS inferior petrosal sinus sampling.

IPV poliovirus vaccine inactivated.

IQ intelligence quotient.

Ir iridium.

ir- see *in-*.

IRB Institutional Review Board.

ir•be•sar•tan (ur″bə-sahr′tan) [USP] an angiotensin II receptor antagonist, used as an antihypertensive; administered orally.

Ires•sa (i-res′ə) trademark for a preparation of gefitinib.

iri•dal•gia (i″rĭ-dal′jə) [*irid-* + *-algia*] pain in the iris.

ir•id•aux•e•sis (ir″id-awk-se′sis) [*irid-* + *auxesis*] thickening of the iris.

iri•dec•tome (ir″ĭ-dek′tōm) [*irid-* + Gr. *ektemnein* to cut out] a cutting instrument for use in iridectomy.

iri•dec•to•me•so•di•al•y•sis (ir″ĭ-dek″to-me″so-di-al′ə-sis) [*irid-* + *-ectomy* + *meso-* + *dialysis*] surgical formation of an artificial iris by excision and separation of adhesions around the inner edge of the iris.

iri•dec•to•mize (ir″ĭ-dek′to-mīz) to remove part of the iris by excision.

iri•dec•to•my (ir″ĭ-dek′tə-me) [*irid-* + *-ectomy*] surgical excision of a full-thickness piece of the iris; called also *corectomy*.

basal i. iridectomy at the base of the iris close to its attachment to the ciliary body.

complete i. surgical excision of a whole radial section of the iris from the root to, and including, the margin. Called also *sector i.* and *total i.*

optic i., optical i. excision of part of the iris as a means of enlarging an abnormally small pupil and improving vision.

peripheral i. a surgical treatment for narrow-angle glaucoma, consisting of a full-thickness excision of a portion of the periphery or root of the iris, with the pupillary margin and sphincter muscle being left intact.

preliminary i., preparatory i. iridectomy performed before removal of the lens in cataract surgery.

sector i. complete i.

therapeutic i. iridectomy performed for the cure of disease of the eye.

total i. complete i.

iri•dec•tro•pi•um (ir″ĭ-dek-tro′pe-əm) ectropion uveae.

iri•de•mia (ir″ĭ-de′me-ə) [*irid-* + *-emia*] hemorrhage from the iris.

iri•den•clei•sis (ir″ĭ-dən-kli′sis) [*irid-* + Gr. *enklein* to lock in] surgical creation of a permanent drain by incarceration of a slip of the iris within a corneal or limbal incision to act as a wick through aqueous humor is filtered from the anterior chamber to the subconjunctival tissues; done to reduce intraocular pressure.

iri•den•tro•pi•um (ir″ĭ-dən-tro′pe-əm) entropion uveae.

iri•de•re•mia (ir″ĭ-də-re′me-ə) aniridia.

iri•des (i′rĭ-dēz, ir′ĭ-dēz) [Gr.] plural of *iris*.

iri•des•cence (ir″ĭ-des′əns) [L. *iridescere* to gleam like a rainbow] the condition of gleaming with bright and changing colors.

iri•des•cent (ir″ĭ-des′ənt) [Gr. *iris* rainbow] having a rainbow-like display of colors in reflected light, as in mother-of-pearl; said of a colony of microorganisms.

irid•e•sis (i-rid′ə-sis) [*irid-* + *-desis*] the operation of repositioning the pupil by bringing a sector of the iris through a corneal or limbal incision and fixing the sector with a suture.

iri•di•ag•no•sis (i″rĭ-di-əg-no′sis) iridodiagnosis.

irid•i•um (Ir) (ĭ-rid′e-əm) [L. *iris* rainbow, from the tints of its salts] a very hard white metal, atomic number 77, atomic weight 192.2.

i. Ir 192 an artificial radioactive isotope of iridium, atomic mass 192, with a half-life of 73.83 days; it emits beta particles (0.67 MeV) and gamma rays (0.296, 0.308, 0.317, 0.468, 0.589, 0.604, 0.612 MeV) and is used in radiotherapy.

iri•di•za•tion (ir″ĭ-dĭ-za′shən) the subjective perception of iridescent halos about lights, occurring in glaucoma.

irid(o)- [Gr. *iris*, gen *iridos* rainbow] a combining form meaning iridescent, or denoting relationship to the iris.

iri•do•avul•sion (ir″ĭ-do-ə-vul′shən) complete tearing away of the iris from its periphery.

iri•do•cap•su•li•tis (ir″ĭ-do-kap-su-li′tis) inflammation of the iris and the capsule of the lens.

iri•do•cele (i-rid′o-sēl) [*irido-* + *-cele*[1]] hernial protrusion of a part of the iris through the cornea.

iri•do•cho•roi•di•tis (ir″ĭ-do-ko″roi-di′tis) inflammation of the iris and the choroid.

iri•do•cil•i•ary (ir″ĭ-do-sil′e-ar″e) [*irido-* + *ciliary*] pertaining to or affecting the ciliary body and iris.

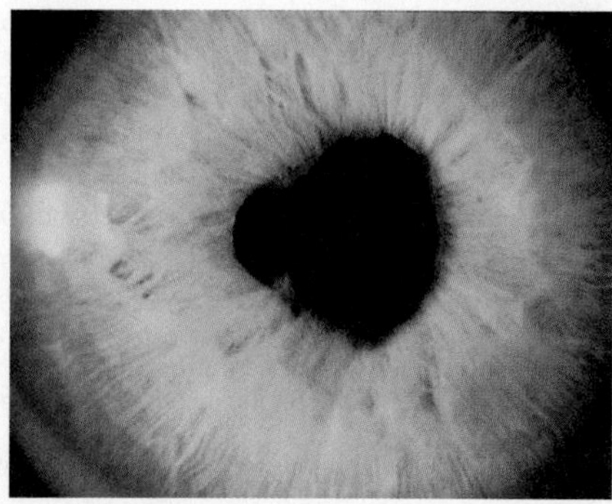

■ Iridocyclitis with an irregular pupil and posterior synechiae in a patient with pauciarticular juvenile rheumatoid arthritis.

iri•do•col•o•bo•ma (ir″ĭ-do-kol″o-bo′mə) [*irido-* + *coloboma*] coloboma of iris.

iri•do•con•stric•tor (ir″ĭ-do-kən-strik′tər) [*irido-* + *constrictor*] a muscle element or an agent that causes constriction of the pupil of the eye.

iri•do•cor•ne•al (ir″ĭ-do-kor′ne-əl) pertaining to the iris and cornea.

iri•do•cor•neo•scle•rec•to•my (ir″ĭ-do-kor″ne-o-sklə-rek′tə-me) surgical excision of a portion of the iris, cornea, and sclera for glaucoma.

iri•do•cy•clec•to•my (ir″ĭ-do-sə-klek′tə-me) [*irido-* + *cyclo-* + *ectomy*] surgical removal of a portion of the iris and of the ciliary body.

iri•do•cy•cli•tis (ir″ĭ-do-sə-kli′tis) [*irido-* + *cyclitis*] inflammation of the iris and of the ciliary body; see also *anterior uveitis*.

Fuchs heterochromic i., heterochromic i. a unilateral, low-grade type of iridocyclitis that leads to loss of pigment of the iris of the affected eye. Called also *heterochromic uveitis*.

recurrent i. periodic ophthalmia.

iri•do•cy•clo•cho•roi•di•tis (ir″ĭ-do-si″klo-ko″roi-di′tis) [*irido-* + *cyclo-* + *choroiditis*] inflammation of the iris, ciliary body, and choroid coat.

iri•do•cys•tec•to•my (ir″ĭ-do-sis-tek′tə-me) [*irido-* + *cyst-* + *ectomy*] an operation to establish an artificial pupil in an eye in which the iris adheres to the residual lens capsule, accomplished by excising a portion of the iris and lens capsule through a corneal incision.

iri•do•cyte (i-rid′o-sīt) [*irido-* + *-cyte*] one of the cells in the scales of fishes that contains crystals of guanine capable of producing iridescence.

irid•od•e•sis (ir″ĭ-dod′ə-sis) iridesis.

iri•do•di•ag•no•sis (ir″ĭ-do-di″əg-no′sis) [*irido-* + *diagnosis*] diagnosis of disease by the appearance of the iris, its color, markings, changes, etc.

iri•do•di•al•y•sis (ir″ĭ-do-di-al′ə-sis) [*irido-* + *dialysis*] separation or loosening of the iris from its root at the ciliary body, either from trauma or from surgical accident.

iri•do•di•as•ta•sis (ir″ĭ-do-di-as′tə-sis) [*irido-* + *diastasis*] a defect of the peripheral border of the iris, but not affecting the pupillary margin, producing the clinical appearance of more than one pupil.

iri•do•di•la•tor (ir″ĭ-do-di′la-tər, -di-la′tər) [*irido-* + *dilator*] 1. the dilator muscle of the pupil. 2. an agent that causes dilation of the pupil of the eye.

iri•do•do•ne•sis (ir″ĭ-do-do-ne′sis) [*irido-* + Gr. *donēsis* tremor] abnormal tremulousness of the iris on movements of the eye, occurring in subluxation of the lens or aphakia that deprives the iris of its usual support.

iri•do•ker•a•ti•tis (ir″ĭ-do-ker″ə-ti′tis) [*irido-* + *keratitis*] inflammation of the iris and cornea.

iri•do•ki•ne•sia (ir″ĭ-do-kĭ-ne′zhə) iridokinesis.

iri•do•ki•ne•sis (ir″ĭ-do-kĭ-ne′sis) [*irido-* + *kinesis*] the contraction and expansion of the iris. **iridokinet′ic** *adj*

iri•do•lep•tyn•sis (ir″ĭ-do-ləp-tin′sis) [*iris* + Gr. *leptynsis* attenuation] thinning or atrophy of the iris.

iri•dol•o•gy (ir″ĭ-dol′ə-je) [*irido-* + *-logy*] a diagnostic technique based on the premise that early pathologic changes elsewhere in the body are reflected in the iris before disease becomes clinically apparent; an analysis of a person's state of health may be made by visual examination of the iris, with the color, density, and position of deposited pigment helping to identify the pathologic process and the organ involved.

iri•do•ma•la•cia (ir″ĭ-do-mə-la′shə) [*irido-* + *malacia*] softening of the iris.

iri•do•me•so•di•al•y•sis (ir″ĭ-do-me″so-di-al′ə-sis) [*irido-* + *meso-* + *dialysis*] surgical loosening of adhesions around the inner edge of the iris.

iri•do•mo•tor (ir″ĭ-do-mo′tər) pertaining to movements of the iris; affecting contraction or dilation of the pupil of the eye.

iri•don•cus (ir″ĭ-dong′kəs) [*irid-* + Gr. *onkos* bulk] tumor or swelling of the iris.

iri•do•pa•ral•y•sis (ir″ĭ-do-pə-ral′ə-sis) iridoplegia.

iri•dop•a•thy (ir″ĭ-dop′ə-the) [*irido-* + *-pathy*] disease of the iris.

iri•do•peri•pha•ki•tis (ir″ĭ-do-per″e-fa-ki′tis) [*irido-* + *peri-* + *phakitis*] inflammation of the capsule of the crystalline lens.

iri•do•ple•gia (ir″ĭ-do-ple′jə) [*irido-* + *-plegia*] paralysis of the sphincter of the iris, with lack of contraction or dilation of the pupil.

accommodation i. failure of the pupil to contract when an accommodative effort is made.

complete i. paralysis of the sphincter of the pupil, with failure to react to any stimulus.

reflex i. failure of the pupil to contract under the influence of light or when skin is stimulated.

sympathetic i. failure of the pupil to dilate when the skin is stimulated.

iri•dop•to•sis (ir″ĭ-dop-to′sis, ir″ĭ-do-to′sis) [*irido-* + *-ptosis*] prolapse of the iris.

iri•do•pu•pil•lary (ir″ĭ-do-pu′pĭ-lar″e) pertaining to the iris and the pupil.

iri•do•rhex•is (ir″ĭ-do-rek′sis) [*irido-* + *-rrhexis*] 1. rupture of the iris. 2. the tearing away of the iris.

iri•dos•chi•sis (ir″ĭ-dos′kĭ-sis) [*irido-* + *-schisis*] splitting of the mesodermal stroma of the iris into two layers so that the anterior section separates and disintegrates into fibrils, the unattached ends of which float freely in the anterior chamber.

iri•do•scle•rot•o•my (ir″ĭ-do-skle-rot′ə-me) [*irido-* + *sclero-* + *-tomy*] a treatment for glaucoma consisting of incision of the sclera and the edge of the iris.

iri•do•ste•re•sis (ir″ĭ-do-stə-re′sis) [*irido-* + Gr. *sterēsis* loss] the absence or loss or removal of part or all of the iris.

iri•dot•o•my (ir″ĭ-dot′ə-me) [*irido-* + *-tomy*] incision of the iris, as in creating an artificial pupil.

Iri•do•vi•ri•dae (ir″ĭ-do-vir′ĭ-de) the iridoviruses: a family of DNA viruses having a virion 125–300 nm in diameter, consisting of a lipid envelope modified by protein subunits surrounding an icosahedral nucleocapsid. The genome consists of a single molecule of linear, double-stranded DNA (MW 100–250×10^6, size 150–350 kbp). Replication and assembly occur in the cytoplasm; virions are released by budding or cell destruction. Most members are insect viruses, but some are pathogenic for fish (*Lymphocystivirus*) and frogs. African swine fever virus was formerly assigned to this family.

iri•do•vi•rus (ir″ĭ-do-vi′rəs) any virus belonging to the family Iridoviridae. **iridovi′ral** *adj*

iri•no•te•can hy•dro•chlo•ride (i″rĭ-no-te′kan) a DNA topoisomerase inhibitor derived from camptothecin, used as an antineoplastic in the treatment of colorectal carcinoma; administered by intravenous infusion.

IRIS International Research Information Service.

Iris (i′ris) a genus of perennial herbs of the family Iridaceae. Some species, such as *I. missourien′sis* Nutt., have been reported to be poisonous to livestock due to an irritant principle in the leaves and rootstalks that causes gastroenteritis.

iris (i′ris) pl. *i′rides* [Gr. "rainbow, halo"] [TA] the circular pigmented membrane behind the cornea, perforated by the pupil; the most anterior portion of the vascular tunic of the eye, it is made up of a flat bar of circular muscular fibers surrounding the pupil, a thin layer of smooth muscle fibers by which the pupil is dilated, thus regulating the amount of light entering the eye, and posteriorly two layers of pigmented epithelial cells. **ir′idal, irid′ial, irid′ic** *adj*

i. bombé a condition in which the iris is bowed forward by the collection of aqueous humor between the iris and lens in total posterior synechia.

detached i. iridodialysis.

i. bicolor heterochromia iridis.

tremulous i. iridodonesis.

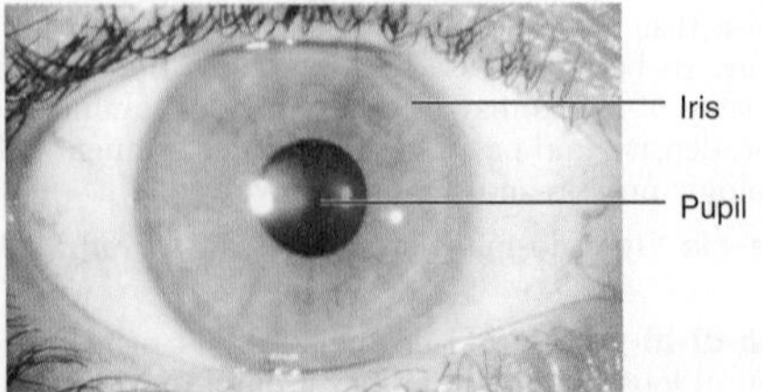

umbrella i. i. bombé.

iris•op•sia (i″ris-op′se-ə) [Gr. *iris* rainbow + *-opsia*] a visual defect in which objects appear surrounded by rings of colored light.

iri•tis (i-ri′tis) [*iris* + *-itis*] inflammation of the iris, usually marked by pain, congestion in the ciliary region, photophobia, contraction of the pupil, and discoloration of the iris. **irit′ic** *adj*

i. catamenia′lis iritis recurring before each menstrual period.

diabetic i. iritis marked by the deposit of glycogen in diabetic patients.

follicular i. iritis marked by multiple small nodules the size of a pinhead.

gouty i. painful iritis occurring in gouty patients; uratic iritis.

i. papulo′sa iritis with papules in the iris; usually syphilitic.

plastic i. iritis in which the exudate consists of fibrinous matter that forms new tissue.

purulent i. iritis in which the exudate is purulent.

serous i. iritis in which the exudate consists of serum.

spongy i. iritis with a fibrinous exudate, forming a spongy mass in the anterior chamber.

sympathetic i. iritis occurring in sympathetic ophthalmoplegia.

uratic i. gouty i.

iri•to•ec•to•my (ir″ĭ-to-ek′tə-me) [*iris* + *-ectomy*] surgical excision of iritic deposits of after-cataract, together with iridectomy, to form an artificial pupil.

irit•o•my (i-rit′ə-me) iridotomy.

IRMA immunoradiometric assay.

iron (Fe) (i′ərn) a metallic element found in certain minerals, in nearly all soils, and in mineral waters: atomic number 26; atomic weight, 55.847; specific gravity, 7.85–7.88. Iron is an essential constituent of hemoglobin, cytochrome, and other components of respiratory enzyme systems; its chief functions are in the transport of oxygen to tissues (in hemoglobin) and in cellular oxidation mechanisms. Dietary sources include muscle meats, eggs, grains, and certain vegetables and fruits. Depletion of iron stores may result in iron-deficiency anemia (q.v.). Excessive consumption of iron causes iron poisoning (q.v.). See also *ferric* and *ferrous.*

i. 55 a radioactive isotope of iron, atomic mass 55, having a half-life of 2.73 years and decaying by electron capture.

i. 59 a radioactive isotope of iron, atomic mass 59, having a half-life of 44.50 days and emitting beta particles (0.273, 0.475 MeV) and gamma rays (1.095, 1.292 MeV); it is used in ferrokinetic studies to determine the rate at which iron is cleared from the plasma and incorporated in red cells.

i. acetate a compound, $Fe(C_2H_3O_2)_3$, used as an astringent.

available i. that portion of iron in the food which can be separated from the total iron content by digestive processes.

carbonyl i. a very pure, finely divided form of elemental iron.

i. chloride either of the binary compounds $FeCl_2$ (ferrous chloride) or $FeCl_3$ (ferric chloride).

i. citrate ferric citrate.

i. dextran [USP] a sterile colloidal solution of ferric hydroxide, $Fe(OH)_3$, complexed with partially hydrolyzed low molecular weight dextran, in water for injection; administered intravenously or intramuscularly as a hematinic.

i. gluconate ferrous gluconate.

heme i. iron occurring in a heme complex, as in hemoglobin and myoglobin. As a dietary source of iron, it is found in meat, fish, and poultry. Cf. *nonheme i.*

nonheme i. iron not occurring as part of a heme complex. As a dietary source of iron, it is found in foods such as eggs, grains, vegetables, and fruits. Cf. *heme i.*

i.-polysaccharide polysaccharide-iron complex.

i. protosulfate ferrous sulfate.

reduced i. finely powdered metallic iron obtained by precipitation with hydrogen from a solution of any soluble salt of iron.

i. sorbitex [USP], **i. sorbitol** a hematinic preparation consisting of a sterile colloidal solution of a complex of trivalent iron, sorbitol, and citric acid, stabilized with dextrin and sorbitol; administered intramuscularly.

i. sucrose a complex of ferric hydroxide, $Fe(OH)_3$, in sucrose; used intravenously as a hematinic in the treatment of iron deficiency anemia in hemodialysis patients receiving supplemental erythropoietin therapy.

i. sulfate ferrous sulfate.

irot•o•my (i-rot′o-me) iridotomy.

ir•ra•di•ate (ĭ-ra′de-āt) to apply ionizing radiation for therapeutic or diagnostic purposes; see *radiotherapy.*

ir•ra•di•a•tion (ĭ-ra″de-a′shən) [*ir-* + *radiation*] 1. radiotherapy. 2. the dispersion of nervous impulse beyond the normal path of conduction. 3. the application of rays, such as ultraviolet rays, to a substance to increase its vitamin efficiency and shelf life. 4. a phenomenon in which, owing to the difference in the illumination of the field of vision, objects appear to be much larger than they really are.

extended field i. irradiation of an extended field (q.v.) in the treatment of malignant lymphomas; called also *extended field radiotherapy.*
external beam i. see under *radiotherapy.*
hemibody i. external beam radiotherapy involving exposure of half the body; called also *hemibody radiotherapy.*
interstitial i. see under *radiotherapy.*
inverted Y field i. irradiation of an inverted Y field (q.v.) in the treatment of malignant lymphoma; called also *inverted* Y *field radiotherapy.*
involved field i. irradiation of only the involved field (q.v.) in the treatment of malignant lymphoma; called also *involved field radiotherapy.*
mantle field i. irradiation of a mantle field (q.v.) as a treatment for malignant lymphoma; called also *mantle field radiotherapy.*
radical i. external beam i.
total body i. (TBI) external beam radiotherapy involving exposure of the entire body; called also *whole-body i.* or *radiotherapy.*
total lymphoid i. (TLI) irradiation of all the lymph node–bearing areas of the body, including the spleen, the thymus, and Waldeyer tonsillar ring; used in the treatment of Hodgkin disease and sometimes to induce immunosuppression prior to transplantation.
ultraviolet blood i. (UBI) a treatment involving removal of blood from a patient, exposing it to ultraviolet radiation, and returning it to the patient's circulation.
whole-body i. total body i.

ir•re•duc•i•ble (ir″e-do͞os′ĭ-bəl) not susceptible to reduction, as a fracture, dislocation, or chemical substance.

ir•reg•u•lar (ĭ-reg′u-lər) [*ir-* + *regular*] not in conformity with the rule of nature; not recurring at regular intervals.

ir•reg•u•lar•i•ty (ĭ-reg″u-lar′ĭ-te) the quality of not conforming with the rule of nature, or of not occurring at regular intervals.
i. of pulse arrhythmia.

ir•re•ver•si•ble (ir″e-vur′sĭ-bəl) incapable of being reversed.

ir•ri•gate (ir′ĭ-gāt) to wash out, as a wound; lavage.

ir•ri•ga•tion (ir″ĭ-ga′shən) [L. *irrigatio*] 1. washing by a stream of water or other fluid; see also *lavage.* 2. a liquid used for such washing.
acetic acid i. [USP] a sterile solution of glacial acetic acid in water for injection; used to irrigate the bladder in the treatment of urinary infections with cystitis.
antegrade colonic i. see under *enema.*
Ringer i. [USP] Ringer injection packaged for irrigation and used as a topical physiologic saline solution.
sodium chloride i. [USP] sodium chloride injection packaged for irrigation; used to irrigate wounds and body cavities and as an enema to flush the colon and promote evacuation.

ir•ri•ga•tor (ir′ĭ-ga″tər) [L. "waterer"] an apparatus for performing irrigation.

ir•ri•go•ra•di•os•co•py (ir″ĭ-go-ra″de-os′ko-pe) fluoroscopy of the intestines during the introduction of a contrast enema.

ir•ri•gos•co•py (ir″ĭ-gos′ko-pe) irrigoradioscopy.

ir•ri•ta•bil•i•ty (ir″ĭ-tə-bil′ĭ-te) 1. the quality or state of being irritable. 2. abnormal responsiveness to slight stimuli.
i. of the bladder see *irritable bladder,* under *bladder.*
chemical i. responsiveness to a chemical stimulus; see *chemoreceptor.*
electric i. responsiveness of nerve or muscle to the stimulus of an electric current passed through it.
mechanical i. responsiveness to a mechanical stimulus; see *mechanoreceptor.*
muscular i. the normal contractile quality of muscular tissue.
myotatic i. the capacity of a muscle to contract in response to stretching.
nervous i. 1. the ability of a nerve to transmit impulses. 2. morbid excitability of the nervous system.

ir•ri•ta•ble (ir′ĭ-tə-bəl) [L. *irritare* to tease] 1. capable of reacting to a stimulus. 2. abnormally sensitive to a stimulus. 3. prone to excessive anger, annoyance, or impatience.

ir•ri•tant (ir′ĭ-tənt) 1. giving rise to irritation. 2. an agent that produces irritation.
primary i. an agent that produces irritation, especially of the skin, on the first exposure to it.

ir•ri•ta•tion (ir″ĭ-ta′shən) [L. *irritatio*] 1. the act of stimulating. 2. a state of overexcitation and undue sensitivity.
direct i. irritation due to direct stimulation of a part.

ir•ri•ta•tive (ir′ĭ-ta″tiv) dependent on or caused by irritation.

Ir•u•kand•ji syndrome (sting) (ir″u-kan′je) [*Irukandji,* an aboriginal tribe in the vicinity of Cairns, Queensland, Australia] see under *syndrome.*

IRV inspiratory reserve volume.

Ir•ving technique (operation) (ur′ving) [F.C. *Irving,* American obstetrician and gynecologist, early 20th century] see under *technique.*

IS insertion sequence; intercostal space.

ISA intrinsic sympathomimetic activity.

Isaacs syndrome (i′zəks) [H. *Isaacs,* American neurologist, 20th century] see under *syndrome.*

I•saacs-Mer•tens syndrome (i′zəks mer′tenz) [H. *Isaacs;* H.G. *Mertens,* German neurologist, 20th century] see under *syndrome.*

isa•tin (i′sə-tin) a crystalline compound, $C_8H_5O_2N$, in the form of yellowish red crystals, soluble in alcohol and ether, slightly soluble in water; used as a reagent.

is•aux•e•sis (is″awk-se′sis) [*iso-* + *auxesis*] growth of a part or parts at the same rate as the growth of the whole.

is•che•mia (is-ke′me-ə) [*isch-* + *emia*] deficiency of blood in a part, usually due to functional constriction or actual obstruction of a blood vessel. **ische′mic** *adj*
brachiocephalic i. Takayasu arteritis.
cerebral i. see under *infarction.*
cold i. ischemia owing to a lowered temperature of the blood, as occurs naturally in hibernating animals; it is a common hazard of organs cryopreserved for transplantation.
colonic i. acute vascular insufficiency of the colon, usually the part supplied by the inferior mesenteric artery; see *ischemic colitis,* under *colitis.*
hepatic i. injury to liver cells resulting from a deficiency of blood or oxygen, usually because of hypotension from decreased cardiac output, shock, or some other cause. Called also *hypoxic* or *ischemic hepatitis* and *shock liver.*
hypoxia-i. see under H.
intestinal i. acute vascular insufficiency of part of the intestine, such as in mesenteric ischemia or colonic ischemia.
mesenteric i. ischemia in an area of the intestine supplied by a mesenteric artery; two types are distinguished, *occlusive* and *nonocclusive mesenteric i.* It may progress to a mesenteric infarction (see under *infarction*).
myocardial i. deficiency of blood supply to the heart muscle, due to obstruction or constriction of the coronary arteries.
nonocclusive mesenteric i. mesenteric ischemia caused by a low rate of blood flow rather than by occlusion; because the subtlety of clinical and radiological signs often delays diagnosis, the risk of intestinal gangrene is high.
occlusive mesenteric i. mesenteric ischemia caused by occlusion of one of the mesenteric arteries, such as by a thrombus or mechanical compression of the artery.
i. re′tinae anemia of the retina; it may occur after profuse hemorrhage in another part of the body or result from arterial embolism or poison.
silent i. cardiac ischemia without pain or other symptoms.
subendocardial i. deficiency of blood supply to the myocardium adjacent to the endocardium.
vertebrobasilar i. see under *insufficiency.*

is•che•sis (is-ke′sis) [Gr. *ischein* to suppress] retention or suppression of a discharge.

is•chia (is′ke-ə) [L.] plural of *ischium.*

is•chi•a•del•phus (is″ke-ə-del′fəs) ischiodidymus.

is•chi•ad•ic (is″ke-ad′ik) 1. sciatic (def. 2). 2. ischial.

is•chi•al (is′ke-əl) pertaining to the os ischii (ischium); called also *ischiadic, ischiatic,* and *sciatic.*

is•chi•al•gia (is″ke-al′jə) [*ischio-* + *-algia*] pain in the os ischii (ischium); called also *ischiodynia.*

is•chi•at•ic (is″ke-at′ik) [L. *ischiaticus*] 1. sciatic (def. 2). 2. ischial.

is•chi•ec•to•my (is″ke-ek′tə-me) surgical removal or excision of the ischium.

ischi(o)- [Gr. *ischion* hip] a combining form denoting relationship to the os ischii (ischium), or to the hip.

is•chio•anal (is″ke-o-a′nəl) pertaining to the ischium and anus.

is•chio•bul•bar (is″ke-o-bul′bər) [*ischio-* + *bulbar*] pertaining to the os ischii (ischium) and the bulb of the urethra.

is•chio•cap•su•lar (is″ke-o-kap′su-lər) [*ischio-* + *capsular*] pertaining to the ischium and the capsular ligament of the hip joint.

is•chio•cele (is′ke-o-sēl″) sciatic hernia.

is•chio•coc•cyg•e•al (is″ke-o-kok-sij′e-əl) pertaining to the ischium and coccyx.

is•chio•coc•cyg•e•us (is″ke-o-kok-sij′e-əs) [*ischio-* + *coccygeus*] ischiococcygeal; see also *musculus ischiococcygeus.*

is•chio•did•y•mus (is″ke-o-did′ĭ-məs) [*ischio-* + *-didymus*] symmetrical conjoined twins united at the pelvis.

is•chio•dym•ia (is″ke-o-dim′e-ə) [*ischio-* + Gr. *didymos* twin + *-ia*] the condition of symmetrical conjoined twins united at the pelvis.

is•chio•dyn•ia (is″ke-o-din′e-ə) [*ischio-* + *-odynia*] ischialgia.

is•chio•fem•o•ral (is″ke-o-fem′o-rəl) pertaining to the ischium and femur.

is•chio•fib•u•lar (is″ke-o-fib′u-lər) pertaining to the ischium and the fibula.

is•chio•glu•te•al (is″ke-o-gloo′te-əl) pertaining to the ischium and the buttocks.

is•chi•om•e•lus (is″ke-om′ə-ləs) [*ischio-* + Gr. *melos* limb] a fetus with an extra limb attached at the base of the vertebral column.

is•chio•ni•tis (is″ke-o-ni′tis) inflammation of the tuberosity of the ischium.

is•chio•pa•gia (is″ke-o-pa′jə) the condition exhibited by an ischiopagus.

is•chi•op•a•gus (is-ke-op′ə-gəs) [*ischio-* + *-pagus*] conjoined twins fused at the ischia, the axes of the two bodies extending in a straight line but in opposite directions; according to the number of lower limbs shared, classified as *bipus, tripus,* and *tetrapus.*

is•chi•op•a•gy (is″ke-op′ə-je) ischiopagia.

is•chio•pu•bic (is″ke-o-pu′bik) pertaining to the ischium and pubis.

is•chio•rec•tal (is″ke-o-rek′təl) pertaining to the ischium and rectum; see also *ischioanal.*

is•chio•sa•cral (is″ke-o-sa′krəl) pertaining to the ischium and sacrum.

is•chio•tho•ra•cop•a•gus (is″ke-o-tho″rə-kop′ə-gəs) iliothoracopagus.

is•chio•vag•i•nal (is″ke-o-vaj′ĭ-nəl) pertaining to the ischium and vagina.

is•chio•ver•te•bral (is″ke-o-vur′tə-brəl) pertaining to the ischium and the vertebral column.

is•chi•um (is′ke-əm) pl. *is′chia* [L., from Gr. *ischion* hip] TA alternative for *os ischii.* See Plate 40.

isch(o)- [Gr. *ischein* to suppress] a combining form denoting relationship to suppression or deficiency.

is•cho•gy•ria (is″ko-ji′re-ə) [*ischo-* + *gyrus*] a condition in which the cerebral convolutions have a jagged appearance, as in bulbar sclerosis.

isch•uria (is-ku′re-ə) [*ischo-* + *-uria*] urinary retention.

i. paradox′a a condition in which the bladder is overdistended with urine, although the patient continues to urinate.

i. spas′tica urinary retention caused by spasm of the sphincter urinae.

ISCP International Society of Comparative Pathology.

-ise see *-ize.*

is•ei•co•nia (i″si-ko′ne-ə) iseikonia. **iseicon′ic** *adj*

is•ei•ko•nia (i″si-ko′ne-ə) [*is-* + Gr. *eikon* image + *-ia*] a condition in which the image of an object is the same in both eyes. Spelled also *iseiconia* and *isoiconia.* **iseikon′ic** *adj*

Isen•tress (i-sen′tres) trademark for a preparation of raltegravir.

is•eth•i•o•nate (i″sə-thi′ə-nāt) USAN contraction for 2-hydroxyethanesulfonate.

is•eth•i•o•nic ac•id (is″eth-i-on′ik) trivial name for 2-hydroxyethanesulfonic acid; used in detergents and surfactants and in synthesis.

ISGE International Society of Gastroenterology; International Society of Gynelogic Endocrinology; International Society of Gynecological Endocrinology.

ISH International Society of Hematology.

Ishi•ha•ra plates, test (e″she-hah′rah) [Shinobu *Ishihara,* Japanese ophthalmologist, 1879–1963] see under *plate* and *test.*

isin•glass (i′sin-glas) a form of gelatin prepared from the swimming bladders of the Russian sturgeon, *Acipenser huso;* used as an adhesive and clarifying agent. Called also *ichthyocolla.*

is•land (i′lənd) 1. something isolated or surrounded. 2. a cluster of cells or an isolated piece of tissue. See also *islet.*

blood i's aggregations of mesenchyme cells in the angioblast of the early embryo, as in the wall of the yolk sac and umbilical vesicle; they subsequently develop into vascular endothelium and blood cells.

bone i. a benign focus of mature cortical bone appearing within trabecular bone on a radiograph.

i's of Calleja discrete collections of pyramidal and polymorphic cells in the caudal part of the anterior perforated substance (olfactory tubercle). Called also *olfactory i's* and *islets of Calleja.*

cartilage i's see *intrachondrial bone,* under *bone.*

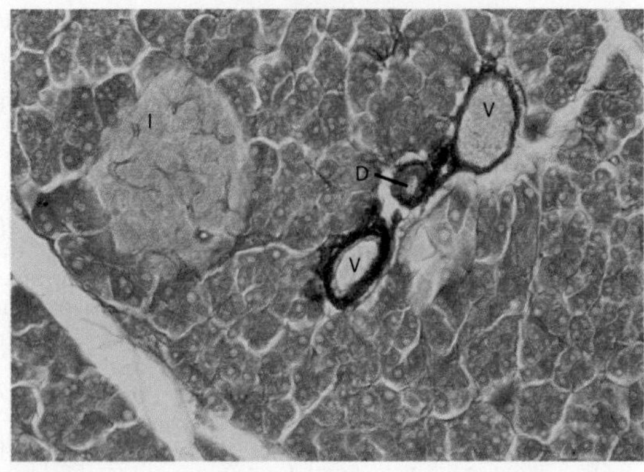

■ Pancreatic islet *(I)*, surrounded by acinar tissue. Blood vessels *(V)* and a small duct *(D)* are also shown.

CpG i's a region of DNA in vertebrate genomes that contains clusters of the dinucleotide 5′-CG-3′ (CpG), which are unmethylated in the germline and in most somatic cells; such regions are located upstream of all housekeeping and some other genes, and appear to play roles in development and regulation of gene expression.

i's of Langerhans see under *islet.*

olfactory i's i's of Calleja.

i's of pancreas pancreatic islets.

Pander i's reddish yellow cords of corpuscular matter in the splanchnopleure of the embryo which develop into blood and blood vessels.

i. of Reil insula (def. 2).

is•let (i′let) a cluster of cells or an isolated piece of tissue; see also *island.*

blood i's see under *island.*

Calleja i's see under *island.*

i's of Langerhans, pancreatic i's irregular microscopic structures scattered throughout the pancreas and comprising its endocrine part (the *endocrine pancreas*). They are composed of at least four types of cells: the *alpha cells,* which secrete glucagon; the *beta cells,* which are the most abundant and secrete insulin; the *delta cells,* which secrete somatostatin; and the *PP cells,* which secrete pancreatic polypeptide. Degeneration of the beta cells, whose secretion (insulin) is important in carbohydrate metabolism, is the major cause of type I diabetes mellitus. Called also *insulae pancreaticae* [TA], *islands of Langerhans,* and *islands of pancreas.*

Walthard i's microscopic inclusions of the germinal epithelium of the ovary, found either in contact with the serosal covering or just below it; they have been implicated in the development of Brenner tumors. Called also *Walthard cell rests* or *inclusions.*

ISM International Society of Microbiologists.

-ism [Gr. *-ismos* noun-forming suffix] a word termination denoting *(a)* a state or condition, particularly a disease state resulting from a specific cause, e.g., alcoholism, *(b)* a process, *(c)* the result of an action, or *(d)* a doctrine or principle, e.g., determinism.

Is•me•lin (is′mə-lin) trademark for a preparation of guanethidine monosulfate.

Is•mo (īs′mo) trademark for a preparation of isosorbide mononitrate.

Is•mot•ic (īs-mot′ik) trademark for a preparation of isosorbide.

ISO International Standards Organization.

is(o)- [Gr. *isos* equal] a prefix or combining form meaning equal, alike, the same, or uniform. In immunology, it indicates *from* a genetically

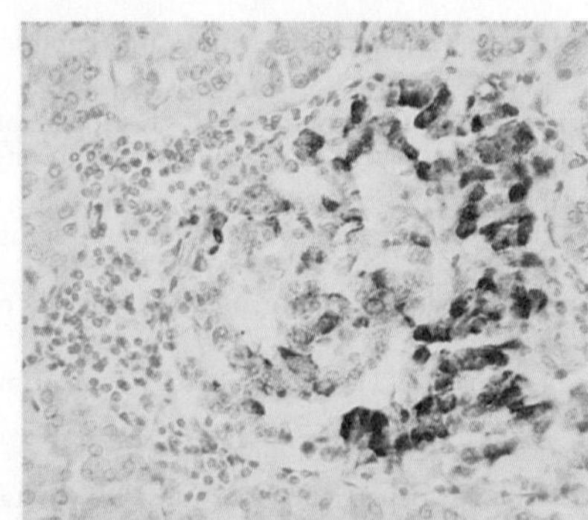

■ Pancreatic islet in early type 1 diabetes mellitus; on the left side it has been infiltrated with T lymphocytes and beta cells are not seen, while on the right the remaining beta cells stain brown with antibody to insulin.

identical individual (as an isograft) or existing in alternate forms in the same species (as an isoantigen). In chemistry it denotes a structural isomer; used in trivial names of alkanes to indicate a one-carbon branch next to the end of the chain, e.g., isohexane is 2-methylpentane; an isoalkyl radical has its free valence at the end of the chain opposite the branch, i.e., isohexyl is 4-methylpentyl.

iso•adre•no•cor•ti•cism (i″so-ə-dre″no-kor′tĭ-siz-əm) euadrenocorticism.

iso•ag•glu•ti•na•tion (i″so-ə-gloo″tĭ-na′shən) agglutination of cells from members of a species by agglutinins originating in genetically dissimilar members of the same species.

iso•ag•glu•ti•nin (i″so-ə-gloo′tĭ-nin) an agglutinin from members of a species that agglutinates cells of genetically different members of the same species.

iso•al•lele (i″so-ə-lēl′) [*iso-* + *allele*] an allele that appears phenotypically identical to another, but that can be distinguished at the protein or DNA level.

iso•al•le•lism (i″so-ə-le′liz-əm) [*iso-* + *allele*] the presence of isoalleles at a locus.

iso•al•lox•a•zine (i″so-ə-lok′sə-zēn) a tricyclic compound comprising a pyrazine ring flanked by a benzene ring and uracil; it is the parent compound of riboflavin and other flavins.

iso•am•yl meth•oxy•cin•na•mate (i″so-am′əl mə-thok″se-sin′ə-māt) amiloxate.

iso•am•yl ni•trite (i″so-am′əl ni′trīt) amyl nitrite.

iso•an•dros•ter•one (i″so-an-dros′tər-ōn) epiandrosterone.

iso•an•ti•body (i-so-an′tĭ-bod″e) an antibody produced by one individual that reacts with antigens (isoantigens) of another individual of the same species; called also *alloantibody*.

iso•an•ti•gen (i″so-an′tĭ-jən) an antigen that induces an immune response when transferred (as by blood transfusion or tissue graft) to a genetically dissimilar individual of the same species.

iso•bar (i′so-bahr) [*iso-* + Gr. *baros* weight] one of two or more chemical species with the same atomic weight but different atomic numbers.

iso•bar•ic (i″so-bar′ik) [*iso-* + *bar-* + *-ic*] 1. having equal or constant pressure or weight across space or time; see also under *solution.* 2. pertaining to an isobar or isobars.

iso•bu•caine hy•dro•chlo•ride (i″so-bu′kān) a local anesthetic, used in combination with epinephrine in dentistry.

iso•bu•tane (i″so-bu′tān) a branched chain configuration of butane, $CH_3CH(CH_3)_2$; cf. *normal butane* and see illustration at *isomerism.*

iso•ca•lo•ric (i″so-kə-lor′ik) containing or providing the same number of calories; equicaloric.

iso•car•box•a•zid (i″so-kahr-bok′sə-zid) a monoamine oxidase inhibitor used as an antidepressant and in the prophylaxis of migraine; administered orally.

iso•cel•lu•lar (i″so-sel′u-lər) [*iso-* + *cellular*] composed of cells of the same kind and size.

iso•cen•ter (i′so-sen′tər) a point at which there is a maximum or minimum of the radiation dose, i.e., the center of the surrounding isodose curves.

iso•cho•les•ter•in (i″so-kə-les′tər-in) isocholesterol.

iso•cho•les•ter•ol (i″so-kə-les′tər-ol) a compound found with cholesterol in wool; apparently a mixture of C_{30} trimethyl cholestanes; a component of lanolin alcohols (see under *alcohol*).

iso•chro•mat•ic (i″so-kro-mat′ik) [*iso-* + *chromatic*] of the same color throughout.

iso•chro•mat•o•phil (i″so-kro-mat′o-fil) [*iso-* + *chromato-* + *-phil*] staining equally with the same dye.

iso•chro•mo•some (i″so-kro′mə-sōm) [*iso-* + *chromosome*] an abnormal chromosome having a median centromere and two identical arms, probably formed by the transverse, rather than the normal longitudinal separation of the centromere of the replicating chromosome. See illustration at *aberration.*

isoch•ro•nal (i-sok′rə-nəl) isochronous.

iso•chron•ic (i″so-kron′ik) isochronous.

isoch•ro•nism (i″sə-kro′niz-əm) [*iso-* + *chrono-* + *-ism*] correspondence between processes with respect to their time, rate, or frequency. Called also *isochrony.*

isoch•ro•nous (i-sok′rə-nəs) [*iso-* + *chrono-* + *-ous*] 1. performed in equal times; said of motions, vibrations, or waves occurring at the same time and being equal in duration. 2. of ciliary beating, occurring in unison; cf *metachronous.* 3. pertaining to or characterized by isochronism; called also *isochronal* and *isochronic.*

isoch•ro•ny (i-sok′rə-ne) isochronism.

isoch•ro•ous (i-sok′ro-əs) [*iso-* + Gr. *chroa* color] isochromatic.

iso•ci•trate (i″so-sĭ′trāt) a fully dissociated (ionized) salt of isocitric acid.

iso•ci•trate de•hy•dro•gen•ase (NAD$^+$) (i″so-sĭ′trāt de-hi′drə-jən-ās) [EC 1.1.1.41] a mitochondrial enzyme that catalyzes the oxidative decarboxylation of isocitrate to form α-ketoglutarate, using NAD^+ as an electron acceptor; the reaction is the key rate-limiting step of the tricarboxylic acid cycle. The enzyme requires Mg^{2+} or Mn^{2+} and is activated by ADP, citrate, and Ca^{2+} and inhibited by NADH, NADPH, and ATP.

iso•ci•trate de•hy•dro•gen•ase (NADP$^+$) (i″so-sĭ′trāt de-hi′drə-jən-ās) [EC 1.1.1.42] an enzyme of the oxidoreductase class that catalyzes the oxidative decarboxylation of isocitrate to form α-ketoglutarate, using $NADP^+$ as an electron acceptor. The enzyme exists as two isozymes, one cytoplasmic and one mitochondrial, requires Mg^{2+} or Mn^{2+}, and occurs in all tissues. The reaction serves to maintain the level of reducing equivalents within the cell.

iso•cit•ric ac•id (i″so-sit′rik) a structural isomer of citric acid, that is an intermediate in the citric (tricarboxylic) acid cycle (q.v.).

iso•co•na•zole (i″so-kon′ə-zōl) an imidazole antifungal used in the treatment of vulvovaginal candidiasis and fungal skin infections; administered topically or intravaginally.

iso•co•ria (i″so-kor′e-ə) [*iso-* + *cor-* + *-ia*] equality in size of the two pupils.

iso•cor•tex (i″so-kor′teks) [*iso-* + *cortex*] [TA] the neocortex as opposed to the allocortex, so called because histologically it consists of six layers and is much more uniform than the allocortex. Called also *homotypical cortex.*

Iso•crin (i′so-krin) trademark for a preparation of oxyphenisatin acetate.

iso•cy•a•nate (i″so-si′ə-nāt) the radical —NCO, often occurring as diisocyanate (q.v.). See also under *asthma.*

iso•cy•a•nide (i″so-si′ə-nīd) one of a class of organic compounds isomeric with the cyanide compounds, containing the N≡C group and characterized by a disagreeable odor; called also *isonitrile.*

iso•cy•clic (i″so-sik′lik, -si′klik) homocyclic.

iso•cy•tol•y•sin (i″so-si-tol′ə-sin) [*iso-* + *cytolysin*] a cytolysin that acts on the cells of animals of the same species as that from which it is derived.

iso•cy•to•sis (i″so-si-to′sis) [*iso-* + *-cyte* + *-osis*] equality of the size of cells, especially red blood corpuscles.

iso•dac•tyl•ism (i-so-dak′təl-iz-əm) [*iso-* + *dactyl-* + *-ism*] a condition in which the fingers are of relatively even length.

iso•dense (i′so-dens″) having the same density as other similar objects, such as an object or area whose density matches that of others on a radiograph.

iso•des•mo•sine (i″so-des′mo-sēn) one of two unusual amino acids found in elastin, the other being desmosine.

iso•di•a•met•ric (i″so-di″ə-met′rik) [*iso-* + *dia-* + *metron* measure] having the same diameter in all directions.

iso•don•tic (i″so-don′tik) [*iso-* + *odontic*] having all the teeth of the same size and shape.

iso•dose (i′so-dōs″) a radiation dose of equal intensity to more than one body area; see also under *curve.*

iso•dy•nam•ic (i″so-di-nam′ik) [*iso-* + *dynamic*] exhibiting equal force or power.

iso•dy•nam•o•gen•ic (i″so-di-nam″o-jen′ik) [*iso-* + *dynamogenic*] producing equal force or power.

iso•ef•fect (i″so-ə-fekt′) an effect midway between two reference points; see under *line.*

iso•ei•co•sa•noid (i″so-i-ko′sə-noid) any of a number of eicosanoid isomers produced from arachidonic acid by the action of free radicals; this group includes the isoprostanes.

iso•elec•tric (i″so-e-lek′trik) [*iso-* + *electric*] showing no variation in electric potential.

iso•en•er•get•ic (i″so-en″ər-jet′ik) exhibiting equal energy.

iso•en•zyme (i″so-en′zīm) isozyme.

Regan i. an isoenzyme of alkaline phosphatase, similar or identical to placental alkaline phosphatase and originating in a variety of tumors, particularly those of the lung. It is occasionally detectable in normal serum.

iso•eth•a•rine (i″so-eth′ə-rēn) a β_2-adrenergic receptor agonist, used as a bronchodilator for the treatment of acute episodes of bronchoconstriction; administered by inhalation.

i. hydrochloride [USP] the hydrochloride salt of isoetharine, having the same actions and uses as the base.

i. mesylate [USP] the mesylate salt of isoetharine, having the same actions and uses as the base.

iso·eu·gen·ol (i″so-u′jən-ol) an aromatic compound used in fragrances; it is a significant cause of sensitization and allergic contact dermatitis.

iso·feb·ri·fu·gine (i″so-feb″rĭ-fu′jēn) an antimalarial alkaloid found in the plant *Dichroa febrifuga* (ch'ang shan).

iso·flu·rane (i″so-floo′rān) [USP] a potent inhalational anesthetic, an isomer of enflurane with similar properties, used for induction and maintenance of general anesthesia.

iso·flu·ro·phate (i″so-flo͞or′o-fāt) [USP] name for diisopropyl flurophosphate (DFP), a potent irreversible anticholinesterase agent, when used as a pharmaceutical; applied topically to the conjunctiva to produce miosis, decrease intraocular pressure, and potentiate accommodation in treatment of glaucoma and accommodative esotropia.

iso·form (i′so-form″) any of a group of two or more different proteins that are produced by different genes and are specific to different tissues but have the same function and a similar sequence.

iso·gam·ete (i″so-gam′ēt) [*iso-* + *gamete*] a gamete of the same size and structure as the gamete with which it unites.

iso·ga·met·ic (i″so-gə-met′ik) characterized by the production of gametes of the same size.

iso·gam·e·ty (i″so-gam′ə-te) production by an individual of one sex of gametes identical with respect to the sex chromosome.

isog·a·my (i-sog′ə-me) [*iso-* + Gr. *gamos* marriage] reproduction resulting from the union of two cells (gametes) that are identical in size and structure, as occurs in protozoa. **isog′amous** *adj*

iso·ge·ne·ic (i″so-jə-ne′ik) syngeneic.

iso·ge·ner·ic (i″so-jə-ner′ik) of the same kind; pertaining to or obtained from individuals of the same genus.

iso·gen·e·sis (i″so-jen′ə-sis) [*iso-* + *-genesis*] similarity in the processes of development.

iso·gen·ic (i″so-jen′ik) syngeneic.

isog·e·nous (i-soj′ə-nəs) developed from the same cell.

iso·graft (i′so-graft″) syngraft.

iso·he·mag·glu·ti·na·tion (i″so-he″mə-gloo″tĭ-na′shən) agglutination of erythrocytes caused by a hemagglutinin from another individual of the same species.

iso·he·mag·glu·ti·nin (i″so-he″mə-gloo′tĭ-nin) a hemagglutinin that agglutinates the erythrocytes of other individuals of the same species.

iso·he·mol·y·sin (i″so-he-mol′ə-sin) [*iso-* + *hemolysin*] a hemolysin that acts on the blood of animals of the same species as that from which it is derived.

iso·he·mol·y·sis (i″so-he-mol′ə-sis) hemolysis of the blood corpuscles of an animal by the lysins in serum from another animal of the same species. **isohemolyt′ic** *adj*

iso·hy·dric (i″so-hi′drik) maintaining a steady pH (concentration of hydrogen ions); see *buffer*.

iso·ico·nia (i″so-i-ko′ne-ə) iseikonia. **isoicon′ic** *adj*

iso·im·mu·ni·za·tion (i″so-im″u-nĭ-za′shən) development of antibodies against an antigen derived from a genetically dissimilar individual of the same species; see also *isoantigen*.

Rh i. development of antibodies against Rh antigens, the antigen involved in almost all cases being the Rh_0 antigen (D antigen). Rh isoimmunization of Rh-negative women may occur after transfusion of Rh-positive blood or during pregnancy with an Rh-positive fetus, when the mother is exposed to fetal blood during delivery, amniocentesis, miscarriage, or abortion, and may result in the development of erythroblastosis fetalis in any subsequent pregnancy with an Rh-positive fetus. See also *Rh_0 (D) immune globulin*, under *globulin*.

iso·in·tense (i″so-in-tens′) having the same intensity as some other object.

Iso·ji·ma test (e″so-je′mah) [S. *Isojima*, Japanese physician, late 20th century] sperm immobilization test; see under *test*.

iso·ki·net·ic (i″so-kĭ-net′ik) maintaining constant torque and tension as muscles shorten or lengthen; see isokinetic exercise, under *exercise*.

iso·late (i′so-lāt) 1. to separate from other persons, materials, or objects. 2. in microbiology, to obtain from a source such as a clinical specimen a pure strain that may have been part of a mixed primary culture. 3. a population that has been obtained by isolation (such as bacteria or other cells obtained in pure culture), or a group of individuals prevented by geographic, ecologic, or social barriers from interbreeding with others of their kind, and thus differentiated by the accumulation of new characteristics.

iso·la·tion (i″so-la′shən) 1. the process of isolating, or the state of being isolated. 2. physical separation of a part, as by tissue culture or by interposition of inert material. 3. the extraction and purification of a chemical substance of unknown structure from a natural source. 4. the separation of infected individuals from those uninfected for the period of communicability of a particular disease; cf. *quarantine* (def. 1). 5. the successive propagation of a growth of microorganisms until a pure culture is obtained. 6. a type of defense mechanism in which emotions are separated from the ideas, impulses, or memories to which they usually connect, so that the idea or impulse enters consciousness detached from its unacceptable feeling. Called also *isolation of affect*.

iso·la·tor (i″so-la′tər) anything that isolates.

surgical i. a large, clear, plastic bag with human-sized pockets that is attached to the patient's body during surgical procedures to prevent contamination by infective agents; the pockets, in which the nurses and surgeons stand, have plastic helmets, earphones and microphones for communication, and closed sleeves leading into the bag through which the surgeons work.

iso·lec·i·thal (i″so-les′ĭ-thəl) [*iso-* + *-lecithal*] having small amounts of yolk evenly distributed throughout the cytoplasm, as in the eggs of mammals and echinoderms.

iso·leu·cine (Ile, I) (i″so-loo′sēn) 1. an essential amino acid, α-amino-β-methylvaleric acid, produced by the hydrolysis of fibrin and other proteins; necessary for optimal growth in infants and for nitrogen equilibrium in human adults. See also table at *amino acid*. 2. [USP] a preparation of isoleucine used as a dietary supplement.

iso·leu·cyl (i″so-loo′səl) the acyl radical of isoleucine.

iso·leu·ko·ag·glu·ti·nin (i″so-loo″ko-ə-gloo′tĭ-nin) a leukocyte agglutinin.

isol·o·gous (i-sol′ə-gəs) characterized by an identical genotype; see *isograft*.

iso·ly·ser·gic ac·id (i″so-li-sur′jik) one of the main cleavage products of the alkaline hydrolysis of the alkaloids characteristic of ergot, and the parent compound of the ergotinine group of alkaloids.

isol·y·sin (i-sol′ə-sin) a lysin that acts on the cells of animals of the same species as that from which it is derived.

isol·y·sis (i-sol′ə-sis) lysis of cells by isolysins. **isolyt′ic** *adj*

iso·mal·tase (i″so-mawl′tās) oligo-1,6-glucosidase; see *α-dextrinase*.

iso·mal·tose (i″so-mawl′tōs) a reducing disaccharide isomeric with maltose, differing in having α-(1,6) rather than α-(1,4) glycosidic linkage; it occurs at branch points of polymers such as glycogen and amylopectin.

iso·mer (i′so-mər) [*iso-* + Gr. *meros* part] any compound exhibiting, or capable of exhibiting, isomerism. An isomer may be structural or stereochemical; see *isomerism*.

isom·er·ase (i-som′ər-ās) [EC 5] a class of enzymes that catalyze geometric or structural changes within a molecule to form a single product. The reactions do not involve a net change in the concentration of compounds other than the substrate and the product. The class includes epimerases, isomerases, mutases, and racemases.

isom·er·ide (i-som′ər-īd) isomer.

isom·e·rism (i-som′ə-riz-əm) [*iso-* + Gr. *meros* part] the relationship that exists between two or more different chemical compounds that have the same molecular formula; it is divided into two broad classes: *constitutional i.* and *stereoisomerism* (q.v.). **isomer′ic** *adj*

chain i. a type of constitutional isomerism in which the compounds differ in regard to the linkages in the basic chain of carbon atoms; see illustration.

***cis-trans* i.** geometric i.

configurational i. stereoisomerism.

conformational i. the relationship between stereoisomers that differ only by rotations about single bonds (conformers).

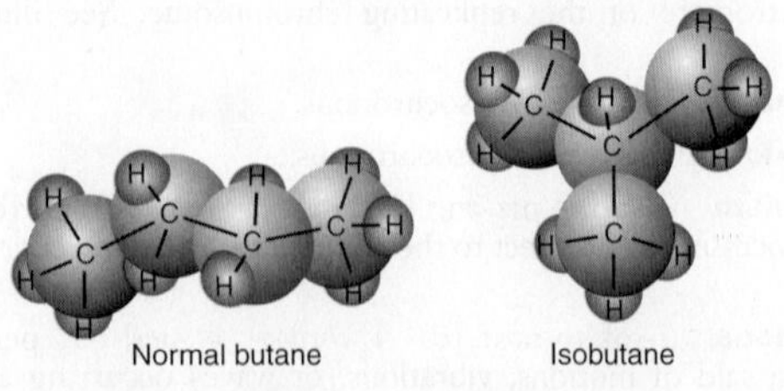

■ Chain isomerism.

constitutional i. the relationship between two or more isomers that have different structures (the same atoms linked in different ways), in contrast to stereoisomerism in which the isomers have the same structure but different configurations (the same linkages but different spatial arrangements). Called also *structural i.*

functional group i. a type of constitutional isomerism dependent upon the presence of different functional groups, such compounds being of distinct chemical types, e.g., ethyl alcohol, C_2H_5OH, and dimethyl ether, CH_3OCH_3.

geometric i. an old division of stereoisomerism that contains isomers that differ in the arrangement of substituents of a rigid structure, such as double-bonded carbon atoms or a ring. The *cis* isomer has two referenced groups on the same side of the ring or double bond; the *trans* isomer on opposite sides. Geometric isomers are thus diastereomers. Called also *cis-trans i.*

optical i. an old division of stereoisomerism that contains isomers that differ in the arrangement of substituents at one or more asymmetric carbon atoms; thus some but not necessarily all are optically active, e.g., *d-*, *l-*, and *meso*-tartaric acid. Some optical isomers are enantiomers (the *d* and *l* forms); some are diastereomers (the *d* and *meso* forms).

position i. a type of constitutional isomerism in which the position occupied by an atom or group differs with reference to the same fundamental carbon chain; for example, *n*-propyl chloride, $CH_3CH_2CH_2Cl$, and isopropyl chloride, $CH_3CHClCH_3$.

spatial i., stereochemical i. stereoisomerism.

structural i. constitutional i.

substitution i. position i.

isom·er·iza·tion (i-som″ər-ĭ-za′shən) the process whereby any isomer, whether structural or stereochemical, is converted into another, usually requiring special conditions of temperature, pressure, or catalysts.

iso·meth·ep·tene mu·cate (i″so-mə-thep′tēn mu′kāt) [USP] an indirect-acting sympathomimetic amine that reduces the stimuli that lead to vascular headaches by constricting dilated carotid and cerebral vessels, used in combination with dichloralphenazone and acetaminophen in the treatment of migraine and tension headache.

iso·met·ric (i″so-met′rik) [*iso-* + Gr. *metron* measure] 1. maintaining the same measurements; of equal dimensions. 2. maintaining uniform length; see under *contraction* and *exercise.*

iso·me·tro·pia (i″so-mə-tro′pe-ə) [Gr. *isometros* of equal measure + *-opia*] equality in the refraction of the two eyes.

isom·e·try (i-som′ə-tre) equality of dimension.

iso·mor·phic (i″so-mor′fik) isomorphous.

iso·mor·phism (i″so-mor′fiz-əm) the quality of being isomorphous.

iso·mor·phous (i″so-mor′fəs) [*iso-* + *-morphous*] being similar in form.

iso·mus·ca·rine (i″so-mus′kə-rēn) a basic substance formed by oxidizing choline; it is isomeric with muscarine, but has different physiologic properties.

iso·neph·ro·tox·in (i″so-nef′ro-tok″sin) [*iso-* + *nephrotoxin*] a nephrotoxin which acts on cells of the animals of the same species from which it is derived.

iso·ni·a·zid (INH) (i″so-ni′ə-zid) [USP] an antibacterial, used as a tuberculostatic, administered orally and intramuscularly.

iso·nic·o·tin·o·yl·hy·dra·zine (i″so-nik″o-tin″o-əl-hi′drə-zēn) isoniazid.

iso·nic·o·tin·yl·hy·dra·zine (i″so-nik″o-tin″əl-hi′drə-zēn) isoniazid.

iso·ni·trile (i″so-ni′trīl) isocyanide.

iso·on·cot·ic (i″so-on-kot′ik) having the same oncotic pressure.

iso·os·mot·ic (i″so-oz-mot′ik) isosmotic.

Iso·paque (i″so-pāk′) trademark for preparations of metrizoate sodium.

Iso·par·or·chis tri·sim·i·li·tu·bis (i″so-pər-or′kis tri-sim″ĭ-lĭ-too′bis) a fluke, commonly parasitic in the air bladder of fish in India and China and sometimes found in humans.

isop·a·thy (i-sop′ə-the) [*iso-* + *-pathy*] the treatment of disease by means of products of the disease or with material from the organ affected, e.g., smallpox by giving minute doses of variolous matter, disease of the liver by giving extract of liver, etc.

isoph·a·gy (i-sof′ə-je) [*iso-* + *-phagy*] autolysis.

iso·pho·ria (i″so-for′e-ə) [*iso-* + *phoria*] equality in the tension of the vertical muscles of each eye; absence of hyperphoria and of hypophoria.

iso·pia (i-so′pe-ə) [*iso-* + *-opia*] equality of vision in the two eyes.

iso·plas·tic (i″so-plas′tik) [*iso-* + *plastic*] syngeneic.

iso·pre·cip·i·tin (i″so-pre-sip′ĭ-tin) a precipitin that is active against antigens of animals of the same species (but of dissimilar genetic makeup) as the animal in which it is formed.

iso·preg·ne·none (i″so-preg′nə-nōn) dydrogesterone.

iso·pren·a·line (i″so-pren′ə-lēn) INN and BAN for *isoproterenol.*

iso·prene (i′so-prēn) an unsaturated branched chain five-carbon hydrocarbon that is the molecular unit of isoprenoid compounds.

CH_3
|
$CH_2 = C — C = CH_2$
|
H

iso·pre·noid (i″so-pre′noid) any compound biosynthesized from or containing isoprene units, including terpenes, carotenoids, fat soluble vitamins, ubiquinone, rubber, and some steroids.

iso·pro·pa·mide io·dide (i″so-pro′pə-mīd) [USP] a long-acting quaternary anticholinergic, used in the treatment of peptic ulcer and other gastrointestinal disorders marked by hyperacidity and hypermotility, administered orally.

iso·pro·pa·nol (i″so-pro′pə-nol) isopropyl alcohol; see under *alcohol.*

iso·pro·pyl (i″so-pro′pəl) the univalent radical, $(CH_3)_2CH—$.

i. alcohol see under *alcohol.*

i. rubbing alcohol see under *alcohol.*

i. meprobamate carisoprodol.

i. myristate [NF] a compound of isopropyl alcohol and saturated high molecular weight fatty acids, principally myristic acid, occurring as a clear, oily liquid; used as an emollient in pharmaceutical preparations.

iso·pro·pyl·ar·te·re·nol (i″so-pro″pəl-ahr″tə-re′nol) isoproterenol.

iso·pros·tane (i″so-pros′tān) any of a group of prostaglandin isomers found in plasma and urine; some are increased in various pathological states.

iso·pro·ter·e·nol (i″so-pro-ter′ə-nol) a synthetic adrenergic, derived from norepinephrine, acting as a nonselective β-adrenergic receptor agonist and having powerful bronchodilator and cardiac stimulant actions.

i. hydrochloride [USP] the hydrochloride salt of isoproterenol, administered intravenously in the treatment of bradycardia and of bronchospasm during anesthesia. It has also been used as a bronchodilator in the treatment of bronchospasm associated with chronic obstructive airway disease, usually administered by oral inhalation.

i. sulfate [USP] the sulfate salt of isoproterenol; administered by oral inhalation as a bronchodilator in the treatment of bronchospasm associated with chronic obstructive airway disease.

isop·ter (i-sop′tər) [*iso-* + Gr. *optēr* observer] a line depicting the area in the field of vision in which the visual acuity is the same.

Isop·tin (īs-op′tin) trademark for preparations of verapamil hydrochloride.

Isop·to-Car·pine (i-sop″to-kahr′pēn) trademark for a preparation of pilocarpine hydrochloride.

iso·pyk·nic (i″so-pik′nik) [*iso-* + *pykn-* + *-ic*] of equal density or thickness; see under *centrifugation.*

Isor·dil (i′sor-dil) trademark for preparations of isosorbide dinitrate.

iso·ri·bo·fla·vin (i″so-ri′bo-fla″vin) an isomer of riboflavin that acts as an antimetabolite to riboflavin and can cause riboflavin deficiency in laboratory animals.

iso·ru·bin (i″so-roo′bin) new fuchsin.

iso·scope (i′so-skōp) [*iso-* + *-scope*] an apparatus for observing the changes of position of the horizontal and vertical lines in the movements of the eyeball.

iso·sen·si·ti·za·tion (i″so-sen″sĭ-tĭ-za′shən) allosensitization.

iso·se·rine (i″so-se′rēn) a compound, isomeric with serine.

iso·sex·u·al (i″so-sek′shoo-əl) [*iso-* + *sexual*] pertaining to or characteristic of the same sex.

isos·mot·ic (i″soz-mot′ik) having the same osmotic pressure.

isos·mo·tic·i·ty (i″soz-mo-tis′ĭ-te) the state or quality of being isosmotic.

iso·sor·bide (i″so-sor′bīd) [USP] a bicyclic ether derivative of glucitol; used as an osmotic diuretic to reduce intraocular pressure.

i. dinitrate [USP] the dinitric acid ester of isosorbide, having coronary and peripheral vasodilating properties; used in the treatment of coronary insufficiency and angina pectoris, administered sublingually and orally.

i. mononitrate an active metabolite of isosorbide dinitrate, having the same actions and uses; administered orally.

Isos·po·ra (i-sos′pə-rə) [*iso-* + *spore*] a genus of coccidian protozoa (suborder Eimeriina, order Eucoccidiida) having two sporocysts in each oocyst and four sporozoites in each sporocyst; found in birds, amphibians, and reptiles. Mammalian parasites formerly classified in this genus have been assigned to the genus *Cystoisospora.*

I. bel′li *Cystoisospora belli.*

I. bige′mina *Cystoisospora burrowsi.*

I. fe′lis *Cystoisospora felis.*

I. ho′minis former name for *Sarcocystis hominis.*

I. laca′zei a species causing intestinal coccidiosis in birds.

I. rivol′ta *Cystoisospora rivolta.*

I. su′is *Cystoisospora suis.*

iso·spore (i′so-spor) [*iso-* + *spore*] 1. an isogamete of organisms that reproduce by spores. 2. an asexual spore produced by a homosporous organism.

isos·po·ri·a·sis (i-sos″pə-ri′ə-sis) 1. infection with protozoa of genus *Isospora.* 2. cystoisosporiasis.

isos·po·rous (i-sos′pə-rəs) having isospores.

iso·stere (i′so-stēr) a compound resembling another compound in electron arrangement but differing in chemical structure.

isos·then·uria (i″sos-thə-nu′re-ə) [*iso-* + *sthen-* + *-uria*] excretion of urine that has not been concentrated by the kidneys and has the same osmolality as that of plasma.

iso·ther·a·py (i″so-ther′ə-pe) [*iso-* + *therapy*] isopathy.

iso·tacho·pho·re·sis (i″so-tak″o-fə-re′sis) [*iso-* + *tacho-* + *phoresis*] a method of zone electrophoresis in which the sample is sandwiched between a lead electrolyte of higher mobility than that of the sample and a trailing electrolyte of lower mobility, in order to eliminate broadening of the zones of separated substances by the carrier electrolytes.

iso·ther·mo·gno·sis (i″so-thur″mo-no′sis) [*iso-* + *therm-* + *gnōsis* recognition] a dysesthesia in which pain, cold, and heat stimuli are all perceived as heat.

iso·thi·o·cy·a·nate (i″so-thi″o-si′ə-nāt) an ester of isothiocyanic acid, R—N═C═S.

allyl i. see under *allyl.*

iso·thi·o·cy·an·ic ac·id (i″so-thi″o-si-an′ik) the molecular species H—N═C═S, which occurs in equilibrium with thiocyanic acid.

iso·throm·bo·ag·glu·ti·nin (i″so-throm″bo-ə-gloo′tĭ-nin) a platelet isoagglutinin.

iso·tone (i′so-tōn″) one of several nuclides having the same number of neutrons, but differing in the number of protons in their nuclei.

iso·to·nia (i″so-to′ne-ə) [*iso-* + *ton-* + *-ia*] 1. a condition of equal tone, tension, or activity. 2. equality of osmotic pressure between two elements of a solution or between two different solutions.

iso·ton·ic (i″so-ton′ik) [*iso-* + *tonic*] 1. denoting a solution in which body cells can be bathed without a net flow of water across the semipermeable cell membrane. 2. denoting a solution having the same tonicity as some other solution with which it is compared, such as physiologic salt solution and the blood serum. 3. maintaining uniform tonus; see under *contraction* and *exercise.*

iso·to·nic·i·ty (i″so-to-nis′ĭ-te) the quality of being isotonic.

iso·tope (i′so-tōp″) [*iso-* + *-tope*] a chemical element having the same atomic number as another (i.e., the same number of nuclear protons) but possessing a different atomic mass (i.e., a different number of nuclear neutrons).

radioactive i. radioisotope.

stable i. an isotope that does not transmute into another element with emission of corpuscular or electromagnetic radiations.

iso·to·pol·o·gy (i″so-to-pol′ə-je) the scientific study of isotopes, and of their uses and applications.

iso·tox·in (i′so-tok″sin) [*iso-* +*toxin*] a toxic substance produced by one animal and poisonous to others of the same species. **isotox′ic** *adj*

iso·trans·plant (i″so-trans′plant) isograft.

iso·trans·plan·ta·tion (i″so-trans″plan-ta′shən) the transplanting of an isograft.

iso·tret·i·noin (i″so-tret′ĭ-no-in, -noin) 13-*cis*-retinoic acid, used systemically for treatment of severe cystic and conglobulate acne; it inhibits the secretion of sebum and alters the lipid composition of the skin surface.

Isot·ri·cha (i-sot′rĭ-kə) [*iso-* + Gr. *thrix, trichos* hair] a genus of ciliate protozoa (suborder Trichostomatina, order Trichostomatida) found in the stomachs of ungulates, and characterized by the presence of an apical cytostome and by dense longitudinal rows of cilia over the entire body surface. Species include *I. prostoma* and *I. intestinalis.*

iso·tri·mor·phism (i″so-tri-mor′fiz-əm) [*iso-* + *tri-* + *morph-* + *-ism*] isomorphism between the three forms of two trimorphous substances. **isotrimor′phous** *adj*

iso·tron (i′so-tron) an apparatus for separating isotopes electromagnetically.

iso·tro·pic (i″so-tro′pik) [*iso-* + *-tropic*] 1. similar in all directions with respect to a property, as in a cubic crystal or a piece of glass. 2. being singly refractive.

isot·ro·py (i-sot′ro-pe) the quality or condition of being isotropic.

iso·type (i′so-tīp) an immunoglobulin heavy or light chain class or subclass characterized by antigenic determinants (isotypic markers) in the constant region. Every normal individual expresses all of the isotypes of its species. Cf. *allotype* and *idiotype.* **isotyp′ic** *adj*

iso·typ·i·cal (i″so-tip′ĭ-kəl) [*iso-* + *typical*] of the same type.

iso·ure·tin (i″so-u-re′tin) formamidoxim, a compound isomeric with urea.

iso·va·ler·ic ac·id (i″so-və-ler′ik) a carboxylic acid occurring in excess in the plasma and urine in isovalericacidemia.

iso·va·ler·ic·ac·i·de·mia (i″so-və-ler″ik-as″ĭ-de′me-ə) an autosomal recessive aminoacidopathy caused by mutation in the *IVD* gene (locus: 15q14-q15), which encodes isovaleryl-CoA dehydrogenase; the resulting enzyme deficiency leads to elevated plasma levels of isovaleric acid and urinary levels of isovaleric acid and isovalerylglycine, causing a characteristic odor of sweaty feet. Clinical signs include severe acidosis and ketosis, lethargy, convulsions, pernicious vomiting, thrombocytopenia, neutropenia, and pancytopenia. Two clinical forms exist: the *acute neonatal form* leads rapidly to coma and death; the *chronic intermittent form* is milder and usually of later onset, with acute episodic attacks and variable psychomotor dysfunction.

iso·va·ler·yl (i″so-və-ler′əl) the radical of isovaleric acid; the thioester formed with coenzyme A, isovaleryl CoA, is an intermediate in the catabolism of leucine.

iso·val·er·yl-CoA de·hy·dro·gen·ase (i″so-və-ler′əl-ko-a′ de-hi′drojən-ās) [EC 1.3.99.10] an enzyme of the oxidoreductase class that catalyzes the dehydrogenation of isovaleryl CoA to 3-methylcrotonyl CoA, using ubiquinone as an electron acceptor. The reaction is a step in the use of leucine as a fuel. Deficiency of the enzyme, an autosomal recessive trait, results in isovalericacidemia.

iso·va·ler·yl·gly·cine (i″so-və-ler″əl-gli′sēn) a conjugate of isovaleric acid and the amide group of glycine; high levels are formed and excreted in the urine in isovalericacidemia.

iso·vo·lu·mic (i″so-və-loo′mik) [*iso-* + *volume*] maintaining the same volume.

Iso·vue (i′so-vu) trademark for preparations of iopamidol.

isox·su·prine hy·dro·chlo·ride (i-sok′su-prēn) [USP] an adrenergic, used as a vasodilator in the treatment of cerebral vascular insufficiency and of peripheral vascular diseases such as arteriosclerosis obliterans, thromboangiitis obliterans, and Raynaud disease. It is administered orally or intramuscularly.

iso·zyme (i′so-zīm) one of various structurally related forms of an enzyme, each having the same mechanism but with differing chemical, physical, or immunologic characteristics. For example, lactate dehydrogenase, a tetramer, exists as five isozymes arising from different combinations of its two kinds of subunits. Called also *isoenzyme.*

is·pa·ghu·la (is″pə-goo′lə) [Persian *ispaghōl* horse's ear, from the shape of the leaves] psyllium.

is·rad·i·pine (is-rad′ĭ-pēn) [USP] a calcium channel blocking agent with actions similar to those of nifedipine, used alone or with a thiazide diuretic for the treatment of hypertension; administered orally.

is·sue (ish′oo) a discharge of pus, blood, or other matter; a suppurating lesion emitting such a discharge.

isth·mec·to·my (is-mek′tə-me) [*isthmus* + *-ectomy*] excision of an isthmus, particularly a thyroid isthmus affected with goiter.

isth·mi (is′mi) [L.] plural of *isthmus.*

isth·mi·tis (is-mi′tis) inflammation of the isthmus of the fauces.

isth·mo·pa·ral·y·sis (is″mo-pə-ral′ə-sis) isthmoplegia.

isth·mo·ple·gia (is″mo-ple′jə) [*isthmus* + *-plegia*] paralysis of the isthmus of the fauces.

isth·mus (is′məs) pl. *isth′mi* [L., from Gr. *isthmos*] a narrow connection between two larger bodies or parts. **isth′mian, isth′mic** *adj*

anterior i. of fauces i. faucium.

i. aor′tae [TA], **aortic i.** a narrowed portion of the aorta, especially noticeable in the fetus, at the point where the ductus arteriosus is attached.

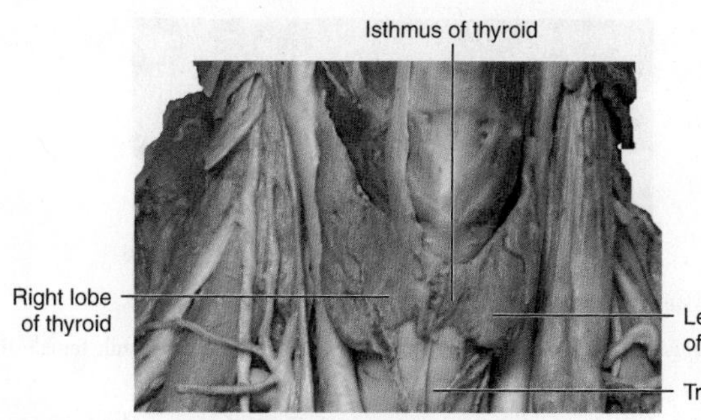

■ Isthmus glandulae thyroideae (isthmus of thyroid gland) connecting the two lobes.

i. of auditory tube i. tubae auditivae.
i. cartila′ginis auricula′ris [TA], **i. cartila′ginis au′ris** isthmus of auricular cartilage: a bridge of cartilage connecting the cartilage of the external acoustic meatus with the main part of the cartilage of the auricle of the external ear.
i. of cingulate gyrus i. gyri cinguli.
i. of eustachian tube i. tubae auditivae.
i. of external auditory meatus a narrowing in the osseous part of the meatus about 2 cm from the internal end of the concha.
i. of fallopian tube i. tubae uterinae.
i. of fauces, i. fau′cium [TA] the constricted aperture between the oral cavity and the pharynx, bounded by the palatoglossal arches and the posterior aspect of the tongue. Called also *oropharyngeal i.*
follicular i. the portion of a hair follicle between the stem and the infundibulum.
i. of gastric gland the part of a gastric gland immediately adjacent to the opening into the gastric pit.
i. glan′dulae thyroi′deae [TA] isthmus of thyroid gland: the band of tissue connecting the lobes of the thyroid gland. Called also *thyroid i.*
i. gy′ri cingula′tus, i. gy′ri cin′guli [TA] isthmus of cingulate gyrus: the constricted portion of the cingulate gyrus, connecting with the parahippocampal gyrus in the region of the splenium of the corpus callosum.
i. gy′ri fornica′ti i. gyri cinguli.
i. of His i. rhombencephali.
i. of limbic lobe i. gyri cinguli.
oropharyngeal i. i. faucium.
i. pro′statae [TA], **i. of prostate** the commissure on the base of the prostate, between the right and the left lateral lobe. Called also *commissura prostatae* [TA alternative] and *commissure of prostate.*
i. rhombence′phali [TA] isthmus of rhombencephalon: a narrow segment of the brain in the fetus, forming the plane of separation between the rhombencephalon and the cerebrum; called also *i. of His.*
thyroid i., i. of thyroid gland i. glandulae thyroideae.
i. tu′bae auditi′vae [TA] isthmus of auditory tube: the narrowest part of the auditory tube, at the junction of the pars ossea and the pars cartilaginea of the tube. Called also *i. tubae auditoriae* [TA alternative].
i. tu′bae audito′riae TA alternative for *i. tubae auditivae.*
i. tu′bae uteri′nae [TA] isthmus of uterine tube: the narrow part of the uterine tube at its junction with the uterus.
i. u′teri [TA] isthmus of uterus: the constricted part of the uterus between the cervix and the body.
i. of Vieussens limbus fossae ovalis.

ISU International Society of Urology.

Isu•prel (i′su-prəl) trademark for preparations of isoproterenol hydrochloride.

itch (ich) 1. any of various skin disorders in which pruritus is a characteristic. 2. pruritus. 3. popular term for *scabies.*
Aujeszky i. pseudorabies.
baker's i. any of several inflammatory dermatoses of the hands seen in bakers; one type is a chronic onychomycosis, and another type is a protein contact dermatitis resulting from proteins in wheat flour.
barber's i. 1. sycosis barbae. 2. tinea barbae.
barn i. sarcoptic mange.
chorioptic i. see under *mange.*
clam digger's i. cercarial dermatitis.
copra i. a dermatitis affecting persons who unload coconuts, caused by the mite *Tyrophagus castellani.*
dew i. ground i.
dhobie i. 1. dhobie mark i. 2. tinea cruris in persons whose clothes have been washed by traditional Indian methods with harsh soaps.
dhobie mark i. a type of urushiol dermatitis seen in laundry workers (dhobies) in India who use a type of marking fluid made from bhilawanol oil and containing urushiols. Called also *dhobie mark dermatitis.*
grain i. a self-limited eruption with wheals and itching, caused by the mite *Pyemotes ventricosus,* which parasitizes the larvae of insects that infest straw, grain, and other plants; it affects persons coming in contact with host plants. Called also *acarodermatitis urticarioides* and *prairie* or *straw i.*
grocer's i. a type of dermatitis with blistering, seen in grocers and caused by mites such as *Glycyphagus domesticus* (which infests stored hides, dried fruits, and grain), or *Tyrophagus* species (which infest copra and cheese).
ground i. the cutaneous manifestations of hookworm disease (see under *disease*), consisting of an itching eruption after larvae enter the skin; seen in humans, cats, and dogs. Called also *hookworm* or *uncinarial dermatitis.*
jock i. tinea cruris.
mad i. pseudorabies.
prairie i. grain i.
Queensland i. *Culicoides* hypersensitivity.
seven-year i. popular term for *scabies.*
straw i. grain i.
sweet i. *Culicoides* hypersensitivity.
swimmer's i. cercarial dermatitis.
winter i. popular term for *asteatotic eczema.*

itch•ing (ich′ing) pruritus.

-ite[1] [Gr. *-itēs* noun and adjective suffix] a suffix denoting a mineral or a rock, or a part of a body or of an organ.

-ite[2] [F., alteration of *-ate*] in chemistry, a suffix denoting a salt or ester of an acid with a name ending in *-ous,* e.g., phosphite. Cf. *-ate*[2].

iter (i′tər) [L.] a way or tubular passage. **i′teral** *adj*
i. chor′dae ante′rius anterior canaliculus for chorda tympani.
i. chor′dae poste′rius canaliculus chordae tympani.

it•ero•par•i•ty (it″ər-o-par′ĭ-te) [L. *iterare* to repeat + *parity*] the state, in an individual organism, of reproducing repeatedly, or more than once in a lifetime.

it•er•op•a•rous (it″ər-op′ə-rəs) [L. *iterare* to repeat + *-parous*] reproducing more than once in a lifetime.

-ites [Gr. *-itēs,* a masculine adjectival termination agreeing with *hydrōps* dropsy (understood)—e.g., tympanites, the windy dropsy] a word termination indicating edema of the part denoted by the word stem to which it is attached.

ith•y•cy•phos (ith″e-si′fōs) ithyokyphosis.

ith•y•lor•do•sis (ith″e-lor-do′sis) [Gr. *ithys* straight + *lordosis*] lordosis without any lateral curvature.

ith•yo•ky•pho•sis (ith″e-o-ki-fo′sis) [Gr. *ithys* straight + *kyphosis*] backward projection of the vertebral column.

-itis pl. *-i′tides* [*-itis,* a feminine adjectival termination agreeing with Gr. *nosos* disease (understood)] a word termination denoting inflammation of the part indicated by the word stem to which it is attached.

Ito hypomelanosis, nevus (e′to) [Minor *Ito,* Japanese dermatologist, 20th century] see under *hypomelanosis* and *nevus.*

ITP idiopathic thrombocytopenic purpura; inosine triphosphate.

it•ra•co•na•zole (it″rə-kon′ə-zōl) a triazole antifungal that inhibits synthesis of ergosterol and so disrupts the fungal cell membrane; used in a variety of infections, administered orally.

ITT insulin tolerance test.

IU International unit *(on the JCAHO "Do Not Use" List).*

IUD intrauterine device.

IUGR intrauterine growth retardation (or restriction).

IUI intrauterine insemination.

IV intravenous; see also under *injection.*

IVC inferior vena cava.

Ivee•gam (i-ve′gam) trademark for a preparation of immune globulin intravenous (human).

Ive•mark syndrome (e′və-mahrk) [Björn Isaac Isaacson *Ivemark,* Swedish pathologist, born 1925] see under *syndrome.*

iver•mec•tin (i″vər-mek′tin) [USP] a semisynthetic member of the avermectin group, most commonly used as an antiparasitic in domestic animals; it is sometimes used to treat human onchocerciasis and as a secondary agent to treat intestinal strongyloidiasis; administered orally.

IVF in vitro fertilization.

IVIC syndrome (e′vēk) [*I*nstituto *V*enezolano de *I*nvestigaciones *C*ientíficas, where it was first observed in 1980] see under *syndrome.*

Ivo•mec (i′vo-mek) trademark for preparations of ivermectin.

Ivor Lew•is esophagectomy (i′vor loo′is) [*Ivor Lewis,* Welsh surgeon, 1895–1982] transthoracic esophagectomy.

ivo•ry (i′vo-re) 1. the bonelike substance (modified dentin) of the tusks of elephants and other large mammals. Called also *ebur.* 2. dentinum.

IVP intravenous pyelogram; intravenous pyelography.

IVRT isovolumic relaxation time.

IVS interventricular septum (of heart).

Ivy loop wiring (i′ve) [Robert Henry *Ivy*, English-born American maxillofacial surgeon, 1881–1974] see under *wiring*.

Ivy test (method) (i′ve) [Andrew Conway *Ivy*, American physiologist, 1893–1978] see under *test*.

Iwan•off (Iwan•ow) cysts (e-vahn′of) [Vladimir P. *Iwanoff* (or *Iwanow*), Russian ophthalmologist, late 19th century] see *Blessig cysts*, under *cyst*.

ixa•bep•i•lone (iks″ə-bep′ĭ-lōn) a microtubule inhibitor used as an antineoplastic alone or in combination with capecitabine for treatment of advanced or metastatic breast cancer that has resisted other drugs; administered by intravenous infusion.

Ix•em•pra (iks-em′prə) trademark for a preparation of ixabepilone.

Ix•o•des (ik-so′dēz) [Gr. *ixōdes* like bird-lime] a genus of parasitic ticks of the family Ixodidae.

I. coo′kei a species found in eastern and midwestern Canada and the United States, attacking dogs and sometimes other mammals; it is the main vector for Powassan encephalitis.

I. dam′mini species name formerly given to a group that is now included in *I. scapularis*.

I. hexa′gonus a species found primarily in Western Europe, attacking wild and domestic carnivores and sometimes humans, and occasionally serving as a vector for borreliosis.

I. holocy′clus a species found in Australia and New Guinea, usually on small marsupials but occasionally on other animals; it is a vector for borreliosis, Queensland tick typhus, and tick paralysis.

I. mar′xi a species most often found on squirrels in the eastern United States and Canada, a vector for Powassan encephalitis.

I. paci′ficus the western black-legged tick, a common species along the Pacific Coast of North America from Mexico to Canada; it usually attacks deer and cattle but sometimes bites humans, and is a vector of Lyme disease, Rocky Mountain spotted fever, and tularemia.

I. persulca′tus the taiga tick, a species found in various parts of Europe and across Asia to Japan, parasitic on ruminants and sometimes other mammals. In humans it is the primary vector for Russian spring-summer encephalitis and sometimes a vector for Lyme disease. In sheep it is a vector for louping ill. In a variety of animals it is a vector for anaplasmosis, babesiosis, and tularemia.

I. rici′nus the castor bean tick, a species found in Europe, Asia, North Africa, and the Americas, parasitic on various mammals. It is a vector for diseases including anaplasmosis, canine babesiosis, louping ill, Lyme disease, erythema chronicum migrans, Russian spring-summer encephalitis, and tularemia.

I. rubicun′dus a species that attacks ruminants in western and southern Africa and causes tick paralysis.

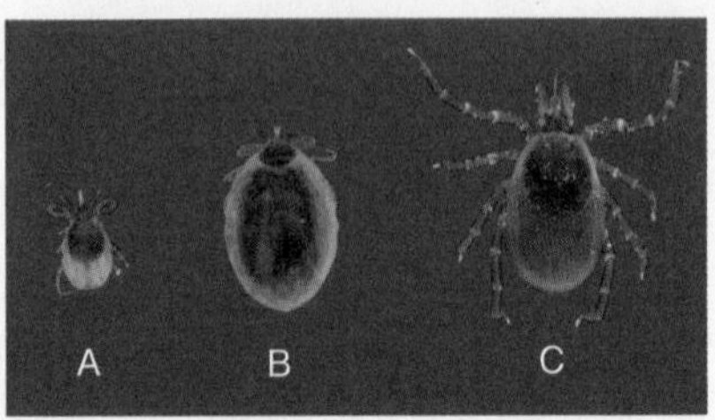

■ *Ixodes scapularis.* Unengaged nymph *(A)*; engorged nymph *(B)*; adult female *(C)*.

I. scapula′ris the eastern black-legged tick, the principal vector of Lyme disease, anaplasmosis, and babesiosis in eastern and midwestern North America, and an occasional vector of tularemia. Its usual reservoirs are mice of the genus *Peromyscus*. Ticks formerly classified as *I. dammini* are now considered a subgroup of this species.

I. spinipal′pus a species that infests rabbits and squirrels in western Canada, and is a vector for Powassan encephalitis.

I. tasma′ni a species found in Australia, usually on small marsupials but occasionally on other mammals; it is a vector for spotted fevers and tick paralysis.

ix•o•di•a•sis (ik″so-di′ə-sis) 1. any disease or lesion due to the bite of an ixodid tick. 2. infestation with ixodid ticks.

ix•od•ic (ik-sod′ik) ixodid (def. 1).

ix•o•did (ik′so-did) 1. pertaining to or caused by ticks of the family Ixodidae. 2. a tick of the family Ixodidae; called also *ixodid* or *hard tick*. 3. pertaining to or caused by ticks of the genus *Ixodes*.

Ix•od•i•dae (ik-sod′ĭ-de) the hard ticks, a family of the superfamily Ixodoidea, distinguished from the soft ticks (Argasidae) by the presence of a scutum. Genera of medical or veterinary interest include *Amblyomma*, *Anocentor*, *Aponomma*, *Boophilus*, *Dermacentor*, *Haemaphysalis*, *Hyalomma*, *Ixodes*, and *Rhipicephalus*.

Ix•od•i•des (ik-sod′ĭ-dēz) the ticks, a suborder of Acarina, including the superfamily Ixodoidea, which comprises the families Ixodidae and Argasidae.

Ix•o•diph•a•gus (ik″so-dif′ə-gəs) a genus of hymenopteran insects. *I. caucur′tei* is a parasite of ixodid ticks.

ix•o•dism (ik′so-diz-əm) ixodiasis.

Ix•o•doi•dea (ik″so-doi′de-ə) a superfamily of the suborder Ixodides, which embraces the families Argasidae and Ixodidae.

Iyen•gar yoga (e-yen′gahr) [Bellur Krishnamachar Sundararaja *Iyengar*, Indian yoga teacher, born 1918] see under *yoga*.

-ize [Gr. *-izein* verb-forming suffix] a word termination meaning *(a)* to cause to be, *(b)* to cause to acquire some quality, *(c)* to become, *(d)* to become similar to, *(e)* to subject to an action or treatment.

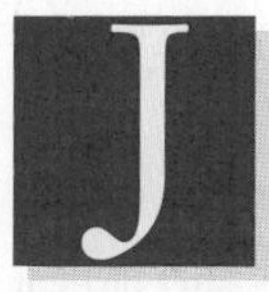

J joule.

jaag·siek·te (yahg-sēk′tə) pulmonary adenomatosis (def. 2).

Ja·bou·lay amputation (operation) (zhah″boo-la′) [Mathieu *Jaboulay*, French surgeon, 1860–1913] hemipelvectomy.

Jac·coud arthropathy (arthritis, syndrome) (zhah-koo′) [Sigismond *Jaccoud*, French physician, 1830–1913] see under *arthropathy*.

jack·et (jak′ət) 1. an enveloping structure or garment, especially a covering for the trunk or for the upper part of the body. 2. jacket crown; see under *crown*.

Minerva j. a plaster-of-Paris jacket that includes both the trunk and the head, with the ears and face left free; used for fractures of the cervical spine and after operations for torticollis.

plaster-of-Paris j. a casing of plaster of Paris enveloping the body for the purpose of correcting deformities.

porcelain j. a jacket crown of porcelain.

Risser j. a combination of plaster, turnbuckles, and hinges, extending from the chin and occiput to one knee, sometimes including one upper limb as far as the elbow; used in scoliosis.

strait j. straitjacket.

jack·screw (jak′skroo″) a threaded device used in orthodontic appliances for the separation or approximation of teeth or jaw segments.

Jack·son appliance, crib (jak′sən) [Victor Hugo *Jackson*, American dentist, 1850–1929] see under *appliance*.

Jack·son's law (rule), syndrome (jak′sənz) [John Hughlings *Jackson*, English neurologist, 1835–1911] see under *law* and *syndrome*.

Jack·son membrane (veil) (jak′sən) [Jabez North *Jackson*, American surgeon, 1868–1935] see under *membrane*.

Jack·son safety triangle (jak′sən) [Chevalier *Jackson*, American laryngologist, 1865–1958] see under *triangle*.

jack·so·ni·an (jak-so′ne-ən) named for John Hughlings *Jackson*, as *jacksonian epilepsy* and *jacksonian march*.

Jacob's ladder (ja′kəb) [from the ladder extending to heaven seen in a dream by the biblical patriarch *Jacob*] 1. an herb of the genus *Polemonium*, especially *P. caeruleum*, a blue-flowered Eurasian species that has astringent, diaphoretic, and hemolytic effects. Called also *Greek valerian*. 2. preparations of *P. caeruleus* herb, used topically for ulcers and internally as an infusion for fever and inflammation.

Ja·cob ulcer (ja′kəb) [Arthur *Jacob*, Irish ophthalmologist, 1790–1874] see under *ulcer*.

ja·co·bine (ja′ko-bin) a poisonous pyrrolizidine alkaloid from the composite-flowered plant *Senecio jacobae;* it causes seneciosis in ruminants.

Ja·cob·son canal, etc. (ja′kəb-sən) [Ludwig Levin *Jacobson*, Danish anatomist, 1783–1843] see *canaliculus tympanicus, cartilago vomeronasalis, nervus tympanicus*, and *organum vomeronasale*.

Ja·cob·son retinitis (yah′kəb-sən) [Julius *Jacobson*, German ophthalmologist, 1828–1889] syphilitic retinitis.

Ja·cod syndrome (triad) (zhah-ko′) [Maurice *Jacod*, French physician, early 20th century] see under *syndrome*.

Jac·quet dermatitis (erythema) (zhah-ka′) [Léonard Marie Lucien *Jacquet*, French dermatologist, 1860–1914] diaper dermatitis.

jac·ta·tio (jak-ta′she-o) [L., from *jactare* to toss about] jactitation.

j. ca′pitis noctur′na rhythmic rolling of the head of a child just before falling asleep.

jac·ta·tion (jak-ta′shən) jactitation.

jac·ti·ta·tion (jak″tĭ-ta′shən) [L. *jactitatio; jactitare* to toss] the tossing to and fro of a patient in acute disease.

Ja·das·sohn anetoderma, nevus (yah′dah-sōn) [Josef *Jadassohn*, German dermatologist in Switzerland, 1863–1936] see under *anetoderma* and see *nevus sebaceus*, under *nevus*.

Ja·das·sohn-Lew·an·dow·sky syndrome (yah′dah-sōn lev-ahn-dov′ske) [J. *Jadassohn;* Felix *Lewandowsky*, German dermatologist, 1879–1921] pachyonychia congenita.

Ja·das·sohn-Pel·li·za·ri anetoderma (yah′dah-sōn pel″e-tsah′re) [J. *Jadassohn;* Pietro *Pellizari*, Italian dermatologist, 1823–1892] see under *anetoderma*.

Ja·das·sohn-Tiè·che nevus (yah′dah-sōn tyĕ′shə) [J. *Jadassohn; Max Tièche*, Swiss physician, 1878–1938] blue nevus; see under *nevus*.

Ja·de·lot lines (furrows) (zhah-də-lo′) [Jean François Nicolas *Jadelot*, physician in Paris, 1791–1830] see under *line*.

Jae·ger test type (ya′gər) [Edward *Jaeger* von Jastthal, Austrian oculist, 1818–1884] see under *test type*.

Jaf·fe reaction, test (yah′fə) [Max *Jaffe*, German physiologic chemist, 1841–1911] see under *reaction* and *test*.

Jaf·fe-Lich·ten·stein disease (jaf′e lik′tən-stīn) [Henry Lewis *Jaffe*, American pathologist, 1896–1979; Louis *Lichtenstein*, American pathologist, 1906–1977] see under *disease*.

jag·siek·te (yahg-sēk′tə) [Afrikaans *jag* hunt + *siekte* sickness] pulmonary adenomatosis (def. 2).

jag·ziek·te (yahg-zēk′tə) pulmonary adenomatosis (def. 2).

JAK [*j*ust *a*nother *k*inase] Janus kinase.

Ja·kob disease (yah′kōb) [Alfons Maria *Jakob*, German psychiatrist, 1884–1931] Creutzfeldt-Jakob disease.

Ja·kob-Creutz·feldt disease (yah′kōb kroits′felt) [A.M. *Jakob;* Hans Gerhard *Creutzfeldt*, German psychiatrist, 1885–1964] Creutzfeldt-Jakob disease.

jal·ap (jal′ap) [Sp. *jalapa*, from the city of *Jalapa*, Veracruz, Mexico] the dried tuberous root of *Exogonium purga* (Hayne) Lindl. Convolvulaceae; its resins possess cathartic properties.

ja·mais vu (zhah′ma voo) [Fr. "never seen"] the sensation that familiar surroundings are strangely unfamiliar; the illusion that one has never seen anything like that before.

Jane·way lesion (jān′wa) [Edward Gamaliel *Janeway*, American physician, 1841–1911] see under *lesion*.

jan·i·ceps (jan′ĭ-seps) [L. *Janus* a two-faced god + *caput* head] conjoined twins with one head and two opposite faces; called also *duplicitas cruciata*.

j. asym′metros conjoined twins with one imperfect and one more complete face.

j. parasi′ticus conjoined twins in which there is partial duplication of the head in the frontal plane.

Jan·net·ta procedure (jə-net′ə) [Peter Joseph *Jannetta*, American neurosurgeon, born 1932] see under *procedure*.

Ja·no·šík embryo (yah′no-shēk) [Jan *Janošík*, Czechoslovakian anatomist, 1856–1927] see under *embryo*.

Jan·sen disease (yahn′sən) [W. Murk *Jansen*, Dutch orthopedic surgeon, 1867–1935] see *metaphyseal dysostosis*, under *dysostosis*.

Jan·ský-Biels·chow·sky disease (yahn′ske byels-chof′ske) [Jan *Janský*, Czech psychiatrist, 1873–1921; Alfred *Bielschowsky*, German ophthalmologist, 1871–1940] see under *disease*.

Jan·thi·no·so·ma (jan″thĭ-no-so′mə) a genus of mosquitoes, sometimes considered to be a subgenus of the genus *Psorophora*. *J. lut′zi* and *J. postica′ta* transport the eggs of botflies *(Dermatobia)* glued to their abdomens.

Janu·met (jan′u-met) trademark for a combination preparation of sitagliptin and metformin hydrochloride.

Ja·nus ki·nase (JAK) (ja′nəs ki′nās) [L. *Janus* god of doorways] a family of non-specific protein-tyrosine kinases (q.v.) activated by binding of cytokines to their plasma membrane receptors; the kinases, bound to the cytoplasmic domains of the receptors, serve as intermediates linking the receptors to activation of the STAT family of transcription factors, which migrate to the nucleus to regulate gene expression. Mutations in JAK3 have been linked to an autosomal recessive form of severe combined immune deficiency.

Ja·nu·via (jə-noo′ve-ə) trademark for a preparation of sitagliptin phosphate.

Ja·quet apparatus (zhah-ka′) [Alfred *Jaquet*, Swiss pharmacologist, 1865–1937] see under *apparatus*.

jar (jahr) a wide-mouthed glass or earthenware container.

bell j. a glass vessel, closed at top, open at bottom, used in laboratory vacuum experiments.

Leyden j. a glass jar partially covered inside and out with tinfoil or other metal, used as a condenser or collector of electricity.

ja·ra·ra·ca (jah″rah-rah′kə) *Bothrops jararaca*, a venomous pit viper found throughout South America.

Jar·cho pressometer (jahr′ko) [Julius *Jarcho*, Russian-born obstetrician in the United States, 1882–1963] see under *pressometer*.

Jar·cho-Lev·in syndrome (jahr′ko lev′in) [Saul Wallenstein *Jarcho*, American physician, mid-20th century; Paul M. *Levin*, American physician, 20th century] see under *syndrome*.

jar·gon (jahr′gən) 1. the technical or specialized language used in a profession or other field of activity. 2. incoherent speech, consisting either of neologisms or of actual words placed in an incoherent order. See also *jargon aphasia*, under *aphasia*.

jar·gon·a·pha·sia (jahr″gon-ə-fa′zhə) jargon aphasia.

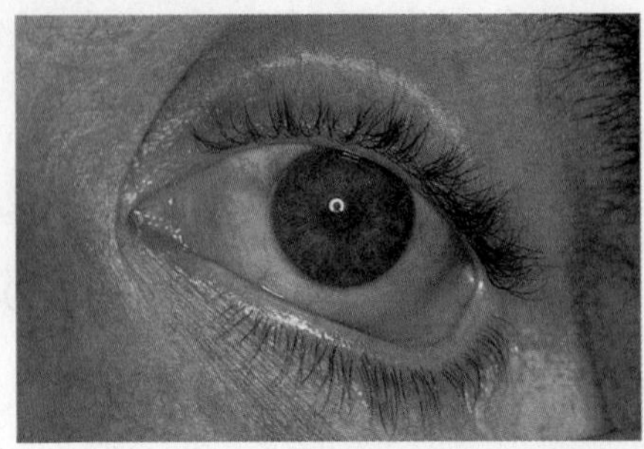

■ Jaundice and subconjunctival hemorrhages in leptospirosis.

Ja•risch-Herx•heim•er reaction (yah′rish herks′hi-mər) [Adolf *Jarisch*, Austrian dermatologist, 1850–1902; Karl *Herxheimer*, German dermatologist, 1861–1944] see under *reaction.*

Jar•ja•vay ligament, muscle (zhahr-zhah-va′) [Jean François *Jarjavay*, French physician, 1815–1868] see under *muscle* and see *ligamentum rectouterinum.*

Jar•vik-7 artificial heart (jahr′vik) [Robert Koffler *Jarvik*, American cardiologist, 20th century] see under *heart.*

Jat•ro•pha (jat′ro-fə) [Gr. *iatros* physician + *trophē* nourishment] a genus of plants of the family Euphorbiaceae, commonly found from Mexico to South America; various species have cathartic, stomachic, febrifuge, and astringent properties. *J. cur′cas* L. and *J. multi′fida* L. (both called *physic nut* or *purging nut*) have seeds containing a cathartic oil and a phytotoxin; when consumed by ruminants they cause diarrhea and damage to various internal organs.

jaun•dice (jawn′dis) [Fr. *jaunisse*, from *jaune* yellow] a condition characterized by hyperbilirubinemia and deposition of bile pigments in the skin, mucous membranes, and sclera, with resulting yellow appearance of the patient; called also *icterus.*

acholuric j. jaundice without choluria or bilirubinuria; seen in hemolytic disease and other forms of unconjugated hyperbilirubinemia as the unconjugated bilirubin is not excreted by the kidneys.

anhepatic j., anhepatogenous j. yellow appearance of the skin and mucous membranes not caused by liver disease.

black j. Winckel disease.

breastfeeding j. jaundice occuring in breastfed infants within the first week of life, most commonly caused by inadequate intake. Cf. *breast milk j.*

breast milk j. jaundice occuring in breastfed infants after the first 3–5 days of life. Serum bilirubin generally peaks at approximately 2 weeks and falls gradually over the next several months; the cause is unknown.

cholestatic j. jaundice resulting from an abnormality in the flow of bile, usually with elevation of serum alkaline phosphatasealkaline phosphatase, retention of bile salts, and variable hypercholesterolemia. The cholestasis may be *extrahepatic* (due to obstruction by a stone, stricture, or neoplasm) or *intrahepatic* (due to liver cell disease such as hepatitis, altered permeability, or obstruction of the intrahepatic biliary system).

congenital familial nonhemolytic j., congenital nonhemolytic j., Crigler-Najjar j. Crigler-Najjar syndrome.

epidemic j. former name for hepatitis A.

familial nonhemolytic j. Gilbert syndrome.

hemolytic j. jaundice caused by increased production of bilirubin from hemoglobin under conditions causing accelerated degradation of erythrocytes.

hepatocellular j. jaundice caused by injury to or disease of the liver cells.

hepatogenic j., hepatogenous j. any jaundice due to a disease or disorder of the liver.

infectious j., infective j. Weil syndrome.

latent j. hyperbilirubinemia without yellow staining of the tissues.

leptospiral j. Weil syndrome.

malignant j. of dogs canine babesiosis.

mechanical j. obstructive j.

neonatal j., j. of the newborn a type of jaundice often seen in newborn infants around the second day of life, due either to excessive bilirubin produced by the accelerated breakdown of erythrocytes seen in most infants, or to inability of the immature liver to conjugate bilirubin efficiently. Most cases are mild (see *physiologic j.*); if it is more severe or does not resolve within a few days, the infant may suffer serious damage such as kernicterus. Called also *neonatal icterus* and *icterus neonatorum*

nonhemolytic j. jaundice caused by an abnormality in metabolism of bilirubin by the liver cells, so that there is excessive unconjugated bilirubin in the blood. The various forms include *Crigler-Najjar, Dubin-Johnson, Gilbert,* and *Rotor syndromes*, as well as *physiologic jaundice.*

nuclear j. kernicterus.

obstructive j. jaundice caused by impediment to the flow of the bile from the liver cells to the duodenum.

physiologic j. mild neonatal jaundice in the first few days after birth; it normally resolves spontaneously as the infant's body systems mature.

picric acid j. jaundice due to picric acid poisoning, usually an occupational illness.

regurgitation j. jaundice attributed to escape of bile from the bile canaliculi into the bloodstream, with urobilinogen in the urine.

retention j. jaundice caused by inability of the liver to dispose of the bilirubin provided by the circulating blood.

spirochetal j. Weil syndrome.

toxemic j., toxic j. jaundice produced by poisons, such as phosphorus, arsine, carbon tetrachloride, or picric acid.

jaw (jaw) either the mandible or the maxilla, the two bony structures in the head of vertebrates; in dentate species they bear the teeth, enabling carnivores to seize their prey and others to bite and chew food.

big j. lumpy j.

bottle j. edema in the mandibular region of a grazing horse or cow, seen secondary to many different edematous conditions; it may clear up if the animal is switched to feeding from a trough.

cleft j. a cleft between the median nasal and maxillary prominences through the alveolus. Called also *gnathoschisis.*

crackling j. noise (crepitation) in the normal or diseased temporomandibular joint associated with jaw movement.

drop j., dropped j. in paralytic rabies in dogs, dropping of the mandible and inability to close the mouth.

Hapsburg j. a mandibular prognathous jaw, often accompanied by a thick overdeveloped lower lip (Hapsburg lip), as seen in many members of the Hapsburg family of European nobility.

lower j. mandibula.

lumpy j. actinomycosis in the mandibular region in cattle; called also *big j.*

overshot j. veterinary term for *retrognathism.*

phossy j. phosphorus necrosis.

pipe j. a painful condition of the jaws caused by carrying a tobacco pipe in the mouth.

rubber j. a type of osteoporosis in dogs and cats with softening of the jaws, resorption, and replacement of the bone by fibrous tissue, occurring in association with renal osteodystrophy.

undershot j. veterinary term for *prognathism;* it is normal in animals such as boxers and bulldogs.

upper j. maxilla.

Ja•wor•ski corpuscles (bodies) (yə-vor′ske) [Walery *Jaworski*, Polish physician, 1849–1924] see under *corpuscle.*

JCAHO (ja′ko) Joint Commission on Accreditation of Healthcare Organizations.

Jean•selme nodules (zhah-selm′) [Antoine Edouard *Jeanselme*, French dermatologist, 1858–1935] see under *nodule.*

Jec•to•fer (jek′to-fər) trademark for a preparation of iron sorbitex.

Jef•fer•son fracture, syndrome (jef′ər-sən) [Sir Geoffrey *Jefferson*, English neurosurgeon, 1886–1961] see under *fracture*, and see *cavernous sinus syndrome*, under *syndrome.*

Jef•fer•so•nia (jef″ər-so′ne-ə) [Thomas *Jefferson*, naturalist and third President of the United States, 1743–1826] a genus of American and Asian herbs of the family Berberidaceae. The root of *J. diphyl′la* (L.) Pers., of North America, is tonic, diuretic, and expectorant; emetic in large doses.

je•ju•nec•to•my (jĕ″joo-nek′tə-me) [*jejun-* + *-ectomy*] surgical removal of the jejunum.

je•ju•ni•tis (jĕ″joo-ni′tis) [*jejun-* + *-itis*] inflammation of the jejunum.

ulcerative j. a rare complication of celiac disease in which there are ulcerations in the wall of the jejunum, with cramping, strictures, and diarrhea.

jejun(o)- [L. *jejunum*, q.v.] a combining form denoting relationship to the jejunum.

je•ju•no•ce•cos•to•my (jə-joo″no-se-kos′tə-me) [*jejuno-* + *ceco-* + *-stomy*] 1. the formation of an anastomosis between the jejunum and cecum. 2. the anastomosis so formed.

je•ju•no•co•los•to•my (jə-joo″no-kə-los′tə-me) [*jejuno-* + *colo-* + *-stomy*] 1. the formation of an anastomosis between the jejunum and the colon. 2. the anastomosis so formed.

je•ju•no•il•e•al (jə-joo″no-il′e-əl) pertaining to or connecting the jejunum and ileum.

je•ju•no•il•e•itis (jə-joo″no-il″e-i′tis) inflammation of the jejunum and ileum together.

ulcerative j. extension of ulcerative jejunitis into the ileum.

je•ju•no•il•e•os•to•my (jə-joo″no-il″e-os′tə-me) [*jejuno-* + *ileo-* + *-stomy*] 1. the formation of an anastomosis between the proximal jejunum and the terminal ileum. 2. the anastomosis so formed. 3. jejunoileal bypass.

je•ju•no•il•e•um (jə-joo″no-il′e-əm) the jejunum and ileum considered as a unit.

je•ju•no•je•ju•nos•to•my (jə-joo″no-jĕ″joo-nos′tə-me) 1. surgical creation of an anastomosis between two portions of the jejunum. 2. the anastomosis so formed.

je•ju•nor•rha•phy (jĕ″joo-nor′ə-fe) [*jejuno-* + *-rrhaphy*] operative repair of the jejunum.

je•ju•nos•to•my (jĕ″joo-nos′tə-me) [*jejuno-* + *-stomy*] 1. the surgical creation of a permanent opening between the jejunum and the surface of the abdominal wall. 2. the opening so formed.

percutaneous endoscopic j. a procedure similar to percutaneous endoscopic gastrostomy but with the tube in the jejunum to allow gastric decompression and avoidance of aspiration.

je•ju•not•o•my (jĕ″joo-not′ə-me) [*jejuno-* + *-tomy*] surgical incision of the jejunum.

je•ju•num (jə-joo′nəm) [L. "empty"] [TA] the second section of the small intestine, extending from the duodenum to the ileum. **jeju′nal** *adj*

jel•ly (jel′e) [L. *gelatina*] a soft substance that is coherent, tremulous, and more or less translucent; generally, a colloidal semisolid mass.

cardiac j. a gelatinous substance found between the endothelium and myocardium of the embryonic heart, which transforms into the connective tissue of the endocardium.

contraceptive j. a nongreasy jelly or cream for introduction into the vagina or onto a diaphragm to prevent conception.

mineral j., petroleum j. petrolatum.

Wharton j. the soft, jellylike, homogeneous intercellular mucoid connective tissue of the umbilical cord; it contains thin collagenous fibers that increase in number with the age of the fetus.

jel•ly•fish (jel′e-fish) 1. the medusa stage, a stage in the life cycle of certain invertebrates of the phylum Cnidaria, class Scyphozoa, when their bodies are transparent and umbrella-shaped and the organisms are free-swimming; the body can vary between species from a few millimeters to two meters in diameter. Genera that inflict poisonous stings include *Aurelia, Carukia, Chironex,* and *Chiropsalmus.* 2. the term is also used for certain other cnidarians that have a medusalike stage, such as members of the genera *Gonionemus* and *Physalia.*

Jen•dras•sik maneuver, sign (yen-drah′sik) [Ernst *Jendrassik,* Hungarian physician, 1858–1921] see under *maneuver* and *sign.*

Jen•est (jen′est) trademark for a therapeutic regimen of norethindrone and ethinyl estradiol.

Jen•ner (jen′ər) Edward, 1749–1823. An English physician who developed the process of producing immunity to smallpox by inoculation (vaccination) with cowpox (vaccinia) vaccine.

Jen•ner method (jen′ər) [Louis Leopold *Jenner,* English physician, 1866–1904] see *Stains and Staining Methods,* under *stain.*

jen•ne•ri•an (jen-e′re-ən) named for Edward *Jenner.*

jen•ner•iza•tion (jen″ər-ĭ-za′shən) production of immunity to a disease by inoculation of an attenuated form of the virus producing the disease.

Jen•sen disease (yen′sən) [Edmund *Jensen,* Danish ophthalmologist, 1861–1950] retinochoroiditis juxtapapillaris.

Jen•sen sarcoma (tumor) (yen′sən) [Carl Oluf *Jensen,* Danish veterinary pathologist, 1864–1934] see under *sarcoma.*

jerk (jurk) a sudden reflex or involuntary movement.

Achilles j., ankle j. triceps surae reflex.

biceps j. biceps reflex.

crossed adductor j. see under *reflex.*

elbow j. triceps reflex.

hypnic j's sudden brief contractions at the onset of sleep, usually in the lower limbs but sometimes also of the head and upper limbs.

jaw j. jaw reflex.

knee j. patellar reflex.

myoclonic j. the jerk seen in myoclonus.

quadriceps j. patellar reflex.

square wave j's inappropriate saccades that interrupt fixation and take the eye off of a stationary or moving object. These occur about 4 to 6 times per minute in normal persons; their frequency may increase in central nervous system conditions that affect eye muscles.

tendon j. see under *reflex.*

triceps surae j. see under *reflex.*

Jer•vell and Lange-Niel•sen syndrome (yer-vel′ lahng′ə-nēl′sən) [Anton *Jervell,* Norwegian cardiologist, 1901–1987; Friedrik *Lange-Nielsen,* Norwegian cardiologist, 20th century] see under *syndrome.*

jet (jet) [L. *iacere* to throw] 1. a stream of fluid projected at high velocity under pressure, or the device for producing such a stream. 2. a high-velocity stream of blood emerging from a stenotic lesion.

j. lag see under *lag.*

ureteral j. the pattern of fluid seen when dense urine from the ureter is expelled into the more dilute urine in the bladder; it can be studied to assess function and patency of the bladder.

water-j. see under *dissector.*

Jeune syndrome (zhoon) [Mathis *Jeune,* French pediatrician, 1910–1983] asphyxiating thoracic dystrophy; see under *dystrophy.*

Je-Vax (je′vaks″) trademark for a preparation of Japanese encephalitis virus vaccine.

Jew•ett brace, nail (joo′ət) [Eugene Lyon *Jewett,* American orthopedic surgeon, 20th century] see under *nail.*

JIA juvenile idiopathic arthritis.

jig•ger (jig′ər) chigoe.

jim•son weed (jim′sən wēd) 1. *Datura stramonium.* 2. stramonium (def. 2).

jing (jing) [Chinese] one of the basic substances that according to traditional Chinese medicine pervade the body, usually translated as "essence"; the body reserves or constitutional makeup, replenished by food and rest, that supports life and is associated with developmental changes in the organism from fetal life through old age and death.

jit•ter (jit′ər) in single fiber electromyography, the variability in interpotential interval as consecutive discharges occur; usually expressed as the mean of consecutive differences (q.v.).

Job syndrome (jōb) [*Job,* character in the Old Testament who suffered from skin disease and other misfortunes] see under *syndrome.*

Jo•bert fossa (zho-bār′) [Antoine Joseph *Jobert* de Lamballe, French surgeon, 1799–1867] see under *fossa.*

jod•bas•e•dow (i″ōd-baz′ə-do) [Ger.] iodine-induced hyperthyroidism.

Joest bodies (yerst) [Ernst *Joest,* German veterinary pathologist, 1873–1926] see under *body.*

Jof•froy reflex (zhof-rwah′) [Alexis *Joffroy,* French physician, 1844–1908] see under *reflex.*

Jo•han•son-Bliz•zard syndrome (jo-han′sən bliz′ərd) [Ann J. *Johanson,* American physician, late 20th century; Robert M. *Blizzard,* American pediatric endocrinologist, late 20th century] see under *syndrome.*

Joh•ne bacillus, disease (yo′nə) [Heinrich Albert *Johne,* German pathologist, 1839–1910] see *Mycobacterium avium* subsp. *paratuberculosis* and see under *disease.*

joh•nin (yo′nin) a filtrate of cultures of *Mycobacterium avium* subsp. *paratuberculosis* (Johne bacillus), similar to tuberculin, used to produce a skin reaction (johnin reaction) in testing cattle for Johne disease.

John•son-Ste•vens disease (jon′sən ste′vənz) [Frank Chambliss *Johnson,* American pediatrician, 1894–1934; Albert Mason *Stevens,* American pediatrician, 1884–1945] Stevens-Johnson syndrome.

joint (joint) [L. *junctio* a joining, connection] the place of union or junction between two or more bones of the skeleton, especially one that allows motion of one or more of the bones. See also entries under *articulatio* and *junctura.*

acromioclavicular j. articulatio acromioclavicularis.

amphidiarthrodial j. amphidiarthrosis.

ankle j. articulatio talocruralis.

apophyseal j's articulationes zygapophysiales.

arthrodial j. articulatio plana.

atlantoaxial j., lateral articulatio atlantoaxialis lateralis.

atlantoaxial j., median articulatio atlantoaxialis mediana.

atlanto-occipital j. articulatio atlantooccipitalis.

j's of auditory ossicles articulationes ossiculorum auditoriorum.

ball-and-socket j. articulatio spheroidea.

biaxial j. a joint that permits movement in two of the assumed three mutually perpendicular axes, or having two degrees of freedom, as the ellipsoidal joint.

bicondylar j. articulatio bicondylaris.

bilocular j. a joint in which the synovial cavity is divided into two compartments by an interarticular cartilage, as the temporomandibular joint.

bleeder's j. hemophilic arthropathy.

bony j's juncturae ossium.

brachioradial j. articulatio humeroradialis.

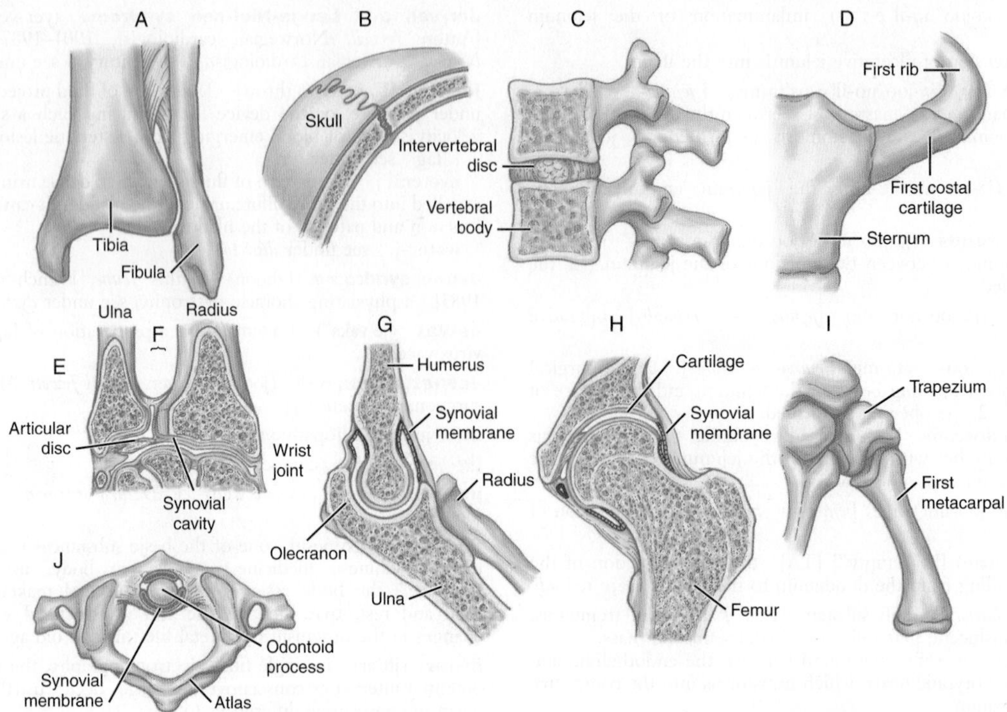

■ Various kinds of joints. *Fibrous: A*, syndesmosis (tibiofibular); *B*, suture (skull). *Cartilaginous: C*, symphysis (vertebral bodies); *D*, synchondrosis (first rib and sternum). *Synovial: E*, condyloid (wrist); *F*, gliding (radioulnar); *G*, hinge or ginglymus (elbow); *H*, ball and socket (hip); *I*, saddle (carpometacarpal of thumb); *J*, pivot (atlantoaxial).

Budin j. a band of cartilage seen at birth between the squamous and the two condylar portions of the occipital bone.
calcaneocuboid j. articulatio calcaneocuboidea.
capitular j. articulatio capitis costae.
carpal j's articulationes carpi.
carpometacarpal j's articulationes carpometacarpales.
carpometacarpal j. of thumb articulatio carpometacarpalis pollicis.
cartilaginous j. junctura cartilaginea.
Charcot j. neuropathic arthropathy.
chondrosternal j's articulationes sternocostales.
Chopart j. articulatio tarsi transversa.
Clutton j. painless symmetrical hydrarthrosis, especially of the knee joints, seen in congenital syphilis.
cochlear j. a type of hinge joint that permits some lateral motion.
coffin j. the second interphalangeal joint of the foot of a horse.
composite j., compound j. articulatio composita.
condylar j., condyloid j. articulatio ellipsoidea.
costocentral j. articulatio capitis costae.
costochondral j's articulationes costochondrales.
costosternal j's articulationes sternocostales.
costotransverse j. articulatio costotransversaria.
costovertebral j's articulationes costovertebrales.
cotyloid j. articulatio cotylica.
coxal j., coxofemoral j. articulatio coxae.
cranial cartilaginous j's juncturae cartilagineae cranii.
cranial fibrous j's juncturae fibrosae cranii.
cranial synovial j's articulationes cranii.
craniovertebral j. articulatio atlantooccipitalis.
cricoarytenoid j. articulatio cricoarytenoidea.
cricothyroid j. articulatio cricothyroidea.
crurotalar j. articulatio talocruralis.
Cruveilhier j. articulatio atlantooccipitalis.
cubital j. articulatio cubiti.
cuboideonavicular j. the articulation between the rounded lateral surface of the navicular bone and the posterior part of the medial surface of the cuboid bone; it is usually fibrous but is occasionally synovial.
cuneonavicular j. articulatio cuneonavicularis.
diarthrodial j. junctura synovialis.
digital j's see *articulationes interphalangeae manus* and *articulationes interphalangeae pedis*, under *articulatio*.
DIP j., distal interphalangeal j. the interphalangeal joint located distally on any digit; see *articulationes interphalangeae manus* and *articulationes interphalangeae pedis*, under *articulatio*.
elbow j. articulatio cubiti.
ellipsoidal j. articulatio ellipsoidea.
enarthrodial j. articulatio spheroidea.
facet j's articulationes zygapophysiales.
false j. pseudarthrosis.
femoral j. articulatio coxae.
fetlock j. either the metacarpophalangeal joint or the metatarsophalangeal joint in an ungulate.
fibrocartilaginous j. symphysis.
fibrous j. junctura fibrosa.
first carpometacarpal j. articulatio carpometacarpalis pollicis.
flail j. a joint that exhibits abnormal mobility.
j's of foot articulationes pedis.
j's of free lower limb juncturae membri inferioris liberi.
freely movable j. junctura synovialis.
j's of free upper limb juncturae membri superioris liberi.
fringe j. a joint affected with chronic villous arthritis.
ginglymoid j. ginglymus.
glenohumeral j. articulatio humeri.
gliding j. articulatio plana.
j's of hand articulationes manus.
j. of head of rib articulatio capitis costae.
hemophilic j. see under *arthropathy*.
hinge j. ginglymus.
hip j. articulatio coxae.
hock j. hock.
humeral j. articulatio humeri.
humeroradial j. articulatio humeroradialis.
humeroulnar j. articulatio humeroulnaris.
iliofemoral j. articulatio coxae.
iliosacral j. articulatio sacroiliaca.
immovable j. synarthrosis.
incudomallear j., incudomalleolar j. articulatio incudomallearis.
incudostapedial j. articulatio incudostapedialis.
intercarpal j's articulationes carpi.
interchondral j's, intercostal j's articulationes interchondrales.
intercuneiform j's articulationes intercuneiformes.
intermetacarpal j's articulationes intermetacarpales.
intermetatarsal j's articulationes intermetatarsales.
interphalangeal j's of fingers articulationes interphalangeae manus.
interphalangeal j's of foot articulationes interphalangeae pedis.
interphalangeal j's of hand articulationes interphalangeae manus.
interphalangeal j's of toes articulationes interphalangeae pedis.
intertarsal j's tarsal j's.
irritable j. a joint subject to attacks of inflammation without discoverable cause.
knee j. articulatio genus.

laryngeal j's see *cartilagines et articulationes laryngis.*
ligamentous j. syndesmosis.
Lisfranc j's articulationes tarsometatarsales.
j's of lower limb juncturae membri inferioris.
lumbosacral j. articulatio lumbosacralis.
j's of Luschka a series of jointlike structures at the lateral edges of the vertebral bodies from vertebra C3 to T1, forming small spurlike lips at the upper surface, covered with cartilage, and containing a capsule filled with fluid. They are considered by some to be true diarthrodial joints, and by others to be degenerative spaces of the intervertebral disks filled with extracellular fluid and lined by a membrane formed by fibrocytes. They are frequent sites of spur formation. Called also *uncovertebral j's.*
mandibular j. articulatio temporomandibularis.
manubriosternal j. symphysis manubriosternalis.
maxillary j. articulatio temporomandibularis.
mediocarpal j. articulatio mediocarpalis.
metacarpophalangeal j's articulationes metacarpophalangeae.
metatarsophalangeal j's articulationes metatarsophalangeae.
midcarpal j. articulatio mediocarpalis.
midtarsal j. articulatio tarsi transversa.
multiaxial j. articulatio spheroidea.
neurocentral j. a synchondrosis between the body (centrum) of a vertebra and either half of the neural arch; it is obliterated by fusion of the vertebral arch and body during the third to sixth years of life.
occipitoatlantal j. articulatio atlantooccipitalis.
open j. a veterinary term for a joint in which the surface of the bones is exposed, as a result of inflammation and sloughing of the tissues.
osseous j's juncturae ossium.
ovoid j. articulatio sellaris.
pastern j. the joint between the short and long pastern bones of a horse, the second most distal of the leg joints.
patellofemoral j. the joint between the articular surface of the patella and the patellar surface of the femur.
j's of pectoral girdle juncturae cinguli pectoralis.
peg-and-socket j. gomphosis.
j's of pelvic girdle juncturae cinguli pelvici.
phalangeal j's see *articulationes interphalangeae manus* and *articulationes interphalangeae pedis,* under *articulatio.*
PIP j. proximal interphalangeal joint.
j. of pisiform bone, pisotriquetral j. articulatio ossis pisiformis.
pivot j. articulatio trochoidea.
plane j. articulatio plana.
polyaxial j. articulatio spheroidea.
proximal interphalangeal j. the interphalangeal joint located proximally on any digit; see *articulationes interphalangeae manus* and *articulationes interphalangeae pedis,* under *articulatio.* Called also *PIP j.*
radiocapitellar j. articulatio humeroradialis.
radiocarpal j. articulatio radiocarpalis.
radioulnar j., distal, radioulnar j., inferior articulatio radioulnaris distalis.
radioulnar j., middle syndesmosis radioulnaris.
radioulnar j., proximal, radioulnar j., superior articulatio radioulnaris proximalis.
rotary j. articulatio trochoidea.
sacrococcygeal j. articulatio sacrococcygea.
sacroiliac j. articulatio sacroiliaca.
saddle j. articulatio sellaris.
scapuloclavicular j. articulatio acromioclavicularis.
sellar j. articulatio sellaris.
shoulder j. articulatio humeri.
j's of shoulder girdle juncturae cinguli pectoralis.
simple j. articulatio simplex.
j's of skull juncturae cranii.
socket j. of tooth syndesmosis dentoalveolaris.
spheroidal j. articulatio spheroidea.
spiral j. cochlear j.
sternoclavicular j. articulatio sternoclavicularis.
sternocostal j's articulationes sternocostales.
stifle j. a joint near the top of the hind leg of a quadruped, homologous to the knee joint of a human being; it actually consists of two joints, that between the femur and tibia, and that between the femur and patella. Called also *stifle* and *knee.*
subtalar j. articulatio subtalaris.
synarthrodial j. synarthrosis.
synovial j. junctura synovialis.
synovial j's of free lower limb articulationes membri inferioris liberi.
synovial j's of free upper limb articulationes membri superioris liberi.
synovial j's of pectoral girdle, synovial j's of shoulder girdle articulationes cinguli pectoralis.
synovial j's of vertebral column articulationes columnae vertebralis.
talocalcaneal j. articulatio subtalaris.
talocalcaneonavicular j. articulatio talocalcaneonavicularis.
talocrural j. articulatio talocruralis.
talonavicular j. the junction between the talus and the navicular bone.
tarsal j's the joints between the various tarsal bones. Called also *intertarsal j's.*
tarsometatarsal j's articulationes tarsometatarsales.
temporomandibular j. articulatio temporomandibularis.
thoracic j's juncturae thoracis.
thoracic synovial j's articulationes thoracis.
tibiofibular j. articulatio tibiofibularis.
tibiofibular j., distal, tibiofibular j., inferior syndesmosis tibiofibularis.
tibiofibular j., proximal, tibiofibular j., superior articulatio tibiofibularis.
transverse tarsal j. articulatio tarsi transversa.
trochoid j. articulatio trochoidea.
j. of tubercle of rib articulatio costotransversaria.
uncovertebral j's j's of Luschka.
uniaxial j. a joint that permits movement in only one of the assumed three mutually perpendicular axes, or having only one degree of freedom, such as a hinge joint or interphalangeal joint.
unilocular j. a synovial joint having only one cavity.
j's of upper limb juncturae membri superioris.
vertebral j's, j's of vertebral column juncturae columnae vertebralis.
vertebral synovial j's articulationes columnae vertebralis.
von Gies j. a chronic syphilitic chondro-osteoarthritis.
wedge-and-groove j. schindylesis.
wrist j. articulatio radiocarpalis.
xiphisternal j. symphysis xiphisternalis.
zygapophyseal j's articulationes zygapophysiales.

Jol·ly bodies (zho-le′) [Justin Marie Jules *Jolly,* French histologist, 1870–1953] Howell-Jolly bodies; see under *body.*

Jol·ly reaction (yol′e) [Friedrich *Jolly,* German neurologist, 1844–1904] see under *reaction.*

Jones brace, fracture, position (jōnz) [Sir Robert *Jones,* English orthopedic surgeon, 1858–1933] see under *brace, fracture,* and *position.*

Jon·nes·co fold, fossa (jo-nes′ko) [Thoma *Jonnesco,* Romanian surgeon, 1860–1926] see *parietoperitoneal fold,* under *fold,* and see *recessus duodenalis superior.*

Jor·dans anomaly (yor′dənz) [Godefridus H.W. *Jordans,* Dutch physician, 1902–1979] see under *anomaly.*

jo·sa·my·cin (jo″sə-mi′sin) a macrolide antibiotic produced by *Streptomyces narbonensis* var. *josamyceticus,* having antibacterial activity similar to that of erythromycin.

Jo·seph clamp, knife, rhinoplasty (yo′səf) [Jacques *Joseph,* German surgeon, 1865–1934] see under *clamp, knife,* and *rhinoplasty.*

Jo·seph disease (zho-sef′) [*Joseph,* an Azorean family affected by the disease] Machado-Joseph disease; see under *disease.*

Jou·bert syndrome (zhoo-bār′) [Marie *Joubert,* Canadian neurologist, 20th century] see under *syndrome.*

joule (J) (jo͞ol) [James Prescott *Joule,* English physicist, 1818–1889] the SI unit of quantity of energy, being the work done by a force of 1 newton acting over a distance of 1 meter in the direction of the force.

JRA juvenile rheumatoid arthritis.

Jud·kins catheter, technique (jud′kinz) [Melvin P. *Judkins,* American radiologist, 1922–1985] see *Judkins coronary catheter* and *Judkins pigtail left vetriculography catheter,* under *catheter,* and see under *technique.*

ju·ga (joo′gə) [L.] plural of *jugum.*

ju·gal (joo′gəl) [L. *jugalis,* from *jugum* yoke] 1. connecting like a yoke. 2. buccal.

ju·ga·le (joo-ga′le) the jugal point; see under *point.*

ju·gate (joo′gāt) 1. locked together. 2. marked by ridges.

Ju·glans (joo′gləns) [L. "Jove's nut," walnut] the walnuts, a genus of trees of the family Juglandaceae. Certain species have parts that have been used medicinally.

ju·go·max·il·lary (joo″go-mak′sĭ-lar″e) zygomaticomaxillary.

jug·u·lar (jug′u-lər) [L. *jugularis,* from *jugulum* neck] 1. cervical (def. 1). 2. pertaining to a jugular vein. 3. a jugular vein.

jug·u·la·tion (jug″u-la′shən) [L. *jugulare* to cut the throat of] the sudden and rapid arrest of disease by therapeutic measures.

ju·gum (joo′gəm) pl. *ju′ga* [L. "a yoke"] yoke: a depression or ridge connecting two structures.
ju′ga alveola′ria mandi′bulae [TA] alveolar yokes of mandible: depressions on the anterior surface of the alveolar process of the mandible, between the ridges caused by the roots of the incisor teeth.

ju′ga alveola′ria maxil′lae [TA] alveolar yokes of maxilla: the depressions on the anterior surface of the alveolar process of the maxilla, between the ridges caused by the roots of the incisor teeth.

ju′ga cerebra′lia TA alternative for *impressiones gyrorum.*

j. sphenoida′le [TA] sphenoidal yoke: the portion of the body of the sphenoid bone that connects its lesser wings.

juice (jo͞os) [L. *jus* broth] any fluid derived from animal or plant tissue; called also *liquor.*

appetite j. gastric juice secreted during eating and varying in character with the appetite for the food which is being eaten.

cherry j. [NF] liquid expressed from the fresh ripe fruit of *Prunus cerasus* (the sour cherry), used as an ingredient in preparing flavored vehicles for pharmaceuticals.

gastric j. the liquid secretion of the gastric glands, consisting primarily of hydrochloric acid and pepsin.

intestinal j. the liquid secreted by the intestinal glands; it contains enzymes that finish the digestion of fats, proteins, and carbohydrates, which started more proximally in the digestive tract.

pancreatic j. the enzyme-containing liquid secretion of the exocrine pancreas, which is discharged into the duodenum.

press j. liquid obtained by submitting finely ground tissue to great pressure.

raspberry j. the liquid expressed from the fresh ripe fruit of varieties of *Rubus idaeus* L. (European red raspberry) or *R. strigosus* Michx. (American red raspberry); used in a syrup as a flavored vehicle for drugs.

jump•ing (jump′ing) 1. the skipping of several steps in a series; moving forward quickly. 2. see under *disease.*

j. the bite correction of crossbite. See also *Kingsley appliance,* under *appliance.*

junc•tio (junk′she-o) pl. *junctio′nes* [L., from *jungere* to join] 1. junction. 2. joint; see also *articulatio.*

j. anorecta′lis [TA] anorectal junction: the site at which the rectum becomes continuous with the anal canal; called also *anorectal line.*

junc•tion (junk′shən) [L. *junctus* past part. of *jungere* to join] the place of meeting or of coming together, as of two different organs or types of tissue. **junc′tional** *adj*

adherens j. a type of adhesive junction that links cell membranes and cytoskeletal elements within and between cells by homophilic interactions between cadherins. Examples include the zonula adherens of epithelial cells and the fascia adherens of cardiac myocytes.

adhesive j. a type of intercellular junction that links cell membranes and cytoskeletal elements within and between cells, connecting adjacent cells mechanically. Examples include adherens junctions and desmosomes.

amelodentinal j. dentinoenamel j.

anomalous pancreaticobiliary j. communication between the common bile duct and the pancreatic duct outside the sphincter of Oddi, allowing pancreatic fluid and bile to mix, resulting in choledochal cysts, biliary tract carcinoma, and obstructive jaundice or pancreatitis secondary to formation of protein plugs.

anorectal j. junctio anorectalis.

atrioventricular j., AV j. part or all of the entire region comprising the atrioventricular node and the bundle of His, with the bundle branches sometimes specifically excluded.

cardioesophageal j. esophagogastric j.

cementodentinal j. dentinocemental j.

cementoenamel j. the line at which the cementum covering the root of a tooth and the enamel covering its crown meet, designated anatomically as the cervical line.

cervicomedullary j. the junction between the spinal cord and the medulla oblongata.

communicating j. gap j.

corneoscleral j. limbus corneae.

craniovertebral j. articulatio atlantooccipitalis.

dentinocemental j. the plane of meeting between the dentin and cementum on the root of a tooth, containing a large amount of protein, particularly collagen, and less inorganic material than either dentin or cementum; it is believed to reduce the mechanical stress and facilitate movement of nutrients between the dentin and cementum. Called also *cementodentinal j.* and *Hopewell-Smith hyaline layer.*

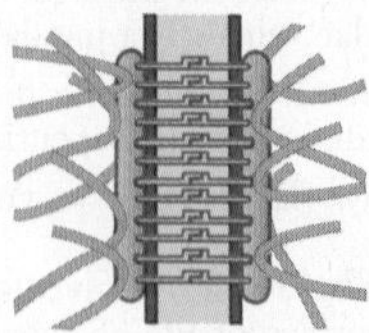

■ Adhesive junction as exemplified by a desmosome.

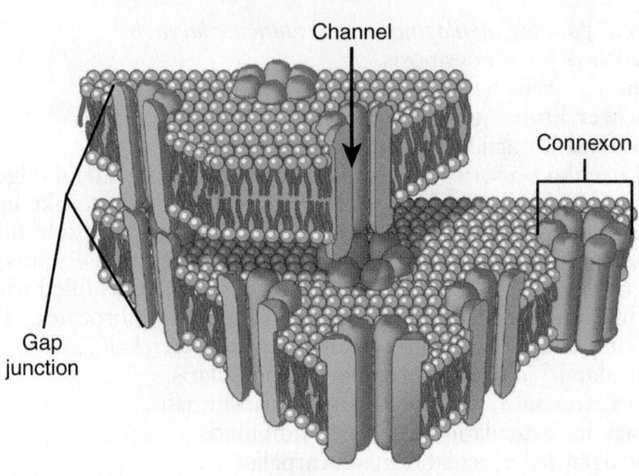

■ Gap junctions providing passageways between the interiors of adjacent cells. Each gap junction consists of two connexons stacked end-to-end, spanning the gap between the membranes, with each connexon comprising six protein subunits arranged around a central channel.

dentinoenamel j. the plane of meeting between the dentin and enamel on the crown of a tooth.

dentogingival j. the zone of meeting of the cementum and the gingiva, consisting of the epithelial attachment and the gingival fibers.

dermal-epidermal j., dermoepidermal j. the plane of meeting between the dermis and epidermis.

esophagogastric j. the site of transition from the stratified squamous epithelium of the esophagus to the simple columnar epithelium of the cardia of the stomach; see also *lower esophageal sphincter,* under *sphincter.* Called also *cardioesophageal j.* and *gastroesophageal j.*

fibromuscular j. a junction between the muscular elements of the wall of the corpus uteri and the fibrous tissue of the cervix.

gap j. a type of intercellular junction comprising a narrowed portion (about 3 nm) of the intercellular space that contains channels or pores (about 2 nm) composed of hexagonal arrays of membrane-spanning proteins around a central lumen *(connexon)* through which pass ions and small molecules such as most sugars, amino acids, nucleotides, vitamins, hormones, and cyclic AMP. In electrically excitable tissues, these gap junctions serve to transmit electrical impulses via ionic currents and are known as *electrotonic synapses;* they are present in such tissues as myocardial tissue and the central nervous system. Called also *nexus.*

gastroesophageal j. esophagogastric j.

ileocecal j. the junction of the ileum and cecum, located at the lower right side of the abdomen and fixed to the posterior abdominal wall.

intercellular j's specialized regions on the borders of cells that provide connections between adjacent cells; they are often divided into adherens, gap, and tight junctions, and desmosomes.

lumbosacral j. articulatio lumbosacralis.

mucocutaneous j. the site of transition between skin and a mucous membrane.

mucogingival j. a sharply scalloped, generally indistinct line running parallel with the free gingival margin, separating the gingival tissue from that of the oral mucosa; visible under the microscope. Called also *mucogingival line.*

myoneural j. neuromuscular j.

myotendinal j. the region where muscle fibers and the collagen of their associated tendons connect and interdigitate.

neuromuscular j. the site of apposition of a motor end plate and the subneural cleft of the skeletal muscle fiber that it innervates. After the nerve is excited, the excitatory neurotransmitter acetylcholine is released from the axon terminal when the nerve is excited, diffuses across the synaptic cleft, and reversibly binds to receptor molecules on the muscle fiber surface, causing the initiation of an action potential that propagates along the muscle fiber and causes it to contract. Called also *myoneural j.*

occluding j. tight j.

pancreaticobiliary j. the junction where the pancreatic duct meets the common bile duct at the hepatopancreatic ampulla. See also *anomalous pancreaticobiliary j.*

pharyngoesophageal j. constrictio pharyngooesophagealis.

sclerocorneal j. limbus corneae.

splice j. see under *site.*

squamocolumnar j. the site of transition between squamous and columnar epithelium, such as occurs between the esophagus and the stomach or within the epithelium of the uterine cervix.

temporoparietal j. the area of the cerebral cortex where the temporal and parietal lobes meet; this area plays a vital role in social interactions and the ability to distinguish the self from others and the environment.

tendinous j's connexus intertendinei.

thoracolumbar j. the part of the vertebral column from the eleventh thoracic vertebra to the first lumbar vertebra; here the spinal curvature changes from kyphosis to lordosis and the orientation of the facet joints changes from coronal to sagittal.

tight j. an intercellular junction between epithelial cells, at which the adjacent plasma membranes are joined tightly together, separated by only 1 to 2 nm and forming a beltlike seal; these junctions occlude the intercellular space and limit intercellular passage of small ions and molecules. Called also *occluding j.* and *zonula occludens.*

ureteropelvic j. the junction of the ureter and kidney at the renal pelvis.

ureterovesical j. the junction where the ureter joins the urinary bladder at one corner of the trigone of the bladder; called also *ureterotrigonal complex.*

junc•tu•ra (junk-too′rə) pl. *junctu′rae* [L. "a joining"] 1. [TA] joint; see also *articulatio.* 2. *(in the pl.)* articular system: official terminology for the joints of the body considered collectively. Called also *systema articulare* [TA alternative].

j. cartilagi′nea [TA] cartilaginous joint: a type of synarthrosis in which the union of the bony elements is by intervening cartilage; the two types are *synchondrosis* and *symphysis.*

junctu′rae cartilagi′neae cra′nii [TA] the cranial cartilaginous joints, comprising the synchondroses cranii.

junctu′rae cin′guli pectora′lis [TA] joints of pectoral girdle: the synovial joints of the pectoral girdle (acromioclavicular and sternoclavicular joints) considered together with the three intrinsic ligaments of the scapula (superior transverse scapular, inferior transverse scapular, and coracoacromial ligaments). Called also *joints of shoulder girdle.*

junctu′rae cin′guli pel′vici [TA] joints of pelvic girdle: the sacroiliac joint and the pubic symphysis.

junctu′rae colum′nae vertebra′lis [TA] joints of vertebral column: the syndesmoses and synovial joints of the vertebral column considered together.

junctu′rae cra′nii [TA] joints of skull: junctions between bones of the skull or between skull bones and other bones. Some are fibrous (juncturae fibrosae cranii), some are cartilaginous (juncturae cartilagineae cranii), and some are synovial (articulationes cranii).

j. fibro′sa [TA] fibrous joint: a type of synarthrosis in which the union of bony elements is by continuous intervening fibrous tissue, which makes little motion possible; the group includes sutures (suturae), gomphoses, and syndesmoses.

junctu′rae fibro′sae cra′nii [TA] cranial fibrous joints: the sutures (suturae cranii) and ligaments connecting the bones of the skull to each other, as well as the syndesmoses holding the teeth in their sockets (syndesmoses dentoalveolares).

junctu′rae mem′bri inferio′ris [TA] joints of lower limb: the joints of the free lower limb and those of the pelvic girdle considered together.

junctu′rae mem′bri inferio′ris li′beri [TA] joints of free lower limb: the synovial joints and syndesmoses of the thigh, leg, and foot. See also *articulationes membri inferioris liberi,* under *articulatio.*

junctu′rae mem′bri superio′ris [TA] joints of upper limb: the joints of the free upper limb and those of the pectoral girdle considered together.

junctu′rae mem′bri superio′ris li′beri [TA] joints of free upper limb: the synovial joints and syndesmoses of the arm, forearm, and hand. See also *articulationes membri superioris liberi,* under *articulatio.*

junctu′rae os′sium [TA] bony joints: the places of junction between two or more bones of the skeleton. It includes fibrous (juncturae fibrosae), cartilaginous (juncturae cartilagineae), and synovial joints (juncturae synoviales). Called also *osseous joints.*

j. synovia′lis [TA] synovial joint: a specialized joint permitting more or less free movement, the union of the bony elements being surrounded by an articular capsule enclosing a cavity lined by synovial membrane; called also *diarthrosis* [TA alternative], *diarthrodial joint,* and *articulatio* [TA alternative]. See illustration at *joint.*

junctu′rae tho′racis [TA] thoracic joints: the joints of the thorax considered as a group, including syndesmoses, synchondroses, and the thoracic synovial joints *(articulationes thoracis).*

junc•tu•rae (junk-too′re) [L.] genitive and plural of *junctura.*

Jung (yoong) Carl Gustav, 1875–1961. Swiss psychiatrist and philosopher. Originally a follower of Freud, Jung soon broke with Freud to become the founder of analytic psychology, hypothesizing two major aspects to the unconscious, the personal or individual and the collective. The striving for harmony between the conscious and the unconscious is seen to be an important lifelong task. Jung introduced new concepts such as *introvert, extrovert, anima,* and *animus,* and expanded ones that Freud had stressed, such as *libido* and *ego.*

Jung muscle (yoong) [Karl Gustav *Jung,* Swiss anatomist, 1794–1864] musculus pyramidalis auriculae.

Ju•nin fever, virus (hoo-nēn′) [*Junín,* Argentina, where the fever and virus have been observed] see under *virus,* and see *Argentine hemorrhagic fever,* under *fever.*

ju•ni•per (joo′nĭ-pər) 1. any tree or shrub of the genus *Juniperus.* 2. a preparation of the berries of *J. communis,* or the volatile oil extracted from them, used for loss of appetite and dyspepsia; it is also used in homeopathy and for a variety of indications in folk medicine.

Ju•nip•er•us (joo-nip′ər-əs) a genus of evergreen coniferous trees and shrubs of the family Cupressaceae.

J. commu′nis a species native to Eurasia and North America, whose berries and the volatile oil extracted from them are used medicinally.

J. oxyce′drus the cade tree, a European species that is the source of juniper tar.

J. sabi′na savin, an evergreen Eurasian shrub that is the source of savin oil.

J. virginia′na the red cedar, an American species occurring chiefly east of the Rocky Mountains, that is the source of cedarwood oil.

jur•is•pru•dence (jo͞or″is-proo′dəns) [L. *juris prudentia* knowledge of law] the scientific study or application of the principles of law and justice.

dental j. the application of the principles of law and justice as they relate to the practice of dentistry, to the obligations of the practitioner to the patient, and to the relations of dentists to each other and to society in general. This term and *forensic dentistry* are sometimes used as synonyms, but some authorities consider the first a branch of law and the second a branch of dentistry. See also *medical j.* and *forensic dentistry.*

medical j. the application of the principles of law as they relate to the practice of medicine, to the obligations of the practitioner to the patient, and to the relations of physicians to each other and to society in general. This term and *forensic medicine* are sometimes used as synonyms, but some authorities consider the first a branch of law and the second a branch of medicine.

jus•to ma•jor (jus′to ma′jər) see *pelvis justo major.*

jus•to mi•nor (jus′to mi′nər) see *pelvis justo minor.*

ju•ve•nile (joo′və-nīl) 1. pertaining to youth or childhood; young or immature. 2. a youth or child; a young animal. 3. a cell or organism intermediate between the immature form and the mature form.

juxta- [L. *juxta* near, close by] a combining form meaning situated near or adjoining.

jux•ta-ar•tic•u•lar (juks″tə-ahr-tik′u-lər) situated near or in the region of a joint.

jux•ta•car•di•ac (juks″tə-kahr′de-ak) paracardiac.

jux•ta•ep•i•phys•e•al (juks″tə-ep-ĭ-fiz′e-əl) [*juxta-* + *epiphyseal*] near to or adjoining an epiphysis.

jux•ta•esoph•a•ge•al (juks″tə-e-sof″ə-je′əl) paraesophageal.

jux•ta•glo•mer•u•lar (juks″tə-glo-mer′u-lər) [*juxta-* + *glomerular*] near or adjoining a renal glomerulus.

jux•tal•lo•cor•tex (juk-stal″o-kor′teks) [*juxta-* + *allocortex*] mesocortex.

jux•ta•med•ul•lary (juks″tə-med′u-lar″e) near the renal medulla.

jux•ta•nu•cle•ar (juks″tə-noo′kle-ər) [*juxta-* + *nuclear*] adjacent to the nucleus.

jux•ta•po•si•tion (juks″tə-pə-zish′ən) apposition.

jux•ta•pul•mo•nary (juks″tə-pool′mo-nar″e) [*juxta-* + *pulmonary*] parapulmonary.

jux•ta•py•lor•ic (juks″tə-pi-lor′ik) near or around the pylorus or the pyloric part of the stomach. Called also *peripyloric.*

jux•ta•spi•nal (juks″tə-spi′nəl) paravertebral.

jux•ta•ves•i•cal (juks″tə-ves′ĭ-kəl) perivesical.

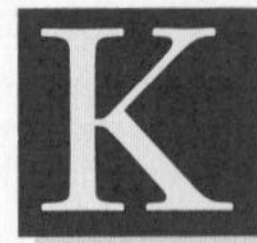

K kelvin; lysine; potassium (L. *ka'lium*).

K equilibrium constant; subscripts may be used to denote the method of measurement, e.g., K_c, K_p.

K_a acid dissociation constant.

K_b base dissociation constant.

K_d dissociation constant.

K_{eq} equilibrium constant.

K_M, K_m Michaelis constant.

K_{sp} solubility product constant.

K_W ion product of water; see under *product.*

k kilo-.

k Boltzmann constant; rate constant.

κ kappa, the tenth letter of the Greek alphabet; symbol for *dielectric constant* and for one of the two types of immunoglobulin light chains (see *immunoglobulin*).

Kab·i·ki·nase (kab″ĭ-ki′nās) trademark for preparations of streptokinase.

Kab·o·lin (kab′ə-lin) trademark for a preparation of nandrolone decanoate.

Ka·di·an (ka′de-ən) trademark for a preparation of morphine sulfate.

Kaes feltwork (line) (kāz) [Theodor *Kaes*, German neurologist, 1852–1913] Kaes-Bekhterev layer; see under *layer.*

Kaes-Bekh·ter·ev layer (kāz′ bek-ter′yev) [T. *Kaes;* Vladimir Mikhailovich *Bekhterev*, Russian neurologist, 1857–1927] see under *layer.*

KAFO knee-ankle-foot orthosis.

Kah·ler's law (kah′lərz) [Otto *Kahler*, German physician, 1849–1893] see under *law.*

kain(o)- see *cen(o)-*[1].

kain·ic ac·id (kān′ik) an excitotoxin found in the seaweed *Diginea simplex;* it is 30 to 100 times as potent as glutamic acid and is used experimentally to study the excitatory mechanisms of glutamate transmitters.

Kai·ser·stuhl disease (ki′zər-shtōōl″) [*Kaiserstuhl* region in Germany, where the disease occurred] see under *disease.*

kak- for words beginning thus, see also those beginning *cac-*.

kak·o·dyl (kak′o-dil) cacodyl.

ka·la-azar (kah′lah-ah-zahr′) [Hindi, "black fever"] visceral leishmaniasis.

kal·a·da·na (kal″ə-da′nə) the dried seeds of *Ipomoea nil* L.; used in India and China for its cathartic and anthelmintic properties.

ka·la·gua (kə-lah′gwə) a drug used in South America in the treatment of tuberculosis.

ka·le·mia (kə-le′me-ə) [L. *kalium* potassium + *-emia*] the presence of potassium in the blood; see *hyperkalemia.*

Ka·le·tra (kə-le′trə) trademark for a combination preparation of lopinavir and ritonavir.

ka·li·e·mia (ka″le-e′me-ə) kalemia.

ka·lim·e·ter (kə-lim′ə-tər) alkalimeter.

ka·lio·pe·nia (ka″le-o-pe′ne-ə) hypokalemia. **kaliope′nic** *adj*

ka·li·ure·sis (ka″le-u-re′sis) [L. *kalium* potassium + *-uresis*] the excretion of potassium in the urine.

ka·li·uret·ic (ka″le-u-ret′ik) 1. pertaining to, characterized by, or promoting kaliuresis. 2. an agent that promotes kaliuresis.

kal·li·din (kal′ĭ-din) lysyl-bradykinin, a decapeptide kinin produced by the action of tissue and glandular kallikreins on low-molecular-weight (LMW) kininogen and having physiologic effects similar to those of bradykinin. Formerly the term was applied to both nona- and decapeptides; bradykinin was called *kallidin I* or *kallidin-9*, and lysyl-bradykinin was called *kallidin II* or *kallidin-10.*

kal·li·kre·in (kal″ĭ-kre′in) any of several serine proteinases that cleave kininogens to form kinins, such as bradykinin and kallidin.

plasma k. [EC 3.4.21.34] a plasma enzyme of the hydrolase class that cleaves HMW kininogen to produce bradykinin; it also activates blood coagulation factors XII and VII and plasminogen. It is formed from prekallikrein by activated coagulation factor XII.

tissue k. [EC 3.4.21.35] an enzyme of the hydrolase class that cleaves LMW kininogen to produce kallidin. It and closely related forms are found in tissues and various glandular secretions including lymph, pancreatic juice, urine, and saliva.

kal·li·kre·in·o·gen (kal″ĭ-kre-in′ə-jən) prekallikrein.

Kall·mann syndrome (kahl′mahn) [Franz Josef *Kallmann*, German-born American psychiatrist, 1897–1965] see under *syndrome.*

Kal·mia (kal′me-ə) a genus of shrubs of the family Ericaceae, whose leaves have been used to treat syphilis, diarrhea, and chronic inflammatory disorders, and are thought to possess cardiac and sedative properties. *K. latifo′lia* L. is mountain laurel; it and related species contain andromedotoxin and are poisonous to livestock.

kal·ure·sis (kal″u-re′sis) kaliuresis.

kal·uret·ic (kal″u-ret′ik) kaliuretic.

ka·ma·la (kah′mə-lə) 1. *Mallotus philippinensis.* 2. the glands and hairs of the capsules of *M. philippinensis*, used as a cathartic and in veterinary medicine as a teniacide. Called also *rottlera.*

Kam·bin triangular working zone (kam′bin) [Parviz *Kambin*, Iranian-born American orthopedist, born 1931] see under *zone.*

Kam·mer·er-Bat·tle incision (kam′ər-ər bat′əl) [Frederic *Kammerer*, American surgeon, 1856–1928; William Henry *Battle*, British surgeon, 1855–1936] see under *incision.*

kam·po (kahm′po) [Japanese] herbal medicine as practiced in Japan, having its origin in traditional Chinese medicine; spelled also *kanpo.*

kan·a·my·cin (kan″ə-mi′sin) an aminoglycoside antibiotic complex derived from *Streptomyces kanamyceticus*, consisting of three components, designated A, B, and C. The form in clinical use is a mixture of kanamycins A and B; it is effective against aerobic gram-negative bacilli and some gram-positive bacteria, including mycobacteria, although its use has declined because of toxicity and limited spectrum of activity.

k. sulfate [USP] the sulfate salt of kanamycin, administered intravenously, intramuscularly, and by inhalation and intraperitoneal infusion in the treatment of a wide variety of infections caused by susceptible gram-negative organisms and orally to suppress bowel flora in the adjunctive treatment of hepatic coma and in preoperative bowel preparation.

Ka·na·vel sign (kə-na′vəl) [Allen Buchner *Kanavel*, American surgeon, 1874–1938] see under *sign.*

Kan·ner syndrome (kah′nər) [Leo *Kanner*, Austrian-born American child psychiatrist, 1894–1981] autistic disorder.

kan·po (kahn′po) kampo.

Kan·tor sign (kan′tər) [John Leonard *Kantor*, American radiologist, 1890–1947] see under *sign.*

Kan·trex (kan′treks) trademark for preparations of kanamycin sulfate.

Ka·o·chlor (ka′o-klor) trademark for a preparation of potassium chloride.

ka·o·lin (ka′o-lin) [*Kao-Ling* or *Gao-Ling*, city in southeastern China where it was first found] 1. a type of hydrated aluminum silicate, found in the form of clay and purified to form the medicinal product. 2. [USP] kaolin that has been purified and pulverized to form a white or light yellow powder with a claylike taste, used as an adsorbent and in the treatment of diarrhea, often in combination with pectin.

ka·o·lin·o·sis (ka″o-lin-o′sis) kaolin pneumoconiosis.

ka·pha (kah′fah) [Sanskrit "phlegm"] according to ayurveda, one of the three doshas, or principles of constitution of the body, condensed from the elements water and earth. Kapha is the principle of stabilizing energy and governs growth in the body and mind and is concerned with structure, stability, lubrication, and fluid balance. It is eliminated from the body through the urine.

Kap·i·dex (kap′ĭ-deks) trademark for a preparation of dexlansoprazole.

Kap·lan-Mei·er survival curve, method (kap′lən mi′ər) [E.L. *Kaplan*, American statistician, 20th century; Paul *Meier*, American statistician, 20th century] see under *curve* and *method.*

Ka·po·si sarcoma, varicelliform eruption (kah′po-she, kap′o-se, kə-po′se) [Moritz *Kaposi* (Moritz Kaposi Kohn), Austrian dermatologist, 1837–1902] see under *eruption* and *sarcoma.*

kap·o·si·form (kap′o-se-form″) resembling Kaposi sarcoma.

kap·pa (kap′ə) [K, κ] 1. the tenth letter of the Greek alphabet. 2. a statistic calculated to quantify the extent to which agreement between observers exceeds that expected on the basis of chance alone.

ka·ra-kurt (kah′rah-koort″) *Latrodectus lugubris*, a venomous Russian spider.

ka·ra·ya (kah′rah-yə) see under *gum.*

Ka·re·nia (ka-re′ne-ə) a genus of plantlike marine and freshwater protozoa of the phylum Dinoflagellata; they produce red tide when present in vast numbers. The species *K. brevis* contains brevetoxins and causes brevetoxicosis in marine animals and neurotoxic shellfish poisoning in humans (see under *poisoning*).

kar·ma (kahr′mə) [Sanskrit "action, deed"] in Indian philosophy, the total effect of a person's actions, both mental and physical, on his or her existence; a person's present state is determined by actions from previous existence, and present actions determine a person's destiny for future existence. According to this concept, one's good or bad actions during prior existence may be manifested as positive or negative effects on health.

Kar•nof•sky scale (kahr-nof′ske) [David A. *Karnofsky*, American clinical oncologist, 1914–1969] see under *scale*.

Kar•plus sign (kahr′ploos) [Johann Paul *Karplus*, Austrian physician and physiologist, 1866–1936] see under *sign*.

Kar•tag•e•ner syndrome (triad) (kahr-tag′ə-nər) [Manes *Kartagener*, Swiss physician, 1897–1975] see under *syndrome*.

Kar•win•skia (kahr-win′ske-ə) a genus of shrubs of the family Rhamnaceae, found mostly in the southwestern United States and Mexico. *K. humboldtia′na* is the buckthorn or coyotillo, a shrub whose fruit causes buckthorn poisoning.

kary•ap•sis (kar″e-ap′sis) [*karyo-* + Gr. *hapsis* joining] union of nuclei in a conjugating cell.

Ka•ry•da•kis flap (kă-re-dah′kis) [George E. *Karydakis*, Greek surgeon, late 20th century] see under *flap*.

kary(o)- [Gr. *karyon* nut, kernel] a combining form denoting relationship to a nucleus; see also words beginning *cary(o)-*.

karyo•chrome (kar′e-o-krōm″) [*karyo-* + *-chrome*] a nerve cell whose nucleus is deeply stainable while its body is not; called also *karyochrome cell* and *caryochrome*.

kary•og•a•my (kar″e-og′ə-me) [*karyo-* + Gr. *gamos* marriage] the union of the nuclei of cells following plasmogamy in fertilization. **karyogam′ic** *adj*

karyo•gram (kar′e-o-gram″) [*karyo-* + *-gram*] an image, prepared by drawing, digitized imaging, or photography, of a systematized array of a chromosome complement; it carries the expanded implication that the chromosomes of a single cell can typify an individual or even a species. See also *karyotype*.

karyo•ki•ne•sis (kar″e-o-kĭ-ne′sis) [*karyo-* + *-kinesis*] the phenomena involved in division of the nucleus of a cell. See *meiosis* and *mitosis*. **karyokinet′ic** *adj*

kary•ol•y•sis (kar″e-ol′ə-sis) [*karyo-* + *-lysis*] 1. the swelling of the nucleus of a necrotic cell and fading of the chromatin as it becomes less basophilic owing to deoxyribonuclease activity. 2. dissolution of the cell nucleus; cf. *karyorrhexis*.

karyo•lyt•ic (kar″e-o-lit′ik) 1. producing or pertaining to karyolysis. 2. destroying cell nuclei.

karyo•mas•ti•gont (kar″e-o-mas′tĭ-gont) [*karyo-* + *mastigont*] a condition characteristic of certain flagellate protozoa in which the mastigont system is associated with a nucleus. Cf. *akaryomastigont*.

karyo•meg•a•ly (kar″e-o-meg′ə-le) [*karyo-* + *-megaly*] abnormal enlargement of the nucleus of a cell, not caused by polyploidy.

kary•om•e•try (kar″e-om′ə-tre) [*karyo-* + *-metry*] measurement of a cell nucleus.

karyo•mi•to•sis (kar″e-o-mi-to′sis) mitosis.

karyo•mor•phism (kar″e-o-mor′fiz-əm) [*karyo-* + *morph-* + *-ism*] the shape of a cell nucleus.

kary•on (kar′e-on) [Gr. *karyon* nucleus] nucleus (def. 2).

karyo•phage (kar′e-o-fāj″) [*karyo-* + *-phage*] a protozoan that exercises phagocytic action on the nucleus of the cell it infects.

karyo•plasm (kar′e-o-plaz″əm) [*karyo-* + *-plasm*] nucleoplasm.

karyo•plast (kar′e-o-plast) a nucleus (def. 2), surrounded by a thin layer of cytoplasm and a plasma membrane, that has been removed from a eukaryotic cell. Cf. *cytoplast*.

karyo•pyk•no•sis (kar″e-o-pik-no′sis) shrinkage of a cell nucleus, with condensation of the chromatin into a solid, structureless mass or masses.

karyo•pyk•not•ic (kar″e-o-pik-not′ik) 1. pertaining to or characterized by karyopyknosis. 2. causing karyopyknosis.

kary•or•rhec•tic (kar″e-o-rek′tik) 1. pertaining to or characterized by karyorrhexis. 2. causing karyorrhexis.

kary•or•rhex•is (kar″e-o-rek′sis) [*karyo-* + *-rrhexis*] fragmentation of a pyknotic cell nucleus in which the chromatin disintegrates into formless granules; it is followed by dissolution (*karyolysis*, def. 2).

karyo•the•ca (kar″e-o-the′kə) [*karyo-* + *theca*] nuclear membrane.

karyo•type (kar′e-o-tīp) [*karyo-* + *type*] formally, the symbolic representation, using numbers, letters, and other symbols, of the chromosomal complement of an individual, tissue, or cell line. In practice, the terms karyotype, idiogram and karyogram are often used interchangeably. karyotyp′ic *adj*

spectral k. (SKY) a colored image of a set of chromosomes, created by adapting fluorescence in situ hybridization (FISH) using combinations of different fluorescent probes to label each of the chromosomes of a metaphase spread uniquely; used particularly to identify chromosome rearrangements.

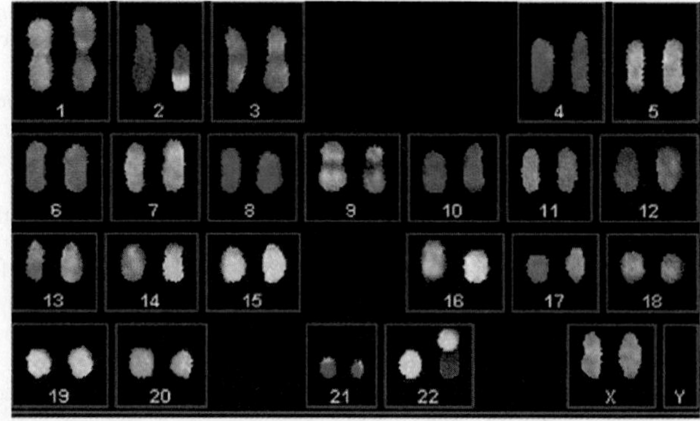

■ Spectral karyotype identifying a rearrangement between chromosomes 2 and 22.

karyo•typ•ing (kar′e-o-tīp″ing) laboratory analysis of an individual's karyotype of chromosomes to find abnormal ones, such as those with missing, extra, or rearranged sequences that might be linked to disease states, birth defects, or other conditions . It can be done on a fetus with cells obtained by amniocentesis or chorionic villus sampling, or on an older person on any kind of tissue. Called also *chromosome analysis*.

karyo•zo•ic (kar″e-o-zo′ik) [*karyo-* + Gr. *zōon* animal] existing in or inhabiting the nuclei of cells, as do certain protozoa.

Kas•a•bach-Mer•ritt syndrome (kas′ə-bahk mer′it) [Haig Haigouni *Kasabach*, American physician, 1898–1943; Katharine Krom *Merritt*, American pediatrician, 20th century] see under *syndrome*.

Ka•sai operation (kah-si′) [Morio *Kasai*, Japanese surgeon, 20th century] portoenterostomy.

ka•sal (ka′sal) chemical name: basic sodium aluminum phosphate; a food additive, with about 30 per cent dibasic sodium phosphate.

Ka•shin-Bek (Ka•schin-Beck) disease (kah′shin bek′) [Nikolai Ivanovich *Kashin* (or *Kaschin*), Russian orthopedist, 1825–1872; E.V. *Bek* (or *Beck*), Russian physician, early 20th century] see under *disease*.

Kast syndrome (kahst) [Alfred *Kast*, German physician, 1856–1903] Maffucci syndrome.

kat katal.

ka•ta (kah′tə) peste des petits ruminants.

kata- [Gr. *kata* down] a prefix meaning down, lower, under, against, along with, very. For words beginning thus, see also those beginning *cata-*.

kata•did•y•mus (kat″ə-did′ə-məs) [*kata-* + *-didymus*] conjoined twins divided in the upper part of the body but single in the lower part. See also *dicephalus*.

kat•al (kat) (kat′əl) a unit of measurement proposed to express activities of all catalysts, including enzymes, being that amount of a catalyst, such as an enzyme, which catalyzes a reaction rate of 1 mole of substrate per second.

kata•ther•mom•e•ter (kat″ə-thər-mom′ə-tər) a pair of alcoholic thermometers, one with a dry bulb and one with a wet bulb. They are heated to 110°F and exposed to the air, and the time is noted that it takes each bulb to fall from 100° to 90°F. From this the temperature as it affects the body can be deduced.

Ka•ta•ya•ma (kah-tah-yah′mah) *Oncomelania*.

Ka•ta•ya•ma fever (disease) (kah-tah-yah′mah) [*Katayama* River Valley, Japan, where it was first reported in the 19th century] see under *fever*.

kath•a•rom•e•ter (kath″ə-rom′ə-tər) an instrument for electrometric determination of basal metabolic rates.

kath•iso•pho•bia (kath″ĭ-so-fo′be-ə) intense, irrational fear of sitting down.

Kath•on (kath′on) trademark for preparations of methylisothiazolinone and methylchloroisothiazolinone.

ka•tine (ka′tin) an alkaloid from *Catha edulis* Forsk. (Celastraceae); its actions on the nervous system are similar to those of cocaine, but it has no local anesthetic properties, and it is used as an appetite depressant and mild euphoriant. The leaves are used as tea and masticatory in Ethiopia, East and South Africa, and Yemen.

kato•pho•ria (kat″ə-for′e-ə) cataphoria.

kato•tro•pia (kat″ə-tro′pe-ə) cataphoria.

Kauff•mann-White classification (kouf′mahn hwīt′) [Fritz *Kauffmann*, German microbiologist, 20th century; P.B. *White*, British microbiologist, 20th century] see under *classification.*

Kauf•man-Mc•Ku•sick syndrome (kouf′man mə-ku′sik) [Robert Lionel *Kaufman*, American physician, born 1937; Victor Almon *McKusick*, American geneticist, born 1921] see under *syndrome.*

ka•va ka•va (kah′və kah′və) [Polynesian *kava* bitter] a preparation of the rhizome of *Piper methysticum*, the kava plant, which is native to the South Pacific islands, having muscle-relaxing, anticonvulsive, anxiolytic, and sedative effects; used for the relief of stress and restlessness, and for sleep induction. It is also used in homeopathy and folk medicine.

Ka•wa•sa•ki disease (kah″wah-sah′ke) [Tomisaku *Kawasaki*, Japanese pediatrician, born 1925] mucocutaneous lymph node syndrome.

Kay Ciel (ka′se-el′) trademark for preparations of potassium chloride.

Kay•ex•a•late (ka-ek′sə-lāt) trademark for a preparation of sodium polystyrene sulfonate.

Kay•ser-Flei•scher ring (ki′zər fli′shər) [Bernhard *Kayser*, German ophthalmologist, 1869–1954; Bruno Richard *Fleischer*, German physician, 1848–1904] see under *ring.*

Ka•zan•ji•an forceps, operation (kah-zahn′je-ən) [Varaztad Hovhannes *Kazanjian*, Armenian-born plastic and maxillofacial surgeon in United States, 1879–1974] see under *forceps* and *operation.*

kb kilobase; sometimes used incorrectly to denote kilobase pairs in double-stranded nucleic acid.

kbp kilobase pairs (1000 base pairs in a nucleic acid).

kcal kilocalorie.

kCi kilocurie.

kD, kDa kilodalton.

K-Dur (kay′door) trademark for a preparation of potassium chloride.

Ke an antigenic marker distinguishing human immunoglobulin λ light chain subtypes. Called also *Kern.*

Kearns-Sayre syndrome (kernz′ sār) [Thomas P. *Kearns*, American ophthalmologist, born 1922; George Pomeroy *Sayre*, American pathologist, born 1911] see under *syndrome.*

kebo•ceph•a•ly (keb″ə-sef′ə-le) cebocephaly.

ked (ked) the sheep tick, *Melophagus ovinus.*

Keen sign (kēn) [William Williams *Keen*, American surgeon, 1837–1932] see under *sign.*

Kef•lex (kef′leks) trademark for preparations of cephalexin.

Kef•lin (kef′lin) trademark for a preparation of cephalothin sodium.

Kef•tab (kef′tab) trademark for a preparation of cephalexin hydrochloride monohydrate.

Kef•ur•ox (kef′u-roks) trademark for a preparation of cefuroxime sodium.

Kef•zol (kef′zol) trademark for a preparation of cefazolin sodium.

Ke•gel exercises (ka′gəl) [Arnold H. *Kegel*, American gynecologist, died 1976] see under *exercise.*

Kehr sign (kār) [Hans *Kehr*, German surgeon, 1862–1916] see under *sign.*

Kehr•er reflex (kār′ər) [Ferdinand *Kehrer*, German neurologist, 1883–1966] see under *reflex.*

Keith node (kēth) [Sir Arthur *Keith*, Scottish-born anatomist in England, 1866–1955] see *nodus sinuatrialis.*

Keith-Flack node (kēth′ flak′) [Sir A. *Keith;* Martin William *Flack*, British physiologist, 1882–1931] nodus sinuatrialis.

Keith-Wag•e•ner-Bar•ker classification (kēth′ wag′ə-nər bahr′kər) [Norman Macdonnell *Keith*, Canadian ophthalmologist in United States, 1885–1976; Henry Patrick *Wagener*, American ophthalmologist, 1890–1961; Nelson W. *Barker*, American physician, 20th century] see under *classification.*

ke•lec•tome (ke′lek-tōm) [Gr. *kēlē* tumor + *-ectomy*] a device used in removing specimens of tissue from tumors.

Kell blood group (kel) [*Kell*, surname of the propositus first observed in 1946] see under *blood group.*

Kel•ler operation (kel′ər) [Col. William Lordan *Keller*, American military surgeon, 1874–1959] see under *operation.*

Kel•lock sign (kel′ək) [T.H. *Kellock*, American physician, late 19th century] see under *sign.*

Kel•ly plication (operation), speculum (kel′e) [Howard Atwood *Kelly*, American surgeon, 1858–1943] see under *plication* and *speculum.*

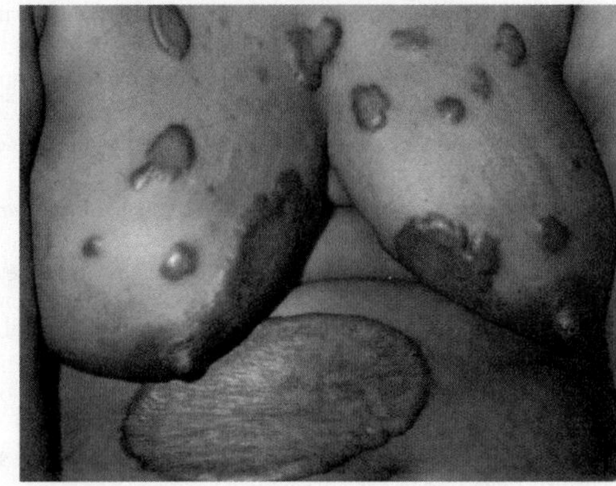

■ Keloids.

ke•loid (ke′loid) [Gr. *kēlis* blemish + *-oid*] a sharply elevated, irregularly shaped, progressively enlarging scar due to formation of excessive amounts of collagen in the dermis during connective tissue repair.

acne k's acne keloidalis.

k. of gums fibromatosis gingivae.

ke•lot•o•my (ke-lot′ə-me) herniotomy.

Kel•vin scale (kel′vin) [William Thomson, Lord *Kelvin*, British physicist, 1824–1907] see under *scale.*

kel•vin (K) (kel′vin) [Lord *Kelvin*] the base SI unit of temperature, equal to 1/273.15 of the absolute temperature of the triple point of water. See also *absolute temperature*, under *temperature*, and *Kelvin scale*, under *scale.*

Kem•a•drin (kem′ə-drin) trademark for a preparation of procyclidine hydrochloride.

Ken•a•cort (ken′ə-kort) trademark for preparations of triamcinolone.

Ken•a•log (ken′ə-log) trademark for preparations of triamcinolone acetonide.

Ken•dall rank correlation coefficient (tau) (ken′dəl) [Maurice George *Kendall*, British statistician, 1907–1983] see under *coefficient.*

Ken•ne•dy classification (ken′ə-de) [Edward *Kennedy*, American dentist, 20th century] see under *classification.*

Ken•ne•dy disease, syndrome (ken′ə-de) [Robert Foster *Kennedy*, American neurologist, 1884–1952] see *spinobulbar muscular atrophy*, under *atrophy*, and see under *syndrome.*

Ken•ny-Caf•fey syndrome (ken′e kaf′e) [Frederic Marshal *Kenny*, American pediatrician, born 1929; John Patrick *Caffey*, American pediatrician, 1895–1978] see under *syndrome.*

ke•no•tox•in (ke′no-tok″sin) [*keno-* + *toxin*] a hypothetical toxin supposedly produced in muscle by muscular contractions, causing fatigue.

Kent bundle (kent) [Albert Frank Stanley *Kent*, English physiologist, 1863–1958] see under *bundle.*

Kent-His bundle (kent′ his′) [A.F.S. *Kent;* Wilhelm *His*, Jr., Swiss physician, 1863–1934] bundle of His.

Ke•pone (ke′pōn) trademark for a preparation of chlordecone.

Kep•pra (kep′rə) trademark for a preparation of levetiracetam.

Ker•an•del sign (ker″ahn-del′) [Jean François *Kerandel*, French physician in Africa, 1873–1934] see under *sign.*

ker•a•phyl•lo•cele (ker″ə-fil′o-sēl) keratoma (def. 2).

ker•a•tal•gia (ker″ə-tal′jə) [*kerat-* + *-algia*] pain in the cornea.

ker•a•tan sul•fate (ker′ə-tan) a glycosaminoglycan found in the cornea, in cartilage, and in the nucleus pulposus and also as the accumulation product in Morquio syndrome. It consists of repeating disaccharide units in specific linkage, each composed of a sulfated *N*-acetylglucosamine residue linked to one of galactose, which is usually sulfated. There are two forms, *keratan sulfate I* and *keratan sulfate II*, which differ in carbohydrate content and localization; the former occurs in the cornea and the latter in skeletal tissues. Called also *keratosulfate.*

ker•a•tec•ta•sia (ker″ə-tek-ta′zhə) [*kerat-* + *ectasia*] protrusion of a thinned, scarred cornea; called also *corneal ectasia.*

ker•a•tec•to•my (ker″ə-tek′tə-me) [*kerat-* + *ectomy*] excision of a portion of the cornea, usually done for anterior staphyloma.

photorefractive k. (PRK) photoablation of the anterior corneal stroma using an excimer laser in order to correct ametropia by the creation of a new radius of curvature.

ke•rat•ic (kə-rat′ik) 1. keratinous (def. 1). 2. horny. 3. corneal.

ker•a•tin (ker′ə-tin) any of a family of scleroproteins that form the primary constituents of epidermis, hair, nails, and horny tissues. Included are the cytokeratins of epithelial tissue and the hard keratins of ectodermally derived structures such as hair and nails. Because it is insoluble in gastric juice, keratin is sometimes used to coat pills designed to pass through the stomach and dissolve in the intestine.

α-k., alpha k. 1. keratin in the form of an α helix, the usual form of hard keratin. 2. hard k.

hard k. one of the two kinds of keratin normally found in human tissues, constituting a family of high-sulfur keratin polypeptides found in hair and nails. Because hard keratin usually occurs as an α helix, it is sometimes called *α-k*.

soft k. cytokeratin.

ker•a•tin•ase (ker′ə-tĭ-nās) an enzyme of the hydrolase class that catalyzes the cleavage of keratin, found in the agent causing tinea pedis, in *Trichophyton mentagrophytes*, and in *Streptomyces*.

ker•a•tin•ic (ker-ə-tin′ik) 1. keratinous (def. 1). 2. horny.

ker•a•tin•iza•tion (ker″ə-tin″ĭ-za′shən) the development of or conversion into keratin.

ker•a•tin•ize (ker′ə-tin-īz) to make or become like keratin.

ke•rat•i•no•cyte (kə-rat′ĭ-no-sīt) an epidermal cell that synthesizes keratin; about 95 per cent of the cells of the epidermis are of this type. They and the melanocytes form the binary cell system of the epidermis. In its successive stages, the keratinocyte is known as basal cell, prickle cell, and granular cell. Called also *malpighian cell*.

ker•a•tin•oid (ker′ə-tin-oid) a form of keratin-coated tablet not soluble in the stomach, but readily soluble in the intestine.

ke•rat•i•no•phil•ic (kə-rat″in-o-fil′ik) keratin-seeking; using keratin as a substrate. Said of fungi.

ke•rat•i•no•some (kə-rat′ĭ-no-sōm″) lamellar body.

ke•rat•i•nous (kə-rat′ĭ-nəs) 1. containing keratin or of the nature of keratin; called also *keratic*. 2. horny.

ker•a•ti•tis (ker″ə-ti′tis) pl. *kerati′tides* [*kerat-* + *-itis*] inflammation of the cornea. Cf. *keratoconjunctivitis* and *keratopathy*.

***Acanthamoeba* k.** amebic keratitis due to infection by *Acanthamoeba* species, usually associated with soft contact lens wear, particularly overnight wear.

acne rosacea k. rosacea k.

actinic k. a type of keratitis caused by the action of ultraviolet light; called also *ultraviolet k*.

alphabet k. striate k.

amebic k. keratitis caused by amebic infections; the most common kind is *Acanthamoeba* keratitis, but other amebae such as *Hartmannella* have occasionally been implicated.

anaphylactic k. interstitial keratitis in one eye, caused by an antibody-antigen reaction to an intracorneal injection of protein in the eye after sensitization from intracorneal injection of protein into the other eye.

annular k. marginal k.

k. arbores′cens dendriform k.

aspergillus k. keratomycosis due to infection by fungi of the genus *Aspergillus*.

bacterial k. bacterial infection of the cornea as a result of contact lens wear, trauma, use of contaminated eye medications, corneal disease, or some other cause; it often progresses rapidly into inflammation, ulceration, and edema that can lead to blindness. Bacteria commonly implicated include species of *Enterobacter*, *Klebsiella*, *Proteus*, *Pseudomonas*, *Serratia*, *Staphylococcus*, and *Streptococcus*.

k. bullo′sa the formation of large or small bullae or blebs on the cornea.

catarrhal ulcerative k. a mild type of keratitis secondary to conjunctivitis.

chronic superficial k. bilateral cellular infiltration and vascularization of the corneas in dogs, usually beginning at the lateral corner and progressing towards the middle so that the cornea becomes pigmented. Since it is limited to German shepherds and a few other breeds, a genetic component is suspected. Called also *degenerative pannus* and *Uberreiter syndrome*.

deep k. interstitial k.

deep pustular k. k. pustuliformis profunda.

dendriform k., dendritic k. herpetic keratitis resulting in a branching ulceration of the cornea.

desiccation k. lagophthalmic k.

Dimmer k. k. nummularis.

disciform k., k. discifor′mis keratitis with the formation of a round or oval, disklike opacity of the cornea.

eosinophilic k. neovascularization and cellular infiltration of the cornea of cats, with formation of an area of pink to white soft plaque beginning at a limbus and progressing towards the center.

epithelial diffuse k. a type of keratitis thought to be due to vitamin B_2 deficiency, generally associated with uveitis, and characterized by minute gray epithelial flecks.

epithelial punctate k. superficial punctate k.

exfoliative k. a type of keratitis sometimes seen with exfoliative dermatitis in a hypersensitive reaction to arsenic, marked by extensive denudation of the corneal epithelium.

exposure k. lagophthalmic k.

fascicular k. a type of keratitis accompanied by formation of a band of blood vessels.

k. filamento′sa keratitis with twisted filaments of mucoid material on the surface of the cornea; called also *filamentary keratopathy*.

fungal k. keratomycosis (def. 1).

furrow k. dendriform k.

***Fusarium* k.** keratomycosis due to infection by fungi of the genus *Fusarium*.

herpetic k. 1. keratitis caused by infection with herpes simplex virus, often with dendritic ulceration (*dendriform* or *dendritic k.*). 2. keratitis occurring as a complication of herpes zoster ophthalmicus.

hypopyon k. suppurative keratitis with purulent infiltration and hypopyon; see *hypopyon ulcer*.

infectious bovine k. see under *keratoconjunctivitis*.

infective k. microbial k.

interstitial k. chronic keratitis with ghost vessels and deep deposits in the substance of the cornea, which becomes hazy with a ground-glass appearance. It usually occurs in children under age 15, associated with congenital syphilis. See also *nonsyphilitic interstitial k*. Called also *parenchymatous k.*, *deep k.*, and *k. profunda*.

interstitial k., nonsyphilitic interstitial keratitis not associated with congenital syphilis; see *Cogan syndrome*.

lagophthalmic k. a type of keratitis that accompanies lagophthalmos because of exposure of the eyeball to the air.

lattice k. bilateral hereditary dystrophy of the cornea with the formation of interwoven filamentous lesions.

marginal k. phlyctenular keratitis in which the papules are arranged around the margin of the cornea; called also *annular k*.

metaherpetic k. keratitis resulting from recurrent herpesvirus infection of the cornea, characterized by shallow ulceration of an anesthetic cornea, accompanied by parenchymatous infiltration and often by persistent iridocyclitis and secondary glaucoma.

microbial k. any of the types of keratitis resulting from infection of the cornea, such as by bacteria, fungi, or amebae (see *amebic k.*, *bacterial k.*, and *keratomycosis*); it is usually associated with soft contact lens wear. Called also *infective k*.

mycotic k. keratomycosis (def. 1).

neuroparalytic k. keratitis characterized by dryness and fissuring of the corneal epithelium as a result of an injury to the trifacial nerve which prevents proper closing of the eyelids; called also *trophic k*.

neurotrophic k. keratitis due to loss of corneal sensation.

k. nummula′ris a slowly developing, benign type of keratitis in which corneal deposits form circular areas with sharply defined edges surrounded by a halo that is less dense; called also *Dimmer k*.

parenchymatous k. interstitial k.

peripheral ulcerative k. a rare type of keratitis with inflammation of the limbal part of the cornea and nearby sclera, which have cellular infiltration, vascular changes, and ulceration that may cause blindness; it may be a complication of rheumatoid arthritis or a bacterial infection but sometimes is idiopathic.

phlyctenular k. see under *keratoconjunctivitis*.

k. profun′da interstitial k.

k. puncta′ta any of various conditions characterized by keratic precipitates.

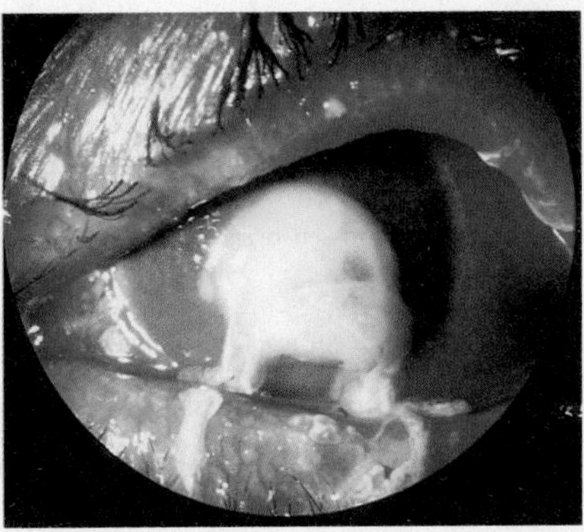

■ Microbial keratitis. Corneal melt caused by bacterial invasion.

k. puncta′ta lepro′sa a type of keratitis occurring with leprosy, consisting of tiny, scattered, white spots.

k. puncta′ta profun′da deep punctate k.

k. puncta′ta subepithelia′lis a type of keratitis in which there are gray areas on the cornea under the Bowman membrane, with an intact superficial epithelium.

punctate k. k. punctata.

punctate k., deep a rare type of keratitis seen in hereditary or acquired syphilitic iritis and marked by sharply defined, pinhead-sized, grayish opacities in the substantia propria; called also *k. punctata profunda.*

punctate k., superficial a type of keratitis usually seen with epidemic keratoconjunctivitis and characterized by small circular epithelial erosions.

purulent k. severe keratitis characterized by a large ulcer with pus in the anterior chamber and purulent disintegration of the cornea.

k. pustulifor′mis profun′da a painful type of keratitis with deep-seated yellow intracorneal spots, hypopyon, and purulent iritis; called also *deep pustular k.*

reaper's k. suppurative keratitis due to the wounding of the cornea by husks or other fragments of grain.

reticular k. a familial type of degeneration of the cornea with reticular areas.

rosacea k. severe keratitis due to involvement of the cornea in rosacea, sometimes leading to ulceration; called also *acne rosacea k.*

sclerosing k. keratitis associated with scleritis, leading to hyperplasia.

scrofulous k. phlyctenular keratoconjunctivitis.

secondary k. keratitis due to disease of some other part of the eye.

serpiginous k. hypopyon ulcer.

k. sic′ca keratoconjunctivitis sicca.

striate k. keratitis marked by parallel and intersecting lines on the corneal epithelium; called also *alphabet k.* Cf. *striate keratopathy.*

suppurative k. keratitis accompanied by suppuration.

trachomatous k. pannus trachomatosus.

trophic k. neuroparalytic k.

ulcerative k. keratitis with ulceration of the corneal epithelium, such as in complication of microbial keratitis. Called also *corneal ulcer.*

ultraviolet k. actinic k.

vascular k. keratitis accompanied by the formation of blood vessels beneath the conjunctiva and outer layers of the cornea.

vesicular k. keratitis with development of small vesicles on the surface of the cornea.

xerotic k. dryness of the cornea, usually preceding keratomalacia.

kerat(o)- [Gr. *keras*, gen. *keratos* horn] a combining form denoting relationship to horny tissue, or to the cornea.

ker•a•to•ac•an•tho•ma (ker″ə-to-ak″an-tho′mə) [*kerato-* + *acanthoma*] a locally destructive epithelial tumor with a superficial crater containing a keratin plug; it closely resembles squamous cell carcinoma clinically and histologically, but is benign and generally undergoes spontaneous regression. Exposure to sunlight is believed to play a role in its etiology.

eruptive k. a manifestation of keratoacanthoma, seen usually in light-skinned, middle-aged adults, consisting of a generalized papular eruption of dome-shaped, skin-colored papules, often sparing the palms and soles.

giant k. a solitary keratoacanthoma more than 2 cm in diameter.

multiple k. a condition almost identical to solitary keratoacanthoma except that it preferentially affects adolescents and young adults and occurs even on areas of skin unexposed to sunlight. See also *self-healing squamous epithelioma*, under *epithelioma.*

solitary k. a manifestation of keratoacanthoma seen primarily in middle-aged to elderly persons, especially white males, consisting of a firm, erythematous papule that enlarges rapidly to form a dome-shaped, skin-colored nodule with an umbilicated center, then slowly involutes and leaves a small focus of scarring. It occurs primarily on sunlight-exposed areas, particularly the face, neck, upper limbs, and backs of the hands.

ker•a•to•can (ker′ə-to-kan″) a leucine-rich repeat protein related to fibromodulin, found in the cornea, where it plays a role in maintenance of corneal transparency.

ker•a•to•cele (ker′ə-to-sēl″) [*kerato-* + *-cele*[1]] herniation of the Descemet membrane.

ker•a•to•cen•te•sis (ker″ə-to-sen-te′sis) [*kerato-* + *-centesis*] aqueous paracentesis.

ker•a•to•con•junc•ti•vi•tis (ker″ə-to-kən-junk″tĭ-vi′tis) [*kerato-* + *conjunctivitis*] inflammation of the cornea and conjunctiva.

epidemic k. a highly infectious disease characterized by scant ocular exudate, round subepithelial corneal opacities associated with the keratitis, and often swelling of regional lymph nodes; there may also be systemic symptoms, especially headache. Adenovirus type 8 has often been isolated from patients with the disease. Called also *shipyard k.*, *viral k.*, and *Sanders disease.*

flash k. actinic conjunctivitis.

infectious k. infectious keratitis with conjunctivitis in cattle, sheep, or goats, characterized by blepharospasm and sometimes corneal or conjunctival opacity. See also *infectious bovine k.*, *infectious caprine k.*, and *infectious ovine k.* Called also *contagious* or *infectious ophthalmia.*

infectious bovine k. infectious keratoconjunctivitis in cattle, usually caused by *Moraxella (Moraxella) bovis*, bovine herpesvirus 1, or *Mycoplasma* species. Called also *infectious bovine keratitis.*

infectious caprine k. infectious keratoconjunctivitis in goats, usually caused by species of *Mycoplasma* or *Moraxella.*

infectious ovine k. infectious keratoconjunctivitis in sheep, caused by *Mycoplasma* species, *Neisseria ovis*, and rickettsiae. Called also *heather blindness.*

phlyctenular k. keratoconjunctivitis marked by the formation of a phlyctenule at the corneal limbus; it has been associated with malnutrition, tuberculosis, and staphylococcus sensitivity. Called also *phlyctenular keratitis*, *phlyctenular ophthalmia*, and *strumous ophthalmia.* See also *phlyctenulosis.*

shipyard k. epidemic k.

k. sic′ca a condition marked by hyperemia of the conjunctiva, lacrimal deficiency, thickening of the corneal epithelium, itching and burning of the eye, and often reduced visual acuity. Called also *dry eye* and *dry eye syndrome.* Cf. *Sjögren syndrome.*

ultraviolet k. actinic conjunctivitis.

vernal k. keratoconjunctivitis caused by allergic reaction, often occurring in the spring but sometimes perennial, characterized by the presence of giant papillae, usually in the upper tarsal conjunctiva, a ropy mucus thread in the inferior fornix, itching, and often ptosis, and may progress to an epithelial defect.

viral k. epidemic k.

ker•a•to•co•nus (ker″ə-to-ko′nəs) [*kerato-* + *conus*] a noninflammatory, usually bilateral protrusion of the cornea, the apex being displaced downward and nasally. It occurs most commonly in females at about puberty. The cause is unknown, but hereditary factors may play a role. Called also *conical cornea.*

ker•a•to•cyst (ker′ə-to-sist) [*kerato-* + *cyst*] an odontogenic cyst lined with a layer of keratinized squamous epithelium and commonly associated with a primordial cyst.

ker•a•to•cyte (ker′ə-to-sīt″) [*kerato-* + *-cyte*] one of the flattened connective tissue cells between the lamellae of fibrous tissue composing the cornea.

ker•a•to•der•ma (ker″ə-to-dur′mə) [*kerato-* + *derma*] 1. a horny skin or covering. 2. hypertrophy of the stratum corneum of the skin; see also *callus* and *hyperkeratosis* (def. 1). Called also *keratodermia.*

acquired k., acquired palmoplantar k. palmoplantar keratoderma secondary to another disease or condition, such as inflammation, a drug reaction, immunodeficiency, internal malignancy, or hormonal changes such as with keratoderma climactericum. Cf. *hereditary palmoplantar k.*

k. blennorrha′gicum a cutaneous manifestation of Reiter syndrome, named for the former idea that it was related to gonorrhea. It usually involves the palms, soles, toes, or glans penis, and is characterized by erythematous macules that form blisters and later develop thick keratotic coverings. The lesions closely resemble those of pustular psoriasis. Called also *keratosis blennorrhagica.*

k. climacte′ricum a type of acquired palmoplantar keratoderma occurring in women about the time of menopause; there is sometimes fissuring of the thickened patches.

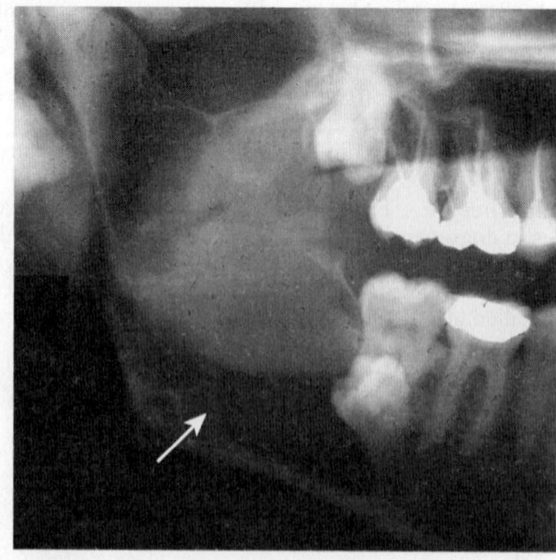

■ Keratocyst visible as a loculated radiolucency extending from the condylar neck to the lower first molar region. There is thinning of the bony cortices but no jaw expansion, and the lower third molar is displaced.

diffuse palmoplantar k. any of several hereditary types of palmoplantar keratoderma; most are autosomal dominant, but a rare type, *mal de Meleda*, is autosomal recessive. They are usually present in infancy but occasionally do not appear until later. The main characteristic is well-demarcated, usually bilateral and symmetrical, confluent areas of scaling on the palms and soles, sometimes spreading to the backs of the hands and feet. Types are now usually distinguished as either *epidermolytic* or *nonepidermolytic palmoplantar keratoderma* depending on whether epidermolysis is present.

epidermolytic palmoplantar k. the most common type of diffuse palmoplantar keratoderma, a genetically heterogeneous, autosomal dominant disorder characterized by epidermolytic hyperkeratosis (q.v.).

k. heredita'rium mu'tilans Vohwinkel syndrome.

hereditary palmoplantar k. any of the types of palmoplantar keratoderma that are passed by autosomal dominant or recessive inheritance. Cf. *acquired palmoplantar k.*

nonepidermolytic palmoplantar k. a rare autosomal dominant type of diffuse palmoplantar keratoderma in which there is hyperkeratosis without epidermolysis and characteristic focal oral, genital, and follicular lesions. Called also *Unna-Thost syndrome.*

k. palma're et planta're, palmoplantar k., k. palmoplanta're, k. of palms and soles a group of mostly inherited disorders characterized by excessive formation of keratin on the palms and soles; this may be localized or diffuse, and sometimes painful lesions result from fissuring of the skin. The condition may occur alone or may accompany or be part of another disorder. Called also *palmoplantar hyperkeratosis* or *keratosis* and *hyperkeratosis* or *keratosis palmaris et plantaris.* See also *diffuse palmoplantar, acquired palmoplantar,* and *hereditary palmoplantar k.*

k. palmoplanta're transgre'diens erythrokeratodermia variabilis.

punctate k., k. puncta'tum an autosomal dominant form of palmoplantar keratoderma in which the lesions are localized in multiple points on the palms and soles; called also *keratosis punctata* and *punctate keratosis.*

ker·a·to·der·ma·to·cele (ker″ə-to-dur'mə-to-sēl) keratocele.

ker·a·to·der·mia (ker″ə-to-dur'me-ə) keratoderma (def. 2).

ker·a·to·ec·ta·sia (ker″ə-to-ek-ta'zhə) kerectasis.

ker·a·to·elas·toi·do·sis (ker″ə-to-e-las″toi-do'sis) [*kerato-* + *elastoidosis*] elastosis with small, firm papules or plaques; see also *acrokeratoelastoidosis.*

k. margina'lis a rare skin condition in which there are collagenous plaques on the hands; it occurs after prolonged sun exposure and thus is considered a variant of solar elastosis.

ker·a·to·gen·e·sis (ker″ə-to-jen'ə-sis) the formation or production of horny material. **keratogenet'ic** *adj*

ker·a·tog·e·nous (ker″ə-toj'ə-nəs) [*kerato-* + *-genous*] giving rise to a growth of horny material.

ker·a·to·glo·bus (ker″ə-to-glo'bəs) megalocornea.

ker·a·to·he·mia (ker″ə-to-he'me-ə) [*kerato-* + *hem-* + *-ia*] the presence of deposits of blood in the cornea.

ker·a·to·hy·a·lin (ker″ə-to-hi'ə-lin) 1. a substance related to keratin, found in the keratohyalin granules of the granular layer of the epidermis. 2. a substance found in granules in the Hassall corpuscles of the thymus.

ker·a·to·hy·a·line (ker″ə-to-hi'ə-līn) 1. both horny and hyaline. 2. pertaining to keratohyalin or to the keratohyalin granules or the keratohyaline layer (stratum granulosum epidermidis). 3. keratohyalin.

ker·a·toid (ker'ə-toid) [*kerato-* + *-oid*] resembling horny or corneal tissue.

ker·a·to·ir·i·do·cyc·li·tis (ker″ə-to-ir″ĭ-do-sik-li'tis) [*kerato-* + *irido-* + *cyclitis*] inflammation of the cornea, iris, and ciliary body.

ker·a·to·i·rid·o·scope (ker″ə-to-ĭ-rid'ə-skōp) [*kerato-* + *irido-* + *-scope*] a form of compound microscope for examining the eye.

ker·a·to·i·ri·tis (ker″ə-to-i-ri'tis) [*kerato-* + *iritis*] inflammation of the cornea and iris.

hypopyon k. hypopyon keratitis.

ker·a·to·lep·tyn·sis (ker″ə-to-lep-tin'sis) [*kerato-* + Gr. *leptynsis* attenuation] removal of the anterior portion of the cornea and covering of the denuded area with bulbar conjunctiva.

ker·a·to·leu·ko·ma (ker″ə-to-loo-ko'mə) [*kerato-* + *leukoma*] a white opacity of the cornea.

ker·a·tol·y·sis (ker″ə-tol'ə-sis) [*kerato-* + *-lysis*] softening and dissolution or peeling of the stratum corneum of the epidermis.

pitted k. a superficial bacterial infection of the skin, usually involving the weightbearing portions of the soles of the feet, characterized by shallow asymptomatic round pits, some of which become confluent to form fissures; it is usually caused by infection with *Kytococcus sedentarius* or *Corynebacterium* species, which produce a proteolytic enzyme that digests the stratum corneum. Called also *keratoma plantare sulcatum.*

k. exfoliati'va a rare, autosomal recessive syndrome in which the skin undergoes superficial peeling over much of the body surface. Called also *deciduous skin* and *peeling skin syndrome.*

ker·a·to·lyt·ic (ker″ə-to-lit'ik) 1. pertaining to, characterized by, or producing keratolysis. 2. an agent that promotes keratolysis.

ker·a·to·ma (ker″ə-to'mə) pl. *keratomas, kerato'mata* [*kerat-* + *-oma*] 1. callus (def. 1). 2. a horny tumor on the inner surface of the wall of a horse's hoof. Called also *keraphyllocele.*

k. heredita'rium mu'tilans Vohwinkel syndrome.

k. palma're et planta're, k. palmoplanta're see under *keratoderma.*

k. planta're sulca'tum *pitted keratolysis.*

ker·a·to·ma·la·cia (ker″ə-to-mə-la'shə) [*kerato-* + *malacia*] a corneal condition, usually bilateral, associated with vitamin A deficiency. It begins with xerotic spots (Bitot spots) on the conjunctiva, while the cornea becomes xerotic and insensitive (xerotic keratitis); as the condition progresses, the haze increases until finally the entire cornea becomes soft, and colliquative necrosis occurs.

ker·a·to·ma·ta (ker″ə-to'mə-tə) plural of *keratoma.*

ker·a·tome (ker'ə-tōm) [*kerato-* + *-tome*] a knife for incising the cornea.

ker·a·tom·e·ter (ker″ə-tom'ə-tər) [*kerato-* + *-meter*] an instrument for measuring the curves of the cornea; called also *ophthalmometer.*

ker·a·to·met·ric (ker″ə-to-met'rik) pertaining to keratometry, or to measurements made with a keratometer.

ker·a·tom·e·try (ker″ə-tom'ə-tre) [*kerato-* + *-metry*] measurement of the anterior curvature of the cornea with a keratometer; called also *ophthalmometry.*

ker·a·to·mi·leu·sis (ker″ə-to-mĭ-loo'sis) [*kerato-* + Gr. *smileusis* carving] keratoplasty in which a slice of the patient's cornea is removed, shaped to the desired curvature on a lathe after freezing, and then sutured back on the remaining cornea to correct optical error.

laser-assisted in-situ k. keratoplasty in which the excimer laser and microkeratome are combined for vision correction; the microkeratome is used to shave a thin slice and create a hinged flap in the cornea, the flap is reflected back, the exposed cornea is reshaped by the laser, and the flap is replaced, without sutures, to heal back into position.

ker·a·to·my·co·sis (ker″ə-to-mi-ko'sis) [*kerato-* + *mycosis*] 1. corneal infection by a fungus; genera commonly implicated include *Aspergillus, Candida, Curvularia,* and *Fusarium.* Causes include trauma such as from contact lens wear or external objects and the spread of fungal endophthalmitis. Called also *fungal* or *mycotic keratitis.* 2. a fungal infection of the stratum corneum.

k. ni'gricans tinea nigra.

ker·a·top·a·thy (ker″ə-top'ə-the) [*kerato-* + *-pathy*] a noninflammatory disease of the cornea.

band k., band-shaped k. a degenerative condition in which a gray band develops axially from the limbus at the level of Bowman membrane into the exposed part of the cornea in the palpebral aperture.

bullous k. corneal degeneration marked by recurring epithelial blebs or bullae that rupture, expose corneal nerves, and cause great pain; it occurs in glaucoma, iridocyclitis, and Fuchs epithelial dystrophy.

climatic k. bilateral, symmetrical corneal degeneration due to extreme heat or cold; called also *Labrador k.*

filamentary k. keratitis filamentosa.

Labrador k. climatic k.

lipid k. deposits of fat in an area of previous corneal vascularization.

striate k. corneal stromal edema causing a network of lines, which is a common, temporary occurrence after cataract surgery. Cf. *striate keratitis.*

vesicular k. corneal epithelial edema with formation of vacuoles. Cf. *vesicular keratitis.*

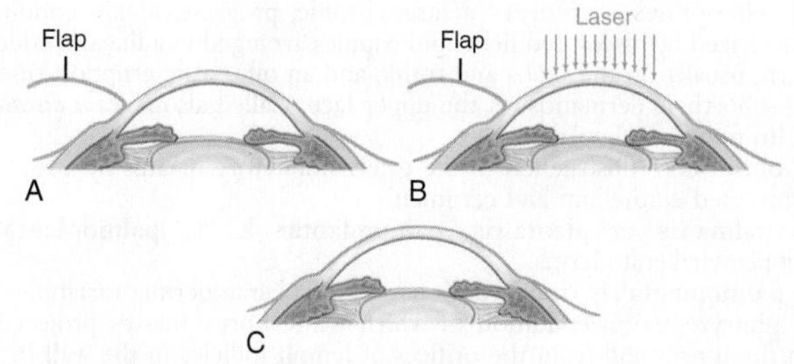

■ Laser-assisted in-situ keratomileusis for treatment of myopia. *(A)*, Creation of flap; *(B)*, laser ablation of the stromal bed, showing the area of tissue removal in blue; *(C)*, flap replaced, with the central cornea flattened

ker•a•to•pha•kia (ker″ə-to-fa′ke-ə) [*kerato-* + *phak-* + *-ia*] a form of keratoplasty in which a slice of donor's cornea is shaped to a desired curvature and inserted between layers of the recipient's cornea to change its curvature.

ker•a•to•plas•ty (ker′ə-to-plas″te) [*kerato-* + *-plasty*] plastic surgery of the cornea; called also *corneal transplantation.* **keratoplast′ic** *adj*

autogenous k. autokeratoplasty.

deep lamellar endothelial k. a type of endothelial keratoplasty involving transplantation of a deep pocket of the cornea. Called also *posterior lamellar endothelial k.*

Descemet stripping endothelial k. a type of endothelial keratoplasty in which the posterior limiting lamina (Descemet membrane) is removed and replaced along with the overlying endothelium.

endothelial k. keratoplasty in which only the diseased inner layers of the cornea are removed and transplanted.

lamellar k. keratoplasty involving the anterior half of the cornea with the anterior chamber remaining intact. See also *deep lamellar endothelial k.*

optic k. keratoplasty with removal and replacement of scar tissue that interferes with vision.

penetrating k. keratoplasty involving a full-thickness section of cornea.

posterior lamellar endothelial k. former name for deep lamellar endothelial k.

refractive k. keratoplasty in which a section of cornea is removed from the patient or a donor, shaped to the desired curvature, and inserted either between layers (keratophakia) or on the cornea (keratomileusis), changing its curvature and correcting optical errors. Called also *keratorefractive* or *lamellar refractive surgery*

tectonic k. keratoplasty to replace corneal tissue that has been lost.

ker•a•to•pro•tein (ker″ə-to-pro′tēn) [*kerato-* + *protein*] the protein of the horny tissues of the body, such as the hair, nails, and epidermis.

ker•a•to•rhex•is (ker″ə-to-rek′sis) [*kerato-* + *rhexis*] rupture of the cornea.

ker•a•tor•rhex•is (ker″ə-to-rek′sis) keratorhexis.

ker•a•to•scle•ri•tis (ker″ə-to-sklə-ri′tis) inflammation of the cornea and sclera.

ker•a•to•scope (ker′ə-to-skōp″) [*kerato-* + *-scope*] a device consisting of alternate black or white concentric circles and used for examining corneal curvature; called also *Placido disk.*

ker•a•tos•co•py (ker″ə-tos′kə-pe) the examination of the cornea; more especially the study of the reflections of light from its anterior surface.

ker•a•to•sis (ker″ə-to′sis) pl. *kerato′ses* [*kerato-* + *-osis*] any horny growth, such as a wart or callus; the most common types are actinic keratosis and seborrheic keratosis.

actinic k. a sharply outlined, red or skin-colored, flat or elevated, verrucous or keratotic growth that sometimes develops into a cutaneous horn or gives rise to a squamous cell carcinoma. It usually affects the middle-aged or elderly, especially those of fair complexion, and is caused by excessive exposure to the sun. Called also *senile* or *solar k.*.

arsenic k., arsenical k. a cutaneous manifestation of chronic arsenic poisoning, which may occur years after arsenic ingestion, characterized by development of discrete hyperkeratotic papules, usually on the palms or soles; sometimes it is associated with premalignant or malignant lesions on other skin areas.

k. blennorrha′gica keratoderma blennorrhagicum.

equine linear k. ridges of hyperkeratotic hairless skin on the sides of the neck and chest of horses, with surface seborrhea; the etiology is unknown.

k. extremita′tum Greither disease.

follicular k., k. follicula′ris Darier disease.

Greither k. see under *disease.*

inverted follicular k. a benign, usually solitary epithelial tumor originating in a hair follicle; it occurs as a flesh-colored papule or nodule, usually on the face, and is characterized histologically by eddies of keratinizing squamous cells adjoining epidermis or follicular epithelium.

k. lichenoi′des chro′nica a rare, chronic, progressive skin condition characterized by discolored lichenoid papules arranged in a linear, reticular pattern, usually on the limbs and trunk, and an oily, scaly eruption resembling seborrheic dermatitis on the upper face. Called also *Nékam disease.*

k. lin′guae leukoplakia.

k. obtu′rans obstruction of the external auditory meatus by a mass of desquamated epithelium and cerumen.

k. palma′ris et planta′ris, palmoplantar k., k. palmoplanta′ris palmoplantar keratoderma.

k. palmoplanta′ris transgre′diens erythrokeratodermia variabilis.

k. pharyn′gea a condition in which white horny masses project out from the tonsils and from the orifices of lymph follicles in the wall of the pharynx.

k. pila′ris a common, benign condition in which hyperkeratosis occurs around hair follicles, usually on the extensor surfaces of the thighs and arms, but sometimes elsewhere; there are discrete follicular papules that reform after removal.

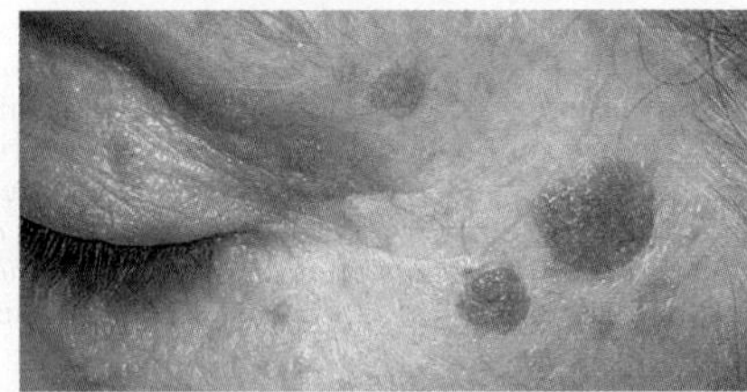

■ Seborrheic keratoses.

k. puncta′ta, k. puncta′ta palma′ris et planta′ris, punctate k. see under *keratoderma.*

radiation k., roentgen k. premalignant keratotic lesions occurring at the site of severe chronic radiodermatitis.

seborrheic k., k. seborrhe′ica a common, usually benign type of skin lesion composed of basaloid cells; it usually first appears after age 30 and presents as a soft, friable plaque with variable pigmentation. The most common sites are the face, trunk, and limbs. Sudden appearance and rapid growth of the lesions is called the *Leser-Trélat sign* and may indicate internal malignancy. Called also *seborrheic wart* and *verruca seborrheica.*

senile k., solar k. actinic k.

k. spinulo′sa lichen spinulosus.

stucco k. a condition seen especially in adults over age 40 who have dry skin, characterized by multiple superficial, gray to light brown lesions resembling a stucco plaster finish on the skin; lesions have a "stuck-on" appearance and can often be removed with minimal bleeding. The usual location is on the feet, ankles, forearms, or backs of the hands. Some authorities consider it a variant of seborrheic keratosis.

tar k. a keratosis caused by exposure to tar; keratotic foci develop and are sometimes followed by formation of keratoacanthomas or intraepidermal, squamous cell, or basal cell carcinoma.

ker•a•to•sul•fate (ker″ə-to-sul′fāt) keratan sulfate.

ker•a•tot•ic (ker″ə-tot′ik) 1. pertaining to or characterized by keratosis. 2. promoting keratosis.

ker•a•to•tome (ker′ə-to-tōm″) keratome.

ker•a•tot•o•my (ker″ə-tot′ə-me) [*kerato-* + *-tomy*] surgical incision of the cornea.

astigmatic k. an operation in which the cornea is relaxed by a series of transverse incisions in order to flatten the meridian in which the incisions are made and increase the curvature in the meridian 90° away; done for the correction of astigmatism.

delimiting k. incision of the cornea in hypopyon ulcer by a cut tangential to the advancing border of the ulcer and made to emerge at a corresponding point in the other side.

radial k. an operation in which a series of incisions is made in the cornea from its outer edge toward its center in spokelike fashion; done to flatten the cornea and thus to correct myopia.

ker•a•to•to•rus (ker″ə-to-to′rəs) [*kerato-* + *torus*] a vaultlike protrusion of the cornea.

Kerck•ring (Kerkring) center (ossicle), folds (valves) (kerk′ring) [Theodorus *Kerckring* (or *Kerkring*), German-born anatomist in the Netherlands, 1640–1693] see under *center* and see *plicae circulares.*

ke•rec•ta•sis (kə-rek′tə-sis) [Gr. *keras* cornea + *ectasis*] a uniform bulging or protrusion of the cornea.

ke•rec•to•my (kə-rek′tə-me) keratectomy.

Ker•ga•ra•dec sign (ker″gah-rah-dek′) [Jean Alexandre le Jameau, Vicomte de *Kergaradec*, French obstetrician and gynecologist, 1788–1877] see *uterine souffle*, under *souffle.*

Ke•ril•ia (kə-ril′e-ə) a genus of poisonous sea snakes. *K. jerdo′ni* is the kerril, a species found in coastal areas of the Indian Ocean.

ke•ri•on (kēr′e-on) [Gr. *kērion* honeycomb] a nodular, boggy, exudative, circumscribed swelling, often covered with pustules, occurring in association with tinea infections, usually tinea barbae or tinea capitis.

Kerk•ring see *Kerckring.*

Ker•ley lines (kur′le) [Sir Peter James *Kerley*, English radiologist, 1900–1979] see under *line.*

Ker•lone (kur′lōn) trademark for a preparation of betaxolol hydrochloride.

ker•ma (kur′mə) [*k*inetic *e*nergy *r*eleased in *ma*terial] a unit of quantity that represents the kinetic energy transferred to charged particles by the uncharged particles per unit mass of an irradiated medium.

Kern (kurn) see *Ke.*

ker•nic•ter•us (kər-nik′tər-əs) [Ger. "nuclear jaundice"] a condition associated with high levels of bilirubin in the blood, nearly always with severe neural symptoms, usually seen in infants as a sequela of icterus gravis neonatorum. It is characterized by deep yellow staining of the basal nuclei, globus pallidus, putamen, caudate nucleus, cerebellar nuclei, bulbar nuclei, and gray substance of the cerebrum, accompanied by widespread destructive changes. Called also *bilirubin encephalopathy.*

Ker•nig sign (ker′nig) [Vladimir Mikhailovich *Kernig*, Russian physician, 1840–1917] see under *sign.*

Ker•no•han notch (kur′nə-han) [James Watson *Kernohan*, Irish-born American pathologist, 1896–1981] see under *notch.*

ker•oid (ker′oid) keratoid.

ker•o•sene (ker′o-sēn) a colorless volatile liquid distilled from petroleum; it is used as a reagent, as engine fuel, and in insecticides, and is irritating to the skin and toxic by inhalation.

ker•o•sine (ker′o-sēn) kerosene.

Kerr sign (kur) [Henry Hyland *Kerr*, American surgeon, 1881–1963] see under *sign.*

ker•ril (ker′il) *Kerilia jerdoni.*

Ker•tes•zia (ker-te′ze-ə) a subgenus of mosquitoes of the genus *Anopheles; K. bella′tor* is a vector of malaria in Brazil.

Ke•shan disease (ke′shan) [*Keshan*, province in China where it is endemic] see under *disease.*

Kes•ling appliance, spring (kes′ling) [Harold D. *Kesling*, American orthodontist, 1901–1979] see under *appliance* and *spring.*

Kes•ten•baum sign (kes′tən-boum) [Alfred *Kestenbaum*, German physician, 20th century] see under *sign.*

ke•tal (ke′təl) [*ket*one + *al*cohol] an acetal derived by a combination of a ketone with two alcohols.

Ke•ta•lar (ke′tə-lər) trademark for a preparation of ketamine hydrochloride.

keta•mine hy•dro•chlo•ride (ke′tə-mēn) [USP] a rapid-acting general anesthetic and anesthesia adjunct, administered intramuscularly and intravenously.

ke•ta•zo•lam (ke-ta′zo-lam) a benzodiazepine used as an antianxiety agent in the treatment of anxiety disorders and for short-term relief of anxiety symptoms; administered orally.

Ke•tek (ke′tek) trademark for a preparation of telithromycin.

ke•tene (ke′tēn) a highly toxic, colorless gas of penetrating odor; also any one of several derivatives from it. It is used industrially as an acetylating agent.

ke•ti•mine (ke′tĭ-mēn) a compound in which the oxygen of a ketone is replaced by the imino group.

ket(o)- a prefix which denotes possession of the carbonyl group, C═O, in a structure in which the other two bonds to carbon are attached to hydrocarbon moieties.

ke•to ac•id (ke′to) a carboxylic acid containing a carbonyl group, such as α-ketoglutaric acid.
 branched-chain k. a. any of the keto acids formed by oxidative decarboxylation of branched-chain amino acids.

3-ke•to•ac•id CoA trans•fer•ase (ke″to-as′id ko-a′ trans′fər-ās) 3-oxoacid CoA-transferase.

ke•to ac•id de•car•box•y•lase (ke′to as′id de″kahr-bok′sə-lās) α-keto acid dehydrogenase.

α-ke•to ac•id de•hy•dro•gen•ase (ke′to as′id de-hi′dro-jən-ās) 1. see under *complex.* 2. the dehydrogenase component of any of the α-keto acid dehydrogenase complexes.

α-ke•to ac•id de•hy•dro•gen•ase de•fi•cien•cy (ke′to as′id de-hi′dro-jən-ās) deficiency of any one of the α-keto acid dehydrogenase complexes.

ke•to•ac•i•de•mia (ke″to-as″id-e′me-ə) the presence of keto acids in the blood.

ke•to•ac•i•do•sis (ke″to-as″ĭ-do′sis) acidosis accompanied by the accumulation of ketone bodies (ketosis) in the body tissues and fluids, as in diabetic ketoacidosis and starvation acidosis.
 diabetic k. (DKA) a type of metabolic acidosis produced by accumulation of ketone bodies resulting from uncontrolled diabetes mellitus. Called also *diabetic acidosis.*
 starvation k. see under *acidosis.*

ke•to•ac•id•uria (ke″to-as″ĭ-du′re-ə) the presence of keto acids in the urine.
 branched-chain k. maple syrup urine disease.

ke•to•acyl (ke″to-a′səl) the acyl radical of a keto acid; the coenzyme A thioesters of 3-keto acids, 3-ketoacyl CoA molecules, are intermediates in fatty acid oxidation.

3-ke•to•ac•yl CoA thi•o•lase (ke″to-a′səl ko-a′ thi′o-lās) acetyl-CoA *C*-acyltransferase.

α-ke•to•adip•ate (ke″to-ə-dip′āt) the anionic form of α-ketoadipic acid.

α-ke•to•adip•ate de•hy•dro•gen•ase (ke″to-ə-dip′āt de-hi′dro-jən-ās) a mitochondrial enzyme activity that catalyzes the decarboxylation and esterification of α-ketoadipic acid, forming glutaryl CoA as a step in the degradation of lysine, hydroxylysine, and tryptophan.

α-ke•to•adip•ic ac•id (ke″to-ə-dip′ik) a dicarboxylic acid formed by transamination of α-aminoadipic acid in the degradation of lysine and hydroxylysine. Written also *2-ketoadipic acid.*

α-ke•to•adip•ic•ac•id•uria (ke″to-ə-dip″ik-as″ĭ-du′re-ə) excretion of α-ketoadipic acid in the urine.

ke•to•a•mi•no•ac•i•de•mia (ke″to-ə-me″no-as″ĭ-de′me-ə) maple syrup urine disease.

β-ke•to•bu•tyr•ic ac•id (ke″to-bu-tēr′ik) acetoacetic acid.

ke•to•co•na•zole (ke″to-kon′ə-zōl) [USP] an imidazole derivative used as a broad-spectrum antifungal agent, administered orally for a wide range of systemic and cutaneous fungal infections and applied topically to the skin in the treatment of various forms of tinea, pityriasis versicolor, cutaneous candidiasis, seborrheic dermatitis, and dandruff; also used as a secondary antiandrogen in the treatment of advanced prostatic carcinoma.

Ke•to-Di•a•stix (ke″to-di′ə-stiks) trademark for a reagent strip for detection of ketones and glucose in the urine.

ke•to•gen•e•sis (ke″to-jen′ə-sis) [*keto-* + *-genesis*] the production of ketone bodies. **ketogenet′ic** *adj*

ke•to•gen•ic (ke″to-jen′ik) 1. forming ketone bodies. 2. capable of being converted into ketone bodies.

α-ke•to•glu•ta•rate (ke″to-gloo′tə-rāt) an anionic form of α-ketoglutaric acid.

α-ke•to•glu•ta•rate de•hy•dro•gen•ase (ke″to-gloo′tə-rāt de-hi′dro-jən-ās) an enzyme of the oxidoreductase class that is a component of the multienzyme α-ketoglutarate dehydrogenase complex (q.v.). The enzyme catalyzes the decarboxylation and oxidation of α-ketoglutarate, forming succinyl bound to the cofactor thiamine pyrophosphate; the succinyl is subsequently transferred to the lipoamide linked to the side chain of a lysine residue of the enzyme dihydrolipoyllysine-residue succinyltransferase, which is also part of the complex. Called *oxoglutarate dehydrogenase (succinyl-transferring)* in EC nomenclature.

α-ke•to•glu•tar•ic ac•id (ke″to-gloo-tar′ik) 2-oxopentanedioic acid, 2-oxoglutaric acid, an intermediate in the tricarboxylic acid cycle (q.v.); α-ketoglutarate is also produced from glutamate in amino group transfer reactions and by oxidative deamination.

ke•to•hep•tose (ke″to-hep′tōs) any ketose containing seven carbon atoms.

ke•to•hexo•ki•nase (ke″to-hek″so-ki′nās) [EC 2.7.1.3] EC nomenclature for *fructokinase.*

ke•to•hex•ose (ke″to-hek′sōs) any ketose containing six carbon atoms, such as fructose. Cf. *aldohexose.*

ke•to•hy•droxy•es•trin (ke″to-hi-drok″se-es′trin) estrone.

α-ke•to•iso•val•er•ate de•hy•dro•gen•ase (ke″to-i″so-val′er-āt de-hi′dro-jən-ās) branched-chain α-keto acid dehydrogenase.

ke•tol (ke′tol) a compound with both a ketone and an alcohol group.

ke•to•lide (ke′to-līd) any of a group of antibacterials structurally related to the macrolides and having a similar mechanism of action, and exhibiting in vitro activity against a number of multidrug-resistant gram-positive organisms; the class includes telithromycin.

ke•tol-isom•er•ase (ke″tol-i-som′ər-ās) a term used in the systematic names of that subset of the isomerases that catalyze the interconversion of aldoses and ketoses [EC 5.3.1].

ke•tol•y•sis (ke-tol′ə-sis) [*ketone* + *-lysis*] the cleavage of ketone bodies. **ketolyt′ic** *adj*

ke•tone (ke′tōn) any of a large class of organic compounds containing the carbonyl group, C═O, whose carbon atom is joined to two other carbon atoms, that is, with the carbonyl group occurring within the carbon chain. See also under *body.*
 dimethyl k. acetone.

ke•to•ne•mia (ke″to-ne′me-ə) an excess of ketone bodies in the blood, as in starvation and diabetes mellitus. See also *ketosis.* Called also *hyperketonemia.*

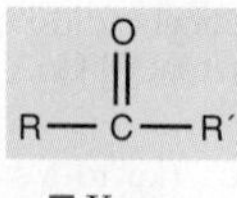

■ Ketone.

ke•ton•ic (ke-to′nik) 1. pertaining to a ketone. 2. developed from a ketone.

ke•to•ni•za•tion (ke″to-nĭ-za′shən) conversion into a ketone.

ke•ton•uria (ke″to-nu′re-ə) ketone bodies in the urine, as in diabetes mellitus; called also *acetonuria* and *hyperketonuria.*

ke•to•pen•tose (ke″to-pen′tōs) any ketose containing five carbon atoms, such as ribulose or xylulose.

ke•to•plas•tic (ke″to-plas′tik) ketogenic.

ke•to•pro•fen (ke″to-pro′fən) [USP] a nonsteroidal antiinflammatory drug derived from propionic acid; used in the treatment of rheumatoid arthritis, osteoarthritis, and other rheumatic and nonrheumatic inflammatory disorders, pain, dysmenorrhea, and vascular headaches; administered orally or rectally.

9-ke•to•re•duc•tase (ke″to-re-duk′tās) prostaglandin-E_2 9-reductase.

β-ke•to•re•duc•tase (ke″to-re-duk′tās) 3-hydroxyacyl-CoA dehydrogenase.

ke•to•ro•lac tro•meth•amine (ke″to-ro′lak) [USP] a nonsteroidal antiinflammatory drug administered intramuscularly, intravenously, or orally for short-term management of pain; also applied topically to the conjunctiva in the treatment of allergic conjunctivitis and of ocular inflammation following cataract surgery.

ke•tose (ke′tōs) one of two subgroups of monosaccharides, being those having a nonterminal carbonyl (keto) group. In all known natural ketoses, the position of the keto group is at the 2 carbon. The class is further divided on the basis of the number of carbon atoms in the sugar, e.g., ketopentose, ketohexose, ketoheptose, etc.

ke•to•side (ke′to-sīd) any glycoside formed from a ketose; e.g., a fructoside.

ke•to•sis (ke-to′sis) abnormally elevated concentration of ketone bodies in the body tissues and fluids when fatty acids are incompletely metabolized, a complication of diabetes mellitus, starvation, and alcoholism. See also *ketoacidosis.*

k. of ruminants ketosis in cows and ewes during times of increased bodily mobilization of fat stores, usually just after they have given birth. See *fat cow syndrome* and *pregnancy toxemia in ewes.*

ke•to•ster•oid (ke″to-ster′oid) a steroid that possesses ketone groups on functional carbon atoms, which are designated in the name. Called also *oxosteroid.*

17-k. (17-KS) any of the C_{19} steroids having a keto group on the 17 carbon, usually denoting the urinary metabolites of androgens secreted by the adrenal cortex and gonads. They are accumulated and excreted abnormally in certain adrenal cortical and ovarian tumors and congenital adrenal hyperplasia.

Ke•to•stix (ke′to-stiks) trademark for a reagent strip for detection of ketone bodies in the urine.

17-ke•to•ster•oid re•duc•tase (ke″to-ster′oid re-duk′tās) 17β-hydroxysteroid dehydrogenase type 3.

ke•tos•uria (ke″tōs-u′re-ə) the presence of a ketose in the urine.

ke•to•tet•rose (ke″to-tet′rōs) a ketose that contains four carbon atoms; see also *erythrulose.*

3-ke•to•thi•o•lase (ke″to-thi′o-lās) acetyl-CoA *C*-acyltransferase.

β-ke•to•thi•o•lase (ke″to-thi′o-lās) acetyl-CoA *C*-acyltransferase.

β-ke•to•thi•o•lase de•fi•cien•cy (ke″to-thi′o-lās) α-methylacetoaceticaciduria.

ke•tot•ic (ke-tot′ik) 1. pertaining to or characterized by ketosis. 2. causing ketosis.

ke•to•ti•fen fu•ma•rate (ke″to-ti′fen) a noncompetitive H_1-receptor antagonist and mast cell stabilizer; administered orally in the chronic treatment of children with mild atopic asthma and topically to the conjunctiva as an antipruritic in the treatment of allergic conjunctivitis.

ke•to•tri•ose (ke″to-tri′ōs) a ketose containing three carbon atoms; see *dihydroxyacetone.*

ke•tox•ime (ke-tok′sīm) the oxime derivative of a ketone.

Ke•ty-Schmidt method (ke′te shmit′) [Seymour Solomon *Kety*, American physiologist, 1915–2000; Carl Frederic *Schmidt*, American physician, 1893–1988] see under *method.*

keV kiloelectron volt; 1000 electron volts.

Kew Gar•dens spotted fever (ku gahr′dənz) [*Kew Gardens*, Queens, New York, where it was first reported in 1946] rickettsialpox.

key (ke) 1. an instrument for opening a lock, or a device similar in appearance or function to such an instrument. 2. by extension, any tool for revealing specific information.

torquing k. an orthodontic instrument used to facilitate the engaging of rectangular arch wires into the edgewise brackets.

key•note (ke′nōt) in homeopathy, the characteristic property of a drug that indicates its use in treating a similar symptom of disease.

Key-Ret•zi•us sheath, foramen (ke′ ret′ze-oos) [Ernst Axel Henrik *Key*, Swedish physician, 1832–1901; Magnus Gustaf *Retzius*, Swedish histologist, 1842–1919] see *sheath of Key and Retzius*, under *sheath*, and see *apertura lateralis ventriculi quarti* under *apertura.*

key•way (ke′wa) the slot into which the male portion of a precision attachment fits.

kg kilogram.

kg-cal large calorie.

kHz kilohertz.

ki (ke) [Japanese] qi.

Ki•brick test (ki′brik) [S. *Kibrick*, American physician, mid-20th century] gelatin agglutination test; see under *test.*

Kidd blood group (kid) [*Kidd*, surname of the propositus first observed in 1951] see under *blood group.*

kid•ney (kid′ne) [Middle English *kidenei*] either of the two organs in the lumbar region that filter the blood, excreting the end-products of body metabolism in the form of urine, and regulating the concentrations of hydrogen, sodium, potassium, phosphate, and other ions in the extracellular fluid. Called also *ren* [TA]. Each human kidney is about 11 cm long, 5–7.5 cm wide, and 2.5 cm thick, and weighs from 120 to 160 g. The kidney is of characteristic shape, with a notch known as the *hilum* on its inner, concave border; renal vessels and nerves and the ureter pass through it, and it communicates with the cavity or sinus of the kidney. The kidney consists of a cortex (see *renal cortex*, under *cortex*) and a medulla (see *renal medulla*, under *medulla*). The medullary substance forms pyramids, whose bases are in the cortex and whose apices, the *renal papillae*, project into the calices of the kidney. The renal pyramids number from 10 to 15. The parenchyma of each kidney is composed of about one million *renal tubules* (nephrons, the functional unit of the kidney), held together by a little connective tissue. Each tubule begins blindly in a renal corpuscle, consisting of a glomerulus and the surrounding glomerular capsule, situated within the cortex. After a neck or constriction below the capsule, it becomes the proximal convoluted tubule, then Henle loop, then the distal convoluted tubule, the connecting tubule, and finally the straight collecting tubule, which opens at the apex of a renal papilla. The straight collecting tubules converge as they descend, forming groups in the center, known as *medullary rays.* See also Plate 20.

abdominal k. an ectopic kidney found above the iliac crest with its hilum adjacent to the second lumbar vertebra.

amyloid k. a kidney with renal amyloidosis.

Armanni-Ebstein k. a kidney that has Armanni-Ebstein lesions (see under *lesion*).

artificial k. popular term for *hemodialyzer.*

Ask-Upmark k. a hypoplastic kidney with fewer lobules than usual and fissures on its surface; most affected persons have severe hypertension, sometimes with hypertensive encephalopathy and retinopathy. The condition may be either congenital or secondary to vesicoureteral reflux with pyelonephritis. Called also *segmental renal hypoplasia.*

atrophic k. a kidney that is reduced in size because of inadequate circulation or loss of nephrons.

cake k. a fused kidney of bizarre shape with irregular lobes, usually found in the pelvis toward the midline but sometimes found in crossed renal ectopia.

cicatricial k. a kidney with irregular areas of scarring from reflux nephropathy or pyelonephritis; see *renal scarring*, under *scarring.*

clump k. cake k.

congested k. an edematous and congested kidney, resulting from inflammation, impaired venous circulation, or urinary obstruction. Called also *large red k.*

contracted k. an atrophic kidney that is scarred and granular.

crossed fused ectopic k. a kidney with crossed renal ectopia (see under *ectopia*).

crush k. the kidney of a person with crush syndrome.

cystic k. a kidney that contains one or more cysts.

definite k., definitive k. metanephros.

disk k. a disk-shaped fused kidney similar to the doughnut kidney but with more fusion at the two poles.

doughnut k. a doughnut-shaped fused kidney resulting from bipolar fusion of the renal anlagen before rotation has begun.

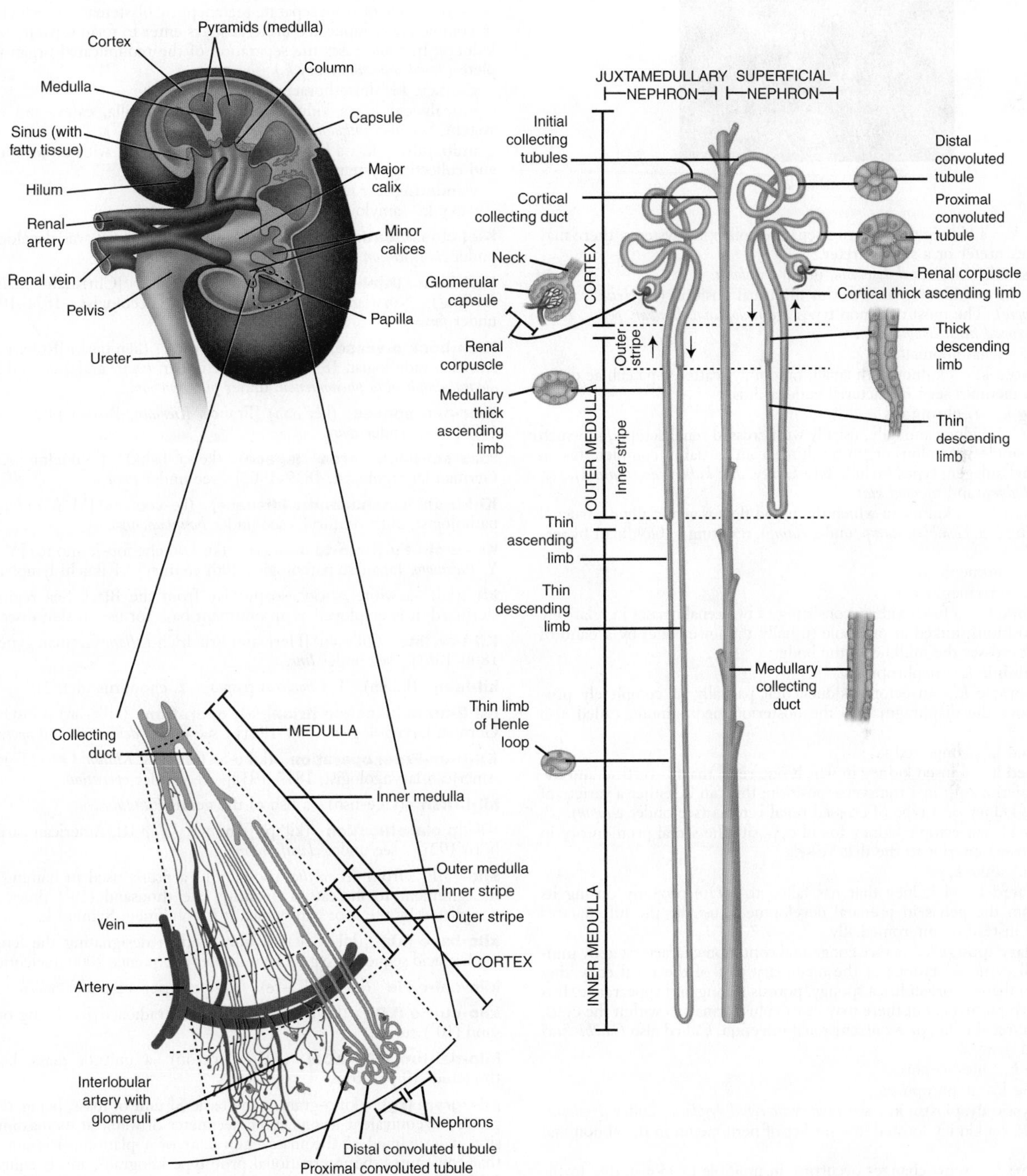

■ **PLATE 20—STRUCTURE OF THE KIDNEY**

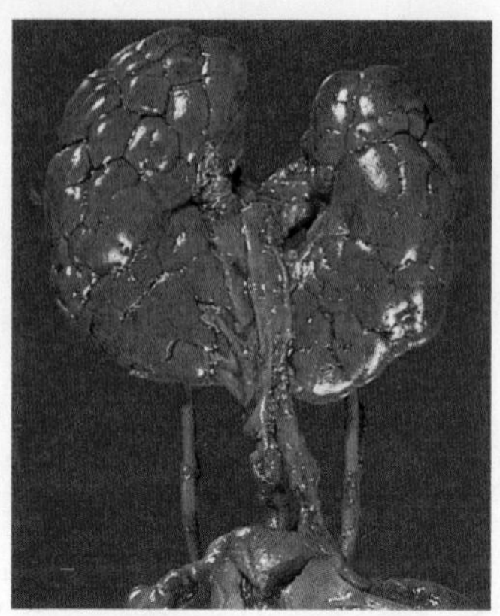

■ Horseshoe kidney.

duplex k. a kidney that has two separate collecting systems; there may be a duplex ureter or a single ureter.

dysplastic k. see *renal dysplasia*, under *dysplasia*.

ectopic k. a kidney that is not in the usual position (see *renal ectopia*, under *ectopia*). The most common types are *abdominal*, *lumbar*, *pelvic*, *thoracic*, and *crossed fused ectopic kidneys*.

fatty k. renal lipomatosis.

flea-bitten k. a kidney with small, randomly scattered petechiae on its surface, sometimes seen in bacterial endocarditis.

floating k. nephroptosis.

fused k. a kidney anomaly, usually with crossed renal ectopia, in which there is a single anomalous organ resulting from partial or complete fusion of the renal anlagen; types include *cake kidney*, *disk kidney*, *doughnut kidney*, *horseshoe kidney*, and *sigmoid kidney*.

Goldblatt k. a kidney in which the blood flow is artificially obstructed by clamping (see *Goldblatt clamp*, under *clamp*), resulting in Goldblatt hypertension.

head k. pronephros.

hind k. metanephros.

horseshoe k. a fused kidney consisting of two renal masses in relatively normal positions, linked at one pole (usually the lower one) by a band of tissue that crosses the midline of the body.

hypermobile k. nephroptosis.

intrathoracic k. an ectopic kidney that partially or completely protrudes above the diaphragm into the posterior mediastinum; called also *thoracic k.*

large red k. congested k.

L-shaped k. a fused kidney in which one renal mass is vertical and the other is inferior to it in a transverse position; this can be either a variety of horseshoe kidney or a type of crossed renal ectopia (see under *ectopia*).

lumbar k. an ectopic kidney found opposite the sacral promontory in the iliac fossa, anterior to the iliac vessels.

lump k. cake k.

malrotated k. a kidney that has failed to rotate properly during its ascent from the pelvis in prenatal development; usually the hilum faces anteriorly instead of anteromedially.

medullary sponge k. a rare congenital condition characterized by multiple small cystic dilatations of the medullary part of the renal collecting tubules, so that the organ has a spongy, porous feeling and appearance. It is usually asymptomatic, but there may be calculus formation within the cysts, hematuria, renal colic, or recurrent renal infection. Called also *Cacchi-Ricci disease* and *sponge k.*

middle k. mesonephros.

movable k. nephroptosis.

multicystic dysplastic k. see *multicystic renal dysplasia*, under *dysplasia*.

mural k. a kidney located in a pocket of peritoneum in the abdominal wall.

myeloma k. renal changes occurring in multiple myeloma, due to filtration of large amounts of Bence Jones protein; they include tubular atrophy with multinucleated giant cells in the tubule walls and interstitium, as well as formation of myeloma casts (see under *cast*); this eventually results in renal failure. Called also *cast* or *myeloma cast nephropathy*.

Page k. compression of a kidney by a hematoma in the subcapsular space, causing hypertension, usually seen after trauma to the abdomen or back.

pancake k. disk k.

pelvic k. an ectopic kidney found opposite the sacrum and below the aortic bifurcation.

polycystic k's see *polycystic kidney disease*, under *disease*.

primordial k. pronephros.

putty k. a complication of renal tuberculosis in which the kidney undergoes massive destruction of the parenchyma and finally autonephrectomy with calcification or caseation of the destroyed parenchyma.

sigmoid k. a fused kidney in which the upper pole of one kidney is fused with the lower pole of the other. Called also *S-shaped k.*

sponge k. medullary sponge k.

S-shaped k. sigmoid k.

supernumerary k. a rare anomaly in which there is another kidney in addition to the usual two; it develops as the result of splitting of the nephrogenic blastema, or from separate metanephric blastemas into which partially or completely reduplicated ureteral stalks enter to form separate capsulated kidneys. In some cases the separation of the reduplicated organ is incomplete (*fused supernumerary k.*).

thoracic k. intrathoracic k.

unicalyceal k. a kidney with a single papilla, calyx, and collecting system. See also *unipapillary k.*

unipapillary k. a kidney with a single papilla, with or without a calyx and collecting system. See also *unicalyceal k.*

wandering k. nephroptosis.

waxy k. amyloid k.

Kiel classification (kēl) [*Kiel*, Germany, where it was developed] see under *classification*.

Kiel•land (Kjel•land) forceps (kyel′ənd) [Christian *Kielland* (or *Kjelland*), Norwegian obstetrician and gynecologist, 1871–1941] see under *forceps*.

Kien•böck disease, phenomenon, unit (kēn′bərk) [Robert *Kienböck*, Austrian radiologist, 1871–1953] see under *disease* and *unit*, and see *paradoxical diaphragm phenomenon*, under *phenomenon*.

Kier•nan spaces (kēr′nən) [Francis *Kiernan*, British physician, 1800–1874] see under *space*.

Kies•sel•bach area (space) (ke′səl-bahk) [Wilhelm *Kiesselbach*, German laryngologist, 1839–1902] see under *area*.

Ki•ku•chi lymphadenitis (disease) (ke-koo′che) [M. *Kikuchi*, Japanese pathologist, 20th century] see under *lymphadenitis*.

Ki•ku•chi-Fu•ji•mo•to disease (ke-koo′che foo-je-mo′to) [M. *Kikuchi*; Y. *Fujimoto*, Japanese pathologist, 20th century] Kikuchi lymphadenitis.

kil (kil) a white, sticky, soapy clay from the Black Sea region; when sterilized, it is employed as an ointment base for use in skin diseases.

Kil•i•an line (kil′e-ən) [Hermann Friedrich *Kilian*, German gynecologist, 1800–1863] see under *line*.

kil•leen (kil′ēn) 1. *Chondrus crispus*. 2. chondrus (def. 2).

Kil•li•an dehiscence (triangle), operation (kil′e-ən) [Gustav *Killian*, German laryngologist, 1860–1921] see under *dehiscence* and *operation*.

Kil•li•an-Freer operation (kil′e-ən frēr′) [G. *Killian*; Otto (Tiger) *Freer*, American laryngologist, 1857–1932] see under *operation*.

kil•li•fish (kil′e-fish) a fish of the genus *Fundulus*.

Kil•lip classification (kil′ip) [Thomas *Killip* III, American cardiologist, born 1927] see under *classification*.

kilo- [Fr., from Gr. *chilioi* thousand] a prefix used in naming units of measurement to indicate a quantity one thousand (10^3) times the unit designated by the root with which it is combined. Symbol k.

kilo•base (kb) (kil′o-bās) a unit used in designating the length of a nucleic acid sequence; e.g., 7 kb indicates a sequence 7000 nucleotides long.

kilo•cal•o•rie (kil′o-kal″ə-re) large calorie; see under *calorie*.

kilo•cu•rie (kCi) (kil″o-ku′re) a unit of radioactivity, being one thousand (10^3) curies.

kilo•dal•ton (kD, kDa) (kil″o-dawl′ton) a unit of mass, being one thousand (10^3) daltons.

kilo•gram (kg) (kil′o-gram) the basic SI unit of mass, being 1000 (10^3) grams, or equivalent to one cubic decimeter of water at its maximum density; it is defined as the mass equivalent of a platinum-iridium cylinder that constitutes the international prototype kilogram, and is equivalent to 2.204623 pounds avoirdupois.

kilo•hertz (kHz) (kil′o-hərtz) one thousand (10^3) hertz.

Ki•loh-Nev•in syndrome (ki′lo nev′in) [Leslie Gordon *Kiloh*, Australian physician, 1917–1997; Samuel *Nevin*, English neurologist, 1905–1979] see under *syndrome*.

ki•lo•me•ter (km) (kĭ-lom′ə-tər, kil′o-me″tər) a unit of linear measurement of the metric system, being 1000 (10^3) meters, or the equivalent of 3280.83 feet, or about five-eighths of a mile.

kilo•unit (kil″o-u′nit) a quantity equivalent to one thousand (10^3) standard units.

kilo•volt (kV) (kil′o-vōlt) one thousand (10^3) volts.

Kim•ber•ley horse disease (kim′bər-le) [*Kimberley*, a district in northeastern Western Australia, where the disease occurs] see under *disease.*

Kim•mel•stiel-Wil•son lesion (nodule), syndrome (kim′əl-stēl wil′sən) [Paul *Kimmelstiel*, German pathologist in the United States, 1900–1970; Clifford *Wilson*, British physician, 1906–1997] see under *lesion* and see *intercapillary glomerulosclerosis*, under *glomerulosclerosis.*

Ki•mu•ra disease (ke-moo′rah) [Tetsuji *Kimura*, Japanese pathologist, 20th century] see under *disease.*

ki•nase (ki′nās) 1. a term used in the recommended and trivial names of the phosphotransferases and diphosphotransferases of the transferase class [EC 2.7.1–6] that catalyze the transfer of a high-energy phosphate group from a donor compound (e.g., ATP or GTP) to an acceptor compound (alcohol, carboxyl, nitrogenous group, or another phosphate group). 2. a suffix used in the trivial names of some enzymes that convert an inactive or precursor form. See also *protein kinase.*

Kind•ler syndrome (kind′lər) [Theresa *Kindler*, British physician, 20th century] see under *syndrome.*

kind•ling (kind′ling) changes in brain physiology caused by repeated subthreshold electrical stimulation; the final result may be epileptogenic changes or less dramatic but chronic behavioral changes. It has been observed in reptiles, amphibians, and a variety of mammals, but its occurrence in humans is controversial.

kine- [Gr. *kinein* to move] a combining form denoting relationship to movement. See also words beginning *cine-.*

kin•e•mat•ics (kin″ə-mat′iks) [Gr. *kinēma* motion] the phase of mechanics that deals with the possible motions of a material body.

kin•e•plas•tics (kin″ə-plas′tiks) kineplasty.

kin•e•plas•ty (kin′ə-plas″te) [*kine-* + *-plasty*] amputation in which the stump is formed in such a way that the muscles are able to produce motion in a prosthesis; called also *kineplastic amputation.* **kineplas′tic** *adj*

Kin•e•ret (kin′ə-ret) trademark for a preparation of anakinra.

kine•sal•gia (kin″ə-sal′jə) [*kinesio-* + *-algia*] pain on muscular exertion.

kine•scope (kin′ə-skōp) [*kine-* + *-scope*] an instrument for measuring ocular refraction, in which the patient observes a fixed object through a slit in a moving disk.

ki•ne•sia (kĭ-ne′zhə) kinetosis.

ki•ne•si•at•rics (kĭ-ne″se-at′riks) kinesitherapy.

ki•ne•sics (kĭ-ne′siks) the study of body movement as a part of the process of communication.

ki•ne•si•es•the•si•om•e•ter (kĭ-ne″se-es-the″ze-om′ə-tər) kinesthesiometer.

ki•ne•si•gen•ic (kĭ-ne″sĭ-jen′ik) [*kinesi-* + *-genic*] caused by movement.

kine•sim•e•ter (kin″ə-sim′ə-tər) [*kinesio-* + *-meter*] an instrument for the quantitative measurement of movements.

ki•ne•sin (ki-ne′sin) any of a family of large cytoplasmic proteins with ATPase activity that bind to vesicles and particles and transport them along microtubules, usually toward the plus end, using energy from ATP hydrolysis. Kinesins are divided into two functional classes: *cytosolic kinesins* are responsible for the transport of vesicles and organelles; *spindle kinesins* are involved in spindle formation and chromosome segregation during cell division. Cf. *dynein.* In EC nomenclature, called *plus-end-directed kinesin ATPase* and *minus-end-directed kinesin ATPase.*

kinesi(o)- [Gr. *kinēsis* movement] a combining form denoting relationship to movement.

ki•ne•si•ol•o•gy (kĭ-ne″se-ol′ə-je) [*kinesio-* + *-logy*] 1. the sum of what is known regarding human motion; the study of motion of the human body. Cf. *biomechanics.* 2. a system of diagnosis based on the theory that muscle dysfunction is secondary to subclinical structural, chemical, or mental dysfunction in other parts of the body; manual muscle testing to help identify the primary dysfunction is an important part of assessment, and treatment aims at correcting the underlying state. Called also *applied kinesiology.*

ki•ne•si•om•e•ter (kĭ-ne″se-om′ə-tər) kinesimeter.

ki•ne•sio•neu•ro•sis (kĭ-ne″se-o-noŏ-ro′sis) [*kinesio-* + *neurosis*] a functional nervous disorder characterized by motor disturbances, such as spasms or tics.

ki•ne•sio•ther•a•py (kĭ-ne″se-o-ther′ə-pe) kinesitherapy.

ki•ne•sis (kĭ-, ki-ne′sis) [Gr.] 1. movement. 2. stimulus-induced motion responsive only to the intensity of the stimulus, not the direction. Cf. *taxis.*

-kinesis a word termination denoting movement or activation, particularly in response to a stimulus specified by the root to which it is attached.

ki•ne•si•ther•a•py (kĭ-ne″sĭ-ther′ə-pe) [*kinesio-* + *therapy*] the treatment of disease by movements or exercise.

kin•es•the•sia (kin″es-the′zhə) [*kine-* + *esthesia*] 1. the awareness of movement, weight, tension, and position of body parts, which is dependent on input from joint and muscle receptors and hair cells. 2. movement sense.

kin•es•the•si•om•e•ter (kin″əs-the″ze-om′ə-tər) [*kinesthesia* + *-meter*] an instrument for testing kinesthesia.

kin•es•the•sis (kin″əs-the′sis) kinesthesia.

kin•es•thet•ic (kin″əs-thet′ik) pertaining to kinesthesia or the muscular sense.

ki•ne•tia (kĭ-ne′she-ə) plural of *kinety.*

ki•net•ic (kĭ-net′ik) [Gr. *kinētikos*] pertaining to or producing motion.

ki•net•i•cist (ki-net′ĭ-sist) a specialist in kinetics.

ki•net•ics (kĭ-net′iks) [Gr. *kinētikos* of or for putting in motion] the branch of dynamics that pertains to the turnover, or rate of change, of a specific factor (e.g., erythrocytes—erythrokinetics, leukocytes—leukokinetics, or iron—ferrokinetics), commonly expressed as units of amount per unit time.

chemical k. the study of the rates and mechanisms of chemical reactions.

urea k. the movement of urea in the body and its excretion through the kidneys or dialysis apparatus. See also *urea kinetic modeling*, under *modeling*, and *urea clearance*, under *clearance.*

ki•ne•tid (kĭ-ne′tid) an elementary, repeating structural unit of ciliate protozoa, consisting of one or more kinetosomes together with various associated organelles.

ki•ne•tin (ki′nə-tin) a highly potent plant-growth factor; used to stimulate the growth of bacterial colonies.

kinet(o)- [Gr. *kinētos* movable] a combining form denoting relationship to motion.

ki•ne•to•car•dio•gram (kĭ-ne″to-kahr′de-o-gram″) [*kineto-* + *cardiogram*] the graphic record obtained by kinetocardiography.

ki•ne•to•car•di•og•ra•phy (kĭ-ne″to-kahr″de-og′rə-fe) [*kineto-* + *cardiography*] the technique of graphically recording the slow vibrations of the anterior chest wall in the region of the heart, the vibrations representing the absolute motion of the heart at a given point on the chest.

ki•ne•to•chore (kĭ-ne′to-kor) [*kineto-* + Gr. *chora* space] a multilayered structure embedded in the surface of the centromere; it is the attachment point for the spindle fibers and directs chromosomal movement in mitosis.

ki•ne•to•des•ma (kĭ-ne″to-des′mə) pl. *kinetodesma′ta* [*kineto-* + Gr. *desmos* band, ligament] one of a bundle of fine, striated fibrils, each of which arises close to the base of a basal body and runs anteriorly parallel to and just beneath the surface of certain ciliate protozoa; the kinetodesmata serve to connect the basal bodies in longitudinal rows. Called also *kinetodesmos.*

ki•ne•to•des•mos (kĭ-ne″to-des′mos) kinetodesma.

ki•ne•to•frag•ment (kĭ-ne″to-frag′mənt) a group of somatic kinetids, not always completely covered with cilia, occurring in the region of the cytosome or oral area in certain ciliate protozoa, many of which are in the class Kinetofragminophorea. See also *frange* and *pseudomembranelle.*

Ki•ne•to•frag•min•o•phor•ea (kĭ-ne″to-frag″min-ə-for′e-ə) [*kineto-* + L. *fragmen* piece + Gr. *phōros* bearing] a class of ciliate protozoa (phylum Ciliophora), characterized by the presence of isolated kinetia in the oral region of the body (kinetofragments) bearing cilia but not compound ciliary organelles; a cytostome and cytopharyngeal apparatus are often present. It comprises four subclasses: Gymnostomatia, Vestibuliferia, Hypostomatia, and Suctoria.

ki•ne•to•gen•ic (kĭ-ne″to-jen′ik) [*kineto-* + *-genic*] causing or producing movement.

ki•ne•to•nu•cle•us (kĭ-ne″to-noo′kle-əs) [*kineto-* + *nucleus*] kinetoplast.

ki•ne•to•plast (kĭ-ne′to-plast) [*kineto-* + *-plast*] a large rod-shaped or cylindrical, DNA-rich, independently replicating cytoplasmic organelle located in close association with the basal body (with which it may seem to be fused) and found within the elongated mitochondrion of protozoa of the order Kinetoplastida. Called also *kinetonucleus.*

Ki•ne•to•plas•tea (kĭ-ne″to-plas′te-ə) a class of protozoa of the phylum Euglenozoa; it includes the medically important order Kinetoplastida.

ki•ne•to•plas•tid (kĭ-ne″to-plas′tid) pertaining or relating to protozoa of the order Kinetoplastida.

Ki•ne•to•plas•ti•da (kĭ-ne″to-plas′tĭ-də) an order of flagellate protozoa of the phylum Euglenozoa; many species are free living, although most are parasites of plants, invertebrates, and vertebrates. They have one or two flagella arising from a depression in the cell body and usually contain a conspicuous kinetoplast located near the flagellar basal bodies. It includes the genus *Trypanosoma* that causes numerous different diseases. Called also *Protomastigida* and *Protomonadina*.

kine·tos·co·py (kin″ə-tos′kə-pe) serial photography which exhibits the motions of the limbs or features; used in diagnosis of disorders of gait and in the study of muscle action.

ki·net·o·sis (kin″ə-to′sis) pl. *kineto′ses* [*kineto-* + *-osis*] any disorder caused by unaccustomed motion; see *motion sickness*.

ki·ne·to·some (kĭ-ne′to-sōm) [*kineto-* + *-some*] basal body.

ki·ne·to·ther·a·py (kĭ-ne″to-ther′ə-pe) kinesitherapy.

ki·ne·ty (ki-ne′te) pl. *kine′tia, kineties* [Gr. *kinetos* movable] a longitudinal unit in the infraciliature of ciliate protozoa, comprising cilia, basal bodies, and kinetodesmata.

King syndrome (king) [J.O. *King*, Australian physician, 20th century] see under *syndrome*.

King unit (king) [Earl Judson *King*, Canadian biochemist, 1901–1962] see under *unit*.

king·dom (king′dəm) [A.S. *cyningdom*] in the traditional classification of living organisms, the highest of the categories. A number of systems have been proposed; the most widely used lists five kingdoms: Monera, Protista, Fungi, Plantae (the plants), and Animalia (the animals). An alternative classification divides all organisms at the highest level into three domains (q.v.).

King·el·la (king-el′ə) [Elizabeth O. *King*, American bacteriologist, 20th century] a genus of gram-negative, aerobic or facultatively anaerobic, rod-shaped bacteria of the family Neisseriaceae, found as natural inhabitants of the human oropharynx. The organisms are potential human pathogens.

K. denitri′ficans a usually nonpathogenic species isolated from the upper respiratory tract and genital tract specimens.

K. indolo′genes *Suttonella indologenes*.

K. kin′gae a species that has been isolated from blood, bone, joint, and throat infections and from cultures of normal mucous membranes.

Kings·ley appliance (plate), splint (kingz′le) [Norman William *Kingsley*, American dentist, 1829–1913] see under *appliance* and *splint*.

kin·ic ac·id (kin′ik) quinic acid.

ki·nin (ki′nin) [Gr. *kinein* to move] any of a group of vasoactive straight-chain polypeptides formed by kallikrein-catalyzed cleavage of kininogens; they cause vasodilation of most vessels but vasoconstriction of the pulmonary bed, and they also alter vascular permeability. Common examples are bradykinin and kallidin.

ki·nin·ase (ki′nin-ās) an enzyme that destroys the activity of circulating kinins.

k. I lysine carboxypeptidase.

k. II peptidyl-dipeptidase A.

ki·nin·o·gen (ki-nin′o-jen″) either of two plasma α_2-globulins that are kinin precursors, called *high-molecular-weight k.* and *low-molecular-weight k.*

high-molecular-weight k. (HMWK) a kininogen of molecular weight 100,000–250,000 that is split by plasma kallikrein to produce bradykinin. Called also *Fitzgerald factor*.

low-molecular-weight k. (LMWK) a kininogen of molecular weight 50,000–75,000 that is split by tissue kallikrein to produce kallidin.

Kin·ni·er Wil·son (kin′e-ər wil′sən) see *Wilson*.

kin(o)- [Gr. *kinein* to move] see *kine-*.

ki·no·cil·i·um (ki″no-sil′e-əm) pl. *kinocil′ia* [*kino-* + *cilium*] a motile filament on the free surface of a cell; see *cilia (def. 2)*. See also *hair cells*, under *cell*, and *stereocilia*.

ki·no·hapt (ki′no-hapt) [*kino-* + Gr. *haptein* to touch] an esthesiometer for making several tactile stimulations at definite intervals of time or space.

ki·nol·o·gy (kĭ-nol′ə-je) kinesiology.

ki·no·mom·e·ter (kĭ″no-mom′ə-ter) [*kino-* + *-meter*] goniometer.

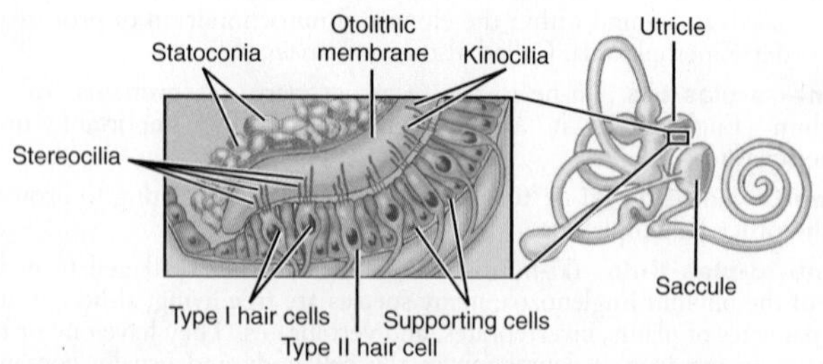

■ Kinocilia and stereocilia on hair cells of the macula utriculi.

Kin·rix (kin′riks) trademark for a combination preparation of diphtheria and tetanus toxoids and acellular pertussis vaccine adsorbed and poliovirus vaccine inactivated.

kin·ship (kin′ship) [A.S. *cynscipe*] the state or fact of descent from a common ancestor.

Kio·nex (ki′o-neks) trademark for a preparation of sodium polystyrene sulfonate.

Kirch·ner diverticulum (kurk′nər) [Wilhelm *Kirchner*, Austrian otologist, 1849–1936] see under *diverticulum*.

Kirk amputation (kurk) [Norman Thomas *Kirk*, Surgeon General of U.S. Army, 1888–1960] see under *amputation*.

Kir·li·an pho·tog·ra·phy (kēr′le-ən) [Semyon *Kirlian*, Russian electrician, 20th century, and Valentina Kirliana, Russian journalist, 20th century] see under *photography*.

Kirsch·ner wire (kursh′nər) [Martin *Kirschner*, German surgeon, 1879–1942] see under *wire*.

Kir·stein method (kir′shtīn) [Alfred *Kirstein*, German physician, 1863–1922] see *direct laryngoscopy*, under *laryngoscopy*.

Kisch reflex (kish) [Bruno *Kisch*, German physiologist, 1890–1966] see under *reflex*.

kiss·pep·tin (kis-pep′tin) 1. a 54–amino acid peptide that suppresses metastasis of cancer cells and plays a role in the onset of puberty. 2. any of various smaller peptides formed by proteolytic cleavage of the 54–amino acid compound, having a variety of functions in various mammals. Defs. 1 and 2 called also *metastin*.

kit·a·sa·my·cin (kit″ə-sə-mi′sin) a macrolide antibiotic produced by *Streptomyces kitasoensis*, active against most gram-positive and some gram-negative bacteria, as well as certain other pathogenic microorganisms. Called also *leucomycin*.

ki·tol (ki′tol) [Gr. *kētos* sea monster, big fish] a substance from whale oil which yields vitamin A on heating.

kj knee jerk.

Kjel·dahl method (test) (kyel′dahl) [Johan Gustav Christoffer *Kjeldahl*, Danish chemist, 1849–1900] see under *method*.

Kjel·land see *Kielland*.

Klar·on (klar′on) trademark for a preparation of sulfacetamide sodium.

Klats·kin tumor (klats′kin) [Gerald *Klatskin*, American internist, 1910–1986] hilar cholangiocarcinoma.

Klebs-Löf·fler bacillus (klebz′ lerf′lər) [Theodor Albrecht Edwin *Klebs*, German bacteriologist, 1834–1913; Friederich A.J. *Löffler*, German bacteriologist, 1852–1915] *Corynebacterium diphtheriae*.

Kleb·si·el·la (kleb″se-el′ə) [T.A.E. *Klebs*] a genus of bacteria of the family Enterobacteriaceae, made up of small, gram-negative, facultatively anaerobic, nonmotile rods, usually occurring singly; they are widely distributed in nature, including in the intestines. They are a frequent cause of nosocomial urinary and pulmonary infections and of wound infections. The type species is *K. pneumo′niae*.

K. granulo′matis a species that is not viable on ordinary media but cultivable on fresh egg-yolk medium and causes granuloma inguinale. Called also *Donovan body*. Formerly called *Calymmatobacterium granulomatis*.

K. mo′bilis a species isolated from feces, sewage, soil, and dairy products; it can cause nosocomial pneumonia in debilitated patients. Called also *Enterobacter aerogenes*.

K. oxyto′ca a species similar to *K. pneumoniae* except that it is indole positive, is found in the mammalian intestinal tract and human clinical specimens, and is a cause of nosocomial infections.

K. ozae′nae *K. pneumoniae* subsp. *ozaenae*.

K. pneumo′niae an encapsulated species found in soil, water, grain, and intestines of animals, as well as associated with infections of the urinary and respiratory tracts. It is the etiologic agent of an acute bacterial pneumonia (see Klebsiella *pneumonia*, under *pneumonia*).

K. pneumo′niae subsp. *ozae′nae* a species occurring in ozena and other chronic respiratory diseases.

K. pneumo′niae subsp. *rhinosclero′matis* a species that causes rhinoscleroma.

K. rhinosclero′matis *K. pneumoniae* subsp. *rhinoscleromatis*.

klee·blatt·schä·del (kla″blaht-sha′dəl) [Ger.] cloverleaf skull; a congenital anomaly in which there is intrauterine synostosis of multiple or all cranial sutures. See *kleeblattschädel syndrome*, under *syndrome*.

Klein-Waar·den·burg syndrome (klīn′ vahr′dən-bərg) [David *Klein*, Swiss ophthalmologist, 1908–1993; Petrus Johannes *Waardenburg*, Dutch ophthalmologist, 1886–1979] Waardenburg syndrome type 3; see under *syndrome*.

Klei•ne-Lev•in syndrome (kli′nə lev′in) [Willi *Kleine*, German psychiatrist, 20th century; Max *Levin*, American neurologist, 20th century] see under *syndrome*.

Kleist sign (klīst) [Karl *Kleist*, German neuropsychiatrist, 1879–1960] see under *sign*.

Klemm sign (klem) [Paul *Klemm*, German surgeon, 1861–1921] see under *sign*.

klept(o)- [Gr. *kleptein* to steal] a combining form denoting relationship to theft or stealing.

klep•to•lag•nia (klep″to-lag′ne-ə) [*klepto-* + Gr. *lagneia* lust] sexual gratification produced by theft.

klep•to•ma•nia (klep″to-ma′ne-ə) [*klepto-* + *-mania*] [DSM-IV] an uncontrollable impulse to steal objects unnecessary for personal use or monetary value, the act being preceded by tension and followed by pleasure or relief, and not caused by anger, delusion, vengeance, or hallucination.

klep•to•ma•ni•ac (klep″to-ma′ne-ak) an individual exhibiting kleptomania.

Kle•stadt cyst (kle′stat) [Walter D. *Klestadt*, American physician, 20th century] nasoalveolar cyst.

Kline•fel•ter syndrome (klīn′fel-tər) [Harry Fitch *Klinefelter*, Jr., American physician, 1912–1990] see under *syndrome*.

Klip•pel-Feil syndrome (klĭ-pel′ fīl′) [Maurice *Klippel*, French neurologist, 1858–1942; André *Feil*, French physician, 20th century] see under *syndrome*.

Klip•pel-Tré•nau•nay syndrome (klĭ-pel′ tra-no-na′) [M. *Klippel;* Paul *Trénaunay*, French physician, 20th century] see under *syndrome*.

Klip•pel-Tré•nau•nay-We•ber syndrome (klĭ-pel′ tra-no-na′ va′ber) [M. *Klippel;* P. *Trénaunay;* Frederick Parkes *Weber*, English physician, 1863–1962] see under *syndrome*.

Klip•pel-Weil sign (klĭ-pel′ vīl′) [M. *Klippel;* Mathieu Pierre *Weil*, French physician, 20th century] see under *sign*.

klis•e•om•e•ter (klis″e-om′ə-tər) cliseometer.

klis•ma•phil•ia (kliz″mə-fil′e-ə) love of enemas; a paraphilia in which sexual excitement depends on the use of enemas.

Klon•o•pin (klon′o-pin) trademark for a preparation of clonazepam.

K-Lor (kay′lor) trademark for a preparation of potassium chloride.

Klor-Con (klor′kon) trademark for preparations containing potassium.

Klos•si•el•la (klos″e-el′ə) a genus of coccidian protozoa (suborder Adeleina, order Eucoccidiida) parasitic in the renal cells of mammals, such as the mouse and guinea pig, characterized by the presence of an oocyst with many spores, each producing many sporozoites.

Klump•ke paralysis (kloomp′kə) [Augusta Dejerine-*Klumpke*, French neurologist, 1859–1927] see under *paralysis*.

Klump•ke-Dej•er•ine paralysis (syndrome) (kloomp′kə dĕ-zhĕ-rēn′) [A. Dejerine-*Klumpke;* Joseph Jules *Dejerine*, French neurologist, 1849–1917] Klumpke paralysis.

Klü•ver-Bu•cy syndrome (kle′vər bu′se) [Heinrich *Klüver*, American psychologist and neurologist, 1897–1979; Paul Clancy *Bucy*, American neurologist, 1904–1992] see under *syndrome*.

Kluy•vera (kli′vər-ə) [Albert Jan *Kluyver*, Dutch microbiologist, 1888–1956] a genus of gram-negative, facultatively anaerobic, rod-shaped bacteria of the family Enterobacteriaceae, occurring in human clinical specimens. It is an occasional opportunistic pathogen, causing respiratory and urinary infections. The type species is *K. ascorba′ta*.

Km see under *allotype*.

km kilometer.

Knapp streaks (striae) (knahp) [Herman Jakob *Knapp*, German-born ophthalmologist in the United States, 1832–1911] see under *streak*.

knead•ing (nēd′ing) pétrissage.

knee (ne) 1. genu (def. 1). 2. any structure bent like the knee. 3. in ungulates, the carpus of the foreleg or the stifle joint of the hind leg.
 back k. genu recurvatum.
 beat k. a subcutaneous cellulitis over the kneecap.
 big k. 1. in cattle, bursitis over the knee. 2. in horses, a tumor of the bony parts of the knee joint. 3. in goats, the adult form of caprine arthritis-encephalitis.
 Brodie k. a chronic synovitis of the knee joint in which the affected parts acquire a soft and pulpy consistency.
 capped k. distention of the synovial bursa over the knee joint of horses or cattle.
 carpet layer's k. prepatellar bursitis.
 floating k. a highly unstable condition of the knee caused by fracture of the ipsilateral femoral and tibial shafts.
 housemaid's k. prepatellar bursitis.
 in k. genu valgum.
 k. of internal capsule genu capsulae internae.
 jumper's k. patellar tendinopathy.
 knock k. genu valgum.
 locked k. inability to extend the lower limb fully as a result of tear of the medial semilunar cartilage.
 out k. genu varum.
 popped k. carpitis.
 rugby k. Osgood-Schlatter disease.
 septic k. a suppurating knee joint.
 sprung k. forward bending of the knee of a horse, due to shortening of the flexor tendons.
 trick k. popular term for a knee joint susceptible to locking in position, most often due to longitudinal splitting of the medial meniscus.

knee•cap (ne′kap) patella.

knee-gall (ne′gawl) thoroughpin.

kneipp•ism (nīp′iz-əm) [Rev. Sebastian *Kneipp*, German priest, 1821–1897, who introduced the practice] a system of hydrotherapy involving applications of cold water, including cold bathing and walking barefoot in the morning dew.

Kne•mi•do•kop•tes (ne″mĭ-do-kop′tēz) a genus of mites. *K. galli′nae*, the depluming mite, causes depluming of fowls. *K. mu′tans* causes the disease called scaly leg in fowls and cage birds.

Knies sign (knēs) [Max *Knies*, German ophthalmologist, 1851–1917] see under *sign*.

Kniest dysplasia (nēst) [Wilhelm *Kniest*, German pediatrician, born 1919] see under *dysplasia*.

knife (nīf) any of various types of cutting instruments.
 Blair k. a knife with a long sharp blade used to cut skin grafts.
 Buck k. a periodontal knife with spear-shaped cutting points, used for interdental incision during gingivectomy.
 button k. a small knife used for the cutting of cartilage.
 cataract k. a knife for cutting the cornea in operations for cataract.
 cautery k. a knife connected with an electric battery, so that the tissues may be seared while being cut, in order to prevent bleeding.
 electric k. a knife-shaped electrode or steel needle which cuts by causing dissolution of tissue when activated by a high-frequency current.
 Gamma K. trademark for an apparatus for producing intracranial lesions by precisely aimed intersecting beams of gamma rays; used in stereotactic radiosurgery.
 Goldman-Fox k. any of a group of knives designed for incision and contouring of gingival tissues in periodontal surgery.
 Graefe k. a slender knife used in linear extraction of cataract.
 Humby k. a knife with a roller attached, used for cutting skin grafts of varying thickness; the distance between the roller and the blade of the knife can be varied by means of a calibration device.
 Joseph k. a double-bladed knife used in corrective rhinoplasty.
 Kirkland k. a periodontal knife that consists of a thin, flattened blade attached to the handle by an angulated shank, the outer edge being elliptical and the inner straight; used for primary gingivectomy.
 Liston k. a long-bladed amputation knife.
 Merrifield k. a periodontal knife with a long narrow triangular blade; used in gingivectomy.
 photon k. an apparatus used in stereotactic surgery, producing intracranial lesions by precisely aimed beams of photons produced by a computer-assisted linear accelerator.

Knight brace (nīt) [James C. *Knight*, American physician, 1810–1887] see under *brace*.

knit•ting (nit′ing) the physiological process of repair of a fractured bone.

knob (nob) a bulbous mass or protuberance.
 aortic k. the hump or knob formed by the aortic arch where it joins the descending thoracic aorta seen in radiographs in anteroposterior projections; called also *aortic knuckle*.
 olfactory k. olfactory vesicle (def. 2).
 surfers' k's see under *nodule*.
 synaptic k. bouton terminal; see under *bouton*.

knock (nok) a sound as of a blow against a firm surface.
 pericardial k. an early diastolic sound resembling an S_3 gallop but earlier and due to sudden deceleration of ventricular filling at capacity in cases of constrictive pericarditis.

knock-knee (nok′ne″) genu valgum.

knock•out (nok′out) the inactivation of a gene by the creation of a mutant allele, either by random mutation or by gene targeting (q.v.); generally used of animals in which specific wild-type alleles are replaced by mutated ones. Spelled also *knock-out*.

Knodt instrumentation, rod (not) [T.H. *Knodt*, American orthopedic surgeon, 20th century] see under *instrumentation* and *rod.*

Knops blood group (nops) [*Knops*, surname of the American propositus first reported on in 1970] see under *blood group.*

knot (not) 1. an intertwining of the ends or parts of one or more threads, sutures, or strips of cloth so they cannot easily be separated.

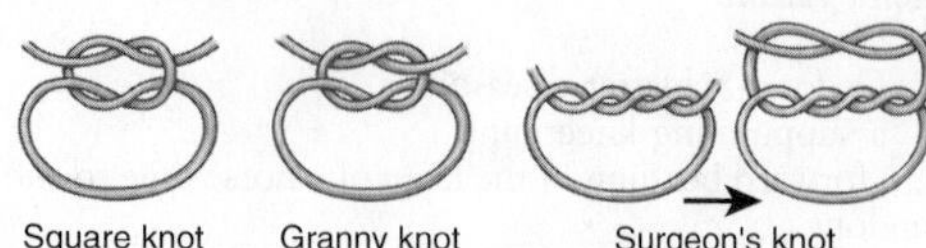

2. in anatomy, a knoblike swelling or protuberance, as a node.

clove-hitch k. a knot consisting of two contiguous loops that are applied around an object, the ends of the cord being toward each other; used for making traction on a part for the reduction of dislocations.

double k. a knot in which the ends of the cord are twisted around each other twice.

enamel k. a small dense group of epithelial cells in the stellate reticulum of a developing tooth, which disappears before enamel formation begins.

false k. 1. a local bulge on the umbilical cord caused by protuberant vessels. Cf. *true k.* 2. granny k.

friction k. double k.

granny k. a double knot in the second loop of which the end of one cord is over, and the other under, its fellow, so that the loops do not lie in the same line and the knot will not hold.

Hensen k., primitive k., protochordal k. primitive node.

reef k. square k.

slip k. a knot so tied as to create a loop that can be opened and closed.

square k. a double knot in which the free ends of the second knot lie in the same plane as the ends of the first knot.

stay k. a knot made with two or more ligatures, each being tied with the first half of a square knot; then all the ends of one side are taken in one hand, and all the ends on the other side in the other hand, and tied as if they formed one single thread.

surfers' k's see under *nodule.*

surgeon's k., surgical k. a knot in which the thread is passed twice through the first loop to prevent slippage.

syncytial k's protuberances of nuclei of the syncytiotrophoblast along the chorionic villi.

true k. a simple knot produced in the looped umbilical cord during pregnancy. Cf. *false k.*

knot•ting (not'ing) formation of a knot or knotlike structure; see also *volvulus.*

ileosigmoid k. a severe type of volvulus consisting of twisting together of the ileum and the sigmoid colon

knuck•le (nuk'əl) the dorsal aspect of any phalangeal joint, especially of the metacarpophalangeal joints of the flexed fingers. By extension sometimes applied to any anatomical structure of similar appearance, such as an extruded loop of intestine in hernia.

aortic k. see under *knob.*

knuck•ling (nuk'ling) a pushing forward and upward of the fetlock joint of a horse, due to shortening of the tendons behind.

Ko•āte (ko'āt) trademark for preparations of antihemophilic factor (human).

Ko•belt tubules (ko'bəlt) [Georg Ludwig *Kobelt*, German physician, 1804–1857] see under *tubule.*

Koch (kawk) Robert, 1843–1910. German physician and bacteriologist; winner of the Nobel prize in physiology or medicine for 1905 for his work and discoveries concerning tuberculosis.

Koch phenomenon, postulate, tuberculin (kawk) [R. *Koch*] see under *phenomenon, postulate,* and *tuberculin.*

Koch-Weeks bacillus (kawk' wēks') [R. *Koch;* John Elmer *Weeks*, American ophthalmologist, 1853–1949] *Haemophilus aegyptius.*

Ko•cher forceps, etc. (ko'kər) [Emil Theodor *Kocher*, Swiss surgeon and Nobel prize winner, 1841–1917] see under *forceps, incision, maneuver, method, reflex,* and *sign.*

Ko•cher-De•bré-Sé•mé•laigne syndrome (ko'kər də-bra' sa-malen'yə) [E.T. *Kocher;* Robert *Debré*, French pediatrician and bacteriologist, 1882–1978; Georges *Sémélaigne*, French pediatrician, 20th century] Debré-Sémélaigne syndrome.

ko•cher•iza•tion (ko″kər-ĭ-za'shən) Kocher maneuver.

Ko•chia (ko'ke-ə) a genus of herbs of the family Chenopodiaceae. *K. scopa'ria* is the summer cypress or fireweed, a shrub of Europe and Asia that has red foliage; when eaten by cattle it causes lacrimation, anorexia, liver damage, and photosensitization.

Kock pouch (kawk) [Nils G. *Kock*, Swedish surgeon, born 1924] see under *pouch.*

Koeb•ner phenomenon (kerb'nər) [Heinrich *Koebner*, German dermatologist, 1838–1904] see under *phenomenon.*

koeb•ner•iza•tion (kerb″nər-ĭ-za'shən) 1. Koebner phenomenon. 2. development of a Koebner phenomenon on an area of skin.

koeb•ner•ize (kerb'nər-īz) to develop a Koebner phenomenon on an area of skin.

Koer•ber-Sa•lus-Elsch•nig syndrome (kur'bər sah'lōōs elsh'nik) [Hermann *Koerber*, German ophthalmologist, 20th century; Robert *Salus*, Austrian ophthalmologist, 20th century; Anton *Elschnig*, Austrian ophthalmologist, 1863–1939] sylvian syndrome; see under *syndrome.*

Ko•ge•nate (ko'jə-nāt) trademark for preparations of antihemophilic factor (recombinant).

Ko•goj spongiform pustule (ko'goi) [Franjo *Kogoj*, Croatian physician, 1894–1983] spongiform pustule; see under *pustule.*

Köh•ler bone disease (ker'lər) [Alban *Köhler*, German physician, 1874–1947] see under *disease.*

Köh•ler-Pel•le•gri•ni-Stie•da disease (ker'lər pel-ə-gre'ne shte'dah) [A. *Köhler;* Augusto *Pellegrini*, Italian physician, 1877–1968; Alfred *Stieda*, German physician, 1869–1945] Pellegrini disease; see under *disease.*

Kohl•rausch folds (kōl'roush) [Otto Ludwig Bernhard *Kohlrausch*, German physician, 1811–1854] plicae transversae recti.

Kohn•stamm phenomenon (kōn'shtahm) [Oskar Felix *Kohnstamm*, German physician, 1871–1917] aftermovement.

koil(o)- [Gr. *koilos* hollow] a combining form meaning hollow or concave.

koi•lo•cyte (koi'lo-sīt″) a concave or hollow cell, such as a normal red blood cell or one of the pyknotic vacuolated epithelial cells with clear cytoplasm seen in koilocytosis.

koi•lo•cy•to•sis (koi″lo-si-to'sis) [*koilo-* + *cyt-* + *-osis*] the presence of abnormal koilocytes that are vacuolated with clear cytoplasm or perinuclear halos and nuclear pyknosis. It is often seen in infections by human papillomavirus of epithelial layers of the uterine cervix or external anal or genital areas. See also *koilocytotic atypia*, under *atypia*, and *condyloma acuminatum.* **koilocytot'ic** *adj*

koi•lo•nych•ia (koi″lo-nik'e-ə) [*koil-* + *onychia*] a type of dystrophy of the fingernails in which they are thin and concave and have raised edges; it is sometimes associated with iron deficiency anemia. Called also *spoon nail.*

koi•lor•rhach•ic (koi″lo-rak'ik) [*koilo-* + *rhachi-* + *-ic*] having a vertebral column in which the lumbar curvature is concave anteriorly. Cf. *kyphosis, kyrtorrhachic,* and *orthorrhachic.*

koi•lo•ster•nia (koi″lo-stur'ne-ə) [*koilo-* + *stern-* + *-ia*] pectus excavatum.

koin(o)- see *cen(o)-*[2].

ko•jic ac•id (ko'jik) a pyrone formed from sugars by a variety of microorganisms, especially species of *Aspergillus;* it has antibiotic and antifungal properties.

Köl•li•ker column, etc. (ker'lĭ-kər) [Rudolf Albert von *Kölliker*, Swiss anatomist in Germany, 1817–1905] see under *granule*, and see *membrana reticularis organi spiralis, nucleus subparabrachialis,* and *sarcostyle.*

Kol•mo•gor•ov-Smir•nov test (kol″mo-gor'of smēr'nof) [Andrei Nicolaievich *Kolmogorov*, Russian mathematician, 1903–1987; Nicolai Vasilievich *Smirnov*, Russian mathematician, 1900–1966] see under *test.*

Kon•do•le•on operation (kon-do'la-ən) [Emmerich (Emmanuel) *Kondoleon*, Greek surgeon, 1879–1939] see under *operation.*

Kö•nig rods (ker'nig) [Charles Joseph *König*, German otologist, late 19th century] see under *rod.*

Kö•nig syndrome (ker'nig) [Franz *König*, German surgeon, 1832–1910] see under *syndrome.*

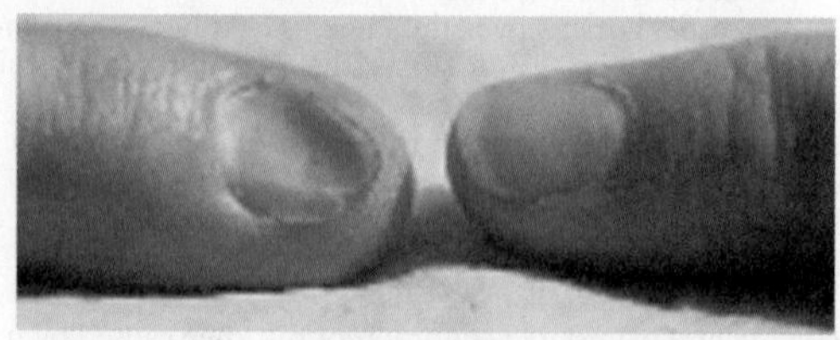

■ Koilonychia *(left).*

ko•nim•e•ter (ko-nim′ə-tər) [Gr. *konis* dust + *metron* measure] an apparatus for counting the number of dust particles in the air. Called also *coniometer* and *konometer*.

ko•nio•cor•tex (ko″ne-o-kor′teks) [Gr. *konis* dust + *cortex*, so called because of the large number and small size of the granular cells] the cortex of the sensory areas of the brain that have particularly many prominent granule cells in layers II and IV; called also *granular cortex*.

ko•ni•ol•o•gy (ko″ne-ol′ə-je) coniology.

ko•nom•e•ter (ko-nom′ə-tər) konimeter.

Kon•syl (kon′səl) a brand of psyllium hydrophilic mucilloid.

Ko•nyne 80 (ko′nīn) trademark for a preparation of factor IX complex.

ko•pi•opia (ko″pe-o′pe-ə) copiopia.

Kop•lik spots (sign) (kop′lik) [Henry *Koplik*, American pediatrician, 1858–1927] see under *spot*.

Ko•rán•yi auscultation (percussion) (ko-rahn′ye) [Baron Friedrich von *Korányi*, Hungarian physician, 1828–1913] see under *auscultation*.

Kor•do•fan gum (kor′də-fan) [*Kordofan* province in the Sudan, where the trees are found] see under *gum*.

ko•ro (ko′ro) a culture-specific acute delusional syndrome occurring in south and east Asia in which the patient believes that the penis or the vulva and nipples are shrinking and may disappear into the abdomen, causing death.

Ko•rot•koff method, sounds, test (kə-rot′kof) [Nicolai Sergeevich *Korotkoff*, Russian physician, 1874–1920] see under *method*, *sound*, and *test*.

Kor•sa•koff (Kor•sa•kov) syndrome (psychosis) (kor′sə-kof) [Sergei Sergeevich *Korsakoff* (or *Korsakov*), Russian neurologist, 1854–1900] see under *syndrome*.

Kör•te-Bal•lance operation (ker′tə bal′əns) [Werner *Körte*, German surgeon, 1853–1937; Sir Charles Alfred *Ballance*, British surgeon, 1856–1936] see under *operation*.

ko•sam (ko′səm) *Brucea sumatrana*, a small evergreen shrub whose seeds are sometimes used locally in the treatment of diarrhea, dysentery, and uterine hemorrhage.

Ko•shev•ni•koff (Ko•schew•ni•kow, Ko•zhev•ni•kov) disease, epilepsy (kə-shef′nĭ-kof) [Alexei Jakovlevich *Koshevnikoff* (or *Koschewnikow* or *Kozhevnikov*), Russian neurologist, 1836–1902] epilepsia partialis continua.

Kost•mann syndrome (neutropenia) (kost′mahn) [Rolf *Kostmann*, Swedish physician, 1909–1982] see under *syndrome*.

Ko•va•lev•sky canal (ko″və-lef′ske) [Alexander Onufrievich *Kovalevsky*, Russian embryologist, 1840–1901] neurenteric canal.

Koy•ter muscle (koi′tər) [Volcherus *Koyter*, Dutch anatomist, 1534–1600] musculus corrugator supercilii.

KP keratic precipitates; see *keratitis punctata*.

K-Phos (ka′fos) trademark for any of several preparations containing monobasic potassium phosphate and sometimes also one or more sodium phosphate salts.

Kr krypton.

Krab•be disease (leukodystrophy) (krah′bə) [Knud H. *Krabbe*, Danish neurologist, 1885–1961] see under *disease*.

Krae•pe•lin (kra′pə-lin) Emil, 1856–1926. German psychiatrist; the father of descriptive psychiatry. He differentiated manic-depressive psychosis from dementia praecox (schizophrenia) and described the basic schizophrenic subtypes: catatonic, hebephrenic, and paranoid. Modern classifications of the psychoses are still essentially kraepelinian.

krait (krāt) any member of the genus *Bungarus*, extremely venomous crotalid snakes found from India across Southeast and East Asia. See table at *snake*.

Kra•me•ria (kra-me′re-ə) [J.G.H. and W.H. *Kramer*, German botanists] a genus of shrubs and herbs of the family Leguminosae. The dried roots of *K. trian′dra* R. et P., or Peruvian rhatany, and of *K. argen′tea* Mart., or Brazilian rhatany, were formerly used as an astringent.

Kras•ke operation (krahs′kə) [Paul *Kraske*, German surgeon, 1851–1930] see under *operation*.

kra•tom•e•ter (krə-tom′ə-tər) a prism-refracting instrument for use in orthoptic training.

krau•ro•sis (kraw-ro′sis) [Gr. *krauros* brittle] a dry, shriveled condition of a part, especially of the vulva (*k. vulvae*).

k. vul′vae *lichen sclerosus* (q.v.) of the vulvar region.

Krau•se end-bulb (krou′zə) [Wilhelm Johann Friedrich *Krause*, German anatomist, 1833–1910] see under *end-bulb*.

Krau•se glands, ligament, valve (krou′zə) [Karl Friedrich Theodor *Krause*, German anatomist, 1797–1868] see *glandulae conjunctivales* and *ligamentum transversum perinei*, and see *Béraud valve*, under *valve*.

Krau•se operation (krou′zə) [Fedor Victor *Krause*, German surgeon, 1857–1937] see under *operation*.

Krau•se-Wolfe graft (krou′zə woolf′) [F.V. *Krause;* John Reissberg *Wolfe*, Scottish ophthalmologist, 1824–1904] see under *graft*.

kre•a•tin (kre′ə-tin) creatine.

kre•bi•o•zen (krə-bi′o-zən) a substance identified as creatine by the Food and Drug Administration, isolated from the blood of horses injected with *Actinomyces bovis*, claimed to be effective in the treatment of cancer; its sale is banned in the United States.

Krebs cycle (krebz) [Sir Hans Adolf *Krebs*, German-born British biochemist and Nobel prize winner, 1900–1981] tricarboxylic acid cycle; see under *cycle*.

Krebs-Hen•se•leit cycle (krebz hen′sə-līt) [Sir H.A. *Krebs;* Kurt *Henseleit*, German biochemist, 1917–1973] urea cycle; see under *cycle*.

Kre•mer test (kra′mər) [Jan A.M. *Kremer*, Dutch physician, late 20th century] SCMC test; see under *test*.

kre(o)- for words beginning thus, see also those beginning *cre(o)-*.

kreso•fuch•sin (kres″o-fo͝ok′sin) a blue-gray powder used as a stain in histology; its aqueous solution is red, the alcoholic solution blue.

Kretsch•mann space (krech′mahn) [Friedrich *Kretschmann*, German otologist, 1858–1934] see under *space*.

Kretsch•mer types (krech′mər) [Ernst *Kretschmer*, German psychiatrist, 1888–1964] see under *type*.

Krey•sik sign (kri′sik) [Friedrich Ludwig *Kreysig*, German physician, 1770–1839] Heim-Kreysig sign.

krimp•siek•te (krimp-zēk′te) [Afrikaans] a disease of cattle in South Africa caused by poisoning with any of several plant species of the genus *Cotyledon*, which contain cotyledontoxin; symptoms include abdominal pain and convulsions that can be fatal.

krin•gle (kring′gəl) see under *domain*.

Kri•sha•ber disease (kre″sah-bār′) [Maurice *Krishaber*, Hungarian physician in France, 1836–1883] see under *disease*.

Kri•sov•ski (Kri•sow•ski) sign (kre-sov′ske) [Max *Krisovski* (or *Krisowski*), German physician, late 19th century] see under *sign*.

Kris•ta•lose (kris′tə-lōs) trademark for a preparation of lactulose.

Kro•may•er lamp (kro′mi-ər) [Ernst Ludwig Franz *Kromayer*, German dermatologist, 1862–1933] see under *lamp*.

Kro•neck•er center, puncture (kro′nek-ər) [Karl Hugo *Kronecker*, German pathologist in Switzerland, 1839–1914] see *cardioinhibitory center*, under *center*, and see under *puncture*.

Krön•lein hernia, operation (krern′līn) [Rudolf Ulrich *Krönlein*, Swiss surgeon, 1847–1910] see *inguinoproperitoneal hernia*, under *hernia*, and see under *operation*.

Kru•ken•berg spindle, tumor (kroo′kən-berg) [Friedrich Ernst *Krukenberg*, German pathologist, 1871–1946] see under *spindle* and *tumor*.

Kru•ken•berg veins (kroo′kən-berg) [Adolph *Krukenberg*, German anatomist, 1816–1877] venae centrales hepatis.

Krus•kal-Wal•lis test (krus′kal wal′is) [William Henry *Kruskal*, American statistician, 1919–2005; Wilson Allen *Wallis*, American statistician, 1912–1998] see under *test*.

kryp•ton (Kr) (krip′ton) [Gr. *kryptos* hidden] an inert gaseous chemical element found in the atmosphere; atomic number 36, atomic weight 83.80.

k. Kr 81m [USP] an unstable radioactive isotope of krypton, atomic mass 81, having a half-life of 13 seconds and emitting gamma rays (0.19 MeV); it is used in pulmonary ventilation studies to evaluate regional function.

KS Kaposi sarcoma.

17-KS 17-ketosteroid.

K-Tab (kay′tab) trademark for a preparation of potassium chloride.

Kt/V in urea kinetics, an expression of the efficiency, or fractional urea clearance, of one hemodialysis session; K is the rate of clearance, t is the amount of time of the session, and V is the urea distribution volume after hemodialysis.

KUB kidney, ureter, and bladder.

ku•bi•sa•ga•ri (koo-be-sah-gah′re) Japanese name for *vestibular neuronitis*.

Kufs disease (koofs) [H. *Kufs*, German psychiatrist, 1871–1955] see under *disease*.

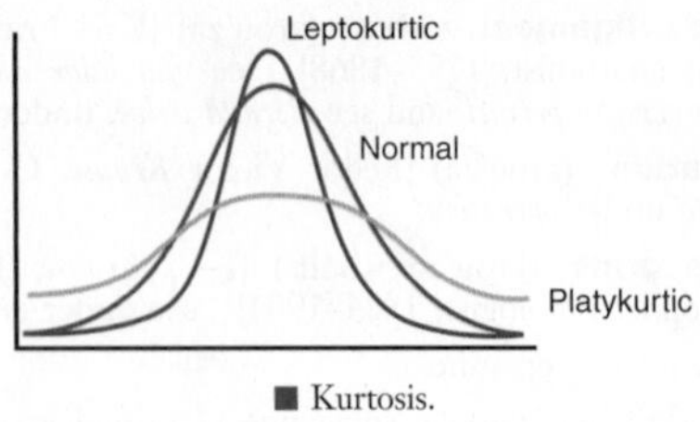

■ Kurtosis.

Ku•gel•berg-We•lan•der syndrome (koo′gəl-berg va′lahn-dər) [Eric Klas Henrik *Kugelberg*, Swedish neurologist, 1913–1983; Lisa *Welander*, Swedish neurologist, 1909–2001] see under *syndrome.*

Kuhl•mann test (ko͞ol′mən) [Frederick *Kuhlmann*, American psychologist, 1876–1941] see under *test.*

Küh•ne terminal plates (ke′nə) [Wilhelm Friedrich (Willy) *Kühne*, German physiologist, 1837–1900] see under *plate.*

Kuhnt-Ju•ni•us disease (ko͞ont′ yoo′ne-us) [Hermann *Kuhnt*, German ophthalmologist, 1850–1925; Paul *Junius*, German ophthalmologist, 1871–1948] disciform macular degeneration; see under *degeneration.*

Kul•chit•sky cells (ko͞ol-chit′ske) [Nicolai K. *Kulchitsky*, Russian histologist, 1856–1925] see under *cell.*

kun•da•li•ni (koon″də-le′ne) [Sanskrit *kundalam* ring, coil] 1. in Hindu tradition, psychospiritual energy that lies dormant in the lowest chakra. 2. see under *yoga.*

Küm•mell disease (spondylitis) (ke′məl) [Hermann *Kümmell*, German surgeon, 1852–1937] see under *disease.*

Küm•mell-Ver•neuil disease (ke′məl vār-nwe′) [H. *Kümmell;* Aristide August Stanislas *Verneuil*, French surgeon, 1823–1895] Kümmell disease.

Kun•kel syndrome (kung′kəl) [Henry George *Kunkel*, American physician, 1916–1983] chronic active hepatitis.

Künt•scher nail (kēnt′shər) [Gerhard *Küntscher*, German surgeon, 1902–1972] see under *nail.*

Kupf•fer cells (koop′fər) [Karl Wilhelm von *Kupffer*, German anatomist, 1829–1902] see under *cell.*

ku•pra•mite (koo′prə-mīt) a gas mask adsorbent for ammonia fumes.

Kur•loff (Kur•lov) bodies (ko͞or′lof) [Mikhail Georgievich *Kurloff* (or *Kurlov*), Russian physician, 1859–1932] see under *body.*

Kur•thia (kur′the-ə) [Heinrich *Kurth*, German bacteriologist, 1860–1901] a genus of bacteria of the family Planococcaceae, consisting of gram-positive, regular, unbranched rods with rounded ends, occurring in chains and of pleomorphic forms. The type species is *K. zop′fii.*

K. zop′fii a species that has been isolated from human feces in mild cases of food poisoning and under normal conditions, as well as from meats and meat products; it is also found in the intestinal contents of chickens and in manure, stagnant water, and milk.

kur•to•sis (kər-to′sis) [Gr. "convexity"] the degree of peakedness or flatness of a probability distribution, relative to the normal distribution with the same variance. See *leptokurtic* and *platykurtic.*

ku•ru (koo′roo) ["shivering" in language of the Fore people of New Guinea] an infectious form of prion disease with a long incubation period, found only among the Fore and neighboring peoples of New Guinea and thought to be associated with ritual cannibalism. It is manifested by truncal and limb ataxia, a shivering-like tremor, and dysarthria and ends invariably in death; strabismus and extrapyramidal symptoms may also be found. Amyloid plaques are present in about two thirds of affected individuals.

Küss experiment (kēs) [Emil *Küss*, German physiologist, 1815–1871] see under *experiment.*

Kuss•maul disease, pulse, etc. (koos′moul) [Adolf *Kussmaul*, German physician, 1822–1902] see *polyarteritis nodosa;* see *paradoxical pulse*, under *pulse*, and *diabetic coma*, under *coma;* and see under *respiration* and *sign.*

Kuss•maul-Kien respiration (koos′moul kēn′) [A. *Kussmaul;* Alphonse Marie Joseph *Kien*, German physician, late 19th century] see under *respiration.*

Kuss•maul-Mai•er disease (koos′moul mi′ər) [A. *Kussmaul;* Rudolf *Maier*, German physician, 1824–1888] polyarteritis nodosa.

Küst•ner's law (kēst′nərz) [Otto Ernst *Küstner*, German gynecologist, 1849–1931] see under *law.*

Ku•trase (ku′trās) trademark for a preparation of pancrelipase.

Ku-Zyme (ku′zīm) trademark for a preparation of pancrelipase.

kV kilovolt.

Kveim test (kvīm) [Morten Ansgar *Kveim*, Norwegian pathologist in Denmark, 1892–1966] see under *test.*

kVp kilovolts peak.

kwash•i•or•kor (kwahsh″e-or′kor) ["condition seen in the displaced child" in the language of the Ga people of Ghana] a form of protein-energy malnutrition produced by severe protein deficiency; caloric intake may be adequate but is usually also deficient. It is characterized by retarded growth, changes in skin and hair pigment, edema, enlarged abdomen, immunodeficiency, and pathologic changes in the liver, including fatty infiltration, necrosis, and fibrosis. Other findings are mental apathy, atrophy of the pancreas, gastrointestinal disorders, anemia, low serum albumin, and dermatoses. The skin of the limbs and back may have dark thickened patches, which may desquamate, leaving pink, almost raw surfaces. Cf. *marasmus.*

marasmic k. a condition in which there is deficiency of both calories and protein, with severe tissue wasting, loss of subcutaneous fat, and usually dehydration.

Ky•a•sa•nur For•est disease (ki-as′ə-no͞or) [*Kyasanur Forest*, in Mysore State, India, where the first cases were reported among forest workers and monkeys in 1957] see under *disease.*

ky•ma•tism (ki′mə-tiz″əm) myokymia.

ky•mog•ra•phy (ki-mog′rə-fe) the recording of variations or undulations, such as of the larynx or the wall of the heart. See also *electrokymography*, *photokymography*, and *videokymography.*

kyn•uren•ic ac•id (kin″u-ren′ik) a bicyclic aromatic compound formed from kynurenine via a transamination reaction and cyclization as a step in one pathway of tryptophan catabolism. It is excreted in the urine in several disorders of tryptophan catabolism.

kyn•ure•nin (kīn″u-re′nin) kynurenine.

kyn•u•ren•i•nase (kīn″u-ren′ĭ-nās) [EC 3.7.1.3] an enzyme of the hydrolase class that catalyzes the cleavage of hydroxykynurenine to hydroxyanthranilic acid and alanine as a step in the metabolism of tryptophan; kynurenine is also a substrate. The enzyme is a pyridoxal phosphate protein, so enzyme activity is reduced in vitamin B_6 deficiency.

kyn•ure•nine (kin-u′rə-nēn″) [Gr. *kyōn* dog + L. *ren* kidney] an aromatic amino acid, first isolated from dog urine; it is formed as an intermediate in the metabolism of tryptophan.

kyn•ure•nine for•mam•i•dase (kīn-u′rə-nēn″ for-mam′ĭ-dās) arylformamidase.

kyn•ure•nine 3-hy•drox•y•lase (kīn-u′rə-nēn″ hi-drok′sĭ-lās) kynurenine 3-monooxygenase.

kyn•ure•nine 3-mono•oxy•gen•ase (kīn-u′rə-nēn″ mon″o-ok′sĭ-jən-ās) [EC 1.14.13.9] an enzyme of the oxidoreductase class that catalyzes the hydroxylation of kynurenine as a step in the metabolism of tryptophan. The enzyme is a flavoprotein, containing FAD, and the reaction requires NADPH.

ky•pho•plas•ty (ki′fo-plas″te) a procedure for adding height to a compressed vertebra in osteoporosis: a balloon is inserted into the fracture through a trocar and expanded, and the resulting space is filled by injection of polymethacrylate cement. **kyphoplas′tic** *adj*

ky•phos (ki′fos) [Gr. "a hump"] the convex prominence of the spine in kyphosis.

ky•pho•sco•li•o•sis (ki″fo-sko″le-o′sis) [*kyphosis* + *scoliosis*] backward and lateral curvature of the vertebral column, as in vertebral osteochondrosis (Scheuermann disease).

ky•pho•sis (ki-fo′sis) [Gr. *kyphōsis* humpback] 1. an area of the vertebral column that is convex. 2. abnormally increased convexity in the curvature of the thoracic vertebral column as viewed from the side. Cf. *lordosis* and *scoliosis.*

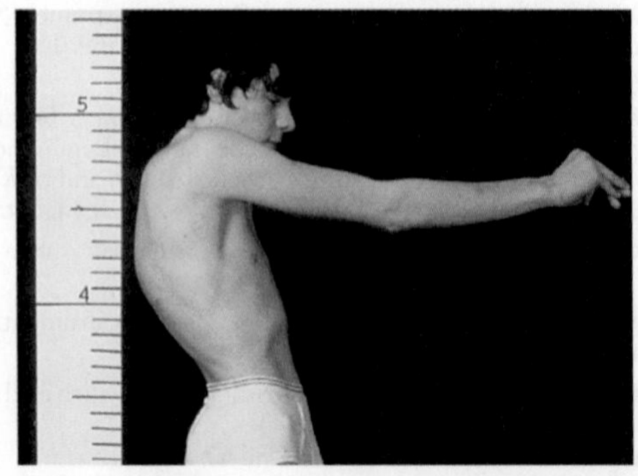

■ Thoracic kyphosis secondary to osteochondrosis; the patient is partially compensating with increased lumbar lordosis.

k. dorsa′lis juveni′lis, juvenile k. see *osteochondrosis.*

sacral k., k. sacra′lis [TA] the dorsally convex curve formed by the sacrum when seen from the side. Called also *pelvic* or *sacral curvature.*

Scheuermann k. see *osteochondrosis.*

thoracic k., k. thora′cica [TA] the dorsally convex curve formed by the thoracic vertebral column when seen from the side. Called also *thoracic curvature.*

ky·phot·ic (ki-fot′ik) affected with or pertaining to kyphosis.

Kyrle disease (kir′lə) [Joseph *Kyrle,* Austrian dermatologist, 1880–1926] see under *disease.*

kyr·tor·rhach·ic (kir″to-rak′ik) [Gr. *kyrtos* curved, convex + *rhachis* spine] having a vertebral column in which the lumbar curvature is convex anteriorly. Cf. *koilorrhachic* and *orthorrhachic.*

Ky·to·coc·cus (ki″to-kok′əs) [Gr. *kytos* skin + *kokkos* berry] a genus of bacteria of the family Dermatophilaceae, consisting of gram-positive, nonencapsulated, coccoid cells; organisms are aerobic, non–spore-forming, nonmotile, mesophilic, chemo-organotrophic, and catalase-positive. The type species is *K. sedenta′rius.*

K. sedenta′rius a species that produces keratin-degrading enzymes and is a cause of pitted keratolysis. Formerly called *Micrococcus sedentarius.*

Ky·tril (ki′tril) trademark for preparations of granisetron hydrochloride.

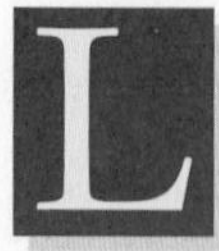

L lambert; left; leucine; light chain (immunoglobulin); liter; lumbar vertebra (L1 through L5); lung.

L. li′bra (pound).

L luminance; self-inductance.

L_0 limes nul; see *L0 dose*, under *dose*.

L+, L_+ limes tod; see *L+ dose*, under *dose*.

L0 limes nul; see *L0 dose*, under *dose*.

L- a chemical prefix (small capital L) that specifies the relative configuration of an enantiomer, the mirror image being specified as D-. Carbohydrates having the same configuration as L-glyceraldehyde at the asymmetric carbon atom most distant from the carbonyl functional group are designated as L (or L_g). Amino acids having the same configuration as L-serine at the α carbon are designated as L (or L_s). See D- for further explanation.

l former symbol for *liter*, now replaced by L.

l. [L.] ligamen′tum (ligament).

l length.

***l*-** [abbreviation for *levo* (left or counterclockwise)] a chemical prefix indicating an enantiomer that rotates the plane of polarization of a beam of light in the counterclockwise direction (levorotatory), the other enantiomer being specified as *d*- (for *dextro*). Largely replaced by (–)-; see note at *d*-.

λ lambda, the eleventh letter of the Greek alphabet; symbol for *wavelength, decay constant*, and one of the two types of immunoglobulin light chains.

L & A light and accommodation (reaction of pupils).

La lanthanum.

La•bar•raque solution (lah-bah-rahk′) [Antoine Germain *Labarraque*, French chemist, 1777–1850] see under *solution*.

Lab•bé triangle, vein (lah-ba′) [Léon *Labbé*, French surgeon, 1832–1916] see under *triangle*, and see *vena anastomotica superior*.

la•bel (la′bəl) 1. a mark, tag, or other characteristic that identifies something. 2. to provide something with such a characteristic.
  radioactive l. a radioisotope that is incorporated into a compound to mark it.

la•bet•a•lol (lə-bet′ə-lol) a beta-adrenergic blocking agent with some alpha-adrenergic blocking activity; used for its antihypertensive effects.
  l. hydrochloride the hydrochloride salt of labetalol, used in the treatment of hypertension; administered orally or intravenously.

la•bia (la′be-ə) [L.] plural of *labium*.

la•bi•al (la′be-əl) [L. *labialis*] 1. pertaining to a lip or labium. 2. in dental anatomy, pertaining to the tooth surface that faces the lip; see under *surface*. 3. bilabial.

la•bi•a•lism (la′be-əl-iz″əm) a speech disorder involving excessive use of bilabial speech sounds.

la•bi•al•ly (la′be-əl-e) toward the lips.

la•bia•plas•ty (la′be-ə-plas″te) plastic surgery of the labia minora, usually to reduce their size; called also *labioplasty*. **labiaplas′tic** *adj*

Lab•i•dog•na•tha (lab″ĭ-dog′nə-thə) a suborder of spiders (order Araneae), including the medically important families Theridiidae and Loxoscelidae.

la•bile (la′bəl, la′bīl) [L. *labilis* unstable, from *labi* to glide] 1. gliding; moving from point to point over the surface; unstable; fluctuating. 2. chemically unstable.
  heat l. thermolabile.

la•bil•i•ty (lə-bil′ə-te) 1. the quality of being labile. 2. in psychiatry, emotional instability; rapidly changing emotions.

labio- [L. *labium* lip] a combining form denoting relationship to a lip, especially to the lips of the mouth.

la•bio•al•ve•o•lar (la″be-o-al-ve′ə-lər) 1. pertaining to the lip and dental alveoli. 2. pertaining to the labial side of a dental alveolus.

la•bio•ax•io•gin•gi•val (la″be-o-ak″se-o-jin′jĭ-vəl) pertaining to or formed by the labial, axial, and gingival walls of a tooth cavity preparation.

la•bio•cer•vi•cal (la″be-o-sur′vĭ-kəl) 1. pertaining to the labial surface of the neck of an anterior tooth. 2. labiogingival.

la•bio•cho•rea (la″be-o-kə-re′ə) [*labio-* + *chorea*] a choreic stiffening of the lips in speech, with stammering.

la•bio•cli•na•tion (la″be-o-klĭ-na′shən) deviation of an anterior tooth from the vertical, in the direction of the lips.

la•bio•den•tal (la″be-o-den′təl) 1. pertaining to the lips and teeth. 2. a speech sound produced by the contact of the lips and teeth, such as *f* and *v*.

la•bio•gin•gi•val (la″be-o-jin′jĭ-vəl) pertaining to or formed by the labial and gingival walls of a tooth cavity. Called also *labiocervical*.

la•bio•glos•so•la•ryn•ge•al (la″be-o-glos″o-lə-rin′je-əl) [*labio-* + *glosso-* + *laryngeal*] pertaining to the lips, tongue, and larynx.

la•bio•glos•so•pha•ryn•ge•al (la″be-o-glos″o-fə-rin′je-əl) pertaining to the lips, tongue, and pharynx.

la•bio•graph (la′be-o-graf″) [*labio-* + *-graph*] an instrument for recording the motions of the lips in speaking.

la•bio•in•ci•sal (la″be-o-in-si′zəl) pertaining to or formed by the labial and incisal surfaces of a tooth.

la•bio•lin•gual (la″be-o-ling′gwəl) 1. pertaining to the lips and the tongue. 2. pertaining to the labial and lingual surfaces of an anterior tooth.

la•bi•ol•o•gy (la″be-ol′ə-je) the study of the movements of the lips. **labiolog′ic** *adj*

la•bio•men•tal (la″be-o-men′təl) pertaining to the lip and chin.

la•bio•na•sal (la″be-o-na′zəl) pertaining to the lip and nose.

la•bio•pal•a•tine (la″be-o-pal′ə-tīn) pertaining to the lip and palate.

la•bio•place•ment (la″be-o-plās′mənt) displacement of a tooth toward the lip.

la•bio•plas•ty (la′be-o-plas″te) 1. cheiloplasty. 2. labiaplasty.

la•bio•te•nac•u•lum (la″be-o-tə-nak′u-ləm) [*labio-* + *tenaculum*] an instrument for holding the lip.

la•bio•ver•sion (la″be-o-vur′zhən) displacement of a tooth labially from the line of occlusion.

la•bi•um (la′be-əm) pl. *la′bia* [L.] 1. lip. 2. a term used in anatomical nomenclature for a liplike structure. 3. *(in the pl.)* the *labia majora* and *minora pudendi*. See also *limbus* and *margo*.
  l. ante′rius os′tii u′teri [TA] anterior lip of external os of uterus: the anterior projection of the cervix into the vagina; it is shorter and thicker than the posterior lip.
  l. ce′rebri an edge of a deep sulcus, e.g., the lips of the calcarine sulcus.
  l. exter′num cris′tae ili′acae [TA] the outer margin or external lip of the iliac crest.
  l. infe′rius o′ris [TA] lower lip: the fleshy margin of the inferior border of the mouth.
  l. inter′num cris′tae ili′acae [TA] the inner margin or internal lip of the iliac crest.
  l. latera′le li′neae as′perae fe′moris [TA] lateral lip of rough line of femur: the distinct outer part of the linea aspera that becomes continuous with the gluteal tuberosity and ends at the greater trochanter above and with the lateral supracondylar line below.
  l. latera′le sul′ci intertubercula′ris TA alternative for *crista tuberculi majoris*.
  l. lim′bi tympa′nicum [TA] tympanic lip of limbus: the lower border of the internal spiral sulcus, formed by the lower extremity of the limbus laminae spiralis.
  l. lim′bi vestibula′re [TA] vestibular lip of limbus: the upper border of the internal spiral sulcus, formed by the upper extremity of the limbus laminae spiralis.
  l. ma′jus puden′di pl. *la′bia majo′ra puden′di* [TA] either of two elongated folds running downward and backward from the mons pubis in the female, one on either side of the median pudendal cleft.
  l. mandibula′re l. inferius oris.
  l. maxilla′re l. superius oris.
  l. media′lis li′neae as′perae fe′moris [TA] medial lip of rough line of femur: the distinct inner part of the linea aspera that becomes continuous with the intertrochanteric line above and the medial supracondylar line below.
  l. media′le sul′ci intertubercula′ris TA alternative for *crista tuberculi minoris*.
  l. mi′nus puden′di pl. *la′bia mino′ra puden′di* [TA] either of two small folds of skin, one on each side, running backward from the clitoris between the labium majus and the opening of the vagina.
  la′bia o′ris [TA] the lips: the fleshy upper and lower margins of the mouth.
  l. poste′rius os′tii u′teri [TA] posterior lip of external os of uterus: the posterior projection of the cervix into the vagina.
  l. supe′rius o′ris [TA] upper lip: the fleshy margin of the superior border of the mouth.
  l. ure′thrae either lateral margin of the external urinary meatus.
  l. voca′le plica vocalis.

la•bor (la′bər) [L. "work"] the function of the female organism by which the product of conception is expelled from the uterus through the vagina to the outside world. Labor may be divided into four stages: The first (the stage of cervical dilatation) begins with the onset of regular uterine contractions and ends when the os is completely dilated. The second stage

(stage of expulsion) extends from the end of the first stage until the expulsion of the infant is completed. The third stage (placental stage) extends from the expulsion of the child until the placenta and membranes are expelled. The fourth stage denotes the hour or two after delivery, when uterine tone is established. See also *labor pains*, under *pain*.

artificial l. induced l.

atonic l. labor protracted because of atony of the uterus.

complicated l. labor in which cephalopelvic disproportion, hemorrhage, or some other untoward event occurs.

delayed l. postponed l.

dry l. labor in which the amniotic fluid escapes before the onset of uterine contractions.

false l. see under *pain*.

habitual premature l. premature labor occurring in at least three successive pregnancies at about the same stage of development and prior to completion of the full gestation period.

induced l. labor brought on by mechanical or pharmacological means.

instrumental l. labor in which birth of the baby is facilitated by the use of instruments.

mimetic l. see *false pains*, under *pain*.

missed l. retention of a dead fetus in the uterus beyond the period of normal gestation.

multiple l. labor in which two or more infants are born.

obstructed l. labor hindered by some mechanical obstruction, such as a contraction in some region of the parturient canal or a tumor.

postmature l., postponed l. labor occurring two weeks or more after the expected date of confinement. See also *postterm pregnancy*, under *pregnancy*.

precipitate l. labor occurring with undue rapidity.

premature l., preterm l. labor that takes place before the normal end of gestation, usually meaning between the twentieth and the thirty-seventh completed weeks after onset of the last menstrual period.

prolonged l., protracted l. labor prolonged beyond the ordinary 18-hour limit.

spontaneous l. labor in which no artificial aid is required.

lab•o•ra•to•ri•an (lab″rə-tor′e-ən) a person devoted to laboratory work, as distinguished from a clinician.

lab•o•ra•to•ry (lab′rə-tor″e) [L. *laboratorium*] a place equipped for performing experimental work or investigative procedures, for the preparation of drugs, chemicals, etc.

clinical l. a laboratory for measurement and examination of materials derived from the human body (e.g., fluids, tissues, cells) for the purpose of providing information on diagnosis, prognosis, prevention, or treatment of disease.

La•borde method (lah-bord′) [Jean Baptiste Vincent *Laborde*, French physician, 1830–1903] see under *method.*

la•bra (la′brə) [L.] plural of *labrum.*

la•bra•le (lə-bra′le) an anthropometric landmark on the border of the lip.

l. infe′rius the lowest point, in the median plane, on the vermilion border of the lower lip.

l. supe′rius the highest point, in the median plane, on the vermilion border of the upper lip.

La•bre•a hepatitis (lah′bre-ə) [Lábrea, Amazonas, Brazil, where it was first observed] see under *hepatitis.*

lab•ro•cyte (lab′ro-sīt) [Gr. *labros* greedy + *-cyte*] mast cell.

la•brum (la′brəm) pl. *la′bra* [L. *lip*] 1. anatomic nomenclature for an edge, brim, or liplike part or structure. 2. the shelflike projection of the head of arthropods that anteriorly covers the mandible and forms the roof of the mouth.

l. acetabula′re, l. aceta′buli [TA] acetabular labrum: a ring of fibrocartilage attached to the rim of the acetabulum of the hip bone, increasing the depth of the cavity; called also *l. glenoidale articulationis coxae.*

l. articula′re [TA] articular labrum: a prominent fibrocartilaginous rim around the periphery of certain joints, such as the acetabulum of the hip bone and the glenoid cavity of the scapula; see also *l. acetabuli* and *l. glenoidale.*

l. glenoida′le [TA] glenoid labrum: a ring of fibrocartilage attached to the rim of the glenoid cavity of the scapula, increasing the depth of the cavity; called also *l. glenoidale articulationis humeri.*

l. glenoida′le articulatio′nis cox′ae l. acetabulare.

l. glenoida′le articulatio′nis hu′meri l. glenoidale.

l. ileocaeca′lis os′tii ilea′lis [TA] ileocecal lip of ileal orifice: the inferior of the two lips forming the ileal orifice. Called also *inferior lip of ileal orifice* and *l. inferius ostii ilealis* [TA alternative].

l. ileoco′licum os′tii ilea′lis [TA] ileocolic lip of ileal orifice: the superior of the two lips forming the ileal orifice. Called also *superior lip of ileal orifice* and *l. superius ostii ilealis* [TA alternative].

l. infe′rius os′tii ilea′lis TA alternative for *l. ileocaecalis ostii ilealis.*

l. supe′rius os′tii ilea′lis TA alternative for *l. ileocolicum ostii ilealis.*

La•bur•num (lə-bur′nəm) a genus of ornamental shrubs with yellow flowers, found in Europe and Asia; its flowers, pods, and seeds contain cystine and cause cysticism when eaten. The most common species is *L. anagyroi′des.*

la•bur•num (lə-bur′nəm) 1. any member of the genus *Laburnum.* 2. *Cytisus laburnum.*

lab•y•rinth (lab′ə-rinth) [Gr. *labyrinthos*] 1. labyrinthus (def. 1). 2. auris interna.

bony l. labyrinthus osseus.

cochlear l. labyrinthus cochlearis.

cortical l. labyrinthus corticis.

endolymphatic l. labyrinthus membranaceus.

ethmoid l., ethmoidal l. labyrinthus ethmoidalis.

Ludwig l. pars convoluta lobuli corticalis renis.

membranous l. labyrinthus membranaceus.

olfactory l. labyrinthus ethmoidalis.

osseous l. labyrinthus osseus.

perilymphatic l. spatium perilymphaticum.

vestibular l. labyrinthus vestibularis.

lab•y•rin•thec•to•my (lab″ə-rin-thek′tə-me) [*labyrinth* + *-ectomy*] surgical removal of the internal ear, done for implacable vestibular dysfunction when severe hearing loss is already present.

transcanal l. labyrinthectomy done through the auditory canals, with removal of the ossicles.

transmastoid l. labyrinthectomy done through the mastoid bone.

lab•y•rin•thi (lab″ə-rin′thi) [L.] genitive and plural of *labyrinthus.*

lab•y•rin•thine (lab″ə-rin′thēn) pertaining to a labyrinth.

lab•y•rin•thi•tis (lab″ə-rin-thi′tis) inflammation of the internal ear; it may be accompanied by hearing loss or vertigo. Called also *otitis interna.*

acute serous l. labyrinthitis caused by invasion of the labyrinth by chemical or toxic irritants, usually from the middle ear. Called also *sterile* or *toxic l.*

acute suppurative l. labyrinthitis in which pus enters the labyrinth, usually either through a fistula after infection of the middle ear (tympanogenic labyrinthitis) or through temporal bone erosion from meningitis (meningogenic labyrinthitis). Occasionally it may be the result of septicemia (hematogenic labyrinthitis). It results in severe and often permanent vertigo and hearing loss. Called also *bacterial l.* and *purulent l.*

bacterial l. acute suppurative l.

circumscribed l. acute serous labyrinthitis in a discrete area, due to erosion of the bony wall of a semicircular canal with exposure of the membranous labyrinth. Called also *labyrinthine fistula* and *perilabyrinthitis.*

hematogenic l. acute suppurative labyrinthitis that results from invasion by bacteria from septicemia.

meningogenic l. acute suppurative labyrinthitis that results from invasion of meningitis through an erosion of the temporal bone.

l. ossi′ficans abnormal ossification in the labyrinth after a trauma or an infection with inflammation.

purulent l. acute suppurative l.

sterile l., toxic l. acute serous l.

tympanogenic l. acute suppurative labyrinthitis that results from invasion from the tympanic cavity.

lab•y•rin•thot•o•my (lab″ə-rin-thot′ə-me) [*labyrinth* + Gr. *temnein* to cut] surgical incision into the internal ear.

lab•y•rin•thus (lab″ə-rin′thəs) gen. and pl. *labyrin′thi* [L., from Gr. *labyrinthos*] 1. labyrinth: a system of intercommunicating cavities or canals. 2. auris interna.

l. cochlea′ris [TA] cochlear labyrinth: the part of the membranous labyrinth that includes the perilymphatic space and the cochlear duct.

l. cor′ticis [TA] cortical labyrinth: a network of tubules and blood vessels in the renal cortex.

l. ethmoida′lis [TA] ethmoidal labyrinth: either of the paired lateral masses of the ethmoid bone, consisting of numerous thin-walled cellular cavities, including the ethmoidal cells and the nasal conchae. Called also *ectethmoid, ectethmoid bone, olfactory labyrinth, lateral mass of ethmoid bone*, and *massa lateralis ossis ethmoidalis.*

l. membrana′ceus [TA] the membranous labyrinth: a system of communicating epithelial sacs and ducts, including the endolymphatic duct, cochlear duct, utricle, saccule, and semicircular ducts, lodged within and attached at certain points to the wall of the osseous labyrinth but separated from the major portion of the bony labyrinth by the perilymphatic space, and containing endolymph; it is divided into vestibular and cochlear parts (see *l. vestibularis* and *l. cochlearis*).

l. os′seus [TA] bony labyrinth: a layer of dense bone in the petrous portion of the temporal bone, in which the membranous labyrinth, the vestibular aqueduct, and the cochlear aqueduct are lodged; it consists of three parts: the vestibule, the semicircular canals, and the cochlea. Called also *osseous labyrinth.*

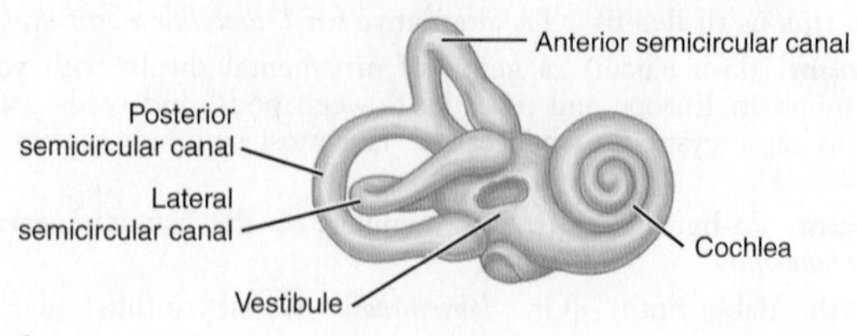

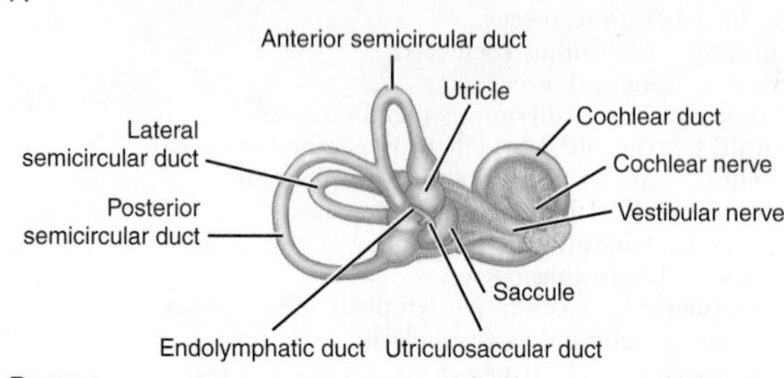

■ Labyrinthus. *(A)*, Anterior view of the labyrinthus osseus (bony labyrinth). *(B)*, Posterior view of the labyrinthus membranaceus (membranous labyrinth), which is contained within the bony labyrinth.

l. vestibula′ris [TA] vestibular labyrinth: the part of the membranous labyrinth that includes the utricle and saccule lodged within the vestibule and the semicircular ducts lodged eccentrically in the corresponding canals.

LAC laparoscopic-assisted colectomy.

lac (lak) gen. *lac′tis* [L.] 1. milk. 2. any milklike medicinal preparation. 3. a resinous material collected from various tropical trees, secreted by an insect, *Laccifer lacca*, and used in the preparation of shellac.

l. femini′num the secretion of the human mammary gland.

l. vacci′num cow's milk.

La•ca•zia (lə-ka′ze-ə) a genus of imperfect fungi of the family Moniliaceae. Formerly called *Loboa.*

L. lo′boi the sole species of the genus; it causes lacaziosis in South America.

la•ca•zi•o•sis (lə-ka′ze-o-sis) an infection seen in tropical areas of South America, caused by *Lacazia loboi*, characterized by red, smooth, hard cutaneous nodules resembling keloids. Called also *Lobo disease* and *lobomycosis.*

Lac•ci•fer (lak′sĭ-fər) a genus of insects of the family Coccidae, order Hemiptera. *L. lac′ca* Kerr (Coccidae) is a source of lac and shellac.

lac•er•a•ble (las′ər-ə-bəl) capable of becoming lacerated.

lac•er•at•ed (las′ər-āt″əd) [L. *lacerare* to tear] torn; mangled; wounded by a jagged instrument.

lac•er•a•tion (las″ər-a′shən) [L. *laceratio*] 1. the act of tearing. 2. a torn, ragged, mangled wound.

la•cer•tus (lə-sur′təs) [L., "lizard," because of a fancied resemblance] a fibrous attachment of a muscle.

l. cor′dis any one of the trabeculae carneae cordis.

l. fibro′sus mus′culi bici′pitis bra′chii TA alternative for *aponeurosis musculi bicipitis brachii.*

l. mus′culi rec′ti latera′lis bul′bi [TA] check ligament of lateral rectus muscle: an extension from the fascia covering the lateral rectus muscle, attaching to the orbital tubercle of the zygomatic bone and limiting the action of the muscle; called also *lateral check ligament.*

Lach•e•sis (lak′ə-sis) [L., from Gr. *Lachesis* one of the three Fates] a genus of venomous pit vipers of the family Crotalidae, found in Central and South America. *L. mu′tus* is the bushmaster or suruçucu.

Lach•no•spi•ra (lak″no-spi′rə) [Gr. *lachnos* woolly hair + Gr. *speira* coil] a genus of gram-negative anaerobic bacteria of the family Bacteroidaceae, made up of curved, rod-shaped cells found in the rumen of cattle. The type species is *L. multipa′ris.*

Lach•no•spi•ra•ceae (lak″no-spi-ra′se-e) a family of bacteria of the order Clostridiales, consisting of gram-negative or weakly gram-positive, anaerobic, motile, curved rods that are isolated from the gastrointestinal tract of mammals. The genera *Butyrivibrio, Lachnospira*, and *Ruminococcus* contain organisms found in the rumens of cattle.

lachry- for words beginning thus, see those beginning *lacri-*.

Lac-Hy•drin (lak-hi′drin) trademark for preparations of ammonium lactate.

la•cis (la′sis) [Fr. "network"] polkissen.

lac•ri•ma (lak′rĭ-mə) pl. *lac′rimae* [L.] see *tears.*

lac•ri•mae (lak′rĭ-me) [L.] plural of *lacrima;* the watery secretion of the lacrimal glands. See *tears.*

lac•ri•mal (lak′rĭ-məl) pertaining to the tears.

lac•ri•ma•tion (lak″rĭ-ma′shən) [L. *lacrimatio*] the secretion and discharge of tears.

lac•ri•ma•tor (lak′rĭ-ma″tər) a substance that increases the flow of tears, such as tear gas.

lac•ri•ma•to•ry (lak′rĭ-mə-tor″e) causing a flow of tears.

lac•ri•mo•na•sal (lak″rĭ-mo-na′zəl) pertaining to the lacrimal sac and the nose.

lac•ri•mo•tome (lak′rĭ-mo-tōm) [*lacrima* + *-tome*] a knife for incising the lacrimal sac or duct.

lac•ri•mot•o•my (lak″rĭ-mot′ə-me) [*lacrima* + *-tomy*] incision of the lacrimal sac or duct.

Lac•ri•sert (lak′rĭ-sert) trademark for a preparation of hydroxypropyl cellulose.

lac•tac•id•emia (lak-tas″ĭ-de′me-ə) excess of lactic acid in the blood; moderate elevations occur during heavy exercise, and severe elevations (lactic acidosis) can occur in diabetes mellitus and in genetic deficiencies of enzymes involved in gluconeogenesis. Called also *lacticacidemia.*

lac•ta•cid•o•gen (lak″tə-sid′o-jən) [*lactic acid* + *-gen*] a term used by Embden to designate the hexose phosphate precursor of lactic acid in muscle contraction.

lac•tac•id•uria (lak-tas″ĭ-du′re-ə) [*lactic acid* + *-uria*] the presence of lactic acid in the urine, as in lactacidemia.

lac•ta•gogue (lak′tə-gog) [*lact-* + *-agogue*] galactagogue.

lac•tal•bu•min (lak″tal-bu′min) any of a group of proteins occurring in milk; the lactalbumins and lactoglobulins constitute the bulk of the proteins in the whey of human milk.

α-l. a milk protein that is a component of lactose synthase; it has no catalytic activity but alters the specificity of the catalytic subunit (glycoprotein 4-β-galactosyltransferase) so that glucose becomes the preferred acceptor substrate and lactose is synthesized.

lac•tam (lak′təm) a cyclic amide formed from aminocarboxylic acids by the elimination of water. They are isomeric with lactims, which are enol forms of lactams.

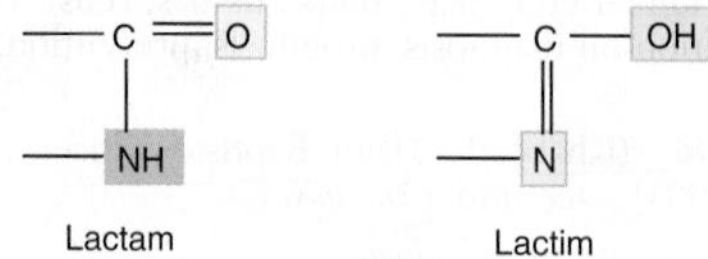

β-l. see under *antibiotic.*

β-lac•ta•mase (lak′tə-mās) [EC 3.5.2.6] any of a group of bacterial enzymes of the hydrolase class, produced by almost all gram-negative species, that catalyze the cleavage of β-lactam rings; such rings occur in penicillins and cephalosporins so that these antibiotics are inactivated by β-lactamases. Individual enzymes are produced by different bacterial species and are called also *penicillinases* or *cephalosporinases* on the basis of their specificities. The enzymes may occur bound to membranes, extracellularly, or in the periplasmic space, may be encoded on the chromosome or on a plasmid, and may be constitutive or inducible.

lac•ta•mide (lak′tə-mīd) the amide of lactic acid.

Lac•ta•ri•us (lak-ta′re-əs) a genus of fungi of the order Agaricales having white spores; it includes both edible and poisonous species. When they are cut or broken, a white or milklike substance is discharged.

lac•tase (lak′tās) 1. a β-galactosidase [EC 3.2.1.23] occurring in the brush border membrane of the intestinal mucosa; together with glycosylceramidase (phlorizin hydrolase), it forms the β-glycosidase complex (q.v.). The enzyme catalyzes the hydrolytic cleavage of lactose to galactose and glucose and also cleaves terminal nonreducing galactose residues from β-glycosides with large hydrophilic aglycons. Reduced or absent enzyme activity (lactase deficiency) may result in symptoms of lactose intolerance. 2. [USP] an official preparation of lactase, derived from the mold *Aspergillus oryzae.*

lac•tase de•fi•cien•cy (lak′tās) the most common disaccharidase deficiency, reduced or absent lactase activity in the intestinal mucosa, usually due to an inherited defect in the enzyme but sometimes secondary to disorders involving the small intestinal mucosa. The hereditary adult form, an autosomal recessive trait, is the normal state in most populations other than white Northern Europeans and may be characterized by abdominal pain, flatulence, and diarrhea after ingestion of milk *(lactose intolerance);* the rare hereditary congenital form *(congenital lactose intolerance)*, an autosomal recessive trait, is characterized by diarrhea, vomiting, and failure to thrive.

lac•tate (lak′tāt) 1. to secrete milk. 2. the anionic form of lactic acid; a salt of lactic acid. For specific salts, see entries under the adjectival form, e.g., for *calcium lactate*, see under *calcium*.

L-lac•tate de•hy•dro•gen•ase (LDH) (lak′tāt de-hi′dro-jən-ās) [EC 1.1.1.27] an enzyme of the oxidoreductase class that catalyzes the reduction of pyruvate to *(S)*-lactate, using NADH as an electron donor. The reaction is the final step in glycolysis (white fibers). The reverse reaction is the first step in the combustion of lactate (heart, red fibers) or its conversion to glucose (liver). The enzyme occurs in the cytoplasm of nearly all cells. It is a tetramer containing M (muscle) and H (heart) subunits; it exists as five distinct isozymes (M_4, M_3H, M_2H_2, MH_3, H_4). Identification of isozyme types in serum is used for clinical diagnosis.

lac•ta•tion (lak-ta′shən) [L. *lactatio*, from *lactare* to suckle] 1. the secretion of milk. 2. the period of secretion of milk.

lac•ta•tion•al (lak-ta′shən-əl) pertaining to lactation.

lac•te•al (lak′te-əl) [L. *lacteus* milky] 1. milky. 2. lactic. 3. any of the intestinal lymphatics that transport chyle; so called because during absorption they are white from absorbed fat. Called also *chyliferous vessel* and *lacteal vessel*.

lac•te•nin (lak′tə-nin) a bacteriostatic substance in milk.

lac•tes•cence (lak-tes′əns) [L. *lactescere* to become milky] resemblance to milk; milkiness.

lac•tic (lak′tik) pertaining to milk; called also *galactic*.

lac•tic ac•id (lak′tik) 1. a metabolic intermediate involved in many biochemical processes; it is the end product of glycolysis, which provides energy anaerobically in skeletal muscle during heavy exercise, and it can be oxidized aerobically in the heart for energy production or can be converted back to glucose (gluconeogenesis). Lactate is also the end product of fermentation in several bacterial species. See also *lacticacidemia*. 2. [USP] a preparation of lactic acid prepared by the lactic fermentation of sugars or prepared synthetically; used as a pharmaceutic necessity.

lac•tic•ac•i•de•mia (lak″tik-as″ĭ-de′me-ə) lactacidemia.

Lac•ti•Care-HC (lak′tĭ-kār″) trademark for preparations of hydrocortisone.

lac•ti•ce•mia (lak″tĭ-se′me-ə) lactacidemia.

lac•tif•er•ous (lak-tif′ər-əs) [L. *lacto-* + *ferre* to bear] 1. conveying milk; called also *galactophorous* and *lactigerous*. 2. galactopoietic.

lac•ti•fuge (lak′tĭ-fūj) [*lact-* + *-fuge*] antigalactic.

lac•tig•e•nous (lak-tij′ə-nəs) [*lacto-* + *-genous*] galactopoietic.

lac•tig•er•ous (lak-tij′ər-əs) [L. *lac* milk + *gerere* to carry] lactiferous.

lac•tim (lak′tim) the enol form of a lactam (q.v.).

lac•ti•nat•ed (lak′tĭ-nāt″əd) prepared with lactose.

Lac•ti•nol (lak′tĭ-nol) trademark for preparations of lactic acid.

lac•ti•tol (lak′tĭ-tol) [NF] a disaccharide analogue of lactulose having an intense sweet taste and used as a bulk sweetener; it also has laxative properties and is used in the management of constipation.

lac•tiv•o•rous (lak-tiv′ə-rəs) [*lact-* + L. *vorare* to devour] feeding or subsisting upon milk.

lact(o)- [L. *lac*, gen. *lactis* milk] a combining form denoting relationship to milk or to lactic acid.

Lac•to•bac•il•la•ceae (lak″to-bas″ĭ-la′se-e) a family of bacteria of the order Lactobacillales, consisting of gram-positive, asporogenous, straight or curved rods occurring singly or in chains. Medically important organisms are contained in the genus *Lactobacillus*.

Lac•to•ba•cil•la•les (lak″to-bas-ĭ-la′lēz) an order of lactic acid–producing bacteria of the class Bacilli; organisms are non–spore-forming, generally nonmotile, and ferment sugars to produce energy. Medically important organisms are included in the families Aerococcaceae, Enterococcaceae, Lactobacillaceae, Leuconostocaceae, and Streptococcaceae.

lac•to•bac•il•li (lak″to-bə-sil′i) [L.] plural of *lactobacillus*.

Lac•to•bac•il•lus (lak″to-bə-sil′əs) [*lacto-* + L. *bacillus* small rod] a genus of bacteria of the family Lactobacillaceae, occurring as large, gram-positive, asporogenous, rod-shaped organisms. They are anaerobic or microaerophilic and occur widely in nature and in the human mouth, vagina, and intestinal tract. In the oral cavity, they are found associated with dental caries but have no known etiologic role. They are separable into two groups, the homofermentative group producing only lactic acid, and the heterofermentative group producing other end products of fermentation.

L. acido′philus a homofermentative lactobacillus producing the fermented product, acidophilus milk; *L. acidophilus* preparations are available for oral consumption as a digestive aid, for the production of B-complex vitamins, and to help prevent infections after antibiotic treatment.

lac•to•bac•il•lus (lak″to-bə-sil′əs) pl. *lactobacil′li*. An organism of the genus *Lactobacillus*.

lac•to•be•zoar (lak″to-be′zor) a concretion in the stomach or intestine consisting of undigested remnants of milk.

lac•to•cele (lak′to-sēl) galactocele.

Lac•to•coc•cus (lak″to-kok′əs) a genus of bacteria of the family Streptococcaceae, found in dairy products and sometimes in opportunistic infections.

L. lac′tis a species with subspecies that ferment milk to specific cheeses and other products. *L. lactis* subsp. *garvi′eae* has been associated with infective endocarditis and skin lesions in humans and nonfatal conditions in other animals.

lac•to•crit (lak′to-krit) [*lacto-* + Gr. *kritēs* judge] an instrument for estimating the amount of fat in milk.

lac•to•den•sim•e•ter (lak″to-den-sim′ə-tər) lactometer.

lac•to•fer•rin (lak′to-fer″in) an iron-binding protein found in the specific granules of neutrophils, where it apparently exerts an antimicrobial activity by withholding iron from ingested bacteria and fungi; it also occurs in many secretions and exudates, such as milk, tears, mucus, saliva, and bile.

lac•to•gen (lak′to-jən) [*lacto-* + *-gen*] any substance that enhances milk production, the principal one being prolactin.

human placental l. (hPL) a polypeptide hormone secreted by the placenta that enters the maternal circulation and disappears from the circulation immediately after delivery. It has growth-promoting activity, is immunologically similar to growth hormone, and inhibits maternal insulin activity during pregnancy. By inhibiting glucose oxidation it can increase the glucose supply to a fetus developing in a malnourished mother. Called also *choriomammotropin*, *chorionic somatomammotropin*, and *placental growth hormone*.

lac•to•gen•e•sis (lak′to-jen′ə-sis) galactopoiesis. **lactogen′ic** *adj*

lac•to•glob•u•lin (lak″to-glob′u-lin) a globulin occurring in milk.

lac•tom•e•ter (lak-tom′ə-tər) [*lacto-* + *meter*] an instrument for ascertaining the specific gravity of milk.

lac•tone (lak′tōn) a cyclic organic compound in which the chain is closed by ester formation between a carboxyl and a hydroxyl group in the same molecule.

lac•to-ovo•ve•ge•ta•ri•an (lak″to-o″vo-vej″ə-tar′e-ən) ovolactovegetarian.

lac•to•pro•tein (lak″to-pro′tēn) a protein derived from milk.

lac•tor•rhea (lak″to-re′ə) galactorrhea.

lac•to•scope (lak′to-skōp) [*lacto-* + *-scope*] a device showing the proportion of cream in milk.

lac•tose (lak′tōs) [L. *lac*, gen. *lactis* milk] a reducing disaccharide occurring as the D-isomer, in both α- and β-configurations, as a major constituent of mammalian milk; on hydrolysis by acids or intestinal lactase, it forms one residue each of galactose and glucose. Cf. *lactose intolerance*, under *intolerance*. Lactose is used as a tablet and capsule diluent, a powder bulking agent, in infant feeding formulas, and as a nutritional supplement.

anhydrous l. [NF] lactose without water of hydration, which may be primarily β-lactose or a mixture of α-lactose and β-lactose.

β-l. anhydrous D-lactose in the β-1 configuration, prepared by crystallizing a heated solution of lactose; sometimes used in pharmaceutical preparations because it is sweeter and more soluble in this configuration.

l. monohydrate [NF] a natural disaccharide obtained from milk and consisting of one glucose and one galactose moiety; it is monohydrated α-lactose.

lac•tose syn•thase (lak′tōs sin′thās) [EC 2.4.1.22] an enzyme of the transferase class that catalyzes the transfer of galactose from UDP-galactose to glucose, forming lactose. The enzyme is a complex of the enzyme glycoprotein 4-β-galactosyltransferase (q.v.) and α-lactalbumin; the latter protein is present in lactating mammary gland cells, where it alters the usual specificity of the former to make lactose synthesis the preferred reaction.

lac•to•side (lak′to-sīd) a glycoside whose sugar constituent is lactose.

lac•tos•uria (lak″to-su′re-ə) elevated levels of lactose, as seen in lactose intolerance or during lactation.

lac•to•syl•cer•a•mide (lak-to″səl-ser′ə-mīd) any of the glycosphingolipids in which the head group on the ceramide is lactose; they occur at low concentrations in all tissues.

lac•to•tox•in (lak′to-tok″sin) a toxic substance formed in milk.

lac•to•trope (lak′to-trōp) lactotroph.

lac•to•troph (lak′to-trōf) an acidophil of the adenohypophysis that stains with an affinity for azocarmine and erythrosin and secretes prolactin. Called also *lactotrope*, *mammatroph*, *mammotroph*, *epsilon acidophil*, *prolactin cell*, and *lactotroph* or *lactotropic cell*.

lac•to•tro•phin (lak′to-tro″fin) prolactin.

lac•to•tro•pin (lak′to-tro″pin) prolactin.

lac•to•veg•e•tar•i•an (lak″to-vej″ə-tar′e-ən) 1. one who practices lactovegetarianism. 2. pertaining to lactovegetarianism.

lac•to•veg•e•tar•i•an•ism (lak″to-vej″ə-tar′e-ən-iz″əm) restriction of the diet to vegetables and dairy products, eschewing other foods of animal origin.

lac•to•yl (lak′to-əl) the radical of lactic acid; $CH_3CH(OH)CO$.

lac•to•yl•glu•ta•thi•one (lak″to-əl-gloo″tə-thi′ōn) glutathione linked to lactic acid; it is an intermediate formed in the conversion of methylglyoxal to lactic acid by glyoxalase.

lac•to•yl•glu•ta•thi•one ly•ase (lak″to-əl-gloo″tə-thi′ōn li′ās) [EC 4.4.1.5] an enzyme of the lyase class that catalyzes the condensation of methylglyoxal and glutathione to form lactoylglutathione as a step in the conversion of methylglyoxal to lactic acid. See also *glyoxalase*.

lac•tu•lose (lak′tu-lōs) a synthetic disaccharide used as a cathartic and to enhance excretion or formation of ammonia in the treatment of portosystemic encephalopathy, including the stages of hepatic precoma and coma.

la•cu•na (lə-ku′nə) gen. and pl. *lacu′nae* [L.] 1. a small pit or hollow cavity, such as one within or between other body structures. 2. a defect or gap, as in the field of vision (scotoma). **lacu′nar** *adj*

absorption l. resorption l.

Blessig lacunae see under *cyst*.

blood l. any one of the blood-filled spaces in the syncytiotrophoblast of the embryo that serve hemotrophic nutrition.

bone l. a small cavity within the bone matrix containing an osteocyte and from which slender canaliculi radiate and penetrate the adjacent lamellae to anastomose with the canaliculi of neighboring lacunae, thus forming a system of cavities interconnected by minute canals. Called also *osseous l.*

cartilage l. any of the small cavities within the cartilage matrix, containing a chondrocyte, or cartilage cell.

cerebral lacunae small areas of cerebral ischemic infarction resulting from occlusion of deep, small end-arterial branches of the middle cerebral, posterior cerebral, and basilar arteries; seen in association with hypertension and arteriosclerosis.

great l. of urethra lacuna magna.

Howship l. resorption l.

intervillous l. one of the blood spaces of the placenta in which the fetal villi are found; called also *trophoblastic l.*

lacu′nae latera′les [TA] lateral lacunae: venous meshworks within the dura mater on either side of, and continuous with, the superior sagittal sinus; arachnoidal granulations project into them. Called also *parasinusoidal lacunae*, *parasinoidal sinuses*, or *spaces*.

l. mag′na great lacuna of urethra: the largest of the urethral lacunae of the male urethra, located on the roof of the fossa navicularis urethrae.

lacunae of Morgagni lacunae urethrales urethrae masculinae.

l. of muscles, muscular l., l. musculo′rum retroinguina′lis [TA] a compartment beneath the inguinal ligament for the passage of the iliopsoas muscle and femoral nerve, separated from the lacuna vasorum by the iliopectineal arch. Called also *muscular compartment* and *iliac canal*.

osseous l. bone l.

parasinusoidal lacunae lacunae laterales.

l. pharyn′gis a depression at the pharyngeal end of the auditory tube.

resorption l. a pit or concavity found in bones undergoing resorption, frequently containing osteoclasts. Similar lacunae also may be found in eroding surfaces of cementum, in which cementoclasts may or may not be located. Called also *absorption l.* and *Howship l.*

trophoblastic l. intervillous l.

lacunae of urethra, urethral lacunae see *lacunae urethrales urethrae femininae* and *lacunae urethrales urethrae masculinae*.

urethral lacunae of female urethra lacunae urethrales urethrae femininae.

urethral lacunae of male urethra, urethral lacunae of Morgagni lacunae urethrales urethrae masculinae.

lacu′nae urethra′les ure′thrae femini′nae [TA] urethral lacunae of female urethra: small depressions or pits in the mucous membrane of the urethra, with their openings usually directed distally; some are openings of ducts of the urethral glands.

lacu′nae urethra′les ure′thrae masculi′nae [TA] urethral lacunae of male urethra: small depressions or pits in the mucous membrane of the urethra, with their openings usually directed distally; some are openings of ducts of the urethral glands. The largest one, at the distal end, is the lacuna magna. Called also *lacunae of Morgagni* and *urethral lacunae of Morgagni*.

vascular l., l. vaso′rum retroinguina′lis [TA] a space for the passage of the femoral vessels into the thigh, separated from the lacuna musculorum by the iliopectineal arch. Called also *vascular compartment*.

la•cu•nae (lə-ku′ne) [L.] genitive and plural of *lacuna*.

la•cune (lə-kūn′) 1. lacuna. 2. lacunar infarct.

la•cu•nule (lə-ku′nūl) [L. *lacunula*] a small lacuna.

la•cus (la′kəs) pl. *la′cus* [L.] lake.

l. lacrima′lis [TA] lacrimal lake: the triangular space at the medial angle of the eye, where the tears collect; called also *lacrimal bay* and *lake*.

LAD 1. left anterior descending (coronary artery); see *ramus interventricularis anterior arteriae coronariae sinistrae*. 2. left axis deviation; leukocyte adhesion deficiency.

Ladd bands, procedure, syndrome (lad) [William Edwards *Ladd*, American physician, 1880–1967] see under *band*, *procedure*, and *syndrome*.

Ladd-Frank•lin's theory (lad′-frangk′linz) [Christine *Ladd-Franklin*, American physician, 1847–1930] see under *theory*.

lad•der•gram (lad′ər-gram″) ladder diagram.

LAE left atrial enlargement; see *atrial enlargement*, under *enlargement*.

lae- for words beginning thus, see also those beginning *le-*.

Lae•laps (le′laps) *Echinolaelaps*.

La•ën•nec cirrhosis, pearls (lah″ĕ-nek′) [René Théophile Hyacinthe *Laënnec*, French physician and inventor of the stethoscope, 1781–1826] see under *cirrhosis* and *pearl*.

La•e•trile (la′ə-tril) trademark for *l*-mandelonitrile-β-glucuronic acid, a semisynthetic derivative of amygdalin; it is alleged to have antineoplastic properties. Cf. *laetrile*.

la•e•trile (la′ə-tril) [*lae*vorotatory + mandeloni*trile*] amygdalin (*l*-mandelonitrile-β-gentiobioside) derived from crushed pits of certain

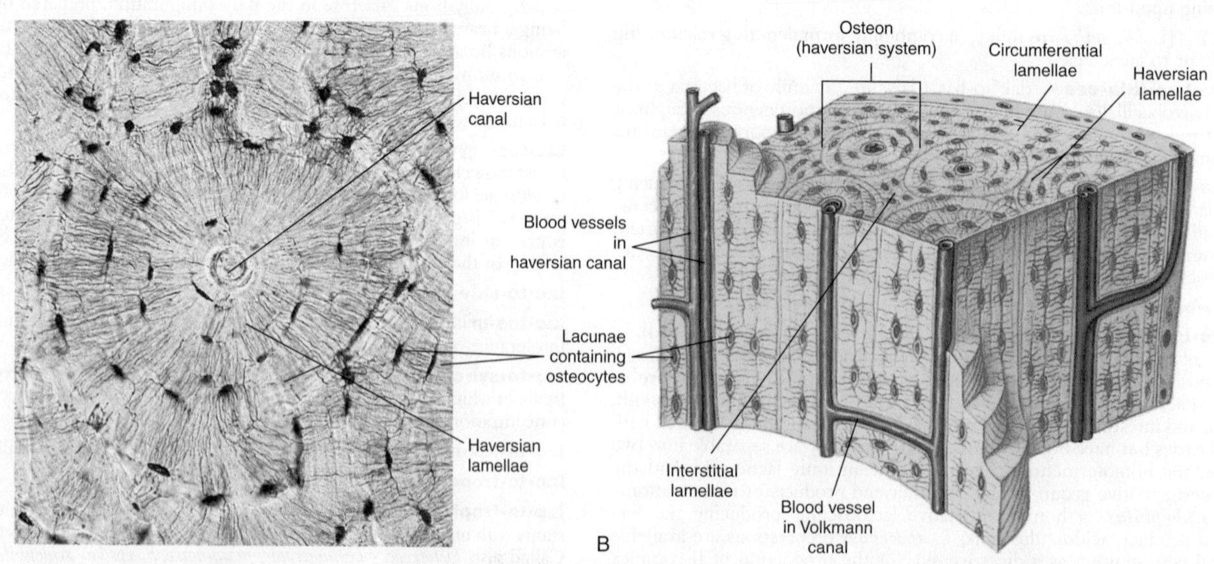

■ Bone lacunae in the shaft of a long bone. *(A)*, Cross section showing an osteon. *(B)*, Diagram of a longitudinal section.

fruits, usually apricots, and alleged to have antineoplastic properties. Cf. *Laetrile.*

lae•ve (le′və) [L. *levis* smooth] nonvillous, as the *chorion laeve.*

laev(o)- for words beginning thus, see those beginning *lev(o)-.*

La•fo•ra bodies, disease (myoclonic epilepsy), sign (lah-fo′rah) [Gonzalo Rodríguez *Lafora,* Spanish neurologist, 1887–1971] see under *body, disease,* and *sign.*

Lag. [L.] lage′na (a flask).

lag (lag) 1. the period of time elapsing between the application of a stimulus and the resulting reaction. 2. see *lag phase,* under *phase.*

l. of accommodation the extent to which the eyes fail to focus accurately.

anaphase l. delayed movement during anaphase of one homologous chromosome in mitosis or of one chromatid in meiosis, so that the chromosome is not incorporated into the nucleus of one of the daughter cells; the result is one normal cell and one cell with monosomy.

extensor l. the amount of drooping at a weakened joint that can extend only passively, no longer actively.

jet l. a condition of desynchrony with disruption of the normal circadian rhythm, caused by rapid travel across several time zones; it is characterized by fatigue, insomnia, and disturbances in body function, and lasts for several days.

lid l. Graefe sign.

nitrogen l. the time that elapses after the administration of a protein before there appears in the urine an amount of nitrogen equivalent to that administered.

la•ge•na (lə-je′nə) [L. "flask"] 1. a part of the upper extremity of the ductus cochlearis. 2. the curved, flask-shaped organ of hearing in vertebrates lower than mammals.

la•gen•i•form (lə-jen′ĭ-form) [*lagena* + *form*] flask-shaped.

Lag•o•chi•las•ca•ris mi•nor (lag″o-kĭ-la′kə-ris mi′nər) a species of parasitic nematodes found in subcutaneous abscesses in Trinidad and Surinam.

lag•o•morph (lag′ə-morf) any mammal of the order Lagomorpha.

Lag•o•mor•pha (lag″ə-mor′fə) [Gr. *lagōs* hare + *-morph*] an order of small mammals having large chisel-shaped incisors, large hind feet, and long ears, including the rabbits, hares, and picas.

lag•oph•thal•mos (lag″of-thal′məs) [Gr. *lagōs* hare + *ophthalmos* eye] a condition in which the eye cannot be completely closed.

lag•oph•thal•mus (lag″of-thal′məs) lagophthalmos.

La•go•vi•rus (la′go-vi″rəs) [Gr. *lagōs* hare + *virus*] a genus of viruses of the family Caliciviridae comprising a wide range of animal pathogens, including rabbit hemorrhagic disease virus, the type species.

La•grange operation (lah-grahzh′) [Pierre Félix *Lagrange,* French ophthalmologist, 1857–1928] sclerectoiridectomy.

LAH left anterior hemiblock; see *hemiblock.*

lai•ose (li′ōs) a pale yellow substance, found in the urine in diabetes mellitus; it is nonfermentable and levorotatory.

LAIV live, attenuated influenza vaccine; see *influenza virus vaccine* (def. 2), under *vaccine.*

lake (lāk) [L. *lacus*] 1. to undergo separation of hemoglobin from the erythrocytes, a phenomenon sometimes occurring in blood. 2. a circumscribed collection of fluid in a hollow or depressed area.

lacrimal l. lacus lacrimalis.

subchorial l. the portion of the placenta, relatively free of villi, just beneath the chorionic plate; at the edge of the placenta it becomes continuous with irregular channels to form the marginal lakes. Called also *subchorial space.*

venous l. a small, blue to purple, sessile, compressible papule or bleb, seen most often on the lips, ears, and face of elderly persons; histologically, they represent dilated capillaries filled with red blood cells and lined with flattened endothelial cells.

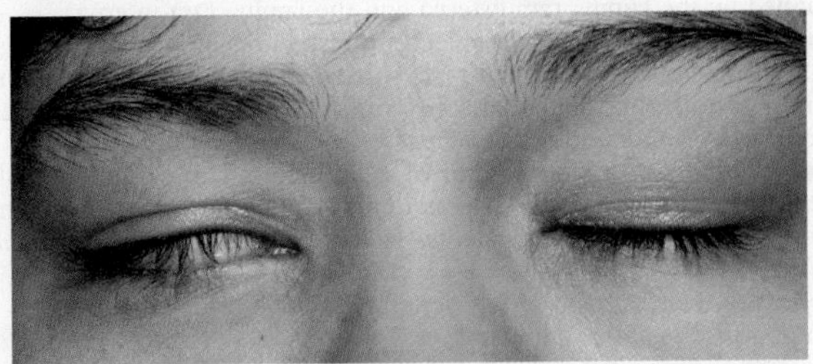

■ Lagophthalmos.

lal•la•tion (lə-la′shən) [L. *lallare* to sing a lullaby] a language disorder consisting of babbling, infantile speech.

Lal•le•mand bodies (lahl-ə-mah′) [Claude François *Lallemand,* French surgeon, 1790–1854] Bence Jones cylinders.

lal(o)- [Gr. *lalein* to babble, speak] a combining form denoting relationship to speech.

lal•og•no•sis (lal″og-no′sis) [*lalo-* + Gr. *gnōsis* knowledge] the understanding of speech.

la•lop•a•thy (lə-lop′ə-the) speech disorder.

lalo•pho•bia (lal″ə-fo′be-ə) irrational fear of speaking.

lal•or•rhea (lal″ə-re′ə) logorrhea.

La•lou•ette pyramid (lah-loo-et′) [Pierre *Lalouette,* French physician, 1711–1792] see under *pyramid.*

LAM lymphangiomyomatosis.

La•marck's theory (lah-mahrks′) [Jean Baptiste Pierre Antoine Monet de *Lamarck,* French naturalist, 1744–1829] see under *theory.*

La•maze method (lə-mahz′) [Fernand *Lamaze,* French obstetrician, 1890–1957] see under *method.*

lamb•da (lam′də) [the eleventh letter of the Greek alphabet, Λ or λ] [TA] the point at the site of the posterior fontanel where the lambdoid and sagittal sutures meet; used as a craniometric landmark.

lamb•da•cism (lam′də-siz-əm) [Gr. *lambdakismos*] 1. a speech disorder consisting of the substitution of *l* for *r.* 2. a speech disorder involving faulty pronunciation of *l.* Called also *paralambdacism.*

lamb•doid (lam′doid) [Gr. *lambda* + *-oid*] shaped like the Greek letter Λ or λ.

Lam•bert's cosine law (lahm′bərts) [Johann Heinrich *Lambert,* German mathematician and physicist, 1728–1777] see under *law.*

Lam•bert-Ea•ton syndrome (myasthenic syndrome) (lam′bərt e′ton) [Edward Howard *Lambert,* American physiologist, 1915–2003; Lealdes McKendree *Eaton,* American neurologist, 1905–1958] see under *syndrome.*

lam•bert (L) (lam′bərt) [J. H. *Lambert*] a unit of luminance, being the luminous intensity of a perfect diffuser emitting one lumen per square centimeter. The unit generally used is one thousandth of this and is called a *millilambert.*

Lam•blia (lam′ble-ə) former name for *Giardia. L. intestina′lis* is a former name for *Giardia lamblia.*

lam•bli•a•sis (lam-bli′ə-sis) giardiasis.

lame (lām) incapable of normal locomotion; deviating from the normal gait. See also *claudication.*

lam•el (lam′əl) lamella (def. 2).

la•mel•la (lə-mel′ə) gen. and pl. *lamel′lae* [L., dim. of *lamina*] 1. a thin leaf or plate, as of bone. 2. a medicated disk or wafer prepared from gelatin, glycerin, and distilled water, and containing a small quantity of an alkaloid, to be inserted under the eyelid. 3. gill (def. 2).

annulate lamellae cytoplasmic organelles of uncertain function, consisting of parallel arrays of cisternae that contain nuclear pore complexes at regular intervals along their length; seen in differentiating and rapidly growing cells, such as oocytes and early embryonic cells of certain species and neoplastic cells.

articular l. the layer of bone to which an articular cartilage is attached.

basic l. circumferential l.

circumferential l. one of the layers of bone that underlie the periosteum *(external circumferential l.)* and endosteum *(internal circumferential l.);* called also *basic l.*

concentric l. haversian l.

cornoid l. a thick column of parakeratotic cells extending outward from a notch in the stratum germinativum of the epidermis, forming the raised border of a lesion of porokeratosis.

enamel lamellae imperfectly calcified areas of enamel located generally in the cervical enamel but also found in the interdigitating surface of the premolars and molars; they are foliaceous structures visible only under the microscope and may extend from the surface to the dentinoenamel junctions and beyond.

endosteal l. one of the bony plates lying beneath the endosteum.

ground l. interstitial l.

haversian l. one of the concentric bony plates surrounding a haversian canal.

intermediate l. interstitial l.

interstitial l. one of the bony plates that fill in between the haversian systems; called also *ground l.* or *intermediate l.*

osseous l. any one of the thin plates into which bone can be divided.

periosteal l., peripheral l. the layer of bone lying next to the periosteum.

posterior border l. of Fuchs the fibrillar layer of the dilator muscle of the iris; called also *Henle membrane.*

triangular l. tela choroidea ventriculi tertii.

la·mel·lae (lə-mel′e) [L.] genitive and plural of *lamella.*

la·mel·lar (lə-mel′ər) 1. pertaining to or resembling lamellae. 2. lamellated (def. 1).

lam·el·lat·ed (lam′ə-lāt″əd) 1. having, composed of, or arranged in lamellae. 2. lamelliform.

la·mel·li·form (lə-mel′ĭ-form) resembling lamellae.

la·mel·li·po·dia (lə-mel″ĭ-po′de-ə) sing. *lamellipo′dium* [*lamella* + *pod-* + *-ia*] delicate sheetlike extensions, composed of cross-linked actin filaments, that form transient adhesions with the cell substrate and wave gently, enabling the cell to move along the substrate.

la·mel·li·po·di·um (lə-mel″ĭ-po′de-əm) singular of *lamellipodia.*

lame·ness (lām′nis) the condition of being lame; see also *gait.*

fescue l., tall fescue l. fescue foot.

La·mic·tal (lə-mik′tahl) trademark for a preparation of lamotrigine.

lam·in (lam′in) any of a group of intermediate filaments that enmesh to form the nuclear lamina. They are structurally similar to keratin filaments. In mammals, three have been described, A–C, with A and C encoded by the same region (*LMNA* gene) and having close sequence homology, but generated by alternative splicing. Mutations affecting *LMNA* have been linked to various disorders, including Emery-Dreifuss muscular dystrophy, limb-girdle muscular dystrophy, dilated cardiomyopathy, familial partial lipodystophy, and progeria.

lam·i·na (lam′ĭ-nə) gen. and pl. *la′minae* [L.] [TA] layer: a thin flat plate or stratum of a composite structure. The term is often used alone to mean the lamina arcus vertebrae.

Lamina

Descriptions of anatomic structures are given on TA terms and include anglicized names of specific layers.

accessory medullary l. of corpus striatum l. medullaris accessoria corporis striati.

l. affix′a [TA] the narrow strip of ependyma overlying the thalamostriate vein and stria terminalis in the central part of the lateral ventricle.

l. ala′ris alar lamina: either of the pair of longitudinal zones of the embryonic neural tube dorsal to the sulcus limitans, from which are developed the dorsal gray columns of the spinal cord and the sensory centers of the brain; called also *alar plate.*

la′minae al′bae cerebel′li white laminae of the cerebellum: the core of white substance that supports a folium of the cerebellar cortex.

l. ante′rior fas′ciae thoracolumba′lis [TA] anterior layer of thoracolumbar fascia: the deepest of the three layers of fascia covering the deep muscles of the lumbosacral region; it is attached below to the iliolumbar ligament and adjoining iliac crest and medially to the transverse processes of the lumbar vertebrae, and above it forms the lateral arcuate ligament. It covers quadratus lumborum and is the origin of transversus abdominis. Called also *l. profunda fasciae thoracolumbalis* [TA alternative], *fascia musculi quadrati lumborum* [TA alternative], and *quadratus lumborum fascia.*

l. ante′rior vagi′nae mus′culi rec′ti abdo′minis [TA] anterior layer of sheath of rectus abdominis muscle: the portion of the muscle sheath lying anterior to the rectus abdominis muscle, formed by aponeuroses of the internal and external oblique muscles superior to the arcuate line and by the aponeuroses of the external oblique, internal oblique, and transversus abdominis muscles inferior to the arcuate line.

l. ar′cus ver′tebrae [TA] lamina of vertebral arch: either of the pair of broad plates of bone flaring out from the pedicles of the vertebral arches and fusing together at the midline to complete the dorsal part of the arch and provide a base for the spinous process.

basal l. 1. the layer of the basement membrane lying next to the basal surface of the adjoining cell layer, composed of an electron-dense lamina densa and an electron-lucent lamina lucida; sometimes used to denote the lamina densa alone. Cf. *reticular l.* 2. basement membrane. 3. l. basalis (def. 1).

basal l. of choroid l. basalis choroideae.

basal l. of ciliary body l. basalis corporis ciliaris.

basal l. of cochlear duct l. basilaris ductus cochlearis.

■ Lamina arcus vertebrae.

l. basa′lis 1. basal lamina: either of the pair of longitudinal zones of the embryonic neural tube ventral to the sulcus limitans, from which are developed the ventral gray columns of the spinal cord and the motor centers of the brain; called also *basal plate.* 2. basal l. (def. 1).

l. basa′lis choroi′deae [TA] basal lamina of choroid: the transparent inner layer of the choroid, which is in contact with the pigmented layer of the retina. Called also *Bruch layer* or *membrane* and *vitreal* or *vitreous lamina.*

l. basa′lis cor′poris cilia′ris [TA] basal lamina of ciliary body: the innermost layer of the ciliary body, continuous with the basal lamina of the choroid.

l. basila′ris duc′tus cochlea′ris [TA] basal lamina of cochlear duct: the wall of the cochlear duct, which separates it from the scala tympani; the spiral organ lies against it.

bony spiral l. l. spiralis ossea.

Bowman l. l. limitans anterior corneae.

capillary l. of choroid l. choroidocapillaris.

l. cartila′ginis cricoi′deae [TA] lamina of cricoid cartilage: the broad posterior part of the cricoid cartilage.

l. cartila′ginis thyroi′deae dex′tra/sinis′tra [TA] lamina of thyroid cartilage: either of the broad plates that form the right and left sides of the cartilage, converging anteriorly to meet at the midline.

l. choriocapilla′ris l. choroidocapillaris.

l. choroidocapilla′ris [TA] choriocapillary layer: the inner layer of the choroid, composed of a single-layered network of small capillaries.

la′minae cor′ticis ce′rebri layers of cerebral cortex.

- l. I l. molecularis.
- l. II l. granularis externa.
- l. III l. pyramidalis externa.
- l. IV l. granularis interna.
- l. V l. pyramidalis interna.
- l. VI l. multiformis.

l. cribro′sa os′sis ethmoida′lis [TA] cribriform plate of ethmoid bone: the horizontal plate of the ethmoid bone that forms the roof of the nasal cavity; it is perforated by many foramina (foramina cribrosa ossis ethmoidalis) for the passage of the olfactory nerves. On its superior surface is a projection called the crista galli.

l. cribro′sa scle′rae [TA] the perforated portion of the sclera through which pass the axons of the ganglion cells of the retina.

l. of cricoid cartilage l. cartilaginis cricoideae.

l. den′sa an electron-dense layer of the basal lamina, consisting mainly of Type IV collagen fibrils and heparan sulfate; it closely follows the plasma membrane of the basal aspect of the adjacent cell layer, from which it is separated by the lamina lucida. In renal glomeruli and pulmonary alveoli, it is bounded by the lamina rara externa and the lamina rara interna.

dental l. a horizontal band projecting perpendicularly from the vestibular lamina and extending into the substance of the embryonic gum, assuming a horseshoe-like shape to conform with the dental arches. Called also *l. dentalis* and *dentogingival l.*

dental l., lateral a lateral band of cells believed to be functionally and structurally similar to the parent dental lamina, which connects the developing tooth germ to the dental lamina. Called also *lateral enamel strand.*

l. denta′lis, dentogingival l. dental l.

l. du′ra see *bundle bone,* under *bone.*

elastic l., external see under *membrane.*
elastic l., internal see under *membrane.*
l. epiphysia′lis [TA] epiphyseal disk: the disk or plate of cartilage interposed between the epiphysis and the shaft of the bone during the period of growth; by its growth the bone increases in length. Called also *epiphyseal plate* and *growth disk* or *plate.*
l. episclera′lis [TA] episcleral lamina: loose connective and elastic tissue covering the sclera and anteriorly connecting it with the conjunctiva. Called also *episcleral layer.*
l. epithelia′lis epithelial lamina: the layer of ependymal cells covering the choroid plexus.
l. exter′na calva′riae [TA] external table of calvaria: the outer compact layer of bone of the flat bones of the skull. Called also *outer table of calvaria.*
l. fibroreticula′ris reticular l. (def. 1).
l. fibro′sa a fibrous layer, as occurs in the cusps of the semilunar valves.
l. fus′ca scle′rae [TA] suprachoroid lamina: a thin layer of loose, pigmented connective tissue on the inner surface of the sclera, connecting it with the choroid; from the point of view of the choroid it is called the *lamina suprachoroidea.*
l. granula′ris exter′na [TA] external granular layer: layer II of the cerebral cortex, composed of many small pyramidal cells and granule cells with short axons.
l. granula′ris inter′na [TA] internal granular layer: layer IV of the cerebral cortex, composed of many densely packed granule cells with short axons and some small pyramidal cells, and traversed by a stria of horizontally arranged fibers (external or outer band or line of Baillarger); it contains neurites derived from cells of other layers and areas of the cerebral cortex and subcortical areas.
l. horizonta′lis os′sis palati′ni [TA] horizontal plate of palatine bone: the horizontal part of the palatine bone, forming the posterior part of the hard palate.
l. inter′na calva′riae [TA] internal table of calvaria: the inner compact layer of bone of the flat bones of the skull. Called also *inner table of calvaria.*
labial l. the ectodermal plate that on splitting separates lip from gum, thus forming the labial groove.
labiodental l. the thickened ectodermal band from which the dental and labial laminae develop.
labiogingival l. labial l.
lateral l. of cartilage of auditory tube, l. latera′lis cartila′ginis tu′bae auditi′vae [TA] the smaller of the two laminae that compose the tubal cartilage; it lies in the lateral wall of the auditory tube.
l. latera′lis proces′sus pterygoi′dei [TA] lateral pterygoid plate: either of a pair of bony plates projecting downward from the roots of the greater wings of the sphenoid bone and forming the medial wall of the ipsilateral infratemporal fossa.
left l. of thyroid cartilage see *l. cartilaginis thyroideae dextra/sinistra.*
l. li′mitans ante′rior cor′neae [TA] anterior limiting lamina: a thin layer of the cornea beneath the outer layer of stratified epithelium, composed of condensed stroma, between it and the substantia propria; called also *Bowman layer* or *membrane.*
l. li′mitans poste′rior cor′neae [TA] posterior limiting lamina: a thin hyaline membrane between the substantia propria and the endothelial layer of the cornea.
limiting l., anterior l. limitans anterior corneae.
limiting l., posterior l. limitans posterior corneae.
l. lu′cida an electron-lucent layer of the basal lamina, composed of laminin, fibronectin, and proteoglycans and lying between the lamina densa and the adjoining cell layer; in the pulmonary alveoli and renal glomeruli, the lamina lucida is split and found on either side of the lamina densa, and called the lamina rara interna and lamina rara externa.
l. me′dia fas′ciae thoracolumba′lis [TA] middle layer of thoracolumbar fascia: the middle of three layers of fascia covering the deep muscles in the lumbosacral region. It is attached above to the twelfth rib and lumbocostal ligament, medially to the transverse processes of the lumbar vertebrae and the intertransverse ligaments, and below to the iliac crest; gives origin to transversus abdominis; and helps to enclose erector spinae.
medial l. of cartilage of auditory tube, l. media′lis cartila′ginis tu′bae auditi′vae [TA] the larger of the two laminae that compose the tubal cartilage; it lies in the medial wall of the auditory tube.
l. media′lis proces′sus pterygoi′dei [TA] medial pterygoid plate: either of a pair of bony plates projecting inferiorly from the roots of the greater wings of the sphenoid bone and forming the lateral boundary of the ipsilateral posterior aperture of the nasal cavity and the most posterior part of the lateral wall of the nasal cavity.
l. medul′laris accesso′ria cor′poris stria′ti [TA] accessory medullary lamina of corpus striatum: a small layer of fibers subdividing the medial segment of the globus pallidus into lateral and medial parts.
l. medul′laris exter′na cor′poris stria′ti TA alternative for *l. medullaris lateralis corporis striati.*
l. medulla′ris inter′na cor′poris stria′ti TA alternative for *l. medullaris medialis corporis striati.*
l. medulla′ris latera′lis cor′poris stria′ti [TA] lateral medullary lamina of corpus striatum: a layer of white substance that separates the lateral globus pallidus from the putamen; called also *external medullary l. of corpus striatum* and *l. medullaris externa corporis striati* [TA alternative].
l. medulla′ris latera′lis tha′lami [TA] external medullary lamina of thalamus: one of two layers of myelinated nerve fibers in the dorsal thalami; it covers the lateral surface of the dorsal thalamus and is separated from the internal capsule by the thalamic reticular nucleus.
l. medulla′ris media′lis cor′poris stria′ti [TA] medial medullary lamina of corpus striatum: a layer of white substance that divides the medial portion of the lentiform nucleus (globus pallidus) into a larger, lateral, and a smaller, medial part; called also *internal medullary l. of corpus striatum* and *l. medullaris interna corporis striati* [TA alternative].
l. medulla′ris media′lis tha′lami [TA] internal medullary lamina of thalamus: one of two layers of myelinated nerve fibers in the dorsal thalami; it is a vertical sheet of white substance which partially splits anterosuperiorly and separates the medial and lateral nuclei. It contains the intralaminar nuclei.
medullary l. of corpus striatum, external l. medullaris lateralis corporis striati.
medullary l. of corpus striatum, internal l. medullaris medialis corporis striati.
medullary l. of corpus striatum, lateral l. medullaris lateralis corporis striati.
medullary l. of corpus striatum, medial l. medullaris medialis corporis striati.
medullary l. of thalamus, external l. medullaris lateralis thalami.
medullary l. of thalamus, internal l. medullaris medialis thalami.
l. membrana′cea cartila′ginis tu′bae auditi′vae [TA], **membranous l. of cartilage of auditory tube** the connective tissue lamina that supports the medial and lateral parts of the auditory tube.
l. modi′oli [TA] lamina of modiolus: a bony plate extending upward toward the cupula as a continuation of the modiolus and of the bony spiral lamina of the cochlea.
l. molecula′ris [TA] molecular layer: layer I of the cerebral cortex, the most superficial of the six layers, composed chiefly of a stria of tangentially oriented myelinated nerve fibers; this layer also contains dendritic terminals from cells of deeper layers, some cortical afferent fibers, sparsely scattered horizontal cells of Cajal, and various other cell types. Called also *plexiform layer of cerebral cortex.*
l. multifor′mis [TA] multiform layer: layer VI of the cerebral cortex, composed of various cell types, chiefly containing irregular fusiform cells, the axons of which project into the white substance of the cerebral cortex hemisphere. Called also *fusiform* or *polymorphic layer of cerebral cortex.*
l. muscula′ris muco′sae muscularis mucosae: the thin layer of smooth muscle fibers usually found as a part of the tunica mucosa deep to the lamina propria mucosae.
l. muscula′ris muco′sae gas′trica [TA] muscularis musosae of stomach: the muscular layer of the mucous membrane (tunica mucosa) of the stomach.
l. muscula′ris muco′sae intesti′ni cras′si [TA] muscularis mucosae of large intestine: the muscular layer of the mucous membrane (tunica mucosa) of the large intestine.
l. muscula′ris muco′sae intesti′ni te′nuis [TA] muscularis mucosae of small intestine: the muscular layer of the mucous membrane (tunica mucosa) of the small intestine.
l. muscula′ris muco′sae oeso′phagi [TA] muscularis mucosae of esophagus: the muscular layer of the mucous membrane (tunica mucosa) of the esophagus.
nuclear l. a tightly woven meshwork composed of lamins that lines the nuclear side of the inner nuclear membrane; it is believed to control

the shape of the nucleus and it mediates interactions of the inner nuclear membrane with chromatin.
l. orbita′lis os′sis ethmoida′lis [TA] orbital plate of ethmoid bone: a thin plate of bone laterally bounding the ethmoid labyrinth on either side and forming part of the medial wall of the orbit; called also *l. papyracea.*
osseous spiral l. l. spiralis ossea.
l. papyra′cea l. orbitalis ossis ethmoidalis.
l. parieta′lis pericar′dii sero′si [TA] parietal layer of serous pericardium: the outer of the two layers of the serous pericardium, lining the fibrous pericardium. Called also *parietal pericardium.*
l. parieta′lis tu′nicae vagina′lis tes′tis [TA] parietal layer of tunica vaginalis of testis: the outer layer of the tunica vaginalis testis, separated from the visceral layer by a cavity.
l. perpendicula′ris os′sis ethmoida′lis [TA] perpendicular plate of ethmoid bone: a thin bony plate that descends from the inferior surface of the cribriform plate of the ethmoid bone and participates in forming the nasal septum.
l. perpendicula′ris os′sis palati′ni [TA] perpendicular plate of palatine bone: the flat, vertical, bony plate that extends superiorly on either side from the palatine bone; it is surmounted by the orbital and sphenoidal processes.
l. pos′terior fas′ciae thoracolumba′lis [TA] posterior layer of thoracolumbar fascia: the outermost of three layers of fascia covering the deep muscles in the lumbosacral region; it is attached to the spines of the lumbar and sacral vertebrae and to the supraspinous ligaments, gives origin to transversus abdominis, and helps to enclose erector spinae. Called also *l. superficialis fasciae thoracolumbalis* [TA alternative].
l. poste′rior vagi′nae mus′culi rec′ti abdo′minis [TA] posterior layer of sheath of rectus abdominis muscle: the portion of the muscle sheath lying posterior to the rectus abdominis muscle, formed by the transversus abdominis muscle and its aponeurosis at the level of the xiphoid process; inferior to the xiphoid process, as far as the arcuate line, it is formed by the aponeuroses of the internal oblique and the transversus abdominis muscles.
l. pretrachea′lis fas′ciae cervica′lis [TA] pretracheal layer of cervical fascia: the layer of deep cervical fascia that is anterior to the trachea and surrounds the thyroid gland; see also *anterior visceral space.* Called also *pretracheal fascia* and *middle layer of deep cervical fascia.*
l. prevertebra′lis fas′ciae cervica′lis [TA] prevertebral layer of cervical fascia: the layer of deep cervical fascia that is anterior to the vertebrae and posterior to the trachea and esophagus; it invests the scalene and levator scapulae muscles and is continuous laterally with the membrana suprapleuralis. Called also *prevertebral fascia.*
l. profun′da fas′ciae tempora′lis [TA] deep layer of temporal fascia: the deep portion of the fascia investing the temporalis muscle.
l. profun′da fas′ciae thoracolumba′lis TA alternative for *lamina anterior fasciae thoracolumbalis.*
l. profun′da mus′culi levato′ris pal′pebrae superio′ris [TA] deep layer of levator palpebrae superioris: the deeper of the two layers of the levator palpebrae superioris muscle, the fibers of which are attached to the tarsus superior palpebrae.
l. pro′pria muco′sae the connective tissue coat of a mucous membrane (tunica mucosa) just deep to the epithelium and basement membrane.
l. pyramida′lis exter′na [TA] external pyramidal layer: layer III of the cerebral cortex, composed of an inner zone of medium-sized pyramidal cells and an outer zone of larger pyramidal cells and other cells whose dendrites and axons extend beyond this layer.
l. pyramida′lis inter′na [TA] internal pyramidal layer: layer V of the cerebral cortex, composed of the largest pyramidal cells, Martinotti cells, and Betz cells, and traversed by a stria of horizontally arranged fibers (Baillarger inner line); the axons of the pyramidal cells leave this layer as either association, projection, or commissural fibers. Called also *ganglionic layer of cerebral cortex.*
l. quadrige′mina TA alternative for *l. tecti mesencephali.*
l. ra′ra exter′na the lamina lucida on the epithelial side of the lamina densa in a renal glomerulus or pulmonary alveolus.
l. ra′ra inter′na the lamina lucida on the endothelial side of the lamina densa in a renal glomerulus or pulmonary alveolus.
reticular l., l. reticula′ris 1. a layer of the basement membrane, adjacent to the connective tissue, seen in some epithelia; it is of variable thickness and is composed of condensed connective tissue with a reticulum of collagen fibers. Cf. *basal l.* 2. membrana reticularis organi spiralis.
Rexed laminae an architectural scheme used to classify the structure of the spinal cord, based on the cytological features of the neurons in different regions of the gray substance. It consists of nine laminae (I–IX) that extend throughout the cord, roughly paralleling the dorsal and ventral columns of the gray substance, and a tenth region (area X) that surrounds the central canal and consists of the dorsal and ventral commissures and the central gelatinous substance.
right l. of thyroid cartilage see *l. cartilaginis thyroideae dextra/sinistra.*
l. rostra′lis rostral lamina: a thin membranous portion of the rostrum of the corpus callosum that passes from the rostrum to the lamina terminalis immediately in front of the anterior commissure.
secondary spiral l. l. spiralis secundaria.
l. sep′ti pellu′cidi [TA] lamina of septum pellucidum: either of the two thin vertical sheets that constitute the septum pellucidum; they may be separated by a cleftlike space.
spinal laminae, lami′nae spina′les I–IX Rexed laminae.
l. spina′lis X [TA] TA alternative for area spinalis X, although it was not named as such by Rexed; see also *Rexed laminae.*
l. spira′lis os′sea [TA] bony spiral lamina: a double plate of bone winding spirally around the modiolus and dividing the spiral canal of the cochlea incompletely into two parts, the scala tympani and the scala vestibuli; called also *spiral plate.*
l. spira′lis secunda′ria [TA] secondary spiral lamina: a bony projection on the outer wall of the osseous spiral lamina in the lower part of the first turn of the cochlea.
l. superficia′lis fas′ciae cervica′lis [TA] investing layer of cervical fascia: the most superficial of the deep layers of cervical fascia, surrounding the neck superficial to the pretracheal layer; it invests the trapezius and sternocleidomastoid muscles and is attached posteriorly to the vertebrae. Called also *investing layer of deep cervical fascia* and *superficial layer of cervical fascia* or *of deep cervical fascia.*
l. superficia′lis fas′ciae tempora′lis [TA] superficial layer of temporal fascia: the superficial portion of the fascia investing the temporalis muscle.
l. superficia′lis fas′ciae thoracolumba′lis TA alternative for *l. posterior fasciae thoracolumbalis.*
l. superficia′lis mus′culi levato′ris pal′pebrae superio′ris [TA] the superficial of the two layers of the levator palpebrae superioris muscle.
suprachoroid l. a thin layer of connective tissue on the inner surface of the sclera; in official terminology it is named *lamina fusca sclerae* or *lamina suprachoroidea* depending on the point from which it is viewed. See *l. fusca sclerae.*
l. suprachoroi′dea [TA] suprachoroid lamina: see *l. fusca sclerae.*
l. supraneuropo′rica the part of lamina terminalis caudal to the anterior neuropore of the embryo; it cannot be delimited accurately in human embryos.
l. tec′ti mesence′phali [TA] tectal plate: the layer of mingled gray and white substance in the tectum of the mesencephalon, from which arise the superior and inferior colliculi. Called also *l. quadrigemina* [TA alternative] and *quadrigeminal plate.*

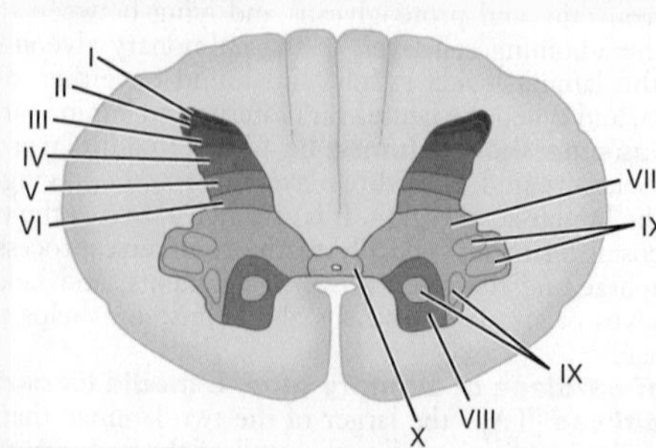

■ Rexed laminae in a cross-section of the spinal cord at approximately the level of the seventh cervical vertebra (C7).

Lamina *Continued*

l. termina'lis [TA] a thin plate derived from the telencephalon extending upward from the optic chiasm and preoptic recess, and forming the anterior wall of the third ventricle.
l. of thyroid cartilage l. cartilaginis thyroideae [dextra/sinistra].
l. tra'gi [TA] tragal lamina: the longitudinal curved lamina of cartilage in the tragus of the auricle, at the beginning of the cartilaginous portion of the external acoustic meatus.
vascular l. of choroid, l. vasculo'sa choroi'deae [TA] the layer of the choroid between the suprachoroid and capillary laminae, containing the largest blood vessels.
l. of vertebra, l. of vertebral arch l. arcus vertebrae.
l. viscera'lis pericar'dii sero'si [TA] visceral layer of serous pericardium: the inner layer of the serous pericardium; it is in contact with the heart and the roots of the great vessels; called also *epicardium* [TA alternative] and *visceral pericardium.*
l. viscera'lis tu'nicae vagina'lis tes'tis [TA] visceral layer of tunica vaginalis testis: the inner part of the tunica vaginalis testis, firmly attached to the testis and epididymis.
l. vi'trea, vitreal l., vitreous l. l. basalis choroideae.
white laminae of cerebellum laminae albae cerebelli.

lam•i•nae (lam'ĭ-ne) [L.] genitive and plural of *lamina.*

lam•i•na•gram (lam'ĭ-nə-gram) tomogram.

lam•i•na•graph (lam'ĭ-nə-graf) an x-ray machine for making radiographs of a layer of tissue at a selected depth.

lam•i•nag•ra•phy (lam″ĭ-nag'rə-fe) [*lamina* + *-graphy*] tomography.

lam•i•na•plas•ty (lam'ĭ-nə-plas″te) [*lamina* + *-plasty*] laminoplasty.

lam•i•nar (lam'ĭ-nər) [L. *laminaris*] 1. pertaining to a lamina or laminae. 2. laminated. 3. of, pertaining to, or being a streamlined, smooth fluid flow.

La•mi•na•ria (lam″ĭ-nar'e-ə) a genus of seaweeds (kelps), various species of which are used as sources of alginates; see *laminarin. L. digita'ta* yields dry stems that are hydrophilic and gradually swell in moist environments, so that they can be used to dilate the uterine cervix in induced abortion.

lam•i•na•rin (lam″ĭ-na'rin) a polysaccharide from seaweed of the genus *Laminaria,* consisting essentially of β-D-glucose residues.
l. sulfate the sulfated form, having antilipemic and anticoagulant properties.

lam•i•nat•ed (lam'ĭ-nāt″ed) having, composed of, or arranged in layers or laminae.

lam•i•nec•to•my (lam″ĭ-nek'tə-me) [*lamina* + *-ectomy*] excision of the posterior arch of a vertebra.

lam•i•nin (lam'ĭ-nin) an adhesive glycoprotein, comprising a number of cell- and tissue-specific isoforms, that is a component of the basement membrane; it binds to heparan sulfate, type IV collagen, and specific cell-surface receptors and is involved in the attachment of epithelial cells to underlying connective tissue.

lam•i•ni•tis (lam″ĭ-ni'tis) 1. inflammation of a lamina. 2. inflammation, congestion, and ischemia of the laminae of a hoof, with breakdown of the union between the horny and sensitive layers; it usually occurs in overweight, overfed animals. Called also *founder.*

lam•i•no•gram (lam'ĭ-no-gram) tomogram.

lam•i•nog•ra•phy (lam″ĭ-nog'rə-fe) tomography.

lam•i•no•plas•ty (lam'in-o-plas″te) incision completely through one lamina of a vertebral arch with creation of a trough in the contralateral lamina; the vertebral arch is then opened like a door, with the trough acting as a hinge; performed to relieve compression of the spinal cord or nerve roots. Called also *open-door l.* **laminoplas'tic** *adj*

Lam•i•no•si•op•tes (lam″ĭ-no-se-op'tēz) a genus of mites of the family Laminosioptidae. *L. cysti'cola* forms nodules in the subcutaneous tissue of chickens and other birds.

Lam•i•no•si•op•ti•dae (lam″ĭ-no-se-op'tĭ-de) a family of mites, some of which infest birds. It includes the genus *Laminosioptes.*

lam•i•not•o•my (lam″ĭ-not'ə-me) [*lamina* + *-tomy*] division of the lamina of a vertebra.

La•mi•sil (lam'ə-sil) trademark for preparations of terbinafine hydrochloride.

la•miv•u•dine (lə-miv'u-dēn) a nucleoside analogue that inhibits reverse transcriptase, used as an antiviral agent in the treatment of chronic hepatitis B infection and, in combination with zidovudine, in the treatment of human immunodeficiency virus infection and acquired immunodeficiency syndrome; administered orally.

la•mo•tri•gine (lə-mo'trĭ-jēn) an anticonvulsant used in the treatment of partial seizures in adult patients formerly treated with an enzyme-inducing anticonvulsant (e.g., carbamazepine) and as an adjunct in the treatment of partial seizures in adults with epilepsy and of generalized seizures associated with Lennox-Gastaut syndrome; it is also used as a mood stabilizer in the treatment of bipolar I disorder. Administered orally.

lamp (lamp) an apparatus for furnishing heat or light.
annealing l. an alcohol lamp for heating and purifying gold foil to be used for filling tooth cavities.
arc l. a source of light consisting of gaseous particles from the electrodes of an electric arc that are raised to a temperature of incandescence by an electric current.
cold quartz l. low pressure mercury arc l.
diagnostic l. a light used for observing subtle shadings in weak fluorescence, for external body examinations, observations of tissue fluorescence, identification of vulvar fluorescence, chromatography, etc.
Eldridge-Green l. an arrangement of lights for testing color vision.
germicidal l. a type of mercury arc lamp whose radiation kills bacteria.
Gullstrand slit l. slit l.
heat l. a lamp held at a distance from the body and used for superficial heating of a part.
high pressure mercury arc l. an ultraviolet radiation lamp having a high vapor pressure with high intensity light because of linear spectral emissions in many wavelength ranges; used as a source of ultraviolet B for treating dermatologic disorders. See also *Goeckerman treatment,* under *treatment.*
hot quartz l. high pressure mercury arc l.
Kromayer l. a type of high pressure mercury arc lamp with a small field of irradiation, used to treat dermatologic disorders in small surface areas of the skin.
low pressure mercury arc l. an ultraviolet radiation lamp having a low vapor pressure, low amperage, high voltage, and a glow discharge; more than 95 per cent of its emission is ultraviolet C in the mercury vapor resonance emission line at 254 nm. In the treatment of skin disorders such as acne, the radiation causes acute erythema followed by desquamation of the affected skin.
mercury arc l., mercury vapor l., quartz l. a lamp in which the arc is struck in mercury and is enclosed in a quartz burner; used in photodynamic therapy. The two most common types are the low pressure or cold quartz type and the high pressure or hot quartz type.
slit l. a lamp having a diaphragm with a slitlike opening through which a narrow flat beam of intense light may be projected into the eye. It gives intense illumination so that microscopic study may be made of the conjunctivae, cornea, iris, lens, and vitreous, the special feature being that it illuminates a section through the substance of these structures. Called also *Gullstrand slit l.* and *slit-lamp biomicroscope.*
sun l. a lamp that gives off radiation, especially ultraviolet, in ranges similar to those of the sun's rays.
ultraviolet l. a lamp that produces ultraviolet rays.
Wood l. a medium-pressure mercury arc lamp containing a nickel oxide filter (Wood filter), used in diagnosis of skin conditions such as erythrasma and fungus infections, as well as for revealing the presence of porphyrins and fluorescent minerals of the skin, scalp, and hair.
xenon arc l. a lamp that produces light of high intensity in a wide continuum of wavelengths; used with optical filters as the most common source of solar-simulating radiation; clinical uses include tests of photosensitivity.

lam•pas (lam'pəs) [Fr.] a swelling and hardening of the mucosa of the hard palate, immediately behind the upper incisors in horses; called also *palatitis.*

lam•ziek•te (lam'zēk-te) [Afrikaans "lame-sickness"] a type of botulism seen in cattle in South Africa after they chew on infected or putrefying bones in an effort to compensate for a phosphorus deficiency.

la•na (lan'ə) gen. and pl. *la'nae* [L.] wool.

la•nat•o•side C (lə-nat'o-sīd) an easily absorbed and stable glycoside obtained from the leaves of *Digitalis lanata,* having the same actions and uses as digitalis; administered orally.

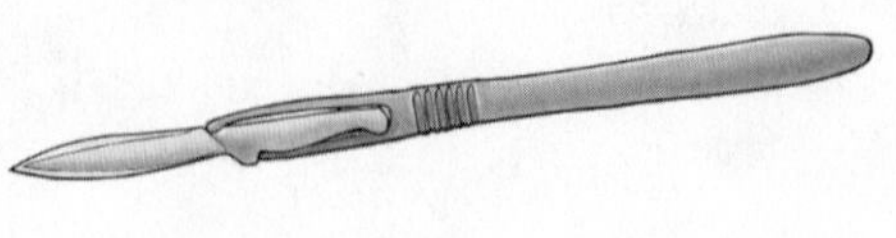

■ Lancet.

lance (lans) [L. *lancea*] 1. lancet. 2. to cut or incise with a lancet.

Lance-Ad·ams syndrome (lans′ ad′əmz) [James W. *Lance*, Australian neurologist, born 1926; Raymond D. *Adams*, American neurologist, 1911–2008] see under *syndrome.*

Lance·field classification, group (lans′fēld) [Rebecca Craighill *Lancefield*, American bacteriologist, 1895–1981] see under *classification* and *group.*

lan·ce·o·late (lan′se-o-lāt) shaped like a lance.

lan·cet (lan′sət) [L. *lancea* lance] a small, pointed, two-edged surgical knife.

abscess l. a wide-bladed lancet with one convex and one concave edge.
acne l. a lancet with a narrow blade for puncturing the papules of acne.
gingival l., gum l. a lancet for incising the gingivae.
spring l. a lancet whose blade is held by a spring.

lan·ci·nat·ing (lan′sĭ-nāt″ing) [L. *lancinas*] tearing, darting, or sharply cutting; see under *pain.*

Lan·ci·si nerves, stria (lahn-che′ze) [Giovanni Maria *Lancisi*, Italian physician, 1654–1720] see *stria longitudinalis lateralis corporis callosi* and *stria longitudinalis medialis corporis callosi.*

Lan·dau-Kleff·ner syndrome (lahn′dou klef′nər) [William M. *Landau*, American neurologist, 20th century; Frank R. *Kleffner*, American speech pathologist, 20th century] see under *syndrome.*

land·mark (land′mark) a readily recognizable anatomical structure used as a point of reference in establishing the location of another structure or in determining certain measurements.

Lan·dolt operation (lahn-do′) [Edmond *Landolt*, French ophthalmologist, 1846–1926] see under *operation.*

Lan·dou·zy muscular dystrophy (lah-doo-ze′) [Louis Théophile Joseph *Landouzy*, French physician, 1845–1917] facioscapulohumeral muscular dystrophy; see under *dystrophy.*

Lan·dou·zy-De·je·rine muscular dystrophy (atrophy) (lah-doo-ze′ dĕ-zhĕ-rēn′) [L.T.J. *Landouzy;* Joseph Jules *Dejerine*, French neurologist, 1849–1917] facioscapulohumeral muscular dystrophy; see under *dystrophy.*

Lan·dry paralysis (syndrome) (lah-dre′) [Jean Baptiste Octave *Landry*, French physician, 1826–1865] Guillain-Barré syndrome.

Land·ström muscle (lahnd′strəm) [John *Landström*, Swedish surgeon, 1869–1910] see under *muscle.*

Land·zert fossa (lahnt′sərt) [T. *Landzert*, German anatomist, 19th century] recessus paraduodenalis.

Lane bands, disease, plate (lān) [Sir William Arbuthnot *Lane*, British surgeon, 1856–1943] see under *band, disease,* and *plate.*

Lan·gen·beck amputation, flap, triangle (lahng′ən-bek) [Bernhard Rudolf Konrad von *Langenbeck*, German surgeon, 1810–1887] see under *amputation* and *triangle,* and see *von Langenbeck bipedicle mucoperiosteal flap,* under *flap.*

Lan·ger axillary arch, lines, muscle (lahng′ər) [Carl Ritter von Edenberg von *Langer*, Austrian anatomist, 1819–1887] see under *arch, line,* and *muscle.*

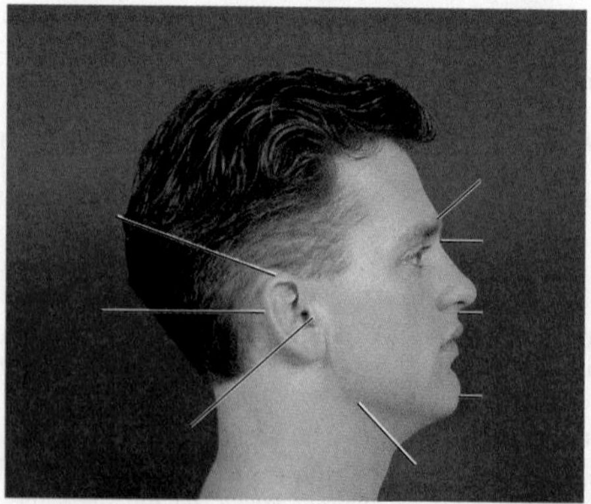

■ Some surface landmarks of the head.

Lang·er mesomelic dysplasia (lang′ər) [Leonard O. *Langer*, Jr., American radiologist, 1928–2008] see under *dysplasia.*

Lang·er-Gie·di·on syndrome (lang′ər zhe-de-aw′) [L.O. *Langer*, Jr.; Andreas *Giedion*, Swiss radiologist, born 1925] see under *syndrome.*

Lan·ger·hans cells, granules, islets (islands) (lahng′ər-hahnz) [Paul *Langerhans*, German pathologist, 1847–1888] see under *cell* and *islet* and see *Birbeck granules,* under *granule.*

Lang·hans cells, layer (stria) (lahng′hahnz) [Theodor *Langhans*, German pathologist, 1839–1915] see under *cell,* and see *cytotrophoblast.*

Lang·ley ganglion, granules, nerves (lang′le) [John Newport *Langley*, English physiologist, 1852–1925] see under *ganglion* and *granule,* and see *pilomotor nerves,* under *nerve.*

lan·i·ary (lan′e-ar″e) [L. *laniare* to tear to pieces] suitable for lacerating, or tearing to pieces; said of canine teeth.

Lan·nois-Gra·de·ni·go syndrome (lah-nwah′ grah-də-ne′go) [Maurice *Lannois*, French physician, late 19th century; Giuseppe *Gradenigo*, Italian physician, 1859–1926] Gradenigo syndrome.

lan·o·lin (lan′o-lin) [*lana* + *oleum*] 1. [USP] the purified waxlike substance from the wool of sheep, cleaned, deodorized, and decolorized, and containing not more than 0.25 per cent water; used in the formulation of water-in-oil creams and ointments. Called also *anhydrous l.* and *refined wool fat.* 2. the same substance, having the same uses, but containing between 25 and 30 per cent water. Called also *hydrous l., hydrous wool fat,* and *wool fat.* When the term is used thus, the anhydrous form of lanolin is usually specified as *anhydrous lanolin.*

anhydrous l. lanolin (def. 1).
hydrous l. lanolin (def. 2).
modified l. [USP] anhydrous lanolin that has been processed to reduce the amount of free lanolin alcohols and detergent and pesticide residues.

la·nos·ter·ol (lə-nos′tər-ol) a tetracyclic sterol formed from squalene; it is the parent steroid in animals, being itself converted in several steps to cholesterol.

La·nox·i·caps (lə-nok′sĭ-kaps) trademark for preparations of digoxin.

La·nox·in (lə-nok′sin) trademark for preparations of digoxin.

lan·re·o·tide ace·tate (lan-re′o-tīd) a synthetic analogue of somatostatin, having actions similar to those of somatostatin but a longer duration of effect; used in treatment of acromegaly. Administered by subcutaneous injection.

lan·so·pra·zole (lan-so′prə-zōl) a substituted benzimidazole that acts as a proton pump inhibitor; used to inhibit the secretion of gastric acid for the symptomatic treatment of duodenal and gastric ulcers and gastroesophageal reflux disease and for the long-term treatment of hyperchlorhydria; administered orally.

Lan·ter·man incisures (clefts) (lan′tər-mən) [A.J. *Lanterman*, American anatomist in Germany, late 19th century] Schmidt-Lanterman incisures; see under *incisure.*

Lan·ter·man-Schmidt incisures (lan′tər-mən shmit′) [A.J. *Lanterman;* Henry D. *Schmidt*, American anatomist, 1823–1888] Schmidt-Lanterman incisures; see under *incisure.*

lan·than·ic (lan′thən-ik) [Gr. *lanthanein* to escape notice, to be concealed] symptom-free; said of a symptomless disease that is undetected, or detected by accident.

lan·tha·num (La) (lan′thə-nəm) [Gr. *lanthanein* to be concealed] a rare metallic element, atomic number 57, atomic weight 138.91.

lan·ti·bi·ot·ic (lan″tĭ-bi-ot′ik) a type of bacteriocin produced by gram-positive bacteria that causes the death of certain other gram-positive bacteria.

Lan·tus (lan′təs) trademark for a preparation of insulin glargine.

la·nu·gi·nous (lə-noo′jĭ-nəs) [L. *lanuginosus*] covered with lanugo.

la·nu·go (lə-noo′go) [L.] [TA] the fine hair on the body of the fetus; called also *down, downy hair, lanugo hair,* and *primary hair.*

LAO left anterior oblique.

LAP leukocyte alkaline phosphatase (see under *alkaline phosphatase*); leukocyte adhesion protein (see β_2 *integrin,* under *integrin*).

lapar(o)- [Gr. *lapara* flank] a combining form denoting relationship to the loin or flank. Sometimes used loosely in reference to the abdomen.

lap·a·ro·cele (lap′ə-ro-sēl″) abdominal hernia.

lap·a·ro·cys·tec·to·my (lap″ə-ro-sis-tek′tə-me) [*laparo-* + *cystectomy*] removal of a cyst by an abdominal incision.

lap·a·ro·cys·tot·o·my (lap″ə-ro-sis-tot′ə-me) [*laparo-* + *cystotomy*] 1. cystotomy through the abdominal wall. 2. laparotomy with removal of the contents of a cyst.

lap·a·ro·hys·ter·ec·to·my (lap″ə-ro-his″tə-rek′tə-me) abdominal hysterectomy.

lap·a·ro·hys·tero·ooph·o·rec·to·my (lap″ə-ro-his″tər-o-o″of-ə-rek′tə-me) [*laparo-* + *hystero-* + *oophorectomy*] hysterectomy and oophorectomy done through an incision in the abdominal wall.

lap·a·ro·hys·tero·sal·pin·go·ooph·o·rec·to·my (lap″ə-ro-his″tər-o-sal-ping″go-o″of-ə-rek′tə-me) removal of the uterus, uterine tubes, and ovaries through an abdominal incision.

lap·a·ro·hys·ter·ot·o·my (lap″ə-ro-his″tər-ot′ə-me) [*laparo-* + *hysterotomy*] abdominal hysterotomy.

lap·a·ro·my·itis (lap″ə-ro-mi-i′tis) [*laparo-* + *my-* + *-itis*] inflammation of the abdominal or lumbar muscles.

lap·a·ro·myo·mec·to·my (lap″ə-ro-mi″o-mek′tə-me) [*laparo-* + *myomectomy*] uterine myomectomy through an abdominal incision.

lap·a·ro·sal·pin·go·ooph·o·rec·to·my (lap″ə-ro-sal-ping″go-o″of-ə-rek′tə-me) salpingo-oophorectomy done through an abdominal incision.

lap·a·ro·scope (lap′ə-ro-skōp″) an instrument, comparable to an endoscope, that is inserted into the peritoneal cavity to inspect it. Called also *celioscope* and *peritoneoscope*.

video l. videolaparoscope.

lap·a·ro·scop·ic (lap″ə-ro-skop′ik) 1. pertaining to a laparoscope. 2. performed using a laparoscope.

lap·a·ros·co·py (lap″ə-ros′kə-pe) [*laparo-* + *-scopy*] examination of the interior of the abdomen by means of a laparoscope. Called also *abdominoscopy*, *celioscopy*, and *peritoneoscopy*.

laser l. introduction of a laser beam into the abdomen through a laparoscope, done to vaporize tissue, as in treating endometriosis or to lyse adhesions. See also *pelviscopy* and *videolaseroscopy*.

lap·a·rot·o·ma·phil·ia (lap″ə-rot″o-mə-fil′e-ə) [*laparotomy* + *-philia*] Munchausen syndrome (q.v.) in which the patient desires abdominal surgery.

lap·a·rot·o·my (lap″ə-rot′ə-me) [*laparo-* + *-tomy*] surgical incision into the abdominal cavity. Called also *celiotomy* and *peritoneotomy*.

staging l. laparotomy for pathologic staging of subdiaphragmatic Hodgkin disease. It always includes splenectomy, wedge and deep needle biopsies of liver lobes, and biopsies of multiple lymph nodes, and it may be accompanied by appendectomy and ovariopexy.

vaginal l. incision into the abdominal cavity through the vagina.

La·picque constant (lah-pēk′) [Louis *Lapicque*, French physiologist, 1866–1952] see under *constant*.

Lap·i·dus operation (lap′ĭ-dəs) [Paul W. *Lapidus*, American orthopedic surgeon, 1893–1981] see under *operation*.

lap·in·iza·tion (lap″in-ĭ-za′shən) [Fr. *lapin* rabbit] passage of a virus through rabbits as a means of modifying its characteristics.

lap·in·ize (lap′in-īz) to attenuate (as a virus or vaccine) by serial passage through rabbits.

La·place's law (lah-plahs′əz) [Pierre Simon de *Laplace*, French mathematician and physicist, 1749–1827] see under *law*.

lap·sus (lap′səs) [L., from *labi* to slip or fall] an error, or slip, thought to be revealing of an unconscious wish or association.

l. ca′lami an unconsciously motivated slip of the pen.

l. lin′guae an unconsciously motivated slip of the tongue.

l. memo′riae an unconsciously motivated lapse of memory.

la·pyr·i·um chlo·ride (lə-pēr′e-əm) a surfactant used in pharmaceutic preparations.

lard (lahrd) [L. *lardum*] the purified internal fat of the abdomen of the hog.

benzoinated l. a preparation of lard containing 1 per cent benzoin; used as a vehicle for medicinal agents and in ointments.

lar·da·ceous (lahr-da′shəs) resembling lard.

Lar·i·am (lar′e-am) trademark for a preparation of mefloquine hydrochloride.

la·rith·mics (lə-rith′miks) [Gr. *laos* people + *arithmos* number] the study which deals with population in its quantitative aspects.

lark·spur (lahrk′spər) 1. any of various species of *Delphinium*, which are highly toxic; see *larkspur poisoning*, under *poisoning*. 2. the dried ripe seeds of *Delphinium ajacis*, used medically as a pediculicide.

Lar·o·do·pa (lar″o-do′pə) trademark for a preparation of levodopa.

La·ron dwarf, syndrome (dwarfism) (lah-rōn′) [Zvi *Laron*, Israeli endocrinologist, born 1927] see under *dwarf* and *syndrome*.

Lar·o·tid (lar′o-tid) trademark for a preparation of amoxicillin.

Lar·rey amputation (operation), cleft, spaces (lah-ra′) [Dominique Jean (Baron de) *Larrey*, French military surgeon, 1766–1842] see under *amputation* and *space*, and see *trigonum sternocostale*.

Lar·sen disease (lahr′sən) [Christian Magnus Falsen Sinding-*Larsen*, Norwegian physician, 1866–1930] see under *disease*.

Lar·sen syndrome (lahr′sən) [Loren Joseph *Larsen*, American orthopedic surgeon, 1914–2002] see under *syndrome*.

Lar·sen-Jo·hans·son disease (lahr′sən yo-hahn′sən) [C.M.F. Sinding-*Larsen*; Sven Christian *Johansson*, Swedish surgeon, 1880–1959] Larsen disease; see under *disease*.

lar·va (lahr′və) gen. and pl. *lar′vae* [L. "ghost"] an independent, motile, sometimes feeding, developmental stage in the life history of an animal. Cf. *imago* (def. 1) and *pupa*.

l. cur′rens a type of rapidly progressive cutaneous larva migrans manifested by an urticarial perianal band, representing autoinoculation of the larvae of *Strongyloides stercoralis* that has migrated to and matured at the anus from an intestinal infection site.

cutaneous l. migrans 1. larva migrans in the skin, characterized by thin, curving, pruritic lines corresponding to the subcutaneous movements of the parasitic larvae. The usual cause is the cat and dog hookworm, *Ancylostoma braziliense*, which burrow beneath the skin but cannot complete their migration to the intestine. Called also *ox-warble* or *sandworm disease* and *creeping eruption*. 2. a similar condition caused by other parasites, such as any of various nematodes (see *gnathostomiasis*) or insect larvae (see *hypodermiasis* and *cutaneous myiasis*).

l. mi′grans 1. a life stage of certain parasitic larvae in which they wander through the body of their host. 2. infestation by such a wandering parasitic larva. 3. cutaneous l. migrans.

ocular l. migrans infection of the eye with nematode larvae, usually *Toxocara canis* or *T. cati*. The larvae may lodge in the choroid or retina or migrate to the vitreous; when they die there, a granulomatous inflammation occurs. The resulting lesion may vary from simply a translucent elevation of the retina to massive retinal detachment and pseudoglioma.

rat-tailed l. see *Eristalis tenax*.

visceral l. migrans a condition caused by prolonged migration of nematode larvae to human tissues other than skin, characterized by persistent hypereosinophilia, hepatomegaly, and frequently by pneumonitis. The most common cause is larvae of *Toxocara canis* or *T. cati*, which do not complete their life cycle in humans. See also *ocular l. migrans*.

lar·va·ceous (lahr-va′shəs) larvate.

lar·vae (lahr′ve) [L.] plural of *larva*.

lar·val (lahr′vəl) 1. pertaining to larvae. 2. larvate.

lar·vate (lahr′vāt) [L. *larva* mask] masked; concealed: said of a disease or a symptom of disease.

lar·vi·cide (lahr′vĭ-sīd) [*larva* + *-cide*] an agent destructive to insect larvae.

lar·vi·pha·gic (lahr″vĭ-fa′jik) larvivorous.

lar·vi·po·si·tion (lahr″vĭ-pə-zish′ən) the act of depositing larvae (living maggots) in the tissues of a host.

lar·viv·o·rous (lahr-viv′ə-rəs) [*larva* + L. *vorare* to eat] feeding on or consuming larvae; said especially of fish which ingest mosquito larvae.

lar·yn·gal·gia (lar″in-gal′jə) [*laryng-* + *-algia*] pain in the larynx.

lar·yn·gec·to·mee (lar″in-jek′tə-me) a person whose larynx has been removed.

lar·yn·gec·to·my (lar″in-jek′tə-me) [*laryng-* + *-ectomy*] surgical removal of the larynx.

la·ryn·ges (lə-rin′jēz) [L.] plural of *larynx*.

lar·yn·gis·mus (lar″in-jiz′məs) [L., from Gr. *laryngismos* a whooping] laryngospasm.

l. paraly′ticus laryngeal hemiplegia.

l. stri′dulus sudden laryngeal spasm with cyanosis and inhalation accompanied by a crowing sound, usually seen in children at night. Called also *false croup*, *spasmodic croup*, and *pseudocroup*.

lar·yn·gi·tis (lar″in-ji′tis) inflammation of the larynx, usually with dryness and soreness of the throat, hoarseness, cough, and dysphagia. **laryngit′ic** *adj*

croupous l. a condition seen mainly in infants or small children and characterized by a resonant barking cough, hoarseness, and stridor. Infection, allergy, a foreign body, or a tumor may be the cause. Laryngeal diphtheria was once a common cause but is now rare.

membranous l. laryngitis attended with the formation of a false membrane.

necrotic l. calf diphtheria in the larynx.

subglottic l. inflammation of the undersurface of the vocal cords. Called also *chorditis vocalis inferior*.

syphilitic l. a chronic form due to syphilitic involvement of the larynx.

tuberculous l. laryngitis due to laryngeal tuberculosis.

vestibular l. viral laryngitis in which edema forms a ring outlining the vestibule of the larynx.

laryng(o)- [L. *larynx*, q.v.] a combining form denoting relationship to the larynx.

la•ryn•go•cele (lə-ring′go-sēl) [*laryngo-* + *-cele*[1]] congenital anomalous filling of the laryngeal saccule with air, sometimes visible as an enlargement on the outside of the neck. There are *internal* and *external* types and mixtures of the two.

external l. a laryngocele that penetrates the thyrohyoid membrane and may be visible as a tumorlike enlargement on the neck, becoming larger with increased intralaryngeal pressure, as from coughing.

internal l. a laryngocele confined within the larynx and not visible on the surface of the neck. Called also *ventricular l.*

ventricular l., l. ventricula′ris internal l.

la•ryn•go•cen•te•sis (lə-ring″go-sen-te′sis) [*laryngo-* + *-centesis*] surgical puncture of the larynx.

la•ryn•go•fis•sure (lə-ring″go-fish′ər) median laryngotomy.

la•ryn•go•gram (lə-ring′go-gram) a radiograph of the larynx.

lar•yn•gog•ra•phy (lar″ing-gog′rə-fe) [*laryngo-* + *-graphy*] radiography of the larynx after instillation of a radiopaque medium into it.

lar•yn•gol•o•gy (lar″ing-gol′ə-je) [*laryngo-* + *-logy*] the branch of medicine that deals with the pharynx, larynx, nasopharynx, and tracheobronchial tree.

la•ryn•go•ma•la•cia (lə-ring″go-mə-la′shə) [*laryngo-* + *malacia*] flaccidity of the epiglottis and aryepiglottic folds, as in congenital laryngeal stridor.

lar•yn•gom•e•try (lar″ing-gom′ə-tre) [*laryngo-* + *-metry*] measurement of the larynx.

la•ryn•go•pa•ral•y•sis (lə-ring″go-pə-ral′ə-sis) laryngeal paralysis.

lar•yn•gop•a•thy (lar-ing-gop′ə-the) [*laryngo-* + *-pathy*] any disorder of the larynx.

la•ryn•go•pha•ryn•ge•al (lə-ring″go-fə-rin′je-əl) pertaining to the larynx and pharynx or to the laryngopharynx.

la•ryn•go•phar•yn•gec•to•my (lə-ring″go-far″ən-jek′tə-me) excision of the larynx and pharynx.

la•ryn•go•pha•ryn•ge•us (lə-ring″go-fə-rin′je-əs) musculus constrictor pharyngis inferior.

la•ryn•go•phar•yn•gi•tis (lə-ring″go-far″ən-ji′tis) inflammation of the larynx and pharynx.

la•ryn•go•phar•ynx (lə-ring″go-far′inks) [*laryngo-* + *pharynx*] pars laryngea pharyngis.

lar•yn•goph•o•ny (lar″ing-gof′ə-ne) [*laryngo-* + Gr. *phōnē* voice] a voice sound heard over the larynx.

la•ryn•go•plas•ty (lə-ring′go-plas″te) [*laryngo-* + *-plasty*] reconstruction of the larynx. **laryngoplas′tic** *adj*

la•ryn•go•ple•gia (lə-ring″go-ple′jə) laryngeal paralysis.

la•ryn•go•pto•sis (lə-ring″gop-to′sis, lə-ring″go-to′sis) [*laryngo-* + *-ptosis*] a lowering and mobilization of the larynx, occurring either congenitally or as part of the aging process.

la•ryn•go•pyo•cele (lə-ring″go-pi′o-sēl) a laryngocele containing pus.

lar•yn•gor•rha•gia (lar″ing-go-ra′jə) [*laryngo-* + *-rrhagia*] hemorrhage from the larynx.

lar•yn•gor•rha•phy (lar″ing-gor′ə-fe) [*laryngo-* + *-rrhaphy*] the operation of suturing the larynx.

la•ryn•gor•rhea (la″ring-go-re′ə) [*laryngo-* + *-rrhea*] excessive secretion of mucus whenever the voice is used.

la•ryn•go•scle•ro•ma (lə-ring″go-sklə-ro′mə) [*laryngo-* + *scleroma*] scleroma of the larynx.

la•ryn•go•scope (lə-ring′go-skōp) [*laryngo-* + *-scope*] an endoscope for use in direct visual examination of the larynx.

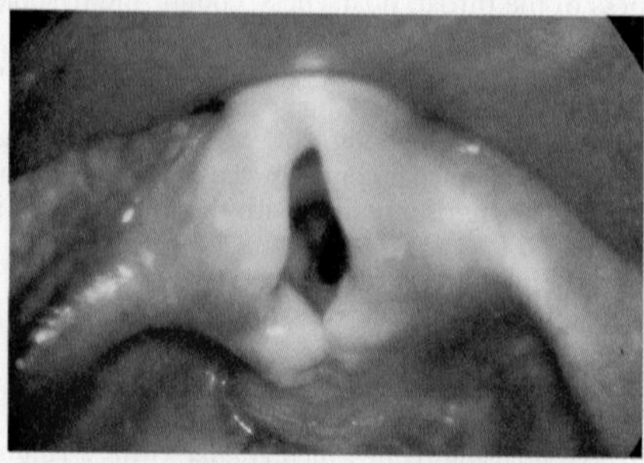

■ Laryngomalacia in an infant.

lar•yn•gos•co•pist (lar″ing-gos′kə-pist) a specialist in laryngoscopy.

lar•yn•gos•co•py (lar″ing-gos′kə-pe) [*laryngo-* + *-scopy*] examination of the interior of the larynx, especially that performed with the laryngoscope (*direct laryngoscopy*). **laryngoscop′ic** *adj*

direct l. direct visual examination of the interior of the larynx performed with a speculum or with a laryngoscope.

indirect l. examination of the interior of the larynx by observation of the reflection of it in a laryngeal mirror.

mirror l. indirect l.

suspension l. examination of the larynx performed with a direct laryngoscope suspended so as to leave both hands of the examiner free.

la•ryn•go•spasm (lə-ring′go-spaz″əm) [*laryngo-* + *spasm*] spasmodic closure of the larynx. Called also *laryngismus* and *glottal, glottic,* or *laryngeal spasm.*

la•ryn•go•stat (lə-ring′go-stat) an appliance for holding a source of radioactive material within the larynx.

la•ryn•go•ste•no•sis (lə-ring″go-stə-no′sis) [*laryngo-* + *stenosis*] narrowing or stricture of the larynx.

lar•yn•gos•to•my (lar″ing-gos′tə-me) [*laryngo-* + *-stomy*] surgical creation of an artificial opening into the larynx.

la•ryn•go•stro•bo•scope (lə-ring″go-stro′bo-skōp″) [*laryngo-* + *stroboscope*] an apparatus for observing the intralaryngeal phenomena with a stroboscopic light.

la•ryn•go•tome (lə-ring′go-tōm) an instrument used in incising the larynx.

lar•yn•got•o•my (lar″ing-got′ə-me) [*laryngo-* + *-tomy*] surgical incision of the larynx.

inferior l. cricothyrotomy.

median l. incision of the larynx through the thyroid cartilage; called also *laryngofissure, thyrofissure,* and *thyrotomy.*

subhyoid l., superior l. incision of the larynx through the thyrohyoid membrane; called also *thyrohyoid l.*

thyrohyoid l. subhyoid l.

la•ryn•go•tra•che•al (lə-ring″go-tra′ke-əl) pertaining to the larynx and trachea.

la•ryn•go•tra•che•itis (lə-ring″go-tra″ke-i′tis) inflammation of the larynx and trachea.

avian l., infectious avian l., infectious l. (ILT) a viral disease of poultry caused by gallid herpesvirus 1, characterized by respiratory distress, an exudate or bleeding, and often death.

la•ryn•go•tra•cheo•bron•chi•tis (lə-ring″go-tra″ke-o-brong-ki′tis) inflammation of the larynx, trachea, and bronchi; an acute form is the most common cause of croup.

la•ryn•go•tra•cheo•bron•chos•co•py (lə-ring″go-tra″ke-o-brong-kos′kə-pe) endoscopic examination of the larynx, trachea, and bronchi.

la•ryn•go•tra•cheo•plas•ty (lə-ring″go-tra′ke-o-plas″te) plastic expansion of the larynx and trachea for the treatment of subglottic stenosis. **laryngotracheoplas′tic** *adj*

la•ryn•go•tra•che•os•co•py (lə-ring″go-tra″ke-os′kə-pe) peroral laryngoscopy and tracheoscopy.

la•ryn•go•tra•che•ot•o•my (lə-ring″go-tra″ke-ot′o-me) [*laryngo-* + *tracheotomy*] incision of the larynx and trachea.

lar•ynx (lar′inks) gen. *laryn′gis,* pl. *laryn′ges* [L., from Gr.] [TA] the musculocartilaginous structure, lined with mucous membrane, connected to the superior part of the trachea and to the pharynx inferior to the tongue and the hyoid bone; the essential sphincter guarding the entrance into the trachea and functioning secondarily as the organ of voice. It is formed by nine cartilages connected by ligaments and eight muscles. **laryn′geal** *adj*

artificial l. an electromechanical device that enables a laryngectomized person to speak. When it is placed against the region of the laryngectomy a buzzing sound is produced, which is converted into simulated speech by movements of the organs of articulation (lips, tongue, glottis).

LAS lymphangioscintigraphy.

la•sal•o•cid (lə-sal′o-sid) an antibiotic produced by *Streptomyces lasaliensis;* used as a coccidiostat in poultry.

La•sègue sign, test (lah-seg′) [Ernest Charles *Lasègue,* French physician, 1816–1883] see under *sign,* and see *straight leg–raising test,* under *test.*

la•ser (la′zər) [*l*ight *a*mplification by *s*timulated *e*mission of *r*adiation] a device that transforms light of various frequencies into an extremely intense, small, and nearly nondivergent beam of monochromatic radiation in the visible region with all the waves in phase. Capable of mobilizing immense heat and power when focused at close range, it is used as a tool in surgical procedures, in diagnosis, and in physiologic studies.

alexandrite l. a laser whose active medium is alexandrite doped with chromium, emitting light in the mid-infrared spectrum and tunable

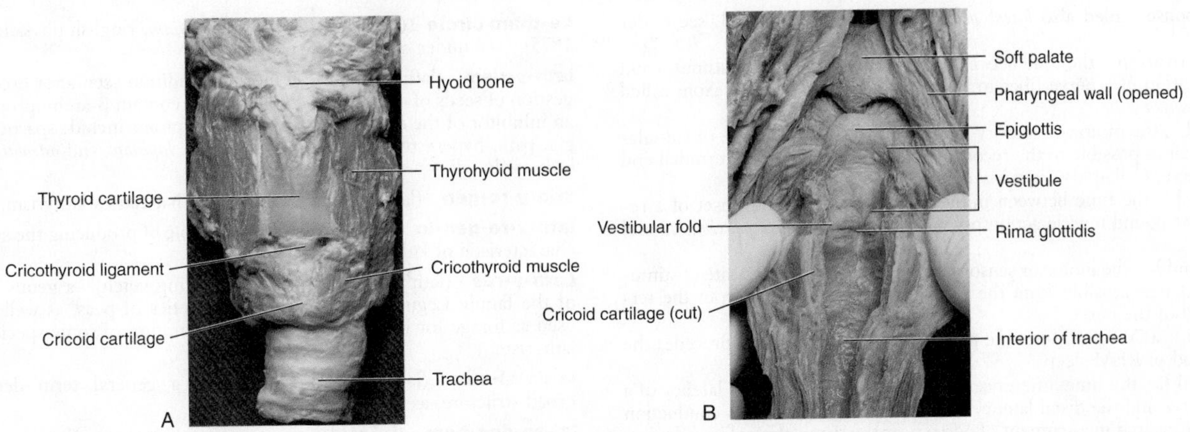

■ *(A)*, Anterior view of the larynx; *(B)*, posterior view of the interior of the pharynx, larynx, and trachea.

between 701 and 826 nm and used usually at 755 nm; used for hair removal and other dermatologic procedures.

argon l. a laser with ionized argon as the active medium whose beam is in the blue and green visible light spectrum, with two energy peaks, at 488 and 514 nm; used for photocoagulation.

carbon-dioxide l. a laser with carbon dioxide gas as the active medium that produces infrared radiation at 10,600 nm; used to excise and incise tissue and to vaporize.

continuous wave l. a laser that continuously emits a beam of coherent light.

dye l. a laser with organic dye dissolved in a solvent as the active medium whose beam is in the visible light spectrum; used in photodynamic therapy.

erbium:YAG l. a laser whose active medium is a crystal of yttrium, aluminum, and garnet doped with erbium ions, and whose beam is in the near infrared spectrum at 2940 nm; used for photoablation and photocoagulation and for a variety of dermatologic procedures.

excimer l. [*exc*ited d*imer*] a laser with rare gas halides as the active medium whose beam is in the ultraviolet spectrum and penetrates tissues only a small distance; the beam breaks chemical bonds instead of generating heat to destroy tissue. Used in ophthalmologic and dermatologic procedures and in laser angioplasty.

helium-neon l. a laser with a mixture of ionized helium and neon gases as the active medium whose beam is in the red visible light spectrum at 633 nm; used as a guiding beam for lasers operating at nonvisible wavelengths.

holmium:YAG l. a laser whose active medium is a crystal of yttrium, aluminum, and garnet doped with holmium ions, and whose beam is in the near infrared spectrum at 2100 nm; used for photocoagulation and photoablation.

ion l. a laser that uses one of the inert gases (argon, helium, neon, or krypton) as the active medium.

krypton l. a laser with krypton ionized by electric current as the active medium whose beam is in the yellow-red visible light spectrum; used for photocoagulation.

KTP l. a laser in which a beam generated from a neodymium:YAG crystal is directed through a potassium titanyl phosphate crystal to produce a beam in the green visible spectrum at 532 nm; its properties are similar to those of the argon laser and it is used for photoablation and photocoagulation.

neodymium:yttrium-aluminum-garnet (Nd:YAG) l. a laser whose active medium is a crystal of yttrium, aluminum, and garnet doped with neodymium ions, and whose beam is in the near infrared spectrum at 1060 nm; used for photocoagulation and photoablation.

potassium titanyl phosphate l. KTP l.

pulsed l. a laser that emits short bursts of energy at fixed intervals rather than a continuous stream of energy.

pulsed dye l. a dye laser in which excitation of the dye by pulses of intense light from a flashlamp produces a beam in the yellow visible light spectrum with a wavelength of 577 or 585 nm, with alternating on and off phases of a few microseconds each; used to decolorize pigmented lesions.

Q-switched l. a laser containing a switching device that causes the laser to produce very high intensity impulses of very short duration.

tunable dye l. a dye laser whose active medium can be altered so that the beam has any of several wavelengths.

LASIK laser-assisted in-situ keratomileusis.

Las•io•he•lea (las″e-o-he′le-ə) a genus of blood-sucking flies of the family Heleidae.

La•six (la′siks) trademark for preparations of furosemide.

Las•sa fever, virus (lah′sə) [*Lassa*, town in Nigeria where the fever was first reported in 1959] see under *fever* and *virus*.

Las•sar paste, plain zinc paste (lahs′ər) [Oskar *Lassar*, German dermatologist, 1849–1908] see under *paste*.

las•si•tude (las′ĭ-to͞od) [L. *lassitudo* weariness] weakness; exhaustion.

la•tah (lah′tah) a culture-specific type of jumping disease seen chiefly among the Malays and other people of Southeast Asia, characterized by hypersuggestibility, echolalia, echopraxis, coprolalia, disorganization, and automatic obedience. It may be identical to myriachit.

la•tan•o•prost (lə-tan′o-prost″) an antiglaucoma agent applied topically to the conjunctiva in the treatment of open-angle glaucoma and ocular hypertension.

La•tar•jet nerve (lah-tahr-zha′) [André *Latarjet*, French anatomist, 1877–1947] see under *nerve*.

Lat. dol. [L.] lat′eri dolen′ti (to the painful side).

lat•e•bra (lat′ə-brə) [L. "hiding place"] a flask-shaped mass of white yolk extending from the blastodisc to the center of eggs such as those of birds.

la•ten•cy (la′tən-se) 1. a state of seeming inactivity or being latent. 2. the time between the instant of stimulation and the beginning

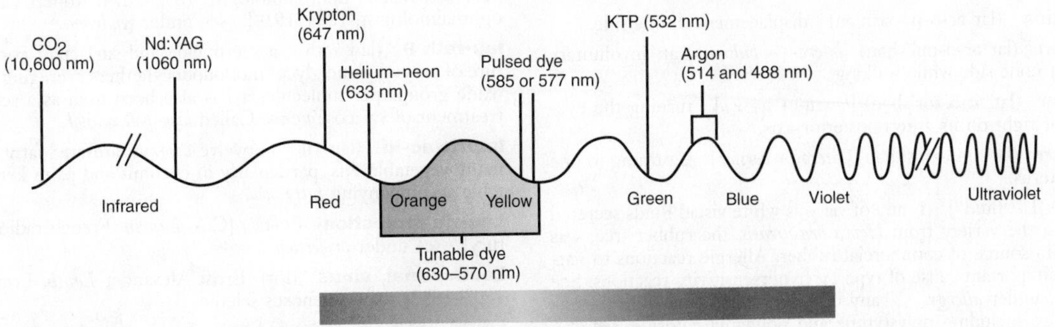

■ Relative positions of various types of lasers on the electromagnetic spectrum.

of a response; called also *latent period* and *conduction time.* 3. see under *stage.*

l. of activation the time between initiation of an electrical stimulus and depolarization of a nerve fiber to begin conduction along the axon; called also *utilization time.*

distal l. the motor or sensory latency measured from a site of stimulation as near as possible to the recording electrodes, i.e., to the terminal end of the nerve. Called also *terminal l.*

motor l. the time between initiation of a stimulus and onset of a resultant compound muscle action potential; see also *distal l., proximal l.,* and *residual l.*

proximal l. the motor or sensory latency measured from a site of stimulation as far as possible from the recording electrodes, i.e., from the terminal end of the nerve.

REM l. a 70- to 100-minute period of NREM sleep that precedes the first period of REM sleep.

residual l. the time difference between the observed distal latency of a motor nerve and the distal latency that was predicted based on conduction velocity measured in a segment of nerve near the stimulating electrode; it is due to factors slowing conduction such as decreased diameter of fine terminal axon branches, synaptic delay at the neuromuscular junction, and presence of unmyelinated segments.

sensory l. the time between initiation of a stimulus and onset of a resultant compound sensory nerve action potential; see also *distal l.* and *proximal l.*

sleep l. the period between the time a person lies down to rest and the onset of sleep.

terminal l. distal l.

la·tent (la′tənt) [L. *latens* hidden] concealed; not manifest; potential; dormant; quiescent.

la·ten·ti·a·tion (la-ten″she-a′shən) the process of making latent; in pharmacology, the chemical modification of a biologically active compound to affect its absorption, distribution, etc., the modified compound being transformed after administration to the active compound by biological processes.

lat·er·ad (lat′ər-ad) toward a side or a lateral aspect.

lat·er·al (lat′ər-əl) [L. *lateralis*] 1. denoting a position farther from the median plane or midline of the body or of a structure. 2. pertaining to a side.

lat·er·a·lis (lat″ər-a′lis) [TA] lateral: a term denoting a structure situated farther from the median plane of the body or the midline of an organ.

lat·er·al·i·ty (lat″ər-al′ĭ-te) either dextrality or sinistrality, a preference to use one side of the body in voluntary motor acts; see also *cerebral dominance* and *lateral dominance,* under *dominance.*

crossed l. the preferential use, in voluntary motor acts, of contralateral members of the different pairs of organs, as the right eye and the left hand.

dominant l. lateral dominance.

latero- [L. *latus,* gen. *lateris* side] a combining form denoting relationship to the side.

lat·ero·ab·do·mi·nal (lat″ər-o-ab-dom′ĭ-nəl) pertaining to the side of the abdomen.

lat·ero·co·nal (lat″ər-o-ko′nəl) [*lateral* + *conal*] lateral to one structure and adjacent to a conus; see under fascia.

lat·ero·de·vi·a·tion (lat″ər-o-de″ve-a′shən) deviation or slight displacement to one side.

lat·ero·dor·sal (lat″ər-o-dor′səl) denoting a position farther from the median plane or midline of the body or of a structure and more toward the back surface.

lat·ero·duc·tion (lat″ər-o-duk′shən) [*latero-* + *duction*] movement of an eye to one side.

lat·ero·flex·ion (lat″ər-o-flek′shən) flexion to either side.

lat·ero·po·si·tion (lat″ər-o-pə-zish′ən) displacement to one side.

lat·ero·pul·sion (lat″ər-o-pul′shən) [*latero-* + *pulsion*] an involuntary tendency to go to one side while walking.

lat·ero·tor·sion (lat″ər-o-tor′shən) [*latero-* + *torsion*] turning the eyeball to the left or right on its anteroposterior axis.

lat·ero·ver·sion (lat″ər-o-vur′zhən) [*latero-* + *version*] a turning to one side, as of the uterus.

la·tex (la′teks) [L. "fluid"] 1. any of various white viscid fluids secreted by certain plants; the variety from *Hevea brasiliensis,* the rubber tree, was formerly the main source of commercial rubber. Allergic reactions to natural latex are an important cause of type IV hypersensitivity reactions. See also *latex allergy,* under *allergy.* 2. any of several synthetic fluids resembling natural latex, including polystyrene and polyvinyl chloride; see also *latex agglutination test* under *tests.*

La·tham circle (la′thəm) [Peter Mere *Latham,* English physician, 1789–1875] see under *circle.*

lath·y·rism (lath′ə-riz-əm) a morbid condition seen after excessive ingestion of seeds of the genus *Lathyrus,* which contain β-aminopropionitrile, an inhibitor of the enzyme lysyl oxidase; symptoms include spastic paraplegia, pain, hyperesthesia, and paresthesia. Cf. *lupinosis* and *osteolathyrism.* **lathyrit′ic** *adj*

lath·y·ro·gen (lath′ə-ro-jən) any agent that causes lathyrism.

lath·y·ro·gen·ic (lath″ə-ro-jen′ik) capable of producing the symptoms characteristic of lathyrism.

Lath·y·rus (lath′ə-rəs) [Gr. *lathyros* chickling vetch] a genus of plants of the family Leguminosae. It includes varieties of peas, as well as herbs used as forage for livestock; excessive consumption of some species causes lathyrism.

la·tis·si·mus (lə-tis′ĭ-məs) [L.] widest: a general term denoting a broad structure, as a muscle.

lat·ro·dec·tism (lat″ro-dek′tiz-əm) [*Latrodectus* + *-ism*] intoxication caused by venom of spiders of the genus *Latrodectus.*

Lat·ro·dec·tus (lat″ro-dek′təs) [L. *latro* robber + Gr. *daknein* to bite] a genus of poisonous spiders. *L. mac′tans* is the black widow spider of the United States; *L. bisho′pi* is found in southern Florida; *L. curarien′sis* in Brazil and Argentina; *L. geomet′ricus* in California and southern Florida; *L. hassel′tii* in New Zealand; *L. lugu′bris* is the kara-kurt of Russia; *L. macula′tus* is found in South Africa; *L. malmigniat′tus* in Europe; and *L. tredecimgutta′tus* in southern Europe and Asiatic Russia.

LATS long-acting thyroid stimulator.

LATS-p [*l*ong-*a*cting *t*hyroid *s*timulator] see under *protector.*

lat·tice (lat′is) 1. a framework of regularly placed, intersecting narrow strips. 2. space l.

crystal l. space l.

space l. the regular, three-dimensional geometrical arrangement of atoms in a crystal; called also *lattice* and *crystal l.*

la·tus[1] (la′təs) [L.] broad, wide.

la·tus[2] (la′təs) gen. *la′teris* pl. *la′tera* [L.] [TA] flank: the side of the body between the ribs and the pelvis. Called also *regio lateralis* [TA alternative].

Latz·ko cesarean section (lahts′ko) [Wilhelm *Latzko,* Austrian obstetrician, 1863–1945] see *cesarean section,* under *section.*

Lau·ber disease (lou′bər) [Hans *Lauber,* Swiss-born ophthalmologist in Austria, 1876–1952] fundus albipunctatus; see under *fundus.*

laud·a·ble (lawd′ə-bəl) [L. *laudabilis*] commendable; healthy; see under *pus.*

lau·da·num (law′də-nəm) opium tincture.

laugh·ter (laf′tər) a series of spasmodic and partly involuntary exhalations with inarticulate vocalization, normally indicative of merriment; it may also be a hysteric manifestation or a reflex result of tickling. See also *gelasmus* and *risus.*

Lau·gier hernia, sign (lo″zhe-a′) [Stanislas *Laugier,* French surgeon, 1799–1872] see under *hernia* and *sign.*

Lau·mo·nier ganglion (lo-mo-nya′) [Jean Baptiste Philippe Nicolas René *Laumonier,* French surgeon, 1749–1818] carotid ganglion.

Lau·nois syndrome (lo-nwah′) [Pierre-Emile *Launois,* French physician, 1856–1914] see under *syndrome.*

Lau·nois-Ben·saude syndrome (lo-nwah′ bah-sōd′) [P.-E. *Launois;* Raoul *Bensaude,* French physician, 1866–1938] multiple symmetric lipomatosis; see under *lipomatosis.*

lau·rate (law′rāt) a salt, ester, or anionic form of lauric acid.

Lau·rence-Moon syndrome (law′rəns mo͞on′) [John Zachariah *Laurence,* British ophthalmologist, 1830–1874; Robert C. *Moon,* American ophthalmologist, 1844–1914] see under *syndrome.*

lau·reth 9 (law′rəth) a spermicide and surfactant consisting of a mixture of polyethylene glycol monododecyl ethers averaging about 9 ethylene oxide groups per molecule; it has also been used as a sclerosing agent in treatment of varicose veins. Called also *polidocanol.*

lau·ric ac·id (law′rik) a twelve-carbon saturated fatty acid occurring in many vegetable fats, particularly in coconut and palm kernel oils. See also table accompanying *fatty acid.*

Lau·rin projection (lo-ră′) [C.A. *Laurin,* French radiologist, 20th century] see under *projection.*

Lauth canal, sinus (lōt) [Ernst Alexander *Lauth,* French physiologist, 1803–1837] sinus venosus sclerae.

Lauth ligament (lōt) [Thomas *Lauth,* French anatomist and surgeon, 1758–1826] ligamentum transversum atlantis.

Lauth violet (lawth) [Charles *Lauth*, English chemist, 1836–1913] thionine.

LAV lymphadenopathy-associated virus; see *human immunodeficiency virus*, under *virus*.

la·vage (lah-vahzh') [Fr.] 1. the irrigation of an organ, such as the stomach or bowel. 2. to wash out, or irrigate.
  bronchoalveolar l. a technique by which cells and fluid from bronchioles and lung alveoli are removed for diagnosis of disease or evaluation of treatment; a bronchoscope is wedged into a bronchus and sterile saline is pumped in and then removed along with the fluid and cells to be analyzed.
  peritoneal l. lavage of the peritoneal cavity for diagnostic purposes or to combat infection.
  pleural l. irrigation of the pleural cavity to assess for presence of malignant or otherwise abnormal cells.

La·van·du·la (lə-van'du-lə) [L.] the lavenders, a genus of Eurasian plants of the family Labiatae, having spicate flowers. *L. angustifo'lia*, subsp. *angustifo'lia* has flowers that contain lavender oil.

lav·en·der (lav'ən-dər) 1. any plant of the genus *Lavandula.* 2. a preparation of the flowers of *L. angustifolia* subsp. *angustifolia* or of the essential oil (lavender oil) extracted from them; used internally for loss of appetite, dyspepsia, nervousness, and insomnia; it is also widely used in folk medicine.

la·veur (lah-voor') [Fr.] an instrument for performing lavage or irrigation.

LAVH laparoscopically assisted vaginal hysterectomy.

law (law) 1. a uniform or constant fact or principle. Cf. *rule.* 2. in statistics, a synonym for *distribution;* for entries not found here, see under *distribution.*

Law

Allen's l. whereas in normal individuals the more sugar is given the more is utilized, the reverse is true in diabetics.
all-or-none l. see *all or none.*
Ångström's l. the wavelengths of the light absorbed by a substance are the same as those given off by it when luminous.
Aran's l. fractures of the base of the skull (except those by contrecoup) result from injuries to the vault, the fractures extending by radiation along the line of shortest circle.
Arndt's l., Arndt-Schulz l. weak stimuli increase physiologic activity, moderate stimuli inhibit activity, and very strong stimuli abolish activity. See also *hormesis.*
l's of articulation a set of rules to be followed in arranging teeth to produce a balanced articulation.
Avogadro's l. equal volumes of all perfect gases at the same temperature and pressure contain the same number of molecules or, in the case of monatomic gases, of atoms.
Baer's l. the more general features common to all members of a group of animals are developed in the embryo earlier than more special features that distinguish members of the group from one another. This concept is the predecessor of the recapitulation theory.
Barfurth's l. the axis of the tissue in a regenerating structure is at first perpendicular to the cut.
Bastian's l., Bastian-Bruns l. if there is a complete transverse lesion in the spinal cord cephalad to the lumbar enlargement, the tendon reflexes of the lower extremities are abolished.
Beer's l., Beer-Lambert l. the absorbance *(A)* of a solution is directly proportional to the length of the light path *(b)* and the concentration *(c);* the proportionality constant is the molar absorptivity (ε); thus $A = \varepsilon bc$. The absorptivity is independent of the concentration and is thus a property of the solute and solvent. Beer's law generally holds only up to a certain concentration, above which the relation between concentration and absorbance becomes nonlinear.
Behring's l. the blood and serum of an immunized person, when transferred to another subject, will render the latter immune.
Bergonié-Tribondeau l. the sensitivity of cells to radiation varies directly with the reproductive capacity of the cells and inversely with their degree of differentiation.
Bowditch's l. all-or-none l.; see *all or none.*
Boyle's l. at a constant temperature the volume of a perfect gas varies inversely as the pressure, and the pressure varies inversely as the volume.
Bunsen-Roscoe l. the photochemical effect produced is equal to the product of the intensity of the illumination and the duration of exposure.
Camerer's l. children of the same weight have the same food requirements regardless of their ages.
Charles' l. at a constant pressure the volume of a given mass of perfect gas varies directly with the absolute temperature.
l. of conservation of energy in any given system the amount of energy is constant; energy is neither created nor destroyed, but only transformed from one form to another.
l. of conservation of mass mass (or matter) can be neither created nor destroyed; this law can be violated on the microscopic level.
Cope's l. genera with little specialization originate many types of organisms; highly specialized genera produce but few biological variations.
Coulomb's l. the force of attraction or repulsion between two electrified bodies is proportional directly to the quantities of electric charge, and inversely as the square of their distance apart.
Courvoisier's l. when the common bile duct is obstructed by a stone, dilatation of the gallbladder is rare; when the duct is obstructed in some other way, dilatation is common. See also under *sign.*
Coutard's l. in radiotherapy, the point of origin of a mucous membrane tumor is the last site to heal following irradiation.
l's of cure in homeopathy, the cure of a disease moves in four general directions: from above downward, from inside outward, from more vital to less vital organs, and in reverse order of symptom appearance.
Curie's l. all substances may be rendered radioactive by the influence of the emanations of radium, and substances thus influenced hold their radioactivity longer when enclosed in some material through which the emanations cannot pass.
Dalton's l. the pressure exerted by a mixture of nonreacting gases is equal to the sum of the partial pressures of the separate components; it holds true only at very low pressures.
Dalton-Henry l. when a fluid absorbs a mixture of gases, it will absorb as much of each gas as it would have absorbed if the gas were present alone.
l. of definite proportions any compound always contains the same kind of elements in the same proportions; called also *Proust's l.*
Descartes' l. the sine of the angle of incidence bears a constant relation to the sine of the angle of refraction for two given media. Called also *l. of sines* and *Snell's l.*
Desmarres' l. when the visual axes are crossed the images are uncrossed; when the axes are uncrossed (diverging) the images are crossed. Useful in determining presence of esophoria and exophoria and of esotropia and exotropia. See also *direct* and *crossed diplopia.*
Dollo's l. phyletic development is irreversible, i.e., reversion to an ancestral peculiarity (atavism) is impossible.
Donders' l. the rotation of the eye around the line of sight is not voluntary; when attention is fixed upon a remote object, the amount of rotation is determined entirely by the angular distance of the object from the median plane and from the horizon.
Draper's l. only the rays that are absorbed by a photochemical substance will produce a chemical change in it.
Dulong and Petit's l. the atomic heat capacity, the product of the atomic weight and the specific heat per gram, is constant for most elements; boron, carbon, and silicon are notable exceptions at normal temperatures.
Einthoven's l. if electrocardiograms are taken simultaneously with the three leads, at any given instant the potential in lead II is equal to the sum of the potentials in leads I and III.
Ewald's l. vestibular nystagmus resulting from endolymph currents in a semicircular canal is in a direction parallel with the plane of that canal and opposite to the current; vestibular nystagmus caused by currents in horizontal canals is primarily from canals whose hair cells are bent towards the utricle.
Fajans' l. the product left after the emission of alpha rays has a valence less by two than that of the parent radioactive substance; the product left after the emission of beta rays has a valence greater by one than that of the parent radioactive substance.
Faraday's l. 1. the amount of a chemical reaction produced by an electric current passed through a cell is proportional to the amount of charge passed. 2. the extent of dissolution or decomposition of electrolytes produced by the same electric current is proportional to their equivalent weights.
Farr's l. "subsidence is a property of all zymotic diseases": the curve that represents the incidence of new cases in an epidemic ascends

rapidly at first, then gradually levels off to a maximum, and finally descends more rapidly than it ascended, thus approximating a bell-shaped curve.
l. of fatigue when the same muscle or group of muscles is kept in constant action until fatigue sets in, the total work done, multiplied by the rate of work, is constant.
Ferry-Porter l. critical fusion frequency is directly proportional to the logarithm of the light intensity.
Fick's first l. of diffusion a substance will diffuse through an area at a rate which is dependent upon the difference in concentration of the substance at two given points.
first l. of thermodynamics see *l's of thermodynamics.*
Flatau's l. the greater the length of the fibers of the spinal cord, the closer are they situated to the periphery.
Flint's l. the ontogeny of an organ is the phylogeny of its blood supply.
Flourens' l. stimulation of the semicircular canal causes nystagmus in the plane of that canal.
Frank-Starling l. Starling's l.
Froriep's l. the skull is developed by the annexation of true vertebrae, the head growing at the expense of the neck.
Galton's l. of regression individuals who exhibit an extreme value of some variable, e.g., extreme tallness, produce offspring who on average tend to exhibit less extreme values of that variable, being somewhat closer to the mean value than are their parents.
gas l. ideal gas l.
Gay-Lussac's l. 1. a modification of Charles' law, adding that, at constant temperature and pressure, the ratio of the volumes of two gases that react with each other is always a small whole number. 2. sometimes used synonymously with *Charles' l.*
Gerhardt-Semon l. various peripheral and central lesions affecting the recurrent laryngeal nerve cause the vocal cord to assume a position between abduction and adduction, the paralysis of the parts being incomplete.
Giraud-Teulon l. binocular retinal images are formed at the intersection of the primary and secondary axes of projection.
Gompertz's l. at advanced ages the risk of dying increases geometrically with age: the death rate at age x may be computed by the formula $q_x = q_0 \cdot e \cdot a^x$, where q_x is the death rate at age x, q_0 is the death rate at age 0, and a is a constant. From middle age on, actual death rates closely approximate the curve that corresponds to this formula.
Goodell's l. see under *sign.*
Graham's l. the rate of diffusion of a gas through porous membranes is in inverse ratio to the square root of their density.
l. of gravitation all bodies attract each other with a force that is directly proportional to their masses and inversely proportional to the square of their distance apart; called also *Newton's l.*
Grotthus' l., Grotthus-Draper l. only those rays of ultraviolet light that are absorbed produce a chemical effect upon the absorbing substance.
Gudden's l. the degeneration of the proximal end of a divided nerve is cellulipetal.
Guldberg and Waage's l. l. of mass action.
Gull-Toynbee l. in otitis media, the lateral sinus and cerebellum are liable to involvement in mastoid disease, and the cerebrum may be attacked when the roof of the tympanum becomes carious. Called also *Toynbee's l.*
Gullstrand's l. in strabismus, if the patient is made to turn the head while fixing a distant object, and the corneal reflex of either eye moves in the direction in which the head is turning, then the movement is toward the weaker muscle.
Haeckel's l. recapitulation theory.
Hanau's l's of articulation a set of purely physical laws that must be observed in the formation of the masticatory surfaces of natural dentition or dentures, to ensure establishment or production of balanced articulation.
Hardy-Weinberg l. the proportions of the three genotypes determined by two alleles (*A* and *a*) occurring with a frequency of p and q, respectively, in a randomly mating population will remain constant from one generation to the next: $AA = p^2$, $Aa = 2pq$, $aa = q^2$. Factors such as mutation, selection, nonrandom mating, migration, and genetic drift can disturb this equilibrium. Called also *Hardy-Weinberg principle* or *rule.*
l. of the heart Starling's l. of the heart.
Heidenhain's l. glandular secretion always involves change in the structure of the gland.
Hellin's l., Hellin-Zeleny l. one in about 89 pregnancies results in the birth of twins; one in 89 × 89, or 7921, of triplets; one in 89 × 89 × 89, or 704,969, of quadruplets.
Henry's l. the solubility of a gas in a liquid solution at constant temperature is proportional to the partial pressure of the gas above the solution.
Hering's l. 1. the principle of bilateral ocular innervation; equal innervation is sent to the muscles of the two eyes so that one eye is never moved independently of the other. 2. the clearness or purity of any sensation depends on the proportion between its intensity and the total of the intensities of all the simultaneous sensations.
Hoff's l. van't Hoff's l.
ideal gas l. the equation of state for an ideal gas: $PV = nRT$, where P is pressure, V volume, n the number of moles of gas, R the gas constant, and T the absolute temperature. It holds approximately for real gases at low pressures and high temperatures.
l. of independent assortment see *Mendel's l's.*
inverse square l. the intensity of radiation is inversely proportional to the square of the distance between a point source and the irradiated surface.
isodynamic l. in the production of heat in the body the different foodstuffs are interchangeable in accordance with their heat-producing values.
Jackson's l. the nerve functions that are latest developed are the first to be lost when the brain is damaged by disease; called also *Jackson's rule.*
Kahler's l. the ascending branches of the posterior roots of the spinal nerves pass within the cord in succession from the root zone toward the mesial plane.
Knapp's l. there should be no difference in retinal image size in the correction of spherical axial anisometropia, provided that the lenses are placed at the anterior focal point of the eye.
Koch's l. see under *postulate.*
Küstner's l. if an ovarian tumor is left-sided, torsion of its pedicle takes place toward the right; if right-sided, toward the left.
Lambert's cosine l. the intensity of radiation on an absorbing surface varies as the cosine of the angle of incidence for parallel rays.
Laplace's l. tension or stress on the cardiac ventricular walls is proportional to the intraventricular pressure and internal radius and inversely proportional to the wall thickness; for a sphere it is most simply expressed as: average circumferential wall stress = (pressure × radius of curvature of the wall) ÷ (2 × wall thickness); more complex equations describe ellipsoidal or other shapes.
l. of large numbers any of several theorems dealing with the convergence of the sample average to the population mean as the sample size is increased.
Listing's l. when the eyeball is moved from a resting position, the rotational angle in the second position is the same as if the eye were turned about a fixed axis perpendicular to the previous and new positions of the visual line (axis opticus; see under *axis*).
malthusian l. the hypothesis that population tends to outrun the means available to sustain it.
Marey's l. as the blood pressure rises, the pulse rate slows. See also *baroreceptor.*
Mariotte's l. Boyle's l.
mass l., l. of mass action the rate of a chemical reaction at constant temperature is proportional to the concentrations of the reacting substances; called also *Guldberg and Waage's l.*
Maxwell-Boltzmann distribution l. a method for calculating the relative number of molecules in a given population which possess a given amount of velocity or energy.
Mendel's l's two laws of inheritance of single-gene traits described by Gregor Mendel, derived from data obtained from his experimental crosses of pea plants; now usually expressed as the *law of segregation* (the members of a pair of allelic genes segregate from one another and pass to different gametes) and the *law of independent assortment* (genes that are not alleles are distributed to the gametes independently of one another).
Mendeleev's (Mendeléef's, Mendeléeff's) l. periodic l.
mendelian l's Mendel's l's.
Meyer's l. the internal structure of fully developed normal bone represents the lines of greatest pressure or traction and affords the greatest possible resistance with the least possible amount of material.
Minot's l. organisms age fastest when young.

Law *Continued*

l. of multiple proportions when two elements combine to form two or more different compounds, the weights of one compound that can combine with a given weight of the second compound form small whole number ratios.
Nernst's l. the current required to stimulate muscle action varies as the square root of its frequency.
Neumann's l. the molecular heat in compounds of analogous constitution is always the same.
Newton's l. l. of gravitation.
Nysten's l. rigor mortis affects first the muscles of mastication, next those of the face and neck, then those of the upper trunk and arms, and last of all those of the legs and feet.
Ohm's l. the strength of an electric current varies directly as the electromotive force and inversely as the resistance.
Ollier's l. in the case of two parallel bones which are joined at their extremities by ligaments, arrest of growth in one of them involves growth disturbance in the other.
Pajot's l. a solid body contained within another body having smooth walls will tend to conform to the shape of those walls; this law governs the rotating movements of the fetus during labor.
Pascal's l. pressure applied to a liquid at any point is transmitted equally in all directions.
periodic l. if the elements are arranged in the sequence of their atomic numbers, they fall into distinctive periods of 2, 8, 8, 18, 18, and 32 elements; see also *periodic table*, under *table.* Called also *Mendeleev's l.*
Petit's l. Dulong and Petit's l.
Pitres' l. in acquired aphasia with a multilingual patient, recovery comes first and most completely in the language most used just before the injury, whether or not it is the patient's mother tongue. Called also *Pitres' rule.* See also *Ribot's l.*
Poiseuille's l. an equation describing the volume flow rate *(F)* of a liquid through a capillary tube:

$$F = \frac{P\pi R^4}{8\eta L},$$

where P is the pressure drop along the tube, R is the radius and L the length of the tube, and η is the viscosity of the fluid.
Prévost's l. in a lateral cerebral lesion the head is turned toward the side involved.
Proust's l. l. of definite proportions.
Raoult's l. the partial pressure of a volatile component of an ideal solution is equal to the mole fraction of that substance in solution times its vapor pressure in the pure state at the temperature of the solution; it is true only for ideal solutions and ideal gases.
l. of reciprocal innervation Sherrington's l. (def. 2).
l. of reciprocal proportions two chemical elements that unite with a third element do so in proportions that are multiples of those in which they unite with each other.
l. of referred pain referred pain only arises from irritation of nerves which are sensitive to those stimuli that produce pain when applied to the surface of the body.
l. of refraction rays of light passing from a rarer to a denser medium are deflected toward a perpendicular to the surface of incidence, whereas rays passing from a denser to a rarer medium are deflected away from the perpendicular. Cf. *Descartes' l.*
l. of regression Galton's l. of regression.
Ribot's l. a law stating that in a multilingual patient with aphasia, recovery comes first in the person's mother tongue. This has been found to be true only in patients who are not truly fluent in the subsequently acquired language or languages. See also *Pitres' l.*
Ricco's l. for small images, the product of the area of illumination and the intensity of illumination is constant for the threshold of detection of a light stimulus, expressed by the formula $LA=C$, where L is the threshold intensity, A is the area of illumination, and C is a constant.
Rosa's l. the possibilities of phyletic variation in an organism decrease in proportion to the extent of its development.
Rubner's l. 1. *(law of constant energy consumption)* the rapidity of growth is proportional to the intensity of the metabolic process. 2. *(law of constant growth quotient)* the same fractional part of the entire energy is utilized for growth; this fractional part is called the *growth quotient.*
Schroeder van der Kolk's l. the sensory fibers of a mixed nerve are distributed to the parts moved by muscles which are stimulated by the motor fibers of the same nerve.
second l. of thermodynamics see *l's of thermodynamics.*
l. of segregation see *Mendel's l's.*
Sherrington's l. 1. every posterior spinal nerve root supplies a special region of the skin, although fibers from adjacent spinal segments may invade such a region. 2. when a muscle receives a nerve impulse to contract, its antagonist receives simultaneously an impulse to relax; see *reciprocal innervation*, under *innervation.*
l. of similars in homeopathy, the principle that a substance that in large doses will produce symptoms of a specific disease will, in extremely small doses, cure the disease.
l. of sines Descartes' l.
Snell's l. Descartes' l.
Spallanzani's l. the law that regeneration is more complete in younger individuals than in older ones.
Starling's l., Starling's l. of the heart the energy liberated with each contraction of the heart is a function of the length of the fibers composing its muscular walls; increased preload causes increased end-diastolic volume (or pressure), which increases the force of ventricular contraction. Called also *Frank-Starling l.* or *mechanism.*
Stokes' l. a muscle situated above an inflamed membrane is often affected with paralysis.
surface l. at constant temperature, the heat production, heat loss, and oxygen consumption in an animal are inversely proportional to the free surface or to the square of a linear dimension.
Talbot's l. when complete fusion occurs and the sensation is uniform, the intensity is the same as would occur were the same amount of light spread uniformly over the disk.
Teevan's l. fractures of bones occur in the line of extension and not in the line of compression.
l's of thermodynamics *zeroth law:* two systems in thermal equilibrium with a third system are in thermal equilibrium with each other. *First law:* energy is conserved in any process; i.e., the energy gained (or lost) by a system is exactly equal to the energy lost (or gained) by the surroundings. *Second law:* there is always an increase in entropy in any naturally occurring (spontaneous) process. *Third law:* absolute zero is unattainable.
third l. of thermodynamics see *l's of thermodynamics.*
Toynbee's l. Gull-Toynbee l.
van der Kolk's l. Schroeder van der Kolk's l.
van't Hoff's l. 1. a substance in solution exerts an osmotic pressure equal to the gas pressure that it would exert if its molecules were in a gaseous state and occupied a volume equal to that of the solution under the same conditions of temperature and pressure. 2. van't Hoff rule.
Virchow's l. the cell elements of tumors are derived from normal and preexisting tissue cells.
Walton's l. l. of reciprocal proportions.
Weigert's l. loss or destruction of elements in the organic world is apt to be followed by overproduction of such elements in the reparative process.
Weigert-Meyer l. see under *rule.*
Wolff's l. a bone, normal or abnormal, develops the structure most suited to resist the forces acting upon it.
Wundt-Lamansky l. the line of vision in moving through a vertical plane parallel to the frontal plane moves in straight lines in the vertical and horizontal directions but in curved paths in all other movements.
Yerkes-Dodson l. as anxiety level increases, task performance is enhanced at first, but after a given point is reached, further anxiety causes declining performance.
zeroth l. of thermodynamics see *l's of thermodynamics.*

lawn (lawn, lahn) an area sown with a thick growth of a living substance.
bacterial l. the confluent blanket of merged colonies resulting from plating a concentrated bacterial solution.

Law·rence-Seip syndrome (law′rəns sīp′) [Robert Daniel *Lawrence*, English physician, 1912–1964; Martin Fredrik *Seip*, Norwegian pediatrician, born 1921] total lipodystrophy; see under *lipodystrophy.*

law•ren•ci•um (Lr) (law-ren′se-əm) [Ernest Orlando *Lawrence*, American physicist, 1901–1958; builder of the first cyclotron for the production of high-energy particles and winner of the Nobel prize for physics in 1939] the chemical element of atomic number 103, atomic weight 257; produced in 1961 by bombardment of californium isotopes of mass 250, 251, and 252.

law•sone (law′sōn) a dye isolated from the leaves of *Lawsonia inermis*, used topically as a sunscreen.

Law•so•nia[1] (law-so′ne-ə) a genus of tropical Old World shrubs of the family Lythraceae. *L. iner′mis* is the source of lawsone and henna.

Law•so•nia[2] (law-so′ne-ə) a genus of gram-negative, rod-shaped bacteria of the family Desulfovibrionaceae; organisms are non–spore-forming, motile, microaerobic, and obligately intracellular. The type species is *L. intracellula′ris*.

L. intracellula′ris a species that is the cause of porcine proliferative enteritis.

lax•a•tion (lak-sa′shən) defecation (def. 2).

lax•a•tive (lak′sə-tiv) [L. *laxativus*] 1. mildly cathartic. 2. an agent that acts to promote defecation; see also *cathartic*. Called also *aperient* and *aperitive*.

bulk l., bulk-forming l. a hydrophilic agent that promotes evacuation of the bowel by absorbing water and expanding, thus increasing the volume of the feces.

contact l. a laxative that increases the motor activity of the intestinal tract; the precise mechanism of action of contact laxatives is unknown, but they produce an accumulation of fluid and electrolytes in the colon and are thought to increase peristalsis by stimulating intramural nerve plexuses. Called also *stimulant l.*

lubricant l. an agent, immiscible with water, that promotes softening of the stool and facilitates the passage of feces through the intestines by its lubricant effect.

saline l. a salt, of which one or both ions are poorly absorbed, administered in hypertonic solution to draw water into the intestinal lumen by osmosis; the resulting distention promotes increased peristalsis and evacuation.

stimulant l. contact l.

lax•i•ty (lak′sĭ-te) [L. *laxare* to loosen] 1. slackness or looseness; a lack of tautness, firmness, or rigidity. 2. slackness or displacement (whether normal or abnormal) in the motion of a joint. Cf. *hypermobility*.

lay•er (la′ər) 1. a stratum or lamina; a sheetlike mass of substance of nearly uniform thickness, several of which may be superimposed, one above another. 2. a female bird of the age when it is laying eggs.

Layer

For descriptions of specific anatomic structures not listed here, see under *lamina* and *stratum*.

adamantine l. dental enamel.
adventitial l. tunica adventitia.
alar l. of deep cervical fascia alar fascia.
ameloblastic l. the inner layer of cells of the enamel organ, created by its invagination, which forms the enamel prisms.
l's of Ammon's horn strata hippocampi.
anterior l. of thoracolumbar fascia lamina anterior fasciae thoracolumbalis.
arachnoid barrier cell l. the outer layer of the cranial and spinal arachnoid mater, immediately internal to the dura mater and loosely attached to the dural border cell layer by occasional cell junctions. Its cells have tightly apposed cell membranes and are connected to each other via numerous tight junctions, effectively forming a barrier to fluid movement.
bacillary l. l. of rods and cones.
basal cell l. stratum basale of epidermis.
basal l. of choroid lamina basalis choroideae.
basal l. of endometrium stratum basale of endometrium.
basal l. of epidermis stratum basale of epidermis.
basement l. see under *membrane*.
Bechterew l., Bekhterev l. Kaes-Bekhterev l.
blastodermic l. germ l.
Bowman l. lamina limitans anterior corneae.
Bruch l. lamina basalis choroideae.
buffy l. see under *coat*.
capillary l. of choroid lamina choroidocapillaris.
l's of cerebral cortex six anatomical divisions of the cerebral cortex (specifically, the *isocortex*), distinguished according to the types of cells and fibers they contain. Numbered from the surface inward, they are: I, molecular layer *(lamina molecularis)*; II, external granular layer *(lamina granularis externa)*; III, external pyramidal layer *(lamina pyramidalis externa)*; IV, internal granular layer *(lamina granularis interna)*; V, internal pyramidal layer *(lamina pyramidalis interna)*; and VI, multiform layer *(lamina multiformis)*. In official terminology, called *strata isocorticis*. See illustration.
Chievitz l. a transient fiber layer separating the inner and outer neuroblastic layers of the optic cup.
choriocapillary l. lamina choroidocapillaris.
circular l. of detrusor stratum circulare musculi detrusoris vesicae.
circular l. of muscular coat of colon stratum circulare tunicae muscularis coli.
circular l. of muscular coat of female urethra stratum circulare tunicae muscularis urethrae femininae.
circular l. of muscular coat of prostatic urethra stratum circulare tunicae muscularis partis prostaticae urethrae.
circular l. of muscular coat of rectum stratum circulare tunicae muscularis recti.
circular l. of muscular coat of small intestine stratum circulare tunicae muscularis intestini tenuis.
circular l. of muscular coat of stomach stratum circulare tunicae muscularis gastricae.
circular l. of tympanic membrane stratum circulare of tympanic membrane.
clear l. of epidermis stratum lucidum of epidermis.
columnar l. mantle l.
compact l. of endometrium the sublayer of the endometrial stratum functionale on the surface facing the interior of the uterus, containing the necks of the uterine glands.
corneal l., cornified l. stratum corneum.
cortical l. the cortex of an organ, as of the brain or kidney.
cutaneous l. of tympanic membrane stratum cutaneum of tympanic membrane.
cuticular l. a striate border of modified cytoplasm at the free end of some columnar cells.
deep l's of cervical fascia, l's of deep cervical fascia the three internal layers of cervical fascia (investing, pretracheal, and prevertebral) and the carotid sheath, considered as one unit.
deep gray l. of superior colliculus stratum griseum profundum colliculi superioris.
deep l. of levator palpebrae superioris lamina profunda musculi levatoris palpebrae superioris.
deep l. of temporal fascia lamina profunda fasciae temporalis.
deep white l. of superior colliculus stratum medullare profundum colliculi superioris.
l's of dentate gyrus strata gyri dentati.

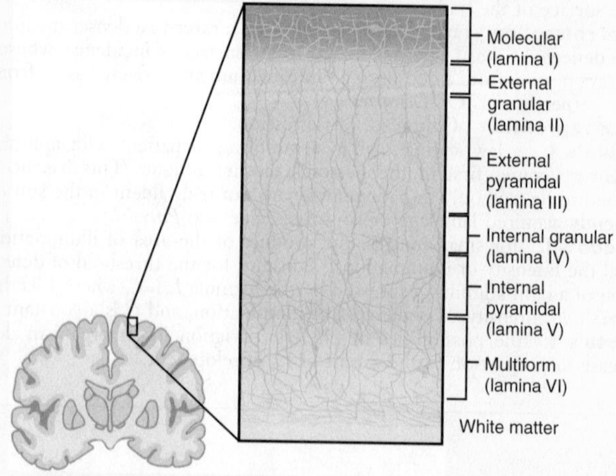

■ Coronal section through the isocortex, showing the six layers.

Dobie l. Z band.
ependymal l. the innermost layer of the wall of the primordial neural tube, bounding the central canal, which differentiates regionally into the roof plate and the floor plate.
episcleral l. lamina episcleralis.
epitrichial l. the most superficial layer of the epidermis of the embryo.
external granular l. of cerebral cortex lamina granularis externa.
external granular l. of olfactory bulb a thin layer between the glomerular layer and the molecular layer, containing periglomerular cells.
external limiting l. of retina external limiting membrane.
external longitudinal l. of detrusor stratum externum longitudinale musculi detrusoris vesicae.
external nuclear l. of retina outer nuclear l. of retina.
external plexiform l. of retina outer plexiform l. of retina.
external pyramidal l. of cerebral cortex lamina pyramidalis externa.
false l. a hen that behaves like a normal layer but does not lay eggs because of defective oviducts.
fatty l. of subcutaneous tissue of abdomen panniculus adiposus telae subcutaneae abdominis.
fibrous l. of articular capsule membrana fibrosa capsulae articularis.
fibrous l. of eyeball tunica fibrosa bulbi.
fibrous l. of fatty l. of subcutaneous tissue stratum fibrosum panniculi adiposi telae subcutaneae.
fibrous l. of tympanic membrane see under *stratum.*
Floegel l. a granular layer in each transparent lateral disk of a muscle fibril.
functional l. of endometrium stratum functionale.
fusiform l. of cerebral cortex lamina multiformis.
ganglion cell l. of retina a layer of the stratum nervosum retinae, situated between the inner plexiform layer and the nerve fiber layer, consisting essentially of the ganglion cells of the retina, and containing also the Müller fibers, neuroglia, and branches of the retinal vessels. In official terminology, called *stratum ganglionicum retinae* [TA]. See illustration at *retina.*
ganglionic l. of cerebellar cortex stratum purkinjense corticis cerebelli.
ganglionic l. of cerebral cortex lamina pyramidalis interna.
ganglionic l. of retina ganglion cell l.
gel l. the more gelatinous part of the tunica mucosa of the airways, overlying the sol layer.
germ l., germ cell l. any of the three primary layers of cells of the embryo (ectoderm, endoderm, and mesoderm), from which the tissues and organs develop. Called also *blastodermic l.*

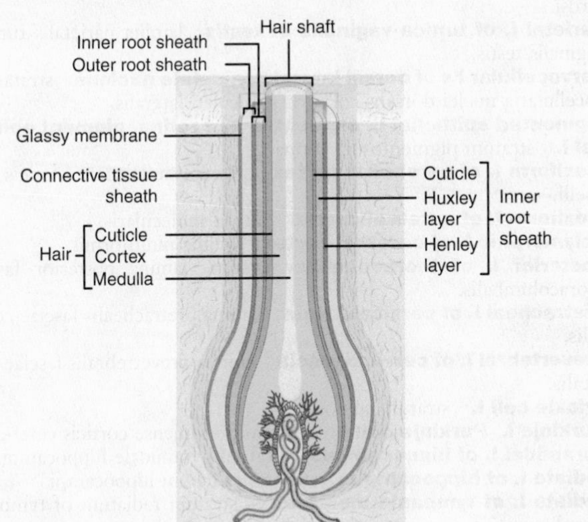

■ Henle and Huxley layers in the inner root sheath in a longitudinal section of a hair follicle.

germinative l. 1. stratum germinativum (def. 2). 2. stratum basale of epidermis.
glomerular l. the layer of the olfactory bulb between the olfactory nerve fiber layer and the external granular layer, containing the olfactory glomeruli.
granular l. of cerebellar cortex stratum granulosum corticis cerebelli.
granular l. of dentate gyrus stratum granulare gyri dentati.
granular l. of epidermis stratum granulosum of epidermis.
granular l. of follicle of ovary stratum granulosum of ovary.
granular l. of Tomes a layer of imperfectly calcified dentin made of small interglobular spaces immediately beneath the dentinocemental junction in the root of a tooth. Called also *Tomes granular l.*
granule l. the granular layer of the cerebral or cerebellar cortex.
half-value l. the thickness of a given substance that will reduce the intensity of a beam of radiation to one half of its initial value; called also *half-value thickness.* Abbreviated HVL.
Haller l. lamina vasculosa choroideae.
Henle l. the outer layer of cells of the inner root sheath of a hair follicle, lying between the outer root sheath and the Huxley layer. See illustration.
Henle fiber l. the outer plexiform layer in the region of the macula lutea; see also *entoretina.*
l's of hippocampus strata hippocampi.
Hopewell-Smith hyaline l. dentinocemental junction.
horny l. stratum corneum.
Huxley l. a layer of the inner root sheath of a hair follicle, lying between the Henle layer and the cuticle of the root sheath. See illustration.
inferior l. of pelvic diaphragm fascia inferior diaphragmatis pelvis.
inner enamel l. the inner, concave wall of the enamel organ.
inner l. of eyeball tunica interna bulbi.
inner l. of glomerular capsule visceral l. of glomerular capsule.
inner limiting l. of retina internal limiting membrane.
inner nuclear l. of retina the layer of the stratum nervosum retinae situated between the inner and outer plexiform layers, consisting essentially of the visual cells. In official terminology, called *stratum nucleare internum retinae* [TA]. See illustration at *retina.*
inner plexiform l. of retina the layer of the stratum nervosum retinae situated between the inner nuclear layer and the ganglion cell layer, consisting primarily of the arborization of the axons of the bipolar cells with the dendrites of the ganglion cells. In official terminology, called *stratum plexiforme internum retinae* [TA]. See illustration at *retina.*
intermediate gray l. of superior colliculus stratum griseum intermedium colliculi superioris.
intermediate white l. of superior colliculus stratum medullare intermedium colliculi superioris.
internal l. a hen whose eggs, usually deformed, are deposited into the abdominal cavity.
internal granular l. of cerebral cortex lamina granularis interna.
internal granular l. of olfactory bulb the innermost layer of the olfactory bulb, adjacent to the beginning of the olfactory tract; it consists of rows of axons from mitral and tufted cells alternating with rows of cell bodies and dendrites of granule cells.
internal limiting l. of retina internal limiting membrane.
internal longitudinal l. of detrusor stratum internum longitudinale musculi detrusoris vesicae.
internal nuclear l. of retina inner nuclear l. of retina.
internal plexiform l. of retina inner plexiform l. of retina.
internal pyramidal l. of cerebral cortex lamina pyramidalis interna.
investing l. fascia investiens.
investing l. of cervical fascia, investing l. of deep cervical fascia lamina superficialis fasciae cervicalis.
l's of isocortex l's of cerebral cortex.
Kaes-Bekhterev l. a thin layer of fibers on the border between the external granular layer and the external pyramidal layer of the cerebral cortex; called also *Bekhterev l.; Kaes feltwork, line,* or *stria; Kaes-Bekhterev stria;* and *Vicq d'Azyr band* or *stripe.*
koniocellular l. of dorsal lateral geniculate nucleus stratum koniocellulare nuclei dorsalis corporis geniculati lateralis.
lacunar-molecular l. of hippocampus stratum moleculare et substratum lacunosum hippocampi.
Langhans l. cytotrophoblast.

Layer *Continued*

longitudinal l. of muscular coat of colon stratum longitudinale tunicae muscularis coli.
longitudinal l. of muscular coat of female urethra stratum longitudinale tunicae muscularis urethrae femininae.
longitudinal l. of muscular coat of membranous urethra stratum longitudinale tunicae muscularis partis intermediae urethrae.
longitudinal l. of muscular coat of prostatic urethra stratum longitudinale tunicae muscularis partis prostaticae urethrae.
longitudinal l. of muscular coat of rectum stratum longitudinale tunicae muscularis recti.
longitudinal l. of muscular coat of small intestine stratum longitudinale tunicae muscularis intestini tenuis.
longitudinal l. of muscular coat of spongy urethra stratum longitudinale tunicae muscularis partis spongiosae urethrae.
longitudinal l. of muscular coat of stomach stratum longitudinale tunicae muscularis gastricae.
magnocellular l's of dorsal lateral geniculate nucleus strata magnocellularia nuclei dorsalis corporis geniculati lateralis.
malpighian l. stratum germinativum (def. 2).
mantle l. the middle layer of the wall of the primordial neural tube, containing primordial nerve cells and later forming the gray matter of the central nervous system.
marginal l. the outermost layer of the wall of the primordial neural tube, a fibrous mesh into which the nerve fibers later grow, forming the white matter of the central nervous system.
membranous l. of subcutaneous tissue stratum membranosum telae subcutaneae.
membranous l. of subcutaneous tissue of abdomen stratum membranosum telae subcutaneae abdominis.
membranous l. of subcutaneous tissue of perineum stratum membranosum telae subcutaneae perinei.
middle l. of deep cervical fascia lamina pretrachealis fasciae cervicalis.
middle l. of thoracolumbar fascia lamina media fasciae thoracolumbalis.
mitral cell l. a thin layer in the olfactory bulb between the molecular layer and the internal granular layer, containing the bodies of the mitral cells.
molecular l. of cerebellar cortex stratum moleculare corticis cerebelli.
molecular l. of cerebral cortex lamina molecularis.
molecular l. of dentate gyrus stratum moleculare gyri dentati.
molecular l. of olfactory bulb a wide layer between the external granular layer and the mitral cell layer, primarily containing dendrites from mitral and tufted cells.
mucous l. of epidermis stratum germinativum (def. 2).
mucous l. of pharynx tunica mucosa pharyngis.
mucous l. of tympanic membrane mucous stratum of tympanic membrane.
multiform l. of cerebral cortex lamina multiformis.
multiform l. of dentate gyrus stratum multiforme gyri dentati.
muscle l. of fatty l. of subcutaneous tissue stratum musculosum panniculi adiposi telae subcutaneae.
muscle l. of pharynx tunica muscularis pharyngis.
muscular l. tunica muscularis.

- **muscular l. of colon** tunica muscularis coli.
- **muscular l. of ductus deferens** tunica muscularis ductus deferentis.
- **muscular l. of esophagus** tunica muscularis oesophagi.
- **muscular l. of female urethra** tunica muscularis urethrae femininae.
- **muscular l. of gallbladder** tunica muscularis vesicae biliaris.
- **muscular l. of large intestine** tunica muscularis intestini crassi.
- **muscular l. of membranous urethra** tunica muscularis partis intermediae urethrae.
- **muscular l. of prostatic urethra** tunica muscularis partis prostaticae urethrae.
- **muscular l. of rectum** tunica muscularis recti.
- **muscular l. of renal pelvis** tunica muscularis pelvis renalis.
- **muscular l. of seminal vesicle** tunica muscularis glandulae vesiculosae.
- **muscular l. of small intestine** tunica muscularis intestini tenuis.
- **muscular l. of spongy urethra** tunica muscularis partis spongiosae urethrae.
- **muscular l. of stomach** tunica muscularis gastrica.
- **muscular l. of ureter** tunica muscularis ureteris.
- **muscular l. of urinary bladder** tunica muscularis vesicae urinariae.
- **muscular l. of uterine tube** tunica muscularis tubae uterinae.
- **muscular l. of vagina** tunica muscularis vaginae.

l's of neocortex l's of cerebral cortex.
nerve fiber l. of retina a layer of the stratum nervosum retinae, situated between the ganglion cell layer and the internal limiting membrane, consisting essentially of the axons of the ganglion cells which pass through the lamina cribrosa to form the optic nerve. In official terminology, called *stratum neurofibrarum retinae* [TA]. See illustration at *retina.*
neural l. of retina stratum nervosum retinae.
neuroepidermal l. ectoderm.
Nitabuch l. an interrupted sheet of fibrinoid in the placenta at the junction of trophoblast and decidua; called also *Nitabuch stria* or *zone.*
odontoblastic l. the epithelioid odontoblastic zone, one to five layers thick, which forms the outer surface of the dental pulp adjacent to the dentin, resting on the Weil basal layer. It produces and maintains the dentin.
olfactory nerve fiber l. the outermost layer of the olfactory bulb, composed of axons of the olfactory cells before they terminate in the adjacent glomerular layer.
Ollier l. osteogenetic l.
optic l. of superior colliculus stratum opticum colliculi superioris.
oriens l. of hippocampus stratum oriens hippocampi.
osteogenetic l. the innermost layer of the periosteum; called also *Ollier l.*
outer enamel l. the outer, convex wall of the enamel organ.
outer l. of glomerular capsule parietal l. of glomerular capsule.
outer limiting l. of retina external limiting membrane.
outer molecular l. outer plexiform l.
outer nuclear l. of retina the layer of the stratum nervosum retinae situated between the external limiting membrane and the outer plexiform layer, consisting essentially of the rod and cone granules (nuclei). Called also *external nuclear l. of retina* and, in official terminology, *stratum nucleare externum retinae* [TA]. See illustration at *retina.*
outer plexiform l. of retina the layer of the stratum nervosum retinae situated between the outer nuclear layer and the inner nuclear layer, consisting essentially of the arborizations of the axons of the rod and cone granules with the dendrites of the bipolar cells. Called also *external plexiform l. of retina* and, in official terminology, *stratum plexiforme externum retinae* [TA]. See illustration at *retina.*
Pander l. the splanchnopleural layer of the mesoblast.
papillary l. stratum papillare dermidis.
parietal l. of glomerular capsule the layer of the glomerular capsule facing outwards, separated from the visceral layer by the urinary space; it is composed of simple squamous epithelium. Called also *outer layer* or *wall of glomerular capsule* and *parietal wall of glomerular capsule.*
parietal l. of pelvic fascia fascia pelvis parietalis.
parietal l. of serous pericardium lamina parietalis pericardii serosi.
parietal l. of tunica vaginalis of testis lamina parietalis tunicae vaginalis testis.
parvocellular l's of dorsal lateral geniculate nucleus strata parvocellularia nuclei dorsalis corporis geniculati lateralis.
pigmented epithelial l., pigmented l. of retina, pigment epithelial l. stratum pigmentosum retinae.
plexiform l. of cerebellar cortex stratum moleculare corticis cerebelli.
plexiform l. of cerebral cortex lamina molecularis.
polymorphic l. of cerebral cortex lamina multiformis.
posterior l. of thoracolumbar fascia lamina posterior fasciae thoracolumbalis.
pretracheal l. of cervical fascia lamina pretrachealis fasciae cervicalis.
prevertebral l. of cervical fascia lamina prevertebralis fasciae cervicalis.
prickle cell l. stratum spinosum.
Purkinje l., Purkinje cell l. stratum purkinjense corticis cerebelli.
pyramidal l. of hippocampus stratum pyramidale hippocampi.
radiate l. of hippocampus stratum radiatum hippocampi.
radiate l. of tympanic membrane stratum radiatum of tympanic membrane.
Rauber l. the most external of the three layers of cells which form the blastodisc or embryonic disc in the young embryo; called also *blastodermic ectoderm* and *primitive ectoderm.*

Layer *Continued*

reticular l. stratum reticulare dermidis.
l. of rods and cones the layer of the stratum nervosum retinae situated between the stratum pigmentosum and the external limiting membrane, comprising the sensitive elements of the retina, the cones, containing a visual pigment, iodopsin, and the rods, containing visual purple, or rhodopsin. In official terminology, called *stratum segmentorum externorum et internorum retinae* [TA]. See also *retina.*
Rohr l. see under *stria.*
Sattler l. the portion of the vascular layer of the choroid that is made up of medium-sized vessels.
sclerotogenous l. the layer of mesoderm cells surrounding the notochord of the embryo and developing into the axial skeleton.
second half-value l. the additional thickness of material needed to reduce the intensity of a radiation beam from one half to one fourth of its original value. Cf. *half-value l.*
serous l. tunica serosa; see specific terms beginning thus under *tunica.*
skeletogenous l. sclerotogenous l.
sol l. a thin layer of the tunica mucosa of the respiratory tract, underlying the gel layer.
somatic l. the external layer of the lateral mesoderm after the coelomic split occurs; the inner component of somatopleure of the embryo.
spinous l., spinous cell l. stratum spinosum.
splanchnic l. the internal layer of the lateral mesoderm after the coelomic split occurs; the component of splanchnopleure outside the entoderm of the embryo.
spongy l. of endometrium the sublayer of the stratum functionale underlying the compact layer; it contains the tortuous portions of the uterine glands.
spongy l. of female urethra tunica spongiosa urethrae femininae.
spongy l. of vagina tunica spongiosa vaginae.
subcallosal l. the layer of nerve fibers on the lower side of the corpus callosum.
subendocardial l. the layer of loose fibrous tissue uniting the endocardium and myocardium; it also contains blood vessels, nerves, and some fibers of the conducting system of the heart. Called also *subendocardium.*
subendothelial l. a middle, fibrous layer of the tunica intima of typical blood vessels, located between the endothelium and internal elastic membrane; it also comprises the bulk of the endocardium, where it lies deep to the lining endothelium. It is composed of varying amounts of collagen and elastic fibers and smooth muscle cells.
subepicardial l. a thin collagenous layer of loose connective tissue uniting the epicardium and myocardium; besides collagen and elastic fibers, it also contains fat cells, nerves, and lymphatic and blood vessels. Called also *subepicardium.*
submantle l. a layer of interglobular dentin usually situated just below the cover (mantle) dentin.
submucosal l. tela submucosa.
submucosal l. of myometrium stratum submucosum of myometrium.
submucous l. tela submucosa.
subodontoblastic l. Weil basal l.
subserosal l. of myometrium stratum subserosum of myometrium.
subserous l. tela subserosa.
subserous l. of bladder tela subserosa vesicae urinariae.
subserous l. of esophagus tela subserosa oesophagi.
subserous l. of gallbladder tela subserosa vesicae biliaris.
subserous l. of large intestine tela subserosa intestini crassi.
subserous l. of liver tela subserosa hepatis.
subserous l. of parietal pleura tela subserosa pleurae parietalis.
subserous l. of pericardium tela subserosa pericardii.
subserous l. of peritoneum fascia extraperitonealis.
subserous l. of small intestine tela subserosa intestini tenuis.
subserous l. of stomach tela subserosa gastrica.
subserous l. of testis tela subserosa testis.
subserous l. of urinary bladder tela subserosa vesicae urinariae.
subserous l. of uterine tube tela subserosa tubae uterinae.
subserous l. of uterus tela subserosa uteri.
subserous l. of visceral pleura tela subserosa pleurae visceralis.
superficial l. of cervical fascia, superficial l. of deep cervical fascia lamina superficialis fasciae cervicalis.
superficial l. of fascia of perineum tela subcutanea perinei.
superficial gray l. of superior colliculus stratum griseum superficiale colliculi superioris.
superficial l. of levator palpebrae superioris lamina superficialis musculi levatoris palpebrae superioris.
superficial l. of temporal fascia lamina superficialis fasciae temporalis.
l's of superior colliculus the seven layers forming the superior colliculus, from outer to inner being the stratum zonale (Layer I), stratum griseum superficiale (Layer II), stratum opticum (Layer III), stratum griseum intermedium (Layer IV), stratum medullare intermedium (Layer V), stratum griseum profundum (Layer VI), and stratum medullare profundum (Layer VII).
superior l. of pelvic diaphragm fascia superior diaphragmatis pelvis.
suprachoroid l. suprachoroid lamina.
supravascular l. of myometrium stratum supravasculare.
synovial l. of articular capsule membrana synovialis capsulae articularis.
Tomes granular l. granular l. of Tomes.
trophic l. endoderm.
vascular l. of eyeball tunica vasculosa bulbi.
vascular l. of myometrium stratum vasculare.
vascular l. of testis tunica vasculosa testis.
vegetative l. endoderm.
visceral l. of glomerular capsule the layer of the glomerular capsule that faces inward toward the capillaries and is composed of podocytes; it is separated from the parietal layer by the urinary space. Called also *inner layer* or *wall of glomerular capsule* and *visceral wall of glomerular capsule.*
visceral l. of pelvic fascia fascia pelvis visceralis.
visceral l. of serous pericardium lamina visceralis pericardii serosi.
visceral l. of tunica vaginalis of testis lamina visceralis tunicae vaginalis testis.
Waldeyer l. the vascular layer of the ovary.
Weil basal l. a clear, relatively cell-free layer, located just inside the odontoblastic layer and overlying the cell-rich zone of the dental pulp, which is visible during the inactive phase of dentinogenesis. It is made up of delicate fibrils embedded in the ground substance; in dentinogenesis the fibrils are incorporated into the matrix. Called also *subodontoblastic l., cell-free* or *cell-poor zone,* and *Weil basal zone.*
white l's of cerebellum laminae albae cerebelli.
zonal l. of superior colliculus stratum zonale colliculi superioris.
zonal l. of thalamus stratum zonale thalami.

La·zer·for·ma·lyde (la″zer-for′mə-līd) trademark for a preparation of dilute formaldehyde in solution.

lb pound (L. *libra*).

LBBB left bundle branch block; see *bundle branch block,* under *block.*

LBP low back pain.

LBW low birth weight; see under *infant.*

LCA left coronary artery; leukocyte common antigens.

LCAD de·fi·cien·cy long-chain acyl-CoA dehydrogenase deficiency; see under *acyl-CoA dehydrogenase.*

LCAT lecithin-cholesterol acyltransferase; see *phosphatidylcholine–sterol O-acyltransferase.*

LCAT deficiency lecithin–cholesterol acyltransferase deficiency.

LCIS lobular carcinoma in situ.

LCM lymphocytic choriomeningitis.

LCR locus control region.

LD lethal dose; light difference.

LD_{50} median lethal dose.

LDA left dorsoanterior (position of the fetus); left displacement of the abomasum.

LDH L-lactate dehydrogenase.

LDL low-density lipoprotein.

LDL-C low-density-lipoprotein cholesterol

L-dopa (el″do′pə) levodopa.

LE left eye; lupus erythematosus (see also under *cell*).

leach·ing (lēch′ing) lixiviation.

lead[1] (Pb) (led) a soft, grayish blue metal with poisonous salts; atomic number 82, atomic weight 207.19. Excessive ingestion causes lead poisoning; see under *poisoning.*

black l. graphite.

l. chloride a compound, $PbCl_2$, used as a reagent and pigment.

l. nitrate a sweet-tasting crystalline agent, $Pb(NO_3)_2$, used as a reagent.

tetra-ethyl l. a highly poisonous organic lead compound used as an antiknock agent in internal combustion motors; it can be absorbed through the skin and may cause mental symptoms and death.

lead[2] (lēd) any of the conductors connected to the electrocardiograph, each comprising two or more electrodes that are attached to specific sites on the body and used to examine electrical activity by monitoring changes in electrical potential between them. See also *electrocardiogram.*

l. I the standard bipolar limb lead attached to the right and left arms.

l. II the standard bipolar limb lead attached to the right arm and left leg.

l. III the standard bipolar limb lead attached to the left arm and left leg.

active fixation l. a pacing lead that attaches to the heart by pins, screws, claws, needles, or similar devices.

augmented unipolar limb l. a unipolar limb lead that has been modified by disconnecting the input of the limb to the central terminal, increasing the voltage output; the three standard leads are designated aV_F, aV_L, and aV_R.

aV_F l. an augmented unipolar limb lead in which the positive (exploratory) electrode is on the left leg.

aV_L l. an augmented unipolar limb lead in which the positive (exploratory) electrode is on the left arm.

aV_R l. an augmented unipolar limb lead in which the positive (exploratory) electrode terminal is on the right arm.

bipolar l. an array involving two electrodes, each of which makes significant contribution to the record, placed at different body sites.

bipolar limb l. any bipolar array in which both electrodes are attached to limbs; usually used to denote one of the three standard limb leads, i.e., lead I, II, or III.

bipolar precordial l. a bipolar array in which both electrodes are attached to the chest; it is often a modification of a standard limb lead.

chest l's precordial l's.

esophageal l. an electrode attached to a wire and inserted in the esophagus.

Frank XYZ l's XYZ l's.

limb l. an array in which any registering electrodes are attached to limbs; it may be unipolar or bipolar.

pacemaker l., pacing l. the connection between the heart and the power source of an artificial cardiac pacemaker, comprising an electrode to contact the heart, a conductor coil, and a terminal pin to connect to the generator.

passive fixation l. a pacing lead that is attached to the heart by flanged areas or tines lodged under trabeculae.

precordial l's leads in which the exploring electrode is placed on the chest and the other is connected to one or more limbs. The term is usually used to denote the V leads (q.v.).

standard l's the 12 leads used in a standard electrocardiogram, comprising the standard bipolar limb leads (I, II and III), the augmented unipolar limb leads (aV_F, aV_L, and aV_R), and the standard precordial leads (V_1 to V_6).

unipolar l. an array of two electrodes, one of which is an exploring electrode attached either to a limb *(unipolar limb l.)* or to the chest *(V l's)* while the other, an indifferent electrode contributing no input, uses a central terminal as reference point.

unipolar limb l. any unipolar array in which the exploring electrode is placed on a limb; designated V_F, V_L, and V_R. In practice, it is usually modified; see *augmented unipolar limb l.*

unipolar precordial l's V l's.

V l's the series of six standard unipolar leads in which the exploring electrode is attached to the chest; their positions are designated V_1 to V_6.

Wilson l's V l's.

XYZ l's leads used in the Frank lead system (q.v.) in spatial vectorcardiography.

leaf (lēf) [A. S. *lēf*] a flattened structure of vascular plants, attached to the plant by a stem and usually green in color, that is the primary site of photosynthesis and transpiration.

belladonna l. [USP] the dried leaves and fruiting tops of *Atropa belladonna* or *A. belladonna* var. *acuminata,* used in the preparation of standardized dosage forms; see under *extract* and *tincture.*

betel l. the dried leaf of *Piper betle,* having expectorant, sialagogic, and stimulant effects; used as a component of the masticatory betel (q.v.).

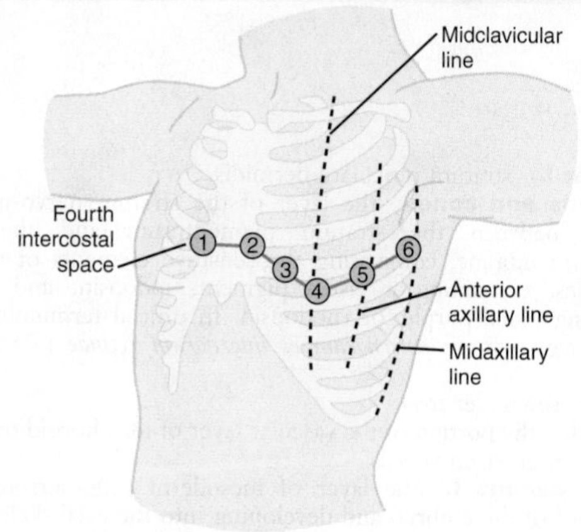

■ Positioning of V leads.

leaf·let (lēf′lət) 1. a small leaf or something resembling one. 2. cusp (def. 2).

Leão spreading depression (la-ah′) [Aristides de Azevedo Pacheco *Leão,* Brazilian physiologist, 1914–1993] see under *depression.*

learn·ing (lur′ning) a relatively long-lasting adaptive behavioral change occurring as a result of experience.

insight l. the highest form of learning, characterized by the ability to evaluate and combine previous experiences to solve a problem or achieve a desired goal.

latent l. learning that occurs without reinforcement, becoming apparent only when a reinforcement or reward is introduced.

observational l. the learning of new behaviors through watching the actions and outcomes of others.

leash (lēsh) a bundle or fasciculus.

Le·ber congenital amaurosis, etc. (la′bər) [Theodor *Leber,* German ophthalmologist, 1840–1917] see *Leber congenital amaurosis,* under *amaurosis, Hassall corpuscles,* under *corpuscle,* and *Hovius plexus,* under *plexus;* and see under *neuropathy.*

Le·bis·tes (lə-bis′tēz) a genus of small fish or minnows. *L. reticula′tus* is the guppy, a top-feeding species also called "millions," cultivated in Barbados to eliminate mosquito larvae.

Le·boy·er method (technique) (lə-bwah-ya′) [Frédéric *Leboyer,* French obstetrician, born 1918] see under *method.*

le·che de hi·gue·rón (la′cha da e-ga-rōn′) [Sp. "milk of fig"] the sap or latex of the wild fig tree *Ficus anthelmintica,* used as a vermifuge.

le·chu·gui·lla (la-choo-ge′yə) [Sp. "little lettuce"] *Agave lecheguilla.*

lec·i·thal (les′ĭ-thəl) [*lecith-* + *-al*[1]] having a yolk.

-lecithal [Gr. *lekithos* yolk] a word termination denoting yolk, affixed to a word stem descriptive of the state of the yolk substance, as *centrolecithal, isolecithal,* etc.

lec·i·thid (les′ĭ-thid) a compound of lecithin with venom hemolysin.

cobra l. a hemolytic compound formed by cobra toxin and the lecithin of the blood.

lec·i·thin (les′ĭ-thin) phosphatidylcholine.

lec·i·thin–cho·les·ter·ol ac·yl·trans·fer·ase (LCAT) (les′ĭ-thin kə-les′tər-ol a″səl-trans′fər-ās) phosphatidylcholine–sterol *O*-acyltransferase.

le·ci·thin–cho·les·ter·ol ac·yl·trans·fer·ase de·fi·cien·cy (les′ĭ-thin kə-les′tər-ol a″səl-trans′fər-ās) an autosomal recessive disorder due to failure of LCAT to esterify plasma cholesterol as the result of mutation in the *LCAT* gene (locus: 16q22.1); cholesterol and phosphatidylcholine accumulate in the plasma and tissues, causing corneal opacities, anemia, and often proteinuria. All classes of lipoproteins show abnormalities. See also *fish eye disease* under *disease.*

lec·i·thin·emia (les″ĭ-thĭ-ne′me-ə) hyperlecithinemia.

lecith(o)- [Gr. *lekithos* yolk] a combining form denoting relationship to the yolk of an egg or ovum.

lec·i·tho·blast (les′ĭ-tho-blast″) [*lecitho-* + *-blast*] the primordial endoderm of a two-layered blastodisc.

lec·i·tho·pro·tein (les″ĭ-tho-pro′tēn) a compound of the protein molecule with a molecule of lecithin; lecithoproteins occur in all cells.

lec·i·tho·vi·tel·lin (les″ĭ-tho-vi-tel′in) a saline extract of egg yolks used in egg yolk agar to test for bacterial lecithinase.

lec•tin (lek′tin) any of a group of hemagglutinating proteins, found primarily in plant seeds, which bind specifically to the branching sugar molecules of glycoproteins and glycolipids on the surface of cells. Certain lectins selectively cause agglutination of erythrocytes of certain blood groups and of malignant cells but not their normal counterparts; others stimulate the proliferation of lymphocytes.

mannose-binding l. (MBL) a protein that is structurally similar to complement component C1 and recognizes many microorganisms, including bacteria, fungi, parasites, and viruses. It initiates the lectin pathway of complement activation, without the presence of antibody, by binding to carbohydrates on the microbial surface and activating C3.

lec•to•type (lek′to-tīp) in bacteriology, a culture taken from the original material to serve as a type culture when the original investigator did not designate a type.

Lec•y•thoph•o•ra (les″ĭ-thof′ə-rə) a genus of imperfect fungi of the form-family Dematiaceae, formerly considered part of the genus *Phialophora*. *L. hoffman′nii* occasionally causes hyalohyphomycosis and *L. muta′bilis* has been found in cases of endocarditis, some fatal.

Led•bän•der (led′bān-der) [Ger.] Büngner bands; see under *band*.

Le Den•tu suture (lə dahn-tu′) [Jean François-Auguste *Le Dentu*, Paris surgeon, 1841–1926] see under *suture*.

Le•Duc technique (implantation) (lə-dūk′) [A. *LeDuc*, French urologist, 20th century] see under *technique*.

Lee ganglion (le) [Robert *Lee*, English obstetrician and gynecologist, 1793–1877] cervical ganglion of uterus; see under *ganglion*.

leech (lēch) [L. *hirudo*] 1. any of the annelids of the class Hirudinea. Some species are bloodsuckers that parasitize various animals. Leeches are sometimes used for drawing blood (see *leeching*). 2. to apply leeches.

American l. *Macrobdella decora*.

artificial l. an apparatus for drawing blood by artificial suction.

horse l. a leech of either genus *Haemopis* or *Limnatis*.

land l. a leech of either genus *Haemadipsa* or *Limnatis*.

medicinal l. *Hirudo medicinalis*.

leeches (lēch′əz) [pl. of *leech*, from the appearance of the lesions] pythiosis.

leech•ing (lēch′ing) the application of a leech for the withdrawal of blood; formerly used extensively in the treatment of various disorders and still used occasionally to reduce postsurgical venous congestion, as in tissue flaps, grafts, or transplants; called also *hirudinization*.

Leeu•wen•hoe•kia (la″wen-hoo′ke-ə) [Anton (Anthony, Antony) van *Leeuwenhoek*, Dutch microscopist, 1632–1723] a genus of mites. *L. australien′sis* is a species found in Australia that causes great irritation by burrowing in the skin.

le•flu•no•mide (lə-floo′no-mīd) an immunomodulator that inhibits pyrimidine synthesis, used as a disease-modifying antirheumatic drug in treatment of rheumatoid arthritis; administered orally.

Le Fort fracture, etc. (lə for′) [Léon-Clément *Le Fort*, French surgeon, 1829–1893] see under *amputation*, *fracture*, *operation*, *sound*, and *suture*.

left-hand•ed (left-hand′əd) using the left hand preferentially, or more skillfully than the right, in voluntary motor acts. See also *handedness* and *laterality*.

leg (leg) 1. the section of the lower limb between the knee and ankle; called also *crus* and *shank*. 2. in common usage, the entire lower limb (in which case, the part below the knee is called the *lower leg*). 3. any of the four limbs of a quadruped.

badger l. inequality in the length of the lower limbs.

baker l. genu valgum.

bandy l. genu varum.

bayonet l. uncorrected backward displacement of the bones of the lower limb at the knee, followed by ankylosis at the joint.

black l. blackleg.

bow l. genu varum.

hind l. the back leg (pelvic limb) of a quadruped. Cf. *foreleg*.

red l. a fatal septicemia in frogs caused by *Aeromonas hydrophila*.

restless l's see under *syndrome*.

rider's l. strain of the adductor muscles of the thigh in horseback riders.

scaly l. a type of mange in fowls in which the legs become enlarged and encrusted due to infestation by species of *Knemidokoptes*.

scissor l. deformity with crossing of the legs in walking, due to spasticity of adductor muscles of the thighs.

splay l's, spraddle l's myofibrillar hypoplasia.

tennis l. a sudden tear at the musculotendinous junction of the medial belly of the gastrocnemius muscle, usually seen in older persons participating in tennis and other sports.

Legg disease (leg) [Arthur Thornton *Legg*, American surgeon, 1874–1939] Legg-Calvé-Perthes disease; see under *disease*.

Legg-Cal•vé-Per•thes disease (leg′ kahl-va′ per′təz) [A.T. *Legg*; Jacques *Calvé*, French orthopedist, 1875–1954; Georg Clemens *Perthes*, German surgeon, 1869–1927] see under *disease*.

Legg-Cal•vé-Per•thes-Wal•den•ström disease (leg′ kahl-va′ per′təz vahl′den-strermz) [A.T. *Legg*; J. *Calvé*; G.C. *Perthes*; Johan Henning *Waldenström*, Swedish orthopedic surgeon, 1877–1972] Legg-Calvé-Perthes disease; see under *disease*.

Le•gio•nel•la (le″jə-nel′ə) [from *legionnaires' disease*] a genus of gram-negative, aerobic, rod-shaped bacteria of the family Legionellaceae, made up of motile, pleomorphic organisms that require cysteine and iron for growth. Their normal habitat is lakes, streams, and moist soil, but they have also been found as contaminants in human habitations, where they can cause legionellosis, a pneumonialike disease spread by the airborne route. The type species is *L. pneumo′phila*.

L. ani′sa a rare species found in water distribution systems and associated with pneumonia and Pontiac fever.

L. bozema′nae a species isolated from lung tissue and associated with pneumonia.

L. dumoff′ii a species isolated from lung tissue and cooling-tower water, and associated with pneumonia.

L. fee′leii a species isolated from coolant-system waters, and associated with Pontiac fever.

L. gorma′nii a species isolated from the banks of rivers and lakes, and associated with pneumonia.

L. jorda′nis a species isolated from the banks of rivers and lakes and from treated sewage.

L. longbeach′ae a species isolated from lung tissue and respiratory secretions and associated with pneumonia.

L. micda′dei a species isolated from lung tissue, respiratory secretions, and pleural fluid, as well as from cooling-tower water, shower heads, tap water, and respiratory therapy equipment; it causes Pittsburgh pneumonia. Called also *Pittsburgh pneumonia agent*.

L. pneumo′phila the cause of legionnaires' disease and Pontiac fever. It was the first species of the genus isolated and characterized, and it has been found in lung tissue, respiratory secretions, pleural fluid, and blood and in numerous environmental sites such as soil from the banks of rivers and streams, cooling-tower water, tap water, shower heads, construction sites, and aerosolized droplets from heat-exchange systems.

L. sainthelen′si a rare species found in ground water in Washington State and in nursing homes in Canada, and causing pneumonia.

L. wadswor′thii a species isolated from pleural tissue and causing pneumonia.

le•gion•el•la (le″jə-nel′ə) pl. *legionel′lae*. Any microorganism of the genus *Legionella*.

Le•gio•nel•la•ceae (le″jə-nel-a′se-e) a family of bacteria of the order Legionellales, consisting of gram-negative, aerobic, chemo-organotrophic, non–spore-forming rods; most are motile by means of one or more flagella. Organisms are facultative intracellular parasites and are pathogenic. It contains the genus *Legionella*.

Le•gio•nel•la•les (le″jə-nel-a′lēz) an order of bacteria of the class Gammaproteobacteria, phylum Proteobacteria, grouped together on the basis of 16S rRNA sequence analysis and consisting of intracellular parasites of invertebrates and vertebrates. It contains the families Legionellaceae and Coxiellaceae.

le•gion•el•lae (le″jə-nel′e) plural of *legionella*.

le•gion•el•lo•sis (le″jə-nel-o′sis) any of several illnesses caused by infection with species of *Legionella*; see *legionnaires' disease*, *Pittsburgh pneumonia*, and *Pontiac fever*. Called also *Legionella pneumonia*.

le•gion•naires disease (le-jən-ārz′) [*legionnaires*, members of the American Legion, whose convention in Philadelphia in 1976 was the scene of a highly publicized epidemic] see under *disease*.

le•gume (leg′ūm, lə-gūm′) 1. the pod, seed, or fruit of a plant of the family Leguminosae, such as a pea or bean. 2. any plant of the family Leguminosae.

leg•u•me•lin (leg″u-me′lin) an albumin from lentils, beans, and other leguminous seeds.

le•gu•min (lə-gu′min) [L. *legumen* pulse] a globulin from the seeds of various plants, chiefly of the legumes.

le•gu•mi•niv•o•rous (lə-gu″mĭ-niv′ə-rəs) feeding on legumes (beans and peas).

Le•gu•mi•no•sae (lə-gu″mĭ-noəse) the pea or legume family, a large family of plants that includes trees, shrubs, and vines; many genera either produce edible seeds or are of medical importance.

le•gu•mi•nous (lə-gu′mĭ-nəs) pertaining to a legume.

lei•as•the•nia (li″əs-the′ne-ə) [*leio-* + *asthenia*] asthenia of smooth muscle.

Leigh disease (le) [Archibald Denis *Leigh*, British neuropathologist, 1915–1998] subacute necrotizing encephalomyelopathy.

Lei•ner disease (li'nər) [Karl *Leiner*, Austrian pediatrician, 1871–1930] see under *disease*.

leio- [Gr. *leios* smooth] a combining form meaning smooth.

leio•dys•to•nia (li″o-dis-to'ne-ə) [*leio-* + *dystonia*] dystonia of smooth muscle.

leio•myo•blas•to•ma (li″o-mi″o-blas-to'mə) epithelioid leiomyoma.

leio•myo•fi•bro•ma (li″o-mi″o-fi-bro'mə) leiomyoma.

leio•myo•ma (li″o-mi-o'mə) pl. *leiomyomas, leiomyo'mata* [*leio-* + *myoma*] a benign tumor derived from smooth muscle; called also *fibroid* and *fibroid tumor*.

bizarre l. epithelioid l.

l. cu'tis a leiomyoma arising from cutaneous or subcutaneous smooth muscle fibers, occurring singly or multiply, usually in the form of lesions arising from arrectores pilorum muscles (piloleiomyoma); it may also occur as a solitary genital lesion arising from dartoic, vulvar, or mammillary muscle or as a solitary angioleiomyoma (q.v.) arising from the muscle of veins. Lesions are smooth, firm, painful, often translucent or waxy nodules, with interlacing bundles of elongated rod- or spindle-shaped cells and finely fibrillar cytoplasm.

epithelioid l. a rare smooth muscle tumor, usually of the stomach, in which the cells are polygonal rather than spindle-shaped; called also *bizarre l.* and *leiomyoblastoma*.

intraligamentous l. a uterine leiomyoma with lateral growth that extends outward between the folds of the broad ligament.

intramural l. a uterine leiomyoma located within the substance of the myometrium in the uterine corpus.

parasitic l. a pedunculated leiomyoma that has partially or completely detached from its site of origin and is attached to the omentum, which now has extended blood vessels into it.

pedunculated l. a submucosal leiomyoma that protrudes into the uterine cavity, forming a bulbous polyp with a firm, round head.

submucosal l. a uterine leiomyoma located next to the endometrium in the corpus of the uterus; this type frequently protrudes into the endometrial cavity, forming a pedunculated leiomyoma.

subserosal l. a uterine leiomyoma located just beneath the tunica serosa of the corpus of the uterus.

l. u'teri, uterine l. a leiomyoma of the uterus, usually occurring in the third and fourth decades of life, characterized by multiple, firm, round, sharply circumscribed, unencapsulated, gray to white tumors that show a whorled pattern on cut section. The majority are within the myometrium of the corpus of the uterus, but they may also occur in the cervix, usually in its posterior wall. Those in the corpus are distinguished by location as either *intramural, submucosal*, or *subserosal leiomyomas*. Called also *fibromyoma uteri, uterine myoma*, and, colloquially, *fibroids*.

vascular l. angioleiomyoma.

leio•my•o•ma•to•sis (li″o-mi″o-mə-to'sis) a condition in which multiple leiomyomas occur throughout the body.

l. cu'tis et u'teri an autosomal dominant condition characterized by small dermal papules, usually on the face, with uterine leiomyomas. Called also *Reed syndrome*.

l. peritonea'lis dissemina'ta abdominal smooth muscle tumors arising as small nodules scattered throughout the peritoneal surfaces, occurring exclusively in women of reproductive age and appearing very similar to low-grade leiomyosarcoma or metastatic carcinoma but usually regressing spontaneously following menopause.

leio•myo•sar•co•ma (li″o-mi″o-sahr-ko'mə) [*leio-* + *myosarcoma*] a sarcoma containing large spindle cells of smooth muscle, most commonly of the uterus, retroperitoneal region, or extremities.

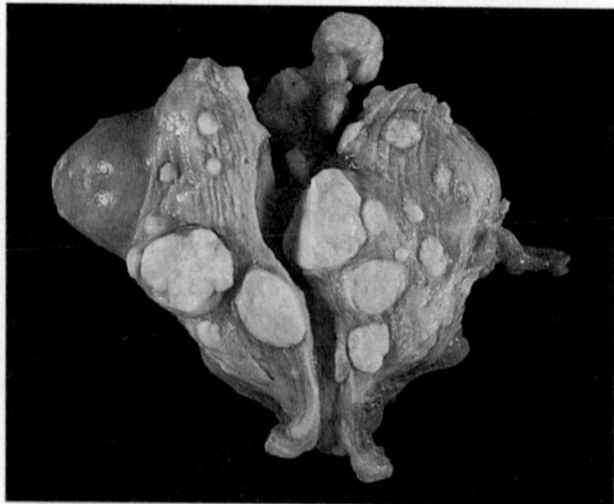

■ Multiple leiomyomas in a sagittal section of the uterus.

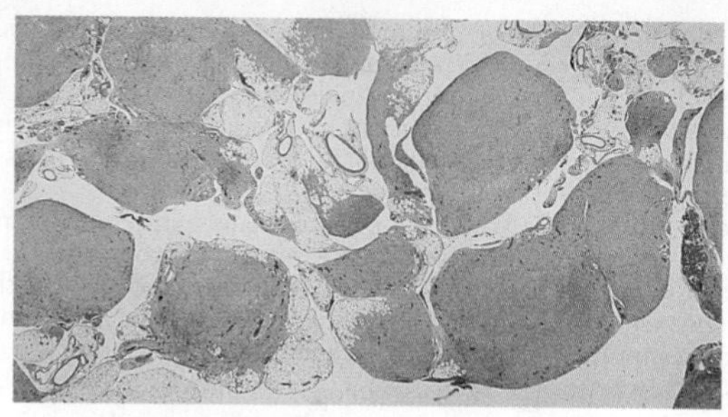

■ Leiomyomatosis peritonealis disseminata.

renal l. a rare leiomyosarcoma in the kidney, usually in the capsule; it occurs more often in women.

leio•myo•sar•co•ma•to•sis (li″o-mi″o-sahr-ko″mə-to'sis) the occurrence of multiple leiomyosarcomas.

leip(o)- for words beginning thus, see those beginning *lip(o)-*.

Leish•man stain (lēsh'mən) [Sir William Boog *Leishman*, English army surgeon and bacteriologist, 1865–1926] see *Stains and Staining Methods*, under *stain*.

Leish•man-Don•o•van body (lēsh'mən don'ə-vən) [Sir W.B. *Leishman;* Charles *Donovan*, Irish physician in India, 1863–1951] amastigote.

Leish•ma•nia (lēsh-ma'ne-ə) [Sir William B. *Leishman*] 1. a genus of flagellate protozoa of the order Kinetoplastida, phylum Euglenozoa, comprising parasites of worldwide distribution; several species are pathogenic. The organisms have two morphologic stages in their life cycle: amastigote, found intracellularly in the vertebrate host; and promastigote, found in the digestive tract of the invertebrate host (i.e., phlebotomine sandfly) and in cultures. The genus is divided into two subgenera, *Leishmania* and *Viannia*, based on the location of development within the sandfly vector; species of the former are present in both the Old and New Worlds, while those of the latter are found only in the New World. The organisms have usually been assigned to complexes and species according to their geographic origin, clinical syndrome produced, and ecologic characteristics, or have been separated on the basis of association with visceral, cutaneous, or mucocutaneous leishmaniasis, but classification increasingly is based on phylogenetic relationships. 2. a subgenus of the genus *Leishmania*, comprising the species that develop in the midgut and foregut.

L. aethio'pica a species, of the subgenus *Leishmania*, causing Ethiopian cutaneous leishmaniasis and diffuse cutaneous leishmaniasis; animal reservoirs are rock and tree hyraxes in the highlands of Ethiopia and Kenya; the vector in Ethiopia is *Phlebotomus longipes* and in Kenya it is *P. pedifer*.

L. amazonen'sis a species, of the subgenus *Leishmania*, transmitted by *Lutzomyia flaviscutellata*, and causing New World cutaneous leishmaniasis in the Amazon region of Brazil and neighboring countries and in Trinidad. *L. amazonensis* is considered by some authorities to be a complex including also the species *L. garnhami;* others consider the two species to be synonymous.

L. ara'bica a species, of the subgenus *Leishmania*, found in Saudi Arabia and causing Old World cutaneous leishmaniasis.

L. brazilien'sis the type species of the subgenus *Viannia*, transmitted by species of *Lutzomyia* and causing cutaneous and mucocutaneous leishmaniasis in Central and South America. It is sometimes described as a complex, in which case it includes also the species *L. peruviana*.

L. chaga'si a species, of the subgenus *Leishmania*, causing American visceral leishmaniasis, usually transmitted by the sandfly *Lutzomyia longipalpis;* now considered to be synonymous with *L. infantum* (q.v.).

L. colombien'sis a species, of the subgenus *Viannia*, transmitted by *Lutzomyia* and causing New World cutaneous leishmaniasis, and occasionally visceral leishmaniasis, in Colombia and Panama.

L. donova'ni the type species of the subgenus *Leishmania*, causing visceral and occasionally Old World cutaneous leishmaniasis in northern and eastern China and an arc surrounding the Indian Ocean from the Indian subcontinent to East Africa. It is transmitted by the sandfly *Phlebotomus*.

L. garnha'mi a species, of the subgenus *Leishmania*, causing cutaneous leishmaniasis in mountainous regions of Venezuela; it is considered by some authorities to be part of the *L. amazonensis* complex; others consider the two species to be synonymous.

L. guyanen'sis a species, of the subgenus *Viannia*, occurring in Guyana, Suriname, and the northern Amazon basin; transmitted chiefly by *Lutzomyia umbratilis;* and causing pian bois (forest yaws). It is sometimes described as a complex, in which case it includes also the species *L. panamensis*.

L. infan'tum a species, of the subgenus *Leishmania*, causing visceral leishmaniasis, and sometimes cutaneous leishmaniasis, from China across the Mediterranean basin to Brazil, transmitted by species of *Phlebotomus* in the Old World and by *Lutzomyia longipalpis* in the New World. Previously, it was considered to be two species: *L. infantum*, predominantly in the Old

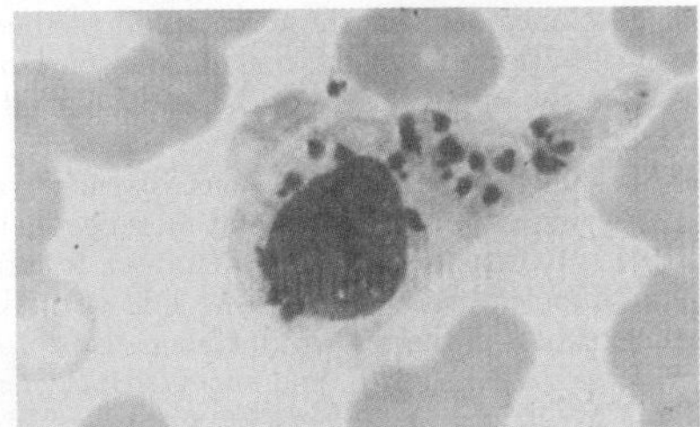

■ *Leishmania donovani* in a stained preparation from bone marrow.

World, and *L. chagasi,* in Central and South America. The two are now considered to be synonymous, although they are still sometimes named separately by geographic region.

L. kil'licki a species, of the subgenus *Leishmania,* found in Tunisia and causing Old World cutaneous leishmaniasis.

L. lainso'ni a species, of the subgenus *Viannia,* transmitted by *Lutzomyia* and causing New World cutaneous leishmaniasis in Brazil.

L. ma'jor a species, of the subgenus *Leishmania,* endemic in dry desert regions in portions of Africa, the Middle East, Asia, India, and southern Russia, and causing Old World cutaneous leishmaniasis, usually as a wet lesion. It is transmitted by *Phlebotomus papatasi* and other *Phlebotomus* species.

L. mexica'na a species, of the subgenus *Leishmania,* found in Central America and southern North America, causing the form of New World cutaneous leishmaniasis called chiclero ulcer and also occasionally causing diffuse cutaneous leishmaniasis. It is transmitted by *Lutzomyia olmeca. L. mexicana* is considered by some authorities to be a complex including also the species *L. pifanoi;* others consider the two species to be synonymous.

L. naif'fi a species, of the subgenus *Viannia,* transmitted by *Lutzomyia* and causing New World cutaneous leishmaniasis in Brazil and French Guyana.

L. panamen'sis a species, of the subgenus *Viannia,* transmitted chiefly by *Lutzomyia trapidoi* and causing New World cutaneous leishmaniasis in Panama and adjacent areas of Central America and Colombia. It is considered to be part of the *L. guyanensis* complex.

L. peruvia'na a species, of the subgenus *Viannia,* found in mountainous areas of Peru and Argentina, probably transmitted by *Lutzomyia verrucarum* and *L. peruensis* and causing uta in humans. It is considered to be part of the *L. braziliensis* complex.

L. pi'fanoi a species, of the subgenus *Leishmania,* causing New World cutaneous leishmaniasis, usually the localized form, in Venezuela. It is considered by some authorities to be part of the *L. mexicana* (q.v.) complex; others consider the two species to be synonymous.

L. sha'wi a species, of the subgenus *Viannia,* transmitted by *Lutzomyia* and causing New World cutaneous leishmaniasis in Brazil.

L. tro'pica a species, of the subgenus *Leishmania,* causing Old World cutaneous leishmaniasis, usually as a dry lesion; it can also cause *leishmaniasis recidivans* or, rarely, visceral leishmaniasis. It is endemic in urban areas of Iran, Iraq, and India, transmitted by *Phlebotomus sergenti,* and in southern France, Italy, and certain Mediterranean islands, transmitted by *P. papatasi.* The principal reservoirs are dogs and humans.

L. venezuelen'sis a species, of the subgenus *Viannia,* transmitted by *Lutzomyia* and causing New World cutaneous leishmaniasis in Venezuela.

leish•ma•nia (lēsh-ma'ne-ə) any protozoan of the genus *Leishmania.*

leish•ma•ni•al (lēsh-ma'ne-əl) pertaining to or caused by leishmanias.

leish•ma•ni•a•sis (lēsh″mə-ni'ə-sis) a protozoal infection caused by *Leishmania;* the principal classification is into cutaneous, mucocutaneous, and visceral types.

acute cutaneous l. zoonotic cutaneous l.

American l. see *New World cutaneous l.* and *American visceral l.*

American cutaneous l. New World cutaneous l.

American visceral l. a type of visceral leishmaniasis seen in South America, Central America, and Mexico, usually caused by *Leishmania chagasi,* and affecting persons of any age. Its major reservoirs are dogs and the usual vector is the sandfly *Lutzomyia longipalpis.*

anergic l., anergic cutaneous l. diffuse cutaneous l.

anthroponotic cutaneous l. a type of Old World cutaneous leishmaniasis found mainly in large urban areas in the Middle East, the Mediterranean region, and the Indian subcontinent; it is caused by *Leishmania tropica* and transmitted by the vectors *Phlebotomus sergenti* and *P. papatasi.* The reservoir may be either human or canine. A slowly developing single lesion that persists for a year or more is typical. Called also *chronic, dry,* or *urban cutaneous l.*

canine l., canine visceral l. 1. visceral leishmaniasis in dogs. 2. infantile visceral l. in which the vector is a dog.

chronic cutaneous l. anthroponotic cutaneous l.

cutaneous l. an endemic type of leishmaniasis characterized by a cutaneous papule that evolves into a nodule, breaks down to form an indolent ulcer, and heals, leaving a depressed scar. Varieties found in Asia and Africa and those found in the Americas are caused by different species of *Leishmania,* have different animal vectors, and are called respectively *Old World cutaneous l.* and *New World cutaneous l.*

diffuse l., diffuse cutaneous l. a rare chronic form of cutaneous leishmaniasis caused by *Leishmania aethiopica* in East Africa, by *L. pifanoi* in Venezuela, and by *L. mexicana* and species of the *Viannia* subgenus in South and Central America. It is characterized by local and hematogenous spread from a primary lesion to produce generalized nodular lesions resembling those of lepromatous leprosy in the skin and sometimes involving the nasal mucosa and laryngopharynx. Individuals with this form of the disease do not develop an effective immune response to it. Called also *anergic* or *anergic cutaneous l.*

disseminated l., disseminated cutaneous l. diffuse cutaneous l.

dry cutaneous l. anthroponotic cutaneous l.

Ethiopian cutaneous l. a form of Old World cutaneous leishmaniasis seen in the highlands of Kenya and Ethiopia, caused by *Leishmania aethiopica;* reservoirs are hyraxes of the genera *Procavia* and *Heterohyrax,* and the vectors are *Phlebotomus pedifer* and *P. longipes.* Lesions are less inflamed and more chronic than those of other Old World forms and generally last for several years; the condition is usually self-limited but may develop into diffuse cutaneous leishmaniasis.

Indian visceral l. a type of visceral leishmaniasis caused by *Leishmania donovani,* usually affecting older children or young adults; humans are the only reservoir hosts and it is transmitted by the sandfly *Phlebotomus argentipes.* It occurs primarily in eastern India and Bangladesh.

infantile visceral l. a type of visceral leishmaniasis caused by *Leishmania infantum,* usually affecting children between ages 1 and 4; reservoirs are dogs, foxes, jackals, and rodents, and vectors are species of *Phlebotomus* sandflies. It occurs in the Mediterranean region, sub-Saharan and East Africa, the Middle East, and China.

lupoid l. l. recidivans.

Mediterranean visceral l. infantile visceral l.

mucocutaneous l., nasopharyngeal l. chronic, progressive metastatic spread of lesions of the variety of New World cutaneous leishmaniasis that is caused by *Leishmania braziliensis* from the skin to the nasal, pharyngeal, and buccal mucosa months to years after appearance of the initial cutaneous lesion, which has usually healed. There may be mutilating destruction of the nasal septum, palate, lips, pharynx, and larynx. Called also *espundia.*

New World l., New World cutaneous l. any of the types of cutaneous leishmaniasis occurring in South America, Central America, or Mexico, zoonoses caused mainly by *Leishmania mexicana, L. amazonensis, L. chagasi,* and *L. braziliensis* and other related species of the *Viannia* subgenus. Their lesions develop and heal similarly to those of the Old World forms but tend to be less nodular and more ulcerative and destructive. Many varieties exist, differing as to animal reservoir, vector, geographical distribution, and clinical and other characteristics; some common forms are mucocutaneous leishmaniasis, chicle or chiclero ulcer, uta, and pian bois. Called also *American cutaneous l.*

Old World l., Old World cutaneous l. any of the types of cutaneous leishmaniasis occurring in Asia, Africa, or the Mediterranean basin. Three separate types are distinguished according to the causative organism: *anthroponotic cutaneous* or *dry cutaneous leishmaniasis, zoonotic cutaneous* or *wet cutaneous leishmaniasis,* and *Ethiopian cutaneous leishmaniasis.* The condition has had many different names, often according to the locality of its occurrence (see under *boil*).

post–kala-azar dermal l. cutaneous symptoms occurring after a person has recovered from visceral leishmaniasis, consisting of hypopigmented or erythematous macules on the face and sometimes the limbs or trunk; the facial lesions gradually progress to papules or nodules that resemble those of lepromatous leprosy. When it occurs soon after recovery, it usually lasts just a short time; when it does not appear until many years later, it may last

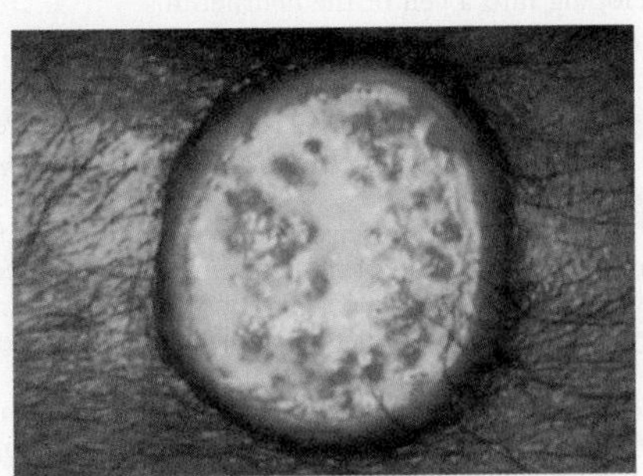

■ Cutaneous leishmaniasis.

much longer. Called also *dermal leishmanoid, leishmanoid,* and *post–kala-azar dermal leishmanoid.*

l. reci′divans a relapsing form of cutaneous leishmaniasis that resembles tuberculosis of the skin and may last for many years. Either the ulcer heals incompletely, scarring centrally but spreading peripherally, or it heals and recurs at the edge of the scar. It is usually caused by *Leishmania tropica* in the Old World and *L. braziliensis* in the New World.

rural l., rural cutaneous l. zoonotic cutaneous l.

urban l., urban cutaneous l. anthroponotic cutaneous l.

visceral l. a chronic infectious disease, highly fatal if untreated, usually caused by *Leishmania donovani, L. infantum,* or *L. chagasi,* found in various tropical and subtropical regions of the world; parasites are found in the cells of the reticuloendothelial system throughout the body, especially in the liver, spleen, bone marrow, lymph nodes, and skin. It is commonly characterized by hepatosplenomegaly, irregular fever, chills, vomiting, emaciation, anemia, leukopenia, hypergammaglobulinemia, and an earth-gray color of the skin. It has traditionally been divided into three different forms according to geographical distribution, vector, and other factors, but such a distinction may prove to be invalid. See *American visceral l., infantile visceral l.,* and *Indian visceral l.* Called also *kala-azar, tropical splenomegaly,* and *black, cachectic, cachexial,* or *Dumdum fever.*

viscerotropic l. a rare type of infection found in northeastern Saudi Arabia; after infection with *Leishmania tropica,* instead of the usual cutaneous symptoms, fever and other systemic symptoms are seen and *Leishmania* can be detected in internal organs.

wet cutaneous l., zoonotic cutaneous l. a type of Old World cutaneous leishmaniasis found mainly in rural areas in parts of the Middle East, Central Asia, and the Indian subcontinent, caused by *Leishmania major;* its reservoirs are desert rodents such as ground squirrels and gerbils (particularly *Rhombomys opimus* and *Meriones* species) and it spreads to humans via the vectors *Phlebotomus papatasi* and *P. duboscqi.* Infection is acute, rapidly evolving, and characterized by multiple sores with inflammation, ulceration, and crusting. Called also *acute* or *rural cutaneous l.*

leish•man•i•ci•dal (lēsh″mən-ĭ-si′dəl) destroying *Leishmania;* see also antileishmanial.

leish•ma•nin (lēsh′mə-nin) a suspension of killed leishmania promastigotes; used in a skin test for cutaneous leishmaniasis; see *leishmanin test,* under *test.*

leish•ma•noid (lēsh′mə-noid) 1. like or resembling leishmaniasis. 2. a lesion of post–kala-azar dermal leishmaniasis.

dermal l., post–kala-azar dermal l. post–kala-azar dermal leishmaniasis.

Lei•u•rus (li-u′rəs) a genus of scorpions of the family Buthidae, found in desert areas throughout Africa and the Middle East. *L. quinquestria′tus* is a common species that has a deadly sting.

Lek•sell apparatus, technique (lek′səl) [Lars *Leksell,* Swedish neurosurgeon, 20th century] see under *apparatus* and *technique.*

Le•laps (le′laps) *Echinolaelaps.*

Lem•bert suture (lahm-bār′) [Antoine *Lembert,* French surgeon, 1802–1851] see under *suture.*

Le•mierre syndrome (lə-myār′) [André Alfred *Lemierre,* French physician, 1875–1956] see under *syndrome.*

Le•mi•eux-Nee•meh syndrome (lə-myoo͝′ na′ma) [Guy *Lemieux,* Canadian physician, 20th century; Jean A. *Neemeh,* Canadian physician, 20th century] see under *syndrome.*

lem•ma (lem′ə) [Gr. "rind," "husk"] a collective term for the three egg membranes.

-lemma a word termination denoting a sheath around another structure.

lem•mo•blast (lem′o-blast) a primordial or immature lemmocyte.

lem•mo•blas•tic (lem″o-blas′tik) forming or developing into neurilemma tissue.

lem•mo•cyte (lem′o-sīt) [*lemma* + *-cyte*] a cell derived from the neural crest and developing into a cell of the neurilemma.

lem•nis•ci (lem-nis′i) plural of *lemniscus.*

lem•nis•cus (lem-nis′kəs) gen. and pl. *lemnis′ci* [L., from Gr. *lēmniskos* ribbon] 1. a ribbon or band. 2. [TA] a band or bundle of sensory fibers in the central nervous system; called also *fillet.* See also *bundle, fasciculus, tract,* and *tractus.*

l. latera′lis [TA] lateral lemniscus: a tract of longitudinal fibers extending upward through the lateral part of the tegmental substance of the pons, formed chiefly by fibers arising from the opposite cochlear nuclei and the trapezoid body, and also some ipsilateral projections, and ascending to terminate in the inferior colliculus and medial geniculate body.

l. media′lis [TA] medial lemniscus: a tract arising from the internal arcuate fibers of the nuclei gracilis and cuneatus, and crossing to the opposite side in the lower part of medulla oblongata to ascend, first between the two olives, and then through the pars dorsalis pontis just dorsal to the pontine nuclei; it continues through the tegmentum of the midbrain and ends in the ventral posterior part of the thalamus. Each lemniscus carries sensory impulses from the opposite side of the body. Called also *sensory l.*

sensory l. l. medialis.

l. spina′lis [TA] spinal lemniscus: the part of each tract containing spinothalamic fibers lying within the pons and mesencephalon, forming a diffuse bundle between the medial and lateral lemnisci. It carries pain, temperature, and tactile impulses from the opposite side of the body and ends in the ventral posterior part of the thalamus. Called also *tractus anterolaterales [TA alternative], anterolateral tracts,* and *anterolateral system.*

l. trigemina′lis [TA] trigeminal lemniscus: a group of fibers conveying sensory impulses from the trigeminal nuclei to the ventral posterior part of the opposite thalamus; it ascends intermingled with the spinal lemniscus and adjacent medial lemniscus. Called also *tractus trigeminothalamicus* [TA alternative] and *trigeminothalamic tract.*

lem•on (lem′ən) 1. *Citrus limon.* 2. the fruit of *C. limon,* which contains citric and ascorbic acids, used as an antiscorbutic, and whose peel contains lemon oil.

Lem•pert fenestration operation (lem′pərt) [Julius *Lempert,* American otologist, 1890–1968] see under *operation.*

LEMS Lambert-Eaton myasthenic syndrome.

lem•ur (lem′ər) any member of the family Lemuridae.

Le•mu•ri•dae (lĕ-mu′rĭ-de) the lemurs, a family of small, arboreal, usually nocturnal primates native to Madagascar and nearby islands; they resemble monkeys but have a sharp, foxlike muzzle and a tail that is long, furry, and never prehensile.

len•a•lid•o•mide (len″ə-lid′o-mīd) an immunomodulator chemically related to thalidomide, used in treatment of a subgroup of myelodysplastic syndrome known as the deletion 5q cytogenetic abnormality; administered orally.

Le•nè•gre disease (lə-neg′rə) [Jean *Lenègre,* French cardiologist, 1904–1972] see under *disease.*

length (*l*) (length) an expression of the longest dimension of an object, or of the measurement between the two ends.

arch l. the length of a line segment within the median plane perpendicular to and extending from the line connecting the first premolars to the most labial point on the anterior arch, usually to the point between the maxillary central incisors. Called also *anterior arch l.*

basialveolar l. the distance from the basion to the lower end of the intermaxillary suture.

basinasal l. the distance from basion to nasion.

crown-heel l. (CHL) the length of an embryo, fetus, or infant from the crown of the head to the heel; used in estimating the age of the embryos during the eighth week and of fetuses. It is the equivalent of *standing height* in older individuals.

crown-rump l. (CRL) the length of an embryo, fetus, or infant from the crown of the head to the breech; used in estimating the age of embryos from the fourth to the eighth week. It is the equivalent of *sitting vertex height* in older individuals.

cycle l. in cardiac pacing, the time interval in milliseconds from one event to the next.

focal l. the distance between a lens and an object from which all rays of light are brought to a focus. Symbol f.

foot l. a heel–great toe measurement useful in estimating the age of fetuses because the foot dimensions are less subject to artifacts of curvature and shrinkage than is the fetus as a whole.

greatest l. a dimension used to express the size of very young human embryos that have not yet developed the structures permitting measurement of crown-rump length, as during the third week.

sitting l. the distance from the crown of the head to the coccyx.

stem l. the distance from the vertex to a line joining the ischial tuberosities.

wave l. see *wavelength.*

len•i•tive (len′ĭ-tiv) [L. *lenire* to soothe] demulcent.

Len•nert classification, lymphoma (len′ərt) [K. *Lennert,* German pathologist, 20th century] see *Kiel Classification* under *classification* and see under *lymphoma.*

Lenn•hoff index (len′hof) [Rudolf *Lennhoff,* German physician, 1866–1933] see under *index.*

Len•nox syndrome (len′əks) [William Gordon *Lennox,* American neurologist, 1884–1960] Lennox-Gastaut syndrome.

Len•nox-Gas•taut syndrome (len′əks gah-sto′) [W.G. *Lennox;* Henri Jean Pascal *Gastaut,* French biologist, 1915–1995] see under *syndrome.*

lens (lenz) [L. "lentil"] 1. a piece of glass or other transparent substance so shaped as to converge or scatter the rays of light, especially the glass used in appropriate frames or other instruments to increase the visual acuity of the human eye. See also *glasses* and *spectacles.* 2. [TA] the transparent

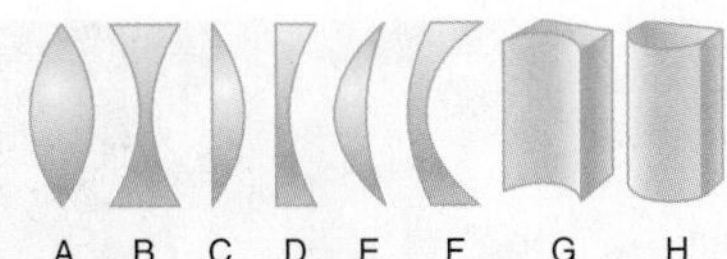

■ Lenses: *(A–F)*, Spherical lenses: *(A)*, biconvex; *(B)*, biconcave; *(C)*, planoconvex; *(D)*, planoconcave; *(E)*, concavoconvex, periscopic convex, converging meniscus; *(F)*, convexoconcave, periscopic concave, diverging meniscus; *(G, H)*, cylindrical lenses, concave and convex.

biconvex body of the eye situated between the posterior chamber and the vitreous body, constituting part of the refracting mechanism of the eye. Called also *l. crystallina* or *crystalline l.*

achromatic l. a lens corrected for chromatic aberration.

acrylic l. a plastic lens used to replace the crystalline lens after cataract surgery.

adherent l. contact l.

anastigmatic l. a lens with spherical surfaces only and no cylindrical ones; called also *stigmatic l.*

aniseikonic l. iseikonic l.

aplanatic l. a lens for correction of spherical aberration and coma.

apochromatic l. a lens corrected for chromatic and spherical aberration.

astigmatic l. cylindrical l.

bandage l. a soft contact lens worn on a diseased or injured cornea to protect or treat it.

biconcave l. a flat lens that has both surfaces concave; called also *concavoconcave l.*

biconvex l. a flat lens that has both surfaces convex.

bicylindrical l. a lens that has both surfaces cylindrical or toroidal.

bifocal l. a lens that has two segments with different refractive powers, ordinarily with the upper for distant and the lower for near vision; used in bifocal glasses.

bispherical l. a lens that is spherical on both sides.

Brücke l. a combination of a double convex and double concave lens so arranged as to give considerable working distance.

cataract l. a powerful lens for glasses to be used after cataract operation.

compound l. a lens made up of two or more segments.

concave l. a lens that has a surface curved like part of the interior of a hollow sphere, so that it diverges rays of light. Called also *diverging l.* and *minus l.*

concave l., double biconcave l.

concave l., periscopic convexoconcave l.

concavoconcave l. biconcave l.

concavoconvex l. a lens that has one concave surface and one convex; the concave surface is of greater curvature than the convex. Called also *periscopic convex l.*, *converging meniscus l.*, and *positive meniscus l.*

condensing l. a large, powerful convex spherical lens to focus available light upon the eye for examination.

contact l. a curved shell of glass or plastic applied directly over the globe or cornea to correct refractive errors; called also *adherent l.*

contact l., corneal a contact lens that rests on the cornea, not on the sclera, and requires no auxiliary liquid; called also *corneal l.*

contact l., gas permeable any contact lens that transmits oxygen and carbon dioxide.

contact l., hard a contact lens that maintains its shape without support and absorbs little or no water; it may be gas permeable or non–gas permeable. Called also *hydrophobic contact l.* and *rigid contact l.*

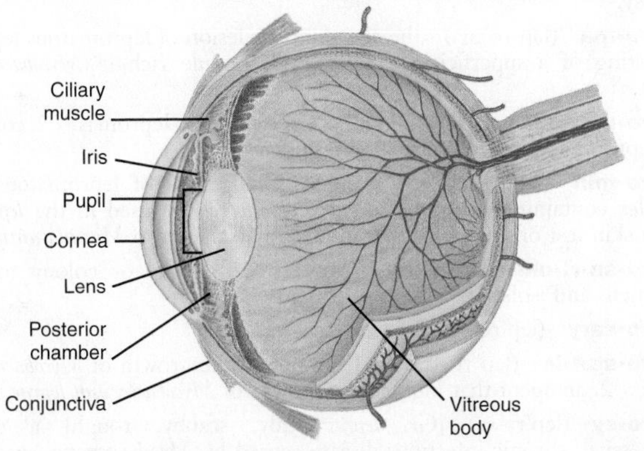

■ Lens of eye.

contact l., hydrophilic soft contact l.

contact l., hydrophobic hard contact l.

contact l., non–gas permeable hard a contact lens, generally formed of polymethyl methacrylate, that transmits little to no oxygen and carbon dioxide to the cornea. Called also *PMMA contact l.*

contact l., PMMA a contact lens made of polymethyl methacrylate; see *non–gas permeable hard contact l.*

contact l., rigid hard contact l.

contact l., scleral a contact lens that covers the cornea and rests on the sclera, with or without an auxiliary liquid between it and the cornea.

contact l., soft a contact lens that when worn is soft, flexible, and water absorbent; called also *hydrophilic contact l.*

converging l., convex l. a lens that is curved like part of the exterior of a hollow sphere, so that it brings light to a focus. Called also *plus l.*

convex l., double biconvex l.

convex l., periscopic concavoconvex l.

convexoconcave l. a lens that has one convex and one concave surface; the convex surface is of greater curvature than the concave. Called also *periscopic concave l.*, *diverging meniscus l.*, and *negative meniscus l.*

corneal l. corneal contact l.

Crookes l. a lens made from glass rendered opaque to ultraviolet and infrared rays but transparent to visible light.

crossed l. a converging lens with minimal spherical aberration.

l. crystalli′na, crystalline l. lens (def. 2).

cylindrical l. a lens used to correct astigmatism, having one plane surface and one cylindrical, or one spherical surface and one toroidal. The meridian along the lens axis has no refractive power, but the meridian at right angles to the axis has maximum refractive power; thus the principal focus is a straight line, not a point. Symbol C. Abbreviated cyl. Called also *astigmatic l.*

decentered l. a lens whose optical axis does not pass through the geometric center.

dispersing l. an incorrect name for *concave l.*

diverging l. concave l.

flat l. a lens with equal curvature on both sides, as opposed to a meniscus lens.

Fresnel l. a thin lens made up of a number of stepped setbacks concentrically arranged; it has the optical properties of a much thicker lens.

honeybee l. a magnifying eyeglass lens designed to resemble the multifaceted eye of the honeybee. It consists of three or six small telescopes mounted in the upper portion of the spectacles and directed toward the center and right and left visual fields. Prisms are included to provide a continuous, unbroken magnified field of view.

immersion l. see under *objective*.

intraocular l. (IOL) an artificial lens inserted into the lens capsule after cataract removal.

iseikonic l. a lens that magnifies but does not refract; it is used to treat aniseikonia because it changes the sizes of the images on the retinas of the eyes. Called also *aniseikonic l.* and *size l.*

meniscus l. a crescent-shaped lens with one concave surface and one convex; the surfaces have different degrees of curvature. See *concavoconvex l.* and *convexoconcave l.*

meniscus l., converging concavoconvex l.

meniscus l., diverging convexoconcave l.

meniscus l., negative convexoconcave l.

meniscus l., positive concavoconvex l.

meter l. a converging lens with a focal length of one meter and a refracting power of one diopter.

minus l. concave l.

omnifocal l. a lens whose power increases continuously and regularly in a downward direction, thereby avoiding the discontinuity in field and power of a bifocal or trifocal lens. Called also progressive l.

orthoscopic l. a lens that gives a very flat and undistorted field of vision, especially at the periphery.

pantoscopic l. bifocal l.

periscopic l. a lens that has a 1.25D base curve.

photochromic l., photosensitive l. a light-sensitive lens that darkens in full light and clears in reduced light.

plane l., plano l. a lens with no curve and no refracting power; light rays enter and leave parallel.

planoconcave l. a lens with one plane and one concave side.

planoconvex l. a lens with one plane and one convex side.

plus l. convex l.

progressive l. omnifocal l.

punktal l. a toric lens that is corrected for astigmatism over the entire field of vision.

safety l. a lens that protects the eye from injury, especially from impact. Impact-resistant lenses may be made by tempering or by using plastic or laminated lenses. See also *safety glasses*.

size l. iseikonic l.

spherical l. (S, sph) a lens that is a segment of a sphere.

spherocylindrical l. a lens with one spherical and one cylindrical surface, and functioning as both a simple spherical lens and a simple cylindrical one.

stigmatic l. anastigmatic l.

toric l. a meniscus lens with a cylindrical curve ground on the outer (convex) surface.

trial l. a lens used in testing the vision.

trifocal l. a lens that has three segments with different refractive powers, ordinarily with the upper for distant, the middle for intermediate, and the lower for near vision; used in trifocal glasses.

lens•om•e•ter (lenz-om′ə-tər) [*lens* + *-meter*] a device for measuring the optical characteristics of lenses; called also *phacometer.*

Len•te Il•e•tin (len′te il′ə-tin) see under *Iletin.*

lenti- [L. *lens*, gen. *lentis* lentil] a combining form meaning shaped like a lentil, or denoting relationship to a lens.

len•ti•cel (len′tĭ-sel) a lens-shaped gland, especially one of those at the base of the tongue.

len•ti•co•nus (len″ti-ko′nəs) [*lenti-* + *conus*] a conical protrusion of the substance of the crystalline lens, covered by capsule or connective tissue, occurring more frequently on the posterior surface, and usually affecting only one eye.

len•tic•u•la (len-tik′u-lə) [L.] nucleus lentiformis.

len•tic•u•lar (len-tik′u-lər) [L. *lenticularis*] 1. pertaining to or shaped like a lens. 2. pertaining to the crystalline lens. 3. pertaining to the lenticular nucleus.

len•tic•u•lo-op•tic (len-tik″u-lo-op′tik) pertaining to the lenticular nucleus and the optic thalamus.

len•tic•u•lo•stri•ate (len-tik″u-lo-stri′āt) pertaining to the lenticular nucleus and the corpus striatum.

len•tic•u•lo•tha•lam•ic (len-tik″u-lo-thə-lam′ik) relating to the lenticular nucleus and the thalamus.

len•ti•form (len′tĭ-form) [*lenti-* + *form*] shaped like a lens; see under *bone* and see *nucleus lentiformis.*

len•tig•i•nes (len-tij′ĭ-nēz) [L.] plural of *lentigo.*

len•tig•i•no•sis (len-tij″ĭ-no′sis) the presence of multiple lentigines.

agminated l. the presence of aggregations of macules up to 1 or 2 cm in diameter on specific body segments.

generalized l., l. profu′sa LEOPARD syndrome.

progressive cardiomyopathic l. Moynahan syndrome (def. 1).

segmental l. the presence of numerous circumscribed lentigines with elongated, prominent rete ridges.

len•tig•i•nous (len-tij′ĭ-nəs) characterized by multiple lentigines; pertaining to or of the nature of a lentigo.

len•ti•glo•bus (len″tĭ-glo′bəs) [*lens* + *globus*] an exaggerated curvation of the crystalline lens, producing a spherical bulging on its anterior surface.

len•ti•go (len-ti′go) pl. *lentig′ines* [L. "freckle"] a small, flat, tan to dark brown or black, macular melanosis on the skin; it resembles a freckle clinically but is histologically distinct because it contains an increased number of normal-appearing melanocytes along the dermal-epidermal junction. Lentigines, unlike freckles, do not darken on exposure to sunlight. Called also *l. simplex.*

l. malig′na a type of lentigo that expands slowly and develops into lentigo maligna melanoma (see under *melanoma*). Called also *Hutchinson freckle* and *melanotic freckle of Hutchinson.*

nevoid l. l. simplex.

senile l., l. seni′lis solar l.

l. sim′plex the most common type of lentigo, a congenital type found on mucous membranes as well as skin, usually associated with a hereditary disorder such as the LEOPARD syndrome or Moynahan syndrome. The rete pegs elongate and the number of melanocytes sharply increases. Single or multiple lesions may occur, and size and configuration vary widely. Called also *nevoid l.*

solar l. a benign, discrete, hyperpigmented macule on chronically sun-exposed skin such as the backs of the hands or the forehead, usually seen in elderly, light-skinned adults. Called also *age spot, liver spot, senile l.,* and *l. senilis.*

Len•ti•vi•ri•nae (len″tĭ-vir-i′ne) the HIV-like viruses: a former subfamily of viruses of the family Retroviridae, containing the genus *Lentivirus.*

Len•ti•vi•rus (len′tĭ-vi″rəs) [L. *lentus* slow + *virus*] a genus of viruses of the family Retroviridae that cause persistent infection that typically results in chronic, progressive, sometimes fatal disease. Species include the human immunodeficiency viruses, caprine arthritis-encephalitis virus, equine infectious anemia virus, simian immunodeficiency virus, and visna/maedi virus.

len•ti•vi•rus (len′tĭ-vi″rəs) any virus of the genus *Lentivirus.* **lentivi′ral** *adj*

len•tu•la (len′chu-lə, len-too′lə) lentulo.

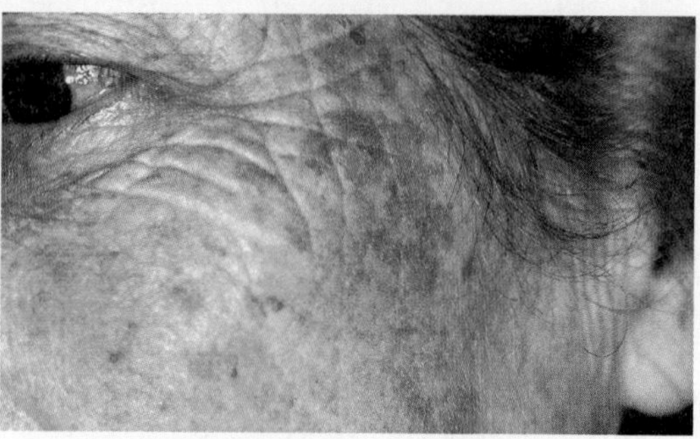

■ Solar lentigines.

len•tu•lo (len′chu-lo, len-too′lo) in root canal therapy, a flexible, spiral, rotating instrument made of stainless steel wire attached to a handpiece, used to place cement into the prepared canal. Called also *lentula* and *paste carrier.*

Lenz syndrome (lents) [Widukind D. *Lenz*, German physician, 1919–1995] see under *syndrome.*

le•on•ti•a•sis (le″on-ti′ə-sis) [Gr. *leōn* lion + *-iasis*] leonine facies.

l. os′sea, l. os′sium leonine facies caused by hypertrophy of the bones of the face and cranium, such as in hyperostosis frontalis interna.

Le•o•pold maneuvers (le′ə-pōld) [Christian Gerhard *Leopold*, German physician, 1846–1911] see under *maneuver.*

le•o•tro•pic (le″o-tro′pik) [Gr. *laios* left + *-tropic*] running spirally from right to left. Cf. *dexiotropic.*

lep•er (lep′ər) a person afflicted with leprosy; a term now in disfavor.

le•pid•ic (lə-pid′ik) scaly.

Lep•i•dop•tera (lep″ĭ-dop′tər -ə) [Gr. *lepis*, gen. *lepidos* flake or scale + *pteron* wing] the butterflies and moths, an order of insects with large wings covered by small transparent scales. The larval form is the caterpillar.

lep•i•dop•ter•ism (lep″ĭ-dop′tər-iz-əm) disease caused by exposure to moths or butterflies (order Lepidoptera), such as caterpillar dermatitis or allergic reactions from inhaling their hairs.

Lep•i•o•ta (lep″e-o′tə) a genus of mushrooms of the family Agaricaceae. They contain amatoxins and can cause mushroom poisoning (see under *poisoning*).

lep•i•ru•din (lep″ĭ-roo′din) a type of direct thrombin inhibitor that is a recombinant form of hirudin, used as an anticoagulant in patients with heparin-induced thrombocytopenia and associated thromboembolic disease; administered intravenously.

Lep•o•ri•pox•vi•rus (lep″ə-rĭ-poks′vi-rəs) [L. *lepus*, gen. *leporis* hare + *poxvirus*] a genus of viruses of the subfamily Chordopoxvirinae (family Poxviridae) with serologic cross-reactivity that infect squirrels and rabbits, including myxoma virus and rabbit fibroma virus.

Le•po•ri•dae (ləpo′rĭ-de) a family of mammals of the order Lagomorpha, including the rabbits and hares.

lep•ra (lep′rə) [Gr. *lepra* leprosy, which makes the skin scaly] leprosy. See also under *reaction.*

lep•re•chaun•ism (lep′rə-kon″iz-əm) Donohue syndrome.

lep•rol•o•gist (lep-rol′ə-jist) a physician specializing in the study and treatment of leprosy.

lep•rol•o•gy (lep-rol′ə-je) a medical specialty, more common through the mid-twentieth century, involving the diagnosis and treatment of leprosy.

lep•ro•ma (ləp-ro′mə) the characteristic lesion of lepromatous leprosy, consisting of a superficial granulomatous nodule rich in *Mycobacterium leprae.*

lep•ro•ma•tous (ləp-ro′mə-təs) 1. pertaining to lepromas. 2. containing lepromas; see *lepromatous leprosy*, under *leprosy.*

lep•ro•min (lep′ro-min) a purified homogenate of lepromatous skin nodules containing heat-killed *Mycobacterium leprae;* used in the *lepromin test*, a skin test of immune status in leprosy. Called also *Mitsuda antigen.*

le•pro•sa•ri•um (lep″ro-sar′e-əm) [L.] a hospital or colony for the treatment and isolation of leprosy patients.

lep•ro•sary (lep′ro-sar″e) leprosarium.

lep•ro•stat•ic (lep″ro-stat′ik) 1. inhibiting the growth of *Mycobacterium leprae.* 2. an agent that inhibits the growth of *Mycobacterium leprae.*

lep•ro•sy (lep′rə-se) [Gr. *lepros* scaly, scabby, rough] a slowly progressive, chronic infectious disease caused by *Mycobacterium leprae* and characterized by granulomatous or neurotrophic lesions in the skin, mucous membranes, nerves, bones, and viscera, with a broad spectrum of clinical symptoms. Two principal types are distinguished: *lepromatous leprosy* and *tuberculoid leprosy*, with gradations between them known as *borderline leprosy*. Called also *Hansen disease*. **leprot′ic, lep′rous** *adj*

borderline l. an immunologically unstable type of leprosy, transitional between the tuberculoid and lepromatous forms and having clinical and histological features of both types; it may evolve toward the former by a reversal reaction or toward the latter by a downgrading reaction. Called also *dimorphous* or *intermediate l.*

borderline lepromatous l. borderline leprosy that is tending toward the lepromatous type, with numerous symmetrical lesions and nerve damage.

borderline tuberculoid l. borderline leprosy that is tending toward the tuberculoid type; lesions are likely to be smaller and more numerous than usual tuberculoid ones.

bovine l. Johne disease.

diffuse lepromatous l., diffuse l. of Lucio Lucio l.

dimorphous l. borderline l.

feline l. a granulomatous skin condition in cats, characterized by nodules that ulcerate and drain, usually on the legs or head; it may be associated with infection by *Mycobacterium lepraemurium*, such as from contact with infected rodents.

histoid l. a rare type of lepromatous leprosy characterized by nodules in the dermis containing whorls or bands of histiocytes.

indeterminate l. early manifestations of leprosy, consisting of a few poorly defined areas of anesthesia or hypoesthesia with hypopigmentation or erythema. Histologically, there are uncharacteristic macules in exposed areas of the skin, which may heal spontaneously or progress and evolve into one of the more definitive forms.

intermediate l. borderline l.

lepromatous l. the more malignant and infectious of the two polar types of leprosy, characterized principally by widespread dissemination of *Mycobacterium leprae* in the tissues (which reflects the poor immune response to infection), and by numerous cutaneous lesions consisting of pale, diffusely and symmetrically distributed macules. The lepromin test is negative. If untreated, the macules gradually progress to form plaques and nodules called lepromas. Infiltrations result in destructive lesions and deformities such as leonine facies, but nerve damage is usually less than that seen in tuberculoid leprosy. Called also *multibacillary l.*

Lucio l. a type of lepromatous leprosy seen especially in Mexico and Central America, characterized by diffuse infiltration of the skin. Advanced cases may be complicated by the Lucio phenomenon (q.v.) with necrosis and ulcers of the skin and scarring. Called also *diffuse lepromatous l.*

multibacillary l. lepromatous l.

murine l. rat l.

paucibacillary l. tuberculoid l.

rat l. a chronic epizootic disease of wild rats caused by *Mycobacterium lepraemurium*, characterized by lesions containing enormous numbers of acid-fast bacilli closely resembling *M. leprae* in size and shape, which may be transmitted to white rats, mice, and guinea pigs by inoculation of infected tissue; a relationship with human leprosy has not been established. Called also *murine l.*

reactional l. leprosy that is complicated by one of the lepra reactions (see under *reaction*).

tuberculoid l. the more benign, less infectious, usually self-limited of the two polar types of leprosy; as a result of well-developed cell-mediated immunity to *Mycobacterium leprae*, acid-fast bacilli usually cannot be identified in the lesions. The lepromin test is positive. It is characterized by asymmetric, sharply defined, anesthetic, discolored, dry macules or plaques with elevated borders; early severe nerve damage; and often muscle atrophy. Called also *paucibacillary l.*

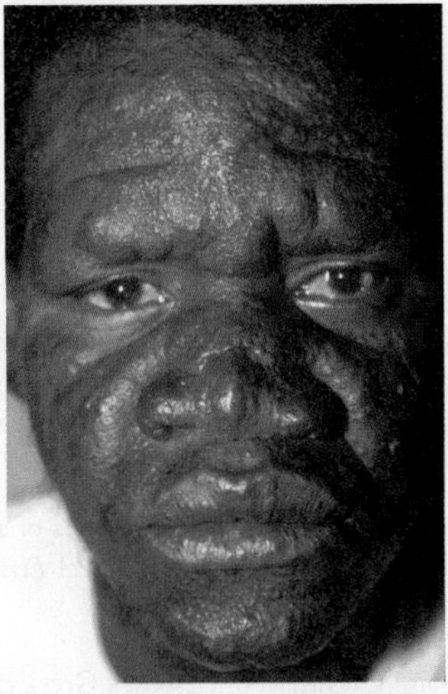

■ Lepromatous leprosy; there is diffuse infiltration of the face with leonine facies and madarosis.

uncharacteristic l. indeterminate l.

lep•tin (lep′tin) a 167 amino acid adipocytokine that is part of a feedback loop that provides information to the brain about the state of nutrient stores. After secretion, it circulates in plasma and interacts with a specific receptor in the hypothalamus, decreasing food intake and increasing energy expenditure. It also increases insulin sensitivity, which is believed to result partly from its effect on the hypothalamus and partly from its action on peripheral tissues.

lep•tin•emia (lep″tin-e′me-ə) hyperleptinemia.

lept(o)- [Gr. *leptos* slender] a combining form meaning slender, thin, or delicate.

lep•to•ceph•a•ly (lep″to-sef′ə-le) abnormal tallness and narrowness of the skull. **leptocephal′ic, leptoceph′alous** *adj*

Lep•to•ci•mex (lep″to-si′meks) *Cimex.*

Lep•to•co•nops (lep″to-ko′nops) a genus of blood-sucking flies of the family Heleidae.

lep•to•cyte (lep′to-sīt) [*lepto-* + *-cyte*] target cell (def. 1).

lep•to•cy•to•sis (lep″to-si-to′sis) the presence of target cells (leptocytes) in the blood.

lep•to•dac•ty•lous (lep″to-dak′tə-ləs) [*lepto-* + *dactyl* + *-ous*] having slender digits.

lep•to•dac•ty•ly (lep″to-dak′tə-le) abnormal slenderness of the digits.

lep•to•don•tous (lep″to-don′təs) [*lepto-* + *odont-* + *-ous*] having slender teeth.

lep•to•kur•tic (lep″to-kur′tik) [*lepto-* + Gr. *kurtos* convex] pertaining to a probability distribution more heavily concentrated around the mean, i.e., having a sharper, narrower peak, than the normal distribution with the same variance. Cf. *platykurtic.*

lep•to•me•nin•ges (lep″to-mə-nin′jēz) (sing. *leptome′ninx*) [*lepto-* + *meninges*] [TA] the pia mater and arachnoid considered together as one functional unit; the pia-arachnoid. **leptomenin′geal** *adj*

lep•to•me•nin•gi•o•ma (lep″to-mə-nin″je-o′mə) a tumor of the leptomeninges.

lep•to•me•nin•gi•tis (lep″to-men″in-ji′tis) [*leptomeninges* + *-itis*] inflammation of the leptomeninges.

sarcomatous l. diffuse sarcomatous infiltration of the pia mater.

lep•to•men•in•gop•a•thy (lep″to-men″in-gop′ə-the) [*leptomeninges* + *-pathy*] any disease of the leptomeninges.

lep•to•men•inx (lep″to-men′inks) [*lepto-* + *meninx*] [TA] singular of leptomeninges. NOTE: In official nomenclature, this term is used as the preferred term when contrasting this structure (arachnoidea mater et pia mater) with the pachymeninx, which is equivalent to the dura mater.

lep•to•mo•nad (lep″to-mo′nad) [*lepto-* + *monad*] 1. pertaining to the genus *Leptomonas.* 2. leptomonas.

Lep•to•mo•nas (lep″to-mo′nəs) [*lepto-* + Gr. *monas* unit, from *monos* single] a genus of parasitic protozoa of the order Kinetoplastida, phylum Euglenozoa, found in the digestive tract of various insects. The organisms are monogenetic, with promastigote forms dominating in the life cycle; amastigotes and cysts also occur.

lep•to•mo•nas (lep″to-mo′nəs) any protozoan of the genus *Leptomonas.*

Lep•to•myx•i•da (lep″to-mik′si-də) [*lepto-* + Gr. *myxa* mucus] an order of ramicristate amebae, protozoa of the class Lobosa, phylum Sarcomastigophora; they typically occur in thin protoplasmic sheets that may be either polyaxial or cylindrical. A genus of medical interest is *Balamuthia.*

lep•to•ne•ma (lep″to-ne′mə) [*lepto-* + Gr. *nēma* thread] leptotene.

lep•to•no•mor•phol•o•gy (lep″to-no-mor-fol′ə-je) the morphology of membranes.

lep•to•pel•lic (lep″to-pel′ik) [*lepto-* + Gr. *pella* bowl] having a narrow pelvis.

lep•to•pho•nia (lep″to-fo′ne-ə) [*lepto-* + *phon-* + *-ia*] hypophonia.

lep•top•ro•sope (lep-top′ro-sōp) an individual exhibiting leptoprosopia.

lep•to•pro•so•pia (lep″to-pro-so′pe-ə) [*lepto-* + *prosop-* + *-ia*] narrowness of the face, with slender features, round, open orbits, long nose, narrow nostrils, and small mouth. **leptoprosop′ic** *adj*

Lep·to·psyl·la (lep″to-sil′ə) a genus of fleas. *L. seg′nis* (also called *L. mus′culi*) is a common flea of the mouse and rat and a vector of plague.

lep·tor·rhine (lep′to-rīn) [*lepto-* + Gr. *rhis* nose] having a nasal index below 48.

lep·to·scope (lep′to-skōp) [*lepto-* + *-scope*] an optical apparatus for measuring the thickness of the plasma membrane of a cell.

Lep·to·sphae·ria (lep″to-sfe′re-ə) a genus of bitunicate fungi of the order Dothideales. *L. senegalen′sis* is an etiologic agent of eumycotic mycetoma in West Africa.

Lep·to·spi·ra (lep″to-spi′rə) [*lepto-* + Gr. *speira* coil] a genus of bacteria of the family Leptospiraceae, consisting of single, finely coiled, motile, aerobic cells with hooked ends that are visible by darkfield microscopy. The type species, which contains all pathogenic strains, is *L. inter′rogans.*

L. austra′lis former name for *L. interrogans* serovar *australis.*

L. autumna′lis former name for *L. interrogans* serovar *autumnalis.*

L. bata′viae former name for *L. interrogans* serovar *bataviae.*

L. biflex′a a species found in both fresh water and sea water; most strains of the genus are saprophytic and nonpathogenic, but occasionally a strain causes mammalian infection.

L. cani′cola former name for *L. interrogans* serovar *canicola.*

L. grippotypho′sa former name for *L. interrogans* serovar *grippotyphosa.*

L. hard′jo former name for *L. interrogans* serovar *hardjo.*

L. hebdo′madis former name for *L. interrogans* serovar *hebdomadis.*

L. hy′os former name for *L. interrogans* serovar *tarassovi.*

L. icterohaemorrha′giae former name for *L. interrogans* serovar *icterohaemorrhagiae.*

L. inter′rogans the species containing all the pathogenic strains of the genus, which cause leptospirosis. It is divided into serological groups that are in turn separated into serovars. A wide range of wild and domestic animals serve as reservoirs and shed the organisms in their urine.

L. inter′rogans **serovar** *austra′lis* a serovar carried by rodents and causing human leptospirosis. Type A, found in Australia, the United States, Europe, Southeast Asia, and Japan, also causes infection in numerous other mammals. Type B, found in Australia, Southeast Asia, and Europe, is not known to cause infection in animals other than humans.

L. inter′rogans **serovar** *autumna′lis* a serovar carried by rodents, causing leptospirosis in Southeast Asia, Japan, and the United States.

L. inter′rogans **serovar** *bata′viae* a serovar carried by rodents, causing leptospirosis in Southeast Asia, Europe, Africa, and Japan.

L. inter′rogans **serovar** *cani′cola* a serovar carried by dogs, causing Stuttgart disease in dogs and other types of leptospirosis in other mammals.

L. inter′rogans **serovar** *grippotypho′sa* a serovar carried by rodents and causing leptospirosis in many different mammals.

L. inter′rogans **serovar** *hard′jo* a serovar carried by rodents and causing leptospirosis in cattle, sheep, and horses.

L. inter′rogans **serovar** *hebdo′madis* a serovar carried by field voles and causing human leptospirosis.

L. inter′rogans **serovar** *hy′os* former name for *L. interrogans* serovar *tarassovi.*

L. inter′rogans **serovar** *icterohaemorrha′giae* a serovar of worldwide distribution that is carried by rodents and is the major cause of Weil syndrome in humans, yellows in dogs, and other diseases in various other mammals.

L. inter′rogans **serovar** *pomo′na* a serovar carried by pigs, cattle, and rodents; the primary cause of swineherd's disease in humans and infection in various other animals.

L. inter′rogans **serovar** *pyro′genes* a serovar carried by rodents and causing human leptospirosis in Japan and Southeast Asia.

L. inter′rogans **serovar** *taras′sovi* a serovar found in pigs, a primary cause of swineherd's disease in humans.

L. pomo′na former name for *L. interrogans* serovar *pomona.*

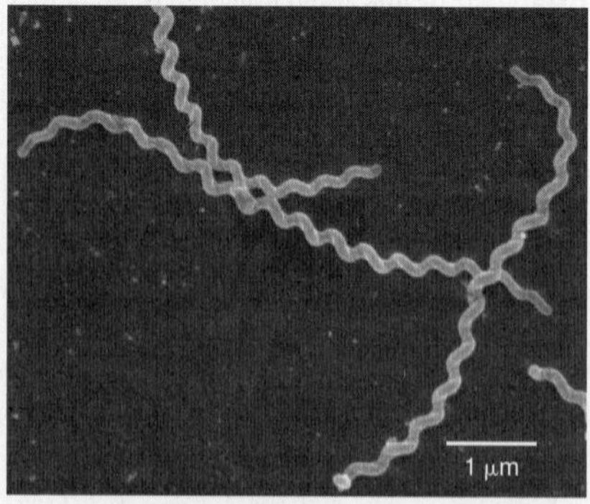

■ Scanning electron micrograph of *Leptospira interrogans,* showing the characteristic tight coils.

L. pyro′genes former name for *L. interrogans* serovar *pyrogenes.*

L. taras′sovi former name for *L. inter′rogans* serovar *tarassovi.*

lep·to·spi·ra (lep″to-spi′rə) an individual organism belonging to the genus *Leptospira.* Called also *leptospire.*

Lep·to·spi·ra·ceae (lep″to-spi-ra′se-e) a family of bacteria of the order Spirochaetales, consisting of flexible helical cells that are aerobic and utilize long-chain fatty acids or alcohols for growth. Medically important organisms are contained in the genus *Leptospira.*

lep·to·spi·ral (lep″to-spi′rəl) of, pertaining to, or caused by leptospiras.

lep·to·spire (lep′to-spīr) leptospira.

lep·to·spi·ro·sis (lep″to-spi-ro′sis) febrile illness caused by infection with one of the serovars of *Leptospira interrogans.* Numerous different mammals shed the organisms in their urine, and others become infected through contact with the urine or tissue of such animals or with contaminated water, soil, or vegetation. All serovars of *L. interrogans* are thought to be able to cause any of the syndromes, which vary from a mild carrier state to a fatal disease. Severe forms, such as Weil syndrome, usually are characterized by jaundice. Different forms of the disease were given different names depending on factors such as clinical features, host animal, geographic distribution, occupation of infected persons, and which serovar of the bacteria was first considered causative.

anicteric l., benign l. a type of leptospirosis in which there is no jaundice and the course and symptoms are relatively mild. Marked meningism and a skin rash may occur. Called also *seven-day fever.*

bovine l. a disease of cattle caused primarily by *Leptospira interrogans* serovar *pomona* and marked by fever, jaundice, anemia, mastitis, and spontaneous abortion.

canine l. leptospirosis in canines; the most common types are Stuttgart disease and yellows (def.1).

l. of cattle bovine l.

equine l. a disease of horses caused by *Leptospira interrogans* and characterized by fever, jaundice, and sometimes spontaneous abortion and iridocyclitis.

l. icterohaemorrha′gica, icterohemorrhagic l. Weil syndrome.

swine l. a disease of pigs, usually caused by *Leptospira interrogans* serovar *pomona.* An acute form in young pigs is marked by fever, jaundice, hemorrhaging, and death. A nonacute form causes abortion in pregnant sows. It may be transmitted to humans and cause swineherd's disease.

lep·to·spir·uria (lep″to-spir-u′re-ə) bacteriuria with *Leptospira* in the urine, due to their invasion of the renal tubules.

lep·to·staph·y·line (lep″to-staf′ə-lēn) [*lepto-* + *staphyline* (def. 2)] pertaining to or characterized by a narrow palate, with a palatal index of 79.9 or less.

lep·to·tene (lep′to-tēn) [*lepto-* + Gr. *tainia* ribbon] the first stage of prophase in meiosis I, during which the chromosomes condense and become visible as slender threads.

Lep·to·trich·ia (lep″to-trik′e-ə) [*lepto-* + Gr. *thrix*, gen. *trichos* hair] a genus of gram-negative, anaerobic bacteria of the family Fusobacteriaceae, found in the human oral cavity, consisting of straight or slightly curved, nonmotile rods with one or both ends rounded or pointed, arranged frequently in pairs or long filaments.

L. bucca′lis a species isolated frequently from the normal oral cavity and occasionally from the vagina and intestinal tract. It is sometimes associated with oral or urogenital infections.

Lep·to·trom·bid·i·um (lep″to-trom-bid′e-əm) a subgenus of the mite genus *Trombicula.*

Lep·tus (lep′təs) [L.] a genus of chiggers, the larval form of mites of the genus *Trombicula.*

Lerch percussion (lurch) [Otto *Lerch*, American physician, 20th century] drop percussion.

Le·redde syndrome (lə-red′) [Emile *Leredde*, French dermatologist, late 19th century] see under *syndrome.*

Lé·ri pleonosteosis, sign (la-re′) [André *Léri*, French physician, 1875–1930] see under *pleonosteosis* and *sign.*

Lé·ri-Weill dyschondrosteosis (syndrome) (la-re′ vīl′) [A. *Léri;* Jean A. *Weill*, French physician, 20th century] see under *dyschondrosteosis.*

Le·riche disease, syndrome (lə-rēsh′) [René *Leriche*, French surgeon, 1879–1955] see *post-traumatic osteoporosis,* under *osteoporosis,* and see under *syndrome.*

Ler·i·tine (ler′ĭ-tīn) trademark for preparations of anileridine.

Ler·mo·yez syndrome (ler″mwah-ya′) [Marcel *Lermoyez*, French otolaryngologist, 1858–1929] see under *syndrome.*

les local excitatory state.

les·bi·an (lez′be-ən) [Gr. *Lesbios* of Lesbos, a Greek island in the Aegean Sea, home of the poetess Sappho and her followers] 1. pertaining to homosexuality between females. 2. a female homosexual.

les•bi•an•ism (lez′be-ən-iz″əm) homosexuality between women; called also *sapphism.*

Lesch-Ny•han syndrome (lesh′ ni′ən) [Michael *Lesch*, American cardiologist, born 1939; William L. *Nyhan*, Jr., American physician, born 1926] see under *syndrome.*

Les•col (les′kol) trademark for preparations of fluvastatin sodium.

Le•ser-Tré•lat sign (la′zär tra-lah′) [Edmund *Leser*, German surgeon, 1853–1916; Ulysse *Trélat*, Jr., French surgeon, 1828–1890] see under *sign.*

le•sion (le′zhən) [L. *laesio; laedere* to hurt] any pathological or traumatic discontinuity of tissue or loss of function of a part.

albopapuloid l's the white scarlike lesions characteristic of one type of dominant epidermolysis bullosa dystrophica.

angiocentric immunoproliferative l. a multisystem disease with adult onset, consisting of invasion and destruction of body structures and tissue by atypical lymphocytoid and plasmacytoid cells resembling a lymphoma; many affected patients develop frank lymphoma. Two subtypes are *lymphomatoid granulomatosis* (involving the lungs, skin, kidneys, nervous system, and gastrointestinal tract) and *polymorphic reticulosis* (involving structures of the nose and face).

Antopol-Goldman l. a hematoma caused by bleeding in the subepithelial tissue of the renal pelvis, usually due to a coagulopathy.

apple core l. a short, well-defined region of the colon that is constricted and has ulcerated mucosa with overhanging margins; seen in various types of cancer.

Armanni-Ebstein l. vacuolation of epithelial cells in the proximal straight tubules of the kidneys (see *Armanni-Ebstein cells*, under *cell*) due to glycogen deposition, a condition seen in untreated diabetes mellitus. Called also *Armanni-Ebstein change* or *degeneration.*

attaching-effacing l. in intestinal infections with enteroadherent or enteropathogenic *Escherichia coli*, an area where the microvilli have been destroyed and bacteria are adherent.

Baehr-Löhlein l. Löhlein-Baehr l.

Bankart l. avulsion of the anterior glenoid labrum following anterior dislocation of the shoulder.

benign lymphoepithelial l. enlargement of the salivary glands, which sometimes become tender, with infiltration of the parenchyma by polyclonal B cells and T cells, atrophy of acini, and formation of lymphoepithelial islands; usually seen in middle-aged women associated with Sjögren syndrome, but also seen in a number of collagen disorders. The lesion is usually benign but may be associated with non-Hodgkin lymphoma. Called also *benign lymphoepithelial sialadenopathy* and formerly called *Mikulicz disease.* When it occurs in combination with lacrimal gland enlargement, it is now called Mikulicz syndrome (q.v.).

Blumenthal l. a proliferative vascular lesion seen in the smaller arteries in diabetes mellitus.

Bracht-Wächter l. see under *body.*

bull's-eye l. 1. a round shadow seen on a radiograph, with a dark circle surrounding a central light circle, thus resembling a bull's eye or target; it is found most often on a view of the duodenal wall and represents tumor metastasis that forms a mass with central ulceration. Called also *target l.* 2. target l. (def. 3).

central l. any lesion of the central nervous system.

coin l. a round or nodular shadow seen on a chest x-ray, due to some disease process, which may be benign or malignant; it is sometimes an artifact.

Dieulafoy l. an abnormally large submucosal artery, usually in the stomach near the gastroesophageal junction but occurring anywhere in the gastrointestinal tract, which can cause pressure erosion of the epithelium, resulting in sudden, massive bleeding that may be recurrent. Called also *Dieulafoy ulcer* and *Dieulafoy vascular malformation.*

Ebstein l. Armanni-Ebstein l.

Ghon primary l. Ghon focus.

gross l. a lesion visible to the naked eye.

Hill-Sachs l. compression fracture of the posteromedial humeral head, sometimes occurring with anterior dislocation of the shoulder, caused by impaction of the humeral head on the anterior rim of the glenoid fossa.

histologic l. a microscopic lesion.

impaction l. an osteopathic term for a lesion of any spinal joint in which there is present abnormal thickening of the intervertebral disk with approximation of all the bony parts.

iris l. target l. (def. 3).

irritative l. a lesion that stimulates activity in the part where it is situated, such as a lesion of the motor cortex that causes seizures by stimulating the excessive firing of neurons.

Janeway l. a small erythematous or hemorrhagic lesion, usually on the palms or soles, in subacute bacterial endocarditis.

jet l. arterial dilatation distal to a stenosis, caused by the turbulence accompanying a poststenotic jet.

Kimmelstiel-Wilson l. a microscopic spherical hyaline mass surrounded by capillaries, found in the kidney glomerulus in the nodular form of intercapillary glomerulosclerosis and virtually pathognomonic of diabetes mellitus. Called also *Kimmelstiel-Wilson nodule.*

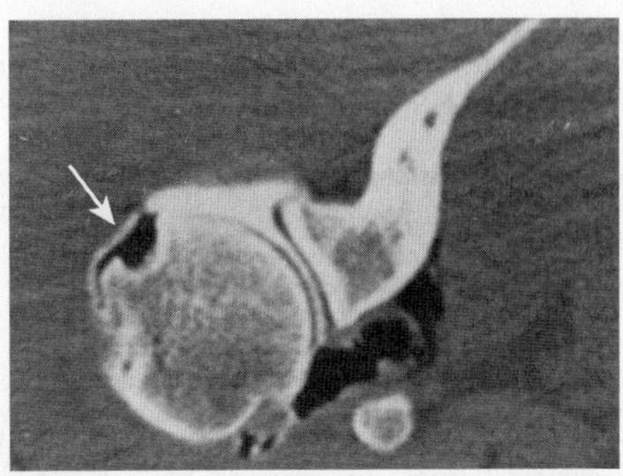

■ Hill-Sachs lesion *(arrow)* of the articular surface of the posterior portion of the humeral head (CT arthrography).

local l. a lesion of the nervous system that gives rise to distinctive local symptoms.

Löhlein-Baehr l. a focal glomerular lesion of necrosis and hyalinization occurring in bacterial endocarditis; the process has been described as focal embolic glomerulonephritis.

molecular l. a lesion not visible even with the aid of a microscope.

onionskin l. 1. the concentric circumvascular fibrosis often found in the spleen and lymph nodes in systemic lupus erythematosus. 2. concentric layers of myointimal cells and collagen, causing luminal narrowing, seen in the interlobular arteries and arterioles of the kidney in malignant hypertension, microangiopathies, and scleroderma. Called also *hyperplastic arteriolitis.*

organic l. structural l.

partial l. a lesion that involves only a part of an organ or of the diameter of a conducting tract.

peripheral l. a lesion of the nerve endings.

precancerous l. a lesion in a tissue in which the cells are likely to become malignant.

primary l. the original lesion manifesting a disease, such as chancre in syphilis or tuberculous granuloma.

ring-wall l. a small ring hemorrhage in the brain that resembles a ring of glia; seen in pernicious anemia.

skip l. a lesion that is discontinuous; the most common occurrence is in two different segments of intestine affected by inflammatory bowel disease.

SLAP l. [*s*uperior *l*abrum *a*nterior-*p*osterior] injury involving the superior glenoid labrum and attachment of the biceps brachii, extending from anterior to posterior, classified into seven types according to the specific features of the injury.

squamous intraepithelial l. abnormal growth of squamous cells in the cervical epithelium; two types are distinguished, *low-grade* and *high-grade*, depending on the malignant potential.

structural l. a lesion that produces an obvious change in a tissue.

systemic l. a lesion limited to a system or set of organs with a common function.

target l. 1. bull's-eye l. 2. a small, circumscribed focus of necrosis with a gray center surrounded by erythema, seen in the lungs in invasive aspergillosis. 3. a skin lesion characteristic of erythema multiforme, consisting of a central zone that has a bulla or crust and is surrounded by one or two concentric zones of changed colors. Called also *bull's-eye l.*

total l. a lesion involving the whole of an organ or of the diameter of a conducting tract.

trophic l. a lesion manifested by a disturbance in the nutrition of a part.

wire-loop l. thickened capillary walls of some parts of a glomerular tuft in disseminated lupus erythematosus.

le•sion•ec•to•my (le″zhən-ek′tə-me) [*lesion* + *-ectomy*] the surgical removal of a discrete lesion within the cerebral cortex while sparing the surrounding tissue; used in the treatment of epilepsy.

Less•haft triangle (space) (les′hahft) [Peter Frantsevich *Lesshaft*, Russian physician, 1836–1909] see under *triangle.*

LET linear energy transfer.

Let•air•is (let′ər-is) trademark for a preparation of ambrisentan.

let-down (let′doun) the transport of milk from the alveoli of the breast to the ducts; called also *milk l.* See also under *reflex.*

le•thal (le′thəl) [L. *lethalis*] 1. fatal. 2. see under *mutation.*

le•thal•i•ty (le-thal′ĭ-te) the capability of an agent or disease of causing death.

leth•ar•gy (leth′ər-je) [Gr. *lēthargia* drowsiness] 1. a lowered level of consciousness marked by listlessness, drowsiness, and apathy; see also *consciousness.* 2. a condition of indifference.

let·ro·zole (let′rə-zōl) a nonsteroidal aromatase inhibitor that inhibits conversion of adrenal androgens to estrogens, used as an antineoplastic in the treatment of advanced breast cancer in postmenopausal women; administered orally.

Let·ter·er-Si·we disease (let′ər-ər se′və) [Erich *Letterer*, German physician, 20th century; Sture August *Siwe*, Swedish pediatrician, 1897–1966] see under *disease.*

Leu leucine.

leu·ce·mia (loo-se′me-ə) leukemia.

leu·cine (Leu, L) (loo′sēn) [Gr. *leukos* white] 1. an essential amino acid, 2-amino-4-methylpentanoic acid, necessary for optimal growth in infants and for nitrogen equilibrium in human adults. It is obtained by the digestion or hydrolytic cleavage of protein. See also table at *amino acid.* 2. [USP] a preparation of leucine used as a dietary supplement.

leu·cine ami·no·pep·ti·dase (LAP) (loo′sēn ə-me″no-pep′tĭ-dās) leucyl aminopeptidase.

leu·cin·im·ide (loo-sin′ĭ-mīd″) the anhydride of leucine, a diketopiperazine; it may be produced by evaporation of leucine solutions.

leu·ci·no·sis (loo″sĭ-no′sis) leucinuria.

leu·cin·uria (loo″sĭ-nu′re-ə) excretion of leucine in the urine, as in some forms of maple syrup urine disease and tyrosinemia. See also *hyperleucinemia.*

leu·ci·tis (loo-si′tis) scleritis.

leuc(o)- see *leuk(o)-.*

leu·co·cyte (loo′ko-sīt) leukocyte.

leu·co·cy·to·sis (loo″ko-si-to′sis) leukocytosis.

Leu·co·cy·to·zo·on (loo″ko-si″to-zo′on) [*leuco-* + *cyte* + Gr. *zōon* animal] a genus of coccidian protozoa (suborder Haemosporina, order Eucoccidiida) parasitic in wild and domestic birds, sometimes causing fatal leucocytozoonosis. Merogony occurs in the hepatocytes and vascular endothelial cells of the host, producing merozoites that invade erythroblasts, erythrocytes, lymphocytes, and monocytes and then develop into gametocytes. Species infecting domestic fowl include *L. simon′di* (called also *L. an′seris*) in ducks and geese; *L. smi′thi* in turkeys; and *L. caulle′ryi, L. andrew′si,* and *L. sabraze′si* in chickens. All are transmitted by black flies (*Simulium* spp.) except *L. caulleryi*, which is transmitted by biting midges (*Culicoides* spp.). Written also *Leukocytozoon.*

leu·co·cy·to·zoo·no·sis (loo″ko-si″to-zo″o-no′sis) an acute malaria-like protozoal disease of domestic fowl, including chickens, ducks, geese, and turkeys, caused by heavy infection with species of *Leucocytozoon*, and characterized by anemia, leukocytosis, and hepatosplenomegaly, which may result in death.

Leu·co·i·um (loo-ko′e-əm) [L., from Gr. *leukos* white + *ion* violet] a genus of Old World plants of the family Amaryllidaceae. *L. aesti′vum* and *L. ver′num*, both called snowflake, are common garden plants that are emetic and poisonous.

leu·co·my·cin (loo″ko-mi′sin) kitasamycin.

Leu·co·nos·toc (loo″ko-nos′tok) [*leuko-* + *Nostoc* a form-genus of cyanobacteria] a genus of nonpathogenic, gram-positive, saprophytic, facultative anaerobes of the family Leuconostocaceae. They are spherical but often lenticular, nonmotile cells, some species of which form dextran. The type species is *L. mesenteroi′des.*

L. mesenteroi′des a dextran-forming species found in slimy sugar solutions, on fruit and vegetables, and in milk and dairy products. It is used in the commercial production of dextran.

Leu·co·nos·to·ca·ceae (loo″ko-nos″tə-ka′se-e) a family of gram-positive, nonmotile, facultatively anaerobic, non–spore-forming bacteria of the order Bacillales; organisms are spherical or lenticular and occur in pairs and chains. Medically important organisms are contained in the genus *Leuconostoc.*

leu·co·sin (loo′ko-sin) an albumin found in the cereal grains.

leu·cot·o·my (loo-kot′ə-me) prefrontal lobotomy.

leu·co·vo·rin (loo″ko-vo′rin) folinic acid.

l. calcium [USP] the calcium salt of folinic acid, used as an antidote for folic acid antagonists, e.g., methotrexate, when there is need to reverse the toxic effects of the latter, in the treatment of megaloblastic anemias due to folic acid deficiency, and as an adjunct in the palliative treatment of colorectal carcinoma; administered orally, intramuscularly, or intravenously.

leu·cyl (loo′səl) the acyl radical of leucine.

leu·cyl ami·no·pep·ti·dase (loo′səl ə-me″no-pep′tĭ-dās) [EC 3.4.11.1] a zinc-containing enzyme of the hydrolase class that catalyzes the removal of the N-terminal amino acid from most L-peptides, particularly those with N-terminal leucine residues but not those with N-terminal lysine or arginine residues. It occurs in tissue cell cytosol, with high activity in the duodenum, liver, and kidney. Abbreviated LAP. Called also *cytosol aminopeptidase.*

Leud·et tinnitus (lo͝o-da′) [Théodor Emile *Leudet*, French physician, 1825–1887] see under *tinnitus.*

leu·en·keph·a·lin (loo″ən-kef′ə-lin) see *enkephalin.*

leu·ka·phe·re·sis (loo″kə-fə-re′sis) [*leuk*ocyte + *apheresis*] the selective separation and removal of leukocytes from withdrawn blood, the remainder of the blood then being retransfused into the donor.

leu·ke·mia (loo-ke′me-ə) [*leuk-* + *-emia*] a progressive, malignant disease of the blood-forming organs, characterized by distorted proliferation and development of leukocytes and their precursors in the blood and bone marrow. It is classified according to degree of cell differentiation as *acute* or *chronic* (terms no longer referring to duration of disease), and according to predominant type of cell involved as *myelogenous* or *lymphocytic.* **leuke′mic** *adj*

Leukemia

acute l. leukemia in which the involved cell line shows little or no differentiation, usually consisting of blast cells; two types are distinguished, acute lymphoblastic leukemia and acute myelogenous leukemia.

acute granulocytic l. acute myelogenous l.

acute lymphoblastic l. (ALL) acute leukemia of the lymphoblastic type, one of the two major categories of acute leukemia, primarily affecting young children. Symptoms include anemia, fatigue, weight loss, easy bruising, thrombocytopenia, granulocytopenia with bacterial infections, bone pain, lymphadenopathy, hepatosplenomegaly, and sometimes spread to the central nervous system (meningismus) or to other organs. Called also *acute lymphocytic l.*

acute lymphocytic l. acute lymphoblastic l.

acute megakaryoblastic l., acute megakaryocytic l. a form of acute myelogenous leukemia in which megakaryocytes are predominant and platelets are increased in the blood, often with fibrosis consisting of reticulin; it can occur at any age. Called also *megakaryoblastic l.* and *megakaryocytic l.*

acute monocytic l. an uncommon form of acute myelogenous leukemia in which the predominating cells are identified as monocytes; it can affect any age group. A few myelocytes may be present, but not as many as in acute myelomonocytic leukemia. Called also *monocytic l.* and *Schilling l.*

acute myeloblastic l. 1. a common kind of acute myelogenous leukemia, in which myeloblasts predominate; it usually occurs in infants and middle-aged to older adults. Two types are distinguished; those that have minimal cell differentiation or maturation and those that have more advanced differentiation. Called also *myeloblastic l.*, and *acute myeloid l.* 2. acute myelogenous l.

acute myelocytic l. acute myelogenous l.

acute myelogenous l. (AML) acute leukemia of the myelogenous type, one of the two major categories of acute leukemia; most types affect primarily middle-aged to elderly people. Symptoms include anemia, fatigue, weight loss, easy bruising, thrombocytopenia, and granulocytopenia that leads to persistent bacterial infections. Several types are distinguished, named according to the stage in which abnormal proliferation begins: *acute undifferentiated l., acute myeloblastic l., acute promyelocytic l., acute myelomonocytic l., acute monocytic l., acute erythroleukemia,* and *acute megakaryocytic l.* Called also *acute myelocytic l.* and *acute nonlymphocytic l.*

acute myeloid l. 1. acute myeloblastic l. (def. 1). 2. acute myelogenous l.

acute myelomonocytic l. one of the more common types of acute myelogenous leukemia, characterized by both malignant monocytes and myeloblasts; it usually affects middle aged to older adults. See also *chronic myelomonocytic l.* Called also *myelomonocytic* or *Naegeli l.*

Leukemia *Continued*

acute nonlymphocytic l. acute myelogenous l.
acute promyelocytic l. acute myelogenous leukemia in which more than half the cells are malignant promyelocytes, often associated with abnormal bleeding secondary to thrombocytopenia, hypofibrinogenemia, and decreased levels of coagulation factor V; it usually occurs in young adults. Called also *promyelocytic l.*
acute undifferentiated l. (AUL) acute myelogenous leukemia in which the predominating cell is so immature and primitive that it cannot be classified. Called also *stem cell l.* and *undifferentiated cell l.*
adult T-cell l. adult T-cell l./lymphoma.
adult T-cell l./lymphoma (ATL) a malignancy of mature T lymphocytes with onset in adulthood, believed to be caused by human T-lymphotropic virus 1 and characterized by circulating pleomorphic malignant lymphocytes, skin lesions, lymphadenopathy, hepatosplenomegaly, hypercalcemia, and lytic bone lesions; its course may be subacute or chronic. Called also *adult T-cell l.* and *adult T-cell lymphoma.*
aleukemic l., aleukocythemic l. leukemia in which the total white blood cell count in the peripheral blood is either normal or below normal; it may be lymphocytic, monocytic, or myelogenous.
basophilic l. a rare type of leukemia in which basophils predominate; both acute and chronic varieties have been observed.
B-cell acute lymphoblastic l. a rare subtype of acute lymphoblastic leukemia consisting of lymphoblasts that express surface immunoglobulins and have a chromosomal translocation similar to that of Burkitt lymphoma.
biphenotypic acute l. (BAL) acute leukemia in which cells of a single population express the markers of more than one cell lineage, usually those of myeloid and either B or T cells, but occasionally those of B and T cells or of all three (B, T, and myeloid) lineages.
blast cell l. acute undifferentiated l.
B-lymphoblastic l. the most common subtype of acute lymphoblastic leukemia, consisting of small uniform lymphoblasts that do not synthesize complete functional immunoglobulins. Called also *pre–B-cell acute lymphoblastic l.*
bovine l. enzootic bovine leukosis.
Burkitt l. the leukemic phase of Burkitt lymphoma.
chronic l. leukemia in which the involved cell line is well-differentiated, usually B lymphocytes, but immunologically incompetent; types distinguished include chronic granulocytic, chronic lymphocytic, chronic myelomonocytic, eosinophilic, and hairy cell leukemia.
chronic granulocytic l. chronic leukemia of the myelogenous type, occurring mainly between the ages of 25 and 60 years, usually associated with a Philadelphia chromosome. The major clinical manifestations of malaise, hepatosplenomegaly, anemia, and leukocytosis are related to abnormal, excessive, unrestrained overgrowth of granulocytes in the bone marrow. Called also *chronic myelocytic l.*, and *chronic myeloid l.*
chronic lymphocytic l. (CLL) chronic leukemia of the lymphocytic type, a common form mainly seen in the elderly; symptoms include lymphadenopathy, fatigue, renal involvement, and pulmonary leukemic infiltrates. Circulating malignant cells are usually differentiated B lymphocytes; a minority of cases have mixed T and B lymphocytes or entirely T lymphocytes.
chronic myelocytic l., chronic myelogenous l., chronic myeloid l. chronic granulocytic l.
chronic myelomonocytic l. a slowly progressing form of chronic leukemia that is myelomonocytic in nature and usually affects the elderly; sometimes it progresses to acute myelomonocytic leukemia. Symptoms include splenomegaly, monocytosis with granulocytosis, and thrombocytopenia.

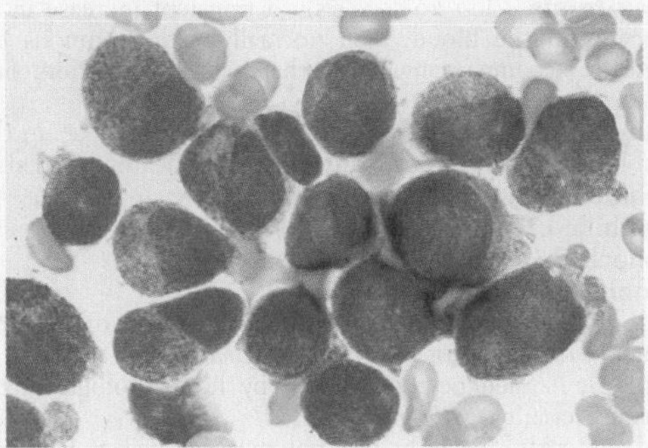
■ Acute promyelocytic leukemia (peripheral blood smear, Wright stain).

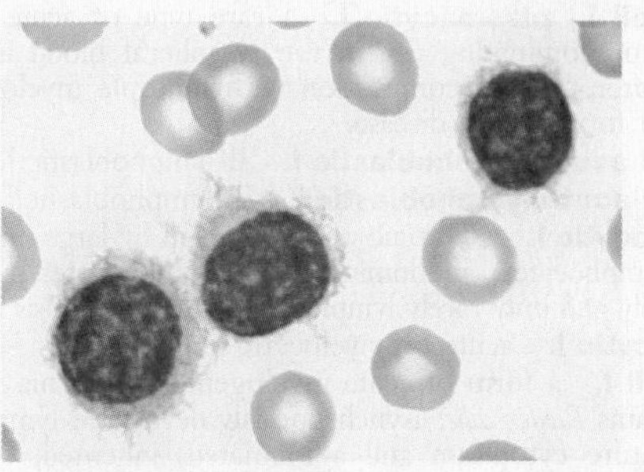
■ Hairy cell leukemia, characterized by lymphoid cells with delicate cytoplasmic projections (peripheral blood smear, Wright-Giemsa stain).

common acute lymphoblastic l. a subclassification of the pre–B-cell type that refers to those showing expression of the common acute lymphoblastic leukemia antigen.
l. cu′tis a cutaneous manifestation of leukemia resulting from infiltration of the skin by malignant leukocytes and occurring as specific or nonspecific lesions, or both coexisting. See also *leukemid.*
eosinophilic l. a form of leukemia in which the eosinophil is the predominating cell. Although resembling chronic granulocytic leukemia in many ways, this form may follow an acute course despite the absence of predominantly blast forms in the peripheral blood.
feline l. a nonspecific term for any of various lymphoid leukemias seen in domestic cats that are infected with the feline leukemia virus; sites most often involved are the gastrointestinal tract, liver, spleen, and thymus.
granulocytic l. myelogenous l.
Gross l. a transmissible murine leukemia, first transmitted to newborn C3H mice by inoculation of filtrate of leukemic tissue from AK2 mice, thus demonstrating its viral etiology.
hairy cell l. a form of chronic leukemia marked by splenomegaly and by an abundance of abnormal large mononuclear cells covered by hairlike villi *(hairy cells)* in the bone marrow, spleen, liver, and peripheral blood. Called also *leukemic reticuloendotheliosis.*
hand mirror–cell l. a rare leukemia characterized by excessive numbers of abnormal, hand mirror–shaped mononuclear cells, usually occurring in females and relatively resistant to treatment. High blast cell counts and central nervous system involvement are common.
hemoblastic l., hemocytoblastic l. acute undifferentiated l.
histiocytic l. acute monocytic l.
leukopenic l. aleukemic l.
lymphatic l. lymphoblastic l.
lymphoblastic l. leukemia associated with hyperplasia and overactivity of the lymphoid tissue; there are increased numbers of circulating malignant lymphocytes and lymphoblasts. See also *acute lymphoblastic l.* and *chronic lymphocytic l.* Called also *lymphatic, lymphocytic, lymphogenous,* and *lymphoid l.*
lymphocytic l., lymphogenous l., lymphoid l. lymphoblastic l.
lymphosarcoma cell l. B-cell type acute lymphoblastic l.
mast cell l. a rare type of leukemia characterized by the presence of overwhelming numbers of tissue mast cells in the peripheral blood.
megakaryoblastic l. acute megakaryocytic l.
megakaryocytic l. 1. acute megakaryocytic l. 2. hemorrhagic thrombocythemia.
micromyeloblastic l. a form of myelogenous leukemia in which the immature, nucleoli-containing cells are small and are distinguishable from lymphocytes only by supravital staining.
monocytic l. acute monocytic l.
myeloblastic l. 1. myelogenous l. 2. acute myeloblastic l.
myelocytic l. myelogenous l.
myelogenous l., myeloid granulocytic l. leukemia arising from myeloid tissue in which the granular, polymorphonuclear leukocytes and their precursors predominate; see also *acute myelogenous l.* and *chronic granulocytic l.* Called also *granulocytic, myeloblastic,* or *myelocytic l.*
myelomonocytic l. acute myelomonocytic l.
Naegeli l. acute myelomonocytic l.

Leukemia *Continued*

plasma cell l., plasmacytic l. a rare type of acute leukemia in which the predominating cell in the peripheral blood is the plasma cell; it is often seen in conjunction with multiple myeloma and may be a variant form of that disease.
pre–B-cell acute lymphoblastic l. B-lymphoblastic l.
pre–T-cell acute lymphoblastic l. T-lymphoblastic l.
prolymphocytic l. a chronic variety marked by large numbers of circulating lymphocytes, predominantly prolymphocytes, with massive splenomegaly and only rarely lymphadenopathy; prognosis is often poor.
promyelocytic l. acute promyelocytic l.
Rieder cell l. a form of acute myelogenous leukemia in which the blood contains *Rieder cells*, asynchronously developed lymphocytes that have immature cytoplasm and a lobulated, indented, comparatively more mature nucleus.
Schilling l. acute monocytic l.
stem cell l. acute undifferentiated l.
subleukemic l. aleukemic l.
T-cell acute lymphoblastic l. acute lymphoblastic leukemia in which cells express surface antigens characteristic of T cells; it is more common in males than in females and affects adults and children equally.
T-lymphoblastic l. acute lymphoblastic leukemia, affecting primarily young men, characterized by uniform lymphoblasts that are morphologically similar to the lymphoblasts seen in B-lymphoblastic leukemia; prognosis is worse than in B-lymphoblastic leukemia. Called also *pre–T-cell acute lymphoblastic l.*
transient l. of infancy transient myeloproliferative disorder.
undifferentiated cell l. acute undifferentiated l.

leu•ke•mid (loo-ke′mid) [*leukemia* + *-id*] any of the polymorphic skin eruptions associated with leukemia; clinically, they may be nonspecific, i.e., papular, macular, purpuric, etc., but histopathologically they may represent true leukemic infiltrations. Cf. *leukemia cutis.*

leu•ke•mo•gen (loo-ke′mo-jən) any substance that causes or produces leukemia.

leu•ke•mo•gen•e•sis (loo-ke″mo-jen′ə-sis) the induction of or development of leukemia.

leu•ke•mo•gen•ic (loo-ke″mo-jen′ik) causing leukemia.

leu•ke•moid (loo-ke′moid) [*leukemia* + *-oid*] having blood and sometimes clinical findings resembling those of leukemia; see under reaction.

leuk•en•ceph•a•li•tis (lo͞ok″ən-sef″ə-li′tis) [*leuko-* + *encephalitis*] inflammation of the white matter of the brain.

Leu•ker•an (loo′kər-ən) trademark for a preparation of chlorambucil.

leu•kin (loo′kin) a thermostable, bactericidal substance extracted from polymorphonuclear leukocytes. See *cationic proteins*, under *protein.*

Leu•kine (loo′kīn) trademark for a preparation of sargramostim.

leuk(o)- [Gr. *leukos* white] a combining form meaning white, or denoting relationship to a leukocyte. Also, *leuc(o)-*.

leu•ko•ag•glu•ti•nin (loo″ko-ə-gloo′tĭ-nin) leukocyte agglutinin.

leu•ko•ar•ai•o•sis (loo″ko-ar″e-o′sis) [*leuko-* + Gr. *araios* thin + *-osis*] areas of hyperintensity of white matter visible on radiographic images of the brain, indicating thinning of those parts; seen particularly in elderly persons and those with Binswanger disease.

leu•ko•blas•to•sis (loo″ko-blas-to′sis) a general term for abnormal proliferation of leukocytes, as seen in certain types of leukemia.

leu•ko•ci•din (loo″ko-si′din) [*leuko-* + L. *caedere* to kill] a substance toxic to leukocytes; specifically, an exotoxin produced by some pathogenic staphylococci and streptococci that destroys leukocytes by lysis of the cytoplasmic granules and is partially responsible for the pathogenicity of the organisms.
  Neisser-Wechsberg l. a leukocidin produced by staphylococci that destroys rabbit but not human leukocytes; it is identical with alpha hemolysin.
  Panton-Valentine (P-V) l. a leukocidin produced by staphylococci that destroys human and rabbit leukocytes by injuring the cell membrane, with subsequent cell degranulation; it is nonhemolytic.

leu•ko•co•ria (loo″ko-kor′e-ə) leukokoria.

leu•ko•crit (loo′ko-krit) [*leuko-* + Gr. *krinein* to separate] the volume percentage of leukocytes in whole blood.

leu•ko•cyte (loo′ko-sīt) [*leuko-* + *-cyte*] a colorless blood cell capable of ameboid movement; there are several different types, classified into the two large groups *granular l's* (basophils, eosinophils, and neutrophils) and *nongranular l's* (lymphocytes and monocytes). Called also *white blood cell* or *corpuscle* and *white cell* or *corpuscle.* **leukocy′tal, leukocyt′ic** *adj*
  agranular l. nongranular l.
  basophilic l. basophil (def. 2).
  eosinophilic l. eosinophil.
  granular l. any leukocyte with abundant granules in the cytoplasm; there are three groups: the basophils, eosinophils, and neutrophils. See also *granulocytic series*, under *series.* Called also *granulocyte.*
  heterophilic l. heterophil (def. 1).
  neutrophilic l. neutrophil (def. 1).
  nongranular l. a leukocyte without specific granules in the cytoplasm, such as a lymphocyte or monocyte. Called also *agranular l.*
  polymorphonuclear l. any fully developed granular leukocyte whose nucleus contains multiple lobes joined by filamentous connections, especially a neutrophil.
  polynuclear neutrophilic l. neutrophil (def. 1).

leu•ko•cyte elas•tase (loo′ko-sīt e-las′tās) [EC 3.4.21.37] a serine endopeptidase that is secreted by certain leukocytes and catalyzes the hydrolysis of proteins, including elastin, and is inhibited by alpha$_1$-antitrypsin. Emphysema resulting from damage to lung tissue by leukocyte elastase occurs in alpha$_1$-antitrypsin deficiency. Called also *neutrophil elastase.*

leu•ko•cy•toc•la•sis (loo″ko-si-tok′lə-sis) degeneration and karyorrhexis of polymorphonuclear neutrophils. **leukocytoclas′tic** *adj*

leu•ko•cy•to•gen•e•sis (loo″ko-si″to-jen′ə-sis) [*leukocyte* + *-genesis*] leukopoiesis.

leu•ko•cy•toid (loo′ko-si″toid) [*leukocyte* + *-oid*] resembling a leukocyte.

leu•ko•cy•tol•o•gy (loo″ko-si-tol′ə-je) the study of leukocytes.

leu•ko•cy•tol•y•sin (loo″ko-si-tol′ə-sin) a lysin that leads to disruption of leukocytes.

leu•ko•cy•tol•y•sis (loo″ko-si-tol′ə-sis) [*leukocyte* + *-lysis*] the breaking down or destruction of leukocytes; called also *leukolysis.*
  venom l. destruction of leukocytes by a leukotoxin in snake venom.

leu•ko•cy•to•lyt•ic (loo″ko-si″to-lit′ik) 1. pertaining to, characterized by, or causing leukocytolysis. 2. an agent that causes leukocytolysis. Called also *antileukocytic* and *leukolytic.*

leu•ko•cy•to•ma (loo″ko-si-to′mə) [*leukocyte* + *-oma*] a tumorlike mass of leukocytes.

leu•ko•cy•to•pe•nia (loo″ko-si″to-pe′ne-ə) leukopenia.

leu•ko•cy•toph•a•gy (loo″ko-si-tof′ə-je) [*leukocyte* + *-phagy*] the ingestion and destruction of leukocytes by histiocytes of the reticuloendothelial system.

leu•ko•cy•to•pla•nia (loo″ko-si″to-pla′ne-ə) [*leukocyte* + Gr. *planē* wandering] the wandering of leukocytes, such as their passage through a membrane.

leu•ko•cy•to•poi•e•sis (loo″ko-si″to-poi-e′sis) leukopoiesis.

leu•ko•cy•to•sis (loo″ko-si-to′sis) a transient increase in the number of leukocytes in the blood; seen normally with strenuous exercise and pathologically accompanying hemorrhage, fever, infection, or inflammation. Cf. *hyperleukocytosis.*
  absolute l. increase in the total number of leukocytes in the blood.
  agonal l. leukocytosis occurring just before death; called also *terminal l.*
  basophilic l. basophilia (def. 1).
  eosinophilic l. eosinophilia (def. 1).
  mononuclear l. mononucleosis (def. 1).
  neutrophilic l. neutrophilia.
  pathologic l. leukocytosis occurring as the result of some morbid condition, such as infection or trauma; cf. *physiologic l.*
  physiologic l. leukocytosis caused by nonpathologic factors such as strenuous exercise; cf. *pathologic l.*
  pure l. increase of only the polymorphonuclear leukocytes of the blood.
  relative l. increase in the proportion of just one type of leukocyte in the blood, without increase of the total number of leukocytes.

terminal l. agonal l.
toxic l. leukocytosis occurring in septicemia and other toxic conditions.

leu•ko•cy•to•sper•mia (loo″ko-si″to-spur′me-ə) [*leukocyte* + *sperm* + *-ia*] excessive leukocytes in the seminal fluid; cf. *pyospermia.* Called also *leukospermia.*

leu•ko•cy•to•tac•tic (loo″ko-si″to-tak′tik) leukotactic.

leu•ko•cy•to•tax•is (loo″ko-si″to-tak′sis) leukotaxis.

leu•ko•cy•to•ther•a•py (loo″ko-si″to-ther′ə-pe) treatment by the administration of leukocytes.

leu•ko•cy•to•tox•ic•i•ty (loo″ko-si″to-tok-sis′ĭ-te) the quality or capability of leukocytolysis; see also *lymphocytotoxicity.*

leu•ko•cy•to•tro•pic (loo″ko-si″to-tro′pik) having a selective affinity for leukocytes.

Leu•ko•cy•to•zo•on (loo″ko-si″to-zo′on) *Leucocytozoon.*

leu•ko•cy•tu•ria (loo″ko-si-tu′re-ə) [*leukocyte* + *-uria*] the discharge of leukocytes in the urine, such as in kidney disease or urinary tract infections.

leu•ko•der•ma (loo″ko-dur′mə) [*leuko-* + *derma*] any of various acquired types of hypomelanosis; called also *leukodermia, leukopathia,* and *leukopathy.* **leukoder′matous, leukodermic** *adj*
l. acquisi′tum centri′fugum halo nevus.
chemical l. leukoderma caused by a skin reaction to a chemical substance; common agents include phenol and catechol derivatives, sulfhydryl compounds, and artificial latex.
l. col′li syphilitic l.
guttate l. leukoderma in which the skin has numerous white drop-shaped spots, a characteristic of some types of tuberous sclerosis.
occupational l. see under *vitiligo.*
postinflammatory l. see under *hypopigmentation.*
syphilitic l. a cutaneous manifestation of secondary syphilis, consisting of round or oval, depigmented spots surrounded by hyperpigmentation on the front and sides of the neck and on the chest. Called also *l. colli.*

leu•ko•der•mia (loo″ko-dur′me-ə) leukoderma.

leu•ko•dys•tro•phy (loo″ko-dis′trə-fe) any of various types of neurodegeneration involving disturbance of the white matter of the brain. See also *adrenoleukodystrophy* and *leukoencephalopathy.*
adult-onset demyelinating l. a progressive, autosomal dominant leukoencephalopathy caused by a tandem repeat at gene locus 5q23.3-q31.1 that results in an extra copy of the lamin B1 gene, characterized by degeneration of the white matter, beginning at the frontal lobes and extending to the centrum semiovale and cerebellum. Symptoms first appear in the fourth or fifth decade and include motor disturbances, bowel and bladder incontinence, and orthostatic hypotension; mental acuity is often retained. Death occurs about 20 years after the appearance of symptoms.
globoid cell l. Krabbe disease.
hereditary cerebral l. Pelizaeus-Merzbacher disease.
Krabbe l. see under *disease.*
metachromatic l. an autosomal recessive disorder due to deficiency of cerebroside-sulfatase (caused by mutation in the *ARSA* gene, locus: 22q13.31-qter) or saposin B (caused by mutation in the *PSAP* gene, locus: 10q22.1). It is characterized by accumulation of sulfatide in neural and nonneural tissues, with a diffuse loss of myelin in the central nervous system. There are three forms due to deficiency of cerebroside sulfatase, with variable age of onset, all initially presenting as mental regression and motor disturbances. The *infantile* form usually begins in the second year of life and is additionally characterized by developmental delay, seizures, optic atrophy, ataxia, weakness, loss of speech, and progressive spastic quadriparesis. The *juvenile* form is clinically similar, but presents between the ages of 4 and 12 years and progresses more slowly; a variant of the juvenile form is caused by deficiency of saposin B. The *adult* form begins after 16 years of age, generally presenting initially as dementia and disturbances in behavior and progressing more slowly to motor and posture disturbances. Called also *sulfatide lipidosis.*
spongiform l. spongy degeneration of central nervous system; see under *degeneration.*
sudanophilic l. a heterogeneous group of diseases, including adrenoleukodystrophy and Pelizaeus-Merzbacher disease, characterized by myelin destruction, with resulting breakdown products that stain bright red with fat stains.
vanishing white matter l. see under *disease.*

leu•ko•ede•ma (loo″ko-ə-de′mə) [*leuko-* + *edema*] a variant condition of the buccal mucosa resembling early leukoplakia, characterized by filmy opalescence of the mucosa in the early stages to a whitish gray cast with a coarsely wrinkled surface in the later stages, associated with intracellular edema of the spinous or malpighian layer.

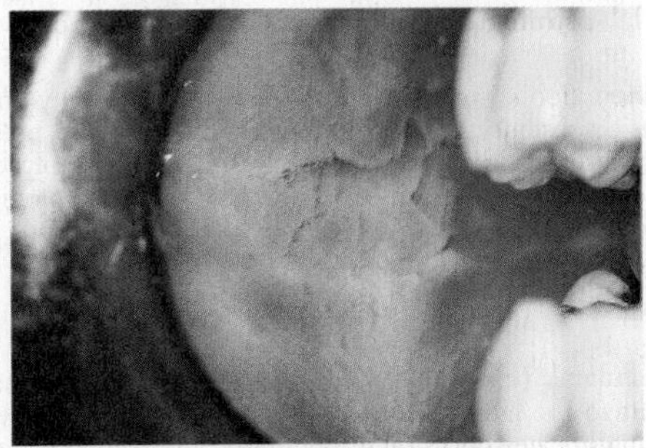

■ Leukoedema.

leu•ko•en•ceph•a•li•tis (loo″ko-ən-sef″ə-li′tis) [*leuko-* + *encephalitis*] 1. inflammation of the white substance of the brain. Cf. *leukoencephalomalacia.* 2. forage poisoning.
acute hemorrhagic l., acute hemorrhagic l. of Weston Hurst acute necrotizing hemorrhagic encephalomyelitis.
l. periaxia′lis concen′trica Baló disease.
van Bogaert sclerosing l. subacute sclerosing panencephalitis.

leu•ko•en•ceph•a•lo•ma•la•cia (loo″ko-en-sef″ə-lo-mə-la′shə) [*leuko-* + *encephalomalacia*] 1. encephalomalacia affecting primarily the white matter. 2. forage poisoning.
mycotoxic l. forage poisoning.

leu•ko•en•ceph•a•lop•a•thy (loo″ko-ən-sef″ə-lop′ə-the) any of a group of diseases affecting the white matter of the brain, especially of the cerebral hemispheres, and occurring as a rule in infants and children. The term *leukodystrophy* is used to denote such disorders due to defect in the formation and maintenance of myelin in infants and children.
metachromatic l. see under *leukodystrophy.*
necrotizing l. a complication sometimes seen after injection of methotrexate intrathecally to treat childhood leukemia of the central nervous system; symptoms include necrosis of white matter of the brain, sometimes with stupor and quadriplegia, and frequently with permanent learning disabilities.
posterior reversible l. reversible posterior leukoencephalopathy syndrome; see under *syndrome.*
progressive multifocal l. opportunistic infection of the central nervous system by the JC virus, seen in immunocompromised persons and sometimes secondary to neoplastic conditions such as lymphosarcoma, lymphoblastic leukemia, or myelogenous leukemia. The demyelination is usually found in the white matter of the cerebral hemispheres but may rarely be seen in the brainstem and cerebellum.
reversible posterior l. see under *syndrome.*
spongiform l. a complication sometimes seen after inhaling vapors of preheated heroin. Pathologically there is demyelination and vacuolization of white matter of the brain, with symptoms including confusion, apathy, and motor restlessness; some patients progress to coma and death.
subacute sclerosing l. subacute sclerosing panencephalitis.

leu•ko•en•ceph•a•ly (loo″ko-ən-sef′ə-le) leukoencephalopathy.

leu•ko•eryth•ro•blas•tic (loo″ko-ə-rith″ro-blas′tik) characterized by the presence of nucleated red cells and immature neutrophils.

leu•ko•eryth•ro•blas•to•sis (loo″ko-ə-rith″ro-blas-to′sis) anemia with space-occupying lesions of the bone marrow that cause bone marrow suppression with immature cells of the erythrocytic and granulocytic series in the circulation. Called also *leukoerythroblastic anemia, myelopathic anemia,* and *myelophthisic anemia.*

leu•ko•ker•a•to•sis (loo″ko-ker″ə-to′sis) [*leuko-* + *keratosis*] oral leukoplakia.

leu•ko•ki•ne•sis (loo″ko-kĭ-ne′sis) the movement of the leukocytes within the circulatory system. **leukokinet′ic** *adj*

leu•ko•ki•net•ics (loo″ko-kĭ-net′iks) [*leukocyte* + *kinetics*] the quantitative, dynamic study of in vivo production, circulation, and destruction of leukocytes.

leu•ko•ki•nin (loo″ko-ki′nin) the parent immunoglobulin molecule from which tuftsin is cleaved.

leu•ko•ko•ria (loo″ko-kor′e-ə) [*leuko-* + Gr. *korē* pupil + *-ia*] a condition characterized by appearance of a whitish reflex or mass in the pupillary area behind the lens; called also *cat's eye reflex.*

leu•ko•krau•ro•sis (loo″ko-kraw-ro′sis) *lichen sclerosus* (q.v.) of the vulvar region.

leu•kol•y•sin (loo-kol′ə-sin) leukocytolysin.

leu•kol•y•sis (loo-kol′ə-sis) leukocytolysis.

leu•ko•lyt•ic (loo″ko-lit′ik) leukocytolytic.

leu•ko•ma (loo-ko′mə) pl. *leuko′mata* [Gr. *leukōma* whiteness] a dense white opacity of the cornea. **leuko′matous** *adj*

adherent l. a white tumor of the cornea enclosing a prolapsed adherent iris.

leu·ko·maine (loo′ko-mān) [Gr. *leukōma* whiteness] any one of a large group of basic substances resembling alkaloids, normally present in the tissues, which are products of metabolism and are probably excrementitious. Some of them may become toxic, and many are physiologically active.

leu·ko·main·ic (loo″ko-mān′ik) pertaining to, caused by, or characterized by a leukomaine.

leu·ko·ma·la·cia (loo″ko-mə-la′shə) softening of the white matter of the brain.

periventricular l. (PVL) bilateral necrosis of the white matter of the brain adjacent to the lateral ventricles, seen in the neonatal period, especially in premature newborns, and manifested by chalky, yellowish-white plaques in the white matter, with proliferation of astrocytes and microglia; cyst formation may lead to multicystic encephalopathy.

leu·ko·ma·ta (loo-ko′mə-tə) plural of *leukoma.*

leu·ko·my·eli·tis (loo″ko-mi″ə-li′tis) [*leuko-* + *myelitis*] inflammation of the white substance of the spinal cord.

leu·ko·my·elop·a·thy (loo″ko-mi″ə-lop′ə-the) [*leuko-* + *myelopathy*] any disease of the white substance of the spinal cord.

leu·kon (loo′kon) the circulating leukocytes and the cells from which they arise; it is the counterpart of *erythron* and *thrombon.*

leu·ko·nych·ia (loo″ko-nik′e-ə) [*leuko-* + *onych-* + *-ia*] opaque, whitish discoloration of the nails, usually partial but occasionally total; there are several different causes. Called also *leukopathia unguium.*

apparent l. white discoloration of the nail that fades when pressure is applied and with maintenance of transparency of the nail plate.

l. puncta′ta, punctate l. the occurrence of white spots on the nails; it can be a normal finding but is sometimes secondary to trauma.

l. stria′ta, striate l. transverse streaks of white occurring on the nail; called also *transverse l.*

l. tota′lis abnormal whiteness of an entire nail.

transverse l. l. striata.

leu·ko·path·ia (loo″ko-path′e-ə) leukoderma.

l. puncta′ta reticula′ris symmet′rica idiopathic guttate hypomelanosis.

l. un′guium leukonychia.

leu·kop·a·thy (loo-kop′ə-the) leukoderma.

leu·ko·pe·de·sis (loo″ko-pə-de′sis) [*leuko*cyte + Gr. *pēdan* to leap] leukocyte emigration.

leu·ko·pe·nia (loo″ko-pe′ne-ə) [*leuko*cyte + *-penia*] reduction in the number of leukocytes in the blood below about 5000 per mm^3. Types are named for the type of cell, such as *agranulocytosis* and *neutropenia;* see also *pancytopenia.* Called also *aleukia, aleukocytosis,* and *leukocytopenia.*

basophil l., basophilic l. basophilopenia.

malignant l., pernicious l. agranulocytosis.

leu·ko·pe·nic (loo″ko-pe′nik) 1. pertaining to or characterized by leukopenia. 2. causing leukopenia.

leu·ko·phago·cy·to·sis (loo″ko-fa″go-si-to′sis) leukocytophagy.

leu·ko·pla·kia (loo″ko-pla′ke-ə) [*leuko-* + Gr. *plax* plate + *-ia*] 1. a white patch on a mucous membrane that will not rub off. 2. oral l.

l. bucca′lis white thickened patches on the mucous membrane of the cheeks. See *oral l.*

hairy l. a white filiform to flat patch (see *oral l.*) occurring on the tongue or, rarely, on the buccal mucosa, caused by infection with Epstein-Barr virus and associated with human immunodeficiency virus infection; it is a predictor of the subsequent development of acquired immunodeficiency syndrome (AIDS). Called also *oral hairy leukoplakia.*

l. lingua′lis white thickened patches on the mucous membrane of the tongue. See *oral l.*

oral l. white, thick patches on the oral mucosa produced by hyperkeratosis of the epithelium, with thickening of stratified squamous epithelium,

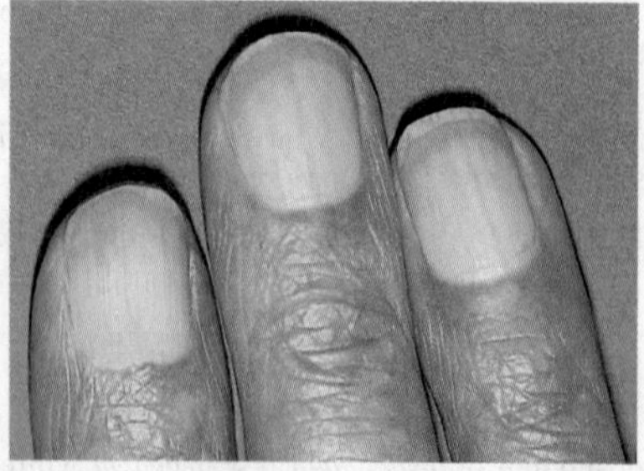

■ Leukonychia.

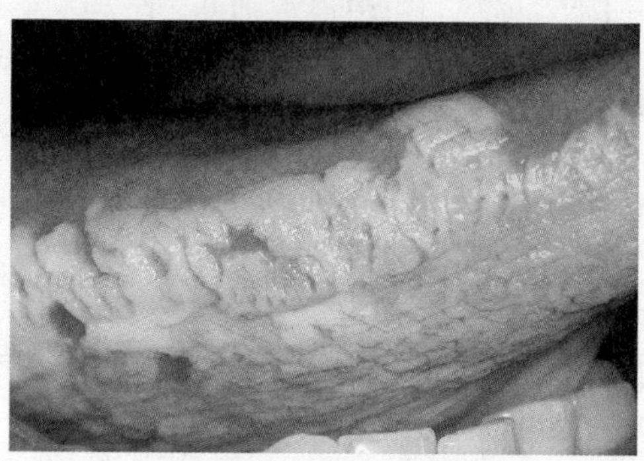

■ Hairy leukoplakia.

hyperkeratosis, hyperplasia, inflammatory infiltration, and degeneration of epithelial cells. It is a benign condition but may predispose to development of epidermoid carcinoma. The etiology is variable, but is mainly associated with tobacco use. Called also *keratosis linguae, leukokeratosis, psoriasis buccalis,* and *psoriasis linguae.*

oral hairy l. hairy l.

speckled l. see under *erythroplakia.*

l. vul′vae 1. former name for lichen sclerosus in females; see under *lichen.* 2. any white-appearing lesion of the vulva.

leu·ko·poi·e·sis (loo″ko-poi-e′sis) the production of leukocytes; called also *leukocytogenesis* and *leukocytopoiesis.*

leu·ko·poi·et·ic (loo″ko-poi-et′ik) 1. pertaining to leukopoiesis. 2. causing leukopoiesis.

leu·ko·poi·e·tin (loo″ko-poi-e′tin) granulopoietin.

leu·ko·pre·cip·i·tin (loo″ko-pre-sip′ĭ-tin) a precipitin specific for leukocyte antigens.

leu·kop·sin (loo-kop′sin) [*leuko-* + *opsin*] visual white; the colorless matter into which rhodopsin is changed by exposure to white light. It is reconvertible into rhodopsin under proper conditions.

leu·ko·re·duc·tion (loo″ko-rə-duk′shən) reduction of the number of leukocytes from a unit of blood prior to transfusion.

leu·kor·rha·gia (loo″ko-ra′jə) [*leuko-* + *-rrhagia*] profuse leukorrhea.

leu·kor·rhea (loo″ko-re′ə) [*leuko-* + *-rrhea*] a whitish, viscid discharge from the vagina and uterine cavity. **leukorrhe′al** *adj*

leu·ko·scope (loo′ko-skōp) [*leuko-* + *-scope*] an instrument that mixes colors to produce white for testing for color blindness.

leu·ko·sis (loo-ko′sis) pl. *leuko′ses.* Proliferation of leukocyte-forming tissue; see *lymphoproliferative disorders, lymphoreticular disorders,* and *myeloproliferative disorders,* under *disorder.*

acute l. Marek disease; see under *disease.*

avian l. a group of viral diseases of chickens, transmitted by related oncoviruses and characterized by proliferation of immature erythroid, myeloid, or lymphoid cells. Leukemic forms include erythroblastosis and myeloblastosis and, rarely, lymphoblastic leukemia. Solid tumors in visceral organs are seen in cases of lymphoid leukosis, erythroblastosis, and myelocytomatosis. Some of the causative viruses induce related neoplasms such as sarcomas, hemangiomas, nephroblastomas, hepatocarcinomas, and osteopetrosis gallinarum, which are now classified as belonging to the leukosis sarcoma group. See also *avian lymphomatosis* and *visceral lymphomatosis,* under *lymphomatosis.*

bovine l. enzootic bovine l.

enzootic bovine l. a progressive fatal lymphosarcoma affecting adult cattle, caused by the bovine leukemia virus, and characterized by infiltration of lymphoid tissue throughout the body by malignant lymphocytes, with enlargement of lymph nodes and spleen. Called also *bovine malignant lymphoma, malignant lymphoma of cattle,* and *bovine leukemia.*

erythroid l. erythroblastosis (def. 2).

fowl l. avian l.

lymphoid l. one of the avian leukosis complex of tumors, involving transformation of B lymphocytes; symptoms include anorexia, emaciation, and an enlarged liver.

myeloblastic l. avian myeloblastosis.

myelocytic l. myelocytomatosis.

skin l. Marek disease when it primarily affects the skin.

sporadic bovine l. a disease similar to enzootic bovine leukosis, with malignant proliferation of lymphoid tissues but no culturable infectious agent; it occurs in three forms that vary in the age of the animal and organ affected: *calf,* seen in animals under six months of age and marked by generalized lymphadenopathy and widespread metastasis; *thymic,* seen in animals 6 to 18 months of age and confined mainly to the thymus; and *cutaneous* or *skin,* the only nonlethal form, affecting young adults and marked by cutaneous tumors that regress spontaneously.

leu·ko·sper·mia (loo″ko-spur′me-ə) leukocytospermia.

leu·ko·sta·sis (loo″ko-sta′sis) increased blood viscosity and hypercoagulability, seen in leukemia that is accompanied by hyperleukocytosis.

leu·ko·tac·tic (loo″ko-tak′tik) 1. able to attract leukocytes. 2. pertaining to leukotaxis; called also *leukocytotactic.*

leu·ko·tax·is (loo″ko-tak′sis) [*leuko-* + *-taxis*] the cytotaxis of leukocytes, tending to collect in regions of injury or inflammation. Called also *leukocytotaxis.*

leu·ko·throm·bin (loo″ko-throm′bin) a fibrin factor formed by leukocytes in the blood.

leu·ko·tome (loo′ko-tōm) [*leuko-* + *-tome*] a neurosurgical tool consisting of a rigid shaft along which runs a thin metallic wire, formed into a loop at one end; the tool is inserted through a bur hole into the skull and rotated about its axis to cut tissue.

leu·kot·o·my (loo-kot′ə-me) prefrontal lobotomy.

transorbital l. see under *lobotomy.*

leu·ko·tox·ic (loo′ko-tok″sik) destructive to leukocytes.

leu·ko·tox·ic·i·ty (loo″ko-tok-sis′ĭ-te) the quality of having a toxic or deleterious effect on leukocytes.

leu·ko·tox·in (loo′ko-tok″sin) [*leukocyte* + *toxin*] a cytotoxin destructive to leukocytes.

leu·ko·trich·ia (loo″ko-trik′e-ə) [*leuko-* + *trich-* + *-ia*] circumscribed depigmentation and whitening of the hair; cf. *poliosis.*

leu·ko·tri·ene (loo″ko-tri′ēn) [from *leuko*cytes + *triene* indicating three double bonds] any of a group of biologically active compounds consisting of straight chain, 20-carbon carboxylic acids with one or two oxygen substituents and three or more conjugated double bonds. They are formed from arachidonic acid by the lipoxygenase pathway and function as regulators of allergic and inflammatory reactions. Leukotrienes are identified by letters A, B, C, D, and E, with subscripts indicating the number of double bonds in the molecule. Some (e.g., LTB_4) stimulate the movement of leukocytes; three others (LTC_4, LTD_4, and LTE_4) together constitute slow-reacting substance of anaphylaxis, which causes bronchial constriction and other allergic reactions.

leu·pro·lide ace·tate (loo-pro′līd) a synthetic gonadotropin-releasing hormone analogue used as an antineoplastic in the palliative treatment of advanced prostatic carcinoma; it is also used in the treatment of endometriosis and central precocious puberty. As an adjunct to iron, it is used preoperatively to improve anemia caused by uterine leiomyomas. Administered subcutaneously and intramuscularly.

leu·pro·rel·in ace·tate (loo″pro-rel′in) INN and BAN for *leuprolide acetate.*

Leu·stat·in (loo-stat′in) trademark for a preparation of cladribine.

Lev disease (lev) [Maurice *Lev,* American pathologist, 1908–1994] see under *disease.*

Lev·a·di·ti method (lev″ə-de′te) [Constantin *Levaditi,* Romanian-born bacteriologist in France, 1874–1953] see *Stains and Staining Methods,* under *stain.*

lev·al·bu·ter·ol hy·dro·chlo·ride (lev″al-bu′tər-ol) *R*-albuterol; a β_2-adrenergic receptor agonist used as a bronchodilator for the treatment and prophylaxis of reversible bronchospasm in reversible obstructive airway disease; administered by inhalation.

lev·al·lor·phan tar·trate (lev″ə-lor′fan) an analogue of levorphanol that acts as an opioid agonist-antagonist, used parenterally for its antagonistic effect in the treatment of respiratory depression caused by opioid analgesics; in the absence of opioid-induced respiratory depression it can itself cause respiratory depression.

le·vam·i·sole hy·dro·chlo·ride (le-vam′ĭ-sōl) [USP] an immunomodulator used orally as an adjunct with fluorouracil in the treatment of Dukes stage C colon cancer following surgical resection of the primary tumor. It is also used as a veterinary anthelmintic, chiefly in the treatment of ascariasis and hookworm infections.

lev·an (lev′an) a homopolysaccharide containing fructose residues in 2,6-glycosidic linkage. Formed from sucrose by the enzyme levansucrase, levan, which is produced by certain species of *Bacillus* and *Leuconostoc,* increases the adhesion of bacteria to surfaces of the teeth and promotes the formation of dental plaque.

lev·an·su·crase (lev″an-soo′krās) [EC 2.4.1.10] an enzyme of the transferase class produced by certain species of *Bacillus* and *Leuconostoc;* it catalyzes the transfer of fructose residues from sucrose to a growing levan polymer, a constituent of dental plaque.

Lev·a·quin (lev′ə-kwin) trademark for preparations of levofloxacin.

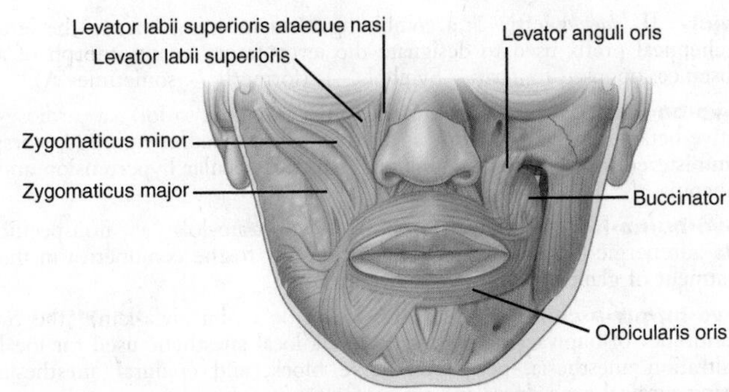

■ Levator muscles acting on the mouth and alae of the nose and adjacent facial muscles.

lev·ar·te·re·nol (lev″ahr-tēr′ə-nol) the levorotatory isomer of norepinephrine, a much more potent pressor agent than the natural dextrorotatory isomer.

l. bitartrate norepinephrine bitartrate.

Lev·a·tol (lev′ə-tol) trademark for a preparation of penbutolol sulfate.

le·va·tor (lə-va′tor) pl. *levato′res* [L. *levare* to raise] 1. a muscle for elevating the organ or structure into which it is inserted; see entries beginning *musculus levator,* under *musculus.* 2. a surgical instrument used to raise depressed osseous fragments in fractures of the skull and other bones.

l. a′ni see under *musculus.*

lev·a·to·res (lev″ə-to′rēz) [L.] plural of *levator.*

Lev·bid (lev′bid) trademark for a preparation of hyoscyamine sulfate.

lev·el (lev′əl) relative position, rank, or concentration.

α l. significance l.

background l. the usual intensity of a chemical or other stimulus in the environment.

confidence l. one minus the confidence coefficient; the probability that a confidence interval does not contain the population parameter. Denoted α. See also *Type I error,* under *error.*

l's of consciousness clinically differentiable degrees of awareness and alertness such as alert wakefulness, lethargy, clouding of consciousness, stupor, and coma.

isoelectric l. see under *line.*

lowest observed adverse effect l. (LOAEL), lowest observed effect l. (LOEL) in studies of the toxicity of chemicals, the lowest dosage level at which chronic exposure to the substance shows adverse effects; usually calculated for laboratory animals.

no observed adverse effect l. (NOAEL), no observed effect l. (NOEL) in studies of the toxicity of chemicals, the highest dosage level at which chronic exposure to the substance shows no adverse effects; usually calculated for laboratory animals.

significance l., l. of significance the probability of incorrectly rejecting the null hypothesis when such a hypothesis is tested. Denoted α. See also *Type I error,* under *error.*

Lev·e·mir (lev′ə-mir) trademark for a preparation of insulin detemir.

le·ve·ti·rac·e·tam (le″və-ti-ras′ə-tam) an anticonvulsant administered orally as an adjunct in the treatment of partial and myoclonic seizures and idiopathic generalized epilepsy.

Lé·vi-Lo·rain dwarfism (syndrome) (la-ve′ lo-rā′) [E. Léopold *Lévi,* French endocrinologist, 1868–1933; Paul Joseph *Lorain,* French physician, 1827–1875] pituitary dwarfism; see under *dwarfism.*

lev·i·ga·tion (lev″ĭ-ga′shən) [L. *levigare* to render smooth] the grinding to a powder of a hard or moistened substance.

Le·vin tube (lə-vin′) [Abraham Louis *Levin,* American physician, 1880–1940] see under *tube.*

lev·i·ta·tion (lev″ĭ-ta′shən) [L. *levis* light] 1. a hallucinatory sensation of floating or rising in the air. 2. a support system for severe burn victims, consisting of a bed in the form of an inflatable chamber containing numerous outlets through which humidified, warm, sterile air is released at a pressure sufficient to raise the patient and give support in a sterile air environment.

Le·vi·tra (lə-ve′trə) trademark for a preparation of tadalafil.

Lev·len (lev′lən) trademark for combination preparations of levonorgestrel and ethinyl estradiol.

Lev·lite (lev-līt′) trademark for combination preparations of levonorgestrel and ethinyl estradiol.

lev·met·am·fet·amine (lev″met-am-fet′ə-mēn) [USP] the *levo* isomer of methamphetamine, used by inhalation as a nasal decongestant.

lev(o)- [L. *laevus* left] 1. a combining form meaning left, to the left. 2. chemical prefix used to designate the levorotatory enantiomorph of a substance; opposed to *dextro-*. Symbol (−)- (formerly *l-;* sometimes Λ).

le•vo•be•tax•o•lol hy•dro•chlo•ride (le″vo-ba-tak′sə-lol) a cardioselective beta-adrenergic blocking agent that acts at β_1-adrenergic receptors; administered topically to the conjunctiva to treat ocular hypertension and glaucoma.

le•vo•bu•no•lol hy•dro•chlo•ride (le″vo-bu′no-lol) a nonspecific beta-adrenergic blocking agent applied topically to the conjunctiva in the treatment of glaucoma and ocular hypertension.

le•vo•bu•piv•a•caine hy•dro•chlo•ride (le″vo-bu-piv′ə-kān) the *S*-enantiomer of bupivacaine hydrochloride; a local anesthetic used for local infiltration anesthesia, peripheral nerve block, and epidural anesthesia during surgical procedures and for postoperative pain management.

le•vo•cab•as•tine hy•dro•chlo•ride (le″vo-kab′ə-stēn) an antihistamine (H_1 receptor antagonist) applied topically to the conjunctiva to treat seasonal allergic conjunctivitis.

le•vo•car•dia (le″vo-kahr′de-ə) [*levo-* + *cardia*] a term denoting the normal position of the heart, used when other viscera are transposed; cf. *dextrocardia.*

isolated l. levocardia associated with transposition (situs inversus) of the abdominal viscera, congenital structural anomaly of the heart, and sometimes with absence of the spleen.

mixed l. corrected transposition of the great vessels; see under *transposition.*

le•vo•car•ni•tine (le″vo-kahr′nĭ-tēn) [USP] a preparation of the biologically active L- isomer of carnitine, used to treat carnitine deficiency, either primary or secondary to an inborn error of metabolism, and to prevent and treat carnitine deficiency associated with hemodialysis in end-stage renal disease; administered orally.

le•vo•ce•ti•ri•zine di•hy•dro•chlo•ride (le″vo-sə-tir′ĭ-zēn) a histamine H_1-receptor antagonist used in treatment of allergic rhinitis and chronic idiopathic urticaria; administered orally.

le•vo•cli•na•tion (le″vo-klĭ-na′shən) [*levo-* + L. *clinatus* leaning] rotation of the upper poles of the vertical meridians of the two eyes to the left. Called also *sinistrotorsion.*

le•vo•cy•clo•duc•tion (le″vo-si″klo-dək′shən) levoduction.

le•vo•do•pa (le″vo-do′pə) [USP] L-dopa, the levorotatory isomer of dopa, used in the treatment of Parkinson disease and other forms of parkinsonism; administered orally.

Le•vo-Dro•mo•ran (le″vo-dro′mə-ran) trademark for preparations of levorphanol tartrate.

le•vo•duc•tion (le″vo-duk′shən) movement of either eye to the left.

le•vo•flox•a•cin (le″vo-flok′sə-sin) a broad-spectrum fluoroquinolone antibacterial agent used in the treatment of infection by susceptible organisms, including bronchitis, community-acquired pneumonia, pyelonephritis, urinary tract infections, acute maxillary sinusitis, and skin and soft tissue infections; administered orally, intravenously, and, in the treatment of bacterial conjunctivitis, applied topically to the conjunctiva.

le•vo•gy•ral (le″vo-ji′rəl) levorotatory.

Le•void (le′void) trademark for a preparation of levothyroxine sodium.

le•vo•me•pro•ma•zine (le″vo-mə-pro′mə-zēn) methotrimeprazine.

le•vo•nor•de•frin (le″vo-nor′də-frin) [USP] an adrenergic, the levo isomer of nordefrin, used as a vasoconstrictor in solutions of local anesthetics, especially in dentistry.

le•vo•nor•ges•trel (le′vo-nor-jes′trel) [USP] the levorotatory form of norgestrel, administered as a subdermal contraceptive implant or in combination with an estrogen component in an oral contraceptive. It is also administered orally as a progestin-only contraceptive for emergency postcoital contraception.

Lev•o•phed (lev′o-fed) trademark for a preparation of norepinephrine bitartrate.

Lev•ora (lə-vor′ə) trademark for combination preparations of levonorgestrel and ethinyl estradiol.

le•vo•ro•ta•ry (le″vo-ro′tə-re) levorotatory.

le•vo•ro•ta•tion (le″vo-ro-ta′shən) a turning to the left.

le•vo•ro•ta•to•ry (le″vo-ro′tə-tor″e) [*levo-* + *rotatory*] turning the plane of polarization of polarized light to the left (counterclockwise).

le•vor•pha•nol tar•trate (le-vor′fə-nol) [USP] a synthetic opioid analgesic with properties and actions similar to those of morphine; used as an analgesic, for moderate to severe pain, and as an adjunct to anesthesia, administered orally, subcutaneously, intramuscularly, or intravenously.

le•vo•si•men•dan (le″vo-sĭ-men′dən) a calcium-sensitizing agent having positive inotropic and vasodilator effects, used in the treatment of heart failure; administered intravenously.

Lev•o•throid (lev′o-throid″) trademark for a preparation of levothyroxine sodium.

le•vo•thy•rox•ine so•di•um (le″vo-thi-rok′sēn) [USP] the monosodium salt of L-thyroxine, the naturally occurring form of thyroxine, obtained from the thyroid gland of domesticated food animals or prepared synthetically. It is used as replacement therapy for hypothyroidism and in the prophylaxis and treatment of goiter and of thyroid carcinoma, administered orally, intramuscularly, or intravenously.

le•vo•tor•sion (le″vo-tor′shən) levoclination.

le•vo•ver•sion (le″vo-vur′zhən) an act of turning to the left; in ophthalmology, movement of the eyes to the left.

Le•vox•yl (lə-vok′sil) trademark for a preparation of levothyroxine sodium.

Lev•ret forceps (ləv-ra′) [André *Levret*, French obstetrician, 1703–1780] see under *forceps.*

Lev•sin (lev′sin) trademark for a preparation of hyoscyamine sulfate.

Lev•si•nex (lev′sin-eks) trademark for a preparation of hyoscyamine sulfate.

Lev•u•gen (lev′u-jən) trademark for a preparation of fructose.

Lev•u•lan (lev′u-lan) trademark for a preparation of aminolevulinic acid hydrochloride.

lev•u•lose (lev′u-lōs) [L. *laevus* left + *-ose*] fructose.

Le•vy-Hol•lis•ter syndrome (le′ve hol′is-tər) [Walter J. *Levy*, South African ophthalmologist, 20th century; David W. *Hollister*, American physician, 20th century] see *lacrimo-auriculo-dento-digital syndrome*, under *syndrome.*

Lé•vy-Rous•sy syndrome (la-ve′ roo-se′) [Gabrielle *Lévy*, French neurologist, 1886–1935; Gustave *Roussy*, French pathologist, 1874–1948] Roussy-Lévy syndrome.

Le•wan•dow•sky nevus elasticus (lev-ahn-dov′ske) [Felix *Lewandowsky*, German dermatologist, 1879–1921] nevus elasticus of Lewandowsky.

Le•wan•dow•sky-Lutz disease (lev-ahn-dov′ske loots′) [F. *Lewandowsky;* Wilhelm *Lutz*, Swiss dermatologist, 1888–1958] epidermodysplasia verruciformis.

Lew•is blood group (loo′is) [*Lewis*, surname of the English propositus first reported on in 1946] see under *blood group.*

Lew•is-Pic•ker•ing test (loo′is pik′ər-ing) [Sir Thomas *Lewis*, English cardiologist, 1881-1945; Sir George White *Pickering*, English scientist, 1904–1980] see under *test.*

Lew•is-Sum•ner syndrome (loo′is sum′nər) [Richard Alan *Lewis*, American neurologist, late 20th century; Austin J. *Sumner*, American neurologist, late 20th century] see under *syndrome.*

lew•i•site (loo′i-sīt) [W. Lee *Lewis*, American chemist, 1879–1943] a lethal war gas; it is a vesicant, lacrimator, and lung irritant.

Le•wy bodies (la′ve) [Frederic H. *Lewy*, German-born neurologist in United States, 1885–1950] see under *body.*

Lex•a•pro (lek′sə-pro) trademark for a preparation of escitalopram oxalate.

Lex•i•va (lek-se′və) trademark for a preparation of fosamprenavir calcium.

Lex•xel (lek′sel) trademark for a combination preparation of enalapril maleate and felodipine.

Ley•den jar (li′dən) [*Leyden*, the Netherlands, where it was invented] see under *jar.*

Ley•den-Mö•bi•us muscular dystrophy, syndrome (li′dən mur′be-əs) [Ernst Viktor von *Leyden*, German physician, 1832–1910; Paul Julius *Möbius*, German neurologist, 1853–1907] limb-girdle muscular dystrophy; see under *dystrophy.*

Ley•dig cells, cylinders (li′dig) [Franz von *Leydig*, German anatomist, 1821–1908] see under *cell* and *cylinder.*

Lf limes flocculating; see *Lf dose*, under *dose.*

LFA left frontoanterior; see *frontoanterior position*, under *position.*

LFA-1 leukocyte function–associated antigen 1.

LFA-2 leukocyte function–associated antigen 2.

LFA-3 leukocyte function–associated antigen 3.

L-form (el′form″) L-phase variant; see under *variant.*

LFP left frontoposterior; see *frontoposterior position,* under *position.*

LFT left frontotransverse; see *frontotransverse position,* under *position.*

LGA large for gestational age; see under *infant.*

LGB laparoscopic gastric banding.

LH luteinizing hormone.

Lher•mitte sign (lār-mēt′) [Jean *Lhermitte,* Paris neurologist, 1877–1959] see under *sign.*

LH-RH luteinizing hormone–releasing hormone.

Li lithium.

LIA leukemia-associated inhibitory activity.

Li•al•da (le-ahl′də) trademark for a preparation of mesalamine.

-liberin [L. *liber* free] a word termination denoting a freeing or releasing; used in names of hormones.

li•bid•i•nal (lĭ-bid′ĭ-nəl) 1. pertaining to or of the nature of libido. 2. erotic.

li•bid•i•nous (lĭ-bid′ĭ-nəs) erotic.

li•bi•do (lĭ-be′do, lĭ-bi′do) pl. *libid′ines* [L.] 1. sexual desire. 2. the psychic energy derived from instinctive biological drives; in early freudian theory it was restricted to the sexual drive, then expanded to include all expressions of love and pleasure, but the concept has evolved to include also the death instinct.

Lib•man-Sacks endocarditis (disease), vegetations (lib′mən saks′) [Emanuel *Libman,* American physician, 1872–1946; Benjamin *Sacks,* American physician, 1873–1939] see under *endocarditis* and *vegetation.*

li•bra (L.) (le′brə, li′brə) pl. *li′brae* [L.] pound.

li•brary (li′brer″e) [L. *libraria*] in genetics, a set of cloned DNA fragments that together represent the entire genome, or the genes transcribed by a particular tissue. Called also *DNA l.*

Lib•rax (lib′raks) trademark for a combination preparation of chlordiazepoxide hydrochloride and clidinium bromide.

Lib•ri•um (lib′re-əm) trademark for preparations of chlordiazepoxide hydrochloride.

lice (līs) plural of *louse.*

li•cense (li′səns) [L. *licere* to be permitted] a permit to perform acts which without it would be illegal.

li•cen•ti•ate (li-sen′she-āt) [L. *licentia* license] one holding a license from an authorized agency giving the right to practice a particular profession.

Lich technique (lik) [R. *Lich, Jr.,* American urologist, 20th century] see under *technique.*

Lich-Gre•goir technique (lik′ grə-gwahr′) [R. *Lich;* W. *Gregoir,* Belgian urologist, 20th century] see under *technique.*

li•chen (li′kən) [Gr. *leichēn* a tree-moss] 1. any of the many thallophytic plants formed by mutualistic combination of an alga and a fungus, the algal component being a green or blue-green alga, and the fungal usually an ascomycete. 2. any of a number of papular skin diseases in which the lesions are small, firm papules set close together.

actinic l. planus l. planus actinicus.

l. amyloido′sus lichen amyloidosis; see under *amyloidosis*

annular l. planus l. planus annularis.

atrophic l. planus l. planus atrophicus.

l. au′reus a rare type of chronic pigmented purpura in which the patient has a single red or rust-colored lesion on the lower limb, usually over a perforating vein.

bullous l. planus lichen planus in which small vesicles and bullae may occur as part of the general papular eruption, or present de novo or on uninvolved skin.

erosive l. planus lichen planus that has developed ulcerations; called also *ulcerative l. planus.*

erythematous l. planus l. planus erythematosus.

follicular l. planus l. planus follicularis.

hypertrophic l. planus l. planus hypertrophicus.

linear l. planus lichen planus that spreads along Blaschko lines; called also *l. planus linearis.*

l. myxedemato′sus a condition resembling myxedema but not associated with thyroid dysfunction, characterized by a fibrocystic proliferation, increased deposition of acid mucopolysaccharides in the skin, and a circulating paraprotein, usually an immunoglobulin G. Manifestations vary: there may be localized or generalized distributions of lichenoid papules and presence or absence of scleroderma; one type has plaques and nodules resembling those of urticaria. The most serious, generalized form with scleroderma is called *scleromyxedema.* Called also *papular mucinosis.*

nail l. planus, l. planus of the nails lichen planus affecting a fingernail or toenail, or several nails, usually with formation of a pterygium that fuses the nail plate to the nail bed and may lead to shedding of the nail. This type may occur with or without lichen planus on the skin.

l. ni′tidus a chronic, usually asymptomatic, inflammatory eruption consisting of discrete, glistening, flat-topped, smooth, tiny papules, located most often on the penis, lower abdomen, inner thighs, flexor aspects of the arms, breasts, or buttocks.

l. obtu′sus cor′neus prurigo nodularis.

oral l. planus lichen planus in the oral cavity, with Wickham striae on the buccal mucous membranes and sides of the tongue; there are often plaques or ulcerations *(erosive l. planus).*

pemphigoid l. planus l. planus pemphigoides.

l. pila′ris l. spinulosus.

l. planopila′ris l. planus follicularis.

l. pla′nus an inflammatory, pruritic disease of the skin or sometimes oral mucosa, genital mucosa, or nails; it may be acute and widespread or chronic and localized. There are numerous different types, named for the configuration or site of the lesions; most resolve spontaneously, leaving residual hyperpigmentation and atrophy. Characteristics include an eruption of violet, umbilicated, flat-topped, scaly papules and white lines called *Wickham striae;* lesions may be discrete or may coalesce to form plaques and other shapes. Similar lesions may be caused by drugs or chemical substances. Called also *l. ruber planus.*

l. pla′nus acti′nicus lichen planus occurring in hot climates or hot weather, especially on sun-exposed areas of the skin, characterized by papular lesions that usually have pale centers and darker borders. Called also *actinic* or *subtropical l. planus.*

l. pla′nus annula′ris lichen planus in which groups of papules form annular configurations, especially on the genitals, lower trunk, and lips, and in the mouth.

l. pla′nus atro′phicus lichen planus characterized by atrophy in the center of preexisting lesions of lichen planus, ultimately leading to atrophic white spots on the skin that aggregate to form small white or purple patches, sometimes with erythematous borders. Called also *atrophic l. planus.*

l. pla′nus bullo′sus bullous l. planus.

l. pla′nus erythemato′sus a rare variant of lichen planus characterized by soft, nonpruritic, erythematous papules.

l. pla′nus follicula′ris lichen planus accompanied by alopecia cicatrisata, with patches of pointed, keratotic lesions around hair follicles, often leading to local atrophy. Called also *l. planopilaris* and *follicular lichen planus.*

l. pla′nus hypertro′phicus lichen planus characterized by verrucous plaques covered with scales, usually located on the shins but sometimes elsewhere on the body. Called also *hypertrophic l. planus* and *l. planus verrucosus.*

l. pla′nus linea′ris linear l. planus.

l. pla′nus pemphigoi′des a condition combining characteristics of both bullous lichen planus and bullous pemphigoid.

l. pla′nus subtro′picus, l. pla′nus tro′picus l. planus actinicus.

l. pla′nus verruco′sus l. planus hypertrophicus.

l. ru′ber monilifor′mis a rare skin condition consisting of discolored papules with a keloidal consistency, arranged in bands and sometimes crisscrossing networks. Some authorities consider the condition to be a variant of lichen simplex chronicus.

l. ru′ber pla′nus l. planus.

l. sclero′sus, l. sclero′sus et atro′phicus a chronic, atrophic skin disease characterized by hard flat white papules with erythematous halos and black follicular keratotic plugs; it is usually around the external genitalia or in the perianal region. In females it is seen in older women or the very young and results in destruction of vulvar architecture, scarring, and shrinkage of the labia with itching, dyspareunia, and dysuria. In males it affects the prepuce and glans penis and may result in stricture of the urethral meatus. Occasionally it may precede squamous cell carcinoma. In females, called also *atrophic* or *leukoplakic vulvitis, leukokraurosis,* and *kraurosis vulvae.* In males, called also *balanitis xerotica obliterans.*

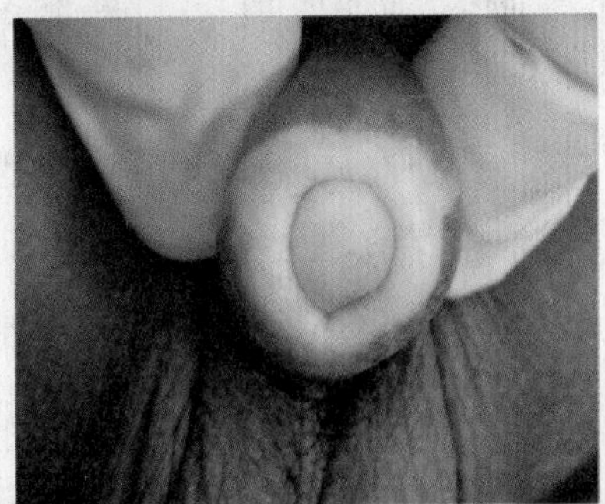

■ Lichen sclerosus et atrophicus in a young boy.

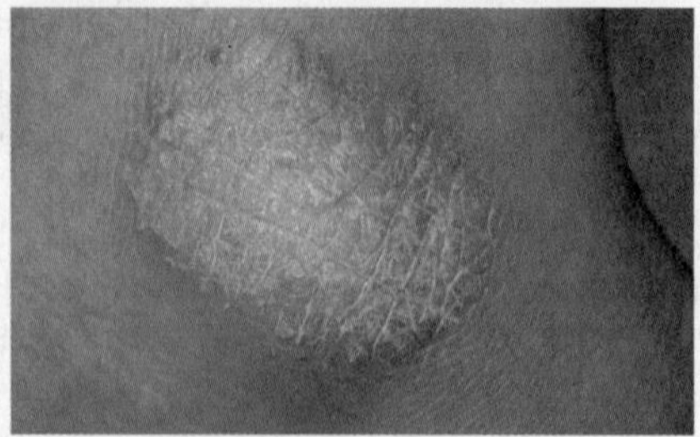

■ Lichen simplex chronicus in an area of chronic excoriation.

l. scrofuloso′rum, l. scrofulo′sus a form of tuberculid manifested as an eruption of clusters of lichenoid papules on the trunk of children and young adults with tuberculous disease.

l. sim′plex chro′nicus eczema caused by repeated itching and rubbing or scratching of the skin; it may arise spontaneously or be associated with other dermatoses. Characteristics are sharply demarcated, circumscribed, scaling patches of thickened, furrowed skin, usually on the face, neck, limbs, or anogenital region. Called also *circumscribed* or *localized neurodermatitis.*

l. spinulo′sus a cutaneous disorder usually seen in children and young adults, characterized by discrete groups of minute, filiform, horny spines protruding from acuminate hair follicle openings; the most common sites are the neck, buttocks, abdominal wall, back of the knee, and extensor surfaces of the arms. Called also *l. pilaris.*

l. stria′tus a self-limited, generally unilateral skin eruption, usually seen in children on the limbs or the sides of the neck; it typically presents as discrete, pink, papular or lichenoid lesions that have an inconspicuous scale and tend to coalesce to form a continuous or interrupted linear patch.

subtropical l. planus l. planus actinicus.

l. syphili′ticus a skin lesion seen in secondary syphilis, consisting of groups of small follicular papules.

l. tro′picus miliaria rubra.

ulcerative l. planus erosive l. planus.

l. urtica′tus papular urticaria.

vesiculobullous l. planus bullous l. planus.

li•chen•i•fi•ca•tion (li-ken″ĭ-fĭ-ka′shən) hypertrophy of the epidermis, with thickening and toughening of the skin to give it a leathery appearance, and exaggeration of its normal markings; this is caused by prolonged rubbing or scratching and may be on seemingly normal skin or on skin that has a pruritic disorder.

li•chen•i•form•in (li-ken″ĭ-form′in) a group of antibiotic substances (licheniformin A, B, and C) isolated from *Bacillus subtilis,* resembling subtilin in their properties.

li•chen•oid (li′kən-oid) resembling the skin lesions known as lichen.

Lich•ten•berg figure (lik′ten-berg) [Georg Christoph *Lichtenberg,* German physicist and humorist, 1742–1799] see under *figure.*

Lich•ten•stein repair (lik′tən-stīn″) [Irving L. *Lichtenstein,* American surgeon, 20th century] see under *repair.*

Licht•heim plaques, sign, etc. (likt′hīm) [Ludwig *Lichtheim,* German physician, 1845–1928] see under *plaque, sign,* and *test,* and see *subacute combined degeneration of spinal cord,* under *degeneration.*

lic•o•rice (lik′ə-ris) 1. *Glycyrrhiza glabra.* 2. [NF] the dried rhizome, roots, and stolons of various species of *Glycyrrhiza,* used as a flavoring and used internally as an expectorant and for the treatment of gastritis. Licorice preparations are also used in traditional Chinese medicine, ayurveda, and folk medicine. Called also *licorice root, liquorice,* and *glycyrrhiza.*

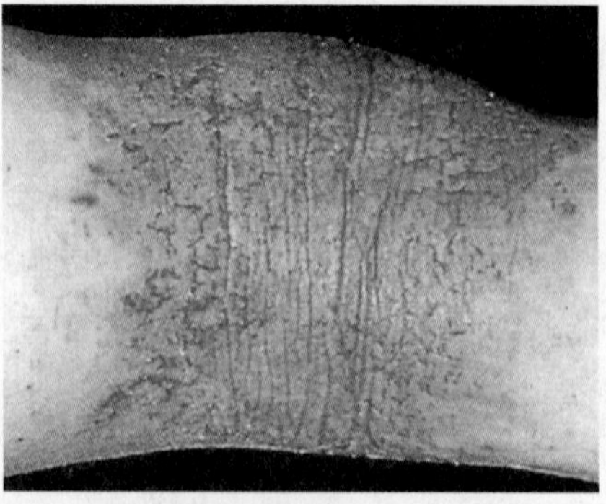

■ Lichenification associated with atopic dermatitis.

lid (lid) [A.S. *hlid*] an eyelid.

granular l's trachoma.

tucked l. of Collier retraction of the upper eyelid in cases of ophthalmoplegia due to a supranuclear lesion in the brainstem.

Lid•dell and Sher•ring•ton reflex (lĭ-del′ sher′ing-tən) [Edward George Tandy *Liddell,* English physiologist, 1895–1981; Sir Charles Scott *Sherrington,* English physiologist, 1857–1952] stretch reflex.

Lid•dle syndrome (lid′əl) [Grant Winder *Liddle,* American physician, born 1921] see under *syndrome.*

Li•dex (li′deks) trademark for preparations of fluocinonide.

li•do•caine (li′do-kān) [USP] a drug having anesthetic, sedative, analgesic, anticonvulsant, and cardiac depressant activities, used as a local anesthetic, applied topically to the skin and mucous membranes.

l. hydrochloride [USP] the monohydrated monohydrochloride salt of lidocaine; used to produce local anesthesia by infiltration injection and by topical application to the skin or mucosa, and to produce caudal, epidural, or retrobulbar anesthesia and peripheral or sympathetic nerve block; also administered intravenously for use as a cardiac antiarrhythmic.

Li•do•derm (li′do-dərm) trademark for a preparation of lidocaine.

li•do•fen•in (HIDA) (li″do-fen′in) a dimethyl-substituted analogue of iminodiacetic acid (IDA); complexed with technetium 99m, it is used for hepatobiliary imaging. See also table at *technetium.*

lie (li) the relation of the long axis of the fetus to that of the mother; see *presentation.*

oblique l. the situation of the fetus when the long axis of its body crosses the long axis of the maternal body at an angle close to 45 degrees; the shoulder usually presents first, but the arm or part of the trunk may instead present first.

transverse l. the situation of the fetus when the long axis of its body crosses the long axis of the maternal body. The shoulder usually presents first, but the arm or any part of the trunk may be the first to appear. Called also *torso, transverse,* or *trunk presentation.* See table at *position.*

Lie•ber•kühn glands (crypts, follicles) (le′ber-kēn) [Johann Nathaniel *Lieberkühn,* German anatomist, 1711–1756] glandulae intestinales.

Lie•ber•mann-Bur•chard test (reaction) (le′bər-mahn burk′hahrd) [Carl Theodore *Liebermann,* German chemist, 1842–1914; H. *Burchard,* German chemist, 19th century] see under *test.*

Lie•ber•meis•ter rule (le′bər-mīs″tər) [Carl von *Liebermeister,* German physician, 1833–1901] see under *rule.*

li•en (li′ən) [L.] TA alternative for *splen.* **lien′al** *adj*

l. accesso′rius splen accessorius.

l. mo′bilis floating spleen.

li•en•ec•to•my (li″ə-nek′tə-me) splenectomy.

li•eni•tis (li″ə-ni′tis) splenitis.

lien(o)- [L. *lien* spleen] a combining form denoting relationship to the spleen.

li•eno•cele (li-e′no-sēl) splenocele.

li•en•og•ra•phy (li″ə-nog′rə-fe) splenography.

li•eno•ma•la•cia (li-e″no-mə-la′shə) splenomalacia.

li•eno•med•ul•lary (li-e″no-med′u-lar″e) splenomedullary.

li•eno•my•elog•e•nous (li-e″no-mi″ə-loj′ə-nəs) splenomedullary (def. 2).

li•eno•pan•cre•at•ic (li-e″no-pan″kre-at′ik) splenopancreatic.

li•en•op•a•thy (li″ə-nop′ə-the) splenopathy.

li•eno•re•nal (li-e″no-re′nəl) pertaining to the spleen and the kidney.

li•eno•tox•in (li-e′no-tok″sin) [*lieno-* + *toxin*] splenotoxin.

li•en•tery (li′ən-ter″e) [Gr. *leienteria; leios* smooth + *enteron* intestine] passage of undigested food in the feces, as seen in some kinds of diarrhea. **lienter′ic** *adj*

Liep•mann apraxia (lēp′mahn) [Hugo Carl *Liepmann,* German neurologist, 1863–1925] see under *apraxia.*

Lie•se•gang phenomenon (striae, waves) (le′zə-gahng) [Raphael Eduard *Liesegang,* German chemist, 1869–1947] see under *phenomenon.*

Lieu•taud triangle (lyoo̅-to′) [Joseph *Lieutaud,* French physician, 1703–1780] see *trigonum vesicae urinariae.*

LIF left iliac fossa; leukocyte inhibitory factor.

life (līf) the aggregate of vital phenomena, a distinctive stimulated condition of organized matter; that principle whereby organized beings are endowed with certain powers and functions not associated with inorganic matter. Generally, living things share, in varying degrees, the following characteristics: organization, irritability, movement, growth, reproduction, and adaptation.

animal l. vegetative life conjoined with the employment of the senses and with spontaneous movements.

mean l. (τ) the average time until decay for a sample of particles of a radionuclide or elementary particle, equal to the reciprocal of the decay constant or 1.443 times the half-life. Called also *lifetime*.

vegetative l. life that is manifested in automatic acts requisite for the maintenance of the individual and the propagation of the species.

life·time (līf′tīm) mean life.

lig. ligament; ligamentum.

lig·a·ment (lig′ə-mənt) 1. a band of tissue that connects bones or supports viscera. Some ligaments are distinct fibrous structures; some are folds of fascia or of indurated peritoneum; still others are relics of fetal vessels or organs. 2. a double layer of peritoneum extending from one visceral organ to another. 3. cordlike remnants of fetal tubular structures that are nonfunctional after birth.

Ligament

For names of specific anatomic structures, see under *ligamentum.*

accessory l. any ligament that strengthens or supports another.
accessory l. of humerus ligamentum coracohumerale.
accessory l's of metacarpophalangeal joints ligamenta collateralia articulationum metacarpophalangealium.
acromioclavicular l. ligamentum acromioclaviculare.
acromiocoracoid l. ligamentum coracoacromiale.
alar l's ligamenta alaria.
alveolodental l. periodontal l.
annular l., external retinaculum musculorum peroneorum superius.
annular l., internal retinaculum musculorum flexorum pedis.
annular l. of radius ligamentum anulare radii.
annular l. of stapes ligamentum anulare stapediale.
annular l's of trachea ligamenta anularia tracheae.
anococcygeal l. corpus anococcygeum.
anterior l. of head of fibula ligamentum capitis fibulae anterius.
anterior l. of head of rib ligamentum capitis costae radiatum.
anterior l. of malleus ligamentum mallei anterius.
anterior l. of neck of rib the anterior portion of the ligamentum costotransversarium superius.
anterior l. of radiocarpal joint ligamentum radiocarpale palmare.
apical l. of dens ligamentum apicis dentis.
appendiculo-ovarian l. a fold of peritoneum extending between the appendix and the broad ligament of the uterus.
Arantius l. ligamentum venosum.
arcuate l's ligamenta flava.
arcuate l., lateral ligamentum arcuatum laterale.
arcuate l., medial ligamentum arcuatum mediale.
arcuate l., median ligamentum arcuatum medianum.
arcuate l. of diaphragm, external ligamentum arcuatum laterale.
arcuate l. of diaphragm, internal ligamentum arcuatum mediale.
arcuate l. of diaphragm, lateral ligamentum arcuatum laterale.
arcuate l. of knee ligamentum popliteum arcuatum.
arcuate pubic l., arcuate l. of pubis, inferior ligamentum pubicum inferius.
arytenoepiglottic l. plica aryepiglottica.
atlanto-occipital l., anterior, atlanto-occipital l., deep ligamentum atlantooccipitale anterius.
atlanto-occipital l., lateral ligamentum atlantooccipitale laterale.
l's of auditory ossicles ligamenta ossiculorum auditoriorum.
l's of auricle, auricular l's ligamenta auricularia.
auricular l., anterior ligamentum auriculare anterius.
auricular l., posterior ligamentum auriculare posterius.
auricular l., superior ligamentum auriculare superius.
Barkow l. the anterior and posterior parts of the elbow joint capsule.
Bellini l. a band passing as part of the capsule of the hip joint to the greater trochanter.
Bérard l. the suspensory ligament of the pericardium, extending to the third and fourth thoracic vertebrae.
Berry l. ligamentum thyrohyoideum laterale.
Bertin l. ligamentum iliofemorale.
Bichat l. the lower bundle of the dorsal sacroiliac ligament.
bifurcate l. ligamentum bifurcatum.
bifurcate l's, deep ligamenta metatarsalia plantaria.
bifurcate l's of Arnold, deep ligamenta tarsometatarsalia plantaria.
bifurcated l. ligamentum bifurcatum.
Bigelow l. ligamentum iliofemorale.
bigeminate l's of Arnold ligamenta tarsometatarsalia dorsalia.
l. of Botallo ligamentum arteriosum.
Bourgery l. ligamentum popliteum obliquum.
brachiocubital l. ligamentum collaterale ulnare.
brachioradial l. ligamentum collaterale radiale.
broad l. of uterus ligamentum latum uteri.
Brodie l. transverse humeral ligament.
Burns l. margo falciformis hiatus saphenus.
calcaneocuboid l. ligamentum calcaneocuboideum.
calcaneocuboid l., plantar ligamentum calcaneocuboideum plantare.
calcaneofibular l. ligamentum calcaneofibulare.
calcaneonavicular l. ligamentum calcaneonaviculare.
calcaneonavicular l., plantar ligamentum calcaneonaviculare plantare.
calcaneotibial l. pars tibiocalcanea ligamenti medialis.
Caldani l. a band passing from the inner border of the coracoid process to the lower border of the clavicle, the first rib, and the tendon of the subclavius.
Campbell l. suspensory l. of axilla.
canthal l's see *ligamentum palpebrale mediale* and *ligamentum palpebrale laterale.*
capitular l., volar deep transverse metacarpal l.
capsular l's ligamenta capsularia.
capsular l., internal ligamentum capitis femoris.
cardinal l. ligamentum cardinale.
carpal l., dorsal ligamenta intercarpalia dorsalia.
carpal l., radiate ligamentum carpi radiatum.
carpal l., transverse retinaculum musculorum flexorum manus.
carpometacarpal l's, anterior ligamenta carpometacarpalia palmaria.
carpometacarpal l's, dorsal ligamenta carpometacarpalia dorsalia.
carpometacarpal l's, palmar ligamenta carpometacarpalia palmaria.
carpometacarpal l's, posterior ligamenta carpometacarpalia dorsalia.
carpometacarpal l's, volar ligamenta carpometacarpalia palmaria.
Casser l., casserian l. ligamentum mallei laterale.
ceratocricoid l. ligamentum ceratocricoideum.
cervical l., lateral ligamentum cardinale.
cervical l., posterior ligamentum nuchae.
cervical l., transverse ligamentum cardinale.
cervical l. of sinus tarsi a strong band behind the bifurcate ligament, extending upward to the neck of the talus.
check l., lateral lacertus musculi recti lateralis bulbi.
check l., medial an extension from the fascia covering the medial rectus muscle, attaching to the lacrimal bone immediately posterior to the posterior lateral crest; called also check ligament of *medial rectus muscle.*
check l's of axis ligamenta alaria.
check l. of lateral rectus muscle lacertus musculi recti lateralis bulbi.
check l. of medial rectus muscle medial check ligament.
chondrosternal l., interarticular ligamentum sternocostale intraarticulare.
l. of Civinini ligamentum pterygospinale.
Clado l. an occasional peritoneal fold connecting the infundibulopelvic ligament and the mesoappendix.
clavicular l., external capsular ligamentum acromioclaviculare.
Cloquet l. vestigium processus vaginalis.
coccygeal l. pars duralis fili terminalis.
coccygeal l., superior ligamentum iliofemorale.
collateral l., fibular ligamentum collaterale fibulare.
collateral l., radial ligamentum collaterale radiale.
collateral l., radial carpal ligamentum collaterale carpi radiale.
collateral l., tibial ligamentum collaterale tibiale.
collateral l., ulnar ligamentum collaterale ulnare.
collateral l., ulnar carpal ligamentum collaterale carpi ulnare.
collateral l. of ankle joint, lateral ligamentum collaterale laterale articulationis talocruralis.
collateral l. of ankle joint, medial ligamentum collaterale mediale articulationis talocruralis.

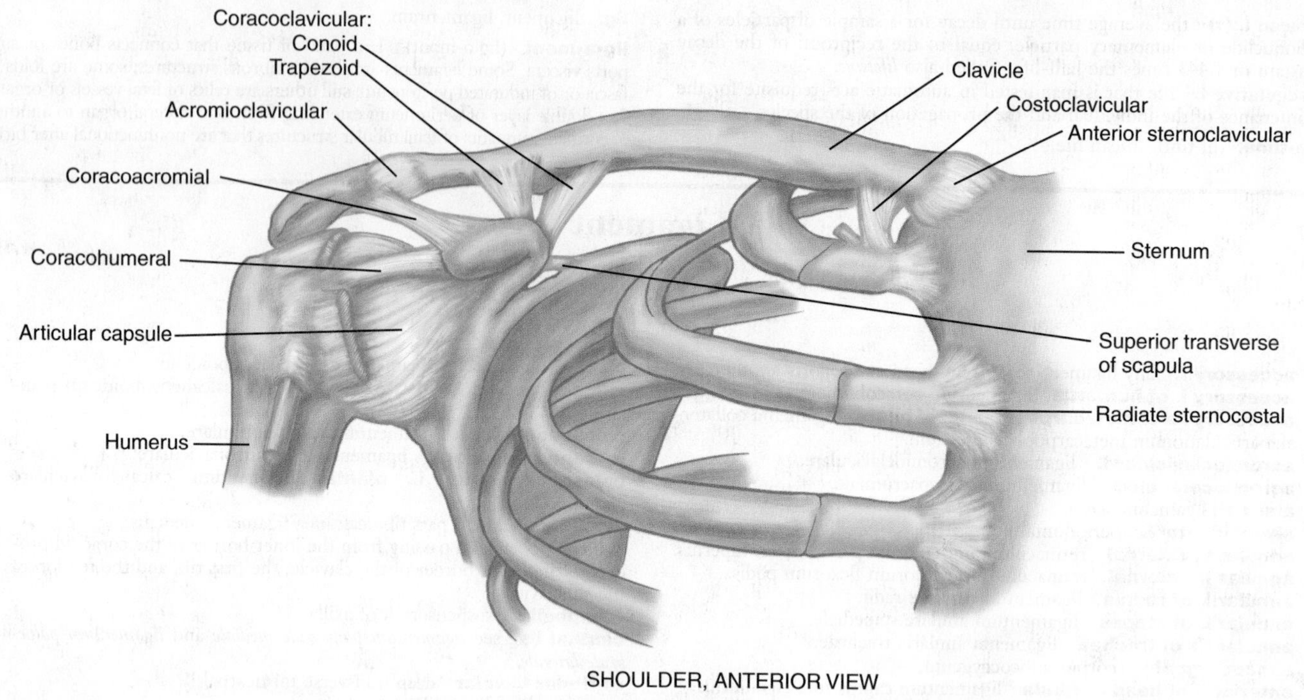

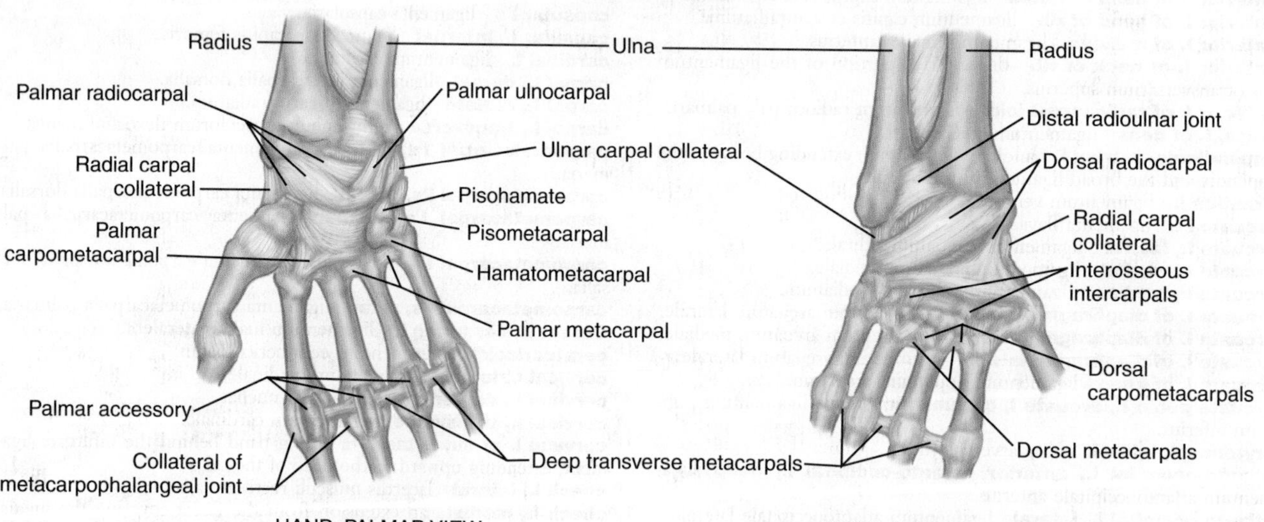

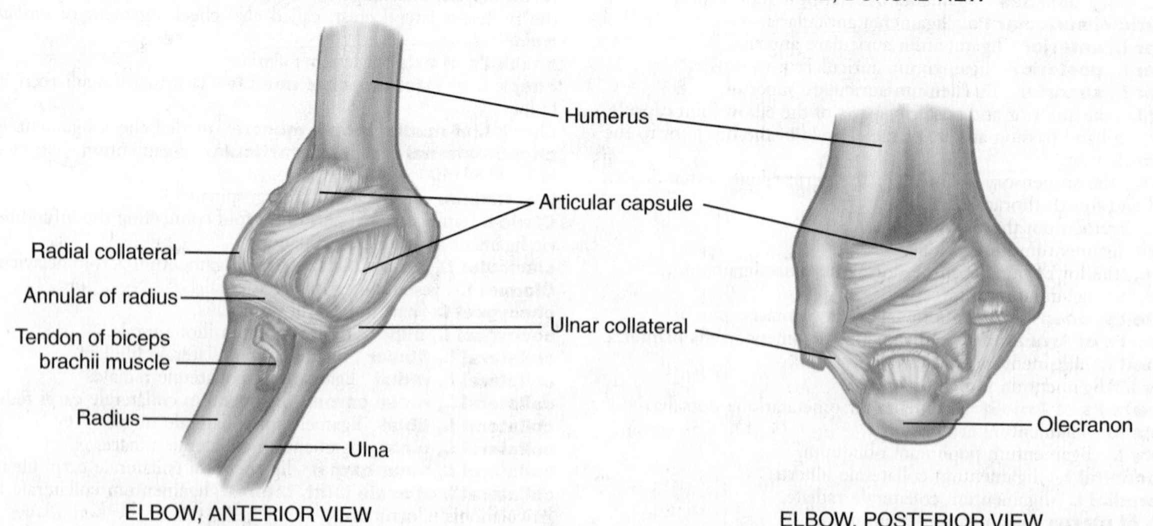

■ **PLATE 21—ARTICULAR LIGAMENTS**

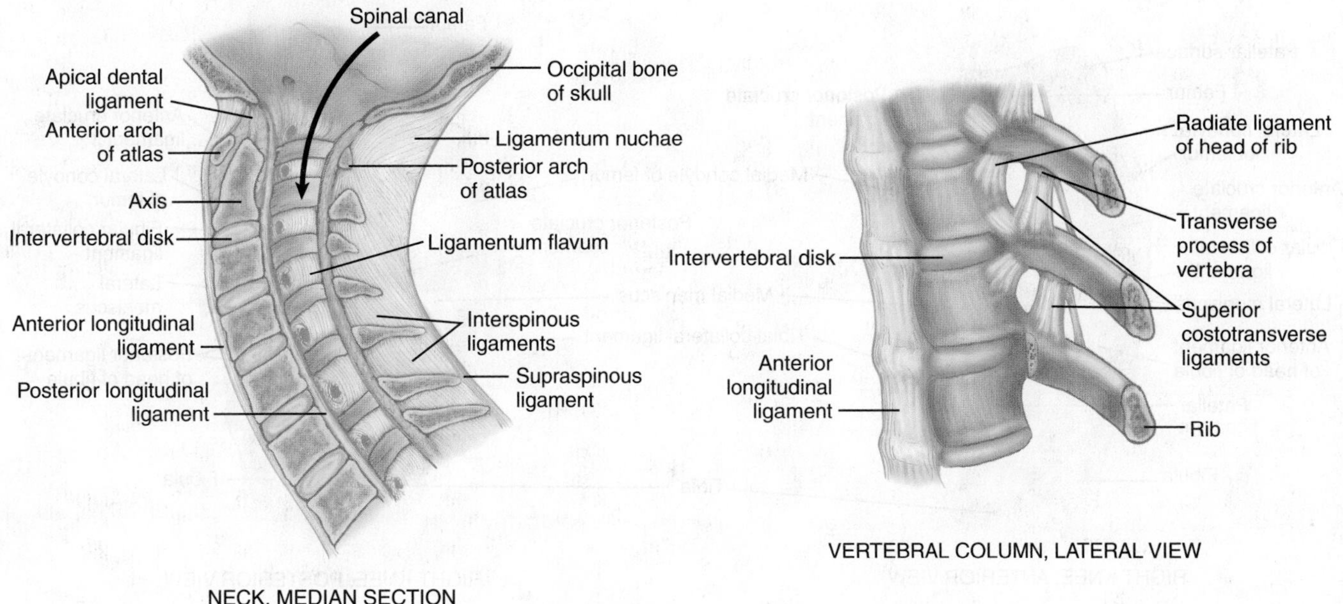

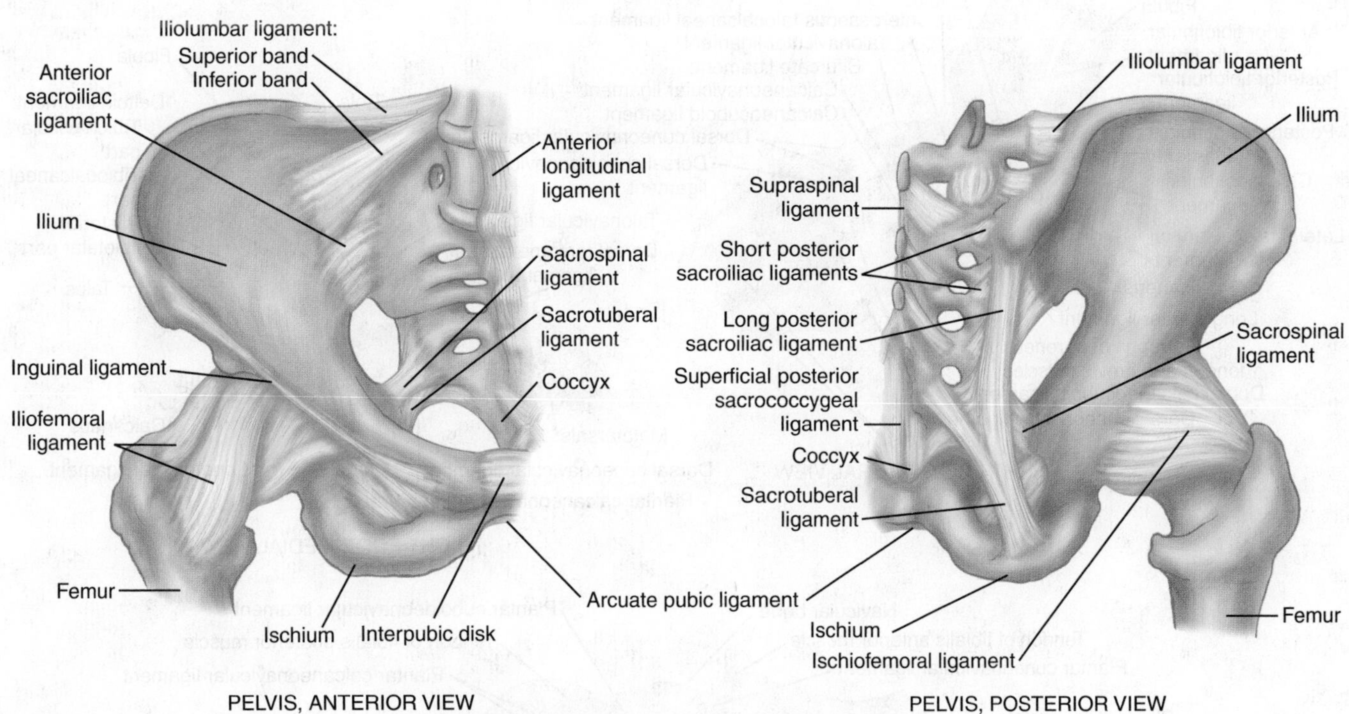

■ PLATE 22—ARTICULAR LIGAMENTS

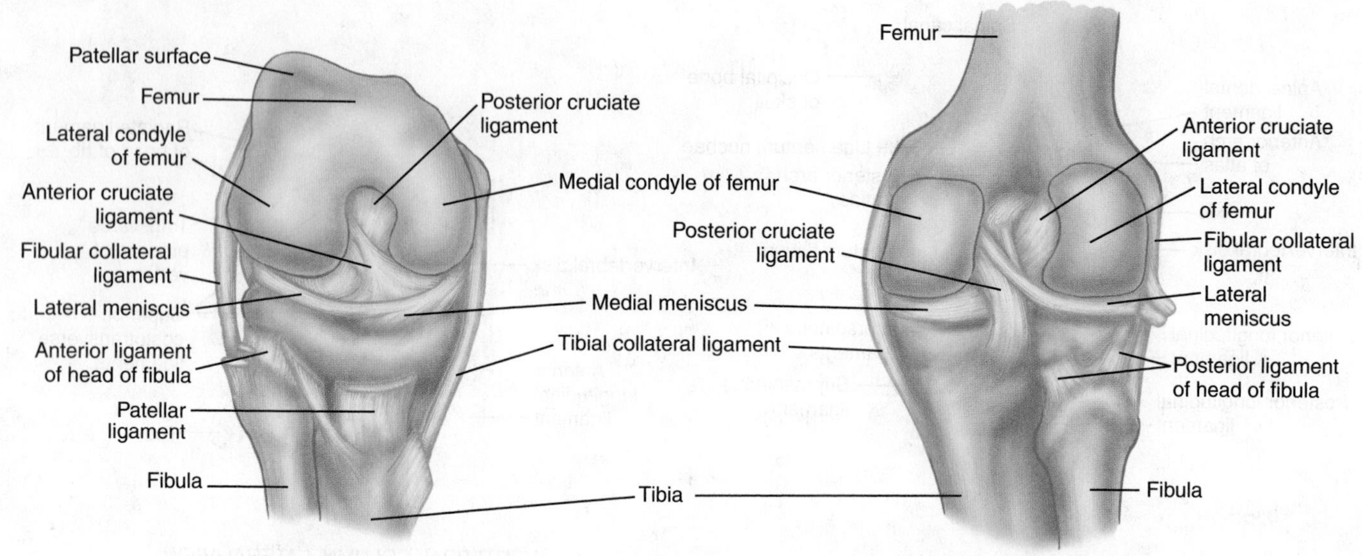

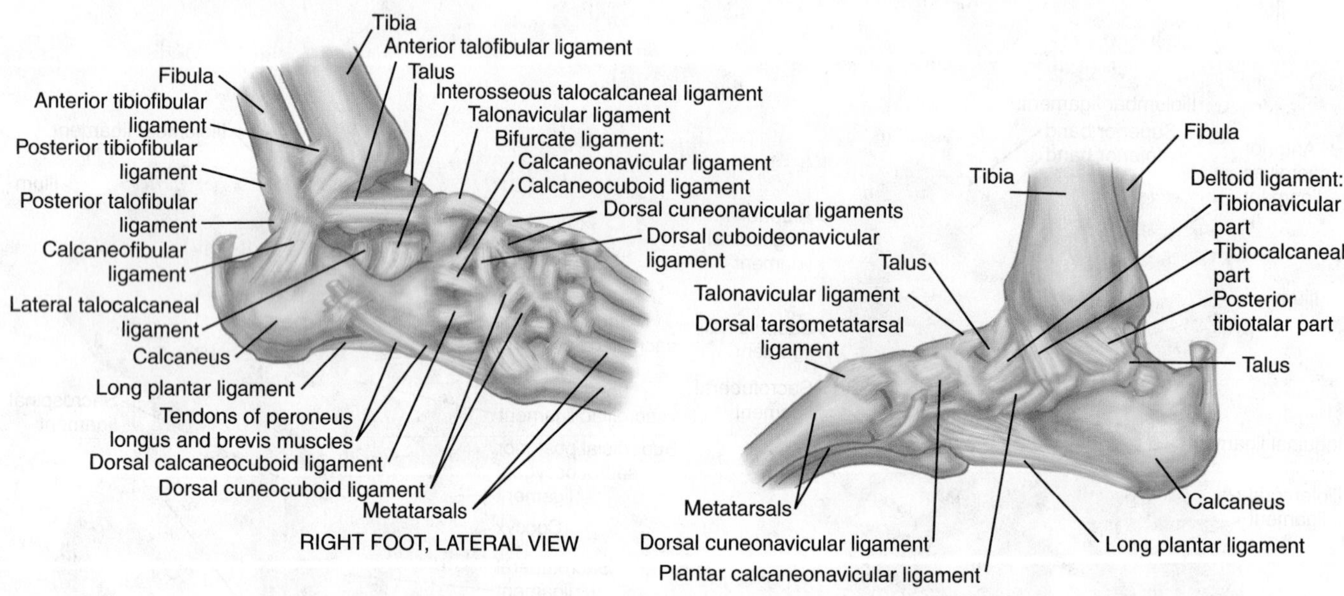

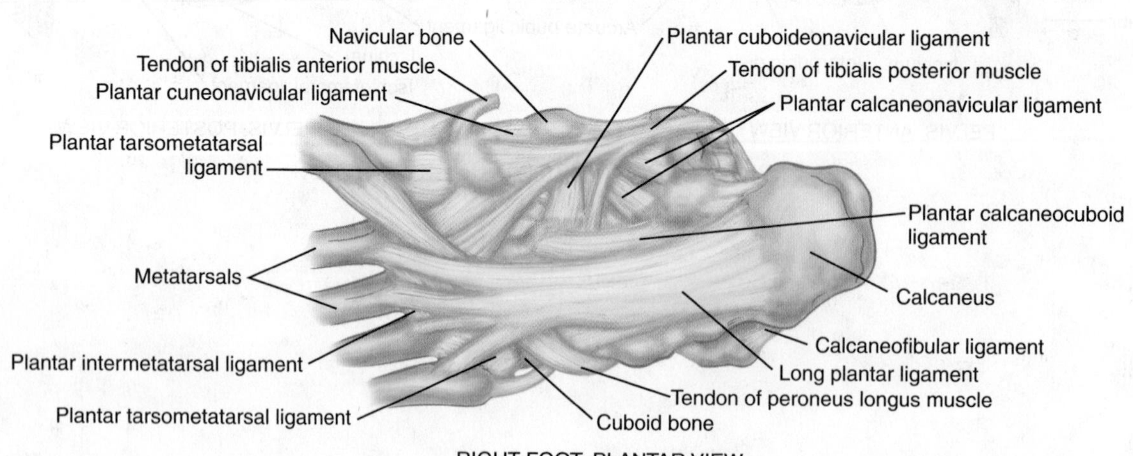

■ **PLATE 23**—ARTICULAR LIGAMENTS

collateral l. of carpus, radial ligamentum collaterale carpi radiale.
collateral l. of carpus, ulnar ligamentum collaterale carpi ulnare.
collateral l's of interphalangeal joints of foot ligamenta collateralia articulationum interphalangealium pedis.
collateral l's of interphalangeal joints of hand ligamenta collateralia articulationum interphalangealium manus.
collateral l's of metacarpophalangeal joints ligamenta collateralia articulationum metacarpophalangealium.
collateral l's of metatarsophalangeal joints ligamenta collateralia articulationum metatarsophalangealium.
Colles l. ligamentum inguinale reflexum.
common l. of knee (of Weber) ligamentum transversum genus.
common l. of wrist joint, deep ligamentum collaterale carpi radiale.
conoid l. ligamentum conoideum.
conus l. tendo infundibuli.
Cooper l. ligamentum pectineum.
Cooper suspensory l's ligamenta suspensoria mammaria.
coracoacromial l. ligamentum coraco-acromiale.
coracoclavicular l. ligamentum coracoclaviculare.
coracoclavicular l., external ligamentum trapezoideum.
coracoclavicular l., internal ligamentum conoideum.
coracohumeral l. ligamentum coracohumerale.
coracoid l. of scapula ligamentum transversum scapulae superius.
cordiform l. of diaphragm centrum tendineum diaphragmatis.
coronary l. of liver ligamentum coronarium hepatis.
coronary l. of radius ligamentum anulare radii.
costocentral l., anterior ligamentum capitis costae radiatum.
costocentral l., interarticular ligamentum capitis costae intraarticulare.
costoclavicular l. ligamentum costoclaviculare.
costocolic l. ligamentum phrenicocolicum.
costocoracoid l. ligamentum transversum scapulae superius.
costopericardiac l. a band of connective tissue joining the upper costosternal articulation with the pericardium.
costosternal l's, radiate ligamenta sternocostalia radiata.
costotransverse l. ligamentum costotransversarium.
costotransverse l., anterior ligamentum costotransversarium superius.
costotransverse l., lateral ligamentum costotransversarium laterale.
costotransverse l., posterior ligamentum costotransversarium superius.
costotransverse l., superior ligamentum costotransversarium superius.
costotransverse l. of Krause, posterior ligamentum costotransversarium laterale.
costovertebral l. ligamentum capitis costae radiatum.
costoxiphoid l's ligamenta costoxiphoidea.
cotyloid l. labrum acetabulare.
Cowper l. pectineal fascia.
cricoarytenoid l., cricoarytenoid l., posterior ligamentum cricoarytenoideum.
cricopharyngeal l., cricosantorinian l. ligamentum cricopharyngeum.
cricothyroid l. the inferior, larger part of the fibroelastic laryngeal membrane, which forms a ligamentous complex consisting of two distinct parts: a median or anterior part (see *ligamentum cricothyroideum medianum*) and paired lateral parts (see *conus elasticus*).
cricothyroid l., anterior ligamentum cricothyroideum medianum.
cricothyroid l., lateral conus elasticus.
cricothyroid l., median ligamentum cricothyroideum medianum.
cricotracheal l. ligamentum cricotracheale.
crucial l's of fingers pars cruciformis vaginae fibrosae digitorum manus.
cruciate l. of atlas ligamentum cruciforme atlantis.
cruciate l's of fingers pars cruciformis vaginae fibrosae digitorum manus.
cruciate l's of knee ligamenta cruciata genus.
cruciate l. of knee, anterior ligamentum cruciatum anterius genus.
cruciate l. of knee, posterior ligamentum cruciatum posterius genus.
cruciate l's of toes pars cruciformis vaginae fibrosae digitorum pedis.
cruciform l. of atlas ligamentum cruciforme atlantis.
crural l. ligamentum inguinale.
Cruveilhier l's ligamenta plantaria articulationum metatarsophalangealium.
cubitoradial l. chorda obliqua membranae interosseae antebrachii.
cubitoulnar l. ligamentum collaterale ulnare.
cuboideometatarsal l's, short ligamenta tarsometatarsalia plantaria.
cuboideonavicular l., dorsal ligamentum cuboideonaviculare dorsale.
cuboideonavicular l., oblique, cuboideonavicular l., plantar ligamentum cuboideonaviculare plantare.
cubonavicular l., cuboscaphoid l., plantar ligamentum cuboideonaviculare plantare.
cuneocuboid l., dorsal ligamentum cuneocuboideum dorsale.
cuneocuboid l., interosseous ligamentum cuneocuboideum interosseum.
cuneocuboid l., plantar ligamentum cuneocuboideum plantare.
cuneometatarsal l's, interosseous ligamenta cuneometatarsalia interossea.
cuneonavicular l's, dorsal ligamenta cuneonavicularia dorsalia.
cuneonavicular l's, plantar ligamenta cuneonavicularia plantaria.
cutaneophalangeal l's ligamentous fibers from the sides of the phalanges near the joints to the skin.
cystoduodenal l. an anomalous fold of peritoneum extending between the gallbladder and the duodenum.
deltoid l. of ankle, deltoid l. of ankle joint ligamentum collaterale mediale articulationis talocruralis.
deltoid l. of elbow ligamentum collaterale ulnare.
dentate l. of spinal cord, denticulate l. ligamentum denticulatum.
Denucé l. a short, wide band connecting the radius and the ulna at the wrist.
diaphragmatic l. the involuting urogenital ridge that becomes the suspensory ligament of the ovary.
dorsal l's, carpal ligamenta intercarpalia dorsalia.
dorsal l., talonavicular ligamentum talonaviculare.
dorsal l's of bases of metacarpal bones ligamenta metacarpalia dorsalia.
dorsal l's of bases of metatarsal bones ligamenta metatarsalia dorsalia.
dorsal l. of radiocarpal joint ligamentum radiocarpale dorsale.
dorsal l's of tarsus ligamenta tarsi dorsalia.
Douglas l. plica rectouterina.
duodenohepatic l. ligamentum hepatoduodenale.
duodenorenal l. an inconstant fold of peritoneum that sometimes extends from the duodenum to the right kidney.
epihyal l. ligamentum stylohyoideum.
external l's of Barkow, plantar ligamenta intercuneiformia plantaria.
external l. of temporomandibular joint ligamentum laterale articulationis temporomandibularis.
fabellofibular l. an occasional ligament apparently replacing the short lateral ligament when the fabella is present; it originates directly from the fabella, passes between the condylar portions of the plantaris and lateral gastrocnemius muscles, and is attached to the apex of the fibula.
falciform l. processus falciformis ligamenti sacrotuberosi.
falciform l. of liver ligamentum falciforme hepatis.

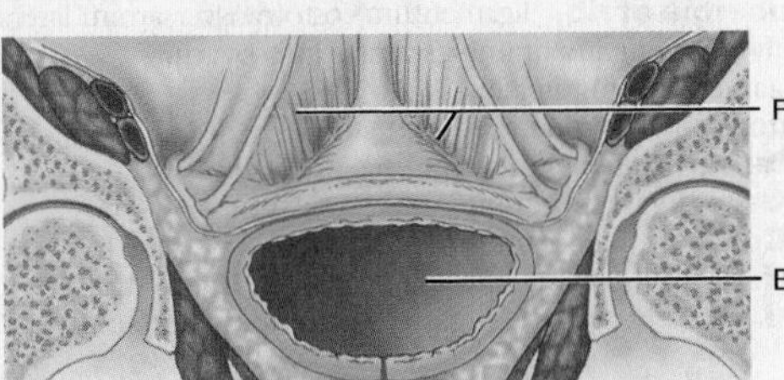

■ False ligaments (peritoneal folds) connecting the bladder to the pelvic walls; shown in frontal section.

fallopian l., l. of Fallopius ligamentum inguinale.
false l. 1. any suspensory ligament that is a peritoneal fold and not of true ligamentous structure. 2. a peritoneal connection between the vertex and sides of the bladder and the walls of the pelvis.
Ferrein l. the thick external part of the capsule of the temporomandibular joint.
fibrous l., anterior ligamentum sternoclaviculare anterius.
fibrous l., posterior ligamentum sternoclaviculare posterius.
flaval l's ligamenta flava.
Flood l. the superior glenohumeral ligament; see *ligamenta glenohumeralia.*
fundiform l. of clitoris ligamentum fundiforme clitoridis.
fundiform l. of penis ligamentum fundiforme penis.
gastrocolic l. ligamentum gastrocolicum.
gastrohepatic l. ligamentum hepatogastricum.
gastrolienal l. ligamentum gastrosplenicum.
gastrophrenic l. ligamentum gastrophrenicum.
gastrosplenic l. ligamentum gastrosplenicum.
genitoinguinal l. ligamentum genitoinguinale.
Gerdy l. suspensory l. of axilla.
Gimbernat l. ligamentum lacunare.
glenohumeral l's ligamenta glenohumeralia.
glenoid l's of Cruveilhier ligamenta plantaria articulationum metatarsophalangealium.
glenoid l. of humerus, glenoid l. of Macalister labrum glenoidale.
Günz l. part of the obturator membrane.
hamatometacarpal l. fibers connecting the hamulus of the hamate bone with the base of the fifth metacarpal bone.
l. of head of femoral bone, l. of head of femur ligamentum capitis femoris.
Helmholtz l. that part of the anterior ligament of the malleus which is attached to the greater tympanic spine.
Henle l. falx inguinalis.
hepatic l's ligamenta hepatis.
hepatocolic l. ligamentum hepatocolicum.
hepatoduodenal l. ligamentum hepatoduodenale.
hepatogastric l. ligamentum hepatogastricum.
hepatophrenic l. ligamentum hepatophrenicum.
hepatorenal l. ligamentum hepatorenale.
Hesselbach l. ligamentum interfoveolare.
Hey l. margo falciformis hiatus saphenus.
Hueck l. reticulum trabeculare.
Humphry l. ligamentum meniscofemorale anterius.
Hunter l. ligamentum teres uteri.
hyaloideocapsular l. the tissue connecting the vitreous body to the peripheral zone of the lens capsule.
hyoepiglottic l. ligamentum hyo-epiglotticum.
iliocostal l. ligamentum lumbocostale.
iliofemoral l. ligamentum iliofemorale.
iliolumbar l. ligamentum iliolumbale.
iliopectineal l. arcus iliopectineus.
iliopubic l. ligamentum inguinale.
iliosacral l., anterior ligamentum sacroiliacum anterius.
iliosacral l., interosseous ligamentum sacroiliacum interosseum.
iliosacral l., long ligamentum sacroiliacum posterius.
iliotibial l. of Maissiat tractus iliotibialis.
iliotrochanteric l. a portion of the articular capsule of the hip joint.
inferior annular l. ligamentum pubicum inferius.
inferior l. of epididymis ligamentum epididymidis inferius.
inferior l. of neck of rib of Henle ligamentum costotransversarium.
inferior l. of tubercle of rib ligamentum costotransversarium laterale.
infundibulopelvic l. ligamentum suspensorium ovarii.
inguinal l. ligamentum inguinale.
inguinal l., external ligamentum inguinale.
inguinal l., internal ligamentum inguinale reflexum.
inguinal l., reflex ligamentum inguinale reflexum.
inguinal l. of Cooper ligamentum pectineum.
interarticular l. any ligament situated within the capsule of a joint.
interarticular l. of head of rib ligamentum capitis costae intraarticulare.
interarticular l. of hip joint ligamentum capitis femoris.
interarticular l. of humeral joint caput longum musculi bicipitis brachii.
intercarpal l's, dorsal ligamenta intercarpalia dorsalia.
intercarpal l's, interosseous ligamenta intercarpalia interossea.
intercarpal l's, palmar, intercarpal l's, volar ligamenta intercarpalia palmaria.
interclavicular l. ligamentum interclaviculare.
intercuneiform l's, dorsal ligamenta intercuneiformia dorsalia.
intercuneiform l's, interosseous ligamenta intercuneiformia interossea.
intercuneiform l's, plantar ligamenta intercuneiformia plantaria.
interfoveolar l. ligamentum interfoveolare.
intermetacarpal l's, anterior proximal ligamenta metacarpalia palmaria.
intermetacarpal l., distal deep transverse metacarpal l.
intermetacarpal l's, dorsal, intermetacarpal l's, dorsal transverse ligamenta metacarpalia dorsalia.
intermetacarpal l's, interosseous ligamenta metacarpalia interossea.
intermetacarpal l's, palmar ligamenta metacarpalia palmaria.
intermetacarpal l's, posterior proximal ligamenta metacarpalia dorsalia.
intermetacarpal l's, volar transverse ligamenta metacarpalia palmaria.
intermetatarsal l., distal plantar deep transverse metatarsal l.
intermetatarsal l's, dorsal proximal, intermetatarsal l's, dorsal transverse ligamenta metatarsalia dorsalia.
intermetatarsal l's, interosseous ligamenta metatarsalia interossea.
intermetatarsal l's, plantar proximal, intermetatarsal l's, plantar transverse ligamenta metatarsalia plantaria.
intermuscular l., fibular septum intermusculare cruris anterius.
intermuscular l. of arm, external septum intermusculare brachii laterale.
intermuscular l. of arm, internal septum intermusculare brachii mediale.
intermuscular l. of arm, lateral septum intermusculare brachii laterale.
intermuscular l. of arm, medial septum intermusculare brachii mediale.
intermuscular l. of thigh, external, intermuscular l. of thigh, lateral septum intermusculare femoris laterale.
intermuscular l. of thigh, medial septum intermusculare femoris mediale.
internal l. of neck of rib ligamentum costotransversarium superius.
interosseous l., radioulnar membrana interossea antebrachii.
interosseous l's, transverse metacarpal ligamenta metacarpalia interossea.
interosseous l's of Barkow, internal ligamenta intercuneiformia plantaria.
interosseous l's of bases of metacarpal bones ligamenta metacarpalia interossea.
interosseous l's of bases of metatarsal bones ligamenta metatarsalia interossea.
interosseous l. of Cruveilhier, costovertebral ligamentum capitis costae intraarticulare.
interosseous l. of Cruveilhier, transversocostal ligamentum costotransversarium.
interosseous l's of knee ligamenta cruciata genus.
interosseous l. of leg membrana interossea cruris.
interosseous l. of pubis discus interpubicus.
interosseous l's of tarsus ligamenta tarsi interossea.
l's of interphalangeal joints of foot, plantar ligamenta plantaria articulationum interphalangealium pedis.
l's of interphalangeal joints of hand, palmar ligamenta palmaria articulationum interphalangealium manus.
interprocess l. a ligament that connects two processes on the same bone.
interpubic l. discus interpubicus.
interspinal l's, interspinous l's ligamenta interspinalia.
intertarsal l's, dorsal ligamenta tarsi dorsalia.
intertarsal l's, interosseous ligamenta tarsi interossea.
intertarsal l's, plantar ligamenta tarsi plantaria.
intertransverse l's ligamenta intertransversaria.
intervertebral l. either of the two longitudinal ligaments of the vertebrae (ligamentum longitudinale anterius and ligamentum longitudinale posterius).

intra-articular l. of head of rib ligamentum capitis costae intraarticulare.
ischiocapsular l., ischiofemoral l. ligamentum ischiofemorale.
ischiosacral l's see *ligamentum sacrospinale* and *ligamentum sacrotuberale.*
Jarjavay l. ligamentum rectouterinum.
Krause l. ligamentum transversum perinei.
laciniate l. retinaculum musculorum flexorum pedis.
laciniate l., external retinaculum musculorum peroneorum superius.
lacunar l., lacunar l. of Gimbernat ligamentum lacunare.
laryngeal l's, extrinsic the ligaments in and around the thyrohyoid membrane, including the lateral and median thyrohyoid, hyoepiglottic, thyroepiglottic, and cricotracheal ligaments.
laryngeal l's, intrinsic the ligaments in and around the fibroelastic membrane of the larynx, including the conus elasticus, the median cricothyroid ligament, and the vocal ligament.
lateral l., short a knee ligament attached to the lowest part of the lateral femoral condyle and extending beyond the dorsum of the semilunar cartilage to the apex of the fibula. See also *fabellofibular l.*
lateral l. of ankle joint ligamentum collaterale laterale articulationis talocruralis.
lateral l. of carpus, radial ligamentum collaterale carpi radiale.
lateral l. of carpus, ulnar ligamentum collaterale carpi ulnare.
lateral l. of colon taenia omentalis.
lateral l's of joints of fingers ligamenta collateralia articulationum interphalangealium manus.
lateral l's of joints of toes ligamenta collateralia articulationum interphalangealium pedis.
lateral l. of knee ligamentum collaterale fibulare.
lateral l. of malleus ligamentum mallei laterale.
lateral meniscofemoral l. ligamentum meniscofemorale posterius.
lateral l's of metacarpophalangeal joints ligamenta collateralia articulationum metacarpophalangealium.
lateral l's of metatarsophalangeal joints ligamenta collateralia articulationum metatarsophalangealium.
lateral l. of rectum ligamentum recti laterale.
lateral l. of temporomandibular joint ligamentum laterale articulationis temporomandibularis.
lateral l. of temporomandibular joint, external ligamentum laterale articulationis temporomandibularis.
lateral l. of temporomandibular joint, internal ligamentum sphenomandibulare.
lateral l. of wrist joint, external ligamentum collaterale carpi radiale.
lateral l. of wrist joint, internal ligamentum collaterale carpi ulnare.
Lauth l. ligamentum transversum atlantis.
l. of left vena cava ligamentum venae cavae sinistrae.
lienophrenic l. ligamentum splenophrenicum.
lienorenal l. ligamentum splenorenale.
Lisfranc l. a fibrous band running from the lower external surface of the medial cuneiform bone to the internal surface of the base of the second metatarsal bone.
Lockwood l. a thickened area of contact between the Tenon capsule and the sheaths of the inferior rectus and inferior oblique muscles.
longitudinal l., anterior ligamentum longitudinale anterius.
longitudinal l., posterior ligamentum longitudinale posterius.
longitudinal l. of abdomen linea alba.
lumbocostal l. ligamentum lumbocostale.
lumbosacral l. the inferior portion of the iliolumbar ligament.
l's of Luschka ligamenta sternopericardiaca.
Mackenrodt l. ligamentum cardinale.
l. of Maissiat tractus iliotibialis.
Mauchart l's ligamenta alaria.
maxillary l., lateral ligamentum laterale articulationis temporomandibularis.
l. of Mayer ligamentum carpi radiatum.
Meckel l. see under *band.*
medial l. of ankle ligamentum collaterale mediale articulationis talocruralis.
medial l. of elbow joint ligamentum collaterale ulnare.
medial l. of temporomandibular joint ligamentum mediale articulationis temporomandibularis.
medial l. of wrist ligamentum collaterale carpi ulnare.
meniscofemoral l., anterior ligamentum meniscofemorale anterius.
meniscofemoral l., posterior ligamentum meniscofemorale posterius.
metacarpal l., deep transverse ligamentum metacarpeum transversum profundum. NOTE: the term may be used to denote any one of the series of bands connecting two adjacent metacarpal bones or may describe the entire series of three bands collectively.
metacarpal l's, dorsal ligamenta metacarpalia dorsalia.
metacarpal l's, interosseous ligamenta metacarpalia interossea.
metacarpal l's, palmar ligamenta metacarpalia palmaria.
metacarpal l., superficial transverse ligamentum metacarpale transversum superficiale.
metacarpophalangeal l's, anterior, metacarpophalangeal l's, palmar ligamenta palmaria articulationum metacarpophalangealium.
l's of metacarpophalangeal joints, palmar ligamenta palmaria articulationum metacarpophalangealium.
metatarsal l., anterior deep transverse metatarsal l.
metatarsal l., deep transverse ligamentum metatarsale transversum profundum. NOTE: the term may be used to denote any of the series of bands connecting two adjacent metatarsal bones or may describe the entire series of four bands collectively.
metatarsal l's, dorsal ligamenta metatarsalia dorsalia.
metatarsal l's, interosseous, metatarsal l's, interosseous transverse ligamenta metatarsalia interossea.
metatarsal l's, lateral ligamenta metatarsalia interossea.
metatarsal l's, lateral proper (of Weber), metatarsal l's, lateral (of Weitbrecht) ligamenta metatarsalia interossea.
metatarsal l's, plantar ligamenta metatarsalia plantaria.
metatarsal l., superficial transverse ligamentum metatarsale transversum superficiale.
metatarsophalangeal l's, inferior, l's of metatarsophalangeal joints, plantar ligamenta plantaria articulationum metatarsophalangealium.
middle l. of neck of rib ligamentum costotransversarium.
mucous l. plica synovialis.
l. of nape ligamentum nuchae.
navicularicuneiform l's, plantar ligamenta cuneonavicularia plantaria.
nephrocolic l. fasciculi from the fatty capsule of the kidney passing inferiorly on the right side to the posterior wall of the ascending colon and on the left side to the posterior wall of the descending colon.
nuchal l. ligamentum nuchae.
oblique l. of Cooper, oblique l. of forearm chorda obliqua membranae interosseae antebrachii.
oblique l's of knee ligamenta cruciata genus.
oblique l. of knee, posterior ligamentum popliteum obliquum.
oblique l. of scapula ligamentum transversum scapulae superius.
oblique l. of superior radioulnar joint chorda obliqua membranae interosseae antebrachii.
occipitoaxial l. membrana tectoria.
occipitoodontoid l's ligamenta alaria.
odontoid l., middle ligamentum apicis dentis.
odontoid l's of axis ligamenta alaria.
orbicular l. of radius ligamentum anulare radii.

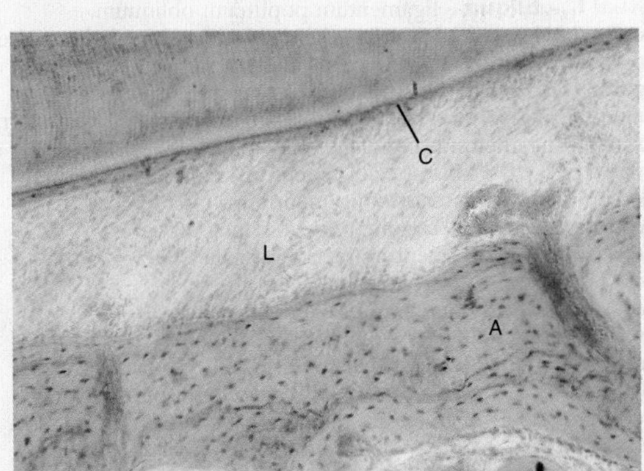

■ Periodontal ligament *(L)* between the cementum *(C)* and the bony alveolus *(A)* in a light micrograph of a tooth socket.

Ligament *Continued*

ovarian l. ligamentum ovarii proprium.
palmar l's 1. see *ligamenta palmaria articulationum interphalangealium manus* and *ligamenta palmaria articulationum metacarpophalangealium.* 2. see *aponeurosis palmaris.*
palmar l., deep transverse deep transverse metacarpal l.
palmar accessory l's see *ligamenta palmaria articulationum metacarpophalangealium* and *ligamenta palmaria articulationum interphalangealium manus.*
palmar l. of carpus ligamentum carpi radiatum.
palmar l. of radiocarpal joint ligamentum radiocarpale palmare.
palpebral l., lateral ligamentum palpebrale laterale.
palpebral l., medial ligamentum palpebrale mediale.
pancreaticocolic l. ligamentum pancreaticocolicum.
pancreaticosplenic l. ligamentum pancreaticosplenicum.
patellar l. ligamentum patellae.
patellar l., internal retinaculum patellae mediale.
patellar l., lateral retinaculum patellae laterale.
pectinate l., pectinate l. of iris reticulum trabeculare.
pectineal l. ligamentum pectineum.
pelvic l., great posterior ligamentum sacrotuberale.
pelvic l., short posterior ligamentum sacrospinale.
pelvic l., transverse ligamentum transversum perinei.
pericardiosternal l's ligamenta sternopericardiaca.
perineal l., transverse, perineal l. of Carcassone ligamentum transversum perinei.
periodontal l. the fibrous connective tissue that surrounds the root of a tooth, separating it from and attaching it to the alveolar bone. It extends from the base of the gingival mucosa to the fundus of the bony socket, and its main function is to hold the tooth in its socket. In official terminology, it may be called *periodontium* [TA]. Called also *alveolodental l.* or *membrane, peridental* or *periodontal membrane.*
Petit l. ligamentum rectouterinum.
petrosphenoid l. 1. synchondrosis sphenopetrosa. 2. synchondrosis spheno-occipitalis.
petrosphenoid l., anterior synchondrosis sphenopetrosa.
phrenicocolic l. ligamentum phrenicocolicum.
phrenicoesophageal l. ligamentum phrenicooesophagealis.
phrenicolienal l., phrenicosplenic l. ligamentum splenorenale.
phrenocolic l. ligamentum phrenicocolicum.
phrenoesophageal l. ligamentum phrenicooesophagealis.
pisimetacarpal l. ligamentum pisometacarpeum.
pisohamate l. ligamentum pisohamatum.
pisometacarpal l. ligamentum pisometacarpeum.
pisounciform l., pisouncinate l. ligamentum pisohamatum.
plantar l's see *ligamenta plantaria articulationum metatarsophalangealium* and *ligamenta plantaria articulationum interphalangealium pedis.*
plantar l., long ligamentum plantare longum.
plantar l., short ligamentum calcaneocuboideum plantare.
plantar accessory l's see *ligamenta plantaria articulationum metatarsophalangealium* and *ligamenta plantaria articulationum interphalangealium pedis.*
plantar l. of second metatarsal bone see *ligamenta tarsometatarsalia plantaria.*
plantar l's of tarsus ligamenta tarsi plantaria.
popliteal l., arcuate ligamentum popliteum arcuatum.
popliteal l., oblique ligamentum popliteum obliquum.
posterior l. of head of fibula ligamentum capitis fibulae posterius.
posterior l. of incus ligamentum incudis posterius.
posterior l. of pinna ligamentum auriculare posterius.
posterior l. of radiocarpal joint ligamentum radiocarpale dorsale.
Poupart l. ligamentum inguinale.
preurethral l. of Waldeyer ligamentum transversum perinei.
prismatic l. of Weitbrecht ligamentum capitis femoris.
pterygomandibular l. raphe pterygomandibularis.
pterygospinal l. ligamentum pterygospinale.
pubic l., inferior ligamentum pubicum inferius.
pubic l., superior ligamentum pubicum superius.
pubic l. of Cowper ligamentum inguinale.
pubic l. of Cruveilhier, anterior discus interpubicus.
pubocapsular l., pubofemoral l. ligamentum pubofemorale.
puboprostatic l. ligamentum puboprostaticum.
puboprostatic l., lateral ligamentum puboprostaticum.
puboprostatic l., medial the ligamentum pubovesicale in the male.
puborectal l. 1. ligamentum puboprostaticum. 2. ligamentum pubovesicale.
pubovesical l. ligamentum pubovesicale.
pubovesical l., lateral ligamentum laterale pubovesicale.
pubovesical l., medial ligamentum pubovesicale mediale.
pulmonary l. ligamentum pulmonale.
quadrate l. ligamentum quadratum.
radial l., lateral, radial l. of cubitocarpal joint ligamentum collaterale carpi radiale.
radiate l. ligamentum capitis costae radiatum.
radiate l., lateral ligamentum collaterale carpi ulnare.
radiate l. of carpus ligamentum carpi radiatum.
radiate l. of head of rib ligamentum capitis costae radiatum.
radiate l. of Mayer ligamentum carpi radiatum.
radiocarpal l., anterior ligamentum radiocarpale palmare.
radiocarpal l., dorsal ligamentum radiocarpale dorsale.
radiocarpal l., palmar, radiocarpal l., volar ligamentum radiocarpale palmare.
rectouterine l. ligamentum rectouterinum.
reflex l. of Gimbernat ligamentum inguinale reflexum.
reinforcing l's ligaments that serve to reinforce joint capsules.
rhomboid l. of clavicle ligamentum costoclaviculare.
rhomboid l. of wrist ligamentum radiocarpale dorsale.
ring l. of hip joint zona orbicularis articulationis coxae.
Robert l. ligamentum meniscofemorale posterius.
round l. of acetabulum ligamentum capitis femoris.
round l. of Cloquet ligamentum capitis costae intraarticulare.
round l. of femur ligamentum capitis femoris.
round l. of forearm chorda obliqua membranae interosseae antebrachii.
round l. of liver ligamentum teres hepatis.
round l. of uterus ligamentum teres uteri.
sacrococcygeal l., anterior ligamentum sacrococcygeum anterius.
sacrococcygeal l., deep dorsal, sacrococcygeal l., deep posterior ligamentum sacrococcygeum posterius profundum.
sacrococcygeal l., lateral ligamentum sacrococcygeum laterale.
sacrococcygeal l., superficial dorsal, sacrococcygeal l., superficial posterior ligamentum sacrococcygeum posterius superficiale.
sacrococcygeal l., ventral ligamentum sacrococcygeum anterius.
sacroiliac l., anterior ligamentum sacroiliacum anterius.
sacroiliac l., dorsal ligamentum sacroiliacum posterius.
sacroiliac l., interosseous ligamentum sacroiliacum interosseum.
sacroiliac l., long posterior see *ligamentum sacroiliacum posterius.*
sacroiliac l., posterior ligamentum sacroiliacum posterius.
sacroiliac l., short posterior see *ligamentum sacroiliacum posterius.*
sacroiliac l., ventral ligamentum sacroiliacum anterius.
sacrosciatic l., anterior ligamentum sacrospinale.
sacrosciatic l., great ligamentum sacrotuberale.
sacrosciatic l., internal, sacrosciatic l., least ligamentum sacrospinale.
sacrospinal l., sacrospinous l. ligamentum sacrospinale.
sacrotuberal l., sacrotuberous l. ligamentum sacrotuberale.
Santorini l. ligamentum cricopharyngeum.
Sappey l. the thicker posterior part of the capsule of the temporomandibular joint.
scaphocuneiform l's, plantar ligamenta cuneonavicularia plantaria.
l. of Scarpa cornu superius marginis falciformis.
Schlemm l's two ligamentous bands strengthening the capsule of the shoulder joint.
scrotal l. of testis gubernaculum testis.
serous l. ligamentum serosum.
skin l's retinacula cutis.
sphenoidal l., external ligamenta intercuneiformia plantaria.
sphenoideotarsal l's ligamenta tarsometatarsalia plantaria.
sphenomandibular l. ligamentum sphenomandibulare.
spinoglenoid l. ligamentum transversum scapulae inferius.
spinosacral l. ligamentum sacrospinale.
spiral l. of cochlea ligamentum spirale ductus cochlearis.
splenocolic l. ligamentum splenocolicum.
splenogastric l. ligamentum gastrosplenicum.
splenophrenic l. ligamentum phrenicosplenicum.
splenorenal l. ligamentum splenorenale.
spring l. ligamentum calcaneonaviculare plantare.
stapedial l. ligamentum anulare stapediale.
stellate l., anterior ligamentum capitis costae radiatum.
sternoclavicular l., anterior ligamentum sternoclaviculare anterius.

Ligament *Continued*

sternoclavicular l., posterior ligamentum sternoclaviculare posterius.
sternocostal l's ligamenta sternocostalia radiata.
sternocostal l., interarticular, sternocostal l., intra-articular ligamentum sternocostale intraarticulare.
sternocostal l's, radiate ligamenta sternocostalia radiata.
sternopericardiac l's ligamenta sternopericardiaca.
l. of Struthers a fibrous band that sometimes extends from the supracondylar process of the humerus to the median epicondyle, enclosing the median nerve and usually the brachial artery and providing an anomalous attachment for the coracobrachialis and part of the pronator teres muscles.
stylohyoid l. ligamentum stylohyoideum.
stylomandibular l., stylomaxillary l. ligamentum stylomandibulare.
subflaval l's ligamenta flava.
subpubic l. ligamentum pubicum inferius.
superficial l. of carpus 1. ligamentum radiocarpale dorsale. 2. ligamentum radiocarpale palmare.
superior l. of epididymis ligamentum epididymidis superius.
superior l. of hip ligamentum iliofemorale.
superior l. of incus ligamentum incudis superius.
superior l. of malleus ligamentum mallei superius.
superior l. of neck of rib, anterior the anterior part of the superior costotransverse ligament.
superior l. of neck of rib, external the posterior part of the superior costotransverse ligament.
superior l. of pinna ligamentum auriculare superius.
suprascapular l. ligamentum transversum scapulae superius.
supraspinal l., supraspinous l. ligamentum supraspinale.
suspensory l., marsupial plica synovialis infrapatellaris.
suspensory l. of axilla a layer ascending from the axillary fascia and ensheathing the pectoralis minor muscle; so called because traction by it during abduction of the upper limb produces the hollow of the armpit *(fossa axillaris)*. Called also *Campbell l.* and *Gerdy l.*
suspensory l. of axis ligamentum apicis dentis.
suspensory l's of breast ligamenta suspensoria mammaria.
suspensory l. of clitoris ligamentum suspensorium clitoridis.
suspensory l. of duodenum musculus suspensorius duodeni.
suspensory l. of humerus ligamentum coracohumerale.
suspensory l. of lens zonula ciliaris.
suspensory l. of liver ligamentum falciforme hepatis.
suspensory l's of mammary gland ligamenta suspensoria mammaria.
suspensory l. of ovary ligamentum suspensorium ovarii.
suspensory l. of penis ligamentum suspensorium penis.
suspensory l. of spleen ligamentum splenorenale.
sutural l. a band of fibrous tissue between the opposed bones of a suture or immovable joint.
synovial l. a large synovial fold.
synovial l. of hip ligamentum capitis femoris.
talocalcaneal l., interosseous ligamentum talocalcaneum interosseum.
talocalcaneal l., lateral ligamentum talocalcaneum laterale.
talocalcaneal l., medial ligamentum talocalcaneum mediale.
l. of talocrural joint, lateral the anterior and posterior talofibular ligaments and the calcaneofibular ligament considered together.
talofibular l., anterior ligamentum talofibulare anterius.
talofibular l., posterior ligamentum talofibulare posterius.
talonavicular l. ligamentum talonaviculare.
talotibial l., anterior pars tibiotalaris anterior ligamenti medialis.
talotibial l., posterior pars tibiotalaris posterior ligamenti medialis.
tarsometatarsal l's, dorsal ligamenta tarsometatarsalia dorsalia.
tarsometatarsal l's, plantar ligamenta tarsometatarsalia plantaria.
l's of tarsus ligamenta tarsi.
temporomandibular l. ligamentum laterale articulationis temporomandibularis.
tendinotrochanteric l. a portion of the capsule of the hip joint.
Teutleben l. ligamentum pulmonale.
thyroepiglottic l. ligamentum thyro-epiglotticum.
thyrohyoid l., lateral ligamentum thyrohyoideum laterale.
thyrohyoid l., median ligamentum thyrohyoideum medianum.
tibiocalcaneal l., tibiocalcanean l. pars tibiocalcanea ligamenti medialis.
tibiofibular l., anterior ligamentum tibiofibulare anterius.
tibiofibular l., posterior ligamentum tibiofibulare posterius.
tibionavicular l. pars tibionavicularis ligamenti medialis.
tracheal l's ligamenta anularia tracheae.
transverse l. ligamentum costotransversarium.
transverse l. of acetabulum ligamentum transversum acetabuli.
transverse l. of atlas ligamentum transversum atlantis.
transverse l. of carpus retinaculum musculorum flexorum manus.
transverse humeral l. a band of fibers bridging the intertubercular groove of the humerus and holding the tendon of the biceps muscle in the groove; called also *Brodie l.*
transverse l. of knee ligamentum transversum genus.
transverse l. of little head of rib ligamentum capitis costae intraarticulare.
transverse l. of pelvis ligamentum transversum perinei.
transverse l. of scapula, inferior ligamentum transversum scapulae inferius.
transverse l. of scapula, superior ligamentum transversum scapulae superius.
transverse l. of wrist retinaculum musculorum flexorum manus.
transverse l's of wrist, dorsal ligamenta intercarpalia dorsalia.
transversocostal l., superior ligamentum costotransversarium superius.
trapezoid l. ligamentum trapezoideum.
l. of Treitz musculus suspensorius duodeni.
triangular l. of abdomen ligamentum inguinale reflexum.
triangular l. of linea alba adminiculum lineae albae.
triangular l. of liver, left ligamentum triangulare sinistrum hepatis.
triangular l. of liver, right ligamentum triangulare dextrum hepatis.
triangular l. of pubis, anterior ligamentum pubicum inferius.
triangular l. of scapula ligamentum transversum scapulae inferius.
triangular l. of thigh ligamentum inguinale reflexum.
trigeminate l's of Arnold ligamenta tarsometatarsalia dorsalia.
triquetral l. of foot ligamentum calcaneofibulare.
triquetral l. of scapula ligamentum transversum scapulae inferius.
trochlear l. deep transverse metacarpal l.
trochlear l's of foot ligamenta plantaria articulationum metatarsophalangealium.
trochlear l's of hand ligamenta palmaria articulationum metacarpophalangealium.
trochlear l. of little heads of metacarpal bones deep transverse metacarpal l.
true l. of bladder, anterior 1. ligamentum puboprostaticum. 2. ligamentum pubovesicale.
tuberososacral l. ligamentum sacrotuberale.
tubopharyngeal l. of Rauber plica salpingopharyngea.
ulnar l., lateral, ulnar l. of carpus ligamentum collaterale carpi ulnare.
ulnocarpal l., palmar ligamentum ulnocarpale palmare.
umbilical l., lateral former name for the medial umbilical ligament, still sometimes used although incorrect and confusing; alternatively, the term is sometimes incorrectly used to denote the lateral umbilical fold.
umbilical l., medial chorda arteriae umbilicalis.
umbilical l., median, umbilical l., middle ligamentum umbilicale medianum.
utero-ovarian l. ligamentum ovarii proprium.
uteropelvic l's expansions of muscular tissue in the broad ligament of the uterus, radiating from the fascia over the obturator internus to the side of the uterus and the vagina.
uterosacral l. ligamentum rectouterinum.
vaginal l's of fingers, l's of vaginal sheaths of fingers vaginae fibrosae digitorum manus.
vaginal l's of toes, l's of vaginal sheaths of toes vaginae fibrosae digitorum pedis.
l's of Valsalva ligamenta auricularia.
venous l. of liver ligamentum venosum.
ventricular l. ligamentum vestibulare.
l. of Vesalius ligamentum inguinale.
vesical l., lateral ligamentum umbilicale medianum.
vesicopubic l. ligamentum pubovesicale.
vesicoumbilical l. ligamentum umbilicale medianum.
vesicouterine l. a ligament that extends from the anterior aspect of the uterus to the bladder.
vestibular l. ligamentum vestibulare.
vocal l. ligamentum vocale.
volar accessory l's see *ligamenta palmaria articulationum metacarpophalangealium* and *ligamenta palmaria articulationum interphalangealium manus.*

Ligament *Continued*

volar l. of carpus, proper, volar l. of wrist, anterior retinaculum musculorum flexorum manus.
Walther oblique l. ligamentum talofibulare posterius.
Weitbrecht l. chorda obliqua membranae interosseae antebrachii.
Winslow l. ligamentum popliteum obliquum.
Wrisberg l. ligamentum meniscofemorale posterius.
xiphicostal l's of Macalister, xiphoid l's ligamenta costoxiphoidea.
Y l. ligamentum iliofemorale.
yellow l's ligamenta flava.
Zinn l. anulus tendineus communis.
zonal l. of thigh zona orbicularis articulationis coxae.

lig·a·men·ta (lig″ə-men′tə) [L.] plural of *ligamentum.*

lig·a·men·to·pexy (lig″ə-men″to-pek′se) ventrosuspension by shortening or suturing the round ligaments of the uterus.

lig·a·men·tous (lig″ə-men′təs) pertaining to or of the nature of a ligament.

lig·a·men·tum (lig″ə-men′təm) pl. *ligamen′ta* [L. "a bandage," from *ligare* to bind] [TA] ligament.

Ligamentum

Descriptions are given on TA terms and include anglicized names of specific ligaments.

l. acromioclavicula′re [TA] acromioclavicular ligament: a dense band that joins the superior surface of the acromion and the acromial extremity of the clavicle together and strengthens the superior part of the articular capsule.
ligamen′ta ala′ria [TA] alar ligaments: two strong bands that pass from the posterolateral part of the tip of the dens of the axis upward and laterally to the condyles of the occipital bone; they limit rotation of the head.
l. anococcy′geum corpus anococcygeum.
l. anula′re ra′dii [TA] annular ligament of radius: a strong fibrous band that encircles the head of the radius and holds it in position; it is attached to the anterior and posterior margins of the radial notch of the ulna, forming, with the notch, a complete ring.
l. anula′re stapedia′le [TA] annular ligament of stapes: a ring of fibrous tissue that attaches the base of the stapes to the fenestra vestibuli of the middle ear.
ligamen′ta anula′ria tra′cheae [TA] annular ligaments of trachea: circular horizontal ligaments that join the tracheal cartilages together; called also *ligamenta trachealia* and *tracheal ligaments.*
l. a′picis den′tis [TA] apical ligament of dens: a cord of tissue extending from the tip of the dens of the axis to the occipital bone, near the anterior margin of the foramen magnum; it is usually delicate but is sometimes well developed.
l. arcua′tum latera′le [TA] lateral arcuate ligament: the ligamentous arch, formed by the fascia of the quadratus lumborum muscle, constituting part of the lumbar portion of the diaphragm; called also *lateral lumbocostal arch* and *lateral Haller arch.*
l. arcua′tum media′le [TA] medial arcuate ligament: the ligamentous arch, formed by the fascia of the psoas muscle, constituting part of the lumbar portion of the diaphragm; called also *medial lumbocostal arch* and *medial Haller arch.*
l. arcua′tum media′num [TA] median arcuate ligament: the ligamentous arch across the anterior surface of the aorta, interconnecting the crura of the diaphragm.
l. arterio′sum [TA] a short, thick, strong fibromuscular cord extending from the pulmonary artery to the arch of the aorta; it is the remains of the ductus arteriosus. Called also *ligament of Botallo.*
l. atlantooccipita′le ante′rius [TA] anterior atlanto-occipital ligament: an inconstant thickening of the middle part of the membrana atlantooccipitalis anterior, forming a median cord that extends from the anterior atlantal tubercle to the basilar occipital bone.
l. atlantooccipita′le latera′le [TA] lateral atlantooccipital ligament: a thickened portion of the articular capsule of the atlantooccipital joint attached to the jugular processes of the occipital bone and to the base of the transverse process of the atlas.
ligamen′ta auricula′ria [TA] ligaments of auricle: the three ligaments (anterior, superior, and posterior) that help attach the auricle to the side of the head. Called also *ligaments of Valsalva.*
l. auricula′re ante′rius [TA] anterior auricular ligament: the auricular ligament that passes from the eminence of the concha to the mastoid part of the temporal bone.
l. auricula′re poste′rius [TA] posterior auricular ligament: the auricular ligament that passes from the eminence of the concha to the mastoid part of the temporal bone.
l. auricula′re supe′rius [TA] superior auricular ligament: the auricular ligament that passes from the spine of the helix to the superior margin of the bony external acoustic meatus.
l. bifurca′tum [TA] bifurcate ligament: a Y-shaped ligament on the dorsum of the foot, comprising the calcaneonavicular and calcaneocuboid ligaments (sometimes referred to as the calcaneonavicular and calcaneocuboid parts).
l. calcaneocuboi′deum [TA] calcaneocuboid ligament: the band of fibers connecting the superior surface of the calcaneus and the dorsal surface of the cuboid bone; together with the calcaneonavicular ligament, it constitutes the bifurcate ligament.
l. calcaneocuboi′deum planta′re [TA] plantar calcaneocuboid ligament: a short, wide, strong band connecting the plantar surfaces of the calcaneus and the cuboid bone; called also *short plantar ligament.*
l. calcaneofibula′re [TA] calcaneofibular ligament: a band of fibers arising from the lateral surface of the lateral malleolus of the fibula just anterior to the apex and passing inferiorly and posteriorly to be attached to the lateral surface of the calcaneus.
l. calcaneonavicula′re [TA] calcaneonavicular ligament: the band of fibers connecting the superior surface of the calcaneus and the lateral surface of the navicular bone; together with the calcaneocuboid ligament, it constitutes the bifurcate ligament.
l. calcaneonavicula′re planta′re [TA] plantar calcaneonavicular ligament: a broad, thick band passing from the anterior margin of the sustentaculum tali to the plantar surface of the navicular bone; it bears on its deep surface a fibrocartilage that helps to support the head of the talus. Called also *spring ligament.*
l. calcaneotibia′le pars tibiocalcanea ligamenti medialis.
l. ca′pitis cos′tae intraarticula′re [TA] intra-articular ligament of head of rib: a horizontal band of fibers attached to the crest separating the two articular facets on the head of the rib, and to the intervertebral disk, thus dividing the joint of the head of the rib into two cavities. It is lacking in the joints of the first, tenth, eleventh, and twelfth ribs.
l. ca′pitis cos′tae radia′tum [TA] radiate ligament of head of rib: fibers that from their attachment on the ventral surface of the head of a rib radiate medially, in a fanlike manner, to attach to the two adjacent vertebrae and to the intervertebral disk between them.
l. ca′pitis fe′moris [TA] ligament of head of femur: a curved triangular or V-shaped fibrous band, attached by its apex to the anterosuperior part of the fovea of the head of the femur and by its base to the sides of the acetabular notch and the intervening transverse ligament of the acetabulum. Called also *l. teres femoris* and *round ligament of femur.*
l. ca′pitis fib′ulae ante′rius [TA] anterior ligament of head of fibula: a band of fibers that passes obliquely superiorly from the anterior part of the head of the fibula to the lateral condyle of the tibia.
l. ca′pitis fib′ulae poste′rius [TA] posterior ligament of head of fibula: a band of fibers that passes obliquely superiorly from the posterior part of the head of the fibula to the lateral condyle of the tibia.

ligamen'ta capsula'ria [TA] capsular ligaments: thickenings of the fibrous membrane of a joint capsule.
l. cardina'le [TA] cardinal ligament: part of a thickening of the visceral pelvic fascia beside the cervix and vagina, passing laterally to merge with the upper fascia of the pelvic diaphragm. Called also *l. transversum cervicis* [TA alternative], *lateral cervical ligament*, and *Mackenrodt ligament*.
l. car'pi radia'tum [TA] radiate carpal ligament: a group of about seven fibrous bands which diverge in all directions on the palmar surface of the mediocarpal joint; the majority radiate from the capitate to the scaphoid, lunate, and triquetral bones.
l. car'pi vola're transverse reinforcing fibers in the antebrachial fascia over the palmar surface of the wrist.
ligamen'ta carpometacarpa'lia dorsa'lia [TA] dorsal carpometacarpal ligaments: a series of bands on the dorsal surface of the carpometacarpal articulations, joining the carpal bones to the bases of the second to fifth metacarpals. The second metacarpal bone is thus joined to the trapezium, trapezoid, and capitate, the third to the capitate, the fourth to the capitate and hamate, and the fifth to the hamate. Called also *posterior carpometacarpal ligaments.*
ligamen'ta carpometacarpa'lia palma'ria [TA] palmar carpometacarpal ligaments: a series of bands on the palmar surface of the carpometacarpal articulations, joining the carpal bones to the second to fifth metacarpals. The second metacarpal bone is thus joined to the trapezium, the third to the trapezium, capitate, and hamate, the fourth to the hamate, and the fifth to the hamate. Called also *anterior* or *volar carpometacarpal ligaments.*
l. ceratocricoi'deum [TA] ceratocricoid ligament: any of the three (anterior, lateral, or posterior) fibrous bands that serve to attach the capsule of the cricothyroid joint on either side.
ligamen'ta collatera'lia articulatio'num digito'rum ma'nus ligamenta collateralia articulationum interphalangealium manus.
ligamen'ta collatera'lia articulatio'num digito'rum pe'dis ligamenta collateralia articulationum interphalangealium pedis.
ligamen'ta collatera'lia articulatio'num interphalangea'lium ma'nus [TA], **ligamen'ta collatera'lia articulatio'num interphalangea'rum ma'nus** collateral ligaments of interphalangeal joints of hand: massive fibrous bands on each side of the interphalangeal joints of the fingers; they are placed diagonally, the proximal ends being near the dorsal, and the distal ends near the palmar margins of the digits. Called also *ligamenta collateralia articulationum digitorum manus.*
ligamen'ta collatera'lia articulatio'num interphalangea'lium pe'dis [TA], **ligamen'ta collatera'lia articulatio'num interphalangea'rum pe'dis** collateral ligaments of interphalangeal joints of foot: fibrous bands, one on either side of each of the interphalangeal joints of the toes. Called also *ligamenta collateralia articulationum digitorum pedis.*
ligamen'ta collatera'lia articulatio'num metacarpophalangea'lium [TA], **ligamen'ta collatera'lia articulatio'num metacarpophalangea'rum** collateral ligaments of metacarpophalangeal joints: massive, strong fibrous bands on either side of each metacarpophalangeal joint, holding the two bones involved in each joint firmly together.
ligamen'ta collatera'lia articulatio'num metatarsophalangea'lium [TA], **ligamen'ta collatera'lia articulatio'num metatarsophalangea'rum** collateral ligaments of metatarsophalangeal joints: strong fibrous bands on either side of each metatarsophalangeal joint, holding the two bones involved in each joint firmly together.
l. collatera'le car'pi radia'le [TA] radial carpal collateral ligament: a short, thick band that passes from the tip of the styloid process of the radius to attach to the scaphoid bone.
l. collatera'le car'pi ulna're [TA] ulnar carpal collateral ligament: a strong fibrous band that passes from the tip of the styloid process of the ulna and is attached to the triquetral and pisiform bones.
l. collatera'le fibula're [TA] fibular collateral ligament: a strong, round fibrous cord on the lateral side of the knee joint, entirely independent of the capsule of the knee joint; it is attached superiorly to the posterior part of the lateral epicondyle of the femur and inferiorly to the lateral side of the head of the fibula just in front of the styloid process.
l. collatera'le latera'le articulatio'nis talocrura'lis [TA] lateral collateral ligament of ankle joint: the three ligamentous fasciculi present on the lateral side of the ankle joint (i.e., the *l. calcaneofibulare, l. talofibulare anterius,* and *l. talofibulare posterius*) considered collectively. Called also *lateral ligament of ankle joint* and *l. laterale articulationis talocruralis.*
l. collatera'le media'le articulatio'nis talocrura'lis [TA] medial ligament of talocrural joint: a large fan-shaped ligament on the medial side of the ankle, passing from the medial malleolus of the tibia down onto the tarsal bones. It comprises four parts: *pars tibionavicularis, pars tibiocalcanea, pars tibiotalaris anterior,* and *pars tibiotalaris posterior.* Called also *l. deltoideum articulationis talocruralis* [TA alternative], *l. mediale articulationis talocruralis, deltoid ligament of ankle,* and *medial ligament of ankle.*
l. collatera'le radia'le [TA] radial collateral ligament: a large bundle of fibers arising from the lateral epicondyle of the humerus and fanning out to be attached to the lateral side of the annular ligament of the radius.
l. collatera'le tibia'le [TA] tibial collateral ligament: a broad, flat, longitudinal band on the medial side of the knee joint; it is attached superiorly to the medial epicondyle of the femur, inferiorly to the medial surface of the body of the tibia, and in between to the medial meniscus.
l. collatera'le ulna're [TA] ulnar collateral ligament: a triangular bundle of fibers attached proximally to the medial epicondyle of the humerus, distally to the coronoid process of the ulna and the medial surface of the olecranon, and to a ridge running between the two.
l. col'li cos'tae l. costotransversarium.
l. conoi'deum [TA] conoid ligament: the conical, posteromedial portion of the coracoclavicular ligament, attached inferiorly by its tip to the base of the coracoid process of the scapula and superiorly by its base to the inferior surface of the clavicle.
l. coracoacromia'le [TA] coracoacromial ligament: one of three intrinsic ligaments of the scapula, a strong broad triangular band that is attached by its base to the lateral border of the coracoid process and by its tip to the summit of the acromion just in front of the articular facet for the clavicle.
l. coracoclavicula're [TA] coracoclavicular ligament: a strong band that joins the coracoid process of the scapula and the acromial extremity of the clavicle; it is divided into two parts, the trapezoid and conoid ligaments.
l. coracohumera'le [TA] coracohumeral ligament: a broad band that arises from the lateral border of the coracoid process of the scapula and passes downward and laterally to be attached to the major tubercle of the humerus.
l. corona'rium he'patis [TA] coronary ligament of liver: the line of reflection of the peritoneum from the diaphragmatic surface of the liver to the undersurface of the diaphragm.
l. costoclavicula're [TA] costoclavicular ligament: a short, powerful ligament that extends from the superior margin of the first costal cartilage to the inferior surface at the sternal end of the clavicle.
l. costotransversa'rium [TA] costotransverse ligament: short fibers that connect the dorsal surface of the neck of a rib with the anterior surface of the transverse process of the corresponding vertebra; called also *l. colli costae* and *l. transversum.*
l. costotransversa'rium latera'le [TA] lateral costotransverse ligament: a fibrous band that passes transversely from the posterior surface of the tip of a transverse process of a vertebra to the nonarticular part of the tubercle of the corresponding rib; called also *l. tuberculi costae.*
l. costotransversa'rium supe'rius [TA] superior costotransverse ligament: a strong band of fibers ascending from the crest of the neck of a rib to the transverse process of the vertebra above; it may be divided into a stronger anterior portion and a weaker posterior portion. It is lacking for the first rib.
ligamen'ta costoxiphoi'dea [TA] costoxiphoid ligaments: inconstant strandlike bands that pass obliquely from the anterior surface of the seventh and sometimes from the sixth costal cartilage to the anterior surface of the xiphoid process of the sternum. Some bands may also be present on the posterior surface.
l. cricoarytenoi'deum [TA], **l. cricoarytenoi'deum poste'rius** cricoarytenoid ligament: the ligament extending from the lamina of the cricoid cartilage to the medial surface of the base and muscular process of the arytenoid cartilage.
l. cricopharyn'geum [TA] cricopharyngeal ligament: a ligament extending from the cricoid lamina to the midline of the pharynx.
l. cricothyroi'deum media'num [TA] median cricothyroid ligament: the median or anterior part of the inferior, larger part of the fibroelastic laryngeal membrane, occurring as a flat band of white tissue continuous medially with the conus elasticus and cranially with the plica vocalis and ligamentum vocale, and connecting the cricoid and thyroid cartilages; called also *anterior cricothyroid ligament.* See also *cricothyroid ligament,* under *ligament.*

Ligamentum *Continued*

l. cricotrachea′le [TA] cricotracheal ligament: a narrow fibrous ring that connects the lower margin of the cricoid cartilage with the upper tracheal cartilage; it is continuous posteriorly with the membranous wall of the trachea.
l. crucia′tum ante′rius ge′nus [TA] anterior cruciate ligament of knee: a strong band that arises from the posteromedial portion of the lateral condyle of the femur, passes anteriorly and inferiorly between the condyles, and is attached to the depression in front of the intercondylar eminence of the tibia.
l. crucia′tum atlan′tis l. cruciforme atlantis.
ligamen′ta crucia′ta digito′rum ma′nus pars cruciformis vaginae fibrosae digitorum manus.
ligamen′ta crucia′ta digito′rum pe′dis pars cruciformis vaginae fibrosae digitorum pedis.
ligamen′ta crucia′ta genua′lia, ligamen′ta crucia′ta ge′nus cruciate ligaments of knee: strong, thick bundles situated in the knee joint between the condyles of the femur, which together form a somewhat cross-shaped structure. See *l. cruciatum anterius genus* and *l. cruciatum posterius genus.*
l. crucia′tum poste′rius ge′nus [TA] posterior cruciate ligament of knee: a strong band that arises from the anterolateral surface of the medial condyle of the femur, passes posteriorly and inferiorly between the condyles, and is inserted into the posterior intercondylar area of the tibia.
l. crucifor′me atlan′tis [TA] cruciform ligament of atlas: a ligament in the form of a cross, of which the transverse ligament of the atlas forms the horizontal bar, and the longitudinal fascicles the vertical bar of the cross; called also *l. cruciatum atlantis.*
l. cuboideonavicula′re dorsa′le [TA] dorsal cuboideonavicular ligament: a fibrous bundle connecting the dorsal surfaces of the cuboid and navicular bones.
l. cuboideonavicula′re planta′re [TA] plantar cuboideonavicular ligament: a fibrous band connecting the plantar surfaces of the cuboid and navicular bones.
l. cuneocuboi′deum dorsa′le [TA] dorsal cuneocuboid ligament: fibers connecting the dorsal surfaces of the cuboid and lateral cuneiform bones.
l. cuneocuboi′deum interos′seum [TA] interosseous cuneocuboid ligament: fibers connecting the central portions of the adjacent surfaces of the cuboid and lateral cuneiform bones, between the articular surfaces.
l. cuneocuboi′deum planta′re [TA] plantar cuneocuboid ligament: a band of fibers connecting the plantar surfaces of the cuboid and lateral cuneiform bones.
ligamen′ta cuneometatarsa′lia interos′sea [TA] interosseous cuneometatarsal ligaments: fibrous bands that join the adjacent surfaces of the cuneiform and the metatarsal bones.
ligamen′ta cuneonavicula′ria dorsa′lia [TA] dorsal cuneonavicular ligaments: bands that join the dorsal surface of the navicular bone to the dorsal surfaces of the three cuneiform bones; called also *ligamenta navicularicuneiformia dorsalia.*
ligamen′ta cuneonavicula′ria planta′ria [TA] plantar cuneonavicular ligaments: bands that join the plantar surface of the navicular bone to the adjacent plantar surfaces of the three cuneiform bones; called also *ligamenta navicularicuneiformia plantaria.*
l. deltoi′deum articulatio′nis talocrura′lis TA alternative for *l. collaterale mediale articulationis talocruralis.*

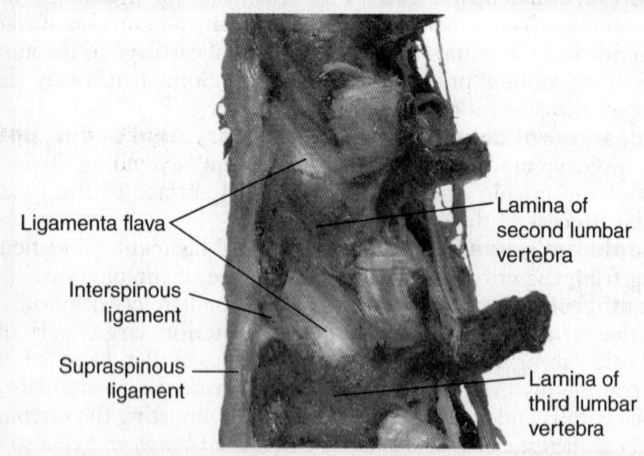

■ Ligamenta flava of several lumbar vertebrae.

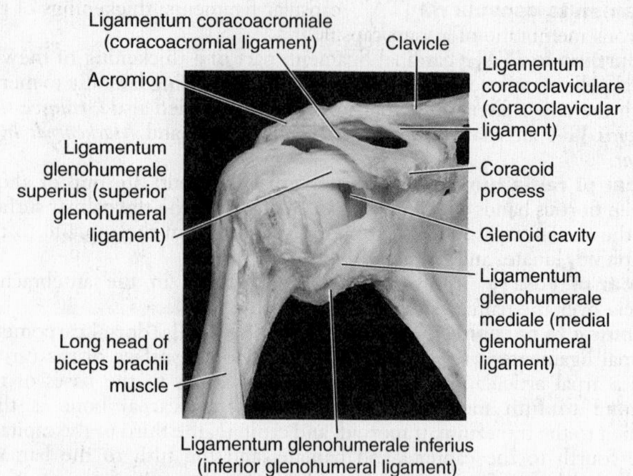

■ Ligamenta glenohumeralia and other ligamenta of the shoulder.

l. denticula′tum [TA] denticulate ligament: either of two symmetrical folds of pia mater of the spinal cord, each beginning in a longitudinal line between the lines of attachment of the anterior and posterior roots. The lateral edge is scalloped and has about 21 pointed processes that extend laterally and fuse with the arachnoid and dura mater. Called also *dentate ligament of spinal cord.*
l. epididy′midis infe′rius [TA] inferior ligament of epididymis: a strand of fibrous tissue, covered with a reflection of the tunica vaginalis, which connects the lower end of the body of the epididymis with the testis.
l. epididy′midis supe′rius [TA] superior ligament of epididymis: a strand of fibrous tissue, covered with a reflection of the tunica vaginalis, which connects the upper end of the body of the epididymis with the testis.
ligamen′ta extracapsula′ria [TA] ligaments of a joint capsule that are outside the capsule.
l. falcifor′me he′patis [TA] falciform ligament of liver: a sickle-shaped sagittal fold of peritoneum that helps to attach the liver to the diaphragm and extends from the coronary ligament of the liver to the umbilicus. In the traditional anatomic conception, it forms the boundary between the right and left lobes.
ligamen′ta fla′va [TA] yellow ligaments: a series of bands of yellow elastic tissue attached to and extending between the ventral portions of the laminae of two adjacent vertebrae, from the junction of the axis and the third cervical vertebra to the junction of the fifth lumbar vertebra and the sacrum. They assist in maintaining or regaining the erect position and serve to close in the spaces between the arches. Called also *arcuate* or *flaval ligaments.*
l. fundifor′me clito′ridis [TA] fundiform ligament of clitoris: a broad elastic band of fascial fibers that arises from the linea alba above the symphysis pubis and then passes down to the clitoris, where it divides and passes around the clitoris and fuses with the fascia of the clitoris.
l. fundifor′me pe′nis [TA] fundiform ligament of penis: a broad elastic band of fascial fibers that arises from the linea alba and from the fibrae intercrurales just above the symphysis pubis and then passes down to the penis, where it divides and passes around the penis and on into the scrotum.
l. gastroco′licum [TA] gastrocolic ligament: a peritoneal fold, part of the greater omentum, that extends from the greater curvature of the stomach to the transverse colon.
l. gastroliena′le TA alternative for *l. gastrosplenicum.*
l. gastrophre′nicum [TA] gastrophrenic ligament: a fold of peritoneum continuous with the gastrosplenic ligament, extending from the right inferior surface of the diaphragm to the cardiac part of the stomach.
l. gastrosple′nicum [TA] gastrosplenic ligament: a peritoneal fold extending from the greater curvature of the stomach to the hilum of the spleen; called also *l. gastrolienale* [TA alternative] and *gastrolienal* or *splenogastric ligament.*
l. genitoinguina′le genitoinguinal ligament: the embryonic precursor of the gubernaculum testis.
ligamen′ta glenohumera′lia [TA] glenohumeral ligaments: bands, usually three, on the inner surface of the articular capsule of the

humerus, attached to the margin of the glenoid cavity and to the anatomical neck of the humerus.
ligamen′ta he′patis [TA] hepatic ligaments: the ligaments of the liver, including the ligamentum coronarium hepatis, ligamentum falciforme hepatis, ligamentum triangulare dextrum hepatis, ligamentum triangulare sinistrum hepatis, and ligamentum hepatorenale.
l. hepatoco′licum [TA] hepatocolic ligament: an occasional fold of peritoneum, an extension of the lesser omentum to the right, passing from the visceral surface of the liver near the gallbladder to the right colic flexure.
l. hepatoduodena′le [TA] hepatoduodenal ligament: a peritoneal fold that passes from the porta hepatis to the superior part of the duodenum. It is continuous on the left with the hepatogastric ligament, and on the right it forms one of the borders of the epiploic foramen. It contains the hepatic artery, portal vein, bile duct, nerves, and lymphatics.
l. hepatogas′tricum [TA] hepatogastric ligament: a peritoneal fold, part of the lesser omentum, that passes from the visceral surface of the liver to the lesser curvature of the stomach.
l. hepatophre′nicum hepatophrenic ligament: a peritoneal fold, part of the lesser omentum, connecting the liver and the diaphragm.
l. hepatorena′le [TA] hepatorenal ligament: a fold of peritoneum that passes from the posterior part of the visceral surface of the liver to the anterior surface of the right kidney; it forms the right margin of the epiploic foramen.
l. hyoepiglot′ticum [TA] hyoepiglottic ligament: a triangular elastic band with its base attached to the upper border of the body of the hyoid bone and its tip to the anterosuperior surface of the epiglottis.
l. iliofemora′le [TA] iliofemoral ligament: a very strong triangular or inverted Y-shaped band that covers the anterior and superior portions of the hip joint. It arises by its apex from the lower part of the anterior inferior iliac spine and is inserted by its base into the intertrochanteric line of the femur.
l. iliolumba′le [TA] iliolumbar ligament: a strong band that passes from the transverse processes of the fourth and fifth lumbar vertebrae to the internal lip of the adjacent portion of the iliac crest.
l. incu′dis poste′rius [TA] posterior ligament of incus: a fibrous band by which the tip of the short crus of the incus is fixed to the fossa incudis.
l. incu′dis supe′rius [TA] superior ligament of incus: a fibrous band that passes from the body of the incus to the roof of the tympanic cavity just back of the superior ligament of the malleus.
l. inguina′le [TA] inguinal ligament: a fibrous band running from the anterior superior spine of the ilium to the spine of the pubis. Called also *inguinal arch* and *arcus inguinalis* [TA alternative].
l. inguina′le reflex′um [TA] reflex inguinal ligament: a triangular band of fibers arising from the lacunar ligament and the pubic bone and passing diagonally upward and medially behind the superficial abdominal ring and in front of the inguinal aponeurotic falx to the linea alba.
ligamen′ta intercarpa′lia dorsa′lia [TA] dorsal intercarpal ligaments: several bands that extend transversely across the dorsal surfaces of the carpal bones, connecting various ones together.
ligamen′ta intercarpa′lia interos′sea [TA] interosseous intercarpal ligaments: short fibrous bands that join the adjacent surfaces of the various carpal bones.
ligamen′ta intercarpa′lia palma′ria [TA] palmar intercarpal ligaments: several bands that extend transversely across the palmar surfaces of the carpal bones, connecting various ones together; called also *volar intercarpal ligaments.*
l. interclavicula′re [TA] interclavicular ligament: a flattened band that passes from the superior surface of the sternal end of one clavicle across the superior margin of the sternum to the same position on the other clavicle.
ligamen′ta intercuneifor′mia dorsa′lia [TA] dorsal intercuneiform ligaments: fibrous bands connecting the dorsal surfaces of the three cuneiform bones.
ligamen′ta intercuneifor′mia interos′sea [TA] interosseous intercuneiform ligaments: short fibrous bands that join the adjacent surfaces of the medial and intermediate, and the intermediate and lateral, cuneiform bones.
ligamen′ta intercuneifor′mia planta′ria [TA] plantar intercuneiform ligaments: fibrous bands that join the plantar surfaces of the cuneiform bones.
l. interfoveola′re [TA] interfoveolar ligament: a thickening in the fascia transversalis on the medial side of the deep inguinal ring; it is connected above to the transversus muscle and below to the inguinal ligament.
ligamenta interspina′lia [TA] interspinal ligaments: several fine fibrous membranes that extend from one vertebral spinous process to the next. They extend obliquely from the yellow ligaments ventrally to the supraspinous ligament dorsally, and contain white fibrous and yellow elastic tissue. They are poorly developed or lacking in the cervical region. Called also *interspinous ligaments.*
ligamenta intertransversa′ria [TA] intertransverse ligaments: several poorly developed fibrous bands that extend from one vertebral transverse process to the next. They consist of fine membranes in the lumbar region and of small cords in the thoracic region, and are lacking in the cervical region.
ligamen′ta intracapsula′ria [TA] intracapsular ligaments: ligaments within a joint capsule.
l. ischiocapsula′re l. ischiofemorale.
l. ischiofemora′le [TA] ischiofemoral ligament: a broad triangular band on the posterior surface of the hip joint. Its base is attached to the ischium posterior and inferior to the acetabulum; its fibers pass superiorly, laterally, and anteriorly across the capsule, bend over the neck, and in part are inserted into the inner side of the trochanteric fossa of the femur and in part blend into the zona orbicularis. Called also *l. ischiocapsulare* and *ischiocapsular ligament.*
l. lacinia′tum retinaculum musculorum flexorum pedis.
l. lacuna′re [TA] lacunar ligament: a small triangular membrane with its base just medial to the femoral ring; one side is attached to the inguinal ligament and the other to the pectineal line of the pubis.
l. later′ale articulatio′nis talocrura′lis l. collaterale laterale articulationis talocruralis.
l. latera′le articulatio′nis temporomandibula′ris [TA] lateral ligament of temporomandibular joint: a strong triangular fibrous band that is attached superiorly by its base to the zygomatic process of the temporal bone, passes down on the lateral side of the joint in contact with the capsule, and is inserted by its apex into the lateral and posterior surfaces of the neck of the condyloid process of the mandible. Called also *l. temporomandibulare* and *temporomandibular ligament.*
l. latera′le puboprosta′ticum TA alternative for l. puboprostaticum.
l. latera′le pubovesica′le [TA] lateral pubovesical ligament: the lateral branch of the pubovesical ligament in the female, extending from the bladder neck to the tendinous arch of the pelvic fascia.
l. la′tum u′teri [TA] broad ligament of uterus: a broad fold of peritoneum extending from the side of the uterus to the wall of the pelvis; it is divided into the mesometrium, mesosalpinx, and mesovarium.
l. lienorena′le TA alternative for *l. splenorenale.*
l. longitudina′le ante′rius [TA] anterior longitudinal ligament: a single long, fibrous band in the midline, attached to the ventral surfaces of the bodies of the vertebrae; it extends from the occipital bone and the anterior tubercle of the atlas down to the sacrum.
l. longitudina′le poste′rius [TA] posterior longitudinal ligament: a single midline fibrous band attached to the dorsal surfaces of the bodies of the vertebrae, extending from the occipital bone to the coccyx.
l. lumbocosta′le [TA] lumbocostal ligament: a strong fascial band that passes from the twelfth rib to the tips of the transverse processes of the first and second lumbar vertebrae.
l. mal′lei ante′rius [TA] anterior ligament of malleus: a fibrous band that extends from the neck of the malleus just above the anterior process to the anterior wall of the tympanic cavity close to the petrotympanic fissure. Some of the fibers pass through the fissure to the spina angulares of the sphenoid bone.
l. mal′lei latera′le [TA] lateral ligament of malleus: a triangular fibrous band that passes from the posterior portion of the incisura tympanica to the head or neck of the malleus.
l. mal′lei supe′rius [TA] superior ligament of malleus: a delicate fibrous strand passing from the roof of the tympanic cavity to the head of the malleus.
l. malle′oli latera′lis ante′rius l. tibiofibulare anterius.
l. malle′oli latera′lis poste′rius l. tibiofibulare posterius.
l. media′le articulatio′nis talocrura′lis l. collaterale mediale articulationis talocruralis.
l. media′le articulatio′nis temporomandibula′ris [TA] the medial ligament of the temporomandibular joint.

l. media′le puboprosta′ticum TA alternative for the ligamentum pubovesicale in the male.
l. media′le pubovesica′le [TA] medial pubovesical ligament: the medial branch of the pubovesical ligament in the female, a forward continuation of the tendinous arch of the pelvic fascia to the pubis.
l. meniscofemora′le ante′rius [TA] anterior meniscofemoral ligament: a small fibrous band of the knee joint, attached to the posterior area of the lateral meniscus and passing superiorly and medially, anterior to the posterior cruciate ligament, to attach to the anterior cruciate ligament.
l. meniscofemora′le poste′rius [TA] posterior meniscofemoral ligament: a small fibrous band of the knee joint, attached to the posterior area of the lateral meniscus and passing superiorly and medially, posterior to the posterior cruciate ligament, to the medial condyle of the femur.
ligamen′ta metacarpa′lia dorsa′lia [TA] dorsal metacarpal ligaments: bands that interconnect the bases of the second to fifth metacarpal bones by passing transversely from bone to bone on their dorsal surfaces.
ligamen′ta metacarpa′lia interos′sea [TA] interosseous metacarpal ligaments: short, strong fibrous bands situated between the adjacent surfaces of the bases of the second to fifth metacarpal bones, just distal to the articular surfaces.
ligamen′ta metacarpa′lia palma′ria [TA] palmar metacarpal ligaments: bands that interconnect the bases of the second to fifth metacarpal bones by passing transversely from bone to bone on their palmar surfaces.
l. metacarpa′le transver′sum profun′dum [TA] deep transverse metacarpal ligament: a narrow fibrous band that extends across and is attached to the palmar surfaces of the heads of the second to fifth metacarpal bones, joining them together.
l. metacarpa′le transver′sum superficia′le [TA] superficial transverse metacarpal ligament: transverse fibers occupying the intervals between the diverging longitudinal bands of the palmar aponeurosis.
ligamen′ta metatarsa′lia dorsa′lia [TA] dorsal metatarsal ligaments: light transverse bands on the dorsal surfaces of the bases of the second to fifth metatarsal bones, similar to the corresponding ligaments on the metacarpal bones.
ligamen′ta metatarsa′lia interos′sea [TA] interosseous metatarsal ligaments: bands between the bases of the second to fifth metatarsal bones, similar to the corresponding ligaments of the hand.
ligamen′ta metatarsa′lia planta′ria [TA] plantar metatarsal ligaments: strong transverse bands on the plantar surfaces of the bases of the second to fifth metatarsal bones.
l. metatarsa′le transver′sum profundum [TA] deep transverse metatarsal ligament: a narrow fibrous band that extends across, is attached to the plantar surfaces of, and thus joins together the heads of all the metatarsal bones.
l. metatarsa′le transver′sum superficia′le [TA] superficial transverse metatarsal ligament: fibers that lie in the superficial fascia of the sole of the foot beneath the heads of the metatarsal bones.
l. muco′sum plica synovialis infrapatellaris.
ligamen′ta navicularicuneifor′mia dorsa′lia ligamenta cuneonavicularia dorsalia.
ligamen′ta navicularicuneifor′mia planta′ria ligamenta cuneonavicularia plantaria.

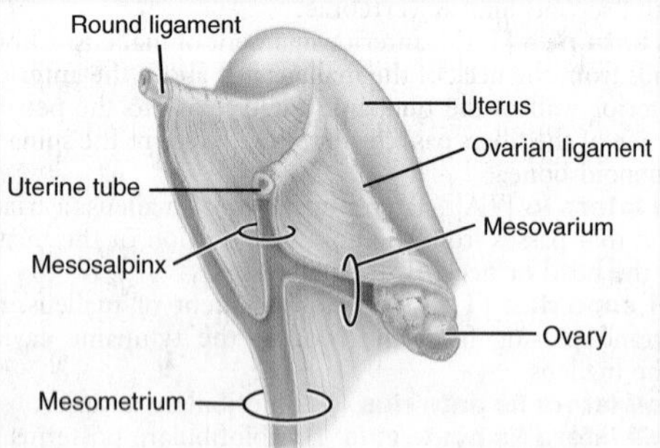

■ Ligamentum latum uteri (broad ligament of uterus), comprising the mesovarium, mesometrium, and mesosalpinx; shown in side view, with the anterior surface of the uterine body facing left.

l. nu′chae [TA] nuchal ligament: a broad, fibrous, roughly triangular sagittal septum in the back of the neck, separating the right and left sides. It extends from the tips of the spinous processes of all the cervical vertebrae to attach to the entire length of the external occipital crest. Caudally it is continuous with the supraspinous ligament.
ligamen′ta ossiculo′rum auditorio′rum TA alternative for *ligamenta ossiculorum auditus.*
ligamen′ta ossiculo′rum audi′tus [TA] ligaments of auditory ossicles: the ligaments of the auditory ossicles, comprising the anterior, lateral, and superior ligaments of the malleus, the posterior and superior ligaments of the incus, and the annular ligament of the stapes.
l. ova′rii pro′prium [TA] ovarian ligament: a musculofibrous cord in the broad ligament, joining the ovary to the upper part of the lateral margin of the uterus just below the attachment of the uterine tube; called also *utero-ovarian ligament* and *ligamentum uteroovaricum* [TA alternative].
ligamen′ta palma′ria articulatio′num interphalangea′lium ma′nus [TA], **ligamen′ta palma′ria articulatio′num interphalangea′rum manus** palmar ligaments of interphalangeal articulations of hand: thick, dense fibrocartilaginous plates on the palmar surfaces of the interphalangeal articulations of the hand, between the collateral ligaments.
ligamen′ta palma′ria articulatio′num metacarpophalangea′lium [TA], **ligamen′ta palma′ria articulatio′num metacarpophalangea′rum** palmar ligaments of metacarpophalangeal articulations: thick dense fibrocartilaginous plates on the palmar surfaces of the metacarpophalangeal articulation, between the collateral ligaments. Called also *anterior* or *palmar metacarpophalangeal ligaments.*
l. palpebra′le latera′le [TA] lateral palpebral ligament: a ligament that anchors the lateral end of the superior and inferior tarsal plates to the margin of the orbit.
l. palpebra′le media′le [TA] medial palpebral ligament: fibrous bands that connect the medial ends of the tarsi to the bones of the orbit, an anterior bundle passing in front of the lacrimal sac and attached to the frontal process of the maxilla, and a posterior bundle passing behind the lacrimal sac and attached to the posterior crest of the lacrimal bone.
l. pancreaticoco′licum [TA] pancreaticocolic ligament: a thickening of the greater omentum that extends from the pancreas to the transverse colon.
l. pancreaticosple′nicum [TA] pancreaticosplenic ligament: a thickening of the greater omentum that extends from the pancreas to the spleen.
l. patel′lae [TA] patellar ligament: the continuation of the central portion of the tendon of the quadriceps femoris muscle distal to the patella; it extends from the patella to the tuberosity of the tibia.
l. pectina′tum an′guli iridocornea′lis reticulum trabeculare.
l. pectinea′le, l. pecti′neum [TA] pectineal ligament: a strong aponeurotic lateral continuation of the lacunar ligament along the pectineal line of the pubis; called also *Cooper ligament.*
l. phrenicoco′licum [TA] phrenicocolic ligament: a peritoneal fold that passes from the left colic flexure to the adjacent costal portion of the diaphragm. Called also *phrenocolic ligament.*
l. phrenicooesophagea′lis [TA] phrenicoesophageal ligament: a cone-shaped expansion of fascia that attaches to the esophagus above the esophagogastric junction and helps attach it to the diaphragm. Called also *phrenoesophageal ligament.*
l. phrenicoliena′le l. phrenicosplenicum.
l. phrenicosple′nicum [TA] phrenicosplenic ligament: a fold in the greater omentum that connects the diaphragm with the concave surface of the spleen; this and the ligamentum splenorenale are the same structure in some persons. Called also *l. phrenicolienale* and *lienophrenic* or *splenophrenic ligament.*
l. pisohama′tum [TA] pisohamate ligament: a fibrous band extending from the pisiform bone to the hook of the hamate bone.
l. pisometacar′peum [TA] pisometacarpal ligament: a fibrous band extending from the pisiform bone to the bases of the fifth, usually the fourth, and sometimes the third metacarpal bone.
ligamen′ta planta′ria articulatio′num interphalangea′lium pe′dis [TA], **ligamen′ta planta′ria articulatio′num interphalangea′rum pe′dis** plantar ligaments of interphalangeal articulations of foot: thick, dense bands on the plantar surfaces of the interphalangeal articulations of the foot, between the collateral ligaments.

Ligamentum *Continued*

ligamen′ta planta′ria articulatio′num metatarsophalangea′lium [TA], **ligamen′ta planta′ria articulatio′num metatarsophalangea′rum** plantar ligaments of metatarsophalangeal articulations: thick, dense bands on the plantar surface of the metatarsophalangeal articulations, between the collateral ligaments. Called also *inferior metatarsophalangeal ligaments.*
l. planta′re lon′gum [TA] long plantar ligament: the longest ligament of the foot, arising from the lower surface of the calcaneus as far back as the lateral and the medial processes, passing forward over the tendon of the peroneus longus, and inserting into the bases of the second through fifth metatarsal bones.
l. popli′teum arcua′tum [TA] arcuate popliteal ligament: a band of variable and ill-defined fibers at the posterolateral part of the knee joint; it is attached inferiorly to the apex of the head of the fibula, arches superiorly and medially over the popliteal tendon, and merges with the articular capsule. Called also *popliteal arch* and *arcuate ligament of knee.*
l. popli′teum obli′quum [TA] oblique popliteal ligament: a broad band of fibers that arises from the medial condyle of the tibia, merges more or less with the tendon of the semimembranosus, and passes obliquely across the back of the knee joint to the lateral epicondyle of the femur. It contains large openings for the passage of vessels and nerves.
l. pterygospina′le [TA] pterygospinal ligament: a band of fibers extending from the superior part of the superior border of the lateral pterygoid plate to the spine of the sphenoid bone.
l. pu′bicum infe′rius [TA] inferior pubic ligament: a thick archlike band of fibers situated along the inferior margin of the symphysis pubis. Its fibers are attached to the medial borders of the inferior rami of the pubic bones and thus it rounds out and forms the summit of the pubic arch.
l. pu′bicum supe′rius [TA] superior pubic ligament: fibers that pass transversely across the superior margin of the symphysis pubis; attached to the bones and to the interpubic disk, they extend laterally as far as the pubic tubercle.
l. pubocapsula′re l. pubofemorale.
l. pubofemora′le [TA] pubofemoral ligament: a band that arises from the entire length of the obturator crest of the pubic bone and passes laterally and inferiorly to merge into the capsule of the hip joint, some fibers reaching to the lower part of the neck of the femur. Called also *l. pubocapsulare.*
l. puboprosta′ticum [TA] puboprostatic ligament: a thickening of the superior fascia of the pelvic diaphragm in the male that, laterally, extends from the prostate to the tendinous arch of the pelvic fascia and, medially, is a forward continuation of the tendinous arch to the pubis. Called also *l. laterale puboprostaticum* [TA alternative].
l. pubovesica′le [TA] pubovesical ligament: a ligament that extends from the bladder neck to the inferior aspect of the pubic bones. In the female it is divided into two distinct parts (see *l. mediale pubovesicale* and *l. laterale pubovesicale*). In the male it is parallel and medial to the puboprostatic ligament and is sometimes called also *medial puboprostatic ligament* or *l. mediale puboprostaticum* [TA alternative].
l. pubovesica′le latera′le l. laterale pubovesicale.
l. pubovesica′le media′le l. mediale pubovesicale.
l. pulmona′le [TA] pulmonary ligament: a vertical pleural fold associated with the lung, extending from the hilus down to the base on the medial surface of the lung; on the left it forms the posterior boundary of the impressio cardiaca.
l. quadra′tum [TA] quadrate ligament: a fibrous bundle connecting the distal margin of the radial notch of the ulna to the neck of the radius.
l. radiocarpa′le dorsa′le [TA] dorsal radiocarpal ligament: a fibrous band that passes obliquely from the posterior border of the distal extremity of the radius to the dorsal surfaces of the proximal row of carpal bones, especially the triquetral and lunate, and to the dorsal intercarpal ligaments.
l. radiocarpa′le palma′re [TA] palmar radiocarpal ligament: several bundles of fibers that pass obliquely from the styloid process and the distal anterior margin of the radius to the lunate, triquetral, capitate, and hamate bones; called also *volar radiocarpal ligament.*
l. rec′ti latera′le [TA] lateral ligament of rectum: either of two thin strands of fascia that are variably present, one on either side of and adjacent to the middle rectal artery and vein. Called also *rectal stalk.*
l. rectouteri′num [TA] rectouterine ligament: a part of the thickening of the visceral pelvic fascia beside the cervix and vagina, passing posteriorly in the rectouterine fold to attach to the front of the sacrum; called also *Jarjavay l.* and *Petit l.*
l. sacrococcy′geum ante′rius [TA] anterior sacrococcygeal ligament: a flat band, homologous with the anterior longitudinal ligament of the vertebral column, that passes from the lower part of the sacrum over onto the anterior part of the coccyx. Called also *l. sacrococcygeum ventrale* [TA alternative] and *ventral sacrococcygeal ligament.*
l. sacrococcy′geum dorsa′le profun′dum TA alternative for *l. sacrococcygeum posterius profundum.*
l. sacrococcy′geum dorsa′le superficia′le TA alternative for *l. sacrococcygeum posterius superficiale.*
l. sacrococcy′geum latera′le [TA] lateral sacrococcygeal ligament: a fibrous band, homologous with the intertransverse ligaments, that passes from the transverse process of the first coccygeal vertebra to the lower lateral angle of the sacrum, thus helping to complete the foramen of the fifth sacral nerve.
l. sacrococcy′geum poste′rius profun′dum [TA] deep posterior sacrococcygeal ligament: the terminal portion of the posterior longitudinal ligament of the vertebral column; it helps to unite the dorsal surfaces of the fifth sacral and the coccygeal vertebrae. Called also *deep dorsal sacrococcygeal ligament* and *l. sacrococcygeum dorsale profundum* [TA alternative].
l. sacrococcy′geum poste′rius superficia′le [TA] superficial posterior sacrococcygeal ligament: a fibrous band continuous with the supraspinous ligament of the vertebral column; attached cranially to the margin of the sacral hiatus, and diverging as it passes caudally to attach to the dorsal surface of the coccyx. Called also *l. sacrococcygeum dorsale superficiale* [TA alternative] and *superficial dorsal sacrococcygeal ligament.*
l. sacrococcy′geum ventra′le TA alternative for *l. sacrococcygeum anterius.*
l. sacroili′acum ante′rius [TA] anterior sacroiliac ligament: any of numerous thin fibrous bands passing from the ventral margin of the auricular surface of the sacrum to the adjacent portions of the ilium; called also *l. sacroiliacum ventralis* and *ventral sacroiliac ligaments.*
l. sacroili′acum dorsa′lis l. sacroiliacum posterius.
l. sacroili′acum interos′seum [TA] interosseous sacroiliac ligament: any of numerous short, strong bundles connecting the tuberosities and adjacent surfaces of the sacrum and the ilium.
l. sacroili′acum poste′rius [TA] posterior sacroiliac ligament: any of numerous strong bands that pass from the ilium to the sacrum. The *long posterior sacroiliac ligament* is more superficial and connects the posterior superior iliac spine with the second, third, and fourth articular tubercles of the sacrum. The *short posterior sacroiliac ligament* is deeper and more nearly horizontal and connects the tuberosity of the ilium with the first and second tubercles on the dorsum of the sacrum. Called also *l. sacroiliacum dorsalis* and *dorsal sacroiliac ligament.*
l. sacroili′acum ventra′lis l. sacroiliacum anterius.
l. sacrospina′le [TA] sacrospinal ligament: one of the long vertical fibrous bands attached by the apex to the spine of the ischium and by the base to the lateral margins of the sacrum. Called also *sacrospinous ligament.*
l. sacrospino′sum l. sacrospinale.
l. sacrotubera′le [TA] sacrotuberal ligament: a large, flat band that is attached below to the ischial tuberosity, spreads out as it ascends, and is attached to the lateral margins of the sacrum and the coccyx and to the posterior inferior iliac spine; called also *l. sacrotuberosum.*
l. sacrotubero′sum l. sacrotuberale.
l. sero′sum serous ligament: a fold of peritoneum or other serous membrane that helps to hold an organ or part in position and transmits blood vessels and nerves.
l. sphenomandibula′re [TA] sphenomandibular ligament: a thin aponeurotic band that extends from the angular spine of the sphenoid bone downward medial to the temporomandibular articulation and attaches to the lingula of the mandible.
l. spira′le duc′tus cochlea′ris [TA] spiral ligament of cochlea: a band of thickened periosteum in the bony cochlea. Cf. *crista basilaris ductus cochlearis.*
l. splenoco′licum [TA] splenocolic ligament: a thickening in the greater omentum that extends from the spleen to the colon.
l. splenorena′le [TA] splenorenal ligament: a fold in the greater omentum that connects the kidney and the concave surface of the spleen; this and the ligamentum phrenicosplenicum are the same structure in some persons. Called also *l. lienorenale* [TA alternative] and *lienorenal ligament.*
l. sternoclavicula′re see *l. sternoclaviculare anterius* and *l. sternoclaviculare posterius.*

Ligamentum *Continued*

l. sternoclavicula're ante'rius [TA] anterior sternoclavicular ligament: a thick reinforcing band on the anterior portion of the articular capsule of the sternoclavicular articulation. It is attached superiorly to the anterior and superior parts of the sternal extremity of the clavicle and inferiorly to the anterior surface of the manubrium of the sternum.

l. sternoclavicula're poste'rius [TA] posterior sternoclavicular ligament: a thick reinforcing band on the posterior portion of the articular capsule of the sternoclavicular articulation. It is attached superiorly to the posterior and superior parts of the sternal extremity of the clavicle and inferiorly to the posterior surface of the manubrium of the sternum.

l. sternocosta'le interarticula're l. sternocostale intraarticulare.

l. sternocosta'le intraarticula're [TA] intra-articular sternocostal ligament: a horizontal fibrocartilaginous plate in the center of the second sternocostal joint, which joins the tip of the costal cartilage to the fibrous junction between the manubrium and the body of the sternum, and thus divides the joint into two parts. Called also *interarticular sternocostal ligament* and *l. sternocostale interarticulare.*

ligamen'ta sternocosta'lia radia'ta [TA] radiate sternocostal ligaments: fibrous bands attached to the sternal end of a costal cartilage, radiating from there out onto the ventral part of the sternum.

ligamen'ta sternopericardi'aca [TA] sternopericardiac ligaments: two (superior and inferior) or more fibrous bands that attach the pericardium to the dorsal surface of the sternum. Called also *ligaments of Luschka.*

l. stylohyoi'deum [TA] stylohyoid ligament: a vertical fibroelastic aponeurotic cord attached superiorly to the tip of the styloid process of the temporal bone and inferiorly to the lesser horn of the hyoid bone.

l. stylomandibula're [TA] stylomandibular ligament: an aponeurotic band attached superiorly to the tip of the styloid process of the temporal bone and inferiorly to the angle and posterior margin of the ramus of the mandible.

l. supraspina'le [TA] supraspinal ligament: a single long, vertical fibrous band passing over and attached to the tips of the spinous processes of the vertebrae from the seventh cervical to the sacrum; it is continuous above with the ligamentum nuchae.

l. suspenso'rium clito'ridis [TA] suspensory ligament of clitoris: a strong fibrous band that comes from the external deep investing fascia and attaches the root of the clitoris to the linea alba, symphysis pubis, and arcuate pubic ligament.

l. suspenso'rium duode'ni TA alternative for *musculus suspensorius duodeni.*

ligamen'ta suspenso'ria mamma'ria [TA] suspensory ligaments of breast: fibrous processes, extending from the corpus mammae to the corium, homologous with the retinacula cutis of other regions of the body.

l. suspenso'rium ova'rii [TA] suspensory ligament of ovary: the portion of the broad ligament lateral to and above the ovary; it contains the ovarian vessels and nerves and passes upward over the iliac vessels.

l. suspenso'rium pe'nis [TA] suspensory ligament of penis: a strong fibrous band that comes from the external deep investing fascia and attaches the root of the penis to the linea alba, symphysis pubis, and arcuate pubic ligament.

l. talocalcanea're interos'seum l. talocalcaneum interosseum.

l. talocalcanea're latera'le l. talocalcaneum laterale.

l. talocalcanea're media'le l. talocalcaneum mediale.

l. talocalca'neum interos'seum [TA] interosseous talocalcaneal ligament: fibrous bands in the sinus tarsi, passing between the opposed surfaces of the calcaneus and the talus; called also *l. talocalcaneare interosseum.*

l. talocalca'neum latera'le [TA] lateral talocalcaneal ligament: a fibrous band passing from the lateral surface of the talus to that of the calcaneus. Called also *l. talocalcaneare laterale.*

l. talocalca'neum media'le [TA] medial talocalcaneal ligament: a fibrous band connecting the medial tubercle of the talus with the sustentaculum tali of the calcaneus. Called also *l. talocalcaneare mediale.*

l. talofibula're ante'rius [TA] anterior talofibular ligament: one or more fibrous bands that pass from the anterior surface of the lateral malleolus of the fibula to the anterior margin of the lateral articular surface of the talus.

l. talofibula're poste'rius [TA] posterior talofibular ligament: a strong fibrous horizontal band passing from the posteromedial face of the lateral malleolus of the fibula to the area of the posterior process of the talus.

l. talonavicula're [TA] talonavicular ligament: a broad, thin fibrous band passing from the dorsal and lateral surfaces of the neck of the talus to the dorsal surface of the navicular bone; called also *talonavicular dorsal ligament.*

l. talotibia'le ante'rius pars tibiotalaris anterior ligamenti medialis.

l. talotibia'le poste'rius pars tibiotalaris posterior ligamenti medialis.

ligamen'ta tar'si [TA] ligaments of tarsus: a general term encompassing the ligaments that connect the bones of the tarsus.

ligamen'ta tar'si dorsa'lia [TA] dorsal ligaments of tarsus: including the bifurcate, dorsal cuboideonavicular, cuneocuboid, cuneonavicular, intercuneiform, and talonavicular ligaments; called also *dorsal intertarsal ligaments.*

ligamen'ta tar'si interos'sea [TA] interosseous ligaments of tarsus, including the interosseous cuneocuboid, intercuneiform, and talocalcaneal ligaments.

ligamen'ta tar'si planta'ria [TA] plantar ligaments of tarsus: the inferior ligaments of the foot, comprising the long plantar and the plantar calcaneocuboid, calcaneonavicular, cuneonavicular, cuboideonavicular, intercuneiform, and cuneocuboid ligaments.

ligamen'ta tarsometatarsa'lia dorsa'lia [TA] dorsal tarsometatarsal ligaments: fibrous bands passing from the dorsal surfaces of the bases of the metatarsal bones to the dorsal surfaces of the cuboid and the three cuneiform bones.

ligamen'ta tarsometatarsa'lia planta'ria [TA] plantar tarsometatarsal ligaments: fibrous bands passing from the plantar surfaces of the bases of the metatarsal bones to the plantar surfaces of the cuboid and the three cuneiform bones.

l. temporomandibula're l. laterale articulationis temporomandibularis.

l. te'res fe'moris l. capitis femoris.

l. te'res he'patis [TA] a fibrous cord, the remains of the left umbilical vein, extending from the porta hepatis (where it is attached to the left branch of the portal vein) out through the fissure for the ligamentum teres and the falciform ligament to the umbilicus.

l. te'res u'teri [TA] round ligament of uterus: a fibromuscular band in the female that is attached to the uterus near the attachment of the uterine tube, passing then along the broad ligament, out through the inguinal ring, and into the labium majus.

l. thyroepiglot'ticum [TA] thyroepiglottic ligament: a fibrous band that attaches the petiolus of the epiglottis to the thyroid cartilage just below the superior notch.

l. thyrohyoi'deum latera'le [TA] lateral thyrohyoid ligament: a round elastic cord that forms the posterior margin of the thyrohyoid membrane; it extends from the tip of the superior horn of the thyroid cartilage upward to the tip of the greater horn of the hyoid bone.

l. thyrohyoi'deum media'num [TA] median thyrohyoid ligament: the central, thicker portion of the thyrohyoid membrane; its broader upper part is attached to the body of the hyoid bone and its narrow lower end to the superior incisure of the thyroid cartilage.

l. tibiofibula're ante'rius [TA] anterior tibiofibular ligament: a flat triangular band that passes diagonally, inferiorly, and laterally from the anterior portion of the lateral surface of the distal end of the tibia to the anterior surface of the distal end of the fibula; called also *l. malleoli lateralis anterius.*

l. tibiofibula're poste'rius [TA] posterior tibiofibular ligament: a fibrous band that passes diagonally, inferiorly, and laterally from the posterior surface of the distal end of the tibia to the adjacent posterior surface of the distal end of the fibula; called also *l. malleoli lateralis posterius.*

l. tibionavicula're pars tibionavicularis ligamenti medialis.

ligamen'ta trachea'lia TA alternative for *ligamenta anularia tracheae.*

l. transver'sum l. costotransversarium.

l. transver'sum aceta'buli [TA] transverse ligament of acetabulum: a fibrous band continuous with the acetabular lip of the hip joint, which bridges the acetabular notch and converts it into a foramen.

l. transver'sum atlan'tis [TA] transverse ligament of atlas: the strong horizontal portion of the cruciform ligament of the atlas. It is attached at each end to the lateral masses of the atlas and curves posteriorly around the dens of the axis. It thus divides the atlantal ring into a smaller anterior division for the dens and a larger posterior division for the spinal cord and related structures. Called also *Lauth ligament.*

l. transver'sum cer'vicis TA alternative for l. cardinale.

l. transver'sum genua'le l. transversum genus.

l. transver'sum ge'nus [TA] transverse ligament of knee: a more or less distinct bundle of fibers in the knee joint, joining together the

Ligamentum *Continued*

anterior convex margin of the lateral meniscus and the anterior concave margin or anterior end of the medial meniscus; called also *l. transversum genuale.*

l. transver′sum pel′vis l. transversum perinei.

l. transver′sum perine′i [TA] transverse perineal ligament: a fibrous band in males that spans the subpubic angle just behind the deep dorsal vein of the penis, formed by thickening of the anterior boundary of the perineal membrane.

l. transver′sum sca′pulae infe′rius [TA] inferior transverse ligament of scapula: one of three intrinsic ligaments of the scapula, composed of more or less distinct fascial fibers that pass from the lateral border of the spine of the scapula to the adjacent margin of the glenoid cavity, thus converting the notch at the base of the spine into a foramen for the passage of the suprascapular vessels and nerves to the infraspinous fossa.

l. transver′sum sca′pulae supe′rius [TA] superior transverse ligament of scapula: one of three intrinsic ligaments of the scapula, a band of fibers that bridges the scapular notch, thus forming a foramen for the passage of the suprascapular nerve. One end is attached to the base of the coracoid process, the other end to the medial border of the scapular notch.

l. trapezoi′deum [TA] trapezoid ligament: a broad, flat band forming the anterolateral portion of the coracoclavicular ligament; it is attached inferiorly to the superior surface of the coracoid process of the scapula and superiorly to the oblique ridge on the inferior surface of the clavicle.

l. triangula′re dex′trum he′patis [TA] right triangular ligament of liver: the pointed right extremity of the coronary ligament of the liver, extending to attach to the diaphragm.

l. triangula′re sinis′trum he′patis [TA] left triangular ligament of liver: a triangular extension of the left extremity of the coronary ligament, which helps to attach the left liver to the diaphragm.

l. tuber′culi cos′tae l. costotransversarium laterale.

l. ulnocarpa′le palma′re [TA] palmar ulnocarpal ligament: bundles of fibers that pass from the styloid process of the ulna to the carpal bones.

l. umbilica′le media′num [TA] median umbilical ligament: a fibrous cord, the remains of the partially obliterated urachus, extending from the urinary bladder to the umbilicus; it is situated in and produces the median umbilical fold.

l. uteroova′ricum TA alternative for *ligamentum ovarii proprium.*

l. ve′nae ca′vae sinis′trae [TA] ligament of left vena cava: a remnant of the embryonic left duct of Cuvier, extending from the left intercostal vein to the oblique vein of left atrium; it is enclosed by the fold of left vena cava.

l. veno′sum [TA] venous ligament of liver: a fibrous cord, the remains of the fetal ductus venosus, lying in the fissure of the venous ligament.

l. ventricula′re l. vestibulare.

l. vestibula′re [TA] vestibular ligament: the membrane that extends from the thyroid cartilage in front to the anterolateral surface of the arytenoid cartilage behind; it lies within the vestibular fold, above the vocal ligament. Called also *l. ventriculare* and *ventricular ligament.*

l. voca′le [TA] vocal ligament: the elastic tissue membrane that extends from the thyroid cartilage in front to the vocal process of the arytenoid cartilage behind; it lies within the vocal fold, below the vestibular ligament.

---

li·gand (li′gand, lig′ənd) [L. *ligare* to tie or bind] 1. a molecule that binds to another molecule, used especially to refer to a small molecule that binds specifically to a larger molecule, e.g., an antigen binding to an antibody, a hormone or neurotransmitter binding to a receptor, or a substrate or allosteric effector binding to an enzyme. 2. a molecule that donates or accepts a pair of electrons to form a coordinate covalent bond with the central metal atom of a coordination complex.

li·gase (li′gās) [EC 6] a class of enzymes that catalyze the formation of a bond between two substrate molecules, coupled with the hydrolysis of a pyrophosphate bond in ATP or a similar energy donor. See also *synthetase.*

li·gate (li′gāt) to tie or bind with a ligature, or otherwise join.

li·ga·tion (li-ga′shən) [L. *ligatio*] 1. the application of a ligature. 2. the process of annealing or joining, such as the DNA ligase–catalyzed joining of two DNA fragments to form a recombinant molecule.

Barron l., elastic l., elastic band l., rubber band l. treatment of hemorrhoids by binding them at the base with rubber bands so that the distal portion sloughs away within several days.

teeth l. the binding together of teeth with wire, thread, or other material for their stabilization and immobilization as a method of tooth movement in orthodontic therapy or following traumatic injury.

tubal l. sterilization of the female by constricting, severing, or crushing the uterine tubes; constriction may be with an encircling plastic ring or other ligature.

lig·a·ture (lig′ə-chər) [L. *ligatura*] 1. any substance, such as surgical gut, cotton, silk, or wire, used to tie a vessel or strangulate a part. 2. see under *wire.*

Barron l., elastic l., elastic band l. rubber band l.

interlacing l., interlocking l. a continuous suture in which the loops interlock.

lateral l. a ligature so applied as to check, but not to interrupt, the distal blood flow.

occluding l. a ligature that occludes the blood supply to distal tissue.

provisional l. a ligature applied at the beginning of an operation but removed before its termination.

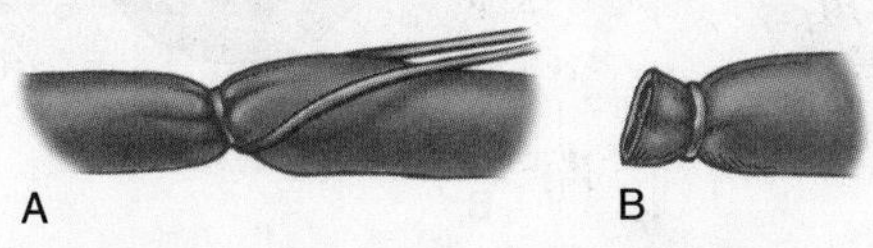

■ *(A),* Occluding ligature; *(B),* terminal ligature.

rubber band l. the rubber band used in rubber band ligation of hemorrhoids; called also *Barron l.*

soluble l. a ligature of prepared animal membrane which is subsequently absorbed, the time of absorption depending upon the method of preparation and the size of the ligature.

suboccluding l. a ligature that obstructs the main blood supply, but leaves unimpaired a portion of tissue capable of establishing capillary anastomosis.

terminal l. a ligature applied to the transected end of a vessel.

thread-elastic l. an elastic thread used for various forms of orthodontic therapy, such as assisting in eruption of impacted teeth, closing spaces, and rotating teeth.

ligg. ligaments; ligamenta.

light (līt) the electromagnetic radiation having a velocity of about 3×10^{10} cm (186,284 miles) per second, and the vibrations in space being at right angles to the direction of transmission. Frequently construed as limited to the range of wavelength between 390 and 770 nanometers, which provides the stimulus for the subjective sensation of sight, but sometimes considered as including part of the ultraviolet and infrared ranges as well.

actinic l. the portion of the spectrum comprising the light rays capable of producing chemical effects.

axial l., central l. light whose rays are parallel to each other and to the optic axis.

coherent l. light of a single wavelength, phase, and frequency that travels in intense, nearly perfect, parallel rays without appreciable divergence.

diffused l. light that has been scattered by reflection and refraction.

idioretinal l. sensation of light that occurs in the complete absence of the electromagnetic waves that ordinarily stimulate the sensation.

infrared l. see under *ray.*

intrinsic l. the dim light always present in the visual field.

l. minimum see under *minimum.*

monochromatic l. one of the colors of the spectrum into which light is divided by a prism; it is light of a single wavelength or a narrow range of wavelengths.

neon l. light from neon gas that has been excited by a high voltage discharge.

oblique l. the light that falls obliquely on a surface.

polarized l. light the vibrations of which are made over one plane or in circles or ellipses.

reflected l. light whose rays have been turned back from an illuminated surface.

refracted l. light whose rays have been bent out of their original course by passing through a transparent membrane.

transmitted l. light the rays of which have passed through an object.

Tyndall l. the light that is reflected or dispersed by particles suspended in a gas or liquid; see *Tyndall phenomenon*, under *phenomenon*.

ultraviolet l. see under *ray*.

white l. a mixture of all wavelengths of electromagnetic energy perceptible as light.

Wood l. filtered ultraviolet radiation from a mercury-vapor source, used in a Wood lamp.

light·en·ing (līt′ən-ing) the sensation of decreased abdominal distention produced by the descent of the uterus into the pelvic cavity, usually occurring from two to three weeks before labor begins.

Light·wood syndrome (līt′wood) [Reginald Cyril *Lightwood*, British pediatrician, 1898–1985] see under *syndrome*.

Lig·nac syndrome (le-nyahk′) [George Otto Emil *Lignac*, Dutch pediatrician, 1891–1954] 1. Fanconi syndrome (def. 2). 2. cystinosis.

Lig·nac-Fan·co·ni syndrome (le-nyahk′ fahn-ko′ne) [G.O.E. *Lignac*; Guido *Fanconi*, Swiss pediatrician, 1892–1979] 1. *Fanconi syndrome* (def. 2), see under *syndrome*. 2. cystinosis.

lig·ne·ous (lig′ne-əs) woody; having a wooden feeling.

lig·no·caine (lig′no-kān) BAN for *lidocaine*.

lig·no·ce·rate (lig″no-sēr′āt) a salt, ester, or anionic form of lignoceric acid.

lig·no·cer·ic ac·id (lig″no-sēr′ik) a saturated 24-carbon fatty acid occurring in sphingomyelin and as a minor constituent of many plant fats. See also table accompanying *fatty acid*.

lig·num (lig′nəm) gen. *lig′ni* [L.] wood.

l. sanc′tum, l. vi′tae the heartwood of *Guaiacum officinale* Linne or of *G. sanctum* Linne.

like·li·hood (līk′le-hood) a function of data that specifies, for each value of an unknown parameter describing a population distribution, the probability of observing the values sampled. See also *maximum likelihood estimate*, under *estimate*.

Lil·ey chart (lil′e) [Sir (Albert) William *Liley*, New Zealand perinatologist, 1929–1983] see under *chart*.

limb (lim) 1. one of the paired appendages of the body used in locomotion or grasping. The terms *arm* and *leg* are commonly used for the human upper and lower limbs, but in technical anatomical terminology those terms refer to only part of their respective limbs. In embryology, the skeleton of each limb is divided into four main parts: the *zonoskeleton*, comprising the scapula and clavicle (as a unit) and the hip bone; the *stylopodium*, comprising the humerus and femur; the *zygopodium*, comprising the radius and ulna and the tibia and fibula; and the *autopodium*, comprising the hand and the foot. Called also *member* and *extremity*. 2. a structure or part resembling an arm or leg.

anacrotic l. ascending l. (def. 2).

anterior l. of internal capsule crus anterius capsulae internae.

anterior l. of stapes crus anterius stapedis.

l's of antihelix crura anthelicis; see under *crus*.

ascending l. 1. the distal part of the loop of Henle (ansa nephroni); see under *ansa*. 2. the ascending portion of a tracing of the pulse wave obtained by the manometer or the sphygmograph; called also *anacrotic l.*

ascending l., thick tubulus rectus distalis.

ascending l., thin any part of the distal end of the thin tubule that is within the ascending limb.

catacrotic l. descending l. (def. 2).

descending l. 1. the proximal part of the loop of Henle (see *ansa nephroni* [TA]). 2. the descending portion of a tracing of the pulse wave obtained by the manometer or the sphygmograph. Called also *catacrotic l.*

hind l. the back leg (pelvic limb) of a quadruped. Cf. *forelimb*.

inferior l. of ansa cervicalis radix inferior ansae cervicalis.

long l. of incus crus longum incudis.

lower l. membrum inferius.

lower l., free the freely movable lower limb from the hip joint to the foot.

pectoral l. thoracic l.

pelvic l. the limb attached to the pelvic girdle; the lower limb of a human or a homologous structure such as a hind limb (q.v.) on another animal.

phantom l. a pseudesthesia after amputation of a limb, consisting of the sensation that the absent part is still present; there may be paresthesias, transient aches, or intermittent or continuous pain (phantom limb pain) perceived as originating in the absent limb. It was formerly thought to be purely psychological, but is now known to have a physical source in the brain.

posterior l. of internal capsule crus posterius capsulae internae.

posterior l. of stapes crus posterius stapedis.

residual l. stump.

retrolenticular l. of internal capsule, retrolentiform l. of internal capsule pars retrolentiformis capsulae internae.

short l. of incus crus breve incudis.

sublenticular l. of internal capsule, sublentiform l. of internal capsule pars sublentiformis capsulae internae.

superior l. of ansa cervicalis radix superior ansae cervicalis.

thoracic l. the limb attached to the thoracic girdle; the upper limb of a human or a homologous structure (wing, foreleg, etc.) in another animal.

upper l. membrum superius.

upper l., free the freely movable upper limb from the acromioclavicular joint to the hand.

lim·bal (lim′bəl) 1. limbic. 2. occurring at the junction of the cornea and conjunctiva.

Lim·berg flap (lim′berg) [Alexander A. *Limberg*, Russian plastic surgeon, 1894–1974] see under *flap*.

lim·ber·neck (lim′bər-nek) a type of botulism in birds, accompanied by flaccid paralysis.

lim·bi (lim′bi) [L.] genitive and plural of *limbus*.

lim·bic (lim′bik) 1. pertaining to a limbus, or margin; forming a border around something. Called also *limbal*. 2. pertaining to a certain region of the rhinencephalon; see *limbic system*, under *system*.

lim·bi·tis (lim-bi′tis) inflammation of the corneal limbus.

Lim·bi·trol (lim′bĭ-trol) trademark for a combination preparation of amitriptyline hydrochloride and chlordiazepoxide.

lim·bus (lim′bəs) gen. and pl. *lim′bi* [L.] a hem, fringe, or border of a structure. See also *border*, *labium*, and *margo*.

l. aceta′buli [TA] acetabular margin: the peripheral margin of the acetabulum to which the labrum acetabulare is attached; called also *acetabular border* or *rim* and *margo acetabuli* [TA alternative].

alveolar l. of mandible arcus alveolaris mandibulae.

alveolar l. of maxilla arcus alveolaris maxillae.

l. alveola′ris mandi′bulae arcus alveolaris mandibulae.

l. alveola′ris maxil′lae arcus alveolaris maxillae.

l. ante′rior pal′pebrae [TA] anterior palpebral margin: the rounded anterior edges of the free margin of the eyelids, from which the eyelashes arise.

l. of bony spiral lamina l. spiralis.

l. conjuncti′vae anulus conjunctivae.

l. cor′neae [TA], **corneal l.** the junctional region between the cornea and the sclera, marked on the outer surface of the eyeball by a slight furrow, the sulcus sclerae; called also *corneoscleral* or *sclerocorneal junction*.

l. fora′minis ova′lis the border of the foramen ovale cordis.

l. fos′sae ova′lis [TA] limbus of fossa ovalis: the prominent rounded margin of the fossa ovalis cordis; it represents the edge of the fetal septum secundum. Called also *annulus ovalis*, *Vieussens annulus*, and *isthmus*, *ring*, or *l. of Vieussens*.

l. la′minae spira′lis os′seae l. spiralis.

l. lu′teus re′tinae macula lutea.

l. membra′nae tym′pani 1. the thickened margin of the tympanic membrane attached to the tympanic sulcus. 2. anulus fibrocartilagineus membranae tympani.

l. palpebra′lis ante′rior l. anterior palpebrae.

l. palpebra′lis poste′rior l. posterior palpebrae.

l. poste′rior pal′pebrae [TA] posterior palpebral margin: the sharp posterior edges of the free margin of the eyelids, closely applied to the eyeball.

l. of sclera l. corneae.

spiral l. 1. labium limbi vestibulare. 2. l. spiralis.

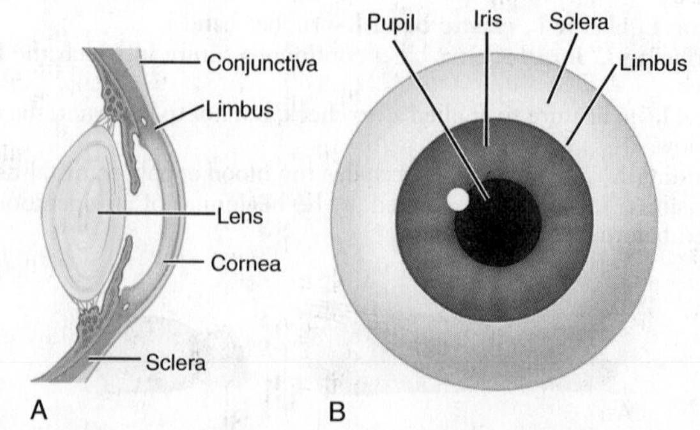

■ Limbus corneae, in a horizontal section *(A)* and anterior view *(B)* of the eye.

l. spira'lis [TA] spiral limbus: the thickened periosteum of the osseous spiral lamina at the attachment of the vestibular membrane. Called also *l. laminae spiralis osseae* and *l. of bony spiral lamina.*

l. of Vieussens l. fossae ovalis.

lime (līm) [L. *calx*] 1. calcium oxide. 2. [USP] a preparation of calcium oxide used as a pharmaceutical necessity. 3. *Citrus aurantifolia.* 4. the acid fruit of *C. aurantifolia,* whose juice contains ascorbic acid; used as an antiscorbutic.

barium hydroxide l. [USP] a mixture of barium hydroxide octahydrate and calcium hydroxide used as a carbon dioxide absorbent in the administration of anesthetic gases and oxygen.

chlorinated l. a bleaching agent and disinfectant.

slaked l. calcium hydroxide.

soda l. see under *soda.*

li•men (li'mən) pl. *li'mina* [L.] 1. threshold (def. 2). 2. in anatomy, the beginning point, boundary, or threshold of a structure.

l. in'sulae [TA] limen of insula: the point at which the cortex of the insula is continuous, on the inferior surface of the cerebral hemisphere, with the cortex of the frontal lobe. Called also *insular threshold.*

l. na'si [TA] the ridge at the junction of the lateral nasal cartilage and the lateral crus of the greater alar cartilage, marking the boundary between the vestibule of the nose and the nasal cavity proper. Called also *nasal valve.*

l. of twoness double point threshold.

li•mes (li'mēz) [L. "boundary"] limit; boundary.

l. dose see *L+ dose, L0 dose, Lf dose,* and *Lr dose,* under *dose.*

lim•i•na (lim'ĭ-nə) [L.] plural of *limen.*

lim•i•nal (lim'ĭ-nəl) [L. *limen* threshold] barely appreciable to the senses; pertaining to a threshold.

lim•i•nom•e•ter (lim"ĭ-nom'ə-tər) [*limen* + *-meter*] an instrument for measuring the strength of a stimulus applied over a tendon and determining the reflex threshold.

lim•it (lim'it) [L. *limes* boundary] a boundary, as one that confines.

assimilation l. saturation l.

audibility l's the extremes of frequency beyond which the human ear perceives no sound: lower limit, 8 Hz; upper, 20,000 Hz. Called also *range of audibility.*

confidence l's the endpoints or boundaries of a confidence interval, delineating the minimum and maximum values of the range expected to contain the parameter.

elastic l. the extent to which elastic material may be deformed without impairing its ability to return to original dimensions. Cf. *proportional l.*

l. of flocculation a term used in expressing the strength of toxin, toxoid, and antitoxin; see *Lf dose,* under *dose.*

Hayflick l. the maximum number of divisions a cell can undergo before cell death, between 50 and 60 in most human cells. Some malignant cell lines escape the limit and undergo immortalization (q.v.).

l. of perception the minimum visual angle below which perception is impossible: an object to be perceived must subtend a visual angle of four or five minutes, thus making its image on the retina about the size of a retinal cone of 3.3–3.6 micrometers in diameter.

proportional l. the highest amount of stress put on a material at which the proportion between stress and strain is linear; beyond this limit, deformation increases more rapidly and is permanent. Cf. *elastic l.*

quantum l. minimum wavelength.

saturation l. the amount of carbohydrate that an organism can metabolize without causing glycosuria; called also *assimilation l.*

lim•i•tans (lim'ĭ-tanz) [L.] limiting; see *membrana limitans.*

lim•i•ta•tion (lim"ĭ-ta'shən) circumscription; the act of limiting, or the state of being limited.

eccentric l. a circumscribed condition of the visual field, more pronounced at some parts of the periphery than at others.

chronic airflow l. chronic obstructive pulmonary disease.

lim•it dex•trin•ase (lim'it dek'strin-ās) oligo-1,6-glucosidase. See *α-dextrinase.*

lim•i•tro•phic (lim"ĭ-tro'fik) controlling nutrition.

Lim•na•tis (lim-na'tis) the land leeches, a genus of the family Gnathobdellidae.

L. nilo'tica a species of North Africa, Central Europe, and the Middle East, commonly used for drawing blood; if large numbers become lodged in the nasal passages, larynx or pharynx of mammals, they may cause anemia and asphyxia (see also *hirudiniasis*). Formerly called *Hirudo aegyptiaca.*

li•moph•thi•sis (li-mof'thĭ-sis) inanition.

li•mo•sis (li-mo'sis) abnormal hunger.

limp (limp) any gait that avoids weight bearing by one leg. Cf. *gait.*

lim•pet (lim'pət) any of various snaillike marine gastropods with cone-shaped shells, of the order Aspidobranchia, subclass Streptoneura.

keyhole l. any member of the genus *Fissurella,* marine gastropods.

lin•a•ma•rin (lin"ə-mah'rin) a toxic cyanogenetic glycoside found in flax *(Linum usitatissimum)* and lima beans *(Phaseolus limensis),* which can cause cyanide poisoning in animals that eat linseed, lima beans, or the plants in large quantities. Called also *phaseolunatin.*

Lin•co•cin (lin-ko'sin) trademark for a preparation of lincomycin hydrochloride.

lin•co•my•cin (lin"ko-mi'sin) a lincosamide antibiotic, effective primarily against gram-positive organisms, produced by a variant of *Streptomyces lincolnensis.*

l. hydrochloride [USP] the monohydrated monohydrochloride salt of lincomycin, used as an antibacterial, mainly in the treatment of infections due to susceptible strains of streptococci, pneumococci, and staphylococci; administered intramuscularly and intravenously.

lin•co•sa•mide (lin-ko'sə-mīd) any in a class of antibiotics originally derived from *Streptomyces lincolnensis,* including lincomycin and clindamycin.

lin•dane (lin'dān) [USP] the gamma isomer of benzene hexachloride, an insecticide more potent than chlorophenothane (DDT); it is used as a pediculicide and scabicide, applied topically to the skin. Called also *gamma benzene hexachloride.*

Lin•dau disease, tumor (lin'dou) [Arvid *Lindau,* Swedish pathologist, 1892–1958] see *von Hippel-Lindau disease,* under *disease,* and see *hemangioblastoma.*

Lin•dau-von Hip•pel disease (lin'dou fōn hip'əl) [Arvid *Lindau;* Eugen *von Hippel,* German ophthalmologist, 1867–1939] von Hippel-Lindau disease; see under *disease.*

Lind•bergh pump (lind'bərg) [Charles A. *Lindbergh,* American aviator, 1902–1974] see under *pump.*

lin•den (lin'dən) any tree of the genus *Tilia* (q.v.).

Lind•ner initial bodies (lind'nər) [Karl D. *Lindner,* Austrian ophthalmologist, 1883–1961] see under *body.*

line (līn) [L. *linea*] 1. a thin straight mark; a stripe, streak, or narrow ridge. 2. in anthropometry, such a mark (often imaginary) traced between different anatomical landmarks. See also *axis* and *plane* (def. 1).

Line

For descriptions of anatomical terms, see also under *linea.*

abdominal l. any imaginary line projected upon the surface of the abdomen, such as one indicating the boundary of a region.

absorption l's dark lines in the spectrum due to absorption of light by the substance (usually an incandescent gas or vapor) through which the light has passed. Cf. *absorption bands.*

accretion l's incremental l's.

acetabular l. a line following the slope of the acetabulum, used in radiographic assessment of the hip joint; with the Hilgenreiner line it forms the acetabular angle.

adrenal l. Sergent white adrenal l.

Aldrich-Mees l's Mees l's.

alveolobasilar l. a line from the basion to the upper alveolar limit.

angular l. collarette.

anococcygeal l., white corpus anococcygeum.

anocutaneous l. linea anocutanea.

anorectal l. junctio anorectalis.

anterior humeral l. on a lateral radiograph of the elbow, a line paralleling the anterior cortex of the humerus; in the normal elbow, it intersects the middle third or the junction of the anterior and middle thirds of the capitellum.

Line *Continued*

arcuate l. of ilium linea arcuata ossis ilii.
arcuate l. of occipital bone, external superior linea nuchalis superior.
arcuate l. of occipital bone, highest linea nuchalis suprema.
arcuate l. of occipital bone, inferior linea nuchalis inferior.
arcuate l. of occipital bone, superior linea nuchalis superior.
arcuate l. of occipital bone, supreme linea nuchalis suprema.
arcuate l. of pelvis linea terminalis pelvis.
arcuate l. of sheath of rectus abdominis muscle linea arcuata vaginae musculi recti abdominis.
auriculobregmatic l. a line from the auricular point to the bregma.
axillary l. linea axillaris.
axillary l., anterior linea axillaris anterior.
axillary l., median linea axillaris media.
axillary l., posterior linea axillaris posterior.
Baillarger external l. stria laminae granularis internae.
Baillarger inner l., Baillarger internal l. stria laminae pyramidalis internae.
Baillarger outer l. stria laminae granularis internae.
base l. 1. a line from the infraorbital ridge to the external acoustic meatus and the middle line of the occiput. 2. baseline.
base-apex l. a line perpendicular to the edge of a prism and bisecting the refracting angle of the prism.
basinasal l. a line from the basion to the nasion. Called also *nasobasal l.*
basiobregmatic l. a line from the basion to the bregma.
Baudelocque l. conjugata externa pelvis.
Beau l's transverse grooves in the nail plate caused by any of various systemic and local traumatic factors; they sometimes advance distally as the nail grows. Deep ones cause onychomadesis.
biauricular l. a line passing over the vertex from one acoustic meatus to the other.
biiliac l. a line joining the most prominent points of the two iliac crests.
bismuth l. a thin blue-black line in the marginal gingiva around the teeth, sometimes confined to the gingival papilla, observed in bismuth poisoning. See also *bismuth stomatitis*, under *stomatitis.*
Blaschko l's a developmental pattern of skin growth seen in functional X-chromosome mosaicism.
blood l. a line of direct descent through several generations.
blue l. see *bismuth l.* and *lead l.*
Blumensaat l. a linear shadow on the lateral radiograph of the knee, representing tangential bone in the intercondylar space.
Brödel bloodless l., Brödel white l. a longitudinal light-colored zone on the anterior surface of the kidney near the convex border, considered to be less vascularized than other areas because it is the border between two areas of arterial distribution.
Brücke l's broad bands alternating with Z bands in the fibrils of the striated muscles.
Bryant l. 1. the vertical side of the iliofemoral triangle. 2. a test line for detecting shortening of the femur.
Burton l. lead l.
calcification l's incremental l's.
Cantlie l. a line extending from the gallbladder to the left side of the inferior vena cava, representing a relatively bloodless area that can be considered to divide the liver into left and right parts.
cell l. a cell culture that is capable of being propagated indefinitely by serial subculture. Cf. *established cell l.*
cement l. a name applied to a line, visible in microscopic examination of bone in cross section, marking the boundary of an osteon (haversian system).
cervical l. an anatomical landmark determined by the junction of the enamel- and the cementum-covered portions of a tooth (the cemento-enamel junction); the dividing line between the crown and root portions of a tooth.
choroid l. taenia choroidea.
Clapton l. a green line on the gums seen in copper poisoning.
clavicular l. a line following the course of the clavicles.
cleavage l's linear clefts in the skin over many parts of the body, indicative of direction of the fibers. They correspond closely to the crease lines in the skin, and assume a characteristic pattern in each body part, although they can vary with body configuration. Called also *Langer* or *tension l's* and *lineae distractiones* [TA].
Conradi l. a line from the base of the xiphoid process to the point on the chest at which the apex beat is felt, indicating the upper limit of percussion dullness of the left liver.

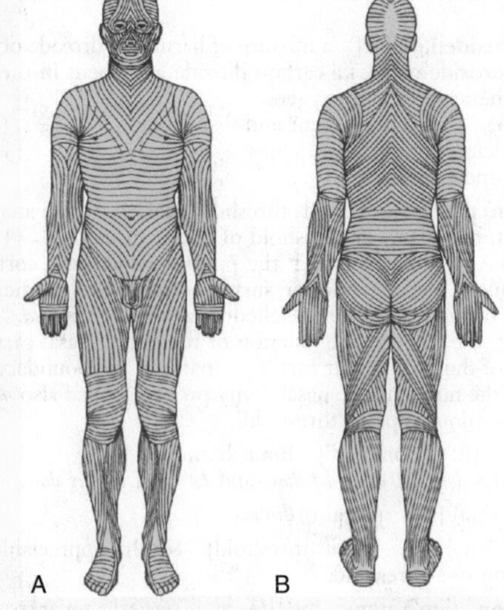

■ Anterior *(A)* and posterior *(B)* views of cleavage lines of the skin.

contour l's l's of Owen.
copper l. a greenish or red line at the border of the gums seen in copper poisoning.
Correra l. a line in the radiograph of the chest, around the outline of the thorax, and bounding the lung fields.
Corrigan l. a purplish line observed on the gums in copper poisoning.
costoarticular l. a line from the sternoclavicular joint to a point on the eleventh rib.
costoclavicular l. linea parasternalis.
costophrenic septal l's see *Kerley l's.*
cricoclavicular l. a line from the cricoid cartilage of the larynx to the point at which the superior projection of the anterior axillary line intersects the clavicle.
cruciate l. eminentia cruciformis.
curved l. of ilium linea arcuata ossis ilii.
curved l. of ilium, inferior linea glutea inferior.
curved l. of ilium, middle linea glutea anterior.
curved l. of ilium, superior linea glutea posterior.
curved l. of occipital bone, highest linea nuchalis suprema.
curved l. of occipital bone, inferior linea nuchalis inferior.
curved l. of occipital bone, superior linea nuchalis superior.
curved l. of occipital bone, supreme linea nuchalis suprema.
Czermak l's spatia interglobularia; see under *spatium.*
Daubenton l. see under *plane.*
Dennie-Morgan l. Morgan fold.
dentate l. linea anocutanea.
De Salle l. nasal l.
developmental l's see under *groove.*
Dobie l. Z band.
Donaldson l. an imaginary line drawn longitudinally through the lateral semicircular canal and bisecting the perpendicular dimension of the posterior canal; in most individuals it will pass just above the endolymphatic sac.
l. of Douglas linea arcuata vaginae musculi recti abdominis.
Duhot l. a line from the superior iliac spine to the apex of the sacrum.
dynamic l's lines in the facial skin that develop as a result of repetitious right-angled pull on the skin by the muscles of expression and are often considered signs of aging; types include laugh lines, glabellar lines, worry lines, and crow's feet.
Eberth l's microscopic broken or scalariform lines at the junction of the cardiac muscle cells.
l's of Ebner delicate lines indicating periods of rest between daily increments of dentin, which are visible on ground sections of a tooth. Called also *incremental l's of Ebner.*
ectental l. the line of junction between the ectoderm and endoderm.

embryonic l. the primitive streak in the center of the germinal area.
epiphyseal l. 1. linea epiphysialis. 2. a strip of lesser density apparent in the radiograph of a long bone, representing the linea epiphysialis.
established cell l. a cell line that has undergone transformation and become immortalized so that it is capable of indefinite proliferation in vitro.
l's of expression relaxed skin tension l's.
external l. of Baillarger stria laminae granularis internae.
facial l. a line connecting the nasion with the pogonion, gnathion, or menton. See also under *height.*
Farre white l. the boundary of the insertion of the mesovarium at the hilus of the ovary.
Feiss l. a line from the medial malleolus to the plantar surface of the first metatarsophalangeal joint.
l. of fixation a straight line extending through the center of rotation of the eye to the object of vision.
focal l., anterior a line whose direction is perpendicular to the meridian of greatest curvature of a refracting surface.
focal l., posterior a line whose direction is perpendicular to the meridian of least curvature of a refracting surface.
forehead l's worry l's.
Frommann l's transverse marks on the axon of a medullated nerve fiber, rendered visible by silver nitrate.
frown l's glabellar l's.
fulcrum l. an axis that extends from one abutment tooth to another, about which a partial denture can rotate during function.
fulcrum l., retentive an imaginary line connecting the retentive points of clasp arms on retaining teeth adjacent to mucosa-borne denture bases, around which a denture tends to rotate when subjected to such forces as the pull of sticky foods.
fulcrum l., stabilizing an imaginary line connecting occlusal rests, around which a denture will rotate under masticatory forces.
Futcher l. Voigt l.
genal l. one of the Jadelot lines, extending from the nasal line near the mouth toward the malar bone.
l. of Gennari the name given to the prominent external band of Baillarger *(stria laminae granularis internae)* in the region of the calcarine sulcus; because it is so highly visible, the region is called the *striate cortex.* Called also *band, stria,* or *stripe of Gennari.*
germ l. germline.
gingival l. 1. a line determined by the level to which the gingiva extends on a tooth; although it tends to follow the curvature of the cervical line, the two rarely coincide. See also *margo gingivalis.* Called also *gum l.* 2. any linear mark visible on the surface of the gingiva, such as a copper line or lead line.
glabellar l's a type of dynamic lines consisting of vertical creases in the skin of the forehead near the glabella that become more prominent when the person frowns. Called also *frown lines.*
gluteal l., anterior linea glutea anterior.
gluteal l., inferior linea glutea inferior.
gluteal l., posterior linea glutea posterior.
Granger l. a curved line seen in radiographs of skulls, indicating the position of the optic groove.
gum l. gingival l. (def. 1).

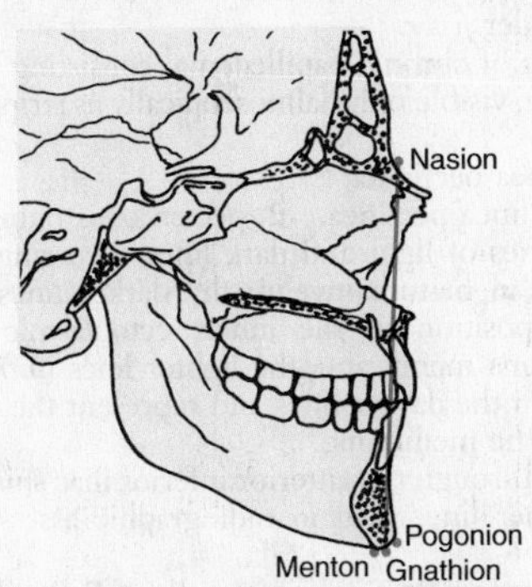

■ Facial line, shown as extending from nasion to gnathion.

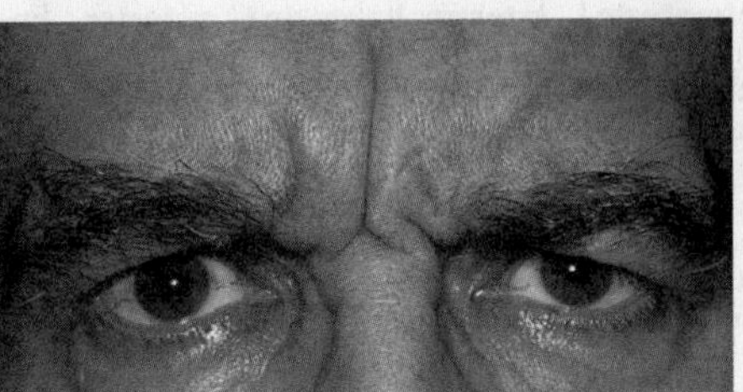
■ Glabellar lines.

Hampton l. a significant radiographic characteristic associated with the niche of the typical benign gastric ulcer in profile.
Harris l's lines of retarded growth seen radiographically at the epiphyses of long bones.
heave l. in an animal with heaves, a groove that appears along the costal arch during the forced contraction of abdominal muscles that follows the normal passive expiratory movement.
Helmholtz l. a line perpendicular to the plane of the axis of rotation of the eyes.
Hensen l. M band.
Hilgenreiner l. a line connecting the superior aspect of the triradiate cartilages of the acetabula, used in radiographic assessment of the hip joint.
Hilton white l. a narrow wavy zone in the anal canal, usually not visible macroscopically but palpable on digital examination, overlying the intersphincteric groove.
Holden l. a sulcus below the inguinal fold, crossing the capsule of the hip joint.
hot l. see under *H.*
Hudson l., Hudson-Stähli l. a linear horizontal brown mark located at about the junction of the middle and lower thirds of the cornea but not reaching the limbus, seen in the normal corneas of approximately 15 per cent of aged individuals. Called also *pigmented l. of the cornea, Stähli pigment l.* and *superficial l. of the cornea.*
Hueter l. a straight line connecting the medial epicondyle of the humerus with the top of the olecranon when the upper limb is in extension.
Hunter l. linea alba.
iliopectineal l. linea arcuata ossis ilii.
imbrication l's of cementum incremental l's of cementum.
imbrication l's of Pickerill lines formed by ends of rod bundles that overlie one another and are arranged in scalariform fashion on the surface of the crown of a tooth; seen on longitudinal sections of a tooth together with the incremental lines, but forming areas not completely contained in the enamel. Called also *Pickerill imbrication l's.* See also *incremental l's.*
incremental l's lines showing the successive layers deposited in a tissue. In the enamel, they are brown striations visible under transmitted light and colorless in reflected light. They may be observed under the microscope in longitudinal sections as oblique lines running inward from the surface and toward the root and in cross sections as rings similar to those in a tree trunk. Dry dentin often shows a series of somewhat parallel lines caused by imperfectly calcified dentin arranged in layers. Called also *accretion, calcification,* or *Retzius l's* and *Retzius parallel striae.* See also *l's of Ebner, imbrication l's of Pickerill,* and *neonatal l.*
incremental l's of cementum very fine dark lines present in longitudinal sections of a tooth, which follow the contour of the root and border with wider light bands, revealing the cyclic activity of cementogenesis. Called also *imbrication l's of cementum.*
incremental l's of Ebner l's of Ebner.
infracostal l. planum subcostale.
infrascapular l. a horizontal line at the level of the inferior angles of the scapulae.
inner l. of Baillarger stria laminae pyramidalis internae.
intercondylar l., intercondyloid l. linea intercondylaris.
intermediate l. of iliac crest linea intermedia cristae iliacae.
internal l. of Baillarger stria laminae pyramidalis internae.
interspinal l. planum interspinale.

Line *Continued*

intertrochanteric l., intertrochanteric l., anterior linea intertrochanterica.
intertrochanteric l., posterior crista intertrochanterica.
intertuberal l. a line drawn between the prominences of the frontal bone.
intertubercular l. planum intertuberculare.
intraperiod l's see *period l's.*
isoeffect l's in radiotherapy, lines on a rectangular graph representing doses of radiation having tumoricidal effects and those having complicating necrotic effects in normal tissues.
isoelectric l. the baseline of the electrocardiogram.
Jadelot l's the genal, labial, nasal, and oculozygomatic lines, lines of the face in young children, formerly thought to indicate specific types of disease. Called also *Jadelot furrows.*
l. of Kaes Kaes-Bekhterev layer.
Kerley l's horizontal linear densities 1 to 2.5 cm long on chest radiographs; they are arranged in stepladder fashion and are believed to represent widening of the interlobular septa, as by edema (in mitral stenosis) or fibrosis (in silicosis). When peripherally situated, particularly at the base of the lungs, they are called *Kerley B lines,* or *costophrenic septal lines.* When centrally situated, they are called *Kerley A lines.*
Kilian l. a prominent line on the promontory of the sacrum.
labial l. one of Jadelot lines, extending laterally from the angle of the mouth, thought to indicate disease of the lungs.
Langer l's cleavage l's.
laugh l's a type of dynamic lines consisting of creases in the facial skin near the mouth that become more prominent when the person laughs.
lead l. a gray or bluish black line at the gingival margin in lead poisoning, seen especially in patients with poor oral hygiene; it is similar to the bismuth line, but is somewhat more diffuse. Called also *blue l.* and *Burton l.* or *sign.*
lip l. a line at the level to which the margin of either lip extends on the teeth.
lip l., high the greatest height to which the maxillary lip is raised.
lip l., low the lowest position of the lower lip during the act of smiling or voluntary retraction.
lower lung l. a horizontal line in radiographs of the upper part of the abdomen, running from the lateral chest wall toward the first lumbar vertebra on each side, and representing the lower posterior boundary of the pleural cavity.
magnetic l's of force lines indicating direction of force in a magnetic field.
major dense l's, major period l's see *period l's.*
mammary l. see under *ridge.*
mammillary l. linea mammillaris.
median l. an imaginary vertical line on the body surface, dividing the surface equally into right and left sides.
median l., anterior linea mediana anterior.
median l., posterior linea mediana posterior.
medioclavicular l. linea medioclavicularis.
Mees l's single or multiple transverse white bands on the fingernails, signifying a change in composition of the nail, seen especially with arsenic poisoning and other trace element poisonings; they have also been reported in leprosy, septicemia, dissecting aortic aneurysm, and acute and chronic renal failure. Called also *Aldrich-Mees l's.*
Meyer l. the axial line of the big toe, which if extended passes through the center of the heel if shoes have never been worn.
midaxillary l. linea axillaris media.
midclavicular l. linea medioclavicularis.
middle l. of scrotum raphe scroti.
midspinal l. a perpendicular line down the middle of the vertebral column.
midsternal l. a line passing through the middle of the sternum from the cricoid cartilage to the xiphoid.
milk l. mammary ridge.
l's of minimal tension relaxed skin tension l's.
Monro l. a line from the umbilicus to the anterior superior iliac spine.
Monro-Richter l. a line from the umbilicus to the left anterior superior iliac spine.
Morgan l. see under *fold.*
Moyer l. a line from the middle of the body of the third sacral vertebra to a point midway between the anterior superior iliac spines.
mucogingival l. see under *junction.*
Muehrcke l's paired, transverse, white bands on the fingernails, signifying an underlying vascular abnormality, seen in various systemic disorders.
muscular l's of scapula lineae musculares scapulae.
mylohyoid l. of mandible, mylohyoidean l. linea mylohyoidea mandibulae.
nasal l. one of the Jadelot lines, extending from the ala nasi in a semicircle around the mouth.
nasobasal l. basinasal l.
nasobasilar l. a line through the basion and nasal point.
nasolabial l. one of the relaxed skin tension lines, extending from the ala nasi to the angle of the mouth along the nasolabial sulcus.
Nélaton l. a line from the anterior superior iliac spine to the most prominent part of the ischial tuberosity.
neonatal l. a line seen on longitudinal sections of a tooth, showing a demarcation between the structures present at birth and those deposited postnatally; in cross sections, the lines are seen as rings *(neonatal rings),* and their variations indicate adaptational changes in tooth formation. See also *l's of Owen.*
nigra l. linea nigra.
nipple l. linea mammillaris.
nuchal l., highest linea nuchalis suprema.
nuchal l., inferior linea nuchalis inferior.
nuchal l., median, nuchal l., middle crista occipitalis externa.
nuchal l., superior linea nuchalis superior.
nuchal l., supreme linea nuchalis suprema.
oblique l. a line that follows an oblique course; see terms beginning *linea obliqua.*
oblique l. of femur linea intertrochanterica.
oblique l. of mandible linea obliqua mandibulae.
oblique l. of mandible, internal linea mylohyoidea mandibulae.
oblique l. of thyroid cartilage linea obliqua cartilaginis thyroideae.
oblique l. of tibia linea musculi solei.
l. of occlusion the alignment of the occluding surfaces of the teeth in a horizontal plane.
oculozygomatic l. one of the Jadelot lines, extending outward from the medial canthus toward the zygoma; thought to indicate a disorder of the nervous system.
omphalospinous l. a line on the abdomen connecting the umbilicus and the anterior superior iliac spine; a guide to the location of the McBurney point.
orthostatic l's natural furrows on the neck, due to physiologic skin excess required at certain areas for the purpose of flexion and extension.
outer l. of Baillarger stria laminae granularis internae.
l's of Owen the sweeping bands seen on longitudinal section that outline the growth of the coronal or radicular dentin, representing a lag of several days between calcification phases, each lasting about 4 days. Called also *contour* or *Salter l's.*
papillary l. linea mammillaris.
pararectal l. linea pararectalis.
parasternal l. linea parasternalis.
paravertebral l. 1. linea paravertebralis. 2. linea vertebralis.
Pastia l's linear striations of hyperpigmentation, seen at the onset of the rash in scarlet fever; they are produced by confluent petechiae in body creases, such as the antecubital fossae and inguinal regions, and they persist after desquamation. Called also *Pastia sign.* See illustration at *scarlet fever,* under *fever.*
Paton l's a sign of chronic papilledema, consisting of thin choroidal folds on the retina, visible ophthalmoscopically as stripes adjacent to the optic disk.
pectinate l. linea pectinata.
pectineal l. 1. linea pectinea. 2. pecten ossis pubis.
period l's a series of light and dark lines occurring in a concentric, repeating pattern in mature myelin: the darker lines *(major dense l's)* represent the apposition of the inner, cytoplasmic surfaces of the Schwann cell plasma membrane; the lighter lines *(intraperiod l's)* bisect the spaces between the darker lines and represent the apposition of the outer surfaces of the membrane.
Perkin l. a line through the anterior inferior iliac spine, perpendicular to the Hilgenreiner line, used in radiographic assessment of the hip joint.
Pickerill imbrication l's imbrication l's of Pickerill.
pigmentary demarcation l. a border in the skin marking an abrupt transition between two areas of differing degrees of pigmentation.

Line *Continued*

pigmented l. of the cornea Hudson l.
Poirier l. a line running from the nasofrontal angle to a point just above the lambda.
popliteal l. of femur linea intercondylaris femoris.
popliteal l. of tibia linea musculi solei.
postaxillary l. linea axillaris posterior.
Poupart l. an imaginary line on the surface of the abdomen, passing perpendicularly through the midpoint of the inguinal ligament (Poupart ligament).
preaxillary l. linea axillaris anterior.
precentral l. a line on the head, extending from a point midway between the inion and glabella downward and forward.
primitive l. see under *streak.*
pupillary l. pupillary axis.
quadrate l. a slight ridge sometimes seen passing vertically downward from the middle of the intertrochanteric crest on the posterior surface of the femur.
radiocapitellar l. a line extending through the axis of the radial head and neck and normally intersecting the middle third of the capitellum in all radiographic views of the elbow.
recessional l's lines or markings on the teeth due to the recession, in the formative period of the teeth, of the soft tissue which gives place to the dentin.
regression l. a regression curve that is a straight line, indicating that two variables are in a simple direct or inverse arithmetic relationship. See also *regression* (def. 5).
Reid base l. base l. (def. 1).
relaxed skin tension l's the natural skin lines and creases of the face and neck, which are the preferred lines of incision in surgery of those areas; called also *l's of expression* and *l's of minimal tension.*
Retzius l's incremental l's.
Richter-Monro l. Monro-Richter l.
Robson l. an imaginary line drawn from the nipple to the umbilicus.
Rolando l. a line on the head marking the position of the central cerebral sulcus (fissure of Rolando) beneath.
Roser l. Nélaton l.
rough l. linea aspera.
Salter l's l's of Owen.
Sampaolesi l. a pigmented, wavy line seen on the cornea in early stages of exfoliation syndrome.
scapular l. linea scapularis.
Schoemaker l. a line connecting the point of the trochanter with the anterior superior iliac spine; the extension of this line normally runs superior to the umbilicus, but runs inferior to it when the trochanter is higher than normal.
segmental l's developmental grooves.
semicircular l's, supreme linea nuchalis suprema.
semicircular l. of Douglas linea arcuata vaginae musculi recti abdominis.
semicircular l. of frontal bone linea temporalis ossis frontalis.
semicircular l. of occipital bone, highest linea nuchalis suprema.
semicircular l. of occipital bone, middle linea nuchalis superior.
semicircular l. of occipital bone, superior linea nuchalis superior.
semicircular l. of parietal bone, inferior linea temporalis inferior ossis parietalis.
semicircular l. of parietal bone, superior linea temporalis superior ossis parietalis.
semilunar l. linea semilunaris.
Sergent white adrenal l. a white line on the abdomen invoked by drawing the fingernail across it; seen in cases of adrenocortical insufficiency; called also *adrenal l.* and *white adrenal l.*
Shenton l. a curved line seen in the radiograph of the normal hip joint, formed by the top of the obturator foramen.
l. of sight a straight line from the center of the pupil to the object viewed.
simian l. see under *crease.*
Skinner l. Shenton l.
soleal l. of tibia linea musculi solei.
Spieghel l., spigelian l., Spigelius l. linea semilunaris.
spiral l. of femur linea intertrochanterica.
Stähli l., Stähli pigment l. Hudson l.
sternal l., sternal l., lateral linea sternalis.
subcostal l. a transverse line on the surface of the abdomen at the level of the inferior edge of the tenth costal cartilage.
subscapular l's lineae musculares scapulae.
superficial l. of the cornea Hudson l.
supracondylar l., lateral linea supracondylaris lateralis.
supracondylar l., medial linea supracondylaris medialis.
supracrestal l., supracristal l. planum supracristale.
supraorbital l. a line across the forehead, just superior to the root of the external angular process of the frontal bone.
survey l. 1. the line indicating the height of a tooth after the cast has been positioned according to the chosen path of insertion. 2. a line produced on a cast of a tooth by a surveyor scriber, marking the greatest height of contour in relation to the chosen path of insertion of the restoration. 3. a line drawn on a tooth or teeth by means of a surveyor for the purpose of determining the positions of the various parts of a clasp or clasps. Called also *clasp guideline.*
suture l. 1. a line of juncture where parts of the body, internal or external, interface or converge. 2. système sécant.
Sydney l. a palmar crease correlated with an increased risk for leukemia and other malignancies in children; like the closely related simian crease, it appears in patients with Down syndrome.
sylvian l. a line on the head extending from the external angular process of the frontal bone to a point three-fourths of an inch inferior to the most prominent point of the parietal bone. It coincides with the direction of the Sylvius fissure (sulcus lateralis cerebri).
temporal l., inferior linea temporalis inferior ossis parietalis.
temporal l., superior linea temporalis superior ossis parietalis.
temporal l. of frontal bone linea temporalis ossis frontalis.
temporal l. of parietal bone, inferior linea temporalis inferior ossis parietalis.
temporal l. of parietal bone, superior linea temporalis superior ossis parietalis.
terminal l. of pelvis linea terminalis pelvis.
tension l's 1. cleavage l's. 2. relaxed skin tension l's.
Topinard l. a line from the glabella to the pogonion.
transverse l's of sacral bone, transverse l's of sacrum lineae transversae ossis sacri.
trapezoid l. linea trapezoidea.
Ullmann l. in cases of spondylolisthesis, a line extended upward at a right angle from the anterior edge of the first sacral vertebra to the superior surface of the sacrum will pass through the last lumbar vertebra.
umbilicoiliac l. a line from the umbilicus to the anterior superior iliac spine.
vertebral l. linea vertebralis.
vibrating l. an imaginary line across the palate that separates its immovable portion, the hard palate, from its movable portion, the soft palate.
Virchow l. a line from the nasion to the lambda.
visual l. see under *axis.*
Voigt l. a dorsoventral pigmentary demarcation line along the lateral edge of the biceps muscle; these usually appear in pairs, one on each arm, and are found in over 20 per cent of black-skinned people but only occasionally in others. Called also *Futcher l.*
Wagner l. a thin whitish line at the junction of the epiphysis and diaphysis of a bone, formed by preliminary calcification.
white l. linea alba.

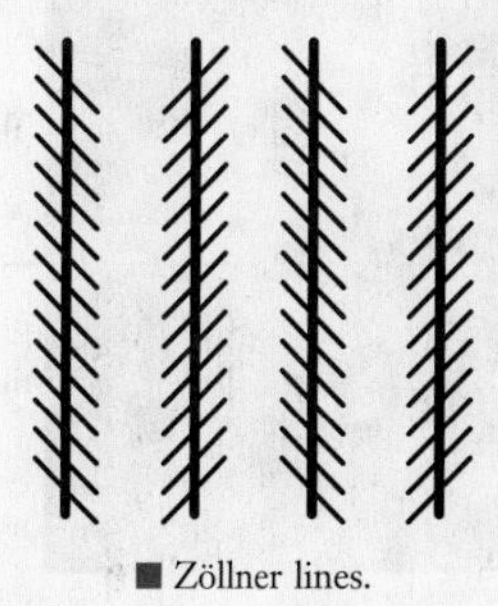

■ Zöllner lines.

Line *Continued*

white adrenal l. Sergent white adrenal l.
white l. of ischiococcygeal muscle corpus anococcygeum.
white l. of pharynx raphe pharyngis.
worry l's a type of dynamic lines consisting of horizontal lines across the forehead that become more prominent when the person is having stress or worry. Called also *forehead l's.*
Z l. Z band.
l's of Zahn laminations visible in antemortem blood clots, caused by alternating layers of gray-white fibrin interspersed with narrow zones of apparent red clot.
Zöllner l's an optical illusion in which long parallel lines seem to converge or diverge owing to their being crossed by a series of short lines parallel to one another but oblique to the long lines and at reverse oblique angles to both adjacent series of intersecting lines, as in a herringbone pattern.

li•nea (lin′e-ə) gen. and pl. *li′neae* [L.] 1. line. 2. [TA] in anatomical terminology, a general term for a streak or narrow ridge on the surface of a structure.

Linea

Descriptions are given on TA terms, and include anglicized names of specific lines.

l. al′ba [TA], **l. al′ba abdo′minis** white line: the tendinous median line on the anterior abdominal wall between the two rectus muscles, formed by the decussating fibers of the aponeuroses of the three flat abdominal muscles.
l. al′ba cervica′lis the blending of the fascial sheaths of the sternothyroid and sternohyoid muscles in the median plane of the neck.
li′neae albican′tes striae albae.
l. anocuta′nea [TA] anocutaneous line: the sinuous line marking the outer end of the pecten analis, the junction where the anal canal lined with stratified squamous epithelium ends and typical external skin begins. Called also *anal verge* and *dentate line.*
l. anorecta′lis junctio anorectalis.
l. arcua′ta os′sis i′lii [TA] arcuate line of ilium: the iliac portion of the terminal line, limiting the ala of the ilium inferiorly on its medial surface.
l. arcua′ta vagi′nae mus′culi rec′ti abdo′minis [TA] arcuate line of sheath of rectus abdominis muscle: a crescentic line marking the termination of the posterior layer of the sheath of the rectus abdominis muscle, just inferior to the level of the iliac crest; called also *semicircular line of Douglas.*
l. as′pera [TA] rough line: the broad, thickened ridge that forms the posterior border of the femur and has distinct lateral and medial lips.
li′neae atro′phicae striae distensae.
l. axilla′ris axillary line: an imaginary vertical line passing through the middle of the axilla, dividing the body into an anterior and a posterior portion.
l. axilla′ris ante′rior [TA] anterior axillary line: an imaginary vertical line continuing the line of the anterior axillary fold with the upper limb in the anatomical position; called also *l. preaxillaris* and *preaxillary line.*
l. axilla′ris me′dia [TA] median axillary line: an imaginary line halfway between the anterior axillary line and the posterior axillary line, passing through the apex of the axilla; called also *l. medio-axillaris* and *midaxillary line.*

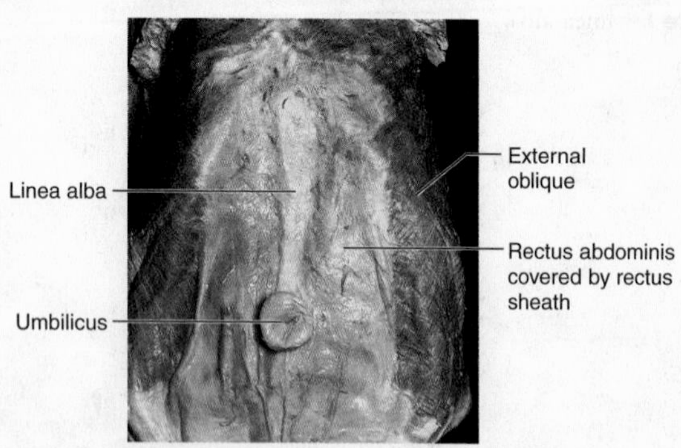

■ Linea alba in a dissection of the superficial muscles of the trunk.

l. axilla′ris poste′rior [TA] posterior axillary line: an imaginary vertical line continuing the line of the posterior axillary fold with the upper limb in the anatomical position; called also *l. postaxillaris* and *postaxillary line.*
li′neae distractio′nes [TA] cleavage lines.
l. epiphysia′lis [TA] epiphyseal line: a plane or plate on a long bone, visible as a line, marking the junction of the epiphysis and diaphysis.
l. glu′tea ante′rior [TA] anterior gluteal line: the middle of three rough curved lines on the gluteal surface of the ala of the ilium; it begins from the iliac crest about 2.5 cm posterior to the anterior superior iliac spine and arches more or less posteriorly to the greater sciatic notch.
l. glu′tea infe′rior [TA] inferior gluteal line: a rough curved line, often indistinct, on the gluteal surface of the ala of the ilium; it runs from the notch between the anterior superior and anterior inferior iliac spines posteriorly to the anterior part of the greater sciatic notch.
l. glu′tea poste′rior [TA] posterior gluteal line: a rough curved line on the gluteal surface of the ala of the ilium; it begins from the iliac crest about 5 cm anterior to the posterior superior iliac spine and runs downward to the greater sciatic notch.
l. iliopecti′nea l. arcuata ossis ilii.
l. innomina′ta l. terminalis pelvis.
l. intercondyla′ris [TA], **l. intercondyloi′dea** intercondylar line: a transverse ridge separating the floor of the intercondylar fossa from the popliteal surface of the femur and giving attachment to the posterior portion of the capsular ligament of the knee.
l. interme′dia cris′tae ili′acae [TA] intermediate line of iliac crest: the area between the inner and outer lips of the iliac crest.
l. intertrochante′rica [TA] intertrochanteric line: a line running obliquely downward and medially from the tubercle of the femur, winding around the medial side of the body of the bone.
l. intertrochante′rica poste′rior crista intertrochanterica.
l. mammilla′ris [TA] mammillary line: an imaginary vertical line on the anterior surface of the body, passing through the center of the nipple.
l. media′na ante′rior [TA] anterior median line: an imaginary vertical line on the anterior surface of the body, dividing the surface equally into right and left sides.
l. media′na poste′rior [TA] posterior median line: an imaginary vertical line on the posterior surface of the body, dividing the surface equally into right and left sides.
l. medio-axilla′ris l. axillaris media.
l. medioclavicula′ris [TA] midclavicular line: an imaginary vertical line on the anterior surface of the body, passing through the midpoint of the clavicle; called also *midclavicular plane.*
li′neae muscula′res sca′pulae muscular lines of scapula: low ridges on the costal surface of the scapula, marking the site of attachment of muscle fibers.
l. mus′culi so′lei [TA] soleal line of tibia: a line extending from the fibular facet downward and inward across the posterior surface of the tibia, giving attachment to fibers of the soleus muscle; called also *l. poplitea tibiae* and *popliteal line of tibia.*
l. mylohyoi′dea mandi′bulae [TA] mylohyoid line of mandible: a ridge on the inner surface of the mandible from the base of the

Linea *Continued*

symphysis to the ascending ramus behind the last molar tooth; it affords attachment to the mylohyoid muscle and superior constrictor of the pharynx.
l. ni′gra a name given the tendinous mesial line of the abdomen (linea alba) when it has become pigmented in pregnancy.
l. nu′chae infe′rior linea nuchalis inferior.
l. nu′chae supe′rior linea nuchalis superior.
l. nu′chae supre′ma linea nuchalis suprema.
l. nucha′lis infe′rior [TA] inferior nuchal line: the most inferior of the three nuchal lines found on the outer surface of the occipital bone, extending laterally from the middle of the external occipital crest to the jugular process.
l. nucha′lis supe′rior [TA] superior nuchal line: a curved line on the outer surface of the occipital bone, extending from the external occipital protuberance toward the lateral angle and giving attachment medially to the trapezius muscle and laterally to the sternocleidomastoid muscle.
l. nucha′lis supre′ma [TA] highest nuchal line: a sometimes indistinct line arching superiorly from the external occipital protuberance and running toward the lateral angle of the occipital bone: the epicranial aponeurosis attaches to it.
l. obli′qua cartila′ginis thyroi′deae [TA] oblique line of thyroid cartilage: a line on the external surface of the lamina of the thyroid cartilage, extending between the two thyroid tubercles.
l. obli′qua mandi′bulae [TA] oblique line of mandible: a ridge on the external surface of the body of the mandible extending from the mental tubercle to the anterior border of the ascending ramus on either side.
l. obli′qua ti′biae l. musculi solei.
l. pararecta′lis pararectal line: an imaginary line corresponding to the lateral margin of the rectus abdominis muscle.
l. parasterna′lis [TA] parasternal line: an imaginary line on the anterior surface of the body midway between the mammillary line and the border of the sternum.
l. paravertebra′lis 1. [TA] paravertebral line: an imaginary line corresponding to the transverse vertebral processes. 2. l. vertebralis.
l. pectina′ta [TA] pectinate line: the wavy line forming the interior end of the pecten analis just below the anorectal junction.
l. pecti′nea [TA] pectineal line: a line running down the posterior surface of the shaft of the femur, giving attachment to the pectineus muscle.
l. popli′tea ti′biae l. musculi solei.
l. postaxilla′ris l. axillaris posterior.
l. preaxilla′ris l. axillaris anterior.
l. scapula′ris [TA] scapular line: an imaginary vertical line on the posterior surface of the body, passing through the inferior angle of the scapula when it is in the anatomical position, i.e., at rest.

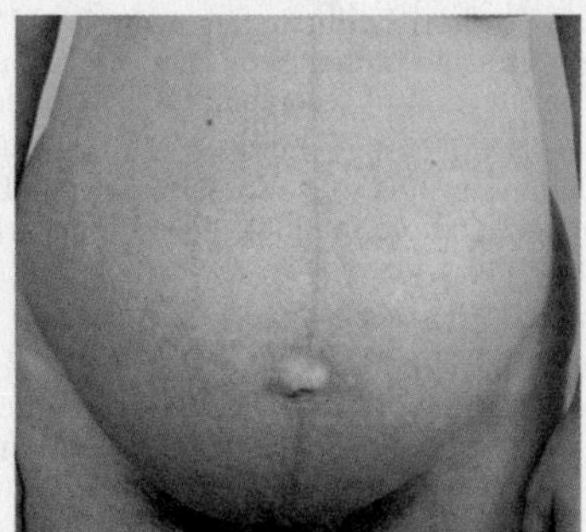

■ Linea nigra in the third trimester of pregnancy.

l. semiluna′ris [TA] semilunar line: a curved line along the lateral border of each rectus abdominis muscle, corresponding to the meeting of the aponeuroses of the internal oblique and transverse abdominal muscles; called also *Spieghel* or *Spigelius line.*
l. splen′dens the sheath for the anterior spinal artery formed by the pia mater in the fissura mediana anterior medullae spinalis.
l. sterna′lis [TA] sternal line: an imaginary vertical line on the anterior surface of the body, corresponding to the lateral border of the sternum.
l. supracondyla′ris latera′lis [TA] lateral supracondylar line: a slight ridge on the lower third of the posterior surface of the femur that is continuous above with the lateral lip of the linea aspera and descends to the lateral epicondyle.
l. supracondyla′ris media′lis [TA] medial supracondylar line: an indistinct ridge on the lower third of the posterior surface of the femur that is continuous above with the medial lip of the linea aspera, being interrupted at its upper end to allow passage of the femoral artery, and descends to the adductor tubercle.
l. tempora′lis infe′rior os′sis parieta′lis [TA] inferior temporal line of parietal bone: a curved line on the external surface of the parietal bone, marking the limit of attachment of the temporal muscle.

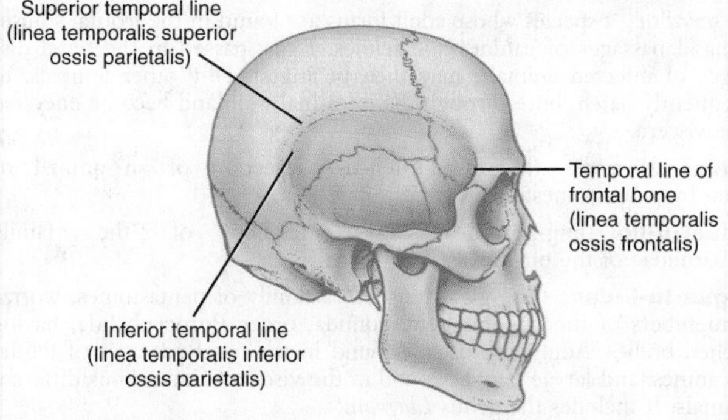

l. tempora′lis os′sis fronta′lis [TA] temporal line of frontal bone: a ridge extending superiorly and posteriorly from the zygomatic process of the frontal bone, dividing into superior and inferior parts that are continuous with corresponding lines on the parietal bone, and giving attachment to the temporal fascia.
l. tempora′lis supe′rior os′sis parieta′lis [TA] superior temporal line of parietal bone: a curved line on the external surface of the parietal bone, superior and parallel to the inferior temporal line, giving attachment to the temporal fascia.
l. termina′lis pel′vis [TA] terminal line of pelvis: a line on the inner surface of either pelvic bone, extending from the sacroiliac joint to the iliopubic eminence anteriorly, and marking the plane separating the false from the true pelvis.
li′neae transver′sae os′sis sa′cri [TA] transverse lines of sacrum: four transverse ridges on the pelvic surface of the sacrum, running between the pairs of pelvic sacral foramina, marking the positions of the former intervertebral disks.
l. trapezoi′dea [TA] trapezoid line: a ridge extending anterolaterally from the conoid tubercle on the inferior surface of the clavicle, giving attachment to the trapezoid portion of the coracoclavicular ligament.
l. vertebra′lis vertebral line: an imaginary vertical line halfway between the scapular and posterior median lines; called also *l. paravertebralis* and *paravertebral line.*

lin•eae (lin′e-e) [L.] genitive and plural of *linea.*

lin•e•age (lin′e-əj) [L. *linea* line] descent traced down from or back to a common ancestor.

cell l. the developmental history of cells as traced from the first division of the original cell or cells.

lin•e•ar (lin′e-ər) 1. pertaining to a line. 2. resembling a line.

lin•er (līn′ər) material applied to the inside of the walls of a cavity or container, for protection or insulation of the surface.

cavity l. an agent used to line a tooth cavity for protection of the pulp from irritation and for neutralization of the free acids of zinc phosphate or silicate cements.

Line•weav•er-Burk equation, plot (līn′wēv-ər burk′) [Hans *Lineweaver,* American chemist, born 1907; Dean *Burk,* American biochemist, 1904–1988] see under *equation* and *plot.*

li•nez•o•lid (lĭ-nez′o-lid) a synthetic antibacterial of the oxazolidinone class, effective against gram-positive organisms; used for the treatment of community-acquired and nosocomial pneumonia, skin and soft tissue infections, and bacteremia, administered orally or intravenously.

lin·gua (ling′gwə) gen. and pl. *lin′guae* [L.] [TA] the tongue: the movable, muscular organ on the floor of the mouth, subserving the special sense of taste and aiding in mastication, deglutition, and the articulation of sound; called also *glossa.* See *tongue.*

l. frena′ta ankyloglossia.
l. geogra′phica benign migratory glossitis.
l. ni′gra black hairy tongue.
l. plica′ta fissured tongue.
l. villo′sa ni′gra black hairy tongue.

lin·guae (ling′gwe) [L.] genitive and plural of *lingua.*

lin·gual (ling′gwəl) [L. *lingualis*] 1. pertaining to or toward the tongue; called also *glossal.* 2. in dental anatomy, pertaining to the tooth surface directed toward the tongue (oral cavity); see *facies lingualis dentis.* Called also *oral.*

lin·gua·le (ling-gwa′le) the point at the upper end of the symphysis of the lower jaw on its lingual surface.

lin·gua·lis (ling-gwa′lis) [L.] relating to the tongue.

lin·gual·ly (ling′gwə-le) toward the tongue.

Lin·guat·u·la (ling-gwă′chə-lə) a genus of wormlike members of the phylum Pentastomida, family Linguatulidae; their adult form inhabits the frontal, nasal, and maxillary sinuses of animals. Their larval form, known as *Porocephalus,* infests the digestive organs and lungs.

L. rhina′ria *L. serrata.*

L. serra′ta a species whose adult forms are found in the frontal sinuses and nasal passages of canines and felines. Eggs, passed in the nasal discharges of infected animals, may then be ingested by other animals, to subsequently hatch, bore through the intestinal wall, and become encysted in the viscera.

lin·guat·u·li·a·sis (ling-gwat″u-li′ə-sis) infection of an animal or human by pentastomes of the genus *Linguatula.*

lin·guat·u·lid (ling-gwat′u-lid) any member of the family Linguatulidae of the phylum Pentastomida.

Lin·gua·tu·li·dae (ling-gwə-tu′lĭ-de) a family of pentastomes, wormlike members of the phylum Pentastomida, order Porocephalida, having flattened bodies. Adults are usually found in the nasal passages of felines and canines, and larvae may be found in the viscera of numerous different mammals. It includes the genus *Linguatula.*

lin·guat·u·lo·sis (ling-gwat″u-lo′sis) linguatuliasis.

lin·gui·form (ling′gwĭ-form) tongue-shaped.

lin·gu·la (ling′gu-lə) gen. and pl. *lin′gulae* [L., dim. of *lingua*] a small tonguelike structure. **lin′gular** *adj*

l. cerebel′li [TA] lingula of cerebellum (I): the most anterior part of the anterior lobe of the cerebellum, where the superior medullary velum attaches. See also *cerebellum.*

l. of left lung l. pulmonis sinistri.

l. of lower jaw l. mandibulae.

l. mandi′bulae [TA] lingula of mandible: the sharp medial boundary of the mandibular foramen, to which is attached the sphenomandibular ligament.

l. pulmo′nis sinis′tri [TA] lingula of left lung: a projection from the lower portion of the upper lobe of the left lung, just beneath the cardiac notch, between the cardiac impression and the inferior margin.

l. of sphenoid, l. sphenoida′lis [TA] sphenoidal lingula: a slender ridge of bone on the lateral margin of the carotid sulcus, projecting posteriorly between the body and greater wing of the sphenoid bone.

lin·gu·lae (ling′gu-le) [L.] genitive and plural of *lingula.*

lin·gu·lec·to·my (ling″gu-lek′tə-me) excision of the lingula of the upper lobe of the left lung.

lingu(o)- [L. *lingua* tongue] a combining form denoting relationship to the tongue.

lin·guo·ax·i·al (ling″gwo-ak′se-əl) pertaining to or formed by the lingual and axial walls of a tooth cavity.

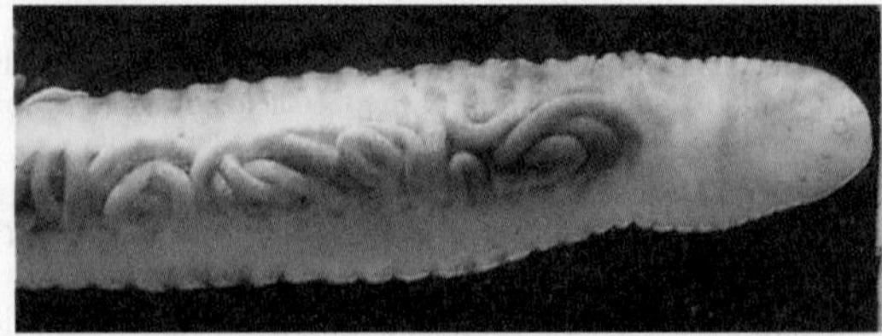

■ *Linguatula serrata;* cephalic third of an adult.

lin·guo·ax·io·gin·gi·val (ling″gwo-ak″se-o-jin′jĭ-vəl) pertaining to or formed by the lingual, axial, and gingival walls of a tooth cavity preparation.

lin·guo·cer·vi·cal (ling″gwo-sur′vĭ-kəl) 1. pertaining to the lingual surface of the neck of a tooth. 2. linguogingival.

lin·guo·cli·na·tion (ling″gwo-klĭ-na′shən) lingual inclination.

lin·guo·clu·sion (ling″gwo-kloo′zhən) lingual occlusion.

lin·guo·den·tal (ling″gwo-den′təl) 1. pertaining to the tongue and teeth. 2. dental (def. 2).

lin·guo·dis·tal (ling″gwo-dis′təl) pertaining to or formed by the lingual and distal surfaces of a tooth, or the lingual and distal walls of a tooth cavity.

lin·guo·gin·gi·val (ling″gwo-jin′ji-vəl) pertaining to the tongue and gingiva; pertaining to or formed by the lingual and gingival walls of a tooth cavity.

lin·guo·in·ci·sal (ling″gwo-in-si′zəl) pertaining to or formed by the lingual and incisal surfaces of a tooth.

lin·guo·me·si·al (ling″gwo-me′ze-əl) pertaining to or formed by the lingual and mesial surfaces of a tooth, or the lingual and mesial walls of a tooth cavity.

lin·guo·oc·clu·sal (ling″gwo-o-kloo′zəl) pertaining to or formed by the lingual and occlusal surfaces of a tooth.

lin·guo·pap·il·li·tis (ling″gwo-pap″ĭ-li′tis) [*linguo-* + *papillitis*] inflammation or ulceration of the papillae of the edges of the tongue.

lin·guo·place·ment (ling″gwo-plās′mənt) lingual placement.

lin·guo·pul·pal (ling″gwo-pul′pəl) pertaining to or formed by the lingual and pulpal walls of a tooth cavity.

lin·guo·ver·sion (ling″gwo-vur′zhən) displacement of a tooth lingually from the line of occlusion.

lin·i·ment (lin′ĭ-mənt) [L. *linimentum; linere* to smear] an oily liquid preparation to be used on the skin.

li·ni·tis (lĭ-ni′tis) [Gr. *linon* thread + *-itis*] inflammation of the gastric cellular tissue.

l. plas′tica diffuse fibrous proliferation of the submucous connective tissue of the stomach, resulting in thickening and fibrosis so that the organ is constricted, inelastic, and rigid (like a leather bottle). It is almost always a manifestation of gastric adenocarcinoma but is occasionally seen in certain benign conditions. Called also *Brinton disease, gastric sclerosis,* and *leather bottle stomach.*

link·age (lingk′əj) 1. the connection between different atoms in a chemical compound, or the symbol representing it in structural formulas; see also *bond.* 2. in genetics, the association of genes having loci on the same chromosome, which results in the tendency of a group of such nonallelic genes to be associated in inheritance.

sex l. the location of a gene responsible for a specific trait on a sex chromosome (usually the X chromosome), resulting in sexually dependent inheritance and expression of the trait.

linked (lingkt) in genetics, pertaining to linkage (def. 2).

link·er (ling′kər) a short synthetic fragment of DNA that contains one or more restriction sites and is used to splice together unrelated nucleic acid sequences in the production of recombinant DNA molecules.

lin·nae·an (lĭ-ne′ən) [Carolus *Linnaeus,* latinized form of Carl von Linné, Swedish botanist, 1707–1778] pertaining to Linnaeus or to the system of taxonomic classification of living organisms, which was originated by Linnaeus. Written also *linnean.*

lin·ne·an (lĭ-ne′ən) linnaean.

Lin·og·na·thus (lin-og′nə-thəs) a genus of sucking lice (order Anoplura). *L. peda′lis,* the foot louse, and *L. ovil′lus* infest sheep; *L. seto′sus* infests dogs and foxes; *L. stenop′sis,* the goat sucking louse, infests goats; *L. africa′nus* infests either sheep or goats; and *L. vitu′li,* the long-nosed cattle louse, infests cattle.

li·no·le·ate (lĭ-no′le-āt) a salt (soap), ester, or anionic form of linoleic acid.

ethyl l. a lipid found on the skin of warm-blooded animals, responsible for its passive water-holding capacity.

lin·o·le·ic ac·id (lin″o-le′ik) a polyunsaturated 18-carbon fatty acid occurring as a major constituent in many vegetable oils. It is an essential fatty acid used in the biosynthesis of prostaglandins and cell membranes. See also table at *fatty acid.*

lin·o·le·in (lin-o′le-in) [*linum* + *oleum*] a neutral fat from linseed oil; the triglyceride of linoleic acid.

li·no·le·nate (lĭ-no′lə-nāt) a salt, ester, or anionic form of linolenic acid.

lin·o·len·ic ac·id (lin″o-len′ik) a polyunsaturated 18-carbon fatty acid occurring in some fish oils (herring, menhaden) and many seed-derived oils.

It is an essential fatty acid that cannot be synthesized by animal tissues and must be obtained in the diet. It is used in the formation of prostaglandins.

lin·o·lic ac·id (lin-o′lik) linoleic acid.

lin·seed (lin′sēd) the dried ripe seed of *Linum usitatissimum*, used topically as a demulcent and emollient and orally as a laxative and as a source of the essential fatty acid α-linolenic acid. It may have antioxidant properties. The seeds are also processed to obtain linseed oil. Linseed contains the cyanogen linamarin, and cyanide poisoning may occur in animals eating large quantities of it. Called also *flaxseed*.

Lin·sto·wi·i·dae (lin-sto-wi′ĭ-de) a family of medium-sized or small tapeworms of the order Cyclophyllidea, subclass Cestoda, which parasitize birds, reptiles, and mammals. Medically important genera are *Oochoristica* and *Inermicapsifer*.

lint (lint) [L. *linteum*, from *linum*, flax] an absorbent surgical dressing material once made by scraping or picking apart old woven linen, but now a specially finished fabric woven in sheets; called also *patent l.* or *sheet l.*

lin·tin (lin′tin) a loose fabric of prepared absorbent cotton used in dressing wounds.

Lin·ton shunt (lin′tən) [Robert Ritchie *Linton*, Scottish-born American surgeon, 1900–1979] splenorenal shunt.

Li·num (li′num) a genus of flowering plants of the family Linaceae. *L. usitatis′simum* L. is the common flax plant, the source of linseed and linseed oil; it also contains the cyanogenetic compound linamarin, which can cause fatal cyanide poisoning in livestock.

lio- for words beginning thus, see also those beginning *leio-*.

Li·or·e·sal (li-or′ə-sal) trademark for preparations of baclofen.

li·o·thy·ro·nine (li″o-thi′ro-nēn) a synthetic pharmaceutical preparation of the levorotatory isomer of triiodothyronine; it is more potent and has a more rapid action than thyroxine.

l. I 125 liothyronine iodinated with ^{125}I; used for the in vitro determination of thyroid function.

l. sodium [USP] the monosodium salt of liothyronine, used as replacement therapy for hypothyroidism and in the prophylaxis and treatment of goiter and of thyroid carcinoma, administered orally or intravenously.

li·o·trix (li′o-triks) a mixture of liothyronine sodium and levothyroxine sodium in a ratio of 1:4 by weight; used as replacement therapy for hypothyroidism and in the prophylaxis and treatment of goiter and of thyroid carcinoma, administered orally.

lip (lip) 1. either the upper or lower fleshy margin of the mouth, together called *labia oris* [TA]. 2. a marginal part; called also *labium*.

anterior l. of cervix of uterus, anterior l. of external os of uterus labium anterius ostii uteri.

cleft l. a congenital cleft or defect in the upper lip, usually due to complete or partial failure of migration and deposit of mesoderm around or over the head in the embryo, with consequent failure of the maxillary prominence to merge with the merged medial nasal prominences. It may be unilateral, bilateral, or median, and may be accompanied by maxillary and palatal defects. Called also *cheiloschisis, harelip*, and *stomatoschisis*.

double l. redundancy of the submucous tissue and mucous membrane of the lip on either side of the median line.

external l. of linea aspera of femur labium laterale lineae asperae femoris.

fibrocartilaginous l. of acetabulum labrum acetabulare.

greater l. of pudendum labium majus pudendi.

Hapsburg l. a thick overdeveloped lower lip that often accompanies a Hapsburg jaw.

ileocecal l. of ileal orifice labrum ileocaecalis ostii ilealis.

ileocolic l. of ileal orifice labrum ileocolicum ostii ilealis.

inferior l. labium inferius oris.

inferior l. of ileal orifice labrum ileocaecalis ostii ilealis.

inferior l. of ileocecal valve the inferior of the two lips of the ileocecal valve of a cadaver, corresponding to the *labrum inferius ostii ilealis* in a living person.

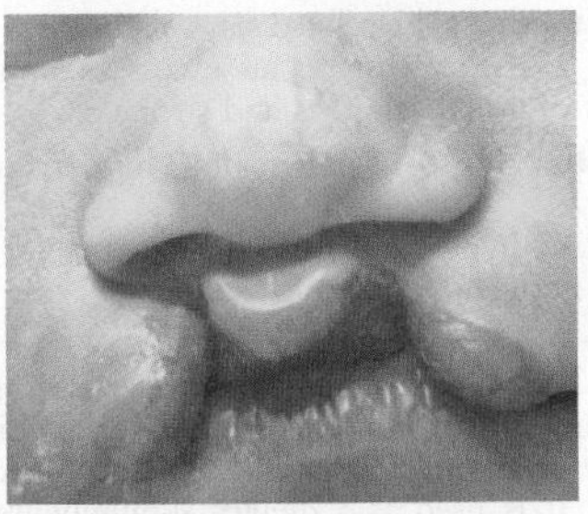

■ Bilateral cleft lip.

internal l. of iliac crest labium internum cristae iliacae.

lateral l. of intertubercular sulcus crista tuberculi majoris.

lateral l. of linea aspera of femur labium laterale lineae asperae femoris.

lesser l. of pudendum labium minus pudendi.

lower l. labium inferius oris.

medial l. of intertubercular sulcus crista tuberculi minoris.

medial l. of linea aspera of femur labium mediale lineae asperae femoris.

posterior l. of cervix of uterus, posterior l. of external os of uterus labium posterius ostii uteri.

posterior l. of pharyngeal opening of auditory tube labium posterius ostii pharyngei tubae auditivae.

rhombic l. the lateral boundary of the rhombencephalon during embryonic life.

superior l. labium superius oris.

superior l. of ileal orifice labrum ileocolicum ostii ilealis.

superior l. of ileocecal valve the superior of the two lips of the ileocecal valve of a cadaver, corresponding to the labrum superius ostii ilealis in a living person.

tympanic l. of limbus labium tympanicum limbi.

upper l. labium superius oris.

vestibular l. of limbus labium vestibulare limbi.

lip·ac·i·de·mia (lip″as-ĭ-de′me-ə) [*lip-* + *acid* + *-emia*] the presence of excessive fatty acids in the blood, as in diabetes mellitus.

lip·ac·i·du·ria (lip″as-ĭ-du′re-ə) [*lip-* + *acid* + *-uria*] the presence of fatty acids in the urine.

lip·a·ro·dysp·nea (lip″ə-ro-disp′ne-ə) the dyspnea of the obese.

lip·ase (lip′ās, li′pās) 1. triacylglycerol lipase. 2. any enzyme that hydrolytically cleaves a fatty acid anion from a triglyceride or phospholipid.

acid l. see under *A*.

hepatic l. a lipase acting at the endothelial surfaces of hepatic tissues (cf. *lipoprotein lipase*) to regulate the levels of plasma lipids. It participates in lipolysis of very-low-density and intermediate-density lipoproteins in the end stages of low-density lipoprotein formation and also in hydrolysis of phospholipids and triglycerides in the metabolism of high-density lipoproteins.

lingual l. a lipase secreted in the mouth and most active in the stomach; it degrades medium- to short-chain triglycerides and appears to prepare ingested lipids for intestinal digestion by facilitating their solubilization.

pancreatic l. the triacylglycerol lipase secreted by the pancreas; it is the major intestinal lipase, digesting ingested fats to fatty acids and monoglycerides. The enzyme requires bile salts and colipase for activity.

lip·as·emia (lip″ās-e′me-ah) hyperlipasemia.

lip·as·uria (lip″ās-u′re-ə) the presence of lipase in the urine, such as in hyperlipasemia.

lip·ec·to·my (lĭ-pek′tə-me) [*lip-* + *-ectomy*] excision of a localized area of subcutaneous adipose tissue, as from the abdominal wall.

suction l., suction-assisted l. surgical removal of localized fat deposits via high-pressure vacuum, which is applied by means of a suction curet or cannula inserted subdermally through one or more small incisions. Called also *liposuction*.

lip·ede·ma (lip″ə-de′mə) [*lip-* + *edema*] an accumulation of excess fat and fluid in subcutaneous tissues.

lip·emia (lĭ-pe′me-ə) hyperlipidemia. **lipe′mic** *adj*

alimentary l. hyperlipidemia after eating, such as carbohydrate-induced, familial fat-induced, and combined fat- and carbohydrate-induced hyperlipemia.

diabetic l. a rare complication of uncontrolled diabetes mellitus consisting of massive increases in plasma triglyceride levels after ingestion of lipid-rich foods, due to deficient metabolism of low-density lipoproteins.

l. retina′lis a milky appearance of the veins and arteries of the retina, occurring when the lipids of the blood exceed 5%, as in diabetes mellitus and leukemia.

lip·id (lip′id) any of a heterogeneous group of fats and fatlike substances characterized by being water-insoluble and being extractable by nonpolar (or fat) solvents such as alcohol, ether, chloroform, benzene, etc. All contain as a major constituent aliphatic hydrocarbons. The lipids, which are easily stored in the body, serve as a source of fuel, are an important constituent of cell structure, and serve other biological functions. Lipids may be considered to include fatty acids, neutral fats, waxes, and steroids. *Compound lipids* comprise the glycolipids, lipoproteins, and phospholipids.

l. A the glycolipid component of lipopolysaccharide (q.v.) that is responsible for its endotoxic activity.

lip·i·de·mia (lip″ĭ-de′me-ə) hyperlipidemia.

lip·id·ic (lip-id′ik) pertaining to or containing lipids.

lip·i·dol·o·gist (lip″ĭ-dol′ə-jist) a specialist in lipidology.

lip•i•dol•o•gy (lip″ĭ-dol′ə-je) the study of lipids.

lip•i•dol•y•sis (lip″ĭ-dol′ĭ-sis) the breaking down of lipids; see also *lipolysis.*

lip•i•do•lyt•ic (lip″ĭ-do-lit′ik) 1. pertaining to or characterized by lipidolysis. 2. causing lipidolysis.

lip•i•dome (lip′ĭ-dōm) [*lipid* + *-ome*] the entire lipid profile of an organism, tissue type, or cell, under particular conditions.

lip•i•do•mics (lip″ĭ-do′miks) the quantitative and qualitative study of the lipids in cells and determination of the molecular mechanisms through which they facilitate cellular function.

lip•i•do•sis (lip″ĭ-do′sis) pl. *lipido′ses.* 1. abnormal accumulations of lipids in the tissues; see also *fatty change*, under *change.* 2. a term for several of the lysosomal storage diseases in which there is an abnormal accumulation of lipids in the reticuloendothelial cells. Called also *lipid storage disease.*
galactosylceramide l. Krabbe disease.
glucosylceramide l. Gaucher disease.
hepatic l. fatty liver.
sphingomyelin l. Niemann-Pick disease.
sulfatide l. metachromatic leukodystrophy.

lip•i•du•ria (lip″ĭ-du′re-ə) the presence of oil or fat in the urine, such as in the nephrotic syndrome or after skeletal trauma; called also *lipuria.*

Lip•i•tor (lip′ĭ-tor) trademark for a preparation of atorvastatin calcium.

lip(o)- [Gr. *lipos* fat] a combining form denoting relationship to fat or to lipids.

lipo•ad•e•no•ma (lip″o-ad″ə-no′mə) a fatty parenchymal cell tumor, especially the parathyroid.

lipo•am•ide (lip″o-am′īd) lipoic acid in amide linkage with lysine side chains of enzymes of the α-ketoglutarate dehydrogenase, branched-chain α-keto acid dehydrogenase, and pyruvate dehydrogenase complexes (q.v.). Its reactive disulfide group and long, flexible chain enable it to transfer intermediates among the enzymes of each complex.

lipo•am•ide de•hy•dro•gen•ase (lip″o-am′īd de-hi′dro-jən″ās) erroneous name for *dihydrolipoyl dehydrogenase.*

lipo•ar•thri•tis (lip″o-ahr-thri′tis) [*lipo-* + *arthritis*] inflammation of the fatty tissue of a joint.

lipo•at•ro•phy (lip″o-at′ro-fe) [*lipo-* + *atrophy*] 1. atrophy of subcutaneous fat. 2. lipodystrophy.
insulin l. localized lipoatrophy occurring at the site of repeated insulin injections.

lipo•blast (lip′o-blast) [*lipo-* + *-blast*] a specialized connective tissue cell that develops into a fat cell. **lipoblas′tic** *adj*

lipo•blas•to•ma (lip″o-blas-to′mə) [*lipo-* + *blastoma*] a benign fatty tumor composed of a mixture of embryonal lipoblastic cells in a myxoid stroma and mature fat cells; the tumor cells are arranged in lobules and occur most often in children.

lipo•blas•to•ma•to•sis (lip″o-blas-to″mə-to′sis) the occurrence of multiple lipoblastomas locally diffused but without a tendency to metastasize.

lipo•car•di•ac (lip″o-kahr′de-ak) [*lipo-* + *cardiac*] relating to a fatty heart.

lipo•cata•bol•ic (lip″o-cat″ə-bol′ik) pertaining to or effecting the destructive metabolism of fat.

lipo•cele (lip′o-sēl) fat hernia.

lipo•cer•a•tous (lip″o-ser′ə-təs) adipoceratous.

lipo•cere (lip′o-sēr) [*lipo-* + *cera*] adipocere.

lipo•chon•dro•ma (lip″o-kon-dro′mə) chondrolipoma.

lipo•chrome (lip′o-krōm) [*lipo-* + *-chrome*] any of a group of fat-soluble pigments, including carotene, lutein, lycopene, and xanthophyll, that are synthesized in plants and on ingestion impart a yellow, yellow-orange, or orange-red color to lipid-containing tissues. Called also *carotenoid*, *lipochrome pigment*, *lipofuscin*, and *wear and tear pigment.*

lipo•chro•me•mia (lip″o-kro-me′me-ə) the presence of an excess of lipochrome in the blood.

lip•o•chro•mo•gen (lip″o-kro′mə-jən) a substance that becomes converted into lipochrome.

lip•o•cor•tin (lip″o-kor′tin) original name for certain proteins now determined to be members of the class of annexins.

lipo•cy•a•nine (lip″o-si′ə-nēn) [*lipo-* + Gr. *kyanos* blue] a blue pigment resulting from the action of strong sulfuric acid on lipochrome.

lipo•cyte (lip′o-sīt) 1. fat cell. 2. hepatic stellate cell.

lip•o•der•ma•to•scle•ro•sis (lip″o-dur″mə-to-sclə-ro′sis) a type of predominantly lobular panniculitis of the lower legs consisting of indurated erythema with scleroderma; it may be either acute and inflammatory or chronic and fibrotic. It primarily affects middle-aged or older women. Called also *hypodermitis sclerodermiformis* and *sclerosing panniculitis.*

lipo•dys•tro•phy (lip″o-dis′trə-fe) [*lipo-* + *dystrophy*] 1. any disturbance of fat metabolism. 2. a group of conditions due to defective metabolism of fat, resulting in the absence of subcutaneous fat; they may be congenital or acquired and partial or total. Called also *lipoatrophy.*
congenital generalized l., congenital progressive l. total l.
generalized l. total l.
intestinal l. Whipple disease.
mesenteric l. see under *panniculitis.*
partial l. a condition usually seen in girls younger than age 10, characterized by a symmetrical loss of subcutaneous fat, generally beginning on the face and gradually extending to the chest, neck, back, and upper extremities, giving the lower part of the body an appearance of adiposity of the buttocks, thighs, and legs. Some affected patients develop insulin-resistant diabetes mellitus, hypertriglyceridemia, and renal disease. Called also *Barraquer* or *Simons disease* and *progressive* or *progressive partial l.*
progressive l. partial l.
progressive congenital l. total l.
progressive partial l. partial l.
total l. a rare, autosomal recessive disorder seen mainly in infant girls, characterized by generalized loss of subcutaneous and extracutaneous adipose tissue with hepatomegaly, hypoglycemia and insulin-resistant nonketotic diabetes, hyperlipemia, elevation of the basal metabolic rate, accelerated somatic growth, advanced bone age, acanthosis nigricans, and hirsutism. Called also *congenital generalized* or *generalized l.*, *Berardinelli-Seip syndrome*, and *lipoatrophic diabetes.*

lipo•fec•tion (lip′o-fek″shən) transfection in which cationic liposomes are the vector for delivery of the nucleic acid, protein, or other negatively charged molecule into the cytoplasm of the foreign cell.

li•pof•er•ous (lĭ-pof′ər-əs) [*lipo-* + *-ferous*] 1. carrying fat. 2. sudanophil.

lipo•fi•bro•ma (lip″o-fi-bro′mə) fibrolipoma.

lipo•fus•cin (lip″o-fu′sin) 1. a yellow to brown, granular, iron-negative lipid pigment found particularly in muscle, heart, liver, and nerve cells undergoing slow, regressive change and accumulating in lysosomes with age, being the product of oxidation and polymerization of the membrane lipids of autophagocytosed organelles. 2. lipochrome.

lipo•fus•cin•o•sis (lip″o-fu″sin-o′sis) any disorder due to abnormal storage of lipofuscins.
ceroid-l., neuronal ceroid-l. a term for several genetic lipidoses of diverse biochemical and clinical characteristics, all characterized by progressive neurodegeneration, loss of vision, and a fatal course; the *infantile type* is Haltia-Santavuori disease; the *late infantile type* is Jansky-Bielschowsky disease; the *juvenile type* is Vogt-Spielmeyer disease; and the *adult type* is Kufs disease.

lipo•gen•e•sis (lip″o-gen′ə-sis) [*lipo-* + *genesis*] the formation of fat; the transformation of nonfat food materials into body fat.

lipo•ge•net•ic (lip″o-jə-net′ik) lipogenic.

lip•o•gen•ic (lip″o-jen′ik) forming, producing, or caused by fat.

li•pog•e•nous (li-poj′ə-nəs) lipogenic.

lipo•gran•u•lo•ma (lip″o-gran″u-lo′mə) [*lipo-* + *granuloma*] a nodule of lipoid material; a foreign body inflammation of adipose tissue containing granulation tissue and oil cysts.

lipo•gran•u•lo•ma•to•sis (lip″o-gran″u-lo-mə-to′sis) a condition of faulty lipid metabolism in which yellow nodules of lipoid matter are deposited in the skin and mucosae, giving rise to granulomatous reactions.
Farber l. see under *disease.*

lipo•hem•ar•thro•sis (lip″o-hem″ahr-thro′sis) [*lipo-* + *hemarthrosis*] the presence of fat-containing blood in a joint, with intra-articular fracture.

lipo•his•tio•di•er•e•sis (lip″o-his″te-o-di-er′ə-sis) [*lipo-* + *histio-* + *dieresis*] disappearance of stored fat from body tissue.

lipo•hy•a•lin (lip″o-hi′ə-lin) the lipid deposited in the beta cells of the pancreas in association with hyalinization in diabetes.

lipo•hy•a•lin•o•sis (lip″o-hi″ə-lin-o′sis) pathologic changes in the intima of cerebral arteries owing to an excess of lipids in the blood; it may be a precursor of atherosclerosis and stroke.

lipo•hy•per•tro•phy (lip″o-hi-pur′trə-fe) hypertrophy of subcutaneous fat.
insulin l. localized hypertrophy of subcutaneous fat at insulin injection sites caused by the lipogenic effect of insulin.

lipo•ic ac•id (lip-o′ik) a necessary cofactor of the pyruvate dehydrogenase, branched-chain α-keto acid dehydrogenase, and α-ketoglutarate dehydrogenase complexes; it contains a reactive disulfide group that can bind and transfer reaction intermediates. In the enzyme complexes it occurs as lipoamide (q.v.). It is used as a dietary supplement for its antioxidant properties. Called also *α-lipoic acid.*

lip•oid (lip′oid) [*lipo-* + Gr. *eidos* form] fatlike; resembling fat; called also *adipoid.*

li•pol•y•sis (lĭ-pol′ə-sis) [*lipo-* + *-lysis*] the decomposition or splitting up of fat; see also *lipidolysis.*

lip•o•lyt•ic (lip″o-lit′ik) 1. pertaining to or characterized by lipolysis. 2. causing lipolysis.

lip•o•ma (lip-o′mə) [*lip-* + *-oma*] a benign, soft, rubbery, encapsulated tumor of adipose tissue, usually composed of mature fat cells; it generally occurs as a solitary lesion in the subcutaneous tissue of the trunk, nucha, or forearms but may occur in deeper soft tissues. **lipo′matous** *adj*

l. annula′re col′li multiple symmetric lipomatosis.

l. arbores′cens an intra-articular tumor usually occurring as a solitary lesion in the knee; it is characterized by numerous swollen treelike synovial villous projections of fatty tissue, and may arise de novo or be associated with disorders such as degenerative joint disease, chronic rheumatoid arthritis, or previous traumatic injury.

l. capsula′re a fatty tumor due to increase of the fat in the capsule of an organ.

l. caverno′sum angiolipoma.

chondroid l. an uncommon benign fatty neoplasm occurring as a well-circumscribed, yellow, sometimes encapsulated, slowly growing mass, typically affecting middle-aged adults, usually women, and most often involving the proximal limbs or the limb girdles; it is characterized by a lobular growth pattern and has large vacuolated cells resembling lipoblasts.

diffuse l. diffuse lipomatosis.

epidural l. an intraspinal lipoma on or outside the spinal dura mater in the thoracic or lumbar region, often causing spinal cord compression; Cushing disease and administration of steroids are common causes.

l. fibro′sum fibrolipoma.

intermuscular l. a slow-growing, infiltrating lesion composed of mature fat cells, occurring in the deeper soft tissues between large muscle groups, predominantly those of the thighs, shoulders, or upper limbs of middle-aged to older adults.

intradural l. an intraspinal lipoma with components within or beneath the dura mater of the spine or sacrum.

intramedullary l. an intraspinal lipoma within the spinal cord.

intramuscular l. a lesion similar to intermuscular lipoma, but occurring within muscle.

intraspinal l. a lipoma within the spinal canal; it may exist entirely within the canal or it may protrude and form part of a lipomyelomeningocele.

l. myxomato′des myxolipoma.

l. ossi′ficans, ossifying l. osteolipoma.

pleomorphic l. a circumscribed, subcutaneous, painless lesion occurring in older adults, particularly men, characterized by mononuclear cells with pleomorphic nuclei, hyperchromatic multinucleated cells, mature fat cells, and thick bands of birefringent collagen.

l. sarcomato′des liposarcoma.

spindle cell l. a rare, benign, circumscribed, painless lesion in the dermis or subcutaneous tissue of the posterior neck or shoulder, usually in middle-aged or older men; it contains fat cells, spindle cells, bundles of birefringent collagen, and a myxoid stroma.

telangiectatic l. angiolipoma.

li•po•ma•toid (lĭ-po′mə-toid) resembling a lipoma.

lip•o•ma•to•sis (lip″o-mə-to′sis) abnormal localized or tumorlike accumulations of fat in the tissues. Called also *liposis.*

l. atro′phicans localized accumulations of fat in certain tissues, associated with emaciation of the rest of the body; see also *partial lipodystrophy.*

benign symmetric l. multiple symmetric l.

congenital l. of pancreas Shwachman-Diamond syndrome.

diffuse l. abnormal increase of subcutaneous fat in the parts above the pelvis, usually in males.

l. doloro′sa see under *adiposis.*

multiple symmetric l. nodular circumscribed lipomatosis in which the fat deposits merge to form a ring around the neck; called also *Madelung disease* or *neck.*

nodular circumscribed l. formation of multiple circumscribed or encapsulated lipomas in subcutaneous tissue. When these are distributed symmetrically around the neck, the condition is called *multiple symmetric lipomatosis* or *Madelung disease.* A variety in which the lipomas press against nerves and become painful is called *adiposis dolorosa.*

pelvic l. deposition of fat around the pelvic cavity, a disorder of unknown etiology; as it progresses, the fat may compress the pelvic organs, causing symptoms such as in the urinary tract or kidneys.

renal l., l. re′nis fatty change in the kidney, as in the nephrotic syndrome, diabetic nephropathy, and other conditions. See also *renal sinus l.* and *renal replacement l.* Called also *fatty kidney.*

renal replacement l. asymmetrical fatty change in the kidney where renal parenchyma has become replaced by fatty tissue, such as with an infection or presence of a calculus. Symptoms include decreased renal function with inflammation, pain, pyuria, and sometimes pyelonephritis.

renal sinus l. increased fat in the renal sinuses. A symmetrical, usually asymptomatic, increase is seen in obesity, steroid therapy, and the atrophy that accompanies the aging process. An asymmetrical increase known as *renal replacement lipomatosis,* which can have severe symptoms, occurs when infection destroys part of the renal parenchyma.

symmetrical l. see *nodular circumscribed l.*

lip•o•mem•brane (lip″o-mem′brān) a thickened, undulating, membrane-like structure seen in certain degenerative conditions, believed to be degenerated cell membranes of lipocytes and macrophages. **lipomem′branous** *adj*

lipo•me•nin•go•cele (lip″o-mə-ning′go-sēl) meningocele associated with an overlying lipoma.

lipo•me•tab•o•lism (lip″o-mə-tab′o-liz-əm) [*lipo-* + *metabolism*] the metabolism of fat; utilization of fat. **lipometabol′ic** *adj*

lipo•my•elo•me•nin•go•cele (lip″o-mi″ə-lo-mə-ning′go-sēl) [*lipoma* + *myelomeningocele*] myelomeningocele with an overlying lipoma.

lipo•myo•he•man•gi•o•ma (lip″o-mi″o-he-man″je-o′mə) [*lipo-* + *myo-* + *hemangioma*] angiomyolipoma.

lipo•my•o•ma (lip″o-mi-o′mə) [*lipo-* + *myoma*] myolipoma.

lipo•myx•o•ma (lip″o-mik-so′mə) [*lipo-* + *myxoma*] myxolipoma.

lipo•ne•phro•sis (lip″o-nə-fro′sis) minimal change disease.

lipo•neu•ro•cy•to•ma (lip″o-noor″o-si-to′mə) a rare type of primitive neuroectodermal tumor that contains adipocytes scattered or clustered between small neoplastic cells; it is nearly always found in the cerebellum *(cerebellar liponeurocytoma).*

Lipo•nys•soi•des (lip″o-nis-oi′dēz) a genus of blood-sucking mites of the family Dermanyssidae. *L. sangui′neus* parasitizes mice and transmits *Rickettsia akari,* which causes rickettsialpox. Formerly called *Allodermanyssus.*

Lipo•nys•sus (lip″o-nis′əs) former name for *Ornithonyssus.*

lipo•ol•i•go•sac•cha•ride (LOS) (lip″o-ol″ĭ-go-sak′ə-rīd) any of a group of substances consisting of a lipid A component linked to an oligosaccharide; they resemble lipopolysaccharides but do not have long polysaccharide side chains. They are found associated with porin on the outer membrane of certain gram-negative bacteria. In some strains of pathogenic bacteria such as *Neisseria gonorrhoeae, Neisseria meningitidis,* and *Moraxella catarrhalis,* they may be biologically active, producing endotoxins or contributing to the cell's resistance to antibiotics.

li•pop•a•thy (lĭ-pop′ə-the) any disorder of lipid metabolism.

lipo•pec•tic (lip″o-pek′tik) 1. pertaining to or characterized by lipopexia. 2. causing lipopexia. Called also *lipopexic.*

lipo•pe•nia (lip″o-pe′ne-ə) [*lipo-* + *-penia*] deficiency of lipids in the body.

lipo•pe•nic (lip″o-pe′nik) 1. pertaining to or characterized by lipopenia. 2. causing lipopenia.

lipo•pep•tide a compound containing both a lipid and a peptide component.

cyclic l. any of various lipopeptides that have cyclic structures; some have pharmaceutic properties.

lipo•pex•ia (lip″o-pek′se-ə) [*lipo-* + *pexia*] the accumulation of fat in the tissues.

lipo•pex•ic (lip″o-pek′sik) lipopectic.

lipo•phage (lip′o-fāj) [*lipo-* + *-phage*] a cell that ingests or absorbs fat.

lipo•pha•gia (lip″o-fa′je-ə) lipolysis. **lipopha′gic** *adj*

li•poph•a•gy (li-pof′ə-je) lipolysis.

lipo•phil (lip′o-fil) [*lipo-* + *-phil*] a substance that has an affinity for lipids.

lipo•phil•ia (lip″o-fil′e-ə) [*lipo-* + *-philia*] 1. affinity for fat. 2. solubility in lipids. 3. a tendency of the obese for fat fixation.

lip•o•phil•ic (lip″o-fil′ik) 1. having an affinity for fat; pertaining to or characterized by lipophilia. 2. absorbing, dissolving, or being dissolved in lipids; used particularly of certain stains or dyes.

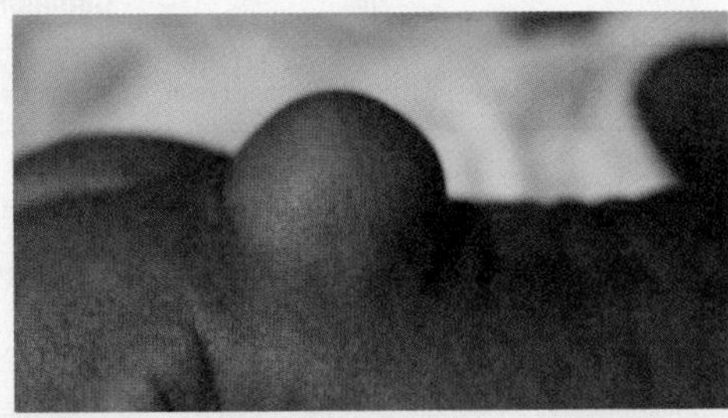

■ Lipomeningocele.

lip•o•phil•in (lip″o-fil′in) proteolipid protein.

lip•o•phore (lip′o-for″) [*lipo-* + *-phore*] a pigment cell containing a lipochrome pigment.

lipo•plas•ty (lip′o-plas″te) suction-assisted lipectomy. **lipoplas′tic** *adj*

lipo•poly•sac•cha•ride (lip″o-pol″e-sak′ə-rīd) 1. a complex of lipid and polysaccharide. 2. a major component of the cell wall of gram-negative bacteria, a type of endotoxin and important group-specific antigen (O antigen). The lipopolysaccharide molecule consists of three parts: lipid A, a glycolipid responsible for the endotoxic activity, which is covalently linked to a heteropolysaccharide chain; the first part of the chain is the core polysaccharide, which is constant within related strains; and the second part of the chain is the O-specific chain, which is highly variable. Lipopolysaccharide from *Escherichia coli* is a commonly used B-cell mitogen (polyclonal activator) in laboratory immunology. Abbreviated LPS.

lipo•pro•tein (lip″o-, li″po-pro′tēn) any of the lipid-protein complexes in which lipids are transported in the blood; lipoprotein particles consist of a spherical hydrophobic core of triglycerides or cholesteryl esters surrounded by an amphipathic monolayer of phospholipids, cholesterol, and apolipoproteins; the four principal classes are high-density, low-density, and very-low-density lipoproteins and chylomicrons.

α-l., alpha l. a lipoprotein belonging to the class of those having the most rapid electrophoretic mobility; the group comprises HDL_2 and HDL_3, the major high-density lipoproteins (q.v.).

l. (a) Lp(a) l.

β-l., beta l. a lipoprotein belonging to the class of those having slower electrophoretic mobility than that of the pre-β lipoproteins, but not remaining at the electrophoretic origin; it comprises the low-density and intermediate-density lipoproteins (qq.v.).

Braun l. in gram-negative bacteria, lipoprotein attached to the peptidoglycan and extending into the lipid bilayer of the outer membrane, anchoring it to the cell wall.

floating beta l's β-VLDL; so called for the abnormally low density of these lipoproteins relative to their electrophoretic mobility.

high-density l. (HDL) any of a class of lipoproteins frequently divided into HDL_2 and HDL_3 (see table) and the minor variant HDL_1 (see *Lp(a) l.*). HDL promotes transport of cholesterol from extrahepatic tissue to the liver for excretion in the bile; synthesized by the liver as discoid "nascent HDL" particles lacking a lipid core, it accumulates a core of cholesteryl esters during reverse cholesterol transport (q.v.) and transfers them to the liver directly or indirectly via other lipoproteins. HDL also shuttles apolipoproteins C-II and E to and from triglyceride-rich lipoproteins during catabolism of the lipoproteins. Serum HDL cholesterol has been negatively correlated with coronary heart disease. Called also (referring to its electrophoretic mobility) *α-l.*

intermediate-density l. (IDL) a class of lipoproteins formed in the degradation of very-low-density lipoproteins; approximately half are cleared rapidly from the plasma into the liver by receptor-mediated endocytosis; the other half are further degraded to form low-density lipoproteins.

low-density l. (LDL) a class of lipoproteins responsible for transport of cholesterol to extrahepatic tissues. It is formed in the circulation when very-low-density lipoproteins are degraded first to intermediate-density lipoproteins and then to LDL by the gain and loss of specific apolipoproteins and the loss of most of their triglycerides. It is taken up and catabolized by both the liver and extrahepatic tissues by specific receptor-mediated endocytosis (see *LDL receptors*, under *receptor*). Called also (referring to its electrophoretic mobility) *β-l.*

Lp(a) l. a lipoprotein particle with a density of 1.05–1.10 g/mL, containing apolipoprotein B-100 as well as an antigenically unique apolipoprotein. It is normally a minor plasma constituent but occurs at vastly elevated levels in some individuals, apparently as an autosomal dominant trait; such elevations have been correlated with increased risk of heart disease. Called also *sinking pre-β-l.* and *HDL_1*.

pre-β-l., pre-beta l. a lipoprotein belonging to the class of those having slower electrophoretic mobility than that of the α-lipoproteins but faster than that of the β-lipoproteins, predominantly comprising the very-low-density lipoproteins (q.v.).

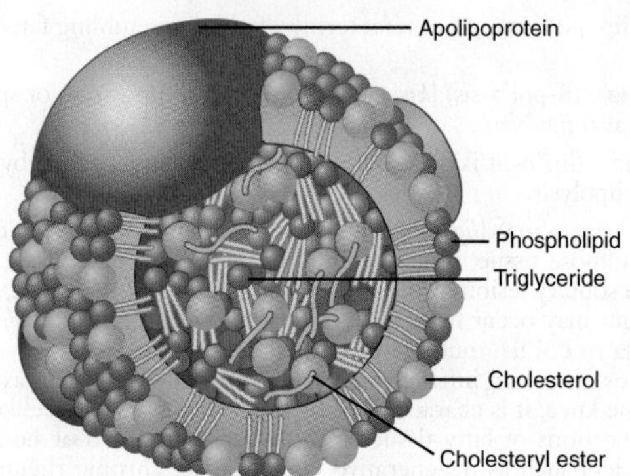

■ Diagram of lipoprotein structure showing the envelope of phospholipids and free cholesterol, core of cholesteryl esters and triglycerides, and apolipoprotein protein component.

sinking pre-β-l. Lp(a) l.

very-high-density l. (VHDL) a class of lipoproteins with density greater than 1.210 g/mL and diameter 15–30 nm; they are composed predominantly of proteins and also contain a high concentration of free fatty acids.

very-low-density l. (VLDL) a class of lipoproteins that transport triglycerides from the intestine and liver to adipose and muscle tissues. Synthesized by the liver, they contain primarily triglycerides in their lipid cores, with some cholesteryl esters; as their triglycerides are cleaved by endothelial lipoprotein lipase and transferred to extrahepatic tissues, the VLDL particles lose most of their apolipoprotein C and become intermediate-density lipoproteins. Called also (referring to electrophoretic mobility) *pre-β-l.*

l. X an abnormal low-density lipoprotein with a high content of free cholesterol and abnormal protein content that occurs in patients with cholestasis.

lipo•pro•tein•emia (lip″o-pro″te-ne′me-ə) hyperlipoproteinemia.

lipo•pro•tein li•pase (lip″o-pro′tēn li′pās) [EC 3.1.1.34] an enzyme of the hydrolase class that catalyzes the hydrolytic cleavage of fatty acyl groups from triglycerides (or di- or monoglycerides) in chylomicrons, very-low-density lipoproteins, and low-density lipoproteins. It occurs on capillary endothelial surfaces, especially in mammary, muscle, and adipose tissue, and requires apolipoprotein C-II as a cofactor.

lipo•pro•tein•o•sis (lip″o-pro″tēn-o′sis) lipoid proteinosis.

lipo•sar•co•ma (lip″o-sahr-ko′mə) [*lipo-* + *sarcoma*] a malignant mesenchymal tumor usually arising from the intermuscular fascia, particularly in the upper thigh, and occurring predominantly in male adults. It is derived from primitive or embryonal lipoblastic cells which exhibit varying degrees of lipoblastic and/or lipomatous differentiation, and is divided into several variant forms.

dedifferentiated l. a highly malignant tumor in which areas of well-differentiated liposarcoma coexist with areas of specific or undifferentiated spindle cell sarcoma.

myxoid l. the most common form of liposarcoma, characterized by primitive mesenchymal cells in a mucopolysaccharide-rich ground substance and a plexiform capillary network; lipoblasts may be scarce. It metastasizes late, if at all.

pleomorphic l. a highly undifferentiated and anaplastic form of liposarcoma with a high metastatic potential; it is characterized by many large tumor giant cells and unusual lipoblasts with frequent, abnormal mitotic figures.

Common Plasma Lipoprotein Classes

Class	Density (g/mL)	Diameter (nm)	Electrophoretic Mobility	Major Apolipoproteins	Predominant Core Lipids
Chylomicrons	0.93	75–1200	Origin	A-I, A-II, B-48, C	Dietary triglycerides
VLDL	0.93–1.006	30–80	Pre-*β*	B-100, C, E	Endogenous triglycerides
IDL	1.006–1.019	25–35	Slow pre-*β*	B-100, E	Endogenous triglycerides, cholesteryl esters
LDL	1.019–1.063	18–25	*β*	B-100	Endogenous cholesteryl esters
HDL_2	1.063–1.125	9–12	*α*	A-I, A-II	Endogenous cholesteryl esters
HDL_3	1.125–1.210	5–9			

VLDL, Very-low-density lipoproteins; IDL, intermediate-density lipoproteins; LDL, low-density lipoproteins; HDL, high-density lipoproteins

round cell l. a highly vascular form of liposarcoma, characterized by small round to oval cells with fine vacuolated cytoplasm and dark central nuclei and by occasional lipoblasts, which are commonly without mitotic figures; it frequently metastasizes.

well-differentiated l. a form of liposarcoma that resembles lipoma, having adult type fat cells and sometimes bizarre, atypical lipoblasts, with infrequent mitoses and tumor giant cells; it may be locally aggressive but rarely metastasizes.

li•po•sis (lĭ-po′sis) [*lipo-* + *-osis*] lipomatosis.

lipo•sol•u•ble (lip″o-sol′u-bəl) [*lipo-* + *soluble*] soluble in fats.

lipo•some (lip′o-sōm) [*lipo-* + *-some*] a spherical particle in an aqueous medium, formed by a lipid bilayer enclosing an aqueous compartment.

lipo•suc•tion (lip′o-suk″shən) suction-assisted lipectomy.

lipo•tei•cho•ic ac•id (lip″o-ti-ko′ik) any of various teichoic acids (q.v.) that are covalently linked to glycolipids of the plasma membrane of gram-positive bacteria. In certain bacteria, they are major antigenic determinants. Cf. *wall teichoic acid.*

lipo•tox•ic•i•ty (lip″o-tok-sis′ĭ-te) the toxic effects on various organs of hyperlipidemia; see *fatty change,* under *change.*

lipo•troph (lip′o-trōf) any of the acidophilic cells of the adenohypophysis that contain β-lipotropin; see *corticotroph.*

lipo•tro•phic (lip″o-tro′fik) 1. pertaining to or characterized by lipotrophy. 2. causing lipotrophy.

li•pot•ro•phy (lĭ-pot′rə-fe) [*lipo-* + *-trophy*] increase of bodily fat.

lipo•tro•pic (lip″o-tro′pik) [*lipo-* + *-tropic*] 1. acting on fat metabolism by hastening the removal of or decreasing the deposit of fat in the liver. 2. an agent that has such effects.

lip•o•tro•pin (lip′o-tro″pin) any of several prohormones that are derivatives of pro-opiomelanocortin and promote lipolysis; the most important one in humans is *β-lipotropin.* Formerly called lipotropic hormone.

β-l. a 91-amino acid polypeptide prohormone that exerts a mild lipolytic action and promotes darkening of the skin by stimulation of melanocytes; it is the precursor molecule of endorphins and melanocyte-stimulating hormones.

li•pot•ro•pism (lĭ-pot′ro-piz″əm) the condition of being lipotropic.

li•pot•ro•py (lĭ-pot′rə-pe) lipotropism.

lipo•vac•cine (lip″o-vak′sēn) [*lipo-* + *vaccine*] a vaccine prepared by suspending microorganisms in vegetable oil for the purpose of delaying absorption of the antigenic substances.

lipo•vi•tel•lin (lip″o-vi-tel′in) [*lipo-* + *vitelline*] a lipoprotein found in the yolk of eggs.

lipo•xan•thine (lip″o-zan′thin) [*lipo-* + Gr. *xanthos* yellow] a yellow lipochrome.

li•pox•i•dase (lĭ-pok′sĭ-dās) lipoxygenase.

li•pox•in (lĭ-pok′sin) any of several conjugated tetraene derivatives of arachidonic acid that oppose the actions of leukotrienes, have potent vasodilating effects, and appear to be toxic to natural killer cells.

li•poxy•ge•nase (lĭ-pok′sĭ-jən-ās) [EC 1.13.11.12] an enzyme of the oxidoreductase class that catalyzes the oxidation of linoleate and related polyunsaturated fatty acids to their hydroperoxide forms. Called also *lipoxidase.*

5-l. arachidonate 5-lipoxygenase.

12-l. arachidonate 12-lipoxygenase.

15-l. arachidonate 15-lipoxygenase.

lipo•yl (lip′o-əl) the acyl radical of lipoic acid.

lip•pa (lip′ə) blepharitis ciliaris.

lip•ping (lip′ing) 1. a wedge-shaped shadow in the radiograph of chondrosarcoma between the cortex and the elevated periosteum. 2. the development of a bony overgrowth in osteoarthritis.

lip•pi•tude (lip′ĭ-to͞od) [L. *lippitudo; lippus* bleareyed] blepharitis ciliaris.

Lip•schütz bodies, ulcer (disease) (lip′shēts) [Benjamin *Lipschütz,* Austrian dermatologist, 1878–1931] see under *body,* and see *ulcus vulvae acutum.*

li•pu•ria (lĭ-pu′re-ə) lipiduria.

Liq. [L.] liquor.

liq•ue•fa•cient (lik″wə-fa′shənt) 1. causing liquefaction. 2. an agent that causes liquefaction.

liq•ue•fac•tion (lik″wə-fak′shən) [L. *liquefactio,* from *liquere* to flow + *facere* to make] the conversion of a material into a liquid form.

gas l. the conversion of gas into a liquid form, brought about by cooling and compression, resulting in a decrease of the average kinetic energy of the molecules sufficiently to allow intermolecular forces of attraction to pull the molecules together. Called also *condensation.*

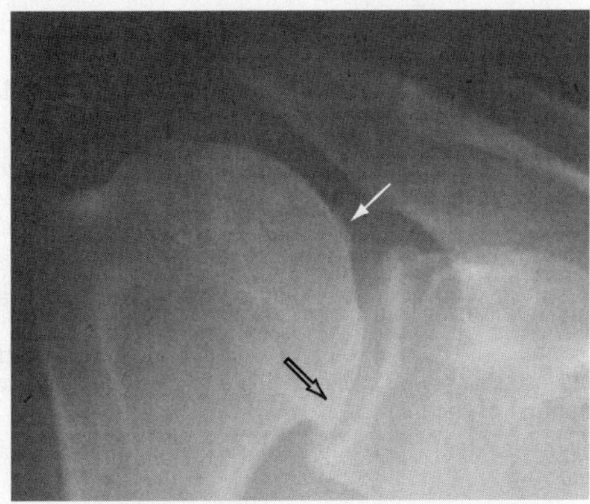

■ Osteophytic lipping *(lower arrow)* from the humeral head in osteoarthritis of the shoulder, including new bone formation deep to the cartilage *(upper arrow).*

liq•ue•fac•tive (lik″wə-fak′tiv) 1. pertaining to or characterized by liquefaction. 2. liquefacient (def. 1).

liq•ue•fy (lik′wə-fi) to become or cause to become liquid; the term includes conversion from both solid and gaseous states.

li•ques•cent (lik-wes′ənt) [L. *liquescere* to become liquid] becoming or tending to become liquid.

liq•uid (lik′wid) [L. *liquidus; liquere* to flow] 1. a substance that flows readily in its natural state. See also *fluid, liquor, mixture,* and *solution.* 2. flowing readily; neither solid nor gaseous. 3. a consonant sound articulated without friction, such as *l* or *r.*

silicone l. see under *oil.*

li•quor (lik′ər, li′kwor) pl. *liquors, liquo′res* [L.] 1. a liquid, especially an aqueous solution containing a medicinal substance. 2. a general term used in anatomical nomenclature for certain fluids of the body. See also *fluid, liquid,* and *solution.*

l. am′nii amniotic fluid.

l. cerebrospina′lis [TA] cerebrospinal fluid: the fluid contained within the four ventricles of the brain, the subarachnoid space, and the central canal of the spinal cord; formed by choroid plexuses and brain parenchyma, it circulates through the ventricles into the subarachnoid space and is absorbed into the venous system.

l. cho′rii a fluid which separates the amnion from the chorion in the early stages of gestation.

l. folli′culi follicular fluid.

l. pu′ris the fluid portion of pus.

l. of Scarpa endolympha.

li•quo•res (li-kwo′rēz) [L.] plural of *liquor.*

li•quor•ice (lik′ər-is) 1. *Glycyrrhiza glabra.* 2. licorice (def. 2).

Lisch nodules (lish) [Karl *Lisch,* Austrian ophthalmologist, 1907–1999] see under *nodule.*

Lis•franc amputation, etc. (lēs-frahngk′) [Jacques *Lisfranc,* French surgeon, 1790–1847] see under *amputation, joint, ligament,* and *tubercle.*

li•sin•o•pril (li-sin′o-pril) [USP] the lysine derivative of the active form of enalapril; an angiotensin-converting enzyme inhibitor used in the treatment of hypertension (alone or in combination with a thiazide diuretic), congestive heart failure, and acute myocardial infarction; administered orally.

lisp•ing (lisp′ing) a form of sigmatism in which *th* sounds are substituted for *s* and *z.*

Lis•sau•er paralysis, tract (column, marginal zone) (lis′ou-ər) [Heinrich *Lissauer,* German neurologist, 1861–1891] see under *paralysis* and see *tractus posterolateralis.*

lis•sen•ce•pha•lia (lis″ən-sə-fa′le-ə) agyria.

lis•sen•ce•phal•ic (lis″ən-sə-fal′ik) 1. having cerebral hemispheres without or with only shallow convolutions, the normal appearance of the brain of many animals (e.g., bats, rodents). Cf. *gyrencephalic.* 2. agyric.

lis•sen•ceph•a•ly (lis″ən-sef′ə-le) agyria.

Walker l. Walker-Warburg syndrome.

lis•sive (lis′iv) [Gr. *lissos* smooth] relieving muscle spasm without interfering with function.

lis•so•sphinc•ter (lis′o-sfingk″tər) [Gr. *lissos* smooth + *sphincter*] musculus sphincter urethrae internus.

Lis•ter (lis′tər) Baron Joseph, 1827–1912. English surgeon who, following Pasteur's theory that bacteria cause infection, introduced to surgery the principle of antisepsis. In 1865 Lister, using carbolic acid as his antiseptic agent together with heat-sterilized instruments, greatly reduced postoperative mortality.

Lis·ter tubercle (lis′tər) [Baron J. *Lister*] tuberculum dorsale radii.

lis·ter·el·lo·sis (lis″tər-ə-lo′sis) listeriosis.

Lis·te·ria (lis-te′re-ə) [Baron Joseph *Lister*] a genus of bacteria of the family Listeriaceae, made up of small, coccoid, gram-positive rods that have a tendency to form chains and palisades; they are found in animal feces, on vegetation, and in silage. The type species is *L. monocyto′genes.*

L. monocyto′genes a species widely distributed in nature, having a striking monocytic action in blood; it is the usual cause of listeriosis.

Lis·te·ri·a·ceae (lis-te″re-a′se-e) a family of gram-positive, non–spore-forming bacteria of the order Bacillales; medically important organisms are contained in the genus *Listeria.*

lis·te·ri·al (lis-ter′e-əl) pertaining to or caused by organisms of the genus *Listeria.*

lis·te·ri·o·sis (lis-te″re-o′sis) 1. human infection caused by *Listeria monocytogenes.* In utero infection occurs transplacentally and results in abortion, stillbirth, or premature birth. Infection acquired by an infant during birth causes cardiorespiratory distress, diarrhea, vomiting, and meningitis. In adults it produces meningitis, endocarditis, febrile gastroenteritis, and disseminated granulomatous lesions. 2. infection of domestic animals by *L. monocytogenes.* In cattle and sheep this causes abortion, encephalitis, and other neurologic signs; nonruminants may suffer from necrosis of the liver. Because affected animals tend to move in circles, it is also known as *circling disease.*

lis·ter·ism (lis′tər-iz″əm) the principles and practice of antiseptic and aseptic surgery.

Lis·ting's law, plane (lis′tingz) [Johann Benedict *Listing,* German physiologist, 1808–1882] see under *law* and *plane.*

Lis·ton knife, splint (lis′tən) [Robert *Liston,* English surgeon, 1794–1847] see under *knife* and *splint.*

Lis·tro·phor·i·dae (lis″tro-for′ĭ-de) a family of mites often found clinging to the hair of mammals. Genera of veterinary interest include *Lynxacarus* and *Myocoptes.*

li·ter (L) (le′tər) [Fr. *litre*] a basic unit of volume used for liquids with the SI system, equal to 1000 cubic centimeters, or 1 cubic decimeter, or to 1.0567 quarts liquid measure.

-lith [Gr. *lithos* stone] a word termination denoting a stone or calculus.

Lith·ane (lith′ān) trademark for a preparation of lithium carbonate.

li·thec·to·my (lĭ-thek′tə-me) lithotomy.

lith·ia (lith′e-ə) see *lithium.*

lith·i·as·ic (lith″e-as′ik) pertaining to lithiasis.

li·thi·a·sis (lĭ-thi′ə-sis) [*lith-* + *-iasis*] 1. the formation or presence of calculi or other concretions. Numerous types are named for the primary ingredient of the calculi formed; see under *calculus.* 2. sometimes used as a synonym for one of the specific types of lithiasis, especially urolithiasis, nephrolithiasis, or cholelithiasis.

appendicular l. appendicolithiasis.

cholecystic l. cholecystolithiasis.

l. conjuncti′vae, conjunctival l. conjunctival concretions.

gallbladder l. cholecystolithiasis.

pancreatic l. pancreatolithiasis.

renal l. nephrolithiasis.

urinary l. urolithiasis.

-lithiasis a word termination signifying calculi or concretions, used following a root designating the site in the body.

lith·ic (lith′ik) 1. calculous. 2. pertaining to lithium.

lith·ic ac·id (lith′ic) uric acid.

lith·i·um (Li) (lith′e-əm) [Gr. *lithos* stone] a white metal; atomic number 3, atomic weight 6.939; its oxide, lithia, Li_2O, is alkaline; its salts are solvents of uric acid to a certain extent in vitro: based on this, it was formerly erroneously thought to be indicated in gout and rheumatic conditions.

l. carbonate [USP] the carbonate salt of lithium, used as a mood stabilizer in treatment of acute manic and hypomanic states in bipolar disorder and in maintenance therapy to reduce the intensity and frequency of subsequent manic episodes; administered orally.

l. citrate [USP] the citrate salt of lithium, having the same actions and uses as the carbonate salt.

lith(o)- [Gr. *lithos* stone] a combining form denoting relationship to stone or to a calculus.

Lith·o·bid (lith′o-bid) trademark for a preparation of lithium carbonate.

litho·cho·late (lith″o-ko′lāt) a salt, ester, or anionic form of lithocholic acid.

litho·cho·lic ac·id (lith″o-ko′lik) a secondary bile acid formed by dehydroxylation of chenodeoxycholic acid in the intestine; some is reabsorbed and forms conjugates with glycine and taurine.

litho·cho·lyl·gly·cine (lith″o-ko″ləl-gli′sēn) a bile salt, the glycine conjugate of lithocholic acid.

litho·cho·lyl·tau·rine (lith″o-ko″ləl-taw′rēn) a bile salt, the taurine conjugate of lithocholic acid.

litho·clast (lith′o-klast) [*litho-* + *-clast*] lithotrite.

litho·gen·e·sis (lith″o-gen′ə-sis) [*litho-* + *-genesis*] the formation of calculi; called also *calculogenesis.*

litho·gen·ic (lith″o-jen′ik) promoting lithogenesis.

li·thog·e·nous (lĭ-thoj′ə-nəs) producing or causing lithogenesis.

litho·kel·y·pho·pe·di·on (lith″o-kel″ĭ-fo-pe′de-on) [*litho-* + Gr. *kelyphos* sheath + *paidion* child] a lithopedion in which both the fetus and the membranes are petrified.

litho·kel·y·phos (lith″o-kel′ĭ-fos) [*litho-* + Gr. *kelyphos* sheath] a dead fetus in which the fetal membranes are calcified.

li·thol·a·paxy (lĭ-thol′ə-pak″se) lithotripsy.

li·thol·y·sis (lĭ-thol′ĭ-sis) [*litho-* + *-lysis*] the dissolution of calculi.

litho·lyt·ic (lith″o-lit′ik) 1. dissolving calculi. 2. an agent that dissolves calculi.

Lith·o·nate (lith′ə-nāt) trademark for a preparation of lithium carbonate.

litho·ne·phri·tis (lith″o-nə-fri′tis) [*litho-* + *nephritis*] inflammation of the kidney due to irritation by calculi.

litho·pe·di·on (lith″o-pe′de-on) [L. *lithopaedium,* from Gr. *lithos* stone + *paidion* child] a dead fetus that has become stony or petrified in utero; called also *calcified fetus.*

Lith·o·stat (lith′o-stat) trademark for a preparation of acetohydroxamic acid.

Lith·o·tabs (lith′o-tabz) trademark for a preparation of lithium carbonate.

litho·tome (lith′o-tōm) a knife for performing lithotomy.

li·thot·o·mist (lĭ-thot′ə-mist) an individual who performs lithotomies.

li·thot·o·my (lĭ-thot′ə-me) [*litho-* + *-tomy*] 1. incision of a duct or organ for removal of a calculus. 2. cystolithotomy.

high l. suprapubic l.

lateral l. cystolithotomy in which the incision is anterior to the rectum and to one side of the raphe.

median l. cystolithotomy in which the incision is made on the raphe of the perineum anterior to the anus.

perineal l. cystolithotomy in which the incision is made in the perineum.

prerectal l. median l.

suprapubic l. cystolithotomy through an incision above the symphysis pubis.

vaginal l. cystolithotomy through an incision within the vagina.

litho·tre·sis (lith″o-tre′sis) [*litho-* + Gr. *trēsis* a boring] the drilling or boring of holes in a calculus.

litho·trip·sy (lith′o-trip″se) [*litho-* + *-tripsy*] the crushing of a urinary calculus or gallstone within the body, followed at once by the washing out of the fragments. It was formerly done surgically but can now also be done by various noninvasive methods. Called also *litholapaxy.*

ballistic l. lithotripsy in which a lithotrite is inserted through an endoscope to bombard a calculus with projectiles, such as tiny metal pellets.

electrohydraulic l. a method used for large calculi; a high-capacity condenser creates a high-voltage spark between two electrodes at the tip of a probe; in a fluid-filled organ this creates a hydraulic shock wave that can be directed toward a calculus, causing it to cavitate and fragment.

extracorporeal shock wave l. a procedure for treating urinary calculi in the upper urinary tract and gallstones: the patient may be either immersed in a large tub of water or placed in contact with a water cushion; a high-energy shock wave generated by a high-voltage spark, electromagnetic impulse, or piezoelectric generator is focused by an ellipsoid reflector on the stone, which disintegrates into particles small enough to be expelled from the organ.

laser l. lithotripsy of urinary calculi or gallstones using any of various lasers.

percutaneous ultrasonic l. ultrasonic lithotripsy done through a probe through a skin incision.

pneumatic l. lithotripsy in which a rigid probe is inserted and pneumatic pressure is applied directly to the calculus.

shock wave l. extracorporeal shock wave l.

ultrasonic l. lithotripsy in which a rigid probe is inserted to the site and high frequency sound waves disintegrate the calculus; it may be either through the skin (percutaneous ultrasonic lithotripsy) or through an endoscope.

litho•trip•ter (lith′o-trip″tər) an instrument for crushing calculi in lithotripsy. Also spelled *lithotriptor.*

litho•trip•tic (lith′o-trip″tik) 1. pertaining to lithotripsy. 2. causing or producing lithotripsy. 3. an agent that causes lithotripsy.

litho•trip•tor (lith′o-trip″tər) lithotripter.

litho•trite (lith′o-trīt) [*litho-* + Gr. *tribein* to rub] an instrument for crushing a urinary calculus; called also *lithoclast.*

li•thot•ri•ty (lĭ-thot′rĭ-te) lithotripsy.

litho•troph (lith′o-trōf) [*litho-* + Gr. *trophē* nutrition] autotroph.

lith•ure•sis (lith″u-re′sis) [*litho-* + *-uresis*] the passage of gravel (q.v.) through the urethra with the urine.

lit•mus (lit′məs) a pigment prepared from *Roccella tinctoria* and other lichens, used as a test for acidity and alkalinity. It has a pH range of 4.5 to 8.3. Crude fractions are *azolitmin, erythrolitmin,* and *erythrolein.*

Lit•o•mo•soi•des (lit″o-mo-soi′dēz) a genus of filarial nematodes. *L. cari′nii* is found in the pleural and peritoneal cavities of the cotton rat, *Sigmodon hispidus*, and is widely used in studies of filariasis.

li•tre (le′tər) [Fr.] liter.

lit•ter (lit′ər) 1. stretcher. 2. the offspring produced at one birth by a multiparous animal.

Lit•tle area (lit′əl) [James Laurence *Little*, American surgeon, 1836–1885] Kiesselbach area; see under *area.*

Lit•tle disease (lit′əl) [William John *Little*, English physician, 1810–1894] see under *disease.*

lit•to•ral (lit′ə-rəl) pertaining to the shore of a large body of water.

Lit•tre glands (crypts), hernia (le′trə) [Alexis *Littre*, French surgeon, 1658–1725] see *glandulae preputiales* and see under *hernia.*

lit•tri•tis (lĭ-tri′tis) inflammation of the urethral glands of the male urethra (Littre glands).

Litz•mann obliquity (litz′mən) [Karl Konrad Theodor *Litzmann*, German gynecologist, 1815–1890] see under *obliquity.*

li•ve•do (lĭ-ve′do) [L.] 1. a discolored spot or patch on the skin, often due to passive congestion. 2. l. reticularis.

idiopathic l. reticularis a type of unknown cause, usually seen in young adults, especially women; it is chronic, characterized by symmetrical diffuse lesions, and more common in winter. Some patients develop ulcerations on the legs or feet, either initially or after edema.

l. racemo′sa 1. l. reticularis. 2. some authorities limit this term to types of livedo reticularis that persist in spite of warming or other environmental changes.

l. reticula′ris a vascular response to any of various disorders, caused by dilation of the subpapillary venous plexus as a result of both increased blood viscosity and blood vessel changes that delay flow away from the skin. Clinical characteristics include reticular, cyanotic skin surrounding pale central areas on the trunk and limbs, becoming more intense on exposure to cold and often disappearing upon warming. The three main types are cutis marmorata, idiopathic livedo reticularis, and secondary livedo reticularis. Called also *l. racemosa.*

secondary l. reticularis, symptomatic l. reticularis types associated with other conditions or disorders, most of which involve blood viscosity changes, embolization, or vessel wall disease; the distribution on the skin is usually asymmetrical and patchy. Associated conditions include vascular diseases such as arteriosclerosis, vascular calcification with hyperparathyroidism, and arteritis; intravascular occlusive conditions such as thrombocytopenia, cryoglobulinemia, emboli, and decompression sickness; and miscellaneous others such as tuberculosis, syphilis, and rheumatic fever.

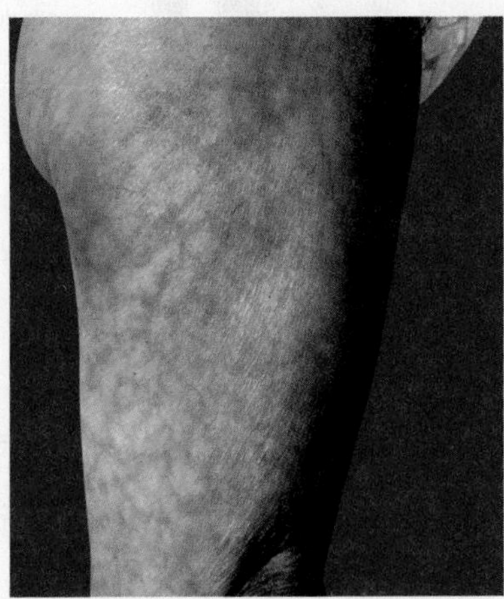

■ Livedo reticularis.

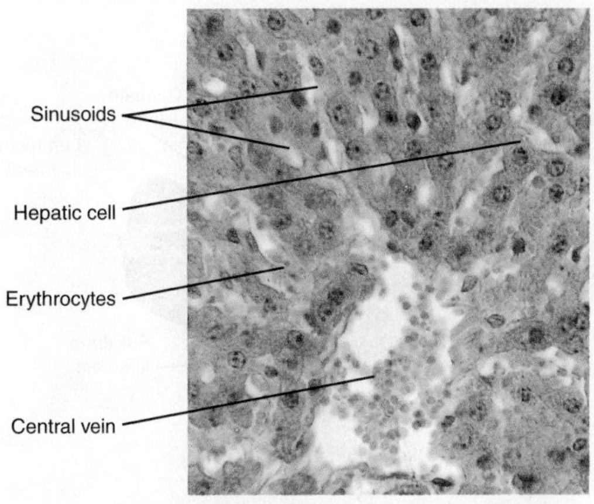

■ Liver tissue (Verhoeff stain).

l. telangiecta′tica cutis marmorata telangiectatica congenita.

liv•e•doid (liv′ə-doid) pertaining to or resembling livedo.

liv•er (liv′ər) [L. *jecur*; Gr. *hēpar*] 1. a large gland of a dark red color found in the upper part of the abdomen on the right side. Its domed upper surface fits closely against and is adherent to the inferior surface of the right diaphragmatic dome, and it has a double blood supply from the hepatic artery and the portal vein. Its traditional anatomic divisions have been four lobes, the left lobe *(lobus hepatis sinister)*, right lobe *(lobus hepatis dexter)*, caudate lobe *(lobus caudatus hepatis)*, and quadrate lobe *(lobus quadratus hepatis)*. Based on the internal blood supply and biliary drainage, a newer anatomic system divides the liver into three regions, the left liver *(pars hepatis sinistra)*, right liver *(pars hepatis dextra)*, and posterior liver *(pars posterior hepatis)*, with the latter being identical to the caudate lobe. The liver is made up of thousands of minute lobules (see *lobuli hepatis*), which are its functional units. Among its many functions are the storage and filtration of blood, secretion of bile, excretion of bilirubin and other substances formed elsewhere in the body, and numerous metabolic functions, including the conversion of sugars into glycogen, which it stores. Called also *hepar* [TA]. 2. the same gland of certain animals, sometimes used as food or from which pharmaceutical products are prepared.

albuminoid l., amyloid l. a liver that has amyloid degeneration; called also *waxy l.*

fatty l. a liver with fatty infiltration, such as from alcohol abuse, jejunoileal bypass surgery, or occasionally diabetes mellitus. Fat is in large droplets and the liver is enlarged but of normal consistency; patients are often asymptomatic, but the condition can progress to hepatitis or cirrhosis if the underlying cause is not removed.

floating l. wandering l.

foamy l. a liver containing gas bubbles from anaerobic bacteria, seen post mortem.

frosted l. perihepatitis chronica hyperplastica.

hobnail l. a liver whose surface is marked by naillike points as a result of cirrhosis.

icing l. perihepatitis chronica hyperplastica.

left l. pars hepatis sinistra.

nutmeg l. a liver that has a mottled appearance when cut, as a result of chronic passive congestion (see under *congestion*).

pigmented l. a liver discolored by pigment, such as in the Dubin-Johnson syndrome.

polycystic l. a liver containing multiple cysts; see *polycystic liver disease*, under *disease.*

posterior l. pars posterior hepatis.

right l. pars hepatis dextra.

shock l. hepatic ischemia.

wandering l. a displaced and movable liver; called also *floating l.*

waxy l. amyloid l.

liv•er phos•phor•y•lase (liv′ər fos-for′ə-lās) the liver isozyme of glycogen phosphorylase.

liv•er phos•phor•y•lase de•fi•cien•cy (liv′ər fos-for′ə-lās) glycogen storage disease, type VI.

liv•er phos•phor•y•lase ki•nase (liv′ər fos-for′ə-lās ki′nās) the liver isozyme of phosphorylase kinase.

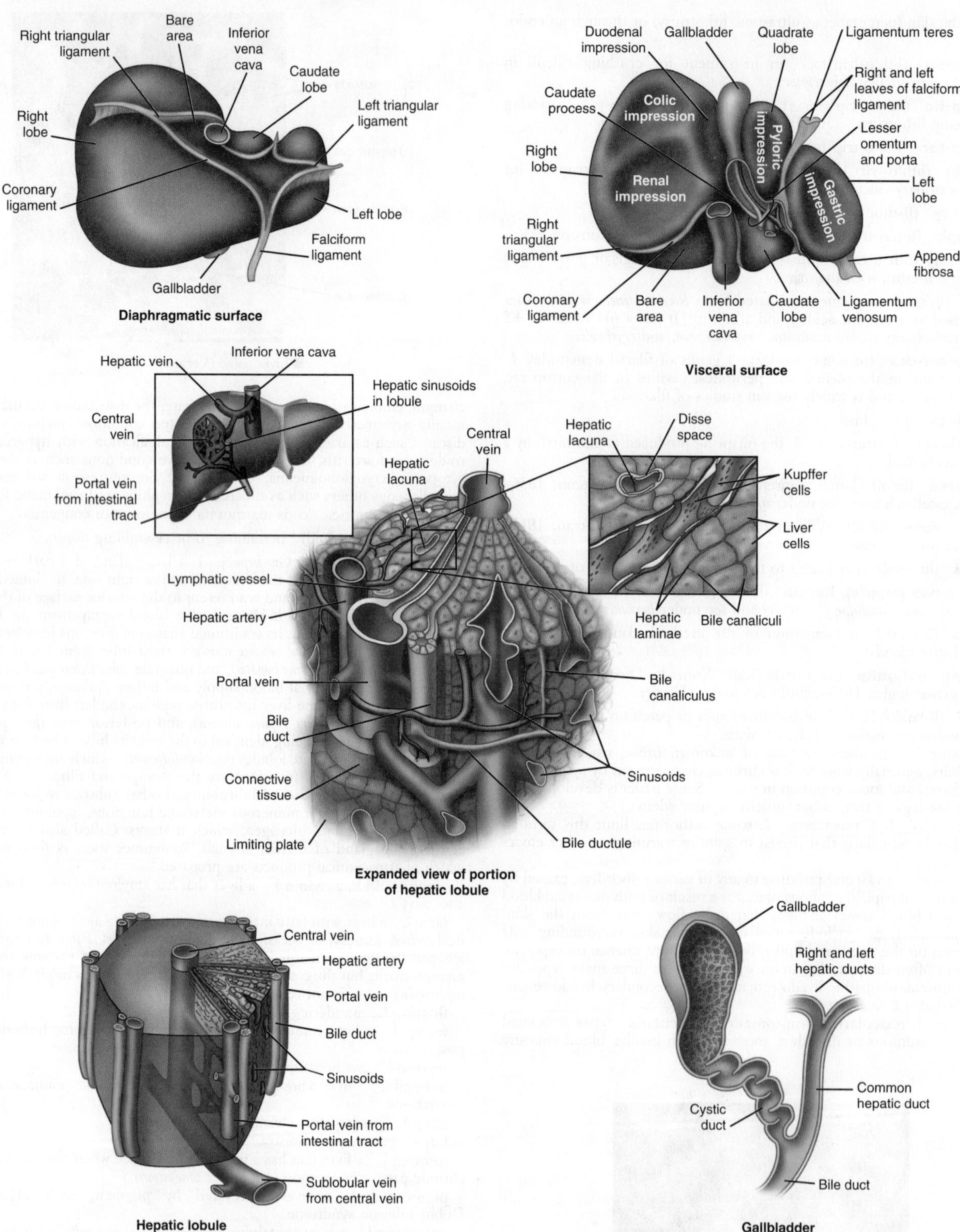

■ **PLATE 24**—STRUCTURE OF THE LIVER

li•ve•tin (li′və-tin) a protein found in yolk of egg.

liv•id (liv′id) [L. *lividus*, lead-colored] discolored, as from the effects of contusion or congestion; black and blue.

li•vid•i•ty (lĭ-vid′ĭ-te) [L. *lividitas*] the quality of being livid; discoloration, as of dependent parts, by the gravitation of the blood.

postmortem l. livor mortis.

Li•vi•e•ra•to sign (le″ve-ə-rah′to) [Panagino *Livierato*, Italian physician, 1860–1936] see under *sign*.

li•vor (li′vor) pl. *livo′res* [L. "bluish color"] 1. lividity. 2. l. mortis.

l. mor′tis discoloration appearing on dependent parts of the body after death, as a result of cessation of circulation, stagnation of blood, and settling of the blood by gravity; called also *postmortem lividity*.

Liv•o•stin (lĭ-vos′tin) trademark for preparations of levocabastine hydrochloride.

lix•iv•i•a•tion (lik-siv″e-a′shən) [L. *lixivia* lye] the separation of soluble from insoluble matter by dissolving out the soluble matter and drawing off the solution; called also *leaching*.

lix•iv•i•um (lik-siv′e-əm) [L.] any alkaline filtrate obtained by leaching ashes or other similar powdered substance; lye.

liz•ard (liz′ərd) any of numerous crawling reptiles with long bodies. One genus, *Heloderma*, has a venomous bite.

beaded l. *Heloderma horridum*, a Mexican species related to the Gila monster, having a venomous bite.

LLL left lower lobe; see *lobus inferior pulmonis sinistri*.

LM light minimum; linguomesial.

lm lumen.

LMA left mentoanterior; see *mentoanterior position*, under *position*.

LMF lymphocyte mitogenic factor.

LMO living modified organism.

LMP left mentoposterior (see *mentoposterior position*, under *position*); last menstrual period; latent membrane protein.

LMT left mentotransverse; see *mentotransverse position*, under *position*.

LMWK low-molecular-weight kininogen.

ln natural logarithm; see *logarithm*.

LNG levonorgestrel.

LNMP last normal menstrual period.

LNPF lymph node permeability factor.

LOA left occipitoanterior; see *occipitoanterior position*, under *position*.

Loa (lo′ə) [Kongo *lowa* eyeworm] a genus of nematodes of the superfamily Filarioidea.

L. lo′a a threadlike species 2.5 to 5 cm long found in West and Central Africa, the cause of loiasis. The immature forms or microfilariae are diurnal, being found in the peripheral circulation in greatest concentrations during the day. Flies of the genus *Chrysops* are the intermediate hosts and vectors.

load (lōd) 1. the quantity of a measurable entity borne by an object or organism. 2. the body content, as of water, salt, or heat, especially as it varies from normal.

allostatic l. term coined as a more precise alternative to the term *stress*, used to refer to environmental challenges that cause an organism to begin efforts to maintain stability (allostasis).

genetic l. 1. the sum of the deleterious genes in a genome. 2. the relative difference between the mean fitness of a population and the fitness of a population composed entirely of individuals with the fittest genotype.

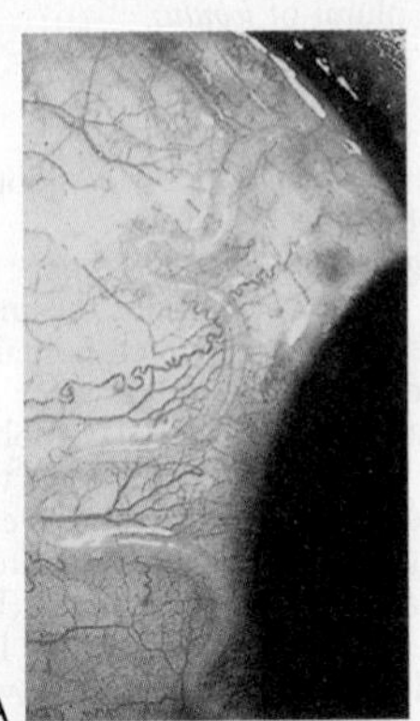

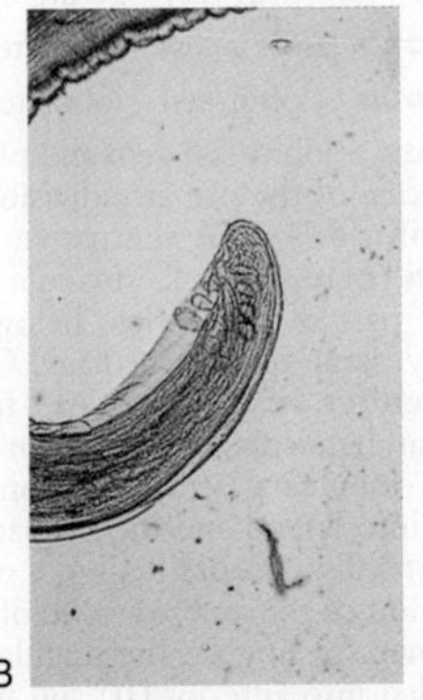

■ *Loa loa. (A)*, Adult worm in eye; *(B)*, tail of adult male, with spicules typical of the species.

occlusal l. the total force exerted on the teeth through the occlusal surfaces during mastication.

viral l. the number of copies of RNA of a given virus per milliliter of blood.

load•ing (lōd′ing) 1. administering sufficient quantities of a substance to test the subject's ability to metabolize it, as in the histidine loading test. 2. the exertion of lengthening force on a body part such as a muscle or ligament.

LOAEL lowest observed adverse effect level.

lo•a•i•a•sis (lo″ə-i′ə-sis) loiasis.

lo•bar (lo′bər) of, pertaining to, or affecting a lobe.

lo•bate (lo′bāt) consisting of or having lobes.

lo•ba•tion (lo-ba′shən) 1. the formation of lobes. 2. the state of having lobes.

renal l. the appearance on x-ray films of small notches along the surface of the kidney, indicating the location of renal lobes.

lobe (lōb) [L. *lobus*, q.v.] 1. a more or less well-defined portion of any organ, especially of the brain, the lungs, or a gland. Lobes are demarcated by fissures, sulci, connective tissue, and shape. Called lobus in official anatomical nomenclature. 2. one of the main divisions of the crown of a tooth, developmentally representing a center of calcification.

anterior l. of cerebellum lobus cerebelli anterior.

anterior l. of hypophysis, anterior pituitary l., anterior l. of pituitary gland adenohypophysis.

appendicular l. Riedel l.

azygos l., l. of azygos vein a small accessory or anomalous lobe at the apex of the right lung, produced when the azygos vein arches over the superior part of the lung and presses deeply into the lung tissue to form the azygos fissure.

caudal l. of cerebellum lobus cerebelli posterior.

caudate l., caudate l. of liver lobus caudatus.

cerebral l's lobi cerebri.

cranial l. of cerebellum lobus cerebelli anterior.

cuneate l. cuneus.

ear l. lobulus auriculae.

flocculonodular l. lobus flocculonodularis.

frontal l. lobus frontalis.

hepatic l's l's of liver.

inferior l., left lobus inferior pulmonis sinistri.

inferior l., right lobus inferior pulmonis dextri.

inferior l. of left lung lobus inferior pulmonis sinistri.

inferior l. of right lung lobus inferior pulmonis dextri.

insular l. insula (def. 2).

intermediate pituitary l., intermediate l. of pituitary gland names often used for the pars intermedia hypophyseos in animals other than humans.

lateral l's of prostate gland lobi prostatae dexter et sinister.

left l. of liver lobus hepatis sinister.

limbic l. lobus limbicus.

l's of liver the four anatomical divisions of the liver; see *lobus hepatis dexter, lobus hepatis sinister, lobus caudatus hepatis*, and *lobus quadratus hepatis*.

lower l., left lobus inferior pulmonis sinistri.

lower l., right lobus inferior pulmonis dextri.

lower l. of left lung lobus inferior pulmonis sinistri.

lower l. of right lung lobus inferior pulmonis dextri.

l's of lung the five anatomic divisions of the lungs; see *lung*. Called also *pulmonary l's*.

l's of mammary gland lobi glandulae mammariae.

median l. of prostate lobus medius prostatae.

middle l., right lobus medius pulmonis dextri.

middle l. of right lung lobus medius pulmonis dextri.

neural l. of hypophysis, neural l. of neurohypophysis, neural l. of pituitary gland lobus nervosus neurohypophysis.

occipital l. the posterior portion of the cerebral hemisphere; see *lobus occipitalis*.

olfactory l. a term applied to the olfactory apparatus on the lower surface of the frontal lobe of the brain. It consists of the olfactory bulb, tract, and trigone.

optic l's corpora bigemina; see under *corpus*.

parietal l. the upper central lobe of the pallium; see *lobus parietalis*.

piriform l. 1. piriform area. 2. in lower mammals, the lateral exposed portion of the olfactory cerebral cortex.

placental l's distinct areas on the uterine surface of the placenta, demarcated by the connective tissue septa.

polyalveolar l. a congenital disorder characterized in early infancy by the presence of far more than the normal number of alveoli in a lobe of the lungs; thereafter, normal multiplication of alveoli does not take place and they become enlarged, i.e., emphysematous.

posterior l. of cerebellum lobus cerebelli posterior.

posterior l. of hypophysis, posterior pituitary l., posterior l. of pituitary gland neurohypophysis.
l's of prostate lobi prostatae dexter et sinister.
pulmonary l's see *lung.*
pyramidal l. of thyroid gland lobus pyramidalis glandulae thyroideae.
pyriform l. piriform l.
quadrate l. of cerebral hemisphere precuneus.
quadrate l. of liver lobus quadratus hepatis.
renal l's lobi renales.
Riedel l. an anomalous tongue-shaped mass of tissue that sometimes projects from the right liver.
right l. of liver lobus hepatis dexter.
rostral l. of cerebellum lobus cerebelli anterior.
spigelian l. lobus caudatus.
superior l., left lobus superior pulmonis sinistri.
superior l., right lobus superior pulmonis dextri.
superior l. of left lung lobus superior pulmonis sinistri.
superior l. of right lung lobus superior pulmonis dextri.
temporal l. lobus temporalis.
l. of thymus lobus thymi.
l. of thyroid gland lobus glandulae thyroideae.
upper l., left lobus superior pulmonis sinistri.
upper l., right lobus superior pulmonis dextri.
upper l. of left lung lobus superior pulmonis sinistri.
upper l. of right lung lobus superior pulmonis dextri.
vagal l. visceral l.
visceral l. the visceral sensory area of fishes.

lo•bec•to•my (lo-bek′tə-me) [*lobe* + *-ectomy*] excision of a lobe, as of the thyroid, liver, brain, or lung. See also *lobotomy.*
occipital l. removal of the occipital lobe, to treat brain cancer or occasionally epilepsy with a focus in the occipital lobe.
sleeve l. excision of a lobe of the lung with removal of a portion of the bronchus and reanastomosis of the resulting ends. Called also *sleeve resection.*
temporal l. excision of part or all of a temporal lobe in the treatment of temporal lobe epilepsy.
thyroid l. removal of all or part of a lobe of the thyroid gland.

Lo•be•lia (lo-be′le-ə) a genus of herbs of the family Campanulaceae; they contain lobeline and other toxic alkaloids and cause mouth ulcerations and diarrhea in ruminants. *L. berlandie′ri* grows in Mexico. *L. infla′ta* is Indian tobacco, which grows in the eastern United States and Canada.

lo•be•lia (lo-be′le-ə) 1. any plant of the genus *Lobelia.* 2. the dried leaves and tops of *Lobelia inflata*, an herb with properties resembling those of nicotine; used in homeopathy to treat asthma.

lo•be•line (lo′bə-lēn) alpha-lobeline, the principal alkaloid found in plants of the genus *Lobelia;* it is responsible for the toxic effects seen in ruminants who ingest the plants. It has been used in antismoking preparations.

lo•ben•da•zole (lo-ben′də-zōl) a veterinary anthelmintic.

lo•bi (lo′bi) [L.] genitive and plural of *lobus.*

lo•bi•tis (lo-bi′tis) inflammation of a lobe, especially of a lobe of the lung.

Lo•bo disease (lo′bo) [Jorge *Lobo*, Brazilian physician, 20th century] lacaziosis.

Lo•boa (lo-bo′ə) [J. *Lobo*] *Lacazia.*

lo•bo•my•co•sis (lo″bo-mi-ko′sis) lacaziosis.

lo•bo•po•di•um (lo″bo-po′de-əm) pl. *lobopo′dia* [*lobe* + *pous* foot] a wide, blunt pseudopodium composed of both ectoplasm and endoplasm. Cf. *axopodium, filopodium,* and *reticulopodium.*

Lo•bo•sa (lo-bo′sə) a class of ameboid protozoa in the subphylum Sarcodina of the phylum Sarcomastigophora; most species have lobopodia, although filopodia and reticulopodia sometimes occur. Orders are grouped into two subclasses: Gymnamoebia or the ramicristate amebae and Testacealobosia or the testate amebae.

Lo•bo•sea (lo-bo′se-ə) [Gr. *lobos* lobe] a former class of ameboid protozoa that was replaced by Lobosa and other classes.

lo•bot•o•my (lo-bot′ə-me) incision into a lobe; in psychosurgery, surgical incision of all the fibers of a lobe of the brain.
frontal l. prefrontal l.
prefrontal l. an operation in which, through holes drilled in the skull, the white matter of the frontal lobe is incised with a leukotome passed through a cannula; called also *leukotomy.*
transorbital l. prefrontal lobotomy performed by way of the orbital plate; called also *transorbital leukotomy.*

Lob•stein ganglion (lōb′shtīn) [Johann Friedrich Georg Christian Martin *Lobstein*, German surgeon, 1777–1835] see under *ganglion.*

lob•u•lat•ed (lob′u-lāt″əd) made up of or divided into lobules.

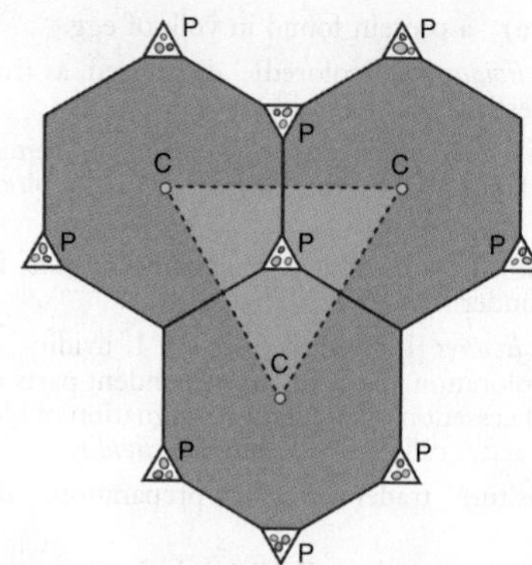

■ Diagram of hepatic *(solid lines)* and portal *(dotted lines)* lobules, showing the portal areas *(P)* and central veins *(C).*

lob•u•la•tion (lob″u-la′shən) the process of becoming or the state of being lobulated.
portal l. the pattern in the liver produced by bands of fibrous tissue interconnecting portal areas.

lob•ule (lob′ūl) a small lobe; see *lobulus.* **lob′ular** *adj*
accessory thymic l's lobuli thymici accessorii.
ansiform l. lobuli semilunares.
anterior quadrangular l. of cerebellum lobulus quadrangularis anterior cerebelli.
l. of auricle lobulus auriculae.
biventral l. lobulus biventer cerebelli.
central l. of cerebellum lobulus centralis cerebelli.
cortical l's of kidney lobuli corticales renis.
l's of epididymis lobuli epididymidis.
gracile l. lobulus gracilis cerebelli.
hepatic l's lobuli hepatis.
inferior parietal l. lobulus parietalis inferior.
inferior semilunar l. lobulus semilunaris inferior.
l's of liver lobuli hepatis.
l's of mammary gland lobuli glandulae mammariae.
l. of pancreas one of the distinct lobules into which the pancreas is divided by extension of septa of the capsule into the gland.
paracentral l. lobulus paracentralis.
paramedian l. lobulus gracilis cerebelli.
portal l. a polygonal mass of liver tissue, larger than a liver acinus, containing portions of three adjacent hepatic lobules, and having a portal vein at its center and a central vein peripherally at each corner.
posterior quadrangular l. of cerebellum lobulus quadrangularis posterior cerebelli.
primary l. of lung terminal respiratory unit.
pulmonary l. lobulus pulmonis.
respiratory l. terminal respiratory unit.
secondary l. of lung an anatomical subdivision of a pulmonary segment, consisting of several branching primary lobules.
semilunar l's lobuli semilunares.
simple l. of cerebellum lobulus simplex cerebelli.
superior parietal l. lobulus parietalis superior.
superior semilunar l. lobulus semilunaris superior.
l's of testis lobuli testis.
l's of thymus lobuli thymi.
l's of thyroid gland lobuli glandulae thyroideae.

lob•u•li (lob′u-li) [L.] genitive and plural of *lobulus.*

lob•u•lose (lob′u-lōs) lobulated.

lob•u•lous (lob′u-ləs) lobulated.

lob•u•lus (lob′u-ləs) gen. and pl. *lo′buli* [L., dim of *lobus*] lobule: a small lobe or one of the primary divisions of a lobe.
l. ansifor′mis TA alternative for *lobuli semilunares.*
l. auri′culae [TA], **l. auricula′ris** lobule of auricle: the inferior, dependent part of the auricle below the antitragus, which contains fibrous and fatty tissue but no cartilage. Called also *earlobe* or *ear lobe.*
l. biven′ter cerebel′li [TA] biventral lobule (HVIII): a lobule of the cerebellar hemisphere, located in the posterior lobe between the tonsilla and the lobulus gracilis and continuous with the pyramis vermis. It is divided into lateral and medial parts by the intrabiventral fissure.
l. centra′lis cerebel′li [TA] central lobule of cerebellum (II and III): the portion of the anterior lobe of the cerebellum between the lingula and the culmen, resting on the lingula and the anterior medullary velum. It is subdivided into anterior (II) and posterior (III) parts.
lo′buli cortica′les re′nis cortical lobules of kidney: more or less distinctly marked small polygonal areas on the surface of a kidney; each area

corresponds to a medullary ray together with its attached renal corpuscles and tubules.

lo′buli epididy′midis [TA] lobules of epididymis: the wedge-shaped parts of the head of the epididymis, each comprising a single efferent ductule of the testis. Called also *coni epididymidis* [TA alternative].

lo′buli glan′dulae mamma′riae [TA] lobules of mammary gland: the smaller subdivisions that make up a lobe of the mammary gland, each drained by a single branch of a lactiferous duct. See also *glandula mammaria*.

lo′buli glan′dulae thyroi′deae [TA] lobules of thyroid gland: irregular areas on the surface of the thyroid gland produced by entrance into the gland of fibrous trabeculae from the sheath.

l. gra′cilis cerebel′li [TA] gracile lobule (HVII B): the portion of the posterior lobe of the cerebellar hemisphere between the semilunar and biventral lobules, anterior to the prebiventral fissure and continuous with the tuber vermis; called also *l. paramedianus cerebelli* [TA alternative] and *paramedian lobule*.

lo′buli he′patis [TA] hepatic lobules: the small vascular units composing the substance of the liver, each of which is polygonal, with a central vein at its center and portal canals peripherally at the corners. See also *liver acinus*, under *acinus*, and see illustration at *portal lobule*, under *lobule*.

l. paracentra′lis [TA] paracentral lobule: a lobe on the medial surface of the cerebral hemisphere, continuous with the precentral and postcentral gyri of the frontal and parietal lobes, and limited below by the cingulate sulcus; it is subdivided into the anterior and posterior paracentral gyri.

l. parafloccula′ris dorsa′lis TA alternative for *pars medialis lobuli biventralis cerebelli*.

l. paramedia′nus cerebel′li TA alternative for *l. gracilis cerebelli*.

l. parieta′lis infe′rior [TA] inferior parietal lobule: the lobule that forms the posterior part of the lateral portion of the parietal lobe of the cerebrum. It lies below the intraparietal sulcus, above the posterior ramus of the lateral cerebral fissure, and behind the postcentral sulcus. It includes the supramarginal and the angular gyri. In the dominant hemisphere, it is concerned with language mechanisms.

l. parieta′lis supe′rior [TA] superior parietal lobule: the posterior part of the upper portion of the parietal lobe of the brain; it lies behind the postcentral sulcus, in front of the parietooccipital fissure, and above the intraparietal sulcus. It comprises association areas concerned with general sensory functions.

l. pulmo′nis [TA] pulmonary lobule: one of the sections into which each bronchopulmonary segment of the lung is subdivided; it is supplied by a single bronchiole and is separated from other lobules by connective tissue septa.

l. quadrangula′ris ante′rior cerebel′li [TA] anterior quadrangular lobule of cerebellum (HIV and HV): the portion of the anterior lobe of the hemisphere of the cerebellum lying between the preculminate and primary fissures, continuous with the culmen; it is divided into anterior (HIV) and posterior (HV) parts.

l. quadrangula′ris poste′rior cerebel′li [TA] posterior quadrangular lobule of cerebellum (HVI): the portion of the posterior lobe of the hemisphere of the cerebellum lying between the primary and posterior superior fissures and continuous with the declive.

lo′buli semiluna′res [TA] semilunar lobules (HVII A): the lobulus semilunaris inferior and lobulus semilunaris superior considered together. Called also *l. ansiformis* [TA alternative].

l. semiluna′ris infe′rior [TA] inferior semilunar lobule (HVII A): a lobule of the cerebellar hemisphere that is continuous with the tuber vermis and is between the superior semilunar lobule and the gracile lobule; called also *crus secundum lobuli ansiformis* [TA alternative] and *second crus of ansiform lobule*.

l. semiluna′ris supe′rior [TA] superior semilunar lobule (HVII A): a lobule of the cerebellar hemisphere that is continuous with the folium vermis and is between the posterior quadrangular lobule and the inferior semilunar lobule; called also *crus primum lobuli ansiformis* [TA alternative] and *first crus of ansiform lobule*.

l. sim′plex cerebel′li [TA] simple lobule of cerebellum (VI and HVI): the large anterior division of the posterior cerebellar lobe, comprising the lobulus quadrangularis cerebelli posterior (HVI) and declive (VI).

lo′buli tes′tis [TA] lobules of testis: the pyramidal subdivisions of the testicular substance, each with its base against the tunica albuginea and its apex at the mediastinum, and composed largely of seminiferous tubules.

lo′buli thy′mi [TA] lobules of thymus: the smaller subdivisions of the lobes of the thymus (q.v.), separated by fibrous trabeculae.

lo′buli thy′mici accesso′rii [TA] accessory thymic lobules: small lobules of ectopic thymus tissue in the neck, representing portions that became detached and left behind in the caudal migration of the gland in embryonic development. Called also *accessory thymic nodules*.

lo·bus (lo′bəs) gen. and pl. *lo′bi* [L., from Gr. *lobos*] lobe: a more or less well-defined portion of an organ, especially the brain, the lungs, or a gland, demarcated by fissures, sulci, or connective tissue septa.

l. ante′rior cerebel′li l. cerebelli anterior.

l. ante′rior hypophy′seos TA alternative for *adenohypophysis*.

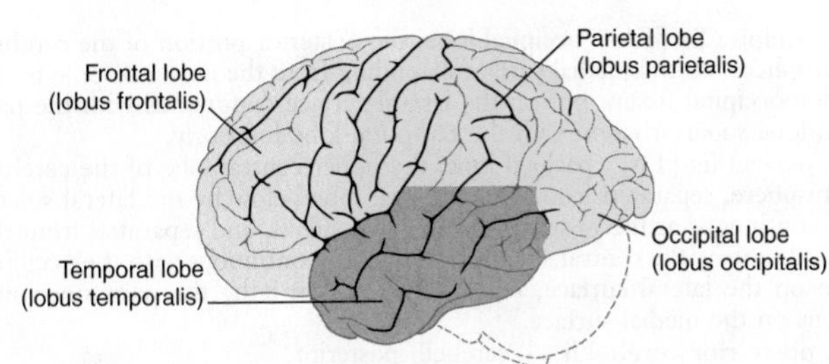

■ Lobi cerebri (lobes of the cerebrum); lateral aspect of left cerebral hemisphere.

l. cauda′lis cerebel′li l. cerebelli posterior.

l. cauda′tus he′patis [TA] caudate lobe of liver: a small lobe of the liver, bounded on the right by the inferior vena cava, which separates it from the right lobe, and on the left by the attachment of the hepatogastric ligament, which separates it from the left lobe. In the newer anatomic classification of the liver (see *segmenta hepatis*, under *segmentum*), this is identical to the posterior part (*pars posterior hepatis*). Called also *spigelian lobe*.

l. cerebel′li ante′rior [TA] anterior lobe of cerebellum: the portion of the cerebellum lying in front of the primary fissure, comprising the lingula, central lobule, alae of central lobules, culmen, and anterior quadrangular lobule; called also *cranial* or *rostral lobe of cerebellum*, *l. cranialis cerebelli*, and *l. rostralis cerebelli*.

l. cerebel′li poste′rior [TA] posterior lobe of cerebellum: the portion of the cerebellum separated from the anterior lobe by the primary fissure and from the flocculonodular lobe by the posterolateral fissure; it comprises the declive, folium vermis, tuber vermis, pyramid, uvula, simple lobule, inferior and superior semilunar lobules, and tonsils. Called also *caudal lobe of cerebellum* and *l. caudalis cerebelli*.

lo′bi cerebra′les, lo′bi ce′rebri [TA] cerebral lobes: the well-defined areas of the cerebral cortex, demarcated by fissures, sulci, and arbitrary lines, including the frontal, temporal, parietal, occipital, limbic, and insular lobes. See illustration.

l. crania′lis cerebel′li l. cerebelli anterior.

l. flocculonodula′ris [TA] flocculonodular lobe: a fundamental subdivision of the cerebellum, located inferiorly, consisting of paired lateral flocculi, their pedunculi, and the nodulus.

l. fronta′lis [TA] frontal lobe: the anterior portion of the cerebral hemisphere, extending from the frontal pole to the sulcus centralis.

lo′bi glan′dulae mamma′riae [TA] lobes of mammary gland: the major subdivisions of the secreting portion of the mammary gland, each drained by a single lactiferous duct and further subdivided into lobules (lobuli glandulae mammariae). See also *glandula mammaria*.

l. glan′dulae thyroi′deae [TA] lobe of thyroid gland: either of the lobes (right or left) of the thyroid gland, located adjacent to either side of the trachea, cricoid cartilage, and thyroid cartilage.

l. glandula′ris hypophy′seos adenohypophysis.

l. he′patis dex′ter [TA] right lobe of liver: in traditional anatomic terminology, the largest of the four lobes of the liver. Anteriorly, it is separated from the left lobe by the falciform ligament. Posteroinferiorly, it is separated from the caudate lobe by the inferior vena cava and from the quadrate lobe by the gallbladder. Sometimes the term has been extended to include the entire caudate and quadrate lobes. See also *pars hepatis dextra*.

l. he′patis sinis′ter [TA] left lobe of liver: in traditional anatomic terminology, the smaller of the two main lobes of the liver. Anteriorly, it is separated from the right lobe by the falciform ligament. Posteroinferiorly, it is separated from the caudate and quadrate lobes by the attachment of the gastrohepatic ligament and the ligamentum teres. See also *pars hepatis sinistra*.

l. infe′rior pulmo′nis dex′tri [TA] inferior lobe of right lung; see *lung*. It has five bronchopulmonary segments (segmenta bronchopulmonalia, q.v.). Called also *right lower lobe* and *lower lobe of right lung*.

l. infe′rior pulmo′nis sinis′tri [TA] inferior lobe of left lung; see *lung*. It has four or five bronchopulmonary segments (segmenta bronchopulmonalia, q.v.). Called also *left lower lobe* and *lower lobe of left lung*.

l. insula′ris TA alternative for *insula* (def. 2).

l. lim′bicus [TA] limbic lobe: a portion of the cerebral cortex at the most medial aspect of the hemisphere, consisting mainly of the subcallosal area, cingulate gyrus, isthmus, and parahippocampal gyrus, and having connections with the limbic system.

l. me′dius pro′statae [TA] median lobe of prostate: an inconstant but normal enlargement of the isthmus of the prostate.

l. me′dius pulmo′nis dex′tri [TA] middle lobe of right lung; see *lung*. It has two bronchopulmonary segments (segmenta bronchopulmonalia, q.v.). Called also *right middle lobe*.

l. nervo′sus neurohypophy′seos [TA] neural lobe of hypophysis: the major portion of the neurohypophysis; called also *neural lobe of neurohypophysis* or *pituitary gland* and *pars nervosa neurohypophyseos* [TA alternative].

l. occipita´lis [TA] occipital lobe: the posterior portion of the cerebral hemisphere, on the medial surface extending from the posterior pole to the parietooccipital fissure but on the lateral surface continuous with the parietal lobe superiorly and with the temporal lobe inferiorly.

l. parieta´lis [TA] parietal lobe: the upper central lobe of the cerebral hemisphere, separated from the temporal lobe below by the lateral sulcus, but continuous at the posterior end of that sulcus, and separated from the frontal lobe by the central sulcus. Behind, it is continuous with the occipital lobe on the lateral surface, but separated from it by the parietooccipital sulcus on the medial surface.

l. poste´rior cerebel´li l. cerebelli posterior.

l. poste´rior hypophy´seos TA alternative for *neurohypophysis.*

lo´bi pro´statae dex´ter et sinis´ter [TA] lobes of prostate: the paired halves (right and left) of the prostate, separated by a more or less distinct median sulcus; called also *lateral lobes of prostate gland.*

l. pyramida´lis glan´dulae thyroi´deae [TA] pyramidal lobe of thyroid gland: an occasional third lobe that extends upward from the isthmus of the gland across the thyroid cartilage to the hyoid bone; it is the residuum of the thyroid stalk of the fetus.

l. quadra´tus he´patis [TA] quadrate lobe of liver: a small lobe of the liver bounded on the right by the gallbladder, which separates it from the right lobe, and on the left by the ligamentum teres, which separates it from the left lobe.

lo´bi rena´les [TA] renal lobes: the units of the kidney, each consisting of a pyramid and its surrounding cortical substance; the division of the kidney into lobes is more distinctly marked in some animals and in infants than in the human adult.

l. rostra´lis cerebel´li l. cerebelli anterior.

l. supe´rior pulmo´nis dex´tri [TA] superior lobe of right lung; see *lung.* It has three bronchopulmonary segments (segmenta bronchopulmonalia, q.v.). Called also *right upper lobe* and *upper lobe of right lung.*

l. supe´rior pulmo´nis sinis´tri [TA] superior lobe of left lung; see *lung.* It has four bronchopulmonary segments (segmenta bronchopulmonalia, q.v.). Called also *left upper lobe* and *upper lobe of left lung.*

l. tempora´lis [TA] temporal lobe: the lower lateral lobe of the cerebral hemisphere, lying below the posterior ramus of the lateral sulcus, lateral to the collateral sulcus, and merging behind with the occipital lobe on the lateral and inferior surfaces.

l. thy´mi [TA] lobe of thymus: either of the two chief parts (right or left) of the thymus, which meet in the midline.

l. va´gi visceral lobe.

lo·cal (lo´kəl) [L. *localis*] restricted to or pertaining to one spot or part; not general.

lo·cal·iza·tion (lo″kəl-ĭ-za´shən) 1. the determination of the site or place of any process or lesion. 2. restriction to a circumscribed or limited area. 3. prelocalization.

cerebral l. the determination of the situation of the various centers of the brain; also the limitation of the various cerebral faculties to a particular center or organ of the brain.

germinal l. the location on a blastoderm of prospective organs; see *fate map,* under *map.*

lo·cal·ized (lo´kəl-īzd) not general; restricted to a limited region or to one or more spots.

lo·cal·iz·er (lo´kəl-īz″ər) 1. an instrument for locating solid particles in the eyeball by radiography. 2. a visual training instrument for establishing correct spatial localization in treating amblyopia ex anopsia.

lo·ca·tor (lo´ka-tər) an instrument or apparatus by which the site of an object is determined.

abutment l. a thin resin base made on a diagnostic denture cast into which holes have been cut to predetermine locations of the cuspid teeth and molar teeth on a subperiosteal implant.

apex l. in root canal therapy, an electronic device used to determine the working length of a canal that has been cleaned out and when a file has reached the apical foramen.

Berman-Moorhead l. an instrument for locating metallic fragments embedded in body tissues.

electroacoustic l. an apparatus that amplifies into an audible click the contact of a probe with a solid object; used in locating foreign objects within the body.

Moorhead foreign body l. Berman-Moorhead l.

Loc. dol. [L.] lo´co dolen´ti (to the painful spot).

lo·chia (lo´ke-ə) [Gr. *lochia*] the vaginal discharge that takes place during the first week or two after childbirth. **lo´chial** *adj*

l. al´ba the final vaginal discharge after childbirth, when the amount of blood is decreased and the leukocytes are increased.

l. ru´bra the vaginal discharge of almost pure blood immediately after childbirth.

l. sanguinolen´ta the thick, maroon-colored vaginal discharge occurring a few days after childbirth.

l. sero´sa the serous vaginal discharge occurring about four or five days after childbirth.

lo·chio·me·tra (lo″ke-o-me´trə) [*lochia* + *metra*] distention of the uterus by retained lochia.

lo·chi·or·rha·gia (lo″ke-o-ra´jə) lochiorrhea.

lo·chi·or·rhea (lo″ke-o-re´ə) [*lochia* + *-rrhea*] an abnormally profuse discharge of lochia.

lo·chi·os·che·sis (lo″ke-os´kə-sis) lochiostasis.

lo·chi·os·ta·sis (lo″ke-os´tə-sis) [*lochia* + *-stasis*] retention of the lochia.

lo·ci (lo´si) [L.] genitive and plural of *locus.*

Locke solution (fluid) (lok) [Frank Spiller *Locke,* British physiologist, 1871–1949] see under *solution.*

lock·jaw (lok´jaw) trismus.

Lock·wood ligament (lok´wood) [Charles Barrett *Lockwood,* English surgeon, 1856–1914] see under *ligament.*

lo·co (lo´ko) [Sp. "insane"] 1. locoweed. 2. locoism. 3. an animal affected with locoism.

loc(o)- [L. *locus* a place] a combining form denoting relationship to place.

Lo·coid (lo´koid) trademark for preparations of hydrocortisone butyrate.

lo·co·ism (lo´ko-iz″əm) a disease of horses, cattle, and sheep caused by poisoning by any of the plants called *locoweed;* it is marked by locomotor disturbances, trembling, depression, and, in pregnant animals, abortion. Called also *loco disease* and *loco poisoning.*

lo·co·mo·tion (lo″kə-mo´shən) [*locus* + *motion*] movement or the ability to move from one place to another. **locomo´tive, locomo´tor, locomo´tory** *adj*

brachial l. brachiation.

lo·co·mo·tor (lo″kə-mo´tər) 1. locomotive. 2. pertaining to or affecting a locomotor system (see under *system*).

lo·co·mo·to·ri·al (lo″ko-mo-tor´e-əl) pertaining to the locomotorium or locomotor system.

lo·co·mo·to·ri·um (lo″ko-mo-tor´e-əm) the structures of an organism concerned with locomotion; in humans, the bones, joints, and muscles of the lower limb, together with their vascular and nerve supplies.

lo·co·re·gion·al (lo″ko-re´jən-əl) limited to a localized area, as contrasted to *systemic* or *metastatic,* such as pertaining to spread of a pathological change beyond the site of origin but only into the nearby region.

lo·co·weed (lo´ko-wēd) [Sp. *loco* insane] any of numerous leguminous plants that grow in arid regions of North America, primarily members of the genera *Astragalus, Hosackia, Oxytropis,* and *Sophora;* they contain a variety of toxins and cause locoism in horses, cattle, and sheep.

loc·u·lar (lok´u-lər) pertaining to a loculus.

loc·u·late (lok´u-lāt) divided into loculi.

loc·u·li (lok´u-li) [L.] plural of *loculus.*

loc·u·lus (lok´u-ləs) pl. *lo´culi* [L., dim. of *locus*] 1. a small space or cavity. 2. a local enlargement of the uterus in some mammals, containing an embryo.

lo·cum (lo´kəm) [L., accusative of *locus*] place.

l. te´nens, l. te´nent a practitioner who temporarily takes the place of another.

lo·cus (lo´kəs) gen. and pl. *lo´ci* [L. "a place"] 1. a place or site, as in the body. 2. in genetics, the position of a gene on a chromosome, different forms of genes (alleles) being found at the same position on homologous chromosomes. The standard method of designating a locus consists of the chromosome number; p (short arm) or q (long arm); region and band number written without separation (11, 12, 13, etc.), moving outward from the centromere; sub-band and sub-sub-band, again written without separation. The centromere is designated by "cen" and the telomere or terminal by "ter."

l. caeru´leus, l. ceru´leus [TA], **l. coeru´leus** a pigmented area in the rostrolateral region of the pontine part of the fourth ventricle floor and extending into the mesencephalon in the lateral portion of the periaqueductal gray substance; cells of this nucleus contain melanin.

complex l. gene complex.

l. mino´ris resisten´tiae a site of lessened resistance; an area, structure, or organ in which there is a weakness, such as potential for breakage of a part or diminished resistance to invasion by microorganisms or their toxins.

operator l. operator.

Lo·dine (lo´dēn) trademark for a preparation of etodolac.

Lo·do·syn (lo´do-sin) trademark for a preparation of carbidopa.

lo·dox·a·mide tro·meth·amine (lo-dok´sə-mīd) a mast cell stabilizer that inhibits type I (immediate) hypersensitivity; applied topically to the eye for the treatment of vernal conjunctivitis, vernal keratitis, and vernal keratoconjunctivitis.

Loeb deciduoma, reaction (lōb) [Leo *Loeb*, American pathologist, 1869–1959] see under *deciduoma* and *reaction*.

Loef·fler see *Löffler*.

LOEL lowest observed effect level.

Lo·es·trin (lo-es′trin) trademark for combination preparations of norethindrone acetate and ethinyl estradiol. When a placebo week of ferrous fumarate tablets are included, the trademark is Loestrin Fe.

Löff·ler alkaline methylene blue stain (lərf′lər) [Friederich August Johannes *Löffler*, German bacteriologist, 1852–1915] see *Stains and Staining Methods*, under *stain*.

Löff·ler endocarditis, syndrome (eosinophilia, pneumonia) (lərf′lər) [Wilhelm *Löffler*, Swiss physician, 1887–1972] see under *endocarditis* and *syndrome*.

Löf·gren syndrome (lərf′grən) [Sven Halvar *Löfgren*, Swedish physician, 20th century] see under *syndrome*.

log·a·dec·to·my (log″ə-dek′tə-me) [Gr. *logades* the whites of the eyes + *-ectomy*] excision of a portion of the conjunctiva.

log·a·graph·ia (log″ə-graf′e-ə) [*log-* + *agraphia*] agraphia.

log·am·ne·sia (log″am-ne′zhə) [*log-* + *amnesia*] 1. receptive aphasia. 2. any condition in which a person cannot remember words.

log·a·pha·sia (log″ə-fa′zhə) [*log-* + *aphasia*] motor aphasia.

log·a·rithm (log′ə-rith-əm) the power to which a number, fixed for a given system and usually called the base number, must be raised to obtain a second number. Logarithms are usually computed in the natural base *e*, and are denoted $\log_e$ (also expressed ln). For example, if $\log_e(y) = x$ then $e^x = y$. See also *e*.

 l. of odds see *lod score*, under *score*.

loge (lōzh) [Fr.] a hut, box, or booth.

 l. de Guyon Guyon canal.

log(o)- [Gr. *logos* word, reason] a combining form denoting relationship to words or speech.

logo·clo·nia (log″o-klo′ne-ə) [*logo-* + *clonus* + *-ia*] spasmodic repetition of words or parts of words, particularly the end syllables, often occurring in Alzheimer disease. Cf. *stuttering* (def. 1). Called also *logospasm*.

logo·gram (log′o-gram) the graphic record of the symptoms and signs exhibited by a specific patient, charted by means of the logoscope.

log·op·a·thy (log-op′ə-the) speech disorder.

logo·pe·dia (log″o-pe′de-ə) logopedics.

logo·pe·dics (log-o-pe′diks) [*logo-* + ortho*pedics*] the study and treatment of speech defects. See also *speech pathology*, under *pathology*. Called also *logopedia*.

log·or·rhea (log″o-re′ə) [*logo-* + *-rrhea*] excessive volubility, with rapid, pressured speech, as seen in manic episodes of bipolar disorder and in some types of schizophrenia. Called also *agitolalia, agitophasia, pressured speech, tachylalia, tachyphasia*, and *verbomania*.

logo·spasm (log′o-spaz″əm) 1. logoclonia. 2. stuttering (def. 1).

log·wood (log′wood) *Haematoxylon campechianum*.

-logy [Gr. *logos* word, reason] a word termination meaning the science or study of, or a treatise on, the subject designated by the stem to which it is affixed.

LOH loss of heterozygosity.

Löh·lein-Baehr lesion (lur′līn bār) [Max Hermann Friedrich *Löhlein*, German physician, 1877–1921; George *Baehr*, American physician, 1887–1978] see under *lesion*.

lo·i·a·sis (lo-i′ə-sis) infection with the nematode eye worm *Loa Loa*, which inhabits subcutaneous connective tissue, especially around the orbit and under the conjunctiva, causing itching, eosinophilia, and occasionally edematous swellings called Calabar swellings. In rare severe cases, worms may migrate farther into the body and cause inflammation of joints or internal organs. Called also *loaiasis*.

loin (loin) regio lumbalis.

Lo·li·um (lo′le-əm) the rye grasses, a genus of plants commonly found in pastures and consumed by livestock.

 L. peren′ne perennial rye grass, a variety that sometimes carries the fungus *Acremonium loliae*, which causes rye grass staggers in ruminants.

 L. ri′gidum Wimmera rye grass, a variety whose seed galls sometimes carry nematodes infected with species of *Corynebacterium*, causing rye grass staggers in ruminants.

 L. temulen′tum darnel, a rye grass whose seeds contain a narcotic that causes darnel poisoning (q.v.) when moldy seeds are eaten.

lo·me·flox·a·cin (lo″mə-flok′sə-sin) a fluoroquinolone antibacterial effective against a wide range of aerobic gram-negative and gram-positive organisms.

 l. hydrochloride the hydrochloride salt of lomefloxacin, administered orally in the treatment of bronchitis and the treatment and prevention of urinary tract infections.

lo·mo·some (lo′mo-sōm) [Gr. *lōma* hem, fringe + *-some*] a spongelike structure in fungi contiguous with the hyphal wall.

Lo·mo·til (lo′mo-til) trademark for combination preparations of diphenoxylate hydrochloride and atropine sulfate.

lo·mus·tine (lo-mus′tēn) a cytotoxic alkylating agent of the nitrosourea (q.v.) group, used as an antineoplastic primarily for treatment of brain tumors and Hodgkin disease; administered orally. Called also *CCNU*.

Lon·cho·car·pus (lon″ko-kahr′pəs) a genus of tropical American woody plants of the family Leguminosae. *L. u′tilis* is the cubé, which yields the toxic insecticide rotenone.

long-chain-fat·ty-ac·id–CoA li·gase (long chān fat′e as′id ko-a′ li′gās) [EC 6.2.1.3] an enzyme of the ligase class that catalyzes the formation of acyl coenzyme A from long chain fatty acids (12 or more carbons) and coenzyme A, using energy derived from ATP hydrolysis. The enzyme occurs in the mitochondrial outer membrane, endoplasmic reticulum, and peroxisome membrane, and it acts on saturated and unsaturated fatty acids as well as some hydroxy acids. Called also *acyl CoA synthetase*.

lon·gev·i·ty (lon-jev′ĭ-te) [L. *longus* long + *aevum* age] the condition or quality of being long lived.

lon·gi·lin·e·al (lon″jĭ-lin′e-əl) built along long, narrow lines; dolichomorphic.

lon·gis·si·mus (lon-jis′ĭ-məs) [L. "longest, very long"] a general term denoting a long structure, as a muscle.

lon·gi·tu·di·nal (lon″jĭ-too′di-nəl) [L. *longitudo* length] lengthwise; parallel to the long axis of the body or an organ.

lon·gi·tu·di·na·lis (lon″ji-too″dĭ-na′lis) [L.] [TA] lengthwise; a term denoting a structure that is parallel to the long axis of the body or an organ.

long·sight·ed·ness (long′sīt-əd-nis) hyperopia.

lon·gus (long′gəs) [L.] long: a general term denoting a long structure, as a muscle.

Loni·ten (lon′ĭ-ten) trademark for a preparation of minoxidil.

Lo·nox (lo′noks) trademark for combination preparations of diphenoxylate hydrochloride and atropine sulfate.

loop (lo͞op) 1. a turn or sharp curve in a cordlike structure; see also *ansa*. 2. something, such as a figure or course, having such a curved or circular shape. 3. an instrument used in microbiology, consisting of a rod-shaped metal handle holding a firm wire of platinum or nichrome, whose free end is formed into a ring that usually has an inside diameter of 4 mm. It is used for the inoculation of cultures of bacteria and fungi.

 amplification l. in positive feedback, the loop through which increased output subsequently increases input and so increases output.

 bulboventricular l. ventricular l.

 capillary l's minute endothelial tubes that carry blood in the papillae of the skin.

 cervical l. peripheral cuboidal cells of the enamel organ that encircle the edge of a developing tooth.

 closed l. a type of feedback in which the input to one or more of the subsystems is affected by its own output.

 feedback l. the circular path seen in a system that has feedback, such that the output of the system participates in the control of the system.

 gamma l. a three-part reflex arc consisting of gamma motoneurons that send impulses along the gamma fibers to the intrafusal fibers, causing the muscle spindle to contract; that in turn excites afferent impulses, which pass through the posterior root to alpha motoneurons in the anterior horn, causing a stretch reflex. Called also *Granit l.*

 Gerdy interatrial l. a small muscular bundle in the interatrial septum of the heart.

 Granit l. gamma l.

 l. of Henle, Henle l. ansa nephroni.

 l. of hypoglossal nerve ansa cervicalis.

 Hyrtl l. an occasional looplike anastomosis between the right and left hypoglossal nerves in the geniohyoid muscle.

 Ivy l. see under *wiring*.

 lenticular l. ansa lenticularis.

 Meyer l., Meyer-Archambault l. a structure formed by some of the fibers of the optic radiation as they loop around the inferior horn of the lateral ventricle before turning posteriorly.

 midgut l. a U-shaped loop of intestine that temporarily forms during the period of rapid elongation and rotation of the midgut in embryonic development. It projects into the proximal part of the umbilical cord, to which it is attached via the yolk stalk; with further development, it retracts into the abdomen, rotating further.

 nephron l. ansa nephroni.

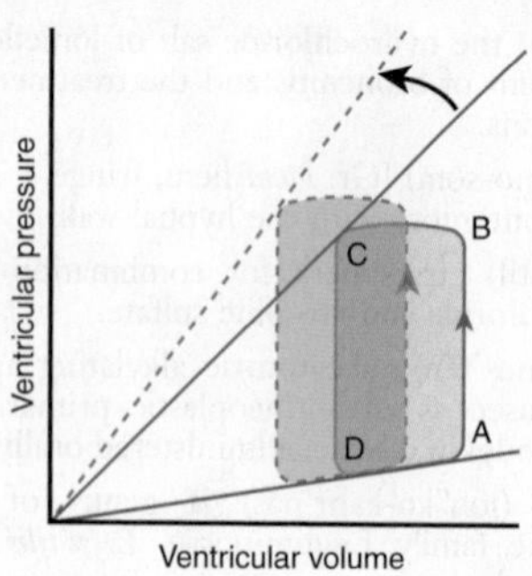

■ Pressure-volume loops comparing a control state *(solid line)* and the addition of a positive inotropic agent *(dotted line)*, assuming constant stroke volume. Beginning with *A*, end-diastole, the period from *A* to *B* represents isovolumetric left ventricular contraction. Ejection occurs from *B*, opening of the aortic valve to *C*, end-systole. The period from *C* to *D*, opening of the mitral valve, represents isovolumetric relaxation, and is followed by ventricular filling in the period from *D* to *A*.

open l. a system in which an input alters the output, but the output has no effect on the input. See also *feedback*.

peduncular l. ansa peduncularis.

pressure-volume l's graphic representations of the pressure within cardiac ventricles as a function of their volumes, recorded over the course of the cardiac cycle under various conditions, such as increased preload or afterload, and used to assess cardiac contractility.

primary intestinal l. midgut l.

sentinel l. a distended loop of small intestine near the pancreas seen on plain films of the abdomen in acute pancreatitis.

Stoerck l. the primitive loop in the embryonic uriniferous tubule which develops into a loop of Henle and a portion of the proximal convoluted tubule.

subclavian l. ansa subclavia.

ventricular l. the early U-shaped loop of the embryonic heart; called also *bulboventricular l.*

l. of Vieussens ansa subclavia.

loop·ful (lo͞op′fəl) the quantity of liquid that can be held within the loop of wire used in transferring microorganisms to other culture media.

loop·ing (lo͞op′ing) the formation of a loop, or bending of something into a loop.

cardiac l. the bending of the tubular embryonic heart to form an S-shaped organ.

loop·o·gram (lo͞op′o-gram″) the radiographic record made in loopography.

loo·pog·ra·phy (loo-pog′rə-fe) a radiological procedure for assessing the integrity of a loop of intestine used as an ileal conduit; the outlet of the conduit is obstructed with a balloon catheter, and contrast medium is injected to flow in a retrograde direction so that the efficiency of its flow up the conduit can be monitored.

loo·sen·ing (loo′sən-ing) freeing from restraint or strictness.

l. of associations in psychiatry, a disorder of thinking in which associations of ideas become so shortened, fragmented, and disturbed as to lack logical relationship; often seen in schizophrenia.

Loo·ser transformation zones (lo′zər) [Emil *Looser*, Swiss surgeon, 1877–1936] see under *zone*.

Loo·ser-Milk·man syndrome (lo′zər milk′man) [Emil *Looser;* Louis Arthur *Milkman*, American radiologist, 1895–1951] Milkman syndrome.

Lo/Ovral (lo-o′vral) trademark for combination preparations of norgestrel and ethinyl estradiol.

LOP left occipitoposterior; see *occipitoposterior position*, under *position*.

lo·per·a·mide hy·dro·chlo·ride (lo-per′ə-mīd) an antiperistaltic that exerts a direct effect on the muscles of the intestinal wall, used in the treatment of acute nonspecific diarrhea, traveler's diarrhea, and chronic diarrhea associated with inflammatory bowel disease, and to reduce the volume of discharge from ileostomies; administered orally.

loph(o)- [Gr. *lophos* ridge, tuft] a combining form denoting a relationship to a ridge or to a tuft.

loph·odont (lof′o-dont) [*lopho-* + Gr. *odous* tooth] having cheek teeth on which the cusps have become connected to form ridges, as in elephants and some rodents.

Lo·phoph·o·ra (lo-fof′ə-rə) [*lopho-* + Gr. *phoros* bearing] a genus of Mexican cacti (family Cactaceae). *L. william′sii* (Lemaire) Coult. is mescal, the source of mescal buttons, which contain peyote and mescaline.

lo·phoph·o·rine (lo-fof′ə-rēn) a poisonous alkaloid from *Lophophora williamsii*, having effects similar to those of mescaline.

lo·phot·ri·chous (lo-fot′rĭ-kəs) [*lopho-* + Gr. *thrix* hair] having two or more flagella at one or both ends; said of a bacterial cell. See *flagellum.*

Lo·pid (lo′pid) trademark for a preparation of gemfibrozil.

lo·pin·a·vir (lo-pin′ə-vir) an HIV protease inhibitor, an antiviral agent used in combination with ritonavir in the treatment of human immunodeficiency virus infection; administered orally.

Lo·pres·sor (lo-pres′or) trademark for preparations of metoprolol tartrate.

Lo·pres·sor HCT (lo-pres′or) trademark for a combination preparation of metoprolol tartrate and hydrochlorothiazide.

Lo·prox (lo′proks) trademark for a preparation of ciclopirox olamine.

Lo·pur·in (lo-pūr′in) trademark for a preparation of allopurinol.

Lor·a·bid (lor′ə-bid) trademark for a preparation of loracarbef.

lor·a·car·bef (lor″ə-kahr′bef) [USP] a carbacephem antibiotic closely related to cefaclor and having similar antibacterial activity, used in the treatment of infections of the urinary and respiratory tracts and of the skin and soft tissues; administered orally.

Lo·rain-Lévi dwarfism (syndrome) (lo-rā′ la-ve′) [Paul Joseph *Lorain*, French physician, 1827–1875; E. Léopold *Lévi*, French endocrinologist, 1868–1933] pituitary dwarfism.

lor·at·a·dine (lə-rat′ə-dēn) [USP] a nonsedating antihistamine (H_1 receptor antagonist) with no significant antimuscarinic effects; used for the treatment of allergic rhinitis and chronic idiopathic urticaria and as a treatment adjunct in asthma, administered orally.

lor·a·ze·pam (lor-az′ə-pam) [USP] a benzodiazepine with anxiolytic and sedative effects, administered orally in the treatment of anxiety disorders and short-term relief of anxiety symptoms and as a sedative-hypnotic agent, and intravenously or intramuscularly for preanesthetic medication; used also intravenously to control status epilepticus and as an antiemetic in cancer chemotherapy.

Lor·cet (lor′set) trademark for combination preparations of hydrocodone bitartrate and acetaminophen.

lor·do·sco·li·o·sis (lor″do-sko″le-o′sis) [*lordosis* + *scoliosis*] lordosis complicated with scoliosis.

lor·do·sis (lor-do′sis) [Gr. *lōrdosis*] 1. a concave portion of the vertebral column as seen from the side. 2. abnormally increased concavity in the curvature of the lumbar vertebral column as viewed from the side; called also *hollow back*, *saddle back*, and *swayback*. Cf. *kyphosis* and *scoliosis*.

cervical l., l. cer′vicis [TA] the dorsally concave curvature of the cervical vertebral column when seen from the side. Called also *cervical curvature.*

l. col′li TA alternative for *l. cervicis.*

l. lumba′lis [TA], **lumbar l.** the dorsally concave curvature of the lumbar vertebral column when seen from the side. Called also *lumbar curvature.*

lor·dot·ic (lor-dot′ik) pertaining to or characterized by lordosis.

Lo·rel·co (lo-rel′ko) trademark for a preparation of probucol.

Lor·enz operation, osteotomy (lor′ənts) [Adolf *Lorenz*, Austrian surgeon, 1854–1946] see under *operation* and *osteotomy*.

Lor·fan (lor′fan) trademark for preparations of levallorphan tartrate.

lo·ri·ca (lo-ri′kə) pl. *lori′cae* [L. "leather cuirass"] a protective rigid encasement or shell, secreted or created by cementing together of various materials, as seen in some invertebrates such as certain protozoa and many rotifers.

lor·i·cate (lor′ĭ-kāt) enclosed in a lorica.

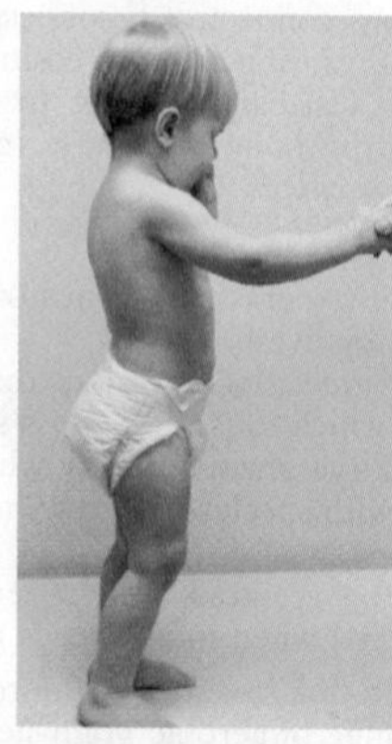

■ Lumbar lordosis and protuberant abdomen characteristic of a toddler.

Lor•tab (lor′tab) trademark for combination preparations of hydrocodone bitartrate and acetaminophen.

LOS lipooligosaccharide.

lo•sar•tan po•tas•si•um (lo-sahr′tan) an angiotensin II receptor antagonist, used as an antihypertensive; administered orally.

loss (laws) escape of something from its proper place.

functional visual l. subnormal vision or altered visual fields without an underlying physical cause, occurring as a manifestation of a number of psychiatric disorders and malingering.

hearing l. see under *H.*

l. of heterozygosity (LOH) loss of the allele from one chromosome of a pair, as by deletion, nondisjunction, mitotic recombination, or suppression of function, so that the locus is converted from heterozygosity to homozygosity or hemizygosity; it is often associated with tumorigenesis.

insensible water l. the amount of fluid lost on a daily basis from the lungs, skin, and respiratory tract, as well as water excreted in the feces; the exact amount cannot be measured, but it is estimated to be between 40 and 600 mL in an adult under normal circumstances.

transient monocular visual l. transient monocular blindness.

LOT left occipitotransverse; see *occipitotransverse position*, under *position.*

Lote•max (lo′tə-maks) trademark for a preparation of loteprednol.

Lo•ten•sin (lo-ten′sin) trademark for a preparation of benazepril hydrochloride.

Lo•ten•sin HCT (lo-ten′sin) trademark for a combination preparation of benazepril hydrochloride and hydrochlorothiazide.

lo•te•pred•nol (lo″tə-pred′nol) a corticosteroid applied topically to the conjunctiva in the treatment of seasonal allergic conjunctivitis, postoperative inflammation, and ocular inflammatory disorders.

lo•tion (lo′shən) [L. *lotio*] a liquid or semiliquid preparation containing one or more active ingredients in a suitable vehicle, for external application to the body; most are suspensions of solids in an aqueous medium, but some are solutions or emulsions.

benzyl benzoate l. [USP] a preparation of benzyl benzoate, triethanolamine, oleic acid, and purified water; used as a topical scabicide.

calamine l. [USP] a preparation of calamine with zinc oxide, glycerin, bentonite magma, and calcium hydroxide topical solution, used as a topical skin protectant.

phenolated calamine l. [USP] a mixture of calamine lotion and liquefied phenol, used as a topical skin protectant.

Lo•trel (lo′trel) trademark for a combination preparation of amlodipine besylate and benazepril hydrochloride.

Lo•trim•in (lo′trĭ-min) trademark for a preparation of clotrimazole.

Lo•tri•sone (lo′trĭ-sōn″) trademark for a combination preparation of betamethasone dipropionate and clotrimazole.

Lo•tro•nex (lo′trə-neks) trademark for a preparation of alosetron hydrochloride.

Lo•tus (lo′tus) a genus of plants of the family Leguminosae, often found in pastures and used for animal feed. *L. america′nus* and *L. cornicula′tus*, both called bird's foot trefoil, contain a cyanogenetic compound that can cause cyanide poisoning in livestock.

Lou Geh•rig disease (loo′ ger′ig) [Lou *Gehrig*, American baseball player, 1903–1941, who died of the disease] see *amyotrophic lateral sclerosis*, under *sclerosis.*

Lou•is angle (loo-e′) [Pierre Charles Alexandre *Louis*, French physician, 1787–1872; the founder of medical statistics] angulus sterni.

Lou•is-Bar syndrome (loo-e′-bahr′) [Denise *Louis-Bar*, Belgian neuropathologist, 20th century] ataxia-telangiectasia; see under *ataxia.*

loupe (lo͞op) [Fr. "magnifying glass"] a convex lens for low magnification of minute objects at very close range; it may be monocular or binocular, held in the hand, set in a headband, or mounted on spectacles.

louse (lous) pl. *lice* [L. *pediculus*] any of various wingless insects parasitic on birds and mammals; they are classified into two orders, Anoplura (the sucking lice) and Mallophaga (the bird lice or biting lice). The causal organisms of typhus, relapsing fever, trench fever, and other diseases are transmitted by louse bites.

bird l. 1. biting l. 2. a biting louse of birds.

biting l. any member of the order Mallophaga; called also *bird l.*

body l. *Pediculus humanus corporis.*

chicken l. any type of biting louse that infests chickens.

clothes l. *Pediculus humanus corporis.*

crab l. *Phthirus pubis.*

foot l. of sheep *Linognathus pedalis.*

goat sucking l. *Linognathus stenopis.*

head l. *Pediculus humanus capitis.*

long-nosed cattle l. *Linognathus vituli.*

pubic l. *Phthirus pubis.*

short-nosed cattle l. *Haematopinus eurysterni.*

sucking l. any member of the order Anoplura.

louse•wort (lous′wort) *Delphinium staphisagria.*

lous•i•cide (lous′i-sīd) pediculicide.

lo•va•stat•in (lo′və-stat″in) [USP] an inhibitor of HMG-CoA reductase, which can lower plasma levels of cholesterol and raise the plasma level of high-density lipoprotein C (HDL-C); used in the treatment of hypercholesterolemia and other forms of dyslipidemia and to reduce the risk of morbidity and mortality associated with atherosclerosis and coronary heart disease; administered orally.

Lo•va•za (lo-va′zə) trademark for a preparation of ethyl esters of omega-3 fatty acids, used to treat hypertriglycerolemia.

Lo•ve•nox (lo′və-noks) trademark for a preparation of enoxaparin sodium.

Lö•we ring (lur′və) [Karl Friedrich *Löwe*, German optician, 1874–1955] see under *ring.*

Lowe syndrome (disease) (lo) [Charles Upton *Lowe*, American pediatrician, born 1921] oculocerebrorenal syndrome.

Lowe-Ter•rey-Mac•Lach•lan syndrome (lo′ ter′e mək-lahk′lən) [C.U. *Lowe;* Mary *Terrey*, American physician, 20th century; Elsie A. *MacLachlan*, American physician, 20th century] oculocerebrorenal syndrome.

Lö•wen•berg scala, forceps (lur′vən-bərg) [Benjamin Benno *Löwenberg*, German otologist in Vienna and Paris, 1836–1905] see under *forceps* and see *ductus cochlearis.*

Lö•wen•thal tract (lur′vən-tahl) [Wilhelm *Löwenthal*, German physician, 1850–1894] tractus tectospinalis.

Low•er rings, tubercle (lo′ər) [Richard *Lower*, English anatomist, 1631–1691] see *anulus fibrosus dexter/sinister cordis* and *tuberculum intervenosum.*

low•er•ing (lo′ər-ing) a decrease.

vapor pressure l. the decrease of the vapor pressure of a solution below that of the pure solvent; the percentage change in vapor pressure is equal to the mole fraction of the solute (osmoles of solute per osmoles of solute plus solvent) and is proportional to the osmolality.

low-grade (lo′grād′) occurring near the low end of a range, as of a fever or malignancy.

Lown-Gan•ong-Le•vine syndrome (loun′ gan′ong lə-vīn′) [Bernard *Lown*, American cardiologist, born 1921; William F. *Ganong*, American physiologist, born 1924; Samuel Albert *Levine*, Polish-born American cardiologist, 1891–1966] see under *syndrome.*

Low-Oges•trel (lo″o-jes′trəl) trademark for a combination preparation of norgestrel and ethinyl estradiol.

Lows•ley operation (louz′le) [Oswald Swinney *Lowsley*, American urologist, 1884–1955] see under *operation.*

lox•a•pine (lok′sə-pēn) a tricyclic dibenzoxazepine derivative with antiemetic, sedative, anticholinergic, and α-antiadrenergic actions; used as an antipsychotic.

l. hydrochloride the hydrochloride salt of loxapine, used as an antipsychotic; administered orally or intramuscularly.

l. succinate [USP] the succinate salt of loxapine, used as an antipsychotic; administered orally.

lox•ar•thron (loks-ahr′thron) [Gr. *loxos* oblique + *arthron* joint] an oblique deformity of a joint without luxation.

lox•ar•thro•sis (loks″ahr-thro′sis) loxarthron.

lox•ia (lok′se-ə) torticollis.

Lox•i•tane (lok′sĭ-tān) trademark for preparations of loxapine.

Lox•os•ce•les (lok-sos′ə-lēz) a genus of six-eyed spiders of the family Loxoscelidae, whose bite causes loxoscelism. *L. lae′ta* is the brown spider of South America and *L. reclu′sa* is the brown recluse spider of North America.

Lox•os•cel•i•dae (lok″so-sel′ĭ-de) a family of spiders (suborder Labidognatha), the false hackled band spinners, which includes the genus *Loxosceles.*

lox•os•ce•lism (lok-sos′ə-liz-əm) a form of arachnidism caused by the bite of *Loxosceles laeta* (the brown spider) or *L. reclusa* (the brown recluse spider), seen from South America to southern North America; it begins with a painful erythematous vesicle and progresses to a gangrenous slough of the affected area.

viscerocutaneous l. a sometimes fatal condition resulting from the bite of the brown spider, with fever and hematuria in addition to the local reaction.

lox•ot•o•my (lok-sot′ə-me) [Gr. *loxos* oblique + *-tomy*] oval amputation.

loz•enge (loz′ənj) [Fr.] 1. a discoid-shaped, solid, medicinal preparation for solution in the mouth, especially for medication of the throat,

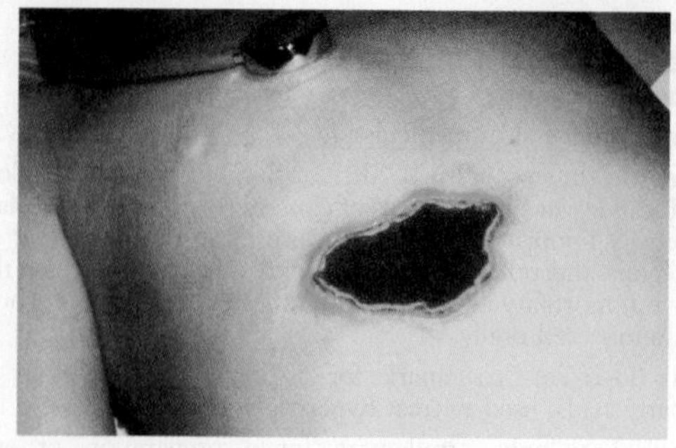

■ Loxoscelism with necrosis in an 8-year-old boy, caused by a bite by a brown recluse spider *(Loxosceles reclusa).*

consisting of an active ingredient incorporated in a suitably flavored base, such as sugar and mucilage, glycerinated gelatin, or a hard sugar candy. Called also *troche.* 2. a triangular area of tissue marked for excision in plastic surgery.

Lo·zol (lo′zol) trademark for a preparation of indapamide.

LP lumbar puncture.

Lp(a) see under *lipoprotein.*

LPF low-power field.

LPH left posterior hemiblock (see *hemiblock*); lipotropic hormone.

LPN licensed practical nurse.

LPR laryngopharyngeal reflux.

LPS lipopolysaccharide (def. 2).

LPV lymphotropic papovavirus.

Lr lawrencium; limes reacting (see *Lr dose,* under *dose.*)

LRD living related donor; see under *transplantation.*

LRR leucine-rich repeat.

LSA left sacroanterior (see *sacroanterior position,* under *position*); Licentiate of Society of Apothecaries.

LScA left scapuloanterior; see *scapuloanterior position,* under *position.*

LScP left scapuloposterior; see *scapuloposterior position,* under *position.*

LSD lysergic acid diethylamide.

LSO lumbosacral orthosis.

LSP left sacroposterior; see *sacroposterior position,* under *position.*

L-spine lumbar spine.

LST left sacrotransverse; see *sacrotransverse position,* under *position.*

LT lymphotoxin.

LTB_4, LTC_4, etc. symbols for various leukotrienes; see *leukotriene.*

LTF lymphocyte-transforming factor.

LTR long terminal repeats.

Lu lutetium.

lubb (lub) a syllable used to represent, or mimic, the first sound of the heart in auscultation. See *lubb-dupp.*

lubb-dupp (ləb-dup′) syllables used to represent the combination of the first and second heart sounds. See *lubb* and *dupp.*

lu·bi·pros·tone (loo″bĭ-pros′tōn) an activator of chloride channels of the apical membrane of the intestine that increases intestinal motility by stimulating the secretion of fluid into the lumen, used in the treatment of chronic idiopathic constipation in adults; administered orally.

lu·bri·cant (loo′brĭ-kənt) a substance that is applied as a surface film to reduce friction between moving parts; see also under *laxative.*

Luc operation (lūk) [Henri *Luc,* French laryngologist, 1855–1925] Caldwell-Luc operation.

Lu·cas sign (loo′kəs) [Richard Clement *Lucas,* English surgeon, 1846–1915] see under *sign.*

Lu·cey-Dris·coll syndrome (loo′se dris′kəl) [J. F. *Lucey,* American physician, 20th century; J. J. *Driscoll,* American physician, 20th century] see under *syndrome.*

lu·cid (loo′sid) [L. *lucidus* clear] clear; not obscure.

lu·cid·i·ty (loo-sid′ĭ-te) the quality or state of having a clear mind; clearness of the mind.

lu·cif·er·ase (loo-sif′ər-ās) trivial name for a variety of monooxygenases that catalyze a reaction producing bioluminescence in certain marine crustaceans, fish, bacteria, and insects [EC 1.13.12.5–8, 1.14.14.3, 1.14.99.21]. The enzyme is a flavoprotein that oxidizes luciferin to an electronically excited compound that emits energy in the form of light. The color of light emitted varies with the organism. The firefly enzyme is a valuable reagent for measurement of ATP concentration.

lu·cif·er·in (loo-sif′ər-in) a heterocyclic phenol which can be reduced and oxidized. It exists in many forms and is present in certain animals capable of bioluminescence; when acted upon by luciferase, in the presence of ATP and molecular oxygen, it produces light.

lu·cif·u·gal (loo-sif′u-gəl) [L. *lux,* gen. *lucis* light + *-fugal*[2]] avoiding, or being repelled by, bright light.

Lu·cil·ia (loo-sil′e-ə) *Phaenicia.*

Lu·cio leprosy, phenomenon (loo′syo) [Rafael *Lucio* Nájera, Mexican physician, 1819–1886] see under *leprosy* and *phenomenon.*

lu·cip·e·tal (loo-sip′ĭ-təl) [*lux* + *-petal*] seeking, or being attracted to, bright light.

lück·en·schä·del (lĕk′en-sha″dəl) [Ger. "skull (with) gaps"] craniolacunia.

Lud·loff sign (lood′lawf) [Karl *Ludloff,* German surgeon, 1864–1945] see under *sign.*

Lud·wig angina (lood′vik) [Wilhelm Friedrich von *Ludwig,* German surgeon, 1790–1865] see under *angina.*

Lud·wig angle (lood′vik) [Daniel *Ludwig,* German anatomist, 1625–1680] angulus sterni.

Lud·wig ganglion, nerve (lood′vik) [Karl Friedrich Wilhelm *Ludwig,* German physiologist, 1816–1895] see under *ganglion,* and see *Cyon nerve* under *nerve.*

Lu·er syringe (loo′ər) [*Luer,* German instrument maker in France, died 1883] see under *syringe.*

lu·es (loo′ēz) [L. "a plague"] syphilis. **luet′ic** *adj*

Luft disease (looft) [Rolf *Luft,* Swedish endocrinologist, 1914–2007] see under *disease.*

Lu·fyl·lin (loo′fə-lin) trademark for preparations of dyphylline.

lug (lug) 1. a projecting part that holds or supports something. 2. the part of a dental casting that projects.

retention l. a piece of metal soldered either to an orthodontic band or to an artificial crown to create greater undercut for retention of a dental prosthesis.

Lu·gol iodine (iodine solution) (loo′gol) [Jean Guillaume Auguste *Lugol,* French physician, 1786–1851] see *strong iodine solution,* under *solution.*

Lukes-Col·lins classification (lo͞oks′ kol′ənz) [L.J. *Lukes,* American pathologist, 20th century; R.D. *Collins,* American pathologist, 20th century] see under *classification.*

LUL left upper lobe; see *lobus superior pulmonis sinistri.*

lu·lib·er·in (loo-lib′ər-in) [*lu*tropin + *-liberin*] luteinizing hormone–releasing hormone.

lum·ba·go (ləm-ba′go) [L. *lumbus* loin] a nonmedical term for any pain in the lower back.

lum·bar (lum′bər, -bahr) pertaining to the loins, the parts of the sides of the back between the thorax and the pelvis.

lum·bar·iza·tion (lum″bər-ĭ-za′shən) a condition in which the first segment of the sacrum is not fused with the second, so that there is one additional articulated vertebra and the sacrum consists of only four segments.

lumb(o)- [L. *lumbus* loin] a combining form denoting relationship to the lumbar region or the lumbar vertebrae.

lum·bo·ab·dom·i·nal (lum″bo-ab-dom′i-nəl) pertaining to the lumbar region and abdomen; pertaining to the sides and the front of the abdomen.

lum·bo·cos·tal (lum″bo-kos′təl) pertaining to the lumbar vertebrae and ribs.

lum·bo·cru·ral (lum″bo-kroo′rəl) pertaining to, affecting, or extending between the lumbar and crural regions.

lum·bo·dor·sal (lum″bo-dor′səl) pertaining to the lumbar region of the back, where the kidneys are located.

lum·bo·dyn·ia (lum″bo-din′e-ə) [*lumbo-* + *-odynia*] lumbago.

lum·bo·il·i·ac (lum″bo-il′e-ak) pertaining to the lumbar vertebrae and ilium.

lum·bo·in·gui·nal (lum″bo-ing′gwĭ-nəl) pertaining to the lumbar and inguinal regions.

lum·bo·sa·cral (lum″bo-sa′krəl) pertaining to the lumbar vertebrae and sacrum, or to the lumbar and sacral regions.

lum·bri·cal (lum′brĭ-kəl) 1. lumbricoid (def. 1). 2. see entries beginning *musculi lumbricales.*

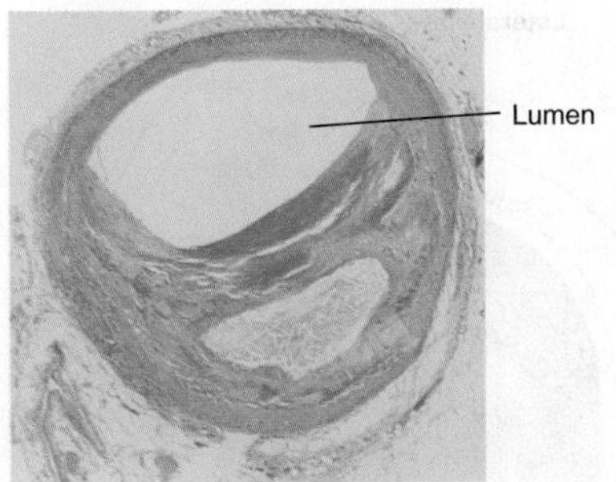

■ Lumen of coronary artery, moderately narrowed by atheromatous plaque.

lum·bri·ci (ləm-bri′si) [L.] plural of *lumbricus.*

lum·bri·cide (lum′brĭ-sīd) [*lumbricus* + *-cide*] ascaricide.

lum·bri·coid (lum′brĭ-koid) [*lumbricus* + *-oid*] pertaining to or resembling an earthworm; said especially of *Ascaris lumbricoides;* called also lumbrical.

lum·bri·co·sis (lum″brĭ-ko′sis) ascariasis.

Lum·bri·cus (ləm-bri′kəs) [L. "earthworm"] a genus of annelids. *L. terres′tris* is the common earthworm, which may act as a host of the nematode *Metastrongylus elongatus,* the intermediate host of the swine influenza virus.

lum·bri·cus (ləm-bri′kəs) pl. *lumbri′ci* [L.] any member of the genus *Lumbricus;* an earthworm.

lu·me·fan·trine (loo″mə-fan′trēn) a schizonticide used in combination with artemether in the treatment of malaria, administered orally.

lu·men (loo′mən) pl. *lu′mina, lumens* [L. "light"] 1. the cavity or channel within a tube or tubular organ. 2. the SI unit of luminous flux; it is the light emitted in a solid angle of 1 steradian by a uniform point source with luminous intensity of 1 candela. Abbreviated lm.

residual l. the remains of the hypophysial pouch (Rathke pouch), located between the pars distalis and pars intermedia of the pituitary gland.

lu·mi·can (loo′mĭ-kan) a leucine-rich repeat protein that is related to fibromodulin and binds collagen; it is found in the cornea, where it plays a role in transparency, as well as in other connective tissues, where it may play a role in the assembly of the extracellular matrix.

lu·mi·chrome (loo′mĭ-krōm) chemical name: 7,8-dimethylalloxazine; a product of the irradiation decomposition of riboflavin.

lu·mi·fla·vin (loo″mĭ-fla′vin) chemical name: 7,8,10-trimethylisoalloxazine; a product of the luminiferous decomposition of riboflavin.

Lu·mi·gan (loo′mĭ-gan) trademark for a preparation of bimatoprost.

lu·mi·na (loo′mĭ-nə) [L.] plural of *lumen.*

Lu·mi·nal (loo′mĭ-nəl) trademark for preparations of phenobarbital.

lu·mi·nal (loo′mĭ-nəl) pertaining to the lumen of a tubular structure.

lu·mi·na·lis (loo″mĭ-na′lis) [TA] luminal.

lu·mi·nance (*L*) (loo′mĭ-nəns) the luminous intensity per unit of projected area of a surface as viewed in a given direction.

lu·mi·nes·cence (loo″mĭ-nes′əns) the property of giving off light without showing a corresponding degree of heat.

lu·mi·nif·er·ous (loo″mĭ-nif′ər-əs) [*lumen* + *-ferous*] conveying light or propagating those vibrations which constitute light.

lu·mi·no·phor (loo′mĭ-nə-for″) [L. *lumen* light + Gr. *phoros* bearing] a chemical group that gives the property of luminescence to organic compounds.

lu·mi·nous (loo′mi-nəs) emitting or reflecting light; glowing with light.

lu·mi·rho·dop·sin (loo″mĭ-ro-dop′sin) a transient intermediate produced upon irradiation of rhodopsin in the visual cycle; see illustration at *visual cycle,* under *cycle.*

lum·pec·to·my (ləm-pek′tə-me) 1. surgical excision of only the palpable lesion in carcinoma of the breast; called also *tylectomy.* 2. surgical removal of a mass. Cf. *excisional biopsy.*

Lums·den center (lumz′dən) [Thomas William *Lumsden,* British physician, 1874–1953] pneumotaxic center.

lu·nar (loo′nər) [L. *luna* moon; in alchemy, silver, for which the moon was the symbol] pertaining to or containing silver, as lunar caustic (silver nitrate).

lu·na·re (loo-na′re) the lunate bone (os lunatum [TA]).

lu·nate (loo′nāt) [L. *luna* moon] moon-shaped, or crescentic; see *os lunatum.*

lu·na·to·ma·la·cia (loo-na″to-mə-la′shə) osteochondrosis of the semilunar (carpal lunate) bone; see *Kienböck disease,* under *disease.*

Lund-Brow·der chart, classification (lund′ brou′dər) [Charles C. *Lund,* American surgeon, 1895–1972; Newton C. *Browder,* American surgeon, 1893–1969] see under *classification.*

Lu·nes·ta (loo-nes′tə) trademark for a preparation of eszopiclone.

lung (lung) [L. *pulmo;* Gr. *pneumōn* or *pleumōn*] either of the pair of organs of respiration, one on the right and one on the left of the thorax (*pulmo dexter* [TA] and *pulmo sinister* [TA]), which are separated from each other by the heart and mediastinal structures. The right lung is composed of upper, middle, and lower lobes, and the left, of upper and lower lobes (see under *lobus*). Pulmonary disorders may be confined to, or localized in, one or more of the segments of the lobes. Each lung consists of an external serous coat (the visceral layer of the pleura), subserous areolar tissue, and lung parenchyma. The latter is made up of lobules, which are bound together by connective tissue. A primary lobule or *terminal respiratory unit* consists of a terminal bronchiole, respiratory bronchioles, and alveolar ducts, which communicate with many alveoli, each alveolus being surrounded by a network of capillary blood vessels. It is between the alveoli and capillaries that gas exchange takes place. See Plates 25 and 43.

accessory l. pulmonary sequestration.

air conditioner l. humidifier l.

arc welder's l. welder's l.

artificial l. oxygenator.

bauxite l. see under *pneumoconiosis.*

bird breeder's l., bird fancier's l., bird handler's l. pigeon breeder's l.

black l. coal workers' pneumoconiosis.

book l., book-l. a lunglike invagination that functions as a gas exchange organ, found on the underside of the abdomen of many arachnids, which opens to the surface by means of a spiracle and contains numerous thin membranous lamellae arranged like book leaves.

brown l. byssinosis.

cadmium l. an occupational disease similar to metal fume fever, caused by inhalation of cadmium dust or fumes; severe cases can be fatal. Cf. *cadmiosis.*

cardiac l. chronic congestion of the lung due to mitral stenosis or left ventricular failure.

cheese handler's l., cheese washer's l. hypersensitivity pneumonitis occurring in workers who wash the mold from cheeses during the aging process, caused by inhalation of spores of *Penicillium* from moldy cheese casings.

coal miner's l. coal workers' pneumoconiosis.

cobalt l. hard metal disease.

corundum smelter's l. bauxite pneumoconiosis.

drowned l. consolidation of the lung with exudation and necrosis, occurring distal to a bronchial obsruction.

epoxy resin l. a type of hypersensitivity pneumonitis caused by inhalation of the fumes of heated epoxy resin that contains phthalic anhydride.

farmer's l. a type of hypersensitivity pneumonitis caused by inhalation of moldy hay dust, characterized by breathlessness with cyanosis or with a dry cough, anorexia, and weight loss. It is most often associated with inhalation of spores of *Saccharopolyspora rectivirgula* or *Thermoactinomyces vulgaris.* Called also *thresher's l.* and *harvester's l.* See also *farmer's lung disease of cattle.*

fibroid l. a lung affected with chronic fibrosis.

grain handler's l. a type of hypersensitivity pneumonitis occurring in those exposed to grain, probably caused by fungal contaminants. See also *grain fever,* under *fever.*

harvester's l. farmer's l.

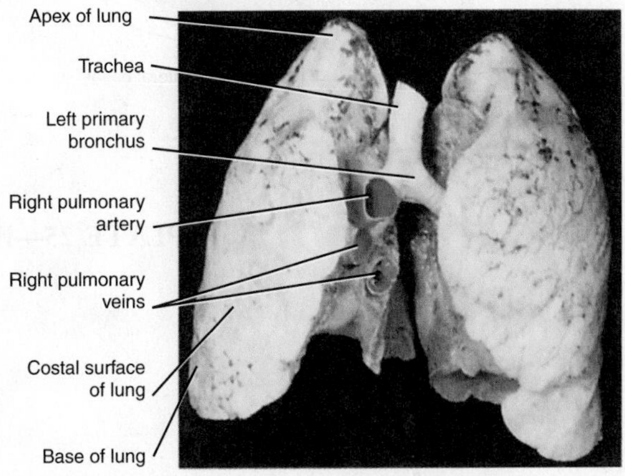

■ Lungs, bronchi, and trachea, which have been separated for clarity.

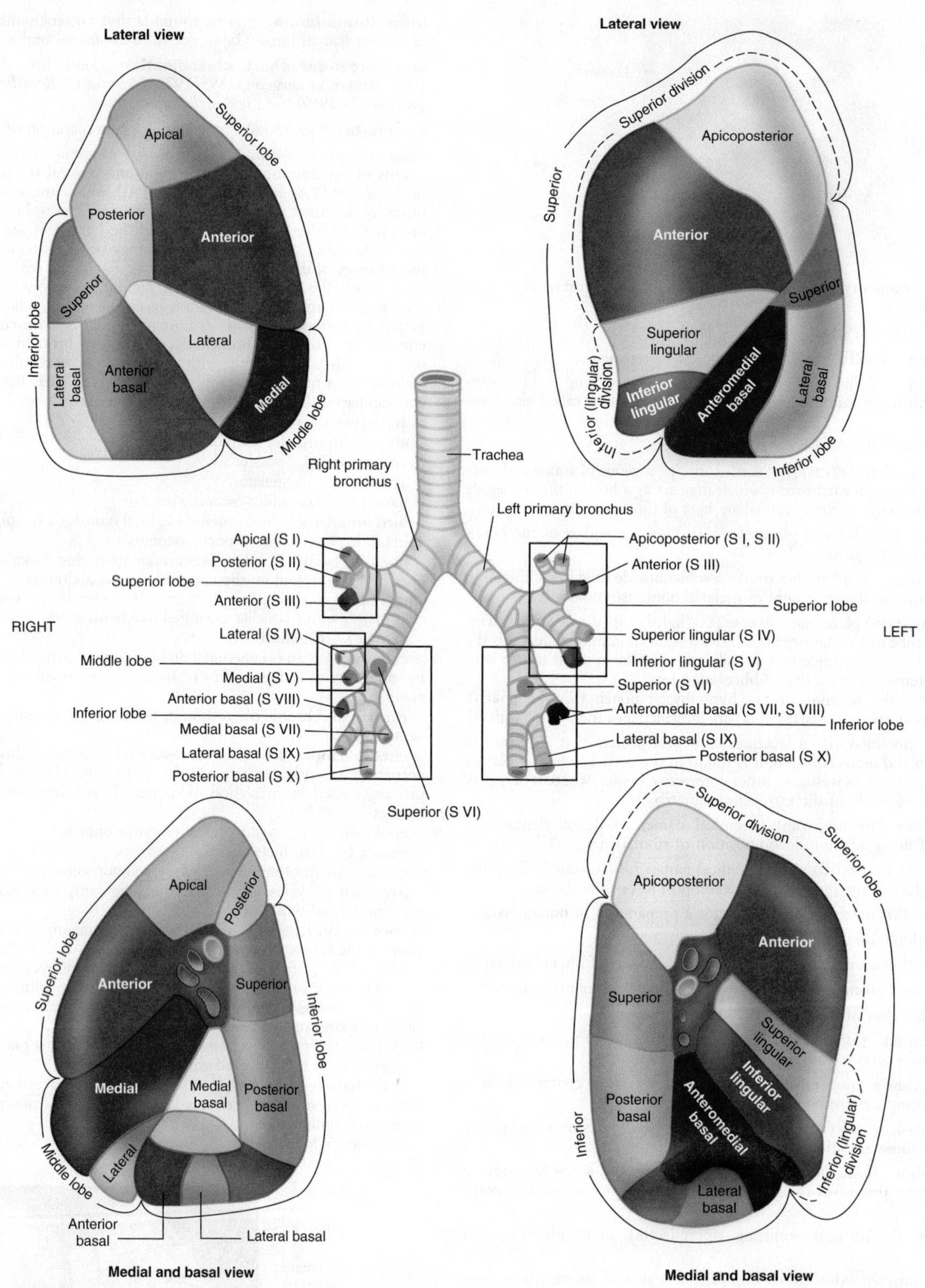

■ PLATE 25—PULMONARY SEGMENTS

honeycomb l. the appearance of multiple small radiolucent shadows on the lung x-ray, representing dilatations of the lung parenchyma, as in idiopathic pulmonary fibrosis; it is also seen with multiple small cysts or cavities.

hot tub l. hypersensitivity pneumonitis associated with indoor hot tub use, caused by inhalation of aerosolized *Mycobacterium avium* complex.

humidifier l. hypersensitivity pneumonitis caused by inhalation of air that has been passed through humidifiers, dehumidifiers, or air conditioners contaminated by any of a variety of fungi, amebas, or thermophilic actinomycetes. See also *humidifier fever*, under *fever.*

hyperlucent l. unilateral emphysema.

iron l. a popular name for the Drinker respirator.

Labrador l. a type of mixed dust pneumoconiosis occurring in iron miners in western Labrador, caused by a mixture of particles of iron, silica, and some anthophyllite (a variety of amphibole asbestos); see also *siderosilicosis.*

left l. see *lung.*

malt worker's l. hypersensitivity pneumonitis in brewery and distillery workers, a form of allergic aspergillosis caused by inhalation of barley dust containing spores of *Aspergillus clavatus* and *A. fumigatus* during the malting process.

mason's l. pneumoconiosis (usually silicosis) in stone masons due to the inhalation of stone dusts.

meat wrapper's l. a type of hypersensitivity pneumonitis seen in meat wrappers, caused by inhalation of fumes of phthalic anhydride contained in the label or the polyvinylchloride wrapping.

miller's l. a type of hypersensitivity pneumonitis seen in those who work with grains or flours contaminated with the wheat weevil *Sitophilus granarius.*

miner's l. coal workers' pneumoconiosis.

mushroom worker's l. a type of farmer's lung seen in those working on mushroom farms, due to inhalation of mold spores from mushroom beds.

pigeon breeder's l. a type of hypersensitivity pneumonitis caused by an acquired sensitivity to bird feces following intimate contact with birds; symptoms include chills, fever, and cough. Pulmonary fibrosis may result. Called also *bird breeder's, bird fancier's,* or *bird handler's l.*

right l. see *lung.*

shock l. acute respiratory distress syndrome.

silo filler's l. a rare type of acute bronchiolitis fibrosa obliterans affecting individuals who inhale high levels of nitrogen oxides, particularly nitrogen dioxide, while working in recently filled silos; death may occur from pulmonary edema. Called also *silo filler's disease.*

silver finisher's l., silver polisher's l. siderosis in silver finishers, caused by inhalation of iron oxide (from jeweler's rouge) and silver particles. The iron oxide particles are phagocytized and the elastic tissue is stained black by the silver; fibrosis does not occur and pulmonary function is not impaired.

thresher's l. farmer's l.

vanishing l. in emphysema, conversion of the lungs into a delicate, fine network of remaining blood vessels among which no alveolar walls survive.

vineyard sprayer's l. hypersensitivity pneumonitis in vineyard workers after spraying vines with a copper sulfate–lime solution.

welder's l. siderosis occurring in welders, caused by the inhalation of iron oxide fumes; the condition is generally asymptomatic, although the presence of other substances in welding fumes may lead to fibrotic lung disease. Called also *arc welder's disease* and *arc welder's l.*

wet l. 1. pulmonary edema. 2. acute respiratory distress syndrome.

white l. pneumonia alba.

lung•worm (lung'wərm) a parasitic worm that invades the lungs, such as the trematode *Paragonimus westermani* in humans, or nematodes of the family Protostrongylidae in other animals. See also *verminous bronchitis, verminous pneumonia,* and *hoose.*

rat l. *Angiostrongylus cantonensis.*

lu•nu•la (loo'nu-lə) gen. and pl. *lu'nulae* [L., dim. of *luna* moon] a small crescent or moon-shaped area.

lunulae of aortic valve, lunulae of cusps of aortic valve lunulae valvularum semilunarium valvae aortae.

lunulae of cusps of pulmonary valve lunulae valvularum semilunarium valvae trunci pulmonalis.

l. of nail l. unguis.

l. un'guis [TA] lunula of nail: the crescentic white area at the base of the nail on a finger or toe.

lunulae of valves of pulmonary trunk, lunulae of pulmonary valves lunulae valvularum semilunarium valvae trunci pulmonalis.

lu'nulae valvula'rum semiluna'rium val'vae aor'tae [TA] lunulae of semilunar cusps of aortic valve: small thinned areas in the cusps of the aortic valve, one on each side of the nodule of the cusp. Called also *lunulae of aortic valve.*

lu'nulae valvula'rum semiluna'rium val'vae trun'ci pulmona'lis [TA] lunulae of semilunar cusps of pulmonary valve: small thinned areas in the cusps of the pulmonary valve, one on each side of the nodule of the cusp. Called also *lunulae of pulmonary valve.*

lu•nu•lae (loo'nu-le) [L.] genitive and plural of *lunula.*

lu•nule (loo'nūl) lunula.

lu•pi•form (loo'pĭ-form) lupoid.

lu•pin•o•sis (loo"pĭ-no'sis) 1. acute atrophy of the liver, often fatal, in ruminants such as cattle, sheep, goats, and horses, due to the ingestion of seeds of plants of the genus *Lupinus* that are contaminated with the fungus *Phomopsis leptostromiformis.* Cf. *lathyrism.* 2. mycotoxic l.

mycotoxic l. poisoning of livestock due to ingestion of *Lupinus* plants contaminated with the fungi *Phomopsis leptostromiformis* or *P. rossiana;* symptoms include liver damage with jaundice and photosensitization.

Lu•pi•nus (loo'pin-us) the lupins, a genus of leguminous herbs. Seeds of mature plants of many species contain toxic alkaloids that cause convulsions in ruminants. Seeds may also be contaminated with a fungus and cause mycotoxic lupinosis. Two species found in western North America, when eaten by pregnant cows, may cause crooked calf disease in fetuses.

lu•poid (loo'poid) [*lupus* + *-oid*] pertaining to or resembling lupus. Called also *lupiform.*

Lu•pron (loo'pron) trademark for preparations of leuprolide acetate.

lu•pus (loo'pəs) [L. "wolf" or "pike"] 1. name formerly given to numerous types of localized destruction or degeneration of the skin caused by cutaneous diseases. 2. l. erythematosus.

chilblain l., chilblain l. erythematosus a chronic unremitting form of lupus erythematosus, caused by microvascular injury secondary to cold exposure; the usual location is on the fingertips, nose, face, ears, hands, calves, or heels. Lesions may at first resemble chilblains or the lesions of lupus pernio, but they eventually assume the appearance of discoid lupus erythematosus. Sometimes this condition is called *l. pernio.*

cutaneous l. erythematosus one of the two main types of lupus erythematosus; it may involve only the skin or may precede involvement of other body systems. A common classification divides it into three groups: the chronic types, including discoid lupus erythematosus and lupus erythematosus profundus; the subacute types, such as neonatal lupus erythematosus; and an acute type with an edematous, erythematous eruption, a facial rash *(butterfly rash),* or an extensive morbilliform eruption, often with systemic exacerbations. The acute type is sometimes the presenting symptom of systemic lupus erythematosus, such as after sun exposure.

discoid l. erythematosus (DLE) a chronic form of cutaneous lupus erythematosus in which the skin lesions mimic those of the systemic form but systemic signs are rare and develop only occasionally after many years. It is characterized by discoid skin plaques with edema, erythema, scaliness, follicular plugging, and skin atrophy surrounded by an elevated erythematous border. The usual location is on the face and scalp, with cicatricial alopecia, but widespread dissemination may occur. See also *l. erythematosus profundus* and *hypertrophic l. erythematosus.*

drug-induced l., drug-induced l. erythematosus lupus erythematosus caused by any of various drugs. Hydralazine, procainamide, and minocycline are the most common ones causing systemic lupus, and various other drugs can cause subacute cutaneous lupus. It usually resolves following withdrawal of the offending drug.

l. erythemato'sus (LE) a group of connective tissue disorders primarily affecting women aged 20 to 40 years, comprising a spectrum of clinical forms in which cutaneous disease may occur with or without systemic involvement. See *cutaneous l. erythematosus* and *systemic l. erythematosus.*

l. erythemato'sus discoi'des discoid l. erythematosus.

l. erythemato'sus hypertro'phicus hypertrophic l. erythematosus.

l. erythemato'sus profun'dus a rare chronic form of cutaneous lupus erythematosus characterized by dermal and subcutaneous inflammatory involvement, with deep, firm nodules, often without surface change. The usual location is on the head, upper arms, chest, buttocks, or thighs, and there may be mild systemic involvement. Lesions heal and leave deeply depressed areas, and the typical lesions of discoid lupus erythematosus

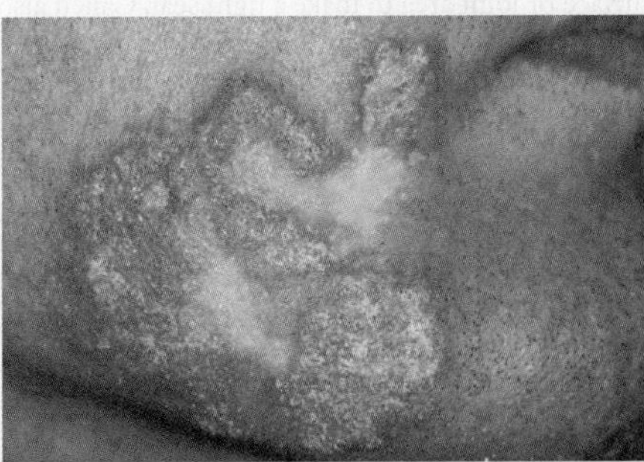

■ Facial lesions of discoid lupus erythematosus, with hyperkeratotic margins and central scarring.

may also be present. Called also *l. profundus* and *LE, lupus,* or *lupus erythematosus panniculitis.*

l. erythemato'sus tu'midus a variant of discoid or systemic lupus erythematosus in which the lesions consist of raised red, purple, or brown plaques that may resemble the lesions of erysipelas or cellulitis.

hypertrophic l. a rare type of lupus vulgaris with lesions consisting of a warty vegetative growth, usually on a moist area near a body orifice.

hypertrophic l. erythematosus a form of discoid lupus erythematosus characterized by verrucous hyperkeratotic lesions that can be mistaken for keratoacanthoma or hypertrophic lichen planus; it often occurs in association with cutaneous lesions, and it has features similar to those of lichen planus.

l. milia'ris dissemina'tus fa'ciei a papular eruption on the central part of the face of adults, which heals spontaneously but leaves scarring. It may be a variant of granulomatous rosacea, or may have an unknown etiology.

neonatal l., neonatal l. erythematosus a condition sometimes seen in infants born to mothers with systemic lupus erythematosus, usually characterized by a rash similar to that of discoid lupus; transiently elevated levels of antinuclear antibodies and LE cells; and sometimes heart block, other cardiac conduction disturbances, hematologic abnormalities, hepatosplenomegaly, or pericarditis. It is usually benign and self-limited, but the discoid skin lesions occasionally persist.

l. per'nio 1. a cutaneous manifestation of sarcoidosis consisting of smooth, shiny, purplish plaques on the ears, forehead, nose, fingers, and toes; it is frequently associated with bone cysts. 2. chilblain l. erythematosus.

l. profun'dus l. erythematosus profundus.

systemic l. erythematosus (SLE) a chronic, inflammatory, often febrile multisystemic disorder of connective tissue that proceeds through remissions and relapses; it may be either acute or insidious in onset and is characterized principally by involvement of the skin *(cutaneous l. erythematosus),* joints, kidneys, and serosal membranes. The etiology is unknown, but it may be a failure of regulatory mechanisms of the autoimmune system, since there are high levels of numerous autoantibodies against nuclear and cytoplasmic cellular components. The condition is marked by a wide variety of abnormalities, including arthritis, arthralgias, nephritis, central nervous system manifestations, pleurisy, pericarditis, leukopenia or thrombocytopenia, hemolytic anemia, an elevated erythrocyte sedimentation rate, and the presence in the blood of distinctive cells called LE cells.

systemic l. erythematosus, ANA-negative antiphospholipid syndrome.

tumid l. 1. l. tumidus. 2. l. erythematosus tumidus.

tumid l. erythematosus l. erythematosus tumidus.

l. tu'midus 1. a type of lupus vulgaris whose lesions consist of localized, soft, edematous patches somewhat resembling keloids. 2. l. erythematosus tumidus.

l. vulga'ris the most common, severe, and variable form of cutaneous tuberculosis, usually of the face and nearby mucous membranes. Usual characteristics include a reddish brown plaque on the skin surrounded by papules and nodules. In time, involved sites may develop extensive atrophy and progressive destruction of cartilage, resulting in disfiguring scars, keloids, lymphedema, and functional impairment from contractures.

Luque instrumentation, rod (loo'ka) [Eduardo Roberto *Luque,* Mexican orthopedic surgeon, 1931–2002] see under *instrumentation* and *rod.*

Lusch·ka crypts, ducts, etc. (lo͞osh'kah) [Hubert von *Luschka,* German anatomist, 1820–1875] see under *crypt, duct, fiber,* and *joint,* and see *apertura lateralis ventriculi quarti, bursa pharyngealis, glomus coccygeum, ligamenta sternopericardiaca,* and *tonsilla pharyngealis.*

lu·si·tro·pic (loo"sĭ-tro'pik) 1. pertaining to lusitropy (relaxation of the ventricles). 2. causing lusitropy.

lu·sit·ro·py (loo-sit'ro-pe) [Gr. *lusis* (variant transliteration of *lysis*) relaxation + *tropē* a turning] the relaxation of the ventricles during diastole.

Lus·tra (lus'trə) trademark for preparations of hydroquinone.

lute (lo͞ot) [L. *lutum* mud] 1. a substance such as cement, wax, or clay that coats a surface or joint area to make a tight seal. Called also *luting agent.* 2. to coat or seal with such a substance.

lu·te·al (loo'te-əl) pertaining to or having the properties of the corpus luteum or its active principle.

lu·te·ec·to·my (loo"te-ek'tə-me) [*lute-* + *-ectomy*] excision of the corpus luteum.

lu·te·in (loo'te-in) [L. *luteus* yellow] 1. a yellow pigment, or lipochrome, from the corpus luteum, from fat cells, and from the yolk of eggs. It is closely related to xanthophyll. 2. any lipochrome.

lu·te·in·ic (loo"te-in'ik) 1. pertaining to lutein. 2. luteal. 3. pertaining to luteinization.

lu·te·in·iza·tion (loo"te-in"ĭ-za'shən) the process by which a postovulatory ovarian follicle transforms into a corpus luteum through vascularization, follicular cell hypertrophy, and lipid accumulation, the latter in some species giving the yellow color indicated by the term.

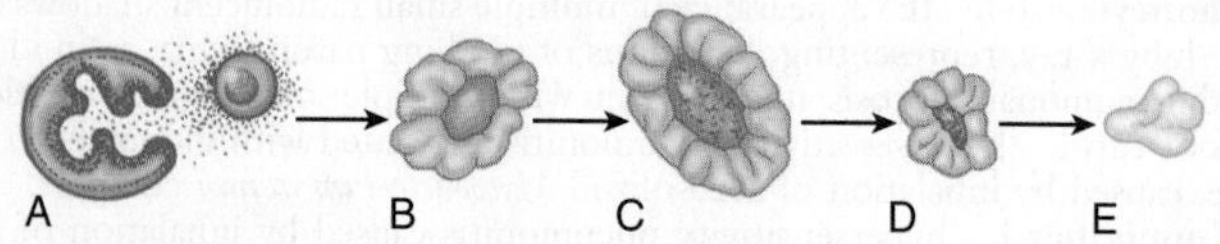

■ Luteinization, beginning after rupture of the ovarian follicle in ovulation *(A)* and progressing through vascularization and hypertrophy of the maturing corpus luteum *(B, C)*; it is followed by regression *(D)* to the corpus albicans *(E)*.

Lu·tem·bach·er syndrome (complex) (loo'təm-bahk"ər) [René *Lutembacher,* French cardiologist, 1884–1968] see under *syndrome.*

lute(o)- [L. *luteus* yellow] a combining form meaning yellow, or denoting relationship to the corpus luteum.

lu·te·ol·y·sin (loo"te-ol'ə-sin) [*luteo-* + *lysin*] a substance that causes degeneration of the corpus luteum.

uterine l. dinoprost.

lu·te·ol·y·sis (loo"te-ol'ə-sis) [*luteo-* + *lysis*] degeneration of the corpus luteum.

lu·teo·lyt·ic (loo"te-o-lit'ik) 1. pertaining to or promoting luteolysis. 2. an agent that promotes luteolysis.

lu·te·o·ma (loo"te-o'mə) [*lute-* + *-oma*] 1. a granulosa-theca cell tumor in which there has been luteinization of the cells. Called also *luteinized granulosa-theca cell tumor.* 2. nodular hyperplasia of ovarian lutein cells sometimes occurring in the last trimester of pregnancy; it may be unilateral or bilateral. Called also *l. of pregnancy* or *pregnancy l.*

lu·teo·tro·pic (loo"te-o-tro'pik) stimulating the formation of the corpus luteum.

lu·te·o·tro·pin (loo'te-o-tro"pin) prolactin.

lu·te·ti·um (Lu) (loo-te'she-əm) the chemical element, atomic number 71, atomic weight 174.97.

Lu·ther·an blood group (loo'thər-ən) [*Lutheran,* surname of the propositus first described in 1945] see under *blood group.*

lu·tro·pin (loo-tro'pin) luteinizing hormone.

Lutz-Splen·do·re-Al·mei·da disease (lo͞ots' splen-do'ra ahl-ma'dah) [Adolfo *Lutz,* Brazilian physician, 1855–1940; Alfonso *Splendore,* Italian physician in Brazil, 1871–1953; Floriano Paulo de *Almeida,* Brazilian physician, 1898–1977] paracoccidioidomycosis.

Lut·zo·my·ia (lo͞ot-zo-mi'ə) a genus of sandflies of the family Psychodidae, the females of which suck blood.

L. flaviscutella'ta the vector of *Leishmania amazonensis.*

L. longipal'pis the vector of *Leishmania chagasi.*

L. olme'ca the vector of *Leishmania mexicana.*

L. peruen'sis a probable vector of *Leishmania peruviana.*

L. tra'pidoi a vector of *Leishmania panamensis.*

L. umbrati'lis the major vector of *Leishmania guyanensis.*

L. verruca'rum a vector of human *bartonellosis* in Peru.

L. wellco'mei the major vector of *Leishmania braziliensis.*

lux (lx) (luks) [L. "light"] the SI unit of illumination, being 1 lumen per square meter.

lux·a·tio (lək-sa'she-o) [L.] dislocation.

l. cox'ae conge'nita congenital dislocation of the hip; see *developmental dysplasia of the hip,* under *dysplasia.*

l. erec'ta dislocation of the shoulder, with the upper limb standing straight up above the head.

l. imperfec'ta sprain.

l. perinea'lis a form of dislocation of the hip in which the head of the femur lies in the perineum.

lux·a·tion (lək-sa'shən) [L. *luxatio*] dislocation.

Malgaigne l. pulled elbow.

Lux·iq (luk'sik) trademark for a preparation of betamethasone valerate.

lux·u·ri·ant (ləg-zhoor'e-ənt) growing freely or excessively.

Luys body syndrome, nucleus (lwe) [Jules Bernard *Luys,* French neurologist, 1828–1895] see *hemiballismus* and *nucleus subthalamicus.*

LVAD left ventricular assist device.

LVEDP left ventricular end-diastolic pressure.

LVEDV left ventricular end-diastolic volume.

LVET left ventricular ejection time.

LVH left ventricular hypertrophy; see *ventricular hypertrophy,* under *hypertrophy.*

LVN licensed vocational nurse.

lx lux.

ly•ase (li'ās) [EC 4] a class of enzymes that catalyze the cleavage of C—C, C—O, C—N, or other bonds without hydrolysis or oxidation to form two molecules, at least one of which contains a double bond. The reverse reaction occurs by the addition of a group to a molecule at a double bond. The class includes aldolases, deaminases, decarboxylases, hydratases or dehydratases, and other cleavage or cyclase enzymes. See also *synthase*.
 17,20-l. 17α-hydroxyprogesterone aldolase.

17,20-ly•ase de•fi•cien•cy (li'ās) a disorder of steroidogenesis caused by mutation in the *CYP17A1* gene (locus: 10q24.3), which encodes steroid 17α-monooxygenase, resulting in deficiency of 17α-hydroxyprogesterone aldolase, an enzyme activity of steroid 17α-monooxygenase that normally catalyzes the conversion of C_{21} to C_9 steroid hormones (androgens and estrogens). The result is a type of congenital adrenal hyperplasia (type V). Males are pseudohermaphroditic and both sexes remain sexually infantile. See also *17α-hydroxylase deficiency* and see table at *hyperplasia*.

ly•can•thro•py (li-kan'thrə-pe) [Gr. *lykos* wolf + *anthrōpos* man] a delusion in which the individual believes that they are a wolf or other animal or that they are able to change into one.

Lych•nis gi•tha•go (lik'nis gĭ-tha'go) *Agrostemma githago.*

ly•cine (li'sēn) betaine.

ly•co•pene (li'ko-pēn) the red carotenoid pigment of tomatoes and various berries and fruits.

ly•co•pe•ne•mia (li"ko-pə-ne'me-ə) a variant of carotenemia resulting from the prolonged and excessive ingestion of tomato juice, which contains lycopene.

Ly•co•per•da•ceae (li"ko-pər-da'se-e) a family of puffballs, fungi of the order Lycoperdales; it includes the genus *Lycoperdon.*

Ly•co•per•da•les (li"ko-pər-da'lēs) the puffballs, an order of perfect fungi of the class Holobasidiomycetes; it includes the family Lycoperdaceae.

Ly•co•per•don (li"ko-pur'don) [Gr. *lykos* wolf + *perdesthai* to break wind] a genus of puffballs, fungi of the family Lycoperdaceae; in folk medicine their dust (spores) is inhaled to treat nosebleeds. See also *lycoperdonosis.*

ly•co•per•do•no•sis (li"ko-pur"do-no'sis) a rare type of hypersensitivity pneumonitis caused by the inhalation of spores from mature *Lycoperdon* mushrooms.

Ly•co•po•di•um (li"ko-po'de-əm) [Gr. *lykos* wolf + *pous* foot] the club mosses, a genus of mosses. *L. clava'tum* and other species are sources of lycopodium.

ly•co•po•di•um (li"ko-po'de-əm) a light dry powder consisting of the spores of species of *Lycopodium*, especially *L. clavatum*, formerly used as a dusting and absorbent powder, and as a coating for pills. Since the spores are uniform in size, they can be used as a measuring unit in microscopy.

lyco•rine (lik'o-rin) a toxic crystalline alkaloid found in the bulbs of species of *Lycoris* and *Narcissus;* it causes vomiting, diarrhea, convulsions, and sometimes death in animals that eat the bulbs. Called also *narcissine.*

Lyc•o•ris (lik'ŏ-ris) a genus of poisonous plants of the family Amaryllidaceae, native to China and Japan, whose bulbs contain the toxin lycorine. *L. radia'ta* Herb. is the source of tazettine, and its bulbs are used in Chinese medicine as an expectorant and emetic.

Ly•co•sa (li-ko'sə) a genus of wolf spiders (family Lycosidae). *L. taren'tula* is the European tarantula.

Ly•co•si•dae (li-ko'sĭ-de) the wolf spiders, a family of venomous ground spiders that chase their prey. Genera include *Lycosa* and *Scaptocosa.*

lyd•i•my•cin (lid"ĭ-mi'sin) an antifungal antibiotic produced by *Streptomyces lydicus*, $C_{10}H_{14}N_2O_3S$.

lye (li) an alkaline percolate from wood ashes; lixivium. Household lye is a crude mixture of sodium hydroxide with some sodium carbonate.

Ly•ell syndrome (li'əl) [Alan *Lyell*, English dermatologist, 20th century] toxic epidermal necrolysis.

ly•ing-in (li"ing-in') 1. puerperal. 2. the puerperium.

Lyme disease (arthritis), borreliosis (līm) [from Old *Lyme*, Connecticut, where the disease was first reported in 1975] see under *disease* and *borreliosis.*

Lym•naea (lim-ne'ə) a genus of pond snails of the order Lymneidae. *L. ollu'la* and *L. bulimoi'des* serve as first intermediate hosts of the liver fluke *Fasciola hepatica;* other species are the hosts of schistosome flukes that cause schistosome dermatitis.

Lym•ne•i•dae (lim-ne'ĭ-de) a family of fresh water snails of the suborder Basommatophora. It includes the genus *Lymnaea.*

lymph (limf) [L. *lympha* water] 1. a transparent, slightly yellow liquid of alkaline reaction, found in the lymphatic vessels and derived from the tissue fluids. It is occasionally of a light-rose color from the presence of red blood corpuscles, and is often opalescent from particles of fat. Under the microscope, lymph is seen to consist of a liquid portion and of cells, most of which are lymphocytes. Lymph is collected from all parts of the body and returned to the blood via the lymphatic system. Called also *lympha* [TA]. See Plate 26. 2. any clear, watery fluid resembling true lymph.
 aplastic l. lymph that contains an excess of leukocytes and does not tend to become organized; called also *corpuscular l.*
 corpuscular l. aplastic l.
 euplastic l., fibrinous l. lymph that tends to coagulate and become organized.
 inflammatory l. the lymph produced by inflammation, as in a wound.
 intercellular l. lymph occupying the intercellular spaces of tissues.
 intravascular l. the lymph of the lymph vessels.
 tissue l. lymph derived from the tissues and not from the blood.

lym•pha (lim'fə) [L. "water"] [TA] the fluid found in the lymphatic vessels; see *lymph.*

lym•phad•e•nec•to•my (lim-fad"ə-nek'tə-me) [*lymphaden* + *-ectomy*] surgical excision of a lymph node or nodes; often accompanied by an adjective referring to which node is removed, such as *axillary l.*, *cervical l.*, or *inguinal l.* Called also *lymph node dissection.*
 retroperitoneal l. surgical removal of lymph nodes in the retroperitoneal space, usually because of cancer metastasis, such as from carcinomas of the genital organs in men. Called also *retroperitoneal lymph node dissection (RPLND).*

lym•phad•e•ni•tis (lim-fad"ə-ni'tis) [*lymphaden* + *-itis*] inflammation of one or more lymph nodes, usually caused by a primary focus of infection elsewhere in the body.
 caseous l. a chronic disease of sheep and goats caused by *Corynebacterium pseudotuberculosis*, characterized by the formation in various lymph nodes of abscesses containing caseous material, sometimes associated with chronic pneumonia and pleurisy. Called also *pseudotuberculosis.*
 cervical l. see under *lymphadenopathy.*
 dermatopathic l. see under *lymphadenopathy.*
 histiocytic necrotizing l., Kikuchi l. a benign, self-limited syndrome of lymphadenopathy, usually in the neck, with a female predominance; characteristics include patchy necrotizing lesions of the paracortex and proliferation of distinctive histiocytes, plasmacytoid monocytes, and immunoblasts surrounded by karyorrhectic debris. Some consider it a self-limited form of systemic lupus erythematosus. Called also *Kikuchi* or *Kikuchi-Fujimoto disease.*
 mediastinal l. see under *lymphadenopathy.*
 mesenteric l. inflammation of the mesenteric lymph nodes, causing pain and swelling resembling that in acute appendicitis. A septal form, which is frequently fatal, and a milder form, which is self-limited, may be caused by either *Yersinia enterocolitica* or *Y. pseudotuberculosis.* Called also *mesenteric adenitis* or *lymphadenopathy.*
 paratuberculous l. caseous l.
 regional l. 1. inflammation of all the lymph nodes that drain a given area. 2. cat-scratch disease.
 regional granulomatous l. cat-scratch disease.
 streptococcal l. of swine streptococcal infection with abscesses in lymph nodes in the necks of pigs; it is often subclinical and discovered when the animal is slaughtered, whereupon the meat may have to be condemned. Called also *jowl abscess* and *cervical abscess.*
 subacute necrotizing l. Kikuchi l.
 tuberculoid l. a condition similar to tuberculous lymphadenitis, caused by disorders such as sarcoidosis, regional enteritis, leprosy, syphilis, or a fungal infection.
 tuberculous l. tuberculosis of lymph nodes, usually cervical ones but sometimes mediastinal ones; see *tuberculous cervical l.* and *tuberculous mediastinal l.* It may be a primary infection or may be caused by lymphatic or

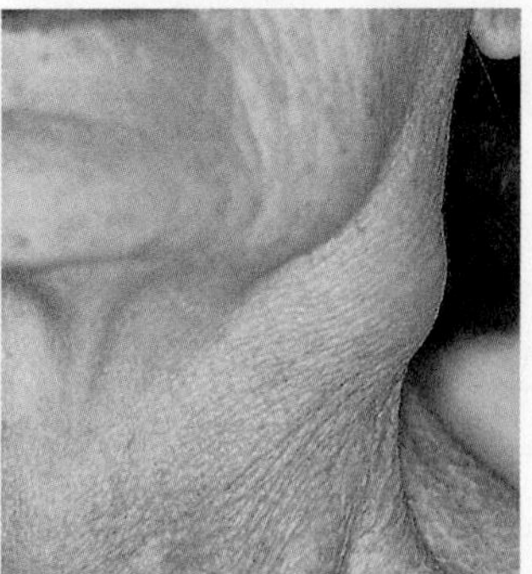

■ Tuberculous lymphadenitis.

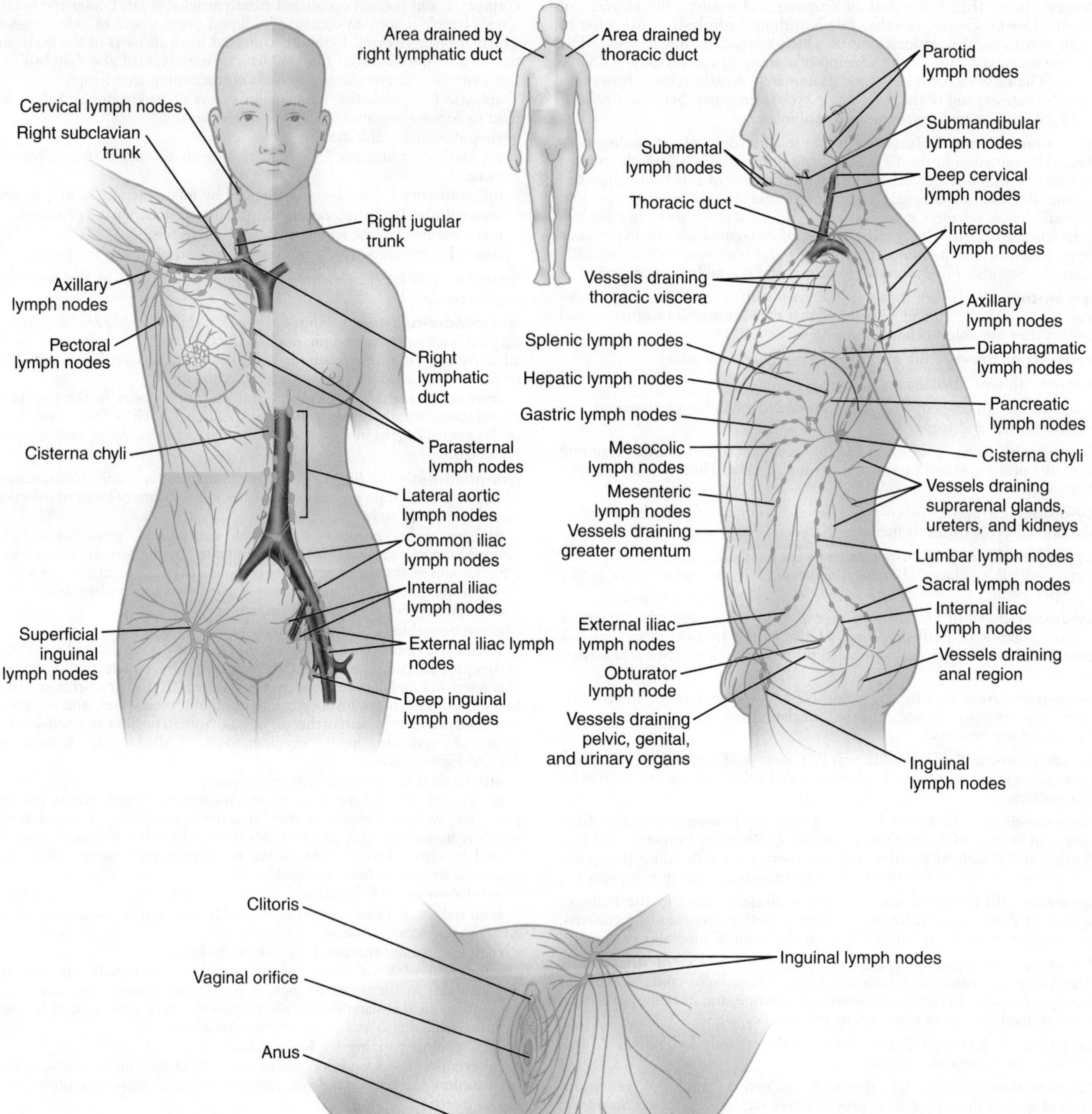

Area drained by right lymphatic duct
Area drained by thoracic duct
Cervical lymph nodes
Right subclavian trunk
Right jugular trunk
Axillary lymph nodes
Pectoral lymph nodes
Right lymphatic duct
Cisterna chyli
Parasternal lymph nodes
Lateral aortic lymph nodes
Common iliac lymph nodes
Internal iliac lymph nodes
Superficial inguinal lymph nodes
External iliac lymph nodes
Deep inguinal lymph nodes
Parotid lymph nodes
Submandibular lymph nodes
Submental lymph nodes
Deep cervical lymph nodes
Thoracic duct
Intercostal lymph nodes
Vessels draining thoracic viscera
Axillary lymph nodes
Splenic lymph nodes
Diaphragmatic lymph nodes
Hepatic lymph nodes
Pancreatic lymph nodes
Gastric lymph nodes
Cisterna chyli
Mesocolic lymph nodes
Vessels draining suprarenal glands, ureters, and kidneys
Mesenteric lymph nodes
Vessels draining greater omentum
Lumbar lymph nodes
Sacral lymph nodes
External iliac lymph nodes
Internal iliac lymph nodes
Vessels draining anal region
Obturator lymph node
Vessels draining pelvic, genital, and urinary organs
Inguinal lymph nodes

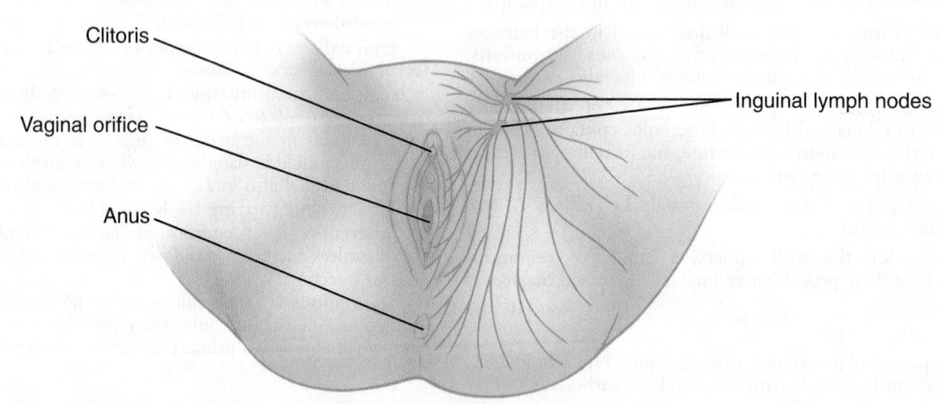

■ **PLATE 26—DIAGRAMMATIC REPRESENTATION OF LYMPHATIC DRAINAGE OF VARIOUS PARTS OF THE BODY**

hematogenous spread from infection elsewhere in the body. Called also *tuberculous lymphadenopathy.*

tuberculous cervical l. tuberculous lymphadenitis involving cervical lymph nodes; called also *tuberculous cervical adenitis* and formerly *scrofula.*

tuberculous mediastinal l. tuberculous lymphadenitis involving mediastinal lymph nodes.

lym•phad•e•no•cele (lim-fad′ə-no-sēl″) a cyst of a lymph node; called also *adenolymphocele.*

lym•phad•e•no•cyst (lim-fad′ə-no-sist″) a degenerated lymph node caused by occlusion of its incoming lymph vessels. By dilatation of the lymph sinuses it becomes a fine-meshed network.

lym•phad•e•no•gram (lim-fad′ə-no-gram″) a radiograph of lymph nodes.

lym•phad•e•nog•ra•phy (lim-fad″ə-nog′rə-fe) radiographic visualization of the lymph nodes, following injection of radiopaque material into a lymphatic vessel.

lym•phad•e•noid (lim-fad′ə-noid) [*lymphaden* + *-oid*] resembling the tissue of lymph nodes; lymphadenoid tissue includes the spleen, bone marrow, tonsils, and the lymphatic tissue of the organs and mucous membranes.

lym•phad•e•no•leu•ko•poi•e•sis (lim-fad″ə-no-loo″ko-poi-e′sis) the production of leukocytes by the lymphadenoid tissue.

lym•phad•e•no•ma (lim-fad″ə-no′mə) lymphoma.

lym•phad•e•nop•a•thy (lim-fad″ə-nop′ə-the) [*lymphaden* + *-pathy*] disease of the lymph nodes, usually with swelling; called also *adenopathy.*

angioimmunoblastic l., angioimmunoblastic l. with dysproteinemia (AILD) a systemic disorder resembling lymphoma, characterized by fever, night sweats, and weight loss; generalized lymphadenopathy with a mixed cellular infiltrate of lymphocytes, immunoblasts, and plasma cells that alters or effaces the nodal architecture; hepatosplenomegaly; maculopapular rash; polyclonal hypergammaglobulinemia; and Coombs-positive hemolytic anemia. It is considered to be a nonmalignant hyperimmune reaction to chronic antigenic stimulation; there is proliferation of B cells accompanied by profound deficiency of T cells. The disease follows a progressive but variable course, with some patients surviving a long time but others developing infections that can be fatal. Called also *immunoblastic l.*

cervical l. enlarged, inflamed, and tender cervical lymph nodes, seen in certain infectious diseases of children, such as acute infections of the throat. See also *tuberculous cervical lymphadenitis*, under *lymphadenitis*. Called also *cervical adenitis* or *lymphadenitis.*

dermatopathic l. regional lymph node enlargement associated with melanoderma or various diseases in which erythroderma is chronically present, such as exfoliative dermatitis or generalized neurodermatitis. Called also *lipomelanotic reticulosis.*

immunoblastic l. angioimmunoblastic l.

mediastinal l. inflammation and swelling of mediastinal lymph nodes, often caused by some underlying condition such as mediastinitis, a cyst, or a tumor that can be malignant such as in leukemia or lymphoma. Called also *mediastinal lymphadenitis.*

mesenteric l. see under *lymphadenitis.*

tuberculous l. see under *lymphadenitis.*

lym•phad•e•no•sis (lim-fad″ə-no′sis) a proliferative process of lymphatic tissue resuulting in enlargement of lymph nodes, as that preceding certain types of leukemia.

l. benig′na cu′tis cutaneous lymphoid hyperplasia; see under *hyperplasia.*

lym•phad•e•not•o•my (lim-fad″ə-not′ə-me) incision into a lymph node.

lym•phad•e•no•va•rix (lim-fad″ə-no-va′riks) enlargement of the lymph nodes from the pressure of dilated lymph vessels.

lym•pha•gogue (lim′fə-gog) an agent promoting the production of lymph.

lym•phan•ge•itis (lim″fan-je-i′tis) lymphangitis.

lym•phan•gi•al (lim-fan′je-əl) pertaining to a lymphatic vessel.

lym•phan•gi•ec•ta•sia (lim-fan″je-ək-ta′zhə) lymphangiectasis.

intestinal l. dilatation of the intestinal lymphatic system, particularly the lacteals in the intestinal villi, characterized by protein-losing enteropathy, steatorrhea, and lymphopenia.

lym•phan•gi•ec•ta•sis (lim-fan″je-ek′tə-sis) [*lymph-* + *angiectasis*] dilatation of lymphatic vessels. **lymphangiectat′ic** *adj*

parapelvic l., peripelvic l. renal sinus cyst.

lym•phan•gi•ec•to•my (lim-fan″je-ek′tə-me) excision of one or more lymphatic vessels.

lym•phan•gi•itis (lim-fan″je-i′tis) lymphangitis.

lym•phan•gio•ad•e•nog•ra•phy (lim-fan″je-o-ad″ə-nog′rə-fe) lymphography.

lym•phan•gio•en•do•the•li•o•ma (lim-fan″je-o-en″do-the″le-o′mə) endothelioma of lymphatic vessels.

lym•phan•gio•fi•bro•ma (lim-fan″je-o-fi-bro′mə) a fibrosing lymphangioma.

lym•phan•gio•gram (lim-fan′je-o-gram″) a radiograph of the lymphatic vessels taken during lymphangiography.

lym•phan•gi•og•ra•phy (lim-fan″je-og′rə-fe) angiography of the lymphatic vessels.

bipedal l., pedal l. radiography of the lymphatic channels of the lower extremity after injection of contrast medium into the first and second interdigital spaces of the foot.

lym•phan•gio•leio•myo•ma•to•sis (lim-fan″je-o-li″o-mi″o-mə-to′sis) lymphangiomyomatosis.

lym•phan•gi•ol•o•gy (lim-fan″je-ol′ə-je) [*lymph-* + *angiology*] the branch of anatomy relating to the lymphatic vessels. Cf. *lymphology.*

lym•phan•gi•o•ma (lim-fan″je-o′mə) a type of vascular malformation of the lymphatic system, made up of newly formed lymph-containing vascular spaces and channels. Called also *angioma lymphaticum*. Cf. *angioma* and *hemangioma.*

capillary l. simple l.

l. caverno′sum, cavernous l. 1. a deeply situated lymphangioma, composed of cavernous lymphatic spaces, and always occurring in the neck or axilla. See also *vascular nevus*, under *nevus*. 2. cystic hygroma.

l. circumscrip′tum a cutaneous and more superficial type of lymphangioma, usually occurring either on the upper portion of the limbs, in the axillary or inguinal folds (usually localized to one region), or on the oral mucosa, especially the tongue; it consists of a grapelike group of thin-walled translucent lymph-filled vesicles that sometimes have a verrucous surface. Some lesions have a deeper component of lymphatic obstruction and lymphedema with localized swelling. See also *vascular nevus*, under *nevus.*

cystic l., l. cys′ticum see under *hygroma.*

fissural l. simple or cavernous lymphangiomas at the site of fetal fissures.

simple l., l. sim′plex a lymphangioma composed of small lymphatic channels that tends to occur subcutaneously in the head and neck region or axilla and sometimes in internal organs. Superficial lesions present as slightly raised or sometimes nodular lesions; deeper lesions are sharply circumscribed, compressible, and gray to pink in color. Called also *capillary l.*

lym•phan•gio•my•o•ma•to•sis (LAM) (lim-fan″je-o-mi″o-mə-to′sis) a progressive disorder of women of child-bearing age, marked by proliferation of atypical smooth muscle cells in the walls of lymphatics of the lower respiratory tract, pleura, mediastinum, and retroperitoneum. Called also *lymphangioleiomyomatosis.*

lym•phan•gi•on (lim-fan′je-on) vas lymphaticum.

lym•phan•gio•phle•bi•tis (lim-fan″je-o-flə-bi′tis) inflammation of the lymph vessels and veins.

lym•phan•gio•sar•co•ma (lim-fan″je-o-sahr-ko′mə) [*lymph-* + *angiosarcoma*] a malignant tumor of vascular endothelial cells arising from lymphatic vessels; it may arise in a limb that is the site of chronic lymphedema, particularly secondary to radical mastectomy.

lym•phan•gio•scin•tig•ra•phy (LAS) (lim-fan″je-o-sin-tig′rah-fe) scintigraphic evaluation of primary and secondary lymphedema using radioactive tracers.

lym•phan•gi•ot•o•my (lim-fan″je-ot′ə-me) [*lymph-* + *angiotomy*] incision into a lymphatic vessel, usually performed for cannulation prior to lymphangiography.

lym•phan•gi•tis (lim″fan-ji′tis) inflammation of a lymphatic vessel or vessels. Acute lymphangitis may result from spread of bacterial infection (most commonly beta-hemolytic streptococci) into the lymphatics, manifested by painful subcutaneous red streaks along the course of the vessels. Called also *angiolymphitis.* **lymphangit′ic** *adj*

l. carcinomato′sa a pseudoinflammatory lesion of the lymphatic vessels of the peritoneum, with edema of the area and proliferation of fibrous tissues around the vessels, due to the infiltration of cancer cells from peritoneal tumors.

epizootic l., l. epizoo′tica a chronic contagious disease of horses, resembling glanders but caused by the yeast fungus *Histoplasma farciminosum;* characteristics include purulent inflammation of subcutaneous lymphatic vessels and regional lymph glands, which form cutaneous ulcers that may take a year to heal. Called also *pseudofarcy, pseudoglanders, African glanders, Japanese farcy* or *glanders,* and *Neapolitan farcy.*

ulcerative l. a chronic contagious disease of horses and other equines, characterized by inflammation of the lymph vessels and a tendency toward ulceration of the skin over the parts affected; called also *ulcerative cellulitis.*

lym•pha•phe•re•sis (lim″fə-fə-re′sis) lymphocytapheresis.

lym•phat•ic (lim-fat′ik) [L. *lymphaticus*] 1. pertaining to lymph or a lymph vessel. 2. a lymphatic vessel. 3. (pl.) the lymphatic system. 4. of a sluggish or phlegmatic temperament.

lym•phat•i•cos•to•my (lim-fat″ĭ-kos′tə-me) [*lymphatic* + *-ostomy*] surgical creation of an opening into a lymphatic duct, usually the thoracic duct.

lym·pha·tism (lim′fə-tiz″əm) 1. status lymphaticus. 2. the lymphatic temperament; a slow or sluggish habit.

lym·pha·ti·tis (lim″fə-ti′tis) inflammation of some part of the lymphatic system.

lym·pha·tog·e·nous (lim″fə-toj′ə-nəs) produced by or derived from the lymph; disseminated by the lymph circulation or through the lymph channels.

lym·pha·tol·o·gy (lim″fə-tol′ə-je) lymphology.

lym·pha·tol·y·sis (lim″fə-tol′ə-sis) [*lymphatic* + *-lysis*] the destruction or solution of lymphatic tissue.

lym·pha·to·lyt·ic (lim″fə-to-lit′ik) [*lymphatic* + *-lytic*] destroying lymphatic tissue.

lym·phec·ta·sia (lim″fek-ta′zhə) [*lymph-* + *ectasia*] distention with lymph.

lym·phe·de·ma (lim″fə-de′mə) [*lymph-* + *edema*] chronic unilateral or bilateral edema of the limbs due to accumulation of interstitial fluid as a result of stasis of lymph, secondary to obstruction of lymph vessels or disorders of lymph nodes.

congenital l. lymphedema occurring at or soon after birth; it may occur as a primary hereditary disorder (Milroy disease) or may be associated with other conditions, such as Turner syndrome.

Meige l. l. praecox.

Milroy l. see under *disease.*

l. prae′cox primary lymphedema of the lower limbs beginning at or near puberty, usually in young women. Called also *Meige l.* or *disease.*

l. tar′da primary lymphedema that manifests after age 35.

lymph·epi·the·li·o·ma (limf″ep-i-the″le-o′mə) lymphoepithelioma.

lym·phi·za·tion (lim″fĭ-za′shən) the formation of lymph.

lymph·no·di·tis (limf″no-di′tis) lymphadenitis.

lymph(o)- [L. *lympha* water] a combining form denoting relationship to lymph, lymphoid tissue, lymphatics, or lymphocytes.

lym·pho·blast (lim′fo-blast) [*lympho-* + *-blast*] a morphologically immature lymphocyte, once thought to represent an early stage in lymphocyte development but now known to be an activated lymphocyte that has been transformed in response to antigenic stimulation. **lymphoblas′tic** *adj*

lym·pho·blas·to·ma (lim″fo-blas-to′mə) [*lymphoblast* + *-oma*] lymphoblastic lymphoma.

lym·pho·blas·to·sis (lim″fo-blas-to′sis) excess of lymphoblasts in the blood, as seen in lymphoblastic leukemia.

lym·pho·cele (lim′fo-sēl) a cyst containing lymph.

lym·pho·ce·ras·tism (lim″fo-sə-ras′tiz-əm) [*lympho-* + Gr. *kerastos* mixed] the formation of cells of the lymphocytic series.

lym·pho·ci·ne·sia (lim″fo-si-ne′zhə) lymphokinesis.

Lym·pho·cryp·to·vi·rus (lim″fo-krip′to-vi″rəs) [*lympho-* + *crypto-* + *virus*] Epstein-Barr–like viruses; a genus of viruses of the subfamily Gammaherpesvirinae (family Herpesviridae) containing both human and animal pathogens, including Epstein-Barr virus and species infecting nonhuman primates.

lym·pho·cyst (lim′fo-sist) lymphocele.

lym·pho·cys·tis (lim″fo-sis′tis) [*lympho-* + *cystis*] a common, chronic, nonfatal disease of marine and freshwater fish, caused by *Lymphocystivirus* and characterized by tumorlike nodules, generally on the skin and fins, consisting of hypertrophied connective tissue cells. Called also *lymphocystis disease.*

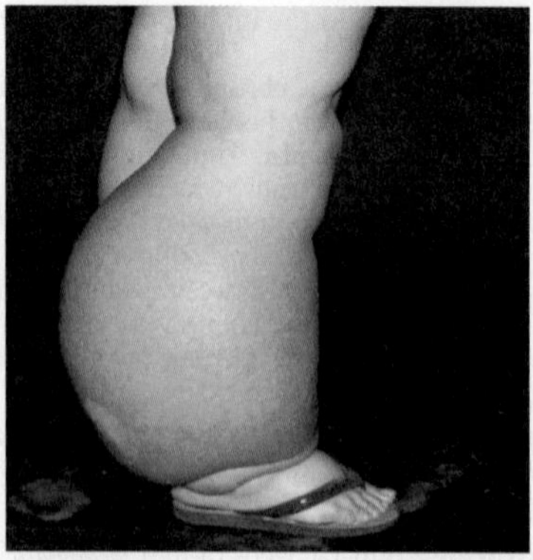

■ Marked lymphedema after inguinal and pelvic lymphadenectomy.

Lym·pho·cys·ti·vi·rus (lim″fo-sis′tĭ-vi″rəs) [*lymphocystis* + *virus*] lymphocystis viruses; a genus of viruses of the family Iridoviridae that cause lymphocystis in marine and freshwater fish.

lym·pho·cy·ta·phe·re·sis (lim″fo-si″tə-fə-re′sis) [*lymphocyte* + *apheresis*] the selective removal of lymphocytes from withdrawn blood, which is then retransfused into the donor. Called also *lymphapheresis.*

lym·pho·cyte (lim′fo-sīt) [*lympho-* + *-cyte*] any of the mononuclear, nonphagocytic leukocytes, found in the blood, lymph, and lymphoid tissues, that are the body's immunologically competent cells and their precursors. They are divided on the basis of ontogeny and function into two classes, B and T lymphocytes, responsible for humoral and cellular immunity, respectively. Most are *small lymphocytes,* 7–10 μm in diameter, with a round or slightly indented heterochromatic nucleus that almost fills the cell and a thin rim of basophilic cytoplasm that contains few granules. When activated by contact with antigen, small lymphocytes begin macromolecular synthesis, the cytoplasm enlarges until the cells are 10–30 μm in diameter, and the nucleus becomes less completely heterochromatic; they are then referred to as *large lymphocytes* or *lymphoblasts.* These cells then proliferate and differentiate into B and T memory cells and into the various effector cell types, B lymphocytes into plasma cells and T cells into helper, cytotoxic, and suppressor cells. Surface markers identifying the lymphocyte types are shown in the accompanying table. See subentries here and under *cell.* **lymphocyt′ic** *adj*

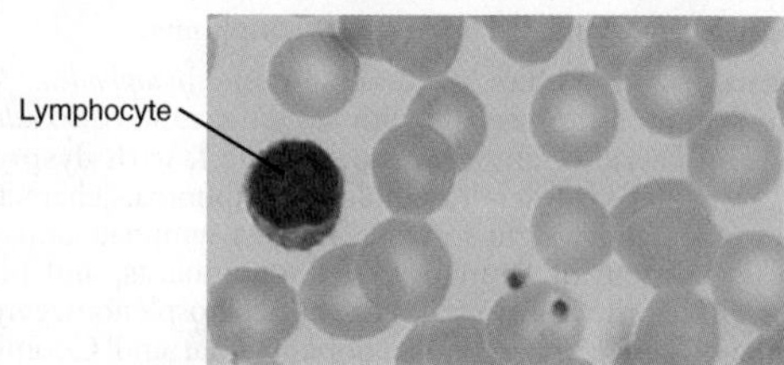

amplifier T l. a T lymphocyte that modifies a developing immune response by releasing nonspecific signals to which other T lymphocytes (either effector or suppressor cells) respond.

B l's bursa-dependent lymphocytes in birds and their counterparts in nonavian vertebrates including human beings, the cells primarily responsible for humoral immunity, the precursors of antibody-producing cells (plasma cells). In birds maturation of these cells takes place in the bursa of Fabricius; the hypothesized analogous tissue in other vertebrates was termed the "bursa-equivalent" tissue. It now appears that B lymphocyte maturation occurs primarily in the bone marrow in mammals. B lymphocytes are characterized by the presence of surface immunoglobulin, monomeric IgM or IgD, which constitutes the B-cell antigen receptors. When stimulated by antigen, a process that requires the cooperation of helper T cells and macrophages, B lymphocytes proliferate and differentiate into plasma cells and memory B cells. The entire clone of cells descended from a single activated B lymphocyte produces immunoglobulins having the same antigen combining site as that in the antigen receptors of the original cell; thus all of the antibody produced and all of the memory cells are specific for the antigen that induced their formation. Called also *B cells.*

CD4 T l's, CD4⁺ T l's CD4 cells.

CD8 T l's, CD8⁺ T l's CD8 cells.

cytotoxic T l's (CTL) differentiated T lymphocytes that can recognize and lyse target cells bearing specific antigens recognized by their antigen receptors. Recognition is MHC restricted; the foreign antigen is recognized only in association with self MHC antigens. The cytotoxic activity requires firm binding of the lymphocyte to the target cell to produce holes in the plasma membrane of the target cell, loss of its cell content, and osmotic lysis. These lymphocytes are important in graft rejection and killing of tumor cells and virus-infected host cells. Murine killer T cells are marked by the Ly-2 and Ly-3 antigens, human cells by the CD4 and CD8 antigens. Called also *killer* or *killer T cells.*

helper T l's helper T cells.

large l. see *lymphocyte.*

large granular l's lymphocytes marked by the presence of large granules visible by light microscopy, responsible for most natural killer cell activity.

plasmacytoid l. a cell morphologically resembling a small lymphocyte but having a well-developed rough endoplasmic reticulum like that of a plasma cell; frequently observed in the blood of patients with plasma cell dyscrasias or hypergammaglobulinemia.

Rieder l. Rieder cell.

small l. see *lymphocyte.*

T l's the cells primarily responsible for cell-mediated immunity; they originate from lymphoid stem cells that migrate from the bone marrow to the thymus and differentiate under the influence of the thymic hormones thymopoietin and thymosin. They are characterized by specific surface

Surface Markers of Lymphocytes

	mIg	CD1	CD3 Thy-1	CD4 Ly-1	CD5, CD8 Ly-2, 3	FcR	CR
B cells	+	–	–	–	–	±	±
T cells							
Helper	–	+	+	+	–	±	–
Killer	–	+	+	–	+	±	–
Suppressor	–	+	+	–	+	±	–
Null cells							
K cells	–	–	–	–	–	+	–
NK cells	–	–	–	–	–	+	–

mIg = membrane immunoglobulin; Thy-1, Ly-1, Ly-2, Ly-3 = mouse T-cell surface antigens; CD1, CD3, CD4, CD5, CD8 = human T-cell surface antigens; FcR = Fc receptors; CR = complement receptors; ± indicates present only on a subset of cells or on cells of certain maturities.

antigens: the pan-T antigens Thy-1 (murine) and CD3 (human) are found on all mature T lymphocytes; other markers characterize T cell subsets. T cell antigen receptors are triggered by antigen only when associated with self MHC antigens, e.g., by antigens processed and presented by macrophages, viral antigens on the surface of host cells, and tumor neoantigens. When activated by antigen, T lymphocytes proliferate and differentiate into T memory cells and the various types of regulatory and effector T cells; see *cytotoxic T l's* and *helper*, *suppressor*, *contrasuppressor*, and *T_{DTH} cells*, under *cell*. Called also *T cells* and *thymus-dependent l's*.

thymus-dependent l's T l's.

thymus-independent l's B l's.

tumor-infiltrating l's (TIL) lymphocytes isolated from the inflammatory infiltrate present in solid tumors and cultured in interleukin-2 (IL-2); they have specific activity against the tumor from which they are derived.

lym·pho·cy·to·blast (lim″fo-si′to-blast) lymphoblast.

lym·pho·cy·to·ma (lim″fo-si-to′mə) [*lymphocyte* + *-oma*] 1. pseudolymphoma. 2. well differentiated lymphocytic lymphoma.

l. cu′tis cutaneous lymphoid hyperplasia.

lym·pho·cy·to·pe·nia (lim″fo-si″to-pe′ne-ə) [*lymphocyte* + *-penia*] reduction in the number of lymphocytes in the blood; called also *lymphopenia*, *hypolymphemia*, and *sublymphemia*.

lym·pho·cy·to·phe·re·sis (lim″fo-si″to-fə-re′sis) lymphocytapheresis.

lym·pho·cy·to·poi·e·sis (lim″fo-si″to-poi-e′sis) [*lymphocyte* + *poiesis*] the development of lymphocytes. **lymphocytopoiet′ic** *adj*

lym·pho·cy·tor·rhex·is (lim″fo-si″to-rek′sis) the rupturing or bursting of lymphocytes.

lym·pho·cy·to·sis (lim″fo-si-to′sis) excess of normal lymphocytes in the blood or in any effusion. **lymphocytot′ic** *adj*

acute infectious l. an acute, benign infectious disease of children characterized by an excess of normal small lymphocytes in the blood without lymphadenopathy or splenomegaly, and with varying degrees of clinical expression and constitutional response.

lym·pho·cy·to·tox·ic·i·ty (lim″fo-si″to-tok-sis′ĭ-te) the quality or capability of lysing lymphocytes, as that of cytotoxic antibodies in the presence of complement or that of primed histoincompatible cytotoxic T lymphocytes.

lym·pho·cy·to·tox·in (lim″fo-si′to-tok″sin) a toxin that has a specific destructive action on lymphocytes.

lym·pho·duct (lim′fo-dəkt) a lymphatic vessel.

lym·pho·epi·the·li·o·ma (lim″fo-ep″ĭ-the″le-o′mə) a pleomorphic, poorly differentiated transitional cell carcinoma arising from modified epithelium overlying the lymphoid tissue of the nasopharynx; it has a high frequency among young adults of East Asian extraction. Called also *lymphoepithelial carcinoma* and *Regaud* or *Schmincke tumor*.

lym·pho·gen·e·sis (lim″fo-jen′ə-sis) the production of lymph.

lym·phog·e·nous (lim-foj′ə-nəs) [*lympho-* + *-genous*] 1. producing lymph. 2. produced from lymph or in the lymphatics.

lym·pho·gram (lim′fo-gram) a radiograph of the lymphatic vessels and lymph nodes.

lym·pho·gran·u·lo·ma (lim″fo-gran″u-lo′mə) 1. Hodgkin disease. 2. a nonspecific term used for any of various granulomatous conditions involving lymph nodes.

l. inguina′le l. venereum.

l. vene′reum a sexually transmitted infection usually seen in warm climates, due to strains of *Chlamydia trachomatis*, characterized by a primary cutaneous or mucosal lesion (papular, ulcerative, herpetiform, or erosive), or urethritis or endocervicitis. This heals spontaneously and may go unnoticed, but is then followed by acute lymphadenopathy. The original infection site determines the later manifestations: in men, the primary lesion is usually on the prepuce, glans, and shaft of the penis, associated with lymphadenitis of inguinal lymph nodes, often with draining buboes *(the inguinal syndrome);* in women, the primary lesion usually involves the posterior vagina, cervix, and labia, associated with hemorrhagic proctocolitis *(the anogenitorectal syndrome)*. Late complications in untreated cases, chiefly in women, include locally destructive ulcerations, rectal strictures, rectovaginal fistulas, and genital elephantiasis. Called also *l. inguinale*.

lym·pho·gran·u·lo·ma·to·sis (lim″fo-gran″u-lo-mə-to′sis) European synonym for Hodgkin disease.

benign l. sarcoidosis.

l. cu′tis the cutaneous manifestation of Hodgkin disease.

lym·phog·ra·phy (lim-fog′rə-fe) radiography of the lymphatic channels and lymph nodes, following injection of radiopaque material in a lymphatic vessel.

bipedal l., pedal l. lymphography of the lower limbs.

lym·pho·his·tio·cyt·ic (lim″fo-his″te-o-sit′ik) involving lymphocytes and histiocytes.

lym·pho·his·tio·cy·to·sis (lim″fo-his″te-o-si-to′sis) lymphocytosis with histiocytosis.

erythrophagocytic l. hemophagocytic l.

familial hemophagocytic l. an autosomal recessive, genetically heterogeneous type of hemophagocytic lymphohistiocytosis; it is characterized by anemia, granulocytopenia, thrombocytopenia, intense phagocytosis of red blood cells, diffuse proliferation of histiocytes of various organs, and enlargement of the liver, spleen, and lymph nodes; it is usually rapidly fatal if untreated.

hemophagocytic l. any of several closely related disorders involving both lymphocytosis and histiocytosis, with excessive hemophagocytosis in the lymphoreticular system or the central nervous system; they are usually seen in children secondary to infection and are often fatal; they can also be secondary to rheumatologic or other conditions, or can be familial (*familial hemophagocytic l.*). Called also *hemophagocytic syndrome* and *macrophage activation syndrome*.

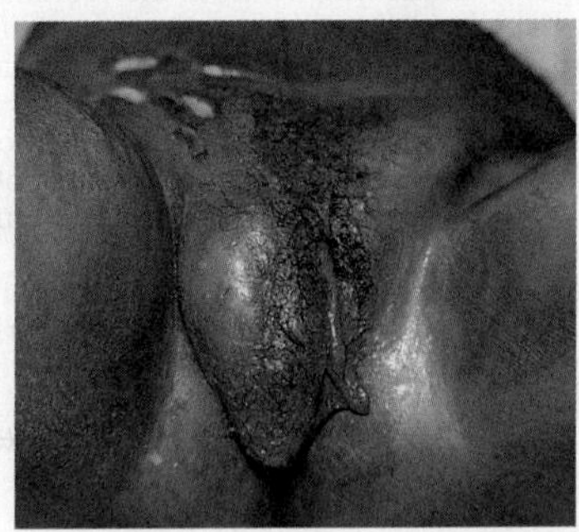

■ Lymphogranuloma venereum causing unilateral vulvar lymphedema and inguinal buboes.

lym·pho·his·tio·plas·ma·cyt·ic (lim″fo-his″te-o-plaz″mə-sit′ik) involving lymphocytes, histiocytes, and plasmacytes.

lym·phoid (lim′foid) [*lymph* + Gr. *eidos* form] resembling or pertaining to lymph or tissue of the lymphoid system.

lym·phoi·dec·to·my (lim″foi-dek′tə-me) excision of lymphoid tissue, such as adenoids and tonsils.

lym·pho·ken·tric (lim″fo-ken′trik) [*lympho-* + Gr. *kentron* a stimulant] stimulating lymphocytopoiesis.

lym·pho·kine (lim′fo-kīn) [*lympho-* + Gr. *kinēsis* movement] a soluble cytokine that mediates immune responses; it is not an antibody or a complement component and is released by sensitized lymphocytes on contact with antigen. Cf. *monokine.*

lym·pho·ki·ne·sis (lim″fo-kĭ-ne′sis) [*lympho-* + *kinesis*] 1. the movement of the endolymph in the semicircular canals. 2. the circulation of lymph in the body.

lym·phol·o·gy (lim-fol′ə-je) [*lympho-* + *-logy*] the study of the lymphatic system. Cf. *lymphangiology.*

lym·phol·y·sis (lym-fol′ĭ-sis) lysis of lymphocytes.

cell-mediated l. (CML) a variation of the mixed lymphocyte culture (MLC) that is a functional test of the ability of cytotoxic T lymphocytes to kill target cells. Lymphocytes from two individuals are cultured together for several days, one population having been prevented from proliferating by treatment with radiation or mitomycin (a "one-way" MLC); they are then cultured for several hours with ^{51}Cr-labeled target cells that are HLA-identical to the stimulator cells. Cytotoxicity is measured as percentage of ^{51}Cr released from specific target cells compared to percentage of ^{51}Cr released from control (nonspecific target) cells.

lym·pho·lyt·ic (lim″fo-lit′ik) causing destruction of lymphocytes.

lym·pho·ma (lim-fo′mə) [*lymph-* + *-oma*] 1. any neoplastic disorder of the lymphoid tissue. 2. malignant l.

Lymphoma

adult T-cell l., adult T-cell leukemia/l. see under *leukemia.*

African l. Burkitt l.

anaplastic large cell l. in a former system of classification, a type of large cell lymphoma in which cells are anaplastic and growth is sinusoidal; called also *Ki-1 l.*

B-cell l. any in a large group of non-Hodgkin lymphomas characterized by malignant transformation of the B lymphocytes; among the many B-cell lymphomas are *Burkitt l., l. cutis, follicular center cell l.,* and *small B-cell l.*

B-cell monocytoid l. a low-grade marginal zone lymphoma in which cells resemble those of hairy cell leukemia.

bovine malignant l. enzootic bovine leukosis.

Burkitt l. a form of small noncleaved cell lymphoma, usually found in central Africa, but also reported from other areas, and manifested most often as a large osteolytic lesion in the jaw or as an abdominal mass. Epstein-Barr virus has been isolated from Burkitt lymphoma and has been implicated as a cause. Called also *Burkitt tumor* and *African l.*

centrocytic l. mantle cell l.

convoluted T-cell l. lymphoblastic lymphoma with markedly convoluted nuclei.

cutaneous T-cell l. a group of lymphomas including a spectrum of disorders, all of which exhibit both clonal expansion of malignant T lymphocytes and malignant infiltration of the skin. The lymphocytes have been arrested at varying stages of differentiation into helper cells, and skin infiltration is often the chief or only manifestation of disease. Mycosis fungoides and Sézary syndrome are the best characterized of these disorders.

l. cu′tis primary skin involvement by B-cell lymphoma without demonstrable systemic disease, most often presenting as a solitary, purple to pink nodule, especially on the head, neck, and face, and usually associated with dissemination to regional lymph nodes and distant hematogenous spread, leading to widespread involvement.

diffuse l. malignant lymphoma in which the neoplastic cells diffusely infiltrate the entire lymph node, without any definite organized pattern. This category from the Rappaport Classification was replaced by some of the cleaved-cell lymphomas in the Lukes-Collins Classification, by the three subtypes of diffuse lymphomas in the Working Formulation of Non-Hodgkin Lymphomas, and by a variety of specific B- and T-cell neoplasms in the Revised European-American Lymphoma Classification. Called also *lymphatic sarcoma* and *lymphosarcoma.*

diffuse, large cell l. a type of non-Hodgkin lymphoma composed of large cleaved and noncleaved cells in a diffuse pattern of infiltration; it is similar to the diffuse mixed variety and has an intermediate grade of malignancy.

diffuse, mixed small and large cell l. a type of lymphoma that mixes the small cleaved cell and large cell varieties; it is similar to the diffuse, large cell type and has an intermediate grade of malignancy.

diffuse, small cleaved cell l. small cleaved cell lymphoma with a diffuse infiltrate of small lymphocytes that have round nuclei and clumped chromatin; this type has an intermediate grade of malignancy.

follicular l. any of several types of non-Hodgkin lymphoma in which the lymphomatous cells are clustered into identifiable nodules or follicles. The cells may be either small cleaved or large (cleaved or uncleaved) cells; tumors in which most or all of the cells are small and cleaved have a better prognosis than those with large cells. Called also *Brill-Symmers disease, giant follicle l.,* and *nodular l.*

follicular center cell l. any of a large group of B-cell lymphomas, comprising four subtypes classified on the basis of the predominant cell type (resembling small cleaved, large cleaved, small noncleaved, and large noncleaved follicular center cells). Because of the wide variety of prognostic levels and the existence of tumors with several types of cells, the original four categories have now been divided up and scattered among several new categories of follicular and diffuse lymphomas.

follicular, mixed small cleaved and large cell l. a type of non-Hodgkin lymphoma with a mixture of small cleaved, large cleaved, and large uncleaved cells; the percentage of large cells is noticeable but less than 50 per cent of the tumor. It has a low grade of malignancy.

follicular, predominantly large cell l. a rare type of follicular lymphoma with large cells that are either cleaved or noncleaved; it has a poorer prognosis than other follicular lymphomas.

follicular, predominantly small cleaved cell l. the most common type of follicular lymphoma; it has a low grade of malignancy and is characterized by the formation of malignant small cleaved follicular center cells. See also *small cleaved cell l.*

giant follicle l., giant follicular l. follicular l.

granulomatous l. Hodgkin disease.

histiocytic l. a rare type of non-Hodgkin lymphoma of intermediate to high malignancy, characterized by large tumor cells that resemble histiocytes morphologically but are considered to be of lymphoid origin. Many tumors formerly placed in this category are now considered to belong in one of the large cell lymphoma groups.

Hodgkin l. see under *disease.*

intermediate lymphocytic l., lymphocytic l., intermediately differentiated mantle cell l.

Ki-1 l. anaplastic large cell l.

large cell l. any of several types of non-Hodgkin lymphoma characterized by formation of malignant large lymphocytes in a diffuse pattern; some varieties contain exclusively one type of cell, such as lymphoblasts or cleaved or uncleaved follicular center cells, and others have a mixture of cells, sometimes including ones that cannot be characterized as to lineage.

large cell, immunoblastic l. a type of non-Hodgkin lymphoma characterized by large lymphoblasts (immunoblasts) that resemble macrophages rather than follicular center cells, and have a diffuse pattern of infiltration; it has a high degree of malignancy and often grows rapidly. The cell population may be exclusively B or T lymphoblasts or a mixture; tumors of predominantly B cells are often associated with a preexisting immunologic disorder such as Sjögren syndrome, systemic lupus erythematosus, or Hashimoto thyroiditis, or with an immunocompromised state.

large cleaved cell l. a type of non-Hodgkin lymphoma characterized by the formation of malignant large cleaved follicular center cells; there are both follicular and diffuse varieties. Because of the wide variety of prognostic levels and the existence of tumors with several types of cells, these tumors have been divided among several different groups of follicular and diffuse lymphomas.

Lymphoma *Continued*

large noncleaved cell l. a type of non-Hodgkin lymphoma characterized by formation of malignant large noncleaved follicular center cells. Because of the wide variety of prognostic levels and the existence of tumors with several types of cells, these tumors have been divided among several different groups of follicular and diffuse lymphomas.
Lennert l. a type of non-Hodgkin lymphoma with a high content of epithelioid histiocytes; bone marrow involvement is common and response to chemotherapy is often poor.
lymphoblastic l. a highly malignant type of non-Hodgkin lymphoma composed of a diffuse, relatively uniform proliferation of cells with round or convoluted nuclei and scanty cytoplasm, which are cytologically similar to the lymphoblasts seen in acute lymphocytic leukemia. See also *convoluted T-cell l.*
lymphoplasmacytic l., lymphoplasmacytoid l. a heterogeneous group of low-grade B-cell lymphomas characterized by a mixture of small lymphocytes and plasmacytoid lymphocytes; it is sometimes associated with Waldenström macroglobulinemia and can involve a number of tissues, including the lymph nodes, spleen, bone marrow, and gastrointestinal tract. Many patients have abnormal local or systemic immune reactions. Called also *immunocytoma.*
malignant l. any of a group of malignant neoplasms characterized by the proliferation of cells native to the lymphoid tissues, i.e., lymphocytes, histiocytes, and their precursors and derivatives. The group is divided into two major clinicopathologic categories: *Hodgkin disease* and *non-Hodgkin lymphoma.*
malignant l. of cattle enzootic bovine leukosis.
MALT l. MALToma.
mantle cell l., mantle zone l. a rare form of non-Hodgkin lymphoma having a usually diffuse pattern with both small lymphocytes and small cleaved cells; it may be a subgroup of diffuse, small cleaved cell lymphoma. It mainly affects people over 50 years of age and runs an indolent course, although it may metastasize to the spleen or liver.
marginal zone l. a group of related B-cell neoplasms that involve the lymphoid tissues in the marginal zone; included are MALTomas and B-cell monocytoid lymphomas.
Mediterranean l. immunoproliferative small intestine disease.
mixed lymphocytic-histiocytic l. non-Hodgkin lymphoma characterized by the presence of a mixed population of cells, with the smaller cells resembling lymphocytes and the larger ones histiocytes. When predominantly follicular it is called *follicular, mixed small cleaved and large cell l.*, and when predominantly diffuse it is called *diffuse, mixed small and large cell l.*
nodular l. follicular l.
non-Hodgkin l. a heterogeneous group of malignant lymphomas, the only common feature being an absence of the giant Reed-Sternberg cells characteristic of Hodgkin disease. They arise from the lymphoid components of the immune system, and present a clinical picture broadly similar to that of Hodgkin disease except the disease is initially more widespread, with the most common manifestation being painless enlargement of one or more peripheral lymph nodes. There have been numerous classifications of the non-Hodgkin lymphomas; the most recent system is the Revised European-American Lymphoma (REAL) Classification (see under *classification*).

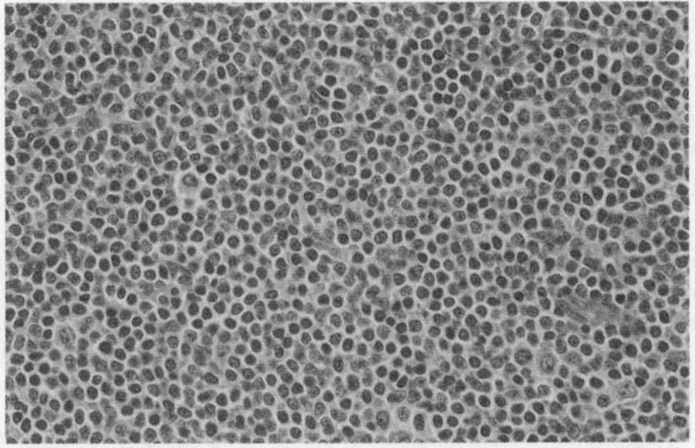
■ Small lymphocytic lymphoma, showing small, well-differentiated lymphocytes.

plasmablastic l. an uncommon, aggressive B-cell lymphoma, occurring mainly in the jaws and oral cavity and chiefly affecting HIV-positive persons, characterized by cells that morphologically resemble those of immunoblastic large B-cell lymphoma but whose immunophenotype shows them to be of plasma cell differentiation.
plasmacytic l., plasmacytoid l. lymphoplasmacytic l.
plasmacytoid lymphocytic l. a rare type of small lymphocytic lymphoma in which the predominant cell type is the plasma cell; it may be the manifestation in lymphoid tissue of Waldenström macroglobulinemia in the blood.
pleomorphic l. small noncleaved cell l.
poorly differentiated lymphocytic l. follicular, predominantly small cleaved cell l.
primary central nervous system l. a large cell lymphoma originating in the central nervous system, with solitary or multifocal foci; their frequency is sharply increased in immunodeficient patients. Formerly called also *microglioma* and *reticulum cell sarcoma of the brain.*
primary cutaneous anaplastic large cell l. a rare type of cutaneous T-cell lymphoma characterized by localized nodules, plaques, or tumors.
primary effusion l. a B-cell lymphoma associated with human herpesvirus 8 infection, characterized by the occurrence of lymphomatous effusions in body cavities without the presence of a solid tumor.
primary intraocular l., primary retinal l. a subgroup of primary central nervous system lymphoma that includes those invading the retina of the eye.
small B-cell l. the usual type of small lymphocytic lymphoma, having predominantly B lymphocytes.
small cleaved cell l. a group of non-Hodgkin lymphoma characterized by the formation of malignant small cleaved follicular center cells; it may have either a follicular or a diffuse pattern. One type, called *follicular, predominantly small cleaved cell lymphoma,* is particularly common. Because of the wide variety of prognostic levels and the existence of tumors with several types of cells, these tumors have now been divided among several different groups of follicular and diffuse lymphomas.
small lymphocytic l. a diffuse form of non-Hodgkin lymphoma with a low grade of malignancy; it represents the neoplastic proliferation of well-differentiated B lymphocytes and may present with either focal lymph node enlargement or generalized lymphadenopathy and splenomegaly. The predominant cell type is a compact, small, normal-appearing lymphocyte with a dark-staining round nucleus, scanty cytoplasm, and little size variation. It nearly always involves the bone marrow, and often malignant cells are found in the blood, so that its clinical picture is similar to that of chronic lymphocytic leukemia. Called also *well-differentiated lymphocytic l.*
small lymphocytic T-cell l. small lymphocytic lymphoma that has predominantly T lymphocytes.
small noncleaved cell l. a highly malignant type of non-Hodgkin lymphoma characterized by the formation of small noncleaved follicular center cells, usually in a diffuse pattern; Burkitt lymphoma is the most common variety. The incidence of all types increases sharply among immunocompromised patients.
T-cell l. any in a heterogenous group of lymphoid tumors involving malignant transformation of T lymphocytes. The category includes *convoluted T-cell l., cutaneous T-cell l., adult T-cell leukemia/lymphoma,* and certain other conditions. Some types of tumors formerly included in this group have been found to be mixtures of T cells and B cell precursors.
U-cell l., undefined l. a category of non-Hodgkin lymphoma comprising those tumors that cannot be classified into a definite type by either morphologic or currently available immunocytochemical markers.
undifferentiated l. small noncleaved cell l.
well-differentiated lymphocytic l. small lymphocytic l.

lym•pho•ma•toid (lim-fo′mə-toid) resembling lymphoma.
lym•pho•ma•to•sis (lim″fo-mə-to′sis) the development of multiple lymphomas in various parts of the body.
  avian l. avian leukosis involving chiefly the lymphocytes. Called also *fowl l.*
  bovine l. enzootic bovine leukosis.
  fowl l., l. of fowls avian l.
  intravascular l. the malignant variant of angioendotheliomatosis.
  neural l. Marek disease in which neurological symptoms are dominant.
  ocular l. Marek disease with ocular symptoms.

visceral l. avian leukosis with solid tumors of the viscera.

lym·pho·ma·tous (lim-fo′mə-təs) pertaining to or of the nature of lymphoma.

lym·pho·myx·o·ma (lim″fo-mik-so′mə) any benign growth consisting of adenoid tissue.

lym·pho·no·di (lim″fo-no′di) [L.] plural of *lymphonodus.*

lym·pho·no·dus (lim″fo-no′dəs) pl. *lymphono′di* [*lympho-* + *nodus*] TA alternative for *nodus lymphoideus.*

lym·phop·a·thy (lim-fop′ə-the) [*lympho-* + *-pathy*] any disease of the lymphatic system.

ataxic l. a sudden swelling of the lymph nodes sometimes accompanying the pain crises of locomotor ataxia.

lym·pho·pe·nia (lim″fo-pe′ne-ə) lymphocytopenia.

lym·pho·pla·sia (lim″fo-pla′zhə) [*lympho-* + *-plasia*] the accumulation of cells of the lymphoreticular system in other tissues.

cutaneous l. cutaneous lymphoid hyperplasia; see under *hyperplasia.*

lym·pho·plas·ma·cyte (lim″fo-plaz′mə-sīt) 1. a small, dense, circulating cell of B-cell lineage, having morphological characteristics of both small lymphocytes and plasma cells and functioning as a memory cell. 2. a term describing the spectrum of lymphocytes and plasma cells that are prominent in lymphoplasmacyte-rich meningioma.

lym·pho·plas·ma·cyt·ic (lim″fo-plaz″mə-sit′ik) containing plasmacytoid lymphocytes and other types of lymphocytes; said of lymphomas.

lym·pho·plas·ma·cy·toid (lim″fo-plaz″mə-si′toid) lymphoplasmacytic.

lym·pho·plas·ma·phe·re·sis (lim″fo-plaz″mə-fə-re′sis) the selective separation and removal of plasma and lymphocytes from withdrawn blood, the remainder of the blood then being retransfused into the donor.

lym·pho·poi·e·sis (lim″fo-poi-e′sis) [*lympho-* + *-poiesis*] 1. the development of lymphatic tissue. 2. lymphocytopoiesis.

lym·pho·poi·et·ic (lim″fo-poi-et′ik) pertaining to, characterized by, or causing lymphopoiesis.

lym·pho·pro·lif·er·a·tive (lim″fo-pro-lif′ər-ə-tiv) pertaining to or characterized by proliferation of the cells of the lymphoreticular system; used to refer to a group of malignant neoplasms. See under *disorder* and see also *lymphoreticular* and *myeloproliferative.*

lym·pho·re·tic·u·lar (lim″fo-rə-tik′u-lər) pertaining to the cells or tissues of both the lymphoid and reticuloendothelial systems; see under *system* and *disorder.*

lym·pho·re·tic·u·lo·sis (lim″fo-rə-tik″u-lo′sis) proliferation of the reticuloendothelial cells of the lymph nodes.

benign l. cat-scratch disease.

lym·phor·rhage (lim′fo-rəj) an accumulation of lymphocytes in a muscle.

lym·phor·rha·gia (lim″fo-ra′jə) [*lympho-* + *-rrhagia*] lymphorrhea.

lym·phor·rhea (lim″fo-re′ə) [*lympho-* + *-rrhea*] a flow of lymph from cut or ruptured lymph vessels.

lym·pho·sar·co·ma (lim″fo-sahr-ko′mə) [*lympho-* + *sarcoma*] a diffuse lymphoma.

lym·pho·scin·tig·ra·phy (lim″fo-sin-tig′rə-fe) scintigraphic detection of metastatic tumor in radioactively labeled lymph nodes, particularly *radiocolloid l.* See also *immunolymphoscintigraphy.*

radiocolloid l., radionuclide l. scintigraphy of the lymph nodes following the administration of radiocolloid, usually labeled with technetium 99m, which migrates to the lymph nodes, where it is retained by phagocytosis; uptake of the tracer is decreased in nodes containing metastatic tumor.

lym·phos·ta·sis (lim-fos′tə-sis) [*lympho-* + *-stasis*] stoppage of the lymph flow.

lym·pho·tax·is (lim″fo-tak′sis) [*lympho-* + *-taxis*] the property of attracting or repulsing lymphocytes.

lym·pho·tism (lim′fo-tiz″əm) a disordered state associated with the development of adenoid tissue.

lym·pho·tox·in (LT) (lim′fo-tok″sin) a lymphokine containing 171 amino acids, one of the tumor necrosis factors, produced by activated T lymphocytes. It inhibits the growth of tumors by causing lysis or stasis of sensitive cells, and also blocks transformation of cells. Called also *tumor necrosis factor β.*

lym·phot·ro·phy (lim-fot′rə-fe) [*lympho-* + *-trophy*] nourishment of cells by lymph in tissues lacking sufficient blood supply.

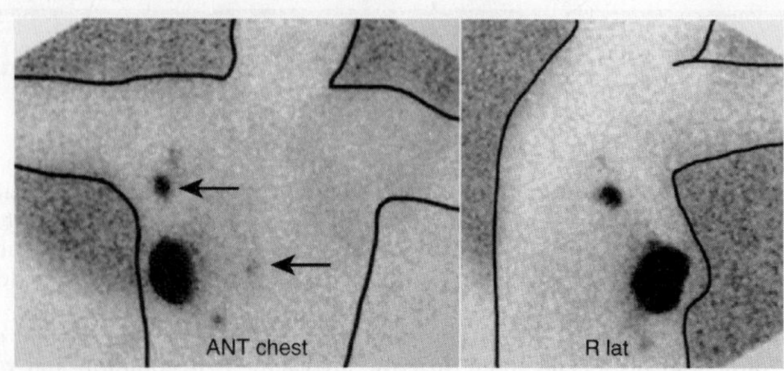

■ Radionuclide lymphoscintigraphy demonstrating multiple routes of lymphatic drainage after injection of radiocolloid around a cancer site in the right breast, including into the right axilla *(upper arrow)*, internal mammary node *(lower arrow)*, and an inframammary node.

lym·pho·tro·pic (lim″fo-tro′pik) [*lympho-* + *-tropic*] having an affinity for lymphatic tissue.

lym·phous (lim′fəs) 1. lymphatic (def. 1). 2. containing lymph.

Lynch incision, operation (linch) [Robert Clyde *Lynch,* American otologist, 1880–1931] see under *incision* and *operation.*

Lynch syndrome (linch) [Henry Thomson *Lynch,* American medical oncologist, born 1928] hereditary nonpolyposis colorectal cancer; see under *cancer.*

Lyn·chia mau·ra (lin′ke-ə maw′rə) *Pseudolynchia canariensis.*

lyn·es·tre·nol (lin-es′trə-nol) a progestational agent used as a component of oral contraceptives.

Lynx·ac·a·rus (lingk-sak′ə-rəs) a genus of mites of the family Listrophoridae. *L. radov′skyi* is found clinging to the hair of domestic cats in Florida, Puerto Rico, and various Pacific islands, causing pruritus and skin lesions.

lyo- [Gr. *lyein* to dissolve] a combining form meaning dissolved or dispersed.

lyo·chrome (li′o-krōm) [*lyo-* + *-chrome*] flavin.

lyo·gel (li′o-jel) [*lyo-* + *gel*] a gel containing much liquid. Cf. *xerogel.*

Ly·on hypothesis (li′ən) [Mary Frances *Lyon,* English geneticist, born 1925] see under *hypothesis.*

ly·on·iza·tion (li″on-ĭ-za′shən) [M.F. *Lyon*] the process by which or condition in which all X chromosomes of the somatic cells in excess of one are inactivated on a random basis. Called also *X-chromosome inactivation.* See also *Lyon hypothesis,* under *hypothesis.*

ly·on·ized (li′o-nīzd) [M.F. *Lyon*] denoting the inactivated X chromosome in a cell, according to the Lyon hypothesis.

lyo·phil (li′o-fil) a lyophilic substance; a material that readily goes into solution.

lyo·phile (li′o-fīl) lyophil.

lyo·phil·ic (li″o-fil′ik) [*lyo-* + *-philic*] having an affinity for, or stable in, solution; denoting a tendency of atoms or groups of atoms to be wetted by a solvent. See also under *colloid.*

ly·oph·i·li·za·tion (li-of″ĭ-lĭ-za′shən) the creation of a stable preparation of a biological substance (blood plasma, serum, etc.), by rapid freezing and dehydration of the frozen product under high vacuum. See also *freeze-drying.*

ly·oph·i·lize (li-of′ĭ-līz) to subject to lyophilization.

lyo·phobe (li′o-fōb) a lyophobic substance; a material that does not readily go into or tends to separate out from solution.

lyo·pho·bic (li″o-fo′bik) [*lyo-* + Gr. *phobein* to fear] not having an affinity for, or unstable in, solution; denoting a tendency of atoms or groups of atoms to avoid being wetted by a solvent. See also under *colloid.*

lyo·sorp·tion (li″o-sorp′shən) the selective adsorption of the solvent portion of a solution.

lyo·tro·pic (li″o-tro′pik) [*lyo-* + *-tropic*] lyophilic; see also under *series.*

Ly·per·o·sia ir·ri·tans (li″pər-o′se-ə ir′ĭ-təns) *Haematobia irritans.*

ly·pres·sin (li-pres′in) [USP] a synthetic preparation of lysine vasopressin, used as an antidiuretic and vasoconstrictor to treat central diabetes insipidus when desmopressin acetate is too potent; administered by intranasal spray.

Lyr·i·ca (lir′ĭ-kə) trademark for a preparation of pregabalin.

Lys lysine.

ly•sate (li′sāt) the material formed by lysis (defs. 1 and 2).

lyse (līz) 1. to cause or produce disintegration of a compound, substance, or cell. 2. to undergo lysis.

ly•ser•gic ac•id (li-sur′jik) a constituent of the ergot alkaloids obtained by hydrolysis.

l. a. diethylamide (LSD) a synthetic ergot alkaloid with psychotomimetic properties and both sympathomimetic and serotoninergic blocking effects; it counteracts barbiturates and is counteracted by suppressants like chlorpromazine. Objective effects include ataxia, fever, hyperreflexia, mydriasis, piloerection, tremor, and sometimes nausea and vomiting. Subjective effects include visual perception disorders and varying degrees of depersonalization, synesthesia, delusions, hallucinations, distortions of thought, sense, time, mood, and body image (which may be extreme). Anxiety may develop into acute panic reactions, and a persistent toxic psychotic state may result. Physical or psychological dependence is rare. Called also *lysergide.*

ly•ser•gide (li-sur′jīd) nonproprietary drug name for lysergic acid diethylamide (LSD).

lys•i•din (lis′ĭ-din) a red crystalline body, methylglyoxalidin, or its yellowish or pinkish, soapy, 50 per cent solution; used as a solvent for uric acid.

l. bitartrate a soluble, white, crystalline powder, of one third the solvent power of pure lysidin.

ly•sin (li′sin) [Gr. *lyein* to dissolve] 1. an antibody that causes complement-dependent lysis of cells; often used with a prefix indicating the target cells, e.g., hemolysin, bacteriolysin. Called also *immune l.* 2. any substance that causes cytolysis.

beta l. beta-lysin.

immune l. lysin (def. 1).

sperm l. any of various enzymatic substances of spermatozoa that dissolve oocyte membranes and permit penetration; most are thought to be produced by the acrosome.

ly•sine (Lys, K) (li′sēn) an essential amino acid, α,ε-diaminocaproic acid, a hydrolytic product of protein first isolated from casein; necessary for optimal growth in infants and for maintenance of nitrogen equilibrium in human adults. See table at *amino acid.*

l. acetate [USP] the monoacetate of L-lysine, used as a dietary supplement.

l. hydrochloride [USP] the monohydrochloride salt of L-lysine, used as a dietary supplement and for the treatment of severe metabolic alkalosis refractory to other treatment.

ly•sine car•boxy•pep•ti•dase (li′sēn kahr-bok″se-pep′tĭ-dās) [EC 3.4.17.3] an enzyme of the hydrolase class that catalyzes the removal of C-terminal basic amino acids from peptides, preferentially removing lysine residues but also removing arginine residues from kinins, inactivating them. The enzyme is found in plasma. Called also *arginine carboxypeptidase* and *kininase I.*

ly•sine de•hy•dro•gen•ase (li′sēn de-hi′dro-jən-ās) an enzyme of the oxidoreductase class that catalyzes the oxidative deamination of lysine, removing the α-amino acid as the first step in a minor pathway of lysine degradation.

ly•sine-ke•to•glu•ta•rate re•duc•tase (li′sēn ke″to-gloo′tə-rāt re-duk′tās) an enzyme activity that catalyzes the condensation of L-lysine and α-ketoglutarate to form saccharopine, using NADPH as an electron donor. The reaction is the initial step in the major route of lysine degradation; the enzyme activity is part of the bifunctional enzyme α-aminoadipic semialdehyde synthase (q.v.). The enzyme activity is absent in hyperlysinemia and substantially reduced in the variant saccharopinuria. In official nomenclature called *saccharopine dehydrogenase ($NADP^+$, L-lysine-forming).*

L-ly•sine:NAD ox•i•do•re•duc•tase (li′sēn ok″sĭ-do-re-duk′tās) lysine dehydrogenase.

ly•sin•o•gen (li-sin′ə-jən) [*lysin* + Gr. *gennan* to produce] an antigenic substance capable of inducing the formation of lysins.

ly•sin•uria (li″sĭ-nu′re-ə) excretion of lysine in the urine.

ly•sis (li′sis) [Gr. "dissolution; a loosing, setting free, releasing"] 1. dissolution or destruction of an organ or structure, such as the destruction of bone by loss of calcium (osteolysis). 2. cytolysis. 3. decomposition, as of a chemical compound by a specific agent. Cf. *degradation.* 4. mobilization of an organ by division of restraining adhesions. 5. gradual abatement of the symptoms of a disease; cf. *crisis* (def. 1).

hot-cold l. lysis that occurs only if the material is incubated as usual and then allowed to stand overnight at room temperature.

-lysis [Gr. "dissolution; a loosing, setting free, releasing"] a word termination denoting dissolution, decomposition, disintegration, or destruction; relief, reduction, or abatement; loosening or setting free.

lys(o)- [Gr. *lysis* dissolution] a combining form denoting relationship to lysis or dissolution.

ly•so•cy•thin (li″so-si′thin) a substance formed by combination between an animal poison and the body tissues and having a cytolytic action.

Ly•so•dren (li′so-drən) trademark for a preparation of mitotane.

ly•so•gen (li′so-jən) [*lyso-* + *-gen*] 1. an agent that induces lysis. 2. lysinogen. 3. a lysogenized bacterium.

ly•so•gen•e•sis (li″so-jen′ə-sis) the production of lysis or lysins.

ly•so•gen•ic (li-so-jen′ik) [*lyso-* + *-genic*] 1. producing lysins or causing lysis. 2. pertaining to lysogeny.

ly•so•ge•nic•i•ty (li″so-jə-nis′ĭ-te) [*lyso-* + Gr. *gennan* to produce + *-ity* condition] 1. the ability to produce lysins or cause lysis. 2. the potentiality of a bacterium to produce phage. 3. the specific association of the phage genome, the prophage, with the bacterial genome in such a way that only a few, if any, phage genes are transcribed.

ly•sog•e•ny (li-soj′ə-ne) the phenomenon in which a bacterium is infected by a temperate bacteriophage, the viral DNA is integrated in the chromosome of the host cell and replicated along with the host chromosome for many generations (the lysogenic cycle), and then production of virions and lysis of host cells (the lytic cycle) begins again. The lytic cycle is initiated spontaneously about once in 10,000 cell divisions or may be induced by ultraviolet radiation or chemical agents.

ly•so•ki•nase (li″so-ki′nās) a substance that activates a proactivator in the fibrinolytic system.

ly•so•phos•pha•ti•date (li″so-fos″fə-ti′dāt) 1. the anionic form of lysophosphatidic acid. 2. any phosphatidic acid–containing phospholipid that lacks one of its fatty acyl groups; the compounds are present as minor constituents of cell membranes as a result of phospholipid metabolism and are so named for their membranolytic qualities at high concentrations.

ly•so•phos•pha•tid•ic ac•id (li″so-fos″fə-tid′ik) phosphatidic acid lacking one of its fatty acyl chains; an intermediate in the synthesis of phosphatidic acid and a component of the lysophosphatidates (def. 2).

ly•so•phos•pho•li•pase (li″so-fos″fo-li′pās) [EC 3.1.1.5] an enzyme of the hydrolase class that catalyzes the hydrolysis of the acyl group from a 2-lysophospholipid, a step in the degradation of dietary and intracellular phospholipids.

ly•so•phos•pho•lip•id (li″so-fos″fo-lip′id) a phospholipid that lacks one of its fatty acyl chains; an intermediate formed during digestion of dietary and biliary phospholipids. The terms lysophospholipid and lysophosphatidate are sometimes used synonymously to denote the monoacyl derivatives of phosphatidic acid–containing compounds.

ly•so•so•mal *α*-glu•co•si•dase (li″so-so′məl gloo-ko′sĭ-dās) glucan 1,4-α-glucosidase.

ly•so•so•mal *α*-glu•co•si•dase de•fi•cien•cy (li″so-so′məl gloo-ko′sĭ-dās) glycogen storage disease, type II.

ly•so•some (li′so-sōm) [*lyso-* + *-some*] a membrane-bound cytoplasmic organelle, generally 250–750 nm in diameter, containing hydrolytic enzymes in an acidic environment and involved in intracellular digestion. Lysosomal enzyme defects result in the progressive accumulation of undigested products within the cell, which leads to lysosomal storage disease (q.v.). See Plate 11. **lysoso′mal** *adj*

primary l. a lysosome that has not yet fused with a phagosome or pinosome.

secondary l. a primary (or another secondary) lysosome that has fused with a phagosome or pinosome, bringing hydrolases in contact with the ingested material and resulting in digestion of the material. See also *autophagy* (def. 2) and *heterophagy.*

ly•so•staph•in (li-so-staf′in) an antibacterial enzyme produced by *Staphylococcus staphylolyticus;* it is specifically active against staphylococci.

ly•so•zyme (li′so-zīm) [EC 3.2.1.17] an enzyme of the hydrolase class that catalyzes the hydrolysis of specific glycosidic linkages in peptidoglycans and in chitin. The enzyme occurs in saliva, tears, egg white, and many animal fluids and catalyzes the breakdown of some bacterial cell walls.

ly•so•zy•mu•ria (li″so-zi-mu′re-ə) urinary excretion of elevated levels of lysozyme.

lys•sa (lis′ə) former name for rabies.

Lys•sa•vi•rus (lis′ə-vi″rəs) [*lyssa* + *virus*] rabies-like viruses; a genus of viruses of the family Rhabdoviridae comprising the rabies virus and other related viruses that infect mammals and arthropods. **lyssavi′ral** *adj*

lys•so•pho•bia (lis″o-fo′be-ə) [Gr. *lyssa* rabies + *-phobia*] irrational fear of going insane.

ly•syl (li′səl) the acyl radical of lysine.

ly•syl hy•drox•y•lase (li′səl hi-drok′sə-lās) an enzyme of the oxidoreductase class that catalyzes the hydroxylation of specific lysine residues in nascent procollagen chains; the hydroxylysine residues act as sites of attachment for disaccharide prosthetic groups and are involved in the formation of strong interchain crosslinks in collagen. The enzyme requires Fe^{2+}, ascorbate, and α-ketoglutarate for activity. Deficiency of enzyme activity, an autosomal recessive trait, results in the kyphoscoliosis type of Ehlers-Danlos syndrome. In EC nomenclature, called *procollagen-lysine 5-dioxygenase.*

ly•syl ox•i•dase (li′səl ok′sĭ-dās) an enzyme of the oxidoreductase class that catalyzes the oxidative deamination of lysine and hydroxylysine residues to the corresponding aldehydes, a step in the formation of covalent crosslinks in collagens and elastins. The reaction requires pyridoxal phosphate and Cu^{2+}.

lyt•ic (lit′ik) [Gr. *lyticos* dissolving, from *lysis* dissolution] 1. pertaining to lysis or to a lysin. 2. producing lysis.

-lytic a word termination denoting lysis of the substance indicated by the stem to which it is affixed.

Lyt•ta (lit′ə) a genus of blister beetles (family Meloidae) that secrete cantharidin and can cause cantharidin poisoning in ruminants. Called also *Russian fly.*

L. vesicato′ria a species whose dried bodies are the source of cantharidin. Called also *Cantharis vesicatoria, blister bug,* and *Spanish fly.*

lyx•ose (lik′sōs) an aldopentose isomeric with ribose at carbons 2 and 3.

lyze (līz) lyse.

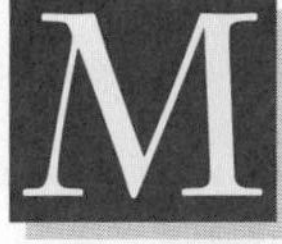

M mega-; methionine; molar[1] (used with a number designating the strength of the solution relative to one molar, e.g., *M/2* or 0.5M for half-molar); molar[2]; morgan; mucoid (see under *colony*); myopia; the low frequency component of the first heart sound (see under *sound*).

M. [L.] mis′ce (mix); mistu′ra (a mixture).

M mutual inductance; molar mass; molar[1].

M_1 mitral valve closure; see *first heart sound*, under *sound*.

M_r relative molecular mass; see *molecular weight*, under *weight*.

m median; meter; milli-.

m. [L.] mus′culus (muscle); minim.

m mass; molal (used with a number designating the strength of the solution relative to one molal).

m- meta- (def. 1).

μ mu, the twelfth letter of the Greek alphabet; symbol for *linear attenuation coefficient*, *population mean*, *micro-*, *electrophoretic mobility*, and the heavy chain of IgM (see *immunoglobulin*).

MA Master of Arts; mental age; meter angle.

mA milliampere.

μA microampere.

MAA macroaggregated albumin; see *aggregated albumin*, under *albumin*. See also table at *technetium*.

MAC membrane attack complex; minimal alveolar concentration; *Mycobacterium avium* complex (see under *disease*).

Mac. [L.] macera′re (macerate).

Mac-1 see under *glycoprotein*.

Ma•ca•ca (mə-kah′kə) the macaques, a genus of monkeys of the family Cercopithecidae. *M. fascicula′ris* is the cynomolgus monkey and *M. mulat′ta* is the rhesus monkey, both used in laboratory research.

ma•caque (mə-kahk′) a member of the genus *Macaca*, short-tailed monkeys; most are native to southern Asia, with one species found in Northwestern Africa and another in South America.
  crab-eating m. cynomolgus monkey.
  rhesus m. see under *monkey*.

Mc•Ar•dle disease (syndrome) (mək-ahr′dəl) [Brian *McArdle*, English neurologist, 1911–2002] see *glycogen storage disease, type V*, under *disease*.

Mc•Bride operation (mək-brīd′) [Earl Duwain *McBride*, American orthopedic surgeon, 1891–1975] see under *operation*.

Mc•Bur•ney incision, point, sign (mək-bur′ne) [Charles *McBurney*, New York surgeon, 1845–1913] see under *incision*, *point*, and *sign*.

Mac•Cal•lum patch, plaques (mə-kal′əm) [William George *MacCallum*, Canadian-born pathologist in the United States, 1874–1944] see under *patch* and *plaque*.

Mc•Car•thy reflex (mə-kahr′the) [Daniel J. *McCarthy*, American neurologist, 1874–1958] see under *reflex*.

Mac•Con•key agar (mə-kong′ke) [Alfred Theodore *MacConkey*, English bacteriologist, 1861–1931] see under *culture medium*.

Mc•Cune-Al•bright syndrome (mə-kūn′ awl′brīt) [Donovan James *McCune*, American pediatrician, 1902–1976; Fuller *Albright*, American physician, 1900–1969] Albright syndrome.

Mc•Don•ald maneuver, rule (mək-don′əld) [Ellice *McDonald*, Canadian gynecologist and pathologist in United States, 1876–1955] see under *maneuver* and *rule*.

Mace (mās) trademark for an aerosol mixture of chloroacetophenone.

mac•er•ate (mas′ər-āt) to soften by wetting or soaking; see *maceration*.

mac•er•a•tion (mas″ər-a′shən) [L. *maceratio*] 1. the softening of a solid by soaking. 2. in histology, the softening of a tissue by soaking, especially in acids, until the connective tissue fibers are so dissolved that the tissue components can be teased apart. 3. in obstetrics, the degenerative changes with discoloration and softening of tissues, and eventual disintegration, of a fetus retained in the uterus after its death.

mac•er•a•tive (mas′ər-ə″tiv) characterized by maceration.

Mac•ew•en sign, triangle (mə-ku′ən) [Sir William *Macewen*, Scottish surgeon, 1848–1924] see under *sign*, and see *foveola suprameatica*.

Mc•Gill operation (mə-gil′) [Arthur Ferguson *McGill*, British surgeon, 1846–1890] suprapubic transvesical prostatectomy.

Mc•Ginn-White sign (mə-gin′ hwīt′) [Sylvester *McGinn*, American cardiologist, 20th century; Paul Dudley *White*, American cardiologist, 1886–1973] see under *sign*.

Ma•cha•do-Gue•rrei•ro test (reaction) (mah-shah′do ga-ra′ro) [Astrogildo *Machado*, Brazilian medical researcher, 1885–1945; Cesar *Guerreiro*, Brazilian medical researcher, 1885–1949] see under *test*.

Ma•cha•do-Jo•seph disease (mah-shah′do zho-sef′) [*Machado* and *Joseph*, Azorean families affected by the disease] see under *disease*.

ma•chine (mə-shēn′) [L. *machina*] a contrivance or apparatus for the production, conversion, or transmission of some form of energy or force.
  heart-lung m. a combination blood pump (artificial heart) and blood oxygenator (artificial lung) used in cardiopulmonary bypass for cardiac surgery.

Mac•Kay-Marg electronic tonometer (mə-ka′ mahrg′) [Ralph Stuart *MacKay*, American biophysicist, born 1924; Elwin *Marg*, American physicist, born 1918] see under *tonometer*.

Mack•en•rodt ligament (mahk′en-rot) [Alwin Karl *Mackenrodt*, German gynecologist, 1859–1925] see *plica rectouterina*.

Mac•ken•zie syndrome (mə-ken′ze) [Sir Stephen *Mackenzie*, London physician, 1844–1909] Jackson syndrome.

Mc•Ku•sick-Kauf•man syndrome (mə-ku′sik kouf′mən) [Victor Almon *McKusick*, American geneticist, 1921–2008; Robert Lionel *Kaufman*, American physician, born 1937] Kaufman-McKusick syndrome.

Mac•Lean-Max•well disease (mə-klān′ maks′wəl) [Charles Murray *MacLean*, English physician in West Africa, 1788–1824; James Laidlaw *Maxwell*, Sr., English physician in China, 1836–1921] see under *disease*.

Mc•Leod phenotype, syndrome (mə-kloud′) [*McLeod*, surname of the propositus first observed in 1961] see under *phenotype* and *syndrome*.

Mac•leod syndrome (mə-kloud′) [William Mathieson *Macleod*, British physician, 1911–1977] see *Swyer-James syndrome*, under *syndrome*.

Mc•Mur•ray test (sign) (mək-mur′e) [Thomas Porter *McMurray*, British orthopedic surgeon, 1887–1949] see under *test*.

Mc•Naugh•ten see *M′Naghten*.

MACOP-B a cancer chemotherapy regimen consisting of methotrexate, folinic acid, Adriamycin (doxorubicin), cyclophosphamide, Oncovin (vincristine), prednisone, and bleomycin.

Mac•ra•can•tho•rhyn•chus (mak″rə-kan″tho-ring′kəs) a genus of acanthocephalans. *M. hirudina′ceus* is parasitic in pigs in the United States, and occasionally humans. *M. in′gens* is a common intestinal parasite of raccoons in North America, and has been found in one human case.

mac•ren•ce•pha•lia (mak-ren″sə-fa′le-ə) macrencephaly.

mac•ren•ceph•a•ly (mak″rən-sef′ə-le) [*macro-* + Gr. *enkephalos* brain] overgrowth of the brain.

macr(o)- [Gr. *makros* large, long] a combining form meaning large, or of abnormal size or length.

mac•ro•abra•sion (mak′ro-ə-bra″zhən) the removal of minute amounts of enamel with a high-speed carbide bur in order to correct tooth discoloration.

mac•ro•ad•e•no•ma (mak″ro-ad″ə-no′mə) a pituitary adenoma over 10 mm in diameter, large enough to be easily visualized by usual radiologic techniques; most are null-cell adenomas and are detected because they exert pressure on surrounding structures. Cf. *microadenoma*.

mac•ro•ag•gre•gate (mak″ro-ag′rə-gāt) an unusually large aggregate of a substance.

mac•ro•aleu•rio•spore (mak″ro-ə-lo͞or′e-o-spor) a large, usually multicellular, aleuriospore; the term is sometimes used interchangeably with *macroconidium*.

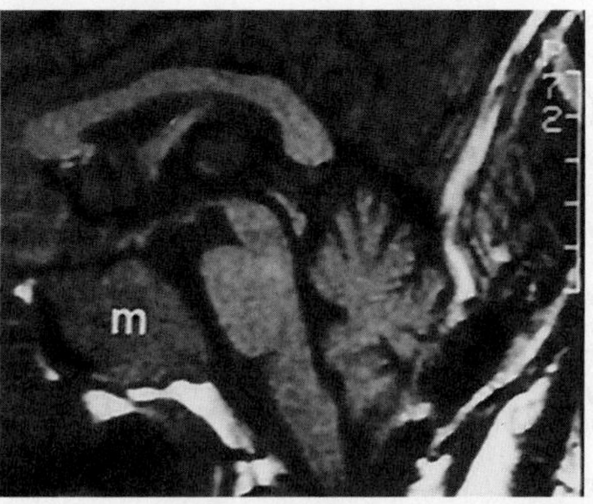

■ Macroadenoma *(m)* arising from the sella turcica and extending upward to fill the suprasellar cistern, in a sagittal MRI scan.

mac·ro·am·y·lase (mac″ro-am′ə-lās) serum amylase bound to a globulin. Because the complex formed (MW 200,000) is too large for renal clearance, its formation results in elevated levels of plasma amylase.

mac·ro·am·yl·a·se·mia (mak″ro-am″əl-ə-se′me-ə) a type of hyperamylasemia due to presence of macroamylase in the blood. **macroamylase′mic** *adj*

mac·ro·anal·y·sis (mak″ro-ə-nal′ə-sis) chemical analysis using 0.1 to 0.2 g of the substance under study.

mac·ro·an·gi·op·a·thy (mak″ro-an″je-op′ə-the) [*macro-* + *angiopathy*] angiopathy involving the large blood vessels, as seen in diabetes mellitus and other conditions.

mac·ro·ar·ray (mak′ro-ə-ra″) an arrangement of DNA samples, consisting of a set of DNA spots, 300 μm or larger in diameter, on a substrate; used for matching of known and unknown DNA samples. Cf. *microarray.*

mac·ro·au·toph·a·gy (mak″ro-aw-toph′ə-je) autophagy in which large volumes of cytoplasm, including proteins, organelles, and ribosomes, are enclosed in a double-membraned vacuole (autophagosome), which fuses with a lysosome. Cf. *microautophagy.*

Mac·rob·del·la (mak″ro-del′ə) a genus of leeches of the family Gnathobdellidae. *M. deco′ra* is a small species widely distributed in the United States and Canada that is sometimes used medicinally.

Mac·ro·bid (mak′ro-bid) trademark for a preparation of nitrofurantoin.

mac·ro·bi·o·ta (mak″ro-bi-o′tə) the macroscopic living organisms of a region; the combined macroflora and macrofauna of a region. **macrobiot′ic** *adj*

mac·ro·blast (mak′ro-blast″) [*macro-* + *-blast*] a large erythroblast resembling a megaloblast. Called also *macroerythroblast* and *macronormoblast.*

mac·ro·ble·pha·ria (mak″ro-blə-far′e-ə) [*macro-* + *blephar-* + *-ia*] abnormal largeness of the eyelid.

mac·ro·bra·chia (mak″ro-bra′ke-ə) [*macro-* + *brachia*] abnormal size or length of the upper limbs.

mac·ro·car·di·us (mak″ro-kahr′de-əs) [*macro-* + Gr. *kardia* heart] a fetus with an extremely large heart.

mac·ro·ce·pha·lia (mak″ro-sə-fa′le-ə) macrocephaly.

mac·ro·ceph·a·lus (mak″ro-sef′ə-ləs) macrocephaly.

mac·ro·ceph·a·ly (mak″ro-sef′ə-le) [*macro-* + *-cephaly*] unusually large size of the head; called also *megalocephaly.* **macrocephal′ic, macroceph′alous** *adj*

mac·ro·chei·lia (mak″ro-ki′le-ə) [*macro-* + *cheil-* + *-ia*] excessive size of the lips.

mac·ro·chei·ria (mak″ro-ki′re-ə) [*macro-* + *cheir-* + *-ia*] megalocheiria.

mac·ro·chem·is·try (mak″ro-kem′is-tre) [*macro-* + *chemistry*] chemistry in which the reactions may be seen with the naked eye. Cf. *microchemistry.* **macrochem′ical** *adj*

mac·ro·chi·lia (mak″ro-ki′le-ə) macrocheilia.

mac·ro·chi·ria (mak″ro-ki′re-ə) macrocheiria.

mac·ro·clit·o·ris (mak″ro-klit′o-ris) clitoromegaly.

mac·ro·cne·mia (mak″ro-ne′me-ə) [*macro-* + Gr. *knēmē* shin + *-ia*] a condition in which the lower limbs are abnormally large below the knees.

mac·ro·co·lon (mak′ro-ko″lən) megacolon.

mac·ro·co·nid·i·um (mak″ro-ko-nid′e-əm) pl. *macroconid′ia* [*macro-* + *conidium*] a large, frequently multicelled conidium or exospore of a fungus that also produces microconidia; the term is sometimes used interchangeably with *macroaleuriospore.*

mac·ro·cor·nea (mak″ro-kor′ne-ə) [*macro-* + *cornea*] megalocornea.

mac·ro·cra·nia (mak″ro-kra′ne-ə) abnormal increase in the size of the skull, the facial area being disproportionately small in comparison, such as with hydrocephalus.

mac·ro·cyc·lic (mak″ro-sik′lik, -si′klik) pertaining to a large cyclic organic compound, usually one containing more than 15 atoms.

mac·ro·cyst (mak′ro-sist) [*macro-* + *cyst*] 1. a large cyst. 2. in mycology, an encysted reproductive cell of certain slime molds. Cf. *microcyst.*

mac·ro·cyte (mak′ro-sīt″) [*macro-* + *-cyte*] an abnormally large erythrocyte, such as those seen in macrocytic anemia. Called also *megalocyte.* **macrocyt′ic** *adj*

mac·ro·cy·the·mia (mak″ro-si-the′me-ə) [*macrocyte* + *hem-* + *-ia*] a condition in which the erythrocytes are larger than normal, such as in macrocytic anemia and some types of liver disease. Called also *macrocytosis* and *megalocytosis.*

mac·ro·cy·to·sis (mak″ro-si-to′sis) macrocythemia.

mac·ro·dac·tyl·ia (mak″ro-dak-til′e-ə) megalodactyly.

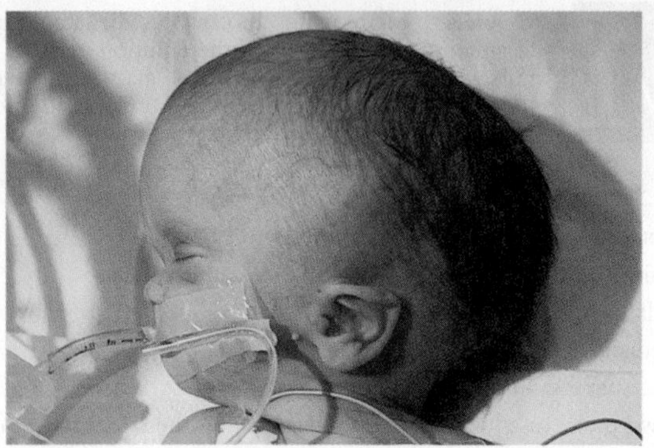

■ Macrocrania.

mac·ro·dac·ty·ly (mak″ro-dak′tə-le) megalodactyly.

Mac·ro·dan·tin (mak″ro-dan′tin) trademark for a preparation of nitrofurantoin.

mac·ro·dont (mak′ro-dont) having large teeth; characterized by macrodontia. Called also *megadont.*

mac·ro·don·tia (mak″ro-don′shə) [*macro-* + *odont* + *-ia*] a developmental disorder characterized by increase in the size of the teeth; it may affect a single tooth or all of the teeth, or teeth of normal size may appear to be abnormally large in proportion to abnormally small jaws. Called also *macrodontism, megadontia,* and *megalodontia.*

mac·ro·don·tic (mak″ro-don′tik) macrodont.

mac·ro·don·tism (mak″ro-don′tiz-əm) macrodontia.

mac·ro·dys·tro·phia (mak″ro-dis-tro′fe-ə) [*macro-* + *dys-* + *troph-* + *-ia*] overgrowth of a part.

m. lipomato′sa progressi′va partial gigantism associated with tumor-like overgrowth of adipose tissue.

mac·ro·el·e·ment (mak″ro-el′ə-mənt) any of the macronutrients that are chemical elements, including calcium, chloride, magnesium, phosphorus, potassium, sodium, and sulfur. Cf. *trace element.*

mac·ro·en·ceph·a·ly (mak″ro-ən-sef′ə-le) macrencephaly.

mac·ro·e·ryth·ro·blast (mak″ro-ə-rith′ro-blast) macroblast.

mac·ro·es·the·sia (mak″ro-es-the′zhə) [*macro-* + *esthesia*] a dysesthesia in which all things touched seem larger than they really are.

mac·ro·fau·na (mak″ro-faw′nə) the animal life, visible to the naked eye, which is present in or characteristic of a special location.

mac·ro·flo·ra (mak″ro-flor′ə) the plant life, visible to the naked eye, which is present in or characteristic of a special location.

mac·ro·fol·lic·u·lar (mak″ro-fə-lik′u-lər) [*macro-* + *follicular*] pertaining to or characterized by large follicles.

mac·ro·gam·ete (mak″ro-gam′ēt) [*macro-* + *gamete*] 1. the larger, less active female anisogamete. 2. the larger of two types of malarial parasites; see *gamete* (def. 2).

mac·ro·ga·me·to·cyte (mak″ro-gə-me′to-sīt) macrogamont.

mac·ro·gam·ont (mak″ro-gam′ont) [*macro-* + *gamont*] a gamont that will produce or become a macrogamete. Called also *macrogametocyte.*

mac·ro·gen·ia (mak″ro-jen′e-ə) [*macro-* + *geni-* + *-ia*] enlargement of the jaw, especially the chin, which may involve only the osseous or soft-tissue components or both the bony and soft tissues.

mac·ro·gen·i·to·so·mia (mak″ro-jen″ĭ-to-so′me-ə) [*macro-* + *genito-* + *soma* + *-ia*] excessive somatic growth, with unusual enlargement of the genital organs.

m. prae′cox epiphyseal syndrome.

mac·ro·gin·gi·vae (mak″ro-jin′jĭ-ve) fibromatosis gingivae.

mac·rog·lia (mak-rog′le-ə) neuroglial cells of ectodermal origin, i.e., the astrocytes and oligodendrocytes considered together. Originally, the term was used for the astrocytes alone.

mac·ro·glob·ule (mak″ro-glob′ūl) a relatively large globule.

melanin m. macromelanosome.

mac·ro·glob·u·lin (mak″ro-glob′u-lin) [*macro-* + *globulin*] a plasma globulin with high molecular weight, such as alpha$_2$-macroglobulin or the IgM M component of Waldenström macroglobulinemia.

α_2-m. a plasma protein that inhibits a wide variety of proteolytic enzymes including trypsin, plasmin, thrombin, kallikrein, and chymotrypsin. It is a tetramer of four identical subunits, M_r between 650,000 and 735,000, and acts by means of a bait region that can entrap proteinases of very different substrate specificities as well as catalytic mechanisms, reducing the accessibility of the proteinase functional sites, particularly to large molecules, but not completely inactivating them. Also written *alpha$_2$-macroglobulin.*

mac•ro•glob•u•lin•emia (mak″ro-glob″u-lĭ-ne′me-ə) [*macroglobulin* + *-emia*] a condition characterized by increased macroglobulins in the blood.

Waldenström m. a plasma cell dyscrasia resembling leukemia, with cells of lymphocytic, plasmacytic, or intermediate morphology, that secrete an IgM M component. There is diffuse infiltration of bone marrow and often the spleen, liver, lymph nodes, or central nervous system (Bing-Neel syndrome). The circulating macroglobulin produces symptoms of hyperviscosity syndrome: weakness, fatigue, bleeding disorders, and visual disturbances; peak incidence is in the sixth and seventh decades.

mac•ro•glos•sia (mak″ro-glos′e-ə) [*macro-* + *gloss-* + *-ia*] excessive size of the tongue.

mac•ro•gna•thia (mak″ro-na′the-ə) [*macro-* + *gnath-* + *-ia*] a condition characterized by abnormally large jaws. See also *prognathism* and *maxillary protrusion*, under *protrusion*.

mac•ro•gol (mak′ro-gol) polyethylene glycol.

mac•ro•graph•ia (mak″ro-graf′e-ə) macrography.

mac•rog•ra•phy (mak-rog′rə-fe) [*macro-* + *-graphy*] a form of dysgraphia in which written letters are larger than the normal writing of the individual. Called also *macrographia*, *megalographia*, and *megalography*.

mac•ro•gy•ria (mak″ro-ji′re-ə) [*macro-* + *gyrus*] moderate reduction in the number of sulci of the cerebrum, sometimes with increase in the brain substance, resulting in excessive size of the gyri.

ma•cro•he•ma•tu•ria (ma″kro-he″mə-tu′re-ə) gross hematuria.

mac•ro•la•bia (mak″ro-la′be-ə) macrocheilia.

mac•ro•lec•i•thal (mak″ro-les′ĭ-thəl) [*macro-* + *-lecithal*] having a large amount of yolk, such as the eggs of fish, birds, reptiles, and monotremes.

mac•ro•lide (mak′ro-līd) 1. a chemical compound characterized by a large lactone ring containing multiple keto and hydroxyl groups. 2. any of a large group of antibacterial antibiotics containing a macrolide ring linked glycosidically to one or more sugars; they are produced by certain species of *Streptomyces* and inhibit protein synthesis by binding to the 50S subunits of 70S ribosomes. Examples include erythromycin, azithromycin, and clarithromycin.

mac•ro•lym•pho•cyte (mak″ro-lim′fo-sīt) an abnormally large lymphocyte.

mac•ro•mas•tia (mak″ro-mas′te-ə) [*macro-* + *mast-* + *-ia*] oversize of the breasts or mammae.

mac•ro•ma•zia (mak″ro-ma′zhə) macromastia.

mac•ro•mel•a•no•some (mak″ro-mel′ə-no-sōm″) a large, spherical melanosome, from one to several μm in diameter, formed in the cytoplasm in disorders affecting melanocytes; called also *melanin macroglobule*.

mac•ro•me•lia (mak″ro-me′le-ə) abnormal largeness of one or more limbs; called also *megalomelia*.

mac•rom•e•lus (mak-rom′ə-ləs) [*macro-* + Gr. *melos* limb] a fetus with abnormally large or long limbs.

mac•ro•mere (mak′ro-mēr″) [*macro-* + *-mere*] one of the large blastomeres formed by unequal cleavage of a zygote as a result of asymmetric positioning of the mitotic spindle. Cf. *micromere*.

mac•ro•meth•od (mak′ro-meth″əd) a chemical method in which the substance to be analyzed is used in customary (not minute) quantity. Cf. *micromethod*.

mac•ro•min•er•al (mak′ro-min″ər-əl) macroelement.

mac•ro•mol•e•cule (mak″ro-mol′ə-kūl) a very large molecule having a polymeric chain structure, as in proteins, polysaccharides, and other natural and synthetic polymers. **macromolec′ular** *adj*

mac•ro•mono•cyte (mak″ro-mon′o-sīt) an abnormally large monocyte.

mac•ro•my•elo•blast (mak″ro-mi′ə-lo-blast) an abnormally large myeloblast.

mac•ro•nem•a•tous (mak″ro-nem′ə-təs) [*macro-* + Gr. *nēma* thread] pertaining to a conidiophore that is noticeably different morphologically from its hypha.

mac•ro•nod•u•lar (mak″ro-nod′u-lər) characterized by large nodules.

mac•ro•nod•ule (mak″ro-nod′ūl) 1. a large nodule. 2. on a radiograph of the lung, a discrete opacity between 3 mm and 30 mm in diameter.

mac•ro•nor•mo•blast (mak″ro-nor′mo-blast) macroblast.

mac•ro•nu•cle•us (mak″ro-noo′kle-əs) [*macro-* + *nucleus*] in ciliate protozoa, the transcriptively active, polyploid nucleus, much larger than the micronucleus, that governs the organism's vegetative processes and is responsible for its phenotype. Called also *trophic nucleus* and *trophonucleus*.

mac•ro•nu•tri•ent (mak″ro-noo′tre-ənt) an essential nutrient required in a relatively large amount, including carbohydrates, fats, proteins, and water. Minerals necessary in relatively large amounts (calcium, chloride, magnesium, phosphorus, potassium, sodium, and sulfur) are sometimes included and sometimes excluded from the definition.

mac•ro•nych•ia (mak″ro-nik′e-ə) [*macro-* + *onych-* + *-ia*] the condition of having unusually large nails; called also *megalonychia*.

mac•ro-or•chi•dism (mak″ro-or′kĭ-diz-əm) [*macro-* + *orchid-* + *-ism*] abnormal enlargement of the testis.

mac•ro•ovalo•cyte (mak″ro-o′və-lo-sīt) an enlarged, oval erythrocyte having a mean corpuscular volume greater than 100 μm^3, seen in megaloblastic anemia. **macro-ovalocyt′ic** *adj*

mac•ro•pa•thol•o•gy (mak″ro-pə-thol′ə-je) [*macro-* + *pathology*] the nonmicroscopical pathologic account of any disease or organ.

mac•ro•pe•nis (mak″ro-pe′nis) excessive size of the penis; called also *macrophallus*, *megalopenis*, and *megalophallus*.

mac•ro•phage (mak′ro-fāj″) [*macro-* + *-phage*] any of the many forms of mononuclear phagocytes found in tissues. They arise from hematopoietic stem cells in the bone marrow, which develop according to the stages of the monocytic series until they are monocytes; these then enter the blood, circulate for about 40 hours, and subsequently enter tissues, where they increase in size, phagocytic activity, and lysosomal enzyme content to become macrophages. Two types, *fixed macrophages* and *free macrophages* (qq.v.) are distinguished. Their morphology varies among different tissues and between normal and pathologic states, and not all macrophages can be identified by morphology alone. However, most are large cells with a round or indented nucleus, a well-developed Golgi apparatus, abundant endocytotic vacuoles, lysosomes, and phagolysosomes, and a plasma membrane covered with ruffles or microvilli. Their functions include nonspecific phagocytosis and pinocytosis, specific phagocytosis of opsonized microorganisms (mediated by Fc receptors and complement receptors); killing of ingested microorganisms; digestion and presentation of antigens to T and B lymphocytes; and secretion of many different products, including enzymes (lysozyme, collagenases, elastase), acid hydrolases, several complement components and coagulation factors, prostaglandins and leukotrienes, and regulatory molecules such as interferon and interleukin-1. Cells now recognized as macrophages include (in normal tissue) interdigitating cells, Kupffer cells, Langerhans cells, microglial cells, osteoclasts, and type A synovial cells, and (in inflamed tissues) epithelioid cells and Langerhans-type and foreign-body–type giant cells. Called also *histiocyte* and *macrophagocyte*.

alveolar m. a rounded granular type, found within the alveoli of the lungs and serving to ingest inhaled particulate matter. Called also *alveolar phagocyte* and *dust cell*.

armed m's macrophages capable of inducing cytotoxicity as a consequence of antigen-binding by cytophilic antibodies on their surfaces or by factors derived from T lymphocytes.

fixed m. a quiescent, sessile macrophage similar to a fibroblast in morphology, found in the lymph nodes, spleen, bone marrow, and connective tissue (where it is called a histiocyte).

free m. an actively motile macrophage, usually having an ameboid shape and highly ruffled surface, found at sites of inflammation.

Hansemann m's von Hansemann cells.

inflammatory m. free m.

mac•ro•phago•cyte (mak″ro-fa′go-sīt) macrophage.

mac•ro•phal•lus (mak″ro-fal′əs) [*macro-* + *phallus*] macropenis.

mac•roph•thal•mia (mak″rof-thal′me-ə) megalophthalmos.

mac•ro•pino•cy•to•sis (mak″ro-pin″o-si-to′sis, -pi″no-si-to′sis) [*macro-* + *pinocytosis*] pinocytosis in which large amounts of extracellular fluid are taken up by extension of the plasma membrane, with the formation of large vesicles (macropinosomes). Cf. *micropinocytosis*.

mac•ro•pino•some (mak″ro-pin′o-sōm, pi′no-sōm) [*macro-* + *pinosome*] the large (up to several hundred nm in diameter) pinocytic vesicle formed by macropinocytosis.

mac•ro•pla•sia (mak″ro-pla′zhə) [*macro-* + *-plasia*] excessive growth of a part or tissue.

mac•ro•po•dia (mak″ro-po′de-ə) [*macro-* + *pod-* + *-ia*] megalopodia.

mac•ro•poly•cyte (mak″ro-pol′e-sīt) a large polymorphonuclear leukocyte with 6 to 14 lobes in the nucleus, seen in conditions such as pancytopenia, vitamin B_{12} or folic acid deficiency. Cf. *polycyte*.

mac•ro•pro•lac•tin (mak″ro-pro-lak′tin) an unusual form of prolactin with high molecular weight and minimal biologic activity; see *macroprolactinemia*.

mac·ro·pro·lac·tin·emia (mak″ro-pro-lak″tĭ-ne′me-ə) the presence in the blood of macroprolactins; this will cause a woman to test positive for hyperprolactinemia, although the macroprolactins have only minimal biologic activity.

mac·ro·pro·lac·ti·no·ma (mak″ro-pro-lak″tĭ-no′mə) a prolactinoma more than 10 mm in diameter, usually associated with serum prolactin levels above 500 ng per ml.

mac·ro·pro·my·elo·cyte (mak″ro-pro-mi′ə-lo-sīt) an abnormally large promyelocyte.

mac·ro·pro·so·pia (mak″ro-pro-so′pe-ə) [*macro-* + *prosop* + *-ia*] excessive size of the face.

ma·crop·sia (mə-krop′se-ə) [*macro-* + *-opsia*] an illusion in which objects are seen as larger than they actually are.

mac·ro·rhin·ia (mak″ro-rin′e-ə) [*macro-* + *rhin-* + *-ia*] excessive size of the nose.

mac·ro·sce·lia (mak″ro-se′le-ə) [*macro-* + Gr. *skelos* leg + *-ia*] excessive size of the lower limbs.

mac·ro·scop·ic (mak″ro-skop′ik) gross (def. 2).

mac·ro·scop·i·cal (mak″ro-skop′ĭ-kəl) 1. pertaining to macroscopy. 2. macroscopic.

ma·cros·co·py (mə-kros′kə-pe) examination with the naked eye.

mac·ro·shock (mak′ro-shok″) a term used in cardiology to denote a moderate to high level of electric current passing across two areas of intact skin; approximately 100 mA can cause ventricular fibrillation. Cf. *microshock.*

mac·ro·sig·moid (mak″ro-sig′moid) megasigmoid.

mac·ro·sis (mə-kro′sis) [*macro-* + *-osis*] increase in size.

mac·ros·mat·ic (mak″roz-mat′ik) [*macr-* + *osmatic*] having the sense of smell strongly or acutely developed.

mac·ro·so·ma·tia (mak″ro-so-ma′she-ə) [*macro-* + *somat-* + *-ia*] macrosomia.

m. adipo′sa conge′nita premature development associated with obesity, attributed to hyperfunction of the adrenal cortex.

mac·ro·so·mia (mak″ro-so′me-ə) [*macro-* + *-somia*] abnormally large size; see also *gigantism* and *megasoma.* Called also *macrosomatia.*

fetal m., neonatal m. excessive birth weight in a neonate, seen most often in children of diabetic mothers or those with cerebral gigantism.

mac·ro·spore (mak′ro-spor) [*macro-* + *spore*] 1. the larger spore form when spores of two sizes are present, as in certain fungi and protozoa. 2. megaspore.

mac·ro·ste·a·to·sis (mak″ro-ste″ə-to′sis) [*macro-* + *steatosis*] macrovesicular steatosis.

mac·ro·ste·reo·gno·sia (mak″ro-ste″re-o-no′zhə) [*macro-* + *stereo-* + *gnosia*] macroesthesia.

mac·ro·sto·mia (mak″ro-sto′me-ə) [*macro-* + *stom-* + *-ia*] greatly exaggerated width of the mouth, resulting from failure of union of the maxillary and mandibular prominences, with extension of the oral orifice toward the ear. The defect may be unilateral or bilateral. See also *lateral facial cleft* and *oblique facial cleft,* under *cleft.*

mac·ro·struc·tur·al (mak″ro-struk′chər-əl) pertaining to gross structure.

Mac·ro·tec (mak′ro-tek) trademark for a kit for the preparation of technetium Tc 99m albumin aggregated.

mac·ro·tia (mak-ro′shə) [*macro-* + *ot-* + *-ia*] abnormal enlargement of the pinna of the ear.

mac·ro·tome (mak′ro-tōm) [*macro-* + *-tome*] an apparatus for cutting large sections of tissue for anatomical study.

mac·ro·tooth (mak′ro-to͞oth) pl. *macroteeth.* An abnormally large tooth.

mac·ro·vas·cu·lar (mac″ro-vas′ku-lər) pertaining to the macrovasculature.

mac·ro·vas·cu·la·ture (mak″ro-vas′ku-lə-chər) the large vessels of the body.

Mac·ro·za·mia (mak″ro-zam′e-ə) a genus of zamia palms that contain macrozamin and other toxic glycosides; animals eating them may develop hepatotoxicity, spinal cord degeneration, and cancer, and ruminants get the condition called zamia staggers.

mac·ro·zam·in (mak″ro-zam′in) a toxic principle from the seeds and leaves of species of the zamia family of palms. In humans it is neoplastic to the liver, kidneys, intestine, and lungs after hydrolysis by intestinal bacteria and yields the breakdown product methylazoxymethanol; in cattle it causes gastrointestinal and liver damage that can be fatal.

mac·u·la (mak′u-lə) gen. and pl. *ma′culae* [L.] 1. in anatomy, a stain, spot, or thickening; an area distinguishable from its surroundings by color or other characteristic. 2. m. lutea. 3. macule. 4. a moderately dense scar of the cornea that can be seen without special optical aids, appreciated as a gray spot intermediate between a nebula and a leukoma.

acoustic maculae the macula sacculi and macula utriculi considered together.

m. adhe′rens desmosome.

ma′culae atro′phicae white patches resembling scars formed on the skin by atrophy.

cerebral m. tache cérébrale.

ma′culae ceru′leae small gray-blue macules found on the chest, abdomen, thighs, or upper arms in pediculosis pubis, especially noticeable in light-skinned individuals. They may be due to altered blood pigments in infested individuals or to an excretion product in the louse's saliva that converts bilirubin to biliverdin.

m. commu′nis a thickened area on the wall of the otic vesicle; it later divides into the macula sacculi and macula utriculi.

ma′culae cribro′sae [TA] see *m. cribrosa inferior, m. cribrosa media,* and *m. cribrosa superior.*

m. cribro′sa infe′rior [TA] the perforated area on the wall of the vestibule through which branches of the vestibulocochlear nerve pass to the crista ampullaris and the posterior semicircular canal.

m. cribro′sa me′dia [TA] the perforated area on the vestibular wall through which branches of the vestibulocochlear nerve pass to the macula of the saccule.

m. cribro′sa supe′rior [TA] the perforated area on the vestibular wall through which branches of the vestibulocochlear nerve pass to the macula of the utricle and to the crista ampullaris of the anterior and lateral semicircular canals.

m. den′sa a zone of compact, heavily nucleated cells, located in the distal straight tubule of the kidney where it makes contact with the vascular end of the glomerulus; it is closely associated anatomically with the juxtaglomerular cells of the afferent arteriole.

false m. the extramacular point on the retina of a squinting eye which receives the same light stimulus as the macula of the fixing eye.

m. fla′va a yellowish nodule visible at one end of a vocal cord.

m. lu′tea [TA] an irregular yellowish depression on the retina, about 3 degrees wide, lateral to and slightly below the optic disk; it is the site of absorption of short wavelengths of light, and it is thought that its variation in size, shape, and coloring may be related to variant types of color vision.

maculae of membranous labyrinth acoustic maculae.

mongolian m. see under *spot.*

m. re′tinae m. lutea.

m. sac′culi [TA] macula of saccule: a thickening in the wall of the saccule where the epithelium contains vestibular hair cells that are stimulated by linear acceleration and deceleration and gravity. This and the macula utriculi together are called *acoustic maculae.*

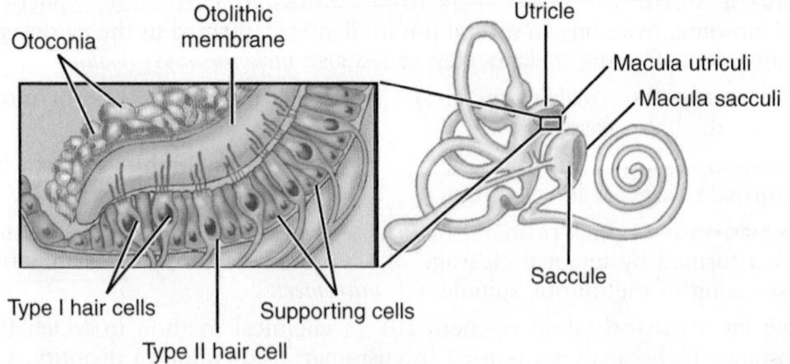

m. utri′culi [TA] macula of utricle: a thickening in the wall of the utricle where the epithelium contains vestibular hair cells that are stimulated by linear acceleration and deceleration and gravity. This and the macula sacculi together are called *acoustic maculae.*

mac·u·lae (mak′u-le) [L.] genitive and plural of *macula.*

mac·u·lar (mak′u-lər) 1. pertaining to or characterized by macules. 2. pertaining to the macula lutea.

mac·u·late (mak′u-lāt) [L. *maculatus* spotted] macular.

mac·ule (mak′ūl) a discolored skin lesion that is not elevated above the surface; see also *patch* and *spot.* Called also *macula.*

ash leaf m. a hypopigmented lesion of the skin occurring in tuberous sclerosis complex, usually 1 to 3 cm in size and having the general shape of an ash leaf, round at one end and pointed at the other. Called also *lance-ovate macule* and *ash leaf spot* or *patch.*

café au lait m's see under *spot.*

coal m. a dark spot seen on the lung in coal workers' pneumoconiosis, representing an aggregation of dust, dust-filled macrophages, and fibroblasts.

lance-ovate m. ash leaf m.

mac·u·lo·cer·e·bral (mak″u-lo-ser′ə-brəl) cerebromacular.

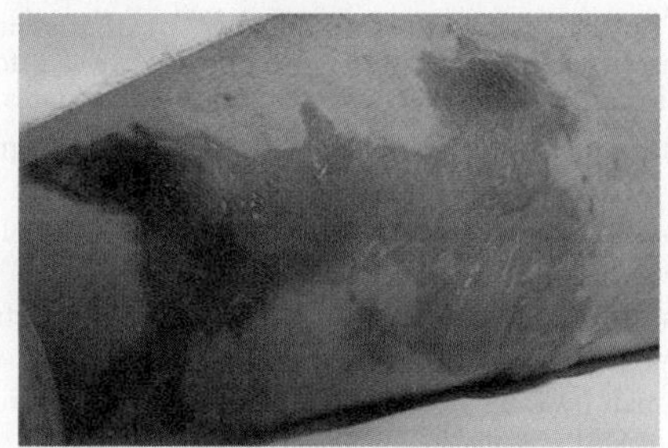

■ Macule.

mac•u•lo•pap•u•lar (mak″u-lo-pap′u-lər) both macular and papular, such as certain types of eruptions.

mac•u•lop•a•thy (mak″u-lop′ə-the) [*macula* + *-pathy*] any pathological condition of the macula lutea. Cf. *retinopathy.*

age-related m. age-related macular degeneration.

bull's eye m. increase in pigment of a circular area of the macula lutea, accompanying degeneration; seen in certain toxic states, macular corneal dystrophy, Stargardt disease, and other conditions.

mac•u•lo•ve•sic•u•lar (mak″u-lo-və-sik′u-lər) both macular and vesicular.

Mc•Vay repair (operation) (mək-va′) [Chester B. *McVay*, American surgeon, 1911–1987] see under *repair.*

mad•a•ro•sis (mad″ə-ro′sis) [Gr. *madaros* bald] loss of the eyelashes or eyebrows or both.

MADD multiple acyl CoA dehydrogenation deficiency; see *glutaricaciduria, type II.*

mad•der (mad′ər) the root of *Rubia tinctoria* L. (Rubiaceae) affording a red dye, mainly alizarin and purpurin.

Mad•dox prism, rods (mad′əks) [Ernest Edmund *Maddox*, English ophthalmologist, 1860–1933] see under *prism* and *rod.*

Ma•de•lung deformity, disease (neck) (mah′də-loong) [Otto Wilhelm *Madelung*, German surgeon, 1846–1926] see under *deformity*, and see *multiple symmetric lipomatosis*, under *lipomatosis.*

mad•ness (mad′nəs) old term for insanity or severe mental disturbance, now considered offensive.

myxedema m. psychiatric disturbances resulting from hypothyroidism and myxedema, ranging from mental slowness and loss of memory to agitation and psychosis.

Ma•du•ra foot (mə-doo′rə) [*Madura*, India, where it was observed in the 1850s] see under *foot.*

Mad•u•rel•la (mad″u-rel′ə) a genus of Fungi Imperfecti of the form-class Hyphomycetes, form-family Dematiaceae. *M. gri′sea* and *M. myceto′matis* (called also *M. myceto′mi*) are etiologic agents of eumycotic mycetoma.

ma•du•ro•my•co•sis (mə-du″ro-mi-ko′sis) mycetoma.

mae•di (mi′the) [Icelandic "dyspnea"] the respiratory form of ovine progressive pneumonia.

m.-visna ovine progressive pneumonia.

MAF macrophage-activating factor; see *interferon-γ*, under *interferon.*

maf•en•ide (maf′ən-īd) an antibacterial homologue of sulfanilamide active against many gram-positive and gram-negative organisms.

m. acetate [USP] the monoacetate salt of mafenide, having the same antibacterial activity as the base; used as a topical antiinfective for adjunctive therapy of patients with second- and third-degree burns.

m. hydrochloride the hydrochloride salt of mafenide, having antibacterial activity similar to that of the acetate salt; used as a topical antiinfective.

Maf•fuc•ci syndrome (mə-foo′che) [Angelo *Maffucci*, Italian physician, 1847–1903] see under *syndrome.*

ma•fil•con A (mə-fil′kon) a hydrophilic contact lens material.

MAG3 mertiatide.

Mag. [L.] mag′nus (large).

mag•al•drate (mag′əl-drāt) [USP] a chemical combination of aluminum and magnesium hydroxides and sulfate; used as an oral antacid.

Mag•an (mag′ən) trademark for magnesium salicylate.

ma•gen•bla•se (mah″gən-blah′zə) [Ger. "stomach bubble"] in the radiograph of the stomach, a dark area above the light shadow of the opaque meal, marking a collection of gas (aerogastria) in the upper part of the stomach.

Ma•gen•die foramen, space (mah-zhah-de′) [François *Magendie*, French physiologist, 1783–1855] see under *space*, and see *apertura mediana ventriculi quarti.*

Ma•gen•die-Hert•wig sign (mah-zhah-de′ hert′vik) [F. *Magendie;* Richard Carl Wilhelm Theodor von *Hertwig*, German zoologist, 1850–1937] skew deviation.

ma•gen•stras•se (mah″gən-strahs′ə) [Ger. "stomach street"] canalis gastricus.

ma•gen•ta (mə-jen′tə) basic fuchsin.

m. 0 pararosaniline.

m. I rosaniline.

m. II triaminoditoylphenylmethane chloride, a component of basic fuchsin.

m. III new fuchsin.

acid m. acid fuchsin.

basic m. basic fuchsin.

mag•got (mag′ət) a soft-bodied larva of an insect, especially a form that usually lives in decaying flesh; sometimes they infest wounds of live animals (see *myiasis*). Families of particular importance are Calliphoridae and Sarcophagidae. The living maggots of *Phaenicia sericata* and *Phormia regina* have been used in the treatment of osteomyelitis and other suppurative infections to clear away dead tissue and promote healing because their secretions contain allantoin.

Congo floor m. the maggot of either *Auchmeromyia luteola* or *A. senegalensis.*

foot m. the larva of *Booponus intonsus.*

rat-tail m., rat-tailed m. a maggot of one of the hover-flies (genera *Eristalis* and *Helophilus);* they cause intestinal and nasal myiasis.

sheep m., wool m. the maggot of any of several species of the family Calliphoridae, which invade the tissues of sheep, causing cutaneous myiasis.

Ma•gill forceps (məgil′) [Sir Ivan Whitehouse *Magill*, British anesthesiologist, 1888–1975] see under *forceps.*

mag•is•tral (maj′is-trəl) [L. *magister* master] pertaining to a master; applied to medicines that are prepared in accordance with a physician's prescription. Cf. *officinal.*

mag•ma (mag′mə) [Gr. *massein* to knead] 1. a thick, viscous, aqueous suspension of finely divided, insoluble, inorganic material. 2. a thin, pastelike substance composed of organic material.

bentonite m. [NF] a suspension of bentonite in purified water; used as a pharmaceutical suspending agent.

magnesia m. milk of magnesia.

m. reticula′re a mesenchymal reticulum within the early chorionic sac.

Mag•na•cort (mag′nə-kort) trademark for a preparation of hydrocortamate hydrochloride.

Mag•nan movement, sign (mah-nyah′) [Valentin Jacques Joseph *Magnan*, French psychiatrist, 1835–1916] see under *movement* and see *formication.*

mag•nes•emia (mag″nə-se′me-ə) hypermagnesemia.

mag•ne•sia (mag-ne′zhə) [the name of a district in ancient Lydia] 1. magnesium oxide. 2. [USP] magnesium hydroxide.

mag•ne•si•um (Mg) (mag-ne′ze-əm) [L.] a light, silvery, metallic element; atomic number 12, atomic weight 24.312, specific gravity 1.74. Its salts are essential in nutrition, being required for the activity of many enzymes, especially those concerned with oxidative phosphorylation. It is a component of both intra- and extracellular fluids and is excreted in the urine and feces. The serum level is approximately 2 mEq/liter. Deficiency causes irritability of the nervous system with tetany, vasodilation, convulsions, tremors, depression, and psychotic behavior. Excessive amounts can be toxic; see *hypermagnesemia.*

m. alginate the magnesium salt of alginic acid; administered orally as a component of an antacid in the treatment of gastroesophageal reflux disease; it combines with gastric acid to form a viscous gel which floats on top of the gastric contents and acts as a physical barrier to reflux.

m. aluminum silicate [NF] a colloid used as a suspending agent for pharmaceuticals, available in Types IA, IB, IC, and IIA, which differ in viscosity and ratio of aluminum content to magnesium content.

m. ammonium phosphate struvite.

m. carbonate [USP] $MgCO_3$, in either the basic hydrated or normal hydrated form; used as an antacid.

m. chloride [USP] an electrolyte replenisher and a treatment and preventative for hypomagnesemia, administered orally or intravenously; also used as a pharmaceutic necessity for hemodialysis and peritoneal dialysis fluids.

m. citrate [USP] a saline laxative used for bowel evacuation before diagnostic procedures or surgery of the colon; administered orally; also used to prevent and treat hypomagnesemia.

m. gluconate [USP] the gluconate salt of magnesium, administered orally in the prevention of hypomagnesemia.

m. hydroxide [USP] $Mg(OH)_2$, an oral antacid and laxative, also used as a preventative for hypomagnesemia.

m. lactate the lactate salt of magnesium, administered orally in the prevention of hypomagnesemia.

m. oxide [USP] a bulky *(light m. oxide)* or relatively dense *(heavy m. oxide)* white powder, MgO; used as a sorbent in pharmaceutical preparations, as an oral antacid and laxative, and as a preventative for hypomagnesemia.

m. phosphate [USP] tribasic magnesium phosphate, $Mg_3(PO_4)_2 \cdot 5H_2O$, used as an antacid.

m. salicylate see under *salicylate.*

m. silicate $MgSiO_3$, a silicate salt of magnesium; the most common hydrated forms occurring in nature are asbestos and talc. See also *silicatosis.*

m. stearate [NF] a compound of magnesium with varying proportions of stearic and palmitic acids, used as a tablet lubricant in pharmaceutical preparations.

m. sulfate [USP] $MgSO_4 \cdot xH_2O$, a salt used as an anticonvulsant in the prophylaxis and treatment of seizures associated with toxemia of pregnancy; also used as an electrolyte replenisher; administered intramuscularly and intravenously. It is administered orally as a laxative; orally, intramuscularly, or intravenously as a treatment or preventative for hypomagnesemia; and locally as an antiinflammatory. Called also *Epsom salt.*

tribasic m. phosphate see *m. phosphate.*

m. trisilicate [USP] a compound of magnesium oxide and silicon dioxide with varying proportions of water, used as a pharmaceutic necessity and an antacid.

mag•ne•su•ria (mag″nə-soo′re-ə) hypermagnesuria.

mag•net (mag′nət) [L. *magnes;* Gr. *magnēs* magnet] an object made of iron oxide or steel that attracts iron and has polarity.

denture m. a magnet made of a nonreactogenic platinum-cobalt alloy or a rare earth element, used for additional retention of dentures. One magnet is implanted into the mandible under the periosteum and the other is attached to the denture, its poles being opposite of those in the mandible. Called also *magnetic implant.*

mag•net•ic (mag-net′ik) pertaining to, derived from, or having the properties of a magnet.

mag•ne•tism (mag′nə-tiz-əm) magnetic attraction or repulsion.

mag•ne•ti•za•tion (mag″nət-ĭ-za′shən) the act or process of rendering an object or substance magnetic.

longitudinal m. the component of a magnetization vector that is parallel to the direction of the magnetic field.

transverse m. the components of a magnetization vector that are in a plane perpendicular to the direction of the magnetic field.

mag•ne•to•car•dio•graph (mag-ne″to-kahr′de-o-graf) a cardiograph that generates electrical signals proportional to magnetic pulses emanating from electrical activity in the heart.

mag•ne•to•elec•tric•i•ty (mag-ne″to-e″lek-tris′ĭ-te) electricity induced by means of a magnet.

mag•ne•to•en•ceph•a•lo•graph (mag-ne″to-ən-sef′ə-lo-graf) an instrument for recording magnetic signals proportional to electroencephalographic waves emanating from electrical activity in the brain.

mag•ne•tol•o•gy (mag″nə-tol′ə-je) the branch of physics that studies magnetics.

mag•ne•tom•e•ter (mag″nə-tom′ə-tər) [*magnetic* + *-meter*] 1. an apparatus for measuring magnetic forces. 2. a device that uses an array of superconductors to detect changes in the magnetic field of the brain, used to diagnose epilepsy, stroke, and deafness.

mag•ne•tron (mag′nə-tron) an electric vacuum tube for generating extremely short electromagnetic waves (microwaves).

mag•net•ro•pism (mag-net′ro-piz-əm) [*magnet* + *tropism*] a growth response in a nonmotile organism under the influence of a magnet.

Mag•ne•vist (mag′nə-vist) trademark for a preparation of gadopentetate dimeglumine.

mag•ni•cel•lu•lar (mag″nĭ-sel′u-lər) composed of large cells, as opposed to *parvicellular.*

mag•ni•fi•ca•tion (mag″nĭ-fĭ-ka′shən) [L. *magnificatio; magnus* great + *facere* to make] 1. apparent increase in size as under the microscope. 2. the process of making something appear larger, as by use of lenses. 3. the ratio of apparent (image) size to real size.

mag•ni•fy (mag′nĭ-fi) to cause to appear larger by the use of lenses or suitable mirrors.

mag•no•cel•lu•lar (mag″no-sel′u-lər) magnicellular.

Mag•no•lia (mag-no′le-ə) [Pierre *Magnol,* French botanist, 1638–1715] a genus of deciduous trees of the family Magnoliaceae. *M. acumina′ta* L., *M. glau′ca* L., and *M. tripeta′la* L. are sources of the medicinal bark called magnolia.

mag•no•lia (mag-no′le-ə) 1. any member of the genus *Magnolia.* 2. the bitter aromatic bark of several species of *Magnolia,* formerly used as a diaphoretic and antifebrile in the southern United States.

mag•num (mag′nəm) [L.] 1. large; great. 2. the os magnum (os capitatum [TA]).

Ma•haim fibers (mah-ă′) [Ivan *Mahaim,* French cardiologist, 1897–1965] see under *fiber.*

Mah•ler sign (mah′ler) [Richter A. *Mahler,* German obstetrician, 1863–1941] see under *sign.*

ma huang (mah hwahng′) [Chinese] any of various species of *Ephedra* used as herbs in Chinese medicine.

Mai•er sinus (mi′ər) [Rudolf *Maier,* German physician, 1824–1888] see under *sinus.*

maim (mām) 1. to disable by a wound; to dismember by violence. 2. a dismemberment or disablement effected by violence.

Mai•mon•i•des (mi-mon′ĭ-dēz) Moses ben Maimon, 1135–1204. Rabbi, physician, and the greatest of the Jewish philosophers, born in Cordoba, Spain. He was the physician to Saladin in Egypt, during which time he wrote many medical works in Arabic, among them a commentary on the aphorisms of Hippocrates and treatises on asthma, diet, poisons, and hygiene. A prayer attributed to him is considered to rank beside the oath of Hippocrates as an ethical guide to the medical profession.

main (mă) [Fr.] hand.

m. d'accoucheur (dah-koo-shoor′) obstetrician's hand.

m. fourchée (fo͞or-sha′) cleft hand.

m. en griffe (ah grēf′) clawhand.

m. en lorgnette (ah lor-nyet′) opera-glass hand.

m. en pince (ah pas′) ["pincer hand"] cleft hand.

m. en singe (ah sazh′) monkey hand.

m. en squelette (ah skə-let′) skeleton hand.

m. succulente (su-ku-laht′) Marinesco succulent hand.

main•tain•er (mān-tān′ər) something that keeps or maintains in another thing existence or continuancy.

space m. 1. an orthodontic appliance, fixed or removable, that maintains the space left by a prematurely lost tooth or the space to be filled by a tooth not yet erupted. See also under *regainer* and *retainer.* 2. separator (def. 2).

main•te•nance (mān′tə-nəns) 1. a term used for procedures or drugs that provide a stable state over a long period as distinguished from a short-term remedial or prophylactic effect. 2. the stable state so provided.

MAIS mild androgen insensitivity syndrome; minimal androgen insensitivity syndrome.

Mai•son•neuve amputation, fracture, sign, urethrotome (ma″zo-noov′) [Jules Germain François *Maisonneuve,* French surgeon, 1809–1897] see under *amputation, fracture, sign,* and *urethrotome.*

Mais•siat band (ligament, tract) (ma″se-ah′) [Jacques Henri *Maissiat,* French anatomist, 1805–1878] tractus iliotibialis.

maize (māz) [Sp. *maíz*] *Zea mays.*

Ma•joc•chi disease (purpura) (mah-zhok′e) [Domenico *Majocchi,* Italian physician, 1849–1929] purpura annularis telangiectodes.

ma•jor (ma′jər) large; significant; great or greatest in scope, effect, number, size, extent, or importance.

makr(o)- for words thus beginning, see those beginning *macr(o)-.*

mal (mahl) [Fr. and Sp., from L. *malum* a bad thing] disease.

m. de caderas (da kah-da′rahs) [Sp. "illness of the hips"] 1. a fatal wasting type of trypanosomiasis seen in horses in South America, associated with weakness, especially of the hindquarters; it is caused by *Trypanosoma equinum* and is transmitted by tabanid flies. 2. South American name for derriengue.

grand m. (grahn) [Fr. "large sickness"] see under *epilepsy.*

haut m. (o) [Fr. "large sickness"] grand mal epilepsy.

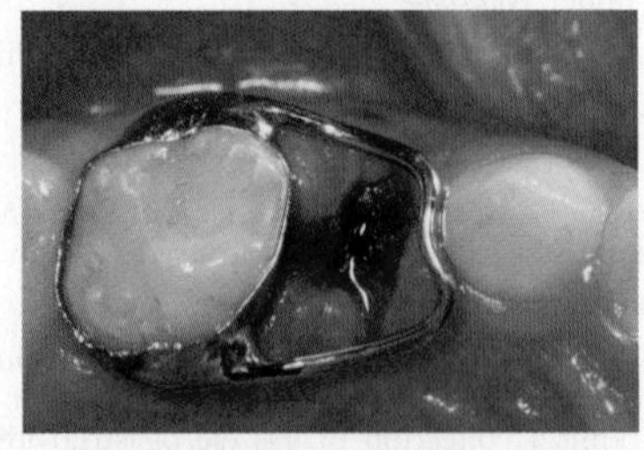

■ Band and loop space maintainer in place after extraction of a primary first molar.

m. de Meleda (də mel′ə-dah) [Fr. "Meleda sickness"] a rare, chronic, autosomal recessive form of diffuse palmoplantar keratoderma in which the hyperkeratosis spreads to involve the backs of the hands and feet, as well as other areas of the body. It is characterized by erythematous, scaling, malodorous cutaneous lesions and sometimes deep fissuring. Called also *Meleda disease.*

m. de mer (də mār′) [Fr.] seasickness.

m. morado (mo-rah′do) [Sp. "purple sickness"] a type of onchodermatitis, seen in Central America, in which the skin has a blue to purple discoloration, especially on the trunk and upper limbs.

m. de ojo (da o′ho) [Sp. "eye sickness"] a Latin American culture-specific syndrome of fever, irritability, headache, and crying, affecting mainly children and considered to be caused by the envious gaze of another.

m. perforant du pied (per-fo-rahn′ du pya′) [Fr. "penetrating disease of the foot"] plantar ulcer.

petit m. (pə-te′) [Fr. "small sickness"] absence epilepsy.

m. rouge (r o͞o zh) [Fr. "red sickness"] a syndrome occurring after inhalation or ingestion of calcium cyanamide followed by drinking an alcoholic beverage, marked by intense flushing, rapid pulse and pounding heart, panting respiration, and perception of the taste and smell of acetaldehyde in the exhaled breath, which may be followed by nausea, vomiting, and a rapid fall in blood pressure. The extent and severity of the symptoms depend on the amount of calcium cyanamide and alcohol in the system. It is due to the inhibition by calcium cyanamide of enzymes required for oxidation of acetaldehyde formed from alcohol, resulting in a buildup of acetaldehyde, which causes altered vascular reactions. A similar syndrome, also due to accumulation of acetaldehyde, occurs on ingestion of disulfiram followed by drinking an alcoholic beverage; this also includes impaired taste, unpleasant breath and perspiration, and lessened sexual potency.

mal- [L. *malus* bad] a prefix meaning bad or abnormal.

ma•la[1] (ma′lə) [L.] 1. bucca. 2. os zygomaticum.

ma•la[2] (mŭ′lə) [Sanskrit] according to ayurveda, waste products of the body formed during metabolism, including urine, feces, mucus, and sweat.

mal•ab•sorp•tion (mal″əb-sorp′shən) impaired intestinal absorption of nutrients; see also *malabsorption syndrome,* under *syndrome.* Sometimes malabsorption is artificially induced as a treatment of morbid obesity, such as with jejunoileal bypass.

congenital lactose m. disaccharide intolerance II.

congenital sucrose-isomaltose m. sucrase-isomaltase deficiency.

glucose-galactose m. an autosomal recessive disorder caused by mutation in the *SLC5A1 (SGLT1)* gene (locus: 22q13.1), which encodes the intestinal sodium/glucose cotransporter, resulting in defective intestinal glucose and galactose transport. It is characterized by neonatal onset of profuse, acidic, watery diarrhea leading to severe dehydration and death if untreated; it can be treated by a glucose- and galactose-free diet.

Ma•la•car•ne pyramid (mah″lah-kahr′na) [Michele Vincenzo Giacintos *Malacarne,* Italian surgeon, 1744–1816] see under *pyramid.*

ma•la•cia (mə-la′shə) [Gr. *malakia*] the morbid softening or softness of a part or tissue. **mala′cic** *adj*

metaplastic m. osteitis fibrosa cystica.

porotic m. softening accompanied by proliferation of connective tissue.

-malacia a word termination denoting abnormal softness or softening in the system designated by the root to which the term is affixed, as *osteomalacia.*

malac(o)- [Gr. *malakos* soft] a combining form denoting a condition of abnormal softness.

mal•a•co•pla•kia (mal″ə-ko-pla′ke-ə) [*malaco-* + Gr. *plax* plaque] the formation of soft patches on the mucous membrane of a hollow organ.

renal m. a variant of malacoplakia of the urinary tract that is confined to the renal parenchyma; it closely resembles xanthogranulomatous pyelonephritis and usually occurs secondary to urinary tract infections or immunocompromised conditions.

m. of the urinary tract a disorder in which there are soft, yellowish raised plaques on the mucous membrane of the bladder and ureters, containing von Hansemann cells with Michaelis-Gutmann bodies, resulting from infection.

m. vesi′cae malacoplakia of the urinary tract when found in the bladder.

mal•a•co•sis (mal″ə-ko′sis) malacia.

mal•a•cot•ic (mal″ə-kot′ik) inclined to malacia; soft; said of teeth.

ma•lac•tic (mə-lak′tik) emollient.

mal•a•die (mahl″ah-de′) [Fr.] disease.

m. des jambes (da zhahmb′) ["disease of the legs"] a disease of rice growers in Louisiana, probably beriberi.

m. de plongeurs (də plaw-zhoor′) ["divers' disease"] inflammation and ulceration in divers in the Mediterranean caused by the stings of sea anemones.

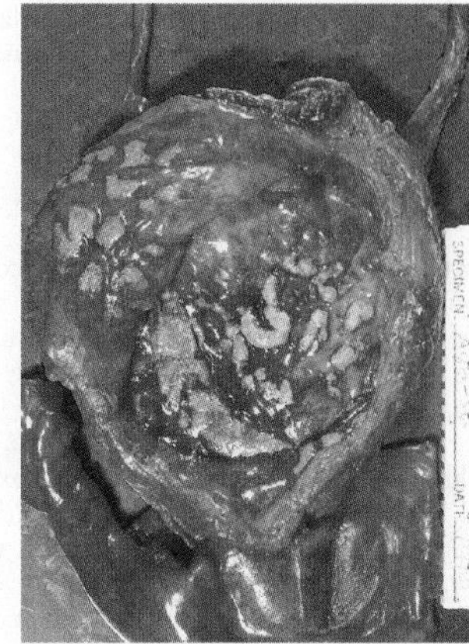

■ Malacoplakia of the urinary tract associated with cystitis, showing inflammatory exudate and broad, flat plaques.

m. de Roger (də ro-ja′) Roger disease.

m. du sommeil (du so-ma′) ["sleeping sickness"] African trypanosomiasis.

m. des tics (da tēk′) ["disease of tics"] Gilles de la Tourette syndrome.

mal•ad•just•ment (mal″ə-just′mənt) in psychiatry, failure to fit one's inner needs to the environment; inability to meet the challenges of daily life.

mal•a•dy (mal′ə-de) [Fr. *maladie*] disease.

ma•lag•ma (mə-lag′mə) [Gr.] an emollient or cataplasm.

mal•aise (mă-lāz′) [Fr.] a vague feeling of bodily discomfort and fatigue.

mal•a•ko•pla•kia (mal″ə-ko-pla′ke-ə) malacoplakia.

mal•align•ment (mal″ə-līn′mənt) displacement out of line, especially displacement of the teeth from their normal relation to the line of the dental arch. Spelled also *malalinement.* See also *malocclusion.*

mal•aline•ment (mal″ə-līn′mənt) malalignment.

ma•lar (ma′lər) [L. *mala* cheek] 1. buccal. 2. zygomatic.

ma•la•ria (mə-lar′e-ə) [It. "bad air"] an infectious disease endemic in many warm regions of the world, caused by obligate intracellular protozoa of the genus *Plasmodium,* usually transmitted by the bites of infected anopheline mosquitoes. It is characterized by prostration with paroxysms of high fever, shaking chills, sweating, anemia, and splenomegaly; death may result from its complications, the most severe of which are cerebral malaria and anemia. After the initial illness, it may follow a chronic or relapsing course. Called also *paludism.* **malar′ial, malar′ious** *adj*

algid m. a severe complication of falciparum malaria caused by a collapse of the vascular system and manifested by shock, syncope, peripheral vascular failure, hypotension, cold, clammy skin, and gastrointestinal symptoms, diarrhea, and vomiting, which is sometimes followed by coma and death.

airport m. malaria transmitted by air traffic when an infected mosquito is carried on an airplane.

benign tertian m. vivax m.

bilious remittent m. a complication of falciparum malaria mainly involving the liver, characterized by continuous vomiting, epigastric and hepatic tenderness, marked jaundice, and high remittent fever.

cerebral m. a severe, often fatal complication of falciparum malaria that primarily involves the brain; characteristics may be either gradual onset of headache, confusion, and psychotic manifestations progressing to delirium, convulsions, and coma, or abrupt rise in temperature sustained at a high level with convulsions and coma.

congenital m. malaria in newborn infants that have been infected transplacentally, usually by *Plasmodium vivax* or *P. malariae.*

falciparum m. malaria due to *Plasmodium falciparum,* in which febrile paroxysms recur irregularly. It is the most severe form of malaria and has the highest levels of parasites in the blood; sometimes it is fatal. It is also the type most likely to be associated with pernicious symptoms, which are the result of sludging and formation in the capillaries of microinfarcts consisting of erythrocytes infected with later stages of *P. falciparum.* Microinfarctions may occur in the brain, liver, adrenal gland, gastrointestinal tract, kidneys, lungs, or other organs. Called also *malignant tertian m.* and *pernicious m.* See also *blackwater fever,* under *fever.*

malariae m. quartan m.

malignant tertian m. falciparum m.

ovale m. malaria caused by *Plasmodium ovale,* seen most often in sub-Saharan Africa. It is clinically similar to but milder than vivax malaria and is often found associated with falciparum malaria. The infected erythrocytes are oblong or oval on a stained blood film.

pernicious m. falciparum m.

***Plasmodium falciparum* m.** falciparum m.

***Plasmodium malariae* m.** quartan m.

***Plasmodium ovale* m.** ovale m.

***Plasmodium vivax* m.** vivax m.

quartan m. malaria in which febrile paroxysms occur every 72 hours (every fourth day counting the day of occurrence as the first day). It is caused by *Plasmodium malariae*, which requires 72 hours for completion of each asexual cycle in the erythrocyte. This is the mildest and most chronic of all human malarial infections. Called also Plasmodium malariae *m.*

quotidian m. malaria in which the febrile paroxysms occur daily, thought to be due to simultaneous infection with two strains of *Plasmodium vivax* or *P. falciparum* that complete their cycles on alternate days. See also *vivax m.*

tertian m. malaria in which febrile paroxysms occur every third day, counting the day of occurrence as the first. Vivax malaria and ovale malaria often follow this pattern.

transfusion m. malaria contracted when a species of *Plasmodium* is transmitted directly from a blood donor, by accidental injection with a contaminated needle, or by intravenous drug users sharing needles.

vivax m. malaria caused by *Plasmodium vivax*. Although this type is less severe than falciparum malaria, it can cause severe symptoms such as anemia. Often there are relapses because of hypnozoites that persist in the liver after cure of the blood stages of the parasite. Febrile paroxysms often recur every other day (tertian malaria), but may recur daily (quotidian malaria). Infected red blood cells often appear enlarged on a stained blood film, because the parasite tends to infect younger erythrocytes. Called also *benign tertian m.*

ma•lar•ia•ci•dal (mə-lar″e-ə-si′dəl) plasmodicidal.

ma•lar•i•ol•o•gist (mə-lar″e-ol′o-jist) a specialist in the study of malaria.

ma•lar•i•ol•o•gy (mə-lar″e-ol′o-je) [*malaria* + *-logy*] the study of malaria.

ma•la•ris (mə-lar′is) [L.] 1. buccal. 2. zygomatic.

Mal•a•rone (mal′ə-rōn) trademark for a combination preparation of proguanil hydrochloride and atovaquone.

Ma•las•sez rest (mah″lah-sa′) [Louis Charles *Malassez*, French physiologist, 1842–1909] see under *rest.*

Mal•as•se•zia (mal″ə-se′zhə) [Louis Charles *Malassez*] a genus of Fungi Imperfecti of the form-family Cryptococcaceae, consisting of yeastlike organisms that produce no mycelium; called also *Pityrosporum.*

M. fur′fur a lipophilic species that forms a part of the normal flora of the human skin but can cause tinea versicolor and has also been associated with other dermatologic conditions. Called also *Pityrosporum orbiculare.*

M. globo′sa a lipophilic species that forms a part of the normal flora of the human skin but can cause tinea versicolor and has also been associated with other dermatologic conditions.

M. ova′lis a cultural variant of *M. furfur.*

M. pachyder′matis a nonlipophilic species that forms a part of the normal flora of various animals and causes otitis externa with seborrheic dermatitis in dogs.

M. restric′ta a lipophilic species that forms a part of the normal flora of the human skin but can cause tinea versicolor and has also been associated with other dermatologic conditions.

M. sympodia′lis a lipophilic species that forms a part of the normal flora of the human skin but can cause tinea versicolor and has also been associated with other dermatologic conditions.

mal•as•sim•i•la•tion (mal″ə-sim″ĭ-la′shən) [L. *malus* ill + *assimilation*] 1. imperfect, faulty, or disordered assimilation. 2. inability of the gastrointestinal tract to transport to the body fluids one or more ingested nutrients, whether due to faulty digestion (maldigestion) or to impaired intestinal mucosal transport (malabsorption).

ma•late (ma′lāt, mal′āt) an ionic form of malic acid.

ma•late de•hy•dro•gen•ase (ma′lāt de-hi′dro-jən-ās) [EC 1.1.1.37] an enzyme of the oxidoreductase class that catalyzes the oxidation of L-malate to oxaloacetate, reducing NAD^+. The enzyme occurs both in the mitochondria and in the cytosol. The reaction is important in the tricarboxylic acid cycle and in the malate-aspartate electron shuttle. See illustration at *tricarboxylic acid cycle*, under *cycle.*

ma•late de•hy•dro•gen•ase (ox•alo•ac•e•tate-de•car•box•y•lat•ing) ($NADP^+$) (ma′lāt de-hi′dro-jən-ās ok-sal″o-as′ə-tāt de-kahr-bok′sə-lāt″ing) an enzyme of the oxidoreductase class that catalyzes the oxidative decarboxylation of L-malate to form pyruvate, reducing $NADP^+$. The cytosolic and mitochondrial forms are isozymes; the cytosolic enzyme is a major source of NADPH for fatty acid synthesis.

mal•a•thi•on (mal″ə-thi′on) an organophosphorus insecticide and topical parasiticide.

mal•ax•ate (mal′ək-sāt) to knead, as in making pills.

mal•ax•a•tion (mal″ək-sa′shən) [Gr. *malaxis* a softening] an act of kneading.

mal•de•scent (mal″də-sent′) failure of an organ or other structure to descend normally during fetal development.

mal•de•vel•op•ment (mal″də-vel′əp-mənt) abnormal growth or development.

mal•di•ges•tion (mal″di-jes′chən) impaired digestion.

male (māl) 1. an organism of the sex that produces spermatozoa. 2. masculine.

mal•e•ate (mal′e-āt) any salt or ester of maleic acid.

ma•le•ic ac•id (mə-le′ik) trivial name for *cis*-butanedioic acid; the *cis* isomer of fumaric acid.

mal•emis•sion (mal″e-mish′ən) anejaculation.

mal•erup•tion (mal″ə-rup′shən) faulty eruption of a tooth, so that it is out of its normal position.

4-ma•le•yl•ace•to•ac•e•tate (ma″le-əl-ə-se″to-as′ə-tāt) an isomer of fumarylacetoacetate, formed by oxidation of homogentisate in the degradation of tyrosine and phenylalanine.

ma•le•yl•ace•to•ac•e•tate isom•er•ase (ma″le-əl-ə-se″to-as′ə-tāt i-som′ər-ās) [EC 5.2.1.2] an enzyme of the isomerase class that catalyzes the interconversion of the isomers 4-maleylacetoacetate and 4-fumarylacetoacetate. The reaction is a step in the use of phenylalanine and tyrosine as fuel.

mal•for•ma•tion (mal″for-ma′shən) [L. *malus* evil + *formation*] 1. a type of anomaly. 2. a morphologic defect of an organ or larger region of the body, resulting from an intrinsically abnormal developmental process.

Arnold-Chiari m. Chiari malformation type II; herniation of the cerebellar tonsils and vermis through the foramen magnum into the spinal canal. It is always associated with lumbosacral myelomeningocele, and hydrocephalus and mental defects are common. Called also *Arnold-Chiari deformity* or *syndrome.*

capillary m. port-wine stain.

cavernous m. see under *hemangioma.*

cerebral arteriovenous m. a congenital anomaly of the brain vasculature composed of arterial and venous channels with many interconnecting shunts without a capillary bed; clinical characteristics include hemorrhage, headache, and focal epileptic seizures. Large malformations may have cranial bruits. Called also *arteriovenous angioma of brain.*

Chiari m. 1. a congenital anomaly in which the cerebellum and medulla oblongata, which is elongated and flattened, protrude into the spinal canal through the foramen magnum. It is classified into three types according to severity: *type I* involves prolapse of the cerebellar tonsils into the spinal canal without elongation of the brainstem; *type II* is the Arnold-Chiari malformation (q.v.); and *type III* consists of complete herniation of the cerebellum to form an occipital encephalocele. It may be accompanied by hydrocephalus, spina bifida, syringomyelia, and mental defects. Called also *Chiari deformity.* 2. Arnold-Chiari m.

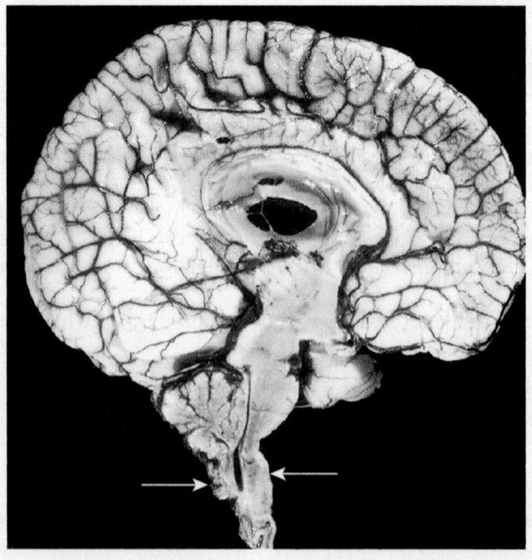

■ Arnold-Chiari malformation in a midsagittal section, showing small posterior fossa contents, downward displacement of the cerebellar vermis, and deformity of the medulla; the arrows indicate the approximate level of the foramen magnum.

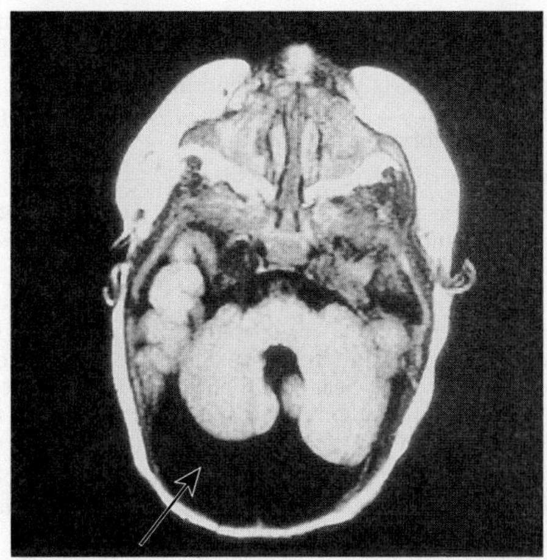

■ Dandy-Walker malformation *(arrow)* in a patient with a large facial segmental hemangioma, characterized by absence of the cerebellar vermis and a large fluid signal intensity in the posterior fossa.

cystic adenomatoid m. a rare variant of congenital cystic disease of the lung, characterized by a mass of interconnecting cysts lined with cuboidal or bronchial epithelium; respiratory distress usually occurs soon after birth and results from compression of normal lung tissue by the cystic lesion.

Dandy-Walker m. a congenital anomaly caused by failure of the roof of the fourth ventricle to develop during embryogenesis, characterized by cystic dilatation of the fourth ventricle, absence or hypoplasia of the vermis, and enlargement of the posterior fossa; hydrocephalus is usually present. Called also *Dandy-Walker deformity* or *syndrome.*

Dieulafoy vascular m. see under *lesion.*

Mondini m. see under *deformity.*

vascular m. an abnormal vascular formation resulting from a developmental anomaly rather than from neoplastic growth; common types include arteriovenous fistulas, some types of hemangiomas and lymphangiomas, nevus anemicus, and nevus flammeus.

mal•func•tion (mal-funk′shən) dysfunction.

Mal•gaigne amputation, luxation, triangle (mahl-gen′yə) [Joseph François *Malgaigne*, French surgeon, 1806–1865] see *subastragalar amputation*, under *amputation*, *pulled elbow*, under *elbow*, and *trigonum caroticum.*

Mal•herbe calcifying epithelioma (mah-lārb′) [Albert *Malherbe*, French surgeon, 1845–1915] pilomatricoma.

mal•ic ac•id (ma′lik, mal′ik) an intermediate in the tricarboxylic acid (Krebs) cycle, formed from fumaric acid and itself oxidized to form oxaloacetic acid; found in apples, pears, and many other fruits; its action is similar to that of tartaric acid, and it is a permitted food additive.

mal•ic en•zyme (ma′lik, mal′ik en′zīm) malate dehydrogenase (oxaloacetate-decarboxylating) ($NADP^+$).

ma•lig•nan•cy (mə-lig′nən-se) [L. *malignare* to act maliciously] 1. a tendency to progress in virulence. 2. the quality of being malignant. 3. a cancer, especially one with the potential to cause death.

ma•lig•nant (mə-lig′nənt) [L. *malignans* acting maliciously] 1. tending to become progressively worse and to result in death. 2. having the properties of anaplasia, invasion, and metastasis; said of tumors.

ma•lin•ger•er (mə-ling′ər-ər) [Fr. *malingre* sickly] an individual who is guilty of malingering.

ma•lin•ger•ing (mə-ling′ər-ing) the willful, deliberate, and fraudulent feigning or exaggeration of the symptoms of illness or injury, done for the purpose of a consciously desired end.

mal•in•ter•dig•i•ta•tion (mal″in-tər-dij″ĭ-ta′shən) failure of interdigitation of parts which are normally so related.

mal•le•a•bil•i•ty (mal″e-ə-bil′ĭ-te) the quality of being malleable.

mal•le•a•ble (mal′e-ə-bəl) [L. *malleare* to hammer] susceptible of being beaten out into a thin plate.

mal•le•al (mal′e-əl) mallear.

mal•le•ar (mal′e-ər) pertaining to the malleus (def. 1); called also *malleal* and *malleolar.*

mal•le•in (mal′e-in) [L. *malleus* glanders] a concentrate prepared from cultures or extracts of *Pseudomonas mallei*, used in the mallein test for glanders.

mal•leo•in•cu•dal (mal″e-o-ing′ku-dəl) incudomalleolar.

mal•le•o•lar (mə-le′o-lər) 1. pertaining to a malleolus. 2. mallear.

mal•le•o•li (mə-le′o-li) [L.] genitive and plural of *malleolus.*

mal•le•o•lus (mə-le′o-ləs) gen. and pl. *malle′oli* [L., dim. of *malleus* hammer] anatomic nomenclature for a rounded process, such as the protuberance on either side of the ankle joint.

external m. m. lateralis.

inner m., internal m. m. medialis.

m. latera′lis [TA] lateral malleolus: the process on the lateral side of the distal end of the fibula, forming, with the malleolus medialis, the mortise in which the talus articulates.

m. media′lis [TA] medial malleolus: the process on the medial side of the distal end of the tibia, forming, with the malleolus lateralis, the mortise in which the talus articulates.

outer m. m. lateralis.

mal•le•ot•o•my (mal″e-ot′ə-me) [*malleus* + Gr. *tomē* a cutting] 1. surgical division of the malleus in cases of ankylosis of the ossicles. 2. surgical separation of the malleoli by division of the ligaments holding them together.

mal•let (mal′ət) a hammerlike tool, usually with a nonmetallic head, for striking something without leaving a mark.

mal•le•us (mal′e-əs) [L. "hammer"] 1. [TA] the outermost of the auditory ossicles, and the one attached to the membrana tympani; its club-shaped head articulates with the incus. Called also *hammer.* See illustration at *ossicula auditus*, under *ossiculum.* 2. glanders.

Mal•loph•a•ga (mal-of′ə-gə) [Gr. *mallos* wool + *phagein* to eat] the biting or bird lice, a large order of insects that feed on the feathers and hair of birds and sometimes attack mammals. Genera include *Damalinia, Felicola, Heterodoxus, Menacanthus*, and *Trichodectes.*

Mal•lo•ry bodies, stain (mal′ə-re) [Frank Burr *Mallory*, American pathologist, 1862–1941] see under *body*, and see *Stains and Staining Methods*, under *stain.*

Mal•lory-Weiss syndrome (mal′ə-re wīs′) [George Kenneth *Mallory*, American pathologist, 1900–1986; Soma *Weiss*, American physician, 1898–1942] see under *syndrome.*

Mal•lo•tus (mə-lo′təs) a genus of trees of the family Euphorbiaceae, native to southern and eastern Asia, the East Indies, and Australia. *M. philippinen′sis* (Lam.) Muell. Arg. is the kamala, source of a medicinal substance, also called kamala.

mal•low (mal′o) [L. *malva*] any plant of the genus *Malva.*

mal•nu•tri•tion (mal″noo-trish′ən) any disorder of nutrition; it may be due to unbalanced or insufficient diet or to defective assimilation or utilization of foods.

malignant m., protein m. kwashiorkor.

protein-calorie m., protein-energy m. (PEM) a class of disorders caused by varying degrees of protein and calorie deficiency, alone or in combination, frequently aggravated by accompanying physiologic and environmental stresses. It may be primary, including such disorders as marasmus, kwashiorkor, and marasmic kwashiorkor, or secondary to other diseases.

mal•oc•clu•sion (mal″ə-kloo′zhən) such malposition and contact of the maxillary and mandibular teeth as to interfere with the highest efficiency during the excursive movements of the jaw that are essential for mastication; originally classified by Angle into four major groups, depending on the anteroposterior jaw relationship as indicated by interdigitation of the first molar teeth, but Class IV is not used (see table).

closed-bite m. closed bite.

open-bite m. open bite.

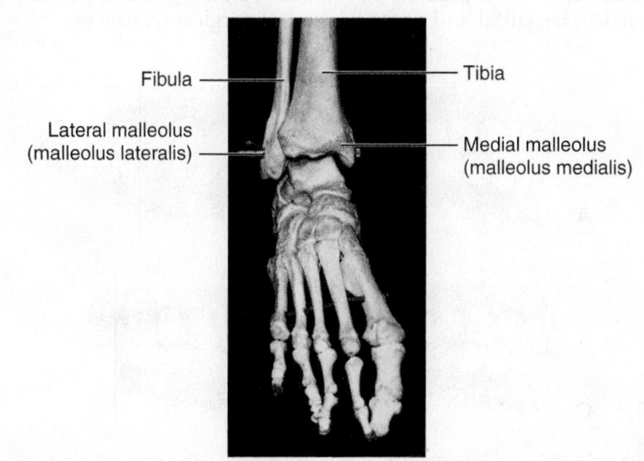

■ Malleolus lateralis (lateral malleolus) and malleolus medialis (medial malleolus), articulating with the talus in the ankle joint.

Angle's Classification of Malocclusion

Class I (Neutroclusion)	Normal anteroposterior relationship of the jaws, as indicated by correct interdigitation of maxillary and mandibular molars, but with crowding and rotation of teeth elsewhere, i.e., a dental dysplasia or an arch length deficiency.
Class II (Distoclusion)	The lower dental arch is posterior to the upper in one or both lateral segments; the lower first molar is distal to the upper first molar.
Division 1	Bilaterally distal with narrow maxillary arch and protruding upper incisors.
Subdivision	Unilaterally distal with other characteristics the same.
Division 2	Bilaterally distal with normal or square-shaped maxillary arch, retruded maxillary central incisors, labially malposed maxillary lateral incisors, and an excessive overbite.
Subdivision	Unilaterally distal with other characteristics the same.
Class III (Mesioclusion)	The lower arch is anterior to the upper in one or both lateral segments; lower first molar is mesial to upper first molar.
Division	Mandibular incisors are usually in anterior cross-bite.
Subdivision	Unilaterally mesial, with other characteristics the same.
Class IV	The dental arches are in distal occlusion upon one lateral half, and in mesial occlusion upon the other half of the mouth.

mal·o·nate-semi·al·de·hyde de·hy·dro·gen·ase (acet·y·lat·ing) (mal′ə-nāt sem″e-al′də-hīd de-hi′dro-jən-ās ə-set′ə-lāt″ing) [EC 1.2.1.18] an enzyme of the oxidoreductase class that catalyzes the decarboxylation of malonate semialdehyde, linking it to coenzyme A to form acetyl coenzyme A; it uses $NAD(P)^+$ as an electron acceptor.

ma·lon·ic ac·id (mə-lon′ik) propanedioic acid, $HOOC\text{-}CH_2COOH$; malonyl coenzyme A is the source of 2-carbon groups transferred to the growing hydrocarbon chain in fatty acid synthesis.

mal·o·nyl (mal′ə-nəl) an acyl radical of malonic acid.

mal·o·nyl CoA (mal′ə-nəl ko-a′) malonyl coenzyme A.

mal·o·nyl co·en·zyme A (mal′ə-nəl ko-en′zīm) the coenzyme A thioester of malonic acid, formed from acetyl coenzyme A by acetyl-CoA carboxylase. It is an intermediate in fatty acid synthesis.

mal·per·fu·sion (mal″pər-fu′zhən) abnormal perfusion.

Mal·pigh·ia (mal-pig′e-ə) [Marcello *Malpighi,* Italian anatomist, 1628–1694] a genus of tropical American fruit-bearing shrubs and trees of the family Malpighiaceae. *M. glab′ra, M. punicifo′lia,* and *M. u′rens* are all called acerola or Barbados cherry and their fruit is rich in vitamin C.

mal·pigh·i·an (mahl-pig′e-ən) named for Marcello *Malpighi,* as *malpighian stigma* and *malpighian tubule.*

mal·posed (mal-pōzd′) not in the normal position.

mal·po·si·tion (mal″pə-zish′ən) [L. *malus* bad + *positio* placement] abnormal or anomalous position of an organ or part; cf. *ectopia.* Called also *allotopia, displacement, dystopia,* and *heterotopia.*

mal·prac·tice (mal-prak′tis) [L. *mal* bad + *practice*] improper or injurious practice; unskillful and faulty medical or surgical treatment.

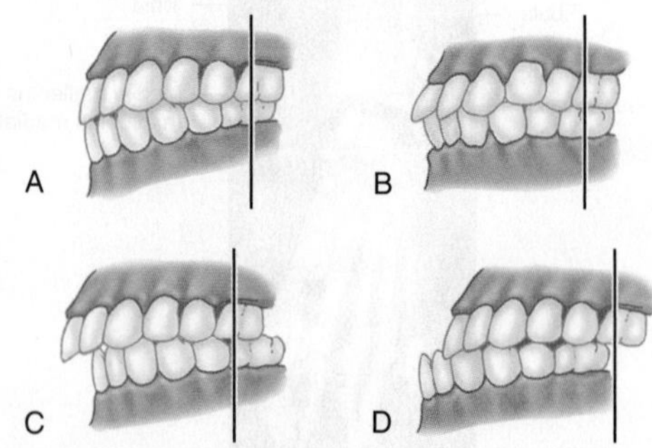

■ *(A),* Normal occlusion; *(B),* Class I malocclusion; *(C),* Class II malocclusion; *(D),* Class III malocclusion. Note the position of the mesial cusp of the maxillary molar relative to the mandibular molar in each type of occlusion.

mal·pres·en·ta·tion (mal″prez-ən-ta′shən) a faulty or abnormal fetal presentation.

mal·ro·ta·tion (mal″ro-ta′shən) 1. abnormal or pathologic rotation, as of the vertebral column. 2. failure of normal rotation of an organ, such as the midgut, during embryonic development.

MALT mucosa-associated lymphoid tissue.

malt (mawlt) grain, for the most part barley, which has been soaked, made to germinate, and then dried; it contains dextrin, maltose, and diastase.

mal·tase (mawl′tās) 1. α-glucosidase. 2. any enzyme with similar glycolytic activity, cleaving α-1,4 or sometimes α-1,6 linked glucose residues from nonreducing termini; in humans there are considered to be four such enzymes. Two are the heat-stable enzymes usually called maltases, constituting the glucoamylase complex (q.v.); the other two are the heat-labile enzymes more commonly called sucrase and α-dextrinase that constitute the sucrase-isomaltase complex (q.v.).

mal·thu·si·an (mal-thoo′se-ən) named for Rev. Thomas Robert *Malthus,* English economist, 1766–1834, as *malthusian law.*

mal·ti·tol (mawl′tĭ-tol) [NF] a hydrogenated, partially hydrolyzed starch used as a bulk sweetener.

mal·to·bi·ose (mawl″to-bi′ōs) maltose.

mal·to·dex·trin (mawl″to-dek′strin) [NF] any polysaccharide of glucose residues in β-(1,4) linkage, such as are formed in incomplete hydrolysis of starch to maltose; used as an excipient in pharmaceutical preparations and a source of carbohydrates in oral dietary supplements and tube feeding.

MALT·oma (mawl-to′mə) a form of extranodal marginal zone lymphoma originating in mucosa-associated lymphoid tissue, particularly that of the gastrointestinal tract; other sites include the larynx, salivary glands, thyroid gland, and lung. It is characterized by small lymphocytes, marginal zone B cells, monocytoid B cells, and plasma cells. Tumors are generally localized and indolent, but may spread or become more aggressive.

mal·tose (mawl′tōs) [NF] a reducing disaccharide composed of two glucose residues in α-(1,4)-glycosidic linkage; it is the fundamental structural unit of glycogen and starch and is used as a nutrient and sweetener.

mal·to·side (mawl′to-sīd) a glycoside composed of maltose residues.

mal·tos·uria (mawl″to-su′re-ə) excessive levels of maltose in the urine.

mal·to·tri·ose (mawl″to-tri′ōs) a reducing disaccharide consisting of three glucose residues in α-(1,4)-glycosidic linkage; it is one of the products of limited digestion of starch or glycogen by α-amylase.

mal·turned (mal-turnd′) turned abnormally; said of teeth twisted on their central axes.

Mal·u·ci·din (mal″u-si′din) trademark for a yeast extract that has abortifacient activity in the dog, cat, and sheep.

mal·un·ion (mal-ūn′yən) union of the fragments of a fractured bone in a faulty position.

Ma·lus (ma′ləs) a genus of flowering trees of the family Rosaceae. *M. sylves′tris* Mill. is the apple (q.v.).

Mal·va (mal′və) [L.] the mallows, a genus of flowering plants of the family Malvaceae. The flowers and leaves of *M. sylves′tris* L. and *M. rotundifo′lia* L. are demulcent and emollient, and are used medicinally in India and other parts of Asia.

mam·ba (mahm′bə) [Zulu *im-amba*] any member of the genus *Dendroaspis,* extremely venomous elapid snakes.

  black m. *Dendroaspis polylepis,* a large black African tree snake whose venom is deadly.

  green m. *Dendroaspis angusticeps,* a large green or black tree snake of eastern and southern Africa whose venom is deadly.

mam·e·lon (mam′ə-lon) [Fr. "nipple"] 1. one of three tubercles sometimes present on the cutting edge of an incisor tooth. 2. the nipple-like elevation in the umbilicus, considered to be the remains of the solid proximal part of the umbilical cord which contained the umbilical arteries and urachus.

ma·mil·la (mə-mil′ə) mammilla.

mam·il·lary (mam′ĭ-lar″e) mammillary.

mam·il·lat·ed (mam″ĭ-lāt′əd) mammillated.

mam·il·la·tion (mam″ĭ-la′shən) mammillation.

ma·mil·li·form (mə-mil′ĭ-form) mammilliform.

mam·il·li·tis (mam″ĭ-li′tis) mammillitis.

mam·ma (mam′ə) gen. and pl. *mam′mae* [L.] [TA] the breast: the modified cutaneous, glandular structure on the anterior aspect of the thorax that contains, in the female, the elements that secrete milk for nourishment of the young. See also *glandula mammaria.* **mam′mary** *adj*

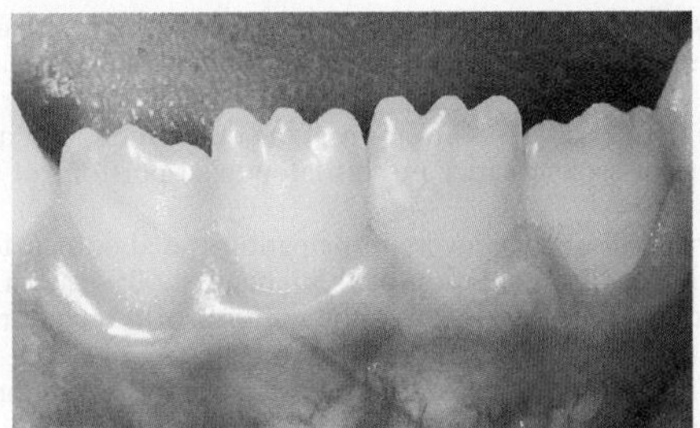
■ Mamelons on mandibular incisors.

m. accesso′ria [TA] accessory mamma: a mammary gland present in excess of the normal number, generally found along the line of the embryonic mammary ridge (crest); called also *accessory mammary gland.*

m. areola′ta a condition of the breast in which there is bulging of the areola of the nipple.

m. masculi′na the rudimentary mammary gland of the male breast; called also *m. virilis.*

supernumerary m. mamma accessoria.

m. vi′rilis m. masculina.

mam•mae (mam′e) [L.] genitive and plural of *mamma.*

mam•mal (mam′əl) an individual belonging to the class Mammalia.

mam•mal•gia (mə-mal′jə) mastalgia.

Mam•ma•lia (mə-mal′e-ə) a class of warm-blooded vertebrate animals, including all that possess hair and suckle their young. It includes three major groups: placentals and marsupials, which are viviparous, and monotremes, which are oviparous.

mam•mal•o•gy (mə-mal′ə-je) [*mammal* + *-logy*] the study of mammals.

mam•ma•plas•ty (mam′ə-plas″te) [*mamma* + *-plasty*] plastic reconstruction of the breast, as may be performed to augment or reduce its size. Spelled also *mammoplasty;* called also *mastoplasty.* **mammaplas′tic** *adj*

Aries-Pitanguy m. a type of reduction mammaplasty to reduce mild to moderate macromastia.

augmentation m. plastic reconstruction of the breast, with increase of its volume by insertion of an autogenous or prosthetic material.

Biesenberger m. a type of reduction mammaplasty with transposition of the nipple, consisting in excision of the lateral portion of the mammary gland, with rotation of the remaining glandular pedicle attached to the nipple and formation of a skin brassiere.

Conway m. a type of reduction mammaplasty for correction of severe macromastia, consisting in partial breast amputation and free transplantation of the nipples and areolae.

reconstructive m. breast reconstruction after mastectomy.

reduction m. plastic reconstruction of the breast with decrease in its volume by excision of tissue.

Strömbeck m. a one-stage type of reduction mammaplasty that includes transposition of the nipple in a medial and lateral pedicle.

mam•ma•troph (mam′ə-trōf) lactotroph.

mam•mec•to•my (mə-mek′tə-me) [*mamm-* + *-ectomy*] mastectomy.

mam•mi•form (mam′ĭ-form) [*mammo-* + *form*] shaped like a breast.

mam•mil•la (mə-mil′ə) gen. and pl. *mammil′lae* [L., dim. of *mamma,* a breast, teat] 1. the nipple (papilla mammaria [TA]). 2. any nipple-like structure; spelled also *mamilla.*

mam•mil•lary (mam′ĭ-lar″e) 1. pertaining to or resembling a nipple; spelled also *mamillary.* 2. pertaining to a nipple. 3. resembling a nipple; spelled also *mamillary.*

mam•mil•lat•ed (mam′ĭ-lāt″əd) having nipple-like projections.

mam•mil•la•tion (mam″ĭ-la′shən) 1. the condition of being mammillated. 2. a nipple-like elevation or projection.

mam•mil•li•form (mə-mil′ĭ-form) [*mammilla* + *form*] shaped like a nipple.

mam•mil•li•plas•ty (mə-mil′ĭ-plas″te) theleplasty.

mam•mil•li•tis (mam″ĭ-li′tis) [*mammilla* + *-itis*] inflammation of the mammilla, or nipple; spelled also *mamillitis.* Called also *thelitis.*

bovine ulcerative m. a herpesviral disease affecting milking cows, characterized by ulcerative lesions on the teats and, less frequently, on the udders.

mam•mil•lo•tha•lam•ic (mam″ĭ-lo″thə-lam′ik) pertaining to or connecting the mammillary body and thalamus.

mam•mi•pla•sia (mam″ĭ-pla′zhə) mammoplasia.

mam•mi•tis (mə-mi′tis) mastitis.

mamm(o)- [L. *mamma,* q.v.] a combining form denoting relationship to the breast, or to a mammary gland; see also words beginning *mast(o)-* and *maz(o)-.*

mam•mo•gen (mam′o-jən) any substance or influence that promotes breast development.

mam•mo•gen•e•sis (mam″o-jen′ə-sis) the development of the mammary glands to the functional state.

mam•mo•gram (mam′ə-gram) a radiograph of the breast.

mam•mog•ra•phy (mə-mog′rə-fe) radiography of the mammary gland.

digital m. a method for breast radiography that converts x-rays into electric signals producing digital images that can be seen on a computer screen and stored; the radiation dose is lower than that of traditional mammography.

Mam•mo•mo•nog•a•mus (mam″o-mon″o-ga′mus) a genus of nematodes of the family Syngamidae. Various species infest the pharynx, larynx, and trachea of cats and other mammals.

mam•mo•pla•sia (mam″o-pla′zhə) [*mammo-* + *-plasia*] the development of breast tissue; called also *mastoplasia.*

adolescent m. the development of breast tissue at adolescence, applied especially to the development and later regression which occurs in males during puberty.

mam•mo•plas•ty (mam′o-plas″te) mammaplasty.

mam•mose (mam′ōs) [L. *mammosus*] 1. having large breasts, or mammae. 2. mammillated.

mam•mo•so•mat•o•trope (mam″o-so-mat′o-trōp) mammosomatotroph.

mam•mo•so•mat•o•troph (mam″o-so-mat′o-trōf) an acidophilic cell of the adenohypophysis that secretes both growth hormone and prolactin.

mam•mot•o•my (mə-mot′ə-me) mastotomy.

mam•mo•troph (mam′o-trōf) lactotroph.

mam•mo•tro•phic (mam″o-tro′fik) mammotropic.

mam•mo•tro•pic (mam″o-tro′pik) [*mammo-* + *-tropic*] having affinity for or a stimulating effect on the mammary gland. Called also *mammotrophic.*

mam•mo•tro•pin (mam′o-tro″pin) prolactin.

Man. [L.] mani′pulus (a handful).

Man•ches•ter operation (man′chəs-tər) [*Manchester,* England, where it was developed] see under *operation.*

man•chette (man-shet′) [Fr. "a cuff"] a cylindrical array of microtubules around the nucleus of a spermatid during spermatogenesis.

man•chi•neel (man″kĭ-nēl′) *Hippomane mancinella,* a tree of tropical America that has a caustic poisonous sap.

Man•del•amine (man-del′ə-mēn″) trademark for a preparation of methenamine mandelate.

man•di•ble (man′dĭ-bəl) mandibula.

man•dib•u•la (man-dib′u-lə) gen. and pl. *mandib′ulae* [L., from *mandere* to chew] [TA] the mandible: the horseshoe-shaped bone forming the lower jaw; the largest and strongest bone of the face, consisting of a body and a pair of rami, which articulate with the skull at the temporomandibular joints. **mandib′ular** *adj*

man•dib•u•lae (man-dib′u-le) [L.] genitive and plural of *mandibula.*

man•dib•u•lec•to•my (man-dib″u-lek′tə-me) surgical removal of the mandible.

man•dib•u•lo•pha•ryn•ge•al (man-dib″u-lo-fə-rin′je-əl) pertaining to the mandible and the pharynx.

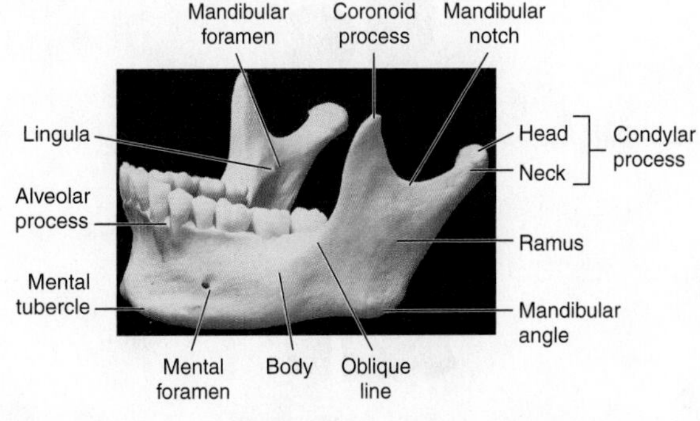

■ Mandibula (mandible).

Man•dol (man′dol) trademark for a preparation of cefamandole.

Man•drag•o•ra (man-drag′o-rə) [L.] a genus of plants of the family Solanaceae. *M. officina′rum* L. is the true European or oriental mandrake, which has the general properties of belladonna and was formerly used as a narcotic and sedative but is now used only in homeopathy. It contains the alkaloids atropine, hyoscyamine, and scopolamine.

man•drake (man′drāk) 1. any plant of the genus *Mandragora.* 2. podophyllum.

man•drel (man′drəl) a shaft in a handpiece that holds a disk, stone, or cup used for grinding or polishing. Called also *mandril.*

man•dril (man′dril) mandrel.

man•drin (man′drin) a stylet or guide for a catheter.

ma•neu•ver (mə-noo′vər) any dexterous procedure. See also entries under *method, operation, procedure, surgery,* and *technique.*

Adson m. see under *test.*

Allen m. with the elbow flexed at a right angle, the arm is extended horizontally and rotated externally at the shoulder, the head being rotated to the contralateral shoulder; obliteration of the radial pulse suggests scalenus anterior syndrome.

Barlow m. a dislocation maneuver used together with the Ortolani maneuver in diagnosing developmental dysplasia of the hip.

Bracht m. (for breech presentation), the breech is allowed to spontaneously deliver up to the umbilicus. The body and extended legs are held together with both hands maintaining the upward and anterior rotation of the fetal body. When the anterior rotation is nearly complete, the fetal body is held against the mother's symphysis. Maintenance of this position can lead to spontaneous completion of delivery.

Brandt-Andrews m. see under *method.*

Catell m. mobilization and reflection superiorly to the left of the right colon, root of the small bowel mesentery, duodenum, and head of the pancreas to expose the retroperitoneal vascular structures.

Credé m. see under *method.*

Dix-Hallpike m. a test for benign positional vertigo: the examiner turns the head of the seated patient to one side and pulls the patient backwards into a supine position with the head hanging over the edge of the examining table; the patient then looks straight ahead and the examiner observes for positional nystagmus, which is indicative of benign positional vertigo. Called also *Dix-Hallpike test* and *Hallpike m.*

forward-bending m. a method of detecting retraction signs in neoplastic changes in the mammae; the patient bends forward from the waist with chin held up and arms extended toward the examiner. If retraction is present, an asymmetry in the breast is seen.

Gowers m. Gowers sign (def. 2).

Hallpike m. Dix-Hallpike m.

Heimlich m. a method of dislodging food or other material from the throat of a choking victim: the rescuer wraps their arms around the victim at the belt line and allows the victim's upper torso to hang forward; the rescuer makes a fist with one hand and grasps it with the other; with both hands placed against the victim's abdomen slightly above the navel and below the rib cage; then forcefully presses into the abdomen with a quick upward thrust. If the victim is sitting, the rescuer stands behind them and performs the same procedure. If the victim is prone, the rescuer turns him or her to lie on their back, kneels astride their torso, places both hands on their abdomen slightly above the navel, and presses forcefully with a sharp upward thrust. The maneuver may be repeated several times if necessary.

Hoguet m. in hernioplasty, conversion of the direct hernial sac to an indirect one by withdrawing the sac from beneath the deep epigastric vessels.

Hueter m. downward and forward pressure on the patient's tongue by the left forefinger of the physician during introduction of a stomach tube.

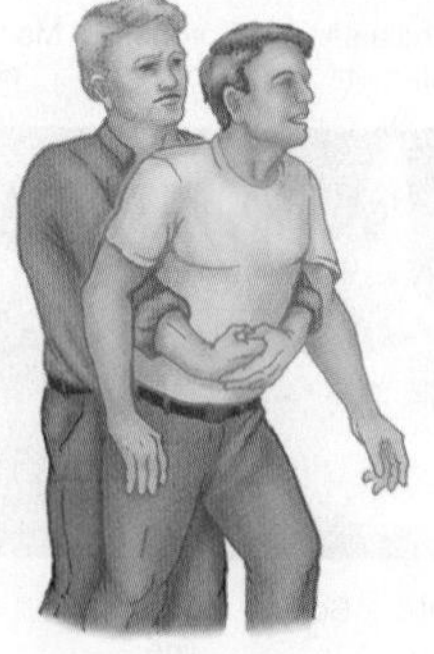

■ Heimlich maneuver.

Jendrassik m. a procedure for emphasizing the patellar reflex: the patient hooks hands together by the flexed fingers and pulls apart as hard as possible.

Kocher m. operative mobilization of the duodenum for exposure of the retroduodenal, intrapancreatic, and intraduodenal portions of the common bile duct.

Leopold m's four maneuvers in palpating the abdomen for ascertaining the position and presentation of the fetus. See illustration.

McDonald m. measurement of the contour of the abdomen to calculate the duration of pregnancy; see also under *rule.*

Mattox m. mobilization and medial reflection of the abdominal viscera to expose the suprarenal aorta for repair of traumatic injury.

Mauriceau m., Mauriceau-Smellie-Veit m. a method of delivering the aftercoming head in cases of breech presentation: the infant's body rests on the physician's palm and forearm with the index and middle fingers over the maxilla to flex the head while the other hand is placed on the infant's shoulders to apply traction. Called also *Smellie method.*

Müller m. an effort to inhale with a closed glottis after exhalation, used during fluoroscopic examination to cause a negative intrathoracic pressure with engorgement of intrathoracic vascular structures, which is helpful in recognizing esophageal varices and distinguishing vascular from nonvascular structures.

Ortolani m. a reduction maneuver used together with the Barlow maneuver in diagnosing developmental dysplasia of the hip.

Osler m. a technique for identifying pseudohypertension: the sphygmomanometer cuff is inflated above systolic blood pressure; if the pulseless radial or brachial artery remains palpable, pseudohypertension may be present.

Pajot m. a maneuver for forceps delivery with traction along the axis of the superior pelvic aperture; one hand over the lock of the forceps pulls downward towards the floor, while the other hand applies horizontal traction.

Phalen m. see under *test.*

Pinard m. a method of bringing down the foot in breech extraction.

Prague m. a method in breech presentation of delivering the head when the fetal back is posterior, by bringing down the breech and making traction on the head with the finger, which is hooked over the nape of the neck.

Pringle m. clamping of the hepatic portal vein to limit hemorrhage during liver surgery.

Ritgen m. delivery of the fetal head by extending it upward and forward through the vulva, between contractions, by pressing with the tips of the fingers upon the perineum behind the anus.

Scanzoni m. a method of forceps rotation of the fetal head when it is in the posterior position of the occiput.

Schreiber m. rubbing of the inner side of the upper part of the thigh while testing for patellar reflex.

Sellick m. the application of pressure to the cricoid cartilage in order to compress the esophagus and prevent passive regurgitation during endotracheal intubation.

Toynbee m. pinching the nostrils and swallowing; if the auditory tube is patent, the tympanic membrane will retract medially. See also *Toynbee test,* under *test.* Called also *Toynbee experiment.*

Valsalva m. 1. forcible exhalation effort against a closed glottis; the resultant increase in intrathoracic pressure interferes with venous return to the heart. Called also *Valsalva experiment.* 2. forcible exhalation effort against occluded nostrils and a closed mouth causes increased pressure in the eustachian tube and middle ear, so that the tympanic membrane moves outward; formerly used as a test of eustachian tube patency. Called also *Valsalva method* or *test.*

Wigand m. see under *version.*

man•ga•fo•di•pir tri•so•di•um (mang″gə-fo′dĭ-pir) [USP] an ionic paramagnetic agent, comprising manganese (II) linked to the chelating agent fodipir; it increases signal intensity of the tissues in magnetic resonance imaging (MRI), enhancing the images obtained, and is used in detection and evaluation of hepatic lesions, administered intravenously.

man•ga•nese (Mn) (mang′gə-nēs) [L. *manganum, manganesium*] a metal resembling iron; atomic number 25, atomic weight 54.938, specific gravity 7.2. It occurs normally throughout the body, concentrated in the mitochondria, chiefly in the pituitary, liver, pancreas, kidney, and bone; it is necessary for the synthesis of mucopolysaccharides and activates a number of enzymes. Clinical deficiency is unknown in humans but may occur in other animals and causes perosis in poultry. Excessive inhalation of manganese dust can cause toxicity; see under *poisoning* and *pneumonitis.*

m. chloride [USP] the tetrahydrated chloride salt of manganese, $MnCl_2 \cdot 4H_2O$, used as a nutritional supplement; administered orally and intravenously as a component of total parenteral nutrition solutions.

m. gluconate [USP] the gluconate salt of manganese, having the same indications and uses as the chloride salt.

m. sulfate [USP] the tetrahydrated sulfate salt of manganese, $MnSO_4 \cdot 4H_2O$, used as a nutritional supplement; administered orally and

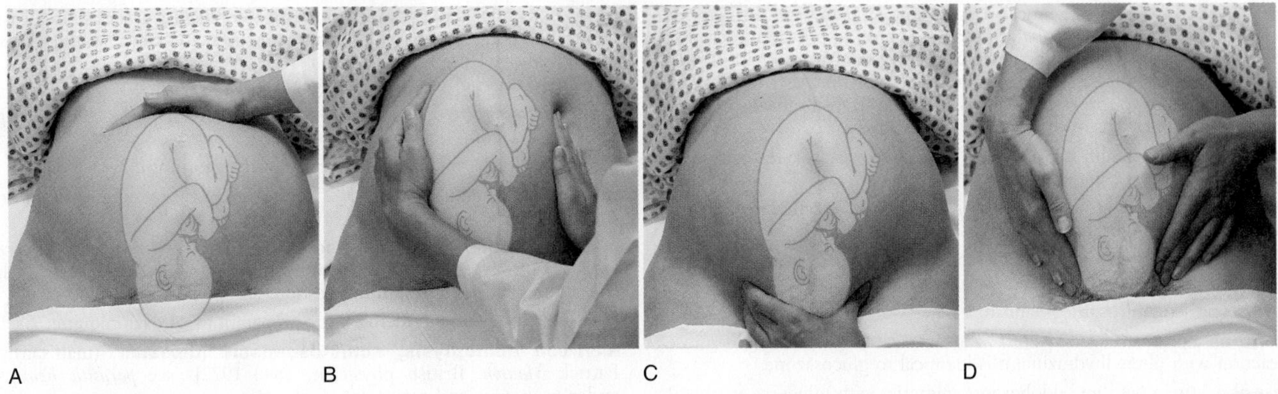

■ Leopold maneuvers. *(A)*, First maneuver. One or both hands are placed over fundus and the fetal part identified. *(B)*, Second maneuver. The palmar surface of one hand is used to locate the back of the fetus and the other hand to feel the irregularities, such as hands and feet. *(C)*, Third maneuver. Thumb and third finger are used to grasp presenting part over the pubic symphysis. *(D)*, Fourth maneuver. Both hands are used to outline the fetal head.

intravenously as a component of total parenteral nutrition solutions. In veterinary medicine, administered to poultry as a source of manganese to prevent perosis.

man•gan•ic (mang-gan′ik) pertaining to manganese as a trivalent element.

man•ga•nism (mang′gə-niz-əm) manganese poisoning; see under *poisoning.*

man•ga•nous (mang′gə-nəs) pertaining to manganese as a divalent element.

mange (mānj) any of several contagious forms of dermatitis caused by the mange mites (q.v.) and affecting many different species of mammals and birds. Although the distribution, manner of spread, and clinical presentation vary with the host and parasite species, mange is typically characterized by cutaneous burrows produced by the mites; scratching associated with deeper lesions, producing crusts and scabs; alopecia; and epidermal hyperplasia with desquamation. Bacterial infection may occur.

chorioptic m. mange caused by infestation with species of *Chorioptes;* it usually occurs on the posterior body of cattle or horses, from the udder and perineum to the hind legs. Called also *chorioptic acariasis* or *itch.*

demodectic m. mange caused by infestation with species of *Demodex,* characterized by folliculitis with pustule formation, usually on the head, neck, or shoulders; it is common in dogs and cattle and occurs sporadically in other species. Called also *demodectic acariasis, demodicosis,* and *follicular m.*

follicular m. demodectic m.

notoedric m. infestation of the ears, head, or neck of a cat by a species of *Notoedres;* it is intensely irritating and serious cases can be fatal.

otodectic m. mange in the ear region from infestation by species of *Otodectes;* see also *otoacariasis.*

psoroptic m. infestation by species of *Psoroptes. P. cuniculi* infests the ears of rabbits and goats, sometimes causing secondary infections of the internal ear or central nervous system. *P. ovis* causes sheep scab, the most common type of mange in sheep, as well as scabies in cattle and horses. *P. equi* infests sheltered areas on horses, such as those covered by hair.

red m. demodectic mange in canines.

sarcoptic m. scabies in animals other than humans.

Man•gif•e•ra (man-jif′ə-rə) a genus of flowering fruit trees of the family Anacardiaceae. *M. indica* is the mango tree; its leaves, bark, and fruit skins cause a type of urushiol dermatitis *(mango dermatitis)* in susceptible persons.

ma•nia (ma′ne-ə) [Gr. "madness"] a phase of bipolar disorder characterized by expansiveness, elation, agitation, hyperexcitability, hyperactivity, and increased speed of thought and speech (flight of ideas); called also *manic syndrome.*

delirious m. hypermania.

unproductive m. a manic episode with some signs and symptoms of depression, such as repression of thought and speech.

-mania a word termination denoting excessive preoccupation with something, as in *erotomania, kleptomania,* and *pyromania.*

ma•ni•a•cal (mə-ni′ə-kəl) manic (def. 2).

man•ic (man′ik) 1. pertaining to mania. 2. suffering from mania.

man•ic-de•pres•sive (man′ik-de-pres′iv) alternating between attacks of mania and depression, as in bipolar disorder.

man•i•fold (man′ĭ-fold) a tube fitting with several outlets on its sides for connecting to other tubes.

Man•i•hot (man′e-hot) [Tupi *manioca*] a genus of herbs and shrubs originally native to tropical regions of the Americas but now also grown in many other tropical regions. *M. esculen′ta* Crantz (Euphorbiaceae) is cassava (q.v.), an important food plant whose root causes cyanide poisoning if eaten raw.

man•i•kin (man′ĭ-kin) a model of the body, usually with movable or removable members and parts; uses include illustrating anatomy; teaching nursing and obstetrics; teaching certain surgical procedures, such as the removal of foreign bodies by bronchoscopy; and teaching cardiopulmonary resuscitation.

man•i•oc (man′e-ok) [Fr., from Tupi *manioca*] cassava.

Manip. [L.] mani′pulus (a handful).

ma•nip•u•la•tion (mə-nip″u-la′shən) [L. *manipulare* to handle] 1. skillful or dextrous treatment. 2. in physical therapy, the forceful passive movement of a joint beyond its active limit of motion. 3. adjustment (def. 5).

conjoined m. an obstetric maneuver done with both hands.

endocrine m. see under *therapy.*

gene m. any process that makes artificial changes in a gene, such as in gene therapy or genetic engineering.

hormonal m. endocrine therapy.

spinal m. adjustment (def. 5).

Mann sign (man) [John Dixon *Mann,* English physician, 1840–1912] see under *sign.*

Mann-Boll•man fistula (man′ bōl′mən) [Frank Charles *Mann,* American physiologist and surgeon, 1887–1962; Jesse Louis *Bollman,* American physiologist, 20th century] see under *fistula.*

Mann-Whit•ney test (man′ hwit′ne) [Henry Berthold *Mann,* Austrian-born American mathematician, 1905–2000; Donald Ransom *Whitney,* American statistician, 1915–2007] rank sum test; see under *test.*

Mann-Wil•liam•son ulcer (man′ wil′yəm-son) [F.C. *Mann;* Carl S. *Williamson,* American surgeon, 1896–1952] see under *ulcer.*

man•na (man′ə) [L.] the dried saccharine exudation from the flowering ash tree, *Fraxinus ornus;* its chief constituents are mannitol, mucilage, and sugar, and it has been used as a laxative.

man•nan (man′an) any polymer consisting solely or mostly of mannose residues, occurring in a variety of plants and as a cell wall constituent of some fungi.

man•ner (man′ər) a way of acting or doing.

m. of death the circumstances under which a death occurs, e.g., suicide or accident; cf. *cause of death,* under *cause.*

man•ner•ism (man′ər-iz-əm) a stereotyped movement or habit peculiar to a given individual.

Mann•hei•mia (man-hi′me-ə) [Walter *Mannheim,* German microbiologist, 20th century] a genus of bacteria of the family Pasteurellaceae, consisting of gram-negative, nonmotile rods or coccobacilli; organisms are mesophilic, non–spore-forming, and facultatively anaerobic or microaerophilic. The type species is *M. haemoly′tica.*

M. haemoly′tica a species that is part of the normal flora of cattle and sheep and is the etiologic agent of hemorrhagic septicemia in sheep and goats, shipping fever in cattle, and a choleralike disease in fowl; it occasionally is found in human infections. Formerly called *Pasteurella haemolytica.*

man•nite (man′īt) mannitol.

man•ni•tol (man′ĭ-tol) 1. a 6-carbon sugar alcohol formed by reduction of mannose or fructose and widely distributed in plants and fungi. 2. [USP] a pharmaceutical preparation of mannitol; an osmotic diuretic used to prevent and treat acute renal failure, to promote excretion of toxic substances, reducing their nephrotoxicity, and to reduce cerebral edema or elevated intracranial or intraocular pressure. Also used as an irrigating solution to prevent hemolysis during transurethral prostatic resection and other transurethral surgical procedures.

Mann•kopf sign (mahn′kopf) [Emil Wilhelm *Mannkopf,* German physician, 1836–1918] see under *sign.*

man•no•py•ra•nose (man″o-pir′ə-nōs) mannose occurring in the cyclic pyranose configuration.

man•no•sa•mine (mə-no′sə-mēn) the amino sugar derivative of mannose at the 2 carbon; it is a component of neuraminic acid.

man•no•san (man′o-sən) mannan.

man•no•sa•zone (mə-no′sə-zōn) the osazone formed from mannose by reaction with phenylhydrazine; it is identical to glucosazone.

man•nose (man′ōs) an aldohexose epimeric with glucose at the 2 carbon; it occurs in oligosaccharides of many glycoproteins and glycolipids.

m. 6-phosphate mannose phosphorylated at the 6 carbon; it is added to lysosomal enzymes during their biosynthesis and, via specific receptors, it serves as a recognition marker to target the enzymes to the lysosomes.

man•nose-1-phos•phate gua•nyl•yl•trans•fer•ase (GDP) (man′ōs fos′fāt gwah″nəl-əl-trans′fər-ās) [EC 2.7.7.22] an enzyme of the transferase class that catalyzes the synthesis of GDP mannose from GDP and mannose 1-phosphate.

man•nose-6-phos•phate isom•er•ase (man′ōs fos′fāt i-som′ər-ās) [EC 5.3.1.8] an enzyme of the isomerase class that catalyzes the interconversion between mannose 6-phosphate and fructose 6-phosphate, a step in the utilization of mannose. Called also *phosphomannose isomerase.*

α-man•no•si•dase (man-ōs′ĭ-dās) [EC 3.2.1.24] an enzyme of the hydrolase class that catalyzes the hydrolysis of terminal, nonreducing, α-linked mannose residues from mannosides, a step in the metabolism of *N*-linked oligosaccharides in glycoproteins. Deficiency of the lysosomal form of the enzyme, an autosomal recessive trait, results in α-mannosidosis.

β-man•no•si•dase (man-ōs′ĭ-dās) [EC 3.2.1.25] an enzyme of the hydrolase class that catalyzes the cleavage of terminal, nonreducing, β-linked mannose residues from mannosides, a step in the metabolism of *N*-linked oligosaccharides of glycoproteins. Deficiency of the enzyme, inherited as an autosomal recessive trait, results in β-mannosidosis.

man•no•side (man′o-sīd) a glycoside of mannose.

α-man•no•si•do•sis (man″o-sĭ-do′sis) an autosomal recessive lysosomal storage disease caused by mutation in the *MAN2B1* gene (locus: 19cen-q12), which encodes lysosomal α-mannosidase; the resulting enzyme defect leads to oligosaccharide accumulation. Characteristics include coarse facies, upper respiratory congestion and infections, profound mental retardation, hepatosplenomegaly, cataracts, radiographic signs of dysostosis multiplex, and kyphosis. There are two types: a severe type I (infantile onset), with death occurring between the ages of 3 and 10 years, and a milder type II (juvenile-adult onset).

β-man•no•si•do•sis (man″o-sĭ-do′sis) an autosomal recessive lysosomal storage disease caused by mutation in the *MANBA* gene (locus: 4q22-q25), which encodes β-mannosidase; the resulting enzyme defect leads to oligosaccharide accumulation. Manifestations, age of onset, and severity vary widely. Characteristics include mental retardation, motor and developmental delay, behavioral problems, hearing loss, speech impairment, seizures, hypotonia, peripheral neuropathy, angiokeratoma, skeletal abnormalities, mild facial dysmorphism, and recurrent infection.

ma•nom•e•ter (mə-nom′ə-tər) [Gr. *manos* thin + *-meter*] an instrument for measuring the pressure or tension of liquids or gases, as of the blood.

aneroid m. a true total-pressure measuring device, which measures pressure by means of an elastic container as compared to that of a vacuum.

mercury m. a manometer that uses changes of height of a column of mercury to measure pressure.

water m. a manometer that uses changes of height of a column of water to measure pressure.

mano•met•ric (man″o-met′rik) 1. pertaining to or ascertained by the manometer. 2. varying with the pressure.

ma•nom•e•try (mə-nom′ə-tre) the measurement of pressure by means of a manometer.

anal m. the measurement of the pressure generated by the anal sphincter; used in the evaluation of fecal incontinence.

anorectal m. measurement of the pressure in the anus and rectum of a severely constipated patient in order to assess physiologic causes.

antroduodenal m. manometry of the gastric antrum and duodenum for the assessment of dysmotility. Called also *gastroduodenal m.*

esophageal m. a diagnostic study to assess the competence of the lower esophageal sphincter. A catheter sheathed with a water-filled balloon is inserted nasally and advanced into the esophagus; a series of measurements reflecting esophageal resting pressures are taken as the catheters are moved.

gastroduodenal m. antroduodenal m.

man•op•to•scope (mə-nop′to-skōp) [*manus* + *opto-* + *-scope*] an apparatus for detecting ocular dominance.

Man. pr. [L.] ma′ne pri′mo (early in the morning).

man•quea (mahn-ka′ah) [Sp.] actinobacillosis of young cattle in South America, marked by formation of abscesses on the legs.

man•sa (man′sə) [Sp.] the root or rhizome of *Anemonopsis californica,* used as a folk remedy in the southwestern United States and northern Mexico to relieve colds and indigestion, and to purify the blood.

Man•sil (man′sil) trademark for preparations of oxamniquine.

Man•son hemoptysis, schistosomiasis (disease) (man′sən) [Sir Patrick *Manson,* British physician, 1844–1922] see *parasitic hemoptysis,* under *hemoptysis,* and see under *schistosomiasis.*

Man•son•el•la (man″sən-el′ə) [Sir Patrick *Manson*] a genus of nematodes of the superfamily *Filarioidea,* characterized by a rounded, enlarged anterior end and a smooth cuticle, found in tropical areas of the Americas and Africa.

M. ozzar′di a parasitic species that causes mansonellosis in Central and South America and the Caribbean; it is transmitted by the biting flies *Culicoides furens* and *Simulium amazonicum.*

M. per′stans a species up to 8 cm long found in tropical regions of the Americas and Africa, transmitted by biting flies of genus *Culicoides.* Adult worms inhabit pleural and peritoneal tissues, while larval forms (microfilariae) are found in the bloodstream. Although considered to be nonpathogenic, they occasionally cause symptoms, including abdominal pain, edema, fever, and hepatosplenomegaly.

M. streptocer′ca a species found in humans and chimpanzees in western and central Africa, transmitted by biting flies of genus *Culicoides.* The microfilariae, which may be found in scarification smears, are sometimes confused with those of *Onchocerca volvulus.* There is a pruritic rash resembling that of onchocerciasis. Formerly classified under the genera *Acanthocheilonema* and *Dipetalonema.*

man•so•nel•li•a•sis (man″so-nəl-i′ə-sis) mansonellosis.

man•so•nel•lo•sis (man″so-nəl-o′sis) infection with nematodes of the genus *Mansonella;* characterized by vague symptoms including headache, coldness of the lower limbs, pruritus, and swollen joints.

Man•so•nia (mən-so′ne-ə) [Sir Patrick *Manson*] a genus of mosquitoes of the tribe Mansoniini, subfamily Culicinae, several species of which transmit *Brugia malayi.* Some species may also transmit viruses such as those causing equine encephalomyelitis.

Man•so•ni•i•ni (man″sə-ne-i′ni) a tribe of mosquitoes of the subfamily Culicinae, including the genera *Coquillettidia* and *Mansonia.*

Man•so•ni•oi•des (man″so-ne-oi′dēz) a subgenus of mosquitoes of the genus *Mansonia. M. annuli′fera* is the chief vector of *Brugia malayi* in India.

man•tle (man′təl) [L. *mantellum* cloak] 1. an enveloping cover or layer. 2. cortex cerebri.

brain m. cortex cerebri.

chordomesodermal m. a continuous epithelial sheet composed of notochordal and mesodermal material during gastrulation.

myoepicardial m. a layer of visceral mesoderm in the early embryo, surrounding the endocardial tube and developing into the myocardium and epicardium.

Man•toux test (reaction) (mahn-too′) [Charles *Mantoux,* French physician, 1877–1947] see under *test.*

man•u•al (man′u-əl) [L. *manualis; manus* hand] 1. of or pertaining to the hand; performed by the hand or hands. 2. a small reference book, particularly one giving instructions or guidelines.

Diagnostic and Statistical M. of Mental Disorders (DSM) see under *D.*

ma•nu•bria (mə-noo′bre-ə) [L.] plural of *manubrium.*

ma•nu•bri•um (mə-noo′bre-əm) pl. *manu′bria* [L.] 1. a handlelike structure or part. 2. m. sterni.

m. mal′lei [TA], m. of malleus the largest process of the malleus; it is attached to the middle layer of the tympanic membrane and has the tendon of the tensor tympani muscle attached to it.

m. ster′ni [TA], m. of sternum the cranial portion of the sternum, which articulates with the clavicles and the first two pairs of ribs.

manu•dy•na•mom•e•ter (man″u-di″nə-mom′ə-tər) [*manus* + *dynamo-* + *-meter*] an apparatus for measuring the force of the thrust of an instrument.

ma•nus (ma′nəs) pl. *ma′nus* [L.] [TA] hand: the distal region of the upper limb, including the carpus, metacarpus, and digits.

m. ca′va a hand deformed by a deep hollowing of the palm.

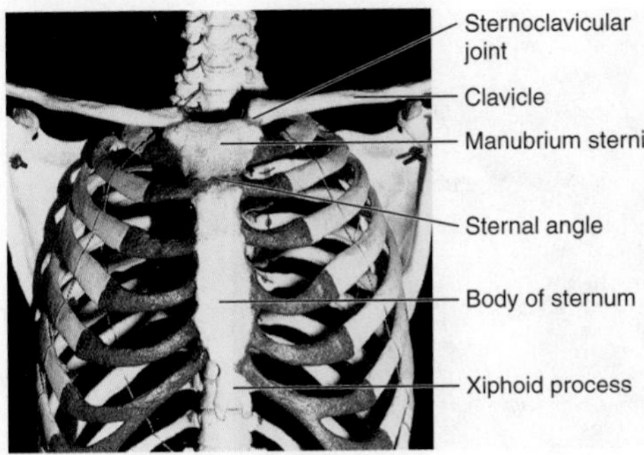

■ Manubrium sterni.

m. exten′sa backward deviation of the hand.
m. flex′a forward deviation of the hand.
m. pla′na flattening of the arch formed normally by the proximal row of the carpal bones; called also *flat hand.*
m. val′ga see *radial clubhand* and *ulnar clubhand,* under *clubhand.*
m. va′ra see *radial clubhand* and *ulnar clubhand,* under *clubhand.*

many·plies (men′ĭ-plīz″) omasum.

man·za·ni·ta (man″zə-ne′ta) [Sp., dim. of *manzana* apple] *Arctostaphylos manzanita.*

MAO maximal acid output; monoamine oxidase (see *amine oxidase [flavin-containing]*).

MAOI monoamine oxidase inhibitor.

MAP mean arterial pressure; microtubule-associated protein.

map (map) a two-dimensional graphic representation of arrangement in space.
chromosome m. a map showing the position of genetic loci on a chromosome, such as a gene map or cytogenetic map.
conjugation m. a gene map used in bacterial genetics, giving the distances between loci based on the time in minutes required to transfer DNA between loci in conjugation.
contig m. a type of physical map composed of overlapping smaller DNA fragments whose order is determined by matching landmarks on the smaller fragments.
cytogenetic m. a map showing the position of gene loci relative to chromosome bands.
fate m. a plan of a blastula or early gastrula stage of an embryo showing areas of prospective significance in normal development.
gene m. a map showing the linear arrangement of genetic loci on a DNA molecule and indicating the distance between them, either in relative or physical units.
genetic m., linkage m. a gene map giving the positions of known genes and markers relative to each other, based on recombination frequencies, rather than as specific physical points; the unit of measurement is the centimorgan. Cf. *physical m.*
genome m. a map that reconstructs the entire set of chromosomes for an organism, giving the relative location of each of the genes, and at its most complete including the entire DNA sequence of all chromosomes.

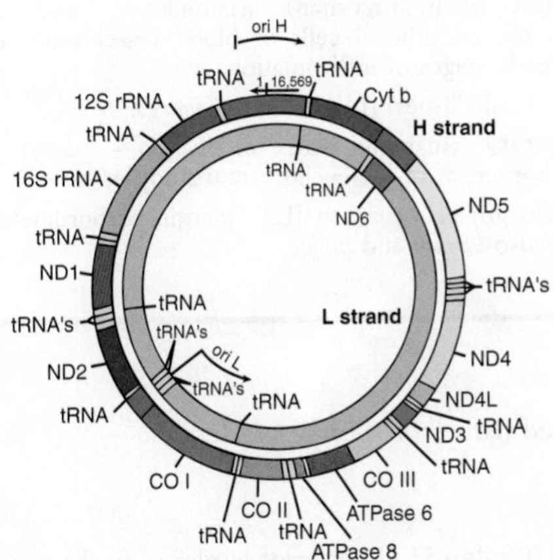

■ Gene map of human mitochondrial DNA, showing the genes transcribed from the heavy (H) and light (L) strands, transcription proceeding counterclockwise on H and clockwise on L. *Ori H, Ori L,* origins of replication; *ND1–6,* NADH dehydrogenase subunits; *Cyt b,* cytochrome b; *CO I–III,* cytochrome oxidase subunits; *tRNA,* transfer RNA; *rRNA,* ribosomal RNA.

physical m. a gene map showing the linear order of genes or markers in the genome, along with the physical distances between them, rather than the frequencies of recombination; measured in base pairs. Cf. *genetic m.*
radiation hybrid m. a physical map created by exposing a cell line containing a human chromosome to radiation, producing breaks in the chromosome; the resulting human chromosome fragments are then fused with rodent chromosomes, and the human fragments identified using amplification techniques; the frequency of breakage between, and subsequent separation of, two loci varies relative to their distance from each other.
restriction m. a physical map indicating restriction enzyme cleavage sites.
STS (sequence-tagged site) m. a physical map indicating the relative order of and distance between sequence-tagged sites (q.v.) within a DNA region.
transduction m. a gene map used in bacterial genetics, giving distances between loci based on relative cotransduction frequencies.

MAPK mitogen-activated protein kinase.

MAP ki·nase (map′ ki′nās) mitogen-activated protein kinase.

ma·ple (ma′pəl) any plant of the genus *Acer.*

map·ping (map′ing) the creation on a flat surface of a representation of an area, showing the relative positions of various features. See also entries under *map.*
body surface m. creation of maps that use contour lines to delineate the isopotential areas of the body surface as determined by electrocardiography, with the potential distributions updated continually during the recording period.
cardiac m. an electrophysiological procedure in which electrical potentials recorded by electrodes placed directly on the heart are processed to give a two-dimensional display of the origin and path of an electrical impulse as it depolarizes the heart.
gene m. determining information about genetic loci on chromosomes, such as relative and absolute positions and DNA sequence; see also under *map.*
intraoperative lymphatic m. sentinel node biopsy.
lymphatic m. the use of dyes or radioactive tracers to identify the first lymph node draining the area of a tumor (sentinel node, q.v.).
peptide m. fingerprinting (q.v.) of a protein.

ma·pro·ti·line (mə-pro′tĭ-lēn) a tetracyclic antidepressant having pharmacological effects similar to those of the tricyclic antidepressants.
m. hydrochloride [USP] the hydrochloride salt of maprotiline, administered orally in the treatment of major depressive disorder; dysthymic disorder; the depressed phase of bipolar disorder; and anxiety associated with depression. It is also used to treat some types of chronic pain.

ma·ran·tic (mə-ran′tik) [Gr. *marantikos* wasting away] marasmic.

ma·ras·moid (mə-raz′moid) resembling marasmus.

ma·ras·mus (mə-raz′məs) [Gr. *marasmos* a dying away] a form of protein-energy malnutrition primarily due to prolonged severe caloric deficit, usually during the first year of life, with growth retardation and progressive wasting of subcutaneous fat and muscle, but usually with retention of the appetite and mental alertness. Infectious diseases may be precipitating factors. Called also *infantile atrophy, athrepsia,* and *pedatrophia.* Cf. *kwashiorkor.* **marasmat′ic, maras′mic** *adj*
enzootic m. a condition of malnutrition in herbivorous animals due to a deficiency of one or more trace elements, especially cobalt or copper. It is marked by progressive emaciation, severe anemia, and finally prostration. See also *bush sickness* and *salt sickness,* under *sickness,* and see *pining.*
nutritional m. marasmic kwashiorkor.

mar·ble·iza·tion (mahr″bəl-ĭ-za′shən) the state of being veined like marble.

Mar·burg disease (hemorrhagic fever), virus (mahr′boork) [*Marburg,* Germany, where the disease was first recognized in 1967] see under *disease* and *virus.*

marc (mahrk) [Fr.] the residue left after maceration of substances used in the preparation of various drugs.

Mar·caine (mahr-kān′) trademark for preparations of bupivacaine hydrochloride.

march (mahrch) the progression of electrical activity through the motor cortex.
cortical m., epileptic m. jacksonian m.
jacksonian m. the spread of abnormal electrical activity from one area of the cerebral cortex to adjacent areas, characteristic of jacksonian epilepsy.

marche (marsh) [Fr.] gait.
m. à petits pas (ah pəte′ pah′) ["gait with little steps"] an abnormal gait in which the patient takes very short steps: seen in some forms of parkinsonism and cerebral arteriosclerosis.

Mar·che·sa·ni syndrome (mahr″kə-sah′ne) [Oswald *Marchesani,* German ophthalmologist, 1900–1952] Weill-Marchesani syndrome.

Mar•chi balls, etc. (mahr′ke) [Vittorio *Marchi*, Italian physician, 1851–1908] see under *ball, globule,* and *reaction,* see *tractus tectospinalis,* and see *Stains and Staining Methods,* under *stain.*

Mar•chi•a•fa•va-Bi•gna•mi disease (mahr″ke-ə-fah′vah be-nyah′me) [Ettore *Marchiafava*, Italian pathologist, 1847–1935; Amico *Bignami*, Italian pathologist, 1862–1929] see under *disease.*

Mar•chi•a•fa•va-Mi•che•li disease (syndrome) (mahr″ke-ə-fah′vah me-ka′le) [E. *Marchiafava;* Ferdinando *Micheli*, Italian physician, 1847–1935] paroxysmal nocturnal hemoglobinuria.

Mar•cus Gunn (mahr′kəs gun) see *Gunn.*

Mar•di•vi•rus (mahr′dĭ-vi″rəs) [*Mar*ek *di*sease + *virus*] a genus of viruses of the subfamily Alphaherpesvirinae (family Herpesviridae); species gallid herpesvirus 1 and gallid herpesvirus 2 cause Marek disease in chickens.

Ma•rek disease (mah′rek) [Josef *Marek*, Hungarian veterinarian, 1867–1952] see under *disease.*

ma•ren•nin (mə-ren′in) [*Marennes,* France, where the oysters are found] a green pigment found in certain oysters, derived from the chlorophyll of a microorganism infesting them.

ma•re•nos•trin (mar″ənos′trin) [L. *Mare Nostrum* our sea (the Mediterranean Sea)] pyrin.

Ma•rey's law (mah-rāz′) [Etienne Jules *Marey*, French physiologist, 1830–1904] see under *law.*

Mar•fan syndrome (mahr′fan) [Antonin Bernard Jean *Marfan*, French pediatrician, 1858–1942] see under *syndrome.*

mar•fan•oid (mahr′fən-oid) having the characteristic symptoms of Marfan syndrome.

mar•gar•i•to•ma (mahr″gər-ĭ-to′mə) cholesteatoma.

mar•gin (mahr′jin) a boundary or edge, such as the boundary of an organ or tumor. Called also *border* and *margo* [TA]. **mar′ginal** *adj*

acetabular m. limbus acetabuli.

acute m. of heart inferior margin of heart.

anal m. the area of the anus just outside the anocutaneous line.

ciliary m. of iris margo ciliaris iridis.

costal m. arcus costalis.

excision m., m. of excision surgical m.

m. of exposure a term proposed to replace the term *m. of safety.*

falciform m. of saphenous opening margo falciformis hiatus saphenus.

free m. of eyelid the conjunctival-lined portion of each eyelid, about 1 mm broad, overlying the eyeball; the anterior border of each bears the eyelashes, and the posterior border is closely applied to the eyeball.

free gingival m., free gum m. margo gingivalis.

frontal m. of greater wing of sphenoid bone margo frontalis alae majoris.

gingival m., gum m. margo gingivalis.

incisal m. margo incisalis.

inferior m. of heart the sharp edge between the sternocostal and diaphragmatic surfaces of the heart, formed mainly by the right ventricle and slightly by the left ventricle, near the apex. Called also *inferior border, acute border,* or *acute m. of heart.*

inferolateral m. of cerebral hemisphere margo inferolateralis hemispherii cerebri.

inferomedial m. of cerebral hemisphere margo inferomedialis hemispherii cerebri.

infraorbital m. of maxilla margo infraorbitalis maxillae.

infraorbital m. of orbit margo infraorbitalis orbitae.

lacrimal m. of maxilla margo lacrimalis maxillae.

lambdoid m. of occipital bone margo lambdoideus ossis occipitalis.

lateral m. of orbit margo lateralis orbitae.

lateral m. of tongue margo linguae.

left m. of heart the rounded margin separating the sternocostal and left surfaces of the heart, formed mainly by the left ventricle but also including a small part of the left atrium and extending obliquely from the left atrium to the apex of the heart in a curve that is convex to the left. Called also *left border, obtuse border* or *obtuse m. of heart.*

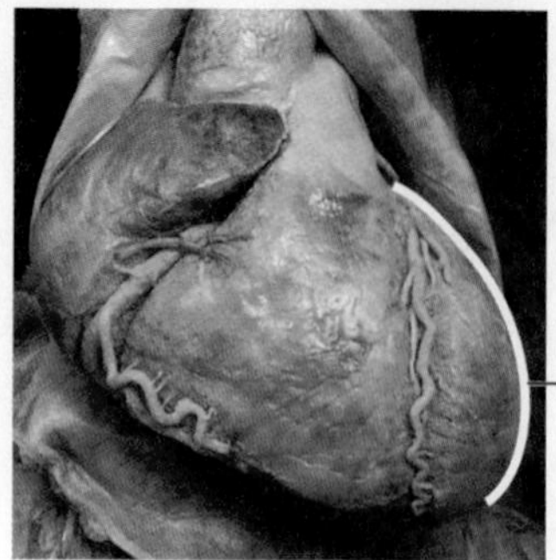

■ Left margin of heart, in an anterior view.

mastoid m. of occipital bone margo mastoideus ossis occipitalis.

medial m. of orbit margo medialis orbitae.

nasal m. of frontal bone margo nasalis ossis frontalis.

obtuse m. of heart left m. of heart.

occipital m. of parietal bone margo occipitalis ossis parietalis.

occipital m. of temporal bone margo occipitalis ossis temporalis.

orbital m. margo orbitalis.

palpebral m., anterior limbus anterior palpebrae.

palpebral m., posterior limbus posterior palpebralis.

parietal m. of frontal bone margo parietalis ossis frontalis.

parietal m. of greater wing of sphenoid bone margo parietalis alae majoris.

parietal m. of squamous part of temporal bone margo parietalis partis squamosae ossis temporalis.

pupillary m. of iris margo pupillaris iridis.

right m. of heart margo dexter cordis.

m. of safety a calculation that takes the highest animal *no observed adverse effect level* (q.v.) and estimates a maximum safe level of exposure for humans. It is now generally superseded by the reference dose.

sphenoidal m. of frontal bone margo sphenoidalis ossis frontalis.

sphenoidal m. of squamous part of temporal bone margo sphenoidalis partis squamosae ossis temporalis.

squamosal m. of greater wing of sphenoid bone margo squamosus alae majoris.

superior m. of cerebral hemisphere margo superior hemispherii cerebri.

superomedial m. of cerebral hemisphere margo superior hemispherii cerebri.

supraorbital m. of frontal bone margo supraorbitalis ossis frontalis.

supraorbital m. of orbit margo supraorbitalis orbitae.

surgical m. the edge of something being surgically removed, such as of skin or other tissue around a lesion.

m. of tongue margo linguae.

zygomatic m. of greater wing of sphenoid bone margo zygomaticus alae majoris.

mar•gi•na•tion (mahr″jĭ-na′shən) accumulation and adhesion of leukocytes to the endothelial cells of blood vessel walls at the site of injury in the early stages of inflammation.

mar•gi•nes (mahr′jĭ-nēs) [L.] plural of *margo.*

mar•gino•plas•ty (mahr-jin′ə-plas″te) [*margin* + *-plasty*] surgical restoration of a border, as of the eyelid. **marginoplas′tic** *adj*

mar•go (mahr′go) pl. *mar′gines* [L.] margin or border; the edge of a structure. See also *labium* and *limbus.*

Margo

Descriptions are given on TA terms, and include anglicized names of specific borders.

m. aceta′buli TA alternative for *limbus acetabuli.*

m. ante′rior cor′poris pancre′atis [TA] anterior border of body of pancreas: the pancreatic border that bounds the anterosuperior and anteroinferior surfaces.

m. ante′rior fi′bulae [TA] anterior border of fibula: the anterolateral border of the body of the fibula.

m. ante′rior pulmo′nis [TA] anterior border of lung: the ventral border of either lung, which descends from behind the sternum,

Margo *Continued*

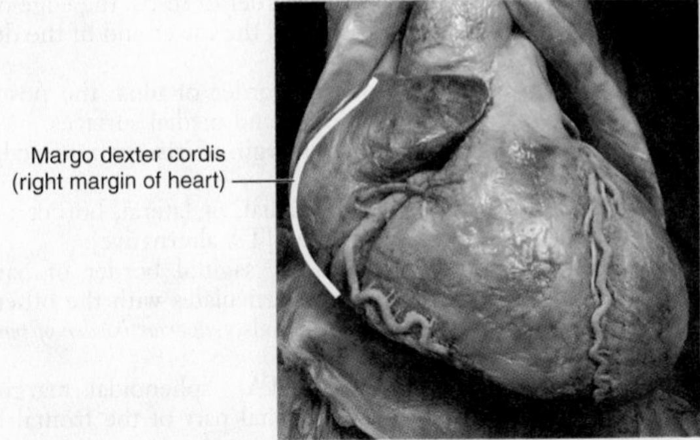

■ Margo dexter cordis (right margin of heart), in an anterior view.

slightly lateral to the midline, and curves laterally to meet the inferior margin.
m. ante′rior ra′dii [TA] anterior border of radius: the edge of the radius that runs obliquely between the radial tuberosity and the styloid process.
m. ante′rior tes′tis [TA] anterior border of testis: the rounded free edge of the testis.
m. ante′rior ti′biae [TA] anterior border of tibia: the prominent anteromedial margin of the body of the tibia, separating the medial and lateral surfaces.
m. ante′rior ul′nae [TA] anterior border of ulna: the volar border of the ulna, separating the medial and posterior surfaces.
m. arcua′tus hia′tus saphe′ni TA alternative for *margo falciformis hiatus sapheni.*
m. cilia′ris i′ridis [TA] ciliary margin of iris: the outer border of the iris, where it is continuous with the ciliary body.
m. dex′ter cor′dis [TA] right margin of heart: the margin of the heart formed by the wall of the profile of the right atrium, running from the apex to the right, and marking the junction of the sternocostal and diaphragmatic cardiac surfaces; seen as a surface except in radiograms and two-dimensional illustrations. Called also *right border of heart.*
m. falcifor′mis hia′tus saphe′ni [TA] falciform margin of saphenous opening: the lateral margin of the saphenous opening; called also *m. arcuatus hiatus sapheni* [TA alternative].
m. fibula′ris pe′dis TA alternative for *m. lateralis pedis.*
m. fronta′lis a′lae majo′ris [TA] frontal margin of greater wing of sphenoid bone: a roughened area on the greater wing where it articulates with the frontal bone; it is at the superolateral margin of the orbital surface of the greater wing at its junction with the cerebral and temporal surfaces.
m. fronta′lis os′sis parieta′lis [TA] frontal border of parietal bone: the edge of the parietal bone that articulates with the frontal bone along the coronal suture.
m. gingiva′lis [TA] gingival margin: the crest of the free gingiva that surrounds the teeth in a collarlike fashion, separated from the adjacent periodontium protectoris by the free gingival groove; it forms the wall of the gingival sulcus. Called also *free gingival margin, free gum margin, gum margin,* and *marginal gingiva.*

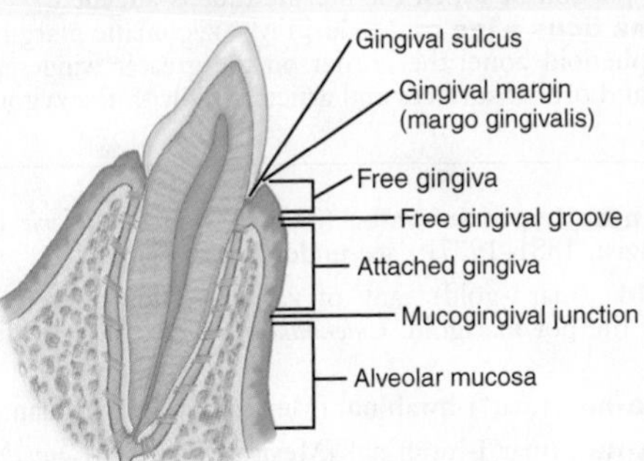

m. incisa′lis [TA] incisal margin: the crest of the biting edge of an incisor tooth.
m. infe′rior cor′poris pancre′atis [TA] inferior border of body of pancreas: the pancreatic border that bounds the anteroinferior and posterior surfaces.
m. infe′rior he′patis [TA] inferior border of liver: the anteroinferior edge of the liver, separating the diaphragmatic and visceral surfaces.
m. infe′rior pulmo′nis [TA] inferior border of lung: the border of the lung that extends in a curve behind the sixth costal cartilage, the upper margin of the eighth rib in the axillary line, the ninth or tenth rib in the scapular line, and passes medially to the eleventh costovertebral joint.
m. infe′rior sple′nis [TA] inferior border of spleen: a straight border of the spleen somewhat less prominent than the superior border, separating the renal surface from the diaphragmatic surface.
m. inferolatera′lis hemisphe′rii ce′rebri [TA] inferolateral margin of cerebral hemisphere: the inferior lateral border of the cerebral hemisphere.
m. inferomedia′lis hemisphe′rii ce′rebri [TA] inferomedial margin of cerebral hemisphere: the inferior medial margin of the cerebral hemisphere.
m. infraorbita′lis maxil′lae [TA] infraorbital margin of maxilla: the short rounded edge of the maxilla where the orbital surface becomes continuous with the anterior surface.
m. infraorbita′lis or′bitae [TA] infraorbital margin of orbit: the inferior edge of the entrance to the orbit, formed by the infraorbital process of the zygomatic bone and the infraorbital margin of the maxilla.
m. interos′seus fi′bulae [TA] interosseous border of fibula: a prominent ridge medial to the anterior border of the fibula, connected with a similar ridge on the tibia by a strong, wide fibrous sheet, the interosseous membrane; called also *interosseous crest of fibula.*
m. interos′seus ra′dii [TA] interosseous border of radius: the prominent medial border of the radius, connected with a similar ridge on the ulna by a strong, wide fibrous sheet, the interosseous membrane; called also *interosseous crest of radius.*
m. interos′seus ti′biae [TA] interosseous border of tibia: the prominent lateral border of the body of the tibia, which separates the posterior and lateral surfaces and gives attachment to the interosseous membrane; called also *interosseous crest of tibia.*
m. interos′seus ul′nae [TA] interosseous border of ulna: the prominent lateral border of the ulna, connected with a similar ridge on the radius by the interosseous membrane; called also *interosseous crest of ulna.*
m. lacrima′lis maxil′lae [TA] lacrimal margin of maxilla: the posterior border of the frontal process of the maxilla where it articulates with the lacrimal bone.
m. lambdoi′deus os′sis occipita′lis [TA] lambdoid border of occipital bone: the edge of the occipital bone that extends from the lateral angle to the superior angle, articulating with the parietal bone to help form the lambdoid suture; called also *lambdoid margin of occipital bone.*
m. latera′lis antebra′chii TA alternative for *m. radialis antebrachii.*
m. latera′lis hu′meri [TA] lateral border of humerus: the edge of the humerus that extends from posteroinferior part of the greater tubercle to the lateral epicondyle.
m. latera′lis or′bitae [TA] lateral margin of orbit: the orbital border formed by the zygomatic process of the frontal bone and the frontal process of the zygomatic bone.
m. latera′lis pe′dis [TA] the lateral, or fibular, border of the foot; called also *m. fibularis pedis* [TA alternative] and *peroneal border of foot.*
m. latera′lis re′nis [TA] lateral border of kidney: the convex narrow border of the kidney.
m. latera′lis sca′pulae [TA] lateral border of scapula: the thick edge of the scapula, extending from the inferior margin of the glenoid cavity to the inferior angle.
m. latera′lis un′guis [TA] lateral border of nail: the edge on either side of the nail; called also *lateral edge of nail.*
m. li′ber ova′rii [TA] free border of ovary: the broad, convex, posterior border of the ovary, opposite the mesovarian margin.
m. li′ber un′guis [TA] free border of nail: the distal overhanging edge of a nail; called also *distal border* or *edge of nail* and *free edge of nail.*
m. lin′guae [TA] margin of tongue: the lateral border of the body of the tongue.
m. mastoi′deus os′sis occipita′lis [TA] mastoid border of occipital bone: the edge of the occipital bone that extends from the jugular process to the lateral angle, articulating with the part of the temporal

Margo *Continued*

bone that bears the mastoid process. Called also *mastoid margin of occipital bone.*
m. media′lis antebra′chii TA alternative for *m. ulnaris antebrachii.*
m. media′lis glan′dulae suprarena′lis [TA] medial border of suprarenal gland: the border that with the superior border divides the anterior from the posterior surface.
m. media′lis hu′meri [TA] medial border of humerus: the edge of the humerus that begins at the lesser tubercle above and continues downward to the medial epicondyle.
m. media′lis or′bitae [TA] medial margin of orbit: the orbital border formed above by the bone and below by the lacrimal crest of the frontal process of the maxilla.
m. media′lis pe′dis [TA] the medial, or tibial, border of the foot; called also *m. tibialis pedis* [TA alternative].
m. media′lis re′nis [TA] medial border of kidney: the concave border of the kidney, which contains the hilum.
m. media′lis sca′pulae [TA] medial border of scapula: the thin edge of the scapula extending from the superior to the inferior angle; called also *vertebral border of scapula.*
m. media′lis ti′biae [TA] medial border of tibia: the border that extends between the medial condyle and medial malleolus of the tibia, separating the medial and posterior surfaces.
m. mesova′ricus ova′rii [TA] mesovarian border of ovary: the border of the ovary that is attached to the broad ligament by means of the mesovarium.
m. nasa′lis os′sis fronta′lis [TA] nasal margin of frontal bone: the articular surface, on each nasal part of the frontal bone, that articulates with the nasal bones and with the frontal processes of the maxilla.
m. occipita′lis os′sis parieta′lis [TA] occipital border of parietal bone: the edge of the parietal bone that articulates with the occipital bone at the lambdoid suture. Called also *occipital margin of parietal bone.*
m. occipita′lis os′sis tempora′lis [TA] occipital margin of temporal bone: the border of the petrous part of the temporal bone that articulates with the occipital bone along the occipitomastoid suture.
m. occul′tus un′guis [TA] hidden border of nail: the proximal buried edge of a nail; called also *proximal border* or *edge of nail.*
m. orbita′lis [TA] orbital margin: the edge of the entrance to the orbit, formed mainly by the frontal and zygomatic bones and the maxilla. See also *m. infraorbitalis orbitae* and *m. supraorbitalis orbitae.*
m. parieta′lis a′lae majo′ris [TA] parietal margin of greater wing of sphenoid bone: the superior edge of the squamous portion of the greater wing, where it articulates with the parietal bone.
m. parieta′lis os′sis fronta′lis [TA] parietal margin of frontal bone: the posterior border of the frontal bone, semicircular in shape, which articulates with the parietal bones.
m. parieta′lis par′tis squamo′sae os′sis tempora′lis [TA] parietal margin of squamous part of temporal bone: the superior border of the squamous part of the temporal bone where it articulates with the parietal bone.
m. poste′rior fi′bulae [TA] posterior border of fibula: the posterolateral ridge of the body of the fibula.
m. poste′rior par′tis petro′sae os′sis tempora′lis [TA] posterior border of petrous part of temporal bone: the border of the petrous part extending from the apex to the jugular notch and articulating with part of the occipital bone.
m. poste′rior ra′dii [TA] posterior border of radius: the edge of the radius that extends from the posterior part of the radial tuberosity to the middle tubercle.
m. poste′rior tes′tis [TA] posterior border of testis: the edge of the testis that is attached to the epididymis and the lower end of the ductus deferens; called also *dorsum of testis.*
m. poste′rior ul′nae [TA] posterior border of ulna: the posterior edge of the ulna, separating the posterior and medial surfaces.
m. pupilla′ris i′ridis [TA] pupillary margin of iris: the inner edge of the iris, surrounding the pupil.
m. radia′lis antebra′chii [TA] the radial, or lateral, border of the forearm; called also *m. lateralis antebrachii* [TA alternative].
m. sagitta′lis os′sis parieta′lis [TA] sagittal border of parietal bone: the edge of the parietal bone that articulates with the other parietal bone along the sagittal suture; called also *superior border of parietal bone.*
m. sphenoida′lis os′sis fronta′lis [TA] sphenoidal margin of frontal bone: the border between the orbital part of the frontal bone and the sphenoid bone.
m. sphenoida′lis par′tis squamo′sae os′sis tempora′lis [TA] sphenoidal margin of squamous part of temporal bone: the anterior border of the temporal bone, articulating with the greater wing of the sphenoid bone.
m. squamo′sus a′lae majo′ris [TA] squamosal margin of greater wing of sphenoid bone: the border of the greater wing of the sphenoid bone that articulates with the squama of the temporal bone.
m. squamo′sus os′sis parieta′lis [TA] squamosal border of parietal bone: the inferior edge of the parietal bone, which articulates with the sphenoid and temporal bones along the squamous suture.
m. supe′rior cor′poris pancre′atis [TA] superior border of body of pancreas: the pancreatic edge that bounds the anterosuperior and posterior surfaces.
m. supe′rior glan′dulae suprarena′lis [TA] superior border of suprarenal gland: the superior edge, which with the medial border divides the anterior from the posterior surface.
m. supe′rior hemisphe′rii cer′ebri [TA] superior margin of cerebral hemisphere: the superior medial margin of the cerebral hemisphere.
m. supe′rior par′tis petro′sae os′sis tempora′lis [TA] superior border of petrous part of temporal bone: the long upper border of the petrosal part; it is grooved by the sulcus for the superior petrosal sinus.
m. supe′rior sca′pulae [TA] superior border of scapula: the thin, short edge of the scapula, extending from the superior angle to the coracoid process.
m. supe′rior sple′nis [TA] superior border of spleen: a somewhat sharp, convex line, sometimes serrated, between the gastric and diaphragmatic surfaces of the spleen.
m. supraorbita′lis or′bitae [TA] supraorbital margin of orbit: the superior edge of the entrance to the orbit, formed by the supraorbital margin of the frontal bone.
m. supraorbita′lis os′sis fronta′lis [TA] supraorbital margin of frontal bone: the anteroinferior edge of the frontal bone, bending down laterally to the zygomatic bone and medially to the frontal process of the maxilla; it marks the junction between the squama and the orbital portion of the bone.
m. tibia′lis pe′dis TA alternative for *m. medialis pedis.*
m. ulna′ris antebra′chii [TA] the ulnar, or medial, border of the forearm; called also *m. medialis antebrachii* [TA alternative].
m. u′teri [TA] border of uterus: the right or left edge of the uterus, at the upper portion of which the uterine tube is attached.
m. zygoma′ticus a′lae majo′ris [TA] zygomatic margin of greater wing of sphenoid bone: the border on the greater wing separating its temporal and orbital surfaces and articulating with the zygomatic bone.

Ma•rie hypertrophy, sign (mah-re′) [Pierre *Marie,* French physician, 1853–1940] see under *hypertrophy* and *sign.*

Ma•rie-Bam•ber•ger disease (mah-re′ bahm′bər-gər) [P. *Marie;* Eugen *Bamberger,* Austrian physician, 1858–1921] hypertrophic pulmonary osteoarthropathy.

Ma•rie-Foix sign (mah-re′ fwah′) [P. *Marie;* Charles *Foix,* French neurologist, 1882–1927] see under *sign.*

Ma•rie-Strüm•pell disease, syndrome (mah-re′ strēm′pəl) [P. *Marie;* Adolf von *Strümpell,* German physician, 1853–1925] rheumatoid spondylitis.

Ma•rie-Tooth disease (mah-re′ to͞oth′) [P. *Marie;* Howard Henry *Tooth,* English physician, 1856–1925] Charcot-Marie-Tooth disease.

Ma•rie Un•na hypotrichosis (mah-re′ oon′ah) [*Marie Unna,* German dermatologist, 1881–1977] see under *hypotrichosis.*

mar•i•gold (mar′ĭ-gōld) any of various yellow-flowered plants; dried flowers of the pot marigold, *Calendula officinalis,* have medicinal uses; see *Calendula.*

mar•i•hua•na (mar″ĭ-hwah′nə) [Mexican Sp.] marijuana.

mar•i•jua•na (mar″ĭ-hwah′nə) [Mexican Sp.] 1. *Cannabis sativa.* 2. a crude preparation of the leaves and flowering tops of *C. sativa,* usually employed in cigarettes and inhaled as smoke for its euphoric properties. See *cannabis.*

Ma•ri•nes•co sign, succulent hand (mah-re-nes′ko) [Georges *Marinesco,* Romanian neurologist, 1863–1938] main succulente.

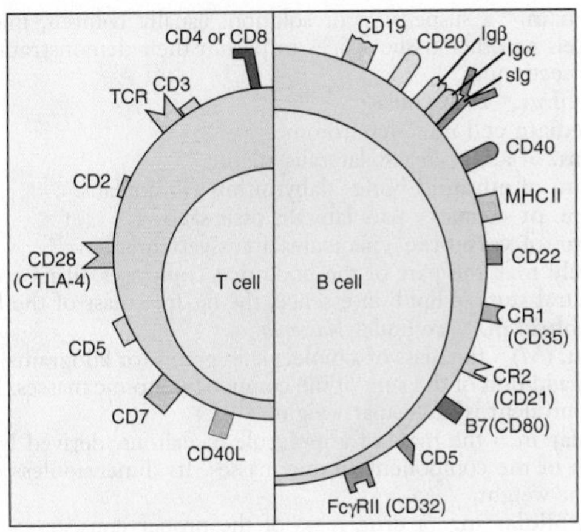

■ Schematic drawing of cell-surface markers on human B and T cells, each marker specific for a different antigen.

Ma•ri•nes•co-Sjö•gren syndrome (mah-re-nes′ko shur′gren) [G. *Marinesco;* Karl Gustav Torsten *Sjögren,* Swedish physician, 1896–1974] see under *syndrome.*

mar•i•no•bu•fa•gin (mar″ĭ-no-bu′fə-jin) a cardiac poison from the skin of the toad, *Bufo marinus.*

Mar•i•nol (mar′ĭ-nol) trademark for a preparation of dronabinol.

Ma•ri•on disease (mah-re-aw′) [Jean Baptiste Camille Georges *Marion,* French urologist, 1869–1960] see under *disease.*

Ma•ri•otte experiment, law, spot (mah-re-ot′) [Edme *Mariotte,* French physicist, 1620–1684] see under *experiment,* and see *Boyle's law,* under *law,* and *blind spot,* under *spot.*

mar•i•tal (mar′ĭ-təl) of or pertaining to marriage.

mar•i•to•nu•cle•us (mar″ĭ-to-noo′kle-əs) [L. *maritus* married + *nucleus*] the nucleus of the oocyte after the spermatozoon has entered it.

Mar•jo•lin ulcer (mahr″zho-lă′) [Jean Nicolas *Marjolin,* French surgeon, 1780–1850] see under *ulcer.*

mark (mahrk) a spot, blemish, or other circumscribed area visible on a surface, particularly on the skin or mucous membrane.
  birth m. see *birthmark.*
  pock m. see *pockmark.*
  Pohl-Pinkus m. see under *constriction.*
  port-wine m. see under *stain.*
  strawberry m. 1. see under *hemangioma.* 2. cavernous hemangioma. 3. vascular nevus.
  stretch m's popular term for *striae distensae;* see under *stria.*

mark•er (mahrk′ər) something that identifies or that is used to identify; cf. *determinant.*
  cell-surface m. an antigenic determinant occurring on the surface of a specific type of cell.
  genetic m. a segment of DNA with a known chromosomal location and an easily detectable phenotype, the inheritance of which can thus be followed.
  surrogate m. a phenomenon whose presence provides indirect evidence for the presence of another phenomenon, such as the viral load as an indicator of the state of the immune system in HIV infection.
  tumor m. a circulating biochemical substance indicative of neoplasia; the most useful being specific, sensitive, and proportional to tumor load. Tumor markers may be used to screen, diagnose, assess prognosis, follow response to treatment, and monitor for recurrence.

Mar•low test (mahr′lo) [Frank William *Marlow,* American ophthalmologist, 1858–1942] see under *test.*

mar•mo•ra•tion (mahr″mo-ra′shən) [L. *marmor* marble] marbleization.

mar•mo•re•al (mahr-mo′re-əl) resembling marble, as bone in osteoporosis.

mar•mot (mahr′mot) any member of the genus *Marmota,* such as the hoary marmot, the yellow-bellied marmot, the woodchuck of North America, and the tarbagan of Asia; several are natural reservoirs of the plague.

Mar•mo•ta (mahr-mo′tə) the marmots, a genus of the family Sciwiidae, terrestrial rodents of North America, Europe, and Asia that are sometimes reservoirs of plague. *M. bo′bak* is the tarbagan of Europe and Asia. *M. mo′max* is the woodchuck of northeastern North America.

Mar•o•gen (mar′ə-jen) trademark for a preparation of epoetin beta.

Ma•ro•teaux acromesomelic dysplasia (mah-ro-to′) [Pierre *Maroteaux,* French physician, born 1926] see under *dysplasia.*

Ma•ro•teaux-La•my syndrome (mah-ro-to′ lah-me′) [P. *Maroteaux;* Maurice Emile Joseph *Lamy,* French physician, 1895–1975] see under *syndrome.*

Mar•plan (mahr′plan) trademark for a preparation of isocarboxazid.

mar•row (mar′o) 1. medulla ossium. 2. any of various soft substances resembling bone marrow (medulla ossium).
  bone m. medulla ossium.
  bone m., red medulla ossium rubra.
  bone m., yellow medulla ossium flava.
  depressed m. bone marrow exhibiting decreased hematopoietic activity. See *bone marrow suppression,* under *suppresssion.*
  fat m. medulla ossium flava.
  gelatinous m. bone marrow that has lost its blood cells and its fat and has acquired a gelatinous appearance.
  red m. medulla ossium rubra.
  spinal m. medulla spinalis.
  yellow m. medulla ossium flava.

mar•ru•bi•in (mə-roo′be-in) a lactone principle, the active ingredient of horehound.

Mar•ru•bi•um (mə-roo′be-əm) a genus of mints of the family Lamiaceae, native to Europe and Asia. *M. vulga′re* (Tourn.) L. is horehound, whose leaves and tops (also called *horehound*) contain marrubiin and are used medicinally.

Mars•de•nia (mahrz-de′ne-ə) a genus of woody vines of the family Asclepiadaceae. *M. conduran′go* Reichb. f. is condurango, a South American species whose bark (also called condurango) is usually poisonous but in small amounts is medicinal.

Marsh disease (mahrsh) [Sir Henry *Marsh,* Irish physician, 1790–1860] Graves disease.

Mar•shall fold, vein (mahr′shəl) [John *Marshall,* English anatomist, 1818–1891] see *plica venae cavae sinistrae* and *vena obliqua atrii sinistri.*

Mar•shall-Mar•chet•ti-Krantz operation (mahr′shəl mahr-ket′e krants′) [Victor F. *Marshall,* American urologist, 1913–2001; Andrew A. *Marchetti,* American obstetrician and gynecologist, 1901–1970; Kermit E. *Krantz,* American obstetrician and gynecologist, born 1923] see under *operation.*

marsh•mal•low (mahrsh′mel″o, -mal″o) 1. a perennial Eurasian herb, *Althaea officinalis,* having clusters of pink flowers and a long, thick, mucilaginous root; the flowers, leaves, syrup, and roots are used medicinally. 2. a preparation of *A. officinalis,* used in the treatment of cough and for irritation of the oral and pharyngeal mucosa; it also has a variety of uses in folk medicine.

mar•su•pia (mahr-soo′pe-ə) [L.] plural of *marsupium.*

mar•su•pi•al (mahr-soo′pe-əl) [L. *marsupium* a pouch] a member of the order Marsupialia.

Mar•su•pi•a•lia (mahr-soo″pe-a′le-ə) an order of the class Mammalia characterized by possession of a marsupium where the young, which are born in an underdeveloped state, are carried and nourished until their development is complete. In some systems of classification, it is considered to be an order of the infraclass or subclass Metatheria. It includes the opossums, kangaroos, wallabies, koalas, and wombats.

mar•su•pi•al•iza•tion (mahr-soo″pe-əl-ĭ-za′shən) [L. *marsupium* pouch] the creation of a pouch; applied especially to surgical exteriorization of a cyst by resection of the anterior wall and suture of the cut edges of the remaining cyst to the adjacent edges of the skin, thereby establishing a pouch of what was formerly an enclosed cyst.

mar•su•pi•um (mahr-soo′pe-əm) pl. *marsu′pia* [L. "a pouch"] 1. an external abdominal pouch or fold of skin for carrying the young; it contains the mammary glands and occurs in marsupials and the spiny anteaters. 2. a similar structure for carrying eggs or the young, as in the male sea horse. 3. scrotum.
  marsu′pia patella′ria plicae alares.

Mar•tin-Bell syndrome (mahr′tin bel′) [James Purdon *Martin,* British physician, 1893–1984; Julia *Bell,* British geneticist, 1879–1979] fragile X syndrome.

Mar•ti•not•ti cells (mahr″te-no′te) [Giovanni *Martinotti,* Italian pathologist, 1857–1928] see under *cell.*

Mar•to•rell syndrome (mahr-to-rel′) [Fernando *Martorell* Otzet, Spanish cardiologist, 1906–1984] Takayasu arteritis; see under *arteritis.*

masc mass concentration.

mas•cu•line (mas′ku-lin″) [L. *masculinus*] 1. pertaining to the male sex. 2. having qualities normally characteristic of males; called also *virile.*

mas·cu·lin·i·ty (mas″ku-lin′ĭ-te) the possession of masculine qualities. Called also *virility.*

mas·cu·lin·iza·tion (mas″ku-lin-ĭ-za′shən) 1. the normal development of primary or secondary sex characters in the male. 2. the induction or development of male secondary sex characters in the female or prepubertal male, such as enlargement of the clitoris or penis, growth of facial and body hair, and deepening of the voice. In females, it is called also *gynandrism.* 3. the condition of having such sex characters. Called also *androgenization.* Cf. *virilescence, virilism,* and *virilization.*

mas·cu·li·nize (mas′ku-lĭ-nīz″) 1. to produce normal secondary sex characters in a male. 2. to produce male secondary sex characters in a female or prepubertal male; see *masculinization* (def. 2).

mas·cu·lin·iz·ing (mas′ku-lin-iz″ing) producing masculinization.

ma·ser (ma′zər) [*m*icrowave *a*mplification by *s*timulated *e*mission of *r*adiation] a device which produces an extremely intense, small, and nearly nondivergent beam of monochromatic radiation in the microwave region with all waves in phase.

mask (mask) 1. a covering for the face, such as a bandage, an apparatus for administering oxygen, or a cloth for prevention of spread of droplets from the nose and mouth. 2. to cover or conceal the true nature of something, such as of a disorder by unrelated symptoms. See *masked.* 3. to interfere with processing of a stimulus; see *masking.* 4. in dentistry, to camouflage metal parts of a prosthesis by covering with opaque material.

BLB m. a face mask that has a combined inspiratory and expiratory valve and a bag for rebreathing, used mainly with oxygen delivery systems at high altitudes, and occasionally for clinical administration of oxygen.

death m. a plaster cast of the face of a dead person.

ecchymotic m. cyanotic discoloration of the head and neck as a result of traumatic asphyxia.

full-face m. a device used in anesthesia to confine the gas to be delivered through the mask into the respiratory tract through the nose or mouth.

Hutchinson m. a sensation as if the skin of the face were compressed by a mask; often a symptom of tabes dorsalis.

meter m. a face mask used with oxygen delivery systems, designed to provide fixed percentage admixtures of air and oxygen.

Parkinson m. see under *facies.*

m. of pregnancy popular term for melasma during pregnancy.

tabetic m. Hutchinson m.

Venturi m. a face mask used in oxygen therapy, delivering a controlled mixture of oxygen and air.

masked (maskt) 1. concealed from view; hidden. 2. not presenting or producing the usual symptoms. 3. blind (def. 2).

mask·ing (mask′ing) 1. in neuropsychology, interference with the processing of one stimulus by accompanying it with a stronger second stimulus; in audiometry, the obscuring of one sound by the presence of another, stronger sound. 2. blinding.

visual m. the most common type of masking used in neuropsychological assessment. It may be either *forward,* with the stronger stimulus coming first, or *backward,* with the stronger stimulus coming second but before the person has processed the initial stimulus.

maso·chism (mas′o-kiz-əm) [Leopold von Sacher-*Masoch,* an Austrian novelist, 1836–1895] the act or instance of gaining pleasure from experiencing physical or psychological pain; the term is usually used to denote *sexual m.* **mas′ochist** *n* **masochis′tic** *adj*

sexual m. [DSM-IV] a paraphilia in which sexual gratification is derived from being hurt, humiliated, or otherwise made to suffer physically or psychologically.

ma·so·pro·col (mə-so′prə-kol) an arachidonate 5-lipoxygenase inhibitor applied topically as an antineoplastic in the treatment of actinic keratoses.

Mas. pil. [L.] mas′sa pilula′rum (pill mass).

mass (mas) [L. *massa*] 1. a lump or body made up of cohering particles; see also *massa.* 2. a cohesive mixture suitable for being made up into pills. 3. the characteristic of matter that gives it inertia; the SI unit for mass is the kilogram. Symbol *m.*

appendiceal m., appendix m. a palpable mass in the right iliac fossa or right loin due to acute appendicitis, usually with abscess secondary to rupture; occasionally caused by adherent omentum and intestine.

atomic m. atomic weight; used particularly when describing a single isotope of a nuclide.

body cell m. the total weight of the cells of the body, including the cell nucleus, cytoplasm, water, salt, protein, and surrounding membrane, but excluding extracellular water and extracellular solids such as collagen, elastin, and bone matrix, constituting in essence the total mass of oxygen-utilizing, carbohydrate-burning, and energy-exchanging cells of the body; regarded as proportional to total exchangeable potassium in the body.

injection m. a suspension or solution, usually colored, injected into blood vessels or other tissue spaces to permit their demonstration on dissection or sectioning.

inner cell m. embryoblast.

intermediate cell m. nephrotome.

lateral m. of atlas massa lateralis atlantis.

lateral m. of ethmoid bone labyrinthus ethmoidalis.

lateral m. of sacrum pars lateralis ossis sacri.

lateral m. of vertebrae pediculus arcus vertebrae.

lean body m. the part of the body that comprises all its components except neutral storage lipid; in essence, the fat-free mass of the body.

metanephric m. see under *blastema.*

molar m. (*M*) the mass of a molecule in grams (or kilograms) per mole, derived by addition of the sum of the component atomic masses. Its dimensionless equivalent is molecular weight.

molecular m. the mass of a molecule in daltons, derived by addition of the sum of the component atomic masses. Its dimensionless equivalent is molecular weight.

pill m., pilular m. a drug mass of the proper consistency for being made into pills.

relative molecular m. (M_r) technically preferable term for *molecular weight.*

Stent m. a plastic resinous material which sets into a very hard substance; used in surgery for making molds shaped to keep grafts in place. See also *stent.*

tigroid m′s Nissl bodies.

ventrolateral m. the portion of the primordial lateral mass of the embryo from which are developed the abdominal, thoracic, and anterior cervical muscles.

mas·sa (mas′ə) gen. and pl. *mas′sae* [L.] mass: anatomic nomenclature for a cohesive lump of material such as tissue or cells.

m. innomina′ta paradidymis.

m. interme′dia adhesio interthalamica.

m. latera′lis atlan′tis [TA] lateral mass of atlas: the thickened lateral portion of the atlas to which the arches are attached and which bears the articulating surfaces and the transverse process.

m. latera′lis os′sis ethmoida′lis labyrinthus ethmoidalis.

m. latera′lis os′sis sa′cri pars lateralis ossis sacri.

m. latera′lis ver′tebrae pediculus arcus vertebrae.

mas·sae (mas′e) [L.] genitive and plural of *massa.*

mas·sage (mə-sahzh′) [Fr., from Gr. *massein* to knead] systematic therapeutic friction, stroking, and kneading of the body.

cardiac m. rhythmic compression of the heart by pressure applied manually over the sternum *(closed cardiac massage)* or directly to the heart through an opening in the chest wall *(open cardiac massage);* done to reinstate and maintain circulation.

carotid sinus m. firm rotatory pressure applied to one side of the neck over the carotid sinus of the supine patient; it causes vagal stimulation, increasing vagal inhibition of sinus and atrioventricular nodes, and it can slow or terminate tachycardia.

classical Western m. methods of massage based on European concepts of anatomy and physiology and using five basic techniques: effleurage, pétrissage, friction, tapotement, and vibration.

deep m. massage techniques whose purpose is to reach structures beneath the superficial tissues, using effleurage, direct pressure, or friction applied perpendicular to the fibers of the affected tissue.

electrovibratory m. massage by means of an electric vibrator.

gingival m. the systematic application of frictional rubbing and stroking to the gingiva.

heart m. cardiac m.

ice m. massage in which ice is rubbed over the body surface for local analgesic effects and relief of muscle spasms.

pneumatic m. pneumomassage.

Swedish m. the most commonly used form of classical Western massage (q.v.), generally performed in the direction of the heart, sometimes with active or passive movement of the joints; used especially for relaxation, relief of muscular tension, and improvement of circulation and range of motion.

vibratory m. electrovibratory m.

mas·sa·sau·ga (mas″ə-saw′gə) [corruption of *Missisauga,* a river in Ontario, Canada] *Sistrurus catenatus,* a small venomous rattlesnake found from New York State to the southwestern United States and northern Mexico. Called also *Massasauga rattlesnake.*

mas·se·ter (mə-se′tər) [Gr. *masētēr* chewer] see *musculus masseter.*

mas·se·ter·ic (mas″ə-ter′ik) pertaining to the masseter muscle.

mas·seur (mə-soor′) [Fr.] 1. a man who performs massage. 2. an instrument for performing massage.

mas·seuse (mə-sooz′) [Fr.] a woman who performs massage.

Human Adenoviruses

Species	Serotype
A	HAdV 12, 18, 31
B	
B1	HAdV 3, 7, 11, 16, 21
B2	HAdV 14, 34, 35, 50
C	HAdV 1, 2, 5, 6
D	HAdV 8, 9, 10, 13, 15, 17, 19, 20, 22–30, 32, 33, 36–39, 42–49, 51
E	HAdV 4
F	HAdV 40, 41

mas•sive (mas′iv) extensive or to a great extent; having a solid bulky form.

Mas•son stain, tumor (mah-saw′) [Claude Laurent Pierre *Masson*, French-born pathologist in Canada, 1880–1959] see *Stains and Staining Methods*, under *stain*, and *intravascular papillary endothelial hyperplasia*, under *hyperplasia*.

mas•so•ther•a•py (mas″o-ther′ə-pe) [Gr. *massein* to knead + *therapy*] the treatment of disease by massage.

MAST [*m*ilitary or *m*edical *a*nti-*s*hock *t*rousers] see *pneumatic antishock garment*, under *garment*.

mas•tad•e•ni•tis (mas″tad-ə-ni′tis) [*mast-* + *aden-* + *-itis*] mastitis.

Mas•tad•e•no•vi•rus (mast-ad′ə-no-vi″rəs) [*mast-* + *adenovirus*] mammalian adenoviruses; a genus of viruses of the family Adenoviridae that infect mammals, causing disease of the respiratory tract, gastrointestinal tract, conjunctiva, central nervous system, and urinary tract; infection may be asymptomatic. Many species induce malignancy. Human viruses are grouped into six species (A–F), including two subspecies of B (B1 and B2), on the basis of structural, immunological, biological, and chemical characteristics and comprise over 50 serotypes. (See accompanying table.) **mastadenovi′ral** *adj*

mas•tal•gia (mas-tal′jə) [*mast-* + *-algia*] pain in the breast; called also *mammalgia* and *mastodynia*.

mas•ta•tro•phia (mas″tə-tro′fe-ə) mastatrophy.

mas•tat•ro•phy (mas-tat′rə-fe) [*mast-* + *atrophy*] atrophy of the mammary gland.

mas•tauxe (mas-tawk′se) [*mast-* + Gr. *auxē* increase] abnormal enlargement of the breast.

mas•tec•to•my (mas-tek′tə-me) [*mast-* + *-ectomy*] excision of the breast; called also *mammectomy*.

extended radical m. radical mastectomy with removal of the ipsilateral half of the sternum and a portion of ribs two through five with the underlying pleura and the internal mammary lymph nodes.

Halsted m. radical m.

Meyer m. radical m.

modified radical m. simple mastectomy together with axillary lymphadenectomy, but with preservation of the pectoral muscles. See illustration.

partial m. removal of only enough breast tissue to ensure that the margins of the resected surgical specimen are free of tumor; called also *segmental m.*

radical m. removal of the breast, pectoral muscles, axillary lymph nodes, and associated skin and subcutaneous tissue in treatment of breast cancer.

segmental m. partial m.

simple m. removal of only the breast tissue and nipple and a small portion of the overlying skin. See illustration.

skin-sparing m., subcutaneous m. excision of breast tissue with preservation of overlying skin, nipple, and areola so that breast form may be reconstructed.

total m. simple m.

Mas•ter "2-step" exercise test (mas′tər) [Arthur Matthew *Master*, American physician, 1895–1973] see under *test*.

mas•tic (mas′tik) [L. *mastiche*; Gr. *mastichē*] 1. *Pistacia lentiscus*. 2. a resinous exudation obtained from *P. lentiscus*, used as a flavored chewing gum base, in plasters, lacquers, and incense, and pharmaceutically in enteric coatings for tablets.

mas•ti•ca•tion (mas″tĭ-ka′shən) [L. *masticare* to chew] chewing; the process of biting and grinding food in preparation for swallowing and digestion.

mas•ti•ca•to•ry (mas′tĭ-kə-tor″e) 1. subserving or pertaining to mastication; affecting the muscles of mastication. 2. a remedy to be chewed but not swallowed.

Mas•ti•go•my•co•ti•na (mas″tĭ-go-mi″ko-ti′nə) [Gr. *mastix* whip + *mykēs* fungus] a grouping of organisms usually considered a subphylum of fungi under the phylum Eumycota; they have a unicellular or mycelial thallus and motile reproductive cells. Animal pathogens are included in the class Oomycetes. In some systems of classification, they are assigned to the Protista rather than the Fungi.

mas•ti•gont (mas′tĭ-gont) [Gr. *mastigoun* to whip] a flagellum; see under *system*.

Mas•ti•goph•o•ra (mas″tĭ-gof′ə-rə) [Gr. *mastix* whip + *phoros* bearing] in older systems of classification, a subphylum of protozoa of the phylum Sarcomastigophora, comprising the flagellates, i.e., all those with one or more flagella in the trophozoite. Mastigophorans have a simple, centrally placed nucleus and reproduce by longitudinal binary fission, and most are free-living but many are parasitic in invertebrates or vertebrates. This group was traditionally divided into the classes Phytomastigophorea and Zoomastigophorea.

mas•ti•goph•o•ran (mas″tĭ-gof′ə-rən) 1. a protozoan of the subphylum Mastigophora. 2. of or belonging to the subphylum Mastigophora; called also *flagellate* and *mastigote*.

mas•ti•goph•o•rous (mas″tĭ-gof′ə-rəs) mastigophoran (def. 2).

Mas•ti•go•proc•tus (mas″tĭ-go-prok′təs) a genus of whip scorpions (order Pedipalpa). *M. gigan′teus* is the vinegaroon, a species with irritating secretions.

mas•ti•gote (mas′tĭ-gōt) mastigophoran.

mas•ti•tis (mas-ti′tis) [*mast-* + *-itis*] inflammation of the mammary gland, or breast.

bovine m. inflammation of the mammary gland of a cow, usually due to an infectious agent such as a bacterium or fungus. Common bacterial pathogens are *Staphylococcus aureus* (see *staphylococcal m.*), *Streptococcus agalactiae*, other species of streptococci, and coliform bacteria (see *coliform m.*). The milk from infected cows may be watery or serous with clots or flakes and clear or brownish in color. Called also *garget*.

chronic cystic m. fibrocystic disease of breast; see under *disease*.

coliform m. bovine mastitis caused by *Escherichia coli*, *Klebsiella* species, or *Enterobacter aerogenes*. The udder becomes inflamed and slightly enlarged and the milk is thin, serous, and brown with flakes. Affected cows may suffer from anorexia, fever, and fatal toxemia.

glandular m. parenchymatous m.

interstitial m. inflammation of the stroma of the mammary gland.

m.-metritis-agalactia lactation failure in swine; see under *failure*.

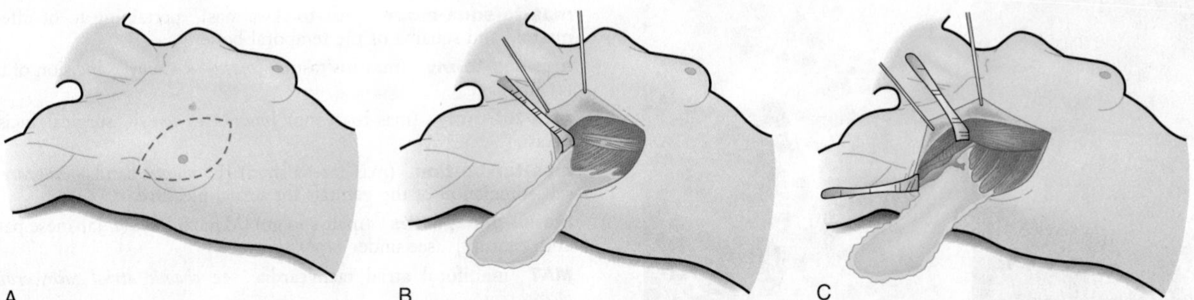

■ *(A, B)*, Simple mastectomy. *(A)*, Skin incisions are generally transverse and surround the central breast and nipple-areolar complex. *(B)*, Skin flaps are raised sharply, separating the gland from the overlying skin and from the underlying muscle. The breast is divided from the axillary contents and dissection stops at the clavipectoral fascia. *(C)*, Modified radical mastectomy. Dissection continues into the axilla and generally up to the axillary vein, removing the level I and sometimes also the level II nodes.

m. neonato´rum a general term applied to an abnormal condition of the breast of the newborn, such as hypertrophy, engorgement and secretion, or inflammation, with or without suppuration.

nocardial m. mastitis in cattle caused by an infection with *Nocardia asteroides* or *N. farcinica.* Characteristics include granulomatous lesions of the udder with fibrosis, inflammation, abscesses, and fever; damage to the udder and milk supply is usually permanent.

parenchymatous m. inflammation of the secreting elements of the mammary gland.

periductal m. inflammation of tissues around the ducts of the mammary gland.

phlegmonous m. inflammation of the breast leading to abscess formation.

plasma cell m. a condition of the breast characterized by infiltration of the breast stroma with plasma cells and proliferation of the cells lining the ducts, possibly related to mammary duct ectasia.

puerperal m. a form of mastitis occurring after delivery.

retromammary m., submammary m. paramastitis.

stagnation m. a local engorgement affecting one or more lobules of the breast and forming a painful lump in the organ; it occurs during early lactation. Called also *caked breast.*

staphylococcal m. bovine mastitis caused by infection with *Staphylococcus aureus;* it may be either subclinical or acute. The acute forms sometimes result in skin sloughing, gangrene, and death. Cf. *udder impetigo.*

suppurative m. mastitis with production of pus.

tuberculous m. mastitis occurring with pulmonary tuberculosis, seen most often in young women.

mast(o)- [Gr. *mastos* breast] a combining form denoting relationship to the breast or to the mastoid process; see also words beginning *mamm(o)-* and *maz(o)-.*

mas•to•cyte (mas´to-sīt″) [Ger. *Mast* food + *-cyte*] mast cell.

mas•to•cy•to•ma (mas″to-si-to´mə) [*masto-* + *cytoma*] a nodular cutaneous mast cell infiltrate, usually present at birth or soon after as a solitary nodule, although three to four lesions may occur. Lesions typical of urticaria pigmentosa may occur later. Called also *mast cell tumor.*

mas•to•cy•to•sis (mas″to-si-to´sis) [*masto-* + *cytosis*] a group of rare diseases characterized by infiltrates of mast cells in the tissues and sometimes other organs. The group includes *diffuse* and *systemic m., mastocytoma, urticaria pigmentosa,* and *telangiectasia macularis eruptiva perstans.*

diffuse m., diffuse cutaneous m. a condition in which the entire skin is thickened, lichenified, and leathery in appearance and accompanied by generalized erythroderma and intense pruritus as a result of widespread infiltration with mast cells. In children, it is often associated with systemic mastocytosis.

systemic m. a condition in which there are mast cell infiltrates in noncutaneous tissues, with or without cutaneous lesions; the most common sites are the liver, spleen, bone, lymph nodes, and gastrointestinal tract. See also *mastocytosis syndrome,* under *syndrome.*

mas•to•dyn•ia (mas″to-din´e-ə) mastalgia.

mas•toid (mas´toid) [*masto-* + *-oid*] 1. breast shaped. 2. mastoid process. 3. pertaining to the mastoid process.

mas•toid•al (mas-toid´əl) mastoid (def. 3).

mas•toi•da•le (mas″toi-da´le) the lowest point of the mastoid process.

mas•toid•al•gia (mas″toid-al´jə) [*mastoid* + *-algia*] pain in the mastoid region.

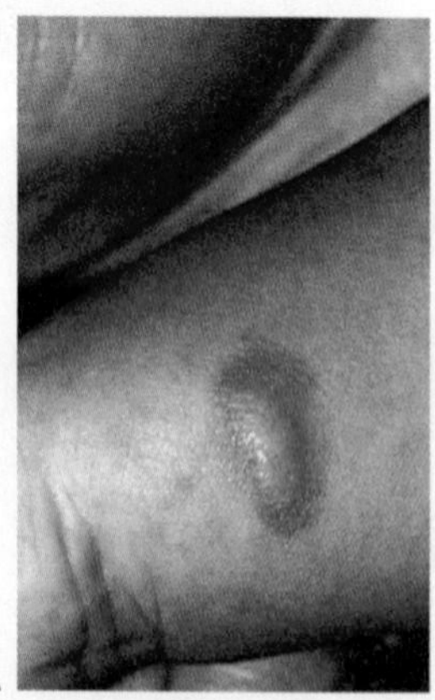

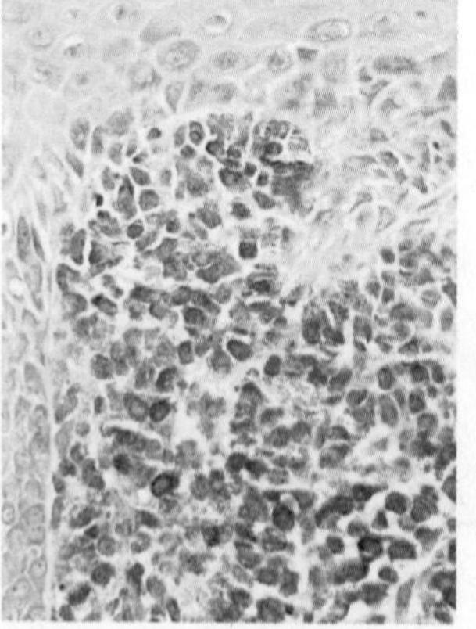

■ Mastocytoma. *(A)*, Solitary mastocytoma in a child; *(B)*, Giemsa stain reveals purple granules characteristic of mast cells in the dermis.

mas•toid•ec•to•my (mas″toid-ek´tə-me) [*mastoid* + *-ectomy*] excision of the mastoid air cells or the mastoid process.

Bondy m. modified radical m.

canal wall down m. open-cavity tympanomastoidectomy.

canal wall up m. closed-cavity tympanomastoidectomy.

closed-cavity m. see under *tympanomastoidectomy.*

cortical m. complete simple m.

intact canal wall m. closed-cavity tympanomastoidectomy.

open-cavity m. see under *tympanomastoidectomy.*

radical m. mastoidectomy with exenteration of air cells, removal of the entire posterior wall of the ear canal, and removal of the tympanic membrane, malleus, and incus, resulting in permanent hearing loss.

radical m., modified mastoidectomy with exenteration of air cells and removal of part of the posterior wall of the ear canal but with preservation of some or all of the ossicles; hearing may be preserved.

simple m. mastoidectomy with exenteration of air cells but no involvement of the wall of the ear canal.

simple m., complete mastoidectomy with exenteration of the air cells and epitympanum but no involvement of the wall of the ear canal. Called also *cortical m.*

mas•toi•deo•cen•te•sis (mas-toi″de-o-sen-te´sis) [*mastoid* + *-centesis*] surgical puncture of the mastoid antrum.

mas•toid•itis (mas″toid-i´tis) inflammation of the mastoid antrum and air cells, sometimes as a result of otitis media.

Bezold m. mastoiditis in which the pus has escaped and formed tracts into the neck; see *Bezold abscess,* under *abscess.*

coalescent m. mastoiditis in which the bony partitions between the air cells erode so that air cells coalesce into large cavities; further erosion of the temporal bone may lead to intracranial abscess.

sclerosing m. mastoiditis attended with hardening and condensation of the bone.

silent m. a progressive destructive mastoiditis with mild systemic and local manifestations.

mas•toid•ot•o•my (mas″toi-dot´ə-me) [*mastoid* + *-tomy*] surgical incision of the mastoid process, usually into the antrum.

Mas•to•mys (mas´tə-mis″) a genus of small African rodents of the family Muridae. *M. natalen´sis* is the multimammate mouse, a species that lives in close proximity to humans in Africa and is the natural host of Lassa virus. An inbred strain is used in cancer research.

mas•to•oc•cip•i•tal (mas″to-ok-sip´ĭ-təl) pertaining to the mastoid process and the occipital bone.

mas•to•pa•ri•e•tal (mas″to-pə-ri´ə-təl) pertaining to the mastoid process and the parietal bone.

mas•to•path•ia (mas″to-path´e-ə) mastopathy.

m. cys´tica a morbid condition of the mammary gland, with the formation of cysts.

mas•top•a•thy (mas-top´ə-the) [*masto-* + *-pathy*] disease of the mammary gland.

cystic m. mastopathia cystica.

mas•to•pexy (mas´to-pek″se) [*masto-* + *-pexy*] mammaplasty performed to correct a pendulous breast.

Mas•toph•o•ra (mas-tof´ə-rə) a genus of spiders; called also *Glyptocranium. M. gasteracanthoi´des* is the cat-headed spider of South America.

mas•to•pla•sia (mas″to-pla´zhə) mammoplasia.

mas•to•plas•ty (mas´to-plas″te) mammaplasty. **mastoplas´tic** *adj*

mas•to•pto•sis (mas″top-to´sis, mas″to-to´sis) [*masto-* + *-ptosis*] pendulous breasts.

mas•tor•rha•gia (mas″to-ra´jə) [*masto-* + *-rrhagia*] hemorrhage from the mammary gland.

mas•to•squa•mous (mas-to-skwa´məs) pertaining to or affecting the mastoid and squama of the temporal bone.

mas•tos•to•my (mas-tos´tə-me) [*masto-* + *-stomy*] incision of the breast for drainage.

mas•tot•o•my (mas-tot´ə-me) [*masto-* + *-tomy*] surgical incision of a breast.

mas•tur•ba•tion (mas″tər-ba´shən) [L. *manus* hand + *stuprare* to rape] self-stimulation of the genitals for sexual pleasure.

Ma•su•gi nephritis (mah-soo´ge) [Matazo *Masugi,* Japanese pathologist, 20th century] see under *nephritis.*

MAT multifocal atrial tachycardia; see *chaotic atrial tachycardia,* under *tachycardia.*

Mat•as operation, test (mat´əs) [Rudolph *Matas,* American surgeon, 1860–1957] see *endoaneurysmorrhaphy,* and see *tourniquet test* (def. 2), under *test.*

match•ing (mach′ing) 1. comparison and selection of objects having similar or identical characteristics. 2. the selection of compatible donors and recipients for transfusion or transplantation. See also *typing.* 3. the selection of subjects for clinical trials or other studies so that the different groups being compared are similar in specified characteristics, e.g., age, sex, or race, in order to reduce bias and error caused by comparison of dissimilar groups. Matching may be on an individual (matched pairs) or a group-wide basis.

cross m. crossmatching.

ma•té (mah-ta′) [Fr., from Sp. *mate*] the dried leaves of *Ilex paraguensis*, used as a source of tea in South America; it contains caffeine and tannins, and has been used as a tonic, diuretic, stomachic, stimulant, and laxative (large doses).

ma•ter (ma′tər) [L.] mother.

arachnoi′dea m. see *arachnoidea mater*, under *A.*

dura m. see *dura mater*, under *D.*

pi′a m. see *pia mater*, under *P.*

ma•te•ria (mə-tēr′e-ə) [L.] matter.

m. al′ba a white to cream-colored, cheesy mass deposited around the necks of the teeth, composed of food debris, mucin, and dead epithelial cells.

m. me′dica pharmacology.

ma•te•ri•al (mə-tēr′e-əl) substance or elements from which a concept may be formulated, or an object constructed.

baseplate m. any dental material used in the construction of a baseplate, including silver, gold, aluminum, platinum, alloys, and plastics.

cross-reacting m. (CRM) a functionally inactive protein, produced by a mutant structural gene, that reacts with antibody to the normal protein.

dental m. any material used in dental practice, particularly a material used in the production of dental bases, restorations, impressions, or prostheses.

impression m. any material used for making dental impressions and impressions of oral structures for restorations, prostheses, and dentures; materials include elastomeric materials, dental plasters, metallic oxide pastes, impression compounds, reversible and irreversible hydrocolloids, silicone base materials, polyethers, polysulfide rubber, and duplicating compounds.

tissue-equivalent m. a material whose absorbing and scattering properties for a given radiation simulate as closely as possible those of a given biological tissue, such as bone, fat, or muscle. Water, for example, is usually the best tissue equivalent material for muscle and soft tissue.

ma•ter•nal (mə-tur′nəl) [L. *maternus; mater* mother] pertaining to the mother.

ma•ter•ni•ty (mə-tur′nĭ-te) [L. *mater* mother] 1. motherhood. 2. a lying-in hospital.

Ma•the•vo•tae•nia (mə-the″vo-te′ne-ə) a genus of tapeworms of the family Anoplocephalidae. The species *M. symme′trica* is a cosmopolitan intestinal parasite of rodents, with insects as intermediate hosts; it has been reported in human infections in Thailand.

Ma•thieu procedure (mah-tyoo′) [P. *Mathieu*, French physician, 20th century] see under *procedure.*

mat•ing (māt′ing) [from Middle Low Ger. *mate* companion] pairing of individuals of opposite sexes, especially for reproduction.

assortative m., assortive m. nonrandom mating in which choice of a mate is influenced by phenotype. *Positive assortative mating* occurs when phenotypically similar mates are chosen, e.g., tall men and tall women; *negative assortative mating* occurs when phenotypically dissimilar mates are chosen, e.g., tall men and short women. Such mating can affect Hardy-Weinberg equilibrium (q.v.) in a population.

backcross m. the mating of a heterozygote and a recessive homozygote; useful in revealing, through the phenotypes of the offspring, the genotype of the heterozygous parent.

nonrandom m. mating in which partner selection is not independent of genotype, such as occurs with assortative mating, inbreeding, or stratification of populations into subgroups.

random m. mating in which partner selection is independent of genotype; for a genotype at any one locus there is a purely random probability of combining with any other genotype at that locus. Called also *panmixis.*

mat•rass (mat′rəs) a glass vessel with a long neck used for treating dry substances in chemical procedures.

mat•ri•cal (mat′rĭ-kəl) of or relating to a matrix.

Ma•tri•ca•ria (mat″rĭ-kar′e-ə) [L.] a genus of flowering herbs of the family Compositae, native to Europe and Asia. *M. recuti′ta* (formerly *M. chamomilla*) is one of two plants called chamomile, whose dried flower heads are used medicinally. *M. nigellaefo′lia* is a type of feverfew and causes hepatic encephalopathy in cattle.

mat•ri•ca•ria (mat″rĭ-kar′e-ə) any plant of the genus *Matricaria*; see also *chamomile.*

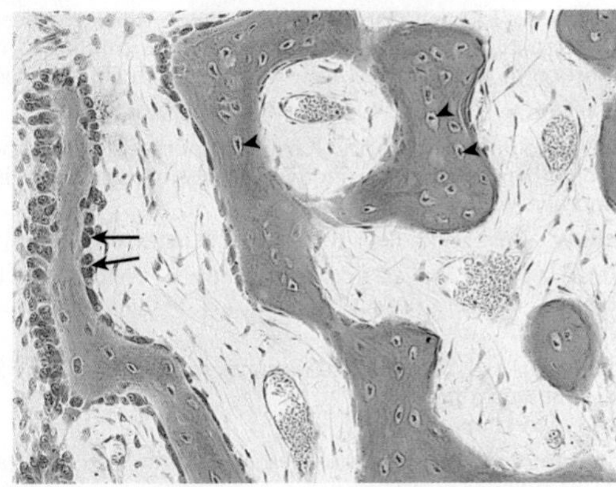

■ Bone matrix, showing intramembranous ossification. Trabeculae of bone are being formed by osteoblasts lining their surface *(arrows)*, osteocytes can be seen trapped in lacunae *(arrowheads)*, and primitive osteons are beginning to form.

ma•tri•cec•to•my (ma″trĭ-sek′tə-me) surgical removal of part of the nail matrix as a treatment for an ingrown toenail; called also *matrixectomy.*

ma•tri•ces (ma′trĭ-sēz) plural of *matrix.*

ma•tri•cial (mə-trish′əl) matrical.

mat•ri•cli•nous (mat′rĭ-kli′nəs) matroclinous.

ma•tri•lin•e•al (ma″trĭ-lin′e-əl) [*mater* + *linea*] descended through the female line.

ma•trix (ma′triks) pl. *ma′trices* [L.] 1. the intracellular substance of a tissue or the tissue from which a structure develops. 2. the groundwork on which anything is cast, or that basic material from which a thing develops. 3. a mold or a form for casting. 4. a plastic or metal strip used to support and shape a plastic restorative material. 5. a piece of gold or platinum foil fitted against the sides and bottom of a cavity, used as a mold in which porcelain for an inlay is baked. 6. resin m. 7. term used for the feldspar component of dental porcelain, which provides a glassy matrix in which quartz particles are dispersed.

amalgam m. matrix band.

bone m. the intercellular substance of bone, consisting of osteocollagenous fibers embedded in an amorphous ground substance and inorganic salts.

capsular m. territorial m.

cartilage m. the intercellular substance of cartilage, consisting of cells and extracellular fibers embedded in an amorphous ground substance; see also *interterritorial m.* and *territorial m.*

cytoplasmic m. the fluid substance of the cytoplasm that fills the spaces between organelles and within the cytoskeleton.

extracellular m. (ECM) any material produced by cells and excreted to the extracellular space within the tissues. It takes the form of both ground substance and fibers and is composed chiefly of fibrous elements, proteins involved in cell adhesion, and glycosaminoglycans and other space-filling molecules. It serves as a scaffolding holding tissues together and its form and composition help determine tissue characteristics. In epithelia, it includes the basement membrane.

functional m. the contiguous and motivating soft tissue organs and tissues in the growth of the craniofacial complex.

germinal m. 1. a gelatinous, highly vascular region of the fetal ependyma that is the source of neurons and glial cells and involutes in the second trimester. 2. an area of reproducing cells, such as a hair matrix or nail matrix.

hair m. the epidermal root of the hair follicle.

interterritorial m. a paler-staining region located among the darker territorial matrices.

mitochondrial m. the dense substance, containing the mitochondrial DNA, ribosomes, and granules, found in the inner chamber (intercristal space) of mitochondria.

nail m., m. of nail m. unguis.

nuclear m. a protein network that fills the nucleus and is associated with a number of nuclear processes, including DNA replication, RNA transcription and processing, and receptor binding. Called also *nucleoskeleton.*

resin m. in a resin matrix composite, the continuous phase (an organic polymer) in which the discrete particles of filler are dispersed. Called also *matrix.*

sarcoplasmic m. the liquid substance which fills muscle cells; it contains the soluble enzymes of the cell.

stem body m. a dense mass of material, appearing at anaphase, that stabilizes the microtubules of the central spindle.

territorial m. basophilic material surrounding groups of cartilage cells.

m. un′guis 1. [TA] nail matrix: the tissue upon which the deep aspect of the nail rests; called also *nail bed.* 2. sometimes limited to only the proximal portion of this structure, from which growth chiefly proceeds.

ma•trix•ec•to•my (ma″trik-sek′tə-me) matricectomy.

mat•ro•cli•nous (mat″ro-kli′nəs) [Gr. *mētēr* mother + *klinein* to incline] inheriting or inherited from the mother; possessing characters inherited from the mother. Cf. *patrocliny.*

mat•ro•cli•ny (mat″ro-kli′ne) the state of being matroclinous.

matte (mat) a term applied to a macroscopic morphology of bacterial colonies that are dull and slightly granular, i.e., neither smooth and glistening nor rough.

mat•ter (mat′ər) 1. anything that occupies space; substance. 2. pus.
gray m. substantia grisea.
white m. substantia alba.

Mat•tox maneuver (mat′əks) [Kenneth L. *Mattox,* American surgeon, born 1938] see under *maneuver.*

Mat•u•lane (mat′u-lān) trademark for a preparation of procarbazine hydrochloride.

mat•u•rate (mach′u-rāt) mature (def. 1).

mat•u•ra•tion (mach″u-ra′shən) [L. *maturatio; maturus* ripe] 1. the stage or process of becoming mature or fully developed. 2. the attainment of emotional and intellectual maturity. 3. in biology, a process of cell division during which the number of chromosomes in the germ cells is reduced to one half the number characteristic of the species. 4. suppuration.

affinity m. the progressive increase in the affinity of antigen for antibody occurring during the immune response, due to selection of B lymphocytes with receptors having high affinity for the antigen.

ma•ture (mə-cho͞or′) [L. *maturus*] 1. to develop to maturity; to ripen. 2. fully developed; ripe.

ma•tur•i•ty (mə-cho͞or′ĭ-te) the period of attainment of maximal development.

Matut. [L.] matuti′nus (in the morning).

ma•tu•ti•nal (mə-too′tĭ-nəl) [L. *matutinalis*] pertaining to or occurring in the morning.

Mau•chart ligament (mou′kahrt) [Burkhard David *Mauchart,* German anatomist, 1696–1751] ligamenta alaria.

Mau•noir hydrocele (mo-nwahr′) [Jean Pierre *Maunoir,* Swiss surgeon, 1768–1861] cervical hydrocele.

Mau•rer dots (clefts, spots), stippling (mou′rer) [Georg *Maurer,* German physician, early 20th century] see under *dot* and *stippling.*

Mau•ri•ac syndrome (mo″re-ahk′) [Pierre *Mauriac,* French physician, 1832–1905] see under *syndrome.*

Mau•ri•ceau maneuver (mo″re-so′) [François *Mauriceau,* French obstetrician, 1637–1709] see under *maneuver.*

Mauth•ner cell, fiber, membrane (sheath) (mout′nər) [Ludwig *Mauthner,* Czech-born Austrian ophthalmologist, 1840–1894] see under *cell* and *fiber,* and see *axolemma.*

mau•ve•in (mo′ve-in) aniline purple, a violet dye used as an indicator, with a pH range of −0.1 to 2.9, being yellow at −0.1 and crimson at 2.9.

Ma•vik (ma′vik) trademark for a preparation of trandolapril.

Max•air (maks′ār) trademark for a preparation of pirbuterol acetate.

Max•alt (maks′awlt) trademark for preparations of rizatriptan benzoate.

Max•a•quin (maks′ə-kwin) trademark for a preparation of lomefloxacin hydrochloride.

MaxEPA (max-e″pe-a′) trademark for a preparation of eicosapentaenoic acid and docosahexaenoic acid.

Max•ib•o•lin (mak-sib′o-lin) trademark for a preparation of ethylestrenol.

Max•i•dex (mak′sĭ-deks″) trademark for a preparation of dexamethasone.

Max•i•done (mak′sĭ-dōn″) trademark for combination preparations of hydrocodone bitartrate and acetaminophen.

Max•i•flor (mak′sĭ-flor″) trademark for preparations of diflorasone diacetate.

max•il•la (mak-sil′ə) gen. *maxil′lae* pl. *maxil′lae, maxillas* [L.] [TA] the irregularly shaped bone that with its fellow forms the upper jaw; it assists in the formation of the orbit, the nasal cavity, and the palate, and lodges the upper teeth. **max′illary** *adj*

max•il•lae (mak-sil′e) [L.] genitive and plural of *maxilla.*

max•il•lec•to•my (mak″sĭ-lek′tə-me) surgical removal of the maxilla.

max•il•li•tis (mak″sĭ-li′tis) inflammation of the maxilla.

max•il•lo•den•tal (mak-sil″o-den′təl) pertaining to the maxilla and the maxillary teeth.

max•il•lo•eth•moi•dec•to•my (mak-sil″o-eth″moi-dek′tə-me) excision of the portion of the maxilla surrounding the maxillary sinus and of the cribriform plate and anterior ethmoid cells.

max•il•lo•fa•cial (mak-sil″o-fa′shəl) pertaining to the maxilla and the face.

max•il•lo•ju•gal (mak-sil″o-joo′gəl) zygomaticomaxillary.

max•il•lo•la•bi•al (mak-sil″o-la′be-əl) pertaining to the maxilla and the lip.

max•il•lo•man•dib•u•lar (mak-sil″o-man-dib′u-lər) pertaining to the maxilla and the mandible.

max•il•lo•pal•a•tine (mak-sil″o-pal′ə-tēn) palatomaxillary.

max•il•lo•pha•ryn•ge•al (mak-sil″o-fə-rin′je-əl) pharyngomaxillary.

max•il•lot•o•my (mak″sĭ-lot′ə-me) surgical sectioning of the maxilla which allows movement of all or a part of the maxilla into the desired position.

max•i•ma (mak′sĭ-mə) [L.] plural of *maximum.*

max•i•mal (mak′sĭ-məl) the greatest possible, allowable, or appreciable; the reverse of *minimal.*

max•i•mum (mak′sĭ-məm) pl. *max′ima* [L. "greatest"] 1. the greatest possible or actual effect or quantity. 2. the acme of a disease or process. 3. largest; utmost. 4. Pirquet's term for the greatest quantity of food an organism can digest.

transport m. (T_m) the highest rate in milligrams per minute at which the renal tubules can transfer a substance either from the tubular luminal fluid to the interstitial fluid or from the interstitial fluid to the tubular luminal fluid, beyond which it may be excreted in the urine. In kidney function tests, it is expressed as T_m with inferior letters representing the substance used in the test, such as $T_{m_{PAH}}$ (transport maximum for *p*-aminohippuric acid).

transport m. for glucose renal threshold for glucose.

tubular m. (T_m) transport m.

Max•i•pime (mak′sĭ-pīm) trademark for a preparation of cefepime.

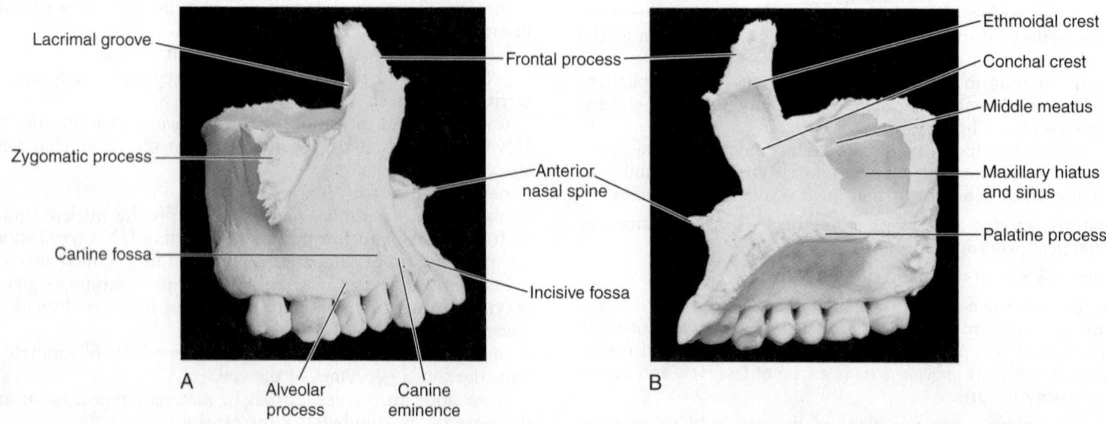

■ Right maxilla. *(A),* Lateral view; *(B),* medial view.

Max·i·vate (mak′sĭ-vāt) trademark for preparations of betamethasone dipropionate.

Max·on (mak′son) trademark for polyglyconate.

Max·zide (maks′īd) trademark for a combination preparation of triamterene and hydrochlorothiazide.

Max·well ring (maks′wel) [Patrick William *Maxwell*, Irish ophthalmologist, 1856–1917] see under *ring*.

May-Hegg·lin anomaly (mi′ heg′lin) [Richard *May*, German physician, 1863–1936; Robert Marquard *Hegglin*, Swiss physician, 1907–1969] see under *anomaly*.

May-White syndrome (ma′ hwīt′) [Duane L. *May*, American physician, 20th century; Harry H. *White*, American physician, born 1934] see under *syndrome*.

May·dl operation (mi′dəl) [Karel *Maydl*, Czech surgeon, 1853–1903] see under *operation*.

May·er hemalum, mucihematein (mi′ər) [Paul *Mayer*, German-born chemist in Italy, 1848–1923] see *Stains and Staining Methods*, under *stain*.

May·er test (ma′yər) [Ferdinand F. *Mayer*, American pharmaceutical chemist, late 19th century] see under *test*.

May·er-Ro·ki·tan·sky-Kü·ster-Hau·ser syndrome (mi′er ro-kĭ-tahn′ske ke′ster hou′zer) [August Franz Josef Karl *Mayer*, German physician, 1787–1865; Karl Freiherr von *Rokitansky*, Austrian pathologist, 1804–1878; Hermann *Küster*, German gynecologist, early 20th century; G.A. *Hauser*, Swiss physician, 20th century] see under *syndrome*.

may·fly (ma′fli) any insect of the order Ephemeroptera.

Ma·yo vein (ma′yo) [William James *Mayo*, American surgeon, 1861–1939] vena prepylorica.

Ma·yo Rob·son see *Robson*.

may·tan·sine (ma-tan′sēn) an antineoplastic derived from species of *Maytenus*, a genus of tropical American shrubs and trees.

may·weed (ma′wēd) *Anthemis cotula*.

Ma·za·braud syndrome (mah-zah-bro′) [André *Mazabraud*, French pathologist, 1921-2006] see under *syndrome*.

maze (māz) a complicated system of intersecting paths used in intelligence tests and in demonstrating learning in experimental animals.

ma·zin·dol (ma′zin-dol) [USP] a sympathomimetic amine having amphetamine-like actions; used as an oral anorectic in the short-term treatment of exogenous obesity.

maz(o)- [Gr. *mazos* breast] a combining form denoting relationship to the breast; see also words beginning *mamm(o)-* and *mast(o)-*.

ma·zo·dyn·ia (ma″zo-din′e-ə) mastodynia.

ma·zo·pexy (ma′zo-pek″se) mastopexy.

ma·zo·pla·sia (ma″zo-pla′zhə) [Gr. *mazos* breast + *-plasia*] degenerative epithelial hyperplasia of the mammary acini.

Maz·zot·ti reaction, test (mah-zo′te) [Luis *Mazzotti*, Mexican parasitologist, 1900–1971] see under *reaction* and *test*.

MB [L.] Medici′nae Baccalau′reus (Bachelor of Medicine).

Mb megabase; myoglobin.

m.b. [L.] mis′ce be′ne (mix well).

MBC minimal bactericidal concentration.

MBP major basic protein; myelin basic protein.

MBL mannose-binding lectin.

MBq megabecquerel.

mbun·du (əm-boon′doo) [Umbundu language of Angola] a poison used in Angola, made from roots of trees of genus *Strychnos*.

MC[1] [L.] Magis′ter Chirur′giae (Master of Surgery).

MC[2] Medical Corps.

mC millicoulomb.

μC microcoulomb.

MCA 3-methylcholanthrene.

MCAD de·fi·cien·cy medium-chain acyl-CoA dehydrogenase deficiency; see under *acyl-CoA dehydrogenase*.

MCD mean of consecutive differences.

MCE myocardial contrast echocardiography.

MCF macrophage chemotactic factor.

MCFA medium-chain fatty acids.

Mcg an antigenic marker distinguishing human immunoglobulin λ light chain subtypes.

mcg microgram.

MCH mean corpuscular hemoglobin.

MCHB Maternal and Child Health Bureau, an agency of the Health Resources and Services Administration.

MCHC mean corpuscular hemoglobin concentration.

MCi megacurie.

mCi millicurie.

μCi microcurie.

MCI/MI abbreviation for a mixture of methylchloroisothiazolinone and methylisothiazolinone; see *methylisothiazolinone*.

MCMI Millon Clinical Multiaxial Inventory.

MCP membrane cofactor protein.

Mcps megacycles per second (million cycles per second); see *megahertz*.

MCS mechanical circulatory support.

M-CSF macrophage colony-stimulating factor.

MCT mean circulation time.

MCV meningococcal conjugate vaccine; mean corpuscular volume.

MCV4 meningococcal conjugate vaccine.

MD [L.] Medici′nae Doc′tor (Doctor of Medicine).

Md mendelevium.

MDA[1] [L.] mento-dextra anterior (right mentoanterior, a position of the fetus; see *position*).

MDA[2] methylenedioxyamphetamine.

MDF myocardial depressant factor.

MDMA 3,4-methylenedioxymethamphetamine.

MDP[1] [L.] mento-dextra posterior (right mentoposterior, a position of the fetus; see *position*).

MDP[2] methylene diphosphonate (medronate, q.v.)

MDR multidrug resistance; multiple drug resistance.

MDS myelodysplasia.

MDT [L.] mento-dextra transversa (right mentotransverse, a position of the fetus; see *position*).

2-ME 2-mercaptoethanol.

Me methyl.

meal (mēl) a portion of food or foods taken at some particular and usually stated or fixed time. Often given with the specific purpose of aiding diagnostic examination. See also *test m.*

barium m. upper gastrointestinal series.

Lundh test m. Lundh test; see under *test*.

opaque m. a test meal containing a substance opaque to x-rays, so that the outline of the stomach and the intestinal tract can be determined.

test m. a meal containing something to aid diagnostic examination of the stomach, as by fluoroscopy or by chemical analysis of stomach contents.

meal·worm (mēl′wərm) 1. the larva of any of various grain beetles of the genus *Tenebrio*, which eat and contaminate grain products such as flour and are also raised as food for insectivorous domestic animals such as birds. Spelled also *meal worm*. 2. the larva of *Asopia farinalis*.

Mean sign (mēn) [James Howard *Mean*, American endocrinologist, 1885–1967] Kocher sign.

mean (mēn) [Old Fr. *meien*, from L. *medianus* middle] 1. an average; a number that in some sense represents the central value of a set of numbers. 2. arithmetic m. 3. in probability and statistics, the expected value (mathematical expectation) of a random variable, the limiting value to which the sample mean converges as the sample size is increased indefinitely (if the limit exists).

arithmetic m. the sum of *n* numbers divided by *n*.

m. of consecutive differences (MCD) the mean value of interpotential intervals when many readings are performed consecutively on the same pair of muscle fibers; see also *jitter*.

geometric m. the *n*th root of the product of *n* numbers, e.g., the geometric mean of [2,8,32] is $(2 \times 8 \times 32)^{1/3} = 8$.

harmonic m. reciprocal of the mean of the reciprocals of the individual values in a given set; e.g., for the set [10, 40, 60] the harmonic mean is $1 \div [\frac{1}{3}(\frac{1}{10} + \frac{1}{40} + \frac{1}{60})] = 21.2$.

population m. (μ) the mean of the probability distribution characterizing a specified population; for a finite population, the arithmetic mean of the population values.

sample m. the arithmetic mean of the observed values of a random sample, conventionally denoted by a barred variable, e.g., $\bar{X}$ (read "X bar").

mea·sles (me′zəlz) 1. a highly contagious viral disease caused by a paramyxovirus, common among children but also seen in the nonimmune of any age. The virus enters the respiratory tract via droplet nuclei, multiplies in the epithelial cells, and spreads throughout the reticuloendothelial system, producing lymphoid hyperplasia, often with characteristic giant cells known as Warthin-Finkeldey cells. The skin eruption is usually preceded by coryza, cervical lymphadenitis, Koplik spots, palpebral conjunctivitis, photophobia, myalgia, malaise, cough, and steadily mounting fever. The typical rash consists of generalized maculopapular lesions that are at first discrete but gradually become confluent, starting behind the ears and on the face and progressing rapidly down the trunk and onto the extremities. Although measles is usually benign, complications may sometimes occur, including secondary bacterial infections such as otitis media, pneumonia, or laryngitis; giant cell pneumonia in immunocompromised children, which does not involve a rash and can be fatal; and rarely, subacute sclerosing panencephalitis years after an initial measles infection. Called also *morbilli* and *rubeola.* 2. name given to some kinds of cysticercosis in domestic animals.

atypical m. a severe form of measles occurring after exposure to wild measles virus in those who previously received inactivated (killed) measles vaccine (a type used in the United States and elsewhere in the mid-1960s), or in some cases live attenuated measles vaccine. It is characterized by fever, headache, myalgia, abdominal symptoms, and cough; this is followed by an atypical rash that may be urticarial, vesicular, petechial, or maculopapular, is found on the wrists and ankles, spreads to the palms, soles, and trunk, and later fades; there may be peripheral edema, interstitial pulmonary infiltrates, and pleural effusion. Koplik spots are absent.

beef m. cysticercosis in cattle.

black m. a rare measleslike condition, formerly more common, possibly from any of various different causes, characterized by hemorrhagic lesions of the skin and mucous membranes, respiratory distress, fever, convulsions, and coma.

German m. rubella.

pork m. cysticercosis in pigs.

sheep m. cysticercosis in sheep.

three-day m. rubella.

mea•sly (me′zle) of meat, having a speckled appearance because of the presence of cysticerci.

meas•ure (mezh′ər) [L. *mensurare*] 1. to determine the extent or quantity of a substance. 2. a specific extent or quantity of a substance. 3. a graduated scale by which the dimensions or mass of an object or substance may be determined. See tables of weights and measures in Appendix 7.

me•a•ti•tis (me″ə-ti′tis) inflammation of the urinary meatus.

me•a•tom•e•ter (me″ə-tom′ə-tər) [L. *meatus* passage + *metrum* measure] an instrument for measuring the urinary meatus.

me•a•to•plas•ty (me-at′o-plas″te) plastic surgery of a meatus. **meatoplas′tic** *adj*

me•a•tos•co•py (me″ə-tos′kə-pe) inspection of a meatus, especially the urinary meatus.

me•ato•tome (me-at′ə-tōm) an instrument for performing meatotomy.

me•a•tot•o•my (me″ə-tot′ə-me) [L. *meatus* passage + Gr. *temnein* to cut] incision of an acoustic or urinary meatus in order to enlarge it.

me•a•tus (me-a′təs) pl. *mea′tus* [L., "a way, path, course"] a passageway in the body, especially one opening on the surface. **mea′tal** *adj*

acoustic m., bony external m. acusticus externus osseus.

acoustic m., bony internal m. acusticus internus.

acoustic m., cartilaginous external m. acusticus externus cartilagineus.

acoustic m., external m. acusticus externus.

acoustic m., internal m. acusticus internus.

m. acus′ticus exter′nus [TA] external acoustic meatus: the passage of the external ear leading to the tympanic membrane, divided into an outer cartilaginous meatus and an inner bony meatus. Called also *external auditory m.* or *canal* and *m. auditorius externus.*

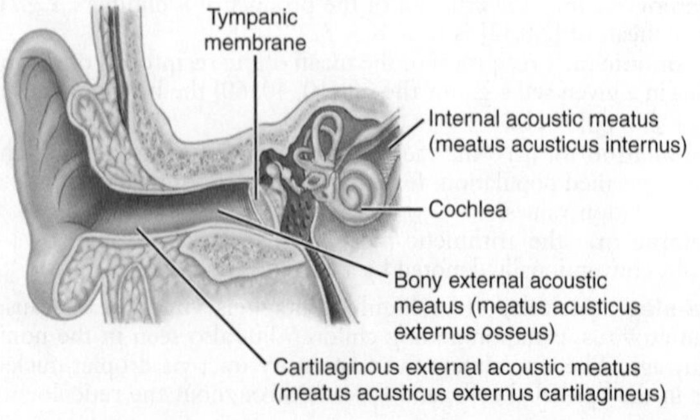

m. acus′ticus exter′nus cartilagi′neus [TA] cartilaginous external acoustic meatus: the cartilaginous part of the external acoustic meatus, found lateral to the bony part.

m. acus′ticus exter′nus os′seus bony external acoustic meatus: the opening in the external surface of the temporal bone, posterior to the condyle of the mandible and anterior to the mastoid air cells.

m. acus′ticus inter′nus [TA] internal acoustic meatus: the passage in the petrous portion of the temporal bone through which the facial, intermediate, and vestibulocochlear nerves and the labyrinthine artery pass. Called also *internal auditory m.* or *canal* and *m. auditorius internus.*

m. acus′ticus inter′nus os′seus m. acusticus internus.

m. audito′rius exter′nus m. acusticus externus.

m. audito′rius exter′nus cartilagi′neus m. acusticus externus cartilagineus.

m. audito′rius exter′nus os′seus m. acusticus externus osseus.

m. audito′rius inter′nus m. acusticus internus.

auditory m., bony external m. acusticus externus osseus.

auditory m., bony internal m. acusticus internus.

auditory m., cartilaginous external m. acusticus externus cartilagineus.

auditory m., external m. acusticus externus.

auditory m., internal m. acusticus internus.

fish-mouth m. a red, swollen, and everted urinary meatus seen in the first stage of acute gonorrhea.

inferior m. of nose m. nasi inferior.

middle m. of nose m. nasi medius.

nasal m., inferior m. nasi inferior.

nasal m., middle m. nasi medius.

nasal m., superior m. nasi superior.

m. na′si infe′rior [TA] inferior meatus of nose: the space beneath the inferior nasal concha, into which the nasolacrimal duct opens.

m. na′si me′dius [TA] middle meatus of nose: the space beneath the middle nasal concha, with which the anterior ethmoidal cells and frontal and maxillary sinuses communicate.

m. na′si supe′rior [TA] superior meatus of nose: the narrow cavity below the superior nasal concha, with which the posterior ethmoidal cells communicate.

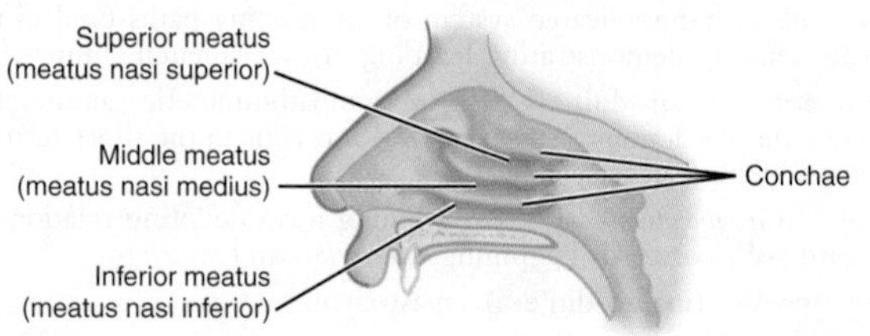

m. nasopharyn′geus [TA] nasopharyngeal meatus: the part of the nasal cavity coinciding with the bony nasopharyngeal cavity.

m. of nose see *m. nasi inferior, m. nasi medius,* and *m. nasi superior.*

superior m. of nose m. nasi superior.

ureteral m., ureteric m. ostium ureteris.

urethral m. m. urinarius.

m. urina′rius, urinary m., urinary m., external the opening of the urethra on the body surface, through which urine is discharged (see *ostium urethrae externum femininae* and *ostium urethrae externum masculinae*). Called also *external urethral orifice.*

urinary m., internal ostium urethrae internum.

Me•ban (me′ban) trademark for a preparation of dehydroemetine.

Meb•a•ral (meb′ə-rəl) trademark for a preparation of mephobarbital.

me•ben•da•zole (mə-ben′də-zōl) [USP] a benzimidazole anthelmintic agent that irreversibly inhibits glucose uptake in the parasite, causing immobilization and death; used in the treatment of infections in humans and dogs by *Ascaris lumbricoides, Enterobius vermicularis, Trichuris trichiura,* hookworm species, and *Capillaria philippinensis.*

me•bev•er•ine hy•dro•chlo•ride (mə-bev′ər-ēn) a smooth muscle relaxant, used as an antispasmodic in the treatment of irritable bowel syndrome; administered orally.

me•bro•fen•in (BrIDA) (me′bro-fen″in) [USP] a trimethyl-bromine–substituted analogue of iminodiacetic acid (IDA); complexed with technetium 99m it is used for hepatobiliary imaging and hepatic function studies; administered intravenously. See table at *technetium.*

Mec•a•dox (mek′ə-doks) trademark for a preparation of carbadox.

mec•amine (mek′ə-mēn) see *mecamylamine hydrochloride.*

mec•a•myl•amine hy•dro•chlo•ride (mek″ə-mil′ə-mēn) [USP] a ganglionic-blocking agent used as an antihypertensive, usually in the treatment of moderate to severe hypertension; administered orally.

MeCbl methylcobalamin.

MeCCNU semustine.

me•chan•i•cal (mə-kan′ĭ-kəl) [Gr. *mēchanikos*] 1. pertaining to or accomplished by physical forces or machinery. 2. performed by means of some artificial mechanism.

me•chan•i•co•re•cep•tor (mə-kan″ĭ-ko-re-sep′tər) mechanoreceptor.

me•chan•ics (mə-kan′iks) the science dealing with the motions of material bodies, including kinematics, dynamics, and statics.
 animal m. biomechanics.
 body m. the application of kinesiology to use of the body in daily life activities and to the prevention and correction of problems related to posture.
 developmental m. embryological mechanisms as revealed mainly by experimentation.

mech•a•nism (mek′ə-niz-əm) [Gr. *mēchanē* machine] 1. a machine or machinelike structure. 2. the manner of combination of parts, processes, etc., which subserve a common function. 3. the theory that the phenomena of life are based on the same physical and chemical laws which operate in the inorganic world; opposed to *vitalism*.
 countercurrent m., countercurrent multiplication m. see under *multiplication*.
 defense m. a usually unconscious mental process that serves to relieve conflict and anxiety arising from one's impulses and drives, e.g., compensation, conversion, denial, rationalization, repression.
 double-displacement m. ping-pong m.
 Duncan m. expulsion of the placenta with the maternal, or rough, surface appearing at the vulva.
 escape m. in the heart, the mechanism of impulse initiation by lower centers, such as the atrioventricular node, in response to lack of impulse propagation by the sinoatrial node.
 Frank-Starling m. Starling's law of the heart.
 m. of labor the factors involved in the expulsion of the fetus, placenta, and membranes through the birth canal in labor.
 leading circle m. see under *model*.
 mental m. an unconscious process, such as a defense mechanism, memory, perception, or thinking, that is a function of the ego and determines behavior.
 oculogyric m. the series of nerve centers concerned in movements of the eye.
 ping-pong m. in an enzyme-catalyzed reaction, the dissociation of one or more products from the enzyme complex before all substrates have been bound; binding may occur in a fixed order or may be random. Cf. *sequential m.*
 reentrant m., reentry m. the mechanism by which a locus of unidirectional block to conduction in cardiac muscle can result in ectopic beats or tachyarrhythmias. In addition to the block, also required are at least areas of slow conduction and refractoriness of the tissue to stimulation. Conduction of a normally initiated impulse is delayed by the block long enough for normal surrounding tissue to repolarize and to be reexcited by the delayed impulse; this may begin a self-perpetuating series of abnormal conduction cycles. See also *ring model, leading circle model*, and *figure-of-eight model*, under *model*, and see *reentry*.
 Schultze m. expulsion of the placenta with the smooth, glistening, fetal surface appearing at the vulva; this is considered normal and is more common than the Duncan mechanism.
 sequential m. in an enzyme-catalyzed reaction, the binding of the enzyme by all substrates, forming a complex, prior to the release of any products; binding may occur in a fixed order or may be random. Cf. *ping-pong m.*
 sliding filament m. the process by which muscle contracts: the thick and thin filaments slide past each other while maintaining a constant length as the result of mechanical forces generated by interaction of cross-bridges (myosin heads) with the actin filaments.
 Starling m. see under *law*.

mech•a•nist (mek′ə-nist) an individual who believes that all phenomena relating to life are based on physical and chemical properties only.

mechan(o)- [Gr. *mēchanē* machine] a combining form meaning mechanical, or denoting relationship to a machine, to physical forces, or to mechanics.

mech•a•no•bul•lous (mek″ə-no-bul′əs) characterized by the eruption of bullae after mechanical trauma such as rubbing or chafing.

mech•a•no•cyte (mek′ə-no-sīt″) [*mechano-* + *-cyte*] fibroblast.

mech•a•nol•o•gy (mek″ə-nol′ə-je) [*mechano-* + *-logy*] the science of mechanics.

mech•a•no•re•cep•tor (mek″ə-no-re-sep′tər) a receptor that is excited by mechanical pressures or distortions, as those responding to sound, touch, and muscular contractions. Specific types are variously

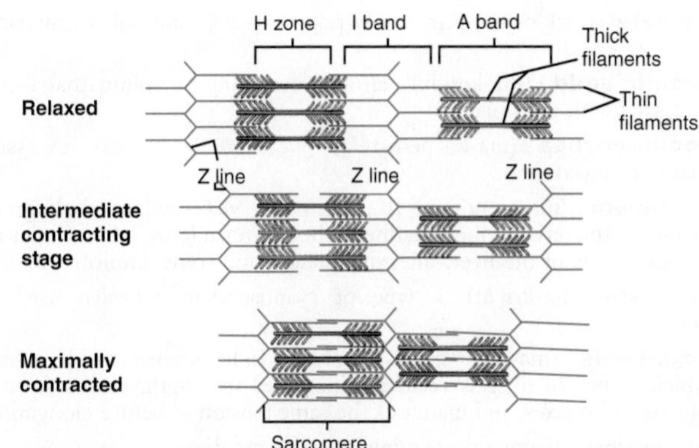

■ Sliding filament mechanism, showing myosin cross-bridges pulling thin filaments toward the center of each sarcomere, shortening the myofibrils.

called *corpuscles, nerve endings*, and *receptors*. See also *rapidly-adapting receptor, slowly-adapting receptor*, and *nonadapting receptor*, under *receptor*.
 high-threshold m. mechanical nociceptor.

mech•a•no•sen•si•tive (mek″ə-no-sen′sĭ-tiv) responding to mechanical distortion; see *mechanosensitive channel*, under *channel*.

me•cha•no•sen•so•ry (mek″ə-no-sen′sə-re) pertaining to sensory activation in response to mechanical pressures or distortions; cf. *mechanoreceptor*.

mech•a•no•ther•a•py (mek″ə-no-ther′ə-pe) [*mechano-* + *-therapy*] the use of mechanical apparatus in the treatment of disease or its results, especially as an aid in performing therapeutic exercises.

mech•a•no•ther•my (mek″ə-no-thur′me) [*mechano-* + Gr. *thermē* heat] therapeutic heat produced by massage, exercise, etc.

mech•lor•eth•amine hy•dro•chlo•ride (mek″lor-eth′ə-mēn) [USP] a cytotoxic alkylating agent of the nitrogen mustard group, used in the treatment of disseminated Hodgkin disease, some non-Hodgkin lymphomas, and mycosis fungoides; administered intravenously. It is also administered intraperitoneally, intrapericardially, and intrapleurally for the palliative treatment of malignant effusions. Called also *HN2* and *nitrogen mustard*.

me•cil•li•nam (mə-sil′ĭ-nəm) INN for *amdinocillin*.

me•cism (me′siz-əm) [Gr. *mēkos* length] abnormal lengthening of a part.

me•cis•to•ce•phal•ic (me-sis″to-sə-fal′ik) [Gr. *mēkistos* tallest + *cephalic*] having a cephalic index less than 71.

me•cis•to•ceph•a•lous (me-sis″to-sef′ə-ləs) mecistocephalic.

Me•cis•to•cir•rus (me-sis″to-sir′əs) a genus of nematodes of the family Trichostrongylidae. *M. digita′lis* is a parasite found in the stomachs of various mammals.

Meck•el band (ligament), ganglion, space (mek′əl) [Johann Friedrich *Meckel* (the elder), German anatomist, 1724–1774] see under *band*, and see *cavum trigeminale, ganglion pterygopalatinum*, and *ganglion submandibulare*.

Meck•el cartilage (rod), diverticulum, plane, syndrome (mek′əl) [Johann Friedrich *Meckel* (the younger) (grandson of J.F. Meckel, the elder), German anatomist, 1781–1833] see under *cartilage, diverticulum, plane*, and *syndrome*.

Mec•lan (mek′lan) trademark for a preparation of meclocycline sulfosalicylate.

mec•li•zine hy•dro•chlo•ride (mek′lĭ-zēn) [USP] an antihistamine used in the management of nausea, vomiting, and dizziness associated with motion sickness and of vertigo associated with disease affecting the vestibular system; administered orally.

mec•lo•cy•cline sul•fo•sal•i•cyl•ate (mek″lo-si′klēn) [USP] a tetracycline antibiotic used for the treatment of acne vulgaris; applied topically.

me•clo•fen•am•ate sodium (mek″lo-fen′ə-māt) [USP] a nonsteroidal antiinflammatory drug used in the treatment of rheumatoid arthritis, osteoarthritis, and other rheumatic and nonrheumatic inflammatory disorders, pain, dysmenorrhea, idiopathic hypermenorrhea, and vascular headaches; administered orally or rectally.

me•co•bal•amine (me″ko-bal′ə-mēn) a naturally occurring hematopoietic vitamin found in the blood, closely related to cyanocobalamin, in which the cyano radical has been replaced by a methyl radical.

me•co•ce•phal•ic (me″ko-sə-fal′ik) [Gr. *mēkos* length + *cephalic*] dolichocephalic.

meco•nate (mek′o-nāt) [Gr. *mēkōn* poppy + *-ate*] any salt of meconic acid.

me•con•ic ac•id (mə-kon′ik) an acid occurring in opium that forms soluble salts with the opiates.

me•co•ni•or•rhea (mə-ko″ne-o-re′ə) [*meconium* + *-rrhea*] excessive discharge of meconium.

me•co•ni•um (mə-ko′ne-əm) [L., from Gr. *mēkōnion*] a dark green mucilaginous material in the intestine of the full-term fetus, being a mixture of the secretions of the liver, intestinal glands, and some amniotic fluid.

me•cryl•ate (mə-kril′āt) a type of cyanoacrylate adhesive used in surgery.

me•cys•ta•sis (mə-sis′tə-sis) [Gr. *mēkynein* to lengthen + *stasis*] a state in which a muscle fiber is relatively increased in length, resists stretch, contracts, and relaxes, and manifests the same tension as before elongation.

MED minimal effective dose; minimal erythema dose.

me•dia (me′de-ə) [L.] 1. plural of *medium.* 2. middle. 3. tunica media vasorum.

me•di•ad (me′de-əd) [*medium* + *-ad*[1]] toward a median line or plane.

me•di•al (me′de-əl) [L. *medialis*] 1. pertaining to the middle; closer to the median plane or the midline of a body or structure. 2. pertaining to the middle layer of structures.

me•di•a•lec•i•thal (me″de-ə-les′ĭ-thəl) [*media-* + *-lecithal*] mesolecithal.

me•di•a•lis (me″de-a′lis) [TA] medial; a general term denoting a structure situated nearer to the median plane or the midline of a body or structure.

me•di•an (me′de-ən) [L. *medianus*] 1. situated in the median plane or in the midline of a body or structure. 2. any value that divides the probability distribution of a random variable in half, i.e., the probability of observing a value above the median and the probability of observing a value below the median are both less than or equal to one half. For a finite population or sample, the median is the middle value of an odd number of values (arranged in ascending order) or any value between the two middle values of an even number of values; in the latter case it is conventional to use the average of the two middle values. Symbol m.

me•di•a•nus (me″de-a′nəs) [L.] [TA] median, or situated in the middle; a general term denoting structures lying in the median plane.

me•di•a•om•e•ter (me″de-ə-om′ə-tər) [*media* + *-meter*] an instrument for detecting and measuring refractive errors of the dioptric media.

me•di•as•ti•na (me″de-ə-sti′nə) [L.] plural of *mediastinum.*

me•di•as•ti•nal (me″de-ə-sti′nəl) of or pertaining to the mediastinum.

me•di•as•ti•ni•tis (me″de-as″tĭ-ni′tis) inflammation of the mediastinum.

acute m. an often fatal inflammation of the mediastinum, with sudden onset of chills, fever, and prostration. Other symptoms are severe chest pain and sometimes tachypnea, tachycardia, pneumomediastinum, and hemomediastinum. It is usually secondary to perforation of the esophagus by forceful vomiting or trauma; less often it may be caused by spread of an infectious process from some adjacent organ or area. There may be obstruction of structures in the area, such as the superior vena cava or the tracheobronchial tree.

chronic m. any of numerous inflammatory conditions of the mediastinum, often secondary to a fungal or tuberculous infection; symptoms may be minimal or the result of obstruction of structures in the area. The most common specific condition is mediastinal fibrosis.

fibrosing m., fibrous m. mediastinal fibrosis.

granulomatous m. mediastinal fibrosis with granulomas.

indurative m. mediastinal fibrosis.

me•di•as•ti•no•gram (me″de-əs-tĭ′no-gram) a radiograph of the mediastinum.

me•di•as•ti•nog•ra•phy (me″de-as″tĭ-nog′rə-fe) radiography of the mediastinum.

me•di•as•ti•no•peri•car•di•tis (me″de-as″tĭ-no-per″e-kahr-di′tis) adhesive pericarditis in which the adhesions extend from the pericardium to the mediastinum. See also *adhesive pericarditis,* under *pericarditis.*

adhesive m. mediastinopericarditis.

me•di•a•sti•no•scope (me″de-ə-sti′no-skōp) a specially designed endoscope used in mediastinoscopy.

me•di•as•ti•no•scop•ic (me″de-as″tĭ-no-skop′ik) pertaining to the mediastinoscope or to mediastinoscopy.

me•di•as•ti•nos•co•py (me″de-as″tĭ-nos′kə-pe) examination of the mediastinum by means of an endoscope inserted through an anterior incision in the suprasternal notch, permitting direct inspection and biopsy of tissue in the anterior superior mediastinum.

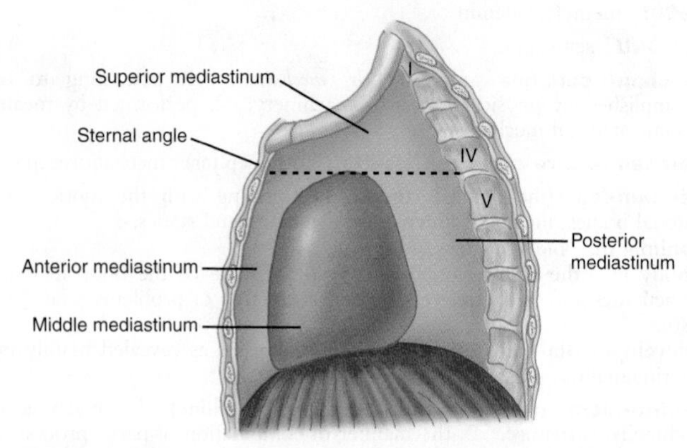

■ Subdivisions of the mediastinum.

me•di•as•ti•not•o•my (me″de-as″tĭ-not′ə-me) [*mediastinum* + *-tomy*] the operation of cutting into the mediastinum. Performed from the front, it is *anterior* or *cervical mediastinotomy;* from the back, *posterior* or *dorsal mediastinotomy.*

me•di•as•ti•num (me″de-ə-sti′nəm) pl. *mediasti′na* [L.] 1. a median septum or partition. 2. [TA] the mass of tissues and organs separating the two pleural sacs, between the sternum anteriorly and the vertebral column posteriorly and from the thoracic inlet superiorly to the diaphragm inferiorly. It contains the heart and pericardium, the bases of the great vessels, the trachea and bronchi, esophagus, thymus, lymph nodes, thoracic duct, phrenic and vagus nerves, and other structures and tissues. The mediastinum is divided into a superior region and an inferior region that comprises anterior, middle, and posterior parts.

m. ante′rius [TA] anterior mediastinum: the division of the mediastinum bounded posteriorly by the pericardium, anteriorly by the sternum, and on each side by the pleura. It contains loose areolar tissue and lymphatic vessels. Called also *anterior mediastinal cavity.*

m. infe′rius [TA] inferior mediastinum: the three inferior portions of the mediastinum, comprising the *m. anterius, m. medium,* and *m. posterius;* see also *mediastinum* (def. 2).

m. me′dium [TA] middle mediastinum: the division of the mediastinum containing the heart enclosed in its pericardium, the ascending aorta, the superior vena cava, the bifurcation of the trachea into bronchi, the proximal portions of the pulmonary arteries and veins, the phrenic nerves, and the arch of the azygos vein. Called also *middle mediastinal cavity.*

m. poste′rius [TA] posterior mediastinum: the division of the mediastinum bounded posteriorly by the vertebral column, anteriorly by the pericardium, and on each side by the pleura. It contains the descending aorta, the azygos, hemiazygos, and accessory hemiazygos veins, the thoracic duct, the esophagus, the vagus nerves, and the greater splanchnic nerves. Called also *posterior mediastinal cavity.*

m. supe′rius [TA] superior mediastinum: the division of the mediastinum extending from the pericardium to the root of the neck, and containing the esophagus and the trachea posteriorly, the thymus or its remains anteriorly, and the great vessels related to the heart and pericardium, the thoracic duct, and the vagus nerves in between. Called also *superior mediastinal cavity.*

m. tes′tis [TA] the partial septum of the testis, formed near its posterior border by fibrous tissue that is continuous with the tunica albuginea; called also *body of Highmore.*

me•di•ate[1] (me′de-ət) indirect; accomplished by the aid of an intervening medium.

me•di•ate[2] (me′de-āt) to convey, intervene, or serve as an intermediary.

me•di•a•tion (me″de-a′shən) the act of intervening or serving as an intermediary.

chemical m. in neurophysiology, the intervention by a chemical substance (neurotransmitter) in the passing of an action potential from a presynaptic to a postsynaptic element.

me•di•a•tor (me′de-a″tər) an object or substance that intervenes on behalf of something else, or transmits or conveys something else, such as (1) a structure of the nervous system that transmits impulses eliciting a specific response; (2) a chemical substance (neurotransmitter) that induces activity in an excitable tissue, such as nerve or muscle; or (3) a substance released from cells as the result of the interaction of antigen with antibody or by the action of antigen with a sensitized lymphocyte.

med•i•ca•ble (med′ĭ-kə-bəl) subject to treatment with reasonable expectation of cure.

Med•i•ca•go (med″ĭ-ka′go) a genus of grasses of the family Leguminosae. *M. polymor′pha* (also called *M. denticula′ta*) is the burr trefoil, which is often used as hay for livestock but sometimes causes the condition called trefoil dermatitis. *M. sati′va* is alfalfa, which is commonly used as hay for livestock; certain strains of it can cause photosensitization, primary ruminal tympany (frothy bloat), or other conditions.

med•i•cal (med′ĭ-kəl) pertaining to medicine or to the treatment of diseases; pertaining to medicine as opposed to surgery.

med•i•cal ex•am•i•ner (med′ĭ-kəl eg-zam′ĭ-nər) a physician who is charged in an official capacity with the investigation and examination of sudden, unexpected, or violent deaths within a given jurisdiction. Cf. *coroner*.

med•i•ca•ment (med′ĭ-kə-mənt, mə-dik′ə-mənt) [L. *medicamentum*] a medicinal substance or agent.

med•i•ca•men•to•sus (med″ĭ-kə-mən-to′səs) [L.] medicamentous.

med•i•ca•men•tous (med″ĭ-kə-men′təs) pertaining to, used in, or caused by a drug or drugs.

Med•i•care (med′ĭ-kār) a program administered by the Social Security Administration which provides medical care for the aged.

med•i•cate (med′ĭ-kāt) [L. *medicatus*] to impregnate or imbue with a medicinal substance.

med•i•cat•ed (med′ĭ-kāt″əd) imbued with a medicinal substance.

med•i•ca•tion (med″ĭ-ka′shən) [L. *medicatio*] 1. a drug or medicine. 2. impregnation with a medicine. 3. administration of a medicine or other remedy.

conservative m. treatment not considered to be aggressive in nature.

hypodermic m. the introduction of remedial agents beneath the skin.

ionic m. iontophoresis.

sublingual m. the administration of medicine by placing it beneath the tongue.

substitutive m. medication for the purpose of causing an acute nonspecific inflammation to overcome a specific one.

transduodenal m. the administration of medicine through a duodenal tube into the intestines without soiling the stomach.

med•i•ca•tor (med′ĭ-ka″tər) an instrument for carrying medicines into a cavity of the body; an applicator.

me•dic•i•nal (mə-dis′ĭ-nəl) [L. *medicinalis*] 1. having healing qualities. 2. pertaining to a medicine or to healing.

med•i•cine (med′ĭ-sin) [L. *medicina*] 1. any drug or remedy. 2. the art and science of the diagnosis and treatment of disease and the maintenance of health. 3. the treatment of disease by nonsurgical means.

alternative m. see *complementary and alternative medicine*.

aviation m. the branch of medicine that deals with physiological, medical, psychological, and epidemiological problems involved in aviation.

behavioral m. a segment of psychosomatic medicine focused on psychological means of influencing physical symptoms, such as biofeedback or relaxation.

Chinese herbal m. a highly complex system of diagnosis and treatment using medicinal herbs, one of the branches of traditional Chinese medicine. Herbs used range from the nontoxic and rejuvenating, such as ginseng, which are used to support the body's healing system, to highly toxic ones, such as aconite, used in the treatment of disease.

clinical m. 1. the study of disease by direct examination of the living patient. 2. the last two years of the usual curriculum in a medical college.

comparative m. the study of phenomena basic to the diseases of all species.

complementary m., complementary and alternative m. (CAM) a large and diverse set of systems of diagnosis, treatment, and prevention based on philosophies and techniques other than those used in conventional Western medicine, often derived from traditions of medical practice used in other, non-Western cultures. Such practices may be described as *alternative*, that is, existing as a body separate from and as a replacement for conventional Western medicine, or *complementary*, that is, used in addition to conventional Western practice. CAM is characterized by its focus on the whole person as a unique individual, on the energy of the body and its influence on health and disease, on the healing power of nature and the mobilization of the body's own resources to heal itself, and on the treatment of the underlying causes, rather than symptoms, of disease. Many of the techniques used are the subject of controversy and have not been validated by controlled studies.

compound m. a preparation that contains a mixture of several drugs.

dosimetric m. the practice of administering medicines by an exact and determinate system of doses.

emergency m. the medical specialty that deals with acutely ill or injured patients who require immediate medical treatment.

emporiac m. travel m.

environmental m. the branch of medicine that considers the effects of the environment on human beings, including such factors as rapid population growth, changes and extremes in temperature, alterations in atmospheric pressure, water pollution, air pollution, radiation, and travel.

evidence-based m. the practice of medicine in which the physician finds, assesses, and implements methods of diagnosis and treatment on the basis of the best available, current research, their clinical expertise, and the needs and preferences of the patient. See also under *practice*.

experimental m. the study of disease based on experimentation in animals.

family m. see under *practice*.

folk m. the use of home remedies and procedures as handed down by tradition.

forensic m. the branch of medicine that deals with the application of medical knowledge to the purposes of law. This term and medical jurisprudence are sometimes used as synonyms, but some authorities consider the first as a branch of medicine and the second as a branch of law. Called also *legal m.*

geographic m. 1. geomedicine. 2. tropical m.

geriatric m. geriatrics.

group m. the practice of medicine by a group of physicians, usually representing various specialties, who are associated together for the cooperative diagnosis, treatment, and prevention of disease. Called also *group practice*.

herbal m. herbalism.

holistic m. a system of medicine that considers the human being as an integrated whole or functioning unit.

hyperbaric m. the treatment of disease in an environment of higher than atmospheric pressure.

internal m. the medical specialty dealing especially with the diagnosis and medical treatment of diseases and disorders of the internal structures of the human body.

ionic m. treatment by electrochemical means, as by cataphoresis and iontophoresis.

laboratory animal m. a specialty of veterinary medicine that deals with the diagnosis, treatment, and prevention of disease in animals used as subjects in biomedical activities.

legal m. forensic m.

maternal-fetal m. a subspecialty of obstetrics concerned with the obstetrical, medical, genetic, and surgical complications of pregnancy and their effects on the mother and fetus. Called also *fetology*.

mind-body m. a holistic approach to medicine that takes into account the effect of the mind on physical processes, including the effects of psychosocial stressors and conditioning, particularly as they affect the immune system; many of the therapeutic techniques used have as their purpose increasing the body's natural resistance to disease by managing the stressors.

molecular m. the study of health and disease at the molecular level, using techniques from molecular biology, gene technology, and other disciplines. Cf. *nanomedicine*.

naturopathic m. naturopathy.

nuclear m. the branch of medicine concerned with the use of radionuclides in the diagnosis and treatment of disease.

occupational m. the branch of medicine that deals with the study, prevention, and treatment of workplace injuries and occupational diseases and with the promotion of optimal health and safety in the workplace.

oral m. dentistry.

orthomolecular m. a system for the prevention and treatment of disease based on the theory that each person's biochemical environment is genetically determined and specific to the individual. Therapy is provided by supplementation with substances naturally present in the body, such as vitamins, minerals, trace elements, and amino acids, in amounts that are optimized for each individual in order to correct nutritional deficiencies and the resulting biochemical abnormalities. Cf. *orthomolecular psychiatry*, under *psychiatry*.

osteopathic m. osteopathy.

patent m. a drug or remedy protected by a trademark, available without prescription. The term was formerly used for quack remedies sold by peddlers.

physical m. physiatry.

podiatric m. podiatry.

preclinical m. 1. the first two years of the usual curriculum in a medical college. 2. preventive m.

preventive m. the branch of medical study and practice that aims at prevention of disease and promotion of health.

proprietary m. a drug or remedy to which the manufacturing pharmaceutical house has exclusive (proprietary) rights, and which is marketed usually under a name that is registered as a trademark.

psychocutaneous m. psychodermatology.

psychosomatic m. a system of medicine that aims at discovering the nature of the relationship of the emotions and bodily function, affirming the principle that the mind and body are one, as well as emphasizing psychosocial aspects of medical care.

rational m. practice of medicine based upon actual knowledge; opposed to *empiricism.*

regenerative m. a field of research that seeks to create living, functional tissues that can be used in the body to repair, replace, restore, or regenerate damaged or diseased tissue; it includes cell-based therapy, tissue engineering, and creation and use of biomaterials.

rehabilitation m. the branch of physiatry concerned with restoration of form and function after injury or illness.

respiratory m. the medical specialty concerned with the anatomy, physiology, and pathology of the respiratory tract and lungs.

sleep m. a medical specialty consisting of the diagnosis and treatment of sleep disorders.

social m. phases of preventive medicine and care of the sick that concern the community as a whole or large groups of persons rather than the individual.

socialized m. a system of medical care regulated and controlled by the government, in which the government assumes responsibility for providing for the health needs and hospital care of the entire population, at no direct cost or at a nominal fee to the individual, by means of subsidies obtained by taxation. Called also *state m.*

space m. the branch of aviation medicine concerned solely with conditions encountered by human beings in space.

sports m. the field of medicine concerned with injuries sustained in athletic endeavors, including their prevention, diagnosis, and treatment.

state m. socialized m.

traditional Chinese m. (TCM) the diverse body of medical theory and practice that has evolved in China, comprising four branches: acupuncture and moxibustion, herbal medicine, qi gong, and tui na. Although TCM encompasses a variety of theory and practice, all of its forms share certain underlying characteristics. The body and mind are considered together as a dynamic system subject to cycles of change and affected by the environment, and emphasis is on supporting the body's self-healing ability. Fundamental to TCM are the yin/yang principle and the concept of basic substances that pervade the body: qi, jing (essence), and shen (spirit), collectively known as the three treasures, and the blood (a fluid and material manifestation of qi) and body fluids (which moisten and lubricate the body). Disease arises from a disturbance of qi within the body, the particular pathological process depending on the location of the disturbance; causes are classified into three groups, external (which are environmental), internal (emotions), and miscellaneous (such as diet, fatigue, or trauma). Diagnosis is by visual assessment, listening and smelling, questioning, and palpation; a single biomedical disease may be associated with a large number of TCM diagnoses, while one TCM diagnosis may encompass a number of biomedical diseases. Once a diagnosis is established, therapy aims at restoring the body's homeostasis by treating the root cause of the disease.

travel m., travelers' m. the subspecialty of tropical medicine consisting of the diagnosis and treatment or prevention of diseases of travelers. Called also *emporiatrics.*

tropical m. medical science as applied to diseases occurring primarily in tropical and subtropical countries. Sometimes called *geographic m.* because diseases of interest to tropical medicine specialists may also occur in developing countries or areas in the temperate climate zones.

veterinary m. a medical specialty consisting of the diagnosis and treatment of diseases of animals other than humans.

med•i•co•chi•rur•gic (med″ĭ-ko-ki-rur′jik) pertaining to medicine and surgery.

med•i•co•den•tal (med″ĭ-ko-den′təl) pertaining to both medicine and dentistry.

med•i•co•le•gal (med″ĭ-ko-le′gəl) pertaining to medicine and law, or to forensic medicine.

med•i•co•me•chan•i•cal (med″ĭ-ko-mə-kan′ĭ-kəl) both medicinal and mechanical.

med•i•co•so•cial (med″ĭ-ko-so′shəl) having both medical and social aspects, as, for example, the prevention and treatment of venereal disease.

med•i•co•topo•graph•i•cal (med″ĭ-ko-top″o-graf′ĭ-kəl) pertaining to topography in its relation to disease.

med•i•co•zoo•log•i•cal (med″ĭ-ko-zo-o-loj′ĭ-kəl) pertaining to zoology in its relation to medicine.

me•di•fron•tal (me″dĭ-fron′təl) median and frontal; pertaining to the middle of the forehead.

medi(o)- [L. *medius* middle] a prefix meaning in the middle or intermediate.

me•dio•car•pal (me″de-o-kahr′pəl) midcarpal.

me•di•oc•cip•i•tal (me″de-ok-sip′ĭ-təl) midoccipital.

me•dio•lat•er•al (me″de-o-lat′ər-əl) [L. *medius* middle + *lateral*] pertaining to the middle and to one side.

me•di•ol•y•sis (me″de-ol′ĭ-sis) destruction of the tunica media of a blood vessel. **mediolyt′ic** *adj*

segmental arterial m. focal destruction of the tunica media of an artery, caused by the disruption of the arterial smooth muscle cells and leading to dissection, aneurysm formation, and hemorrhage.

me•dio•ne•cro•sis (me″de-o-nə-kro′sis) necrosis of the tunica media of a blood vessel, often leading to its rupture.

m. of aorta cystic medial necrosis.

me•dio•tar•sal (me″de-o-tahr′səl) [L. *medius* middle + *tarsal*] pertaining to the middle of the tarsus.

Med•i•pren (med′ĭ-pren″) trademark for a preparation of ibuprofen.

me•di•sca•le•nus (me″de-skə-le′nəs) musculus scalenus medius.

me•di•sect (me′dĭ-sekt) [L. *medius* middle + *secare* to cut] to divide or dissect medially.

med•i•ta•tion (med″ĭ-ta′shən) an intentional and self-regulated focusing of attention, originally used primarily in religious and spiritual practice, whose purpose is to relax and calm the mind and body.

mindfulness m. a technique of meditation in which distracting thoughts and feelings are not ignored but are rather acknowledged and observed nonjudgmentally as they arise in order to create a detachment from them and gain insight and awareness.

transcendental m. a technique for attaining a state of physical relaxation and psychological calm by the regular practice of a relaxation procedure (generally two 20-minute periods a day) that entails the repetition of a mantra that blocks distracting thoughts from entering the mind.

me•di•um (me′de-əm) pl. *mediums, me′dia* [L. "middle"] 1. a substance that transmits impulses. 2. culture medium, see under *C.* 3. a preparation used in treating histologic specimens.

active m. the aggregated atoms, ions, or molecules, contained in a laser's optical cavity, in which stimulated emission will occur under the proper excitation.

clearing m. a substance used for rendering histologic specimens transparent.

contrast m. a substance that is introduced into or around a structure or tissues and has a significant difference from the structure or tissues in the extent of absorption of x-rays, thus allowing radiographic visualization. See *radiopaque m.* and *radiolucent m.* Called also *contrast agent.*

culture m. see under *C.*

dioptric media refracting media.

disperse m., dispersion m., dispersive m. the continuous or external portion of a colloid system in which the particles of the disperse phase are distributed; it is analogous to the solvent in a true solution. Cf. *disperse phase.*

mounting m. mountant.

nutrient m. see *nutrient culture* under *culture medium.*

radiocontrast m. contrast m.

radiolucent m. a contrast medium that permits the passage of x-rays.

radiopaque m. a contrast medium that blocks the passage of x-rays.

refracting media the transparent tissues and fluids in the eye through which light rays pass and by which they are refracted and brought to a focus on the retina; the structures include the cornea, aqueous humor, crystalline lens, and vitreous body. Called also *dioptric media.*

separating m. any substance which facilitates separation, such as a coating used upon a surface that serves to prevent adherence to it of another surface; in dentistry, a substance applied to the investment surface of a denture flask to protect the resin from the surfaces in the mold space to avoid incorporation of water in the resin from the gypsum and to prevent adherence of the investing material and the resin.

Wickersheimer m. see under *fluid.*

me•di•us (me′de-əs) [L.] [TA] in the middle; a term used in reference to a structure lying between two other structures that are anterior and posterior, superior and inferior, or internal and external in position.

MEDLARS (med′lahrz) [*Med*ical *L*iterature *A*nalysis and *R*etrieval *S*ystem] a computerized bibliographic system of the National Library of Medicine, from which the *Index Medicus* is produced.

MEDLINE (med′līn) [from *MED*LARS on *line*] a computerized bibliographic retrieval system, an on-line segment of MEDLARS.

Med•rol (med′rol) trademark for preparations of methylprednisolone.

med•ro•nate (med′ro-nāt) MDP; a methylene-substituted diphosphonate compound with an affinity for sites of osteoid mineralization; complexed with technetium 99m it is used in bone imaging. Called also *methylene diphosphonate.* See table at *technetium.*

med•roxy•pro•ges•ter•one ac•e•tate (məd-rok″se-pro-jes′tər-ōn) [USP] a progestin administered orally for treatment of secondary amenorrhea and dysfunctional uterine bleeding, induction of menses, prevention and treatment of endometrial hyperplasia in postmenopausal hormone replacement therapy, and testing for endogenous estrogen production; administered orally or intramuscularly as an antineoplastic in treatment of metastatic endometrial, breast, and renal carcinoma; and administered intramuscularly as a long-acting contraceptive.

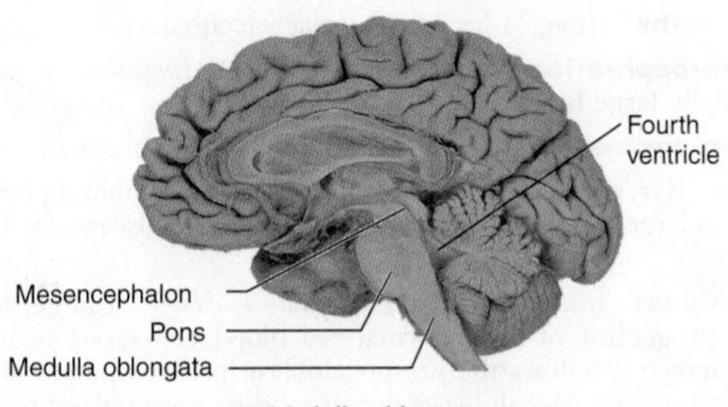

■ Medulla oblongata.

med•ry•sone (med′rə-sōn″) a synthetic glucocorticoid used topically in the treatment of corticosteroid-responsive allergic and inflammatory conditions of the eye.

me•dul•la (mə-dul′ə) gen. and pl. *medul′lae* [L.] 1. the most interior portion of an organ or structure. 2. m. oblongata. 3. m. ossium.

adrenal m., m. of adrenal gland m. glandulae suprarenalis.

m. of bone m. ossium.

m. glan′dulae suprarena′lis [TA] medulla of suprarenal or adrenal gland: the inner, reddish brown, soft part of the adrenal gland; it synthesizes, stores, and releases catecholamines. Called also *adrenal m.* and *suprarenal m.*

hair m., m. of hair, m. of hair shaft a tiny area of material in some hairs, running up the middle of the hair cortex.

inner m. of kidney inner zone of renal medulla.

m. of kidney m. renalis.

m. of lymph node m. nodi lymphoidei.

m. no′di lympha′tici TA alternative for *m. nodi lymphoidei.*

m. no′di lymphoi′dei [TA] medulla of lymph node: the central part of a lymph node, comprising cords and sinuses; called also *m. nodi lymphatici* [TA alternative].

m. oblonga′ta TA alternative for *myelencephalon;* the truncated cone of nerve tissue continuous above with the pons and below with the spinal cord. It lies anterior to the cerebellum, and the upper part of its posterior surface forms the floor of the lower part of the fourth ventricle; it contains ascending and descending tracts, and important collections of nerve cells that deal with vital functions, such as respiration, circulation, and special senses. Called also *bulb of rhombencephalon,* and *bulbus rhombencephali* [TA alternative]. See also *brainstem.*

m. os′sium [TA] bone marrow: the soft material filling the cavities of the bones, made up of a meshwork of connective tissue containing branching fibers, the meshes being filled with marrow cells, which consist variously of fat cells, large nucleated cells or myelocytes, and giant cells called megakaryocytes. See also *m. ossium flava* and *m. ossium rubra.*

m. os′sium fla′va [TA] yellow bone marrow: ordinary bone marrow of the kind in which the fat cells predominate.

m. os′sium ru′bra [TA] red bone marrow: marrow of developing bone, of the ribs, vertebrae, and many of the smaller bones; it is the site of production of erythrocytes and granular leukocytes.

outer m. of kidney outer zone of renal medulla.

m. ova′rii [TA] medulla of ovary: the loose fibroelastic tissue and mass of contorted blood vessels that forms the core of the ovary.

renal m., m. rena′lis [TA], **m. re′nis** the inner part of the substance of the kidney, composed chiefly of collecting tubule elements, loops of Henle, and vasa recta, organized grossly into renal pyramids.

m. spina′lis [TA] spinal cord: that part of the central nervous system that is lodged in the vertebral canal. It extends from the foramen magnum, where it is continuous with the medulla oblongata, to the upper part of the lumbar region, ending between the twelfth thoracic and third lumbar vertebrae, often at or near the first and second lumbar vertebrae. It is composed of an inner core of *gray substance,* in which nerve cells predominate, and an outer layer of *white substance,* in which myelinated nerve fibers predominate, and is enclosed in three protective membranes, or *meninges*: the *dura mater, arachnoid,* and *pia mater.* Thirty-one *spinal nerves* originate from the spinal cord: 8 cervical, 12 thoracic, 5 lumbar, 5 sacral, and 1 coccygeal. It conducts impulses to and from the brain, and controls many automatic muscular activities (reflexes). See also *Rexed laminae,* under *lamina,* and Plates 9 and 42.

suprarenal m., m. of suprarenal gland m. glandulae suprarenalis.

m. thy′mi [TA] medulla of thymus: the central portion of each lobule of the thymus; it contains many more reticular cells and far fewer lymphocytes than does the surrounding cortex.

me•dul•lae (mə-dul′e) [L.] genitive and plural of *medulla.*

med•ul•lary (med′ə-lar″e, mə-dul′ə-re) [L. *medullaris*] 1. pertaining to a medulla. 2. pertaining to bone marrow. Called also *myeloid.* 3. pertaining to the spinal cord. Called also *myeloid.*

med•ul•lat•ed (med′ə-lāt″əd) myelinated.

med•ul•la•tion (med″ə-la′shən) 1. myelinization. 2. myelopoiesis. 3. the formation of a medulla.

med•ul•lec•to•my (med″ə-lek′tə-me) [*medull-* + *-ectomy*] excision of a medulla, such as the adrenal medulla.

med•ul•li•tis (med″ə-li′tis) 1. osteomyelitis. 2. myelitis.

med•ul•li•za•tion (med″ə-lĭ-za′shən) 1. the enlargement of the haversian canals in rarefying osteitis, followed by their conversion into marrow channels. 2. replacement of bone by marrow cells.

medull(o)- a combining form denoting relationship to marrow or to a medulla.

me•dul•lo•adre•nal (mə-dul″o-ə-dre′nəl) adrenomedullary.

me•dul•lo•ar•thri•tis (mə-dul″o-ahr-thri′tis) [*medullo-* + *arthritis*] inflammation of the marrow spaces of the articular extremities of bones.

me•dul•lo•blast (mə-dul′o-blast) an undifferentiated cell of the embryonic neural tube that may develop into either a neuroblast or a spongioblast.

me•dul•lo•blas•to•ma (mə-dul″o-blas-to′mə) a malignant, highly radiosensitive cerebellar tumor composed of undifferentiated neuroglial cells and usually considered a type of primitive neuroectodermal tumor. Most medulloblastomas occur in children and arise in or adjacent to the roof of the fourth ventricle.

me•dul•lo•epi•the•li•o•ma (mə-dul″o-ep″ĭ-the″le-o′mə) a rare type of neuroepithelial tumor, usually found in the brain or retina, composed of primitive neuroepithelial cells lining the tubular spaces; called also *neurocytoma* and *neuroepithelioma.* Cf. *diktyoma.*

me•dul•lo•ther•a•py (mə-dul″o-ther′ə-pe) Pasteur's preventive treatment of rabies with emulsions of fixed virus in rabbit spinal cord.

me•du•sa (mə-doo′sə) [Gr. *Medusa* one of the three mythological gorgons] 1. the bell-shaped stage in the life cycle of certain members of the phylum Cnidaria, especially the jellyfish. 2. jellyfish.

Mees lines (māz) [R.A. *Mees,* Dutch scientist, 20th century] see under *line.*

me•fe•nam•ic ac•id (mef″ə-nam′ik) [USP] a nonsteroidal antiinflammatory drug administered orally in the short-term treatment of pain, inflammation, dysmenorrhea, and vascular headaches, and the prophylaxis of menstruation-associated migraines.

mef•lo•quine hy•dro•chlo•ride (mef′lo-kwin) [USP] a synthetic 4-quinolone methanol compound used as an antimalarial, effective against chloroquine-resistant strains of *Plasmodium falciparum* and *P. vivax;* administered orally for the treatment of falciparum and vivax malaria, as well as for prophylaxis of the falciparum type.

Me•fox•in (mə-fok′sin) trademark for a preparation of cefoxitin sodium.

MEG magnetoencephalograph.

mega- [Gr. *megas* big, great] a prefix *(a)* meaning large, enlarged, or of abnormally large size; see also words beginning *megal(o)-*, and *(b)* used in naming units of measurement to indicate a quantity one million (10^6) times the unit designated by the root with which it is combined (symbol M).

mega•base (Mb) (meg′ə-bās) a unit of length corresponding to one million bases of DNA.

mega•bec•que•rel (MBq) (meg″ə-bək-ə-rel′) a unit of radioactivity, being one million (10^6) becquerels.

mega•blad•der (meg″ə-blad′ər) megacystis.

mega•bow•el (meg″ə-bow′əl) megacolon.

mega•cal•y•co•sis (meg″ə-kal″ĭ-ko′sis) [*mega-* + *calix* + *-osis*] nonobstructive dilatation of the renal calices due to malformation of the renal papillae; called also *megapolycalicosis.* Spelled also *megacalicosis.*

mega•ca•lyx (meg″ə-ka′liks) an abnormally large renal calyx; see *megacalycosis.*

mega•caryo•blast (meg″ə-kar′e-o-blast) megakaryoblast.

mega•caryo•cyte (meg″ə-kar′e-o-sīt″) megakaryocyte.

Me•gace (mə-gās′) trademark for preparations of megestrol acetate.

mega•ce•cum (meg″ə-se′kəm) [*mega-* + *cecum*] abnormal enlargement of the cecum.

mega•ceph•a•ly (meg″ə-sef′ə-le) macrocephaly.

mega•cho•led•o•chus (meg″ə-ko-led′o-kəs) abnormal dilatation of the common bile duct.

mega•co•lon (meg″ə-ko′lən) an abnormally large or dilated colon; the condition may be congenital or acquired, acute or chronic. Called also *macrocolon.*

acquired m., acquired functional m. any type associated with chronic constipation but normal ganglionic innervation; sometimes the cause is

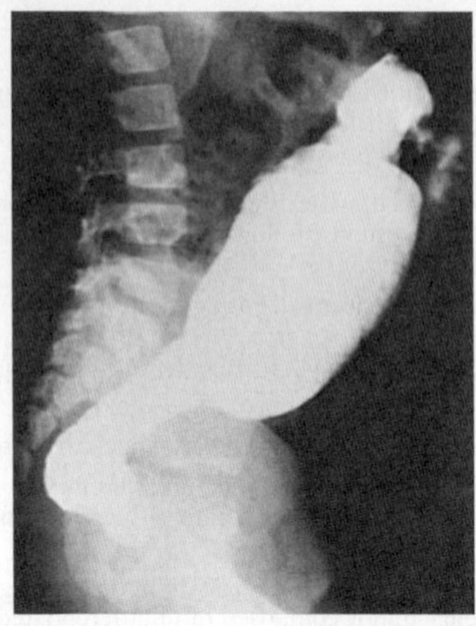

■ Congenital megacolon; lateral view of barium enema in a three-year-old girl.

simply faulty bowel habits, such as in mentally retarded children or adults with mental illness. Called also *idiopathic m.*

acute m. toxic m.

aganglionic m. congenital m.

chagasic m. the megacolon seen with Chagas disease.

congenital m. megacolon in a section of the colon due to congenital absence of intrinsic ganglion cells in the myenteric and submucosal plexuses of the next distal segment; the aganglionic part is abnormally narrow, and its loss of motor function causes massive hypertrophic dilatation of more proximal segments. The condition appears soon after birth, is more common in males, and causes extreme constipation, abdominal distention, and sometimes vomiting; when severe, it may result in growth retardation. It is sometimes divided into short-segment and long-segment forms, may occur as an isolated trait or in conjunction with other congenital anomalies, and may show dominant, recessive, or multigenic patterns of inheritance, with gender-dependent penetrance. It has been associated with mutations in one or a combination of several genes, including genes encoding either a protein-tyrosine kinase receptor *(RET)* or one of its ligands, and genes encoding either endothelin-3 *(EDN3)* or its receptor *(EDNRB)*. Called also *Hirschsprung disease, aganglionic m.,* and *pelvirectal achalasia.*

idiopathic m. acquired m.

toxic m. acute dilatation of the colon associated with amebic or ulcerative colitis; it may precede perforation of the colon. Called also *acute m.*

mega·cu·rie (MCi) (meg″ə-ku′re) a unit of radioactivity, being one million (10^6) curies.

mega·cys·tis (meg″ə-sis′tis) an abnormally enlarged urinary bladder; called also *megabladder* and *megalocystis.*

mega·dont (meg′ə-dont) macrodont.

mega·don·tia (meg″ə-don′shə) macrodontia.

mega·du·o·de·num (meg″ə-doo″o-de′nəm) an abnormally large or dilated duodenum; it may be congenital or acquired (as in systemic scleroderma), and is usually due to a disorder of motor function.

mega·dyne (meg′ə-dīn″) [*mega-* + *dyne*] one million (10^6) dynes.

mega·esoph·a·gus (meg″ə-ə-sof′ə-gəs) pathologic dilatation of the esophagus; see *esophageal achalasia,* under *achalasia.*

chagasic m. the megaesophagus seen with Chagas disease.

mega·ga·me·to·phyte (meg″ə-gə-me′to-fīt) [*mega-* + *gameto-* + *-phyte*] the female gametophyte in heterosporous plants, developed from the megaspore.

mega·hertz (MHz) (meg′ə-hərtz) one million (10^6) hertz, or one million cycles per second; typically applied to the frequency of electromagnetic waves.

mega·karyo·blast (meg″ə-kar′e-o-blast) the earliest cytologically identifiable precursor in the thrombocytic series, a large cell that matures to form a promegakaryocyte. Spelled also *megacaryoblast.*

mega·karyo·cyte (meg″ə-kar′e-o-sīt) [*mega-* + *karyo-* + *-cyte*] a giant cell 50 to 100 µm in diameter, with a greatly lobulated nucleus, found in the bone marrow; mature blood platelets are released from its cytoplasm. Called also *megalokaryocyte;* spelled also *megacaryocyte.*

mega·karyo·cy·to·poi·e·sis (meg″ə-kar″e-o-si′to-poi-e′sis) [*megakaryocyte* + *-poiesis*] the production of megakaryocytes.

mega·karyo·cy·to·sis (meg″ə-kar″e-o-si-to′sis) the presence of megakaryocytes in the blood or of excessive numbers in the bone marrow, as in polycythemia vera.

mega·lec·i·thal (meg″ə-les′ĭ-thəl) macrolecithal.

meg·al·en·ceph·a·lon (meg″əl-ən-sef′ə-lon) [*megalo-* + *encephalon*] an abnormally large brain.

meg·al·en·ceph·a·ly (meg″əl-ən-sef′ə-le) macrencephaly.

megal(o)- [Gr. *megas,* gen. *megalou* big, great] a combining form meaning large, enlarged, or of abnormally large size; see also words beginning *mega-.*

meg·a·lo·blast (meg′ə-lo-blast″) [*megalo-* + *-blast*] a large, nucleated, immature progenitor of an abnormal red blood cell series seen in some types of anemia; it follows the promegaloblast in development and retains some of its features. Megaloblasts correspond to normoblasts (see *erythroblast*) of the normal red cell maturation series and are correspondingly classified as basophilic, polychromatophilic, and orthochromatic. See also *megaloblastic anemia,* under *anemia.*

meg·a·lo·blas·toid (meg″ə-lo-blas′toid) resembling a megaloblast.

meg·a·lo·ce·pha·lia (meg″ə-lo-sə-fa′le-ə) macrocephaly.

meg·a·lo·ceph·a·ly (meg″ə-lo-sef′ə-le) macrocephaly. **megalocephal′ic** *adj*

meg·a·loc·e·ros (meg″ə-los′ə-rəs) [*megalo-* + *keras* horn] a fetus having projections from the forehead resembling horns.

meg·a·lo·chei·ria (meg″ə-lo-ki′re-ə) [*megalo-* + *cheir-* + *-ia*] abnormal largeness of the hands; called also *cheiromegaly* and *macrocheiria.*

meg·a·lo·clit·o·ris (meg″ə-lo-klit′o-ris) clitoromegaly.

meg·a·lo·cor·nea (meg″ə-lo-kor′ne-ə) [*megalo-* + *cornea*] a usually bilateral developmental anomaly of the cornea, which is of abnormal size at birth, sometimes reaching a diameter of more than 18 mm in the adult. It may be inherited as an X-linked recessive or as an autosomal dominant trait. Called also *macrocornea.*

meg·a·lo·cys·tis (meg″ə-lo-sis′tis) megacystis.

meg·a·lo·cyte (meg′ə-lo-sīt″) macrocyte.

meg·a·lo·cy·to·sis (meg″ə-lo-si-to′sis) macrocythemia.

meg·a·lo·dac·tyl·ia (meg″ə-lo-dak-til′e-ə) megalodactyly.

meg·a·lo·dac·ty·lism (meg″ə-lo-dak′tə-liz-əm) megalodactyly.

meg·a·lo·dac·ty·ly (meg″ə-lo-dak′tə-le) [*megalo-* + Gr. *daktylos* finger] abnormal largeness of fingers or toes. **megalodac′tylous** *adj*

meg·a·lo·don·tia (meg″ə-lo-don′shə) macrodontia.

meg·a·lo·esoph·a·gus (meg″ə-lo-ə-sof′ə-gəs) *megaesophagus.*

meg·a·lo·gas·tria (meg″ə-lo-gas′tre-ə) gastromegaly.

meg·a·lo·glos·sia (meg″ə-lo-glos′e-ə) macroglossia.

meg·a·lo·graph·ia (meg″ə-lo-graf′e-ə) macrography.

meg·a·log·ra·phy (meg″ə-log′rə-fe) macrography.

meg·a·lo·he·pat·ia (meg″ə-lo-he-pat′e-ə) hepatomegaly.

meg·a·lo·kary·o·cyte (meg″ə-lo-kar′e-o-sīt″) megakaryocyte.

meg·a·lo·ma·nia (meg″ə-lo-ma′ne-ə) [*megalo-* + *-mania*] unreasonable conviction of one's own extreme greatness, goodness, or power; the ideas in megalomania are known as *delusions of grandeur.*

meg·a·lo·ma·ni·ac (meg″ə-lo-ma′ne-ak) an individual exhibiting megalomania.

meg·a·lo·me·lia (meg″ə-lo-me′le-ə) macromelia.

meg·a·lo·nych·ia (meg″ə-lo-nik′e-ə) macronychia.

meg·a·lo·pe·nis (meg″ə-lo-pe′nis) macropenis.

meg·a·lo·phal·lus (meg″ə-lo-fal′əs) macropenis.

meg·a·loph·thal·mos (meg″ə-lof-thal′mos) [*megalo-* + Gr. *ophthalmos* eye] abnormally large size of the eyes; called also *macrophthalmia.*

anterior m. megalocornea.

meg·a·loph·thal·mus (meg″ə-lof-thal′məs) megalophthalmos.

meg·a·lo·pia (meg″ə-lo′pe-ə) macropsia.

meg·a·lo·po·dia (meg″ə-lo-po′de-ə) [*megalo-* + *pod-* + *-ia*] excessive size of the feet; called also *macropodia.*

Meg·a·lo·pyge (meg″ə-lo-pij′e) [*megalo-* + Gr. *pygē* rump] a genus of hairy moths. *M. opercula′ris* is the flannel moth or puss moth, whose caterpillar has stinging hairs that cause a form of insect dermatitis.

meg·a·lo·sple·nia (meg″ə-lo-sple′ne-ə) splenomegaly.

meg·a·lo·spore (meg′ə-lo-spor″) a macrospore.

meg·a·lo·syn·dac·ty·ly (meg″ə-lo-sin-dak′tə-le) [*megalo-* + *syndactyly*] a condition in which the digits are very large and more or less completely grown together.

meg·a·lo·thy·mus (meg″ə-lo-thi′məs) an enlarged thymus.

meg·a·lo·ure·ter (meg″ə-lo″u-re′tər) megaureter.

meg•a•lo•ure•thra (meg″ə-lo″u-re′thrə) congenital dilation of the urethra, due usually to abnormal development of the corpus spongiosum but occasionally to some abnormality of the corpus cavernosum.

fusiform m. a huge diverticulum of the anterior urethra, owing to absence of an entire section of the corpus spongiosum.

scaphoid m. a large diverticulum on one side of the anterior urethra, owing to a defect in the corpus spongiosum.

-megaly [Gr. *megas*, gen. *megalou* big, great] a word termination denoting abnormal enlargement of the structure signified by the root to which it is attached, as splenomegaly.

mega•poly•cal•i•co•sis (meg″ə-pol″e-kal″ĭ-ko′sis) megacalycosis.

mega•pros•o•pous (meg″ə-pros′o-pəs) [*mega-* + *prosopo-* + *-ous*] having a large face.

mega•rec•tum (meg″ə-rek′təm) megacolon confined to the rectum.

Mega•rhi•ni•ni (meg″ə-ri′nĭ-ne) in some systems of classification, a tribe of tropical non-bloodsucking mosquitoes; they fly by day, feed on flowers, and are usually highly colored. Their large larvae are predaceous and have been used to control the breeding of bloodsucking mosquitoes.

Mega•rhi•nus (meg″ə-ri′nəs) a genus of large, showy, but harmless mosquitoes of tropical and subtropical countries.

mega•seme (meg′ə-sēm) [*mega-* + Gr. *sēma* sign] having an orbital index of 89 or more.

mega•sig•moid (meg″ə-sig′moid) [*mega-* + *sigmoid*] megacolon confined to the sigmoid colon; called also *macrosigmoid.*

mega•so•ma (meg″ə-so′mə) [*mega-* + *soma*] great size and stature, not amounting to gigantism.

mega•spo•ran•gi•um (meg″ə-spə-ran′je-əm) pl. *megasporan′gia* [*mega-* + *sporangium*] the sporangium in which megaspores develop.

mega•spore (meg′ə-spor) [*mega-* + *spore*] 1. macrospore. 2. macroconidium. 3. one of four haploid spores, usually larger than the microspore, formed in the megasporangium from a megaspore mother cell, and from which the megagametophyte, or female gametophyte, develops.

mega•throm•bo•cyte (meg″ə-throm′bo-sīt) an abnormally large platelet, usually newly formed; seen in greater numbers during an increase in platelet production.

Mega•tryp•a•num (meg″ə-trip′ə-nəm) [*mega-* + Gr. *trypanon* borer] in some systems of classification, a subgenus of *Trypanosoma* that includes usually nonpathogenic species found in domestic animals.

mega•unit (meg′ə-u″nit) a quantity one million (10^6) times that of a standard unit.

mega•ure•ter (meg″ə-u-re′tər) [*mega-* + *ureter*] congenital dilatation of the ureter; it may be either a primary condition or secondary to something else. Called also *megaloureter.* See also *ureterectasis* and *hydroureter.*

congenital m. megaureter.

obstructive m. megaureter in the segment proximal to an obstruction, such as that caused by aperistalsis that interferes with passage of urine.

reflux m. dilatation of the ureter secondary to vesicoureteral reflux.

mega•vi•ta•min (meg′ə-vi″tə-min) a dose of vitamin(s) vastly exceeding the amount recommended for nutritional balance.

mega•volt (MV) (meg′ə-vōlt″) [*mega-* + *volt*] one million (10^6) volts.

mega•vol•tage (meg′ə-vōl″təj) in radiotherapy, voltage greater than 1 megavolt. Cf. *orthovoltage* and *supervoltage.*

me•ges•trol ac•e•tate (mə-jes′trol) [USP] a synthetic progestational agent used as an antineoplastic in the palliative treatment of recurrent, inoperable, or metastatic carcinoma of the breast or endometrium and for the treatment of anorexia, cachexia, and significant weight loss in patients with cancer or acquired immunodeficiency syndrome; administered orally.

meg•lu•mine (meg′loo-mēn) [USP] a crystalline base used in the preparation of certain radiopaque media. Called also *methylglucamine.* See also under *diatrizoate* and *iodipamide.*

m. antimonate a compound of pentavalent antimony and meglumine, used in treatment of leishmaniasis; administered by intramuscular or intravenous injection.

meg•ohm (meg′ōm) [*mega-* + *ohm*] one million (10^6) ohms.

meg•oph•thal•mos (meg″of-thal′mos) hydrophthalmos.

MEGX monoethylglycinexylidide.

Mehl•nähr•scha•den (māl″nār-shah′dən) [Ger.] a nutritional deficiency syndrome similar to kwashiorkor, due to inadequate protein intake and overabundance of carbohydrate; the clinical characteristics include growth failure, preservation of subcutaneous fat with wasting of muscle, edema, and psychomotor abnormalities.

mei•bo•mi•an (mi-bo′me-ən) named for Heinrich *Meibom*, German anatomist, 1638–1700, as *meibomian stye.*

mei•bo•mi•a•ni•tis (mi-bo″me-ə-ni′tis) inflammation of the meibomian (tarsal) glands; cf. *tarsadenitis.*

mei•bo•mi•tis (mi″bo-mi′tis) meibomianitis.

Meige lymphedema (disease), syndrome (māzh) [Henri *Meige*, French physician, 1866–1940] see under *syndrome*, and see *lymphedema praecox.*

Meigs capillaries (megz) [Arthur V. *Meigs*, American physician, 1850–1912] see under *capillary.*

Meigs syndrome (megz) [Joe Vincent *Meigs*, American surgeon, 1892–1963] see under *syndrome.*

Meigs-Sal•mon syndrome (megz′ să′mən) [J.V. *Meigs;* Udall J. *Salmon*, American obstetrician, 20th century] see under *syndrome.*

mei(o)- see *mio-.*

mei•o•sis (mi-o′sis) [Gr. *meiōsis* diminution] a special type of cell division occurring in the maturation of germ cells, consisting of two successive cell divisions (meiosis I and meiosis II) without an interval of DNA replication, by means of which diploid germ cells (primary spermatocytes and oocytes) give rise to haploid gametes. During meiosis I, homologous chromosomes are paired and segregated, resulting in a haploid number of paired chromatids; during meiosis II the paired chromatids are separated. See illustration. Cf. *mitosis.* **meiot′ic** *adj*

Mei•row•sky phenomenon (mi-rov′ske) [Emil *Meirowsky*, German-American dermatologist, 1876–1960] see under *phenomenon.*

Meiss•ner corpuscle, ganglion, plexus (mīs′ner) [Georg *Meissner*, German physiologist, 1829–1905] see *plexus submucosus* and see under *corpuscle* and *ganglion.*

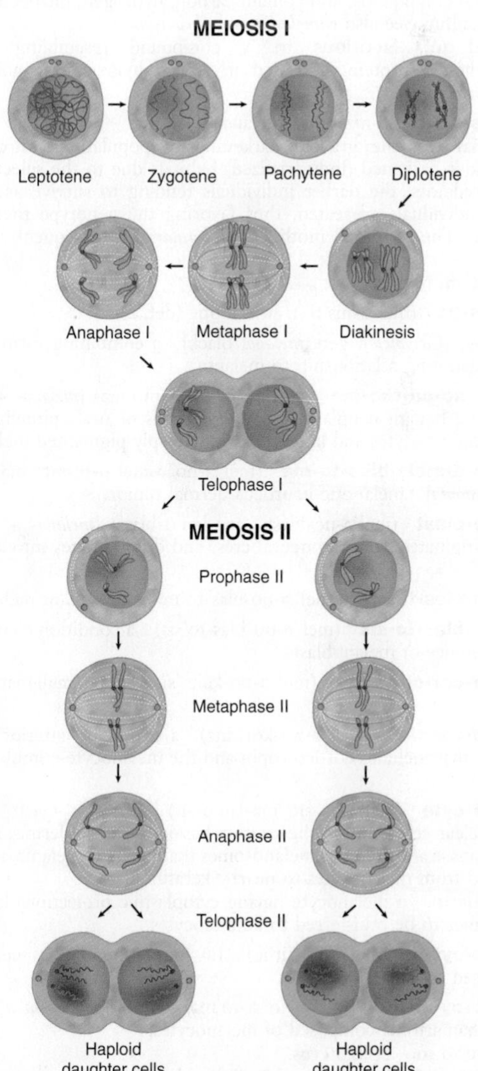

■ Meiosis (only two of the 23 human chromosome pairs are shown, the chromosomes from one parent in blue, those from the other parent in pink).

mel (mel) [L.] 1. honey. 2. a compound of honey with some medicinal agent.

mel·ag·ra (məl-ag′rə) [*mel-* + *-agra*] muscular pain in the extremities.

Mel·a·leu·ca (mel″ə-loo′kə) a genus of trees of the family Myrtaceae, native to Australia and the East Indies. *M. leucaden′dron* is the cajeput or cajuput tree, whose fresh leaves and twigs yield cajeput oil; *M. alternifo′lia* is the tea tree, which is the source of tea tree oil.

mel·al·gia (məl-al′jə) [*mel-* + *-algia*] pain in the limbs.

mel·an·cho·lia (mel″an-ko′le-ə) [*melan-* + *chol-* + *-ia*] former name for *depression;* in modern psychiatric terminology it refers especially to severe forms of major depressive disorder. **melanchol′ic** *adj*

m. agita′ta, agitated m. agitated depression.

involutional m. former name for a mood disorder now subsumed under the category of major depressive disorder.

mel·an·choly (mel′ən-kol″e) melancholia.

mel·a·nem·e·sis (mel″ə-nem′ə-sis) black vomit.

mel·a·ne·mia (mel″ə-ne′me-ə) [*melan-* + *-emia*] the presence of black, pigmentary masses in the blood, as in hemochromatosis.

Mel·a·nex (mel′ə-neks) trademark for a preparation of hydroquinone.

Me·la·nia (mə-la′ne-ə) *Thiara.*

mel·a·nic·ter·us (mel″ə-nik′tər-əs) Winckel disease.

mel·a·nif·er·ous (mel″ə-nif′ər-əs) [*melanin* + *-ferous*] containing melanin or other black pigment.

mel·a·nin (mel′ə-nin) [Gr. *melas* black] any of several closely related dark, amorphous pigments of the skin, hair, and various tumors, of the choroid coat of the eye and of the brain (neuromelanin, q.v.). Melanins are produced by polymerization of oxidation products of tyrosine and dihydroxyphenyl compounds, and contain carbon, hydrogen, nitrogen, oxygen, and often sulfur. See also *eumelanin* and *pheomelanin.*

artificial m., factitious m. a compound resembling melanin, formed when a protein is heated in strong hydrochloric acid; called also *melanoid.*

mel·a·nism (mel′ə-niz″əm) melanosis.

industrial m. the gradual darkening of populations of organisms living in soot-darkened (industrialized) habitats due to the selective pressure of predators, the darker individuals tending to survive as the conspicuous individuals are eaten, thus favoring the genotype that darkens their color. The peppered moth, *Biston betularia,* is a frequently used example.

metallic m. argyria.

mel·a·nis·tic (mel″ə-nis′tik) melanotic (def. 2).

melan(o)- [Gr. *melas,* gen. *melanos* black] a combining form meaning black, or denoting relationship to melanin.

mel·a·no·ac·an·tho·ma (mel″ə-no-ak″ən-tho′mə) [*melano-* + *acanthoma*] a rare, benign neoplasm of the epidermis or oral epithelium, composed of keratinocytes and large dendritic, deeply pigmented melanocytes.

mel·a·no·a·melo·blas·to·ma (mel″ə-no″ə-mel″o-blas-to′mə) [*melano-* + *ameloblastoma*] melanotic neuroectodermal tumor.

mel·a·no·blast (mel′ə-no-blast″, mə-lan′o-blast) [*melano-* + *-blast*] a cell that originates from the neural crest and differentiates into a melanocyte.

mel·a·no·blas·to·ma (mel″ə-no-blas-to′mə) malignant melanoma.

mel·a·no·blas·to·sis (mel″ə-no-blas-to′sis) a condition characterized by the presence of melanoblasts.

mel·a·no·car·ci·no·ma (mel″ə-no-kahr″sĭ-no′mə) malignant melanoma.

mel·a·no·cor·tins (mel″ə-no-kor′tinz) a group of anterior pituitary hormones that includes corticotropin and the melanocyte-stimulating hormones.

mel·a·no·cyte (mel′ə-no-sīt, mə-lan′o-sīt) [*melano-* + *-cyte*] a type of dendritic clear cell found in the stratum basale of the epidermis; it synthesizes tyrosinase and contains melanosomes that produce melanin and can be transferred from melanocytes to nearby keratinocytes.

dendritic m. a melanocyte having cytoplasmic projections laden with melanosomes to be transferred to keratinocytes.

mel·a·no·cyt·ic (mel″ə-no-sit′ik) 1. pertaining to melanocytes. 2. composed of melanocytes.

mel·a·no·cy·to·ma (mel″ə-no″si-to′mə) [*melanocyte* + *-oma*] a neoplasm or hamartoma composed of melanocytes.

compound m. Spitz nevus.

dermal m. 1. blue nevus. 2. cellular blue nevus.

m. of optic disk a nonmalignant pigmented tumor of the optic disk, usually asymptomatic but sometimes causing blurred vision.

mel·a·no·cy·to·sis (mel″ə-no″si-to′sis) [*melanocyte* + *-osis*] excessive melanocytes in the tissues.

congenital dermal m. mongolian spot.

oculodermal m. nevus of Ota.

mel·a·no·der·ma (mel″ə-no-dur′mə) [*melano-* + *derma*] abnormally increased melanin in the skin, with hyperpigmented patches; it may be due either to increased production by the melanocytes that are normally present or to increased absolute numbers of melanocytes.

parasitic m. vagabond's disease.

mel·a·no·der·ma·ti·tis (mel″ə-no-dur″mə-ti′tis) [*melano-* + *dermatitis*] dermatitis associated with an increased deposit of melanin in the skin.

lichenoid m. lichen planus actinicus.

m. tox′ica lichenoi′des tar melanosis.

me·lan·o·gen (mə-lan′o-jən) [*melano-* + *-gen*] a colorless chromogen, convertible into melanin, which may occur in the urine in certain diseases, e.g., malignant melanoma.

mel·a·no·gen·e·sis (mel″ə-no-jen′ə-sis) [*melano-* + *-genesis*] the production of melanin.

mel·a·no·gen·ic (mel″ə-no-jen′ik) causing the production of melanin.

mel·a·no·glos·sia (mel″ə-no-glos′e-ə) [*melano-* + *gloss-* + *-ia*] black hairy tongue.

mel·a·noid (mel′ə-noid″) [*melan-* + *-oid*] 1. resembling melanin; of a dark color. 2. artificial melanin.

Mel·a·no·les·tes (mel″ə-no-les′tēz) the corsairs, a genus of biting insects of the family Reduviidae. *M. pi′cipes* is the black corsair, a species whose bite resembles a severe wasp sting.

mel·a·no·ma (mel″ə-no′mə) [*melan-* + *-oma*] 1. a tumor arising from melanocytes of the skin or other organs. 2. malignant m. **melano′matous** *adj*

acral-lentiginous m. (ALM) the most common type of melanoma in nonwhite individuals, but uncommon in light-skinned persons, found chiefly on the palms and soles, especially on the distal phalanges of the fingers and toes. It typically presents as an irregular, enlarging black macule and has a prolonged noninvasive stage. When on the nail fold or bed it is called a *subungual melanoma.* Less often it may be found on a mucosal surface, such as the vulva or vagina.

amelanotic m. an unpigmented malignant melanoma.

benign juvenile m. Spitz nevus.

canine limbal m. a type of uveal melanoma in dogs, arising from the junction between the cornea and sclera; most are benign but tumor expansion may cause loss of vision.

choroidal m. uveal melanoma that involves the choroid.

Cloudman m. S91 a firm, black subcutaneous tumor originally found at the base of the tail of a female DBA mouse, and proven to be transplantable to, and invariably metastatic in, other DBA mice and BALB/c mice.

desmoplastic m. a rare type of malignant melanoma characterized by white patches containing spindle cells, usually on sun-exposed areas of the body. Called also *spindle cell m.*

Harding-Passey m. a transplantable, nonmetastasizing melanoma originally found on the ear of a brown mouse.

intraocular m. ocular m.

juvenile m. Spitz nevus.

lenti′go malig′na m. a cutaneous malignant melanoma found most often on sun-exposed areas of the skin, especially the face. It begins as a circumscribed macular patch of mottled pigmentation, showing shades of dark brown, tan, or black *(lentigo maligna* or *melanotic freckle of Hutchinson);* later it enlarges by lateral growth before dermal invasion occurs. This type is the slowest growing, has the least tendency to metastasize, and seems to be the least aggressive form of malignant melanoma.

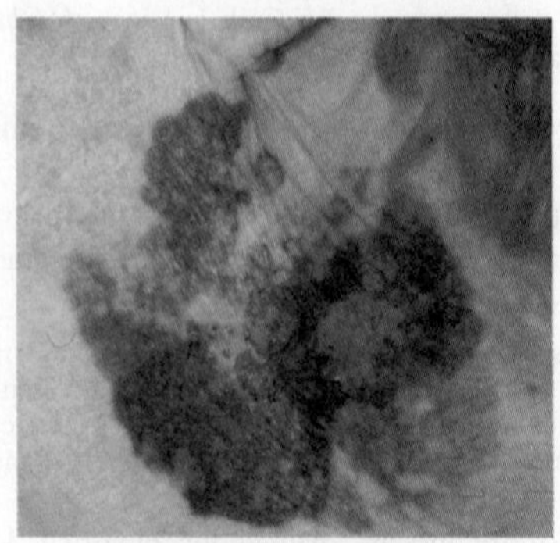

■ Lentigo maligna melanoma.

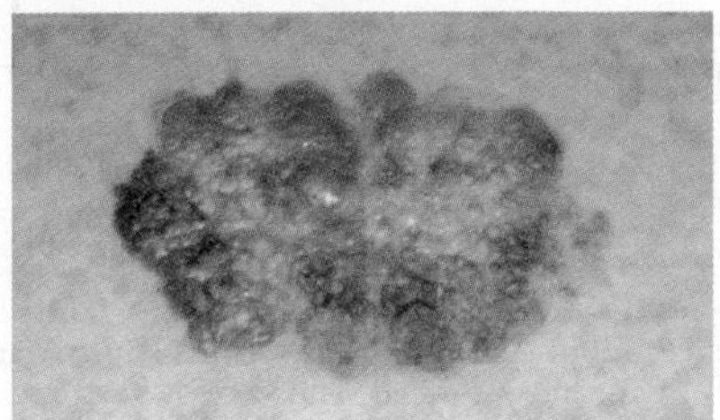

■ Superficial spreading melanoma.

malignant m. a malignant neoplasm of melanocytes, arising de novo or from a preexisting benign nevus or lentigo maligna, occurring most often in the skin but sometimes in the oral cavity, esophagus, anal canal, vagina, leptomeninges, conjunctivae, or eye. These tumors are classified into four clinical types: *superficial spreading m.*, *lentigo maligna m.*, *acral-lentiginous m.*, and *nodular m.* Called also *melanotic carcinoma*, *melanoblastoma*, and *melanocarcinoma*.

mucosal m. melanoma on a mucous membrane, chiefly the palate but also elsewhere on the head and neck, genitalia, and esophagus, usually in older women; most are lentiginous, but nodular and superficial spreading melanomas also occur.

nodular m. a type of malignant melanoma arising without a perceptible radial growth phase, most often occurring on the head, neck, and trunk, typically presenting as a uniformly pigmented, elevated, bizarrely colored nodule that enlarges rather rapidly and commonly ulcerates, which may arise de novo or from a preexisting malignant melanoma of a different type.

nontumorigenic m. melanoma in the stage of radial growth, when the risk of metastasis is slight; cf. *tumorigenic m.*

ocular m., ocular malignant m. malignant melanoma arising from the structures of the eye, usually the choroid, ciliary body, or iris, and occurring most often in the fifth and sixth decades of life. The most common site of metastasis is the liver; if this occurs, the condition is usually rapidly fatal.

spindle cell m. desmoplastic m.

subungual m. acral-lentiginous melanoma occurring in the nail fold or bed; called also *melanotic whitlow*.

superficial spreading m. the most common type of malignant melanoma, characterized by a period of radial growth atypical of melanocytes in the epidermis, usually with a lymphocytic cellular host response that may be accompanied by partial or complete regression of the radial growth phase; deeply invasive growth (vertical growth) is superimposed on the radial phase. It occurs most often on the lower leg or back, usually presenting as a small pigmented macule to a slightly palpable flat lesion that assumes an irregular outline on enlargement.

tumorigenic m. melanoma in the stage of vertical growth, when the risk of metastasis becomes significant; cf. *nontumorigenic m.*

uveal m., uveal malignant m. the most common type of ocular malignant melanoma, consisting of overgrowth of uveal melanocytes and often preceded by a uveal nevus.

mel•a•no•ma•to•sis (mel″ə-no″mə-to′sis) the formation of melanomas in various parts of the body.

mel•a•no•nych•ia (mel″ə-no-nik′e-ə) [*melan-* + *onychia*] blackening of the nail by melanin pigmentation.

mel•a•no•phage (mel′ə-no-fāj″) [*melano-* + *-phage*] a histiocyte laden with phagocytosed melanin.

mel•a•no•phore (mel′ə-no-for″) [*melano-* + *-phore*] a type of chromatophore containing melanin, found especially in the dermis of fishes, amphibians, and reptiles.

mel•a•no•pla•kia (mel″ə-no-pla′ke-ə) [*melano-* + Gr. *plax* plate + *-ia*] the presence of pigmented patches on the oral mucosa.

mel•a•nop•ty•sis (mel″ə-nop′tĭ-sis) [*melano-* + Gr. *ptyein* to spit] the expectoration of black sputum, as in coal workers' pneumoconiosis.

mel•a•no•sis (mel″ə-no′sis) [*melan-* + *-osis*] excessive pigmentation of part of the body owing to a disturbance in melanin pigmentation; called also *melanism*.

Becker m. see under *nevus*.

m. bul′bi m. oculi.

circumscribed precancerous m. lentigo maligna melanoma.

m. co′li black or brown discoloration of the mucous membrane of the colon due to pigment from certain cathartics that has leaked into the lamina propria.

Dubreuilh m. lentigo maligna melanoma.

m. i′ridis, m. of iris abnormal pigmentation of the iris by infiltration of melanoblasts.

neurocutaneous m. giant hairy nevus accompanied by malignant melanomas of the meninges.

m. o′culi a usually congenital condition in which there is a diffuse increase in pigmentation of the uveal tract and often of the more superficial ocular tissues. Called also *m. bulbi*.

oculocutaneous m., oculodermal m. nevus of Ota.

primary acquired m. appearance on the conjunctiva of flat, brown pigmentation, seen primarily in persons over age 40; many cases are benign, but if it is aplastic or contains nodules it may be premalignant, sometimes developing into melanoma.

Riehl m. patchy melanoderma with light to dark brown pigmentation, most intensely on the forehead and cheeks, behind the ears, on the sides of the neck, and on other sun-exposed areas. It is seen most often in women and may be an inflammatory photosensitivity or phototoxic reaction.

m. scle′rae congenital flecks of pigmentation in the sclera.

tar m. a dermatosis representing photosensitivity or phototoxicity induced by exposure to tar or other hydrocarbons, usually occupationally, most often involving the face or back of the hands, and characterized by pruritus associated with the development of reticular pigmentation, telangiectases, and small, dark, lichenoid, follicular papules. Called also *melanodermatitis toxica lichenoides*.

transient neonatal pustular m. a congenital skin condition usually seen in babies of African descent, characterized by pigmented macules and vesicopustules that may rupture and leave a scaly collar. It usually resolves completely within a few weeks to two years.

mel•a•no•some (mel′ə-no-sōm″) [*melano-* + *-some*] any of the granules within the melanocytes that contain tyrosinase and synthesize melanin, and can be transferred from the melanocytes to keratinocytes.

mel•a•not•ic (mel″ə-not′ik) 1. pertaining to or characterized by the presence of melanin. 2. characterized by melanosis.

mel•a•no•trich•ia (mel″ə-no-trik′e-ə) [*melano-* + *trich-* + *-ia*] abnormal hyperpigmentation of the hair.

m. lin′guae black hairy tongue.

mel•a•no•troph (mel′ə-no-trōf″) [*melano-* + Gr. *trophē* nourishment] a pituitary cell type that elaborates melanocyte-stimulating hormone and β-endorphins. Melanotrophs are abundant in animals that have a pars intermedia adenohypophyseos; humans have very few.

mel•a•no•tro•pic (mel″ə-no-tro′pik) [*melano-* + *-tropic*] having an affinity for melanin; influencing the deposit of melanin.

mel•a•no•tro•pin (mel′ə-no-tro″pin) melanocyte-stimulating hormone.

me•lan•thin (mə-lan′thin) an amorphous and poisonous glycoside or saponin from the seeds of *Nigella sativa*.

mel•an•u•re•sis (mel″ən-u-re′sis) melanuria.

mel•an•uria (mel″ə-nu′re-ə) [*melan-* + *uria*] excretion of urine that is darkly stained or turns dark on standing. **melanu′ric** *adj*

me•lar•so•prol (mə-lahr′so-prol) an antiprotozoal effective against *Trypanosoma*, used in the treatment of advanced cases of African trypanosomiasis, administered intravenously.

me•las•ma (mə-laz′mə) [Gr. *melas* black] melanosis with sharply demarcated brown macules, usually symmetrically on the face or neck, seen most often during pregnancy, at menopause, and in those taking oral contraceptives, and occasionally in other women or in men. It affects persons with light brown skin much more often than those with light skin. A similar condition is sometimes seen in chronic liver disease. Called also *chloasma* and *mask of pregnancy*.

mel•a•to•nin (mel″ə-to′nin) a hormone synthesized by the pineal gland in many species of animals; its secretion increases during exposure to light. In adult amphibians it produces lightening of the dermal pigmentation by promoting aggregation of melanosomes. In mammals it influences

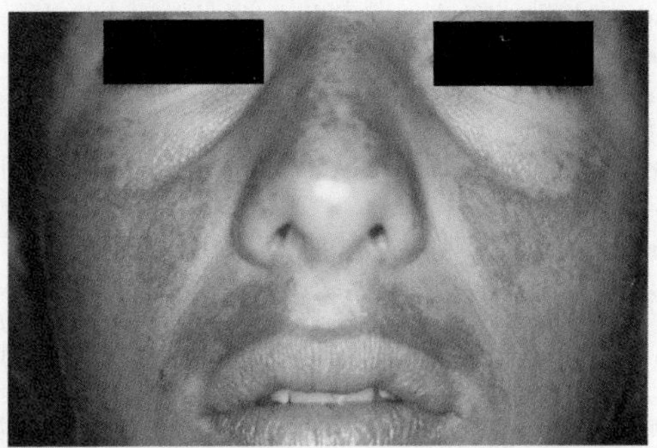

■ Melasma.

hormone production and in many species it regulates seasonal changes such as reproductive pattern and fur color. In humans it is implicated in the regulation of sleep, mood, puberty, and ovarian cycles. It has been tried therapeutically for a number of conditions, including insomnia and jet lag.

Me·le·da disease (mel′ə-dah) [*Meleda* (Serbo-Croat *Mljet*), an island in the eastern Adriatic Sea, part of Croatia, where the condition is prevalent because of intermarriage] mal de Meleda.

me·le·na (mə-le′nə) [Gr. *melaina*, feminine of Gr. *melas* black] the passage of dark-colored feces stained with blood pigments or with altered blood. **mele′nic** *adj*

m. neonato′rum melena of the newborn, due to the extravasation of blood into the alimentary canal.

m. spu′ria melena in a nursing infant in which the blood comes from the fissured nipple of the mother.

m. ve′ra true melena; as distinguished from melena spuria.

Me·le·ney ulcer (gangrene), synergistic gangrene (mə-le′ne) [Frank Lamont *Meleney*, American surgeon, 1889–1963] see under *ulcer*, and see *progressive synergistic gangrene*, under *gangrene*.

mel·en·ges·trol ac·e·tate (mel-ən-jes′trol) [USP] a progestin and antineoplastic, commonly administered as a feed additive to cattle to suppress estrus and promote growth.

me·lez·i·tose (mə-lez′ĭ-tōs) a reducing trisaccharide composed of glucose and turanose, an isomer of sucrose. It occurs in poplars and conifers, and in the honey produced by bees that have collected from these trees.

meli- [Gr. *meli*, gen. *melitos* honey] a combining form meaning sweet, or denoting relationship to honey or to sugar.

-melia [Gr. *melos* limb + *-ia*] a word termination denoting a limb.

Me·lia (mel′e-ə) a genus of deciduous trees of the family Meliaceae, native to Indonesia and Australia, having pinnate or bipinnate leaves, fragrant white or purplish flowers, and small fruits.

M. aze′darach the azedarach, chinaberry, or umbrella tree, a common shade tree whose seeds are used as beads, whose root bark is an anthelmintic, and whose leaf juice is a diuretic and emmenagogue. Its fruit is poisonous, causing severe local irritation, neurological symptoms, cardiotoxicity, and dyspnea.

meli·bi·ase (mel″ĭ-bi′ās) α-galactosidase.

meli·bi·ose (mel″ĭ-bi′ōs) a disaccharide composed of galactose in α-(1,6) linkage with glucose; it is a constituent of the trisaccharide raffinose.

meli·ce·ra (mel″i-se′rə) [*meli-* + *cera*] 1. a cyst filled with honeylike fluid. 2. viscid, syrupy.

meli·ce·ris (mel″ĭ-se′ris) melicera.

Mel·i·lo·tus (mel″ĭ-lo′tus) the sweet clovers, a genus of leguminous herbs with trifoliate leaves; they are commonly consumed by livestock, but because they contain dicumarol, when they spoil they are the cause of the hemorrhagic condition called *sweet clover disease*.

me·li·oi·do·sis (me″le-oi-do′sis) [Gr. *mēlis* a distemper of asses + *-oid* + *-osis*] an infection, usually of rodents, which can spread to other animals and is caused by *Burkholderia pseudomallei*. Most cases are seen in Southeast Asia, but it has also been seen in temperate regions. Human disease, usually acquired through contamination of a break in the skin with soil or water, may range from a dormant infection to localized abscesses, benign pneumonia, or fatal septicemia; late activation of inapparent disease or recrudescence of previous symptoms may also occur. In other animals the syndrome varies considerably and usually involves caseous or suppurative lesions of the lymph nodes or viscera. Called also *pseudoglanders*.

Me·lis·sa (mə-lis′ə) [Gr. "bee"] a genus of plants of the family Lamiaceae. The tops and leaves of *M. officina′lis*, or lemon balm, contain tannin and a volatile oil and are a cooling stimulant and diaphoretic.

mel·is·so·pho·bia (mə-lis″o-fo′be-ə) apiphobia.

me·lis·so·ther·a·py (mə-lis″o-ther′ə-pe) [Gr. *melissa* bee + *therapy*] apiotherapy.

me·li·tis (mə-li′tis) [Gr. *mēlon* cheek + *-itis*] inflammation of the cheek.

melit(o)- see *meli-*.

mel·i·tose (mel′ĭ-tōs) former name for *raffinose*.

mel·i·tu·ria (mel″ĭ-tu′re-ə) [*melit-* + *-uria*] sugar in the urine; specific types are named for the sugar in question, such as *fructosuria*, *galactosuria*, *glycosuria*, *lactosuria*, *maltosuria*, *sucrosuria*, and so on. Spelled also *mellituria*.

Mel·kers·son syndrome (mel′kər-son) [Ernst Gustaf *Melkersson*, Swedish physician, 1898–1932] see under *syndrome*.

Mel·kers·son-Ro·sen·thal syndrome (mel′kər-son ro′zen-tahl) [E.G. *Melkersson;* Curt *Rosenthal*, German psychiatrist, 20th century] Melkersson syndrome.

mel·li·tum (mə-li′təm) pl. *melli′ta* [L.] a pharmaceutical preparation made with honey.

mel·li·tu·ria (mel″ĭ-tu′re-ə) melituria.

Mel·nick-Fra·ser syndrome (mel′nik fra′zər) [Michael *Melnick*, American geneticist, 20th century; Frank Clarke *Fraser*, Canadian geneticist, born 1930] branchio-oto-renal syndrome.

Mel·nick-Nee·dles syndrome (mel′nik ne′dəlz) [John Charles *Melnick*, American radiologist, 1928–2008; Carl F. *Needles*, American pediatrician, born 1935] see under *syndrome.*

mel(o)-[1] [Gr. *melos* limb] a combining form denoting relationship to a limb.

mel(o)-[2] [Gr. *mēlon* cheek] a combining form denoting relationship to the cheek.

Me·lo·chia py·ram·i·da·ta (mə-lo′ke-ə pĭ-ram″ĭ-da′tə) a shrub found in Central America; ingestion by cattle causes derrengue.

melo·did·y·mus (mel″ə-did′ə-məs) [*melo-*[1] + *-didymus*] an individual with a supernumerary limb.

Me·lo·i·dae (məlo′ĭ-de) the blister beetles, a family of beetles whose dried bodies raise blisters when rubbed on human skin and are sometimes used as counterirritants. Genera include *Epicauta* and *Lytta* (which contain cantharidin), *Paederus* (which contains pederin), *Psalydolytta*, and *Sessinia*. See also *cantharidin poisoning*, under *poisoning*.

melo·la·bi·al (mel″o-la′be-əl) buccolabial.

me·lono·plas·ty (mə-lon′o-plas″te) meloplasty.

Me·loph·a·gus (mə-lof′ə-gəs) a genus of wingless flies of the family Hippoboscidae. *M. ovi′nus*, the sheep ked, is a common ectoparasite of sheep and goats.

melo·plas·ty (mel′o-plas″te) [*melo-*[2] + *-plasty*] plastic surgery of the cheek. **meloplas′tic** *adj*

Mel·o·psit·ta·cus (mel″o-sit′ə-kəs) a genus of psittacine birds. *M. undula′tus* is the budgerigar (q.v.).

melo·rhe·os·to·sis (mel″o-re″os-to′sis) [*melo-*[1] + *rheo-* + *ostosis*] a form of osteosclerosis or hyperostosis extending in a linear track through one of the long bones of an extremity, and consisting of proliferated ivory-like new bone. See *rheostosis.*

me·los·chi·sis (mə-los′kĭ-sis) [*melo-*[2] + *-schisis*] oblique facial cleft.

me·lo·tia (mə-lo′shə) [*mel-*[2] + *ot-* + *-ia*] a developmental anomaly characterized by displacement of the ear onto the cheek.

mel·ox·i·cam (mə-lok′sĭ-kam) a nonsteroidal antiinflammatory drug used in the treatment of osteoarthritis; administered orally.

mel·pha·lan (mel′fə-lan) [USP] a cytotoxic alkylating agent that is the L-phenylalanine derivative of mechlorethamine, used as an antineoplastic, primarily for treatment of multiple myeloma, administered orally or intravenously; it is also used in regional limb perfusion for melanoma of the extremity, administered by arterial infusion. Called also *L-sarcolysin* and *L-phenylalanine mustard (L-PAM)*.

melt·ing (mel′ting) 1. undergoing or causing to undergo the transition from solid to liquid, as by the application of heat or pressure. 2. in molecular biology, the disruption of secondary structure in molecules or parts of molecules, such as the heat-induced general or localized separation of a double-stranded nucleic acid to form a single-stranded molecule or region.

corneal m. dissolution of part or all of the cornea, usually referring to its occurrence with something other than an infection; it is seen most often as a complication of advanced Sjögren syndrome with keratoconjunctivitis sicca. Cf. *keratolysis*.

mem·an·tine (mem′an-tēn) an *N*-methyl-D-aspartate (NMDA) antagonist used in the treatment of symptoms of moderate to severe Alzheimer disease. It protects the brain's nerve cells against glutamate, which is released in excess amounts by cells damaged by Alzheimer disease and which overstimulates the NMDA receptors; administered orally.

mem·ber (mem′bər) [L. *membrum*] 1. a part of the body distinct from the rest in function or position. 2. a limb; see *membrum inferius* and *membrum superius*.

mem·ber·ment (mem′bər-mənt) the manner of arrangement of parts in a body.

mem·bra (mem′brə) [L.] plural of *membrum*.

mem·bra·na (mem-bra′nə) gen. and pl. *membra′nae* [L.] a membrane: anatomic nomenclature for a thin layer of tissue covering a surface, lining a cavity, or dividing a space or organ.

Membrana

Descriptions are given on TA terms, and include anglicized names of specific membranes.

m. atlantooccipita′lis ante′rior [TA] anterior atlanto-occipital membrane: a single midline ligamentous structure that passes from the anterior arch of the atlas to the anterior margin of the foramen magnum, and corresponds in position with the anterior longitudinal ligament of the vertebral column.
m. atlantooccipita′lis poste′rior [TA] posterior atlanto-occipital membrane: a single midline ligamentous structure that passes from the posterior arch of the atlas to the posterior margin of the foramen magnum, and corresponds in position with the ligamenta flava.
m. basa′lis basement membrane.
m. capsula′ris capsular membrane.
m. epipapilla′ris an abnormal fibrous membrane on the optic disk.
m. fibroelas′tica laryn′gis [TA] fibroelastic membrane of larynx: the fibroelastic layer beneath the mucous coat of the larynx, comprising the quadrangular membrane and the conus elasticus. See also *intrinsic laryngeal ligaments*, under *ligament*.
m. fibro′sa cap′sulae articula′ris [TA] fibrous membrane of articular capsule: the outer of the two layers of the articular capsule of a synovial joint, composed of dense white fibrous tissue; called also *stratum fibrosum capsulae articularis* [TA alternative].
m. flac′cida pars flaccida membranae tympanicae.
m. germinati′va blastoderm.
m. granulo′sa layers of cuboidal epithelial cells at the periphery of an ovarian follicle and surrounding the antrum or fluid-filled cavity.
m. granulo′sa exter′na the external granular layer of the retina.
m. granulo′sa inter′na the internal granular layer of the retina.
m. hyaloi′dea m. vitrea.
m. intercosta′lis exter′na [TA] external intercostal membrane: any of the aponeurotic bands parallel with, and perhaps replacing, the fibers of the external intercostal muscles in the spaces between the costal cartilages, from the ventral tips of the ribs medially to the sternum.
m. intercosta′lis inter′na [TA] internal intercostal membrane: any of the aponeurotic bands parallel with, and perhaps replacing, the fibers of the internal intercostal muscles in the spaces between the ribs, from the angles of the ribs medially to the vertebral column.
m. interos′sea [TA] interosseous membrane: a dense fibrous membrane that stretches between and unites the bones in a syndesmosis.
m. interos′sea antebra′chii [TA] interosseous membrane of forearm: a thin fibrous sheet that connects the bodies of the radius and ulna, passing from the interosseous margin of the radius to that of the ulna.
m. interos′sea cru′ris [TA] interosseous membrane of leg: a thin aponeurotic lamina attached to the interosseous borders of the tibia and fibula, deficient for a short distance at the proximal end of the bones; it separates the muscles on the anterior and posterior parts of the leg.
m. li′mitans 1. one of the limiting membranes of the retina; see *external* and *internal limiting membrane* (def. 1), under *membrane*. 2. the limiting membrane of glia fibrils and perivascular feet separating the parenchyma of the central nervous system from the pia and blood vessels. It is sometimes considered together with the pia mater as the *pia-glia*.
m. nic′titans 1. plica semilunaris conjunctivae. 2. nictitating membrane.
m. obturato′ria [TA] obturator membrane: a strong membrane that fills the obturator foramen except superiorly at the obturator groove, where a deficiency is left, the obturator canal.
m. perfora′ta a term sometimes used to designate the first appearance of dentin in the fetus, manifested as a thick limiting line between the ameloblasts and odontoblasts.
m. perine′i [TA] perineal membrane: the triangular fibrous membrane stretched horizontally between the ischiopubic rami, attached at its base to the perineal body; its apex thickens to form the transverse perineal ligament.
m. pupilla′ris [TA] pupillary membrane: the portion of the tunica vasculosa lentis that is in front of the pupil; it is a mesodermal layer attached to the rim or front of the iris during embryonic development, sometimes persisting in the adult. Called also *Wachendorf membrane*.

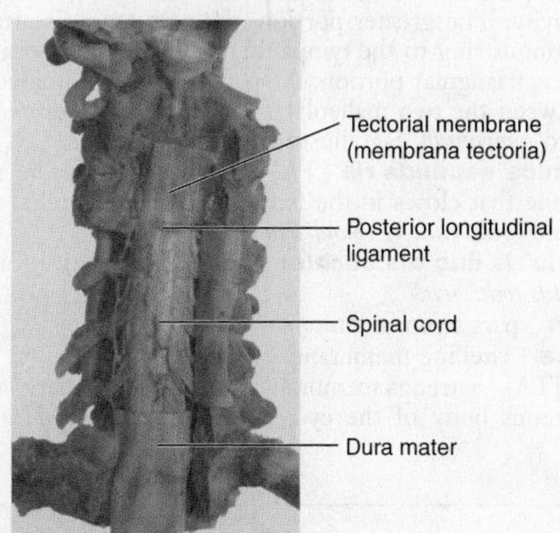

■ Membrana tectoria (tectorial membrane) in a posterior view of a dissection of the vertebral column. The vertebral arches, brainstem, and upper part of the spinal cord have been removed.

m. quadrangula′ris [TA] quadrangular membrane: the upper part of the fibroelastic membrane of the larynx.
m. reticula′ris or′gani spira′lis [TA] reticular membrane of spiral organ: a netlike membrane over the spiral organ; the free ends of the outer hair cells pass through its apertures. Called also *reticular lamina*.
m. spira′lis duc′tus cochlea′ris TA alternative for *paries tympanicus ductus cochlearis*.
m. stapedia′lis [TA] stapedial membrane: a membrane filling the arch formed by the crura and base of the stapes.
m. statoconio′rum [TA] otolithic membrane: the gelatinous membrane surmounting the maculae, containing the statoconia, and having special sensory hairs projecting into it.
m. ster′ni [TA] sternal membrane: the thick fibrous membrane that envelopes the sternum; it is formed by the intermingling of fibers of the radiate sternocostal ligaments, the periosteum, and the tendinous origin of the pectoralis major.
m. suprapleura′lis [TA] suprapleural membrane: the strengthened portion of the endothoracic fascia attached to the inner part of the first rib and the transverse process of the seventh cervical vertebra.
m. synovia′lis cap′sulae articula′ris [TA] synovial membrane of articular capsule: the inner of the two layers of the articular capsule of a synovial joint, composed of loose connective tissue and having a free smooth surface that lines the joint cavity. It secretes the synovial fluid. Called also *stratum synoviale capsulae articularis* [TA alternative].
m. synovia′lis infe′rior articulatio′nis temporomandibula′ris [TA] inferior synovial membrane of temporomandibular joint: the synovial membrane that lines the articular capsule of the joint below the articular disk.
m. synovia′lis supe′rior articulatio′nis temporomandibula′ris [TA] superior synovial membrane of temporomandibular joint: the synovial membrane that lines the articular capsule of the joint above the articular disk.
m. tecto′ria [TA] tectorial membrane: a strong fibrous band connected cranially with the basilar part of the occipital bone and caudally with the dorsal surface of the bodies of the second and third cervical vertebrae. It is actually the cranial prolongation of the deeper portion of the posterior longitudinal ligament of the vertebral column.
m. tecto′ria duc′tus cochlea′ris [TA] tectorial membrane of cochlear duct: a delicate gelatinous mass extending from the limbus and resting on the spiral organ of the ear and connected with the hairs of the hair cells; called also *Corti membrane*.
m. ten′sa pars tensa membranae tympanicae.
m. thyrohyoi′dea [TA] thyrohyoid membrane: a broad fibroelastic sheet attached above to the upper margin of the posterior surface of the hyoid bone and below to the upper border of the thyroid cartilage. See also *extrinsic laryngeal ligaments*, under *ligament*.

Membrana *Continued*

m. tympa′nica [TA] tympanic membrane: the obliquely placed, thin membranous partition between the external acoustic meatus and the tympanic cavity. The greater portion, the pars tensa, is attached by a fibrocartilaginous ring to the tympanic plate of the temporal bone; the much smaller, triangular portion, the pars flaccida, is situated anterosuperiorly between the two malleolar folds. Called also *drumhead, drum, eardrum,* and *tympanum.* See illustration and Plate 14.
m. tympa′nica secunda′ria [TA] secondary tympanic membrane: the membrane that closes in the fenestra cochlearis; called also *Scarpa membrane* and *membrane of round window.*
m. vestibula′ris duc′tus cochlea′ris TA alternative for *paries vestibularis ductus cochlearis.*
m. vi′brans pars tensa membranae tympanicae.
m. vitelli′na vitelline membrane.
m. vi′trea [TA] vitreous membrane: a delicate boundary layer investing the vitreous body of the eye; called also *m. hyaloidea* or *hyaloid membrane.*

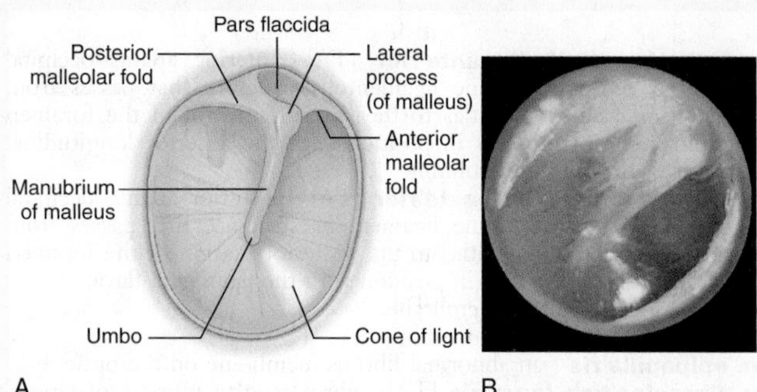

■ Diagram *(A)* and otoscopic view *(B)* of normal membrana tympanica (tympanic membrane).

mem•bra•nae (mem-bra′ne) [L.] genitive and plural of *membrana.*

mem•bra•nate (mem′brə-nāt) having the character of a membrane.

mem•brane (mem′brān) a thin layer of tissue that covers a surface, lines a cavity, or divides a space or organ; see also *membrana.* **membrana′ceous, mem′branous** *adj*

Membrane

For names of specific anatomic structures not found here, see under *membrana.*

abdominal m. peritoneum.
adamantine m. cuticula dentis.
alveolar-capillary m., alveolocapillary m. a thin tissue barrier between pulmonary alveoli and adjacent capillaries, the site of gas exchange between alveolar air and capillary blood. Called also *alveolar-capillary* or *alveolocapillary barrier* and *blood-air* or *blood-gas barrier.*
alveolodental m. periodontal ligament.
anal m. the dorsal part of the cloacal membrane after its division by the urorectal septum.
antral m. a congenital abnormal membrane in the pyloric antrum, partially or completely blocking the gastric outlet. See also *prepyloric atresia.* Called also *antral diaphragm* or *web.*
apical m. the layer of plasma membrane on the apical side (the side towards the lumen) of the epithelial cells in a body tube or cavity, separated from the basolateral membrane by the tight junction.
aponeurotic m. aponeurosis.
arachnoid m. arachnoidea.
Ascherson m. the covering of casein enclosing the milk globules.
asphyxial m. hyaline m. (def. 2); so called because of its interference with gaseous exchange in the lungs.
atlanto-occipital m., anterior membrana atlantooccipitalis anterior.
atlanto-occipital m., posterior membrana atlantooccipitalis posterior.
basal m. of semicircular duct the basement membrane underlying the epithelium of a semicircular duct.
basement m. a sheet of amorphous extracellular material upon which the basal surfaces of epithelial cells rest; other cells associated with basement membranes are muscle cells, Schwann cells, fat cells, and capillaries. The membrane is interposed between the cellular elements and the underlying connective tissue. It comprises two layers, the basal lamina and the reticular lamina, and is composed of Type IV collagen (which is unique to basement membranes), laminin, fibronectin, and heparan sulfate proteoglycans.
basilar m. of cochlear duct lamina basilaris ductus cochlearis.
basolateral m. the layer of plasma membrane of epithelial cells that is adjacent to the basement membrane and separated from the apical membrane by the zonula occludens.
Bichat m. fenestrated m.
birth m′s the amnion and chorion.
Bowman m. lamina limitans anterior corneae.
Bruch m. lamina basalis choroideae.
Brunn m. the epithelium of the olfactory region of the nose.
bucconasal m. oronasal m.
buccopharyngeal m. oropharyngeal m.
capsular m. the portion of the tunica vasculosa lentis that lies posterior to the lens.
capsulopupillary m. the part of the tunica vasculosa lentis that is around the edges of the lens.
cell m. plasma m.
chorioallantoic m. chorioallantois.
cloacal m. the thin, temporary barrier between the hindgut and the exterior, formed by the endoderm of the hindgut and the ectoderm of the cloaca of the embryo; its dorsal part forms the *anal membrane.*
complex m. a membrane made up of several layers differing in structure.
compound m. a membrane consisting of two distinct layers, such as the tympanic membrane.
Corti m. membrana tectoria ductus cochlearis.
cricothyroid m., cricovocal m. conus elasticus.

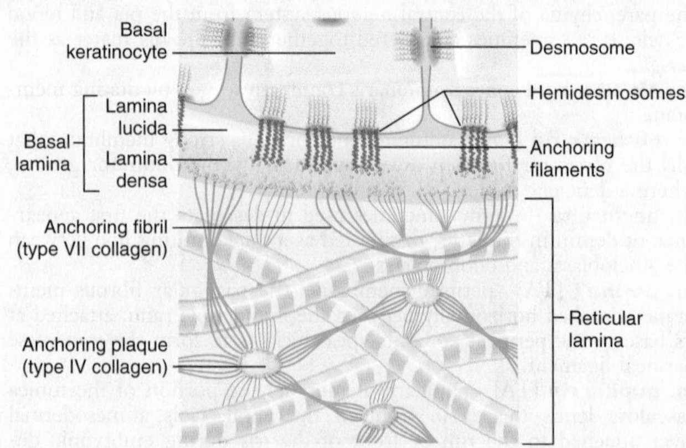

■ Basement membrane, comprising the lamina lucida and lamina densa, which together constitute the basal lamina, and the collagen-containing reticular lamina beneath, in a diagram of a section through epithelial tissue.

croupous m. false m.
cyclitic m. a false membrane which sometimes covers the vitreous body in cyclitis.
cytoplasmic m. plasma m.
Debove m. the delicate layer between the epithelium and the tunica propria of the bronchial, tracheal, and intestinal mucous membranes.
decidual m., deciduous m. decidua.
dentinoenamel m. a continuous thin membrane laid down by ameloblasts adjoining the basement membrane separating them from the dentin in an early developing tooth.
Descemet m. lamina limitans posterior corneae.
diphtheritic m. a type of pseudomembrane characteristic of diphtheria, resulting from coagulation necrosis.
drum m. membrana tympanica.
egg m. any of several investments surrounding the oocyte: if derived from the oocyte itself, as the vitelline membrane, it is called *primary;* if from the follicular cells, as the zona pellucida, it is called *secondary;* if from the oviduct, as the albumen around rabbit's egg or the albumen and shell of hen's egg, it is called *tertiary.* Called also *egg envelope* and, collectively, *lemma.*
elastic m. 1. a membrane composed largely of elastic fibers. 2. see *external elastic m.* and *internal elastic m.*
enamel m. 1. cuticula dentis. 2. the inner layer of cells within the enamel organ of the dental germ in the fetus; called also *Hannover intermediate m.*
endoneural m. neurilemma.
endoral m. paroral m.
epiretinal m. a pathologic membrane partially covering the surface of the retina, probably originating chiefly from the cells of the pigment epithelium and glia; membranes peripheral to the macula are generally asymptomatic, while those involving the macula or adjacent to it may cause reduction in vision, visual distortion, and diplopia.
excitable m. the membrane of an excitable cell.
exocoelomic m. a layer of flattened cells that develops as a lining of the blastocyst or chorionic cavity just after implantation. Together with the hypoblast, it forms the covering layer of the primary yolk sac. Called also *Heuser m.*
external elastic m. a fenestrated elastic membrane that constitutes the innermost component of the tunica adventitia of arteries. Called also *external elastic lamina.*
external intercostal m. membrana intercostalis externa.
external limiting m. 1. a thin fenestrated layer of the stratum nervosum retinae adjacent to the outer nuclear layer and through which extend the visual rods and cones. Called also *outer limiting m., external* or *outer limiting layer,* and, in official terminology, *stratum limitans externum retinae* [TA]. See illustration at *retina.* 2. a membrane investing the external surface of the embryonic neural tube. Called also *outer limiting m.*
extraembryonic m's the trophoblastic parts of the conceptus that provide for the support of the embryo or fetus by attachment, mechanical protection, endocrine action, and the mediation of chemical exchange with the maternal circulation. They include the yolk sac (umbilical vesicle), allantois, amnion, umbilical cord, and chorion, including the placenta. Called also *fetal m's.*
false m. pseudomembrane.
fenestrated m. 1. a membrane that has tiny pores or fenestrae. 2. either of the elastic membranes of arteries; see *internal elastic m.* and *external elastic m.*
fertilization m. a strong membrane formed around the fertilized oocyte in some species of animals by adhesion of part of the contents of the cortical granules to the inner surface of the vitelline membrane; it prevents the entry of additional spermatozoa.
fetal m's extraembryonic m's.
fibroelastic m. of larynx membrana fibroelastica laryngis.
fibrous m. of articular capsule membrana fibrosa capsulae articularis.
filtration slit m. slit diaphragm.
germinal m. blastoderm.
glassy m. 1. the basement membrane of a vesicular ovarian follicle; in cross section it appears as a distinct brilliant line, and it persists in the ovary long after its follicle has degenerated. 2. lamina basalis choroideae. 3. hyaline m. (def. 1).
glomerular m., glomerular basement m. (GBM), glomerular capillary m. the fenestrated basement membrane of the visceral layer of the glomerular capsule, lying adjacent to glomerular capillaries and consisting of the lamina rara interna, lamina densa, and lamina rara externa. On its outer surface is the layer of podocytes and the slit diaphragm. See also *filtration barrier,* under *barrier.*
gradocol m's thin membranes made of collodion or similar substances and graded as to porosity; used in ultrafiltration and sometimes to estimate the diameters of viruses or other small particles.
ground m. inophragma.
Hannover intermediate m. enamel m. (def. 2).
hemodialyzer m. the semipermeable membrane that filters the blood in a hemodialyzer, commonly made of cuprophane, cellulose acetate, polyacrylonitrile, polymethyl methacrylate, or polysulfone.
Henle m. posterior border lamella of Fuchs; see under *lamella.*
Henle elastic m. external elastic m.
Henle fenestrated m. fenestrated m.
Heuser m. exocoelomic m.
high efficiency m. a hemodialyzer membrane that has clearance characteristics that increase progressively with increases in dialysis blood flow rates; this usually implies that the membrane is not a high flux membrane.
high flux m. a hemodialyzer membrane that has a high permeability to fluids and solutes and thus a high rate of clearance of fluids and solutes composed of large molecules.
hyaline m. 1. the membrane between the outer root sheath and the inner fibrous layer of a hair follicle. Called also *glassy m.* 2. a layer of eosinophilic hyaline material lining the alveoli, alveolar ducts, and bronchioles, found at autopsy in infants who have died of neonatal respiratory distress syndrome. Similar changes may be seen in adults who have died of viral respiratory infections. Called also *asphyxial m.* and *vernix m.*
hyaloid m. membrana vitrea.
hymenal m. hymen.
hyoglossal m. a fibrous lamina connecting the undersurface of the tongue with the hyoid bone.
hyothyroid m. membrana thyrohyoidea.
inferior synovial m. of temporomandibular joint membrana synovialis inferior articulationis temporomandibularis.
inner limiting m. internal limiting m.
internal elastic m. a fenestrated elastic membrane that constitutes the outermost component of the tunica intima of arteries. Called also *internal elastic lamina.*
internal intercostal m. membrana intercostalis interna.
internal limiting m. 1. the basal lamina of the Müller fibers in the retina; it is the layer of the stratum nervosum retinae located just internal to the nerve fiber layer and separates the inner, conical ends of the cells from the vitreous body. Called also *inner* or *internal limiting layer* and, in official terminology, *stratum limitans internum retinae* [TA]. See illustration at *retina.* 2. a membrane lining the internal surface of the embryonic neural tube.
interosseous m. membrana interossea.
interosseous m. of forearm membrana interossea antebrachii.
interosseous m. of leg membrana interossea cruris.
interspinal m's see *ligamenta interspinalia.*
intersutural m. the pericranium lying between the cranial sutures.
ion-selective m. a membrane that is more permeable to particular types of ions than to other types, e.g., K^+-selective glass membrane. Many biological membranes exhibit ion-selective behavior.
Jackson m. a delicate curtain or web of adhesions (regarded by some as a sheet of peritoneum), which may extend from the lateral abdominal wall to the cecum, covering the cecum and producing obstruction. Called also *Jackson veil.*
keratogenous m. 1. matrix unguis. 2. a similar structure in the hoof of an animal, from which horny tissue grows.
Kölliker m. membrana reticularis organi spiralis.
limiting m. a membrane that constitutes the border of some tissue or structure.
Mauthner m. axolemma.
medullary m. endosteum.
mucocutaneous m. a membrane that is partly mucous and partly cutaneous, such as the tympanic membrane.
mucous m. tunica mucosa.
- **mucous m. of auditory tube** tunica mucosa tubae auditivae.
- **mucous m. of bronchi** tunica mucosa bronchiorum.
- **mucous m. of ductus deferens** tunica mucosa ductus deferentis.
- **mucous m. of esophagus** tunica mucosa oesophagi.

mucous m. of female urethra tunica mucosa urethrae femininae.
mucous m. of gallbladder tunica mucosa vesicae biliaris.
mucous m. of large intestine tunica mucosa intestini crassi.
mucous m. of larynx tunica mucosa laryngis.
mucous m. of membranous urethra tunica mucosa partis intermediae urethrae.
mucous m. of mouth tunica mucosa oris.
mucous m. of nose tunica mucosa nasi.
mucous m. of pharynx tunica mucosa pharyngis.
mucous m. of prostatic urethra tunica mucosa partis prostaticae urethrae.
mucous m. of renal pelvis tunica mucosa pelvis renalis.
mucous m. of seminal vesicle tunica mucosa glandulae vesiculosae.
mucous m. of small intestine tunica mucosa intestini tenuis.
mucous m. of spongy urethra tunica mucosa partis spongiosae urethrae.
mucous m. of stomach tunica mucosa gastrica.
mucous m. of tongue tunica mucosa linguae.
mucous m. of trachea tunica mucosa tracheae.
mucous m. of tympanic cavity tunica mucosa cavitatis tympanicae.
mucous m. of ureter tunica mucosa ureteris.
mucous m. of urinary bladder tunica mucosa vesicae urinariae.
mucous m. of uterine tube tunica mucosa tubae uterinae.
mucous m. of uterus tunica mucosa uteri.
mucous m. of vagina tunica mucosa vaginae.

Nasmyth m. primary (enamel) cuticle.

nictitating m. a transparent fold of skin lying deep to the other eyelids at the mesial side, which may be drawn over the front of the eyeball; found in reptiles and birds generally and in many mammals. See also *haw.* Called also *third eyelid* and *membrana nictitans.*

nuclear m. 1. either of the membranes, inner and outer, comprising the nuclear envelope. 2. nuclear envelope.

oblique m. of forearm chorda obliqua membranae interosseae antebrachii.

obturator m. membrana obturatoria.

olfactory m. the olfactory portion of the mucous membrane lining the nasal fossa.

oral m. oropharyngeal m.

oronasal m. a thin epithelial plate separating the nasal pits from the oral cavity of the embryo. Called also *bucconasal m.*

oropharyngeal m. a transient embryonic septum at the cranial limit of the foregut, in the depths of the stomodeum; it temporarily separates the mouth cavity from the pharynx. Called also *buccopharyngeal m.* and *pharyngeal septum.*

otolithic m. membrana statoconiorum.

outer limiting m. external limiting m.

ovular m. vitelline m.

palatine m. the membrane covering the roof of the mouth.

pansporoblastic m. a surface membrane surrounding the sporoblasts in a pansporoblast; characteristic of microsporidian protozoa of the suborder Pansporoblastina.

paroral m. in certain ciliate protozoa, a movable membrane-like sheet(s) formed by fusion of the bases of a longitudinal row of cilia that borders the right side of the buccal cavity; it serves to gather food and push it toward the cytostome. Called also *endoral m.* and *undulating m.* Cf. *membranelle.*

pericolic m. occasional bands of peritoneum extending between the abdominal wall and the serosa of the colon. See *pericolic membrane syndrome*, under *syndrome.*

peridental m. periodontal ligament.

perineal m. membrana perinei.

periodontal m. see under *ligament.*

periorbital m. periorbita.

peritrophic m. a delicate, cylindrical sheath of chitin continuously secreted from the posterior edge of the foregut of insects and millipedes that ingest solid food, which surrounds the food as it passes through the midgut.

pharyngeal m. in the embryo, one of the thin membranes, consisting of ectoderm, mesoderm, and endoderm, that separate the pharyngeal pouches from the pharyngeal grooves; the first pharyngeal membrane, with its associated mesenchyme, becomes the tympanic membrane.

pituitary m. of nose tunica mucosa nasi.

placental m. the semipermeable membrane that separates the fetal from the maternal blood in the placenta. In the human (hemochorial) placenta, it is composed of fetal vascular endothelium, connective tissue, cytotrophoblast, and syncytiotrophoblast, and it becomes thinner as pregnancy progresses. Sometimes inappropriately called the *placental barrier*; there are only a few substances that cannot pass through the membrane.

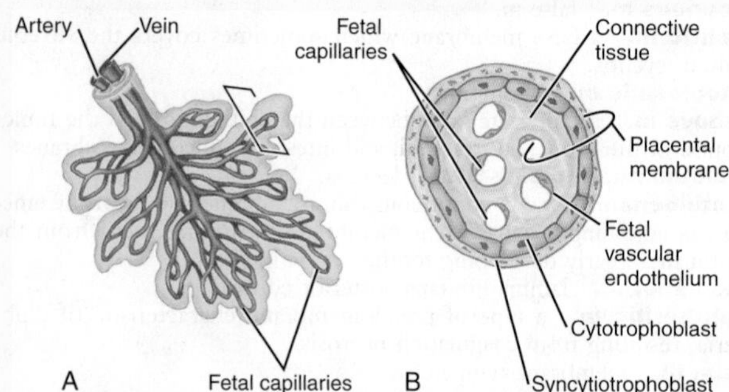

■ Placental membrane separating the blood in the fetal capillaries from the maternal blood in the intervillous space. *(A)*, Chorionic villus containing the fetal vessels and surrounded by maternal blood in the intervillous space; *(B)*, cross-section through a villus, showing the layers of the placental membrane separating the fetal blood from the maternal blood surrounding the villus.

plasma m. the structure enveloping a cell, enclosing the cytoplasm and forming a selective permeability barrier; it consists of a lipid bilayer with integral and peripheral proteins and contains channels and pumps to transport substances across the membrane, as well as receptors to receive stimuli from the external environment and transduce them into intracellular signals. See Plate 12. Called also *cell m.*, *cytoplasmic m.*, and *plasmalemma.*

platelet demarcation m. a more or less tridimensional system of paired membranes that serve to partition the megakaryocyte cytoplasm, each partition containing azurophilic granules and representing a future blood platelet.

pleuropericardial m's a pair of partitions in the embryo that separate the pericardial cavity from the pleural cavities; formed by enlargement of the pleuropericardial folds and containing the common cardinal veins and phrenic nerves.

pleuroperitoneal m's a pair of partitions in the embryo that close off the pericardioperitoneal canals and separate the pleural cavities from the peritoneal cavity; formed by enlargement of the pleuroperitoneal folds; they develop into the posterolateral portions of the diaphragm.

postsynaptic m. the area of plasma membrane of a postsynaptic cell, either a muscle fiber or a neuron, that is within the synapse and has areas especially adapted for receiving neurotransmitters.

presynaptic m. the area of plasma membrane of a presynaptic axon that is within the synapse and has sites (active zones) especially adapted for the release of neurotransmitters.

proper m. of semicircular duct the outer, loose, connective tissue layer of a semicircular duct.

pseudoserous m. a membrane resembling serous membrane, but differing from it in structure.

pupillary m. membrana pupillaris.

pupillary m., persistent a congenital defect in dogs in which remnants of the tunica vasculosa lentis are found on the surface of the iris or cornea, sometimes with a corneal opacity.

pyloric m. a congenital abnormal membrane in the pylorus, partially or completely blocking the gastric outlet. See also *prepyloric atresia.* Called also *pyloric diaphragm* and *pyloric web.*

pyogenic m. a membrane which produces pus.

pyophylactic m. a fibrinous membrane lining a pus cavity and tending to prevent reabsorption of injurious materials.

quadrangular m. membrana quadrangularis.

radioulnar interosseous m. membrana interossea antebrachii.

Reissner m. paries vestibularis ductus cochlearis.

reticular m. of spiral organ membrana reticularis organi spiralis.

Rivinus m. pars flaccida membranae tympanicae.

m. of round window membrana tympanica secundaria.

Ruysch m., ruyschian m. the capillary layer of the choroid in addition to the pigmented layer of the retina and Bruch membrane (the basal complex of the choroid).

Membrane *Continued*

Scarpa m. membrana tympanica secundaria.
schneiderian m. tunica mucosa nasi.
Schwann m. neurilemma.
secondary tympanic m. membrana tympanica secundaria.
semipermeable m. a membrane that is freely traversed by solvent, such as water, but which permits the passage of only certain solutes.
serous m. tunica serosa.
shell m. a double fibrous layer lining the shell of the egg of some animals, such as birds.
Shrapnell m. pars flaccida membranae tympanicae.
slit m. see under *diaphragm.*
spiral m. of cochlear duct paries tympanicus ductus cochlearis.
stapedial m. membrana stapedialis.
sternal m. membrana sterni.
striated m. see *zona pellucida* (def. 1).
subepithelial m. basement m.
superior synovial m. of temporomandibular joint membrana synovialis superior articulationis temporomandibularis.
suprapleural m. membrana suprapleuralis.
synaptic m. the part of the plasma membrane of a neuron that is within a synapse; see *postsynaptic m.* and *presynaptic m.*
synovial m. of articular capsule membrana synovialis capsulae articularis.
tarsal m. orbital septum.
tectorial m. membrana tectoria.
tectorial m. of cochlear duct membrana tectoria ductus cochlearis.
tendinous m. aponeurosis.
Tenon m. vagina bulbi.
thyrohyoid m. membrana thyrohyoidea.
Toldt m. the part of the renal fascia anterior to the kidney.
tympanic m. membrana tympanica.
undulating m. 1. in certain flagellate protozoa, a delicate finlike cytoplasmic membrane along the lateral aspect of the body; its outer margin is formed by a flagellum that may continue free beyond the end of the body. It serves a locomotor function; when it vibrates it produces undulating movements. 2. paroral m.
unit m. the trilaminar membrane common to all cells, consisting of a lipid bilayer with an intercalated protein layer; see illustration at bilayer.
vernix m. hyaline m. (def. 2); so called because it was originally thought to be the result of aspiration of vernix by the fetus in utero.
vestibular m. of cochlear duct paries vestibularis ductus cochlearis.
vitelline m. the cytoplasmic, noncellular membrane surrounding an oocyte.
vitreous m. 1. membrana vitrea. 2. lamina basalis choroideae. 3. lamina limitans posterior corneae. 4. hyaline m. (def. 1).
Wachendorf m. membrana pupillaris.
yolk m. vitelline m.
Zinn m. zonula ciliaris.

mem•bra•nec•to•my (mem″brə-nek′tə-me) excision of a membrane.

mem•bra•nelle (mem″brə-nel′) a triangular or fan-shaped organelle bordering the left side of the buccal cavity or peristomial area in certain ciliate protozoa, formed by fusion of the bases of short, transverse rows (up to three) of cilia; it serves in locomotion and to gather and push food toward the cytostome. Cf. *paroral membrane.*

mem•bra•ni•form (məm-bra′nĭ-form) membranoid.

mem•bra•no•car•ti•lag•i•nous (mem″brə-no-kahr″tĭ-laj′ĭ-nəs) 1. developed in both membrane and cartilage. 2. partly cartilaginous and partly membranous.

mem•bra•noid (mem′brə-noid) resembling a membrane.

mem•bran•ol•y•sis (mem″brān-ol′ĭ-sis) disruption of any membrane.

mem•brum (mem′brəm) pl. *mem′bra* [L.] limb.
m. infe′rius [TA] lower limb: the limb extending from the gluteal region to the foot; see also *leg*, and see *regiones membri inferioris*, under *regio.* It is specialized for weight-bearing and locomotion.
m. supe′rius [TA] upper limb: the limb of the body extending from the superior part of the deltoid region to the hand; see also *arm*, and see *regiones membri superioris*, under *regio.* It is specialized for functions requiring great mobility, such as grasping and manipulating.

mem•o•ry (mem′ə-re) [L. *memoria*] the mental faculty by which sensations, impressions, and ideas are recalled.
anterograde m. remote m.
echoic m. the part of the sensory storage system that holds auditory stimuli.
eye m. visual m.
iconic m. the part of the sensory storage system that holds visual stimuli.
immediate m. short-term m.
immunologic m. the capacity of the immune system to respond more rapidly and strongly to subsequent antigenic challenge than to the first exposure. Called also *anamnesis.* See *memory cells*, under *cell*, and *primary* and *secondary immune response*, under *response.*
kinesthetic m. motor m.
long-term m. memory that is retained over long periods of time.
motor m. the memory of movements in the limbs and other parts of the body.
physiological m. the physical storage of engrams in the brain by means of RNA.
remote m. a memory serviceable for events long past, but not able to acquire new recollections; called also *anterograde m.* and *palinmnesis.*
replacement m. the replacing of one memory with a different one; cf. *screen m.*
screen m. a consciously tolerable memory serving to "screen" or conceal another memory that might be disturbing or emotionally painful if recalled.
short-term m. memory that is lost within a brief period (from a few seconds to a maximum of about 30 minutes) unless reinforced.
visual m. memory for visual impressions.

MEN multiple endocrine neoplasia.

Mena•can•thus (men″ə-kan′thus) a genus of parasitic biting lice (order Mallophaga). *M. palli′dulus* and *M. strami′neus* attack chickens and turkeys.

me•nac•me (mə-nak′me) [*men-* + Gr. *akmē* highest point] 1. the height of menstrual activity. 2. that period of a woman's life which is marked by menstrual activity.

Me•nac•tra (mə-nak′trə) trademark for a preparation of meningococcal conjugated vaccine.

men•a•di•ol (men″ə-di′ol) the reduced, dihydro form of menadione.
m. sodium diphosphate [USP] a synthetic, water-soluble derivative of menadione (vitamin K_3), to which it is converted in the body; used as a prothrombinogenic vitamin for the same purposes as menadione (q.v.); administered orally, intravenously, or subcutaneously.

men•a•di•one (men″ə-di′ōn) vitamin K_3. 1. [USP] a synthetic fat-soluble provitamin that can be chemically converted in the body to active vitamin K by addition of a long side chain; used as a source of vitamin K in the treatment of hypoprothrombinemia associated with vitamin K deficiency, as occurs in hepatic or biliary disease and malabsorption syndromes, or after administration of salicylates, anticoagulants, or certain antibiotics; administered orally or intramuscularly. 2. the basic double ring quinone structure that is the parent structure of the related compounds with vitamin K activity, which can be formed by addition of long side chain substituents.
m. sodium bisulfite a water-soluble derivative of menadione having the same actions and uses as the base.

men•al•gia (mən-al′jə) [*men-* + *-algia*] pain accompanying menstruation.

men•aph•thone (mən-af′thōn) menadione.

men•a•quin•one (men″ə-kwin′ōn) any of a series of compounds in which the phytyl side chain of phytonadione (vitamin K_1) is replaced by a side chain of prenyl units and which have vitamin K activity. This form of the vitamin is usually available to the human body even in cases of dietary deficiency because menaquinones are synthesized by the intestinal flora. Called also *vitamin K_2.*

me•nar•che (mə-nahr′ke) [*men-* + Gr. *archē* beginning] the establishment or beginning of menstruation. **menar′chal, menar′cheal, menar′chial** *adj*

Men•del's laws (men′dəlz) [Gregor Johann *Mendel*, Austrian monk and naturalist, 1822–1884] see under *law.*

Men•del reflex (men′dəl) [Kurt *Mendel*, German neurologist, 1874–1946] Mendel-Bekhterev reflex; see under *reflex.*

Men·del-Bekh·ter·ev reflex, sign (men′dəl bek-ter′yev) [K. *Mendel;* Vladimir Mikhailovich *Bekhterev,* Russian neurologist, 1857–1927] see under *reflex* and *sign.*

Men·de·le·ev's law, table (men″də-la′efs) [Dimitri Ivanovich *Mendeleev* (or *Mendeléef* or *Mendeléeff*), Russian chemist, 1834–1907] see *periodic law,* under *law* and *periodic table,* under *table.*

men·de·le·vi·um (Md) (men″də-le′ve-əm) [Dimitri Ivanovich *Mendeléeff*] the radioactive chemical element of atomic number 101, atomic weight 256, originally discovered in debris from a thermonuclear explosion in 1952.

men·de·li·an (mən-de′le-ən) named for Gregor Johann *Mendel,* as *mendelian law.*

men·del·ism (men′dəl-iz″əm) the principles of heredity derived from Mendel's laws.

men·del·iz·ing (men′dəl-iz″ing) exhibiting the simple patterns of inheritance of single gene traits elaborated by Gregor Mendel; see *Mendel's laws,* under *law.*

Men·del·son syndrome (men′dəl-sən) [Curtis Lester *Mendelson,* American obstetrician and gynecologist, 1913–2002] see under *syndrome.*

Men·des da Cos·ta syndrome (mān′dās dah kōs′tah) [Samuel *Mendes da Costa,* Dutch dermatologist, early 20th century] erythrokeratodermia variabilis.

Men·est (men′əst) trademark for a preparation of esterified estrogens.

Mé·né·trier disease (ma-na″tre-a′) [Pierre *Ménétrier,* French physician, 1859–1935] hypertrophic gastritis.

Menge pessary (meng′gə) [Karl *Menge,* German gynecologist, 1864–1945] see under *pessary.*

Men·go encephalomyelitis, virus (men′go) [*Mengo* district in Uganda, where the disease was first seen in 1948] see under *encephalomyelitis* and *virus.*

Me·niere disease (mĕ-nyār′) [Prosper *Meniere,* French physician, 1799–1862. The spelling *Meniere* appears on his birth certificate, *Menière* and *Ménière* on his works. Ménière was the choice of his son] see under *disease.*

me·nin·gem·a·to·ma (mə-nin″jem-ə-to′mə) epidural hematoma.

me·nin·geo·cor·ti·cal (mə-nin″je-o-kor′tĭ-kəl) meningocortical.

me·nin·ge·o·ma (mə-nin″je-o′mə) meningioma.

me·nin·ge·or·rha·phy (mə-nin″je-or′ə-fe) [*meningo-* + *-rrhaphy*] suture of the meninges.

me·nin·ges (mə-nin′jēz) [Gr., pl. of *mēninx* membrane] [TA] the three membranes that envelop the brain and spinal cord: the dura mater, pia mater, and arachnoid. **menin′geal** *adj*

me·ning·hem·a·to·ma (mə-ninj″hem-ə-to′mə) epidural hematoma.

me·nin·gi·o·ma (mə-nin″je-o′mə) [*meninges* + *-oma*] a benign, slow-growing tumor of the meninges, usually next to the dura mater, probably arising from cells associated with arachnoid villi. It may erode the skull or cause hyperostosis, and increased intracranial pressure is common. Meningiomas are now usually classified according to anatomic location; an older classification by histologic features exists, but histologic features have not been shown to influence clinical behavior.

angioblastic m., angiomatous m. a meningioma with many blood vessels, which may vary in size from capillary to cavernous; called also *angioblastoma.*

cerebellopontine angle m. a posterior fossa meningioma located in the cerebellopontine angle; it may cause symptoms like those of an acoustic neuroma or may compress any of the first five cranial nerves.

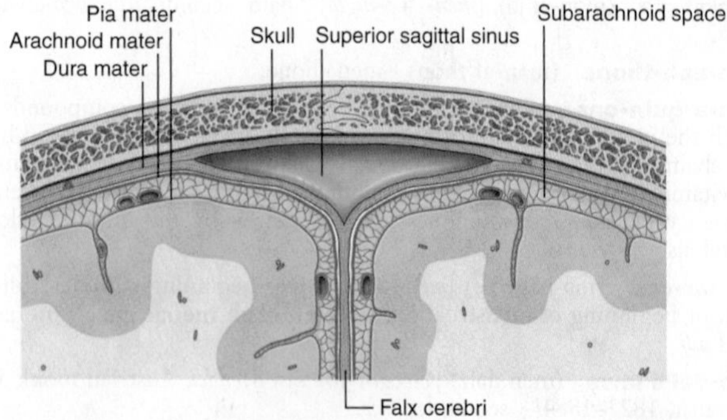

■ Cranial meninges, comprising the dura mater, arachnoid mater, and pia mater, in a superior coronal view.

chordoid m. a rare, moderately malignant type of meningioma characterized histologically by cells in lobules and chains resembling those of a chordoma.

clear cell m. a rare, moderately malignant type of meningioma characterized histologically by clear cells.

clival m. a posterior fossa meningioma located over the middle or rostral part of the clivus; symptoms include palsy of the fifth, seventh, or eighth cranial nerve and gait ataxia.

convexity m's a diverse group of meningiomas located within the sulci of the brain, usually anterior to the central sulcus; they may be silent for long periods. Symptoms include seizures, weakness of the arm and face, and personality changes.

cystic m. a meningioma containing or adjacent to cysts; cf. *microcystic m.*

falcine m., falx m. a meningioma in or near the falx cerebri; symptoms are similar to those of a parasagittal meningioma.

fibroblastic m., fibrous m. a meningioma characterized by fibrous tissue with bundles of spindle cells; called also *meningofibroblastoma.*

lymphoplasmacyte-rich m. a rare type of meningioma characterized by a polyclonal infiltrate of lymphocytes and plasma cells.

meningothelial m., meningotheliomatous m. a meningioma composed of characteristic uniform tumor cells that form lobules surrounded by thin collagenous septa; cells with the lobules have poorly defined boundaries, resembling a syncytium; called also *syncytial m.* and *meningothelioma.*

microcystic m. a rare, benign type of meningioma characterized by small cysts and a wet, glistening surface when cut; the fluid may contain plasma proteins.

m. of the olfactory groove a meningioma located in the ethmoid fossa (olfactory groove); symptoms include anosmia, visual defects including Kennedy syndrome, and psychic disturbances.

orbital m. a meningioma that enters the orbit, arising either in the meninges of the optic nerve or within the brain; symptoms include loss of visual acuity and sometimes paralysis of eye muscles.

papillary m. a rare, malignant type of meningioma characterized by cells in a papillary configuration, often with necrosis or cyst formation.

parasagittal m. a meningioma located next to the superior sagittal sinus, often growing into the sinus; symptoms are variable according to location and may include seizures, weakness or paresthesias in the lower limbs, and visual field defects. See also *falx m.*

posterior fossa m. a meningioma in the posterior cranial fossa; these include tentorial, clival, and cerebellopontine angle meningiomas.

psammomatous m. a transitional meningioma that contains many psammoma bodies; called also *psammoma.*

rhabdoid m. a rare, malignant type of meningioma characterized histologically by rhabdoid cells with eccentric nuclei; these are most often seen as recurrences of formerly benign meningiomas.

secretory m. a rare, benign type of meningioma characterized by the formation of glands, inclusions, and intraluminal hyalin; small, dark cells form around blood vessels and may cause edema.

m. of the sphenoid ridge a meningioma located along the sphenoid ridge; symptoms commonly include trigeminal neuralgia, unilateral exophthalmos progressing to blindness, Kennedy syndrome, and Tolosa-Hunt syndrome.

spinal m. a meningioma adjacent to the spinal cord, usually beginning intradurally but sometimes extending through the dura mater; the most common locations are near the foramen magnum and in the thoracic region.

suprasellar m. a meningioma located above the sella turcica near its tuberculum; because of its proximity to the optic chiasm, it pushes against the optic nerve and causes bitemporal hemianopia and other visual deficits. Called also *m. of the tuberculum sellae.*

syncytial m. meningothelial m.

tentorial m. a posterior fossa meningioma located on the tentorium cerebelli; it may cause seizures, visual hallucinations, and visual field deficits.

transitional m. a meningioma histologically intermediate between the meningothelial and fibroblastic types; calcification of whorls of cells often causes psammoma bodies. See also *psammomatous m.*

m. of the tuberculum sellae suprasellar m.

me·nin·gi·o·ma·to·sis (mə-nin″je-o″mə-to′sis) a condition characterized by the formation of multiple meningiomas.

me·nin·gism (mə-nin′jiz-əm) the symptoms and signs of meningeal irritation associated with acute febrile illness or dehydration without actual infection of the meninges. Called also *meningismus* and *pseudomeningitis.*

men·in·gis·mus (men″in-jis′məs) meningism.

men·in·gi·tis (men″in-ji′tis) pl. *meningi′tides* [*mening-* + *-itis*] inflammation of the meninges, usually by either a bacterium *(bacterial m.)* or a virus *(viral m.).* **meningit′ic** *adj*

acute aseptic m. aseptic m.

anthrax m. a rare, highly fatal condition resembling typical hemorrhagic meningitis, caused by hematogenous spread of the anthrax bacillus from a primary focus of infection; manifestations include hemorrhagic cerebrospinal fluid and neurological signs and symptoms.

aseptic m. any of several mild types of meningitis, most of which are caused by viruses; see *viral m.* Called also *acute aseptic m.* and *sterile m.*

***Aspergillus* m.** fungal meningitis caused by a species of *Aspergillus;* some cases are iatrogenic and others occur in immunocompromised persons.

bacterial m. meningitis caused by bacteria, usually characterized by fever, headache, a stiff neck, and altered mental status. Common pathogens are *Haemophilus influenzae* (see *Haemophilus influenzae m.*), *Neisseria meningitidis* (see *meningococcal m.*), *Streptococcus pneumoniae* (see *pneumococcal m.*), and *Mycobacterium tuberculosis* (see *tuberculous m.*). Called also *purulent* or *pyogenic m.* Cf. *viral m.*

basilar m. that which affects the meninges at the base of the brain.

benign lymphocytic m. lymphocytic choriomeningitis.

***Candida* m., candidal m.** fungal meningitis caused by spread of a case of candidiasis into the central nervous system.

m. carcinomato′sa, carcinomatous m. a misnomer for meningeal carcinoma, a condition that is not inflammatory.

cerebral m. inflammation of the meninges of the brain.

cerebrospinal m. any inflammation of the membranes of the brain and spinal cord; see *bacterial m.* and *viral m.*

chronic m. a variable syndrome of fever, headache, lethargy, stiff neck, confusion, nausea, and vomiting, with pleocytosis and with or without hypoglycorrachia, which fails to improve over a period of 4 weeks; it may be produced by any of a large number of infectious agents and noninfectious conditions.

coccidioidal m. fungal meningitis resulting from coccidioidomycosis that has invaded the central nervous system.

cryptococcal m. the most common type of fungal meningitis, caused by *Cryptococcus neoformans.*

eosinophilic m. meningitis characterized by an increase in lymphocytes and a high percentage of eosinophils in the cerebrospinal fluid; it usually results from infection with the rat lungworm, *Angiostrongylus cantonensis.* Called also *eosinophilic meningoencephalitis.*

epidemic cerebrospinal m. meningococcal m.

external m. external pachymeningitis.

fungal m. meningitis caused by invasion of the nervous system by a fungus, usually as an opportunistic infection in an immunocompromised person. Common fungi causing this are *Cryptococcus neoformans, Coccidioides immitis,* and species of *Candida* and *Aspergillus.*

gummatous m. meningitis during the tertiary stage of syphilis in which there are many small gummata in the membranes.

***Haemophilus influenzae* m.** bacterial meningitis caused by infection with *Haemophilus influenzae,* seen most often in young children and the elderly.

internal m. internal pachymeningitis.

lymphocytic m. see under *choriomeningitis.*

lymphomatous m. metastasis of non-Hodgkin lymphoma to the meninges; symptoms include headaches, altered mental status, seizures, cranial neuropathies, and radiculopathies; some cases are asymptomatic.

meningococcal m. an acute type of bacterial meningitis caused by infection with *Neisseria meningitidis.* It usually appears in epidemics, and symptoms are those of acute cerebral and spinal meningitis, usually with seropurulent meningeal irritation and an eruption of cutaneous erythematous, herpetic, or hemorrhagic spots. A hemorrhagic complication that sometimes occurs is called Waterhouse-Friderichsen syndrome (see under *syndrome*). Called also *cerebrospinal fever* and *epidemic cerebrospinal m.*

Mollaret m. recurrent febrile attacks, malaise, headache, and meningeal signs accompanied by a marked polymorphonuclear inflammatory reaction in the cerebrospinal fluid.

mumps m. an aseptic meningitis secondary to mumps; see also *mumps meningoencephalitis,* under *meningoencephalitis.*

neoplastic m. meningitis resulting from cancer metastasis to the leptomeninges or subarachnoid space.

occlusive m. leptomeningitis of children which leads to the closure of the lateral and median apertures of the fourth ventricle.

m. ossi′ficans ossification of the cerebral meninges.

otitic m. meningitis occurring as a complication of otitis media.

plague m. meningitis occurring as a rare complication of bubonic plague as a result of hematogenous spread of the infection from a bubo to involve the meninges, or less often as a primary infection without antecedent bubo formation. Called also *meningeal plague.*

pneumococcal m. bacterial meningitis caused by pneumococcus *(Streptococcus pneumoniae),* a potentially fatal type seen most often in young children or the elderly. Up to half the cases are secondary to other infections, such as those of the lungs, ears, or paranasal sinuses, and reinfection may occur. The incidence is increased in asplenic or immunocompromised patients, such as those with sickle cell disease or lymphocytic leukemia.

purulent m., pyogenic m. bacterial m.

m. sero′sa circumscrip′ta chronic adhesive arachnoiditis.

spinal m. inflammation of the meninges of the spinal cord.

sterile m. aseptic m.

streptococcal m. meningitis in piglets caused by *Streptococcus suis;* characteristics include incoordination, tremors, convulsions, and sometimes paralysis that can be fatal.

m. sympa′thica a condition of the cerebrospinal fluid caused by inflammation in the neighborhood of the meninges. It is marked by increase in the pressure of the fluid and increase in its albumin and cellular content. The fluid is sterile and there may be symptoms of meningitis.

syphilitic m. general paresis.

tubercular m., tuberculous m. a severe type of bacterial meningitis caused by *Mycobacterium tuberculosis,* usually spreading from a primary infection in the lungs.

viral m. meningitis due to any of various viruses, such as the coxsackieviruses, mumps virus, or the virus of lymphocytic choriomeningitis; characteristics include malaise, fever, headache, stiffness of neck and back, nausea, and cerebrospinal fluid pleocytosis (principally lymphocytic); it usually has a short uncomplicated course. See also *aseptic m.*

mening(o)- [Gr. *mēninx,* gen. *mēningos* membrane] a combining form denoting relationship to a membrane, especially relationship to the meninges.

me·nin·go·ar·ter·i·tis (mə-ning″go-ahr″tər-i′tis) inflammation of the meningeal arteries.

me·nin·go·cele (mə-ning′go-sēl″) [*meningo-* + *-cele*[1]] hernial protrusion of the meninges through a bony defect; the two types are *cranial m.* and *spinal m.* See also *spina bifida cystica.*

anterior m. a rare type of meningocele that protrudes anteriorly from the vertebral column, usually in the sacral region; symptoms often are mild and go unnoticed.

cranial m. hernial protrusion of the meninges through a defect in the cranium (cranium bifidum), usually forming a fluid-filled sac; called also *craniomeningocele.* See also *encephalocele.*

sacral m. a meningocele in the sacral region; symptoms may remain occult until adulthood and include neurologic deficits and abdominal masses with pressure. Both posterior and anterior types have been observed; see also *anterior m.*

spinal m. hernial protrusion of the meninges through a defect in the vertebral column (spina bifida), usually posteriorly, forming a fluid-filled sac; locations are almost always in the thoracic or lumbar region although cervical and sacral meningoceles do occur. See also *myelomeningocele.*

spurious m., traumatic m. a condition resembling cranial meningocele, but caused by trauma; meninges herniate through a skull defect after tearing of the arachnoid. Called also *Billroth disease* and *cephalhydrocele traumatica.*

me·nin·go·ceph·a·li·tis (mə-ning″go-sef″ə-li′tis) meningoencephalitis.

me·nin·go·coc·ce·mia (mə-ning″go-kok-se′me-ə) invasion of the bloodstream by meningococci.

me·nin·go·coc·ci (mə-ning″go-kok′si) plural of *meningococcus.*

me·nin·go·coc·co·sis (mə-ning″go-kŏ-ko′sis) any infection caused by meningococci, such as meningitis or pneumonia.

me·nin·go·coc·cus (mə-ning″go-kok′əs) pl. *meningococ′ci* [*meningo-* + *coccus*] an individual organism of the species *Neisseria meningitidis.*

me·nin·go·cor·ti·cal (mə-ning″go-kor′tĭ-kəl) pertaining to or affecting the meninges and cortex of the brain.

me·nin·go·cyte (mə-ning′go-sīt″) a histiocyte of the meninges.

me·nin·go·en·ceph·a·li·tis (mə-ning″go-ən-sef″ə-li′tis) [*meningo-* + *encephalo-* + *-itis*] inflammation of the brain and meninges. Called also *cerebromeningitis* and *encephalomeningitis.*

amebic m. primary amebic m.

eosinophilic m. see under *meningitis.*

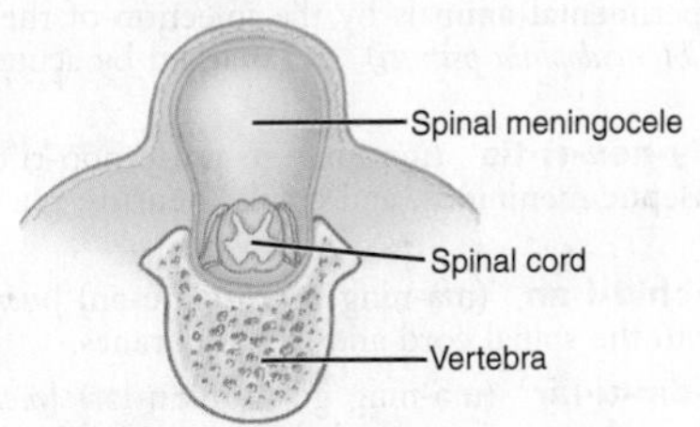

■ Cross-section of a spinal meningocele.

granulomatous m. an inflammatory disease of the central nervous system of dogs, of unknown etiology, characterized by granulomatous accumulations of histiocytes, lymphocytes, and plasma cells around blood vessels in the white matter and meninges. Onset is acute, with subsequent seizures, dementia, and sometimes paralysis and blindness. Most animals die within two months. Called also *granulomatous meningoencephalomyelitis* and *inflammatory reticulosis*.

mumps m. a usually benign type of meningoencephalitis seen in children, caused by the mumps virus, and characterized by fever, vomiting, nuchal rigidity, lethargy, parotitis, headache, convulsions, abdominal pain, diarrhea, and delirium.

primary amebic m. (PAM) a rare, acute, often fatal type of meningoencephalitis caused by infection with the usually free-living soil and water ameba *Naegleria fowleri.* It is characterized by suppuration and fever and is most often seen in young persons who have bathed in contaminated fresh water. Pathogens gain access to the central nervous system through the nasal mucosa and cribriform plate and then follow the olfactory bulbs and nerves to the brain and meninges. Similar but more subacute or chronic infections by species of *Acanthamoeba* and *Balamuthia* are called granulomatous amebic encephalitis.

thromboembolic m. an acute type of septicemia of cattle, characterized by fever, ataxia, blindness, coma, and death within hours, caused by infection with *Haemophilus somnus.* Called also *sleeper syndrome.* See also *Haemophilus septicemia of cattle.*

toxoplasmic m. the meningoencephalitis that sometimes occurs in toxoplasmosis, characterized by seizures and mental confusion, followed by coma and death if untreated. Pathologically, the brain may contain cysts and necrotic areas, with occasional hydrocephalus caused by blockage of aqueducts by sloughed material. There is a sharply increased incidence, often with recurring attacks, in immunocompromised patients. Called also *toxoplasmic encephalitis* or *encephalomyelitis.*

syphilitic m. general paresis.

me•nin•go•en•ceph•a•lo•cele (mə-ning″go-ən-sef′ə-lo-sēl″) encephalocele.

me•nin•go•en•ceph•a•lo•my•eli•tis (mə-ning″go-ən-sef″ə-lo-mi″ə-li′tis) inflammation of the meninges, brain, and spinal cord.

granulomatous m. see under *meningoencephalitis.*

me•nin•go•en•ceph•a•lo•my•elop•a•thy (mə-ning″go-ən-sef″ə-lo-mi″ə-lop′ə-the) disease involving the meninges, brain, and spinal cord.

me•nin•go•en•ceph•a•lop•a•thy (mə-ning″go-ən-sef″ə-lop′ə-the) noninflammatory disease of the cerebral meninges and the brain. Called also *encephalomeningopathy.*

me•nin•go•fi•bro•blas•to•ma (mə-ning″go-fi″bro-blas-to′mə) fibroblastic meningioma.

me•nin•go•gen•ic (mə-ning″go-jen′ik) [*meningo-* + *-genic*] arising in the meninges.

men•in•go•ma (men″in-go′mə) meningioma.

me•nin•go•ma•la•cia (mə-ning″go-mə-la′shə) [*meningo-* + *-malacia*] softening of a membrane.

me•nin•go•my•eli•tis (mə-ning″go-mi″ə-li′tis) [*meningo-* + *myelo-* + *-itis*] inflammation of the spinal cord and its membranes. Called also *myelomeningitis.*

syphilitic m. Erb spastic paraplegia.

me•nin•go•my•elo•cele (mə-ning″go-mi′ə-lo-sēl″) myelomeningocele.

me•nin•go•my•elo•en•ceph•a•li•tis (mə-ning″go-mi″ə-lo-en-sef″ə-li′tis) meningoencephalomyelitis.

me•nin•go•my•elo•ra•dic•u•li•tis (mə-ning″go-mi″ə-lo″rə-dik″u-li′tis) [*meningo-* + *myelo-* + *radiculitis*] inflammation of the meninges, spinal cord, and roots of the spinal nerves. Called also *rhizomeningomyelitis.*

me•nin•go•os•teo•phle•bi•tis (mə-ning″go-os″te-o-flə-bi′tis) [*meningo-* + *osteo-* bone + *phleb-* + *-itis*] periostitis with inflammation of the veins of a bone.

men•in•gop•a•thy (men″in-gop′ə-the) [*meningo-* + *-pathy*] any disease of the meninges.

me•nin•go•pneu•mo•ni•tis (mə-ning″go-noo-mo-ni′tis) a disease produced in experimental animals by the injection of the etiologic agent of psittacosis *(Chlamydophila psittaci)*, and marked by acute meningitis and pneumonitis.

me•nin•go•poly•neu•ri•tis (mə-ning″go-pol″e-nŏŏ-ri′tis) the triad of radiculopathy, aseptic meningitis, and cranial neuritis; see also *neuroborreliosis.*

me•nin•go•ra•chid•i•an (mə-ning″go-rə-kid′e-ən) [*meningo-* + *rachidian*] pertaining to the spinal cord and its membranes.

me•nin•go•ra•dic•u•lar (mə-ning″go-rə-dik′u-lər) [*meningo-* + *radicular*] pertaining to the meninges and the roots of the cranial and spinal nerves.

me•nin•go•ra•dic•u•li•tis (mə-ning″go-rə-dik″u-li′tis) inflammation of the meninges and roots of the spinal nerves.

me•nin•go•re•cur•rence (mə-ning″go-re-kur′əns) syphilitic meningitis induced in a syphilitic patient by antisyphilitic treatment.

me•nin•gor•rha•gia (mə-ning″go-ra′jə) [*meningo-* + *-rrhagia*] hemorrhage from the cerebral or spinal membranes; see *subarachnoid hemorrhage* and *subdural hemorrhage.* Called also *meningorrhea.*

me•nin•gor•rhea (mĕ-ning″go-re′ə) meningorrhagia.

men•in•go•sis (men″in-go′sis) the membranous attachment of bones to each other.

me•nin•go•the•li•o•ma (mə-ning″go-the″le-o′mə) meningothelial meningioma.

me•nin•go•vas•cu•lar (mə-ning″go-vas′ku-lər) pertaining to the meninges and blood vessels.

me•ninx (me′ninks) [Gr. *mēninx* membrane] singular of *meninges* (q.v.).

m. primiti′va, primitive m. loose embryonic mesenchyme surrounding the brain and spinal cord in the embryo; from it the three layers of the meninges are formed.

me•nis•cal (mə-nis′kəl) of or pertaining to a meniscus.

men•is•cec•to•my (men″ĭ-sek′tə-me) excision of an intra-articular meniscus, as in the knee joint.

me•nis•ci (mə-nis′i) [L.] genitive and plural of *meniscus.*

men•is•ci•tis (men″ĭ-si′tis) inflammation of a meniscus of the knee joint.

me•nis•co•fem•o•ral (mə-nis″ko-fem′or-əl) pertaining to or connecting the femur and a meniscus.

me•nis•co•syn•o•vi•al (mə-nis″ko-sə-no′ve-əl) pertaining to a meniscus and the synovial membrane.

me•nis•cus (mə-nis′kəs) gen. and pl. *menis′ci* [L., from Gr. *mēniskos*, crescent] 1. a crescent-shaped structure appearing at the surface of a liquid column, as in a pipet or buret, made concave or convex by the influence of capillarity. 2. a crescent-shaped structure of the body. Often used alone to designate one of the menisci of the knee joint; see *m. lateralis articulationis genus* and *m. medialis articulationis genus.*

m. of acromioclavicular joint discus articularis articulationis acromioclavicularis.

m. articula′ris [TA] articular meniscus: a pad, commonly a wedge-shaped crescent of fibrocartilage or dense fibrous tissue, found in some synovial joints; one side forms a marginal attachment at the articular capsule and the other two sides extend into the joint, ending in a free edge.

converging m. a concavoconvex lens.

discoid m., discoid lateral m. a semilunar lateral meniscus of the knee that has been transformed into a thickened, irregular discoid mass as a result of excess motion of the meniscus, which in turn results from congenital absence of attachment of the posterior horn of the meniscus to the tibial plateau. The excess motion also causes a clicking sound on flexion and extension of the knee. Occasionally, a discoid medial meniscus is observed. Called also *congenital discoid meniscus.*

diverging m. a convexoconcave lens.

m. of inferior radioulnar joint discus articularis articulationis radioulnaris distalis.

joint m. articular m.

Kuhnt m. the lining of the physiologic cup of the optic disk, composed of a thick accumulation of neuroglia.

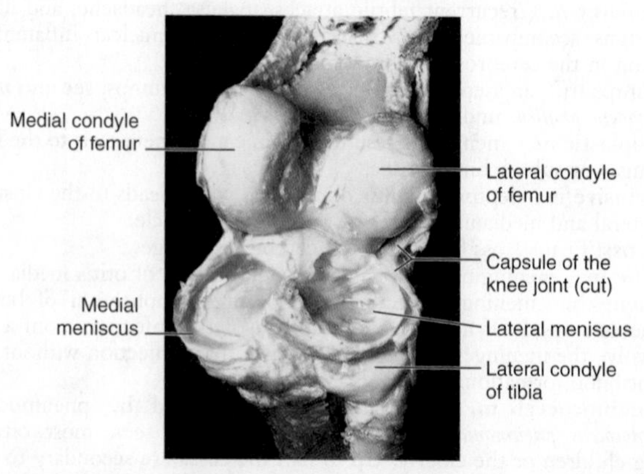

■ Articular menisci, exemplified by the lateral and medial menisci of the knee joint; shown in a posterior view of the right knee.

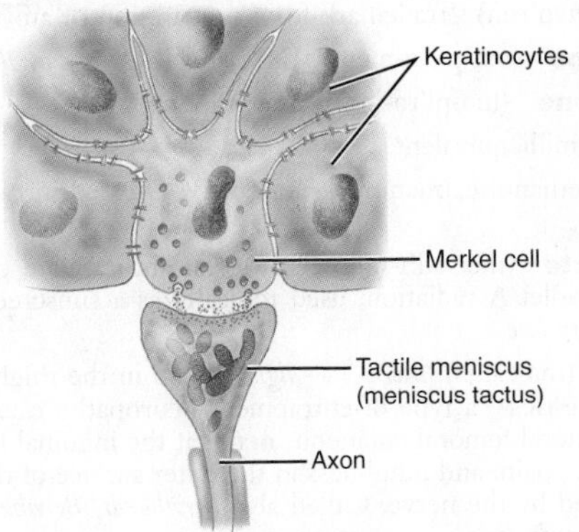

■ Schematic diagram of the meniscus tactus (tactile meniscus) of a nerve fiber in contact with a Merkel cell of the epithelium.

m. latera′lis articulatio′nis ge′nus [TA] lateral meniscus of knee joint: a crescent-shaped disk of fibrocartilage, but nearly circular in form, attached to the lateral margin of the superior articular surface of the tibia.

m. media′lis articulatio′nis ge′nus [TA] medial meniscus of knee joint: a crescent-shaped disk of fibrocartilage attached to the medial margin of the superior articular surface of the tibia.

negative m. a convexoconcave lens.

positive m. a concavoconvex lens.

m. of sternoclavicular joint discus articularis articulationis sternoclavicularis.

tactile m., m. tac′tus one of the small, cup-shaped, tactile nerve endings within the skin; many of them are formed by branches of a single nerve fiber, and each one is in contact with a single, modified epithelial cell called a Merkel cell. These are found in the deep epidermis, in hair follicles, and in the hard palate, and function as tactile receptors. Called also *tactile disk.*

m. of temporomandibular joint discus articularis articulationis temporomandibularis.

Men•i•sper•mum (men″ĭ-spur′məm) [Gr. *mēnē* moon + *sperma* seed] a genus of plants of the family Menispermaceae. *M. canaden′se* L. is the moonseed or yellow parilla, whose root was formerly used medicinally; the plant and its fruit resemble a grapevine and grapes and have been the cause of poisoning of children, sometimes fatal.

Men•kes disease (meng′kəz) [John H. *Menkes*, American physician, born 1928] see under *disease.*

Men•nell sign (men′əl) [James Beaver *Mennell*, English physician, 1880–1957] see under *sign.*

men(o)- [Gr. *mēn* month] a combining form denoting relationship to the menses.

meno•lip•sis (men″ə-lip′sis) temporary cessation of the menses.

meno•met•ror•rha•gia (men″o-me″tro-ra′jə) excessive and prolonged uterine bleeding occurring at irregular, frequent intervals.

Meno•mune (men′o-mūn) trademark for a preparation of meningococcal polysaccharide vaccine.

meno•pause (men′ə-pawz″) [*meno-* + *pause*] cessation of menstruation in the human female, occurring usually around the age of 50. See also *climacteric.* **menopau′sal** *adj*

artificial m. cessation of menstruation produced by artificial means, such as surgical operation or irradiation.

m. prae′cox, premature m. premature cessation of ovulation and menstrual cycles, occurring before age 40, sometimes caused by primary germ cell deficiency, acquired refractoriness to pituitary gonadotropin, or autoimmunization. Called also *premature ovarian failure.*

meno•pla•nia (men″ə-pla′ne-ə) [*meno-* + Gr. *planē* deviation] vicarious menstruation.

men•or•rha•gia (men″ə-ra′jə) [*meno-* + *-rrhagia*] hypermenorrhea.

men•or•rhal•gia (men″ə-ral′jə) [*menorrhea* + *-algia*] dysmenorrhea.

men•or•rhea (men″ə-re′ə) [*meno-* + *-rrhea*] 1. the normal discharge of the menses. 2. profuse menstruation.

men•or•rhe•al (men″o-re′əl) pertaining to menorrhea.

me•nos•che•sis (mə-nos′kə-sis) [*meno-* + *-schesis*] retention of the menses.

meno•stax•is (men″ə-stak′sis) [*meno-* + *staxis*] excessively prolonged menstruation.

meno•tro•pins (men′o-tro″pinz) [USP] an extract of human postmenopausal urine containing both follicle-stimulating hormone and luteinizing hormone. In females, it has the property of stimulating growth and maturation of ovarian follicles. In males, it has the properties of maintaining and stimulating testicular Leydig cells related to testosterone production and of being responsible for full development and maturation of spermatozoa in the seminiferous tubules. It is used to treat male hypogonadism, to induce ovulation and pregnancy in anovulatory women in whom the anovulation is not due to primary ovarian failure, and to increase the numbers of oocytes for patients attempting conception using assisted reproductive technologies such as gamete intrafallopian transfer (GIFT) or in vitro fertilization; administered intramuscularly. Called also *human menopausal gonadotropin.*

meno•uria (men″o-u′re-ə) [*meno-* + *-uria*] the flowing of menstrual blood through a fistula into the bladder.

Men•ri•um (men′re-əm) trademark for preparations of chlordiazepoxide and esterified estrogens.

men•ses (men′sēz) [L., pl. of *mensis* month] the monthly flow of blood from the genital tract of women; see *menstruation.*

men•stru•al (men′stroo-əl) [L. *menstrualis*] pertaining to the menses or to menstruation; called also *catamenial* and *emmenic.*

men•stru•ant (men′stroo-ənt) a woman or girl who is menstruating or is capable of menstruating.

men•stru•ate (men′stroo-āt) [L. *menstruare*] to undergo the monthly changes of menstruation (q.v.).

men•stru•a•tion (men″stroo-a′shən) the cyclic, physiologic discharge through the vagina of blood and mucosal tissues from the nonpregnant uterus; it is under hormonal control and normally recurs, usually at approximately four-week intervals, in the absence of pregnancy during the reproductive period (puberty through menopause) of the female of the human and a few species of primates. It is the culmination of the menstrual cycle; see illustration under *cycle.*

anovular m., anovulatory m. periodic uterine bleeding without preceding ovulation.

delayed m. menstruation the first appearance of which is delayed beyond the sixteenth year.

difficult m. dysmenorrhea.

infrequent m. oligomenorrhea.

nonovulational m. anovular m.

profuse m. hypermenorrhea.

regurgitant m., retrograde m. a back flow through the uterine tubes by which epithelial cells and other materials may be discharged through the tubal ostia and deposited on the ovaries and adjacent organs, as in endometriosis.

scanty m. hypomenorrhea.

supplementary m. menstrual discharge from the uterus and also from some other part.

suppressed m. amenorrhea.

vicarious m. discharge of blood from an extragenital source at the time a menstrual period is normally expected; thought to result from generally increased capillary permeability related to the menstrual cycle.

men•stru•ous (men′stroo-əs) menstrual.

men•stru•um (men′stroo-əm) [L. *menstruus* menstruous: it was long believed that the menstrual fluid had a peculiar solvent quality] a solvent medium.

men•su•al (men′su-əl) [L. *mensis* month] monthly.

men•su•ra•tion (men″su-ra′shən) [L. *mensuratio; mensura* measure] the act or process of measuring.

men•tal[1] (men′təl) [L. *mens* mind] pertaining to the mind; called also *phrenic* and *psychic.*

men•tal[2] (men′təl) [L. *mentum* chin] pertaining to the chin; called also *genial* and *genian.*

men•ta•lis (men-ta′lis) [L.] relating to the chin; see under *musculus.*

men•tal•i•ty (men-tal′ĭ-te) 1. mental power or capacity. 2. way of thought; mental set.

Men•tas•tics (men-tas′tiks) [shortened from *mental gymnastics*] service mark for a component of the Trager Approach (q.v.).

men•ta•tion (men-ta′shən) mental activity.

Men•tax (men′taks) trademark for a preparation of butenafine hydrochloride.

Men•tha (men′thə) [L.] the mints, a widely distributed genus of aromatic perennial herbs of the family Lamiaceae.

M. cardi′aca Scotch spearmint, a source of spearmint oil.

M. piperi′ta peppermint, the source of peppermint oil.

M. pule′gium European pennyroyal; see *pennyroyal.*

M. spica′ta common spearmint, a source of spearmint oil.

men•thol (men′thol) [USP] an alcohol obtained from the oils of various species of *Mentha* or prepared synthetically, used as a topical antipruritic, and as an inhalation for treatment of upper respiratory disorders.

men·thyl (men′thəl) the monovalent radical, $C_{10}H_{19}$.
  m. anthranilate meradimate.

men·ti·cide (men′tĭ-sīd) [*mental*[1] + *-cide*] brainwashing.

ment(o)- [L. *mentum* chin] a combining form denoting relationship to the chin. See also words beginning *geni(o)-*.

men·to·an·te·ri·or (men″to-an-tēr′e-ər) [*mento-* + *anterior*] see under *position.*

men·to·la·bi·al (men″to-la′be-əl) [*mento-* + *labial*] pertaining to the chin and lip.

men·ton (men′ton) a craniometric landmark, being the most inferior point on the mandibular symphysis on a lateral jaw projection.

men·to·plas·ty (men′to-plas″te) [*mento-* + *-plasty*] plastic surgery of the chin; surgical correction of deformities and defects of the chin. **mentoplas′tic** *adj*

men·to·pos·te·ri·or (men″to-pos-tēr′e-ər) [*mento-* + *posterior*] see under *position.*

men·to·trans·verse (men″to-trans-vərs′) [*mento-* + *transverse*] see under *position.*

men·tum (men′təm) [L.] [TA] the chin.

Men·y·an·thes (men″e-an′thēz) [perhaps from Gr. *mēn* month + *anthos* flower] a genus of plants of the family Gentianaceae. *M. trifolia′ta* L., or buckbean, is a bitter tonic and has febrifuge properties.

MEP maximum expiratory pressure.

mep·a·crine hy·dro·chlo·ride (mep′ə-krēn) quinacrine hydrochloride.

me·par·tri·cin (mə-pahr′trĭ-sin) an antifungal and antiprotozoal, used chiefly in the treatment of vaginal and cutaneous candidiasis, applied topically.

me·pen·zo·late bro·mide (mə-pen′zo-lāt) a quaternary ammonium compound with anticholinergic and antimuscarinic effects, used as an adjunct in the treatment of peptic ulcers and in the treatment of disorders in which hypermotility of the colon is a feature; administered orally.

Mep·er·gan (mep′er-gan) trademark for a combination preparation of meperidine hydrochloride and promethazine hydrochloride.

me·per·i·dine hy·dro·chlo·ride (mə-per′ĭ-dēn) [USP] a synthetic opioid analgesic, used as an analgesic to relieve moderate to severe pain, including during childbirth, and as an adjunct to anesthesia; administered orally, intramuscularly, subcutaneously, or intravenously. Abuse of this drug may lead to dependence. Called also *pethidine hydrochloride.*

Meph·a·quin (mef′ə-kwin) trademark for a preparation of mefloquine hydrochloride.

me·phen·amine (mə-fen′ə-mēn) orphenadrine.

me·phen·e·sin (mə-fen′ə-sin) a centrally acting skeletal muscle relaxant, used for the treatment of painful muscle spasm; administered orally.

me·phen·ter·mine sul·fate (mə-fen′tər-mēn) an adrenergic, used for its vasopressor effects in the treatment of certain hypotensive states, administered orally, intramuscularly, or intravenously. It is also applied topically to the nasal mucosa as a decongestant.

me·phen·y·to·in (mə-fen′ə-to-in) [USP] an anticonvulsant used for the suppression and control of generalized tonic-clonic and simple and complex partial epileptic seizures that are refractory to other drugs; administered orally.

me·phi·tis (mə-fi′tis) [L.] a foul exhalation. **mephit′ic** *adj*

meph·o·bar·bi·tal (mef″o-bahr′bĭ-təl) [USP] a long-acting barbiturate, used as an anticonvulsant in grand mal and petit mal epilepsy, administered orally.

Meph·y·ton (mef′ĭ-ton) trademark for preparations of phytonadione (vitamin K_1).

me·piv·a·caine hy·dro·chlo·ride (mə-piv′ə-kān) [USP] a local anesthetic, an analogue of lidocaine; used for infiltration anesthesia, peripheral nerve block, Bier block, and epidural block. It is also used for infiltration and nerve block in dental procedures.

me·pred·ni·sone (mə-pred′nĭ-sōn) [USP] a synthetic glucocorticoid used in the treatment of inflammatory, allergic, rheumatic, and other corticosteroid-responsive diseases, such as certain endocrine, respiratory, neoplastic, and collagen diseases, administered orally.

me·pro·ba·mate (mə-pro′bə-māt, mep″ro-bam′āt) [USP] a carbamate derivative, having tranquilizing and muscle relaxant actions. It is used as an oral sedative for the relief of anxiety and tension, as an adjunct in the treatment of conditions in which anxiety and tension are manifested, and to promote sleep in anxious, tense patients; it has also been used in the treatment of painful musculoskeletal disorders.
  isopropyl m. carisoprodol.

Mep·ron (mep′ron) trademark for a preparation of atovaquone.

me·pyr·amine (mə-pir′ə-mēn) INN and BAN for *pyrilamine.*

me·py·ra·pone (mə-pi′rə-pōn) metyrapone.

mEq, meq milliequivalent.

MER the methanol extraction residue of BCG; used in cancer immunotherapy.

mer·ad·i·mate (mer-ad′ĭ-māt) [USP] an anthranilate compound that absorbs ultraviolet A radiation; used topically as a sunscreen. Called also *menthyl anthranilate.*

me·ral·gia (mə-ral′jə) [*mero-*[2] + *-algia*] pain in the thigh.
  m. paresthe′tica a type of entrapment neuropathy caused by entrapment of the lateral femoral cutaneous nerve at the inguinal ligament, causing paresthesia, pain, and numbness in the outer surface of the thigh in the region supplied by the nerve. Called also *Bernhardt, Bernhardt-Roth, Roth,* or *Roth-Bernhardt disease.*

mer·bro·min (mər-bro′min) a mercurial antiseptic that has been used topically for the disinfection of skin and wounds.

mer·cap·tan (mər-kap′tan) [L. *mercurium captans* seizing or combining with mercury] thiol (def. 2).

2-mer·cap·to·eth·a·nol (2-ME) (mər-kap″to-eth′ə-nol) a foul-smelling sulfhydryl compound that acts as a reducing agent; used to differentiate between IgG and IgM in a mixture by disrupting the disulfide bonds of IgM so that only IgG is measurable. See also under *tests.*

β-mer·cap·to·eth·yl·amine (mər-kap″to-eth′əl-ə-mēn″) cysteamine.

mer·cap·tol (mər-kap′tol) a compound formed from a ketone by introducing two thio-alkyl (—SR) groups in place of the bivalent oxygen.

mer·cap·to·pu·rine (6-MP) (mər-kap″to-pu′rēn) [USP] a thiopurine that can be incorporated into the nucleotide 6-thiol MP, an analogue of inosine monophosphate (IMP), which then inhibits new purine synthesis in two places, by serving as a pseudofeedback inhibitor of the first step in the pathway and also by inhibiting the conversion of IMP to adenine and guanine nucleotides. Mercaptopurine is administered orally as an antineoplastic, primarily for treatment of acute lymphoblastic leukemia, and has also been used as an immunosuppressant in treatment of Crohn disease, ulcerative colitis, and severe psoriatic arthritis. Called also *6-mercaptopurine.*

mer·cap·tur·ic ac·id (mər-kap-tūr′ik) a cysteine conjugate of an aromatic compound formed initially as a glutathione conjugate in the liver and excreted in the urine.

Mer·chant projection (mur′chənt) [A.C. *Merchant,* American radiologist, 20th century] see under *projection.*

Mer·cier bar (mer-sya′) [Louis Auguste *Mercier,* French urologist, 1811–1882] plica interureterica.

mer·co·cre·sols (mur″ko-kre′solz) a combination of cresol derivatives and an organic mercury, used for its germicidal, fungicidal, and bacteriostatic properties.

mer·cu·ra·mide (mər-kūr′ə-mīd) mersalyl.

mer·cu·ri·al (mər-kūr′e-əl) [L. *mercurialis*] 1. pertaining to mercury. 2. a preparation of mercury.

mer·cu·ri·al·ism (mər-kūr′e-əl-iz″əm) mercury poisoning; see under *poisoning.*

mer·cur·ic (mər-kūr′ik) pertaining to mercury as a bivalent element.
  m. chloride mercury bichloride.

Mer·cu·ro·chrome (mər-ku′rə-krōm) trademark for preparations of merbromin.

mer·cu·rous (mur′kūr-əs) pertaining to mercury as a monovalent element.

mer·cu·ry (Hg) (mur′kūr-e) a metallic element, liquid at ordinary temperatures; atomic number, 80; atomic weight 200.59, specific gravity 13.546. It is insoluble in ordinary solvents, partially soluble in boiling hydrochloric acid, and soluble in nitric acid. It forms two sets of compounds: *mercurous,* in which a single atom of mercury combines with a monovalent radical, and *mercuric,* in which a single atom of mercury combines with a bivalent radical. The mercuric salts are more soluble and irritant than the mercurous ones. Mercury and its salts have been used medicinally, but because of the risk of mercury poisoning (see under *poisoning*) their use has diminished.
  m. 197 a radioactive isotope of mercury, atomic mass 197, having a half-life of 2.67 years and decaying by electron capture with emission of gamma rays (0.077 MeV); it has been used in renal imaging.
  m. 203 a radioactive isotope of mercury, atomic mass 203, having a half-life of 46.60 days and emitting beta particles (0.214 MeV) and gamma rays (0.279 MeV); it has been used in renal imaging.
  ammoniated m. [USP] a topical anti-infective, $HgNH_2Cl$.

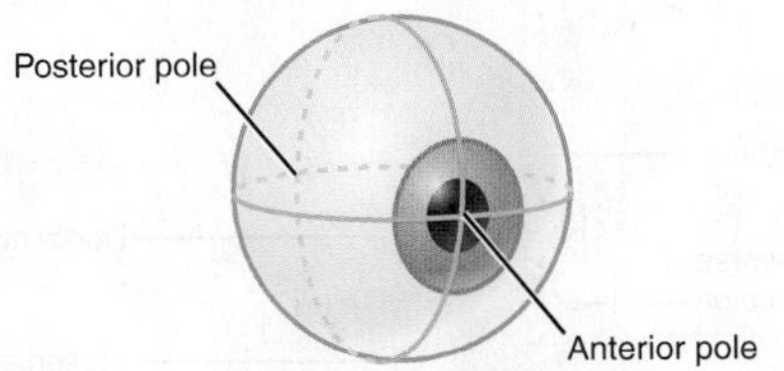

■ Meridiani bulbi oculi (meridians of eyeball).

m. bichloride, m. perchloride an extremely poisonous compound, $HgCl_2$, used formerly in the treatment of syphilis and now as a disinfectant. Called also *mercuric chloride*.

methyl m. a highly toxic compound formed by methylation of mercury, formerly used as a fungicide and disinfectant and for other industrial purposes; it is one of the most common causes of mercury poisoning (see under *poisoning*). Also written *methylmercury*.

-mere [Gr. *meros* part] a word termination denoting a segment or a part.

Me·rid·ia (mə-rid′e-ə) trademark for a preparation of sibutramine hydrochloride.

me·rid·i·an (mə-rid′e-ən) 1. an imaginary line on the surface of a spherical body, marking the intersection with the surface of a plane passing through its axis. Called also *meridianus*. 2. in acupuncture, a system of 20 lines (12 principal and 8 collateral) connecting acupoints and regarded as channels through which qi flows.

m. of cornea an imaginary line marking the intersection with its surface of an anteroposterior plane passing through the apex of the cornea.

m's of eyeball meridiani bulbi oculi.

me·rid·i·a·ni (mə-rid″e-a′ne) [L.] plural of *meridianus*.

me·rid·i·a·nus (mə-rid″e-a′nəs) pl. *meridia′ni* [L., from *medius* middle + *dies* day] meridian.

meridia′ni bul′bi o′culi [TA] meridians of eyeball: imaginary lines encircling the eyeball, marking the intersection with its surface of planes passing through its anteroposterior axis.

me·rid·i·o·nal (mə-rid′e-o-nəl) pertaining to a meridian or made along a meridian; as *meridional section*.

Mer·i·o·nes (mer-e-o′nēz) a genus of gerbil-like rodents found in desert areas of Central Asia; several species are common reservoirs for *Leishmania major*, which causes cutaneous leishmaniasis.

mer·i·sis (mer′ĭ-sis) growth in size due to cell division.

mer·ism (mer′iz-əm) [Gr. *meros* a part] the repetition of parts in an organism so as to form a regular pattern. **meris′tic** *adj*

mer·i·stem (mer′ĭ-stem) [Gr. *merizein* to divide] the undifferentiated embryonic tissue of plants.

mer·i·ste·mat·ic (mer″ĭ-stə-mat′ik) 1. pertaining to meristem. 2. composed of meristem.

Mer·kel cell (corpuscle, disk, tactile cell) (mur′kəl) [Friedrich Sigmund *Merkel*, German anatomist, 1845–1919] see under *cell*.

Mer·kel filtrum, muscle (mur′kəl) [Karl Ludwig *Merkel*, German anatomist, 1812–1876] see *filtrum ventriculi* and *musculus ceratocricoideus*.

Mer·kel-Ran·vier cells (mur′kəl rah-vya′) [F.S. *Merkel;* Louis Antoine *Ranvier*, French pathologist, 1835–1922] see under *cell*.

mer·lin (mur′lin) a cytoskeletal protein that acts as a tumor suppressor; a defect in the gene that codes for this protein is the cause of neurofibromatosis 2. Called also *schwannomin*.

mer·mi·thid (mer′mĭ-thid) pertaining to or of the family Mermithidae.

Mer·mith·i·dae (mər-mith′ĭ-de) a family of nematodes of the superfamily Mermithoidea; the cabbage snakes.

Mer·mith·oi·dea (mer″mith-oi′de-ə) a superfamily of aphasmids including the cabbage snakes (family Mermithidae), the larvae of which may accidentally occur in the human digestive tract as contaminants of food or water.

mer(o)-[1] [Gr. *meros* part] a combining form meaning part.

mer(o)-[2] [Gr. *mēros* thigh] a combining form denoting relationship to the thigh.

mero·acra·nia (mer″o-ə-kra′ne-ə) [*mero-*[1] + *a-*[1] + Gr. *kranion* skull] congenital absence of part of the cranium.

mero·an·en·ceph·a·ly (mer″o-an″ən-sef′ə-le) [*mero-*[1] + *anencephaly*] congenital absence of part of the brain, usually the forebrain and midbrain. Cf. *anencephaly*.

mero·blas·tic (mer″o-blas′tik) [*mero-*[1] + *blast-* + *-ic*] partially dividing; undergoing cleavage in which only part of the zygote participates; see under *cleavage*.

mero·cox·al·gia (me″ro-kok-sal′jə) [*mero-*[2] + *coxalgia*] pain in the thigh and hip.

mero·crine (mer′o-krin) [*mero-*[1] + Gr. *krinein* to separate] partly secreting; denoting that type of glandular secretion in which the secreting cell remains intact throughout the process of formation and discharge of the secretory products; as in the salivary and pancreatic glands. Cf. *apocrine* and *holocrine*.

mero·cyst (mer′o-sist) [*mero-*[1] + *cyst*] a large schizont seen in certain hemosporidian protozoa from which merozoites are released to invade the host's erythrocytes, where they develop into gametocytes.

mero·cyte (mer′o-sīt) [*mero-*[1] + *-cyte*] a supernumerary sperm nucleus in the oocyte in cases of polyspermy.

me·rog·a·my (mə-rog′ə-me) microgamy.

mero·gen·e·sis (mer″o-jen′ə-sis) [*mero-*[1] + *-genesis*] cleavage of a zygote. **merogenet′ic, merogen′ic** *adj*

mero·gon·ic (mer″o-gon′ik) pertaining to or resulting from merogony.

me·rog·o·ny (mə-rog′ə-ne) [*mero-*[1] + Gr. *gonos* procreation] 1. the development of a fragment of a disrupted oocyte. 2. schizogony resulting in the production of merozoites.

diploid m. development of a portion of an oocyte containing the fused male and female pronuclei.

parthenogenetic m. development, as a result of artificial stimulation, of a part of an oocyte containing the nucleus.

mero·me·lia (mer″o-me′le-ə) [*mero-*[1] + *-melia*] congenital absence of any part of a limb, as in adactyly, hemimelia, or phocomelia; cf. *amelia*.

mero·mi·cro·so·mia (mer″o-mi″kro-so′me-ə) [*mero-*[1] + *microsomia*] unusual smallness of some part of the body.

mero·mor·pho·sis (mer″o-mor-fo′sis) [*mero-*[1] + *morphosis*] incomplete restoration or regeneration of a lost part.

mero·my·ar·i·an (mer″o-mi-ar′e-ən) [*mero-*[1] + Gr. *mys* muscle] designating a type of nematode musculature in which there are only a few muscle cells in a given area, the cells being platymyarian in type.

mero·myo·sin (mer″o-mi′o-sin) a fragment of the myosin molecule isolated by treatment with proteolytic enzymes; there are two types, heavy (H-meromyosin) and light (L-meromyosin). *L-meromyosin* makes up the major part of the rodlike backbone of the molecule; *H-meromyosin* contains the subfragment responsible for the ATPase activity of myosin. See Plate 32.

mer·ont (mer′ont) [*mero-*[1] + *ontos* being] the asexual stage in the development of certain protozoa, especially nonsporozoa, that gives rise to merozoites. See also *schizont* and *segmenter*.

mer·o·pen·em (mer″o-pen′əm) [USP] a broad-spectrum antibiotic of the carbapenem group, similar to imipenem in structure and activity and used in the treatment of intra-abdominal infections and bacterial meningitis; administered intravenously. It is not as susceptible to metabolism in the kidneys as imipenem and need not be administered with cilastatin.

me·ro·pia (mə-ro′pe-ə) [*mero-*[1] + *-opia*] partial blindness.

mero·ra·chis·chi·sis (me″ro-rə-kis′kĭ-sis) [*mero-*[1] + *rachi-* + *schisis*] fissure of a part of the vertebral column; called also *mesorachischisis* and *rachischisis partialis*. Cf. *spina bifida*.

mero·spo·ran·gi·um (mer″o-spə-ran′je-əm) a small sporangium, usually cylindrical, containing a few spores in a chain or row.

mer·os·tot·ic (mer″os-tot′ik) [*mero-*[1] + L. *os* bone] pertaining to or affecting only a part of a bone.

mero·zo·ite (mer″o-zo′īt) [*mero-*[1] + *zo-* + *-ite*[1]] a stage in the life cycle of certain sporozoan protozoa resulting from merogony. Called also *schizozoite*.

mero·zy·gote (mer″o-zi′gōt) [*mero-*[1] + *zygote*] the partially diploid bacterial zygote that results from the transfer of a portion of the genetic information of a donor cell to the total genetic information of the recipient. See also *heterogenote* and *homogenote*.

Mer·phen·yl (mur′fən-əl) trademark for preparations of phenylmercuric compounds.

Mer·rem (mer′əm) trademark for a preparation of meropenem.

MERRF myoclonic epilepsy with ragged red fibers; see *MERRF syndrome*, under *syndrome*.

mer·sa·lyl (mur′sə-ləl) a mercurial diuretic that has been used in combination with theophylline in the treatment of edema secondary to such conditions as cardiorenal diseases, nephrosis, and cirrhosis, administered intramuscularly and intravenously.

mer·ti·a·tide (mur′te-ə-tīd″) a carboxylated, diamido-, disulfur-containing compound; complexed with technetium Tc 99m it is used in functional and anatomical renal imaging. See table at *technetium*. Called also *MAG3*.

Mer·thi·o·late (mər-thi′o-lāt) trademark for preparations of thimerosal.

Mer·u·vax (mer′u-vaks″) trademark for preparations of rubella virus vaccine live.

mer·y·cism (mer′ĭ-siz″əm) rumination.

Merz·bach·er-Pel·i·zae·us disease (merts′bah-ker pa″le-tsa′oos) [Ludwig *Merzbacher*, German physician 1875–1942; Friedrich *Pelizaeus*, German neurologist, 1850–1917] Pelizaeus-Merzbacher disease; see under *disease*.

MESA microsurgical epididymal sperm aspiration.

me·sad (me′sad) mesiad.

me·sal (me′səl) mesial.

me·sal·amine (mə-sal′ə-mēn) [USP] 5-aminosalicylic acid, an active metabolite of sulfasalazine, used in the prophylaxis and treatment of inflammatory bowel disease and ulcerative proctitis; administered orally or rectally.

me·sal·a·zine (mə-sal′ə-zēn) INN and BAN for *mesalamine*.

mes·an·gio·cap·il·lary (mes-an″je-o-kap′ĭ-lar″e) pertaining to or affecting the mesangium and the associated capillaries.

mes·an·gi·ol·y·sis (mes-an″je-ol′ĭ-sis) degenerative changes to the mesangium, starting with loosening and detachment of its matrix and progressing to dissolution with degeneration of mesangial cells.

mes·an·gi·um (mes-an′je-əm) the thin membrane that helps support the capillary loops in a renal glomerulus. **mesan′gial** *adj*

extraglomerular m. collective term for the lacis cells.

Me·san·to·in (mə-san′toin) trademark for a preparation of mephenytoin.

mes·a·ra·ic (mes″ə-ra′ik) [Gr. *mesaraion* mesentery] mesenteric.

mes·ar·ter·itis (mes″ahr-tər-i′tis) [*mes-* + *arteritis*] inflammation of the tunica media of an artery.

Mönckeberg m. see under *arteriosclerosis*.

me·sati·ce·phal·ic (mə-sat″ĭ-sə-fal′ik) [Gr. *mesatos* medium + *cephal-* + *-ic*] mesocephalic.

me·sati·ker·kic (mə-sat″ĭ-ker′kik) [Gr. *mesatos* medium + *kerkis* the radius of the arm] having a radiohumeral index of 75 to 80.

me·sati·pel·lic (mə-sat″ĭ-pel′ik) [Gr. *mesatos* medium + *pella* bowl] having a transverse diameter of the pelvic inlet almost the same as that of the true conjugated diameter.

me·sati·pel·vic (mə-sat″ĭ-pel′vik) mesatipellic.

mes·ax·on (mes-ak′son) a pair of parallel membranes marking the line of edge-to-edge contact of the Schwann cell encircling the axon.

mes·cal (mes-kahl′) [Nahuatl *metl ixcalli* concoction or stew of the maguey plant] 1. *Lophophora williamsii.* 2. a Mexican alcoholic beverage made from the maguey plant.

mes·ca·line (mes′kə-lēn) a poisonous hallucinogenic alkaloid found in mescal buttons; it produces an intoxication with delusions of color and music.

mes·cal·ism (mes′kə-liz″əm) intoxication caused by mescal buttons or mescaline.

mes·ec·to·derm (mez-ek′to-dərm) embryonic migratory cells, derived from the neural crest of the head, that contribute to the formation of the meninges and become pigment cells.

mes·en·ce·phal·ic (mez-en″sə-fal′ik) pertaining to the mesencephalon.

mes·en·ceph·a·li·tis (mez″en-sef″ə-li′tis) inflammation of the mesencephalon.

mes·en·ceph·a·lo·hy·po·phys·e·al (mez″en-sef″ə-lo-hi″po-fiz′e-əl) mesencephalohypophysial.

mes·en·ceph·a·lo·hy·po·phys·i·al (mez″en-sef″ə-lo-hi″po-fiz′e-əl) pertaining to the mesencephalon and the pituitary gland (hypophysis). Spelled also *mesencephalohypophyseal.*

mes·en·ceph·a·lon (mez″en-sef′ə-lon) [*meso-* + *encephalon*] 1. [TA] the part of the brain developed from the middle of the three primary vesicles of the embryonic neural tube; it comprises the tectum, midbrain tegmentum, and basis pedunculi; see Plate 9. See also *brainstem.* 2. the middle of the three primary brain vesicles in the embryo, lying between the prosencephalon and the rhombencephalon. Called also *midbrain.*

mes·en·ceph·a·lot·o·my (mez″en-sef″ə-lot′ə-me) [*mesencephalon* + Gr. *tomē* a cutting] production of lesions in the midbrain, especially in the pain-conducting pathways for the relief of intractable pain. Formerly performed directly with a surgical incision, it is now done stereotactically with current from inserted electrodes.

mes·en·chy·ma (mez-eng′kĭ-mə) mesenchyme.

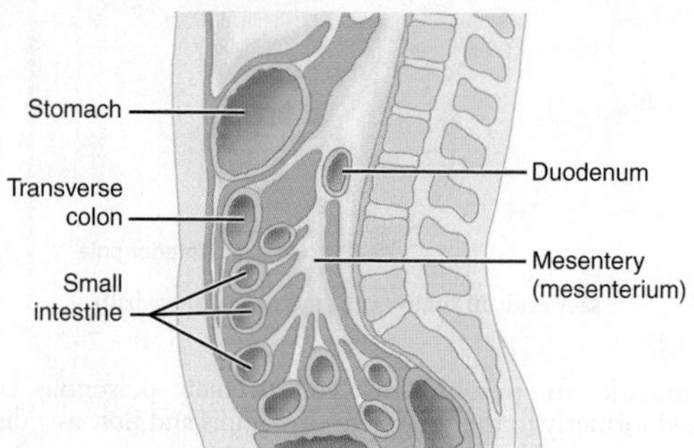

■ Mesenterium (mesentery) in a median sagittal section.

mes·en·chyme (mez′əng-kīm″) [*mes-* + Gr. *enchyma* infusion] the meshwork of loosely organized embryonic connective tissue in the mesoderm from which are formed the connective tissues of the body, and also the blood vessels and lymphatic vessels. **mesen′chymal** *adj*

mes·en·chy·mo·ma (mez″ən-ki-mo′mə) a tumor of mixed mesenchymal tissues with two or more cellular elements not commonly associated, not counting fibrous tissue as one of the elements.

benign m. a benign tumor composed of two or more clearly recognizable mesenchymal elements in addition to fibrous tissue.

malignant m. a sarcoma composed of two or more cellular elements (excluding fibrous tissue); called also *mixed cell sarcoma.*

mes·en·ter·ec·to·my (mez″ən-tə-rek′tə-me) [*mesentery* + *-ectomy*] resection of mesentery.

mes·en·ter·i·o·lum (mes″ən-tər-i′o-ləm) a small mesentery.

m. appen′dicis vermifor′mis mesoappendix.

mes·en·ter·io·pexy (mez″ən-ter′e-o-pek″se) [*mesentery* + *-pexy*] fixation or suspension of the mesentery.

mes·en·ter·i·or·rha·phy (mez″ən-ter″e-or′ə-fe) [*mesentery* + *-rrhaphy*] suture or repair of the mesentery.

mes·en·ter·i·pli·ca·tion (mez″ən-ter″ĭ-plĭ-ka′shən) [*mesentery* + *plication*] shortening the mesentery by plication.

mes·en·ter·itis (mez″en-tə-ri′tis) inflammation of the mesentery.

retractile m., sclerosing m. inflammation and variable fibrosis of the mesentery producing thickening, sclerosis, and retraction, sometimes resulting in distortion or obstruction of intestinal loops. Some authorities consider this a fibrotic variant of mesenteric panniculitis.

mes·en·ter·i·um (mez″ən-ter′e-əm) [TA] mesentery: a membranous fold attaching any of various organs to the body wall, especially the folds of peritoneum that attach the intestines to the abdominal wall.

m. commu′ne, m. dorsa′le commu′ne dorsal common mesentery: the primordial embryonic mesentery, a double-layered median partition formed by association of the splanchnic mesoderm with the endoderm, extending from the roof of the coelom toward the midventral wall, and dividing the coelom into halves; it contains the primordial gut, and encloses the heart, lungs, and liver as they develop.

mes·en·tero·ax·i·al (mez-en″tər-o-ak′se-əl) pertaining to the mesenteric axis of part of the gastrointestinal tract.

mes·en·ter·on (mez-en′tər-on) [*meso-* + *enteron*] midgut.

mes·en·tery (mez′ən-ter″e) mesenterium. **mesenter′ic** *adj*

m. of ascending part of colon mesocolon ascendens.

caval m. a ridge at the right of the embryonic mesogastrium, in which a hepatic segment of the inferior vena cava develops.

common m., common m., dorsal mesenterium dorsale commune.

m. of descending part of colon mesocolon descendens.

dorsal m. mesenterium dorsale commune.

primitive m., primordial m. mesenterium dorsale commune.

m. of rectum mesorectum.

m. of sigmoid colon mesocolon sigmoideum.

m. of transverse part of colon mesocolon transversum.

ventral m. the embryonic mesentery attaching the stomach and the proximal duodenal region of the primordial intestine to the ventral body wall.

m. of vermiform appendix mesoappendix.

mes·epi·the·li·um (mes″ep-ĭ-the′le-əm) mesothelium.

MeSH (mesh) [*Me*dical *S*ubject *H*eadings] a thesaurus published by the National Library of Medicine for use in MEDLARS.

mesh·work (mesh′wərk) a network or reticulum.

trabecular m. reticulum trabeculare.

me·si·ad (me′ze-ad) [Gr. *mesos* middle] toward the middle; called also *mesad.*

me·si·al (me′ze-əl) [Gr. *mesos* middle] on the side towards the center line of the dental arch.

me·si·al·ly (me′ze-al″e) mesiad.

mesi(o)- [Gr. *mesos* in the middle] in dentistry, a combining form denoting relationship to the middle; specifically, the mesial surface of a tooth or the mesial wall of a tooth cavity.

me·sio·buc·cal (me″ze-o-buk′əl) pertaining to or formed by the mesial and buccal surfaces of a tooth, or the mesial and buccal walls of a tooth cavity preparation.

me·sio·buc·co·oc·clu·sal (me″ze-o-buk″o-ə-kloo′zəl) pertaining to or formed by the mesial, buccal, and occlusal surfaces of a tooth.

me·sio·buc·co·pul·pal (me″ze-o-buk″o-pul′pəl) pertaining to or formed by the mesial, buccal, and pulpal walls of a tooth cavity.

me·sio·cer·vi·cal (me″ze-o-sur′vi-kəl) 1. pertaining to the mesial surface of the neck of a tooth. 2. mesiogingival.

me·sio·cli·na·tion (me″ze-o-klĭ-na′shən) deviation of a tooth from the vertical, in the direction of the tooth next mesial (anterior) to it in the dental arch.

me·sio·clu·sion (me″ze-o-kloo′zhən) [*mesio-* + L. *cludere* to close] malocclusion in which the mandibular arch is in an anterior position in relation to the maxillary arch (prognathism). Generally considered as identical with Class III in Angle classification of malocclusion (see *malocclusion*). Called also *anterior occlusion, anteroclusion,* and *protrusive occlusion.*

me·sio·dens (me′ze-o-denz″) pl. *mesioden′tes* [*mesio-* + *dens*] the most common supernumerary tooth, appearing singly or in pairs as a small tooth with a cone-shaped crown and a short root between the maxillary central incisors; it may be erupted, impacted, or even inverted.

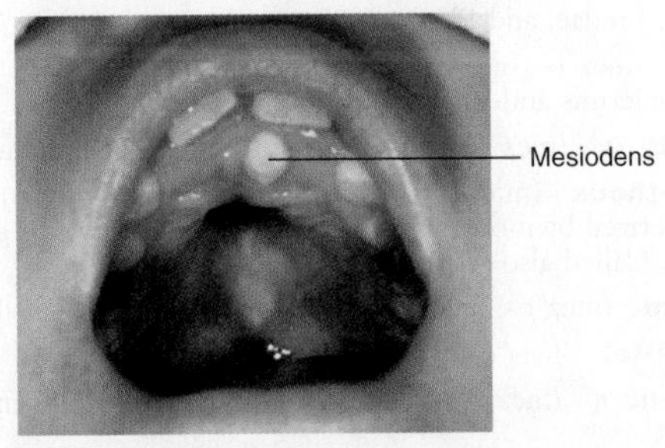

me·sio·den·tes (me″ze-o-den′tēz) plural of *mesiodens.*

me·sio·dis·tal (me″ze-o-dis′təl) pertaining to the mesial and distal surfaces of a tooth.

me·sio·gin·gi·val (me″ze-o-jin′jĭ-vəl) pertaining to or formed by the mesial and gingival walls of a tooth cavity.

me·sio·in·ci·so·dis·tal (me″ze-o-in-si″zo-dis′təl) pertaining to the mesial, incisal, and distal surfaces of an anterior tooth.

me·sio·la·bi·al (me″ze-o-la′be-əl) pertaining to or formed by the mesial and labial surfaces of a tooth, or the mesial and labial walls of a tooth cavity preparation.

me·sio·la·bio·in·ci·sal (me″ze-o-la″be-o-in-si′zəl) pertaining to or formed by the mesial, labial, and incisal surfaces of a tooth.

me·sio·lin·gual (me″ze-o-ling′gwəl) pertaining to or formed by the mesial and lingual surfaces of a tooth, or the mesial and lingual walls of a tooth cavity preparation.

me·sio·lin·guo·in·ci·sal (me″ze-o-ling″gwo-in-si′zəl) pertaining to or formed by the mesial, lingual, and incisal surfaces of a tooth.

me·sio·lin·guo·oc·clu·sal (me″ze-o-ling″gwo-ə-kloo′zəl) pertaining to or formed by the mesial, lingual, and occlusal surfaces of a tooth.

me·sio·lin·guo·pul·pal (me″ze-o-ling″gwo-pul′pəl) pertaining to or formed by the mesial, lingual, and pulpal walls of a tooth cavity preparation.

me·si·on (me′se-on) planum medianum.

me·si·o·oc·clu·sal (me″ze-o-ŏ-kloo′zəl) pertaining to or formed by the mesial and occlusal surfaces of a tooth, or the mesial and occlusal walls of a tooth cavity.

me·si·o·oc·clu·sion (me″ze-o-ŏ-kloo′zhən) mesioclusion.

me·si·o·oc·clu·so·dis·tal (me″ze-o-ŏ-kloo″zo-dis′təl) pertaining to the mesial, occlusal, and distal surfaces of a posterior tooth.

me·sio·pul·pal (me″ze-o-pul′pəl) pertaining to or formed by the mesial and pulpal walls of a tooth cavity preparation.

me·sio·pul·po·la·bi·al (me″ze-o-pul″po-la′be-əl) pertaining to or formed by the mesial, pulpal, and labial walls of a tooth cavity preparation.

me·sio·pul·po·lin·gual (me″ze-o-pul″po-ling′gwəl) pertaining to or formed by the mesial, pulpal, and lingual walls of a tooth cavity preparation.

me·sio·ver·sion (me″ze-o-vur′zhən) deviation of a tooth from the vertical, in the direction of the tooth next mesial (anterior) to it in the dental arch.

me·sit·y·lene (mə-sit′ə-lēn) a triply methylated derivative of benzene occurring in petroleum and coal tar or synthesized from acetone; used as a solvent.

mes·na (mez′nə) a sulfhydryl compound given orally or intravenously together with a urotoxic antineoplastic agent such as ifosfamide because it inactivates some of the urotoxic metabolites and thus helps prevent hemorrhagic cystitis.

mes(o)- [Gr. *mesos* middle] a prefix meaning in the middle, intermediate, or moderate.

meso- [Gr. *mesos* middle] a prefix signifying 1. inactive or without effect on polarized light even though the molecule has asymmetric carbon atoms, because the two halves are mirror images. 2. an intermediate hydrated form of an inorganic acid. 3. a middle position, as in certain cyclic organic compounds.

meso·ac·cum·bens (mez″o-, me″zo-ă-kum′bens) projecting from the ventral tegmental area of the mesencephalon to the nucleus accumbens; said of nerve fibers. See under *pathway.*

meso·aor·ti·tis (mez″o-, me″zo-a″or-ti′tis) inflammation of the tunica media of the aorta.

m. syphili′tica inflammation of the middle coat of the aorta due to syphilis.

meso·ap·pen·dix (mez″o-, me″zo-ə-pen′dix) [*meso-* + *appendix*] [TA] the peritoneal fold attaching the appendix to the mesentery of the ileum.

meso·bi·lin (mez″o-, me″zo-bi′lin) a compound found in the urine as a derivative of bilirubin via enterohepatic circulation.

meso·bil·i·ru·bin (mez″o-, me″zo-bil″ĭ-roo′bin) a compound formed by the reduction of bilirubin.

meso·bil·i·ru·bin·o·gen (mez″o-, me″zo-bil″ĭ-roo-bin′o-jən) a reduced form of bilirubin, formed in the intestine; on oxidation it forms stercobilin.

meso·bil·i·ver·din (mez″o-, me″zo-bil″ĭ-vur′din) an oxidation product of mesobilirubinogen.

meso·blast (mez′o-, me′zo-blast″) [*meso-* + *-blast*] mesoderm, especially in the early undifferentiated stages. **mesoblas′tic** *adj*

meso·blas·te·ma (mez″o-, me″zo-blas-te′mə) the cells composing the mesoblast.

meso·car·dia (mez″o-, me″zo-kahr′de-ə) [*meso-* + *cardia*] atypical location of the heart with the apex in the middle line of the thorax.

meso·car·di·um (mez″o-, me″zo-kahr′de-əm) [*meso-* + Gr. *kardia* heart] the part of the embryonic mesentery that connects the heart with the body wall ventrally and the foregut dorsally.

arterial m. the part of the lamina visceralis pericardii serosi (visceral pericardium) that encloses the aorta and pulmonary artery.

dorsal m. the temporary dorsal mesentery of the heart in the embryo; its site in adults is represented by the transverse sinus of the pericardium.

venous m. the part of the lamina visceralis pericardii serosi (visceral pericardium) that encloses the venae cavae and pulmonary veins.

ventral m. a mesentery attaching the heart to the ventral body wall; it is scarcely represented in human development.

meso·car·pal (mez″o-, me″zo-kahr′pəl) midcarpal.

meso·ca·val (mez″o-, me″zo-ka′vəl) pertaining to or connecting the superior mesenteric vein and inferior vena cava.

meso·ce·cum (mez″o-, me″zo-se′kəm) [*meso-* + *cecum*] the occasionally occurring mesentery of the cecum. **mesoce′cal** *adj*

meso·ce·phal·ic (mez″o-, me″zo-sĕ-fal′ik) [*meso-* + *cephalic*] characterized by or pertaining to a skull having an average breadth-length index, with a cephalic index of 75.0 to 79.9.

Meso·ces·toi·des (mez″o-ses-toi′dēz) a genus of tapeworms of the family Mesocestoididae, whose larvae are often found in the coelom or peritoneum of many different vertebrates; the adult form is found most often in the intestines of carnivorous mammals and birds.

Meso·ces·toi·di·dae (mez″o-ses-toi′dĭ-de) a family of medium-sized to large tapeworms of the order Cyclophyllidea, subclass Cestoda, which parasitize carnivorous birds and mammals. *Mesocestoides* is the type genus.

meso·chon·dri·um (mez″o-, me″zo-kon′dre-əm) [*meso-* + Gr. *chondros* cartilage] the matrix in which are embedded the cellular elements of hyaline cartilage.

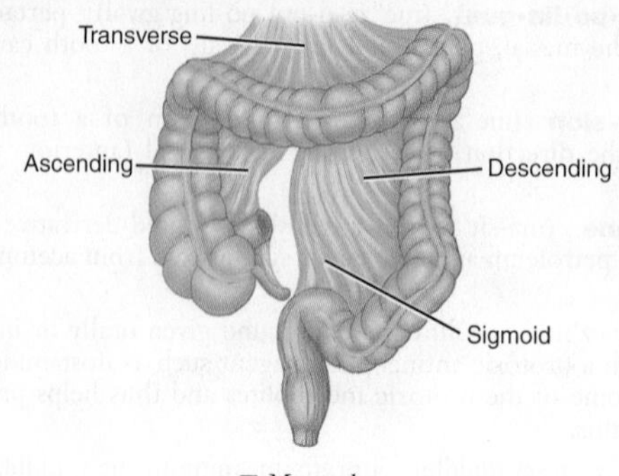

■ Mesocolon.

meso•cho•roi•dea (mez″o-, me″zo-ko-roi′de-ə) the middle coat of the choroid.

meso•co•lon (mez′o-, me′zo-ko″lən) [*meso-* + *colon*] [TA] the process of the peritoneum by which the colon is attached to the posterior abdominal wall. It is divided into ascending, transverse, descending, and sigmoid or pelvic portions, according to the segment of the colon to which it gives attachment. **mesocol′ic** *adj*

m. ascen′dens [TA], **ascending m.** the peritoneum attaching the ascending colon to the posterior abdominal wall, usually obliterated when the ascending colon becomes retroperitoneal.

m. descen′dens [TA], **descending m.** the peritoneum attaching the descending colon to the posterior abdominal wall; it is usually absent because the descending colon is ordinarily retroperitoneal.

iliac m. m. sigmoideum.

left m. m. descendens.

pelvic m. m. sigmoideum.

right m. m. ascendens.

sigmoid m., m. sigmoi′deum [TA] the peritoneum attaching the sigmoid colon to the posterior abdominal wall; called also *iliac* or *pelvic m.*

transverse m., m. transver′sum [TA] the peritoneum attaching the transverse colon to the posterior abdominal wall.

meso•co•lo•pexy (mez″o-, me″zo-ko′lo-pek″se) [*mesocolon* + *-pexy*] suspension or fixation of the mesocolon.

meso•cord (mez′o-, me′zo-kord) an umbilical cord adherent to the placenta by a connecting fold of the amnion; more correctly, the connecting fold itself.

meso•cor•nea (mez″o-, me″zo-kor′ne-ə) substantia propria corneae.

meso•cor•tex (mez″o-, me″zo-kor′teks) [*meso-* + *cortex*] [TA] the cortex of the cingulate gyrus, which is intermediate in form between the allocortex and the isocortex and has four or five distinct layers; called also *juxtallocortex*. **mesocor′tical** *adj*

meso•cor•ti•cal (mez″o-, me″zo-kor′tĭ-kəl) 1. pertaining to the mesocortex. 2. projecting from the ventral tegmental area of the midbrain to the frontal cortex; said of nerve fibers. See under *system*.

meso•cra•nic (mez″o-, me″zo-kra′nik) having a cranial index between 75.0 and 79.9.

Meso•cri•ce•tus (mes″o-kri-se′təs) a genus of rodents of the family Muridae, one of several genera of hamsters. *M. aura′tus* is the Syrian or golden hamster.

meso•cu•nei•form (mez″o-, me″zo-ku′ne-ĭ-form) os cuneiforme intermedium.

meso•cyst (mez′o-, me′zo-sist) [*meso-* + *cyst*] the layer of peritoneum attaching the gallbladder to the liver.

meso•derm (mez′o-, me′zo-dərm″) [*meso-* + *-derm*] the middle layer of the three primary germ layers of the embryo, lying between the ectoderm and the endoderm. From it are derived the connective tissue, bone and cartilage, muscle, blood and blood vessels, lymphatics and lymphoid organs, notochord, pleura, pericardium, peritoneum, kidney, and gonads. Cf. *ectoderm* and *endoderm*. **mesoder′mal, mesoder′mic** *adj*

cardiogenic m. splanchnic mesoderm in the cardiogenic region where the embryonic heart develops; it gives rise to the paired endocardial tubes.

extraembryonic m. mesoderm that is located outside the embryo and belonging to fetal accessory organs, covering for example the amnion and yolk sac.

gastral m. mesoderm that is infolded with the endoderm during gastrulation.

head m. loose mesoderm, cranial to the somites.

lateral m. the lateral sheets of mesoderm within which the embryonic coelom arises.

paraxial m. mesoderm lying alongside the notochord and neural tube.

peristomal m. mesoderm derived from the ventral lip of the blastopore or from the primitive streak.

somatic m. the outer of the two layers into which the embryonic mesoderm divides; associated with ectoderm to constitute the somatopleure.

splanchnic m. the inner of the two layers into which the embryonic mesoderm divides; associated with endoderm to constitute splanchnopleure.

mes•odont (mez′o-, me′zo-dont) [*meso-* + Gr. *odous* tooth] having a dental index between 42 and 44.

mes•odon•tic (mez″o-, me″zo-don′tik) having medium sized teeth.

mes•odon•tism (mez″o-, me″zo-don′tiz-əm) the state of having medium sized teeth, or a dental index between 42 and 44.

meso•du•o•de•nal (mez″o-, me″zo-doo″o-de′nəl) pertaining to the mesoduodenum.

meso•du•o•de•num (mez″o-, me″zo-doo″o-de′nəm) [*meso-* + *duodenum*] 1. the mesenteric fold that encloses the duodenum in early fetal life. 2. the mesentery of the duodenum.

meso•epi•did•y•mis (mez″o-, me″zo-ep″ĭ-did′ĭ-mis) a fold of the tunica vaginalis testis that sometimes connects the epididymis with the testicle.

meso•esoph•a•gus (mez″o-, me″zo-ə-sof′ə-gəs) the portion of the primordial mesentery that encloses the developing esophagus.

meso•gas•ter (mez″o-, me″zo-gas′tər) [*meso-* + *gaster*] mesogastrium.

meso•gas•tri•um (mez″o-, me″zo-gas′tre-əm) [*meso-* + Gr. *gastēr* belly] the portion of the primordial mesentery that encloses the stomach, and from which the greater omentum is developed. **mesogas′tric** *adj*

Meso•gas•trop•o•da (mez″o-gas″trop″ə-də) an order of marine and fresh water snails of the subclass Streptoneura; it includes a number of intermediate hosts of parasitic trematodes, such as the families Hydrobiidae, Pilidae, and Pleuroceridae.

meso•glea (mez″o-, me″zo-gle′ə) [*meso-* + Gr. *gloia* glue] the layer between the epidermis and gastrodermis of cnidarians.

mes•og•nath•ic (mez″og-, me″zog-nath′ik) mesognathous.

me•sog•na•thous (mə-zog′nə-thəs) [*meso-* + *gnath-* + *-ous*] pertaining to or characterized by moderate protrusion of the jaw, with a gnathic index of 98 to 103. Called also *mesognathic*.

meso•ile•um (mez″o-, me″zo-il′e-əm) the mesentery of the ileum.

***meso*-ino•si•tol** (mes″o-in-o′sĭ-tol) *myo*-inositol.

meso•je•ju•num (mez″o-, me″zo-jə-joo′nəm) the mesentery of the jejunum.

meso•lec•i•thal (mez″o-, me″zo-les′ĭ-thəl) [*meso-* + *-lecithal*] having a medium amount of yolk, such as the eggs of amphibians.

meso•lim•bic (mez″o-, me″zo-lim′bik) projecting from the ventral tegmental area of the midbrain to the structures of the limbic system; said of nerve fibers. See under *system*.

meso•mel•ic (mez″o-, me″zo-mel′ik) [*meso-* + *mel-* + *-ic*] pertaining to the midportion of the upper or lower limb.

meso•mere (mez′o-, me′zo-mēr) [*meso-* + *-mere*] 1. a blastomere of size intermediate between a macromere and a micromere. 2. a midzone of the mesoderm between the epimere and hypomere.

meso•mer•ic (mez″o-, me″zo-mer′ik) exhibiting mesomerism.

me•som•er•ism (mə-som′ər-iz″əm) the existence of organic chemical structures that can not be accurately represented by a single structural formula, the actual formula lying intermediate between several possible representations that differ only in the position of electrons.

meso•me•tri•um (mez″o-, me″zo-me′tre-əm) [*meso-* + Gr. *mētra* uterus] 1. [TA] the portion of the broad ligament below the mesovarium, composed of the layers of peritoneum that separate to enclose the uterus. 2. tunica muscularis uteri.

meso•morph (mez′o-, me′zo-morf″) [*meso*derm + Gr. *morphē* form] an individual having a type of body build in which tissues derived from the mesoderm predominate: there is a relative preponderance of muscle, bone, and connective tissue, usually with heavy, hard physique of rectangular outline, a somatotype classified between ectomorph and endomorph. **mesomor′phic** *adj*

meso•mor•phy (mez′o-, me′zo-mor″fe) the condition of being a mesomorph.

mes•on (mez′on, me′zon) [Gr. *mesos* middle] a short-lived subatomic particle of a mass usually less than that of a proton but more than that of an electron; it may carry either a positive, a negative, or a neutral electric charge.

meso•na•sal (mez″o-, me″zo-na′zəl) situated in the middle of the nose.

meso•neph•roi (mez″o-, me″zo-nef′roi) plural of *mesonephros*.

mes•o•ne•phro•ma (mez″o-, me″zo-nə-fro′mə) clear cell adenocarcinoma.

meso•neph•ron (mez″o-, me″zo-nef′ron) mesonephros.

meso•neph•ros (mez″o-, me″zo-nef′ros) pl. *mesoneph′roi* [*meso-* + Gr. *nephros* kidney] the excretory organ of the embryo, arising caudad to the pronephros or pronephric rudiments and using its duct; it consists of a long tube in the lower part of the body cavity, running parallel with the vertebral axis and joined at right angles by a row of twisting tubes. See also *metanephros*. Called also *mesonephron*, *middle kidney*, and *wolffian body*. **mesoneph′ric** *adj*

meso•omen•tum (mez″o-, me″zo-o-men′təm) the fold by which the omentum is attached to the abdominal wall.

meso•phile (mez′o-, me′zo-fīl″) an organism which grows best at temperatures between 20° and 45° C.

meso•phil•ic (mez″o-, me″zo-fil′ik) [*meso-* + *-philic*] fond of moderate temperature; said of bacteria which develop best at temperatures between 20° and 45° C. Cf. *psychrophilic* and *thermophilic*.

meso•phle•bi•tis (mez″o-, me″zo-flə-bi′tis) inflammation of the tunica media of a vein.

meso•phrag•ma (mez″o-, me″zo-frag′mə) [*meso-* + Gr. *phragmos* a fencing in] a name given to the M band. Cf. *inophragma*, and *Z band*, under *band*.

me•soph•ry•on (mə-sof′re-on) [*meso-* + *ophryon*] the glabella or its central point.

meso•phyll (mez′o-, me′zo-fil) [*meso-* + Gr. *phyllon* leaf] the tissue of the inner part of a leaf.

me•so•pia (mə-so′pe-ə) the condition of having mesopic vision.

me•sop•ic (mə-sop′ik) [*meso-* + Gr. *ōpsis* sight] pertaining to vision at intermediate levels of illumination, e.g., at twilight.

meso•pneu•mon (mez″o-, me″zo-noo′mon) [*meso-* + Gr. *pneumon* lung] the union of the two layers of the pleura at the hilum of the lung.

meso•por•phy•rin (mez″o-, me″zo-por′fĭ-rin) a porphyrin (q.v.) in which two pyrrole rings each have one methyl and one propionate side chain and the other two pyrrole rings each have one methyl and one ethyl side chain.

meso•pro•sop•ic (mez″o-, me″zo-pro-sop′ik) [*meso-* + *prosop-* + *-ic*] having a face of moderate width.

meso•pul•mo•num (mez″o-, me″zo-pəl-mo′nəm) the portion of the embryonic mesentery that encloses the laterally expanding lung.

meso•ra•chis•chi•sis (mez″o-, me″zo-rə-kis′kĭ-sis) merorachischisis.

mes•or•chi•um (məz-or′ke-əm) [*meso-* + Gr. *orchis* testis] the portion of the primordial mesentery that encloses the fetal testis, represented in the adult by a fold between the testis and epididymis. **mesor′chial** *adj*

meso•rec•tum (mez″o-, me″zo-rek′təm) [*meso-* + *rectum*] the fold of peritoneum connecting the upper portion of the rectum with the sacrum. **mesorec′tal** *adj*

meso•rid•a•zine (mez″o-rid′ə-zēn) a phenothiazine antipsychotic that is a metabolite of thioridazine, having properties similar to those of chlorpromazine.

m. besylate [USP] the besylate salt of mesoridazine; an antipsychotic agent which has been used in the treatment of alcoholism, schizophrenia, psychoneurotic manifestations, and certain behavioral problems, administered orally and intramuscularly.

meso•rop•ter (mez″o-, me″zo-rop′tər) [*meso-* + *horopter*] the normal position of the eyes with their muscles at rest.

mes•or•rhine (mez′o-, me′zo-rīn) [*meso-* + Gr. *rhis* nose] having a nasal index between 48 and 53.

meso•sal•pinx (mez″o-, me″zo-sal′pinks) [*meso-* + *salpinx*] [TA] the part of the broad ligament of the uterus above the mesovarium, composed of layers that enclose the uterine tube.

meso•scap•u•la (mez″o-, me″zo-skap′u-lə) spina scapulae.

meso•seme (mez′o-, me′zo-sēm) [*meso-* + Gr. *sēma* sign] having an orbital index between 83 and 89.

meso•sig•moid (mez″o-, me″zo-sig′moid) the peritoneal fold by which the sigmoid flexure is attached to the posterior abdominal wall.

meso•sig•moi•di•tis (mez″o-, me″zo-sig″moi-di′tis) inflammation of the mesosigmoid.

meso•sig•moido•pexy (mez″o-, me″zo-sig-moi′do-pek″se) [*mesosigmoid* + *-pexy*] suspension or fixation of the mesosigmoid in the treatment of rectal prolapse.

meso•some (mez′o-, me′zo-sōm″) [*meso-* + *-some*] an invagination of the cell membrane occurring in certain bacteria. Various mesosomes are associated with DNA replication, with cell secretion, and with electron transport of the organism.

meso•staph•y•line (mez″o-, me″zo-staf′ə-lēn) [*meso-* + *staphyline* (def. 2)] pertaining to or characterized by a palate with a moderate width, with a palatal index of 80.0 to 84.9.

meso•ster•num (mez″o-, me″zo-stur′nəm) corpus sterni.

meso•stri•a•tal (mez″o-, me″zo-stri-a′təl) nigrostriatal.

meso•stro•ma (mez″o-, me″zo-stro′mə) the embryonic fibrillar tissue analogous to the vitreous, which develops into Bowman and Descemet membranes.

meso•tar•sal (mez″o-, me″zo-tahr′səl) midtarsal.

meso•tau•ro•don•tism (mez″o-, me″zo-taw″ro-don′tiz-əm) [*meso-* + *taurodontism*] taurodontism in which the tooth roots branch only in the middle.

meso•ten•din•e•um (mez″o-, me″zo-tən-din′e-əm) [L.] [TA] the delicate connective tissue sheath attaching a tendon to its fibrous sheath.

meso•ten•don (mez″o-, me″zo-ten′don) mesotendineum.

meso•ten•on (mez″o-, me″zo-ten′on) mesotendineum.

meso•the•li•o•ma (mez″o-, me″zo-the″le-o′mə) a tumor derived from mesothelial tissue (peritoneum, pleura, pericardium); both benign and malignant varieties exist. Malignant varieties are often the result of excessive exposure to asbestos.

benign fibrous m. a localized tumor of the pleura, firm and encapsulated and sometimes vascular; size ranges from small to enormous. It has not been linked to asbestos exposure. Called also *localized fibrous m.*

diffuse m. malignant m.

localized fibrous m. solitary fibrous tumor.

malignant m. a malignant tumor of the pleura, peritoneum, or pericardium, appearing as broad sheets of cells; some regions contain spindle-shaped, sarcoma-like cells and others show adenomatous patterns. Many of these tumors, particularly in the pleura and peritoneum, have been linked to excessive exposure to asbestos. Called also *diffuse m.*

peritoneal m. a malignant mesothelioma in the peritoneum, a form linked to heavy asbestos exposure and sometimes accompanying the pleural variety; it may spread to involve the intestines and cause obstruction. Symptoms include ascites, pain, and a mass in the abdomen.

pleural m. a malignant mesothelioma of the pleural space, often spreading widely and invading other thoracic structures; patients are often older men who present with dyspnea, chest pain, and extensive pleural effusions. It is usually fatal within one year.

m. of testis, m. of tunica vaginalis a malignant mesothelioma of the tunica vaginalis testis, usually first manifesting as a hydrocele; sometimes it is metastatic from the lungs, but not all cases have been linked to asbestos exposure. It often follows a more indolent course than the pleural or peritoneal varieties.

meso•the•li•um (mez″o-, me″zo-the′le-əm) [*meso-* + *epithelium*] the layer of flat cells, derived from the mesoderm, that line the coelom or body cavity of the embryo. In the adult, it forms the simple squamous epithelium that covers all true serous membranes (peritoneum, pericardium, pleura). **mesothe′lial** *adj*

meso•the•nar (mez″o-, me″zo-the′nər) [*meso-* + *thenar*] musculus adductor pollicis.

mes•o•tro•pic (mez″o-, me″zo-tro′pik) situated in the middle of a cavity, as the abdomen.

meso•tym•pa•num (mez″o-, me″zo-tim′pə-nəm) the portion of the middle ear medial to the tympanic membrane.

meso•va•ri•um (mez″o-, me″zo-var′e-əm) [L.] [TA] the portion of the broad ligament of the uterus between the mesometrium and mesosalpinx; it is drawn out to enclose and hold the ovary in place. **mesova′rian** *adj*

me•squite (mə-skēt′) [Nahuatl *mizquitl*] any plant of the genus *Prosopis*. Called also *algaroba* or *algarroba*.

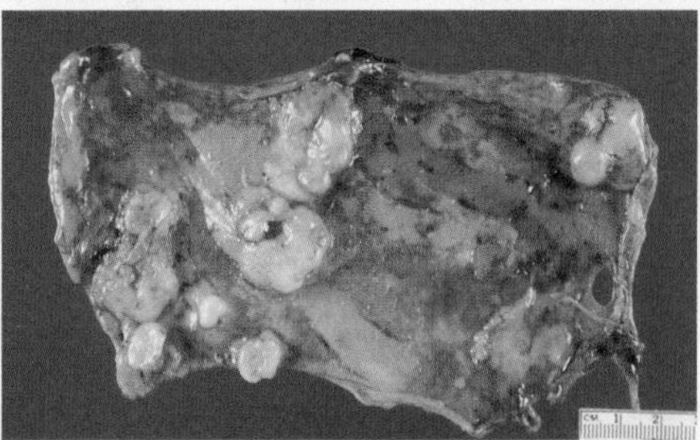

■ Malignant mesothelioma present as multiple nodules on the parietal pleura.

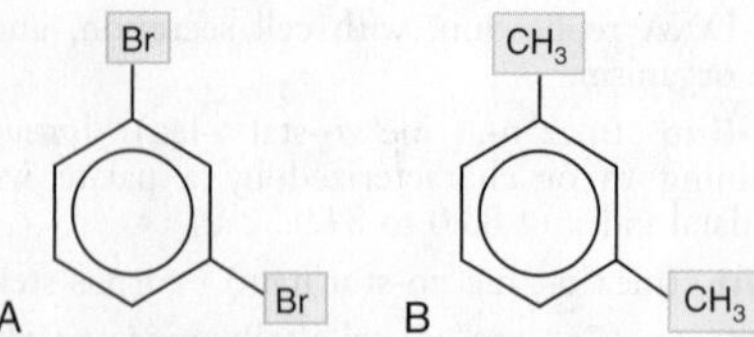

■ Two examples of disubstituted benzene derivatives with substituents in the *meta*-position. *(A)*, 1,3-dibromobenzene; *(B)*, *meta*-xylene (1,3-dimethylbenzene).

mes•sen•ger (mes′ən-jər) an information carrier such as a hormone or an electrical impulse.

first m. a factor or hormone that binds to a receptor on the external surface of a cell and sets off a series of reactions that eventually convert a precursor into a second messenger.

second m. any of several classes of intracellular signals that act at or are situated within the plasma membrane and translate electrical or chemical messages from the environment (first messengers) into cellular responses; such messengers include changes in membrane potential, calcium ions, cyclic nucleotides, and products of phosphatidylinositol turnover.

mes•ter•o•lone (məs-ter′ə-lōn) an androgen with actions and uses similar to those of testosterone.

Mes•ti•non (mes′tĭ-non) trademark for preparations of pyridostigmine bromide.

mes•tra•nol (mes′trə-nol) [USP] the 3-methyl ether of ethinyl estradiol, used in combination with a progestational agent as an oral contraceptive.

mes•uran•ic (mez″u-ran′ik) [*meso-* + *uran-* + *-ic*] having a maxilloalveolar index between 110.0 and 114.9.

mes•y•late (mes′ə-lāt) USAN contraction for *methanesulfonate.*

Met methionine.

met(a)- [Gr. *meta* after, beyond, over] a prefix indicating *(a)* change, transformation, or exchange or *(b)* after or next.

meta- 1. symbol *m-;* in organic chemistry, a prefix indicating a 1,3-substituted benzene ring, e.g., *m*-xylene (1,3-dimethylbenzene) or *m*-nitrophenol (3-nitrophenol). 2. in inorganic chemistry, a prefix indicating a polymeric acid anhydride, e.g., metaphosphoric acid.

meta-anal•y•sis (met″ə-ə-nal′ə-sis) [*meta-* + *analysis*] any systematic method that uses statistical analysis to integrate the data from a number of independent studies.

me•tab•a•sis (mə-tab′ə-sis) [*meta-* + Gr. *bainein* to go] 1. a change in the manifestations or course of a disease. 2. metastasis, or change in the site of a morbid process from one region of the body to another.

meta•bi•o•sis (met″ə-bi-o′sis) [*meta-* + *biosis*] the dependence of one organism upon another for its existence; commensalism.

met•a•bol•ic (met″ə-bol′ik) pertaining to or of the nature of metabolism.

met•a•bo•lim•e•ter (met″ə-bo-lim′ə-tər) [*metabolism* + *-meter*] an apparatus for measuring basal metabolism.

met•a•bo•lim•e•try (met″ə-bə-lim′ə-tre) the measurement of basal metabolism.

me•tab•o•lism (mə-tab′ə-liz″əm) [Gr. *metaballein* to turn about, change, alter] 1. the sum of all the physical and chemical processes by which living organized substance is produced and maintained (anabolism), and also the transformation by which energy is made available for the uses of the organism (catabolism). 2. biotransformation.

basal m. the minimal energy expended for the maintenance of respiration, circulation, peristalsis, muscle tonus, body temperature, glandular activity, and the other vegetative functions of the body. The rate of basal metabolism (basal metabolic rate) is measured by means of a calorimeter, in a subject at absolute rest, 14 to 18 hours after eating, and is expressed in calories per hour per square meter of body surface.

drug m. biotransformation of drugs.

endogenous m. metabolism of the proteins of the body tissues.

energy m. the metabolic processes by which energy is released.

excess m. of exercise the amount by which the oxygen consumed or the carbon dioxide eliminated during exercise and recovery exceeds the corresponding amounts during sleep.

exogenous m. metabolism of ingested foodstuffs.

inborn error of m. see under *error.*

intermediary m. the various chemical reactions involved in the transformation of food molecules into essential cellular building blocks.

me•tab•o•lite (mə-tab′ə-līt) any substance produced by metabolism or by a metabolic process.

essential m. a necessary constituent of normal metabolic processes.

me•tab•o•liz•a•ble (mə-tab′o-līz″ə-bəl) capable of being transformed by metabolism.

me•tab•o•lome (mə-tab′ə-lōm) [*metabolite* + *-ome*] the entire pool of low-molecular-weight molecules present in cells, or other biological samples, in a particular physiological or developmental state.

me•tab•o•lo•mics (mə-tab″ə-lo′miks) the qualitative and quantitative study of the endogenous metabolites in a particular cell or other biological sample.

me•tab•o•re•cep•tor (mə-tab″o-re-sep′tər) a type of receptor found in skeletal muscle that responds to an increase in metabolic products and stimulates an increase in circulation in response to exercise.

meta•bu•teth•amine hy•dro•chlo•ride (met″ə-bu-teth′ə-mēn) a local anesthetic used in dentistry to produce infiltration and nerve block anesthesia.

meta•car•pal (met″ə-kahr′pəl) 1. pertaining to the metacarpus. 2. a bone of the metacarpus; one of the ossa metacarpi.

meta•car•pec•to•my (met″ə-kahr-pek′tə-me) excision or resection of a metacarpal bone.

meta•car•pe•us (met″ə-kahr′pe-əs) [*meta-* + *carpus*] metacarpal.

meta•car•po•pha•lan•ge•al (met″ə-kahr″po-fə-lan′je-əl) pertaining to the metacarpus and phalanges.

meta•car•pus (met″ə-kahr′pəs) [*meta-* + *carpus*] [TA] the part of the hand between the wrist and the fingers, its skeleton being five cylindric bones (metacarpals) extending from the carpus to the phalanges. See also *ossa metacarpi,* under *os*[2].

met•a•cele (met′ə-sēl) metacoeloma.

meta•cen•tric (met″ə-sen′trik) [*meta-* + *center* (def. 1)] having the centromere near the middle, so that the arms of the chromosome are approximately equal in length. Cf. *acrocentric* and *submetacentric.*

meta•cer•ca•ria (met″ə-sər-kar′e-ə) pl. *metacerca′riae.* The encysted resting or maturing stage of a trematode parasite in the tissues of an intermediate host (mollusks, aquatic arthropods, fishes, or amphibia) or on vegetation; in some cases these are the infective or transfer stage of parasites.

meta•chro•ma•sia (met″ə-kro-ma′zhə) [*meta-* + Gr. *chrōma* color] 1. a condition in which tissues do not stain true with a given stain. 2. staining in which the same stain colors different tissues in different tints. 3. the change of color produced by staining.

meta•chro•mat•ic (met″ə-kro-mat′ik) [*meta-* + *chromatic*] staining differently with the same dye; said of tissues in which different elements take on different colors when a certain dye is applied. By extension, said of dyes by which different tissues are stained differently.

meta•chro•ma•tin (met″ə-kro′mə-tin) the basophil element in chromatin.

meta•chro•ma•tism (met″ə-kro′mə-tiz″əm) metachromasia.

meta•chro•mato•phil (met″ə-kro-mat′o-fil) a cell that does not stain in the usual manner with a given stain.

meta•chro•mia (met″ə-kro′me-ə) metachromasia.

meta•chro•mic (met″ə-kro′mik) metachromatic.

meta•chro•mo•phil (met″ə-kro′mo-fil) [*meta-* + *chromo-* + *-phil*] staining in an abnormal manner with a given stain.

meta•chro•mo•phile (met″ə-kro′mo-fīl) metachromophil.

me•tach•ro•nous (mə-tak′rə-nəs) [*meta-* + *chrono-* + *-ous*] 1. of ciliary beating, occurring in waves; cf *isochronous.* 2. term used in oncology to refer to neoplasms that develop later in patients who have had a previous tumor. Cf. *asynchronous.*

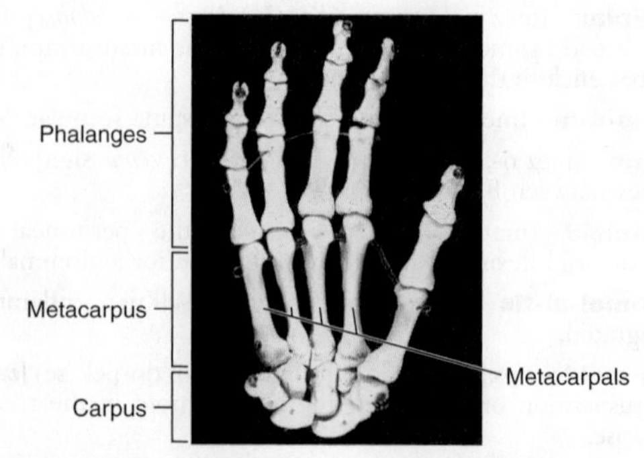

■ Metacarpus, comprising the metacarpal bones, which extend between the carpus and phalanges and are numbered lateromedially.

meta·chro·sis (met″ə-kro′sis) [*meta-* + Gr. *chrōsis* coloring] change of color in animals.

meta·coele (met′ə-sēl) metacoeloma.

meta·coe·lo·ma (met″ə-se-lo′mə) the part of the embryonic coelom that develops into the pleuroperitoneal cavity; called also *metacele* and *metacoele.*

meta·cone (met′ə-kōn) [*meta-* + *cone*] the distobuccal cusp of an upper molar tooth.

meta·con·id (met″ə-kon′id) [*meta-* + *con(o)-* + *-id*] the mesiolingual cusp of a lower molar tooth.

meta·con·ule (met″ə-kon′ūl) the small intermediate cusp between the metacone and the protocone of the upper molar teeth of various mammals.

meta·cor·tan·dra·lone (met″ə-kor-tan′drə-lōn) prednisolone.

meta·cre·sol (met″ə-kre′sol) [USP] *m*-cresol; one of the three isomeric forms of cresol, and the most strongly antiseptic of the group; used as a disinfectant.

m. purple, m. sulfonphthalein a triphenylmethane compound which is a brilliant indicator, being red at pH 1.2, blue at pH 2.8, yellow at pH 7.4, and purple at pH 9.0.

Meta·date (met′ə-dāt) trademark for preparations of methylphenidate hydrochloride.

meta·fe·male (met″ə-fe′māl) [*meta-* + *female*] a sex chromosome abnormality, XXX karyotype, among females.

meta·gas·ter (met″ə-gas′tər) [*meta-* + *gaster*] the permanent intestinal canal of the embryo.

meta·gas·tru·la (met″ə-gas′troo-lə) [*meta-* + *gastrula*] a gastrula with a cleavage differing from that of the standard type.

meta·gel·a·tin (met″ə-jel′ə-tin) a substance produced by treating gelatin with oxalic acid.

meta·gen·e·sis (met″ə-jen′ə-sis) [*meta-* + *-genesis*] alternation of generations used specifically to denote the regular alternation of sexual and asexual modes of reproduction in the life cycle, as in certain fungi.

met·a·ger·ia (met″ə-je′re-ə) acrogeria.

meta·go·ni·mi·a·sis (met″ə-go″nĭ-mi′ə-sis) infection of the intestine of a human or other animal by flukes of the genus *Metagonimus.*

Meta·gon·i·mus (met″ə-gon′ĭ-məs) [*meta-* + Gr. *gonimos* productive] a genus of flukes of the family Heterophyidae. *M. yokoga′wai (M. ova′tus)* is found in the small intestines of mammals in East Asia, Indonesia, Israel, and the Balkans.

meta·he·mo·glo·bin (met″ə-he′mo-glo″bin) methemoglobin.

Meta·hy·drin (met″ə-hi′drin) trademark for a preparation of trichlormethiazide.

meta·ic·ter·ic (met″ə-ik-ter′ik) posticteric.

meta·iodo·ben·zyl·guan·i·dine (MIBG) (met″ə-i″o-do-ben″zəl-gwahn′ĭ-dēn) iobenguane.

met·al (met′əl) [L. *metallum;* Gr. *metallon*] any element marked by luster, malleability, ductility, and conductivity of electricity and heat and which will ionize positively in solution.

alkali m. one of a group of monovalent metals including lithium, sodium, potassium, rubidium, and cesium.

alkaline earth m's a group of grayish white, malleable metals that are easily oxidized in air, comprising beryllium, magnesium, calcium, strontium, barium, and radium.

base m. a metal that oxidizes or corrodes relatively easily; cf. *noble m.*

colloidal m. a colloidal solution of a metal; see *electrosol.*

fusible m. an alloy that melts at a relatively low temperature, as at or around the boiling point of water. Bismuth, lead, and tin are usually the principal constituents.

heavy m. a metal with a high specific gravity, usually defined as being above 5.0.

noble m. a metal that is highly resistant to oxidation and corrosion; cf. *base m.*

met·al·de·hyde (met-al′də-hīd) a molluscacide commonly used in gardens, mixed with bran to form flakes or pellets; animals eating it suffer neurotoxicity with tremors, dyspnea, and sometimes convulsions that can be fatal.

me·tal·lic (mə-tal′ik) 1. pertaining to, consisting of, or of the nature of metal. 2. made of metal.

met·al·lized (met′əl-īzd) treated with metals.

met·al·liz·ing (met′əl-īz-ing) making something metallic, as when treating the surface of impression material with metals so that it will conduct electricity before electroplating.

me·tal·lo·car·boxy·pep·ti·dase (mə-tal″o-kahr-bok″se-pep′tĭ-dās) [EC 3.4.17] any of a group of carboxypeptidases containing a tightly bound metal or metal ion that participates in catalysis.

me·tal·lo·cy·a·nide (mə-tal″o-si′ə-nīd) a compound of cyanogen with a metal.

me·tal·lo·en·do·pep·ti·dase (mə-tal″o-en″do-pep′tĭ-dās) [EC 3.4.24] any of a group of endopeptidases containing a tightly bound metal or metal ion that participates in catalysis.

me·tal·lo·en·zyme (mə-tal″o-en′zīm) an enzyme containing a tightly bound metal atom (e.g., cobalt, copper, iron, molybdenum, or zinc) as an integral part of its structure.

me·tal·lo·fla·vo·pro·tein (mə-tal″o-fla″vo-pro′tēn) a flavoprotein that contains a bound metal ion as part of its structure, e.g., xanthine oxidase.

met·al·loid (met′əl-oid) [*metal* + *-oid*] 1. any element with both metallic and nonmetallic properties, as silicon, boron, or arsenic. 2. resembling a metal.

me·tal·lo·phil·ic (mə-tal″o-fil′ik) having an affinity for metal-containing stains; said of cells.

me·tal·lo·por·phy·rin (mə-tal″o-por′fə-rin) a combination of a metal with porphyrin, e.g., heme (iron).

me·tal·lo·pro·tein (mĕ-tal″o-pro′tēn) a protein that has one or more tightly bound metal ions forming part of its structure.

me·tal·lo·pro·tein·ase (mĕ-tal″o-pro′tēn-ās) any of the endopeptidases or carboxypeptidases that have divalent cations as part of their active structure.

matrix m. (MMP) any of a group of endopeptidases that hydrolyze proteins of the extracellular matrix; faulty regulation of MMP activity resulting in excessive matrix degradation contributes to degenerative diseases such as arthritis and to tumor metastasis.

met·al·los·co·py (met″əl-os′kə-pe) [*metal* + *-scopy*] observation of the effects of applying metal to the body.

me·tal·lo·ther·a·py (mə-tal″o-ther′ə-pe) [*metal* + *therapy*] the treatment of disease by applying metals to the skin.

met·al·lur·gy (met′əl-ur″je) [*metal* + Gr. *ergon* work] the science and art of using metals.

meta·mer (met′ə-mər) a compound exhibiting, or capable of exhibiting, metamerism.

meta·mere (met′ə-mēr) [*meta-* + *-mere*] one of a series of homologous segments of the body of an animal. Cf. *antimere.*

meta·mer·ic (met″ə-mer′ik) pertaining to or characterized by metamerism.

me·tam·er·ism (mə-tam′ər-is″əm) 1. isomerism, particularly a type of structural isomerism in which different radicals of the same chemical type are attached to the same polyvalent element and yet give rise to compounds possessing identical molecular formulas, for example, diethylamine, $(C_2H_5)_2NH$, and methyl propylamine, $CH_3NHC_3H_7$. 2. arrangement into metameres by the serial repetition of a structural pattern.

meta·mo·nad (met″ə-mo′nad) [*meta-* + *monad*] a group of protozoa comprising all the zooflagellates except those in the orders Choanoflagellida and Kinetoplastida, most of which are symbionts in the insect gut.

meta·mor·phop·sia (met″ə-mor-fop′se-ə) [*meta-* + *morph-* + *-opsia*] a disturbance of vision in which objects are seen as distorted in shape.

meta·mor·pho·sis (met″ə-mor′fə-sis) [*meta-* + *morphosis*] change of shape or structure, particularly a transition from one developmental stage to another, as from larva to adult form. **metamorph′ic** *adj*

fatty m. fatty change.

retrograde m., retrogressive m. degeneration; usually, a retrograde metabolic change.

tissue m. any change in tissues, either normal or pathologic.

Met·a·mu·cil (met″ə-mu′sil) trademark for a preparation of psyllium hydrophilic mucilloid.

meta·my·elo·cyte (met″ə-mi′ə-lo-sīt″) a precursor in the granulocytic series, being a cell intermediate in development between a promyelocyte and the mature segmented and granular polymorphonuclear leukocyte. The protein synthesis seen in earlier stages decreases or stops; the nucleus becomes indented and its chromatin becomes coarse and clumped; and the cytoplasm becomes pink like that of a mature granulocyte. Called also *juvenile neutrophil, cell,* or *form.*

Me·tan·dren (mə-tan′drən) trademark for preparations of methyltestosterone.

meta·neph·rine (met″ə-nef′rin) a methylated metabolite of epinephrine excreted in the urine and found in certain tissues.

met·a·neph·ro·gen·ic (met″ə-nef″ro-jen′ik) [*metanephros* + *-genic*] capable of giving rise to the metanephros.

meta·neph·roi (met″ə-nef′roi) plural of *metanephros.*

meta·neph·ron (met″ə-nef′ron) metanephros.

meta·neph·ros (met″ə-nef′ros) pl. *metaneph′roi* [*meta-* + Gr. *nephros* kidney] the primordium of the permanent kidney, developing later than and caudal to the mesonephros, from the mesonephric duct and nephrogenic cord. Called also *definite, definitive,* or *hind kidney.* **metaneph′ric** *adj*

meta·neu·tro·phil (met″ə-noo′tro-fil) [*meta-* + *neutrophil*] staining abnormally with neutral stains.

meta·phase (met′ə-fāz″) [*meta-* + *phase*] the stage of cell division following prometaphase, during which the asters move further apart and the chromosomes move along the spindle microtubules to the center of the cell and line up to form the equatorial or metaphase plate. In meiosis I, the kinetochores of homologous chromosome pairs become directed at opposite poles.

Met·a·phen (met′ə-fən) trademark for preparations of nitromersol.

meta·phos·phor·ic ac·id (met″ə-fos-for′ik) a glassy solid polymer of phosphoric acid, soluble in water; used as a reagent for chemical analysis and as a test for albumin in the urine. Called also *glacial phosphoric acid.*

me·taph·y·ses (mə-taf′ə-sēz) plural of *metaphysis.*

meta·phys·i·al (met″ə-fiz′e-əl) metaphyseal.

me·taph·y·sis (mə-taf′ə-sis) pl. *metaph′yses* [*meta-* + *physis*] [TA] the wider part at the extremity of the shaft of a long bone, adjacent to the epiphyseal disk. During development it contains the growth zone and consists of spongy bone; in the adult it is continuous with the epiphysis. **metaphys′eal** *adj*

meta·phys·itis (met″ə-fis-i′tis) inflammation of the metaphysis of a long bone.

meta·pla·sia (met″ə-pla′zhə) [*meta-* + *-plasia*] the change in the type of adult cells in a tissue to another form of adult cells that are not normal for that tissue.

agnogenic myeloid m. the primary or idiopathic form of myeloid metaplasia, which is often accompanied by myelofibrosis; it is considered one of the myeloproliferative disorders. Called also *aleukemic* or *nonleukemic myelosis.*

myeloid m. a syndrome characterized by myeloid tissue in extramedullary sites with nucleated erythrocytes and immature granulocytes in the circulating blood and extramedullary hematopoiesis in the liver and spleen, as well as anemia and splenomegaly. Both a primary form *(agnogenic myeloid m.)* and secondary forms are known.

nephrogenic m. a rare benign neoplasm of the mucosa of the urinary bladder or the urethra, consisting of tubular structures resembling those of the nephron; called also *nephrogenic adenoma.*

primary myeloid m. agnogenic myeloid m.

pseudopyloric m. gastric metaplasia in which the gastric glands disappear and are replaced by tubules that closely resemble normal pyloric glands.

m. of pulp transformation of the usual types of cells normally found in the pulp tissue into entirely different types.

secondary myeloid m. myeloid metaplasia secondary to some other condition, such as carcinoma, tuberculosis, leukemia, leukoerythroblastosis, or polycythemia vera.

squamous m. transformation of other types of epithelium, such as glandular, mucosal, or pseudostratified, into stratified squamous epithelium, seen in certain pathologic conditions or produced experimentally. Called also *epidermalization* and *epidermidalization.*

me·tap·la·sis (mə-tap′lə-sis) the stage in which the organism has attained completed growth.

meta·plasm (met′ə-plaz″əm) [*meta-* + *plasm*] deuteroplasm.

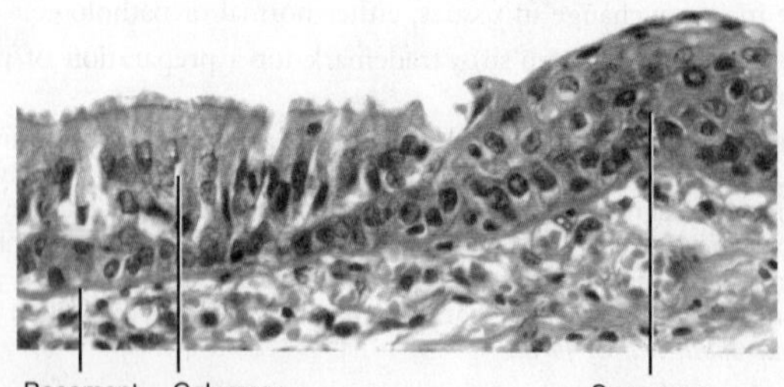

■ Metaplasia of columnar epithelium *(left)* to squamous epithelium *(right)* in a bronchus.

meta·plas·tic (met″ə-plas′tik) 1. pertaining to or characterized by metaplasia. 2. formed by or of the nature of metaplasm (deuteroplasm).

meta·pneu·mon·ic (met″ə-noo-mon′ik) [*meta-* + *pneumonic*] succeeding or following pneumonia.

Meta·pneu·mo·vi·rus (met″ə-noo′mo-vi″rəs) a genus of viruses of the subfamily Pneumovirinae (family Paramyxoviridae) that cause respiratory infections; it includes the avian and human metapneumoviruses.

meta·pneu·mo·vi·rus (met″ə-noo′mo-vi″rəs) any virus belonging to the genus *Metapneumovirus.*

avian m. a species that causes upper respiratory infection in turkeys and chickens.

human m. a species that causes respiratory infection in humans that is clinically similar to, but less severe than, that caused by respiratory syncytial virus.

meta·poph·y·sis (met″ə-pof′ə-sis) [*meta-* + *apophysis*] the mammillary process on the superior articular or prearticular processes of certain vertebrae.

Met·a·prel (met′ə-prəl) trademark for preparations of metaproterenol sulfate.

meta·pro·ter·e·nol sul·fate (met″ə-pro-ter′ə-nol) [USP] a β_2-adrenergic receptor agonist with significant β_1-adrenergic activity, having bronchodilator and cardiac stimulant actions; used as a bronchodilator in the treatment of asthma-associated bronchospasm and the treatment and prophylaxis of reversible bronchospasm associated with chronic obstructive airway disease, administered orally and by inhalation.

meta·psy·chol·o·gy (met″ə-si-kol′ə-je) a term applied to various philosophical theories about mental functions and mental "structures" which are justifiable on logical grounds but not verifiable by experiment or observation; in psychoanalysis such theories concern the topography (id, ego, superego) and economics (quantities of psychic energy or excitation) of mental processes.

meta·py·rone (met″ə-pi′rōn) metyrapone.

meta·ram·i·nol bi·tar·trate (met″ə-ram′ĭ-nol) [USP] a sympathomimetic agent acting mainly as an α-adrenergic agonist but also stimulating the β_1-adrenergic receptors of the heart and having potent vasopressor activity, used especially for the prevention and treatment of acute hypotensive states occurring with spinal anesthesia and for adjunctive therapy of hypotension due to hemorrhage, reactions to medications, surgical complication, and shock associated with brain damage due to trauma or tumor; administered intramuscularly and intravenously.

met·ar·chon (mət-ahr′kon) an agent which, without being toxic, so changes the behavior of a pest that its persistence is diminished, e.g., a confusing sex attractant.

meta·rho·dop·sin (met″ə-ro-dop′sin) a transient intermediate produced upon irradiation of rhodopsin in the visual cycle and existing in two forms, metarhodopsins I and II. The latter dissociates to form opsin and all-*trans* retinal. See illustration at *visual cycle,* under *cycle.*

met·ar·te·ri·ole (met″ahr-tēr′e-ōl) arterial capillary.

meta·ru·bri·cyte (met″ə-roo′brĭ-sīt) orthochromatic erythroblast.

meta·sta·ble (met′ə-sta″bəl) 1. a condition differing from stable in that, although the substance is stable in small perturbations, it can be transformed to a more stable condition by relatively large perturbations. 2. subject to inevitable change or destruction eventually, but apparently stable owing to slowness of change.

me·tas·ta·sec·to·my (mə-tas″tə-sek′tə-me) [*metastasis* + *-ectomy*] excision of one or more metastases.

me·tas·ta·ses (mə-tas′tə-sēz) plural of *metastasis* (def. 2).

me·tas·ta·sis (mə-tas′tə-sis) [*meta-* + Gr. *stasis* stand] 1. the transfer of disease from one organ or part to another not directly connected with it. It may be due either to the transfer of pathogenic microorganisms (e.g., tubercle bacilli) or to transfer of cells, as in malignant tumors. The capacity to metastasize is a characteristic of all malignant tumors. 2. pl. *metastases.* A growth of pathogenic microorganisms or of abnormal cells distant from the site primarily involved by the morbid process. **metastat′ic** *adj*

calcareous m. the formation of bone salts in the kidneys and elsewhere in softening of bone.

contact m. transfer from one surface to another with which the former is in contact.

crossed m. passage of material from the venous to the arterial circulation without going through the lungs.

direct m. metastasis in the direction of the blood or lymph stream.

metachronous m. a metastasis found at a later time than the condition at the primary site; cf. *synchronous m.*

paradoxical m., retrograde m. metastasis taking place in a direction opposite to that of the blood stream.

synchronous m. a metastasis found at the same time as the condition at the primary site; cf. *metachronous m.*

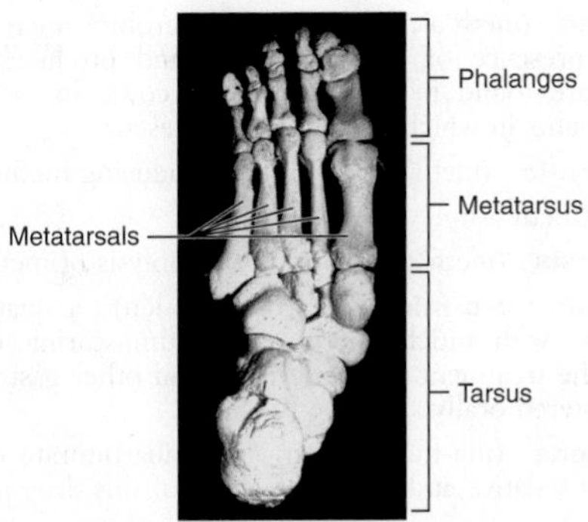

■ Metatarsus, comprising the metatarsal bones, which extend between the tarsus and phalanges and are numbered mediolaterally.

me•tas•ta•size (mə-tas′tə-sīz) to form new foci of disease in a distant part by metastasis.

meta•ster•num (met″ə-stur′nəm) [*meta-* + *sternum*] processus xiphoideus.

me•tas•tin (mə-tas′tin) kisspeptin.

Meta•stron (met′ə-stron) trademark for a preparation of strontium chloride Sr 89.

Meta•stron•gyl•i•dae (met″ə-stron-jil′ĭ-de) a family of nematodes of the superfamily Strongyloidea, consisting of lungworms; it includes the genus *Metastrongylus.*

Meta•stron•gy•lus (met″ə-stron′jə-ləs) a genus of nematodes of the family Metastrongylidae, usually found as lungworms in pigs and sometimes causing verminous bronchitis. *M. elonga′tus* is a species that may also infect humans and ruminants but has little pathogenic effect.

meta•tar•sal (met″ə-tahr′səl) 1. pertaining to the metatarsus. 2. a bone of the metatarsus; one of the ossa metatarsi.

meta•tar•sal•gia (met″ə-tahr-sal′jə) [*meta-* + *tars-* + *-algia*] pain and tenderness in the metatarsal region.

Morton m. see under *neuralgia.*

meta•tar•sec•to•my (met″ə-tahr-sek′tə-me) excision or resection of the metatarsus.

meta•tar•se•us (met″ə-tahr′se-əs) metatarsal.

meta•tar•so•pha•lan•ge•al (met″ə-tahr″so-fə-lan′je-əl) pertaining to the metatarsus and the phalanges of the toes.

meta•tar•sus (met″ə-tahr′səs) [*meta-* + *tarsus*] [TA] the part of the foot between the tarsus and the toes, its skeleton being the five long bones (the metatarsals) extending from the tarsus to the phalanges. See also *ossa metatarsi,* under *os*[2].

m. adductoca′vus a deformity of the foot in which metatarsus adductus is associated with pes cavus.

m. adductova′rus a deformity of the foot in which metatarsus adductus is associated with metatarsus varus.

m. adduc′tus a congenital deformity of the foot in which the fore part of the foot deviates toward the midline.

m. ata′vicus abnormal shortness of the first metatarsal bone.

m. bre′vis a condition in which the first metatarsal bone is shorter than normal and often abducted.

m. la′tus a broadened foot due to spreading of the anterior part of the foot resulting from separation of the heads of the metatarsal bones from each other; called also *broad foot* and *spread foot.*

m. pri′mus va′rus angulation of the first metatarsal bone toward the midline of the body, producing an angle sometimes of 20 degrees or more between its base and that of the second metatarsal bone.

m. va′rus a congenital deformity of the foot in which its inner border is off the ground with the sole turned inward, the patient walking on the outer border of the foot.

meta•thal•a•mus (met″ə-thal′ə-məs) [*meta-* + *thalamus*] [TA] the part of the diencephalon inferior to the caudal end of the dorsal thalamus, comprising the lateral and medial geniculate bodies.

Meta•the•ria (met″ə-the′re-ə) [*meta-* + Gr. *thērion* beast, animal] in some systems of classification a subclass of the Mammalia, and in others an infraclass of the subclass Theria, including the pouched mammals or marsupials.

meta•the•ri•an (met″ə-the′re-ən) any member of the Metatheria.

me•tath•e•sis (mə-tath′ə-sis) [*meta-* + Gr. *thesis* placement] 1. the artificial transfer of a morbid process. 2. a chemical reaction in which an element or radical in one compound exchanges places with another element or radical in another compound.

meta•thet•ic (met″ə-thet′ik) pertaining to or of the nature of metathesis.

meta•throm•bin (met″ə-throm′bin) [*meta-* + *thrombin*] the inactive combination of thrombin and antithrombin.

meta•troph (met′ə-trōf) a metatrophic organism.

meta•tro•phia (met″ə-tro′fe-ə) 1. atrophy from malnutrition. 2. a change in diet.

meta•tro•phic (met″ə-tro′fik) utilizing organic matter for food. Cf. *paratrophic.*

me•tat•ro•phy (mə-tat′rə-fe) [*meta-* + *-trophy*] 1. the state of being metatrophic; metatrophic nutrition. 2. metatrophia.

meta•typ•ic (met″ə-tip′ik) metatypical.

meta•typ•i•cal (met″ə-tip′ĭ-kəl) composed of the elements of the tissue on which it develops, but having those elements arranged in an atypical manner; said of tumors.

meta•van•a•date (met″ə-van′ə-dāt) any salt of vanadic acid.

sodium m. a highly poisonous salt having a variety of industrial applications.

me•tax•a•lone (mə-taks′ə-lōn) a centrally acting skeletal muscle relaxant used in the treatment of painful musculoskeletal conditions, administered orally.

Meta•zoa (met″ə-zo′ə) [*meta-* + Gr. *zōon* animal] that division of the animal kingdom which includes all multicellular animals whose cells become differentiated to form tissues. It comprises all animals except Protozoa.

met•a•zoa (met″ə-zo′ə) plural of *metazoon.*

meta•zo•al (met″ə-zo′əl) 1. belonging to the Metazoa. 2. pertaining to or caused by metazoa.

meta•zo•an (met″ə-zo′ən) 1. pertaining to metazoa; metazoal. 2. a metazoon.

meta•zo•nal (met″ə-zo′nəl) situated after or below a sclerozone.

meta•zo•on (met″ə-zo′on) pl. *metazo′a.* An individual of the Metazoa.

Metch•ni•koff's theory (mech′nĭ-kofs) [Elie *Metchnikoff* (Ilia Ilich Mechnikov), Russian-born zoologist in France and Nobel prize winner, 1845–1916] see under *theory.*

Metch•ni•ko•vel•li•da (mech″nĭ-ko-vel′ĭ-də) an order of parasitic protozoa (class Rudimicrosporea, phylum Microspora) having characters of the class.

me•te•cious (mə-te′shəs) heterecious.

met•en•ce•phal•ic (met″ən-sə-fal′ik) pertaining to the metencephalon.

met•en•ceph•a•lon (met″en-sef′ə-lon) [*met-* + *encephalon*] 1. [TA] the rostral portion of the rhombencephalon, comprising the cerebellum and the pons. See Plate 9. 2. the anterior of the two brain vesicles formed by specialization of the rhombencephalon in the developing embryo.

met•en•ceph•a•lo•spi•nal (met″ən-sef″ə-lo-spi′nəl) pertaining to the metencephalon (cerebellum and pons) and the spinal cord.

met•en•keph•a•lin (met″en-kef′ə-lin) see *enkephalin.*

me•te•or•ism (me′te-ə-riz″əm) [Gr. *meteōrizein* to raise up] tympanites.

me•te•oro•pa•thol•o•gy (me″te-ə-ro-pə-thol′ə-je) the pathology of conditions caused by atmospheric conditions.

me•te•orop•a•thy (me″te-ə-rop′ə-the) [Gr. *meteōros* high in the air + *pathos* disease] any disorder due to conditions of climate.

me•te•oro•tro•pic (me″te-ə-ro-tro′pik) responding to influence by meteorological factors; pertaining to or characterized by meteorotropism.

me•te•orot•ro•pism (me″te-ə-rot′rə-piz″əm) the response to influence by meteorological factors noted in certain biological events, such as sudden death, attacks of angina, joint pain, insomnia, and traffic accidents.

me•ter (me′tər) [Gr. *metron* measure] 1. the base SI unit of linear measure, approximately equivalent to 39.37 inches; currently defined as the distance that light will travel in a vacuum in 1/299,792,458 of a second. Symbol m. 2. an apparatus for measuring the quantity of something passing through it, such as a gas or an electric current.

dosage m. dosimeter.

flow m. see *flowmeter.*

light m. an instrument for measuring light in foot candles.

peak flow m. an instrument for measuring the flow of air in the early part of forced exhalation.

rate m. a radiation detector whose output is proportional to instantaneous radiation intensity (rate of radioactive emissions).

-meter [Gr. *metron* measure] a word termination denoting an instrument used in measuring.

met·er·ga·sis (met″ər-ga′sis) [*meta-* + *erg-* + *-asis*] change of function.

me·tes·trum (mə-tes′trəm) metestrus.

me·tes·trus (mə-tes′trəs) [*meta-* + *estrus*] in female mammals that have estrous cycles, the period of subsiding follicular function or rest following estrus. Called also *metestrum*.

met·for·min hy·dro·chlo·ride (mət-for′min) [USP] a biguanide antihyperglycemic agent that potentiates the action of insulin, used in the treatment of type 2 diabetes mellitus; administered orally.

meth·a·cho·line (meth″ə-ko′lēn) a cholinergic agonist, having a longer duration of action than acetylcholine and predominantly muscarinic effects; it has vasodilator and cardiac vagomimetic effects but has largely been replaced by other drugs. It is also used in bronchial challenge testing.

m. chloride [USP] the chloride salt of methacholine, used as a cholinergic, especially in the treatment of Raynaud disease, scleroderma, vascular spasm due to cold, and chronic varicose ulcers, administered orally, subcutaneously, and by iontophoresis.

me·thac·e·tin (mə-thas′ə-tin) the methyl derivative of phenacetin, measured in a liver function test; see *methacetin breath test*, under *test*. Called also *p-acetanisidine*.

meth·ac·ry·late (meth-ak′rə-lāt) an ester of methacrylic acid, or the resin derived from polymerization of the ester. See also *acrylic resins*, under *resin*.

meth·a·cryl·ic ac·id (meth″ə-kril′ik) an organic acid, 2-methylpropenoic acid, that polymerizes easily to form a ceramic-like mass. Its esters, methyl and polymethyl methacrylate, are used in the manufacture of acrylic resins and plastics.

meth·a·cy·cline (meth″ə-si′klēn) a semisynthetic broad-spectrum antibiotic of the tetracycline group.

m. hydrochloride [USP] the monohydrochloride salt of methacycline, used as an antibacterial, administered orally.

meth·a·done hy·dro·chlo·ride (meth′ə-dōn) [USP] a synthetic opioid analgesic, possessing pharmacologic actions similar to those of morphine and heroin and similar potential for addiction; used as an analgesic and as a narcotic abstinence syndrome suppressant in the treatment of heroin addiction (see also *narcotic blockade*, under *blockade*), administered orally, intramuscularly, and subcutaneously.

Meth·adose (meth′ə-dōs) trademark for preparations of methadone hydrochloride.

me·thal·li·bure (mə-thal′ĭ-būr) an anterior pituitary activator used to prevent estrus in swine.

meth·am·phet·amine (meth″am-fet′ə-mēn) a sympathomimetic amine closely related chemically to both amphetamine and ephedrine, having actions similar to those of amphetamine. Abuse of this drug may lead to dependence; see *amphetamine* (def. 1).

m. hydrochloride [USP] the sulfate salt of the dextrorotatory isomer of methamphetamine, having the same actions as the base; used orally in the treatment of attention-deficit/hyperactivity disorder. It has been used as an anorectic in the treatment of obesity but is no longer recommended for this purpose.

meth·a·nal (meth′ə-nal) formaldehyde.

meth·an·di·e·none (meth″ən-di′ə-nōn) an anabolic-androgenic steroid used in veterinary medicine.

meth·an·dro·sten·o·lone (məth-an″dro-sten′ə-lōn) an anabolic-androgenic steroid used especially in the adjunctive treatment of senile and postmenopausal osteoporosis and in selected cases of pituitary dwarfism, administered orally.

meth·ane (meth′ān) a colorless, odorless, flammable gas, CH_4, produced by decomposition of organic matter, which may explode when mixed with air or oxygen; it is the first member of a homologous series of saturated hydrocarbons including butane, ethane, hexane, pentane, and propane.

meth·ane·sul·fo·nate (meth″ān-sul′fo-nāt) any salt or ester of methanesulfonic acid; called also *mesylate*.

meth·ane·sul·fon·ic ac·id (meth″ān-səl-fon′ik) a corrosive, toxic acid, used as a catalyst and as a solvent.

■ Methane.

meth·a·no·gen (meth′ə-no-jen″) an anaerobic microorganism that grows in the presence of carbon dioxide and produces methane gas. Methanogens are found in the stomach of cows, in swamp mud, and other environments in which oxygen is not present.

meth·a·no·gen·ic (meth″ə-no-jen′ik) producing methane.

meth·a·nol (meth′ə-nol) methyl alcohol.

meth·a·nol·y·sis (meth″ə-nol′ə-sis) alcoholysis of methyl alcohol.

me·than·the·line bro·mide (mə-than′thə-lēn) a quaternary ammonium compound with anticholinergic and antimuscarinic effects; used as an adjunct in the treatment of peptic ulcer and other gastrointestinal disorders, administered orally.

me·thaq·ua·lone (mə-thak′wə-lōn) a nonbarbiturate compound formerly used as a sedative and hypnotic; abuse of this drug may lead to dependence.

me·thar·bi·tal (mə-thahr′bĭ-təl) a long-acting barbiturate used as an anticonvulsant for the control of generalized tonic-clonic and simple partial seizures in epilepsy; administered orally.

meth·a·zo·la·mide (meth″ə-zo′lə-mīd) [USP] a carbonic anhydrase inhibitor used as an adjunct to reduce intraocular pressure in the treatment of glaucoma; administered orally.

meth·di·la·zine (məth-di′lə-zēn) an antihistamine derived from phenothiazine, having sedative and antimuscarinic effects; used in the symptomatic treatment of hypersensitivity reactions, particularly pruritic dermatoses; administered orally.

m. hydrochloride [USP] the monohydrochloride salt of methdilazine, having the same actions and uses as the base; administered orally.

met·hem·al·bu·min (met″he-mal-bu′min) a brown pigment formed by the binding of albumin with heme; this occurs only when the serum has been depleted of unsaturated haptoglobin and is indicative of intravascular hemolysis.

met·hem·al·bu·min·emia (met″hēm-al-bu″min-e′me-ə) the presence of methemalbumin in the blood.

met·heme (met′hēm) [*met-* + *heme*] heme in which the iron is in the ferric (Fe^{3+}) state.

met·he·mo·glo·bin (met-he′mo-glo″bin) [*met-* + *hemoglobin*] a brown pigment formed from hemoglobin by oxidation of the ferrous to the ferric state with essentially ionic bonds. A small amount is present in the blood normally, but injury or toxic agents convert a larger proportion of hemoglobin into methemoglobin, which does not function reversibly as an oxygen carrier.

met·he·mo·glo·bin·emia (met″he-mo-glo″bĭ-ne′me-ə) [*methemoglobin* + *-emia*] the presence of excessive methemoglobin in the blood, resulting in cyanosis and headache, dizziness, fatigue, ataxia, dyspnea, tachycardia, nausea, vomiting, and drowsiness, which can progress to stupor, coma, and occasionally death.

acquired m. methemoglobinemia caused by exposure to a toxic chemical or drug; many different agents have been implicated, including nitrate and nitrite compounds, sulfonamides, and aniline dyes. Called also *toxic m.*

congenital m., hereditary m. any of several rare types caused by inherited conditions. Deficiency of cytochrome-b_5 reductase is an autosomal recessive condition that may be either confined to the erythrocytes and relatively symptom-free or generalized to the leukocytes and sometimes the brain, muscle, and fibroblasts, in which case the individual may be mentally retarded. Abnormalities of hemoglobin M are autosomal dominant conditions that cause cyanosis in infancy but usually few other symptoms.

toxic m. acquired m.

met·he·mo·glo·bin·emic (met″he-mo-glo″bĭ-ne′mik) 1. pertaining to or causing methemoglobinemia. 2. an agent that causes methemoglobinemia.

met·he·mo·glo·bin re·duc·tase (NADH) (met-he″mə-glo′bin re-duk′tās) cytochrome-b_5 reductase.

met·he·mo·glo·bin re·duc·tase (NADPH) (met-he″mo-glo′bin re-duk′tās) NADPH methemoglobin reductase.

met·he·mo·glo·bin·uria (met″he-mo-glo-bĭ-nu′re-ə) the occurrence of methemoglobin in the urine.

meth·en·amine (meth-en′ə-mēn) [USP] a compound that hydrolyzes formaldehyde in acidic urine to provide mild antiseptic activity, used as a urinary antibacterial; administered orally.

m. hippurate [USP] a compound of methenamine and hippuric acid, used orally as a urinary antibacterial.

m. mandelate [USP] a salt of methenamine and mandelic acid, used orally as a urinary antibacterial.

m. silver a solution of methenamine and silver nitrate, used as a histopathological stain to demonstrate fungal cell walls, Donovan bodies, and *Klebsiella pneumoniae rhinoscleromatis*.

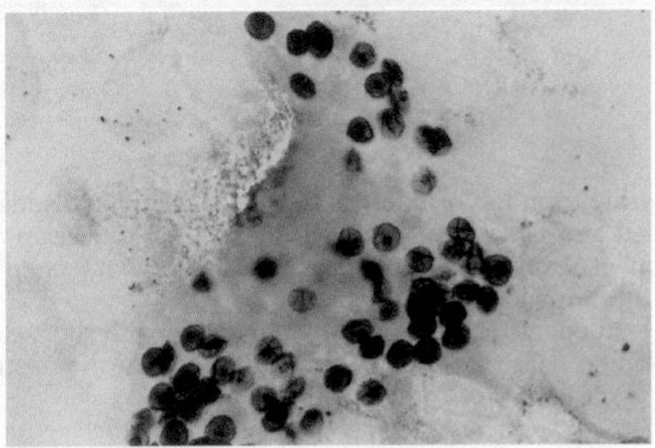

■ Methenamine silver used to demonstrate a cluster of *Pneumocystis jiroveci* cysts.

meth•ene (meth′ēn) methylene.

meth•en•o•lone en•an•thate (meth-en′ə-lōn ə-nan′thāt) an anabolic-androgenic steroid used in veterinary medicine.

5,10-meth•e•nyl•tet•ra•hy•dro•fo•late (meth″ə-nəl-tet′rə-hi″dro-fo′lāt) a substituted derivative of tetrahydrofolate, carrying a methylidyne group; it is formed in histidine degradation and in the interconversion of various folates, linking the flow of activated one-carbon units from serine and thymidylate synthesis with purine synthesis and the liver enzyme system for discarding excess single carbons.

meth•e•nyl•tet•ra•hy•dro•fo•late cy•clo•hy•dro•lase (meth″ə-nəl-tet″rə-hi″dro-fo′lāt si″klo-hi′drə-lās) [EC 3.5.4.9] an enzyme activity of the hydrolase class that catalyzes the cleavage of 5,10-methenyltetrahydrofolate to 10-formyltetrahydrofolate, a step in the system of folate-mediated one-carbon transfer reactions. The enzyme activity is part of a trifunctional enzyme that also includes methylenetetrahydrofolate dehydrogenase ($NADP^+$) and formate–tetrahydrofolate ligase activities.

5,10-meth•e•nyl•tet•ra•hy•dro•fo•late syn•the•tase (meth″ə-nəl-tet″rə-hi″dro-fo′lāt sin′thə-tās) 5-formyltetrahydrofolate cyclo-ligase.

Meth•er•gine (meth′ər-jin) trademark for preparations of methylergonovine maleate.

meth•i•cil•lin so•di•um (meth″ĭ-sil″in) a semisynthetic penicillin, used intravenously or intramuscularly as an antibacterial in resistant staphylococcal infections. Called also *dimethoxyphenyl penicillin sodium.*

meth•im•a•zole (meth-im′ə-zōl) [USP] a thyroid inhibitor, used in the treatment of hyperthyroidism, administered orally. Called also *thiamazole.*

meth•ine (meth′īn) methylidyne.

me•thi•o•carb (mə-thi′o-kahrb) an organophosphorus molluscacide; larger animals that ingest it may suffer diarrhea, ataxia, and pulmonary edema that can be fatal.

me•thi•o•nine (Met, M) (mə-thi′o-nēn) 1. chemical name: α-amino-γ-methylmercaptobutyric acid; a naturally occurring essential amino acid furnishing both methyl groups and sulfur necessary for normal metabolism. See also table at *amino acid.* 2. [USP] a preparation of methionine used as a dietary supplement.

m. C 11 [USP] L-methionine in which a portion of the molecules have been labeled with carbon 11, used as a tracer in positron emission tomography for the detection of malignant neoplasms; administered intravenously.

me•thi•o•nine ad•eno•syl•trans•fer•ase (mə-thi′o-nēn ə-den″o-səl-trans′fər-ās) [EC 2.5.1.6] an enzyme of the transferase class that catalyzes the formation of *S*-adenosylmethionine from methionine and ATP, occurring in several isozymes. Deficiency of the hepatic isozyme causes hypermethioninemia, but is otherwise benign.

me•thi•o•nine syn•thase (mə-thi′o-nēn syn′thās) [EC 2.1.1.13] an enzyme of the transferase class that catalyzes the remethylation of homocysteine to form methionine, using 5-methyltetrahydrofolate as a methyl donor and requiring methylcobalamin as a coenzyme; the reaction also regenerates tetrahydrofolate. Deficiency of enzyme activity can result from any of several defects, including deficiency of the apoenzyme, inability to convert cobalamin specifically to methylcobalamin or, more generally, to either of the cobalamin-containing coenzymes, deficiency of 5,10-methylenetetrahydrofolate reductase activity, familial megaloblastic anemia or other defect in absorption or transport of vitamin B_{12}, or nutritional deficiency of vitamin B_{12} or folate; it results in homocystinuria, with developmental delay and neurologic abnormalities, and hypomethioninemia. Defects in cobalamin metabolism are characterized additionally by hematologic abnormalities and some also by methylmalonicacidemia (q.v.).

me•thi•o•nyl (mə-thi′o-nəl) the acyl radical of methionine.

me•this•a•zone (mə-this′ə-zōn) an antiviral agent; it has been used to provide short-term protection against smallpox and the severe complications of vaccination.

meth•o•car•ba•mol (meth″o-kahr′bə-mol) [USP] a skeletal muscle relaxant, administered orally, intramuscularly, or intravenously in the treatment of painful musculoskeletal conditions.

Meth•o•cel (meth′o-sel) trademark for preparations of cellulose ethers, including Methocel A (methylcellulose) and Methocel E, F, J, and K (hydroxypropyl methylcellulose).

meth•od (meth′əd) [Gr. *methodos*] the manner of performing any act or operation. See also under *maneuver, operation, procedure, technique, treatment, stain, test,* etc.

Method

Abbott m. treatment of scoliosis by lateral pulling and counterpulling on the vertebral column by means of wide bandages and pads until the deformity is overcorrected, and then applying a plaster jacket to produce pressure, counterpressure, and fixation of the spine in its corrected position.

absorption m. the separate and selective removal of agglutinins from specific immune sera by the addition of homologous particulate antigen(s) (e.g., bacterial cells or red blood cells) to the immune sera, or by the passage of specific immune sera through columns containing antigen on an insoluble support (immunosorbent) with which the homologous antibody combines and is thereby removed from the serum.

acid hematin m. a formerly common method of estimating hemoglobin: the hemoglobin was converted into acid hematin by adding hydrochloric acid and the resulting color was compared to a standard color scale.

agar dilution m. a dilution method of antibiotic susceptibility testing done in a series of test tubes containing agar.

Altmann-Gersh m. a method of preparing tissue for histologic study by freeze drying.

autoclave m. see *Clark-Collip m.* (def. 2).

back pressure–arm lift m. Holger Nielsen m.

Barger m. a method for determining osmotic pressure from vapor pressure.

Barraquer m. phacoerysis.

Bethea m. see under *sign.*

Bivine m. treatment of strychnine poisoning by administration of chloral hydrate.

Bobath m. a system of therapeutic exercise designed to inhibit spasticity and to aid in the development of new reflex responses and equilibrium reactions by modifying postures that progress from simple movements to more complex ones in a sequence based on the neurological development of an infant.

Brandt-Andrews m. a method of expressing the placenta from the uterus in the third stage of labor: the left hand grasps the umbilical cord while the right is placed on the maternal abdomen with the fingers over the anterior uterine surface. The right hand is gently pressed backward and slightly upward as the left applies gentle traction on the cord. Called also *Brandt-Andrews maneuver* and *controlled cord traction.*

brine flotation m. *(for concentration of eggs)* a portion of the feces is suspended in a saturated solution of sodium chloride and let stand for a time; then eggs are collected from the surface.

broth dilution m. a dilution method of antimicrobial susceptibility testing done in a series of test tubes containing broth; it is now usually done as the broth microdilution method.

broth microdilution m. a variant of the broth dilution method that uses microscopic amounts of the antimicrobial and inoculum.

Brunnstrom m. a system of therapeutic exercise designed to inhibit spasticity through the sensory stimulation of synergetic movements; to the degree that the synergies subside, the voluntary isolated movements

that remain can be emphasized so that motor control is gradually increased.
buffy coat m. *(for detecting* Leishmania, *microfilariae, and trypanosomes)* a blood sample is centrifuged in a hematocrit tube and the buffy coat is examined for parasites.
calcium, m's for see specific methods, including *Clark-Collip m.* (def. 1).
caliper m. a method for approximating fat content in the body by measuring the thickness of folds of the skin at stated areas of the body by means of specially designed calipers.
Callahan m. 1. in root canal therapy, a filling method in which the canal is first flooded with a chloroform-rosin solution and then gutta-percha is dissolved in the solution. 2. a method of tracing and opening up a root canal by destroying the pulp tissue with a 50 per cent sulfuric acid solution.
Castaneda m. *(for rickettsiae in smears)* a thin smear is made in a phosphate buffer (pH 7.6) and air-dried, stained with methylene blue solution for 3 minutes, counterstained with safranine solution, and washed, blotted, and dried. Rickettsiae appear pale blue; cell nuclei and protoplasm are red.
chest pressure–arm lift m. Silvester m.
Chick-Martin m. see under *test.*
chloropercha m. in root canal therapy, a method of filling the canal with gutta-percha dissolved in a chloroform-rosin solution; see *Callahan m.* (def. 1) and *Johnson m.*
Ciaccio m. treatment of tissue for the purpose of rendering visible the intracellular lipids; they are fixed with acid chromate solution and stained with Sudan III.
Clark-Collip m. 1. *(for calcium in serum)* dilute the serum and add ammonium oxalate; wash the precipitate, dissolve with sulfuric acid, and titrate with potassium permanganate. 2. *(for urea in blood)* to 5 mL of blood filtrate add 1 mL of NH_4Cl and heat in autoclave at 150°C for ten minutes. Make alkaline, distill into acid, and titrate, using methyl red as indicator.
Clauss m. a type of fibrinogen assay similar to the test for thrombin time, estimating the functional fibrinogen level by adding fibrin reagent to plasma and noting the time until fibrinogen converts to fibrin; it differs from the thrombin time by using plasma diluted with Owren buffer and using a much stronger concentration of thrombin reagent. Called also *Clauss assay.*
Converse m. reconstruction of the ear lobe by raising a flap of skin below the auricle with a superior base about one third larger than the proposed lobe; a full-thickness skin graft covers the defect at the site of the flap except for the last third of the medial aspect of the pedicle.
Couette m. a method for measuring viscosity by calculating the rate of movement of an inner cylinder separated from an outer cylinder by a thin layer of the fluid whose viscosity is being tested.
Coutard m. a method of x-ray irradiation by protracted and fractionated dosage.
creatine, m's for see specific methods, including *Folin m.* (defs. 4, 5) and *Folin and Wu m.* (def. 2).
creatinine, m's for see specific methods, including *Folin m.* (def. 6) and *Folin and Wu m.* (defs. 1, 2), and see under *test.*
Credé m. 1. method of expressing the placenta by forcing the uterus down into the pelvis and at the same time squeezing the uterus from all sides so that its contents are expelled. 2. a similar method for expressing urine from the bladder, especially in paralytic bladder. Defs. 1 and 2 called also *Credé maneuver.* 3. the placing of a drop of 2 per cent solution of silver nitrate in each eye of a newborn child for the prevention of ophthalmia neonatorum.

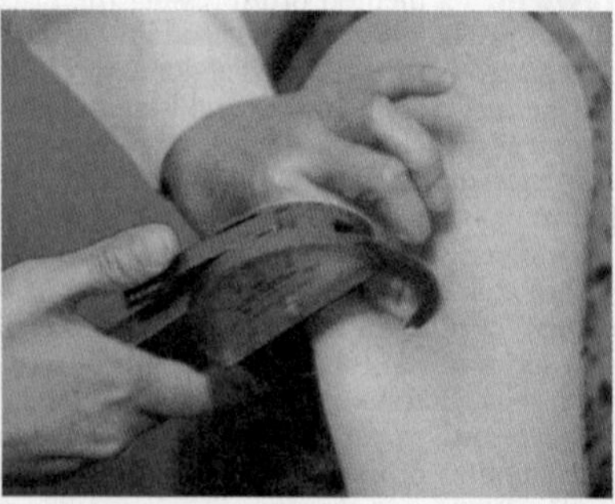

■ Caliper method being used to measure the thickness of the skinfold over the triceps muscle.

Cronin m. an operation to correct a flat nasal tip with short columella by using bilateral flaps of skin elevated in the floor of the nostrils.
cup plate m. see *ring test* (def. 1), under *tests.*
Denis-Leche m. *(for total sulfate)* add acid and autoclave to decompose protein, then precipitate with barium chloride, dry, and weigh.
Dickinson m. a method of controlling postpartum hemorrhage: the entire uterus is grasped through the abdominal wall, lifted out of the pelvis, and compressed against the vertebral column.
dilution m. any of various antimicrobial susceptibility tests in which a given microorganism is inoculated into a series of tubes or wells containing different concentrations of a particular antibiotic and the minimal inhibitory concentration and the minimal bactericidal concentration are determined.
direct m. ophthalmoscopy in which the ophthalmoscope is held close to the eye being examined and an erect virtual image of the fundus is obtained.
direct centrifugal flotation m. Lane m.
disk diffusion m. see *disk diffusion test,* under *test.*
Domagk m. *(for demonstration of reticuloendothelial cells)* a culture of gram-positive staphylococci in physiologic salt solution is injected into the femoral vein of a rat which is then killed in fifteen to thirty minutes. In formalin-fixed sections stained by cresyl violet or by Gram stain followed by alum-carmine, Kupffer cells and other cells of the reticuloendothelial system stand out strikingly.
Duke m. see under *test.*
dye dilution m. a type of indicator dilution method for assessing flow through the circulatory system; the indicator is a dye, usually indocyanine green.
egg concentration, m. for see *brine flotation m.*
Eicken m. examination of the hypopharynx, with the cricoid cartilage drawn forward.
Ellinger m. *(for indican)* precipitate the urine with basic lead acetate and filter. To the filtrate add Obermayer reagent. Shake out the indigo with chloroform, evaporate off the chloroform, and titrate the residue with potassium permanganate.
Eskimo m. closed reduction of an anterior shoulder dislocation by having the patient lie on the unaffected side and applying traction against gravity by lifting the patient by the affected arm.
external rotation m. closed reduction of anterior shoulder dislocation by adducting the arm to the patient's side with the elbow flexed to 90 degrees as the patient lies supine, then rotating the arm externally using the forearm as a lever.
Fahraeus m. the original (1918) method that was used to determine the erythrocyte sedimentation rate.
Faust m. a method of diagnosing helminth and protozoan infections by centrifugation of washed feces with zinc sulfate of a specific gravity of 1.180, after which eggs and protozoan cysts may be removed from the supernatant layer.
Fay m. a system of therapeutic exercise for overcoming spasticity; the central nervous system is reeducated according to a theory of hierarchical development starting with the performance of simple reflex movements and progressing to more advanced patterns of coordination.
Feldenkrais M. a proprietary system that uses an exploratory technique to enable patients to relearn dysfunctional movement patterns. Therapy takes two forms: *awareness through movement,* in which the patient is guided verbally through increasingly complex structured movements, and *functional integration,* in which the practitioner introduces new motion patterns to the patient by gentle manipulation.
fibrinogen, m. for see *fibrinogen assay,* under *assay.*
Fick m. a method for measuring cardiac output based on the Fick principle applied to pulmonary blood flow: the rate of oxygen consumption by the lungs, when divided by the arteriovenous oxygen difference (the difference in oxygen concentration between the arterial and venous systems), gives the rate of blood flow across the pulmonary capillaries and the cardiac output. See also *indicator dilution m.*
Fishberg m. a method for determining specific gravity of the urine, which serves as a concentration test of renal function.
Fiske and Subbarow's m. 1. *(for acid-soluble phosphorus in blood)* destroy organic matter by heating with sulfuric and nitric acids, precipitate the phosphates as magnesium ammonium phosphate, and reduce

the precipitate with para-amino-naphthol-sulfonic acid. Compare the blue color with a standard phosphate solution. 2. *(for inorganic phosphates)* the phosphates are precipitated as ammonium phosphomolybdate. This is then reduced by para-amino-naphthol-sulfonic acid and the blue color compared colorimetrically with a standard solution.
flash m. see *pasteurization.*
flotation m. any method for separating cysts and eggs from the heavier component of the feces; this requires use of a solution intermediate in density between the parasitic material (which floats) and the bulk of the feces (which remains as sediment after centrifugation).
Folin m. 1. *(for acetone)* aerate the acetone into a solution of sodium bisulfite and then determine the amount of nephelometric comparison with a standard acetone solution using Scott and Wilson reagent. 2. *(for amino acids in blood)* make 10 mL of protein-free blood filtrate slightly alkaline to phenolphthalein. Add 2 mL of beta-naphthaquinone solution and place in the dark. The next day add 2 mL of acetic acid–acetate solution and 2 mL of 4 per cent thiosulfate solution. Dilute to 25 mL and compare the blue color with a standard amino-acid solution similarly treated. 3. *(for ammonia nitrogen)* sodium carbonate is added to the urine to free the ammonia, which is aerated into standard acid and titrated. 4. *(for creatine)* precipitate the proteins of the blood with picric acid and filter. To the filtrate add sodium hydroxide and compare color with a standard solution of creatine. 5. *(for creatine in urine)* change creatine into creatinine by heating at 90°C for three hours in the presence of third normal HCl. Determine creatinine by picric acid and alkali and deduct the preformed creatinine. 6. *(for creatinine in urine)* to the urine add picric acid and sodium hydroxide and compare the red color with a half normal solution of potassium bichromate. 7. *(for ethereal sulfates)* remove the inorganic sulfates with barium chloride and then the conjugated sulfates after hydrolyzing with boiling dilute hydrochloric acid. 8. *(for inorganic sulfates)* acidify the urine with hydrochloric acid, precipitate with barium chloride, filter, dry, ignite, and weigh. 9. *(for protein in urine)* add acetic acid and heat, wash, dry, and weigh the precipitate. 10. *(for total acidity)* add potassium oxalate to the urine to precipitate the calcium which should otherwise precipitate at the neutral point, and titrate with tenth normal sodium hydroxide, using phenolphthalein as an indicator. 11. *(for total sulfates)* boil the urine for thirty minutes with dilute hydrochloric acid, precipitate with barium chloride, filter, dry, ignite, and weigh. 12. *(for urea and allantoin)* decompose the urea by heating with magnesium chloride and hydrochloric acid, distill off the ammonia, and titrate.
Folin and Wu m. 1. *(for creatinine)* the color produced by the unknown (protein-free blood filtrate or urine) in an alkaline solution of picric acid is compared in a colorimeter with the color produced by a known solution of creatinine or with a standard solution of potassium bichromate. 2. *(for creatine plus creatinine)* the creatine of a protein-free blood filtrate is changed to creatinine by heating with dilute hydrochloric acid in an autoclave, and the creatinine thus produced together with the preformed creatinine is determined colorimetrically after adding an alkaline picrate solution. 3. *(nonprotein nitrogen)* the total nonprotein nitrogen in the protein-free blood filtrate is determined by setting free the nitrogen as ammonia by the Kjeldahl process, nesslerizing this ammonia, and comparing with a standard. 4. *(for protein-free blood filtrate)* lake the blood with distilled water, add sodium tungstate and sulfuric acid, and filter. 5. *(for urea)* change the urea to ammonia by means of urease, and nesslerize. 6. *(for uric acid)* uric acid is precipitated from the protein-free blood filtrate or from urine by silver lactate, treated with phosphotungstic acid, and the blue color compared with the color produced by known amounts of uric acid.
Fülleborn m. *(for parasite eggs in feces)* 1 g of feces is ground and mixed with 20 mL of a saturated solution of sodium chloride; the mixture is allowed to stand for at least one hour, and then coverglasses are floated on the surface and transferred without draining to slides.
Gerota m. injection of the lymphatics with a dye, such as Prussian blue, which is soluble in chloroform or ether, but not in water.
glucose, m's for See *glucose test,* under *test.*
Gram m. see *Stains and Staining Methods,* under *stain.*
Hamilton m. *(in postpartum hemorrhage),* compress the uterus between a fist in the vagina and a hand pressing down the abdominal wall.
Heublein m. ionizing irradiation of the whole body with low-dose increments protracted for ten to twenty hours per day over several days.
hippocratic m. closed reduction of anterior shoulder dislocation by abduction of the arm with longitudinal traction and gentle external rotation; countertraction is provided by the placing of the physician's foot against the chest wall.
Hirschberg m. measurement of the deviation of a strabismic eye by observing the reflection of a candle from the cornea.
holding m. see *pasteurization.*
Holger Nielsen m. a nonmechanical method of emergency artificial respiration: with victim prone, rescuer alternately extends victim's arms to aid inhalation and presses down on victim's scapulae to aid exhalation. Called also *Nielsen m.* and *back pressure–arm lift m.*
indican, m's for see *Ellinger m.*
indicator dilution m. any of several methods for assessing flow through the circulatory system by injection of a known quantity of an indicator, such as a dye, radionuclide, or chilled liquid, into the system and monitoring its concentration over time at a specific point in the system. See also *dye dilution m.* and *thermodilution.*
indirect m. ophthalmoscopy that uses a high diopter condensing lens to form an image of the retina anterior to the eye.
Ivy m. see under *test.*
Jendrassik-Grof m. 1. *(for conjugated bilirubin)* a fasting sample of serum or plasma is collected and acidified by the addition of hydrochloric acid. Ehrlich's diazo reagent is added so that the conjugated bilirubin begins forming blue azobilirubin. After 10 minutes the reaction is stopped and the amount of azobilirubin in the sample is measured. 2. *(for total bilirubin)* to an acidified fasting sample as in the previous method, caffeine benzoate is added as an accelerator for the unconjugated bilirubin to form azobilirubin. When the reaction is stopped, the azobilirubin in the sample thus represents the total of both conjugated and unconjugated bilirubin.
Johnson m. a modification of the Callahan method (def. 1) of root canal therapy; the canal is first flooded with alcohol, allowing diffusion of the chloroform component of the chloroform-rosin solution; alcohol deep in the dentin facilitates rosin dissolved in the chloroform to be diffused into the dentin.
Kaplan-Meier m. the analysis of survival data to create a Kaplan-Meier survival curve (q.v.). Called also *product-limit m.* or *estimate.*
Kety-Schmidt m. a method of measuring perfusion flow of blood through brain tissue.
Kirby-Bauer m. disk diffusion test.
Kirstein m. direct laryngoscopy.
Kjeldahl m. (1883), a method of determining the amount of nitrogen in an organic compound. It consists in heating the material to be analyzed with strong sulfuric acid. The nitrogen is thereby converted to ammonia, which is distilled off and caught in tenth normal solution of sulfuric acid. By titration the amount of ammonia is determined, and from this the amount of nitrogen is estimated.
Klüver-Barrera m. a histologic staining method in which myelin sheaths are stained blue-green and the cells purple.
Kocher m. closed reduction of anterior shoulder dislocation by applying traction and external rotation of the arm, then bringing the arm across the patient's chest to effect reduction, and finally internally rotating the arm.
Korotkoff m. the auscultatory method of determining blood pressure.
Laborde m. the making of rhythmic traction movements on the tongue in order to stimulate the respiratory centers in asphyxiation.
Lamaze m. a psychoprophylactic method of preparing for delivery, involving education of the prospective mother in the physiology of pregnancy and parturition as well as in techniques such as breathing exercises and bearing down for the easing of delivery.
Lane m. a method of diagnosing hookworm infection by centrifugation of 1 mL of washed feces mixed with brine, the tube being covered with a cover slip on which the eggs can be counted. Called also *direct centrifugal flotation m.,* or *DCF.*
lateral condensation m. a method of root canal therapy in which the main portion of the canal is filled with a primary gutta-percha cone or silver point and sealer cement or paste and the remaining space is packed with auxiliary gutta-percha cones. Spreader sites and pluggers are used to force gutta-percha into the canal laterally and sometimes vertically. Called also *multiple cone m.*
Leboyer m. a method of delivery of the infant based upon the theory that the violence associated with birth causes emotional trauma to the infant, which will affect the child's personality throughout life. The concepts of this method emphasize that the delivery should be gentle

and controlled, without unnecessary intervention; the infant should be handled gently, with the head, neck, and sacrum supported; the infant should not be overstimulated and should be allowed to breathe spontaneously, without painful stimuli such as spanking. Called also *Leboyer technique.*
Milch m. closed reduction of anterior shoulder dislocation by traction on the arm, which is abducted overhead with the patient in the supine position, external rotation, and pressure on the head of the humerus; in some modifications of this technique the patient lies prone.
Monte Carlo m. artificial replication, usually by computer, of a sampling experiment; used to estimate a probability.
mouth-to-mouth m. see under *resuscitation.*
multiple cone m. lateral condensation m.
Nielsen m. Holger Nielsen m.
Nikiforoff m. a method of fixing blood films by placing them for from five to fifteen minutes in absolute alcohol, pure ether, or equal parts of alcohol and ether.
Ogino-Knaus m. rhythm method.
optical density m. the measuring of growth rates of cells by taking the optical density or turbidity of a dense population and comparing this with optical densities of known dilutions of the sample.
Orsi-Grocco m. palpatory percussion of the heart.
panoptic m. see *Giemsa stain,* at *Stains and Staining Methods,* under *stain.*
Pap silver m. a method for demonstrating reticulum.
point source m. a method of intracavitary irradiation of the bladder wall utilizing a small point source of radiation at the center of a Foley catheter balloon inflated with a radiopaque solution containing methylene blue or indigo carmine.
Politzer m. an imprecise test for patency of the auditory tube: with the mouth closed and one nostril occluded, air is forced into the other nostril through a rubber tube; this should cause positive pressure in the middle ear so that the tympanic membrane bulges outward. Called also *Politzer test.*
Ponseti m. a technique for correcting clubfoot by weekly manipulation and casting, lasting 5–6 weeks, followed by maintenance with a foot abduction orthosis to prevent recurrence; a percutaneous tenotomy is usually performed before the final casting to lengthen the Achilles tendon and prevent development of a rocker-bottom foot deformity.
potassium hydroxide concentration m. *(for oocysts of* Cyclospora *in a stool sample):* a fecal suspension is mixed with potassium hydroxide and saline, filtered, and centrifuged; the sediment is then examined on a slide.
product-limit m. Kaplan-Meier m.
proprioceptive neuromuscular facilitation m. see under *facilitation.*
radioactive balloon m. a method of intracavitary irradiation of the bladder wall utilizing a Foley catheter balloon filled with a radioactive solution.
retrofilling m. see *retrofilling.*
rhythm m. a method of preventing conception by restricting coitus to the so-called safe period, avoiding the days just before and after the expected time of ovulation. Called also *periodic abstinence.*
Rideal-Walker m. a method for calculating the phenol coefficient of a disinfectant; cultures of *Salmonella enterica* subsp. *enterica* serovar Typhi are incubated with serial dilutions of the test compound, with dilutions of phenol as standards. Samples are removed at intervals, transferred to sterile broth, and the resulting cultures incubated and examined for bacterial growth.

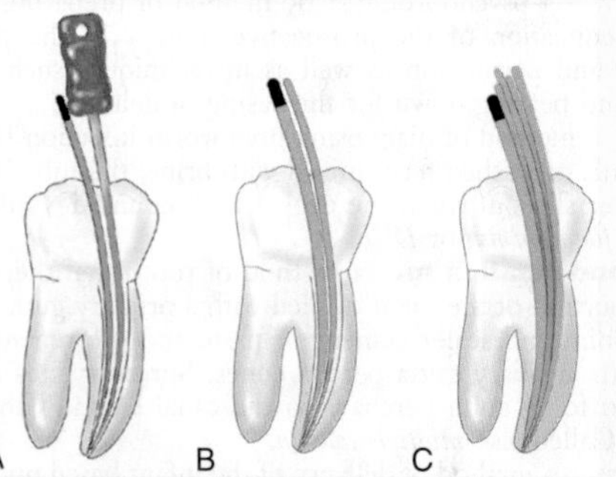

■ Lateral condensation method. *(A),* Primary cone in place with filling spreader. *(B),* Auxiliary cone placed in space created by spreader. *(C),* All auxiliary cones in place.

Ritchie formalin–ethyl acetate m. *(for detecting parasites in the feces):* the feces are diluted and centrifuged; formalin and ethyl acetate are added to the sample; it is recentrifuged; and the final sediment is examined as a wet mount. Called also *Ritchie formalin–ethyl acetate sedimentation.*
Ritgen m. see under *maneuver.*
Romanowsky (Romanovsky) m. see *Stains and Staining Methods,* under *stain.*
Rood m. a technique for overcoming spasticity, based on the theory that stimulation of a specific area of the skin will promote the contraction of underlying muscles and lead to the reciprocal relaxation of related antagonistic muscles; stimulation is done by stroking with a special brush or with ice.
Rosen m. a bodywork technique based on the premise that there is a connection between chronic muscular tension and suppressed emotions or trauma; using gentle touch and verbal support and guided by careful attention to changes in muscle tension and breathing patterns, the therapist helps the patient to relax the muscular tension and so to bring the underlying repressed memories to the surface and release them.
Sahli m. acid hematin m.
Schafer m. a nonmechanical method of emergency artificial respiration: patient is prone with forehead on one arm; rescuer's knees are on either side of patient's hips; pressure is exerted on patient's back using two hands over the lower ribs; rescuer rises up slowly and simultaneously relaxes the pressure on patient's back; procedure is repeated every 5 seconds.
sectional m. in root canal therapy, filling of the canal by packing in 2- to 3-mm cut sections of gutta-percha cones until it is filled.
Sheather sugar flotation m., modified a method for detecting oocysts of *Cryptosporidium* in a stool sample; a fecal suspension is mixed with a boiled sugar solution, phenol, and sugar flotation solution and then examined on a slide.
sib-pair m. see under *analysis.*
silver cone m., silver point m. in root canal therapy, a method of filling the canal in which a prefitted silver point is sealed into the canal apex and irregularities in the canal that are not sealed with the point are obliterated by gutta-percha through lateral condensation or segmentation, or by a root canal paste or sealer.
Silvester m. a nonmechanical method of emergency artificial respiration: with patient supine, rescuer pulls patient's arms firmly over head to raise the ribs and aid inhalation; the arms are then brought down and pressed against the chest to aid exhalation; procedure is repeated 16 times per minute. Called also *chest pressure–arm lift m.*
single cone m. in root canal therapy, a method of filling the canal with a single well-fitting gutta-percha cone or silver point in conjunction with a sealer cement or paste.
Sluder m. a method formerly used for tonsillectomy; the tonsils were removed with a small guillotine-like apparatus.
Smellie m. Mauriceau maneuver.
Somogyi m. *(for amylase activity)* a method based on the disappearance of the blue color given by iodine and amylose (linear fraction of starch) after amylase in serum, urine, etc., is allowed to act on starch.
sperm swim-up m. see under *technique.*
split cast m. 1. a procedure for placing indexed casts on a dental articulator to facilitate their removal and replacement on the instrument. 2. the procedure of checking the ability of a dental articulator to receive or be adjusted to a maxillomandibular relation record. Called also *split cast mounting.*
Stimson m. 1. closed reduction of anterior shoulder dislocation by using a small weight to exert traction on the affected arm, which hangs over the edge of the table with the patient in the prone position. 2. a method for closed reduction of posterior hip dislocation: the patient lies prone with the distal pelvis overhanging the bed and the hip, knee and ankle flexed to 90°. Reduction is accomplished by grasping the leg just distal to the knee and applying downward force, with gentle rotation of the hip and, if necessary, pressure on the femoral head.
sugar, m's for see *sugar test,* under *test.*
sulfosalicylic acid m. *(for proteinuria)* sulfosalicylic acid is added to urine and the mixture is left standing for 10 minutes; the degree of turbidity is then compared to a known scale to estimate the amount of protein in the urine.

Method *Continued*

sulfur, total, m's for see specific methods, including *Denis-Leche m.*
Sumner m. *(for glucose in urine)* heat 1 mL of urine and 3 mL of Sumner dinitrosalicylic acid reagent, dilute to 25 mL and compare the color with that of a standard glucose solution similarly treated.
suspension m. a method of intracavitary irradiation of the bladder wall by instilling a radioactive solution or suspension directly into the bladder by means of a catheter.
template m. a bleeding time test in which a template with a standard-sized slit is laid on the patient's forearm and an incision is made through the slit with a standard-sized knife.
thermal dilution m. thermodilution.
traction-countertraction m. closed reduction of anterior shoulder dislocation by longitudinal traction on the arm with external rotation; countertraction is provided by a sheet passed around the chest under the axilla of the affected shoulder and held by an assistant.

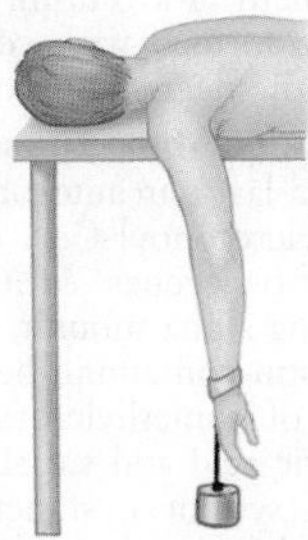

■ Stimson method for reduction of anterior shoulder dislocation.

urea, m's for see specific methods, including *Clark-Collip m.* (def. 2), *Folin m.* (def. 12), and *Folin and Wu m.* (def. 5). See also *urea test*, under *test.*
Valsalva m. Valsalva maneuver (def. 2).
van Gehuchten m. fixing of a histologic tissue in a mixture of glacial acetic acid 10 parts, chloroform 30 parts, and alcohol 60 parts.
Van Slyke m. see under *test.*
vertical condensation m. in root canal therapy, a method of filling the canal by alternately heating and vertically condensing gutta-percha until the apical third of the canal is filled; the coronal portion of the canal is then filled with warmed 2- to 4-mm sections of gutta-percha cones.
Welcker m. determination of the total blood volume by bleeding and then washing out the blood vessels.
Westergren m. the most common method for testing the erythrocyte sedimentation rate; four volumes of whole blood are mixed with one volume of sodium citrate anticoagulant-diluent solution and placed in a Westergren tube graduated in millimeters from 0 to 200, filling to the 0 mark; the tube is placed in a vertical position for 1 hour and the fall of the level of red cells is recorded in mm/hr.
Whipple m. the use of liver in pernicious anemia.
Wintrobe m. *(for erythrocyte sedimentation rate)* EDTA-anticoagulated whole blood is placed in a Wintrobe hematocrit tube, the tube is left standing undisturbed in a vertical position, and the fall of the level of red cells in one hour is recorded in mm/hr. The volume of packed red cells can then be determined using the same tube.
Wynn m. a procedure for repair of bilateral cleft lips by means of a long, narrow triangular flap.
Yuzpe m. a regimen for postcoital contraception, consisting of a combination of 200 μg ethinyl estradiol and 2 mg norgestrel in two divided doses 12 hours apart.
Ziehl-Neelsen m. see *Stains and Staining Methods*, under *stain.*

meth•od•ol•o•gy (meth″ə-dol′ə-je) the science of method; the science which deals with the principles of procedure in research and study.

meth•o•hex•i•tal (meth″o-hek′sĭ-təl) [USP] an ultrashort-acting barbiturate used as a pharmaceutic necessary in the preparation of the sodium salt for injection.

m. sodium [USP] the monosodium salt of methohexital, used as a general anesthetic, as an adjunct to general or local anesthesia, and as a sedative for certain diagnostic procedures performed in children; administered intravenously, intramuscularly, or rectally.

meth•o•trex•ate (MTX) (meth″o-trek′sāt) [USP] a folic acid antagonist that acts by inhibiting synthesis of DNA, RNA, thymidylate, and protein; used as an antineoplastic in treatment of a wide variety of malignancies, including acute lymphocytic, meningeal, and acute myelocytic leukemia; gestational choriocarcinoma; chorioadenoma destruens; hydatidiform mole; carcinoma of the breast, lung, and head and neck; non-Hodgkin lymphomas; mycosis fungoides; and osteosarcoma; administered orally. It is also used as an antipsoriatic and antiarthritic in the treatment of severe, recalcitrant, disabling psoriasis and severe rheumatoid and psoriatic arthritis.

m. sodium [USP] the sodium salt of methotrexate, having the same actions and uses as the base; administered intrathecally, intramuscularly, intravenously, and intra-arterially.

meth•o•tri•mep•ra•zine (meth″o-tri-mep′rə-zēn) [USP] a phenothiazine derivative used as an antipsychotic, antiemetic, analgesic, preoperative sedative, and adjunct to anesthesia. Called also *levomepromazine.*

me•thox•amine hy•dro•chlo•ride (mə-thok′sə-mēn) a selective α_1-adrenergic agonist used for its vasopressor effect in the treatment of acute hypotensive states, particularly during anesthesia, and in the treatment of paroxysmal supraventricular tachycardia, administered intramuscularly or intravenously.

me•thox•sa•len (mə-thok′sə-lən) [USP] a psoralen occurring in *Ammi majus* and other plants; used orally and topically in conjunction with exposure to ultraviolet radiation to facilitate repigmentation in idiopathic vitiligo, to produce a phototoxic reaction in psoriasis, and to treat mycosis fungoides. It is also used in the treatment of cutaneous T-cell lymphoma, administered as part of photopheresis.

me•thoxy•chlor (mə-thok′sə-klor) a chlorinated hydrocarbon insecticide effective against mosquito larvae and houseflies.

meth•oxy•flu•rane (mə-thok″se-floo′rān) [USP] a highly potent inhalational anesthetic agent, used primarily to produce analgesia during the first stage of labor; its use in surgery is limited by a dose-related nephrotoxicity to procedures of short duration; it produces profound analgesia and good muscle relaxation; induction and recovery are slower than with halothane or enflurane.

me•thox•yl (mə-thok′səl) the chemical group, CH_3O—.

meth•oxy•phen•amine hy•dro•chlo•ride (mə-thok″se-fen′ə-mēn) [USP] an adrenergic used mainly as a bronchodilator in the treatment of bronchial asthma, administered orally.

8-me•thoxy•psor•a•len (mə-thok′se-sor′ə-lən) methoxsalen.

meth•sux•i•mide (meth-suk′sĭ-mīd) [USP] an anticonvulsant used in the treatment of seizures in absence epilepsy, administered orally.

meth•y•clo•thi•a•zide (meth″ĭ-klo-thi′ə-zīd) [USP] a thiazide diuretic used for treatment of hypertension and edema; administered orally.

meth•yl (meth′əl) [Gr. *methy* wine + *hylē* wood] the chemical group or radical —CH_3, sometimes abbreviated Me.

m. benzene toluene.

m. benzylidene camphor enzacamene.

m. bromide a colorless gas soluble in alcohol and benzene, used in ionization chambers and fire extinguishers and as a reagent and fumigant; it is also found in automobile exhaust. If inhaled in excessive amounts it is neurotoxic, and if a solution touches the skin it causes blistering.

m. ethyl-pyrrole a substituted pyrrole obtained from, and probably a constituent of, bilirubin.

m. hydride methane.

m. hydroxy-furfural the furfural that is produced from the hexose in the Molisch test and causes the color.

m. iodide a colorless liquid that turns brown on exposure to light, used in microscopy and in testing for pyridine. It is irritating to skin and mucous membranes and is a suspected carcinogen. Called also *iodomethane.*

m. isobutyl ketone [NF] a transparent, colorless, mobile, volatile liquid used as an alcohol denaturant in pharmaceutical preparations.

m. methacrylate a methyl ester of methacrylic acid, which polymerizes to form polymethyl methacrylate; used in the manufacture of acrylic resins (q.v.) and plastics.

m. salicylate [NF] a volatile oil with a characteristic wintergreen odor and taste; used as a counterirritant in ointments or liniments for muscle pain and also as a flavoring agent. Called also *betula oil, gaultheria oil, sweet birch oil,* and *wintergreen oil.*

m. ***tert*****-butyl ether** a solvent used to dissolve cholesterol calculi in the gallbladder; infused and aspirated cyclically via catheter over a period of several hours.

meth·yl·ace·tic ac·id (meth″əl-ə-se′tik) propionic acid.

α-meth·yl·ac·e·to·ace·tic ac·id (meth″əl-ə-se″to-ə-se′tik) acetoacetic acid methylated at the second carbon; attached to coenzyme A, it is an intermediate in isoleucine degradation. It is excreted in excess in the urine in α-methylacetoaceticaciduria.

α-meth·yl·ac·e·to·ace·tic·ac·id·uria (meth″əl-ə-se″to-ə-se″tik-as″ĭ-du′re-ə) an autosomal recessive aminoacidopathy due to deficiency of α-methylacetoacetyl CoA thiolase, the β-ketothiolase catalyzing the final step in isoleucine catabolism; it is characterized by episodes of severe metabolic ketoacidosis and urinary excretion of several intermediates of isoleucine catabolism, including α-methylacetoacetic acid.

α-meth·yl·ac·e·to·ac·e·tyl (meth″əl-ə-se″to-as′ə-tēl″) the acyl radical of α-methylacetoacetic acid; the thioester formed with coenzyme A, α-methylacetoacetyl CoA, is an intermediate in the catabolism of isoleucine.

α-meth·yl·ac·e·to·ac·e·tyl CoA thi·o·lase (meth″əl-ə-se″to-as′ə-tēl ko-a′ thi′o-lās) an acetyl-CoA *C*-acyltransferase (β-ketothiolase) specifically catalyzing the final step in isoleucine catabolism, the cleavage of α-methylacetoacetyl CoA to form acetyl CoA and propionyl CoA. Deficiency of the enzyme, an autosomal recessive trait, results in α-methylacetoaceticaciduria.

meth·yl·amine (meth′əl-ə-mēn″) a flammable, explosive gas, CH_3NH_2, used in tanning and in organic synthesis and produced naturally in some decaying fish, certain plants, and crude methanol; it is irritating to the eyes.

N**-meth·yl-D-as·par·tate (NMDA)** (meth′əl as′pahr-tāt) a neurotransmitter similar to glutamate, found in the central nervous system; a synthetic preparation is used experimentally to study the excitatory mechanisms of glutamate transmitters.

meth·yl·ate (meth′əl-āt) 1. a compound of methyl alcohol and a base. 2. to add a methyl group to a substance.

meth·yl·at·ed (meth′əl-āt″əd) containing or combined with a methyl group.

meth·yl·a·tion (meth″əl-a′shən) addition of one or more methyl groups to a substance.

DNA m. the postsynthetic addition of methyl groups to specific sites on DNA molecules; the reaction is catalyzed by DNA methyltransferases specific for nucleotide and position of methylation, and methylation of sites is passed down to daughter strands at mitosis. In eukaryotes, the C5 position of cytosine is methylated; in animal cells, at 5′-CG-3′ doublets. Methylation is involved in gene expression, and plays a role in a variety of epigenetic mechanisms, including development, X chromosome inactivation, genomic imprinting, mutability of DNA, and uncontrolled cell growth in cancer. In prokaryotes, the N6 position of adenosine is also a site of methylation, and methylation of bacterial DNA protects it from cleavage by the restriction enzymes that inactivate bacteriophage DNA and plays a role in the DNA repair process.

meth·yl·at·ro·pine ni·trate (meth″əl-at′tro-pēn) a quaternary ammonium derivative of atropine, having the same actions and uses as atropine (q.v.), but with much less effect on the central nervous system and with strong ganglionic blocking activity. Called also *atropine methonitrate* and *atropine methylnitrate.*

meth·yl·az·oxy·meth·a·nol (meth″əl-əz-ok″se-meth′ə-nol) a substance that is formed after hydrolysis of cycasin or macrozamin by intestinal bacteria and is carcinogenic to the liver, kidneys, intestine, and lungs.

meth·yl·ben·ze·tho·ni·um chlo·ride (meth″əl-ben″zə-tho′ne-əm) [USP] a disinfectant quaternary compound which is bacteriostatic for urea-splitting organisms that may cause ammonia dermatitis. It is applied topically to areas of the skin coming in contact with urine, feces, or perspiration, and is used in a rinse for diapers, bed linen, and undergarments of incontinent adults and children.

meth·yl·cel·lu·lose (meth″əl-sel′u-lōs) [USP] a methyl ether of cellulose, supplied in differing degrees of viscosity; used as a suspending and viscosity-increasing agent and tablet excipient in pharmaceutical preparations, administered orally as a laxative, and applied topically to the conjunctiva to protect the cornea during certain ophthalmic procedures and to lubricate the cornea.

hydroxypropyl m. see under *H.*

meth·yl·chlo·ro·for·mate (meth″əl-klor″o-for′māt) a lacrimatory gas used as a warning agent in fumigations with hydrogen cyanide.

meth·yl·chlo·ro·iso·thi·a·zo·li·none (meth″əl-klor″o-i″so-thi-ə-zōl′ĭ-nōn) see *methylisothiazolinone.*

3-meth·yl·cho·lan·threne (meth″əl-ko-lan′thrēn) a highly carcinogenic polycyclic aromatic hydrocarbon synthesized by pyrolytic degradation of cholic acid, deoxycholic acid, or cholesterol. It is a procarcinogen that requires metabolic activation to exert a mutagenic effect and is widely used in laboratory studies of chemical carcinogenesis. Abbreviated MCA.

meth·yl·co·bal·a·min (meth″əl-ko-bal′ə-min) a cobalamin derivative in which the substituent is a methyl group. It is one of two metabolically active forms synthesized upon ingestion of vitamin B_{12} and is the predominant form in the serum; it acts as a coenzyme in the reaction catalyzed by 5-methyltetrahydrofolate-homocysteine methyltransferase. Abbreviated MeCbl.

3-meth·yl·cro·ton·ic ac·id (meth″əl-kro-ton′ik) crotonic acid methylated at the 3 carbon; it is excreted at elevated levels in urine when 3-methylcrotonoyl-CoA carboxylase activity is impaired.

meth·yl·cro·ton·o·yl-CoA car·box·y·lase (meth″əl-kro-ton′o-əl ko-a′ kahr-bok′sə-lās) [EC 6.4.1.4] a biotin-containing enzyme of the ligase class that catalyzes the ATP-driven carboxylation of 3-methylcrotonyl CoA to form 3-methylglutaconyl CoA as a step in the use of leucine as a fuel. Deficiency of the enzyme, an autosomal recessive trait, results in 3-methylcrotonyl carboxylase deficiency; enzyme activity is also absent in multiple carboxylase deficiency (q.v.). Written also *methylcrotonyl CoA carboxylase.*

3-meth·yl·cro·ton·yl (meth″əl-kro′tə-nil″) the radical of 3-methylcrotonic acid; the thioester formed with coenzyme A, 3-methylcrotonyl CoA, is an intermediate in the degradation of leucine.

3-meth·yl·cro·to·nyl CoA car·box·y·lase de·fi·cien·cy (meth″əl-kro′tə-nil″ ko-a′ kahr-bok′sə-lās) an autosomal recessive aminoacidopathy due to deficiency of methylcrotonoyl-CoA carboxylase, which can result from mutation in either of two genes: *MCCC1* (locus: 3q25-q27), which encodes the biotin-containing alpha subunit, or *MCCC2* (locus: 5q12-q13), which encodes the non–biotin-containing beta subunit. It is characterized by increased urine levels of 3-methylcrotonylglycine, 3-methylcrotonic acid, and 3-hydroxyisovaleric acid and variable presentation of mental retardation, central nervous system dysfunction, and muscular atrophy. Written also *β-methylcrotonyl CoA carboxylase deficiency.*

3-meth·yl·cro·ton·yl·gly·cine (meth″əl-kro″to-nəl-gli′sēn) a conjugate of 3-methylcrotonic acid and glycine, formed and excreted in excess in the urine when 3-methylcrotonoyl-CoA carboxylase activity is impaired.

β-meth·yl·cro·to·nyl·gly·cin·u·ria (meth″əl-kro″to-nəl-gli″sĭ-nu′re-ə) 1. 3-methylcrotonyl CoA carboxylase deficiency. 2. excretion of 3-methylcrotonylglycine in the urine, as occurs in 3-methylcrotonyl CoA carboxylase deficiency or multiple carboxylase deficiency.

meth·yl·cy·to·sine (meth″əl-si′to-sēn) a pyrimidine occurring in deoxyribonucleic acid.

meth·yl·di·chlor·ar·sin (meth″əl-di″klor-ahr′sin) a lethal and vesicating war gas.

meth·yl·do·pa (meth″əl-do′pə) [USP] a phenylalanine derivative administered orally or intravenously in the treatment of hypertension, including that caused by renal disease.

meth·yl·do·pate hy·dro·chlo·ride (meth″əl-do′pāt) [USP] the ethyl ester hydrochloride of methyldopa, used as an antihypertensive, administered by intravenous infusion.

meth·y·lene (meth′ə-lēn) the bivalent hydrocarbon radical —CH_2— or CH_2═. Called also *methene.*

m. blue see under *blue.*

m. diphosphonate medronate.

meth·y·lene·di·oxy·am·phet·amine (MDA) (meth″ə-lēn-di-ok″se-am-fet′ə-mēn) a compound chemically related to amphetamine and mescaline that has hallucinogenic properties; it is widely abused and causes dependence.

3,4-meth·y·lene·di·oxy·meth·am·phet·amine (MDMA) (meth″ə-lēn″di-ok″se-meth″am-fet′ə-mēn) a compound chemically related to amphetamine and having hallucinogenic properties; it is widely abused. Popularly called *Ecstasy.*

5,10-meth·y·lene·tet·ra·hy·dro·fo·late (meth″ə-lēn-tet″rə-hi″dro-fo′lāt) a doubly methylated, reduced derivative of folic acid occurring as an intermediate in the transfer of methyl groups to methionine, receiving them from formaldehyde, serine, and glycine.

meth·y·lene·tet·ra·hy·dro·fo·late de·hy·dro·gen·ase (NADP⁺) (meth″ə-lēn-tet″rə-hi″dro-fo′lāt de-hi′dro-jən-ās) [EC 1.5.1.5] an enzyme activity of the oxidoreductase class that catalyzes the oxidation of 5,10-methylenetetrahydrofolate to 5,10-methenyltetrahydrofolate, using $NADP^+$ as an electron acceptor. The reaction occurs in the system of folate-mediated one-carbon transfer reactions. The enzyme activity is part of a trifunctional enzyme that also includes methenyltetrahydrofolate cyclohydrolase and formate–tetrahydrofolate ligase activities.

meth•y•lene•tet•ra•hy•dro•fo•late re•duc•tase [NAD(P)H] (meth″ə-lēn-tet″rə-hi″dro-fo′lāt re-duk′tās) [EC 1.5.1.20] an enzyme of the oxidoreductase class that catalyzes the reduction of 5,10-methylenetetrahydrofolate to 5-methyltetrahdyrofolate, using $FADH_2$ and NADH as primary and secondary electron donors, respectively. The reaction is the means by which methyl groups are generated de novo for methylation reactions. Deficiency of the enzyme, an autosomal recessive trait, results in homocystinuria due to deficiency of methionine synthase; hypomethioninemia and neurologic abnormalities are present but megaloblastic anemia is absent.

meth•y•lene•tet•ra•hy•dro•fo•late re•duc•tase (MTHFR) de•fi•cien•cy (meth″ə-lēn-tet″rə-hi″dro-fo′lāt re-duk′tās) a common, autosomal recessive, inborn error of folate metabolism caused by mutation in the *MTHFR* gene (locus: 1p36.3), which encodes the enzyme. The chief biochemical finding is homocystinuria with normal levels of plasma methionine. Clinical manifestations, age of onset, and severity are highly variable; characteristics include signs of neurologic damage ranging from psychiatric symptoms to fatal developmental delay, microcephaly, ectopia lentis, and thrombosis. Some patients are asymptomatic.

meth•y•len•o•phil (meth″ə-len′o-fil) 1. an element easily stainable with methylene blue. 2. methylenophilous.

meth•y•len•oph•i•lous (meth″ə-lən-of′ĭ-ləs) [*methylene* + Gr. *philein* to love] stainable with methylene blue.

meth•yl•er•go•no•vine mal•e•ate (meth″əl-ur″go-no′vēn) [USP] an oxytocic used especially to prevent or combat postpartum or postabortion hemorrhage and atony; administered orally, intramuscularly, and intravenously.

meth•yl•glu•ca•mine (meth″əl-gloo′kə-mēn) meglumine.

3-meth•yl•glu•ta•con•ic ac•id (meth″əl-gloo″tə-kon′ik) a dicarboxylic acid occurring at elevated levels in 3-methylglutaconicaciduria and 3-hydroxy-3-methylglutaricaciduria.

3-meth•yl•glu•ta•con•ic•ac•id•uria (meth″əl-gloo″tə-kon″ik-as″ĭ-dure-ə) 1. a genetically heterogeneous group of inherited branched-chain aminoacidopathies characterized by excessive urinary excretion of 3-methylglutaconic acid. 2. urinary excretion of 3-methylglutaconic acid.

3-m. type I an autosomal recessive disorder of leucine catabolism caused by mutation in the *AUH* gene on chromosome 9, which encodes methylglutaconyl-CoA hydratase, characterized by increased urinary excretion of 3-methylglutaconic, 3-hydroxyisovaleric, and 3-methylglutaric acids, delayed speech development, choreoathetosis, optic atrophy, and mild psychomotor delay.

3-m. type II Barth syndrome.

3-m. type III an autosomal recessive neuroophthalmologic syndrome caused by mutation in the *OPA3* gene (locus: 19q13.2-q13.3), which encodes a ubiquitously expressed protein of unknown function. It is characterized by early-onset optic atrophy and later development of choreoathetosis, spasticity, cerebellar ataxia, nystagmus, and cognitive deficits; urinary excretion of 3-methylglutaconic acid is mildly increased. Called also *Costeff optic atrophy syndrome.*

3-m. type IV a clinically heterogeneous group of autosomal recessive disorders otherwise unclassified and characterized by mildly increased urinary excretion of 3-methylglutaconic acid; characteristics are variable and include psychomotor retardation, hypotonia, neonatal respiratory distress, inguinal hernia, subaortic stenosis, simian crease, and hepatic dysfunction.

3-m. type V an autosomal recessive disorder caused by mutation in the *DNAJC19* gene (locus: 3q26.3), which encodes a mitochondrial transport protein, characterized by early-onset dilated cardiomyopathy, ataxia, growth failure, and urinary excretion of 3-methylglutaconic acid. Called also *dilated cardiomyopathy with ataxia.*

3-meth•yl•glu•ta•con•yl (meth″əl-gloo″tə-kon′əl) a radical of 3-methylglutaconic acid; the thioester formed with coenzyme A, 3-methylglutaconyl CoA, is an intermediate in the catabolism of leucine.

meth•yl•glu•ta•con•yl-CoA hy•dra•tase (meth″əl-gloo″tə-kon′əl ko-a′ hi′drə-tās) [EC 4.2.1.18] an enzyme of the lyase class that catalyzes the hydration of 3-methylglutaconyl CoA to form 3-hydroxy-3-methylglutaryl CoA, a step in the catabolism of leucine. Deficiency of the enzyme, an autosomal recessive trait, causes 3-methylglutaconicaciduria.

3-meth•yl•glu•tar•ic ac•id (meth″əl-gloo-tar′ik) a dicarboxylic acid occurring at elevated levels in the urine in one form of 3-methylglutaconicaciduria and in 3-hydroxy-3-methylglutaricaciduria.

meth•yl•gly•ox•al (meth″əl-gli-ok′səl) the compound CH_3—CO—CHO, the aldehyde of pyruvic acid; it is formed from dihydroxyacetone phosphate in the liver and is a substrate for glyoxalase.

meth•yl•gly•ox•a•lase (meth″əl-gli-ok′sə-lās) lactoylglutathione lyase.

meth•yl•gly•ox•al•i•din (meth″əl-gli″ok-sal′ĭ-din) lysidin.

3-meth•yl•his•ti•dine (meth″əl-his′tĭ-dēn) an amino acid occurring in myofibrillar proteins that is released by catabolism and excreted in the urine; the rate of urinary excretion has been proposed as an indicator of muscle protein breakdown. Abbreviated 3MH.

meth•yl•hy•dan•to•in (meth″əl-hi-dan′to-in) a crystalline compound found in fresh meat and formed by the decomposition of creatine.

me•thyl•ic (mə-thil′ik) containing methyl.

me•thyl•i•dyne (mə-thil′ĭ-dīn) the trivalent hydrocarbon radical —CH═ or CH≡. Called also *methine.*

Meth•yl•in (meth′ə-lin) trademark for preparations of methylphenidate hydrochloride.

meth•yl•in•dol (meth″əl-in′dol) skatole.

meth•yl•iso•thi•a•zo•li•none (meth″əl-i″so-thi-ə-zo′lĭ-nōn) a preservative used in conjunction with methylchloroisothiazolinone as a broad-spectrum antifungal and antibiotic agent in cosmetics, in swimming pool biocides, and in various industrial preparations. It is a common cause of contact allergy and can cause chemical burn at high concentrations.

meth•yl•ma•lon•ic ac•id (meth″əl-mə-lon′ik) a carboxylic acid occurring in excess in the blood and other body fluids in methylmalonicacidemia.

meth•yl•ma•lon•ic•ac•i•de•mia (meth″əl-mə-lon″ik-as″ĭ-de′me-ə) 1. a genetically heterogeneous, autosomal recessive aminoacidopathy characterized by an excess of methylmalonic acid in the blood and urine, with metabolic ketoacidosis, hyperglycinemia, hyperglycinuria, and hyperammonemia, and presenting in infancy as failure to thrive, persistent vomiting and dehydration, respiratory distress, and hypotonia. It results from any of several defects that cause deficiency of methylmalonyl-CoA mutase (q.v.) activity, including defects in the apoenzyme, in the biosynthesis of adenosylcobalamin (see *cob(I)alamin adenosyltransferase* and *cobalamin reductase*), in the transport of cobalamin, or in the pathway of biosynthesis common to both cobalamin-containing coenzymes; the last two defects also cause homocystinuria due to deficiency of methionine synthase (q.v.). Called also *methylmalonicaciduria.* 2. excess of methylmalonic acid in the blood.

meth•yl•ma•lon•ic•ac•id•uria (meth″əl-mə-lon″ik-as″ĭ-du′re-ə) 1. excess of methylmalonic acid in the urine. 2. methylmalonicacidemia.

meth•yl•mal•o•nyl (meth″əl-mal′ə-nəl) the radical of methylmalonic acid; the thioester it forms with coenzyme A, methylmalonyl CoA, is an intermediate in the catabolism of certain amino acids and odd-number chain length fatty acids.

meth•yl•mal•o•nyl-CoA epim•er•ase (meth″əl-mal′ə-nəl ko-a′ ə-pim′ər-ās) [EC 5.1.99.1] an enzyme of the isomerase class that catalyzes the equilibration of D- and L- isomers of methylmalonyl CoA. The reaction is part of the route by which three-carbon compounds from some amino acids and from odd-number chain length fatty acids are used as fuels. Called also *methylmalonyl-CoA racemase.*

meth•yl•mal•o•nyl-CoA mu•tase (meth″əl-mal′ə-nəl ko-a′ mu′tās) [EC 5.4.99.2] an enzyme of the isomerase class that catalyzes the isomerization of L-methylmalonyl coenzyme A to succinyl coenzyme A, requiring adenosylcobalamin as a coenzyme. The reaction is a step in the use of isoleucine, threonine, valine, propionate, and other odd-number chain length fatty acids as fuels. Deficiency of enzyme activity, which may be caused by defects in the apoenzyme, in the coenzyme, or in cobalamin metabolism, results in methylmalonicacidemia.

meth•yl•mal•o•nyl-CoA ra•ce•mase (meth″əl-mal′ə-nəl ko-a′ ra′sə-mās) methylmalonyl-CoA epimerase.

meth•yl•mer•cap•tan (meth″əl-mər-kap′tən) a gas formed in the intestines by the decomposition of proteins; said to impart to the urine the odor noticed after eating asparagus, and to the breath the characteristic odor of fetor hepaticus.

meth•yl•mer•cu•ry (meth″əl-mur′kūr-e) methyl mercury; see under *mercury.*

meth•yl•meth•ac•ry•late (meth″əl-meth-ak′rə-lāt) see under *methyl.*

meth•yl•mor•phine (meth″əl-mor′fēn) codeine.

Meth•yl•o•bac•te•ri•a•ceae (meth″ə-lo-bak-tēr″e-a′se-e) a family of gram-negative or gram-variable bacteria of the order Rhizobiales. The one genus of medical importance is *Methylobacterium.*

Meth•yl•o•bac•te•ri•um (meth″ə-lo-bak-tēr′e-əm) a genus of rose-colored, gram-negative, aerobic, rod-shaped bacteria of the family Methylobacteriaceae that can facultatively use methane or methanol as sources of carbon and energy; some species have occasionally been found in opportunistic infections such as bacteremia or those in the respiratory tract or urinary tract.

3-meth•yl-2-oxo•bu•ta•no•ate de•hy•dro•gen•ase (2-meth•yl•pro•pa•no•yl-trans•fer•ring) (meth′əl ok″so-bu″tə-no′āt de-hi′dro-jən-ās meth″əl-pro″pəno′əl trans′fər-ing) [EC 1.2.4.4] official nomenclature for *branched-chain α-keto acid dehydrogenase.*

meth·yl·par·a·ben (meth″əl-par′ə-bən) [NF] an antifungal compound, closely related to butylparaben, ethylparaben, and propylparaben; used as a preservative in pharmaceutic preparations.

m. sodium [NF] the sodium salt of methylparaben, having the same actions and uses as the base.

meth·yl·pen·tose (meth″əl-pen′tōs) a hexose derivative in which carbon 6 exists in reduced form, as a methyl group; e.g., *fucose.* See also *deoxyhexose.*

meth·yl·phen·i·date hy·dro·chlo·ride (meth″əl-fen′ĭ-dāt) [USP] a central stimulant used in the treatment of attention-deficit/hyperactivity disorder, narcolepsy, and certain forms of depression associated with medical conditions which would preclude treatment with conventional antidepressants; administered orally.

meth·yl·pred·nis·o·lone (meth″əl-pred-nis′ə-lōn) [USP] a synthetic glucocorticoid derived from progesterone, used in replacement therapy for adrenocortical insufficiency and as an antiinflammatory and immunosuppressant in a wide variety of disorders; administered orally.

m. acetate [USP] the 21-acetate ester of methylprednisolone, administered topically as an antiinflammatory, by intramuscular injection in replacement therapy for adrenocortical insufficiency, and by intra-articular, intramuscular, intralesional, or soft-tissue injection as an antiinflammatory and immunosuppressant in a wide variety of disorders.

m. hemisuccinate [USP] the hemisuccinate salt of methylprednisolone, having actions and uses similar to those of the base.

m. sodium succinate [USP] the 21-succinate sodium salt of methylprednisolone, having actions and uses similar to those of the base; it is highly soluble in water and is chiefly used for the rapid achievement of high blood levels of methylprednisolone in short-term emergency treatment; administered by intramuscular or intravenous injection.

meth·yl·pu·rines (meth″əl-pu′rēnz) see under *purine.*

meth·yl·py·ra·pone (meth″əl-pi′rə-pōn) metyrapone.

4-meth·yl-1H-py·ra·zole (meth″əl-pi′rə-zōl) fomepizole.

meth·yl·py·ri·dine (meth″əl-pi′rĭ-dēn) a basic substance oxidized in the body to pyridine-carboxylic acid.

meth·yl·ro·san·i·line chlo·ride (meth″əl-ro-zan′ĭ-lēn) gentian violet; see under *gentian.*

meth·yl·tes·tos·te·rone (meth″əl-tes-tos′tə-rōn) [USP] a synthetic anabolic-androgenic steroid derived from cholesterol, having actions similar to those of testosterone (q.v.); used in males in the treatment of primary and secondary hypogonadism and delayed puberty, and in postmenopausal females in the palliation of metastatic breast carcinoma; administered orally.

5-meth·yl·tet·ra·hy·dro·fo·late (meth″əl-tet″rə-hi″dro-fo′lāt) a substituted, reduced derivative of folic acid, occurring as a source of methyl groups for the regeneration of methionine; it is formed by reduction of 5,10-methylenetetrahydrofolate and is the principal form of folic acid during transport and storage in the body.

meth·yl·the·o·bro·mine (meth″əl-the″o-bro′mēn) caffeine.

meth·yl·thi·o·nine chlo·ride (meth″əl-thi′o-nēn) methylene blue; see under *blue.*

meth·yl·trans·fer·ase (meth″əl-trans′fər-ās) [EC 2.1.1] any member of the sub-subclass of enzymes of the transferase class that catalyzes the transfer of a methyl group from one compound to another. Called also *transmethylase.*

5-meth·yl·ura·cil (meth″əl-ūr′ə-sil) thymine.

meth·yl·xan·thine (meth″əl-zan′thēn) any of the methylated derivatives of xanthine, including caffeine, theobromine, and theophylline and their derivatives. Methylxanthines relax smooth muscle, stimulate the central nervous system and cardiac muscle, and produce diuresis; they are used clinically as bronchodilators.

meth·y·ser·gide (meth″ĭ-sur′jīd) a potent serotonin antagonist having direct vasoconstrictor effects.

m. maleate [USP] the maleate salt of methysergide, having the same actions as the base; used in the prophylaxis of vascular (e.g., migraine, cluster) headache, administered orally.

Met·i·cor·ten (met″ĭ-kor′tən) trademark for a preparation of prednisone.

met·i·pran·o·lol hy·dro·chlo·ride (met″ĭ-pran′ə-lol) a nonselective beta-adrenergic blocking agent, applied topically to the conjunctiva in the treatment of glaucoma and ocular hypertension.

met·myo·glo·bin (mət-mi″o-glo′bin) a compound formed from myoglobin by oxidation of the ferrous to the ferric state.

met·o·clo·pra·mide hy·dro·chlo·ride (met″o-klo′prə-mīd) [USP] a prokinetic dopamine receptor antagonist that stimulates gastric motility, used as an antiemetic, as an adjunct in gastrointestinal radiology and intestinal intubation, and in the treatment of gastroparesis and gastroesophageal reflux; administered orally, intramuscularly, and intravenously.

met·o·cu·rine io·dide (met″o-ku′rēn) a nondepolarizing neuromuscular blocking agent, used as an anesthesia adjunct to induce skeletal muscle relaxation and to reduce the intensity of muscle contractions in convulsive therapy; administered intravenously.

me·to·la·zone (mə-to′lə-zōn) [USP] a sulfonamide derivative that has a different chemical structure from but the same pharmacologic actions as the thiazide diuretics, used in the treatment of hypertension and edema; administered orally.

me·ton·y·my (mə-ton′ĭ-me) [*meta-* + Gr. *onyma* name] a disturbance of language seen in schizophrenic disorders in which an inappropriate but related term is used instead of the correct one.

me·top·a·gus (mə-top′ə-gəs) metopopagus.

me·top·ic (me-top′ik) frontal (def. 1).

me·to·pi·on (mə-to′pe-on) the craniometric point on the median line of the forehead, midway between the frontal eminences.

Met·o·pi·rone (met′o-pi′rōn) trademark for preparations of metyrapone.

met·o·pism (met′o-piz″əm) the persistence of the frontal suture.

metop(o)- [Gr. *metōpon* forehead] a combining form denoting relationship to the forehead.

met·o·pop·a·gus (met″o-pop′ə-gəs) [*metopo-* + *-pagus*] a craniopagus in which the fusion is in the region of the forehead.

met·o·pro·lol (met″o-pro′lol) a cardioselective β_1-adrenergic blocking agent.

m. succinate [USP] the succinate salt of metoprolol, used for the treatment of angina pectoris and hypertension; administered orally.

m. tartrate [USP] the tartrate salt of metoprolol, used in the treatment of hypertension, angina pectoris, and myocardial infarction; administered orally and intravenously.

Met·or·chis (met-or′kis) [*meta-* + Gr. *orchis* testicle] a genus of trematodes of the family Opisthorchiidae. *M. al′bidus* and *M. conjunc′tus* parasitize cats, dogs, and other mammals.

met·o·ser·pate hy·dro·chlo·ride (met″o-sur′pāt) a veterinary sedative used in chickens.

me·tra (me′trə) [Gr. *metra* womb] uterus.

me·tra·term (me′trə-tərm) [*metr-* + L. *terminus* boundary] the external opening of the uterus in some tapeworms (Diphyllobothriidae).

me·tra·to·nia (me″trə-to′ne-ə) [*metr-* + *atonia*] uterine atony.

me·tre (me′tər) meter.

met·re·chos·co·py (met″rə-kos′kə-pe) [Gr. *metron* measure + *ēchō* sound + *-scopy*] combined mensuration, auscultation, and inspection.

me·trec·to·pia (me″trek-to′pe-ə) [*metr-* + *ectopia*] uterine displacement.

me·treu·ryn·ter (me″troo-rin′tər) [*metr-* + Gr. *eurynein* to stretch] an inflatable bag for dilating the cervical canal.

met·ric (met′rik) [Gr. *metron* measure] 1. pertaining to measures based on the meter; see Appendix 7. 2. having the meter as a basis.

met·ri·fo·nate (met″rĭ-fo′nāt) [USP] an organophosphorus insecticide having potent anticholinesterase activity; especially effective against *Schistosoma haematobium.* Administered topically or sometimes orally to kill parasites on the skin or inside the body. In veterinary medicine it is most often administered orally as an anthelmintic. Overdosage can cause organophosphorus compound poisoning (q.v.). Called also *trichlorfon* and *trichlorphon.*

met·rio·ce·phal·ic (met″re-o-sə-fal′ik) [Gr. *metrios* moderate + *cephal-* + *-ic*] having a skull with a vertical index between 72 and 77.

met·ri·pho·nate (met′rĭ-fo′nāt) metrifonate.

me·tri·tis (mə-tri′tis) [*metr-* + *-itis*] inflammation of the uterus. Several varieties are named, according to the part of the organ affected—cervical, corporeal, interstitial, and parenchymatous.

contagious equine m. (CEM) a highly contagious venereal disease of horses caused by infection with *Taylorella equigenitalis;* symptoms may include endometritis and salpingitis with a profuse purulent discharge, but sometimes infection is subclinical with only a lowered conception rate.

m. dis′secans, dissecting m. metritis characterized by the passage of fragments or large masses of the necrotic uterine wall.

mastitis-m.-agalactia lactation failure in swine; see under *failure.*

puerperal m. infection of the uterus of the puerperal woman.

me·triz·a·mide (mə-triz′ə-mīd) a water-soluble, non-ionic, iodinated derivative of benzoic acid used as a radiopaque medium in radiography and computed tomography.

met·ri·zo·ate so·di·um (met″rĭ-zo′āt) an iodinated ionic compound used as a radiopaque medium.

metr(o)- [Gr. *mētra* uterus] a combining form denoting relationship to the uterus; see also *hyster(o)-*.

me•tro•cele (me′tro-sēl) uterine hernia.

Met•ro•Cream (met′ro-krēm″) trademark for a preparation of metronidazole.

me•tro•cys•to•sis (me″tro-sis-to′sis) formation of cysts in the uterus.

me•tro•en•do•me•tri•tis (me″tro-en″do-me-tri′tis) combined inflammation of the uterus and its mucous membranes.

me•tro•fi•bro•ma (me″tro-fi-bro′mə) [*metro-* + *fibroma*] uterine leiomyoma.

Met•ro•Gel (met′ro-jel) trademark for preparations of metronidazole.

me•trog•e•nous (mə-troj′ə-nəs) derived from the uterus.

me•trog•ra•phy (mə-trog′rə-fe) hysterography.

Met•ro I.V. (met′ro) trademark for a preparation of metronidazole.

me•tro•leu•kor•rhea (me″tro-loo″ko-re′ə) leukorrhea of uterine origin.

me•trol•o•gy (mə-trol′ə-je) [Gr. *metron* measure + *-logy*] the science which deals with measurement.

Met•ro•Lo•tion (met′ro-lo″shən) trademark for a preparation of metronidazole.

me•tro•lym•phan•gi•tis (me″tro-lim″fan-ji′tis) inflammation of the uterine lymphatic vessels.

me•tro•men•or•rha•gia (me″tro-men″o-ra′jə) menometrorrhagia.

met•ro•ni•da•zole (met″ro-ni′də-zōl) [USP] an antiprotozoal and antibacterial effective against obligate anaerobes; administered orally and intravaginally in bacterial vaginosis and *Trichomonas vaginalis* infection in females and orally in *T. vaginalis* infection in males and intestinal amebiasis. It is used orally or intravenously in extraintestinal amebiasis and infection by obligate anaerobic bacteria and intravenously for the prophylaxis of colonic perioperative infection. It is also used topically in the treatment of rosacea.

m. **benzoate** [USP] the benzoate salt of metronidazole, having the same uses as the base; administered orally.

m. **hydrochloride** the hydrochloride salt of metronidazole, administered intravenously for the same indications for which the base is used intravenously.

me•trono•scope (mə-tron′ə-skōp) an instrument for giving exercises in rhythmic reading to correct poorly coordinated ocular movements.

me•trop•a•thy (mə-trop′ə-the) [*metro-* + *-pathy*] hysteropathy.

me•tro•peri•to•ne•al (me″tro-per″ĭ-to-ne′əl) pertaining to or communicating between the uterus and peritoneum or peritoneal cavity.

me•tro•peri•to•ni•tis (me″tro-per″ĭ-to-ni′tis) [*metro-* + *peritonitis*] inflammation of the peritoneum about the uterus, or peritonitis resulting from infection after metritis.

me•tro•phle•bi•tis (me″tro-flə-bi′tis) [*metro-* + *phlebo-* + *-itis*] inflammation of the veins of the uterus.

me•tro•plas•ty (me′tro-plas″te) plastic surgery on the uterus; called also *uteroplasty*. **metroplas′tic** *adj*

me•trop•o•lis (mə-trop′ə-lis) [Gr. *mētropolis* mother-state, as opposed to her colonies] the area in which a particular species of organisms commonly occurs.

me•tro•pto•sis (me″trop-to′sis, me″tro-to′sis) uterine prolapse.

me•tror•rha•gia (me″tro-ra′jə) [*metro-* + *-rrhagia*] uterine bleeding, usually of variable amount, occurring at completely irregular but frequent intervals; sometimes the period of flow is prolonged.

me•tror•rhea (me″tro-re′ə) [*metro-* + *-rrhea*] a free or abnormal uterine discharge.

me•tror•rhex•is (me″tro-rek′sis) [*metro-* + *-rrhexis*] rupture of the uterus.

me•tro•sal•pin•gi•tis (me″tro-sal″pin-ji′tis) [*metro-* + *salping-* + *-itis*] inflammation of the uterus and uterine tubes.

me•tro•scope (me′tro-skōp) hysteroscope.

me•tros•ta•sis (mə-tros′tə-sis) [Gr. *metron* measure + *-stasis*] a state in which the length of a muscle fiber is relatively fixed, and at which length it contracts and relaxes.

me•tro•stax•is (me″tro-stak′sis) [*metro-* + *staxis*] a slight but persistent escape of blood from the uterus.

me•tro•ste•no•sis (me″tro-stə-no′sis) [*metro-* + *stenosis*] contraction or stenosis of the cavity of the uterus, as in Asherman syndrome.

-metry [Gr. *metrein* to measure] a word termination denoting the measurement of, or the science of measuring, an object specified by the word stem to which the termination is affixed.

M. et sig. [L.] mi′sce et sig′na (mix and write a label).

met•u•la (met′u-lə) [L., dim. of *meta* cone] a flask-shaped branch of the conidiophore of certain fungi, which has phialides; seen in *Aspergillus*, *Penicillium*, and other genera. Called also *sterigma*. See illustration at *mold*.

me•tyr•a•pone (mə-tēr′ə-pōn) [USP] an inhibitor of the enzyme steroid 11β-hydroxylase; used in a test of hypothalamic-pituitary function. See *metyrapone test*, under *tests*.

me•ty•ro•sine (mə-ti′ro-sēn) [USP] an inhibitor of tyrosine 3-monooxygenase, which catalyzes the first step in catecholamine synthesis, used to control hypertensive attacks in pheochromocytoma; administered orally.

MeV megaelectron volt (one million electron volts).

Mev•a•cor (mev′ə-kor) trademark for a preparation of lovastatin.

me•val•o•nate (mə-val′o-nāt) a salt, ester, or anionic form of mevalonic acid.

me•val•o•nate ki•nase (mə-val′o-nāt ki′nās) [EC 2.7.1.36] an enzyme of the transferase class that catalyzes the ATP-dependent phosphorylation of mevalonate as a step in the biosynthesis of cholesterol and other isoprenoids. Deficiency of the enzyme causes mevalonicaciduria.

mev•a•lon•ic ac•id (mev-ə-lon′ik) a carboxylic acid precursor of sterols and other isoprenoids; it accumulates abnormally in mevalonicaciduria.

me•va•lon•ic•ac•id•uria (mev-ə-lon″ik-as″ĭ-du′re-ə) an autosomal recessive aminoacidopathy caused by mutation in the *MVK* gene (locus: 12q24), which encodes mevalonate kinase; the resulting deficiency of the enzyme is characterized by excessive urinary excretion of mevalonic acid, with variable clinical symptoms including developmental delay, hypotonia, hepatosplenomegaly, and failure to thrive.

mex•il•e•tine hy•dro•chlo•ride (mek′sĭ-lə-tēn) an oral antiarrhythmic agent, similar to lidocaine in structure and action, used in the treatment of life-threatening ventricular arrhythmias.

Mex•i•til (mek′sĭ-til) trademark for a preparation of mexiletine hydrochloride.

Mey•en•burg complexes (mi′ən-boorg) [Hans von *Meyenburg*, German-born pathologist in Switzerland, 20th century] see under *complex*.

Mey•er disease (mi′ər) [Hans Wilhelm *Meyer*, Danish physician, 1824–1895] see under *disease*.

Mey•er line, organ, sinus (mi′ər) [Georg Hermann von *Meyer*, German anatomist, 1815–1892] see under *line*, *organ*, and *sinus*.

Mey•er loop (mi′ər) [Adolf B. *Meyer*, American psychiatrist, 1866–1950] see under *loop*.

Mey•er-Ar•cham•bault loop (mi′ər ahr-shahm-bo′) [A.B. *Meyer*; La Salle *Archambault*, American neurologist, 1879–1940] Meyer loop.

Mey•er-Betz disease (mi′ər-betz′) [Friedrich *Meyer-Betz*, German physician, early 20th century] see under *disease*.

Mey•er-Schwick•er•ath and Wey•ers syndrome (mi′ər-shvik′ə-raht vi′ərz) [Gerhard Rudolph Edmund *Meyer-Schwickerath*, German ophthalmologist, born 1920; Helmut *Weyers*, German pediatrician, 20th century] oculodentodigital dysplasia; see under *dysplasia*.

Mey•nert cells, commissure, etc. (mi′nərt) [Theodor Herman *Meynert*, German neurologist and psychiatrist in Vienna, 1833–1892] see under *cell* and *commissure*, and see *nucleus basalis telencephali* and *tractus habenulointerpeduncularis*.

me•ze•re•in (mə-ze′re-in) a toxic glycoside found in *Daphne mezereum*, causing severe or even fatal irritation of the alimentary tract when the plant is eaten.

me•ze•re•um (me-ze′re-əm) [L.] the dried bark of *Daphne mezereum*, formerly used as a diaphoretic, diuretic, and stimulant; it is highly irritating to the gastrointestinal tract and produces vesication when rubbed on the skin.

Mez•lin (mez′lin) trademark for a preparation of mezlocillin sodium.

mez•lo•cil•lin so•di•um (mez″lo-sil′in) [USP] a semisynthetic, broad-spectrum penicillin of the ureidopenicillin group, effective against a wide range of gram-positive and gram-negative aerobic and anaerobic bacteria; especially useful in treating mixed infections; administered intramuscularly or intravenously.

μF microfarad.

MFR monthly fecundity rate.

M. ft. [L.] mistu′ra fi′at (let a mixture be made).

Mg magnesium.

mg milligram.

μg microgram *(on The JCAHO "Do Not Use" List)*.

MGUS monoclonal gammopathy of undetermined significance; see *benign monoclonal gammopathy*, under *gammopathy*.

3MH 3-methylhistidine.

MHA-TP microhemagglutination assay–*Treponema pallidum.*

MHC major histocompatibility complex.

mho (mo) [*ohm* spelled backwards, because it is a reciprocal ohm] former name for *siemens.*

MHz megahertz.

MI myocardial infarction.

Mi·a·cal·cin (mi″ə-kal′sin) trademark for a preparation of calcitonin-salmon.

Mi·an·eh bug (me′ə-na) [the city of *Mianeh*, Iran] see under *bug.*

mi·an·ser·in hy·dro·chlo·ride (me-an′sər-in) a tetracyclic antidepressant with antihistaminic effects; administered orally.

Mi·bel·li porokeratosis (me-bel′e) [Vittorio *Mibelli*, Italian dermatologist, 1860–1910] see under *porokeratosis.*

MIBG, mIBG iobenguane (*m*-iodobenzylguanidine).

MIBI sestamibi.

MIC minimal inhibitory concentration.

mi·ca (mi′kə) [L.] any of a group of complex aluminum silicate compounds; see also *mica pneumoconiosis*, under *pneumoconiosis.*

mi·ca·ceous (mi-ka′shəs) 1. pertaining to mica. 2. resembling mica, or occurring in silvery gray flakes.

mi·ca·fun·gin so·di·um (mi″kə-fun′jin) an antifungal agent used in treatment of candidiasis; administered by intravenous infusion.

Mi·ca·nol (mi′kə-nol) trademark for a preparation of anthralin.

Mi·car·dis (mi-kahr′dis) trademark for a preparation of telmisartan.

Mi·ca·tin (mi′kə-tin) trademark for preparations of miconazole nitrate.

mi·ca·tion (mi-ka′shən) any quick motion, such as winking.

mi·ca·to·sis (mi″kə-to′sis) pneumoconiosis due to inhalation of and tissue reaction to mica particles.

mi·cel·la (mi-sel′ə) see *micelle.*

mi·celle (mi-sel′) a colloid particle formed by an aggregation of small molecules.

Mi·chae·lis constant (mĭ-ka′lis) [Leonor *Michaelis*, German-born American biochemist, 1875–1949] see under *constant.*

Mi·chae·lis rhomboid (mĭ-ka′lis) [Gustav Adolf *Michaelis*, German obstetrician, 1798–1848] see under *rhomboid.*

Mi·chae·lis-Gut·mann bodies (mĭ-ka′lis goot′mahn) [L. *Michaelis;* C. *Gutmann*, German physician, 20th century] see under *body.*

Mi·chae·lis-Men·ten equation (mĭ-ka′lis men′tən) [L. *Michaelis;* Maude Lenore *Menten*, American physician, 1879–1960] see under *equation.*

Mi·chel aplasia, deafness (me-shel′) [E.M. *Michel*, French physician, 19th century] see under *aplasia* and *deafness.*

mi·con·a·zole (mi-kon′ə-zōl) [USP] an imidazole derivative used as a broad-spectrum antifungal agent; administered by intravenous infusion in the treatment of systemic fungal infections and topically in the treatment of various forms of tinea and cutaneous candidiasis.

m. nitrate [USP] the nitrate salt of miconazole; used topically in the treatment of various forms of tinea and cutaneous candidiasis, and intravaginally in the treatment of vulvovaginal candidiasis.

Mi·cra·nin (mi′krə-nin″) trademark for a combination preparation of meprobamate and aspirin.

mi·cren·ce·pha·lia (mi″krən-sə-fa′le-ə) micrencephaly.

mi·cren·ceph·a·lon (mi″krən-sef′ə-lon) [*micr-* + *encephalon*] a small brain.

mi·cren·ceph·a·lous (mi″krən-sef′ə-ləs) having a small brain.

mi·cren·ceph·a·ly (mi″krən-sef′ə-le) [*micr-* + Gr. *enkephalos* brain] abnormal smallness of the brain.

MIC·Rho·GAM (mi′kro-gam″) trademark for a preparation of $Rh_0(D)$ immune globulin.

micr(o)- [Gr. *mikros* small] a prefix denoting small size; also used in naming units of measurement (symbol μ) to indicate one millionth (10^{-6}) of the unit designated by the root with which it is combined.

mi·cro·abra·sion (mi′kro-ə-bra″zhən) removal of minute amounts of dental enamel using an abrasive compound in order to correct enamel defects.

mi·cro·ab·scess (mi″kro-ab′ses) a small, localized collection of pus.

Munro m. a small focal collection of pyknotic polymorphonuclear leukocytes within the parakeratotic portion of the stratum corneum. It is a cardinal sign of active psoriasis and is also found in other dermatoses such as seborrheic dermatitis. Called also *Munro abscess.* Cf. *spongiform pustule.*

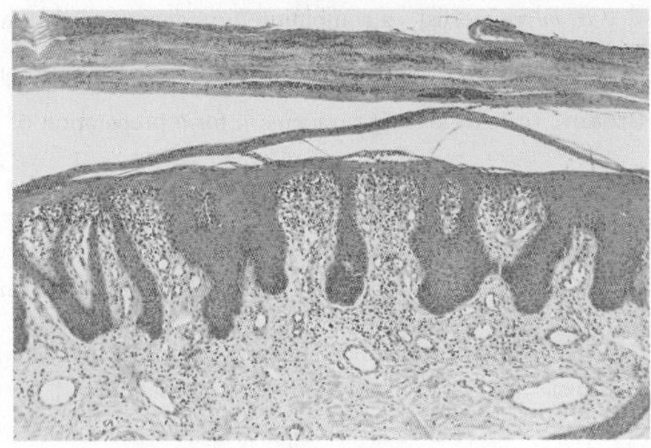

■ Munro microabscesses, together with marked epidermal hyperplasia and parakeratotic scale, within the superficial epidermal layers in psoriasis.

Pautrier m. one of the well-defined collections of atypical mononuclear cells found in nonspongiotic intraepidermal vesicles in T-cell lymphomas and mycosis fungoides. Called also *Pautrier abscess.*

mi·cro·ad·e·nec·to·my (mi″kro-ad″ə-nek′tə-me) microadenomectomy.

mi·cro·ad·e·no·ma (mi″kro-ad″ə-no′mə) 1. any adenoma too small to be easily visualized by usual radiographic techniques. 2. specifically, a pituitary adenoma less than 10 mm in diameter and not visible by usual radiographic techniques; most endocrine-active adenomas are this size and are detected because of their hormone activities. Cf. *macroadenoma.*

mi·cro·ad·e·no·mec·to·my (mi″kro-ad″ə-no-mek′tə-me) surgical removal of a microadenoma; called also *microadenectomy.*

mi·cro·aero·bic (mi-kro-ār-o′bik) microaerophilic.

mi·cro·aero·phile (mi″kro-ār′o-fīl) a microaerophilic microorganism.

mi·cro·aero·phil·ic (mi″kro-ār′o-fil″ik) [*micro-* + *aero-* + *-philic*] requiring oxygen for growth but at lower concentration than is present in the atmosphere; said of bacteria.

mi·cro·aer·oph·i·lous (mi″kro-ār-of′ĭ-ləs) microaerophilic.

mi·cro·aero·to·nom·e·ter (mi″kro-ār″o-to-nom′ə-tər) an instrument for measuring the volume of gases in the blood.

mi·cro·ag·gre·gate (mi″kro-ag′rə-gət) a collection of microscopic particles, such as that of platelets, leukocytes, and fibrin in stored blood.

mi·cro·al·bu·min·uria (mi″kro-al-bu″min-u′re-ə) urinary excretion of albumin in quantities that are above the reference interval but too low to be measured by conventional dipstick tests; it is an early indicator of glomerulopathy.

mi·cro·aleu·rio·spore (mi″kro-ə-loo′re-o-spor) a small aleuriospore; the term is sometimes used interchangeably with *microconidium.*

mi·cro·am·me·ter (mi″kro-am′me-tər) an instrument for measuring currents in the microampere range.

mi·cro·am·pere (μA) (mi″kro-am′pēr) one millionth (10^{-6}) of an ampere.

mi·cro·anal·y·sis (mi″kro-ə-nal′ə-sis) [*micro-* + *analysis*] the chemical analysis of minute quantities of material.

mi·cro·an·as·to·mo·sis (mi″kro-ən-as″tə-mo′sis) anastomosis between very small tubular structures.

mi·cro·anat·o·my (mi″kro-ə-nat′ə-me) histology, especially organology.

mi·cro·an·eu·rysm (mi″kro-an′u-riz″əm) a microscopic aneurysm, a characteristic feature of diabetes mellitus.

mi·cro·an·gi·op·a·thy (mi″kro-an″je-op′ə-the) [*micro-* + *angiopathy*] angiopathy involving the small blood vessels. **microangiopath′ic** *adj*

diabetic m. the presence of generalized basement membrane thickening of capillaries throughout many vascular beds as a complication of diabetes mellitus.

thrombotic m. the formation of thrombi in the arterioles and capillaries; some authorities propose this as a name for a single syndrome that would include both thrombotic thrombocytopenic purpura and hemolytic uremic syndrome.

mi·cro·an·gi·os·co·py (mi″kro-an″je-os′kə-pe) capillaroscopy.

mi·cro·ar·ray (mi′kro-ə-ra″) an arrangement of DNA samples, consisting of a set of DNA spots, typically 200 μm or less in diameter, on a substrate; used for automated high-throughput matching of known and unknown DNA samples. Cf. *macroarray.*

mi·cro·au·toph·a·gy (mi″kro-aw-toph′ə-je) autophagy in which small amounts of cytoplasm or individual organelles are engulfed, either by invagination of a lysosomal membrane or by invagination of the endosomal membrane during the formation of multivesicular bodies. Cf *macroautophagy.*

Mi•cro•as•ca•ceae (mi″kro-as-ka′se-e) a family of fungi of the order Microascales, subdivision Ascomycotina, which are mostly saprobes; pathogenic genera include *Microascus* and *Pseudallescheria.*

Mi•cro•as•ca•les (mi″kro-as-ka′lēz) [*micro-* + *ascus*] an order of perfect fungi of the subphylum Ascomycotina, consisting mainly of saprobes from soil and dung and characterized by prototunicate asci; it includes the family Microascaceae.

Mi•cro•as•cus (mi″kro-as′kəs) a genus of fungi of the family Microascaceae. *M. cine′reus* has been isolated from onychomycosis and other human infections.

mi•cro•bac•te•ria (mi″kro-bak-tēr′e-ə) [L.] plural of *microbacterium.*

Mi•cro•bac•te•ri•a•ceae (mi″kro-bak-tēr″e-a′se-e) a family of bacteria of the suborder Micrococcineae, order Actinomycetales, grouped together on the basis of 5S ribosomal RNA sequence analysis; pathogenic organisms are included in the genus *Microbacterium.*

Mi•cro•bac•te•ri•um (mi″kro-bak-tēr′e-əm) [*micro-* + *bacterium*] a genus of bacteria of the family Microbacteriaceae, consisting of small diphtheroid, motile or nonmotile, gram-positive rods, found in dairy products; organisms are obligately aerobic, non–spore-forming, and catalase-positive and are characterized by resistance to heat. It is an opportunistic pathogen, causing nosocomial infections in debilitated and immunocompromised patients. The type species is *M. lac′ticum.*

mi•cro•bac•te•ri•um (mi″kro-bak-tēr′e-əm) pl. *microbacte′ria* [L.] 1. an organism belonging to the genus *Microbacterium.* 2. a microorganism.

mi•cro•bal•ance (mi′kro-bal″əns) a balance for measuring minute quantities.

mi•cro•bar (mi′kro-bahr) one millionth (10^{-6}) of a bar.

mi•crobe (mi′krōb) [*micro-* + Gr. *bios* life] 1. microorganism. 2. sometimes restricted to microorganisms that cause disease.

mi•cro•bi•al (mi-kro′be-əl) of or pertaining to or caused by microbes.

mi•cro•bi•an (mi-kro′be-ən) microbial.

mi•cro•bic (mi-kro′bik) microbial.

mi•cro•bi•ci•dal (mi-kro″bĭ-si′dəl) lethal to microbes; cf. *antimicrobial.*

mi•cro•bi•cide (mi-kro′bĭ-sīd″) [*microbe* + *-cide*] 1. a substance that destroys microbes; see also *antimicrobial.* 2. a substance that destroys infectious agents, including also viruses; sometimes used specifically for that used to prevent transmission of sexually transmitted diseases, such as HIV.

mi•cro•bio•as•say (mi″kro-bi″o-as′a) the determination of minute quantities of an active substance or nutrient factor by a biologic method.

mi•cro•bi•ol•o•gist (mi″kro-bi-ol′ə-jist) a specialist in microbiology.

mi•cro•bi•ol•o•gy (mi″kro-bi-ol′ə-je) [*micro-* + *biology*] the science that deals with the study of microorganisms, including algae, bacteria, fungi, protozoa, and viruses. **microbiolog′ical** *adj*

mi•cro•bio•pho•tom•e•ter (mi″kro-bi″o-fo-tom′ə-tər) an instrument for measuring the growth of bacterial cultures by the turbidity of the medium.

mi•cro•bi•o•ta (mi″kro-bi-o′tə) the microscopic living organisms of a region; the combined microflora and microfauna of a region. **microbiot′ic** *adj*

mi•cro•blast (mi′kro-blast″) [*micro-* + *-blast*] an abnormally small erythroblast.

mi•cro•ble•pha•ria (mi″kro-blə-far′e-ə) [*micro-* + *blephar-* + *-ia*] a developmental anomaly characterized by abnormal shortness of the vertical dimensions of the eyelids.

mi•cro•bleph•a•rism (mi″kro-blef′ə-riz″əm) microblepharia.

mi•cro•bleph•a•ry (mi″kro-blef′ə-re) microblepharia.

mi•cro•body (mi′kro-bod″e) any of a group of related ovoid or spherical, granular, membrane-bound organelles containing oxidative enzymes and other substances, assembled from proteins synthesized in the cytoplasm on free ribosomes. Types include *peroxisomes* (found in animals and some plants), *glycosomes* (protozoa), and *glyoxysomes* (plants and microorganisms).

mi•cro•bra•chia (mi″kro-bra′ke-ə) [*micro-* + *brachia*] abnormal smallness of the arms.

mi•cro•bra•chi•us (mi″kro-bra′ke-əs) [*micro-* + Gr. *brachiōn* arm] a fetus with abnormally small arms.

mi•cro•bren•ner (mi″kro-bren′ər) [*micro-* + Ger. *Brenner* burner] a needle-pointed electric cautery.

mi•cro•bub•bles (mi′kro-bub″əlz) very small bubbles that can be burst by sufficiently intense ultrasound, used as contrast agents in ultrasonography and therapeutically to dissolve blood clots and to deliver therapeutic agents such as drugs.

mi•cro•bu•ret (mi″kro-bu-ret′) a buret with a capacity of the order of 0.1 to 10 mL, with graduated intervals of 0.001 to 0.02 mL.

mi•cro•cal•ci•fi•ca•tion (mi″kro-kal″sĭ-fĭ-ka′shən) a minute area of calcification in the tissues.

mi•cro•cal•ci•fi•cec•to•my (mi″kro-kal″sĭ-fĭ-sek′tə-me) surgical excision of microcalcifications.

mi•cro•ca•lix (mi″kro-ka′liks) a very small renal calix arising by caliceal branching, usually at the side of a calix of normal size. Spelled also *microcalyx.*

mi•cro•ca•lyx (mi″kro-ka′liks) microcalix.

mi•cro•can•nu•la (mi′kro-kan″u-lə) a cannula of extremely small caliber.

mi•cro•car•ci•no•ma (mi″kro-kahr″sĭ-no′mə) a carcinoma that is at a very small or preclinical stage.

papillary m. of thyroid, papillary thyroid m. a papillary thyroid carcinoma that measures less than 1 cm in diameter; called also *occult papillary thyroid carcinoma* and *occult papillary carcinoma of thyroid gland.*

mi•cro•car•dia (mi″kro-kahr′de-ə) [*micro-* + *cardia*] smallness of the heart.

mi•cro•ce•pha•lia (mi″kro-sə-fa′le-ə) microcephaly.

mi•cro•ceph•a•lus (mi″kro-sef′ə-ləs) microcephaly.

mi•cro•ceph•a•ly (mi″kro-sef′ə-le) [*micro-* + *cephaly*] abnormal smallness of the head, usually associated with mental retardation. Called also nanocephaly. **microcephal′ic, microceph′alous** *adj*

mi•cro•chei•lia (mi″kro-ki′le-ə) [*micro-* + *cheil-* + *-ia*] abnormal smallness of the lips.

mi•cro•chei•ria (mi″kro-ki′re-ə) [*micro-* + *cheir-* + *-ia*] abnormal smallness of the hands, as a result of hypoplasia of all the skeletal elements.

mi•cro•chem•is•try (mi″kro-kem′is-tre) [*micro-* + *chemistry*] the study of chemical reactions using quantities invisible to the naked eye; chemistry which deals with minute quantities (a few milligrams) of substances, using apparatus of small size. Cf. *macrochemistry.* **microchem′ical** *adj*

mi•cro•chi•mer•ism (mi″kro-ki-mēr′iz-əm) the presence in an individual of small numbers of cells or small amounts of DNA derived from another genetically distinct individual, as of donor cells in a graft recipient or of cells transferred between mother and fetus during pregnancy.

fetal m. persistence in the mother of cells derived from the fetus.

maternal m. persistence of cells derived from the mother in her offspring.

mi•cro•cin•e•ma•tog•ra•phy (mi″kro-sin″ə-mə-tog′rə-fe) [*micro-* + Gr. *kinēma* movement + *graphein* to write] the making of moving picture photographs of microscopic subjects. Called also *microkinematography.* See also *cinemicrography.*

mi•cro•cir•cu•la•tion (mi″kro-sur″ku-la′shən) the flow of blood in the microvasculature of the body. **microcirculato′ry** *adj*

mi•cro•cli•mate (mi″kro-kli′mət) the immediate climatic environment, as that of a vector insect.

mi•cro•cne•mia (mi″kro-ne′me-ə) [*micro-* + Gr. *knēmē* tibia] abnormal shortness of the lower limb.

Mi•cro•coc•ca•ceae (mi″kro-kə-ka′se-e) a family of gram-positive, aerobic or facultatively anaerobic bacteria of the suborder Micrococcineae, order Actinomycetales, consisting of spherical cells that divide primarily in two or three planes, which sometimes remain in contact after division to form clusters or packets. Genera of medical interest include *Arthrobacter, Micrococcus,* and *Rothia.*

mi•cro•coc•ci (mi″kro-kok′si) plural of *micrococcus.*

Mi•cro•coc•ci•neae (mi″kro-kok-sin′e-e) a suborder of bacteria of the order Actinomycetales comprising a highly diverse group of organisms; medically important members are included in the families Brevibacteriaceae, Cellulomonadaceae, Dermabacteraceae, Dermatophilaceae, Microbacteriaceae, and Micrococcaceae.

Mi•cro•coc•cus (mi″kro-kok′əs) [*micro-* + Gr. *kokkos* berry] a genus of bacteria of the family Micrococcaceae, consisting of spherical, gram-positive, aerobic cells, usually occurring in irregular masses. Saprophytic and nonpathogenic forms are found in soil, water, dust, and dairy products; it is an uncommon cause of infective endocarditis. The type species is *M. lu′teus.*

M. sedenta′rius *Kytococcus sedentarius.*

mi•cro•coc•cus (mi″kro-kok′əs) pl. *micrococ′ci.* 1. an organism of the genus *Micrococcus.* 2. a spherical microorganism of extremely small size.

mi•cro•co•lon (mi″kro-ko′lən) an abnormally small colon.

mi•cro•col•o•ny (mi′kro-kol″ə-ne) a microscopic colony of bacteria.

mi•cro•co•me•do (mi″kro-ko′mə-do) a type of tiny comedo seen in early stages of acne.

mi•cro•co•me•done (mi″kro-ko′mə-dōn) microcomedo.

mi•cro•con•cen•tra•tion (mi″kro-kon″sən-tra′shən) a minute amount of solute, less than 0.05 per cent of the solution.

mi•cro•co•nid•i•um (mi″kro-ko-nid′e-əm) pl. *microconid′ia.* A small, usually single-celled conidium or exospore in a fungus that also produces macroconidia; the term is sometimes used interchangeably with *microaleuriospore.*

mi•cro•co•ria (mi″kro-ko′re-ə) [*micro-* + *coro-* + *-ia*] congenital, usually hereditary, smallness of the pupil.

mi•cro•cor•nea (mi″kro-kor′ne-ə) [*micro-* + *cornea*] a usually bilateral developmental anomaly, in which the cornea is unusually small (less than 11 mm after one year of age), due to arrest of development. It may be associated with other ocular abnormalities, such as microphthalmia, hydrophthalmia, multiple defects of the anterior chamber, cataract, and glaucoma, and may be inherited as an X-linked recessive or as an autosomal dominant trait.

mi•cro•cou•lomb (μC) (mi″kro-koo′lom) one millionth (10^{-6}) of a coulomb.

mi•cro•cra•nia (mi″kro-kra′ne-ə) abnormal smallness of the cranium, the cranial cavity being reduced in all diameters, and the facial area being disproportionately large in comparison.

mi•cro•crys•tal (mi′kro-kris″təl) an extremely minute crystal.

mi•cro•crys•tal•line (mi″kro-kris′tə-lin) made up of minute crystals.

mi•cro•cu•rie (μCi) (mi′kro-ku″re) a unit of radioactivity, being one millionth (10^{-6}) of a curie.

mi•cro•cyst (mi′kro-sist) [*micro-* + *cyst*] 1. a very small cyst. 2. in bacteriology, a type of resting cell developed from the vegetative cells of certain species of Myxobacterales and Nocardiaceae. 3. in mycology, a resting cell produced by certain slime molds. Cf. *macrocyst.*

Mi•cro•cys•tis (mi″kro-sis′tis) a genus of cyanobacteria that sometimes contaminates water and can cause cyanobacteria poisoning. Called also *Anacystis.*

mi•cro•cyte (mi′kro-sīt″) [*micro-* + *-cyte*] 1. an abnormally small erythrocyte, i.e., one 5 μm or less in diameter. Called also *microerythrocyte.* 2. microglial cell.

hypochromic m. a small erythrocyte with less than the usual coloring, as seen in iron deficiency anemia.

mi•cro•cy•the•mia (mi″kro-si-the′me-ə) [*microcyte* + *hem-* + *-ia*] a condition in which the erythrocytes are smaller than normal; see also *microcytic anemia,* under *anemia.* Called alse *microcytosis.*

mi•cro•cyt•ic (mi″kro-sit′ik) pertaining to or characterized by microcytes.

mi•cro•cy•to•sis (mi″kro-si-to′sis) microcythemia.

mi•cro•cy•to•tox•ic•i•ty (mi″kro-si″to-tok-sis′ĭ-te) [*micro-* + *cytotoxicity*] the capability of lysing or damaging cells by procedures that use extremely minute amounts of material such as target cells, antibody, and complement (e.g., lymphotoxicity procedures).

mi•cro•dac•tyl•ia (mi″kro-dak-til′e-ə) microdactyly.

mi•cro•dac•ty•ly (mi″kro-dak′tə-le) [*micro-* + Gr. *daktylos* finger] abnormal smallness of the digits.

mi•cro•de•le•tion (mi″kro-də-le′shən) a chromosomal deletion too small to be detected with the light microscope.

mi•cro•dens•i•tom•e•ter (mi″kro-dens″ĭ-tom′ə-tər) an instrument used in spectroscopy to measure lines in a spectrum by light transmission measurement.

mi•cro•derm•abra•sion (mi″kro-dur″mə-bra′zhən) superficial dermabrasion using a mechanical abrader or a stream of particles, done primarily to treat acne scars or other mild lesions or to stimulate and remodel skin collagen.

mi•cro•der•ma•tome (mi″kro-dur′mə-tōm) an instrument for cutting very thin skin sections.

mi•cro•de•ter•mi•na•tion (mi″kro-de-tur″mĭ-na′shən) a chemical examination in which minute quantities of the substance to be examined are used.

mi•cro•di•lu•tion (mi″kro-di-loo′shən) a dilution method of antimicrobial susceptibility testing that uses only microscopic amounts of pathogens and antimicrobials.

mi•cro•dis•kec•to•my (mi″kro-dis-kek′tə-me) debulking of a herniated nucleus pulposus using an operating microscope or loupe for magnification.

arthroscopic m. microdiskectomy performed with instruments introduced into the area of herniation through an arthroscope.

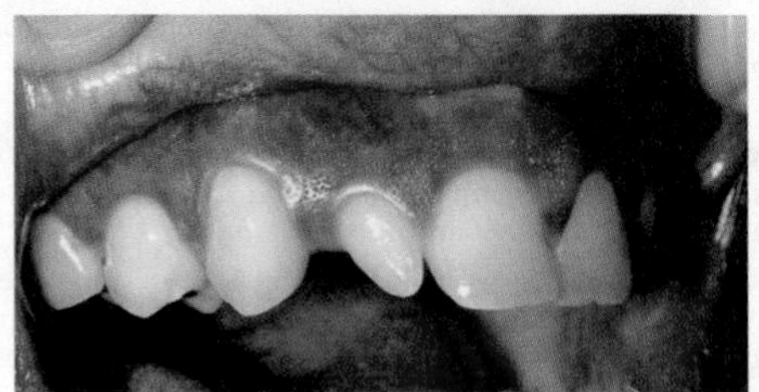

■ Microdontia of a maxillary lateral incisor.

mi•cro•dis•sec•tion (mi″kro-dĭ-sek′shən) dissection of tissue or cells under the microscope.

mi•cro•dont (mi′kro-dont) [*micro-* + Gr. *odous* tooth] having an abnormally small tooth or teeth.

mi•cro•don•tia (mi″kro-don′shə) [*micro-* + *odont-* + *-ia*] a developmental disorder characterized by abnormal smallness of the teeth; it may affect a single tooth or all of the teeth, or teeth of normal size may appear abnormally small in proportion to abnormally large jaws. Called also *microdontism.* **microdon′tic** *adj*

mi•cro•don•tism (mi″kro-don′tiz-əm) microdontia.

mi•cro•do•sage (mi′kro-do″səj) dosage in small quantities.

mi•cro•dose (mi′kro-dōs) a very small dose.

mi•cro•drep•a•no•cyt•ic (mi″kro-drep″ə-no-sit′ik) containing microcytic and drepanocytic elements, as in sickle cell–thalassemia disease.

mi•cro•drep•a•no•cy•to•sis (mi″kro-drep″ə-no-si-to′sis) sickle cell–thalassemia disease.

mi•cro•dys•ge•ne•sia (mi″kro-dis-jə-ne′zhə) subtle abnormalities of neurons in the area surrounding the hippocampus and cerebellum, seen in cases of epilepsy.

mi•cro•ecol•o•gy (mi″kro-ĕ-kol′ə-je) the branch of ecology of parasites concerned with the relationships of the organisms and the environment provided by the hosts.

mi•cro•eco•sys•tem (mi″kro-ĕ″ko-sis′təm) a miniature ecological system, occurring naturally or produced in the laboratory for experimental purposes.

mi•cro•elec•trode (mi″kro-ə-lek′trōd) an electrode with an extremely small tip, used in a voltage clamp or other apparatus to stimulate or record bioelectric potentials of single cells intracellularly or extracellularly.

mi•cro•elec•tro•pho•re•sis (mi″kro-e-lek″tro-fə-re′sis) electrophoresis in which migrating particles are observed by light microscopy. **microelectrophoret′ic** *adj*

mi•cro•em•bo•lus (mi″kro-em′bo-ləs) pl. *microem′boli.* An embolus of microscopic size.

mi•cro•en•ceph•a•ly (mi″kro-ən-sef′ə-le) micrencephaly.

mi•cro•en•vi•ron•ment (mi″kro-ən-vi′ron-mənt) the environment at the microscopic or cellular level.

mi•cro•eryth•ro•cyte (mi″kro-ə-rith′ro-sīt) microcyte (def. 1).

mi•cro•es•ti•ma•tion (mi″kro-es″tĭ-ma′shən) microdetermination.

mi•cro•far•ad (μF) (mi″kro-far′əd) a unit of electrical capacitance, being one millionth (10^{-6}) of a farad.

mi•cro•fau•na (mi″kro-faw′nə) the animal life, visible only under the microscope, which is present in or characteristic of a special location.

mi•cro•fi•bril (mi″kro-fi′bril) 1. an extremely small fibril, often a unit of a compound fiber. 2. the basic structural unit of the plant cell wall; composed of cellulose in higher plants and most algae, chitin in some fungi, and mannan or xylan in some algae.

mi•cro•fil•a•ment (mi″kro-fil′ə-mənt) a cytoplasmic structure, 5–7 nm in diameter, composed of two chains of G-actin coiled around each other to form an F-actin filament and having a plus-minus polarity. Microfilaments are components of the cytoskeleton and participate in the formation of adherens junctions and tight junctions.

mi•cro•fil•a•re•mia (mi″kro-fil″ə-re′me-ə) the presence of microfilariae in the circulating blood.

mi•cro•fi•la•ria (mi″kro-fĭ-lar′e-ə) pl. *microfila′riae.* the prelarval stage of Filarioidea in the blood of humans and in the tissues of the vector. This term is sometimes incorrectly used as a genus and is then spelled with a capital M.

m. bancrof′ti the microfilaria of *Wuchereria bancrofti.*

m. diur′na the microfilaria of *Loa loa.*

m. lo′a the microfilaria of *Loa loa.*

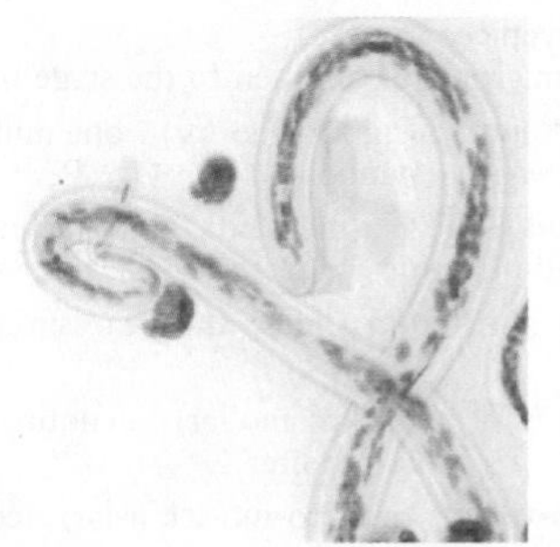

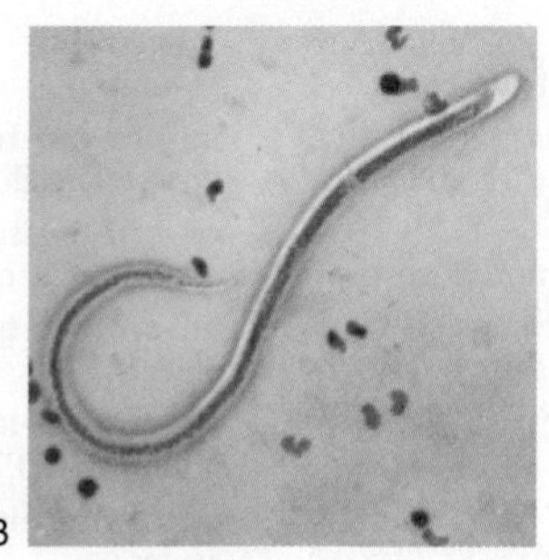

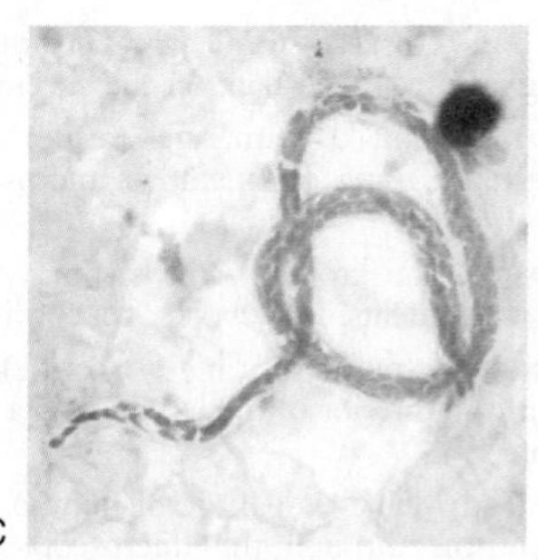

■ Microfilariae of *(A), Loa loa; (B), Wuchereria bancrofti; (C), Mansonella perstans. A* and *B* have sheaths covering the body and tapered tails; *A* and *C* have nuclei extending to their tail tips.

m. streptocer′ca the microfilaria of *Mansonella streptocerca*, found in the subcutaneous tissues.

m. vol′vulus the prelarval form of *Onchocerca volvulus*, found in skin snips taken from infected persons.

mi•cro•fil•a•ri•der•mia (mi″kro-fil″ə-rĭ-der′me-ə) the presence of microfilariae under the skin.

mi•cro•film (mi′kro-film) 1. a trade term for 16- or 35-millimeter film to be used in high-speed automatic machines for the photographic reproduction, in greatly reduced size, of books, documents, forms, or other record files. 2. to photographically reproduce, in greatly reduced size, on film specially designed for the purpose.

mi•cro•fil•ter (mi′kro-fil″tər) a filter that removes particles with diameters of 0.1–10.0 µm; used, for example, to remove microbubbles and microaggregates from the blood in cardiopulmonary bypass.

mi•cro•flo•ra (mi″kro-flor′ə) the entire population of microorganisms present in or characteristic of a specific location.

mi•cro•flu•or•om•e•try (mi″kro-flo͞o-rom′ə-tre) cytophotometry.

mi•cro•fol•lic•u•lar (mi″kro-fə-lik′u-lər) [*micro-* + *follicular*] pertaining to or characterized by small follicles.

mi•cro•frac•ture (mi″kro-frak′chər) 1. a minute break or crack, as in a dental restoration. 2. a minute, incomplete break or area of discontinuity in a bone. 3. an arthroscopic procedure for the repair of articular cartilage defects: the damaged cartilage is débrided and small holes are made in the subchondral bone; the clot formed by bleeding through the holes forms the basis for cartilage regeneration.

mi•cro•gam•ete (mi″kro-gam′ēt) [*micro-* + *gamete*] 1. the smaller, often flagellated, actively motile male anisogamete. 2. the smaller of two types of malarial parasites; see *gamete* (def. 2).

mi•cro•ga•me•to•cyte (mi″kro-gə-me′to-sīt) microgamont.

mi•cro•ga•me•to•phyte (mi″kro-gə-me′to-fīt) [*micro-* + *gameto-* + *-phyte*] the male gametophyte in heterosporous plants, developed from the microspore.

mi•cro•gam•ont (mi″kro-gam′ont) [*micro-* + *gamont*] a gamont that produces microgametes by fission. Called also *microgametocyte*.

mi•crog•a•my (mi-krog′ə-me) conjugation or fusion when the gametes are smaller than the somatic cells.

mi•cro•gas•tria (mi″kro-gas′tre-ə) [*micro-* + *gastr-* + *-ia*] abnormal smallness of the stomach; one variety is a rare congenital anomaly in which the stomach consists of a narrow tube.

mi•cro•gen•e•sis (mi″kro-jen′ə-sis) [*micro-* + *-genesis*] abnormally small development of a part.

mi•cro•gen•ia (mi″kro-jen′e-ə) [*micro-* + *geni-* + *-ia*] an extremely small chin, caused by underdevelopment of the mandibular symphysis or malocclusion with excessive prominence of alveolar structures. See also *micrognathia*.

mi•cro•gen•i•tal•ism (mi″kro-jen′ĭ-təl-iz-əm) [*micro-* + *genitalism*] abnormal smallness of the external genitals.

Mic•ro•ges•tin Fe (mi″kro-jes′tin) trademark for a therapeutic regimen of norethindrone acetate and ethinyl estradiol, which contains also a placebo week of ferrous fumarate tablets.

mi•crog•lia (mi-krog′le-ə) [*micro-* + *-glia*] the small, nonneural, interstitial cells of mesodermal origin that form part of the supporting structure of the central nervous system. They are of various forms and may have slender branched processes. They are migratory and act as phagocytes to waste products of nerve tissue. See also *microglial cell* and *gitter cell*. **microg′lial** *adj*

mi•crog•lia•cyte (mi-krog′le-ə-sīt) microglial cell.

mi•crog•lio•cyte (mi-krog′le-o-sīt) microglial cell.

mi•cro•gli•o•ma (mi″kro-gli-o′mə) former name for *primary central nervous system lymphoma*.

mi•cro•glob•u•lin (mi″kro-glob′u-lin) any globulin or fragment of a globulin that has low molecular weight.

β_2-m., beta$_2$-m. a small (mol. wt. 12,000), nonpolymorphic protein, homologous to the C3 domain of IgG, that is one subunit of class I major histocompatibility antigens.

mi•cro•glos•sia (mi″kro-glos′e-ə) [*micro-* + *gloss-* + *-ia*] undersize of the tongue.

mi•cro•gna•thia (mi″kro-na′the-ə) [*micro-* + *gnath-* + *-ia*] 1. abnormal smallness of the mandible; see also *vertical overlap* (def. 1). Called also *micromandible*, and *brachygnathia*. 2. micromaxilla.

mi•cro•go•nio•scope (mi″kro-go′ne-o-skōp) [*micro-* + *gonioscope*] a magnifying gonioscope.

mi•cro•gram (µg) (mi′kro-gram″) a unit of mass, being one millionth (10^{-6}) of a gram.

mi•cro•graph (mi′kro-graf″) 1. an instrument for recording extremely minute movements. It acts by making a greatly magnified record on a photographic film of the minute motions of a diaphragm. 2. the photograph of a minute object or specimen (tissue, etc.) as seen through a microscope.

electron m. the photograph of an object through an electron microscope.

mi•cro•graph•ia (mi″kro-graf′e-ə) [*micro-* + *graph-* + *-ia*] a dysgraphia in which handwriting is tiny or decreases in size from normal to minute, seen in parkinsonism.

mi•crog•ra•phy (mi-krog′rə-fe) [*micro-* + *-graphy*] 1. an account of microscopic objects. 2. microscopy.

mi•cro•grav•i•ty (mi′kro-grav′ĭ-te) the minute amount of gravitational force existing in outer space; it results in a weightless condition and enhances the likelihood of certain diseases.

mi•cro•gy•ria (mi″kro-ji′re-ə) [*micro-* + *gyr-* + *-ia*] polymicrogyria.

mi•cro•gy•rus (mi″kro-ji′rəs) pl. *microgy′ri* [*micro-* + *gyrus*] an abnormally small, malformed convolution of the brain, as seen in polymicrogyria.

mi•cro•he•mat•o•crit (mi″kro-he-mat′ə-krit) a hematocrit determination done on an extremely small quantity of blood, by use of a capillary tube and a high speed centrifuge.

mi•cro•he•ma•tu•ria (mi″kro-he″mə-tu′re-ə) microscopic hematuria.

mi•cro•he•pat•ia (mi″kro-hə-pat′e-ə) [*micro-* + *hepat-* + *-ia*] smallness of the liver.

mi•cro•his•tol•o•gy (mi″kro-his-tol′ə-je) histology.

mi•cro•in•cin•er•a•tion (mi″kro-in-sin″ər-a′shən) the incineration of minute specimens of tissue or other substance, for identification from the ash of the elements composing it.

mi•cro•in•farct (mi″kro-in′fahrkt) a very small infarct due to obstruction of circulation in capillaries, arterioles, or small arteries.

mi•cro•in•jec•tor (mi″kro-in-jek′tər) an instrument for infusion of very small amounts of fluids or drugs.

mi•cro•in•ter•lock (mi″kro-in′tər-lok″) the growth of mineralized bone into the porous surface of a specially constructed prosthesis, anchoring the prosthesis into place.

mi•cro•in•va•sion (mi″kro-in-va′zhən) microscopic extension of malignant cells into adjacent tissue in carcinoma in situ. **microinva′sive** *adj*

Mi•cro-K (mi″kro-ka′) trademark for a preparation of potassium chloride.

mi•cro•kin•e•ma•tog•ra•phy (mi″kro-kin″ə-mə-tog′rə-fe) microcinematography.

mi•cro•ker•a•tome (mi″kro-ker′ə-tōm) an instrument for removing a thin slice, or creating a thin hinged flap, on the surface of the cornea.

mi•cro•lam•i•nec•to•my (mi″kro-lam″ĭ-nek′tə-me) excision of the posterior arch of a vertebra using an operative microscope or loupe for magnification.

mi•cro•lap•a•ros•co•py (mi″kro-lap″ə-ros′kə-pe) minilaparoscopy using extremely small instruments. **microlaparoscop′ic** *adj*

mi•cro•lar•yn•gos•co•py (mi″kro-lar″ing-gos′kə-pe) [*micro-* + *laryngo-* + *scopy*] examination of the interior of the larynx with a laryngoscope with binocular magnification.

mi•cro•leak•age (mi″kro-le′kəj) leakage of minute amounts of fluids, debris, and microorganisms through the microscopic space between a dental restoration or its cement and the adjacent surface of the cavity preparation; it may progress through the dentin into the pulp.

mi•cro•lec•i•thal (mi″kro-les′ĭ-thəl) [*micro-* + *-lecithal*] containing little yolk, such as the eggs of mammals and echinoderms.

mi•cro•le•sion (mi″kro-le′zhən) a minute lesion.

mi•cro•leu•ko•blast (mi″kro-loo′ko-blast) myeloblast.

Mi•cro•lite (mi′kro-līt) trademark for a kit for the preparation of technetium Tc 99m albumin colloid.

mi•cro•li•ter (μL) (mi′kro-le″tər) one millionth (10^{-6}) of a liter.

mi•cro•lith (mi′kro-lith) [*micro-* + *-lith*] a minute concretion or calculus.

mi•cro•li•thi•a•sis (mi″kro-lĭ-thi′ə-sis) [*micro-* + *lithiasis*] the formation of minute concretions in an organ.

m. alveola′ris pulmo′num, pulmonary alveolar m. a condition caused by deposition in the alveoli of the lungs of minute calculi, which appear radiographically as fine, sandlike mottling.

testicular m. the presence of tiny calcifications in the seminiferous tubules; in some cases this precedes development of a tumor.

mi•crol•o•gy (mi-krol′ə-je) [*micro-* + *-logy*] the science dealing with the handling and preparation of materials for microscopic study.

mi•cro•man•di•ble (mi″kro-man′dĭ-bəl) micrognathia (def. 1).

mi•cro•ma•nip•u•la•tion (mi″kro-mə-nip″u-la′shən) 1. surgery, injection, dissection, or other procedures done with a micromanipulator. 2. in male factor infertility, the processing of gametes, such as by partial removal of the zona pellucida or direct injection of sperm into the egg.

mi•cro•ma•nip•u•la•tor (mi″kro-mə-nip′u-la″tər) an attachment to a microscope for manipulating tiny instruments used in examination and dissection of minute objects under the microscope.

mi•cro•ma•nom•e•ter (mi″kro-mə-nom′ə-tər) an apparatus for indicating gas or vapor pressure from a very small sample, as of blood or other fluid.

mi•cro•mano•met•ric (mi″kro-man″o-met′rik) relating to gas or vapor pressure from very small samples, as of blood or other fluid.

mi•cro•mas•tia (mi″kro-mas′te-ə) abnormal smallness of the mamma.

mi•cro•max•il•la (mi″kro-mək-sil′ə) abnormal smallness of the maxilla; called also *micrognathia.*

mi•cro•ma•zia (mi″kro-ma′ze-ə) [*micro-* + *maz-* + *-ia*] micromastia.

mi•cro•meg•a•lop•sia (mi″kro-meg″ə-lop′se-ə) [*micro-* + *megal-* + *-opsia*] the condition in which objects appear too small or too large, or too small and too large by turns.

mi•cro•me•lia (mi″kro-me′le-ə) [*micro-* + *-melia*] a developmental anomaly characterized by abnormal smallness or shortness of the limbs.

mi•crom•e•lus (mi-krom′ə-ləs) an individual exhibiting micromelia.

mi•cro•mere (mi′kro-mēr) [*micro-* + *-mere*] one of the small blastomeres formed by unequal cleavage of a fertilized oocyte as the result of asymmetric positioning of the mitotic spindle. Cf. *macromere.*

mi•cro•me•tab•o•lism (mi″kro-mə-tab′ə-liz-əm) metabolism as studied by micromethods.

mi•cro•me•tas•ta•sis (mi″kro-mə-tas′tə-sis) the spread of cancer cells from the primary tumor to distant sites, where they form microscopic secondary tumors.

mi•cro•meta•stat•ic (mi″kro-met″ə-stat′ik) 1. pertaining to or caused by micrometastasis. 2. clinically undetectable; said of a metastatic tumor.

mi•crom•e•ter[1] (mi-krom′ə-tər) [*micro-* + *-meter*] an instrument for measuring objects seen through the microscope.

eyepiece m. a micrometer that is used in connection with the eyepiece of a microscope.

filar m. an eyepiece micrometer in which the micrometer screw acts upon a slide carrying a movable wire: one revolution of the screw moves the wire 1 mm across the field.

ocular m. eyepiece m.

stage m. a micrometer fastened to the stage of a microscope.

mi•cro•me•ter[2] **(μm)** (mi′kro-me″tər) one millionth (10^{-6}) of a meter. Formerly called *micron* (symbol μ).

mi•cro•meth•od (mi″kro-meth′əd) any technique involving use of exceedingly small quantities of material. Cf. *macromethod.*

mi•crom•e•try (mi-krom′ə-tre) the measurement of microscopic objects.

mi•cro•mo•lar (μM) (mi″kro-mo′lər) denoting a concentration of one millionth (10^{-6}) of a mole per liter.

mi•cro•mo•lec•u•lar (mi″kro-mo-lek′u-lər) composed of small molecules.

Mi•cro•mo•nas (mi″kro-mo′nəs) [*micro-* + Gr. *monas* unit, from *monos* single] a genus of obligately anaerobic, gram-positive bacteria of the family Peptostreptococcaceae, consisting of non–spore-forming, nonmotile cocci occurring in chains or clusters. The type species is *M. mi′cros.*

M. mi′cros a species that is part of the normal flora of the mouth and probably of the gastrointestinal and female genitourinary tracts; it is occasionally isolated from pathological specimens. Called also *Peptostreptococcus micros.*

Mi•cro•mo•no•spo•ra (mi″kro-mon″o-spor′ə) [*micro-* + Gr. *monos* single + *sporos* seed] a genus of bacteria of the family Micromonosporaceae, made up of gram-positive, spore-forming, generally aerobic organisms that form a branched mycelium; they occur as saprophytic forms in soil and water. Various species are sources of aminoglycoside antibiotics. The type species is *M. chal′cea.*

M. echinospo′ra a species that produces gentamicin. Formerly called *M. purpurea.*

M. inyoen′sis a species that produces sisomicin.

M. purpu′rea *M. echinospora.*

Mi•cro•mo•nos•po•ra•ceae (mi″kro-mon″o″spə-ra′se-e) a phenotypically diverse family of bacteria of the suborder Micromonosporineae, order Actinomycetales, consisting of aerobic, gram-positive, non–acid-fast, sporogenic soil organisms that form nonfragmenting, branched, and septate hyphae. Some species in the genera *Actinoplanes* and *Micromonospora* produce antibiotics.

Mi•cro•mo•no•spo•ri•neae (mi″kro-mon″o-spə-rin′e-e) a phenotypically diverse suborder of gram-positive bacteria of the order Actinomycetales, grouped together on the basis of 16S rRNA sequence analysis. It contains the single family Micromonosporaceae.

mi•cro•my•elia (mi″kro-mi-e′le-ə) [*micro-* + *myel-* + *-ia*] abnormal smallness of the spinal cord.

mi•cro•my•elo•blast (mi″kro-mi′ə-lo-blast) a small, immature myelocyte, observed in micromyeloblastic leukemia.

mi•cron (μ) (mi′kron) [Gr. *mikros* small] former name for *micrometer* (μm).

Mi•cro•nase (mi′kro-nās) trademark for a preparation of glyburide.

mi•cro•nee•dle (mi′kro-ne″dəl) a fine glass needle for use in microsurgery.

Mi•cro•ne•ma (mi″kro-ne′mə) *Halicephalobus.*

mi•cro•nem•a•tous (mi″kro-nem′ə-təs) [*micro-* + Gr. *nēma* thread] pertaining to a conidiophore morphologically similar to its hypha.

mi•cro•neme (mi″kro-nēm) [*micro-* + Gr. *nēma* thread] any of the electron-dense, convoluted tubular organelles forming part of the apical complex in apicomplexan protozoa, often associated with or giving rise to rhoptries. Called also *sarconeme.*

mi•cro•neu•rog•ra•phy (mi″kro-noo͝-rog′rə-fe) the study of conduction in individual nerve fibers or bundles of fibers using a microelectrode.

mi•cro•neu•ro•sur•gery (mi″kro-noor″o-sur′jər-e) surgery conducted under high magnification with miniaturized instruments on microscopic vessels and structures of the nervous system.

mi•cro•nize (mi′kro-nīz) [Gr. *micron* a small thing] to reduce to a fine powder; to reduce to particles a micron in diameter.

mi•cro•nod•u•lar (mi″kro-nod′u-lər) pertaining to or characterized by very small nodules.

mi•cro•nod•ule (mi″kro-nod′ūl) 1. a very small nodule. 2. on a radiograph of the lung, a discrete opacity less than 3 mm in diameter.

Mi•cro•nor (mi′kro-nor) trademark for a preparation of norethindrone.

mi•cro•nor•mo•blast (mi″kro-nor′mo-blast) an abnormal red cell precursor in which there has been defective hemoglobin synthesis, characterized by a narrow rim of cytoplasm and an overdeveloped pyknotic nucleus.

mi•cro•nu•cle•us (mi″kro-noo′kle-əs) [*micro-* + *nucleus*] in ciliate protozoa, the transcriptively inert, diploid nucleus, much smaller than the macronucleus, that is involved in reproduction.

mi•cro•nu•tri•ent (mi″kro-noo′tre-ənt) any essential dietary element required only in small quantities, e.g., trace minerals.

mi•cro•nych•ia (mi″kro-nik′e-ə) [*micr-* + *onych-* + *-ia*] abnormal smallness of the nails of fingers or toes.

mi•cro•or•chi•dism (mi″kro-or′kĭ-diz-əm) [*micro-* + *orchid-* + *-ism*] abnormal smallness of the testis; called also *microrchidia.*

mi•cro•or•gan•ism (mi″kro-or′gən-iz-əm) [*micro-* + *organism*] a microscopic organism; those of medical interest include bacteria, fungi, and protozoa. Viruses are often classified as microorganisms, although they are sometimes excluded because they are not cellular and they are unable to replicate without a host cell. **microorgan′ic, microorganis′mal** *adj*

mi•cro•pan•nus (mi-kro-pan′əs) a small area of pannus on the cornea.

mi•cro•par•a•site (mi″kro-par′ə-sīt) a parasitic microorganism.

mi•cro•pa•thol•o•gy (mi″kro-pə-thol′ə-je) [*micro-* + *pathology*] 1. the sum of what is known regarding minute pathologic changes. 2. the pathology of diseases caused by microorganisms.

mi•cro•pe•nis (mi″kro-pe′nis) abnormal smallness of the penis; called also *microphallus.*

mi•cro•per•fu•sion (mi″kro-pər-fu′zhən) perfusion of a minute amount of a substance.

mi•cro•phage (mi′kro-fāj″) [*micro-* + *-phage*] a small phagocyte, such as a type of actively motile neutrophil. Called also *microphagocyte.*

mi•cro•phago•cyte (mi″kro-fa′go-sīt) [*micro-* + *phagocyte*] microphage.

mi•cro•pha•kia (mi″kro-fa′ke-ə) [*micro-* + *phak-* + *-ia*] abnormal smallness of the crystalline lens.

mi•cro•phal•lus (mi″kro-fal′əs) [*micro-* + *phallus*] micropenis.

mi•cro•phone (mi′kro-fōn) a device for converting an acoustic signal into an electric signal for purposes of amplification or transmission.

cardiac catheter-m. phonocatheter.

mi•cro•pho•nia (mi″kro-fo′ne-ə) [*micro-* + *-phonia*] hypophonia.

mi•cro•phon•ic (mi″kro-fon′ik) 1. serving to amplify sound. 2. cochlear m.

cochlear m. the electrical potential generated in the auditory hair cells of the organ of Corti in response to acoustic stimulation; called also *cochlear potentials* and *Wever-Bray phenomenon.*

mi•cro•pho•to•graph (mi″kro-fo′tə-graf) [*micro-* + *photograph*] a photograph of small size. Cf. *photomicrograph.*

mi•croph•thal•mia (mi″krof-thal′me-ə) microphthalmos.

mi•croph•thal•mos (mi″krof-thal′mos) [*micro-* + Gr. *ophthalmos* eye] a developmental defect causing moderate or severe reduction in size of the eye. Opacities of the cornea and lens, scarring of the retina and choroid, and other abnormalities may also be present. Cf. *nanophthalmos.*

mi•croph•thal•mo•scope (mi″krof-thal′mə-skōp) [*micro-* + *ophthalmoscope*] an instrument for performing fundus microscopy.

mi•cro•phyte (mi′kro-fīt) [*micro-* + *-phyte*] a microscopic vegetable organism. Cf. *microzoon.*

mi•cro•pig•men•ta•tion (mi″kro-pig″mən-ta′shən) the implantation of minute amounts of pigment into the skin for treatment of hypopigmentation, as in vitiligo.

mi•cro•pino•cy•to•sis (mi″kro-pin″o-si-to′sis) the taking up into a cell of specific macromolecules by invagination of the plasma membrane which is then pinched off, resulting in small vesicles in the cytoplasm; cf. *macropinocytosis.*

mi•cro•pi•pet (mi″kro-pi-pet′) a pipet for handling small quantities of liquids (up to 1 mL).

mi•cro•pi•tu•i•cyte (mi″kro-pĭ-too′ĭ-sīt) see *pituicyte.*

mi•cro•pla•sia (mi″kro-pla′zhə) [*micro-* + *-plasia*] dwarfism.

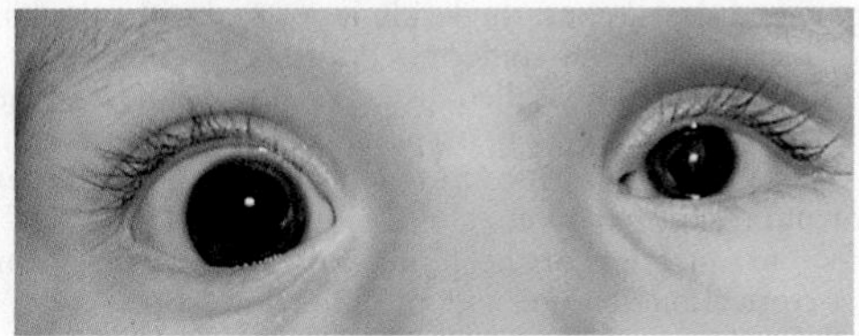

■ Microphthalmos and microcornea of the left eye.

mi•cro•pleth•ys•mog•ra•phy (mi″kro-pleth″is-mog′rə-fe) [*micro-* + *plethysmography*] the recording of minute changes in the size of a part as produced by the circulation of blood in it.

mi•cro•po•dia (mi″kro-po′de-ə) [*micro-* + *pod-* + *-ia*] abnormal smallness of the feet.

mi•cro•po•lar•i•scope (mi″kro-po-lar′ĭ-skōp) a microscope with a polariscope attached.

mi•cro•poly•gy•ria (mi″kro-pol″e-ji′re-ə) polymicrogyria.

Mi•cro•po•lys•po•ra (mi″kro-pol″e-spor′ə) [*micro-* + Gr. *poly* many + *sporos* seed] in former systems of classification, a genus of bacteria of the family Micromonosporaceae; species have been assigned to other genera.

M. fae′ni *Saccharopolyspora rectivirgula.*

mi•cro•pore (mi′kro-por) [*micro-* + *pore*] an ultrastructural organelle in the side of the body of apicomplexan protozoa, consisting of a cytoplasmic ring or cylinder formed by invagination of the outer membrane of the pellicle at the site of a disruption of the inner membrane. Formerly called *micropyle.*

mi•cro•pre•cip•i•ta•tion (mi″kro-pre-sip″ĭ-ta′shən) precipitation with a very small amount of reagent, observed under the microscope.

mi•cro•pre•da•tion (mi″kro-prə-da′shən) the derivation by an organism of elements essential for its existence from larger organisms of other species which it does not destroy.

mi•cro•pred•a•tor (mi″kro-pred′ə-tər) [*micro-* + *predator*] an organism, e.g., the mosquito, that derives elements essential for its existence from other species of organisms, larger than itself, without causing their destruction.

mi•cro•probe (mi′kro-prōb″) a minute probe, as one used in microsurgery.

laser m. a laser beam utilized to vaporize a minute area of tissue, as in a biopsy specimen, which is then subjected to emission spectrography.

mi•cro•pro•jec•tion (mi″kro-pro-jek′shən) [*micro-* + *projection*] the throwing of the image of a microscopic object on a screen.

mi•cro•pro•jec•tor (mi″kro-pro-jek′tər) a projector that fits the viewing stage of a microscope and enlarges the image on an illuminated viewing screen.

mi•cro•pro•lac•ti•no•ma (mi″kro-pro-lak″tĭ-no′mə) a prolactinoma less than 10 mm in diameter, usually associated with serum prolactin levels of 100 to 500 ng per milliliter.

mi•cro•pro•so•pus (mi″kro-pro-so′pəs) [*micro-* + Gr. *prosōpon* face] a fetus with an abnormally small or poorly developed face.

mi•cro•pro•tein (mi″kro-pro′tēn) a protein present in only microscopic amounts.

mi•cro•pro•tein•uria (mi″kro-pro″te-nu′re-ə) proteinuria at a level too subtle to be measured by conventional means, often seen with the hyperfiltration of diabetes mellitus; cf. *microalbuminuria.*

mi•crop•sia (mi-krop′se-ə) [*micr-* + *-opsia*] a visual disorder in which objects appear smaller than their actual size. **microp′tic** *adj*

mi•cro•punc•ture (mi′kro-punk″chər) 1. the creation of minute openings by piercing. 2. in renal physiology, the process by which nephron segments are pierced.

mi•cro•pus (mi-kro′pəs) a person with micropodia.

mi•cro•pyle (mi′kro-pīl) [*micro-* + Gr. *pylē* gate] 1. a minute opening in the ovum of certain invertebrates, such as arthropods, that permits entrance of a sperm. 2. a minute opening in the apex of the ovule of a seed plant that admits the pollen tube. 3. former name for *micropore.*

mi•cro•ra•dio•gram (mi″kro-ra′de-o-gram) a picture produced by microradiography.

mi•cro•ra•di•og•ra•phy (mi″kro-ra″de-og′rə-fe) [*micro-* + *radiography*] a process by which a radiograph of a small or very thin object is produced on fine-grained photographic film under conditions which permit subsequent microscopic examination or enlargement of the radiograph at linear magnifications of up to several hundred and with a resolution approaching the resolving power of the photographic emulsion (about 1000 lines per millimeter).

mi•cror•chid•ia (mi″kror-kid′e-ə) micro-orchidism.

mi•cro•re•frac•tom•e•ter (mi″kro-re″frak-tom′ə-tər) a refractometer for the discovery of variations in minute structures, such as of blood corpuscles.

mi•cro•res•pi•rom•e•ter (mi″kro-res″pĭ-rom′ə-tər) an apparatus for investigating the oxygen utilization of isolated tissues.

mi•cro•rhin•ia (mi″kro-rin′e-ə) [*micro-* + *rhin-* + *-ia*] abnormal smallness of the nose.

micro•RNA (miRNA) (mi″kro-ahr′en-a) any of a number of very small (20–22 nucleotides) RNA molecules that act as negative regulators of gene expression by binding to specific segments of messenger RNA, thus interfering with translation. MicroRNAs are important in the regulation of cellular development, differentiation, proliferation, apoptosis, and stress response; abnormalities of miRNA expression are involved in the development of malignancies.

mi•cro•roent•gen (μR) (mi″kro-rent′gen) one millionth (10^{-6}) of a roentgen.

mi•cro•sat•el•lite (mi″kro-sat′ə-līt) a stretch of DNA consisting of tandem repeating units of two, three, or four nucleotides; they occur throughout the genome, rarely within coding sequences, and are highly polymorphic, with codominant mendelian inheritance. See also under *polymorphism.*

mi•cros•ce•lous (mi-kros′kə-ləs) [*micro-* + Gr. *skelos* leg] having short lower limbs.

mi•cro•scope (mi′kro-skōp″) [*micro-* + *-scope*] an instrument used to obtain an enlarged image of small objects and reveal details of structure not otherwise distinguishable.

acoustic m. a microsocpe in which very high frequency sound waves (close to one billion cycles per second [one gigahertz]) are focused on the object and the reflected beam is processed electronically and stored for display on a television screen.

beta ray m. a microscope that reveals emission of beta particles from a microscopic specimen by means of a scintillator.

binocular m. a microscope with two eyepieces, making possible simultaneous viewing with both eyes.

capillary m. an instrument for giving an enlarged image of capillaries, often used for viewing the capillaries of the nail bed.

centrifuge m. a microscope built into a high-speed centrifuge, by which a magnified image of a specimen undergoing centrifugal force may be produced.

color-contrast m. Rheinberg m.

comparison m. a microscope that allows simultaneous viewing of parts of images of two separate specimens; it may have either two microscopes bridged together with a comparison eyepiece, or one microscope with two body tubes and lens systems.

compound m. a microscope that consists of two lens systems, one above the other, in which the image formed by the system nearer the object (objective) is further magnified by the system nearer the eye (eyepiece).

corneal m. a specially designed instrument with lenses of high magnifying power, for observing minute changes in the cornea and iris.

darkfield m. a microscope that has a central stop in the condenser, so that light rays are diverted to the side and the object is illuminated from the side, so that details appear light against a dark background. See also *ultramicroscope.*

electron m. a microscope in which an electron beam, instead of light, forms an image for viewing, allowing much greater magnification and resolution. The image may be viewed on a fluorescent screen or may be photographed. Types include the *scanning* and the *transmission electron microscope.*

fluorescence m. a microscope used for the examination of specimens stained with fluorochromes or fluorochrome complexes, e.g., a fluorescein-labeled antibody, which fluoresces in ultraviolet light.

hypodermic m. a combination of a fiberoptic probe (housed in a hypodermic needle) and a microscope for examining cell structure in tissue and muscle without a cutaneous incision.

infrared m. a microscope in which radiation of 800 μm or longer wavelength is used as the image-forming energy.

integrating m. a microscope in which a special mechanical stage permits recording of the sizes of the components of the specimen.

interference m. a microscope for observing the same kind of refractile detail as that observed with the phase microscope, but utilizing two separate beams of light which are sent through the specimen and combined with each other in the image plane.

ion m. an electron microscope modified to use ions (e.g., of lithium), instead of electrons.

laser m. see *laser microprobe.*

light m. a microscope in which the specimen is viewed under visible light.

opaque m. a microscope with vertical illumination or with the condenser built around the objective (epimicroscope) for viewing opaque specimens.

operating m. a specially designed magnifying instrument employed in the performance of delicate microsurgical procedures, as in operations on the middle ear, on small blood vessels, or on a vocal cord. Called also *surgical m.*

phase m., phase-contrast m. a microscope that converts variations of the refracting index in the object into variations of intensity in the image. Altering the phase relationship of light passing through and that passing around the object allows details of living cells to be seen without the fixation and staining that are normally necessary.

polarizing m. a microscope equipped with a polarizer, analyzer, and means for measurement of the alteration of the polarized light by the specimen.

polarizing m., rectified a polarizing microscope corrected for depolarization from curved lens surfaces so that full apertures can be used.

projection x-ray m. a microscope using soft x-radiation for high resolution; the images may be photographed or observed directly on a fluorescent viewing screen.

reflecting m. a microscope that uses mirrors instead of lenses to form the image.

Rheinberg m. a type of darkfield microscope whose condenser is modified by having a colored instead of an opaque stop, with the annulus in a complementary color. Called also *color-contrast m.*

scanning m., scanning electron m. an electron microscope in which a beam of electrons scans over a specimen point by point, causing the emission of a secondary beam that makes an image on the fluorescent screen of a cathode ray tube; differences in depth over the surface may be imaged in three dimensions.

schlieren m. a microscope in which light is deviated by the insertion of one or two diaphragms in the optical system, to reveal differences in refractive index in a specimen.

simple m. a microscope that consists of a single lens; a magnifying glass.

slit lamp m. see *slit lamp,* under *lamp.*

stereoscopic m. a binocular biobjective microscope, or a binocular monobjective microscope modified to give a three-dimensional view of the specimen.

stroboscopic m. a microscope using flashing illumination, permitting analysis of motion in the specimen.

surgical m. operating m.

transmission electron m. (TEM) an electron microscope that transmits a beam of electrons through the object, forming an image on a screen behind it.

trinocular m. a binocular microscope with a third eyepiece tube for photomicrography or other use.

ultra-m. see *ultramicroscope.*

ultrasonic m. a microscope that uses the reflection of ultrasonic or mechanical vibration to reveal the detail of the specimen.

ultraviolet m. a microscope using reflecting optics or quartz and other ultraviolet-transmitting lenses, having ultraviolet radiation as the image-forming energy.

x-ray m. a microscope in which a beam of x-rays is used instead of light, the image usually being reproduced on film.

mi•cro•scop•ic (mi″kro-skop′ik) 1. of extremely small size; visible only by the aid of the microscope. 2. pertaining or relating to a microscope or to microscopy.

mi•cro•scop•i•cal (mi″kro-skop′ĭ-kəl) microscopic.

mi•cros•co•pist (mi-kros′kə-pist) a person skilled in using the microscope.

mi•cros•co•py (mi-kros′kə-pe) [*micro-* + *-scopy*] examination under or observation by means of the microscope.

clinical m. employment of the microscope in making clinical diagnoses.

confocal m. a form of light microscopy, usually using fluorescence, that uses point illumination and a spatial pinhole to eliminate out-of-focus information and increase contrast in specimens that are thicker than the focal plane. By incrementally adjusting the focal point, serial thin sections of a specimen can be obtained; the images taken at different depths can be combined to produce three-dimensional views.

cryoelectron m. electron microscopy of a specimen that has been rapidly frozen so that it is embedded in a thin film of noncrystalline ice; the specimen is held on a stage cooled to liquid nitrogen temperatures.

electron m. examination by means of the electron microscope.

epifluorescence m. a type of fluorescence microscopy that uses two filters; only light of short wavelengths is allowed to illuminate the specimen and only its longer wavelength emissions are allowed to reach the examiner's eye.

epiluminescence m., epiluminescent m. a technique for the examination of pigmented skin lesions: the lesion is covered with an oil immersion and a glass slide to make the epidermis translucent and then is examined with a binocular microscope. Called also *dermatoscopy* and *dermoscopy.*

fluorescence m. microscopy of natural fluorescent materials or of specimens stained with fluorochromes, which emit light when exposed to blue light or ultraviolet radiation.

fundus m. examination of the fundus of the eye with an instrument combining a corneal microscope and an ophthalmoscope.

immunofluorescence m. fluorescence microscopy using immunofluorescence (q.v.) staining methods.

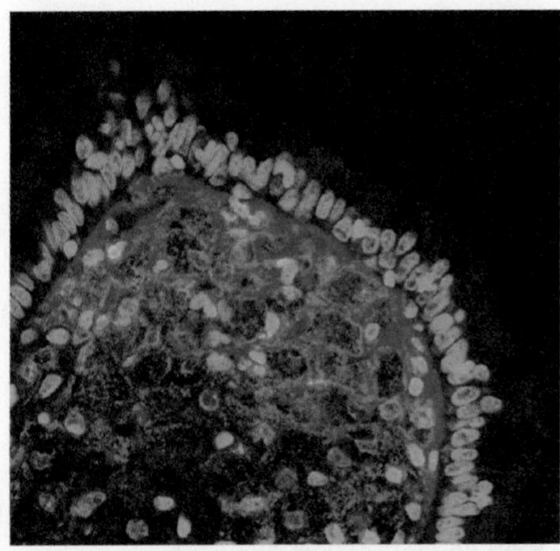

■ Confocal microscopy used to examine fluorescent in situ hybridization of a small intestinal biopsy specimen in a patient with Whipple disease. The intestinal villus shows ribosomal RNA (rRNA) of the infecting bacteria *Tropheryma whipplei (blue)*, as well as human cell nuclei *(green)*, and vimentin *(red)*.

television m. projection on a television screen of the image obtained by use of a flying spot, or scanning, microscope, or by use of a television camera over a microscope.

mi•cro•sec•ond (μs) (mi′kro-sek″ənd) one millionth (10^{-6}) of a second.

mi•cro•sec•tion (mi″kro-sek′shən) an extremely thin section for examination with the microscope.

mi•cro•seme (mi′kro-sēm) [*micro-* + Gr. *sēma* sign] having an orbital index of 83 or less.

mi•cro•shock (mi′kro-shok″) a term used in cardiology to denote a low level of electric current applied directly to myocardial tissue; as little as 0.1 mA causes ventricular fibrillation. Cf. *macroshock.*

mi•cro•slide (mi′kro-slīd) the slide on which objects for microscopic examination are mounted.

mi•cros•mat•ic (mi″kros-mat′ik) [*micro-* + *osmatic*] having the sense of smell, but of relatively feeble development, as in humans.

mi•cro•some (mi′kro-sōm″) [*micro-* + *-some*] any of the vesicular fragments of endoplasmic reticulum formed after disruption and centrifugation of cells. **microso′mal** *adj*

mi•cro•so•mia (mi″kro-so′me-ə) [*micro-* + *-somia*] small body size; see also *dwarfism.*

m. feta′lis abnormally small size of the fetus.

hemifacial m. a craniofacial malformation consisting of unilateral mandibular hypoplasia, macrostomia, and ear deformities, often associated with ocular and vertebral anomalies (*oculoauriculovertebral spectrum*, for which this term is sometimes used synonymously). Most cases are sporadic, but instances of autosomal dominant or recessive inheritance have been reported.

mi•cro•spec•tro•pho•tom•e•ter (mi″kro-spek″tro-fo-tom′ə-tər) a system combining a microscope with a spectrophotometer.

mi•cro•spec•tro•scope (mi″kro-spek′trə-skōp) [*micro-* + *spectroscope*] a spectroscope to be used in connection with a microscope for the examination of the spectra of microscopic objects.

mi•cro•spheres (mi′kro-sfērz″) small, uniform, spherical particles, often labeled with a radioisotope or a chemical marker, used for the study of blood flow and the occlusion of blood vessels in the treatment of hypervascular tumors such as uterine leiomyomas.

mi•cro•sphe•ro•cyte (mi″kro-sfe′ro-sīt) spherocyte.

mi•cro•sphero•cy•to•sis (mi″kro-sfe″ro-si-to′sis) spherocytosis.

mi•cro•sphero•lith (mi″kro-sfēr′o-lith) a type of particle sometimes found in bile, resembling a miniature gallstone.

mi•cro•sphyg•mia (mi″kro-sfig′me-ə) [*micro-* + *sphygm-* + *-ia*] a pulse that is difficult to perceive by the finger.

mi•cro•sphyg•my (mi″kro-sfig′me) microsphygmia.

mi•cro•sple•nia (mi″kro-sple′ne-ə) [*micro-* + *splen-* + *-ia*] smallness of the spleen. **microsple′nic** *adj*

Mi•cros•po•ra (mi-kros′pə-rə) [*micro-* + *spore*] a phylum of protozoa found as obligatory intracellular parasites in nearly all major animal groups, being especially common in insects, sometimes causing economically important disease. The spore phase is characterized by the presence of minute unicellular spores, each with an imperforate wall containing one nucleus or a dinucleate sporoplasm and a simple or complex extrusion apparatus with a polar tube or polar cap always present; mitochondria are absent. It comprises two classes: Rudimicrosporea and Microsporea.

mi•cro•spo•ran•gi•um (mi″kro-spə-ran′je-əm) pl. *microsporan′gia* [*micro-* + *sporangium*] the sporangium in which microspores develop.

mi•cro•spore (mi′kro-spor) [*micro-* + *spore*] 1. the smaller spore form when spores of two sizes are present, as in certain fungi and protozoa. 2. in heterogenous plants, one of four haploid spores, usually smaller than the megaspore, formed in the microsporangium from a microspore mother cell, and from which the microgametophyte, or male gametophyte, develops. See also *pollen.*

Mi•cro•spor•ea (mi″kro-spor′e-ə) a class of parasitic protozoa (phylum Microspora), the spores of which have a complex extrusion apparatus of Golgi origin, often including a polaroplast and posterior vacuole and a typically filamentous polar tube extending backward from the polar cap and coiling around inside of the three-layered spore wall; a sporocyst may or may not be present. It comprises two orders: Minisporida and Microsporida.

Mi•cro•spor•i•da (mi″kro-spor′ĭ-də) [*micro-* + *spore*] an order of parasitic protozoa (class Microsporea, phylum Microspora), usually found in invertebrates such as arthropods; human infection occurs in immunocompromised persons. Organisms in this group tend toward maximum development and varied specialization of accessory spore organelles accompanied by a reduction of sporocysts. There are two suborders: Pansporoblastina and Apansporoblastina. Called also *Cnidosporidia* and *Microsporidia.*

mi•cro•spor•i•dan (mi″kro-spor′ĭ-dən) 1. pertaining to protozoa of the phylum Microspora. 2. any protozoan of the phylum Microspora. 3. microsporidian (def. 2).

Mi•cro•spo•rid•ia (mi″kro-spə-rid′e-ə) Microsporida.

mi•cro•spo•rid•ia (mi″kro-spə-rid′e-ə) a nontaxonomic group comprising protozoa of the order Microsporida.

mi•cro•spo•rid•i•al (mi″kro-spə-rid′e-əl) pertaining to or caused by microsporidia.

mi•cro•spo•rid•i•an (mi″kro-spo-rid′e-ən) 1. microsporidial. 2. any protozoan of the order Microsporida. 3. microsporidan.

mi•cro•spo•rid•i•o•sis (mi″kro-spo-rid″e-o′sis) infection with protozoa of the order Microsporida. Human infection is usually restricted to immunocompromised patients, with symptoms including diarrhea and wasting. Types include encephalitozoonosis and nosematosis.

Mi•cros•po•ron (mi-kros′pə-ron) *Microsporum.*

mi•cro•spo•ro•sis (mi-kro″spə-ro′sis) infection with a fungus of genus *Microsporum.*

Mi•cros•po•rum (mi-kros′pə-rəm) [*micro* + Gr. *sporos* seed] a genus of Fungi Imperfecti, family Moniliaceae, mostly small-spored ectothrix ringworm fungi (dermatophytes); numerous species are causes of diseases of the skin and hair. As the perfect (sexual) stages are identified, they are classified in the genus *Arthroderma.* Called also *Microsporon.*

M. audoui′nii a small-spored ectothrix that is the most common cause of prepuberal tinea capitis in Europe and of about half the cases in the United States.

M. ca′nis a small-spored ectothrix that commonly causes ringworm in cats and dogs and can be transmitted to children, in whom it causes tinea capitis and tinea corporis. It is also probably the cause of a dermatomycosis in horses. It has perfect (sexual) stages in genus *Arthroderma.* Called also *M. felineum* and *M. lanosum.*

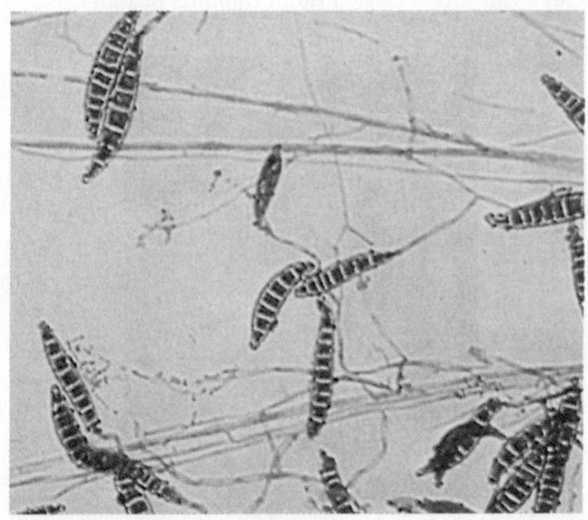

■ *Microsporum canis*, showing characteristic spindle-shaped, echinulate macroconidia with thick walls and tapered ends.

M. coo'kei a common geophilic species that sometimes causes dermatophytosis in rodents, dogs, and humans. Its perfect (sexual) stage is *Arthroderma cajetani.*

M. feli'neum *M. canis.*

M. ferrugi'neum a small-spored ectothrix that is anthropophilic and causes tinea capitis, mainly in children. Called also *Trichophyton ferrugineum.*

M. ful'vum a geophilic species that can be a large-spored ectothrix and cause tinea corporis or tinea capitis.

M. galli'nae *Trichophyton gallinae.*

M. gyp'seum a common geophilic species that can be a large-spored ectothrix and cause tinea capitis and tinea corporis. Its perfect (sexual) stage is *Arthroderma gypsea.*

M. lano'sum *M. canis.*

M. na'num a geophilic species that can be a large-spored ectothrix and cause ringworm in pigs and occasionally in humans. It has perfect (sexual) stages in genus *Arthroderma.*

M. persi'color a geophilic species that usually infects small rodents but occasionally causes tinea capitis or tinea corporis in humans. Its perfect (sexual) stage is *Arthroderma persicolor.*

M. vanbreuseghe'mii a large-spored ectothrix that causes dermatophytosis. It has perfect (sexual) stages in genus *Arthroderma.*

mi•cro•ste•a•to•sis (mi″kro-ste″ə-to′sis) [*micro-* + *steatosis*] microvesicular steatosis.

Mi•cro•stix-3 (mi′kro-stiks) trademark for a reagent strip with a chemical test area for recognition of nitrite in urine, which turns pink on contact with nitrite, and two culture areas for semiquantification of bacterial growth after 18–24 hours of incubation. One culture area supports both gram-negative and gram-positive organisms; the other, only gram-negative organisms.

mi•cro•sto•mia (mi″kro-sto′me-ə) [*micro-* + *stom-* + *-ia*] unusually small size of the mouth.

mi•cro•stra•bis•mus (mi″kro-strə-biz′məs) [*micro-* + *strabismus*] strabismus of such slight degree that the deviation is undetectable by the usual methods.

mi•cro•sur•gery (mi′kro-sur″jər-e) dissection of minute structures under the microscope by means of instruments held in the hand, such as for the ear or larynx. **microsur′gical** *adj*

transanal endoscopic m. (TEM) a technique of endoscopic microsurgery that allows direct visualization and removal of tumors of the distal half of the rectum.

mi•cro•syr•inge (mi″kro-sə-rinj′) a syringe fitted with a screw-thread micrometer head for the accurate control of minute measurements.

mi•cro•tech•nic (mi″kro-tek′nik) micrology.

mi•cro•tech•nique (mi″kro-tek-nēk′) a procedure or technique done at the microscopic level, such as microchemistry, micromanipulation, or microsurgery.

mi•cro•the•lia (mi″kro-the′le-ə) [*micro-* + *thel-* + *-ia*] unusual smallness of the nipples.

mi•cro•throm•bo•sis (mi″kro-throm-bo′sis) presence of many small thrombi in the capillaries and other small blood vessels.

mi•cro•throm•bus (mi″kro-throm′bəs) pl. *microthrom′bi.* a small thrombus located in a capillary or other small blood vessel.

mi•cro•tia (mi-kro′shə) [*micro-* + *ot-* + *-ia*] gross hypoplasia or aplasia of the auricle of the ear, with a blind or absent external acoustic meatus.

mi•cro•ti•ter (mi″kro-ti′tər) a titer of minute quantity.

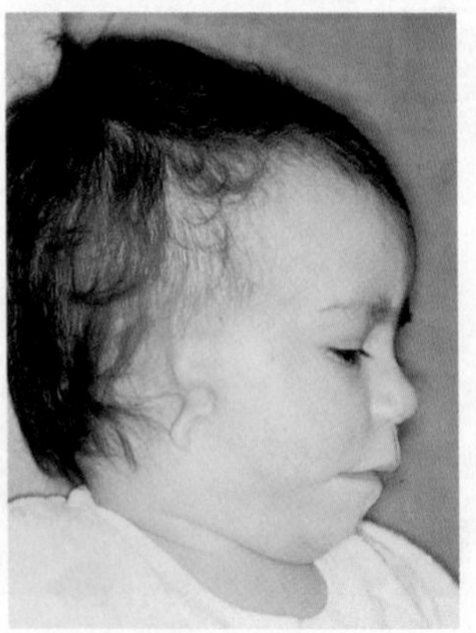

■ Microtia.

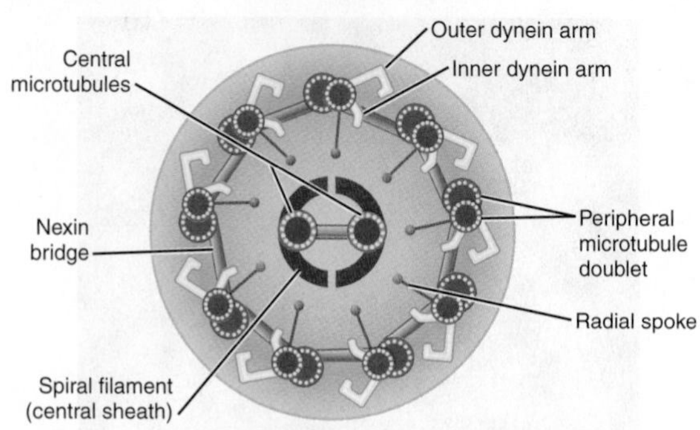

■ Microtubules in a 9 + 2 array in a cross-section of the axoneme of a cilium.

mi•cro•tome (mi′kro-tōm) [*micro-* + *-tome*] an instrument for cutting thin slices of tissue for microscopical study.

freezing m. a microtome for cutting frozen sections.

rocking m. a microtome in which the specimen is held in the end of a lever which passes up and down over a stationary knife.

rotary m. a microtome in which a wheel action is translated into a back-and-forth movement of the specimen being sectioned.

sliding m. a microtome in which the specimen being sectioned is made to slide on a track.

mi•crot•o•my (mi-krot′ə-me) [*micro-* + *-tomy*] the cutting of thin sections; called also *histotomy.*

mi•cro•to•nom•e•ter (mi″kro-to-nom′ə-tər) a small tonometer for measuring the oxygen and carbon dioxide tension in arterial blood.

mi•cro•trans•fu•sion (mi″kro-trans-fu′zhən) introduction into the circulation of a small quantity of blood of another individual, as sometimes occurs with transplacental passage of a small amount of fetal blood into the maternal circulation.

mi•cro•trau•ma (mi″kro-traw′mə) a slight trauma or lesion; a microscopic lesion.

Mi•cro•trom•bid•i•um aka•mu•shi (mi″kro-trom-bid′e-əm ah″kah-moo′she) *Trombicula akamushi.*

mi•cro•tro•pia (mi″kro-tro′pe-ə) microstrabismus.

mi•cro•tu•bule (mi″kro-too′būl) a tubular cytoplasmic structure, 25 nm in diameter and of variable length, composed of α- and β-tubulin dimers, whose orientation imparts polarity; microtubules are involved in maintenance of cell shape and in the movements of organelles and inclusions and form the spindle fibers of mitosis. In cilia and flagella, they are constantly arranged with two single microtubules in the center and nine pairs of doublets arrayed around the central two.

astral m's microtubules that radiate outward from the mitotic spindle pole, forming the aster; they interact with the cellular cortex to orient the spindle in the cell.

interpolar m's microtubules of the mitotic spindle whose minus ends terminate near the pole and whose plus ends extend beyond the chromosomes so that they interdigitate with microtubules extending from the opposite pole. Called also *polar m's.*

kinetochore m's microtubules of the mitotic spindle, organized into bundles (kinetochore fibers), that attach to the kinetochore, oriented so that their plus ends are embedded in the kinetochore and their minus ends are at or near the spindle pole.

polar m's interpolar m's.

subpellicular m's the microtubules (24 to 26) radiating posteriorly from the polar rings, directly beneath the pellicle, forming part of the apical complex in certain protozoa.

Mi•cro•tus (mi-kro′təs) [*micro-* + Gr. *ous, ōtos,* ear] a genus of voles, rodents of the family Muridae. *M. agres′tis* and *M. montebel′li* are field voles found in the Arctic and are reservoirs of *Leptospira interrogans* serovar *hebdomadis.*

mi•cro•tus (mi-kro′təs) an individual with microtia.

mi•cro•unit (μU) (mi′kro-u″nit) one millionth (10^{-6}) of a standard unit.

mi•cro•vas•cu•lar (mi″kro-vas′ku-lər) pertaining to the microvasculature.

mi•cro•vas•cu•la•ture (mi″kro-vas′ku-lə-chər) the portion of the vasculature of the body comprising the finer vessels, sometimes described as those with an internal diameter of 100 microns or less.

mi•cro•vas•cu•li•tis (mi″kro-vas″ku-li′tis) inflammation of the microvasculature.

mi•cro•vas•cu•lop•a•thy (mi″kro-vas″ku-lop′ə-the) any disorder affecting the microvasculature.

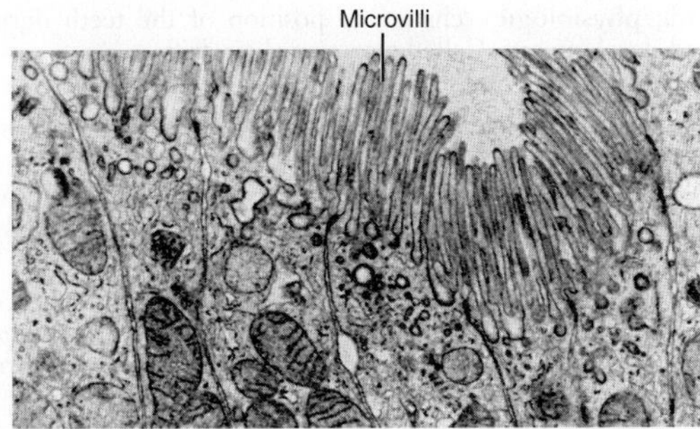

■ Microvilli forming the brush border of the proximal tubule pars convoluta from a normal human kidney.

retinal m. HIV-associated retinopathy.

mi•cro•ves•sel (mi'kro-ves"əl) any of the finer vessels of the body; cf. *microvasculature.*

mi•cro•vil•li (mi"kro-vil'i) [pl. of L. *microvillus* a tuft of hair] minute cylindrical processes on the free surface of a cell, organized around a core of cross-linked actin filaments anchored to the terminal web, which increase the surface size of the cell; found especially in cells of the proximal convolution of the renal tubules and of the intestinal epithelium; see also *brush border*, under *border.*

mi•cro•vil•lus (mi"kro-vil'əs) a minute process or protrusion from the free surface of a cell; see *microvilli.*

mi•cro•vis•co•sim•e•ter (mi"kro-vis"ko-sim'ə-tər) a viscosimeter for measuring the viscosity of blood plasma, using a small quantity of blood.

mi•cro•volt (μV) (mi'kro-volt) [*micro-* + *volt*] one millionth (10^{-6}) of a volt.

mi•cro•vol•tom•e•ter (mi"kro-vol-tom'ə-tər) an instrument for detecting minute changes of electric potential in the body.

mi•cro•watt (μW) (mi'kro-waht) [*micro-* + *watt*] one millionth (10^{-6}) of a watt.

mi•cro•wave (mi'kro-wāv) a wave typical of electromagnetic radiation between far infrared and radio waves, generally regarded as extending from 300,000 to 100 megacycles (wavelength of 1 mm to 30 cm).

Mi•crox (mi'kroks) former name for Mykrox.

Mi•cro•zide (mi'kro-zīd) trademark for a preparation of hydrochlorothiazide.

mi•croxy•cyte (mi-krok'sĭ-sīt) [*micr-* + *oxy-* + *-cyte*] any finely granular oxyphil cell.

mi•croxy•phil (mi-krok'sĭ-fil) microxycyte.

mi•cro•zoa (mi"kro-zo'ə) plural of *microzoon.*

mi•cro•zo•on (mi"kro-zo'on) pl. *microzo'a* [*micro-* + Gr. *zōon* animal] a microscopic animal organism. Cf. *microphyte.*

Mi•cru•roi•des (mi"kroo-roi'dēz) a genus of venomous snakes of the family Elapidae. *M. euryxan'thus* is the Arizona or Sonoran coral snake of Mexico and the southwestern United States.

Mi•cru•rus (mi-kroo'rəs) a genus of venomous snakes of the family Elapidae. *M. ful'vius* is the Eastern or Texas coral snake, a species found in the southern United States and tropical America whose body is marked with bright red, yellow, and black bands. Called also *Elaps.* See table at *snake.*

mic•tion (mik'shən) urination.

mic•tu•rate (mik'tu-rāt) urinate.

mic•tu•ri•tion (mik"tu-rĭ'shən) [L. *micturire* to urinate] urination.

MID minimum infective dose.

Mi•da•mor (mi'də-mor) trademark for preparations of amiloride hydrochloride.

mid•ax•il•la (mid"ak-sil'ə) the center of the axilla.

mid•azo•lam (mid'a-zo-lam") a benzodiazepine used as an antianxiety agent and muscle relaxant. It is stronger than diazepam but otherwise similar in actions and properties; administered intravenously or intramuscularly.
m. maleate a tranquilizer used for sedation and in the induction of anesthesia, administered intravenously.

mid•body (mid'bod"e) 1. a thin, dense intercellular bridge, consisting of the remnants of spindle fibers with a dense knob derived from the stem body matrix at its center, that results from the constriction of the cleavage furrow in cytokinesis; although it usually disappears by the end of cytokinesis, in some tissues it persists as a ring canal connecting adjacent cells. 2. the middle region of the trunk.

mid•brain (mid'brān") mesencephalon.

mid•car•pal (mid-kahr'pəl) between the two rows of bones of the carpus.

mid•di•as•tol•ic (mid"di-ə-stol'ik) occurring in the middle third of diastole.

mid•dle•piece (mid'əl-pēs) middle piece; see under *piece.*

mid•face (mid'fās") the middle of the face, including the nose, nasion, and glabella.

mid•foot (mid'foot") the middle portion of the foot, comprising the region of the navicular, cuboid, and cuneiform bones.

mid•fron•tal (mid-fron'təl) pertaining to the middle of the forehead.

midge (mij) 1. a small dipterous insect of the family Chironomidae; many species give painful bites, and some are vectors of *Mansonella ozzardi* and *Dipetalonema perstans.* 2. any of several small biting insects resembling the Chironomidae, such as various members of Ceratopogonidae and Culicoides.
owl m. *Phlebotomus.*

mid•gut (mid'gut") 1. the region of the embryonic digestive tract into which the yolk sac opens; it gives rise to most of the intestines. Ahead of it is the foregut and caudal to it is the hindgut. 2. the middle endodermal portion of the digestive tract of invertebrates, such as arthropods, comprising a stomach and sometimes a midintestine. Called also *mesenteron.*

mid•kine (mid'kīn) a multifunctional, low-molecular-weight heparin-binding growth factor that is a mediator of organogenesis during the embryonic period. It is important in cell growth, survival and migration; neurogenesis; and carcinogenesis.

mid•oc•cip•i•tal (mid"ok-sip'ĭ-təl) pertaining to or located in the middle of the occiput.

mi•do•drine hy•dro•chlo•ride (mi'do-drēn) a direct-acting sympathomimetic agent, which stimulates the α-adrenergic receptors of the arteriolar and venous vasculature; used as a vasopressor in the treatment of orthostatic hypotension, administered orally.

mid•pain (mid'pān") intermenstrual pain.

mid•pe•riph•e•ry (mid"pə-rif'ə-re) the middle zone of the fundus.

mid•piece (mid'pēs) middle piece.

mid•plane (mid'plān") the median plane of a bilateral structure.

mid•riff (mid'rif) 1. diaphragma (def. 1). 2. the middle region of the torso; the region between the inferior border of the breast and the waistline.

Mid•rin (mid'rin) trademark for a combination preparation of isometheptene mucate, dichloralphenazone, and acetaminophen.

mid•sec•tion (mid-sek'shən) a cut through the middle of any organ or part.

mid•ster•num (mid-stur'nəm) corpus sterni.

mid•tar•sal (mid-tahr'səl) between the two rows of bones of the tarsus.

mid•teg•men•tum (mid"təg-men'təm) the median or central part of the tegmentum.

mid•wife (mid'wīf") an individual who practices midwifery; see *nurse-midwife.*

mid•wi•fery (mid'wif-re, mid'wi-fər-e) the practice of assisting in childbirth. See *nurse-midwife* and *obstetrics.*

Mie•scher granuloma, granulomatous cheilitis (me'sher) [Guido *Miescher*, Swiss dermatologist, 1877–1961] see *granulomatous cheilitis*, under *cheilitis*, and *actinic granuloma*, under *granuloma.*

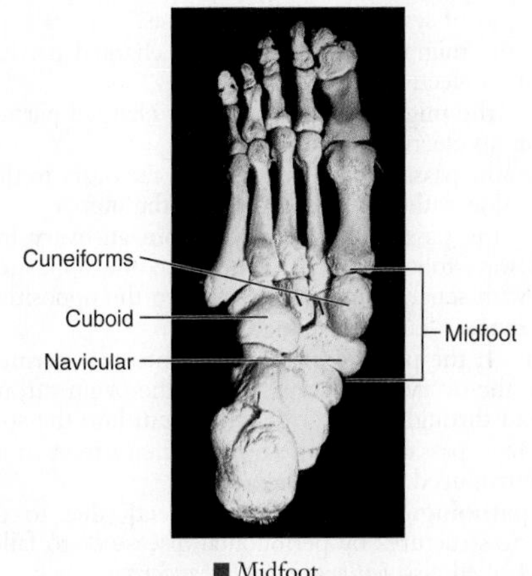

■ Midfoot.

MIF migration inhibition (or inhibitory) factor.

Mif•e•prex (mif′ə-preks) trademark for a preparation of mifepristone.

mif•e•pris•tone (mif″ə-pris′tōn) an antiprogestin used in combination with misoprostol or other prostaglandin as a postcoital contraceptive, terminating pregnancy in the first trimester; administered orally. Called also *RU-486.*

Mi•ger•got (mi′gər-got) trademark for combination preparations of ergotamine tartrate and caffeine.

mig•li•tol (mig′lĭ-tol) an α-glucosidase inhibitor used in treatment of type 2 diabetes, administered orally.

mi•graine (mi′grān) [Fr., from Gr. *hemikrania* an affection of half of the head] an often familial symptom complex of periodic attacks of vascular headache, usually temporal and unilateral in onset, commonly associated with irritability, nausea, vomiting, constipation or diarrhea, and often photophobia. Attacks are preceded by constriction of the cranial arteries, often with resultant prodromal sensory (especially ocular) symptoms and the spreading depression of Leão; the migraines themselves commence with the vasodilation that follows. Two primary types are distinguished, *m. with aura* and *m. without aura;* the variety without an aura is more common.

abdominal m. migraine in which abdominal symptoms (nausea and vomiting) are prominent.

acute confusional m. a rare variant of classic migraine occurring in children, marked by attacks of confusion and disorientation, with agitation manifested as a mixture of apprehension and combativeness; headache may not appear at first but always develops eventually.

m. with aura migraine that is preceded by a prodrome of neurologic symptoms, often visual ones such as teichopsia; called also *classic m.*

m. without aura migraine of sudden onset, without a prodrome; called also *common m.*

basilar m., basilar artery m. a type of ophthalmic migraine whose aura fills both visual fields and which may be accompanied by dysarthria and problems of equilibrium such as vertigo and incoordination; the symptoms are in the area supplied by the basilar and posterior cerebral arteries. Called also *Bickerstaff m.*

Bickerstaff m. basilar m.

classic m. m. with aura.

common m. m. without aura.

complicated m. migrainous infarction.

familial hemiplegic m. a rare type of hemiplegic migraine that is passed on as an autosomal dominant trait.

hemiplegic m. migraine associated with varying degrees of transient hemiplegia or hemiparesis.

neurologic m. classic m.

ocular m. ophthalmic m.

ophthalmic m. migraine accompanied by amblyopia, teichopsia, or other visual disturbance; see also *basilar m.*, *ophthalmoplegic m.*, and *retinal m.* Called also *ocular m.*

ophthalmoplegic m. periodic migraine accompanied by ophthalmoplegia; called also *Möbius disease.*

retinal m. a type of ophthalmic migraine with retinal symptoms such as monocular visual loss or blurring, probably because of constriction of one or more retinal arteries.

mi•grain•eur (me″gran-oor′) [Fr.] a person who suffers from migraine.

mi•grain•oid (mi′grən-oid) [*migraine* + *-oid*] resembling migraine.

mi•grain•ous (mi′grən-əs) resembling, or of the nature of migraine.

Mi•gra•nal (mi′grə-nal″) trademark for a preparation of dihydroergotamine mesylate.

mi•gra•tion (mi-gra′shən) [L. *migratio*] 1. an apparently spontaneous change of place, as of symptoms. 2. diapedesis.

anodic m. the migration of a negatively charged particle toward the positive pole in an electrical field.

cathodic m. the migration of a positively charged particle toward the negative pole in an electrical field.

external m. the passage of an oocyte from the ovary to the uterine tube of the opposite side without passing through the uterus.

internal m. the passing of an oocyte from an ovary into the uterus in the normal way, followed by its entry into the opposite uterine tube or, in animals with separate uterine horns, into the opposite horn.

m. of leukocytes leukocyte emigration.

m. of ovum 1. the passage of the ovum into the uterine tube after its discharge from the ovary. 2. the passage of the ovum through the reproductive tract and through the uterine epithelium into the stroma.

retrograde m. passage into the upper urinary tract of a substance or foreign body introduced through the urethra.

tooth m., pathologic drifting of the teeth due to destruction of tooth-supporting structures by periodontal disease or to failure to replace missing teeth. Called also *pathologic tooth wandering.*

tooth m., physiologic change of position of the teeth during their growth and development. Called also *physiologic drift.*

transperitoneal m. external m.

mi•gra•to•ry (mi′grə-tor″e) 1. roving or wandering. 2. of, pertaining to, or characterized by migration; undergoing periodic migration.

Mi•ka•nia (mĭ-ka′ne-ə) [J.G. *Mikan*, Czech botanist, 19th century] a genus of tropical American vines of the family Compositae. *M. gua′co* Humb. & Bonpl. is the medicinal plant guaco.

Mi•ku•licz angle, cells, etc. (me′koo-lich″) [Johann von *Mikulicz-*Radecki, Polish surgeon, 1850–1905] see under *angle*, *cell*, *clamp*, *disease*, *drain*, *operation*, *pack*, and *syndrome*, and see *periadenitis mucosa necrotica recurrens.*

Milch method (milch) see under *method.*

mil•dew (mil′doo) 1. any of various fungi that grow on vegetable or other material, divided into *downy* and *powdery* types. 2. the condition caused by such a fungus.

downy m., false m. a mildew of the family Peronosporaceae.

powdery m. a mildew of the order Erysiphales.

Miles operation (mīlz) [William Ernest *Miles*, British surgeon, 1869–1947] see under *operation.*

mil•ia (mil′e-ə) [L.] plural of *milium.*

mi•li•a•ria (mil″e-ar′e-ə) [L. *milium* millet] 1. a skin condition associated with obstruction of sweat ducts, resulting in sweat retention, rupture of ducts below the level of the obstruction, and extravasation of sweat within the skin. The three most common types are miliaria crystallina, miliaria rubra, and miliaria profunda, distinguished according to the level of obstruction; they are seen primarily in infants, although they sometimes occur in adults in hot, humid conditions. 2. m. rubra.

m. al′ba m. crystallina.

apocrine m. Fox-Fordyce disease.

m. crystalli′na the most superficial type of miliaria; sweat escapes in or just beneath the stratum corneum, producing noninflammatory vesicles that look like droplets because of the thinness of the layer covering them. Called also *m. alba* and *sudamina.*

m. profun′da the deepest type of miliaria, with occlusion of the ducts at the dermoepidermal junction. It occurs following severe, recurrent miliaria rubra and is seen primarily in hot, humid climates. Because large numbers of sweat glands are inactivated, it can lead to heat intolerance or heat stress, as in tropical anhidrotic asthenia.

m. pustulo′sa a variant of miliaria rubra in which pustules develop.

m. ru′bra a condition resulting from obstruction of sweat ducts deep in the epidermis, with rupture producing pruritic erythematous papular vesicles. The itching and vesicle formation may be due to vasodilatation and stimulation of itch receptors in the epidermis. The severity of the symptoms fluctuates with the heat load of the individual. Called also *heat rash* and *prickly heat.*

mil•i•ary (mil′e-ar-e) [L. *miliaris* like a millet seed] 1. resembling a millet seed. 2. characterized by minute lesions resembling millet seeds.

mi•lieu (mēl-yoo′) [Fr.] surroundings; environment.

m. extérieur (eks-ta″re-oor′) the external environment.

m. intérieur (ă-ta″re-oor′) interior environment; the blood and lymph that bathe the cells of the body.

mil•i•um (mil′e-əm) pl. *mil′ia* [L. "millet seed"] a tiny epidermal cyst that is a round, smooth, firm, white to yellow papule just under the skin. These occur in groups and are usually found in the pilosebaceous units of the eyelids, cheeks, or forehead; they occur in all age groups, including babies, and may arise de novo or in association with skin diseases or trauma to the skin. Called also *whitehead.* See also *Epstein pearls*, under *pearl.*

colloid m. a small, discrete, translucent, white to yellow, firm papule containing an amorphous colloid; these occur in profuse eruptions, usually on the face or back of the hands during middle age.

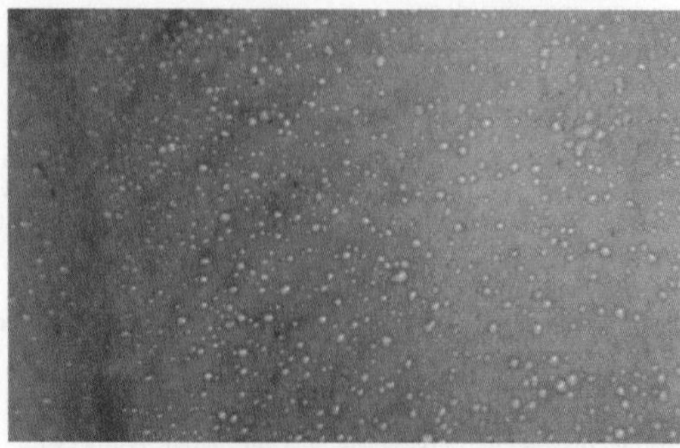

■ Miliaria crystallina.

multiple eruptive milia a type of colloid milia seen in children, transmitted by autosomal dominant inheritance.

milk (milk) [L. *lac*] 1. the fluid secretion of the mammary gland forming the natural food of young mammals. 2. any whitish milklike substance, e.g., coconut milk or plant latex. 3. a liquid (emulsion or suspension) resembling the secretion of the mammary gland.

acidophilus m. milk fermented with cultures of *Lactobacillus acidophilus;* used in gastrointestinal disorders in attempts to modify the bacterial flora of the intestinal tract.

condensed m. milk which has been partly evaporated and sweetened with sugar.

evaporated m. milk prepared by evaporation of half its water content.

fortified vitamin D m. vitamin D m.

homogenized m. milk so treated that the fats become intimately combined with the general body of the milk, the emulsified particles of fat being made so minute that the cream does not separate.

litmus m. see *litmus-milk culture medium*, under *culture medium.*

lowfat m. milk having 1 to 2 per cent fat content.

m. of magnesia [USP] a suspension of magnesium hydroxide, used as an antacid and laxative.

modified m. milk in which the constituents have been made to correspond in amount to the composition of human milk.

nonfat m. milk having no greater than 0.5 per cent fat content.

pasteurized m. milk that has been specially heat treated to kill bacteria; see *pasteurization.*

skim m. milk from which some or all of the cream has been removed; see *lowfat m.* and *nonfat m.*

soy m. a liquid made from soybeans, used as a milk substitute and a source of calcium for those unable or unwilling to ingest dairy products.

m. of sulfur precipitated sulfur.

uterine m. a white milky substance in the gravid uterus of some species, presumably for nourishment of the embryo.

vegetable m. synthetic milk made from vegetable sources (such as soy).

vitamin D m. cow's milk supplemented with 400 IU of vitamin D per quart.

witch's m. milk secreted in the breast of the newborn child; hexenmilch.

milk•ing (milk′ing) the pressing out of the contents of a tubular part, such as the urethra, by running the finger along it.

Milk•man syndrome (milk′man) [Louis Arthur *Milkman*, American radiologist, 1895–1951] see under *syndrome.*

milk•weed (milk′wēd) any plant of the genus *Asclepias.*

milk•wort (milk′wort) any plant of the genus *Polygala.*

milky (mil′ke) 1. having the appearance of milk; whitish, cloudy, and fluid. 2. filled with or consisting of milk or a milklike fluid. 3. chylous.

Mil•lard-Gub•ler syndrome (paralysis) (me-yahr′ goo-bla′) [Auguste L.J. *Millard*, French physician, 1830–1915; Adolphe Marie *Gubler*, French physician, 1821–1879] see under *syndrome.*

Mil•le•po•ra (mil″ə-po′rə) the fire corals, a genus of invertebrates of the phylum Cnidaria, class Hydrozoa. Several species found in the Caribbean have stings that are toxic or cause skin irritation.

Mil•ler syndrome (mil′ər) [Marvin *Miller*, American pediatrician, 1911–1999] see under *syndrome.*

Mil•ler-Ab•bott tube (mil′ər ab′ət) [T. Grier *Miller*, American physician, 1886–1981; William Osler *Abbott*, American physician, 1902–1943] see under *tube.*

Mil•ler-Diek•er syndrome (mil′ər de′kər) [James Quinter *Miller*, American neurologist, born 1926; H. *Dieker*, American physician, 20th century] see under *syndrome.*

Mil•ler Fish•er syndrome (mil′ər fish′ər) [Charles Miller Fisher, Canadian neurologist, born 1913] Fisher syndrome.

milli- [L. *mille* thousand] a prefix indicating one thousand (e.g., millipede); also used in naming units of measurement (symbol m) to indicate one thousandth (10^{-3}) of the unit designated by the root with which it is combined.

mil•li•am•me•ter (mil″e-am′me-tər) an ammeter that registers a current in milliamperes.

mil•li•am•pere (mA) (mil″e-am′pēr) one thousandth (10^{-3}) of an ampere.

mil•li•bar (mil′ĭ-bahr) one thousandth (10^{-3}) of a bar.

mil•li•cou•lomb (mC) (mil″ĭ-koo′lom) one thousandth (10^{-3}) of a coulomb.

mil•li•cu•rie (mCi) (mil″ĭ-ku′re) a unit of radioactivity, being one thousandth (10^{-3}) of a curie.

mil•li•equiv•a•lent (mEq) (mil″e-e-kwiv′ə-lənt) one thousandth (10^{-3}) of the equivalent weight of an element, radical, or compound.

mil•li•gram (mg) (mil′ĭ-gram) one thousandth (10^{-3}) of a gram.

Mil•li•kan-Sie•kert syndrome (mil′ĭ-kən se′kərt) [Clark Harold *Millikan*, American neurologist, born 1915; Robert George *Siekert*, American neurologist, born 1924] vertebrobasilar insufficiency.

mil•li•lam•bert (mil″i-lam′bərt) one thousandth (10^{-3}) of a lambert.

mil•li•li•ter (mL) (mil′ĭ-le″tər) a unit of volume, being one thousandth (10^{-3}) of a liter.

mil•li•me•ter (mm) (mil′ĭ-me″tər) a unit of linear measure, being one thousandth (10^{-3}) of a meter.

mil•li•mo•lar (mM) (mil′ĭ-mo″lər) denoting a concentration of 1 millimole per liter.

mil•li•mole (mmol) (mil′ĭ-mōl) one thousandth (10^{-3}) of a mole (see *mole*[1]).

Mil•lin operation (mil′in) [Terence John *Millin*, British urologist, 20th century] see under *operation.*

mill•ing-in (mil′ing-in) correction of occlusal disharmonies of natural or artificial teeth by the use of abrasives between their occluding surfaces while they are rubbed together in the mouth or on the articulator. See also *grinding-in; occlusal adjustment*, under *adjustment;* and *selective grinding*, under *grinding.*

mil•lions (mil′yənz) a name applied to various small fish that devour mosquito larvae, such as *Lebistes reticulatus.*

mil•li•os•mole (mOsm) (mil″e-os′mōl) one thousandth (10^{-3}) of an osmole.

mil•li•pede (mil′ĭ-pēd) any arthropod of the class Diplopoda.

mil•li•rad (mrad) (mil′ĭ-rad) one thousandth (10^{-3}) of a rad.

mil•li•rem (mrem) (mil′ĭ-rem) one thousandth (10^{-3}) of a rem.

mil•li•roent•gen (mR) (mil′ĭ-rent″gən) one thousandth (10^{-3}) of a roentgen.

mil•li•sec•ond (ms) (mil′ĭ-sek″ənd) one thousandth (10^{-3}) of a second.

mil•li•unit (mU) (mil′ĭ-u″nit) one-thousandth (10^{-3}) of a standard unit.

mil•li•volt (mV) (mil′ĭ-vōlt) one thousandth (10^{-3}) of a volt.

Mil•lon test (reaction, reagent) (me-yaw′) [Auguste Nicolas Eugène *Millon*, French chemist, 1812–1867] see under *test.*

mil•pho•sis (mil-fo′sis) [Gr. *milphōsis*] loss of the eyelashes.

mil•ri•none (mil′rĭ-nōn) [USP] a cardiotonic used in the treatment of congestive heart failure; administered intravenously.

Mil•roy disease (lymphedema) (mil′roi) [William Forsyth *Milroy*, American physician, 1855–1942] see under *disease.*

mil•tef•o•sine (mil-tef′o-sēn) a phospholipid derivative that disrupts certain types of cell membranes and is used in treatment of visceral leishmaniasis; administered orally.

Mil•town (mil′toun) trademark for a preparation of meprobamate.

Mil•wau•kee brace, shoulder syndrome (mil-waw′ke) [*Milwaukee*, Wisconsin, USA] see under *brace* and *syndrome.*

mi•me•sis (mĭ-me′sis) [Gr. *mimēsis* imitation] 1. the simulation of one disease by another. 2. mimicry (def. 2).

mi•met•ic (mĭ-met′ik) [Gr. *mimētikos*] 1. pertaining to or exhibiting mimicry. 2. marked by simulation of another disease.

-mimetic a word termination indicating simulation of a function, process, etc., designated by the root to which it is affixed, as *sympathomimetic.*

mim•ic (mim′ik) 1. mimetic (def. 1). 2. one who imitates, or that which imitates. 3. to imitate or simulate.

genetic m. genocopy.

mim•ic•ry (mim′ik-re″) [Gr. *mimos* to imitate] 1. imitation or simulation. 2. an adaptation for survival in which an organism takes on a resemblance to some other organism or a nonliving object.

mim•ma•tion (mĭ-ma′shən) mytacism.

mi•mo•sis (mi-mo′sis) mimesis.

min. [L.] min′imum (a minim).

Mi•na•ma•ta disease (me″nah-mah′tah) [*Minamata* Bay, Japan, source of poisoned seafood that caused the disease in the 1950s] see under *disease.*

mind (mīnd) [from A.S. *gemynd*] 1. the organ or seat of consciousness; the faculty, or function of the brain, by which an individual becomes aware of the surroundings and of their distribution in space and time; by which feelings, emotions, and desires are experienced; and which gives the ability to attend, to remember, to learn, to reason, and to decide. 2. the organized totality of an organism's mental and psychological processes, conscious and unconscious. 3. the characteristic thought process of a person or group.

min•er•al (min′ər-əl) [L. *minerale*] a nonorganic homogeneous solid substance, usually a constituent of the earth's crust.
  trace m. a mineral that is a trace element.

min•er•alo•cor•ti•coid (min″ər-al″o-kor′tĭ-koid) any of the group of C21 corticosteroids that are involved in the regulation of electrolyte and water balance through their effects on ion transport in epithelial cells; the most important one is aldosterone. They promote retention of sodium, loss of potassium, and the secondary retention of water; some also have varying degrees of glucocorticoid activity.

Mi•ner•va jac•ket (mĭ-nur′və) [*Minerva*, Roman goddess of wisdom, because of its resemblance to her armor] see under *jacket.*

mini- [*mini*ature] a combining form denoting something smaller than is usual for objects in a given class.

mini•chro•mo•some (min″e-kro′mə-sōm) [*mini-* + *chromosome*] 1. a chromatin structure resembling a small chromosome, formed by certain viruses when they infect eukaryotic cells and composed of viral DNA complexed with host histones. 2. a plasmid that contains a chromosomal origin of replication.

min•i•fy (min′ĭ-fi) [L. *minus* less] to render less or diminish; the opposite of magnify.

mini•lap•a•ros•co•py (min″e-lap″ə-ros′kə-pe) laparoscopy using very small instruments. **minilaparoscop′ic** *adj*

mini•lap•a•rot•o•my (min″e-lap″ə-rot′ə-me) [*mini-* + *laparotomy*] a very short laparotomy incision.

min•im (m.) (min′im) [L. *minimum* least] a unit of capacity (liquid measure) equal to one sixtieth of a fluid dram, or the equivalent of 0.0616 milliliter.

min•i•ma (min′ĭ-mə) [L.] plural of *minimum.*

min•i•mal (min′ĭ-məl) [L. *minimus* least] smallest or least; the smallest possible. In some terms, *minimal* and *minimum* are used interchangeably.

min•i•mum (min′ĭ-məm) pl. *min′ima* [L. "smallest"] 1. the smallest amount or lowest limit. 2. minimal.
  m. audi′bile, m. audible auditory threshold.
  m. cognosci′bile the threshold of visual recognition of complicated shapes or contours.
  m. legi′bile the threshold of visible recognition of form, as of test letters or numbers.
  light m. (LM) the smallest degree of light perceived by the eye.
  m. sensi′bile threshold of consciousness.
  m. separa′bile resolution threshold.
  m. visi′bile light m.

min•i•pill (min′e-pil) progestin-only contraceptive.

mini•plate (min′e-plāt) a small bone plate.

Mini•press (min′e-pres) trademark for a preparation of prazosin hydrochloride.

mini•sat•el•lite (min″e-sat′ə-līt) any of a series of short (usually 1000 to 5000 base pairs) lengths of DNA dispersed throughout the genome, comprising tandemly repeated nucleotide sequences, each repeating unit composed of approximately 10 to 60 base pairs. Within a genome, different minisatellites may differ in their repeating unit, but the repeating unit within a minisatellite is relatively constant, and the number of repeating units in a given minisatellite varies between individuals in a species. Because of this length polymorphism, minisatellites are sometimes called *variable number tandem repeats* or *variable number of tandem repeats.*

Mini•spor•i•da (min″e-spor′ĭ-də) [*mini-* + *spore*] an order of parasitic protozoa (class Microsporea, phylum Microspora) having a general tendency toward minimum development of accessory spore organelles accompanied by maximum development of sporocysts, and characterized by spores without a well-developed polaroplast, usually with a relatively short polar tube, with little or no endospore.

Mini•tran (min′e-tran) trademark for a preparation of nitroglycerin.

Mini•zide (min′e-zīd) trademark for a combination preparation of prazosin hydrochloride and polythiazide.

Min•kow•ski figure (min-kof′ske) [Oskar *Minkowski*, Lithuanian physician in Germany, 1858–1931] see under *figure.*

Min•kow•ski-Chauf•fard syndrome (min-kof′ske sho-fahr′) [O. *Minkowski;* Anatole-Marie-Emile *Chauffard*, French physician, 1855–1932] hereditary spherocytosis.

Mi•no•cin (mĭ-no′sin) trademark for preparations of minocycline hydrochloride.

mi•no•cy•cline (mĭ-no-si′klēn) a semisynthetic broad-spectrum antibiotic of the tetracycline group.
  m. hydrochloride [USP] the monohydrochloride salt of minocycline, used in the treatment of a wide variety of infections, administered orally or intravenously.

Mi•nor disease, sign (me′nor) [Lazar Salomonovich *Minor*, Russian neurologist, 1855–1942] see under *disease* and *sign.*

mi•nor (mi′nər) insignificant; small or least in scope, effect, number, size, extent, or importance.

Mi•not-von Wil•le•brand syndrome (mi′not fon vil′ə-brahnt) [Francis *Minot*, American physician, 1821–1899; Erick Adolf *von Willebrand*, Finnish physician, 1870–1949] see *von Willebrand disease*, under *disease.*

mi•nox•i•dil (mĭ-nok′sĭ-dil) [USP] a potent, long-acting orally effective vasodilator, acting primarily on arterioles, used as an antihypertensive; also applied topically in the treatment of androgenetic alopecia.

mint (mint) 1. any plant of the genus *Mentha.* 2. any of certain other plants resembling those of genus *Mentha.*
  mountain m. a plant of the genus *Pycnanthemum.*

Min•te•zol (min′tə-zol) trademark for a preparation of thiabendazole.

mi•nute (mi-no͞ot′) [L. *minuere* to diminish] extremely small.
  double m's acentric chromosomal fragments created by gene amplification and newly integrated into the chromosome; they are tumor markers indicative of solid neoplasms with poor prognosis.

MIO minimal identifiable odor.

mi(o)- [Gr. *meiōn* smaller] a combining form meaning less, or denoting relationship to contraction.

Mio•chol (mi′o-kol) trademark for a preparation of acetylcholine chloride.

mio•did•y•mus (mi″o-did′ĭ-məs) [*mio-* + *-didymus*] asymmetrical conjoined twins in which a smaller head is joined to the larger one at the occiput.

mio•lec•i•thal (mi″o-les′ĭ-thəl) microlecithal.

mio•pra•gia (mi″o-pra′je-ə) hypofunction.

mi•o•pus (mi′o-pəs) [*mio-* + Gr. *ōps* face] a fetus with two fused heads, one face being rudimentary.

mi•o•sis (mi-o′sis) [Gr. *meiōsis* diminution] contraction of the pupil.
  irritative m. spastic m.
  paralytic m. miosis due to paralysis of the dilator of the iris.
  spastic m. miosis due to spasm of the sphincter pupillae.
  spinal m. miosis occurring in spinal diseases.

mi•ot•ic (mi-ot′ik) 1. an agent that causes the pupil to contract. 2. meiotic.

MIP maximum inspiratory pressure.

mi•ra•cid•ia (mi-rə-sid′e-ə) plural of *miracidium.*

mi•ra•cid•i•um (mi-rə-sid′e-əm) pl. *miraci′dia* [Gr. *meirakidion* boy, young man] the first stage larva of a trematode which undergoes further development in the body of a snail.

mir•ac•u•lin (mir-ak′u-lin) a glycoprotein from the fruit of the tropical plant *Synsepalum dulcificum* which, after it is tasted, is able to change the perception of the taste of acids from sour to sweet.

Mir•a•don (mir′ə-don) trademark for a preparation of anisindione.

Mira•Lax (mir′ə-laks) trademark for a preparation of polyethylene glycol 3350.

Mira•pex (mir′ə-peks) trademark for a preparation of pramipexole dihydrochloride.

Mir•cette (mər-set′) trademark for a therapeutic regimen of desogestrel and ethinyl estradiol.

mire (mēr) [Fr., from L. *mirari* to look at] one of the figures on the arm of an ophthalmometer whose images are reflected on the cornea. The measurement of their variations determines the amount of corneal astigmatism.

Mi•re•na (mĭ-rĕ′nə) trademark for a preparation of levonorgestrel.

Mi•riz•zi syndrome (me-rēt′se) [Pablo Luis *Mirizzi*, Argentine surgeon, 1893–1964] see under *syndrome.*

MIRL membrane inhibitor of reactive lysis; see *protectin.*

miRNA microRNA.

mir•ror (mir′ər) [Fr. *miroir*] a polished surface that reflects sufficient light to yield images of objects in front of it.
  concave m. a mirror with a concave reflecting surface.

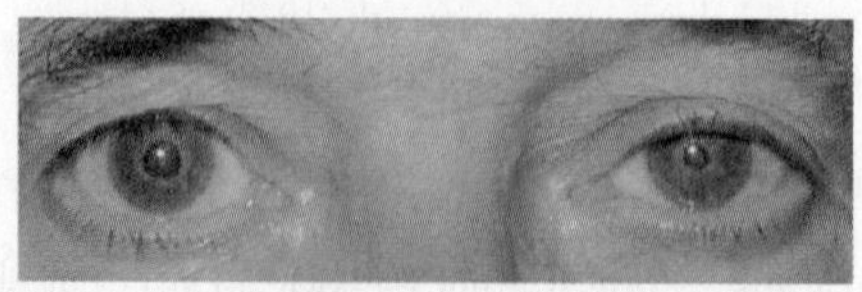

■ Miosis and eyelid ptosis of the left eye in Horner syndrome.

convex m. a mirror with a convex reflecting surface.
dental m. mouth m.
frontal m. head m.
Glatzel m. a mirror held below the nose for receiving moist breath to assess nasal patency; see also *pneumatype*.
head m. a circular mirror strapped to the head of the examiner to reflect light into a cavity, especially the nose, pharynx, or larynx. Called also *frontal m.*
mouth m. a small mirror, magnifying or nonmagnifying, used to reflect the operating field in the oral cavity, to retract the tissues and tongue, and to protect the tissues from injury during operation. Called also *dental m.* See also *dental reflector*, under *reflector*.
nasographic m. Glatzel m.
plane m. a mirror with a flat reflecting surface.

mir•taz•a•pine (mir″taz-ə-pēn) an antidepressant compound unrelated to any of the classes of antidepressants; administered orally.

mir•ya•chit (mir-yah′chit) myriachit.

MIS müllerian-inhibiting substance; see *antimüllerian hormone*.

mis•an•thro•py (mis-an′thrə-pe) [*miso-* + *anthrop-* + *-ia*] hatred of human beings.

mis•car•riage (mis′kar-əj) popular term for *spontaneous abortion*.

mis•ce (M.) (mis′e) [L.] mix.

mis•ci•ble (mis′ĭ-bəl) susceptible of being mixed.

mis•clas•si•fi•ca•tion (mis″klas-ĭ-fĭ-ka′shən) assignment of subjects, values, or attributes to inappropriate groups or categories. In *nondifferential m.* the probability or direction of misclassification error is constant across all study groups while in *differential m.* it varies across the groups.

mis•i•den•ti•fi•ca•tion (mis″i-den″tĭ-fĭ″ka′shən) failure to identify correctly persons or objects known to the subject, caused by confusion or memory loss.
delusional m. misidentification due to the mistaken belief that a person or object has been transformed physically or mentally. See also *Capgras syndrome*, under *syndrome*, and *Frégoli phenomenon*, under *phenomenon*.

mis(o)- [Gr. *misos* hatred] a combining form meaning hatred of.

mi•sog•a•my (mĭ-sog′ə-me) [*miso-* + Gr. *gamos* marriage] hatred of or aversion to marriage.

mi•sog•y•ny (mĭ-soj′ĭ-ne) [*miso-* + Gr. *gynē* woman] hatred of women.

mi•so•nid•a•zole (mi″so-nid′ə-zōl) a compound structurally related to metronidazole, formerly used as an antitrichomonal and antiprotozoal but now primarily used as a radiosensitizer. Administered orally.

mi•so•pro•stol (mi-so-pros′tol) a synthetic prostaglandin E_1 analogue administered orally to prevent gastric ulcer associated with long-term therapy with nonsteroidal antiinflammatory drugs. It is also used orally in combination with mifepristone to terminate pregnancy, acting to soften and ripen the cervix and induce uterine contractions.

mis•pair•ing (mis-pār′ing) incorrect pairing of entities or objects.
slipped strand m. incorrect pairing of DNA strands during replication caused by misalignment of the two strands in regions containing tandem repeats.

mis•sense (mis′sens) in genetics, pertaining to a mutation in which a codon is altered so that it encodes a different amino acid from that found in the wild type.

mist. [L.] mistu′ra (a mixture).

mis•tle•toe (mis′əl-to) any of several parasitic shrubs of the family Loranthaceae. European mistletoe is *Viscum album;* it contains small amounts of toxins such as pressor amines, beta-phenylethylamine, and tyramine and is used for rheumatism and as an adjunct in cancer therapy; it is also used in traditional Chinese medicine and homeopathy.

MIT monoiodotyrosine.

Mit. [L.] mit′te (send).

Mitch•ell disease (mich′əl) [Silas Weir *Mitchell*, American neurologist, 1829–1914] erythromelalgia.

Mitch•ell operation (mich′əl) [Charles L. *Mitchell*, American orthopedic surgeon, 20th century] see under *operation*.

Mit•chel•la (mĭ-chel′ə) [John *Mitchell*, American botanist, 18th century] a genus of creeping perennial evergreen herbs of the family Rubiaceae. *M. re′pens* L. is the partridge berry or deerberry, a North American species that when dried is the medicinal herb called *mitchella*.

mitch•el•la (mĭ-chel′ə) 1. any plant of the genus *Mitchella*. 2. the dried plant *Mitchella repens*, used as a diuretic, astringent, and antidiarrheal, and formerly as a uterine tonic.

mite (mīt) any arachnid arthropod of the order Acarina except the ticks. Most mites are minute and have transparent or semitransparent bodies; many are parasitic, causing skin irritation (acariasis). Families that have genera that attack humans include Acaridae, Cheyletiellidae, Demodicidae, Dermanyssidae, Glycyphagidae, Sarcoptidae, Tetranychidae, and Trombiculidae. Other genera that attack nonhuman mammals and birds are found in the families Halarachnidae, Listrophoridae, and Myobiidae.
auricular m. see *Otodectes*.
bird m. *Dermanyssus gallinae.*
burrowing m. *Sarcoptes scabiei.*
cheese m. *Tyrophagus longior.*
chicken m. *Dermanyssus gallinae.*
chigger m. trombiculid.
citrus red m. *Panonychus citri.*
clover m. *Bryobia praetiosa.*
copra m. *Tyrophagus castellani.*
depluming m. *Knemidokoptes gallinae.*
face m. either *Demodex brevis* or *D. folliculorum.*
flour m. *Tyrophagus farinae.*
follicle m. either *Demodex brevis* or *D. folliculorum.*
food m. *Glycyphagus domesticus.*
fowl m. *Dermanyssus gallinae.*
hair follicle m. either *Demodex brevis* or *D. folliculorum.*
harvest m. chigger.
house dust m. either *Dermatophagoides pteronyssinus* or *D. farinae.*
itch m. 1. *Sarcoptes scabiei.* 2. *Notoedres cati.*
kedani m. *Trombicula akamushi.*
louse m. *Pyemotes.*
mange m. any of various mites that cause mange; such as species of *Chorioptes*, *Demodex*, *Knemidokoptes*, *Notoedres*, *Otodectes*, *Psoroptes*, and *Sarcoptes.*
meal m. *Tyrophagus.*
mouse m. *Liponyssoides sanguineus.*
mower's m. chigger.
nasal m. *Pneumonyssus caninum.*
northern fowl m. *Ornithonyssus sylviarum.*
onion m. *Acarus rhyzoglypticus hyacinthi.*
poultry m. *Dermanyssus gallinae.*
rat m. see *Ornithonyssus.*
red m. chigger.
scab m. see *Psoroptes.*
scabies m. *Sarcoptes scabiei.*
spinning m. *Bryobia praetiosa.*
straw m., straw itch m. either *Pyemotes tritici* or *P. ventricosus.*
tropical fowl m. *Ornithonyssus bursa.*
tropical rat m. *Ornithonyssus bacoti.*
two-spotted spider m. *Tetranychus urticae.*

mi•tel•la (mi-tel′ə) [L.] a sling for the upper limb.

Mith•ra•cin (mith′rə-sin) trademark for a preparation of plicamycin.

mith•ra•my•cin (mith″rə-mi′sin) former name for *plicamycin.*

mith•ri•da•tism (mith′rĭ-da″tiz-əm) [*Mithridates*, died 63 B.C., king of Pontus, who reportedly took poisons so as to become immunized against them] the acquisition of immunity to the effects of a poison by ingestion of gradually increasing amounts of it.

mi•ti•ci•dal (mi″tĭ-si′dəl) destructive to mites.

mi•ti•cide (mi′tĭ-sīd) an agent that is destructive to mites.

mit•i•gate (mit′ĭ-gāt) [L. *mitigara* to soften] to moderate; to render milder.

mi•tis (mi′tis) [L.] mild.

mit(o)- [Gr. *mitos* thread] a combining form meaning threadlike, or denoting relationship to a thread, or to mitosis.

mi•to•car•cin (mi″to-kahr′sin) an antineoplastic antibiotic derived from *Streptomyces* species.

mi•to•chon•dria (mi″to-kon′dre-ə) (sing. *mitochon′drion*) [*mito-* + *chondri-* + *-ia*] small spherical to rod-shaped cytoplasmic organelles, consisting of inner and outer bilayer membranes with a space between them. The inner membrane is infolded to form a series of projections (cristae), and the space between the cristae is filled by the mitochondrial matrix, which contains DNA, RNA, ribosomes, and granules. Mitochondria generate energy (in the form adenosine triphosphate [ATP] synthesis) by the oxidation of nutrients, and they contain the enzymes of the tricarboxylic acid (Krebs) cycle and for fatty acid oxidation and oxidative phosphorylation. In response to toxic insults they release enzymes that cause apoptosis. Mitochondria can replicate independently and code for the synthesis of some of their proteins; inheritance of mitochondrial DNA is maternal, and mitochondrial DNA defects cause a variety of diseases. See illustration and Plates 11 and 12. **mitochon′drial** *adj*

mi•to•chon•dri•al ATP•ase (mi-tə-kon′dre-əl a-te-pe′ase) H^+-transporting ATP synthase.

mi•to•chon•dri•on (mi″to-kon′dre-on) singular of *mitochondria.*

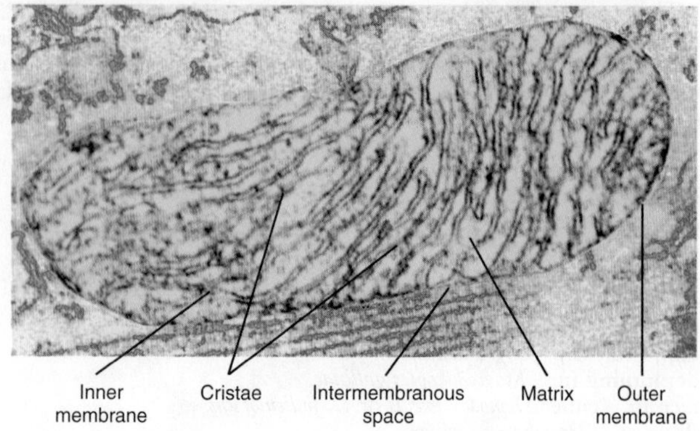

■ Transmission electron micrograph of a mitochondrion.

mi•to•cro•min (mi″to-kro′min) an antineoplastic antibiotic produced by *Streptomyces viridochromogenes.*

mi•to•gen (mi′to-jən) a substance that induces blast transformation; DNA, RNA, and protein synthesis; and proliferation of lymphocytes, e.g., concanavalin A, phytohemagglutinin, pokeweed mitogen, or lipopolysaccharide.

pokeweed m. a lectin isolated from pokeweed *(Phytolacca americana)*; it is a mitogen that stimulates both B and T lymphocytes. Abbreviated PWM.

mi•to•gen-ac•ti•vat•ed pro•tein ki•nase (MAPK) (mi′to-jən ak′tĭ-vāt-əd pro′tēn ki′nās) [EC 2.7.11.24] any of a group of protein-serine/threonine kinases that when activated enter the cell nucleus and catalyze the phosphorylation of serine and threonine residues in transcription factors that regulate gene expression; it is the final member of a signal transduction cascade of three protein kinases that is initiated by stimulation of a wide variety of membrane receptors and is important in the regulation of cell growth and differentiation. Called also *MAP kinase.*

mi•to•gen•e•sis (mi″to-jen′ə-sis) [*mito-* + *-genesis*] the production, or causation, of mitosis in or transformation of a cell.

mi•to•ge•net•ic (mi″to-jə-net′ik) 1. pertaining to or characterized by mitogenesis. 2. causing mitogenesis.

mi•to•gen•ic (mi″to-jen′ik) causing or inducing mitogenesis.

mi•to•lac•tol (mi″to-lak′tol) an alkylating agent that has been used as an antineoplastic in the treatment of invasive ovarian carcinoma; administered orally.

mi•to•mal•cin (mi″to-mal′sin) an antineoplastic antibiotic produced by *Streptomyces malayensis.*

mi•to•my•cin (mi″to-mi′sin) 1. any of a group of antitumor antibiotics (e.g., mitomycin A, B, C) produced by *Streptomyces caespitosus.* 2. [USP] mitomycin C, which acts as a bifunctional or trifunctional alkylating agent causing cross-linking of DNA and inhibition of DNA synthesis and is relatively phase-specific for the late G_1 and early S phases of the cell cycle. It has activity against many types of carcinoma as well as chronic myelogenous leukemia, but because of its severe toxicity and myelosuppression it is usually used only for palliation in patients who have not responded to other treatment. Administered intravenously.

mi•to•sis (mi-to′sis) pl. *mito′ses* [*mito-* + *-osis*] a complex of processes by which two daughter nuclei receive identical complements of the number of chromosomes characteristic of the somatic cells of the species. It is the means by which the body grows and replaces cells and is divided into five phases: *prophase, prometaphase, metaphase, anaphase,* and *telophase* (qq.v.). NOTE: The term *mitosis* is used interchangeably with cell division, but strictly speaking it refers to nuclear division, whereas *cytokinesis* refers to division of the cytoplasm. Cf. *meiosis.* **mitot′ic** *adj*

closed m. mitosis in which the formation of the spindle and separation of chromosomes occurs with the nuclear envelope intact; common in single-celled eukaryotes. Cf. *open m.*

multipolar m. abnormal mitosis in which the spindle has more than two poles, resulting in the formation of more than two daughter cells.

open m. mitosis in which the nuclear envelope disassembles before the separation of the chromosomes; the normal type of mitosis in higher plants and animals. Cf. *closed m.*

pathologic m. atypical, asymmetrical mitosis indicative of malignancy.

mi•to•sper (mi′to-spər) an antineoplastic substance derived from *Aspergillus glaucus.*

mi•to•spore (mi′to-spor) an asexual spore, so called because it is produced by mitosis; when motile it is called a *zoospore.*

mi•to•tane (mi′to-tān) [USP] a cytotoxic compound related to the insecticides DDT and TDE (DDD) that causes severe damage to the adrenal cortex, causing a rapid decrease in adrenocorticosteroid production; used for palliation in inoperable adrenocortical carcinoma of both functional and nonfunctional types, administered orally.

mi•to•xan•trone hy•dro•chlo•ride (mi″to-zan′trōn) [USP] a DNA-intercalating agent of the anthracenedione family that causes cross-links and strand breaks and is a topoisomerase inhibitor; used as an antineoplastic agent for the treatment of acute myelogenous leukemia and the palliative treatment of advanced hormone-refractory prostate cancer. It is also used to reduce the frequency and severity of relapses in patients with secondary multiple sclerosis. Administered intravenously.

mi•tral (mi′trəl) 1. shaped like a miter (tall pointed hat worn by a Roman Catholic bishop). 2. pertaining to the left atrioventricular valve.

mi•tral•iza•tion (mi″trəl-ĭ-za′shən) straightening of the left border and prominence of the pulmonary salient of the cardiac shadow, a configuration commonly seen radiographically in mitral stenosis.

Mi•tro•fa•noff procedure (me-tro′fah-nof) [Paul *Mitrofanoff,* French pediatric surgeon, born 1934] appendicovesicostomy.

Mit•su•da antigen, reaction, test (mit′soo-dah″) [Kensuke *Mitsuda,* Japanese physician, 1876–1964] see under *reaction;* see *lepromin;* and see *lepromin test,* under *test.*

mit•tel•schmerz (mit′əl-shmərtz) [Ger. *mittel* mid, middle, + *schmerz* pain, suffering] pain associated with ovulation, usually occurring in the middle of the menstrual cycle.

Mi•va•cron (mi′və-kron″) trademark for a preparation of mivacurium chloride.

mi•va•cu•rium chlo•ride (mi″və-ku′re-əm) a nondepolarizing neuromuscular blocking agent of short duration administered intravenously as an adjunct to general anesthesia, facilitating endotracheal intubation and inducing skeletal muscle relaxation.

mixed (mikst) affecting various parts at once; showing two or more different characteristics.

mixo•sco•pia (mik″so-sko′pe-ə) [Gr. *mixis* intercourse + *skopein* to examine] a paraphilia in which gratification is obtained by the sight of the object of one's desire engaged in sexual intercourse with another.

mixo•troph (mik′so-trōf) in bacterial physiology, the ability to use alternative sources for metabolism and energy, as being capable of growth in either the absence or presence of light, or with either organic or inorganic compounds for nutrition.

mixo•tro•phic (mik″so-tro′fik) having the nutritional characters of both animals and plants.

Mix•tard (miks′tərd) trademark for a mixture of 30 per cent insulin (def. 3) and 70 per cent isophane insulin suspension.

mix•ture (miks′chər) [L. *mixtura, mistura*] a combination of different drugs or ingredients, as a fluid resulting from mixing a fluid with other fluids, or with solids, or a suspension of a solid in a liquid.

Gunning m. a mixture used in estimating the nitrogen in the urine, consisting of 15 mL of concentrated sulfuric acid, 10 g of potassium sulfate, and 0.5 g of copper sulfate.

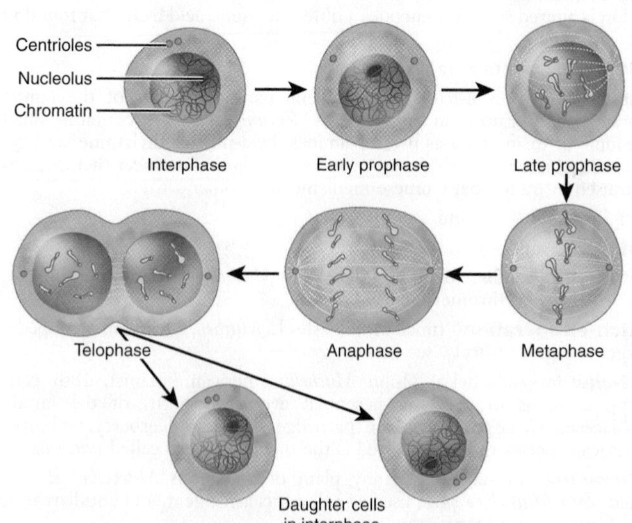

■ Mitosis shown as occurring in a cell of a hypothetical animal with a diploid chromosome number of six (haploid number three); one pair of chromosomes is short, one pair is long and hooked, and one pair is long and knobbed.

Mayer glycerin-albumin m. a mixture of equal parts of white of egg and glycerin, with a small amount of sodium salicylate, for affixing paraffin sections to slides.

racemic m. racemate.

Ringer m. see under *injection* and *irrigation*.

MJD Machado-Joseph disease.

MK monkey lung (cell culture).

MKS meter-kilogram-second system.

mL, ml milliliter.

μL microliter.

MLA[1] [L.] mento-laeva anterior (left mentoanterior, a position of the fetus; see *position*).

MLA[2] Medical Library Association.

MLBW moderately low birth weight; see under *infant*.

MLC mixed lymphocyte culture; minimal lethal concentration.

MLD median lethal dose; minimum lethal dose.

MLNS mucocutaneous lymph node syndrome.

MLP [L.] mento-laeva posterior (left mentoposterior, a position of the fetus; see *position*).

MLR mixed lymphocyte reaction; see *mixed lymphocyte culture*, under *culture*.

MLT [L.] mento-laeva transversa (left mentotransverse, a position of the fetus; see *position*).

MM mucous membrane.

mM millimolar.

mm millimeter.

μM micromolar.

μm micrometer.

MMF mycophenolate mofetil.

mm Hg millimeter of mercury, a unit of pressure equal to that exerted by a column of mercury at 0°C one millimeter high at standard gravity. It is equal to 1 torr, or 133.3 pascals.

MMIHS megacystis-microcolon–intestinal hypoperistalsis syndrome.

mmol millimole.

MMP matrix metalloproteinase.

MMPI Minnesota Multiphasic Personality Inventory.

MMR measles-mumps-rubella (vaccine); see *measles, mumps, and rubella vaccine live*, under *vaccine*.

M-M-R trademark for preparations of measles, mumps, and rubella virus vaccine live.

MMRV measles, mumps, rubella and varicella virus vaccine live.

MMSE Mini-Mental State Examination.

Mn manganese.

M'Nagh•ten (Mc•Naugh•ten) rule (mək-naw'tən) [Daniel *M'Naghten*, died 1865; acquitted of murder in 1843 by a British court on the grounds of insanity] see under *rule*.

mne•mic (ne'mik) mnemonic.

mne•mon•ic (ne-mon'ik) [Gr. *mnēmonikos* pertaining to memory] pertaining to, characterized by, or promoting recollection, or memory.

mne•mon•ics (ne-mon'iks) the cultivation or improvement of memory by special methods or techniques.

MNGIE mitochondrial neurogastrointestinal encephalomyopathy.

MO Medical Officer.

Mo molybdenum.

Mo•ban (mo'bən) trademark for a preparation of molindone hydrochloride.

Mo•bic (mo'bik) trademark for a preparation of meloxicam.

Mo•bi•li•na (mo"bĭ-li'nə) [L. *mobilis* mobile] a suborder of ciliate protozoa of the order Peritrichida, subclass Peritrichia, which are mobile; usually conical, cylindrical, or discoidal; and orally and aborally flattened. They characteristically have a ciliary girdle and a complex thigmotactic apparatus at the aboral end, often with a highly distinctive denticulate ring of "teeth." All species are ectoparasites or endoparasites of fresh water or marine vertebrates and invertebrates, and those found on the gills of fish are pathogenic.

mo•bil•i•ty (mo-bil'ĭ-te) [L. *mobilis* mobile] 1. capability of movement, of being moved, or of flowing freely. 2. rate of movement of a charged particle in an applied electric field.

electrophoretic m. 1. the rate of migration (usually in cm/s) per unit electric field strength (usually V/cm) of a charged particle in electrophoresis. Symbol μ. 2. any measure of the rate of migration of an ionic species in electrophoresis, e.g., β electrophoretic mobility, designating the electrophoretic mobility of a beta globulin.

tooth m. physiologic movement of a tooth, varying in degree for different teeth and different times of day; that exceeding a normal range is pathological.

mo•bi•li•za•tion (mo"bĭ-lĭ-za'shən) the process of making a fixed part or stored substance mobile, as by separating a part from surrounding structures to make it accessible for an operative procedure or by causing release into the circulation for body use of a substance stored in the body.

stapes m. surgical correction of immobility of the stapes, in treatment of deafness resulting from otosclerosis.

mo•bil•om•e•ter (mo"bil-om'ə-tər) an instrument for measuring the consistency of liquids such as oil, cream, liquid foods, etc.

Mo•bi•lun•cus (mo"bĭ-lung'kəs) [L. *mobilis* motile + *uncus* hook] a genus of gram-negative, anaerobic, small, curved, rod-shaped bacteria of the family Actinomycetaceae, frequently isolated from women with bacterial vaginosis.

Mo•bin-Ud•din filter (mo'bin-ud'in) [Kazi *Mobin-Uddin*, Indian-born American vascular surgeon, 1930–1999] see under *filter*.

Mo•bitz type I block, type II block (mo'bits) [Woldemar *Mobitz*, Russian-born cardiologist in Germany, 1889–1951] see under *block*.

Mö•bi•us disease, sign, syndrome (mur'be-əs) [Paul Julius *Möbius*, German neurologist, 1853–1907] see under *sign* and *syndrome* and see *ophthalmoplegic migraine*, under *migraine*.

moc•ca•sin (mok'ə-sin) any of several species of snakes of the genus *Agkistrodon*.

highland m. copperhead (def. 1).

water m. *Agkistrodon piscivorus*, a venomous semiaquatic crotalid snake with an olive or brown back, found in the southern United States. Called also *cottonmouth*.

mo•daf•i•nil (mo-daf'ĭ-nil") a central nervous system stimulant used in the treatment of narcolepsy, obstructive sleep apnea, and sleep disorders associated with shift work; administered orally.

mo•dal•i•ty (mo-dal'ĭ-te) 1. a method of application of, or the employment of, any therapeutic agent, especially a physical agent. 2. in homeopathy, a condition that modifies drug action; a condition under which symptoms develop, becoming better or worse. 3. a specific sensory entity, such as taste.

mode (mōd) [L. *modus* measure, manner] 1. a manner, way, or method of acting; a particular condition of functioning. 2. in statistics, the most frequently occurring value or item in a distribution; when data are grouped, it is the midpoint of the grouping with the highest frequency. A distribution with two peaks is bimodal. 3. the manner of interaction between a ventilator and the person being ventilated, usually defined in terms of what the stimulus is that starts the ventilation.

assist m. a mode of positive pressure ventilation in which the patient initiates and terminates all or most breaths and the ventilator gives some amount of support. Cf. *control m.* and *assist-control m.* Called also *assisted m.*

assist-control m. a mode of positive pressure ventilation in which the ventilator is in assist mode unless the patient's respiration rate falls below a certain amount, in which case the ventilator switches to a control mode. When the strength or rate of respiration increases again, the ventilator goes back into assist mode.

assisted m. assist m.

control m., controlled m. a mode of positive pressure ventilation in which the ventilator controls the initiation and volume of breaths. Cf. *assist m.* and *assist-control m.*

pacing m. in cardiac pacing, the manner of stimulation of a cardiac chamber by an artificial pacemaker, referring to whether or not sensed cardiac signals (events) are used to inhibit or trigger stimulation.

pressure control m. a mode of positive pressure ventilation in which each breath is augmented by air at a fixed rate and amount of pressure, with tidal volume not being fixed. See also under *ventilation*.

pressure support m. a mode of positive pressure ventilation similar to the assist mode; the patient breathes spontaneously and breathing is augmented by air at a preset amount of pressure. See also under *ventilation*.

mod•el (mod'əl) 1. something that represents or simulates something else; a replica. 2. a reasonable facsimile of the body or any of its parts; used for demonstration and teaching purposes. 3. cast (def. 5). 4. to imitate another's behavior; see *modeling*. 5. a hypothesis or theory.

animal m. any condition found in an animal that is of value in studying a biological phenomenon, e.g., a pathological mechanism of an animal disorder useful in studying human disease.

Cox proportional hazards m. a method of analysis of multiple factors (variables) that influence an actuarial curve of the risk of a given negative outcome such as disease occurrence or death. A hazard rate is computed for each separate variable (e.g., among those patients with that factor who had not previously suffered a negative outcome, how many subsequently suffered the negative outcome during a short interval) and cumulative hazard rates are computed for the combinations of variables that exist in actual situations.

figure-of-eight m. in cardiology, a variation of the leading circle model of reentry in which the interface of refractory tissue is a curved barrier, with the result that the wavefronts split, proceed around each edge of the arc, and return centrally to describe a figure eight configuration.

fluid mosaic m. the generally accepted theory that cell membranes are composed of bilayers made up of external phospholipids and a central hydrophobic region, with membrane proteins floating in the phospholipids and held in position by various chemical and physical bonding mechanisms. See Plate 12.

leading circle m. in cardiology, a multidimensional model of reentry that describes the cycle of alternating tissue activation and refractoriness in terms of a functional, rather than anatomical, intertissue interface acting as a barrier around which the wavefronts circle. In the model, their pathway is the smallest circuit in which the head of each wavefront is just within the tail of that preceding and thus is able to excite tissue still in its relative refractory period.

proportional hazards m. Cox proportional hazards m.

ring m. in cardiology, a model describing the mechanism of anatomical reentry, based on a circuit that is formed around an impenetrable barrier to propagation and contains a locus of slow conduction. The locus blocks the initial normal impulse but is traversed by later impulses from the opposite direction that reexcite normal cardiac fibers, which can occur repetitively. There must exist either a segment of slow conduction or overall slow conduction with a locus of unidirectional block, and total conduction time in the circuit must exceed the refractory period of the fibers so that an excitable gap exists between a wavefront head and the tail of that preceding. See also *reentrant mechanism*, under *mechanism*.

mod·el·ing (mod′əl-ing) 1. learning vicariously by observation and imitation, which can be used as a form of behavior therapy. 2. developing or using a hypothesis or theory.

urea kinetic m. the tracing of urea kinetics during hemodialysis, considering urea as a representative medium-sized molecule whose clearance is similar to that of other more toxic substances. A series of mathematical equations are used, taking measured serum urea concentrations and using them to develop other parameters such as dialyzer clearance, urea generation rate of the body, protein catabolic rate, and urea distribution volume.

Mod·er·il (mod′ər-il) trademark for a preparation of rescinnamine.

Mo·di·con (mo′dĭ-kon) trademark for combination preparations of norethindrone and ethinyl estradiol.

mod·i·fi·ca·tion (mod″ĭ-fĭ-ka′shən) the process or result of changing the form or characteristics of an object or substance.

behavior m. see under *therapy*.

effect m. the alteration of the association between two variables under study as a function of a third variable.

genetic m. see under *engineering*.

racemic m. racemate.

mod·i·fi·er (mod′ĭ-fi″ər) an agent that changes the form or characteristics of an object or substance.

biologic response m. (BRM), biological response m. a method or agent, such as a cytokine, monoclonal antibody, or vaccine, that alters host-tumor interaction, usually by amplifying the antitumor mechanisms of the immune system, but also by various mechanisms directly or indirectly affecting host or tumor cell characteristics. Called also *biomodulator*.

leukotriene m. any of a group of antiasthmatic agents that act by inhibiting the formation or activity of leukotrienes; the major types are the leukotriene receptor antagonists and the leukotriene pathway modifiers.

leukotriene pathway m. a type of leukotriene modifier that acts by interfering with leukotriene formation on the leukotriene pathway.

mo·di·o·li·form (mo″de-o′lĭ-form) shaped like the hub of a wheel.

mo·di·o·lus (mo-di′o-ləs) [L. "nave," "hub"] [TA] the central pillar or columella of the cochlea; called also *columella cochleae*.

Mod. praesc. [L.] mo′do praescrip′to (in the way directed).

mod·u·la·tion (mod″u-la′shən) [L. *modulare* to measure] 1. the act of tempering or toning down. 2. alteration in a cell in response to environmental stimuli. 3. embryologic induction in a specific region.

antigenic m. alteration or loss of reactivity of cell surface antigens resulting from redistribution of antigenic sites due to the presence of bound antibody.

biochemical m. in combination chemotherapy, the use of one substance to modulate negative side effects of the primary agent, increasing the effectiveness or allowing a higher dose of the primary agent.

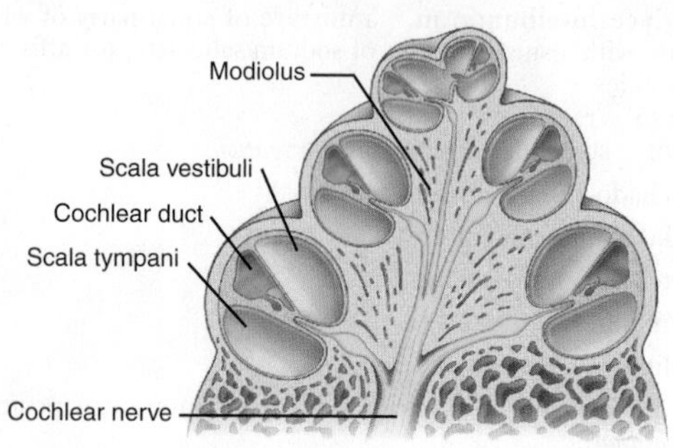

■ Modiolus in a cross-section through the axis of the cochlea.

mod·u·la·tor (mod′u-la″tər) a specific inductor that brings out characteristics peculiar to a definite region.

selective estrogen receptor m. (SERM) an agent that activates some estrogen receptors but not others, thereby having estrogenlike effects on target tissues (such as bone) without affecting other tissues that have estrogen receptors.

mod·u·lus (mod′u-ləs) pl. *mo′duli* [L., dim. of *modus* quantity] a coefficient that indicates by a numerical value the extent to which a substance has a given property.

elastic m., m. of elasticity a coefficient indicating the ratio between deforming stress to a unit of area of a substance and the extent of resulting deformation.

Mod·uret·ic (mod″u-ret′ik) trademark for preparations of amiloride hydrochloride with hydrochlorothiazide.

MODY maturity-onset diabetes of youth.

Moe plate (mo) [John Howard *Moe*, American orthopedic surgeon, 1905–1988] see under *plate*.

Moe·bi·us see *Möbius*.

Moel·ler glossitis (mur′ler) [Julius Otto Ludwig *Moeller*, German surgeon, 1819–1887] see under *glossitis*.

Moel·ler-Bar·low disease (mur′ler bahr′lo) [J.O.L. *Moeller*; Sir Thomas *Barlow*, London physician, 1845–1945] see under *disease*.

Moen·cke·berg see *Mönckeberg*.

mo·e·no·my·cins (mo″ə-no-mi′sinz) bambermycins.

mo·e·sin (mo′ə-sin) an actin-binding protein, related to ezrin and radixin, see *ERM proteins*, under *protein*.

mo·ex·i·pril hy·dro·chlo·ride (mo-ek′sĭ-pril″) an angiotensin-converting enzyme inhibitor used as an antihypertensive, alone or in combination with a thiazide diuretic; administered orally.

mo·fe·til (mo′fə-til) USAN contraction for 2-(4-morpholinyl)ethyl.

mogi·ar·thria (moj-e-ahr′thre-ə) [Gr. *mogis* with difficulty + *arthr-*[2] + *-ia*] dysarthria due to defective muscular coordination.

mogi·pho·nia (moj-ĭ-fo′ne-ə) dysphonia.

Mohr syndrome (mor) [Otto Lous *Mohr*, Norwegian geneticist, 1886–1967] see under *syndrome*.

Moh·ren·heim fossa (triangle), space (mo′ren-hīm) [Baron Joseph Jacob Freiherr von *Mohrenheim*, Austrian surgeon, 1759–1799] see *fossa infraclavicularis* and see under *space*.

Mohs chemosurgery, surgery (micrographic surgery, technique) (mōz) [Frederic Edward *Mohs*, American surgeon, 1910–2002] see under *chemosurgery* and *surgery*.

moi·e·ty (moi′ə-te) [Fr. *moitié*, from L. *medietas*, *medius*, middle] any equal part; a half; also any part or portion.

carbohydrate m. a carbohydrate-derived portion of the structure of a molecule.

mol (mol) mole[1].

mo·lal (*m*) (mo′ləl) containing one mole of solute per kilogram of solvent. NOTE: *molal* refers to the weight of the solvent, *molar* to the volume of the solution.

mo·lal·i·ty (mo-lal′ĭ-te) the number of moles of a solute per kilogram of pure solvent. NOTE: *molality* refers to the weight of the solvent, *molarity* to the volume of the solution.

mo·lar[1] (M, *M*) (mo′lər) 1. pertaining to a mole of a substance, such as molar mass or molar absorptivity, i.e., the quantity of some property associated with a mole of the substance. 2. a measure of the concentration of a solute, expressed as the number of moles of solute per liter of solution, e.g., 0.25M = 0.25 mole per liter (mol/L). The latter notation is used in the SI system.

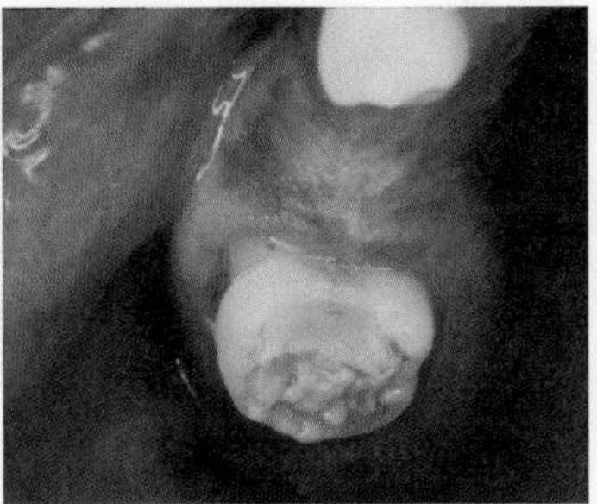

■ Mulberry molar of congenital syphilis.

mo·lar[2] **(M)** (mo′lər) [L. *molaris* belonging to a mill, from *mola* millstone] 1. see under *tooth*. 2. pertaining to a molar tooth.

Moon m's see under *tooth*.

mulberry m. a malformed first molar tooth characterized by dwarfing of the cusps and hypertrophy of the enamel surrounding the cusp with agglomeration of masses of globules, giving it the appearance of a mulberry; seen in congenital syphilis and certain other diseases. Called also *mulberry tooth*.

sixth-year m. the permanent first molar tooth, so called because it usually erupts at the age of 6 years just posterior to the last molar of the deciduous dentition.

supernumerary m. paramolar.

third m. see under *tooth*.

twelfth-year m. the permanent second molar tooth, so called because it usually erupts at the age of 12 years.

mo·lar·i·form (mo-lar′ĭ-form) shaped like a molar tooth; showing molarlike characteristics.

mo·la·ris (mo-lar′is) [L. "millstone, grinder, molar tooth"] 1. adapted for grinding. 2. one of the molar teeth (dentes molares [TA]).

m. ter′tius wisdom tooth (dens serotinus [TA]).

mo·lar·i·ty (mo-lar′ĭ-te) the number of moles of a solute per liter of solution. Cf. *molality*.

mold (mōld) [Middle English *moulde*] 1. an imprecise term used to refer to any member of one of the two largest groupings of fungi (the other being the *yeasts*); molds are parasitic and saprobic, and most exist as multicellular filamentous colonies. Common molds are *Mucor*, *Penicillium*, *Rhizopus*, and *Aspergillus*. See illustration. 2. the deposit or growth produced by such a fungus. 3. a form in which an object is given shape; see also *cast*. 4. an object so shaped. 5. the act of so forming or shaping.

slime m. any member of the fungal class Myxomycetes.

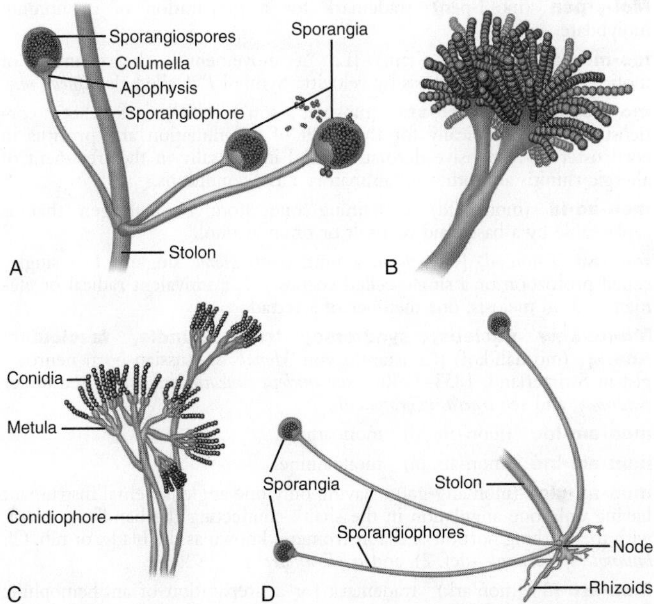

■ Characteristic structures of common molds. *(A)*, Sporangia of *Absidia* arising from a stolon; *(B)*, conidiophores and conidia of *Aspergillus; (C)*, brushlike conidiophores and parallel chains of conidia of *Penicillium; (D)*, sporangiophores of *Rhizopus* arising from a node above the rhizoids.

white m. white or slightly gray patches that form on the surface of meat in cold storage and other products due to the growth of fungi.

mold·ing (mōld′ing) [L. *modulus* mold, form] 1. the creation of shape, or fashioning of an object. 2. the shaping of the fetal head in adjustment to the size and shape of the birth canal.

border m. the shaping of dental impression material by the manipulation or action of the tissues and structures adjacent to the borders of an impression. Called also *tissue m.*

compression m. a method of molding in which compression is used to pack the material in and to express its excess from the mold.

injection m. the act or process of forcing a plastic material, such as a softened resin, into the mold space under pressure.

tissue m. border m.

mole[1] **(mol)** (mōl) [Ger. *Mol*, short for *Molekulargewicht* molecular weight] the base SI unit of amount of matter, being that amount of substance (in a system) that contains as many elementary entities (e.g., atoms, ions, molecules, or radicals) as there are carbon atoms in 0.012 kg of carbon 12 (^{12}C); thus one mole equals 6.023×10^{23} (Avogadro's number) elementary entities. Formerly, the connotation of mole was gram molecular weight (q.v.) and the two terms were sometimes used synonymously.

mole[2] (mōl) [A.S. *māl* spot] 1. melanocytic nevus. 2. sometimes applied loosely to any blemish of the skin, especially a pigmented one.

atypical m., dysplastic m. dysplastic nevus.

pigmented m. see under *nevus*.

mole[3] (mōl) [L. *mola* millstone, mole] a fleshy mass or tumor formed in the uterus by the degeneration or abnormal development of a zygote.

blood m. a mass in the uterus made up of blood clots, the placenta, and fetal membranes retained after fetal death.

Breus m. a pathologic change in the placenta found in abortion consisting of accumulation of masses of intervillous hematomas that project into the chorionic space.

cystic m. hydatidiform m.

fleshy m. blood m.

hydatid m., hydatidiform m. an abnormal pregnancy characterized by placental abnormality involving swollen chorionic villi, which form a large, grapelike mass of vesicles, by trophoblastic hyperplasia, and by loss of fetal blood vessels in the villi, with proliferation of the epithelial covering of the villi and dissolution and cystic cavitation of the avascular stroma. It is designated *complete* when all villi are swollen and fetal tissues are absent, and *partial* when only some villi are swollen and fetal tissues are present. Complete moles usually possess only paternal chromosomes, the result of fertilization of an oocyte lacking an active nucleus; partial moles are usually triploid and possess both maternal and paternal chromosomes. Called also *cystic* or *vesicular m.*

invasive m., malignant m. chorioadenoma destruens.

tubal m. the mass of blood clot and chorionic villi found after death of the conceptus in a tubal pregnancy.

vesicular m. hydatidiform m.

mol·e·cule (mol′ə-kūl) [L. *molecula* little mass] a very small mass of matter; the smallest amount of a substance which can exist alone; an aggregation of atoms; specifically, a chemical combination of two or more atoms which form a specific chemical substance. To break up the molecule into its constituent atoms is to change its character. The number and kind of atoms in a molecule vary with the compound. **molec′ular** *adj*

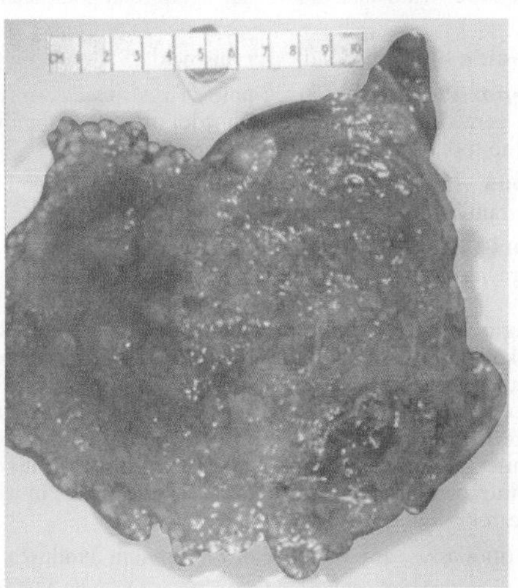

■ Complete hydatidiform mole.

cell adhesion m's (CAM) cell surface glycoproteins that mediate intercell adhesion in vertebrates; most can be grouped into four large classes: cadherins, immunoglobulins, integrins, and selectins.

cell interaction m's, CI m's products of cell interaction genes (q.v.).

diatomic m. a molecule containing two atoms.

hexatomic m. a molecule containing six atoms.

intercellular adhesion m. 1 (ICAM-1) a type of cell adhesion molecule that contains five immunoglobulin-like domains and is expressed on a variety of cells, including B and T lymphocytes, fibroblasts, keratinocytes, and endothelial cells. It functions as a ligand for leukocyte function–associated antigen 1 (LFA-1) and glycoprotein Mac-1 and as a specific receptor for rhinoviruses and *Plasmodium*.

intercellular adhesion m. 2 (ICAM-2) a type of cell adhesion molecule containing two immunoglobulin-like domains and having a tissue distribution similar to that of ICAM-1; it serves as a ligand for leukocyte function–associated antigen 1 (LFA-1).

junctional adhesion m. any of a subfamily of immunoglobulins that are expressed by leukocytes and platelets and by endothelial and epithelial cells; they regulate interactions among leukocytes, platelets, and endothelial cells and participate in the formation of tight junctions.

messenger m. a molecule that carries a messenger from one cell to another, usually itself not binding to the receptor site.

middle m. any molecule that has an atomic mass between 350 and 2000 daltons; these accumulate in the body fluids of patients with uremia.

monatomic m. a molecule consisting of a single atom.

nonpolar m. a molecule in which the electrical potential is symmetrically distributed over the molecule.

polar m. a molecule in which the electrical potential is not symmetrically distributed.

tetratomic m. a molecule made up of four atoms.

triatomic m. a molecule composed of three atoms.

mo•lin•done hy•dro•chlo•ride (mo-lin′dōn) [USP] a dihydroindolone antipsychotic agent, used especially in the treatment of schizophrenia, brief reactive psychosis, and schizophreniform disorders; administered orally.

Mo•lisch test (reaction) (mo′lish) [Hans *Molisch*, Czech botanist in Vienna, 1856–1937] see under *test.*

Moll glands (mol) [Jacob Antonius *Moll*, Dutch ophthalmologist, 1832–1914] glandulae ciliares.

Mol•la•ret meningitis (mo-lah-ra′) [Pierre *Mollaret*, French neurologist, 1898–1987] see under *meningitis.*

Mol•li•cu•tes (mol″ĭ-ku′tēz) [L. *mollis* soft + *cutis* skin] a class of generally parasitic bacteria of the phylum Firmicutes, consisting of pleomorphic, coccoid, or filamentous cells that are bounded by a triple-layered membrane and lack a cell wall but have an internal cytoskeleton. The class comprises the smallest and simplest microorganisms capable of self-replication. Medically important organisms are included in the orders Acholeplasmatales and Mycoplasmatales, as well as the family Erysipelotrichaceae (incertae sedis).

Mol•lus•ca (mo-lus′kə) [L. *molluscus* soft] a large phylum of invertebrates that have a soft unsegmented body often protected by a calcareous shell; it includes snails, slugs, mussels, oysters, clams, octopuses, nautiluses, squids, cuttlefish, and others.

mol•lusc•a•ci•dal (mo-lusk″ə-si′dəl) destructive to snails and other mollusks.

mol•lusc•a•cide (mo-lusk′ə-sīd) an agent that kills snails and other mollusks.

mol•lusc•i•cide (mo-lus′ĭ-sīd) molluscacide.

Mol•lus•ci•pox•vi•rus (mə-lus′kĭ-poks-vi″rəs) [*molluscum contagiosum* + *poxvirus*] a genus of the subfamily Chordopoxvirinae (family Poxviridae) containing the molluscum contagiosum virus.

mol•lus•cous (mo-lus′kəs) 1. pertaining to or resembling a mollusk. 2. pertaining to molluscum.

mol•lus•cum (mo-lus′kəm) [L. *molluscus* soft] 1. any of various skin diseases characterized by soft, rounded, cutaneous lesions. 2. m. contagiosum.

m. contagio′sum a common, benign, usually self-limited viral infection of the skin and occasionally the conjunctivae by a poxvirus, transmitted by autoinoculation, close contact, or fomites. It primarily affects children but may also be seen (often sexually transmitted) in adolescents and adults. The characteristic lesion is a flesh-colored or gray umbilicated papule that becomes white, has a caseous core, and can be expressed; it contains pathognomonic intracytoplasmic inclusions *(molluscum bodies)*, in which replicating virions can be found.

mol•lusk (mol′əsk) any member of the phylum Mollusca.

Mo•lo•ney test (reaction) (mə-lo′ne) [Peter Joseph *Moloney*, Canadian immunochemist, 20th century] see under *test.*

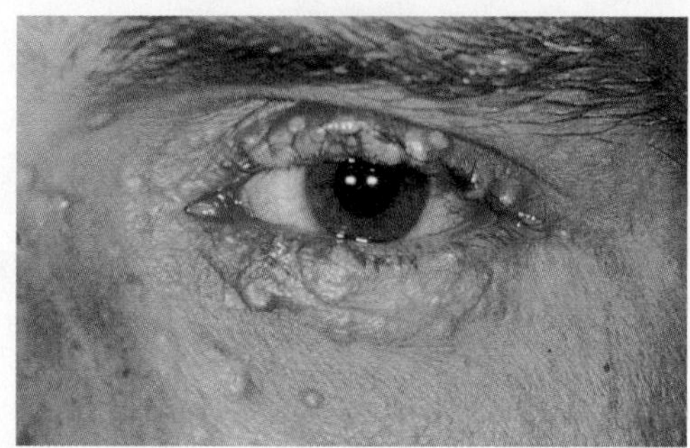

■ Molluscum contagiosum.

molt•ing (mōlt′ing) ecdysis.

Mol wt, mol wt molecular weight.

mo•lyb•date (mə-lib′dāt) any salt of molybdic acid; some are used in tests, especially for the detection of heavy metal ions.

mo•lyb•de•no•sis (mə-lib″də-no′sis) molybdenum poisoning.

mo•lyb•den•um (Mo) (mə-lib′də-nəm) [Gr. *molybdos* lead] a hard, silvery-white, metallic element; atomic number, 42; atomic weight, 95.94; specific gravity, 10.2. It is an essential trace element, being a component of the enzymes xanthine oxidase, aldehyde oxidase, and nitrate reductase. Livestock grazing in certain types of pasture may suffer from molybdenum poisoning.

mo•lyb•dic (mə-lib′dik) containing molybdenum as a hexavalent element.

mo•lyb•dic ac•id (mə-lib′dik) an inorganic acid existing only in solution; commercial molybdic acid is either ammonium molybdate or molybdenum trioxide.

mo•lyb•do•en•zyme (mə-lib″do-en′zīm) any enzyme containing a molybdenum cofactor, such as aldehyde oxidase, sulfite oxidase, and xanthine dehydrogenase. Molybdenum is part of the redox system for electron transport in all of these enzymes that are currently known.

mo•lyb•do•fla•vo•pro•tein (mə-lib″do-fla′vo-pro″tēn) a molybdoenzyme that is also a flavoprotein, such as aldehyde oxidase or xanthine oxidase.

mo•lyb•do•pro•tein (mə-lib″do-pro′tēn) a protein containing molybdenum.

mo•lyb•dop•ter•in (mə″lib-dop′tər-in) the nonmetal portion of a molybdenum cofactor; it is a pterin derivative with an aliphatic side chain that can attach to molybdenum by its two sulfhydryl groups.

mo•lyb•dous (mə-lib′dəs) containing molybdenum as a tetravalent element.

Mol•y•pen (mol′ĭ-pen) trademark for a preparation of ammonium molybdate.

mo•men•tum (mo-men′təm) [L. "a movement"] the quantity of motion; the product of mass by velocity. Symbol *P.* Called also *linear m.*

mo•met•a•sone fu•ro•ate (mo-met′ə-sōn″) [USP] a synthetic corticosteroid used topically for the relief of inflammation and pruritus in corticosteroid-responsive dermatoses and intranasally in the treatment of allergic rhinitis and other inflammatory nasal conditions.

mon•ac•id (mon-as′id) containing one atom of hydrogen that is replaceable by a base; said of a salt or of an alcohol.

mon•ad (mon′əd) [Gr. *monas* a unit, from *monos* single] 1. a single-celled protozoon or a single-celled coccus. 2. a univalent radical or element. 3. in meiosis, one member of a tetrad.

Mo•na•kow nucleus, syndrome, tract (bundle, fasciculus, fibers) (mo-nah′kof) [Constantin von *Monakow*, Russian-born neurologist in Switzerland, 1853–1930] see *nucleus cuneatus accessorius*, see under *syndrome*, and see *tractus rubrospinalis.*

mon•am•ide (mon-am′id) monoamide.

mon•am•ine (mon-am′in) monoamine.

mon•an•gle (mon′ang-gəl) having only one angle; a dental instrument having only one angulation in the shank connecting the handle, or shaft, with the working portion of the instrument, known as the blade, or nib. Cf. *binangle*, *quadrangle* (def. 2), and *triple-angle.*

Mon•arc-M (mon′ark) trademark for a preparation of antihemophilic factor (human).

mon•ar•thric (mon-ahr′thrik) pertaining to or affecting a single joint.

mon•ar•thri•tis (mon″ahr-thri′tis) [*mono-* + *arthritis*] inflammation of a single joint.

m. defor′mans arthritis deformans of a single joint.

mon•ar•tic•u•lar (mon″ahr-tik′u-lər) monarthric.

mon•ath•e•to•sis (mon″ath-ə-to′sis) [*mon-* + *athetosis*] athetosis of one limb.

mon•atom•ic (mon″ə-tom′ik) [*mon-* + *atomic*] 1. monovalent (def. 1). 2. monobasic. 3. consisting of monatomic molecules.

mon•auch•e•nos (mon-awk′ə-nəs) a dicephalic fetus with one neck.

mon•au•ral (mon-aw′rəl) [*mon-* + *aural*[1]] pertaining to one ear. Called also *monotic* and *uniaural.*

mon•avi•ta•min•o•sis (mon″ə-vi″tə-min-o′sis) a deficiency disease in which only one vitamin is lacking in the diet.

Mön•cke•berg arteriosclerosis (calcification, degeneration, mesarteritis, sclerosis) (murng′kə-bərg) [Johann Georg *Mönckeberg*, German pathologist, 1877–1925] see under *arteriosclerosis.*

Mon•di•ni cochlea, deafness, deformity (malformation) (monde′ne) [C. *Mondini*, Italian physician, 1729–1803] see under *cochlea, deafness,* and *deformity.*

Mon•dor disease (maw-dor′) [Henri *Mondor*, French surgeon, 1885–1962] see under *disease.*

mo•ne•cious (mo-ne′shəs) monoecious.

mo•nen•sin (mo-nen′sin) [USP] a veterinary antibiotic, antifungal, and coccidiostat produced by *Streptomyces cinnamonensis;* used as a coccidiostat in poultry, cattle, and sheep.

m. sodium [USP] the sodium salt of monensin, having the same uses as the base.

Mo•ne•ra (mo-ne′rə) [Gr. *monērēs* single] in the traditional five-kingdom system of classification, a kingdom comprising unicellular organisms without true nuclei, i.e., the prokaryotes, including the bacteria and cyanobacteria (formerly blue-green algae). Organisms formerly placed in this kingdom are now classified in the domains Archaea and Bacteria.

mo•ner•u•la (mo-ner′u-lə) pl. *moner′ulae* [Gr. *monērēs* single] an impregnated oocyte before it has a cleavage nucleus.

mon•es•thet•ic (mon″əs-thet′ik) [*mon-* + *esthetic*] pertaining to or affecting a single sense or sensation.

mon•es•trous (mon-es′trəs) completing only one estrous cycle in each sexual season.

Mon•ge disease (mōn′ha) [Carlos *Monge*, Peruvian pathologist, 1884–1970] chronic mountain sickness.

mon•go•lism (mong′go-liz-əm) term formerly used for *Down syndrome;* now considered offensive.

Mon•i•e•zia (mon″ĭ-e′zhə) a genus of cestodes of the family Anoplocephalidae. *M. benedi′ni* and *M. expan′sa* are found in the small intestines of young cattle, goats, and sheep; heavy infestations may cause diarrhea and wasting.

mo•nil•e•thrix (mo-nil′ə-thriks) [L. *monile* necklace + *-thrix*] an autosomal dominant condition in which the hairs are brittle and have multiple constrictions, rarely reaching 1 to 2 cm before breaking.

Mo•nil•ia (mo-nil′e-ə) [L. *monile* necklace] 1. former name for *Candida.* 2. a genus of imperfect fungi of the family Moniliaceae; its perfect (sexual) stage is *Sclerotinia.*

Mo•nil•i•a•ceae (mo-nil″e-a′se-e) in some systems of classification, a form-family of colorless or light-colored Fungi Imperfecti of the form-order Moniliales; genera of medical importance include *Acremonium, Aspergillus, Beauveria, Blastomyces, Botrytis, Coccidioides, Epidermophyton, Fusarium, Histoplasma, Paecilomyces, Paracoccidioides, Penicillium, Scedosporium, Sporothrix, Trichoderma, Trichophyton, Trichothecium,* and *Verticillium.*

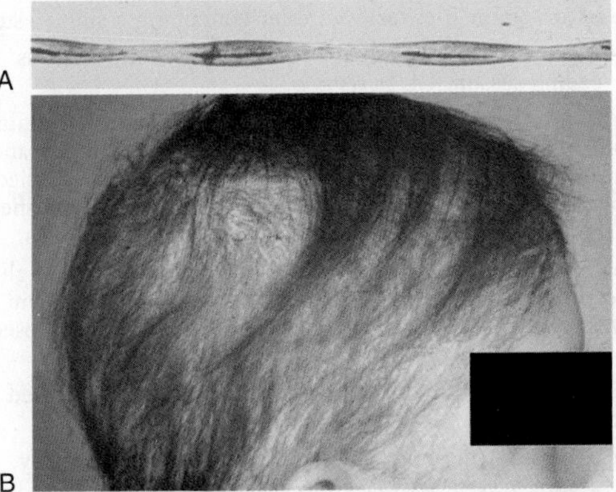

■ Monilethrix. *(A)*, Ultrastructure of a hair, showing alternating elliptical nodes and constrictions; *(B)*, clinical presentation.

mo•nil•i•al (mo-nil′e-əl) 1. candidal. 2. pertaining to or caused by *Monilia.*

Mo•nil•i•a•les (mo-nil″e-a′lēz) in some systems of classification, a form-order of Fungi Imperfecti of the form-class Hyphomycetes, consisting of fungi whose conidiophores are not organized on conidiomata. It includes the form-families Dematiaceae, Moniliaceae, and Tuberculariaceae. Some authorities call this form-order *Hyphomycetales.*

mon•i•li•a•sis (mon-ĭ-li′ə-sis) candidiasis.

mo•nil•i•form (mo-nil′ĭ-form) [L. *monile* necklace + *form*] shaped like a necklace or string of beads.

Mo•nil•i•for•mis (mo-nil″ĭ-for′mis) a genus of acanthocephalans. *M. monilifor′mis* (formerly *Echinorhynchus moniliformis*) is a parasite of rats, mice, and dogs, and a facultative parasite in humans.

Mon•i•stat (mon′ĭ-stat) trademark for preparations of miconazole.

mon•i•tor (mon′ĭ-tər) [L. "one who reminds," from *monere* to remind, admonish] 1. to check constantly on a state or condition, as on the vital signs of a patient under anesthesia and undergoing surgery, or to determine the amount of exposure to radiation. 2. an apparatus used to observe or record such physiological signs as respiration, pulse, and blood pressure in a patient.

ambulatory ECG m. a portable continuous electrocardiograph recorder, typically monitoring two channels for 24 hours; it is used to detect the frequency and duration of cardiac rhythm disturbances and to assess pacemaker programming. The term is sometimes used synonymously with *Holter monitor.*

Holter m. a type of ambulatory ECG monitor.

mon•key (mung′ke) any member of several families of nonhuman primates, usually distinguished as *New World monkeys* (see superfamily Platyrrhina) or *Old World monkeys* (see superfamily Cercopithecoidea).

cynomolgus m. *Macaca fascicularis*, a macaque native to South America, much used in laboratory research. Called also *crab-eating macaque.*

rhesus m. *Macaca mulatta*, a light brown macaque native to India, much used in physiological research. See also *Rh factor*, under *factor.* Called also *rhesus macaque* and *rhesus.*

mon•key•pox (mung′ke-poks) a mild, epidemic, exanthematous disease occurring in captive monkeys and other mammals; it can be transmitted to humans, in whom it causes a disease clinically similar to smallpox.

monks•hood (mungks′hood) 1. aconite. 2. Aconitum.

mon(o)- [Gr. *monos* single] 1. a combining form meaning one or single, or limited to one part. 2. in chemistry, combined with one atom, group, or radical.

mono•ac•yl•glyc•er•ol (mon″o-a″səl-glis′ər-ol) monoglyceride.

mono•ac•yl•glyc•er•ol lip•ase (mon″o-a″səl-glis′ə-rol li′pās) acylglycerol lipase.

mono•am•ide (mon″o-am′īd) an amide containing one amide group.

mono•amine (mon″o-ə-mēn′) an amine molecule containing one amino group; biogenic amines in this group include serotonin, dopamine, epinephrine, and norepinephrine.

mono•amine ox•i•dase (MAO) (mon″o-ə-mēn′ ok′sĭ-dās) amine oxidase (flavin-containing).

mono•am•in•er•gic (mon″o-am″in-ur′jik) of or pertaining to neurons that secrete monoamine neurotransmitters.

mono•am•ni•on•ic (mon″o-am″ne-on′ik) having or developing within a single amniotic cavity, such as monoamnionic twins.

mono•am•ni•ot•ic (mon″o-am″ne-ot′ik) monoamnionic.

mono•ar•thri•tis (mon″o-ahr-thri′tis) monarthritis.

mono•ar•tic•u•lar (mon″o-ahr-tik′u-lər) monarthric.

mon•o•bac•tam (mon″o-bak′tam) a class of synthetic antibiotics having a monocyclic β-lactam nucleus.

mono•ba•sic (mon″o-ba′sik) [*mono-* + *basic*] having but one base; a term applied to an acid having only one replaceable atom of hydrogen and therefore yielding only one series of salts, as HCl.

mono•ben•zone (mon″o-ben′zōn) [USP] a melanin-inhibiting agent structurally related to hydroquinone; used as a topical depigmenting agent in vitiligo.

mono•blast (mon′o-blast) [*mono-* + *-blast*] the earliest precursor in the monocytic series, which matures to develop into the promonocyte; it has a fine chromatin structure and nucleoli are usually visible. Monoblasts are not normally seen in the bone marrow or peripheral blood, but may be seen in myelogenous leukemia.

mono·blas·to·ma (mon″o-blas-to′mə) a neoplasm containing monoblasts and monocytes; see *acute monocytic leukemia*, under *leukemia.*

mono·blep·sia (mon″o-blep′se-ə) [*mono-* + Gr. *blepsis* sight + *-ia*] 1. a condition of the vision in which it is more distinct when only one eye is used. 2. a variety of color blindness in which only one color is perceived. See also *monochromatism.*

mono·bra·chia (mon″o-bra′ke-ə) [*mono-* + *brachi-* + *-ia*] a developmental anomaly characterized by the presence of a single upper limb.

mono·bra·chi·us (mon″o-bra′ke-əs) an individual exhibiting monobrachia.

mono·bro·mat·ed (mon″o-bro′māt-əd) [L. *monobromatus*] having a single atom of bromine in each molecule.

mono·cal·cic (mon″o-kal′sik) containing one atom of calcium in the molecule.

mono·car·box·yl·ic ac·id (mon″o-kahr″bok-sil′ik) a carboxylic acid containing a single carboxyl group.

mono·car·di·an (mon″o-kahr′de-ən) [*mono-* + Gr. *kardia* heart] possessing a heart with a single atrium and ventricle, as that of a shark.

mono·celled (mon′o-səld) [*mono-* + *cell*] unicellular.

mono·cel·lu·lar (mon″o-sel′u-lər) unicellular.

mono·ceph·a·lus (mon″o-sef′ə-ləs) [*mono-* + *-cephalus*] a fetus with one head but with some duplication of its parts.

m. tet′rapus dibra′chius conjoined twins with one head, two upper limbs, and partial or complete duplication of the pelvis, with four lower limbs, the pair belonging to one member often being fused in a single limb.

m. tri′pus dibra′chius conjoined twins with one head, two upper limbs, and partial duplication of the pelvis, with a median whole or rudimentary third lower limb.

mono·cho·rea (mon″o-kə-re′ə) [*mono-* + *chorea*] chorea affecting but one limb.

mono·cho·ri·al (mon″o-kor′e-əl) monochorionic.

mono·cho·ri·on·ic (mon″o-kor″e-on′ik) [*mono-* + *chorionic*] having or developing in a common chorionic sac, such as monozygotic twins.

mono·chro·ic (mon″o-kro′ik) monochromatic (def. 1).

mono·chro·ma·cy (mon″o-kro′mə-se) monochromatic vision.

mono·chro·ma·sy (mon″o-kro′mə-se) monochromatic vision.

mono·chro·mat (mon″o-kro′mat) a person who has monochromatic vision; called also *achromat.*

mono·chro·mat·ic (mon″o-kro-mat′ik) 1. existing in or having only one color. 2. pertaining to or having monochromatic vision. 3. staining with only one dye at a time. Cf. *polychromatic.*

mono·chro·ma·tism (mon″o-kro′mə-tiz″əm) monochromatic vision.

cone m. monochromatism in which there is some cone function and normal visual acuity and which is not associated with nystagmus and photophobia.

rod m. monochromatism in which there is complete absence of cone function and which is accompanied by poor vision, photophobia, and nystagmus.

mono·chro·mato·phil (mon″o-kro-mat′ə-fil) [*mono-* + *chromato-* + *-phil*] 1. stainable with only one kind of stain. 2. any cell or other element that will take only one stain.

mono·chro·ma·top·sia (mon″o-kro″mə-top′se-ə) monochromatic vision.

mono·chro·mo·phil·ic (mon″o-kro″mo-fil′ik) stainable with only one kind of stain.

Mono·cid (mon′o-sid) trademark for a preparation of cefonicid sodium.

Mono·clate-P (mon′o-klāt″) trademark for a preparation of antihemophilic factor (human).

mono·clin·ic (mon″o-klin′ik) [*mono-* + Gr. *klinein* to incline] a term applied to crystals in which the vertical axis is inclined to one lateral axis, but is at right angles to the other.

mono·clo·nal (mon″o-klo′nəl) derived from or pertaining to a single clone.

mono·con·tam·i·nat·ed (mon″o-kən-tam′ĭ-nāt″əd) infected by a single species of microorganism, or by a single type of contaminating agent; see *monoxenic.*

mono·con·tam·i·na·tion (mon″o-kən-tam″ĭ-na′shən) experimental infection of a previously germ-free animal by a single infectious agent. See *monoxenic.*

mono·cor·di·tis (mon″o-kor-di′tis) inflammation of one vocal cord.

mono·cra·ni·us (mon″o-kra′ne-əs) monocephalus.

mono·cro·ta·line (mon″o-kro′tə-lēn) a poisonous pyrrolizidine alkaloid found in various species of *Crotalaria*, the cause of crotalism.

mo·noc·ro·tism (mə-nok′rə-tiz-əm) [*mono-* + Gr. *krotos* beat] presence of a monocrotic pulse, with neither an anacrotic nor a dicrotic notch. **monocrot′ic** *adj*

mon·oc·u·lar (mon-ok′u-lər) [*mono-* + *ocular*] 1. pertaining to or having but one eye. 2. having but one eyepiece, as in a microscope.

mon·oc·u·lus (mon-ok′u-ləs) [*mono-* + *oculus*] 1. a bandage for covering one eye. 2. cyclops.

mono·cy·clic (mon″o-sik′lik, -si′klik) pertaining to one cycle. In chemistry, having a molecular structure containing only one ring.

mono·cyte (mon′o-sīt) [*mono-* + *-cyte*] a mononuclear phagocytic leukocyte, 13 to 25 μm in diameter, with an ovoid or kidney-shaped nucleus, containing lacy, linear chromatin and abundant gray-blue cytoplasm filled with fine reddish and azurophilic granules. Formed in the bone marrow from promonocytes, monocytes are transported to tissues such as the lung and liver, where they develop into macrophages. See also *monocytic series*, under *series.*

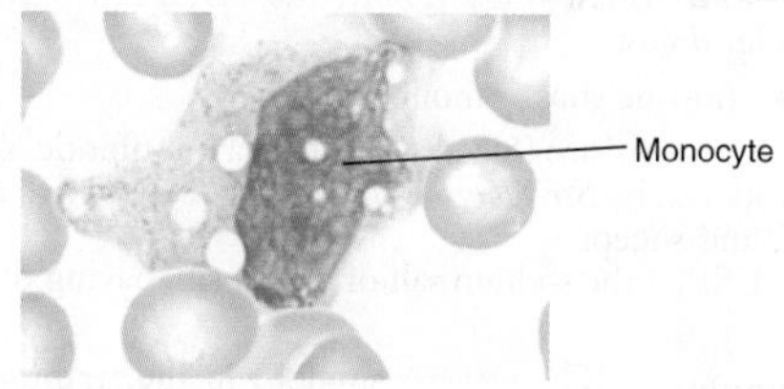

mono·cyt·ic (mon″o-sit′ik) 1. pertaining to, characterized by, or of the nature of monocytes. 2. pertaining to the monocytic series; see under *series.*

mono·cy·toid (mon″o-si′toid) resembling a monocyte.

mono·cy·to·pe·nia (mon″o-si″to-pe′ne-ə) [*monocyte* + *-penia*] abnormal decrease in the proportion of monocytes in the blood.

mono·cy·to·poi·e·sis (mon″o-si″to-poi-e′sis) [*monocyte* + *-poiesis*] the formation of monocytes.

mono·cy·to·sis (mon″o-si-to′sis) increase in the proportion of monocytes in the blood; see also *mononucleosis.*

mono·dac·tyl·ia (mon″o-dak-til′e-ə) monodactyly.

mono·dac·tyl·ism (mon″o-dak′təl-iz-əm) monodactyly.

mono·dac·ty·ly (mon″o-dak′tə-le) [*mono-* + Gr. *daktylos* finger] a developmental anomaly characterized by the presence of only one digit on a hand or foot.

mono·dal (mon-o′dəl) [*mono-* + Gr. *hodos* road] having connection with one terminal of a resonator or of a grounded solenoid, so that the patient is a capacitor for entrance and exit of high frequency currents.

mono·der·mal (mon″o-dur′məl) pertaining to or possessing just one germ cell layer; said of tumors.

mono·der·mo·ma (mon″o-dər-mo′mə) a tumor that has developed from one germ layer.

mono·di·plo·pia (mon″o-dĭ-plo′pe-ə) [*mono-* + *diplopia*] double vision in one eye only.

Mono·don·tus (mon″o-don′təs) *Bunostomum.*

Mono·dox (mon′o-doks″) trademark for a preparation of doxycycline.

mo·noe·cious (mo-ne′shəs) [*mono-* + Gr. *oikos* house] having reproductive organs typical of both sexes in a single individual.

mono·es·ter (mon″o-es′tər) an ester containing a single ester group.

mon·o·es·trous (mon″o-es′trus) having just one estrous cycle per annual breeding season. Cf. *polyestrous.*

mono·eth·a·nol·amine (mon″o-eth″ə-nōl′ə-mēn) 1. 2-aminoethanol; an amino alcohol occurring in phosphatidylethanolamines and derived metabolically by decarboxylation of serine. Its oleate salt is called ethanolamine oleate (q.v.). Called also *ethanolamine.* 2. [NF] a purified preparation of this substance, used as a surfactant in pharmaceuticals.

mono·eth·yl·gly·cine·xy·li·dide (MEGX) (mon″o-eth″əl-gli″sēn-zi′lĭ-dīd) the principal active metabolite of lidocaine, produced in the liver; measurement of the conversion of lidocaine to MEGX is used in liver function tests.

mono·film (mon′o-film) a monomolecular layer transferred to a prepared plate.

mo·nog·a·mous (mə-nog′ə-məs) pertaining to monogamy.

mo·nog·a·my (mə-nog′ə-me) [*mono-* + Gr. *gamos* marriage] 1. marriage to a single spouse. 2. the animal mating system in which each individual mates with just one partner for the entire breeding season. Cf. *polygamy.*

mono·gan·gli·al (mon″o-gang′gle-əl) affecting a single ganglion.

mono·gas·tric (mon″o-gas′trik) [*mono-* + *gastr-* + *-ic*] having just one stomach, as opposed to ruminants and certain other animals.

mono·gen (mon′o-jən) 1. a monovalent chemical element which combines in only one proportion. 2. an antiserum produced by the use of one antigen (i.e., immunogen).

mono·gen·e·sis (mon″o-jen′ə-sis) [*mono-* + *-genesis*] 1. asexual reproduction. 2. oneness of origin.

mono·ge·net·ic (mon″o-jə-net′ik) 1. pertaining to or exhibiting monogenesis. 2. having a single host in the life cycle; said of certain parasitic protozoa.

mono·gen·ic (mon″o-jen′ik) pertaining to or influenced by a single gene.

mono·ger·mi·nal (mon″o-jur′mĭ-nəl) monozygotic.

mono·glyc·er·ide (mon″o-glis′ər-īd) a compound consisting of one molecule of fatty acid esterified to glycerol, usually occurring as an intermediate in triglyceride metabolism. Called also *monoacylglycerol*.

mono·glyc·er·ide ac·yl·trans·fer·ase (mon″o-glis′ər-īd a″səl-trans′fər-ās) 2-acylglycerol *O*-acyltransferase.

mono·graph (mon′o-graf) [*mono-* + *-graph*] an essay or treatise on one subject.

mono·hor·mo·nal (mon″o-hor-mo′nəl) secreting a single hormone.

mono·hy·brid (mon″o-hi′brid) [*mono-* + *hybrid*] 1. an individual heterozygous at a single locus, produced by parents each of whom is homozygous for a different allele at that single locus. 2. pertaining to such an individual.

mono·hy·drat·ed (mon″o-hi′drāt-əd) united with a single molecule of water or a single hydroxyl group.

mono·hy·dric (mon″o-hi′drik) containing one atom of replaceable hydrogen.

mono·in·fec·tion (mon″o-in-fek′shən) infection with a single kind of organism.

mono·io·do·ty·ro·sine (mon″o-i-o″do-ti′ro-sēn) an iodinated amino acid that is an intermediate in the thyroidal biosynthesis of thyroxine and triiodothyronine. Abbreviated MIT.

mono·kary·on (mon″o-kar′e-on) [*mono-* + *karyon*] a growth stage in the mycelium of fungi, especially Basidiomycetes, in which each cell has one haploid nucleus. **monokaryot′ic** *adj*

Mono·ket (mon′o-ket″) trademark for a preparation of isosorbide mononitrate.

mono·kine (mon′o-kīn) a soluble cytokine that mediates immune responses; it is not an antibody or a complement component and is produced by mononuclear phagocytes (monocytes or macrophages). Cf. *lymphokine*.

mono·lay·er (mon″o-la′ər) 1. a single layer, used especially of the growth of cells in culture or of uniformly oriented polar (especially lipid) molecules. 2. pertaining to or consisting of such a layer.

mono·loc·u·lar (mon″o-lok′u-lər) [*mono-* + *loculus*] unilocular.

mono·ma·nia (mon″o-ma′ne-ə) [*mono-* + *-mania*] a form of mental disorder characterized by preoccupation with one subject or idea.

mono·max·il·lary (mon″o-mak′sĭ-lar″e) pertaining to or affecting one maxilla.

mono·mel·ic (mon″o-mel′ik) [*mono-* + *mel-* + *-ic*] affecting one limb.

mono·mer (mon′o-mər) [*mono-* + Gr. *meros* part] 1. a simple molecule of a compound of relatively low molecular weight, consisting of simple unrepeated structural units, which can react to form a dimer, trimer, polymer, etc. 2. some basic unit of a molecule, either the molecule itself or some structural or functional subunit of it, e.g., an individual polypeptide chain in a multi-subunit protein.

fibrin m. the material resulting from the highly specific and orderly cleavage of fibrinogen by thrombin; through polymerization, these monomers form macromolecular fibrin.

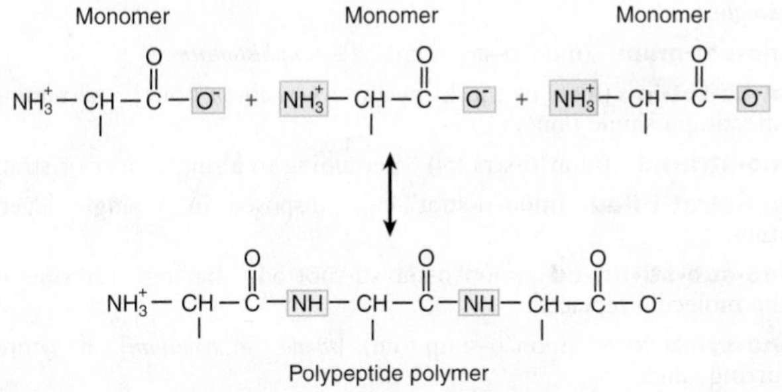

Monomer Monomer Monomer

$NH_3^+-CH-C(=O)-O^- + NH_3^+-CH-C(=O)-O^- + NH_3^+-CH-C(=O)-O^-$

↕

$NH_3^+-CH-C(=O)-NH-CH-C(=O)-NH-CH-C(=O)-O^-$

Polypeptide polymer

■ Monomer. Individual amino acids constitute the monomeric building blocks of (polymeric) polypeptides.

mono·mer·ic (mon″o-mer′ik) pertaining to, made up of, or affecting a single segment, as distinguished from dimeric, polymeric, etc.

mono·me·tal·lic (mon″o-mə-tal′ik) having one atom of a metal in the molecule.

mono·meth·yl·hy·dra·zine (mon″o-meth″əl-hi′drə-zēn) a toxin found in many species of *Gyromitra* mushrooms, acting as an antagonist to pyridoxine; six or more hours after ingestion, patients develop headache, dizziness, malaise, and vomiting, occasionally progressing to delirium, coma, and convulsions.

mono·mi·cro·bi·al (mon″o-mi-kro′be-əl) marked by the presence of a single species of microorganisms.

mono·mo·lec·u·lar (mon″o-mo-lek′u-lər) pertaining to or involving one molecule.

mono·mor·phic (mon″o-mor′fik) [*mono-* + *morph-* + *-ic*] existing in only one form; maintaining the same form throughout all stages of development.

mono·mor·phism (mon″o-mor′fiz-əm) the quality or condition of being monomorphic.

mono·mor·phous (mon″o-mor′fəs) composed of lesions all of the same age, form, and shape.

mon·om·pha·lus (mon-om′fə-ləs) omphalopagus.

mono·myo·ple·gia (mon″o-mi′o-ple′jə) [*mono-* + *myo-* + *-plegia*] paralysis restricted to a single muscle.

mono·myo·si·tis (mon″o-mi″o-si′tis) [*mono-* + *myositis*] a myositis of the biceps muscle occurring periodically.

Mo·non·chus (mo-nong′kəs) a genus of nematodes living in fresh water or moist soil, reportedly found in human urine, probably representing a case of spurious parasitosis.

mono·neu·ral (mon″o-noor′əl) [*mono-* + *neural*] 1. pertaining to or receiving branches from a single nerve. 2. having only one neuron.

mono·neur·ic (mon″o-noor′ik) mononeural.

mono·neu·ri·tis (mon″o-nŏŏ-ri′tis) [*mono-* + *neur-* + *-itis*] disease of a single nerve.

m. mul′tiplex see under *mononeuropathy*.

mono·neu·rop·a·thy (mon″o-nŏŏ-rop′ə-the) disease affecting a single nerve.

cranial m. see under *neuropathy*.

multifocal m., multiple m., m. multiplex mononeuropathy of several different nerves simultaneously. Called also *mononeuritis multiplex* and *multiple neuropathy*.

Mono·nine (mon′o-nīn″) trademark for a preparation of coagulation factor IX (human).

mono·nu·cle·ar (mon″o-noo′kle-ər) [*mono-* + *nuclear*] 1. having but one nucleus; called also *mononucleate* and *uninuclear*. 2. a cell having a single nucleus, especially a monocyte of the blood or tissues.

mono·nu·cle·ate (mon″o-noo′kle-āt) mononuclear (def. 1).

mono·nu·cle·o·sis (mon″o-noo″kle-o′sis) 1. excessive numbers of circulating monocytes (see *monocytosis*), usually referring to abnormal types. 2. infectious m.

chronic m. chronic fatigue syndrome.

cytomegalovirus m. a type of acquired cytomegalic inclusion disease that resembles infectious mononucleosis, with fever, splenomegaly, hepatic involvement, atypical lymphocytes, and a negative heterophil antibody test, but without pharyngitis or cervical adenopathy. It may occur as an opportunistic infection in immunocompromised persons or after multiple blood transfusions (see *postperfusion syndrome*, under *syndrome*).

infectious m. a common, acute, usually self-limited infectious disease caused by the Epstein-Barr virus, characterized by fever, membranous pharyngitis, lymph node and splenic enlargement, lymphocyte proliferation, and atypical lymphocytes; it gives rise to various immune reactions, such as development of transient heterophile antibodies and persistent Epstein-Barr virus antibodies. Potential complications include hepatitis and encephalomeningitis. It affects primarily adolescents and young adults, being spread by saliva transfer and possibly other modes; in children the infection is largely subclinical. Called also *glandular fever* and *kissing disease*.

mono·nu·cle·o·tide (mon″o-noo′kle-o-tīd) a product obtained by the digestion or hydrolytic decomposition of nucleic acid. It is a compound of phosphoric acid and a pentoside. The latter is a combination of a pentose

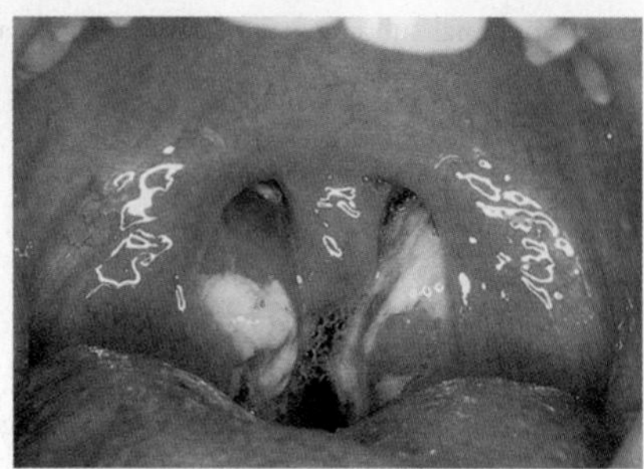

■ Severe pharyngotonsillitis, with uvular erythema and edema, in infectious mononucleosis.

(ribose or 2-deoxyribose) with one of the following bases: adenine, cytosine, guanine, thymine, or uracil.

mono·oc·ta·no·in (mon″o-ok″tə-no′in) a semisynthetic glycerol derivative used to dissolve cholesterol stones in the common and intrahepatic bile ducts; administered as a continuous perfusion via catheter.

mono-os·te·it·ic (mon″o-os″te-it′ik) denoting a type of osteitis which affects a single bone.

mono-ov·u·lar (mon″o-ov′u-lər) monovular.

mono·oxy·gen·ase (mon″o-ok′sĭ-jə-nās″) a term used in the recommended names of some enzymes of the oxidoreductase class; it denotes any enzyme catalyzing the incorporation of one atom from molecular oxygen into a compound while reducing the other atom of oxygen to water; this includes those in which the oxygen acceptor acts also as the hydrogen donor [EC 1.13.12] as well as those in which a second compound acts as the hydrogen donor in a coupled reaction [EC 1.14.13 to 1.14.18 and 1.14.99]. Called also *mixed function oxidase.*

mono·par·e·sis (mon″o-pə-re′sis) [*mono-* + *paresis*] paresis of a single limb.

mono·par·es·the·sia (mon″o-par″es-the′zhə) [*mono-* + *paresthesia*] paresthesia of a single limb.

mo·nop·a·thy (mə-nop′ə-the) [*mono-* + *-pathy*] a disease affecting a single part.

mono·pe·nia (mon″o-pe′ne-ə) monocytopenia.

mono·pha·gia (mon″o-fa′je-ə) [*mono-* + *-phagia*] 1. desire for one kind of food only. 2. the eating of only one meal a day.

mo·noph·a·gism (mə-nof′ə-jiz-əm) monophagia.

mono·pha·sia (mon″o-fa′zhə) [*mono-* + *-phasia*] aphasia with ability to utter but one word or phrase.

mono·pha·sic (mon″o-fa′zik) exhibiting only one phase or variation. Cf. *diphasic* and *triphasic.*

mono·phe·nol mono·oxy·gen·ase (mon″o-fe′nol mon″o-ok′sĭ-jən-ās″) [EC 1.14.18.1] any of a group of enzymes of the oxidoreductase class that catalyze the hydroxylation of tyrosine to dopa and the oxidation of dopa to dopaquinone. They are copper proteins that also act on catechols and substituted catechols (i.e., act as catechol oxidases). The reaction is a step in the formation of melanin pigments from tyrosine. Cf. *catechol oxidase.*

mono·phos·phate (mon″o-fos′fāt) a salt containing a single phosphate radical.

mon·oph·thal·mus (mon″of-thal′məs) cyclops.

mono·phy·let·ic (mon″o-fi-let′ik) [*mono-* + Gr. *phylē* tribe] arising or descended from a single cell type; see *monophyletic theory,* under *theory.*

mono·phy·le·tism (mon″o-fi′lə-tiz-əm) monophyletic theory; see under *theory.*

mono·phy·le·tist (mon″o-fi′lə-tist) an adherent of the monophyletic theory; see under *theory.*

mono·phy·odont (mon″o-fi′o-dont) [*mono-* + Gr. *phyein* to grow + *odous* tooth] having only one set of teeth, and those permanent. Cf. *diphyodont* and *polyphyodont.*

mon·o·pia (mon-o′pe-ə) cyclopia.

mono·plas·mat·ic (mon″o-plaz-mat′ik) [*mono-* + *plasmatic*] made up of a single substance.

mono·plast (mon′o-plast) [*mono-* + *-plast*] a single constituent cell.

mono·ple·gia (mon″o-ple′jə) [*mono-* + *-plegia*] paralysis of a limb. **monople′gic** *adj*

mono·po·dia (mon″o-po′de-ə) [*mono-* + *pod-* + *-ia*] monopodial symmelia.

mono·po·di·al (mon″o-po′de-əl) having a single median foot; see *symmelia.*

mono·poi·e·sis (mon″o-poi-e′sis) monocytopoiesis.

mono·po·lar (mon′o-po″lər) of an electrical apparatus, having a single pole, with the ground acting as the second pole. Called also *uniterminal.*

Mono·pril (mon′o-pril) trademark for a preparation of fosinopril sodium.

Mono·psyl·lus (mon″o-sil′əs) [*mono-* + Gr. *psylla* flea] a genus of fleas. *M. ani′sus* is a rat flea found in Japan and northern China.

mono·pty·chi·al (mon″o-ti′ke-əl) [*mono-* + Gr. *ptychē* fold] arranged in a single layer; said of glands whose cells are arranged on the basement membrane in a single layer. Cf. *polyptychial.*

mono·pus (mon′o-pəs) 1. monopodial. 2. sympus monopus.

mon·or·chia (mon-or′ke-ə) monorchism.

mon·or·chid (mon-or′kid) 1. having just one testis in the scrotum; see *monorchism.* 2. an individual with monorchism.

mon·or·chid·ic (mon″or-kid′ik) [*mono-* + *orchid-* + *-ic*] monorchid (def. 1).

mon·or·chid·ism (mon-or′kid-iz-əm) monorchism.

mon·or·chism (mon′or-kiz″əm) the condition of having only one testis in the scrotum; called also *monorchidism.*

Mon·or·cho·tre·ma (mon-or″ko-tre′mə) [*mono-* + Gr. *orchis* testicle + *trēma* aperture] a genus of flukes of the family Heterophyidae, found in birds and mammals in the Middle East and Taiwan, and characterized by having only a single testis. They have as invertebrate host an operculate snail, and as first vertebrate host an edible fish.

mono·rhin·ic (mon″o-rin′ik) pertaining to or possessing one nasal cavity.

mono·sac·cha·ride (mon″o-sak′ə-rīd) a simple sugar; a carbohydrate that cannot be decomposed by hydrolysis. The monosaccharides are colorless crystalline substances with a sweet taste and all have the general formula $C_nH_{2n}O_n$. They are classified according to the number of carbon atoms in the chain into dioses ($C_2H_4O_2$), trioses ($C_3H_6O_3$), etc., and are further classified as aldoses or ketoses.

mon·ose (mon′ōs) monosaccharide.

mono·sex·u·al (mon″o-sek′shoo-əl) showing the traits of one sex only.

mono·so·di·um glu·ta·mate (mon″o-so′de-əm gloo′tə-māt) the monosodium salt of L-glutamic acid, used as a pharmaceutic necessity and also to enhance the flavor of foods. See also *Chinese restaurant syndrome,* under *syndrome.*

mono·some (mon′o-sōm) [*mono-* + *-some*] 1. the chromosome lacking a homologue in monosomy. 2. a single ribosome complexed with a strand of messenger RNA (mRNA). Cf. *polysome.* 3. a single ribosome that has dissociated from a polysome.

mono·so·my (mon′o-so″me) absence of one chromosome of a homologous pair in the complement of an otherwise diploid cell (2n−1), as seen in Turner syndrome and various other conditions. **monoso′mic** *adj*

mono·spasm (mon′o-spaz″əm) [*mono-* + *spasm*] spasm of a single limb or part. Different varieties are distinguished according to the part affected or to the site of the causal lesion; as, brachial, facial, lateral, peripheral, etc.

mono·spe·cif·ic (mon″o-spə-sif′ik) having an effect only on a particular kind of cell or tissue, or reacting with a single antigen, as a monospecific antiserum.

mono·sper·my (mon′o-spur″me) [*mono-* + Gr. *sperma* seed] fertilization in which only one spermatozoon enters the oocyte.

Mono·spo·ri·um (mon″o-spor′e-əm) former name for *Scedosporium.*

Mono·sto·ma (mon″o-sto′mə) [Gr. *monos* single + *stoma* mouth] *Paramphistomum.*

Mono·sto·mum (mon″o-sto′məm) *Paramphistomum.*

mon·os·tot·ic (mon″os-tot′ik) [*mono-* + Gr. *osteon* bone] pertaining to or affecting a single bone.

mono·stra·tal (mon″o-stra′təl) pertaining to a single layer or stratum.

mono·strat·i·fied (mon″o-strat′ĭ-fīd) disposed in a single layer or stratum.

mono·sub·sti·tut·ed (mon″o-sub′stĭ-to͞ot″əd) having only one atom in the molecule replaced.

mono·symp·tom (mon″o-simp′tom) [*mono-* + *symptom*] a symptom occurring singly.

mono·symp·to·mat·ic (mon″o-simp″tə-mat′ik) expressed by a single symptom.

mono·syn·ap·tic (mon″o-sĭ-nap′tik) pertaining to or relayed through only one synapse.

mono·ther·a·py (mon″o-ther′ə-pe) treatment of a condition by means of a single drug.

mono·ther·mia (mon″o-thur′me-ə) [*mono-* + *therm-* + *-ia*] a condition in which the body temperature remains the same throughout the day.

mono·thet·ic (mon″o-thet′ik) [*mono-* + Gr. *thetikos* fit for placing] denoting a taxonomic group classified on the basis of a single character, as opposed to polythetic.

mono·thio·glyc·er·ol (mon″o-thi″o-glis′ər-ol) [NF] a clear, colorless, moderately viscous liquid used as a preservative in pharmaceutical preparations.

mon·o·tic (mon-o′tik) [*mono-* + *ot-* + *-ic*] 1. monaural. 2. possessing a single ear.

mo·not·o·cous (mo-not′ə-kəs) [*mono-* + *toc-* + *-ous*] giving birth to but one offspring at a time.

Mono·tre·ma·ta (mon″o-tre′mə-tə) the lowest order of mammals, including animals which lay eggs similar to those of reptiles, and nourish their young by a mammary gland which has no nipple, in a shallow pouch developed only during lactation. The only living representatives are the spiny anteater and duck-billed platypus. In some systems of classification, considered to be an order of subclass Prototheria, class Mammalia.

mono·treme (mon′o-trēm) a member of the order Monotremata.

mono·trich·ic (mon″o-trik′ik) monotrichous.

mon·ot·ri·chous (mə-not′rĭ-kəs) [*mono-* + *trich-* + *-ous*] having a single polar flagellum; said of a bacterial cell. See *flagellum*.

mon·o·tro·pic (mon″o-tro′pik) [*mono-* + *-tropic*] affecting only one particular kind of bacterium, virus, or tissue. Cf. *polytropic*.

mono·un·sat·u·rat·ed (mon″o-ən-sach′ər-āt″əd) of a chemical compound, containing one double or triple bond; used particularly of fatty acids, such as oleic acid.

mono·ure·ide (mon″o-u′re-id) see *ureide*.

mono·va·lent (mon″o-va′lənt) 1. having a valence of one. Called also *univalent*. 2. denoting an antiserum, vaccine, or antitoxin specific for a single antigen or organism.

mono·vi·sion (mon′o-vizh″ən) vision resulting from the correction of one eye for near and the other eye for far vision, especially with contact lenses, as a substitute for bifocal glasses.

mon·ov·u·lar (mon-ov′u-lər) pertaining to or derived from a single oocyte; as monozygotic twins.

mon·ov·u·la·to·ry (mon-ov′u-lə-tor″e) ordinarily discharging only one oocyte in one ovarian cycle.

mono·xen·ic (mon″o-zen′ik) [*mono-* + *xen-* + *-ic*] associated with a single species of microorganisms; said of otherwise germ-free animals contaminated by a single type of organism.

mo·nox·e·nous (mə-nok′sə-nəs) [*mono-* + Gr. *xenos* host] homoxenous.

mon·ox·ide (mon-ok′sīd) an oxide containing but one atom of oxygen; vernacularly applied to carbon monoxide.

mono·zy·gos·i·ty (mon″o-zi-gos′ĭ-te) [*mono-* + *-zygosity*] the state of being monozygotic.

mono·zy·got·ic (mon″o-zi-got′ik) pertaining to or derived from a single zygote, as monozygotic twins.

mono·zy·gous (mon″o-zi′gəs) monozygotic.

Mon·ro bursa, foramen, line, sulcus (mən-ro′) [Alexander *Monro* (Secundus), Scottish anatomist and surgeon, 1733–1817] see *bursa intratendinea olecrani*, *foramen interventriculare*, and *sulcus hypothalamicus*, and see under *line*.

Mon·ro-Kel·lie doctrine (mən-ro′ kel′e) [A. *Monro* (Secundus); George *Kellie*, Scottish anatomist, late 18th century] see under *doctrine*.

Mon·ro-Rich·ter line (mən-ro′ rik′ter) [A. *Monro* (Secundus); August Gottlieb *Richter*, German surgeon, 1742–1812] see under *line*.

mons (monz) pl. *mon′tes* [L. "mountain"] an elevation or eminence.

m. pu′bis [TA] the rounded fleshy prominence over the symphysis pubis.

$$\mathrm{CH_3(CH_2)_5}\backslash\ /\mathrm{(CH_2)_7COOH}\quad \mathrm{C{=}C}\quad \mathrm{H}/\ \backslash\mathrm{H}$$

■ A monounsaturated fatty acid, palmitoleic acid (*cis*-9-hexadecenoic acid).

m. ure′teris a papilla-like elevation of the mucosa of the bladder at its junction with the ureter.

m. ve′neris m. pubis.

Mon·son curve (mon′sən) [George S. *Monson*, American dentist, 1869–1933] see under *curve*.

Mon·so·nia (mon-so′ne-ə) a genus of African and Asian plants of the family Geraniaceae; certain species are used in medicine as astringents or in the treatment of dysentery.

mon·ster (mon′stər) [L. *monstrum*] 1. an animal whose appearance is considered strange or frightening. 2. a term formerly used to denote a fetus or infant with such pronounced developmental anomalies as to be grotesque and usually nonviable.

Gila m. *Heloderma suspectum*, a venomous lizard found especially in Arizona and New Mexico.

mon·stros·i·ty (mon-stros′ĭ-te) [L. *monstrositas*] monster (def. 2).

mon·strum (mon′strəm) pl. *mon′stra* [L.] monster (def. 2).

mon·tage (mon-tahzh′) an arrangement of electrodes on the scalp for several simultaneous electroencephalographic recordings at multiple sites over a given area or over the entire brain.

Mon·teg·gia dislocation, fracture (mon-tej′ə) [Giovanni Battista *Monteggia*, Italian surgeon, 1762–1815] see under *dislocation* and *fracture*.

mon·te·lu·kast so·di·um (mon″tə-loo′kast) a leukotriene receptor antagonist used as an antiasthmatic agent; administered orally.

mon·tes (mon′tēz) [L.] plural of *mons*.

Mont·gom·ery follicles, glands, tubercles (mont-gum′ər-e) [William Fetherstone *Montgomery*, Irish obstetrician, 1797–1859] see under *tubercle*, and see *Naboth follicles*, under *follicle*, and *glandulae areolares*.

mon·tic·u·lus (mon-tik′u-ləs) gen. and pl. *monti′culi* [L., dim. of *mons*] a small eminence.

m. cerebel′li the projecting or central part of the superior vermis.

Mon·u·rol (mon′u-rol) trademark for a preparation of fosfomycin tromethamine.

mood (mo͞od) [A.S. *mōd* disposition] a pervasive and sustained emotion that, when extreme, can color one's whole view of life and markedly affect behavior. Mood is generally used to refer to either elation or depression. See also *mood disorders*, under *disorder*.

dysphoric m. a mood that is unpleasant.

elevated m. a mood characterized by an exaggerated sense of well-being, cheerfulness, or elation.

euthymic m. a mood that is neither elevated nor depressed.

expansive m. a mood characterized by a lack of restraint in expressing one's feelings, often with an overestimation of self-importance or significance.

irritable m. a mood that is easily annoyed or provoked to anger.

mood-con·gru·ent (mo͞od kong′groo-ənt) consistent with one's mood. The term is used particularly in the classification of mood disorders: in those disorders with psychotic features, *mood-congruent psychotic features* are grandiose delusions or related hallucinations occurring in a manic episode or depressive delusions or related hallucinations in a major depressive episode, while *mood-incongruent psychotic features* are delusions or hallucinations that either contradict or are inconsistent with the prevailing emotions, such as delusions of persecution or of thought insertion in either a manic or a depressive episode.

mood-in·con·gru·ent (mo͞od in″kong′groo-ənt) not mood-congruent (q.v.).

Moon teeth (molars) (mo͞on) [Henry *Moon*, English surgeon, 1845–1892] see under *tooth*.

Moore fracture (mo͞or) [Edward Mott *Moore*, American surgeon, 1814–1902] see under *fracture*.

Moore lightning streaks (mo͞or) [Robert Foster *Moore*, British ophthalmologist, 1878–1963] see under *streak*.

Moore syndrome (mo͞or) [Matthew T. *Moore*, American neuropsychiatrist, 1901–1997] abdominal epilepsy.

Moor·en ulcer (mo′rən) [Albert *Mooren*, German ophthalmologist, 1828–1899] see under *ulcer*.

Moor·head foreign body locator (mo͞or′hed) [John J. *Moorhead*, American surgeon, 20th century] Berman-Moorhead locator.

8-MOP trademark for a preparation of methoxsalen.

MOPP a cancer chemotherapy regimen consisting of mechlorethamine, Oncovin (vincristine), procarbazine, and prednisone.

mo·ran·tel tar·trate (mo-ran′təl) an anthelmintic used in sheep and cattle.

Mor·ax-Ax·en·feld bacillus, conjunctivitis, diplococcus (mor′ahks ahk′sen-felt″) [Victor *Morax*, Swiss ophthalmologist in Paris, 1866–1935;

Theodor *Axenfeld*, German ophthalmologist, 1867–1930] see under *conjunctivitis*, and see *Moraxella (Moraxella) lacunata*.

Mo•rax•el•la (mo″rak-sel′ə) [Victor *Morax*] a genus of bacteria of the family Moraxellaceae, consisting of gram-negative, short, aerobic, oxidase-positive, nonpigmented organisms found as parasites and pathogens on the mucous membranes of mammals. The genus includes two subgenera: *M. (Moraxella)* occurring as rods, and *M. (Branhamella)* occurring as cocci.

M. anatipes′tifer *Riemerella anatipestifer*.

M. bo′vis *M. (Moraxella) bovis*.

M. (Branhamel′la) catarrha′lis a normal inhabitant of the human nasal cavity and nasopharynx, occasionally causing otitis media or respiratory disease (see Moraxella catarrhalis *pneumonia*, under *pneumonia*). Called also *Branhamella catarrhalis*.

M. lacuna′ta *M. (Moraxella) lacunata*.

M. liquefa′ciens *M. (Moraxella) lacunata*.

M. (Moraxel′la) bo′vis the etiologic agent of infectious bovine keratoconjunctivitis.

M. (Moraxel′la) lacuna′ta an etiologic agent of conjunctivitis and corneal infections; called also *M. liquefaciens*.

Mo•rax•el•la•ceae (mo″rak-sel-a′se-e) a family of gram-negative, rod-shaped, coccoid, or coccal bacteria, of the order Pseudomonadales; organisms are nonmotile, chemo-organotrophic, aerobic, and usually catalase-positive. Medically important organisms are contained in the genera *Acinetobacter* and *Moraxella*.

mor•bid (mor′bid) [L. *morbidus* sick] 1. pertaining to, affected with, or inducing disease; diseased. 2. unhealthy or unwholesome. 3. characterized by preoccupation with gloomy or unwholesome feelings or thoughts.

mor•bid•i•ty (mor-bid′ĭ-te) 1. a diseased condition or state. 2. the incidence or prevalence of a disease or of all diseases in a population. See *morbidity rate*, under *rate*.

mor•bil•li (mor-bil′i) [L.] measles.

mor•bil•li•form (mor-bil′ĭ-form) [*morbilli* + *form*] like measles; resembling the eruption of measles.

Mor•bil•li•vi•rus (mor-bil′ĭ-vi″rəs) [L. *morbilli* measles + *virus*] measles-like viruses; a genus of viruses of the subfamily Paramyxovirinae (family Paramyxoviridae) comprising the agents of measles, canine distemper, rinderpest, and peste des petits ruminants. **morbillivi′ral** *adj*

mor•bil•lous (mor-bil′əs) pertaining to measles.

MORC Medical Officers Reserve Corps.

mor•cel•la•tion (mor″səl-a′shən) [Fr. *morcellement*, from *morceau*, a piece or morsel] the division of solid tissue (such as a tumor) into pieces, which can then be removed.

mor•celle•ment (mor″səl-maw′) morcellation.

mor•dant (mor′dənt) [L. *mordere* to bite] 1. a substance capable of intensifying or deepening the reaction of a specimen to a stain; the chief mordants are alum, aniline, oil, and phenol. 2. to subject to the action of a mordant preliminary to staining.

Mor. dict. [L.] mo′re dic′to (in the manner directed).

Mo•rel ear, syndrome (mo-rel′) [Augustin Benoit *Morel*, French psychiatrist, 1809–1873] see under *ear*, and see *hyperostosis frontalis interna*.

mo•res (mo′rēz) [L., pl. of *mos* custom] the traditions and habits which are generally regarded as conducive to social welfare.

Mor•ga•gni caruncle, foramen, etc. (mor-gah′nye) [Giovanni Battista *Morgagni*, Italian anatomist and pathologist, 1682–1771; professor at Padua, and the founder of pathological anatomy, whose clinicopathological reports were published in 1761 under the title *De sedibus et causis morborum* ("The Seats and Causes of Disease")] see under *caruncle*, *foramen*, *fossa*, *globule*, *hernia*, *lacuna*, and *prolapse*, and see *appendix testis*, *columnae anales*, *fossa navicularis urethrae*, *glandulae urethrales urethrae masculinae*, *sinus anales*, and *ventriculus laryngis*.

Mor•ga•gni-Ad•ams-Stokes syndrome (mor-gah′nye ad′əmz stōks′) [G.B. *Morgagni;* Robert *Adams*, Irish physician, 1791–1875; William *Stokes*, Irish physician, 1804–1878] Adams-Stokes syndrome; see under *syndrome*.

mor•ga•gni•an (mor-gah′nye-ən) named for Giovanni Battista *Morgagni*.

mor•gan (M) (mor′gən) [Thomas Hunt *Morgan*, American zoologist and Nobel prize winner, 1866–1945] a unit of distance on a linkage map; see *centimorgan*.

Mor•ga•nel•la (mor″gə-nel′ə) [Harry de Reimer *Morgan*, British physician, 1863–1931] a genus of gram-negative, facultatively anaerobic, rod-shaped bacteria of the family Enterobacteriaceae, made up of motile, pleomorphic organisms found in the feces of many mammals. The organisms resemble *Proteus*, except that they do not produce hydrogen sulfide or liquefy gelatin.

M. morga′nii the single species of the genus. It is a primary cause of urinary tract infections and is an opportunistic pathogen, causing secondary infections of blood, respiratory tract, and wounds. Called also *Proteus morganii*.

morgue (morg) [Fr.] a place where dead bodies may be temporarily kept, for identification or until claimed for burial.

mo•ria (mo′re-ə) [Gr. *mōria* folly] an abnormal tendency to joke, particularly inappropriately.

mor•i•bund (mor′ĭ-bund″) [L. *moribundus*] in a dying state.

mor•i•ci•zine hy•dro•chlo•ride (mor-ĭ′sĭ-zēn) [USP] a phenothiazine derivative used as an antiarrhythmic in the treatment of ventricular arrhythmias; administered orally.

Mo•rin•ga (mo-ring′gə) a genus of trees of the family Moringaceae, native to southern Asia and tropical Africa. *M. oli′fera* is the horseradish tree, whose root tastes like horseradish and whose nuts yield an oil that was formerly used in the treatment of rheumatism and dyspepsia.

Mor•i•son pouch (mor′ĭ-sən) [James Rutherford *Morison*, British surgeon, 1853–1939] see under *pouch*.

Mo•ri•ta therapy (mo-re′tah) [Shomei *Morita*, Japanese physician, 20th century] see under *therapy*.

mor•ning glo•ry (mor′ning glo′re) 1. any of various species of *Ipomoea*, which are toxic to humans and can be fatal to ruminants. 2. any of various other plants of the family Convolvulaceae that resemble those of the genus *Ipomoea*.

Mo•ro reflex (mo′ro) [Ernst *Moro*, Austrian pediatrician, 1874–1951] see under *reflex*.

-morph [Gr. *morphē* form] a word termination denoting relationship to form or shape, especially an individual or substance possessing a certain form, indicated by the preceding root, as *mesomorph*.

mor•phal•lax•is (mor″fə-lak′sis) [Gr. *morphē* form + *allaxis* exchange] the renewal of lost tissue or a part by reorganization of the remaining part of the body of an animal. **morphallac′tic** *adj*

mor•phea (mor-fe′ə) [Gr. *morphē* form] a localized form of scleroderma having one or more supple, nonindurated, pink to purple macules and later discrete, yellow to white patches or plaques in which the skin is hard, dry, and smooth. The lesions may remain localized or become generalized. Called also *circumscribed* or *localized scleroderma*. Cf. *systemic scleroderma*.

deep m. morphea that involves the deep dermis, subcutaneous tissue, and sometimes underlying muscle and bone; the tissue collapses to form a hard plaque that may interfere with motility. Called also *m. profunda* and *subcutaneous m.*

generalized m. extensive morphea over large sections of a body part, sometimes becoming so extensive as to involve all layers of the skin; it may lead to progressive disability, contractures of the limbs, and progressive atrophy.

guttate m. morphea characterized by small, rounded, atrophic macules, arranged in clusters or lines and sometimes surrounded by a purplish zone. This type is difficult to distinguish from lichen sclerosus, and some authorities believe the two conditions are the same. Called also *white spot disease*.

linear m., m. linea′ris see under *scleroderma*.

plaque m., plaque-type m. the most common form of morphea, with lesions arranged in plaques.

m. profun′da, subcutaneous m. deep m.

mor•phe•a•form (mor′fe-ə-form″) resembling morphea.

mor•pheme (mor′fēm) a meaningful unit of sound.

mor•phine (mor′fēn) [L. *morphina*, *morphinum*] the principal and most active opioid alkaloid of opium (q.v.), an opioid analgesic having powerful analgesic action and some central stimulant action. In the United States, it is

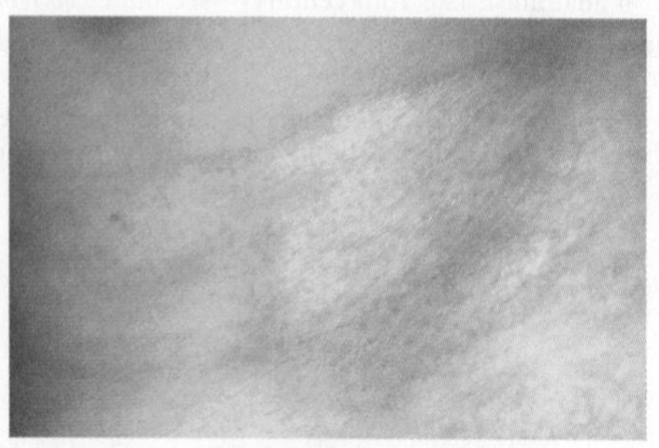

■ Morphea.

usually used in the form of the sulfate salt, while in Germany and Great Britain, the hydrochloride salt is usually preferred. It is used as an analgesic for relief of severe pain, antitussive, adjunct to anesthesia, and as an adjunct to treatment of pulmonary edema secondary to left ventricular failure. Abuse of morphine and its salts leads to dependence. **morphin′ic** *adj*

dimethyl m. thebaine.

m. hydrochloride the trihydrate hydrochloride salt of morphine, having the same actions as the base; it is the form usually preferred in Germany and Great Britain.

m. sulfate [USP] the pentahydrate sulfate salt of morphine, having the same actions as the base; used as an opioid analgesic, administered orally, parenterally, or rectally. It is the form usually preferred in the United States.

mor•phin•ism (mor′fin-iz″əm) 1. a pathologic state due to the habitual misuse of morphine. 2. morphine addiction.

mor•phin•iza•tion (mor″fin-ĭ-za′shən) subjection to the influence of morphine.

morph(o)- [Gr. *morphē* form] a combining form denoting relationship to form or structure.

mor•pho•dif•fer•en•ti•a•tion (mor″fo-dif″ər-en″she-a′shən) arrangement of formative cells in development of tissues or organs, which leads to production of the ultimate shape of the structure.

mor•pho•gen (mor′fo-jən) a substance in embryonic tissue that forms a concentration gradient and influences morphogenesis.

mor•pho•gen•e•sis (mor″fo-jen′ə-sis) [*morpho-* + *-genesis*] the evolution and development of form, as the development of the shape of a particular organ or part of the body, or the development undergone by individuals who attain the type to which the majority of the individuals of the species approximate.

mor•pho•ge•net•ic (mor″fo-jə-net′ik) producing growth; producing form or shape.

mor•phog•e•ny (mor-foj′ə-ne) morphogenesis.

mor•pho•log•i•cal (mor″fo-loj′ĭ-kəl) pertaining to morphology.

mor•phol•o•gy (mor-fol′ə-je) [*morpho-* + *-logy*] 1. the science of the forms and structure of organisms. 2. the form and structure of a particular organism, organ, or part.

mor•phol•y•sis (mor-fol′ĭ-sis) [*morpho-* + *-lysis*] destruction of form.

mor•phom•e•try (mor-fom′ə-tre) [*morpho-* + *-metry*] the measurement of the forms or structures of organisms. **morphomet′ric** *adj*

mor•phon (mor′fon) [Gr. *morphōn* forming] an individual organism or structural unit.

mor•phoph•y•ly (mor-fof′ə-le) [*morpho-* + Gr. *phylon* tribe] the branch of phylogenesis dealing with the evolutionary development of form.

mor•pho•phys•ics (mor″fo-fiz′iks) the study of the physical and chemical causes of development.

mor•pho•sis (mor-fo′sis) [Gr. *morphōsis* a shaping, bringing into shape] the process of formation of a part or organ. **morphot′ic** *adj*

morpho•type (mor′fo-tīp) 1. a group of individuals within a species that are differentiated by morphological characteristics. 2. a variant strain of a bacterial species, differentiated by morphological characteristics. Called also *morphovar*.

morpho•var (mor′fo-vahr, mor′fo-var) morphotype.

Mor•quio syndrome (mor′kyo) [Luis *Morquio*, Uruguayan pediatrician, 1867–1935] see under *syndrome*.

Mor•quio-Ull•rich disease (mor′kyo ool′rik) [L. *Morquio;* Otto *Ullrich*, German physician, 1894–1957] Morquio syndrome; see under *syndrome*.

mor•rhua (mor′u-ə) [L.] *Gadus morrhua*.

mor•rhu•ate (mor′u-āt) a salt, ester, or anionic form of morrhuic acid.

m. sodium [USP] the sodium salts of the fatty acids of cod liver oil; used as a sclerosing agent, especially for the treatment of varicose veins and hemorrhoids, injected in solution into varicosities.

mor•rhu•ic ac•id (mor′u-ik) a mixture of fatty acids occurring in cod liver oil.

Mor•ris syndrome (mor′is) [John McLean *Morris*, American surgeon, 1914–1993] complete androgen insensitivity syndrome; see under *syndrome*.

mors (morz) [L.] death.

m. thy′mica a type of sudden infant death syndrome or death of a child formerly thought to occur in thymic asthma and status lymphaticus.

mor•sal (mor′səl) [L. *morsus* bite] taking part in mastication; a term applied to the masticating surface of a bicuspid or molar.

Mor. sol. [L.] mo′re so′lito (in the usual way).

mor•sus (mor′səs) [L.] bite; sting.

m. huma′nus a bite by a human being.

mor•tal (mor′təl) [L. *mortalis*] 1. subject to death, or destined to die. 2. fatal.

mor•tal•i•ty (mor-tal′ĭ-te) 1. the quality of being mortal. 2. death rate. 3. in life insurance, the ratio of actual deaths to expected deaths.

mor•tar (mor′tər) [L. *mortarium*] a bell-shaped or urn-shaped vessel of glass, iron, porcelain, or other material, in which drugs are beaten, crushed, or ground with a pestle.

mor•ti•cian (mor-tish′ən) [L. *mors* death] an undertaker; a person trained to care for the dead.

Mor•ti•e•rel•la (mor″te-ə-rel′ə) a genus of fungi of the family Mortierellaceae, characterized by the lack of a columella and branched, tapering sporangiophores. It occasionally causes indolent human mucormycosis.

M. wol′fii a species, first isolated from soil in India, that causes pneumonia and mycotic abortion in cattle in Australia, New Zealand, England, and the United States.

Mor•ti•e•rel•la•ceae (mor″te-ə-rel-a′se-e) a family of fungi of the order Mucorales, having a rudimentary or absent columella and occurring mainly as a soil saprophyte; it includes one pathogenic genus, *Mortierella*.

mor•ti•fi•ca•tion (mor″tĭ-fĭ-ka′shən) gangrene.

Mor•ton neuralgia (disease, foot, metatarsalgia, toe), neuroma, test (mor′tən) [Thomas George *Morton*, American surgeon, 1835–1903] see under *neuralgia*, *neuroma*, and *test*.

mor•tu•ary (mor′choo-ar″e) [L. *mortuarium* tomb] 1. pertaining to death. 2. a place where dead bodies are kept until burial or cremation.

mor•u•la (mor′u-lə) [L. *morus* mulberry] 1. the solid mass of blastomeres formed by cleavage of a zygote. 2. an inclusion body seen in circulating blood cells in anaplasmosis and ehrlichiosis, consisting of a membrane-bound cluster of organisms that is formed by binary fission.

mor•u•lar (mor′u-lər) 1. pertaining to a morula. 2. resembling a mulberry.

mor•u•la•tion (mor″u-la′shən) the process of formation of the morula.

mor•u•loid (mor′u-loid) [*morula* + *-oid*] 1. shaped like a mulberry. 2. a bacterial colony in the form of a mulberry-like mass.

Mor•van syndrome (mor-van′) [Augustin Marie *Morvan*, French physician, 1819–1897] see under *syndrome* and see *syringomyelia*.

mo•sa•ic (mo-za′ik) [Gr. *mouseion*, from *mousa*, Muse] 1. a pattern made of numerous small pieces fitted together. 2. in genetics, an individual composed of two or more cell lines that are karyotypically or genotypically distinct but are derived from a single zygote. Cf. *chimera*. 3. in embryology, the condition in the fertilized eggs of some species, such as the sea urchin, whereby the cells of early stages have developed cytoplasm which determines the parts that are to develop. 4. in plant pathology, a viral disease characterized by mottling of the foliage.

mo•sa•i•cism (mo-za′ĭ-siz″əm) in genetics, the presence in an individual of two or more cell lines that are karyotypically or genotypically distinct and are derived from a single zygote. Cf. *chimerism*.

erythrocyte m. the mixture of two blood types in each of nonidentical twins as a result of anastomosis of placental blood vessels.

confined placental m. mosaicism in which a chromosomal abnormality (usually trisomy) is restricted to the placenta; it occurs in about 2 per cent of viable pregnancies and is a possible cause of intrauterine growth retardation.

gonadal m. mosaicism that results from mosaicism within the gonad so that some of the germ cells are mutants. More than one offspring of a gonadal mosaic for a dominant trait may show the trait although it is not manifested in the parent.

mo•sa•ic•plas•ty (mo-za′ik-plas″te) an arthroscopic technique for repair of articular cartilage defects by means of small autografts of osteochondral tissue implanted to fill defects in nearby articular cartilage. **mosaicplas′tic** *adj*

Mosch•co•witz disease (mosh′ko-wits) [Eli *Moschcowitz*, American physician, 1879–1964] thrombotic thrombocytic purpura; see under *purpura*.

Mos•ler sign (mōz′lər) [Karl Friedrich *Mosler*, German physician, 1831–1911] see under *sign*.

mOsm milliosmole.

mos•qui•to (məs-ke′to) pl. *mosquitoes* [Sp. "little fly"] any of the gnatlike insects of the family Culicidae; many are bloodsucking and are vectors of human and animal diseases; others are venomous.

anautogenous m. a mosquito that requires a blood meal in the adult stage for the production of viable eggs.

arygamous m. a mosquito that requires large or outdoor spaces for breeding.

Asian tiger m. *Aedes albopictus.*
autogenous m. 1. a mosquito that can produce viable eggs without a blood meal. 2. *Aedes albopictus.*
forest day m. *Aedes albopictus.*
house m. either *Culex pipiens* or *C. quinquefasciatus.*
steyogamous m. a mosquito that can breed in captivity in limited spaces.
yellow fever m. *Aedes aegypti.*

mos•qui•to•ci•dal (məs-ke″to-si′dəl) destructive to mosquitoes.

mos•qui•to•cide (mos-ke′to-sīd) [*mosquito* + *-cide*] an agent that is destructive to mosquitoes.

moss (mos) 1. any plant of the class Musci. 2. material composed of or derived from a plant of the class Musci.
Ceylon m. *Gracilaria lichenoides.*
club m. 1. any moss of the genus *Lycopodium;* some species have their spores inside small club-shaped structures. 2. any of various other mosses of genera related to *Lycopodium.*
Iceland m. 1. *Cetraria islandica,* a lichen native to Iceland. 2. a preparation of the dried thallus of *C. islandica,* used for cough and bronchitis, dyspepsia, loss of appetite, and inflammation of the oropharyngeal mucosa.
Irish m. 1. *Chondrus crispus.* 2. chondrus (def. 2).
pearl m., salt rock m. 1. *Chondrus crispus.* 2. chondrus (def. 2).

Mosse syndrome (maw′sə) [Max *Mosse,* German physician, 20th century] see under *syndrome.*

Mos•so ergograph (mo′so) [Angelo *Mosso,* Italian physiologist, 1846–1910] see under *ergograph*

Mo•tais operation (mo-ta′) [Ernest *Motais,* French ophthalmologist, 1845–1913] see under *operation.*

moth (mawth) any of numerous flying insects of the order Lepidoptera. See also *insect dermatitis,* under *dermatitis.*
brown-tail m. *Euproctis chrysorrhoea.*
flannel m. *Megalopyge opercularis.*
io m. *Automeris io.*
meal m. a moth that infests grain and meal, such as *Asopia farinalis* or *Pyralis farinalis.*
peppered m. *Biston betularia.*
puss m. *Megalopyge opercularis.*
silkworm m. *Bombyx mori.*
tussock m. *Hemerocampa leukostigma.*

moth•er (muth′ər) [L. *mater*] 1. the female parent. 2. something from which another thing is derived, as a *mother cell.*
genetic m. the woman whose contribution to the child was the oocyte, and hence genes. Sometimes a woman who cannot carry a fetus can nevertheless be a genetic mother via in vitro fertilization with implantation in a gestational surrogate mother.
gestational m. the woman who carries the fetus in her uterus; she may be the natural mother or a gestational surrogate mother.
gestational surrogate m. a surrogate mother who is carrying a fetus produced by in vitro fertilization and is not the genetic mother of the fetus.
surrogate m. a woman who carries a pregnancy for another woman or couple, usually because the latter suffers from infertility.

mo•tif (mo-tēf′) a structural element of a protein that is smaller than a domain and has a specific function.

mo•tile (mo′təl, mo′tīl) having spontaneous but not conscious or volitional movement.

mo•til•in (mo-til′in) a polypeptide hormone (2698 daltons, 22 amino acids) secreted by the enterochromaffin cells of the intestine; it increases motility of several portions of the gastrointestinal tract and stimulates pepsin secretion. Its release is stimulated by the presence of acid or fat in the duodenum; its physiologic role in gastrointestinal function is not yet known.

mo•til•i•ty (mo-til′ĭ-te) 1. spontaneous movement. 2. the ability to move spontaneously.
gastric m. the spontaneous movements of the stomach muscles that grind food and mix it with gastric secretions, and move the products into the duodenum.
intestinal m. the muscular movements of the various segments of the intestines to process digested food and move it along.

mo•tion (mo′shən) movement.
brownian m. see under *movement.*
continuous passive m. (CPM) a technique for promoting healing of articular cartilage.

mo•ti•va•tion (mo″tĭ-va′shən) in psychology, any of the forces that activate behavior toward satisfying needs or achieving goals.

mo•tive (mo′tiv) in psychology, any state that affects an individual's goal-directed behavior.

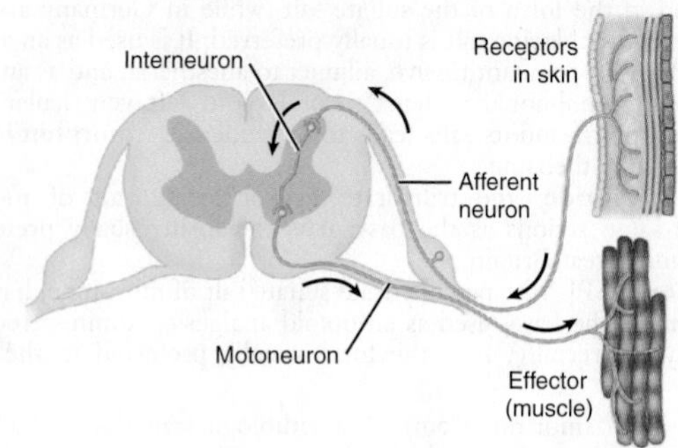

■ Motoneuron shown as the efferent neuron in a three-neuron reflex arc.

achievement m. the desire to achieve for the sake of achievement per se.
aroused m. a motive that is actively influencing behavior, or that can be inferred from actual behavior.

mo•to•fa•cient (mo″to-fa′shənt) producing motion; a term applied to that phase of muscular activity by which the muscle produces actual motion, in contradistinction to the *nonmotofacient* phase in which the muscle is contracting without producing motion.

Mo•to•fen (mo′to-fen) trademark for a combination preparation of difenoxin hydrochloride and atropine sulfate.

mo•to•neu•ron (mo″to-noor′on) an efferent neuron conveying motor impulses. Called also *motor neuron.*
alpha m's neurons of the anterior spinal cord that give rise to the alpha fibers which innervate the skeletal muscle fibers. Cf. *anterior horn cell.*
beta m's neurons of the anterior spinal cord that give rise to the beta fibers that innervate extrafusal and intrafusal muscle fibers.
gamma m's neurons of the anterior spinal cord that give rise to the gamma (fusimotor) fibers which innervate intrafusal fibers of the muscle spindle. Cf. *anterior horn cell* and *gamma loop.*
heteronymous m's motoneurons supplying muscles other than the one from which the afferent impulses originate.
homonymous m's motoneurons supplying the muscle from which the afferent impulses originate.
lower m. a peripheral neuron whose cell body lies in the ventral gray columns of the spinal cord and whose termination is in a skeletal muscle.
peripheral m. in a reflex arc, a motoneuron that receives impulses from interneurons. Cf. *peripheral sensory neuron.*
upper m. a neuron in the cerebral cortex that conducts impulses from the motor cortex to a motor nucleus of one of the cerebral nerves or to a ventral gray column of the spinal cord.

mo•tor (mo′tər) [L., from *movēre,* past part. *motus,* to move] 1. a muscle, nerve, or center that effects or produces movement. 2. producing or subserving motion.
plastic m. the tissues of an amputation stump used to secure motion in an artificial limb.

mo•tor•ic•i•ty (mo″tər-is′ĭ-te) the faculty of performing movement; power of movement.

Mo•trin (mo′trin) trademark for preparations of ibuprofen.

MOTT mycobacteria other than tubercle bacilli. See *nontuberculous mycobacteria,* under *mycobacterium.*

mot•tle (mot′əl) unevenness of density or texture on a recorded radiographic image.
quantum m. mottle caused by quantum noise.

mot•tled (mot′ld) marked by spots or blotches of different colors or shades.

mot•tling (mot′ling) a condition of spotting with patches of color.

mou•lage (moo-lahzh′) [Fr. "molding"] the making of molds or models in wax or plaster, as of a structure or a lesion; also such a mold or model.

mould (mōld) mold.

mould•ing (mōld′ing) molding.

mound•ing (mound′ing) myoedema (def. 1).

Mou•nier-Kuhn syndrome (moo-nya′-kūn′) [Pierre *Mounier-Kuhn,* French physician, 20th century] tracheobronchomegaly.

Mount syndrome (mount) [Lester Adrian *Mount,* American neurosurgeon, 1910–1999] Mount-Reback syndrome.

Mount-Re•back syndrome (mount′ re′bak) [L.A. *Mount;* S. *Reback,* American physician, 20th century] see under *syndrome.*

mount (mount) 1. to fix on or in a support. 2. a support, backing, setting, or the like, on which something may be fixed. 3. to prepare specimens and slides for study. 4. a specimen on a slide prepared for study.

wet m. a temporary preparation in which a fluid specimen or suspension of a specimen is placed on a slide for microscopic examination and covered with a coverslip to keep it moist instead of being dehydrated and imbedded in a permanent mounting medium.

mount•ant (mount′ənt) a medium, such as natural resins, polymers, or glycerol, in which objects are embedded for study, especially with the microscope; called also *mounting medium.*

mount•ing (mount′ing) the preparation of specimens and slides for study.

split cast m. 1. a dental cast with key grooves on its base, mounted on an articulator for the purpose of easy removal and accurate replacement. Split remounting metal plates may be used instead of grooves in casts. 2. see under *method.*

mourn•ing (mor′ning) 1. the normal psychological processes that follow the loss of a loved one; grief is the accompanying emotional state. Four phases have been described: a short phase of numbness and denial, followed by a phase of yearning and protest marked by intense pining for the dead, followed by a phase of disorganization marked by pain and despair, ending in a phase of detachment and reorganization of love relationships that completes the work of mourning. 2. social expressions of grief, such as funeral and burial services, prayers, the wearing of black or other specific garments, or other rituals.

mouse (mous) 1. any of numerous small rodents of the family Muridae; some are household pests around the world and others are used as experimental animals. 2. a small weight, or movable structure.

CFW m. [*c*ancer-*f*ree *w*hite] a mouse belonging to a strain bred for use in research laboratories.

deer m. *Peromyscus maniculatus.*

house m. 1. any of several species that live in dwellings of humans. 2. *Mus musculus.*

joint m. one of the portions of the fringes in the synovial membrane of joints in osteoarthritis which are changed into cartilage and become free in the joints. Cf. *arthrolith* and *arthrophyte.*

knockin m. a mouse that has had a specific gene artificially inserted into its genome.

knockout m. a mouse that has had a specific gene artificially deleted from its genome.

meadow m. vole.

multimammate m. *Mastomys natalensis.*

New Zealand black m. NZB m.

nude m., ***nu/nu*** **m.** a mouse homozygous for the *nu* gene; these mice are hairless and congenitally athymic and thus lack T lymphocytes.

NZB m. [*N*ew *Z*ealand *b*lack] a mouse belonging to a strain bred to develop autoimmune disease closely resembling human systemic lupus erythematosus.

peritoneal m. a free body in the peritoneal cavity, such as a small mass of omentum or epiploic appendage that has twisted off and become coated with fibrin; it may appear as a soft density on the radiograph.

pleural m. a fibrinous body sometimes seen in the pleural space on a radiograph.

red-backed m. any of several vole species of the genus *Clethrionomys.*

SCID m. [*s*evere *c*ombined *i*mmuno*d*eficiency] a mouse belonging to a strain lacking T and B lymphocytes and immunoglobulins, used as a model for studies of the immune system.

vesper m. any member of the species *Calomys,* reservoirs for various disease-causing viruses.

white-footed m. *Peromyscus leucopus.*

wood m. 1. *Apodemus sylvaticus,* a European species that serves as a reservoir of *Leptospira interrogans* serovar *grippotyphosa.* 2. any of several vole species of the genus *Clethrionomys.*

mouse•pox (mous′poks) infectious ectromelia.

mouth (mouth) [L. *os, oris*] 1. oral cavity; see *cavitas oris.* 2. any aperture or opening.

broken m. a condition in aging sheep in which teeth are broken or missing, especially incisors, so that the animals have trouble grazing.

denture sore m. denture stomatitis.

dry m. xerostomia.

glass-blowers' m. swelling of the parotid gland in glass-blowers; see also *parotid pneumatocele,* under *pneumatocele.*

parrot m. brachygnathia in a horse.

sore m. contagious ecthyma.

tapir m. a condition in which the mouth resembles that of a tapir, with the orbicularis oris muscle atrophied and the lips thickened and separated; seen in facioscapulohumeral muscular dystrophy.

trench m. necrotizing ulcerative gingivitis; so called because it occurred in the troops in the trenches in World War I.

watery m. a disease of newborn lambs in the British Isles in which they cannot nurse, have excessive abdominal fluid and fluid dripping from the mouth, and soon become comatose and die; the cause is thought to be infection with a strain of *Escherichia coli.*

white m. thrush (def. 1).

mouth•wash (mouth′wahsh″) a solution for rinsing the mouth, e.g., the official [NF] preparation of potassium bicarbonate, sodium borate, thymol, eucalyptol, methyl salicylate, amaranth solution, alcohol, glycerin, and purified water.

move•ment (mo͞ov′mənt) 1. an act of changing position; called also *motion.* 2. defecation (def. 2).

active m. voluntary movement produced by the person's own muscles, as opposed to *passive movement.*

ameboid m. movement characteristic of amebae and leukocytes by extension of the plasma membrane to form a balloonlike pseudopodium that attaches to the substrate and into which the cytosol flows, moving the cell forward. Movement is accompanied by cyclic changes in the viscosity of the cytosol that result from the assembly and severing of actin filaments, with the leading edge of the pseudopodium being a gel and the cytoplasm flowing into the pseudopod being a sol.

angular m. a movement which changes the angle between two bones.

associated m. 1. a movement of parts that act together, as of the eyes. 2. contralateral associated m. 3. synkinesis.

automatic m. any involuntary movement, such as a reflex, a synkinesia, or a spasm.

ballistic m's a rapid series of related movements, such as saccadic movements of the eyes, set into motion by one complex command from the brain, with no feedback on individual segments before the entire series is finished.

Bennett m. the lateral shift of the mandibular condyles and articular disks in the direction of the working bite as the lower jaw swings in preparation for mastication.

border m. any extreme compass of mandibular movement limited by bone, ligaments, or soft tissues; usually applied to horizontal mandibular movements.

border tissue m's movements produced by action of the muscles and other tissues adjoining the borders of a denture.

bowel m. defecation (def. 2).

brownian m. the random zigzag or dancing motion of minute solute particles suspended in a solvent, due to bombardment by rapidly moving solvent molecules.

choreic m's, choreiform m's irregular, jerky movements of muscles or groups of muscles.

ciliary m. the lashing motion of cilia occurring in certain tissues.

circus m. 1. a peculiar circular gait; an involuntary rolling or tumbling movement, the result of lesions of the brain and basal nerve centers. 2. continuous cycling of an excitatory wavefront in a ring or circuit around muscle, such as around a region of cardiac tissue in reentry (q.v.).

contralateral associated m. a movement on the paralyzed side in hemiplegia associated with active movement of the corresponding part on the unaffected side. Called also *associated m.* and *spasmodic synkinesis.*

dystonic m. a large slow, amplified athetoid movement.

euglenoid m. a wormlike writhing movement, usually nonprogressive, resulting from local expansion and contraction of the body, seen in flagellates with thin pellicles and very plastic bodies, as in certain species of the order Euglenida and certain other protozoa.

excursive m's excursion.

fetal m. movement of a fetus in the uterus, usually observable at 18 to 20 weeks in a primigravida and 16 to 18 weeks in a multipara.

forced m. 1. passive m. 2. involuntary m.

free mandibular m. any unhampered movement of the mandible.

Frenkel m's see under *exercise.*

functional mandibular m's movements of the mandible that occur in the performance of some function, as mastication, swallowing, articulation of vocal sounds, and yawning.

gliding m. a translatory movement in which one surface glides over another, without any angular or rotary movements, being the simplest kind of motion of a joint.

hinge m. movement occurring in a single plane, as that occurring in opening or closing of the mouth.

intermediary m's, intermediate m's mandibular movements between the extremes of mandibular excursions.

involuntary m. movement of a limb or other body part caused by involuntary contraction of muscles; common types are athetosis, ballismus, chorea, myoclonus, seizure, tic, and tremor. Called also *forced m.*

jaw m. mandibular m.

Magnan m. forward and backward movement of the tongue when it is drawn out; observed in general paresis.

mandibular m. any movement of which the mandible is capable; see also *free mandibular m.* and *functional mandibular m's.* Called also *jaw m.*

masticatory m's functional mandibular movements seen in mastication of food.

molecular m. brownian m.

morphogenetic m. a flowing of cell groups concerned with the formation of germ layers or of organ primordia.

nucleopetal m. the movement of a male pronucleus toward the female pronucleus in the ootid.

opening m. a mandibular movement seen during jaw separation.

passive m. any movement of the body caused by a force entirely outside of the organism, such as in passive exercise (see under *exercise*).

pendular m. one of the movements of the small intestine in digestion, consisting of a gentle swinging to and fro of the different loops, ascribed to rhythmical contractions of the longitudinal muscles. See also *segmentation m.*

posterior opening m. the opening movement of the mandible about the terminal hinge axis.

rapid eye m. (REM) the rapid conjugate movement of the eyes that occurs during REM sleep (see under *sleep*).

reflex m. reflex (def. 2).

saccadic m. the quick movement of the eye in going from one fixation point to another; see also *saccade.*

scissors m. a movement of the pupillary reflex seen with a retinoscope, resembling the opening and shutting of scissors; it is indicative of irregular astigmatism.

segmentation m. one of the movements of the small intestine in digestion, consisting of small, irregular or rhythmic, circular contractions that segment a portion of the intestine into evenly spaced parts resembling a string of sausages. See also *pendular m.*

spontaneous m. automatic m.

Swedish m. see under *gymnastics.*

synkinetic m. synkinesis.

vermicular m. peristalsis.

mov•er (mo̅o̅v′ər) something that moves.

prime m. a muscle that acts directly to bring about a desired movement.

moxa (mok′sə) [Japanese] the dried leaves of *Artemisia vulgaris*, burned on or near acupoints in moxibustion.

mox•a•lac•tam (mok″sə-lak′tam) a semisynthetic antibiotic chemically related to the third-generation cephalosporins, having a broad spectrum of antibacterial activity and reported to be effective against some β-lactamase producing organisms.

m. disodium the disodium salt of moxalactam, used to treat a wide variety of infections caused by susceptible organisms; administered intramuscularly and intravenously.

mox•i•bus•tion (mok″sĭ-bus′chən) the stimulation of an acupoint by the burning of a cone or cylinder of moxa placed at or near the point. The cone may be burned on the skin, either directly or placed on a mediating substance, or at a short distance from the skin on a cigarlike moxa pole. It may also be burned on the handle of an acupuncture needle, the heat being transmitted through the needle to the acupuncture site.

mox•i•flox•a•cin (mok″sĭ-flok′sə-sin) a fluoroquinolone antibacterial effective against many gram-positive and gram-negative bacteria.

m. hydrochloride the hydrochloride salt of moxifloxacin, administered orally in the treatment of bacterial exacerbation of chronic bronchitis, acute sinusitis, community-acquired pneumonia, and skin and skin structure infections due to susceptible organisms.

Moy•na•han syndrome (moi′nə-han) [E.J. *Moynahan*, British physician, 20th century] see under *syndrome.*

Mo•zart ear (mōt′sahrt) [Wolfgang Amadeus *Mozart*, Austrian composer, 1756–1791, who was reported to have this ear deformity] see under *ear.*

6-MP 6-mercaptopurine; see *mercaptopurine.*

mp melting point.

MPD maximum permissible dose; see under *dose.*

MPH Master of Public Health.

MPI DMSA Kid•ney Re•a•gent (kid′ne re-a′jənt) trademark for a kit for the preparation of technetium Tc 99m succimer.

MPI MDP trademark for a kit for the preparation of technetium Tc 99m medronate.

MPI Py•ro•phos•phate (pi″ro-fos′fāt) trademark for a preparation of technetium Tc 99m pyrophosphate.

MPI Tc 99m DTPA trademark for a kit for the preparation of technetium Tc 99m pentetate.

MPO myeloperoxidase.

MPS mononuclear phagocyte system; mucopolysaccharidosis.

MPSV meningococcal polysaccharide vaccine.

MR mitral regurgitation.

mR milliroentgen.

μR microroentgen.

MRA Medical Record Administrator; magnetic resonance angiography.

MRACP Member of Royal Australasian College of Physicians.

mrad millirad.

MRC Medical Reserve Corps.

MRCP Member of the Royal College of Physicians.

MRCPE Member of the Royal College of Physicians of Edinburgh.

MRCP (Glasg) Member of the Royal College of Physicians and Surgeons of Glasgow *qua* Physician.

MRCPI Member of the Royal College of Physicians of Ireland.

MRCS Member of the Royal College of Surgeons.

MRCSEd Member of the Royal College of Surgeons of Edinburgh.

MRCSI Member of the Royal College of Surgeons of Ireland.

MRCVS Member of the Royal College of Veterinary Surgeons.

MRD minimum reacting dose.

MRDM malnutrition-related diabetes mellitus.

mrem millirem.

MRI magnetic resonance imaging.

MRL Medical Record Librarian; now called Medical Record Administrator.

mRNA messenger RNA.

MRSA methicillin-resistant *Staphylococcus aureus.*

MS Master of Science; Master of Surgery; mitral stenosis; multiple sclerosis.

ms millisecond.

MSA multiple system atrophy.

MSA-C multiple system atrophy with predominant cerebellar ataxia.

MSA-P multiple system atrophy with predominant parkinsonism.

μs microsecond.

MS Con•tin (kon′tin) trademark for a preparation of morphine sulfate.

MSE Mental Status Examination.

msec millisecond.

Mse•le•ni joint disease (əm-sə-le′ne) [*Mseleni* Mission Station, South Africa, where the condition was first observed in 1970] see under *disease.*

MSG monosodium glutamate.

MSH melanocyte-stimulating hormone.

MSI microsatellite instability.

MSIR trademark for preparations of morphine sulfate.

MSL midsternal line.

MSLT multiple sleep latency test.

MS/MS tandem mass spectrometry.

MSUD maple syrup urine disease.

MT Medical Technologist.

MTC medullary thyroid carcinoma.

MTD maximum tolerated dose.

mtDNA mitochondrial DNA.

MTHFR methylenetetrahydrofolate reductase; see *methylenetetrahydrofolate reductase deficiency.*

MTOC microtubule organizing center.

MTP microsomal triglyceride transfer protein.

MTX methotrexate.

mU milliunit.

mu (mu) [M, μ] the twelfth letter of the Greek alphabet.

m.u. mouse unit.

μU microunit.

MUAP motor unit action potential.

MUC maximum urinary concentration.

Muc. [L.] mucila′go (mucilage).

Much granules (mook) [Hans Christian R. *Much*, German physician, 1880–1932] see under *granule.*

Mu•cha disease (moo′kah) [Viktor *Mucha*, Austrian dermatologist, 1877–1919] pityriasis lichenoides et varioliformis acuta.

Mu•cha-Ha•ber•mann disease (moo′kah hah′ber-mahn) [V. *Mucha;* Rudolf *Habermann*, German dermatologist, 1884–1941] pityriasis lichenoides et varioliformis acuta.

mu•ci- [L. *mucus*] a combining form denoting relationship to mucus, or to mucin.

mu•ci•car•mine (mu″sĭ-kahr′min) a specific stain for mucin containing carmine and aluminum chloride; used to detect mucin-secreting tissues or tumors and to identify certain fungi.

mu•ci•car•mi•no•phil•ic (mu″sĭ-kahr″mĭ-no-fil′ik) pertaining to a cell or other element that stains readily with mucicarmine.

mu•cif•er•ous (mu-sif′ər-əs) [*muci-* + *-ferous*] muciparous.

mu•ci•fi•ca•tion (mu″sĭ-fĭ-ka′shən) the mucus-producing changes in the vaginal epithelium of laboratory animals during the progestational stage of the ovarian cycle.

mu•ci•form (mu′sĭ-form″) [*muci-* + *form*] mucoid (def. 1).

mu•ci•gen (mu′sĭ-jən) [*muci-* + *-gen*] the substance from which mucin is derived.

mu•cig•e•nous (mu-sij′ə-nəs) muciparous.

mu•ci•gogue (mu′sĭ-gog) [*muci-* + *-agogue*] 1. stimulating the secretion of mucus. 2. an agent that stimulates the secretion of mucus.

mu•ci•he•ma•tein (mu″sĭ-he′mə-tēn) a hematein-based staining fluid for mucins.

Mayer m. see *Stains and Staining Methods*, under *stain*.

mu•ci•lage (mu′sĭ-ləj) [L. *mucilago*] 1. an artificial viscid paste of gum or dextrin used in pharmacy as a vehicle or excipient, or in therapy as a demulcent. 2. a naturally formed viscid principle in a plant, consisting of a gum dissolved in the juices of the plant.

acacia m. a preparation of acacia and benzoic acid in purified water, used as a suspending agent for drugs.

tragacanth m. [NF] a preparation of tragacanth, benzoic acid, and glycerin in distilled water, used as a skin protective.

mu•ci•lag•i•nous (mu″sĭ-laj′ĭ-nəs) of the nature of mucilage; slimy and adhesive.

mu•cil•loid (mu′sĭ-loid) a preparation of a mucilaginous substance.

psyllium hydrophilic m. a powdered preparation of the mucilaginous portion of the seeds of blond psyllium *(Plantago ovata)*, used in the treatment of simple constipation resulting from lack of bulk.

mu•cin (mu′sin) 1. any of a group of protein-containing glycoconjugates with high sialic acid or sulfated polysaccharide content that compose the chief constituent of mucus. 2. more generally, any of a wide variety of glycoconjugates such as mucoproteins, glycoproteins, glycosaminoglycans, and glycolipids.

mu•ci•no•blast (mu-sin′o-blast) [*mucin* + *-blast*] the progenitor of a mucous cell.

mu•ci•noid (mu′sĭ-noid) [*mucin* + *-oid*] resembling or pertaining to mucin. Called also *mucoid.*

mu•ci•no•lyt•ic (mu″sĭ-no-lit′ik) [*mucin* + *-lytic*] dissolving or splitting up mucin.

mu•ci•no•sis (mu″sĭ-no′sis) any of a large group of conditions characterized by abnormal deposits of mucins (a type of mucopolysaccharide) in the skin; they may be primary conditions or secondary to an underlying condition.

acral persistent papular m. a type of dermal mucinosis characterized by flesh-colored papules on the lower arms and hands, seen in women more often than in men.

cutaneous focal m. a type of dermal mucinosis in which there is a solitary nodule on the skin.

cutaneous lupus m. a variant of systemic and discoid lupus erythematosus in which mucin deposits in the dermis cause papules and nodules to appear on the skin, usually on the chest, back, upper arms, or thighs. Called also *papulonodular m.*

dermal m. any of the types caused by deposition of mucin in the dermis, with nodules, papules, or plaques on the skin surface.

focal m., focal cutaneous m. cutaneous focal m.

follicular m. a disease of the pilosebaceous unit, usually on the scalp, face, or neck, caused by mucinous infiltration of tissues; it presents clinically as grouped follicular papules or plaques with associated hair loss and may be either a primary condition or secondary to lymphoma or occasionally other conditions. Called also *alopecia mucinosa.*

papular m. lichen myxedematosus.

papular and nodular m., papulonodular m. cutaneous lupus m.

plaquelike m., plaquelike cutaneous m. reticular erythematous m.

reticular erythematous m. (REM) a type of dermal mucinosis characterized by erythematous papules or plaques in a reticular pattern, usually in the midline of the back; it is most often seen in women after sun exposure.

self-healing juvenile cutaneous m. a type of dermal mucinosis usually seen in children, characterized by mucinous plaques or nodules on the face, the neck, or a limb.

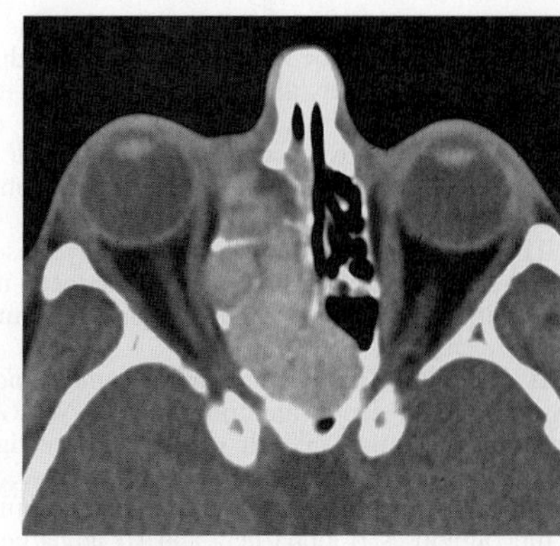

■ Axial CT image showing a large mucocele of the ethmoidal and sphenoidal sinuses in a patient with allergic fungal rhinosinusitis.

mu•ci•nous (mu′sĭ-nəs) resembling or marked by the formation of mucin.

mu•cin•uria (mu″sin-u′re-ə) [*mucin* + *-uria*] the occurrence of mucin in the urine; it may suggest vaginal contamination.

mu•cip•a•rous (mu-sip′ə-rəs) [*muci-* + *-parous*] producing or secreting mucus. Called also *blennogenic, blennogenous, muciferous,* and *mucigenous.*

mu•ci•tis (mu-si′tis) mucositis.

Muck•le-Wells syndrome (muk′əl welz′) [Thomas James *Muckle*, Canadian pediatrician, 20th century; Michael Vernon *Wells*, English physician, 20th century] see under *syndrome.*

muc(o)- [L. *mucus*] a combining form denoting relationship to mucus, or to a mucous membrane.

mu•co•car•ti•lage (mu″ko-kahr′tĭ-ləj) a soft cartilage the cells of which are in a mucuslike matrix.

mu•co•cele (mu′ko-sēl) [*muco-* + *-cele*[1]] 1. dilatation of a cavity with accumulated mucous secretion. 2. mucus retention cyst. 3. mucus extravasation phenomenon.

suppurating m. mucopyocele.

mu•co•cil•i•ary (mu″ko-sil′e-ar-e) [*muco-* + *ciliary*] pertaining to mucus and to the cilia of the epithelial cells in the respiratory system.

mu•coc•la•sis (mu-kok′lə-sis) [*muco-* + Gr. *klasis* a breaking] surgical destruction of the mucous lining of any organ.

mu•co•col•pos (mu″ko-kol′pos) [*muco-* + Gr. *kolpos* vagina] accumulation of mucus in the vaginal canal.

mu•co•cu•ta•ne•ous (mu″ko-ku-ta′ne-əs) [*muco-* + *cutaneous*] pertaining to or affecting the mucous membrane and the skin.

mu•co•cyst (mu′ko-sist) [*muco-* + *cyst*] any of the paracrystalline, saccular or rod-shaped, subpellicular cystic organelles seen in certain ciliate protozoa, which contain a mucoid material that is expelled through a pore in the pellicle; its function is uncertain but it may be involved in the formation of cysts or protective coverings.

mu•co•ep•i•der•moid (mu″ko-ep″ĭ-dur′moid) composed of mucus-producing and epithelial cells; see under *carcinoma.*

mu•co•fi•brous (mu″ko-fi′brəs) composed of mucus and fibrous tissue.

mu•co•floc•cu•lent (mu″ko-flok′u-lənt) containing threads of mucus.

mu•co•gin•gi•val (mu″ko-jin′jĭ-vəl) pertaining to the oral mucosa and gingiva, or to the line of demarcation between them (mucogingival junction).

mu•co•gin•gi•vi•tis (mu″ko-jin″jĭ-vi′tis) inflammation of the gingiva, particularly at the mucogingival junction.

mu•coid (mu′koid) [*muc-* + *-oid*] 1. resembling mucus. Called also *blennoid, muciform,* and *myxoid.* 2. mucinoid.

mu•co•lem•ma (mu″ko-lem′ə) mucin coat, a noncellular envelope secreted around the rabbit egg and its oolemma by the oviduct.

mu•co•lip•i•do•sis (mu″ko-lip″ĭ-do′sis) pl. *mucolipido′ses.* any of a group of lysosomal storage diseases in which both glycosaminoglycans (mucopolysaccharides) and lipids accumulate in tissues but without excess of glycosaminoglycans in the urine.

m. I sialidosis.

m. II, m. II alpha/beta a rapidly progressing disease of young children, characterized histologically by abnormal fibroblasts containing a large number of dark inclusions which fill the central part of the cytoplasm except for the juxtanuclear zone (I-cells), and clinically by severe growth impairment, minimal hepatomegaly, extreme mental and motor retardation, and clear corneas. It is an autosomal recessive disorder due to mutation in the *GNPTAB* gene (locus: 12q23.3), which encodes the alpha and beta subunits of UDP-*N*-acetylglucosamine–lysosomal-enzyme *N*-acetylglucosamine-phosphotransferase, resulting in failure of lysosomal enzymes to be incorporated into lysosomes. Called also *I-cell disease.*

m. III a term usually used to denote mucolipidosis III alpha/beta; it can be used to include mucolipidosis III gamma.

m. IIIA, m. III alpha/beta an autososmal recessive disorder due to mutation in the same gene as in mucolipidosis II alpha/beta; more residual enzyme activity remains and the clinical characteristics are milder. Called also *pseudo-Hurler polydystrophy.*

m. IIIC, m. III gamma a rare variant form of mucolipidosis; it is an autososmal recessive disorder due to mutation in the *GNPTG* gene (locus: 16p), which encodes the gamma subunit of UDP-*N*-acetylglucosamine–lysosomal-enzyme *N*-acetylglucosamine-phosphotransferase, resulting in failure of lysosomal enzymes to be incorporated into lysosomes. It is clinically similar to mucolipidoses II alpha/beta and III alpha/beta but is less severe.

m. IV an autosomal recessive neurodegenerative lysosomal storage disorder caused by mutation in the *MCOLN1* gene (locus: 19p13.3-p13.2), which encodes a membrane protein important in endocytosis and lysosomal transport. It is characterized by psychomotor retardation and severe visual impairment, initially manifest in infancy or childhood as corneal clouding.

mu•co•lyt•ic (mu″ko-lit′ik) 1. capable of reducing the viscosity of mucus. 2. an agent that reduces the viscosity of mucus.

mu•co•mem•bra•nous (mu″ko-mem′brə-nəs) mucosal.

Mu•co•myst (mu′ko-mist) trademark for a preparation of acetylcysteine.

mu•co•peri•chon•dri•um (mu″ko-per″e-kon′dre-əm) perichondrium having a mucosal surface, as that of the nasal septum. **mucoperichon′drial** *adj*

mu•co•peri•os•te•al (mu″ko-per″e-os′te-əl) consisting of mucous membrane and periosteum.

mu•co•peri•os•te•um (mu″ko-per″e-os′te-əm) periosteum having a mucous surface, as in parts of the auditory apparatus.

mu•co•poly•sac•cha•ride (mu″ko-pol″e-sak′ə-rīd) 1. glycosaminoglycan. 2. less frequently, any polysaccharide with a high hexosamine content, including the glycosaminoglycans, which are acidic, as well as neutral polysaccharides such as chitin.

mu•co•poly•sac•cha•ri•do•sis (mu″ko-pol″e-sak″ə-ri-do′sis) pl. *mucopolysaccharido′ses.* Any of a group of lysosomal storage diseases resulting from defects in degradation of the glycosaminoglycans dermatan sulfate, heparan sulfate, keratan sulfate, chondroitin sulfate or a combination of them, which are then excreted in the urine and accumulate in tissues, affecting the bony skeleton, joints, liver, spleen, eyes, ears, skin, teeth, and the cardiovascular, respiratory, and central nervous systems. The prototype for mucopolysaccharidosis is Hurler syndrome (q.v.).

m. I (MPS I) originally, Hurler syndrome; the term now encompasses any of the forms characterized by deficiency of L-iduronidase and excretion in the urine of dermatan sulfate and heparan sulfate.

m. IH (MPS I H) Hurler syndrome.

m. IH/S (MPS I H/S) Hurler-Scheie syndrome.

m. IS (MPS I S) Scheie syndrome.

m. II (MPS II) Hunter syndrome.

m. III (MPS III) Sanfilippo syndrome.

m. IV (MPS IV) Morquio syndrome.

m. V former name for Scheie syndrome, now classified as *m. IS.*

m. VI (MPS VI) Maroteaux-Lamy syndrome.

m. VII (MPS VII) Sly syndrome.

mu•co•poly•sac•cha•ri•du•ria (mu″ko-pol″e-sak″ə-rĭ-du′re-ə) an excess of mucopolysaccharides in the urine.

mu•co•pro•tein (mu″ko-pro′tēn) a covalently linked conjugate of protein and polysaccharide, the latter containing many hexosamine residues and constituting approximately 4 to 30 per cent of the weight of the compound; mucoproteins occur mainly in mucous secretions. Cf. *glycoprotein.*

Tamm-Horsfall m. see under *protein.*

mu•co•pu•ru•lent (mu″ko-pu′roo-lənt) containing both mucus and pus.

mu•co•pus (mu′ko-pus″) [*muco-* + *pus*] a mixture of mucus and pus.

mu•co•pyo•cele (mu″ko-pi′o-sēl″) an infected or purulent mucocele.

Mu•cor (mu′kor) [L., "bread mold"] a genus of fungi of the family Mucoraceae, order Mucorales, which form delicate, white tubular filaments and spherical, black sporangia; it produces no stolons or rhizoids, and sporangiophores arise at all parts of the thallus. A number of species cause mucormycosis.

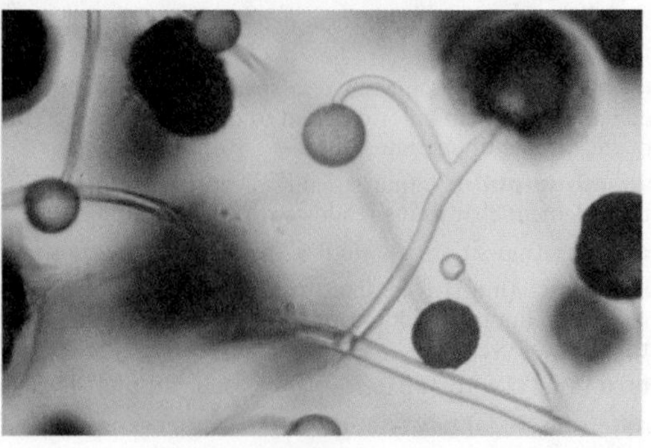

■ *Mucor.*

M. circinelloi′des a species found as normal flora in various warm-blooded animals, and sometimes causing opportunistic mucormycosis.

M. corym′bifer *Absidia corymbifera.*

M. hiema′lis a species that is a normal inhabitant of the soil but occasionally causes cutaneous mucormycosis.

M. muce′do a species of common soil saprobes causing rotting of fruit, baked goods, and insects; it is sometimes isolated from human feet and skin but has not been found to be pathogenic.

M. pusil′lus *Rhizomucor pusillus.*

M. racemosis′simus a species that grows on decaying vegetation and bread, and sometimes causes otomycosis and mucormycosis.

M. ramo′sus *Absidia corymbifera.*

M. rhizopodifor′mis *Rhizopus rhizopodiformis.*

Mu•co•ra•ceae (mu″kə-ra′se-e) a family of fungi of the order Mucorales, characterized by having the thallus not segmented or ramified; pathogenic genera include *Absidia, Apophysomyces, Mucor, Rhizomucor,* and *Rhizopus.*

mu•co•ra•ceous (mu″kə-ra′shəs) pertaining to fungi of the order Mucorales.

Mu•co•ra•les (mu″kə-ra′lēz) an order of perfect fungi of the class Zygomycetes made up of bread molds and related fungi, the majority of which are saprobes; pathogenic species are included in the families Cunninghamellaceae, Mortierellaceae, Mucoraceae, and Saksenaeaceae and cause mainly opportunistic infections such as mucormycosis.

mu•cor•my•co•sis (mu″kor-mi-ko′sis) [*Mucor* + *-mycosis*] 1. fungal infection by members of the order Mucorales, such as species of *Rhizopus, Mucor,* or *Absidia,* usually an opportunistic infection in immunocompromised or debilitated patients. Organisms enter through the respiratory tract, digestive tract, or a skin lesion, and then invade blood vessel walls and are disseminated in the blood; spread along nerve trunks also occurs. The disease may affect the head and neck, the respiratory tract, the digestive tract, or occasionally the skin. Clinical manifestations range from chronic to fulminant. Fungi of class Entomophthorales cause a similar condition called *entomophthoromycosis.* Called also *phycomycosis* and *zygomycosis.* 2. a similar infection in domestic animals, causing abortion or placentitis in cows and rumenitis in ruminants.

cerebral m. fulminant, usually fatal mucormycosis affecting the brain; it may be caused by dissemination of fungi from a distant site or by direct extension from the nasopharynx (rhinocerebral mucormycosis).

cutaneous m. mucormycosis affecting the skin, resulting from either contamination of a wound or spread outward of rhinocerebral mucormycosis. The infecting agent is usually a species of *Rhizopus* or occasionally *Saksenaea vasiformis.*

pulmonary m. mucormycosis type affecting the lung; symptoms include bronchitis, cavitation, and hemoptysis; it has a grave prognosis, often with death within a month.

rhinocerebral m. cerebral mucormycosis in which the original site of infection is in the ethmoid, sphenoid, or maxillary sinuses, the palate, or the pharynx.

mu•co•sa (mu-ko′sə) [L. "mucus"] tunica mucosa. **muco′sal** *adj*

alveolar m. the mucosal lining of the dental alveoli; a thin, soft, fragile continuation of the mucous membrane of the cheek, lips, and floor of the mouth.

m. of auditory tube tunica mucosa tubae auditivae.

m. of bronchi tunica mucosa bronchiorum.

m. of ductus deferens tunica mucosa ductus deferentis.

m. of esophagus tunica mucosa oesophagi.

m. of female urethra tunica mucosa urethrae femininae.

m. of gallbladder tunica mucosa vesicae biliaris.

m. of large intestine tunica mucosa intestini crassi.

m. of larynx tunica mucosa laryngis.

m. of membranous urethra tunica mucosa partis intermediae urethrae.
m. of mouth tunica mucosa oris.
m. of nose tunica mucosa nasi.
m. of pharynx tunica mucosa pharyngis.
m. of prostatic urethra tunica mucosa partis prostaticae urethrae.
redundant supraglottic m. see under *syndrome.*
m. of renal pelvis tunica mucosa pelvis renalis.
m. of seminal vesicle tunica mucosa glandulae vesiculosae.
m. of small intestine tunica mucosa intestini tenuis.
m. of spongy urethra tunica mucosa partis spongiosae urethrae.
m. of stomach tunica mucosa gastrica.
m. of tongue tunica mucosa linguae.
m. of trachea tunica mucosa tracheae.
m. of tympanic cavity tunica mucosa cavitatis tympanicae.
m. of ureter tunica mucosa ureteris.
m. of urinary bladder tunica mucosa vesicae urinariae.
m. of uterine tube tunica mucosa tubae uterinae.
m. of uterus tunica mucosa uteri.
m. of vagina tunica mucosa vaginae.

mu•co•san•guin•e•ous (mu″ko-sang-gwin′e-əs) composed of mucus and blood.

mu•co•sec•to•my (mu-ko-sek′tə-me) [*mucosa* + *-ectomy*] excision of the tunica mucosa, such as in the colon in the treatment of inflammatory bowel disease.
circumferential m. stapled hemorrhoidopexy.

mu•co•se•rous (mu″ko-se′rəs) pertaining to or producing both mucus and serum.

mu•co•sin (mu-ko′sin) a form of mucin peculiar to the more tenacious varieties of mucus, as that of the nasal and uterine cavities.

mu•co•si•tis (mu″ko-si′tis) inflammation of a mucous membrane.

mu•co•stat•ic (mu″ko-stat′ik) 1. arresting the secretion of mucus. Called also *blennostatic.* 2. denoting the normal relaxed condition of the tissues of the mucosa of the jaws.

mu•co•sul•fa•ti•do•sis (mu″ko-sul″fə-tĭ-do′sis) multiple sulfatase deficiency.

mu•co•tome (mu′ko-tōm) a dermatome for removing mucous membrane for transplantation; see *Castroviejo dermatome*, under *dermatome.*

mu•cous (mu′kəs) [L. *mucosus*] 1. pertaining to or relating to mucus. 2. covered with mucus. 3. secreting, producing, or containing mucus.

mu•co•vis•ci•do•sis (mu″ko-vis″ĭ-do′sis) cystic fibrosis, so called because of the abnormally viscous mucoid secretions observed in the disease.

mu•cro (mu′kro) pl. *mucro′nes* [L. "a sharp point"] the pointed end of a part or organ.

mu•cro•nate (mu′kro-nāt) [*mucro* + *-ate*] 1. having a spinelike tip. 2. xiphoid (def. 1).

Mu•cu•na (mu-ku′nə) [L., from Portuguese] a genus of plants of the family Leguminosae. *M. pru′riens* is cowage, an herb native to the East Indies whose seeds contain L-dopa; its pods bear the medicinal but allergenic hairs also called cowage (q.v.).

mu•cus (mu′kəs) [L.] the free slime of the mucous membranes, composed of secretion of the glands, along with various inorganic salts, desquamated cells, and leukocytes.
cervical m. mucus secreted by the mucous membrane of the uterine cervix; it undergoes chemical and physical changes owing to hormone stimulation during the menstrual cycle and plays an important role in helping spermatozoa travel inwards after coitus.

Muehr•cke lines (mūr′ke) [Robert C. *Muehrcke*, American physician, 1921–2003] see under *line.*

Muel•ler (me′ler) see *Müller.*

Muel•le•ri•us (mu-ler′e-əs) a genus of nematodes of the family Protostrongylidae. *M. capilla′ris* is a lungworm that causes hoose in sheep and goats.

muf•fle (muf′əl) a part of a furnace, usually removable or replaceable, in which material may be placed for processing, without exposing it to the direct action of the heat source.

MUGA multiple gated acquisition (scanning); see *equilibrium radionuclide angiocardiography*, under *angiocardiography.*

mug•wort (mug′wort) [A.S. *mucgwyrt*, from *mycg* midge + *wyrt* plant] 1. any of several plants of the genus *Artemisia*, particularly *A. vulgaris.* 2. a preparation of *A. vulgaris*, used internally for gastrointestinal complaints and as a tonic; it is also used in homeopathy and traditional Chinese medicine. See also *moxa.*

Muir-Tor•re syndrome (mūr′ tor′e) [Edward G. *Muir*, British physician, 1906-1973; Douglas Paul *Torre*, American dermatologist, 1919–1996] Torre syndrome; see under *syndrome.*

Mul•der angle (mool′der) [Johannes *Mulder*, Dutch anatomist, 1769–1810] see under *angle.*

Mul•der sign (click) (mul′dər) [J. D. *Mulder*, Dutch orthopedist, mid-20th century] see under *sign.*

Mül•ler capsule, duct, etc. (me′ler) [Johannes Peter *Müller*, German physiologist, 1801–1858, the founder of scientific medicine in Germany] see *capsula glomeruli* and *ganglion superius nervi glossopharyngei;* see *paramesonephric duct*, under *duct;* and see under *maneuver* and *tubercle.*

Mül•ler fibers (cells, radial cells), muscle (me′ler) [Heinrich *Müller*, German anatomist, 1820–1864] see under *fiber* and *muscle.*

Mül•ler fluid (me′ler) [Hermann Franz *Müller*, German histologist, 1866–1898] see under *fluid.*

Mül•ler sign (me′ler) [Friedrich von *Müller*, German physician, 1858–1941] see under *sign.*

mull•er (mul′er) a kind of pestle, flat at the bottom, used for grinding drugs upon a slab of similar material.

mül•le•ri•an (meu-ler′e-ən) named for Johannes Peter *Müller.*

Mül•le•ri•us (mu-ler′e-əs) Muellerius.

mul•tan•gu•lar (məl-tang′gu-lər) having many angles or corners.

multi- [L. *multus* many, much] a combining form meaning many or much; see also words beginning *poly-.*

mul•ti•al•le•lic (mul″te-ə-le′lik) pertaining to or having many alleles at a single gene locus.

mul•ti•ar•tic•u•lar (mul″te-ahr-tik′u-lər) pertaining to or affecting many joints.

mul•ti•ax•ial (mul″te-ak′se-əl) having several axes, or able to revolve around several different axes.

mul•ti•bac•il•lary (mul″te-bas′ĭ-lar″e) pertaining to or made up of a number of bacilli.

mul•ti•cap•su•lar (mul″te-cap′su-lər) having many capsules, as a lamellar (pacinian) corpuscle.

mul•ti•cell (mul′te-sel) any organ made up of many cells; any group of functionally active cells.

mul•ti•cel•lu•lar (mul″te-sel′u-lər) [*multi-* + *cellular*] 1. composed of many cells. 2. containing many hollow spaces.

mul•ti•cel•lu•lar•i•ty (mul″te-sel″u-lar′ĭ-te) the state of being composed of many cells; the state of being multicellular.

mul•ti•cen•tric (mul″te-sen′trik) [*multi-* + *center*] polycentric.

mul•ti•cen•tric•i•ty (mul″te-sən-tris′ĭ-te) polycentricity.

mul•ti•con•tam•i•nat•ed (mul″te-kən-tam′ĭ-nāt″əd) infected by several different species of microorganisms or other types of contaminating agents.

mul•ti•cus•pid (mul″te-kus′pid) [*multi-* + *cuspid*] having many cusps, such as a tooth with many cusps. Called also *multicuspidate.*

mul•ti•cus•pi•date (mul″te-kus′pĭ-dāt) multicuspid.

mul•ti•cys•tic (mul″te-sis′tik) polycystic.

mul•ti•den•tate (mul″te-den′tāt) [*multi-* + *dentate*] having many teeth or toothlike processes.

mul•ti•elec•trode (mul-te-e-lek′trōd) multilead electrode.

mul•ti•fac•to•ri•al (mul″te-fak-tor′e-əl) 1. of or pertaining to, or arising through the action of many factors. 2. in genetics, arising as the result of the interaction of several genes and usually, to some extent, of nongenetic factors. Cf. *polygenic.*

mul•ti•fid (mul′tĭ-fid) cleft into many parts.

mul•tif•i•dus (məl-tif′ĭ-dəs) [L., from *multus* many + *findere* to split] cleft into many parts, as the musculus multifidus.

mul•ti•fo•cal (mul″te-fo′kəl) arising from or pertaining to many foci.

mul•ti•form (mul′tĭ-form) polymorphic.

mul•ti•gan•gli•on•ic (mul″te-gang″gle-on′ik) pertaining to, affecting, or possessing many ganglia.

mul•ti•glan•du•lar (mul″te-glan′du-lər) pluriglandular.

mul•ti•grav•i•da (mul″te-grav′ĭ-də) [*multi-* + *gravida*] a woman who has been pregnant several times. Also written gravida II, III, etc., according to the number of pregnancies.
grand m. a woman who has had five or more previous pregnancies.

mul•ti•hal•lu•cal•ism (mul″te-hal′u-kəl-iz-əm) [*multi-* + *hallucal* + *-ism*] a developmental anomaly characterized by the presence of more than one great toe on one foot.

mul•ti•hal•lu•cism (mul″te-hal′u-siz-əm) multihallucalism.

mul•ti•in•fec•tion (mul″te-in-fek′shən) mixed infection.

mul•ti•lo•bar (mul″te-lo′bər) having numerous lobes.

mul•ti•lob•u•lar (mul″te-lob′u-lər) [*multi-* + *lobular*] having many lobules.

mul•ti•loc•u•lar (mul″te-lok′u-lər) [*multi-* + *locular*] having many cells or compartments (loculi). Called also *plurilocular*.

mul•ti•mam•mae (mul″te-mam′e) [*multi-* + *mammae*] the condition of having more than two breasts.

mul•ti•mer (mul′tĭ-mər) a protein molecule made up of more than one polypeptide chain. Cf. *polymer*.

mul•ti•mo•dal (mul″te-mo′dəl) 1. having more than one mode. 2. of a graph, having several maxima (peaks). 3. multisensory.

mul•ti•nod•u•lar (mul″te-nod′u-lər) composed of many nodules.

mul•ti•nu•cle•ar (mul″te-noo′kle-ər) multinucleated; polynuclear.

mul•ti•nu•cle•ate (mul″te-noo′kle-āt) multinucleated.

mul•ti•nu•cle•at•ed (mul″te-noo′kle-āt″əd) of cells, having more than one nucleus.

mul•tip•a•ra (məl-tip′ə-rə) [*multi-* + *para*] a woman who has had two or more pregnancies which resulted in viable fetuses, whether or not the offspring were alive at birth. Also written para II, III, IV, etc., according to the number of offspring.

grand m. a woman who has had five or more pregnancies which resulted in viable fetuses.

mul•ti•par•i•ty (mul″te-par′ĭ-te) 1. the condition of being a multipara. 2. the production of several offspring in one gestation.

mul•tip•a•rous (məl-tip′ə-rəs) [*multi-* + *-parous*] 1. having had two or more pregnancies which resulted in viable fetuses. 2. producing several offspring or eggs at one time.

mul•ti•ple (mul′tĭ-pəl) [L. *multiplex*] manifold; occurring in or affecting various parts of the body at once.

mul•tip•let (mul′tĭ-plet) multiple discharge.

mul•ti•pli•ca•tion (mul″tĭ-plĭ-ka′shən) a process of increasing.

countercurrent m. the mechanism in the loops of Henle of the renal tubules by which urine is concentrated; it is dependent upon unique solute transport processes at different parts of the loops of Henle and the vasa recta.

mul•ti•plic•i•tas (mul″tĭ-plis′ĭ-təs) a multiplication; a developmental anomaly characterized by the presence of an abnormal multiplicity of organs, or of a specific organ.

m. cor′dis a developmental anomaly characterized by the presence of a number of separate hearts.

mul•ti•po•lar (mul″te-po′lər) [*multi-* + *polar*] having more than two poles or processes.

mul•ti•pol•li•cal•ism (mul″te-pol′ĭ-kəl-iz-əm) [*multi-* + *pollical* + *-ism*] a developmental anomaly characterized by the presence of more than one thumb on one hand.

mul•ti•root•ed (mul″te-ro͞ot′əd) having many roots; said of molar teeth.

mul•ti•sen•si•tiv•i•ty (mul″te-sen″sĭ-tiv′ĭ-te) the condition of being sensitive (allergic) to more than one antigen (allergen).

mul•ti•sen•so•ry (mul″te-sen′sə-re) capable of responding to more than one kind of sensory input; said of certain neurons in the central nervous system.

mul•ti•syn•ap•tic (mul″te-sĭ-nap′tik) polysynaptic.

mul•ti•ter•mi•nal (mul″te-tur′mĭ-nəl) having several sets of terminals so that several electrodes may be used.

mul•ti•tu•ber•cu•late (mul″te-too-bur′ku-lət) having many tubercles.

mul•ti•va•lent (mul″te-va′lənt) [*multi-* + L. *valere* to have value] 1. having a valence of two or more. 2. denoting an antiserum, vaccine, or antitoxin specific for more than one antigen or an organism. Called also *polyvalent*.

mul•ti•va•ri•ate (mul″te-var′e-āt) involving more than one variable.

mul•ti•vis•cer•al (mul″te-vis′ər-əl) pertaining to, affecting, or consisting of several viscera.

mum•mi•fi•ca•tion (mum″ĭ-fĭ-ka′shən) conversion into a state resembling that of a mummy, such as occurs in dry gangrene, or the shriveling and drying up of a dead fetus.

mumps (mumps) an acute infectious disease caused by a paramyxovirus called mumps virus, spread by direct contact, airborne droplet nuclei, fomites contaminated by infectious saliva, and perhaps urine; it is usually seen in children under the age of 15, but sometimes in adults. Many cases are subclinical, but in those that are clinically apparent the principal manifestation is parotitis, usually associated with painful swelling of one or both parotid glands and sometimes other salivary glands. Occasionally there may be infection of other organs, with complications such as epididymo-orchitis in males, oophoritis in females, meningoencephalitis, or pancreatitis. Called also *epidemic parotitis*.

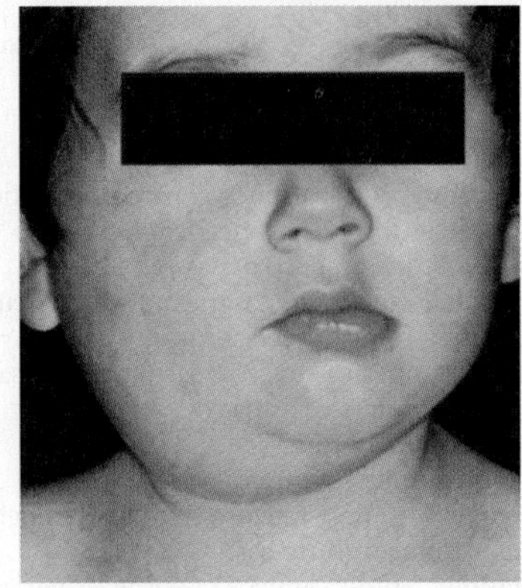

■ Mumps.

iodine m. swelling of the salivary and lacrimal glands as a toxic reaction to iodine therapy.

Mumps•vax (mumps′vaks) trademark for a preparation of mumps virus vaccine live.

Mun•chau•sen syndrome (moon′chou-zən) [Baron Karl Friedrich Hieronymus *Münchhausen*, German soldier and traveler, 1720–1797, a reputed teller of exaggerated tales] see under *syndrome*.

Münch•mey•er disease (mēnch′mi-ər) [Ernst *Münchmeyer*, German physician, 1846–1880] see under *disease*.

Mun•ro microabscess (abscess) (mən-ro′) [William John *Munro*, English dermatologist, 19th century] see under *microabscess*.

Mun•ro point (mən-ro′) [John Cummings *Munro*, American surgeon, 1858–1910] see under *point*.

Mun•ro Kerr cesarean section, incision (mən-ro′ kər′) [John Martin *Munro Kerr*, Scottish gynecologist and obstetrician, 1868–1955] see under *incision* and *section*.

Mun•son sign (mun′sən) [Edward Sterling *Munson*, American ophthalmologist, born 1933] see under *sign*.

MUP motor unit potential.

Mu•pap•il•lo•ma•vi•rus (mu-pap″ĭ-lo′mə-vi″rəs) a genus of the family Papillomaviridae that contains a few of the human papillomaviruses.

mu•pir•o•cin (mu-pir′o-sin) [USP] an inhibitor of bacterial protein synthesis, produced by fermentation of *Pseudomonas fluorescens* and effective against staphylococci and non-enteric streptococci; applied topically in the treatment of impetigo.

m. calcium the calcium salt of mupirocin, applied intranasally for the treatment of nasal colonization with methicillin-resistant *Staphylococcus aureus*.

mu•ral (mu′rəl) [L. *muralis*, from *murus* wall] pertaining to or occurring in the wall of a cavity.

mu•ra•li•um (mu-ra′le-əm) pl. *mura′lia* [L., from *murus* wall] a histologic structure comprising a complex system of interconnected walls, such as that formed by the hepatic cords.

mu•ram•ic ac•id (mu-ram′ik) a compound consisting of glucosamine and lactic acid joined by an ether linkage; it occurs naturally as the *N*-acetyl derivative (MurNAc) in peptidoglycan, the characteristic polysaccharide composing bacterial cell walls.

mu•ram•i•dase (mu-ram′ĭ-dās) lysozyme.

Mur•chi•son-Pel-Eb•stein fever (mur′chĭ-sən pel′ eb′shtīn) [Charles *Murchison*, British physician, 1830–1879; Pieter Klaases *Pel*, Dutch physician, 1852–1919; Wilhelm *Ebstein*, German physician, 1836–1912] Pel-Ebstein fever.

Mu•rex (mu′reks) a genus of whelks of the family Muricidae. *M. purpu′rea* is a Mediterranean species from which murexine (or purpurine) is obtained.

mu•rex•ine (mu-rek′sin) [*Murex* + *-ine*] a neurotoxic substance derived from the median zone of the hypobranchial gland of gastropods of the genus *Murex* and related species; the substance is called *purpurine* when derived from snails of the genus *Purpura*.

Mu•ric•i•dae (mu-ris′ĭ-de) a family of marine snails of the order Neogastropoda, including the genera *Murex* and *Purpura*.

Mu•ri•dae (mu′rĭ-de) a large family of rodents including many types of mice and rats, as well as gerbils, hamsters, and voles. Some are used as laboratory animals or pets and others are household pests and reservoirs of disease. Genera of medical or laboratory interest include *Apodemus, Calomys, Clethrionomys, Cricetulus, Cricetus, Gerbillus, Mastomys, Mesocricetus, Microtus, Mus, Neotoma, Oryzomys, Peromyscus, Rattus, Rhombomys*, and *Sigmodon*.

mu•ri•form (mu′rĭ-form) [L. *murus* wall + *form*] wall-like, used in mycology and bacteriology to describe a spore having both transverse and longitudinal septa.

mu•rine (mu′rin) [L. *mus, muris* mouse] pertaining to or affecting mice or rats.

mur•mur (mur′mər) [L.] an auscultatory sound, benign or pathologic, particularly a periodic sound of short duration of cardiac or vascular origin.

amphoric m. see under *resonance*.

anemic m. a cardiac murmur heard in anemic patients.

aneurysmal m. a vascular murmur heard over an aneurysm.

aortic m. a sound generated by blood flowing through a diseased aorta or aortic valve.

apex m., apical m. one heard at the apex of the heart.

apical diastolic m. a diastolic murmur heard at the apex of the heart, indicative of mitral stenosis or another condition causing altered flow through the mitral valve; it consists essentially of low-frequency vibrations, which account for its rumbling quality.

arterial m. a murmur (bruit) over an artery, sometimes aneurysmal and sometimes constricted.

attrition m. pericardial friction rub.

Austin Flint m. a presystolic or mid-diastolic murmur heard at the cardiac apex in aortic regurgitation, originating at the mitral valve when blood enters simultaneously from both the aorta and the left atrium.

basal diastolic m's diastolic murmurs at the base of the heart, due to aortic or pulmonic regurgitation.

bellows m. to-and-fro m.

brain m. a murmur produced over a vascular abnormality in the brain.

cardiac m. a sound of finite length generated by turbulence of blood flow through the heart; often classified as systolic, diastolic, or continuous, and further divided on the basis of its timing within systole or diastole. Murmurs are graded from 1 to 6 on the basis of increasing loudness.

cardiopulmonary m., cardiorespiratory m. a sound generated within lung tissue and related to movement of the heart.

Carey Coombs m. a rumbling apical mid-diastolic cardiac murmur occurring in the acute phase of rheumatic fever and disappearing afterward.

continuous m. a humming cardiac murmur extending throughout systole into late diastole or to the end of diastole; it is due to conditions characterized by connections between the aorta and the pulmonary artery or its branches (such as patent ductus arteriosus), by arteriovenous fistulas, or by altered blood flow in arteries or veins. Cf. *systolic m.* and *diastolic m.*

cooing m. a type of musical murmur, resembling the cooing of a bird.

crescendo m. a murmur marked by progressively increasing loudness and abrupt cessation, e.g., the presystolic murmur in mitral stenosis with sinus rhythm.

Cruveilhier-Baumgarten m. a venous murmur heard at the abdominal wall over veins connecting the portal and caval systems.

deglutition m. a murmur heard over the esophagus during swallowing.

diamond-shaped m. a cardiac murmur with a characteristic crescendo-decrescendo pattern of intensity on the phonocardiogram; it is almost always a systolic ejection murmur caused by aortic stenosis.

diastolic m. cardiac murmurs occurring during diastole and usually due to semilunar valve regurgitation or to altered blood flow through atrioventricular valves; they are frequently divided into early and mid-diastolic murmurs.

Duroziez m. a double murmur over the femoral or other large peripheral artery, due to aortic insufficiency.

early diastolic m. a high frequency cardiac murmur beginning immediately after the second heart sound and progressively diminishing in intensity; it results from semilunar valve regurgitation.

early systolic m. a regurgitant cardiac murmur beginning at the first heart sound and diminishing and ending well before the second heart sound; it results from abbreviation of pansystolic murmurs due to special circumstances such as acute mitral regurgitation or ventricular septal defect that is associated with pulmonary hypertension.

ejection m. a type of systolic murmur occurring predominantly in midsystole, at the time of maximal ejection volume and blood flow velocity, such as that heard in aortic or pulmonary stenosis; it is due to ejection of blood into the root of the aorta or pulmonary artery, is diamond-shaped, and ends before the second heart sound. Cf. *regurgitant m.*

extracardiac m. a murmur heard over the heart originating from another structure, such as a cardiopulmonary murmur.

Flint m. Austin Flint m.

flow m. hemic murmur.

friction m. see under *rub*.

functional m. a cardiac murmur generated in the absence of organic cardiac disease. Called also *innocent m., inorganic m.*, and *physiologic m.*

Gibson m. a long rumbling sound occupying most of systole and diastole, usually localized in the second left interspace near the sternum, and usually indicative of patent ductus arteriosus. Called also *machinery m.*

Graham Steell m. a high-pitched diastolic murmur caused by pulmonary regurgitation secondary to severe pulmonary hypertension; it is heard at the left sternal edge, level with the second or third costal cartilage.

Hamman m. see under *sign*.

heart m. cardiac m.

hemic m. a murmur due to an abnormal, usually anemic, condition of the blood.

holosystolic m. pansystolic m.

hourglass m. a cardiac murmur characterized by two periods of maximum loudness joined by a period of decreasing, then increasing, loudness, with the point of lowest intensity midway between the two peaks.

humming-top m. venous hum.

innocent m., inorganic m. functional m.

late systolic m. a regurgitant murmur beginning in the middle or last third of systole and continuing until the second heart sound; it is often associated with a midsystolic click and mitral valve prolapse.

machinery m. Gibson m.

mid-diastolic m. a mainly low-frequency cardiac murmur beginning a short time after the second heart sound; it is associated with early ventricular filling and is caused by turbulence in the ventricle due to altered flow of blood through one or both atrioventricular valves, such as occurs in mitral or tricuspid stenosis.

midsystolic m. a cardiac murmur, usually an ejection murmur, beginning a short time after the first heart sound and ending before the second heart sound; it is almost always a functional murmur or the result of obstruction to ventricular outflow, such as occurs in aortic or pulmonary stenosis.

mitral m. cardiac murmur due to disease of the mitral valve.

musical m. a cardiac murmur, usually systolic, resulting when the responsible vibrations have a periodic harmonic pattern.

organic m. a murmur due to a lesion in the organ or organ system being examined.

pansystolic m. a regurgitant murmur that extends throughout systole and is due to blood flow between two chambers normally of very different pressures in systole; the most common causes are mitral or tricuspid regurgitation and ventricular septal defects. Called also *holosystolic m.*

pericardial m. see under *rub*.

physiologic m. functional m.

pleuropericardial m. a pleural friction sound heard in the pericardial region and resembling a pericardial rub.

prediastolic m. early diastolic m.

presystolic m. (PSM) a cardiac murmur occurring immediately prior to ventricular ejection, usually associated with atrial contraction and the acceleration of blood flow through a narrowed atrioventricular valve.

pulmonary m., pulmonic m. a murmur due to disease of the pulmonary valve or artery.

regurgitant m. a cardiac murmur due to regurgitation of blood through an abnormal valvular orifice, usually occurring throughout systole. Cf. *ejection m.*

Roger m. bruit de Roger.

seagull m. a raucous murmur with musical qualities resembling the call of a seagull, such as that heard occasionally in aortic insufficiency, and attributed specifically to eversion or retroversion of the right anterior aortic cusp.

seesaw m. to-and-fro m.

Steell m. Graham Steell m.

stenosal m. a sound produced in an artery by artificial pressure or by a stenosis.

Still m. a functional low-frequency, vibratory or buzzing, cardiac murmur of childhood, occurring in midsystole and usually of maximal intensity at the lower left sternal border.

systolic m. a cardiac murmur occurring during systole; usually due to mitral or tricuspid regurgitation or to aortic or pulmonary obstruction. These are often distinguished as either ejection or regurgitant murmurs, and on the basis of cardiac cycle timing, they may be classified as early systolic, midsystolic, late systolic, or pansystolic murmurs.

to-and-fro m. a friction rub or murmur heard with both systole and diastole.

tricuspid m. a cardiac murmur caused by disease of the tricuspid valve.

vascular m. a murmur heard over a blood vessel; see *arterial m.* and *venous m.*

venous m. a murmur heard over a vein.

vesicular m. vesicular breath sounds; see under *sound*.

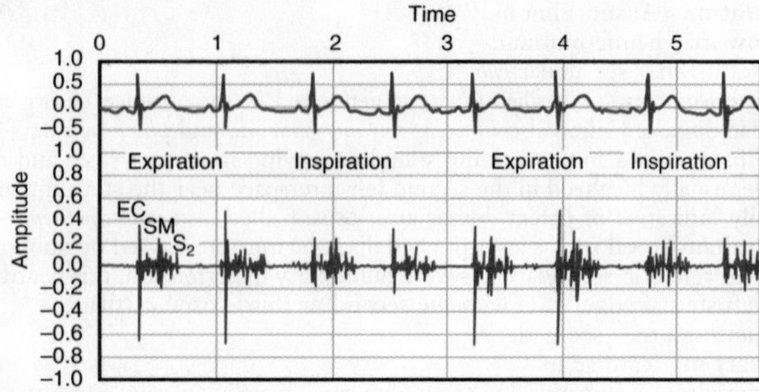

■ Systolic murmur *(SM)* in a child with valvular pulmonary stenosis. The phonocardiogram is recorded at the left upper sternal border and also shows an intermittent systolic ejection click *(EC)* occurring in the expiratory phase of the respiratory cycle. *(S_2)*, Second heart sound.

mu•ro•mo•nab-CD3 (mu″ro-mo′nab) a murine monoclonal antibody to the CD3 antigen of human T cells that functions as an immunosuppressant in the treatment of acute allograft rejection of renal, hepatic, and cardiac transplants; administered intravenously.

Mur•phy percussion, sign (mur′fe) [John Benjamin *Murphy*, American surgeon, 1857–1916] see under *percussion* and *sign.*

Mur•ray Val•ley encephalitis (disease), virus (mur′e val′e) [*Murray Valley*, Australia, where the disease occurred in epidemics in 1950 and 1951] see under *encephalitis* and *virus.*

mur•ri•na (moo-re′nə) [Sp. *morriña*] surra in horses in Central and South America.

Mus (mus) [L. "mouse"] a genus of rodents of the family Muridae, including several species of mice.

M. mus′culus the house mouse, a small, usually gray species that is the most common one around the world in human dwellings; it is an important cause of food destruction and sometimes a carrier of disease.

M. norve′gicus former name for *Rattus norvegicus.*

Mus•ca (mus′kə) [L. "fly"] a genus of flies of the family Muscidae whose mouth parts are adapted for suction only.

M. autumna′lis the face fly, a species commonly found in Europe, the Americas, and parts of Asia and Africa, often crawling on the faces of large mammals such as cattle and horses.

M. domes′tica the common house fly. It may act as a mechanical carrier of the microorganisms of typhoid fever, cholera, dysentery, plague, anthrax, tetanus, trachoma, leprosy, and encephalitis, and of pyogenic bacteria, cysts of some protozoa, and helminth ova. The larvae may cause myiasis.

M. domes′tica ne′bulo a subspecies of *M. domestica* found in India.

M. domes′tica vici′na a subspecies of *M. domestica* common in Egypt and India.

M. lute′ola see *Auchmeromyia.*

M. sor′bens a species of bush flies found in Ethiopia, East Asia, Indonesia, and Australia, believed to transmit conjunctivitis, trachoma, and other infections.

M. vomito′ria *Calliphora vomitoria.*

mus•ca (mus′kə) pl. *mus′cae* [L.] a fly.

mus′cae hispa′nicae cantharides.

mus′cae volitan′tes [L. "flitting flies"] specks seen floating before the eyes; see *floaters.*

mus•ca•cide (mus′kə-sīd) [*musca* + *-cide*] 1. destructive to flies. 2. any agent that destroys flies.

mus•cae (mus′e) [L.] plural of *musca.*

mus•car•dine (mus′kər-din) a fungal infection of silkworms caused by *Beauveria bassiana.*

mus•ca•rine (mus′kə-rēn) a cholinomimetic alkaloid occurring in the mushrooms *Amanita muscaria* and various species of the genera *Inocybe* and *Clitocybe;* ingestion causes *muscarinism*, a type of mushroom poisoning characterized by parasympathetic effects such as decrease in heart rate and contractility; bronchoconstriction; dilation of arterioles; increase in motility, tone, and secretion of the stomach and intestines; stimulation of the urinary bladder; and stimulation of the salivary, lacrimal, and sweat glands. See also *muscarinic receptors*, under *receptor.*

mus•ca•rin•ic (mus″kə-rin′ik) denoting the effects of muscarine or acetylcholine at muscarinic receptors (q.v.).

mus•ca•rin•ism (mus′kə-rin-iz-əm) a type of mushroom poisoning caused by the ingestion of mushrooms containing muscarine.

mus•ce•ge•net•ic (mus″e-jə-net′ik) giving rise to muscae volitantes.

Mus•ci (mus′ke) [L.] the mosses, a class of lower plants that are cryptogams.

mus•ci•cide (mus′ĭ-sīd) muscacide.

Mus•ci•dae (mus′ĭ-de) a family of flies of the order Diptera. It includes the genera *Fannia, Haematobia, Glossina, Musca, Muscina*, and *Stomoxys.*

mus•ci•mol (mus′kĭ-mol) a neurotoxin similar in chemical structure and activity to ibotenic acid, found in species of *Amanita* mushrooms.

Mus•ci•na (mə-si′nə) the nonbiting stable flies, a genus of the family Muscidae that breeds in feces and frequents dwellings; it is closely related to the house fly.

mus•cle (mus′əl) [L. *musculus* (q.v.)] an organ which by contraction produces the movements of an animal organism; there are two varieties: *striated*, including the skeletal muscles, in which contraction is voluntary, and the cardiac muscle; and *smooth*, or *nonstriated*, including all the involuntary muscles except the heart. Striated muscles are covered with a thin layer of connective tissue *(epimysium)* from which septa *(perimysium)* pass, dividing the muscle into *fasciculi* containing parallel fibers separated by connective tissue septa *(endomysium).* Each fiber consists of sarcoplasm composed of alternate light and dark portions (whence the name *striated muscle*); each contains embedded in it the *myofibrils* and is surrounded by *sarcolemma.* Smooth muscles are composed of elongated, spindle-shaped, nucleated cells arranged parallel to one another and to the long axis of the muscle, and these cells are often grouped into bundles of varying size. The muscles, bundles, and cells are enclosed in an indifferent connective tissue material much as is found in striated muscles. Called also *musculus* [TA].

Muscle

Muscles are often referred to by their Latin names with the omission of the word *musculus*, e.g., *rectus abdominis* for *musculus rectus abdominis*. For muscles so called, see under *musculus.*

abductor digiti minimi m. of hand musculus abductor digiti minimi manus.

abductor digiti minimi m. of foot musculus abductor digiti minimi pedis.

abductor m. of great toe, abductor hallucis m. musculus abductor hallucis.

abductor m. of little finger musculus abductor digiti minimi manus.

abductor m. of little toe musculus abductor digiti minimi pedis.

abductor pollicis brevis m. musculus abductor pollicis brevis.

abductor pollicis longus m. musculus abductor pollicis longus.

abductor m. of thumb, long musculus abductor pollicis longus.

abductor m. of thumb, short musculus abductor pollicis brevis.

adductor m., great musculus adductor magnus.

adductor m., long musculus adductor longus.

adductor m., short musculus adductor brevis.

adductor m., smallest musculus adductor minimus.

adductor brevis m. musculus adductor brevis.

adductor m. of great toe musculus adductor hallucis.

adductor hallucis m. musculus adductor hallucis.

adductor longus m. musculus adductor longus.

adductor magnus m. musculus adductor magnus.

adductor minimus m. musculus adductor minimus.

adductor pollicis m. musculus adductor pollicis.

adductor m. of thumb musculus adductor pollicis.

Aeby m. musculus depressor labii inferioris.

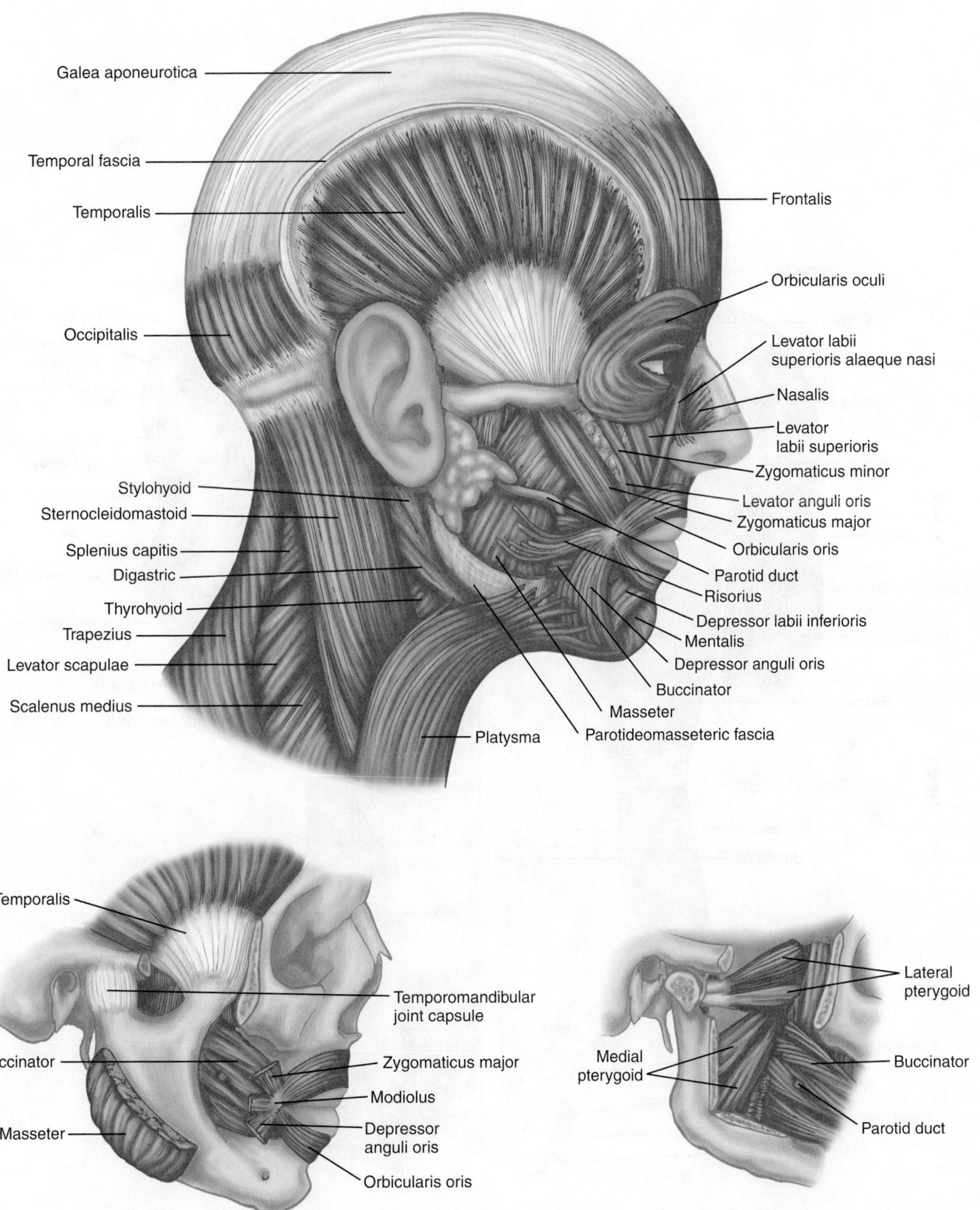

■ **PLATE 27**—MUSCLES OF THE HEAD AND NECK

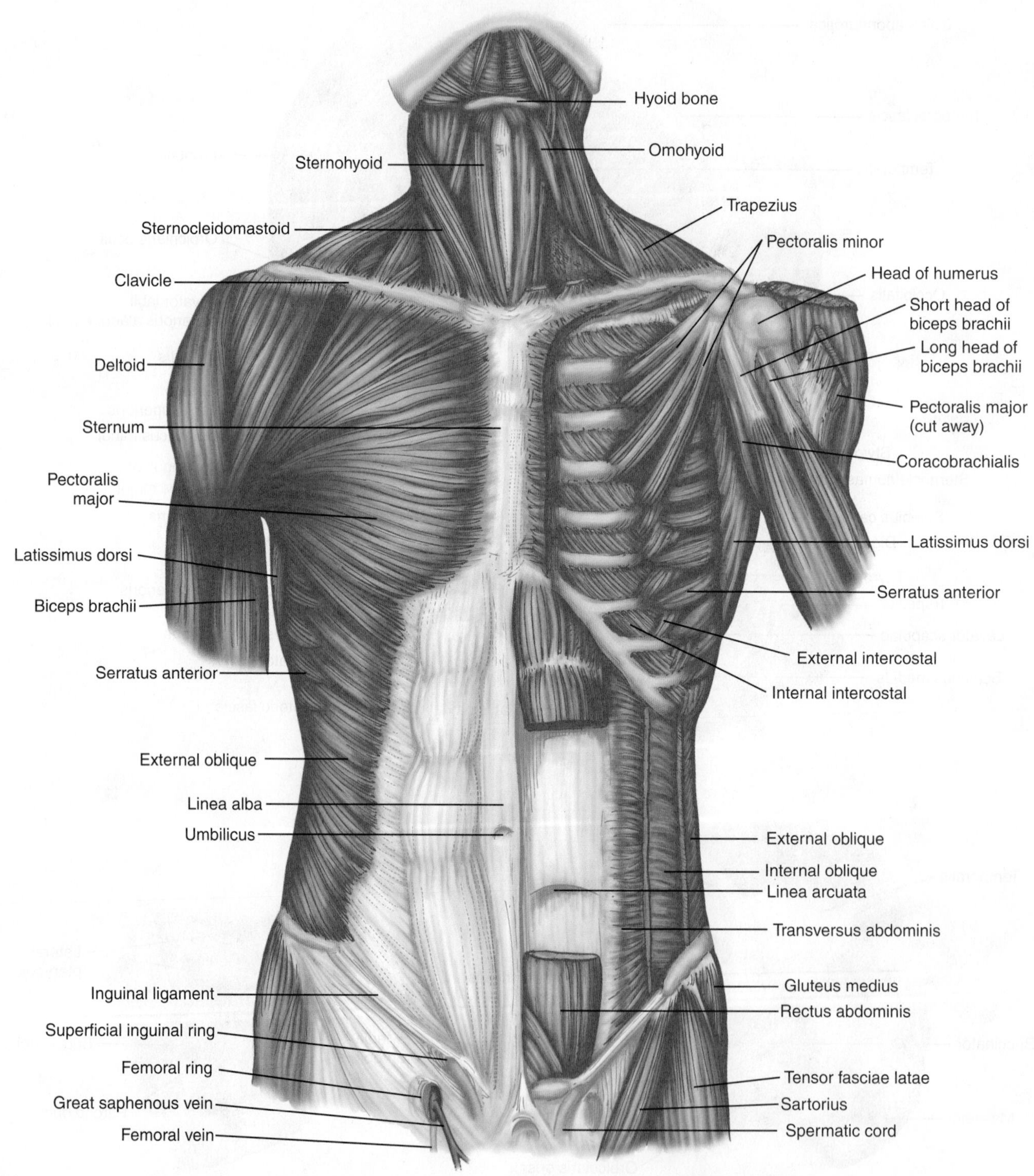

■ **PLATE 28**—MUSCLES OF THE TRUNK, ANTERIOR VIEW

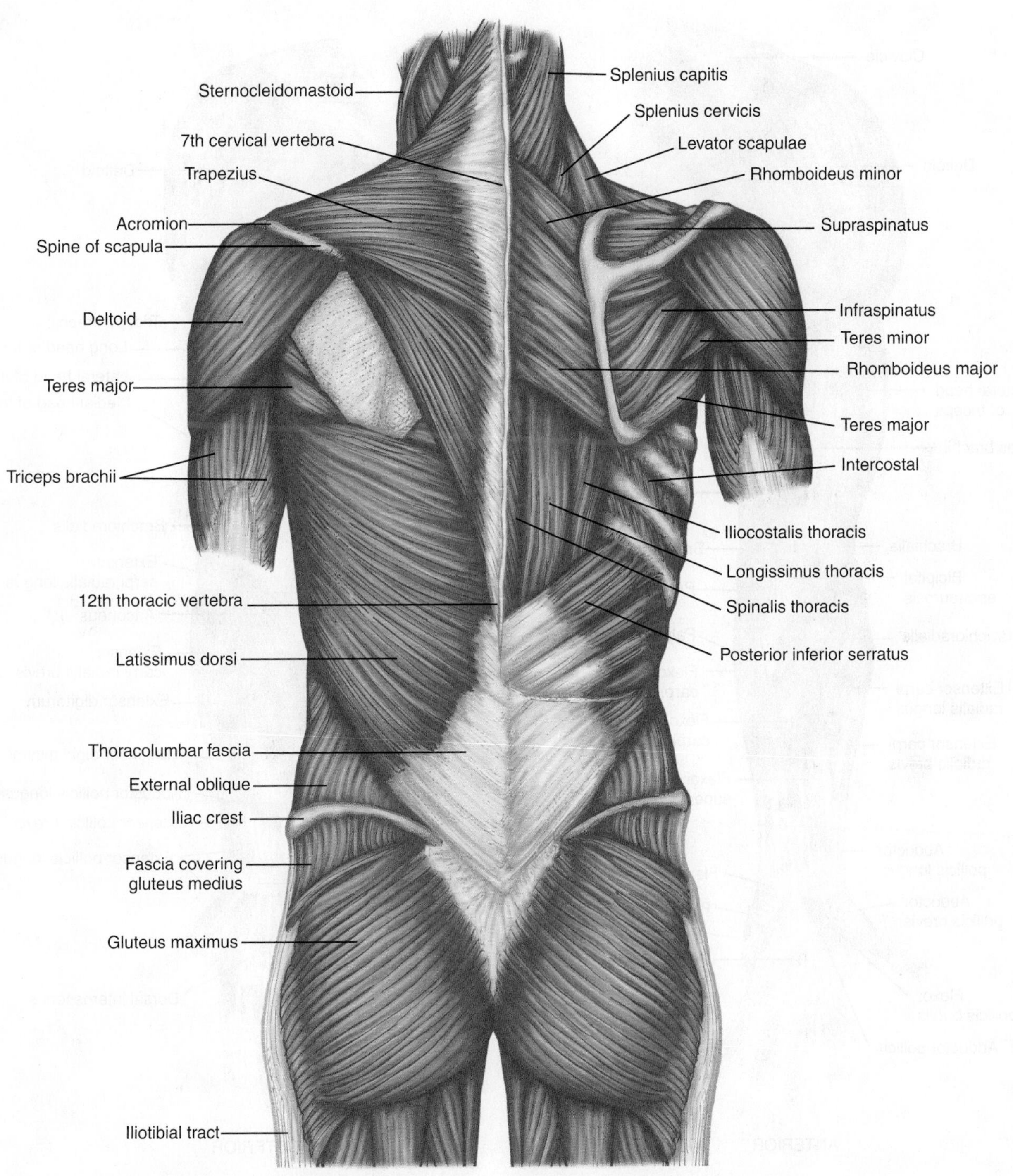

■ **PLATE 29**—MUSCLES OF THE TRUNK, POSTERIOR VIEW

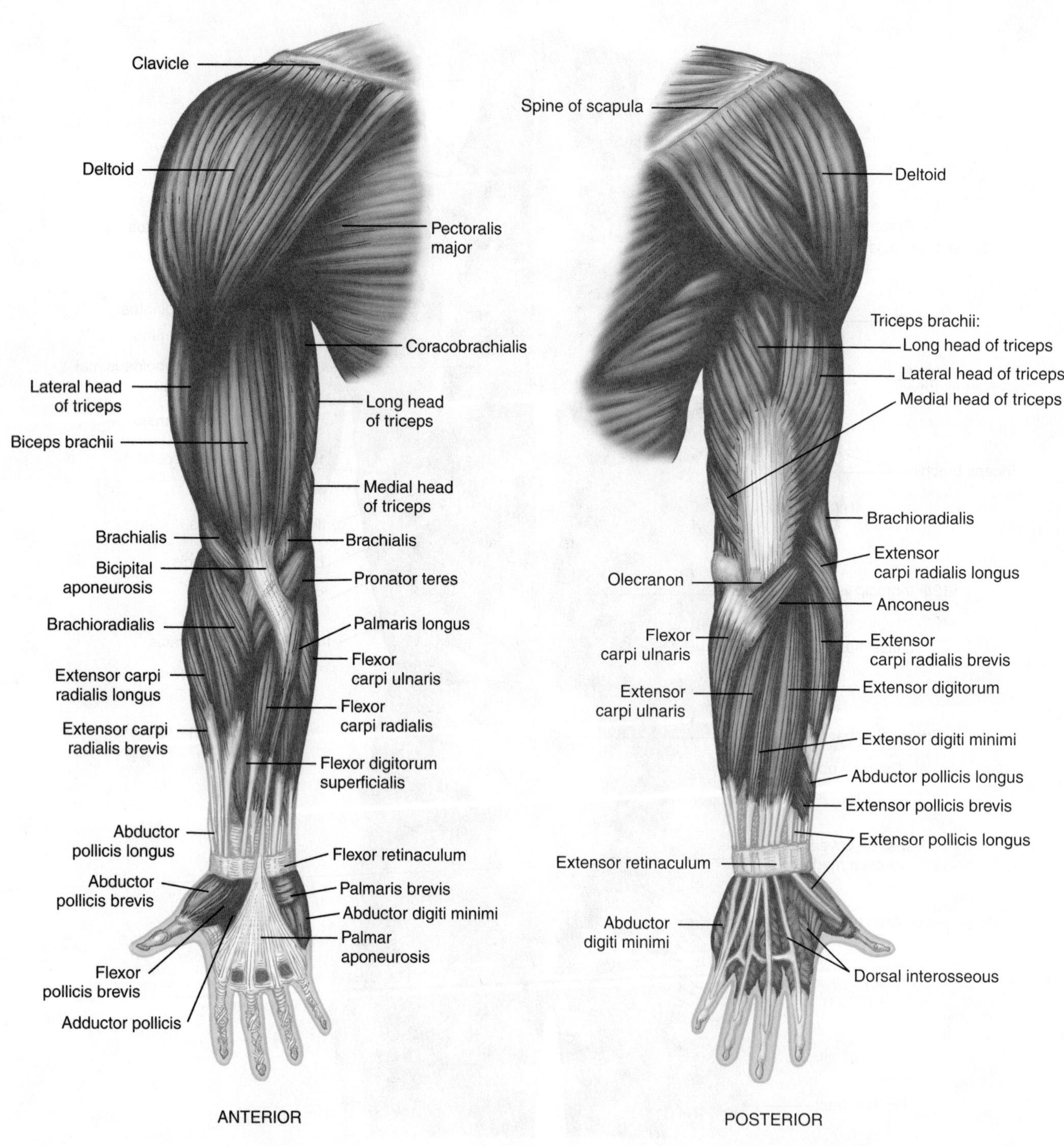

■ **PLATE 30**—SUPERFICIAL MUSCLES OF THE UPPER LIMB

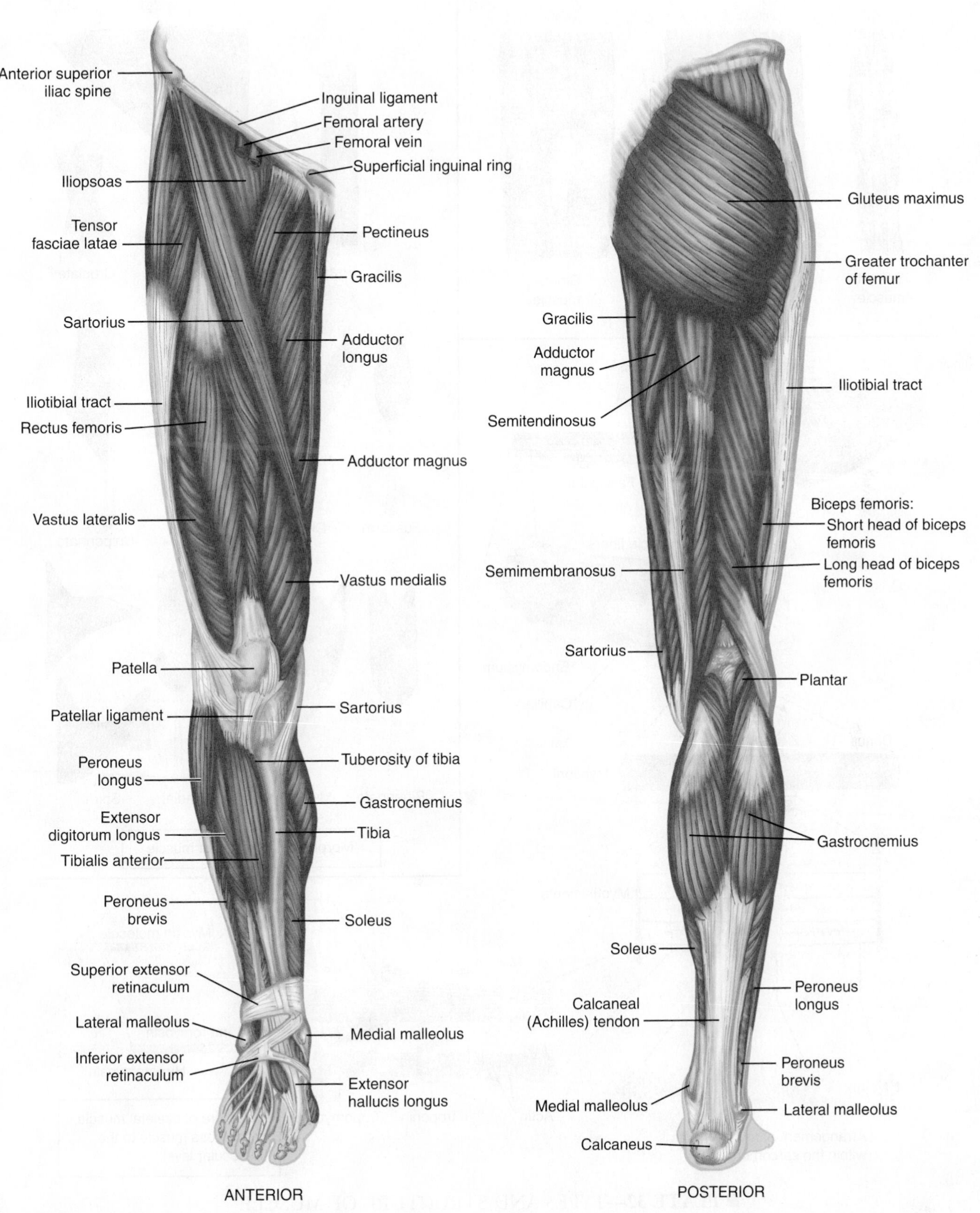

■ **PLATE 31**—SUPERFICIAL MUSCLES OF THE LOWER LIMB

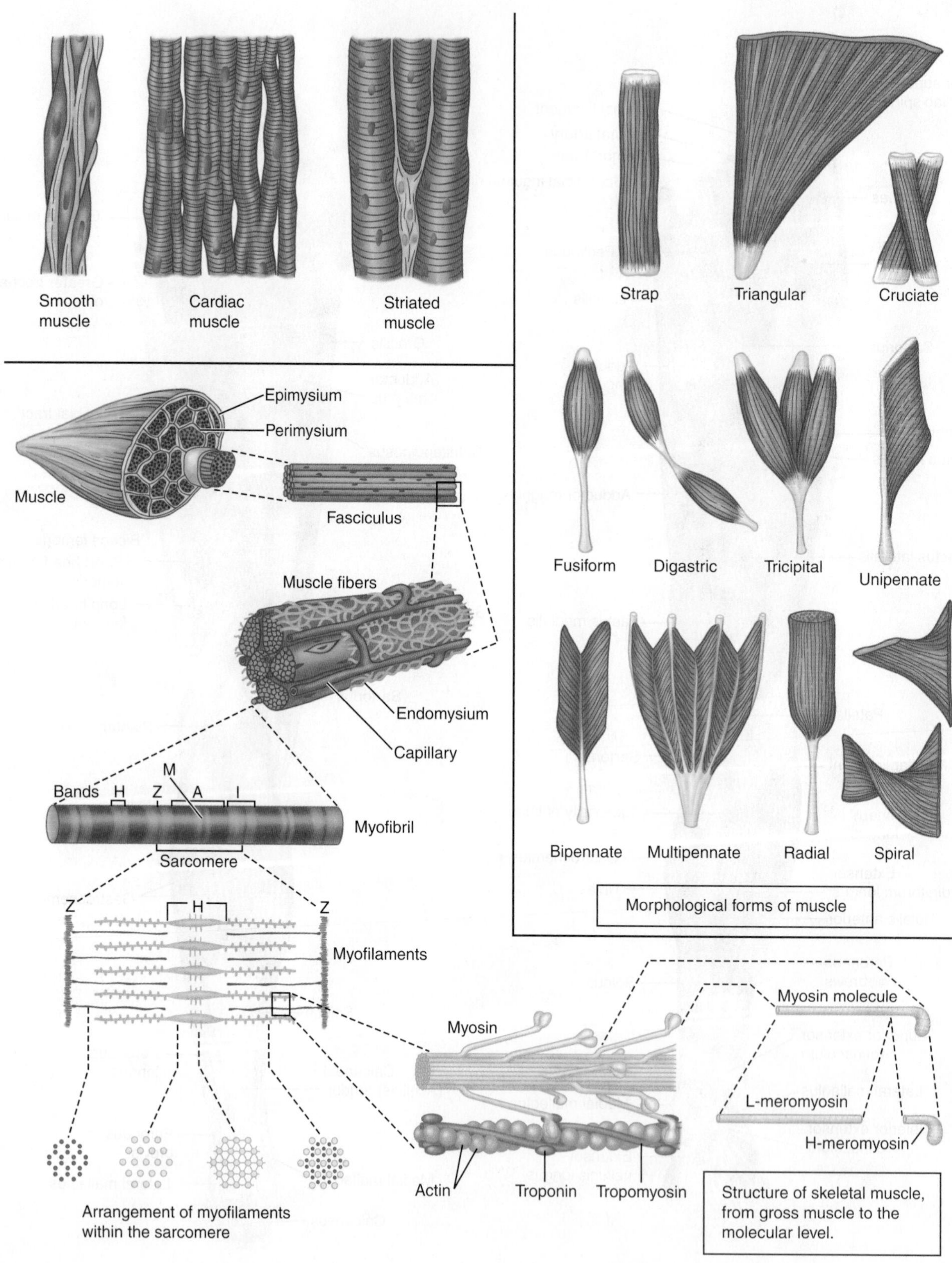

■ **PLATE 32**—TYPES AND STRUCTURE OF MUSCLE

agonistic m. a muscle opposed in action by another muscle (the *antagonistic muscle*). Called also *agonist.*
Albinus m. 1. musculus risorius. 2. musculus scalenus medius.
anconeus m. musculus anconeus.
anconeus m., lateral caput laterale musculi tricipitis brachii.
anconeus m., medial caput mediale musculi tricipitis brachii.
anconeus m., short caput laterale musculi tricipitis brachii.
anorectoperineal m's musculi anorectoperineales.
antagonistic m. a muscle that counteracts the action of another muscle (the *agonistic muscle*). Called also *antagonist.*
antigravity m's the muscles, mainly extensors of the knees, hips, and back, that by their tone resist the constant pull of gravity in the maintenance of normal posture.
antitragicus m., m. of antitragus musculus antitragicus.
appendicular m's the muscles of a limb.
arrector m. of hair, arrector pili m. musculus arrector pili.
articular m. musculus articularis.
articular m. of elbow musculus articularis cubiti.
articular m. of knee musculus articularis genus.
articularis cubiti m. musculus articularis cubiti.
articularis genus m. musculus articularis genus.
aryepiglottic m. pars aryepiglottica musculi arytenoidei obliqui.
arytenoid m., oblique musculus arytenoideus obliquus.
arytenoid m., transverse musculus arytenoideus transversus.
m's of auditory ossicles musculi ossiculorum auditoriorum.
auricular m's 1. the extrinsic auricular muscles; see *musculus auricularis anterior, posterior,* and *superior.* 2. musculi auriculares.
auricular m., anterior musculus auricularis anterior.
auricular m., oblique musculus obliquus auriculae.
auricular m., posterior musculus auricularis posterior.
auricular m., superior musculus auricularis superior.
auricular m., transverse musculus transversus auriculae.
Bell m. muscular strands between the ureteral orifices and the uvula vesicae in the male, marking the boundary of the trigone of the urinary bladder. Called also *ureteric bridge.*
biceps m. of arm, biceps brachii m. musculus biceps brachii.
biceps femoris m., biceps m. of thigh musculus biceps femoris.
bipennate m. musculus pennatus.
Bowman m. musculus ciliaris.
brachial m., brachialis m. musculus brachialis.
brachioradial m., brachioradialis m. musculus brachioradialis.
Braune m. musculus puborectalis.
bronchoesophageal m., bronchoesophageus m. musculus bronchooesophageus.
Brücke m. the longitudinal fibers of the ciliary muscle.
buccinator m. musculus buccinator.
buccopharyngeal m. pars buccopharyngea musculi constrictoris pharyngis superioris.
bulbocavernosus m., bulbocavernous m., bulbospongiosus m. musculus bulbospongiosus.
canine m. musculus levator anguli oris.
cardiac m. the muscle of the heart, comprising the chief component of the myocardium and lining the walls of the large vessels joined to the heart; it is composed of fibers of striated but involuntary muscle. The composition and organization of its fibers resemble those of skeletal muscle, but instead of forming a syncytium, its branched, mononucleate cells are linked end to end by intercalated disks that provide both mechanical and ionic coupling for coordination of the entire muscle. See Plate 32.
Casser m., casserian m. ligamentum mallei anterius.
ceratocricoid m. musculus ceratocricoideus.
ceratopharyngeal m. pars ceratopharyngea musculi constrictoris pharyngis medii.
cervical m's musculi colli.
Chassaignac axillary m. an occasional muscle bundle extending from the lower edge of the latissimus dorsi across the hollow of the axilla to the brachial fascia or to the lower border of the pectoralis minor.
chondroglossus m. musculus chondroglossus.
chondropharyngeal m. pars chondropharyngea musculi constrictoris pharyngis medii.
ciliary m. musculus ciliaris.
cleidohyoid m. a slip of muscle sometimes seen augmenting the sternohyoid muscle, extending from the hyoid bone to the clavicle.
coccygeal m. musculus ischiococcygeus.
compressor naris m., compressor m. of naris pars transversa musculi nasalis.
compressor urethrae m. musculus compressor urethrae.
congenerous m's muscles having a common action or function.
constrictor m. of pharynx, inferior musculus constrictor pharyngis inferior.
constrictor m. of pharynx, middle musculus constrictor pharyngis medius.
constrictor m. of pharynx, superior musculus constrictor pharyngis superior.
coracobrachial m., coracobrachialis m. musculus coracobrachialis.
corrugator m., superciliary, corrugator supercilii m. musculus corrugator supercilii.
Crampton m. the anterior portion of the ciliary muscle in birds.
cremaster m. musculus cremaster.
cricoarytenoid m., lateral musculus cricoarytenoideus lateralis.
cricoarytenoid m., posterior musculus cricoarytenoideus posterior.
cricopharyngeal m., cricopharyngeus m. pars cricopharyngea musculi constrictoris pharyngis inferioris.
cricothyroid m. musculus cricothyroideus.
cruciate m. a muscle in which the fiber bundles are arranged in the shape of an X. Called also musculus cruciatus.
cutaneous m. musculus cutaneus.
dartos m. musculus dartos; the term is also used more broadly to denote the tunica dartos (q.v.).
deltoid m. musculus deltoideus.
depressor m., superciliary musculus depressor supercilii.
depressor m. of angle of mouth, depressor anguli oris m. musculus depressor anguli oris.
depressor labii inferioris m., depressor m. of lower lip musculus depressor labii inferioris.
depressor m. of nasal septum musculus depressor septi nasi.
depressor septi nasi m., depressor m. of septum of nose musculus depressor septi nasi.
depressor supercilii m. musculus depressor supercilii.
detrusor m. of bladder, detrusor urinae m. musculus detrusor vesicae urinariae.
diaphragmatic m. diaphragma (def. 1).
digastric m. musculus digastricus.
dilator m. musculus dilatator.
dilator naris m., dilator m. of naris pars alaris musculi nasalis.
dilator m. of pupil, dilator pupillae m. musculus dilatator pupillae.
dorsal m's musculi dorsi.
double m. myofiber hyperplasia.
emergency m's muscles that ordinarily are not required to do something but that aid the prime movers when something is done that requires great force.
epicranial m., epicranius m. musculus epicranius.
epimeric m. a muscle derived from an epimere and innervated by a posterior ramus of a spinal nerve.
epitrochleoanconeus m. musculus epitrochleoanconaeus.
erector m. of penis musculus ischiocavernosus.
erector spinae m., erector m. of spine musculus erector spinae.
eustachian m. musculus tensor tympani.
m's of expression musculi faciei.
extensor carpi radialis brevis m. musculus extensor carpi radialis brevis.
extensor carpi radialis longus m. musculus extensor carpi radialis longus.
extensor carpi ulnaris m. musculus extensor carpi ulnaris.
extensor digiti minimi m. musculus extensor digiti minimi.
extensor digitorum m. musculus extensor digitorum.
extensor digitorum brevis m. musculus extensor digitorum brevis.
extensor digitorum longus m. musculus extensor digitorum longus.
extensor m. of digits, common, extensor m. of fingers musculus extensor digitorum.
extensor m. of fifth digit, proper musculus extensor digiti minimi.
extensor m. of great toe, long musculus extensor hallucis longus.
extensor m. of great toe, short musculus extensor hallucis brevis.
extensor hallucis brevis m. musculus extensor hallucis brevis.

extensor hallucis longus m. musculus extensor hallucis longus.
extensor m. of index finger, extensor indicis m. musculus extensor indicis.
extensor m. of little finger musculus extensor digiti minimi.
extensor pollicis brevis m. musculus extensor pollicis brevis.
extensor pollicis longus m. musculus extensor pollicis longus.
extensor m. of thumb, long musculus extensor pollicis longus.
extensor m. of thumb, short musculus extensor pollicis brevis.
extensor m. of toes, long musculus extensor digitorum longus.
extensor m. of toes, short musculus extensor digitorum brevis.
extensor m. of wrist, long radial musculus extensor carpi radialis longus.
extensor m. of wrist, short radial musculus extensor carpi radialis brevis.
extensor m. of wrist, ulnar musculus extensor carpi ulnaris.
extraocular m's musculi externi bulbi oculi.
extrinsic m. a muscle that does not originate in the same limb or part in which it is inserted.
m's of eye musculi externi bulbi oculi.
facial m's, m's of facial expression musculi faciei.
facial and masticatory m's musculi faciales et masticatores.
fast m. white m.
m's of fauces see *musculi palati mollis et faucium.*
femoral m. musculus vastus intermedius.
fibular m., long musculus fibularis longus.
fibular m., short musculus fibularis brevis.
fibular m., third musculus fibularis tertius.
fibularis brevis m. musculus fibularis brevis.
fibularis longus m. musculus fibularis longus.
fibularis tertius m. musculus fibularis tertius.
fixation m's, fixator m's accessory muscles that serve to steady a part.
flexor m., accessory musculus quadratus plantae.
flexor carpi radialis m. musculus flexor carpi radialis.
flexor carpi ulnaris m. musculus flexor carpi ulnaris.
flexor digiti minimi brevis m. of hand musculus flexor digiti minimi brevis manus.
flexor digiti minimi brevis m. of foot musculus flexor digiti minimi brevis pedis.
flexor digitorum brevis m. musculus flexor digitorum brevis.
flexor digitorum longus m. musculus flexor digitorum longus.
flexor digitorum profundus m. musculus flexor digitorum profundus.
flexor digitorum superficialis m. musculus flexor digitorum superficialis.
flexor m. of fingers, deep musculus flexor digitorum profundus.
flexor m. of fingers, superficial musculus flexor digitorum superficialis.
flexor m. of great toe, long musculus flexor hallucis longus.
flexor m. of great toe, short musculus flexor hallucis brevis.
flexor hallucis brevis m. musculus flexor hallucis brevis.
flexor hallucis longus m. musculus flexor hallucis longus.
flexor m. of little finger, short musculus flexor digiti minimi brevis manus.

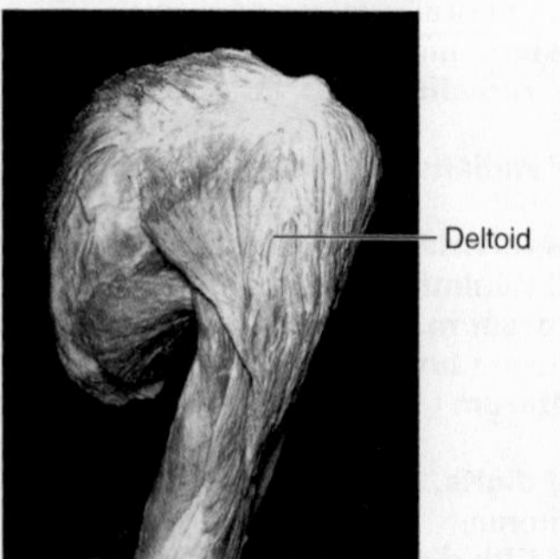

■ Extrinsic muscle exemplified by the deltoid muscle, which originates at the clavicle, acromion, and spine of the scapula and inserts into the deltoid tuberosity of the humerus.

flexor m. of little toe, short musculus flexor digiti minimi brevis pedis.
flexor pollicis brevis m. musculus flexor pollicis brevis.
flexor pollicis longus m. musculus flexor pollicis longus.
flexor m. of thumb, long musculus flexor pollicis longus.
flexor m. of thumb, short musculus flexor pollicis brevis.
flexor m. of toes, long musculus flexor digitorum longus.
flexor m. of toes, short musculus flexor digitorum brevis.
flexor m. of wrist, radial musculus flexor carpi radialis.
flexor m. of wrist, ulnar musculus flexor carpi ulnaris.
Folius m. ligamentum mallei laterale.
frontal m. venter frontalis musculi occipitofrontalis.
fusiform m. musculus fusiformis.
gastrocnemius m. musculus gastrocnemius.
gastrocnemius m., lateral caput laterale musculi gastrocnemii.
gastrocnemius m., medial caput mediale musculi gastrocnemii.
Gavard m. the oblique fibers of the muscular coat of the stomach (see *tunica muscularis gastrica*).
gemellus m., inferior musculus gemellus inferior.
gemellus m., superior musculus gemellus superior.
genioglossus m. musculus genioglossus.
geniohyoid m. musculus geniohyoideus.
glossopalatine m. musculus palatoglossus.
glossopharyngeal m. pars glossopharyngea musculi constrictoris pharyngis superioris.
gluteal m., greatest musculus gluteus maximus.
gluteal m., least musculus gluteus minimus.
gluteal m., middle musculus gluteus medius.
gluteus maximus m. musculus gluteus maximus.
gluteus medius m. musculus gluteus medius.
gluteus minimus m. musculus gluteus minimus.
gracilis m. musculus gracilis.
Guthrie m. see *musculus sphincter urethrae externus urethrae femininae* and *musculus sphincter urethrae externus urethrae masculinae.*
hamstring m's the muscles of the back of the thigh, including the biceps femoris, the semitendinosus, and the semimembranosus.
helicis major m. musculus helicis major.
helicis minor m. musculus helicis minor.
m. of helix, greater musculus helicis major.
m. of helix, lesser musculus helicis minor.
Hilton m. musculus aryepiglotticus.
Horner m. pars profunda partis palpebralis musculi orbicularis oculi.
Houston m. fibers of the bulbocavernosus muscle compressing the dorsal vein of the penis.
hyoglossal m., hyoglossus m. musculus hyoglossus.
m's of hyoid bone see *musculi infrahyoidei* and *musculi suprahyoidei.*
hypaxial m's the musculus longus capitis, musculus longus colli, the vertebral portion of the diaphragm, and the musculus sacrococcygeus anterior; called also *subvertebral m's.*
hypomeric m. a muscle derived from a hypomere and innervated by an anterior ramus of a spinal nerve.
hypothenar m's the intrinsic muscles of the little finger; flexing, abducting, and opposing it, and comprising the palmaris brevis, abductor digiti minimi, flexor digiti minimi brevis, and opponens digiti minimi.
iliac m., iliacus m. musculus iliacus.
iliococcygeal m., iliococcygeus m. musculus iliococcygeus.
iliocostal m. musculus iliocostalis.
iliocostal m. of neck musculus iliocostalis cervicis.
iliocostalis m. musculus iliocostalis.
iliocostalis cervicis m. musculus iliocostalis cervicis.
iliocostalis lumborum m. 1. musculus iliocostalis lumborum. 2. pars lumbalis musculi iliocostalis lumborum.
iliocostalis thoracis m. pars thoracica musculi iliocostalis lumborum.
iliopsoas m. musculus iliopsoas.
incisive m's of inferior lip musculi incisivi labii inferioris.
incisive m's of lower lip musculi incisivi labii inferioris.
incisive m's of superior lip musculi incisivi labii superioris.
incisive m's of upper lip musculi incisivi labii superioris.
infrahyoid m's musculi infrahyoidei.
infraspinatus m., infraspinous m. musculus infraspinatus.
inspiratory m's the muscles that act during inhalation, such as the diaphragm and the intercostal and pectoral muscles.

intercostal m's, external musculi intercostales externi.
intercostal m's, innermost musculi intercostales intimi.
intercostal m's, internal musculi intercostales interni.
interfoveolar m. ligamentum interfoveolare.
interossei m's, palmar musculi interossei palmares.
interossei m's, plantar musculi interossei plantares.
interossei m's of foot, dorsal musculi interossei dorsales pedis.
interossei m's of hand, dorsal musculi interossei dorsales manus.
interosseous m's, palmar musculi interossei palmares.
interosseous m's, plantar musculi interossei plantares.
interosseous m's, volar musculi interossei palmares.
interosseous m's of foot, dorsal musculi interossei dorsales pedis.
interosseous m's of hand, dorsal musculi interossei dorsales manus.
interspinal m's musculi interspinales.
interspinal m's, lumbar musculi interspinales lumborum.
interspinal m's of neck musculi interspinales cervicis.
interspinal m's of thorax musculi interspinales thoracis.
interspinales m's musculi interspinales.
interspinales cervicis m's musculi interspinales cervicis.
interspinales lumborum m's musculi interspinales lumborum.
interspinales thoracis m's musculi interspinales thoracis.
intertransversarii m's musculi intertransversarii.
intertransversarii m's, anterior cervical musculi intertransversarii anteriores cervicis.
intertransversarii m's, lateral lumbar musculi intertransversarii laterales lumborum.
intertransversarii m's, lateral posterior cervical musculi intertransversarii posteriores laterales cervicis.
intertransversarii m's, medial lumbar musculi intertransversarii mediales lumborum.
intertransversarii m's, medial posterior cervical musculi intertransversarii posteriores mediales cervicis.
intertransversarii m's, thoracic musculi intertransversarii thoracis.
intertransverse m's musculi intertransversarii.
intertransverse m's, lateral lumbar musculi intertransversarii laterales lumborum.
intertransverse m's, medial lumbar musculi intertransversarii mediales lumborum.
intertransverse m's of neck, anterior musculi intertransversarii anteriores cervicis.
intertransverse m's of neck, lateral posterior musculi intertransversarii posteriores laterales cervicis.
intertransverse m's of neck, medial posterior musculi intertransversarii posteriores mediales cervicis.
intertransverse m's of thorax musculi intertransversarii thoracis.
intra-auricular m's the stapedius and tensor tympani muscles.
intraocular m's the intrinsic muscles of the eyeball.
intrinsic m. a muscle that is contained (origin, belly, and insertion) in the same limb or structure.
involuntary m. a muscle that is not under the control of the will; the term includes both smooth muscle, composed of nonstriated fibers, as well as cardiac muscle, composed of striated fibers.
iridic m's the muscles controlling the iris.

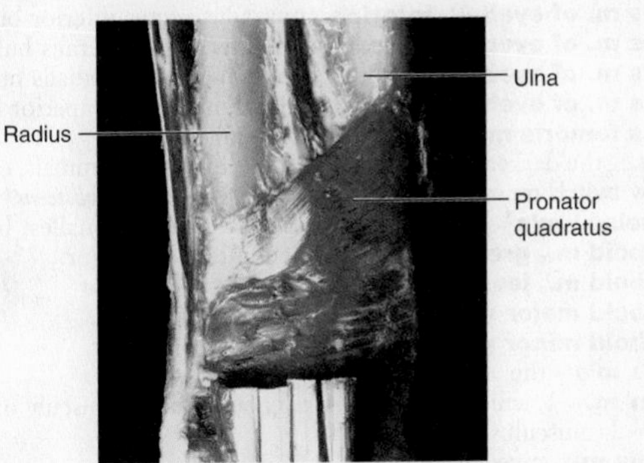

■ Intrinsic muscle exemplified by the pronator quadratus, which originates at the ulna and inserts into the radius.

ischiocavernosus m., ischiocavernous m. musculus ischiocavernosus.
ischiococcygeal m., ischiococcygeus m. musculus ischiococcygeus.
Jarjavay m. a muscle arising from the ramus of the ischium and inserting in the constrictor muscle of the vagina, which acts to depress the urethra.
Jung m. musculus pyramidalis auriculae.
Koyter m. musculus corrugator supercilii.
Landström m. minute muscle fibers in the fascia around and behind the eyeball, attached in front to the anterior orbital fascia and eyelids.
Langer m. muscular fibers from the insertion of the pectoralis major muscle over the bicipital groove to the insertion of the latissimus dorsi.
m's of larynx musculi laryngis.
latissimus dorsi m. musculus latissimus dorsi.
levator m. of angle of mouth, levator anguli oris m. musculus levator anguli oris.
levator ani m. musculus levator ani.
levatores costarum m's musculi levatores costarum.
levatores costarum breves m's musculi levatores costarum breves.
levatores costarum longi m's musculi levatores costarum longi.
levator glandulae thyroideae m. musculus levator glandulae thyroideae.
levator labii superioris m. musculus levator labii superioris.
levator labii superioris alaeque nasi m. musculus levator labii superioris alaeque nasi.
levator palpebrae superioris m. musculus levator palpebrae superioris.
levator m. of prostate musculus puboprostaticus.
levator m's of ribs musculi levatores costarum.
levator m's of ribs, long musculi levatores costarum longi.
levator m's of ribs, short musculi levatores costarum breves.
levator m. of scapula, levator scapulae m. musculus levator scapulae.
levator m. of thyroid gland musculus levator glandulae thyroideae.
levator m. of upper eyelid musculus levator palpebrae superioris.
levator m. of upper lip musculus levator labii superioris.
levator m. of upper lip and ala of nose musculus levator labii superioris alaeque nasi.
levator veli palatini m. musculus levator veli palatini.
lingual m's musculi linguae.
long m. of head musculus longus capitis.
long m. of neck musculus longus colli.
longissimus m. musculus longissimus.
longissimus m. of back musculus longissimus thoracis.
longissimus capitis m. musculus longissimus capitis.
longissimus cervicis m. musculus longissimus cervicis.
longissimus m. of head musculus longissimus capitis.
longissimus m. of neck musculus longissimus cervicis.
longissimus thoracis m., longissimus m. of thorax musculus longissimus thoracis.
longitudinal m. of tongue, inferior musculus longitudinalis inferior linguae.
longitudinal m. of tongue, superior musculus longitudinalis superior linguae.
longus capitis m. musculus longus capitis.
longus colli m. musculus longus colli.
m's of lower limb musculi membri inferioris.
lumbrical m's of foot musculi lumbricales pedis.
lumbrical m's of hand musculi lumbricales manus.
masseter m. musculus masseter.
m's of mastication, masticatory m's musculi masticatorii.
mentalis m. musculus mentalis.
Merkel m. musculus ceratocricoideus.
mesothenar m. musculus adductor pollicis.
Müller m. 1. fibrae circulares musculi ciliaris. 2. musculus orbitalis. 3. musculus tarsalis superior.
multifidus m's musculi multifidi.
multipennate m. musculus multipennatus.
mylohyoid m. musculus mylohyoideus.
mylopharyngeal m. pars mylopharyngea musculi constrictoris pharyngis superioris.
nasal m., nasalis m. musculus nasalis.

Muscle *Continued*

m's of neck musculi colli.
nonstriated m., nonstriated involuntary m. smooth m.
oblique m. of abdomen, external musculus obliquus externus abdominis.
oblique m. of abdomen, internal musculus obliquus internus abdominis.
oblique m. of auricle musculus obliquus auriculae.
oblique m. of eyeball, inferior musculus obliquus inferior bulbi.
oblique m. of eyeball, superior musculus obliquus superior bulbi.
oblique m. of head, inferior musculus obliquus capitis inferior.
oblique m. of head, superior musculus obliquus capitis superior.
obliquus capitis inferior m. musculus obliquus capitis inferior.
obliquus capitis superior m. musculus obliquus capitis superior.
obturator m., external, obturator externus m. musculus obturatorius externus.
obturator m., internal, obturator internus m. musculus obturatorius internus.
occipital m. venter occipitalis musculi occipitofrontalis.
occipitofrontal m., occipitofrontalis m. musculus occipitofrontalis.
ocular m's, oculorotatory m's musculi externi bulbi oculi.
Oddi m. musculus sphincter ampullae hepatopancreaticae.
Oehl m. muscle fibers in the chordae tendineae of the left atrioventricular valve.
omohyoid m. musculus omohyoideus.
opponens digiti minimi m. musculus opponens digiti minimi.
opponens pollicis m. musculus opponens pollicis.
opposing m. of little finger musculus opponens digiti minimi.
opposing m. of thumb musculus opponens pollicis.
orbicular m. musculus orbicularis.
orbicular m. of eye musculus orbicularis oculi.
orbicular m. of mouth musculus orbicularis oris.
orbicularis oculi m. musculus orbicularis oculi.
orbicularis oris m. musculus orbicularis oris.
orbital m., orbitalis m. musculus orbitalis.
organic m. visceral m.
m's of palate and fauces see *musculi palati mollis et faucium.*
palatine m's musculi palati mollis et faucium.
palatoglossus m. musculus palatoglossus.
palatopharyngeal m., palatopharyngeus m. musculus palatopharyngeus.
palmar m., long musculus palmaris longus.
palmar m., short musculus palmaris brevis.
palmaris brevis m. musculus palmaris brevis.
palmaris longus m. musculus palmaris longus.
papillary m's musculi papillares.
papillary m. of conus arteriosus a septal papillary muscle arising near the septal end of the supraventricular crest and attached to the anterior and septal cusps of the tricuspid valve.
papillary m. of left ventricle, anterior musculus papillaris anterior ventriculi sinistri.
papillary m. of left ventricle, posterior musculus papillaris posterior ventriculi sinistri.
papillary m. of right ventricle, anterior musculus papillaris anterior ventriculi dextri.
papillary m. of right ventricle, posterior musculus papillaris posterior ventriculi dextri.
papillary m's of right ventricle, septal several small papillary muscles in the right ventricle of the heart, arising from the interventricular septum and attaching to adjacent cusps of the tricuspid valve via chordae tendineae.
pectinate m's of left atrium musculi pectinati atrii sinistri.
pectinate m's of right atrium musculi pectinati atrii dextri.
pectineal m., pectineus m. musculus pectineus.
pectoral m., greater musculus pectoralis major.
pectoral m., smaller musculus pectoralis minor.
pectoralis major m. musculus pectoralis major.
pectoralis minor m. musculus pectoralis minor.
m's of pelvic diaphragm musculi diaphragmatis pelvis.
pennate m., penniform m. musculus pennatus.
perineal m's, m's of perineum musculi perinei.
peroneal m., long musculus fibularis longus.
peroneal m., short musculus fibularis brevis.
peroneal m., third musculus fibularis tertius.
pharyngeal m's musculi pharyngis.
pharyngopalatine m. musculus palatopharyngeus.
Phillips m. a muscular slip from the radial collateral ligament of the wrist and the styloid process of the radius to the phalanges.
piriform m., piriformis m. musculus piriformis.
plantar m., plantaris m. musculus plantaris.
platysma m. see *platysma.*
pleuroesophageal m., pleuroesophageus m. musculus pleurooesophageus.
popliteal m., popliteus m. musculus popliteus.
postaxial m. a muscle on the dorsal side of a limb.
preaxial m. a muscle on the ventral side of a limb.
procerus m. musculus procerus.
pronator m., quadrate musculus pronator quadratus.
pronator m., round musculus pronator teres.
pronator quadratus m. musculus pronator quadratus.
pronator teres m. musculus pronator teres.
psoas m., greater musculus psoas major.
psoas m., smaller musculus psoas minor.
psoas major m. musculus psoas major.
psoas minor m. musculus psoas minor.
pterygoid m., external musculus pterygoideus lateralis.
pterygoid m., internal musculus pterygoideus medialis.
pterygoid m., lateral musculus pterygoideus lateralis.
pterygoid m., medial musculus pterygoideus medialis.
pterygopharyngeal m. pars pterygopharyngea musculi constrictoris pharyngis superioris.
puboanal m., puboanalis m. musculus puboanalis.
pubococcygeal m., pubococcygeus m. musculus pubococcygeus.
puboperineal m., puboperinealis m. musculus puboperinealis.
puboprostatic m., puboprostaticus m. musculus puboprostaticus.
puborectal m., puborectalis m. musculus puborectalis.
pubovaginal m., pubovaginalis m. musculus pubovaginalis.
pubovesical m., pubovesicalis m. musculus pubovesicalis.
pyloric sphincter m. musculus sphincter pyloricus.
pyramidal m. musculus pyramidalis.
pyramidal m. of auricle musculus pyramidalis auriculae.
pyramidalis m. musculus pyramidalis.
quadrate m. musculus quadratus.
quadrate m. of sole musculus quadratus plantae.
quadrate m. of thigh, quadratus femoris m. musculus quadratus femoris.
quadratus lumborum m. musculus quadratus lumborum.
quadratus plantae m. musculus quadratus plantae.
quadriceps femoris m., quadriceps m. of thigh musculus quadriceps femoris.
rectococcygeal m., rectococcygeus m. musculus rectococcygeus.
rectourethral m's musculi anorectoperineales.
rectouterine m., rectouterinus m. musculus rectouterinus.
rectovesical m., rectovesicalis m. musculus rectovesicalis.
rectus abdominis m. musculus rectus abdominis.
rectus capitis anterior m. musculus rectus capitis anterior.
rectus capitis lateralis m. musculus rectus capitis lateralis.
rectus capitis posterior major m. musculus rectus capitis posterior major.
rectus capitis posterior minor m. musculus rectus capitis posterior minor.
rectus m. of eyeball, inferior musculus rectus inferior bulbi.
rectus m. of eyeball, lateral musculus rectus lateralis bulbi.
rectus m. of eyeball, medial musculus rectus medialis bulbi.
rectus m. of eyeball, superior musculus rectus superior bulbi.
rectus femoris m. musculus rectus femoris.
red m. the darker-colored muscle tissue of some mammals, composed of slow twitch muscle fibers. Called also *slow m.* Cf. *white m.*
Reisseisen m's the smooth muscle fibers of the smallest bronchi.
rhomboid m., greater musculus rhomboideus major.
rhomboid m., lesser musculus rhomboideus minor.
rhomboid major m. musculus rhomboideus major.
rhomboid minor m. musculus rhomboideus minor.
rider's m's the adductor muscles of the thigh.
Riolan m. 1. ciliary bundle of pars palpebralis musculi orbicularis oculi. 2. musculus cremaster.
risorius m. musculus risorius.
rotator m's musculi rotatores.
rotator m's, long musculi rotatores longi.

Muscle *Continued*

rotator m's, short musculi rotatores breves.
rotator m's of neck musculi rotatores cervicis.
rotator m's of thorax musculi rotatores thoracis.
rotatores m's musculi rotatores.
rotatores cervicis m's musculi rotatores cervicis.
rotatores lumborum m's musculi rotatores lumborum.
rotatores thoracis m's musculi rotatores thoracis.
Rouget m. the circular portion of the ciliary muscle.
Ruysch m. the muscular tissue of the fundus uteri.
sacrococcygeal m., anterior musculus sacrococcygeus ventralis.
sacrococcygeal m., dorsal musculus sacrococcygeus dorsalis.
sacrococcygeal m., posterior musculus sacrococcygeus dorsalis.
sacrococcygeal m., ventral musculus sacrococcygeus ventralis.
sacrospinal m. musculus erector spinae.
salpingopharyngeal m., salpingopharyngeus m. musculus salpingopharyngeus.
Santorini m. musculus risorius.
sartorius m. musculus sartorius.
scalene m., anterior musculus scalenus anterior.
scalene m., middle musculus scalenus medius.
scalene m., posterior musculus scalenus posterior.
scalene m., smallest musculus scalenus minimus.
scalenus anterior m. musculus scalenus anterior.
scalenus medius m. musculus scalenus medius.
scalenus minimus m. musculus scalenus minimus.
scalenus posterior m. musculus scalenus posterior.
Sébileau m. the deeper fibers of the musculus dartos.
semimembranosus m., semimembranous m. musculus semimembranosus.
semipennate m. musculus semipennatus.
semispinal m. musculus semispinalis.
semispinal m. of head musculus semispinalis capitis.
semispinal m. of neck musculus semispinalis cervicis.
semispinal m. of thorax musculus semispinalis thoracis.
semispinalis m. musculus semispinalis.
semispinalis capitis m. musculus semispinalis capitis.
semispinalis cervicis m. musculus semispinalis cervicis.
semispinalis thoracis m. musculus semispinalis thoracis.
semitendinosus m., semitendinous m. musculus semitendinosus.
serratus m., anterior musculus serratus anterior.
serratus m., inferior posterior musculus serratus posterior inferior.
serratus m., superior posterior musculus serratus posterior superior.
serratus anterior m. musculus serratus anterior.
serratus posterior inferior m. musculus serratus posterior inferior.
serratus posterior superior m. musculus serratus posterior superior.
Sibson m. musculus scalenus minimus.
skeletal m. any of the striated muscles that are attached to bones and typically cross at least one joint; they are under voluntary control and facilitate movement of the skeleton.
slow m. red m.
smooth m., smooth involuntary m. a type of muscle without transverse striations in its constituent fibers; it is found in the walls of the viscera and blood vessels and in the dermis and is not under voluntary control. See *muscle* and see Plate 32.
m's of soft palate and fauces musculi palati mollis et faucium.
soleus m. musculus soleus.
somatic m. skeletal m.
sphincter m. musculus sphincter.
sphincter m. of anus, external musculus sphincter ani externus.
sphincter m. of anus, internal musculus sphincter ani internus.
sphincter m. of bile duct musculus sphincter ductus choledochi.
sphincter m. of female urethra, external musculus sphincter urethrae externus urethrae femininae.
sphincter m. of hepatopancreatic ampulla musculus sphincter ampullae hepatopancreaticae.
sphincter m. of male urethra, external, sphincter m. of membranous urethra musculus sphincter urethrae externus urethrae masculinae.
sphincter m. of pancreatic duct musculus sphincter ductus pancreatici.
sphincter m. of pupil musculus sphincter pupillae.
sphincter m. of pylorus musculus sphincter pyloricus.
sphincter m. of urethra, sphincter urethrae m. see *musculus sphincter urethrae externus urethrae femininae* and *musculus sphincter urethrae externus urethrae masculinae.*
sphincter m. of urethra, internal, sphincter m. of urinary bladder musculus sphincter urethrae internus.
sphincter urethrovaginalis m. musculus sphincter urethrovaginalis.
spinal m. musculus spinalis.
spinal m. of head musculus spinalis capitis.
spinal m. of neck musculus spinalis cervicis.
spinal m. of thorax musculus spinalis thoracis.
spinalis m. musculus spinalis.
spinalis capitis m. musculus spinalis capitis.
spinalis cervicis m. musculus spinalis cervicis.
spinalis thoracis m. musculus spinalis thoracis.
splenius capitis m. musculus splenius capitis.
splenius cervicis m. musculus splenius cervicis.
splenius m. of head musculus splenius capitis.
splenius m. of neck musculus splenius cervicis.
stapedius m. musculus stapedius.
sternal m., sternalis m. musculus sternalis.
sternocleidomastoid m. musculus sternocleidomastoideus.
sternohyoid m. musculus sternohyoideus.
sternomastoid m. musculus sternocleidomastoideus.
sternothyroid m. musculus sternothyroideus.
strap m's musculi infrahyoidei.
striated m., striped m. a muscle whose fibers are divided by transverse bands into striations, including cardiac and skeletal muscle; the term is often used as a synonym for skeletal muscle. See *muscle* and see Plate 32.
striated involuntary m. cardiac m.
striated voluntary m. skeletal m.
styloglossus m. musculus styloglossus.
stylohyoid m. musculus stylohyoideus.
stylopharyngeal m., stylopharyngeus m. musculus stylopharyngeus.
subclavius m. musculus subclavius.
subcostal m's, subcostales m's musculi subcostales.
suboccipital m's musculi suboccipitales.
subscapular m., subscapularis m. musculus subscapularis.
subvertebral m's hypaxial m's.
supinator m. musculus supinator.
suprahyoid m's musculi suprahyoidei.
supraspinatus m., supraspinous m. musculus supraspinatus.
suspensory m. of duodenum musculus suspensorius duodeni.
synergic m's, synergistic m's muscles that assist one another in action.
tarsal m., inferior musculus tarsalis inferior.
tarsal m., superior musculus tarsalis superior.
temporal m., temporalis m. musculus temporalis.
temporoparietal m., temporoparietalis m. musculus temporoparietalis.
tensor m. of fascia lata, tensor fasciae latae m. musculus tensor fasciae latae.
tensor tympani m., tensor m. of tympanic membrane musculus tensor tympani.
tensor veli palatini m., tensor m. of velum palatinum musculus tensor veli palatini.
teres major m. musculus teres major.
teres minor m. musculus teres minor.
m. of terminal notch musculus incisurae terminalis.
Theile m. musculus transversus perinei superficialis.
thenar m's the abductor and flexor muscles of the thumb.
thyroarytenoid m. musculus thyroarytenoideus.
thyroepiglottic m. pars thyroepiglottica musculi thyroarytenoidei.
thyrohyoid m. musculus thyrohyoideus.
thyropharyngeal m., thyropharyngeus m. pars thyropharyngea musculi constrictoris pharyngis inferioris.
tibial m., anterior musculus tibialis anterior.
tibial m., posterior musculus tibialis posterior.
tibialis anterior m. musculus tibialis anterior.
tibialis posterior m. musculus tibialis posterior.
m's of tongue musculi linguae.
tracheal m., trachealis m. musculus trachealis.

Muscle *Continued*

trachelomastoid m. musculus longissimus capitis.
tragicus m., m. of tragus musculus tragicus.
transverse abdominal m. musculus transversus abdominis.
transverse m. of auricle musculus transversus auriculae.
transverse m. of chin musculus transversus menti.
transverse m. of nape musculus transversus nuchae.
transverse perineal m., deep musculus transversus perinei profundus.
transverse perineal m., superficial musculus transversus perinei superficialis.
transverse m. of thorax musculus transversus thoracis.
transverse m. of tongue musculus transversus linguae.
transversospinal m's, transversospinales m's musculi transversospinales.
transversus abdominis m. musculus transversus abdominis.
transversus menti m. musculus transversus menti.
transversus nuchae m. musculus transversus nuchae.
transversus thoracis m. musculus transversus thoracis.
trapezius m. musculus trapezius.
m. of Treitz musculus suspensorius duodeni.
triangular m. musculus triangularis.
triceps m. of arm, triceps brachii m. musculus triceps brachii.
triceps m. of calf, triceps surae m. musculus triceps surae.
trigonal m's musculi trigoni vesicae urinariae.
trigonal m., deep musculus trigoni vesicae urinariae profundus.
trigonal m., superficial musculus trigoni vesicae urinariae superficialis.
unipennate m. musculus semipennatus.
unstriated m. smooth m.
m's of upper limb musculi membri superioris.
m's of urogenital diaphragm the muscles considered to participate in the urogenital diaphragm (see under *diaphragm*).
m. of uvula musculus uvulae.
vastus intermedius m. musculus vastus intermedius.
vastus lateralis m. musculus vastus lateralis.
vastus medialis m. musculus vastus medialis.
vertical m. of tongue musculus verticalis linguae.
vestigial m. a muscle that was once well developed but through evolution has become rudimentary.
visceral m. muscle fibers associated chiefly with the hollow viscera and largely of splanchnic mesodermal origin; except for the striated fibers in the wall of the heart, they are smooth muscle fibers bound together by reticular fibers.
vocal m., vocalis m. musculus vocalis.
voluntary m. any muscle that normally is under the control of the will, i.e., a skeletal muscle (q.v.).
white m. the paler-colored muscle tissue of some mammals, composed of fast twitch muscle fibers. Called also *fast m.* Cf. *red m.*
Wilson m. see *musculus sphincter urethrae externus urethrae femininae* and *musculus sphincter urethrae externus urethrae masculinae.*
yoked m's muscles that normally act simultaneously and equally, as in moving the eyes.
zygomatic m., zygomatic m., greater musculus zygomaticus major.
zygomatic m., lesser musculus zygomaticus minor.
zygomaticus major m. musculus zygomaticus major.
zygomaticus minor m. musculus zygomaticus minor.

mus•cle phos•pho•fruc•to•ki•nase (mus′əl fos″fo-frook″to-ki′nās) the muscle isozyme of 6-phosphofructokinase.

mus•cle phos•pho•fruc•to•ki•nase de•fi•cien•cy (mus′əl fos″fo-frook″to-ki′nās) glycogen storage disease, type VII.

mus•cle phos•phor•y•lase (mus′əl fos-for′ə-lās) the muscle isozyme of glycogen phosphorylase.

mus•cle phos•phor•y•lase de•fi•cien•cy (mus′əl fos-for′ə-lās) glycogen storage disease, type V.

mus•cu•lam•ine (mus″ku-lam′in) a base isolated from hydrolyzed calf's muscle; it is the same as spermine.

mus•cu•lar (mus′ku-lər) [L. *muscularis*] 1. pertaining to, composed of, or composing muscle. 2. having a well-developed musculature.

mus•cu•la•ris (mus″ku-lar′is) [L.] 1. muscular. 2. pertaining to a muscular layer or coat; see *tunica muscularis* and *lamina muscularis mucosae.*
  m. exter′na tunica muscularis.
  m. muco′sae lamina muscularis mucosae.
  m. mucosae of esophagus lamina muscularis mucosae oesophagi.
  m. mucosae of large intestine lamina muscularis mucosae intestini crassi.
  m. mucosae of small intestine lamina muscularis mucosae intestini tenuis.
  m. mucosae of stomach lamina muscularis mucosae gastrica.

mus•cu•lar•i•ty (mus″ku-lar′ĭ-te) the condition or quality of being muscular.

mus•cu•lar•ize (mus′ku-lər-īz) to change into muscle tissue.

mus•cu•la•ture (mus′ku-lə-chər) the muscular apparatus of the body, or of any part of it.

mus•cu•li (mus′ku-li) [L.] genitive and plural of *musculus.*

mus•cu•lo•apo•neu•rot•ic (mus″ku-lo-ap′o-nōō-rot′ik) pertaining to a muscle and its aponeurosis.

mus•cu•lo•cu•ta•ne•ous (mus″ku-lo″ku-ta′ne-əs) pertaining to, composed of, or supplying both muscles and skin. Called also *myocutaneous.*

mus•cu•lo•der•mic (mus″ku-lo-dur′mik) musculocutaneous.

mus•cu•lo•elas•tic (mus″ku-lo-e-las′tik) composed of muscular and elastic tissue.

mus•cu•lo•in•tes•ti•nal (mus″ku-lo-in-tes′tĭ-nəl) pertaining to the muscles and the intestines.

mus•cu•lo•mem•bra•nous (mus″ku-lo-mem′brə-nəs) [*musculus* + *membranous*] both muscular and membranous.

mus•cu•lo•phren•ic (mus″ku-lo-fren′ik) [*muscular* + *phrenic*] pertaining to or supplying both the diaphragm and the adjoining muscles.

mus•cu•lo•skel•e•tal (mus″ku-lo-skel′ə-təl) pertaining to or comprising the skeleton and the muscles, as musculoskeletal system.

mus•cu•lo•spi•ral (mus″ku-lo-spi′rəl) [*musculus* + *spiral*] pertaining to muscles and having a spiral direction, as the nervus radialis.

mus•cu•lo•ten•di•nous (mus″ku-lo-ten′dĭ-nəs) pertaining to or composed of muscle and tendon.

mus•cu•lus (mus′ku-ləs) gen. and pl. *mus′culi* [L., dim. of *mus* mouse, because of a fancied resemblance to a mouse moving under the skin] 1. muscle. 2. [TA] *(in the pl.)* muscular system: in official terminology, the muscles (generally restricted to the skeletal muscles), bursae, and synovial sheaths considered collectively. Called also *systema musculare* [TA alternative].

Musculus

The names occurring here are often used without the word *musculus,* e.g., *rectus abdominis* for *musculus rectus abdominis.*

mus′culi abdo′minis [TA] the muscles of the abdomen.
m. abduc′tor dig′iti min′imi ma′nus [TA] abductor muscle of little finger: *origin,* pisiform bone, flexor carpi ulnaris tendon; *insertion,* medial surface of base of proximal phalanx of little finger; *innervation,* ulnar; *action,* abducts little finger.
m. abduc′tor dig′iti min′imi pe′dis [TA] abductor muscle of little toe: *origin,* medial and lateral tubercles of calcaneus, plantar fascia; *insertion,* lateral surface of base of proximal phalanx of little toe; *innervation,* superficial branch of lateral plantar; *action,* abducts little toe.

Musculus *Continued*

m. abduc′tor hal′lucis [TA] abductor muscle of great toe: *origin*, medial tubercle of calcaneus, plantar fascia; *insertion*, medial surface of base of proximal phalanx of great toe; *innervation*, medial plantar; *action*, abducts, flexes great toe.
m. abduc′tor pol′licis bre′vis [TA] short abductor muscle of thumb: *origin*, scaphoid, ridge of trapezium, flexor retinaculum of hand; *insertion*, lateral surface of base of proximal phalanx of thumb; *innervation*, median; *action*, abducts thumb.
m. abduc′tor pol′licis lon′gus [TA] long abductor muscle of thumb: *origin*, posterior surfaces of radius and ulna; *insertion*, radial side of base of first metacarpal bone; *innervation*, posterior interosseous; *action*, abducts, extends thumb.
m. adduc′tor bre′vis [TA] short adductor muscle: *origin*, outer surface of body and inferior ramus of pubis; *insertion*, upper part of linea aspera of femur; *innervation*, obturator; *action*, adducts, rotates, flexes thigh.
m. adduc′tor hal′lucis [TA] adductor muscle of great toe (2 heads): *origin*, OBLIQUE HEAD—bases of second, third, and fourth metatarsals, and sheath of peroneus longus, TRANSVERSE HEAD—capsules of metatarsophalangeal joints of three lateral toes; *insertion*, lateral side of base of proximal phalanx of great toe; *innervation*, lateral plantar; *action*, adducts great toe.
m. adduc′tor lon′gus [TA] long adductor muscle: *origin*, crest and symphysis of pubis; *insertion*, linea aspera of femur; *innervation*, obturator; *action*, adducts, rotates, flexes thigh.
m. adduc′tor mag′nus [TA] great adductor muscle (2 parts): *origin*, DEEP PART—inferior ramus of pubis, ramus of ischium, SUPERFICIAL PART—ischial tuberosity; *insertion*, DEEP PART—linea aspera of femur, SUPERFICIAL PART—adductor tubercle of femur; *innervation*, DEEP PART—obturator, SUPERFICIAL PART—sciatic; *action*, DEEP PART—adducts thigh, SUPERFICIAL PART—extends thigh.
m. adduc′tor mi′nimus [TA] smallest adductor muscle: a name given the anterior portion of the adductor magnus muscle; *insertion*, ischium, body and ramus of pubis; *innervation*, obturator and sciatic; *action*, adducts thigh.
m. adduc′tor pol′licis [TA] adductor muscle of thumb (2 heads): *origin*, CAPUT OBLIQUUM—sheath of flexor carpi radialis, palmar ligaments of carpus, capitate bone, and bases of second and third metacarpals, CAPUT TRANSVERSUM—lower two thirds of anterior surface of third metacarpal; *insertion*, medial surface of base of proximal phalanx of thumb; *innervation*, ulnar; *action*, adducts, opposes thumb.
m. ancone′us [TA] anconeus muscle: *origin*, back of lateral epicondyle of humerus; *insertion*, olecranon and posterior surface of ulna; *innervation*, radial; *action*, extends forearm.
mus′culi anorectoperinea′les [TA] anorectoperineal muscles: bands of smooth muscle fibers extending from the perineal flexure of the rectum to the membranous urethra in the male. Called also *musculi rectourethrales* [TA alternative].
m. antitra′gicus [TA] antitragicus muscle: *origin*, outer part of antitragus; *insertion*, caudate process of helix and antihelix; *innervation*, temporal and posterior auricular.
m. arrec′tor pi′li [TA] arrector pili muscle: a type of tiny smooth muscle of the skin whose contraction causes the hair to stand erect with cutis anserina (goose flesh). *origin*, papillary layer of dermis; *insertion*, a hair follicle; *innervation*, sympathetic; *action*, elevate a hair on the skin.
m. articula′ris articular muscle: a muscle that is attached at one end to the synovial capsule of a joint.
m. articula′ris cu′biti [TA] articular muscle of elbow: a few fibers of the deep surface of the triceps brachii that insert into the posterior ligament and synovial membrane of the elbow joint.
m. articula′ris ge′nus [TA] articular muscle of knee: *origin*, distal fourth of anterior surface of shaft of femur; *insertion*, synovial membrane of knee joint; *innervation*, femoral; *action*, lifts capsule of knee joint.
m. aryepiglot′ticus pars aryepiglottica musculi arytenoidei obliqui.
m. arytenoi′deus obli′quus [TA] oblique arytenoid muscle: one of the intrinsic muscles of the larynx; *origin*, dorsal aspect of muscular process of arytenoid cartilage; *insertion*, apex of opposite arytenoid cartilage; *innervation*, recurrent laryngeal; *action*, closes inlet of larynx.
m. arytenoi′deus transver′sus [TA] transverse arytenoid muscle: one of the intrinsic muscles of the larynx; *origin*, dorsal aspect of muscular process of arytenoid cartilage; *insertion*, dorsal aspect of muscular process of opposite arytenoid cartilage; *innervation*, recurrent laryngeal; *action*, approximates arytenoid cartilages.
mus′culi auricula′res auricular muscles: the intrinsic auricular muscles that extend from one part of the auricle to another, including the helicis major and minor, tragicus, antitragicus, transversus auricularis, and obliquus auricularis.
m. auricula′ris ante′rior [TA] anterior auricular muscle: *origin*, superficial temporal fascia; *insertion*, cartilage of ear; *innervation*, facial; *action*, draws the auricle forward.
m. auricula′ris poste′rior [TA] posterior auricular muscle: *origin*, mastoid process; *insertion*, cartilage of ear; *innervation*, facial; *action*, draws auricle backward.
m. auricula′ris supe′rior [TA] superior auricular muscle: *origin*, galea aponeurotica; *insertion*, cartilage of ear; *innervation*, facial; *action*, raises auricle.
m. bi′ceps bra′chii [TA] biceps muscle of arm (2 heads): *origin*, CAPUT LONGUM—upper border of glenoid cavity, CAPUT BREVE—apex of coracoid process; *insertion*, radial tuberosity and fascia of forearm; *innervation*, musculocutaneous; *action*, flexes forearm, supinates hand.
m. bi′ceps fe′moris [TA] biceps muscle of thigh (2 heads): *origin*, LONG HEAD—ischial tuberosity, SHORT HEAD—linea aspera of femur; *insertion*, head of fibula, lateral condyle of tibia; *innervation*, LONG HEAD—tibial, SHORT HEAD—peroneal, popliteal; *action*, flexes leg, extends thigh.
m. bipenna′tus TA alternative for *musculus pennatus*.
m. brachia′lis [TA] brachial muscle: *origin*, anterior surface of humerus; *insertion*, coronoid process of ulna; *innervation*, radial, musculocutaneous; *action*, flexes forearm.
m. brachioradia′lis [TA] brachioradial muscle: *origin*, lateral supracondylar ridge of humerus; *insertion*, lower end of radius; *innervation*, radial; *action*, flexes forearm.
m. bronchoesopha′geus [TA] bronchoesophageal muscle: a name given muscular fasciculi that arise from the wall of the left bronchus and reinforce muscles of the esophagus.
m. buccina′tor [TA] buccinator muscle: *origin*, buccinator ridge of mandible, alveolar process of maxilla, pterygomandibular ligament; *insertion*, orbicularis oris at angle of mouth; *innervation*, buccal branch of facial; *action*, compresses cheek and retracts angle of the mouth.
m. buccopharyn′geus pars buccopharyngea musculi constrictoris pharyngis superioris.
mus′culi bul′bi musculi externi bulbi oculi.
m. bulbocaverno′sus m. bulbospongiosus.
m. bulbospongio′sus [TA] bulbospongiosus muscle: *origin*, central point of perineum, median raphe of bulb; *insertion*, fascia of penis (male) or clitoris (female); *innervation*, pudendal; *action*, constricts spongy urethra in males and vaginal orifice in females, contributes to erection of penis or clitoris. Called also *bulbocavernosus* or *bulbocavernous muscle*.
mus′culi ca′pitis [TA] the muscles of the head.
m. ceratocricoi′deus [TA] ceratocricoid muscle: a name given a muscular fasciculus arising from the cricoid cartilage and inserted on the inferior cornu of the thyroid cartilage, considered one of the intrinsic muscles of the larynx.
m. ceratopharyn′geus pars ceratopharyngea musculi constrictoris pharyngis medii.
mus′culi cer′vicis TA alternative for *musculi colli*.
m. chondroglos′sus [TA] chondroglossus muscle: *origin*, medial side and base of lesser cornu of hyoid bone; *insertion*, substance of tongue; *innervation*, hypoglossal; *action*, depresses, retracts tongue.
m. chondropharyn′geus pars chondropharyngea musculi constrictoris pharyngis medii.
m. cilia′ris [TA] ciliary muscle: *origin*, scleral spur; *insertion*, outer layers of choroid and ciliary processes; *innervation*, oculomotor, parasympathetic; *action*, affects shape of lens in visual accommodation.
m. coccy′geus TA alternative for *m. ischiococcygeus*.
mus′culi col′li [TA] the muscles of the neck, including the sternocleidomastoid and the longus colli, and the suprahyoid, infrahyoid, and scalene muscles. Called also *cervical muscles* and *musculi cervicis* [TA alternative].
m. compres′sor na′ris pars transversa musculi nasalis.
m. compres′sor ure′thrae [TA] compressor muscle of urethra (occurs only in females): *origin*, ischiopubic ramus on each side; *insertion*, blends with its partner on the other side anterior to the urethra below the external urethral sphincter; *innervation*, perineal branches of pudendal; *action*, accessory urethral sphincter.
m. constric′tor pharyn′gis infe′rior [TA] inferior constrictor muscle of pharynx: *origin*, undersurfaces of cricoid and thyroid

cartilages; *insertion*, median raphe of posterior wall of pharynx; *innervation*, glossopharyngeal, pharyngeal plexus, rami of superior laryngeal and recurrent laryngeal; *action*, constricts pharynx. It is divided into a cricopharyngeal part and a thyropharyngeal part (*pars cricopharyngea* and *pars thyropharyngea*).

m. constric′tor pharyn′gis me′dius [TA] middle constrictor muscle of pharynx: *origin*, cornua of hyoid and stylohyoid ligament; *insertion*, median raphe of posterior wall of pharynx; *innervation*, pharyngeal plexus of vagus and glossopharyngeal; *action*, constricts pharynx. It is divided into a ceratopharyngeal part and a chondropharyngeal part (*pars ceratopharyngea* and *pars chondropharyngea*).

m. constric′tor pharyn′gis supe′rior [TA] superior constrictor muscle of pharynx: *origin*, medial pterygoid plate, pterygomandibular raphe, mylohyoid ridge of mandible, and mucous membrane of floor of mouth; *insertion*, median raphe of posterior wall of pharynx; *innervation*, pharyngeal plexus of vagus; *action*, constricts pharynx. It is divided into buccopharyngeal, glossopharyngeal, mylopharyngeal, and pterygopharyngeal parts (*pars buccopharyngea, pars glossopharyngea, pars mylopharyngea*, and *pars pterygopharyngea*).

m. coracobrachia′lis [TA] coracobrachial muscle: *origin*, coracoid process of scapula; *insertion*, medial surface of shaft of humerus; *innervation*, musculocutaneous; *action*, flexes, adducts arm.

m. corruga′tor superci′lii [TA] superciliary corrugator muscle: *origin*, medial end of superciliary arch; *insertion*, skin of eyebrow; *innervation*, facial; *action*, draws eyebrow downward and medially. Called also *Koyter muscle*.

m. cremas′ter [TA] cremaster muscle: *origin*, inferior margin of internal oblique muscle of abdomen; *insertion*, pubic tubercle; *innervation*, genital branch of genitofemoral; *action*, elevates testis.

m. cricoarytenoi′deus latera′lis [TA] lateral cricoarytenoid muscle: one of the intrinsic muscles of the larynx; *origin*, lateral surface of cricoid cartilage; *insertion*, muscular process of arytenoid cartilage; *innervation*, recurrent laryngeal; *action*, approximates vocal folds.

m. cricoarytenoi′deus poste′rior [TA] posterior cricoarytenoid muscle: one of the intrinsic muscles of the larynx; *origin*, back of cricoid cartilage; *insertion*, muscular process of arytenoid cartilage; *innervation*, recurrent laryngeal; *action*, separates vocal folds.

m. cricopharyn′geus TA alternative for *pars cricopharyngea musculi constrictoris pharyngis inferioris*.

m. cricothyroi′deus [TA] cricothyroid muscle: one of the intrinsic muscles of the larynx; *origin*, front and side of cricoid cartilage; *insertion*, lamina of thyroid cartilage; *innervation*, external ramus of superior laryngeal; *action*, tenses vocal folds.

m. crucia′tus cruciate muscle.

m. cuta′neus [TA] cutaneous muscle: striated muscle that inserts into the skin, such as the platysma.

m. dar′tos dartos muscle: the nonstriated muscle fibers of the tunica dartos, the deeper layers of which help to form the septum of the scrotum. Called also *dartos*.

m. deltoi′deus [TA] deltoid muscle: *origin*, clavicle, acromion, spine of scapula; *insertion*, deltoid tuberosity of humerus; *innervation*, axillary; *action*, abducts, flexes, extends arm.

m. depres′sor an′guli o′ris [TA] depressor muscle of angle of mouth: *origin*, lower border of mandible; *insertion*, angle of mouth; *innervation*, facial; *action*, pulls down angle of mouth.

m. depres′sor la′bii inferio′ris [TA] depressor muscle of lower lip: *origin*, anterior portion of lower border of mandible; *insertion*, orbicularis oris and skin of lower lip; *innervation*, facial; *action*, depresses lower lip.

m. depres′sor sep′ti na′si [TA] depressor muscle of nasal septum: *origin*, incisor fossa of maxilla; *insertion*, ala and septum of nose; *innervation*, facial; *action*, contracts nostril and depresses ala. Called also *depressor muscle of septum of nose* and *depressor septi nasi muscle*.

m. depres′sor superci′lii [TA] superciliary depressor muscle: a name given a few fibers of the orbital part of the orbicularis oculi muscle that are inserted in the eyebrow, which they depress.

m. detru′sor vesi′cae urina′riae detrusor muscle of bladder: the bundles of smooth muscle fibers forming the muscular coat of the urinary bladder, which are arranged in a longitudinal and a circular layer and, on contraction, serve to expel urine. Called also *detrusor urinae* and *detrusor urinae muscle*.

mus′culi diaphrag′matis pel′vis the muscles of the pelvic diaphragm.

m. digas′tricus [TA] digastric muscle: *origin*, VENTER ANTERIOR—digastric fossa on deep surface of inferior border of mandible near symphysis, VENTER POSTERIOR—mastoid notch of temporal bone; *insertion*, intermediate tendon on hyoid bone; *innervation*, VENTER ANTERIOR—mylohyoid, VENTER POSTERIOR—digastric branch of facial; *action*, elevates hyoid bone, lowers jaw.

m. dilata′tor [TA] dilator muscle: a general term for a muscle that dilates; called also *dilator*.

m. dilata′tor pupil′lae [TA] dilator pupillae muscle: a name given to fibers extending radially from the sphincter pupillae to the ciliary margin; *innervation*, sympathetic; *action*, dilates iris.

m. dila′tor na′ris pars alaris musculi nasalis.

mus′culi dor′si [TA] dorsal muscles: the muscles of the back.

m. epicra′nius [TA] epicranial muscle: a name given the muscular covering of the scalp, including the occipitofrontalis and temporoparietalis muscles, and the galea aponeurotica.

m. epitrochleoancone′us epitrochleoanconeus muscle: an occasional band of fibers originating at the back of the medial condyle of the humerus and inserting on the medial side of the olecranon process, innervated by a branch of the ulnar nerve.

m. erec′tor spi′nae [TA] erector muscle of spine: a name given the fibers of the more superficial of the deep muscles of the back, originating from the sacrum, spines of the lumbar and the eleventh and twelfth thoracic vertebrae, and the iliac crest, which split and insert as the musculi iliocostalis, longissimus, and spinalis (qq.v.).

m. exten′sor car′pi radia′lis bre′vis [TA] short radial extensor muscle of wrist: *origin*, lateral epicondyle of humerus, *insertion*, base of third metacarpal bone; *innervation*, deep branch of radial; *action*, extends and abducts wrist joint.

m. exten′sor car′pi radia′lis lon′gus [TA] long radial extensor muscle of wrist: *origin*, lateral supracondylar ridge of humerus; *insertion*, base of second metacarpal bone; *innervation*, radial; *action*, extends and abducts wrist joint.

m. exten′sor car′pi ulna′ris [TA] ulnar extensor muscle of wrist (2 heads): *origin*, CAPUT HUMERALE—lateral epicondyle of humerus, CAPUT ULNARE—posterior border of ulna; *insertion*, base of fifth metacarpal bone; *innervation*, deep branch of radial; *action*, extends and adducts wrist joint.

m. exten′sor di′giti mi′nimi [TA] extensor muscle of little finger: *origin*, common extensor tendon and adjacent intermuscular septa; *insertion*, extensor expansion of little finger; *innervation*, deep branch of radial; *action*, extends little finger.

m. exten′sor di′giti quin′ti pro′prius m. extensor digiti minimi.

m. exten′sor digito′rum [TA] extensor muscle of fingers: *origin*, lateral epicondyle of humerus; *insertion*, extensor expansion of each (nonthumb) finger; *innervation*, posterior interosseus; *action*, extends wrist joint and phalanges.

m. exten′sor digito′rum bre′vis [TA] short extensor muscle of toes: *origin*, superior surface of calcaneus; *insertion*, tendons of extensor digitorum longus of first, second, third, and fourth toes; *innervation*, deep peroneal; *action*, extends toes.

m. exten′sor digito′rum lon′gus [TA] long extensor muscle of toes: *origin*, anterior surface of fibula, lateral condyle of tibia, interosseous membrane; *insertion*, extensor expansion of each of the four lateral toes; *innervation*, deep peroneal; *action*, extends toes.

m. exten′sor hal′lucis bre′vis [TA] short extensor muscle of great toe: a name given the portion of the extensor digitorum brevis muscle that goes to the great toe.

m. exten′sor hal′lucis lon′gus [TA] long extensor muscle of great toe: *origin*, front of fibula and interosseous membrane; *insertion*, dorsal surface of base of distal phalanx of great toe; *innervation*, deep peroneal; *action*, dorsiflexes ankle joint, extends great toe.

m. exten′sor in′dicis [TA] extensor muscle of index finger: *origin*, posterior surface of body of ulna, interosseous membrane; *insertion*, extensor expansion of index finger; *innervation*, posterior interosseous; *action*, extends index finger.

m. exten′sor in′dicis pro′prius m. extensor indicis.

m. exten′sor pol′licis bre′vis [TA] short extensor muscle of thumb: *origin*, posterior surface of radius and interosseous membrane; *insertion*, dorsolateral base of proximal phalanx of thumb; *innervation*, posterior interosseous; *action*, extends thumb.

m. exten′sor pol′licis lon′gus [TA] long extensor muscle of thumb: *origin*, posterior surface of ulna and interosseous membrane; *insertion*,

base of distal phalanx of thumb; *innervation*, posterior interosseous; *action*, extends thumb, adducts and rotates thumb laterally.
mus′culi exter′ni bul′bi o′culi [TA] extraocular muscles: the six voluntary muscles that move the eyeball, including the superior, inferior, middle, and lateral recti, and the superior and inferior oblique muscles. Called also *musculi bulbi*, *muscles of eye*, and *ocular muscles*.
mus′culi extremita′tis inferio′ris musculi membri inferioris.
mus′culi extremita′tis superio′ris musculi membri superioris.
mus′culi facia′les, mus′culi facie′i [TA] facial muscles: a group of cutaneous muscles of the facial structures, which includes the muscles of the scalp, ear, eyelids, nose, and mouth, and the platysma; called also *muscles of expression* and *muscles of facial expression*.
m. fibula′ris bre′vis [TA] short peroneal muscle: *origin*, lateral surface of fibula; *insertion*, tuberosity on base of fifth metatarsal bone; *innervation*, superficial peroneal; *action*, everts, abducts, plantar flexes foot. Called also *m. peroneus brevis* [TA alternative].
m. fibula′ris lon′gus [TA] long peroneal muscle: *origin*, lateral condyle of tibia, head and lateral surface of fibula; *insertion*, medial cuneiform, first metatarsal; *innervation*, superficial peroneal; *action*, abducts, everts, plantar flexes foot. Called also *m. peroneus longus* [TA alternative].
m. fibula′ris ter′tius [TA] third peroneal muscle: *origin*, anterior surface of fibula, interosseous membrane; *insertion*, base of fifth metatarsal; *innervation*, deep peroneal; *action*, everts, dorsiflexes foot. Called also *m. peroneus tertius* [TA alternative].
m. flex′or accesso′rius TA alternative for *m. quadratus plantae*.
m. flex′or car′pi radia′lis [TA] radial flexor muscle of wrist: *origin*, medial epicondyle of humerus; *insertion*, base of second metacarpal; *innervation*, median; *action*, flexes and abducts wrist joint.
m. flex′or car′pi ulna′ris [TA] ulnar flexor muscle of wrist (2 heads): *origin*, CAPUT HUMERALE—medial epicondyle of humerus, CAPUT ULNARE—olecranon, ulna, intermuscular septum; *insertion*, pisiform, hook of hamate, proximal end of fifth metacarpal; *innervation*, ulnar; *action*, flexes and adducts wrist joint.
m. flex′or di′giti mi′nimi bre′vis ma′nus [TA] short flexor muscle of little finger: *origin*, hook of hamate bone, palmar surface of flexor retinaculum; *insertion*, medial side of proximal phalanx of little finger; *innervation*, ulnar; *action*, flexes little finger.
m. flex′or di′giti mi′nimi bre′vis pe′dis [TA] short flexor muscle of little toe: *origin*, base of fifth metatarsal, sheath of peroneus longus muscle; *insertion*, lateral surface of base of proximal phalanx of little toe; *innervation*, lateral plantar; *action*, flexes little toe.
m. flex′or di′giti quin′ti bre′vis ma′nus m. flexor digiti minimi brevis manus.
m. flex′or di′giti quin′ti bre′vis pe′dis m. flexor digiti minimi brevis pedis.
m. flex′or digito′rum bre′vis [TA] short flexor muscle of toes: *origin*, medial tuberosity of calcaneus, plantar fascia; *insertion*, middle phalanges of four lateral toes; *innervation*, medial plantar; *action*, flexes four lateral toes.
m. flex′or digito′rum lon′gus [TA] long flexor muscle of toes: *origin*, posterior surface of shaft of tibia; *insertion*, distal phalanges of four lateral toes; *innervation*, posterior tibial; *action*, flexes toes and plantar flexes foot.
m. flex′or digito′rum profun′dus [TA] deep flexor muscle of fingers: *origin*, shaft of ulna, coronoid process, interosseous membrane; *insertion*, bases of distal phalanges of fingers; *innervation*, ulnar and anterior interosseous; *action*, flexes distal phalanges.
m. flex′or digito′rum subli′mis m. flexor digitorum superficialis.
m. flex′or digito′rum superficia′lis [TA] superficial flexor muscle of fingers (2 heads): *origin*, HUMEROULNAR HEAD—medial epicondyle of humerus, coronoid process of ulna, RADIAL HEAD—oblique line of radius, anterior border; *insertion*, sides of middle phalanges of four (nonthumb) fingers; *innervation*, median; *action*, primarily flexes middle phalanges.
m. flex′or hal′lucis bre′vis [TA] short flexor muscle of great toe: *origin*, undersurface of cuboid, lateral cuneiform; *insertion* (2 heads): LATERAL HEAD—lateral side of base of proximal phalanx of toe; MEDIAL HEAD—medial side of base of proximal phalanx of toe; *innervation*, medial plantar; *action*, flexes great toe.
m. flex′or hal′lucis lon′gus [TA] long flexor muscle of great toe: *origin*, posterior surface of fibula; *insertion*, base of distal phalanx of great toe; *innervation*, tibial; *action*, flexes great toe.
m. flex′or pol′licis bre′vis [TA] short flexor muscle of thumb (2 heads): *origin*, CAPUT SUPERFICIALE—flexor retinaculum, distal part of tubercle of trapezium, CAPUT PROFUNDUM—trapezoid and capitate bones and palmar ligaments of distal row of carpal bones; *insertion*, radial side of base of proximal phalanx of thumb; *innervation*, median, ulnar; *action*, flexes and adducts thumb. The deep head varies considerably in size and may be absent.
m. flex′or pol′licis lon′gus [TA] long flexor muscle of thumb: *origin*, anterior surface of radius, interosseous membrane, and medial epicondyle of humerus or coronoid process of ulna; *insertion*, base of distal phalanx of thumb; *innervation*, anterior interosseous; *action*, flexes thumb.
m. fronta′lis venter frontalis musculi occipitofrontalis.
m. fusifor′mis [TA] fusiform muscle: a spindle-shaped muscle in which the fibers are approximately parallel to the long axis of the muscle but converge upon a tendon at either end.
m. gastrocne′mius [TA] gastrocnemius muscle (2 heads): *origin*, CAPUT MEDIALE—popliteal surface of femur, upper part of medial condyle, and capsule of knee, CAPUT LATERALE—lateral condyle and capsule of knee; *insertion*, aponeurosis unites with tendon of soleus to form calcaneal tendon (Achilles tendon); *innervation*, tibial; *action*, plantar flexes ankle joint, flexes knee joint.
m. gemel′lus infe′rior [TA] inferior gemellus muscle: *origin*, tuberosity of ischium; *insertion*, greater trochanter of femur; *innervation*, nerve to quadratus femoris; *action*, rotates thigh laterally.
m. gemel′lus supe′rior [TA] superior gemellus muscle: *origin*, spine of ischium; *insertion*, greater trochanter of femur; *innervation*, nerve to internal obturator; *action*, rotates thigh laterally.
m. genioglos′sus [TA] genioglossus muscle: *origin*, superior mental spine; *insertion*, hyoid bone and inferior surface of tongue; *innervation*, hypoglossal; *action*, protrudes and depresses tongue.

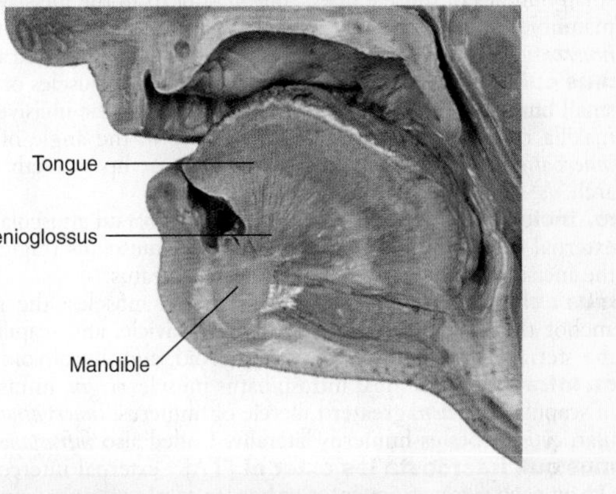

m. geniohyoi′deus [TA] geniohyoid muscle: *origin*, inferior mental spine; *insertion*, body of hyoid bone; *innervation*, a branch of first cervical nerve through hypoglossal; *action*, elevates and draws hyoid forward, or depresses mandible when hyoid is fixed by its depressors.
m. glossopalati′nus m. palatoglossus.
m. glossopharyn′geus pars glossopharyngea musculi constrictoris pharyngis superioris.
m. glu′teus max′imus [TA] gluteus maximus muscle: *origin*, posterior aspect of ilium, posterior surface of sacrum and coccyx, sacrotuberous ligament, fascia covering gluteus medius; *insertion*, iliotibial tract of fascia lata, gluteal tuberosity of femur; *innervation*, inferior gluteal; *action*, extends, abducts, and rotates thigh laterally.
m. glu′teus me′dius [TA] gluteus medius muscle: *origin*, lateral surface of ilium between anterior and posterior gluteal lines; *insertion*, greater trochanter of femur; *innervation*, superior gluteal; *action*, abducts and rotates thigh medially.
m. glu′teus mi′nimus [TA] gluteus minimus muscle: *origin*, lateral surface of ilium between anterior and inferior gluteal lines; *insertion*, greater trochanter of femur; *innervation*, superior gluteal; *action*, abducts, rotates thigh medially.
m. gra′cilis [TA] gracilis muscle: *origin*, lower half of body and entire inferior ramus of pubis; *insertion*, medial surface of shaft of tibia; *innervation*, obturator; *action*, adducts thigh, flexes knee joint.
m. he′licis ma′jor [TA] helicis major muscle: *origin*, spine of helix; *insertion*, anterior border of helix; *innervation*, auriculotemporal and posterior auricular; *action*, tenses skin of auditory canal.
m. he′licis mi′nor [TA] helicis minor muscle: *origin*, anterior rim of helix; *insertion*, concha; *innervation*, temporal, posterior auricular.

Musculus *Continued*

m. hyoglos′sus [TA] hyoglossal muscle: *origin,* body and greater cornu of hyoid bone; *insertion,* side of tongue; *innervation,* hypoglossal; *action,* depresses and retracts tongue.
m. ili′acus [TA] iliac muscle: *origin,* iliac fossa and base of sacrum; *insertion,* greater psoas tendon and lesser trochanter of femur; *innervation,* femoral; *action,* flexes thigh, trunk on limb.
m. iliococcy′geus [TA] iliococcygeal muscle: the posterior portion of the levator ani, which originates as far anteriorly as the obturator canal and inserts on the side of the coccyx and the anococcygeal ligament; *innervation,* third and fourth sacral; *action,* helps to support pelvic viscera and resist increases in intra-abdominal pressure.
m. iliocosta′lis [TA] iliocostalis muscle: the lateral division of the erector spinae, which includes the *musculus iliocostalis cervicis* and *musculus iliocostalis lumborum.*
m. iliocosta′lis cer′vicis [TA] iliocostalis cervicis muscle: *origin,* angles of third, fourth, fifth, and sixth ribs; *insertion,* transverse processes of fourth, fifth, and sixth cervical vertebrae; *innervation,* branches of cervical; *action,* extends cervical spine. Called also *m. iliocostalis colli* [TA alternative].
m. iliocosta′lis col′li TA alternative for *m. iliocostalis cervicis.*
m. iliocosta′lis lumbo′rum [TA] iliocostalis lumborum muscle: the iliocostalis muscle acting on the thoracic and lumbar regions; it is subdivided into a lumbar part *(pars lumbalis musculi iliocostalis lumborum)* and a thoracic part *(pars thoracica musculi iliocostalis lumborum).*
m. iliopso′as [TA] iliopsoas muscle: a compound muscle consisting of the iliacus and the psoas major.
mus′culi incisi′vi la′bii inferio′ris incisive muscles of inferior lip: small bundles of muscle fibers, one arising from the incisive fossa of the mandible on each side and passing laterally to the angle of the mouth; *innervation,* facial; *action,* closely apply lower lip to teeth and alveolar arch.
mus′culi incisi′vi la′bii superio′ris incisive muscles of superior lip: small bundles of muscle fibers, one arising from the incisive fossa of the maxilla on each side and passing laterally to the angle of the mouth; *innervation,* facial; *action,* closely apply upper lip to teeth and alveolar arch.
m. incisu′rae termina′lis [TA] an inconstant muscular slip in the external ear, continuing forward from the musculus tragicus to bridge the incisure of the cartilaginous external meatus.
mus′culi infrahyoi′dei [TA] infrahyoid muscles: the muscles that anchor the hyoid bone to the sternum, clavicle, and scapula, including the sternohyoid, omohyoid, sternothyroid, and thyrohyoid muscles.
m. infraspina′tus [TA] infraspinatus muscle: *origin,* infraspinous fossa of scapula; *insertion,* greater tubercle of humerus; *innervation,* suprascapular; *action,* rotates humerus laterally. Called also *infraspinous muscle.*
mus′culi intercosta′les exter′ni [TA] external intercostal muscles (11 on each side): *origin,* inferior border of rib; *insertion,* superior border of rib below; *innervation,* intercostal; *action,* primarily elevate ribs in inspiration, also active in expiration.
mus′culi intercosta′les inter′ni [TA] internal intercostal muscles (11 on each side): *origin,* inferior border of rib and costal cartilage; *insertion,* superior border of rib and costal cartilage below; *innervation,* intercostal; *action,* draw ribs together in respiration and expulsive movements, also act in inspiration.
mus′culi intercosta′les in′timi [TA] innermost intercostal muscles: the layer of muscle fibers separated from the internal intercostal muscles by the intercostal nerves.
mus′culi interos′sei dorsa′les ma′nus [TA] dorsal interosseous muscles of hand (4): *origin,* by two heads from adjacent sides of metacarpal bones; *insertion,* bases of proximal phalanges and corresponding extensor expansions of second, third, and fourth fingers; *innervation,* ulnar; *action,* abduct fingers, flex proximal phalanges, extend middle and distal phalanges.
mus′culi interos′sei dorsa′les pe′dis [TA] dorsal interosseous muscles of foot (4): *origin,* adjacent surfaces of metatarsal bones; *insertion,* base of proximal phalanges of second, third, and fourth toes and their extensor expansions; *innervation,* lateral plantar; *action,* abduct, flex toes.
mus′culi interos′sei palma′res [TA] palmar interosseous muscles (3): *origin,* sides of second, fourth, and fifth metacarpal bones; *insertion,* bases of proximal phalanges and corresponding extensor expansions of second, fourth, and fifth fingers; *innervation,* ulnar; *action,* adduct fingers, flex proximal phalanges, extend middle and distal phalanges.
mus′culi interos′sei planta′res [TA] plantar interosseous muscles (3): *origin,* medial surfaces of third, fourth, and fifth metatarsal bones; *insertion,* medial side of base of proximal phalanges of third, fourth, and fifth toes and their extensor expansions; *innervation,* lateral plantar; *action,* adduct, flex toes.
mus′culi interos′sei vola′res musculi interossei palmares.
mus′culi interspina′les [TA] interspinal muscles: short bands of muscle fibers between spinous processes of contiguous vertebrae, including the *musculi interspinales cervicis, musculi interspinales thoracis,* and *musculi interspinales lumborum.*
mus′culi interspina′les cer′vicis [TA] interspinal muscles of neck: paired bands of muscle fibers extending between spinous processes of contiguous cervical vertebrae, innervated by spinal nerves, and acting to extend the vertebral column. Called also *musculi interspinales colli* [TA alternative].
mus′culi interspina′les col′li TA alternative for *musculi interspinales cervicis.*
mus′culi interspina′les lumbo′rum [TA] lumbar interspinal muscles: paired bands of muscle fibers extending between spinous processes of contiguous lumbar vertebrae, innervated by spinal nerves, and acting to extend the vertebral column.
mus′culi interspina′les thora′cis [TA] interspinal muscles of thorax: paired bands of muscle fibers extending between spinous processes of contiguous thoracic vertebrae, innervated by spinal nerves, and acting to extend the vertebral column.
mus′culi intertransversa′rii [TA] intertransverse muscles: small muscles passing between the transverse processes of contiguous vertebrae, including the lateral and medial lumbar intertransverse muscles, the intertransverse muscles of the thorax, and the anterior, lateral posterior, and medial posterior intertransverse muscles of the neck.
mus′culi intertransversa′rii anterio′res cer′vicis [TA] anterior intertransverse muscles of neck: small muscles passing between the anterior tubercles of adjacent cervical vertebrae, innervated by anterior primary rami of spinal nerves, and acting to bend the vertebral column laterally. Called also *musculi intertransversarii anteriores colli* [TA alternative].
mus′culi intertransversa′rii anterio′res col′li TA alternative for *musculi intertransversarii anteriores cervicis.*
mus′culi intertransversa′rii latera′les lumbo′rum [TA] lateral lumbar intertransverse muscles: small muscles passing between the transverse processes of adjacent lumbar vertebrae, innervated by anterior primary rami of spinal nerves, and acting to bend the vertebral column laterally.
mus′culi intertransversa′rii media′les lumbo′rum [TA] medial lumbar intertransverse muscles: small muscles passing from the accessory process of one lumbar vertebra to the mammillary process of the contiguous lumbar vertebra, innervated by posterior primary rami of spinal nerves, and acting to bend the vertebral column laterally.
mus′culi intertransversa′rii posterio′res latera′les cer′vicis [TA] lateral posterior intertransverse muscles of neck: small muscles passing between the posterior tubercles of adjacent cervical vertebrae, lateral to the intertransversarii posteriores mediales cervicis, innervated by anterior primary rami of spinal nerves, and acting to bend the vertebral column laterally. Called also *musculi intertransversarii posteriores laterales colli* [TA alternative].
mus′culi intertransversa′rii posterio′res latera′les col′li TA alternative for *musculi intertransversarii posteriores laterales cervicis.*
mus′culi intertransversa′rii posterio′res media′les cer′vicis [TA] medial posterior intertransverse muscles of neck: small muscles passing between the posterior tubercles of adjacent cervical vertebrae, close to the vertebral body, innervated by posterior primary rami of spinal nerves, and acting to bend the vertebral column laterally. Called also *musculi intertransversarii posteriores mediales colli* [TA alternative].
mus′culi intertransversa′rii posterio′res media′les col′li TA alternative for *musculi intertransversarii posteriores mediales cervicis.*
mus′culi intertransversa′rii thora′cis [TA] intertransverse muscles of thorax: poorly developed muscle bundles extending between the anterior tubercles of adjacent thoracic vertebrae, innervated by posterior primary rami of spinal nerves, and acting to bend the vertebral column laterally.
m. ischiocaverno′sus [TA] ischiocavernous muscle: *origin,* ramus of ischium; *insertion,* crus penis (crus clitoridis); *innervation,* perineal; *action,* maintains erection of penis (clitoris).
m. ischiococcy′geus [TA] ischiococcygeal muscle: *origin,* ischial spine; *insertion,* lateral border of lower part of sacrum, upper coccyx; *innervation,* third and fourth sacral; *action,* supports and raises coccyx. Called also *coccygeal muscle* and *m. coccygeus* (TA alternative).

mus′culi laryn′gis [TA] muscles of larynx: the intrinsic and extrinsic muscles of the larynx, including the oblique and transverse arytenoid, ceratocricoid, lateral and posterior cricoarytenoid, cricothyroid, thyroarytenoid, and vocal muscles.
m. latis′simus dor′si [TA] *origin*, spines of lower thoracic vertebrae, lumbar and sacral vertebrae through attachment to thoracolumbar fascia, iliac crest, lower ribs, inferior angle of scapula; *insertion*, floor of intertubercular sulcus of humerus; *innervation*, thoracodorsal; *action*, adducts, extends, and rotates humerus medially.
m. leva′tor an′guli o′ris [TA] levator muscle of angle of mouth: *origin*, canine fossa of maxilla; *insertion*, orbicularis oris and skin at angle of mouth; *innervation*, facial; *action*, raises angle of mouth.
m. leva′tor a′ni [TA] levator ani muscle: a name applied collectively to important muscular components of the pelvic diaphragm, including the pubococcygeus, puborectalis, and iliococcygeus muscles.
mus′culi levato′res costa′rum [TA] levator muscles of ribs (12 on each side): originating from the transverse processes of the seventh cervical and first to eleventh thoracic vertebrae and inserting medial to the angle of a lower rib (see *musculi levatores costarum breves* and *musculi levatores costarum longi*); innervated by intercostal nerves and aiding in elevation of the ribs in respiration.
mus′culi levato′res costa′rum bre′ves [TA] short levator muscles of ribs: the levatores costarum muscles of each side that insert medial to the angle of the rib next below the vertebra of origin.
mus′culi levato′res costa′rum lon′gi [TA] long levator muscles of ribs: the lower levatores costarum muscles of each side, which have fascicles extending down to the second rib below the vertebra of origin.
m. leva′tor glan′dulae thyroi′deae [TA] levator muscle of thyroid gland: an inconstant muscle originating on the isthmus or pyramid of the thyroid gland and inserting on the body of the hyoid bone.
m. leva′tor la′bii superio′ris [TA] levator muscle of upper lip: *origin*, lower orbital margin; *insertion*, muscle of upper lip; *innervation*, facial nerve; *action*, raises upper lip.
m. leva′tor la′bii superio′ris alae′que na′si [TA] levator muscle of upper lip and ala of nose: *origin*, upper part of frontal process of maxilla; *insertion*, cartilage and skin of ala nasi, and upper lip; *innervation*, infraorbital branch of facial; *action*, raises upper lip and dilates nostril.
m. leva′tor pal′pebrae superio′ris [TA] levator muscle of upper eyelid: *origin*, sphenoid bone above optic canal; *insertion*, tarsal plate and skin of upper eyelid; *innervation*, oculomotor; *action*, raises upper lid.
m. leva′tor pro′statae TA alternative for *m. puboprostaticus.*
m. leva′tor sca′pulae [TA] levator muscle of scapula: *origin*, transverse processes of four upper cervical vertebrae; *insertion*, medial border of scapula; *innervation*, third and fourth cervical; *action*, raises scapula.
m. leva′tor ve′li palati′ni [TA] *origin*, apex of petrous portion of temporal bone and cartilaginous part of auditory tube; *insertion*, aponeurosis of soft palate; *innervation*, pharyngeal plexus of vagus; *action*, raises and draws back soft palate.
mus′culi lin′guae [TA], **mus′culi lingua′les** muscles of tongue: the extrinsic and intrinsic muscles that move the tongue; called also *lingual muscles.*
m. longis′simus [TA] longissimus muscle: the largest element of the erector spinae, which includes the *musculus longissimus capitis, musculus longissimus cervicis,* and *musculus longissimus thoracis.*
m. longis′simus ca′pitis [TA] longissimus muscle of head: *origin*, transverse processes of four or five upper thoracic vertebrae, articular processes of three or four lower cervical vertebrae; *insertion*, mastoid process of temporal bone; *innervation*, branches of cervical; *action*, draws head backward, rotates head.
m. longis′simus cer′vicis [TA] longissimus muscle of neck: *origin*, transverse processes of four or five upper thoracic vertebrae; *insertion*, transverse processes of second to sixth cervical vertebrae; *innervation*, lower cervical and upper thoracic; *action*, extends cervical vertebrae. Called also *m. longissimus colli* [TA alternative].
m. longis′simus col′li TA alternative for *m. longissimus cervicis.*
m. longis′simus thora′cis [TA] longissimus muscle of thorax: *origin*, transverse and articular processes of lumbar vertebrae and thoracolumbar fascia; *insertion*, transverse processes of all thoracic vertebrae, nine or ten lower ribs; *innervation*, lumbar and thoracic; *action*, extends thoracic vertebrae. The portion in the lumbar region is sometimes denoted separately *(pars lumbalis musculi longissimus thoracis).*
m. longitudina′lis infe′rior lin′guae [TA] inferior longitudinal muscle of tongue: *origin*, inferior surface of tongue at base; *insertion*, tip of tongue; *innervation*, hypoglossal; *action*, changes shape of tongue in mastication and deglutition.
m. longitudina′lis supe′rior lin′guae [TA] superior longitudinal muscle of tongue: *origin*, submucosa and septum of tongue; *insertion*, margins of tongue; *innervation*, hypoglossal; *action*, changes shape of tongue in mastication and deglutition.
m. lon′gus ca′pitis [TA] long muscle of head: *origin*, transverse processes of third to sixth cervical vertebrae; *insertion*, basilar part of occipital bone; *innervation*, branches from first, second, and third cervical; *action*, flexes head.
m. lon′gus cer′vicis TA alternative for *m. longus colli.*
m. lon′gus col′li [TA] long muscle of neck: *origin*, SUPERIOR OBLIQUE PORTION—transverse processes of third to fifth cervical vertebrae; INFERIOR OBLIQUE PORTION—bodies of first to third thoracic vertebrae; VERTICAL PORTION—bodies of three upper thoracic and three lower cervical vertebrae; *insertion*, SUPERIOR OBLIQUE PORTION—tubercle of anterior arch of atlas; INFERIOR OBLIQUE PORTION—transverse processes of fifth and sixth cervical vertebrae; VERTICAL PORTION—bodies of second to fourth cervical vertebrae; *innervation*, anterior cervical; *action*, flexes and supports cervical vertebrae. Called also *m. longus cervicis* [TA alternative].
mus′culi lumbrica′les ma′nus [TA] lumbrical muscles of hand: *origin*, tendons of flexor digitorum profundus; *insertion*, extensor expansions of the four nonthumb fingers; *innervation*, median and ulnar; *action*, flex metacarpophalangeal joint and extend middle and distal phalanges.
mus′culi lumbrica′les pe′dis [TA] lumbrical muscles of foot: *origin*, tendons of flexor digitorum longus; *insertion*, extensor expansions of four lateral toes; *innervation*, medial and lateral plantar; *action*, flex metatarsophalangeal joints, extend distal phalanges.
m. masse′ter [TA] masseter muscle: *origin*, PARS SUPERFICIALIS—zygomatic process of maxilla and inferior border of zygomatic arch, PARS PROFUNDA—inferior border and medial surface of zygomatic arch; *insertion*, PARS SUPERFICIALIS—angle and ramus of mandible, PARS PROFUNDA—superior half of ramus and lateral surface of coronoid process of mandible; *innervation*, masseteric, from mandibular division of trigeminal; *action*, raises mandible, closes jaws.
mus′culi masticato′rii [TA] masticatory muscles: a group of muscles responsible for the movement of the jaws during mastication, including the masseter, temporal, and medial and lateral pterygoid muscles; called also *muscles of mastication.*
mus′culi mem′bri inferio′ris [TA] muscles of lower limb: the muscles acting on the thigh, leg, and foot.
mus′culi mem′bri superio′ris [TA] muscles of upper limb: the muscles acting on the arm, forearm, and hand.
m. menta′lis [TA] *origin*, incisive fossa of mandible; *insertion*, skin of chin; *innervation*, facial; *action*, wrinkles skin of chin.
mus′culi multi′fidi [TA] multifidus muscles: *origin*, sacrum, sacroiliac ligament, mammillary processes of lumbar, transverse processes of thoracic, and articular processes of cervical vertebrae; *insertion*, spines of contiguous vertebrae above; *innervation*, posterior rami of spinal nerves; *action*, extend, rotate vertebral column.
m. multipenna′tus [TA] multipennate muscle: a muscle in which the fiber bundles converge to several tendons.
m. mylohyoi′deus [TA] mylohyoid muscle: *origin*, mylohyoid line of mandible; *insertion*, body of hyoid bone and median raphe; *innervation*, mylohyoid branch of inferior alveolar; *action*, elevates hyoid bone, supports floor of mouth.
m. mylopharyn′geus pars mylopharyngea musculi constrictoris pharyngis superioris.
m. nasa′lis [TA] nasal muscle: *origin*, maxilla; *insertion*, PARS ALARIS—ala nasi, PARS TRANSVERSA—by aponeurotic expansion with fellow of opposite side; *innervation*, facial; *action*, PARS ALARIS—aids in widening nostril, PARS TRANSVERSA—depresses cartilage of nose.
m. obli′quus auri′culae [TA] oblique muscle of auricle: *origin*, cranial surface of concha; *insertion*, cranial surface of auricle above concha; *innervation*, temporal and posterior auricular (branches of facial).
m. obli′quus ca′pitis infe′rior [TA] inferior oblique muscle of head: *origin*, spinous process of axis; *insertion*, transverse process of atlas; *innervation*, posterior rami of spinal nerves; *action*, rotates atlas and head.
m. obli′quus ca′pitis supe′rior [TA] superior oblique muscle of head: *origin*, transverse process of atlas; *insertion*, occipital bone;

innervation, posterior rami of spinal nerves; *action*, extends and moves head laterally.
m. obli′quus exter′nus abdo′minis [TA] external oblique muscle of abdomen: *origin*, lower eight ribs at costal cartilages; *insertion*, crest of ilium, linea alba through rectus sheath; *innervation*, seventh to twelfth intercostal; *action*, flexes and rotates vertebral column, increases intra-abdominal pressure, acts as accessory respiratory muscle.
m. obli′quus infe′rior bul′bi [TA] inferior oblique muscle of eyeball: *origin*, orbital surface of maxilla; *insertion*, sclera; *innervation*, oculomotor; *action*, rotates eyeball upward and outward.
m. obli′quus infe′rior o′culi m. obliquus inferior bulbi.
m. obli′quus inter′nus abdo′minis [TA] internal oblique muscle of abdomen: *origin*, inguinal ligament, iliac crest, thoracolumbar fascia; *insertion*, inferior three or four costal cartilages, linea alba, conjoined tendon to pubis; *innervation*, seventh to twelfth intercostal, first lumbar; *action*, flexes and rotates vertebral column, increases intra-abdominal pressure, acts as accessory respiratory muscle.
m. obli′quus supe′rior bul′bi [TA] superior oblique muscle of eyeball: *origin*, lesser wing of sphenoid above optic canal; *insertion*, sclera; *innervation*, trochlear; *action*, rotates eyeball downward and outward.
m. obli′quus supe′rior o′culi m. obliquus superior bulbi.
m. obturato′rius exter′nus [TA] obturator externus muscle: *origin*, pubis, ischium, and external surface of obturator membrane; *insertion*, trochanteric fossa of femur; *innervation*, obturator; *action*, rotates thigh laterally.
m. obturato′rius inter′nus [TA] obturator internus muscle: *origin*, pelvic surface of hip bone and obturator membrane, margin of obturator foramen, ramus of ischium, inferior ramus of pubis; *insertion*, greater trochanter of femur; *innervation*, fifth lumbar, first and second sacral; *action*, rotates thigh laterally.
m. occipita′lis venter occipitalis musculi occipitofrontalis.
m. occipitofronta′lis [TA] occipitofrontal muscle: *origin*, VENTER FRONTALIS—galea aponeurotica, VENTER OCCIPITALIS—highest nuchal line of occipital bone; *insertion*, VENTER FRONTALIS—skin of eyebrows and root of nose, VENTER OCCIPITALIS—galea aponeurotica; *innervation*, VENTER FRONTALIS—temporal branch of facial, VENTER OCCIPITALIS—posterior auricular branch of facial; *action*, VENTER FRONTALIS—raises eyebrows, VENTER OCCIPITALIS—draws scalp posteriorly.
mus′culi o′culi musculi externi bulbi oculi.
m. omohyoi′deus [TA] omohyoid muscle, comprising two bellies (superior and inferior) connected by a central tendon that is bound to the clavicle by a fibrous expansion of the cervical fascia; *origin*, superior border of scapula; *insertion*, lateral border of hyoid bone; *innervation*, upper cervical through ansa cervicalis; *action*, depresses hyoid bone.
m. oppo′nens di′giti mi′nimi [TA] opposing muscle of little finger: *origin*, hook of hamate bone, flexor retinaculum; *insertion*, ulnar margin of fifth metacarpal; *innervation*, eighth cervical through ulnar; *action*, rotates, abducts, and flexes fifth metacarpal.
m. oppo′nens pol′licis [TA] opposing muscle of thumb: *origin*, tubercle of trapezium, flexor retinaculum; *insertion*, radial side of first metacarpal; *innervation*, sixth and seventh cervical through median; *action*, flexes and opposes thumb.
m. orbicula′ris [TA] orbicular muscle: a muscle that encircles a body opening, such as the eye or mouth.
m. orbicula′ris o′culi [TA] orbicular muscle of eye: the oval sphincter muscle surrounding the eyelids, consisting of three parts: *origin*, PARS ORBITALIS—medial margin of orbit, including frontal process of maxilla, PARS PALPEBRALIS—medial palpebral ligament, PARS LACRIMALIS—posterior lacrimal crest; *insertion*, PARS ORBITALIS—near origin after encircling orbit, PARS PALPEBRALIS—fibers intertwine to form lateral palpebral raphe, PARS LACRIMALIS—lateral palpebral raphe, upper and lower tarsi; *innervation*, facial; *action*, closes eyelids, wrinkles forehead, compresses lacrimal sac.

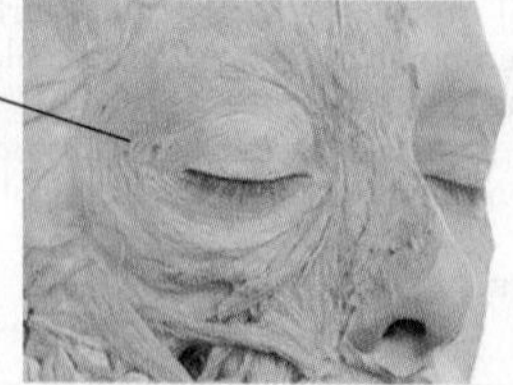

m. orbicula′ris o′ris [TA] orbicular muscle of mouth, comprising a *pars labialis*, fibers restricted to the lips, and a *pars marginalis*, fibers blending with those of adjacent muscles; *innervation*, facial; *action*, closes and protrudes lips.
m. orbita′lis [TA] orbital muscle: a thin layer of nonstriated muscle that bridges the inferior orbital fissure; *innervation*, sympathetic branches.
mus′culi ossiculo′rum auditorio′rum [TA] muscles of auditory ossicles: the two muscles of the middle ear, the tensor tympani and the stapedius.
mus′culi os′sis hyoi′dei muscles of the hyoid bone; see *musculi infrahyoidei* and *musculi suprahyoidei.*
mus′culi pala′ti see *musculi palati mollis et faucium.*
mus′culi pala′ti mol′lis et fau′cium [TA] muscles of soft palate and fauces: the intrinsic and extrinsic muscles that act upon the soft palate *(musculi palati)* and the adjacent pharyngeal wall.
m. palatoglos′sus [TA] palatoglossus muscle: *origin*, undersurface of soft palate; *insertion*, side of tongue; *innervation*, pharyngeal plexus of vagus; *action*, elevates tongue, constricts fauces.
m. palatopharyn′geus [TA] palatopharyngeal muscle: one of the intrinsic muscles of the larynx; *origin*, soft palate; *insertion*, aponeurosis of pharynx, posterior border of thyroid cartilage; *innervation*, pharyngeal plexus of vagus; *action*, aids in deglutition.
m. palma′ris bre′vis [TA] short palmar muscle: *origin*, palmar aponeurosis; *insertion*, skin of medial border of hand; *innervation*, ulnar; *action*, assists in deepening hollow of palm.
m. palma′ris lon′gus [TA] long palmar muscle: *origin*, medial epicondyle of humerus; *insertion*, flexor retinaculum, palmar aponeurosis; *innervation*, median; *action*, flexes wrist joint, anchors skin and fascia of hand.
mus′culi papilla′res [TA] papillary muscles: conical muscular projections from the walls of the cardiac ventricles, attached to the cusps of the atrioventricular valves by the chordae tendineae. There is an anterior and a posterior papillary muscle in each ventricle, as well as a group of small papillary muscles on the septum in the right ventricle.
m. papilla′ris ante′rior ventri′culi dex′tri [TA] anterior papillary muscle of right ventricle: the papillary muscle arising from the sternocostal wall of the right ventricle.
m. papilla′ris ante′rior ventri′culi sinis′tri [TA] anterior papillary muscle of left ventricle: the papillary muscle arising from the anterior wall of the left ventricle.
m. papilla′ris poste′rior ventri′culi dex′tri [TA] posterior papillary muscle of right ventricle: the papillary muscle arising from the diaphragmatic wall of the right ventricle.
m. papilla′ris poste′rior ventri′culi sinis′tri [TA] posterior papillary muscle of left ventricle: the papillary muscle arising from the posterior wall of the left ventricle.
mus′culi pectina′ti a′trii dex′tri [TA] pectinate muscles of right atrium: small ridges of muscle fibers projecting from the inner walls of the right auricle of the heart and extending in the right atrium to the crista terminalis.
mus′culi pectina′ti a′trii sinis′tri [TA] pectinate muscles of left atrium: small ridges of muscle fibers projecting from the inner walls of the left auricle of the heart.
m. pectin′eus [TA] pectineal muscle: *origin*, pectineal line of pubis; *insertion*, pectineal line of femur; *innervation*, obturator and femoral; *action*, flexes, adducts thigh.
m. pectora′lis ma′jor [TA] greater pectoral muscle: *origin*, clavicle, sternum, six upper costal cartilages, aponeurosis of obliquus externus abdominis. These origins are reflected in the subdivision of the muscle into clavicular, sternocostal, and abdominal parts; *insertion*, crest of intertubercular groove of humerus; *innervation*, medial and lateral pectoral; *action*, adducts, flexes, rotates arm medially.
m. pectora′lis mi′nor [TA] smaller pectoral muscle: *origin*, third, fourth, and fifth ribs; *insertion*, coracoid process of scapula; *innervation*, lateral and medial pectoral; *action*, draws shoulder forward and downward, raises third, fourth, and fifth ribs in forced inspiration.
m. penna′tus [TA] pennate muscle: a muscle in which the fibers approach the tendon of insertion from a wide area and are inserted through a large segment of its circumference. Called also *m. bipennatus* [TA alternative] and *bipennate* or *penniform muscle.*
mus′culi perinea′les, mus′culi perine′i [TA] muscles of perineum: the muscles participating in formation of the perineum.

Musculus *Continued*

m. perone′us bre′vis TA alternative for *m. fibularis brevis.*
m. perone′us lon′gus TA alternative for *m. fibularis longus.*
m. perone′us ter′tius TA alternative for *m. fibularis tertius.*
mus′culi pharyn′gis [TA] pharyngeal muscles: the muscular coat of the pharynx, consisting of the three constrictor muscles and the stylopharyngeal, salpingopharyngeal, and palatopharyngeal muscles.
m. pharyngopalati′nus m. palatopharyngeus.
m. pirifor′mis [TA] piriform muscle: *origin,* ilium, second to fourth sacral vertebrae; *insertion,* upper border of greater trochanter of femur; *innervation,* first and second sacral; *action,* rotates thigh laterally.
m. planta′ris [TA] plantar muscle: *origin,* oblique popliteal ligament, lateral supracondylar line of femur; *insertion,* posterior part of calcaneus; *innervation,* tibial; *action,* plantar flexes foot; flexes knee.
m. pleurooesopha′geus [TA] pleuroesophageal muscle: a bundle of smooth muscle fibers usually connecting the esophagus with the left mediastinal pleura.
m. popli′teus [TA] popliteal muscle: *origin,* lateral condyle of femur, lateral meniscus; *insertion,* posterior surface of tibia; *innervation,* tibial; *action,* flexes leg, rotates leg medially.
m. proce′rus [TA] procerus muscle: *origin,* fascia over nasal bone; *insertion,* skin of forehead; *innervation,* facial; *action,* draws medial angle of eyebrows down.
m. prona′tor quadra′tus [TA] *origin,* anterior surface and border of distal third or fourth of shaft of ulna; *insertion,* anterior surface and border of distal fourth of shaft of radius; *innervation,* anterior interosseous; *action,* pronates forearm.
m. prona′tor te′res [TA] (2 heads): *origin,* CAPUT HUMERALE—medial epicondyle of humerus, CAPUT ULNARE—coronoid process of ulna; *insertion,* lateral surface of radius; *innervation,* median; *action,* flexes elbow and pronates forearm.
m. pso′as ma′jor [TA] greater psoas muscle: *origin,* lumbar vertebrae; *insertion,* lesser trochanter of femur; *innervation,* second and third lumbar; *action,* flexes thigh or trunk.
m. pso′as mi′nor [TA] smaller psoas muscle: *origin,* last thoracic and first lumbar vertebrae; *insertion,* pectineal line, iliopectineal eminence, iliac fascia; *innervation,* first lumbar; *action,* flexes trunk. Absent in 40 to 50 per cent of persons.
m. pterygoi′deus latera′lis [TA] lateral pterygoid muscle (2 heads): *origin,* CAPUT SUPERIUS—infratemporal surface of greater wing of sphenoid and infratemporal crest; CAPUT INFERIUS—lateral surface of lateral pterygoid plate; *insertion,* neck of condyle of mandible, temporomandibular joint capsule; *innervation,* mandibular; *action,* protrudes mandible, opens jaws, moves mandible from side to side.
m. pterygoi′deus media′lis [TA] medial pterygoid muscle: *origin,* medial surface of lateral pterygoid plate, tuberosity of maxilla; *insertion,* medial surface of ramus and angle of mandible; *innervation,* mandibular; *action,* closes jaws.
m. pterygopharyn′geus pars pterygopharyngea musculi constrictoris pharyngis superioris.
m. puboana′lis [TA] puboanal muscle: fibers from the medial part of the pubococcygeus muscle that decussate and blend with the longitudinal muscle layer and fascia of the rectum.
m. pubococcy′geus [TA] pubococcygeal muscle: the anterior portion of the levator ani, originating anterior to the obturator canal; *insertion,* anococcygeal body and side of coccyx; *innervation,* pudendal; *action,* helps support pelvic viscera and resist increases in intraabdominal pressure.
m. puboperinea′lis [TA] puboperineal muscle: fibers from the medial part of the pubococcygeus muscle that insert into the perineal body.
m. puboprosta′ticus [TA] puboprostatic muscle: a part of the anterior portion of the pubococcygeus muscle, inserted in the prostate and the tendinous center of the perineum; innervated by the pudendal nerve, it supports and compresses the prostate and is involved in control of micturition. Called also *levator muscle of prostate* or *m. levator prostatae* (TA alternative).
m. puborecta′lis [TA] puborectal muscle: a portion of the levator ani having a more lateral origin from the pubic bone, and continuous posteriorly with the corresponding muscle of the opposite side; *innervation,* third and fourth sacral; *action,* helps support pelvic viscera and resist increases in intra-abdominal pressure, maintains perineal flexure at anorectal junction. Called also *Braune muscle.*
m. pubovagina′lis [TA] pubovaginal muscle: a part of the anterior portion of the pubococcygeus muscle, which is inserted into the urethra and vagina; innervated by the pudendal nerve, it is involved in control of micturition.
m. pubovesica′lis [TA] pubovesical muscle: smooth muscle fibers extending from the neck of the urinary bladder to the pubis.
m. pyramida′lis [TA] pyramidal muscle: *origin,* anterior aspect of pubis, anterior pubic ligament; *insertion,* linea alba; *innervation,* last thoracic; *action,* tenses abdominal wall.
m. pyramida′lis auri′culae [TA] pyramidal muscle of auricle: a prolongation of the fibers of the tragicus to the spina helicis.
m. quadra′tus [TA] quadrate muscle: a square-shaped muscle.
m. quadra′tus fe′moris [TA] *origin,* upper part of lateral border of tuberosity of ischium; *insertion,* quadrate tubercle of femur, intertrochanteric crest; *innervation,* fourth and fifth lumbar and first sacral; *action,* adducts, rotates thigh laterally.
m. quadra′tus lumbo′rum [TA] *origin,* iliac crest, thoracolumbar fascia; *insertion,* twelfth rib, transverse processes of four upper lumbar vertebrae; *innervation,* first and second lumbar and twelfth thoracic; *action,* flexes lumbar vertebrae laterally, fixes last rib.
m. quadra′tus plan′tae [TA] *origin,* calcaneus and plantar fascia; *insertion,* tendons of flexor digitorum longus; *innervation,* lateral plantar; *action,* aids in flexing toes. Called also *m. flexor accessorius* [TA alternative] or *accessory flexor muscle.*
m. quad′riceps fe′moris [TA] quadriceps muscle of thigh: a name applied collectively to the rectus femoris, vastus intermedius, vastus lateralis, and vastus medialis, inserting by a common tendon that surrounds the patella and ends on the tuberosity of the tibia, and acting to extend the leg upon the thigh. See individual components.
m. rectococcy′geus [TA] rectococcygeal muscle: smooth muscle fibers originating on the anterior surface of the second and third coccygeal vertebrae and inserting on the posterior surface of the rectum, innervated by autonomic nerves, and acting to retract and elevate the rectum.
mus′culi rectourethra′les TA alternative for musculi anorectoperineales.
m. rectouteri′nus [TA] rectouterine muscle: a band of fibers in the female, running between the cervix of the uterus and the rectum, in the rectouterine fold.
m. rectovesica′lis [TA] rectovesical muscle: a band of fibers in the male, connecting the longitudinal musculature of the rectum with the external muscular coat of the bladder.
m. rec′tus abdom′inis [TA] *origin,* pubic crest and symphysis; *insertion,* xiphoid process, cartilages of fifth, sixth, and seventh ribs; *innervation,* branches of lower thoracic; *action,* flexes lumbar vertebrae, supports abdomen.
m. rec′tus ca′pitis ante′rior [TA] *origin,* lateral mass of atlas; *insertion,* basilar part of occipital bone; *innervation,* first and second cervical; *action,* flexes, supports head.
m. rec′tus ca′pitis latera′lis [TA] *origin,* upper surface of transverse process of atlas; *insertion,* jugular process of occipital bone; *innervation,* first and second cervical; *action,* flexes, supports head.
m. rec′tus ca′pitis poste′rior ma′jor [TA] *origin,* spinous process of axis; *insertion,* occipital bone; *innervation,* suboccipital and greater occipital; *action,* extends head.
m. rec′tus ca′pitis poste′rior mi′nor [TA] *origin,* posterior tubercle of atlas; *insertion,* occipital bone; *innervation,* suboccipital and greater occipital; *action,* extends head.
m. rec′tus fe′moris [TA] *origin,* anterior inferior iliac spine, rim of acetabulum; *insertion,* base of patella, tuberosity of tibia; *innervation,* femoral; *action,* extends knee, flexes thigh at hip.
m. rec′tus infe′rior bul′bi [TA] inferior rectus muscle: *origin,* anulus tendineus communis; *insertion,* underside of sclera; *innervation,* oculomotor; *action,* adducts, rotates eyeball downward and medially.
m. rec′tus latera′lis bul′bi [TA] lateral rectus muscle: *origin,* anulus tendineus communis; *insertion,* lateral side of sclera; *innervation,* abducens; *action,* abducts eyeball.
m. rec′tus media′lis bul′bi [TA] medial rectus muscle: *origin,* anulus tendineus communis; *insertion,* medial side of sclera; *innervation,* oculomotor; *action,* adducts eyeball.
m. rec′tus supe′rior bul′bi [TA] superior rectus muscle: *origin,* anulus tendineus communis; *insertion,* upper aspect of sclera; *innervation,* oculomotor; *action,* adducts, rotates eyeball upward and medially.
m. rhomboi′deus ma′jor [TA] rhomboid major muscle: *origin,* spinous processes of second, third, fourth, and fifth thoracic vertebrae;

insertion, medial margin of scapula; *innervation*, dorsal scapular; *action*, retracts, elevates scapula.
m. rhomboi′deus mi′nor [TA] rhomboid minor muscle: *origin*, spinous processes of seventh cervical to first thoracic vertebrae, lower part of ligamentum nuchae; *insertion*, medial margin of scapula at root of the spine; *innervation*, dorsal scapular; *action*, adducts, elevates scapula.
m. riso′rius [TA] risorius muscle: *origin*, fascia over masseter; *insertion*, skin at angle of mouth; *innervation*, buccal branch of facial; *action*, draws angle of mouth laterally.
mus′culi rotato′res [TA] rotator muscles: a series of small muscles deep in the groove between the spinous and transverse processes of the vertebrae, including the *musculi rotatores cervicis*, *musculi rotatores thoracis*, and *musculi rotatores lumborum*.
mus′culi rotato′res bre′ves short rotator muscles: a name given the musculi rotatores that insert on the lamina of the vertebra next above the vertebra of origin.
mus′culi rotato′res cer′vicis [TA] rotator muscles of neck: *origin*, transverse processes of cervical vertebrae; *insertion*, base of spinous process of superjacent vertebrae; *innervation*, spinal nerves; *action*, extend vertebral column and rotate it toward the opposite side. Called also *musculi rotatores colli* [TA alternative].
mus′culi rotato′res col′li TA alternative for *musculi rotatores cervicis*.
mus′culi rotato′res lon′gi long rotator muscles: a name given the musculi rotatores that cross one or two segments of the vertebral column and insert into the spine of the vertebra next above.
mus′culi rotato′res lumbo′rum [TA] *origin*, transverse processes of lumbar vertebrae; *insertion*, base of spinous process of superjacent vertebrae; *innervation*, spinal nerves; *action*, extend vertebral column and rotate it toward the opposite side.
mus′culi rotato′res thora′cis [TA] rotator muscles of thorax: *origin*, transverse processes of thoracic vertebrae; *insertion*, base of spinous process of superjacent vertebrae; *innervation*, spinal nerves; *action*, extend vertebral column and rotate it toward the opposite side.
m. sacrococcy′geus ante′rior m. sacrococcygeus ventralis.
m. sacrococcy′geus dorsa′lis dorsal sacrococcygeal muscle: a muscular slip passing from the dorsal aspect of the sacrum to the coccyx.
m. sacrococcy′geus poste′rior m. sacrococcygeus dorsalis.
m. sacrococcy′geus ventra′lis ventral sacrococcygeal muscle: a musculotendinous slip passing from the lower sacral vertebrae to the coccyx.
m. sacrospina′lis m. erector spinae.
m. salpingopharyn′geus [TA] salpingopharyngeal muscle: *origin*, auditory tube near its orifice; *insertion*, posterior part of palatopharyngeus; *innervation*, pharyngeal plexus of vagus; *action*, elevates upper lateral wall of pharynx.
m. sarto′rius [TA] sartorius muscle: *origin*, anterior superior iliac spine; *insertion*, proximal part of medial surface of tibia; *innervation*, femoral; *action*, flexes leg at knee and thigh at pelvis.
m. scale′nus ante′rior [TA] anterior scalene muscle: *origin*, transverse processes of third to sixth cervical vertebrae; *insertion*, scalene tubercle of first rib; *innervation*, fourth to sixth cervical; *action*, raises first rib, flexes cervical vertebrae forward and laterally and rotates to opposite side.
m. scale′nus me′dius [TA] middle scalene muscle: *origin*, transverse processes of second to seventh cervical vertebrae and often atlas; *insertion*, upper surface of first rib; *innervation*, third to eighth cervical; *action*, raises first rib, flexes cervical vertebrae forward and laterally and rotates to opposite side.
m. scale′nus mi′nimus [TA] smallest scalene muscle: a band occasionally found between the musculi scalenus anterior and scalenus medius; *origin*, transverse process of seventh cervical vertebra; *insertion*, first rib, suprapleural membrane; *innervation*, seventh cervical; *action*, raises first rib, flexes and rotates cervical vertebrae, supports suprapleural membrane. Called also *Sibson muscle*.
m. scale′nus poste′rior [TA] posterior scalene muscle: *origin*, posterior tubercles of transverse processes of fourth to sixth cervical vertebrae; *insertion*, second rib; *innervation*, sixth to eighth cervical; *action*, raises second rib, flexes cervical vertebrae laterally.
m. semimembrano′sus [TA] semimembranous muscle: *origin*, tuberosity of ischium; *insertion*, medial condyle and border of tibia, lateral condyle of femur; *innervation*, tibial; *action*, flexes and rotates leg medially, extends thigh at hip.
m. semipenna′tus [TA] semipennate muscle: a muscle in which the fiber bundles approach the tendon of insertion from only one direction and are inserted through only a small segment of its circumference. Called also *m. unipennatus* [TA alternative] and *unipennate muscle*.
m. semispina′lis [TA] semispinal muscle: a muscle composed of fibers extending obliquely from the transverse processes of the vertebrae to the spine, except for the semispinalis capitis; it includes the *m. semispinalis capitis*, *m. semispinalis cervicis*, and *m. semispinalis thoracis*.
m. semispina′lis ca′pitis [TA] semispinal muscle of head: *origin*, transverse processes of five or six upper thoracic and four lower cervical vertebrae; *insertion*, between superior and inferior nuchal lines of occipital bone; *innervation*, suboccipital, greater occipital, and other branches of cervical; *action*, extends head and rotates to opposite side.
m. semispina′lis cer′vicis [TA] semispinal muscle of neck: *origin*, transverse processes of five or six upper thoracic vertebrae; *insertion*, spinous processes of second to fifth cervical vertebrae; *innervation*, branches of cervical; *action*, extends, rotates vertebral column.
m. semispina′lis dor′si m. semispinalis thoracis.
m. semispina′lis thora′cis [TA] semispinal muscle of thorax: *origin*, transverse processes of sixth to tenth thoracic vertebrae; *insertion*, spinous processes of two lower cervical and four upper thoracic vertebrae; *innervation*, spinal nerves; *action*, extends, rotates vertebral column.
m. semitendino′sus [TA] semitendinous muscle: *origin*, tuberosity of ischium; *insertion*, upper part of medial surface of tibia; *innervation*, tibial; *action*, flexes and rotates leg medially, extends thigh.
m. serra′tus ante′rior [TA] anterior serratus muscle: *origin*, eight or nine upper ribs; *insertion*, medial border of scapula; *innervation*, long thoracic; *action*, draws scapula forward; rotates scapula to raise shoulder in abduction of arm.
m. serra′tus poste′rior infe′rior [TA] inferior posterior serratus muscle: *origin*, spines of two lower thoracic and two or three upper lumbar vertebrae; *insertion*, inferior border of four lower ribs; *innervation*, ninth to twelfth thoracic; *action*, lowers ribs in expiration.
m. serra′tus poste′rior supe′rior [TA] superior posterior serratus muscle: *origin*, ligamentum nuchae, spinous processes of upper thoracic vertebrae; *insertion*, second, third, fourth, and fifth ribs; *innervation*, first four thoracic; *action*, raises ribs in inspiration.
m. so′leus [TA] soleus muscle: *origin*, fibula, tibia, tendinous arch between tibia and fibula and passing over popliteal vessels; *insertion*, calcaneus by tendo calcaneus; *innervation*, tibial; *action*, plantar flexes foot.
m. sphinc′ter [TA] sphincter muscle: a ringlike muscle that closes a natural orifice; it may be either of smooth muscle or striated muscle. Called also *sphincter*.
m. sphinc′ter ampul′lae hepatopancrea′ticae [TA] sphincter of hepatopancreatic ampulla: muscle fibers investing the hepatopancreatic ampulla in the wall of the duodenum; called also *Oddi muscle*, *sphincter of Oddi*, and *Glisson sphincter*.
m. sphinc′ter a′ni exter′nus [TA] external anal sphincter: *origin*, tip of coccyx, anococcygeal ligament; *insertion*, tendinous center of perineum; *innervation*, inferior rectal and perineal branch of fourth sacral; *action*, closes anus.
m. sphinc′ter a′ni inter′nus [TA] internal anal sphincter: a thickening of the circular lamina of the tunica muscularis at the caudal end of the rectum.
m. sphinc′ter duc′tus bilia′ris TA alternative for *m. sphincter ductus choledochi*.
m. sphinc′ter duc′tus chole′dochi [TA] sphincter of bile duct: an annular sheath of muscle that invests the bile duct within the wall of the duodenum.
m. sphinc′ter duc′tus pancrea′tici [TA] sphincter muscle of pancreatic duct: a sphincter that surrounds the pancreatic duct just above the hepatopancreatic ampulla. Called also *pancreatic sphincter* and *sphincter of pancreatic duct*.
m. sphinc′ter pupil′lae [TA] sphincter muscle of pupil: circular fibers of the iris, innervated by the ciliary nerves (parasympathetic), and acting to contract the pupil.
m. sphinc′ter pylo′ricus [TA] pyloric sphincter muscle: a thickening of the circular muscle of the stomach around its opening into the duodenum; called also *pyloric sphincter* and *sphincter muscle of pylorus*.
m. sphinc′ter supracollicula′ris TA alternative for m. sphincter urethrae internus.
m. sphinc′ter ure′thrae 1. m. sphincter urethrae externus urethrae femininae. 2. m. sphincter urethrae externus urethrae masculinae.
m. sphinc′ter ure′thrae exter′nus ure′thrae femini′nae [TA] external sphincter muscle of female urethra: *origin*, ramus of

Musculus *Continued*

pubis; *insertion,* median raphe behind and in front of urethra; *innervation,* perineal; *action,* compresses the central part of the urethra. Called also *striated sphincter, external sphincter of female urethra* and *external urethral sphincter of female urethra.*
m. sphinc′ter ure′thrae exter′nus ure′thrae masculi′nae [TA] external sphincter muscle of male urethra: *origin,* ramus of pubis; *insertion,* median raphe behind and in front of urethra; *innervation,* perineal; *action,* compresses the membranous part of the urethra. Called also *striated sphincter, external sphincter of male urethra, external urethral sphincter of male urethra,* and *m. sphincter urethrae membranaceae.*
m. sphinc′ter ure′thrae inter′nus [TA] internal sphincter muscle of urethra: a circular layer of smooth muscle fibers surrounding the internal urethral orifice in males, innervated by the vesical nerve, and acting to close the internal orifice of the urethra. No such structure exists in females. Called also *internal sphincter of urethra; internal urethral sphincter; preprostatic, smooth,* or *supracollicular sphincter; m. sphincter supracollicularis* [TA alternative]; and *m. sphincter vesicae urinariae.*
m. sphinc′ter ure′thrae membrana′ceae m. sphincter urethrae externus urethrae masculinae.
m. sphinc′ter urethrovagina′lis [TA] sphincter urethrovaginalis muscle: *origin,* perineal body; *insertion,* passes lateral to the vagina on either side and blends with its partner anterior to the urethra below the compressor urethrae muscle; *innervation,* perineal branches of the pudendal nerve; *action,* accessory urethral sphincter and may facilitate closing the vagina.
m. sphinc′ter vesi′cae urina′riae m. sphincter urethrae internus.
m. spina′lis [TA] spinal muscle: the medial division of the erector spinae, including the *m. spinalis capitis, m. spinalis cervicis,* and *m. spinalis thoracis.*
m. spina′lis ca′pitis [TA] spinal muscle of head: *origin,* spines of upper thoracic and lower cervical vertebrae; *insertion,* occipital bone; *innervation,* branches of cervical; *action,* extends head.
m. spina′lis cer′vicis [TA] spinal muscle of neck: *origin,* lower part of ligamentum nuchae, spinous processes of seventh cervical and sometimes two upper thoracic vertebrae; *insertion,* spinous processes of axis and sometimes of second to fourth cervical vertebrae; *innervation,* branches of cervical; *action,* extends vertebral column.
m. spina′lis dor′si m. spinalis thoracis.
m. spina′lis thora′cis [TA] spinal muscle of thorax: *origin,* spinous processes of two upper lumbar and two lower thoracic; *insertion,* spines of upper thoracic vertebrae; *innervation,* branches of thoracic and lumbar; *action,* extends vertebral column.
m. sple′nius ca′pitis [TA] splenius muscle of head: *origin,* lower half of ligamentum nuchae, spinous processes of seventh cervical and three or four upper thoracic vertebrae; *insertion,* mastoid part of temporal bone, occipital bone; *innervation,* middle and lower cervical; *action,* extends, rotates head.
m. sple′nius cer′vicis [TA] splenius muscle of neck: *origin,* spinous processes of third to sixth thoracic vertebrae; *insertion,* transverse processes of two or three upper cervical vertebrae; *innervation,* posterior rami of lower cervical; *action,* extends, rotates head and neck.
m. stape′dius [TA] stapedius muscle: *origin,* interior of pyramidal eminence of tympanic cavity; *insertion,* posterior surface of neck of stapes; *innervation,* stapedial branch of facial; *action,* dampens stapedial movement.
m. sterna′lis [TA] sternal muscle: a band occasionally found parallel to the sternum on the sternocostal origin of the pectoralis major.
m. sternocleidomastoi′deus [TA] sternocleidomastoid muscle (2 heads): *origin,* STERNAL HEAD—manubrium sterni, CLAVICULAR HEAD—superior surface of medial third of clavicle; *insertion,* mastoid process and superior nuchal line of occipital bone; *innervation,* accessory nerve and cervical plexus; *action,* flexes vertebral column, rotates head upward and to opposite side.
m. sternohyoi′deus [TA] sternohyoid muscle: *origin,* manubrium sterni, posterior sternoclavicular ligament, clavicle; *insertion,* body of hyoid bone; *innervation,* upper ansa cervicalis; *action,* depresses hyoid bone and larynx.
m. sternothyroi′deus [TA] sternothyroid muscle: *origin,* manubrium sterni; *insertion,* lamina of thyroid cartilage; *innervation,* ansa cervicalis; *action,* depresses thyroid cartilage.
m. styloglos′sus [TA] styloglossus muscle: *origin,* styloid process; *insertion,* margin of tongue; *innervation,* hypoglossal; *action,* raises and retracts tongue.
m. stylohyoi′deus [TA] stylohyoid muscle: *origin,* styloid process; *insertion,* body of hyoid bone; *innervation,* facial; *action,* draws hyoid and tongue superiorly and posteriorly.
m. stylopharyn′geus [TA] stylopharyngeal muscle: one of the intrinsic muscles of the larynx; *origin,* styloid process; *insertion,* thyroid cartilage and pharyngeal constrictors; *innervation,* pharyngeal plexus, glossopharyngeal; *action,* raises and dilates pharynx.
m. subcla′vius [TA] subclavius muscle: *origin,* first rib and its cartilage; *insertion,* lower surface of clavicle; *innervation,* fifth and sixth cervical; *action,* depresses lateral end of clavicle.
mus′culi subcosta′les [TA] subcostal muscles: *origin,* inner surface of ribs: *insertion,* inner surface of first, second, and third ribs below; *innervation,* intercostal; *action,* draw adjacent ribs together, depress ribs.
mus′culi suboccipita′les [TA] suboccipital muscles: the muscles situated just below the occipital bone, including the recti capitis posteriores major and minor, the obliquus capitis inferior and superior, the recti capitis anterior and lateral, the splenius capitis, and the longus capitis muscles.
m. subscapula′ris [TA] subscapular muscle: *origin,* subscapular fossa of scapula; *insertion,* lesser tubercle of humerus; *innervation,* subscapular; *action,* rotates humerus medially.
m. supina′tor [TA] supinator muscle: *origin,* lateral epicondyle of humerus, ulna, elbow joint fascia; *insertion,* radius; *innervation,* deep radial; *action,* supinates forearm.
mus′culi suprahyoi′dei [TA] suprahyoid muscles: the muscles that attach the hyoid bone to the skull, including the digastric, stylohyoid, mylohyoid, and geniohyoid muscles.
m. supraspina′tus [TA] supraspinous muscle: *origin,* supraspinous fossa of scapula; *insertion,* greater tubercle of humerus; *innervation,* suprascapular; *action,* abducts humerus.
m. suspenso′rius duode′ni [TA] suspensory muscle of duodenum: a flat band of smooth muscle originating from the left crus of the diaphragm, and continuous with the muscular coat of the duodenum at its junction with the jejunum. Called also *ligamentum suspensorius duodeni* [TA alternative].
m. tarsa′lis infe′rior [TA] inferior tarsal muscle: *origin,* m. rectus inferior bulbi; *insertion,* tarsal plate of lower eyelid; *innervation,* sympathetic; *action,* widens palpebral fissure.
m. tarsa′lis supe′rior [TA] superior tarsal muscle: *origin,* m. levator palpebrae superioris; *insertion,* tarsal plate of upper eyelid; *innervation,* sympathetic; *action,* widens palpebral fissure. Called also *Müller muscle.*
m. tempora′lis [TA] temporal muscle: *origin,* temporal fossa and fascia; *insertion,* coronoid process of mandible; *innervation,* mandibular; *action,* closes jaws.
m. temporoparieta′lis [TA] temporoparietal muscle: *origin,* temporal fascia above ear; *insertion,* galea aponeurotica; *innervation,* temporal branches of facial; *action,* tightens scalp.
m. ten′sor fas′ciae la′tae [TA] tensor muscle of fascia lata: *origin,* iliac crest; *insertion,* iliotibial tract of fascia lata; *innervation,* superior gluteal; *action,* flexes, rotates thigh medially.
m. ten′sor tym′pani [TA] tensor muscle of tympanic membrane: *origin,* cartilaginous portion of auditory tube; *insertion,* manubrium of malleus; *innervation,* mandibular; *action,* tenses tympanic membrane.
m. ten′sor ve′li palati′ni [TA] *origin,* scaphoid fossa at base of medial pterygoid plate, wall of auditory tube, spine of sphenoid; *insertion,* aponeurosis of soft palate, horizontal part of palatine bone; *innervation,* mandibular; *action,* tenses soft palate, opens auditory tube.
m. te′res ma′jor [TA] teres major muscle: *origin,* inferior angle of scapula; *insertion,* lip of intertubercular sulcus of humerus; *innervation,* lower subscapular; *action,* adducts, extends, rotates arm medially.
m. te′res mi′nor [TA] teres minor muscle: *origin,* lateral margin of scapula; *insertion,* greater tubercle of humerus; *innervation,* axillary; *action,* rotates arm laterally.
mus′culi thora′cis [TA] the muscles of the thorax.
m. thyroarytenoi′deus [TA] thyroarytenoid muscle: one of the intrinsic muscles of the larynx; *origin,* lamina of thyroid cartilage; *insertion,* muscular process of arytenoid cartilage; *innervation,* recurrent laryngeal; *action,* relaxes, shortens vocal folds.

Musculus *Continued*

m. thyrohyoi′deus [TA] thyrohyoid muscle: *origin,* lamina of thyroid cartilage; *insertion,* greater cornu of hyoid bone; *innervation,* first cervical; *action,* raises and changes form of larynx.

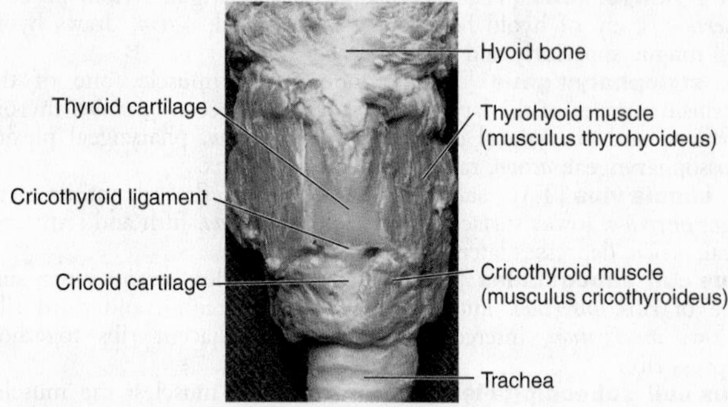

m. thyropharyn′geus TA alternative for *pars thyropharyngea musculi constrictoris pharyngis inferioris.*

m. tibia′lis ante′rior [TA] anterior tibial muscle: *origin,* lateral condyle and lateral surface of tibia, interosseous membrane; *insertion,* medial cuneiform and base of first metatarsal; *innervation,* deep peroneal; *action,* dorsiflexes and inverts foot.

m. tibia′lis poste′rior [TA] posterior tibial muscle: *origin,* tibia, fibula, interosseous membrane; *insertion,* bases of second to fourth metatarsals and tarsals, except talus; *innervation,* tibial; *action,* plantar flexes and inverts foot.

m. trachea′lis [TA] tracheal muscle: a transverse layer of smooth fibers in the dorsal portion of the trachea; *insertion,* tracheal cartilages; *innervation,* autonomic fibers; *action,* lessens caliber of trachea.

m. tra′gicus [TA] muscle of tragus: a short, flattened vertical band on the lateral surface of the tragus, innervated by the auriculotemporal and posterior auricular nerves.

mus′culi transversospina′les [TA] a general term including the semispinalis and multifidus muscles and the rotatores.

m. transver′sus abdo′minis [TA] transverse abdominal muscle: *origin,* cartilages of six lower ribs, thoracolumbar fascia, iliac crest, inguinal ligament; *insertion,* linea alba through rectus sheath, conjoined tendon to pubis; *innervation,* lower intercostals, iliohypogastric, ilioinguinal; *action,* increases intra-abdominal pressure, acts as accessory respiratory muscle.

m. transver′sus auri′culae [TA], **m. transver′sus auricula′ris** transverse muscle of auricle: *origin,* cranial surface of auricle; *insertion,* circumference of auricle; *innervation,* posterior auricular; *action,* retracts helix.

m. transver′sus lin′guae [TA] transverse muscle of tongue: *origin,* median septum of tongue; *insertion,* dorsum and margins of tongue; *innervation,* hypoglossal; *action,* changes shape of tongue in mastication and deglutition.

m. transver′sus men′ti [TA] transverse muscle of chin: superficial fibers of the depressor anguli oris which turn back and cross to the opposite side.

m. transver′sus nu′chae [TA] transverse muscle of nape: a small muscle often present, passing from the occipital protuberance to the posterior auricular muscle; it may be either superficial or deep to the trapezius.

m. transver′sus perine′i profun′dus [TA] deep transverse perineal muscle: *origin,* ramus of ischium; *insertion,* tendinous center of perineum; *innervation,* perineal; *action,* fixes tendinous center of perineum.

m. transver′sus perine′i superficia′lis [TA] superficial transverse perineal muscle: *origin,* ramus of ischium; *insertion,* tendinous center of perineum; *innervation,* perineal; *action,* fixes tendinous center of perineum. Called also *Theile muscle.*

m. transver′sus thora′cis [TA] transverse muscle of thorax: *origin,* mediastinal surface of sternum and of xiphoid process; *insertion,* cartilages of second to sixth ribs; *innervation,* intercostal; *action,* draws ribs downward.

m. trape′zius [TA] trapezius muscle: *origin,* occipital bone, ligamentum nuchae, spinous processes of seventh cervical and all thoracic vertebrae; *insertion,* clavicle, acromion, spine of scapula; *innervation,* accessory nerve and cervical plexus; *action,* elevates shoulder, rotates scapula to raise shoulder in abduction of arm, draws scapula backward.

m. triangula′ris 1. [TA] triangular muscle: a muscle that is triangular in shape. 2. m. depressor anguli oris.

m. tri′ceps bra′chii [TA] triceps muscle of arm (3 heads): *origin,* CAPUT LONGUM—infraglenoid tubercle of scapula, CAPUT LATERALE—posterior surface of humerus, lateral border of humerus, lateral intermuscular septum, CAPUT MEDIALE—posterior surface of humerus below radial groove, medial border of humerus, medial intermuscular septum; *insertion,* olecranon of ulna; *innervation,* radial; *action,* extends forearm, long head adducts and extends arm.

m. tri′ceps su′rae [TA] the gastrocnemius and soleus considered together.

mus′culi trigo′ni vesi′cae urina′riae [TA] trigonal muscles: a submucous sheet of smooth muscle at the bladder trigone, continuous with ureteral muscles above and with those of the proximal urethra below. Its superficial and deep layers are morphologically distinct.

m. trigo′ni vesi′cae urina′riae profun′dus [TA] deep trigonal muscle: the deep layer of trigonal muscles, which is continuous with the musculus detrusor vesicae urinariae.

m. trigo′ni vesi′cae urina′riae superficia′lis [TA] the superficial layer of the trigonal muscles, continuous proximally with the muscles of the ureteral wall.

m. unipenna′tus TA alternative for *m. semipennatus.*

m. u′vulae [TA] muscle of uvula: *origin,* posterior nasal spine of palatine bone and aponeurosis of soft palate; *insertion,* uvula; *innervation,* pharyngeal plexus of vagus; *action,* raises uvula.

m. vas′tus interme′dius [TA] *origin,* anterior and lateral surfaces of femur; *insertion,* patella, common tendon of quadriceps femoris; *innervation,* femoral; *action,* extends leg.

m. vas′tus latera′lis [TA] *origin,* lateral aspect of femur; *insertion,* patella, common tendon of quadriceps femoris; *innervation,* femoral; *action,* extends leg.

m. vas′tus media′lis [TA] *origin,* medial aspect of femur; *insertion,* patella, common tendon of quadriceps femoris; *innervation,* femoral; *action,* extends leg.

m. ventricula′ris a name applied to fibers of the thyroarytenoid muscle running into the vestibular folds.

m. vertica′lis lin′guae [TA] vertical muscle of tongue: *origin,* dorsal fascia of tongue; *insertion,* sides and base of tongue; *innervation,* hypoglossal; *action,* changes shape of tongue in mastication and deglutition.

m. voca′lis [TA] vocal muscle: one of the intrinsic muscles of the larynx; *origin,* angle between laminae of thyroid cartilage; *insertion,* vocal process of arytenoid cartilage; *innervation,* recurrent laryngeal; *action,* shortens and relaxes vocal folds.

m. zygoma′ticus m. zygomaticus major.

m. zygoma′ticus ma′jor [TA] greater zygomatic muscle: *origin,* zygomatic bone in front of temporal process; *insertion,* angle of mouth; *innervation,* facial; *action,* draws angle of mouth backward and upward.

m. zygoma′ticus mi′nor [TA] lesser zygomatic muscle: *origin,* zygomatic bone near maxillary suture; *insertion,* orbicularis oris and levator labii superioris; *innervation,* facial; *action,* draws upper lip upward and laterally.

Muse (mūz) trademark for a suppository form of alprostadil.

mush·room (mush′rōōm) the fruiting body (basidiocarp) of any of a variety of basidiomycetous fleshy fungi of the order Agaricales, especially one that is edible. Poisonous species are popularly called *toadstools.* See also *agaric.*

mu·si·co·gen·ic (mu″zĭ-ko-jen′ik) caused by or in reaction to musical sounds.

Mus·set sign (mu-sa′) [Louis Charles Alfred de *Musset,* French poet, 1810–1857, who died of aortic insufficiency] see under *sign.*

mus·si·ta·tion (mus″ĭ-ta′shən) [L. *mussitare* to mutter] the moving of the lips with no utterance of articulate sounds.

Mus·tard operation (mus′tərd) [William Thornton *Mustard,* Canadian surgeon, 1914–1987] see under *operation.*

mus·tard (mus′tərd) [L. *sinapis*] 1. any of several plants of the genus *Brassica.* 2. the ripe seeds of black mustard or white mustard; when they are crushed and moistened, volatile oils are liberated that are responsible for the counterirritant, stimulant, and emetic properties of mustard.

3. resembling, or something resembling, mustard in one or more of its properties; e.g., mustard gas, named for its odor.

black m., brown m. *Brassica nigra* (L.) Koch, a source of volatile oil of mustard and used internally as an emetic and externally as a counterirritant (see *mustard plaster*, under *plaster*); it is also used in homeopathy to treat upper respiratory irritation and the gastrointestinal tract. Since the plant contains sinigrin, animals consuming large quantities of it may develop fatal gastroenteritis.

nitrogen m. 1. mechlorethamine hydrochloride. 2. any of a group of cytotoxic alkylating agents (q.v.) having the general formula $R—N(CH_2CH_2Cl_2)_2$; they are homologous with the vesicant war gas dichlorodiethyl sulfide (mustard gas). Those used as antineoplastic and immunosuppressive agents include chlorambucil, cyclophosphamide, ifosfamide, mechlorethamine, melphalan, and uracil mustard.

L-phenylalanine m. melphalan.

uracil m. a cytotoxic alkylating agent that is the uracil derivative of nitrogen mustard, used as an antineoplastic in the treatment of chronic lymphocytic and chronic granulocytic leukemia, non-Hodgkin lymphoma, mycosis fungoides, and polycythemia vera; now generally replaced by more effective agents.

white m., yellow m. *Brassica alba* (L.) Rabenh., which has been used as an emetic and counterirritant. Since the plant contains sinigrin, animals consuming large quantities of it may develop fatal gastroenteritis.

Mus·tar·gen (mus′tər-jən) trademark for a preparation of mechlorethamine hydrochloride.

mu·ta·cism (mu′tə-siz-əm) mytacism.

mu·ta·gen (mu′tə-jən) [*muta*tion + *gen*esis] a chemical or physical agent that induces or increases genetic mutations above the spontaneous background level.

mu·ta·gen·e·sis (mu″tə-jen′ə-sis) [*muta*tion + *-genesis*] the induction of genetic mutation.

site-directed m., site-specific m. a method for producing a defined DNA mutation; a sequence alteration is made in vitro at a specific nucleotide or region and the altered DNA is reintroduced into cells.

mu·ta·gen·ic (mu″tə-jen′ik) inducing genetic mutation.

mu·ta·ge·nic·i·ty (mu″tə-jə-nis′ĭ-te) the ability to induce genetic mutation.

Mu·ta·my·cin (mu″tə-mi′sin) trademark for a preparation of mitomycin.

mu·tant (mu′tənt) [L. *mutare* to change] 1. something, as an organism, cell, virus, or gene, that has undergone genetic mutation. 2. produced by mutation.

mu·ta·ro·tase (mu″tə-ro′tās) aldose 1-epimerase.

mu·ta·ro·ta·tion (mu″tə-ro-ta′shən) a change in the optical activity of a freshly prepared solution of a pure compound that occurs because of the formation of diastereoisomers of the original compound having different optical activity, e.g., the equilibration of the α and β anomers of glucose.

mu·tase (mu′tās) [EC 5.4] any member of a subclass of enzymes of the isomerase class that act as intramolecular transferases, catalyzing the intramolecular shift of an acyl, amino, phosphate, or other chemical group.

mu·ta·tion (mu-ta′shən) [L. *mutatio*, from *mutare* to change] 1. in genetics, a permanent transmissible change in the genetic material, usually in a single gene, although the term is sometimes used to include gross alterations in chromosomal structure. 2. a cell, virus, or organism exhibiting such a change.

amber m. see *nonsense m.*

auxotrophic m. a mutation resulting in the inability of bacteria to grow on minimal media.

back m. reverse m.

biochemical m. a mutation that affects the metabolism of the organism.

chromosomal m. a mutation affecting large regions of a chromosome and caused by breakage, e.g., by *deletion*, *inversion*, or *translocation*. See also *genomic m.* and *point m.*

cold-sensitive m. a conditional mutation producing a gene functional at high temperatures and nonfunctional at low.

conditional m. a mutation affecting an organism's phenotype under restrictive growth conditions but not under permissive growth conditions, the wild type being expressed equivalently under both growth conditions.

conditional lethal m. a mutation lethal only under certain environmental or genetic conditions; see also *lethal m.*

constitutive m. a mutation that causes a gene usually under regulatory control to be expressed constantly, independent of regulation.

dominant negative m. a mutation whose gene product adversely affects the normal, wild-type gene product in the same cell, usually by combining with it and disabling or inactivating it.

dynamic m. a mutation acting on tandemly arrayed DNA repeat sequences, leading to their intergenerational instability and allelic expansion.

forward m. a mutation causing a change in a gene away from the wild type form, sometimes specifically one producing an altered (mutant) phenotype; cf. *reverse m.*

frameshift m. a mutation resulting from an insertion or deletion in a coding sequence that is not an exact multiple of 3 base pairs, so that from the point of mutation onwards, the codons are read out of phase; the reading frame of the gene is changed, and a completely different set of amino acids is made into protein.

gain-of-function m. a mutation that alters the gene product so that it is increased in quantity or possesses a new function or other new pattern of gene expression.

genomic m. a mutation affecting the number of chromosomes present, e.g., aneuploidy, in which the genome gains or loses one or more chromosomes, and polyploidy, in which the overall chromosome number is doubled or tripled. See also *chromosomal m.* and *point m.*

germinal m., germline m. a mutation in a germ cell, altering the gametes and thus transmitted to progeny. Cf. *somatic m.*

heat-sensitive m. a conditional mutation producing a gene functional at low temperatures and nonfunctional at high.

heterozygous m. mutation occurring on only one allele of a pair.

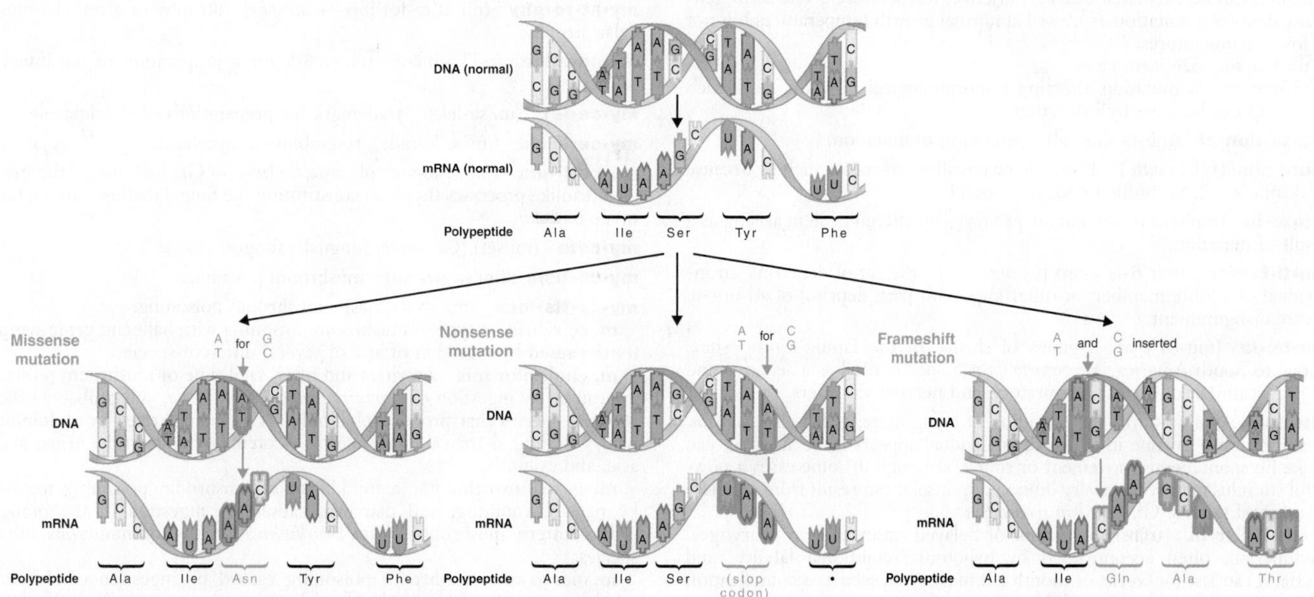

■ Diagram showing the effects on translation of missense, nonsense, and frameshift mutations to a DNA segment.

induced m. a mutation caused by external factors which are experimentally or accidentally produced; see also *spontaneous m.*
leaky m. a gene mutation that reduces but does not abolish the activity of the gene product.
lethal m. a mutation that results in the premature death of the organism; see also *conditional lethal m.*
loss-of-function m. a mutation that alters the gene product so that it is decreased in quantity or lacks one or more normal functions.
missense m. a mutation that changes a codon so that it codes for a different amino acid; cf. *nonsense m.*
natural m. spontaneous m.
nonsense m. a mutation in which one of the three termination codons in the mRNA (UAG, *amber;* UAA, *ochre;* UGA, *umber* or *opal*), used to signal the end of a polypeptide, appears in the middle of a genetic message, causes premature termination of transcription, and results in the production of an incomplete, generally nonfunctional polypeptide. See also *missense m.*
null m. a mutation that entirely eliminates the function of a gene so that there is no gene product.
nutritional m. a mutation affecting an organism's ability to produce a molecule, e.g., an amino acid, essential for growth.
ochre m. see *nonsense m.*
opal m. see *nonsense m.*
point m. a mutation resulting from a change in a single base pair in the DNA molecule, caused by the substitution of one nucleotide for another. See also *chromosomal m.* and *genomic m.*
private m. a mutation observed in a single family or a very small group.
reading frameshift m. frameshift m.
reverse m. specifically, a mutation that restores the original nucleotide sequence of the wild-type gene and thus its phenotype; however, the term is often extended to include any mutation that causes reversion (q.v.) to a wild type phenotype. Cf. *forward m.*
silent m. 1. a mutation that does not affect function or production of the gene product. 2. more specifically, a change in the DNA sequence of a coding region that does not change the amino acid sequence of the polypeptide product, and so does not affect the phenotype.
somatic m. a mutation in a somatic cell, rather than a germ cell; it provides the basis for mosaicism, but is not transmitted to progeny. Somatic mutations have been implicated in the development of many forms of cancer. Cf. *germline m.*
spontaneous m. one of the mutations occurring at a low but measurable rate in all organisms, presumably because of the inherent rates of error in the replication and transmission of a genome. Called also *natural m.* See also *induced m.*
suppressor m. a mutation that partially or completely masks phenotypic expression of another (primary) mutation but occurs at a different site from it (i.e., causes suppression); it may be intragenic or intergenic. The term is used particularly to describe a secondary mutation that restores the ability of a transfer RNA to recognize a nonsense codon that was created by the primary mutation.
synonymous m. silent m., def. 2.
temperature-sensitive m., t-s m. a conditional mutation producing a protein product with a temperature-dependent instability; thus the phenotype is normal at some (permissive) temperatures, but expression of the mutation can be elicited at other (restrictive) temperatures. The term generally denotes a mutation expressed at normal growth temperatures but not at lower temperatures.
umber m. see *nonsense m.*
visible m. a mutation affecting a morphological trait and for which screening can be done by inspection.

mu•ta•tion•al (mu-ta′shən-əl) pertaining to mutation.

mute (mūt) [L. *mutus*] 1. unable or unwilling to speak, such as because of deafness. 2. to muffle or soften a sound.

mu•te•in (mu′tēn) [from *mu*tant-pro*tein*] an altered protein arising as a result of mutation.

mu•ti•la•tion (mu″tĭ-la′shən) [L. *mutilatio*] the act of depriving an individual of a limb, member, or other important part; deprival of an organ; severe disfigurement.

Mu•tis•ia (mu-tiz′e-ə) a genus of shrubs of the family Compositae, native to South America. *M. viciaefo′lia* is a species used as a sedative and in the treatment of cardiac, respiratory, and nervous disorders.

mu•tism (mu′tiz-əm) the condition of being mute; called also *aphonia.*
akinetic m. a state in which the individual appears to be alert but can make no spontaneous movement or sound, although in some cases a powerful stimulus may evoke a very limited response; it can result from a variety of cerebral lesions. Cf. *locked-in syndrome.*
cerebellar m. transient mutism of delayed onset and oropharyngeal dysfunction, often accompanied by hypotonia, emotional lability, and ataxia; it can last for weeks or months. It most often seen as a complication of posterior fossa surgery in children.
elective m. selective m.
selective m. [DSM-IV] a mental disorder of childhood characterized by continuous refusal to speak in social situations by a child who is able and willing to speak to selected persons.

mu•tu•al•ism (mu′choo-əl-iz-əm) symbiosis in which both populations (or individuals) gain from the association and are unable to survive without it.

mu•tu•al•ist (mu′tu-əl-ist) any organism or species associated with another in a relationship which is beneficial to both.

muz•zle (muz′əl) the most anterior region of the face of various animals, consisting of the nose, jaws, and surrounding structures.

MV[1] [L.] Med′icus Veterina′rius (veterinary physician).

MV[2] megavolt; minute volume.

mV millivolt.

μV microvolt.

M-VAC a cancer chemotherapy regimen consisting of methotrexate, vinblastine, Adriamycin (doxorubicin), and cisplatin.

MVP mitral valve prolapse.

MVV maximal (or maximum) voluntary ventilation.

MW molecular weight.

μW microwatt.

My myopia.

my•al•gia (mi-al′jə) [*my-* + *algia*] pain in a muscle or muscles. Called also *myodynia.*
epidemic m. see under *pleurodynia.*
pelvic tension m. levator ani syndrome.

My•am•bu•tol (mi-am′bu-tol) trademark for a preparation of ethambutol hydrochloride.

My•an•e•sin (mi-an′ə-sin) trademark for a preparation of mephenesin.

my•a•sis (mi-a′sis) myiasis.

my•as•the•nia (mi″əs-the′ne-ə) [*my-* + *asthenia*] muscular weakness; any constitutional anomaly of muscle. **myasthen′ic** *adj*
familial infantile m. gravis choline acetyltransferase deficiency.
m. gra′vis an autoimmune disease of neuromuscular function due to the presence of antibodies to acetylcholine receptors at the neuromuscular junction; characteristics include muscle fatigue and exhaustion that fluctuates in severity, without sensory disturbance or atrophy. It may be restricted to one muscle group or become generalized with severe weakness and sometimes respiratory insufficiency. It may affect any muscle of the body, but especially those of the eyes, face, lips, tongue, throat, and neck. Called also *Erb-Goldflam, Goldflam,* or *Goldflam-Erb disease.*
m. gra′vis pseudoparaly′tica m. gravis.
m. laryn′gis phonasthenia.
neonatal m. a transient myasthenia (lasting from a week to a month) affecting offspring of myasthenic women, characteristically marked by difficulty in sucking and swallowing.

my•a•to•nia (mi″ə-to′ne-ə) [*my-* + *atonia*] amyotonia.

my•at•o•ny (mi-at′ə-ne) amyotonia.

my•at•ro•phy (mi-at′rə-fe) [*my-* + *atrophy*] atrophy of a muscle; muscular atrophy.

My•ca•mine (mi′kə-mēn) trademark for a preparation of micafungin sodium.

My•ce•lex (mi′sə-leks) trademark for preparations of clotrimazole.

my•ce•li•oid (mi-se′le-oid) resembling a mycelium.

my•ce•li•um (mi-se′le-əm) pl. *myce′lia* [*myc-* + Gr. *hēlos* nail] the mass of threadlike processes (hyphae) constituting the fungal thallus. **myce′lial, myce′lian** *adj*

my•cete (mi′sēt) [Gr. *mykēs* fungus] fungus.

my•ce•tism (mi′sə-tiz-əm) mushroom poisoning.

my•ce•tis•mus (mi″sə-tiz′məs) mushroom poisoning.
m. ce′rebris a type of mushroom poisoning with hallucinogenic symptoms, caused by ingestion of any of several different species.
m. cholerifor′mis a serious and often fatal type of mushroom poisoning caused by ingestion of *Amanita phalloides, A. verna,* and probably other *Amanita* species that produce phalloidin; it is characterized by abdominal pain, vomiting, diarrhea, bloody stools, protein and casts in the urine, malaise, and cyanosis.
m. gastrointestina′lis a mild form of mushroom poisoning marked by nausea, vomiting, and diarrhea, caused by ingestion of the orange jack-o-lantern mushroom *(Clitocybe illudens)* or any of numerous other species.
m. nervo′sus mushroom poisoning caused by ingestion of *Amanita pantherina* or *A. muscaria,* which elaborate muscarine. It is marked by such symptoms as tearing, sweating, salivation, persistent peristalsis,

Selected Etiologic Agents of Mycetoma

Agent	Grain Color
Actinomycotic	
Actinomadura madurae	White to yellow or pink
Actinomadura pellitieri	Red
Actinomyces israelii	White to yellow
Nocardia asteroides	White (when present)
Nocardia brasiliensis	White
Nocardia otitidis-caviarum	White to yellow
Nocardiopsis dassonvillei	Cream color
Streptomyces somaliensis	Yellow to brown
Eumycotic	
Acremonium falciforme	White to yellow
Acremonium kiliense	White
Acremonium recifei	White
Aspergillus nidulans	White
Corynespora cassicola	Black
Curvularia geniculata	Black
Curvularia lunata	Black
Exophiala jeanselmei	Black
Fusarium moniliforme	White
Fusarium oxysporum	White
Fusarium solani	White
Leptosphaeria senegalensis	Black
Leptosphaeria tompkinsii	Black
*Madurella grisea**	Black
Madurella mycetomatis	Black
Neotestudina rosatii	White
Phialophora cyanescens	White
Plenodomus avramii	Black
Pseudallescheria boydii	White
Pseudochaetosphaeronema larense	Black
Pyrenochaeta mackinnonii	Black
*Pyrenochaeta romeroi**	Black

*Believed to be related if not identical.

retching and vomiting, contraction of the pupil and ciliary muscles, acute excitement, delirium, and coma.

m. sanguina′rius a type of mushroom poisoning caused by ingestion of *Helvella esculenta* or other species of *Helvella;* symptoms include hemoglobinuria, abdominal pain, and jaundice.

mycet(o)- [Gr. *mykēs*, gen. *mykētos* fungus] a combining form denoting relationship to fungus. See also *myc(o)-*.

my•ce•to•gen•ic (mi″sə-to-jen′ik) mycetogenous.

my•ce•tog•e•nous (mi″sə-toj′ə-nəs) [*myceto-* + *-genous*] caused by fungous growths; called also *mycetogenic.*

my•ce•to•ma (mi″sə-to′mə) [*myceto-* + *-oma*] a slowly progressive, destructive infection of the cutaneous and subcutaneous tissues, fascia, and bone caused by certain actinomycetes *(actinomycotic m.)* or fungi *(eumycotic m.)*, acquired by traumatic implantation of the fungus or bacterium. It usually involves the foot *(Madura foot)* or leg, although the hand or any other site may be inoculated. The primary lesion is a tumefaction, with granulomas, suppurating abscesses, and sinuses discharging grains or granules representing microcolonies of the pathogen. Called also *maduromycosis.* See illustration and table.

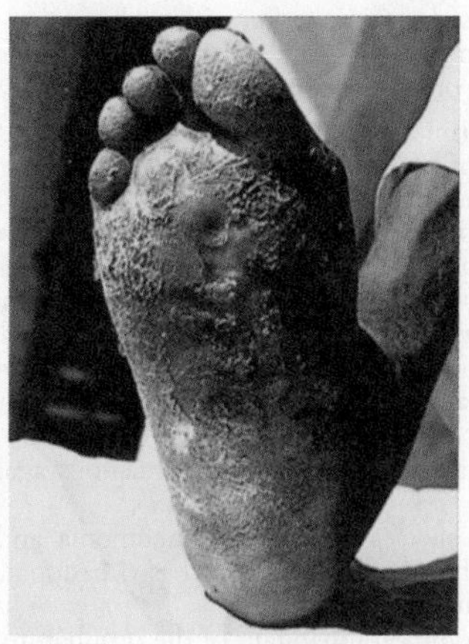

■ Mycetoma affecting the foot (Madura foot).

actinomycotic m. mycetoma caused by infection with actinomycetes; see table. Called also *actinomycetoma.*

eumycotic m. mycetoma caused by infection with Eumycota (true fungi); see table. Called also *eumycetoma.*

My•ce•to•zoa (mi-se″to-zo′ə) former name for Myxomycetes when it was considered a group of protozoa.

My•ci•guent (mi′sĭ-gwent″) trademark for preparations of neomycin sulfate.

myc(o)- [Gr. *mykēs*, fungus] a combining form denoting relationship to fungus. Also, *mycet(o)-*.

my•co•bac•te•ria (mi″ko-bak-tēr-eə) plural of *mycobacterium.*

My•co•bac•te•ri•a•ceae (mi″ko-bak-tēr″e-a′se-e) a family of bacteria of the suborder Corynebacterineae, order Actinomycetales, made up of slightly curved or straight, rod-shaped, gram-positive, aerobic, mesophilic cells, sometimes branching. They are found in soil, water, and dairy products and also as parasites. The family contains the genus *Mycobacterium.*

my•co•bac•te•ri•o•sis (mi″ko-bak-tēr-eo′sis) a disease caused by a mycobacterium, usually excluding *Mycobacterium tuberculosis;* see *nontuberculous mycobacteria,* under *mycobacterium.* Immunocompromised patients are particularly susceptible. See also *atypical tuberculosis.*

My•co•bac•te•ri•um (mi″ko-bak-tēr′e-əm) [*myco-* + Gr. *baktērion* little rod] a large genus of bacteria of the family Mycobacteriaceae, consisting of aerobic, acid-fast, nonmotile, curved or straight rods; it includes the highly pathogenic organisms that cause tuberculosis *(M. tuberculosis)* and leprosy *(M. leprae).* The type species is *M. tuberculo′sis.*

M. absces′sus a species closely related to, and formerly classified as a subspecies of, *M. chelonae*, occurring widely in the environment and causing skin and soft tissue infections.

M. africa′num a species that resembles *M. bovis* and *M. tuberculosis* and causes disease in tropical Africa.

M. asia′ticum a slow-growing species that has occasionally been found in bronchopulmonary infections.

M. a′vium the avian type of tubercle bacillus, causing tuberculosis in chickens and swine, and lung disease in humans. See also *Mycobacterium avium-intracellulare complex* under *complex.*

M. a′vium* subsp. *paratuberculo′sis the cause of Johne disease, a chronic enteritis of cattle, sheep, and goats. Called also *Johne bacillus.* Formerly called *M. paratuberculosis.*

M. bal′nei *M. marinum.*

M. boenic′kei a rapid-growing, nonpigmented species that has been isolated from skin, soft tissue, and bone infections.

M. bohe′micum a slow-growing, pigmented species that has been found in cases of lymphadenitis.

M. bo′vis a virulent species, isolated originally from tuberculous tubercles in cattle, that causes tuberculosis; in humans, disease is usually acquired by children from infected milk. An attenuated strain of *M. bovis* is used to prepare BCG vaccine.

M. brande′ri a slow-growing, nonpigmented species that has been found in cases of bronchopulmonary disease.

M. cela′tum a slow-growing, pigmented species that has been found in cases of bronchopulmonary disease, as well as in disseminated infections of immunocompromised persons.

M. chelo′nae a rapid-growing, nonphotochromogenic species that is an opportunistic pathogen, found in soil and soft tissue abscesses; it produces synovial lesions, gluteal abscesses, and gross lesions in various organs.

M. conspi′cuum a slow-growing, pigmented species that has been found in disseminated infections in immunocompromised persons.

M. elephan′tis a rapid-growing, pigmented species found in cases of lymphadenitis.

M. flaves′cens a scotochromogenic species isolated from drug-treated tuberculous guinea pigs but considered nonpathogenic for humans.

M. fortu′itum a rapid-growing, nonphotochromogenic species that is potentially pathogenic, producing lesions of lung, bone, or soft tissue following trauma. It has been found in soil and in injection sites of humans, cattle, and cold-blooded animals.

M. gas′tri a species found in soil and human gastric and sputum specimens; it is usually nonpathogenic but has occasionally been associated with respiratory infections.

M. genaven′se a slow-growing, nonpigmented species that has been found in cases of enteritis, skin and soft tissue infections, and opportunistic infections.

M. goo′dii a rapid-growing species that has been isolated from bronchopulmonary and bone infections.

M. gordo′nae a scotochromogenic species found in tap water and soil and in human sputum and gastric lavage; it is usually nonpathogenic, but sometimes causes systemic disease in immunocompromised patients.

M. haemo′philum a nonphotochromogenic, pathogenic species that requires hemin for growth; it is a rare cause of ulcerative skin lesions and pulmonary and joint disease in immunocompromised patients.

M. heckeshornen'se a slow-growing, pigmented species that has been found in bronchopulmonary infections.

M. heidelbergen'se a slow-growing, pigmented species that has been found in cases of lymphadenitis.

M. houstonen'se a rapid-growing, nonpigmented species that has been isolated from skin, soft tissue, and bone infections.

M. immunoge'num a rapid-growing, nonpigmented species that has been isolated from skin, soft tissue, and bone infections.

M. interjec'tum a slow-growing, pigmented species that has been found in cases of lymphadenitis.

M. intracellula're a species associated with human lung infections. See also *Mycobacterium avium-intracellulare complex* under *complex*.

M. kansa'sii a slow-growing, photochromogenic species that is the etiologic agent of a tuberculosis-like disease and is often isolated from lung secretions or tubercles; the incidence of infection is sharply increased among immunocompromised persons. See also *photochromogen*.

M. la'cus a rapid-growing, pigmented species found in skin and soft tissue infections.

M. lentifla'vum a slow-growing, pigmented species that has been found in cases of lymphadenitis.

M. lep'rae the cause of human leprosy, not yet cultivated in vitro, isolated from suspect lesions as acid-fast bacilli, typically in intracellular clumps or in groups of bacilli side by side.

M. lepraemu'rium a noncultivable species resembling *M. leprae* in size and shape, which causes a chronic epizootic disease in wild rats; see also *rat leprosy*, under *leprosy*.

M. mageriten'se a rapid-growing, nonpigmented species that has been isolated from skin, soft tissue, and bone infections.

M. malmoen'se a slow-growing, nonphotochromogenic species associated with lung disease.

M. mari'num a moderate-growing, photochromogenic species found in aquariums, diseased fish, and swimming pools, the cause of skin lesions and swimming pool granuloma in humans. Called also *M. balnei* and *M. platypoecilus*.

M. micro'ti a species producing generalized tuberculosis in field mice and also infecting guinea pigs, rabbits, and calves. It is not virulent for humans and has been used for the preparation of experimental vaccines. Called also *vole bacillus* and *M. tuberculosis* var. *muris*.

M. mucoge'nicum a rapid-growing, nonpigmented species that has been isolated from skin, soft tissue, and bone infections.

M. neworleansen'se a rapid-growing, nonpigmented species that has been isolated from skin, soft tissue, and bone infections.

M. nonchromoge'nicum a slow-growing, nonphotochromogenic, nonpathogenic species found in soil; it is occasionally associated with infections of the skin, soft tissue, or bone.

M. novocastren'se a rapid-growing, pigmented species that has been found in skin and soft tissue infections.

M. palus'tre a slow-growing, pigmented species that has been found in cases of lymphadenitis.

M. paratuberculo'sis *M. avium* subsp. *paratuberculosis*.

M. peregri'num a rapid-growing, nonpigmented species that has been isolated from skin, soft tissue, and bone infections.

M. platypoe'cilus *M. marinum*.

M. porci'num a rapid-growing, nonpigmented species that has been isolated from skin, soft tissue, and bone infections.

M. scrofula'ceum a slow-growing, scotochromogenic species found in human secretions, particularly pus from suppurating cervical lymphadenitis in children, as well as in sputum and gastric lavage, sometimes in association with lung disease.

M. senegalen'se a rapid-growing, nonpigmented species that has been isolated from skin, soft tissue, and bone infections.

M. sep'ticum a rapid-growing, nonpigmented species that has been isolated from skin, soft tissue, and bone infections.

M. si'miae a slow-growing, photochromogenic species that sometimes causes lung disease or opportunistic infections.

M. smeg'matis a rapid-growing, nonphotochromogenic species originally isolated from human smegma and found also in soil and water; it has been associated with chronic bronchopulmonary disease and infections of the skin and bone. Called also *smegma bacillus*.

M. szul'gai a slow-growing, pathogenic species that behaves as a scotochromogen at 37°C and as a photochromogen at 25°C. It is associated with pulmonary infections but may be found in nonpulmonary sites.

M. ter'rae a slow-growing, nonpigmented species normally found in soil, water, and human sputum and gastric lavage specimens; it is occasionally associated with infections of the skin, soft tissue, or bone.

M. tri'plex a slow-growing, nonpigmented species that has been found in bronchopulmonary infections.

M. tuberculo'sis a slow-growing, nonphotochromogenic, pathogenic species that causes tuberculosis in numerous species of mammals. Human infection is commonly in the lung; rates of both pulmonary and nonpulmonary disease are sharply increased among immunocompromised individuals. Strains of low virulence have also been isolated from cases of lupus erythematosus, scrofuloderma, and urogenital tuberculosis. Called also *tubercle bacillus*.

M. tus'ciae a slow-growing, pigmented species that has been found in cases of lymphadenitis.

M. ul'cerans a slow-growing, nonphotochromogenic species that causes Buruli ulcer.

M. wolinskyi a rapid-growing species that has been linked to bone infections.

M. xeno'pi a slow-growing, scotochromogenic species found in human secretions; it is usually harmless but is occasionally associated with chronic pulmonary disease.

my·co·bac·te·ri·um (mi″ko-bak-tēr′e-əm) pl. *mycobacte'ria*. an organism of the genus *Mycobacterium*.

anonymous mycobacteria, atypical mycobacteria nontuberculous mycobacteria.

Group I–IV mycobacteria nontuberculous mycobacteria.

nontuberculous mycobacteria mycobacteria other than *M. tuberculosis* or *M. bovis*. They are divided into four groups (Runyon groups) based on pigmentation and rate of growth, each containing several species. Group I includes slow-growing photochromogens; group II slow-growing scotochromogens; group III slow-growing nonphotochromogens; and group IV rapidly growing mycobacteria. Called also *anonymous* or *atypical mycobacteria*.

my·co·bac·tin (mi″ko-bak′tin) a complex lipophilic compound found in the cell envelope of certain species of *Mycobacterium;* it is also required for growth by at least one species. Mycobactin chelates iron and facilitates iron transport into the cell.

My·co-Bio·tic II (mi′ko-bi-ot′ik) trademark for a combination preparation of nystatin and triamcinolone acetonide.

My·co·bu·tin (mi″kə-bu′tin) trademark for a preparation of rifabutin.

My·co·cen·tros·po·ra (mi″ko-sen-tros′pə-rə) a genus of imperfect fungi of the form-class Hyphomycetes. *M. aceri'na* has been identified as the cause of verrucose skin lesions.

My·co·der·ma (mi″ko-dur′mə) a former genus of imperfect fungi whose species are now included in *Candida, Blastomyces, Coccidioides,* and *Paracoccidioides. M. ace'ti* is a misnomer for a combination of yeasts that produce acetic acid from fermentation of alcohol.

my·co·flo·ra (mi″ko-flor′ə) the number and varieties of fungi present in or characteristic of a specific location.

My·co·gen II (mi′ko-jən″) trademark for a combination preparation of nystatin and triamcinolone acetonide.

my·co·lic ac·ids (mi-ko′lik) α-alkyl, β-hydroxy substituted long chain fatty acids found in the cell walls of bacteria in the genera *Mycobacterium, Nocardia,* and *Corynebacterium;* they may be responsible for the acid-fast staining properties of these organisms.

My·co·log II (mi′ko-log) trademark for a combination preparation of nystatin and triamcinolone acetonide.

my·col·o·gist (mi-kol′ə-jist) a specialist in mycology.

my·col·o·gy (mi-kol′ə-je) [*myco-* + *-logy*] the science and study of fungi.

my·co·pa·thol·o·gy (mi″ko-pə-thol′ə-je) the scientific study of the pathologic changes caused by fungi.

my·co·phage (mi′ko-fāj) [*myco-* + *-phage*] a virus that infects fungi and may cause their lysis.

my·coph·a·gy (mi-kof′ə-je) ingestion of mushrooms and other fungi.

my·co·pheno·late mo·fe·til (MMF) (mi″ko-fen′ə-lāt) an immunosuppressive agent used in conjunction with cyclosporine and corticosteroids to prevent rejection of allogeneic renal, hepatic, and cardiac transplants; administered orally or intravenously.

My·co·plas·ma (mi′ko-plaz″mə) [*myco-* + Gr. *plasma* anything formed or molded] a genus of bacteria of the family Mycoplasmataceae, made up of round, highly pleomorphic, gram-negative cells that are bounded by a single triple-layered membrane and lack a true cell wall. Cholesterol or another sterol is required for growth. *M. mycoi'des* causes pleuropneumonia in cattle, and other species comprise the pleuropneumonialike organisms (see under *organism*). The organisms are parasites and pathogens widely distributed on the mucous membranes of mammals and birds, and are common contaminants of animal cell cultures. The type species is *M. mycoi'des*.

M. agalac'tiae a species that causes contagious agalactia in sheep and goats.

M. argini'ni a species that causes pneumonia and other respiratory diseases in cattle, sheep, and goats, and has occasionally infected humans who worked with infected animals.

M. bucca'le a common inhabitant of the oropharynx of nonhuman primates. Called also *M. orale type 2*.

M. ca′nis a nonpathogenic species commonly found in the throat and respiratory and genital tracts of dogs.
M. conjunc′tivae a species that causes keratoconjunctivitis in sheep and goats.
M. fau′cium a species found in the oropharynx of primates. Called also *M. orale type 3*.
M. fermen′tans a species occasionally isolated from the human genital tract and oropharynx, and causing serious infections in immunocompromised persons.
M. gallisep′ticum a pathogen for poultry, causing respiratory disease, encephalitis, and infectious arthritis.
M. genita′lium a species that has been found in urinary tract infections.
M. granula′rum *Acholeplasma granularum.*
M. haemoca′nis a nonpathogenic species found in dogs. Formerly called *Haemobartonella canis.*
M. haemofe′lis a species that causes feline infectious anemia and can be transmitted from cat to cat by biting during fights. Formerly called *Haemobartonella felis.*
M. haemomu′ris a common parasite of laboratory rats, in which the infection is activated by splenectomy. Formerly called *Haemobartonella muris.*
M. ho′minis a common inhabitant of the human vagina and cervix that may cause infections of the male and female reproductive tracts, respiratory disease, or pharyngitis.
M. hyorhi′nis a common inhabitant of the nasal cavity in swine that can also cause mycoplasmal polyarthritis or polyserositis.
M. hyosyno′viae a common inhabitant of the nasopharynx of swine that can also cause mycoplasmal polyarthritis.
M. laidla′wii *Acholeplasma laidlawii.*
M. mycoi′des the type species of *Mycoplasma*, which is the etiologic agent of pleuropneumonia in cattle and goats.
M. neuroly′ticum a species of which some strains elaborate a neurolytic exotoxin that causes rolling disease in mice.
M. ora′le a species found in the upper respiratory tract of primates. Called also *M. orale type 1* and *M. pharyngis.*
M. ora′le **type 1** *M. orale.*
M. ora′le **type 2** *M. buccale.*
M. ora′le **type 3** *M. faucium.*
M. pe′netrans a species that has been found in urinary tract infections.
M. pharyn′gis *M. orale.*
M. pi′rum a species that has been found in urinary tract infections.
M. pneumo′niae a species that often causes inapparent infections or mild respiratory tract disease but can also cause mycoplasmal pneumonia (q.v.). Called also *Eaton agent.*
M. saliva′rium a nonpathogenic species found as part of the normal flora of the human oral cavity and upper respiratory tract.
M. syno′viae a species that causes infectious synovitis in birds.

my•co•plas•ma (mi′ko-plaz″mə) pl. *mycoplasmas, mycoplas′mata.* A bacterium of the class Mollicutes.
T-strain m. *Ureaplasma.*

my•co•plas•mal (mi″ko-plaz′məl) of, pertaining to, or caused by *Mycoplasma.*

My•co•plas•ma•ta•ceae (mi″ko-plaz″mə-ta′se-e) a family of bacteria of the order Mycoplasmatales, made up of organisms that require a sterol for growth. It contains the genera *Eperythrozoon, Haemobartonella, Mycoplasma,* and *Ureaplasma.*

My•co•plas•ma•ta•les (mi″ko-plaz″mə-ta′ləs) an order of bacteria of the class Mollicutes, containing a single family, the Mycoplasmataceae.

my•co•plas•mo•sis (mi″ko-plaz-mo′sis) infection with *Mycoplasma*; see also *mycoplasmal pneumonia, polyarthritis,* and *polyserositis.*

my•cose (mi′kōs) trehalose.

my•co•side (mi′ko-sīd) a glycolipid that contains mycolic acid and a polysaccharide moiety. A distinctive mycoside found in the cell walls confers immunologic cross-reactivity on cells of *Corynebacterium, Mycobacteria,* and *Nocardia.*

my•co•sis (mi-ko′sis) [*myc-* + *-osis*] 1. any disease caused by a fungus. 2. any of various other diseases that were originally thought to be caused by fungi.
m. fungoi′des a chronic or rapidly progressive form of cutaneous T-cell lymphoma; its name arose from the erroneous belief that it was of fungal origin. It may evolve into generalized lymphoma with a tendency for nodal, hematogenous, and visceral involvement. Its course has three successive stages: the *premycotic stage*, associated with intensely pruritic erythematous, eczematous, or psoriasiform eruptions; the *mycotic stage*, or *stage of infiltrated plaques*, characterized by the presence of abnormal lymphocytes called *Sézary cells;* and the *tumor stage*, characterized by mushroomlike tumors that often ulcerate. In a variant type of tumor stage called *mycosis fungoides d'emblée*, the tumors may develop without preceding lesions or prodromal symptoms. Called also *granuloma fungoides.*

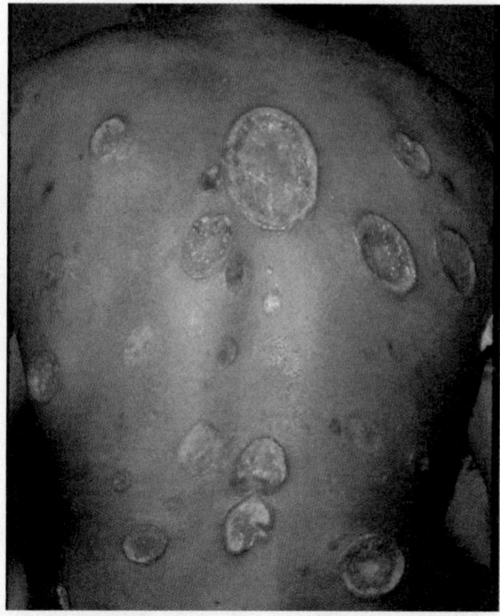
■ Mycosis fungoides, with ulcerated plaques and tumors.

m. fungoides d'emblée see *m. fungoides.*
m. lepto′thrica a benign condition of the tonsils and pharynx produced by the bacterium *Leptotrichia buccalis.*
splenic m. siderotic splenomegaly.

-mycosis a word termination denoting a fungal disease or infection.

my•cos•ta•sis (mi-kos′tə-sis) fungistasis.

my•co•stat (mi′ko-stat) fungistat.

My•co•stat•in (mi′ko-stat″in) trademark for preparations of nystatin.

my•cos•ter•ol (mi-kos′tə-rol) any of the sterols isolated from fungi.

my•cot•ic (mi-kot′ik) 1. pertaining to mycosis. 2. caused by a fungus. 3. pertaining to or caused by any microorganism; obsolete except in the phrase *mycotic aneurysm.*

My•co•tor•u•loi•des (mi″ko-tor″u-loi′dēz) *Candida.*

my•co•tox•i•co•sis (mi″ko-tok″sĭ-ko′sis) 1. poisoning caused by a fungal or bacterial toxin. 2. poisoning resulting from ingestion of fungi. See table, and see also *mushroom poisoning.* Called also *mycetism* and *mycetismus.*

my•co•tox•in (mi′ko-tok″sin) a fungal toxin.

my•co•tox•in•iza•tion (mi″ko-tok″sin-ĭ-za′shən) inoculation with a mycotoxin.

My•co-Tri•acet II (mi′ko-tri′ə-set) trademark for a combination preparation of nystatin and triamcinolone acetonide.

Myd•frin (mid′frin) trademark for preparations of phenylephrine hydrochloride.

My•dri•a•cyl (mĭ-dri′ə-səl) trademark for a preparation of tropicamide.

my•dri•a•sis (mĭ-dri′ə-sis) [Gr.] 1. physiologic dilatation of the pupil. 2. abnormal dilatation of the pupil. 3. dilatation of the pupil caused by a drug.
alternating m. varying inequality of the pupils, with mydriasis first on one side and then on the other; called also *bounding* or *springing m.*
bounding m. alternating m.
paralytic m. dilation of the pupil caused by paralysis of the oculomotor nerve.
spasmodic m., spastic m. dilation of the pupil due to spasm of the dilator pupillae muscle or to overaction of the sympathetic pathway.
spinal m. dilation of the pupil due to lesion of the ciliospinal center of the spinal cord.
springing m. alternating m.

myd•ri•at•ic (mid″re-at′ik) 1. dilating the pupil. 2. any drug that dilates the pupil.

my•ec•to•my (mi-ek′tə-me) [*my-* + *-ectomy*] excision of a portion of muscle.

my•ec•to•pia (mi-ek-to′pe-ə) [*myo-* + *ectopia*] displacement of a muscle.

my•ec•to•py (mi-ek′tə-pe) myectopia.

my•elal•gia (mi″ə-lal′jə) [*myel-* + *-algia*] pain in the spinal cord.

my•el•ate•lia (mi″el-ə-te′le-ə) myelodysplasia.

my•el•at•ro•phy (mi″əl-at′rə-fe) [*myel-* + *atrophy*] atrophy of the spinal cord.

Types of Mycotoxicosis

Fungus	Condition(s) Caused	Toxin
Acremonium coenophialum	Fescue foot	Unknown
Acremonium lolii	Rye grass staggers	Unknown
Alternaria species	Alternariatoxicosis	Unknown
Aspergillus (any species)	Aspergillustoxicosis	Various
(1) *A. clavatus, A giganteus, A. terreus*	(Neurotoxicity)	Patulin
(2) *A. flavus* et al.	Aflatoxicosis	Aflatoxin
(3) *A. ochraceus*	Ochratoxicosis	Ochratoxin
Claviceps paspali	Paspalum staggers	Unknown
Claviceps purpurea	Ergotism	Ergot alkaloids
Dendrodochium toxicum	Dendrodochiotoxicosis	Unknown
Diplodia species	Diplodiosis	Unknown
Endoconidium temulentum	Darnel poisoning (endoconidiotoxicosis)	Unknown
Fusarium culmorum, F. roseum	(Vulvovaginitis)	Zearalenone
Fusarium culmorum, F. roseum, F. moniliforme, F. sporotrichioides	Forage poisoning (fusariotoxicosis)	T-2 toxin, deoxynivalenol, diacetoxyscirpenol
Myrothecium roridum, M. verrucaria	Myrotheciotoxicosis	Roridin, verrucarin
Penicillium citrinum	(Nephrotoxicity)	Citrinin
Penicillium claviforme, P. expansum, P. patulum, et al.	(Neurotoxicity)	Patulin
Phomopsis leptostromiformis, P. rossiana	Mycotoxic lupinosis	Phomopsin
Pithomyces chartarum	Facial eczema of ruminants (pithomycotoxicosis)	Sporidesmin
Rhizoctonia leguminicola	Slobbers	Slaframine
Stachybotrys atra	Stachybotryotoxicosis	Roridin, satratoxin, verrucarin

my•el•emia (mi″ə-le′me-ə) [*myel-* + *-emia*] myelocytosis.

my•el•en•ceph•a•li•tis (mi″əl-en-sef″ə-li′tis) encephalomyelitis.

my•el•en•ceph•a•lon (mi″əl-en-sef′ə-lon) [*myel-* + *encephalon*] 1. [TA] medulla oblongata. 2. the posterior of the two brain vesicles formed by specialization of the rhombencephalon in the developing embryo.

my•el•en•ceph•a•lo•spi•nal (mi″əl-en-sef″ə-lo-spi′nəl) pertaining to the myelencephalon and spinal cord.

my•elin (mi′ə-lin) [Gr. *myelos* marrow] the substance of the cell membrane of Schwann cells that coils to form the myelin sheath (see under *sheath*); it has a high proportion of lipid to protein and serves as an electrical insulator. **myelin′ic** *adj*

my•eli•nat•ed (mi′ə-lĭ-nāt″əd) having a myelin sheath.

my•elin•a•tion (mi″ə-lĭ-na′shən) myelinization.

my•eli•ni•za•tion (mi″ə-lin″ĭ-za′shən) the act of furnishing with or taking on myelin; formation of a myelin sheath. Called also *medullation*, *myelination*, and *myelinogenesis*.

my•eli•noc•la•sis (mi″ə-lĭ-nok′lə-sis) demyelination.

acute perivascular m. acute disseminated encephalomyelitis.

postinfection perivenous m. postinfection encephalomyelopathy.

my•elino•gen•e•sis (mi″ə-lin″o-jen′ə-sis) myelinization.

my•elino•ge•net•ic (mi″ə-lin″o-jə-net′ik) 1. producing myelin. 2. producing or causing myelinization.

my•eli•nog•e•ny (mi″əl-ĭ-noj′ə-ne) [*myelin* + *-geny*] myelogeny.

my•elin•ol•y•sis (mi″ə-lin-ol′ə-sis) demyelination.

central pontine m. symmetric demyelination affecting the base and tegmentum of the pons, possibly caused by rapid correction of hyponatremia, and characterized by rapidly progressing paraparesis or quadriparesis, dysarthria, dysphagia, and impaired consciousness; areas of demyelination may also occur outside the pons. It is associated with a variety of conditions, including alcoholism, malignancies, burns, and liver transplantation.

osmotic m. central pontine myelinolysis, so called because of the frequency of extrapontine demyelination.

my•eli•nop•a•thy (mi″ə-lĭ-nop′ə-the) any disease of the myelin; degeneration of the white matter of the brain.

my•eli•no•sis (mi″ə-lĭ-no′sis) demyelinating disease.

central pontine m. central pontine myelinolysis.

my•elino•tox•ic (mi′ə-lin-o-tok″sik) having a deleterious effect on myelin; causing demyelination.

my•elino•tox•ic•i•ty (mi″ə-lin-o-tok-sis′ĭ-te) the property of being myelinotoxic.

my•elit•ic (mi″ə-lit′ik) pertaining to myelitis.

my•eli•tis (mi″ə-li′tis) pl. *myeli′tides* [*myel-* + *-itis*] 1. inflammation of the spinal cord, often part of a more specifically defined disease process. One group of diseases is named according to whether primarily white matter or gray matter is affected (see *leukomyelitis* and *poliomyelitis*); another group is defined by whether there is coexistent disease of the meninges *(meningomyelitis)* or the brain *(encephalomyelitis)*. In practice, the term is also used to denote noninflammatory lesions of the spinal cord; see *myelopathy*. 2. inflammation of the bone marrow; see *osteomyelitis*.

acute m. any type that develops rapidly.

ascending m. see under *myelopathy*.

bulbar m. myelitis involving the medulla oblongata.

cavitary m. syringomyelia.

central m. myelitis affecting chiefly the gray substance of the spinal cord; see *poliomyelitis* and *syringomyelia*.

chronic m. any type that progresses slowly, taking between six weeks and two years to progress to full manifestation of the disease.

compression m. see under *myelopathy*.

concussion m. see under *myelopathy*.

cornual m. myelitis affecting the horns of gray matter of the spinal cord; see also *poliomyelitis*.

diffuse m. disseminated m.

disseminated m. myelitis with several distinct foci of inflammation in the spinal cord.

hemorrhagic m. hematomyelitis.

neuro-optic m. neuromyelitis optica.

periependymal m. myelitis surrounding the central canal of the spinal cord.

postinfectious m. myelitis occurring after a viral infection; see also *acute disseminated encephalomyelitis*.

postvaccinal m. myelitis occurring after vaccination; see also *acute disseminated encephalomyelitis*. Called also *m. vaccinia*.

subacute m. myelitis that develops over a period of a few weeks; cf. *acute m.* and *chronic m.*

subacute necrotic m. Foix-Alajouanine syndrome.

syphilitic m. myelitis occurring as part of meningovascular neurosyphilis.

transverse m. myelitis in which the functional effect of the lesions spans the width of the entire cord at a given level.

m. vacci′nia postvaccinal m.

viral m. myelitis due to infection of the spinal cord by a virus, such as poliovirus, herpesvirus, or human immunodeficiency virus.

myel(o)- [Gr. *myelos* marrow] a combining form denoting relationship to marrow, to the spinal cord, or to myelin.

my•elo•ab•la•tion (mi″ə-lo-ab-la′shən) [*myelo-* + *ablation*] severe or complete bone marrow suppression (q.v.), such as by administration of high doses of chemotherapy or radiation therapy prior to bone marrow transplantation. **myeloab′lative** *adj*

my•elo•ar•chi•tec•ture (mi″ə-lo-ahr′kĭ-tek″chər) 1. the arrangement of nerve fibers in the cerebral and cerebellar cortices. 2. the organization of the nerve tracts in the spinal cord and brainstem.

my•elo•blast (mi′ə-lo-blast) [*myelo-* + *-blast*] an immature cell found in the bone marrow and not normally in the peripheral blood, the most primitive precursor in the granulocytic series, which develops into the promyelocyte. Myeloblasts have fine, evenly distributed chromatin, several nucleoli, and a nongranular basophilic cytoplasm.

my•elo•blas•te•mia (mi″ə-lo-blas-te′me-ə) [*myeloblast* + *-emia*] the presence of myeloblasts in the blood, as in acute myeloblastic leukemia.

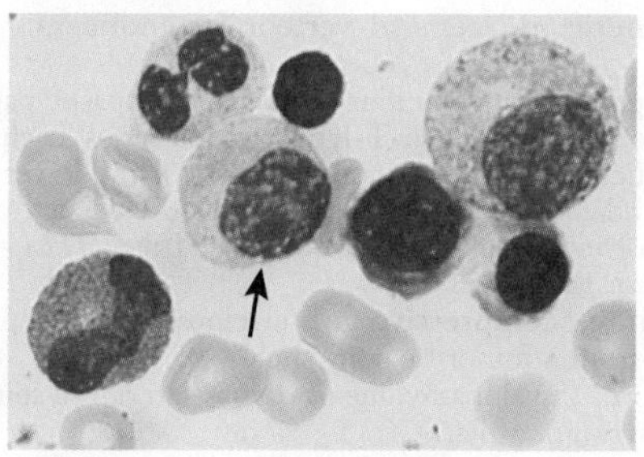

■ Neutrophilic myelocyte *(arrow).*

my•elo•blas•to•ma (mi″ə-lo-blas-to′mə) [*myeloblast* + *-oma*] a focal malignant tumor, observed in acute myelogenous leukemia, composed of myeloblasts or early myeloid precursors occurring outside of the bone marrow.

my•elo•blas•to•ma•to•sis (mi″ə-lo-blas″to-mə-to′sis) the presence of multiple myeloblastomas.

my•elo•blas•to•sis (mi″ə-lo-blas-to′sis) 1. the presence of an excess of myeloblasts in the blood, as in acute myeloblastic leukemia. 2. avian m.

avian m. a neoplastic viral disease of chickens, one of the avian leukosis complex, with proliferation of malignant myeloblasts in the bone marrow, liver, spleen, and kidneys, as well as spontaneous hemorrhages. Called also *myeloblastic leukosis.*

my•elo•cele (mi′ə-lo-sēl) [*myelo-* + *-cele*[1]] protrusion of the substance of the spinal cord through a defect in the vertebral arch, with varying degrees of protective covering; cf. *myelomeningocele*.

my•elo•clast (mi′ə-lo-klast) [*myelo-* + *-clast*] a cell which splits up myelin sheaths.

my•elo•cyst (mi′ə-lo-sist) [*myelo-* + *cyst*] a benign cyst developed from rudimentary medullary canals.

my•elo•cys•tic (mi″ə-lo-sis′tik) both myeloid and cystic in structure.

my•elo•cys•to•cele (mi″ə-lo-sis′to-sēl) myelomeningocele.

my•elo•cys•to•me•nin•go•cele (mi″ə-lo-sis″to-mə-ning′go-sēl) myelomeningocele.

my•elo•cyte (mi′ə-lo-sīt) [*myelo-* + *-cyte*] a precursor in the granulocytic series, being a cell intermediate in development between a promyelocyte and a metamyelocyte; in this stage, differentiation of cytoplasmic granules has begun, so that they are specifically basophilic, eosinophilic, or neutrophilic. **myelocyt′ic** *adj*

my•elo•cy•the•mia (mi″ə-lo-si-the′me-ə) myelocytosis.

my•elo•cy•to•ma (mi″ə-lo-si-to′mə) 1. chronic granulocytic leukemia. 2. myeloma.

my•elo•cy•to•ma•to•sis (mi″ə-lo-si″to-mə-to′sis) a neoplastic viral disease of fowl, one of the avian leukosis complex, marked by bone tumors composed of myeloid cells, and sometimes increased numbers of myeloid cells in the circulating blood.

my•elo•cy•to•sis (mi″ə-lo-si-to′sis) the presence of an excessive number of myelocytes in the blood; see also *myelodysplasia* (def. 1). Called also *myelocythemia* and *myelosis.*

my•elo•dys•pla•sia (mi″ə-lo-dis-pla′zhə) [*myelo-* + *dysplasia*] 1. a neural tube defect (q.v.) causing defective development of any part of the spinal cord, especially the lower segments. Called also *myelatelia.* 2. dysplasia of myelocytes and other elements in bone marrow, which may take the form of myelosuppression or of abnormal proliferation; in the latter case it may precede myelogenous leukemia. See also *myelodysplastic syndrome,* under *syndrome.*

my•elo•dys•plas•tic (mi″ə-lo-dis-plas′tik) pertaining to myelodysplasia.

my•elo•en•ce•phal•ic (mi″ə-lo-en″sə-fal′ik) cerebrospinal.

my•elo•en•ceph•a•li•tis (mi″ə-lo-en-sef″ə-li′tis) [*myelo-* + *encephal-* + *-itis*] inflammation of the spinal cord and brain; called also *encephalomyelitis.*

eosinophilic m. neurologic symptoms caused by invasion of the central nervous system by *Gnathostoma spinigerum,* including severe nerve root pain, paralysis of limbs, sudden sensory impairment, and eosinophilic, bloody, or yellow-stained spinal fluid.

equine protozoal m. a condition in horses consisting of myelitis and encephalitis from central nervous system infection with an unknown protozoan, possibly a species of *Sarcocystis*; symptoms include lameness and ataxia, usually asymmetric, progressing to paresis and sometimes blindness, facial paralysis, and dysphagia.

my•elo•en•ceph•a•lop•a•thy (mi″ə-lo-en-sef″ə-lop′ə-the) encephalomyelopathy.

equine degenerative m. a disease of young horses with degeneration of axons and myelin in the spinal cord and medulla oblongata; spasticity, defective proprioception, and ataxia develop progressively, sometimes ending as paraplegia or paralysis. It may be either hereditary or due to a vitamin E deficiency.

my•elo•fi•bro•sis (mi″ə-lo-fi-bro′sis) replacement of the bone marrow by fibrous tissue, occurring in association with a myeloproliferative disorder such as agnogenic myeloid metaplasia or secondary to another unrelated condition. Called also *myelosclerosis.*

m. with myeloid metaplasia myelofibrosis associated with extramedullary hematopoiesis; generally restricted to agnogenic myeloid metaplasia (with which it is often used synonymously) and myeloid metaplasia secondary to polycythemia vera or essential thrombocythemia.

osteosclerosis m. myelosclerosis (def. 2).

my•elof•u•gal (mi″ə-lof′u-gəl) [*myelo-* + *-fugal*[2]] spinifugal.

my•elo•gen•e•sis (mi″ə-lo-jen′ə-sis) 1. myelinization. 2. myelopoiesis.

my•elo•gen•ic (mi″ə-lo-jen′ik) 1. myelogenous. 2. myelopoietic.

my•elog•e•nous (mi″ə-loj′ə-nəs) [*myelo-* + *-genous*] 1. produced in the bone marrow; called also *myelogenic.* 2. myelinogenetic.

my•elog•e•ny (mi″ə-loj′ə-ne) the maturation of the myelin sheaths of nerve fibers in the development of the central nervous system. Cf. *myelinization.*

my•elo•gone (mi′ə-lo-gōn″) a white blood cell of the myeloid series having a reticulate violaceous nucleus, well-stained nucleolus, and a deep blue rim of cytoplasm.

my•elo•gram (mi′ə-lo-gram) 1. a radiograph of the spinal cord. 2. a graphic representation of the differential count of cells found in a stained preparation of bone marrow.

my•elog•ra•phy (mi″ə-log′rə-fe) [*myelo-* + *-graphy*] radiography of the spinal cord after injection of a contrast medium into the subarachnoid space.

oxygen m. myelography in which oxygen is used as the contrast medium.

my•eloid (mi′ə-loid) [*myelo-* + *-oid*] 1. resembling bone marrow. 2. having the appearance of myelocytes, but not derived from bone marrow. 3. medullary (def. 2). 4. medullary (def. 3).

my•eloi•din (mi″ə-loi′din) [*myelin* + Gr. *eidos* form] a substance resembling myelin, occurring in the pigmented cells of the retina.

my•eloi•do•sis (mi″ə-loi-do′sis) the development of myeloid tissue, especially hyperplastic development of such tissue.

my•elo•ken•tric (mi″ə-lo-ken′trik) [*myeloid* + Gr. *kentron* stimulus] stimulating myelopoiesis.

my•elo•li•po•ma (mi″ə-lo-lĭ-po′mə) a rare benign tumor of the adrenal gland, several centimeters in diameter, composed in varying proportions of adipose tissue, lymphocytes, and primitive myeloid cells, probably a developmental abnormality.

my•elol•y•sis (mi″ə-lol′ĭ-sis) demyelination.

my•elo•ma (mi″ə-lo′mə) [*myelo-* + *-oma*] 1. a tumor composed of cells of the type normally found in the bone marrow. 2. multiple m.

giant cell m. giant cell tumor of bone.

indolent m. a variant of multiple myeloma in which the tumor cells are hypoproliferative; an M component and bone marrow plasmacytosis are present, but significant bone marrow destruction, hypercalcemia, and Bence Jones proteinuria are absent.

localized m. solitary m.

multiple m. a disseminated type of plasma cell dyscrasia characterized by multiple bone marrow tumor foci and secretion of an M component, associated with widespread osteolytic lesions resulting in bone pain, pathologic fractures, hypercalcemia, and normochromic normocytic anemia; spread to extraosseous sites occurs frequently in advanced disease. Depression of immunoglobulin levels results in increased susceptibility to infection. Bence Jones proteinuria is present in many cases and may result in systemic amyloidosis. Renal failure from calcium nephropathy or extensive cast formation may also occur. Called also *plasma cell m.* See also *myeloma cell,* under *cell.*

plasma cell m. multiple m.

sclerosing m. myeloma associated with osteosclerosis, most often manifested by peripheral neuropathy; the myeloma involved may be localized or a part of multiple myeloma; POEMS syndrome (q.v.) may be present.

solitary m. a variant of multiple myeloma in which there is a single localized tumor focus. Called also *localized m.*

my•elo•ma•la•cia (mi″ə-lo-mə-la′shə) [*myelo-* + *-malacia*] morbid softening of the spinal cord.

my•elo•ma•toid (mi″ə-lo′mə-toid) resembling myeloma.

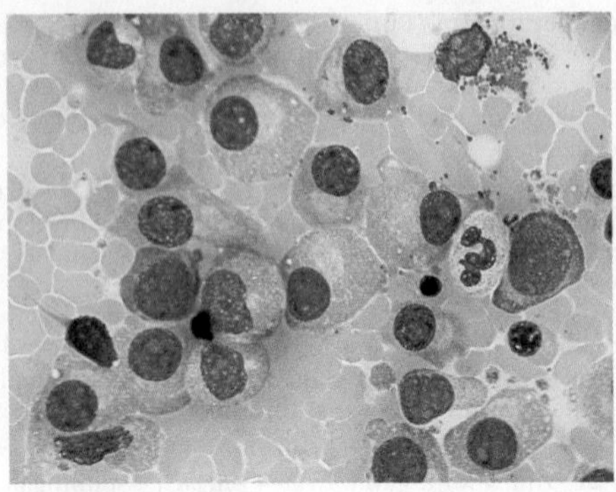

■ Multiple myeloma in bone marrow, showing large plasma cells with nucleoli.

my•elo•ma•to•sis (mi″ə-lo-mə-to′sis) multiple myeloma.

my•elo•me•nia (mi″ə-lo-me′ne-ə) [*myelo-* + *men-* + *-ia*] vicarious menstruation into the spinal cord, associated with plaques of endometriosis in the spinal canal.

my•elo•men•in•gi•tis (mi″ə-lo-men″in-ji′tis) meningomyelitis.

my•elo•me•nin•go•cele (mi″ə-lo-mə-ning′go-sēl″) [*myelo-* + *meningo-cele*] hernial protrusion of the spinal cord and its meninges through a defect in the vertebral arch (spina bifida); cf. *spinal meningocele.* Called also *meningomyelocele* and *myelocystocele.*

my•elo•mere (mi′ə-lo-mēr) [*myelo-* + *-mere*] one of the segments of the developing brain and spinal cord.

my•elo•mono•cyt•ic (mi″ə-lo-mon″o-sit′ik) characterized by both myelocytes and monocytes; said of leukemia.

my•elo•neu•ri•tis (mi″ə-lo-noŏ-ri′tis) neuromyelitis.

my•elo•neu•rop•a•thy (mi″ə-lo-noŏ-rop′ə-the) symptoms of damage to the spinal cord and nerves in the lower limbs, with weakness, spasticity, and dysesthesias, caused by long-term exposure to nitrous oxide.

my•elo•op•ti•co•neu•rop•a•thy (mi″ə-lo-op″tĭ-ko-noo-rop′ə-the) a disorder affecting the spinal cord and optic nerve.

subacute m. (SMON) a clinical syndrome reported from Japan affecting the spinal cord, optic nerve, and peripheral nerves, preceded by diarrhea. Symptoms include paresthesia in both lower limbs, gait disturbances, visual disturbances, abnormalities of deep tendon reflexes, and psychic disorders. The hydroxyquinolones (especially clioquinol), taken for gastrointestinal disorders, have been implicated as an etiologic factor.

my•elo•path•ic (mi″ə-lo-path′ik) pertaining to or characterized by myelopathy.

my•elop•a•thy (mi″ə-lop′ə-the) [*myelo-* + *-pathy*] 1. any of various functional disturbances or pathological changes in the spinal cord, often referring to nonspecific lesions in contrast to the inflammatory lesions of myelitis. 2. a pathological condition of the bone marrow; see also *myelodysplasia* (def. 2).

anterior m. anterior spinal artery syndrome.

ascending m. myelopathy that progresses cephalad along the spinal cord.

carcinomatous m. a rapidly progressive, paraneoplastic myelopathy, most often associated with carcinoma of the lung, but also seen with other carcinomas. It is characterized by a rapidly developing myelopathic syndrome due to necrosis of both the gray and white matter of the spinal cord. Called also *paraneoplastic m.* and *paracarcinomatous m.*

cervical m. compression myelopathy of the cervical spinal cord, a complication that occasionally arises from rheumatoid arthritis or osteoarthritis.

cervical spondylotic m. spondylotic cervical m.

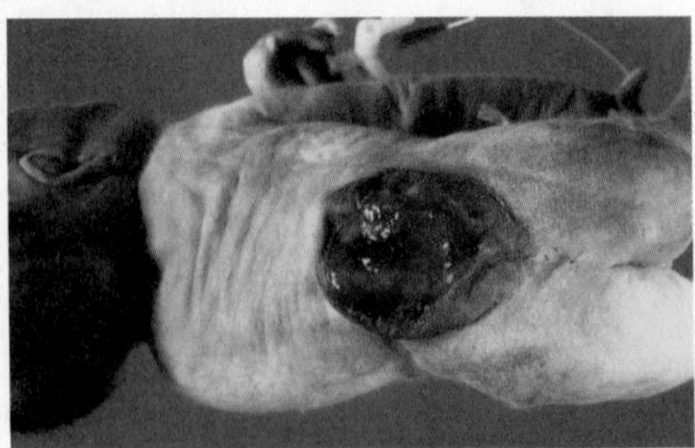

■ Myelomeningocele.

cervical stenotic m., cervical vertebral stenotic m. wobbler syndrome (def. 2).

chronic progressive m. gradually progressive spastic paraparesis associated with infection by human T-lymphotropic virus 1, characterized by progressive difficulty in walking and weakness of the lower limb, sensory disturbances, and urinary incontinence, with no evidence of spinal compression or involvement of motoneurons. Called also *HTLV-1–associated m.* and *tropical spastic paraparesis.*

compression m., compressive m. myelopathy due to pressure on the spinal cord, as from a tumor or bony spur.

concussion m. myelopathy due to concussion of the spinal cord (q.v.).

cystic m. syringomyelia.

descending m. myelopathy that progresses caudad along the spinal cord.

focal m. myelopathy affecting a small area only, or several small areas.

funicular m. leukomyelopathy.

hemorrhagic m. myelopathy associated with hemorrhage; see also *hematomyelia.*

hereditary m. an autosomal recessive disease seen in young Afghan hounds, characterized by cavitation and necrosis of the white matter of the spinal cord, with pelvic limb paralysis before the age of one year.

HIV-associated m. degeneration of the spinal cord in persons infected with the human immunodeficiency virus (HIV), usually in late stages of the disease; there is vacuolization of the cord with symptoms including leg weakness, gait problems, paresthesias, and sometimes bowel and bladder incontinence.

HTLV-1 m., HTLV-1–associated m. chronic progressive m.

necrotizing m. myelopathy marked by necrosis of the spinal cord.

paracarcinomatous m., paraneoplastic m. carcinomatous m.

radiation m. a slowly progressive myelopathy occurring six months or longer after excessive exposure of the spinal cord to radiation, usually in the form of radiation therapy.

spondylotic cervical m. myelopathy secondary to encroachment by cervical spondylosis on the spinal cord within the spinal canal, often in those with a congenitally small spinal canal; called also *cervical spondylotic m.*

systemic m. myelopathy which affects distinct tracts in the spinal cord.

transverse m. myelopathy that extends across the spinal cord.

traumatic m. myelopathy which follows injury to the spinal cord.

vacuolar m. loss of myelin and spongy degeneration of the spinal cord with microscopic vacuolation, similar to that of subacute combined degeneration of the spinal cord, caused by infection with human immunodeficiency virus. Symptoms include spastic paraparesis, sensory ataxia in the lower limbs, and unsteadiness of gait.

my•elo•per•ox•i•dase (MPO) (mi″ə-lo-pər-ok′sĭ-dās) peroxidase (def. 2).

my•elo•per•ox•i•dase (MPO) de•fi•cien•cy (mi″ə-lo-pər-ok′sĭ-dās) an autosomal recessive disorder caused by mutation in the myeloperoxidase gene (*MPO*, locus:17q23.1), characterized by the complete absence of MPO in azurophil granules of neutrophils and monocytes; the deficiency is usually clinically insignificant although candidiasis may occur, especially in persons with diabetes mellitus.

my•elop•e•tal (mi″ə-lop′ə-təl) [*myelo-* + *-petal*] spinipetal.

my•elo•phage (mi′ə-lo-fāj″) [*myelo-* + *-phage*] a macrophage which digests or breaks down myelin.

my•elo•phthis•ic (mi″ə-lo-tiz′ik) 1. myelosuppressive. 2. causing wasting of the spinal cord.

my•e•loph•thi•sis (mi″ə-lof′thĭ-sis) [*myelo-* + *phthisis*] 1. wasting of the spinal cord. 2. bone marrow suppression secondary to marrow infiltration by tumor with local production of myelosuppressive cytokines.

my•elo•plast (mi′ə-lo-plast″) [*myelo-* + *-plast*] any leukocyte of the bone marrow.

my•elo•ple•gia (mi″ə-lo-ple′jə) [*myelo-* + *-plegia*] spinal paralysis.

my•elo•poi•e•sis (mi″ə-lo-poi-e′sis) [*myelo-* + *-poiesis*] the formation of bone marrow or the cells that arise from it. See also *hematopoiesis.* Called also *medullation* and *myelogenesis.* **myelopoiet′ic** *adj*

ectopic m., extramedullary m. the formation of myeloid tissue outside the bone marrow.

my•elo•pore (mi′ə-lo-por) [*myelo-* + *pore*] a canal or opening in the spinal cord.

my•elo•pro•lif•er•a•tive (mi″ə-lo-pro-lif′ər-ə-tiv) pertaining to or characterized by medullary and extramedullary proliferation of bone marrow constituents, including erythroblasts, granulocytes, megakaryocytes, and fibroblasts. See under *disorder* and see also *lymphoproliferative.*

my•elo•ra•dic•u•li•tis (mi″ə-lo-rə-dik″u-li′tis) [*myelo-* + *radiculitis*] inflammation of the spinal cord and the posterior nerve roots.

my•elo•ra•dic•u•lo•dys•pla•sia (mi″ə-lo-rə-dik″u-lo-dis-pla′zhə) developmental abnormality of the spinal cord and spinal nerve roots.

my•elo•ra•dic•u•lop•a•thy (mi″ə-lo-rə-dik″u-lop′ə-the) disease of the spinal cord and spinal nerve roots; called also *radiculomyelopathy*.

my•elor•rha•gia (mi″ə-lo-ra′jə) [*myelo-* + *-rrhagia*] hematomyelia.

my•elo•sar•co•ma (mi″ə-lo-sahr-ko′mə) a sarcomatous growth made up of myeloid tissue or bone marrow cells; see also *myeloma*.

my•elo•sar•co•ma•to•sis (mi″ə-lo-sahr-ko″mə-to′sis) multiple myeloma.

my•elos•chi•sis (mi″ə-los′kĭ-sis) [*myelo-* + *-schisis*] a developmental anomaly characterized by a cleft spinal cord, owing to failure of the neural plate to fuse and form a complete neural tube, or to rupture of the neural tube after closure. Cf. *diastematomyelia* and *spina bifida*.

my•elo•scle•ro•sis (mi″ə-lo-sklə-ro′sis) 1. sclerosis of the spinal cord, such as in multiple sclerosis. 2. obliteration of the normal marrow cavity by small spicules of bone; the pathogenesis may be similar to that of myelofibrosis. Called also *osteosclerosis myelofibrosis*. 3. myelofibrosis.

my•elo•scope (mi′əlo-skōp″) an ultrathin fiberoptic neuroendoscope for examination of the spinal canal.

my•elos•co•py (mi″ə-los′kə-pe) examination of the spinal canal by means of a myeloscope.

my•elo•sis (mi″ə-lo′sis) 1. myelocytosis. 2. the formation of a tumor of the spinal cord.

aleukemic m., chronic nonleukemic m. agnogenic myeloid metaplasia.

erythremic m. erythroleukemia.

nonleukemic m. agnogenic myeloid metaplasia.

my•elo•spon•gi•um (mi″ə-lo-spun′je-əm) [*myelo-* + Gr. *spongos* sponge] the network from which the neuroglial tissue is developed: it pervades the embryonic neural tube, and is composed of the spongioblasts and their branching processes.

my•elo•sup•pres•sion (mi″ə-lo-sə-presh′ən) bone marrow suppression.

my•elo•sup•pres•sive (mi″ə-lo-sə-pres′iv) 1. causing bone marrow suppression. 2. an agent causing bone marrow suppression.

my•elo•syph•i•lis (mi″ə-lo-sif′ĭ-lis) spinal syphilis.

my•elo•ther•a•py (mi″ə-lo-ther′ə-pe) [*myelo-* + *therapy*] the therapeutic use of bone marrow. Cf. *bone marrow transplantation*.

my•elo•tome (mi′ə-lo-tōm) [*myelo-* + *-tome*] 1. an instrument for making sections of the spinal cord. 2. an instrument used for cutting the spinal cord squarely across in removing the brain in postmortem examinations.

my•elot•o•my (mi″ə-lot′o-me) the operation of severing tracts in the spinal cord.

Bischof m. surgical division of the spinal cord longitudinally through the lumbar region to relieve spasticity.

commissural m. longitudinal division of the spinal cord, to sever crossing sensory fibers and produce localized analgesia.

my•elo•tox•ic (mi′ə-lo-tok″sik) [*myelo-* + *toxic*] 1. destructive to bone marrow. 2. myelosuppressive. 3. arising from diseased bone marrow.

my•elo•tox•ic•i•ty (mi″ə-lo-tok-sis′ĭ-te) the quality of being myelotoxic.

my•en•ter•on (mi-en′tər-on) [*my-* + *enteron*] the muscular coat of the intestines; see *tunica muscularis intestini crassi* and *tunica muscularis intestini tenuis*. **myenter′ic** *adj*

My•er•son sign (mi′ər-sən) [Abraham *Myerson*, American neurologist, 1881–1948] see under *sign*.

my•es•the•sia (mi″es-the′zhə) [*my-* + *esthesia*] muscle sense (def. 1).

my•i•a•sis (mi-i′ə-sis) [Gr. *myia* fly + *-iasis*] a condition caused by infestation of the body by fly maggots.

creeping m. larva migrans caused by fly larvae.

cutaneous m. 1. infestation of an animal by maggots, found in areas of thick hair or wool and on nearby skin, usually when the area is chronically wet or fouled by feces or urine. Sheep are particularly susceptible, and serious cases may result in skin breakdown and death. The maggots are usually larvae of *Phaenicia*, *Phormia*, *Chrysomyia*, or *Calliphora* species. Several different types are distinguished according to the part of the body infested; see under *strike*. 2. cutaneous larva migrans in humans caused by fly larvae. Called also *dermatomyiasis* and *m. linearis*.

cutaneous blowfly m. cutaneous myiasis in animals caused by blowflies. Called also *blowfly strike* and *fly strike*.

dermal m. 1. cutaneous m. 2. cutaneous larva migrans (def. 1).

intestinal m. the presence of living fly larvae in the intestines.

m. linea′ris cutaneous m. (def. 2).

nasal m. myiasis in the nasal passages.

ocular m. ophthalmomyiasis.

traumatic m., wound m. cutaneous myiasis at the site of a wound or ulcer. In animals it is called also *wound strike*.

my•io•des•op•sia (mi-i″o-dəs-op′se-ə) [Gr. *myiōdes* flylike + *-opsia*] the appearance of muscae volitantes.

my•io•sis (mi″i-o′sis) myiasis.

my•itis (mi-i′tis) myositis.

myk(o)- for words beginning thus, see those beginning *myc(o)-*.

My•krox (mi′kroks) trademark for a preparation of metolazone.

My•ler•an (mi′lər-an) trademark for a preparation of busulfan.

My•lo•cel (mi′lo-sel) trademark for a preparation of hydroxyurea.

my•lo•hy•oid (mi″lo-hi′oid) [Gr. *mylai* molar teeth + *hyoid*] pertaining to molar teeth and the hyoid bone.

my•lo•pha•ryn•ge•al (mi″lo-fə-rin′je-əl) [Gr. *mylai* molar teeth + *pharyngeal*] pertaining to molar teeth and the pharynx.

My•lo•targ (mi′lo-tahrg) trademark for a preparation of gemtuzumab ozogamicin.

My•meth•a•sone (mi-meth′ə-sōn″) trademark for a preparation of dexamethasone.

my(o)- [Gr. *mys*, gen. *myos* muscle] a combining form denoting relationship to muscle.

myo•ad•en•yl•ate de•am•i•nase (mi″o-ad′ən-əl-āt de-am′ĭ-nās) the muscle isozyme of AMP deaminase; it is the isoenzyme A of AMP deaminase (q.v.).

myo•ad•en•yl•ate de•am•i•nase de•fi•cien•cy (mi″o-ad′ən-əl-āt de-am′ĭ-nās) a mild autosomal recessive disorder caused by mutation in the *AMPD1* gene (locus: 1p21-p13), which encodes the muscle isoform of AMP deaminase, characterized by fatigue, cramps, and myalgia after exercise.

myo•al•bu•min (mi″o-al-bu′min) an albumin constituting about one per cent of the protein of muscle.

myo•ar•chi•tec•ton•ic (mi″o-ahr″kĭ-tek-ton′ik) [*myo-* + *architectonic*] pertaining to the structure of muscle.

myo•at•ro•phy (mi″o-at′rə-fe) myatrophy.

Myo•bia (mi-o′be-ə) a genus of mites of the family Myobiidae; *M. mus′culi* causes dermatitis in laboratory mice.

Myo•bi•i•dae (mi″o-be′ĭ-de) a family of parasitic mites, including the genera *Myobia* and *Radfordia*.

myo•blast (mi′o-blast) [*myo-* + *-blast*] an embryonic cell that becomes a muscle cell or fiber; called also *sarcoblast*. **myoblas′tic** *adj*

myo•blas•to•ma (mi″o-blas-to′mə) a benign circumscribed tumorlike lesion of soft tissue, possibly consisting of myoblasts.

granular cell m. see under *tumor*.

myo•blas•to•my•o•ma (mi″o-blas″to-mi-o′mə) myoblastoma.

Myo•bloc (mi′o-blok) trademark for a preparation of botulinum toxin type B.

myo•bra•dia (mi″o-bra′de-ə) [*myo-* + *brady-* + *-ia*] a slow, sluggish reaction of muscle to electric stimulation.

myo•car•di•op•a•thy (mi″o-kahr″de-op′ə-the) cardiomyopathy.

myo•car•di•or•rha•phy (mi″o-kahr″de-or′ə-fe) [*myocardium* + *-rrhaphy*] suture of the myocardium.

myo•car•di•tis (mi″o-kahr-di′tis) [*myo-* + *carditis*] inflammation of the muscular walls of the heart. **myocardit′ic** *adj*

acute isolated m. an acute type of interstitial myocarditis of unknown etiology, marked by sudden onset, absence of endocarditis or pericarditis, and frequently death. Called also *Fiedler* or *idiopathic m.*

bacterial m. myocarditis associated with bacterial infection; it may be caused either by the presence of the organisms in the myocardium or by toxins released from a distant infection.

chronic m. chronic myocardial inflammatory disease; formerly used loosely to indicate any myocardial deficiency.

diphtheritic m. myocarditis due to bacterial toxin production in diphtheria; primary lesions are degenerative and necrotic, with a secondary inflammatory response. It is usually subclinical but can cause permanent cardiac damage.

fibrous m. a term formerly used frequently to describe focal or diffuse fibrosis of the myocardium caused by chronic inflammation.

Fiedler m. acute isolated m.

giant cell m. a subtype of acute isolated myocarditis characterized by multinucleate giant cells and other inflammatory cells including lymphocytes, plasma cells, and macrophages, and by ventricular dilatation, mural thrombi, and widespread areas of necrosis. The term is sometimes used synonymously with *granulomatous m.* or may be distinguished from it as not including granuloma formation.

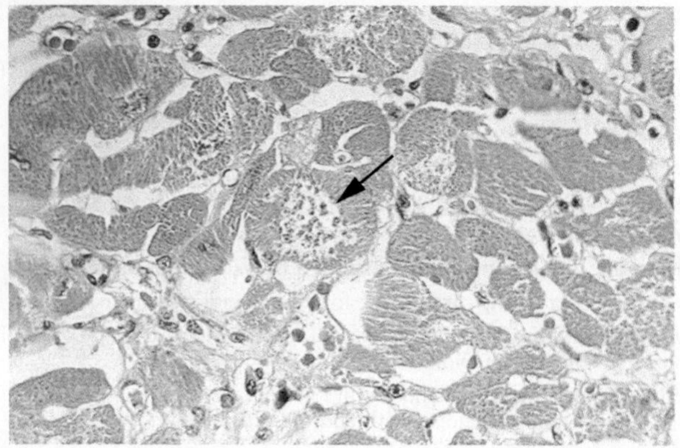

■ Infectious myocarditis in Chagas disease. A myofiber is distended with trypanosomes *(arrow)* and surrounded by an inflammatory reaction and necrosis of individual myofibers.

granulomatous m. see *giant cell m.*

hypersensitivity m. myocarditis due to allergic reactions caused by hypersensitivity to various agents, particularly sulfonamides, penicillins, and methyldopa. It is characterized by interstitial infiltration, principally perivascular, by lymphocytes, plasma cells, macrophages, and eosinophils.

idiopathic m. acute isolated m.

infectious m. myocarditis due to infectious agents, including bacteria, viruses, rickettsiae, protozoa, spirochetes, and fungi; they may damage the myocardium by direct invasion, production of toxins, or mediation of an immunological response.

interstitial m. myocarditis affecting chiefly the interstitial fibrous tissue.

parenchymatous m. myocarditis affecting chiefly the muscle substance itself.

protozoal m. myocarditis due to protozoal infection, occurring particularly in Chagas disease and toxoplasmosis.

rheumatic m. a common sequela of rheumatic fever characterized histologically by Aschoff bodies in the interstitial tissues of the heart.

rickettsial m. myocarditis associated with infection by rickettsiae; it is frequently subclinical and occurs particularly in Q fever and scrub typhus.

toxic m. degeneration and focal necrosis of myocardial fibers caused by drugs, chemicals, physical agents such as radiation, animal or insect toxins, or other agents or situations causing trauma to the myocardium.

tuberculous m. granulomatous inflammation of the myocardium in tuberculosis, usually resulting from infection elsewhere in the body.

viral m. myocarditis due to viral infection, particularly by enteroviruses; it most often occurs in infants, pregnant women, and immunosuppressed patients.

myo•car•di•um (mi″o-kahr′de-əm) [*myo-* + Gr. *kardia* heart] [TA] the middle and thickest layer of the heart wall, composed of cardiac muscle. **myocar′dial** *adj*

hibernating m. see *myocardial hibernation*, under *hibernation.*

stunned m. see *myocardial stunning*, under *stunning.*

myo•cele (mi′o-sēl) [*myo-* + *-cele*[1]] hernia of muscle; protrusion of a muscle through its ruptured sheath.

myo•ce•li•tis (mi″o-se-li′tis) [*myo-* + *celi-* + *-itis*] inflammation of the muscles of the abdomen.

myo•cel•lu•li•tis (mi″o-sel″u-li′tis) myositis conjoined with cellulitis.

myo•cho•sis (mi″o-ko′sis) [*myo-* + Gr. *chōsis* a piling up] shortening of the circular muscle and taeniae of the colon, resulting in a corrugated appearance and a narrowing of the lumen, caused by the deposition of elastin in contracted form; seen in diverticulosis and some prediverticular conditions.

Myo•chry•sine (mi″o-kri′sin) trademark for a preparation of gold sodium thiomalate.

myo•clo•nia (mi″o-klo′ne-ə) any disorder characterized by myoclonus.

m. conge′nita congenital tremor syndrome.

m. epilep′tica myoclonic epilepsy.

m. fibrilla′ris mul′tiplex myokymia.

fibrillary m. the twitching of the fibrils of a muscle; see *fibrillation* (def. 2).

pseudoglottic m. hiccup.

my•oc•lo•nus (mi-ok′lo-nəs) [*myo-* + *clonus*] shocklike contractions of a portion of a muscle, an entire muscle, or a group of muscles, restricted to one area of the body or appearing synchronously or asynchronously in several areas. It may be part of a disease process (e.g., epileptic or post-anoxic myoclonus) or be a normal physiological response (e.g., nocturnal myoclonus). **myoclon′ic** *adj*

action m. intention m.

Baltic m. myoclonus occurring as part of Unverricht-Lundborg disease; it is often photosensitive.

cortical m. myoclonus caused by an electrical discharge in the cerebral cortex; it may be a precursor of epilepsia partialis continua.

cortical reflex m. cortical myoclonus caused by an external stimulus.

epileptic m. myoclonus occurring as part of an epileptic aura or seizure; see *myoclonic epilepsy* under *epilepsy.*

essential m. myoclonus of unknown etiology; it may involve single or multiple muscles and may be initiated by excitement or an attempt at voluntary movement. A few cases have been found to be autosomal dominant.

intention m. myoclonus that occurs when voluntary muscle activity is initiated; called also *action m.*

m. mul′tiplex paramyoclonus multiplex.

negative m. myoclonus caused by sudden muscle relaxation; cf. *positive m.*

nocturnal m. myoclonic jerks of the limbs occurring as a person is falling asleep or is asleep; in the latter case they may disrupt sleep. Called also *periodic leg* or *limb movement disorder.*

ocular m. rapid oscillations of eye muscles, often seen with palatal myoclonus.

opsoclonus-m. see under *syndrome.*

palatal m. rapid, rhythmic, up-and-down movements of one side or both sides of the palate, often with ipsilateral synchronous clonic movements of muscles of the face, tongue, pharynx, and diaphragm. Called also *palatal nystagmus* or *tremor.*

positive m. myoclonus caused by a sudden muscle contraction; cf. *negative m.*

postanoxic m., posthypoxic m. myoclonus in patients who have had hypoxia or anoxia with heart failure and have gone through cardiopulmonary resuscitation. An acute form with status epilepticus is life-threatening. A chronic form occurs in patients with a relatively normal level of consciousness and is called *Lance-Adams syndrome.*

propriospinal m. a type of spinal myoclonus characterized by jerking of thoracic and abdominal muscles. It often occurs when a person is falling asleep, and some cases are psychogenic.

reflex m. myoclonus in response to an external stimulus; see also *cortical reflex m.* and *reflex epilepsy.*

spinal m. myoclonus having its origin in the spinal cord.

stimulus-sensitive m. reflex m.

tardive m. a variant of tardive dyskinesia characterized by myoclonic movements of the face, neck, and upper limbs.

myo•coele (mi′o-sēl) [*myo-* + *-coele*] the cavity within a myotome (def. 2).

myo•col•pi•tis (mi″o-kol-pi′tis) [*myo-* + *colp-* + *-itis*] inflammation of the muscular layers of the vaginal wall.

myo•com•ma (mi″o-kom′ə) [*myo-* + Gr. *komma* cut] 1. a myotome or muscle segment, as in a fish. 2. the septum between two adjacent myotomes.

Myo•cop•tes (mi″o-kop′tēz) a genus of mites of the family Listrophoridae. *M. musculi′nus* is found clinging to the hair of guinea pigs and mice and may cause dermatitis and hair loss.

my•oc•to•nine (mi-ok′to-nin) [*myo-* + Gr. *kteinein* to kill] a poisonous alkaloid from *Aconitum lycoctonum.*

my•oc•u•la•tor (mi-ok′u-la″tər) [*myo-* + L. *oculus* eye] an ocular instrument, on the principle of the orthoptoscope, which allows fusion and movement laterally, vertically, and in rotation. Cf. *myoscope.*

my•o•cu•ta•ne•ous (mi″o-ku-ta′ne-əs) musculocutaneous.

myo•cyte (mi′o-sīt) [*myo-* + *-cyte*] muscle cell.

Anichkov (Anitschkow) m. see under *cell.*

myo•cy•tol•y•sis (mi″o-si-tol′ĭ-sis) [*myo-* + *cytolysis*] disintegration of muscle fibers.

focal m. of heart a miliary lesion characterized by loss of muscular syncytium, preservation of stroma, absence of inflammatory reaction, and eventual necrosis.

myo•cy•to•ma (mi″o-si-to′mə) [*myocyte* + *-oma*] a tumor made up of myocytes.

myo•de•gen•er•a•tion (mi″o-de-jen″ər-a′shən) [*myo-* + *degeneration*] degeneration of muscle.

myo•des•op•sia (mi″o-dəs-op′se-ə) myiodesopsia.

myo•di•as•ta•sis (mi″o-di-as′tə-sis) [*myo-* + *diastasis*] separation of a muscle.

myo•di•op•ter (mi″o-di-op′tər) the force of ciliary muscle contraction necessary to raise the refraction of the emmetropic eye by 1 diopter from a state of rest.

myo•dy•nam•ic (mi″o-di-nam′ik) relating to muscular force.

myo•dy•nam•ics (mi″o-di-nam′iks) the physiology of muscular action.

myo•dy•na•mom•e•ter (mi″o-di″nə-mom′ə-tər) dynamometer.

my•odyn•ia (mi″o-din′e-ə) [*myo-* + *-odynia*] myalgia.

myo•dys•to•nia (mi″o-dis-to′ne-ə) [*myo-* + *dys-* + *ton-* + *-ia*] disorder of muscular tone.

my•o•dys•tro•phia (mi″o-dis-tro′fe-ə) 1. muscular dystrophy. 2. myotonic dystrophy.

m. feta′lis amyoplasia congenita.

myo•dys•tro•phy (mi″o-dis′trə-fe) 1. muscular dystrophy. 2. myotonic dystrophy.

myo•ede•ma (mi″o-ə-de′mə) [*myo-* + *edema*] 1. the rising in a lump by a wasting muscle when struck; called also *mounding*. 2. edema of a muscle.

myo•elas•tic (mi″o-e-las′tik) composed of elastic fibers associated with smooth muscle cells.

myo•elec•tric (mi″o-e-lek′trik) pertaining to the electric or electromotive properties of muscle.

myo•elec•tri•cal (mi″o-e-lek′trĭ-kəl) myoelectric.

myo•en•do•car•di•tis (mi″o-en″do-kahr-di′tis) [*myo-* + *endocarditis*] combined myocarditis and endocarditis.

myo•epi•the•li•al (mi″o-ep″ĭ-the′le-əl) 1. pertaining to myoepithelium. 2. composed of myoepithelium.

myo•epi•the•li•o•ma (mi″o-ep″ĭ-the″le-o′mə) [*myoepithelium* + *-oma*] a benign tumor predominantly composed of myoepithelial cells; a pure myoepithelial neoplasm is rare.

myo•epi•the•li•um (mi″o-ep″ĭ-the′le-əm) [*myo-* + *epithelium*] a specialized type of epithelium that has contractile qualities; see *myoepithelial cells*, under *cell*.

myo•fas•ci•al (mi″o-fash′e-əl) pertaining to or involving the fascia surrounding and associated with muscle tissue.

myo•fas•ci•i•tis (mi″o-fas″e-i′tis) [*myo-* + *fasciitis*] inflammation of a muscle and its fascia, particularly of the fascial insertion of muscle to bone. Called also *myofascitis*.

myo•fas•ci•tis (mi″o-fə-si′tis) myofasciitis.

myo•fi•ber (mi′o-fi″bər) muscle fiber.

myo•fi•bril (mi″o-fi′bril) muscle fibril: one of the slender threads that can be made visible in a muscle fiber by maceration in certain acids. They run parallel with the long axis of the fiber, and are composed of numerous myofilaments (q.v.). See Plate 32. **myofi′brillar** *adj*

myo•fi•bril•la (mi″o-fi-bril′ə) pl. *myofibril′lae*. myofibril.

myo•fi•bro•blast (mi″o-fi′bro-blast) an atypical fibroblast combining the ultrastructural features of a fibroblast and a smooth muscle cell; it has a highly irregular nucleus, a large amount of rough endoplasmic reticulum, and a dense collection of myofilaments.

myo•fi•bro•ma (mi″o-fi-bro′mə) leiomyoma.

myo•fi•bro•ma•to•sis (mi″o-fi″bro-mə-to′sis) fibromatosis in which there is proliferation of muscle tissue, presenting as solitary or multiple nodules that may involve any organ and almost always occurring in children; it is usually benign, but multifocal lesions involving vital organs may be lethal.

infantile m. a condition present at birth or occurring soon after, characterized by solitary or multiple, firm, rubbery, spherical or ovoid nodules in the skin and subcutaneous tissues. The nodules are composed of myofibroblasts and may undergo ulceration and calcification. In about half of patients, skeletal fibromas also occur; when lesions are limited to the skin and bones (a condition sometimes known as *congenital multiple fibromatosis*), prognosis is good and lesions resolve spontaneously. Visceral involvement may also occur (*congenital generalized fibromatosis*, q.v.) and is highly lethal.

myo•fi•bro•sis (mi″o-fi-bro′sis) [*myo-* + *fibrosis*] replacement of muscle tissue by fibrous tissue.

m. cor′dis myofibrosis of the heart.

myo•fila•ment (mi″o-fil′ə-mənt) [*myo-* + *filament*] any of the numerous ultramicroscopic threadlike structures occurring in bundles in the myofibrils of striated muscle fibers. The thick *myosin filaments* and the thin *actin filaments* are together responsible for the contractile properties of muscle. Also present are *intermediate filaments*, of uncertain function, composed of desmin and vimentin. See Plate 32.

myo•func•tion•al (mi″o-funk′shən-əl) 1. pertaining to muscular function. 2. pertaining to the use of muscles as an adjunct in orthodontic therapy.

myo•ge•lo•sis (mi″o-jə-lo′sis) [*myo-* + L. *gelare* to freeze] an area of hardening in a muscle, especially in the gluteus muscle.

myo•gen•e•sis (mi″o-jen′ə-sis) the development of muscle tissue, especially its embryonic development. **myogenet′ic** *adj*

my•o•gen•ic (mi″o-jen′ik) 1. myogenetic. 2. originating in myocytes or muscle tissue.

my•og•e•nous (mi-oj′ə-nəs) originating in muscle tissue.

my•og•lia (mi-og′le-ə) [*myo-* + *-glia*] a fibrillar substance formed by muscle cells, and present only during early embryogenesis of muscle fibers; called also *border fibrils*.

myo•glo•bin (Mb) (mi′o-glo″bin) the oxygen-transporting pigment of muscle, a type of hemoprotein resembling a single subunit of hemoglobin, composed of one globin polypeptide chain and one heme group (containing one iron atom); it combines with oxygen released by erythrocytes, stores it, and transports it to the mitochondria of muscle cells, where it generates energy by combustion of glucose to carbon dioxide and water.

myo•glo•bin•uria (mi″o-glo″bĭ-nu′re-ə) the presence of myoglobin in the urine, as in deficiency of muscle phosphorylase, in crush injuries, and after vigorous and prolonged exercise in susceptible persons.

familial m., idiopathic m. Meyer-Betz disease.

paralytic m. azoturia (def. 2).

spontaneous m. Meyer-Betz disease.

myo•glob•u•lin (mi″o-glob′u-lin) [*myo-* + *globulin*] a globulin found in muscle.

myo•glob•u•lin•uria (mi″o-glob″u-lĭ-nu′re-ə) the presence of myoglobulin in the urine.

my•og•na•thus (mi-og′nə-thəs) [*myo-* + Gr. *gnathos* jaw] a fetus with a supernumerary lower jaw attached to the normally placed lower jaw. See also *dignathus*.

myo•gram (mi′o-gram) [*myo-* + *-gram*] the record or tracing made by a myograph.

myo•graph (mi′o-graf) [*myo-* + *-graph*] an apparatus for recording the effects of a muscular contraction.

myo•graph•ic (mi″o-graf′ik) pertaining to a myograph or to myography.

my•og•ra•phy (mi-og′rə-fe) [*myo-* + *-graphy*] 1. the use of the myograph. 2. a description of the muscles. 3. radiography of muscle tissue after injection of an opaque medium. **myograph′ic** *adj*

myo•he•mo•glo•bin (mi″o-he′mo-glo″bin) myoglobin.

my•oid (mi′oid) [*my-* + *-oid*] 1. resembling or like a muscle. 2. a substance resembling muscle.

visual cell m. the basophilic inner region of the inner segment of the dendritic process of a retinal rod or cone, lying between the ellipsoid and the soma, and containing agranular endoplasmic reticulum and free ribosomes.

***myo*-ino•si•tol** (mi″o-in-o′sĭ-tol) see under *inositol*.

***myo*-ino•si•tol-1 (or 4)-mono•phos•pha•tase** (mi″o-in-o′sĭ-tol mon″o-fos′fə-tās) former official name for *inositol-phosphate phosphatase*.

myo•is•che•mia (mi″o-is-ke′me-ə) [*myo-* + *ischemia*] local deficiency of blood supply in muscle.

myo•ki•nase (mi″o-ki′nās) adenylate kinase.

myo•ki•ne•sis (mi″o-kĭ-ne′sis) [*myo-* + *-kinesis*] movement of muscles, especially displacement of muscle fibers in operation. **myokinet′ic** *adj*

myo•kym•ia (mi″o-ki′me-ə) [*myo-* + Gr. *kyma* wave] a benign condition marked by brief spontaneous tetanic contractions of motor units or groups of muscle fibers, usually adjacent groups of fibers contracting alternately. Called also *myoclonia fibrillaris multiplex*.

myo•lem•ma (mi″o-lem′ə) [*myo-* + *-lemma*] the sarcolemma.

myo•li•po•ma (mi″o-lĭ-po′mə) [*myo-* + *lip-* + *-oma*] a benign mesenchymoma containing fatty or lipomatous elements.

my•ol•o•gy (mi-ol′ə-je) [*myo-* + *-logy*] the scientific study of muscles, and the body of knowledge relating to muscles.

my•ol•y•sis (mi-ol′ĭ-sis) [*myo-* + *-lysis*] disintegration or degeneration of muscle tissue.

m. cardiotox′ica degeneration of the heart muscle occurring in systemic infection.

my•o•ma (mi-o′mə) pl. *myomas, myo′mata* [*my-* + *-oma*] a benign tumor made up of muscular elements. See also *leiomyoma*. **myo′matous** *adj*

m. striocellula′re rhabdomyoma.

uterine m. see under *leiomyoma*.

my•o•ma•gen•e•sis (mi″o-mə-jen′ə-sis) the production or causation of myoma.

my•o•ma•la•cia (mi″o-mə-la′shə) [*myo-* + *-malacia*] morbid softening of a muscle.

my•o•ma•ta (mi-o′mə-tə) plural of *myoma*.

my•o•ma•tec•to•my (mi″o-mə-tek′tə-me) myomectomy (def. 1).

my•o•ma•to•sis (mi″o-mə-to′sis) the formation of multiple myomas.

my•o•mec•to•my (mi″o-mek′tə-me) [*myoma* + *-ectomy*] 1. surgical removal of a myoma (leiomyoma). 2. myectomy.

abdominal m. uterine myomectomy using an abdominal approach. Called also *laparomyomectomy.*

uterine m. surgical excision of a uterine myoma (leiomyoma); called also *fibroidectomy* and *fibromectomy.*

vaginal m. uterine myomectomy using a vaginal approach; called also *colpomyomectomy.*

myo•mel•a•no•sis (mi″o-mel″ə-no′sis) [*myo-* + *melanosis*] melanosis, or black pigmentation of a portion of the muscular substance.

myo•mere (mi′o-mēr) [*myo-* + *-mere*] myotome (def. 2).

my•om•e•ter (mi-om′ə-tər) [*myo-* + *-meter*] an apparatus for measuring muscle contraction.

myo•me•tri•tis (mi″o-me-tri′tis) [*myo-* + *metritis*] inflammation of the muscular substance, or myometrium, of the uterus.

myo•me•tri•um (mi-o-me′tre-əm) [*myo-* + Gr. *mētra* uterus] TA alternative for *tunica muscularis uteri.*

myo•mot•o•my (mi″o-mot′ə-me) incision into a myoma.

my•on (mi′on) [*myo-* + *-on* neuter ending] a muscular unit.

myo•ne•cro•sis (mi″o-nə-kro′sis) necrosis or death of individual muscle fibers.

clostridial m. gas gangrene.

myo•neme (mi′o-nēm) [*myo-* + Gr. *nēma* thread] any of various fibrillar organelles, known or believed to have contractile properties, commonly seen in the cytoplasm of stalked ciliate protozoa, but also occurring in certain nonciliates and certain nonprotozoans.

myo•neph•ro•path•ic (mi″o-nef″ro-path′ik) pertaining to kidney disease caused by muscle breakdown.

myo•neu•ral (mi″o-noor′əl) [*myo-* + *neural*] pertaining to both muscle and nerve; said of the nerve terminations in muscles.

my•on•y•my (mi-on′ĭ-me) [*myo-* + Gr. *onoma* name] nomenclature of the muscles.

myo•pal•mus (mi″o-pal′məs) muscle twitching.

myo•path•ia (mi″o-path′e-ə) myopathy.

m. infraspina′ta a condition marked by the sudden development of pain in the shoulder with tenderness in the infraspinatus muscle.

myo•path•ic (mi″o-path′ik) of the nature of a myopathy.

my•op•a•thy (mi-op′ə-the) [*myo-* + *-pathy*] any disease of a muscle.

acute quadriplegic m. critical illness m.

alcoholic m. myopathy affecting alcoholics, commonly characterized by acute myoglobinuria and sometimes by proximal limb weakness.

amyloid m. a rare manifestation of certain forms of amyloidosis, characterized by stiffness, proximal or diffuse weakness, generalized enlargement of muscles, a woody consistency of the limbs, and macroglossia.

Bethlem m. a genetically heterogeneous, autosomal dominant myopathy with onset in early infancy, caused by mutation in any of the three genes that encode collagen VI subunits. It is characterized by slowly progressive weakness of the upper arm and pelvic girdle muscles; hypotonia; delayed motor milestones; talipes; torticollis; and contractures of the ankles, hips, knees, and elbows.

capture m. a form of exertional rhabdomyolysis seen in wild animals that are captured and put under restraint.

central core m. see under *disease.*

centronuclear m. myotubular m.

critical illness m. severe muscle weakness, hypotonia, and depressed tendon reflexes of many different muscles in patients in intensive care units; in some it may be a complication of therapy with corticosteroids or neuromuscular blocking agents, but in others the cause is unknown. Called also *acute quadriplegic m.*

deep pectoral m., degenerative m. degeneration and necrosis of areas of the pectoral muscles in turkeys owing to increased pressure on blood vessels and resultant ischemia; in some breeds it is hereditary. Muscles become greenish, resulting in loss of value of the meat. Called also *green muscle disease.*

desmin m., desmin-related m. myofibrillar m.

distal m. any of numerous forms of muscular dystrophy, varying in mode of inheritance and age of onset, that affect first the feet and hands and progress to involve more proximal muscle groups. Among the disorders included here are *Welander distal m.* and the *hereditary inclusion body myopathies.* Called also *distal muscular dystrophy.*

fibrotic m. fibrosis with adhesions in the thigh muscles of working horses; the muscles eventually become hard and ossified. Called also *ossifying m.*

hereditary inclusion body m. any of a group of distal myopathies characterized by inclusion bodies with rimmed vacuoles. An autosomal recessive type is due to mutation in the *GNE* gene (locus: 9p13.3), which encodes a key enzyme in sialic acid biosynthesis. It has onset between the ages of 20 and 40 and affects primarily the lower limbs but spares the quadriceps muscles until late in the course. An autosomal dominant type is due to mutation in the *MYHC2A* gene (locus: 17p13.1), which encodes a myosin heavy chain. It affects the quadriceps muscles first. A rare third type, allelic with the autosomal recessive type, is Nonaka distal myopathy.

infectious m. see under *myositis.*

inflammatory m. myositis.

late distal hereditary m. Welander distal m.

lipid m. any metabolic myopathy caused by a defect in fatty acid oxidation, with the accumulation of triglycerides in muscle; manifestations depend on the specific enzyme deficiency and include limb and respiratory weakness, cardiomyopathy, encephalopathy, and myoglobinuria.

metabolic m. myopathy due to disordered metabolism, usually caused by genetic defects or hormonal dysfunction.

mitochondrial m. any of a group of myopathies associated with an increased number of enlarged, often abnormal, mitochondria in muscle fibers, manifested by exercise intolerance, generalized weakness, lactic acidosis, infantile quadriparesis, ophthalmoplegia, and cardiac abnormalities. Underlying metabolic defects include defects in substrate utilization, defects in the coupling of mitochondrial respiration to phosphorylation, and deficiencies in mitochondrial respiratory chain components.

myofibrillar m. any of several hereditary muscle conditions characterized by abnormal desmin in the myofibrils; affected persons have muscle weakness in distal parts of the limbs and cardiomyopathy. Both autosomal dominant and recessive types have been observed. Called also *desmin m.* and *desmin-related m.*

myotubular m. a genetically heterogenous, often fatal myopathy characterized by myofibers resembling those of early fetal muscle, i.e., with the nucleus located centrally and surrounded by a halo of apparently empty space. The *X-linked* form is most common and is caused by mutation in the *MTM1* gene (locus: Xq28), which encodes a protein required for muscle cell differentiation. The *autosomal dominant* form is caused by mutation in any of several genes. The *autosomal recessive* form is caused by mutation in the *BIN1* gene (locus: 2q14), which encodes a tumor suppressor protein. Called also *centronuclear m.*

nemaline m. a genetically and clinically heterogeneous, mainly congenital myopathy, characterized histologically by the presence of small, rodlike particles in the muscle fibers. Inheritance can be either autosomal dominant or autosomal recessive. The most common form presents as hypotonia and muscle weakness in infancy and is nonprogressive or slowly progressive. A more severe form is characterized by profound hypotonia and respiratory distress, arthrogryposis, and death in the first few months of life. A late-onset form, marked by mild proximal weakness beginning in early adulthood, has been reported, and rare sporadic cases are also seen.

Nonaka m., Nonaka distal m. a rare, autosomal recessive myopathy due to mutation in the *GNE* gene (locus: 9p13.3), which encodes a key enzyme in sialic acid biosynthesis; it is allelic with autosomal recessive hereditary inclusion body myopathy. It is characterized by rimmed vacuoles in the muscles of the legs, usually sparing the gastrocnemius muscles.

nutritional m. myopathy in domestic animals, usually young ones, caused by dietary deficiencies; two common types are enzootic muscular dystrophy and vitamin E–selenium deficiency syndrome.

ocular m. progressive external ophthalmoplegia.

ossifying m. fibrotic m.

rod m. nemaline m.

steroid m. muscle weakness and atrophy, usually in proximal limb muscles, after prolonged use of steroids.

thyrotoxic m. weakness and wasting of skeletal muscles, especially in the pelvic and shoulder girdles, accompanying hyperthyroidism.

Welander m., Welander distal m. an autosomal dominant distal myopathy with onset usually after age 40 and not affecting life span; it first affects the small muscles of the hands and feet and then spreads proximally. Called also *late distal hereditary m.*

my•ope (mi′ōp) [Gr. *myein* to shut + *ōps* eye] a nearsighted person; one affected with myopia.

myo•pec•tin•e•al (mi″o-pek-tin′e-əl) [*myo-* + *pectineal*] pertaining to the muscles of the inguinal region and the pectineal (Cooper) ligament.

myo•peri•car•di•tis (mi″o-per″ĭ-kahr-di′tis) [*myo-* + *pericarditis*] myocarditis combined with pericarditis.

myo•phage (mi′o-fāj) a phagocyte which destroys the contractile substance of muscle.

my•oph•a•gism (mi-of′ə-jiz-əm) [*myo-* + *phag-* + *-ism*] wasting of muscle tissue.

myo•phone (mi′o-fōn) [*myo-* + Gr. *phōnē* voice] a device which renders audible the sound of a muscular contraction.

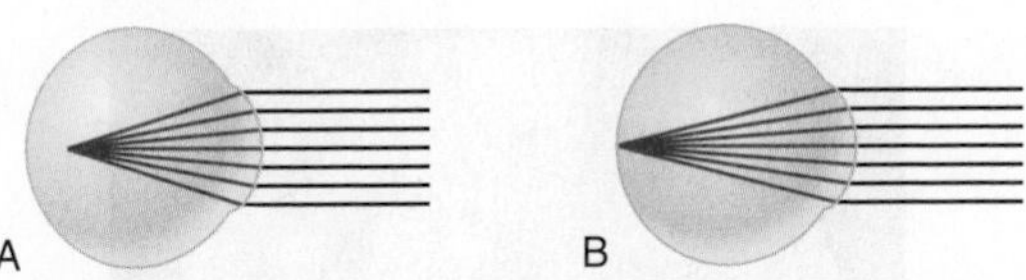

■ Myopia: error of refraction in a myopic eye *(A)*, contrasted with normal refraction in an emmetropic eye *(B)*.

myo•phos•phor•y•lase (mi″o-fos-for′ə-lās) the muscle isozyme of glycogen phosphorylase.

myo•phos•phor•y•lase de•fi•cien•cy (mi″o-fos-for′ə-lās) glycogen storage disease, type V.

my•o•pia (M) (mi-o′pe-ə) [Gr. *myein* to shut + *-opia*] an error of refraction in which rays of light entering the eye parallel to the optic axis are brought to a focus in front of the retina, as a result of the eyeball being too long from front to back *(axial m.)* or of an increased strength in refractive power of the media of the eye *(index m.)* Called also *nearsightedness*, because the near point is less distant than it is in emmetropia with an equal amplitude of accommodation. **myop′ic** *adj*

curvature m. myopia due to changes or increases in the curvature of the refracting surfaces of the eye, especially of the cornea.

index m. myopia due to variations in the index of refraction of the media of the eye.

malignant m., pernicious m. progressive myopia, associated with grave disease of the choroid and leading to retinal detachment and blindness.

primary m. simple m.

prodromal m. a condition marked by the return of the ability to do close work without eyeglasses; sometimes seen in incipient cataract.

progressive m. myopia that continues to increase abnormally rapidly in adult life.

simple m. 1. myopia due to normal growth of the healthy eyeball. It stops increasing at maturity and may be corrected to normal visual acuity. 2. myopia without astigmatism.

myo•plasm (mi′o-plaz″əm) [*myo-* + *-plasm*] the contractile part of the muscle cell, or myofibril.

myo•plas•tic (mi″o-plas′tik) 1. pertaining to myoplasty. 2. pertaining to the use of muscle tissue in plastic surgery.

myo•plas•ty (mi′o-plas″te) plastic surgery on muscle; an operation in which portions of partly detached muscle are utilized, especially in the field of defects or deformities.

Myo•po•rum (mi″o-po′rəm) a genus of shrubs and trees of Australia and New Zealand, many species of which are poisonous to livestock. *M. lae′tum*, the ngaio, causes photosensitization and sometimes fatal hemorrhaging.

myo•pro•tein (mi″o-pro′tēn) a protein obtained from muscle tissue.

my•op•sis (mi-op′sis) myiodesopsia.

my•o•rhyth•mia (mi″o-rith′me-ə) abnormal, regular, repetitive muscle contractions.

oculofacioskeletal m. synchronous movements of the ocular, facial, and limb muscles, seen in some persons with Whipple disease.

oculomasticatory m. synchronous movements of the ocular and pharyngeal muscles, seen in some persons with Whipple disease.

my•or•rha•phy (mi-or′ə-fe) [*myo-* + *-rrhaphy*] suture of divided muscle; called also *myosuture.*

my•or•rhex•is (mi″o-rek′sis) [*myo-* + *-rrhexis*] the rupture of a muscle.

myo•sal•gia (mi″o-sal′jə) myalgia.

myo•sal•pin•gi•tis (mi″o-sal″pin-ji′tis) [*myo-* + *salpingitis*] inflammation of the muscular tissue of the uterine tube.

myo•sal•pinx (mi″o-sal′pinks) the muscular tissue of the uterine tube.

my•o•san (mi′o-sən) a denatured and insoluble form of myosin.

myo•sar•co•ma (mi″o-sahr-ko′mə) [*myo-* + *sarcoma*] a malignant tumor derived from muscle tissue; see also *leiomyosarcoma* and *rhabdomyosarcoma.*

myo•schwan•no•ma (mi″o-shwah-no′mə) schwannoma.

myo•scle•ro•sis (mi″o-sklə-ro′sis) [*myo-* + *sclero-* + *-sis*] hardening, or sclerosis, of muscle tissue.

myo•scope (mi′o-skōp) [*myo-* + *-scope*] an ocular instrument, on the principle of the orthoptoscope, which allows fusion and movement laterally, vertically, and in rotation. Cf. *myoculator.*

myo•sep•tum (mi″o-sep′təm) myocomma.

my•o•sin (mi′o-sin) any of a family of proteins with ATPase activity, existing in a number of isoforms; it moves along actin filaments (F-actin) using the energy from ATP hydrolysis. Myosin consists of a *head* that produces motion by "walking" along the actin filament and is joined by a neck domain to a *tail* that contains binding sites determining specific activity. Within cells, myosins are involved in transport of vesicles and organelles. *Myosin II*, made up of two heavy and four light chains, is the main constituent of the thick filaments of muscle fibers, is responsible for the contraction and relaxation of muscle, and is the motor that drives cytokinesis. Cf. *actomyosin.* See Plate 32.

my•o•sin ATP•ase (mi′o-sin a-te-pe′ās) [EC 3.6.4.1] a specialized enzyme activity of myosin heads that couples the energy derived from the hydrolysis of ATP with motion by the successive making and breaking of cross-bridges between actin and myosin filaments. It is actin-activated: in the absence of actin, ATP hydrolysis occurs at a low rate, increasing to the maximum only when myosin is bound to actin.

my•o•sin•uria (mi″o-sĭ-nu′re-ə) the presence of myosin in the urine.

my•o•sis (mi-o′sis) miosis.

myo•si•tis (mi″o-si′tis) [*myo-* + *-itis*] inflammation of a voluntary muscle; called also *inflammatory myopathy.* **myosit′ic** *adj*

acute progressive m. a rare disease in which the inflammation gradually involves the whole muscular system, causing death by asphyxia and pneumonia.

m. a frigo′re fibrositis resulting from cold or chilling.

eosinophilic m. 1. a rare disorder characterized by proximal muscle weakness, myalgia, elevated muscle enzyme levels in the serum, electromyographic abnormalities, and eosinophilic infiltration of skeletal muscle and sometimes the viscera. It is occasionally associated with eosinophilic fasciitis or hypereosinophilic syndrome. Called also eosinophilic polymyositis. 2. inflammation of the muscles of mastication in dogs, especially large breeds such as German shepherds; it may be an autoimmune disorder. As the muscles swell, the animal has increased difficulty swallowing. Facial edema may also cause exophthalmos. 3. myositis of facial muscles in cattle, usually subclinical and found as a greenish discolored lesion of the meat after the animal is slaughtered.

m. fibro′sa myositis in which there is a formation of connective tissue within the muscle substance.

inclusion body m. a progressive type of myositis that primarily involves muscles of the pelvic region and lower limbs, usually seen in older people; the muscles are infiltrated by mononuclear inflammatory cells, sarcoplasmic vacuoles, masses of filaments and filamentous microtubules, and sometimes eosinophilic bodies.

infectious m., interstitial m. inflammation of the connective and septal elements of muscular tissue.

orbital m. see under *pseudotumor.*

m. ossi′ficans myositis with formation of bony deposits or ossification of muscles.

m. ossi′ficans circumscrip′ta myositis with formation of a muscular osteoma, such as rider's bone.

m. ossi′ficans progressi′va fibrodysplasia ossificans progressiva.

m. ossi′ficans trauma′tica myositis ossificans due to injury.

parenchymatous m. myositis affecting the essential substance of a muscle.

primary multiple m. an acute febrile disease characterized by edema and inflammation of the skin and muscles in various parts of the body.

progressive ossifying m. fibrodysplasia ossificans progressiva.

proliferative m. a benign, rapidly growing, reactive, nodular lesion similar to nodular fasciitis but characterized by fibroblast proliferation within skeletal muscle; histologically it resembles sarcoma.

rheumatoid m. fibrositis.

m. sero′sa myositis with a serous exudate.

spontaneous bacterial m. pyomyositis.

suppurative m. myositis due to bacteremia and associated with suppuration and gangrene. Cf. *pyomyositis.*

myo•spasm (mi′o-spaz″əm) spasm (def. 1).

myo•spher•u•lo•sis (mi″o-sfēr″u-lo′sis) an inflammatory giant cell reaction linked to topical use of tetracycline in oil-based ointment on wounds.

myo•stat•in (mi″o-stat′in) a member of the transforming growth factor-β family that acts as a negative regulator to inhibit muscle growth.

my•os•te•o•ma (mi-os″te-o′mə) [*my-* + *osteoma*] a muscle tumor containing bony deposits or areas.

my•os•then•ic (mi″os-then′ik) [*myo-* + *sthen-* + *-ic*] pertaining to strength of muscle.

my•os•then•om•e•ter (mi″os-thən-om′ə-tər) [*myo-* + *stheno-* + *-meter*] dynamometer.

myo•stro•ma (mi″o-stro′mə) [*myo-* + *stroma*] the stroma or framework of muscle tissue.

myo•stro•min (mi″o-stro′min) a protein occurring in muscle stroma.

myo•su•ria (mi″o-su′re-ə) [*myo-* + *-uria*] myosinuria.

myo•su•ture (mi″o-soo′chər) myorrhaphy.

myo•syn•i•ze•sis (mi″o-sin″ĭ-ze′sis) [*myo-* + Gr. *synizēsis* a sinking down] adhesion of muscles.

myo•tac•tic (mi″o-tak′tik) [*myo-* + L. *tactus* touch] pertaining to the proprioceptive sense of muscles.

my•ot•a•sis (mi-ot′ə-sis) [*myo-* + Gr. *tasis* stretching] stretching of muscle.

myo•tat•ic (mi″o-tat′ik) performed or induced by stretching or extending a muscle.

myo•ten•on•to•plas•ty (mi″o-tən-on′to-plas″te) tenomyoplasty.

myo•teno•si•tis (mi″o-ten″o-si′tis) [*myo-* + *teno-* + *-itis*] inflammation of a muscle and its tendon.

myo•te•not•o•my (mi″o-tə-not′ə-me) [*myo-* + *tenotomy*] surgical division of the tendon of a muscle.

myo•ther•a•py (mi′o-ther″ə-pe) a bodywork technique whose purpose is the relief of muscle spasm and muscle-related pain by the application of pressure at specific trigger points, using the fingers, knuckles, and elbows, together with corrective exercise.

myo•ther•mic (mi″o-thur′mik) [*myo-* + *therm-* + *-ic*] pertaining to temperature changes in muscle produced by its activity.

myo•til•in (mi″o-til′in) a cytoskeletal protein expressed in skeletal and cardiac muscle. It binds to α-actinin and is localized in the Z band of sarcomeres. Mutation in the gene encoding myotilin has been linked to an autosomal dominant subtype of limb-girdle muscular dystrophy.

myo•tome (mi′o-tōm) [*myo-* + *-tome*] 1. an instrument for performing myotomy. 2. the muscle plate or portion of a somite that develops into noncardiac striated muscle; called also *myomere.* 3. a group of muscles innervated from a single spinal segment.

myo•tom•ic (mi″o-tom′ik) pertaining to or derived from a myotome.

my•ot•o•my (mi-ot′ə-me) [*myo-* + *-tomy*] the cutting or dissection of a muscle or of muscular tissue.

cricopharyngeal m. resection of the cricopharyngeal muscle as treatment for intractable dysphagia or pharyngoesophageal diverticulum.

Heller m. esophagocardiomyotomy.

Livaidatis circular m. a surgical treatment for esophageal atresia consisting of anastomosis of the upper and lower pouches and lengthening of the upper pouch by circumferential esophagomyotomy.

Myo•ton•a•chol (mi″o-tōn′ə-kol) trademark for preparations of bethanechol chloride.

myo•to•nia (mi″o-to′ne-ə) [*myo-* + *ton-* + *-ia*] dystonia involving increased muscular irritability and contractility with decreased power of relaxation; cf. *tetanus* (def. 2). **myoton′ic** *adj*

m. atro′phica myotonic dystrophy.

chondrodystrophic m. Schwartz-Jampel syndrome.

m. conge′nita tonic spasm and rigidity of certain muscles when an attempt is made to move them after a period of rest or when mechanically stimulated; the stiffness disappears as the muscles are used. There are autosomal dominant and autosomal recessive forms; both are due to mutation in the *CLCN1* gene (locus: 7q35), which encodes a skeletal muscle chloride channel. The autosomal dominant form is called also *Thomsen disease;* the autosomal recessive form, which is more severe, appears later in childhood, and is often also characterized by muscle weakness, is called also *Becker disease.*

m. dystro′phica myotonic dystrophy.

m. fluc′tuans a rare autosomal dominant myotonia characterized by fluctuating degrees of muscle stiffness, aggravated by potassium intake, but not associated with muscle weakness. Like myotonia permanens and several other disorders, it is due to mutation in the *SCNA4A* gene (locus: 17q23.1-q25.3), which encodes a subunit of a voltage-gated sodium channel.

m. heredita′ria m. congenita.

m. le′vior a rare mild form of autosomal dominant myotonia congenita.

m. per′manens a rare autosomal dominant myotonia characterized by severe myotonia and hypertrophy of muscles around the neck and shoulders, aggravated by potassium intake, but not associated with muscle weakness. Like myotonia fluctuans and several other disorders, it is due to mutation in the *SCNA4A* gene (locus: 17q23.1-q25.3), which encodes a subunit of a voltage-gated sodium channel.

my•ot•o•noid (mi-ot′ə-noid) [*myo-* + *ton-* + *-oid*] resembling myotonia; said of reactions in muscle which are marked by slow contraction or relaxation.

my•ot•o•nus (mi-ot′ə-nəs) tonic spasm (physiological tetanus) of a muscle or of a group of muscles.

myo•tro•phic (mi″o-tro′fik) 1. increasing the weight of muscle. 2. pertaining to myotrophy.

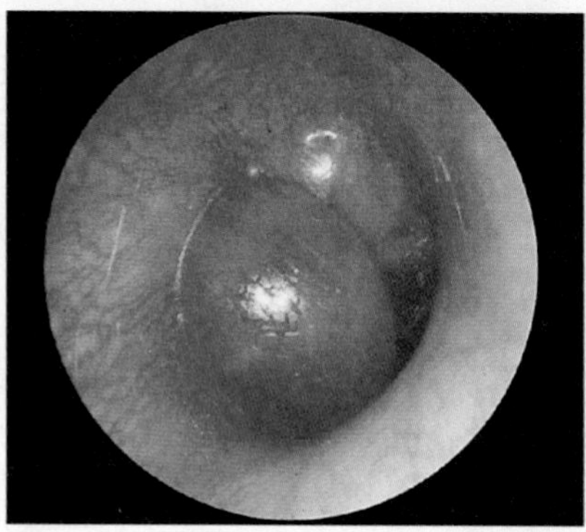

■ Bullous myringitis.

my•ot•ro•phy (mi-ot′rə-fe) [*myo-* + *-trophy*] nutrition of muscle.

my•o•tro•pic (mi″o-tro′pik) [*myo-* + *-tropic*] having an affinity for muscle, as myotropic organisms.

myo•tube (mi′o-tōōb″) myotubule.

myo•tu•bule (mi″o-too′būl) a developing muscle cell or fiber with a centrally, rather than peripherally, located nucleus. **myotu′bular** *adj*

myo•vas•cu•lar (mi″o-vas′ku-lər) [*myo-* + *vascular*] pertaining to a muscle and its blood vessels.

Myo•view (mi′o-vu″) trademark for a kit for the preparation of technetium Tc 99m tetrofosmin.

Myo•zyme (mi′o-zīm) trademark for a preparation of alglucosidase alfa.

myria- [Gr. *myrios* numberless] a combining form meaning a great number.

myr•ia•chit (mir-yah′chit) [Russ.] a variety of jumping disease seen in Siberia, possibly identical to latah. Spelled also *miryachit.*

Myr•i•an•gi•a•les (mir″e-an″je-a′lēz) former name for Dothideales.

myr•ia•pod (mir′e-ə-pod) a member of the Myriapoda; a centipede or millipede.

Myr•i•ap•o•da (mir″e-ap′ə-də) [*myria-* + Gr. *pous* foot] a superclass of arthropods, including the classes Chilopoda (centipedes) and Diplopoda (millipedes).

myr•i•cyl (mir′ĭ-cəl) the radical occurring in beeswax and other waxes.

my•rin•ga (mĭ-ring′gə) membrana tympanica.

my•rin•gec•to•my (mir″in-jek′tə-me) [*myring-* + *-ectomy*] tympanectomy.

my•rin•gi•tis (mir″in-ji′tis) [*myring-* + *-itis*] inflammation of the tympanic membrane.

m. bullo′sa, bullous m. a form of viral otitis media in which serous or hemorrhagic blebs appear on the membrana tympani and often on the adjacent wall of the auditory meatus.

myring(o)- [L. *myringa,* tympanic membrane] a combining form denoting relationship to the membrana tympani.

my•rin•go•der•ma•ti•tis (mĭ-ring″go-dur″mə-ti′tis) [*myringo-* + *dermatitis*] inflammation of the outer layer of the tympanic membrane, with the formation of blebs.

my•rin•go•plas•ty (mĭ-ring′go-plas″te) [*myringo-* + *-plasty*] surgical restoration of a perforated tympanic membrane by grafting. See also *tympanoplasty.* **myringoplas′tic** *adj*

my•rin•go•sta•pe•dio•pexy (mĭ-ring″go-stə-pe′de-o-pek″se) fixation of the pars tensa of the membrana tympani to the head of the stapes.

my•rin•go•tome (mĭ-ring′go-tōm) a knife used in operations on the tympanic membrane.

my•rin•got•o•my (mir″ing-got′o-me) [*myringo-* + *-tomy*] the creation of a hole in the tympanic membrane, as for tympanocentesis. Called also *tympanostomy* and *tympanotomy.*

my•rinx (mi′rinks) membrana tympanica.

myr•is•tate (mir′is-tāt) a salt, ester, or anionic form of myristic acid.

isopropyl m. see under *isopropyl.*

My•ris•ti•ca (mə-ris′tĭ-kə) [Gr. *myrizein* to anoint] a genus of tropical trees of the family Myristicaceae. *M. fra′grans* is the nutmeg, source of nutmeg oil. See also *nutmeg poisoning,* under *poisoning.*

my•ris•tic ac•id (mĭ-ris′tik) a saturated 14-carbon fatty acid occurring in most animal and vegetable fats, particularly butterfat and coconut, palm, and nutmeg oils. See also table accompanying *fatty acid.*

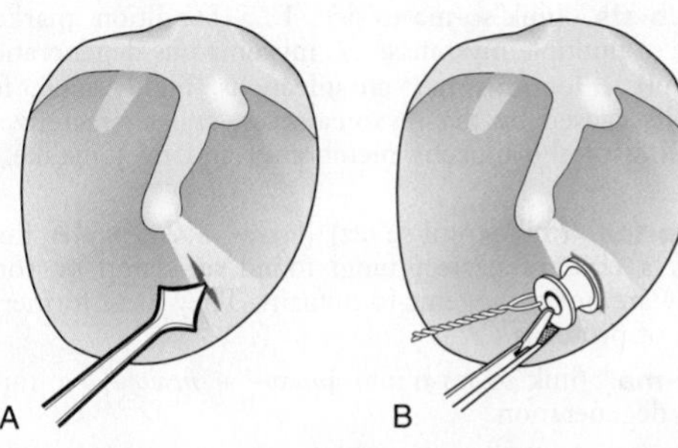

■ Myringotomy incision *(A)* and grommet insertion *(B)*.

myr•me•cia (mir-me′se-ə) [L.] a type of deep palmoplantar wart that protrudes above the skin surface and is caused by a human papillomavirus.

My•roi•da•ceae (mi″roi-da′se-e) in some systems of classification, a family of bacteria of the phylum Bacteroidetes; organisms of medical interest are contained in the genus *Myroides.*

My•roi•des (mi-roi′dēz) [Gr. *myros* perfume + *-oeidēs* resembling] a genus of gram-negative bacteria of the family Flavobacteriaceae, consisting of nonmotile, non–spore-forming, rod-shaped organisms that produce a yellow pigment and a fruity odor. Members were formerly included in the genus *Flavobacterium.* The type species is *M. odora′tus.*

M. odoratimi′mus a species, formerly classified in *Flavobacterium odoratum,* that is a cause of nosocomial infections.

M. odora′tus a species, formerly classified in *Flavobacterium odoratum,* that causes nosocomial bacteremia and soft tissue infection.

my•ro•the•cio•tox•i•co•sis (mi″ro-the″se-o-tok″sĭ-ko′sis) mycotoxicosis in ruminants caused by eating grass or feed contaminated with fungi of the species *Myrothecium,* which contain roridins and verrucarins. In its chronic form animals have intestinal ulcerations and weight loss. In the acute form, characteristics include diarrhea, hepatitis, and pulmonary congestion and edema that can be fatal.

My•ro•the•ci•um (mi″ro-the′se-um) a genus of imperfect fungi of the form-class Hyphomycetes that contaminates grasses and contains roridins and verrucarins, causing myrotheciotoxicosis. Certain species contain trichothecenes and can cause alimentary toxic aleukia. Species include *M. ro′ridum* and *M. verruca′ria.*

My•rox•i•lon (mi-rok′sə-lon) a genus of tropical American trees of the family Leguminosae. *M. perei′rae* Klotzsch yields balsam of Peru and *M. bal′samum* yields tolu balsam.

myrrh (mər) [Gr. *murrha*] [USP] the oleo-gum-resin obtained from species of *Commiphora;* it is applied topically in the treatment of mild inflammations of the oral and pharyngeal mucosa.

myr•te•nol (mur′tə-nol) a terpene alcohol from the volatile oil distilled from the leaves of *Myrtus communis.*

myr•ti•form (mir′tĭ-form) shaped like myrtle or myrtle berries.

Myr•tus (mur′təs) [L., from Gr. *myrtos*] a genus of shrubs of the family Myrtaceae that have white or pink flowers. *M. commu′nis* L. is a European species of myrtle whose leaves are antiseptic and astringent.

My•so•line (mi′so-lēn) trademark for preparations of primidone.

my•so•phil•ia (mi″so-fil′e-ə) [Gr. *mysos* uncleanness of body or mind + *-philia*] abnormal interest in dirt or filth, with a desire for contact with it that may encompass a paraphilia.

my•so•pho•bia (mi″so-fo′be-ə) [Gr. *mysos* uncleanness of body or mind + *-phobia*] irrational fear of dirt and contamination. **mysopho′bic** *adj*

my•ta•cism (mi′tə-siz-əm) [Gr. *mytakismos*] a speech disorder consisting of too free use of *m* sounds; called also *mimmation* and *mutacism.*

My•te•lase (mi′tə-lās) trademark for a preparation of ambenonium chloride.

mytho•pho•bia (mith″o-fo′be-ə) [Gr. *mythos* myth + *-phobia*] irrational fear of myths or of stating an untruth.

My•trex (mi′treks) trademark for a combination preparation of nystatin and triamcinolone acetonide.

myx•ad•e•ni•tis (miks″ad-ə-ni′tis) [*myx-* + *aden-* + *-itis*] inflammation of a mucous gland.

m. labia′lis cheilitis glandularis.

myx•ame•ba (miks″ə-me′bə) [*myx-* + *ameba*] a uninucleate, naked, free-living ameboid cell without either cilia or flagella produced from a spore, which aggregates and fuses with other myxamebas to form a plasmodium or aggregates without fusion to form a pseudoplasmodium.

myx•an•gi•tis (miks″ən-ji′tis) [*myx-* + *angitis*] inflammation of the ducts of mucous glands.

myx•as•the•nia (miks″əs-the′ne-ə) [*myxo-* + *asthen-* + *-ia*] deficiency in the secretion of mucus.

myx•ede•ma (miks″ə-de′mə) [*myxo-* + *edema*] dry, waxy swelling of the skin with abnormal deposits of glycosaminoglycans in the skin or other tissues; it is considered to be a type of mucinosis and is usually associated with primary hypothyroidism. The edema is nonpitting, and there are distinctive facial changes including swollen lips and a thickened nose. Cf. *lichen myxedematosus.* **myxedem′atous** *adj*

circumscribed m. pretibial m.

congenital m., infantile m. cretinism.

nodular m. pretibial m.

operative m. myxedema developing after thyroidectomy.

papular m. lichen myxedematosus.

pituitary m. myxedema associated with hypothyroidism caused by thyroid stimulating hormone deficiency.

pretibial m. localized myxedema associated with hyperthyroidism and exophthalmos, typically found on the anterior (pretibial) surface of the legs; the mucin deposits appearing as both plaques and papules. Called also *Graves, infiltrative,* or *thyroid dermopathy* and *circumscribed* or *nodular m.*

primary m. atrophic thyroiditis.

secondary m. pituitary m.

myx•edem•a•toid (miks″ə-dem′ə-toid) [*myxedema* + *-oid*] resembling myxedema.

myx•i•o•sis (mik″se-o′sis) a discharge of mucus.

myx(o)- [Gr. *myxa* mucus] a combining form denoting relationship to mucus, or to slime.

myxo•blas•to•ma (mik″so-blas-to′mə) myxoma.

myxo•chon•dro•fi•bro•sar•co•ma (mik″so-kon″dro-fi″bro-sahr-ko′mə) [*myxo-* + *chondro-* + *fibro-* + *sarcoma*] a malignant mesenchymoma containing myxoid, chondroid, and fibrous elements.

myxo•chon•dro•ma (mik″so-kon-dro′mə) [*myxo-* + *chondroma*] chondroma with a stroma resembling primitive mesenchymal tissue.

myxo•chon•dro•sar•co•ma (mik″so-kon″dro-sahr-ko′mə) chondromyxosarcoma.

myxo•cys•ti•tis (mik″so-sis-ti′tis) [*myxo-* + *cystitis*] inflammation of the mucosa of the bladder.

myxo•cys•to•ma (mik″so-sis-to′mə) [*myxo-* + *cyst-* + *-oma*] myxoma with cystic degeneration.

myxo•cyte (mik′so-sīt) [*myxo-* + *cyte*] one of the characteristic cells of mucous tissue.

myxo•en•chon•dro•ma (mik″so-en″kon-dro′mə) [*myxo-* + *enchondroma*] a chondroma in which some of the elements have undergone mucous degeneration.

myxo•en•do•the•li•o•ma (mik″so-en″do-the″le-o′mə) hemangioendothelioma with myxomatous degeneration.

myxo•fi•bro•ma (mik″so-fi-bro′mə) [*myxoma* + *fibroma*] a fibroma containing myxomatous tissue.

odontogenic m. odontogenic myxoma, particularly one containing large amounts of collagen.

myxo•fi•bro•sar•co•ma (mik″so-fi″bro-sahr-ko′mə) [*myxo-* + *fibro-* + *sarcoma*] the myxoid subtype of malignant fibrous histiocytoma.

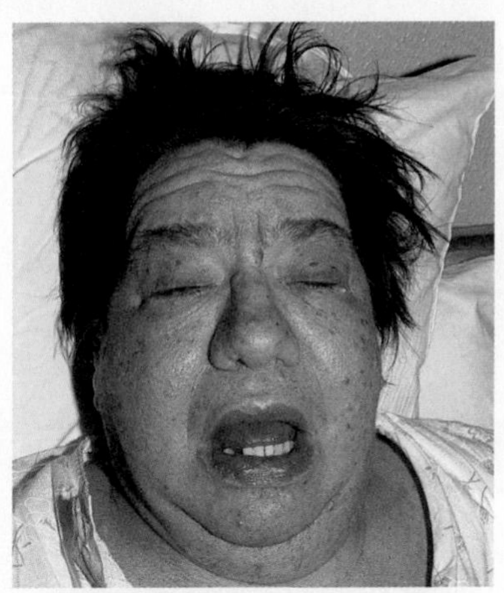
■ Myxedema in adult hypothyroidism.

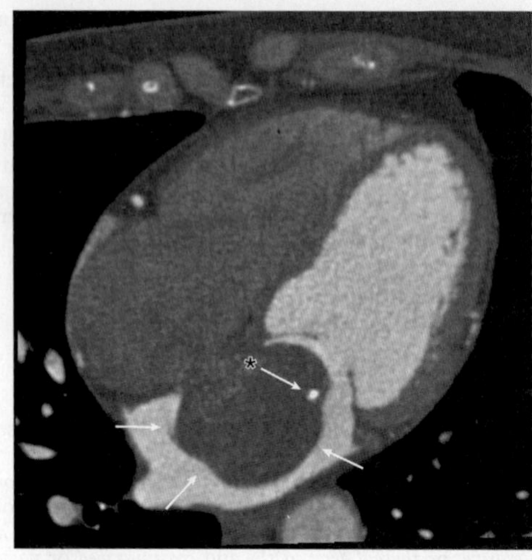

■ Large left atrial myxoma *(arrows)* with attachment to the interatrial septum; it contains a small calcification *(asterisk)*.

myxo•gli•o•ma (mik″so-gli-o′mə) a glioma which has undergone myxomatous degeneration.

myxo•glob•u•lo•sis (mik″so-glob″u-lo′sis) [*myxo-* + *globule* + *-osis*] a morphological variant of mucocele in which the mucus forms globoid bodies resembling pearls, occurring mainly in the vermiform appendix but also seen in the oral cavity.

myx•oid (mik′soid) [*myxo-* + *-oid*] mucoid (def. 1).

myxo•li•po•ma (mik″so-lĭ-po′mə) [*myxo-* + *lipoma*] lipoma with foci of myxomatous degeneration.

myx•o•ma (mik-so′mə) pl. *myxomas, myxo′mata* [*myx-* + *-oma*] a benign tumor composed of primitive connective tissue cells and stroma resembling mesenchyme. Called also *colloid tumor, gelatinous tumor,* and *mucous tumor.* myxo′matous *adj*

atrial m. a benign gelatinous growth usually pedunculated and usually arising from the interatrial septum of the heart in the region of the fossa ovalis; symptoms may include effort dyspnea, loss of weight, fatigue, low-grade fever, polyneuritis, nausea, and palpitations, and sometimes sudden syncopal attacks related to obstruction.

cystic m. myxocystoma.

enchondromatous m. a myxoma containing cartilage in the intercellular substance.

m. fibro′sum myxofibroma.

infectious m. myxomatosis cuniculi.

lipomatous m. myxolipoma.

nerve sheath m. neurothekeoma.

odontogenic m. an uncommon odontogenic tumor of the jaw, apparently arising from the mesenchymal portion of the tooth germ, and possibly produced by myxomatous degeneration of an odontogenic fibroma.

m. sarcomato′sum myxosarcoma.

vascular m. a myxoma containing many blood vessels.

myx•o•ma•to•sis (mik″so-mə-to′sis) 1. a condition marked by the development of multiple myxomas. 2. myxomatous degeneration.

m. cuni′culi, infectious m. an infectious, highly fatal, febrile disease of rabbits caused by the myxoma virus, and characterized by edematous swelling of the mucous membranes and myxomalike tumors of the skin.

Myxo•my•ce•tes (mik″so-mi-se′tēz) [*myxo-* + Gr. *mykēs* fungus] the slime molds, a class of perfect fungi found on damp or rotting plant material; they are not pathogenic to humans. They were formerly thought to be groups of protozoa.

myxo•my•o•ma (mik″so-mi-o′mə) [*myxo-* + *myoma*] a myoma with myxomatous degeneration.

myxo•pap•il•lo•ma (mik″so-pap″ĭ-lo′mə) myxoma combined with papilloma.

myxo•poi•e•sis (mik″so-poi-e′sis) [*myxo-* + *-poiesis*] the formation of mucus.

myxo•sar•co•ma (mik″so-sahr-ko′mə) [*myxo-* + *sarcoma*] a sarcoma containing myxomatous tissue. myxosarco′matous *adj*

odontogenic m. a rare form of odontogenic myxoma characterized by hypercellularity, atypical cytological features, and locally aggressive behavior.

Myxo•so•ma (mik″so-so′mə) [*myxo-* + Gr. *soma* body] a genus of parasitic protozoa (suborder Platysporina, order Bivalvulida), having a mucoid envelope around the spore. *M. cerebra′lis* infects salmonid fishes, causing whirling disease.

myxo•spor•an (mik″so-spor′ən) any protozoan of the class Myxosporea.

Myxo•spor•ea (mik″so-spor′e-ə) [*myxo-* + *spore*] a class of histozoic or celozoic parasitic protozoa (phylum Myxozoa) found in cold-blooded vertebrates, having spores with one or two sporoplasms and one to six (typically two) polar capsules, each capsule with a coiled polar tube, the probable function of which is anchorage to the host's tissues. The spore membrane usually has two, sometimes up to six, valves. It comprises two orders: Bivalvulida and Multivalvulida.

myxo•vi•rus (mik′so-vi″rəs) [*myxo-* + *virus*] a group of RNA viruses characterized by special affinities for mucopolysaccharides and glycoproteins, similarities in virion structure, neuraminidase activity, and hemagglutination. Myxoviruses are divided into the families Orthomyxoviridae and Paramyxoviridae. myxovi′ral *adj*

Myxo•zoa (mik″so-zo′ə) [*myxo-* + Gr. *zōon* animal] a phylum of chiefly histozoic or celozoic parasitic protozoa having spores of multicellular origin, with one or more polar capsules and one, two, or three, rarely more, valves, and usually found in fishes but also in amphibians and reptiles. It comprises two classes: Myxosporea and Actinosporea.

myxo•zo•an (mik″so-zo′ən) 1. any protozoan of the phylum Myxozoa. 2. pertaining to protozoa of the phylum Myxozoa.

My•zo•my•ia (mi″zo-mi′ə) [Gr. *myzan* to suck + *myia* fly] a series of mosquitoes, part of the subgenus *Cellia* of the genus *Anopheles.*

My•zo•rhyn•chus (mi″zo-ring′kəs) [Gr. *myzan* to suck + *rhynchos* snout] a series of mosquitoes, part of the subgenus *Anopheles* of the genus *Anopheles.* Several species are carriers of malarial parasites in Asia and Africa.

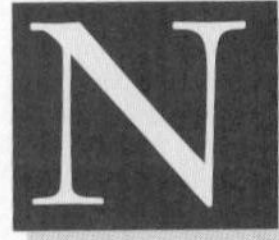

N newton; nitrogen; normal (solution), used with a number designating the strength of the solution relative to the normal, e.g., N/2 or 0.5 N for half-normal.

N normal (see N); number; Avogadro's number; neutron number; (in statistics) population size.

***N*-** in chemical nomenclature, a prefix indicating that the group or groups named immediately after the symbol are joined to the molecule via its nitrogen atoms.

N_A Avogadro's number.

n nano-; refractive index; neutron.

n. [L.] ner'vus (nerve).

n (haploid) chromosome number; refractive index; (in statistics) sample size.

***n*-** normal (def. 2b).

n_D refractive index.

ν nu, the thirteenth letter of the Greek alphabet; symbol for *degrees of freedom*, *frequency* (def. 1), *neutrino*, and *kinematic viscosity*.

NA *Nomina Anatomica*; numerical aperture.

Na sodium (L. *na'trium*).

NAAT nucleic acid amplification test.

Na•bi-HB (nah'be-āch"be") trademark for a preparation of human hepatitis B immune globulin.

nab•i•lone (nab'ĭ-lōn) a synthetic cannabinoid with antianxiety and antiemetic actions; used for the prevention of chemotherapy-associated nausea and vomiting.

Na•both follicles (cysts, glands) (nah'bot) [Martin *Naboth*, German anatomist, 1675–1721] see under *follicle*.

na•bo•thi•an (nə-bo'the-ən) named for Martin *Naboth*, as *nabothian follicle*.

na•bu•me•tone (nə-bu'mə-tōn") a nonsteroidal antiinflammatory drug used in the treatment of osteoarthritis and rheumatoid arthritis; administered orally.

na•cre•ous (na'kre-əs) [Fr. *nacre* mother of pearl] having a grayish-white, translucent color, with a pearl-like luster; said of bacterial colonies.

NAD nicotinamide adenine dinucleotide; no appreciable disease.

NAD^+ the oxidized form of nicotinamide adenine dinucleotide.

NADH the reduced form of nicotinamide adenine dinucleotide.

NADH cy•to•chrome b_5 re•duc•tase (si'to-krōm re-duk'tās) cytochrome-b_5 reductase.

NADH de•hy•dro•ge•nase (ubi•quin•one) (de-hi'dro-jən-ās u-bik'win-ōn) [EC 1.6.5.3] an enzyme complex of the inner mitochondrial membrane that catalyzes the transfer of electrons from NADH to ubiquinone, oxidizing the former and reducing the latter in a reaction of the electron transport chain (q.v.). The enzyme complex contains flavoprotein (FMN) and iron-sulfur prosthetic groups and is associated with proton translocation and the resultant synthesis of ATP.

NADH met•he•mo•glo•bin re•duc•tase (met-he'mo-glo-bin re-duk'tās) cytochrome-b_5 reductase.

NADH ox•i•dase (ok'sĭ-dās) NADH peroxidase.

NADH per•ox•i•dase (pər-ok'sĭ-dās) [EC 1.11.1.1] an enzyme of the oxidoreductase class that catalyzes the transfer of electrons from NADH to hydrogen peroxide, reducing the latter to water. The enzyme contains FAD.

NADH-Q re•duc•tase (re-duk'tās) NADH dehydrogenase (ubiquinone).

na•di (nah'de) in ayurveda, any of the channels that carry vital energy through the body.

NAD^+ ki•nase (ki'nās) [EC 2.7.1.23] an enzyme of the transferase class that catalyzes the phosphorylation of NAD^+ to form $NADP^+$.

na•do•lol (na-do'lol) [USP] a nonselective beta-adrenergic blocking agent, administered orally in the treatment of angina pectoris and hypertension.

Nad•o•stine (nad'o-stēn) trademark for preparations of nystatin.

NADP nicotinamide adenine dinucleotide phosphate.

$NADP^+$ the oxidized form of nicotinamide adenine dinucleotide phosphate.

NADPH the reduced form of nicotinamide adenine dinucleotide phosphate.

NADPH–cy•to•chrome P-450 re•duc•tase (si'to-krōm re-duk'tās) NADPH–hemoprotein reductase.

NADPH–he•mo•pro•tein re•duc•tase (he'mo-pro"tēn re-duk'tās) [EC 1.6.2.4] an enzyme of the oxidoreductase class that catalyzes the transfer of electrons to cytochromes via oxidation of NADPH. It is a flavoprotein (FMN, FAD) occurring in the endoplasmic reticulum and serving as the initial electron donor in reactions catalyzed by cytochrome P-450 monooxygenases (e.g., unspecific monooxygenase). It can also transfer electrons to cytochromes *b* and *c*. Called also *NADPH–cytochrome P-450 reductase*. Formerly called *NADPH–ferrihemoprotein reductase*.

NADPH met•he•mo•glo•bin re•duc•tase (met-he'mo-glo"bin re-duk'tās) an enzyme of the erythrocytes that catalyzes the reduction of methemoglobin to hemoglobin via oxidation of NADH. The physiological significance of the enzyme is uncertain; no endogenous intermediate electron carrier has been found, although the enzyme can be activated if methylene blue or other artificial electron acceptor is introduced. Called also *methemoglobin reductase (NADPH)*.

NADPH ox•i•dase (ok'sĭ-dās) a plasma membrane–associated enzyme complex that catalyzes the univalent reduction of oxygen using NADPH as an electron donor; the superoxide anion formed acts as an oxidant in the phagocyte microbicidal system, proceeding through a series of electron transfer reactions that form the respirator burst. Various genetic defects in the system result in chronic granulomatous disease.

$NAD(P)^+$ trans•hy•dro•gen•ase (AB-spe•ci•fic) (trans-hi'dro-jən-ās spə-sif'ik) [EC 1.6.1.2] an enzyme of the inner mitochondrial membrane that uses the energy generated by proton translocation to catalyze the reaction $NADH + NADP^+ = NAD^+ + NADPH$. The enzyme is regulated by the relative concentrations of NAD and NADP and by the energy state of the membrane, becoming activated in the presence of excess ATP and electrons from the electron transport chain. The enzyme from heart is A specific with respect to NAD^+ and B specific with respect to $NADP^+$.

nad•ro•pa•rin cal•ci•um (nad-ro-pa'rin) a low molecular weight heparin used in treatment and prophylaxis of thromboembolism and unstable angina, and in prevention of clotting during extracorporeal circulation; administered subcutaneously.

NAD^+ syn•thase (glu•ta•mine-hy•dro•lys•ing) (sin'thās gloo'tə-mēn hi'dro-līz"ing) [EC 6.3.5.1] an enzyme of the transferase class that catalyzes the transfer of an amino group from glutamine to desamido-NAD^+ to form NAD^+.

Nae•ge•li's leukemia (na'gĕ-le) [Otto *Naegeli*, Swiss hematologist, 1871–1938] acute myelomonocytic leukemia.

Nae•ge•li syndrome (na'gĕ-le) [Oskar *Naegeli*, Swiss dermatologist, 1885–1959] Franceschetti-Jadassohn syndrome.

Nae•gle•ria (na-glēr'e-ə) a genus of free-living protozoa (order Schizopyrenida, subclass Gymnamoebia) found in fresh water, soil, and sewage; they have both an ameboid and a flagellate stage in their life cycles, with two flagella present in the latter stage. Infection is usually acquired by swimming in contaminated water. Certain species, especially *N. fow'leri*, are capable of facultative parasitism; some strains are highly pathogenic and may cause fatal primary amebic meningoencephalitis.

nae•gle•ri•a•sis (na"glə-ri'ə-sis) infection with protozoa of the genus *Naegleria*, usually in the form of primary amebic meningoencephalitis.

naev(o)- for words beginning thus, see those beginning *nev(o)-*.

na•fam•o•stat mes•y•late (nə-fam'o-stat) a proteinase inhibitor used in treatment of acute pancreatitis and as an anticoagulant in hemofiltration.

naf•a•rel•in ace•tate (naf'ə-rel"in) a synthetic preparation of gonadotropin-releasing hormone, used in the treatment of central precocious puberty and of endometriosis; administered by nasal spray.

naf•cil•lin so•di•um (naf-sil'in) [USP] a semisynthetic, acid- and penicillinase-resistant penicillin, used as an antibacterial in severe staphylococcal infections caused by penicillinase-positive organisms; administered orally, intramuscularly, or intravenously.

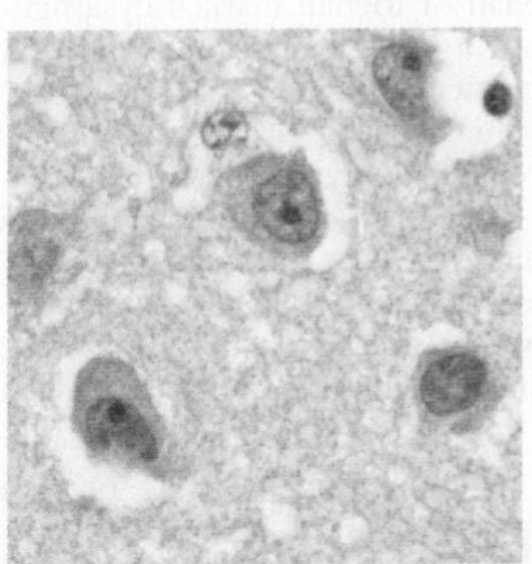

■ *Naegleria fowleri* trophozoites in brain tissue.

Naff·zig·er operation, syndrome (naf′zig-ər) [Howard Christian *Naffziger*, American surgeon, 1884–1961] see under *operation*, and see *scalenus syndrome*, under *syndrome*.

naf·ro·nyl ox·a·late (naf′ro-nəl) a vasodilator which has been used in the treatment of peripheral and cerebral vascular disorders.

naf·ta·lo·fos (naf′tə-lo-fos) a veterinary anthelmintic.

naf·ti·fine hy·dro·chlo·ride (naf′tĭ-fēn) [USP] a broad-spectrum antifungal agent, chemically related to allylamines, applied topically to the skin.

Naf·tin (naf′tin) trademark for preparations of naftifine hydrochloride.

na·ga·na (nah-gah′nah) [Zulu, from *ngana* feeble, weak] any of various tsetse fly–transmitted types of trypanosomiasis in domestic animals in Africa, including cattle, horses, sheep, goats, dogs, pigs, and camels. It may be acute or chronic and its pathogenicity and symptoms vary according to factors such as the trypanosome involved and the species infected. Anemia, fever, and emaciation occur in many species, corneal opacities in horses and dogs, and abortion in cows.

Na·geotte bracelets, nodule (nah-zhot′) [Jean *Nageotte*, Paris histologist, 1866–1948] see under *bracelet* and *nodule*.

Na·ger acrofacial dysostosis (syndrome) (nah-zher′) [Félix Robert *Nager*, Swiss otorhinolaryngologist, 1877–1959] see under *dysostosis*.

Na·ger-de Rey·nier syndrome (nah-zher′ də ra-nya′) [F.R. *Nager;* Jean Pierre *de Reynier*, Swiss otologist, born 1914] Nager acrofacial dysostosis; see under *dysostosis*.

Na·gla·zyme (na′glə-zīm) trademark for a preparation of galsulfase.

Na·gler effect (nah′glər) [Joseph *Nagler*, Austrian radiologist, 20th century] see under *effect*.

Na·gler reaction (test) (na′glər) [F.P.O. *Nagler*, Australian bacteriologist, 20th century] see under *reaction*.

nai·ad (ni′ad) [Gr. *nan* to flow] an aquatic, gill-breathing nymph (q.v.) of certain arthropods.

nail (nāl) 1. unguis. 2. a rod of metal, bone, or other material used for fixation of the ends or the fragments of fractured bones.

brittle n's fragilitas unguium.

eggshell n. a fingernail that is thin and curved upward at its distal edge.

half-and-half n. a fingernail or toenail with a distinct border between a white proximal part and a darker, pink to brown, distal part, sometimes seen in chronic renal disease.

hippocratic n. the markedly convex nail seen on a clubbed finger; see also *clubbing*. Called also *watch crystal n.*

ingrown n. see under *toenail*.

Jewett n. a nail for internal fixation of a trochanteric fracture; the nail is fastened to a plate for fixing the head and neck of the bone to the shaft.

Küntscher n. a tubular metal nail for the intramedullary fixation of fractures.

Neufeld n. a device for internal fixation of intertrochanteric fracture of the femur, the V nail section being set at an angle of about 130 degrees to the plate portion.

parrot beak n. a fingernail or toenail that curves around the end of the digit and is shaped like a parrot's beak.

pincer n. a nail, usually a toenail, that curves outward excessively distally and pinches the nailbed; called also *trumpet n.*

pitted n. a nail with surface pits, usually under 1 mm in diameter, seen most often in psoriasis, and less frequently in alopecia areata and a few other conditions.

Plummer n's onycholysis with discoloration of the nails in thyrotoxicosis.

racket n. a thumbnail, or occasionally other nail, that is much shorter than it is wide; this is usually inherited as an autosomal dominant trait. In the most common form, the distal phalanx is shortened as well.

ram's horn n. onychogryphosis.

reedy n. a fingernail or toenail marked by longitudinal furrows.

Smith-Petersen n. a flanged nail for fixing the head of the femur in fracture of the femoral neck.

spoon n. koilonychia.

Terry n's apparent leukonychia in which the white discoloration affects the entire nail except for 1–2 mm at the distal margin; it is frequently seen in cirrhosis, congestive heart failure, and certain other conditions.

trumpet n. pincer n.

watch crystal n., watch glass n. hippocratic n.

yellow n. the thick, yellow to green nail seen in the yellow nail syndrome.

nail·ing (nāl′ing) the operation of fixing or fastening of a fractured bone with a nail.

intramedullary n., marrow n., medullary n. the fixation of a fractured long bone by insertion of a steel rod into the marrow cavity of the bone.

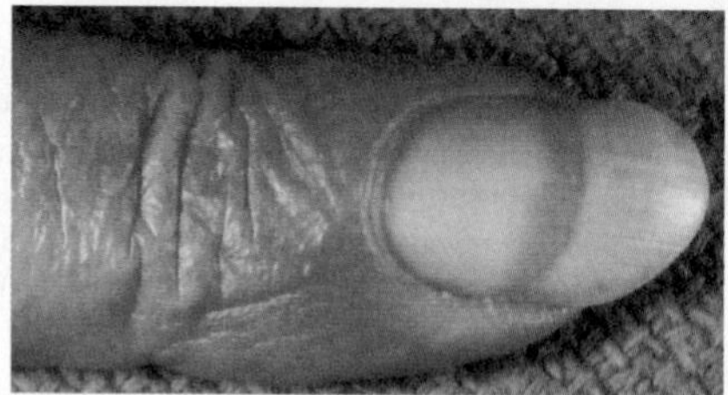

■ Terry nail.

Nai·ro·bi sheep disease (ni-ro′be) [*Nairobi*, Kenya, where it is particularly prevalent] see under *disease*.

Nai·ro·vi·rus (ni′ro-vi″rəs) [*Nairobi* sheep disease + *virus*] a genus of viruses of the family Bunyaviridae, containing at least 33 species in seven serogroups; it includes Crimean-Congo hemorrhagic fever virus and Nairobi sheep disease virus. The chief vectors are ticks of the genera *Amblyomma* and *Hyalomma*.

na·ïve (nah-ēv′) [Fr. "ingenuous, unaffected"] not previously exposed to therapy or treatment.

Na·ja (na′jə) a genus of venomous snakes of the family Elapidae found in Asia and Africa, including most of the cobras. *N. ha′je* is the Egyptian cobra; *N. mossambi′ca* is the Mozambique cobra; *N. na′ja* is the Asian cobra; *N. nigricol′lis* is the black-necked cobra; and *N. ni′vea* is the Cape cobra. See table at *snake*.

na·ja (nah′jə) [Ar.] 1. Asian cobra. 2. a homeopathic preparation made from the venom of *Naja naja*.

Na^+,K^+-ATP·ase (a-te-pe′ās) an enzyme that spans the plasma membrane and hydrolyzes ATP to maintain the gradients of sodium (Na^+) and potassium (K^+) across the cell membrane; for each ATP hydrolyzed, three sodium ions are extruded from the cell and two potassium ions are brought in. The gradients are necessary for protein biosynthesis, maintenance of osmotic equilibrium, propagation of nerve impulses, and secondary transport of some molecules (e.g., glucose) across cell membranes. See also *adenosinetriphosphatase*. Called also *Na^+-K^+*, *sodium*, or *sodium-potassium pump*. In EC nomenclature, called *Na^+/K^+-exchanging ATPase*.

Na^+/K^+-ex·chang·ing ATP·ase (eks-chānj′ing a-te-pe′ās) [EC 3.6.3.9] EC nomenclature for *Na^+,K^+-ATPase*.

Na^+/K^+-trans·port·ing ATP·ase (trans-port′ing a-te-pe′ās) Na^+,K^+-ATPase.

nal·bu·phine hy·dro·chlo·ride (nal′bu-fēn) an opioid analgesic, used in the treatment of moderate to severe pain and as an anesthesia adjunct; administered intravenously, intramuscularly, and subcutaneously.

na·led (nah′led) dimethyl phosphate, an insecticide used on plants and to control mosquitoes; accidental overexposure can cause irritation to the skin and respiratory tract, convulsions, and sometimes death.

Nal·fon (nal′fon) trademark for a preparation of fenoprofen calcium.

nal·i·dix·ic ac·id (nal″ĭ-dik′sik) [USP] a quinolone antibacterial used orally in the treatment of urinary infections caused by gram-negative organisms, especially those caused by *Proteus* species.

Nall·pen (nawl′pen) trademark for preparations of nafcillin sodium.

nal·me·fene hy·dro·chlo·ride (nal′mə-fēn″) a derivative of naltrexone that acts as an opioid antagonist, used in the treatment of opioid toxicity and overdose and of postoperative opioid depression; administered parenterally.

nal·ox·one hy·dro·chlo·ride (nal-ok′sōn) an opioid antagonist structurally related to oxymorphone, used in the diagnosis and treatment of opioid toxicity, to reverse opioid-induced respiratory depression, and as an adjunct in the treatment of hypotension associated with septic shock; administered parenterally.

nal·trex·one hy·dro·chlo·ride (nal-trek′sōn) [USP] a synthetic congener of oxymorphone, chemically related to naloxone, that acts as an opioid antagonist; administered orally or intramuscularly in the treatment of opioid or alcohol abuse.

name (nām) a word or words used to designate a unique entity and distinguish it from others.

British Approved N. (BAN) an official nonproprietary name approved by the British Pharmacopoeia Commission.

generic n. 1. in chemistry, a name applied to a class of compounds, e.g., alkane or halide. 2. nonproprietary n. 3. in biology, the name applied to a genus.

International Nonproprietary N. (INN) the nonproprietary designation recommended by the World Health Organization for any pharmaceutical preparation.

nonproprietary n. a short name coined for a drug or chemical not subject to proprietary (trademark) rights and recommended or recognized by an official body, e.g., USAN, INN, or BAN.

pharmacy equivalent n. (PEN) a shortened name for a drug or combination of drugs, used by pharmacists or practitioners when it may be impractical to use the full official term; when used for a combination of drugs, the term usually consists of the prefix *co-* plus an abbreviation for each drug in the combination.

proprietary n. a brand name or trademark under which a proprietary product is marketed. See *proprietary.*

public n. nonproprietary n.

systematic n. in chemical nomenclature, a name of a substance based on the chemical structure of a compound.

trivial n. in chemical nomenclature, a name of a substance that does not reflect its chemical structure; many trivial names are semisystematic, e.g., the *-ol* in glycerol indicates that it is an alcohol.

United States Adopted N. (USAN) a nonproprietary designation for any compound used as a drug, established by negotiation between the manufacturer of the compound and a nomenclature committee known as the USAN Council, which is sponsored jointly by the American Medical Association, the American Pharmaceutical Association, and The United States Pharmacopeial Convention. A liaison representative of the United States Food and Drug Administration sits on the USAN Council. The term is currently limited to names adopted by the Council since June, 1961. These names will appear as the monograph titles in the official compendia, USP and NF, when and if the respective drugs are admitted to either compendium.

Na•men•da (nə-men′də) trademark for a preparation of memantine.

NAMI National Alliance for the Mentally Ill.

NAN *N*-acetylneuraminic acid.

NANBH non-A, non-B hepatitis.

nan•dro•lone (nan′dro-lōn) an anabolic-androgenic steroid that differs from testosterone in lacking a methyl group attached to carbon 10 of the steroid nucleus; it has anabolic effects that are more pronounced than its androgenic effects.

n. decanoate [USP] an ester of nandrolone having a long duration of action, used in the treatment of severe growth retardation in children and as an adjunct in the treatment of chronic wasting diseases and anemia associated with renal insufficiency; administered intramuscularly.

n. phenpropionate [USP] an ester of nandrolone having a moderate duration of action, used in the treatment of metastatic breast cancer and of severe growth retardation in children; administered intramuscularly.

na•nism (na′niz-əm) [L. *nanus* dwarf] dwarfism.

mulibrey n. [*mu*scle, *li*ver, *br*ain, and *ey*es] a rare autosomal recessive disorder due to mutation in the *TRIM37*gene (locus: 17q22-q23), which encodes a peroxisomal protein; marked by dwarfism and constrictive pericarditis. Affected infants have a triangular face often with hypocephaloid skull, muscular hypotonia, squeaky voice, and yellowish dots and pigment dispersion in the ocular fundus.

pituitary n. see under *dwarfism.*

Nan•niz•zia (nə-niz′e-ə) a genus of fungi, classified in the family Gymnoascaceae but later found to be the same as *Arthroderma.*

nann(o)- see *nan(o)-.*

Nan•no•mo•nas (nan″o-mo′nəs) [*nanno-* + Gr. *monas* unit] in some systems of classification, a salivarian subgenus of the genus *Trypanosoma,* including *T. congolense, T. dimorphon,* and *T. simiae.*

nan(o)- [Gr. *nanos* dwarf] a combining form designating small size; also used in naming units of measurement (symbol n) to indicate one billionth (10^{-9}) of the unit designated by the root with which it is combined.

nano•ce•pha•lia (nan″o-sə-fa′le-ə) microcephaly.

nano•ceph•a•ly (nan″o-sef′ə-le) microcephaly. **nanoceph′alous** *adj*

nano•cor•mia (nan″o-kor′me-ə) [*nano-* + Gr. *kormos* trunk + *-ia*] a developmental anomaly characterized by abnormal smallness of the body, or trunk.

nano•cu•rie (nCi) (nan″o-ku′re) a unit of radioactivity, being one billionth (10^{-9}) of a curie.

nano•gram (ng) (nan′o-gram) one billionth (10^{-9}) of a gram.

nan•oid (nan′oid) [*nano-* + *-oid*] 1. dwarfish. 2. dwarfed.

nano•li•ter (nL) (nan′o-le″tər) a unit of capacity equal to one billionth (10^{-9}) of a liter.

nano•ma•te•ri•al (nan″o-mə-te′re-əl) a tiny amount of a substance that has at least one dimension that is 1.0 to 100.0 nm across; cf. *nanoparticle.*

nano•med•i•cine (nan″o-med′ĭ-sin) molecular medicine at the nanometer level.

nano•me•lia (nan″o-me′le-ə) micromelia.

nan•om•e•lus (nan-om′ə-ləs) micromelus.

nano•me•ter (nm) (nan′o-me″tər) one billionth (10^{-9}) of a meter.

nano•par•ti•cle (nan″o-pahr′tĭ-kəl) a tiny particle of a biological unit, 50 nm or less in diameter; spherical or capsule-shaped ones can be examined to see if they interact as desired with drugs or other substances. Cf. *nanomaterial.*

nan•oph•thal•mia (nan″of-thal′me-ə) nanophthalmos.

nan•oph•thal•mos (nan″of-thal′məs) [*nan-* + Gr. *ophthalmos* eye] microphthalmos in an eye that is otherwise normal; a nanophthalmic eye is very hyperopic and prone to angle-closure glaucoma.

nano•phy•e•ti•a•sis (nan″o-fi″ə-ti′ə-sis) infection by the fluke *Nanophyetus salmincola* after ingestion of contaminated fish. Human infection is usually mild, with bloating, cramping, and diarrhea. In dogs it causes salmon poisoning (q.v.), with rickettsiosis and a high fever that can be fatal.

Nano•phy•e•tus (nan″o-fi′ə-təs) a genus of trematodes of the family Troglotrematidae; called also *Troglotrema. N. salmin′cola* is found in the kidney and under the skin of fish, especially salmon and trout, and serves as a vector of *Neorickettsia helminthoeca,* the etiologic agent of salmon poisoning (q.v.). It can then be transmitted to any animal that eats infected raw fish.

nano•plank•ton (na″no-plank′ton) plankton of extremely minute size.

nan•o•scale (nan′o-skāl) a tiny (submicroscopic) scale; see *nanotechnology.*

nano•sec•ond (ns) (nan′o-sek″ond) one billionth (10^{-9}) of a second.

nano•so•ma (nan″o-so′mə) dwarfism.

nano•so•mia (nan″o-so′me-ə) dwarfism.

nano•tech•nol•o•gy (nan″o-tek-nol′ə-je) technology at the level of atoms, molecules, and molecular fragments, including manipulating them and creating new structures.

nano•unit (nU) (nan′o-u″nit) one billionth (10^{-9}) of a standard unit.

nan•ous (nan′əs) 1. dwarfish. 2. dwarfed.

na•nu•ka•ya•mi (nah″noo-kah-yah′me) a type of leptospirosis seen in Japan; called also *nanukayami fever.*

na•nus (nă′nəs) [L., from Gr. *nanos*] a dwarf.

NAP [*n*asion, point *A*, *p*ogonion] see *angle of convexity.*

nape (nāp) the back of the neck (nucha [TA]).

na•pex (na′peks) the region of the scalp just inferior to the occipital protuberance.

naph•az•o•line hy•dro•chlo•ride (naf-az′o-lēn) [USP] an adrenergic used as a vasoconstrictor, applied topically to the nasal or ocular mucous membranes.

naph•tha (naf′thə) [L., from Arabic] any of various volatile, often flammable, liquid hydrocarbon mixtures from petroleum, natural gas, or coal tar, sometimes specifically petroleum benzoin or ligroin; specific fractions are used as solvents, dry cleaning fluids, in synthesis, in varnishes and paints, and as fuels.

naph•tha•lene (naf′thə-lēn) a silvery, crystalline hydrocarbon from coal tar oil, used as an intermediate, moth repellent, fungicide, and preservative and formerly used as an antiseptic in diarrhea of typhoid fever; it is toxic by ingestion, inhalation, and skin absorption.

chlorinated n. any of a group of compounds resulting from chlorination of naphthalene; their uses include wood preservatives, varnishes, and machine lubricating oils. Excessive exposure can cause halogen acne in humans, and contamination of cattle feed during harvesting or processing can cause hyperkeratosis in the animals. Called also *chloronaphthalene.*

naph•thol (naf′thol) a crystalline, antiseptic substance from coal tar occurring in two forms, α- or 1-naphthol and β- or 2-naphthol, used in dyes, organic synthesis, perfumes, insecticides, and formerly in pharmaceutical compounds; it is toxic by ingestion and skin absorption. See also under *poisoning.*

naph•tho•late (naf′tho-lāt″) a naphthol compound in which a base takes the place of hydrogen in the hydroxyl.

naph•thol•ism (naf′thol-iz-əm) naphthol poisoning.

naph•thyl (naf′thəl) the radical, $C_{10}H_7$.

naph•thyl•amine (naf-thil′ə-mēn) a nitrogen-substituted arylamine, existing as two different isomers, *α-* or *1-naphthylamine* and *β-* or *2-naphthylamine.* Both isomers are used in dyes and are carcinogenic.

na•pi•form (na′pĭ-form) [L. *napus* turnip + *forma* shape] having the shape or form of a turnip.

NAPNES National Association for Practical Nurse Education and Services.

nap•ra•path (nap′rə-path) a practitioner of naprapathy.

na•prap•a•thy (nə-prap′ə-the) [Czech *napravit* to correct + *-pathy*] a system of therapy employing manipulation of connective tissue (ligaments, muscles, and joints) and dietary measures; said to facilitate the recuperative and regenerative processes of the body. **naprapath′ic** *adj*

Nap•re•lan (nap′rə-lan) trademark for a preparation of naproxen sodium.

Na•pro•syn (nap′rə-sin) trademark for preparations of naproxen.

na•prox•en (nə-prok′sən) [USP] a nonsteroidal antiinflammatory drug that is a propionic acid derivative, used in the treatment of pain, inflammation, osteoarthritis, rheumatoid arthritis, gout, calcium pyrophosphate deposition disease, fever, and dysmenorrhea and in the prophylaxis and suppression of vascular headache; administered orally or rectally.
  n. sodium [USP] the sodium salt of naproxen, having the same actions and uses as the base.

nap•sy•late (nap′sə-lāt) USAN contraction for 2-naphthalenesulfonate.

NAPT National Association for Poetry Therapy.

Na•qua (na′kwə) trademark for a preparation of trichlormethiazide.

nar•a•sin (nar′ə-sin) [USP] a veterinary coccidiostat and growth stimulant.

nar•a•trip•tan hy•dro•chlo•ride (nar″ə-trip′tan) [USP] a selective serotonin receptor agonist used in the acute treatment of migraine; administered orally.

Nar•can (nahr′kan) trademark for a preparation of naloxone hydrochloride.

nar•cis•sine (nahr-sis′ēn) lycorine.

nar•cis•sism (nahr′sĭ-siz-əm) [from *Narcissus,* a character in Greek mythology who fell in love with his own image reflected in water] dominant interest in oneself; self-love; the state in which the ego is invested in oneself, rather than in another person. **narcissis′tic** *adj*
  primary n. narcissism occurring in the early infantile phase of object relationship development, when the child has not differentiated him or herself from the outside world and regards all sources of pleasure as originating from within.
  secondary n. narcissism in which the libido, once attached to external love objects, is redirected back to the self.

Nar•cis•sus (nahr-sis′əs) a genus of flowering plants of the family Amaryllidaceae, whose bulbs contain the toxin lycorine. *N. pseudonarcis′sus* L. is the daffodil. *N. tazet′ta* contains the alkaloid tazettine.

nar•cis•sus (nahr-sis′əs) any plant of the genus *Narcissus.*

narc(o)- [Gr. *narkē* numbness] a combining form denoting relationship to stupor, to a stuporous state, or to narcosis.

nar•co•anal•y•sis (nahr″ko-ə-nal′ĭ-sis) a controversial method of psychotherapy that uses administration of medications to release suppressed or repressed thoughts or affect-laden and unacceptable ideas. **narcoanalyt′ic** *adj*

nar•co•hyp•no•sis (nahr″ko-hip-no′sis) hypnotic suggestions made while the patient is under the influence of a narcotic drug.

nar•co•lep•sy (nahr′ko-lep″se) [*narco-* + Gr. *lepsis* a taking hold, a seizure] [DSM-IV] recurrent, uncontrollable, brief episodes of sleep, often associated with hypnagogic or hypnopompic hallucinations, cataplexy, and sleep paralysis. Called also *Gélineau syndrome* and *paroxysmal sleep.*

nar•co•lep•tic (nahr″ko-lep′tik) 1. pertaining to, characterized by, or producing narcolepsy. 2. an agent that produces narcolepsy. 3. a person with narcolepsy.

nar•co•ma (nahr-ko′mə) a stuporous state produced by narcotics.

nar•cose (nahr′kōs) stuporous.

nar•co•sine (nahr′ko-sēn) noscapine.

nar•co•sis (nahr-ko′sis) [Gr. *narkōsis* a benumbing] a nonspecific and reversible depression of function of the central nervous system marked by stupor or insensibility, produced by opioid drugs and certain other substances.
  basal n. narcosis marked by complete unconsciousness, amnesia, and analgesia.
  carbon dioxide n. respiratory acidosis.
  nitrogen n. a state resembling drunkenness, with euphoria and disorientation, seen in divers below about 30 meters (100 feet) who are breathing compressed air, because of the high nitrogen content of air; some of the nitrogen enters the bloodstream and acts as a narcotic. Sometimes popularly called *rapture of the deep.*

nar•co•stim•u•lant (nahr″ko-stim′u-lənt) having both narcotic and stimulant properties.

nar•cot•ic (nahr-kot′ik) [Gr. *narkōtikos* benumbing, deadening] 1. pertaining to or producing narcosis. 2. an agent that produces insensibility or stupor, applied especially to the opioids, i.e., to any natural or synthetic drug that has actions like those of morphine.

nar•cot•i•co•ac•rid (nahr-kot″ĭ-ko-ak′rid) both narcotic and acrid.

nar•co•tine (nahr′ko-tēn) noscapine.

nar•co•tize (nahr′ko-tīz) to put under the influence of a narcotic.

nar•cous (nar′kəs) stuporous.

Nar•dil (nahr′dil) trademark for a preparation of phenelzine sulfate.

na•res (na′rēz) (sing. *na′ris*) [L.] [TA] the external orifices of the nose; called also *nostrils.*
  anterior n., external n. nares.
  posterior n. the paired choanae; see *choana* (def. 2).

na•ris (na′ris) [L.] singular of *nares.*

Na•ro•pin (nă′ro-pin) trademark for a preparation of ropivacaine hydrochloride.

Nar•the•ci•um (nahr-the′se-əm) a genus of herbs of the family Liliaceae, which have yellow flowers. *N. ossifra′gum* is the bog asphodel, a species that can cause yellows, a form of hepatogenous photosensitization, in ruminants that eat it.

na•sal (na′zəl) [L. *nasalis*] 1. pertaining to the nose; called also *rhinal.* 2. a speech sound produced by having air flow through the nose, such as *n, ng,* or *m.*

Na•sa•cort AQ (na′zə-kort) trademark for a preparation of triamcinolone acetonide.

Na•sal•ide (na′zəl-īd″) trademark for a preparation of flunisolide.

na•sa•lis (na-za′lis) [L., from *nasus* nose] nasal.

Na•sa•rel (na′zə-rel) trademark for a preparation of flunisolide.

nas•cent (nas′ənt, na′sənt) [L. *nascens*] 1. just born; just coming into existence. 2. just liberated from a chemical combination, and hence more reactive because uncombined.

Nas•co•bal (nas′ko-bal) trademark for a preparation of cyanocobalamin.

NASH nonalcoholic steatohepatitis.

na•sio•in•i•ac (na″ze-o-in′e-ak) pertaining to the nasion and the inion.

na•si•on (na′ze-on) [L. *nasus* nose] [TA] a cephalometric landmark located where the internasal and nasofrontal sutures meet; it corresponds roughly to the depression at the root of the nose just inferior to the level of the eyebrows.

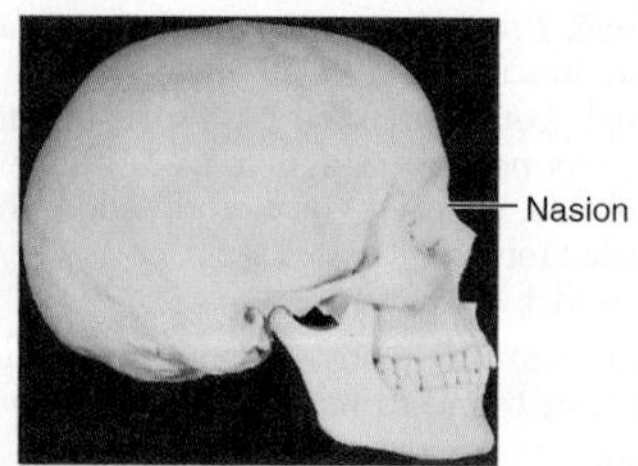

Nas•myth membrane (nas′mith) [Alexander *Nasmyth,* Scottish dental surgeon in London, died 1847] primary (enamel) cuticle.

NAS–NRC National Academy of Sciences–National Research Council.

nas(o)- [L. *nasus* nose] a combining form denoting relationship to the nose.

na•so•an•tral (na″zo-an′trəl) pertaining to the nose and the maxillary antrum (sinus).

na•so•an•tri•tis (na″zo-an-tri′tis) rhinoantritis.

na•so•an•tros•to•my (na″zo-an-tros′tə-me) surgical formation of a nasoantral window for drainage of an obstructed maxillary sinus.

na•so•bron•chi•al (na″zo-brong′ke-əl) pertaining to the nasal cavities and the bronchi.

na•so•cil•i•ary (na″zo-sil′e-ar″e) pertaining to or affecting the eyes, brow, and root of the nose, as the nasociliary nerve.

na•so•eth•moi•dal (na″zo-eth-moi′dəl) ethmonasal.

na•so•fron•tal (na″zo-fron′təl) pertaining to the nose or other nasal structures and the forehead or the frontal bone; called also *frontonasal.*

na•so•gas•tric (na″zo-gas′trik) pertaining to the nose and stomach, as in (nasogastric) aspiration of the stomach's contents.

na•so•la•bi•al (na″zo-la′be-əl) [*naso-* + *labial*] pertaining to the nose and lip.

na·so·lac·ri·mal (na″zo-lak′rĭ-məl) pertaining to the nose and lacrimal apparatus.

na·so·ma·nom·e·ter (na″zo-mə-nom′ə-tər) rhinomanometer.

Na·so·nex (na′zo-neks) trademark for a preparation of mometasone furoate.

na·so-oral (na″zo-or′əl) oronasal.

na·so·pal·a·tine (na″zo-pal′ə-tīn) [*naso-* + *palatine*] pertaining to the nose and palate.

na·so·pha·ryn·ge·al (na″zo-fə-rin′je-əl) 1. pertaining to the nose and the pharynx. 2. pertaining to the nasopharynx.

na·so·phar·yn·gi·tis (na″zo-far″in-ji′tis) inflammation of the nasopharynx. Called also *epipharyngitis* and *rhinopharyngitis.*

na·so·pha·ryn·go·la·ryn·go·scope (na″zo-fə-ring″go-lə-ring′go-skōp) a flexible fiberscope for examining the nasopharynx and larynx.

na·so·pha·ryn·go·scope (na″zo-fə-ring′go-skōp) a lighted, telescopic endoscope for use in examination of the nasopharynx and the pharyngeal end of the auditory tube.

na·so·phar·ynx (na″zo-far′inks) [*naso-* + *pharynx*] pars nasalis pharyngis.

na·so·ros·tral (na″zo-ros′trəl) pertaining to the nose and the rostrum of the sphenoid bone.

na·so·scope (na′zo-skōp) [*naso-* + *-scope*] rhinoscope.

na·so·sep·tal (na″zo-sep′təl) pertaining to the nasal septum.

na·so·sep·ti·tis (na″zo-sep-ti′tis) inflammation of the nasal septum.

na·so·si·nus·itis (na″zo-si″nə-si′tis) rhinosinusitis.

na·so·spi·na·le (na″zo-spi-na′le) the point at which a horizontal line tangential to the inferior margins of the nasal aperture is intersected by the median plane.

na·so·tra·che·al (na″zo-tra′ke-əl) pertaining to the nose and the trachea.

na·so·tur·bi·nal (na″zo-tur′bĭ-nəl) pertaining to the nose and a turbinate bone.

na·sus (na′səs) [L.] [TA] nose: the specialized structure of the face that serves as the organ of the sense of smell and as part of the respiratory system. See also *n. externus* and *cavitas nasi.*

n. exter′nus the external nose: the part of the nose that protrudes on the face; made up of an osteocartilaginous framework, covered externally by muscles and skin and lined internally by mucous membrane; it has two apertures that open into the nasal cavity and is separated into two halves by the nasal septum.

NAT nucleic acid test.

na·tal[1] (na′təl) [L. *nates* buttocks] gluteal.

na·tal[2] (na′təl) [L. *natus* birth] pertaining to birth.

na·tal·i·ty (na-tal′ĭ-te) [L. *natalis* pertaining to birth] birth rate.

nat·al·iz·u·mab (nat″ə-liz′u-mab) a recombinant humanized IgG4κ monoclonal antibody, produced in murine myeloma cells, that binds to α4-integrin, which is expressed on the surface of all leukocytes except neutrophils, preventing transmigration of leukocytes into inflamed parenchymal tissue. It is used in the treatment of patients with relapsing forms of multiple sclerosis, to delay the accumulation of physical disability and reduce the frequency of clinical exacerbations; administered intravenously.

nat·a·my·cin (nat″ə-mi′sin) a polyene antibiotic used in topical treatment of fungal keratitis, blepharitis, and conjunctivitis.

na·teg·li·nide (nə-teg′lĭ-nīd) an antidiabetic agent that lowers blood glucose concentrations by stimulating the release of insulin from the beta cells of the islets of Langerhans; administered orally in the treatment of type 2 diabetes, either alone or in combination with metformin.

na·tes (na′tēz) (sing., *na′tis*) [L.] [TA] buttocks: the prominences formed by the gluteal muscles on the lower part of the back; called also *breech* and *clunes* [TA alternative].

na·ti·mor·tal·i·ty (na″tĭ-mor-tal′ĭ-te) fetal death rate.

Na·tion·al For·mu·lary (NF) a book of standards for certain pharmaceuticals and preparations that are not included in the USP *(United States Pharmacopeia).* It is recognized as a book of official standards by the Pure Food and Drugs Act of 1906.

na·tis (na′tis) [L. "rump"] singular of *nates.*

na·tive (na′tiv) [L. *nativus*] normal to a location; unaltered from its natural state.

Nat·o·lone (nat′o-lōn) trademark for a preparation of pregnenolone.

Na·tre·cor (na′trə-kor) trademark for a preparation of nesiritide.

na·tre·mia (nə-tre′me-ə) hypernatremia.

na·tri·ure·sis (na″tre-u-re′sis) [L. *natrium* sodium + *-uresis*] the excretion of sodium in the urine, particularly in excessive amounts; see also *salt-losing syndrome*, under *syndrome.*

pressure n. increased urinary excretion of sodium along with water when there is an increase of arterial pressure, a compensatory mechanism to maintain blood pressure within the normal range. See also *pressure diuresis*, under *diuresis.*

na·tri·uret·ic (na″tre-u-ret′ik) 1. pertaining to, characterized by, or promoting natriuresis. 2. an agent that promotes natriuresis.

nat·ru·re·sis (nat″roo-re′sis) natriuresis. **natruret′ic** *adj*

nat·u·ral (nach′ə-rəl) [L. *naturalis*, from *natura* nature] neither artificial nor pathologic.

Nat·ure·tin (nat″u-re′tin) trademark for a preparation of bendroflumethiazide.

na·turo·path (na′chər-o-path″) a practitioner of naturopathy.

na·tur·op·a·thy (na″chər-op′ə-the) a drugless system of health care, making use of a wide variety of therapies, such as hydrotherapy, heat, massage, and herbal medicine, whose purpose is to treat the whole person to stimulate and support the person's own innate healing capacity. Naturopathic philosophy is summarized in six principles: the healing power of nature, first do no harm, identify and treat the cause, treat the whole person, prevention, and the physician as teacher. **naturopath′ic** *adj*

nau·sea (naw′ze-ə) [L., from Gr. *nausia* seasickness] a sensation of wanting to vomit, vaguely referred to the epigastrium and abdomen, and often culminating in vomiting.

n. gravida′rum morning sickness.

nau·se·ant (naw′ze-ənt) 1. inducing nausea. 2. an agent that causes nausea.

nau·se·ate (naw′ze-āt) to affect with nausea.

nau·seous (naw′shəs) 1. pertaining to nausea. 2. producing nausea.

Nav·ane (nav′ān) trademark for preparations of thiothixene.

na·vel (na′vəl) umbilicus.

blue n. Cullen sign.

enamel n. either of two depressions between the lateral dental lamina and the developing tooth germ, one pointing distally *(distal enamel n.)* and the other mesially *(mesial enamel n.).*

Na·vel·bine (na-vel′bēn) trademark for a preparation of vinorelbine tartrate.

na·vi·cu·la (nə-vĭ′ku-lə) [L. "boat"] frenulum labiorum pudendi.

na·vic·u·lar (nə-vik′u-lər) scaphoid.

Nax·os disease (nahk′sōs) [*Naxos*, Greek island in the Aegean Sea where the condition was first observed] see under *disease.*

Nb niobium.

NBT nitroblue tetrazolium; see under *test.*

NBTE nonbacterial thrombotic endocarditis.

NCF neutrophil chemotactic factor.

NCHS National Center for Health Statistics.

NCI National Cancer Institute.

nCi nanocurie.

NCMH National Committee for Mental Hygiene.

NCN National Council of Nurses.

NCRP National Committee on Radiation Protection and Measurements.

NCV nerve conduction velocity.

ND Doctor of Naturopathy.

Nd neodymium.

NDA National Dental Association.

nDNA nuclear DNA; see under *DNA.*

NDV Newcastle disease virus.

Nd:YAG neodymium:yttrium-aluminum-garnet; see under *laser.*

Ne neon.

near-sight (nēr′sīt) myopia. **near′sighted** *adj*

near-sight·ed·ness (nēr′sīt″əd-nis) myopia.

ne·ar·thro·sis (ne″ahr-thro′sis) [*ne-* + *arthrosis* (def. 1)] 1. a false joint; pseudarthrosis. 2. an artificial joint inserted in total joint replacement.

Neb·cin (neb′sin) trademark for preparations of tobramycin sulfate.

ne·ben·kern (na-ben′kərn) [Ger. *neben* near, beside + *kern* kernel, nucleus] a large mitochondrial mass around the axial filament in the flagellum of the spermatozoon, formed by coalescence of smaller mitochondria during spermatogenesis.

ne•biv•o•lol (nĕ-biv′ə-lol) a β-adrenergic blocking agent used as an antihypertensive; administered orally.

neb•ra•my•cin (neb″rə-mi′sin) an aminoglycoside antibacterial complex produced by *Streptomyces tenebrarius,* consisting of eight components; factor 6 (tobramycin) is used clinically as an antibiotic and factor 2 (apramycin) is used as an antibiotic in veterinary medicine.

neb•u•la (neb′u-lə) gen. and pl. *ne′bulae* [L. "mist"] 1. a slight corneal opacity or scar that can be seen only by oblique illumination; it seldom interferes with vision. 2. a preparation, particularly an oily preparation, for use in a nebulizer.

neb•u•lar•ine (neb-u-lar′in) an antibiotic substance isolated from the juice of the fungus *Clitocybe nebularis,* which has tuberculostatic and antimitotic activity, and in high dilutions preferentially inhibits growth of some cancer cells.

neb•u•lin (neb′u-lin) a giant (600–800kD) actin-binding protein occurring in the sarcomere; it is believed to maintain the lattice of thin filaments and may regulate their length; mutations in the gene encoding nebulin result in nemaline myopathy.

neb•u•li•za•tion (neb″u-lĭ-za′shən) [L. *nebula* mist] 1. conversion into an aerosol or spray. 2. treatment by an aerosol. Called also *atomization.*

neb•u•liz•er (neb′u-li″zər) a device for creating and throwing an aerosol spray. Called also *atomizer.*

Neb•u•Pent (neb′u-pent) trademark for preparations of pentamidine isethionate.

Ne•ca•tor (ne-ka′tor) [L. "murderer"] a genus of nematode parasites of the family Ancylostomatidae.

N. america′nus the American or New World hookworm, which can cause hookworm disease in humans and occasionally pigs. It resembles *Ancylostoma duodenale* but is shorter and more slender. Its buccal cavity contains four plates, four pharyngeal lancets, and a dorsal conic tooth. Called also *Ancylostoma americanum* and *Uncinaria americana.*

ne•ca•to•ri•a•sis (ne-ka″to-ri′ə-sis) hookworm disease in humans or pigs caused by infection with species of *Necator.*

ne•ces•si•ty (nə-ses′ĭ-te) something necessary or indispensable.

pharmaceutic n., pharmaceutical n. a substance having slight or no value therapeutically, but used in the preparation of various pharmaceuticals, including preservatives, solvents, ointment bases, and flavoring, coloring, diluting, emulsifying, and suspending agents; called also *pharmaceutic* or *pharmaceutical aid.*

neck (nek) 1. cervix (def. 1). 2. a constricted part; see also *collum.*

anatomical n. of humerus collum anatomicum humeri.

n. of ankle bone collum tali.

bladder n. cervix vesicae.

bull n. marked edema of the anterior neck and submandibular region associated with massive cervical lymphadenopathy.

n. of condyloid process of mandible collum mandibulae.

dental n. cervix dentis.

n. of dorsal horn of spinal cord cervix cornus posterioris medullae spinalis.

false n. of humerus collum chirurgicum humeri.

femoral n., n. of femur collum femoris.

n. of fibula collum fibulae.

n. of gallbladder collum vesicae biliaris.

n. of gastric gland a constricted area of a gastric gland just interior to the isthmus.

n. of glans penis collum glandis penis.

n. of humerus collum anatomicum humeri.

lateral n. of vertebra pediculus arcus vertebrae.

Madelung n. multiple symmetric lipomatosis.

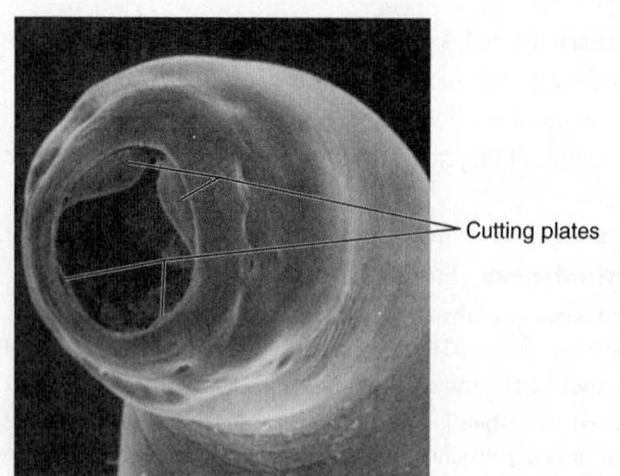

■ *Necator americanus,* showing dorsal and ventral pairs of cutting plates in the head.

n. of malleus collum mallei.

n. of mandible collum mandibulae.

n. of pancreas collum pancreatis.

n. of posterior horn of spinal cord cervix cornus posterioris medullae spinalis.

n. of radius collum radii.

n. of rib collum costae.

n. of scapula collum scapulae.

n. of spermatozoon a short portion of the tail of a spermatozoon, just posterior to the head, anterior to the middle piece. Called also *connecting piece.* See illustration at *spermatozoon.*

surgical n. of humerus collum chirurgicum humeri.

n. of talus collum tali.

n. of tooth cervix dentis.

true n. of humerus collum anatomicum humeri.

turkey gobbler n. submental vertical skin folds due to aging.

n. of urinary bladder cervix vesicae.

uterine n., n. of uterus cervix uteri.

n. of vertebra, n. of vertebral arch pediculus arcus vertebrae.

webbed n. pterygium colli.

wry n. torticollis.

neck•lace (nek′ləs) a band encircling the neck.

Casal n. an area of erythema and pigmentation around the neck in pellagra; called also *Casal collar.*

Ne•con (ne′kon) trademark for oral contraceptive therapeutic regimens containing norethindrone as the progestational agent and either ethinyl estradiol or mestranol as the estrogen component.

nec•rec•to•my (nek-rek′tə-me) [*necro-* + *-ectomy*] excision of necrotic tissue.

nec•ren•ceph•a•lus (nek″ren-sef′ə-ləs) encephalomalacia.

necr(o)- [Gr. *nekros* dead] a combining form denoting relationship to death or to a dead body, cells, or tissue.

nec•ro•bac•il•lo•sis (nek″ro-bas″ĭ-lo′sis) any of various infections with *Fusobacterium necrophorum,* such as foot rot and calf diphtheria in cattle, gangrenous dermatitis in horses, and Schmorl disease in hogs, cattle, and rabbits. Called also *bacillary necrosis.*

interdigital n. foot rot of cattle.

nec•ro•bi•o•sis (nek″ro-bi-o′sis) [*necro-* + *biosis*] swelling, basophilia, and distortion of collagen bundles in the dermis, sometimes with obliteration of normal structure, but without actual necrosis, such as in granuloma annulare and necrobiosis lipoidica. Cf. *gangrene* and *necrosis.* **necrobiot′ic** *adj*

equine nodular n. crops of firm cutaneous nodules on the sides of the neck and trunk of a horse, filled with degenerated collagen and eosinophils. Called also *collagenolytic granuloma.*

n. lipoi′dica a degenerative disease of dermal connective tissue, characterized by erythematous papules or nodules in the lower leg and sometimes elsewhere, forming shiny yellow to red plaques that are covered with telangiectatic vessels and have a depressed center. More than half of affected patients have diabetes mellitus, although the condition appears the same in both diabetic and nondiabetic patients. See also *diabetic dermopathy,* under *dermopathy.*

n. lipoi′dica diabetico′rum necrobiosis lipoidica in diabetics.

nec•ro•cy•to•sis (nek″ro-si-to′sis) [*necro-* + *cyt-* + *-osis*] death and decay of cells.

nec•ro•gen•ic (nek″ro-jen′ik) [*necro-* + *-genic*] productive of necrosis or death.

ne•crog•e•nous (nə-kroj′ə-nəs) originating or arising from dead matter.

nec•ro•in•flam•ma•tion (nek″ro-in″flə-ma′shən) inflammation accompanied by death of the affected tissue; called also *necrotic* or *necrotizing inflammation.*

ne•crol•o•gist (nə-krol′ə-jist) a specialist in necrology.

ne•crol•o•gy (nə-krol′ə-je) [*necro-* + *-logy*] the statistics or records of deaths. **necrolog′ic** *adj*

ne•crol•y•sis (nə-krol′ĭ-sis) [*necro-* + *-lysis*] separation or exfoliation of tissue due to necrosis.

toxic epidermal n. an exfoliative skin disease seen primarily in adults as a severe reaction to a drug, although it may rarely be caused by infection, neoplastic disease, or chemical exposure. There is full-thickness epidermal necrosis that results in subepidermal separation, bulla formation, and inflammatory changes in the dermis; the widespread loss of epidermis leaves raw areas where the skin surface looks scalded. Called also *Lyell syndrome* and *nonstaphylococcal scalded skin syndrome.* Cf. *staphylococcal scalded skin syndrome.*

nec•ro•ma•nia (nek″ro-ma′ne-ə) [*necro-* + *-mania*] pathological preoccupation with dead bodies.

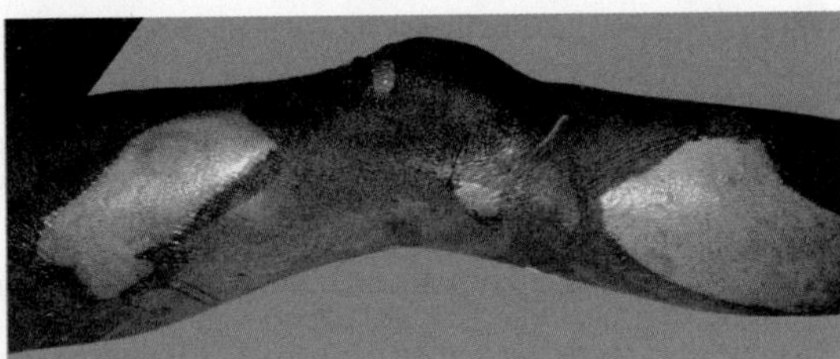

■ Toxic epidermal necrolysis.

nec•ro•mi•me•sis (nek″ro-mi-me′sis) [*necro-* + *mimesis*] a delusion in which individuals act as if dead because they believe themselves to be so.

nec•ro•nec•to•my (nek″ro-nek′tə-me) [*necro-* + *-ectomy*] necrectomy.

ne•croph•a•gous (nə-krof′ə-gəs) [*necro-* + *phag-* + *-ous*] devouring or subsisting on dead bodies.

nec•ro•phil•ia (nek″ro-fil′e-ə) [*necro-* + *-philia*] fascination or obsession with death, usually specifically sexual attraction to or sexual contact with dead bodies. Called also *necrophilism*.

nec•ro•phil•ic (nek″ro-fil′ik) 1. pertaining to or characterized by necrophilia. 2. showing preference for dead tissue, as necrophilic bacteria.

ne•croph•i•lism (nə-krof′ĭ-liz-əm) necrophilia.

ne•croph•i•lous (nə-krof′ĭ-ləs) necrophilic.

ne•croph•i•ly (nə-krof′ĭ-le) necrophilia.

nec•ro•pho•bia (nek″ro-fo′be-ə) [*necro-* + *-phobia*] irrational fear of death or of dead bodies.

nec•rop•sy (nek′rop-se) [Gr. *nekros* dead + *opsis* view] examination of a body after death; see *autopsy*.

nec•ro•sa•dism (nec″ro-sa′diz-əm) [*necro-* + *sadism*] mutilation of a corpse for the purpose of exciting or gratifying sexual feelings.

nec•rose (nek′rōs) to become necrotic or to undergo necrosis.

nec•ro•ses (nə-kro′sēz) [Gr.] plural of *necrosis*.

ne•cro•sis (nə-kro′sis) pl. *necro′ses* [Gr. *nekrōsis* deadness] the sum of the morphological changes indicative of cell death and caused by the progressive degradative action of enzymes; it may affect groups of cells or part of a structure or an organ. **necrot′ic** *adj*

acute pancreatic n. acute necrotizing pancreatitis.

acute retinal n. (ARN) a syndrome of necrotizing retinitis with uveitis, retinal periarteritis, vasculitis, and hyalitis, caused by herpesvirus infection. It is characterized by retinal vascular narrowing and obstruction, exudates from the peripheral retina, patches of vitreous opacification, severe loss of vision, and often retinal detachment. Called also *acute retinal necrosis syndrome* and *ARN syndrome*.

acute tubular n. acute renal failure with mild to severe damage or necrosis of tubule cells, usually secondary to either nephrotoxicity, ischemia after major surgery, trauma (crush syndrome), severe hypovolemia, sepsis, or burns.

arteriolar n. arteriolonecrosis.

aseptic n. increasing sclerosis and cystic changes in the head of the femur which sometimes follow traumatic dislocation of the hip. A similar condition sometimes develops in the head of the humerus after shoulder dislocation.

avascular n. coagulation n.

avascular n. of bone osteonecrosis.

bacillary n. necrobacillosis.

ballooning n. see under *degeneration*.

bridging n. septa of confluent necrosis bridging adjacent central veins and portal triads of hepatic lobules, a characteristic of subacute hepatic necrosis.

caseation n., caseous n. caseation (def. 2).

central n. necrosis of the central portion of a cell, a bone, or a lobule of the liver.

cerebrocortical n. polioencephalomalacia.

cheesy n. caseation (def. 2).

coagulation n., coagulative n. necrosis in which tissue becomes a dry, opaque, eosinophilic mass containing the outlines of anucleated cells, resulting from the denaturation of proteins following hypoxic injury, such as that caused by ischemia in infarction. Called also *avascular n.* and *ischemic n.*

colliquative n. liquefactive n.

contraction band n. a cardiac lesion seen in patients with neurologically induced cardiographic changes, in myocardial biopsy specimens, and in cocaine or epinephrine toxicity, characterized by hypercontracted myofibrils with contraction bands and mitochondrial damage; it is caused by calcium ion influx into dying cells, which results in the arrest of cells in the contracted state, following severe ischemia and subsequent reperfusion.

cystic medial n. changes in the medial layer of the aorta, consisting of degeneration and necrosis of elastic and muscle fibers, mucoid infiltration, and cyst formation, often resulting in dissecting aneurysm; called also *Erdheim disease* and *medionecrosis of aorta*.

dietary hepatic n. hepatosis dietetica.

epiphyseal ischemic n. degeneration and eventual replacement of the osseous nucleus of an epiphysis, which collapses under pressure and causes distortion of the surrounding healthy tissue; attributed to interference with the blood supply of the epiphysis. It may affect the femur, tibia, tarsal navicular head, humerus, etc. Called also *osteochondrosis*.

Erdheim cystic medial n. changes in the medial layer of the aorta, consisting of degeneration and necrosis of elastic and muscle fibers, mucoid infiltration, and cyst formation, often resulting in dissecting aneurysm; called also *medionecrosis of aorta*.

exanthematous n. an acute necrotizing process involving the gingivae, jaw bones, and contiguous soft tissues, which primarily affects children; it resembles gangrenous stomatitis, except that there is slight odor, a tendency to be self-limited, a low mortality rate, and a normal leukocyte count.

fat n. a condition in which the neutral fats in the cells of adipose tissue are split by enzymatic action into fatty acids and glycerol, producing minute, chalky white areas where the released fatty acids react with calcium, magnesium, and sodium ions to form soaps; it usually affects the pancreas and peripancreatic fat in acute hemorrhagic pancreatitis. Called also *steatonecrosis*.

fibrinoid n. deposition of fibrin and other plasma proteins in the walls of afferent renal arterioles in malignant hypertension, often accompanied by an inflammatory infiltrate within the walls and thrombosis of the vessel lumen. Called also *necrotizing arteriolitis*.

focal n. the presence of small foci of necrosis, such as in bone, the lung, or the liver in the course of an infection.

gangrenous n. cell death caused by a combination of ischemia and superimposed bacterial infection, combining the features of coagulation and liquefactive necrosis.

gangrenous pulp n. necrosis of the pulp tissue due to ischemia with superimposed bacterial infection, representing an advanced stage of untreated pulpitis. Called also *pulp gangrene*. See also *necrotic pulp*, under *pulp*.

hyaline n. Zenker degeneration.

infectious bulbar n. heel abscess.

infectious pancreatic n. an acute disease affecting fry and young fish, originally seen in salmonids, but also affecting non-salmonids and shellfish, caused by the infectious pancreatic necrosis virus. It is characterized by darkened pigmentation, whirling about the long axis, and massive necrosis of the pancreas, pylorus, and anterior intestine, with the formation of a white exudate.

ischemic n. coagulation n.

ischemic n. of bone osteonecrosis.

labial n. of rabbits a fatal necrobacillosis of rabbits that begins in the lower lip and extends down to the thorax.

liquefaction n., liquefactive n. necrosis in which the necrotic material becomes softened and liquefied; called also *colliquative n.*

massive hepatic n. extensive necrosis of the liver, a rare, usually fatal complication of fulminant hepatitis, exposure to hepatotoxins, or drug hypersensitivity. A lobe or the entire liver shrinks, becoming soft, flabby, and yellow to green in color with a wrinkled capsule; there is confluent necrosis of liver cells, often with fatty change.

medial n. medionecrosis.

mercurial n. necrosis due to mercury poisoning.

mummification n. dry gangrene.

Paget quiet n. a process of local necrosis and sequestrum formation in the superficial layers of the shaft of a long bone with a minimal amount of suppuration around the sequestrum and without sinus formation.

peripheral n. necrosis of the peripheral portion of an organ, such as of a liver lobule in puerperal eclampsia.

phosphorus n. necrosis of the jaw, sometimes associated with deposition of new subperiosteal bone, occurring in workers exposed to yellow phosphorus fumes. Called also *phosphonecrosis* and *phossy jaw*.

piecemeal n. interface hepatitis.

postpartum pituitary n. necrosis of the pituitary during the postpartum period, often associated with shock and excessive uterine bleeding during delivery, and leading to variable patterns of hypopituitarism; called also *Sheehan syndrome*.

pressure n. necrosis due to insufficient local blood supply, as in pressure ulcers.

radiation n. radionecrosis.

radium n. necrosis of bones due to exposure to radium, formerly common in workers in radium plants.

renal cortical n. necrosis of the renal cortex due to ischemia, often following acute tubular necrosis; it is usually seen as a complication of an obstetric condition such as abruptio placentae, septic abortion, preeclampsia, retained fetus, or amniotic fluid embolism.

n. of renal papillae, renal papillary n. an accompaniment of acute pyelonephritis, most often seen in diabetics, characterized by necrosis of the renal papillae of one or both kidneys, with sharp demarcation between necrotic and living tissue. Called also *necrotizing papillitis* and *necrotizing renal papillitis.*

septic n. necrosis resulting from bacterial infection.

subacute hepatic n. any of a small group of viral hepatitis cases characterized by bridging necrosis and an increased incidence of progression to chronic active hepatitis, cirrhosis, or liver failure. Called also *submassive hepatic n.*

subcutaneous fat n. of newborn a rare type of predominantly lobular panniculitis seen in neonates, with nodules and indurated patches at various places on the skin, which usually resolve spontaneously within a few months. Called also *adiponecrosis subcutanea neonatorum.*

submassive hepatic n. subacute hepatic n.

n. ustilagi′nea dry gangrene from ergotism.

Zenker n. see under *degeneration.*

nec•ro•sper•mia (nek″ro-spur′me-ə) [*necro-* + *sperm-* + *-ia*] a condition in which the spermatozoa of the semen are either motionless or dead. **necrosper′mic** *adj*

nec•ro•tiz•ing (nek′ro-tīz″ing) causing necrosis.

ne•crot•o•my (nə-krot′ə-me) [*necro-* + *-tomy*] 1. dissection of a dead body. 2. sequestrectomy.

osteoplastic n. removal of a sequestrum from a bone after first lifting a flap of the bone, which is replaced after the operation.

nec•ro•tox•in (nek′ro-tok″sin) a toxin that kills tissue cells, such as one of the exotoxins secreted by species of *Clostridium* or by *Staphylococcus aureus.*

nec•ro•zoo•sper•mia (nek″ro-zo″o-spur′me-ə) necrospermia.

Nec•tria (nek′tre-ə) a genus of fungi of the family Hypocreaceae, usually found on wood or various fruits. It contains the perfect (sexual) stage of several species of *Acremonium* and *Fusarium.*

Nec•tu•rus (nek-tu′rəs) a genus of salamanders having large external gills; employed in physiologic research.

NED no evidence of disease.

ned•o•cro•mil (ned″o-kro′mil) a nonsteroidal antiinflammatory drug administered by inhalation for the prevention of airway inflammation and bronchoconstriction in the treatment of bronchial asthma.

n. sodium the sodium salt of nedocromil; administered topically to the conjunctiva in the treatment of allergic conjunctivitis.

nee•dle (ne′dəl) [L. *acus*] 1. a sharp instrument for suturing or puncturing. 2. to puncture with a needle, as in discission of the lens for treatment of cataract.

Abrams n. a biopsy needle designed to reduce the danger of introducing air into tissues, as in pleural biopsy.

aneurysm n. a needle with a handle, used in ligating blood vessels.

aspirating n. a long, hollow needle for removing fluid from a cavity.

atraumatic n. an eyeless surgical needle with the suture attached to a hollow end.

Brockenbrough n. a curved steel transseptal needle within a Brockenbrough transseptal catheter; used to puncture the interatrial septum.

butterfly n. a phlebotomy needle with tabs like the wings of a butterfly that provide a firm anchor for taping.

cataract n. a needle used in removing a cataract.

Chiba n. fine n.

Cope n. a blunt-ended hooklike needle with a concealed cutting edge and snare, used in biopsy of the pleura, pericardium, peritoneum, and synovium.

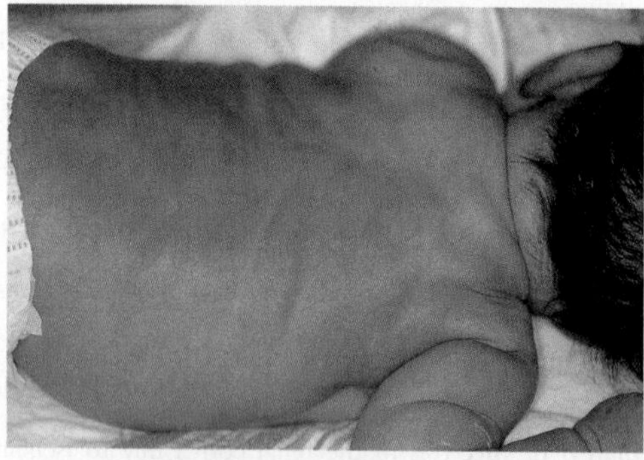

■ Subcutaneous fat necrosis of newborn.

Deschamps n. a needle with the eye near the point, and a long handle attached; used in ligating deep-seated arteries.

discission n. a special form of cataract needle.

fine n. a very thin, highly flexible steel needle with a narrow inner core used to cannulate very small bile ducts to perform percutaneous (or fine needle) transhepatic cholangiography (see under *cholangiography*). Called also *Chiba n.* and *skinny n.*

Hagedorn n′s surgical needles that are flat from side to side, with a straight cutting edge near the point and a large eye.

hypodermic n. a short, slender, hollow needle used in injecting drugs beneath the skin.

knife n. a slender knife with a needlelike point, used in discission of a cataract and other ophthalmic operations, as in goniotomy and goniopuncture.

ligature n. a slender steel needle with a long handle and an eye in its curved end, used for passing a ligature underneath an artery.

Menghini n. a needle that does not require rotation to cut loose the tissue specimen in a biopsy of the liver.

Reverdin n. a surgical needle having an eye which can be opened and closed by means of a slide.

scalp vein n. a short rigid needle with flexible wings on each side; used to infuse IV fluids for short periods of time, in patients with small veins or in children.

Seldinger n. a needle with a blunt, tapered external cannula with a sharp obturator; used for the initial percutaneous insertion characteristic of the Seldinger technique for arterial or venous access.

Silverman n. an instrument for taking tissue specimens, consisting of an outer cannula, an obturator, and an inner split needle with longitudinal grooves in which the tissue is retained when the needle and cannula are withdrawn.

skinny n. fine n.

spatula n. a minute needle with a flat or slightly curved concave surface that does not cut or pierce, used in ophthalmic surgery.

stop n. a needle with a shoulder that prevents it from being inserted beyond a certain distance.

swaged n. a needle permanently attached to the suture material.

transseptal n. a needle used to puncture the interatrial septum in transseptal catheterization.

Tuohy n. a needle in which the opening at the end is angled 45 degrees so that a catheter or endoscope through its lumen exits at an angle; used for examination or treatment of the epidural space or subarachnoid space.

Veress n. a hollow needle consisting of a sharp trocar with a slanted end surrounding an inner cylinder with a blunt end; after the trocar is introduced into a body cavity the blunt cylinder is advanced outward so that internal organs are not injured by the sharp edge; used for insufflation of a body cavity, such as for pneumoperitoneum in minimally invasive surgery.

Vim-Silverman n. a needle used in needle biopsy.

nee•dle•scop•ic (nee″dəl-skop′ik) done with a minilaparoscopic technique in which tiny instruments are passed through the lumen of a hollow needle such as the Veress needle.

neem (nēm) [Hindi *nīm*] *Azadirachta indica,* a large evergreen tree native to India and Sri Lanka, with compound leaves and small white flowers and having antifungal, antibacterial, antiviral, and antimalarial activity. All of its parts have long been used medicinally for a wide variety of indications, and its oil is used as an insecticide.

NEFA nonesterified fatty acids.

ne•fa•zo•done hy•dro•chlo•ride (nə-fa′zo-dōn) [USP] a compound structurally related to trazodone, used as an antidepressant; administered orally.

ne•flu•o•ro•pho•tom•e•ter (nə-floor″o-fo-tom′ə-tər) fluoronephelometer.

nef•o•pam hy•dro•chlo•ride (nef′o-pam) a non-opioid analgesic, used for the relief of mild to moderate pain; administered intramuscularly and orally.

neg•a•tive (neg′ə-tiv) [L. *negativus*] 1. having a value less than zero. 2. indicating absence, as of a condition or organism. 3. characterized by refusal, denial, resistance, or opposition.

neg•a•tiv•ism (neg′ə-tĭ-viz″əm) resistance or opposition to advice, suggestions, or commands; e.g., in catatonic schizophrenia patients may lower their arms if asked to raise them or may resist efforts to move them.

neg•a•tron (neg′ə-tron) the negative electron; see *positron* and *electron.*

Neg•Gram (neg′ram) trademark for preparations of nalidixic acid.

ne•glect (nə-glekt′) [L. *neglegere* to disregard] disregard of or failure to perform some task or function.

hemispatial n. failure to respond to stimuli on one side, usually opposite the side of a lesion in a cerebral hemisphere. Cf. *unilateral n.*

sensory n. unilateral n.

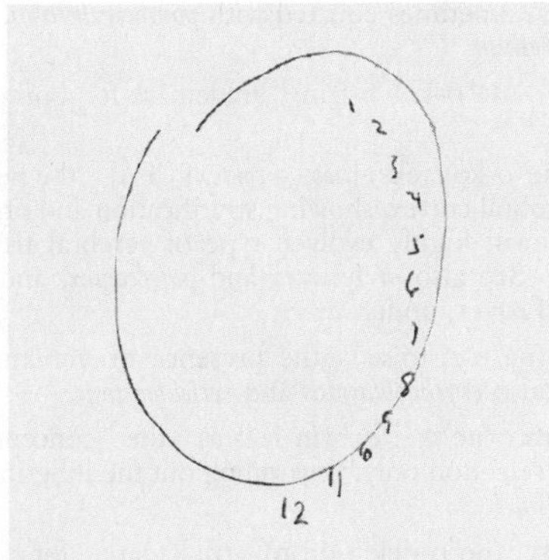

■ Clock drawn by a patient with hemispatial neglect, showing absence of attention to detail on the left and crowding of detail to the right.

unilateral n. hemiapraxia with failure to pay attention to bodily grooming and stimuli on one side but not on the other, usually due to a lesion in the central nervous system, as after a stroke. Called also *hemineglect* and *selective inattention.* Cf. *dressing apraxia.*

Ne•gri bodies (na′gre) [Adelchi *Negri,* Italian physician, 1876–1912] see under *body.*

Ne•gri-Ja•cod syndrome (na′gre zhah-ko′) [Silvio *Negri,* Italian physician, 20th century; Maurice *Jacod,* French physician, 20th century] Jacod syndrome.

Ne•gro phenomenon (sign) (na′gro) [Camillo *Negro,* Italian neurologist, 1861–1927] see *cogwheel rigidity,* under *rigidity.*

NEI National Eye Institute.

Neis•ser diplococcus (ni′sər) [Albert Ludwig Siegmund *Neisser,* German physician, 1855–1916] see *Neisseria gonorrhoeae.*

Neis•ser-Wechs•berg phenomenon (ni′sər veks′berg) [Max *Neisser,* German physician, 1869–1938; Friedrich *Wechsberg,* German physician, 1873–1929] see *complement deviation,* under *deviation.*

Neis•se•ria (ni-se′re-ə) [A.L.S. *Neisser*] a genus of bacteria of the family Neisseriaceae, consisting of gram-negative, oxidase-positive cocci characteristically coffee bean–shaped and paired. The organisms are aerobic or facultatively anaerobic and are part of the normal flora of the oropharynx, nasopharynx, and genitourinary tract. The genus includes the gonococcus, the several meningococcus types, pigmented forms occasionally associated with meningitis, and a number of saprophytic or parasitic but nonpathogenic species. The type species is *N. gonorrhoe′ae.*

N. cine′rea a species that causes eye infections in children and occasional infections, sometimes invasive, in adults.

N. flaves′cens a species characterized by the production of yellow pigmented colonies. It is sometimes found in the body fluids of patients with meningitis and septicemia.

N. gonorrhoe′ae the specific etiologic agent of gonorrhea, occurring typically as pairs of flattened cells, found primarily in purulent venereal discharges.

N. lacta′mica a species that ferments lactose, found frequently in throat and nasopharyngeal cultures of infants and young children; it occasionally causes endocarditis and meningitis in humans.

N. meningi′tidis a prominent cause of meningitis and the specific etiologic agent of meningococcal meningitis; it can also cause meningococcal pneumonia, a type of bacterial pneumonia (see under *pneumonia*). Species can be differentiated serologically into at least 13 groups (A, B, C, D, E, H, I, K, L, W-135, X, Y, and Z); groups A, B, and C are responsible for most cases of disease, with B and C being predominant in Europe and the Americas and A and C predominant in Asia and Africa.

N. muco′sa a species that produces mucoid colonies that are often adherent; it is found in the nasopharynx and occasionally causes pneumonia.

N. polysaccha′rea a species that is usually only commensal in the upper respiratory tract but can cause opportunistic infections in susceptible persons.

N. sic′ca a species that forms dry gray, slimy white, or yellow colonies and is part of the normal flora of the nasopharynx, saliva, and sputum; it occasionally causes infections in susceptible persons.

N. subfla′va a species that produces smooth, yellow-pigmented colonies, found in the nasopharynx and occasionally in the cerebrospinal fluid of persons with meningitis.

N. wea′veri a species that is part of the normal oropharyngeal flora of dogs and causes infection in persons bitten by dogs.

Neis•se•ri•a•ceae (ni-se″re-a′se-e) a family of gram-negative, aerobic cocci and rod-shaped bacteria of the order Neisseriales, occurring singly or in pairs, short chains, or masses. The organisms are parasitic or saprophytic, and some produce pigment. Medically important organisms are included in the genera *Chromobacter, Eikenella, Kingella,* and *Neisseria.*

Neis•se•ri•a•les (ni-se″re-a′lēz) an order of bacteria of the class Betaproteobacteria, phylum Proteobacteria, consisting of gram-negative, aerobic, coccal, coccoid, or rod-shaped organisms occurring singly, in pairs, or in masses. It contains a single family, the Neisseriaceae.

neis•se•ri•al (ni-se′re-əl) of, relating to, or caused by *Neisseria.*

Né•kam disease (na-kahm′) [L. *Nékam,* French dermatologist, 20th century] keratosis lichenoides chronica.

nek•ton (nek′ton) [Gr. *nēktos* swimming] collective term for marine organisms that swim actively, as contrasted with plankton.

Né•la•ton catheter, line, sphincter (na-lah-taw′) [Auguste *Nélaton,* French surgeon, 1807–1873] see under *catheter, line,* and *sphincter.*

nel•ar•a•bine (nel-ar′ə-bēn) a prodrug of a purine nucleoside analog, used as an antimetabolite antineoplastic in treatment of T-cell acute lymphoblastic leukemia and lymphoma that is relapsed or refractory to other regimens.

nel•fin•a•vir mesy•late (nel-fin′ə-vir) an HIV protease inhibitor that causes the formation of immature, noninfectious viral particles, used in the treatment of human immunodeficiency virus infection; administered orally.

Nel•ova (nə-lo′və) trademark for oral contraceptive therapeutic regimens containing norethindrone as the progestational agent and either ethinyl estradiol or mestranol as the estrogen component.

Nel•son syndrome (nel′sən) [Don H. *Nelson,* American internist, born 1925] see under *syndrome.*

nem•a•line (nem′ə-lēn) [Gr. *nēma* thread] threadlike or rod-shaped.

nem•a•thel•minth (nem″ə-thel′minth) [*nemat-* + *helminth*] a worm of the phylum Nemathelminthes.

Nem•a•thel•min•thes (nem″ə-thəl-min′thēz) in some systems of classification, a phylum that includes Acanthocephala and Nematoda.

ne•mat•i•cide (nə-mat′ĭ-sīd) nematocide.

nem•a•ti•za•tion (nem″ə-tĭ-za′shən) nematodiasis.

nemat(o)- [Gr. *nēma* thread, gen. *nēmatos*] a combining form denoting relationship to a nematode, or to a threadlike structure.

nem•a•to•blast (nem′ə-to-blast) [*nemato-* + *-blast*] spermatid.

Nem•a•toc•era (nem″ə-tos′ər-ə) [Gr. *nēma* thread + *keras* horn] a suborder of insects of the order Diptera, characterized by having antennae of many segments; it includes the gnats, mosquitoes, midges, black flies, craneflies, gallflies, and others.

nem•a•to•cide (nem′ə-to-sīd″) [*nemato-* + *-cide*] 1. destructive to nematode worms. 2. an agent that destroys nematodes.

nem•a•to•cyst (nem′ə-to-sist″) a minute stinging structure, found in the cnidoblasts of jellyfish and other coelenterates, used for anchorage, for defense, and for the capture of prey.

Nem•a•to•da (nem″ə-to′də) [Gr. *nēma* thread + *eidos* form] the roundworms, a class of the phylum Aschelminthes, tapered cylindrical helminths, of which many species are parasites. They are characterized by longitudinally oriented muscles and by a triradiate esophagus. In some systems of classification, they are considered to be a separate phylum. Sometimes called *Nemathelminthes,* or a class under that phylum.

nem•a•tode (nem′ə-tōd) any member of the class Nematoda; called also *roundworm* or *round worm* and *eelworm* or *eel worm.*

nem•a•to•des•ma (nem″ə-to-dez′mə) pl. *nematodesma′ta* [*nemato-* + Gr. *desmos* band, ligament] a bundle of parallel microtubules serving to support the cytostome and cytopharyngeal apparatus and associated organelles of certain ciliate protozoa; also seen in certain flagellate groups. Called also *trichite.*

nem•a•to•di•a•sis (nem″ə-to-di′ə-sis) infection by nematode parasites.

Nem•a•to•di•rus (nem″ə-to′dĭ-rəs) a genus of nematodes of the family Trichostrongylidae, found as parasites in the duodenum of ruminants.

nem•a•toid (nem′ə-toid) resembling a thread; pertaining to a nematode parasite.

nem•a•tol•o•gist (nem″ə-tol′ə-jist) a specialist in nematology.

nem•a•tol•o•gy (nem″ə-tol′ə-je) the branch of zoology which deals with nematode worms.

Nem•a•to•mor•pha (nem″ə-to-mor′fə) [Gr. *nēma* thread + *morphē* form] a class of the phylum Aschelminthes, consisting of long, slender, cylindrical worms; commonly called *hairworms, horse hairs,* or *hair eels.* They are parasitic as juveniles. In some systems of classification, they are considered to be a separate phylum. Called also *Gordiacea.*

nem•a•to•sis (nem″ə-to′sis) nematodiasis.

nem•a•to•sper•mia (nem″ə-to-spur′me-ə) [*nemato-* + *sperm-* + *-ia*] spermatozoa having elongated tails, as seen in mammals and various other animals.

Nem•bu•tal (nem′bu-tal) trademark for preparations of pentobarbital sodium.

nem•ic (nem′ik) nematoid.

Nem•o•rhi•na (nem″o-ri′nə) a subgenus of the genus *Glossina* (tsetse flies) that cause West African trypanosomiasis.

ne(o)- [Gr. *neos* new] 1. a combining form meaning new or recent, or denoting an immature form. 2. in chemistry, a prefix denoting a new chemical compound related in some way to an older one, to whose name it is added.

neo•ad•ju•vant (ne″o-aj′oo-vənt) denoting preliminary cancer therapy that precedes a necessary second modality of treatment. See under *therapy.*

neo•an•ti•gen (ne″o-an′tĭ-jən) a new antigenic determinant, such as a tumor-associated antigen, that is formed when a protein is modified by metabolic processes or that emerges when a conformational change exposes a previously unexpressed epitope.

neo•ar•thro•sis (ne″o-ahr-thro′sis) nearthrosis.

neo•bio•gen•e•sis (ne″o-bi″o-jen′ə-sis) [*neo-* + *biogenesis*] biopoiesis.

neo•blad•der (ne″o-blad′ər) an artificial reservoir for urine created as continent urinary diversion to replace the bladder following cystectomy, constructed from a detubularized bowel segment or from a segment of the stomach, with implantation of the ureters and urethra. Called also *continent urinary reservoir.*

Camey n. a formerly widely used type of ileal neobladder made from a U-shaped section of ileum.

Hautmann n. a type of orthotopic ileal neobladder constructed from a W-shaped section of ileum.

ileal n. a neobladder made from a section of ileum; called also *continent ileal reservoir.*

orthotopic n. a neobladder that is in the normal anatomical position of the bladder, with discharge of urine through the urethra.

Studer n. a low pressure type of orthotopic ileal neobladder.

neo•blas•tic (ne″o-blas′tik) [*neo-* + *blast-* + *-ic*] originating in or of the nature of new tissue.

Neo-Cal•glu•con (ne″o-kal′gloo-kon) trademark for a preparation of calcium glubionate.

neo•cer•e•bel•lum (ne″o-ser″ə-bel′əm) [*neo-* + *cerebellum*] [TA] the phylogenetically newest part of the cerebellum, considered to correspond to its lateral parts, including the cerebellar hemispheres and the middle portion of the vermis. Because the hemispheres are the primary site of termination of the projections from the pons, the corticopontocerebellar fibers, the term is sometimes equated with *pontocerebellum.* Cf. *archicerebellum* and *paleocerebellum.*

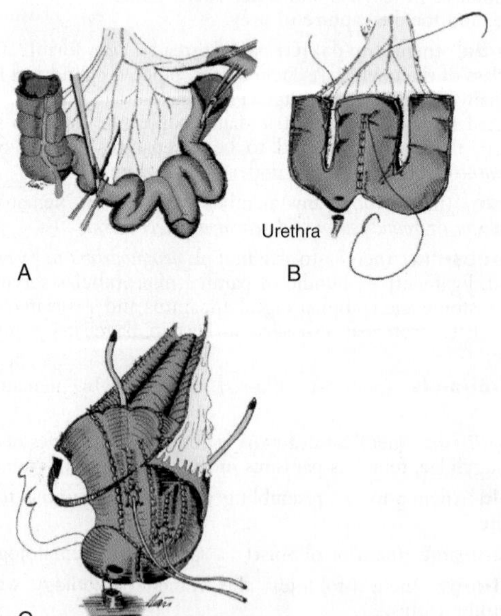

■ Construction of Hautmann neobladder. *(A),* A segment of terminal ileum is isolated and incised on the antimesenteric border. *(B),* The ileum is arranged into an M or W configuration with the limbs sutured to one another. *(C),* A buttonhole of ileum is removed on an antimesenteric portion of the ileum and the urethra and ileum are anastomosed. The ureters are implanted and stented, and the reservoir is closed in a side-to-side manner.

Neo-Cob•e•frin (ne″o-kob′ə-frin) trademark for a preparation of levonordefrin.

neo•cor•tex (ne″o-kor′teks) [*neo-* + *cortex*] [TA] the newer, six-layered portion of the cerebral cortex, showing stratification and organization characteristic of the most highly evolved type of cerebral tissue. Called also *nonolfactory cortex.* See also *archicortex* and *paleocortex*, and see illustration at *layers of cerebral cortex*, under *layer.*

neo•cy•to•sis (ne″o-si-to′sis) the presence of immature erythrocytes in the blood; see also *erythroblastosis* and *reticulocytosis.*

neo•dar•win•ism (ne″o-dahr′win-iz-əm) the concept that species evolve by natural selection only, thus ruling out the inheritance of acquired traits; see *darwinism.*

Neo•Dec•a•dron (ne″o-dek′ə-dron) trademark for a combination preparation of dexamethasone sodium phosphate and neomycin sulfate.

neo•dym•i•um (Nd) (ne″o-dim′e-əm) a rare element of atomic number, 60; atomic weight, 144.24.

neo•en•dor•phin (ne″o-en-dor′fin; -en′dor-fin) either of a pair of opioid peptides, designated α and β, closely related to and derived from the same precursor as the dynorphins.

neo•fe•tal (ne″o-fe′təl) pertaining to the transitional period between the embryonic and fetal stages of human prenatal development.

neo•fe•tus (ne″o-fe′təs) the human embryo at the end of the eighth week after fertilization.

neo•for•ma•tion (ne″o-for-ma′shən) a new growth of tissue or neoplasm. **neofor′mative** *adj*

Neo•frin (ne′o-frin″) trademark for preparations of phenylephrine hydrochloride.

ne•og•a•la (ne-og′ə-lə) [*neo-* + Gr. *gala* milk] the first milk developed after childbirth; see also *colostrum.*

Neo•gas•trop•o•da (ne″o-gas-trop′ə-də) an order of marine-dwelling gastropods of the subclass Streptoneura; it includes the family Conidae, which contains some poisonous species, and the genus *Murex.*

neo•gen•e•sis (ne″o-jen′ə-sis) [*neo-* + *-genesis*] regeneration. **neogenet′ic** *adj*

neo•glot•tis (ne″o-glot′is) a surgically constructed glottis created by suturing the pharyngeal mucosa over the superior end of the transected trachea above the primary tracheostoma, making a permanent stoma in the mucosa; it is created to permit phonation after laryngectomy. Called also *pseudoglottis.* **neoglot′tic** *adj*

neo•in•ti•ma (ne″o-in′tĭ-mə) a new layer of endothelial cells formed on the intimal surface of a blood vessel graft or vascular prosthesis. Cf. *pseudointima.*

neo•lal•ia (ne″o-lal′e-ə) [*neo-* + *lal-* + *-ia*] speech into which many neologisms are incorporated, as in schizophrenia.

neo•lal•ism (ne″o-lal′iz-əm) neolalia.

ne•ol•o•gism (ne-ol′ə-jiz″əm) [*neo-* + *log-* + *-ism*] a newly coined word; in psychiatry, a new word whose meaning may be known only to the person using it and may be related to the person's conflicts.

Ne•o•loid (ne′o-loid) trademark for a preparation of castor oil.

neo•mem•brane (ne″o-mem′brān) pseudomembrane.

neo•morph (ne′o-morf) [*neo-* + *-morph*] a part or organ recently acquired in the course of evolution.

neo•mor•phism (ne″o-mor′fiz-əm) the development of new form in the course of evolution.

neo•mort (ne′o-mort) a corpse immediately after death.

neo•my•cin (ne″o-mi′sin) [USP] an aminoglycoside antibiotic complex derived from *Streptomyces fradiae*, consisting of three components designated A, B, and C. The form in clinical use is a mixture of neomycins B and C; it is effective against a wide range of aerobic gram-negative bacilli and some gram-positive bacteria.

n. sulfate [USP] the sulfate salt of neomycin, used for urinary tract irrigation, administered orally in preoperative bowel preparation, and applied topically to the skin, conjunctiva, and ears in the treatment of infections due to susceptible organisms; in topical preparations it is often combined with other antibiotics or antiinflammatory steroids.

ne•on (Ne) (ne′on) [Gr. *neos* new] an inert gaseous element discovered in the air in 1898; atomic weight, 20.183; atomic number, 10.

neo•na•tal (ne″o-na′təl) [*neo-* + *natal* (def. 1)] pertaining to the first four weeks after birth.

neo•nate (ne′o-nāt) 1. newborn infant. 2. newborn (def. 1).

neo•na•tol•o•gist (ne″o-na-tol′ə-jist) a physician specializing in neonatology.

neo•na•tol•o•gy (ne″o-na-tol′ə-je) the art and science of diagnosis and treatment of disorders of the newborn infant.

neo•pal•li•um (ne″o-pal′e-əm) [*neo-* + *pallium*] neocortex.

neo•pla•sia (ne″o-pla′zhə) the formation of a neoplasm, i.e., the progressive multiplication of cells under conditions that would not elicit, or would cause cessation of, multiplication of normal cells.

biliary intraepithelial n. any of several premalignant lesions in the bile ducts that have varying degrees of severity, with flat pseudopapillae or micropapillae, and commonly develop into cholangiocarcinoma. Called also *biliary dysplasia.*

cervical intraepithelial n. (CIN) dysplasia of the cervical epithelium, often premalignant, characterized by various degrees of hyperplasia, abnormal keratinization, and presence of condylomata.

gestational trophoblastic n. (GTN) a group of neoplastic disorders that originate in the placenta, including the benign *hydatidiform mole* and the malignant *chorioadenoma destruens* and *choriocarcinoma.* Called also *gestational trophoblastic disease* and *trophoblastic disease.*

lobular n. lobular carcinoma in situ.

multiple endocrine n. (MEN) a group of rare genetic disorders characterized by hyperplasia and hyperfunction of two or more components of the endocrine system. Several types have been distinguished; all are transmitted as autosomal dominant traits with varying penetrance. Called also *multiple endocrine adenomatosis, polyendocrine adenomatosis,* and *polyendocrinoma.*

type 1 that due to mutation in the tumor suppressor gene *MEN1* (locus: 11q13); it is characterized by tumors of the anterior pituitary, parathyroid glands, and pancreatic islet cells in association with a high incidence of peptic ulcers and sometimes the Zollinger-Ellison syndrome. Called also *Wermer syndrome.*

type 2 that due to mutation in the *RET* oncogene (locus: 10q11.2), characterized by tendency to medullary carcinoma of the thyroid; it is divided into three subtypes distinguished on the characteristic tissues involved: 2A, 2B, and familial medullary thyroid carcinoma (q.v.).

type 2A a subtype of type 2 characterized additionally by pheochromocytoma (often bilateral and multiple), and parathyroid hyperplasia. Called also *Sipple syndrome.*

type 2B a subtype of type 2 resembling type 2A except that parathyroid hyperplasia is rare, mean survival time is shorter, a marfanoid body habitus may occur, and there may be disfiguring neuromas of the lips, buccal mucosa, and tongue, neurofibromas of the skin, ganglioneuromas of the gastrointestinal tract, thickened corneal nerves, and café au lait spots. Called also *mucosal neuroma syndrome.*

penile intraepithelial n. dysplasia of epithelium of the penis, usually on the prepuce or glans, ranging from mild disorientation of epithelial cells with cellular pleomorphism to carcinoma in situ or invasive carcinoma. It is characterized by a slowly growing, circumscribed, erythematous, moist, velvety, shiny patch. Called also *erythroplasia of Queyrat.*

prostatic intraepithelial n. neoplastic changes in epithelial cells of prostatic ducts and acini showing some morphologic features of cancer but not involving stromal invasion; these are sometimes precursors of carcinoma or adenocarcinoma.

vaginal intraepithelial n. a rare precancerous lesion of the vaginal epithelium, having a squamous cell origin. Various degrees of hyperplasia are distinguished according to the extent of epithelium involved.

vulval intraepithelial n., vulvar intraepithelial n. a precancerous lesion of the vulva, having a squamous cell origin. Various degrees of hyperplasia are distinguished according to the extent of epithelium involved; low-grade lesions show acetowhitening, whereas higher-grade ones have papule formation and sharp demarcation from surrounding tissue.

neo•plasm (ne′o-plaz″əm) [*neo-* + *-plasm*] any new and abnormal growth; specifically a new growth of tissue in which the growth is uncontrolled and progressive (see *neoplasia*). Malignant neoplasms are distinguished from benign in that the former show a greater degree of anaplasia and have the properties of invasion and metastasis. Called also *tumor.*

intraductal papillary mucinous n. a benign tumor of the pancreatic duct that secretes excessive mucin and may be a type of mucinous cystic neoplasm; called also *intraductal papillary mucinous tumor.*

neo•plas•tic (ne″o-plas′tik) 1. pertaining to or like a neoplasm. 2. pertaining to neoplasia.

neo•plas•ti•gen•ic (ne″o-plas″tĭ-jen′ik) tumorigenic.

Ne•op•syl•la (ne-op′səl-ə) a genus of fleas.

ne•op•ter•in (ne-op′tər-in) a pteridine derivative excreted in the urine at low levels; urinary excretion is elevated in some disorders of tetrahydrobiopterin biosynthesis, certain malignant diseases, viral infection, and graft rejection. The term is also used to denote the class of related compounds.

Ne•or•al (ne-or′əl) trademark for preparations of cyclosporine.

neo•rec•tum (ne″o-rek′təm) ileoanal reservoir.

Neo•rick•ett•sia (ne″o-rĭ-ket′se-ə) [*neo-* + *rickettsia*] a genus of bacteria of the family Anaplasmataceae, consisting of gram-negative, nonmotile, coccoid or pleomorphic cells, occurring in cytoplasmic vacuoles in monocytes and macrophages. Organisms are transmitted by flukes and cause disease in canids, horses, and humans. The type species is *N. helminthoe′ca.*

N. helminthoe′ca the etiologic agent of salmon poisoning in dogs and other canids; it lives inside the salmon fluke, *Nanophyetus salmincola,* and if this parasitizes a fish, animals that eat the fish will become infected. Horizontal transmission can also occur.

N. risti′cii a species that causes equine monocytic ehrlichiosis. Formerly called *Ehrlichia risticii.*

N. sennet′su a species that is the etiologic agent of sennetsu fever. Formerly called *Ehrlichia sennetsu.*

neo•rick•ett•si•o•sis (ne″o-rĭ-ket″se-o′sis) infection with *Neorickettsia.*

sennetsu n. see under *fever.*

Neo•scan (ne′o-skan″) trademark for a preparation of gallium Ga 67 citrate.

Neo•schoen•gas•tia (ne″o-shān-gas′te-ə) a genus of mites of the family Trombiculidae. *N. america′na* infests chickens in the southern United States.

neo•sphinc•ter (ne″o-sfingk′ter) a surgically created anal sphincter, such as for treatment of severe incontinence or imperforate anus.

Ne•os•po•ra (ne-os′pə-rə) a genus of protozoa of the phylum Apicomplexa, morphologically similar to *Toxoplasma. N. cani′num* is parasitic in dogs and other mammals, causing neosporosis.

Neo•spor•in (ne″o-spo′rin) trademark for combination preparations of neomycin sulfate, polymyxin B sulfate, and (in some preparations) either bacitracin zinc or gramicidin.

neo•spo•ro•sis (ne″o-spə-ro′sis) infection of dogs and other mammals by *Neospora caninum*; characteristics are similar to those of toxoplasmosis, with neurologic and ophthalmic symptoms predominating.

neo•stig•mine (ne″o-stig′mēn) a cholinesterase inhibitor and prokinetic agent, which acts by inhibiting destruction of acetylcholine and so facilitating transmission of impulses across the neuromuscular junction. Effects include miosis, bradycardia, increased intestinal and skeletal muscle tone, increased salivary and sweat gland secretion, and constriction of bronchi and ureters. It also has direct effects on skeletal muscle fibers.

n. bromide [USP] the bromide salt of neostigmine, used as a cholinergic in the symptomatic control of myasthenia gravis, and to produce miosis in certain forms of glaucoma in patients who have developed tolerance to other miotics; administered orally and applied to the conjunctiva.

n. methylsulfate [USP] the methylsulfate salt of neostigmine, used as a cholinergic in the symptomatic treatment of myasthenia gravis, as a diagnostic test for myasthenia gravis, in the prevention and treatment of postoperative stasis and atony of the gastrointestinal tract or urinary bladder, and for reversal of the effects of nondepolarizing neuromuscular blocking agents such as tubocurarine after surgery; administered intravenously, intramuscularly, or subcutaneously.

ne•os•to•my (ne-os′tə-me) [*neo-* + *-stomy*] surgical creation of an artificial opening into an organ or between two organs.

neo•stri•a•tum (ne″o-stri-a′təm) [*neo-* + *striatum*] the later developed portion of the corpus striatum, represented by the caudate nucleus and the putamen; called also *striatum.* Cf. *paleostriatum.*

Neo•stron•gy•lus (ne″o-stron′jĭ-ləs) a genus of parasitic nematodes of the family Protostrongylidae, some species of which are lungworms of sheep and goats.

ne•ot•e•ny (ne-ot′ə-ne) [*neo-* + Gr. *teinein* to extend] 1. the tendency to remain in the larval state, although gaining sexual maturity. 2. the retention in an adult organism of some of its ancestor's larval characteristics.

Neo•tes•tu•di•na (ne″o-tes″too-di′nə) a genus of bitunicate fungi of the order Dothideales. *N. rosa′tii* is an etiologic agent of eumycotic mycetoma in tropical Africa and Australia.

neo•thal•a•mus (ne″o-thal′ə-məs) [*neo-* new + *thalamus*] new thalamus; the phylogenetically new part of the thalamus, i.e., the part connected to the neocortex. Cf. *paleothalamus.*

Ne•ot•o•ma (ne-ot′ə-mə) a genus of rodents of western North America, the wood or pack rats.

Neo•tri•zine (ne″o-tri′zēn) trademark for preparations of trisulfapyrimidenes.

Neo•trom•bic•u•la (ne″o-trom-bik′u-lə) a genus of mites. *N. autumna′lis* is a European species whose larva is a type of chigger that causes trombiculiasis of the skin.

neo•type (ne′o-tīp) a strain of bacteria that replaces a type culture which no longer exists, and that agrees with the original description of the taxon and is accepted by international agreement.

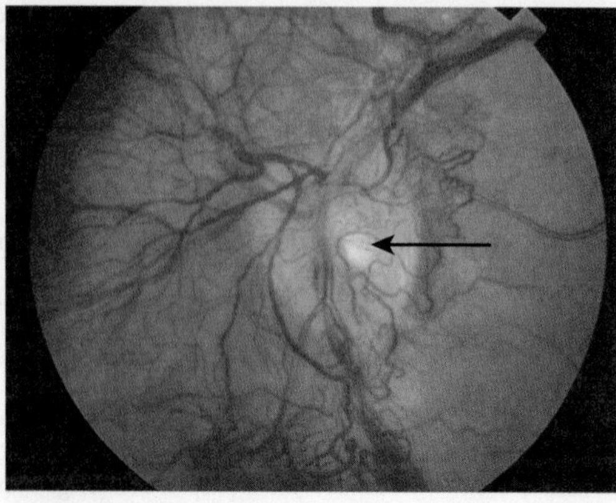

■ Neovascularization on the optic disk *(arrow)* in a patient with proliferative diabetic retinopathy.

neo•u•re•thra (ne″o-u-re′thrə) a surgically created urethra, such as in urethroplasty for hypospadias.

neo•va•gi•na (ne″o-və-ji′nə) [*neo-* + *vagina*] a surgically created vagina, as after vaginectomy or in male-to-female transsexual surgery.

neo•vas•cu•lar (ne″o-vas′ku-lər) pertaining to or characterized by neovascularization.

neo•vas•cu•lar•iza•tion (ne″o-vas″ku-lər-ĭ-za′shən) 1. new blood vessel formation in abnormal tissue or in abnormal positions. 2. revascularization. Cf. *angiogenesis* (def. 2).

Nep•e•ta (nep′ə-tə) a genus of mints of the family Labiatae, found in parts of Europe and Asia. *N. cata′ria* L. is catnip, a plant that contains the volatile aromatic oil nepetalactone, an attractant to cats; its leaves and tops, called *cataria*, are carminative and stimulant for humans.

nep•e•ta•lac•tone (nep″ə-tə-lak′tōn) the chief constituent of the aromatic volatile oil from the leaves and tops of *Nepeta cataria*, an attractant to cats.

nephel(o)- [Gr. *nephelē* cloud or mist] a combining form denoting relationship to clouds or cloudiness.

neph•e•lom•e•ter (nef″ə-lom′ə-tər) an instrument that measures the turbidity of a solution by measuring the amount of light that is scattered at an angle from a beam of light passing through the solution. Cf. *turbidimeter.*

neph•e•lom•e•try (nef″ə-lom′ə-tre) [*nephelo-* + *-metry*] measurement of the concentration of a suspension by means of a nephelometer.

neph•rad•e•no•ma (nef″rad-ə-no′mə) [*nephr-* + *adenoma*] adenoma of the kidney.

ne•phral•gia (nə-fral′jə) [*nephr-* + *-algia*] pain in a kidney. **nephral′gic** *adj*

neph•rec•ta•sia (nef″rek-ta′zhə) [*nephr-* + *ectasia*] distention of the kidney.

ne•phrec•ta•sis (nə-frek′tə-sis) nephrectasia.

ne•phrec•to•mize (nə-frek′tə-mīz) to deprive of one or both kidneys by surgical removal.

ne•phrec•to•my (nə-frek′tə-me) [*nephr-* + *-ectomy*] surgical excision of a kidney.

abdominal n., anterior n. nephrectomy through an incision in the abdominal wall.

laparoscopic n. a minimally invasive type of nephrectomy using laparoscopic techniques.

lumbar n. nephrectomy through an incision in the lumbar region; called also *posterior n.*

paraperitoneal n. nephrectomy done through an incision in the side along the twelfth rib.

posterior n. lumbar n.

radical n. removal of a kidney with its fascia after prior ligation of the renal artery and vein, as well as removal of the adjacent adrenal gland and all lymph nodes in the region; done for treatment of renal cell carcinoma.

neph•re•de•ma (nef″rə-de′mə) congestion or edema of the kidney; called also *nephremia.*

neph•rel•co•sis (nef″rəl-ko′sis) [*nephr-* + *elcosis*] ulceration of the kidney.

ne•phre•mia (nə-fre′me-ə) [*nephr-* + *-emia*] nephredema.

neph•ric (nef′rik) renal.

ne•phrid•i•um (nə-frid′e-əm) one of the segmentally arranged, paired, tubular excretory organs in invertebrates, analogous to the vertebrate kidney.

neph•rin (nef′rin) a transmembrane protein found in strands in the slit diaphragm of the renal glomerulus, chemically related to the immunoglobulin family of cell adhesion molecules.

ne•phri•tis (nə-fri′tis) pl. *nephri′tides* [*nephr-* + *-itis*] inflammation of the kidney; a focal or diffuse proliferative or destructive process that may involve the glomerulus, tubule, or interstitial renal tissue. See also *glomerulonephritis.* Cf. *nephrosis.* **nephrit′ic** *adj*

acute n. see under *glomerulonephritis.*

acute focal bacterial n. acute pyelonephritis.

acute interstitial n. a type of interstitial nephritis usually seen as a complication of a systemic infection, especially by beta-hemolytic streptococci, although it sometimes has an allergic etiology. The kidneys may be normal in size and appearance, or may be enlarged, soft, and discolored. It often resolves if the infection is treated or the offending drug or allergen is removed.

acute tubulointerstitial n. an early stage of tubulointerstitial nephritis similar to acute pyelonephritis but with involvement further into the renal medulla to involve the tubules.

allergic interstitial n. acute interstitial nephritis that is part of an allergic reaction, such as to medication.

anti-GBM n., anti–GBM antibody n., anti–glomerular basement membrane n. glomerulonephritis, usually the rapidly progressive type (q.v.), marked by circulating anti-GBM antibodies and linear deposits of immunoglobulin and complement along the glomerular basement membrane. When associated with pulmonary hemorrhage the condition is called *Goodpasture syndrome.* Called also *anti-GBM disease* or *glomerulonephritis* and *anti–glomerular basement membrane disease* or *glomerulonephritis.*

arteriosclerotic n. a type of nephritis resulting either from the aging process, with hyaline changes of the large and small arterioles, or from hypertension, with hyaline or muscular changes of the small arterioles in the glomerular hilum. Renal damage occurs primarily through ischemic atrophy of the tubules with resultant focal or diffuse fibrosis of interstitial tissue.

bacterial n. renal inflammation caused by bacterial infection, usually in the form of pyelonephritis; it may be focal or diffuse.

Balkan n. Balkan nephropathy.

n. caseo′sa, caseous n. nephritis with caseation of renal cells, such as in renal tuberculosis.

chronic n. see under *glomerulonephritis.*

chronic interstitial n. the more common type of interstitial nephritis, which progresses to the point where there is interstitial fibrosis with atrophic, shrunken kidneys, a lowered glomerular filtration rate, and danger of renal failure.

chronic tubulointerstitial n. tubulointerstitial nephritis that has progressed to the point where there is interstitial fibrosis with shrunken kidneys, a lowered glomerular filtration rate, and danger of renal failure.

congenital n. nephritis existing at birth, such as in congenital syphilitic nephritis or Alport syndrome.

fibrous n. nephritis in which there is fibrosis of interstitial tissue, such as in chronic interstitial or chronic tubulointerstitial nephritis.

glomerular n. glomerulonephritis.

n. gravida′rum n. of pregnancy.

hemorrhagic n. nephritis with hemorrhage and gross hematuria.

Henoch-Schönlein purpura n. a type of glomerulonephritis sometimes seen with Henoch-Schönlein purpura; clinical characteristics usually resemble those of IgA nephropathy, and a rapidly progressive form can lead to renal failure.

hereditary tubulointerstitial n. familial juvenile nephronophthisis (def. 1).

Heymann n. an experimental model of membranous glomerulonephritis, induced in rats by injection of an antigen preparation derived from tubule brush borders, which causes an autoimmune reaction by the native tubules.

interstitial n. primary or secondary disease of the renal interstitial tissue. Causes include arterial, arteriolar, glomerular, or tubular disease that destroys individual nephrons; toxic involvement of interstitial cells and tubules by systemic diseases such as gout *(gouty nephropathy);* drug exposure such as overuse of phenacetin *(analgesic nephropathy);* and mercury poisoning. Clinically, it may be manifested by loss of concentrating capacity, hyponatremia, hyperkalemia, acidosis, non-nephrotic proteinuria, and abnormal urine sediment. See *acute interstitial n.* and *chronic interstitial n.*

lupus n. glomerulonephritis (diffuse, focal, or membranous) associated with systemic lupus erythematosus, marked by deposition of antigen-antibody complexes in the mesangium and basement membrane. The clinical course is highly variable and depends in part on the morphological findings, which have been classified into five subgroups by the World Health Organization.

Masugi n. an animal model of antibody-mediated glomerulonephritis produced by injection of heterologous antibody against renal antigens. It occurs in two phases. The *heterologous phase*, occurring within a few hours, consists of the inflammatory response triggered by the nephrotoxic antibody binding to antigens in the glomerular basement membrane and resembles anti–GBM antibody nephritis. The *autologous phase*, occurring 4–6 days later, consists of the host response to the foreign antibody and does not correspond to a human disease.

megalocytic interstitial n. an early stage of malacoplakia of the urinary tract in which there are no Michaelis-Gutmann bodies.

nephrotoxic serum n. Masugi n.

parenchymatous n. nephritis that affects mainly the renal parenchyma; see *tubulointerstitial n.*

pneumococcal n., pneumococcus n. nephritis or glomerulonephritis from infection with *Streptococcus pneumoniae*, usually as a complication of pneumonia or empyema. See also *poststreptococcal glomerulonephritis*, under *glomerulonephritis.*

potassium-losing n. see under *nephropathy.*

n. of pregnancy nephritis occurring during pregnancy, such as a glomerulonephritis or pyelonephritis (pyelonephritis of pregnancy).

radiation n. kidney damage caused by ionizing radiation; symptoms include glomerular and tubular damage, hypertension, and proteinuria, sometimes leading to renal failure. It may be acute or chronic, and some varieties do not manifest until years after the radiation exposure.

salt-losing n. see under *nephropathy.*

scarlatinal n. nephritis or glomerulonephritis due to scarlet fever. See also *poststreptococcal glomerulonephritis*, under *glomerulonephritis.*

suppurative n. pyonephritis.

syphilitic n. nephritis that accompanies syphilis, either the congenital variety or an advanced stage of the acquired disease, characterized by inflammation in the area of the renal medulla.

transfusion n. a nephropathy following blood transfusion from a donor whose blood is incompatible with that of the recipient.

tuberculous n. interstitial nephritis caused by infection with *Mycobacterium tuberculosis.*

tubular n., tubulointerstitial n. nephritis of the tubules and interstitial tissues of the kidney, usually seen secondary to a drug sensitization, systemic infection, graft rejection, or autoimmune disease; characteristics include lymphocytes in interstitial infiltrate and within tubules, mild hematuria, and pyuria. See also *acute tubulointerstitial n.* and *chronic tubulointerstitial n.*

ne·phrit·o·gen·ic (nə-frit″o-jen′ik) giving rise to nephritis.

nephr(o)- [Gr. *nephros* kidney] a combining form denoting relationship to the kidney.

neph·ro·ab·dom·i·nal (nef″ro-ab-dom′ĭ-nəl) pertaining to or communicating between the kidney and the abdominal wall. Cf. *nephrocutaneous.*

neph·ro·an·gio·scle·ro·sis (nef″ro-an″je-o-sklə-ro′sis) hypertension with renal lesions of arterial origin.

neph·ro·blas·to·ma (nef″ro-blas-to′mə) Wilms tumor.

cystic n., differentiated n. multilocular cyst of kidney.

neph·ro·blas·to·ma·to·sis (nef″ro-blas-to″mə-to′sis) clusters of microscopic blastema cells, tubules, and stromal cells at the periphery of renal lobes of infants, thought to be a precursor of Wilms tumor.

neph·ro·bron·chi·al (nef″ro-brong′ke-əl) pertaining to or connecting a kidney and a bronchus.

neph·ro·cal·ci·no·sis (nef″ro-kal″si-no′sis) [*nephro-* + *calcinosis*] a condition characterized by precipitation of calcium salts such as calcium phosphate and calcium oxalate in the renal tubules, sometimes resulting in nephrolithiasis, renal insufficiency, and polyuria.

neph·ro·car·di·ac (nef″ro-kahr′de-ak) cardiorenal.

neph·ro·cele (nef′ro-sēl) [*nephro-* + *-cele*[1]] hernial protrusion of a kidney.

neph·ro·col·ic (nef″ro-kol′ik) [*nephro-* + *colic*] renocolic.

neph·ro·co·lon·ic (nef″ro-kə-lon′ik) renocolic.

neph·ro·cu·ta·ne·ous (nef″ro-ku-ta′ne-əs) pertaining to or communicating between the kidney and the skin.

neph·ro·cys·ti·tis (nef″ro-sis-ti′tis) [*nephro-* + *cyst-* + *-itis*] inflammation of the kidney and bladder.

neph·ro·cys·to·sis (nef″ro-sis-to′sis) [*nephro-* + *cyst-* + *-osis*] any cystic disease of the kidney; see also *polycystic kidney disease.*

neph·ro·gas·tric (nef″ro-gas′trik) gastrorenal.

neph·ro·gen·ic (nef″ro-jen′ik) [*nephro-* + *-genic*] forming kidney tissue.

ne·phrog·e·nous (nə-froj′ə-nəs) originating or arising in the kidney.

neph·ro·gram (nef′ro-gram) renogram.

ne·phrog·ra·phy (nə-frog′rə-fe) [*nephro-* + *-graphy*] renography.

neph·ro·hy·dro·sis (nef″ro-hi-dro′sis) hydronephrosis.

neph·roid (nef′roid) [*nephro-* + *-oid*] kidney-shaped, or resembling a kidney.

neph·ro·lith (nef′ro-lith) [*nephro-* + *-lith*] renal calculus.

neph·ro·li·thi·a·sis (nef″ro-lĭ-thi′ə-sis) 1. the formation of renal calculi (see under *calculus*). 2. the diseased condition associated with the presence of renal calculi. Called also *renal lithiasis.*

neph·ro·li·thot·o·my (nef″ro-lĭ-thot′ə-me) [*nephrolith* + *-tomy*] the removal of renal calculi by an incision through the kidney.

percutaneous n. nephrolithotomy using an endoscope that penetrates the skin.

ne·phrol·o·gist (nə-frol′ə-jist) a specialist in nephrology.

ne·phrol·o·gy (nə-frol′ə-je) [*nephro-* + *-logy*] scientific study of the kidney, its anatomy, physiology, pathology, and pathophysiology.

ne·phrol·y·sis (nə-frol′ə-sis) [*nephro-* + *-lysis*] 1. solution of kidney substance. 2. the operation of separating the kidney from paranephric adhesions.

neph·ro·lyt·ic (nef″ro-lit′ik) pertaining to, characterized by, or producing nephrolysis.

ne·phro·ma (nə-fro′mə) [*nephr-* + *-oma*] a tumor of the kidney or of kidney tissue.

benign cystic n. multilocular cyst of kidney.

congenital mesoblastic n. mesoblastic n.

embryonal n. Wilms tumor.

mesoblastic n. a renal tumor similar to Wilms tumor but appearing earlier in infancy and with more infiltration of surrounding tissue.

multilocular cystic n. multilocular cyst of kidney.

neph·ro·ma·la·cia (nef″ro-mə-la′shə) [*nephro-* + *-malacia*] softening of the kidney.

neph·ro·meg·a·ly (nef″ro-meg′ə-le) [*nephro-* + *-megaly*] enlargement of the kidney, such as in compensatory hypertrophy.

neph·ro·mere (nef′ro-mēr) [*nephro-* + *-mere*] nephrotome.

neph·ron (nef′ron) [Gr. *nephros* kidney + *-on* neuter ending] the anatomical and functional unit of the kidney, consisting of the renal corpuscle, the proximal convoluted tubule, the descending and ascending limbs of the loop of Henle (see *ansa nephroni* [TA]), the distal convoluted tubule, and the collecting tubule. See Plate 20.

juxtamedullary n. a nephron whose proximal convoluted tubule is close to the corticomedullary border and whose loop of Henle extends deep into the renal medulla.

superficial n. a nephron whose proximal convoluted tubule is in the outer part of the renal cortex and whose loop of Henle goes only a short way into the renal medulla.

neph·ro·nia (nə-fro′ne-ə) nephropathy.

lobar n. acute pyelonephritis.

neph·ron·oph·thi·sis (nef″ron-of′thĭ-sis) [*nephron* + *phthisis*] wasting disease of the kidney substance.

familial juvenile n. 1. a progressive hereditary disease of the kidneys characterized clinically by anemia, polyuria, and renal loss of sodium, progressing to chronic renal failure; pathological characteristics include tubular atrophy, interstitial fibrosis, glomerular sclerosis, and medullary cysts. Called also *medullary cystic disease, medullary cystic kidney disease,* and *juvenile nephronophthisis–medullary cystic disease complex.* 2. according to some authorities, just one variant of the juvenile nephronophthisis–medullary cystic disease complex, of autosomal recessive inheritance with onset in childhood.

neph·ro·path·ia (nef″ro-path′e-ə) nephropathy.

n. epide′mica a mild, usually asymptomatic form of epidemic hemorrhagic fever with renal manifestations, caused by Puumala virus. Proteinuria, elevated creatine levels, and leukocytosis may occur; it is occasionally hemorrhagic but seldom fatal.

ne·phrop·a·thy (nə-frop′ə-the) [*nephro-* + *-pathy*] any disease of the kidneys; see also *nephritis.* Called also *nephrosis.* **nephropath′ic** *adj*

acute urate n., acute uric acid n. rapidly progressive nephropathy caused by the precipitation of uric acid crystals in the renal tubules, leading to obstruction and acute renal failure, seen especially in patients with lymphoproliferative or myeloproliferative diseases, usually after the induction of chemotherapy.

AIDS n. former name for *HIV-associated n.*

amyloid n. renal amyloidosis.

analgesic n. interstitial nephritis with renal papillary necrosis, seen with excessive use of analgesics, usually aspirin, phenacetin, or acetaminophen alone or in combination.

Balkan n., Balkan endemic n. a slowly progressive type of chronic interstitial nephritis seen in only in farming villages along the Danube river in the Balkan republics. The cause is unknown and has been attributed to chronic heavy metal poisoning such as with lead or cadmium, poisoning by grains containing the mycotoxins citrinin and ochratoxin A, or other factors. Called also *Balkan nephritis.*

BK polyomavirus n., BK virus n. a type of interstitial nephritis caused by infection with BK polyomavirus, seen in kidney transplant recipients owing to immunosuppression; it usually results in transplant loss.

cadmium n. chronic tubulointerstitial nephritis caused by prolonged low-level cadmium poisoning.

cast n. myeloma kidney.

cholemic n. renal disease associated with hepatic or biliary dysfunction, especially types that are accompanied by obstructive jaundice.

chronic urate n., chronic uric acid n. gouty n.

contrast n., contrast-induced n., contrast medium n., contrast medium–induced n. kidney damage by a contrast medium. usually seen in patients already weakened by some other condition such as diabetes mellitus, proteinuria, hypovolemia, multiple myeloma, or preexisting renal insufficiency; there is usually a sharp decline in the glomerular filtration rate after administration of the agent, sometimes with acute renal failure, followed in a few days by return to the patient's previous level of function. Called also *contrast, contrast-induced,* or *contrast medium nephrotoxicity.*

C1q n. a type of immune complex glomerulonephritis with deposits of complement component C1q; signs and symptoms are similar to those of minimal change disease or mild focal segmental glomerulosclerosis.

diabetic n. the nephropathy that commonly accompanies later stages of diabetes mellitus; it begins with hyperfiltration, renal hypertrophy, microalbuminuria, and hypertension; in time, proteinuria develops, with other signs of renal failure leading to end-stage renal disease.

familial juvenile hyperuricemic n. autosomal dominant nephropathy of juvenile onset, with hyperuricemia that may cause gout, decreased glomerular filtration, hypertension, and eventual renal failure. It can be caused by mutation in the *UMOD* gene (locus: 16p12.3), which encodes Tamm-Horsfall protein (also called uromodulin) or can be caused by mutation in the *REN* gene (locus: 1q32), which encodes the enzyme renin.

gouty n. any of a group of chronic kidney diseases associated with the abnormal production and excretion of uric acid; called also *chronic urate* or *uric acid n.*

heavy metal n. the kidney damage resulting from any of various forms of heavy metal poisoning, usually in the form of tubulointerstitial nephritis. See *cadmium n., lead n.,* and *mercury n.*

HIV-associated n., human immunodeficiency virus–associated n. renal pathology in patients infected with the human immunodeficiency virus, similar to focal segmental glomerulosclerosis, with proteinuria, enlarged kidneys, and dilated tubules containing proteinaceous casts; it may progress to end-stage renal disease within weeks.

hypokalemic n. nephropathy with hypokalemia, interstitial nephritis, swelling and vacuolation of proximal renal tubules, and progressive renal failure, resulting from long-term conditions such as oncotic overloading of the kidney filtration mechanisms by sugars. Cf. *potassium-losing n.*

IgA n. a common, chronic form of glomerulonephritis marked by hematuria and proteinuria and by deposits of immunoglobulin A in the mesangial areas of the renal glomeruli, with subsequent reactive hyperplasia of mesangial cells. Called also *Berger disease* and *IgA glomerulonephritis.*

IgM n. mesangial proliferative glomerulonephritis.

immunoglobulin A n. IgA n.

immunoglobulin M n. IgM n.

ischemic n. nephropathy resulting from partial or complete obstruction of a renal artery and the accompanying ischemia; there is a significant reduction in the glomerular filtration rate.

kaliopenic n. hypokalemic n.

lead n. the kidney damage that accompanies lead poisoning; lead deposits appear in the epithelium of the proximal tubules and as nuclear inclusions in cells. In time this leads to chronic tubulointerstitial nephritis with chronic renal failure and other symptoms.

light chain n. nephropathy caused by deposition of abnormal light chains (usually kappa chains but sometimes lambda chains) in renal basement membranes, often with glomerulosclerosis; it may be associated with a plasma cell dyscrasia such as multiple myeloma (see *myeloma kidney*, under *kidney*).

membranous n. see under *glomerulonephritis.*

mercury n. acute tubular necrosis caused by mercury poisoning after ingestion of inorganic mercury salts.

minimal change n. see under *disease.*

mycotoxic n. kidney damage in livestock, usually pigs, due to ochratoxins or citrinin contaminating their food, usually produced by *Penicillium.* Symptoms include edema around the kidneys with degeneration of proximal tubules, fibrosis, polyuria, and enlarged kidneys. Called also *mycotic* or *mold nephrosis.*

myeloma cast n. myeloma kidney.

obstructive n. nephropathy caused by obstruction of the urinary tract (usually the ureter), with hydronephrosis, slowing of the glomerular filtration rate, and tubular abnormalities.

polyomavirus type BK n. BK virus n.

potassium-losing n. hypokalemic nephropathy after persistent potassium loss; it may be seen in metabolic alkalosis, adrenocortical hormone excess, or in intrinsic renal disease such as renal tubular acidosis or juxtaglomerular cell hyperplasia. Called also *potassium-losing nephritis.*

radiocontrast n. contrast n.

reflux n. childhood pyelonephritis in which the renal scarring results from vesicoureteral reflux, with radiological appearance of intrarenal reflux.

salt-losing n. any intrinsic renal disease causing salt wasting; it usually affects the renal medulla (e.g., medullary cystic disease, polycystic kidney disease, pyelonephritis), resulting in volume depletion and hypotension. See also *salt-losing syndrome,* under *syndrome.* Called also *salt-losing nephritis* and *Thorn syndrome.*

saturnine n. lead n.

sickle cell n. chronic kidney pathology seen with sickle cell disease, including microangiopathy with capillary obstruction, dilated or obliterated vasa recta, enlarged glomeruli, interstitial fibrosis, and an increased glomerular filtration rate.

sodium-losing n. salt-losing n.

thin basement membrane n. a rare, autosomal dominant, usually benign disorder characterized by abnormal thinning of the basement membranes of the glomerular capillaries and persistent hematuria; at least some cases are due to mutation in the *COL4A3* or *COL4A4* genes (both at locus 2q36-q37), which each encode an alpha subunit chain of type IV collagen. Called also *benign familial hematuria.*

toxic n. kidney damage caused by the effects of a nephrotoxin; the most common symptoms are dysfunction and then necrosis of the proximal tubules, sometimes progressing to renal failure.

urate n., uric acid n. any of a group of kidney diseases occurring in patients with hyperuricemia, including an acute form (see *acute urate n.*), a chronic form (see *gouty n.*), and nephrolithiasis with formation of uric acid calculi.

vasomotor n. renal dysfunction owing to impairment of blood flow to the kidney that is not severe enough to cause infarction.

neph•ro•pexy (nef′ro-pek″se) [*nephro-* + *-pexy*] the fixation or suspension of a floating kidney.

ne•phroph•thi•sis (nə-frof′thĭ-sis) [*nephro-* + *phthisis*] 1. renal tuberculosis. 2. nephronophthisis.

neph•ro•poi•et•ic (nef″ro-poi-et′ik) [*nephro-* + Gr. *poiein* to make] nephrogenic.

neph•rop•to•sia (nef″rop-to′se-ə) nephroptosis.

neph•rop•to•sis (nef″rop-to′sis, nef″ro-to′sis) [*nephro-* + *-ptosis*] downward displacement of the kidney; called also *floating, hypermobile, movable,* or *wandering kidney.*

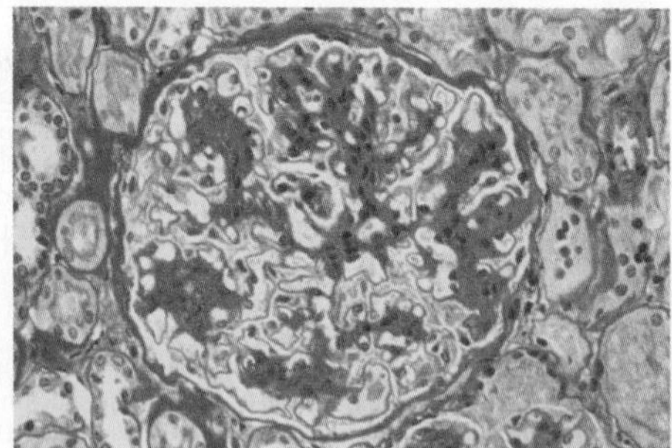

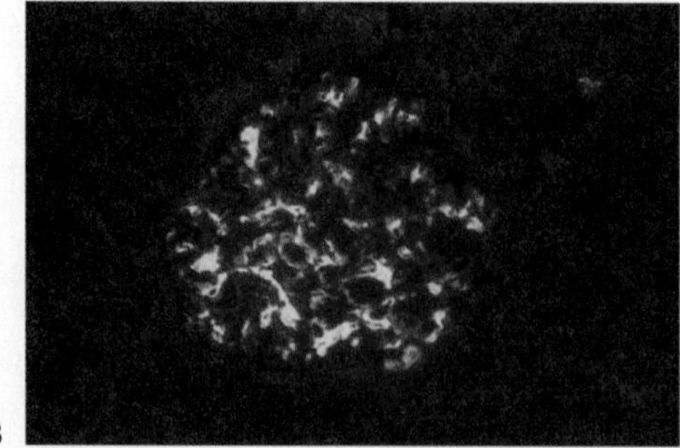

■ IgA nephropathy. *(A)*, Light microscopy showing mesangial proliferation and matrix increase; *(B)*, characteristic immunofluorescence deposition of IgA, principally in mesangial regions.

neph•ro•py•eli•tis (nef″ro-pi″ə-li′tis) [*nephro-* + *pyelitis*] pyelonephritis.

neph•ro•py•elog•ra•phy (nef″ro-pi″ə-log′rə-fe) radiography of the kidney and renal pelvis.

neph•ro•py•elo•li•thot•o•my (nef″ro-pi″ə-lo-lĭ-thot′ə-me) [*nephro-* + *pyelo-* + *lithotomy*] removal of a calculus from the renal pelvis by an incision through the kidney substance.

neph•ror•rha•gia (nef″ro-ra′jə) [*nephro-* + *-rrhagia*] renal hemorrhage.

neph•ror•rha•phy (nef-ror′ə-fe) [*nephro-* + *-rrhaphy*] nephropexy with suturing of the kidney.

neph•ro•scle•ro•sis (nef″ro-sklə-ro′sis) [*nephro-* + *sclerosis*] sclerosis or hardening of the kidney, usually due to renovascular disease.

arteriolar n. nephrosclerosis of arterioles; it usually has an insidious onset and is often associated with hypertension, cylindruria, edema, hypertrophy of the heart, degeneration of renal tubules, and glomerulonephritis, resulting in renal insufficiency, congestive heart failure, and cerebral hemorrhage. Two types are distinguished: *benign* and *malignant* (q.v.). Called also *intercapillary n.* and *glomerulosclerosis.*

benign n., benign arteriolar n. a type of arteriolar nephrosclerosis usually seen in patients over 60 years old and associated with benign hypertension and hyaline arteriolosclerosis; in younger persons it may occur in diabetics with a predisposition to arteriosclerosis and in those with hypertension resulting from an apparent underlying disease such as pheochromocytoma. Called also *hyaline arteriolar n.*

hyaline arteriolar n. benign n.

hyperplastic arteriolar n. malignant n.

hypertensive n. the most common kind of arteriolar nephrosclerosis, due to hypertension of the renal arterioles.

intercapillary n. arteriolar n.

malignant n., malignant arteriolar n. a rare form of arteriolar nephrosclerosis affecting all the vessels of the body, especially small renal arteries and arterioles, often associated with malignant hypertension and hyperplastic arteriolosclerosis. It may occur without previous hypertension or superimposed on benign hypertension or primary renal disease, especially glomerulonephritis, benign nephrosclerosis, or pyelonephritis. Called also *hyperplastic arteriolar n.* and *Fahr-Volhard disease.*

neph•ro•scope (nef′ro-skōp) an endoscope inserted into an incision in the renal pelvis for viewing the inside of the kidney; there are both rigid types and flexible types with three channels (for telescope, fiberoptic light input, and irrigation).

neph•ros•co•py (nə-fros′kə-pe) visualization of the kidney with a nephroscope. Called also *renoscopy.*

ne•phro•ses (nə-fro′sēz) plural of *nephrosis.*

ne•phro•sis (nə-fro′sis) pl. *nephro′ses* [*nephr-* + *-osis*] 1. nephropathy. 2. any disease of the kidneys that includes purely degenerative lesions of the tubules.

amyloid n. renal amyloidosis.

infectious avian n. infectious bursal disease.

lipid n., lipoid n. minimal change disease.

mold n., mycotic n. mycotoxic nephropathy.

necrotizing n. renal disease characterized by necrosis of the tubular epithelium.

neph•ro•so•ne•phri•tis (nə-fro″so-nə-fri′tis) [*nephrosis* + *nephritis*] renal disease with nephrotic and nephritic components.

hemorrhagic n., Korean hemorrhagic n. epidemic hemorrhagic fever.

neph•ro•so•nog•ra•phy (nef″ro-so-nog′rə-fe) ultrasonic scanning of the kidney.

ne•phros•to•gram (nə-fros′to-gram) [*nephrostomy* + *-gram*] radiographic inspection of a nephrostomy after injection of contrast material into the kidney.

ne•phros•to•li•thot•o•my (nə-fros″to-lĭ-thot′ə-me) [*nephrostomy* + *lithotomy*] removal of renal calculi through a nephrostomy tube inserted through the abdominal wall into the renal pelvis.

ne•phros•to•ma (nə-fros′tə-mə) [*nephro-* + *stoma*] one of the funnel-shaped and ciliated orifices of excretory tubules that open into the coelom in the embryo, best seen in lower vertebrates.

neph•ro•stome (nef′ro-stōm) nephrostoma.

ne•phros•to•my (nə-fros′tə-me) [*nephro-* + *-stomy*] insertion of a catheter from the surface of the skin through the renal parenchyma into the renal pelvis, under the sonographic or fluoroscopic guidance, as for urinary diversion or insertion of a catheter, or to gain access to the upper urinary tract as for dilation of a stricture or removal of a calculus. Called also *percutaneous n.*

ne•phrot•ic (nə-frot′ik) pertaining to, resembling, or caused by nephrosis.

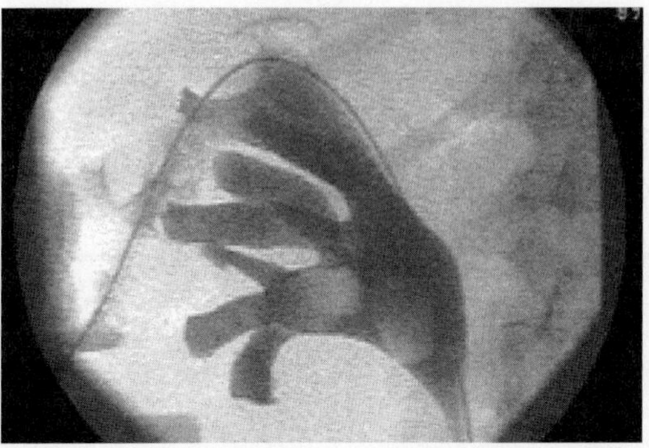

■ Nephrostomy, with a subcostal point of entry and the guidewire advanced into the ureter.

neph•ro•tome (nef′ro-tōm) one of the segmented divisions of the mesoderm connecting the somite with the lateral plates of unsegmented mesoderm; it is the source of much of the urogenital system. Called also *intermediate cell mass* and *middle plate.*

neph•ro•to•mo•gram (nef″ro-to′mo-gram) the sectional radiograph of the kidney obtained by nephrotomography.

neph•ro•to•mog•ra•phy (nef″ro-to-mog′rə-fe) radiologic visualization of the kidney by tomography after intravenous introduction of contrast medium as a bolus or by infusion. **nephrotomograph′ic** *adj*

ne•phrot•o•my (nə-frot′ə-me) [*nephro-* + *-tomy*] a surgical incision into the kidney.

abdominal n. nephrotomy performed through an incision into the abdomen.

anatrophic n. incision into the kidney between its vascular segments, to minimize bleeding and parenchymal injury and to prevent atrophy.

lumbar n. nephrotomy performed through an incision in the lumbar region.

neph•ro•tox•ic (nef′ro-tok″sik) toxic or destructive to kidney cells.

neph•ro•tox•ic•i•ty (nef″ro-tok-sis′ĭ-te) the quality of being toxic or destructive to kidney cells.

contrast n., contrast agent n., contrast-induced n., contrast medium n. see under *nephropathy.*

neph•ro•tox•in (nef′ro-tok″sin) [*nephro-* + *toxin*] a toxin that has a specific destructive effect on kidney cells.

neph•ro•tro•pic (nef″ro-tro′pik) renotropic (def. 1).

neph•ro•tu•ber•cu•lo•sis (nef″ro-too-bur″ku-lo′sis) [*nephro-* + *tuberculosis*] renal tuberculosis.

neph•ro•ure•ter•ec•to•my (nef″ro-u-re″tər-ek′tə-me) [*nephro-* + *ureterectomy*] excision of a kidney and all or part of the ureter; called also *ureteronephrectomy.*

neph•ro•ure•tero•cys•tec•to•my (nef″ro-u-re″tər-o-sis-tek′tə-me) [*nephro-* + *uretero-* + *cystectomy*] excision of the kidney, ureter, and part or all of the bladder.

neph•ro•u•re•ter•os•co•py (nef″ro-u-re″tər-os′kə-pe) ureterorenoscopy.

Nep•ta•zane (nep′tə-zān) trademark for a preparation of methazolamide.

nep•tu•ni•um (Np) (nep-too′ne-əm) [from planet *Neptune*] a radioactive element of atomic number 93 and atomic weight 237, occurring in certain earths and obtained by splitting the uranium atom with neutrons. It is unstable and changes into plutonium.

ne•quin•ate (nə-kwin′āt) a coccidiostat for poultry.

NER nucleotide excision repair.

Ne•ri sign (na′re) [Vincenzo *Neri*, Italian neurologist, early 20th century] see under *sign.*

Ne•ri•um (ne′re-əm) a genus of evergreen shrubs of the family Apocynaceae, native to the Mediterranean region and Asia, including the oleanders; most species contain toxic glycosides (see *oleandrism*). Common species include *N. olean′der* and *N. in′dicum.*

N. olean′der L., the common oleander, a popular ornamental flowering garden plant; its roots, flowers, seeds, and bark contain toxic cardiac glycosides. See *oleandrism.*

Nernst equation, potential (nernst) [Walther Hermann *Nernst*, German physical chemist, 1864–1941] see under *equation* and *potential.*

nerve (nurv) [L. *nervus*] a cordlike structure made up of a collection of fibers that convey impulses between a part of the central nervous system and some other region of the body. A nerve consists of a connective tissue sheath (epineurium) enclosing bundles of fibers (funiculi or fasciculi); each bundle is in turn surrounded by its own sheath of connective tissue (perineurium), the inner surface of which is formed by a membrane of flattened mesothelial cells. Very small nerves may consist of only one funiculus derived from the parent nerve. Within each such bundle, the individual nerve fibers, which are microscopic in size, are surrounded by interstitial connective tissue (endoneurium). An individual nerve fiber (an axon with its covering sheath) consists of formed elements in a matrix of protoplasm (axoplasm), the entire structure being enclosed in a thin membrane (axolemma). Each nerve fiber is enclosed by a cellular sheath (neurilemma), from which it may or may not be separated by a lipid layer (myelin sheath) derived from neurilemmal cells. In official terminology called *nervus.*

Nerve

For names and descriptions of specific nerves, see under *nervus.*

abducens n., abducent n. nervus abducens.
n. to abductor digiti minimi of foot Baxter n.
accelerator n's the cardiac sympathetic nerves, which, when stimulated, accelerate the action of the heart.
accessory n., accessory n., spinal nervus accessorius.
accessory n., vagal ramus internus nervi accessorii.
acoustic n. nervus vestibulocochlearis.
afferent n. any nerve that transmits impulses from the periphery toward the central nervous system, as a sensory nerve; cf. *efferent n.*
alveolar n., inferior nervus alveolaris inferior.
alveolar n's, superior nervi alveolares superiores.
ampullary n., anterior nervus ampullaris anterior.
ampullary n., inferior nervus ampullaris posterior.
ampullary n., lateral nervus ampullaris lateralis.
ampullary n., posterior nervus ampullaris posterior.
ampullary n., superior nervus ampullaris anterior.
anal n's, inferior nervi anales inferiores.
Andersch n. nervus tympanicus.
anococcygeal n. nervus anococcygeus.
antebrachial cutaneous n., lateral nervus cutaneus antebrachii lateralis.
antebrachial cutaneous n., medial nervus cutaneus antebrachii medialis.
antebrachial cutaneous n., posterior nervus cutaneus antebrachii posterior.
aortic n. Cyon n.
Arnold n. ramus auricularis nervi vagi.
articular n. any mixed peripheral nerve that supplies a joint and its associated structures. See also *rami articulares,* under *ramus.*
auditory n. nervus vestibulocochlearis.
auricular n's, anterior nervi auriculares anteriores.
auricular n., great nervus auricularis magnus.
auricular n., internal ramus posterior nervi auricularis magni.
auricular n., posterior nervus auricularis posterior.
auricular n. of vagus n. ramus auricularis nervi vagi.
auriculotemporal n. nervus auriculotemporalis.
autonomic n. nervus autonomicus.
axillary n. nervus axillaris.
Baxter n. the first branch of the lateral plantar nerve, arising near the bifurcation of the tibial nerve (or sometimes from the tibial nerve itself), passing deep to the abductor hallucis muscle, and ending on the abductor digiti minimi muscle; it sends small sensory branches to the skin of the lateral sole and motor branches to the abductor the abductor digiti minimi, flexor digitorum brevis, and quadratus plantae muscles. Called also *n. to abductor digiti minimi of foot.*
Bell n. nervus thoracicus longus.
brachial cutaneous n., inferior lateral nervus cutaneus brachii lateralis inferior.
brachial cutaneous n., medial nervus cutaneus brachii medialis.
brachial cutaneous n., posterior nervus cutaneus brachii posterior.
brachial cutaneous n., superior lateral nervus cutaneus brachii lateralis superior.
buccal n., buccinator n. nervus buccalis.
cardiac n., inferior nervus cardiacus cervicalis inferior.
cardiac n., middle nervus cardiacus cervicalis medius.
cardiac n., superior nervus cardiacus cervicalis superior.
cardiac n's, supreme rami cardiaci cervicales superiores nervi vagi.
cardiac n's, thoracic rami cardiaci thoracici.
caroticotympanic n's nervi caroticotympanici.
caroticotympanic n., inferior see *nervi caroticotympanici.*
caroticotympanic n., superior see *nervi caroticotympanici.*
carotid n's, external nervi carotici externi.
carotid n., internal nervus caroticus internus.
cavernosal n's see *nervi cavernosi clitoridis* and *nervi cavernosi penis,* under *nervus.*
cavernous n's of clitoris nervi cavernosi clitoridis.
cavernous n's of penis nervi cavernosi penis; see also *greater* and *lesser cavernous n's of penis.*
cavernous n. of penis, greater a cavernous nerve on the dorsum penis running forward from the plexus prostaticus to supply erectile tissue of the corpus cavernosum penis and the corpus spongiosum.
cavernous n's of penis, lesser cavernous nerves that pierce the proximal tunic of the corpus spongiosum penis and supply the urethra and erectile tissue in the corpus spongiosum.
celiac n's rami coeliaci nervi vagi.
centrifugal n. efferent n.
centripetal n. afferent n.
cerebral n's nervi craniales.
cervical n's nervi cervicales.
cervical n., descending radix inferior ansae cervicalis.
cervical n., transverse nervus transversus colli.
cervical cardiac n., inferior nervus cardiacus cervicalis inferior.
cervical cardiac n., middle nervus cardiacus cervicalis medius.
cervical cardiac n., superior nervus cardiacus cervicalis superior.
chorda tympani n. see *chorda tympani.*
ciliary n's, long nervi ciliares longi.
ciliary n's, short nervi ciliares breves.
circumflex n. nervus axillaris.
cluneal n's, inferior nervi clunium inferiores.
cluneal n's, middle nervi clunium medii.
cluneal n's, superior nervi clunium superiores.
coccygeal n. nervus coccygeus.
cochlear n. nervus cochlearis.
n. of Cotunnius nervus nasopalatinus.
cranial n's nervi craniales.
cranial n., first nervus olfactorius.
cranial n., second nervus opticus.
cranial n., third nervus oculomotorius.
cranial n., fourth nervus trochlearis.
cranial n., fifth nervus trigeminus.
cranial n., sixth nervus abducens.
cranial n., seventh nervus facialis.
cranial n., eighth nervus vestibulocochlearis.
cranial n., ninth nervus glossopharyngeus.
cranial n., tenth nervus vagus.
cranial n., eleventh nervus accessorius.
cranial n., twelfth nervus hypoglossus.
crural interosseous n. nervus interosseus cruris.
cubital n. nervus ulnaris.
cutaneous n. any mixed peripheral nerve that supplies a region of the skin. See also *rami cutanei,* under *ramus.*
cutaneous n's, femoral see *cutaneous n. of thigh, intermediate; cutaneous n. of thigh, medial; nervus cutaneus femoris lateralis;* and *nervus cutaneus femoris posterior.*
cutaneous n., perforating nervus cutaneus perforans.
cutaneous n. of abdomen, anterior ramus cutaneus anterior [pectoralis/abdominalis] ramorum ventralium nervorum thoracicorum.
cutaneous n. of arm, inferior lateral nervus cutaneus brachii lateralis inferior.
cutaneous n. of arm, medial nervus cutaneus brachii medialis.
cutaneous n. of arm, posterior nervus cutaneus brachii posterior.
cutaneous n. of arm, superior lateral nervus cutaneus brachii lateralis superior.
cutaneous n. of calf, lateral nervus cutaneus surae lateralis.
cutaneous n. of calf, medial nervus cutaneus surae medialis.

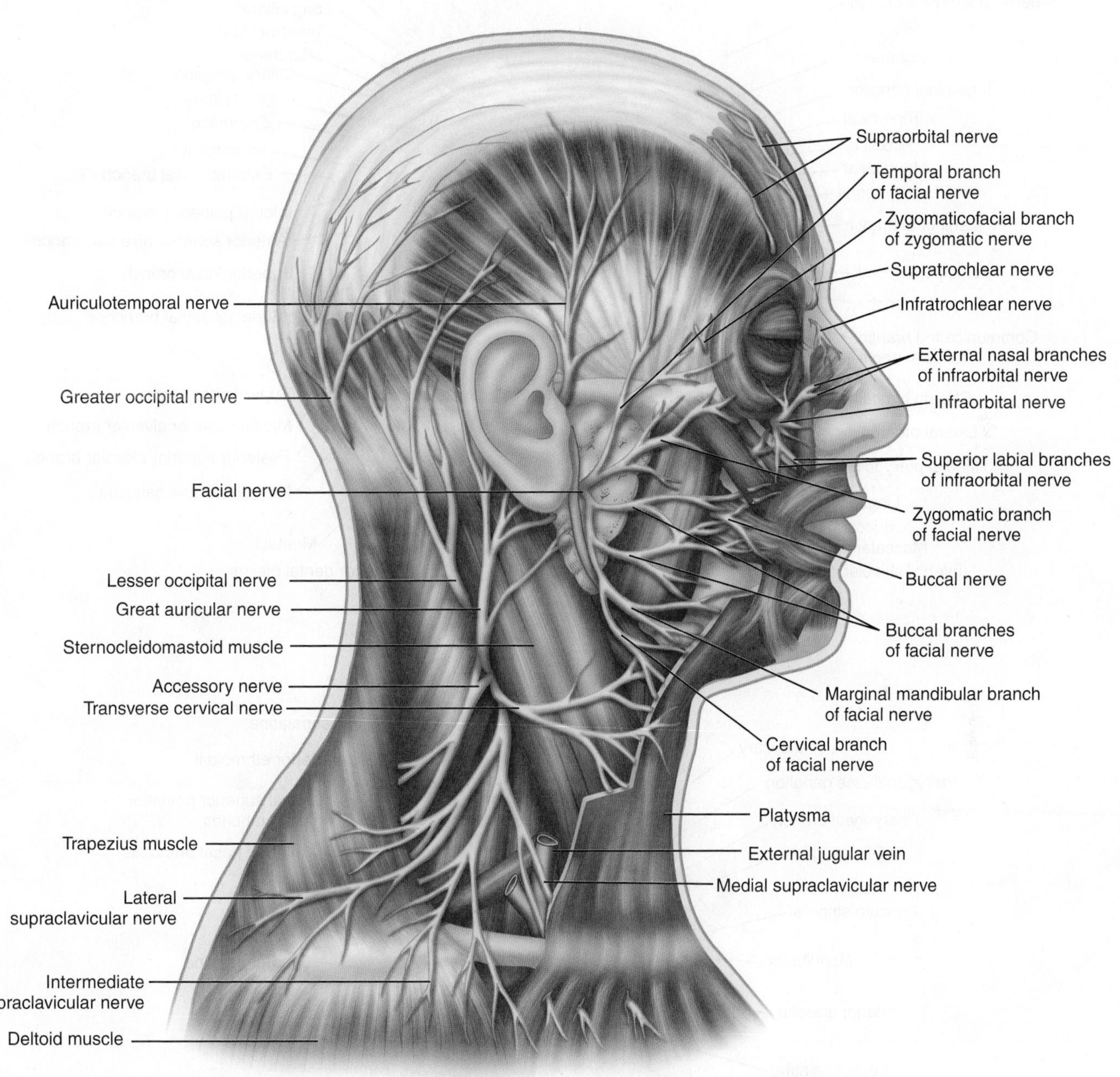

■ **PLATE 33**—SUPERFICIAL NERVES AND MUSCLES OF THE HEAD AND NECK

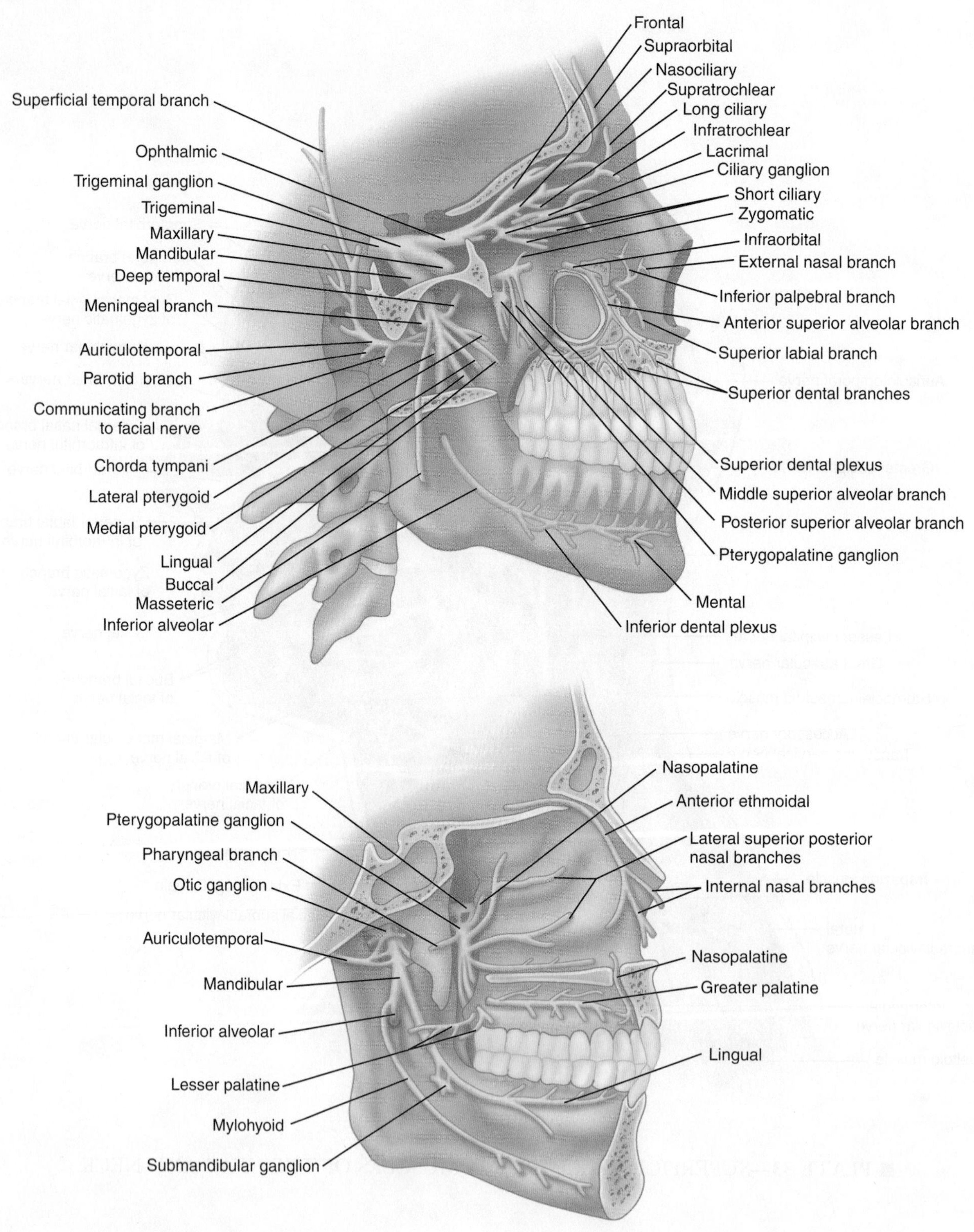

■ **PLATE 34**—DEEP NERVES SHOWN IN RELATION TO BONES OF THE FACE

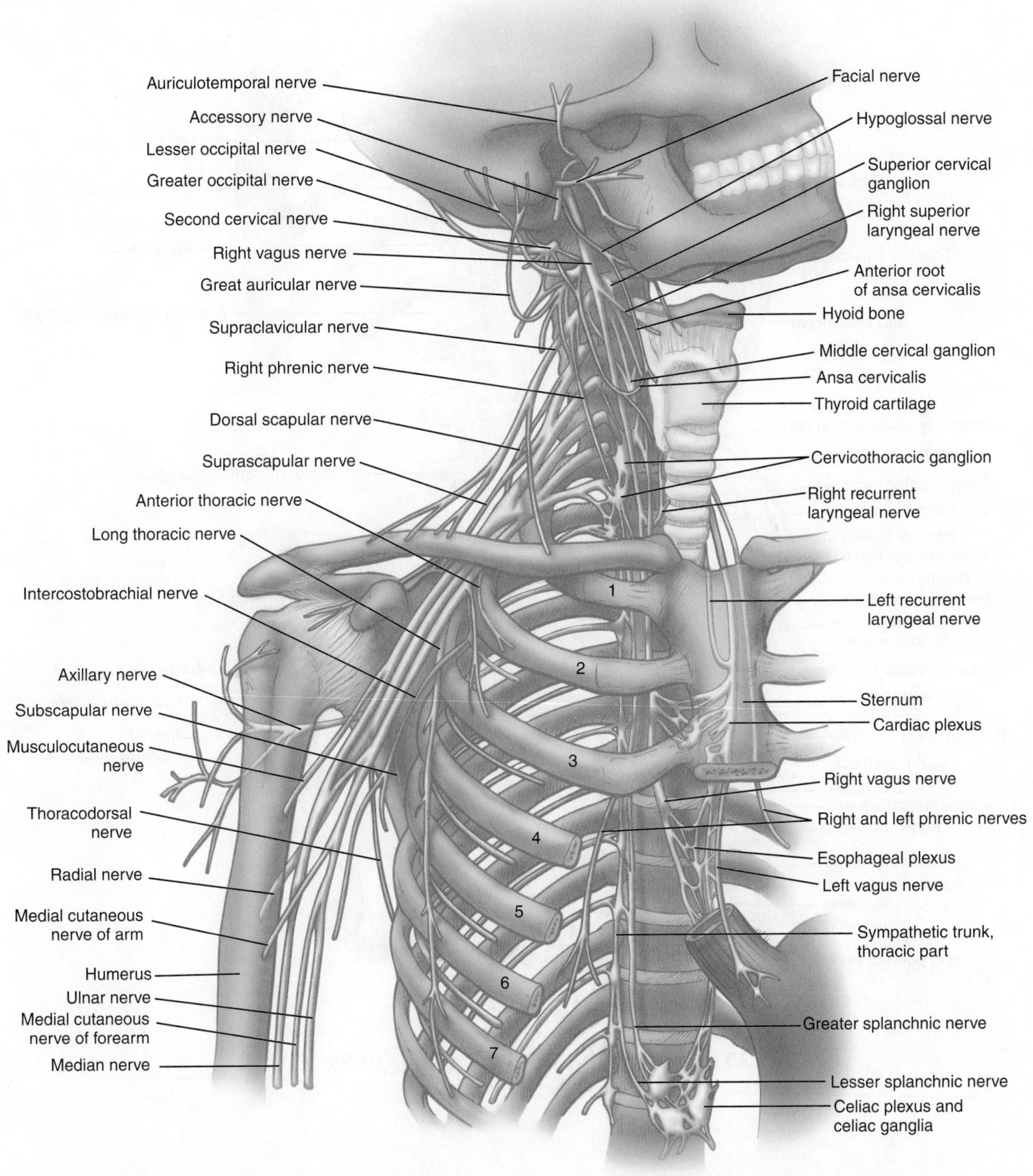

■ **PLATE 35**—DEEP NERVES OF THE NECK, AXILLA, AND UPPER THORAX

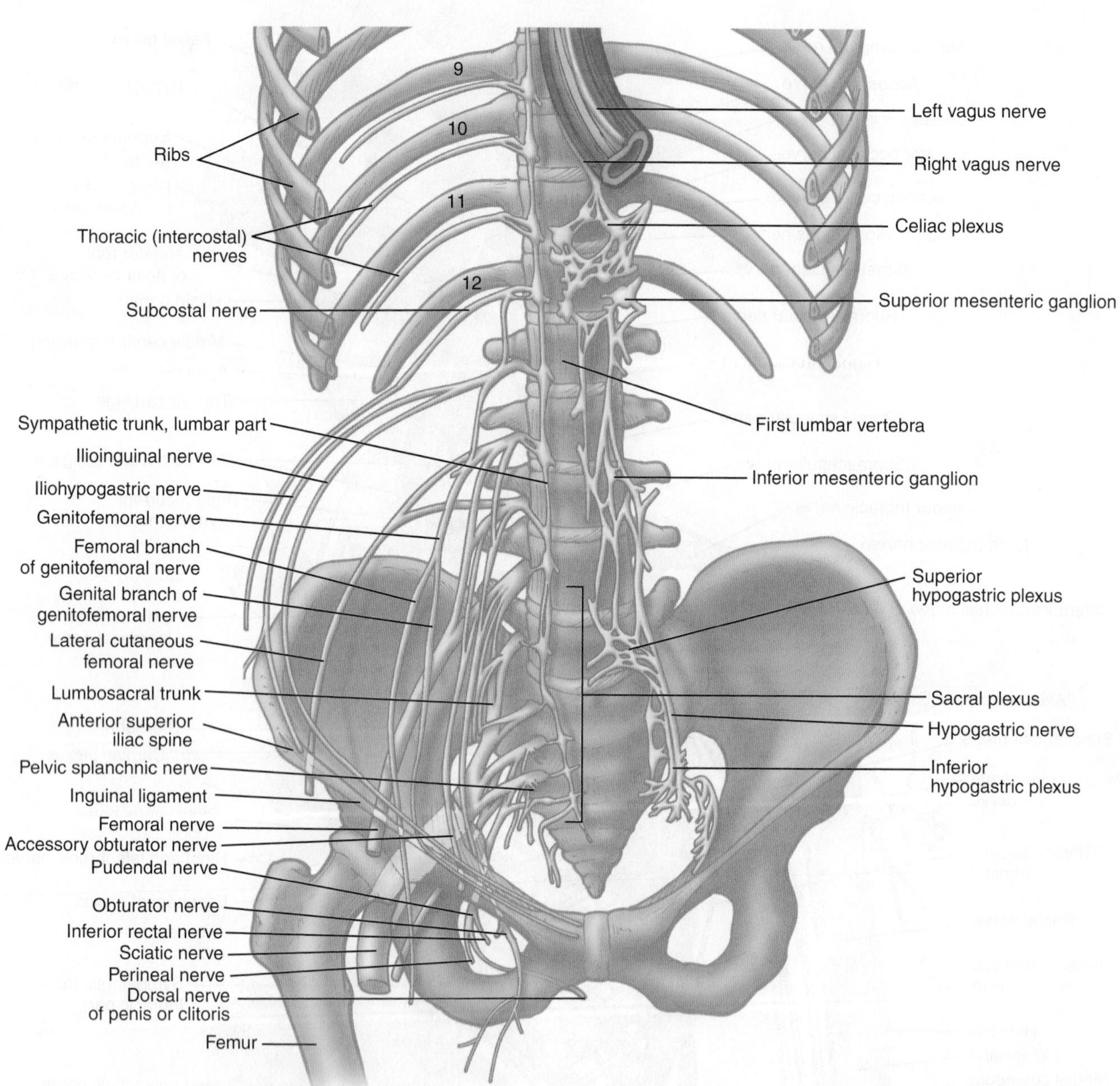

■ **PLATE 36**—DEEP NERVES OF THE LOWER TRUNK

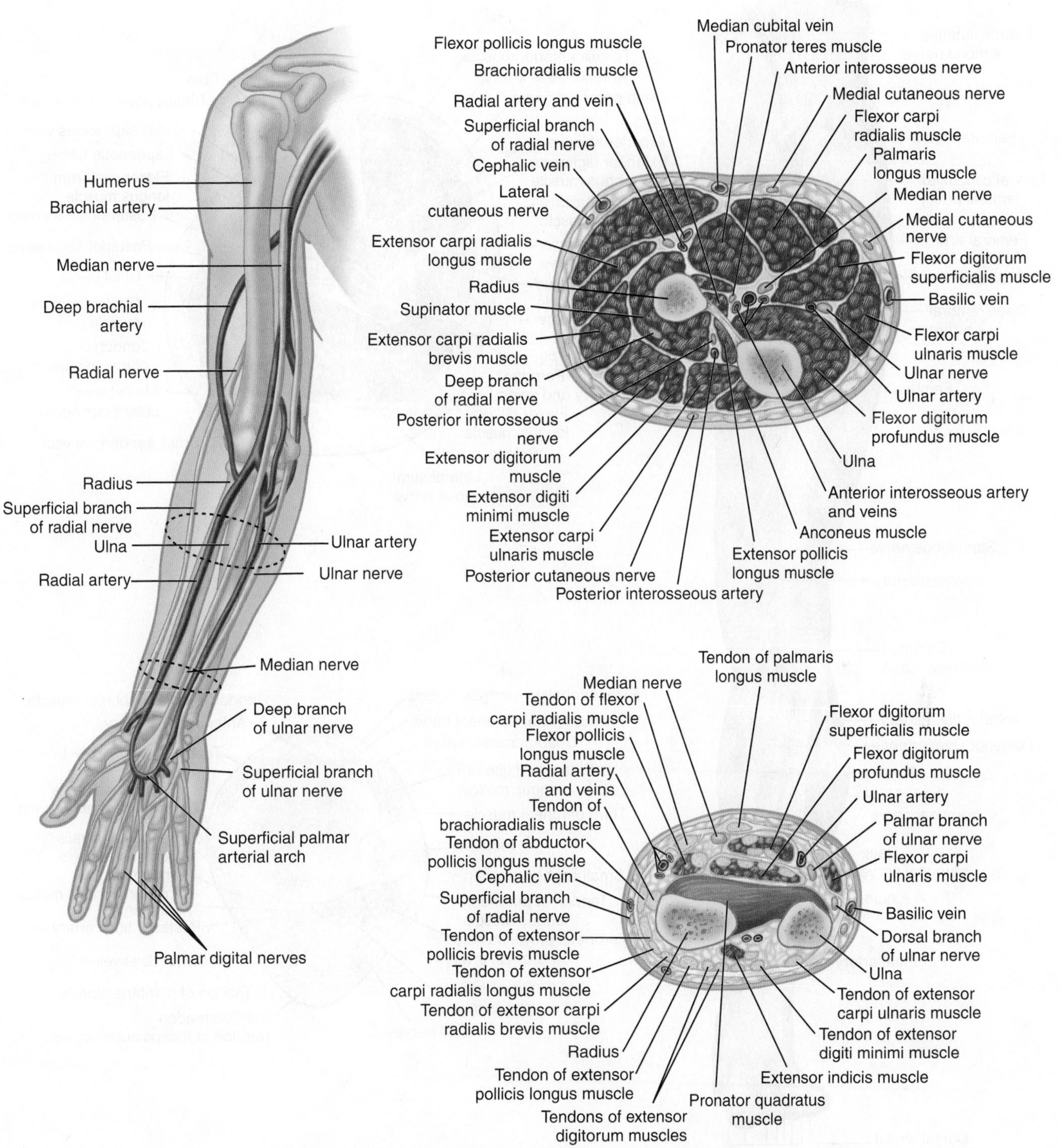

■ **PLATE 37**—NERVES OF THE UPPER LIMB

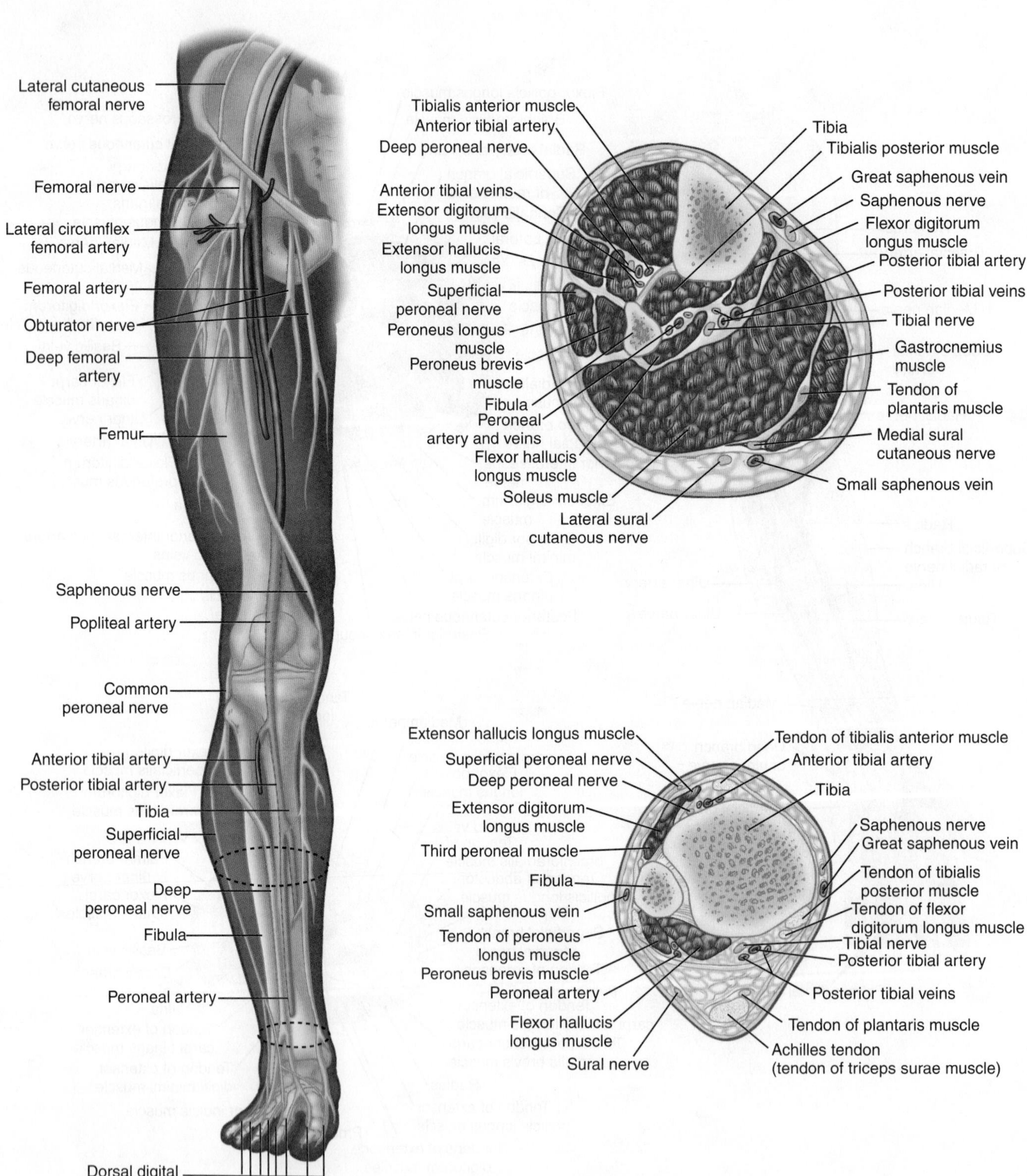

■ **PLATE 38**—NERVES OF THE LOWER LIMB

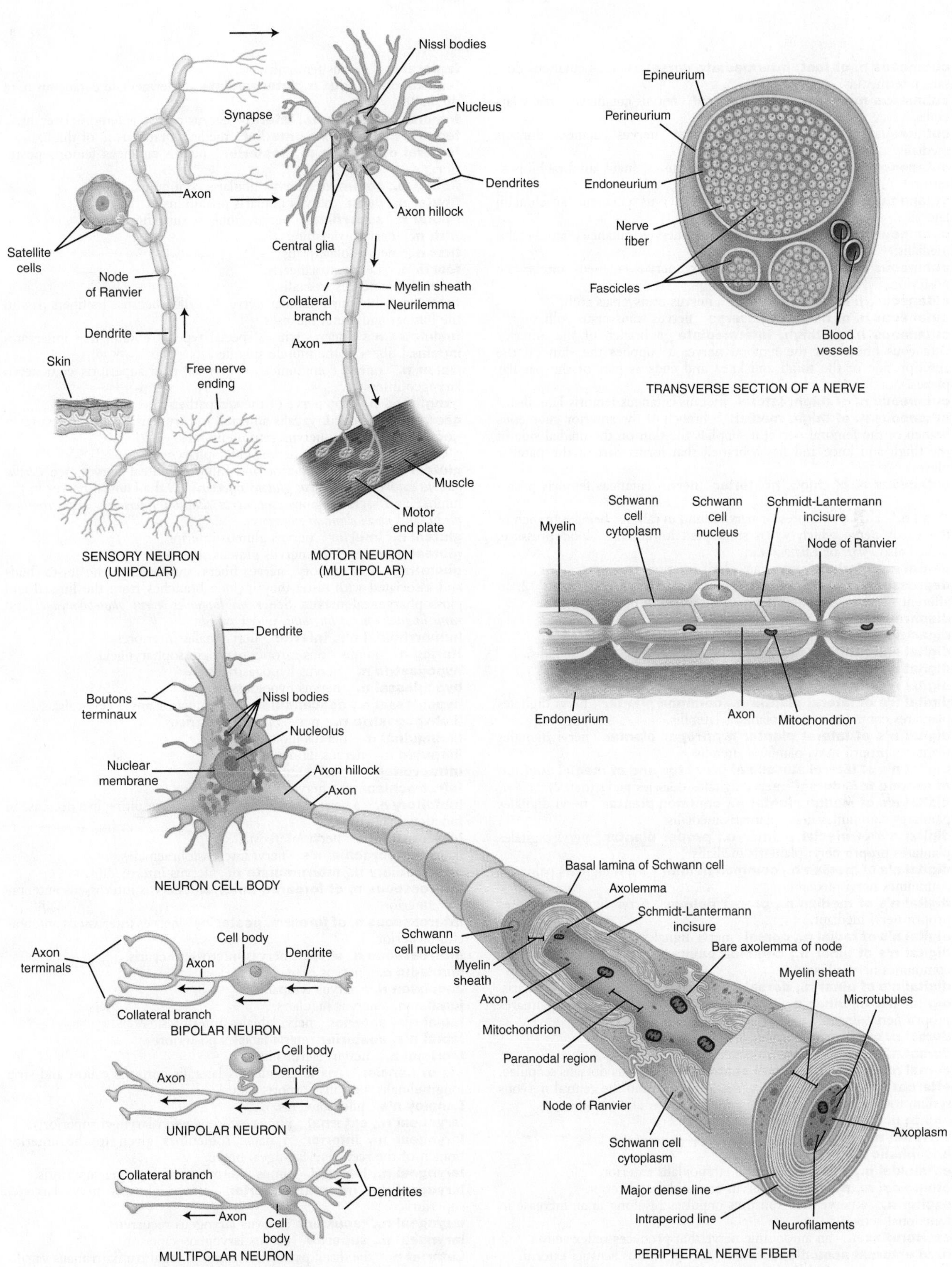

■ **PLATE 39—STRUCTURE OF NERVE TISSUE**

Nerve *Continued*

cutaneous n. of foot, intermediate dorsal nervus cutaneus dorsalis intermedius.
cutaneous n. of foot, lateral dorsal nervus cutaneus dorsalis lateralis.
cutaneous n. of foot, medial dorsal nervus cutaneus dorsalis medialis.
cutaneous n. of forearm, dorsal nervus cutaneus antebrachii posterior.
cutaneous n. of forearm, lateral nervus cutaneus antebrachii lateralis.
cutaneous n. of forearm, medial nervus cutaneus antebrachii medialis.
cutaneous n. of forearm, posterior nervus cutaneus antebrachii posterior.
cutaneous n. of neck, anterior nervus transversus colli.
cutaneous n. of neck, transverse nervus transversus colli.
cutaneous n. of thigh, intermediate a branch of the anterior cutaneous branch of the femoral nerve; it supplies the skin on the anterior side of the thigh and knee and ends as part of the patellar plexus.
cutaneous n. of thigh, lateral nervus cutaneus femoris lateralis.
cutaneous n. of thigh, medial a branch of the anterior cutaneous branch of the femoral nerve; it supplies the skin on the medial side of the thigh and knee and has a branch that forms part of the patellar plexus.
cutaneous n. of thigh, posterior nervus cutaneus femoris posterior.
Cyon n. a type of depressor nerve found in rabbits, being a branch of the vagus nerve which when stimulated lowers the blood pressure. Called also *aortic* or *Ludwig n.*
dental n., inferior nervus alveolaris inferior.
depressor n. 1. a nerve that lessens the activity of an organ. 2. an afferent nerve whose stimulation causes a fall in blood pressure.
diaphragmatic n. nervus phrenicus.
digastric n. ramus digastricus nervi facialis.
digital n's, radial dorsal nervi digitales dorsales nervi radialis.
digital n's, ulnar dorsal nervi digitales dorsales nervi ulnaris.
digital n's of foot, dorsal nervi digitales dorsales pedis.
digital n's of lateral plantar n., common plantar nervi digitales plantares communes nervi plantaris lateralis.
digital n's of lateral plantar n., proper plantar nervi digitales plantares proprii nervi plantaris lateralis.
digital n's of lateral surface of great toe and of medial surface of second toe, dorsal nervi digitales dorsales pedis (def. 2).
digital n's of medial plantar n., common plantar nervi digitales plantares communes nervi plantaris medialis.
digital n's of medial plantar n., proper plantar nervi digitales plantares proprii nervi plantaris medialis.
digital n's of median n., common palmar nervi digitales palmares communes nervi mediani.
digital n's of median n., proper palmar nervi digitales palmares proprii nervi mediani.
digital n's of radial n., dorsal nervi digitales dorsales nervi radialis.
digital n's of ulnar n., common palmar nervi digitales palmares communes nervi ulnaris.
digital n's of ulnar n., dorsal nervi digitales dorsales nervi ulnaris.
digital n's of ulnar n., proper palmar nervi digitales palmares proprii nervi ulnaris.
dorsal n. of clitoris nervus dorsalis clitoridis.
dorsal n. of penis nervus dorsalis penis.
dorsal n. of scapula, dorsal scapular n. nervus dorsalis scapulae.
efferent n. any nerve that carries impulses from the central nervous system toward the periphery, as a motor nerve; cf. *afferent n.*
eighth n. nervus vestibulocochlearis.
eleventh n. nervus accessorius.
encephalic n's nervi craniales.
ethmoidal n., anterior nervus ethmoidalis anterior.
ethmoidal n., posterior nervus ethmoidalis posterior.
excitor n. a nerve that transmits impulses resulting in an increase in functional activity.
excitoreflex n. an autonomic nerve that produces reflex action.
n. of external acoustic meatus nervus meatus acustici externi.
facial n. nervus facialis.
facial n., temporal see *rami temporales nervi facialis.*
femoral n. nervus femoralis.
femoral cutaneous n., intermediate intermediate cutaneous n. of thigh.
femoral cutaneous n., lateral nervus cutaneus femoris lateralis.
femoral cutaneous n., medial medial cutaneous n. of thigh.
femoral cutaneous n., posterior nervus cutaneus femoris posterior.
fibular n., common nervus fibularis communis.
fibular n., deep nervus fibularis profundus.
fibular n., superficial nervus fibularis superficialis.
fifth n. nervus trigeminus.
first n. nervus olfactorius.
fourth n. nervus trochlearis.
frontal n. nervus frontalis.
furcal n. the fourth lumbar nerve, so called because its fibers pass to the lumbar and sacral plexuses.
fusimotor n's nerves with a special type of ending that innervates intrafusal fibers of the muscle spindle.
Galen n. ramus communicans nervi laryngei superioris cum nervo laryngeo inferiore.
gangliated n. any nerve of the sympathetic nervous system.
gastric n's truncus vagalis anterior and truncus vagalis posterior.
genitofemoral n. nervus genitofemoralis.
glossopharyngeal n. nervus glossopharyngeus.
gluteal n's 1. the superior and inferior gluteal nerves; see *nervus gluteus superior* and *nervus gluteus inferior.* 2. the cluneal nerves in the lumbar and sacral regions; see *nervi clunium inferiores, nervi clunium medii,* and *nervi clunium superiores.*
gluteal n., inferior nervus gluteus inferior.
gluteal n., superior nervus gluteus superior.
gustatory n's sensory nerve fibers innervating the taste buds and associated with taste; they include branches from the lingual and glossopharyngeal nerves. See *rami linguales nervi glossopharyngei* and *rami linguales nervi lingualis,* under *ramus.*
hemorrhoidal n's, inferior nervi anales inferiores.
Hering n. ramus sinus carotici nervi glossopharyngei.
hypogastric n. nervus hypogastricus.
hypoglossal n. nervus hypoglossus.
hypoglossal n., descending radix superior ansae cervicalis.
iliohypogastric n. nervus iliohypogastricus.
ilioinguinal n. nervus ilioinguinalis.
iliopubic n. nervus iliohypogastricus.
infraorbital n. nervus infraorbitalis.
infratrochlear n. nervus infratrochlearis.
inhibitory n. a nerve that transmits impulses resulting in a decrease in functional activity.
intercostal n's nervi intercostales.
intercostobrachial n's nervi intercostobrachiales.
intermediary n., intermediate n. nervus intermedius.
interosseous n. of forearm, anterior nervus interosseus antebrachii anterior.
interosseous n. of forearm, posterior nervus interosseus antebrachii posterior.
interosseous n. of leg nervus interosseus cruris.
ischiadic n. nervus ischiadicus.
Jacobson n. nervus tympanicus.
jugular n. nervus jugularis.
labial n's, anterior nervi labiales anteriores.
labial n's, posterior nervi labiales posteriores.
lacrimal n. nervus lacrimalis.
n's of Lancisi stria longitudinalis lateralis corporis callosi and stria longitudinalis medialis corporis callosi.
Langley n's pilomotor n's.
laryngeal n., external ramus externus nervi laryngei superioris.
laryngeal n., inferior a name sometimes given to the anterior branch of the recurrent laryngeal nerve.
laryngeal n., internal ramus internus nervi laryngei superioris.
laryngeal n., internal superior ramus internus nervi laryngei superioris.
laryngeal n., recurrent nervus laryngeus recurrens.
laryngeal n., superior nervus laryngeus superior.
Latarjet n. the distal part of the anterior vagal trunk (truncus vagalis anterior), which runs along the lesser curvature of the stomach.
n. to lateral pterygoid nervus pterygoideus lateralis.

Nerve *Continued*

n. to levator ani a branch of the sacral plexus that innervates the levator ani muscle.
lingual n. nervus lingualis.
longitudinal n's of Lancisi stria longitudinalis lateralis corporis callosi and stria longitudinalis medialis corporis callosi.
Ludwig n. Cyon n.
lumbar n's nervi lumbales.
lumboinguinal n. ramus femoralis nervi genitofemoralis.
n. of Luschka 1. ramus meningeus nervorum spinalium. 2. nervus ethmoidalis posterior.
mandibular n. nervus mandibularis.
masseteric n. nervus massetericus.
maxillary n. nervus maxillaris.
n. to medial pterygoid nervus pterygoideus medialis.
median n. nervus medianus.
meningeal n. ramus meningeus nervi maxillaris.
mental n. nervus mentalis.
mixed n., n. of mixed fibers nervus mixtus.
motor n. nervus motorius.
motor n. of tongue nervus hypoglossus.
musculocutaneous n. nervus musculocutaneus.
musculocutaneous n. of leg nervus fibularis superficialis.
musculospiral n. nervus radialis.
myelinated n. a nerve, especially a peripheral nerve, whose fibers (axons) are encased in a myelin sheath, which in turn is enclosed by a neurilemma. Cf. *unmyelinated n.*
mylohyoid n., n. to mylohyoid nervus mylohyoideus.
nasociliary n. nervus nasociliaris.
nasopalatine n. nervus nasopalatinus.
ninth n. nervus glossopharyngeus.
obturator n. nervus obturatorius.
obturator n., accessory nervus obturatorius accessorius.
obturator n., internal nervus musculi obturatorii interni.
n. to obturator internus, n. to obturator internus and gemellus superior nervus musculi obturatorii interni.
occipital n., greater nervus occipitalis major.
occipital n., least nervus occipitalis tertius.
occipital n., lesser, occipital n., smaller nervus occipitalis minor.
occipital n., third nervus occipitalis tertius.
oculomotor n. nervus oculomotorius.
olfactory n. 1. nervus olfactorius. 2. *(in the pl.)* fila olfactoria.
ophthalmic n. nervus ophthalmicus.
optic n. nervus opticus.
pain n. a sensory nerve that conducts stimuli producing the sensation of pain.
palatine n., anterior nervus palatinus major.
palatine n., greater nervus palatinus major.
palatine n's, lesser nervi palatini minores.
palatine n., medial, palatine n., middle see *nervi palatini minores.*
palatine n., posterior see *nervi palatini minores.*
parasympathetic n. any of the nerves of the parasympathetic nervous system (see under *system*).
parotid n's rami parotidei nervi auriculotemporalis.
n. to pectineus a branch of the femoral nerve that begins just below the inguinal ligament and innervates the pectineus muscle.
pectoral n., lateral nervus pectoralis lateralis.
pectoral n., medial nervus pectoralis medialis.
perforating cutaneous n. nervus cutaneus perforans.
perineal n's nervi perineales.
peripheral n. any nerve outside the central nervous system.
peroneal n., accessory deep nervus peroneus profundus accessorius.
peroneal n., common nervus fibularis communis.
peroneal n., deep nervus fibularis profundus.
peroneal n., superficial nervus fibularis superficialis.
petrosal n., deep nervus petrosus profundus.
petrosal n., greater, petrosal n., greater superficial nervus petrosus major.
petrosal n., lesser, petrosal n., lesser superficial nervus petrosus minor.
pharyngeal n. nervus pharyngeus.
phrenic n. nervus phrenicus.
phrenic n's, accessory nervi phrenici accessorii.
phrenicoabdominal n's rami phrenicoabdominales nervi phrenici.
pilomotor n's the nerves that supply the arrectores pilorum muscles.
pineal n. nervus pinealis.
piriform n., n. to piriformis nervus musculi piriformis.
plantar n., lateral nervus plantaris lateralis.
plantar n., medial nervus plantaris medialis.
pneumogastric n. nervus vagus.
popliteal n., lateral nervus fibularis communis.
popliteal n., medial nervus tibialis.
presacral n. plexus hypogastricus superior.
pressor n. any afferent nerve whose irritation stimulates a vasomotor center and increases intravascular tension.
pterygoid n., external nervus pterygoideus lateralis.
pterygoid n., internal nervus pterygoideus medialis.
pterygoid n., lateral nervus pterygoideus lateralis.
pterygoid n., medial nervus pterygoideus medialis.
n. of pterygoid canal nervus canalis pterygoidei.
pterygopalatine n's rami ganglionares nervi maxillaris ad ganglion pterygopalatinum.
pudendal n. nervus pudendus.
n. to quadratus femoris, n. to quadratus femoris and gemellus inferior nervus musculi quadrati femoris.
radial n. nervus radialis.
radial n., deep ramus profundus nervi radialis.
radial n., superficial ramus superficialis nervi radialis.
rectal n's, inferior nervi anales inferiores.
recurrent n. nervus laryngeus recurrens.
recurrent n., ophthalmic ramus meningeus recurrens nervi ophthalmici.
saccular n. nervus saccularis.
sacral n's nervi sacrales.
saphenous n. nervus saphenus.
n. to sartorius a branch of the femoral nerve that arises in common with the intermediate cutaneous nerve and innervates the sartorius muscle.
scapular n., dorsal nervus dorsalis scapulae.
Scarpa n. nervus nasopalatinus.
sciatic n. nervus ischiadicus.
sciatic n., small nervus cutaneus femoris posterior.
scrotal n's, anterior nervi scrotales anteriores.
scrotal n's, posterior nervi scrotales posteriores.
second n. nervus opticus.
secretomotor n. secretory n.
secretory n. any efferent nerve whose stimulation increases glandular activity.
sensory n. nervus sensorius.
seventh n. nervus facialis.
sinus n. ramus sinus carotici nervi glossopharyngei.
sinu-vertebral n. ramus meningeus nervorum spinalium.
sixth n. nervus abducens.
somatic n's the motor and sensory nerves that supply skeletal muscle and somatic tissues.
spermatic n., external ramus genitalis nervi genitofemoralis.
sphenopalatine n's rami ganglionares nervi maxillaris ad ganglion pterygopalatinum.
n. to sphincter ani a branch of the sacral plexus that innervates the sphincter ani muscle.
spinal n's nervi spinales.
splanchnic n's the nerves of the blood vessels and viscera, especially the visceral branches of the thoracic, abdominal (lumbar), and pelvic parts of the sympathetic trunks.
splanchnic n., greater nervus splanchnicus major.
splanchnic n., inferior nervus splanchnicus minor.
splanchnic n., least nervus splanchnicus imus.
splanchnic n., lesser nervus splanchnicus minor.
splanchnic n., lowest nervus splanchnicus imus.
splanchnic n's, lumbar nervi splanchnici lumbales.
splanchnic n's, pelvic radix parasympathica gangliorum pelvicorum.
splanchnic n's, sacral nervi splanchnici sacrales.
stapedial n., stapedius n., n. to stapedius nervus stapedius.
stylohyoid n. ramus stylohyoideus nervi facialis.
stylopharyngeal n. ramus musculi stylopharyngei nervi glossopharyngei.
subclavian n., n. to subclavius nervus subclavius.

Nerve *Continued*

subcostal n. nervus subcostalis.
sublingual n. nervus sublingualis.
suboccipital n. nervus suboccipitalis.
subscapular n's nervi subscapulares.
sudomotor n's the nerves that innervate the sweat glands.
supraclavicular n's nervi supraclaviculares.
supraclavicular n's, anterior nervi supraclaviculares mediales.
supraclavicular n's, intermediate nervi supraclaviculares intermedii.
supraclavicular n's, lateral nervi supraclaviculares laterales.
supraclavicular n's, medial nervi supraclaviculares mediales.
supraclavicular n's, middle nervi supraclaviculares intermedii.
supraclavicular n's, posterior nervi supraclaviculares laterales.
supraorbital n. nervus supraorbitalis.
suprascapular n. nervus suprascapularis.
supratrochlear n. nervus supratrochlearis.
sural n. nervus suralis.
sural cutaneous n., lateral nervus cutaneus surae lateralis.
sural cutaneous n., medial nervus cutaneus surae medialis.
sympathetic n. 1. truncus sympathicus. 2. one of the nerves of the sympathetic nervous system (see under *system*).
temporal n., anterior deep see *nervi temporales profundi.*
temporal n's, deep nervi temporales profundi.
temporal n., middle deep see *nervi temporales profundi.*
temporal n., posterior deep see *nervi temporales profundi.*
temporal n's, subcutaneous rami temporales superficiales nervi auriculotemporalis.
n. to tensor tympani nervus musculi tensoris tympani.
n. to tensor veli palatini nervus musculi tensoris veli palatini.
tenth n. nervus vagus.
tentorial n. ramus meningeus recurrens nervi ophthalmici.
terminal n. nervus terminalis.
third n. nervus oculomotorius.
thoracic n's nervi thoracici.
thoracic n., long nervus thoracicus longus.
thoracic splanchnic n., greater nervus splanchnicus major.
thoracic splanchnic n., lesser nervus splanchnicus minor.
thoracic splanchnic n., lowest nervus splanchnicus imus.
thoracodorsal n. nervus thoracodorsalis.
tibial n. nervus tibialis.
Tiedemann n. a name given to a plexus of sympathetic nerve fibrils surrounding the central artery of the retina.
tonsillar n's rami tonsillares nervi glossopharyngei.
transverse n. of neck nervus transversus colli.
trigeminal n. nervus trigeminus.
trochlear n. nervus trochlearis.
twelfth n. nervus hypoglossus.
tympanic n. nervus tympanicus.
ulnar n. nervus ulnaris.
unmyelinated n. a nerve whose fibers (axons) are not encased in a myelin sheath, and which may or may not be enclosed by a neurilemma. Cf. *myelinated n.*
utricular n. nervus utricularis.
utriculoampullary n. nervus utriculoampullaris.
vaginal n's nervi vaginales.
vagus n. nervus vagus.
Valentin n. a nerve sometimes observed connecting the pterygopalatine ganglion and the abducent nerve.
vascular n's nervi vasorum.
vasoconstrictor n. a nerve whose stimulation causes contraction of the blood vessels.
vasodilator n. a nerve whose stimulation causes dilation of the blood vessels.
vasomotor n. any nerve concerned in controlling the caliber of vessels, whether as a vasodilator or a vasoconstrictor.
vasosensory n. any nerve supplying sensory fibers to the vessels.
vertebral n. nervus vertebralis.
vestibular n. nervus vestibularis.
vestibulocochlear n. nervus vestibulocochlearis.
vidian n. nervus canalis pterygoidei.
visceral n. nervus autonomicus.
n. of Willis nervus accessorius.
Wrisberg n. 1. nervus intermedius. 2. nervus cutaneus brachii medialis.
zygomatic n. nervus zygomaticus.
zygomaticofacial n. ramus zygomaticofacialis nervi zygomatici.
zygomaticotemporal n. ramus zygomaticotemporalis nervi zygomatici.

ner·vi (nur'vi) [L.] genitive and plural of *nervus.*

ner·vi·mo·til·i·ty (nur″vĭ-mo-til′ĭ-te) susceptibility to nervimotion.

ner·vi·mo·tion (nur″vĭ-mo′shən) motion effected through the agency of a nerve.

ner·vi·mo·tor (nur″vĭ-mo′tər) pertaining to a motor nerve.

ner·vi·mus·cu·lar (nur″vĭ-mus′ku-lər) pertaining to the nerve supply of muscles.

ner·vo·mus·cu·lar (nur″vo-mus′ku-lər) nervimuscular.

ner·von·ate (nər-von′āt) a salt, ester, or anionic form of nervonic acid.

ner·vone (nur′vōn) a cerebroside isolated from nerve tissue.

ner·von·ic ac·id (nər-von′ik) a polyunsaturated 24-carbon fatty acid occurring in cerebrosides and sphingomyelin. See also table accompanying *fatty acid.*

ner·vous (nur′vəs) [L. *nervosus,* from *nervus*] 1. neural (def. 1). 2. unduly excitable or easily agitated.

ner·vous·ness (nur′vəs-nis) excessive excitability and irritability, with mental and physical unrest.

ner·vus (nur′vəs) gen. and pl. *ner′vi* [L.] [TA] nerve.

Nervus

Descriptions are given on TA terms, and include anglicized names of specific nerves.

n. abdu′cens [TA] abducens nerve: sixth cranial nerve; *origin,* a nucleus in the pons, immediately internal to the facial colliculus in the floor of the fourth ventricle, emerging from the brainstem anteriorly between the pons and medulla oblongata; *distribution,* lateral rectus muscle of eye; *modality,* motor.
n. accesso′rius [TA] accessory nerve: eleventh cranial nerve; *origin,* by spinal roots from the side of the spinal cord (cervical segments C1 to C5); the roots briefly unite with what is sometimes called the cranial root of accessory nerve (although it is now known to be part of the vagus nerve), forming the trunk of the accessory nerve. Upon exiting the jugular foramen, the spinal and cranial roots separate again to form the external branch (ramus externus nervi accessorii) and internal branch (ramus internus nervi accessorii), respectively; *modality,* motor.
n. acus′ticus n. vestibulocochlearis.
n. alveola′ris infe′rior [TA] inferior alveolar nerve: *origin,* mandibular nerve; *branches,* inferior dental plexus, mylohyoid and mental nerves; *distribution*—see individual branches, under *plexus* and in this table; *modality,* motor and general sensory.
ner′vi alveola′res superio′res [TA] superior alveolar nerves: a term denoting collectively the alveolar branches arising from the maxillary and infraorbital nerves, innervating the teeth and gums of the upper jaw and the maxillary sinus, and forming the superior dental

plexus, viz., *rami alveolares superiores anteriores nervi infraorbitalis, ramus alveolaris superior medius nervi infraorbitalis,* and *rami alveolares superiores posteriores nervi maxillaris.*

n. ampulla′ris ante′rior [TA] anterior ampullary nerve: the branch of the vestibular nerve that innervates the ampulla of the anterior semicircular duct, ending around the hair cells of the ampullary crest.

n. ampulla′ris latera′lis [TA] lateral ampullary nerve: the branch of the vestibular nerve that innervates the ampulla of the lateral semicircular duct, ending around the hair cells of the ampullary crest.

n. ampulla′ris poste′rior [TA] posterior ampullary nerve: the branch of the vestibular nerve that innervates the ampulla of the posterior semicircular duct, ending around the hair cells of the ampullary crest.

ner′vi ana′les inferio′res [TA] inferior anal nerves: *origin,* pudendal nerve, or independently from sacral plexus; *distribution,* sphincter ani externus muscle, skin around anus, and lining of anal canal up to pectinate line; *modality,* general sensory and motor. Called also *inferior rectal nerves* and *nervi rectales inferiores* [TA alternative].

n. anococcy′geus [TA] anococcygeal nerve: *origin,* coccygeal plexus; *distribution,* sacrococcygeal joint, coccyx, skin over the coccyx; *modality,* general sensory.

n. articula′ris articular nerve.

ner′vi auricula′res anterio′res [TA] anterior auricular nerves: *origin,* auriculotemporal nerve; *distribution,* skin of anterosuperior part of external ear; *modality,* general sensory.

n. auricula′ris mag′nus [TA] great auricular nerve: *origin,* cervical plexus—C2–C3; *branches,* anterior and posterior rami; *distribution,* skin over parotid gland and mastoid process, and both surfaces of auricle; see individual branches under *ramus; modality,* general sensory.

n. auricula′ris poste′rior [TA] posterior auricular nerve: *origin,* facial nerve; *branches,* occipital ramus; *distribution,* auricularis posterior and occipitofrontalis muscles and skin of external acoustic meatus; *modality,* motor and general sensory.

n. auriculotempora′lis [TA] auriculotemporal nerve: *origin,* by two roots from the mandibular nerve; *branches,* anterior auricular nerve, nerve of external acoustic meatus, parotid branches, branch to tympanic membrane, and branches communicating with facial nerve; its terminal branches are superficial temporal to the scalp; *distribution*—see individual branches, in this table and under *ramus; modality,* general sensory.

n. autono′micus [TA] autonomic nerve: any of the parasympathetic or sympathetic nerves of the autonomic nervous system; called also *n. visceralis* and *visceral nerve.*

n. axilla′ris [TA] axillary nerve: *origin,* posterior cord of brachial plexus (C5–C6); *branches,* lateral superior cutaneous nerve of arm and muscular rami; *distribution,* deltoid and teres minor muscles, skin on back of arm; *modality,* motor and general sensory.

n. bucca′lis [TA] buccal nerve: *origin,* mandibular nerve; *distribution,* skin and mucous membrane of cheeks, gums, and perhaps the first two molars and the premolars; *modality,* general sensory.

n. cana′lis pterygoi′dei [TA] nerve of pterygoid canal: *origin,* union of deep and greater petrosal nerves; *distribution,* pterygopalatine ganglion and branches; *modality,* parasympathetic and sympathetic. Called also *radix facialis.*

n. cardi′acus cervica′lis infe′rior [TA] inferior cervical cardiac nerve: *origin,* cervicothoracic ganglion; *distribution,* heart via cardiac plexus; *modality,* sympathetic (accelerator) and visceral afferent (chiefly pain).

n. cardi′acus cervica′lis me′dius [TA] middle cervical cardiac nerve: *origin,* middle cervical ganglion; *distribution,* heart; *modality,* sympathetic (accelerator) and visceral afferent (chiefly pain).

n. cardi′acus cervica′lis supe′rior [TA] superior cervical cardiac nerve: *origin,* superior cervical ganglion; *distribution,* heart; *modality,* sympathetic (accelerator).

ner′vi cardi′aci thora′cici rami cardiaci thoracici.

ner′vi caroticotympa′nici [TA] caroticotympanic nerves: *origin,* internal carotid plexus; inferior and superior nerves can be distinguished; together with tympanic nerve, they form the tympanic plexus; *distribution,* tympanic region and parotid gland; *modality,* sympathetic.

ner′vi caro′tici exter′ni [TA] external carotid nerves: *origin,* superior cervical ganglion; *distribution,* cranial blood vessels and glands via the external carotid plexus; *modality,* sympathetic.

n. caro′ticus inter′nus [TA] internal carotid nerve: *origin,* superior cervical ganglion; *distribution,* cranial blood vessels and glands via internal carotid plexus; *modality,* sympathetic.

ner′vi caverno′si clito′ridis [TA] cavernous nerves of clitoris: *origin,* uterovaginal plexus; *distribution,* erectile tissue of clitoris; *modality,* parasympathetic, sympathetic, and visceral afferent.

ner′vi caverno′si pe′nis [TA] cavernous nerves of penis: *origin,* prostatic plexus; *distribution,* erectile tissue of penis; *modality,* sympathetic, parasympathetic, and visceral afferent. See also *greater* and *lesser cavernous nerves of penis,* under *nerve.*

ner′vi cervica′les [TA] cervical nerves: the eight pairs of nerves (C1–C8) that arise from the cervical segments of the spinal cord and, except for the last pair, leave the vertebral column above the correspondingly numbered vertebra. The anterior rami of the upper four, on either side, unite to form the cervical plexus, and those of the lower four, together with the anterior branch of the first thoracic nerve, form most of the brachial plexus.

ner′vi cilia′res bre′ves [TA] short ciliary nerves: *origin,* ciliary ganglion; *distribution,* smooth muscle and tunics of eye; *modality,* parasympathetic, sympathetic, and general sensory.

ner′vi cilia′res lon′gi [TA] long ciliary nerves: *origin,* nasociliary nerve, from ophthalmic nerve; *distribution,* dilator pupillae, uvea, cornea; *modality,* sympathetic and general sensory.

ner′vi clu′nium inferio′res [TA] inferior cluneal nerves: general sensory nerve branches of the posterior femoral cutaneous nerve, innervating the skin of the lower part of the buttocks.

ner′vi clu′nium me′dii [TA] middle cluneal nerves: general sensory nerve branches of the plexus formed by the lateral branches of posterior rami of the first four sacral nerves, innervating ligaments of the sacrum and the skin over the posterior buttocks.

ner′vi clu′nium superio′res [TA] superior cluneal nerves: general sensory nerve branches of the posterior rami of the upper lumbar nerves, innervating the skin of the upper part of the buttocks.

n. coccy′geus [TA] coccygeal nerve: either of the thirty-first pair of spinal nerves (Co), arising from the coccygeal segment of the spinal cord.

n. cochlea′ris [TA] cochlear nerve: the part of the vestibulocochlear nerve concerned with hearing, consisting of fibers that arise from the bipolar cells in the spiral ganglion and have their receptors in the spiral organ of the cochlea.

ner′vi crania′les [TA] cranial nerves: the twelve pairs of nerves that are connected with the brain, including the nervi olfactorii (I), and the opticus (II), oculomotorius (III), trochlearis (IV), trigeminus (V), abducens (VI), facialis (VII), vestibulocochlearis (VIII), glossopharyngeus (IX), vagus (X), accessorius (XI), and hypoglossus (XII). Called also *cerebral nerves, encephalic nerves,* and *nervi encephalici.*

n. cuta′neus cutaneous nerve.

n. cuta′neus antebra′chii latera′lis [TA] lateral cutaneous nerve of forearm: *origin,* continuation of musculocutaneous nerve; *distribution,* skin over radial side of forearm and sometimes an area of skin of dorsum of hand; *modality,* general sensory. Called also *lateral antebrachial cutaneous nerve.*

n. cuta′neus antebra′chii media′lis [TA] medial cutaneous nerve of forearm: *origin,* medial cord of brachial plexus (C8, T1); *branches,* anterior and posterior; *distribution,* skin of front, medial, and posteromedial aspects of forearm; *modality,* general sensory. Called also *medial antebrachial cutaneous nerve.*

n. cuta′neus antebra′chii poste′rior [TA] posterior cutaneous nerve of forearm: *origin,* radial nerve; *distribution,* skin of dorsal aspect of forearm; *modality,* general sensory. Called also *posterior antebrachial cutaneous nerve.*

n. cuta′neus bra′chii latera′lis infe′rior [TA] inferior lateral cutaneous nerve of arm: *origin,* radial nerve; *distribution,* skin of lateral surface of lower part of arm; *modality,* general sensory. Called also *inferior lateral brachial cutaneous nerve.*

n. cuta′neus bra′chii latera′lis supe′rior [TA] superior lateral cutaneous nerve of arm: *origin,* axillary nerve; *distribution,* skin of back of arm; *modality,* general sensory. Called also *superior lateral brachial cutaneous nerve.*

n. cuta′neus bra′chii media′lis [TA] medial cutaneous nerve of arm: *origin,* medial cord of brachial plexus (T1); *distribution,* skin on medial and posterior aspects of arm; *modality,* general sensory. Called also *medial brachial cutaneous nerve.*

n. cuta′neus bra′chii poste′rior [TA] posterior cutaneous nerve of arm: *origin*, radial nerve in the axilla; *distribution*, skin on back of arm; *modality*, general sensory. Called also *posterior brachial cutaneous nerve*.

n. cuta′neus dorsa′lis interme′dius [TA] intermediate dorsal cutaneous nerve: *origin*, superficial peroneal nerve; *branches*, dorsal digital nerves of foot; *distribution*, skin of front of lower third of leg and dorsum of foot, and skin and joints of adjacent sides of third and fourth, and of fourth and fifth toes; *modality*, general sensory.

n. cuta′neus dorsa′lis latera′lis [TA] lateral dorsal cutaneous nerve: *origin*, continuation of sural nerve; *distribution*, skin and joints of lateral side of foot and fifth toe; *modality*, general sensory.

n. cuta′neus dorsa′lis media′lis [TA] medial dorsal cutaneous nerve: *origin*, superficial peroneal nerve; *distribution*, skin and joints of medial side of foot and big toe, and adjacent sides of second and third toes; *modality*, general sensory.

n. cuta′neus femora′lis latera′lis n. cutaneus femoris lateralis.

n. cuta′neus femora′lis poste′rior n. cutaneus femoris posterior.

n. cuta′neus fe′moris latera′lis [TA] lateral femoral cutaneous nerve: *origin*, lumbar plexus—L2–L3; *distribution*, skin of lateral and anterior aspects of thigh; *modality*, general sensory. Called also *lateral cutaneous nerve of thigh*.

n. cuta′neus fe′moris poste′rior [TA] posterior femoral cutaneous nerve: *origin*, sacral plexus—S1–S3; *branches*, inferior cluneal nerves and perineal rami; *distribution*, skin of buttock, external genitalia, and back of thigh and calf; *modality*, general sensory. Called also *posterior cutaneous nerve of thigh*.

n. cuta′neus per′forans [TA] perforating cutaneous nerve: one arising from the posterior surface of the second and third sacral nerves, piercing the sacrotuberous ligament, and supplying the skin over the inferomedial gluteus maximus; it is absent in one third of the population.

n. cuta′neus su′rae latera′lis [TA] lateral sural cutaneous nerve: *origin*, common peroneal nerve; *distribution*, skin of lateral side of back of leg, rarely may continue as the sural nerve; *modality*, general sensory. Called also *lateral cutaneous nerve of calf*.

n. cuta′neus su′rae media′lis [TA] medial sural cutaneous nerve: *origin*, tibial nerve; usually joins sural communicating branch of common peroneal nerve to form the sural nerve; *distribution*, may continue as the sural nerve; *modality*, general sensory. Called also *medial cutaneous nerve of calf*.

ner′vi digita′les dorsa′les hal′lucis latera′lis et dig′iti secun′di media′lis nervi digitales dorsales pedis (def. 2).

ner′vi digita′les dorsa′les ner′vi radia′lis [TA] dorsal digital nerves of radial nerve: *origin*, superficial branch of radial nerve; *distribution*, skin and joints of back of thumb, index finger, middle finger, and medial aspect of ring finger, as far distally as the distal phalanx; *modality*, general sensory.

ner′vi digita′les dorsa′les ner′vi ulna′ris [TA] dorsal digital nerves of ulnar nerve: *origin*, dorsal branch of ulnar nerve; *distribution*, skin and joints of medial side of little finger, dorsal aspects of adjacent sides of little and ring fingers; *modality*, general sensory.

ner′vi digita′les dorsa′les pe′dis dorsal digital nerves of foot: 1. [TA] nerves supplying the third, fourth, and fifth toes; *origin*, intermediate dorsal cutaneous nerve; *distribution*, skin and joints of adjacent sides of third and fourth, and of fourth and fifth toes; *modality*, general sensory. 2. [TA] nerves supplying the first and second toes; *origin*, medial terminal division of deep peroneal nerve; *distribution*, skin and joints of adjacent sides of great and second toes; *modality*, general sensory.

ner′vi digita′les palma′res commu′nes ner′vi media′ni [TA] common palmar digital nerves of median nerve: *number*, four; *origin*, lateral and medial divisions of median nerve; *branches*, proper palmar digital nerves; *distribution*, thumb, index, middle, and ring fingers, and first two lumbrical muscles—see individual branches, in this table; *modality*, motor and general sensory.

ner′vi digita′les palma′res commu′nes ner′vi ulna′ris [TA] common palmar digital nerves of ulnar nerve: *number*, two; *origin*, superficial branch of ulnar nerve; *branches*, proper palmar digital nerves; *distribution*, little and ring fingers—see individual branches, in this table; *modality*, general sensory.

ner′vi digita′les palma′res pro′prii ner′vi media′ni [TA] proper palmar digital nerves of median nerve: *origin*, common palmar digital nerves; *distribution*, first two lumbrical muscles, skin and joints of both sides and palmar aspect of thumb, index, and middle fingers, radial side of ring finger, and back of distal aspect of these digits; *modality*, general sensory and motor.

ner′vi digita′les palma′res pro′prii ner′vi ulna′ris [TA] proper palmar digital nerves of ulnar nerve: *origin*, the lateral of the two common palmar digital nerves from the superficial branch of the ulnar nerve; *distribution*, skin and joints of adjacent sides of fourth and fifth fingers; *modality*, general sensory.

ner′vi digita′les planta′res commu′nes ner′vi planta′ris latera′lis [TA] common plantar digital nerves of lateral plantar nerve: *number*, two; *origin*, superficial branch of lateral plantar nerve; *branches*, the medial nerve gives rise to two proper plantar digital nerves; *distribution*, the lateral one to the musculus flexor digiti minimi brevis pedis and to skin and joints of lateral side of sole and little toe; the medial one to adjacent sides of fourth and fifth toes—see individual branches, in this table; *modality*, motor and general sensory.

ner′vi digita′les planta′res commu′nes ner′vi planta′ris media′lis [TA] common plantar digital nerves of medial plantar nerve: *number*, four; *origin*, medial plantar nerve; *branches*, muscular branches and proper plantar digital nerves; *distribution*, flexor hallucis brevis muscle and first lumbrical muscles, skin and joints of medial side of foot and great toe, and adjacent sides of great and second, second and third, and third and fourth toes—see individual branches, in this table; *modality*, motor and general sensory.

ner′vi digita′les planta′res pro′prii ner′vi planta′ris latera′lis [TA] proper plantar digital nerves of lateral plantar nerve: *origin*, common plantar digital nerves; *distribution*, flexor digiti minimi brevis muscle, skin and joints of lateral side of sole and little toe, and adjacent sides of fourth and fifth toes; *modality*, motor and general sensory.

ner′vi digita′les planta′res pro′prii ner′vi planta′ris media′lis [TA] proper plantar digital nerves of medial plantar nerve: *origin*, common plantar digital nerves; *distribution*, skin and joints of medial side of great toe, and adjacent sides of great and second, second and third, and third and fourth toes; the nerves extend to the dorsum to supply nail beds and tips of toes; *modality*, general sensory.

n. dorsa′lis clito′ridis [TA] dorsal nerve of clitoris: *origin*, pudendal nerve; *distribution*, transversus perinei profundus and sphincter urethrae muscles; corpus cavernosum clitoridis; and skin, prepuce, and glans of clitoris; *modality*, general sensory and motor.

n. dorsa′lis pe′nis [TA] dorsal nerve of penis: *origin*, pudendal nerve; *distribution*, transversus perinei profundus and sphincter urethrae muscles; corpus cavernosum penis; and skin, prepuce, and glans of penis; *modality*, general sensory and motor.

n. dorsa′lis sca′pulae [TA] dorsal scapular nerve: *origin*, brachial plexus—anterior ramus of C5; *distribution*, rhomboid muscles and occasionally the levator scapulae muscle; *modality*, motor.

ner′vi encepha′lici nervi craniales.

ner′vi erigen′tes radix parasympathica gangliorum pelvicorum.

n. ethmoida′lis ante′rior [TA] anterior ethmoidal nerve: *origin*, continuation of nasociliary nerve, from ophthalmic nerve; *branches*, internal, external, lateral, and medial nasal rami; *distribution*, mucosa of upper and anterior nasal septum, lateral wall of nasal cavity, skin of lower bridge and tip of nose; *modality*, general sensory.

n. ethmoida′lis poste′rior [TA] posterior ethmoidal nerve: *origin*, nasociliary nerve, from ophthalmic nerve; *distribution*, mucosa of posterior ethmoid cells and of sphenoidal sinus; *modality*, general sensory.

n. facia′lis [TA] facial nerve: seventh cranial nerve, consisting of two roots: a large motor root, which supplies the muscles of facial expression, and a smaller root, the nervus intermedius (q.v.). *Origin*, inferior border of pons, between olive and inferior cerebellar peduncle; *branches* (of motor root), stapedius and posterior auricular nerves, parotid plexus, digastric, stylohyoid, temporal, zygomatic, buccal, lingual, marginal mandibular, and cervical rami, and a communicating ramus with the tympanic plexus; *distribution*: see individual branches, in this table and under *ramus; modality*, motor, parasympathetic, general sensory, special sensory. See also *n. intermediofacialis*.

n. femora′lis [TA] femoral nerve: *origin*, lumbar plexus (L2–L4); descending behind the inguinal ligament to the femoral triangle; *branches*, saphenous nerve, muscular and anterior cutaneous rami; *distribution*, skin of thigh and leg, muscles of front of thigh, and hip and knee joints; see individual branches, in this table and under *ramus; modality*, general sensory and motor.

n. fibula′ris commu′nis [TA] common peroneal nerve: *origin*, sciatic nerve in lower part of thigh; *branches and distribution*, supplies short head of biceps femoris muscle (while still incorporated in sciatic nerve), gives off lateral sural cutaneous nerve and sural communicating branch as it descends in popliteal fossa, supplies knee and superior tibiofibular joints and tibialis anterior muscle, and divides into superficial and deep peroneal nerves; *modality*, general sensory and motor. Called also *n. peroneus communis* [TA alternative].

n. fibula′ris profun′dus [TA] deep peroneal nerve: *origin*, a terminal branch of common peroneal nerve; *branches and distribution*, winds around the neck of the fibula and descends on the interosseous membrane to the front of the ankle; gives off muscular rami, an articular branch, and lateral and medial terminal branches (see individual branches under *ramus* and *branch*); *modality*, general sensory and motor. Called also *n. peroneus profundus* [TA alternative].

n. fibula′ris superficia′lis [TA] superficial peroneal nerve: *origin*, a terminal branch of common peroneal nerve; *branches and distribution*, descends in front of the fibula, supplies peroneus longus and brevis muscles and, in the lower part of the leg, divides into the muscular rami, medial and intermediate dorsal cutaneous nerves; see also individual branches, in this table and under *ramus; modality*, general sensory and motor. Called also *n. peroneus superficialis* [TA alternative].

n. fronta′lis [TA] frontal nerve: *origin*, ophthalmic division of trigeminal nerve; enters the orbit through the superior orbital fissure; *branches*, supraorbital and supratrochlear nerves; *distribution*, chiefly to the forehead and scalp—see individual branches, in this table; *modality*, general sensory.

n. genitofemora′lis [TA] genitofemoral nerve: *origin*, lumbar plexus (L1–L2); *branches*, genital and femoral rami; *distribution*, see individual branches, under *ramus; modality*, general sensory and motor.

n. glossopharyn′geus [TA] glossopharyngeal nerve: ninth cranial nerve; *origin*, several rootlets from lateral side of upper part of medulla oblongata, between the olive and the inferior cerebellar peduncle; *branches*, tympanic nerve, pharyngeal, stylopharyngeal, carotid, tonsillar, and lingual rami, and rami communicating with the auricular and meningeal rami of the vagus nerve, with the chorda tympani, and with the auriculotemporal nerve; *distribution*, it has two enlargements (superior and inferior ganglia) and supplies the tongue, pharynx, and parotid gland—see individual branches, in this table and under *ramus; modality*, motor, parasympathetic, and general, special, and visceral sensory.

n. glu′teus infe′rior [TA] inferior gluteal nerve: *origin*, sacral plexus (L5–S2); *distribution*, gluteus maximus muscle; *modality*, motor.

n. glu′teus supe′rior [TA] superior gluteal nerve: *origin*, sacral plexus (L4–S1); *distribution*, gluteus medius and minimus muscles, tensor fasciae latae, and hip joint; *modality*, motor and general sensory.

n. hypogas′tricus [TA] hypogastric nerve: a nerve trunk situated on either side (right and left), interconnecting the superior and inferior hypogastric plexuses.

n. hypoglos′sus [TA] hypoglossal nerve: twelfth cranial nerve; *origin*, several rootlets in the anterolateral sulcus between the olive and the pyramid of the medulla oblongata; it passes through the hypoglossal canal to the tongue; *branches*, lingual rami; *distribution*, styloglossus, hyoglossus, and genioglossus muscles and intrinsic muscles of the tongue; *modality*, motor.

n. iliohypogas′tricus [TA] iliohypogastric nerve: *origin*, lumbar plexus—L1 (sometimes T12); *branches*, lateral and anterior cutaneous rami; *distribution*, the skin above the pubis and over the lateral side of the buttock, and occasionally the pyramidalis; *modality*, motor and general sensory. Called also *n. iliopubicus* [TA alternative] and *iliopubic nerve*.

n. ilioinguina′lis [TA] ilioinguinal nerve: *origin*, lumbar plexus—L1 (sometimes T12); accompanies the spermatic cord through the inguinal canal; *branches*, anterior scrotal or labial rami; *distribution*, skin of scrotum or labia majora, and adjacent part of thigh; *modality*, general sensory.

n. iliopu′bicus TA alternative for *n. iliohypogastricus*.

n. infraorbita′lis [TA] infraorbital nerve: *origin*, continuation of the maxillary nerve, entering the orbit through the inferior orbital fissure, and occupying in succession the infraorbital groove, canal, and foramen; *branches*, middle and anterior superior alveolar, inferior palpebral, internal and external nasal, and superior labial rami; *distribution*—see individual branches, under *ramus; modality*, general sensory.

n. infratrochlea′ris [TA] infratrochlear nerve: *origin*, nasociliary nerve from ophthalmic nerve; *branches*, palpebral rami; *distribution*, skin of root and upper bridge of nose and lower eyelid, conjunctiva, lacrimal duct; *modality*, general sensory.

ner′vi intercosta′les [TA] intercostal nerves: anterior rami of the first eleven thoracic spinal nerves, situated between the ribs. The first three send branches to the brachial plexus as well as to the thoracic wall; the fourth, fifth, and sixth supply only the thoracic wall; and the seventh through eleventh are thoracoabdominal in distribution. Called also *rami anteriores nervorum thoracicum* [TA alternative] and *rami ventrales nervorum thoracicorum* [TA alternative]. The primary anterior division of the twelfth thoracic nerve is subcostal rather than intercostal in position and is known as the subcostal nerve (see *nervus subcostalis*). It differs in course and relationship from the other anterior branches and so is classified separately.

ner′vi intercostobrachia′les [TA] intercostobrachial nerves: two nerves arising from the intercostal nerves and supplying the skin of the upper limb. The first is constant: *origin*, second intercostal nerve; *distribution*, skin on back and medial aspect of arm; *modality*, general sensory. A second intercostobrachial nerve is often present; *origin*, third intercostal nerve; *distribution*, skin of axilla and medial aspect of arm; *modality*, general sensory.

n. intermediofacia′lis the nervus facialis and the nervus intermedius considered together; so called because they are two radices of the same cranial nerve and, even though they usually occur as separate trunks, they form a common trunk.

n. interme′dius [TA] intermediate nerve: the smaller root of the facial nerve, lying between the main root and the vestibulocochlear nerve; it joins the main root at, or merges with, the geniculate ganglion at the geniculum of the facial nerve; *branches*, chorda tympani and greater petrosal nerve; *distribution*, lacrimal, nasal, palatine, submandibular, and sublingual glands, and anterior two-thirds of tongue; *modality*, parasympathetic and special sensory. Called also *Wrisberg nerve*. See also *n. intermediofacialis*.

n. interos′seus antebra′chii ante′rior [TA] anterior interosseous nerve of forearm: *origin*, median nerve; *distribution*, flexor pollicis longus, flexor digitorum profundus, and pronator quadratus muscles, wrist and intercarpal joints; *modality*, motor and general sensory.

n. interos′seus antebra′chii poste′rior [TA] posterior interosseous nerve of forearm: *origin*, continuation of deep branch of radial nerve; *distribution*, abductor pollicis longus, extensors of the thumb and second finger, and wrist and intercarpal joints; *modality*, motor and general sensory.

n. interos′seus cru′ris [TA] interosseous nerve of leg: *origin*, tibial nerve; *distribution*, interosseous membrane and tibiofibular syndesmosis; *modality*, general sensory. Called also *crural interosseous nerve*.

n. ischia′dicus [TA] sciatic nerve, the largest nerve of the body: *origin*, sacral plexus (L4–S3); it leaves the pelvis through the greater sciatic foramen; *branches*, divides into the tibial and common peroneal nerves, usually in lower third of thigh; *distribution*—see individual branches, in this table; *modality*, general sensory and motor. Called also *n. sciaticus*.

n. jugula′ris [TA] jugular nerve: a branch of the superior cervical ganglion that communicates with the vagus and glossopharyngeal nerves.

ner′vi labia′les anterio′res [TA] anterior labial nerves: *origin*, ilioinguinal nerve; *distribution*, skin of anterior labial region of labia majora, and adjacent part of thigh; *modality*, general sensory.

ner′vi labia′les posterio′res [TA] posterior labial nerves: *origin*, perineal nerves; *distribution*, labium majus; *modality*, general sensory.

n. lacrima′lis [TA] lacrimal nerve: *origin*, ophthalmic division of trigeminal nerve, entering the orbit through the superior orbital fissure; *distribution*, lacrimal gland, conjunctiva, lateral commissure of eye, and skin of upper eyelid; *modality*, general sensory.

n. laryngea′lis recur′rens n. laryngeus recurrens.

n. laryngea′lis supe′rior n. laryngeus superior.

n. laryn′geus recur′rens [TA] recurrent laryngeal nerve: *origin*, vagus nerve (chiefly the cranial part of the accessory nerve): *branches*, inferior laryngeal nerve and tracheal, esophageal, pharyngeal, and inferior cardiac rami; *distribution*—see individual branches, in this table and under *ramus; modality*, parasympathetic, visceral afferent, and motor. Called also *n. laryngealis recurrens*.

n. laryn′geus supe′rior [TA] superior laryngeal nerve: *origin*, inferior ganglion of vagus nerve; *branches*, external, internal, and communicating rami; *distribution*, inferior constrictor of pharynx and cricothyroid muscles, and mucosa of epiglottis, base of tongue, and larynx; *modality*, motor, general sensory, visceral afferent, and parasympathetic. Called also *n. laryngealis superior*.

n. lingua′lis [TA] lingual nerve: *origin*, mandibular nerve, descending to the tongue, first medial to the mandible and then under cover of the mucous membrane of the mouth; *branches*, sublingual nerve, lingual rami, rami to isthmus of fauces, and rami communicating with the hypoglossal nerve and chorda tympani; *distribution*—see individual branches, in this table and under *ramus; modality*, general sensory.

ner′vi lumba′les [TA] lumbar nerves: the five pairs of nerves (L1–L5) that arise from the lumbar segments of the spinal cord, each pair leaving the vertebral column below the correspondingly numbered vertebra. The anterior rami of these nerves participate in the formation of the lumbosacral plexus.

n. lumboinguina′lis ramus femoralis nervi genitofemoralis.

n. mandibula′ris [TA] mandibular nerve, one of three terminal divisions of the trigeminal nerve, passing through the foramen ovale to the infratemporal fossa. *Origin*, trigeminal ganglion; *branches*, meningeal ramus, masseteric, deep temporal, lateral and medial pterygoid, buccal, auriculotemporal, lingual, and inferior alveolar nerves; *distribution*, extensive distribution to muscles of mastication, skin of face, mucous membrane of mouth, and teeth; see individual branches, in this table and under *ramus; modality*, general sensory and motor.

n. massete′ricus [TA] masseteric nerve: *origin*, mandibular division of trigeminal nerve; *distribution*, masseter muscle and temporomandibular joint; *modality*, motor and general sensory.

n. maxilla′ris [TA] maxillary nerve, one of the three terminal divisions of the trigeminal nerve, passing through the foramen rotundum, and entering the pterygopalatine fossa. *Origin*, trigeminal ganglion; *branches*, meningeal ramus, zygomatic, superior alveolar, and infraorbital nerves, ganglionic branches to pterygopalatine ganglion, and, indirectly, the branches of the pterygopalatine ganglion; *distribution*, extensive distribution to skin of face and scalp, mucous membrane of maxillary sinus and nasal cavity, and teeth—see individual branches, in this table and under *ramus; modality*, general sensory.

n. mea′tus acus′tici exter′ni [TA] nerve of external acoustic meatus: *origin*, auriculotemporal nerve; *distribution*, skin lining external acoustic meatus, and tympanic membrane; *modality*, general sensory.

n. media′nus [TA] median nerve: *origin*, lateral and medial cords of brachial plexus—C6–T1; *branches*, anterior interosseous nerve of forearm, common palmar digital nerves, muscular and palmar rami, and a communicating branch with the ulnar nerve; *distribution*, the elbow, wrist, and intercarpal joints, anterior muscles of the forearm, muscles of the digits, skin of the palm, thenar eminence, and digits—see also individual branches, in this table and under *ramus; modality*, general sensory.

n. menin′geus me′dius ramus meningeus nervi maxillaris.

n. menta′lis [TA] mental nerve: *origin*, inferior alveolar nerve; *branches*, mental, gingival, and inferior labial rami; *distribution*, skin of chin, and lower lip; *modality*, general sensory.

n. mix′tus [TA] mixed nerve: a nerve composed of both sensory (afferent) and motor (efferent) fibers.

n. moto′rius [TA] motor nerve: a peripheral efferent nerve that conducts impulses from the spinal cord or brain to motor end plates or other terminals, resulting in stimulation of muscle contractions.

n. mus′culi obturato′rii inter′ni [TA] nerve to obturator internus: *origin*, anterior branches of anterior rami of L5, S1–S2; *distribution*, gemellus superior and obturator internus muscles; *modality*, general sensory and motor. Called also *n. obturatorius internus* and *internal obturator nerve.*

n. mus′culi pirifor′mis [TA] nerve to piriformis: *origin*, posterior branches of anterior rami of S1–S2; *distribution*, piriformis muscle; *modality*, general sensory and motor. Called also *n. piriformis* and *piriform nerve.*

n. musculi quadra′ti fe′moris [TA] nerve to quadratus femoris: *origin*, anterior branches of anterior rami of L4–L5; *distribution*, gemellus inferior, anterior quadratus femoris muscle, hip joint; *modality*, general sensory and motor. Called also *n. quadratus femoris.*

n. mus′culi tenso′ris tym′pani [TA] nerve to tensor tympani: *origin*, nerve to medial pterygoid; *distribution*, tensor tympani muscle; *modality*, motor.

n. mus′culi tenso′ris ve′li palati′ni [TA] nerve to tensor veli palatini: *origin*, nerve to medial pterygoid; *distribution*, tensor veli palatini muscle; *modality*, motor. Called also *n. tensoris veli palatini.*

n. musculocuta′neus [TA] musculocutaneous nerve: *origin*, lateral cord of brachial plexus—C5–C7; *branches*, lateral cutaneous nerve of forearm, and muscular branches (see *rami musculares nervi musculocutanei*, under *ramus*); *distribution*, coracobrachialis, biceps brachii, and brachialis muscles; elbow joint; skin of radial side of forearm; *modality*, general sensory and motor.

n. mylohyoi′deus [TA] mylohyoid nerve: *origin*, inferior alveolar nerve; *distribution*, mylohyoid muscle, anterior belly of digastric muscle; *modality*, motor. Called also *nerve to mylohyoid.*

n. nasocilia′ris [TA] nasociliary nerve: *origin*, ophthalmic division of trigeminal nerve; *branches*, long ciliary, posterior ethmoidal, anterior ethmoidal, and infratrochlear nerves, and a communicating branch to the ciliary ganglion; *distribution*—see individual branches, in this table; *modality*, general sensory.

n. nasopalati′nus [TA] nasopalatine nerve: *origin*, pterygopalatine ganglion; *distribution*, mucosa and glands of most of nasal septum and anterior part of hard palate; *modality*, parasympathetic and general sensory.

n. nervo′rum a small nerve supplying the epineurium of a larger nerve.

n. obturato′rius [TA] obturator nerve: *origin*, lumbar plexus—L3–L4; *branches*, anterior, posterior, and muscular rami; *distribution*, adductor muscles and gracilis muscle, skin of medial part of thigh, and hip and knee joints—see individual branches, under *ramus; modality*, general sensory and motor.

n. obturato′rius accesso′rius [TA] accessory obturator nerve: *origin*, anterior branches of anterior rami of L3–L4; *distribution*, pectineus muscle, hip joint, communicates with obturator nerve; *modality*, general sensory and motor.

n. obturato′rius inter′nus n. musculi obturatorii interni.

n. occipita′lis ma′jor [TA] greater occipital nerve: *origin*, medial branch of posterior ramus of C2; *distribution*, semispinalis capitis muscle and skin of scalp as far forward as the vertex; *modality*, general sensory and motor.

n. occipita′lis mi′nor [TA] lesser occipital nerve: *origin*, superficial cervical plexus (C2–C3); *distribution*, ascends behind the auricle and supplies some of the skin on the side of the head and on the cranial surface of the auricle; *modality*, general sensory.

n. occipita′lis ter′tius [TA] third occipital nerve: *origin*, medial branch of posterior ramus of C3; *distribution*, skin of upper part of back of neck and head; *modality*, general sensory.

n. octa′vus [L. "eighth nerve"] n. vestibulocochlearis.

n. oculomoto′rius [TA] oculomotor nerve: third cranial nerve; *origin*, brainstem, emerging medial to cerebral peduncles and running forward in the cavernous sinus; *branches*, superior and inferior rami; *distribution*, entering the orbit through the superior orbital fissure, the branches supply the levator palpebrae superioris, all extrinsic eye muscles except the lateral rectus and superior oblique, and carry parasympathetic fibers for the ciliaris and sphincter pupillae muscles; *modality*, motor and parasympathetic.

n. olfacto′rius [TA] olfactory nerve: first cranial nerve, the central processes of the olfactory receptor cells, or fila olfactoria, considered collectively.

n. ophthal′micus [TA] ophthalmic nerve, one of the three terminal divisions of the trigeminal nerve. *Origin*, trigeminal ganglion; *branches*, recurrent meningeal (tentorial) ramus, frontal, lacrimal, and nasociliary nerves; *distribution*, eyeball and conjunctiva, lacrimal gland and sac, nasal mucosa and frontal sinus, external nose, upper eyelid, forehead, and scalp; see individual branches, in this table and under *ramus; modality*, general sensory.

n. op′ticus [TA] optic nerve: second cranial nerve, the so-called nerve of sight, actually part of the central nervous system throughout its course, misnamed as a nerve because of its cordlike appearance; it consists chiefly of axons and central processes of cells of the ganglionic layer of the retina, which leave each orbit through the optic canal, joining with those of the opposite side to form the optic chiasm (the medial fibers of each nerve crossing over to the opposite side), then continuing on each side as the optic tract.

n. palati′nus ma′jor [TA] greater palatine nerve: *origin*, pterygopalatine ganglion; *branches*, posterior inferior (lateral) nasal branches; *distribution*, emerges through the greater palatine foramen and supplies the palate; *modality*, parasympathetic, sympathetic, and general sensory.

ner′vi palati′ni mino′res [TA] lesser palatine nerves: *origin*, pterygopalatine ganglion; *distribution*, emerge through the lesser palatine foramen and supply the soft palate and tonsil; *modality*, parasympathetic, sympathetic, and general sensory.

n. pectora′lis latera′lis [TA] lateral pectoral nerve: *origin*, lateral cord of brachial plexus or anterior divisions of upper and middle trunks (C5–C7); *distribution*, usually several nerves supplying the musculus

pectoralis minor and acromioclavicular and shoulder joints; *modality*, motor and general sensory.
n. pectora′lis media′lis [TA] medial pectoral nerve: *origin*, medial cord or lower trunk of brachial plexus (C8, T1); *distribution*, usually several nerves supplying the musculus pectoralis major and musculus pectoralis minor; *modality*, motor.
ner′vi perinea′les [TA] perineal nerves: *origin*, pudendal nerve in the pudendal canal; *branches*, muscular branches and posterior scrotal or labial nerves; *distribution*, muscular branches supply the bulbospongiosus, ischiocavernosus, superficial transversus perinei muscles and bulb of the penis and, in part, the sphincter ani externus and levator ani; the scrotal (labial) nerves supply the scrotum or labium majus; *modality*, general sensory and motor.
n. perone′us commu′nis TA alternative for *n. fibularis communis*.
n. perone′us profun′dus TA alternative for *n. fibularis profundus*.
n. perone′us profun′dus accesso′rius accessory deep peroneal nerve: a branch of the superficial peroneal nerve that sometimes occurs supplying the musculus peroneus brevis, often extending to the lateral malleolus, and ending in twigs to the musculus extensor digitorum brevis and adjacent joints.
n. perone′us superficia′lis TA alternative for *n. fibularis superficialis*.
n. petro′sus ma′jor [TA] greater petrosal nerve: *origin*, intermediate nerve via geniculate ganglion; *distribution*, running forward from the geniculate ganglion, it joins the deep petrosal nerve of the pterygoid canal, and reaches lacrimal, nasal, and palatine glands and nasopharynx, via pterygopalatine ganglion and its branches; *modality*, parasympathetic and general sensory. Called also *radix parasympathica ganglii pterygopalatini* [TA alternative] (which is the term preferred in the official nomenclature when the ganglia of the pars parasympathica are being considered), *radix intermedia ganglii pterygopalatini* [TA alternative], and *parasympathetic root of pterygopalatine ganglion*.
n. petro′sus mi′nor [TA] lesser petrosal nerve: *origin*, tympanic plexus; *distribution*, parotid gland via otic ganglion and auriculotemporal nerve; *modality*, parasympathetic. Called also *radix parasympathica ganglii otici* [TA alternative]. NOTE: radix is the term preferred in the official nomenclature when considering the ganglia of the pars parasympathica.
n. petro′sus profun′dus [TA] deep petrosal nerve: *origin*, internal carotid plexus; *distribution*, joins greater petrosal nerve to form nerve of pterygoid canal, and supplies lacrimal, nasal, and palatine glands via pterygopalatine ganglion and its branches; *modality*, sympathetic. Called also *radix sympathica ganglii pterygopalatini* [TA alternative]. NOTE: radix is the term preferred in the official nomenclature when considering the ganglia of the pars parasympathica.
n. pharyn′geus [TA] pharyngeal nerve: a nerve running from the posterior part of the pterygopalatine ganglion, through the pharyngeal canal with the pharyngeal branch of the maxillary artery, to the mucous membrane of the nasal part of the pharynx posterior to the auditory tube.
n. phre′nicus [TA] phrenic nerve: *origin*, cervical plexus (C4–C5); *branches*, pericardial and phrenicoabdominal rami; *distribution*, pleura, pericardium, diaphragm, peritoneum, and sympathetic plexuses; *modality*, general sensory and motor.
ner′vi phre′nici accesso′rii [TA] accessory phrenic nerves: an inconstant contribution of the fifth cervical nerve to the phrenic nerve; when present, they run a separate course to the root of the neck or into the thorax before joining the phrenic nerve.
n. pinea′lis [TA] pineal nerve: postganglionic fibers that arise in the superior cervical ganglion and terminate in the pineal gland.
n. pirifor′mis n. musculi piriformis.
n. planta′ris latera′lis [TA] lateral plantar nerve: *origin*, the smaller of terminal branches of tibial nerve; *branches*, muscular, superficial, and deep rami; *distribution*, lying between first and second layers of muscles of sole, it supplies the quadratus plantae, abductor digiti minimi, flexor digiti minimi brevis, adductor hallucis, interossei, and second, third, and fourth lumbrical muscles, and gives off cutaneous and articular twigs to lateral side of sole and fourth and fifth toes—see individual branches, under *ramus; modality*, general sensory and motor.
n. planta′ris media′lis [TA] medial plantar nerve: *origin*, the larger of the terminal branches of tibial nerve; *branches*, common plantar digital nerves and muscular rami; *distribution*, abductor hallucis, flexor digitorum brevis, flexor hallucis brevis, and first lumbrical muscles, and cutaneous and articular twigs to the medial side of the sole, and to the first to fourth toes—see individual branches, in this table and under *ramus; modality*, general sensory and motor.
n. presacra′lis TA alternative for *plexus hypogastricus superior*.
n. pterygoi′deus latera′lis [TA] lateral pterygoid nerve: *origin*, mandibular nerve; *distribution*, lateral pterygoid muscle; *modality*, motor.
n. pterygoi′deus media′lis [TA] medial pterygoid nerve: *origin*, mandibular nerve; *branches*, nerve to tensor tympani, nerve to tensor veli palatini; *distribution*, medial pterygoid, tensor tympani, and tensor veli palatini muscles; *modality*, motor.
n. puden′dus [TA] pudendal nerve: *origin*, sacral plexus (S2–S4); *branches*, enters the pudendal canal, gives off the inferior anal nerve, and then divides into the perineal nerve and dorsal nerve of the penis (clitoris); *distribution*, muscles, skin, and erectile tissue of perineum—see individual branches; *modality*, general sensory, motor, and parasympathetic.
n. quadra′tus fe′moris n. musculi quadrati femoris.
n. radia′lis [TA] radial nerve: *origin*, posterior cord of brachial plexus (C6–C8, and sometimes C5 and T1); *branches*, posterior cutaneous and inferior lateral cutaneous nerves of arm, posterior cutaneous nerve of forearm, muscular, deep, and superficial rami; *distribution*, descending in the back of arm and forearm, it is ultimately distributed to skin on back of arm, forearm, and hand, extensor muscles on back of arm and forearm, and elbow joint and many joints of hand; see individual branches, in this table and under *ramus; modality*, general sensory and motor.
ner′vi recta′les inferio′res TA alternative for *nervi anales inferiores*.
n. saccula′ris [TA] saccular nerve: the branch of the vestibular nerve that innervates the macula of the saccule.
ner′vi sacra′les [TA] sacral nerves: the five pairs of nerves (S1–S5) that arise from the sacral segments of the spinal cord; the anterior rami of the first four pairs participate in the formation of the sacral plexus.
ner′vi sacra′les et n. coccy′geus [TA] see *nervi sacrales* and *n. coccygeus*.
n. saphe′nus [TA] saphenous nerve: *origin*, termination of femoral nerve, descending first with femoral vessels and then on medial side of leg and foot; *branches*, infrapatellar and medial crural cutaneous rami; *distribution*, knee joint, subsartorial and patellar plexuses, skin on medial side of leg and foot; see individual branches, under *ramus; modality*, general sensory.
n. scia′ticus n. ischiadicus.
ner′vi scrota′les anterio′res [TA] anterior scrotal nerves: *origin*, ilioinguinal nerve; *distribution*, skin of anterior scrotal region; *modality*, general sensory.
ner′vi scrota′les posterio′res [TA] posterior scrotal nerves: *origin*, perineal nerves; *distribution*, skin of scrotum; *modality*, general sensory.
n. senso′rius [TA] sensory nerve: a peripheral afferent nerve that conducts impulses from receptors on a sense organ to the termination of its axon in the spinal cord or brain.
ner′vi spina′les [TA] spinal nerves: the thirty-one pairs of nerves that arise from the spinal cord and pass out between the vertebrae, including the eight pairs of cervical, twelve of thoracic, five of lumbar, five of sacral, and one pair of coccygeal nerves.
n. spino′sus TA alternative for *ramus meningeus nervi mandibularis*.
n. splanch′nicus i′mus [TA] least splanchnic nerve: *origin*, last ganglion of sympathetic trunk or lesser splanchnic nerve; *distribution*, aorticorenal ganglion and adjacent plexus; *modality*, sympathetic and visceral afferent. Called also *lowest thoracic splanchnic nerve* and *n. splanchnicus thoracicus imus*.
ner′vi splanch′nici lumba′les [TA] lumbar splanchnic nerves: *origin*, lumbar ganglia or sympathetic trunk; *distribution*, upper nerves join celiac and adjacent plexuses, middle ones go to intermesenteric and adjacent plexuses, and lower ones descend to superior hypogastric plexus; *modality*, preganglionic sympathetic and visceral afferent. Called also *nervi splanchnici lumbares* [TA alternative].
ner′vi splanch′nici lumba′res nervi splanchnici lumbales.
n. splanch′nicus ma′jor [TA] greater splanchnic nerve: *origin*, thoracic sympathetic trunk and fifth through tenth thoracic ganglia; *distribution*, descending through the diaphragm or its aortic openings, ends in celiac ganglia and plexuses, with a splanchnic ganglion commonly occurring near the diaphragm; *modality*, preganglionic sympathetic and visceral afferent. Called also *greater thoracic splanchnic nerve* and *n. splanchnicus thoracicus major*.
n. splanch′nicus mi′nor [TA] lesser splanchnic nerve: *origin*, ninth and tenth thoracic ganglia of sympathetic trunk; *branches*, renal ramus;

distribution, pierces the diaphragm, joins the aorticorenal ganglion and celiac plexus, and communicates with the renal and superior mesenteric plexuses; *modality*, preganglionic sympathetic and visceral afferent. Called also *lesser thoracic splanchnic nerve* and *n. splanchnicus thoracicus minor.*

ner′vi splanch′nici pelvi′ci TA alternative for *radix parasympathica gangliorum pelvicorum.*

ner′vi splanch′nici sacra′les [TA] sacral splanchnic nerves: *origin*, sacral part of sympathetic trunk; *distribution*, pelvic organs and blood vessels via inferior hypogastric plexus; *modality*, preganglionic sympathetic and visceral afferent.

n. splanch′nicus thora′cicus i′mus n. splanchnicus imus.

n. splanch′nicus thora′cicus ma′jor n. splanchnicus major.

n. splanch′nicus thora′cicus mi′nor n. splanchnicus minor.

n. stape′dius [TA] stapedius nerve: *origin*, facial nerve; *distribution*, stapedius muscle; *modality*, motor.

n. statoacus′ticus n. vestibulocochlearis.

n. subcla′vius [TA] subclavian nerve: *origin*, upper trunk of brachial plexus (C5); *distribution*, subclavius muscle and sternoclavicular joint; *modality*, motor and general sensory.

n. subcosta′lis [TA] subcostal nerve: *origin*, anterior ramus of twelfth thoracic nerve; *distribution*, skin of lower abdomen and lateral side of gluteal region, parts of transversus, oblique, and rectus muscles, and usually the pyramidalis muscle, and adjacent peritoneum; *modality*, general sensory and motor.

n. sublingua′lis [TA] sublingual nerve: *origin*, lingual nerve; *distribution*, sublingual gland and overlying mucous membrane; *modality*, parasympathetic and general sensory.

n. suboccipita′lis [TA] suboccipital nerve: *origin*, posterior ramus of first cervical nerve; *distribution*, emerges above posterior arch of atlas and supplies muscles of suboccipital triangle and semispinalis capitis muscle; *modality*, motor.

ner′vi subscapula′res [TA] subscapular nerves: *origin*, posterior cord of brachial plexus (C5); *distribution*, usually two or more nerves, upper and lower, supplying subscapularis and teres major muscles; *modality*, motor.

ner′vi supraclavicula′res [TA] supraclavicular nerves: a term denoting collectively the common trunk, which is a branch of the cervical plexus (C3–C4) and which emerges under cover of the posterior border of the sternocleidomastoid muscle and divides into the nervi supraclaviculares intermedii, nervi supraclaviculares laterales, and nervi supraclaviculares mediales.

ner′vi supraclavicula′res interme′dii [TA] intermediate supraclavicular nerves: *origin*, cervical plexus (C3–C4); *distribution*, descend in the posterior triangle, cross the clavicle, and supply the skin over pectoral and deltoid regions; *modality*, general sensory.

ner′vi supraclavicula′res latera′les [TA] lateral supraclavicular nerves: *origin*, cervical plexus (C3–C4); *distribution*, descend in the posterior triangle, cross the clavicle, and supply the skin of superior and posterior parts of shoulder; *modality*, general sensory. Called also *nervi supraclaviculares posteriores.*

ner′vi supraclavicula′res media′les [TA] medial supraclavicular nerves: *origin*, cervical plexus (C3–C4); *distribution*, descend in posterior triangle, cross the clavicle, and supply the skin of medial infraclavicular region; *modality*, general sensory.

ner′vi supraclavicula′res posterio′res nervi supraclaviculares laterales.

n. supraorbita′lis [TA] supraorbital nerve: *origin*, continuation of frontal nerve, from ophthalmic nerve; *branches*, lateral and medial rami; *distribution*, leaves orbit through supraorbital notch or foramen, and supplies the skin of upper eyelid, forehead, anterior scalp (to vertex), mucosa of frontal sinus; *modality*, general sensory.

n. suprascapula′ris [TA] suprascapular nerve: *origin*, brachial plexus (C5–C6); *distribution*, descends through suprascapular and spinoglenoid notches and supplies acromioclavicular and shoulder joints, and supraspinatus and infraspinatus muscles; *modality*, motor and general sensory.

n. supratrochlea′ris [TA] supratrochlear nerve: *origin*, frontal nerve, from ophthalmic nerve; *distribution*, leaves orbit at medial end of supraorbital margin and supplies the forehead and upper eyelid; *modality*, general sensory.

n. sura′lis [TA] sural nerve: *origin*, medial sural cutaneous nerve and communicating branch of common peroneal nerve; *branches*, lateral dorsal cutaneous nerve and lateral calcaneal rami; *distribution*, skin on back of leg, and skin and joints on lateral side of heel and foot; see individual branches, in this table and under *ramus; modality*, general sensory.

ner′vi tempora′les profun′di [TA] deep temporal nerves, usually two in number, anterior and posterior, with a third middle one often seen: *origin*, mandibular nerve; *distribution*, temporalis muscle; *modality*, motor.

n. tenso′ris ve′li palati′ni n. musculi tensoris veli palatini.

n. termina′lis [TA] terminal nerve: the collection of nerve filaments found in the pia mater between the olfactory bulb and the crista galli, and passing through the cribriform plate to the nasal mucosa; ganglion cells occur along their course.

ner′vi thora′cici [TA] thoracic nerves: the twelve pairs of spinal nerves (T1–T12) that arise from the thoracic segments of the spinal cord, each pair leaving the vertebral column below the correspondingly numbered vertebra. They innervate the body wall of the thorax and upper abdomen.

n. thora′cicus lon′gus [TA] long thoracic nerve: *origin*, brachial plexus (anterior rami of C5–C7); *distribution*, descends behind brachial plexus to serratus anterior muscle; *modality*, motor.

n. thoracodorsa′lis [TA] thoracodorsal nerve: *origin*, posterior cord of brachial plexus (C7–C8); *distribution*, latissimus dorsi muscle; *modality*, motor.

n. tibia′lis [TA] tibial nerve: *origin*, sciatic nerve in lower part of thigh; *branches*, interosseous nerve of leg, medial sural cutaneous and sural nerves, medial and lateral plantar nerves, and muscular and medial calcaneal branches; *distribution*, while still incorporated in the sciatic nerve, it supplies the semimembranosus and semitendinosus muscles, long head of biceps, and adductor magnus muscle; it supplies the knee joint as it descends in the popliteal fossa and, continuing into the leg, supplies the muscles and skin of the calf and sole of the foot, and the toes; see individual branches, in this table and under *ramus; modality*, general sensory and motor.

n. transver′sus cervica′lis TA alternative for *n. transversus colli.*

n. transver′sus col′li [TA] transverse cervical nerve: *origin*, cervical plexus (C2–C3); *branches*, superior and inferior rami; *distribution*, skin on side and front of neck; *modality*, general sensory. Called also *cutaneous* or *transverse nerve of neck* and *n. transversus cervicalis* [TA alternative].

n. trige′minus [TA] trigeminal nerve: fifth cranial nerve, which emerges from the lateral surface of the pons as a motor and a sensory root, together with some intermediate fibers. The sensory root expands into the trigeminal ganglion, which contains the cells of origin of most of the sensory fibers, and from which the three divisions of the nerve arise. See *n. mandibularis, n. maxillaris*, and *n. ophthalmicus.* The trigeminal nerve is sensory in supplying the face, teeth, mouth, and nasal cavity, and motor in supplying the muscles of mastication.

n. trochlea′ris [TA] trochlear nerve: fourth cranial nerve; *origin*, the fibers of each trochlear nerve (one on either side) decussate across the median plane and emerge from the back of the brainstem below the corresponding inferior colliculus; *distribution*, runs forward in lateral

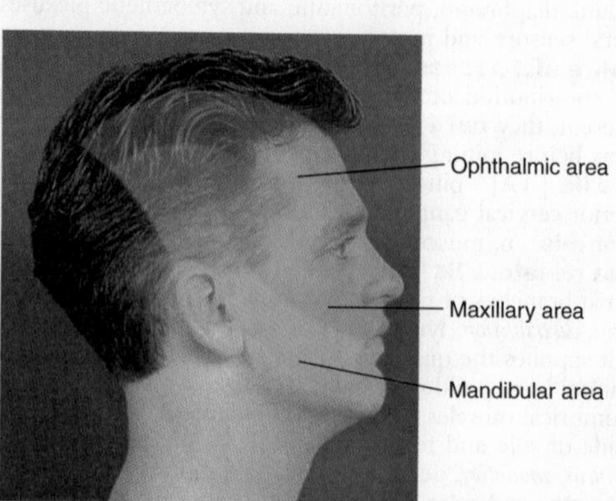

■ Diagram of the general distribution of the nervus trigeminus (trigeminal nerve). Shown are the three areas, ophthalmic, maxillary, and mandibular, supplied by its three main divisions, the nervi ophthalmicus, maxillaris, and mandibularis, respectively.

Nervus *Continued*

wall of cavernous sinus, traverses the superior orbital fissure, and supplies superior oblique muscle of eyeball; *modality*, motor.

n. tympa′nicus [TA] tympanic nerve: *origin*, inferior ganglion of glossopharyngeal nerve; *branches*, helps form tympanic plexus; *distribution*, mucous membrane of tympanic cavity, mastoid air cells, auditory tube, and, via lesser petrosal nerve and otic ganglion, the parotid gland; *modality*, general sensory and parasympathetic. Called also *Jacobson nerve*.

n. ulna′ris [TA] ulnar nerve: *origin*, medial and lateral cords of brachial plexus (C7–T1); *branches*, muscular, dorsal, palmar, superficial, and deep rami; *distribution*, ultimately to skin on front and back of medial part of hand, some flexor muscles on front of forearm, many short muscles of hand, elbow joint, many joints of hand; see individual branches, under *ramus; modality*, general sensory and motor.

n. utricula′ris [TA] utricular nerve: the branch of the vestibular nerve that innervates the macula of the utricle.

n. utriculoampulla′ris [TA] utriculoampullary nerve: a nerve that arises by peripheral division of the vestibular nerve, and supplies the utricle and ampullae of the semicircular ducts.

ner′vi vagina′les [TA] vaginal nerves: *origin*, uterovaginal plexus; *distribution*, vagina; *modality*, sympathetic and parasympathetic.

n. va′gus [TA] vagus nerve: tenth cranial nerve; *origin*, by numerous rootlets from lateral side of medulla oblongata in the groove between the olive and the inferior cerebellar peduncle; *branches*, superior and recurrent laryngeal nerves, meningeal, auricular, pharyngeal, cardiac, bronchial, gastric, hepatic, celiac, and renal rami, pharyngeal, pulmonary, and esophageal plexuses, and anterior and posterior trunks; *distribution*, descending through the jugular foramen, it presents as a superior and an inferior ganglion, and continues through the neck and thorax into the abdomen. It supplies sensory fibers to the ear, tongue, pharynx, and larynx, motor fibers to the pharynx, larynx, and esophagus, and parasympathetic and visceral afferent fibers to thoracic and abdominal viscera; see individual branches, in this table and under *ramus; modality*, parasympathetic, visceral afferent, motor, general sensory.

ner′vi vaso′rum [TA] vascular nerves: the nerve branches that supply the adventitia of the blood vessels.

n. vertebra′lis [TA] vertebral nerve: *origin*, cervicothoracic and vertebral ganglia; *distribution*, ascends with vertebral artery and gives fibers to spinal meninges, cervical nerves, and posterior cranial fossa; *modality*, sympathetic.

n. vestibula′ris [TA] vestibular nerve: the posterior part of the vestibulocochlear nerve, which is concerned with the sense of equilibrium. It consists of fibers arising from bipolar cells in the vestibular ganglion, and divides peripherally into a superior and an inferior part. The sensory receptors, located in the ampullae of the semicircular canals, the utricle, and the saccule, are called vestibular hair cells.

n. vestibulocochlea′ris [TA] vestibulocochlear nerve: eighth cranial nerve; it emerges from the brain between the pons and the medulla oblongata, at the cerebellopontine angle and behind the facial nerve. It divides near the lateral end of the internal acoustic meatus into two functionally distinct and incompletely united components, the vestibular nerve and the cochlear nerve, and is connected with the brain by corresponding roots, the vestibular and the cochlear roots. Called also *n. acusticus, n. octavus*, and *acoustic nerve*.

n. viscera′lis n. autonomicus.

n. zygoma′ticus [TA] zygomatic nerve: *origin*, maxillary nerve, entering the orbit through the inferior orbital fissure; *branches*, zygomaticofacial and zygomaticotemporal rami; *distribution*, communicates with the lacrimal nerve and supplies the skin of the temple and adjacent part of the face; see individual branches, under *ramus*; *modality*, general sensory.

Nes·a·caine (nes′ə-kān) trademark for preparations of chloroprocaine hydrochloride.

ne·sid·i·ec·to·my (ne-sid″e-ek′tə-me) [Gr. *nēsidion* islet + *-ectomy*] excision of the pancreatic islets.

ne·sid·io·blast (ne-sid′e-o-blast″) [Gr. *nēsidion* islet + *-blast*] any of the cells that mature to become islet cells.

ne·sid·io·blas·to·ma (ne-sid″e-o-blas-to′mə) islet cell tumor.

ne·sid·io·blas·to·sis (ne-sid″e-o-blas-to′sis) diffuse proliferation of islet cells.

ne·sir·i·tide (nə-sir′ĭ-tīd) a preparation of recombinant human brain natriuretic peptide, used in the treatment of acutely decompensated congestive heart failure; administered intravenously.

Ne·so·kia (nə-so′ke-ə) a genus of burrowing rodents found in southern Asia. *N. bengalen′sis* is the bandicoot (def. 1).

Ness·ler reagent (solution) (nes′ler) [Julius *Nessler*, German chemist, 1827–1905] see under *reagent*.

ness·ler·iza·tion (nes″lər-ĭ-za′shən) treatment with Nessler reagent.

nest (nest) a small mass of cells, usually foreign to the area in which they are found.

Brunn epithelial n′s solid or branched glandlike clusters of transitional epithelium occurring in the lamina propria mucosae of the lower urinary tract.

cell n. a mass of closely packed epithelial cells surrounded by a stroma of connective tissue.

junctional n. a nest of dysplastic cells seen at the dermoepidermal junction as part of a junctional nevus.

Walthard cell n′s Walthard islets.

nest·ed (nes′təd) located within something else, such as a nested variable.

net (net) a meshlike structure of interlocking fibers or strands; see also *network, plexus*, and *rete*.

Neth·er·ton syndrome (neth′ər-tən) [Earl Weldon *Netherton*, American dermatologist, 20th century] see under *syndrome*.

net·il·mi·cin (net″il-mi′sin) a semisynthetic aminoglycoside antibiotic derived from sisomicin, effective against aerobic gram-negative bacilli and some gram-positive organisms.

n. sulfate [USP] the sulfate salt of netilmicin, administered intramuscularly and intravenously in the treatment of severe systemic infections for which less toxic antibiotics are ineffective or contraindicated.

Net·ro·my·cin (net″ro-mi′sin) trademark for a preparation of netilmicin sulfate.

net·tle (net′əl) any plant of the genus *Urtica*.

stinging n. 1. *Urtica dioica*. 2. [USP] a preparation of *U. dioica*. The root is used to treat urinary problems associated with benign prostatic hyperplasia. The fresh or dried flowering plant is used for urinary tract infections, kidney and bladder stones, and rheumatism and also has a wide variety of use in folk medicine.

Net·tle·ship-Falls ocular albinism (net′əl-ship fawlz′) [Edward *Nettleship*, English ophthalmologist and dermatologist, 1845–1913; Harold Francis *Falls*, American ophthalmologist and geneticist, 1909–2006] see under *albinism*.

net·work (net′wurk″) a meshlike structure of interlocking fibers, strands, or tubules; see also *net, plexus*, and *rete*.

acromial n. rete acromiale.

arterial n. rete arteriosum.

arterial n., cutaneous rete arteriosum dermidis.

arterial n., subpapillary rete arteriosum subpapillare.

arterial n. of dermis rete arteriosum dermidis.

articular n. of elbow rete articulare cubiti.

articular n. of knee rete articulare genus.

articular vascular n. rete vasculosum articulare.

calcaneal n. rete calcaneum.

Chiari n. a network of fine fibers which sometimes extend across the interior of the right atrium of the heart from the valve of coronary sinus and the valve of inferior vena cava to the crista terminalis; it is believed to represent incomplete resorption of the septum spurium. It may act as a nucleus for thrombus formation.

***cis*-Golgi n.** a branched reticulum on the side of the Golgi complex closest to the nucleus that receives proteins and lipids synthesized in the endoplasmic reticulum for further processing in the Golgi complex.

dorsal carpal n. rete carpale dorsale.

idiotype–anti-idiotype n. a regulatory mechanism mounted in response to the unique or idiotypic determinants of lymphocytes or antibodies upon antigenic stimulation. Activation of a B cell results in a clone of plasma cells producing immunoglobulin of a single idiotype, which, because it was previously present in very small quantities, can be recognized as "nonself" and results in the production of anti-idiotypic antibodies directed against its idiotypic determinants. There can also be anti–anti-idiotypic antibodies directed against the second antibodies, antibodies directed against them, and so forth. These antibodies react with antigen receptors on B cells and T helper and suppressor cells, as well as with circulating antibodies, to enhance or suppress production of the initial antibody by various mechanisms.

lymphocapillary n. rete lymphocapillare.

malleolar n., lateral rete malleolare laterale.

malleolar n., medial rete malleolare mediale.

neurofibrillar n. the network formed by the neurofibrils of a nerve cell.

patellar n. rete patellare.

peritarsal n. a set of lymphatics in the eyelid.

Purkinje n., subendocardial terminal n. rami subendocardiales.

subpapillary n. rete arteriosum subpapillare.

***trans*-Golgi n. (TGN)** a network of membranous tubules and associated vesicles on the cytoplasmic side of the Golgi complex in which proteins processed through the Golgi complex are packaged and distributed to their various destinations.

venous n. rete venosum.

venous n., plantar, venous n., plantar cutaneous rete venosum plantare.

venous n. of foot, dorsal rete venosum dorsale pedis.

venous n. of hand, dorsal rete venosum dorsale manus.

Neu·bau·er artery (noi′bou-ər) [Johann Ernst *Neubauer*, German anatomist, 1742–1777] arteria thyroidea ima.

Neu·berg ester (noi′berk) [Carl *Neuberg*, German biochemist, 1877–1956] see *fructose 6-phosphate.*

Neu·feld nail (noo′feld) [Alonzo John *Neufeld*, American orthopedic surgeon, 1906–1984] see under *nail.*

Neu·feld reaction (test) (noi′felt) [Fred *Neufeld*, German bacteriologist, 1861–1945] see under *reaction.*

Neu·las·ta (noo-las′tə) trademark for a preparation of pegfilgrastim.

Neu·mann's law (noi′mahnz) [Franz Ernst *Neumann*, German physicist, 1798–1895] see under *law.*

Neu·mann sheath (noi′mahn) [Ernst *Neumann*, German pathologist, 1834–1918] see under *sheath.*

Neu·me·ga (noo-ma′gə) trademark for a preparation of oprelvekin.

Neu·po·gen (noo′po-jən) trademark for a preparation of filgrastim.

neu·rag·mia (noo͝-rag′me-ə) [*neur-* + Gr. *agmos* break] the tearing of a nerve trunk.

neu·ral (noor′əl) [L. *neuralis*] 1. pertaining to a nerve or to the nerves. 2. situated in the region of the spinal axis, as the neural arch; cf. *hemal.*

neu·ral·gia (noo͝-ral′jə) [*neur-* + *-algia*] pain extending along the course of one or more nerves. Many varieties of neuralgia are distinguished according to the part affected, as brachial, facial, occipital, or supraorbital, or to the cause, as anemic, diabetic, gouty, malarial, or syphilitic. **neural′gic** *adj*

cervicobrachial n. cervicobrachialgia.

cervico-occipital n. neuralgia in the upper cervical nerves, especially the posterior division of the second cervical nerve.

cranial n. neuralgia along the course of a cranial nerve. Cf. *glossopharyngeal n., trigeminal n.*, and *Ramsay Hunt syndrome* (def. 1).

geniculate n. Ramsay Hunt syndrome (def. 1).

glossopharyngeal n. neuralgia affecting the petrosal and jugular ganglia of the glossopharyngeal nerve, marked by severe paroxysmal pain originating on the side of the throat and occasionally extending to the ear. Rarely, attacks may be associated with cardiac slowing or arrest, and syncope.

hallucinatory n. a mental impression of pain without any actual peripheral stimulus.

Hunt n. Ramsay Hunt syndrome (def. 1).

intercostal n. neuralgia of the intercostal nerves.

mandibular joint n. vertex and occipital pain, otalgia, glossodynia, and pain about the nose and eyes, associated with disturbed function of the temporomandibular joint.

migrainous n. cluster headache.

Morton n. a form of foot pain, metatarsalgia caused by compression of a branch of the plantar nerve by the metatarsal heads; chronic compression may lead to formation of a neuroma. Called also *Morton disease, foot, metatarsalgia*, or *toe.*

nasociliary n. Charlin syndrome.

occipital n. pain in the distribution of the occipital nerves, due to pressure or trauma to the nerve. Called also *occipital headache.*

peripheral n. pain along the course of a peripheral sensory nerve.

postherpetic n. persistent burning pain and hyperesthesia along the distribution of a cutaneous nerve following an attack of herpes zoster, especially Ramsay Hunt syndrome or herpes zoster ophthalmicus.

red n. erythromelalgia.

reminiscent n. a mental impression of neuralgic pain persisting after the actual pain has ceased.

sciatic n. sciatica.

Sluder n., sphenopalatine n. neuralgia of the territory supplied by the sphenopalatine ganglion, causing a burning and boring pain in the area of the superior maxilla and a radiation of the pain into the neck and shoulder.

stump n. neuralgia at the site of an amputation.

trifacial n., trifocal n. trigeminal n.

trigeminal n. severe, episodic pain in the area supplied by the trigeminal nerve, often precipitated by stimulation of well-defined trigger points. Called also *trifacial n., trifocal n.*, and *tic douloureux.*

Vail n., vidian n. neuralgia affecting the vidian nerve (nervus canalis pterygoidei), usually secondary to inflammation of the sphenoid sinus, with pain in the face, neck, and shoulders.

neu·ral·gi·form (noo͝-ral′ji-form) resembling neuralgia.

neu·ra·min·ic ac·id (noor″ə-min′ik) a nine carbon amino sugar formed from mannosamine and pyruvate, mostly important as its *N*-acyl derivatives (sialic acids).

neu·ra·min·i·dase (noor″ə-min′ĭ-dās) an enzyme of the hydrolase class that catalyzes the cleavage of glucosidic linkages between a sialic acid residue and a hexose or hexosamine residue at the nonreducing terminal of oligosaccharides in glycoproteins, glycolipids, and proteoglycans. Cytosolic, plasma membrane, and lysosomal forms of the enzyme exist; deficiency of the latter, an autosomal recessive trait, causes sialidosis; enzyme activity is also lacking in galactosialidosis. Viral neuraminidase found on the surface of influenza viruses enables viral release from the host cell. In EC nomenclature, called *exo-α-sialidase.* Called also *sialidase.*

neu·rana·gen·e·sis (noor″an-ə-jen′ə-sis) [*neur-* + Gr. *anagennan* to regenerate] regeneration or renewal of nerve tissue.

neu·ra·poph·y·sis (noor″ə-pof′ə-sis) [*neur-* + *apophysis*] the structure forming either side of the neural arch.

neu·ra·prax·ia (noor″ə-prak′se-ə) [*neur-* + *apraxia*] failure of conduction in a nerve in the absence of structural changes, due to blunt injury, compression, or ischemia; return of function normally ensues. Called also *axonapraxia.* Cf. *axonotmesis* and *neurotmesis.*

neu·rar·chy (noor′ahr-ke) [*neur-* + Gr. *archē* rule] the control of the cerebrospinal system over the body.

neu·rar·throp·a·thy (noor″ahr-throp′ə-the) neuroarthropathy.

neu·ras·the·nia (noor″əs-the′ne-ə) [*neur-* + *asthenia*] a syndrome of chronic mental and physical weakness and fatigue, thought to be caused by exhaustion of the nervous system; no longer used in Western diagnosis but still used in traditional Chinese medicine.

neu·rax·is (noo͝-rak′sis) [*neur-* + *axis*] the central nervous system. **neurax′ial** *adj*

neu·rec·ta·sia (noor″ək-ta′zhə) [*neur-* + *ectasia*] neurotony.

neu·rec·to·my (noo͝-rek′tə-me) [*neur-* + *-ectomy*] the excision of a part of a nerve.

neu·rec·to·pia (noor″ək-to′pe-ə) [*neur-* + *ectopia*] displacement of a nerve or abnormal situation of a nerve.

neu·rec·to·py (noo͝-rek′tə-pe) neurectopia.

neu·reg·u·lin (noo͝-reg′u-lin) any of a group of proteins thought to be regulators of nerve and muscle development and of oncogenic transformation of epithelial cells.

neu·ren·ter·ic (noor″ən-ter′ik) [*neur-* + *enteric*] pertaining to the neural tube and archenteron of the embryo, applied especially to the canal interconnecting them.

neur·epi·the·li·al (noor″ep-ĭ-the′le-əl) neuroepithelial.

neur·epi·the·li·um (noor″ep-i-the′le-əm) neuroepithelium.

neu·rer·gic (noo͝-rur′jik) [*neur-* + *erg-* + *-ic*] pertaining to or dependent on nerve action.

neur·ex·er·e·sis (noor″ek-ser′ə-sis) [*neur-* + *exeresis*] nerve avulsion.

neu·ri·dine (noor′ĭ-dēn) a base isolated from fresh human brain, identical with spermine.

neu·ri·lem·ma (noor″ĭ-lem′ə) [*neur-* + *-lemma*] the thin membrane spirally enwrapping the myelin layers of certain fibers, especially of peripheral nerves, or the axons of certain unmyelinated nerve fibers. Called also *neurolemma, Schwann membrane, sheath of Schwann*, and *endoneural membrane.* **neurilem′mal** *adj*

neu·ri·lem·mi·tis (noor″ĭ-lem-i′tis) inflammation of the neurilemma.

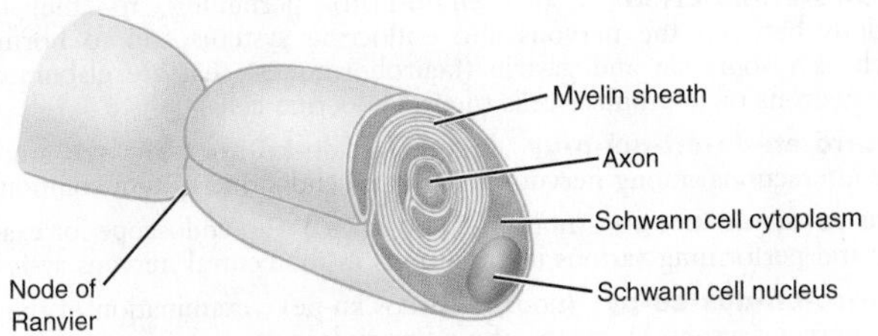

■ Neurilemma enclosing axon in a peripheral nerve fiber.

neu•ri•lem•mo•ma (noor″ĭ-lem-o′mə) neurilemoma.

neu•ri•lem•o•ma (noor″ĭ-lem-o′mə) a tumor of a neurilemma, the most common type of neurogenic tumor, usually isolated and encapsulated. Most are benign but occasionally they become malignant. Cf. *neurofibroma.* Called also *schwannoma.*

acoustic n. acoustic neuroma.

neu•ril•i•ty (nōō-ril′ĭ-te) the sum of the attributes and functions of nerve tissue.

neu•ri•mo•til•i•ty (noor″ĭ-mo-til′ĭ-te) nervimotility.

neu•ri•mo•tor (noor″ĭ-mo′tər) nervimotor.

neu•rine (noor′ēn) a poisonous ptomaine with a fishy odor, formed by dehydration of choline during putrefaction and found in decaying fish, fungi, and also in the brain and in many other normal tissues; used in biochemical research.

neu•ri•no•ma (noor″ĭ-no′mə) schwannoma.

acoustic n. acoustic neuroma.

acoustic n., bilateral neurofibromatosis 2.

neu•rite (noor′īt) any of the branched processes extending from the cell body of a neuron; it includes axons, dendrites, and undifferentiated processes such as those seen in immature neurons and in vitro.

neu•rit•ic (nōō-rit′ik) 1. pertaining to or affected with neuritis. 2. pertaining to a neurite.

neu•ri•tis (nōō-ri′tis) [*neur-* + *-itis*] inflammation of a nerve, with pain and tenderness, anesthesia and paresthesias, paralysis, wasting, and disappearance of the reflexes. See also *neuropathy.*

alcoholic n. see under *neuropathy.*

brachial n. neuralgic amyotrophy.

cauda equina n. inflammation of the nerve roots of the cauda equina of a horse or dog, usually seen in adults; symptoms include paralysis of the tail and certain abdominal muscles, with incoordination of the hind limbs and often fecal and urinary incontinence. Called also *cauda equina syndrome.*

dietetic n. beriberi.

fallopian n. neuritis of the facial nerve in the fallopian canal.

Gombault n. progressive hypertrophic neuropathy.

hereditary optic n. Leber hereditary optic neuropathy.

interstitial hypertrophic n. progressive hypertrophic interstitial neuropathy.

intraocular n., intraocular optic n. papillitis (def. 2).

lead n. see under *neuropathy.*

leprous n. see under *polyneuritis.*

n. mi′grans, migrating n. neuritis affecting first one nerve and then another.

multiple n. polyneuritis.

n. mul′tiplex ende′mica beriberi.

optic n. inflammation of the optic nerve; the two principal types, named according to the part of the nerve affected, are *intraocular optic n.* (or *papillitis*) and *retrobulbar optic n.*

orbital optic n. retrobulbar optic n.

periaxial n. segmental neuropathy.

peripheral n. neuritis of one or more peripheral nerves; cf. *polyneuritis.*

postfebrile n. neuritis following fever, such as in Guillain-Barré syndrome.

postocular optic n. retrobulbar optic n.

radiation n. radioneuritis.

radicular n. radiculitis.

retrobulbar n., retrobulbar optic n. optic neuritis in the portion of the optic nerve that is posterior to the eyeball; called also *postocular optic n.*

n. saturni′na lead neuropathy.

segmental n. see under *neuropathy.*

serum n. see under *neuropathy.*

shoulder-girdle n. neuralgic amyotrophy.

syphilitic n. neuritis due to neurosyphilis.

toxic n. see under *neuropathy.*

vestibular n. see under *neuronitis.*

neur(o)- [Gr. *neuron* nerve] a combining form denoting relationship to a nerve or nerves, or to the nervous system.

neu•ro•acan•tho•cy•to•sis (noor″o-ə-kan″tho-si-to′sis) choreoacanthocytosis.

neu•ro•al•ler•gy (noor″o-al′ər-je) allergy in nervous tissue.

neu•ro•anas•to•mo•sis (noor″o-ə-nas″tə-mo′sis) surgical formation of an anastomosis between nerves.

neu•ro•anat•o•my (noor″o-ə-nat′ə-me) [*neuro-* + *anatomy*] the branch of neurology that is concerned with the anatomy of the nervous system.

neu•ro•ar•throp•a•thy (noor″o-ahr-throp′ə-the) [*neuro-* + *arthropathy*] any disease of joint structures associated with disease of the central or peripheral nervous system.

neu•ro•as•per•gil•lo•sis (noor″o-as″pər-jil-o′sis) cerebral aspergillosis.

neu•ro•as•tro•cy•to•ma (noor″o-as″tro-si-to′mə) [*neuro-* + *astrocytoma*] a glioma composed mainly of astrocytes, closely resembling an astrocytoma and most commonly found in the floor of the third ventricle and the temporal lobes, although it may arise in almost any part of the central nervous system.

neu•ro•be•hav•ior•al (noor″o-be-hāv′u-rəl) relating to neurologic status as assessed by observation of behavior.

neu•ro•bi•ol•o•gist (noor″o-bi-ol′ə-jist) a specialist in neurobiology.

neu•ro•bi•ol•o•gy (noor″o-bi-ol′ə-je) the biology of the nervous system, including its anatomy, physiology, biochemistry, and so on.

neu•ro•bio•tax•is (noor″o-bi″o-tak′sis) [*neuro-* + *biotaxis*] the theory that nerve cell bodies have a tendency during development to migrate in the direction from which they habitually receive their stimuli.

neu•ro•blast (noor′o-blast) [*neuro-* + *-blast*] any embryonic cell that develops into a nerve cell or neuron.

sympathetic n. sympathoblast.

neu•ro•blas•to•ma (noor″o-blas-to′mə) sarcoma consisting of malignant neuroblasts, usually arising in the autonomic nervous system (sympathicoblastoma) or in the adrenal medulla; it is considered a type of neuroepithelial tumor and affects mostly infants and children up to 10 years of age.

olfactory n. a rare, slow-growing, malignant tumor of neuroectodermal origin that begins in neuroepithelial cells of the olfactory membrane. The tumor appears primarily in the nasal cavity and nasopharynx of adults as a painful swelling and eventually may spread to the sinuses, palate, orbit, and brain. Called also *esthesioneuroblastoma.*

neu•ro•bor•rel•i•o•sis (noor″o-bə-rel″e-o′sis) borreliosis affecting the nervous system, most commonly manifested by meningitis, cranial neuritis, or radiculopathy, or a combination of these; severity ranges from mild neuritis to severe meningopolyneuritis (Bannwarth syndrome).

neu•ro•car•di•ac (noor″o-kahr′de-ak) [*neuro-* + *cardiac*] pertaining to the nervous system and the heart.

neu•ro•cen•tral (noor″o-sen′trəl) pertaining to the body (centrum) of a vertebra and the pedicles of the vertebral arch.

neu•ro•cen•trum (noor″o-sen′trəm) one of the embryonic vertebral elements from which the spinous processes of the vertebrae develop.

neu•ro•cep•tor (noor′o-sep″tər) [*neuro-* + *-ceptor*] the postsynaptic area of a dendrite or effector organ; see also *postsynaptic membrane*, under *membrane.*

neu•ro•chem•is•try (noor″o-kem′is-tre) the branch of neurology that is concerned with the chemistry of the nervous system.

neu•ro•chon•drite (noor″o-kon′drīt) [*neuro-* + *chondr-* + *-ite*[1]] one of the embryonic cartilaginous elements that develop into the vertebral arch of a vertebra.

neu•ro•cho•rio•ret•i•ni•tis (noor″o-kor″e-o-ret″ĭ-ni′tis) [*neuro-* + *chorioretinitis*] inflammation of the optic nerve, choroid, and retina.

neu•ro•cho•roi•di•tis (noor″o-kor″oi-di′tis) inflammation of the choroid coat and optic nerves.

neu•ro•cir•cu•la•to•ry (noor″o-sur′ku-lə-tor″e) pertaining to the nervous and circulatory systems.

neu•roc•la•dism (nōō-rok′lə-diz″əm) [*neuro-* + Gr. *klados* branch] the formation of new branches by the process of a neuron; especially the force by which, in regeneration of divided nerves, the newly formed axons of the proximal stump become attracted by the peripheral stump so as to form a bridge between the two ends. Called also *odogenesis.*

neu•ro•cog•ni•tive (noor″o-kog′nĭ-tiv) said of those aspects of cognition that are most closely connected to specific areas of the brain; cf. *neuropsychology.*

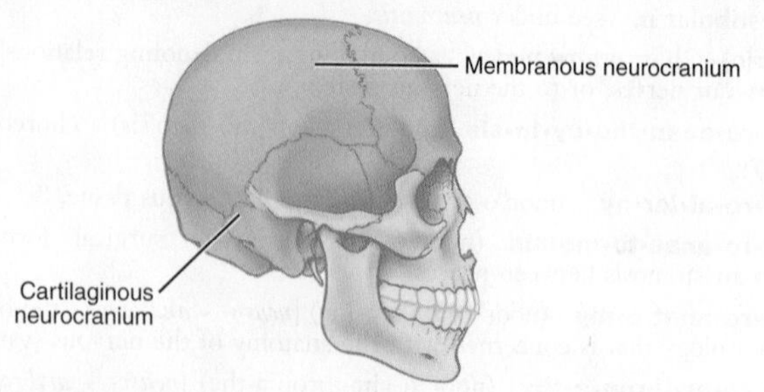

■ Neurocranium, comprising membranous and cartilaginous portions; the former, the calvaria, includes the frontal and parietal and portions of the temporal, occipital, and sphenoid bones; the latter, the chondrocranium, includes the ethmoid and portions of the occipital, temporal, and sphenoid bones.

neu•ro•com•mu•ni•ca•tions (noor″o-kə-mu″nĭ-ka′shənz) the branch of neurology dealing with the transfer and integration of information within the nervous system.

neu•ro•cra•ni•um (noor″o-kra′ne-əm) [TA] brain box; the portion of the cranium that encloses the brain; cf. *viscerocranium.* **neurocra′nial** *adj*
cartilaginous n. chondrocranium.
membranous n. the part of the neurocranium formed by intramembranous ossification and comprising the bones of the calvaria.

neu•ro•cris•top•a•thy (noor″o-kris-top′ə-the) [*neuro-* + *crista* + *-pathy*] any disease arising from maldevelopment of the neural crest.

neu•ro•crit•i•cal (noor″o-krit′ĭ-kəl) said of intensive care for neurologic conditions; called also *neurointensive.*

neu•ro•cu•ta•ne•ous (noor″o-ku-ta′ne-əs) pertaining to the nerves and the skin; pertaining to the cutaneous nerves.

neu•ro•cys•ti•cer•co•sis (noor″o-sis″tĭ-sər-ko′sis) [*neuro-* + *cysticercosis*] infection of the central nervous system with the larval forms (cysticerci) of *Taenia solium;* manifestations are highly variable, depending on the location and number of cysts, and may include seizures, hydrocephalus, and other neurologic dysfunctions, often with distinctive lesions visible by computed tomography or magnetic resonance imaging.

neu•ro•cy•tol•o•gy (noor″o-si-tol′ə-je) the branch of neurology that is concerned with the cellular components of the nervous system.

neu•ro•cy•tol•y•sin (noor″o-si-tol′ĭ-sin) a constituent of the venom of certain snakes (rattlesnake, coral snake, cobra), which lyses nerve cells.

neu•ro•cy•to•ma (noor″o-si-to′mə) 1. medulloepithelioma. 2. ganglioneuroma.

neu•ro•de•gen•er•a•tion (noor″o-de-jen″ər-a′shən) degeneration of nerve tissue; see types under *degeneration.* **neurodegen′erative** *adj*

neu•ro•den•drite (noor″o-den′drīt) dendrite.

neu•ro•den•dron (noor″o-den′dron) dendrite.

neu•ro•derm (noor′o-dərm) that portion of the ectoderm which develops into the neural tube; called also *neural ectoderm.*

neu•ro•der•ma•ti•tis (noor″o-dur″mə-ti′tis) [*neuro-* + *dermatitis*] name given to various types of eczema presumed to be cutaneous responses to prolonged scratching, rubbing, or pinching to relieve pruritus; there may be polymorphic lesions at the same or different times. Some authorities consider this a psychogenic disorder.
circumscribed n., n. circumscrip′ta lichen simplex chronicus.
disseminated n. atopic dermatitis.
exudative n. nummular eczema.
localized n. lichen simplex chronicus.
nummular n. see under *eczema.*

neu•ro•de•vel•op•men•tal (noor″o-de-vel″op-men′təl) [*neuro-* + *developmental*] pertaining to the development of the nervous system.

neu•ro•dyn•ia (noor″o-din′e-ə) neuralgia.

neu•ro•ec•to•derm (noor″o-ek′to-dərm) the portion of the ectoderm of the early embryo that gives rise to the central and peripheral nervous systems, including some glial cells. Cf. *neuroderm.* **neuroectoder′mal** *adj*

neu•ro•ef•fec•tor (noor″o-ə-fek′tər) of or relating to the junction between a neuron and the effector organ it innervates.

neu•ro•elec•tric•i•ty (noor″o-e″lek-tris′ĭ-te) the electrical signals, currents, or voltages generated by the nervous system.

neu•ro•en•ceph•a•lo•my•elop•a•thy (noor″o-en-sef″ə-lo-mi″ə-lop′ə-the) [*neuro-* + *encephalo-* + *myelopathy*] disease involving the brain, spinal cord, and nerves.
optic n. neuromyelitis optica.

neu•ro•en•do•crine (noor″o-en′do-krin) pertaining to the interactions between the nervous and endocrine systems and to hormones such as vasopressin and gastrin (neurohormones) that are elaborated in the neurons or neuronlike cells (neuroendocrine cells).

neu•ro•en•do•cri•nol•o•gy (noor″o-en″do-krĭ-nol′ə-je) the study of the interactions among nervous system and endocrine system components.

neu•ro•en•do•scope (noor″o-en′do-skōp″) an endoscope for examining and performing various interventions in the central nervous system.

neu•ro•en•dos•co•py (noor″o-en-dos′kə-pe) examination of the central nervous system by means of a neuroendoscope.

neu•ro•en•do•vas•cu•lar (noor″o-en″do-vas′ku-lər) within a cerebral artery.

neu•ro•en•ter•ic (noor″o-en-ter′ik) neurenteric.

neur•o•ep•i•de•mi•ol•o•gy (noor″o-ep″ĭ-de″me-ol′ə-je) the epidemiology of neurologic conditions.

neu•ro•epi•der•mal (noor″o-ep″ĭ-dur′məl) [*neuro-* + *epidermal*] pertaining to or giving origin to the nervous and epidermal tissues.

neu•ro•epi•the•li•al (noor″o-ep″ĭ-the′le-əl) 1. pertaining to neuroepithelium. 2. composed of neuroepithelium.

neu•ro•epi•the•li•o•ma (noor″o-ep″ĭ-the″le-o′mə) medulloepithelioma.
peripheral n. peripheral neuroectodermal tumor.

neu•ro•epi•the•li•um (noor″o-ep″ĭ-the′le-əm) [*neuro-* + *epithelium*] 1. simple columnar epithelium made up of cells specialized to serve as sensory cells for the reception of external stimuli, such as the sensory cells of the cochlea, vestibule, nasal mucosa, and tongue. Called also *neurepithelium* and *sensory epithelium.* 2. the epithelium of the ectoderm, from which the central nervous system is developed.
n. cris′tae ampulla′ris neuroepithelium of ampullary crest: the specialized epithelium of the ampullary crest of the labyrinth, containing vestibular hair cells that project into the cupula and serve as sensory receptors.
n. macula′rum neuroepithelium of maculae: the specialized epithelium of the maculae of the labyrinth, containing vestibular hair cells that project into the otolithic membrane and serve as sensory receptors.

neu•ro•fi•ber (noor″o-fi′bər) neurofibra.

neu•ro•fi•bra (noor″o-fi′brə) pl. *neurofi′brae* [L.] [TA] nerve fiber or neurofiber: a slender process of a neuron; the term is often synonymous with axon. Nerve fibers are classified on the basis of the presence or absence of a myelin sheath as myelinated or unmyelinated. In the terminology for types of nerve fibers, the word *nerve* is frequently dropped; e.g., *myelinated f's, unmyelinated f's,* etc. For bundles or tracts of nerve fibers, see under *bundle, fasciculus, lemniscus, tract,* and *tractus.* Called also *fiber* and *fibra.*
neurofi′brae afferen′tes [TA] afferent nerve fibers: nerve fibers that convey sensory impulses from the periphery to the central nervous system; classified according to function as somatic afferent and visceral afferent fibers. Called also *sensory fibers.*
n. associatio′nis fibra associationis.
neurofi′brae autono′micae [TA] autonomic nerve fibers: nerve fibers that innervate smooth muscle, cardiac muscle, and glandular epithelium. They either stimulate and activate the muscle or tissue *(autonomic efferent fibers)* or receive sensory impulses from them *(autonomic afferent fibers).* Called also *neurofibrae viscerales* and *visceral nerve fibers.*
n. commissura′lis fibra commissuralis.
neurofi′brae efferen′tes [TA] efferent nerve fibers: nerve fibers that convey motor impulses away from the central nervous system toward the periphery; classified according to function as somatic efferent and visceral efferent fibers. Called also *motor fibers.*
neurofi′brae postgangliona′res, neurofi′brae postganglio′nicae [TA] postganglionic nerve fibers: the axons of postganglionic neurons.
neurofi′brae pregangliona′res, neurofi′brae preganglio′nicae [TA] preganglionic nerve fibers: the axons of preganglionic neurons.
n. projectio′nis fibra projectionis.
neurofi′brae soma′ticae [TA] somatic nerve fibers: nerve fibers that innervate skeletal muscles and somatic tissues. They either stimulate and activate the muscle or tissue *(somatic efferent fibers)* or receive sensory impulses from them *(somatic afferent fibers).* Called also *somatic fibers.*
neurofi′brae tangentia′les [TA] tangential fibers: tangentially oriented nerve fibers arranged in striae in the superficial layers of the hippocampus and cerebral cortex.
neurofi′brae viscera′les neurofibrae autonomicae.

neu•ro•fi•bril (noor″o-fi′bril) any of the fibrils visible in the perikaryon, dendrites, and axon of a neuron in light microscopy after staining with silver; the fibrils are believed to be neurofilament bundles, and perhaps also neurotubules, that have become coated with silver particles. **neurofi′brillar** *adj*

neu•ro•fi•bril•la (noor″o-fi-bril′ə) pl. *neurofibril′lae.* Neurofibril.

neu•ro•fi•bro•ma (noor″o-fi-bro′mə) [*neuro-* + *fibroma*] a usually benign tumor of peripheral nerves caused by abnormal proliferation of Schwann cells; called also *fibroneuroma*. Cf. *neurilemoma*.

cutaneous n., dermal n. a neurofibroma arising within the skin, occurring as a small, fleshy nodule that may become pedunculated, overlying a palpable subcutaneous lesion.

plexiform n. a fusiform, ropelike enlargement of a nerve, consisting of Schwann cells, fibroblasts, and inflammatory cells in a loose myxoid ground, usually occurring as multiple lesions in neurofibromatosis 1, although occasionally arising as a solitary, spontaneous lesion. Called also *plexiform* or *Verneuil neuroma*.

solitary n. a neurofibroma arising along a nerve trunk, occurring as spontaneous lesion without internal manifestations.

neu•ro•fi•bro•ma•to•sis (noor″o-fi-bro″mə-to′sis) either of two familial conditions characterized by developmental changes in the nervous system and other structures, with formation of neurofibromas. Called also *multiple neuroma* and *neuromatosis*.

n. 1 (NF1) an autosomal dominant disorder due to mutation in the *NF1* gene (locus: 17q11.2), which encodes the tumor suppressor neurofibromin; it is marked by developmental changes in the nervous system, muscles, bones, and skin with café au lait spots, intertriginous freckling, Lisch nodules, and multiple pedunculated neurofibromas over much of the body. Called also *von Recklinghausen disease* and *peripheral n.*

n. 2 (NF2) an autosomal dominant disorder due to mutation in the *NF2* gene (locus: 22q12.2), which encodes the cytoskeletal protein merlin (also called neurofibromin-2), which acts as a tumor suppressor. It is characterized by usually bilateral acoustic neuromas (q.v.), sometimes with skin changes like those seen in neurofibromatosis 1, central and peripheral nerve tumors, and presenile lens opacities. Called also *bilateral acoustic neurinoma, neuroma*, or *neurofibromatosis*, and *central n.*

bilateral acoustic n. n. 2.

central n. n. 2.

peripheral n. n. 1.

neu•ro•fi•bro•min (noor″ro-fi′bro-min) a GTPase-activating protein that functions as a tumor suppressor; a defect in the gene that codes for this protein is the cause of neurofibromatosis 1.

neu•ro•fi•bro•sar•co•ma (noor″o-fi″bro-sahr-ko′mə) malignant peripheral nerve sheath tumor.

neu•ro•fil•a•ment (noor″o-fil′ə-ment) a type of intermediate filament occurring with neurotubules in the neurons; it has a cytoskeletal function and may be involved in the intracellular transport of metabolites.

neu•ro•gan•gli•itis (noor″o-gang″gle-i′tis) ganglionitis.

neu•ro•gan•gli•on (noor″o-gang′gle-on) ganglion (def. 2).

neu•ro•gas•tric (noor″o-gas′trik) involving the innervation of the stomach.

neuro•gas•tro•en•ter•ol•o•gy (noor″o-gas″tro-en″tər-ol′ə-je) a medical subspecialty that deals with the function and dysfunction of the gastrointestinal tract and its innervation.

neu•ro•gen (noor′o-jən) the chemical substance by means of which the primary organizer causes the development of the neural plate.

neu•ro•gen•e•sis (noor″o-jen′ə-sis) [*neuro-* + *-genesis*] the development of nervous tissue.

neu•ro•ge•net•ic (noor″o-jə-net′ik) 1. pertaining to neurogenesis. 2. neurogenic.

neu•ro•ge•net•ics (noor″o-jə-net′iks) [*neuro-* + *genetics*] the study of genetic influences on the nervous system, including embryonic

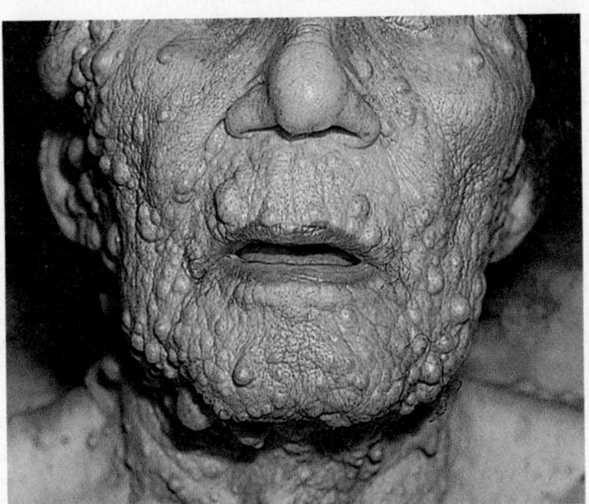

■ Multiple neurofibromas on the face of a patient with neurofibromatosis.

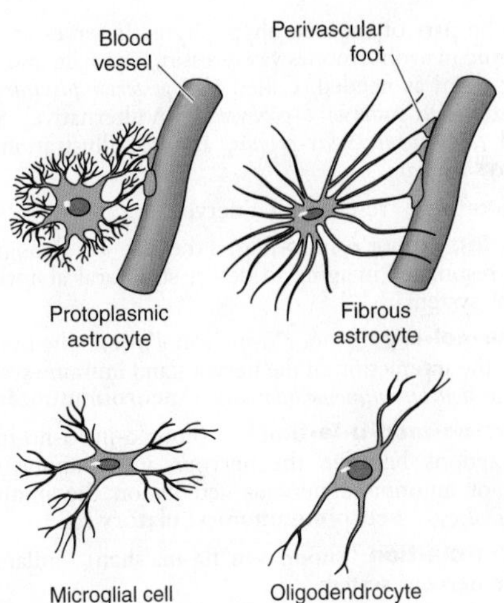

■ Neuroglia, showing various types of neuroglial cells.

development of the nervous system and neurological disorders that have a genetic basis.

neu•ro•gen•ic (noor″o-jen′ik) [*neuro-* + *-genic*] 1. forming nervous tissue. 2. originating in the nervous system or from a lesion in the nervous system.

neu•rog•e•nous (nōō-roj′ə-nəs) neurogenic.

neu•rog•lia (nōō-rog′le-ə) [*neuro-* + *-glia*] [TA] the supporting structure of nervous tissue. It consists of a fine web of tissue made up of modified ectodermal elements, in which are enclosed peculiar branched cells known as *neuroglial cells* or *glial cells*. The neuroglial cells are of three types: astrocytes and oligodendrocytes (astroglia and oligodendroglia), which appear to play a role in myelin formation, transport of material to neurons, and maintenance of the ionic environment of neurons; and microglial cells, which phagocytize waste products of nerve tissue. Called also *glia*. **neurog′lial** *adj*

interfascicular n. oligodendroglia of white matter along the myelin sheaths.

peripheral n. the neurilemma, Schwann cells, and satellite cells of the peripheral nervous system.

neu•rog•lio•cyte (nōō-rog′le-o-sīt″) [*neuroglia* + *-cyte*] a cell of the neuroglia.

neu•rog•lio•cy•to•ma (nōō-rog″le-o-si-to′mə) glioma.

neu•rog•li•o•ma (nōō-rog″le-o′mə) glioma.

n. gangliona′re ganglioglioma.

neu•rog•li•o•ma•to•sis (nōō-rog″le-o-mə-to′sis) gliomatosis.

neu•rog•li•o•sis (nōō-rog″le-o′sis) gliomatosis.

neu•ro•gly•co•pe•nia (noor″o-gli″ko-pe′ne-ə) [*neuro-* + *glycopenia*] chronic hypoglycemia of a degree sufficient to impair brain function, resulting in personality changes and intellectual deterioration that may progress to convulsions, coma, and occasionally even death.

neu•ro•gram (noor′o-gram″) [*neuro-* + *-gram*] residua of past cerebral activities which make up the brain disposition and thus take part in the formation of personality.

neu•ro•his•tol•o•gy (noor″o-his-tol′ə-je) the histology of the nervous system.

neu•ro•hor•mone (noor′o-hor″mōn) a hormone secreted by a specialized neuron into the bloodstream, the cerebrospinal fluid, or the intercellular spaces of the nervous system; examples are neuropeptides and other types of neuromodulators. Cf. *neuroendocrine*. **neurohormo′nal** *adj*

neu•ro•hu•mor (noor″o-hu′mər) neurohormone.

neu•ro•hu•mor•al (noor″o-hu′mər-əl) 1. mediated by neurohormones. 2. neurohormonal. 3. mediated by neurohormones.

neu•ro•hy•po•phys•e•al (noor″o-hi″po-fiz′e-əl) neurohypophysial.

neu•ro•hy•po•phys•ec•to•my (noor″o-hi″po-fiz-ek′tə-me) [*neuro-* + *hypophysectomy*] surgical removal of the neurohypophysis.

neu•ro•hy•poph•y•sis (noor″o-hi-pof′ə-sis) [*neuro-* + *hypophysis*] [TA] the posterior lobe of the hypophysis (pituitary gland), which originates as an evagination from the floor of the embryonic diencephalon and is the neural portion of the gland. It consists of the infundibulum or neural stalk, which is continuous with the hypothalamus, and the neural lobe, which is its main body. The median eminence is sometimes considered to be part of the neurohypophysis. It serves as a reservoir for the hypothalamic neurohormones vasopressin, oxytocin, and the neurophysins, releasing them as needed. Called also *posterior pituitary*, *posterior lobe of hypophysis*, and *lobus posterior hypophyseos* [TA alternative]. See also *adenohypophysis* and *circumventricular organs*, and see illustration at *hypophysis*. **neurohypophys′ial** *adj*

neu•roid (noor′oid) resembling a nerve.

neu•ro•imag•ing (noor′o-im″ə-jing) the use of radiographic studies and magnetic resonance imaging to detect structural abnormalities in the central nervous system.

neu•ro•im•mu•nol•o•gy (noor″o-im″u-nol′ə-je) the branch of science that deals with the interaction of the nervous and immune systems in health and disease (see *neuroimmunomodulation*). **neuroimmunolog′ic** *adj*

neu•ro•im•mu•no•mod•u•la•tion (noor″o-im″u-no-mod″u-la′shən) complex interactions between the nervous and immune systems, such as the effects of autonomic nervous activity on the immune response. Cf. *neuroimmunology*. **neuroimmunomod′ulatory** *adj*

neu•ro•in•flam•ma•tion (noor″o-in″flə-ma′shən) inflammation of a nerve or of the nervous system.

neu•ro•in•ten•sive (noor″o-in-ten′siv) neurocritical.

neu•ro•in•ten•siv•ist (noor″o-in-ten′siv-ist) a neurologist who specializes in the provision of neurologic intensive care; see *intensive care unit*, under *unit*.

neu•ro•in•ter•ven•tion (noor″o-in″tər-ven′shən) treatment of neurologic diseases using interventional neurology. **neurointerven′tional** *adj*

neu•ro•in•ter•ven•tion•al•ist (noor″o-in″tər-ven′shən-əl-ist) a specialist in interventional neurology.

neu•ro•in•ter•ven•tion•ist (noor″o-in″tər-ven′shən-ist) neurointerventionalist.

neu•ro•in•va•sive (noor″o-in-va′siv) having a tendency to attack the central nervous system.

neu•ro•ker•a•tin (noor″o-ker′ə-tin) proteinaceous material left after the myelin of a myelin sheath is dissolved away during fixation; it forms a network that probably does not exist in vivo.

neu•ro•ki•nin (noor″o-ki′nin) [*neuro-* + *kinin*] a kinin that stimulates nerve receptors.

neu•ro•lab•y•rin•thi•tis (noor″o-lab″ĭ-rin-thi′tis) inflammation of the neural structures of the labyrinth.

neu•ro•lath•y•rism (noor″o-lath′ĭ-riz-əm) lathyrism.

neu•ro•lem•ma (noor″o-lem′ə) neurilemma.

neu•ro•lep•tan•al•ge•sia (noor″o-lep″tan-əl-je′ze-ə) [*neuroleptic* + *analgesia*] a state of quiescence, altered awareness, and analgesia produced by the administration of a combination of an opioid analgesic and a neuroleptic agent.

neu•ro•lep•tan•al•ge•sic (noor″o-lep″tan-əl-je′zik) 1. pertaining to or producing neuroleptanalgesia. 2. an agent that produces neuroleptanalgesia.

neu•ro•lep•tan•es•the•sia (noor″o-lep″tan-es-the′zhə) [*neuroleptic* + *anesthesia*] a state of neuroleptanalgesia and unconsciousness, produced by the combined administration of an opioid analgesic and a neuroleptic agent, together with the inhalation of nitrous oxide and oxygen.

neu•ro•lep•tan•es•thet•ic (noor″o-lep″tan-əs-thet′ik) 1. pertaining to or producing neuroleptanesthesia. 2. an agent that produces neuroleptanesthesia.

neu•ro•lep•tic (noor″o-lep′tik) [*neuro-* + Gr. *lēpsis* a taking hold] a term coined to refer to the effects on cognition and behavior of the original antipsychotic agents, which produced a state of apathy, lack of initiative, and limited range of emotion and in psychotic patients caused a reduction in confusion and agitation and normalization of psychomotor activity. The term is still used to refer to agents used to produce such effects as part of anesthesia or analgesia; however, it is outdated as a synonym for antipsychotic agents because newer agents do not necessarily have such effects. See *antipsychotic*.

neu•ro•leu•kin (noor″o-loo′kin) glucose-6-phosphate isomerase.

neu•ro•lin•guis•tics (noor″o-ling-gwis′tiks) the study of language acquisition, processing, and production at the neurological level.

neu•ro•li•po•ma•to•sis (noor″o-lĭ-po″mə-to′sis) lipomatosis with neurologic complications.

n. doloro′sa see under *adiposis*.

Neu•ro•lite (noor′o-līt″) trademark for a kit for the preparation of technetium Tc 99m bicisate.

neu•ro•lo•gia (noor″o-lo′jə) neurology.

neu•rol•o•gist (noo͝-rol′ə-jist) a physician whose practice focuses on neurology.

neu•rol•o•gy (noo͝-rol′ə-je) [*neuro-* + *-logy*] the medical specialty that deals with the nervous system, both normal and in disease. **neurolog′ic** *adj*

clinical n. the specialty concerned with the diagnosis and treatment of disorders of the nervous system.

interventional n. a subspecialty of neurology concerned with the use of minimally invasive procedures for the diagnosis and treatment of vascular diseases of the central nervous system.

vascular n. a subspecialty of neurology concerned with the diagnosis and treatment of cerebrovascular conditions such as stroke syndrome.

neu•ro•lu•es (noor″o-loo′ēz) neurosyphilis.

neu•ro•lym•pho•ma•to•sis (noor″o-lim″fo-mə-to′sis) lymphoblastic infiltration of a nerve.

n. gallina′rum Marek disease in which neurological symptoms are dominant.

neu•rol•y•sin (noo͝-rol′ĭ-sin) a cytolysin which has a specific destructive action upon nerve cells.

neu•rol•y•sis (noo͝-rol′ĭ-sis) [*neuro-* + *lysis*] 1. release of a nerve sheath by cutting it longitudinally. 2. the operative breaking up of perineural adhesions. 3. the relief of tension upon a nerve obtained by stretching. 4. destruction or dissolution of nerve tissue; sometimes done as a temporary or permanent measure for the relief of pain or spasticity. See also *rhizotomy*. Called also *nerve block*.

alcohol n. intrathecal neurolysis in which dehydrated alcohol is injected at the point where the dorsal root emerges from the spinal cord.

celiac plexus n. lysis of the nerves originating in the celiac plexus, done for intractable pain in the stomach, pancreas, gallbladder, or other organs of the upper abdomen.

chemical n. neurolysis (def. 4) by injection of a neurolytic chemical such as glycerol, phenol, or alcohol adjacent to a nerve; see also *chemical rhizotomy*.

intramuscular n. motor point block.

intrathecal n. chemical neurolysis in which a substance is injected under the dura mater of the spinal cord.

phenol n. intrathecal neurolysis in which a solution of 5 to 7.5 per cent phenol in glycerol is injected into a dorsal root ganglion.

trigeminal n. see under *rhizotomy*.

neu•ro•lyt•ic (noor″o-lit′ik) pertaining to neurolysis.

neu•ro•ma (noo͝-ro′mə) [*neur-* + *-oma*] a tumor growing from a nerve or made up largely of nerve cells and nerve fibers. Many lesions formerly called neuromas are now given more specific names such as *ganglioneuroma*, *neurilemoma*, or *neurofibroma*. **neuro′matous** *adj*

acoustic n. a progressively enlarging, benign tumor, usually within the internal auditory canal arising from Schwann cells of the vestibular division of the eighth cranial nerve; the symptoms, which vary with the size and location of the tumor, may include hearing loss, headache, disturbances of balance and gait, facial numbness or pain, and tinnitus. It may be unilateral or bilateral (neurofibromatosis 2). Called also *acoustic neurilemoma*, *neurinoma*, or *schwannoma*, and *acoustic nerve tumor*.

amputation n. traumatic n.

amyelinic n. a neuroma containing only nonmedullated nerve fibers.

n. cu′tis neuroma seated in the skin.

false n. 1. something that looks like a neuroma but does not contain nerve cells. 2. traumatic n.

ganglionar n., ganglionated n., ganglionic n. ganglioneuroma.

interdigital n., intermetatarsal n. Morton n.

medullated n. myelinic n.

Morton n. the neuroma that results from Morton neuralgia.

multiple n. 1. neurofibromatosis. 2. neuromatosis.

myelinic n. a neuroma that contains myelinated nerve fibers; called also *medullated n.*

nevoid n. n. telangiectodes.

plantar n. Morton n.

plexiform n. see under *neurofibroma*.

stump n. amputation n.

n. telangiecto′des a neuroma that contains an excess of blood vessels; called also *nevoid n.*

traumatic n. a non-neoplastic unorganized bulbous or nodular mass of nerve fibers and Schwann cells produced by hyperplasia of nerve fibers and their supporting tissues after accidental or purposeful sectioning of the nerve. Called also *amputation n.*, *false n.*, and *pseudoneuroma*.

true n. a neuroma made up of nerve tissue; see also *ganglioneuroma*.

Verneuil n. plexiform neurofibroma.

neu•ro•ma•la•cia (noor″o-mə-la′shə) [*neuro-* + *malacia*] necrosis and softening of the nerves.

neu•ro•ma•la•kia (noor″o-mə-la′ke-ə) neuromalacia.

neu•ro•ma•to•sis (noo-ro″mə-to′sis) 1. any disease characterized by multiple neuromas. 2. neurofibromatosis.

neu•ro•mech•a•nism (noor′o-mek′ə-niz-əm) the structure and arrangement of the nervous system in relation to function.

neu•ro•me•di•a•tor (noor″o-me′de-a-tər) a mediator in the nervous system; see *mediator.*

neu•ro•mel•a•nin (noor″o-mel′ə-nin) a modified melanin present in neurons of the brain, particularly of the substantia nigra and locus caeruleus, which owe their pigmentation to its presence; the mechanism of its formation, as well as its function and effects, is uncertain.

neu•ro•me•nin•ge•al (noor″o-mə-nin′je-əl) pertaining to or affecting nervous tissue and the meninges.

neu•ro•mere (noor′o-mēr) [*neuro-* + *-mere*] any of the series of transitory segmental elevations in the wall of the neural tube of the developing embryo; those specific to the rhombencephalon may be called rhombomeres. Called also *neural segment.*

neu•ro•met•rics (noor″o-met′riks) a computer-assisted method for evaluating brain functions by quantitative analysis of the results of tests such as the electroencephalogram or measurements of evoked potentials. Data from patients with similar signs or symptoms are compared with a normative data base to identify links between patterns of electrical activity and of behavioral or other symptomatic abnormalities.

neu•ro•mi•met•ic (noor″o-mĭ-met′ik) 1. eliciting a response in effector organs that simulates that elicited by nervous impulses. 2. an agent that elicits such a response.

neu•ro•mod•u•la•tion (noor″o-mod″u-la′shən) 1. electrical stimulation of a peripheral nerve, the spinal cord, or the brain for relief of pain; it may be done transcutaneously or with an implanted stimulator. 2. the effect of a neuromodulator on another neuron. **neuromod′ulatory** *adj*

neu•ro•mod•u•la•tor (noor″o-mod′u-la″tər) a substance other than a neurotransmitter, released by a neuron and conveying information to adjacent or distant neurons, either enhancing or damping their activities. Neuropeptides are often neuromodulators.

neu•ro•mon•i•tor•ing (noor″o-mon′ĭ-tər-ing) intraoperative monitoring of nerves and neural tissue by processes such as evoked potentials, electroencephalography, and electromyography, with notification of the surgeon if significant changes occur.

neu•ro•mor•phom•e•try (noor″o-mor-fom′ə-tre) the determination of the size and shape of brain structures. **neuromorphomet′ric** *adj*

neu•ro•mo•tor (noor″o-mo′tər) 1. involving both nerves and muscles. 2. pertaining to nervous impulses to muscles.

neu•ro•mus•cu•lar (noor″o-mus′ku-lər) pertaining to muscles and nerves, or to the relationship between them.

neu•ro•mus•cu•lo•skel•e•tal (noor″o-mus″ku-lo-skel′ə-təl) pertaining to or affecting the nervous, muscular, and skeletal systems.

neu•ro•my•al (noor″o-mi′əl) neuromuscular.

neu•ro•my•as•the•nia (noor″o-mi″es-the′ne-ə) [*neuro-* + *myasthenia*] muscular weakness associated with emotional lability.

epidemic n. chronic fatigue syndrome.

neu•ro•my•eli•tis (noor″o-mi″ə-li′tis) [*neuro-* + *myelitis*] inflammation of nervous and medullary substance; myelitis attended with neuritis.

n. op′tica combined, but not usually clinically simultaneous, demyelination of the optic nerve and the spinal cord; it is marked by diminution of vision and possibly blindness, flaccid paralysis of the extremities, and sensory and genitourinary disturbances. Called also *Devic disease, optic neuroencephalomyelopathy, neuro-optic myelitis,* and *ophthalmoneuromyelitis.*

neu•ro•my•op•a•thy (noor″o-mi-op′ə-the) any disease of both muscles and nerves, especially a muscular disease of nervous origin. **neuromyopath′ic** *adj*

carcinomatous n. a paraneoplastic syndrome of neuromyopathy in patients having carcinoma, usually of the lung. Cf. *carcinomatous polyneuropathy.*

neu•ro•myo•si•tis (noor″o-mi″o-si′tis) [*neuro-* + *myositis*] neuritis complicated with myositis.

neu•ro•myo•to•nia (noor″o-mi″o-to′ne-ə) [*neuro-* + *myotonia*] myotonia caused by electrical activity of a peripheral nerve, characterized by stiffness, delayed relaxation, fasciculations, and myokymia.

acquired n. Isaacs syndrome.

neu•ron (noor′on) [Gr. "nerve"] [TA] any of the conducting cells of the nervous system. A typical neuron consists of a cell body, containing the nucleus and the surrounding cytoplasm (perikaryon); several short radiating processes (dendrites); and one long process (the axon), which terminates in twiglike branches (telodendrons) and may have branches (collaterals) projecting along its course. The axon together with its covering or sheath forms the nerve fiber. See illustration and Plate 39. Called also *nerve cell.* **neu′ronal** *adj*

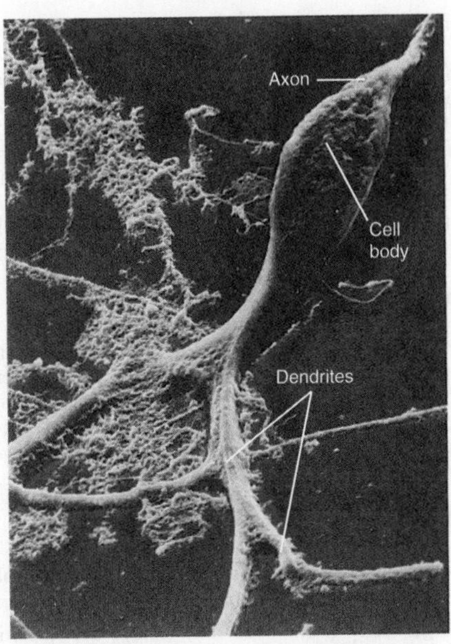

■ Scanning electron micrograph of a neuron.

afferent n. any neuron conducting a nerve impulse that originated at a receptor and is proceeding towards the center. See also *sensory n.,* and see *afferent fibers,* under *fiber.*

bipolar n. a neuron having two processes, one projecting from each end of the cell body; these may be either one axon and one dendrite or two dendrites.

central n. a neuron which belongs entirely to the central nervous system.

connector n. interneuron.

efferent n. any neuron conducting a nerve impulse that originated at the center and is proceeding towards the periphery. See also *efferent fibers,* under *fiber.*

fusimotor n's gamma motoneurons.

Golgi type I n's pyramidal neurons with very long axons, that leave the gray matter of the central nervous system, traverse the white matter, and terminate in the periphery; called also *Golgi type I cells.*

Golgi type II n's stellate neurons with short axons that do not pass out of the gray matter in which the cell body lies, and are especially numerous in the cerebral and cerebellar cortices and in the retina. Called also *Golgi type II cells.*

intercalary n., intercalated n., internuncial n. interneuron.

local circuit n. Golgi type II n.

motor n. motoneuron.

multiform n. multipolar n.

multimodal n. multisensory n.

multipolar n. a neuron with several to many processes; such neurons vary in shape, depending on the arrangement of the processes, with pyramidal and stellate (star) shapes being common. Called also *polymorphic n.*

multisensory n. a neuron in the cerebral cortex or subcortical regions that can receive input from more than one sensory modality; the inputs may be simultaneous, reinforcing each other.

peripheral sensory n. in a reflex arc, a sensory neuron whose fibers end at synapses with interneurons. Cf. *peripheral motoneuron.*

piriform n's Purkinje cells.

polymorphic n. multipolar n.

postganglionic n's neurons in the autonomic nervous system whose cell bodies are situated in the autonomic ganglia and whose purpose is to relay impulses beyond the ganglia. See also *pars parasympathetica divisionis autonomici systematis nervosi,* under *pars.*

postsynaptic n. any neuron located distal to a specified synaptic cleft.

preganglionic n's neurons in the autonomic nervous system whose cell bodies lie in the central nervous system and whose efferent fibers terminate in the autonomic ganglia. See also *pars parasympathica divisionis autonomici systematis nervosi,* under *pars.*

premotor n's upper motoneurons.

presynaptic n. any neuron located proximal to a specified synaptic cleft.

primary sensory n. a sensory neuron that is the first in an afferent pathway, beginning at the receptor and ending at a synapse with a secondary sensory neuron, often within a nucleus of the central nervous system. One common type is the pseudounipolar neuron.

projection n. a neuron that serves for the transmission of nervous impulses, whether motor or sensory, between the cerebral cortex and other parts of the nervous system. See also *projection fibers*, under *fiber*.

pseudounipolar n. a unipolar neuron, almost always a primary sensory neuron, that was originally bipolar but whose two processes fused during development to form a single process that bifurcates at a distance from the cell body. One branch is structurally an axon with a myelin sheath but functions as a dendrite, with afferent conduction originating in a nerve ending.

Purkinje n's see under *cell*.

pyramidal n. see under *cell*.

secondary sensory n. a sensory neuron that is the second in an afferent pathway, being stimulated at a synapse by a primary sensory neuron and often extending some distance into the central nervous system.

sensory n. any neuron with a sensory function; an afferent neuron conveying sensory impulses. Cf. *primary sensory n.* and *secondary sensory n.* See Plate 39.

spiny n. a neuron whose dendrites have many spines (gemmules), such as a Golgi type I neuron.

tuberohypophysial n's hypothalamic neurons, located primarily in the arcuate nucleus, whose axons form the tuberohypophysial tract.

unipolar n. a neuron with one process only; see also *pseudounipolar n.*

neu·ro·nav·i·ga·tion (noor″o-nav″i-ga′shən) the use of computer-assisted technology during surgery to aid in precise navigation within the central nervous system.

neu·rone (noor′ōn) neuron.

neu·ro·neph·ric (noor″o-nef′rik) pertaining to the innervation of the kidneys.

neu·ro·ne·vus (noor″o-ne′vəs) [*neuro-* + *nevus*] an intradermal nevus in which the nevus cells differentiate into nervelike structures and may clinically resemble neurofibroma or have the clinical aspect of a giant pigmented nevus. Called also *neural nevus*.

neu·ro·ni·tis (noor″o-ni′tis) inflammation of one or more neurons.

vestibular n. a disturbance of vestibular function consisting of a single attack of severe vertigo, usually accompanied by nausea and vomiting but without auditory symptoms; it attacks mainly young to middle-aged adults and usually improves within a few days. Called also *endemic paralytic vertigo*, *epidemic vertigo*, *paralytic vertigo*, and *vestibular neuritis*.

neu·ro·nop·a·thy (noor″on-op′ə-the) polyneuropathy involving destruction of the cell bodies of neurons.

sensory n. degeneration of peripheral sensory neurons in the dorsal root ganglia, with inflammation and infiltration by lymphocytes, characterized by pain and numbness that begins in the limbs and may advance to the trunk and face. It may be a complication of an autoimmune condition, heavy metal poisoning, or certain cancers, especially small cell lung carcinoma.

neu·rono·phage (nōō-ron′o-fāj) [*neuron* + *-phage*] a phagocyte that ingests nerve cells.

neu·rono·pha·gia (noor″on-o-fa′jə) the ingestion of nerve cells by phagocytic action.

neu·rono·tro·pic (noor″on-o-tro′pik) [*neuron* + *-tropic*] having a special affinity for neurons.

Neu·ron·tin (nōō-ron′tin) trademark for preparations of gabapentin.

neu·ro·on·col·o·gy (noor″o-on-kol′ə-je) the field of specialization dealing with tumors of the nervous system.

neu·ro·oph·thal·mol·o·gy (noor″o-of″thəl-mol′ə-je) [*neuro-* + *ophthalmology*] a medical specialty that combines neurology and ophthalmology, dealing with neurological aspects of vision, the eye, and its adnexa.

neu·ro·otol·o·gy (noor″o-o-tol′ə-je) a medical specialty that combines neurology and otology, dealing especially with portions of the nervous system related to the ear.

neu·ro·pace·mak·er (noor″o-pās′māk-ər) an implant device that relieves pain due to nerve injury.

neu·ro·pap·il·li·tis (noor″o-pap″ĭ-li′tis) papillitis (def. 2).

neu·ro·par·a·lyt·ic (noor″o-par″ə-lit′ik) affected with or pertaining to paralysis of a nerve or nerves.

neu·ro·patho·gen·e·sis (noor″o-path″o-jen′ə-sis) development of disease of the nervous system.

neu·ro·patho·ge·nic·i·ty (noor″o-path″o-jə-nis′ĭ-te) the quality of producing or the ability to produce pathologic changes in nerve tissue.

neu·ro·pa·thol·o·gy (noor″o-pə-thol′ə-je) the branch of medicine dealing with morphological and other aspects of disease of the nervous system.

neu·rop·a·thy (nōō-rop′ə-the) [*neuro-* + *-pathy*] a functional disturbance or pathological change in the peripheral nervous system, sometimes limited to noninflammatory lesions as opposed to those of neuritis; the etiology may be known or unknown. Known etiologies include complications of other diseases (such as diabetes or porphyria), or of toxicity states (such as poisoning with arsenic, isoniazid, lead, or nitrofurantoin). The terms *mononeuropathy* and *polyneuropathy* may be used to denote whether one nerve or several are involved. A number of conditions may be called either neuropathies or polyneuropathies; if not found here, see under *polyneuropathy*. **neuropath′ic** *adj*

acute autonomic n. a rare subtype of Guillain-Barré syndrome characterized by malfunction of peripheral nerves of the autonomic nervous system, with manifestations such as orthostatic hypotension, anhidrosis, and problems associated with lack of intestinal motility. Called also *acute pandysautonomia*.

acute motor axonal n. (AMAN) a subtype of Guillain-Barré syndrome seen in China, caused by infection with *Campylobacter jejuni*.

acute motor-sensory axonal n. a rare subtype of Guillain-Barré syndrome involving primarily large sensory nerve fibers in the limbs, with paresthesias and weakness but not paralysis.

alcoholic n. neuropathy due to thiamine deficiency in chronic alcoholism.

amyloid n. see under *polyneuropathy*.

angiopathic n. neuropathy caused by arteritis of the blood vessels supplying the nerves. It is usually a systemic complication of diseases such as Wegener granulomatosis, temporal arteritis, systemic lupus erythematosus, rheumatoid arthritis, systemic scleroderma, and polyarteritis nodosa; occasional nonsystemic cases occur in the form of a mononeuropathy that is more indolent than the systemic forms.

arsenic n., arsenical n. see under *polyneuropathy*.

ascending n. neuropathy that progresses from the feet upwards to affect the thigh, hip, trunk, and so on.

auditory n. neuropathy in the eighth cranial nerve with apparently normal function of the outer hair cells but dysfunction of the inner hair cells or cochlear nerve; it is seen most often in young children, who have partial sensorineural hearing loss.

autonomic n. any neuropathy of the autonomic nervous system, causing symptoms such as orthostatic hypotension, disordered bowel, bladder, or sexual functions, or abnormal pupillary reflexes; it is a complication of many diseases including Adie syndrome, chronic alcoholism, diabetes mellitus, dysautonomia, and Shy-Drager syndrome.

axonal n. axonopathy.

brachial plexus n. brachial plexopathy.

common peroneal n. neuropathy caused by a lesion of the common peroneal nerve, with symptoms such as ankle drop and sensory loss in the foot.

compression n., compressive n. entrapment n.

cranial n. neuropathy due to a lesion of one of the cranial nerves, such as in Bell palsy, optic neuritis, or trigeminal neuralgia.

critical illness n. see under *polyneuropathy*.

Dejerine-Sottas n. progressive hypertrophic n.

descending n. neuropathy that starts proximally (shoulder, hip) and spreads distally toward the limb extremities (hands, feet).

diabetic n. any of several clinical types of polyneuropathy seen with diabetes mellitus; there are sensory, motor, autonomic, and mixed varieties. The most common kind is a chronic condition called symmetrical sensory polyneuropathy; it affects first the nerves of the lower limbs and often autonomic nerves; pathologically, there is segmental demyelination of peripheral nerves. An uncommon acute form is the ischemic variety, accompanied by severe pain, weakness, and wasting of proximal and distal muscles, peripheral sensory impairment, and loss of tendon reflexes. With autonomic involvement there may be orthostatic hypotension, nocturnal diarrhea, retention of urine, impotence, and small diameter of the pupils with sluggish reaction to light. Called also *diabetic polyneuropathy*.

entrapment n. any of a group of neuropathies, often overuse injuries, in which a peripheral nerve is injured by compression in its course through a fibrous or osseofibrous tunnel or at a point where it abruptly changes its course through deep fascia over a fibrous or muscular band. Examples include *carpal tunnel syndrome*, *cubital tunnel syndrome*, *meralgia paresthetica*, *Morton neuralgia*, *musculospiral paralysis*, *pronator syndrome*, and *tarsal tunnel syndrome*. Called also *compression* or *pressure n.* and *nerve compression syndrome*.

femoral n. neuropathy due to injury to the femoral nerve, characterized by a variety of sensory and motor deficits in the lower limb; the most common causes are diabetes mellitus, anticoagulant-induced retroperitoneal hemorrhage, and trauma during surgery.

giant axonal n. an autosomal recessive neuropathy of childhood due to mutation in the *GAN* gene (locus: 16q24.1), which encodes gigaxonin, a protein involved in the ubiquitin-proteasome system targeting damaged proteins for destruction. There are central and peripheral nervous system

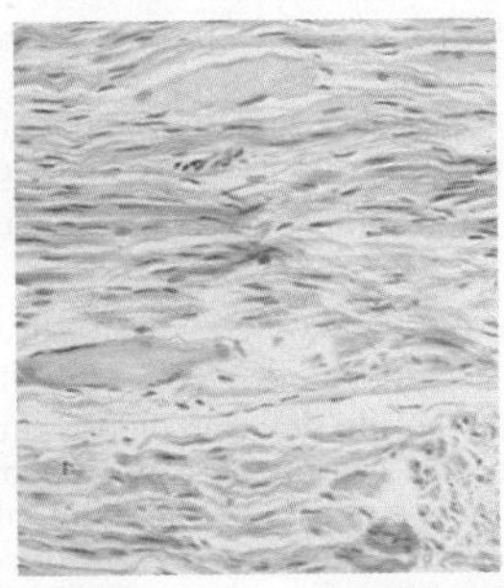
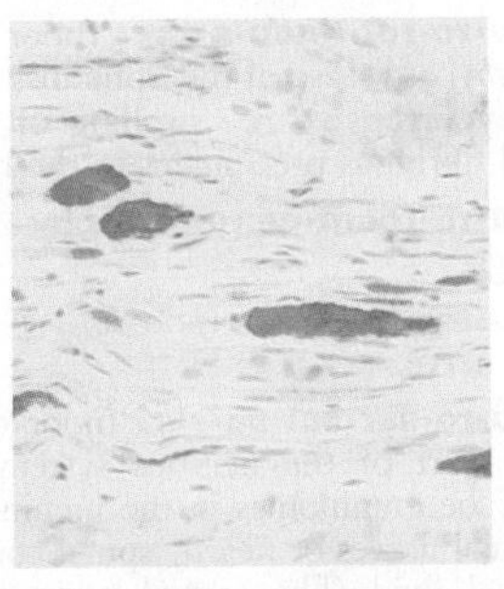

■ Giant axonal neuropathy. *(A)*, Prominent eosinophilic enlarged axons are randomly distributed and occasionally surrounded by rings of Schwann cells. *(B)*, Immunohistochemical staining demonstrating neurofilaments in axonal spheroids.

symptoms and enlarged axons made up of masses of tightly woven neurofilaments.

hepatic n. neuropathy caused by liver disease, particularly one of three varieties: an asymptomatic or mild demyelinating polyneuropathy, often seen with chronic liver failure; a polyneuritis similar to acute idiopathic polyneuritis, sometimes seen with viral hepatitis; and a painful sensory neuropathy, sometimes seen with biliary cirrhosis.

hereditary hypertrophic n. progressive hypertrophic n.

hereditary n. with liability to pressure palsies (HNPP) an autosomal dominant neuropathy due to deletion of the *PMP22* gene (locus: 17p11.2), which encodes a specific myelin protein; it is allelic with Charcot-Marie-Tooth disease type IA , which is caused by duplication of that gene. It is characterized by pain, weakness, and pressure palsy in the arms and hands with onset in childhood or adolescence; myelin sheaths become swollen and sausage-shaped but there is neither demyelination nor damage to axons. Called also *tomaculous n.*

hereditary motor and sensory n. (HMSN) any of a group of hereditary polyneuropathies involving muscle weakness, atrophy, sensory deficits, and vasomotor changes in the lower limbs. Some diseases in this group have been numbered: types I and II are varieties of Charcot-Marie-Tooth disease and type III is progressive hypertrophic neuropathy. Called also *hereditary sensory and motor n.*

hereditary optic n. Leber hereditary optic n.

hereditary sensory n. see *hereditary sensory and autonomic n.*, types I and II.

hereditary sensory and autonomic n. (HSAN) any of a genetically and clinically heterogeneous group of inherited neuropathies characterized by sensory loss and variable autonomic disturbances without significant motor involvement.

type I an autosomal dominant disorder caused by mutations in the *SPTLC1* gene (locus:9q22.1-q22.3), which encodes a subunit of serine *C*-palmitoyltransferase. It is characterized by signs of radicular sensory loss affecting mainly the feet and legs; shooting pains; chronic, indolent, trophic ulceration of the feet; and sometimes deafness. Onset is in the second to fourth decades of life.

type II a slowly progressive autosomal recessive polyneuropathy caused by mutations in the *HSN2* isoform of the *WNK1* gene (locus:12p13), which encodes a protein that may play a role in the development or maintenance of sensory neurons. It is characterized by sensory loss in the distal upper and lower limb and, to a lesser degree, in the trunk and face; trophic ulceration of the extremities; few autonomic symptoms; and loss of tendon reflexes. Onset is almost in infancy or early childhood.

type III familial dysautonomia.

type IV an autosomal recessive disorder with onset in infancy, caused by mutations in the *NTRK1* gene (locus: 1q21-q22), which encodes the tyrosine kinase receptor for nerve growth factor. It is characterized by insensitivity to pain, anhidrosis, episodes of fever, self-mutilation, mild mental retardation, emotional lability, and hyperactivity. Small unmyelinated axons are absent or nearly so, the number of myelinated axons is decreased, and sweat gland innervation is absent.

type V an autosomal recessive disorder caused by mutations in the *NGFB* gene (locus: 1p13.1), which encodes the β subunit of nerve growth factor. It is clinically similar to, but less severe than, type IV, without significant anhidrosis; intelligence is normal. There are a mild loss of unmyelinated axons and a selective loss of myelinated axons.

hereditary sensory and motor n. hereditary motor and sensory n.

hereditary sensory radicular n. see *hereditary sensory and autonomic n.*, types I and II.

hip pocket n. popular term for levator ani syndrome.

hypertrophic interstitial n. progressive hypertrophic n.

ischemic n. an injury to a peripheral nerve caused by a reduction in blood supply; the most common variety is diabetic neuropathy.

ischemic monomelic n. ischemic neuropathy in just one limb.

isoniazid n. polyneuropathy seen in some patients on isoniazid therapy, consisting of symmetrical numbness and paresthesias of the lower extremities.

lead n. a form of segmental (demyelination) neuropathy seen with chronic lead poisoning; see under *poisoning*.

Leber hereditary optic n., Leber optic n. a rare hereditary disorder due to mutation in any of multiple genes encoded by the mitochondrial genome, showing variable penetrance, and in Caucasians preferentially expressed in males. It is characterized by degeneration of the optic nerve and papillomacular bundle, resulting in a progressive loss of central vision and scotoma. Called also *hereditary optic n.* or *atrophy, Leber optic atrophy*, and *Leber disease*.

leprous n. the asymmetric polyneuropathy that accompanies leprosy.

long thoracic n. long thoracic nerve palsy.

lumbar plexus n. lumbar plexopathy.

lumbosacral plexus n. lumbosacral plexopathy.

lumbosacral radiculoplexus n. a syndrome of pain, muscle weakness, and mild sensory deficits, generally worsening at night, that affects the lower limb. It is caused by ischemic injury to the lumbosacral plexus and nerve roots secondary to microvasculitis and occurs most commonly as a complication of diabetes mellitus. Called also *lumbosacral radiculoplexopathy*.

median n. neuropathy due to a lesion of the median nerve or one of its branches; see *anterior interosseous syndrome* and *pronator teres syndrome*, under *syndrome*.

motor n. neuropathy or polyneuropathy involving only motor nerves.

multifocal motor n. a variant of chronic inflammatory demyelinating polyneuropathy characterized by conduction blocks at multiple sites on motor nerves without significant change in sensory nerves in the area; muscles innervated by the affected nerves undergo slow atrophy.

multiple n. 1. polyneuropathy. 2. mononeuropathy multiplex.

nitrofurantoin n. neuropathy seen in some patients being treated with nitrofurantoin; it consists of symmetrical pain and paresthesias in the feet, which may in time spread to the hands.

nutritional n. see under *polyneuropathy*.

paraneoplastic n. see under *polyneuropathy*.

periaxial n. segmental n.

peripheral n. polyneuropathy.

porphyric n. see under *polyneuropathy*.

pressure n. entrapment n.

progressive hypertrophic n. a condition characterized by hyperplasia of the interstitial connective tissue, causing thickening of peripheral nerve trunks and posterior roots, and by sclerosis of the posterior columns of the spinal cord. It is a slowly progressive familial disease beginning in early life, marked by atrophy of distal parts of the lower limbs, and by diminution of tendon reflexes and of sensation. Called also *Dejerine disease, Dejerine-Sottas atrophy, disease*, or *n., interstitial hypertrophic neuritis, hereditary hypertrophic n.*, and *hypertrophic interstitial n.* See also *hereditary motor and sensory n.*

radial n. entrapment neuropathy of any part of the radial nerve, usually with paralysis of the extensor muscles of the wrist and fingers. Common types include crutch paralysis, cheiralgia paresthetica, and radial tunnel syndrome. Called also *musculospiral paralysis, Saturday night palsy, radial palsy* or *paralysis*, and *radial nerve palsy* or *paralysis*.

radiculoplexus n. radiculoplexopathy.

sacral plexus n. sacral plexopathy.

sarcoid n. a polyneuropathy seen with sarcoidosis, characterized by either cranial polyneuritis or spinal nerve deficits and sometimes large areas of sensory loss on the trunk.

sciatic n. sciatica.

segmental n. neuropathy in which there is loss of myelin segments; called also *periaxial* or *segmental neuritis* and *periaxial n.*

senile n. mild neuropathy occurring in the elderly, especially in nerves of the upper and lower limbs.

sensorimotor n. neuropathy or polyneuropathy involving both sensory and motor nerves.

sensory n. neuropathy or polyneuropathy of sensory nerves.

serum n., serum sickness n. a neurologic disorder, usually involving the cervical nerves or brachial plexus, occurring two to eight days after the injection of foreign protein, such as an antiserum or antitoxin of animal origin, characterized by local pain followed by sensory disturbances and paralysis. Called also *serum neuritis*.

suprascapular n. a type of entrapment neuropathy caused by a lesion of the suprascapular nerve at the scapular notch, characterized by pain and weakness at the shoulder joint upon external rotation of the upper arm.

tomaculous n. hereditary n. with liability to pressure palsies.

toxic n. neuropathy caused by ingestion of a toxin; substances commonly implicated are *n*-hexane solvents, organophosphorus insecticides, acrylamide, heavy metals, and a variety of drugs.

traumatic n. neuropathy resulting from trauma.

trigeminal n. neuropathy from a lesion of the trigeminal nerve, marked by sensory loss in the face and weakness of the muscles of mastication.

tropical ataxic n. a type of myelopathy with neuropathy, seen most often in a region of Nigeria where the diet is high in cassava, owing to incomplete processing of the cassava so that not all of its cyanide is removed. This results in cyanide poisoning with paraparesis and burning pain in the limbs; some patients have ocular symptoms such as amblyopia.

ulnar n. any neuropathy of the ulnar nerve. Those in the elbow region are usually entrapment neuropathies *(cubital tunnel syndrome)*; those in the wrist region may cause only muscle weakness in the hand or weakness accompanied by sensory deficits in the area of the little finger.

vasculitic n. angiopathic n.

neu•ro•pep•tide (noor″o-pep′tīd) any of several types of molecules found in brain tissue, composed of short chains of amino acids; they include endorphins, enkephalins, vasopressin, and others. They are often localized in axon terminals at synapses and are classified as putative neurotransmitters, although some are also hormones.

n. Y a 36–amino acid peptide found in neurons supplying blood vessels, as well as in the basal ganglia, thalamus, hypothalamus, and dorsal horn of the spinal cord; it is a vasoconstrictor and is believed to play a role in regulation of feeding behavior.

neu•ro•phar•ma•col•o•gy (noor″o-fahr″mə-kol′ə-je) the branch of pharmacology that deals especially with the action of drugs upon various parts and elements of the nervous system. **neuropharmacolog′ic** *adj*

neu•ro•phil•ic (noor″o-fil′ik) neurotropic.

neu•roph•thal•mol•o•gy (noor″of-thəl-mol′ə-je) neuro-ophthalmology.

neu•ro•phy•sin (noor″o-fi′sin) any of a group of soluble proteins (molecular weights 9500–10,500) derived from the precursors of vasopressin, oxytocin, and related hormones, secreted in the hypothalamus. They serve as transport proteins for vasopressin and oxytocin.

neu•ro•phys•i•ol•o•gy (noor″o-fiz″e-ol′ə-je) [*neuro-* + *physiology*] the physiology of the nervous system.

neu•ro•pil (noor′o-pil) [*neuro-* + Gr. *pilos* felt] a dense feltwork of interwoven cytoplasmic processes of nerve cells (dendrites and axons) and of neuroglial cells in the gray matter of the central nervous system.

neu•ro•pile (noor′o-pīl) neuropil.

neu•ro•plasm (noor′o-plaz″əm) [*neuro-* + *-plasm*] the undifferentiated basophilic protoplasm of a nerve cell. **neuroplas′mic** *adj*

neu•ro•plas•ty (noor′o-plas″te) [*neuro-* + *-plasty*] plastic surgery of a nerve. **neuroplas′tic** *adj*

neu•ro•plex•us (noor″o-plek′səs) a plexus of nerves.

neu•ro•pore (noor′o-por) [*neuro-* + *pore*] the open anterior end (rostral neuropore) or the open posterior end (caudal neuropore) of the neural tube of the early embryo. These openings gradually close during the fourth week as the primordial spinal cord develops.

anterior n. rostral n.

caudal n., posterior n. the embryonic opening at the caudal end of the neural tube, which closes by the 25-somite stage (about 27 days).

rostral n. the embryonic opening at the rostral end of the neural tube, which closes at the 20-somite stage (about 25 days).

neu•ro•prax•ia (noor″ə-prak′se-ə) neurapraxia.

neu•ro•pro•ba•sia (noor″o-pro-ba′zhə) [*neuro-* + Gr. *pro* forward + *basis* walking] advance along the nerves; said of the action of certain viruses.

neu•ro•pro•tec•tion (noor″o-pro-tek′shən) protection against neurotoxicity. **neuroprotec′tant, neuroprotec′tive** *adj*

neu•ro•psy•chi•a•trist (noor″o-si-ki′ə-trist) a physician who specializes in neuropsychiatry.

neu•ro•psy•chi•a•try (noor″o-si-ki′ə-tre) [*neuro-* + *psychiatry*] the branch of medicine which includes both neurology and psychiatry. **neuropsychiat′ric** *adj*

neu•ro•psy•chol•o•gy (noor″o-si-kol′ə-je) [*neuro-* + *psychology*] a discipline combining neurology and psychology to study the relationship between the functioning of the brain and cognitive processes or behavior, using psychological testing and assessment to assay central nervous system function and diagnose specific behavioral or cognitive deficits or disorders. **neuropsycholog′ical** *adj*

neu•ro•psy•cho•met•ric (noor″o-si″ko-met′rik) pertaining to the quantitative testing of neurological processes underlying cognitive processes and behaviors.

neu•ro•psy•cho•phar•ma•col•o•gy (noor″o-si″ko-fahr″mə-kol′ə-je) psychopharmacology.

neu•ro•ra•di•ol•o•gy (noor″o-ra″de-ol′ə-je) radiology of the nervous system.

neu•ro•re•ha•bil•i•ta•tion (noor″o-re″hə-bil″ĭ-ta′shən) rehabilitation after damage to some part of the nervous system.

neu•ro•ret•i•ni•tis (noor″o-ret″ĭ-ni′tis) inflammation of the optic nerve and retina.

neu•ro•ret•i•nop•a•thy (noor″o-ret″ĭ-nop′ə-the) [*neuro-* + *retina* + *-pathy*] a disease of the optic disk and retina.

hypertensive n. swelling of the optic disk and formation of serous and fibrinous precipitates in the retina, occurring in severe hypertension.

neu•ro•roent•gen•og•ra•phy (noor″o-rent″gən-og′rə-fe) neuroradiology.

neu•ror•rha•phy (no͝o-ror′ə-fe) [*neuro-* + *-rrhaphy*] the suturing of a cut nerve.

neu•ro•sar•coi•do•sis (noor″o-sahr″koi-do′sis) sarcoidosis involving any part of the nervous system. In the central nervous system there may be granulomas in the meninges near the base of the brain, affecting cranial nerves or nearby spinal cord or obstructing the outflow of cerebrospinal fluid. The cranial nerve most often affected is the facial nerve, resulting in Heerfordt syndrome. The optic nerve, trigeminal nerve, and vestibulocochlear nerve are affected less often. In some patients granulomas affect the hypothalamus and cause endocrine symptoms.

neu•ro•sar•co•ma (noor″o-sahr-ko′mə) a sarcoma with neural elements.

neu•ro•schis•to•so•mi•a•sis (noor″o-skis″to-so-mi′ə-sis) schistosomiasis affecting the central nervous system, most often caused by *Schistosoma japonicum*.

neu•ro•sci•ence (noor′o-si″əns) any of the branches of science dealing with the embryology, anatomy, physiology, biochemistry, or other aspects of the nervous system.

neu•ro•sci•en•tist (noor″o-si′ən-tist) a specialist in any of the branches of the neurosciences.

neu•ro•se•cre•tion (noor″o-sə-kre′shən) [*neuro-* + *secretion*] 1. the secretory activities of nerve cells, as the secretion of releasing hormones, vasopressin, neurotransmitters, etc. 2. the product of such activities; a neurosecretory substance.

neu•ro•se•cre•to•ry (noor″o-sə-kre′tə-re) pertaining to neurosecretion.

neu•ro•seg•men•tal (noor″o-seg-men′təl) [*neuro-* + *segmental*] of or pertaining to a pair of spinal dorsal and ventral roots or to the area which they supply.

neu•ro•sen•so•ry (noor″o-sen′sə-re) sensorineural.

neu•ro•ses (no͝o-ro′sēz) plural of *neurosis.*

neu•ro•sis (no͝o-ro′sis) pl. *neuro′ses* [*neur-* + *-osis*] 1. former name for a category of mental disorders characterized by anxiety and avoidance behavior. In general, the term refers to disorders in which the symptoms are distressing to the person, reality testing is intact, behavior does not violate gross social norms, and there is no apparent organic etiology. Classified in DSM-IV under *anxiety disorders, dissociative disorders, mood disorders, sexual disorders,* and *somatoform disorders.* 2. in psychoanalytic theory, the specific etiological process that gives rise not only to neuroses as defined above but also to personality disorders (formerly called character neuroses to emphasize this) and some psychotic disorders. Unconscious conflicts involving opposing wishes or forbidden infantile wishes give rise to an unconscious anticipation of danger (experienced as anxiety) in situations that activate a conflict, and anxiety serves as a signal to trigger unconscious defense mechanisms, the operation of which is visible to the conscious mind and to observers in the form of neurotic symptoms or pathological personality traits.

cardiac n. neurocirculatory asthenia.

character n. a type of character or personality disorder with some neurotic characteristics, particularly one of a predominantly obsessive-compulsive or hysterical nature; see also *neurosis.*

compensation n. persistent physical and psychological symptoms following an injury, for which the patient feels deserving of financial or other compensation.

compulsion n. obsessive-compulsive disorder.

conversion n. see under *disorder.*

depersonalization n. see under *disorder.*

experimental n. a state produced in an experimental animal, usually by exposure to frustration or conflict, that resembles human neuroses.

hypochondriacal n. hypochondriasis.

hysterical n. former name for a group of conditions now divided between *conversion disorder* and *dissociative disorders.* See also *hysteria.*

obsessional n. obsessive-compulsive disorder.

obsessive-compulsive n. see under *disorder.*

phobic n. phobic disorder; see *phobia.*

prison n. chronophobia occurring in prisoners having trouble adjusting to a long prison sentence, characterized by feelings of restlessness, panic, anxiety, and claustrophobia.

transference n. a phenomenon occurring during psychoanalysis, in which transference causes the patient to undergo, with the analyst as the object, an intense repetition of childhood conflicts and traumas,

reexperiencing impulses, feelings, and fantasies that originally developed in relation to the parents.
  traumatic n. posttraumatic stress disorder.
  vegetative n. acrodynia.

neu·ro·skel·e·tal (noor″o-skel′ə-təl) pertaining to the nervous tissues and the skeletal muscular tissue.

neu·ro·skel·e·ton (noor″o-skel′ə-ton) endoskeleton.

neu·ro·some (noor′o-sōm) [*neuro-* + *-some*] 1. perikaryon. 2. any of the minute particles found in the protoplasm of a neuron.

neu·ro·spasm (noor′o-spaz″əm) [*neuro-* + *spasm*] a spasm caused by a disorder in the motor nerve supplying the muscle.

neu·ro·splanch·nic (noor″o-splangk′nik) pertaining to the cerebrospinal and sympathetic nervous systems; neurovisceral.

neu·ro·spon·gi·o·ma (noor″o-spon″je-o′mə) glioma.

Neu·ros·po·ra (nōō-ros′pə-rə) a genus of usually saprobic fungi of the family Sordariaceae, comprising the bread molds; they are capable of converting tryptophan to nicotinic acid and are extensively used in genetic and enzyme research.

neu·ro·ste·roid (noor″o-ster′oid) a steroid produced in the brain.

neu·ro·sta·tus (noor″o-sta′təs) the state or condition of neural symptoms in a case history.

neu·ro·stim·u·la·tion (noor″o-stim-u-la′shən) stimulation of nerves or neural tissue for therapeutic purposes. **neurostim′ulatory** *adj*

neu·ro·sur·geon (noor′o-sur″jən) a physician who specializes in neurosurgery.

neu·ro·sur·gery (noor′o-sur″jər-e) surgery of the nervous system.
  functional n. 1. neurosurgery designed to restore physiological activity of nerves, such as by enhancing conductivity of nerve fibers or improving blood flow to nerve tissue. 2. psychosurgery.
  stereotactic n. the use of stereotactic surgical techniques in the treatment of disease of the central nervous system.

neu·ro·su·ture (noor″o-soo′chər) neurorrhaphy.

neu·ro·syph·i·lis (noor″o-sif′ĭ-lis) [*neuro-* + *syphilis*] the central nervous system manifestations of syphilis, which may be divided into two groups: asymptomatic and symptomatic; the latter includes meningovascular and parenchymatous neurosyphilis (see *general paresis*, under *paresis*, and *tabes dorsalis*).
  asymptomatic n. neurosyphilis diagnosed when there is a positive VDRL test in the cerebrospinal fluid in the absence of the signs and symptoms of neurologic disease.
  meningovascular n. neurosyphilis at the stage of extensive meningeal involvement, secondarily investing and then occluding vessels in their course through the subarachnoid space, resulting in focal or widespread cerebrovascular disease. Called also *meningovascular syphilis*.
  parenchymatous n. neurosyphilis that causes widespread parenchymal damage; called also *parenchymatous syphilis*. See *general paresis*, under *paresis*, and *tabes dorsalis*.
  paretic n. general paresis.
  tabetic n. tabes dorsalis.

neu·ro·ten·di·nous (noor″o-ten′dĭ-nəs) pertaining to both nerve and tendon.

neu·ro·ten·sin (noor″o-ten′sin) a tridecapeptide found in the small intestine and brain; it induces vasodilatation and hypotension and in the brain it is a neurotransmitter.

neu·ro·ter·mi·nal (noor″o-tur′mĭ-nəl) end-organ.

neur·o·the·ke·o·ma (noor″o-the″ke-o′mə) [*neuro-* + Gr. *thēkē* sheath + *-oma*] a type of nerve sheath tumor that secretes excessive mucin, usually seen on the heads of adults. Called also *nerve sheath myxoma*.

neu·ro·thele (noor″o-the′le) [*neuro-* + Gr. *thele* nipple] a sensory papilla located in the papillary layer of the dermis; called also *nerve papilla* and *nervous papilla*.

neu·rot·ic (nōō-rot′ik) 1. pertaining to or characterized by neurosis. 2. a person affected with a neurosis.

neu·rot·iza·tion (nōō-rot″ĭ-za′shən) the regeneration of a nerve after its division.

neu·rot·me·sis (noor″ot-me′sis) [*neuro-* + Gr. *tmēsis* cutting apart] partial or complete severance of a nerve, with disruption of the axon and its myelin sheath and the connective tissue elements; regeneration does not occur. Cf. *axonotmesis* and *neurapraxia*.

neu·ro·tome (noor′o-tōm) [*neuro-* + *-tome*] 1. a needlelike knife for dissecting the nerves. 2. neuromere.

neu·ro·to·mog·ra·phy (noor″o-to-mog′rə-fe) tomography of the central nervous system.

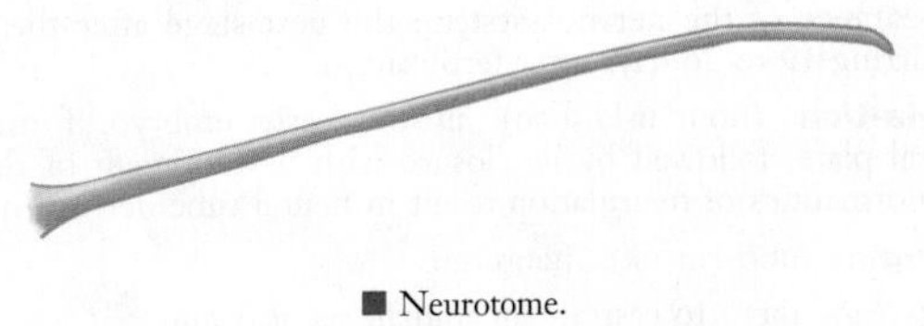

■ Neurotome.

neu·rot·o·my (nōō-rot′ə-me) [*neuro-* + *-tomy*] interruption of a nerve through surgical cutting or production of artificial lesions.
  radiofrequency n. percutaneous radiofrequency rhizotomy.
  retrogasserian n. trigeminal rhizotomy.

neu·rot·o·ny (nōō-rot′ə-ne) [*neuro-* + Gr. *teinein* to stretch] the stretching of a nerve; called also *neurectasia*.

neu·ro·tox·ic (noor′o-tok″sik) poisonous or destructive to nerve tissue.

neu·ro·tox·ic·i·ty (noor″o-tok-sis′ĭ-te) the quality of exerting a destructive or poisonous effect upon nerve tissue.

neu·ro·tox·in (noor′o-tok″sin) a toxin that is poisonous to or destroys nerve tissue, especially the exotoxins secreted by *Clostridium botulinum*, *C. tetani*, *Corynebacterium diphtheriae*, and *Shigella dysenteriae*.

neu·ro·trans·duc·er (noor″o-trans-dōōs′ər) a neuron that synthesizes and releases hormones which serve as the functional link between the nervous system and the pituitary gland.

neu·ro·trans·mis·sion (noor″o-trans-mish′ən) the process by which a neurotransmitter is released, crosses the synapse, and affects the action of the target cell.

neu·ro·trans·mit·ter (noor″o-trans′mit-ər) any of a group of substances that are released on excitation from the axon terminal of a presynaptic neuron of the central or peripheral nervous system and travel across the synaptic cleft to either excite or inhibit the target cell. Among the many substances that have the properties of a neurotransmitter are acetylcholine, norepinephrine, epinephrine, dopamine, glycine, γ-aminobutyrate, glutamic acid, substance P, enkephalins, endorphins, and serotonin.
  false n. an amine, e.g., octopamine, that can be stored in and released from presynaptic vesicles but that has little effect on postsynaptic receptors.

neu·ro·trau·ma (noor″o-traw′mə) [*neuro-* + *trauma*] mechanical injury of a nerve.

neu·ro·tro·phic (noor″o-tro′fik) pertaining to neurotrophy.

neu·ro·tro·phin (noor′o-tro″fin) any of a family of growth factors that block apoptosis in neurons and thus promote nerve growth; the best-known example is nerve growth factor.

neu·rot·ro·phy (nōō-rot′rə-fe) [*neuro-* + *-trophy*] 1. the nutrition and maintenance of tissues as regulated by nervous influence. 2. the nutrition and maintenance of nervous tissue.

neu·ro·tro·pic (noor″o-tro′pik) having a selective affinity for nervous tissue, or exerting its principal effect on the nervous system.

neu·rot·ro·pism (nōō-rot′ro-piz″əm) [*neuro-* + *tropism*] 1. the quality of having a special affinity for nervous tissue. 2. the alleged tendency of regenerating nerve fibers to grow toward specific portions of the periphery.

neu·rot·ro·py (nōō-rot′rə-pe) neurotropism.

neu·ro·tu·bule (noor″o-too′būl) a microtubule occurring in a neuron.

neu·ro·vac·cine (noor″o-vak-sēn′) vaccinia virus prepared by growing the virus in the brain of a rabbit.

neu·ro·var·i·co·sis (noor″o-var″ĭ-ko′sis) a varicose state of the fibers of a nerve.

neu·ro·va·ri·o·la (noor″o-və-ri′ə-lə) neurovaccine.

neu·ro·vas·cu·lar (noor″o-vas′ku-lər) pertaining to both nervous and vascular elements; pertaining to the nerves that control the caliber of blood vessels.

neu·ro·veg·e·ta·tive (noor″o-vej′ə-ta″tiv) pertaining to the vegetative (autonomic) nervous system.

neur·o·vi·rol·o·gy (noor″o-vi-rol′ə-je) the study of the effects of viruses on the nervous system.

neu·ro·vir·u·lence (noor″o-vir′u-ləns) the competence of an infectious agent to produce pathologic effects on the nervous system. **neurovir′ulent** *adj*

neu·ro·vi·rus (noor′o-vi″rəs) a vaccine virus which has been modified by passing into nervous tissue.

neu·ro·vis·cer·al (noor″o-vis′ər-əl) neurosplanchnic.

neu·ru·la (noor′u-lə) [*neuro-* + dim. *-ula*] the early embryo during the development of the neural tube from the neural plate, marking the first appearance of the nervous system; the next stage after the gastrula, and occurring 19 to 26 days after fertilization.

neu•ru•la•tion (noor″u-la′shən) in the early embryo, formation of the neural plate, followed by its closure with development of the neural tube; abnormalities of neurulation result in neural tube defects (q.v.).

neu•rur•gic (noo-rur′jik) neurergic.

neu•ter (noo′tər) to castrate an animal; see *spay* and *geld.*

neu•tral (noo′trəl) [L. *neutralis,* from *neuter,* neither] in chemistry, neither acid nor basic.

neu•tral•ism (noo′trəl-iz-əm) the absence of interaction between coexisting organisms of different species.

neu•tral•i•ty (noo-tral′ĭ-te) the state of being neutral.

neu•tral•iza•tion (noo″trəl-ĭ-za′shən) the act or process of rendering neutral.

viral n. the process by which antibody alone or antibody plus complement neutralizes the infectivity of a virus. The antibody may coat the virus forming a stable complex or may cause conformational changes in viral structural proteins on binding; either process may interfere with binding of the virion to cellular receptor sites and entry into the cell. Enveloped viruses may be lysed by complement.

neu•tral•ize (noo′trəl-īz) to render neutral.

Neu•tra•pen (noo′trə-pən) trademark for a lyophilized preparation of penicillinase.

neu•tri•no (noo-tre′no) [It. "little neutron"] an elementary particle that has no electric charge and no mass, and that very rarely reacts with matter; it is a product of beta decay. Symbol ν.

neutr(o)- [L. *neuter* neither] a combining form meaning neither.

neu•tro•clu•sion (noo″trŏ-kloo′zhən) [*neutro-* + L. *cludere* to close] malocclusion characterized by irregularities of individual teeth, but with normal mesiodistal or normal anteroposterior relation of the mandibular to the maxillary dental arch. Generally regarded as identical with class I in the Angle classification of malocclusion.

neu•tro•cyte (noo′tro-sīt) neutrophil (def. 1).

neu•tron (noo′tron) [*neutr-* + *-on*] an electrically neutral or uncharged particle of matter existing along with protons in the atoms of all elements except the mass 1 isotope of hydrogen. Symbol n.

epithermal n. a neutron having an energy level of a few hundredths of an electron volt to 100 electron volts.

fast n. a neutron having an energy level exceeding 10^5 electron volts.

intermediate n. a neutron having an energy level of 100 to 100,000 electron volts.

slow n. 1. thermal n. 2. any neutron having an energy level up to 100 electron volts.

thermal n. a neutron having an energy level of about 0.025 electron volt; called also *slow n.*

neu•tro•pe•nia (noo″tro-pe′ne-ə) [*neutrophil* + *-penia*] an abnormal decrease in the number of neutrophils in the blood, with the absolute neutrophil count being less than 1500/μL.

alloimmune neonatal n. neutropenia in the newborn due to in utero incompatibility between its immunoglobulin G antigens and those of the mother's blood; the mother's blood produces IgG antineutrophil antibodies that cross the placenta and sensitize fetal neutrophils. Affected infants may have fever, pneumonia, septicemia, and other infections that can be fatal. The condition eventually resolves itself as the infant's immunoglobulin replaces that from the mother.

autoimmune n. neutropenia caused by autoantibodies against the neutrophils; it may occur in isolation, in association with other autoimmune conditions, or secondary to malignancy, infection, or a drug complication. The most common type is alloimmune neonatal neutropenia.

chronic benign n., chronic familial n. a rare autosomal dominant peripheral neutropenia, related to but less severe than agranulocytosis. It is usually seen in children and is characterized by hyperglobulinemia, recurrent infections, oral ulcerations, hyperplastic gingivitis, periodontitis and early tooth loss, and finger clubbing. Called also *familial benign chronic n.*

cyclic n. 1. a chronic type of neutropenia that abates and recurs, accompanied by malaise, fever, stomatitis, and various types of infections. Called also *periodic n.* 2. a rare autosomal recessive disorder of gray collie dogs in which there is a bone marrow stem cell defect with periodic fluctuations in numbers of circulating neutrophils, platelets, and reticulocytes; during the episodes animals have lethargy, fever, arthralgias, and bacterial infections that can be fatal. Called also *cyclic hematopoiesis* and *gray collie syndrome.*

drug-induced n. neutropenia caused by medications; the most common mechanisms are immunologic (formation of antibodies destructive to neutrophils or of immune complexes that bind to neutrophils), followed by inhibition of granulopoiesis and direct damage to bone marrow or precursor cells of the granulocytic series.

familial benign chronic n. chronic benign n.

hypersplenic n. primary splenic n.

idiopathic n. agranulocytosis.

isoimmune neonatal n. alloimmune neonatal n.

Kostmann n. see under *syndrome.*

malignant n. agranulocytosis.

periodic n. cyclic n.

peripheral n. decrease in the number of neutrophils in the circulating blood.

primary splenic n. a syndrome characterized by splenomegaly, hypercellular bone marrow, profound leukopenia and neutropenia, and susceptibility to infection, occasionally with anemia and thrombocytopenia. Called also *hypersplenic n.*

severe congenital n. (SCN) a heterogeneous disorder of hematopoiesis characterized by maturation arrest of granulopoiesis at the promyelocyte stage, an absolute neutrophil count below 500/μL, often with monocytosis and eosinophilia, and severe bacterial infections that begin in infancy. Four forms, with different genetic defects and modes of inheritance, have been identified.

SCN1 an autosomal dominant or sporadic form (gene locus: 19p13.3) caused by mutation in the gene that encodes leukocyte elastase.

SCN2 an autosomal dominant form (gene locus: 1p22) caused by a mutation that disables activity of a transcriptional repressor that targets the leukocyte elastase gene.

SCN3 Kostmann syndrome.

SCN4 an autosomal recessive form (gene locus: 17q21) caused by expression of a defective catalytic subunit of glucose-6-phosphatase.

neu•tro•phil (noo′tro-fil) [*neutro-* + *-phil*] 1. a mature granular leukocyte that is polymorphonuclear (its nucleus having three to five lobes connected by slender threads of chromatin, and cytoplasm containing fine granules); neutrophils have the properties of chemotaxis, adherence to immune complexes, and phagocytosis. The counterpart in nonhuman mammals is the heterophil. Called also *neutrocyte* and *neutrophilic leukocyte.* 2. any cell, structure, or histologic element readily stainable by neutral dyes.

band n. see under *cell.*

giant n. macropolycyte.

juvenile n. metamyelocyte.

polymorphonuclear n. (PMN) the usual type of mature neutrophil, which has a multilobar nucleus; see also *polymorphonuclear leukocyte,* under *leukocyte.*

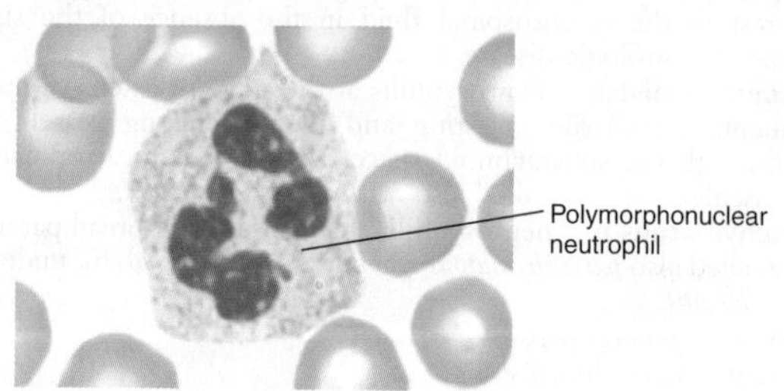

rod n., stab n. band cell.

neu•tro•phil elas•tase (noo′tro-fil e-las′tās) leukocyte elastase.

neu•tro•phil•ia (noo″tro-fil′e-ə) increase in the number of neutrophils in the blood; it is the most common form of leukocytosis and can have any of numerous causes, including acute infections, intoxications, hemorrhage, and rapidly growing malignant neoplasms. Called also *neutrophilic leukocytosis.*

neu•tro•phil•ic (noo″tro-fil′ik) 1. stainable by neutral dyes. 2. neither anthropophilic nor zoophilous; said of certain mosquitoes.

neu•tro•pism (noo′tro-piz-əm) neurotropism.

neu•tro•tax•is (noo″tro-tak′sis) [*neutrophil* + *-taxis*] the attractive or repellent influence exerted by neutrophils.

ne•vi (ne′vi) [L.] plural of *nevus.*

ne•vir•a•pine (nə-vir′ə-pēn) a nonnucleoside reverse transcriptase inhibitor, used in combination with other antiretroviral agents in the treatment of human immunodeficiency virus type 1 (HIV-1) infection; administered orally.

nev(o)- [L. *naevus* mole] a combining form denoting relationship to a nevus, or mole.

ne•vo•cel•lu•lar (ne″vo-sel′u-lər) pertaining to or composed of nevus cells; called also *nevocytic.*

ne•vo•cyte (ne′vo-sīt) nevus cell. **nevocyt′ic** *adj*

ne•void (ne′void) resembling a nevus.

ne•vo•li•po•ma (ne″vo-lĭ-po′mə) lipomatous nevus.

ne•vus (ne′vəs) pl. *ne′vi* [L. *naevus*] 1. any congenital lesion of the skin; see also *birthmark*. 2. a type of hamartoma representing a circumscribed stable malformation of the skin or occasionally the oral mucosa, which is not due to external causes and therefore presumed to be of hereditary origin. The excess (or deficiency) of tissue may involve epidermal, connective tissue, adnexal, nervous, or vascular elements.

Nevus

achromic n. n. depigmentosus.

acquired n. a nevus that is not present at birth but appears later in life.

amelanotic n. a melanocytic nevus that contains no pigment. Cf. *n. depigmentosus.*

n. ane′micus a congenital disorder characterized by pale, round, well-defined macules with irregular borders that may have a normal or decreased amount of melanin, thought to be due to a functional incapacity of the blood vessels to dilate as a result of increased sensitivity to catecholamines. It is often adjacent to areas of vascular malformation in the capillaries.

n. ara′neus spider angioma.

n. with architectural disorder new name proposed for *dysplastic nevus.*

atypical n., atypical melanocytic n. dysplastic n.

balloon cell n. a type of intradermal nevus, usually brown with a yellow halo, consisting of balloon cells with pale cytoplasm that contains large vacuoles formed of altered melanosomes; it is sometimes confused with a melanoma.

bathing trunk n. a giant hairy nevus on the area of the lower trunk that is usually covered by bathing trunks.

Becker n. a usually acquired but occasionally hereditary nevus seen mostly in males in the second and third decades of life, consisting of epidermal melanosis with segmental, uniform, light hyperpigmentation, followed several years later by growth of long dark hairs from the lesions. The usual location is on one shoulder or side of the upper trunk, and the lesion may spread over time. Called also *Becker melanosis* and *pigmented hairy epidermal n.*.

blue n. a benign, usually solitary type of melanocytic nevus, representing a localized proliferation of melanocytes in the dermis. It is a dark blue to black, moderately firm, rounded, sharply defined nodule containing spindle-shaped melanocytes with slender cytoplasmic processes, and is generally seen in association with melanin-laden macrophages in a sclerotic dermis. Called also *dermal melanocytoma* and *Jadassohn-Tièche n.*

blue rubber bleb n. a rare type of nevus characterized by bluish hemangiomas with soft, elevated, nipple-like centers, found on the skin surface, in the gastrointestinal tract, and sometimes on mucous membranes; it may be accompanied by pain, hyperhidrosis, or gastrointestinal bleeding. Some are inherited as autosomal dominant traits. See also *blue rubber bleb nevus syndrome*, under *syndrome.*

cellular n. melanocytic n.

cellular blue n. a usually congenital type of large blue nevus found in the dermis or subcutaneous tissue around the buttocks or sacrococcygeal region. It consists of deeply pigmented, dendritic, spindle-shaped melanocytes alternating with cellular islands of spindle cells with pale cytoplasm. Occasionally one may undergo malignant transformation to melanoma. Called also *dermal melanocytoma.*

CHILD n. a type of hyperkeratotic epidermal nevus seen in plaques or bands in the CHILD syndrome.

choroidal n. a flat or slightly raised uveal nevus of the choroid, usually brown to gray in color.

Clark n. dysplastic n.

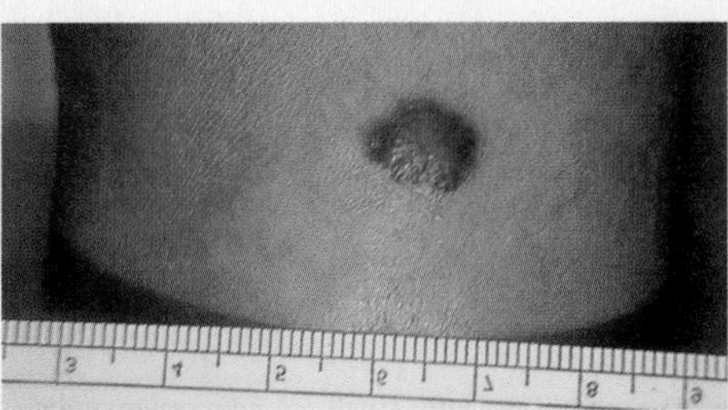

■ Cellular blue nevus.

comedo n., n. comedo′nicus a rare type of epidermal nevus characterized by aggregations of dilated keratin-filled hair follicles, producing large cutaneous patches covered with comedo-like lesions. The usual location is on the trunk, an upper limb, or the neck, and it may be in a linear or zosteriform pattern. It is occasionally associated with other conditions such as ichthyosis, certain carcinomas, vascular nevi, or cataracts.

compound n. a type of melanocytic nevus, clinically indistinguishable from an intradermal nevus, with nests of nevus cells in the epidermis as well as newly forming ones in the dermis.

congenital n. a nevus present at birth, generally larger than acquired nevi; larger lesions are associated with an increased risk of melanoma.

congenital hairy n., congenital melanocytic n., congenital pigmented n. a type of melanocytic nevus that is present at birth and is usually hairy and darkly pigmented; it may be either small or large. See also *giant hairy n.*

connective tissue n. any of several types of hamartomas involving components of connective tissue, usually present at or soon after birth; they may be inherited or acquired and may be associated with other diseases. There may be single or multiple nodules, papules, or plaques; the most common type is a plaque of firm, flat or cobblestoned, closely set, skin-colored papules. Called also *collagenoma, juvenile elastoma,* and *n. elasticus.*

n. depigmento′sus a developmental anomaly in which the skin has irregular areas, bands, or streaks of hypomelanosis, usually unilaterally on the trunk or a limb. Called also *achromic n.*

dermal n. intradermal n.

dysplastic n., dysplastic melanocytic n. a type of acquired, atypical melanocytic nevus with an irregular border, indistinct margin, and mixed coloring, characterized by dysplastic melanocytes in the epidermis. Particularly in patients with other family who have these lesions, they may be precursors of malignant melanoma. See also *dysplastic nevus syndrome*, under *syndrome.* Called also *atypical* or *atypical melanocytic n., atypical* or *dysplastic mole*, and *Clark n.*

n. elas′ticus 1. pseudoxanthoma elasticum. 2. connective tissue n.

n. elasticus of Lewandowsky connective tissue n.

epidermal n., epithelial n. any of various types of hamartoma of the epidermis representing developmental anomalies that produce faulty mature or nearly mature cutaneous structures as a result of overproduction of surface or adnexal epithelium. Many patients with these lesions have involvement of other organ systems; see *epidermal nevus syndrome*, under *syndrome.*

fatty n. lipomatous n.

n. flam′meus a common congenital vascular malformation involving mature capillaries, presenting as a sharply demarcated, flat, irregularly shaped patch, sometimes flesh colored and sometimes orange *(salmon patch)* or dark red to purple *(port-wine stain)*; the usual location is on the face or neck. The ones closer to flesh color tend to involute during childhood, while discolored ones usually are persistent.

n. fuscoceru′leus acromiodeltoi′deus n. of Ito.

n. fuscoceru′leus ophthalmomaxilla′ris n. of Ota.

giant congenital hairy n., giant congenital pigmented n., giant hairy n., giant pigmented n. a type of congenital hairy nevus that is particularly large (usually over 20 cm in diameter); this type is present at birth, usually bilaterally symmetric, and located on the trunk or distal part of the limbs. It may be associated with other cutaneous and subcutaneous lesions such as neurofibromas, other developmental anomalies, and occasionally malignant melanoma.

hair follicle n. trichofolliculoma.

halo n. a melanocytic nevus surrounded by a halo of depigmentation that may be an immune response to the nevus cells. A minority may be related to development of melanoma. Called also *leukoderma acquisitum centrifugum* and *Sutton n.*

ichthyosiform n. CHILD n.

inflammatory linear verrucous epidermal n. (ILVEN) a congenital type of epidermal nevus characterized by tiny, pruritic, wartlike lesions in a linear distribution, usually on one lower limb, with a clinical resemblance to psoriasis or eczema.

Nevus *Continued*

intradermal n. a type of melanocytic nevus, clinically indistinguishable from a compound nevus, in which the nests of nevus cells lie exclusively within the dermis. Called also *dermal n.*

n. of Ito a lesion similar to nevus of Ota except for its location; this type is in the region of the shoulder and upper arm in areas of distribution of the posterior supraclavicular and lateral cutaneous brachial nerves. Called also *n. fuscoceruleus acromiodeltoideus.*

Jadassohn n., Jadassohn sebaceous n. n. sebaceus.

Jadassohn-Tièche n. blue n.

junction n., junctional n. a type of melanocytic nevus in which the nests of nevus cells are confined to the dermal-epidermal junction; it usually presents clinically as a small, discrete, flat or slightly raised macule.

kissing n. a congenital condition in which matching nevi are on the upper and lower eyelids, so that they appear to be one lesion when the eye is closed.

linear epidermal n. n. unius lateris.

n. lipomato′sus lipomatous n.

n. lipomato′sus cuta′neus superficia′lis, n. lipomato′sus superficia′lis a usually congenital type of connective tissue nevus, characterized by ectopic, mature adipocytes in the dermis and single or multiple soft, skin-colored or yellowish papules, nodules, and plaques, usually located on the lower trunk, gluteal region, or thigh.

lipomatous n. a nevus containing a large amount of fibrofatty tissue. Called also *fatty n., n. lipomatosus,* and *nevolipoma.*

melanocytic n. any of numerous acquired or inherited skin lesions composed of nests of nevus cells (altered melanocytes), usually presenting as tan to brown macules or papules with well-defined, rounded borders. There are three principal types, based on histologic pattern and location; see *compound n., intradermal n.,* and *junction n.* Called also *cellular, nevocellular, nevocytic,* and *nevus cell n.*

nape n. nuchal n.

neural n., neuroid n. neuronevus.

nevocellular n., nevocytic n., nevomelanocytic n., nevus cell n. melanocytic n.

nuchal n. a type of nevus flammeus found on the nape of the neck, lateral to the midline and between the occipital protuberance and the fifth cervical vertebra. Called also *nape* or *Unna n.*

organoid n. n. sebaceus.

n. of Ota, Ota n. a persistent lesion resembling a mongolian spot, involving the conjunctiva, skin around the eye, and adjacent structures; it is seen primarily in babies and in young people around the time of puberty, and in East Asians and people of African descent much more than in light-skinned people. The skin lesions are manifested as macular blue to brown patchy areas of pigmentation that grow slowly and become deeper in color. Called also *oculodermal melanocytosis* and *n. fuscoceruleus ophthalmomaxillaris.*

pigmented n. 1. any nevus containing melanin, such as a Becker nevus, melanocytic nevus, or nevus spilus. Called also *n. pigmentosus.* 2. melanocytic n.

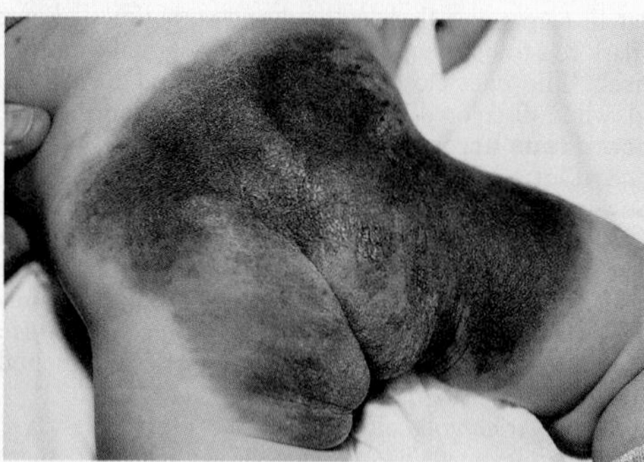

■ Giant congenital pigmented nevus.

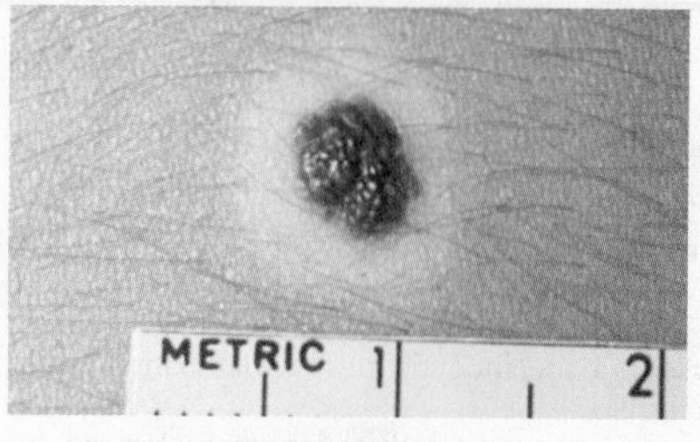

■ Halo nevus.

pigmented hairy epidermal n. Becker n.

n. pigmento′sus pigmented n.

port-wine n. see under *stain.*

sebaceous n., n. seba′ceus, n. sebaceus of Jadassohn a type of circumscribed, alopecic, yellow to brown epidermal nevus, present at birth, with hyperplastic sebaceous glands and hair follicles; the size can vary considerably. The usual location is on the scalp, face, or neck, and it persists throughout life. Called also *Jadassohn* or *Jadassohn sebaceous n.* See also *sebaceous nevus syndrome,* under *syndrome.*

n. sim′plex salmon patch (def. 2).

speckled lentiginous n. n. spilus.

spider n. see under *angioma.*

n. spi′lus a type of melanocytic nevus that is tan to brown, has a smooth surface, and is speckled with smaller, darker macules. Called also *speckled lentiginous n.*

n. spi′lus tar′dus Becker n.

spindle cell n., spindle and epithelioid cell n., Spitz n. a benign compound nevus usually seen in children before puberty, composed of spindle cells and epithelioid cells and presenting as a smooth to slightly scaly pink to red papule or nodule, often with surface telangiectasia. It is usually located in the dermis and is sometimes associated with large atypical cells and multinucleate cells. Because it has a close resemblance to malignant melanoma, it has sometimes been given the misnomers *benign juvenile* and *juvenile melanoma.*

n. spongio′sus al′bus muco′sae white sponge n.

stellar n. spider angioma.

strawberry n. 1. see under *hemangioma.* 2. cavernous hemangioma.

Sutton n. halo n.

systematized n. a type of nevus in which lesions are diffuse or extensive, often forming a pattern.

n. uni′us la′teris a congenital, verrucous type of epidermal nevus, ranging from pink to dark colored, occurring in a linear, unilateral pattern. On the limbs the lesions usually follow the long axis and may be arranged in continuous or broken spiral streaks, bands, or patches; on the trunk, they usually have a transverse orientation, as if along the distribution of the intercostal nerves.

Unna n. nuchal n.

uveal n. a nevus of the uvea, often bilateral and sometimes premalignant; it may be present at birth but more often becomes clinically evident at puberty due to increased pigmentation.

vascular n., n. vascula′ris, n. vasculo′sus 1. any nevus caused by a vascular malformation (see under *malformation*). 2. strawberry hemangioma.

n. verruco′sus, verrucous n. an epidermal nevus with a warty appearance.

white sponge n. a benign autosomal dominant disorder characterized by exuberant, spongy whiteness of mucous membranes, especially of the oral mucosa, with gray-white, soft, sometimes friable lesions with fissures and folds; it reaches maximal severity at adolescence or early adulthood without further progression. Called also *familial white folded mucosal dysplasia* and *n. spongiosus albus mucosae.*

---

new•born (noo′born) 1. recently born. 2. newborn infant; see under *infant.*

New•cas•tle disease (noo′kas-əl) [*Newcastle,* England, near which it was first observed in 1926] see under *disease.*

newt (no͞ot) any of various small, slender salamanders belonging to several genera, including *Taricha;* they have an aquatic larval stage but vary in whether the adult stage is aquatic, terrestrial, or some combination.

New·ton's law (noo'tənz) [Sir Isaac *Newton*, English mathematician, physicist, and astronomer, 1643–1727] see under *law*.

new·ton (N) (noo'tən) [Sir Isaac *Newton*] the SI unit of force, being that when applied in a vacuum to a body having a mass of one kilogram accelerates it at the rate of one meter per second squared.

nex·a·var (neks'ə-var) trademark for a preparation of sorafenib.

Nex·i·um (nek'se-əm) trademark for a preparation of esomeprazole magnesium.

nex·us (nek'səs) pl. *nex'us* [L. "bond"] 1. a bond, especially one between members of a series or group. 2. gap junction.

Ne·ze·lof syndrome (nĕ-zə-lof') [Christian *Nezelof*, French pediatrician, born 1922] see under *syndrome*.

NF *National Formulary*.

NF1 neurofibromatosis 1.

NF2 neurofibromatosis 2.

NFLPN National Federation of Licensed Practical Nurses.

ng nanogram.

NGF nerve growth factor.

NHC National Health Council.

NHGRI National Human Genome Research Institute, a division of the National Institutes of Health.

NHLBI National Heart, Lung, and Blood Institute.

NHMRC National Health and Medical Research Council.

NHS National Health Service (British).

NH_2-ter·mi·nal (tur'mĭ-nəl) N-terminal.

Ni nickel.

NIA National Institute on Aging.

NIAAA National Institute on Alcohol Abuse and Alcoholism.

Nia-Bid (ni'ə-bid) trademark for a preparation of niacin.

ni·a·cin (ni'ə-sin) 1. nicotinic acid, a member of the vitamin B complex that is a constituent of the redox coenzymes nicotinamide adenine dinucleotide (NAD) and nicotinamide adenine dinucleotide phosphate (NADP). 2. [USP] a preparation of niacin, used in the prophylaxis and treatment of niacin deficiency and the treatment of hyperlipidemia; administered orally, intramuscularly, or intravenously.

ni·a·cin·a·mide (ni″ə-sin'ə-mīd) [USP] nicotinamide, a B complex vitamin used in the prophylaxis and treatment of pellagra; administered orally, intravenously, or intramuscularly.

Nia·cor (ni'ə-kor) trademark for a preparation of niacin.

NIAID National Institute of Allergy and Infectious Diseases.

NIAMSD National Institute of Arthritis and Musculoskeletal and Skin Diseases.

Nia·span (ni'ə-span) trademark for a preparation of niacin.

nib (nib) the working part of a dental condenser, which corresponds to the blade in an excavating or cutting instrument. Called also *condenser point*.

ni·car·ba·zin (ni-kahr'bə-zin) a coccidiostat used in poultry.

ni·car·di·pine hy·dro·chlo·ride (ni-kahr'dĭ-pēn) a calcium channel blocking agent structurally related to nifedipine that acts as a vasodilator; administered orally in the treatment of angina pectoris and hypertension.

nic·co·lum (nik'o-ləm) [L.] nickel.

NICHD National Institute of Child Health and Human Development.

niche (nich) [Fr. "recess"] a defect in an otherwise even surface, especially a depression or recess in the wall of an organ as seen on a radiograph or by the unaided eye.

Barclay n. a deformity of the duodenal cap in a duodenal ulcer, seen as a projection on the radiograph.

ecologic n. the place of an organism within its community or ecosystem.

Haudek n. see under *sign*.

n. of round window fossula fenestrae cochleae.

nick (nik) a break in just one strand of a double-stranded nucleic acid.

nick·el (Ni) (nik'əl) [L. *niccolum*] a silver-white metallic element; specific gravity, 8.9; atomic number, 28; atomic weight, 58.71. Long-term excessive exposure to metallic nickel, as in jewelry, can cause contact dermatitis *(nickel dermatitis)*; excessive exposure to nickel fumes can cause nasal and lung cancers.

n. carbonyl a combination of nickel and carbonyl ions, produced in the refining of nickel; it is extremely toxic, causing pulmonary edema and dyspnea, and carcinogenic, causing lung and nasal cancers.

n. sulfate the sulfate salt of nickel, used in electroplating and as a mordant in dyeing; skin exposure causes allergic contact dermatitis.

nick·ing (nik'ing) localized constrictions in the retinal blood vessels seen in arterial hypertension.

ni·clo·sa·mide (nĭ-klo'sə-mīd) a salicylanilide anthelmintic effective against the tapeworms *Diphyllobothrium latum*, *Hymenolepis nana*, *Taenia saginata*, and the adults of *Taenia solium;* administered orally to humans, cats, and dogs.

Nico-400 (nik'o) trademark for a preparation of niacin.

Nic·ol prism (nik'ol) [William *Nicol*, Scottish physicist, 1768–1851] see under *prism*.

Ni·co·la·do·ni sign (ne-ko-lə-do'ne) [Carl *Nicoladoni*, German surgeon, 1847–1902] Branham sign; see under *sign*.

Ni·co·las-Fa·vre disease (ne-ko-lah' fahv'rə) [Joseph *Nicolas*, French physician, 1868–1960; Maurice Jules *Favre*, French physician, 1876–1954] lymphogranuloma venereum.

Ni·co·nyl (ni'ko-nəl) trademark for a preparation of isoniazid.

Nic·o·ti·a·na (nik″o-she-a'nə) [Jean *Nicot* de Villemain, 1530–1600, who introduced tobacco chewing to the queen of France] a genus of annual plants of the family Solanaceae, native to tropical America. *N. taba'cum* L. and certain other species are sources of tobacco.

nic·o·tin·a·mide (nik″o-tin'ə-mīd) INN for *niacinamide*.

n. adenine dinucleotide (NAD) a coenzyme composed of nicotinamide mononucleotide (NMN) coupled to adenosine monophosphate (AMP) by pyrophosphate linkage. It is found widely in nature and is involved in numerous enzymatic reactions in which it serves as an electron carrier by being alternately oxidized (NAD^+) and reduced (NADH).

n. adenine dinucleotide phosphate (NADP) a coenzyme composed of nicotinamide mononucleotide (NMN) coupled by pyrophosphate linkage to the 5′-phosphate of adenosine 2′,5′-bisphosphate. It serves as an electron carrier in numerous reactions, being alternately oxidized ($NADP^+$) and reduced (NADPH). Formerly called also *triphosphopyridine nucleotide (TPN)*.

n. mononucleotide (NMN) a nucleotide containing covalently linked nicotinamide and ribose 5-phosphate. It is a constituent of NAD and NADP.

nic·o·tin·ate (nik″o-tin'āt) the dissociated form of nicotinic acid.

n. ribonucleotide nicotinic acid coupled to ribose 5′-phosphate via an amino linkage; it is an intermediate in the synthesis of NAD.

nic·o·tine (nik'o-tēn, nik'o-tin) [L. *nicotiana* tobacco] 1. a very poisonous, colorless, soluble fluid alkaloid with a pyridine-like odor and a burning taste, obtained from tobacco or produced synthetically. It is used as an agricultural insecticide and in pharmacological and physiological studies for its neurological effects (see also *nicotinic*) 2. [USP] a preparation of nicotine, administered orally, intranasally, by inhalation, or as a transdermal patch as an aid to smoking cessation; also used in veterinary medicine as an external parasiticide.

n. polacrilex [USP] nicotine bound to a cation exchange resin; used in nicotine chewing gum as an aid to smoking cessation.

n. sulfate the sulfate salt of nicotine, formerly a component of veterinary vermifuges; it can cause poisoning in lambs and calves. See *nicotine sulfate poisoning*, under *poisoning*.

nic·o·tin·ic (nik″o-tin'ik) denoting the effect of nicotine and other drugs in initially stimulating and subsequently, in high doses, inhibiting neural impulses at autonomic ganglia and the neuromuscular junction. See also *nicotinic receptors*, under *receptor*.

nic·o·tin·ic ac·id (nik″o-tin'ik) niacin.

nic·o·tin·ism (nik'o-tin-iz″əm) nicotine poisoning.

nic·o·tino·lyt·ic (nik″o-tin-o-lit'ik) [*nicotine* + *-lytic*] destroying or suppressing the toxic action of nicotine.

Nic·o·trol (nik'o-trol) trademark for preparations of nicotine.

ni·cou·ma·lone (ni-koo'mə-lōn) BAN for *acenocoumarol*.

Nic·o·zide (nik'o-zīd) trademark for preparations of isoniazid.

nic·ta·tion (nik-ta'shən) winking.

nic·ti·ta·tion (nik″tĭ-ta'shən) [L. *nictitare* to wink] winking.

NIDA National Institute on Drug Abuse.

ni·dal (ni'dəl) pertaining to a nidus.

ni·da·tion (ni-da'shən) [L. *nidus* nest] implantation (def. 1).

NIDCR National Institute of Dental and Craniofacial Research.

NIDD non–insulin-dependent diabetes mellitus; see *type 2 diabetes mellitus*, under *diabetes*.

NIDDK National Institute of Diabetes and Digestive and Kidney Diseases.

NIDDM non–insulin-dependent diabetes mellitus; see *type 2 diabetes mellitus*, under *diabetes*.

ni·di (ni'di) [L.] plural of *nidus*.

ni·do·gen (ni′də-jen) a sulfated 150-kD adhesive glycoprotein that links collagen IV to laminin in the basement membrane. Called also *entactin.*

ni·dus (ni′dəs) pl. *ni′di* [L. "nest"] 1. the point of origin or focus of a morbid process. 2. nucleus (def. 2).

n. a′vis a depression in the cerebellum between the posterior velum and the uvula, the location of the tonsil of the cerebellum.

NIEHS National Institute of Environmental Health Sciences.

Niel·sen method (nēl′sen) [Holger *Nielsen,* Danish army officer, 1866–1955] Holger Nielsen method; see under *method.*

Nie·mann disease (ne′mahn) [Albert *Niemann,* German pediatrician, 1880–1921] Niemann-Pick disease; see under *disease.*

Nie·mann-Pick cells, disease (ne′mahn pik′) [A. *Niemann;* Ludwig *Pick,* German physician, 1868–1944] see under *cell* and *disease.*

ni·fed·i·pine (ni-fed′ĭ-pēn) [USP] a calcium channel blocking agent used as a coronary vasodilator in the treatment of coronary insufficiency and stable angina pectoris, and as an antihypertensive; administered orally.

ni·fur·sem·i·zone (ni″fūr-sem′ĭ-zōn) an antiprotozoal effective against *Histomonas;* used in poultry.

ni·fur·sol (ni′fūr-sol) an antiprotozoal effective against *Histomonas;* used in poultry.

night·mare (nīt′mār″) a terrifying dream; an anxiety attack during dreaming, accompanied by mild autonomic reactions and usually awakening the dreamer, who recalls the dream but is oriented.

night·shade (nīt′shād″) 1. any of several flowering plants of the genus *Solanum.* 2. deadly n.; see *belladonna* (def. 1).

deadly n. belladonna (def. 1).

NIGMS National Institute of General Medical Sciences.

ni·gra (ni′grə) [L. "black"] the substantia nigra. **ni′gral** *adj*

ni·gri·cans (ni′grĭ-kəns) [L.] blackish.

ni·gri·ti·es (ni-grish′e-ēz) [L.] blackness.

n. lin′guae black hairy tongue.

ni·gro·pal·li·dal (ni″gro-pal′ĭ-dəl) pertaining to the substantia nigra and the globus pallidus.

ni·gro·sin (ni′gro-sin) an aniline dye having a special affinity for ganglion cells, used to stain tissues from the central nervous system for study under the microscope.

ni·gro·stri·a·tal (ni″gro-stri-a′təl) projecting from the substantia nigra to the corpus striatum; said of a bundle of nerve fibers.

NIH National Institutes of Health.

ni·hil·ism (ni′il-iz″əm) [L. *nihil* nothing + *-ism*] 1. an attitude of skepticism regarding traditional values and beliefs or their frank rejection. 2. a delusion of nonexistence of part or all of the self or the world.

therapeutic n. skepticism regarding the therapeutic value of drugs or treatment procedures.

ni·keth·a·mide (nĭ-keth′ə-mīd) a central and respiratory stimulant used to counteract respiratory and central nervous system depression and circulatory failure, administered intramuscularly and intravenously.

Ni·ki·fo·roff method (ne-ke′fə-rof) [Mikhail *Nikiforoff,* Russian dermatologist, 1858–1915] see under *method.*

Ni·kol·sky sign (nĭ-kol′ske) [Petr Vasilyevich *Nikolsky,* Russian dermatologist, 1858–1940] see under *sign.*

Ni·lan·dron (nĭ-lan′drən) trademark for a preparation of nilutamide.

Ni·le·var (ni′lə-vahr) trademark for preparations of norethandrolone.

Nil·stat (nil′stat) trademark for preparations of nystatin.

ni·lu·ta·mide (ni-loo′tə-mīd) a nonsteroidal antiandrogen used as an antineoplastic, in combination with measures to lower testosterone levels such as bilateral orchiectomy, in treatment of prostatic carcinoma; administered orally.

Nim·bex (nim′beks) trademark for a preparation of cisatracurium besylate.

NIMH National Institute of Mental Health.

nim·i·dane (nim′ĭ-dān) a veterinary acaricide.

ni·mo·di·pine (ni-mo′dĭ-pēn) [USP] a calcium channel blocking agent structurally related to nifedipine, used as a vasodilator to reduce the incidence and severity of ischemic deficits following subarachnoid hemorrhage from a ruptured intracranial aneurysm; administered orally.

Ni·mo·top (ni′mo-top) trademark for a preparation of nimodipine.

NINDS National Institute of Neurological Disorders and Stroke.

Nin·hy·drin (nin-hi′drin) trademark for a preparation of triketohydrindene hydrate.

NINR National Institute for Nursing Research.

ni·o·bi·um (Nb) (ni-o′be-əm) [*Niobe,* of Greek mythology, who was turned into stone] chemical element, atomic number, 41; atomic weight, 92.906.

NIOSH National Institute for Occupational Safety and Health.

Ni·pah encephalitis, virus (ne′pə) [*Nipah,* village in Malaysia, from where the virus was first isolated] see under *encephalitis* and *virus.*

Ni·pent (ni′pent) trademark for a preparation of pentostatin.

ni·per·yt (ni′pər-it) pentaerythritol tetranitrate.

NIPHS noninsulinoma pancreatogenous hypoglycemia syndrome.

nip·pers (nip′ərz) pincers (def. 2).

nip·ple (nip′əl) 1. papilla mammae. 2. any structure shaped like the papilla mammae.

Nip·po·stron·gy·lus (nip″o-stron′jə-ləs) a genus of hookworms of the family Trichostrongylidae. *N. brasilien′sis* (called also *N. mu′ris*) parasitizes rats.

Ni·ra·vam (ni′rə-vam) trademark for a preparation of alprazolam.

ni·rid·a·zole (nĭ-rid′ə-zōl) an antischistosomal also used in the treatment of intestinal and extraintestinal amebiasis and in dracunculiasis, administered orally.

ni·sin (ni′sin) a polypeptide antibiotic produced by *Streptococcus lactis* and occurring naturally in certain cheeses. Nisin is active against certain streptococci, *Mycobacterium tuberculosis,* and several other bacteria and is used as a preservative in food processing.

ni·sol·di·pine (ni-sol′dĭ-pēn) a calcium channel blocking agent used in the treatment of hypertension; administered orally.

Nis·sen fundoplication (operation) (nis′en) [Rudolf *Nissen,* Swiss surgeon, 1896–1981] see under *fundoplication.*

Nis·sl bodies (granules, substance), degeneration, method of staining (nis′əl) [Franz *Nissl,* German neurologist, 1860–1919] see under *body and degeneration,* and see *Stains and Staining Methods,* under *stain.*

NIST National Institute of Standards and Technology (formerly the National Bureau of Standards).

ni·sus (ni′səs) [L., from *niti* to strive] an effort, strong tendency, or endeavor to achieve an outcome or aim.

nit (nit) the egg of a louse.

Ni·ta·buch layer (stria, zone) (ne′tah-book) [Raissa *Nitabuch,* German physician, 19th century] see under *layer.*

ni·tar·sone (nĭ-tahr′sōn) an antiprotozoal effective against *Histomonas;* used in poultry.

ni·ta·zox·a·nide (ni″tə-zok′sə-nīd) an antiprotozoal used in the treatment of cryptosporidiosis in patients with HIV infection and acquired immunodeficiency syndrome.

ni·ti·nol (ni′tĭ-nol) [*ni*ckel *ti*tanium *N*aval *O*rdnance *L*aboratory (where it was developed)] any of several alloys of nickel and titanium that are resistant to fatigue, have low moduli of elasticity, and return to their original shape after deformation if they are heated; used in orthodontic materials.

ni·tram·ine (ni-tram′in) a nitro derivative of an amine, having the group —NNO_2.

ni·trate (ni′trāt) any salt or ester of nitric acid or the NO_3^- anion; organic nitrates, e.g., nitroglycerin, are used as coronary vasodilators in the treatment of angina pectoris.

ni·trate re·duc·tase (ni′trāt re-duk′tās) any of several enzymes occurring in plants and some bacteria and catalyzing the reduction of nitrate to nitrite. The reaction allows plants to use the nitrogen from nitrate for protein synthesis and allows some bacteria, under certain conditions, to use nitrate as a terminal electron acceptor in respiration. A test for nitrate reduction in a bacterial culture is useful in identification of Enterobacteriaceae, mycobacteria, and certain anaerobic bacteria.

ni·traz·e·pam (ni-traz′ə-pam) a benzodiazepine used as a sedative and anticonvulsant; administered orally.

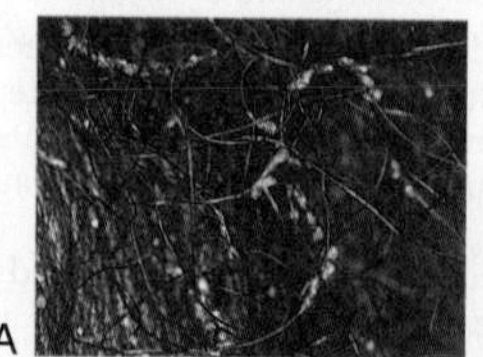

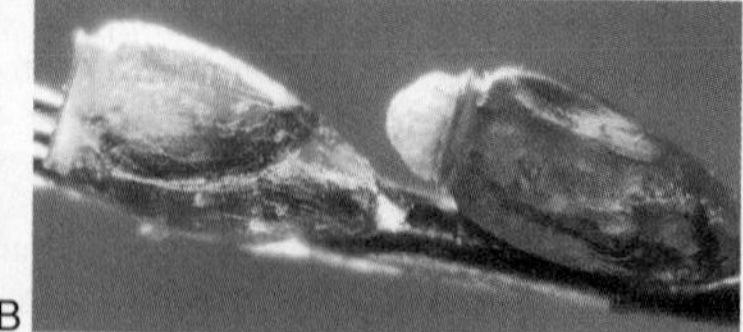

■ Nits of *Phthirus pubis. (A),* Clinical appearance of nits on hair; *(B),* microscopic appearance of nits attached to hair shaft.

ni•tren•di•pine (ni-tren′dĭ-pēn) a calcium channel blocking agent related to nifedipine, administered orally as an antihypertensive; its predominant effects are in the peripheral circulation, reducing both systolic and diastolic blood pressures.

ni•tric (ni′trik) pertaining to or containing nitrogen, applied especially to compounds containing nitrogen with a higher valence than that contained in the nitrous compounds.

n. oxide 1. NO, a naturally occurring gas that in the body is a short-lived dilator substance released from vascular endothelial cells in response to the binding of vasodilators to endothelial cell receptors; it causes activation of guanylate cyclase in vascular smooth muscle, leading to an increase in cyclic GMP, which inhibits muscular contraction and produces relaxation. Excess nitric oxide is toxic to cells of the central nervous system and causes the hypotension seen in septic shock. Called also *endothelial-* or *endothelium-derived relaxing factor*. 2. a preparation of nitric oxide used in conjunction with ventilatory support or other agents as a pulmonary antihypertensive in the treatment of hypoxic respiratory failure due to persistent fetal circulation in term or near-term neonates; administered by inhalation.

ni•tric ac•id (ni′trik) a strong mineral acid, HNO_3, an extremely corrosive liquid with a characteristic suffocating odor; it is a strong oxidizing agent that is highly toxic by inhalation and corrosive to skin and mucous membranes.

fuming n. a. nitric acid containing dissolved oxides of nitrogen; it is a very strong oxidizing agent.

ni•tri•da•tion (ni″trĭ-da′shən) combination with nitrogen to form a nitride.

ni•tride (ni′trīd) a binary compound of nitrogen with a metal.

ni•tri•fi•ca•tion (ni″trĭ-fĭ-ka′shən) [*nitric acid* + L. *facere* to make] oxidation of the nitrogen in ammonia and organic compounds to nitrites and to nitrates, carried out by soil bacteria of the family Nitrobacteraceae.

ni•tri•fi•er (ni′trĭ-fi″ər) a nitrifying microorganism.

ni•tri•fy•ing (ni′trĭ-fi″ing) oxidizing ammonia to nitrite (nitrosification) and then to nitrate.

ni•trile (ni′tril) an organic compound containing trivalent nitrogen attached to one carbon atom, —C≡N.

ni•trilo•tri•ace•tic ac•id (ni″tril-o-tri-ə-se′tik) a chelating agent found in synthetic detergents; in excessive amounts it is an epigenetic carcinogen for kidney and bladder cancer.

ni•trite (ni′trīt) any salt or ester of nitrous acid or the NO_2^- anion; organic nitrites, e.g., amyl nitrite, have been used as coronary vasodilators in the treatment of angina pectoris.

ni•tri•toid (ni′trĭ-toid) resembling a nitrite or the reaction caused by a nitrite.

ni•tri•tu•ria (ni″trĭ-tu′re-ə) the presence of nitrites in the urine, indicating bacteriuria with bacteria that reduce nitrates to nitrites.

nitro- a prefix indicating presence of the group $—NO_2$.

ni•tro-amine (ni′tro-ə-mēn″) nitramine.

ni•tro•an•i•line (ni″tro-an′ĭ-līn) a dye used in paints, paint removers, inks, and solvents; excessive exposure can cause nitroaniline poisoning.

ni•tro•bac•te•ria (ni″tro-bak-te′re-ə) plural of *nitrobacterium*.

ni•tro•bac•te•ri•um (ni″tro-bak-tēr′e–əm) pl. *nitrobacte′ria* [*nitro-* + *bacterium*] a bacterium that oxidizes nitrites to nitrates.

ni•tro•ben•zene (ni″tro-ben′zēn) a poisonous benzene derivative used in the manufacture of aniline. Called also *nitrobenzol* and *oil of mirbane*.

ni•tro•ben•zol (ni″tro-ben′zol) nitrobenzene.

ni•tro•blue tet•ra•zo•li•um (ni′tro-bloo tet″rə-zo′le-əm) a yellow water-soluble dye that on reduction is converted to a dark blue water-insoluble formazan; see also under *test*.

ni•tro•cel•lu•lose (ni″tro-sel′u-lōs) pyroxylin.

Ni•tro•disc (ni′tro-disk″) trademark for a preparation of nitroglycerin.

Ni•tro-Dur (ni′tro-dur″) trademark for a preparation of nitroglycerin.

ni•tro•fu•ran (ni″tro-fu′ran) any of a group of antibacterials, including furazolidone, nitrofurazone, nitrofurantoin, and related compounds, which are effective against a wide range of bacteria.

ni•tro•fu•ran•to•in (ni″tro-fu-ran′to-in) [USP] a synthetic broad-spectrum antibacterial effective against many gram-negative and gram-positive organisms, including *Escherichia coli*, *enterococci*, *Staphylococcus aureus*, *Staphylococcus saprophyticus*, and *Klebsiella* and *Enterobacter* species; used in the treatment of urinary tract infections due to susceptible bacteria, administered orally.

ni•tro•fu•ra•zone (ni″tro-fu′rə-zōn) [USP] an antibacterial effective against a wide variety of gram-negative and gram-positive organisms. It is used topically as a local antiinfective in skin lesions including wounds, burns, skin infections, and ulcers and to aid healing and prevent infection of skin grafts.

Ni•tro•gard (ni′tro-gahrd″) trademark for a preparation of nitroglycerin.

ni•tro•gen (N) (ni′tro-jən) [Gr. *nitron* niter + *-gen*] 1. a colorless, gaseous element found free in the air; specific gravity, 0.9713; atomic number, 7; atomic weight, 14.007. It forms about four fifths of common air. Chemically it is almost inert, but it forms by combination of nitric acid and ammonia. It is important biologically, being a constituent of protein and nucleic acids and thus present in all living cells. It will not support respiration; although not a poison, it is fatal if breathed alone, because of the lack of oxygen. It is soluble in the blood and body fluids and when released as bubbles of gas by reduction of atmospheric pressure it causes serious or even fatal symptoms (see *decompression sickness*, under *sickness*). 2. [NF] an official preparation, not less than 99 per cent N_2 by volume; used to replace air in pharmaceutical preparations.

n. 13 a radioactive isotope of nitrogen, atomic mass 13, having a half-life of 9.97 minutes; it decays by positron emission (1.190 MeV) and is used as a tracer in positron emission tomography.

amide n. the portion of the nitrogen in protein that exists in the form of acid amides.

blood urea n. see *urea nitrogen*, under *urea*.

n. dioxide a brownish, irritant gas, NO_2, generated by the decomposition of nitrogen tetroxide or the reaction of metals with concentrated nitric acid. Exposure to heavy concentrations causes lung damage with coughing, dyspnea, and acute bronchiolitis. See also *silo filler's lung*, under *lung*.

n. mustard see under *mustard*.

nomadic n. free nitrogen from the air which enters into plant and animal growth.

nonprotein n. the nitrogenous constituents of the blood exclusive of the protein bodies. It consists of the nitrogen of urea, uric acid, creatine, creatinine, amino acids, polypeptides, and an undetermined part known as *rest nitrogen*.

n. pentoxide a crystalline compound, N_2O_5, or nitric anhydride, which combines with water to form nitric acid.

n. peroxide n. tetroxide.

rest n. see *nonprotein n.*

n. tetroxide a poisonous volatile liquid, N_2O_4; at room temperature it decomposes to nitrogen dioxide (q.v.). Called also *n. peroxide*.

urea n. see under *urea*.

ni•tro•gen•ase (ni′tro-jən-ās) an enzyme system of nitrogen-fixing bacteria and blue-green algae that catalyzes the reduction of molecular nitrogen (N_2) to ammonia (NH_3).

ni•tro•gen-fix•ing (ni′tro-jən-fik′sing) accomplishing nitrogen fixation (see under *fixation*); said of certain bacteria.

ni•trog•e•nous (ni-troj′ə-nəs) containing nitrogen.

ni•tro•glyc•er•in (ni″tro-glis′ər-in) 1. a colorless to yellow liquid formed by the action of nitric and sulfuric acids on glycerin. It explodes on concussion, but is safe if diluted with inert excipients. Exposure to excessive amounts causes headache, blurred vision, vomiting, hypotension, and syncope, and possibly cyanosis and methemoglobinemia. Prolonged exposure causes tolerance, and abrupt discontinuation can cause withdrawal symptoms. 2. [USP] a pharmaceutical preparation of nitroglycerin, diluted with lactose, dextrose, alcohol, propylene glycol, or other excipient for safety and officially called *diluted nitroglycerin*; it has antianginal, antihypertensive, and vasodilator properties and is used in medicine for the prophylaxis and treatment of angina pectoris, the treatment of congestive heart failure, as an adjunct in the treatment of myocardial infarction, and for blood pressure control or controlled hypotension during surgery. Administered by absorption through the oral mucous membranes, orally, intravenously, topically, or with a transdermal patch.

ni•tro•hy•dro•chlo•ric ac•id (ni″tro-hi″dro-klor′ik) aqua regia.

Ni•tro•lin•gual (ni″tro-ling′gwəl) trademark for a preparation of nitroglycerin.

ni•tro•mer•sol (ni″tro-mur′sol) [USP] a mercurial compound that has been used as a topical antiinfective agent and for disinfection of surgical and dental instruments and equipment.

ni•trom•e•ter (ni-trom′ə-tər) [*nitrogen* + *-meter*] an apparatus for measuring the quantity of nitrogen given off in a reaction.

ni•tro•naph•tha•lene (ni″tro-naf′thə-lēn) a compound, used in the alpha form to mask fluorescence in mineral oils and in dye manufacture; its vapors may cause vesication and opacity of the cornea. The beta form is highly toxic by ingestion.

ni•tro•naph•tha•lin (ni″tro-naf′thə-lin) nitronaphthalene.

ni•tro•phe•nol (ni″tro-fe′nol) an indicator with a pH range of 5 to 7, being colorless at 5 and yellow at 7.

Ni·tro·press (ni′tro-pres) trademark for a preparation of sodium nitroprusside.

2-ni·tro·pro·pane (ni″tro-pro′pān) a flammable yellow liquid prepared by the reaction of propane with nitric acid under pressure; used as a solvent, rocket propellant, and gasoline additive. It is carcinogenic.

ni·tro·pro·tein (ni″tro-pro′tēn) a nitrated protein made by treating serum protein with nitric acid.

ni·tro·prus·side (ni″tro-prus′īd) the anion $[Fe(CN_5)NO]^{2-}$; see *sodium nitroprusside,* under *sodium.*

ni·tros·amine (ni-trōs′ə-mēn) any of a group of *N*-nitroso derivatives of secondary amines (R_2N—NO), formed by the combining of nitrates with amines; some nitrosamines show carcinogenic activity. Under certain conditions, nitrite-containing foods can form nitrosamines in the mammalian stomach, causing hepatotoxicity and other symptoms.

ni·tro·sate (ni′tro-sāt) to convert into a nitroso compound.

ni·tro·sa·tion (ni″tro-sa′shən) conversion into a nitroso compound.

ni·tro·scan·ate (ni″tro-skan′āt) an anthelmintic used in dogs.

ni·trose (ni′trōs) a term used to include nitric and nitrous acids.

ni·tro·si·fi·ca·tion (ni-tro″sĭ-fĭ-ka′shən) the oxidation of ammonia into nitrites.

ni·tro·si·fy·ing (ni-tro′sĭ-fi″ing) oxidizing ammonia into nitrites; said of certain bacteria of the family Nitrobacteraceae.

nitroso- a prefix indicating presence of the group —NO.

ni·tro·so·bac·te·ria (ni-tro″so-bak-te′re-ə) plural of *nitrosobacterium.*

ni·tro·so·bac·te·ri·um (ni-tro″so-bak-te′re-əm) pl. *nitrosobacte′ria.* A bacterium that oxidizes ammonia to nitrites.

***N*-ni·tro·so·di·meth·yl·amine** (ni-tro″so-di-meth′əl-ə-mēn″) a yellow liquid nitrosamine formerly used in rocket fuels, as an antioxidant, and for other purposes; it is sometimes found as a contaminant in fish meal, causing hepatotoxicity and carcinogenesis. Called also *dimethylnitrosamine.*

***N*-ni·tro·so·di·phen·yl·amine** (ni-tro″so-di-fen′əl-ə-mēn″) a bicyclic nitrosamine used as an accelerator in the vulcanization of rubber; it is carcinogenic. Called also *diphenylnitrosamine.*

Ni·tro·so·mo·na·da·les (ni-tro″so-mo″nə-da′lēz) [L. *nitrosus* nitrous + Gr. *monas* unit, from *monos* single] a morphologically, metabolically, and ecologically diverse order of bacteria of the class Betaproteobacteria, phylum Proteobacteria, grouped together on the basis of 16S rRNA sequence analysis. Organisms of medical interest are contained in the family Spirillaceae.

ni·tro·so·sub·sti·tu·tion (ni-tro″so-sub″stĭ-too′shən) the substitution of the radical nitryl for some other radical or atom in a compound.

ni·tro·so·urea (ni-tro″so-u′re-ə) any of several chemically related antineoplastic agents including carmustine, lomustine, semustine, and the antibiotic streptozocin. Carmustine, lomustine, and semustine are closely related chemically, are highly lipid-soluble, cross the blood-brain barrier, and are used against brain tumors; they act by alkylation, carbamoylation, and inhibition of DNA repair; they are not cross-resistant with other alkylating agents and are highly effective against resting (G_0) cells; the major side effect is dose-limiting bone marrow suppression. Streptozocin differs from the others in that it is not cross-resistant with them, is not myelosuppressive, and does not act by carbamoylation.

Ni·tro·stat (ni′tro-stat″) trademark for a preparation of nitroglycerin.

ni·tro·sug·ars (ni″tro-shoog′ərz) a class of substances which have been used in the treatment of angina pectoris.

ni·tro·syl (ni′tro-səl) the univalent radical NO.

ni·trous (ni′trəs) pertaining to nitrogen in its lowest valency.

n. oxide [USP] dinitrogen monoxide, N_2O, a colorless, odorless gas that is a weak inhalational anesthetic. It is nonflammable but supports combustion and is primarily used in combination with a potent halogenated inhalational anesthetic (halothane, isoflurane, or enflurane) to produce general anesthesia. Use as a sole agent requires high concentrations that may cause hypoxia. Popularly called *laughing gas.*

ni·trous ac·id (ni′trəs) a weak acid, HNO_2, existing only in aqueous solution.

ni·tro·vaso·di·la·tor (ni″tro-va″zo-di′la-tər, -vas″o-) any of a class of vasodilators, such as nitroglycerin, that mimic the activity of nitric oxide.

ni·tro·xan·thic ac·id (ni″tro-zan′thik) trinitrophenol.

ni·trox·yl (ni-trok′səl) nitryl.

ni·tryl (ni′trəl) the radical NO_2.

Nitzs·chia (nich′e-ə) a genus of marine diatoms. *N. pun′gens* is a source of the neurotoxin domoic acid, the cause of amnesic shellfish poisoning (see under *poisoning*).

Nix (niks) trademark for preparations of permethrin.

ni·za·ti·dine (nĭ-za′tĭ-dēn) [USP] a histamine H_2 receptor antagonist, used to inhibit gastric acid secretion in the prophylaxis and treatment of gastric and duodenal ulcers, gastroesophageal reflux disease, and conditions that cause gastric hypersecretion; administered orally.

Ni·zo·ral (ni′zor-al) trademark for preparations of ketoconazole.

nL nanoliter.

NLN National League for Nursing.

nm nanometer.

NMA National Medical Association.

NMDA *N*-methyl-D-aspartate.

NMN nicotinamide mononucleotide.

NMR nuclear magnetic resonance.

NMRI Naval Medical Research Institute, part of the National Naval Medical Center.

NMS neuroleptic malignant syndrome.

N-Mul·ti·stix (mul′te-stiks) trademark for a reagent strip for testing urine specimens for protein, glucose, ketones, bilirubin, occult blood, urobilinogen, and nitrite, and to indicate urinary pH.

NNRTI non-nucleoside reverse transcriptase inhibitor.

nn. [L.] nervi (nerves).

No nobelium.

No. [L.] nu′mero (to the number of).

No·ack syndrome (no′ahk) [Margot *Noack,* German physician, 20th century] Pfeiffer syndrome; see under *syndrome.*

NOAEL no observed adverse effect level.

no·bel·i·um (No) (no-bel′e-əm) [Alfred Bernhard *Nobel*] the chemical element of atomic number 102, atomic weight 253, obtained in 1958 by bombardment of ^{246}Cm with ^{12}C ions in a heavy ion linear accelerator.

No·car·dia (no-kahr′de-ə) [Edmond Isidore Etienne *Nocard,* French veterinarian, 1850–1903] a large genus of bacteria of the family Nocardiaceae, consisting mainly of soil saprophytes; a few are pathogenic. Organisms are gram-positive and aerobic, with branching filaments that break into bacillary or coccal forms, and produce chains of spores by simple fragmentation of hyphal branches. The type species is *N. asteroi′des.*

N. asteroi′des an acid-fast filamentous actinomycete, the most common cause of nocardiosis, especially pulmonary nocardiosis; it can also cause actinomycotic mycetoma in humans and nocardial mastitis in cattle.

N. brasilien′sis an acid-fast pathogenic species that produces yellow to brown mycelium with branching filaments, usually found in the tropics in soil; it can cause nocardiosis and actinomycotic mycetoma. Called also *Actinomyces brasiliensis.*

N. coeli′aca a species that produces the antibiotic substance nocardin.

N. farci′nica a species of acid-fast, filamentous actinomycetes of uncertain classification, which causes farcy and nocardial mastitis in cattle and actinomycotic mycetoma in humans; it may be identical to *N. asteroides.*

N. orienta′lis former name for *Amycolatopsis orientalis.*

N. oti′tidiscavia′rum a species of widespread distribution that sometimes causes nocardiosis and actinomycotic mycetoma in which the granules secreted in the pus are white.

No·car·di·a·ceae (no-kahr″de-a′se-e) a family of bacteria of the suborder Corynebacterineae, order Actinomycetales, consisting of nonmotile, gram-positive microorganisms that form branching hyphae that fragment into rod-shaped to coccoid elements; organisms are aerobic, chemoorganotrophic, and catalase-positive. It includes the genera *Nocardia* and *Rhodococcus.*

no·car·di·al (no-kahr′de-əl) pertaining to or caused by *Nocardia.*

no·car·di·a·sis (no″kahr-di′ə-sis) nocardiosis.

no·car·din (no-kahr′din) an antibiotic substance from *Nocardia coeliaca,* active against tubercle bacilli.

no·car·dio·form (no-kahr′de-o-form″) characterized by a fugacious mycelium that breaks into bacillary or coccal forms.

No·car·di·op·sa·ceae (no-kahr″de-op-sa′se-e) a family of gram-positive, aerobic, non–acid-fast, filament-forming bacteria of the suborder Streptosporangineae, order Actinomycetales; organisms of medical interest are contained in the genus *Nocardiopsis.*

No·car·di·op·sis (no-kahr″de-op′sis) a genus of soil bacteria of the family Nocardiopsaceae, consisting of gram-positive, aerobic, non–acid-fast organisms that form filaments. The organisms differ in cell wall type and are not resistant to lysozymes. They are potential pathogens, causing abscesses and pulmonary lesions. The type species is *N. dassonvil′lei.*

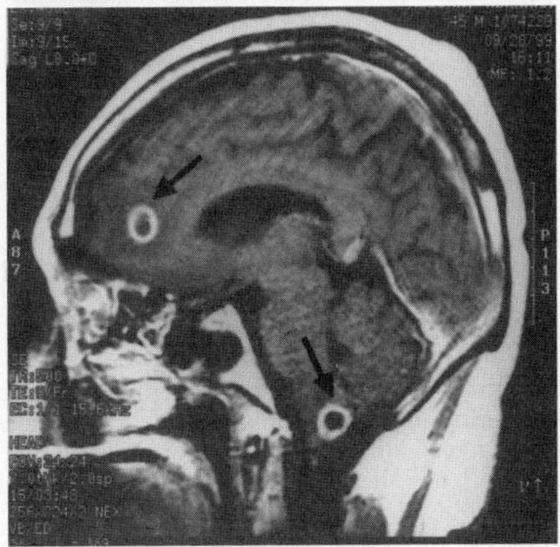

■ Nocardiosis. Multiple gadolinium-enhanced brain lesions *(arrows)* on MRI scan.

N. dassonvil'lei a species, separable into a number of subspecies, that is a cause of human infection, including actinomycotic mycetoma, conjunctivitis, skin infections, and hypersensitivity pneumonitis.

no•car•di•o•sis (no-kahr″de-o′sis) infection with a species of *Nocardia*, usually *N. asteroides*, but occasionally *N. brasiliensis*, *N. farcinica*, or *N. otitidiscaviarum*. There is usually an acute or chronic suppurative lung infection *(pulmonary n.)* with abscesses, but there is a marked tendency to spread to other organs such as the brain, skin, or subcutaneous tissues, sometimes with a fatal outcome. Called also *nocardiasis*.

bovine n. infection of cattle with species of *Nocardia*; see *bovine farcy* and *nocardial mastitis*.

pulmonary n. lung infection with a species of *Nocardia*; it ranges from subclinical to a type of pneumonia with necrosis, cavitation, and abscess formation; it is most common in debilitated or immunocompromised patients. See also *Nocardia pneumonia*.

no•ce•bo (no-se′bo) [L. "I will harm"] an adverse, nonspecific side effect occurring in conjunction with a medication but not directly resulting from the pharmacologic action of the medication.

Noch•tia (nok′te-ə) a genus of small nematode worms. *N. noch′ti* infests the stomach of an Indonesian monkey, causing tumors.

noci- [L. *nocēre* to injure] a combining form denoting relationship to injury or to a noxious or deleterious agent or influence.

no•ci•as•so•ci•a•tion (no″se-ə-so″se-a′shən) the unconscious discharge of nervous energy under the stimulus of trauma, as in surgical shock.

no•ci•cep•tin (no″sĭ-sep′tin) a 17–amino acid neuropeptide that binds to orphan opioid receptors but not to regular opioid receptors and has analgesic properties Called also *orphanin FQ*.

no•ci•cep•tion (no″sĭ-sep′shən) the ability to feel pain (q.v.), caused by stimulation of a nociceptor; called also *pain sense*, *algesia*, *algesthesia*, and *nociperception*.

no•ci•cep•tor (no″sĭ-sep′tər) [*noci-* + *-ceptor*] a receptor for pain caused by injury to body tissues; the injury may be from physical stimuli such as mechanical, thermal, or electrical stimuli, or from chemical stimuli such as the presence of a toxin or an excess of a nontoxic substance. Most nociceptors are in either the skin *(cutaneous n's)* or the walls of viscera *(visceral n's)*. **nocicep′tive** *adj*

C-fiber n. polymodal n.

cutaneous n's nociceptors in the skin, responding to stimuli such as heat, chemicals, and mechanical displacement; the two most common kinds are *polymodal nociceptors* and *mechanical nociceptors*.

mechanical n. a nociceptor of myelinated nerve fibers, activated primarily by strong mechanical displacement of the skin; called also *high-threshold mechanoreceptor*.

polymodal n. a nociceptor of unmyelinated nerve fibers, activated by several different types of stimuli such as heat, mechanical pressure, or chemical mediators of inflammation as a result of tissue injury. Called also *C-fiber n.*

no•ci•fen•sor (no″sĭ-fen′sər) [*noci-* + L. *fendere* to defend] protecting against injury; said of a system of nerves in the skin and mucous membranes which are concerned with local defense against injury.

no•ci•in•flu•ence (no″se-in′floo-əns) injurious or traumatic influence.

no•ci•per•cep•tion (no″sĭ-pər-sep′shən) nociception.

Noct. [L.] noc′te (at night).

noc•tal•bu•min•uria (nok″tal-bu″mĭ-nu′re-ə) [L. *nox* night + *albuminuria*] albuminuria in urine secreted at night.

noc•tam•bu•la•tion (nok″tam-bu-la′shən) somnambulism.

noc•ti•pho•bia (nok″tĭ-fo′be-ə) [L. *nox* night + *-phobia*] irrational fear of night and darkness.

Noct. maneq. [L.] noc′te mane′que (at night and in the morning).

noc•tu•ria (nok-tu′re-ə) [L. *nox* night + *-uria*] urinary frequency at night; called also *nycturia*.

noc•tur•nal (nok-tur′nəl) [L. *nocturnus*] pertaining to, occurring at, or active at night.

node (nōd) [L. *nodus* knot] 1. a small mass of tissue in the form of a swelling, knot, or protuberance, either normal or pathological. 2. in fungi, a swelling on a stolon where the rhizomes arise. See illustration at *mold*. **no′dal** *adj*

Node

For descriptions of specific anatomic structures not found here, see under *nodus*.

abdominal lymph n's nodi lymphoidei abdominis.
accessory lymph n's nodi lymphoidei accessorii.
anorectal lymph n's nodi lymphoidei pararectales.
anterior axillary lymph n's nodi lymphoidei axillares pectorales.
anterior cervical lymph n's nodi lymphoidei cervicales anteriores.
anterior jugular lymph n's nodi lymphoidei cervicales anteriores superficiales.
anterior mediastinal lymph n's lymph nodes along the great vessels of the superior mediastinum and on the anterior part of the diaphragm, receiving lymph from adjacent structures.
anterior tibial lymph n. nodus lymphoideus tibialis anterior.
apical axillary lymph n's nodi lymphoidei axillares apicales.
appendicular lymph n's nodi lymphoidei appendiculares.
Aschoff n., n. of Aschoff and Tawara nodus atrioventricularis.
atrioventricular n., AV n. (AVN) nodus atrioventricularis.
axillary lymph n's nodi lymphoidei axillares.
Babès n's see under *nodule*.
Bouchard n's cartilaginous and bony enlargements of the proximal interphalangeal joints of the fingers in degenerative joint disease. Such nodules in the distal interphalangeal joints are called *Heberden n's*.
brachial lymph n's nodi lymphoidei brachiales.
brachiocephalic lymph n's nodi lymphoidei brachiocephalici.
bronchopulmonary lymph n's nodi lymphoidei bronchopulmonales.
buccal lymph n., buccinator lymph n. nodus lymphoideus buccinatorius.
celiac lymph n's nodi lymphoidei coeliaci.
central axillary lymph n's nodi lymphoidei axillares centrales.

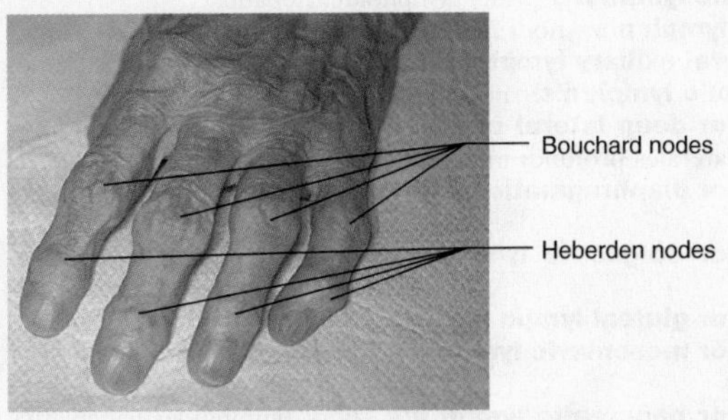

■ Bouchard and Heberden nodes in a patient with osteoarthritis.

Node *Continued*

central superior mesenteric lymph n's nodi lymphoidei mesenterici superiores centrales.
Cloquet n. nodus lymphoideus ingunalis profundus proximalis.
colic lymph n's nodi lymphoidei colici dextri/medii/sinistri.
common iliac lymph n's nodi lymphoidei iliaci communes.
cubital lymph n's nodi lymphoidei cubitales.
cystic lymph n. nodus lymphoideus cysticus.
deep anterior cervical lymph n's nodi lymphoidei cervicales anteriores profundi.
deep inguinal lymph n's nodi lymphoidei inguinales profundi.
deep lateral cervical lymph n's a chain of lymph nodes situated in the posterior cervical triangle; the chain is subdivided into smaller chains of lymph nodes, including a superior group (lateral, anterior, and jugulodigastric nodes) and an inferior group (lateral, anterior, and jugulo-omohyoid nodes).
deep lymph n's of upper limb nodi lymphoidei profundi membri superioris.
deep parotid lymph n's nodi lymphoidei parotidei profundi.
deep popliteal lymph n's nodi lymphoidei poplitei profundi.
delphian n. a lymph node encased in the fascia in the midline, just anterior to the thyroid isthmus, so called because it is exposed first at surgery and, if diseased, is indicative of disease in the thyroid gland, but not of a specific disease process.
deltopectoral lymph n's nodi lymphoidei deltopectorales.
distal deep inguinal lymph n. nodus lymphoideus inguinalis profundus distalis.
epicolic lymph n's minute lymph nodes situated on the wall of the colon and sometimes in the epiploic appendices.
epitrochlear lymph n's nodi lymphoidei cubitales.
external iliac lymph n's nodi lymphoidei iliaci externi.
facial lymph n's nodi lymphoidei faciales.
fibular lymph n. nodus lymphoideus fibularis.
Flack n. nodus sinuatrialis.
foraminal lymph n. nodus lymphoideus foraminalis.
gastric lymph n's nodi lymphoidei gastrici dextri/sinistri.
gastroepiploic lymph n's, gastro-omental lymph n's nodi lymphoidei gastroomentales dextri/sinistri.
gluteal lymph n's nodi lymphoidei gluteales.
gouty n. a nodule produced by gouty inflammation.
Heberden n's small hard nodules, formed usually at the distal interphalangeal joints of the fingers, produced by calcific spurs of the articular cartilage and associated with interphalangeal osteoarthritis. Heredity is an important etiologic factor. Such nodules in the proximal interphalangeal nodes are called *Bouchard nodes.* Called also *Heberden sign.*
hemal n's nodes found in certain mammals, especially ruminants, having a rich content of erythrocytes within sinuses and an organization much like a lymph node but with no lymphatic supply. They are located near the spleen, the kidney, and large blood vessels along the ventral side of the vertebrae, and their functions are probably like those of the spleen. A special type *(hemolymph nodes)* are found in the pig. The presence of hemal nodes in humans is doubtful. Called also *hemal glands, hemolymph n's,* and *vascular glands.*
hemolymph n's 1. hemal n's. 2. special types of hemal nodes found in the pig, having characteristics midway between those of ordinary lymph nodes and typical hemal nodes, containing both blood and lymphatic vessels, the contents of both of which mix in the sinuses; called also *hemolymph glands.*
Hensen n. primitive n.
hepatic lymph n's nodi lymphoidei hepatici.
hilar lymph n's nodi lymphoidei bronchopulmonales.
humeral axillary lymph n's nodi lymphoidei axillares humerales.
ileocolic lymph n's nodi lymphoidei ileocolici.
inferior deep lateral cervical lymph n's nodi lymphoidei cervicales laterales profundi inferiores.
inferior diaphragmatic lymph n's nodi lymphoidei phrenici inferiores.
inferior epigastric lymph n's nodi lymphoidei epigastrici inferiores.
inferior gluteal lymph n's nodi lymphoidei gluteales inferiores.
inferior mesenteric lymph n's nodi lymphoidei mesenterici inferiores.
inferior pancreatic lymph n's nodi lymphoidei pancreatici inferiores.
inferior pancreaticoduodenal lymph n's nodi lymphoidei pancreaticoduodenales inferiores.
inferior phrenic lymph n's nodi lymphoidei phrenici inferiores.
inferior superficial inguinal lymph n's nodi lymphoidei inguinales superficiales inferiores.
inferior tracheobronchial lymph n's nodi lymphoidei tracheobronchiales inferiores.
infra-auricular lymph n's nodi lymphoidei infraauriculares.
infraclavicular lymph n's nodi lymphoidei deltopectorales.
infrahyoid lymph n's nodi lymphoidei infrahyoidei.
inguinal lymph n's nodi lymphoidei inguinales.
intercostal lymph n's nodi lymphoidei intercostales.
interiliac lymph n's nodi lymphoidei interiliaci.
intermediate common iliac lymph n's nodi lymphoidei iliaci communes intermedii.
intermediate deep inguinal lymph n. nodus lymphoideus inguinalis profundus intermedius.
intermediate external iliac lymph n's nodi lymphoidei iliaci externi intermedii.
intermediate lacunar lymph n. nodus lymphoideus lacunaris intermedius.
intermediate lumbar lymph n's nodi lymphoidei lumbales intermedii.
internal iliac lymph n's nodi lymphoidei iliaci interni.
interpectoral lymph n's nodi lymphoidei interpectorales.
intraglandular parotid lymph n's nodi lymphoidei intraglandulares.
intrapulmonary lymph n's nodi lymphoidei intrapulmonales.
jugulodigastric lymph n. nodus lymphoideus jugulodigastricus.
jugulo-omohyoid lymph n. nodus lymphoideus juguloomohyoideus.
juxtaintestinal mesenteric lymph n's nodi lymphoidei juxtaintestinales.
Keith n., Keith-Flack n. nodus sinuatrialis.
lateral aortic lymph n's nodi lymphoidei aortici laterales.
lateral axillary lymph n's nodi lymphoidei axillares humerales.
lateral caval lymph n's nodi lymphoidei cavales laterales.
lateral cervical lymph n's nodi lymphoidei cervicales laterales.
lateral common iliac lymph n's nodi lymphoidei iliaci communes laterales.
lateral external iliac lymph n's nodi lymphoidei iliaci externi laterales.
lateral jugular lymph n's a group of deep lateral cervical lymph nodes found next to the internal jugular vein, emptying into the jugular trunk.
lateral lacunar lymph n. nodus lymphoideus lacunaris lateralis.
lateral pericardial lymph n's nodi lymphoidei pericardiaci laterales.
lateral vesical lymph n's nodi lymphoidei vesicales laterales.
left colic lymph n's see *nodi lymphoidei colici dextri/medii/sinistri.*
left gastric lymph n's see *nodi lymphoidei gastrici dextri/sinistri.*
left gastro-omental lymph n's see *nodi lymphoidei gastroomentales dextri/sinistri.*
left lumbar lymph n's nodi lymphoidei lumbales sinistri.
lumbar lymph n's numerous large lymph nodes extending from the aortic bifurcation to the aortic hiatus of the diaphragm, as three parallel chains: left, intermediate, and right.
lymph n. nodus lymphoideus.
lymph n. of anterior border of omental foramen nodus lymphoideus foraminalis.
lymph n. of arch of azygos vein nodus lymphoideus arcus venae azygos.
lymph n. of ligamentum arteriosum nodus lymphoideus ligamenti arteriosi.
lymph n's of lower limb nodi lymphoidei membri inferioris.
lymph n. of omental foramen nodus lymphoideus foraminalis.
lymph n's of upper limb nodi lymphoidei membri superioris.
malar lymph n. nodus lymphoideus malaris.
mandibular lymph n. nodus lymphoideus mandibularis.
mastoid lymph n's nodi lymphoidei mastoidei.
medial common iliac lymph n's nodi lymphoidei iliaci communes mediales.
medial external iliac lymph n's nodi lymphoidei iliaci externi mediales.

medial lacunar lymph n. nodus lymphoideus lacunaris medialis.
mesenteric lymph n's nodes that lie at the root of the mesentery, receiving lymph from parts of the small intestine, cecum, appendix, and large intestine; they are subdivided into superior and inferior groups.
mesocolic lymph n's nodi lymphoidei mesocolici.
middle colic lymph n's see *nodi lymphoidei colici dextri/medii/sinistri.*
milker's n's 1. milker's nodules (def. 1). 2. paravaccinia (def. 1).
nasolabial lymph n. nodus lymphoideus nasolabialis.
obturator lymph n's nodi lymphoidei obturatorii.
occipital lymph n's nodi lymphoidei occipitales.
Osler n's small, raised, swollen tender areas, about the size of a pea, usually bluish but sometimes pink or red or having a blanched center, seen most commonly in the pads of the fingers or toes, the thenar or hypothenar eminences, or the soles of the feet; these are practically pathognomonic of subacute bacterial endocarditis.
pancreatic lymph n's nodi lymphoidei pancreatici.
pancreaticoduodenal lymph n's nodi lymphoidei pancreaticoduodenales.
paracardial lymph n's a group of small lymph nodes that often form a chain or ring (anulus lymphaticus cardiae) around the cardiac opening of the stomach.
paracolic lymph n's nodi lymphoidei paracolici.
paramammary lymph n's nodi lymphoidei paramammarii.
pararectal lymph n's nodi lymphoidei pararectales.
parasternal lymph n's nodi lymphoidei parasternales.
paratracheal lymph n's nodi lymphoidei paratracheales.
parauterine lymph n's nodi lymphoidei parauterini.
paravaginal lymph n's nodi lymphoidei paravaginales.
paravesical lymph n's nodi lymphoidei paravesicales.
parietal abdominal lymph n's nodi lymphoidei abdominis parietales.
parietal lymph n's nodi lymphoidei parietales.
parietal pelvic lymph n's nodi lymphoidei pelvis parietales.
Parrot n's Parrot sign (def. 2).
pectoral axillary lymph n's nodi lymphoidei axillares pectorales.
pelvic lymph n's nodi lymphoidei pelvis.
peroneal lymph n. nodus lymphoideus fibularis.
popliteal lymph n's nodi lymphoidei poplitei.
postaortic lymph n's nodi lymphoidei retroaortici.
postcaval lymph n's nodi lymphoidei retrocavales.
posterior axillary lymph n's nodi lymphoidei axillares subscapulares.
posterior mediastinal lymph n's a group of lymph nodes situated behind the pericardium in relation to the esophagus and thoracic aorta, which receive lymph from the esophagus, pericardium, diaphragm, and lungs and pass efferent vessels mainly to the thoracic duct and sometimes to the tracheobronchial lymph nodes.
posterior tibial lymph n. nodus lymphoideus tibialis posterior.
postvesical lymph n's nodi lymphoidei retrovesicales.
preaortic lymph n's nodi lymphoidei preaortici.
preauricular lymph n's nodi lymphoidei preauriculares.
precaval lymph n's nodi lymphoidei precavales.
prececal lymph n's nodi lymphoidei precaecales.
prelaryngeal cervical lymph n's nodi lymphoidei prelaryngei.
prepericardial lymph n's nodi lymphoidei prepericardiaci.
pretracheal lymph n's nodi lymphoidei pretracheales.
prevertebral lymph n's nodi lymphoidei prevertebrales.
prevesical lymph n's nodi lymphoidei prevesicales.
primitive n. a mass of cells at the cranial end of the primitive streak, related to the organization of an embryo. Called also *primitive knot.*
promontorial lymph n's nodi lymphoidei promontorii.
proximal deep inguinal lymph n. nodus lymphoideus ingunalis profundus proximalis.
pulmonary juxtaesophageal lymph n's nodi lymphoidei juxtaoesophageales pulmonales.
pulmonary lymph n's nodi lymphoidei intrapulmonales.
pyloric lymph n's nodi lymphoidei pylorici.
n's of Ranvier constrictions occurring on myelinated nerve fibers at regular intervals of about 1 mm; at these sites the myelin sheath is absent and the axon is enclosed only by Schwann cell processes. See illustration and Plate 39.
retroaortic lymph n's nodi lymphoidei retroaortici.
retroauricular lymph n's nodi lymphoidei mastoidei.
retrocaval lymph n's nodi lymphoidei retrocavales.

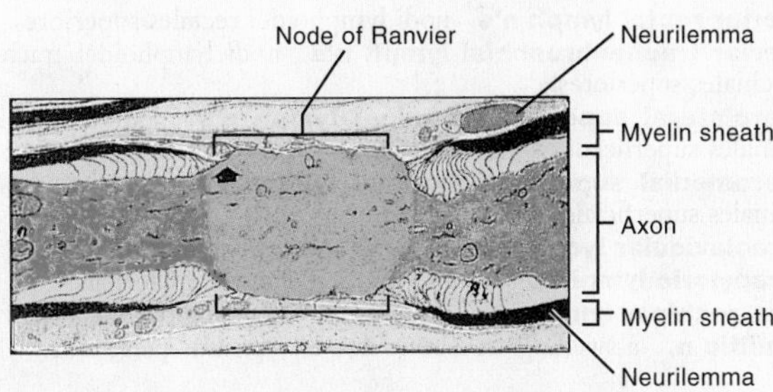

■ Node of Ranvier (transmission electron micrograph).

retrocecal lymph n's nodi lymphoidei retrocaecales.
retropharyngeal lymph n's nodi lymphoidei retropharyngeales.
retropyloric n's nodi lymphoidei retropylorici.
retrovesical lymph n's nodi lymphoidei retrovesicales.
right colic lymph n's see *nodi lymphoidei colici dextri/medii/sinistri.*
right gastric lymph n's see *nodi lymphoidei gastrici dextri/sinistri.*
right gastro-omental lymph n's see *nodi lymphoidei gastroomentales dextri/sinistri.*
right lumbar lymph n's nodi lymphoidei lumbales dextri.
Rosenmüller n. nodus lymphoideus inguinalis profundus proximalis.
Rotter n's nodi lymphoidei interpectorales.
n. of Rouvière the most superior of the lateral group of the retropharyngeal lymph nodes, located at the base of the skull.
SA n. nodus sinuatrialis.
sacral lymph n's nodi lymphoidei sacrales.
Schmorl n. an irregular or hemispherical bone defect in the upper or lower margin of the body of the vertebra.
sentinel n. 1. the first lymph node to receive drainage from a tumor, used to determine whether there is regional lymph node metastasis in certain types of cancer; lack of metastasis to the sentinel node indicates a very low risk of metastasis to more distal nodes. 2. signal n.
sigmoid lymph n's nodi lymphoidei sigmoidei.
signal n. an enlarged supraclavicular lymph node that is often the first sign of an abdominal tumor; called also *sentinel n., Troisier n.,* and *Virchow n.*
singer's n's vocal cord nodules.
sinoatrial n., sinuatrial n., sinus n. nodus sinuatrialis.
splenic lymph n's nodi lymphoidei splenici.
subaortic lymph n's nodi lymphoidei subaortici.
submandibular lymph n's nodi lymphoidei submandibulares.
submental lymph n's nodi lymphoidei submentales.
subpyloric n's nodi lymphoidei subpylorici.
subscapular axillary lymph n's nodi lymphoidei axillares subscapulares.
superficial anterior cervical lymph n's nodi lymphoidei cervicales anteriores superficiales.
superficial inguinal lymph n's nodi lymphoidei inguinales superficiales.
superficial lateral cervical lymph n's nodi lymphoidei cervicales laterales superficiales.
superficial lymph n's of upper limb nodi lymphoidei superficiales membri superioris.
superficial parotid lymph n's nodi lymphoidei parotidei superficiales.
superficial popliteal lymph n's nodi lymphoidei poplitei superficiales.
superior deep lateral cervical lymph n's nodi lymphoidei cervicales laterales profundi superiores.
superior diaphragmatic lymph n's nodi lymphoidei phrenici superiores.
superior gluteal lymph n's nodi lymphoidei gluteales superiores.
superior mesenteric lymph n's nodi lymphoidei mesenterici superiores.
superior pancreatic lymph n's nodi lymphoidei pancreatici superiores.
superior pancreaticoduodenal lymph n's nodi lymphoidei pancreaticoduodenales superiores.
superior phrenic lymph n's nodi lymphoidei phrenici superiores.

Node *Continued*

superior rectal lymph n's nodi lymphoidei rectales superiores.
superior tracheobronchial lymph n's nodi lymphoidei tracheobronchiales superiores.
superolateral superficial inguinal lymph n's nodi lymphoidei inguinales superficiales superolaterales.
superomedial superficial inguinal lymph n's nodi lymphoidei inguinales superficiales superomediales.
supraclavicular lymph n's nodi lymphoidei supraclaviculares.
suprapyloric lymph n. nodus lymphoideus suprapyloricus.
supratrochlear lymph n's nodi lymphoidei supratrochleares.
syphilitic n. a swelling on a bone due to syphilitic periostitis.
n. of Tawara nodus atrioventricularis.
teacher's n's vocal cord nodules.
thoracic lymph n's nodi lymphoidei thoracis.
thyroid lymph n's nodi lymphoidei thyroidei.
tracheal lymph n's nodi lymphoidei paratracheales.
tracheobronchial lymph n's nodi lymphoidei tracheobronchiales.
Troisier n., Virchow n. signal n.
visceral abdominal lymph n's nodi lymphoidei abdominis viscerales.
visceral lymph n's nodi lymphoidei viscerales.
visceral pelvic lymph n's nodi lymphoidei pelvis viscerales.

no•di (no′di) [L.] genitive and plural of *nodus.*

no•dose (no′dōs) [L. *nodosus*] having nodes or projections.

no•dos•i•ty (no-dos′ĭ-te) [L. *nodositas*] 1. the quality or condition of having nodes or nodules. 2. node.

no•do•ven•tric•u•lar (no″do-ven-trik′u-lər) connecting the atrioventricular node to the ventricle.

nod•u•lar (nod′u-lər) 1. like a nodule or node. 2. marked with nodules.

Nod•u•la•ria (nod″u-la′re-ə) a genus of cyanobacteria; certain species, such as *N. spumi′gena*, sometimes contaminate water and can cause cyanobacteria poisoning.

nod•u•lat•ed (nod′u-lāt″əd) nodular.

nod•u•la•tion (nod″u-la′shən) the presence of nodules.

nod•ule (nod′ūl) [L. *nodulus* little knot] 1. a small boss or node that is solid and can be detected by touch. 2. on a radiograph of the lung, a discrete opacity less than 30 mm in diameter. 3. nodulus.

accessory thymic n's lobuli thymici accessorii.

aggregated lymphoid n's of small intestine noduli lymphoidei aggregati intestini tenuis.

aggregated lymphoid n's of vermiform appendix noduli lymphoidei aggregati appendicis vermiformis.

Albini n's gray nodules of the size of small grains, sometimes seen on the free edges of the atrioventricular valves of infants; they are remains of fetal structures.

apple jelly n's minute translucent nodules of a distinctive yellow to reddish brown color, visible on diascopic examination of the lesions of lupus vulgaris.

n's of Arantius noduli valvularum semilunarium valvae aortae.

Aschoff n's Aschoff bodies.

Babès n's collections of microglial cells around neurons in the central nervous system, seen in rabies and other types of viral encephalitis; called also *Babès nodes* or *tubercles.*

Bohn n's inclusion cysts found in the mouths of newborns along the buccal and lingual aspects of the dental ridges and on the palate away from the raphe; they are considered to be remnants of mucous-gland tissue trapped during fetal development. Called also *Bohn pearls.*

Brenner n's nodular masses of tumor in the cyst wall in cases of Brenner tumor.

Busacca n's an accumulation of epithelioid cells and lymphocytes occurring in chronic inflammation of the iris, usually on its anterior surface around the region of the ciliary zone.

n. of cerebellum nodulus vermis.

cirrhotic n. a regenerative nodule surrounded by fibrous septa.

coal n. a palpable lesion of the lung seen in coal workers' pneumoconiosis, containing coal dust, dust-filled macrophages, and collagen fibers; it is larger than and develops from a coal macule.

cold n. a thyroid nodule that is less detectable than surrounding tissues on a radionuclide scan because of low uptake of the tracer; up to one in four may be malignant.

cortical n's nodules of closely packed lymphocytes in the cortical portion of a lymph gland.

Dalen-Fuchs n's small hemispherical mounds principally composed of epithelioid cells and cells of the retinal epithelium, seen in sympathetic ophthalmia and certain other disorders.

dysplastic n. a cluster, at least 1 mm in diameter, of dysplastic hepatocytes, occurring as a precancerous lesion of the liver; called also *adenomatous hyperplasia.*

Gamna n's, Gandy-Gamna n's brown or yellow pigmented nodules seen in the spleen in certain cases of enlargement, such as Banti disease and siderotic splenomegaly.

Hoboken n's dilatations of the outer surface of the umbilical arteries.

hot n. a thyroid nodule that is more detectable than surrounding tissues on a radionuclide scan because of high uptake of the tracer; most are nonmalignant causes of hyperthyroidism, but a small number may be malignant.

Jeanselme n's, juxtaarticular n's gummata of tertiary syphilis and of nonvenereal treponemal diseases, located on joint capsules, bursae, or tendon sheaths.

Kimmelstiel-Wilson n. see under *lesion.*

Koeppe n's white to gray nodules observed at the pupillary border in chronic inflammation of the iris, and consisting of accumulations of epithelioid cells and lymphocytes.

large regenerative n. macroregenerative nodule (def. 2).

Lisch n's hamartomas of the iris, occurring in neurofibromatosis.

Lutz-Jeanselme n's Jeanselme n's.

lymphatic n., lymphoid n. a small, dense accumulation of lymphocytes expressing tissue cytogenetic and defense functions; it may be encapsulated within lymph node cortex or may be dispersed in epithelial tissue, as in the intestine and tonsils.

lymphoid n's of lingual tonsil noduli lymphoidei tonsillae lingualis.

lymphoid n's of pharyngeal tonsil noduli lymphoidei tonsillae pharyngealis.

macroregenerative n. 1. dysplastic n. 2. a multiacinar regenerative nodule that is over 5 mm in diameter; called also *large regenerative n.*

microglial n's nodules seen in the central nervous system in a variety of infectious diseases.

milker's n's 1. paravaccinia in humans, contracted during milking of infected cows; it consists of purple nodules on the fingers and adjacent areas, which later break down, crust, and heal without scarring. Called also *milker's nodes.* 2. paravaccinia (def. 1).

monoacinar regenerative n. a benign type of regenerative nodule that has a single portal tract.

multiacinar regenerative n. a benign type of regenerative nodule that has multiple portal tracts; when over 5 mm in diameter it is called a *large regenerative* or *macroregenerative n.*

Nageotte n. a cluster of satellite cells in a ganglion, resulting from satellite cell proliferation following the degeneration of a ganglion cell body in neuropathy.

pearly n. one of the nodules of bovine tuberculosis.

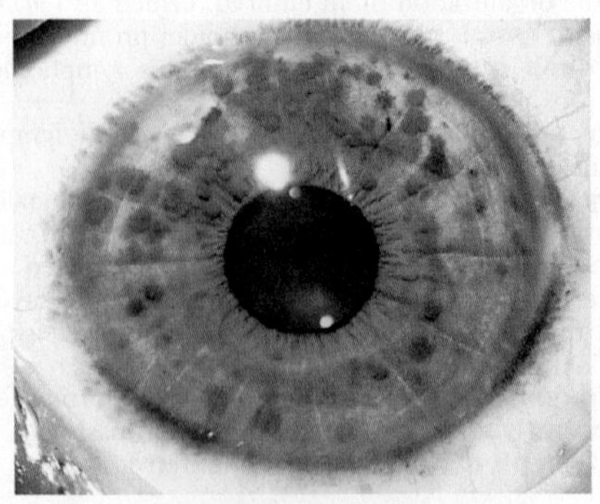

■ Lisch nodules.

primary lymphoid n. a lymphoid nodule that has not been exposed to antigen and lacks a germinal center; upon activation of B lymphocytes it develops into a secondary lymphoid nodule.

pulp n. denticle (def. 2).

regenerative n. a region of localized proliferation of hepatocytes and associated stroma arising in response to liver injury. There are several different types; some are premalignant and some are not. See also *nodular hyperplasia of the liver*, under *hyperplasia*.

rheumatic n's small, round or oval, mostly subcutaneous nodules resembling Aschoff bodies, seen in cases of rheumatic fever.

rheumatoid n's subcutaneous nodules consisting of central foci of necrosis surrounded by palisade-like coronas of fibroblasts, often seen in patients with rheumatoid arthritis.

Schmorl n. a nodule seen in radiographs of the spine, due to prolapse of a nucleus pulposus into an adjoining vertebra.

secondary lymphoid n. a lymphoid nodule that has been exposed to antigen and contains a germinal center with actively proliferating B lymphocytes, developing from a primary lymphoid nodule.

n's of semilunar cusps of aortic valve noduli valvularum semilunarium valvae aortae.

n's of semilunar cusps of pulmonary valves noduli valvularum semilunarium valvae trunci pulmonalis.

siderotic n's focal fibrotic lesions with crystals of iron on the degenerated elastic tissue fibers, seen in the spleen in Banti disease.

singer's n's vocal cord n's.

Sister Mary Joseph n. a nodule deep in the subcutis in the umbilical area associated with metastasizing intra-abdominal cancer, usually of gastric, ovarian, colorectal, or pancreatic origin.

solitary n's, solitary lymphoid n's noduli lymphoidei solitarii.

splenic lymphoid n's noduli lymphoidei splenici.

surfers' n's hyperplastic, fibrosing, sometimes ulcerated granulomas 1 to 3 cm in diameter, occurring over bony prominences of the feet and legs of surfers as a result of repeated trauma from kneeling on surfboards. Called also *surfers' knobs*.

teacher's n's vocal cord n's.

thyroid n's pathological nodules in the thyroid gland, often filled with colloid; some are indicative of adenoma or carcinoma. See *cold n.*, *hot n.*, and *warm n.*

triticeous n. cartilago triticea.

typhoid n. a mass of macrophages and other necrotic cells observed in the liver in typhoid fever.

typhus n's minute nodules, originally described in typhus, produced by perivascular infiltration of polymorphonuclear leukocytes and mononuclear cells in rickettsial disease.

n. of vermis nodulus vermis.

vocal n's, vocal cord n's, vocal fold n's small white nodules appearing on the vocal cords in chorditis tuberosa. Called also *singer's n's* or *nodes* and *teacher's n's* or *nodes*.

warm n. a nodule in the thyroid gland that can concentrate radioiodine; usually not carcinomatous.

weathering n's asymptomatic white papules on the helices of the ears, usually seen in elderly light-skinned men who have spent considerable time outdoors.

Wohlbach n's typhus n's.

nod•u•li (no'du-li) [L.] genitive and plural of *nodulus*.

nod•u•lo•sis (nod″u-lo'sis) the development of nodules, usually on fingers, toes, or other parts of the extremities.

rheumatoid n. a rare syndrome of polyarthralgia with swelling, subchondral bone cysts, and subcutaneous rheumatoid nodules; it usually follows a benign course, although progression to rheumatoid arthritis has been seen.

nod•u•lous (nod'u-ləs) 1. nodular. 2. nodose.

nod•u•lus (nod'u-ləs) gen. and pl. *no'duli* [L., dim. of *nodus*] 1. nodule: a small knot or node; used in anatomical terminology to designate a comparatively minute collection of tissue. Cf. *granuloma*. 2. n. vermis.

n. lymphoi'deus lymphoid nodule.

no'duli lymphoi'dei aggrega'ti appen'dicis vermifor'mis [TA] aggregated lymphoid nodules of vermiform appendix: oval elevated areas of lymphoid tissue occupying the greater part of the submucosa of the vermiform appendix.

no'duli lymphoi'dei aggrega'ti intesti'ni te'nuis [TA] aggregated lymphoid nodules of small intestine: oval elevated areas of lymphoid tissue on the mucosa of the small intestine, composed of many lymphoid follicles closely packed together; called also *Peyer glands*, or *patches*.

no'duli lymphoi'dei liena'les TA alternative for *noduli lymphoidei splenici*.

no'duli lymphoi'dei solita'rii [TA] solitary lymphoid nodules: small concentrations of lymphoid tissue scattered throughout the mucosa and submucosa of the small and large intestines. Called also *solitary lymphatic* or *lymphoid follicles*.

no'duli lymphoi'dei sple'nici [TA] splenic lymphoid nodules: aggregations of B lymphocytes that occur at intervals along the periarteriolar lymphoid sheaths in the white pulp of the spleen. Called also *noduli lymphoidei lienales* [TA alternative], and *malpighian bodies* or *corpuscles*.

no'duli lymphoi'dei tonsil'lae lingua'lis [TA] lymphoid nodules of lingual tonsil: aggregations of lymphoid tissue embedded in the submucosa of the posterior part of the tongue; together they constitute the lingual tonsil. Called also *lingual follicles*.

no'duli lymphoi'dei tonsil'lae pharyngea'lis [TA] lymphoid nodules of pharyngeal tonsil: aggregations of lymphoid tissue that constitute the parenchyma of the pharyngeal tonsil.

no'duli valvula'rum semiluna'rium val'vae aor'tae [TA] nodules of semilunar cusps of aortic valve: small fibrous tubercles, one at the center of the free margin of each semilunar cusp of the valve.

no'duli valvula'rum semiluna'rium val'vae trun'ci pulmona'lis [TA] nodules of semilunar cusps of pulmonary valve: small fibrous tubercles, one at the center of the free margin of each semilunar cusp.

n. ver'mis [TA] nodule of vermis (X): the most anterior lobule of the inferior surface of the vermis, connected on each side to the inferior medullary velum, and forming the central part of the flocculonodular lobe; called also *nodule of cerebellum*.

no•dus (no'dəs) gen. and pl. *no'di* [L.] a node or knot; used in anatomical terminology to denote a small mass of tissue.

Nodus

Descriptions of anatomic structures are given on TA terms, and include anglicized names of specific nodes.

n. atrioventricula'ris [TA] atrioventricular node: a small area of specialized cardiac muscle cells and fibers that receives the cardiac impulses from the sinoatrial node and passes them on toward the ventricles, introducing a delay in impulse conduction. It is located in the right atrium between the tricuspid valve and the orifice of the coronary sinus, is composed of a meshwork of (Purkinje) fibers continuous with the atrial muscle fibers and the bundle of His, and is supplied by a branch of the right coronary artery. The node is sometimes subdivided on the basis of electrophysiology into atrionodal (AN), nodal (N), and nodal-His (NH) regions. See illustration at *nodus sinuatrialis*.

n. lympha'ticus TA alternative for *n. lymphoideus*.

n. lymphoi'deus [TA] lymph node: any of the accumulations of lymphoid tissue organized as definite lymphoid organs, varying from 1 to 25 mm in diameter, situated along the course of lymphatic vessels, and consisting of an outer cortical and an inner medullary part. The lymph nodes are the main source of lymphocytes of the peripheral blood and, as part of the reticuloendothelial system, serve as a defense mechanism by removing noxious agents, such as bacteria and toxins, and probably play a role in antibody production. See illustration and Plate 26. Called also *lymphonodus* and *n. lymphaticus* [TA alternatives].

no'di lymphoi'dei abdo'minis [TA] abdominal lymph nodes: the lymph nodes that drain the abdomen; subdivided into parietal (nodi lymphoidei abdominis parietales) and visceral lymph nodes nodi lymphoidei abdominis viscerales .

no'di lymphoi'dei abdo'minis parieta'les [TA] parietal abdominal lymph nodes: the lymph nodes that drain the abdominal walls, comprising the left, intermediate, and lumbar lymph nodes, inferior phrenic lymph nodes, and inferior epigastric lymph nodes.

no'di lymphoi'dei abdo'minis viscera'les [TA] visceral abdominal lymph nodes: the numerous lymph nodes that drain the abdominal viscera.

no′di lymphoi′dei acces′sorii [TA] accessory lymph nodes: a chain of lymph nodes of the inferior deep lateral cervical group that follow the spinal accessory nerve and receive lymph from the occipital, postauricular, and suprascapular nodes and from the scalp, neck, and shoulder.
no′di lymphoi′dei anorecta′les TA alternative for *nodi lymphoidei pararectales.*
no′di lymphoi′dei aor′tici latera′les [TA] lateral aortic lymph nodes: two chains (right and left) of the left lumbar group that are on the left side of the aorta and drain the suprarenal glands, kidneys, ureters, testes, ovaries, pelvic viscera (except the intestines), and posterior abdominal wall.
no′di lymphoi′dei appendicula′res [TA] appendicular lymph nodes: lymph nodes situated along the appendicular artery and in the mesoappendix that drain into the ileocolic lymph nodes.
n. lymphoi′deus ar′cus ve′nae a′zygos [TA] lymph node of arch of azygos vein: a lymph node sometimes present on the azygos vein at the point where it arches over the root of the lung.
no′di lymphoi′dei axilla′res [TA] axillary lymph nodes: the 20 to 30 lymph nodes of the axilla, which receive lymph from all the lymph vessels of the upper limb, most of those of the breast, and the cutaneous vessels from the trunk above the level of the umbilicus. They are divided into groups: apical, central, humeral (lateral), pectoral (anterior), and subscapular (posterior).
no′di lymphoi′dei axilla′res anterio′res TA alternative for *nodi lymphoidei axillares pectorales.*
no′di lymphoi′dei axilla′res apica′les [TA] apical axillary lymph nodes: six to twelve axillary lymph nodes partly posterior to the superior part of the pectoralis minor muscle and partly in the apex of the axilla, receiving afferent vessels that accompany the cephalic vein and draining all other axillary nodes; their efferent vessels unite to form the subclavian trunk.
no′di lymphoi′dei axilla′res centra′les [TA] central axillary lymph nodes: three or four axillary lymph nodes embedded in adipose tissue near the base of the axilla; they receive lymph from the lateral, pectoral, and subscapular nodes and drain into the apical nodes.
no′di lymphoi′dei axilla′res humera′les [TA] humeral axillary lymph nodes: a group of four to six axillary lymph nodes lying posteromedial to the axillary vein and receiving most of the lymphatic drainage from the upper limb. Called also *nodi lymphoidei axillares laterales* [TA alternative] and *lateral axillary lymph nodes.*
no′di lymphoi′dei axilla′res latera′les TA alternative for *nodi lymphoidei axillares humerales.*
no′di lymphoi′dei axilla′res pectora′les [TA] pectoral axillary lymph nodes: four or five axillary lymph nodes along the inferior border of the pectoralis minor muscle near the lateral thoracic artery; they receive lymph from the skin and muscles of the anterior and lateral thoracic walls and mammary gland and drain into the central and apical nodes. Called also *nodi lymphoidei axillares anteriores* [TA alternative] and *anterior axillary lymph nodes.*
no′di lymphoi′dei axilla′res posterio′res TA alternative for *nodi lymphoidei axillares subscapulares.*

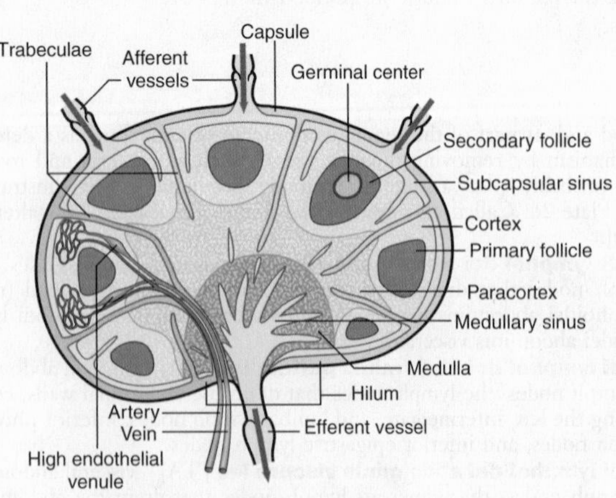

■ Nodus lymphoideus (lymph node).

no′di lymphoi′dei axilla′res subscapula′res [TA] subscapular axillary lymph nodes: six or seven axillary lymph nodes along the inferior margins of the posterior axillary wall along the course of the subscapular artery; they receive lymph from the skin and superficial muscles of the posterior part of the neck and the posterior thoracic wall and drain into the apical and central nodes. Called also *nodi lymphoidei axillares posteriores* [TA alternative] and *posterior axillary lymph nodes.*
no′di lymphoi′dei brachia′les [TA] brachial lymph nodes: isolated lymph nodes, varying in number and position, located along the brachial vessels between the humeral axillary and the supratrochlear lymph nodes.
no′di lymphoi′dei brachiocepha′lici [TA] brachiocephalic lymph nodes: thoracic lymph nodes located in the superior mediastinum, anterior to the brachiocephalic veins, receiving drainage from the thymus, thyroid gland, and pericardium and uniting with parasternal nodes to form the bronchomediastinal trunk.
no′di lymphoi′dei bronchopulmona′les [TA] bronchopulmonary lymph nodes: lymph nodes embedded in the root of the lung, mainly at the hilum that drain into the tracheobronchial lymph nodes; called also *hilar lymph nodes.*
n. lymphoi′deus buccinato′rius [TA] buccinator lymph node: one of a variable number of facial lymph nodes lying on a line between the angle of the mandible and the mouth, receiving the afferent vessels draining the temporal and infratemporal fossae and nasopharynx; their efferent vessels drain into the superior deep cervical nodes. Called also *buccal lymph node.*
no′di lymphoi′dei cava′les latera′les [TA] lateral caval lymph nodes: a group of lymph nodes of the right lumbar group that are on the right side of the inferior vena cava.
no′di lymphoi′dei cervica′les anterio′res [TA] anterior cervical lymph nodes: a group of lymph nodes ventral to the larynx and trachea, consisting of superficial vessels on the anterior jugular vein *(nodi lymphoidei cervicales anteriores superficiales)* and deep vessels *(nodi lymphoidei cervicales anteriores profundi)* on the middle cricothyroid ligament as well as ventral to the trachea. Called also *nodi lymphoidei colli anteriores* [TA alternative].
no′di lymphoi′dei cervica′les anterio′res profun′di [TA] deep anterior cervical lymph nodes: a group of numerous large lymph nodes that form a chain along the internal jugular vein, extending from the base of the skull to the root of the neck, situated near the pharynx, esophagus, and trachea; they receive lymph from both superficial and deep structures.
no′di lymphoi′dei cervica′les anterio′res superficia′les [TA] superficial anterior cervical lymph nodes: lymph nodes along the external jugular vein as it emerges from the parotid gland, being superficial to the sternocleidomastoid muscle; they receive afferent vessels from the auricle and parotid region. Called also *nodi lymphoidei jugulares anteriores* [TA alternative] and *anterior jugular lymph nodes.*
no′di lymphoi′dei cervica′les latera′les [TA] lateral cervical lymph nodes: the superficial and deep groups of lymph nodes of the lateral cervical region; the latter are generally subdivided into superior and inferior groups. Called also *nodi lymphoidei colli laterales* [TA alternative].
no′di lymphoi′dei cervica′les latera′les profun′di inferio′res [TA] inferior deep lateral cervical lymph nodes: a group of lymph nodes adjacent to the carotid sheath, partly deep to the sternocleidomastoid muscle and extending into the subclavian triangle. They receive lymph from the back of the scalp and neck, the tongue, the superficial pectoral region, and part of the arm and drain into the jugular trunk.
no′di lymphoi′dei cervica′les latera′les profun′di superio′res [TA] superior deep lateral cervical lymph nodes: a group of lymph nodes adjacent to the carotid sheath deep to the sternocleidomastoid muscle; they receive lymph from a number of structures of the head and neck and drain into the inferior deep cervical nodes or the jugular trunk.
no′di lymphoi′dei cervica′les latera′les superficia′les [TA] superficial lateral cervical lymph nodes: lymph nodes situated along the external jugular vein that send efferent vessels to the deep lateral cervical lymph nodes.
no′di lymphoi′dei coeli′aci [TA] celiac lymph nodes: a few nodes along the celiac trunk, which receive lymph from the stomach, spleen, duodenum, liver, and pancreas.
no′di lymphoi′dei co′lici dex′tri/me′dii/sinis′tri [TA] colic lymph nodes: a subgroup of the mesocolic lymph nodes, situated along the right, middle, and left colic arteries.

no′di lymphoi′dei col′li anterio′res TA alternative for *nodi lymphoidei cervicales anteriores.*
no′di lymphoi′dei col′li latera′les TA alternative for *nodi lymphoidei cervicales laterales.*
no′di lymphoi′dei cubita′les [TA] cubital lymph nodes: lymph nodes occurring in the elbow region, mainly comprising the supratrochlear lymph nodes (nodi lymphoidei supratrochleares) but also including scattered isolated nodes, as in the cubital fossa near the bifurcation of the brachial artery; called also *epitrochlear lymph nodes.*
n. lymphoi′deus cys′ticus [TA] cystic lymph node: a hepatic lymph node situated in the curve of the neck of the gallbladder at the junction of the cystic and common hepatic ducts.
no′di lymphoi′dei deltopectora′les [TA] deltopectoral lymph nodes: one or two lymph nodes in the groove between the pectoralis major and deltoid muscles, just inferior to the clavicle, which drain into the apical lymph nodes. Called also *nodi lymphoidei infraclaviculares* [TA alternative] and *infraclavicular nodes.*
no′di lymphoi′dei epigas′trici infe′riores [TA] inferior epigastric lymph nodes: lymph nodes along the deep epigastric vessels, receiving lymph from the lower abdominal wall.
no′di lymphoi′dei facia′les [TA] facial lymph nodes: lymph nodes situated along the course of the facial artery and vein, which receive afferent vessels draining the eyelids, conjunctiva, nose, cheeks, lips, and gums, and send efferent vessels to the submandibular nodes.
n. lymphoi′deus fibula′ris [TA] fibular lymph node: a lymph node situated along the peroneal artery; called also *peroneal lymph node.*
n. lymphoi′deus foramina′lis [TA] lymph node of anterior border of omental foramen: a hepatic lymph node situated along the upper part of the common bile duct; called also *lymph node of omental foramen.*
no′di lymphoi′dei gas′trici dex′tri/sinis′tri [TA] gastric lymph nodes: a few nodes along the right and left gastric arteries that receive lymph from the stomach, spleen, duodenum, liver, and pancreas.
no′di lymphoi′dei gastroomenta′les dex′tri/sinis′tri [TA] gastro-omental lymph nodes: lymph nodes situated in the greater omentum along the pyloric half of the greater curvature of the stomach in association with the right and left gastroepiploic arteries; called also *gastroepiploic lymph nodes.*
no′di lymphoi′dei glutea′les [TA] gluteal lymph nodes: internal iliac lymph nodes situated along the gluteal arteries; subdivided into superior and inferior groups.
no′di lymphoi′dei glutea′les inferio′res [TA] inferior gluteal lymph nodes: the internal iliac lymph nodes situated along the inferior gluteal artery.
no′di lymphoi′dei glutea′les superio′res [TA] superior gluteal lymph nodes: the internal iliac lymph nodes situated along the superior gluteal artery.
no′di lymphoi′dei hepa′tici [TA] hepatic lymph nodes: a variable number of lymph nodes situated along the proper and common hepatic arteries and the bile ducts that receive lymph from the stomach, spleen, duodenum, liver, and pancreas; two are fairly common: the cystic node and the foraminal node.
no′di lymphoi′dei ileoco′lici [TA] ileocolic lymph nodes: nodes in the region of the ileocolic junction, draining adjacent structures and draining into the superior mesenteric lymph node.
no′di lymphoi′dei ili′aci commu′nes [TA] common iliac lymph nodes: the four to six lymph nodes grouped at the sides and dorsal to the common iliac vessels, comprising five groups: medial, intermediate, lateral, subaortic, and promontory; they receive afferent vessels from the lateral and internal iliac lymph nodes and send efferent vessels to the lateral aortic lymph nodes.
no′di lymphoi′dei ili′aci commu′nes interme′dii [TA] intermediate common iliac lymph nodes: the common iliac lymph nodes situated between the common iliac vessels.
no′di lymphoi′dei ili′aci commu′nes latera′les [TA] lateral common iliac lymph nodes: the common iliac lymph nodes situated on the lateral aspect of the common iliac vessels.
no′di lymphoi′dei ili′aci commu′nes media′les [TA] medial common iliac lymph nodes: the common iliac lymph nodes situated on the medial aspect of the common iliac vessels.
no′di lymphoi′dei ili′aci exter′ni [TA] external iliac lymph nodes: the eight to ten nodes along the external iliac vessels, comprising five groups: medial, intermediate, lateral, interiliac, and obturator lymph nodes; they receive afferent vessels from the inguinal lymph nodes, deep part of the abdominal wall below the umbilicus, and some pelvic viscera and send efferent vessels to the common iliac lymph nodes.
no′di lymphoi′dei ili′aci exter′ni interme′dii [TA] intermediate external iliac lymph nodes: the external iliac lymph nodes situated between the external iliac vessels.
no′di lymphoi′dei ili′aci exter′ni latera′les [TA] lateral external iliac lymph nodes: the external iliac lymph nodes situated on the lateral aspect of the external iliac vessels.
no′di lymphoi′dei ili′aci exter′ni media′les [TA] medial external iliac lymph nodes: the external iliac lymph nodes situated on the medial aspect of the external iliac vessels.
no′di lymphoi′dei ili′aci inter′ni [TA] internal iliac lymph nodes: nodes grouped around the origins of the branches of the internal iliac vessels, comprising two groups: superior and inferior gluteal and sacral lymph nodes; they receive afferent vessels from the pelvic viscera, perineum, and buttocks and send efferent vessels to the common iliac lymph nodes.
no′di lymphoi′dei infraauricula′res [TA] infra-auricular lymph nodes: deep parotid lymph nodes situated below the ear.
no′di lymphoi′dei infraclavicula′res TA alternative for *nodi lymphoidei deltopectorales.*
no′di lymphoi′dei infrahyoi′dei [TA] infrahyoid lymph nodes: lymph nodes lying beneath the deep cervical fascia anterior to the thyrohyoid membrane that receive lymph from the anterior cervical nodes and epiglottic region and drain into the deep cervical nodes.
no′di lymphoi′dei inguina′les [TA] inguinal lymph nodes: lymph nodes situated along the course of the inguinal ligament; they are subdivided into superficial (nodi lymphoidei inguinales superficiales) and deep (nodi lymphoidei inguinales profundi) groups of nodes.
no′di lymphoi′dei inguina′les profun′di [TA] deep inguinal lymph nodes: one to three nodes deep to the fascia lata along the femoral vein; they receive lymph from the deep structures of the lower limb and from the penis or clitoris, and superficial inguinal lymph nodes and drain into the external iliac lymph nodes.
n. lymphoi′deus inguina′lis profun′dus dista′lis [TA] distal deep inguinal lymph node: the most inferior of the deep inguinal lymph nodes, located just distal to the junction of the great saphenous and femoral veins.
n. lymphoi′deus inguina′lis profun′dus interme′dius [TA] intermediate deep inguinal lymph node: the central and most inconstant of the deep inguinal lymph nodes, lying in the femoral canal.
n. lymphoi′deus inguina′lis profun′dus proxima′lis [TA] proximal deep inguinal lymph node: the most superior of the deep inguinal lymph nodes; it is inconstant and when present usually lies laterally in the femoral ring. Called also *Cloquet* or *Rosenmüller node.*
no′di lymphoi′dei inguina′les superficia′les [TA] superficial inguinal lymph nodes: lymph nodes situated in the subcutaneous tissue inferior to the inguinal ligament on either side of the proximal part of the greater saphenous vein, comprising two upper (supermedial and superolateral) groups and one lower (inferior) group; they drain the skin of the lower abdominal wall, penis, scrotum or labia majora, perineum, and buttocks.
no′di lymphoi′dei inguina′les superficia′les inferio′res [TA] inferior superficial inguinal lymph nodes: the lower superficial inguinal lymph nodes situated below the opening of the saphenous vein.
no′di lymphoi′dei inguina′les superficia′les superolatera′les [TA] superolateral superficial inguinal lymph nodes: the upper superficial inguinal nodes situated on the lateral side of the opening of the saphenous vein.
no′di lymphoi′dei inguina′les superficia′les superomedia′les [TA] superomedial superficial inguinal lymph nodes: the upper superficial inguinal lymph nodes situated on the medial side of the opening of the saphenous vein.
no′di lymphoi′dei intercosta′les [TA] intercostal lymph nodes: lymph nodes in the back of the thorax, along the intercostal vessels.
no′di lymphoi′dei interili′aci [TA] interiliac lymph nodes: the external iliac lymph nodes situated between the external and internal iliac vessels and the obturator artery.
no′di lymphoi′dei interpectora′les [TA] interpectoral lymph nodes: small inconstant lymph nodes that may occur between the pectoralis major and minor muscles, draining into the axillary nodes.
no′di lymphoi′dei intraglandula′res [TA] intraglandular parotid lymph nodes: deep parotid lymph nodes situated within the substance of the parotid gland.

Nodus *Continued*

no′di lymphoi′dei intrapulmona′les [TA] intrapulmonary lymph nodes: nodes located along the larger bronchi within the lung substance, through which lymph from the lung drains. Called also *pulmonary lymph nodes.*

no′di lymphoi′dei jugula′res anterio′res TA alternative for *nodi lymphoidei cervicales anteriores superficiales.*

n. lymphoi′deus jugulodigas′tricus [TA] jugulodigastric lymph node: one of the deep lateral cervical lymph nodes lying on the internal jugular vein at the level of the greater cornu of the hyoid bone, i.e., just below the posterior belly of the digastric muscle.

n. lymphoi′deus juguloomohyoi′deus [TA] jugulo-omohyoid lymph node: one of the inferior deep lateral cervical lymph nodes lying on the internal jugular vein just above the tendon of the omohyoid muscle.

no′di lymphoi′dei juxtaintestina′les [TA] juxtaintestinal mesenteric lymph nodes: the mesenteric lymph nodes situated close to the wall of the intestine between the branches of the jejunal and ileal arteries; they drain into the superior mesenteric lymph node.

no′di lymphoi′dei juxtaoesophagea′les [TA] juxtaesophageal lymph nodes: posterior mediastinal lymph nodes situated on both sides of the esophagus.

n. lymphoi′deus lacuna′ris interme′dius [TA] intermediate lacunar lymph node: a lymph node situated between the external iliac vessels at the lacuna vasorum.

n. lymphoi′deus lacuna′ris latera′lis [TA] lateral lacunar lymph node: a lymph node situated on the lateral aspect of the external iliac vessels at the lacuna vasorum.

n. lymphoi′deus lacuna′ris media′lis [TA] medial lacunar lymph node: a lymph node situated on the medial aspect of the external iliac vessels at the lacuna vasorum.

no′di lymphoi′dei liena′les TA alternative for *nodi lymphoidei splenici.*

n. lymphoi′deus ligamen′ti arterio′si [TA] lymph node of ligamentum arteriosum: the lowest anterior mediastinal lymph node situated anterior to the ligamentum arteriosum.

no′di lymphoi′dei lingua′les [TA] small lymph nodes situated on the hyoglossus, receiving afferent vessels from the tongue and draining into the superior deep cervical lymph nodes.

no′di lymphoi′dei lumba′les dex′tri [TA] right lumbar lymph nodes: the chain of lumbar lymph nodes situated partly in front of the vena cava and partly behind it on the psoas major muscle, comprising three groups: lateral caval, precaval, and retrocaval (postcaval) lymph nodes.

no′di lymphoi′dei lumba′les interme′dii [TA] intermediate lumbar lymph nodes: the chain of lumbar lymph nodes that lie in the median plane, between the left and right lumbar lymph nodes.

no′di lymphoi′dei lumba′les sinis′tri [TA] left lumbar lymph nodes: the chain of lumbar lymph nodes situated at the side of the abdominal aorta on the psoas major muscle, comprising three groups: right and left lateral aortic, preaortic, and retroaortic (postaortic) lymph nodes.

n. lymphoi′deus mala′ris [TA] malar lymph node: one of a variable number of facial lymph nodes situated in the region of the zygomatic minor muscle.

n. lymphoi′deus mandibula′ris [TA] mandibular lymph node: one of a variable number of facial lymph nodes situated near the angle of the mandible, into which lymph from some of the superficial tissues of the head and neck is drained.

no′di lymphoi′dei mastoi′dei [TA] mastoid lymph nodes: lymph nodes, two or three on each side, that are superficial to the mastoid attachment of the sternocleidomastoid muscle and deep to the posterior auricular muscle; they drain the nasal fossae and paranasal sinuses, hard and soft palate, middle ear, and nasopharynx and oropharynx. Called also *retroauricular lymph nodes.*

no′di lymphoi′dei mem′bri inferio′ris [TA] lymph nodes of lower limb: the groups of lymph nodes occurring in and draining the lower limb; most occur in the inguinal region, subdivided into superficial and deep groups, and in the popliteal fossa.

no′di lymphoi′dei mem′bri superio′ris [TA] lymph nodes of upper limb: the lymph nodes of the hand, forearm, arm, and axilla; the former three groups draining into those of the axilla. They are subdivided into superficial (nodi lymphoidei superficiales membri superioris) and deep nodes (nodi lymphoidei profundi membri superioris).

no′di lymphoi′dei mesente′rici inferio′res [TA] inferior mesenteric lymph nodes: nodes situated along the inferior mesenteric vessels and receiving lymph from the adjacent region; they comprise two groups: the sigmoid and superior rectal lymph nodes.

no′di lymphoi′dei mesente′rici superio′res [TA] superior mesenteric lymph nodes: mesenteric lymph nodes situated along the superior mesenteric artery and draining various other groups of nodes in the region.

no′di lymphoi′dei mesente′rici superio′res centra′les [TA] central superior mesenteric lymph nodes: the middle group of superior mesenteric nodes, situated along the ileal and jejunal branches of the superior mesenteric artery.

no′di lymphoi′dei mesocol′ici [TA] mesocolic lymph nodes: lymph nodes situated in the mesocolon, comprising two groups: paracolic and colic (right, middle, and left colic); they drain through the superior mesenteric lymph nodes.

n. lymphoi′deus nasolabia′lis [TA] nasolabial lymph node: one of a variable number of facial lymph nodes situated near the junction of the superior labial and facial arteries, which drains the upper lip and external nose into the submandibular node.

no′di lymphoi′dei obturato′rii [TA] obturator lymph nodes: the external iliac lymph nodes situated in the obturator canal.

no′di lymphoi′dei occipita′les [TA] occipital lymph nodes: several small nodes near the occipital insertion of the semispinalis capitis muscle.

no′di lymphoi′dei pancrea′tici [TA] pancreatic lymph nodes: nodes found along the pancreatic arteries that drain lymph from the pancreas to the pancreaticosplenic lymph nodes.

no′di lymphoi′dei pancrea′tici inferio′res [TA] inferior pancreatic lymph nodes: lymph nodes associated with the inferior pancreatic artery.

no′di lymphoi′dei pancrea′tici superio′res [TA] superior pancreatic lymph nodes: lymph nodes associated with the superior pancreatic artery.

no′di lymphoi′dei pancreaticoduodena′les [TA] pancreaticoduodenal lymph nodes: small lymph nodes located between the head of the pancreas and the duodenum, subdivided into superior and inferior groups.

no′di lymphoi′dei pancreaticoduodena′les inferio′res [TA] inferior pancreaticoduodenal lymph nodes: lymph nodes situated along the inferior pancreaticoduodenal artery.

no′di lymphoi′dei pancreaticoduodena′les superio′res [TA] superior pancreaticoduodenal lymph nodes: lymph nodes situated along the superior pancreaticoduodenal artery.

no′di lymphoi′dei paracol′ici [TA] paracolic lymph nodes: a subgroup of the mesocolic lymph nodes, situated along the medial borders of the ascending and descending colon and along the mesenteric borders of the transverse and sigmoid colon.

no′di lymphoi′dei paramamma′rii [TA] paramammary lymph nodes: lymph nodes on the lateral mammary gland that drain into the axillary lymph nodes.

no′di lymphoi′dei pararecta′les [TA] pararectal lymph nodes: lymph nodes situated around the rectum, embedded in its muscular coat; they drain into the inferior mesenteric, sacral, internal iliac, common iliac, and superficial inguinal nodes. Called also *nodi lymphoidei anorectales* [TA alternative] and *anorectal lymph nodes.*

no′di lymphoi′dei parasterna′les [TA] parasternal lymph nodes: nodes located along the course of the internal thoracic artery, which drain the mammary gland, abdominal wall, and diaphragm.

no′di lymphoi′dei paratrachea′les [TA] paratracheal lymph nodes: lymph nodes on either side of the esophagus and trachea, extending upward into the neck, which receive lymph from the esophagus, trachea, and tracheobronchial lymph nodes.

no′di lymphoi′dei parauteri′ni [TA] parauterine lymph nodes: lymph nodes situated around the uterus, consisting of superficial (beneath the peritoneum) and deep (in the substance of the uterine wall) nodes: they drain into the lumbar, external and internal iliac, sacral, and superficial inguinal lymph nodes.

no′di lymphoi′dei paravagina′les [TA] paravaginal lymph nodes: lymph nodes situated around the vagina; they drain into the external and internal iliac, common iliac, and superficial inguinal lymph nodes.

no′di lymphoi′dei paravesica′les [TA] paravesical lymph nodes: lymph nodes situated around the urinary bladder, comprising three groups: prevesical, postvesical, and lateral vesical lymph nodes; they drain into the external and internal iliac lymph nodes and, in association with some lymph nodes from the prostate, into the sacral and common iliac lymph nodes.

no′di lymphoi′dei parieta′les parietal lymph nodes: lymph nodes that receive lymph from the walls of a body cavity; see *nodi lymphoidei abdominis parietales* and *nodi lymphoidei pelvis parietales.* Cf. *nodi lymphoidei viscerales.*

no′di lymphoi′dei paroti′dei profun′di [TA] deep parotid lymph nodes: lymph nodes on the lateral wall of the pharynx lying deep to or embedded in the deep substance of the parotid gland, through which lymph drains from the external acoustic meatus, auditory tube, tympanum, soft palate, and posterior nasal cavity.

no′di lymphoi′dei paroti′dei superficia′les [TA] superficial parotid lymph nodes: lymph nodes lying in the subcutaneous tissue of the parotid gland directly in front of the tragus.

no′di lymphoi′dei pel′vis [TA] pelvic lymph nodes: the lymph nodes that drain the pelvis; subdivided into parietal (nodi lymphoidei pelvis parietales) and visceral lymph nodes nodi lymphoidei pelvis viscerales .

no′di lymphoi′dei pel′vis parieta′les [TA] parietal pelvic lymph nodes: the lymph nodes that drain the wall of the pelvis, including the common iliac, external iliac, and internal iliac lymph nodes.

no′di lymphoi′dei pel′vis viscera′les [TA] visceral pelvic lymph nodes: the lymph nodes that drain the pelvic viscera, including the paravesicular, parauterine, paravaginal, and pararectal lymph nodes.

no′di lymphoi′dei pericardi′aci latera′les [TA] lateral pericardial lymph nodes: lymph nodes accompanying the pericardiacophrenic artery.

no′di lymphoi′dei phre′nici inferio′res [TA] inferior diaphragmatic lymph nodes: parietal lymph nodes accompanying the inferior vessels of the diaphragm; called also *inferior phrenic lymph nodes.*

no′di lymphoi′dei phre′nici superio′res [TA] superior diaphragmatic lymph nodes: several nodes on the thoracic surface of the diaphragm, receiving lymph from the intercostal spaces, pericardium, diaphragm, and liver; called also *superior phrenic lymph nodes.*

no′di lymphoi′dei popli′tei [TA] popliteal lymph nodes: lymph nodes embedded in the fat of the popliteal fossa, comprising superficial and deep groups; their efferent vessels accompany the femoral vessels to the deep inguinal lymph nodes.

no′di lymphoi′dei popli′tei profun′di [TA] deep popliteal lymph nodes: the popliteal lymph nodes situated at the sides of the popliteal vessels.

no′di lymphoi′dei popli′tei superficia′les [TA] superficial popliteal lymph nodes: the popliteal lymph nodes situated at the termination of the small saphenous vein.

no′di lymphoi′dei postaor′tici TA alternative for *nodi lymphoidei retroaortici.*

no′di lymphoi′dei postcava′les TA alternative for *nodi lymphoidei retrocavales.*

no′di lymphoi′dei postvesica′les TA alternative for *nodi lymphoidei retrovesicales.*

no′di lymphoi′dei preaor′tici [TA] preaortic lymph nodes: a group of lymph nodes of the left lumbar group that is in front of the aorta and drains the abdominal part of the alimentary canal and its derivatives.

no′di lymphoi′dei preauricula′res [TA] preauricular lymph nodes: deep parotid lymph nodes situated in front of the ear.

no′di lymphoi′dei precaeca′les [TA] prececal lymph nodes: lymph nodes situated in front of the cecum that drain into the anterior ileocolic lymph nodes.

no′di lymphoi′dei precava′les [TA] precaval lymph nodes: a group of lymph nodes of the right lumbar group that is in front of the inferior vena cava.

no′di lymphoi′dei prelaryn′gei [TA] prelaryngeal lymph nodes: deep anterior cervical lymph nodes situated in front of the larynx that help drain the thyroid gland.

no′di lymphoi′dei prepericardi′aci [TA] prepericardial lymph nodes: lymph nodes situated between the pericardium and sternum.

no′di lymphoi′dei pretrachea′les [TA] pretracheal lymph nodes: deep anterior cervical lymph nodes situated in front of the trachea near the inferior thyroid veins.

no′di lymphoi′dei prevertebra′les [TA] prevertebral lymph nodes: lymph nodes situated in back of the thoracic aorta.

no′di lymphoi′dei prevesica′les [TA] prevesical lymph nodes: the paravesical lymph nodes situated in front of the urinary bladder.

no′di lymphoi′dei profun′di mem′bri superio′ris [TA] deep lymph nodes of upper limb: the lymph nodes situated internal to the deep fascia of the upper limb, most of which are grouped in the axilla; they accompany the radial, ulnar, interosseous, and brachial arteries and end in the brachial axillary lymph nodes.

no′di lymphoi′dei promonto′rii [TA] promontorial lymph nodes: the common iliac lymph nodes situated in front of the sacral promontory.

no′di lymphoi′dei pylo′rici [TA] pyloric lymph nodes: lymph nodes found anterior to the head of the pancreas, receiving lymph from the pyloric part of the stomach. They are subdivided into three groups: suprapyloric, subpyloric, and retropyloric nodes.

no′di lymphoi′dei recta′les superio′res [TA] superior rectal lymph nodes: a group of lymph nodes of the inferior mesenteric group, situated along the superior rectal artery.

no′di lymphoi′dei retroaor′tici [TA] retroaortic lymph nodes: a group of lymph nodes of the left lumbar group, situated behind the aorta and formed by peripheral nodes of the right and left lateral aortic lymph nodes. Called also *postaortic lymph nodes* and *nodi lymphoidei postaortici* [TA alternative].

no′di lymphoi′dei retrocaeca′les [TA] retrocecal lymph nodes: lymph nodes situated in back of the cecum that drain into the posterior ileocecal lymph nodes.

no′di lymphoi′dei retrocava′les [TA] retrocaval lymph nodes: a group of lymph nodes of the right lumbar group situated behind the inferior vena cava. Called also *postcaval lymph nodes* and *nodi lymphoidei postcavales* [TA alternative].

no′di lymphoi′dei retropharyngea′les [TA] retropharyngeal lymph nodes: deep cervical lymph nodes, one median and two lateral groups, situated behind the upper part of the pharynx, especially concerned with drainage of the nasal fossae, paranasal sinuses, hard and soft palates, middle ear, nasopharynx, and oropharynx.

no′di lymphoi′dei retropylo′rici [TA] retropyloric lymph nodes: pyloric lymph nodes situated posterior to the pylorus.

no′di lymphoi′dei retrovesica′les [TA] postvesical lymph nodes: the paravesical lymph nodes situated in back of the urinary bladder. Called also *nodi lymphoidei postvesicales* [TA alternative].

no′di lymphoi′dei sacra′les [TA] sacral lymph nodes: the internal iliac lymph nodes situated along the lateral and median sacral vessels; they receive lymph from the rectum and posterior pelvic wall.

no′di lymphoi′dei sigmoi′dei [TA] sigmoid lymph nodes: a group of lymph nodes of the inferior mesenteric group, situated along the sigmoid arteries.

no′di lymphoi′dei sple′nici [TA] splenic lymph nodes: lymph nodes in the capsule and larger trabeculae of the spleen that drain into adjacent lymph nodes; called also *nodi lymphoidei lienales* [TA alternative].

no′di lymphoi′dei subaor′tici [TA] subaortic lymph nodes: the common iliac lymph nodes situated below the bifurcation of the aorta.

no′di lymphoi′dei submandibula′res [TA] submandibular lymph nodes: the three to six nodes alongside the submandibular gland, through which lymph drains from the adjacent skin and mucous membrane.

no′di lymphoi′dei submenta′les [TA] submental lymph nodes: nodes under the chin into which the lymph from some of the superficial tissues of the head and neck is drained.

no′di lymphoi′dei subpylo′rici [TA] subpyloric lymph nodes: pyloric lymph nodes located inferior to the pylorus.

no′di lymphoi′dei superficia′les mem′bri superio′ris [TA] superficial lymph nodes of upper limb: the lymph nodes of the upper limb that are superficially placed, such as the cubital lymph nodes; all except those in the hand and on the back of the forearm converge toward and accompany the superficial veins.

no′di lymphoi′dei supraclavicula′res [TA] supraclavicular lymph nodes: the deep lateral cervical lymph nodes situated inferior to the omohyoid muscle, extending into the omoclavicular portion of the posterior triangle of the neck.

n. lymphoi′deus suprapylo′ricus [TA] suprapyloric lymph node: a pyloric lymph node located superior to the duodenum on the right gastric artery.

no′di lymphoi′dei supratrochlea′res [TA] supratrochlear lymph nodes: one or two lymph nodes superficial to the deep fascia proximal to the medial epicondyle and medial to the basilic vein and draining into the deep lymph vessels.

Nodus *Continued*

no′di lymphoi′dei tho′racis [TA] thoracic lymph nodes: the lymph nodes that drain the thoracic wall together with those draining the deeper thoracic tissues.
no′di lymphoi′dei thyroi′dei [TA] thyroid lymph nodes: deep anterior cervical lymph nodes situated around the thyroid gland.
n. lymphoi′deus tibia′lis ante′rior [TA] anterior tibial lymph node: a lymph node situated along the anterior tibial artery.
n. lymphoi′deus tibia′lis poste′rior [TA] posterior tibial lymph node: a lymph node situated along the posterior tibial artery.
no′di lymphoi′dei tracheobronchia′les [TA] tracheobronchial lymph nodes: thoracic lymph nodes located around the roots of lobar and main bronchi and along the sides of the trachea, draining the lungs; they are subdivided into superior and inferior groups.
no′di lymphoi′dei tracheobronchia′les inferio′res [TA] inferior tracheobronchial lymph nodes: nodes in the angle of the bifurcation of the trachea, receiving lymph from adjacent structures.
no′di lymphoi′dei tracheobronchia′les superio′res [TA] superior tracheobronchial lymph nodes: nodes between the trachea and the bronchus on either side, receiving lymph from adjacent structures.
no′di lymphoi′dei vesica′les latera′les [TA] lateral vesical lymph nodes: the paravesical lymph nodes situated in relation to the lateral umbilical ligament.
no′di lymphoi′dei viscera′les visceral lymph nodes: lymph nodes that receive lymph from the viscera in a body cavity; see *nodi lymphoidei abdominis viscerales* and *nodi lymphoidei pelvis viscerales.* Cf. *nodi lymphoidei parietales.*
n. sinuatria′lis [TA] sinoatrial node: a microscopic collection of atypical cardiac muscle fibers (Purkinje fibers) at the superior end of the sulcus terminalis, at the junction of the superior vena cava and the right atrium. The cardiac rhythm normally takes its origin in this node, which thus is known also as the *cardiac pacemaker.* See illustration. Called also *sinuatrial* or *sinus node.*

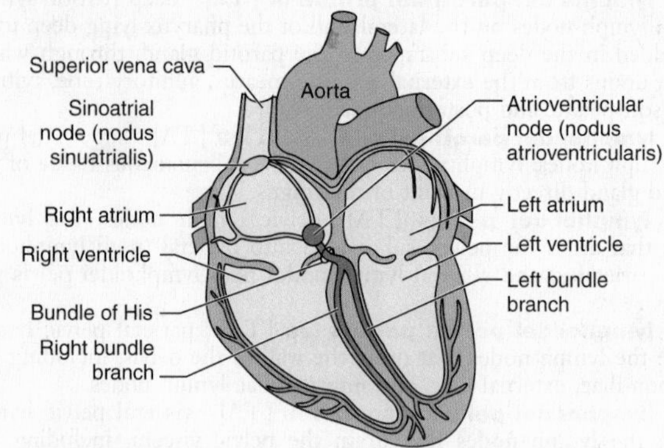

■ Diagram of the conduction system of the heart, showing the nodus sinuatrialis (sinoatrial node) and nodus atrioventricularis (atrioventricular node).

NOEL no observed effect level.

no•e•ma•tacho•graph (no-e″mə-tak′o-graf) [Gr. *noēma* thought + *tacho-* + *-graph*] a device for registering the time required in a mental operation.

no•e•ma•ta•chom•e•ter (no-e″mə-tə-kom′ə-tər) [Gr. *noēma* thought + *tacho-* + *-meter*] a device for measuring the time required in a mental operation.

no•e•mat•ic (no″e-mat′ik) pertaining to thought or the operation of the mind.

no•e•sis (no-e′sis) [Gr. *noēsis* thought] the operation of the intellect; cognition. **noet′ic** *adj*

no•gal•a•my•cin (no-gal″ə-mi′sin) an antineoplastic antibiotic produced by a variant of *Streptomyces nogalater.*

noise (noiz) unwanted variations in a signal that result from imperfections in the transmission of the signal, e.g., electrical signals in electrodiagnosis other than those being studied (most often originating within the electrical apparatus). See also *signal-to-noise ratio,* under *ratio.*
  end-plate n. the monophasic type of end-plate activity.
  quantum n. in radiology, randomness of image or projection measurements owing to defective counting of the number of photons emitted.

Nol•va•dex (nol′və-deks″) trademark for a preparation of tamoxifen citrate.

no•ma (no′mə) [Gr. *nomai* eating sores] 1. a gangrenous process of the mouth and face, usually seen in debilitated or malnourished children; it begins as a small vesicle or ulcer on the gingiva, rapidly becomes necrotic, and spreads to destroy large areas of the oral mucosa and tissues of the face, resulting in severe disfigurement and sometimes even death. Bacteria implicated in the etiology include fusiform bacilli, *Treponema vincentii,* and *Bacteroides melaninogenicus.* Called also *cancrum oris* and *gangrenous stomatitis.* 2. a rare condition with gangrenous erosions similar to those of noma of the face but involving the genitalia; see *erosive balanitis,* under *balanitis,* and *erosive vulvitis,* under *vulvitis.*
  n. neonato′rum noma (def. 1) presenting within the first month of life, usually in infants who are premature and malnourished; the most common infecting organism is *Pseudomonas aeruginosa.*
  n. vul′vae erosive vulvitis.

no•mad•ic (no-mad′ik) wandering; unsettled; free.

no•men (no′mən) pl. *no′mina* [L.] a name.
  no′mina genera′lia [TA] general terminology: terms that denote a general structure type to which a number of specific structures belong.

no•men•cla•ture (no′mən-kla″chər) [*nomen* + *calare* to call] a classified system of names, as of anatomical structures, organisms, etc. See *Terminologia Anatomica.*
  binomial n. the nomenclature used in scientific classification of living organisms in which each organism is designated by two latinized names (genus and species), both of which must always be used because species names are not necessarily unique. NOTE: The genus name is always capitalized, the species name is not, and both are italicized, e.g., *Escherichia coli.* When a name is repeated the genus name may be abbreviated by its initial, e.g., *E. coli.*

NOMID neonatal-onset multisystem inflammatory disease.

No•mi•na Ana•to•mi•ca (NA) (no′mĭ-nə an″ə-tom′ĭ-kə) [L. "anatomical names"] a former official body of anatomical nomenclature, applied specifically to that revised by the International Anatomical Nomenclature Committee appointed by the Fifth International Congress of Anatomists held at Oxford in 1950, and approved by the Sixth International Congress of Anatomists (Paris, 1955) with revisions approved by the Seventh (New York, 1960), Eighth (Wiesbaden, 1965), Tenth (Tokyo, 1975), Eleventh (Mexico City, 1980), and Twelfth (London, 1985) International Congresses of Anatomists. It has been superseded by *Terminologia Anatomica* [TA] (1998).

nom•i•nal (nom′ĭ-nəl) [L. *nominalis,* from *nomen* name] pertaining to a name or names.

nom(o)- [Gr. *nomos* custom, law] a combining form denoting relationship to usage or law.

no•mo•gen•e•sis (no″mo-jen′ə-sis) [*nomo-* + *-genesis*] the theory of evolution according to which the course of evolution is fixed and predetermined by law, no place being left for chance.

nom•o•gram (nom′o-gram) [*nomo-* + *-gram*] a figure consisting of three or more straight or curved lines, each graduated for a different variable and aligned in such a way that a straightedge crossing all of the scales cuts the scales at values of the variable that have a specified mathematical or empirical relationship. Called also *nomograph.*

no•mo•graph (nom′o-graf) nomogram.

no•mo•top•ic (no″mo-top′ik) [*nomo-* + *top-* + *-ic*] occurring at a normal place; occurring normally.

non- [L. *non* not] a combining form meaning not.

non(a)- [L. *nona* nine] a combining form meaning nine.

non•ad•her•ent (non″ad-hēr′ənt) not adherent to or connected with adjacent structures.

non•an•ti•gen•ic (non″an-tĭ-jen′ik) not antigenic; not eliciting an immune response in a particular animal.

non•a•pep•tide (non″ə-pep′tīd) [*nona-* + *peptide*] a peptide containing nine amino acids.

non com•pos men•tis (non kom′pos men′tis) [L.] not of sound mind, and so not legally responsible.

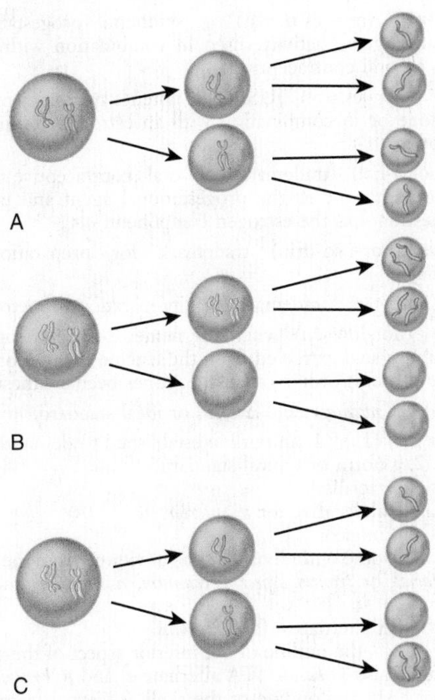

■ Nondisjunction. Normal meiosis *(A)* is contrasted with failure of homologous chromosomes to separate in meiosis I *(B)* or of sister chromatids to separate in meiosis II *(C)*.

non·con·duc·tor (non″kən-duk′tər) any substance that does not readily transmit electricity, light, or heat.

non·de·po·lar·iz·er (non″de-po′lər-īz-ər) a muscle relaxant that produces striate muscle paralysis by competitive interference with the transmission of nerve impulses from nerve ending to muscle receptor.

non·di·a·bet·ic (non″di-ə-bet′ik) not caused by or affected with diabetes.

non·dis·junc·tion (non″dis-junk′shən) failure *(a)* of two homologous chromosomes to pass to separate cells during the first division of meiosis, or *(b)* of the two chromatids of a chromosome to pass to separate cells during mitosis or during the second meiotic division. As a result, one daughter cell has an extra chromosome and the other has one too few. If this happens in meiosis, after fertilization an *aneuploid* individual may develop, e.g., a child with trisomy 21 (Down syndrome).

non·elec·tro·lyte (non″e-lek′tro-līt) a substance that does not dissociate into ions; in solution it is a nonconductor of electricity.

non·flag·el·lat·ed (non-flaj′ə-lāt″ed) not having flagella.

non·heme (non′hēm) not bound within a porphyrin ring; said of iron so contained within a protein.

non·ho·mo·ge·ne·i·ty (non-ho″mo-jə-ne′ĭ-te) the lack of homogeneity; the state of not being homogeneous.

no·ni·grav·i·da (no″nĭ-grav′ĭ-də) [*nona-* + *gravida*] a woman pregnant for the ninth time. Written gravida IX.

non·in·fec·tious (non″in-fek′shəs) not infectious; not spread by contact, inhalation, etc.; not able to spread disease.

non·in·vo·lu·tion (non″in-vo-loo′shən) failure of a part to return to normal size and condition after enlargement from functional activity, as noninvolution of the uterus after pregnancy.

no·nip·a·ra (no-nip′ə-rə) [*nona-* + *para*] a woman who has had nine pregnancies which resulted in viable offspring. Written para IX.

non·med·ul·lat·ed (non-med′u-lāt″əd) unmyelinated.

non·met·al (non-met′əl) any chemical element that is not a metal or a metalloid.

non·mo·tor (non-mo′tər) said of symptoms other than the obvious motor ones in a neurologic condition affecting primarily motor neurons.

non·my·eli·nat·ed (non-mi′ə-lĭ-nāt″əd) unmyelinated.

Non·ne-Mil·roy disease (non′ə mil′roi) [Max *Nonne*, German neurologist, 1861–1939; William Forsyth *Milroy*, American physician, 1855–1942] see under *disease*.

Non·ne-Mil·roy-Meige syndrome (non′ə mil′roi māzh) [M. *Nonne;* W. F. *Milroy;* Henri *Meige*, French physician, 1866–1940] see under *syndrome*.

non·neu·ro·nal (non″noo͝-ro′nəl) pertaining to or composed of nonconducting cells of the nervous system, e.g., neuroglial cells.

non·nu·cle·at·ed (non-noo′kle-āt″əd) without a nucleus; cf. *anucleate*.

non·oc·clu·sion (non″o-cloo′zhən) open bite.

non·ol·i·gu·ric (non-ol″ĭ-gu′rik) not pertaining to, characterized by, or conducive to oliguria.

non·on·co·gen·ic (non″on-ko-jen′ik) not giving rise to tumors or causing tumor formation.

non·opaque (non″o-pāk′) not opaque, such as a radiolucent medium.

non·ose (non′ōs) a monosaccharide containing nine atoms of carbon in the molecule.

non·ox·y·nol (non-ok′sĭ-nol) nonylphenoxypolyethoxyethanol. Any of a group of compounds of the general composition $C_{15}H_{24}O(C_2H_4O)_n$, which are assigned numbers according to the approximate value of *n*: *nonoxynol 4* is $C_{15}H_{24}O(C_2H_4O)_4$, or $C_{23}H_{40}O_5$; *nonoxynol 9* is $C_{33}H_{60}O_{10}$; *nonoxynol 15* is $C_{45}H_{84}O_{16}$; *nonoxynol 30* is $C_{75}H_{144}O_{31}$. Nonoxynol 4, 15, and 30 are nonionic surfactants, and nonoxynol 9 is used as a spermicide. Nonoxynol 10, in which *n* varies from 6 to 16, is used as a pharmaceutical surfactant.

non·para·met·ric (non″par-ə-met′rik) denoting statistical methods or tests requiring neither parameters nor distributional assumptions.

non·par·ous (non-par′əs) nulliparous.

non·pen·e·trance (non-pen′ə-trəns) in genetics, lack of phenotypic expression of a particular genotype by an individual. Cf. *penetrance*.

non·pho·to·chro·mo·gen (non″fo-to-kro′mə-jən) a microorganism that does not produce pigment in the presence of light. The term is specifically applied to mycobacteria that do not produce carotenoid pigmentation; included in this group is the common pathogen *Mycobacterium avium–intracellulare*.

non·po·lar (non-po′lər) not having poles; not exhibiting dipole characteristics.

non·pro·pri·e·tary (non″pro-pri′ə-tar-e) not protected against free competition by patent, trademark, or other means; see also *generic* and see under *name*.

non repetat. [L.] non repeta′tur (do not repeat).

non·re·spond·er (non″re-spon′dər) a person or animal that after vaccination against a given virus does not show any immune response when challenged with the virus.

non·ro·ta·tion (non″ro-ta′shən) [*non-* + L. *rotare* to turn] failure of rotation of a part to its proper position.

n. of the intestine failure of rotation of the intestine during embryonic development, so that the small intestine lies on the right side of the abdomen and the large intestine on the left.

non·sa·pon·i·fi·a·ble (non-sə-pon″ĭ-fi′ə-bəl) incapable of being hydrolyzed to give a fatty acid salt and an alcohol; said of lipids.

non·se·cre·tor (non″se-kre′tər) an individual with A or B type blood whose saliva and other body secretions do not contain the A or B blood group antigens; see also *secretor*.

non·self (non′self″) in immunology, pertaining to foreign antigens. Cf. *self*.

non·sep·tate (non-sep′tāt) without a septum or septa.

non·spe·cif·ic (non″spə-sif′ik) not specific or definite; not having a specific cause or target.

non·spe·cif·ic pro·tein-ty·ro·sine ki·nase (non″spə-sif′ik pro′tēn ti′ro-sēn ki′nās) [EC 2.7.10.2] a group comprising those protein-tyrosine kinases that lack a transmembrane domain. They are further divided into families (e.g., JAK kinases), which differ structurally but which are involved in signaling pathways important in processes such as cell growth, differentiation, and adhesion, in lymphocyte activation, and in oncogenesis. Cf. *receptor protein-tyrosine kinase*.

non·spe·cif·ic ser·ine/thre·o·nine pro·tein ki·nase (non″spə-sif′ik sēr′ēn thre′o-nēn pro′tēn ki′nās) [EC 2.7.11.1] a group comprising those protein-serine/threonine kinases that do not have a transmembrane domain, do not have an activating compound, and have either no or unknown specificity. Cf. *receptor protein serine/threonine kinase*.

non·syn·dro·mal (non″sin-dro′məl) nonsyndromic.

non·syn·drom·ic (non″sin-drom′ik) not occurring as part of a syndrome.

non·union (non-ūn′yən) failure of the ends of a fractured bone to unite.

non·va·lent (non-va′lənt) [*non-* + L. *valere* to be able] having no chemical valency: not capable of entering into chemical composition; said of argon, helium, and the other inert gases.

non•vi•a•ble (non-vi′ə-bəl) [*non-* + *viable*] not capable of living.

no•nyl (no′nəl) the monovalent radical C_9H_{19}.

Noo•nan syndrome (noo′nən) [Jacqueline Anne *Noonan*, American pediatrician, born 1928] see under *syndrome.*

noo•tro•pic (no″o-tro′pik) [Gr. *noos, nous* mind + *-tropic*] having positive effects on organically impaired cognition or nervous system function; said of certain drugs.

NOPHN National Organization for Public Health Nursing.

NOR nucleolar organizing region.

nor- chemical prefix denoting *(a)* a compound (e.g., norleucine) of normal structure (having an unbranched chain of carbon atoms) that is isomeric with one (e.g., leucine) having a branched chain, or *(b)* a compound (e.g., norepinephrine) whose chain or ring contains one less methylene (CH_2) group than does that of its homologue (e.g., epinephrine).

nor•adren•a•line (nor″ə-dren′ə-lin) norepinephrine.

nor•ad•ren•er•gic (nor″ad-rən-ur′jik) activated by or secreting norepinephrine.

Nor•co (nor′ko) trademark for combination preparations of hydrocodone bitartrate and acetaminophen.

Nor•cu•ron (nor-kūr′on) trademark for a preparation of vecuronium bromide.

nor•def•rin hy•dro•chlo•ride (nor-def′rin) an adrenergic agent isomeric with epinephrine, having significant central stimulant action and almost no vasoconstrictor action; the levo-isomer, *levonordefrin* (q.v.), is usually used when vasoconstriction is desired. Called also *homoarterenol hydrochloride.*

Nor•dette (nor-det′) trademark for a combination preparation of levonorgestrel and ethinyl estradiol.

Nor•di•tro•pin (nor′dĭ-tro″pin) trademark for a preparation of somatropin.

no•re•flow (no-re′flo) see under *phenomenon.*

nor•el•ges•tro•min (nor″el-jes′trə-min) a progestational agent used in contraceptive patches in combination with ethinyl estradiol.

nor•epi•neph•rine (nor″ep-ĭ-nef′rin) 1. one of the naturally occurring catecholamines, a neurohormone released by the postganglionic adrenergic nerves and some brain neurons; it is a major neurotransmitter that acts on α- and $β_1$-adrenergic receptors. It is also secreted by the adrenal medulla in response to splanchnic stimulation and is stored in the chromaffin granules. It is a powerful vasopressor and is released in the body usually in response to hypotension or stress. Called also *noradrenaline.* 2. a pharmaceutical preparation of the same substance, usually used in the form of the bitartrate salt.

n. bitartrate [USP] the bitartrate salt of the levorotatory isomer of norepinephrine, having the vasoconstrictor actions of the parent compound; used to restore the blood pressure in certain cases of acute hypotension, and to improve cardiac function during decompensation associated with congestive heart failure or cardiovascular surgery, administered intravenously. Called also *levarterenol bitartrate.*

nor•epi•neph•rin•er•gic (nor-ep″ĭ-nef-rin″ur′jik) 1. pertaining to neurons that release norepinephrine, or to the effects of such release. 2. pertaining to tissues or organs affected by norepinephrine.

nor•eth•an•dro•lone (nor″əth-an′drə-lōn) a synthetic anabolic-androgenic steroid equal to testosterone in anabolic activity, but having less androgenic activity, used in the treatment of anemia; administered orally.

nor•eth•in•drone (nor-eth′in-drōn) [USP] a progestational agent having some anabolic, estrogenic, and androgenic properties; used as an oral contraceptive, alone or in combination with an estrogen component.

n. acetate [USP] the acetate salt of norethindrone, used in the treatment of secondary amenorrhea, dysfunctional uterine bleeding, and endometriosis, administered orally; also used in combination with an estrogen component as an oral contraceptive.

nor•eth•is•ter•one (nor″əth-is′tər-ōn) INN and BAN for *norethindrone.*

nor•ethy•no•drel (nor″ə-thi′no-drəl) [USP] a progestin used in combination with an estrogen component as an oral contraceptive, to control endometriosis, for the treatment of hypermenorrhea, and to produce cyclic withdrawal bleeding.

Nor•flex (nor′fleks) trademark for a preparation of orphenadrine citrate.

nor•flox•a•cin (nor-flok′sə-sin) a fluoroquinolone antibacterial effective against penicillin-resistant *Neisseria gonorrhoeae;* administered orally.

Nor•ge•sic (nor-je′zik) trademark for combination preparations of orphenadrine citrate, aspirin, and caffeine.

nor•ges•ti•mate (nor-jes′tĭ-māt) a synthetic progestational agent having little androgenic activity; used in combination with an estrogen component as an oral contraceptive.

nor•ges•trel (nor-jes′trəl) [USP] a potent synthetic progestational agent used, alone or in combination with an estrogen component, as an oral contraceptive.

Nor•i•nyl (nor′ə-nəl) trademark for oral contraceptive preparations containing norethindrone as the progestational agent and either ethinyl estradiol or mestranol as the estrogen component.

Nor•iso•drine (nor-i′so-drin) trademark for preparations of isoproterenol sulfate.

Nor•i•tate (nor′ĭ-tāt) trademark for a preparation of metronidazole.

nor•leu•cine (nor-loo′sēn) chemical name: 2-aminohexanoic acid. A nonessential amino acid extracted from the leucine fraction of the decomposition of the proteins of nervous tissue. It has been synthesized.

norm (norm) [L. *norma* rule] a fixed or ideal standard.

nor•ma (nor′mə) [L.] 1. an outline established to define the aspects of the cranium. 2. a norm or typical standard.

n. ante′rior n. facialis.

n. basa′lis TA alternative for *n. inferior.*

n. basila′ris n. inferior.

n. facia′lis [TA] the outline of the skull as viewed from the front; called also *anterior, facial,* or *frontal aspect of cranium, n. anterior,* and *n. frontalis* [TA alternative].

n. fronta′lis TA alternative for *n. facialis.*

n. infe′rior [TA] the outline of the inferior aspect of the skull, viewed from above; called also *n. basalis* [TA alternative] and *n. basilaris.*

n. latera′lis [TA] the outline of the skull as viewed from either side; called also *temporal aspect of cranium* and *n. temporalis.*

n. occipita′lis [TA], n. poste′rior the outline of the skull as viewed from behind; called also *occipital aspect of cranium.*

n. sagitta′lis the outline of a sagittal section through the skull.

n. supe′rior [TA] the outline of the superior surface of the skull; called also *superior* or *vertical aspect of cranium* and *n. verticalis* [TA alternative].

n. tempora′lis n. lateralis.

n. ventra′lis basis cranii externa.

n. vertica′lis TA alternative for *n. superior.*

nor•mal (nor′məl) [L. *norma* rule] 1. agreeing with the regular and established type. 2. in chemistry, *(a)* denoting a solution containing in each 1000 mL 1 g equivalent weight of the active substance, symbol N or *N*; *(b)* denoting aliphatic hydrocarbons in which no carbon atom is combined with more than 2 other carbon atoms, symbol *n-*; *(c)* denoting salts formed from acids and bases in such a way that no acidic hydrogen of the acid remains nor any of the basic hydroxyl of the base.

nor•mal•i•ty (nor-mal′ĭ-te) 1. the state of being normal. 2. the number of gram-equivalent weights of solute per liter of solution.

nor•mal•iza•tion (nor″məl-ĭ-za′shən) 1. the process of bringing or restoring to the normal standard. 2. in statistics, the process of transforming data so that it has no units but is expressed in terms of standard deviations from the mean.

nor•meta•neph•rine (nor-met″ə-nef′rin) a methylated metabolite of norepinephrine excreted in the urine and found in certain tissues.

norm(o)- [L. *norma* rule] a combining form meaning conforming to the rule; normal or usual.

nor•mo•al•bu•mi•nu•ria (nor″mo-al-bu″mĭ-nu′re-ə) a normal level of albumin in the blood.

nor•mo•bar•ic (nor″mo-bar′ik) isobaric (def. 1).

nor•mo•blast (nor′mo-blast) [*normo-* + *-blast*] 1. a term often used as a synonym of erythroblast, but sometimes specifically denoting nucleated

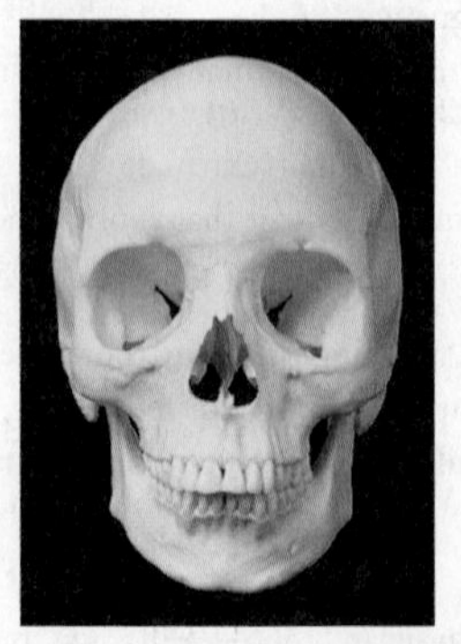

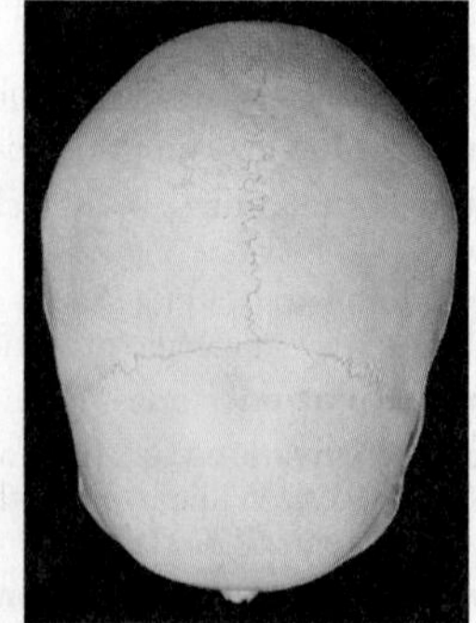

■ *(A),* Norma facialis; *(B),* norma superior.

cells in a normal course of erythrocyte maturation, as distinguished from megaloblasts (q.v.); when the term is used with this meaning, the developmental stages of the nucleated cells of the erythrocytic series (q.v.) are generally named pronormoblasts *(proerythroblasts)* and basophilic, polychromatophilic, and orthochromatic normoblasts (see under *erythroblast*). 2. orthochromatic erythroblast.

acidophilic n. orthochromatic erythroblast.

basophilic n. a nucleated immature erythrocyte, having cytoplasm generally similar to that of the earlier proerythroblast but sometimes even more basophilic, and usually regular in outline. The nucleus is still relatively large, but the chromatin strands are thicker and more deeply staining, giving a coarser appearance; the nucleoli have disappeared. Called also *prorubricyte*, *early n.*, and *basophilic* or *early erythroblast*.

early n. basophilic erythroblast.

eosinophilic n. orthochromatic erythroblast.

intermediate n. polychromatophilic erythroblast.

late n., orthochromatic n., oxyphilic n. see under *erythroblast*.

polychromatic n., polychromatophilic n. see under *erythroblast*.

nor·mo·blas·tic (nor″mo-blas′tik) relating to or having the character of a normoblast.

nor·mo·blas·to·sis (nor″mo-blas-to′sis) excessive production of normoblasts by the bone marrow.

nor·mo·cal·ce·mia (nor″mo-kal-se′me-ə) a normal level of calcium in the blood. **normocalce′mic** *adj*

nor·mo·cap·nia (nor″mo-kap′ne-ə) eucapnia. **normocap′nic** *adj*

nor·mo·cho·les·ter·ol·emia (nor″mo-kə-les″tər-ol-e′me-ə) a normal level of cholesterol in the blood.

nor·mo·cho·les·ter·ol·emic (nor″mo-kə-les″tər-ol-e′mik) 1. pertaining to or characterized by normocholesterolemia. 2. tending to produce normocholesterolemia.

nor·mo·chro·ma·sia (nor″mo-kro-ma′zhə) [*normo-* + Gr. *chrōma* color] 1. a normal staining reaction in a cell or tissue. 2. normochromia.

nor·mo·chro·mia (nor″mo-kro′me-ə) normal color; indicating the color of erythrocytes having a normal hemoglobin content; see also *normochromic anemia*, under *anemia*. **normochro′mic** *adj*

nor·mo·crin·ic (nor″mo-krin′ik) pertaining to normal secretion or to normal endocrine action.

nor·mo·cyte (nor′mo-sīt) [*normo-* + *-cyte*] an erythrocyte that is normal in size, shape, and color. Called also *normoerythrocyte*. **normocyt′ic** *adj*

nor·mo·cy·to·sis (nor″mo-si-to′sis) a normal state of the blood in respect to the erythrocytes.

Nor·mo·dyne (nor′mo-dīn) trademark for a preparation of labetalol hydrochloride.

nor·mo·eryth·ro·cyte (nor″mo-ə-rith′ro-sīt) normocyte.

nor·mo·gly·ce·mia (nor″mo-gli-se′me-ə) euglycemia. **normoglyce′mic** *adj*

nor·mo·ka·le·mia (nor″mo-kə-le′me-ə) [*normo-* + L. *kalium* potassium + *-emia*] a normal level of potassium in the blood. **normokale′mic** *adj*

nor·mo·lip·i·de·mic (nor″mo-lip″ĭ-de′mik) pertaining to or characterized by normal levels of lipids in the blood.

nor·mo·or·tho·cy·to·sis (nor″mo-or″tho-si-to′sis) [*normo-* + *orthocytosis*] an increase in total numbers of leukocytes in the blood but with a normal proportion between the different varieties; see also *absolute leukocytosis*.

nor·mo·skeo·cy·to·sis (nor″mo-ske″o-si-to′sis) [*normo-* + Gr. *skaios* left + *-cyte* + *-osis*] a condition of the leukocytes of the blood in which the number is normal, but there are many immature forms (deviation to the left).

nor·mos·mia (nor-mos′me-ə) a normal state of the sense of smell. **normos′mic** *adj*

nor·mo·sper·mia (nor″mo-spur′me-ə) production of spermatozoa normal in number and motility. **normosperm′ic** *adj*

nor·mo·sthen·uria (nor″mo-sthən-u′re-ə) [*normo-* + *stheno-* + *-uria*] 1. the secretion of urine of varying specific gravity within the normal range. 2. normally active urination.

nor·mo·ten·sion (nor″mo-ten′shən) normal tone, tension, or pressure.

nor·mo·ten·sive (nor″mo-ten′siv) 1. characterized by normal tone, tension, or pressure, as by normal blood pressure. 2. a person with normal blood pressure.

nor·mo·ther·mia (nor″mo-thur′me-ə) [*normo-* + *therm-* + *-ia*] a normal state of temperature, especially normal body temperature (37°C or 98.6°F). **normother′mic** *adj*

nor·mo·to·nia (nor″mo-to′ne-ə) normal tone or tension. **normoton′ic** *adj*

nor·mo·tro·phic (nor″mo-tro′fik) of normal development; exhibiting neither hypertrophy nor hypotrophy.

nor·mo·uri·ce·mia (nor″mo-u″rĭ-se′me-ə) a normal value of uric acid in the blood. **normourice′mic** *adj*

nor·mo·vo·le·mia (nor″mo-vo-le′me-ə) [*normo-* + *volume* + *-emia*] normal blood volume. **normovole′mic** *adj*

Nor·o·vi·rus (nor′o-vi″rəs) the noroviruses, a genus of the family Caliciviridae that causes acute foodborne gastroenteritis, with nausea and vomiting lasting from 12 to 60 hours; the type species is Norwalk virus. Called also Norwalk-like viruses.

nor·o·vi·rus (nor′o-vi″rəs) any virus of the genus *Norovirus*. **norovi′ral** *adj*

Nor·ox·in (nor-ok′sin) trademark for a preparation of norfloxacin.

Nor·pace (nor′pās) trademark for preparations of disopyramide phosphate.

Nor·plant (nor′plant) trademark for a preparation of levonorgestrel.

Nor·pram·in (nor′prə-min) trademark for a preparation of desipramine hydrochloride.

nor·pseu·do·ephed·rine (nor-soo″do-ə-fed′rēn) a nervous system stimulant chemically related to ephedrine, extracted from the leaves of the shrub *Catha edulis*.

Nor-QD trademark for a preparation of norethindrone.

Nor·rie disease (nor′e) [Gordon *Norrie*, Danish ophthalmologist, 1855–1941] see under *disease*.

Nor·ris corpuscles (nor′is) [Richard *Norris*, English physiologist, 1831–1916] see under *corpuscle*.

North·ern blot (blot analysis, blot hybridization) (nor′thərn) [facetious coinage by analogy with *Southern blot*] see under *blot*.

nor·trip·ty·line hy·dro·chlo·ride (nor-trip′tə-lēn) [USP] a tricyclic antidepressant of the dibenzocycloheptadiene class, also used to treat panic disorder and to relieve chronic, severe pain; administered orally.

Nor·vasc (nor′vask) trademark for a preparation of amlodipine besylate.

Nor·vir (nor′vir) trademark for preparations of ritonavir.

Nor·walk gastroenteritis, virus (nor′wawk) [*Norwalk*, Ohio, location of the outbreak from which the virus was isolated] see under *gastroenteritis* and *virus*.

nos·ca·pine (nos′kə-pēn) an alkaloid of opium used as an antitussive, administered orally.

n. hydrochloride the hydrochloride salt of noscapine, having the same actions, uses, and route of administration as the base.

nose (nōz) [L. *nasus;* Gr. *rhis*] 1. nasus. 2. nasus externus.

cleft n. a developmental anomaly resulting from incomplete union of the paired nasal primordia.

collie n. nasal solar dermatitis.

external n. nasus externus.

saddle n., saddle-back n., swayback n. concavity of the contour of the bridge of the nose due to collapse of cartilaginous or bony support, or both; it was once most often due to congenital syphilis, but is now more commonly the result of trauma, surgery, a congenital epidermal defect, or leprosy. Called also *saddle nose deformity*.

nose·bleed (nōz′blēd″) epistaxis.

nose·gay (nōz′ga) a name applied to an anatomical structure resembling a small bunch of flowers.

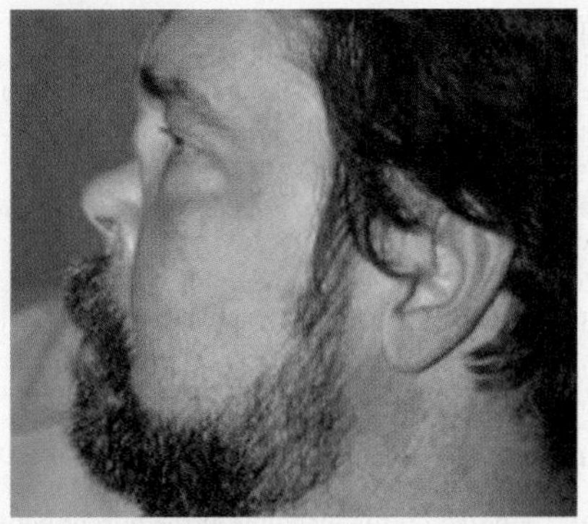

■ Saddle nose in a patient with Wegener granulomatosis.

Riolan n. the group of muscles that take their origin from the styloid process of the temporal bone.

No·se·ma (no-se′mə) [Gr. *nosēma* sickness] a genus of intracellular protozoa (suborder Apansporoblastina, order Microsporida), formerly thought to be identical to *Encephalitozoon;* many are parasitic in invertebrates, especially insects, and a few species cause human infection.

N. al′gerae *Brachiola algerae.*

N. a′pis the etiologic agent of the bee condition called nosema disease.

N. bomby′cis the etiologic agent of the disease pébrine in silkworms.

N. conno′ri a species that causes corneal and disseminated infections in humans.

N. cuni′culi *Encephalitozoon cuniculi.*

N. ocula′rum a species that causes corneal infections in humans.

no·se·ma·to·sis (no-se″mə-to′sis) 1. infection of insects or other invertebrates with protozoa of the genus *Nosema.* 2. former name for *encephalitozoonosis.*

nose·piece (nōz′pēs″) the portion of a microscope nearest to the stage, which bears the objective or objectives, constructed so as to permit change of the objective without disturbing the focus of the instrument.

quick-change n. a nosepiece bearing a single objective, which may be quickly attached to or removed from a microscope.

rotating n. a nosepiece bearing more than one objective, designed to permit the one selected to be rotated into place, with its axis coincident with the optical axis of the microscope.

nos·eti·ol·o·gy (nos″e-te-ol′ə-je) [*nos-* + *etiology*] the study of the causation of disease.

no·si·hep·tide (no″sĭ-hep′tīd) a veterinary growth stimulant.

nos(o)- [Gr. *nosos* disease] a combining form denoting relationship to disease.

noso·co·mi·al (nos″o-ko′me-əl) [*noso-* + Gr. *komeion* to take care of] pertaining to or originating in the hospital, usually referring to a disease or other pathologic condition.

noso·gen·e·sis (nos″o-jen′ə-sis) pathogenesis.

noso·gen·ic (nos″o-jen′ik) pathogenic.

no·sog·e·ny (no-soj′ə-ne) [*noso-* + *-geny*] pathogenesis.

noso·ge·og·ra·phy (nos″o-je-og′rə-fe) geomedicine.

no·sog·ra·phy (no-sog′rə-fe) [*noso-* + *-graphy*] a written account or description of diseases.

no·sol·o·gy (no-sol′ə-je) [*noso-* + *-logy*] the science of the classification of diseases; called also *nosonomy.* **nosolog′ic** *adj*

no·som·e·try (no-som′ə-tre) [*noso-* + *-metry*] the measurement of the morbidity rate.

no·son·o·my (no-son′ə-me) nosology.

noso·pho·bia (nos″o-fo′be-ə) [*noso-* + *-phobia*] irrational dread of sickness or of some particular disease.

noso·poi·et·ic (nos″o-poi-et′ik) [*noso-* + Gr. *poiein* to make] causing or producing disease.

Noso·psyl·lus (nos″o-sil′əs) [*noso-* + Gr. *psylla* flea] a genus of fleas. *N. fascia′tus,* the rat flea of North America and Europe, is a vector of murine typhus and probably of plague.

noso·tox·ic (nos′o-tok″sik) pertaining to nosotoxicosis or nosotoxins.

noso·tox·i·co·sis (nos″o-tok″sĭ-ko′sis) [*noso-* + *toxicosis*] toxicosis.

noso·tox·in (nos′o-tok″sin) [*noso-* + *toxin*] a toxin that causes disease.

noso·tro·pic (nos″o-tro′pik) [*noso-* + *-tropic*] directed against or opposed to a disease; cf. *prophylactic.*

nos·tril (nos′tril) naris; see *nares.*

nos·trum (nos′trəm) [L.] a quack, patent, or secret remedy.

no·tal·gia (no-tal′jə) [*not-* + *-algia*] dorsalgia.

n. paresthe′tica intense itching and pain on the back at the medial scapular borders, often with paresthesias and skin hyperpigmentation.

no·tan·ce·pha·lia (no″tən-sə-fa′le-ə) [*not-* + *an-* + *cephal-* + *-ia*] congenital absence of the posterior aspect of the cranium.

no·tan·en·ce·pha·lia (no″tən-ən-sə-fa′le-ə) [*not-* + *anencephalia*] absence of the cerebellum.

no·ta·tion (no-ta′shən) [L. *notare* to note] a system of characters or symbols used to express technical facts or quantities.

Palmer n. Palmer tooth notation system.

notch (noch) an indentation or depression, especially one on the edge of a bone or other organ. See also *incisura.*

acetabular n. incisura acetabuli.

angular n. incisura angularis.

antegonial n. a notch on the mandible at the border between the body and ramus.

anterior n. of auricle incisura anterior auriculae.

aortic n. dicrotic n.

auricular n. incisura anterior auriculae.

n. of cardiac apex incisura apicis cordis.

cardiac n. of left lung incisura cardiaca pulmonis sinistri.

cardiac n. of stomach, cardial n. incisura cardialis.

n. in cartilage of acoustic meatus incisura cartilaginis meatus acustici.

cerebellar n., anterior a wide notch on the anterior surface of the cerebellum, occupied by the inferior colliculi and superior cerebellar peduncles.

cerebellar n., posterior a notch between the cerebellar hemispheres posteriorly, containing the falx cerebelli.

clavicular n. of sternum incisura clavicularis sterni.

coracoid n. incisura scapulae.

costal n's of sternum incisurae costales sterni.

cotyloid n. incisura acetabuli.

dicrotic n. a small downward deflection in the arterial pulse or pressure contour immediately following closure of the aortic valve and preceding the dicrotic wave; sometimes used as a marker for the end of systole or the ejection period.

digastric n. of temporal bone incisura mastoidea ossis temporalis.

ethmoidal n. of frontal bone incisura ethmoidalis ossis frontalis.

fibular n. of tibia incisura fibularis tibiae.

frontal n. incisura frontalis.

gastric n. incisura angularis.

greater ischial n., greater ischiatic n. incisura ischiadica major.

greater sciatic n. incisura ischiadica major.

interarytenoid n. incisura interarytenoidea.

interclavicular n. incisura jugularis sterni.

intercondylar n. of femur fossa intercondylaris femoris.

intertragic n. incisura intertragica.

intervertebral n., inferior incisura vertebralis inferior.

intervertebral n., superior incisura vertebralis superior.

jugular n. of occipital bone incisura jugularis ossis occipitalis.

jugular n. of sternum incisura jugularis sterni.

jugular n. of temporal bone incisura jugularis ossis temporalis.

Kernohan n. a groove in the cerebral peduncle caused by displacement of the brainstem against the tentorium in some cases of transtentorial herniation.

lacrimal n. of maxilla incisura lacrimalis maxillae.

lesser ischial n., lesser ischiatic n. incisura ischiadica minor.

lesser sciatic n. incisura ischiadica minor.

n. for ligamentum teres incisura ligamenti teretis.

mandibular n. incisura mandibulae.

mastoid n. of temporal bone incisura mastoidea ossis temporalis.

nasal n. of frontal bone margo nasalis ossis frontalis.

nasal n. of maxilla incisura nasalis maxillae.

pancreatic n. incisura pancreatis.

parietal n. of temporal bone incisura parietalis ossis temporalis.

popliteal n. fossa intercondylaris femoris.

preoccipital n. incisura preoccipitalis.

presternal n. incisura jugularis sterni.

pterygoid n. incisura pterygoidea.

radial n., radial n. of ulna incisura radialis ulnae.

rivinian n., Rivinus n. incisura tympanica.

sacrosciatic n. incisura ischiadica major.

scapular n. incisura scapulae.

semilunar n. of ulna incisura trochlearis ulnae.

Sibson n. an inward bend of the left upward limit of precordial dullness in acute pericardial effusion.

sigmoid n. incisura mandibulae.

sphenopalatine n. of palatine bone incisura sphenopalatina ossis palatini.

sternal n. incisura jugularis sterni.

supraorbital n. incisura supraorbitalis.

suprascapular n. incisura scapulae.

suprasternal n. incisura jugularis sterni.

tentorial n. incisura tentorii cerebelli.

terminal n. of auricle incisura terminalis auricularis.

thyroid n., inferior incisura thyroidea inferior.

thyroid n., superior incisura thyroidea superior.

trigeminal n. a notch in the superior border of the petrosal portion of the temporal bone, near the apex, for transmission of the trigeminal nerve.

trochlear n. incisura trochlearis ulnae.

tympanic n. incisura tympanica.

ulnar n. of radius incisura ulnaris radii.

umbilical n. incisura ligamenti teretis.

vertebral n., inferior incisura vertebralis inferior.

vertebral n., superior incisura vertebralis superior.

No·tech·is (no-tek′is) a genus of extremely venomous Australian snakes of the family Elapidae. *N. scuta′tus* is the tiger snake, whose body is chiefly brown with dark bands. See table at *snake*.

no·ten·ceph·a·lo·cele (no″ten-sef′ə-lo-sēl″) [*not-* + *encephalocele*] occipital encephalocele.

no·ten·ceph·a·lus (no″ten-sef′ə-ləs) [*noto-* + Gr. *enkephalos* brain] a fetus affected with notencephalocele.

Noth·na·gel syndrome (not′nah-gəl) [Carl Wilhelm Hermann *Nothnagel*, Austrian physician, 1841–1905] see under *syndrome*.

no·ti·fi·a·ble (no″tĭ-fi′ə-bəl) necessary to be reported to a government health agency.

not(o)- [Gr. *nōton* back] a combining form denoting relationship to the back.

no·to·chord (no′to-kord) [*noto-* + *chord*] the rod-shaped body, composed of cells derived from the mesoblast of the primitive node of the embryo, defining the primitive axis of the body and acting as the center of development of the axial skeleton; it is the common factor of all species of the phylum Chordata. Called also *chorda dorsalis*.

no·to·chor·do·ma (no″to-kor-do′mə) chordoma.

No·to·ed·res (no″to-ed′rēz) a genus of mange mites of the family Sarcoptidae. *N. ca′ti* is the itch mite, which causes a persistent, sometimes fatal, mange in cats and may also infest rabbits and humans.

no·to·ed·ric (no″to-ed′rik) pertaining to or caused by *Notoedres*.

no·to·gen·e·sis (no″to-jen′ə-sis) [*noto-* + *-genesis*] development of the notochord.

no·tom·e·lus (no-tom′ə-ləs) [*noto-* + Gr. *melos* limb] a fetus with accessory limbs on the back.

not-self (not′self″) nonself.

no·tum (no′təm) [Gr. *nōton* back] 1. back. 2. the dorsal element of each segment of an arthropod.

nou·me·nal (noo′mə-nəl) [Gr. *noumenon* a thing thought] pertaining to rational intuition independent of sensory perception.

No·van·trone (no-van′trōn) trademark for a preparation of mitoxantrone hydrochloride.

No·va·rel (no′və-rel) trademark for a preparation of chorionic gonadotropin.

no·vo·bio·cin (no″vo-bi′o-sin) an antibiotic obtained from *Streptomyces niveus* and other *Streptomyces* species, effective chiefly against staphylococci and other gram-positive organisms.

n. calcium the calcium salt of novobiocin, having the same actions as the base; used in the treatment of infections in children due to susceptible bacteria resistant to other antibiotics; administered orally.

n. sodium the sodium salt of novobiocin, having the same appearance, actions, uses, and mode of administration as the calcium salt; usually used in adults.

No·vo·cain (no′və-kān) trademark for preparations of procaine hydrochloride.

No·vo·lin (no′vo-lin) trademark for preparations of insulin human produced by recombinant DNA technology; different forms are identified by letters following the trademark; e.g., Novolin L denotes insulin human zinc suspension, or by numerals, e.g., Novolin 70/30 denotes a preparation of isophane insulin human suspension and regular insulin human in a 7:3 ratio.

No·vo·Log (no′vo-log) trademark for a preparation of insulin aspart.

No·vo·Sev·en (no″vo-sev′en) trademark for a preparation of coagulation factor VII.

noxa (nok′sə) pl. *nox′ae* [L. "harm"] an injurious agent, act, or influence.

nox·ious (nok′shəs) [L. *noxius*] hurtful, pernicious, or damaging to tissue.

nox·o·fil (nok′sə-fil) trademark for a preparation of posaconazole.

NP-59 iodomethylnorcholesterol.

Np neptunium.

NPA National Perinatal Association.

NPH Il·e·tin (il′ə-tin) see under *Iletin*.

Nplate trademark for a preparation of romiplostim.

NPN nonprotein nitrogen.

NPO [L.] nil per os (nothing by mouth).

NRC normal retinal correspondence.

NREM non–rapid eye movement; see under *sleep*.

NRI selective norepinephrine reuptake inhibitor.

NS normal saline.

ns nanosecond.

NSAIA nonsteroidal antiinflammatory analgesic (or agent); see under *drug*.

NSAID nonsteroidal antiinflammatory drug.

NSCLC non–small cell lung carcinoma.

nsec nanosecond.

NSIAD nephrogenic syndrome of inappropriate antidiuresis.

NSILA nonsuppressible insulin-like activity.

NSNA National Student Nurses' Association.

NSR normal sinus rhythm.

NST nonstress test.

N-ter·mi·nal (tur′mĭ-nəl) the amino (NH_2) end of a polypeptide chain, conventionally written to the left; called also *NH_2-terminal*.

NTP normal temperature and pressure; National Toxicology Program.

nU nanounit.

nu (noo) [N, ν] the thirteenth letter of the Greek alphabet.

Nu·bain (nu′bān) trademark for a preparation of nalbuphine hydrochloride.

nu·bec·u·la (noo-bek′u-lə) [L., dim. of *nubes* cloud] nebula (def. 1).

nu·cha (noo′kə) [L.] the nape, or posterior aspect of the neck. **nu′chal** *adj*

Nuck canal, diverticulum (nook) [Anton *Nuck*, Dutch anatomist, 1650–1692] see under *canal* and see *processus vaginalis peritonei*.

nu·cle·ar (noo′kle-ər) pertaining to a nucleus.

nu·cle·ase (noo′kle-ās) a general term for enzymes of the hydrolase class that catalyze the cleavage of phosphodiester linkages in nucleic acids to form nucleotides or oligonucleotides [EC 3.1.11–31]. The nucleases are classified in subgroups on the basis of their substrate specificity; they may be endonucleases or exonucleases, each of which may be specific for the ribonucleic acids (ribonucleases) or deoxyribonucleic acids (deoxyribonucleases).

nu·cle·at·ed (noo′kle-āt″əd) [L. *nucleatus*] having a nucleus or nuclei.

nu·clei (noo′kle-i) [L.] genitive and plural of *nucleus*.

nu·cle·ic ac·id (noo-kle′ik) a high-molecular-weight nucleotide polymer. There are two types: *deoxyribonucleic acid* (DNA) and *ribonucleic acid* (RNA) (q.v.).

infectious n. a. viral nucleic acid capable of infecting a cell and inducing the production of viruses.

nu·cle·ide (noo′kle-īd) any compound of nucleic acid with a metallic element.

nu·cle·i·form (noo′kle-ĭ-form) shaped like a nucleus.

nucle(o)- [L. *nucleus*, q.v.] a combining form denoting relationship to a nucleus.

nu·cleo·cap·sid (noo″kle-o-kap′sid) a unit of viral structure, consisting of a capsid (protein coat) with the enclosed nucleic acid; some simple viruses are naked nucleocapsids, while in others the nucleocapsids form part of a more complex structure.

nu·cleo·cy·to·plas·mic (noo″kle-o-si″to-plaz′mik) pertaining to the nucleus and cytoplasm.

nu·cle·of·u·gal (noo″kle-of′u-gəl) [*nucleo-* + *-fugal*[2]] moving away from a nucleus.

nu·cleo·glu·co·pro·tein (noo″kle-o-gloo″ko-pro′tēn) a combination of a nucleoprotein with a carbohydrate.

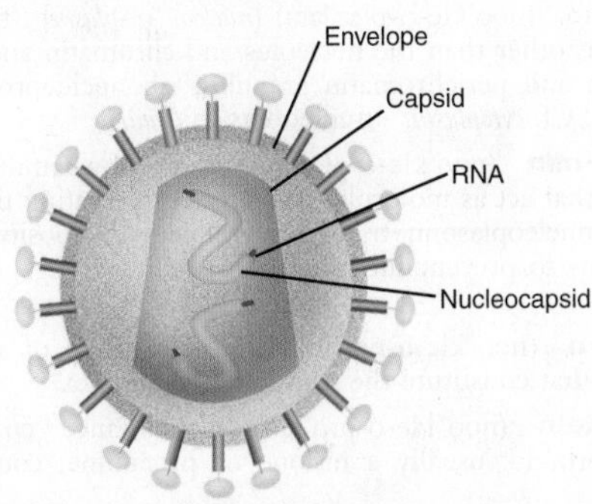

■ Nucleocapsid in a schematic diagram of HIV-1; molecules of protease, integrase, and reverse transcriptase, which also occur within the capsid, are omitted for simplicity.

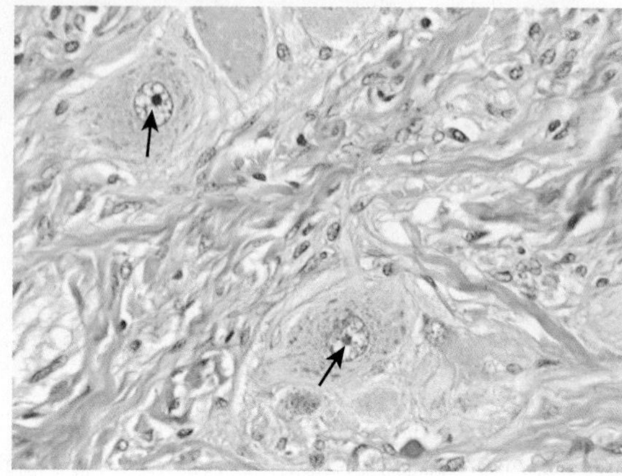

■ Prominent nucleoli *(arrows)* in the eccentric nuclei of ganglion cells.

nu•cleo•his•tone (noo″kle-o-his′tōn) a complex nucleoprotein composed of deoxyribonucleic acid (DNA) and histone.

nu•cle•oid (noo′kle-oid) 1. resembling a nucleus. 2. a DNA-containing region lacking a surrounding nuclear membrane, occurring in prokaryotes, mitochondria, and chloroplasts; it is analagous to the eukaryotic cell nucleus. 3. the core of nucleic acid surrounded by the protein capsid in some viruses.

nu•cle•o•li (noo-kle′o-li) [L.] plural of *nucleolus.*

nu•cle•o•li•form (noo″kle-o′lĭ-form) resembling a nucleolus; called also *nucleoloid.*

nu•cle•o•lin (noo-kle′o-lin) a 100-kD nucleolar protein that acts as a multifunctional shuttle between the nucleus and cytoplasm and also occurs on the cell surface.

nu•cle•o•loid (noo′kle-o-loid) nucleoliform.

nu•cleo•lo•ne•ma (noo″kle-o″lo-ne′mə) [*nucleolus* + Gr. *nēma* thread] a network of strands formed by organization of fine ribonucleoprotein granules in the nucleolus of a cell.

nu•cle•o•lus (noo-kle′ə-ləs″) gen. and pl. *nucle′oli* [L., dim. of *nucleus*] a rounded, dense body, present in the nucleus of eukaryotic cells during interphase, that is the site of ribosomal RNA (rRNA) synthesis and ribosomal subunit assembly. It consists of *(a)* a fibrillar center, containing the rRNA genes, surrounded by *(b)* the pars fibrosa, a dense fibrillar component where transcription occurs, and *(c)* the pars granulosa, a granular component where the ribosomal subunits are assembled. Multiple nucleoli occur in some cells. **nucle′olar** *adj*

nu•cle•on (noo′kle-on) a particle of the atomic nucleus, a proton or a neutron.

nu•cle•on•ic (noo″kle-on′ik) nuclear.

nu•cle•on•ics (noo″kle-on′iks) nuclear physics.

nu•cle•op•e•tal (noo″kle-op′ə-təl) [*nucleo-* + *-petal*] moving toward a nucleus.

nu•cleo•phago•cy•to•sis (noo″kle-o-fa″go-si-to′sis) the engulfing of the nuclei of other cells by phagocytes; see *tart cell,* under *cell.*

nu•cleo•phile (noo′kle-o-fīl″) an electron donor in chemical reactions involving covalent catalysis in which the donated electrons bond other chemical groups (electrophiles).

nu•cleo•phil•ic (noo″kle-o-fil′ik) being or serving as a nucleophile.

nu•cleo•plasm (noo′kle-o-plaz″əm) [*nucleo-* + *-plasm*] the contents of the cell nucleus other than the nucleolus and chromatin and consisting of interchromatin and perichromatin granules, ribonucleoproteins, and the nuclear matrix. Cf. *cytoplasm.* **nucleoplas′mic** *adj*

nu•cleo•plas•min (noo′kle-o-plaz″min) any of a family of acidic nuclear proteins that act as molecular chaperones, mediating the assembly of nucleosomes; nucleoplasmin transiently reduces the positive charges on histone proteins to prevent incorrect nonspecific aggregation of histones and DNA.

nu•cleo•po•rin (noo″kle-o-por′in) any of a group of structurally diverse proteins that constitute the nuclear pore complex.

nu•cleo•pro•tein (noo″kle-o-pro′tēn) a substance composed of a simple basic protein, usually a histone or protamine, combined with a nucleic acid.

deoxyribose n. a deoxyribonucleic acid–protein complex.

ribose n. a ribonucleic acid–protein complex.

nu•cleo•si•dase (noo″kle-o-si′dās) a term used in the recommended names of some glycosidases hydrolyzing *N*-glycosyl linkages [EC 3.2.2] to denote those catalyzing the cleavage of a nucleoside to form a purine or pyrimidine base and a sugar.

nu•cleo•side (noo′kle-o-sīd″) a heterocyclic nitrogenous base, particularly a purine or pyrimidine, in *N*-glycosidic linkage with a sugar, particularly a pentose; it is often used specifically to denote a compound obtained by hydrolysis of nucleic acids, a purine or pyrimidine linked to ribose or deoxyribose, e.g., adenosine or cytidine.

nu•cleo•side-di•phos•phate ki•nase (noo′kle-o-sīd di′fos-fāt ki′nās) [EC 2.7.4.6] an enzyme of the transferase class with broad specificity that catalyzes the reversible transfer of a phosphate from ATP to a nucleoside diphosphate to form a nucleoside triphosphate. The reaction is part of the mechanism that regenerates high-energy nucleotides for metabolic processes and conserves the purine-pyrimidine pool.

nu•cleo•side-phos•phate ki•nase (noo′kle-o-sīd fos′fat ki′nās) [EC 2.7.4.4] any enzyme of the transferase class that catalyzes the transfer of a phosphate from ATP to a nucleoside phosphate to form a nucleoside diphosphate. The reaction is part of the mechanism that regenerates high energy nucleotides for metabolic processes and conserves the purine-pyrimidine pool. Specific enzymes exist for individual nucleosides (e.g., adenylate kinase).

nu•cleo•side phos•phor•y•lase (noo′kle-o-sīd″ fos-for′ə-lās) any of the enzymes of the sub-subclass pentosyltransferases [EC 2.4.2] that catalyze the phosphorolysis of a nucleoside to form the free base and a ribose (or deoxyribose) 1-phosphate as a step in the degradation of nucleic acids and nucleotides. See also *purine-nucleoside phosphorylase* and *pyrimidine-nucleoside phosphorylase.*

nu•cle•o•sis (noo″kle-o′sis) nuclear proliferation; abnormal increase in the production of nuclei, such as occurs in the subsarcolemmal nuclei of muscle following injury.

nu•cleo•skel•e•ton (noo″kle-o-skel′ə-tən) nuclear matrix.

nu•cleo•some (noo′kle-o-sōm) [*nucleo-* + *-some*] the primary structural unit of eukaryotic chromatin; a complex of histone and DNA seen with the electron microscope as one of the "beads on a string" characteristic of the partially unfolded chromatin in low ionic strength buffer. It comprises a segment of approximately 146 base pairs of DNA wrapped twice around an octamer core of two each of the histones H2A, H2B, H3, and H4, and is connected to each adjacent nucleosome by a short linker DNA segment. The nucleosomes are further compacted into a 30-nm diameter fiber, the structure of which remains controversial; the classic model describes it as a helical solenoid (q.v.).

nu•cleo•ti•dase (noo″kle-o-ti′dās) 1. [EC 3.1.3.31] an enzyme of the hydrolase class that catalyzes the cleavage of a nucleotide to a nucleoside and orthophosphate. 2. any of several enzymes catalyzing this reaction, individual enzymes being named for their specificities (e.g., 5′-nucleotidase, polynucleotide 3′-phosphatase).

5′-nu•cleo•ti•dase (noo″kle-o-ti′dās) [EC 3.1.3.5] a membrane-bound, cytoplasmic nucleotidase specifically cleaving phosphate from the 5′ position of nucleotides to yield nucleosides. The enzyme acts on a wide range of 5′-nucleotides and the reaction is part of the main nucleotide degradation pathway.

nu•cleo•tide (noo′kle-o-tīd) a phosphate ester of a nucleoside, particularly the 5′-phosphate of a pyrimidine or purine in *N*-glycosidic linkage with ribose or deoxyribose, as occurs in nucleic acid.

cyclic n's nucleotides in which the phosphate group forms a ring, as in AMP and GMP.

nu•cleo•tid•yl (noo″kle-o-tid′əl) a nucleotide residue.

nu•cleo•tid•yl•trans•fer•ase (noo″kle-o-tid′əl-trans′fər-ās) [EC 2.7.7] any member of a sub-subclass of enzymes of the transferase class that catalyze the transfer of a nucleotidyl group from a nucleoside di- or triphosphate donor group to an acceptor group.

nu•cleo•tox•in (noo′kle-o-tok″sin) 1. a toxin from cell nuclei. 2. a toxin that affects cell nuclei.

nu•cle•us (noo′kle-əs) gen. and pl. *nu′clei* [L., dim. of *nux* nut] 1. the central core of a body or object. 2. cell nucleus: a spheroid body within a eukaryotic cell, separated from the cytoplasm by the nuclear envelope (which is penetrated by pores to allow communication with the cytoplasm), and containing chromatin, a nucleolus or nucleoli, and nucleoplasm. In the nucleus the cell's genetic information is stored on the chromosomes and RNA transcription and processing occur. 3. [TA] a group of nerve cells ordinarily located within the central nervous system and bearing a direct relationship to the fibers of a particular tract or system. 4. in organic chemistry, the combination of atoms forming the central element or basic framework of the molecule of a specific compound or class of compounds. 5. see *atomic n.* See illustration on page 1304.

Nucleus

Descriptions of anatomic structures are given on TA terms, and include anglicized names of specific nuclei.

abducens n., n. abdu′cens n. nervi abducentis.
n. of abducens nerve n. nervi abducentis.
nu′clei accesso′rii ner′vi oculomoto′rii [TA] accessory nuclei of oculomotor nerve: a collection of small cells located dorsal to the upper part of the somatic groups of the oculomotor nuclear complex, comprising the parasympathetic outflow via the ciliary ganglion to the ciliary muscle and sphincter pupillae of the eye; called also *Edinger* or *Edinger-Westphal nuclei.*
accessory n. of anterior column of spinal cord n. nervi accessorii.
accessory basal amygdaloid n. a nucleus in the basolateral part of the amygdaloid body.
accessory cuneate n. n. cuneatus accessorius.
n. of accessory nerve n. nervi accessorii.
accessory oculomotor nuclei, accessory nuclei of oculomotor nerve nuclei accessorii nervi oculomotorii.
accessory olivary n., dorsal n. olivaris accessorius posterior.
accessory olivary n., medial n. olivaris accessorius medialis.
accessory olivary n., posterior n. olivaris accessorius posterior.
accessory n. of ventral column of spinal cord n. nervi accessorii.
n. accum′bens [TA], **n. accum′bens sep′ti** a collection of pleomorphic cells in the caudal part of the base of the anterior horn of the lateral ventricle internal to the olfactory tubercle, lying between the head of the caudate nucleus and the anterior perforated substance.
acoustic nuclei, nuclei of acoustic nerve vestibulocochlear nuclei.
n. ambi′guus [TA] ambiguous nucleus: the nucleus of origin of motor fibers of the vagus and glossopharyngeal nerves that supply the striated muscles of the larynx and pharynx. It consists of an intermittent cell column in the middle of the lateral funiculus of the medulla oblongata, between the caudal end of the medulla and the level of exit of the glossopharyngeal nerve.
n. amyg′dalae corpus amygdaloideum.
n. amyg′dalae centra′lis [TA] central amygdaloid nucleus: a nucleus in the corticomedial part of the amygdaloid body, providing the major relay for projections from the amygdala to the brainstem and also receiving numerous return projections.
n. amyg′dalae cortica′lis [TA] cortical amygdaloid nucleus: a nucleus in the corticomedial part of the amygdaloid body.
n. amyg′dalae latera′lis [TA] lateral amygdaloid nucleus: a nucleus in the basolateral part of the amygdaloid body.
n. amyg′dalae media′lis [TA] medial amygdaloid nucleus: a nucleus in the corticomedial part of the amygdaloid body.
amygdaloid n. corpus amygdaloideum.
amygdaloid n., basal a nucleus in the basolateral part of the amygdaloid body.
amygdaloid n., central n. amygdalae centralis.
amygdaloid n., cortical n. amygdalae corticalis.
amygdaloid n., lateral n. amygdalae lateralis.
amygdaloid n., medial n. amygdalae medialis.
n. an′sae lenticula′ris [TA], **n. of ansa lenticularis** a collection of neurons in the ansa lenticularis as it curves around the medial edge of the globus pallidus.
n. ante′rior hypotha′lami [TA] anterior hypothalamic nucleus: a group of neuron cell bodies in the anterior hypothalamic region.
anterior medial n. of oculomotor nerve n. anteromedialis nervi oculomotorii.
anterior olfactory n. n. olfactorius anterior.
anterior nuclei of thalamus, nu′clei anterio′res tha′lami [TA] the three nuclei in the anterior part of the thalamus: the *nucleus anteroventralis, nucleus anterodorsalis,* and *nucleus anteromedialis.* Together, they receive connections from the mammillary body and fornix and project fibers to the cingulate cortex.
n. anterodorsa′lis tha′lami [TA] anterodorsal nucleus of thalamus: one of the three anterior nuclei of the thalamus.
anterolateral n. of spinal cord, n. anterolatera′lis medul′lae spina′lis [TA] a group of nerve cells in the gray substance of the anterolateral region of the anterior column of the spinal cord; called also *ventrolateral n. of spinal cord.*
anteromedial n. of spinal cord n. anteromedialis medullae spinalis.
anteromedial n. of thalamus n. anteromedialis thalami.
n. anteromedia′lis medul′lae spina′lis [TA] anteromedial nucleus of spinal cord: a group of nerve cells in the gray matter of the anteromedial region of the anterior column of the spinal cord; called also *ventromedial n. of spinal cord.*
n. anteromedia′lis ner′vi oculomoto′rii [TA] anterior medial nucleus of oculomotor nerve: ventrally placed cells in the lateral part of the oculomotor nuclear complex *(nucleus nervi oculomotorii);* they are distinct from the dorsally placed cells in the middle third of the complex and have a somatic motor function. Called also *ventral medial n. of oculomotor nerve* and *ventromedial n. of oculomotor nuclear complex.*
n. anteromedia′lis tha′lami [TA] anteromedial nucleus of thalamus: one of the three anterior nuclei of the thalamus.
n. anteroventra′lis tha′lami [TA] anteroventral nucleus of thalamus: one of the three anterior nuclei of the thalamus.
arcuate n. of hypothalamus n. arcuatus hypothalami.
arcuate n. of medulla oblongata n. arcuatus medullae oblongatae.
n. arcua′tus hypotha′lami [TA] arcuate nucleus of hypothalamus: a nucleus of nerve cells in the posterior hypothalamic region, extending into the median eminence and almost entirely surrounding the base of the infundibulum. Called also *infundibular n., n. infundibularis* [TA alternative] and *n. semilunaris* [TA alternative].
n. arcua′tus medul′lae oblonga′tae [TA] arcuate nucleus of medulla oblongata: one of the group of small, irregular areas of gray substance found on the ventromedial aspect of the pyramid of the medulla oblongata.
nu′clei a′reae H, H_1, H_2 nuclei campi perizonalis.
atomic n. the central core of an atom, constituting almost all of its mass but only a small part of its volume, and composed of protons and neutrons, the protons being positively charged and their number (atomic number) being fixed for all the atoms of each element and equal to the number of the orbiting electrons. The neutrons, which bear no charge, may vary in number, accounting for the isotopes of an element.
auditory nuclei, nuclei of auditory nerve strictly speaking, the cochlear nuclei (nuclei cochleares), although the term is often used more loosely to denote the entire group of vestibulocochlear nuclei.
autonomic oculomotor nuclei nuclei accessorii nervi oculomotorii.
Balbiani n. yolk n.
Barrington n. pontine micturition center.
basal nuclei nuclei basales.
basal n. of Meynert, basal n. of telencephalon n. basalis telencephali.
nu′clei basa′les [TA] basal nuclei: subcortical nuclei in the inferior part of the cerebral hemispheres, lying in close relation to the internal capsule. Although various subcortical nuclei have traditionally been considered to be part of the basal nuclei, in official anatomical terminology the term is now restricted to the corpus striatum (nucleus caudatus and nucleus lentiformis). Called also *basal ganglia.*
n. basalis of Meynert n. basalis telencephali.
n. basa′lis telence′phali [TA] basal nucleus of telencephalon: a group of neurons in the basal forebrain that has wide projections to the neocortex and is rich in acetylcholine and choline acetyltransferase. It undergoes degeneration in paralysis agitans and Alzheimer disease. Called also *Meynert n.*
Béclard n. a vascular lentil-shaped center of ossification seen in the cartilage of the lower epiphysis of the femur during the latter part of fetal life.
bed n. of stria terminalis n. striae terminalis.
Bekhterev (Bechterew) n. n. vestibularis superior.
Blumenau n. n. cuneatus accessorius.
n. of Burdach column n. cuneatus.
n. caeru′leus [TA] a compact aggregation of pigmented neurons subjacent to the locus caeruleus; it is sometimes considered one of the medial reticular nuclei. Rostrally, it ends in the vicinity of the mesencephalic nucleus of the trigeminal nerve. Written also *n. ceruleus* and *n. coeruleus.*
n. cam′pi dorsa′lis [TA] nucleus of dorsal field: the group of nerve cell bodies among the fibers of field H_1 of Forel. See also *nuclei campi perizonalis.*

Nucleus *Continued*

n. cam′pi media′lis [TA] nucleus of medial field: any of the groups of neurons scattered along the caudomedial border of the zona incerta in field H of Forel (prerubral field). Called also *n. of prerubral field* and *n. of tegmental field.* See also *nuclei campi perizonalis.*
nu′clei cam′pi perizona′lis [TA] nuclei of perizonal field: the group of nuclei in the ventral thalamus comprising the nucleus of the prerubral field (field H of Forel) and neurons scattered along the thalamic and lenticular fasciculi in fields H_1 and H_2 of Forel.
n. cam′pi ventra′lis [TA] nucleus of ventral field: the group of nerve cell bodies among the fibers of field H_2 of Forel. See also *nuclei campi perizonalis.*
caudal n., central n. caudalis centralis.
nuclei of caudal colliculus nuclei colliculi inferioris.
n. cauda′lis centra′lis central caudal nucleus: an unpaired collection of cells in the caudal third of the oculomotor nuclear complex (nucleus nervi oculomotorii [TA]), located in the median raphe somewhat dorsal to the lateral nuclei.
caudate n., n. cauda′tus [TA] an elongated, arched gray mass closely related to the lateral ventricle throughout its entire extent and consisting of a head, body, and tail. The caudate nucleus and putamen form a functional unit (the neostriatum) of the corpus striatum.
cell n., cellular n. nucleus (def. 2).
central n. of spinal cord n. centralis medullae spinalis.
central lateral n. of thalamus n. centralis lateralis thalami.
central medial n. of thalamus n. centralis medialis thalami.
n. centra′lis latera′lis tha′lami [TA] central lateral nucleus of thalamus: one of the smaller intralaminar nuclei of the dorsal thalamus, situated in the dorsal part of the internal medullary lamina.
n. centra′lis media′lis tha′lami [TA] medial central nucleus of thalamus: one of the smaller intralaminar nuclei, situated medially in the internal medullary lamina.
n. centra′lis medul′lae spina′lis [TA] central nucleus of spinal cord: a group of nerve cells in the gray substance in the central region of the anterior column of the spinal cord.
n. centromedia′nus tha′lami [TA] centromedian nucleus of thalamus: the largest and most caudal of the intralaminar nuclei of the dorsal thalamus; its main connections are with the corpus striatum.
cerebellar n., lateral n. lateralis cerebelli. See also *n. dentatus.*
cerebellar n., medial n. medialis cerebelli.
nu′clei cerebel′li [TA] cerebellar nuclei: four accumulations of gray substance embedded in the white substance of the cerebellum, comprising the nucleus dentatus, nucleus emboliformis, nucleus globosus, and nucleus fastigii; called also *intracerebellar nuclei* and *roof nuclei* (q.v.).
n. ceru′leus n. caeruleus.
cervical n., lateral n. cervicalis lateralis.
n. cervica′lis latera′lis [TA] lateral cervical nucleus: a small group of cells in the lateral funiculus of the first and second cervical segments of the spinal cord, comprising a relay station in a spinocervicothalamic path.
cholane n. a cyclopentenophenanthrene structure forming the basis of certain compounds found in bile acids; sterols; toad poisons; heart glycones such as digitalis, strophanthus, and ouabain; sex hormones; and various carcinogenic hydrocarbons.

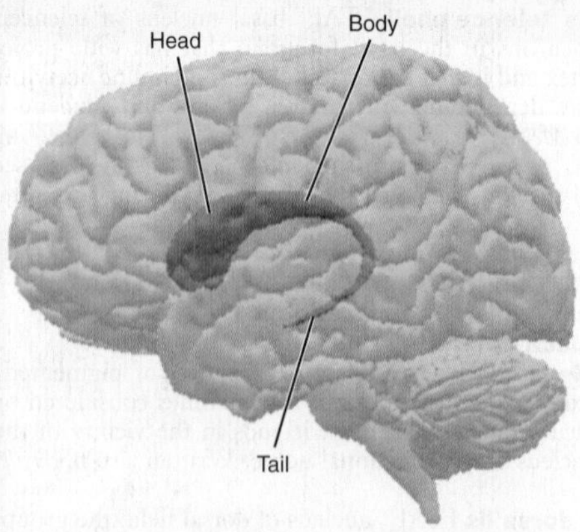

■ Nucleus caudatus (caudate nucleus) in a lateral view of the left side of the brain.

Clarke n. n. thoracicus posterior.
cleavage n. segmentation n.
cochlear nuclei nuclei cochleares.
cochlear n., anterior n. cochlearis anterior.
cochlear n., dorsal, cochlear n., posterior n. cochlearis posterior.
cochlear n., ventral n. cochlearis anterior.
nuclei of cochlear nerve nuclei cochleares.
nu′clei cochlea′res [TA] cochlear nuclei: the two nuclei, *anterior* and *posterior,* partly encircling the restiform body at the junction of the medulla oblongata and the pons, in which the fibers of the cochlear part of the vestibulocochlear nerve terminate; called also *nuclei of cochlear nerve.*
n. cochlea′ris ante′rior [TA] anterior cochlear nucleus: the anterior of the two cochlear nuclei; located on the anterolateral aspect of the restiform body; it receives the larger, ascending branches of the cochlear nerve. Called also *ventral cochlear n.*
n. cochlea′ris poste′rior [TA] posterior cochlear nucleus: the posterior of the two cochlear nuclei, located on the dorsal aspect of the restiform body; it forms an eminence (the *auditory tubercle*) on the lateral part of the vestibular area of the floor of the fourth ventricle. Called also *dorsal cochlear n.*
n. coeru′leus n. caeruleus.
nu′clei colli′culi inferio′ris [TA] nuclei of inferior colliculus: the large oval-shaped group of nerve cells that make up most of the substance of the inferior colliculus. Called also *nuclei of caudal colliculus.*
n. commis′surae posterio′ris [TA] nucleus of posterior commissure: a nucleus of the rostral midbrain tegmentum, located adjacent to the posterior commissure and near the oculomotor nucleus.
n. commissura′lis ner′vi va′gi [TA] commissural nucleus of vagus nerve: a group of noradrenergic neurons that encloses the dorsolateral aspect of the nucleus of the hypoglossal nerve and approaches the ependymal floor of the fourth ventricle.
n. commissura′lis rhomboida′lis [TA] rhomboid nucleus: one of the median nuclei of the thalamus, bordering the third ventricle and ventral to the central medial nucleus; see *nuclei mediani thalami.* Called also *n. rhomboidalis.*
conjugation n. fertilization n.
nu′clei cor′poris genicula′ti media′lis [TA] medial geniculate nuclei: nuclei within the medial geniculate body, composed of ventral *(n. ventralis corporis geniculati medialis),* medial *(n. medialis magnocellularis corporis geniculati medialis),* and dorsal *(n. dorsalis corporis geniculati medialis)* nuclei that receive ascending auditory and some nonauditory fibers and project to the auditory cortex. Called also *nuclei of medial geniculate body.*
nu′clei cor′poris trapezoi′dei [TA] nuclei of trapezoid body: groups of nerve cell bodies of the superior olivary complex, lying within the fibers of the trapezoid body. The posterior receive cochlear fibers and contribute to the formation of the trapezoid body and lateral lemniscus while the anterior are mingled with the fibers of the trapezoid body and contribute to the lateral lemniscus.
n. of cranial nerve n. nervi cranialis.
cuneate n. n. cuneatus.
cuneate n., lateral n. cuneatus accessorius.
n. cunea′tus [TA] cuneate nucleus: a nucleus in the medulla oblongata at the rostral end of the fasciculus cuneatus, in which the fibers of this fasciculus synapse; the cells project to the thalamus via the medial lemniscus.
n. cunea′tus accesso′rius [TA] accessory cuneate nucleus: a group of nerve cells lying lateral to the nucleus cuneatus that relay impulses from upper limb fibers in the fasciculus cuneatus to the cerebellum (rostral spinocerebellar tract) via posterior external arcuate fibers and the inferior cerebellar peduncle; called also *lateral cuneate n.*
n. cuneifor′mis [TA] cuneiform nucleus: a large nucleus in the mesencephalon representing a widening and continuation of the tracts from the medial column reticular nuclei.
Darkshevich n. a small nucleus dorsal to the medial longitudinal fasciculus in the central gray matter at the rostral end of the cerebral aqueduct; it is believed to receive fibers from the fasciculus and from the superior colliculus.
daughter n. a new cell nucleus arising from an existing nucleus by division.

Deiters n. n. vestibularis lateralis.
dental n. pulpa dentis.
dentate n. n. dentatus. See also *n. lateralis cerebelli.*
n. denta′tus [TA] dentate nucleus: the largest and most lateral of the cerebellar nuclei, lying in the white matter of the cerebellum just lateral to the emboliform nucleus, and receiving Purkinje cell fibers primarily from the lateral cortical zone; its axons form most of the superior cerebellar peduncle and project chiefly to the contralateral red nucleus and thalamus, and also to the reticular and vestibular nuclei and inferior olive. It is the term preferred in official terminology when considering humans, and is frequently also used to describe nonhuman primates. Called also *lateral cerebellar n.* See also *n. lateralis cerebelli.*
diploid n. a cell nucleus containing the number of chromosomes typical of the somatic cells of the particular species.
dorsal n. of Clarke n. thoracicus posterior.
dorsal column nuclei the nucleus cuneatus and nucleus gracilis, which are at the upper end of the dorsal column of the spinal cord. Called also *posterior column nuclei.*
n. of dorsal field n. campi dorsalis.
dorsal lateral n. of thalamus n. dorsalis lateralis thalami.
dorsal n. of medial geniculate body n. dorsalis corporis geniculati medialis.
dorsal medial n. of thalamus n. mediodorsalis thalami.
dorsal n. of oculomotor nerve n. dorsalis nervi oculomotorii.
dorsal raphe n. n. raphes posterior.
dorsal nuclei of thalamus nuclei dorsales thalami.
dorsal n. of vagus nerve n. posterior nervi vagi.
n. dorsa′lis cor′poris genicula′ti latera′lis [TA] dorsal lateral geniculate nucleus: the large dorsal part of the lateral geniculate nucleus, consisting of six concentrically arranged cell layers in a dome-shaped mound, which receive crossed and uncrossed fibers of the optic tract that are connected with the visual cortex. See also *n. ventralis corporis geniculati lateralis.*
n. dorsa′lis cor′poris genicula′ti media′lis [TA] dorsal nucleus of medial geniculate body: the larger, dorsal part of the medial geniculate nucleus, receiving ascending auditory fibers from the inferior colliculus as well as afferent projections from some nonauditory areas of the brainstem, and projecting to the auditory cortex.
n. dorsa′lis hypotha′lami [TA] dorsal hypothalamic nucleus: a nerve cell nucleus situated in the dorsal portion of the intermediate hypothalamic region.
n. dorsa′lis latera′lis tha′lami [TA] lateral dorsal nucleus of thalamus: a nucleus in the dorsal part of the thalamus and slightly medial to the internal medullary lamina and having extensive connections with the cerebral cortex.
n. dorsa′lis ner′vi oculomoto′rii [TA] dorsal nucleus of oculomotor nerve: a group of dorsally placed cells in the lateral part of the oculomotor nuclear complex (nucleus nervi oculomotorii); they are distinct from the ventrally placed cells in the middle third of the complex and have a somatic motor function. Called also *posterior n. of oculomotor nerve.*
n. dorsa′lis ner′vi va′gi TA alternative for *n. posterior nervi vagi.*
nu′clei dorsa′les tha′lami [TA] dorsal nuclei of thalamus: the nuclei forming the posterior end of the dorsal thalamus, including the nucleus dorsalis lateralis and nucleus lateralis posterior.
dorsolateral n. of oculomotor nuclear complex n. dorsalis nervi oculomotorii.
dorsolateral n. of spinal cord, n. dorsolatera′lis medul′lae spina′lis n. posterolateralis medullae spinalis.
dorsomedial n. of intermediate hypothalamus n. dorsomedialis hypothalamicae intermediae.
dorsomedial n. of thalamus n. mediodorsalis thalami.
dorsomedial n. of spinal cord n. posteromedialis medullae spinalis.
n. dorsomedia′lis hypothala′micae interme′diae [TA] dorsomedial nucleus of intermediate hypothalamus: a group of nerve cell bodies found in the dorsal part of the intermediate hypothalamic region.
droplet nuclei small pathogen-containing particles of respiratory secretions expelled into the air by coughing, which are reduced by evaporation to small, dry particles that can remain airborne for long periods; this is one mechanism for airborne infection (droplet infection) of disease.
drumstick n. a leukocyte nucleus that has a drumstick.
Edinger nuclei, Edinger-Westphal nuclei nuclei accessorii nervi oculomotorii.
egg n. n. of oocyte.
n. embolifor′mis [TA] emboliform nucleus: a small cerebellar nucleus that lies between the dentate nucleus and globose nucleus and contributes to the superior cerebellar peduncles. It is the term preferred in official terminology when considering humans, and is frequently also used to describe nonhuman primates. Cf. *n. interpositus inferior.*
enamel n. in the cap stage of odontogenesis, a slight indentation in the outer dental epithelium of a developing tooth, in the end of the enamel cord; a temporary structure that disappears before enamel formation begins.
n. endopeduncula′ris [TA] endopeduncular nucleus: a small nucleus in the internal capsule of the hypothalamus adjacent to the medial edge of the globus pallidus.
n. of facial nerve n. nervi facialis.
fastigial n. n. fastigii.
n. fasti′gii [TA] fastigial nucleus: the most medial of the cerebellar nuclei, near the midline in the roof of the fourth ventricle; it projects to the pons and medulla oblongata, chiefly to the vestibular nuclei. It is the term preferred in official terminology when considering humans, and is frequently also used to describe nonhuman primates. Cf. *n. medialis cerebelli.*
fertilization n. the nucleus produced by fusion of the male and female pronuclei in the fertilized oocyte; called also *conjugation n., zygote n.,* and *synkaryon.*
n. gelatino′sus n. pulposus.
geniculate n., dorsal lateral n. dorsalis corporis geniculati lateralis.
geniculate n., lateral a nucleus within the lateral geniculate body, composed of a small ventral part (n. ventralis corporis geniculati lateralis) and large dorsal part (n. dorsalis corporis geniculati lateralis).
geniculate nuclei, medial nuclei corporis geniculati medialis.
geniculate n., ventral lateral n. ventralis corporis geniculati lateralis.
n. genicula′tus latera′lis lateral geniculate nucleus.
nu′clei genicula′ti media′les nuclei corporis geniculati medialis.
germ n., germinal n. pronucleus.
gigantocellular n., n. gigantocellula′ris [TA] either of a symmetrical pair of large medial column reticular nuclei located in the superior part of the medulla oblongata and the posterior part of the pons, lateral to the nucleus raphes magnus and inferior to the caudal pontine reticular nucleus; its neurons are serotoninergic. Called also *gigantocellular intermediate reticular n.* and *gigantocellular reticular n.*
gingival n. a part of the cerebellum in the third and fourth months of fetal life.
n. globo′sus [TA] globose nucleus: a cerebellar nucleus that lies between the emboliform nucleus and the nucleus fastigii and projects its fibers via the superior cerebellar peduncle (brachium conjunctivum). It is the term preferred in official terminology when considering

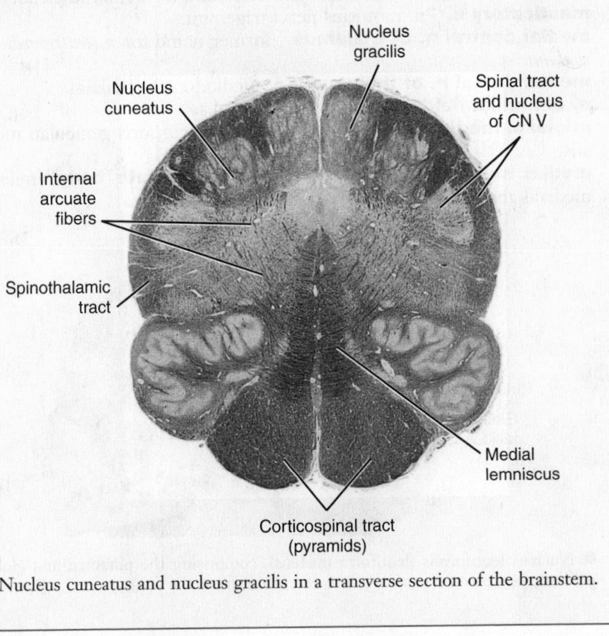

■ Nucleus cuneatus and nucleus gracilis in a transverse section of the brainstem.

humans, and is frequently also used to describe nonhuman primates. Cf. *n. interpositus posterior.*
nuclei of glossopharyngeal nerve nuclei nervi glossopharyngei.
Goll n. n. gracilis.
gonad n. micronucleus.
n. gra′cilis [TA] gracile nucleus: a nucleus in the medulla oblongata at the rostral end of the fasciculus gracilis of the cord, in which the fibers of the fasciculus gracilis synapse; the cells project to the thalamus via the medial lemniscus. Called also *Goll n.* See illustration at *nucleus cuneatus.*
habenular n., lateral n. habenularis lateralis.
habenular n., medial n. habenularis medialis.
n. habenula′ris latera′lis [TA] lateral habenular nucleus: the more dispersed of the two nerve cell groups situated deep to the habenular trigone; it receives fibers from the stria medullaris thalami and projects to the raphe nuclei, reticular formation of mesencephalon, pars compacta of substantia nigra, and hypothalamus and basal forebrain.
n. habenula′ris media′lis [TA] medial habenular nucleus: the more densely packed of the two nerve cell groups situated deep to the habenular trigone; it receives fibers from the stria medullaris thalami and projects to the interpeduncular nucleus of the midbrain.
haploid n. a cell nucleus containing half of the number of chromosomes typical of the somatic cells of a particular species.
hypoglossal n., n. of hypoglossal nerve n. nervi hypoglossi.
hypothalamic n., anterior n. anterior hypothalami.
hypothalamic n., dorsal n. dorsalis hypothalami.
hypothalamic n., dorsomedial n. dorsomedialis hypothalamicae intermediae.
hypothalamic n., posterior n. posterior hypothalami.
hypothalamic n., ventrolateral, hypothalamic n., ventromedial n. ventromedialis hypothalami.
nuclei of inferior colliculus nuclei colliculi inferioris.
inferior n. of trigeminal nerve n. spinalis nervi trigemini.
infundibular n. nucleus arcuatus hypothalami.
n. infundibula′ris TA alternative for *n. arcuatus hypothalami.*
n. intercala′tus [TA] intercalated nucleus: a group of nerve cells between the dorsal nucleus of the vagus nerve and the nucleus of the hypoglossal nerve, forming part of the perihypoglossal nuclear complex; called also *Staderini n.*
n. intermediolatera′lis medul′lae spina′lis [TA] intermediolateral nucleus of spinal cord: a nucleus situated in the substantia intermedia lateralis of thoracic and upper lumbar levels of the spinal cord, within the lateral horn, and whose cells give rise to the preganglionic sympathetic outflow.
n. intermediomedia′lis medul′lae spina′lis [TA] intermediomedial nucleus of spinal cord: a nucleus composed of scattered cells in the substantia intermedia centralis, medial to the nucleus intermediolateralis; it is most prominent in the cervical spinal cord and is thought to be propriospinal in its connections.
n. interpeduncula′ris [TA] interpeduncular nucleus: a nucleus situated between the cerebral peduncles immediately dorsal to the interpeduncular fossa, which receives the fasciculus retroflexus.
interposed n., anterior n. interpositus anterior.
interposed n., posterior n. interpositus posterior.
n. interpo′situs ante′rior [TA] n. emboliformis; the term is preferred in official terminology when considering nonprimate mammals, and is occasionally used to refer to primates.
n. interpo′situs poste′rior [TA] n. globosus; the term is preferred in official terminology when considering nonprimate mammals, and is occasionally used to refer to primates.
interstitial n. of Cajal nucleus interstitialis.
n. interstitia′lis [TA] interstitial nucleus: a nucleus at the rostral end of the medial longitudinal fasciculus in the mesencephalic tegmentum; its chief connections are reciprocal with vestibular nuclei and it also projects to the spinal cord.
intracerebellar nuclei nuclei cerebelli.
intralaminar nuclei of thalamus, nu′clei intralamina′res tha′lami [TA] the nuclei within the internal medullary lamina of the thalamus, lying between the medial dorsal nucleus above and the lateral posterior nucleus below; included are the centromedian, paracentral, parafascicular, central lateral, and central medial nuclei.
Kölliker-Fuse n. n. subparabrachialis.
lateral dorsal n. of thalamus n. dorsalis lateralis thalami.
n. of lateral geniculate body lateral geniculate nucleus.
nuclei of lateral lemniscus nuclei lemnisci lateralis.
lateral n. of mammillary body n. mammillaris lateralis.
n. of lateral olfactory stria a nucleus in the corticomedial part of the amygdaloid body.
lateral posterior n. of thalamus n. lateralis posterior thalami.
lateral ventral nuclei of thalamus nuclei ventrales laterales thalami.
n. latera′lis cerebel′li [TA] n. dentatus; the term is preferred in official terminology when considering nonprimate mammals, and is occasionally used to refer to primates. Called also *dentate n.*
n. latera′lis dorsa′lis tha′lami [TA] n. dorsalis lateralis thalami.
n. latera′lis poste′rior tha′lami [TA] lateral posterior nucleus of thalamus: a nucleus in the ventral lateral part of the thalamus having major connections with the cingulate gyrus.
nu′clei lemnis′ci latera′lis [TA] nuclei of lateral lemniscus: several diffuse cell groups interposed in the course of the lateral lemniscus through the pons.
n. of lens n. lentis.
lenticular n. n. lentiformis.
n. lentifor′mis [TA] lentiform nucleus: the part of the corpus striatum somewhat resembling a biconvex lens, divided into an external, larger, lateral part (putamen) and an internal, smaller, medial part (globus pallidus). The globus in turn is divided into lateral and medial segments by the internal medullary lamina; the medial segment may be subdivided into lateral and medial parts by the accessory medullary lamina. Called also *lenticular n.*
n. len′tis [TA] nucleus of lens: the harder internal part of the lens of the eye.
linear n., inferior n. linearis inferioris.
linear n., intermediate n. linearis intermedius.
linear n., superior n. linearis superior.
n. linea′ris inferio′ris [TA] inferior linear nucleus: a raphe nucleus located in the mesencephalon.
n. linea′ris interme′dius [TA] intermediate linear nucleus: a raphe nucleus located in the mesencephalon.
n. linea′ris supe′rior [TA] superior linear nucleus: a raphe nucleus located in the mesencephalon.
n. of Luys n. subthalamicus.
magnus raphe n. n. raphes magnus.
n. mammilla′ris latera′lis [TA] lateral nucleus of mammillary body: the smaller of the two main nuclei of the mammillary body, which receive fibers from the basal olfactory areas and the fornix, and project to the thalamus and midbrain via mammillothalamic and mammillotegmental fasciculi.
n. mammilla′ris media′lis [TA] medial nucleus of mammillary body: the larger, predominant mass of cells, forming the medial of the two main nuclei of the mammillary body, which receive fibers from the basal olfactory areas and the fornix, and project to the thalamus and midbrain via mammillothalamic and mammillotegmental fasciculi.
masticatory n. n. motorius nervi trigemini.
medial central n. of thalamus former name for *n. centromedianus thalami.*
medial dorsal n. of thalamus n. mediodorsalis thalami.
n. of medial field nucleus campi medialis.
nuclei of medial geniculate body nuclei corporis geniculati medialis.
medial magnocellular n. of medial geniculate body nucleus medialis magnocellularis corporis geniculati medialis.

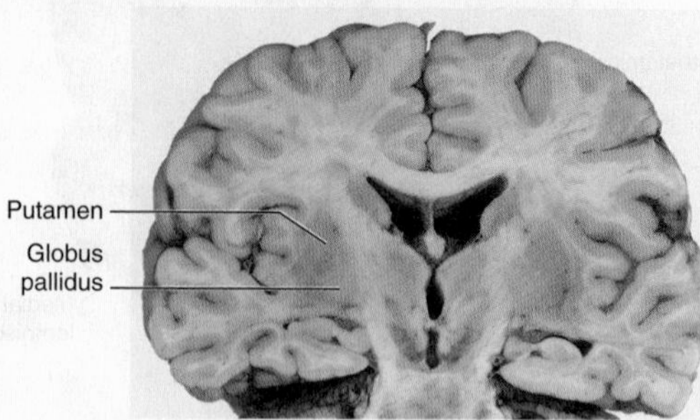

■ Nucleus lentiformis (lentiform nucleus), comprising the putamen and globus pallidus, in a coronal section of the cerebrum, from the front.

medial n. of mammillary body n. mammillaris medialis.
medial nuclei of thalamus nuclei mediales thalami.
n. media′lis cerebel′li [TA] n. fastigii; the term is preferred in official terminology when considering nonprimate mammals, and is occasionally used to refer to primates.
n. media′lis magnocellula′ris cor′poris genicula′ti media′lis [TA] the medial of the medial geniculate nuclei; it receives afferent projections from both auditory and nonauditory neurons of the brainstem, from the fibers of the inferior colliculus and deep layers of the superior colliculus, and projects to the auditory cortex and adjacent insular and opercular fields.
nu′clei media′les tha′lami [TA] medial nuclei of thalamus: groups of nerve cells lying between the internal medullary lamina laterally and projecting toward the ependymal lining of the third ventricle medially; included are the large nucleus mediodorsalis and a series of smaller nuclei of uncertain significance and connections.
median raphe n. n. raphes medianus.
median nuclei of thalamus nuclei mediani thalami.
nu′clei media′ni tha′lami [TA] median nuclei of thalamus: small groups of nonspecific nerve cells scattered in the periventricular gray substance, separating the medial part of the thalamus from the ependyma of the third ventricle, and partly forming the interthalamic adhesion when this structure is present; included in the group are the anterior and posterior paraventricular nuclei, nucleus parataenialis, nucleus commissuralis rhomboidalis, and nucleus reuniens.
n. mediodorsa′lis tha′lami [TA] medial dorsal nucleus of thalamus: the largest of the medial nuclei of the thalamus, having a rostral magnocellular part and a caudolateral parvocellular part, both of which make extensive intrathalamic connections with most of the other thalamic nuclei and with the frontal and temporal lobes. Called also *dorsomedial n. of thalamus.*
n. of mesencephalic tract of trigeminal nerve, mesencephalic trigeminal n., mesencephalic n. of trigeminal nerve n. mesencephalicus nervi trigemini.
n. mesencepha′licus ner′vi trige′mini [TA] mesencephalic n. of trigeminal nerve: one of the nuclei of the trigeminal nerve, consisting of a slender column of cells in the lateral central gray matter of the superior part of the fourth ventral and cerebral aqueduct. It is the only central nervous system site of primary sensory neurons; its cells resemble posterior root ganglion cells. The peripheral processes of the cells, which form the mesencephalic tract, carry proprioceptive impulses; the central processes have widespread cerebellar and brainstem connections, including the motor nucleus of the trigeminal nerve.
Meynert n. n. basalis telencephali.
midline nuclei of thalamus nuclei mediani thalami.
Monakow n. n. cuneatus accessorius.
motor n. any collection of cells of the central nervous system giving origin to motor fibers of a nerve.
motor n. of facial nerve n. nervi facialis.
n. moto′rius ner′vi trige′mini [TA] motor nucleus of trigeminal nerve: the nucleus of origin of the motor fibers of the trigeminal nerve, located in the dorsolateral part of the pons, just medial to the principal sensory nucleus and the entering sensory root.
n. ner′vi abducen′tis [TA] nucleus of abducens nerve: the nucleus of origin of the abducens nerve; it lies in the lower part of the pons internal to the facial colliculus in the floor of the fourth ventricle; fibers from the facial nucleus form a caudal-to-rostral loop about the nucleus. Called also *abducens n.* and *n. abducens.*
n. ner′vi accesso′rii [TA] nucleus of accessory nerve: an irregularly shaped group of nerve cells giving rise to the accessory nerve; found in the upper six cervical spinal cord segments, at the anterior border of the anterior column of the spinal cord in an intermediate or central position. Called also *accessory n. of anterior column of spinal cord.*
n. ner′vi crania′lis [TA] nucleus of cranial nerve: any of the nerve cells in the central nervous system that give rise to, or transmit or receive impulses from, the motor and sensory components of the cranial nerves.
n. ner′vi facia′lis [TA] nucleus of facial nerve: the nucleus of origin of the motor fibers of the facial nerve, which innervate the muscles of facial expression; the nucleus lies in the ventrolateral part of the lower pons, and its emerging fibers form a caudal-to-rostral loop about the nucleus of the abducens nerve. Called also *motor n. of facial nerve.*
nu′clei ner′vi glossopharyn′gei nuclei of glossopharyngeal nerve: the nuclei of origin and termination of the glossopharyngeal nerve, located in the medulla oblongata, comprising the inferior salivatory nucleus, the rostral part of the nucleus ambiguus, and the nuclei of solitary tract.
n. ner′vi hypoglos′si [TA] nucleus of hypoglossal nerve: the nucleus of origin of the hypoglossal nerve, forming a column in the central gray matter internal to the hypoglossal trigone from below the level of the inferior olive to the upper part of the medulla oblongata. Called also *hypoglossal n.*
n. ner′vi oculomoto′rii [TA] nucleus of oculomotor nerve: a nuclear complex that is the origin of the fibers of the oculomotor nerve, situated in the tegmentum of the mesencephalon immediately ventral to the central gray matter, between the medial longitudinal fasciculi. The complex comprises larger paired dorsolateral and ventromedial somatic groups (see *n. dorsalis nervi oculomotorii* and *n. anteromedialis nervi oculomotorii*) as well as scattered small nuclei that have a parasympathetic function. Innervation of the superior rectus of one eye originates in the contralateral oculomotor nucleus; the other elements of the nucleus supply ipsilateral eye muscles via the oculomotor nerve.
n. ner′vi phre′nici [TA] nucleus of phrenic nerve: a centrally positioned group of nerve cells in the gray substance of the anterior column of the spinal cord, extending from the third to the fifth cervical segments, which innervate the diaphragm; called also *phrenic n.*
n. ner′vi puden′di [TA] nucleus of pudendal nerve: a group of somatomotor neurons in the ventral horns of the spinal cord at the S1 and S2 levels, innervating the musculature of the pelvic floor and the external urethral and external anal sphincters. Called also *Onuf n.*
n. ner′vi trochlea′ris [TA] nucleus of trochlear nerve: the nucleus of origin of the motor fibers of the trochlear nerve; it lies in the central gray matter on the dorsal surface of the medial longitudinal fasciculus in the lower part of the mesencephalon. Called also *trochlear nucleus.*
obscurus raphe n. n. raphes obscurus.
oculomotor n., n. of oculomotor nerve n. nervi oculomotorii.
n. olfacto′rius ante′rior [TA] anterior olfactory nucleus: scattered groups of neurons intermingled with the olfactory tract that run caudally from the end of the olfactory bulb; some of them receive synaptic stimuli from the fibers of the olfactory tract.
n. oliva′ris accesso′rius media′lis [TA] medial accessory olivary nucleus: the band of gray substance that lies medial to the principal olivary nucleus and projects fibers to the opposite side of the cerebellum, especially to the vermis.
n. oliva′ris accesso′rius poste′rior [TA] posterior accessory olivary nucleus: the band of cells that lies posterior to the principal olivary nucleus and projects fibers to the opposite side of the cerebellum, especially to the vermis. Called also *dorsal accessory olivary n.*
nu′clei oliva′res inferio′res TA alternative for *complexus olivaris inferior.*
n. oliva′ris principa′lis [TA] principal olivary nucleus: the convoluted nucleus constituting the main portion of the inferior olivary complex; it comprises dorsal, ventral, and lateral lamellae.
n. oliva′ris supe′rior [TA] superior olivary nucleus: a band of gray substance located laterally at the level of the pontomedullary junction superior to the inferior olivary nucleus; its fibers form the olivocochlear tract. Called also *superior olivary complex* and *cranial* or *rostral olivary n.*
olivary n. 1. complexus olivaris inferior. 2. oliva.
olivary nuclei, caudal complexus olivaris inferior.
olivary n., cranial n. oliva′ris supe′rior.
olivary n., dorsal accessory n. olivaris accessorius posterior.
olivary nuclei, inferior complexus olivaris inferior.
olivary n., posterior accessory n. olivaris accessorius posterior.
olivary n., rostral, olivary n., superior n. olivaris superior.
Onuf n., n. of Onufrowicz n. nervi pudendi.
n. of oocyte the structure within the oocyte that becomes the female pronucleus after fertilization has occurred.
n. ori′ginis [TA] nucleus of origin: any of the groups of nerve cells in the central nervous system from which arise the motor, or efferent, fibers of the cranial nerves.
pallidal raphe n. n. raphes pallidus.
parabrachial nuclei nuclei parabrachiales.
parabrachial n., lateral n. parabrachialis lateralis.
parabrachial n., medial n. parabrachialis medialis.
nu′clei parabrachia′les [TA] the nucleus parabrachialis lateralis, nucleus parabrachialis medialis, and nucleus subparabrachialis considered collectively.

n. parabrachia′lis latera′lis [TA] lateral parabrachial nucleus: either of a pair of reticular nuclei located symmetrically on the lateral aspect of the superior cerebellar peduncle in the rostral pons, extending to the level of exit of the trochlear nerve.
n. parabrachia′lis media′lis [TA] medial parabrachial nucleus: either of a pair of reticular nuclei located symmetrically on the medial aspect of the superior cerebellar peduncle in the rostral pons.
n. paracentra′lis tha′lami [TA] paracentral nucleus of thalamus: one of the smaller reticular nuclei of the dorsal thalamus, situated ventrolateral to the dorsal medial nucleus and medial to the central lateral nucleus.
n. parafascicula′ris tha′lami [TA] parafascicular nucleus of thalamus: one of the smaller reticular nuclei of the dorsal thalamus, situated medial to the centromedian nucleus and ventral to the dorsal medial nucleus.
paragigantocellular n., lateral, n. paragigantocellula′ris latera′lis [TA] either of a pair of lateral column reticular nuclei located symmetrically at the level of the facial nucleus, rostral to the nucleus retroambiguus.
paramedian n., dorsal, paramedian n., posterior n. paramedianus posterior.
n. paramedia′nus poste′rior [TA] posterior paramedian nucleus: a group of nerve cells near the posterior surface of the medulla oblongata, forming part of the perihypoglossal nuclear complex; called also *dorsal paramedian n.*
n. parasolita′rius [TA] parasolitary nucleus: an aggregation of nerve cells situated ventrolateral to the solitary nucleus.
nu′clei parasympa′thici sacra′les [TA] sacral parasympathetic nuclei: a group of nerve cells in the second through the fourth sacral segments of the spinal cord, located lateral to the central canal and central gelatinous substance, between the bases of the anterior and posterior gray columns; the cells are the source of the pelvic or sacral outflow of parasympathetic preganglionic fibers.
n. parataenia′lis tha′lami [TA], **paratenial n. of thalamus** one of the median nuclei of the thalamus, situated ventral and medial to the stria medullaris; see *nuclei mediani thalami.*
paraventricular n. of hypothalamus n. paraventricularis hypothalami.
paraventricular nuclei of thalamus nuclei paraventriculares thalami.
paraventricular n. of thalamus, anterior n. paraventricularis anterior thalami.
paraventricular n. of thalamus, posterior n. paraventricularis posterior thalami.
n. paraventricula′ris ante′rior tha′lami [TA] anterior paraventricular nucleus of thalamus: the anterior of the two nuclei paraventriculares thalami (q.v.).
n. paraventricula′ris hypotha′lami [TA] paraventricular nucleus of hypothalamus: a sharply defined band of cells in the wall of the third ventricle in the anterior hypothalamic region; many of its cells are neurosecretory in function, secreting oxytocin, which is carried to the neurohypophysis (posterior pituitary) by the fibers of the paraventriculohypophysial tract.
n. paraventricula′ris poste′rior tha′lami [TA] posterior paraventricular nucleus of thalamus: the posterior of the two nuclei paraventriculares thalami (q.v.).
nu′clei paraventricula′res tha′lami [TA] paraventricular nuclei of thalamus: the *nucleus paraventricularis anterior thalami* and *nucleus paraventricularis posterior thalami,* two of the nuclei mediani thalami (q.v.); they are situated on the dorsomedial wall of the thalamus, juxtaposed to the third ventricle.
pedunculopontine tegmental n. n. tegmentalis pedunculopontinus.
perifornical n., n. perifornica′lis [TA] a group of nerve cells in the lateral hypothalamic area.
perihypoglossal nuclei, nu′clei perihypoglossa′les [TA] a group of nerve cells immediately adjacent to the nucleus of the hypoglossal nerve in the gray substance of the medulla oblongata, all of which contain cells with characteristics suggestive of reticular connections; the complex includes the nucleus intercalatus, the nucleus paramedianus dorsalis, the nucleus prepositus, and the sublingual nucleus. Called also *perihypoglossal nuclear complex.*
nu′clei perioliva′res [TA], **periolivary nuclei** a diffuse group of nuclei forming a large part of the superior olivary complex in the tegmentum of the caudal pons; they may be subdivided into medial and lateral groups.
n. periventricula′ris poste′rior [TA] posterior periventricular nucleus: a nucleus of nerve cells in the intermediate hypothalamic area, lying in the posterior part of the third ventricle.
nuclei of perizonal field nuclei campi perizonalis.
Perlia n. a group of cells in the midline of the oculomotor nuclear complex, thought to be associated with ocular convergence.
phenanthrene n. cholane n.
phrenic n., n. of phrenic nerve n. nervi phrenici.
polymorphic n. a cell nucleus that assumes an irregular form or splits up into more or less completely separated lobes, such as the nuclei of polymorphonuclear leukocytes.
nuclei of pons, pontine nuclei nuclei pontis.
pontine raphe n., pontine n. of raphe n. raphes pontis.
pontine reticular n., caudal, pontine reticular n., inferior intermediate n. reticularis pontis caudalis.
pontine reticular nuclei, intermediate see *n. reticularis pontis caudalis* and *n. reticularis pontis rostralis.*
pontine reticular n., oral, pontine reticular n., superior intermediate n. reticularis pontis rostralis.
pontine reticular n., tegmental n. reticularis tegmenti pontis.
pontine n. of trigeminal nerve n. principalis nervi trigemini.
nu′clei pon′tis [TA] nuclei of pons: masses of nerve cells scattered throughout the ventral part of the pons, in which the longitudinal fibers of the pons terminate; the majority of axons arising from these cells cross to the opposite side and form the middle cerebellar peduncle, which projects to the cerebellar cortex and nuclei.
posterior column nuclei dorsal column nuclei.
n. of posterior commissure n. commissurae posterioris.
n. poste′rior hypotha′lami [TA], **posterior n. of hypothalamus** posterior hypothalamic nucleus: a nucleus of nerve cells in the posterior hypothalamic region, above the lateral and medial nuclei of the mammillary body; it has major brainstem connections via periventricular fibers and the dorsal longitudinal fasciculus.
n. poste′rior ner′vi va′gi [TA] posterior nucleus of vagus nerve: the nucleus of origin of the parasympathetic fibers of the vagus nerve, situated in the trigone of the vagus nerve in the floor of the fourth ventricle, lateral to the nucleus of the hypoglossal nerve; called also *dorsal vagal n., dorsal n. of vagus nerve,* and *n. dorsalis nervi vagi* [TA alternative].
posterior n. of oculomotor nerve n. dorsalis nervi oculomotorii.
posterior periventricular n. n. periventricularis posterior.
posterior raphe n. n. raphes posterior.
posterior nuclei of thalamus nuclei posteriores thalami.
posterior n. of vagus nerve n. posterior nervi vagi.
nu′clei posterio′res tha′lami [TA] posterior nuclear complex of thalamus: groups of nerve cells anterior to the pulvinar, forming an ill-defined complex that receives afferents from spinothalamic fibers and superior and inferior colliculi.
n. posterolatera′lis medul′lae spina′lis [TA] posterolateral nucleus of spinal cord: a group of nerve cells in the posterolateral gray substance of the anterior column of the spinal cord; called also *dorsolateral n. of spinal cord.*
n. posteromedia′lis medul′lae spina′lis [TA] posteromedial nucleus of spinal cord: a group of nerve cells in the posteromedial gray substance of the anterior column of the spinal cord; called also *dorsomedial n. of spinal cord.*
pregeniculate n. n. ventralis corporis geniculati lateralis.
n. pregenicula′tus TA alternative for *n. ventralis corporis geniculati lateralis.*
preoptic n., lateral n. preopticus lateralis.
preoptic n., medial n. preopticus medialis.
preoptic n., median n. preopticus medianus.
preoptic n., periventricular n. preopticus periventricularis.
n. preop′ticus latera′lis [TA] lateral preoptic nucleus: a nucleus of nerve cells in the preoptic area of the basal forebrain.
n. preop′ticus media′lis [TA] medial preoptic nucleus: a nucleus of nerve cells in the preoptic area of the basal forebrain, ventral to the anterior commissure.
n. preop′ticus media′nus [TA] median preoptic nucleus: a nucleus of nerve cells in the preoptic area of the basal forebrain.
n. preop′ticus periventricula′ris [TA] periventricular preoptic nucleus: a nucleus of nerve cells in the preoptic area of the basal

forebrain; the nucleus is situated adjacent to the wall of the preoptic recess of the third ventricle.
n. prepo′situs [TA] prepositus nucleus: a group of nerve cells rostral to the hypoglossal nucleus and nucleus intercalatus and caudal to the abducent nucleus; it forms part of the perihypoglossal nuclei.
n. of prerubral field n. campi medialis.
nu′clei pretecta′les [TA] pretectal nuclei: various groups of nerve cells in the pretectal area which receive impulses chiefly from the optic tract; they project to the nucleus accessorius of the oculomotor nerve and constitute the midbrain center for the pupillary light reflex.
principal olivary n. n. olivaris principalis.
principal sensory n. of trigeminal nerve, n. principa′lis ner′vi trige′mini [TA] the nucleus of termination of afferent fibers of the trigeminal nerve, carrying impulses for sensations of touch and pressure, located in the dorsolateral part of the middle of the pons, just lateral to the trigeminal motor nucleus. Called also *pontine n. of trigeminal nerve.*
n. pro′prius [TA] a column of large neurons that extends throughout the posterior column of the spinal cord, ventral to the gelatinous substance; it corresponds to some of the cell constituents of Rexed laminae III and IV.
n. of pudendal nerve n. nervi pudendi.
n. pulpo′sus [TA] a semifluid mass of fine white and elastic fibers that forms the central portion of an intervertebral disk; it has been regarded as the persistent remains of the embryonic notochord.
nu′clei pulvina′res tha′lami [TA] pulvinar nuclei: a subgroup of the dorsal thalamic nuclei consisting of those that form the prominent, cushion-like medial portion of the posterior extremity of the thalamus (the pulvinar).
raphe nuclei, nu′clei ra′phes [TA] the median column reticular nuclei, a subgroup of the reticular nuclei of the brainstem, found in narrow longitudinal sheets along the raphae of the medulla oblongata, pons, and mesencephalon; they include many neurons that synthesize serotonin. Their ascending fibers project to parts of the limbic system and their descending fibers project to other brainstem nuclei, the medulla oblongata, and the pons. In the group are the *nucleus raphes magnus, nucleus raphes obscurus, nucleus raphes pallidus, nucleus raphes pontis, nucleus raphes posterior, nucleus raphes medianus, nucleus linearis inferioris, nucleus linearis intermedius,* and *nucleus linearis superior.*
n. ra′phes dorsa′lis n. raphes posterior.
n. ra′phes mag′nus [TA] magnus raphe nucleus: a raphe nucleus partially overlapping the nucleus pallidus and nucleus obscurus in the medulla oblongata and projecting upward into the caudal pons; its neurons are serotoninergic.
n. ra′phes media′nus [TA] median raphe nucleus: a raphe nucleus in the anterior part of the pons; its neurons are serotoninergic. Called also *superior central n.*
n. ra′phes obscu′rus [TA] obscurus raphe nucleus: a raphe nucleus of the medulla oblongata closely associated with the nucleus pallidus raphes; its neurons are serotoninergic.
n. ra′phes pal′lidus [TA] pallidal raphe nucleus: a raphe nucleus of the medulla oblongata closely associated with the nucleus raphes obscurus; its neurons are serotoninergic.
n. ra′phes pon′tis [TA] pontine raphe nucleus: a raphe nucleus in the central part of the pons; its neurons are serotoninergic.
n. ra′phes poste′rior [TA] posterior raphe nucleus: a large raphe nucleus extending from the anterior part of the pons through the mesencephalon; its neurons are serotoninergic. Called also *dorsal raphe n.* and *n. raphes dorsalis.*

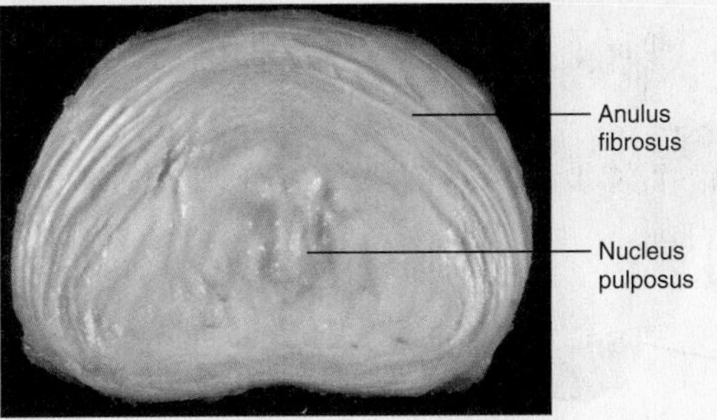

■ Intervertebral disk in transverse section, showing the nucleus pulposus and the anulus fibrosus.

red n. n. ruber.
reproductive n. micronucleus.
reticular nuclei nuclei reticulares.
reticular n., caudal pontine n. reticularis pontis caudalis.
reticular n., gigantocellular, reticular n., gigantocellular intermediate n. gigantocellularis.
reticular n., lateral 1. n. reticularis lateralis medullae oblongatae. 2. see *lateral column reticular nuclei.*
reticular nuclei, lateral column a pair of symmetrical groups of scattered small reticular nuclei of the brainstem, each arranged in a column lateral to the medial column reticular nuclei; most of their neurons are associative in nature. Included are the nucleus reticularis lateralis medullae oblongatae, nucleus tegmenti pedunculopontinus, nucleus reticularis parvocellularis, nucleus paragigantocellularis lateralis, nucleus parabrachialis lateralis, nucleus parabrachialis medialis, and nucleus subparabrachialis.
reticular n., magnocellular n. gigantocellularis.
reticular nuclei, medial column two groups of reticular nuclei of the brainstem, located symmetrically in the central parts of the two halves of the tegmentum; their neurons are often large, with long axons, and have dendrites and preterminal axons at right angles to the long axis of the brainstem. Included are the nucleus gigantocellularis, nucleus reticularis tegmenti pontis, nucleus reticularis pontis caudalis, nucleus reticularis pontis rostralis, nucleus cuneiformis, and nucleus subcuneiformis.
reticular nuclei, median column nuclei raphes.
reticular n., oral pontine n. reticularis pontis rostralis.
reticular n., paramedian n. reticularis paramedianus.
reticular n., parvocellular nucleus reticularis parvocellularis.
reticular nuclei, pontine 1. any of the reticular nuclei located in the pons. 2. see *n. reticularis pontis caudalis, n. reticularis pontis rostralis,* and *n. reticularis tegmenti pontis.*
reticular n., tegmental pontine n. reticularis tegmenti pontis.
reticular nuclei of brainstem, nuclei of the reticular formation nuclei reticulares.
reticular n. of medulla oblongata, intermediate n. reticularis intermedius medullae oblongatae.
reticular n. of medulla oblongata, lateral n. reticularis lateralis medullae oblongatae.
reticular nuclei of raphe nuclei raphes.
reticular n. of tegmentum n. reticularis tegmenti pontis.
reticular n. of thalamus n. reticularis thalami.
nu′clei reticula′res [TA] reticular nuclei: nuclei found in the reticular formation of the brainstem, occurring primarily in longitudinal columns in three groups: the *median column reticular nuclei* (see *nuclei raphes*), *medial column reticular nuclei* (q.v.), and *lateral column reticular nuclei* (q.v.). The term also encompasses several other nuclei that are not in any of the three columns, e.g., the nucleus reticularis thalami.
n. reticula′ris interme′dius medul′lae oblonga′tae [TA] intermediate reticular nucleus of medulla oblongata: either of a symmetrical pair of small medial column reticular nuclei in the medulla oblongata lateral to the nucleus raphes obscurus.
n. reticula′ris latera′lis medul′lae oblonga′tae [TA] lateral reticular nucleus: either of a symmetrical pair of lateral column reticular nuclei, each in a lateral funiculus of the medulla oblongata adjacent to a nucleus ambiguus.
n. reticula′ris paramedia′nus [TA] paramedian reticular nucleus: a small nucleus in the ventromedial medulla oblongata near the nucleus of the hypoglossal nerve.
n. reticula′ris parvocellula′ris [TA] parvocellular reticular nucleus: either of a pair of principal lateral column reticular nuclei, lying lateral to the nucleus gigantocellularis and adjacent to the nucleus ambiguus.
n. reticula′ris pon′tis cauda′lis [TA] caudal pontine reticular nucleus: a medial column reticular nucleus in the pons, located next to the nucleus reticularis tegmenti pontis and superior to the gigantocellular nucleus. Called also *inferior intermediate pontine reticular n.*
n. reticula′ris pon′tis ora′lis, n. reticula′ris pon′tis rostra′lis [TA] oral pontine reticular nucleus: either of a symmetrical pair of medial column reticular nuclei in the central part of the pons, one on either side of the superior central nucleus. Called also *superior intermediate pontine reticular n.*

Nucleus *Continued*

n. reticula′ris tegmen′ti pon′tis [TA] tegmental pontine reticular nucleus: either of a pair of medial column reticular nuclei located in the inferomedial pontine tegmentum medial to the medial lemniscus at levels between the levels of the genu of facial nerve and the rostral pons. Called also *reticulotegmental n.*
n. reticula′ris tha′lami [TA] reticular nucleus of thalamus: a thin layer of cells on the lateral surface of the thalamus, located within the external medullary lamina and between this lamina and the internal capsule.
reticulate n. of thalamus n. reticularis thalami.
reticulotegmental n. n. reticularis tegmenti pontis.
n. retroambi′guus [TA] retroambiguus nucleus: a nucleus near the nucleus ambiguus, with motor fibers that control muscles of both inhalation and exhalation.
retrodorsal lateral n. of spinal cord n. retroposterolateralis medullae spinalis.
retrofacial n., n. retrofacia′lis [TA] a small nucleus between the nucleus ambiguus and the facial nucleus, believed to be a source of vagal efferent visceral fibers.
retro-olivary nuclei a group of nuclei in the dorsal region of the superior olivary complex in the tegmentum of the caudal pons.
retroposterior lateral n. of spinal cord, n. retroposterolatera′lis medul′lae spina′lis [TA] a group of nerve cells in the gray substance of the retroposterolateral region of the anterior column of the spinal cord, which innervates the digital muscles.
n. reu′niens [TA] one of the median nuclei of the thalamus; it is situated adjacent to, and extending into, the massa intermedia when this structure is present; see *nuclei mediani thalami.*
rhomboid n., n. rhomboida′lis n. commissuralis rhomboidalis.
Roller n. 1. sublingual n. 2. a small nucleus located immediately inferior to the hypoglossal nucleus.
roof nuclei a term sometimes used to refer to the nuclei cerebelli (particularly the fastigial nucleus) because some of them are situated in close proximity to the roof of the fourth ventricle of the brain.
n. ru′ber [TA] red nucleus: a distinctive oval nucleus (pink in fresh specimens because of an iron-containing pigment in many of the cells) centrally placed in the upper mesencephalic reticular formation; it receives fibers from the cerebellar nuclei and cerebral cortex and projects fibers to the cerebellum, brainstem, and spinal cord. See also *pars magnocellularis nuclei rubri* and *pars parvocellularis nuclei rubri.*
sacral parasympathetic nuclei nuclei parasympathici sacrales.
salivary n., inferior n. salivatorius inferior.
salivary n., superior n. salivatorius superior.
n. salivato′rius infe′rior [TA] inferior salivatory nucleus: a short column of cells in the posterolateral part of the reticular formation in the lower pons and upper medulla oblongata; they comprise the parasympathetic outflow of the glossopharyngeal nerve for the supply of the parotid gland. Called also *inferior salivary n.*
n. salivato′rius supe′rior [TA] superior salivatory nucleus: a cluster of cells in the posterolateral pons near the internal genu of the facial nerve and generally continuous with the inferior salivatory nucleus; its cells comprise the parasympathetic outflow of the facial nerve for the supply of the lacrimal, nasal, palatine, submandibular, and sublingual glands. Called also *superior salivary n.*
salivatory n., caudal n. salivatorius inferior.
salivatory n., inferior n. salivatorius inferior.
salivatory n., rostral, salivatory n., superior n. salivatorius superior.
sanded n. a type of cell nucleus seen in hepatocytes of persons with chronic hepatitis B; it has a characteristic appearance caused by the presence of large amounts of hepatitis B antigen. A similar phenomenon is seen in hepatitis D.
Schwalbe n. n. vestibularis medialis.
Schwann n. the nucleus of a Schwann cell.
segmentation n. the fertilization nucleus after cleavage has begun. Called also *cleavage n.*
n. semiluna′ris TA alternative for *n. arcuatus hypothalami.*
sensory n. the nucleus of termination of the afferent (sensory) fibers of a peripheral nerve.
sensory n. of trigeminal nerve, inferior n. spinalis nervi trigemini.
sensory n. of trigeminal nerve, principal n. principalis nervi trigemini.
septal n., lateral n. septalis lateralis.
septal n., medial n. septalis medialis.
n. septa′lis latera′lis [TA] lateral septal nucleus: a nucleus in the septal area, continuous with the gray lamina of the septum pellucidum; it has afferent and cholinergic efferent connections with a variety of forebrain and brainstem areas including the hippocampus, the lateral hypothalamus, the tegmentum, and the amygdaloid bodies.
n. septa′lis media′lis [TA] medial septal nucleus: a nucleus in the septal area, coextensive with the diagonal band of Broca; it has afferent and cholinergic efferent connections with a variety of forebrain and brainstem areas including the hippocampus, the lateral hypothalamus, the tegmentum, and the amygdaloid bodies.
shadow n. a cell nucleus that does not stain and appears as a faint shadow under the microscope.
Siemerling n. one of the subdivisions of the nucleus nervi oculomotorius.
solitary nuclei, nuclei of solitary tract nuclei tractus solitarii.
somatic n. macronucleus.
sperm n. the structure within the head of the spermatozoon that becomes the male pronucleus after the spermatozoon fertilizes the oocyte.
spherical n. n. globosus.

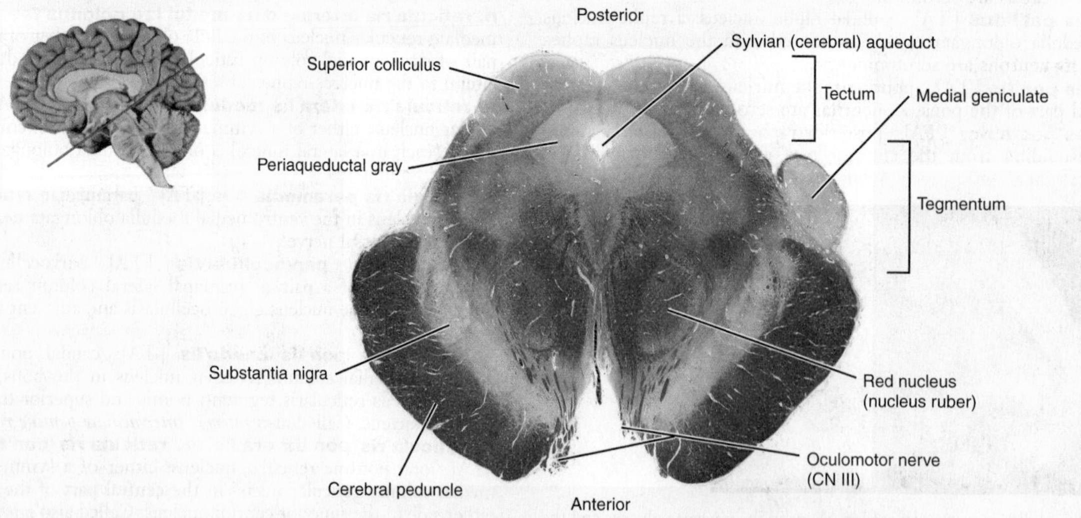

■ Nucleus ruber (red nucleus) in a transverse slice through the midbrain.

Nucleus *Continued*

spinal n. of trigeminal nerve, n. spina′lis ner′vi trige′mini [TA] a column of cells that lies along the medial aspect of the spinal tract, extending from the level of entry of the trigeminal nerve to the second cervical segment of the spinal cord, where it is continuous with the dorsal gray column. The nucleus has several cytoarchitectonic subdivisions and the fibers of the spinal tract end in it. Called also *inferior n. of trigeminal nerve*, and *inferior sensory n. of trigeminal nerve.*
Spitzka n. Perlia n.
Staderini n. n. intercalatus.
Stilling n. n. thoracicus posterior.
n. stri′ae termina′lis [TA] bed nucleus of stria terminalis: the collection of scattered groups of neurons between the fibers near the anterior end of the stria terminalis; they serve a relay function.
striate n. a term loosely applied to the neostriatum, to a nucleus of the corpus striatum, or to the corpus striatum itself.
n. subcaeru′leus [TA], **n. subceru′leus** a group of neurons subjacent to the nucleus caeruleus in the anterior part of the pons; sometimes considered part of the medial column reticular nuclei.
n. subcuneifor′mis [TA] subcuneiform nucleus: a nucleus in the mesencephalon adjacent to and closely associated with the cuneiform nucleus.
sublingual n. a sharply defined nucleus immediately ventral to the nucleus of the hypoglossal nerve, forming part of the perihypoglossal nuclear complex; called also *Roller n.*
subparabrachial n., n. subparabrachia′lis [TA] either of a pair of parabrachial nuclei that constitute part of the lateral column reticular nuclei; it is a pneumotaxic center lying ventral to the medial and lateral parabrachial nuclei in the pons. Called also *Kölliker-Fuse n.*
subthalamic n., n. subthala′micus [TA] a biconvex mass of gray matter on the medial side of the junction of the internal capsule and the crus cerebri; its chief connections are with the globus pallidus. Called also *n. of Luys* and *Luys body.*
superior central n., superior central raphe n. n. raphes medianus.
n. of superior olive n. olivaris superior.
suprachiasmatic n., n. suprachiasma′ticus [TA] a small nucleus in the supraoptic region of the hypothalamus, just above the optic chiasm; it influences rhythmical aspects of hypothalamic functions in many vertebrate species, including humans.
n. supraop′ticus [TA] supraoptic nucleus: a sharply defined nucleus of nerve cells in the anterior hypothalamic region, immediately above the lateral part of the optic chiasm; many of its cells are neurosecretory in function, secreting vasopressin, which is carried to the neurohypophysis (posterior pituitary) by the fibers of the supraopticohypophysial tract; other cells are osmoreceptors, which respond to increased osmotic pressure to signal the release of vasopressin by the neurohypophysis.
n. tec′ti n. fastigii.
tegmental nuclei, anterior nuclei tegmentales anteriores.
tegmental n., laterodorsal, tegmental n., lateroposterior n. tegmentalis posterolateralis.
tegmental nuclei, ventral nuclei tegmentales anteriores.
n. of tegmental field n. campi medialis.
tegmental pedunculopontine reticular n. n. tegmentalis pedunculopontinus.
nu′clei tegmenta′les anterio′res [TA] anterior tegmental nuclei: several masses of neurons of the mesencephalic tegmentum, situated ventral to the medial longitudinal fasciculus. Called also *ventral tegmental nuclei.*
n. tegmenta′lis pedunculoponti′nus [TA] tegmental pedunculopontine nucleus: a nucleus at the posterior end of the mesencephalon, sometimes considered one of the lateral column reticular nuclei. It merges anteriorly into the cuneiform and subcuneiform nuclei.
n. tegmenta′lis posterolatera′lis [TA] lateroposterior tegmental nucleus: a nucleus of nerve cells in the mesencephalic tegmentum, situated dorsal to the nucleus of the trochlear nerve. Called also *laterodorsal tegmental n.*
terminal n., n. terminatio′nis [TA] any of the groups of nerve cells within the central nervous system upon which the axons of primary afferent neurons of various cranial nerves synapse.
thalamic nuclei nuclei of thalamus.
thalamic nuclei, anterior nuclei anteriores thalami.
thalamic nuclei, medial nuclei mediales thalami.
thalamic nuclei, median nuclei mediani thalami.
thalamic nuclei, posterior nuclei posteriores thalami.
thalamic n., reticular n. reticularis thalami.
thalamic nuclei, ventral nuclei ventrales thalami.
nuclei of thalamus the nuclei and nuclear groups in the thalamus. Groups are the *nuclei anteriores thalami, nuclei dorsales thalami, nuclei mediales thalami, nuclei mediani thalami, nuclei intralaminares thalami, nuclei posteriores thalami,* and *nuclei ventrales thalami.* The *nucleus reticularis thalami* and *nucleus subthalamicus* are also thalamic nuclei.
thoracic n., thoracic n., dorsal, thoracic n., posterior n. thoracicus posterior.
n. thora′cicus dorsa′lis TA alternative for *n. thoracicus posterior.*
n. thora′cicus poste′rior [TA] posterior thoracic nucleus: a well-defined column of cells in the medial part of the intermediate zone (lamina VII) of the spinal gray matter, medial to the intermediolateral cell column, usually extending from the eighth cervical segment caudally to the second or third lumbar segment; it gives rise to the ipsilateral posterior spinocerebellar tract. Called also *thoracic column, Clarke column* or *nucleus, dorsal thoracic nucleus, nucleus thoracicus dorsalis* [TA alternative], and *Stilling column* or *nucleus.*
nu′clei trac′tus solita′rii [TA] nuclei of solitary tract: any of various nuclei of termination of the visceral afferent fibers of the facial, glossopharyngeal, and vagus nerves, which enter the tractus solitarius. The nuclei surround the tractus solitarius and their caudal ends join with the caudal ends of the corresponding nuclei of the opposite side. Called also *solitary nuclei.*
nuclei of trapezoid body nuclei corporis trapezoidei.
triangular n. 1. n. vestibularis medialis. 2. n. triangularis septi.
triangular septal n. n. triangularis septi.
n. triangula′ris sep′ti [TA] triangular septal nucleus: a nucleus of nerve cells of the caudal region of the septum pellucidum.
trigeminal nuclei nuclei of trigeminal nerve.
trigeminal mesencephalic n. n. mesencephalicus nervi trigeminalis.
trigeminal motor n. n. motorius nervi trigemini.
nuclei of trigeminal nerve four nuclei associated with the trigeminal nerve, located in the midbrain, pons, and medulla oblongata and extending as far caudally as the upper cervical spinal cord. See *n. mesencephalicus nervi trigemini, n. motorius nervi trigemini, n. principalis nervi trigemini,* and *n. spinalis nervi trigemini.*
trochlear n., n. of trochlear nerve n. nervi trochlearis.
trophic n. macronucleus.
nu′clei tubera′les latera′les [TA] lateral tuberal nuclei: nerve cell nuclei situated ventrally in the intermediate hypothalamic region, mainly in the lateral hypothalamic area.
vagal n., dorsal n. posterior nervi vagi.
nuclei of vagus nerve the nuclei of origin and termination of the vagus nerve, situated in the medulla oblongata, comprising the posterior nucleus of the vagus nerve, the nucleus ambiguus, and the nuclei tractus solitarii.
ventral anterior n. of thalamus n. ventralis anterior thalami.
n. of ventral field n. campi ventralis.
ventral intermediate n. of thalamus n. ventralis intermedius thalami.
ventral lateral nuclei of thalamus nuclei ventrales laterales thalami.
ventral medial nuclei of thalamus nuclei ventrales mediales thalami.
ventral medial n. of oculomotor nerve n. anteromedialis nervi oculomotorii.
ventral posterior nuclei of thalamus nuclei ventrobasales thalami.
ventral posterolateral n. of thalamus n. ventralis posterolateralis thalami.
ventral posteromedial n. of thalamus n. ventralis posteromedialis thalami.
ventral principal n. of medial geniculate body n. ventralis corporis geniculati medialis.
ventral nuclei of thalamus nuclei ventrales thalami.
n. ventra′lis ante′rior tha′lami [TA] ventral anterior nucleus of thalamus: a nucleus anteriorly located within the ventral nuclei of the thalamus, anterior to the ventral lateral nucleus, and lateral and medial to the internal and external medullary laminae, respectively; it is subdivided into magnocellular and principal divisions.
n. ventra′lis cor′poris genicula′ti latera′lis [TA] ventral lateral geniculate nucleus: the smaller, ventral part of the lateral geniculate

Nucleus *Continued*

nucleus, projecting toward the zona incerta of the ventral thalamus. Called also *pregeniculate n.* and *n. pregeniculatus* [TA alternative].
n. ventra′lis cor′poris genicula′ti media′lis [TA] ventral principal nucleus of medial geniculate body: the principal relay nucleus of the medial geniculate nuclei, receiving ascending auditory fibers from the inferior colliculus and relaying information on sound intensity and frequency and its binaural properties to the auditory cortex.
n. ventra′lis interme′dius tha′lami [TA] ventral intermediate nucleus of thalamus: a nucleus medially located within the ventral nuclei of the thalamus.
nu′clei ventra′les latera′les tha′lami [TA] ventral lateral nuclei of thalamus: nuclei ventrolaterally located within the ventral thalamic nuclei, subdivided into anterior and posterior nuclei; called also *ventral lateral complex of thalamus.*
nu′clei ventra′les media′les tha′lami [TA] ventral medial complex of thalamus: a group of nuclei located in the medial portion of the ventral thalamic nuclei.
n. ventra′lis posterolatera′lis tha′lami [TA] ventral posterolateral nucleus of thalamus: the more lateral of the two posterior ventral nuclei of the thalamus; it is the terminus of spinothalamic fibers and the medial lemniscus and it projects to the postcentral and posterior paracentral gyri.
n. ventra′lis posteromedia′lis tha′lami [TA] ventral posteromedial nucleus of thalamus: the more medial of the two posterior ventral nuclei of the thalamus; it is the terminus of trigeminothalamic fibers and projects to the face area of the postcentral gyrus.
nu′clei ventra′les tha′lami [TA] ventral nuclei of thalamus: a large group of nuclei lying between the internal medullary lamina and the internal capsule; it includes ventral anterior, ventral intermediate, ventral lateral, ventral medial, ventrobasal and other nuclei, which relay impulses to various specific areas of the cerebral cortex.
nu′clei ventrobasa′les tha′lami [TA] ventrobasal complex of thalamus: the nuclei that form the posterior ventral part of the ventral nuclei of the thalamus, comprising a posterolateral nucleus and a posteromedial nucleus; see *n. ventralis posterolateralis thalami* and *n. ventralis posteromedialis thalami.* Called also *ventral posterior nuclei of thalamus.*
ventrolateral nuclei of thalamus nuclei ventrales thalami.
ventrolateral n. of spinal cord n. anterolateralis medullae spinalis.
ventromedial n. of hypothalamus n. ventromedialis hypothalami.
ventromedial n. of oculomotor nuclear complex n. anteromedialis nervi oculomotorii.
ventromedial n. of spinal cord n. anteromedialis medullae spinalis.
n. ventromedia′lis hypotha′lami [TA] ventromedial hypothalamic nucleus: a group of nerve cell bodies found in the ventral portion of the intermediate hypothalamic region; it is involved in diverse functions, e.g., food intake and sexual behavior.
vesicular n. a form of cell nucleus, the membrane of which stains deeply, while the central part is rather pale.
vestibular nuclei nuclei vestibulares.
vestibular n., caudal n. vestibularis inferior.
vestibular n., cranial n. vestibularis superior.
vestibular n., inferior n. vestibularis inferior.
vestibular n., lateral n. vestibularis lateralis.
vestibular n., medial, vestibular n., middle n. vestibularis medialis.
vestibular n., rostral, vestibular n., superior n. vestibularis superior.
nu′clei vestibula′res [TA] vestibular nuclei: the four cellular masses in the lateral floor of the fourth ventricle: the *superior, lateral, medial,* and *inferior vestibular nuclei,* in which the short ascending and longer descending branches of the vestibular nerve terminate and in which cerebellar projections are received. The nuclei give rise to widely dispersed projections to motor nuclei in the brainstem and cervical cord via the medial longitudinal fasciculi from all the vestibular nuclei to the cerebellum (chiefly from the inferior and medial nuclei), and to motor cells throughout the spinal cord (from the lateral nucleus). Additional connections of the nuclei provide for conscious perception of, and autonomic reactions to, labyrinthine stimulation. Called also *acoustic nuclei* and *nuclei of acoustic nerve.*
n. vestibula′ris cauda′lis n. vestibularis inferior.
n. vestibula′ris infe′rior [TA] inferior vestibular nucleus: a vestibular nucleus that lies lateral to the medial vestibular nucleus and medial to the restiform body.
n. vestibula′ris latera′lis [TA] lateral vestibular nucleus: a vestibular nucleus composed of large multipolar nerve cells that lies immediately superior to the inferior vestibular nucleus; its upper end becomes continuous with the superior vestibular nucleus. Called also *Deiters n.*
n. vestibula′ris media′lis [TA] medial vestibular nucleus: a vestibular nucleus that lies in the floor of the fourth ventricle and extends upward from the medulla oblongata into the caudal pons; called also *triangular n.* and *Schwalbe n.*
n. vestibula′ris supe′rior [TA] superior vestibular nucleus: a small vestibular nucleus that lies above the lateral vestibular nucleus. Called also *Bekhterev (Bechterew) n.* and *cranial* or *rostral vestibular n.*
vestibulocochlear nuclei, nuclei of vestibulocochlear nerve the vestibular and cochlear nuclei considered together; see *nuclei vestibulares* and *nuclei cochleares.*
Voit n. a cerebellar nucleus accessory to the dentate nucleus.
Westphal nuclei nuclei accessorii nervi oculomotorii.
yolk n. a special area of the cytoplasm of an oocyte in which the synthetic activities leading to the accumulation of food supplies in the oocyte are apparently initiated; called also *vitelline body* and *Balbiani n.* or *body.*
zygote n. fertilization n.

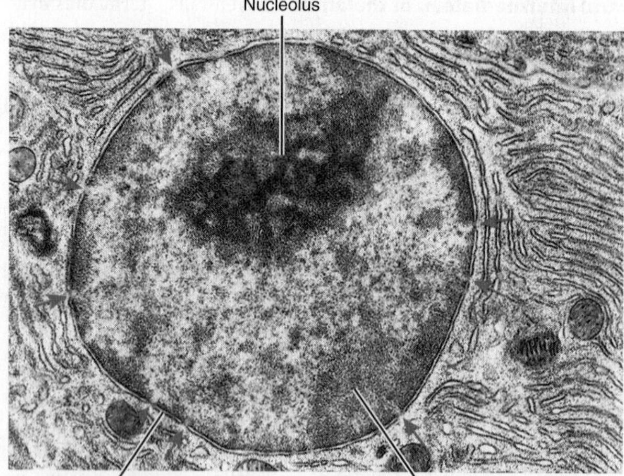

■ Electron micrograph of a cell, showing the chromatin-rich nucleus bounded by the double-membraned nuclear envelope, the inner and outer membranes of which enclose the perinuclear space. The arrows point to nuclear pores.

nu•clide (noo′klīd) a species of atom characterized by the atomic number, mass number, and quantum state of its nucleus, and capable of existing for a measurable lifetime (generally greater than 10^{-10} sec). Thus nuclear isomers are separate nuclides, but promptly decaying excited nuclear states and unstable intermediates in nuclear reactions are not so considered.
radioactive n. radionuclide.

nu•do•pho•bia (noo″do-fo′be-ə) [L. *nudus* unclothed, bare + *-phobia*] an abnormal aversion to being unclothed.

Nu•el spaces (ne-el′) [Jean Pierre *Nuel,* Belgian oculist, 1847–1920] see under *space.*

NUG necrotizing ulcerative gingivitis.

Nuhn glands (nōōn) [Anton *Nuhn,* German anatomist, 1814–1889] anterior lingual glands, see under *gland.*

Nu•Lev (noo′lev) trademark for a preparation of hyoscyamine sulfate.

null (nul) 1. insignificant; having no consequence or value. 2. absent or nonexistent. 3. zero; nothing.

nul•lip•a•ra (nə-lip′ə-rə) [L. *nullus* none + *para*] a woman who has never borne a viable child. Also written para 0.

nul•li•par•i•ty (nul″ĭ-par′ĭ-te) the condition or fact of being nulliparous.

nul•lip•a•rous (nə-lip′ə-rəs) [*null* + *-parous*] having never given birth to a viable infant.

nul·li·som·ic (nul″ĭ-som′ik) lacking one pair of chromosomes (2n − 2).

Nu·LYTELY (noo-līt′le) trademark for combination preparations of polyethylene glycol 3350 and electrolytes (sodium bicarbonate, sodium chloride, and potassium chloride).

numb (num) [A.S. *niman*] anesthetic (def. 1).

num·ber (num′bər) [Fr. *nombre*, from L. *numerus*] a symbol, as a figure or word, expressive of a certain value or of a specified quantity determined by count.

acetyl n. the number of milligrams of potassium hydroxide necessary to neutralize the acetic acid saponified from 1 gram of acetylated fat; it represents the extent to which hydroxyl groups are present.

acid n. the number of milligrams of potassium hydroxide necessary to neutralize the free fatty acids in 1 gram of fat; it represents a measure of the amount of free fatty acids in the fat.

atomic n. (*Z*) the number of protons in the nucleus of a nuclide; all the atoms of a chemical element have the same atomic number; sometimes indicated by a subscript preceding the symbol of a chemical element (e.g., $_{1}H$).

Avogadro's n. (*N*, N_A) the number of molecules in one mole of a substance: 6.023×10^{23}.

Brinell hardness n. a number indicative of the degree of relative hardness of a material, calculated after measuring the diameter of the impression made by a steel ball pressed under a known load into the surface of the material being tested; equal to the load in kilograms divided by the surface area of the indentation in square millimeters.

chromosome n. the number of chromosomes present in the somatic cells of an organism; the normal individual receives, at conception, one set of chromosomes (the haploid number, symbol *n*) from each of the gametes forming the zygote, thus acquiring the diploid number (2*n*). In humans, *n* equals 23.

copy n. 1. the number of times a given gene or chromosome is physically represented in the genome. 2. the average number of times a specific plasmid occurs in a bacterial cell.

CT n. the attenuation value determined for each pixel in a CT scan on a scale in which water is 0, compact bone +1000, and air −1000. See *Hounsfield unit* under *unit*.

dibucaine n. an expression of the percentage of inhibition of the enzyme cholinesterase in a serum sample by dibucaine; used to differentiate between normal and abnormal serum cholinesterase phenotypes. Normal or usual is about 80; intermediate is about 60; abnormal or atypical is about 20. Abbreviated DN.

hardness n. a number indicative of the degree of relative hardness of materials. See *Brinell*, *Knoop*, *Rockwell*, and *Vickers hardness n.*

Hehner n. the percentage of water insoluble fatty acids obtainable from a fat or oil.

Hittorf n. the fraction of the total electric current passing through an electrolytic solution that is carried by a given ion species; called also *transference n.* and *transport n.*

hydrogen n. the amount of hydrogen that one gram of a fat can absorb; it represents the quantity of unsaturated fatty acids in the fat.

iodine n. the amount of iodine in grams which 100 grams of a fat or oil can absorb; it is inversely related to the amount of unsaturated fatty acids present in the fat or oil.

isotopic n. the number which when added to twice the atomic number gives the atomic weight.

Knoop hardness n. a number indicative of the degree of relative hardness of a material, calculated from the load employed and the length of the long axis of the impression made by the rhomboidal pyramid of a diamond pressed into the surface of the material being tested. It is the test most commonly used in dental practice to test the hardness of teeth.

linking n. in topology (def. 3), the total number of times one strand of the DNA double helix winds around the other in a right-hand direction, given a DNA molecule with constrained ends. Two molecules differing only in linking number are topoisomers.

Loschmidt n. the number of molecules per unit volume of an ideal gas at standard temperature and pressure; Avogadro's number divided by 22.4 liters per mole.

mass n. (*A*) the number of nucleons (protons plus neutrons) in the atom of a nuclide; generally indicated by a superscript preceding the symbol of a chemical element (e.g., ^{131}I) to denote a specific isotope.

neutron n. (*N*) the number of neutrons in a nucleus, representing the difference between the mass number and the atomic number.

oxidation n. a number assigned to each atom in a molecule or ion that represents the number of electrons theoretically gained (positive oxidation numbers) or lost (negative numbers) in converting the atom to the elemental form. Oxidation numbers are assigned according to the following rules. The oxidation number of atoms in an elemental form is zero, and the oxidation number of a monatomic ion equals the ionic charge. Group I and Group II metals always have oxidation numbers of +1 and +2, respectively. Fluorine always has an oxidation number of −1; oxygen always of −2, except in peroxides and superoxides (where it is −1) and in compounds containing O—F bonds. Hydrogen always has an oxidation number of +1, except in metal hydrides (where it is −1). Oxidation numbers are assigned to other atoms so that the sum for all atoms in a neutral compound equals zero and the sum for all atoms in a polyatomic ion equals the ionic charge. Called also *oxidation state*.

polar n. the number of valences (positive or negative) possessed by an atom in any particular compound.

Polenske n. the number of milliliters of tenth normal potassium hydroxide required to neutralize the insoluble, volatile fatty acids from 5 g of the fat.

Reichert-Meissl n. the number of milliliters of tenth normal potassium hydroxide (KOH) required to neutralize the soluble volatile fatty acids distilled from 5 g of fat after it has been saponified with KOH and then made acid with orthophosphoric acid or sulfuric acid.

Reynolds n. (R_e) the velocity of flow of a fluid multiplied by the diameter of the vessel and divided by the kinematic viscosity of the circulating fluid. It is lower for turbulent flow and higher for laminar flow, and is used for characterizing the conditions for the onset of turbulence.

Rockwell hardness n. a number indicative of the degree of relative hardness of materials, determined by measuring the depth of the impression made by a steel or diamond penetrator pressed into the surface of the material being tested. There are a number of Rockwell hardness tests and scales, using various combinations of loads and penetrators; the load and penetrator combination must always be specified when stating a Rockwell hardness number.

saponification n. the number of milligrams of potassium hydroxide required to saponify the fatty acids in 1 gram of a fat or oil; it is inversely related to the average molecular weight of the fatty acid molecules.

tooth n. a number or letter assigned to each of the primary or permanent teeth to denote its position in the dentition; see *Fédération Dentaire Internationale tooth numbering system*, *Palmer tooth notation system*, *Universal Numbering System*, and *International Standards Organization System for Teeth*, under *system*. See illustration.

transference n., transport n. Hittorf n.

triangulation n. (T) a number expressing the multiple of 60 subunits that a viral capsid with icosahedral symmetry contains, so called because it expresses the number of subtriangles into which each face of the capsid is divided.

turnover n. the number of molecules of substrate acted upon by one molecule of enzyme per minute.

twisting n. (*T*) in topology (def. 3), the number of ordinary (Watson-Crick) helical turns in a DNA molecule with constrained ends.

variable n. of tandem repeats (VNTR) see under *repeat*.

Vickers hardness n. a number indicative of the degree of relative hardness of materials, determined by measuring the long diagonals of indentation made by pressing the pyramidal point of a diamond into the surface of the material being tested; equal to the load in kilograms divided by the area, in square millimeters, of the recovered indentation; called also *diamond pyramid hardness*.

wave n. in light waves, the reciprocal of the wavelength expressed as a fraction of a centimeter.

writhing n. (*W*) in topology (def. 3), the number of superhelical turns in a DNA molecule with constrained ends.

numb·ness (num′nis) anesthesia (def. 1).

num·mu·lar (num′u-lər) [L. *nummularis*] 1. coin-sized and coin-shaped. 2. made up of round, flat disks. 3. piled, like coins, in a rouleau.

Nu·mor·phan (noo-mor′fən) trademark for preparations of oxymorphone hydrochloride.

nun·na·tion (nən-a′shən) [Heb. *nun* letter N] 1. a speech disorder consisting of too frequent use of *n* sounds. 2. hypernasality.

Nu·per·cain·al (noo″pər-kān′əl) trademark for preparations of dibucaine.

Nu·prin (noo′prin) trademark for a preparation of ibuprofen.

N-Uri·stix (u′rĭ-stiks) trademark for a reagent strip designed for testing for nitrite, glucose, and protein in urine.

nurse (nurs) 1. a person who is especially prepared in the scientific basis of nursing and who meets certain prescribed standards of education and clinical competence. 2. to provide services that are essential to or helpful in the promotion, maintenance, and restoration of health and well-being. See also *nursing*. 3. suckle.

advanced practice n. (APN), advanced practice registered n. (APRN) a registered nurse having education beyond the basic nursing education and certified by a nationally recognized professional organization in a nursing specialty, or meeting other criteria established by a Board of Nursing.

clinical n. specialist a registered nurse with a high degree of knowledge, skill, and competence in a specialized area of nursing. These skills are made directly available through the provision of nursing care to clients and are indirectly available through guidance and planning of care with other nursing personnel. Clinical nurse specialists hold a master's degree in

	Molars			Premolars		Canine	Incisors				Canine	Premolars		Molars		
	Maxillary Arch															
I	1	2	3	4	5	6	7	8	9	10	11	12	13	14	15	16
II	18	17	16	15	14	13	12	11	21	22	23	24	25	26	27	28
III	8┘	7┘	6┘	5┘	4┘	3┘	2┘	1┘	└1	└2	└3	└4	└5	└6	└7	└8
III	8┐	7┐	6┐	5┐	4┐	3┐	2┐	1┐	┌1	┌2	┌3	┌4	┌5	┌6	┌7	┌8
II	48	47	46	45	44	43	42	41	31	32	33	34	35	36	37	38
I	32	31	30	29	28	27	26	25	24	23	22	21	20	19	18	17
	Mandibular Arch															
	Right								Left							

■ Tooth number. Diagram comparing the numbering of the teeth using the Universal *(I)*, International Standards Organization *(II)*, and Palmer *(III)* tooth numbering systems.

nursing, preferably with an emphasis in clinical nursing. Called also *n. specialist.*

n. clinician a registered nurse who is working in clinical practice. Generally, minimal preparation for this role is the baccalaureate degree.

community n. the name given in Great Britain to a public health nurse, from the fact that such a nurse was placed in charge of each one of the districts into which the city or community was divided. See also *public health n.*

community health n. public health n.

general duty n. a registered nurse, usually one who has not undergone training beyond the basic nursing program, who sees to the general nursing care of patients in a hospital or other health agency.

graduate n. a graduate of a school of nursing; often used to designate one who has not been registered or licensed to practice. Called also *trained n.*

hospital n. a nurse employed by a hospital.

licensed practical n. (LPN), licensed vocational n. a graduate of a school of practical nursing whose qualifications have been examined by a state board of nursing and who has been legally authorized to practice as a licensed practical or vocational nurse, under the supervision of a physician or registered nurse.

occupational health n. an especially prepared registered nurse employed by an institution to apply nursing principles and procedures for the promotion, restoration, and maintenance of optimal health of its employees as compared to a nurse who performs normal nursing functions in an occupational setting.

office n. a registered nurse employed by a physician in his office to perform or to assist him in the performance of certain procedures.

practical n. a person who has had practical experience in nursing care but who is not a graduate of any kind of nursing school; not to be confused with a licensed practical nurse.

n. practitioner a registered nurse with advanced education and clinical training in a specialized area of health care; nurse practitioners can diagnose, prescribe, and perform procedures as regulated by the state employing them.

private n., private duty n. a nurse who attends an individual patient, usually on a fee-for-service basis, and who may specialize in a specific class of diseases.

probationer n. a person who has entered a school of nursing and is under observation to determine her fitness for the nursing profession; applied principally to nursing students enrolled in hospital schools of nursing.

public health n. (PHN) an especially prepared registered nurse employed in a community agency to safeguard the health of persons in the community, giving care to the sick in their homes, promoting health and well-being by teaching families how to keep well, and assisting in programs for the prevention of disease. Called also *community health n.* and *visiting n.*

Queen's N. in Great Britain, a district nurse who has been trained at or in accordance with the regulations of the Queen Victoria Jubilee Institute for Nurses.

registered n. a graduate nurse who has been legally authorized (registered) to practice after examination by a state board of nurse examiners or similar regulatory authority, and who is legally entitled to use the designation RN.

school n. an especially prepared registered nurse employed in a school system or public health agency to assist in safeguarding the health of students and to teach health practices.

scrub n. a nurse who directly assists the surgeon in the operating room.

special n. 1. a private nurse. 2. a nurse who specializes in a particular class of cases.

n. specialist clinical n. specialist.

student n. a person enrolled in a basic program of nursing education.

trained n. graduate n.

visiting n. see *public health n.*

wet n. a woman who breast-feeds the infant of another.

nurse-mid·wife (nurs-mid′wīf) an individual educated in the two disciplines of nursing and midwifery, who possesses evidence of certification according to the requirements of the American College of Nurse-Midwives. Abbreviated CNM (Certified Nurse-Midwife).

nurse-mid·wi·fery (nurs-mid′wi-fər-e) the independent management of care of essentially normal newborns and women, antepartally, intrapartally, postpartally, and/or gynecologically, occurring within a health care system which provides for medical consultation, collaborative management, or referral, and is in accord with the functions, standards, and qualifications as defined by the American College of Nurse-Midwives.

nur·se·ry (nur′sə-re) the department in a hospital where newborn infants are cared for.

day n., day care n. an institution devoted to the care of young children during the day.

nurs·ing (nurs′ing) 1. the provision, at various levels of preparation, of services that are essential to or helpful in the promotion, maintenance, and restoration of health and well-being or in the prevention of illness, as of infants, of the sick and injured, or of others for any reason unable to provide such services for themselves. Sometimes designated according to the age of the patients being cared for (e.g., pediatric or geriatric nursing), or their particular health problems (e.g., gynecologic, medical, obstetrical, orthopedic, psychiatric, surgical, urological nursing, or the like), or the setting in which the services are provided (e.g., office, school, or occupational health nursing). See also *nurse.* 2. breastfeeding.

evidence-based n. the practice of nursing in which the nurse makes clinical decisions on the basis of the best available, current research evidence, their own clinical expertise, and the needs and preferences of the patient. See also under *practice.*

Nuss·baum experiment (noos′boum) [Moritz *Nussbaum*, German histologist, 1850–1915] see under *experiment.*

nut (nut) [L. *nux;* Gr. *karyon*] a seed element, as of various trees, usually enclosed in a coating of variable hardness.

areca n., betel n. areca (def 2).

ground n. peanut.

physic n., purging n. 1. *Jatropha curcas.* 2. *J. multifida.* 3. the seed of either of these trees, which contains a cathartic oil and a phytotoxin that is poisonous, sometimes causing death.

nu·ta·tion (noo-ta′shən) [L. *nutatio*] the act of nodding, especially involuntary nodding. **nu′tatory** *adj*

nut·gall (nut′gawl) [L. *galla*] an excrescence growing on oak trees (genus *Quercus*), especially *Q. alba* (the white oak), produced by insect eggs and larvae embedded in the plant tissues; it is a source of gallic and tannic acids, which are used in various pharmaceuticals for their astringent properties. Called also *gall, Aleppo gall,* and *gallnut.*

nut·meg (nut′meg) 1. *Myristica fragrans.* 2. the seed of *M. fragrans;* see also under *oil* and *poisoning.*

Nu·tra·cort (noo′trə-kort″) trademark for preparations of hydrocortisone.

nu·tra·ceu·ti·cals (noo″trə-soo′tĭ-kəlz) functional foods.

nu·tri·ceu·ti·cals (noo″trĭ-soo′tĭ-kəlz) nutraceuticals.

nu·tri·ent (noo′tre-ənt) [L. *nutriens*] 1. nourishing; providing nutrition. 2. a food or other substance that provides energy or building material for the survival and growth of a living organism; called also *nutriment.*

conditionally essential n's nutrients that must be supplied to the body only under special conditions, such as stress, illness, or aging.

essential n's nutrients (proteins, minerals, carbohydrates, fats, vitamins) necessary for growth, normal functioning, and maintaining life; they must be supplied by food, since they cannot be synthesized by the body.

secondary n. a substance that stimulates the intestinal microflora to synthesize other nutrients.

nu·tri·ge·no·mics (noo″trĭ-je-no′miks) [*nutrition* + *genomics*] a field of study combining nutrition and genomics, examining how foods affect genes and how individual genetic differences can influence the response to particular nutrients, or other naturally occurring compounds in foods.

nu·tri·lite (noo′trĭ-līt) a substance essential in minute amounts in the nutrition of a microorganism.

nu·tri·ment (noo′trĭ-mənt) [L. *nutrimentum*] nutrient (def. 2).

nu·tri·ol·o·gy (noo″tre-ol′ə-je) the science of nutrition; the study of foods and their use in diet and therapy.

nu·tri·tion (noo-trĭ′shən) [L. *nutritio*] the taking in and metabolism of nutrients (food and other nourishing material) by an organism so that life is maintained and growth can take place. **nutri′tional** *adj*

adequate n. see under *diet.*

enteral n. the delivery of nutrients in liquid form directly into the stomach, duodenum, jejunum; used when the patient's condition precludes oral intake.

parenteral n. administration of nutriment intravenously.

total parenteral n. (TPN) the intravenous administration of the total nutrient requirements of the patient with gastrointestinal dysfunction, accomplished via a central venous catheter, usually inserted in the superior vena cava via a subclavian vein. Called also *parenteral hyperalimentation* and *total parenteral alimentation.*

nu·tri·tion·ist (noo-trĭ′shən-ist) a specialist in food and nutrition; see also *dietitian.*

nu·tri·tious (noo-trĭ′shəs) [L. *nutritius*] affording nourishment or nutrition.

nu·tri·tive (noo′trĭ-tiv″) 1. nutritional. 2. nutritious.

nu·tri·ture (noo′trĭ-chur″) the status of the body in relation to nutrition, generally or in regard to a specific nutrient, such as protein.

Nu·tro·pin (noo′trə-pin) trademark for a preparation of somatropin.

Nu·va·Ring (noo′və-ring) trademark for a combination preparation of etonogestrel and ethinyl estradiol.

nux (nuks) gen. *nu′cis* [L.] nut.

n. vo′mica the dried ripe seed of *Strychnos nux-vomica* L. (Loganiaceae), containing several alkaloids, principally strychnine and brucine. It has been used as a bitter tonic and central nervous system stimulant, and in veterinary medicine it is used as a bitter tonic and in the treatment of inappetence, atony of the rumen, and chronic indigestion.

nvCJD new variant Creutzfeldt-Jakob disease.

NVS nutritionally variant streptococci.

Ny·a·derm (ni′ə-dərm) trademark for preparations of nystatin.

nyc·tal·gia (nik-tal′jə) [*nyct-* + *-algia*] pain that occurs in sleep only.

nyc·ta·lope (nik′tə-lōp) a person affected with nyctalopia.

nyc·ta·lo·pia (nik″tə-lo′pe-ə) [*nyct-* + Gr. *alaos* blind + *-opia*] night blindness; failure or imperfection of vision at night or in a dim light, with good vision only on bright days.

nyc·ta·pho·nia (nik″tə-fo′ne-ə) [*nyct-* + *aphonia*] elective mutism with loss of voice during the night.

nyc·tero·hem·er·al (nik″tər-o-hem′ər-əl) nyctohemeral.

nyct(o)- [Gr. *nyx,* gen. *nyctos* night] a combining form denoting relationship to night or to darkness.

nyc·to·hem·er·al (nik″to-hem′ər-əl) [*nycto-* + Gr. *hēmera* day] pertaining to both night and day.

nyc·to·phil·ia (nik″to-fil′e-ə) [*nycto-* + *-philia*] an abnormal preference for darkness or for night; called also *scotophilia.*

nyc·to·pho·bia (nik″to-fo′be-ə) [*nycto-* + *phobia*] irrational fear of darkness.

nyc·to·pho·nia (nik″to-fo′ne-ə) [*nycto-* + *phon-* + *-ia*] elective mutism with loss of voice during the day but not at night.

nyc·tu·ria (nik-tu′re-ə) [*nyct-* + *-uria*] 1. nocturia. 2. passage of more urine at night than during the day.

NYD not yet diagnosed.

Ny·dra·zid (ni′drə-zid) trademark for preparations of isoniazid.

Ny·hus classification (ni′həs) [Lloyd M. *Nyhus,* American surgeon, born 1923] see under *classification.*

nyl·i·drin hy·dro·chlo·ride (nil′ĭ-drin) a synthetic adrenergic used as a peripheral vasodilator; administered orally, intramuscularly, and subcutaneously.

ny·lon (ni′lon) a synthetic polymerized plastic which in fiber form is used as a nonabsorbable suture material.

nymph (nimf) [Gr. *nymphē* a bride] a stage in the life cycle of certain arthropods, such as ticks, between the larva and the adult; it somewhat resembles the adult but is small, sexually immature, and wingless. Cf. *naiad.*

nym·pha (nim′fə) gen. and pl. *nym′phae* [L., from Gr. *nymphē* a bride] labium minus pudendi.

n. of Krause clitoris.

nym·phec·to·my (nim-fek′tə-me) [*nymph-* + *-ectomy*] excision of the labia minora.

nym·phi·tis (nim-fi′tis) inflammation of the labia minora.

nymph(o)- [Gr. *nymphē* bride] a combining form denoting relationship to the nymphae, or labia minora.

nym·pho·ca·run·cu·lar (nim″fo-kə-rung′ku-lər) pertaining to the labia minora and the caruncula hymenalis.

nym·pho·hy·me·ne·al (nim″fo-hi″mə-ne′əl) pertaining to the labia minora and the hymen.

nym·pho·ma·nia (nim″fo-ma′ne-ə) [*nympho-* + *-mania*] abnormal, excessive, insatiable sexual desire in the female. Cf. *satyriasis.*

nym·pho·ma·ni·ac (nim″fo-ma′ne-ak) 1. affected with nymphomania. 2. one who is affected with nymphomania.

nym·phot·o·my (nim-fot′ə-me) [*nympho-* + *-tomy*] surgical incision of the labia minora or clitoris.

Nys·sen-van Bo·gaert syndrome (ni′sen vahn bo′gärt) [René *Nyssen,* Belgian neurologist, 1891–1972; Ludo *van Bogaert,* Belgian neurologist, 1897–1989] metachromatic leukodystrophy (adult form); see under *leukodystrophy.*

Nyss·o·rhyn·chus (nis″o-ring′kəs) [Gr. *nyssa* prick + *rhynchos* snout] a subgenus of mosquitoes of the genus *Anopheles;* several species act as carriers of the malarial parasite in tropical America.

nys·tag·mi·form (nis-tag′mĭ-form) nystagmoid.

nys·tag·mo·graph (nis-tag′mo-graf) [*nystagmus* + *-graph*] an instrument for recording the movements of the eyeball in nystagmus.

nys·tag·moid (nis-tag′moid) resembling nystagmus.

nys·tag·mus (nis-tag′məs) [Gr. *nystagmos* drowsiness, from *nystazein* to nod] an involuntary, rapid, rhythmic movement of the eyeball, which may be horizontal, vertical, rotatory, or mixed, i.e., of two varieties. **nystag′mic** *adj*

amaurotic n. nystagmus in the blind or in those with defects of central vision; called also *ocular n.*

amblyopic n. nystagmus caused by a lesion interfering with central vision.

ataxic n. unilateral nystagmus in multiple sclerosis, marked by impaired lateral conjugate gaze.

aural n. vestibular n.

caloric n. rotatory nystagmus induced by irrigating the ears with warm or cold water or air; see *caloric test,* under *test.*

central n. jerk nystagmus caused by a lesion somewhere in the neurologic pathways regulating gaze.

congenital n., congenital hereditary n. nystagmus usually present at birth; it is most often horizontal and pendular, but occasionally jerky and pendular. It may be caused by or associated with optic atrophy, coloboma, albinism, bilateral macular lesions, congenital cataract, severe astigmatism, or glaucoma.

convergence n. a rhythmic oscillation of the eyes, in which they have a rapid adduction movement relative to each other alternating with a slow abduction movement; usually caused by a tumor of the aqueduct of Sylvius, third ventricle, or midbrain. It is often accompanied by retraction nystagmus.

disjunctive n. nystagmus in which the eyes swing toward and away from each other.

dissociated n. nystagmus in which the movements in the two eyes are dissimilar.

downbeat n. a type of vertical nystagmus in which the fast phase is downward; seen in lesions at the cervicomedullary junction.

electrical n. galvanic n.

end-position n. nystagmus seen at extremes of gaze in normal individuals; called also *pseudonystagmus.*

fixation n. nystagmus that occurs only when a person gazes fixedly at an object.

galvanic n. vestibular nystagmus caused by electrical stimulation of the labyrinth of the internal ear; called also *electrical n.*

gaze n. nystagmus made apparent by looking to the right or to the left.

gaze paretic n. a type of gaze nystagmus seen in patients recovering from central nervous system lesions: If the eyes fail to stay fixed to one side only, that is the affected side of a cerebral or pontine lesion; if the defect is in vertical gaze, it usually signifies a lesion in the pretectal area.

jerk n., jerky n. nystagmus consisting of slow movement in one direction followed by a rapid return movement in the opposite direction; called also *resilient* or *rhythmical n.*

labyrinthine n. vestibular n.

latent n. nystagmus that occurs only when one eye is covered.

lateral n. nystagmus in which the eye movements are from side to side.

miner's n. an occupational disease of coal miners consisting of abnormal eye movements associated with other signs and symptoms; it is considered by some to be related to poor lighting and by others as a functional disorder.

ocular n. amaurotic n.

opticokinetic n., optokinetic n. the normal nystagmus occurring when looking at objects passing across the field of vision, as in viewing from a moving railroad car or automobile. It can be induced for testing purposes to check ocular and vestibular functioning.

oscillating n. pendular n.

palatal n. see under *myoclonus.*

paretic n. a false nystagmus occurring when there is a weakness of the ocular muscles.

pendular n. nystagmus in which the eye oscillations have an equal rate, amplitude, direction, and type of movement; called also *oscillating n., undulatory n.,* and *vibratory n.*

periodic alternating n. a rare type of jerk nystagmus that has rhythmic changes in amplitude and direction with intervals of quiet between periods.

positional n. nystagmus that occurs, or changes its form or intensity, when a person puts the head into specific positions.

railroad n. optokinetic n.

resilient n. jerk n.

retraction n., n. retracto'rius 1. a spasmodic retraction of the eyeball backward into the orbit, occurring on attempted movement of the eye; it is a sign of disease of the midbrain. 2. sylvian syndrome; see under *syndrome.*

rhythmical n. jerk n.

rotatory n. nystagmus in which the movement is about the visual axis.

secondary n. nystagmus seen after abrupt cessation of rotation of the head, caused by the labyrinthine fluid continuing to move.

see-saw n. nystagmus in which one eye moves up as the other moves down.

spontaneous n. nystagmus that does not have specific stimulation of the vestibular system.

undulatory n. pendular n.

unilateral n. nystagmus in only one eye.

upbeat n. a vertical nystagmus with the fast phase upward, occurring in lesions of the vermis cerebelli.

vertical n. an up-and-down movement of the eyes.

vestibular n. nystagmus due to disturbance of the vestibular system; eye movements are rhythmic, with a slow and a fast component. Called also *aural n.* and *labyrinthine n.* Cf. *vestibular vertigo.*

vibratory n. pendular n.

voluntary n. rapid rhythmic eye movements, up to 80 a second, that can be produced at will by some normal individuals.

nys·tag·mus-my·oc·lo·nus (nis-tag'məs-mi-ok'lə-nəs) a rare congenital condition in which there is nystagmus together with abnormal involuntary movements of the extremities and trunk.

ny·sta·tin (ni-stat'in) [USP] a polyene antifungal agent produced by the growth of *Streptomyces noursei,* effective against *Candida albicans* and other *Candida* species; used in the treatment of vaginal, intestinal, oropharyngeal, and cutaneous candidal infections, administered orally and topically. Called also *fungicidin.*

nys·tax·is (nis-tak'sis) [Gr.] nystagmus.

Ny·sten's law (ne-stawz') [Pierre Hubert *Nysten,* Belgian pediatrician in France, 1771–1818] see under *law.*

Ny·stex (ni'steks) trademark for preparations of nystatin.

Ny·stop (ni'stop) trademark for preparations of nystatin.

nyx·is (nik'sis) [Gr. "pricking"] puncture, or paracentesis.

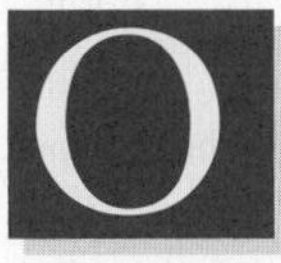

O ohne Hauch; oxygen.

O. [L.] o'culus (eye).

o- ortho- (def. 2).

Ω the Greek capital letter omega; symbol for *ohm.*

ω omega, the twenty-fourth letter of the Greek alphabet.

ω- a prefix designating (1) the carbon atom farthest from the principal functional group, as in ω-oxidation; and (2) the last in a series of related entities or terms.

OA ocular albinism.

OAE otoacoustic emissions.

OAF osteoclast activating factor.

oak (ōk) 1. any tree of the genus *Quercus.* 2. any of certain trees that resemble those of *Quercus.*

poison o. 1. either of two species of *Rhus; R. diversiloba* is the western poison oak and *R. toxicodendron* is the eastern poison oak. A variant of the latter, called *Atlantic poison oak,* is found in the southeastern United States. 2. name sometimes given to *Rhus radicans* (poison ivy) when it is freestanding and shrublike.

white o. *Quercus alba,* a source of nutgall.

OAP a cancer chemotherapy regimen consisting of Oncovin (vincristine), ara-C (cytarabine), and prednisone.

oa•sis (o-a'sis) pl. *oa'ses* [Gr. "a fertile islet in a desert"] an island or spot of healthy tissue in a diseased area.

OAT ornithine aminotransferase.

oath (ōth) a solemn declaration or affirmation.

o. of Hippocrates, hippocratic o. see under *H.*

oat•meal (ōt'mēl) meal made from oats *(Avena sativa),* used in the preparation of a bland, nutritious food.

colloidal o. [USP] a colloidal extract from oatmeal, used as an emollient in dermatologic preparations.

OB obstetrics.

OBA Office of Biotechnology Activities, a division of the National Institutes of Health.

ob•duc•tion (ob-duk'shən) [L. *obductio*] a medicolegal autopsy.

O'Beirne sphincter (o-birn') [James *O'Beirne,* Irish surgeon, 1786–1862] rectosigmoid sphincter.

obe•li•ad (o-be'le-ad) toward the obelion.

obe•li•on (o-be'le-on) [Gr., dim. of *obelos* a spit] a point on the sagittal suture where it is crossed by a line which connects the parietal foramina. obe'liac *adj*

Ober operation, test (sign) (o'bər) [Frank Roberts *Ober,* American orthopedic surgeon, 1881–1960] see under *operation* and *test.*

obese (o-bēs') [L. *obesus*] excessively fat.

obes•i•ty (o-bēs'ĭ-te) [L. *obesus* fat] an increase in body weight beyond the limitation of skeletal and physical requirement, as the result of an excessive accumulation of fat in the body. Called also *adiposity, adiposis,* and *corpulency.*

abdominal o. android o.

adult-onset o. obesity beginning in adulthood and characterized by increase in size (hypertrophy) of adipose cells with no increase in their number; called also *hypertrophic o.*

alimentary o. exogenous o.

android o. obesity in which fat is localized around the waist and in the upper body, most frequently seen in men and having a poorer prognosis for morbidity and mortality than the gynoid type. Called also *abdominal* or *visceral o.* Cf. *gynoid o.*

clinically severe o. morbid o.

endogenous o. obesity due to metabolic (endocrine) abnormalities or genetic defects that affect the synthesis of enzymes involved in intermediate metabolism.

exogenous o. obesity due to overeating; called also *alimentary o.* and *simple o.*

gynecoid o., gynoid o. obesity in which fat is localized in the lower half of the body, most frequently seen in women, and having a better prognosis for morbidity and mortality than the android type. Cf. *android o.*

hyperinsulinar o. obesity due to excessive insulin secretion, associated with hypoglycemia and increased appetite.

hyperplastic-hypertrophic o. lifelong o.

hypertrophic o. adult-onset o.

hypogonadal o. obesity associated with hypogonadism.

hypothyroid o. obesity associated with hypothyroidism.

lifelong o. obesity beginning in childhood and characterized by an increase both in number (hyperplasia) and in size (hypertrophy) of adipose cells; called also *hyperplastic-hypertrophic o.*

morbid o. obesity severe enough to endanger the health of a person, often associated with serious or even life-threatening disorders such as diabetes mellitus, atherosclerosis, hypertension, or the pickwickian syndrome. Many authorities define this as when the person is 45 kg (100 pounds) over ideal weight or has a body mass index of 40 or more. Called also *clinically severe o.*

simple o. exogenous o.

visceral o. android o.; so called from the theory that deep intra-abdominal (visceral) fat plays a large role in the associated morbidity and mortality.

obes•og•e•nous (o″bēs-oj'ə-nəs) producing or causing obesity.

obex (o'beks) [L. "barrier"] [TA] the ependyma-lined junction of the taeniae of the fourth ventricle of the brain at the inferior angle.

obi•dox•ime chlo•ride (o″bĭ-dok'sēm) a cholinesterase reactivator which has been used to counter organophosphorus poisoning.

ob•jec•tive (ob-jek'tiv) [L. *objectivus*] 1. perceptible to the external senses. 2. a result for whose achievement an effort is made. 3. the lens or system of lenses in a microscope (or telescope) that is nearest to the object under examination.

achromatic o. a microscope objective in which the chromatic aberration is corrected for two colors and the spherical aberration is corrected for one color.

apochromatic o. a microscope objective in which the chromatic aberration is corrected for three colors and the spherical aberration is corrected for two colors.

dry o. a microscope objective designed to be used without a liquid between its tip and the cover glass over the specimen.

flat field o. a microscope objective that provides an image in which all parts of the field are simultaneously in focus.

fluorite o. a microscope objective in which some of the lenses are made from fluorite instead of glass.

immersion o. a microscope objective designed to have its tip and the cover glass over the specimen connected by a liquid instead of by air. The liquid may be water (water immersion) or a specially prepared oil (oil immersion).

semiapochromatic o. a type of microscope objective in which spherical aberration and chromatic aberration are both corrected for two colors.

ob•li•gate (ob'lĭ-gāt) [L. *obligatus*] not facultative; necessary; compulsory; capable of survival only under particular conditions, as an obligate aerobe.

ob•lig•a•to•ry (əb-lig'ə-tor″e) obligate.

oblique (o-blēk') [L. *obliquus*] slanting; inclined; between a horizontal and a perpendicular direction.

external o. musculus obliquus externus abdominis.

internal o. musculus obliquus internus abdominis.

obliq•ui•ty (o-blik'wĭ-te) the state of being oblique, or slanting.

Litzmann o. inclination of the fetal head so that the posterior parietal bone presents to the parturient canal; called also *posterior asynclitism.*

Nägele o. the position of the fetal head in which the anterior parietal bone presents to the parturient canal, the biparietal diameter being oblique in relation to the brim of the pelvis; called also *anterior asynclitism.*

o. of pelvis inclination of the pelvis.

obli•quus (o-bli'kwəs) [L.] oblique.

oblit•er•a•tion (ob-lit″ər-a'shən) [L. *obliteratio*] complete removal, whether by disease, degeneration, surgical procedure, irradiation, or otherwise.

cortical o. a condition in which the cerebral cortex is marked by areas in which the ganglion cells have disappeared.

ob•lon•ga•ta (ob″long-gah'tə) [L.] oblong, sometimes used informally to refer to the medulla oblongata.

ob•nu•bi•la•tion (ob-noo″bĭ-la'shən) clouding of consciousness.

O'Bri•en akinesia (o-bri'ən) [Cecil Starling *O'Brien,* American ophthalmologist, 1889–1977] see under *akinesia.*

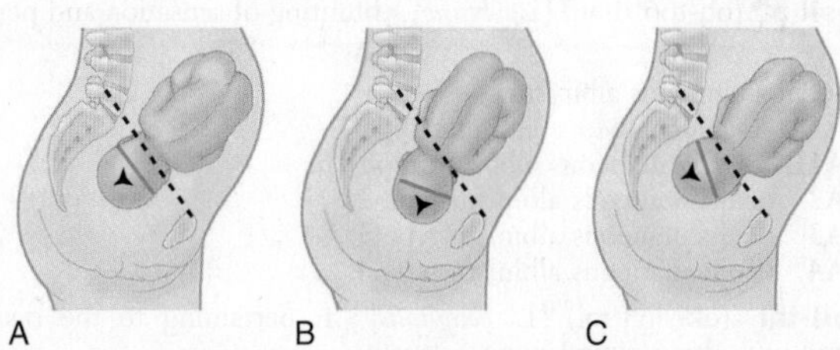

■ Obliquity. *(A),* Concordance of the fetal and pelvic planes, synclitism; *(B),* Litzmann obliquity (posterior asynclitism); *(C),* Nägele obliquity (anterior asynclitism).

ob·serv·er (ob-sur′vər) one who takes note of or watches.
participant o. in certain psychoanalytic theory, the role of the therapist; not merely examining the overt and covert behavior of the patient but also participating by analyzing his or her own reactions as well as their relevance to the therapy.

ob·ses·sion (ob-sesh′ən) [L. *obsessio*] a recurrent, persistent thought, image, or impulse that is unwanted and distressing (ego-dystonic) and comes involuntarily to mind despite attempts to ignore or suppress it. Common obsessions involve thoughts of violence, contamination, and self-doubt. **obses′sive** *adj*

ob·ses·sive-com·pul·sive (əb-ses′iv-kəm-pul′siv) pertaining to obsessions and compulsions, to obsessive-compulsive disorder, or to obsessive-compulsive personality disorder.

ob·so·les·cence (ob″so-les′əns) [L. *obsolescere* to grow old] the cessation or the beginning of the cessation of any physiologic process.

ob·ste·tri·cian (ob″stə-trĭ′shən) [L. *obstetrix* midwife] one who practices obstetrics.

ob·stet·rics (ob-stet′riks) [L. *obstetrix* midwife] the branch of surgery that deals with the management of pregnancy, labor, and the puerperium. **obstet′ric, obstet′rical** *adj*

ob·sti·pa·tion (ob″stĭ-pa′shən) [L. *obstipatio*] intractable constipation.

ob·struc·tion (ob-struk′shən) [L. *obstructio*] 1. the act of blocking or clogging. 2. the state or condition of being clogged. Cf. *atresia.* Called also *blockage, closure,* and *occlusion.*
bladder outlet o. any of various blockages in the outflow of urine from the bladder; causes include benign prostatic hyperplasia, bladder neck dyssynergia, prostate cancer or another tumor that presses against the urethra, and a variety of other conditions.
chronic airflow o., chronic airway o. name given to a group of disorders in which the upper or lower airways are chronically obstructed; it includes chronic bronchitis, emphysema, and other types of chronic obstructive pulmonary disease.
closed-loop o. intestinal obstruction caused by the closing off of both ends of a segment, such as in volvulus.
congenital nasolacrimal duct o. obstruction of the nasolacrimal duct of an infant as a result of incomplete canalization; affected children have tears and debris on the cheek below the duct.
false colonic o. Ogilvie syndrome; see under *syndrome.*
gastric outlet o. obstruction of the gastric (pyloric) outlet, usually resulting from deformity or scarring with ulceration; symptoms include weight loss, nausea, and vomiting. Called also *pyloric outlet o.* and *pyloroduodenal o.*
intestinal o. blockage of the intestine due to a mechanical cause (such as volvulus) or a nonmechanical cause (such as ileus).
membranous o. of inferior vena cava an occasional cause of Budd-Chiari syndrome in which there is a congenital membrane obstructing the inferior vena cava and blocking outflow from the hepatic veins.
pyloric outlet o., pyloroduodenal o. gastric outlet o.

ob·stru·ent (ob′stroo-ənt) [L. *obstruens*] 1. causing obstruction or blocking. 2. any agent or agency that causes obstruction.

ob·tund (ob-tund′) [L. *obtundere* to make dull] 1. to render dull or blunt. 2. to render a sensation less acute. 3. to reduce the level of alertness.

ob·tun·da·tion (ob″tən-da′shən) mental blunting with mild to moderate reduction in alertness and a diminished sensation of pain.

ob·tun·dent (ob-tun′dənt) [L. *obtundere* to make dull] 1. pertaining to or causing obtundation. 2. having the power to soothe pain. 3. an agent that blunts irritation or soothes pain.

ob·tu·ra·tion (ob″tə-ra′shən) obstruction.
canal o., root canal o. in root canal therapy, filling of the canal completely and densely with a nonirritating hermetic sealing agent. Called also *root canal filling.*

ob·tu·ra·tor (ob′tə-ra′tər) [L.] 1. any structure, natural or artificial, that closes an opening. 2. speech-aid prosthesis.

ob·tu·sion (ob-too′zhən) [L. *obtusio*] blunting of sensation and perception.

OCA oculocutaneous albinism.
OCA1A oculocutaneous albinism type 1.
OCA1B oculocutaneous albinism type 1b.
OCA2 oculocutaneous albinism type 2.
OCA3 oculocutaneous albinism type 3.
OCA4 oculocutaneous albinism type 4.

oc·cip·i·tal (ok-sip′ĭ-təl) [L. *occipitalis*] 1. pertaining to the occiput. 2. located near the occipital bone.

oc·cip·i·ta·lis (ok-sip″ĭ-ta′lis) [L., from *occiput,* q.v.] 1. [TA] occipital. 2. the posterior part of the occipitofrontalis muscle.

oc·cip·i·tal·iza·tion (ok-sip″ĭ-təl-ĭ-za′shən) synostosis of the atlas with the occipital bone.

oc·cip·i·to·an·te·ri·or (ok-sip″ĭ-to-an-tēr′e-ər) having the occiput directed forward toward the pubis (designating the position of the fetus in relation to the maternal pelvis).

oc·cip·i·to·at·loid (ok-sip″ĭ-to-at′loid) pertaining to the occipital bone and the atlas.

oc·cip·i·to·ax·oid (ok-sip″ĭ-to-ak′soid) pertaining to the occipital bone and the axis.

oc·cip·i·to·bas·i·lar (ok-sip″ĭ-to-bas′ĭ-lər) pertaining to the occiput and the base of the skull.

oc·cip·i·to·breg·mat·ic (ok-sip″ĭ-to-breg-mat′ik) pertaining to the occiput and the bregma.

oc·cip·i·to·cal·car·ine (ok-sip″ĭ-to-kal′kar-īn) both occipital and calcarine.

oc·cip·i·to·cer·vi·cal (ok-sip″ĭ-to-sur′vĭ-kəl) pertaining to the occiput and the neck.

oc·cip·i·to·fa·cial (ok-sip″ĭ-to-fa′shəl) pertaining to the occiput and the face.

oc·cip·i·to·fron·tal (ok-sip″ĭ-to-frun′təl) pertaining to the occiput and the forehead.

oc·cip·i·to·fron·ta·lis (ok-sip″ĭ-to-fron-ta′lis) occipitofrontal; see under *musculus.*

oc·cip·i·to·mas·toid (ok-sip″ĭ-to-mas′toid) pertaining to the occipital bone and the mastoid process.

oc·cip·i·to·men·tal (ok-sip″ĭ-to-men′təl) pertaining to the occiput and the chin.

oc·cip·i·to·pa·ri·e·tal (ok-sip″ĭ-to-pə-ri′ə-təl) pertaining to the occipital and parietal bones or lobes of the brain.

oc·cip·i·to·pos·te·ri·or (ok-sip″ĭ-to-pos-tēr′e-ər) having the occiput directed toward the back, or turned toward the sacrum (designating the position of the fetus in relation to the maternal pelvis).

oc·cip·i·to·tem·po·ral (ok-sip″ĭ-to-tem′pə-rəl) pertaining to the occipital and the temporal bones.

oc·cip·i·to·tha·lam·ic (ok-sip″ĭ-to-thə-lam′ik) pertaining to the occipital lobe and the thalamus.

oc·ci·put (ok′sĭ-pət) [L.] [TA] the posterior part of the head.

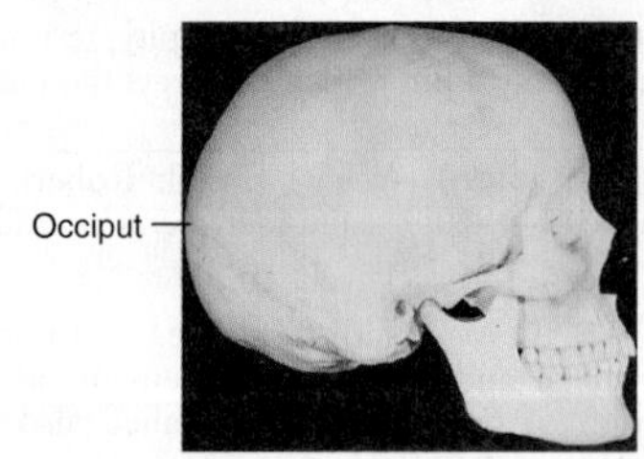

oc·clude (ə-klōōd′) 1. to fit close together. 2. to close tight, as to bring the mandibular teeth into contact with the teeth in the maxilla. 3. obstruct.

oc·clud·er (ə-klōōd′ər) a type of dental articulator.

oc·clu·din (ə-klōō′din) any of a family of transmembrane proteins, consisting of two hydrophobic extracellular loops and four transmembrane domains, that associate with occludins in adjacent plasma membranes in the formation of tight junctions.

oc·clu·sal (ə-kloo′zəl) 1. occlusive. 2. pertaining to the contacting surfaces of opposing teeth or of opposing occlusion rims, or to the masticating surfaces of the premolar and molar teeth.

oc·clu·sion (ə-kloo′zhən) [L. *occlusio*] 1. obstruction. 2. the trapping of a liquid or gas within cavities in a solid or on its surface. 3. the relationship between the teeth as components of the masticatory system in normal function, dysfunction, and parafunction. See also *bite* and *malocclusion.* 4. momentary closure of part of the vocal tract, which produces a plosive.
abnormal o. malocclusion.
acentric o. a condition in which the habitual voluntary closure pattern of the mandible does not coincide with centric relation, producing primary premature tooth contacts in the centric path of closure.
anatomic o. occlusion in which the arrangement of natural teeth in the same arch and in opposing arches is defined by dental or skeletal landmarks rather than functional criteria.

anterior o. mesioclusion.

balanced o. occlusion in which the occlusal contact of the teeth on the working side of the jaw is accompanied by the harmonious contact of the teeth of the opposite (balancing) side. The occlusion of artificial teeth may be *mechanically balanced*, as on an articulator, without reference to physiologic considerations, or *physiologically balanced*, functioning in harmony with the temporomandibular joint and the neuromuscular system.

buccal o. the position of a posterior tooth when it is outside (buccal to) the line of occlusion.

central o., centric o. occlusion in the vertical and horizontal position of the mandible in which the cusps of the mandibular and maxillary teeth interdigitate maximally. Ideally, the lingual cusps of the maxillary bicuspids make contact with the marginal ridges of the mandibular bicuspids and the marginal ridges of the second bicuspid and first molar. The mesial lingual cusps of the maxillary molar occlude in the central fossae of the mandibular molars, while the distal cusps of the maxillary molars occlude on the marginal ridges of the mandibular molars. Similarly, the supporting cusps of the mandibular teeth occlude on the marginal ridges and fossae of the maxillary molars and bicuspids.

coronary o., coronary artery o. complete obstruction of one of the coronary arteries, usually from progressive atherosclerosis (sometimes complicated by thrombosis), rarely from embolism, arteritis, or dissecting aneurysm.

distal o. the position of a lower tooth when it is distal to its opposite number in the maxilla. Called also *postnormal o.*

eccentric o. acentric o.

edge-to-edge o., end-to-end o. occlusion in which the anterior maxillary and mandibular teeth meet along their incisal edges when the mandible is in centric position. Called also *edge-to-edge bite* and *end-to-end bite.*

enteromesenteric o. obstruction of blood vessels in both the mesentery and the wall of the intestine.

functional o. such contact of the maxillary and mandibular teeth as will provide the highest efficiency in the centric position and during all excursive movements of the jaw that are essential to mastication, without producing trauma.

habitual o. the consistent relationship of the teeth in the maxilla to those of the mandible when the teeth in both jaws are brought into maximum contact, such relationship varying from individual to individual; the ideal habitual occlusion is centric occlusion, but it is seldom attained without corrective dental treatment.

hyperfunctional o. traumatic o.

ideal o. perfect interdigitation of the upper and lower teeth.

labial o. the position of an anterior tooth when it is outside (labial to) the line of occlusion.

lateral o. the occlusion of the teeth when the lower jaw is moved to the right or left of centric position.

lingual o. malocclusion in which the tooth is lingual to the line of the normal dental arch. Called also *linguoclusion.*

mechanically balanced o. see *balanced o.*

mesial o. the position of a lower tooth when it is mesial to its opposite number in the maxilla. Called also *prenormal o.*

neutral o. normal o.

normal o. the contact of the upper and lower teeth in the centric relationship.

pathogenic o. an occlusal relationship that is capable of producing pathologic changes in the supporting tissues. See also *traumatic o.*

physiologically balanced o. see *balanced o.*

posterior o. distoclusion.

postnormal o. distal o.

prenormal o. mesial o.

protrusive o. mesioclusion.

retrusive o. distoclusion.

spherical form of o. an arrangement of teeth that places their occlusal surfaces on the surface of an imaginary sphere, about 8 inches in diameter, with its center above the level of the teeth; see also *Monson curve*, under *curve.*

terminal o. the relationship of opposing occlusal surfaces that provides the maximum natural or planned contact and/or intercuspation.

traumatic o. progressive injury to the supporting structure of the teeth as a result of occlusal dysfunction. Called also *hyperfunctional o.* See also *traumatogenic o.*

traumatogenic o. abnormal occlusion capable of producing injury to the teeth, residual ridges, and periodontal structures. See *traumatic o.*

venous o. the blocking of venous return; it occurs naturally in the penis during an erection or it may be induced artificially in a part such as in the arm during venous occlusion plethysmography.

working o. the contact made between the teeth on the side toward which the mandible is moved.

oc•clu•sive (ə-kloo′siv) pertaining to or causing occlusion.

oc•clu•so•cer•vi•cal (ŏ-kloo″so-ser′vĭ-kəl) pertaining to the occlusal surface and the neck of a tooth.

oc•clu•som•e•ter (ok″loo-som′ə-tər) gnathodynamometer.

oc•clu•so•re•ha•bil•i•ta•tion (o-kloo″zo-re″hə-bil″ĭ-ta′shən) the bringing about or restoration of proper occlusal relations of teeth.

oc•cult (ə-kult′) [L. *occultus*] obscure; concealed from observation; difficult to understand.

oc•cu•pan•cy (ok′u-pən-se) the period of time during which a unit quantity of a substance, administered in a specified way, is present in, or occupies, a part of the body before it is excreted or broken down.

OCD obsessive-compulsive disorder.

ocel•lus (o-sel′əs) [L., dim. of *oculus* eye] 1. a rudimentary eye with photosensitive pigmented cells, such as a small simple eye or eyespot of some insects and other invertebrates. 2. a roundish, eyelike patch of color.

Ochoa syndrome (o-cho′ah) [Bernardo *Ochoa* Arismendi, Colombian pediatric surgeon, 20th century] urofacial syndrome.

ochra•tox•i•co•sis (o″krə-tok″sĭ-ko′sis) a type of mycotoxicosis in pigs and sometimes other animals that have eaten grain or flour products contaminated by ochratoxin-producing molds such as *Aspergillus ochraceus* or *Penicillium viridicatum.* Characteristics include kidney damage with anorexia, prostration, and sometimes death. Balkan nephritis is closely related and may be a rare form of ochratoxicosis in humans. See also *mycotoxic nephropathy.*

ochra•tox•in (o′krə-tok″sin) any of a group of mycotoxins produced by *Aspergillus ochraceus* and certain species of *Penicillium*, sometimes found contaminating grains, peanuts, and green coffee beans. It has been implicated in cases of hepatic carcinoma and Balkan nephritis. The most common and the most toxic is ochratoxin A, which causes ochratoxicosis.

Ochro•bac•trum (o″kro-bak′trəm) [Gr. *ōchros* pale + *baktron* staff] a widely distributed genus of bacteria of the family Brucellaceae, consisting of gram-negative, motile rods; organisms are obligately aerobic, chemoorganotrophic, oxidase-positive, and catalase-negative. The type species is *O. anthropi.*

O. anthro′pi a species that causes nosocomial bacteremia and soft tissue infections, particularly in critically ill or immunocompromised patients; it is most often associated with infected intravenous catheters.

O. interme′dium a species that is a rare opportunistic pathogen, causing nosocomial infections.

Ochro•co•nis (o″krə-co′nis) [Gr. *ōchros* pale + *konis* dust] a genus of Fungi Imperfecti of the form-family Dematiaceae.

O. gallopa′vum a thermophilic species that causes encephalitis in chickens and turkeys, sometimes in epidemics, and has been found in opportunistic infections of humans. Called also *Dactylaria gallopava.*

ochrom•e•ter (o-krom′ə-tər) [Gr. *ōchros* pale + *-meter*] an instrument for measuring the capillary blood pressure by registering the force necessary to compress a finger by a rubber balloon until blanching of the skin occurs.

Ochro•my•ia (o″kro-mi′ə) *Cordylobia.*

ochro•no•sis (o″krə-no′sis) [Gr. *ōchros* pale + *nos-* + *-sis*] generalized deposition of dark pigment in the connective tissues, usually secondary to alkaptonuria (q.v.). It is characterized by urine that darkens on standing and visible dusky discoloration of the sclerae and ears. The pigment is a sequela of accumulation of homogentisic acid in the connective tissues. **ochronot′ic** *adj*

exogenous o. ochronosis induced by exposure to chemicals such as phenolic compounds or hydroquinone.

Ochro•phy•ta (o″kro-fi′tə) Phaeophyta.

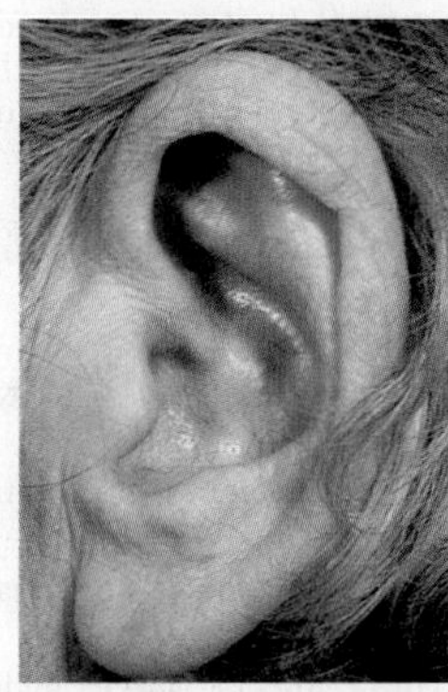

■ Dark pigmentation of ear cartilage in ochronosis.

Oci•mum (os′ĭ-məm) [L., from Gr. *ōkimon*] a genus of plants of the family Labiatae, comprising the basils; *O. sanc′tum*, or tulsi, is considered sacred in India and is used in ayurvedic medicine.

oc•ry•late (ok′rə-lāt) a type of cyanoacrylate adhesive used in surgery.

OCT optical coherence tomography; ornithine carbamoyltransferase; oxytocin challenge test.

oct(a)- [Gr. *oktō*, L. *octo* eight] a combining form meaning eight.

oc•ta•dec•a•no•ate (ok″tə-dek″ə-no′āt) stearate.

oc•ta•de•ca•no•ic ac•id (ok″tə-dek″ə-no′ik) systematic name for *stearic acid;* see also table at *fatty acid.*

oc•ta•meth•yl pyro•phos•phor•a•mide (ok″tə-meth′əl pir″o-fos-for′ə-mīd″) an organophosphorus compound used as a systemic insecticide for plants. Called also *schradan.* Abbreviated OMPA.

Oc•ta•mide (ok′tə-mīd) trademark for preparations of metoclopramide hydrochloride.

oc•tane (ok′tān) an oily hydrocarbon occurring in petroleum.

oc•ta•no•ic ac•id (ok″tə-no′ik) systematic name for *caprylic acid.* See also table accompanying *fatty acid.*

oc•ta•pep•tide (ok″tə-pep′tīd) a peptide which on hydrolysis yields eight amino acids.

oc•ta•va•lent (ok″tə-va′lənt) [*octa-* + L. *valens* able] having a valence of eight.

oc•tet (ok-tet′) a group of eight identical or similar objects or entities, as the group of eight electrons (four pairs) in the outer, or valence, shell of an atom, which pairs may or may not be shared with another atom.

oc•ti•ci•zer (ok″tĭ-si′zər) a plasticizer for pharmaceuticals.

oc•ti•grav•i•da (ok″tĭ-grav′ĭ-də) [*octa-* + *gravida*] a woman pregnant for the eighth time; also written gravida VIII.

oc•tin•ox•ate (ok-tin′ok-sāt) [USP] a cinnamate compound that absorbs ultraviolet B; used topically as a sunscreen.

oc•tip•a•ra (ok-tip′ə-rə) [*octa-* + *para*] a woman who has had eight pregnancies which resulted in viable offspring; also written para VIII.

oc•ti•sal•ate (ok″tĭ-sal′āt) [USP] a substituted salicylate that absorbs ultraviolet B radiation; used as a sunscreen. Called also *octyl salicylate.*

oc•to•cryl•ene (ok′to-kril″ēn) [USP] a cinnamate compound that absorbs ultraviolet B; used topically as a sunscreen.

oc•to•pam•ine (ok″to-pam′ēn) a sympathomimetic amine thought to result from inability of the diseased liver to metabolize tyrosine; it is called a false neurotransmitter, since it can be stored in presynaptic vesicles, replacing norepinephrine, but has little effect on postsynaptic receptors. It is used as the hydrochloride salt in treatment of hypotension.

oc•to•pus (ok′tə-pəs) any of numerous carnivorous marine mollusks having eight tentacles.

blue-ringed o. *Hapalochlaena maculosa*, a venomous species found along the coast of Australia that when excited bites its enemy and secretes tetrodotoxin. See *tetrodotoxism.*

oc•tose (ok′tōs) a monosaccharide containing eight carbon atoms in the molecule.

oc•tox•y•nol 9 (ok-toks′ĭ-nol) [NF] a clear, pale yellow, viscous liquid used as a surfactant in pharmaceutical preparations. Called also *octylphenoxy polyethoxyethanol.*

Oc•treo•scan (ok-tre′o-skan″) trademark for a preparation of indium In 111 pentetreotide.

oc•tre•o•tide (ok-tre′o-tīd) an eight–amino acid synthetic analogue of somatostatin, having actions similar to those of somatostatin but having a prolonged duration of effect.

o. acetate the acetate salt of octreotide, used as a treatment adjunct for the palliative treatment of diarrhea associated with gastrointestinal endocrine tumors, such as carcinoid tumors and VIPomas, and to decrease the secretion of growth hormone in acromegaly; administered subcutaneously, intragluteally, or intravenously.

oc•tyl (ok′təl) a general term for any 8-carbon radical having the formula C_8H_{17}.

o. methoxycinnamate octinoxate.

o. salicylate octisalate.

oc•tyl•phe•noxy poly•eth•oxy•eth•a•nol (ok″təl-fə-nok′se pol″e-əth-ok″se-eth′ə-nol) octoxynol 9.

Ocu•coat (ok′u-kōt) trademark for a preparation of hydroxypropyl methylcellulose.

Oc•u•fen (ok′u-fen) trademark for a preparation of flurbiprofen sodium.

oc•u•fil•con (ok″u-fil′kon) any of three hydrophilic contact lens materials, designated A, B, or C.

Ocu•flox (ok′u-floks) trademark for a preparation of ofloxacin.

oc•u•lar (ok′u-lər) [L. *ocularis*, from *oculus* eye] 1. of, pertaining to, or affecting the eye; called also *ophthalmic* and *optic.* 2. eyepiece.

oc•u•len•tum (ok″u-len′təm) pl. *oculen′ta* [L. *oculus* eye] an eye ointment.

oc•u•li (ok′u-li) [L.] genitive and plural of *oculus.*

oc•u•list (ok′u-list) ophthalmologist.

ocul(o)- [L. *oculus* eye] a combining form denoting relationship to the eye.

oc•u•lo•ceph•a•lo•gyr•ic (ok″u-lo-sef″ə-lo-gi′rik) [*oculo-* + *cephalo-* + *gyr-* + *-ic*] pertaining to the movements of the head in connection with vision.

oc•u•lo•cu•ta•ne•ous (ok″u-lo-ku-ta′ne-əs) pertaining to or affecting both the eyes and the skin.

oc•u•lo•fa•cial (ok″u-lo-fa′shəl) pertaining to the eyes and the face.

oc•u•lo•gen•e•sis (ok″u-lo-jən′ə-sis) [*oculo-* + *-genesis*] development of the eye of a fetus from part of the neural tube.

oc•u•lo•gy•ra•tion (ok″u-lo-ji-ra′shən) movement of the eye about the anteroposterior axis. **oculogy′ric** *adj*

oc•u•lo•man•dib•u•lo•dys•ceph•a•ly (ok″u-lo-man-dib″u-lo-dis-sef′ə-le) [*oculo-* + *mandibulo-* + *dyscephaly*] malformation of the cranium and facial bones with optic abnormalities; see *oculomandibulofacial syndrome*, under *syndrome.*

oc•u•lo•met•ro•scope (ok″u-lo-met′rə-skōp) [*oculo-* + *metro-* + *-scope*] an instrument for performing retinoscopy in which the trial lenses are rotated before the eyes without effort on the part of the examiner.

oc•u•lo•mo•tor (ok″u-lo-mo′tər) [*oculo-* + *motor*] 1. pertaining to or effecting movements of the eye. 2. pertaining to the oculomotor nerve.

oc•u•lo•my•co•sis (ok″u-lo-mi-ko′sis) [*oculo-* + *mycosis*] any disease of the eye caused by a fungus.

oc•u•lo•na•sal (ok″u-lo-na′səl) pertaining to the eye and the nose.

oc•u•lop•a•thy (ok″u-lop′ə-the) ophthalmopathy.

oc•u•lo•pu•pil•lary (ok″u-lo-pu′pĭ-lar-e) pertaining to the pupil of the eye.

oc•u•lo•spi•nal (ok″u-lo-spi′nəl) pertaining to the eye and the spinal cord.

oc•u•lo•zy•go•mat•ic (ok″u-lo-zi″go-mat′ik) pertaining to the eye and the zygomatic arch (zygoma).

oc•u•lus (ok′u-ləs) gen. and pl. *o′culi* [L.] [TA] the organ of vision; see *eye.* Symbol O.

Oc•u•press (ok′u-pres″) trademark for a preparation of carteolol hydrochloride.

Oc•u•sert (ok′u-sərt) trademark for a drug delivery system placed in the cul-de-sac of the eyes and providing a sustained release of pilocarpine.

Oc•u•sulf (ok′u-sulf″) trademark for preparations of sulfacetamide sodium.

OD[1] [L.] o′culus dex′ter (right eye).

OD[2] optical density; Doctor of Optometry; outside diameter; popular term for *overdose.*

ODA [L.] occipitodextra anterior (right occipitoanterior, a position of the fetus; see *position*).

odax•es•mus (o″dak-sez′məs) [Gr. *odaxēsmos* an itching] the biting of the tongue or cheek in an epileptic seizure.

odax•et•ic (o″dak-set′ik) [Gr. *odaxētikos*] causing a biting or itching sensation.

ODC orotidine 5′-phosphate decarboxylase.

Od•di sphincter (muscle) (od′e) [Ruggero *Oddi*, Italian physician, 1864–1913] musculus sphincter ampullae hepatopancreaticae.

ODDD oculodentodigital dysplasia.

od•di•tis (od-i′tis) inflammation of the sphincter of Oddi.

odds (odz) the ratio of a part to the remainder; it is a means of expressing the chance that a particular event will occur. See also under *ratio.*

odo•gen•e•sis (od″o-jen′ə-sis) [Gr. *hodos* pathway + *-genesis*] neurocladism.

odon•tal•gia (o-don-tal′jə) [*odont-* + *-algia*] toothache. **odontal′gic** *adj*

odon•tec•to•my (o″don-tek′tə-me) [*odont-* + *-ectomy*] excision or removal of a tooth; tooth extraction.

odon•ti•at•ro•gen•ic (o-don″te-at″ro-jen′ik) [*odont-* + *iatro-* + *-genic*] occurring as a result of treatment by a dentist.

odon•tic (o-don′tik) dental.

odont(o)- [Gr. *odous*, gen. *odontos* tooth] a combining form denoting relationship to a tooth or to the teeth.

odon•to•am•e•lo•blas•to•ma (o-don″to-am″ə-lo-blas-to′mə) ameloblastic odontoma.

odon•to•blast (o-don′to-blast) [*odonto-* + *-blast*] one of the columnar connective tissue cells which deposit dentin and form the outer surface of the dental pulp adjacent to the dentin.

odon•to•blas•to•ma (o-don″to-blas-to′mə) a tumor made up of odontoblasts.

odon•to•both•ri•tis (o-don″to-both-ri′tis) alveolitis.

odon•to•cla•mis (o-don″to-kla′mis) [*odonto-* + Gr. *klamys* cloak] dental operculum.

odon•to•clast (o-don′to-klast) [*odonto-* + *-clast*] cementoclast.

odon•to•gen (o-don′to-jen) [*odonto-* + *-gen*] the substance which develops into the dentin of the teeth.

odon•to•gen•e•sis (o-don″to-jen′ə-sis) [*odonto-* + *genesis*] the development and formation of the teeth; it has been divided into three stages: the *lamina-bud stage*, *cap stage*, and *bell stage*. **odontogenet′ic** *adj*

o. imperfec′ta dentinogenesis imperfecta.

odon•to•gen•ic (o-don″to-jen′ik) 1. forming teeth. 2. arising in tissues which give origin to the teeth.

odon•tog•e•nous (o″don-toj′ə-nəs) 1. arising or originating in the teeth. 2. originating in a dental condition.

odon•to•gram (o-don′to-gram) [*odonto-* + *-gram*] the tracing made by an odontograph.

odon•to•graph (o-don′to-graf) [*odonto-* + *-graph*] an instrument for recording the unevenness of surface of tooth enamel.

odon•tog•ra•phy (o″don-tog′rə-fe) [*odonto-* + *-graphy*] 1. a description of the teeth. 2. the use of the odontograph. Called also *dentography*.

odon•to•iat•ria (o-don″to-i-at′re-ə) [*odonto-* + Gr. *iatreia* cure] dental therapeutics.

odon•toid (o-don′toid) [*odont-* + *-oid*] toothlike; resembling a tooth.

odon•to•lith (o-don′to-lith) [*odonto-* + *-lith*] dental calculus.

odon•to•li•thi•a•sis (o-don″to-lĭ-thi′ə-sis) [*odonto-* + *lith-* + *-iasis*] a condition marked by the presence of dental calculus.

odon•tol•o•gist (o″don-tol′ə-jist) dentist.

odon•tol•o•gy (o″don-tol′ə-je) [*odonto-* + *-logy*] 1. the sum of knowledge regarding the teeth. 2. dentistry.

odon•tol•y•sis (o-don-tol′ĭ-sis) [*odonto-* + *-lysis*] tooth resorption.

odon•to•ma (o-don-to′mə) [*odont-* + *-oma*] 1. odontogenic tumor. 2. a specific type of mixed odontogenic tumor, in which both the epithelial and mesenchymal cells exhibit complete differentiation, resulting in formation of tooth structures.

o. adamanti′num ameloblastic o.

ameloblastic o. a rare, slow-growing, mixed odontogenic tumor that combines the characteristics of composite odontoma and ameloblastoma, and occurs more commonly on the mandible than on the maxilla.

complex composite o. a common type of composite odontoma, with calcified dental tissues in an irregular mass, and without morphologic similarity to even rudimentary teeth.

composite o. an odontogenic tumor of the jaws, most commonly of the molar region, composed of both ectodermal and mesodermal tooth components. The two types are *compound composite odontoma* and *complex composite odontoma*.

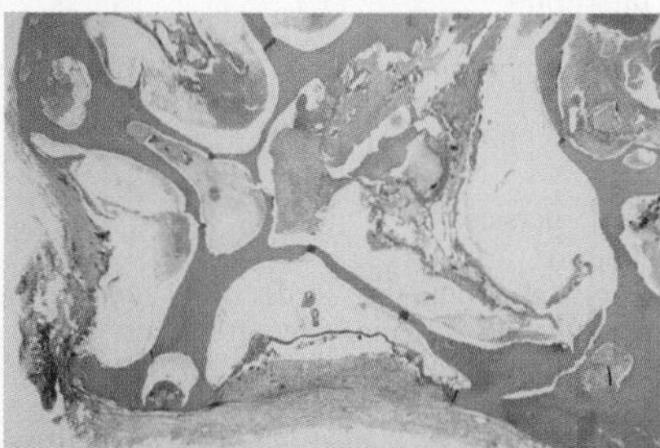

■ Complex composite odontoma, characterized microscopically by irregular spaces containing residual elements of enamel matrix surrounded by septa of dentin interspersed with occasional areas of pulpal tissue. A fibrous connective tissue capsule is present in the periphery.

compound composite o. a composite odontoma in which the enamel and dentin are laid down so that the structure bears a superficial anatomic resemblance to normal teeth.

coronal o., coronary o. an odontoma associated with the crown of a tooth or formed when the crown of the tooth was developing.

dilated o. dens in dente.

embryoplastic o. a soft odontoma formed in the period that precedes the formation of the dental tissues.

fibrous o. an odontoma that contains fibrous elements.

mixed o. an odontoma that contains different elements of the tooth structure.

radicular o. an odontoma associated with the root of a tooth, or one formed at the time when the root of the tooth was developing.

odon•ton•o•my (o″don-ton′ə-me) [*odonto-* + Gr. *onoma* name] the nomenclature of dentistry; a system of terminologies in all branches of dentistry and related fields. Called also *dentonomy*.

odon•top•a•thy (o″don-top′ə-the) [*odonto-* + *-pathy*] any disease of the teeth. **odontopath′ic** *adj*

odon•to•peri•os•te•um (o-don″to-per″e-os′te-əm) periodontium (def. 1).

odon•to•pho•bia (o-don″to-fo′be-ə) [*odonto-* + *-phobia*] an irrational fear associated with teeth, as that aroused by the sight of teeth, or abnormal dread of dental operations.

odon•to•plas•ty (o-don′to-plas″te) recontouring of a tooth surface, such as to enhance calculus and plaque control and morphology of the gingiva. **odontoplas′tic** *adj*

odon•to•pri•sis (o-don″to-pri′sis) [*odonto-* + Gr. *prisis* sawing] bruxism.

odon•to•ra•dio•graph (o-don″to-ra′de-o-graf) a radiograph of a tooth or of the teeth.

odon•to•schism (o-don′to-skiz-əm) [*odonto-* + Gr. *schisma* cleft] fissure of a tooth.

odon•tos•co•py (o″don-tos′kə-pe) [*odonto-* + *-scopy*] the taking of dental impressions.

odon•to•sis (o″don-to′sis) [*odont-* + *-osis*] the formation or eruption of the teeth.

odon•tot•o•my (o″don-tot′ə-me) [*odonto-* + *-tomy*] the operation of cutting into a tooth, especially incision into an occlusal groove.

odon•to•trip•sis (o-don″to-trip′sis) [*odonto-* + *tripsis*] wearing away of the teeth.

odor (o′dər) [L.] a volatile emanation that is perceived by the sense of smell.

minimal identifiable o., minimum perceptible o. the lowest concentration of a substance in air, or in another medium, which still permits its identification by the sense of smell, see also *olfact*.

odor•ant (o′dər-ənt) any substance capable of eliciting olfactory excitation, i.e., of stimulating the sense of smell.

odor•if•er•ous (o″dər-if′ər-əs) [*odor* + *-ferous*] fragrant; emitting an odor.

odor•im•e•ter (o″dər-im′ə-tər) an instrument for performing odorimetry.

odor•im•e•try (o″dər-im′ə-tre) measurement of the strength of olfactory stimuli.

odor•i•phore (o-dor′ĭ-for) osmophore.

odor•i•vec•tor (o″dər-ĭ-vek′tər) a substance which gives off an odor.

ODP [L.] occipito-dextra posterior (right occipitoposterior, a position of the fetus; see *position*).

ODT [L.] occipito-dextra transversa (right occipitotransverse, a position of the fetus; see *position*).

odyn•acu•sis (o″din-ə-ku′sis) [*odyno-* + *acou-* + *-sis*] painful hearing.

-odynia [Gr. *odynē* pain] a word ending denoting a painful condition.

odyn(o)- [Gr. *odynē* pain] a combining form meaning pain.

odyn•om•e•ter (o″din-om′ə-tər) [*odyno-* + *-meter*] algesimeter.

od•y•no•pha•gia (od″ĭ-no-fa′jə) [*odyno-* + *-phagia*] a dysphagia in which swallowing causes pain.

oe- for words beginning thus, see also those beginning with *e-*.

Oeci•a•cus (e-si′ə-kəs) a genus of insects related to bedbugs but having hairy bodies covered by long silklike coats; they are found on birds and in their nests. *O. hiru′dinis* is found on barn swallows in Europe and sometimes invades homes and attacks humans, causing severe irritation. *O. vica′rius* is found on swallows in North America.

oed•i•pism (ed′ĭ-piz-əm) [from *Oedipus*, King of Thebes, who blinded himself after unknowingly killing his father and marrying his mother] intentional injury of one's own eyes.

Oed·i·pus complex (e′dĭ-pəs) [*Oedipus,* character in Greek legend who was raised by a foster parent and later unwittingly killed his father and married his mother] see under *complex.*

Oehl muscle (url) [Eusebio *Oehl,* Italian anatomist, 1827–1903] see under *muscle.*

Oeh·ler symptom (ur′lər) [Johannes *Oehler,* German physician, early 20th century] see under *symptom.*

Oenan·the (e-nan′the) the dropworts, a genus of umbelliferous plants that grow in wet places in the British Isles. The roots of several species contain poisonous alcohols that can cause fatal convulsions and opisthotonos in ruminants.

Oeno·the·ra (e-nə-thēr′ə, e-noth′ə-rə) [Gr. *oinothēras,* a plant, possibly of the genus *Epilobium*] a genus of mainly North American annual or biennial herbs having nocturnal yellow flowers, including the medicinal species *O. bien′nis.*

Oer·sko·via (er-sko′ve-ə) [Jeppe *Ørskov,* Danish microbiologist, 20th century] a genus of bacteria of the family Cellulomonadaceae, consisting of branching hyphae that break up into motile flagellate rods; organisms are gram-positive, mesophilic, and facultatively anaerobic. It is an opportunistic human pathogen. The type species is *O. turba′ta.*

oer·sted (ur′sted) [Hans Christian *Oersted,* Danish physicist, 1777–1851] an older unit of magnetic field strength, largely replaced by the SI unit amperes per meter.

oesophag(o)- for words beginning thus, see those beginning *esophag(o)-.*

Oesoph·a·go·don·tus (e-sof″ə-go-don′təs) a genus of nematodes of the family Strongylidae. *O. robus′tus* is a blood-sucking parasite in the colon of the horse.

oesoph·a·go·sto·mi·a·sis (ə-sof″ə-go-sto-mi′ə-sis) infection of a human or other animal with nematodes of the genus *Oesophagostomum.* See *nodular worm disease,* under *disease.*

Oesoph·a·gos·to·mum (ə-sof″ə-gos′to-məm) [*Oesophagus* + Gr. *stoma* mouth] the nodular worms, a genus of nematodes of the family Strongylidae, parasitic in the intestines of various animals; the larvae often encyst in the intestinal wall, while the adults are mostly free in the lumen. See *nodular worm disease,* under *disease.*

O. bifur′cum a parasite that forms tumors in the large intestine of monkeys and occasionally of humans in Africa and the Philippines.

O. brevicau′dum a species that causes nodular worm disease in pigs.

O. columbia′num a species that causes nodular worm disease in sheep and goats in the southern United States.

O. denta′tum a species that causes nodular worm disease in pigs.

O. radia′tum a species that causes nodular worm disease in cattle.

O. stephanos′tomum a species, normally parasitic in gorillas; a single human case has been recorded from Brazil.

O. venulo′sum a species that causes nodular worm disease in ruminants.

oesoph·a·gus (ə-sof′ə-gəs) [Gr. *oisophagos,* gullet, related to *phagein* to eat] [TA] official terminology for *esophagus.*

oestr- for words beginning thus, see also those beginning *estr-.*

oes·tri·a·sis (es-tri′ə-sis) infestation with larvae of flies of the genus *Oestrus.*

Oes·tri·dae (es′trĭ-de) a family of flies, including the bot, heel, and warble flies. They are very hairy diptera with rudimentary mouth parts and with the antennae inserted into round pits. Genera include *Cuterebra, Dermatobia, Gasterophilus, Hypoderma, Oestrus,* and *Rhinoestrus.*

Oes·trus (es′trəs) [Gr. *oistros* gadfly] a genus of botflies of the family Oestridae. *O. o′vis (O. ho′minis)* is a species whose larvae infest nasal cavities and sinuses of sheep and sometimes cause ophthalmomyiasis in humans.

OFD oral-facial-digital; see under *syndrome.*

of·fi·cial (ə-fish′əl) [L. *officialis; officum* duty] recognized by the current U. S. Pharmacopeia or National Formulary, and meeting the standards established by the respective authority.

of·fic·i·nal (o-fis′ĭ-nəl) [L. *officinalis; officina* shop] denoting pharmaceutical preparations that are regularly kept at pharmacies. Cf. *magistral.*

oflox·a·cin (o-flok′sə-sin) [USP] a broad-spectrum fluoroquinolone antibacterial with actions similar to those of norfloxacin, effective against a wide variety of aerobic gram-negative and gram-positive organisms; administered orally in the treatment of prostatitis, sexually transmitted diseases, and infections of the lower respiratory tract, urinary tract, and skin and soft tissues, and applied topically in the treatment of bacterial corneal ulcers, otitis externa, and otitis media.

Ofu·ji disease, papuloerythroderma (o-foo′je) [Shigeo *Ofuji,* Japanese dermatologist, 20th century] see *eosinophilic pustular folliculitis,* under *folliculitis,* and see under *papuloerythroderma.*

Ogen (o′jən) trademark for preparations of estropipate.

Oges·trel (o-jes′trəl) trademark for a combination preparation of norgestrel and ethinyl estradiol.

Og·il·vie syndrome (o′gil-ve) [Sir William Heneage *Ogilvie,* English surgeon, 1887–1971] see under *syndrome.*

Ogi·no-Knaus method (o-ge′no knous′) [Kusaka *Ogino,* Japanese gynecologist, 1882–1975; Hermann *Knaus,* Austrian gynecologist, 1892–1970] rhythm method; see under *method.*

OGTT oral glucose tolerance test.

Ogu·chi disease (o-goo′che) [Chuta *Oguchi,* Japanese ophthalmologist, 1875–1945] see under *disease.*

Oha·ra disease (o-hah′rah) [Shoichiro *Ohara,* Japanese physician, 20th century] see under *disease.*

OH-Cbl hydroxocobalamin.

17-OHCS 17-hydroxycorticosteroid.

Ohm's law (ōmz) [George Simon *Ohm,* German physicist, 1787–1854] see under *law.*

ohm (Ω) (ōm) [George S. *Ohm*] the SI unit of electrical resistance, being equivalent to the resistance of a circuit in which a current of one ampere is maintained by an electromotive force of one volt.

ohm·am·me·ter (ōm″am′me″tər) an ohmmeter and ammeter combined.

ohm·me·ter (ōm′me-tər) an instrument for measuring electric resistance in ohms.

ohne Hauch (o′nə houkh) [Ger. "without breath" cf. *Hauch*] see *O antigen,* under *antigen,* and *O colony,* under *colony.* Symbol O.

OI osteogenesis imperfecta; oxygenation index.

-oid [Gr. *-oeidēs,* from *eidos* form] a word termination denoting resemblance to the thing specified by the stem to which it is affixed, as ovoid.

Oid·i·um (o-id′e-əm) [dim. of Gr. *ōon* egg] 1. the imperfect (asexual) stage of powdery mildews (order Erysiphales), which cause many plant diseases. 2. a former genus of fungi, now divided between the genera *Candida, Geotrichum,* and *Olpitrichum.*

oid·i·um (o-id′e-əm) a short cylindrical asexual spore formed by the fragmentation of a hypha.

OIH orthoiodohippurate; see *iodohippurate sodium.*

oil (oil) [L. *oleum*] 1. an unctuous, combustible substance that is liquid, or easily liquefiable, on warming, and is soluble in ether but insoluble in water. Such substances, depending on their origin, are classified as animal, mineral, or vegetable oils. Depending on their behavior on heating, they are classified as volatile or fixed. 2. a fat that is liquid at room temperature.

Oil

almond o. 1. [NF] a preparation of the fixed oil obtained by expression from the seed of *Prunus dulcis* (the almond), used as an emollient, perfume, and oleaginous vehicle. It may be derived from either *P. dulcis* var. *dulcis,* (the sweet almond) or *P. dulcis* var. *amara* (the bitter almond). It is not the same as the volatile oil distilled from the bitter almond; see *bitter almond o.* (def. 2). Called also *expressed almond o.* 2. bitter almond o. (def. 2).

anise o. [NF] a volatile oil distilled from the dried, ripe fruit of *Pimpinella anisum* or of *Illicium verum;* used as a flavoring agent for drugs.

apricot kernel o. persic o.

arachis o. peanut o.

argemone o. an oil from the seeds of *Argemone mexicana*; it contains the toxic alkaloid sanguinarine. In certain countries it may be found as a contaminant of cooking oil and may cause epidemic dropsy.

aromatic castor o. [USP] a mixture of castor oil and suitable flavoring agents, containing at least 95 per cent castor oil; used as a cathartic.

banana o. amyl acetate.

Oil *Continued*

bergamot o. a volatile oil obtained by expression from the rind of the fresh fruit of bergamot *(Citrus bergamia)*. It is used in perfumes but can cause photosensitivity.
betula o. methyl salicylate.
bhilawanol o. the oil extracted from the seed of the Indian tree *Semecarpus anacardium*, traditionally used for marking laundry; it contains urushiols and causes the dermatitis called *dhobie mark itch*.
birch tar o. a pyroligneous oil obtained by dry distillation of the bark and wood of various birches (genus *Betula*), especially *B. alba*, rectified by steam distillation; used topically in the treatment of eczema and other dermatitides.
bitter almond o. 1. the fixed oil expressed from *Prunus dulcis* var. *amara* (the bitter almond). Cf. *almond o.* (def. 1). 2. the volatile oil distilled from *Prunus dulcis* var. *amara*, or from other kernels containing amygdalin; it is predominantly benzaldehyde, but also contains hydrogen cyanide and so has been replaced by benzaldehyde as a pharmaceutical flavoring agent.
bitter orange o. a volatile oil obtained from the peel or flowers of the bitter orange *(Citrus aurantium)*; used as a flavoring agent.
borage o. the oil extracted from the seeds of borage *(Borago officinalis)*; used for the treatment of neurodermatitis and as a food supplement.
cade o. juniper tar.
cajeput o. a volatile oil from the fresh leaves and twigs of *Melaleuca leucadendron* and other species of *Melaleuca;* used as a stimulant and rubefacient in rheumatism and other muscle and joint pain, and in veterinary medicine as a rubefacient and parasiticide in the treatment of ringworm. Spelled also *cajuput o.*
canola o. rapeseed oil, specifically that prepared from plants bred to contain lowered amounts of erucic acid.
caraway o. [NF] a volatile oil distilled from the dried ripe fruit of *Carum carvi*, yielding at least 50 per cent by volume of carvone; used as a flavoring agent for drugs and as a carminative.
cardamom o. [NF] a volatile oil distilled from the seed of the cardamom plant *(Elettaria cardamomum)*, used as a flavoring agent in pharmaceutical preparations.
cassia o. cinnamon oil derived from *Cinnamomum cassia.*
castor o. [USP] a fixed oil obtained from the seed of the castor bean plant, *Ricinus communis;* a topical emollient for certain dermatoses and a powerful cathartic; because of its strength as a cathartic, other agents are now preferred for treatment of digestive disorders.
cedar o., cedarwood o., o. of cedar wood a volatile oil from the wood of the red cedar, *Juniperus virginiana*, used as a clearing agent in microscopical techniques; the thicker fraction is used as the immersion medium with oil-immersion objectives.
chloriodized o. an iodine monochloride addition product of vegetable oil, a radiopaque medium.
cinnamon o. a volatile oil distilled with steam from the leaves and twigs of *Cinnamomum cassia* or *Cinnamomum zeylanicum;* used as a flavoring agent for pharmaceuticals.
citronella o. a fragrant oil extracted from *Cymbopogon nardus*, used as an insect repellent.
clove o. [NF] a volatile oil, consisting chiefly of eugenol, distilled from the dried flower buds of *Syzygium aromaticum* (clove); used as a flavor in pharmaceutical preparations, and used externally in the treatment of colds and headache and as a dental antiseptic and analgesic. It also has a variety of uses in Indian medicine.
coconut o. the fixed oil obtained by expression or extraction from the kernels of seeds of *Cocos nucifera;* used as an ointment base and edible oil.
cod liver o. [USP] the partially destearinated fixed oil obtained from fresh livers of *Gadus morrhua* and other species of the family Gadidae; used as a source of vitamin A and vitamin D. In veterinary medicine, it is also used topically to promote wound healing and in abscesses, burns, and dermatoses.
coriander o. a volatile oil distilled with steam from the dried ripe fruit of *Coriandrum sativum;* used as a flavoring agent.
corn o. [NF] a refined fixed oil obtained from the embryo of *Zea mays;* used as a solvent and vehicle for various medicinal agents and as a vehicle for injections. It has also been promoted as a source of polyunsaturated fatty acids in special diets.
cottonseed o. [NF] the fixed oil obtained by expression from the seeds of cultivated varieties of cotton (genus *Gossypium*). It is used in soaps, oleomargarine, lubricants, and salad and cooking oils, and as a solvent and vehicle for injections. In veterinary medicine, it is used as a delousing agent, usually combined with two parts of pine tar for ear ticks of horses, and as a mild emollient and laxative for small animals.
croton o. the thick, fixed oil of the seeds of *Croton tiglium;* it is a drastic purgative and counterirritant, unsafe for human use, and is used as a standard irritant in pharmacological research.
distilled o. volatile o.
drying o. a type of fixed oil which thickens and hardens on exposure to the air, especially when spread out in a thin layer, being converted to a solid by absorption and reaction with oxygen.
dwarf pine needle o. pine needle o.
empyreumatic o. a volatile oil formed by the destructive distillation of organic material.
essential o., ethereal o. volatile o.
ethiodized o. [USP] an iodine addition product of the ethyl ester of the fatty acids of poppyseed oil, used as a radiopaque medium in various diagnostic procedures.
eucalyptus o. a volatile oil distilled with steam from the fresh leaf of *Eucalyptus globulus* and other species of *Eucalyptus;* used as a pharmaceutical flavoring agent and as an expectorant and local antiseptic. It is also used externally for rheumatism and has a large number of uses in folk medicine. See also *eucalyptol.*
evening primrose o. oil produced by cold extraction from the ripe seeds of *Oenothera biennis*, the evening primrose; used internally in the treatment of mastalgia, premenstrual syndrome, and atopic eczema.
expressed o. fixed o.
expressed almond o. almond o. (def. 1).
fatty o. fixed o.
fennel o. [NF] a volatile oil distilled from fennel (the seeds of *Foeniculum vulgare*), used as a flavoring agent for pharmaceuticals; also used internally for cough, bronchitis, and dyspepsia.
fixed o. an oil that does not evaporate on warming. Such oils, consisting of a mixture of fatty acids and their esters, are classified as *solid* (chiefly stearin), *semisolid* (chiefly palmitin), and *liquid* (chiefly olein). They are also classified as *drying*, *semidrying*, and *nondrying*, depending on their tendency to solidify when exposed, in a thin film, to air. Called also *expressed o.* and *fatty o.*
flaxseed o. linseed o.
gaultheria o. methyl salicylate.
groundnut o. peanut o.
iodized o. an iodine addition product of vegetable oil; used as diagnostic radiopaque medium.
lavender o., lavender flowers o. a volatile oil distilled with steam from the fresh flowering tops of *Lavandula angustifolia* subsp. *angustifolia* or prepared synthetically; used as a perfume in pharmaceutical preparations. It is also used internally for loss of appetite, dyspepsia, nervousness, and insomnia, and externally in balneotherapy for functional circulatory disorders; it is also widely used in folk medicine.
lemon o. [NF] the volatile oil obtained by expression without heat from the fresh peel of the fruit of *Citrus limon;* used as a flavoring agent.
light mineral o. [NF], **light white mineral o.** a mixture of liquid hydrocarbons obtained from petrolatum, with a specific gravity of 0.818–0.880; used similarly to mineral oil. Called also *light liquid paraffin* and *light liquid petrolatum.*
linseed o. the fixed oil obtained from the dried ripe seed of *Linum usitatissimum;* used as an emollient in various topical preparations, and in veterinary medicine as a laxative. Called also *flaxseed o.*
o. of male fern a dark green oleoresin from the root of the male fern, *Dryopteris filix-mas;* it has been used as an anthelmintic but is highly toxic.
mineral o. [USP] a mixture of liquid hydrocarbons obtained from petroleum, with a specific gravity of 0.845–0.905; used as a cathartic, as a skin emollient and cleanser, and as a solvent and oleaginous vehicle in pharmaceutical preparations. Called also *heavy liquid petrolatum, liquid petrolatum, liquid paraffin*, and *white mineral o.*
o. of mirbane nitrobenzene.
o. of mustard see *volatile o. of mustard.*
myristica o. nutmeg o.
nondrying o. a type of fixed oil that does not harden but rather remains sticky to the touch indefinitely when exposed in a thin film to air.
nutmeg o. the volatile oil distilled with steam from the dried kernels of the ripe seeds of *Myristica fragrans;* used as a flavoring agent in pharmaceutical preparations. Called also *myristica o.*
olive o. [NF] the fixed oil obtained from the ripe fruit of *Olea europaea;* used as a setting retardant for dental cements, a topical emollient,

Oil *Continued*

and a pharmaceutic necessity, and has been used as a laxative. Called also *sweet o.*

orange o. [NF] the volatile oil obtained by expression from the fresh peel of the ripe fruit of *Citrus sinensis;* used as a flavoring agent in pharmaceuticals. Called also *sweet orange o.* Cf. *bitter orange o.*

peach kernel o. persic o.

peanut o. [NF] the refined fixed oil obtained from peanuts *(Arachis hypogaea)*; used as a solvent and oleaginous vehicle for drugs, and as a laxative in veterinary medicine. Called also *arachis o.* and *groundnut o.*

pennyroyal o. an essential oil derived from pennyroyal (q.v.); its use as an abortifacient has caused death.

peppermint o. [NF] the volatile oil distilled from the fresh above-ground parts of the flowering plant of peppermint *(Mentha piperita);* used as a flavor in pharmaceutical preparations, and as a gastric stimulant and carminative.

persic o. an oil expressed from the kernels of varieties of *Prunus armeniaca* (the apricot) and *P. persica* (the peach); used as a vehicle for drugs.

pine o. the volatile oil obtained by steam distillation of the wood of *Pinus palustris* and other species of *Pinus;* used as a deodorant and disinfectant. It is a gastrointestinal and central nervous system toxin.

pine needle o. the volatile oil distilled with steam from the fresh leaf of the Swiss mountain pine, *Pinus mugo,* and its variety *P. mugo,* var. *pumilio;* used as a perfume and flavoring agent, and has been used to relieve cough and nasal congestion.

pine tar o. rectified tar o.

rapeseed o. the oil expressed from seeds of *Brassica napus,* used in the manufacture of soaps, margarines, and lubricants. An edible variety is called canola oil (q.v.).

rectified tar o. the volatile oil from pine tar rectified by steam distillation; in veterinary medicine, administered internally as a stimulant expectorant and externally as an antipruritic, antiseptic, and stimulant for skin diseases. Also used as a disinfectant and deodorizer.

ricinus o. castor o.

rose o. [NF] the volatile oil distilled with steam from the fresh flowers of *Rosa alba, R. centifolia, R. damascena,* or *R. gallica,* used as a perfuming agent and flavoring agent. Called also *attar of roses.*

rosemary o. the volatile oil distilled with steam from the fresh flowering tops of *Rosmarinus officinalis,* used as a flavoring or perfuming agent.

safflower o. an oily liquid extracted from the seeds of the safflower, *Carthamus tinctorius,* containing predominantly linoleic acid; used as a pharmaceutic aid, as a component of total parenteral nutrition solutions, and in the diet in the management of hypercholesterolemia.

sandalwood o., santal o. a viscid oily liquid with a characteristic odor and taste, distilled with steam from the dried heartwood of *Santalum album* (sandalwood); a common essential oil potentially toxic to the kidneys.

sassafras o. the volatile oil distilled from the root of *Sassafras albidum;* it contains safrole and is toxic and carcinogenic.

savin o. an acrid oil from the fresh tops of *Juniperus sabina,* the chief constituent of which is sabinol. It has been used in folk medicine, but may cause hematuria and violent gastrointestinal irritation when administered internally; fatal poisoning has resulted from its use as an abortifacient.

semidrying o. a fixed oil that dries incompletely or slowly when exposed in a thin film to air.

sesame o. [NF] the refined fixed oil obtained from the seed of *Sesamum indicum;* it is used as a solvent and oleaginous vehicle for drugs.

silicone o. any of various long-chain fluid silicone polymers; those of medical interest being polydimethylsiloxanes. Various silicone oils, particularly of viscosity between 5000 and 5400 centistokes, are injected into the vitreous to serve as a vitreous substitute during or after vitreoretinal surgery, such as to maintain retinal tamponade in the management of complicated retinal detachment.

spearmint o. the volatile oil distilled with steam from the fresh overground parts of *Mentha spicata* or *M. cardiaca,* yielding at least 55 per cent by volume of carvone; used as a flavor for pharmaceutical preparations.

sweet o. olive o.

sweet almond o. the fixed oil expressed from *Prunus dulcis* var. *dulcis* (the sweet almond). Cf. *almond o.* (def. 1).

sweet birch o. methyl salicylate.

sweet orange o. orange o.

tea tree o. an essential oil obtained by steam distillation from the leaves and branch tips of *Melaleuca alternifolia,* having bacteriostatic and weak antiviral and antimycotic properties, used topically for skin infections; it is also used internally and externally in folk medicine for a variety of indications.

theobroma o. cocoa butter.

thyme o. the volatile oil from fresh, flowering *Thymus vulgaris;* used as a flavoring agent for drugs, and as an antitussive and expectorant.

turpentine o. the volatile oil distilled from turpentine; its chief constituent is pinene, which is used in the synthetic production of camphor. It is used as a counterirritant and rubefacient.

volatile o. an oil that evaporates readily; such oils are usually found in aromatic plants, to which they give odor and other characteristics. Most consist of a mixture of two or more terpenes. Called also *distilled, essential,* or *ethereal o.*

volatile o. of mustard a volatile oil distilled from the seeds of black mustard *(Brassica nigra);* it consists predominantly of allyl isothiocyanate and is used as a strong counterirritant and rubefacient.

white mineral o. mineral o.

wintergreen o. methyl salicylate.

---

oint•ment (oint′mənt) [L. *unguentum*] a semisolid preparation for external application to the skin or mucous membranes, usually containing a medicinal substance. Called also *unguent* and *salve.*

benzoic and salicylic acids o. [USP] a preparation of benzoic acid and salicylic acid in a ratio of about 2:1 in a suitable ointment, used topically as an antifungal and keratolytic agent in the treatment of tinea pedis; called also *Whitfield o.*

bland lubricating ophthalmic o. [USP] an ointment for use in the eye, composed of white petrolatum and mineral oil; it may also contain lanolin, modified lanolin, or lanolin alcohols.

coal tar o. [USP] a preparation of coal tar, polysorbate 80, and zinc oxide paste, used as a topical antieczematic and antipsoriatic.

compound resorcinol o. [USP] a preparation of resorcinol, zinc oxide, bismuth subnitrate, juniper tar, yellow wax, petrolatum, anhydrous lanolin, and glycerin, used as a topical antifungal and keratolytic.

hydrophilic o. [USP] a water-in-oil emulsion consisting of methylparaben, propylparaben, sodium lauryl sulfate, propylene glycol, stearyl alcohol, white petrolatum, and purified water; used as an ointment base.

PEG o., polyethylene glycol o. [NF] a mixture of polyethylene glycol 4000 and polyethylene glycol 400, used as a water-soluble ointment base.

rose water o. [USP] a preparation of cetyl esters wax, white wax, almond oil, sodium borate, stronger rose water, purified water, and rose oil, used as an emollient and ointment base.

simple o. white o.

white o. [USP] an oleaginous ointment base prepared from white wax and white petrolatum.

Whitfield o. benzoic and salicylic acids o.

yellow o. [USP] an oleaginous ointment base prepared from yellow wax and petrolatum.

oja (o′jə) according to ayurveda, the imprint of self in the physical body, which arises from the strength of the metabolism and balance a body maintains in knowing itself, thus governing the immune system.

oka•da•ic ac•id (o-kə-dā′ik) a polyether fatty acid that inhibits protein phosphatase and promotes tumor formation; it is found in protozoa of the genera *Dinophysis* and *Prorocentrum,* and is the toxin responsible for diarrhetic shellfish poisoning (see under *poioning*).

Oka•za•ki fragments (o-kah-zah′ke) [Reiji *Okazaki,* Japanese molecular biologist, 1930–1975] see under *fragment.*

Oken body (corpus) (o′kən) [Lorenz *Oken,* German physiologist, 1779–1851] see *mesonephros.*

OL [L.] o′culus lae′vus (left eye).

Ol. [L.] o′leum (oil).

-ol suffix indicating that the substance is an alcohol or a phenol, i.e., a hydroxyl derivative of a hydrocarbon.

OLA [L.] occipitolaeva anterior (left occipitoanterior, a position of the fetus; see *position*).

ol•amine (ol′ə-mēn) USAN contraction for *ethanolamine*.

o•lan•za•pine (o-lan′zə-pēn) a monoaminergic agent used as an antipsychotic in the management of schizophrenia and for short-term treatment of manic episodes in bipolar disorder; administered orally.

Old•field syndrome (ōld′fēld) [Michael C. *Oldfield*, British physician, 20th century] see under *syndrome*.

Olea (o′le-ə) a genus of small trees or shrubs of the family Oleaceae, which have drupaceous fruit. *O. europae′a* L. is the commonly cultivated olive tree, source of olive oil.

olea[1] (o′le-ə) [L. "olive"] olive (def. 1).

olea[2] (o′le-ə) [L.] plural of *oleum*.

ole•ag•i•nous (o″le-aj′ĭ-nəs) [L. *oleaginus*] oily; greasy; unctuous.

ole•an•der (o″le-an′dər) *Nerium oleander*.

ole•an•drism (o″le-an′driz-əm) poisoning by oleander, which contains cardiac glycosides. Characteristics include gastroenteritis with vomiting and diarrhea, increased pulse rate, and increased respiration, sometimes ending fatally.

ole•ate (o′le-āt) 1. a salt, anion, or ester of oleic acid. 2. a solution of an alkaloid or other basic drug in oleic acid, used as an ointment.

olec•ra•non (o-lek′rə-non) pl. *olec′rana* [Gr. *ōlekranon*] [TA] the proximal bony projection of the ulna at the elbow, its anterior surface forming part of the trochlear notch. **olec′ranal** *adj*

ole•fin (o′lə-fin) [*oleo-* + L. *facere* to make] any of a class of unsaturated aliphatic hydrocarbons having one or more double bonds; those with one double bond are called alkenes.

ole•ic ac•id (o-le′ik) 1. a monounsaturated 18-carbon fatty acid, liquid at room temperature and occurring in most animal fats and vegetable oils. See also table accompanying *fatty acid*. 2. [NF] a preparation consisting mainly of oleic acid with some palmitic and stearic acids, manufactured from fats and oils that are derived from edible sources unless the mixture is for external use only; used as an emulsifying agent and to assist absorption of some drugs by the skin.

ole•in (o′le-in) the triglyceride formed from oleic acid, occurring in most fats and oils.

ole(o)- [L. *oleum* oil] a combining form denoting relationship to oil.

oleo•chryso•ther•a•py (o″le-o-kris″o-ther′ə-pe) [*oleo-* + *chrysotherapy*] therapeutic administration of gold salts in oily suspensions.

oleo•gran•u•lo•ma (o″le-o-gran″u-lo′mə) paraffinoma.

oleo•in•fu•sion (o″le-o-in-fu′zhən) a preparation made by infusing a drug in oil.

ole•o•ma (o″le-o′mə) [*oleo-* + *-oma*] paraffinoma.

ole•om•e•ter (o″le-om′ə-tər) [*oleo-* + *-meter*] an instrument for testing the purity of oil.

oleo•pal•mi•tate (o″le-o-pal′mĭ-tāt) an oleate and a palmitate of the same base.

oleo•peri•to•ne•og•ra•phy (o″le-o-per″ĭ-to-ne-og′rə-fe) radiography of the peritoneum following the injection of iodized oil.

oleo•res•in (o″le-o-rez′in) [*oleo-* + *resin*] 1. any natural combination of a resin and a volatile oil, such as exudes from pines and other plants. 2. a compound prepared by exhausting a drug, containing both volatile oil and resin, by percolation with a volatile solvent, such as acetone, alcohol, or ether, and concentrating the percolate until the solvent has been dissipated.
 aspidium o. oil of male fern.
 capsicum o. an alcoholic extract of the dried ripe fruits of various species of *Capsicum*; used as an irritant and carminative.

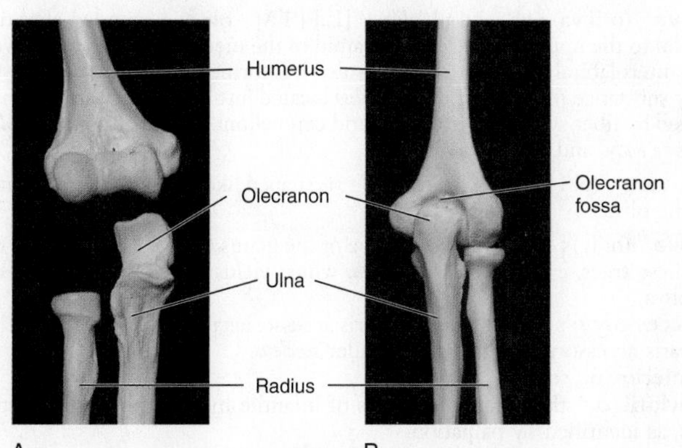

■ Olecranon in *(A)*, anterior view of the humerus, radius, and ulna and *(B)*, posterior view of the articulated elbow joint.

oleo•sac•cha•rum (o″le-o-sak′ə-rəm) [*oleo-* + Gr. *sakcharon* sugar] a triturate of sugar with a volatile oil; used as a flavoring agent in pharmaceutical preparations.

oleo•ste•ar•ate (o″le-o-ste′ər-āt) an oleate and a stearate of the same base.

oleo•ther•a•py (o″le-o-ther′ə-pe) [*oleo-* + *therapy*] treatment with oil, particularly treatment by the injection of oil.

oleo•tho•rax (o″le-o-tho′raks) a method of collapse therapy in which oil or paraffin was inserted into part of the thoracic cavity.

oleo•vi•ta•min (o″le-o-vi′tə-min) a preparation of fish liver oil or edible vegetable oil containing one or more fat-soluble vitamins or their derivatives.
 o. A and D [USP] an oily preparation containing vitamin A and natural or synthetic vitamin D; used as a dietary supplement.

oleo•yl (o-le′o-əl) the acyl radical of oleic acid.

ole•um (o′le-əm) gen. *o′lei* pl. *o′lea* [L. "oil"] oil.

ol•fact (ol′fakt) a unit of odor, the minimum perceptible odor, being the minimum concentration of a substance in solution which can be perceived by a large number of normal individuals, expressed in terms of grams per liter.

ol•fac•tant (ol-fak′tənt) odorant.

ol•fac•tion (ol-fak′shən) [L. *olfacere* to smell] 1. the sense of smell; the ability to perceive and distinguish odors. 2. the act of perceiving and distinguishing odors.

ol•fac•tism (ol-fak′tiz-əm) a sensation of smell produced by other than olfactory stimuli.

ol•fac•tol•o•gy (ol″fak-tol′ə-je) the science of the sense of smell. Called also *osmics*, *osmology*, and *osphresiology*.

ol•fac•tom•e•ter (ol″fak-tom′ə-tər) [*olfactus* + *-meter*] an apparatus for testing the sensitiveness of perception of odors.

ol•fac•tom•e•try (ol″fak-tom′ə-tre) the measurement of the sense of smell.

ol•fac•to•ry (ol-fak′tə-re) [L. *olfacere* to smell] pertaining to olfaction, or the sense of smell.

ol•fac•tus (ol-fak′təs) gen. *olfac′tus*. Olfaction (def. 1); see also *organum olfactus*.

Oli•gel•la (ol″ĭ-gel′ə) [*olig-* + L. *-ella* diminutive ending] a genus of aerobic, gram-negative bacteria of the family Alcaligenaceae, consisting of non–spore-forming, chemo-organotrophic small rods or coccobacilli, often occurring in pairs; some are motile by means of peritrichous flagella. The type species is *O. urethra′lis*.
 O. ureoly′tica a species, most strains of which are motile, isolated primarily from the urine of persons with indwelling urinary catheters, in whom it associated with the development of urinary calculi; it may also cause bacteremia.
 O. urethra′lis a nonmotile species that is a commensal of the genitourinary tract; most infections are asymptomatic, but bacteremia, septic arthritis, and peritonitis may occur.

ol•i•ge•mia (ol″ĭ-je′me-ə) hypovolemia.

olig(o)- [Gr. *oligos* little, few] a combining form meaning *(a)* few, little, or scanty, *(b)* less than normal, or *(c)* deficient. Cf. *pauci-*.

ol•i•go•am•ni•os (ol″ĭ-go-am′ne-os) [*oligo-* + *amnios*] oligohydramnios.

ol•i•go•an•al•ge•sia (ol″ĭ-go-an″əl-je′ze-ə) the use of analgesics too infrequently or at doses insufficient to relieve pain.

ol•i•go•an•u•ria (ol″ĭ-go-an-u′re-ə) oliguria in which there is a temporary complete cessation of urinary flow.

ol•i•go•ar•thri•tis (ol″ĭ-go-ahr-thri′tis) arthritis of a small number of joints.

ol•i•go•as•then•o•sper•mia (ol″ĭ-go-as″thə-no-spur′me-ə) [*oligospermia* + *asthenospermia*] oligospermia with decreased sperm motility.

ol•i•go•as•tro•cy•to•ma (ol″ĭgo-as″tro-si-to′mə) a mixed glioma consisting of elements derived from astrocytes and elements derived from oligodendrocytes.
 anaplastic o. a malignant type of oligoastrocytoma characterized histopathologically by pleomorphism, atypical nuclei, and high mitotic activity.

ol•i•go•blast (ol′ĭ-go-blast″) a primitive oligodendrocyte.

ol•i•go•chro•ma•sia (ol″ĭ-go-kro-ma′se-ə) hypochromia (def. 1).

ol•i•go•clo•nal (ol″ĭ-go-klo′nəl) pertaining to or derived from a few clones. Cf. *polyclonal*.

ol·i·go·cys·tic (ol″ĭ-go-sis′tik) [*oligo-* + *cystic*] containing only a few cysts.

ol·i·go·dac·ty·ly (ol″ĭ-go-dak′tə-le) [*oligo-* + Gr. *daktylos* finger] the presence of less than the usual number of fingers or toes; called also *hypodactyly.*

ol·i·go·den·dria (ol″i-go-den′dre-ə) oligodendroglia.

ol·i·go·den·dro·blas·to·ma (ol″ĭ-go-den″dro-blas-to′mə) oligodendroglioma.

ol·i·go·den·dro·cyte (ol″ĭ-go-den′dro-sīt) [*oligodendro*glia + *-cyte*] a cell of the oligodendroglia.

ol·i·go·den·drog·lia (ol″ĭ-go-den-drog′le-ə) [*oligo-* + *dendro-* + *neuroglia*] 1. the non-neural cells of ectodermal origin forming part of the adventitial structure (neuroglia) of the central nervous system; projections of the surface membrane of each of these cells (oligodendrocytes) fan out and coil around the axon of many neurons to form myelin sheaths in the white matter. With microglia, they form the perineuronal satellites in the gray matter. 2. the tissue composed of such cells. **oligodendrog′lial** *adj*

ol·i·go·den·dro·gli·o·ma (ol″ĭ-go-den″dro-gli-o′mə) a usually benign neoplasm derived from and composed of oligodendrocytes in varying stages of differentiation; the majority are seen in adults in the white matter of the brain. Called also *oligodendroblastoma.*

anaplastic o. a malignant type of oligodendroglioma characterized histopathologically by increased cell density, atypical nuclei anaplasia, increased mitotic activity, and necrosis.

ol·i·go·dip·sia (ol″ĭ-go-dip′se-ə) [*oligo-* + *dipsia*] hypodipsia.

ol·i·go·don·tia (ol″ĭ-go-don′shə) [*olig-* + *odont-* + *-ia*] absence of many teeth, usually associated with small size of the existing teeth and other anomalies.

ol·i·go·dy·nam·ic (ol″ĭ-go-di-nam′ik) [*oligo-* + *dynamic*] active in very minute quantities; said especially of heavy metal ions (Hg^{2+}, Ag^{+}) to describe toxic effect on cells and organisms.

ol·i·go·en·ceph·a·lon (ol″ĭ-go-ən-sef′ə-lon) micrencephalon.

ol·i·go·ga·lac·tia (ol″ĭ-go-gə-lak′she-ə) hypogalactia.

ol·i·go·gen·ic (ol″ĭ-go-jen′ik) [*oligo-* + *genic*] produced or influenced by the action of a few different genes.

ol·i·gog·lia (ol″ĭ-gog′le-ə) oligodendroglia.

ol·i·go-1,4-1,4-glu·can·trans·fer·ase (ol″ĭ-go-gloo″kan-trans′fər-ās) an enzyme activity catalyzing the transfer of short α-1,4 linked glucose chains from side chains of limit dextrins to new α-1,4 linkages on main chains or glucose, thereby exposing α-1,6 branch points for debranching and further degradation. The enzyme activity is the transferase activity of amylo-1,6-glucosidase (q.v.).

ol·i·go-1,6-glu·co·si·dase (ol″ĭ-go-gloo-ko′sĭ-dās) [EC 3.2.1.10] EC nomenclature for *α-dextrinase.*

ol·i·go·glu·co·side (ol″ĭ-go-gloo′ko-sīd) an oligosaccharide composed of glucose residues. Cf. *polyglucoside.*

ol·i·go·hy·dram·ni·os (ol″ĭ-go-hi-dram′ne-os) [*oligo-* + *hydro-* + *amnion*] the presence of less than the normal amount of amniotic fluid, defined as 500 mL or less at term and smaller amounts at earlier gestational ages. See also *oligohydramnios sequence*, under *sequence.*

ol·i·go·hy·dru·ria (ol″ĭ-go-hi-droo′re-ə) [*oligo-* + *hydruria*] hypersthenuria.

Ol·i·go·hy·me·no·phor·ea (ol″ĭ-go-hi″mə-no-for′e-ə) [*oligo-* + *hymen* + Gr. *phoros* bearing] a class of ciliate protozoa (phylum Ciliophora), characterized by the presence of an oral apparatus that is usually well developed and situated at least partially in a buccal cavity and by oral ciliature that is clearly distinct from the somatic ciliature, consisting of a paraoral membrane on the right side and a few compound organelles on the left. Some species are loricate, and colony formation is common in some groups. It comprises two subclasses: Hymenostomatia and Peritrichia.

ol·i·go·hy·per·men·or·rhea (ol″ĭ-go-hi″pər-men″o-re′ə) oligomenorrhea with excessive menstrual flow.

ol·i·go·hy·po·men·or·rhea (ol″ĭ-go-hi″po-men″o-re′ə) oligomenorrhea with diminished menstrual flow.

ol·i·go·lec·i·thal (ol″ĭ-go-les′ĭ-thəl) [*oligo-* + *-lecithal*] microlecithal.

ol·i·go·meg·a·ne·phro·nia (ol″ĭ-go-meg″ə-nə-fro′ne-ə) [*oligo-* + *mega-* + *nephron* + *-ia*] congenital renal hypoplasia in which there is a reduced number of lobes and nephrons, with hypertrophy of the nephrons. **oligomeganephron′ic** *adj*

ol·i·go·men·or·rhea (ol″ĭ-go-men″ə-re′ə) [*oligo-* + *meno-* + *-rrhea*] menstrual flow happening less often than normal, defined as at intervals of 35 days to 6 months; called also *infrequent menstruation.*

ol·i·go·mer (ol′ĭ-go-mər) [*oligo-* + Gr. *meros* part] a polymer formed by the combination of relatively few monomers.

ol·i·go·me·tal·lic (ol″ĭ-go-mə-tal′ik) containing only small quantities of metals.

ol·i·go·mor·phic (ol″ĭ-go-mor′fik) [*oligo-* + *morph-* + *-ic*] passing through only a few forms of growth; said of microorganisms.

ol·i·go·nec·ro·sper·mia (ol″ĭ-go-nek″ro-spur′me-ə) [*oligo-* + *necro-* + *sperm-* + *-ia*] decreased live spermatozoa, and some dead, in the spermatic fluid.

ol·i·go·neph·ro·nia (ol″ĭ-go″nə-fro′ne-ə) renal hypoplasia.

ol·i·go·ni·tro·phil·ic (ol″ĭ-go-ni″tro-fil′ik) [*oligo-* + *nitrogen* + *-philic*] absorbing nitrogen from the air and from media containing combined nitrogen; said of microorganisms.

ol·i·go·nu·cle·o·tide (ol″ĭ-go-noo′kle-o-tīd) [*oligo-* + *nucleotide*] a single-stranded nucleic acid segment of a few (usually fewer than 20) nucleotides, particularly one produced by recombinant technology and used as a probe or primer.

ol·i·go·ov·u·la·tion (ol″ĭ-go-ov″u-la′shən) maturation and discharge of oocytes from the ovaries at a lesser frequency than normal.

ol·i·go·pep·tide (ol″ĭ-go-pep′tīd) the structure formed by the linkage of a few amino acids.

ol·i·gop·nea (ol″ĭ-gop-ne′ə) [*oligo-* + *-pnea*] hypopnea.

ol·i·go·sac·cha·ride (ol″ĭ-go-sak′ə-rīd) a carbohydrate that on hydrolysis yields a small number of monosaccharides (from two to four, or according to some definitions up to ten). Cf. *polysaccharide.*

N-linked o. an oligosaccharide that in glycoproteins is attached to the amide nitrogen of asparagine.

O-linked o. an oligosaccharide that in glycoproteins is attached to the oxygen of the hydroxyl group of serine or threonine and in collagen is attached via galactose to the hydroxyl group of hydroxylysine.

ol·i·go·sac·cha·ryl·trans·fer·ase (ol″ĭ-go-sak″ə-ril-trans′fər-ās) an enzyme of the transferase class that catalyzes the transfer of the assembled oligosaccharide precursor from the dolichol phosphate carrier to the asparagine residue of a polypeptide chain in *N*-linked glycosylation. In EC nomenclature called *dolichyl-diphosphooligosaccharide–protein glycotransferase.*

ol·i·go·sper·ma·tism (ol″ĭ-go-spur′mə-tiz-əm) oligospermia.

ol·i·go·sper·mia (ol″ĭ-go-spur′me-ə) [*oligo-* + *sperm-* + *-ia*] a decreased number of spermatozoa in the semen; called also *oligozoospermia.*

ol·i·go·syn·ap·tic (ol″ĭ-go-sin-ap′tik) [*oligo-* + *synaptic*] involving a few synapses in series and therefore a sequence of only a few neurons; called also *paucisynaptic.* Cf. *polysynaptic.*

ol·i·go·troph (ol′ĭ-go-trōf) an oligotrophic organism.

ol·i·go·tro·phic (ol″ĭ-go-tro′fik) [*oligo-* + *-trophic*] able to live in a nutrient-poor environment; said of bacteria and other microorganisms.

ol·i·go·typ·ing (ol′ĭ-go-tīp″ing) a process based on the polymerase chain reaction, typing different strains of bacteria using oligonucleotide probes.

ol·i·go·zo·o·sper·ma·tism (ol″ĭ-go-zo″o-spur′mə-tiz-əm) oligospermia.

ol·i·go·zo·o·sper·mia (ol″ĭ-go-zo″o-spur′me-ə) oligospermia.

ol·i·gu·ria (ol″ĭ-gu′re-ə) [*oligo-* + *-uria*] diminished urine production and excretion as compared with fluid intake, usually defined as less than 500 mL per 24 hours. Called also *hypouresis.* **oligu′ric** *adj*

olis·the (o-lis′the) olisthy.

olis·thy (o-lis′the) [Gr. *olisthanein* to slip] a slipping, as the slipping of the bones of a joint from their normal relation in the joint. **olisthet′ic** *adj*

oli·va (o-li′və) gen. and pl. *oli′vae* [L.] [TA] olive: a rounded elevation, lateral to the upper part of each pyramid of the medulla oblongata, between the anterolateral and posterolateral sulci; it is formed by an irregular mass of gray substance *(nucleus olivaris caudalis)* located just beneath its surface and is linked by fiber systems to the pons and cerebellum. Called also *inferior olive, olivary body*, and *olivary nucleus.*

ol·i·vary (ol′ĭ-var″e) [L. *olivarius*] 1. shaped like an olive. 2. pertaining to the oliva.

ol·ive (ol′iv) [L. *oliva*] 1. any tree of the genus *Olea.* 2. the fruit of one of these trees, especially *O. europaea*, which yields olive oil (see under *oil*). 3. oliva.

accessory o′s the nucleus olivaris accessorius posterior and the nucleus olivaris accessorius medialis; see under *nucleus.*

inferior o. oliva.

pyloric o. the enlarged pylorus of infantile hypertrophic pyloric stenosis, as identified by palpation.

spurge o. mezereum.

Ol·i·ver sign (ol′ĭ-vər) [William Silver *Oliver*, English physician, 1836–1908] tracheal tugging.

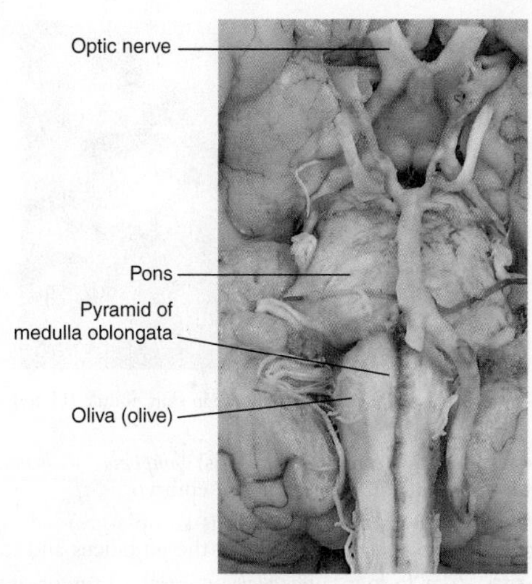

■ Oliva (olive) shown in an anterior (inferior) view of the brain.

ol·i·vif·u·gal (ol″ĭ-vif′u-gəl) [*oliva* + *-fugal*²] moving or conducting away from the oliva.

ol·i·vip·e·tal (ol″ĭ-vip′ə-təl) [*oliva* + *-petal*] passing or conducting toward the oliva.

ol·i·vo·pon·to·cer·e·bel·lar (ol″ĭ-vo-pon″to-ser″ə-bel′ər) pertaining to the olivae, the middle peduncles, and the cortex of the cerebellum.

Ol·lier disease, law, layer (o-le-a′) [Léopold Louis Xavier Edouard *Ollier*, French surgeon, 1830–1900] see *enchondromatosis*, and see under *law* and *layer*.

Ol·lier-Thiersch graft (o-le-a′ tērsh′) [L.L.X.E. *Ollier*; Karl *Thiersch*, German surgeon, 1822–1895] see under *graft*.

Ol·lu·la·nus (ol″u-lan′us) a genus of nematodes. *O. tricus′pis* is a small worm found in the stomachs of pigs and cats that causes gastritis.

ol·me·sar·tan me·dox·o·mil (ol″mə-sahr′tan mə-dok′so-mil) a selective angiotensin receptor antagonist used as an antihypertensive, administered orally.

Olm·sted syndrome (olm′sted) [H.C. *Olmsted*, American physician, early 20th century] see under *syndrome*.

olo·pa·ta·dine hy·dro·chlo·ride (o″lo-pat′ə-dēn) an antihistamine (H_1 receptor antagonist) used in the treatment of allergic conjunctivitis, applied topically to the conjunctiva.

OLP [L.] occipitolaeva posterior (left occipitoposterior, a position of the fetus; see *position*).

Ol·pi·trich·um (ol-pĭ-trik′əm) a genus of Fungi Imperfecti of the form-family Moniliaceae, which contains species of the former genera *Oidium* and *Acladium;* they are found in soil, and are sometimes isolated from infected wounds.

ol·sal·a·zine so·di·um (ol-sal′ə-zēn) a compound consisting of two molecules of mesalamine linked by an azo bond, used in treatment of ulcerative colitis; administered orally.

Ols·hau·sen operation (olz′hou-zen) [Robert von *Olshausen*, German obstetrician, 1835–1915] see under *operation*.

OLT [L.] occipitolaeva transversa (left occipitotransverse, a position of the fetus; see *position*).

Olux (o′luks) trademark for a preparation of clobetasol propionate.

o.m. [L.] om′ni ma′ne (every morning).

-oma [Gr. *ōma*, noun-forming suffix] a word termination meaning tumor or neoplasm of the part indicated by the stem to which it is attached.

oma·ceph·a·lus (o″mə-sef′ə-ləs) omocephalus.

Oma·cor (o′mə-kor) trademark for a preparation of ethyl esters of ω-3 fatty acids.

oma·gra (o-ma′grə) [*om-* + *-agra*] gout in the shoulder.

omal·gia (o-mal′jə) [*om-* + *-algia*] pain in the shoulder.

oma·liz·u·mab (o″mə-liz′ə-mab) a recombinant, DNA-derived monoclonal antibody that binds selectively to immunoglobulin E, prevents IgE from binding to mast cells and basophils, and thus decreases allergic reactions; used in treatment of asthma and administered by injection.

omar·thri·tis (o″mahr-thri′tis) [*om-* + *arthr-* + *-itis*] inflammation of the shoulder joint.

oma·si·tis (o″mə-si′tis) inflammation of the omasum.

oma·sum (o-ma′səm) [L.] the third stomach of a ruminant; its walls are lined with many folia that have rough surfaces, serving to grind up food. Called also *manyplies* and *psalterium*. **oma′sal** *adj*

Om·bré·danne operation (ōm-bra-dahn′) [Louis *Ombrédanne*, French surgeon, 1871–1956] see under *operation*.

OMD Doctor of Oriental Medicine.

-ome [by analogy with gen*ome*] a word termination denoting the complete set of substances or entities of a specified type, such as proteins, in a cell or organism.

omega (o-ma′gə) [Ω, ω] the twenty-fourth, and final, letter of the Greek alphabet. See also ω-.

ome·ga pep·ti·dase (o-ma′gə pep′tĭ-dās) [EC 3.4.19] any of a group of exopeptidases that catalyze the cleavage of a substituted N- or C-terminal amino acid residue from a peptide chain.

Omenn syndrome (o′mən) [Gilbert Stanley *Omenn*, American internist, born 1941] see under *syndrome*.

omen·ta (o-men′tə) [L.] plural of *omentum*.

omen·tec·to·my (o″mən-tek′tə-me) [*omentum* + *-ectomy*] excision of all or a portion of the omentum.

omen·tin (o-men′tin) an adipocytokine important in insulin resistance and energy homeostasis. Plasma and adipose tissue levels are reduced in diabetic and obese persons.

omen·ti·tis (o″mən-ti′tis) inflammation of the omentum.

omen·to·cele (o-men′to-sēl) omental hernia.

omen·to·fix·a·tion (o-men″to-fik-sa′shən) omentopexy.

omen·to·pexy (o-men′to-pek″se) [*omentum* + *-pexy*] any of various operations in which omentum is fastened to some other tissue, especially when the omentum is used as a circulatory bridge to reduce congestion or provide vascular nutrition.

omen·to·plas·ty (o-men′to-plas″te) [*omentum* + *-plasty*] the use of omental grafts to cover raw surfaces in abdominal surgery. **omentoplas′tic** *adj*

omen·to·por·tog·ra·phy (o-men″to-por-tog′rə-fe) radiography of the hepatic portal veins after injection of a contrast medium into the gastroepiploic vein in the base of the omentum.

omen·tor·rha·phy (o″mən-tor′ə-fe) [*omentum* + *-rrhaphy*] suture or repair of the omentum.

omen·tot·o·my (o″mən-tot′ə-me) [*omentum* + Gr. *temnein* to cut] incision of the omentum.

omen·to·vol·vu·lus (o-men″to-vol′vu-ləs) volvulus of the omentum.

omen·tum (o-men′təm) pl. *omen′ta* [L. "fat skin"] a fold of peritoneum extending from the stomach to adjacent organs in the abdominal cavity; see *o. majus* and *o. minus*. Called also *epiploon*. **omen′tal** *adj*

colic o., gastrocolic o. o. majus.

gastrohepatic o. o. minus.

gastrosplenic o. ligamentum gastrosplenicum.

greater o. o. majus.

lesser o. o. minus.

o. ma′jus [TA] greater omentum: a prominent peritoneal fold suspended from the greater curvature of the stomach and passing inferiorly a variable distance in front of the intestines; it is attached to the anterior surface of the transverse colon.

o. mi′nus [TA] lesser omentum: a peritoneal fold joining the lesser curvature of the stomach and the first part of the duodenum to the porta hepatis.

splenogastric o. ligamentum gastrosplenicum.

omen·tum·ec·to·my (o-men″təm-ek′tə-me) [*omentum* + *-ectomy*] omentectomy.

omep·ra·zole (o-mep′ra-zōl) [USP] a proton pump inhibitor used in the treatment of dyspepsia, gastroesophageal reflux disease, and gastric hypersecretory conditions including Zollinger-Ellison syndrome, and peptic ulcer, and in conjunction with antibiotics in the treatment of peptic ulcer associated with *Helicobacter pylori* infection; administered orally.

om·i·cron (om′ĭ-kron) [O, o] the fifteenth letter of the Greek alphabet.

omi·tis (o-mi′tis) [*omo-* + *-itis*] inflammation of the shoulder.

om·ma·tid·i·um (om″ə-tid′e-əm) pl. *ommatid′ia* [Gr. dim. of *omma* eye] one of the units of the compound eye of arthropods, itself complete with all the functional and structural elements of the eye (including lens, retina, photoreceptor cells).

Om·ma·ya reservoir (o-mi′yə) [Ayub Khan *Ommaya*, Pakistani neurosurgeon in the United States, born 1930] see under *reservoir*.

Om·nar·is (om-nār′is) trademark for a preparation of ciclesonide.

Omn. bih. [L.] om'ni biho'ra (every two hours).

Omn. hor. [L.] om'ni ho'ra (every hour).

Om•ni•cef (om'nĭ-sef″) trademark for a preparation of cefdinir.

Om•ni•paque (om'nĭ-pāk) trademark for preparations of iohexol.

Om•ni•pen (om'nĭ-pen″) trademark for preparations of ampicillin.

om•nip•o•tence (om-nip'ə-tens) fantasies of special abilities and power and superiority to others; occurring in infancy and sometimes later in life as a defense mechanism or as an expression of delusional thinking.

Om•ni•scint (om'nĭ-sint″) trademark for a preparation of indium In 111 satumomab pendetide.

Om•ni•scan (om'nĭ-skan) trademark for a preparation of gadodiamide.

om•niv•o•rous (om-niv'ə-rəs) [L. *omnis* all + *vorare* to eat] subsisting upon both plants and animals.

Omn. noct. [L.] om'ni noc'te (every night).

om(o)- [Gr. *ōmos* shoulder] a combining form denoting relationship to the shoulder.

omo•ceph•a•lus (o″mo-sef'ə-ləs) [*omo-* + *-cephalus*] a fetus with no upper limbs and an incomplete head.

omo•cla•vic•u•lar (o″mo-klə-vik'u-lər) pertaining to the shoulder and the clavicle.

omo•dyn•ia (o″mo-din'e-ə) [*omo-* + *-odynia*] omalgia.

omo•hy•oid (o″mo-hi'oid) pertaining to the shoulder and the hyoid bone.

omo•pha•gia (o″mo-fa'je-ə) [Gr. *ōmos* raw + *-phagia*] the eating of raw food.

omo•ster•num (o″mo-stur'nəm) the interarticular cartilage at the joint between the sternum and clavicle.

OMPA octamethyl pyrophosphoramide.

om•pha•lec•to•my (om″fə-lek'tə-me) [*omphalo-* + *-ectomy*] excision of the umbilicus.

Om•pha•lia (om-fa'le-ə) a genus of mushrooms of the family Agaricaceae. *O. lapides'cens* is dried and used as an anthelmintic called *raigan* in Chinese medicine.

om•phal•ic (om-fal'ik) [Gr. *omphalikos*] umbilical.

om•pha•li•tis (om″fə-li'tis) [*omphalo-* + *-itis*] inflammation of the umbilicus.

o. of birds infection of the yolk sac with bacteria normally found in the alimentary tract and on the skin of the hen, leading to death of the embryo or of the chick up to ten days after hatching; called also *mushy chick disease.*

omphal(o)- [Gr. *omphalos* navel] a combining form denoting relationship to the umbilicus.

om•pha•lo•an•gi•op•a•gous (om″fə-lo-an″je-op'ə-gəs) allantoidoangiopagous.

om•pha•lo•an•gi•op•a•gus (om″fə-lo-an″je-op'ə-gəs) allantoidoangiopagus.

om•pha•lo•cele (om'fə-lo-sēl″) [*omphalo-* + *-cele*[1]] protrusion at birth of part of the intestine through a large defect in the abdominal wall at the umbilicus, the protruding bowel being covered only by a thin transparent membrane composed of amnion and peritoneum. Cf. *umbilical hernia.* Called also *amniocele, exomphalos, exumbilication,* and *umbilical eventration.*

om•pha•lo•cho•ri•on (om″fə-lo-kor'e-on) choriovitelline placenta.

om•pha•lo•did•y•mus (om″fə-lo-did'ĭ-məs) gastrodidymus.

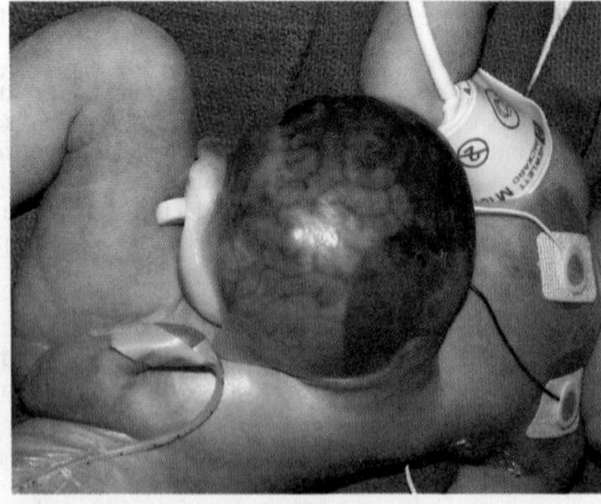

■ Omphalocele.

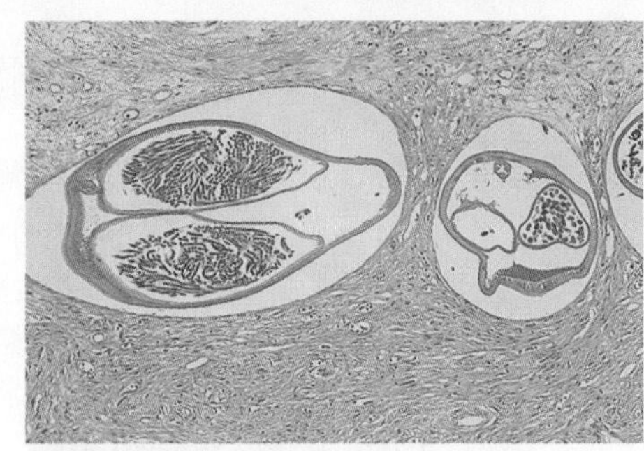

■ Cross-section of adult *Onchocerca volvulus* in skin nodule (H & E stain).

om•pha•lo•gen•e•sis (om″fə-lo-jen'ə-sis) [*omphalo-* + *-genesis*] development of the umbilicus or yolk sac in the embryo.

om•pha•lo•is•chi•op•a•gus (om″fə-lo-is-ke-op'ə-gəs) [*omphalo-* + *ischio-* + *-pagus*] conjoined twins united at the umbilicus and the ischia.

om•pha•lo•ma (om″fə-lo'mə) [*omphalo-* + *-oma*] a tumor of the umbilicus.

om•pha•lo•mes•en•ter•ic (om″fə-lo-mes″ən-ter'ik) pertaining to the umbilicus and mesentery.

om•pha•lop•a•gus (om″fə-lop'ə-gəs) [*omphalo-* + *-pagus*] conjoined twins united in the region of the umbilicus.

om•pha•lo•phle•bi•tis (om″fə-lo-flə-bi'tis) [*omphalo-* + *phlebitis*] 1. inflammation of the umbilical veins. 2. infection with suppurative lesions of the umbilicus in young animals; see also *navel ill,* under *ill.*

om•pha•lor•rha•gia (om″fə-lo-ra'jə) [*omphalo-* + *-rrhagia*] hemorrhage from the umbilicus.

om•pha•lor•rhea (om″fə-lo-re'ə) [*omphalo-* + *-rrhea*] an effusion of lymph at the navel.

om•pha•lor•rhex•is (om″fə-lo-rek'sis) [*omphalo-* + *-rrhexis*] rupture of the umbilicus.

om•pha•lo•site (om'fə-lo-sīt″) [*omphalo-* + Gr. *sitos* food] an underdeveloped member of allantoidoangiopagous twins, which is joined to the more developed member (autosite) by the vessels of the umbilical cord.

om•pha•lot•o•my (om″fə-lot'ə-me) [*omphalo-* + *-tomy*] the cutting of the umbilical cord.

om•pha•lus (om'fə-ləs) [Gr. *omphalos*] umbilicus.

Om. quar. hor. [L.] om'ni quadran'te ho'ra (every quarter of an hour).

-on [from *ion* (q.v.)] a word termination denoting a unit or quantum.

o.n. [L.] om'ni noc'te (every night).

onan•ism (o'nə-niz″əm) [*Onan,* son of Judah] 1. coitus interruptus. 2. masturbation.

ona•ye (o-nah'ye) an extremely strong poison from the seeds of *Strophanthus hispidus.*

On•ca•spar (on'kə-spar) trademark for a preparation of pegaspargase.

onch(o)- see *onc(o)-*[2].

On•cho•cer•ca (ong″ko-sur'kə) [*oncho-* + Gr. *kerkos* tail] a genus of nematode parasites of the superfamily Filarioidea that infect humans and ruminants. The adults live and breed in subcutaneous fibroid nodules; the young (the microfilariae) are carried by the lymph and are found chiefly in the skin, subcutaneous connective tissues, and eyes.

O. caecu'tiens *O. volvulus.*

O. cervica'lis a species found in the cervical ligament of horses and mules, usually not causing symptoms.

O. gibso'ni a species that produces subcutaneous nodular swellings on the legs of cattle and zebras.

O. vol'vulus a common parasite whose insect vector breeds in fast-flowing rivers and streams in tropical regions of the Americas and Africa, particularly West Africa. It is the etiologic agent of human onchocerciasis and is transmitted by the bites of buffalo gnats of the genus *Simulium,* in which the parasite passes part of its life cycle.

on•cho•cer•ci•a•sis (ong″ko-sər-ki'ə-sis) [*Onchocerca* + *-iasis*] infection with nematodes of the genus *Onchocerca.* Human infection is caused by *O. volvulus,* with heavy infestations usually characterized by the firm subcutaneous nodules called *onchocercomas;* persistent dermatitis with a pruritic papular rash and sometimes edema, lichenification, thickening, wrinkling, skin atrophy, and areas of leukoderma; lymphadenitis; and ocular lesions. The latter are caused by invasion by microfilariae (eye worms), which die and cause irritation with punctate or sclerosing keratitis that may progress to opacification of the cornea and blindness. Called also *onchocercosis, volvulosis,* and numerous local names.

on·cho·cer·co·ma (ong″ko-sər-ko′mə) [*Onchocerca* + *-oma*] a firm, usually freely movable and nontender subcutaneous nodule containing a tangled mass of adult *Onchocerca volvulus* worms; seen in onchocerciasis.

on·cho·cer·co·sis (ong″ko-sər-ko′sis) onchocerciasis.

on·cho·der·ma·ti·tis (ong″ko-dur-mə-ti′tis) the cutaneous manifestations of onchocerciasis, beginning with a pruritic rash with papules and later developing into extensive atrophic and pigmentary changes.

On·ci·co·la (on-sik′ə-lə) a genus of parasitic acanthocephalans. *O. ca′nis* has been found in the intestines of dogs in the midwestern United States.

onc(o)-[1] [Gr. *onkos* mass, bulk] a combining form denoting relationship to a tumor, swelling, or mass.

onc(o)-[2] [Gr. *onkos* barb, hook] a combining form denoting relationship to a barb or hook.

On·co·cer·ca (ong″ko-sur′kə) *Onchocerca.*

on·co·cyte (ong′ko-sīt) a large epithelial cell with an extremely acidophilic, granular cytoplasm, containing huge numbers of mitochondria; these cells undergo neoplastic transformation. **oncocyt′ic** *adj*

on·co·cy·to·ma (ong″ko-si-to′mə) [*oncocyte* + *-oma*] 1. a usually benign adenoma composed of oncocytes, often referring specifically to a tumor of the salivary glands. Called also *oncocytic adenoma*, *oxyphilic adenoma*, and *oxyphil cell tumor*. 2. Hürthle cell adenoma.

renal o. a benign neoplasm of the kidney that resembles a renal cell carcinoma but is encapsulated and not invasive; most patients are middle-aged and have few overt symptoms from the tumor.

on·co·cy·to·sis (on″ko-si-to′sis) metaplasia of oncocytes.

on·co·fe·tal (ong″ko-fe′təl) [*onco-*[1] + *fetal*] occurring both in tumor tissue and during fetal development; see under *antigen.*

on·co·gene (ong′ko-jēn) a gene capable under certain conditions of causing the initial and continuing conversion of normal cells into cancer cells. The term may be used to denote such a gene occurring in a viral genome (v-*onc*) or a cellular gene derived from alteration of a proto-oncogene (c-*onc*).

viral o. an oncogene carried by a virus into a cell, where it becomes incorporated into the DNA of the cell.

on·co·gen·e·sis (ong″ko-jen′ə-sis) tumorigenesis. **oncogenet′ic** *adj*

on·co·gen·ic (ong″ko-jen′ik) giving rise to tumors (either benign or malignant) or causing tumor formation; said especially of tumor-inducing viruses. Cf. *tumorigenic.*

on·co·ge·nic·i·ty (ong″ko-jə-nis′ĭ-te) the quality or property of being able to cause tumor formation.

on·co·ge·no·mics (ong″ko-je-no′miks) cancer genomics.

on·cog·e·nous (ong-koj′ə-nəs) arising in or originating from a tumor.

on·coi·des (ong-koi′dēz) [*onco-*[1] + Gr. *eidos* form] turgid swelling; intumescence.

on·co·lip·id (ong″ko-lip′id) [*onco-*[1] + *lipid*] a structurally altered lipid moiety of a lipoprotein molecule found in the plasma of cancer patients.

on·col·o·gy (ong-kol′ə-je) [*onco-*[1] + *-logy*] the sum of knowledge concerning tumors; the study of tumors.

radiation o. the study and treatment of cancers using radiation therapy.

on·col·y·sate (ong-kol′ĭ-sāt) any agent that lyses or destroys tumor cells. Cf. *cytotoxicity.*

on·col·y·sis (ong-kol′ĭ-sis) [*onco-*[1] + *-lysis*] the lysis or destruction of tumor cells; see also *cytotoxicity.* **oncolyt′ic** *adj*

on·co·ma (ong-ko′mə) [Gr. *onkōma*] tumor.

On·co·me·la·nia (ong″ko-mə-la′ne-ə) a genus of fresh water snails of the family Bulimidae, found in eastern Asia and nearby Pacific islands; some species transmit schistosomiasis japonica. Formerly called *Katayama.*

on·com·e·ter (ong-kom′ə-tər) an instrument for measuring oncotic pressure.

On·co·Scint CR/OV (on′ko-sint″) trademark for a preparation of indium In 111 satumomab pendetide.

on·co·sis (ong-ko′sis) [*onco-*[1] + *-osis*] a morbid condition characterized by the development of tumors.

on·co·sphere (ong′ko-sfēr) [*onco-*[2] + *sphere*] the larva of the tapeworm contained within the external embryonic envelope and armed with six hooks; it may be found in the feces.

on·co·ther·a·py (ong″ko-ther′ə-pe) [*onco-*[1] + *therapy*] the treatment of tumors.

on·cot·ic (ong-kot′ik) 1. pertaining to, caused by, or marked by swelling. 2. see under *pressure.*

on·cot·o·my (ong-kot′ə-me) [*onco-*[1] + *-tomy*] the incision of a tumor or swelling.

on·co·tro·pic (ong″ko-tro′pik) [*onco-*[1] + *-tropic*] having a special affinity or attraction for tumor cells; called also *tumoraffin.*

On·co·vin (ong′ko-vin) trademark for a preparation of vincristine sulfate.

On·co·vi·ri·nae (on″ko-vir-i′ne) a former subfamily of the Retroviridae that included members causing certain types of tumors.

on·co·vi·rus (ong′ko-vi″rəs) [*onco-*[1] + *virus*] any of the tumor-producing retroviruses that were in the former subfamily called Oncovirinae. **oncovi′ral** *adj*

on·dan·se·tron hy·dro·chlo·ride (on-dan′sə-tron) [USP] an antiemetic used for prevention of nausea and vomiting occurring after surgery or in conjunction with cancer chemotherapy or radiotherapy; administered orally or intravenously.

On·dine curse (on-dēn′) [*Ondine*, sea nymph in German mythology who cursed an unfaithful human lover by abolishing the automaticity of his bodily functions] primary alveolar hypoventilation.

-one a suffix used in chemistry to indicate *(a)* quintivalent nitrogen, and *(b)* a compound having two hydrocarbon radicals attached to the carbonyl group; a ketone.

onei·rism (o-ni′riz-əm) an abnormal dreamlike state of consciousness. **onei′ric** *adj*

oneir(o)- [Gr. *oneiros* dream] a combining form denoting relationship to a dream.

onei·ro·gen·ic (o″ni-ro-jen′ik) producing a dreamlike state; capable of causing dreams.

onei·roid (o′ni-roid) resembling a dream.

onei·rol·o·gy (o″ni-rol′ə-je) [*oneiro-* + *-logy*] the science of dreams and their interpretation.

onei·ro·phre·nia (o-ni″ro-fre′ne-ə) [*oneiro-* + *phren-* + *-ia*] a form of schizophrenia characterized by clouding of consciousness.

oni·um (o′ne-əm) a term applied to a cation in which nitrogen has its maximum covalency, as in the ammonium ion NH_4^+. The compounds include betaines, cholines, and amine oxides.

on·lay (on′la″) 1. a graft applied or laid on the surface of an organ or structure. 2. a cast metal restoration that overlays cusps, thus lending strength to the restored tooth.

epithelial o. an epithelial graft whose edges are not completely approximated to the edges of the wound, thus permitting new epithelium to grow out around the margin; see also under *inlay.*

on·o·mato·ma·nia (on″ə-mat″ə-ma′ne-ə) [Gr. *onoma* name + *-mania*] irresistible preoccupation with specific words or names.

on·o·mato·pho·bia (on″ə-mat″ə-fo′be-ə) [Gr. *onoma* name + *-phobia*] irrational fear of hearing a particular word or name.

on·o·mat·o·poe·ia (on″ə-mat″ə-pe′ə) [Gr. *onoma* name + *poiein* to make] the formation of meaningless words that imitate sounds, such as may occur to excess in some cases of schizophrenia.

on·o·mato·poi·e·sis (on″ə-mat″ə-poi-e′sis) onomatopoeia.

On·tak (on′tak) trademark for a preparation of denileukin diftitox.

on·to·gen·e·sis (on″to-jen′ə-sis) ontogeny.

on·tog·e·ny (on-toj′ə-ne) [Gr. *ōn* existing + *-geny*] the development of the individual organism. Cf. *phylogeny.* **ontogenet′ic, ontogen′ic** *adj*

Onu·fro·wicz nucleus (o-noo′fro-vich) [Bronislaw *Onufrowicz*, Swiss anatomist, late 19th century] see under *nucleus.*

ony·al·ai (o″ne-al′a-e) a nutritional disorder seen in Central Africa, marked by the formation on the palatal and buccal mucous membranes of blebs containing semicoagulated blood; there are no signs of constitutional disorder. It is a form of thrombocytopenic purpura.

on·y·cha·tro·phia (on″ĭ-kə-tro′fe-ə) [*onych-* + *atrophia*] atrophy of a nail or nails.

on·y·chat·ro·phy (on″ĭ-kat′rə-fe) onychatrophia.

on·y·chaux·is (on″ĭ-kawk′sis) [*onych-* + Gr. *auxein* to increase] simple hypertrophy of a nail without deformity; called also *hyperonychia.* Cf. *onychogryphosis* and *pachyonychia.*

on·y·chec·to·my (on″ĭ-kek′tə-me) [*onych-* + *-ectomy*] 1. excision of a nail or nail bed. 2. removal of the claws of an animal; called also *declawing.*

onych·ia (o-nik′e-ə) [*onych-* + *-ia*] inflammation of the matrix of the nail resulting in shedding of the nail. Called also *onychitis.* See also *paronychia.*

on·y·chi·tis (on″ĭ-ki′tis) onychia.

onych(o)- [Gr. *onyx*, gen. *onychos* nail] a combining form denoting relationship to the nails.

on·y·choc·la·sis (on″ĭ-kok′lə-sis) onychorrhexis.

on·y·cho·cryp·to·sis (on″ĭ-ko-krip-to′sis) ingrown toenail.

on·y·cho·cyte (on′ĭ-ko-sīt″) one of the tightly packed keratinized cells arranged in layers to make up the nail plate.

on·y·cho·dys·tro·phy (on″ĭ-ko-dis′trə-fe) nail dystrophy.

on·y·cho·gen·ic (on″ĭ-ko-jen′ik) [*onycho-* + *-genic*] producing or forming nail substance.

on·y·cho·gram (o-nik′o-gram) a tracing made by the onychograph.

on·y·cho·graph (o-nik′o-graf″) [*onycho-* + *-graph*] an instrument for observing and recording the nail pulse and capillary circulation.

on·y·cho·gry·pho·sis (on″ĭ-ko-grə-fo′sis) [*onycho-* + *gryphosis*] long-term hypertrophy of a nail, producing a hooked or incurved clawlike deformity. Called also *ram's horn n.* and *onychogryposis.* Cf. *onychauxis.*

on·y·cho·gry·po·sis (on″ĭ-ko-grə-po′sis) onychogryphosis.

on·y·cho·het·ero·to·pia (on″ĭ-ko-het″ər-o-to′pe-ə) [*onycho-* + *heterotopia*] abnormal placement of the nails.

on·y·chol·y·sis (on″ĭ-kol′ĭ-sis) [*onycho-* + *-lysis*] separation of the nail plate from the nail bed, usually beginning at the free margin and progressing proximally.

on·y·cho·ma·de·sis (on″ĭ-ko-mə-de′sis) [*onycho-* + Gr. *madēsis* loss of hair] separation of the nail plate from the nail bed and shedding distally to a groove that has formed; it may be due to a systemic condition or trauma. See also *Beau line*, under *line.* Called also *defluvium unguium* and *onychoptosis.*

on·y·cho·ma·la·cia (on″ĭ-ko-mə-la′shə) [*onycho-* + *malacia*] softening of a nail or nails.

on·y·cho·ma·tri·co·ma (on″ĭ-ko-ma″trĭ-ko′mə) a rare type of benign tumor of the nail matrix in which the nail is thickened, discolored, and excessively curved and has hollows that contain digitated tumor substance.

on·y·cho·my·co·sis (on″ĭ-ko-mi-ko′sis) fungal infection of the toenails or fingernails. It usually is seen first as white patches or pits on the surface or around the edges of the nails, followed by infection beneath the nail plate. Called also *dermatophytic o.*, *tinea unguium*, and *ringworm of the nail.*

on·y·cho-os·teo·dys·pla·sia (on″ĭ-ko-os″te-o-dis-pla′zhə) [*onycho-* + *osteo-* + *dysplasia*] 1. osteo-onychodysplasia (def. 1). 2. nail-patella syndrome.

on·y·cho·pachy·der·mo·peri·os·to·sis (on″ĭ-ko-pak″e-dur″mo-per″e-os-to′sis) periostitis in a digit with nail and soft tissue involvement.

psoriatic o. a rare complication of psoriatic arthritis in one or more terminal phalanges, with nail dystrophy, swelling of soft tissues, and periostitis.

on·y·cho·pa·thol·o·gy (on″ĭ-ko-pə-thol′ə-je) [*onycho-* + *pathology*] the study of diseases of the nails.

on·y·chop·a·thy (on″ĭ-kop′ə-the) [*onycho-* + *-pathy*] disease or deformity of the nails. Called also *onychosis.* **onychopath′ic** *adj*

on·y·cho·pha·gia (on″ĭ-ko-fa′jə) [*onycho-* + *-phagia*] the habit of biting the nails.

on·y·choph·a·gy (on″ĭ-kof′ə-je) onychophagia.

on·y·cho·pho·sis (on″ĭ-ko-fo′sis) [*onycho-* + Gr. *phōs* light + *-osis*] a callus in a nail groove, such as one occurring with an ingrown toenail.

on·y·chop·to·sis (on″ĭ-kop-to′sis, on″ĭ-ko-to′sis) onychomadesis.

on·y·chor·rhex·is (on″ĭ-ko-rek′sis) [*onycho-* + *-rrhexis*] striation, brittleness, and breakage of the nail plate in a longitudinal direction.

on·y·cho·schi·zia (on″ĭ-ko-skiz′e-ə) [*onycho-* + *schiz-* + *-ia*] splitting of the nail plate, sometimes into layers, usually in a transverse (horizontal) direction at the free edge.

on·y·cho·sis (on″ĭ-ko′sis) onychopathy.

on·y·cho·til·lo·ma·nia (on″ĭ-ko-til″o-ma′ne-ə) compulsive picking or tearing at the nails.

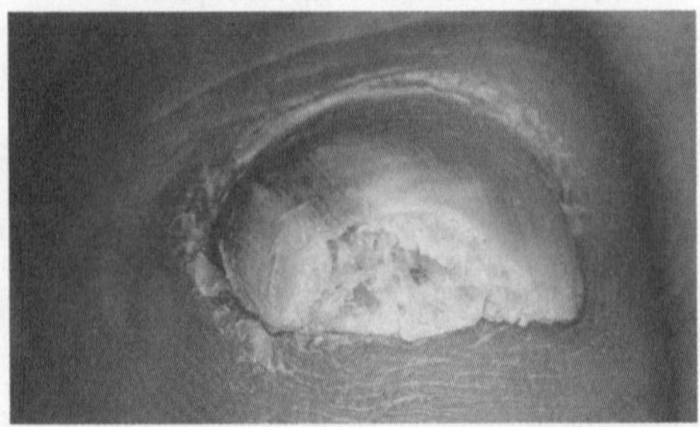

■ Onychomycosis and lifting of the nail plate.

on·y·chot·o·my (on″ĭ-kot′ə-me) [*onycho-* + *-tomy*] incision of a nail.

Ony·ge·na·les (on″ĭ-jə-na′lēz) an order of keratinophilic perfect fungi of the subphylum Ascomycotina, series Prototunicatae; medically important genera include *Ajellomyces* and *Arthroderma.*

o′nyong-nyong (o-nyong′nyong) ["severe joint pain" in the language of the Acholi people of East Africa] an acute, nonfatal febrile disease due to an alphavirus, transmitted by anopheline mosquitoes, occurring in Uganda, Kenya, Tanzania, Malawi, and Senegal, and clinically resembling dengue and chikungunya; it is characterized by lymphadenitis, joint pains, and an extremely pruritic morbilliform skin rash. Called also *o′nyong-nyong fever.*

on·yx (on′iks) [Gr. "nail"] 1. unguis. 2. a type of hypopyon.

on·yx·is (ə-nik′sis) ingrown toenail.

oo- [Gr. *ōon* egg] a combining form denoting relationship to an oocyte or egg; see also words beginning *ov(o)-.*

oo·blast (o′o-blast) [*oo-* + *-blast*] a primordial cell from which an oocyte ultimately is developed.

Oo·cho·ris·ti·ca (o″o-ko-ris′tĭ-kə) a large genus of tapeworms, family Linstowiidae, which are parasitic in birds, reptiles, and mammals.

oo·cy·e·sis (o″o-si-e′sis) [*oo-* + *-cyesis*] ovarian pregnancy.

oo·cyst (o′o-sist) [*oo-* + *cyst*] the encysted or encapsulated zygote in the life cycle of sporozoan protozoa, which by the process of sporogony develops into a sporozoite or a sporocyst containing sporozoites.

oo·cyte (o′o-sīt) [*oo-* + *-cyte*] the immature female reproductive cell prior to fertilization, derived from an oogonium and occurring in two stages, primary and secondary oocytes.

primary o. an oocyte that has begun but not completed the first maturation division; it is derived from an oogonium by differentiation near the time of birth.

primordial o. an oocyte very early in its development.

secondary o. an oocyte in the period between the first and second maturation division; it is derived from a primary oocyte shortly before ovulation by a division that splits off the first polar body. If fertilized, it divides into an ootid and the second polar body; otherwise it perishes. In humans, it is a round cell about 0.1 mm in diameter, and consists of protoplasm that contains some yolk, enclosed by a thin cell wall, the vitelline membrane. It is surrounded by the zona pellucida and corona radiata.

oog·a·my (o-og′ə-me) in the most restrictive sense, fertilization of a large nonmotile female gamete by a small, motile male gamete or sperm, as in certain algae; the term is often used more generally to mean the sexual union of two dissimilar gametes (heterogamy). **oog′amous** *adj*

oo·gen·e·sis (o″o-jen′ə-sis) [*oo-* + *-genesis*] the process of formation of female gametes (oocytes).

oo·ge·net·ic (o″o-jə-net′ik) 1. pertaining to oogenesis. 2. producing oocytes. Called also *oogenic, ovogenetic*, and *ovogenic.*

oo·gen·ic (o″o-jen′ik) oogenetic.

oo·go·ni·um (o″o-go′ne-əm) pl. *oogo′nia* [*oo-* + Gr. *gonē* generation] 1. a primordial oocyte during fetal development; it is derived from a primordial germ cell, multiplies rapidly, then becomes encapsulated in primordial follicle cells and, near the time of birth, becomes a primary oocyte by entering into prophase of the first maturation division. 2. in certain fungi and algae, the female gametangium containing one or more eggs (oospheres).

oo·ki·ne·sis (o″o-kĭ-ne′sis) [*oo-* + *-kinesis*] the mitotic movements of the oocyte during maturation and fertilization.

oo·ki·nete (o″o-ki′nēt, o″o-kĭ-net′) [*oo-* + Gr. *kinetos* movable] the motile, worm-shaped zygote of certain protozoa, such as *Plasmodium*, which is found in the insect vector.

oo·lem·ma (o″o-lem′ə) [*oo-* + *-lemma*] zona pellucida (def. 1).

Oo·my·ce·tes (o″o-mi-se′tēz) [*oo-* + Gr. *mykēs* fungus] a class of funguslike chromists of the phylum Oomycota. The subclass Saprolegniomycetidae includes animal pathogens.

oo·my·co·sis (o-o-mi-ko′sis) infection by fungi of the class Oomycetes; it does not occur in humans. *Pythium* species infect horses and *Saprolegnia* species infect fish.

Oo·my·co·ta (o″o-mi-ko′tə) [*oo-* + Gr. *mykēs* fungus, from the large round oogonium] the water molds, a phylum of funguslike, filamentous organisms belonging to the Chromista and formerly classified with the fungi. They differ from the fungi in having a cell wall that consists of cellulose, reproducing sexually by biflagellate spores, and possessing diploid nuclei in the vegetative state. It includes plant and animal parasites and comprises the class Oomycetes and a number of organisms incertae sedis.

oo·pha·gia (o″o-fa′je-ə) oophagy.

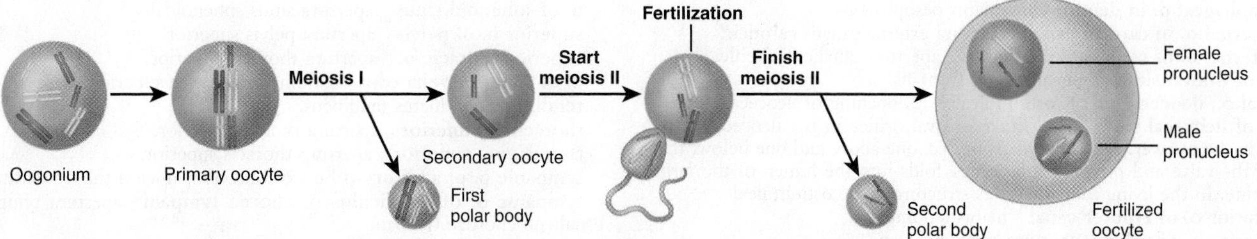

■ Oogenesis, depicting only six of the 46 double-stranded chromosomes (oogonium, primary oocyte), three of the 23 double-stranded chromosomes (secondary oocyte, first polar body), and three of the 23 single-stranded chromosomes (second polar body, spermatozoon, and female and male pronuclei) in human oogenesis, and showing random assortment of homologous chromosome pairs. Crossing over, which may occur in meiosis I, has been omitted. Progression through meiosis II is only completed if fertilization occurs; the spermatozoon and male pronucleus are depicted out of scale for clarity.

ooph•a•gy (o-of′ə-je) [Gr. *ōophagein* to eat eggs] the eating of eggs; said of insects whose diet consists largely of eggs.

ooph•or•al•gia (o″of-ər-al′jə) [*oophor-* + *-algia*] pain in an ovary.

ooph•o•rec•to•mize (o″of-ə-rek′tə-mīz) to surgically remove one or both of the ovaries; See also *castrate* and *spay*.

ooph•o•rec•to•my (o″of-ə-rek′tə-me) [*oophor-* + *-ectomy*] the removal of an ovary or ovaries; if done bilaterally, the individual is incapable of reproduction (see *castration*). Called also *ovariectomy*.

ooph•o•ri•tis (o″of-ə-ri′tis) [*oophor-* + *-itis*] inflammation of an ovary.
  o. paroti′dea oophoritis occurring in association with infection by the virus causing mumps.

oophor(o)- [Gr. *ōophoros* bearing eggs] a combining form denoting relationship to the ovary.

ooph•o•ro•cys•tec•to•my (o-of″ə-ro-sis-tek′tə-me) [*oophoro-* + *cyst-* + *-ectomy*] excision of an ovarian cyst.

ooph•o•ro•cys•to•sis (o-of″ə-ro-sis-to′sis) [*oophoro-* + *cyst* + *-osis*] the formation of ovarian cysts.

ooph•o•rog•e•nous (o-of″ə-roj′ə-nəs) derived from the ovary.

ooph•o•ro•hys•ter•ec•to•my (o-of″ə-ro-his″tər-ek′tə-me) [*oophoro-* + *hysterectomy*] surgical removal of the uterus and ovaries.

ooph•o•ron (o-of′ə-ron) [Gr. *ōon* egg + *pherein* to bear] ovarium.

ooph•o•rop•a•thy (o-of″ə-rop′ə-the) [*oophoro-* + *-pathy*] any disease of the ovaries. Called also *ovariopathy*.

ooph•o•ro•pexy (o-of′ə-ro-pek″se) the operation of elevating and fixing an ovary to the abdominal wall.

ooph•o•ro•plas•ty (o-of′ə-ro-plas″te) plastic surgery of the ovary.

ooph•o•ro•sal•pin•gec•to•my (o-of″ə-ro-sal″pin-jek′tə-me) [*oophoro-* + *salpingectomy*] salpingo-oophorectomy.

ooph•o•ro•sal•pin•gi•tis (o-of″ə-ro-sal″pin-ji′tis) salpingo-oophoritis.

ooph•o•ros•to•my (o-of″ə-ros′tə-me) [*oophoro-* + *-stomy*] the making of an opening into an ovarian cyst.

ooph•o•rot•o•my (o-of″ə-rot′ə-me) incision of an ovary.

ooph•or•rha•gia (o-of″ə-ra′jə) [*oophoro-* + *-rrhagia*] severe hemorrhage from an ovary.

oo•phyte (o′o-fīt) [*oo-* + *-phyte*] any member of the generation in the life history of mosses, ferns, etc., in which the sexual organs are produced.

oo•plasm (o′o-plaz″əm) the cytoplasm of an oocyte.

oo•sphere (o″o-sfēr) 1. an unfertilized female gamete of certain fungi; when fertilized by an antheridium it becomes an oospore. 2. the large, nonmotile, fertile gamete of certain algae and fungi.

Oos•po•ra (o-os′pə-rə) [*oo-* + Gr. *sporos* seed] a genus of Fungi Imperfecti of the form-family Moniliaceae that is associated with disease of citrus trees and potatoes. *O. lac′tis* is now called *Geotrichum candidum* and *O. tozeu′ri* is now called *Madurella mycetomi*.

oo•spo•ran•gi•um (o″o-spə-ran′je-əm) oosphere (def. 1).

oo•spore (o′o-spor) [*oo-* + *spore*] 1. in certain fungi that have sexual spores, the final developmental stage after fusion of sexually differentiated gametes. 2. the thick-walled, resting zygote formed from a fertilized oosphere.

oo•the•ca (o″o-the′kə) [*oo-* + *theca*] 1. an egg case, such as is found in certain animals. 2. ovarium.

oothec(o)- [Gr. *ōon* egg +*thēkē* case] for words beginning thus, see those beginning *oophor(o)-* and *ovari(o)-*.

oo•tid (o′o-tid) a mature oocyte; one of four cells derived from the two consecutive divisions of the primary oocyte, and corresponding to the spermatids that are derived from division of the primary spermatocyte. In mammals, the second maturation division is not completed unless fertilization occurs; hence the ootid has male as well as female pronuclear (haploid) elements.

oo•type (o′o-tīp) [*oo-* + Gr. *typos* impression] in some trematodes, a dilated portion of the uterus into which the oviduct opens and where the ovum is fertilized, provided with the yolk, and invested with a shell.

oo•zo•oid (o″o-zo′oid) [*oo-* + *zo-* + *-oid*] an individual developed from an oocyte, that is, as a result of sexual reproduction. Cf. *blastozooid*.

opac•i•fi•ca•tion (o-pas″ĭ-fĭ-ka′shən) 1. the development of opacity, as of the cornea or lens. 2. the rendering of a tissue or organ opaque to radiation by introduction of a contrast medium.

opac•i•ty (o-pas′ĭ-te) [L. *opacitas*] 1. the condition of being opaque. 2. an opaque spot or area. See also *cataract*.

opal•es•cent (o″pəl-es′ənt) showing a milky iridescence, like an opal.

Opa•li•na (o″pə-li′nə) [L. *opalus* opal] a genus of ciliate parasitic protozoa (order Opalinida, class Opalinatea) found as endocommensals in the colon of frogs and toads. The life cycle of *O. rana′rum* involves asexual reproduction in adult frogs and sexual reproduction in tadpoles.

Opa•li•na•ta (o″pə-lĭ-na′tə) in older classifications of protozoa, a subphylum of the phylum Sarcomastigophora, including parasitic, flat, leaflike, multinucleate species; they are usually found as endocommensals in anurans and less often in fish, salamanders, and reptiles. They have cilia arranged in multiple oblique longitudinal rows over the entire body surface, but differ from the Ciliophora in having only one type of nucleus (i.e., no differentiated micronuclei and macronuclei) and in reproducing sexually. This group contains just the single class of Opalinatea.

Opa•li•na•tea (o″pə-lĭ-na′te-ə) a class of parasitic ciliated protozoa of the phylum Sarcomastigophora, comprising the single order of Opalinida.

opa•line (o′pə-lēn) [L. *opalus* opal] having the appearance of an opal.

opa•lin•id (o″pə-lin′id) 1. pertaining or referring to protozoa of the subphylum Opalinata. 2. any protozoan of the subphylum Opalinata.

Opa•lin•i•da (o″pə-lin′ĭ-də) an order of ciliated parasitic protozoa of the class Opalinatea, phylum Sarcomastigophora, with characteristics of the class. *Opalina* is a representative genus.

Opana (o-pan′ə) trademark for a preparation of oxymorphone hydrochloride.

opaque (o-pāk′) [L. *opacus* dark] impervious to light rays, or by extension to x-rays or other electromagnetic radiations; neither transparent nor translucent.

open (o′pən) 1. exposed to the air; not covered by unbroken skin. 2. interrupted (as a circuit) so that an electric current cannot pass. 3. not obstructed or closed. 4. pertaining to a clinical trial or other experiment that is not blind; i.e., the subjects and the persons administering the test know which treatment is administered to which subject.

open•ing (o′pən-ing) an aperture, orifice, or open space; see also *inlet* and *outlet*. Anatomic nomenclature for various types of openings includes *aditus*, *apertura*, *foramen*, *fossa*, *hiatus*, and *ostium*.
  o. in adductor magnus muscle hiatus tendineus.
  aortic o. ostium aortae.
  aortic o. in diaphragm hiatus aorticus.
  atrioventricular o., left ostium atrioventriculare sinistrum.
  atrioventricular o., right ostium atrioventriculare dextrum.
  cardiac o., cardial o. ostium cardiacum.
  caval o. foramen venae cavae.
  o. of cochlear canaliculus apertura canaliculi cochleae.
  o. of coronary artery see under *ostium*.
  o. of coronary sinus ostium sinus coronarii.
  cutaneous o. of male urethra ostium urethrae externum masculinae.

duodenal o. of stomach ostium pyloricum.
esophageal o. in diaphragm hiatus oesophageus.
external o. of carotid canal apertura externa canalis carotici.
external o. of cochlear canaliculus apertura canaliculi cochleae.
o. of frontal sinus apertura sinus frontalis.
ileal o., ileocecal o. 1. ostium ileale. 2. opening of ileocecal valve.
o. of ileocecal valve the slitlike or oval orifice in the ileocecal valve, seen in the cadaver. It has two flaps or lips, one above and one below, that form the valve and project at thickened folds into the lumen of the large intestine. In the living individual this structure is the ostium ileale.
inferior o. of Hunter canal hiatus tendineus.
inferior o. of pelvis apertura pelvis inferior.
inferior thoracic o. apertura thoracis inferior.
o. of inferior vena cava ostium venae cavae inferioris.
internal o. of carotid canal apertura interna canalis carotici.
internal o. of cochlear canal apertura interna canaliculi cochleae.
internal o. of vestibular canaliculus apertura interna canaliculi vestibuli.
nasal o. of facial skeleton apertura piriformis.
o. of nasolacrimal duct apertura ductus nasolacrimalis.
orbital o., o. of orbital cavity, anterior aditus orbitalis.
ovarian o. of uterine tube ostium abdominale tubae uterinae.
o's of papillary ducts foramina papillaria renalis.
pharyngeal o. of auditory tube ostium pharyngeum tubae auditivae.
piriform o. apertura piriformis.
o. of pulmonary trunk ostium trunci pulmonalis.
o's of pulmonary veins ostia venarum pulmonalium.
pyloric o. ostium pyloricum.
saphenous o. hiatus saphenus.
o. of sphenoid sinus apertura sinus sphenoidalis.
superior o. of pelvis apertura pelvis superior.
superior thoracic o. apertura thoracis superior.
o. of superior vena cava ostium venae cavae superioris.
tendinous o. hiatus tendineus.
thoracic o., inferior apertura thoracis inferior.
thoracic o., superior apertura thoracis superior.
tympanic o. of auditory tube ostium tympanicum tubae auditivae.
tympanic o. of canaliculus of chorda tympani apertura tympanica canaliculi chordae tympani.
uterine o. of uterine tube ostium uterinum tubae uterinae.
o. of vermiform appendix ostium appendicis vermiformis.
vesicourethral o. ostium urethrae internum.
o. of vestibular canaliculus apertura canaliculi vestibuli.

op•er•a•ble (op'ər-ə-bəl) subject to being operated upon with a reasonable degree of safety; appropriate for surgical removal.

op•er•ant (op'ər-ənt) in psychology, any response that is not elicited by specific external stimuli but that recurs at a given rate in a particular set of circumstances. See also *conditioning.*

op•er•ate (op'ər-āt) 1. to perform an operation. 2. an individual that has undergone a specific experimental surgical procedure, in contrast to the normal control.

op•er•a•tion (op″ər-a'shən) [L. *operatio*] 1. any act performed with instruments or by the hands of a surgeon; a surgical procedure. 2. the process or act of functioning, doing, or performing.

Operation

For terms not found here, see also *method, procedure, repair, surgery, technique,* or the specific type of operation such as *amputation.*

Abbe o. attachment of a triangular, full-thickness flap from the median portion of the lower lip to fill a defect in the upper lip.
Adams o. 1. subcutaneous intracapsular division of the neck of the femur for ankylosis of the hip. 2. subcutaneous division of the palmar fascia at various points for Dupuytren contracture. 3. excision of a wedge-shaped piece from the eyelid for relief of ectropion.
Akin o. resection of the medial prominence of the first metatarsal head and cuneiform osteotomy of the proximal phalanx of the great toe, done for hallux valgus.
Albee o. operation for ankylosis of the hip, consisting of cutting off the upper surface of the head of the femur and freshening a corresponding point on the acetabulum, and permitting the two freshened surfaces to rest in contact.
Albee-Delbet o. an operation for fracture of the neck of the femur, done by drilling a hole through the trochanter and the neck and head of the femur and inserting a bone peg in this hole.
Albert o. surgical removal of part of the knee to cause ankylosis and treat a flail joint.
Alexander o., Alexander-Adams o. shortening of the round ligaments to repair displacement of the uterus.
Alouette o. see under *amputation.*
Ammon o. 1. blepharoplasty by a flap from the cheek. 2. dacryocystotomy. 3. for epicanthus: resection of a spindle-shaped piece of skin over the bridge of the nose, undermining the flaps of the epicanthal fold, and closing with sutures.
Aries-Pitanguy o. see under *mammaplasty.*
Baldy o., Baldy-Webster o. Webster o.
Barkan o. goniotomy.
Barker o. 1. an excision of the hip joint by an anterior cut. 2. a special method of excising the astragalus by an incision extending from just above the external malleolus forward and inward to the dorsum of the foot.
Barraquer o. phacoerysis.
Barsky o. an operation for repair of a cleft hand with a missing central ray and a deep central V-shaped cleft, consisting of closing the cleft, bringing the ring and index fingers closer together, and correcting the associated syndactyly, if present.
Barton o. an operation for ankylosis consisting of sawing through the bone and removing a V-shaped piece.
Basset o. a method of dissecting the inguinal glands in radical operations for cancer of the vulva.
Bassini o. see under *repair.*
Belsey Mark IV o. fundoplication for gastroesophageal reflux with the fundus being wrapped 270 degrees around the circumference of the esophagus, leaving its posterior wall free; done through a thoracic incision. Called also *Belsey Mark IV fundoplication.*
Berger o. interscapulothoracic amputation.
Berke o. 1. a modification of the Blaskovics operation for ptosis of the upper eyelid, with resection of the levator muscle through a skin incision and excision of excess muscle. 2. a modification of the Motais operation for ptosis of the upper eyelid, with suspension of the ptotic lid from the superior rectus muscle.
Bier o. see under *amputation.*
Biesenberger o. see under *mammaplasty.*
Billroth o. either of two operations with partial resection of the stomach and anastomosis of the remaining stomach to either the duodenum (Billroth I) or the jejunum (Billroth II). Called also *Billroth gastrectomy* or *gastroenterostomy.*
Blair-Brown o. repair of a cleft lip by the use of a lateral flap one-half the length of the lip.
Blalock-Hanlon o. a palliative operation for transposition of the great vessels, consisting of the creation of an interatrial septal defect.
Blalock-Taussig o. the side-to-side anastomosis of the left subclavian artery to the left pulmonary artery (sometimes the right subclavian to the right pulmonary artery) in order to shunt some of the systemic circulation into the pulmonary circulation; performed as

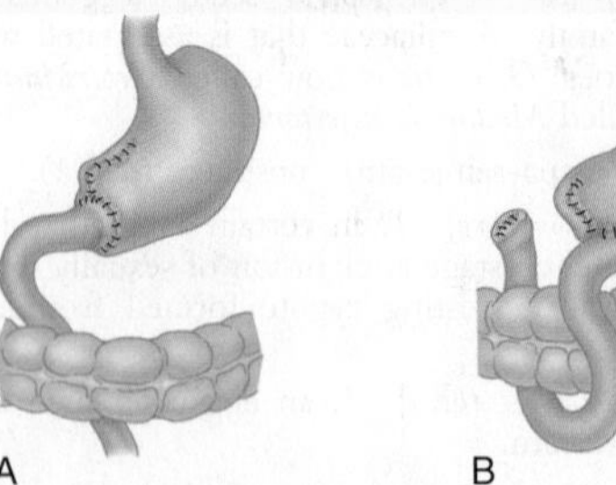

■ *(A),* Billroth I operation; *(B),* Billroth II operation.

palliative treatment of tetralogy of Fallot or other congenital anomalies associated with insufficient pulmonary arterial flow.
Blaskovics o. an operation for ptosis of the upper eyelid, consisting of excision of the levator muscle and the tarsus through a conjunctival approach.
Bricker o. see under *technique.*
Brock o. transventricular closed valvotomy.
Browne o. a type of urethroplasty for repair of hypospadias; an intact strip of epithelium is left on the ventral surface of the penis to form the roof of the urethra, and the floor of the urethra is formed by epithelialization from the lateral wound margins. Called also *Denis Browne o.*
Brunschwig o. pelvic exenteration.
Buck o. cuneiform excision of the patella and the ends of tibia and fibula.
Burow o. a method of excising triangles of skin at the base of the pedicle of a skin flap to facilitate advancement.
Caldwell-Luc o. 1. antrostomy in which an opening is made into the maxillary sinus by way of an incision through the roof of the mouth opposite the premolar teeth, usually done to remove tooth roots or abnormal tissue from the sinus. 2. in fractures of the zygomatic bone and maxilla, the packing of the maxillary sinus by approaching the antrum through the canine fossa of the maxilla above the tooth apices, thus allowing reduction of displaced fragments of the zygoma by upward and outward pressure. Called also *Luc o.*
Carpue o. Indian rhinoplasty.
Cecil o. a two-stage urethroplasty for hypospadias repair, with construction of a new urethral segment buried in the scrotum, and later by separation of the new urethra from the scrotum. Called also *Cecil urethroplasty.*
Charles o. treatment of elephantiasis and other types of massive lymphedema of the lower limb by excision of subcutaneous tissue followed by skin grafting.
Chopart o. see under *amputation.*
Colonna o. 1. a reconstruction operation for intracapsular fracture of the femoral neck. 2. a common type of capsular arthroplasty of the hip.
Commando o. an operation for management of oral cancer, consisting in resection of the primary lesion and the regional lymphatic nodes.
concrete o's a stage in reasoning or functioning usually seen in children between the ages of approximately 7 and 11, following the stage of preoperational thinking and preceding that of formal operations; it is characterized by comprehension of relational terms, decrease in egocentricity and increase in the ability to appreciate the perspective of others, understanding of the reversibility of events and ideas as well as of conservation of volume and quantity, and the beginning of logical thought, although it is initially restricted to objects immediately present.
Conway o. see under *mammaplasty.*
Cooper ligament o. McVay repair.
cosmetic o. a surgical procedure intended to remove or correct a deformity in an esthetically acceptable manner.
Cotte o. removal of the presacral nerve.
Dandy o. trigeminal rhizotomy using an approach through the posterior cranial fossa.
Daviel o. one of the first operations for cataract extraction, which consisted of lens extraction through a corneal incision without cutting the iris.
Denis Browne o. Browne o.
Denonvilliers o. plastic correction of a defective ala nasi by transferring a triangular flap from the adjacent side of the nose.
Dieffenbach o. plastic closure of triangular defects by displacing a quadrangular flap toward one side of the triangle.
Duhamel o. the treatment of congenital megacolon by a modification of the pull-through operation and establishment of a longitudinal anastomosis between the proximal ganglionated segment of colon and the rectum, leaving the rectum in situ.
Dührssen o. vaginofixation of the uterus.
Dupuy-Dutemps o. blepharoplasty of the lower lid with tissue from the opposing lid.
Dupuytren o. shoulder disarticulation.
Emmet o. 1. a method of repairing a lacerated perineum. 2. trachelorrhaphy. 3. surgical creation of a vesicovaginal fistula to secure drainage of the bladder in cystitis.
equilibrating o. tenotomy of the direct antagonist of a paralyzed eye muscle.
Esser o. epithelial inlay.
Estes o. implantation of an ovary into a uterine cornu; performed to establish fertility when the uterine tubes are absent.
Estlander o. 1. resection of one or more ribs in empyema so as to allow the chest wall to collapse and close the abnormal cavity; of historical interest. 2. rotation of a triangular flap from the side of the lower lip to fill a defect in the lateral upper lip.
Eversbusch o. an operation for ptosis of the upper eyelid, consisting of resection of the levator muscle through a skin incision.
exploratory o. surgical incision into an area of the body followed by inspection and palpation of organs and tissues to determine the cause of unexplained symptoms.
Fergusson o. removal of the maxilla through an incision running along the junction of the nose with the cheek, around the ala of the nose to the median line, and then down to bisect the upper lip. Called also *Fergusson incision.*
Finney o. see under *pyloroplasty.*
flap o. 1. any operation involving the raising of a flap of tissue. 2. in periodontics, an operation to secure greater access to granulation tissue and osseous defects, consisting of detachment of the gingivae, the alveolar mucosa, and/or a portion of the palatal mucosa. 3. see under *amputation.*
formal o's a form of thinking following the stage of concrete operations and representing the final, most mature state of thinking; usually occurring after the age of 11 and characterized by the emergence of true logical thought, with the capability for deductive reasoning, abstract thinking, formulation and testing of hypotheses, appreciation for multiple perspectives on an issue, and the manipulation of ideas and concepts.
Fothergill o. Manchester o.
Frazier-Spiller o. trigeminal rhizotomy using an approach through the middle cranial fossa.
Fredet-Ramstedt o. pyloromyotomy.
Gifford o. delimiting keratotomy.
Gilliam o. an operation for retroversion of the uterus by drawing a loop of each round ligament through the abdominal wall and fixing the loops to the abdominal fascia.
Gillies o. 1. operation for correction of ectropion using a split-thickness skin graft and a mold. 2. a technique for reducing fractures of the zygoma and zygomatic arch through an incision in the temporal region above the hairline.
Girdlestone o. see under *resection.*
Glenn o. an operation for congenital cyanotic heart disease, consisting of anastomosis of the superior vena cava to the right pulmonary artery.
Graefe o. an early, pioneering operation for cataract, which consisted of removal of the lens by an incision in the sclera, with laceration of the capsule and iridectomy.
Gritti o. see under *amputation.*
Guyon o. see under *amputation.*
Halsted o. radical mastectomy.
Hancock o. see under *amputation.*
Hartley-Krause o. excision of the gasserian ganglion and its roots to relieve trigeminal neuralgia; of historical interest.
Hartmann o. see under *procedure.*
Haultain o. a modification of the Huntington operation for replacement of a chronically inverted uterus, involving a posterior incision in the uterus through the cervical ring.
Heineke-Mikulicz o. see under *pyloroplasty.*
Heller o. esophagocardiomyotomy.
Hey o. see under *amputation.*
Hibbs o. a spinal fusion operation done by fracturing the spinous processes of the vertebrae and pressing the tip of each downward to rest in the denuded area caused by the fracture of its elbow below.
Hoffa o., Hoffa-Lorenz o. Lorenz o.
Homans o. a formerly common treatment for elephantiasis and other types of massive edema of the lower limb, consisting of excision of subcutaneous tissue and redundant skin on the lateral and medial aspects.
Horsley o. excision of an area of motor cortex for relief of athetoid and convulsive movements of an upper extremity; of historical interest.
Huntington o. transabdominal repair of a chronically inverted uterus. It is done by grasping the invaginated portion of the uterus with forceps; as the uterus is pulled up, additional forceps are placed sequentially

lower down, and upward traction is applied. After the uterus is in place, the position is maintained by packing through the vagina.
Indian o. see under *rhinoplasty.*
interval o. an operation performed during the interval between two acute attacks of a disease, as in appendicitis.
Irving o. see under *technique.*
Italian o. tagliacotian rhinoplasty.
Jaboulay o. hemipelvectomy.
Jatene o. a type of arterial switch procedure (q.v.).
Kasai o. portoenterostomy.
Kazanjian o. 1. a technique of surgical extension of the buccal vestibular sulcus of edentulous ridges to increase their height and to improve denture retention. 2. the use of extraskeletal fixation for support in fractures of the zygomatic bone and maxilla: a small hole is drilled through the infraorbital rim, and a stainless steel wire is inserted with both ends brought out through the wound, where they are twisted together into a loop or hook. Rubber band traction between the suspension wire and an outrigger on a head cap provides support for the zygomatic fragments.
Keller o. sagittal resection of the medial prominence of the first metatarsal head and excision of the base of the proximal phalanx of the great toe; done for hallux valgus.
Kelly o. see under *plication.*
Killian o. excision of the anterior wall of the frontal sinus, removal of the diseased tissue, and formation of a permanent communication with the nose.
Killian-Freer o. submucous resection of the nasal septum, including the septal cartilage, vomer, and perpendicular plate of the ethmoid.
King o. arytenoidopexy.
Kondoleon o. a formerly common treatment for elephantiasis and other types of lymphedema by the removal of strips of subcutaneous tissue; it was later modified to the Homans operation.
Körte-Ballance o. anastomosis of the facial and hypoglossal nerves.
Kraske o. removal of the coccyx and part of the sacrum for access to rectal carcinoma.
Krause o. extradural excision of the gasserian ganglion for trigeminal neuralgia; of historical interest.
Krönlein o. resection of the outer wall of the orbit for the removal of an orbital tumor without excising the eye.
Küstner o. replacement of an inverted uterus through an incision made in the cervix and uterus along the posterior surface.
Lagrange o. sclerectoiridectomy.
Landolt o. the formation of a lower eyelid with a double pedicle or bridge flap of eyelid skin taken from the upper lid.
Lapidus o. a procedure for correction of hallux valgus, involving wedge resection and fusion of the innermost cuneometatarsal joint and establishment of a bridge between the bases of the first and second metatarsals.
Larrey o. see under *amputation.*
Latzko o. 1. Latzko cesarean section. 2. a method of repairing a vesicovaginal fistula by using mucosa denuded from the posterior wall of the vagina as a flap to cover the fistula.
Le Fort o., Le Fort-Neugebauer o. the operation of uniting the anterior and posterior vaginal walls along the middle line for the repair or prevention of prolapse of the uterus.
Lempert fenestration o. an operation for otosclerosis, consisting of drilling a small window into the lateral semicircular canal and then placing a flap of skin over the fistula.
Lisfranc o. 1. see under *amputation.* 2. shoulder disarticulation.
Lorenz o. an operation for developmental dysplasia of the hip, consisting of reduction of the dislocation, and keeping the head of the femur fixed against the rudimentary acetabulum until a socket is formed.
Lowsley o. an operation for repair of simple epispadias, consisting of closing the cleft urethra, splitting the glans, and burying the repaired urethra deep in the soft tissue so that its orifice will be at the normal site.
Luc o. Caldwell-Luc o.
Lynch o. incision of the frontal sinus and removal of its floor and contents; done in cases of expanding mucoceles, pyoceles, and tumors of the sinus.
McBride o. resection of the medial prominence of the first metatarsal head, medial capsulorrhaphy, resection of the fibular sesamoid, and transfer of the adductor tendon to the neck of the first metatarsal; done for hallux valgus.
McDonald o. an operation for incompetent cervix, in which the cervical os is closed with a purse-string suture.
McGill o. suprapubic transvesical prostatectomy.
McVay o. see under *repair.*
magnet o. removal of a fragment of steel or iron from the eyeball by means of a powerful magnet.
major o. an operation of major surgery (q.v.).
Manchester o. an operation for uterine prolapse comprising dilation and curettage, anterior repair, amputation of the vaginal portion of the cervix, shortening of the cardinal ligaments, and posterior colpoperineorrhaphy.
Marshall-Marchetti-Krantz o. an operation for the correction of stress incontinence; the anterior portion of the urethra, vesical neck, and bladder are sutured to the posterior surface of the pubic bone.
Matas o. endoaneurysmorrhaphy.
Maydl o. one of the pioneering treatments for exstrophy of bladder, attaching the ureters to the rectum (see *ureterorectostomy*).
Mikulicz o. 1. Heineke-Mikulicz pyloroplasty. 2. Vladimiroff-Mikulicz amputation.
Miles o. surgical treatment for cancer of the lower sigmoid and rectum, with removal of the pelvic colon, mesocolon, and adjacent lymph nodes, and wide perineal excision of the rectum and anus, and a permanent colostomy.
Millin o. a formerly common method of radical retropubic prostatectomy.
minor o. an operation of minor surgery (q.v.).
Mitchell o. a procedure for correction of hallux valgus, involving distal osteotomy of the first metatarsal.
Motais o. an operation for ptosis, consisting of transplanting the middle portion of the tendon of the superior rectus muscle of the eyeball into the upper lid.
Mustard o. correction of transposition of great vessels by construction of a small barrier inside the atrium, composed of pericardial tissue or synthetic material, to direct the systemic and pulmonary venous blood into the left and right ventricles, respectively.
Naffziger o. excision of the superior and lateral walls of the orbit for exophthalmos.
Nissen o. see under *fundoplication.*
Ober o. medial subtalar syndesmotomy for clubfoot.
Olshausen o. the operation of fixing or suturing the uterus to the abdominal wall for the cure of retroversion.
Ombrédanne o. transscrotal orchiopexy.
open o. an operation in which the tissues and organs are exposed to view through a surgical incision.
Partsch o. a technique for marsupialization of dental cyst.
Patey o. modified radical mastectomy.
Péan o. hip joint amputation in which the vessels are ligated during the course of the operation.
Phelps o. an open and direct incision through the sole and inner side of the foot, done for talipes.
Phemister o. use of an onlay graft of cancellous bone without internal fixation, for treatment of a stable but ununited fracture.
plastic o. an operation in which the shape of a part or the character of its covering is altered by transplantation of tissue or other means.
Polya o. subtotal gastrectomy with anastomosis of the transected end of the stomach to the side of the jejunum.
Pomeroy o. see under *technique.*
Potts o. anastomosis between the descending aorta and left pulmonary artery as palliative treatment of congenital pulmonary stenosis. Called also *Potts anastomosis* or *shunt.*
pull-through o. surgery on the intestine in which a diseased segment is removed and a proximal segment is pulled down and through the part just beyond the removed part. See *ileoanal pull-through anastomosis, Duhamel o., Soave o.,* and *Swenson o.*
radical o. see under *surgery.*
Ramstedt o. pyloromyotomy.
Rastelli o. an operation for correction of large ventricular septal defects with pulmonary stenosis and infundibular stenosis; an intraventricular patch is placed so that blood flows through the septal defect and out the aorta, and a prosthesis is placed to establish continuity between the right ventricle and the pulmonary artery.

Operation *Continued*

Regnoli o. excision of the tongue through a median opening below the lower jaw, reaching from the chin to the hyoid bone.
Ridell o. obliteration of the frontal sinus by removal of the anterior wall and floor and sometimes posterior walls of the sinus; for treatment of malignant tumors.
Roux-en-Y o. see under *anastomosis.*
Saemisch o. transfixion of the cornea and of the base of the ulcer for the cure of hypopyon.
Scanzoni o. see under *maneuver.*
Schauta o. radical hysterectomy by the vaginal route.
Schede o. 1. incision into the thorax for chronic empyema. 2. in cases of necrotic bone, excision of dead bone and diseased tissue, after which the cavity is permitted to fill with a blood clot that is kept moist and aseptic and eventually becomes organized.
Scheie o. 1. scleral cauterization with peripheral iridectomy for treatment of glaucoma. 2. a technique for needling and aspiration of cataract.
Sédillot o. a flap operation for restoring the upper lip.
Senning o. a surgical technique for correction of transposition of the great vessels, consisting of the creation of two channels that connect the atria and cross the systemic and pulmonary venous circulations.
Shirodkar o. an operation for incompetent cervix in which the cervical os is closed with a surrounding purse-string suture.
Silver o. resection of the medial prominence of the first metatarsal head, medial capsulorrhaphy of the first metatarsophalangeal joint, and sectioning of the adductor tendon; done for hallux valgus.
Sistrunk o. a surgical procedure for removal of thyroglossal cysts and sinuses.
Soave o. treatment of congenital megacolon by an endorectal pull-through operation, with normal colon connected to the anus through a rectum denuded of mucosa.

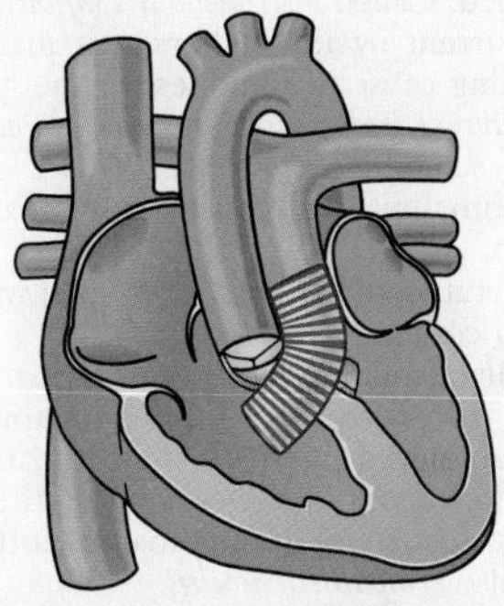

■ Rastelli operation, showing the prosthesis placed to connect the right ventricle and pulmonary artery.

Spinelli o. the operation of splitting the anterior wall of the prolapsed inverted uterus, reversing the organ, and restoring it to the correct position.
Stein o. an operation for reconstruction of the lower lip with flaps taken from the upper lip.
Steindler o. surgical correction of pes cavus by stripping muscle and fascia from the plantar calcaneal surface.
Stokes o. Gritti-Stokes amputation.
Strömbeck o. see under *mammaplasty.*
Sturmdorf o. conical excision of the diseased endocervix.
Swenson o. an operation for congenital megacolon, consisting of removal of the rectum and the aganglionic segment of the intestine and an ileoanal pull-through anastomosis with preservation of the anal sphincters.
Syme o. see under *amputation.*
tagliacotian o. see under *rhinoplasty.*
Teale o. see under *amputation.*
Thiersch o. removal of thin split-thickness skin grafts by means of a razor, skin-graft cutting knife, or a dermatome.
Thompson o. a formerly common treatment for elephantiasis and other types of massive lymphedema of the lower limb, consisting of excision of some subcutaneous tissue and burying of a dermal flap among the underlying muscles.
Torek o. one of the pioneering operations for esophageal cancer, consisting of removal of the thoracic part of the esophagus.
Torkildsen o. ventriculocisternal shunt.
Toupet o. see under *fundoplication.*
Trendelenburg o. 1. synchondroseotomy. 2. transthoracic pulmonary embolectomy.
van Hook o. ureteroureterostomy.
Vineberg o. implantation of the internal mammary artery into the myocardium to enhance the growth of collateral circulation.
von Burow o. Burow o.
Waters o. a form of extraperitoneal cesarean section.
Waterston o. anastomosis between the ascending aorta and right pulmonary artery as palliative treatment of congenital pulmonary stenosis. Called also *Waterston anastomosis* or *shunt.*
Webster o. for retrodisplacement of the uterus: the round ligaments are passed through the perforated broad ligaments and fixed to the back of the uterus.
Wertheim o. radical hysterectomy; removal of the uterus, tubes, parametrium, tissues surrounding the upper vagina, and pelvic lymphatics.
Whipple o. see under *procedure.*
Whitehead o. a treatment for hemorrhoids consisting of surgical removal.
Witzel o. see under *gastrostomy.*
Young o. 1. an operation for penile epispadias, with formation of a new urethral tube. 2. perineal prostatectomy.
Ziegler o. V-shaped iridectomy for forming an artificial pupil.

op•er•a•tive (op′ər-ə-tiv) [L. *operativus*] 1. pertaining to an operation. 2. effective; not inert.

op•er•a•tor (op′ər-a-tər) [L. *operari* to work] a DNA sequence preceding the coding sequence of a structural gene in an operon, to which a regulator protein binds to control transcription of the structural genes in that operon.

op•er•a•tory (op′ər-ə-tor″e) the working area of a dental office, in which treatment is provided to patients.

oper•cu•la (o-pur′ku-lə) [L.] plural of *operculum.*

oper•cu•lar (o-pur′ku-lər) pertaining to an operculum.

oper•cu•late (o-pur′ku-lāt) having an operculum; said of an ascus.

oper•cu•lec•to•my (o-per″ku-lek′tə-me) the surgical removal of a mucosal flap partially or completely covering an unerupted tooth.

oper•cu•li•tis (o-per″ku-li′tis) pericoronitis.

oper•cu•lum (o-pur′ku-ləm) pl. *oper′cula* [L.] 1. a lid or covering structure. 2. one of the insular opercula (q.v.). 3. in fungi, a small cap on an ascus that pops open when the mature organism is ready to eject its spores.

cartilaginous o. discus articularis articulationis temporomandibularis.

dental o. the hood of gingival tissue overlying the crown of an erupting tooth; called also *odontoclamis* and *tooth hood.*

frontal o., o. fronta′le 1. [TA] the portion of the insular opercula within the frontal lobe; it corresponds to the pars orbitalis, pars triangularis, and pars opercularis of the inferior frontal gyrus together with the lower end of the precentral gyrus. 2. the portion of the insular opercula lying between the anterior and ascending rami of the lateral sulcus, corresponding to the pars opercularis gyri frontalis inferioris; when used this way, the term is contrasted with the operculum frontoparietale. It may also be expanded to include the pars orbitalis gyri frontalis inferioris, in which case the frontal operculum is said to have two parts: frontal and orbital. 3. the anterior portion of the operculum frontoparietale, corresponding to the pars opercularis gyri frontalis inferior.

frontoparietal o., o. frontoparieta′le the part of the cerebrum that covers the upper portion of the insula; from anterior to posterior, it consists of the part of the inferior frontal gyrus behind the ascending branch of the lateral sulcus (corresponding to the pars opercularis gyri frontalis inferioris), the lower ends of the precentral and postcentral gyri, and the anterior and lower part of the inferior parietal lobule. The term is used in contrast with operculum frontale (def. 2) (q.v.), although its frontal, as opposed to parietal, portion may itself be called *operculum frontale* (see *o. frontale,* def. 3).

opercula of insula, insular opercula the areas of the cerebral cortex overlapping above and below the insula, forming part of the lips of the lateral sulcus, and separated by the rami of the lateral sulcus; see *o. frontale*, *o. frontoparietale*, and *o. temporale*.

occipital o. a part of the occipital lobe of the brain demarcated by the sulcus lunatus, when the latter structure is present.

parietal o., o. parieta'le [TA] the portion of the insular opercula within the parietal lobe, corresponding to the lower end of the postcentral gyrus and the anterior and lower part of the inferior parietal lobule. It has often been considered as a portion of the operculum frontoparietale (q.v.).

temporal o., o. tempora'le [TA] the parts of the superior temporal gyrus and transverse temporal gyri that cover the lower portion of the insula.

trophoblastic o. the plug of trophoblast that helps close the gap in the endometrium made by the implanting blastocyst.

op•er•on (op'ər-on) [L. *opera* work + Gr. *-on* neuter ending] in prokaryotes, a chromosomal segment constituting a functional unit of transcription and so of genetic regulation. It comprises one or more structural genes, their promoter, and an operator region that through interaction with a regulator protein controls the structural genes.

OPG osteoprotegerin.

ophi•a•sis (o-fi'ə-sis) [Gr. *ophis* snake] a form of alopecia areata of long duration, involving the temporal and occipital margins of the scalp in a continuous band.

Ophid•ia (o-fid'e-ə) [Gr. *ophidion* serpent] a suborder of Reptilia, the snakes. See table at *snake*.

ophi•di•a•sis (o″fi-di'ə-sis) ophidism.

ophid•ic (o-fid'ik) pertaining to, caused by, or derived from snakes.

ophi•dism (o'fi-diz-əm) poisoning by snake venom.

Oph•i•oph•a•gus (of″e-of'ə-gəs) [Gr. *ophis* snake + *phagein* to eat] a genus of venomous snakes of the family Elapidae. *O. han'nah* is the king cobra. See also table at *snake*.

ophi•o•tox•emia (o″fe-o-tok-se'me-ə) [Gr. *ophis* snake + *toxemia*] poisoning by snake venom.

ophi•tox•emia (o″fe-tok-se'me-ə) ophiotoxemia.

Oph•ry•o•gle•ni•na (of″re-o-glə-ni'nə) [Gr. *ophrys* eyebrow + *glēnē* socket] a suborder of large, chiefly freshwater, histophagous ciliate protozoa of the order Hymenostomatida, characterized by a polymorphous life cycle and an oral apparatus including three ciliary organelles on the left and an associated watchglass organelle on the right. Several species cause disease in marine and freshwater fish, resulting in great economic loss. *Ichthyophthirius* is a representative genus.

oph•ry•on (of're-on) [Gr. *ophrys* eyebrow + *-on* neuter ending] the middle point of the transverse supraorbital line.

oph•ry•o•sis (of″re-o'sis) [Gr. *ophrys* eyebrow] spasm of the eyebrow.

Oph•thaine (of'thān) trademark for a preparation of proparacaine hydrochloride.

oph•thal•mag•ra (of″thəl-mag'rə) [*ophthalm-* + *-agra*] sudden pain in the eye.

oph•thal•mal•gia (of″thəl-mal'jə) [*ophthalm-* + *-algia*] pain in the eye.

oph•thal•ma•tro•phia (of″thəl-mə-tro'fe-ə) [*ophthalm-* + *atrophia*] atrophy of the eye.

oph•thal•mec•to•my (of″thəl-mek'tə-me) [*ophthalm-* + *-ectomy*] the surgical removal of an eye; enucleation of the eyeball.

oph•thal•men•ceph•a•lon (of″thəl-men-sef'ə-lon) [*ophthalm-* + *encephalon*] the retina, optic nerve, and visual apparatus of the brain.

oph•thal•mia (of-thal'me-ə) [Gr., from *ophthalmos* eye] severe inflammation of the eye or of the conjunctiva or deeper structures of the eye.

actinic ray o. actinic conjunctivitis.

Brazilian o. keratomalacia.

catarrhal o. a severe form of simple conjunctivitis.

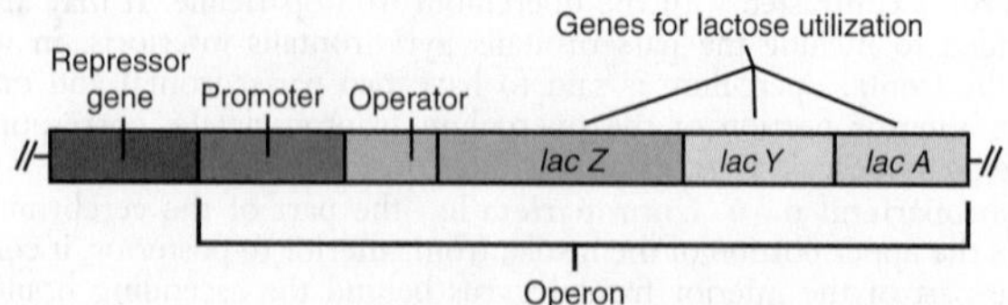

■ *Escherichia coli lac* operon. In the absence of lactose, the product of the repressor gene binds the operator region and prevents transcription of genes involved in lactose utilization by blocking movement of the RNA polymerase from promoter to structural gene region; the operon is repressed. If lactose is added, an inducer binds the repressor protein, lessening its affinity for the operator. The RNA polymerase can then proceed from promoter to structural genes, so that the operon is derepressed, or expressed.

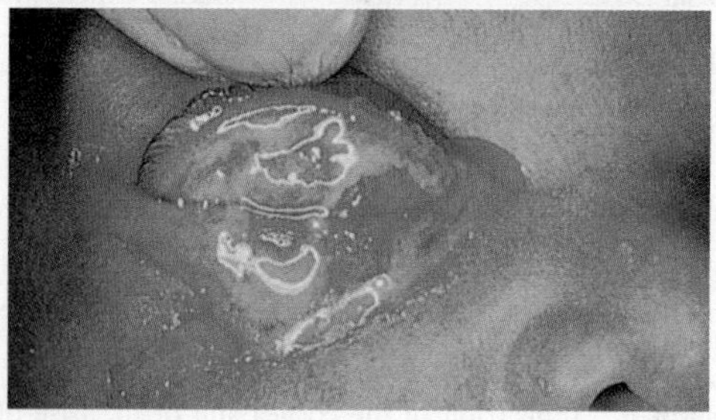

■ Ophthalmia neonatorum in an infant with gonococcal infection.

caterpillar o. o. nodosa.

contagious o. infectious keratoconjunctivitis.

o. eczemato'sa phlyctenulosis.

Egyptian o. trachoma.

electric o., flash o. actinic conjunctivitis.

gonorrheal o. acute and severe purulent ophthalmia due to gonorrheal infection.

granular o. trachoma.

hepatic o. retinochoroidal degeneration with nyctalopia due to liver disease.

infectious o. infectious keratoconjunctivitis.

metastatic o. choroiditis due to metastasis or to pyemia.

mucous o. catarrhal o.

o. neonato'rum any hyperacute purulent conjunctivitis occurring during the first ten days of life, usually contracted during birth from infected vaginal discharge of the mother; it formerly referred only to gonorrheal infections. An iatrogenic form sometimes occurs after administration of silver nitrate. Called also *neonatal conjunctivitis*.

neuroparalytic o. keratitis due to lesion of branches of the fifth nerve or of the gasserian ganglion.

o. nivia'lis snow blindness.

o. nodo'sa inflammation of the conjunctiva produced by caterpillar hairs, and marked by the formation of a round, gray swelling where each hair is embedded. Called also *nodular conjunctivitis*.

periodic o. recurrent uveitis in horses; it may occur in one or both eyes and is the leading cause of blindness in the horse. Called also *equine recurrent uveitis*, *recurrent iridocyclitis*, and *moon blindness*.

phlyctenular o. see under *keratoconjunctivitis*.

purulent o. ophthalmia with purulent discharge, commonly due to gonorrheal infection.

scrofulous o. keratoconjunctivitis associated with tuberculosis.

spring o. vernal conjunctivitis.

strumous o. phlyctenular keratoconjunctivitis.

sympathetic o., transferred o. granulomatous inflammation of the uveal tract of the uninjured eye (the sympathizing eye) following some weeks after a wound involving the uveal tract of the other eye (the exciting eye). The end result is bilateral granulomatous inflammation of the entire uveal tract. Called also *sympathetic uveitis*.

ultraviolet ray o. actinic conjunctivitis.

oph•thal•mic (of-thal'mik) ocular (def. 1).

oph•thal•mi•tis (of″thəl-mi'tis) [*ophthalm-* + *-itis*] inflammation of the eye. **ophthalmit'ic** *adj*

ophthalm(o)- [Gr. *ophthalmos* eye] a combining form denoting relationship to the eye.

oph•thal•mo•blen•nor•rhea (of-thal″mo-blen″o-re'ə) [*ophthalmo-* + *blennorhea*] gonorrheal or purulent ophthalmia.

oph•thal•mo•cele (of-thal'mo-sēl) exophthalmos.

oph•thal•mo•des•mi•tis (of-thal″mo-dez-mi'tis) [*ophthalmo-* + *desmitis*] inflammation of the ocular tendons.

oph•thal•mo•di•a•phan•o•scope (of-thal″mo-di-ə-fan'o-skōp) [*ophthalmo-* + *diaphanoscope*] an instrument to examine the interior or the retina of the eye by transillumination.

oph•thal•mo•di•as•tim•e•ter (of-thal″mo-di″əs-tim'ə-tər) [*ophthalmo-* + *diastema* + *-meter*] an instrument for determining the proper distance at which to place lenses for the two eyes.

oph•thal•mo•do•ne•sis (of-thal″mo-də-ne'sis) [*ophthalmo-* + Gr. *donēsis* trembling] a trembling motion of the eyes.

oph•thal•mo•dy•na•mom•e•ter (of-thal″mo-di″nə-mom'ə-tər) [*ophthalmo-* + *dynamo-* + *-meter*] 1. an instrument for measuring the retinal arterial pressure. 2. an instrument for determining the near point of convergence.

oph•thal•mo•dy•na•mom•e•try (of-thal″mo-di″nə-mom'ə-tre) 1. determination of retinal arterial pressure by ophthalmodynamometer.

2. determination of the near point of convergence by an ophthalmodynamometer.

oph·thal·mo·dyn·ia (of-thal″mo-din′e-ə) ophthalmalgia.

oph·thal·mo·ei·ko·nom·e·ter (of-thal″mo-i″kə-nom′ə-tər) [*ophthalmo-* + Gr. *eikōn* image + *-meter*] an instrument used to determine both the refraction of the eye and the relative size and shape of the ocular images.

oph·thal·mo·graph (of-thal′mo-graf) [*ophthalmo-* + *-graph*] an instrument for photographing the movements of the eye during reading.

oph·thal·mog·ra·phy (of″thəl-mog′rə-fe) [*ophthalmo-* + *-graphy*] description or photography of the eyes.

oph·thal·mo·gy·ric (of-thal″mo-ji′rik) oculogyric.

oph·thal·mo·leu·ko·scope (of-thal″mo-loo′ko-skōp) [*ophthalmo-* + *leukoscope*] an apparatus for testing color perception by means of colors produced by polarized light.

oph·thal·mo·lith (of-thal′mo-lith) dacryolith.

oph·thal·mol·o·gist (of″thəl-mol′ə-jist) a physician who specializes in the diagnosis and medical and surgical treatment of diseases and defects of the eye and related structures.

oph·thal·mol·o·gy (of″thəl-mol′ə-je) [*ophthalmo-* + *-logy*] the medical specialty that deals with the eye, including its anatomy, physiology, and pathology. **ophthalmolog′ic** *adj*

oph·thal·mo·ma·la·cia (of-thal″mo-mə-la′shə) [*ophthalmo-* + *malacia*] abnormal softness of the eye.

oph·thal·mom·e·ter (of″thəl-mom′ə-tər) keratometer.

oph·thal·mo·met·ro·scope (of-thal″mo-met′rə-skōp) [*ophthalmo-* + *metro-* + *-scope*] an ophthalmoscope with an attachment for measuring the refraction of the eye.

oph·thal·mom·e·try (of″thəl-mom′ə-tre) keratometry.

oph·thal·mo·my·ia·sis (of-thal″mo-mi-i′ə-sis) [*ophthalmo-* + *myiasis*] infection of the eye by insect larvae, most commonly of the botfly *Oestrus ovis*. Called also *ocular myiasis*.

oph·thal·mo·my·itis (of-thal″mo-mi-i′tis) [*ophthalmo-* + *myitis*] inflammation of the muscles that move the eyeball.

oph·thal·mo·myo·si·tis (of-thal″mo-mi″o-si′tis) [*ophthalmo-* + *myositis*] inflammation of the eye muscles.

oph·thal·mo·my·ot·o·my (of-thal″mo-mi-ot′ə-me) [*ophthalmo-* + *myotomy*] surgical division of the muscles of the eye.

oph·thal·mo·neu·ri·tis (of-thal″mo-noo͝-ri′tis) optic neuritis.

oph·thal·mo·neu·ro·my·eli·tis (of-thal″mo-noor″o-mi″ə-li′tis) neuromyelitis optica.

oph·thal·mo·pa·re·sis (of-thal″mo-pə-re′sis) ophthalmoplegia.

oph·thal·mop·a·thy (of″thəl-mop′ə-the) [*ophthalmo-* + *-pathy*] any disease of the eye.

dysthyroid o. see under *orbitopathy*.

external o. any disease of the eyelids, cornea, conjunctiva, or eye muscles.

Graves o. see under *orbitopathy*.

infiltrative o. ocular changes, most often seen in thyroid disorders, caused by increased water content of the orbital contents, including discomfort, lacrimation, exophthalmos, edema, chemosis, and conjunctival infection; if the changes are severe, malignant exophthalmos results.

internal o. any disease of the deep or more essential parts of the eye.

oph·thal·mo·pha·com·e·ter (of-thal″mo-fa-kom′ə-tər) [*ophthalmo-* + *phacometer*] an ophthalmometer used to determine the refractive power of the lens.

oph·thal·mo·phle·bot·o·my (of-thal″mo-flə-bot′ə-me) [*ophthalmo-* + *phlebotomy*] phlebotomy to relieve congestion of the conjunctival veins.

oph·thal·moph·thi·sis (of″thəl-mof′thĭ-sis) ophthalmomalacia.

oph·thal·mo·plas·ty (of-thal′mo-plas″te) [*ophthalmo-* + *-plasty*] plastic surgery of the eye or of its appendages. **ophthalmoplas′tic** *adj*

oph·thal·mo·ple·gia (of-thal″mo-ple′jə) [*ophthalmo-* + *-plegia*] paralysis of the eye muscles. **ophthalmople′gic** *adj*

basal o. ophthalmoplegia due to a lesion at the base of the brain.

chronic progressive external o. progressive external o.

exophthalmic o. external ocular paresis and exophthalmos of Graves disease.

external o. paralysis of the external ocular muscles.

fascicular o. ophthalmoplegia due to lesion in the pons varolii.

internal o. paralysis of the iris and ciliary apparatus.

internuclear o. a horizontal ocular motor disturbance due to a lesion of the medial longitudinal fasciculus.

nuclear o. ophthalmoplegia caused by a lesion of the nuclei of the motor nerves of the eye.

orbital o. ophthalmoplegia due to lesion in the orbit.

partial o. paralysis of either one or two of the eye muscles.

o. plus Kearns-Sayre syndrome.

progressive external o. a slowly progressing, bilateral myopathy often affecting only the extraocular muscles, but sometimes also the orbicularis oculi. The levators of the upper lids are usually affected first, with ptosis resulting, followed by progressive, total ocular paresis. Called also *ocular myopathy*.

supranuclear o. ophthalmoplegia caused by a lesion above the nuclei of the motor nerves of the eye.

total o., o. tota′lis ophthalmoplegia that affects both the extrinsic and intrinsic muscle structures of the eye.

oph·thal·mop·to·sis (of-thal″mop-to′sis, of-thal″mo-to′sis) exophthalmos.

oph·thal·mor·rha·gia (of-thal″mo-ra′jə) [*ophthalmo-* + *-rrhagia*] hemorrhage from the eye.

oph·thal·mor·rhea (of-thal″mo-re′ə) [*ophthalmo-* + *-rrhea*] oozing of blood from the eye.

oph·thal·mor·rhex·is (of-thal″mo-rek′sis) [*ophthalmo-* + *rhexis*] rupture of the eyeball.

oph·thal·mo·scope (of-thal′mo-skōp) [*ophthalmo-* + *-scope*] an instrument containing a perforated mirror and lenses used to examine the interior of the eye; called also *funduscope*.

binocular o. an ophthalmoscope by which the fundus of the eye is viewed with both eyes through two eyepieces; called also *stereo-ophthalmoscope*.

direct o. an ophthalmoscope that produces an upright, or unreversed, image of approximately 15 times magnification.

indirect o. an ophthalmoscope that produces an inverted, or reversed, direct image of 2 to 5 times magnification, depending on the dioptric power to the examining lens.

scanning laser o. (SLO) an instrument for retinal imaging in which light from a low-power laser beam that scans the retina is reflected back to a sensor; the light detected by the sensor is used to create a full-color composite digital image.

oph·thal·mos·co·py (of″thəl-mos′kə-pe) the examination of the interior of the eye with the ophthalmoscope. Called also *funduscopy*.

direct o. direct, close-range ophthalmoscopic observation of the fundus; the image is virtual, erect, and magnified.

indirect o. ophthalmoscopic examination of the fundus with the interposition of a strong convex lens between the observer and the patient; the image is real and inverted.

medical o. ophthalmoscopy performed to diagnose local or systemic diseases such as diabetes mellitus, hypertension, and cerebral tumor.

metric o. ophthalmoscopy performed for the measurement of refraction.

oph·thal·mo·spec·tro·scope (of-thal″mo-spek′tro-skōp) an instrument used in ophthalmospectroscopy.

oph·thal·mo·spec·tros·co·py (of-thal″mo-spek-tros′kə-pe) [*ophthalmo-* + *spectroscopy*] ophthalmoscopic and spectroscopic examination of the ocular fundus.

oph·thal·mos·ta·sis (of″thəl-mos′tə-sis) [*ophthalmo-* + *stasis*] fixation of the eye with the ophthalmostat.

oph·thal·mo·stat (of-thal′mo-stat″) [*ophthalmo-* + Gr. *histanai* to halt] an instrument for holding the eye steady during operation.

oph·thal·mo·sta·tom·e·ter (of-thal″mo-stə-tom′ə-tər) exophthalmometer.

oph·thal·mo·syn·chy·sis (of-thal″mo-sin′kĭ-sis) [*ophthalmo-* + *synchysis*] effusion into the eye.

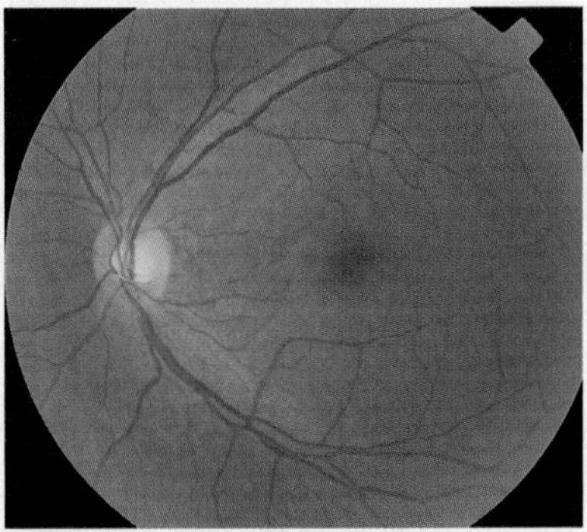

■ Normal fundus viewed by ophthalmoscopy.

oph·thal·mo·ther·mom·e·ter (of-thal″mo-thər-mom′ə-tər) [*ophthalmo-* + *thermometer*] an apparatus for recording the temperature of the eye.

oph·thal·mot·o·my (of″thəl-mot′ə-me) [*ophthalmo-* + *-tomy*] the operation of incising the eyeball.

oph·thal·mo·to·nom·e·ter (of-thal″mo-tə-nom′ə-tər) tonometer (def. 2).

oph·thal·mo·tox·in (of-thal′mo-tok″sin) [*ophthalmo-* + *toxin*] a toxin acting on the eye.

oph·thal·mo·trope (of-thal′mo-trōp) [*ophthalmo-* + Gr. *trepein* to turn] a mechanical eye that moves like a real eye, used for demonstrating the action of the ocular muscles.

oph·thal·mo·tro·pom·e·ter (of-thal″mo-tro-pom′ə-tər) strabismometer.

oph·thal·mo·tro·pom·e·try (of-thal″mo-tro-pom′ə-tre) strabismometry.

oph·thal·mo·vas·cu·lar (of-thal″mo-vas′ku-lər) pertaining to the blood vessels of the eye.

oph·thal·mo·xe·ro·sis (of-thal″mo-ze-ro′sis) xerophthalmia.

Oph·thet·ic (of-thet′ik) trademark for a preparation of proparacaine hydrochloride.

Oph·tho·chlor (of′tho-klor) trademark for a preparation of chloramphenicol.

-opia [Gr. *ōps* eye] a combining form denoting condition or a defect of the eye, or of vision.

opi·an (o′pe-ən) noscapine.

opi·a·nine (o-pi′ə-nin) noscapine.

opi·ate (o′pe-ət) 1. a drug derived from opium, or a semisynthetic drug derived an opium component. 2. hypnotic (def. 2).

endogenous o's endorphins and enkephalins that are released by the body as a defense against pain or during physical exercise, deep relaxation, sexual activity, crying, and laughing.

Opie paradox (o′pe) [Eugene Lindsay *Opie*, American pathologist, 1873–1971] see under *paradox.*

opi·oid (o′pe-oid) 1. any synthetic narcotic that has opiate-like analgesic activity but is not derived from opium. 2. more broadly, any compound with opiate-like activity. Included here are the opiates; synthetic agents not derived from opium; and naturally occurring peptides that bind at or otherwise influence the opiate receptors of cell membranes, including the dynorphins, endorphins, and enkephalins.

opip·ra·mol hy·dro·chlo·ride (o-pip′rə-mol) a tricyclic antidepressant with mild tranquilizing properties; administered orally.

Opi·so·cros·tis (o″pĭ-so-kros′tis) a genus of fleas. *O. bru′neri* is a squirrel flea that may be a vector of sylvatic plague.

opis·the (o-pis′the) [Gr. *opisthen* behind] the posterior daughter organism after transverse division of a ciliate protozoan; cf. *proter.*

opis·the·nar (o-pis′the-nər) [*opistho-* + *thenar*] the dorsum of the hand.

opis·thi·o·ba·si·al (o-pis″the-o-ba′se-əl) pertaining to or connecting the opisthion and basion.

opis·thi·on (o-pis′the-on) [Gr. *opisthion* rear, posterior] [TA] a craniometric landmark located at the midpoint of the posterior border of the foramen magnum.

opis·thio·na·si·al (o-pis″the-o-na′ze-əl) connecting the opisthion and nasion.

opisth(o)- [Gr. *opisthen* behind, at the back] a combining form meaning backward or denoting relationship to the back.

opis·tho·cra·ni·on (o-pis″tho-kra′ne-on) [*opistho-* + Gr. *kranion* the upper part of the head] a craniometric landmark determined instrumentally to indicate the posterior end of the maximum cranial length measured along the midline of the glabella.

opis·tho·ge·nia (o-pis″tho-je′ne-ə) defective development of the jaws following ankylosis of the jaw. Cf. *retrognathism.*

opis·thog·na·thism (o″pis-thog′nə-thiz-əm) retrognathism.

opis·tho·mas·ti·gote (o″pis-tho-mas′tĭ-gōt) [*opistho-* + Gr. *mastix* whip] a morphologic stage in the life cycle of certain trypanosomatid protozoa in which the kinetoplast and basal body are posterior to the nucleus, the flagellum runs through the body of the cell to emerge anteriorly as a free-flowing structure, and an undulating membrane is absent. Cf. *amastigote, choanomastigote, epimastigote, promastigote,* and *trypomastigote.*

opis·thor·chi·a·sis (o″pis-thor-ki′ə-sis) infection of the biliary tract by liver flukes of the genus *Opisthorchis.* In heavy infections there is local injury to the distal bile capillaries and surrounding liver tissue; this may ultimately develop into cirrhosis of the liver with areas of necrosis and fatty degeneration. See also *clonorchiasis.* Called also *opisthorchosis.*

Opis·thor·chi·i·dae (o″pis-thor-ki′ĭ-de) a family of trematodes; it includes the genera *Metorchis, Opisthorchis, Parametorchis,* and *Pseudamphistomum.*

Opis·thor·chis (o″pis-thor′kis) [*opistho-* + *orchis*] a genus of trematodes of the family Opisthorchiidae, characterized by having the testes near the posterior end of the body.

O. feli′neus the Siberian liver fluke found in the liver of various mammals; infection (see *opisthorchiasis*) comes from eating infected fish, such as *Leuciscus rutilis, Idus melanotus,* and related species.

O. nover′ca *Amphimerus noverca.*

O. sinen′sis the common liver fluke of China, Japan, Korea, Taiwan, and Indochina, found in the bile ducts of mammals that eat fresh water fish containing the larvae. Larval development requires two intermediate hosts, the first a snail of the genus *Parafossarulus* or *Bithynia,* the second a fresh water fish of the carp family. Called also *Clonorchis sinensis.*

O. tenuicol′lis a species found in the bile ducts and sometimes the intestines of mammals.

O. viver′rini a species that causes opisthorchiasis in the civet cat and sometimes humans in Thailand.

opis·thor·cho·sis (o″pis-thor-ko′sis) opisthorchiasis.

opis·thot·o·noid (o″pis-thot′ə-noid) resembling opisthotonos.

opis·thot·o·nos (o″pis-thot′ə-nəs) [*opistho-* + Gr. *tonos* tension] a form of spasm consisting of extreme hyperextension of the body; the head and the heels are bent backward and the body bowed forward. **opisthoton′ic** *adj*

o. feta′lis an exaggerated deflection attitude of the fetus during labor, which may persist during the neonatal period, but which gradually changes to a more normal posture.

opis·thot·o·nus (o″pis-thot′ə-nəs) opisthotonos.

Opitz disease (o′pits) [Hans *Opitz,* German pediatrician, 20th century] see under *disease.*

Opitz syndrome (o′pits) [John Marius *Opitz,* German-born pediatrician in the United States, born 1935] see under *syndrome.*

Opitz-Fri·as syndrome (o′pits fre′ahs) [J.M. *Opitz;* Jaime L. *Frías,* Chilean pediatrician, 20th century] see under *syndrome.*

opi·um (o′pe-əm) [L., from Gr. *opion*] [USP] the air-dried milky exudate obtained from the unripe capsules of *Papaver somniferum* or *P. album.* Various principles and derivatives of opium, including some 20 alkaloids, notably morphine, codeine, papaverine, and thebaine, are used for their narcotic and analgesic effects. Because it is highly addictive, the production of opium is restricted, and the cultivation of the plants from which it is obtained is prohibited by most nations under an international agreement. Called also *crude o.* and *gum o.*

crude o. opium.

denarcotized o., deodorized o. powdered opium freed from certain nauseating constituents by extraction with purified petroleum benzin.

gum o. opium.

opo·ceph·a·lus (o″po-sef′ə-ləs) [Gr. *ōps* face + *-cephalus*] a fetus with the ears fused to the head, one orbit, no mouth, and no nose.

opo·did·y·mus (o″po-did′ĭ-məs) [Gr. *ōps* face + *-didymus*] a fetus with two fused heads and with the sense organs partially fused.

opod·y·mus (o-pod′ĭ-məs) opodidymus.

opos·sum (o-pos′əm) [Algonquian] a member of any of several genera of marsupial mammals; see *Didelphis.*

Op·pen·heim reflex (sign) (op′en-hīm) [Hermann *Oppenheim,* German neurologist, 1858–1919] see under *reflex.*

op·po·nens (o-po′nənz) [L.] opposing; said of an opposing structure, as musculus opponens.

op·por·tu·nist (op″ər-too′nist) an opportunistic organism.

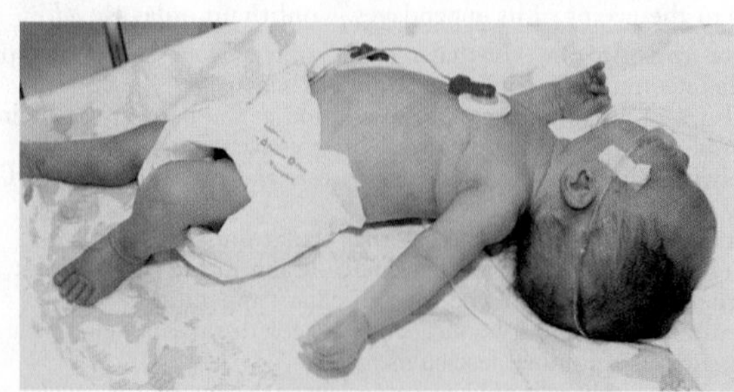

■ Opisthotonos.

op·por·tu·nis·tic (op″ər-too-nis′tik) 1. denoting a microorganism that does not ordinarily cause disease but that becomes pathogenic under certain circumstances, such as in immunodeficiency conditions. 2. denoting a disease or infection caused by such an organism.

oprel·ve·kin (o-prel′və-kin″) a recombinant derivative of interleukin-11, used as a hematopoietic stimulator to prevent thrombocytopenia following myelosuppressive chemotherapy in patients with nonmyeloid malignancies; administered subcutaneously.

OPRT orotate phosphoribosyltransferase.

-opsia [Gr. *opsis* sight] a combining form denoting a condition or a defect of vision.

op·sin (op′sin) a protein of the retinal rods (scotopsin) and cones (photopsin) that combines with 11-*cis*-retinal (q.v.) to form visual pigments. The opsins are also named according to the color of pigment: iodopsin (violet), rhodopsin (purple), etc. See illustration at *visual cycle*, under *cycle*.

op·si·om·e·ter (op″se-om′ə-tər) optometer.

op·si·uria (op″se-u′re-ə) [Gr. *opse* late + *-uria*] the condition in which more urine is excreted during fasting than during digestion.

op·so·clo·nia (op″so-klo′ne-ə) opsoclonus.

op·so·clo·nus (op″so-klo′nəs) a condition characterized by nonrhythmic horizontal and vertical oscillations of the eyes, observed in various disorders of the brainstem or cerebellum.

o.-myoclonus see under *syndrome*.

paraneoplastic o. opsoclonus occurring as part of the paraneoplastic type of opsoclonus-myoclonus syndrome (see under *syndrome*).

op·so·nin (op′sə-nin) [Gr. *opsōnein* to buy victuals] any substance that binds to particulate antigens and induces their phagocytosis by macrophages and neutrophils. In current usage the term is used to refer to substances of two types, opsonizing antibodies (IgM, IgG1, and IgG3, immunoglobulins specific for the antigen) and certain complement fragments (C3b, C3d, and C4b, which become bound to the antigen during complement activation), both of which trigger phagocytosis by binding to specific cell-surface receptors, Fc receptors, and complement receptors on neutrophils and macrophages. **opson′ic** *adj*

immune o. opsonizing antibody.

op·so·ni·za·tion (op″sə-nĭ-za′shən) the rendering of bacteria and other cells subject to phagocytosis by the action of an opsonin.

op·so·nize (op′sə-nīz) to function as an opsonin.

op·so·no·cy·to·phag·ic (op″sə-no-si″to-faj′ik) denoting the phagocytic activity of blood in the presence of serum opsonins and homologous leukocytes.

op·so·no·pha·go·cy·to·sis (op″so-no-fa″go-si-to′sis) phagocytosis by macrophages and monocytes in the presence of specific serum opsonins.

op·so·no·phil·ia (op″sə-no-fil′e-ə) [*opsonin* + *-philia*] affinity for opsonins. **opsonophil′ic** *adj*

op·tic (op′tik) [Gr. *optikos* of or for sight] ocular (def. 1).

Op·ti·caine (op′tĭ-kān″) trademark for a preparation of tetracaine hydrochloride.

op·ti·cal (op′tĭ-kəl) [L. *opticus;* Gr. *optikos*] visual.

op·ti·cian (op-tish′ən) an expert in opticianry.

op·ti·cian·ry (op-tish′ən-re) the science of optics as applied to filling and adapting of ophthalmic prescriptions and products.

op·ti·co·chi·as·mat·ic (op″tĭ-ko-ki″az-mat′ik) pertaining to the optic nerves and chiasma.

op·ti·co·cil·i·ary (op″tĭ-ko-sil′e-ar-e) pertaining to the optic and ciliary nerves.

op·ti·co·ki·net·ic (op″tĭ-ko-kĭ-net′ik) optokinetic.

op·ti·co·na·si·on (op″tĭ-ko-na′se-on) the distance from the posterior edge of the optic foramen to the nasion.

op·ti·co·pu·pil·lary (op″tĭ-ko-pu′pĭ-lar-e) pertaining to the optic nerve and the pupil.

Op·ti·crom (op′tĭ-krom) trademark for preparations of cromolyn sodium.

op·tics (op′tiks) [Gr. *optikos* of or for sight] the science of light and of vision.

fiber o. see *fiberoptics*.

op·ti·mal (op′ti-məl) the best; the most favorable.

Op·ti·MARK (op′tĭ-mahrk) trademark for a preparation of gadoversetamide.

op·tim·e·ter (op-tim′ə-tər) optometer.

Op·ti·mine (op′tĭ-mēn″) trademark for a preparation of azatadine maleate.

op·ti·mum (op′tĭ-məm) [L. "best"] that condition of surroundings which is conducive to the most favorable activity or function.

Op·ti·pran·o·lol (op″tĭ-pran′ə-lol) trademark for a preparation of metipranolol hydrochloride.

Op·ti·son (op′tĭ-son) trademark for a preparation of albumin microspheres sonicated.

Op·ti·var (op′tĭ-vahr) trademark for a preparation of azelastine hydrochloride.

opt(o)- [Gr. *optos* seen] a combining form denoting relationship to vision or sight.

op·to·chi·as·mic (op″to-ki-az′mik) opticochiasmatic.

op·to·chin (op′to-kin) a derivative of cupreine that has a specific bactericidal effect on *Streptococcus pneumoniae* and is used in the optochin susceptibility test; called also ethylhydrocupreine.

op·to·gram (op′to-gram) [*opto-* + *-gram*] the retinal image formed by the bleaching of the visual purple under the influence of light.

op·to·ki·net·ic (op″to-kĭ-net′ik) [*opto-* + *kinetic*] pertaining to movement of the eyes and of objects in the visual field, as in nystagmus.

op·to·me·ninx (op″to-me′ningks) [*opto-* + Gr. *mēninx* membrane] the retina.

op·tom·e·ter (op-tom′ə-tər) [*opto-* + *-meter*] an instrument formerly used to measure ocular refraction; called also *opsiometer*, *optimeter*, and *refractometer*.

op·tom·e·trist (op-tom′ə-trist) a health care provider who examines, diagnoses, treats, and manages diseases and disorders of the visual system, the eye, and associated structures, as well as diagnosing related systemic conditions. See *optometry*.

op·tom·e·try (op-tom′ə-tre) [*opto-* + *-metry*] the professional practice consisting of examination of the eyes to evaluate health and visual abilities, diagnosis of eye diseases and conditions of the eye and visual system, and provision of treatment by such means as the prescription of eyeglasses and contact lenses and the use of vision therapy, low-vision aids, drugs (in most states), and certain surgical procedures.

op·to·my·om·e·ter (op″to-mi-om′ə-tər) [*opto-* + *myometer*] a device used in measuring the power of the extrinsic ocular muscles.

op·to·phone (op′tə-fōn) [*opto-* + Gr. *phōnē* voice] an instrument by means of which light and darkness are made discernible to the blind through their sense of hearing, the light waves being transformed into sound waves.

op·to·type (op′to-tīp) test type.

Opun·tia (o-pun′she-ə) the prickly pears, a large genus of cacti. *O. ficus-indica* has edible fruit called the Indian fig or sabra, but its spines cause sabra dermatitis. *O. vulga′ris* is used as a remedy in homeopathy.

OPV poliovirus vaccine live oral.

OR operating room.

ora[1] (o′rə) gen. and pl. *o′rae* [L.] an edge or margin.

o. serra′ta re′tinae [TA] the irregular anterior margin of the pars optica of the retina, lying internal to the junction of the choroid and the ciliary body.

ora[2] (o′rə) [L.] plural of *os*[1].

orad (o′rad) [*ora-* + *-ad*[1]] toward the mouth.

orae (o′re) [L.] genitive and plural of *ora*[1].

Or·a·graf·in (or″ə-graf′in) trademark for a preparation of ipodate calcium or ipodate sodium.

oral (or′əl) [L. *oralis*] 1. pertaining to the mouth; taken through or applied in the mouth. 2. lingual (def. 2).

ora·le (o-ra′le) a craniometric landmark, being the point in the midline of the maxillary suture just lingual to the central incisors in the alveolar process.

oral·i·ty (o-ral′ĭ-te) in psychoanalytic theory, the psychic organization of all the sensations, impulses, and personality traits derived from the oral stage of psychosexual development.

oral·o·gy (o-ral′ə-je) [*oral* + *-logy*] stomatology.

Ora·morph (or′ə-morf″) trademark for a preparation of morphine sulfate.

or·ange (or′ənj) [L. *aurantium*] 1. any of several species of *Citrus*, particularly *Citrus aurantium*, the bitter orange, and *Citrus sinensis*, the sweet orange. 2. the fruit of *C. aurantium* or *C. sinensis*; used in pharmaceutical preparations. 3. a color between red and yellow, produced by energy of wavelengths between 590 and 630 nm. 4. a dye or stain with this color. 5. of or relating to the fruit of *Citrus aurantium.*

o. III methyl o.

acid o. 10 o. G.

acridine o. a substituted acridine derivative that acts as a fluorescent basic dye; sometimes used for vital and supravital staining, including detection of nucleic acids, differentiation of DNA and RNA, and detection of malignant cells.

bitter o. *Citrus aurantium*, or its fruit; its peel and flowers are used in pharmaceutical preparations.

o. G an acid azo dye used as a counterstain in histology and cytology and as a component of Mallory acid fuchsin, orange G, and aniline blue stain.

gold o., methyl o., Poirier o. an orange-yellow aniline dye, used as an indicator with a pH range of 3.2 to 4.4 and a color change from pink to yellow. Called also *helianthin* and *o. III.*

sweet o. *Citrus sinensis*, or its fruit; its peel is used in pharmaceutical preparations.

wool o. o. G.

or•an•ge•o•phil (or-an′je-o-fĭl) [*orange* + *-phil*] 1. staining readily with orange dyes. 2. a cell or other histologic element that stains readily with orange dyes. 3. somatotroph.

orang•u•tan (ə-rang′ə-tan″) [Malayan "wild man"] *Pongo pygmaeus*, an anthropoid ape native to Indonesia, used for laboratory studies because it is susceptible to some human diseases.

Or•ap trademark for a preparation of pimozide.

Ora•sone (or′ə-sōn″) trademark for preparations of prednisone.

or•bic•u•lar (or-bik′u-lər) [L. *orbicularis*] circular, or rounded.

or•bic•u•la•re (or-bik″u-la′re) [L.] processus lenticularis incudis.

or•bic•u•li (or-bik′u-li) genitive and plural of *orbiculus.*

or•bic•u•lus (or-bik′u-ləs) gen. and pl. *orbic′uli* [L., dim. of *orbis* orb, circle] a small circular or disk-shaped structure.

o. cilia′ris [TA] ciliary disk: the thin part of the ciliary body extending between its crown and the ora serrata retinae; called also *pars plana corporis ciliaris.*

or•bit (or′bit) orbita.

or•bi•ta (or′bĭ-tə) gen. and pl. *or′bitae* [L. "mark of a wheel, circuit"] [TA] orbit: the bony cavity that contains the eyeball and its associated muscles, vessels, and nerves; the ethmoid, frontal, lacrimal, nasal, palatine, sphenoid, and zygomatic bones, and the maxilla contribute to its formation.

or•bi•tae (or′bĭ-te) [L.] genitive and plural of *orbita.*

or•bi•tal (or′bĭ-təl) 1. pertaining to the orbit. 2. in an atom, the wave function describing the probability of occurrence of an electron of a particular energy level of an atom or molecule; each orbital can hold two electrons of opposing spin.

hybrid o. a type of atomic orbital occurring in covalently bonded atoms, representing distortion or hybridization of dissimilar individual orbitals characteristic of the isolated atom such that all bonding orbitals become functionally equivalent.

or•bi•ta•le (or″bĭ-ta′le) an anthropometric landmark, the lowest point on the inferior margin of the orbit.

or•bi•ta•lis (or″bĭ-ta′lis) [L.] pertaining to the orbit.

or•bi•tog•ra•phy (or″bĭ-tog′rə-fe) [*orbit* + *-graphy*] visualization of the orbit and its contents using radiography or computed tomography.

or•bi•to•na•sal (or″bĭ-to-na′zəl) pertaining to the orbit and the nose.

or•bi•to•nom•e•ter (or″bĭ-to-nom′ə-tər) [*orbit* + *tonometer*] an instrument for measurement of the backward displacement of the eyeball produced by a given pressure exerted against its anterior aspect; called also *piezometer.*

or•bi•to•nom•e•try (or″bĭ-to-nom′ə-tre) the measurement of the backward displacement of the eyeball under varying pressures.

or•bi•top•a•gus (or″bĭ-top′ə-gəs) [*orbit* + *-pagus*] conjoined twins in which the smaller parasitic fetus is attached to the orbit of the larger twin.

or•bi•top•a•thy (or″bĭ-top′ə-the) [*orbit* + *-pathy*] disease affecting the orbit and its contents.

dysthyroid o. the ocular changes associated with thyroid dysfunction, most often Graves disease, including endocrine exophthalmos, malignant exophthalmos, and infiltrative ophthalmopathy; called also *dysthyroid ophthalmopathy.*

Graves o. dysthyroid orbitopathy occurring in Graves disease. Called also *Graves ophthalmopathy.*

or•bi•to•stat (or′bĭ-to-stat) [*orbit* + Gr. *statos* placed] an instrument for measuring the axis of the orbit.

or•bi•to•tem•po•ral (or″bĭ-to-tem′pə-rəl) pertaining to the orbital and temporal regions.

or•bi•tot•o•my (or″bĭ-tot′ə-me) [*orbit* + *-tomy*] the operation of incising or opening into the orbit through the orbital margin.

Or•bi•vi•rus (or′bĭ-vi″rəs) [L. *orbis* circle + *virus*] orbiviruses; a genus of viruses of the family Reoviridae, separable into at least 14 antigenically distinct groups. They infect a variety of vertebrates and include the human pathogens Orungo virus and Kemerovo virus, as well as the agents of bluetongue and African horse sickness. Mosquitoes, sandflies, and ticks are vectors.

or•bi•vi•rus (or′bĭ-vi″rəs) any virus of the genus *Orbivirus.* **orbivi′ral** *adj*

or•ce•in (or-se′in) a brown coloring matter, derived from orcinol and soluble in alcohol; used as a specific stain for elastic tissue.

or•chal•gia (or-kal′jah) orchialgia.

or•chec•to•my (or-kek′tə-me) orchiectomy.

or•chel•la (or-shel′ə) a histologic stain composed of 5 mL of acetic acid and 40 mL each of alcohol and water, colored to a dark red with archil from which excess of ammonia has been driven off.

or•chi•al•gia (or″ke-al′jə) [*orchi-* + *-algia*] pain in a testis. Called also *orchiodynia* and *testalgia.*

or•chi•dec•to•my (or″kĭ-dek′tə-me) orchiectomy.

or•chid•ic (or-kid′ik) testicular.

or•chi•di•tis (or″kĭ-di′tis) orchitis.

orchid(o)- [Gr. *orchidion*, dim. of *orchis* testis] a combining form denoting relationship to the testes.

or•chi•do•epi•did•y•mec•to•my (or″kĭ-do-ep″ĭ-did″ĭ-mek′tə-me) epididymo-orchidectomy.

or•chi•dom•e•ter (or″kĭ-dom′ə-tər) an instrument for measuring the testis.

Prader o. a string of plastic models of testes, marked according to their volume in cubic centimeters; used for measuring the size of the

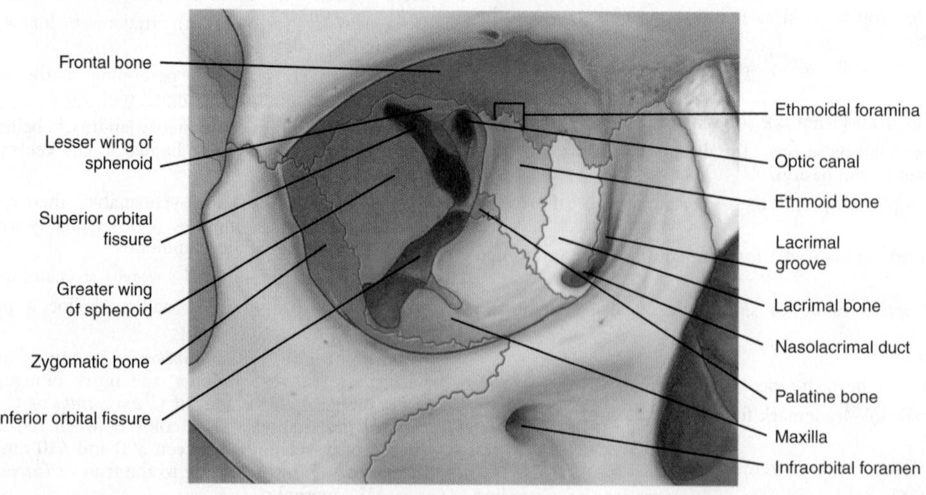

■ Orbita (orbit).

testes either in growing boys or in men who have an abnormal condition or have had a procedure done.

or•chi•dop•a•thy (or″kĭ-dop′ə-the) orchiopathy.

or•chi•do•pexy (or′kĭ-do-pek″se) orchiopexy.

or•chi•do•plas•ty (or′kĭ-do-plas″te) orchioplasty.

or•chi•dot•o•my (or″kĭ-dot′ə-me) orchiotomy.

or•chi•ec•to•my (or″ke-ek′tə-me) [*orchio-* + Gr. *-ectomy*] excision of one or both testes; if it is bilateral, the individual is incapable of reproduction (see *castration*).

radical inguinal o. surgical removal of a testis and of the spermatic cord up to the internal inguinal ring.

or•chi•epi•did•y•mi•tis (or″ke-ep″ĭ-did″ə-mi′tis) epididymo-orchitis.

orchi(o)- [Gr. *orchis*, gen. *orchios* testis] a combining form denoting relationship to the testes.

or•chio•blas•to•ma (or″ke-o-blas-to′mə) yolk sac tumor.

or•chio•cele (or′ke-o-sēl″) [*orchio-* + *-cele*[1]] 1. protrusion of a testis due to a hernia. 2. scrotal hernia.

or•chio•dyn•ia (or″ke-o-din′e-ə) orchialgia.

or•chio•neu•ral•gia (or″ke-o-noo̅-ral′jə) [*orchio-* + *neuralgia*] orchialgia.

or•chi•op•a•thy (or″ke-op′ə-the) [*orchio-* + *-pathy*] any disease of the testis. Called also *orchidopathy* and *testopathy*.

or•chio•pexy (or′ke-o-pek″se) [*orchio-* + *-pexy*] surgical fixation in the scrotum of an undescended testis; called also *orchidopexy*.

or•chio•plas•ty (or′ke-o-plas″te) [*orchio-* + *-plasty*] plastic surgery of the testis. **orchioplas′tic** *adj*

or•chi•or•rha•phy (or″ke-or′ə-fe) [*orchio-* + *-rrhaphy*] orchiopexy.

or•chi•ot•o•my (or″ke-ot′ə-me) [*orchio-* + *-tomy*] an incision into a testis, such as for drainage; called also *orchidotomy*.

Or•chis (or′kis) [Gr. *orchis* testicle, so called because the roots or rhizomes of certain species resemble testicles] a genus of orchids, flowering plants of the family Orchidaceae; some species are medicinal.

or•chis (or′kis) [Gr.] TA alternative for testis.

or•chi•tis (or-ki′tis) [*orchi-* + *-itis*] inflammation of a testis, marked by pain, swelling, and a feeling of weight, often seen accompanying epididymitis (see *epididymo-orchitis*). It may occur idiopathically or be associated with conditions such as mumps, gonorrhea, filarial disease, syphilis, or tuberculosis. **orchit′ic** *adj*

filarial o. orchitis caused by lymphatic obstruction due to filariasis; see also *elephantiasis scroti*.

mumps o. orchitis seen as a complication of mumps.

spermatogenic granulomatous o. orchitis in which the normal structure of the testis has been replaced by gray-white granulomatous tissue without evident necrosis; it is thought to be in some way a reaction to spermatozoa.

traumatic o. orchitis following trauma, vas ligation, or surgical manipulation, without evidence of previous disease.

or•cin (or′sin) orcinol.

or•ci•nol (or′sĭ-nol) an antiseptic principle derived mainly from lichens, used as a reagent in various tests; called also *orcin*.

or•der (or′dər) [L. *ordo* a line, row, or series] a taxonomic category subordinate to a class and superior to a family; see *taxon*.

or•der•ly (or′dər-le) an attendant in a hospital who works under the direction of a nurse.

or•di•nal (or′dĭ-nəl) being of a specified position in a ranked, often numbered, series (e.g., first, second, third, etc.).

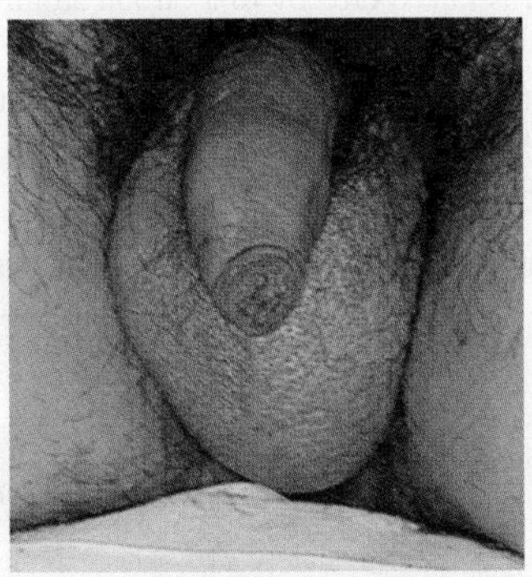

■ Mumps orchitis.

or•di•nate (or′dĭ-nət) [L. *ordinare* to arrange in order] in a two-dimensional coordinate system, the distance of a point from the horizontal *(x)* axis, measured along a line parallel to the *y*-axis. Denoted by *y*. Cf. *abscissa*.

orel•la•nine (o-rel′ə-nēn) a toxic chemical found in certain species of *Cortinarius* mushrooms in Europe and Japan; ingestion causes gastritis, chills, headaches, myalgias, and occasionally renal tubular necrosis progressing to renal failure.

orel•line (or′ə-lēn) a toxic chemical found in certain species of *Cortinarius* mushrooms in Europe and Japan; ingestion causes gastritis, chills, headaches, myalgias, and occasionally renal tubular necrosis progressing to renal failure.

Oren•cia (o-ren′se-ə) trademark for a preparation of abatacept.

ore•o•se•li•num (o″re-o-se-li′num) [L.] *Peucedanum oreoselinum*, a plant used in homeopathy as a diuretic.

Oret•ic (o-ret′ik) trademark for a preparation of hydrochlorothiazide.

orex•i•gen•ic (o-rek″sĭ-jen′ik) [Gr. *orexis* appetite + *-genic*] increasing or stimulating the appetite.

orex•in (ə-rek′sin) either of two neuropeptides (orexin A and orexin B) produced in the hypothalamus and regulating feeding behavior as well as the sleep-wake cycle. Called also *hypocretin*.

ORF open reading frame; see *reading frame*, under *frame*.

orf (orf) contagious ecthyma.

ORFeome (orf′e-ōm) the totality of DNA sequences in a genome that are open reading frames and thus could code for protein products.

or•gan (or′gən) [L. *organum* (q.v.)] organum.

acoustic o. organum spirale.

Bidder o. an anterior portion of the gonad of male toads, ovarian in character.

cement o. the embryonic tissue that develops into the cement layer of the tooth.

Chievitz o. an embryonic outgrowth behind the parotid gland; sometimes it merges into the gland and sometimes it disappears.

circumventricular o's several small structures located around the edges of the third and fourth ventricles, lacking the regular blood-brain barrier and thus serving as significant sites for neural-endocrine interaction. They include the area postrema, median eminence, subcommissural organ, subfornical organ, and vascular organ of lamina terminalis. Sometimes also included are the funiculus separans, neurohypophysis, and pineal body.

o. of Corti organum spirale.

critical o. the organ or organ system in which a specific radioactive material tends to concentrate, and thus the organ receiving the highest level of exposure to the radioactivity.

digestive o's the organs concerned with the ingestion, digestion, and assimilation of food (*systema digestorium* [TA]).

effector o. effector (def. 2).

enamel o. a circumscribed knoblike mass of ectodermal cells arising from the dental lamina; it produces the enamel cap from which the dental enamel develops.

end o. end-organ; see under *E*.

extraperitoneal o. any of the abdominal viscera, e.g., the kidneys, lying on the abdominal wall and invested by peritoneum only on the anterior surface; called also *retroperitoneal o.*

genital o's the various internal and external structures of the female and male genitalia; see terms beginning *organa genitalia*, under *organum*.

o. of Giraldés paradidymis.

Golgi tendon o. an encapsulated nerve ending found in tendons of mammalian muscles and acting as a mechanoreceptor; arranged in series with the muscle, it is sensitive to mechanical distortion induced by either passive stretch of the tendon or isometric contraction of the muscle and thus signals muscle tension, being the receptor responsible for the lengthening reaction, or clasp-knife reflex. Called also *Golgi corpuscle*, *tendon o.* or *spindle*, and *neurotendinous o.* or *spindle*.

gustatory o. organum gustatorium.

holdfast o. holdfast.

intraperitoneal o. any of the abdominal viscera suspended in the peritoneal cavity by a mesentery.

intromittent o. any male copulatory organ (one used to transfer sperm to the female reproductive tract), such as the human penis or the claspers seen especially in male insects and cartilaginous fishes.

Jacobson o. organum vomeronasale.

lateral line o's a system of sense organs arranged in longitudinal canals in the skin of fishes and amphibians; they contain mechanoreceptors that are sensitive to changes in pressure and current and to vibrations of low frequency and thus aid in localizing objects.

o's of mastication masticatory apparatus.

Meyer o. an area of circumvallate papillae on either side of the posterior part of the tongue.

neurotendinous o. Golgi tendon o.
olfactory o. organum olfactorium.
parapineal o. a median dorsal outgrowth of the pineal body in certain lower vertebrates such as tailless amphibians, primitive fishes, and lizards; its principal cell type is an apparent photoreceptor. In some species it may specialize to form an extracranial epiphyseal eye. Called also *parietal o.*
parietal o. parapineal o.
primary lymphoid o's organa lymphoidea primaria.
primitive fat o. brown adipose tissue.
reproductive o's the various internal and external structures involved in reproduction in the female and male; see terms beginning *organa genitalia*, under *organum.*
retroperitoneal o. extraperitoneal o.
Rosenmüller o. epoöphoron.
rudimentary o. 1. a primordium. 2. an imperfectly or incompletely developed organ.
secondary lymphoid o's organa lymphoidea secundaria.
segmental o. the pronephros, mesonephros, and metanephros together.
sense o's, sensory o's organa sensuum. See under *organum.*
o. of shock, shock o. an organ that reacts in anaphylactic shock; these organs have responses that determine the nature and, to a large extent, the outcome of a given anaphylactic reaction.
o's of special sense organa sensuum.
spiral o. organum spirale.
subcommissural o. organum subcommissurale.
subfornical o. organum subfornicale.
target o. an organ that is affected by a specific hormone, as the adrenal cortex by corticotropin.
tendon o. Golgi tendon o.
terminal o. the organ at either end of a reflex arc.
urinary o's the organs of the urinary system; see *systema urinarium.*
vascular o. of lamina terminalis organum vasculosum of lamina terminalis.
vestibulocochlear o. organum vestibulocochleare.
vestigial o. an undeveloped organ that, in the embryo or in some more or less remote ancestor, was well developed and functional.
vomeronasal o. organum vomeronasale.
Weber o. utriculus prostaticus.
o's of Zuckerkandl corpora paraaortica.

or·ga·na (or'gə-nə) plural of *organum.*

or·ga·nel·la (or″gə-nel'ə) pl. *organel'lae* [L., dim. of *organum*] organelle.

or·ga·nelle (or″gə-nel') [L. *organella,* dim. of *organum* organ] any of the membrane-bound organized cytoplasmic structures of distinctive morphology, biochemical composition, and function present in all eukaryotic cells, including such structures as the nucleus, mitochondria, lysosomes, peroxisomes, Golgi apparatus, and endoplasmic reticulum, as well as chloroplasts in plants and cilia, flagella, and the cytopharynx in protozoa. See Plates 11 and 12.
holdfast o. holdfast.

or·gan·ic (or-gan'ik) 1. pertaining to or arising from an organ or the organs; cf. *functional* (def. 2). 2. having an organized structure. 3. arising from an organism. 4. pertaining to substances derived from living organisms. 5. denoting chemical substances containing covalently bound carbon atoms. 6. pertaining to or cultivated by the use of animal or vegetable fertilizers, rather than synthetic chemicals.

Or·gan·i·din NR (or-gan'ĭ-din) trademark for a preparation of guaifenesin.

or·gan·i·fi·ca·tion (or-gan″ĭ-fĭ-ka'shən) the incorporation of iodide into tyrosyl residues in the thyroid by thyroid peroxidase, resulting in the formation of mono- and diiodotyrosines.

or·gan·ism (or'gə-niz″əm) any individual living thing, whether animal or plant.
consumer o's the organisms of an ecosystem, plants or animals, that eat other plants or animals.
genetically modified o. (GMO), living modified o. (LMO) a living organism that has a novel combination of genetic material acquired through genetic engineering.
nitrifying o's nitrogen bacteria that are capable of oxidizing ammonia to nitrites and nitrates.
nitrosifying o's nitrogen bacteria that are capable of oxidizing ammonia to nitrites.
pleuropneumonialike o's (PPLO) originally, a group of filtrable microorganisms similar to *Mycoplasma mycoides,* which causes pleuropneumonia in cattle. They are now classified as bacteria and have been assigned to various species of the genus *Mycoplasma.*

or·ga·ni·za·tion (or″gə-nĭ-za'shən) 1. the process of organizing or of becoming organized. 2. an organized body, group, or structure. 3. the replacement of blood clots by fibrous tissue.
health maintenance o. (HMO) a broad term encompassing a variety of health care delivery systems utilizing group practice and providing alternatives to the fee-for-service private practice of medicine and allied health professions. They are essentially prepaid, organized systems for providing comprehensive health care within a geographic area to all persons under contract and they emphasize preventive medicine.
Peer Review O., Professional Review O. (PRO) an organization of health care professionals, in a designated area, state, or community, established to monitor health care services paid for through Medicare, Medicaid, and Maternal and Child Health programs to assure that services provided are medically necessary, meet professional standards, and are provided in the most economic medically appropriate health care agency or institution.
Professional Standards Review O. (PSRO) former name for *Professional Review O.*

or·ga·nize (or'gə-nīz″) 1. to provide with an organic structure. 2. to form into organs.

or·ga·niz·er (or'gə-nīz″ər) a part of an embryo that so influences some other part as to bring about and direct its histological and morphological differentiation. Parts developing as a result of induction, and inducing in their turn are classified as organizers of the second grade, third grade, and so on. Cf. *activator* (def. 2) and *inductor.*
nucleolar o., nucleolus o. nucleolar organizing region.
primary o. the mesodermal cells of the dorsal lip region of the blastopore in amphibians, or similar region in other vertebrates, which triggers gastrulation.
secondary o. an organizer of second grade, such as the optic cup, which exerts influence on the developing lens.
tertiary o. an organizer of third grade, such as the tympanic ring, which exerts influence on the tympanic membrane.

organ(o)- [Gr. *organon* organ] a combining form meaning organic, or denoting relationship to an organ.

or·ga·no·ax·i·al (or″gə-no-ak'se-əl) pertaining to the longitudinal axis of an organ.

or·ga·no·chlo·rine (or″gə-no-klor'ēn) any compound of chlorine and organic elements, such as the chlorinated hydrocarbons.

or·ga·no·fac·tion (or″gə-no-fak'shən) organogenesis.

or·ga·no·fer·ric (or″gə-no-fer'ik) containing iron and some organic compound.

or·ga·no·gel (or-gan'o-jəl) a gel in which an organic liquid takes the place of water.

or·ga·no·gen·e·sis (or″gə-no-jen'ə-sis) [*organo-* + *-genesis*] the origin and development of organs. **organogenet'ic** *adj*

or·ga·no·gen·ic (or″gə-no-jen'ik) originating in an organ.

or·ga·nog·e·ny (or″gə-noj'ə-ne) organogenesis.

or·ga·noid (or'gə-noid) [*organ* + *-oid*] 1. resembling an organ. 2. a structure which resembles an organ.

or·ga·no·lep·tic (or″gə-no-lep'tik) [*organo-* + Gr. *lambanein* to seize] 1. making an impression on an organ of special sense. 2. capable of receiving a sense impression.

or·ga·nol·o·gy (or″gə-nol'ə-je) [*organo-* + *-logy*] the sum of what is known regarding the organs of the body.

or·ga·no·meg·a·ly (or″gə-no-meg'ə-le) [*organo-* + *-megaly*] enlargement of an internal organ or organs; called also *visceromegaly.*

or·ga·no·mer·cu·ri·al (or″gə-no-mər-ku're-əl) any mercury-containing organic compound.

or·ga·no·me·tal·lic (or″gə-no-mə-tal'ik) consisting of a metal in combination with an organic radical; used particularly for a compound in which the metal is linked directly to a carbon atom.

or·ga·nop·a·thy (or″gə-nop'ə-the) [*organo-* + *-pathy*] organic disease.

or·ga·no·pexy (or″gə-no-pek'se) [*organo-* + *-pexy*] the surgical fixation of an organ, especially of the uterus.

Organochlorine Insecticides (Chlorinated Hydrocarbons)

Aldrin	Endrin
Chlordane	Heptachlor
Chlordecone	Lindane
DDT (dichlorodiphenyltri-chloroethane)	Methoxychlor
Dieldrin	TDE (tetradichlorodiphenylethane; DDD)
Endosulfan	Toxophene (camphochlor)

Organophosphorus Insecticides

Acephate	Malathion
Azinphos-methyl	Methyl demeton
Chlorfenvinphos	Methyl parathion
Chlorothion	Mevinphos
Chlorpyrifos	Naled
Coumaphos	Parathion
Demeton	Phorate
Diazinon	Ronnel
Dichlorvos	Octamethyl pyrophosphoramide
Dicrotophos	Temephos
Dimethoate	Tetraethyl pyrophosphate (TEPP)
Dioxathion	Trichlorfon
Disulfoton	
Ethyl *p*-nitrophenyl benzenethiophosphonate (EPN)	

or·ga·noph·i·lism (or-gə-nof′ĭ-liz-əm) organotropism. **organophil′ic** *adj*

or·ga·no·phos·phate (or″gə-no-fos′fāt) phosphate esterified to organic compounds such as glucose or sorbitol; see *organophosphorus.*

or·ga·no·phos·pho·rus (or″gə-no-fos′for-əs) a compound containing phosphorus bound to an organic molecule; several organophosphorus compounds are used as insecticides, and they are highly toxic cholinesterase inhibitors. See *organophosphorus compound poisoning*, under *poisoning.*

or·ga·no·tax·is (or″gə-no-tak′sis) [*organo-* + *-taxis*] a tendency to selective migration to some particular organ.

or·ga·no·ther·a·py (or″gə-no-ther′ə-pe) [*organo-* + *therapy*] the treatment of disease by the administration of animal organs or their extracts, or synthetic versions of these.

or·ga·no·trope (or′gə-no-trōp″) an organotropic element or agent.

or·ga·no·tro·phic (or″gə-no-tro′fik) [*organo-* + *-trophic*] heterotrophic.

or·ga·not·ro·pism (or″gə-not′rə-piz″əm) [*organo-* + *tropism*] the special affinity of chemical compounds or of pathogenic agents for particular tissues or organs of the body. **organotrop′ic** *adj*

or·ga·not·ro·py (or″gə-not′rə-pe) organotropism.

or·ga·num (or′gə-nəm) pl. *or′gana* [L., from Gr. *organon* tool, instrument] organ: a somewhat independent part of the body that is arranged according to a characteristic structural plan, and performs a special function or functions; it is composed of various tissues, one of which is primary in function.

or′gana genita′lia femini′na exter′na [TA] female external genitalia: the pudendum femininum, clitoris, and urethra. See Plate 44.

or′gana genita′lia femini′na inter′na [TA] female internal genitalia: the ovaries, uterine tubes, uterus, and vagina. See Plate 44.

or′gana genita′lia masculi′na exter′na [TA] male external genitalia: the penis, scrotum, and urethra. See Plate 44.

or′gana genita′lia masculi′na inter′na [TA] male internal genitalia: the testis, epididymis, ductus deferens, seminal vesicle, ejaculatory duct, prostate, and bulbourethral gland. See Plate 44.

o. gustato′rium [TA] gustatory organ: the organ of taste, comprising the taste buds, most of which are found within the epithelial covering of the tongue; called also *o. gustus* [TA alternative].

o. gus′tus TA alternative for *o. gustatorium.*

or′gana lymphoi′dea prima′ria [TA] primary lymphoid organs: those organs of the lymphatic system that are involved in lymphocyte generation from stem cells, comprising the bone marrow and thymus.

or′gana lymphoi′dea secunda′ria [TA] secondary lymphoid organs: those organs of the lymphatic system in which mature lymphocytes are activated and the immune response initiated, including the lymph nodes, spleen, and accessory lymphoid tissue (e.g., tonsils).

o. olfacto′rium [TA] olfactory organ: the specialized structures subserving the function of the sense of smell, including the olfactory region of the nasal mucosa containing the bipolar cells of origin of the olfactory nerves, together with the olfactory glands; called also *o. olfactus* [TA alternative].

o. olfac′tus TA alternative for *o. olfactorium.*

or′gana sen′suum [TA] sense organs: organs that receive stimuli that give rise to sensations, i.e., organs that translate certain forms of energy into nerve impulses that are perceived as special sensations; they are characterized by highly specialized neuroreceptors and relationships, and include the visual, vestibulocochlear, olfactory, and gustatory organs. Called also *organs of special sense.*

o. spira′le [TA] spiral organ: the organ, resting on the basilar membrane of the cochlear duct, that contains the auditory hair cells, special sensory receptors for hearing, as well as several types of supporting cells, such as the inner and outer pillar cells, inner and outer phalangeal cells, border cells, and Hensen cells. Called also *organ of Corti.*

o. subcommissura′le [TA] subcommissural organ: a group of tall columnar ciliated ependymal cells lining the dorsal aspect of the cerebral aqueduct, situated dorsoventral to the commissure of the epithalamus; it is one of the circumventricular organs and may have neuroendocrine and neurosecretory functions.

o. subfornica′le [TA] subfornical organ: a group of specialized ependymal cells, similar to those of the subcommissural organ, projecting toward the cavity of the third ventricle from its anterior wall between the columns of the fornix; it is one of the circumventricular organs. Called also *intercolumnar tubercle.*

or′gana urina′ria, or′gana uropoë′tica the organs of the urinary system; see *systema urinarium.*

o. vasculo′sum lam′inae termina′lis [TA] vascular organ of lamina terminalis: an area of the lamina terminalis where many neurons pass through a double-layered capillary bed and the blood-brain barrier is modified; it has a superficial capillary layer that receives blood from nearby arteries and drains into a deeper layer, from which blood passes to the cerebral veins. It is one of the *circumventricular organs.*

o. vestibulocochlea′re [TA] vestibulocochlear organ: a collective term in official anatomical terminology applied to those structures outside the central nervous system that are concerned with balance and hearing, and comprising the internal, middle, and external ear. See Plate 14.

o. vomeronasa′le [TA] vomeronasal organ: a short rudimentary canal just above the vomeronasal cartilage, opening in the side of the nasal septum and passing from there blindly upward and backward; called also *Jacobson organ.*

Or·ga·ran (or′gə-ran) trademark for a preparation of danaparoid sodium.

or·gasm (or′gaz-əm) [Gr. *orgasmos* swelling, or *organ* to swell, to be lustful] the apex and culmination of sexual excitement.

or·go·tein (or′go-tēn) a group of water-soluble congeners derived from red blood cells, liver, and other tissues, of molecular weight about 33,000 with compact conformation maintained by about 4 gram-atoms of divalent metal; produced from beef liver as a copper-zinc mixed chelate having superoxide dismutase activity. It has antiinflammatory properties and has been injected locally in the treatment of degenerative joint disorders.

ori·en·ta·tion (or″e-ən-ta′shən) 1. awareness of one's environment, with reference to place, time, and people. 2. the relative positions of atoms or groups in chemical compounds.

Ori·en·tia (or″e-en′she-ə) [L. *oriens* east] a genus of bacteria of the family Rickettsiaceae that includes organisms formerly classified in the genus *Rickettsia.* It comprises small rod-shaped to coccoid, often pleomorphic microorganisms. The cells have typical cell walls, possess no flagella, are gram-negative, and multiply only inside host cells. The type species is *O. tsutsugamu′shi.*

O. tsutsugamu′shi the etiologic agent of scrub typhus, transmitted by larval mites of the genus *Trombicula,* from rodent reservoirs of infection. Called also *Rickettsia tsutsugamushi.*

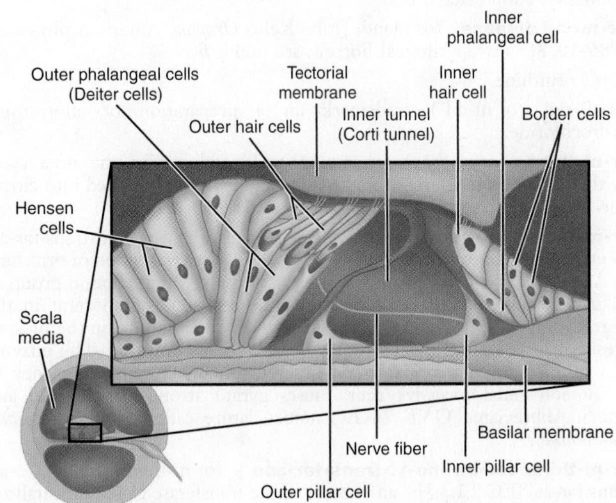

■ Detail of the organum spirale (spiral organ) in the cochlear duct in the internal ear.

or·i·fice (or′ĭ-fis) [L. *orificium*] 1. the entrance or outlet of a body cavity. Called also *ostium* [TA]. 2. any foramen, meatus, or opening. Called also *ostium* [TA] and *orificium*. **orific′ial** *adj*

abdominal o. of uterine tube ostium abdominale tubae uterinae.

aortic o. ostium aortae.

cardiac o., cardial o. ostium cardiacum.

o. of coronary sinus ostium sinus coronarii.

duodenal o. of stomach ostium pyloricum.

external o. of urethra, external urethral o. urinary meatus.

external o. of uterus ostium uteri.

follicular o., o. of hair follicle the opening of a hair follicle on the skin surface, giving egress to the secretion of the sebaceous glands, and to the hairs; called also *pilosebaceous o.*

hymenal o. ostium vaginae.

ileal o. 1. ostium ileale. 2. opening of ileocecal valve.

o. of ileal papilla ostium ileale.

ileocecal o. 1. ostium ileale. 2. opening of ileocecal valve.

o. of ileocecal valve see under *opening*.

o. of inferior vena cava ostium venae cavae inferioris.

internal o. of urethra, internal urethral o. ostium urethrae internum.

left atrioventricular o. ostium atrioventriculare sinistrum.

mitral o. ostium atrioventriculare sinistrum.

myopectineal o., myopectineal o. of Fruchaud a region of the groin bounded superiorly by the internal oblique and transversus abdominis muscles, medially by the rectus abdominis muscle, laterally by the iliopsoas muscle, and inferiorly by Cooper ligament and the pubis. It transmits the spermatic cord and femoral vessels; all inguinal hernias begin as weak areas in this orifice.

pharyngeal o. of auditory tube ostium pharyngeum tubae auditivae.

pilosebaceous o. follicular o.

pulmonary o., o. of pulmonary trunk ostium trunci pulmonalis.

o. of pulp canal foramen apicis dentis.

pyloric o. ostium pyloricum.

reticulo-omasal o. a sphincter between the reticulum and the omasum of a ruminant.

right atrioventricular o. ostium atrioventriculare dextrum.

o. of superior vena cava ostium venae cavae superioris.

tricuspid o. ostium atrioventriculare dextrum.

tympanic o. of auditory tube ostium tympanicum tubae auditivae.

o. of ureter, ureteral o. ostium ureteris.

uterine o. of uterine tube ostium uterinum tubae uterinae.

vaginal o. ostium vaginae.

o. of vermiform appendix ostium appendicis vermiformis.

vesicourethral o. ostium urethrae internum.

or·i·fi·cia (or″ĭ-fish′e-ə) [L.] plural of *orificium*.

or·i·fi·ci·um (or″ĭ-fish′e-əm) pl. *orifi′cia* [L.] orifice.

or·i·gin (or′ĭ-jin) [L. *origo* beginning] the source or beginning of anything, especially the more proximal, fixed end or attachment of a muscle (as distinguished from its insertion), or the site of emergence of a peripheral nerve from the central nervous system.

Or·i·nase (or′ĭ-nās) trademark for a preparation of tolbutamide.

ori·no·ther·a·py (o-ri″no-ther′ə-pe) [Gr. *oreinos* pertaining to mountains + *therapy*] treatment by living in high, mountainous regions.

or·li·stat (or′lĭ-stat) a pancreatic lipase inhibitor that prevents the digestion, and therefore absorption, of dietary fat, used in the treatment of obesity; administered orally.

Or·mond disease (or′mənd) [John Kelso *Ormond*, American physician, 1886–1978] retroperitoneal fibrosis; see under *fibrosis*.

Orn ornithine.

Or·ni·dyl (or′nĭ-dil″) trademark for a preparation of eflornithine hydrochloride.

or·ni·thine (or′nĭ-thēn) an amino acid produced in the urea cycle by the splitting off of urea from arginine and is itself converted into citrulline. On decomposition, it gives rise to putrescine.

or·ni·thine ami·no·trans·fer·ase (or′nĭ-thēn ə-me″no-trans′fər-ās) an enzyme of the transferase class that catalyzes the conversion of ornithine to Δ^1-pyrroline 5-carboxylate via transfer of the ornithine amino group to an α-keto acid (e.g., α-ketoglutarate). The reaction is important in the degradation of ornithine from excess dietary tissue arginine, in the biosynthesis of proline, and in the de novo synthesis of ornithine. The enzyme is a mitochondrial matrix protein occurring in most cells; deficiency of it, an autosomal recessive trait, causes gyrate atrophy of choroid and retina. Abbreviated OAT. In EC nomenclature called *ornithine–oxo-acid transaminase*.

or·ni·thine car·ba·mo·yl·trans·fer·ase (or′nĭ-thēn kahr-bam″o-əl-trans′fər-ās) [EC 2.1.3.3] an enzyme of the transferase class that catalyzes the carbamoylation of ornithine by carbamoyl phosphate to form citrulline. The reaction occurs in liver mitochondria as part of the urea cycle (see illustration at *urea cycle*, under *cycle*). Called also *ornithine transcarbamoylase (OTC)*. Abbreviated OCT.

or·ni·thine car·ba·mo·yl·trans·fer·ase (OCT) de·fi·cien·cy (or′nĭ-thēn kahr-bam″o-əl-trans′fər-ās) an aminoacidopathy due to mutation in the *OTC* gene (locus: Xp21.1), which encodes ornithine carbamoyltransferase, an enzyme of the urea cycle; most hemizygous males show complete deficiency and do not survive the neonatal period; heterozygous females show varying degrees of deficiency and age of onset. Characteristic signs include hyperammonemia, neurologic abnormalities, and oroticaciduria. Called also *ornithine transcarbamoylase (OTC) deficiency*.

or·ni·thine de·car·box·y·lase (or′nĭ-thēn de″kahr-bok′sə-lās) [EC 4.1.1.17] a cytosolic enzyme of the lyase class that catalyzes the decarboxylation of ornithine to form putrescine; the reaction occurs in the conversion of arginine to spermine and spermidine and in the synthesis of γ-aminobutyric acid via putrescine. The enzyme requires pyridoxal phosphate as a cofactor and is concentrated in rapidly proliferating cells.

or·ni·thin·emia (or″nĭ-thĭ-ne′me-ə) hyperornithinemia.

or·ni·thine–oxo-ac·id trans·am·i·nase (or′nĭ-thēn ok′so as′id trans-am′ĭ-nās″) [EC 2.6.1.13] EC nomenclature for *ornithine aminotransferase*.

or·ni·thine trans·car·ba·mo·yl·ase (OTC) (or′nĭ-thēn trans″kahr-bə-mo′əl-ās) ornithine carbamoyltransferase.

or·ni·thine trans·car·bam·y·lase (OTC) (or′nĭ-thēn trans″kahr-bam′ə-lās) ornithine carbamoyltransferase.

Or·ni·thod·o·ros (or″nĭ-thod′ə-rəs) [Gr. *ornis, ornithos* bird + *doros* bag] a genus of argasid ticks with species found in many parts of the world, parasitic on many different mammals and often serving as reservoirs and vectors of *Borrelia* species or other infectious agents. Medically important vector species include *O. gur′neyi* in Australia; *O. as′perus, O. tartakov′skyi, O. tholoza′ni*, and *O. verruco′sus* in Russia, the Middle East, and other parts of Asia; *O. erra′ticus* in Spain and North Africa; *O. herm′sii, O. par′keri, O. ru′dis, O. tala′je*, and *O. turica′ta* in Mexico, Central America, and the western United States; and *O. mouba′ta* and *O. savi′gnyi* in parts of Africa and Asia. *O. coria′ceus* of the western United States and Mexico is the pajaroello tick, notorious for its painful bite owing to a toxin in its saliva.

Or·ni·tho·nys·sus (or″nĭ-tho-nis′əs) a genus of mites of the family Dermanyssidae; formerly called *Liponyssus*.

O. baco′ti the rat mite or tropical rat mite, a species whose bite may cause rat mite dermatitis; it also experimentally transmits murine typhus.

O. bur′sa the tropical fowl mite, commonly found on chickens and wild birds or in their nests.

O. sylvia′rum the northern fowl mite, commonly a parasite of many domestic and wild fowl.

or·ni·tho·sis (or″nĭ-tho′sis) [Gr. *ornis, ornithos* bird + *-osis*] 1. psittacosis in nonpsittacine birds or humans. 2. any kind of psittacosis.

oro-[1] [L. *os*, gen. *oris* mouth] a combining form denoting relationship to the mouth.

oro-[2] [Gr. *oros* whey, serum] see *orrho-*.

oro·dyn·ia (o″ro-din′e-ə) stomatalgia.

oro·lin·gual (or″o-ling′gwəl) [*oro-*[1] + *lingual*] pertaining to the mouth and tongue.

oro·man·dib·u·lar (o″ro-man-dib′u-lər) [*oro-*[1] + *mandibular*] pertaining to the mouth and mandible.

oro·max·il·lary (or″o-mak′sĭ-lar″e) pertaining to the mouth and the maxillary region.

oro·men·in·gi·tis (or″o-men″in-ji′tis) orrhomeningitis.

oro·na·sal (or″o-na′zəl) [*oro-*[1] + *nasal*] pertaining to the mouth and nose.

oro·pha·ryn·ge·al (or″o-fə-rin′je-əl) 1. pertaining to the mouth and the pharynx; called also *pharyngo-oral*. 2. pertaining to the pars oralis pharyngis (oropharynx).

oro·phar·ynx (or″o-far′inks) [*oro-*[1] + *pharynx*] pars oralis pharyngis.

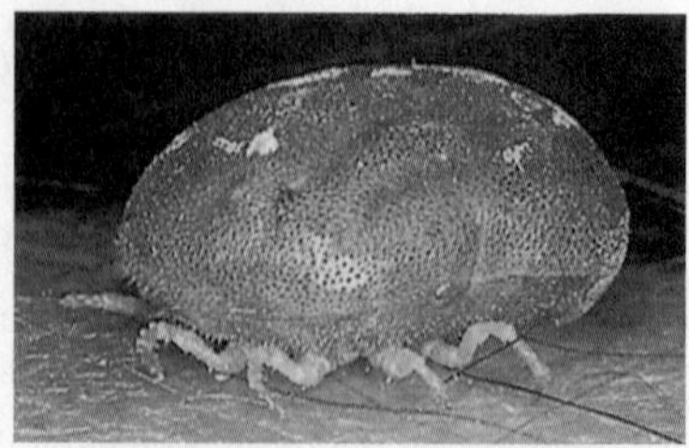

■ Fully engorged *Ornithodoros moubata*.

Orop·syl·la (o″rop-sil′ə) a genus of fleas.

O. idahoen′sis a rodent flea of the western United States, implicated in the transmission of sylvatic plague.

O. monta′na former name for *Diamanus montanus*.

O. silantie′wi a flea of the Manchuria marmot or tarbagan, capable of transmitting plague.

or·o·so·mu·coid (or″o-so-mu′koid) α1-acid glycoprotein; see under *glycoprotein*.

or·o·tate (or′o-tāt) a dissociated form of orotic acid.

or·o·tate phos·pho·ri·bo·syl·trans·fer·ase (OPRT) (or′o-tāt fos″fo-ri″bo-səl-trans′fər-ās) [EC 2.4.2.10] an enzyme activity of the transferase class that catalyzes the transfer to orotate of a ribosyl group from phosphoribosylpyrophosphate (PRPP) to form orotidine 5′-phosphate as a step in the synthesis of pyrimidine nucleotides. The catalytic sites for this activity and for orotidine 5′-phosphate decarboxylase (ODC) activity occur on a single protein, called *UMP synthase;* deficiency of both activities, an autosomal recessive trait, results in hereditary oroticaciduria, type I.

orot·ic ac·id (ə-rot′ik) uracil-6-carboxylic acid, an intermediate in the biosynthesis of the pyrimidine nucleotides.

orot·ic·ac·i·du·ria (ə-rot″ik-as″ĭ-du′re-ə) 1. excess of orotic acid in the urine. 2. an autosomal recessive defect of pyrimidine metabolism due to deficiency of orotate phosphoribosyltransferase (OPRT) or orotidine-5′-phosphate decarboxylase (ODC), two activities contained on the single multifunctional enzyme UMP synthase, which is encoded by the *UMPS* gene (locus: 3q13). Manifestations include crystalluria and excessive excretion of orotic acid in the urine, megaloblastic anemia with hypochromic, microcytic circulating erythrocytes, and physical and mental growth retardation. There are two biochemical types: *type I* is due to deficiency of both OPRT and ODC activities; *type II* is due to deficiency of ODC activity only.

orot·i·dine (ə-rot′ĭ-dēn) a nucleoside, orotic acid linked by its N1 nitrogen to the C1 carbon of ribose; a phosphorylated derivative, orotidine 5′-phosphate, is an intermediate in pyrimidine nucleotide biosynthesis.

orot·i·dine-5′-phos·phate de·car·box·y·lase (ODC) (ə-rot′ĭ-dēn fos′fāt de″kahr-bok′sə-lās) [EC 4.1.1.23] an enzyme of the lyase class that catalyzes the decarboxylation of orotidine 5′-phosphate to form uridine monophosphate in the synthesis of pyrimidine nucleotides. The catalytic sites for this activity and for the orotate phosphoribosyltransferase (OPRT) activity reside on a single protein, called UMP synthase. Deficiency of ODC activity only, an autosomal recessive trait, results in oroticaciduria, type II.

orot·i·dyl·ate (ə-rot″ĭ-dil′āt) a dissociated form of orotidylic acid.

orot·i·dyl·ate de·car·box·y·lase (ə-rot″ĭ-dil′āt de″kahr-bok′sə-lās) orotidine-5′-phosphate decarboxylase.

orot·i·dyl·ic ac·id (ə-rot″ĭ-dil′ik) phosphorylated orotidine, usually referring to orotidine 5′-phosphate (see *orotidine*).

oro·tra·che·al (or″o-tra′ke-əl) pertaining to the mouth (os) and the trachea.

Oroya fever (o-roi′ə) [La *Oroya*, Peru, where the earliest cases were reported in 1885] see under *fever*.

or·pha·nin FQ (or′fə-nin) nociceptin.

or·phen·a·drine (or-fen′ə-drēn) the *ortho*-methyl analogue of diphenhydramine, having anticholinergic, antihistaminic, antispasmodic, and euphoric actions. Called also *mephenamine*.

o. citrate [USP] the citrate salt of orphenadrine, used as a skeletal muscle relaxant in acute spasm of voluntary muscles, regardless of location, especially posttraumatic, discogenic, and tension spasms, administered orally, intramuscularly, or intravenously.

o. hydrochloride the hydrochloride salt of orphenadrine, having the same actions and uses as the citrate salt; also used in the symptomatic treatment of parkinsonism. Administered orally.

Or·phen·ge·sic (or″fən-je′zik) trademark for combination preparations of orphenadrine citrate, aspirin, and caffeine.

orrho- [Gr. *orrhos* whey, serum] a combining form denoting relationship to serum.

or·rho·men·in·gi·tis (or″o-men″in-ji′tis) [*orrho-* + *meningitis*] inflammation of a serous membrane.

ORS oral rehydration salts.

Or·si-Groc·co method (or′se grok′o) [Francesco *Orsi*, Italian physician, 1828–1890; Pietro *Grocco*, Italian physician, 1857–1916] see under *method*.

ORT oral rehydration therapy.

or·the·sis (or-the′sis) pl. *orthe′ses*. Orthosis. **orthet′ic** *adj*

or·thet·ics (or-thet′iks) orthotics.

or·the·tist (or′thə-tist) orthotist.

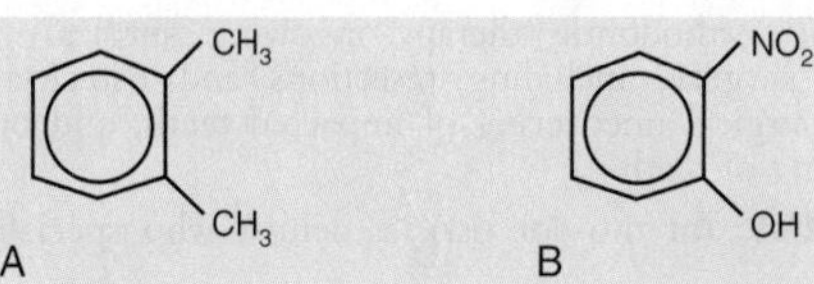

■ Two examples of disubstituted benzene derivatives with substituents in the *ortho*-position. *(A)*, *o*-xylene (1,2-dimethylbenzene); *(B)*, *o*-nitrophenol.

orth(o)- [Gr. *orthos* straight] a combining form meaning straight, normal, or correct.

ortho- 1. symbol *o*-; in organic chemistry, a prefix indicating a 1,2-substituted benzene ring, e.g., *o*-xylene (1,2-dimethylbenzene) or *o*-nitrophenol (2-nitrophenol). 2. in inorganic chemistry, a prefix indicating the common form of an acid as opposed to dimeric or polymeric anhydrides indicated by the prefixes *pyro-* and *meta-*, respectively.

or·tho·ac·id (or″tho-as′id) an acid containing as many hydroxyl groups as the valence of the acidulous element.

or·tho·bi·o·sis (or″tho-bi-o′sis) [*ortho-* + *biosis*] proper living; living in accordance with all the laws of health.

Or·tho·bun·ya·vi·rus (or″tho-bun′yə-vi″rəs) a widespread genus of viruses of the family Bunyaviridae, containing at least 161 species in 18 serogroups and 4 unclassified species; human pathogens of this genus cause febrile disease and encephalitis. Important pathogenic species include Bunyamwera, Bwamba, California encephalitis, Guama, Jamestown Canyon, La Crosse, Oropouche, and Tahyna viruses. The usual mode of transmission is by the bite of infected mosquitoes, although a few species are tick-borne. Formerly called *Bunyavirus*.

or·tho·ce·phal·ic (or″tho-sə-fal′ik) [*ortho-* + *cephalic*] having a head with a vertical index of 70.1 to 75.

or·tho·ceph·a·lous (or″tho-sef′ə-ləs) orthocephalic.

Or·tho-Cept (or′tho-sept′) trademark for combination preparations of desogestrel and ethinyl estradiol.

or·tho·cho·rea (or″tho-kə-re′ə) [*ortho-* + *chorea*] choreic movements in the erect posture.

or·tho·chro·mat·ic (or″tho-kro-mat′ik) 1. staining normally. 2. denoting a photographic emulsion sensitive to all colors except red.

or·tho·chro·mic (or″tho-kro′mik) orthochromatic.

or·tho·chro·mo·phil (or″tho-kro′mo-fil) [*ortho-* + *chromo-* + *-phil*] staining normally with neutral stains.

Or·tho·clone OKT3 (or′tho-klōn) trademark for a preparation of muromonab-CD3.

or·tho·cre·sol (or″tho-kre′sol) one of the three isomeric forms of cresol.

Or·tho-Cyc·len (or′tho-si′klən) trademark for combination preparations of norgestimate and ethinyl estradiol.

or·tho·cy·to·sis (or″tho-si-to′sis) [*ortho-* + *-cyte* + *-osis*] the presence of mature cells only in the blood.

or·tho·dac·ty·lous (or″tho-dak′tə-ləs) [*ortho-* + *dactyl-* + *-ous*] having straight digits.

or·tho·den·tin (or″tho-den′tin) [*ortho-* + *dentin*] straight-tubed dentin, as seen in the teeth of mammals.

or·tho·de·ox·ia (or″tho-de-ok′se-ə) accentuation of arterial hypoxemia in the erect position, improved by assumption of a recumbent position.

or·tho·di·chlo·ro·ben·zene (or″tho-di-klor″o-ben′zēn) *o*-dichlorobenzene.

Or·tho Di·en·es·trol (or′tho di″ən-es′trol) trademark for a preparation of dienestrol.

or·tho·dig·i·ta (or″tho-dij′ĭ-tə) [*ortho-* + *digitus*] the art of correcting deformities of the toes and fingers.

or·tho·don·tia (or″tho-don′shə) orthodontics.

or·tho·don·tics (or″tho-don′tiks) [*ortho-* + *odont-* + *-ic*] the branch of dentistry concerned with the supervision, guidance, and correction of the growing or mature dentofacial structures. Called also *dentofacial orthopedics* and *orthodontology*. **orthodon′tic** *adj*

corrective o. the phase of orthodontics concerned with the reduction or elimination of an existing malocclusion and its attendant sequelae.

interceptive o. the phase of orthodontics concerned with elimination of a condition that might lead to the development of malocclusion.

preventive o., prophylactic o. the phase of orthodontics concerned with preservation of the integrity of proper occlusion through the use of orthodontic procedures and devices.

surgical o. orthodontic therapy involving surgical procedures or orthognathic surgery, including resections and ostectomies, cosmetic surgery, the surgical uncovering of impacted teeth, and positioning and transpositioning of teeth.

or·tho·don·tist (or″tho-don′tist) a dentist who specializes in orthodontics.

or·tho·don·tol·o·gy (or″tho-don-tol′ə-je) orthodontics.

or·tho·dro·mic (or″tho-dro′mik) [Gr. *orthodromein* to run straight forward] conducting impulses in the normal direction; said of nerve fibers. Cf. *antidromic.*

Or·tho-Est (or″tho-est′) trademark for preparations of estropipate.

Or·tho Ev·ra (or′tho ev′rə) trademark for a contraceptive patch containing norelgestromin and ethinyl estradiol.

or·tho·gly·ce·mic (or″tho-gli-se′mik) euglycemic.

Or·thog·na·tha (or-thog′nə-thə) a suborder of spiders (order Araneae) of temperate and tropical areas of the world; Theraphosidae and Dipluridae are families of medical importance.

or·thog·nath·ia (or″thog-nath′e-ə) [*ortho-* + *gnath-* + *-ia*] the branch of oral medicine dealing with the cause and treatment of malposition of the bones of the jaw.

or·thog·na·thic (or″thog-nath′ik) 1. pertaining to orthognathia. 2. orthognathous.

or·thog·na·thous (or-thog′nə-thəs″) [*ortho-* + *gnath-* + *-ous*] pertaining to or characterized by minimal protrusion of the mandible or minimal prognathism, with a gnathic index of 98 or less. Called also *orthognathic.*

or·tho·grade (or′tho-grād″) [*ortho-* + L. *gradi* to walk] characterized by walking with the body upright, such as the bipeds. Cf. *pronograde.*

Or·tho·hep·ad·na·vi·rus (or″tho-hep-ad′nə-vi″rəs) [*ortho-* + hepadnavirus] hepatitis B viruses that infect mammals; a genus of the family Hepadnaviridae that includes hepatitis B virus and species infecting ground squirrels and woodchucks.

or·tho·io·do·hip·pu·rate (or″tho-i″o-do-hip′ūr-āt) see *iodohippurate sodium.*

or·tho·ker·a·to·sis (or″tho-ker″ə-to′sis) thickening of the stratum corneum without parakeratosis, i.e., without the abnormal retention of keratinocyte nuclei.

or·thol·i·dine (or-thol′ĭ-dēn) *o*-tolidine.

or·thol·o·gous (or-thol′ə-gəs) [*ortho-* + *homologous*] related by phylogenetic descent and diverging after speciation; see under *gene.*

or·tho·me·lic (or″tho-me′lik) [*ortho-* + *mel-* + *-ic*] correcting deformities of the limbs.

or·thom·e·ter (or-thom′ə-tər) exophthalmometer.

or·tho·mo·lec·u·lar (or″tho-mo-lek′u-lər) [*ortho-* + *molecular*] relating to or aimed at restoring the optimal concentrations and functions at the molecular level of the substances (e.g., vitamins) normally present in the body. See also under *medicine* and *psychiatry.*

or·tho·mor·phia (or″tho-mor′fe-ə) [*ortho-* + *morph-* + *-ia*] the surgical and mechanical correction of deformities.

Or·tho·myxo·vi·ri·dae (or″tho-mik″so-vir′ĭ-de) [*ortho-* + *myxo-* + *virus* + *-idae*] the influenzaviruses: a family of RNA viruses having a pleomorphic virion that may be roughly spherical and 80–120 nm in diameter or filamentous and up to several microns long, consisting of a lipid bilayer envelope with large peplomers, surrounding a helical nucleocapsid. The genome consists of seven (influenza C virus) or eight (influenza A virus and influenza B virus) molecules of linear negative-sense single-stranded RNA (total MW approximately 5×10^6, total size 10.0–13.6 kb). Viruses contain seven to nine major polypeptides, including a transcriptase and a neuramidase, and are sensitive to lipid solvents, radiation, and disinfectants. Replication occurs in the nucleus and cytoplasm, and assembly is by budding on the plasma membrane. Genera include *Influenzavirus A, Influenzavirus B, Influenzavirus C,* and the Thogoto-like viruses.

or·tho·myxo·vi·rus (or″tho-mik′so-vi″rəs) any virus belonging to the family Orthomyxoviridae. **orthomyxovi′ral** *adj*

or·tho·neu·tro·phil (or″tho-noo′tro-fil) orthochromophil.

Or·tho-No·vum (or″tho-no′vəm) trademark for oral contraceptive therapeutic regimens containing norethindrone as the progestational agent and either ethinyl estradiol or mestranol as the estrogen component.

or·tho·pae·dic (or″tho-pe′dik) orthopedic.

or·tho·pae·dics (or″tho-pe′diks) orthopedics.

or·tho·pan·to·graph (or″tho-pan′to-graf″) panoramic radiograph.

Or·tho·pan·to·mo·graph (or″tho-pan-to′mo-graf) trademark for the equipment used in pantomography.

or·tho·pe·dic (or″tho-pe′dik) [*ortho-* + *ped-*[1] + *-ic*] pertaining to the correction of deformities of the musculoskeletal system; pertaining to orthopedics.

or·tho·pe·dics (or″tho-pe′diks) the branch of surgery that is specially concerned with the preservation and restoration of the function of the skeletal system, its articulations, and associated structures.

dentofacial o. orthodontics.

functional jaw o. the use of muscle force to effect changes in jaw position and tooth alignment with a removable orthodontic appliance.

or·tho·pe·dist (or″tho-pe′dist) an orthopedic surgeon.

or·tho·per·cus·sion (or″tho-pər-kush′ən) [*ortho-* + *percussion*] percussion in which the distal phalanx of the pleximeter finger is held perpendicularly to the chest wall.

or·thoph·o·ny (or-thof′ə-ne) [*ortho-* + Gr. *phōnē* voice] the direct and correct production of sound.

or·tho·pho·ria (or″tho-fo′re-ə) [*ortho-* + *phoria*] the absence of heterophoria; the normal condition in which the visual axes remain parallel after the visual fusional stimuli have been partially or entirely eliminated. **orthophor′ic** *adj*

or·tho·phos·phate (or″tho-fos′fāt) an anion or salt of orthophosphoric acid or of any of its esters; it is the major intracellular anion. Abbreviated P_i. Called also *inorganic phosphate.*

or·tho·phos·phor·ic ac·id (or″tho-fos-for′ik) a strong mineral acid, H_3PO_4, the monomeric form of phosphoric acid.

or·tho·pia (or-tho′pe-ə) [*orth-* + *-opia*] the prevention or correction of strabismus.

or·tho·ples·sim·e·ter (or″tho-plə-sim′ə-tər) an instrument used to take the place of the pleximeter finger in orthopercussion.

or·thop·nea (or″thop-ne′ə) [*ortho-* + *-pnea*] dyspnea that is relieved by assuming an upright position. Cf. *platypnea.* **orthopne′ic** *adj*

two-pillow o. orthopnea that is relieved by elevating the head and chest from the recumbent position by the use of two pillows; see also *orthopnea position,* under *position.*

or·tho·pod (or′tho-pod) orthopedist.

Or·tho·pox·vi·rus (or′tho-poks-vi″rəs) [*ortho-* + *poxvirus*] a genus of viruses of the subfamily Chordopoxvirinae (family Poxviridae) with nucleic acid homology and serologic cross-reactivity that cause generalized infections with a rash in mammals, including camelpox, cowpox, ectromelia, monkeypox, and vaccinia viruses. The virtually extinct agent of smallpox, variola virus, belongs to this genus.

or·tho·pox·vi·rus (or′tho-poks-vi″rəs) a virus of the genus *Orthopoxvirus.* **orthopoxvi′ral** *adj*

or·tho·prax·is (or″tho-prak′sis) orthopraxy.

or·tho·praxy (or′tho-prak″se) [*ortho-* + Gr. *prassein* to make] the mechanical correction of deformities.

Or·tho-Pre·fest (or″tho-pre′fest) trademark for a therapeutic regimen of estradiol and norgestimate.

or·tho·psy·chi·a·try (or″tho-si-ki′ə-tre) [*ortho-* + *psychiatry*] an interdisciplinary field that combines psychiatry with principles of psychology, sociology, social work, and other fields in the study and practice of maintaining or restoring mental health, emphasizing a prophylactic approach to mental disease.

Or·thop·tera (or-thop′tər-ə) [*ortho-* + Gr. *pteron* wing] an order of biting insects that do not undergo metamorphosis; they include the grasshoppers, locusts, crickets, and cockroaches.

or·thop·tic (or-thop′tik) correcting obliquity of one or both visual axes.

or·thop·tics (or-thop′tiks) a technique of eye exercises designed to correct the visual axes of eyes not properly coordinated for binocular vision.

or·thop·tist (or-thop′tist) a specialist in orthoptics.

or·thop·to·scope (or-thop′to-skōp) [*ortho-* + *opto-* + *-scope*] an instrument for orthoptic or exercise treatment in anomalies of the ocular muscles, strabismus, or amblyopia.

Or·tho·reo·vi·rus (or″tho-re′o-vi″rəs) [*ortho-* + *r*espiratory *e*nteric *o*rphan + *virus*] a genus of viruses of the family Reoviridae, formerly classed as echoviruses, separable into three serotypes. No causative relationship to any disease has been proved in humans, although reoviruses have been isolated from both healthy individuals and patients with a variety of diseases. In other mammals reoviruses are associated with respiratory and enteric disease, and in chickens and turkeys, with arthritis.

or·tho·rhom·bic (or″tho-rom′bik) having three unequal axes intersected at right angles.

or·thor·rhach·ic (or″tho-rak′ik) [*ortho-* + *rhachi-* + *-ic*] having a vertebral column with practically no curvature in the lumbar region; cf. *koilorrhachic* and *kyrtorrhachic.*

or·tho·scope (or′tho-skōp) [*ortho-* + *-scope*] an apparatus that neutralizes the corneal refraction by means of a layer of water; it is used in examining the eye.

or·tho·scop·ic (or″tho-skop′ik) 1. pertaining to orthoscopy or an orthoscope. 2. having normal, undistorted vision. 3. pertaining to an optical system that produces undistorted images.

or·thos·co·py (or-thos′kə-pe) examination of the eye by means of the orthoscope.

or·tho·sis (or-tho′sis) pl. *ortho′ses* [Gr. *orthōsis* making straight] an orthopedic appliance or apparatus used to support, align, prevent, or correct deformities or to improve the function of movable parts of the body. See also *brace* and *splint*. **orthot′ic** *adj*

ankle o. (AO) an orthosis designed for a disorder affecting the ankle only.

ankle-foot o. (AFO) any orthotic device for the lower limb that encloses the ankle and foot and does not extend above the knee; often there is a cuff or other device in the region of the knee or upper calf to take weight off the limb.

balanced forearm o. a forearm orthosis for persons with severe weakness or paralysis of the elbow or forearm, consisting of a trough to support the forearm and a mechanism such as a Bowden cable linking it to the shoulder region, so that small movements of the shoulder girdle or trunk produce motion at the elbow.

CASH o. see under *brace*.

cervical o. (CO) a rigid plastic orthosis that encircles the neck and supports the chin and the back of the head; used in the treatment of injuries to the cervical spine.

dynamic o. an orthosis that not only supports and protects but also aids in initiating and performing motion of the part or adjacent parts; it usually also helps the part deal with the forces resulting from the action, and supports movements necessary for activities of daily living.

elbow-wrist-hand o. (EWHO) an orthosis designed for treatment of disorders of the upper limb below the shoulder; there may or may not be a finger or thumb component.

Engen extension o. an orthosis for extension contracture of the knee or elbow that provides three points of pressure: one over the apex of the deformity and two on the opposite side of the limb at a distance.

flexor hinge o. see under *splint*.

floor reaction o. a type of ankle-foot orthosis that allows full plantar flexion but stops at a 90° angle so that the foot component in the shoe can aid push-off.

foot o. an orthosis only for the foot, without an ankle component, used to reposition an abnormal foot or redistribute weight bearing.

forearm o. an orthosis that supports a weakened forearm, with or without a wrist component; there are two types, the trough or gutter type that go around halfway or less and the circumferential type that wrap completely around.

fracture o. an orthosis designed to hold bones in place after a fracture; see also *fracture splint*, under *splint*.

functional o. dynamic o.

halo o. see under *device*.

hand o. (HO) see under *splint*.

hip o. (HO) an orthosis that supports and protects primarily structures in the hip area.

hip abduction o. any of various specialized hip orthoses designed to abduct the legs and correct developmental dysplasia of the hip in infants.

hip-knee-ankle-foot o. (HKAFO) any orthotic device for the lower limb that encloses the knee, ankle, and foot and extends to the hip, often being attached by means of a strap in the pelvic region; used for patients with paralysis of the lower limbs for whom walking is unlikely.

hyperextension o. a type of thoracolumbosacral orthosis that maintains hyperextension of the spine following compression fractures in the lower thoracic or upper lumbar regions.

ischial weight-bearing o. a hip-knee-ankle-foot orthosis that transmits weight from the ischium to the ground; there is usually a large cuff in the ischial region to absorb weight and provide attachment for the upright bars; the knee and ankle may be either allowed movement with hinges or kept rigid.

knee-ankle-foot o. (KAFO) any orthotic device for the lower limb that extends from above the knee to the ankle and foot.

lumbosacral o. (LSO) a spinal orthosis that encircles the body in the lumbosacral region; different types vary in width, from belts to corsets, as well as in rigidity.

opponens o. a static type of hand splint that holds the thumb metacarpal in maximal abduction and the thumb phalanges in extension to treat adduction contracture of the thumb.

patellar tendon-bearing o. an ankle-foot orthosis designed to take weight off the heel and ankle by means of a cuff in the lower knee region and metal uprights to the shoe sole. Called also *PTB o.*

pneumatic o. a plastic garment with inflatable tubes that surround the trunk or limbs; inflation of a tube provides stabilization and rigidity for the enclosed body part.

poster o. a cervical orthosis with rigid upright posts, sometimes adjustable in length, extending from flat plates in the chin and occipital regions down to plates or a jacket on the chest and back.

PTB o. patellar tendon-bearing o.

reciprocating gait o. (RGO) a type of hip-knee-ankle-foot orthosis with links between the two hips so that a paralyzed person can walk step over step, usually with the aid of crutches.

resting o. static o.

serial stretch o's a series of static orthoses to keep a body part with a flexion contracture on gentle passive stretch; at each therapy session the joint is extended as far as it will comfortably go and a splint is shaped to hold it at that angle; eventually an optimal position of extension is reached.

shoulder-elbow-wrist-hand o. (SEWHO) one for treatment of weakness or paralysis of the entire upper limb from shoulder to hand.

SOMI o. sternal-occipital-mandibular immobilizer.

spinal o. a corset or other orthosis that surrounds part or all of the trunk to support or align the vertebral column or to prevent movement following trauma; see *lumbosacral o.* and *thoracolumbosacral o.*

standing o. see under *frame*.

static o. an orthosis that does not allow motion of the part and is primarily for support only.

supramalleolar o. (SMO) an ankle-foot orthosis that extends just above the malleolus.

tenodesis o. any of numerous types of wrist-hand orthosis with hinge mechanisms to reinforce normal tenodesis and support flexion and extension. Called also *tenodesis splint*.

therapeutic o. dynamic o.

thoracolumbar o. a spinal orthosis that supports the thoracic and lumbar regions; there is usually also a sacral component. See *thoracolumbosacral o.*

thoracolumbosacral o. (TLSO) a spinal orthosis that goes over the lumbar, sacral, and thoracic regions and thus limits movement of the thorax; different types vary in rigidity and in the kind of support given to the thorax.

Toronto Legg-Perthes o. a type of knee-ankle-foot orthosis that treats or prevents deformities resulting from conditions such as Legg-Calvé-Perthes disease by holding the hips abducted at 45° while permitting hip flexion, knee flexion, and ambulation.

UCBL o. [*U*niversity of *C*alifornia *B*iomechanics *L*aboratory] a common type of foot orthosis that provides arch support and is made of thermoplastic or thermoset material.

wrist o. see under *splint*.

wrist-hand o. (WHO) any of numerous types of orthoses that support and protect the lower forearm, wrist, and hand; they may be either dynamic or static, and they may have finger or thumb components. See also *hand splint* and *wrist splint*.

or·tho·stat·ic (or″tho-stat′ik) [*ortho-* + *-static*] pertaining to or caused by standing erect.

or·tho·stat·ism (or′tho-stat″iz-əm) an erect standing position of the body.

or·tho·ster·eo·scope (or″tho-ster′e-o-skōp) an apparatus for stereoradiography.

or·tho·ther·a·py (or″tho-ther′ə-pe) [*ortho-* + *therapy*] treatment of disorders by correction of posture.

or·thot·ics (or-thot′iks) the field of knowledge relating to orthoses and their use.

or·thot·ist (or-thot′ist) [Gr. *orthōtēr* a restorer or preserver] a person skilled in orthotics and practicing its application in individual cases.

or·tho·tol·u·eno-azo-be·ta-naph·thol (or″tho-tol″u-ēn″o-az″o-ba″tə-naf′thol) a poisonous dye used in processing citrus fruits.

or·thot·o·nos (or-thot′ə-nəs) [*ortho-* + Gr. *tonos* tension] tetanic fixation of the head, body, and limbs in a rigid straight line.

or·thot·o·nus (or-thot′ə-nəs) orthotonos.

or·tho·top·ic (or″tho-top′ik) [*ortho-* + *top-* + *-ic*] occurring at the normal place or upon the proper part of the body; pertaining to a tissue transplant grafted into its normal place in the body.

Or·tho Tri-Cyc·len (or′tho tri-si′klən) trademark for therapeutic regimens of norgestimate and ethinyl estradiol.

or·tho·tro·pia (or″tho-tro′pe-ə) 1. absence of strabismus. 2. a condition of the eye in which there is no deviation of the visual axis with respect to a given meridian of the eye, e.g., hypotropia without lateral deviation.

or·tho·tro·pic (or″tho-tro′pik) pertaining to or characterized by orthotropia.

Ortho•visc (or′tho-visk) trademark for a preparation of hyaluronan.

or•tho•vol•tage (or′tho-vōl″təj) in radiotherapy, voltage in the range of 140 to 400 kilovolts, as contrasted to *supervoltage* and *megavoltage.*

Or•thox•ine (or-thok′sēn) trademark for preparations of methoxyphenamine hydrochloride.

Ort•ner syndrome (ort′ner) [Norbert *Ortner*, Austrian physician, 1865–1935] see under *syndrome.*

Or•to•la•ni sign (click) (or-to-lah′ne) [Marius *Ortolani*, Italian orthopedic surgeon, 20th century] see under *sign.*

Oru•dis (o-roo′dis) trademark for preparations of ketoprofen.

Or•u•vail (or′oo-vāl) trademark for a preparation of ketoprofen.

Ory•za (o-ri′zə) [L., from Gr. *oryza* rice] a genus of cereal plants of the grass family (Gramineae). *O. sati′va* is rice.

Ory•zo•mys (o″rĭ-zo′mis) [Gr. *oryza* rice + *mys* mouse] the rice rats, a genus of rodents of the family Muridae, found in warm regions of the Americas. *O. palus′tris* is a vector for hantavirus pulmonary syndrome.

OS [L.] o′culus sinis′ter (left eye).

Os osmium.

os[1] (os) gen. *o′ris* pl. *o′ra* [L. "an opening, or mouth"] 1. any orifice of the body. 2. [TA] oral cavity (mouth); see *cavitas oris.*

external o. of uterus ostium uteri.

internal o. of uterus ostium uteri internum.

internal o. of uterus, anatomical ostium anatomicum uteri internum.

internal o. of uterus, histological ostium histologicum uteri internum.

os[2] (os) gen. *os′sis* pl. *os′sa* [L.] 1. bone (q.v.). 2. [TA] *(in the pl.)* skeletal system: official terminology for the bones and cartilages of the body considered collectively. Called also *systema skeletale* [TA alternative].

Os

Descriptions are given on TA terms, and include anglicized names of specific bones.

o. aceta′buli acetabulum.

o. acromia′le a movable joint between the spine of the scapula and the epiphysis of the acromion.

o. basila′re basioccipital bone.

o. bre′ve [TA] short bone: one whose main dimensions are approximately equal, e.g., one of the bones of the carpus or tarsus.

o. cal′cis calcaneus.

o. capita′tum [TA] capitate bone: the bone in the distal row of carpal bones lying between the trapezoid and hamate bones.

o. carpa′le dista′le pri′mum o. trapezium.

o. carpa′le dista′le quar′tum o. hamatum.

o. carpa′le dista′le secun′dum o. trapezoideum.

o. carpa′le dista′le ter′tium o. capitatum.

os′sa carpa′lia TA alternative for *ossa carpi.*

os′sa car′pi [TA] carpal bones: the eight bones of the wrist (carpus), including the *o. capitatum, o. hamatum, o. lunatum, o. pisiforme, o. scaphoideum, o. trapezium, o. trapezoideum,* and *o. triquetrum.* Called also *ossa carpalia* [TA alternative].

o. centra′le [TA] central bone: an accessory bone sometimes found on the back of the carpus.

o. centra′le tar′si o. naviculare.

o. coc′cygis [TA] coccygeal bone: the small bone caudad to the sacrum in humans, formed by union of four (sometimes five or three) rudimentary vertebrae, and forming the caudal extremity of the vertebral column; called also *coccyx* [TA alternative] and *tail bone.*

o. coro′nae small pastern bone; see *pastern bone,* under *bone.*

o. cos′tae, o. costa′le costa (def. 2).

o. cox′ae [TA] the hip bone, which comprises the ilium, ischium, and pubis. Called also *o. pelvicum* and *pelvic bone.*

os′sa crania′lia ossa cranii.

os′sa cra′nii [TA] cranial bones: the bones of the cranium, including the occipital, temporal, parietal, frontal, ethmoid, sphenoid, lacrimal, and nasal bones; the concha nasalis; and the vomer. Some authorities also include the maxilla, the palatine bone, and the zygomatic bone. Called also *ossa cranialia.*

o. cuboi′deum [TA] cuboid bone: a bone on the lateral side of the tarsus between the calcaneus and the fourth and fifth metatarsal bones.

o. cuneifor′me interme′dium [TA] intermediate cuneiform bone: the intermediate and smallest of the three wedge-shaped tarsal bones located medial to the cuboid and between the navicular and the first three metatarsal bones; called also *o. cuneiforme secundum.*

o. cuneifor′me latera′le [TA] lateral cuneiform bone: the most lateral of the three wedge-shaped tarsal bones located medial to the cuboid and between the navicular and the first three metatarsal bones; called also *o. cuneiforme tertium.*

o. cuneifor′me media′le [TA] medial cuneiform bone: the medial and largest of the three wedge-shaped tarsal bones located medial to the cuboid and between the navicular and the first three metatarsal bones; called also *o. cuneiforme primum.*

o. cuneifor′me pri′mum o. cuneiforme mediale.

o. cuneifor′me secun′dum o. cuneiforme intermedium.

o. cuneifor′me ter′tium o. cuneiforme laterale.

o.′sa digito′rum ma′nus [TA] bones of digits of hand: the 14 bones that compose the skeleton of the fingers—two for the thumb and three for each finger. Called also *phalanges digitorum manus* [TA alternative] and *phalanges of fingers.*

o.′sa digito′rum pe′dis [TA] bones of digits of foot: the bones that compose the skeleton of the toes—two for the great toe and often the fifth toe and three for each of the other toes. Called also *phalanges digitorum pedis* [TA alternative] and *phalanges of toes.*

o. epitympa′nicum a bone of very early fetal life that becomes the posterior portion of the squama that aids in forming the mastoid cells.

o. ethmoida′le [TA] ethmoid bone: the cubical bone located between the orbits and consisting of the lamina cribrosa, the lamina perpendicularis, and the paired lateral masses.

o.′sa facia′lia, o.′sa facie′i facial bones.

o. femora′le femur (def. 1).

o. fe′moris TA alternative for *femur* (def. 1).

os′sa fonticulo′rum a type of sutural bones (ossa suturalia [TA]) that are often found next to the fontanelles of infants.

o. fronta′le [TA] frontal bone: a single bone that closes the anterior part of the cranial cavity and forms the skeleton of the forehead; it is developed from two halves, the line of separation (the frontal or metopic suture) sometimes persisting in adult life.

o. hama′tum [TA] hamate bone: the medial bone in the distal row of carpal bones; called also *fourth carpal* or *unciform bone.*

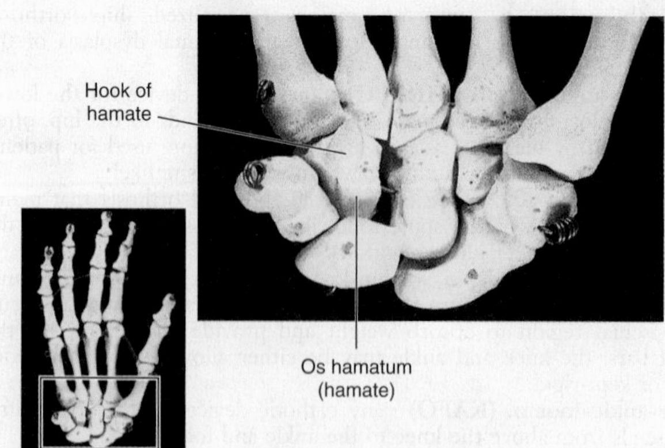

o. hyoi′deum [TA] hyoid bone: a horseshoe-shaped bone situated at the base of the tongue, just superior to the thyroid cartilage.

o. ilia′cum o. ilium.

Os *Continued*

o. i'lii, o. i'lium [TA] iliac bone: the expansive superior portion of the os coxae (hip bone); it is a separate bone in early life. Called also *ilium* and *o. iliacum* [TA alternatives]. See Plate 40.
o. in'cae o. interparietale.
o. incisi'vum [TA] incisive bone: the portion of the maxilla that bears the incisor teeth. In humans, the embryonic bone called the premaxilla fuses with the maxilla proper to form the adult bone. In most other vertebrates it persists as an independent bone. Called also *premaxilla* [TA alternative].
o. innomina'tum o. coxae.
o. intercuneifor'me an occasionally occurring bone situated between the medial and intermediate cuneiform bones.
o. interme'dium o. lunatum.
o. intermetatar'seum an occasionally occurring accessory bone situated between the proximal ends of the first and second metatarsal bones.
o. interparieta'le [TA] interparietal bone: the portion of the squamous part of the occipital bone that lies superior to the highest nuchal line when this portion remains separate throughout life.
o. irregula're [TA] irregular bone: a bone that is not readily classified as long, short, or flat; e.g., skull, hip bones, vertebrae.
o. is'chii [TA] ischial bone: the inferior dorsal portion of the os coxae (hip bone); it is a separate bone in early life. Called also *ischium* [TA alternative]. See Plate 40.
o. lacrima'le [TA] lacrimal bone: a thin scalelike bone at the anterior part of the medial wall of the orbit, articulating with the frontal and ethmoid bones and the maxilla and inferior nasal concha. Called also *o. unguis.*
o. lon'gum [TA] long bone: a bone that has a longitudinal axis of considerable length, consisting of a body or shaft (the diaphysis) and an expanded portion (the epiphysis) at each end that is usually articular; typically found in the limbs.
o. luna'tum [TA] lunate bone: the bone in the proximal row of carpal bones lying between the scaphoid and triquetral bones.
o. mag'num o. capitatum.
os'sa ma'nus [TA] the bones of the hand: the carpals, metacarpals, and phalanges.
os'sa mem'bri inferio'ris [TA] bones of inferior limb: the os coxae, pelvis, patella, tibia, fibula, tarsus, metatarsus, and digits of the foot.
os'sa mem'bri superio'ris [TA] bones of superior limb: the humerus, radius, ulna, carpus, metacarpus, and digits of the hand.
os'sa metacarpa'lia TA alternative for *ossa metacarpi.*
o. metacarpa'le ter'tium TA alternative for *o. metacarpi tertium.*
os'sa metacar'pi [TA] metacarpal bones: the five cylindrical bones of the hand (metacarpals), which articulate proximally with the bones of the carpus and distally with the proximal phalanges of the fingers; numbered from that articulating with the proximal phalanx of the thumb to the most lateral one articulating with the proximal phalanx of the little finger. Called also *metacarpals* and *ossa metacarpalia* [TA alternative]. See also *o. metacarpi tertium.*
o. metacar'pi ter'tium [TA] third metacarpal bone: the middle metacarpal bone, which presents the styloid process on the dorsal surface of the radial side of its base. Called also *o. metacarpale tertium* [TA alternative].
os'sa metatarsa'lia TA alternative for *ossa metatarsi.*
os'sa metatar'si [TA] metatarsal bones: the five bones (metatarsals) extending from the tarsus to the phalanges of the toes, being numbered in the same sequence from the most medial to the most lateral. Called also *ossa metatarsalia* [TA alternative].
o. multan'gulum ma'jus o. trapezium.
o. multan'gulum mi'nus o. trapezoideum.
o. nasa'le [TA] nasal bone: either of the two small, oblong bones that together form the bridge of the nose.
o. navicula're [TA] navicular bone: the ovoid-shaped tarsal bone that is situated between the talus and the three cuneiform bones; called also *o. naviculare pedis.*
o. navicula're ma'nus o. scaphoideum.
o. navicula're pe'dis o. naviculare.
o. navicula're pe'dis retarda'tum Köhler bone disease (def. 1).
o. occipita'le [TA] occipital bone: a single trapezoid-shaped bone situated at the posterior and inferior part of the cranium, articulating with the two parietal and two temporal bones, the sphenoid bone, and the atlas; it contains a large opening, the foramen magnum.
o. odontoi'deum an anomalous bone that replaces all or part of the dens axis and is not attached to the atlas.
o. orbicula're processus lenticularis incudis.
o. in o. a radiation-induced injury appearing on radiographs as a vertebra within a vertebra.
o. palati'num [TA] palatine bone: the irregularly shaped bone forming the posterior part of the hard palate, the lateral wall of the nasal fossa between the medial pterygoid plate and the maxilla, and the posterior part of the floor of the orbit.
o. parieta'le [TA] parietal bone: either of the two quadrilateral bones forming part of the superior and lateral surfaces of the skull, and joining each other in the midline at the sagittal suture.
o. pe'dis coffin bone.
os'sa pe'dis [TA] the bones of the foot: the bones making up the skeleton of the foot, including the tarsal and metatarsal bones and the phalanges.
o. pel'vicum o. coxae.
o. pe'nis baculum.
o. perone'um a sesamoid bone sometimes formed in the tendon of the peroneus longus muscle.
o. pisifor'me [TA] pisiform bone: the medial bone of the proximal row of carpal bones.
o. pla'num 1. [TA] flat bone: any bone whose thickness is slight, sometimes consisting of only a thin layer of compact bone, or two layers with intervening spongy bone and marrow; usually bent or curved, rather than flat. 2. lamina orbitalis ossis ethmoidalis.
o. pneuma'ticum [TA] pneumatic bone: a bone that contains air-filled cavities or sinuses.
o. pri'api baculum.
o. pu'bis [TA] pubic bone: the anterior inferior part of the os coxae (hip bone) on either side, articulating with its fellow in the anterior midline at the pubic symphysis; it is a separate bone in early life. Called also *pubis* [TA alternative].
o. radia'le o. scaphoideum.
o. sa'crum [TA] sacrum: the wedge-shaped bone formed usually by five fused vertebrae that are lodged dorsally between the two hip bones (ossa coxae).
o. scaphoi'deum [TA] scaphoid bone: the most lateral bone of the proximal row of carpal bones; called also *o. naviculare manus.*
os'sa sesamoi'dea ma'nus [TA] sesamoid bones of hand, usually located in the palmar region in the tendons of the flexor pollicis brevis and adductor pollicis muscles. See *sesamoid bones,* under *bone.*
os'sa sesamoi'dea pe'dis [TA] sesamoid bones of foot, usually located in the metatarsal region, particularly in the tendon of the flexor hallucis brevis muscle. See *sesamoid bones,* under *bone.*
o. sphenoida'le [TA] sphenoid bone: a single irregular, wedge-shaped bone at the base of the skull, forming a part of the floor of the anterior, middle, and posterior cranial fossae.
o. subtibia'le an occasionally occurring bone found over the tip of the medial malleolus.
os'sa suprasterna'lia [TA] suprasternal bones: ossicles occasionally occurring in the ligaments of the sternoclavicular articulation.
o. sutura'le pl., os'sa sutura'lia [TA] sutural bone: any of the small irregular bones in the sutures between the bones of the skull, most frequently in the course of the lambdoid suture and often at the fontanelles *(ossa fonticulorum);* called also *epactal bone* and *wormian bone.*

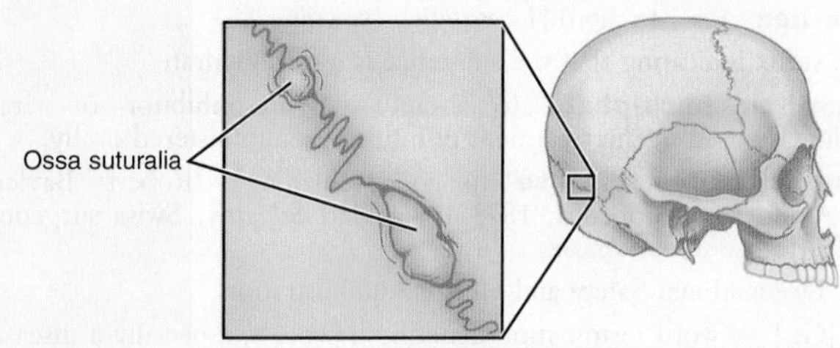

Os *Continued*

os′sa tarsa′lia TA alternative for *ossa tarsi.*
o. tarsa′le dista′le pri′mum o. cuneiforme mediale.
o. tarsa′le dista′le quar′tum o. cuboideum.
o. tarsa′le dista′le secun′dum o. cuneiforme intermedium.
o. tarsa′le dista′le ter′tium o. cuneiforme laterale.
os′sa tar′si [TA] tarsal bones: the seven bones of the ankle (tarsus), including the calcaneus, o. cuboideum, ossa cuneiforme intermedium, laterale, and mediale, o. naviculare, and talus. Called also *ossa tarsalia* [TA alternative].
o. tar′si fibula′re calcaneus.
o. tar′si tibia′le talus.
o. tempora′le [TA] temporal bone: one of the two irregular bones forming part of the lateral surfaces and base of the skull, and containing the organs of hearing. It is divided anatomically into three parts: the *petrous, squamous,* and *tympanic parts (pars petrosa, pars squamosa,* and *pars tympanica)* and the styloid process.
os′sa tho′racis the bones of the thorax; see *skeleton thoracis.*
o. tibia′le exter′num a small anomalous bone situated in the angle between the navicular bone and the head of the talus.
o. trape′zium [TA] trapezium bone: the most lateral bone of the distal row of carpal bones; called also *o. multangulum majus.*
o. trapezoi′deum [TA] trapezoid bone: the bone in the distal row of carpal bones lying between the trapezium and capitate bones; called also *o. multangulum minus.*
o. trigo′num [TA] an external tubercle at the back of the talus, sometimes occurring as a separate bone.
o. trique′trum [TA] triquetral bone: the bone in the proximal row of carpal bones lying between the lunate and pisiform bones; called also *triangular bone.*
o. un′guis o. lacrimale.
o. vesalia′num pe′dis vesalian bone: the proximal and external part of the tuberosity of the fifth metatarsal bone.
o. wor′mi o. suturale.
o. zygoma′ticum [TA] zygomatic bone: the quadrangular bone of the cheek, articulating with the frontal bone, the maxilla, the zygomatic process of the temporal bone, and the greater wing of the sphenoid bone.

OSA obstructive sleep apnea.

OSAHS obstructive sleep apnea–hypopnea syndrome.

OSAS obstructive sleep apnea syndrome; see *sleep apnea.*

osa•zone (o′sə-zōn) any of a series of compounds obtained by heating a sugar with phenylhydrazine and an acid; the resulting crystals are characteristic of specific sugars and have been used to identify them. See also individual compounds; e.g., *glucosazone.*

os•cil•la•tion (os″ĭ-la′shən) [L. *oscillare* to swing] a backward and forward motion, like a pendulum; see also *vibration, fluctuation,* and *variation.*

os•cil•la•tor (os′ĭ-la″tər) an apparatus for producing oscillations; an electric circuit designed to generate alternating current at a particular frequency.

Os•cil•la•to•ria (ə-sil″ə-to′re-ə) a genus of cyanobacteria that sometimes contaminate water and can cause cyanobacteria poisoning.

oscill(o)- [L. *oscillare* to swing] a combining form denoting relationship to oscillation.

os•cil•lo•gram (ŏ-sil′o-gram) [*oscillo-* + *-gram*] the graphic record made by an oscillograph or a permanent record of the display on the oscilloscope.

os•cil•lo•graph (ŏ-sil′o-graf) [*oscillo-* + *-graph*] an instrument for producing a permanent record of variations in electrical voltage over time.

os•cil•lom•e•ter (os″ĭ-lom′ə-tər) [*oscillo-* + *-meter*] an instrument for measuring oscillations of any kind, such as changes in the volume of the arteries accompanying the heart beat. See also *sphygmo-oscillometer.* **oscillomet′ric** *adj*

os•cil•lop•sia (os″ĭ-lop′se-ə) [*oscillo-* + *-opsia*] a symptom in which objects appear to wiggle, jerk, or move back and forth; it sometimes accompanies nystagmus, especially the downbeat type. Called also *oscillating vision.*

os•cil•lo•scope (ə-sil′ə-skōp) [*oscillo-* + *-scope*] an instrument that displays a visual representation of electrical variations on the fluorescent screen of a cathode-ray tube.

Os•ci•nis pal•li•pes (os′ĭ-nis pal′ĭ-pēz) *Hippelates pallipes.*

os•ci•tate (os′ĭ-tāt) to yawn.

os•ci•ta•tion (os″ĭ-ta′shən) [L. *oscitatio*] yawning.

-ose a suffix indicating that the substance is a carbohydrate.

osel•tam•i•vir phos•phate (o″səl-tam′ĭ-vir) an inhibitor of viral neuraminidase used in the treatment of influenza, administered orally.

Os•good-Schlat•ter disease (oz′good shlah′tər) [Robert Bayley *Osgood,* American orthopedist, 1873–1956; Carl *Schlatter,* Swiss surgeon, 1864–1934] see under *disease.*

OSHA Occupational Safety and Health Administration.

-osis [Gr.] a word termination denoting a process, especially a disease or morbid process, and sometimes conveying the meaning of abnormal increase. See also *-sis.*

Os•ler disease, maneuver, nodes, etc. (ōs′lər) [Sir William *Osler,* Canadian-born physician, 1849–1919; successively professor of medicine in McGill University, the University of Pennsylvania, Johns Hopkins University, and the University of Oxford] see *hereditary hemorrhagic telangiectasia,* under *telangiectasia;* see *polycythemia vera;* and see under *maneuver, node, sign,* and *triad.*

Os•ler-Va•quez disease (ōs′lər vah-ka′) [Sir W. *Osler;* Louis Henri *Vaquez,* French physician, 1860–1936] polycythemia vera.

Os•ler-We•ber-Ren•du disease (ōs′lər va′bər ron-du′) [Sir W. *Osler;* Frederick Parkes *Weber,* British physician, 1863–1962; Henri Jules Louis Marie *Rendu,* French physician, 1844–1902] hereditary hemorrhagic telangiectasia.

os•mate (oz′māt) a salt containing the OsO_4^{2-} anion, e.g., potassium osmate K_2OsO_4.

os•mat•ic (oz-mat′ik) [Gr. *osmasthai* to smell] 1. olfactory. 2. having a sense of smell; applied to a category of animals subdivided further into macrosmatic and microsmatic. Cf. *anosmatic.*

os•me•sis (oz-me′sis) olfaction (def. 2).

os•mic (oz′mik) containing osmium.

os•mic ac•id (oz′mik) 1. osmium tetroxide. 2. the hypothetical acid, H_2OsO_4, which forms osmate salts.

os•mi•cate (oz′mĭ-kāt) to stain or impregnate with osmium tetroxide (osmic acid).

os•mics (oz′miks) [Gr. *osmē* odor] olfactology.

os•mi•dro•sis (oz″mĭ-dro′sis) bromhidrosis.

os•mi•fi•ca•tion (oz″mĭ-fĭ-ka′shən) treatment with osmium or osmic acid, as in histologic technique.

os•mi•oph•i•lic (oz″me-o-fil′ik) [*osmic* acid + *-philic*] staining easily with osmium or osmium tetroxide.

os•mio•pho•bic (oz″me-o-fo′bik) [*osmic* acid + *phobia*] resistant to staining with osmium or osmium tetroxide.

Os•mi•trol (os′mĭ-trol) trademark for a preparation of mannitol.

os•mi•um (Os) (oz′me-əm) [Gr. *osmē* odor; so named because of the odor of the vapor, OsO_4, produced by oxidation of the element] 1. a very hard, gray, toxic, and nearly infusible metal; atomic number, 76; atomic weight, 190.2. 2. a homeopathic trituration of metallic osmium.

o. **tetroxide** OsO_4, a colorless or light yellow crystalline compound with a pungent odor, used as a fixative in preparing histologic specimens; if splashed in the eyes it can cause conjunctivitis, corneal damage, and in severe cases blindness. Called also *osmic acid.*

osm(o)-[1] [Gr. *osmē* odor] a combining form denoting relationship to odors.

osm(o)-[2] [Gr. *ōsmos* impulse] a combining form denoting relationship to osmosis.

os•mol (oz′mōl) osmole.

os•mo•lal•i•ty (oz″mo-lal′ĭ-te) the concentration of osmotically active particles in solution expressed in terms of osmoles of solute per kilogram of solvent. The osmolality is directly proportional to the colligative properties of solutions: osmotic pressure, boiling point elevation, freezing point depression, and vapor pressure lowering.

os•mo•lar (oz-mo′lər) pertaining to the concentration of osmotically active particles in solution.

os•mo•lar•i•ty (oz″mo-lar′ĭ-te) the concentration of osmotically active particles in solution expressed in terms of osmoles of solute per liter of solution.

os•mole (oz′mōl) the amount of substance that dissociates in solution to form one mole of osmotically active particles, e.g., 1 mole of glucose, which is not ionizable, forms 1 osmole of solute, but 1 mole of sodium chloride forms 2 osmoles of solute. Symbol Osm. Abbreviated *osmol.*

os•mol•o•gy[1] (oz-mol′ə-je) [*osmo-*[1] + *-logy*] olfactology.

os•mol•o•gy[2] (oz-mol′ə-je) [*osmo-*[2] + *-logy*] the branch of physical chemistry that deals with osmosis.

os•mo•lute (oz′mo-lo͞ot″) an osmotically active solute.

os•mom•e•ter (oz-mom′ə-tər) [*osmo-*[2] + *-meter*] a device for measuring osmotic concentration or pressure.

freezing-point o. an osmometer using freezing-point depression measurement for analysis of osmotic pressure (number of particles, molecules, or ions) of solutions.

Hepp o. an osmometer in which very small quantities of material can be used and a direct reading of the osmotic pressure may be made.

membrane o. an osmometer in which diffusion through a semipermeable membrane indicates the osmotic pressure of macromolecules (number of molecules or ions) in a solution.

os•mo•phil•ic (oz″mo-fil′ik) [*osmo-*[2] + *-philic*] having an affinity for solutions with a high osmotic pressure.

os•mo•pho•bia (oz″mo-fo′be-ə) [*osmo-*[1] + *-phobia*] irrational fear of odors.

os•mo•phore (oz′mo-for″) [*osmo-*[1] + *-phore*] the group of atoms in a molecule of a compound that is responsible for its characteristic odor.

os•mo•re•cep•tor[1] (oz″mo-re-sep′tər) [*osmo-*[1] + *receptor*] olfactory receptor.

os•mo•re•cep•tor[2] (oz″mo-re-sep′tər) [*osmo-*[2] + *receptor*] any of a group of specialized neurons in the supraoptic nuclei of the hypothalamus that are stimulated by increased osmolality (chiefly, increased sodium concentration) of the extracellular fluid; their excitation promotes the release of vasopressin by the neurohypophysis.

os•mo•reg•u•la•tion (oz″mo-reg″u-la′shən) maintenance of osmolarity by a simple organism or body cell relative to the surrounding medium. **osmoreg′ulatory** *adj*

os•mose (oz′mōs) to pass through a membrane by osmosis.

os•mo•sis (oz-mo′sis, os-mo′sis) [Gr. *ōsmos* impulsion] the diffusion of pure solvent across a membrane in response to a concentration gradient, usually from a solution of lesser to one of greater solute concentration. **osmot′ic** *adj*

reverse o. the passage of solvent across a semipermeable membrane going from a solution of greater to one of lesser solute concentration, i.e., in the opposite direction from the usual; it is caused by application of hydrostatic pressure to the solution with greater concentration.

os•mo•sol•o•gy (oz″mo-sol′ə-je) the science of osmosis.

os•mo•stat (oz′mo-stat″) the regulatory centers that control the osmolality of the extracellular fluid.

reset o. an osmostat that is set abnormally low, so that too much antidiuretic hormone is released and the person has hyponatremia; this is seen most often in malignancies, cachexia, malnutrition, and pregnancy.

os•mo•tax•is (oz″mo-tak′sis) [*osmo-*[2] + *-taxis*] directional movement of a cell in response to changes in osmotic pressure.

os•mo•ther•a•py (oz″mo-ther′ə-pe) [*osmo-*[2] + *therapy*] treatment by the intravenous injection of hypertonic solutions to produce dehydration.

os•phre•si•ol•o•gy (os″fre-ze-ol′ə-je) olfactology.

os•phre•sis (os-fre′sis) olfaction (def. 1).

os•sa (os′ə) [L.] plural of *os*[2] (q.v.).

os•sa•ture (os′ə-chər) the arrangement of bones in the body or in a part.

os•se•in (os′e-in) the collagen of bone.

os•se•let (os′ə-let) an exostosis on the inner aspect of a horse's knee or on the lateral aspect of the fetlock.

osse(o)- [L. *osseus* bony, from *os* bone] pertaining to bone or containing a bony element.

os•seo•al•bu•moid (os″e-o-al′bu-moid) a protein derived from bone after hydration of the collagen.

os•seo•apo•neu•rot•ic (os″e-o-ap″o-no͝o-rot′ik) pertaining to bone and the aponeurosis of a muscle.

os•seo•car•ti•lag•i•nous (os″e-o-kahr″tĭ-laj′ĭ-nəs) osteochondral.

os•seo•fi•brous (os″e-o-fi′brəs) made up of fibrous tissue and bone.

os•seo•in•te•gra•tion (os″e-o-in″tə-gra′shən) [*osseo-* + *integration*] direct anchorage of an implant by the formation of bony tissue around it without growth of fibrous tissue at the bone-implant interface. See also *osseointegrated implant,* under *implant.*

os•seo•mu•cin (os″e-o-mu′sin) the homogeneous ground substance that binds together the collagen and elastic fibrils of bony tissue.

os•seo•mu•coid (os″e-o-mu′koid) a mucin existing in bone.

os•se•ous (os′e-əs) [L. *osseus*] of the nature or quality of bone; bony.

os•si•cle (os′ĭ-kəl) [L. *ossiculum*] ossiculum; a small bone. **ossic′ular** *adj*

Andernach o's the ossa suturalia; see *os suturale.*

auditory o's ossicula auditus; see under *ossiculum.*

o. of Bertin concha sphenoidalis.

epactal o. os suturale.

episternal o's ossa suprasternalia.

intercalcar o. os suturale.

Kerckring (Kerkring) o. see under *center.*

Riolan o's small bones occasionally seen in the suture between the mastoid portion of the temporal bone and the occipital bone.

sphenoturbinal o. concha sphenoidalis.

wormian o's the ossa suturalia; see *os suturale.*

os•sic•u•la (o-sik′u-lə) [L.] plural of *ossiculum.*

os•sic•u•lec•to•my (os″ĭ-ku-lek′tə-me) [*ossiculum* + *-ectomy*] surgical removal of an ossicle, or of the ossicles, of the ear.

os•si•cu•lot•o•my (os″ĭ-ku-lot′ə-me) [*ossiculum* + *-tomy*] surgical incision of the ossicles of the ear.

os•sic•u•lum (ə-sik′u-ləm) pl. *ossi′cula* [L.] ossicle; a small bone.

ossi′cula audito′ria TA alternative for *ossicula auditus.*

ossi′cula audi′tus [TA] auditory ossicles: the malleus, incus, and stapes, the small bones of the middle ear, which transmit vibrations from the tympanic membrane to the oval window. Called also *ossicula auditoria* [TA alternative] and *ossicular chain.*

os•si•des•mo•sis (os″ĭ-dəs-mo′sis) osteodesmosis.

os•sif•er•ous (ə-sif′ər-əs) [*os*[2] + *-ferous*] producing bone.

os•sif•ic (ə-sif′ik) [L. *os* bone + *facere* to make] forming or becoming bone.

os•si•fi•ca•tion (os″ĭ-fĭ-ka′shən) [L. *ossificatio*] the formation of bone or of a bony substance; the conversion of fibrous tissue or of cartilage into bone or a bony substance.

cartilaginous o. endochondral o.

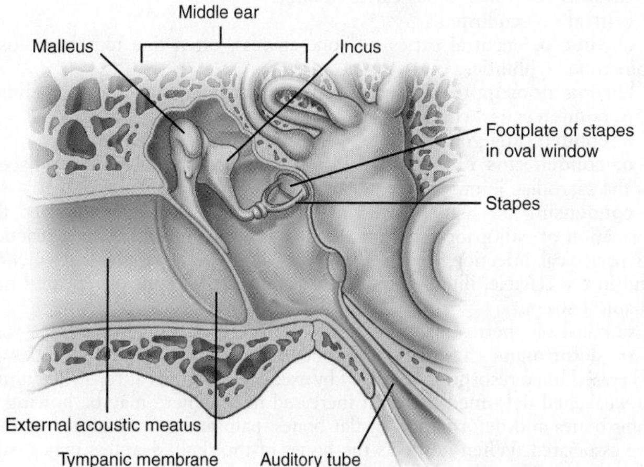

■ Auditory ossicles (ossicula auditus) and adjacent structures.

ectopic o. a pathological condition in which bone arises in tissues not in the osseous system and in connective tissues usually not manifesting osteogenic properties.
endochondral o. ossification that occurs in and replaces cartilage.
extraskeletal o. a general term encompassing ectopic and heterotopic ossification.
heterotopic o. the formation of bone in abnormal locations, secondary to pathology either at the local site or elsewhere.
intramembranous o. ossification that occurs in and replaces connective tissue, as occurs in the calvaria and in periosteal bone formation.
metaplastic o. the development of bony substance in normally soft structures.
perichondral o. ossification that occurs in a layered manner beneath the perichondrium or, later, the periosteum.
periosteal o. a type of intramembranous bone formation.

os•si•form (os'ĭ-form) resembling bone.

os•si•fy•ing (os'ĭ-fi″ing) changing or developing into bone.

os•si•phone (os'ĭ-fōn) [L. *os*, pl. *ossa* bone + Gr. *phōnē* voice] an early type of hearing aid that used bone conduction.

os•tal•gia (os-tal'jə) ostealgia.

os•tar•thri•tis (os″tahr-thri'tis) osteoarthritis.

os•te•al (os'te-əl) bony; osseous.

os•te•al•bu•moid (os″te-al'bu-moid) osseoalbumoid.

os•te•al•gia (os″te-al'jə) [*oste-* + *-algia*] pain in a bone or in the bones; called also *osteodynia.*

os•te•ana•gen•e•sis (os″te-an″ə-jen'ə-sis) osteoanagenesis.

os•te•anaph•y•sis (os″te-ə-naf'ĭ-sis) [*osteo-* + Gr. *anaphyein* to reproduce] reproduction of bone.

os•te•ar•thri•tis (os″te-ahr-thri'tis) osteoarthritis.

os•te•ar•throt•o•my (os″te-ahr-throt'ə-me) [*osteo-* + *arthro-* + *-tomy*] excision of an articular end of a bone.

os•tec•to•my (os-tek'tə-me) [*osteo-* + *-ectomy*] the excision of a bone or a portion of a bone.

os•te•ec•to•my (os″te-ek'tə-me) ostectomy.

os•te•ec•to•pia (os″te-ek-to'pe-ə) [*osteo-* + *-ectopia*] displacement of a bone.

os•te•ec•to•py (os″te-ek'tə-pe) osteectopia.

os•te•in (os'te-in) ossein.

os•te•ite (os'te-īt) an independent bony element or center of ossification.

os•te•itis (os″te-i'tis) [*osteo-* + *-itis*] inflammation of a bone, involving the haversian spaces, canals, and their branches, and generally the medullary cavity, and marked by enlargement of the bone, tenderness, and a dull, aching pain. See also *osteomyelitis.*
acute o. osteomyelitis, usually of septic origin.
o. albumino'sa osteitis with accumulation of a sticky, albuminous liquid.
alveolar o. dry socket.
carious o. osteomyelitis.
o. carno'sa o. fungosa.
caseous o. tuberculous caries of bone.
central o. endosteitis.
chronic o. central caries or bone abscess; often due to tuberculosis, sometimes syphilitic.
chronic nonsuppurative o. sclerosing nonsuppurative osteomyelitis.
o. conden'sans condensing o.
o. conden'sans generalisa'ta osteopoikilosis.
o. conden'sans i'lii condensing osteitis affecting the ilium adjacent to the sacroiliac joint.
condensing o. a focal inflammatory reaction of bone marked by the formation of radiopaque sclerotic lesions; it occurs in the jaw as a reaction to periapical infection (see *focal sclerosing osteomyelitis*, under *osteomyelitis*) and in the clavicle, ilium, or pubis, probably as the result of repeated mechanical stress.
cortical o. periostitis.
o. defor'mans a disease of bone marked by repeated episodes of increased bone resorption followed by excessive attempts at repair, resulting in weakened deformed bones of increased mass. There may be bowing of long bones and deformation of flat bones; pain and pathological fractures are associated. When it affects the bones of the skull, deafness may result. Called also *Paget disease of bone.*
o. fibro'sa cys'tica, o. fibro'sa cys'tica generalisa'ta rarefying osteitis with fibrous degeneration and formation of cysts, and with the presence of fibrous nodules on the affected bones; it is due to marked osteoclastic activity secondary to hyperfunction of the parathyroid gland. Called also *Recklinghausen* or *von Recklinghausen disease.*
o. fibro'sa dissemina'ta polyostotic fibrous dysplasia.
o. fibro'sa localisa'ta monostotic fibrous dysplasia.
o. fibro'sa osteoplas'tica o. fibrosa cystica.
o. fungo'sa chronic osteitis in which the haversian canals are dilated and filled with granulation tissue.
Garré o. sclerosing nonsuppurative osteomyelitis.
o. granulo'sa o. fungosa.
gummatous o. a chronic form associated with syphilis.
necrotic o. osteomyelitis.
parathyroid o. o. fibrosa cystica.
pedal o. inflammation of the pedal (coffin) bone of the forefoot of a horse, due to overwork, corns, or repeated trauma such as that due to an irregular conformation of the hoof surface. Called also *peditis.*
o. pu'bis a symptom-producing inflammatory condition of the pubic bones in the region of the symphysis, which may be associated with surgical procedures on pelvic structures or with pregnancy, infection of the urinary tract, degenerative changes, rheumatic disease, or other conditions.

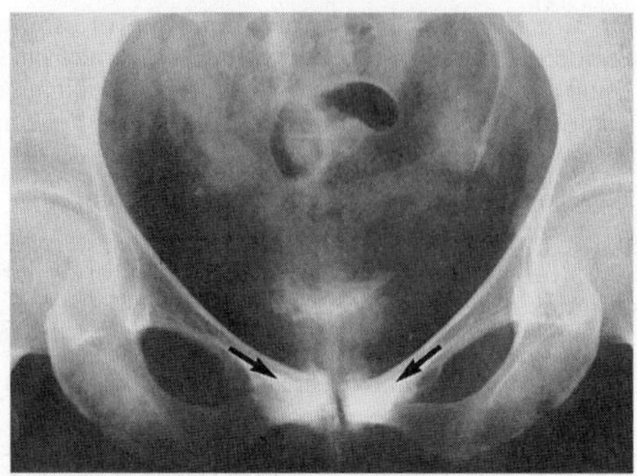

■ Osteitis pubis with sclerosis along both sides of the pubic symphysis *(arrows)* in a woman.

rarefying o. a bone disease in which the inorganic matter is lessened and the hard bone becomes cancellated.
sclerosing o. sclerosing nonsuppurative osteomyelitis.
secondary hyperplastic o. hypertrophic pulmonary osteoarthropathy.
vascular o. rarefying osteitis in which the spaces formed become occupied by blood vessels.

os•tem•py•e•sis (os″təm-pi-e'sis) [*osteo-* + *empyesis*] suppuration within a bone.

oste(o)- [Gr. *osteon* bone] a combining form denoting relationship to a bone or to the bones.

os•teo•acu•sis (os″te-o-ə-ku'sis) [*osteo-* + Gr. *akousis* hearing] bone conduction.

os•teo•ad•he•rin (os″te-o-ad-hēr'in) a leucine-rich repeat protein related to fibromodulin, containing keratan sulfate and found in extracellular matrix; it plays a role in the mineralization of bones and teeth. Called also *osteomodulin.*

os•teo•ana•gen•e•sis (os″te-o-an'ə-jen'ə-sis) [*osteo-* + Gr. *anagenesis*] regeneration of bone.

os•teo•an•es•the•sia (os″te-o-an″es-the'zhə) the insensitiveness of bone.

os•teo•an•eu•rysm (os″te-o-an'u-riz-əm) aneurysm in a bone.

os•teo•ar•thri•tis (os″te-o-ahr-thri'tis) [*osteo-* + *arthr-* + *-itis*] a noninflammatory degenerative joint disease seen mainly in older persons, characterized by degeneration of the articular cartilage, hypertrophy of bone at the margins, and changes in the synovial membrane. It is accompanied by pain, usually after prolonged activity, and stiffness, particularly in the morning or with inactivity. Called also *degenerative arthritis, hypertrophic arthritis,* and *degenerative joint disease.* **osteoarthrit'ic** *adj*
o. defor'mans, o. defor'mans ende'mica, endemic o. Kashin-Bek disease.
facet o., facet joint o. a type of spondylarthritis centered in facet joints, with disk degeneration and pain; it is most common in the lumbar region and also occurs in the cervical region. Called also *facet* or *facet joint arthritis* and *facet* or *facet joint arthropathy.*
hyperplastic o. hypertrophic pulmonary osteoarthropathy.

interphalangeal o. a localized form of arthritis involving the finger joints, characterized by the formation of nodosities (Bouchard nodes and Heberden nodes) and degenerative changes with intermittent inflammatory episodes, and leading eventually to deformities and ankyloses.

os·teo·ar·throp·a·thy (os″te-o-ahr-throp′ə-the) [*osteo-* + *arthropathy*] any disease of the joints and bones.

familial o. of fingers Thiemann disease.

hypertrophic pulmonary o. symmetrical osteitis of the four limbs, chiefly localized to the phalanges and the terminal epiphyses of the more distal long bones, sometimes extending to the proximal ends of the limbs and the flat bones, and accompanied by dorsal kyphosis and joint abnormalities. It is often secondary to chronic conditions of the lungs and heart. Called also *hyperplastic osteoarthritis, Marie-Bamberger disease* or *syndrome, pulmonary o.*, and *secondary hypertrophic o.*

idiopathic hypertrophic o., primary hypertrophic o. pachydermoperiostosis.

pulmonary o., secondary hypertrophic o. hypertrophic pulmonary o.

os·teo·ar·thro·sis (os″te-o-ahr-thro′sis) osteoarthritis.

o. juveni′lis Köhler bone disease (def. 1).

os·teo·ar·throt·o·my (os″te-o-ahr-throt′ə-me) ostearthrotomy.

os·teo·ar·tic·u·lar (os″te-o-ahr-tik′u-lər) pertaining to or affecting bones and joints.

os·teo·blast (os′te-o-blast″) [*osteo-* + *-blast*] a cell that arises from a fibroblast and that, as it matures, is associated with the production of bone. **osteoblas′tic** *adj*

os·teo·blas·to·ma (os″te-o-blas-to′mə) [*osteoblast* + *-oma*] a benign, painful, rather vascular tumor of bone characterized by the formation of osteoid tissue and primitive bone; called also *giant osteoid osteoma.*

os·teo·ca·chex·ia (os″te-o-kə-kek′se-ə) cachexia due to chronic bone disease; also chronic disease of bone. **osteocachec′tic** *adj*

os·teo·cal·cin (os″te-o-kal′sin) a vitamin K–dependent, calcium-binding bone protein, the most abundant noncollagen protein in bone; increased serum concentrations are a marker of increased bone turnover in disease states. Called also *bone Gla protein.*

os·teo·camp·sia (os″te-o-kamp′se-ə) [*osteo-* + Gr. *kamptein* to bend] curvature or bending of a bone, as in rickets.

os·teo·camp·sis (os″te-o-kamp′sis) osteocampsia.

os·teo·car·ti·lag·i·nous (os″te-o-kahr″tĭ-laj′ĭ-nəs) pertaining to or composed of bone and cartilage.

os·teo·ce·men·tum (os″te-o-se-men′təm) [*osteo-* + *cementum*] a hard bonelike secondary cementum, typically arranged in concentric layers around the root and frequently showing numerous resting lines, such as that occurring in hypercementosis.

os·teo·chon·dral (os″te-o-kon′drəl) pertaining to or composed of bone and cartilage; pertaining to a bone and its articular cartilage. Called also *osseocartilaginous.*

os·teo·chon·dri·tis (os″te-o-kon-dri′tis) [*osteo-* + *chondr-* + *-itis*] inflammation of both bone and cartilage.

o. defor′mans juveni′lis Legg-Calvé-Perthes disease.

o. defor′mans juveni′lis dor′si osteochondrosis of vertebrae; see *osteochondrosis.*

o. dis′secans osteochondritis with splitting of pieces of cartilage into the joint, particularly in the knee joint or shoulder joint.

o. ischiopu′bica a condition observed in the radiograph, consisting of granular-looking bodies at the junction of the ischium and os pubis in children.

juvenile deforming metatarsophalangeal o. Köhler bone disease (def. 2).

o. necro′ticans necrosis and destruction in the cartilage of the sesamoid bone of the great toe.

o. os′sis metacar′pi et metatar′si Thiemann disease (q.v.) affecting both the fingers and toes.

os·teo·chon·dro·dys·pla·sia (os″te-o-kon″dro-dis-pla′zhə) [*osteo-* + *chondro-* + *dys-* + *-plasia*] any of a large, heterogeneous group of hereditary intrinsic disorders of bone and cartilage, characterized by abnormalities in the size and shape of bones of the limbs, spine, and skull and radiologic abnormalities of the bones.

os·teo·chon·dro·dys·tro·phia (os″te-o-kon″dro-dis-tro′fe-ə) Morquio syndrome.

o. defor′mans Morquio syndrome.

os·teo·chon·dro·dys·tro·phy (os″te-o-kon″dro-dis′trə-fe) Morquio syndrome.

familial o. Morquio syndrome.

os·teo·chon·dro·fi·bro·ma (os″te-o-kon″dro-fi-bro′mə) fibrosing osteochondroma.

os·teo·chon·drol·y·sis (os″te-o-kon-drol′ə-sis) osteochondritis dissecans.

os·teo·chon·dro·ma (os″te-o-kon-dro′mə) [*osteo-* + *chondroma*] a benign tumor consisting of projecting adult bone capped by cartilage projecting from the lateral contours of endochondral bones. Called also *chondrosteoma, osteocartilaginous exostosis*, and *osteoenchondroma.*

fibrosing o. a tumor containing the elements of osteoma, chondroma, and fibroma.

os·teo·chon·dro·ma·to·sis (os″te-o-kon-dro″mə-to′sis) a condition marked by the presence of multiple osteochondromas, such as occurs in multiple cartilaginous exostoses or enchondromatosis; the term is sometimes used to denote one of the two conditions specifically, usually the former.

multiple o. osteochondromatosis.

synovial o. a rare condition in which cartilage bodies are formed in the synovial membrane of the joints, tendon sheaths, or bursae, later undergoing secondary calcification and ossification; some of the bodies may become detached and remain as viable, growing structures in the synovial spaces.

os·teo·chon·dro·myx·o·ma (os″te-o-kon″dro-mik-so′mə) [*osteochondroma* + *myxoma*] osteochondroma containing myxoid elements.

os·teo·chon·drop·a·thy (os″te-o-kon-drop′ə-the) [*osteo-* + *chondro-* + *-pathy*] any morbid condition affecting both bone and cartilage, or marked by abnormal enchondral ossification.

polyglucose (dextran) sulfate–induced o. an experimentally produced disorder of enchondral ossification characterized by a deficient formation of bone matrix in the metaphyses of long bones.

os·teo·chon·dro·sar·co·ma (os″te-o-kon″dro-sahr-ko′mə) [*osteo-* + *chondrosarcoma*] chondrosarcoma occurring in bone; used for those tumors including cartilaginous foci but not neoplastic foci of bone.

os·teo·chon·dro·sis (os″te-o-kon-dro′sis) a disease of the growth or ossification centers in children that begins as degeneration or necrosis and is followed by regeneration or recalcification. Called also *epiphyseal ischemic necrosis.* It can occur in any of numerous bones: in the calcaneus (os calcis) it is sometimes called *apophysitis;* in the capitular head of the femur it is called *Legg-Calvé-Perthes, Perthes*, or *Waldenström disease* and *coxa plana;* in the lunate bone it is called *Kienböck disease;* in the head of the second metatarsal it is called *Freiberg infraction;* in the tibial tuberosity it is called *Osgood-Schlatter* or *Schlatter disease;* in the vertebrae it is called *Scheuermann* or *juvenile kyphosis;* and in the capitellum of the humerus it is called *Panner disease.*

o. defor′mans ti′biae aseptic necrosis of the medial condyle of the tibia, producing genu varum; called also *Blount disease* and *tibia vara.*

os·teo·chon·drous (os″te-o-kon′drəs) osteochondral.

os·teo·cla·sia (os″te-o-kla′zhə) [*osteo-* + Gr. *klasis* a breaking + *-ia*] the absorption and destruction of bone tissue.

os·te·oc·la·sis (os″te-ok′lə-sis) [*osteo-* + Gr. *klasis* a breaking] the surgical fracture or refracture of bones.

os·teo·clast (os′te-o-klast″) [*osteo-* + *-clast*] 1. a large multinuclear cell associated with the absorption and removal of bone; osteoclasts become highly active in the presence of parathyroid hormone, causing increased bone resorption and release of bone salts (phosphorus and, especially, calcium) into the extracellular fluid. 2. an instrument for use in the surgical fracture or refracture of bones.

os·teo·clas·tic (os″te-o-klas′tik) pertaining to or of the nature of an osteoclast; destructive to bone.

os·teo·clas·to·ma (os″te-o-klas-to′mə) [*osteoclast* + *-oma*] giant cell tumor of bone.

os·teo·clas·ty (os′te-o-klas″te) osteoclasis.

os·teo·com·ma (os″te-o-kom′ə) [*osteo-* + Gr. *komma* fragment] any of the pieces or members of a series of bony structures, as a vertebra.

os·teo·con·duc·tion (os″te-o-kən-duk′shən) in bone restoration or bone grafts, the ability of certain substances to act as scaffolding for growth of bone. **osteoconduc′tive** *adj*

os·teo·cra·ni·um (os″te-o-kra′ne-əm) [*osteo-* + *cranium*] the fetal cranium during its stage of ossification.

os·teo·cys·to·ma (os″te-o-sis-to′mə) [*osteo-* + *cystoma*] a bone cyst.

os·teo·cyte (os′te-o-sīt″) an osteoblast that has become embedded within the bone matrix, occupying a flat oval cavity (bone lacuna, q.v.) and sending, through the canaliculi, slender cytoplasmic processes that make contact with processes of other osteocytes.

os•teo•den•tin (os″te-o-den′tin) [*osteo-* + *dentin*] dentin that resembles bone: seen in the teeth of certain fish and pathologically in other species, in which it is produced by rapid formation of secondary dentin, with entrapment of cells.

os•teo•den•ti•no•ma (os″te-o-den″tĭ-no′mə) an odontoma composed of bone and dentin.

os•teo•der•mia (os″te-o-dur′me-ə) osteoma cutis.

os•teo•des•mo•sis (os″te-o-des-mo′sis) [*osteo-* + *desmo-* + *-sis*] 1. the formation of bone and tendon. 2. ossification of tendon.

os•teo•di•as•ta•sis (os″te-o-di-as′tə-sis) [*osteo-* + *diastasis*] the separation of two adjacent bones.

os•te•odyn•ia (os″te-o-din′e-ə) ostealgia.

os•teo•dys•plas•ty (os′te-o-dis-plas″te) [*osteo-* + *dys-* + *-plasty*] abnormal development of bone.

Melnick-Needles o., o. of Melnick and Needles see under *syndrome.*

os•teo•dys•tro•phia (os″te-o-dis-tro′fe-ə) osteodystrophy.

o. cys′tica osteitis fibrosa cystica.

o. fibro′sa osteitis fibrosa cystica.

os•teo•dys•tro•phy (os″te-o-dis′trə-fe) defective bone formation.

Albright hereditary o. pseudohypoparathyroidism.

renal o. a condition resulting from chronic kidney disease and renal failure, characterized by elevated serum phosphorus with low or normal serum calcium levels and stimulation of parathyroid function. Bone disease includes a variable mixture of osteitis fibrosa cystica, osteomalacia, osteoporosis, and sometimes osteosclerosis. Onset is usually in childhood, resulting in renal dwarfism.

os•teo•ec•ta•sia (os″te-o-ek-ta′zhə) [*osteo-* + *ectasia*] bowing of the bones.

familial o. hyperostosis corticalis deformans juvenilis.

os•teo•ec•to•my (os″te-o-ek′tə-me) ostectomy.

os•teo•en•chon•dro•ma (os″te-o-en″kon-dro′mə) osteochondroma.

os•teo•epiph•y•sis (os″te-o-ə-pif′ə-sis) [*osteo-* + *epiphysis*] any bony epiphysis.

os•teo•fi•bro•ma (os″te-o-fi-bro′mə) [*osteo-* + *fibroma*] a benign tumor containing both osseous and fibrous elements.

os•teo•fi•bro•ma•to•sis (os″te-o-fi″bro-mə-to′sis) polyostotic form of fibrous dysplasia of bone.

cystic o. Jaffe-Lichtenstein disease.

os•teo•flu•o•ro•sis (os″te-o-floo-ro′sis) skeletal changes, usually consisting of osteomalacia and osteosclerosis, caused by the chronic intake of excessive quantities of fluorides. See also *fluorosis* (def. 2).

os•teo•gen (os′te-o-jen″) [*osteo-* + *-gen*] the substance composing the inner layer of the periosteum, from which bone is formed.

os•teo•gen•e•sis (os″te-o-jen′ə-sis) [*osteo-* + *-genesis*] formation of bone; the development of the bones. **osteogenet′ic** *adj*

o. imperfec′ta (OI) a group of inherited connective tissue disorders characterized by brittle, easily fractured bones and sometimes other manifestations, including blue sclerae, wormian bones, shortened limbs and limb deformities, fragile skin, muscle weakness, lax joints, bleeding and easy bruising, hearing loss, dyspnea, and dentinogenesis imperfecta. It is subdivided into eight types, I–VIII, on the basis of clinical features, course, and radiographic findings, but phenotypes vary greatly within types. Most cases are caused by autosomal dominant mutations in *COL1A1* or *COL1A2*, genes that encode the a1 chain of type I collagen; the mutations may result in production of abnormal collagen or in decreased production of normal collagen. There are several rarer types caused by autosomal recessive mutations of the cartilage-associated protein *(CRTAP)* or prolyl 3-hydroxylase 1 *(LEPRE1)* genes, both of which are involved in processing of the a1 chain of type I collagen. *Type I,* the most common, is also the mildest, and accounts for approximately 50 per cent of cases. *Type II* is the most severe, and is usually lethal in infancy.

os•teo•gen•ic (os″te-o-jen′ik) [*osteo-* + *-genic*] derived from or composed of any tissue that is concerned in the growth or repair of bone.

os•te•og•e•nous (os″te-oj′ə-nəs) osteogenic.

os•te•og•e•ny (os″te-oj′ə-ne) osteogenesis.

os•te•og•ra•phy (os″te-og′rə-fe) [*osteo-* + *-graphy*] a description of the bones.

os•teo•ha•lis•ter•e•sis (os″te-o-hə-lis″tər-e′sis) [*osteo-* + *hal-* + *sterein* to deprive] loss or deficiency of the mineral elements of bones.

os•teo•he•ma•chro•ma•to•sis (os″te-o-he″mə-kro″mə-to′sis) [*osteo-* + *hema-* + *chromato-* + *-sis*] discoloration of the bone by blood pigment, such as occurs in congenital erythropoietic porphyria in cattle.

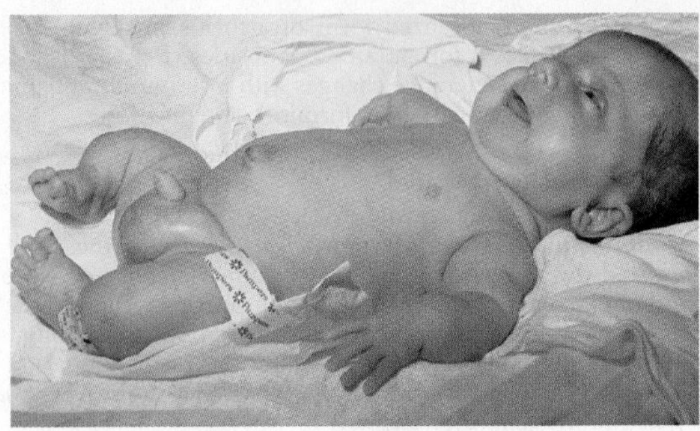

■ Osteogenesis imperfecta type II. The infant was born with multiple fractures and limb deformities and had dark bluish-gray sclerae.

os•teo•hy•da•tid•o•sis (os″te-o-hi″də-tid-o′sis) hydatid disease of bone.

os•te•oid (os′te-oid) [*osteo-* + *-oid*] 1. resembling bone. 2. the organic matrix of bone; young bone that has not undergone calcification.

os•teo•in•duc•tion (os″te-o-in-duk′shən) the act or process of stimulating osteogenesis. **osteoinduc′tive** *adj*

os•teo•lath•y•rism (os″te-o-lath′ĭ-riz-əm) a skeletal disorder produced in laboratory animals by diets containing the sweet pea *(Lathyrus odoratus)* or its active principle, β-aminopropionitrile, or other aminonitriles. In rats it is characterized by hernias, dissecting aortic aneurysms, lameness of the hind legs, exostoses, and kyphoscoliosis and other skeletal deformities, apparently as the result of defective aging of collagen tissue.

os•teo•lipo•chon•dro•ma (os″te-o-lip″o-kon-dro′mə) [*osteo-* + *lipo-* + *chondroma*] a benign cartilaginous tumor containing osseous and fatty elements.

os•teo•li•po•ma (os″te-o-lĭ-po′mə) [*osteo-* + *lipoma*] a lipoma with osseous metaplasia; called also *ossifying lipoma.*

Os•teo•lite (os′te-o-līt″) trademark for a kit for the preparation of technetium Tc 99m medronate.

os•teo•lo•gia (os″te-o-lo′jə) osteology; the nomenclature relating to the bones.

os•te•ol•o•gist (os″te-ol′ə-jist) a specialist in osteology.

os•te•ol•o•gy (os″te-ol′ə-je) [*osteo-* + *-logy*] the scientific study of the bones; applied also to the body of knowledge relating to the bones.

os•te•ol•y•sis (os″te-ol′ə-sis) [*osteo-* + *-lysis*] dissolution of bone; applied especially to the removal or loss of the calcium of bone. **osteolyt′ic** *adj*

os•te•o•ma (os″te-o′mə) [*oste-* + *-oma*] a benign, slow-growing tumor composed of well-differentiated, densely sclerotic, compact bone, usually arising in membrane bones, particularly the skull and facial bones.

compact o. a small, dense, compact tumor of mature lamellar bone with little medullary space, usually occurring in the craniofacial or nasal bones.

o. cu′tis progressive dermal ossification during childhood, with hard, round to irregular nodules representing islands of heterotopic bone within the dermis or subcutis, followed by coalescence of the lesions into plaques, and later by invasion of deep connective tissues. It may be sporadic or inherited as an autosomal dominant trait; the affected gene encodes a subunit of the G protein stimulating adenylyl cyclase. Called also *progressive osseous heteroplasia.*

o. du′rum, o. ebur′neum compact o.

giant osteoid o. osteoblastoma.

ivory o. compact o.

o. medulla′re an osteoma containing marrow spaces.

osteoid o. a small, benign but painful, circumscribed tumor of spongy bone occurring especially in the bones of the extremities and vertebrae, most often in young persons.

o. spongio′sum, spongy o. osteoma containing cancellated bone.

trabecular o. o. spongiosum.

os•teo•ma•la•cia (os″te-o-mə-la′shə) [*osteo-* + *-malacia*] inadequate or delayed mineralization of osteoid in mature cortical and spongy bone; it is the adult equivalent of rickets and accompanies that disorder in children. The etiology of osteomalacia and its clinical and biochemical manifestations are as described for rickets (q.v.). **osteomala′cic** *adj*

antacid-induced o. osteomalacia in which the combination of low dietary phosphorus intake and chronic excessive consumption of aluminum hydroxide–containing antacids has led to phosphate depletion;

characteristics include hypophosphatemia, nephrolithiasis, anorexia, muscle weakness, and bone loss.

anticonvulsant o. 1. osteomalacia occurring in anticonvulsant rickets of children. 2. anticonvulsant rickets in adults.

familial hypophosphatemic o. osteomalacia occurring in familial hypophosphatemic rickets.

hepatic o. osteomalacia as a complication of cholestatic liver disease, which may lead to severe bone pain and multiple fractures.

oncogenic o., oncogenous o. osteomalacia occurring in association with usually benign mesenchymal neoplasms. The tumors appear to produce a substance that impairs renal tubular functions such as phosphate transport and hydroxylation of 25-hydroxyvitamin D; hypophosphatemia secondary to reduced renal resorption of phosphate is a major cause of the bone disease. Called also *tumor-induced o.*

puerperal o. osteomalacia resulting from exhaustion of skeletal stores of calcium and phosphorus by repeated pregnancies and lactation.

renal tubular o. osteomalacia resulting from acidosis and hypercalciuria when deficient renal tubular activity has caused inability to produce acid urine or ammonia.

senile o. softening of bones in old age due to vitamin D deficiency.

tumor-induced o. oncogenic o.

os•teo•mal•a•co•sis (os″te-o-mal″ə-ko′sis) osteomalacia.

os•teo•ma•toid (os″te-o′mə-toid) resembling an osteoma.

os•teo•ma•to•sis (os″te-o-mə-to′sis) the formation of multiple osteomas.

os•teo•mere (os′te-o-mēr″) [*osteo-* + *-mere*] one of a series of similar bony structures, such as the vertebrae.

os•te•om•e•try (os″te-om′ə-tre) [*osteo-* + *-metry*] the measurement of bones.

os•teo•mi•o•sis (os″te-o-mi-o′sis) [*osteo-* + *mio-* + *-sis*] disintegration of bone.

os•teo•mod•u•lin (os″te-o-mod′u-lin) osteoadherin.

os•teo•my•eli•tis (os″te-o-mi″ə-li′tis) [*osteo-* + *myelitis*] inflammation of bone caused by infection, usually by a pyogenic organism, although any infectious agent may be involved. It may remain localized or may spread through the bone to involve the marrow, cortex, cancellous tissue, and periosteum. **osteomyelit′ic** *adj*

acute hematogenous o. osteomyelitis resulting from localization of blood-borne bacteria in bone, usually seen in the long bones of children following blunt trauma or adjacent infection; the most common infecting organism is *Staphylococcus aureus.* When it spreads to the joints it is known as *septic* or *bacterial arthritis.*

conchiolin o. a condition seen in workers in mother-of-pearl, probably due to the inhaled dust being deposited in the bone marrow. Cf. *coniosis.*

diffuse sclerosing o. a chronic diffuse inflammatory response of bone to low-grade infection, with inflammatory cell infiltrate, fibrous replacement of marrow, and dense sclerotic masses of trabecular bone. Polymorphonuclear leukocytes, plasma cells, and focal osteoblasts may be present. Oral lesions occur predominantly in the mandible of older persons and are often sequelae of chronic periodontal disease.

focal sclerosing o. a chronic confined inflammatory response of bone to low-grade infection, with formation of dense trabecular bony masses with little interstitial marrow tissue. It occurs particularly in the mandible of children and young adults, adjacent to the apex of a tooth with long-term pulpitis. Called also *osteitis condensans.* and *condensing osteitis.*

Garré o. sclerosing nonsuppurative o.

salmonella o. osteomyelitis due to salmonella organisms; it occurs more frequently than normal in sickle cell disease.

sclerosing nonsuppurative o. chronic idiopathic osteomyelitis involving the long bones, particularly the tibia and femur, and characterized by a diffuse inflammatory reaction, increased density and spindle-shaped sclerotic thickening of the cortex, and an absence of suppuration; called also *Garré o., osteitis,* or *disease,* and *chronic nonsuppurative osteitis.*

typhoid o. a type of osteomyelitis that usually occurs in the late convalescent stage of typhoid fever.

os•teo•my•elo•dys•pla•sia (os″te-o-mi″ə-lo-dis-pla′zhə) [*osteo-* + *myelo-* + *dys-* + *-plasia*] a condition characterized by thinning of the osseous tissue of bones and increase in size of the marrow cavities, accompanied by leukopenia and fever.

os•teo•my•elog•ra•phy (os″te-o-mi″ə-log′rə-fe) radiographic visualization of bone marrow.

os•teo•myxo•chon•dro•ma (os″te-o-mik″so-kon-dro′mə) osteochondromyxoma.

os•te•on (os′te-on) [Gr. "*bone*"] the basic unit of structure of compact bone, comprising a haversian canal and its concentrically arranged lamellae, of which there may be 4 to 20, each 3 to 7 microns thick, in a single (haversian) system; such units are directed mainly in the long axis of the bone.

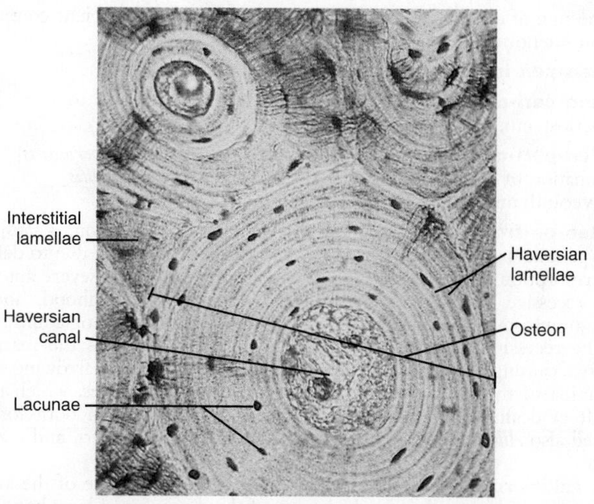

■ Osteons in photomicrograph of a section of a flat bone.

os•te•one (os′te-ōn) osteon.

os•teo•ne•cro•sis (os″te-o-nə-kro′sis) [*osteo-* + *necrosis*] necrosis of bone due to obstruction of its blood supply. Called also *avascular* or *ischemic necrosis of bone.*

os•teo•nec•tin (os″te-o-nek′tin) [*osteo-* + L. *nectere* to fasten] a phosphoprotein that binds both collagen and calcium and serves as a regulator of mineralization, found in bone and platelets.

os•teo•neu•ral•gia (os″te-o-nōō-ral′jə) [*osteo-* + *neuralgia*] neuralgia of a bone.

os•teo•odon•to•ma (os″te-o-o″don-to′mə) ameloblastic odontoma.

os•teo•on•y•cho•dys•pla•sia (os″te-o-on″ĭ-ko-dis-pla′zhə) [*osteo-* + *onycho-* + *dysplasia*] 1. abnormal development of nails and bones; called also *onycho-osteodysplasia.* 2. nail-patella syndrome.

hereditary o. nail-patella syndrome.

os•teo•path (os′te-o-path″) a practitioner of osteopathy.

os•teo•path•ia (os″te-o-path′e-ə) osteopathy (def. 1).

o. conden′sans myelosclerosis (def. 2).

o. conden′sans dissemina′ta osteopoikilosis.

o. hemorrha′gica infan′tum Moeller-Barlow disease.

o. hyperosto′tica conge′nita melorheostosis.

o. hyperosto′tica mul′tiplex infan′tilis diaphyseal dysplasia.

o. stria′ta multiple condensations of cancellous bone beginning at the epiphyseal line and extending into the diaphysis, an abnormality seen only on radiographic examination.

os•teo•path•ic (os″te-o-path′ik) pertaining to osteopathy.

os•teo•pa•thol•o•gy (os″te-o-pə-thol′ə-je) any disease of bone.

os•te•op•a•thy (os″te-op′ə-the) [*osteo-* + *-pathy*] 1. any disease of a bone. 2. a system of therapy founded by Andrew Taylor Still (1828–1917), based on the theory that the body can make its own remedies against disease and other toxic conditions when it is in normal structural relationship and has favorable environmental conditions and adequate nutrition. It uses generally accepted physical, medicinal, and surgical methods of diagnosis and therapy, while placing chief emphasis on maintenance of normal body mechanics and on manipulative methods of detecting and correcting faulty structure.

alimentary o. hunger o.

amyloid o. local osteoarticular lytic lesions often found in patients with hemodialysis-associated amyloidosis.

hunger o. disturbances of the skeletal system observed in famine areas, characterized by a reduction in the amount of normally calcified bone, and attributed to dietary deficiencies and associated hormonal dysfunction.

hypertrophic o. a condition in dogs similar to the hypertrophic pulmonary osteoarthropathy of humans; characteristics include hyperostosis of the limbs and later other skeletal regions, sometimes associated with tumors, tuberculosis, or other pulmonary conditions. Called also *acropachia.*

myelogenic o. any bone disease due to the impaired relation between the medullary and osseous tissues.

os•teo•pe•nia (os″te-o-pe′ne-ə) [*osteo-* + *-penia*] 1. any decrease in bone mass below the normal. 2. reduced bone mass due to a decrease in the rate of osteogenesis to the extent that there is insufficient compensation for normal bone lysis.

os•teo•pen•ic (os″te-o-pen′ik) pertaining to osteopenia.

os•teo•peri•os•te•al (os″te-o-per″e-os′te-əl) pertaining to bone and its periosteum.

os•teo•peri•os•ti•tis (os″te-o-per″e-os-ti′tis) [*osteo-* + *periostitis*] inflammation of a bone and its periosteum. Called also *periosteitis.*

alveolodental o. periodontitis.

os•teo•pe•tro•sis (os″te-o-pe-tro′sis) [*osteo-* + Gr. *petra* stone + *-osis*] a rare genetic disease characterized by abnormally dense bone, due to defective resorption of immature bone. It occurs in two forms: a severe autosomal recessive form occurring in utero, infancy, or childhood, and a benign autosomal dominant form occurring in adolescence or adulthood. In the recessive form, the proliferation of bone obliterates the marrow cavity, causing anemia and hepatosplenomegaly, and narrowing the foramina of the skull, causing compression of cranial nerves, which may result in deafness and blindness. Fractures are common in both forms. Called also *Albers-Schönberg* or *marble bones disease, ivory bones,* and *marble bones.*

o. gallina′rum a neoplastic viral disease of chickens, one of the avian leukosis complex, marked by thickening of the diaphyses of long bones.

infantile malignant o. the autosomal recessive type of osteopetrosis.

os•teo•phage (os′te-o-fāj) [*osteo-* + *-phage*] osteoclast (def. 1).

os•teo•pha•gia (os″te-o-fa′je-ə) [*osteo-* + *-phagia*] the eating of bone due to a craving for phosphorus.

os•teo•phle•bi•tis (os″te-o-flə-bi′tis) [*osteo-* + *phleb-* + *-itis*] inflammation of the veins of a bone.

os•te•oph•o•ny (os″te-of′ə-ne) bone conduction.

os•teo•phy•ma (os″te-o-fi′mə) osteophyte.

os•teo•phyte (os′te-o-fīt″) [*osteo-* + *-phyte*] a bony excrescence or osseous outgrowth. Called also *osteophyma.*

os•teo•phy•to•sis (os″te-o-fi-to′sis) a condition characterized by the formation of osteophytes.

os•teo•plaque (os′te-o-plak) a layer of bone.

os•teo•plast (os′te-o-plast) [*osteo-* + *-plast*] osteoblast.

os•teo•plas•tic (os″te-o-plas′tik) 1. osteogenic. 2. pertaining to osteoplasty.

os•teo•plas•ti•ca (os″te-o-plas′tĭ-kə) osteitis fibrosa cystica.

os•teo•plas•ty (os′te-o-plas″te) [*osteo-* + *-plasty*] plastic surgery of the bones.

os•teo•poi•ki•lo•sis (os″te-o-poi″kĭ-lo′sis) [*osteo-* + *poikil-* + *-osis*] an autosomal dominant trait due to mutation in the *LEMD3* gene (locus: 12q14), which encodes an inner nuclear membrane protein. It is characterized by multiple sclerotic foci in the ends of long bones and scattered stippling in round and flat bones, usually without symptoms and diagnosed fortuitously by x-ray examination. **osteopoikilot′ic** *adj*

os•teo•pon•tin (os″te-o-pon′tin) an acidic calcium-binding phosphoprotein with a high affinity for hydroxyapatite, involved in bone mineralization and in dystrophic calcification.

os•teo•po•ro•sis (os″te-o-pə-ro′sis) [*osteo-* + *por-*[1] + *-osis*] reduction in bone mineral density, leading to fractures after minimal trauma. **osteoporot′ic** *adj*

age-related o. senile o.

o. circumscrip′ta cra′nii demineralization of the bones of the skull, characteristic of the destructive or osteolytic phase of Paget disease; called also *Schüller disease.*

o. of disuse decrease in bone substance as a result of lack of re-formation of laminae because there is not the functional stress that ordinarily leads to replacement of laminae in new stress lines.

involutional o. senile o.

juvenile o. any of several rare types of osteoporosis seen in children and adolescents; they are usually due to an underlying medical condition such as juvenile idiopathic arthritis, diabetes mellitus, hyperparathyroidism, or a malabsorption syndrome, but some cases are idiopathic.

postmenopausal o. osteoporosis occurring in women within 3 to 20 years after menopause, affecting trabecular bone more than cortical bone, and manifested mainly by vertebral fractures of the painful crush type, hip fracture, Colles fracture, and increased tooth loss.

posttraumatic o. loss of bone substance following an injury in which there is damage to a nerve, sometimes due to an increased blood supply caused by the neurogenic insult, or to disuse secondary to pain. It is one component of complex regional pain syndrome, type 1. Called also *Sudeck atrophy.*

senile o. osteoporosis in men and women over 70, manifested mainly by hip and vertebral fractures of the painless multiple wedge type leading to kyphosis. Called also *age-related* or *involutional o.*

os•te•o•pro•teg•er•in (OPG) (os″te-o-pro-teg′ər-in) a protein secreted in the body that inhibits maturation of osteoclasts.

os•teo•ra•dio•ne•cro•sis (os″te-o-ra″de-o-nə-kro′sis) necrosis of bone following irradiation.

os•te•or•rha•gia (os″te-o-ra′jə) [*osteo-* + *-rrhagia*] hemorrhage from bone.

os•te•or•rha•phy (os″te-or′ə-fe) [*osteo-* + *-rrhaphy*] the suturing or wiring of bones.

os•teo•sar•co•ma (os″te-o-sahr-ko′mə) [*osteo-* + *sarcoma*] a malignant primary neoplasm of bone composed of a malignant connective tissue stroma with evidence of malignant osteoid, bone, or cartilage formation. Classical osteosarcoma is a poorly differentiated tumor affecting mainly young adults, most often involving the long bones, and is classified as *osteoblastic, chondroblastic,* or *fibroblastic* according to which histologic component predominates. Called also *osteogenic sarcoma.* **osteosarco′matous** *adj*

chondroblastic o. see *osteosarcoma.*

classical o. see *osteosarcoma.*

extraosseous o. a rare neoplasm occurring in the soft tissues of the body, generally in the thighs, composed of sarcomatous tissue that produces malignant osteoid and bone; it is histologically identical to osteosarcoma occurring in bone.

fibroblastic o. see *osteosarcoma.*

gnathic o. o. of jaw.

high-grade surface o. a highly malignant osteosarcoma histologically identical to classical osteosarcoma but located on the surface of a bone.

intracortical o. a rare form of osteosarcoma affecting mainly young adults, consisting of an osteolytic lesion confined within the cortex of a bone with a surrounding area of cortical sclerosis.

intraosseous low-grade o. a well-differentiated osteosarcoma of low malignancy arising within a bone, composed of spindle cells arranged in interlacing bundles separated by collagen fibers, with invasion of fatty marrow or extraosseous soft tissue.

o. of jaw a variant of osteosarcoma occurring in the mandible or maxilla, having a slightly older age of onset than classical osteosarcoma, with less tendency to metastasize than other osteosarcomas.

juxtacortical o. parosteal o.

multicentric o. the occurrence of osteosarcomas in more than one bone or in different sites on the same bone; lesions may be synchronous or metachronous.

osteoblastic o. see *osteosarcoma.*

parosteal o. a variant of osteosarcoma consisting of a slowly growing tumor that arises from the cortex of a bone and grows outward, eventually surrounding the bone; it resembles cancellous bone and is characterized histologically by a fibrous stroma containing bony spicules and trabeculae. It affects adults in the second through fifth decades of life and is less malignant than classical osteosarcoma. Called also *juxtacortical o.* and *parosteal sarcoma.*

periosteal o. a variant of osteochondroma consisting of a soft, lobulated tumor arising from the periosteum of a long bone and growing outward from the bone; histologically it is a chondroblastic osteosarcoma.

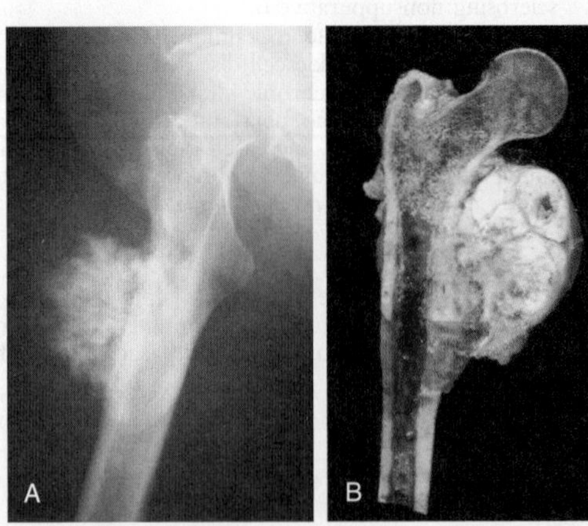

■ *(A),* Lateral radiograph of periosteal osteosarcoma of the proximal femur in a 67-year-old woman. *(B),* Cut specimen showing lesion arising from surface of bone, without involvement of marrow cavity.

small-cell o. a variant of osteosarcoma resembling Ewing sarcoma, composed of small round to spindle-shaped cells arranged in sheets or separated into lobules by fibrous septa, and having areas of osteoid and sometimes chondroid formation; called also *polyhistiocytoma* and *multipotential primary sarcoma of bone.*

telangiectatic o. an aggressive, lytic form occurring as a soft, cystic tumor containing aneurysmally dilated blood-filled spaces lined by pleomorphic cells producing osteoid foci.

os•teo•sar•co•ma•to•sis (os″te-o-sahr-ko″mə-to′sis) the simultaneous occurrence of multiple osteosarcomas; synchronous multicentric osteosarcoma.

os•teo•scle•ro•sis (os″te-o-sklə-ro′sis) [*osteo-* + *sclerosis*] the hardening or abnormal density of bone, as in eburnation and condensing osteitis. **osteosclerot′ic** *adj*

o. conge′nita achondroplasia.

o. fra′gilis osteopetrosis.

o. myelofibrosis myelosclerosis (def. 2).

os•teo•sep•tum (os″te-o-sep′təm) pars ossea septi nasi.

os•te•o•sis (os″te-o′sis) the formation of bony tissue, especially the infiltration of connective tissue with bone.

o. cu′tis osteoma cutis.

o. ebur′nisans monome′lica melorheostosis.

parathyroid o. osteitis fibrosa cystica.

os•teo•su•ture (os′te-o-soo″chər) [*osteo-* + *suture*] osteorrhaphy.

os•teo•syn•o•vi•tis (os″te-o-sin″o-vi′tis) synovitis together with osteitis of the neighboring bones.

os•teo•syn•the•sis (os″te-o-sin′thə-sis) [*osteo-* + *synthesis*] surgical fastening of the ends of a fractured bone by sutures, rings, plates, or other mechanical means.

os•teo•ta•bes (os″te-o-ta′bēz) [*osteo-* + *tabes*] a disease, chiefly of infants, in which the cells of the bone marrow are destroyed and the marrow disappears.

os•teo•throm•bo•phle•bi•tis (os″te-o-throm″bo-flə-bi′tis) inflammation extended through intact bone by a progressive thrombophlebitis of small venules, such as sometimes occurs in the mastoid bone.

os•teo•throm•bo•sis (os″te-o-throm-bo′sis) [*osteo-* + *thrombosis*] thrombosis of the veins of a bone.

os•teo•tome (os′te-o-tōm″) [*osteo-* + *-tome*] a chisel-like knife for cutting bone.

os•te•ot•o•my (os″te-ot′ə-me) [*osteo-* + *-tomy*] the surgical cutting of a bone.

angulation o. in midhumeral amputation, the bending of a small terminal of the humerus at a right angle to the bone shaft so as to provide a projection that locks the prosthesis to the bone.

block o. osteotomy in which a section of bone is removed.

cuneiform o. the removal of a wedge of bone.

cup-and-ball o. osteotomy in which the distal fragment is pointed and the proximal fragment is recessed.

displacement o. surgical division of a bone and shifting of the divided ends to change the alignment of the bone or to alter weight-bearing stresses.

innominate o. pelvic osteotomy to deepen the acetabulum in developmental dysplasia of the hip.

inverted L o. a type of osteotomy performed on the mandible to correct prognathism, the cut being an inverted L shape made in the ramus just below the condyle.

Le Fort o. transverse sectioning and repositioning of the maxilla; the incision for each of the three types *(Le Fort I, II,* and *III o's)* is placed along the line defined by the corresponding Le Fort fracture (q.v.).

linear o. the sawing or linear cutting of a bone.

Lorenz o. osteotomy of the neck of the femur by a V-shaped cutting of the femur so as to prevent displacement of the shaft.

pelvic o. pubiotomy.

sagittal ramus o. sagittal split o.

sagittal split o. sagittal splitting of mandible; see under *splitting.*

sandwich o. a surgical technique for augmenting an atrophic mandible; it is similar to a visor osteotomy (q.v.) but the split is a horizontal one confined between the mental foramina so that only the anterior portion of the cranial fragment is lifted upward.

total maxillary o. Le Fort I o.; see *Le Fort o.*

vertical ramus o. a type of osteotomy performed to correct prognathism; the ramus is resected in a vertical line proceeding from the sigmoid notch to the angle area of the lower border of the mandible.

visor o. a surgical technique for augmenting an atrophic mandible, performed by splitting the mandible sagittally and sliding the cranial fragment upward, then supporting the structure with interposed grafts. Cf. *sandwich o.*

visor/sandwich o. a combination of the visor and sandwich osteotomies in which the cut is in the vertical plane posterior to the mental foramina and at a 45° angle in the anterior region.

os•teo•tribe (os′te-o-trīb″) [*osteo-* + Gr. *tribein* to rub] an instrument for rasping carious bone.

os•teo•trite (os′te-o-trīt″) osteotribe.

os•te•ot•ro•phy (os″te-ot′rə-fe) [*osteo-* + *-trophy*] nutrition of bone.

os•te•ot•y•lus (os″te-ot′ə-ləs) [*osteo-* + Gr. *tylos* callus] the callus enclosing the end of a broken bone.

Os•ter•ta•gia (os″tər-ta′jə) [Robert von *Ostertag*, German veterinarian, 1864–1940] a genus of attenuated nematode stomach worms of the family Trichostrongylidae, found mostly in cysts on the wall of the abomasum of cattle and other ruminants. It closely resembles *Teladorsagia.*

os•ter•ta•gi•a•sis (os″tər-tə-ji′ə-sis) infection of the abomasum of a ruminant by nematodes of the genus *Ostertagia.* In lambs and calves, if there are large numbers of adult worms the host may suffer from anorexia and diarrhea. In older animals, when the resident worm population yields large numbers of larvae, the result is edema and thickening of the abomasal mucosa, with chronic diarrhea and emaciation that can be fatal.

os•ter•tag•i•o•sis (os″tər-taj″e-o′sis) ostertagiasis.

os•tia (os′te-ə) [L.] plural of *ostium.*

os•ti•ole (os′te-ōl) a pore, such as in a perithecium or pycnidium.

os•tio•me•a•tal (os″te-o-me-a′təl) [*ostium* + *meatal*] pertaining to an opening (ostium) and a meatus, especially in the nasal cavity.

os•ti•tis (os-ti′tis) osteitis.

os•ti•um (os′te-əm) pl. *os′tia* [L.] an opening, aperture, or orifice. **os′tial** *adj*

o. abdomina′le tu′bae uteri′nae [TA] abdominal orifice of uterine tube: the funnel-shaped opening by which the uterine tube communicates with the pelvic cavity.

o. anato′micum u′teri inter′num [TA] anatomical internal os of uterus: the internal orifice of the uterine cervix, marking the anatomical point at which the cervix opens into the corpus uteri; it may not correspond to the histological internal os *(o. histologicum uteri internum).*

o. aor′tae [TA] aortic opening: the opening between the left ventricle and the ascending aorta; guarded by the aortic valve. Called also *aortic orifice.*

o. appen′dicis vermifor′mis [TA] opening of vermiform appendix: the orifice between the vermiform appendix and the cecum.

o. atrioventricula′re dex′trum [TA] right atrioventricular opening: the opening between the right atrium and the right ventricle of the heart, guarded by the right atrioventricular valve; called also *tricuspid orifice* and *right atrioventricular orifice.*

o. atrioventricula′re sinis′trum [TA] left atrioventricular opening: the opening between the left atrium and the left ventricle of the heart, guarded by the left atrioventricular valve; called also *mitral orifice* and *left atrioventricular orifice.*

o. cardi′acum [TA] cardiac opening: the orifice between the esophagus and the cardia (cardiac part of stomach). Called also *cardiac orifice.*

coronary o., o. of coronary artery either of the two openings in the aortic sinuses that mark the origins of the left and right coronary arteries.

ethmoid o., ethmoidal o., o. of ethmoidal sinus, o. of ethmoid sinus any of various small openings connecting an ethmoidal sinus or air cell to the nasal cavity.

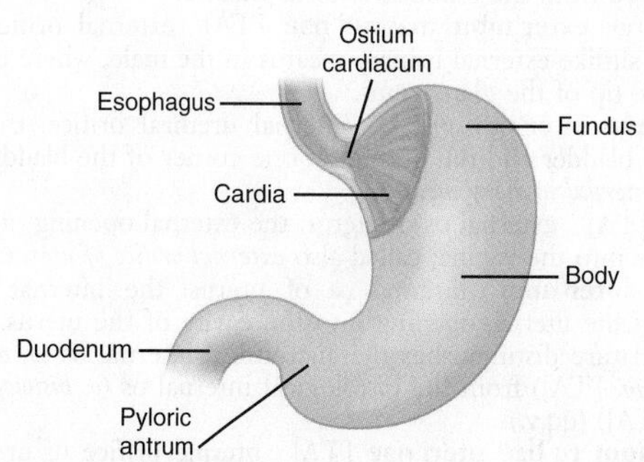

■ Ostium cardiacum (cardiac opening) in a cutaway view of the stomach and esophagus.

follicular o. see under *orifice.*
frontal o., frontal sinus o., o. of frontal sinus apertura sinus frontalis.
o. histolo′gicum u′teri inter′num [TA] histological internal os of uterus: the histological lower limit of the isthmus uteri, which is the level of transition between endometrium undergoing menstrual changes above and cervical mucosa not undergoing such changes below; it may not correspond to the anatomical internal os *(o. anatomicum uteri internum).*
o. ilea′le [TA] ileal orifice: the opening at the junction of the ileum and cecum, which is rounded at the left (anterior) end and pointed at the right (posterior) end. It has two lips, one above and one below (TA, *labrum ileocaecale* and *labrum ileocolicum*). In a cadaver this is the site of the so-called ileocecal valve; in the living individual the ileum here forms a conical projection called the *papilla ilealis.* Called also *o. ileocaecale* or *ileocecale, ileal opening,* and *ileocecal opening* or *orifice.*
o. ileocaeca′le, o. ileoceca′le 1. o. ileale. 2. term formerly used as a synonym for *opening of ileocecal valve.*
o. inter′num u′teri o. uterinum tubae uterinae.
maxillary o., maxillary sinus o. hiatus maxillaris.
o. pharyn′geum tu′bae auditi′vae [TA] pharyngeal opening of auditory tube: the opening at the inferior end of either auditory tube, located on each of the lateral walls of the pharynx, posterior and inferior to the posterior end of the inferior nasal concha. Called also *o. pharyngeum tubae auditoriae* [TA alternative] and *pharyngeal orifice of auditory tube.*
o. pharyn′geum tu′bae audito′riae TA alternative for *o. pharyngeum tubae auditivae.*
o. pri′mum an opening in the lowest aspect of the septum primum of the embryonic heart, posteriorly near the primordial atrioventricular valves. Called also *interatrial foramen primum.*
o. primum, persistent an endocardial cushion defect characterized by a cleft in the basal portion of the atrial septum, usually associated with cleft mitral valve.
o. pylo′ricum [TA] pyloric orifice or opening: the orifice between the pylorus of the stomach and the duodenum. Called also *gastric* or *pyloric outlet.*
o. secun′dum an opening high in the septum primum of the embryonic heart, approximately where the foramen ovale will develop. Called also *interatrial foramen secundum.*
o. si′nus corona′rii [TA] opening of coronary sinus: an opening in the wall of the right atrium, situated between the opening of the inferior vena cava and the atrioventricular opening, the lower part of which is covered by the valve of the coronary sinus. Called also *orifice of coronary sinus.*
sinusoidal o. any of the openings of the anterior cardiac veins into the right atrium of the heart.
sphenoid o., sphenoid sinus o., o. of sphenoid sinus apertura sinus sphenoidalis.
o. trun′ci pulmona′lis [TA] opening of pulmonary trunk: the opening between the right ventricle and the pulmonary trunk, guarded by the pulmonary valve; called also *pulmonary orifice.*
o. tympa′nicum tu′bae auditi′vae [TA] tympanic opening of auditory tube: the opening of the auditory tube on the carotid wall of the tympanic cavity. Called also *o. tympanicum tubae auditoriae* [TA alternative] and *tympanic orifice of auditory tube.*
o. tympa′nicum tu′bae audito′riae TA alternative for *o. tympanicum tubae auditivae.*
o. ure′teris [TA] orifice of ureter: the opening of a ureter into the bladder; the two orifices are at the lateral angles of the trigone of the bladder. Called also *ureteral orifice* or *meatus.*
o. ure′thrae exter′num femini′nae [TA] external orifice of female urethra: the external urinary meatus in the female, where the urethra opens into the vestibule; it is surrounded by a sphincter of striated muscle derived from the bulbocavernosus muscle.
o. ure′thrae exter′num masculi′nae [TA] external orifice of male urethra: the slitlike external urinary meatus in the male, where the urethra opens on the tip of the glans penis.
o. ure′thrae inter′num [TA] internal urethral orifice: the opening between the bladder and the urethra at one corner of the bladder trigone; called also *internal urinary meatus.*
o. u′teri [TA] external os of uterus: the external opening of the cervix of the uterus into the vagina; called also *external orifice of uterus.*
o. u′teri inter′num internal os of uterus: the internal orifice of the cervix of the uterus, opening into the cavity of the uterus. The official nomenclature distinguishes the anatomical internal os (*o. anatomicum uteri internum,* [TA]) from the histological internal os (*o. histologicum uteri internum,* [TA]) (qq.v.).
o. uteri′num tu′bae uteri′nae [TA] uterine orifice of uterine tube: the point at which the cavity of the uterine tube becomes continuous with that of the uterus.
o. vagi′nae [TA] vaginal orifice: the external opening of the vagina, situated just posterior to the external urethral orifice.
o. val′vae ilea′lis, o. val′vae ileocaeca′lis opening of ileocecal valve.
o. ve′nae ca′vae inferio′ris [TA] the opening of the inferior vena cava into the right atrium of the heart; it is accompanied by a valve that, in the adult, is usually rudimentary.
o. ve′nae ca′vae superio′ris [TA] the opening of the superior vena cava into the right atrium of the heart; it is unaccompanied by a valve.
os′tia vena′rum pulmona′lium [TA] the openings of the pulmonary veins (in the human, usually four) into the left atrium of the heart; they are unaccompanied by valves.

os·to·mate (os′tə-māt) one who has undergone enterostomy or ureterostomy.

os·to·my (os′tə-me) a general term referring to any operation in which an artificial opening is formed between two hollow organs or between one or more such viscera and the abdominal wall for discharge of intestinal contents or of urine.

-ostomy [Gr. *stoma* mouth] a word termination denoting an operation in which an artificial opening is formed, with the organ into which the opening is made denoted by the combining form to which the word termination is attached.

os·to·sis (os-to′sis) osteogenesis.

os·tra·ceous (os-tra′shəs) [Gr. *ostrakon* shell] shaped like or resembling an oyster shell.

os·tra·co·sis (os″trə-ko′sis) [Gr. *ostrakon,* shell] bone change that takes on the consistency of oyster shell.

os·treo·tox·ism (os″tre-o-tok′siz-əm) [Gr. *ostreon* oyster + *toxikon* poisoning] poisoning caused by the eating of contaminated oysters.

Os·trum-Furst syndrome (os′trəm furst′) [Herman William *Ostrum,* American physician, 1893–1970; William *Furst,* American physician, 20th century] see under *syndrome.*

Os·wal·do·cru·zia (oz-wahl″do-kroo′ze-ə) [G. *Oswaldo Cruz,* Brazilian physician, 1872–1917] a genus of nematodes of the family Trichostrongylus, inhabiting the lungs and intestines of reptiles and amphibians.

OT Old tuberculin; *(in anatomy)* old term.

Ota nevus (o′tah) [Masao T. *Ota,* Japanese dermatologist, 1885–1945] see under *nevus.*

otal·gia (o-tal′jə) [Gr. *ōtalgia*] pain in the ear; called also *earache* and *otodynia.*
o. denta′lis reflex pain in the ear due to dental disease.
o. intermit′tens otalgia of an intermittent type.
reflex o. referred pain (q.v.) in the ear, usually from a lesion of the buccal cavity or nasopharynx.
secondary o. otalgia due to inflammation of the geniculate ganglion.
tabetic o. otalgia in tabes dorsalis owing to degeneration of the intermediate nerve.

otal·gic (o-tal′jik) 1. pertaining to earache. 2. an earache remedy.

OTC 1. over the counter; applied to drugs not required by law to be sold on prescription only. 2. ornithine transcarbamoylase; see *ornithine carbamoyltransferase.*

OTD organ tolerance dose.

otic (o′tik) [Gr. *ōtikos*] pertaining to the ear; called also *aural.*

Oti·o·bi·us (o″te-o′be-əs) *Otobius.*

oti·tis (o-ti′tis) [*ot-* + *-itis*] inflammation of the ear, often with pain, fever, hearing loss, tinnitus, and vertigo. See also *o. externa, o. media,* and *o. interna.* **otit′ic** *adj*
aviation o. barotitis media.
o. desquamati′va otitis externa or media in which there are overdevelopment and desquamation of the cutaneous or mucous epithelium.
o. exter′na inflammation of the external auditory canal.
o. externa, acute acute infection of the cartilaginous external auditory meatus, caused by either a fungus *(otomycosis)* or a bacteria *(acute bacterial otitis externa).* It is common in swimmers and in hot, humid weather. Symptoms include pain and swelling, sometimes with formation of a circumscribed furuncle *(circumscribed otitis externa).* Called also *swimmer's ear* and *tank ear.*
o. externa, acute bacterial acute otitis externa caused by a bacterial infection, usually with a species of *Pseudomonas* and less often with *Staphylococcus* and formation of a furuncle. See also *circumscribed o. externa.*
o. externa, acute fungal otomycosis.
o. externa, circumscribed acute bacterial otitis externa in a limited area with formation of a furuncle, which may obstruct the canal; usually due to a staphylococcal infection. Cf. *diffuse o. externa.* Called also *furuncular o. externa* and *furuncular o.*
o. externa, diffuse otitis externa involving a relatively wide area, without formation of a furuncle. Cf. *circumscribed o. externa.*
o. externa, fungal otomycosis.
o. externa, furuncular circumscribed o. externa.

o. externa, malignant a progressive, necrotizing, frequently fatal infection of the external auditory canal and base of the skull, caused by *Pseudomonas aeruginosa;* it affects chiefly elderly diabetic and immunocompromised patients. Called also *necrotizing o. externa.*
o. externa, necrotizing malignant o. externa.
external o. o. externa.
furuncular o. circumscribed o. externa.
o. inter′na labyrinthitis.
o. me′dia inflammation of the middle ear; subtypes are distinguished by length of time from onset *(acute* versus *chronic)* and by type of discharge *(serous* versus *suppurative).*
o. media, adhesive tympanic membrane atelectasis.
o. media, atelectatic tympanic membrane atelectasis.
o. media, catarrhal serous o. media.
o. media, mucoid serous otitis media in which the secretion is particularly viscous.
o. media, purulent suppurative o. media.
o. media, secretory serous o. media.
o. media, serous chronic otitis media marked by serous effusion into the middle ear. Called also *secretory* or *catarrhal o. media.*
o. media, suppurative otitis media with a discharge of pus (otorrhea); infecting bacteria are usually *Streptococcus* species, *Haemophilus influenzae,* or *Staphylococcus aureus.* It may be either acute or chronic. See also *Gradenigo syndrome.* Called also *purulent o. media.*
parasitic o. otoacariasis.

ot(o)- [Gr. *ous,* gen. *ōtos* ear] a combining form denoting relationship to the ear.

oto•ac•a•ri•a•sis (o″to-ak″ə-ri′ə-sis) [*oto-* + *acariasis*] infection of the ears of cats, dogs, and domestic rabbits with the mite *Otodectes;* see also *otodectic mange.* Called also *otocariasis* and *parasitic otitis.*

oto•bi•o•sis (o″to-bi-o′sis) infestation of an animal by ticks of the genus *Otobius.*

Oto•bi•us (o-to′be-əs) [*oto-* + Gr. *bios* manner of living] a genus of argasid ticks, originally native to the western United States and Canada but now found around the world. The nymphs of *O. megni′ni,* the spinose ear tick of cattle and other domestic animals, may also attack human ears but is not a vector for disease.

oto•ca•ri•a•sis (o″to-kə-ri′ə-sis) otoacariasis.

Oto•cen•tor (o″to-sen′tor) *Anocentor.*

oto•ceph•a•lus (o″to-sef′ə-ləs) otocephaly.

oto•ceph•a•ly (o″to-sef′ə-le) [*oto-* + *-cephaly*] a congenital anomaly characterized by lack of a lower jaw and by ears that are united inferior to the face.

oto•cer•e•bri•tis (o″to-ser″ə-bri′tis) otoencephalitis.

oto•co•nia (o″to-ko′ne-ə) [*oto-* + *coni-* + *-ia*] plural of otoconium.

otoc•o•nite (o-tok′o-nīt) statoconium.

oto•co•ni•um (o″to-ko′ne-əm) [L.] statoconium.

oto•cra•ni•um (o″to-kra′ne-əm) [*oto-* + *cranium*] the area of the petrous part of the temporal bone surrounding the osseous labyrinth. **otocra′nial** *adj*

oto•cyst (o′to-sist″) [*oto-* + *cyst*] 1. the auditory vesicle of the embryo, the primordium of the internal ear. 2. the auditory sac of certain animals.

Oto•dec•tes (o″to-dek′tēz) [*oto-* + Gr. *dēktēs* a biter] a genus of mange mites of the family Psoroptidae. *O. cyno′tis* infests the external ear canal of cats, dogs, foxes, and ferrets, causing otodectic mange and otoacariasis.

oto•dec•tic (o″to-dek′tik) pertaining to or caused by *Otodectes.*

oto•dyn•ia (o″to-din′e-ə) [*oto-* + *-odynia*] otalgia.

oto•en•ceph•a•li•tis (o″to-ən-sef″ə-li′tis) [*oto-* + *encephalitis*] inflammation of the brain due to an extension from an inflamed middle ear. See also *otitis media.*

oto•gen•ic (o″to-jen′ik) otogenous.

otog•e•nous (o-toj′ə-nəs) [*oto-* + *-genous*] originating within the ear.

otog•ra•phy (o-tog′rə-fe) [*oto-* + *-graphy*] a description of the ear.

oto•lar•yn•gol•o•gy (o″to-lar″ing-gol′ə-je) [*oto-* + *laryngo-* + *-logy*] the branch of medicine concerned with medical and surgical treatment of the head and neck, including the ears, nose, and throat. Called also *otorhinolaryngology.*

oto•lite (o′to-līt) 1. statoconium. 2. otolith (def. 2).

oto•lith (o′to-lith″) [*oto-* + *-lith*] 1. statoconium. 2. a calcareous mass in the internal ear of vertebrates or in the otocyst of invertebrates.

otol•o•gist (o-tol′ə-jist) a physician who specializes in otology.

otol•o•gy (o-tol′ə-je) [*oto-* + *-logy*] the branch of medicine that deals with the medical treatment and surgery of the ear, and its anatomy, physiology, and pathology. **otolog′ic** *adj*

oto•mas•toid•itis (o″to-mas″toid-i′tis) mastoiditis combined with otitis media, usually of the suppurative type.

oto•mi•cro•scope (o″to-mi′kro-skōp) a microscope for examination of structures inside the ear.

oto•mi•cros•co•py (o″to-mi-kros′kə-pe) examination of structures inside the ear with an otomicroscope.

oto•my•co•sis (o″to-mi-ko′sis) [*oto-* + *-mycosis*] fungal infection of the external auditory meatus, usually by a species of *Aspergillus,* marked by pruritus and exudative inflammation; there may be secondary bacterial infection. It is more common in hot weather and tropical climates. Called also *fungal* or *acute fungal otitis externa.*
***Aspergillus* o.** otomycosis caused by a species of *Aspergillus,* usually *A. niger.* Called also *aural aspergillosis.*

oto•my•ia•sis (o″to-mi-i′ə-sis) infestation of the ear by larvae.

oto•neu•ral•gia (o″to-no͝o-ral′jə) [*oto-* + *neuralgia*] neuralgic pain in the ear.

oto•neu•ro•log•ic (o″to-noo″ro-loj′ik) pertaining to those portions of the nervous system relating to the ear.

oto•neu•rol•o•gy (o″to-no͝o-rol′ə-je) neuro-otology.

oto•pha•ryn•ge•al (o″to-fə-rin′je-əl) pertaining to the ear and pharynx.

oto•plas•ty (o′to-plas″te) [*oto-* + *-plasty*] plastic surgery of the ear, done to correct deformities and defects. **otoplas′tic** *adj*

oto•py•or•rhea (o″to-pi″o-re′ə) [*oto-* + *pyorrhea*] otorrhea that is purulent.

oto•rhi•no•lar•yn•gol•o•gy (o″to-ri″no-lar″ing-gol′ə-je) [*oto-* + *rhino-* + *laryngo-* + *-logy*] otolaryngology.

oto•rhi•nol•o•gy (o″to-ri-nol′ə-je) [*oto-* + *rhino-* + *-logy*] the branch of medicine that deals with the nose and ear and their diseases.

otor•rhea (o″to-re′ə) [*oto-* + *-rrhea*] a discharge from the ear, especially a purulent one.
cerebrospinal fluid o. escape of cerebrospinal fluid through the external auditory meatus due to fracture or other pathology of the temporal bone; cf. *cerebrospinal fluid fistula.*

oto•sal•pinx (o″to-sal′pinks) [*oto-* + *salpinx*] tuba auditiva.

oto•scle•ro•sis (o″to-sklə-ro′sis) [*oto-* + *sclerosis*] otospongiosis of the bony labyrinth, especially adjacent to the footplate of the stapes; it may cause bony ankylosis of the stapes, resulting in conductive hearing loss. Cochlear otosclerosis may also develop, resulting in sensorineural hearing loss. **otosclerot′ic** *adj*

oto•scope (o′to-skōp″) [*oto-* + *-scope*] an instrument for inspecting or auscultating the ear; called also *auriscope.*
Siegle o. an otoscope which gives a view of the drum membrane when subjected to condensed or rarefied air.

otos•co•py (o-tos′kə-pe) examination of the ear by means of the otoscope.

oto•sis (o-to′sis) a false impression of sounds uttered by others.

oto•spon•gi•o•sis (o″to-spun″je-o′sis) the formation of spongy bone in the bony labyrinth of the ear; see *otosclerosis.*

oto•tox•ic (o′to-tok″sik) causing damage to the vestibulocochlear nerve or the organs of hearing and balance. See also *ototoxicity.*

oto•tox•ic•i•ty (o″to-tok-sis′ĭ-te) the quality of causing damage to the vestibulocochlear nerve or the organs of hearing and balance. See also *ototoxic hearing loss,* under *hearing loss.*

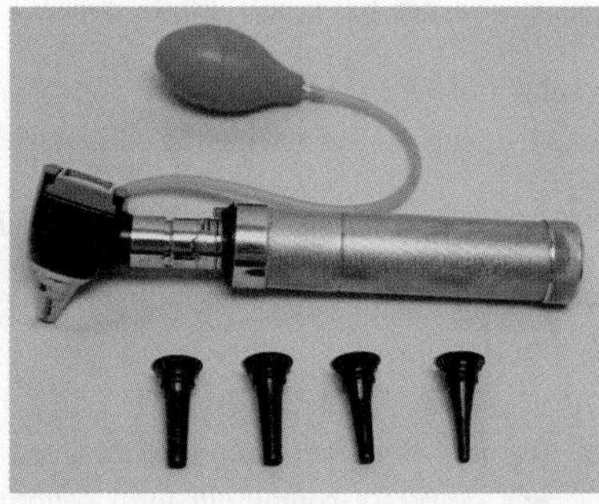

■ Otoscope with specula of various sizes and pneumatic attachment.

Ot·to disease, pelvis (ot′o) [Adolph Wilhelm *Otto*, German surgeon, 1786–1845] see *protrusio acetabuli* and see under *pelvis.*

OU [L.] o′culus uter′que (each eye).

oua·ba·in (wah-ba′in) a cardiac glycoside consisting of a molecule of rhamnose linked to a steroid nucleus, obtained principally from the seeds of *Strophanthus gratus* (Wall & Hock.) Baill. (Apocynaceae), having the same actions as digitalis but producing digitalization more rapidly; used in the emergency treatment of acute congestive heart failure, administered intravenously. Called also *G-strophanthin* or *strophanthin-G.*

Ouch·ter·lo·ny technique (test) (ok′tər-lo″ne) [Orjan Thomas Gunnarson *Ouchterlony,* Swedish bacteriologist, 1914–2004] double diffusion in two dimensions; see under *diffusion.*

ounce (oz) (ouns) [L. *uncia*] a measure of weight in both the avoirdupois and apothecaries' systems. The ounce *avoirdupois* is one sixteenth of a pound, or 437.5 grains (28.3495 g). The *apothecaries'* ounce, symbol ℥, is one twelfth of a pound, or 480 grains (31.103 g).

fluid o. (fl oz) a unit of capacity (liquid measure) of the apothecaries' system, in the United States being 8 fluid drams, one sixteenth of a pint, or the equivalent of 29.57 mL. In Great Britain, it is an *imperial ounce* and is 8 (imperial) fluid drams but is one twentieth of an (imperial) pint, or 28.41 mL.

-ous 1. a suffix meaning possessing, having, or full of, e.g., cancerous. 2. in chemistry, a suffix used to indicate an ion or acid exhibiting the lower of two oxidation states, the other being indicated by the suffix *-ic.*

out·breed·ing (out′brēd-ing) the breeding of genetically unrelated plants or animals; called also *crossbreeding.*

out·let (out′lət) a means or route of exit or egress.

bladder o. ostium urethrae internum.
gastric o. ostium pyloricum.
pelvic o. apertura pelvis inferior.
pyloric o. ostium pyloricum.
thoracic o. apertura thoracis inferior. NOTE: the term is used differently clinically in "thoracic outlet syndrome"; see note at *apertura thoracis superior.*

out·li·er (out′li-ər) in statistics, an observation so distant from the central mass of the data that it noticeably influences results; it is often considered an error and removed from the data, although not necessarily appropriately so.

out·pa·tient (out′pa-shənt) a patient who comes to the hospital, clinic, or dispensary for diagnosis and/or treatment but does not occupy a bed.

out·pock·et·ing (out-pok′ət-ing) evagination.

out·pouch·ing (out′pouch-ing) evagination.

out·put (out′poot″) the yield; the total of anything produced by any functional system of the body.

basal acid o. (BAO) on the pentagastrin test, the output of gastric acid for one hour with minimal stimulation in a fasting patient, expressed as mmol/hr.

cardiac o. (CO) the effective volume of blood expelled by either ventricle of the heart per unit of time (usually volume per minute); it is equal to the stroke volume multiplied by the heart rate.

energy o. the energy a body is able to manifest in work or activity.

maximal acid o. (MAO) on the pentagastrin test, the output of gastric acid for one hour after administration of pentagastrin, expressed as mmol/hr.

peak acid o. (PAO) on the pentagastrin test, after administration of pentagastrin, the sum of the two highest 15-minute outputs of gastric acid multiplied by 2, expressed as mmol/hr.

stroke o. see under *volume.*

urinary o. the amount of urine excreted by the kidneys.

work o. of the heart the amount of energy that the heart converts to work; usually expressed per heart beat *(stroke work o.)* or per minute *(minute work o.).*

ova (o′və) [L.] plural of *ovum.*

oval (o′vəl) [L. *ovalis*] egg-shaped; having the outline of the long section of an egg.

ov·al·bu·min (ōv″al-bu′min) [*ovum* + *albumin*] an albumin obtainable from the whites of eggs.

ovalo·cyte (o′və-lo-sīt) elliptocyte.

ovalo·cy·to·sis (o-val″o-si-to′sis) elliptocytosis.

ovar·i·al·gia (o-var″e-al′jə) oophoralgia.

ovar·i·ec·to·my (o-var″e-ek′tə-me) oophorectomy.

ovari(o)- [L. *ovarium* ovary] a combining form denoting relationship to the ovary.

ovar·io·cele (o-var′e-o-sēl) [*ovario-* + *-cele*[1]] ovarian hernia.

ovar·io·cen·te·sis (o-var″e-o-sen-te′sis) [*ovario-* + *-centesis*] surgical puncture of an ovary.

ovar·io·cy·e·sis (o-var″e-o-si-e′sis) [*ovario-* + *-cyesis*] ovarian pregnancy.

ovar·io·gen·ic (o-var″e-o-jen′ik) arising in the ovary.

ovar·io·hys·ter·ec·to·my (o-var″e-o-his″tər-ek′tə-me) oophorohysterectomy.

ovar·i·op·a·thy (o-var″e-op′ə-the) [*ovario-* + *-pathy*] oophoropathy.

ovar·io·pexy (o-var″e-o-pek′se) [*ovario-* + *-pexy*] oophoropexy.

ovar·i·or·rhex·is (o-var″re-o-rek′sis) [*ovario-* + *-rrhexis*] rupture of an ovary.

ovar·io·sal·pin·gec·to·my (o-var″e-o-sal″pin-jek′tə-me) salpingo-oophorectomy.

ovar·i·os·to·my (o-var″e-os′tə-me) oophorostomy.

ovar·io·tes·tis (o-var″e-o-tes′tis) ovotestis.

ovar·i·ot·o·my (o-var″e-ot′ə-me) [*ovario-* + *-tomy*] 1. oophorectomy. 2. removal of an ovarian tumor.

abdominal o. ovariotomy performed through the abdominal wall.
vaginal o. ovariotomy performed through the vagina.

ovar·io·tu·bal (o-var″e-o-too′bəl) tubo-ovarian.

ova·ri·tis (o″və-ri′tis) oophoritis.

ova·ri·um (o-var′e-əm) pl. *ova′ria* [L.] [TA] ovary: the female gonad, one of the two sexual glands in which the oocytes are formed. It is a flat oval body along the lateral wall of the pelvic cavity, attached to the posterior surface of the broad ligament. It consists of a cortex and medulla; the former is composed of stroma and ovarian follicles in various stages of maturation, and the latter, occupying a small area in the hilar region, receives the vessels and nerves. The ovarium is covered by specialized epithelium continuous with the peritoneum at the mesovarium.

o. masculi′num appendix testis.

ova·ry (o′və-re) ovarium. **ova′rian** *adj*

polycystic o's 1. ovaries containing multiple, small follicular cysts filled with yellow or blood-stained, thin serous fluid, characteristic of polycystic ovary syndrome. 2. polycystic ovary syndrome.

Ov·con (ov′kon) trademark for combination preparations of norethindrone and ethinyl estradiol.

OVD occlusal vertical dimension.

over·ac·tiv·i·ty (o″vər-ak-tiv′ĭ-te) hyperactivity (def. 1).

detrusor o. involuntary contractions of the detrusor urinae muscle from any cause; see *detrusor hyperreflexia* and *detrusor instability.* Called also *detrusor hyperactivity.*

over·bite (o′vər-bīt″) vertical overlap (def. 1).

deep o. closed bite.
horizontal o. see under *overlap.*
vertical o. see under *overlap.*

over·clo·sure (o″vər-klo′zhər) the loss of occlusal vertical dimension.

reduced interarch distance o. the loss of occlusal or contact vertical dimension.

over·com·pen·sa·tion (o″vər-kom″pən-sa′shən) conscious or unconscious exaggerated correction for a real or imagined physical or psychological deficiency.

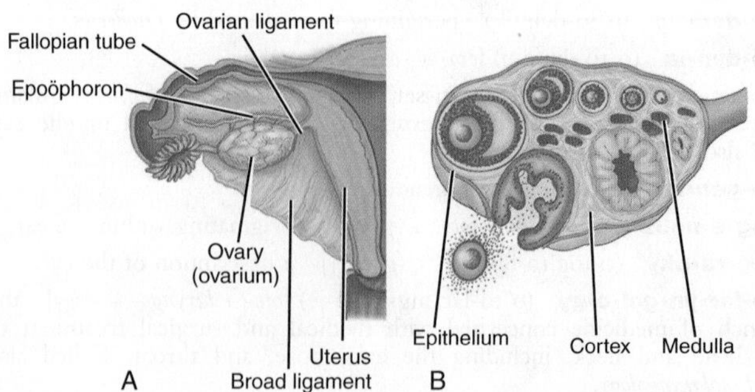

■ Ovarium (ovary). *(A),* Reproductive organs. *(B),* Ovarian microstructure, with the stages of ovarian follicle development depicted counterclockwise from the top right, showing follicles progressively more mature: from primordial to primary, secondary, then tertiary, followed by ovulation, and finally corpora lutea from maturation to degeneration.

over·cor·rec·tion (o″vər-kə-rek′shən) the use of too powerful lenses in correcting defect of vision.

over·den·ture (o″vər-den′chər) overlay denture.

over·de·ter·mi·na·tion (o″vər-de-ter″mĭ-na′shən) in psychoanalytic theory, the concept that every dream, disorder, aspect of behavior, or other emotional reaction or symptom has multiple causative factors.

over·do·sage (o″vər-do′səj) 1. the administration of an excessive dose. 2. the condition resulting from an excessive dose.

over·dose (o′vər-dōs″) 1. to administer an excessive dose. 2. an excessive dose.

over·drive (o′vər-drīv″) in cardiology, a more rapid heart rate produced in the correction of an underlying pathologic rhythm; see also under *pacing*.

over·erup·tion (o″vər-e-rup′shən) supraclusion.

over·ex·ten·sion (o″vər-ek-sten′shən) extension, as of a limb, beyond the normal limit.

over·flow (o′vər-flo) the continuous escape of a fluid, as of the tears or the urine.

motor o. contralateral associated movement.

over·graft·ing (o″vər-graft′ing) the application of a second skin graft over a previously healed graft from which the epithelium has been removed, as a means of reinforcing split-thickness grafts.

over·growth (o′vər-grōth) 1. excessive growth, as of plants, fungi, or bacteria. 2. in particular, excessive growth of a part, due either to increase in size of the constituent cells (hypertrophy) or to an increase in their number (hyperplasia).

small intestinal bacterial o. stasis syndrome.

over·hang (o′vər-hang) the extension, over the margins of a tooth cavity, of an excessive amount of filling material.

over·hy·dra·tion (o″vər-hi-dra′shən) hyperhydration.

over·in·fla·tion (o″vər-in-fla′shən) hyperinflation.

congenital lobar o. see under *emphysema*.

nonobstructive pulmonary o. compensatory emphysema.

obstructive pulmonary o. localized obstructive emphysema.

over·jet (o′vər-jet″) horizontal overlap.

over·jut (o′vər-jət) horizontal overlap.

over·lap (o′vər-lap) 1. to cover and extend beyond a certain point. 2. anything that lies or extends over and partially covers something.

horizontal o. extension of the incisal or buccal cusp ridges of the maxillary teeth labially or buccally to the incisal margins and ridges of the mandibular teeth when the jaws are in habitual occlusion. Called also *horizontal overbite*, *overjet*, and *overjut*.

vertical o. 1. extension of the incisal ridges of the maxillary anterior teeth below the incisal ridges of the mandibular anterior teeth when the jaws are in centric occlusion. Cf. *micrognathia*. Called also *overbite* or *over bite* and *vertical overbite*. 2. the distance that the teeth lap over their antagonists. 3. the relationship of the maxillary incisors to the mandibular incisors when the incisal edges pass each other in centric occlusion.

over·lay (o′vər-la) an increment; a later addition superimposed upon an already existing mass, state, or condition.

emotional o. psychogenic o.

psychogenic o. the emotionally determined increment to an existing organic symptom or disability.

over·load (o′vər-lōd) excess.

African iron o. genetic predisposition to iron loading that is exacerbated by excessive intake of dietary iron; seen in persons of African descent. Called also *Bantu siderosis*.

iron o. an excess of iron in the body; see *hemochromatosis*, *hemosiderosis*, and *siderosis*.

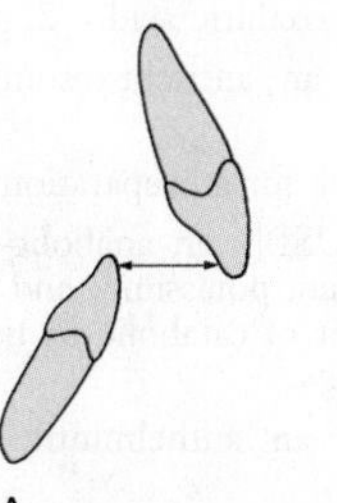

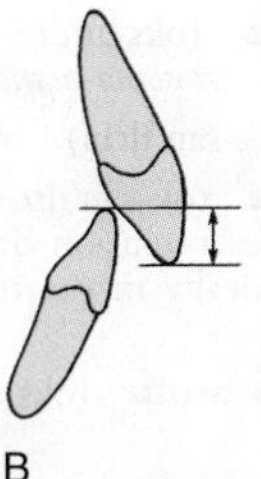

■ *(A)*, Horizontal overlap (overjet); *(B)*, vertical overlap (overbite).

sensory o. a condition in which an individual receives an excessive or intolerable amount of sensory stimuli; the effects of sensory overload are similar to those of sensory deprivation, including confusion and hallucination.

over·match·ing (o″vər-mach′ing) in statistics, matching of too many variables or matching variables too closely when selecting cases and controls for study, so that true causal relationships between variables may be obscured, irrelevant variables may be included, or the study may become too complex and specific for appropriate controls to be reasonably obtained.

over·nu·tri·tion (o″vər-noo-trĭ′shən) hyperalimentation (def. 1).

over·reach·ing (o″vər-rēch′ing) an error of gait in the horse, in which the toe of the hind hoof strikes the heel of the forefoot.

over·re·sponse (o″vər-re-spons′) abnormally intense response or reaction to a stimulus.

over·rid·ing (o″vər-rīd′ing) 1. the slipping of either part of a fractured bone past the other. 2. extending beyond the usual position.

over·sens·ing (o′vər-sens″ing) inappropriate sensing of electrical signals by an artificial cardiac pacemaker, either extracardiac signals or cardiac signals other than those it is set to detect; in demand pacemakers the result is slowed or irregular pacemaker output.

over·stain (o′vər-stān) to stain a tissue excessively, so that certain elements may be properly stained when the excess of stain is washed out.

over·strain (o′vər-strān) an abnormal degree of fatigue brought about by activity; it is intermediate between fatigue and actual exhaustion.

over·stress (o′vər-stres) excessive activity resulting in overstrain.

over·toe (o′vər-to) hallux valgus in which the great toe overlies its fellows.

over·tone (o′vər-tōn) any whole number multiple of a fundamental tone.

psychic o. the consciousness of a fringe or halo of associated relations that surrounds every image presented to the mind.

over·trans·fu·sion (o″vər-trans-fu′zhən) overloading of the circulation by excessive transfusion of blood or other fluid; see *hypervolemia*.

over·ven·ti·la·tion (o″vər-ven″tĭ-la′shən) hyperventilation.

over·weight (o′vər-wāt) excessive increase in adipose tissue (obese overweight) or in muscle and skeletal tissue (muscular overweight).

ovi- see *ov(o)-*.

ovi·cide (o′vĭ-sīd) an agent destructive to the eggs of certain organisms.

Ovide (o′vīd) trademark for a preparation of malathion.

Ovi·drel (ov′ĭ-drel) trademark for a preparation of choriogonadotropin alfa.

ovi·du·cal (o′vĭ-doo-kəl) oviductal.

ovi·duct (o′vĭ-dukt″) [*ovi-* + *duct*] 1. tuba uterina. 2. in nonmammals, a passage through which ova leave the maternal organism or pass to an organ that communicates with the exterior of the body.

ovi·duc·tal (o″vĭ-duk′təl) 1. pertaining to an oviduct. 2. pertaining to a uterine tube (oviduct); see *tubal*.

ovif·er·ous (o-vif′ər-əs) [*ovi-* + *-ferous*] producing ova.

ovi·form (o′vĭ-form) [*ovi-* + *form*] oval.

ovi·gen·e·sis (o″vĭ-jen′ə-sis) [*ovi-* + *-genesis*] oogenesis.

ovi·ge·net·ic (o″vĭ-jə-net′ik) oogenetic.

ovi·gen·ic (o″vĭ-jen′ik) oogenetic.

ovig·e·nous (o-vij′ə-nəs) oogenetic.

ovig·er·ous (o-vij′ər-əs) [*ovi-* + L. *gerere* to bear] producing or containing ova.

ovine (o′vīn) [L. *ovinus* of a sheep] pertaining to, characteristic of, or derived from sheep.

ovi·par·i·ty (o″vĭ-par′ĭ-te) the quality of being oviparous.

ovip·a·rous (o-vip′ə-rəs) [*ovi-* + *-parous*] capable of producing eggs from which the young are hatched outside the body of the maternal organism. Cf. *ovoviviparous* and *viviparous*.

ovi·po·si·tion (o″vĭ-pə-zĭ′shən) [*ovi-* + L. *ponere* to place] the act of laying or depositing eggs.

ovi·pos·i·tor (o″vĭ-poz′ĭ-tər) a specialized organ by means of which many female insects deposit their eggs in various plant structures or in the soil.

ovi·sac (o′vĭ-sak) [*ovi-* + *sac*] an egg-containing capsule, such as a vesicular ovarian follicle.

ov(o)- [L. *ovum* egg] a combining form denoting relationship to an egg, or to ova. Also, *ovi-*. See also words beginning *oo-*.

ovo·cyte (o′vo-sīt) oocyte.

ovo·gen·e·sis (o″vo-jen′ə-sis) oogenesis.

ovo·glob·u·lin (o″vo-glob′u-lin) a globulin found in the white of an egg.

ovo·go·ni·um (o″vo-go′ne-əm) oogonium.

ovoid (o′void) [*ovo-* + *-oid*] 1. oval. 2. an egg-shaped structure.
myelin o's small oval compartments containing myelin that are formed by the breaking up of the myelin sheath in wallerian degeneration.

ovo·lac·to·veg·e·tar·i·an (o″vo-lak″to-vej″ə-tar′e-ən) 1. pertaining to ovolactovegetarianism. 2. one who practices ovolactovegetarianism.

ovo·lac·to·veg·e·tar·i·an·ism (o″vo-lak″to-vej″ə-tar′e-ən-iz″əm) restriction of the diet to vegetables, dairy products, and eggs, eschewing other foods of animal origin.

ovo·lyt·ic (o″vo-lit′ik) splitting up egg albumin.

ovo·mu·cin (o″vo-mu′sin) a glycoprotein from the white of egg.

ovo·mu·coid (o″vo-mu′koid) [*ovo-* + *mucoid*] a glycoprotein derivable from egg white.

ovo·plasm (o′vo-plaz″əm) [*ovo-* + *-plasm*] ooplasm.

ovo·tes·tis (o″vo-tes′tis) an abnormal gonad containing both testicular and ovarian tissue, seen in hermaphroditism. Called also *ovariotestis.*

ovo·trans·fer·rin (o″vo-trans-fer′in) an iron-binding protein in egg white having the same properties as transferrin.

ovo·veg·e·tar·i·an (o″vo-vej″ə-tar′e-ən) 1. pertaining to ovovegetarianism. 2. one who practices ovovegetarianism.

ovo·veg·e·tar·i·an·ism (o″vo-vej″ə-tar′e-ən-iz″əm) restriction of the diet to vegetables and eggs, eschewing other foods of animal origin.

ovo·vi·tel·lin (o″vo-vi-tel′in) vitellin.

ovo·vivi·par·i·ty (o″vo-viv″ĭ-par′ĭ-te) the quality of being ovoviviparous.

ovo·vi·vip·a·rous (o″vo-vi-vip′ə-rəs) [*ovo-* + *vivi-* + *-parous*] bearing living young that hatch from large, yolk-filled eggs inside the body of the maternal organism, the embryo being nourished by food stored in the egg; said of lizards, etc. Cf. *oviparous* and *viviparous.*

Ov·ral (ōv′ral) trademark for combination preparations of norgestrel and ethinyl estradiol.

Ov·rette (ōv-ret′) trademark for a preparation of norgestrel.

ovu·lar (ov′u-lər) 1. pertaining to an ovule. 2. pertaining to an oocyte.

ovu·la·tion (ov″u-la′shən) the discharge of a secondary oocyte from a vesicular ovarian follicle. **ov′ulatory** *adj*
amenstrual o. ovulation that occurs in the absence of menstrual bleeding.
anestrous o. ovulation that occurs in animals unaccompanied by other events of estrus.
paracyclic o., supplementary o. an extra ovulation in a particular estrous cycle.

ovule (o′vūl) [L. *ovulum*] 1. the oocyte within the ovarian (graafian) follicle. 2. any small, egglike structure. 3. the megasporangium enclosed within one or more integuments that, after fertilization, becomes a plant seed.

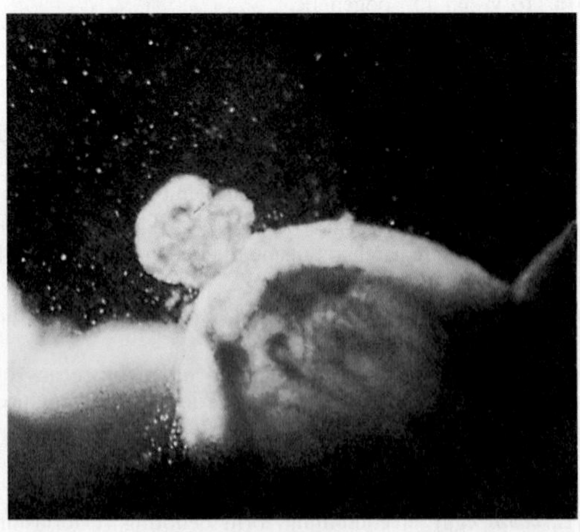

■ Ovulation.

primordial o. a rudimentary oocyte within the ovary.

ovu·log·e·nous (ov″u-loj′ə-nəs) producing or developing from an ovule or oocyte.

ovum (o′vəm) gen. *o′vi* pl. *o′va* [L.] 1. the female reproductive cell which, after fertilization, becomes a zygote that develops into a new member of the same species. 2. imprecise term for *oocyte.* 3. formerly, any of various stages from the primary oocyte to the implanting blastocyst. 4. in some species (e.g., insects, birds, reptiles), any stage from the unfertilized female reproductive cell, through the developing embryo surrounded by nutrient material and protective covering, up to the point when the young emerge.
blighted o. a zygote (not actually an ovum) in which development has ceased at an early stage, and abnormality or degeneration is evident.
Hertig-Rock ova 34 embryos, ranging from 1 to 17 days of age, 21 of which were normal, and 13 abnormal to one degree or another; isolated between 1938 and 1953, they constitute the only series of such early human conceptuses in existence.

Owen lines (o′ən) [Sir Richard *Owen*, English anatomist and paleontologist, 1804–1892] see under *line.*

Ow·ren disease (o′ren) [Paul Arnor *Owren*, Norwegian hematologist, 1905–1990] parahemophilia.

ox- see *oxy-.*

ox·ac·id (oks-as′id) oxyacid.

ox·a·cil·lin so·di·um (oks″ə-sil′in) [USP] a semisynthetic penicillinase-resistant isoxazolyl penicillin, used primarily in the treatment of infections due to penicillin-resistant staphylococci; administered orally, intramuscularly, or intravenously.

ox·al·al·de·hyde (ok″səl-al′də-hīd) glyoxal.

ox·a·late (ok′sə-lāt) a salt of oxalic acid; see also *oxalate poisoning,* under *poisoning.*
balanced o. a mixture of ammonium and potassium oxalates in a 3:2 ratio, used as an anticoagulant in the collection of blood for laboratory examination.

ox·a·lat·ed (ok′sə-lāt″əd) treated with oxalate solution.

ox·a·la·tion (ok″sə-la′shən) treatment with or exposure to oxalates.

ox·a·le·mia (ok″sə-le′me-ə) [*oxalate* + *-emia*] an excess of oxalates in the blood.

ox·al·ic ac·id (ok-sal′ik) HOOC•COOH, a strong dicarboxylic acid found in foods such as spinach and rhubarb or produced in the body by metabolism of glyoxylic acid or ascorbic acid; it is not metabolized but excreted in the urine. Ingestion of a diet rich in oxalates or a genetic disorder of glycine metabolism (primary hyperoxaluria) may lead to the formation of oxalate calculi in the urinary tract. See also *oxalate poisoning,* under *poisoning.*

ox·a·li·plat·in (ok′sə-le-plat″in) a platinum-based compound chemically related to cisplatin and carboplatin, used as an antineoplastic in treatment of stage III colon cancer after the primary tumor has been removed; administered by intravenous injection.

ox·al·ism (ok′səl-iz″əm) oxalate poisoning.

ox·a·lo·ac·e·tate (ok″sə-lo-as′ə-tāt) an anionic form of oxaloacetic acid.

ox·a·lo·ace·tic ac·id (ok″sə-lo-ə-se′tik) an intermediate in the tricarboxylic acid cycle (q.v.); it is convertible to aspartic acid by a transamination reaction.

ox·a·lo·sis (ok″sə-lo′sis) generalized deposition of calcium oxalate in renal and extrarenal tissues, as may occur in primary hyperoxaluria.

ox·al·uria (ok″səl-u′re-ə) hyperoxaluria.

ox·al·ur·ic ac·id (ok″səl-ūr′ik) the amide of oxalic acid and urea, which occurs in urine.

ox·a·lyl (ok′sə-ləl) the divalent group, $(C{:}O)_2$, formed from oxalic acid by the loss of two hydroxyl groups.

ox·a·lyl·urea (ok″sə-ləl-u′re-ə) 1. oxaluric acid. 2. parabanic acid.

ox·am·ni·quine (oks-am′nĭ-kwin) an antischistosomal especially effective against *Schistosoma mansoni.*

Ox·an·drin (ok-san′drin) trademark for a preparation of oxandrolone.

ox·an·dro·lone (ok-san′dro-lōn) [USP] an anabolic-androgenic steroid that promotes retention of nitrogen, potassium, and phosphorus, and is administered orally in the treatment of catabolic or tissue-wasting diseases or states.

ox·an·tel pam·o·ate (oks′ən-təl) an anthelmintic effective against *Trichuris.*

ox·a·pro·zin (ok″sə-pro′zin) [USP] a nonsteroidal antiinflammatory drug, used in the treatment of rheumatoid arthritis and osteoarthritis.

ox•az•e•pam (ok-saz′ə-pam) [USP] a benzodiazepine used as an antianxiety agent in the treatment of anxiety disorders and anxiety associated with depression, for short-term relief of anxiety symptoms, especially in the elderly, and for the treatment of the symptoms of acute alcohol withdrawal; administered orally.

oxa•zo•lid•in•one (ok″sə-zo-lid′ĭ-nōn) any of a class of synthetic, heterocyclic antibacterial agents effective against gram-positive organisms; they bind to the bacterial 50S ribosomal subunit and prevent formation of the 70S ribosomal initiation complex, thus preventing bacterial RNA translation and protein synthesis.

ox•car•baz•e•pine (oks″kahr-baz′ə-pēn) an anticonvulsant used in the treatment of partial seizures; administered orally.

ox•et•o•rone fu•mar•ate (ok-set′o-rōn) an analgesic specific in migraine.

ox•fen•da•zole (oks-fen′də-zōl) [USP] a benzimidazole anthelmintic used to treat ruminant infestatations by either roundworms or tapeworms.

ox•i•ben•da•zole (ok″sĭ-ben′də-zōl) a benzimidazole anthelmintic used to treat roundworm and lungworm infestations in horses and other ruminants.

ox•i•con•a•zole ni•trate (ok″sĭ-kon′ə-zōl) an imidazole antifungal used topically in the treatment of tinea pedis, tinea corporis, and tinea cruris; it inhibits biosynthesis of ergosterol, a component of the fungal cell membrane.

ox•i•dant (ok′sĭ-dənt) the electron acceptor in an oxidation-reduction (redox) reaction.

ox•i•dase (ok′sĭ-dās) a term used in the recommended names of some oxidoreductases to denote those in which molecular oxygen is the hydrogen acceptor.

mixed function o. monooxygenase.

ox•i•da•tion (ok″sĭ-da′shən) the act of oxidizing or state of being oxidized. Chemically it consists of the increase of positive charges on an atom or the loss of negative charges. Most biological oxidations are accomplished by the removal of a pair of hydrogen atoms (dehydrogenation) from a molecule. Such oxidations must be accompanied by reduction of an acceptor molecule. *Univalent o.* indicates loss of one electron; *divalent o.*, the loss of two electrons.

alpha o. oxidation of a fatty acid at the alpha carbon, that adjacent to the carboxyl group, as occurs in the metabolism of phytanic acid. Written also *α-oxidation.*

beta o. oxidation of a fatty acid at the beta carbon atom, the second carbon from the carboxyl group, with the result that the two end carbons are split off as acetic acid (acetyl coenzyme A) and with the formation of a fatty acid containing two fewer carbon atoms. Written also *β-oxidation.*

biological o. the enzymatic process by which food is metabolized, resulting in the release of energy. See also *oxidation.*

coupled o. the enzymatic oxidation of two donor molecules, with the incorporation of oxygen into one of the donors.

omega o. a minor pathway of fatty acid oxidation in which the ω-carbon is oxidized, forming an α,ω-dicarboxylic acid. Written also *ω-oxidation.*

ox•i•da•tion-re•duc•tion (ok″sĭ-da′shən re-duk′shən) the chemical reaction whereby electrons are removed (oxidation) from atoms of the substance being oxidized and transferred to atoms being reduced (reduction). Called also *redox.*

ox•i•da•tive (ok′sĭ-da-tiv) 1. pertaining to oxidation. 2. capable of oxidation.

ox•ide (ok′sīd) [L. *oxidum*] any compound of oxygen with an element or radical.

ox•i•dize (ok′sĭ-dīz″) to combine or cause to combine with oxygen, or to lose electrons. See *oxidation.*

ox•i•do•re•duc•tase (ok″sĭ-do-re-duk′tās) [EC 1] any member of a class of enzymes that catalyze the reversible transfer of electrons from a substrate that becomes oxidized (hydrogen or electron donor) to a substrate that becomes reduced (hydrogen or electron acceptor). The class includes dehydrogenases, hydroxylases, oxidases, oxygenases, peroxidases, and reductases.

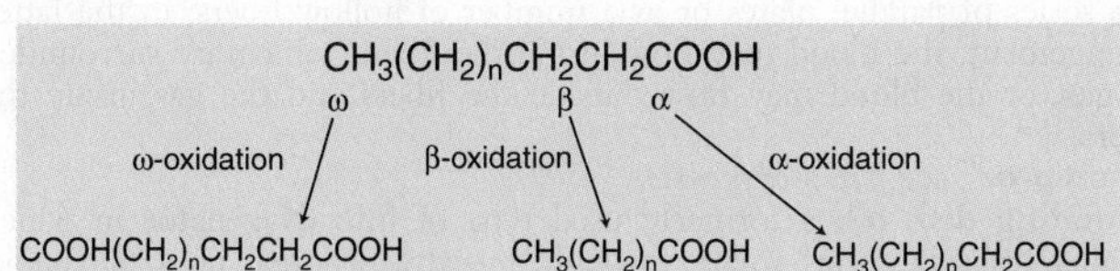

■ Oxidation of a saturated fatty acid having (n + 4) carbon atoms; α-oxidation yields a saturated fatty acid of one fewer carbons, β-oxidation a saturated fatty acid of two fewer carbon atoms, and ω-oxidation a dicarboxylic acid with no loss of carbon atoms.

ox•i•do•sis (ok″sĭ-do′sis) acidosis.

ox•i•dro•nate (HDP, HMDP) (ok″sĭ-dro′nāt) a hydroxymethylene-substituted diphosphonate compound having an affinity for sites of osteoid mineralization; complexed with technetium 99m it is used in bone imaging. See table at *technetium.*

ox•im (ok′sim) oxime.

ox•ime (ok′sēm) any of a series of compounds containing the CH(═NOH) group, formed by the action of hydroxylamine on an aldehyde or a ketone.

ox•im•e•ter (ok-sim′ə-tər) a photoelectric device for determining the oxygen saturation of the blood.

CO-o. a device that uses spectrophotometry to measure relative blood concentrations of oxyhemoglobin, carboxyhemoglobin, methemoglobin, and reduced hemoglobin.

ear o. a pulse oximeter for attachment to the ear, by which oxygen saturation of the blood flowing through the ear can be determined.

finger o. a pulse oximeter whose sensor is attached to a finger, so that the oxygenation of blood flowing through the finger can be determined.

intracardiac o. an instrument for measuring the concentration of oxygen or dye in blood within the heart; see also *oxygen gas analyzer*, under *analyzer.*

pulse o. an oximeter that measures the oxygen saturation of arterial blood by passing a beam of red and infrared light through a pulsating capillary bed, the ratio of red to infrared transmission varying with the oxygen saturation of the blood; because it responds only to pulsatile objects, it does not detect nonpulsating objects like skin and venous blood.

whole blood o. an oximeter for determination of oxygen saturation of removed specimens of blood.

ox•im•e•try (ok-sim′ə-tre) determination of the oxygen saturation of arterial blood using an oximeter.

pulse o. a noninvasive method of indicating the arterial oxygen saturation of functional hemoglobin, using a pulse oximeter.

ox•ine (ok-sēn′) oxyquinoline.

ox•ir•ane (ok′sĭ-rān) ethylene oxide.

Ox•i•stat (ok′sĭ-stat) trademark for preparations of oxiconazole nitrate.

oxo- the approved prefix in formal nomenclature for *keto-*, as in *oxoglutarate* for *ketoglutarate.* Terms prefixed with *keto-* are the common forms in the United States.

3-oxo•ac•id CoA-trans•fer•ase (ok″so-as′id ko-a′ trans′fər-ās) [EC 2.8.3.5] an enzyme of the transferase class that catalyzes the shift of coenzyme A (CoA) from succinyl CoA to acetoacetic acid to form acetoacetyl CoA; the reaction is part of a mechanism by which free β-hydroxybutyrate can be converted to acetyl CoA and used as fuel. The enzyme is present in muscle and nerve tissue but absent from liver, and it can also act on some related keto acids. Called also *3-ketoacid CoA transferase.*

oxo-ac•id-ly•ase (ok″so-as″id-li′ās) [EC 4.1.3] any member of a sub-subclass of enzymes of the lyase class that catalyze the cleavage of a C—C bond of a 3-hydroxy acid.

oxo•glu•ta•rate de•hy•dro•gen•ase (suc•ci•nyl-trans•fer•ring) (ok″so-gloo′tə-rāt de-hi′dro-jən-ās suk′sĭ-nəl trans′fər-ing) [EC 1.2.4.2] EC nomenclature for *α-ketoglutarate dehydrogenase.*

2-oxo•glu•tar•ic ac•id (ok″so-gloo-tar′ik) α-ketoglutaric acid.

2-oxo•iso•val•er•ate de•hy•dro•gen•ase (ok″so-i″so-val′er-āt de-hi′dro-jən-ās) branched-chain α-keto acid dehydrogenase.

oxo•lin•ic ac•id (ok-so-lin′ik) a synthetic antibacterial used orally in the treatment of urinary tract infections caused by gram-negative organisms, including *Escherichia coli, Proteus* species, and *Klebsiella* species.

oxo•ni•um (ok-so′ne-əm) containing tetravalent basic oxygen.

oxo•phen•ar•sine hy•dro•chlo•ride (ok″so-fən-ahr′sēn) an arsenical with antispirochetal and antitrypanosomal properties; rarely used in the treatment of syphilis and trypanosomiasis.

5-oxo•pro•li•nase (ATP-hy•dro•lyz•ing) (ok″so-pro′lĭ-nās hi′dro-li-zing) [EC 3.5.2.9] an enzyme of the hydrolase class that catalyzes the ATP-dependent linearization of 5-oxoproline to form glutamate; the reaction is a part of the mechanism of transport of amino acids into tissue cells by the γ-glutamyl cycle.

5-oxo•pro•line (ok″so-pro′lēn) a ninhydrin-negative, acidic lactam of glutamic acid occurring at the N-terminus of several peptides and proteins. Called also *pyroglutamic acid* or *pyroglutamate.*

5-oxo•pro•lin•u•ria (ok″so-pro″lin-u′re-ə) 1. excess of 5-oxoproline in the urine. 2. generalized deficiency of glutathione synthetase; see *glutathione synthetase deficiency*.

oxo•ste•roid (ok″so-ster′oid) ketosteroid.

ox•pen•tif•yl•line (oks″pən-tif′ə-lēn) BAN for pentoxifylline.

ox•pren•o•lol hy•dro•chlo•ride (oks-pren′ə-lol) [USP] a nonselective beta-adrenergic blocking agent, administered orally in the treatment of hypertension, hypertrophic cardiomyopathy, cardiac arrhythmias, and myocardial infarction.

Ox•sor•a•len (ok-sor′ə-lən) trademark for preparations of methoxsalen.

ox•triph•yl•line (oks-trif′ə-lēn) [USP] the choline salt of theophylline, used as a bronchodilator in the prevention and treatment of symptoms of asthma and of reversible airway obstruction associated with chronic bronchitis, emphysema, or other chronic obstructive pulmonary disease; administered orally.

oxy- [Gr. *oxys* keen] a combining form *(a)* meaning sharp, quick, or sour, *(b)* denoting relationship to acid, or *(c)* denoting the presence of oxygen in a compound. Also, *ox-*.

oxy•ac•id (ok″se-as′id) an acid containing both oxygen and hydrogen atoms. When there are two common oxyacids of the same element, that with the higher oxidation state is designated by the suffix *-ic*, that with the lower by *-ous*. When additional oxidation states occur, the prefix *hypo-* may be used to indicate a lower state and *per-* to indicate a higher state; see accompanying table. Called also *oxo acid* and *oxacid*.

oxy•ben•zene (ok″se-ben′zēn) phenol (def. 1).

oxy•ben•zone (ok″se-ben′zōn) [USP] a benzophenone compound used as a topical sunscreen; it absorbs UVB and some UVA rays.

oxy•blep•sia (ok″se-blep′se-ə) [*oxy-* + Gr. *blepsis* vision + *-ia*] oxyopia.

oxy•bu•ty•nin chlo•ride (ok″se-bu′tĭ-nin) an anticholinergic that has a direct antispasmodic effect on smooth muscle; used in the treatment of uninhibited neurogenic bladder and reflex neurogenic bladder, administered orally or transdermally.

oxy•bu•tyr•ia (ok″se-bu-tir′e-ə) the presence of hydroxybutyric acid in urine.

oxy•bu•tyr•ic ac•id (ok″se-bu-tir′ik) hydroxybutyric acid.

oxy•bu•tyr•ic•ac•i•de•mia (ok″se-bu-tir″ik-as″ĭ-de′me-ə) oxybutyria.

Oxy•cel (ok′sĭ-sel) trademark for preparations of oxidized cellulose.

oxy•ce•pha•lia (ok″se-sə-fa′le-ə) oxycephaly.

oxy•ceph•a•ly (ok″se-sef′ə-le) [*oxy-* + *-cephaly*] a condition in which the top of the head is pointed or conical owing to premature closure of the coronal and lambdoid sutures. Called also *acrocephaly*, *hypsicephaly*, *turricephaly*, *steeple head* or *skull*, and *tower head* or *skull*. **oxycephal′ic, oxyceph′alous** *adj*

oxy•chlo•ride (ok″se-klor′īd) an element or radical combined with oxygen and chlorine.

oxy•chlo•ro•sene (ok″se-klor′o-sēn) the hypochlorous acid complex of a mixture of the phenyl sulfonate derivatives of aliphatic hydrocarbons, having actions similar to those of chlorine; used as a topical anti-infective.

o. sodium the sodium salt of oxychlorosene, used like the base.

oxy•cho•line (ok″se-ko′lin) muscarine.

oxy•chro•mat•ic (ok″se-kro-mat′ik) acidophilic (def. 1).

oxy•clo•za•nide (ok″se-klo′zə-nīd) a salicylanilide anthelmintic used against adult liver flukes in cattle and sheep.

oxy•co•done (ok″se-ko′dōn) an opioid agonist analgesic derived from morphine.

o. hydrochloride [USP] the hydrochloride salt of oxycodone, used as an analgesic; administered orally or rectally.

o. terephthalate [USP] a salt of oxycodone used as an analgesic, administered orally.

Oxyacids of Chlorine

Hypochlorous acid	$HClO$
Chlorous acid	$HClO_2$
Chloric acid	$HClO_3$
Perchloric acid	$HClO_4$

Oxy•Con•tin (ok″se-kon′tin) trademark for a preparation of oxycodone hydrochloride.

oxy•cy•a•nide (ok″se-si′ə-nīd) the oxide of any binary compound of cyanogen.

Oxy•Fast (ok″se-fast′) trademark for a preparation of oxycodone hydrochloride.

ox•y•gen (O) (ok′sĭ-jən) [Gr. *oxys* sour + *gennan* to produce] a gaseous element existing free in the air and in combination in most nonelementary solids, liquids, and gases; atomic number, 8; atomic weight, 15.999. There are three naturally occurring isotopes, with atomic weights of 16, 17, and 18 (heavy oxygen). Oxygen constitutes 20 per cent by weight of the atmospheric air; it is the essential agent in the respiration of plants and animals and, although nonflammable, is necessary to support combustion. It forms the characteristic constituent of ternary acids. It is administered by inhalation in some pulmonary and cardiac disorders.

o. 15 an artificial radioactive isotope of oxygen, atomic mass 15, having a half-life of 2.04 minutes; it decays by positron emission (1.70 MeV) and is used as a tracer in the measurement of regional blood volume and flow and oxygen metabolism by positron emission tomography.

heavy o. an isotope of oxygen of atomic weight 18.

high pressure o. hyperbaric o.

hyperbaric o. oxygen under greater than atmospheric pressure. Called also *high pressure o.*

molecular o. dioxygen, O_2.

singlet o. a highly reactive, dimagnetic, excited state ($^1O_2$) of dioxygen that rapidly decays with the emission of visible light to the paramagnetic (triplet) ground state. Singlet oxygen is thought to be involved in the oxidative killing of ingested microorganisms by neutrophils; it is produced during the respiratory burst by spontaneous reactions of hydrogen peroxide with superoxide and hypochlorite ions.

ox•y•gen•ase (ok′sĭ-jən-ās) [EC 1.13] any member of a subclass of enzymes of the oxidoreductase class that catalyze the oxidation of a single substrate (hydrogen donor) with incorporation of one or both atoms of oxygen from molecular oxygen into the substance oxidized.

ox•y•gen•ate (ok′sĭ-jə-nāt) to add oxygen to.

ox•y•gen•a•tion (ok″sĭ-jə-na′shən) 1. the act or process of adding oxygen to something. 2. saturation with oxygen.

extracorporeal membrane o. (ECMO) extracorporeal life support.

hyperbaric o. exposure of a patient to oxygen under pressure greater than normal atmospheric pressure, done for individuals who need more oxygen than they can take in by breathing in the normal atmosphere or with an oxygen mask.

ox•y•gen•a•tor (ok′sĭ-jə-na″tər) a device that mechanically oxygenates venous blood extracorporeally. It is used in combination with one or more pumps for maintaining circulation during open heart surgery and for assisting the circulation in patients seriously ill with some cardiac and pulmonary disorders. Called also *artificial lung*.

bubble o. a device in which a stream of pure oxygen is broken up into small bubbles that diffuse through a column of blood, with gas exchange occurring on the bubbles' surface; the oxygenated blood is defoamed and collected in a reservoir for return to the patient's circulatory system.

disk o. rotating disk o.

film o. a device, encased in a container of oxygen, that makes possible the production of a thin film of blood to facilitate the exchange of gases; see *rotating disk o.* and *screen o.*

intravascular o. a device consisting of hundreds of hollow fibers through which oxygen is drawn by a vacuum pump; it is implanted in the vena cava, where gas exchange occurs as blood flows over the fibers. Used to provide part of the gas exchange needs of patients with acute respiratory failure, allowing mechanical ventilation to be performed at reduced pressures, thus reducing or preventing oxygen toxicity and barotrauma.

membrane o. a device in which blood and oxygen are separated by a semipermeable membrane, generally of Teflon or polypropylene, across which gas exchange occurs. The membrane may be arranged as a series of parallel plates or as a number of hollow fibers; in the latter arrangement, the blood may flow inside the fibers, which are surrounded by gas, or the blood may flow outside the fibers and the gas inside the fibers.

pump-o. see *pump-oxygenator*.

rotating disk o. a formerly used type of film oxygenator in which parallel disks in series rotate through an extracorporeal pool of venous blood in a container of oxygen; gaseous exchange occurs between the thin film of blood on the exposed surfaces of the disks and the oxygen in the container.

screen o. a formerly used type of film oxygenator in which the venous blood is passed over a series of screens in a container of oxygen, gaseous exchange taking place in the thin film of blood produced on the screens.

ox·y·gen·ic (ok″sĭ-jen′ik) containing oxygen.

oxy·hem·a·to·por·phy·rin (ok″se-hem″ə-to-por′fĭ-rin) a pigment sometimes found in the urine, closely allied to hematoporphyrin.

oxy·heme (ok′se-hēm) heme.

oxy·he·mo·chro·mo·gen (ok″se-he″mo-kro′mo-jən) heme.

oxy·he·mo·cy·a·nine (ok″se-he″mo-si′ə-nēn) hemocyanin charged with oxygen.

oxy·he·mo·glo·bin (ok″se-he′mo-glo″bin) hemoglobin that contains bound O_2, a compound formed from hemoglobin on exposure to alveolar gas in the lungs, with formation of a covalent bond with oxygen and without change of the charge of the ferrous state.

oxy·hy·per·gly·ce·mia (ok″se-hi″pər-gli-se′me-ə) a condition in which there is slight glycosuria and an oral glucose tolerance curve that rises about 180–200 mg per 100 mL but returns to fasting values 2.5 hours after ingestion of the glucose.

oxy·io·dide (ok″se-i′o-dīd) an element or radical combined with oxygen and iodine.

OxyIR (ok′se-i-ahr″) trademark for a preparation of oxycodone hydrochloride.

Oxy·lo·bi·um (ok″se-lo′be-um) a genus of leguminous plants, many of which contain fluoroacetates and can cause fatal fluoroacetate poisoning in livestock.

oxy·met·az·o·line hy·dro·chlo·ride (ok″se-mət-az′o-lēn) [USP] an adrenergic, used topically as a vasoconstrictor to reduce swelling and congestion of the nasal mucosa and to relieve redness associated with minor irritations of the eye.

oxy·meth·o·lone (ok″se-meth′ə-lōn) [USP] an anabolic-androgenic steroid used in the treatment of anemia and for the prophylaxis and treatment of hereditary angioedema; administered orally.

ox·ym·e·try (ok-sim′ə-tre) oximetry.

Oxy·mo·nad·i·da an order of protozoa of the phylum Sarcomastigophora

oxy·mor·phone hy·dro·chlo·ride (ok″se-mor′fōn) [USP] a semisynthetic opioid analgesic, used as an analgesic for relief of moderate to severe pain and as an adjunct to anesthesia; administered intramuscularly, subcutaneously, intravenously, or rectally.

oxy·myo·glo·bin (ok″se-mi′o-glo″bin) a compound formed from myoglobin on exposure to atmospheric conditions, with formation of a covalent bond with oxygen and without change of the charge of the ferrous state.

oxy·myo·he·ma·tin (ok″se-mi″o-he′mə-tin) oxidized myohematin from muscle.

oxy·ner·von (ok″se-nur′von) a cerebroside isolated from the brain.

oxy·neu·rine (ok″se-noor′in) betaine.

ox·yn·tic (ok-sin′tik) [Gr. *oxynō* to make acid] secreting acid.

ox·yn·to·mod·u·lin (ok-sin″to-mod′u-lin) a common enteroglucagon, secreted in the intestinal tract and having glycogenolytic activity.

oxy·opia (ok″se-o′pe-ə) [*oxy-* + *-opia*] acuteness of vision; called also *oxyblepsia.*

oxy·op·ter (ok″se-op′tər) [*oxy-* + Gr. *optēr* observer] a unit of measurement of visual acuity, being the reciprocal value of the visual angle expressed in degrees. An oxyopter (1 degree) is equivalent to 60 Snellen units (60′) and corresponds to the counting of fingers at 1 meter.

oxy·para·plas·tin (ok″se-par″ə-plas′tin) the oxyphilic part of paraplastin.

oxy·phen·bu·ta·zone (ok″se-fən-bu′tə-zōn) a nonsteroidal antiinflammatory drug derived from phenylbutazone, which has been administered orally in the treatment of arthritis, gout, and similar conditions.

oxy·phen·cy·cli·mine hy·dro·chlo·ride (ok″se-fən-si′klĭ-mēn) an anticholinergic, having antispasmodic, antisecretory, and antimotility activities; used especially in the treatment of peptic ulcer and spasm of the gastrointestinal tract, administered orally.

oxy·phe·ni·sa·tin (ok″se-fə-ni′sə-tin) a cathartic, administered as an enema to cleanse the bowel before surgery or colon examination.

o. acetate the diacetyl derivative of oxyphenisatin, used as a cathartic, administered orally.

oxy·phen·yl·eth·yl·amine (ok″se-fen″əl-eth″əl-am′ēn) tyramine.

oxy·phil (ok′se-fil) 1. *(in the pl.)* oxyphil cells. 2. *(in the pl.)* Askanazy cells. 3. acidophilic (def. 1).

oxy·phil·ic (ok″se-fil′ik) [*oxy-* + *-philic*] acidophilic (def. 1).

ox·yph·i·lous (ok-sif′ĭ-ləs) acidophilic (def. 1).

oxy·pho·nia (ok″se-fo′ne-ə) [Gr. *oxyphōnia*] an abnormally sharp quality or pitch of the voice.

oxy·plasm (ok′se-plaz″əm) the oxyphil part of the cytoplasm.

oxy·pu·rine (ok″se-pu′rēn) a purine containing oxygen. The oxypurines include hypoxanthine or monoxypurine, xanthine or dioxypurine, and uric acid or trioxypurine.

oxy·pur·i·nol (ok″se-pūr′ĭ-nol) the active metabolite of allopurinol, a xanthine oxidase inhibitor responsible for much of the activity of allopurinol against gout.

oxy·quin·o·line (ok″se-kwin′o-lēn) a dicyclic aromatic compound used as a bacteriostatic and fungistatic in the preparation of fungicides and as a disinfectant; it is also used as a chelating agent.

o. sulfate [NF] the sulfate salt of oxyquinoline, used as a complexing agent for pharmaceuticals; it is also used as a topical antiseptic and disinfectant.

oxy·rhine (ok′se-rīn) [*oxy-* + Gr. *rhis* nose] having a sharp-pointed nose.

oxy·salt (ok′se-sawlt) any salt of an oxoacid.

Oxy·spi·ru·ra (ok″se-spi-roo′rə) a genus of nematodes of the family Thelaziidae. *O. manso′ni* is found under the nictitating membrane of chickens and other fowl.

oxy·ster·ol (ok″se-ster′ol) any of various oxidation products of cholesterol; many are biologically active.

ox·yt·a·lan (ok-sit′ə-lən) a connective tissue fiber that is found in humans, monkeys, and certain other animals and is resistant to acid hydrolysis. It occurs in structures subjected to mechanical stress including tendons, ligaments, adventitia, connective tissue sheaths surrounding skin appendages, and the periodontal membranes. On electron microscopic examination, fibrillar and amorphous components are revealed. Called also *oxytalan fiber.*

ox·yt·a·lan·ol·y·sis (ok-sit″ə-lən-ol′ĭ-sis) destruction of oxytalan fibers.

oxy·tet·ra·cy·cline (ok″se-tet″rə-si′klēn) [USP] a broad-spectrum antibiotic of the tetracycline group produced by *Streptomyces rimosus,* effective against a wide range of both gram-positive and gram-negative organisms, used as an antibacterial and as an adjunct in the treatment of amebiasis; administered orally or intramuscularly.

o. calcium [USP] the calcium salt of oxytetracycline, used as an antibacterial; administered orally.

o. hydrochloride [USP] the monohydrochloride salt of oxytetracycline, used as an antibacterial and antirickettsial; administered orally or intramuscularly.

oxy·to·cia (ok-se-to′se-ə) [*oxy-* + *toc-* + *-ia*] rapid labor.

oxy·to·cic (ok-se-to′sik) 1. pertaining to, characterized by, or promoting oxytocia. 2. an agent that hastens evacuation of the uterus by stimulating contractions of the myometrium.

oxy·to·cin (ok″se-to′sin) 1. a nonapeptide secreted by the magnocellular neurons of the hypothalamus and stored as a posterior pituitary hormone along with vasopressin. It promotes uterine contractions and milk ejection and contributes to the second stage of labor. 2. [USP] a preparation of this substance obtained from the neurohypophyses of domestic food animals or produced synthetically; it is administered intramuscularly or intravenously to induce labor, increase the force of uterine contractions, contract uterine muscle after delivery of the placenta, and control postpartum hemorrhage, and intranasally to stimulate milk ejection. In veterinary medicine it is used to stimulate letdown of milk in cows with agalactia.

oxy·to·ci·nase (ok″se-to′sĭ-nās) cystinyl aminopeptidase.

Oxy·trol (ok′e-trol) trademark for a preparation of oxybutynin chloride.

Oxy·tro·pis (ok″se-tro′pis) a genus of leguminous plants, related botanically to *Astragalus;* like *Astragalus,* it is one of the groups called *locoweed* that causes locoism in grazing animals.

Oxy·u·ra·nus (ok″se-u-ra′nəs) a genus of venomous snakes of the family Elapidae. *O. scutella′tus* is the taipan of Australia and New Guinea.

oxy·uri·a·sis (ok″se-u-ri′ə-sis) 1. infection of a human or other animal with oxyurids. 2. enterobiasis.

oxy·urid (ok-se-u′rid) any nematode of the superfamily Oxyuroidea. Called also *pinworm* and *seatworm.*

Oxy•uri•dae (ok″se-u′rĭ-de) a family of nematodes, many of which are intestinal parasites. Genera of medical or veterinary interest are *Enterobius*, *Oxyuris*, and *Syphacia*.

oxy•uri•o•sis (ok″se-u″re-o′sis) oxyuriasis.

Oxy•uris (ok″se-u′ris) [Gr. *oxys* sharp + *oura* tail] a genus of intestinal nematodes of the family Oxyuridae. *O. e′qui*, the largest known pinworm, is found in the cecum, colon, and rectum of the horse. *O. vermicula′ris* has been renamed *Enterobius vermicularis*.

oxy•uroid (ok-se-u′roid) oxyurid.

Oxy•uroi•dea (ok″se-u″roi-de′ə) the oxyurids, a superfamily of small nematode phasmids with a bulbous esophagus, usually found as parasites in the cecum and colon of vertebrates, but sometimes found in insects and other invertebrates. The single family of medical or veterinary interest is *Oxyuridae*. In some systems of classification, Oxyuroidea is considered to be an order.

Oz (oz) an antigenic marker distinguishing immunoglobulin human λ light chain subtypes.

oz ounce (It. *onza*).

oze•na (o-ze′nə) [Gr. *ozaina* a fetid polypus in the nose] a late stage of atrophic rhinitis with a thick mucopurulent discharge, mucosal crusting, and fetor, often associated with the presence of *Klebsiella pneumoniae* subsp. *ozaenae*. **oze′nous** *adj*

ozone (o′zōn) [Gr. *ozē* stench] a bluish explosive gas or blue liquid, an allotropic and more active form of oxygen, O_3 that is formed when oxygen is exposed to the silent discharge of electricity. It is an antiseptic and disinfectant. Ozone is a major air pollutant and is irritating and toxic to the respiratory system.

ozo•nom•e•ter (o″zo-nom′ə-tər) [*ozone* + *-meter*] an instrument for estimating the ozone in the air.

ozo•sto•mia (o″zo-sto′me-ə) halitosis.

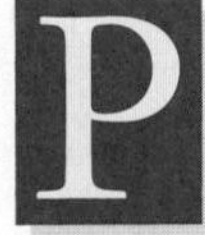

P para; peta-; phosphate (group); phosphorus; poise; posterior; premolar; proline; pupil.

P power; pressure; probability.

P_1 parental generation.

P_2 pulmonic second sound.

Pco_2 the partial pressure of carbon dioxide (carbon dioxide tension); also written PCO_2.

P_i orthophosphate.

P_{O_2} the partial pressure of oxygen (oxygen tension).

p pico-; proton; the short arm of a chromosome.

p momentum; (in statistics) the probability that a specific event will occur. Cf. *q*.

***p*-** para- (def. 2).

p53 see under *gene* and *protein.*

p150,95 glycoprotein p150,95; see *complement receptor 4 (CR4)*, under *receptor.*

Π the Greek capital letter pi, used in mathematics to indicate a product;

$$\Pi_{i=1}^{n} x_i = x_1 \times x_2 \times \ldots \times x_n.$$

π pi, the sixteenth letter of the Greek alphabet; mathematical symbol for the ratio of the circumference to the diameter of a circle, approximately 3.1415926536; symbol for *osmotic pressure.*

Φ the Greek capital letter phi, used as the symbol for magnetic flux.

φ phi, the twenty-first letter of the Greek alphabet.

ψ psi, the twenty-third letter of the Greek alphabet; symbol in molecular biology for *pseudouridine.*

PA physician assistant; posteroanterior; pulmonary artery.

Pa pascal; protactinium.

PAB, PABA *p*-aminobenzoic acid.

PAC premature atrial complex; see *atrial premature complex*, under *complex.*

pa•ca (pă′kə) [Sp., from Tupi] *Cuniculus paca*, a large nocturnal burrowing rodent of Central and South America; it is sometimes a reservoir for parasites such as *Echinococcus vogeli.*

pac•chi•o•ni•an (pah″ke-o′ne-ən) named for Antonio *Pacchioni*, Italian anatomist, 1665–1726.

Pace sign (pās) [J. Blair *Pace*, American physician, 1916–1994] see under *sign.*

pace•mak•er (pās′ma-kər) 1. an object or substance that influences the rate at which a certain phenomenon occurs. 2. the natural cardiac pacemaker or an artificial cardiac pacemaker. 3. in biochemistry, a substance whose rate of reaction sets the pace for a series of interrelated reactions.

Pacemaker

AAI p. atrial demand inhibited p.

AAIR p. an atrial demand inhibited pacemaker that is responsive to the patient's respiratory rate and thus to exercise and metabolic needs.

AAT p. atrial demand triggered p.

antitachycardia p. an implanted pacemaker that terminates tachycardia by delivering one or more pacing stimuli; it may require arrhythmia detection and device activation by the patient or may detect arrhythmias and deliver stimuli automatically.

AOO p. atrial asynchronous p.

artificial p., artificial cardiac p. a device that uses electrical impulses to reproduce or regulate the rhythms of the heart. Battery-driven and connected to the heart by leads and electrodes, it may be temporary or permanent and is inserted transvenously, transcutaneously, epicardially, or via the esophagus or coronary artery. Most pacemakers are either triggered or inhibited to modify output by sensing the intracardiac potential of one or more cardiac chambers; they have some degree of programmability and may also have antitachycardia functions. A five letter code is used to categorize pacemakers by their combinations of these features; see table. Popularly called *pacemaker.*

asynchronous p. an artificial cardiac pacemaker that delivers stimuli at a fixed rate, independent of any atrial or ventricular activity.

asynchronous atrial p. atrial asynchronous p.

asynchronous ventricular p. ventricular asynchronous p.

atrial asynchronous p. an artificial cardiac pacemaker that stimulates the atrium at a constant rate, without sensing atrial or ventricular activity; now rarely used except to initiate or terminate some tachycardias. Called also *AOO p.*

atrial demand inhibited p. an artificial cardiac pacemaker that delivers stimuli to the atrium at a fixed rate in the absence of sensed atrial activity; spontaneous cardiac activity causes inhibition of pacemaker output, termination of the current stimulation cycle, and initiation of a new cycle. Called also *AAI p.*

atrial demand triggered p. an artificial cardiac pacemaker that delivers stimuli to the atrium at a fixed rate in the absence of sensed atrial activity; spontaneous cardiac activity triggers pacemaker output, which

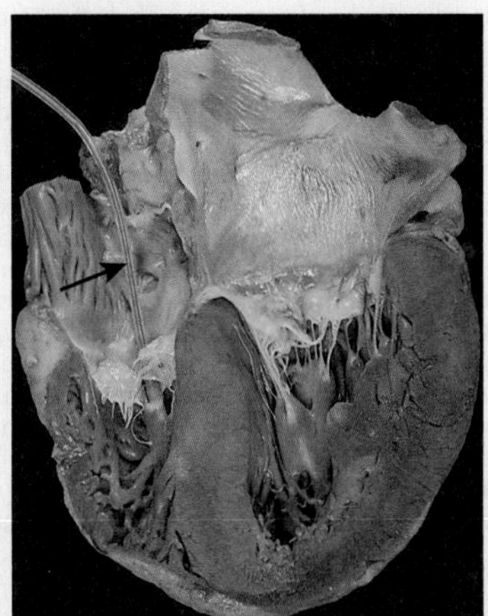

■ Pacemaker lead *(arrow)* terminating in the right ventricle.

NASPE/BPEG* Generic (NBG) Pacemaker Code

Position† Category	I Chamber(s) Paced	II Chamber(s) Sensed	III Response to Sensing	IV Programmability, Rate Modulation	V Antitachyarrhythmia Function(s)
	O = None	O = None	O = None	O = None	O = None
	A = Atrium	A = Atrium	T = Triggers pacing	P = Simple programmable	P = Pacing (antitachyarrhythmia)
	V = Ventricle	V = Ventricle	I = Inhibits pacing	M = Multiprogrammable	S = Shock
	D = Dual (A + V)	D = Dual (A + V)	D = Dual (T + I)	C = Communicating	D = Dual (P + S)
Manufacturer's Designation Only	S = Single (either A or V)	S = Single (either A or V)		R = Rate modulation	

*NASPE, North American Society of Pacing and Electrophysiology; BPEG, British Pacing and Electrophysiology Group.
†Positions I through III describe only antibradyarrhythmia functions of the pacemaker.

Pacemaker *Continued*

falls ineffectively in the myocardial refractory period and initiates a new pacemaker stimulation cycle. Called also *AAT p.*

atrial synchronous ventricular p. a dual chamber cardiac pacemaker that senses atrial activity and delivers a ventricular stimulus after a preset interval; used in patients with impaired atrioventricular conduction but normal sinus node function. Called also *VAT p.* See also *atrial synchronous ventricular inhibited p.*

atrial synchronous ventricular inhibited p. a dual chamber cardiac pacemaker similar to an atrial synchronous ventricular pacemaker but able to sense ventricular as well as atrial activity. Called also *VDD p.*

atrioventricular junctional p. an ectopic pacemaker occurring in the atrioventricular junction.

atrioventricular (AV) sequential p. an artificial cardiac pacemaker used in patients with abnormal sinus node function and impaired AV conduction; it senses ventricular, and sometimes atrial, activity and in addition to stimulating the atrium also stimulates the ventricle after an appropriate delay. Committed versions invariably deliver the ventricular stimulus while noncommitted versions deliver it only in the absence of interim ventricular activity. See also *DVI p.*, *DDD p.*, and *DDI p.*

automatic p. universal p.

bipolar p. an implanted pacemaker in which the lead contains both electrodes, anode and cathode, and is thus a complete circuit.

cardiac p. the group of cells rhythmically initiating the heartbeat, characterized physiologically by a slow loss of membrane potential during diastole. Usually the pacemaker site is the sinoatrial node. See also *artificial cardiac p.*

cilium p. the biological regulator that controls the frequency of the beat of the cilia of cells by determining the rate of contraction and excitation.

DDD p. an artificial cardiac pacemaker that can sense and pace both the atria and ventricles; it is capable of operating in both triggered and inhibited modes as necessary.

DDDR p. a universal pacemaker that is responsive to the patient's respiratory rate and thus to exercise and metabolic needs.

DDI p. a type of atrioventricular sequential pacemaker that delivers impulses to the atrium and ventricles on the basis of sensed ventricular and atrial activity, although the latter can only inhibit atrial impulses and cannot trigger ventricular stimulation. Cf. *DVI p.* and *DDD p.*

demand p. an implanted pacemaker whose generator stimulus is inhibited for a set interval (refractory period) by a signal derived from depolarization (normal or ectopic), thus minimizing the risk of pacemaker-induced ventricular fibrillation.

diaphragmatic p. electrophrenic p.

dual chamber p. a pacemaker having two leads, one in the atrium and one in the ventricle, so that electromechanical synchrony between the chambers can be approximated.

DVI p. a type of atrioventricular sequential pacemaker that delivers impulses to the atrium and ventricle on the basis of sensed ventricular activity only. Cf. *DDI p.* and *DDD p.*

ectopic p. any biological cardiac pacemaker other than the sinoatrial node; under normal conditions it is not active.

electronic p. artificial p.

electrophrenic p. the device used in electrophrenic respiration; it converts radiofrequency signals into electrical impulses that stimulate the phrenic nerve, resulting in descent and flattening of the diaphragm and improved inhalation of air. Called also *diaphragmatic* or *phrenic p.*

escape p. an ectopic pacemaker that assumes control of cardiac impulse propagation because of failure of the sinoatrial node to generate one or more normal impulses.

external p., external cardiac p. an artificial cardiac pacemaker located outside the body with output wires connected to circular chest electrodes, with a wire sewn directly into the heart, or with an electrode inserted through an intravenous catheter.

fixed-rate p. an artificial cardiac pacemaker set to pace at only a single rate.

fully automatic p. universal p.

gastric p. a saddle-shaped area of the greater curvature of the stomach at the junction of its proximal and middle thirds, where electric potentials originate that regulate the frequency of gastric contractions.

p. of heart cardiac p.

implantable p., implanted p., internal p. an artificial cardiac pacemaker completely implanted into the subcutaneous tissue.

junctional p. atrioventricular junctional p.

latent p. ectopic p.

phrenic p. electrophrenic p.

radiofrequency p. an artificial cardiac pacemaker consisting of an antenna coil on the skin and a subcutaneously implanted receiving coil with an electrode inserted into the ventricular myocardium. Pulses from a lightweight radio transmitter carried by the patient are transmitted to the pacemaker.

rate responsive p. an artificial cardiac pacemaker that can deliver stimuli at a rate adjustable to some parameter independent of atrial activity, such as respiratory rate, physical activity level, blood temperature, or mixed venous oxygen saturation level.

runaway p. a malfunctioning artificial cardiac pacemaker that abruptly accelerates its pacing rate, resulting in pacemaker-induced ventricular tachycardia.

secondary p. ectopic p.

single chamber p. an implanted pacemaker having only one lead, which is placed in either the atrium or the ventricle.

synchronous p. an implanted pacemaker that synchronizes the electromechanical events in the atrium with those of the ventricle by delivering stimuli in response to sensed activity in the atrium, ventricle, or both.

transthoracic p. an external cardiac pacemaker that delivers stimuli through the chest wall, such as one connected to the heart by percutaneous pacing wires introduced through a transthoracic needle or one in which large electrodes are placed on the skin over the heart.

transvenous p. an artificial cardiac pacemaker, either external or implantable, that is connected to the heart by pacing leads passed through the venous circulation.

unipolar p. an implanted pacemaker in which the lead has a single stimulating electrode, the cathode, with the anode connected to an indifferent electrode, usually the outer surface of the pulse generator.

universal p. a term sometimes used to describe a DDD pacemaker, emphasizing that because it can be programmed to operate in one of numerous possible pacemaker modes under specific circumstances, it can be made to most closely approximate normal electrophysiologic functioning under a variety of conditions.

VAT p. atrial synchronous ventricular p.

VDD p. atrial synchronous ventricular inhibited p.

ventricular p. an ectopic pacemaker occurring in a ventricle.

ventricular asynchronous p. an artificial cardiac pacemaker that stimulates the ventricle at a constant rate, without sensing atrial or ventricular activity; now rarely used except to initiate or terminate some tachycardias. Called also *VOO p.*

ventricular demand inhibited p. an artificial cardiac pacemaker that delivers stimuli to the ventricle at a fixed rate in the absence of sensed ventricular activity; spontaneous cardiac activity causes inhibition of pacemaker output, termination of the current stimulation cycle, and initiation of a new cycle. Called also *VVI p.*

ventricular demand triggered p. an artificial cardiac pacemaker that delivers stimuli to the ventricle at a fixed rate in the absence of sensed ventricular activity; spontaneous cardiac activity triggers pacemaker output, which falls ineffectively in the myocardial refractory period and initiates a new cycle of pacemaker stimulation. Called also *VVT p.*

VOO p. ventricular asynchronous p.

VVI p. ventricular demand inhibited p.

VVIR p. a ventricular demand inhibited pacemaker that is responsive to the patient's respiratory rate and thus to exercise and metabolic needs.

VVT p. ventricular demand triggered p.

wandering atrial p. a condition in which the site of origin of the impulses controlling the heart rate shifts from one point to another within the atria, including the sinus node, changing with almost every beat. P waves and PR intervals vary, and the rate of impulse formation is somewhat irregular. It occurs when the rate of sinus impulses falls below a critical level or fails.

Pace•rone (pās′ə-rōn) trademark for preparations of amiodarone hydrochloride.

pachy- [Gr. *pachys* thick] a combining form meaning thick.

pachy•bleph•a•ron (pak″e-blef′ə-ron) [*pachy-* + Gr. *blepharon* eyelid] a thickening of the eyelid, chiefly near the border.

pachy•bleph•a•ro•sis (pak″e-blef″ə-ro′sis) pachyblepharon.

pachy·ce·pha·lia (pak″e-sə-fa′le-ə) pachycephaly.

pachy·ceph·a·ly (pak″e-sef′ə-le) [*pachy-* + *-cephaly*] abnormal thickness of the bones of the skull, as in acromegaly. **pachycephal′ic, pachyceph′alous** *adj*

pachy·chei·lia (pak″e-ki′le-ə) [*pachy-* + *cheil-* + *-ia*] thickening of the lips.

pachy·der·ma (pak″e-dur′mə) [*pachy-* + *derma*] abnormal thickening of the skin. See also *pachydermoperiostosis.* **pachyder′matous, pachyder′mic** *adj*

pachy·der·ma·to·cele (pak″e-dər-mat′o-sēl) [*pachy-* + *dermato-* + *-cele*[1]] a plexiform neuroma that has grown so large that it resembles elephantiasis.

pachy·der·mia (pak″e-dur′me-ə) pachyderma.

pachy·der·mo·peri·os·to·sis (pak″e-dur″mo-per″e-os-to′sis) [*pachy-* + *dermo-* + *periostosis*] a rare syndrome characterized by pachyderma with deep folds and furrows on the forehead, cheeks, and scalp *(cutis verticis gyrata)*, as well as seborrhea, hyperhidrosis, periostosis of long bones, digital clubbing, and spadelike enlargement of the hands and feet. It is more prevalent in males and usually first appears during adolescence. Some forms are hereditary and others are secondary to cardiopulmonary diseases or malignancies. Called also *idiopathic* or *primary hypertrophic osteoarthropathy* and *Touraine-Solente-Golé syndrome.*

pachy·glos·sia (pak″e-glos′e-ə) [*pachy-* + *gloss-* + *-ia*] abnormal thickness of the tongue.

pa·chyg·na·thous (pə-kig′nə-thəs) [*pachy-* + *gnath-* + *-ous*] having a large jaw. See also *macrognathia* and *prognathism.*

pachy·gy·ria (pak″e-ji′re-ə) macrogyria.

pachy·lep·to·men·in·gi·tis (pak″e-lep″to-men″in-ji′tis) [*pachy-* + *lepto-* + *mening-* + *-itis*] inflammation of the dura and pia together.

pachy·men·in·ges (pak″e-mə-nin′jēz) plural of *pachymeninx.*

pachy·men·in·gi·tis (pak″e-men″in-ji′tis) [*pachy-* + *mening-* + *-itis*] inflammation of the dura mater; the symptoms of the disease resemble those of meningitis. Cf. *leptomeningitis.*

cerebral p. inflammation of the dura of the brain.

circumscribed p. pachymeningitis limited to a definite area of the dura.

external p. inflammation of the outer layers of the dura.

hypertrophic cervical p. hypertrophic spinal pachymeningitis in the cervical region.

hypertrophic spinal p. a diffuse fibrosing form of pachymeningitis in the spinal canal; it may be due to tuberculosis, syphilis, or other causes.

internal p. inflammation of the inner layer of the dura.

p. intralamella′ris intradural abscess.

purulent p. abscess on the dura mater; see *extradural, intradural,* and *subdural abscess,* under *abscess.*

spinal p. inflammation of the dura of the vertebral column.

syphilitic p. pachymeningitis that is caused by syphilis; see also *hypertrophic spinal p.*

pachy·men·in·gop·a·thy (pak″e-men″in-gop′ə-the) [*pachymeninx* + *-pathy*] any noninflammatory disease of the dura mater.

pachy·me·ninx (pak″e-me′ninks) pl. *pachymenin′ges* [*pachy-* + *meninx*] [TA] the dura mater. NOTE: In official nomenclature, this term is used as the preferred term when contrasting this structure with the leptomeninx, which comprises the arachnoidea mater and the pia mater (arachnoidea mater et pia mater).

pachy·me·ter (pə-kim′ə-tər) [*pachy-* + *meter*] an instrument used to determine thickness.

pa·chyn·sis (pə-kin′sis) [Gr.] a thickening, especially an abnormal thickening. **pachyn′tic** *adj*

pachy·onych·ia (pak″e-o-nik′e-ə) [*pachy-* + *onych-* + *-ia*] hypertrophy and thickening of the nails.

p. conge′nita a genetically heterogeneous syndrome characterized by increased thickness of the nails that progresses to onychogryphosis; hyperkeratosis of the palms, soles, knees, and elbows; widespread tiny cutaneous horns; leukoplakia of the mucous membranes; and usually hyperhidrosis of the hands and feet. Bullae may develop on the palms and soles following trauma. It is usually an autosomal dominant disorder caused by mutations affecting any of several genes encoding various keratins; inheritance may rarely be autosomal recessive. Called also *Jadassohn-Lewandowsky syndrome.*

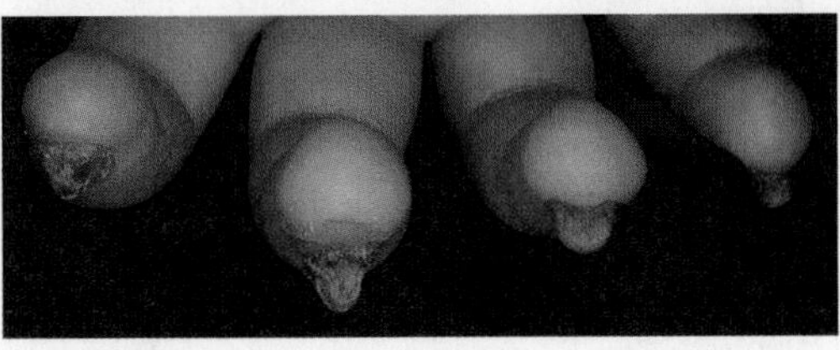

■ Pachyonychia.

pachy·peri·os·ti·tis (pak″e-per″e-os-ti′tis) periostitis of long bones resulting in abnormal thickness of the bones.

pachy·peri·to·ni·tis (pak″e-per″ĭ-to-ni′tis) sclerosing peritonitis.

pachy·pleu·ri·tis (pak″e-plo͝o-ri′tis) [*pachy-* + *pleuritis*] 1. fibrothorax. 2. pleural fibrosis.

pachy·sal·pin·gi·tis (pak″e-sal″pin-ji′tis) [*pachy-* + *salping-* + *-itis*] chronic interstitial inflammation of the muscular coat of a uterine tube, producing thickening; called also *mural salpingitis* and *parenchymatous salpingitis.*

pachy·sal·pin·go·ova·ri·tis (pak″e-sal-ping″go-o″və-ri′tis) chronic parenchymatous inflammation of the ovary and uterine tube.

pachy·tene (pak′e-tēn) [Gr. *pachytēs* thickness] the third stage of prophase in meiosis I, during which synapsis is complete, forming pairs of homologous chromosomes known as bivalents, and genetic material may be exhanged by crossing over.

pachy·vag·i·nal·itis (pak″e-vaj″ĭ-nəl-i′tis) [*pachy-* + *vaginalitis*] inflammatory thickening of the tunica vaginalis testis.

pach·y·vag·i·ni·tis (pak″e-vaj″ĭ-ni′tis) [*pachy-* + *vaginitis*] chronic vaginitis with thickening of the vaginal walls.

cystic p. emphysematous vaginitis.

pac·ing (pās′ing) setting of the pace, or regulation of the rate of something.

antitachycardia p. cardiac pacing with stimuli timed to terminate a tachyarrhythmia.

asynchronous p. cardiac pacing in which impulse generation by the pacemaker occurs at a fixed rate, independent of underlying cardiac activity.

atrial p. cardiac pacing by means of an intracardiac electrode inserted in the atrium or by temporary placement of an esophageal electrode.

bipolar p. cardiac pacing in which both electrodes contact the cardiac tissue; inappropriate sensing of electromagnetic interference and extracardiac stimulation are less frequent than in unipolar pacing.

biventricular p. cardiac resynchronization therapy.

burst p. overdrive p.

cardiac p. regulation of the rate of contraction of the heart muscle by an artificial cardiac pacemaker.

competitive p. underdrive p.

continuous p. continuous delivery of cardiac pacing stimuli, either at a normal or overdrive rate, to prevent tachycardias.

coupled p. a variation of paired pacing in which the patient's natural depolarization serves as the first of the two stimuli, with the second induced by an artificial cardiac pacemaker.

diaphragm p., diaphragmatic p. electrophrenic respiration.

dual chamber p. cardiac pacing using an artificial pacemaker that paces, senses, or does both in the atria and in the ventricles.

epicardial p. a method for temporary cardiac pacing or sensing of the atria or ventricles by attaching pacing leads to the epicardial surface; usually used in the diagnosis and treatment of postoperative dysrhythmias.

esophageal p. transesophageal p.

overdrive p. cardiac pacing that increases the heart rate with an artificial cardiac pacemaker in order to suppress certain arrhythmias.

paired p. cardiac pacing in which two impulses are delivered to the heart in close succession, the second generally just at the end of the refractory period induced by the first; used to slow tachyarrhythmias and to improve cardiac performance.

phrenic p. electrophrenic respiration.

physiologic p. cardiac pacing in which the pacemaker stimulates cardiac activity such that it duplicates as closely as possible the normally conducted sinus rhythm.

ramp p. cardiac pacing in which stimuli are delivered at a rapid but continually altering rate, either from faster to slower *(rate decremental* or *tune down)*, from fast to faster *(cycle length decremental* or *ramp up)*, or in some cyclic combination of increasing and decreasing rates; it is used to terminate tachyarrhythmias.

single chamber p. cardiac pacing in which the artificial pacemaker paces and senses in either atria or ventricles, usually in the latter.

synchronous p. cardiac pacing in which information about sensed activity in one or more cardiac chambers is used to set timing of impulse generation by the artificial pacemaker.

transcutaneous p. a temporary method for cardiac pacing, in which large surface, high impedance electrodes are applied to the anterior and posterior chest walls to deliver high current stimuli of long duration for pacing of the ventricles.

transesophageal p. a temporary method for cardiac pacing using leads placed within the esophagus to effect temporary atrial pacing in the diagnosis and treatment of dysrhythmias.

transthoracic p. a temporary method for cardiac pacing in which a hooked pacing lead is attached to the ventricular endocardium by insertion through the chest wall or epigastric area and then the ventricular wall; it is used in emergency situations, usually cardiac arrest, as an alternative to transcutaneous pacing.

transvenous p. a permanent or temporary method for cardiac pacing in which the pacing leads, inserted by means of a catheter, are connected to the endocardium via the venous circulation; the pulse generator may be implanted or external.

ultrafast train p., ultrarapid p. a form of overdrive pacing in which a short series of pacing stimuli is delivered at a rate equivalent to 3000 to 6000 beats per minute to terminate a tachyarrhythmia.

underdrive p. a method of cardiac pacing for terminating certain slow ventricular or supraventricular tachycardias by means of slow asynchronous pacing, with stimuli delivered at a rate that is not an even fraction of the tachycardia rate, in order to capture the heart rate.

unipolar p. cardiac pacing that uses only a single electrode in contact with the cardiac tissue, with the indifferent electrode generally part of the pulse generator metal housing.

ventricular p. cardiac pacing in which the stimulus from the pacemaker is delivered to the ventricle.

Pa·ci·ni corpuscle (pah-che′ne) [Filippo *Pacini*, Italian anatomist, 1812–1883] see under *corpuscle*.

pa·cin·i·an (pə-sin′e-ən) named for Filippo *Pacini*.

pack (pak) 1. treatment by wrapping a patient in blankets or sheets or a limb in towels, wet or dry and either hot or cold. 2. the blankets, sheets, or towels used for this purpose. 3. a tampon.

cold p. blankets, sheets, or towels that have been dipped in cold water, for wrapping a limb or the entire body.

dry p. dry, hot blankets or towels for wrapping a limb or the entire body.

full p. a pack that encloses the entire body.

half p. a pack applied from the axillae to below the knees.

hot p. hot blankets or towels, wet or dry, for wrapping a limb or the entire body.

Hydrocollator p. trademark for a hot pack containing silicate gel in a porous bag that is soaked in hot water and laid over cloth over a body part.

ice p. a folded towel filled with crushed ice, often used in place of an icebag.

Mikulicz p. layers of mesh or gutta-percha sewn together at the edges, packed with strips of gauze, often placed in a denuded pelvic area to wall off the unperitonealized surfaces; also used for packing off abdominal viscera to improve operative exposure.

partial p. a wet pack covering only a portion of the body.

periodontal p. a surgical dressing applied over the surgical wound following periodontal operations to provide a matrix for the regeneration of tissue and enhance healing processes.

salt p. a type of wet pack consisting of sheets or blankets wrung out after immersion in salt water.

three-quarters p. a wet pack that extends from the toes to the axillae.

throat p. a moistened gauze pack used as a posterior pharyngeal seal around a noncuffed endotracheal tube.

wet p., wet-sheet p. wet blankets or sheets, hot or cold, for wrapping a limb or the entire body.

pack·er (pak′ər) an instrument for introducing dressing into the uterus or vagina, or into another body cavity or wound.

pack·ing (pak′ing) 1. the act of filling a wound or cavity with gauze, sponges, pads, or other material. 2. the material used for filling a cavity.

pac·li·tax·el (pak″lĭ-tak′səl) an antineoplastic agent that acts by promoting and stabilizing the polymerization of microtubules, isolated from the Pacific yew tree *(Taxus brevifolia);* used in the treatment of advanced ovarian or breast carcinoma, non–small cell lung carcinoma, and AIDS-related Kaposi sarcoma. Administered intravenously.

PACU postanesthesia care unit; see under *unit*.

pad (pad) a cushionlike mass of soft material.

abdominal p. a pad for the absorption of discharges from abdominal wounds; also for packing off abdominal viscera to improve exposure during surgical procedures. Called also *laparotomy p.*

abdominal fat p. the subcutaneous fat in the abdomen.

buccal fat p. corpus adiposum buccae.

calcaneal fat p. heel p. (def. 1).

dinner p. a pad placed over the abdomen before a plaster jacket is applied. The pad is then removed, leaving space under the jacket to provide for expansion of the abdomen after eating.

grounding p. an inactive electrode, part of a monopolar electrocautery, that is attached to the patient and returns the current distributed from the active electrode to the generator through an attached cable to complete the electrical circuit.

gum p's edentulous segments of the maxilla and the mandible that correspond to the underlying primary teeth.

heating p. a hollow pad with an electric mechanism inside that can be adjusted to a variety of temperatures; used for superficial warming of body parts.

heel p. 1. a specialized collection of fibrous and adipose tissue underlying the calcaneus to form a cushion for the heel; called also *calcaneal fat p.* and *heel fat p.* 2. a soft pad inserted in a shoe to cushion the heel.

heel fat p. heel p. (def. 1).

infrapatellar fat p. corpus adiposum infrapatellare.

knuckle p's small fibrous nodules on the dorsal surface of the interphalangeal joints, with thickening of the dermis and epidermis, thought to be hereditary; they may be associated with camptodactyly or Dupuytren contracture.

laparotomy p. abdominal pad.

metatarsal p. 1. a specialized collection of fibrous and adipose tissue underlying the metatarsal bones to form a cushion for the anterior part of the foot. 2. a soft pad inserted in a shoe to cushion the metatarsal region.

occlusal p. a pad which covers the occlusal surface of a tooth.

Passavant p. crista palatopharyngea.

plantar fat p. either of two specialized collections of fibrous and adipose tissue on the plantar surface of the foot, serving as cushions to absorb pressure, such as when a person walks. See *heel p.* (def. 1) and *metatarsal p.* (def. 1).

retromolar p. a mass of tissue, often pear-shaped, located at the distal termination of the mandibular residual ridge, and made up of the retromolar papilla and the retromolar glandular prominence.

retropatellar fat p. corpus adiposum infrapatellare.

sucking p., suctorial p. corpus adiposum buccae.

Pad·gett dermatome (paj′ət) [Earl Calvin *Padgett*, American surgeon, 1893–1946] see under *dermatome*.

pad·i·mate A (pad′ĭ-māt) a substituted aminobenzoate having properties similar to those of *p*-aminobenzoic acid, used as a sunscreen.

pad·i·mate O (pad′ĭ-māt) a substituted aminobenzoate having properties similar to those of *p*-aminobenzoic acid, used as a sunscreen.

pae- for words beginning thus, see also those beginning *pe-*.

Pae·cil·o·my·ces (pe-sil″o-mi′sēz) a genus of soil-inhabiting Fungi Imperfecti of the form-class Hyphomycetes, form-family Moniliaceae, which morphologically resembles Penicillium; see paecilomycosis. *P. lilaci′nus* infection in humans is most often oculomycosis; both *P. lilaci′nus* and *P. vario′ti* cause human mycotic endocarditis that can be fatal. Various species cause systemic infections in cats and dogs.

pae·ci·lo·my·co·sis (pe″sĭ-lo-mi-ko′sis) a fungal infection with species of *Paecilomyces*.

Pae·der·us (pe′dər-əs) a genus of blister beetles (family Meloidae), native to South America, Asia, and Africa, from which pederin has been isolated.

paed(o)- see *ped(o)-*[1].

Pae·ni·ba·cil·lus (pe″nĭ-bə-sil′əs) [L. *paene* almost + *Bacillus*] a genus of bacteria of the family Paenibacillaceae, consisting of gram-positive or gram-negative, motile, spore-producing, aerobic or facultatively anaerobic rods. Almost all species are positive for catalase; most are soil saprophytes, but some are pathogenic for insects. Many species were formerly assigned to the genus *Bacillus*.

P. al′vei the etiologic agent of European foulbrood of honeybees. Formerly called *Bacillus alvei*.

P. lar′vae the etiologic agent of American foulbrood of honeybees. Formerly called *Bacillus larvae*.

P. polymyx′a a saprophytic soil and water microorganism that produces the antibiotic polymyxin. Formerly called *Bacillus polymyxa*.

Pae·ni·ba·cil·la·ceae (pe″nĭ-bas″ĭ-la′se-e) a family of bacteria of the order Bacillales; medically important organisms are contained in the genera *Brevibacillus* and *Paenibacillus*.

PAF platelet-activating factor.

PAF-ac·e·ther (əs-e′thər) platelet-activating factor.

Page kidney (pāj) [Irwin H. *Page*, American physician, 20th century] see under *kidney*.

PAGE polyacrylamide gel electrophoresis.

Pag·et cell, disease, necrosis, test (paj′ət) [Sir James *Paget*, English surgeon, 1814–1899] see under *cell, disease, necrosis,* and *test*.

Pag·et-Schroet·ter syndrome (paj′ət shrur′tər) [Sir J. *Paget;* Kristelli Leopold von *Schroetter*, Austrian physician, 1837–1908] see under *syndrome*.

pa·get·ic (pə-jet′ik) affected with or relating to Paget disease.

pag·et·oid (paj′ə-toid) resembling or characteristic of Paget disease.

Pag•i•tane (paj′ĭ-tān) trademark for a preparation of cycrimine hydrochloride.

pa•go•pha•gia (pa″go-fa′je-ə) [Gr. *pagos* frost + *-phagia*] the ingestion of extraordinary amounts of ice, a type of pica often related to iron deficiency.

-pagus [Gr. *pagos* that which is fixed] a word termination denoting a symmetrical pair of twins conjoined at the site indicated by the stem to which it is affixed, as *craniopagus, pygopagus, thoracopagus.*

PAH *p*-aminohippuric acid; phenylalanine hydroxylase.

PAHA *p*-aminohippuric acid.

Pah•vant Val•ley fever (pah′vant val′e) [*Pahvant Valley*, Utah, where some of the first cases were reported] tularemia.

PAI plasminogen activator inhibitor.

pain (pān) [L. *poena, dolor;* Gr. *algos, odynē*] a more or less localized sensation of discomfort, distress, or agony, resulting from the stimulation of specialized nerve endings. It serves as a protective mechanism insofar as it induces the sufferer to remove or withdraw from the source.

axial p., axial back p. low back pain limited to the middle (spinal axis) of the lumbar region.

baseline p. the average intensity of pain experienced for 12 or more hours in a 24-hour period.

bearing-down p. pain accompanying uterine contractions during the second stage of labor.

boring p. a sensation as of being pierced with a long, slender, twisting object; called also *terebrant p.*

breakthrough p. a transient increase in pain intensity from a baseline pain level of no greater than moderate.

central p. pain due to a lesion in the central nervous system.

chest p. see *pectoralgia, pleurodynia,* and *thoracalgia.*

chronic functional abdominal p. (CFAP) a type of abdominal pain that may be severe, lasts for more than six months, and has no known physical cause (not being accompanied by change in bowel habits); causes proposed include psychogenic causes and abnormal sensitivity to nerve impulses in the region.

dilating p's labor pains during the first stage of labor.

expulsive p's labor pains during the second stage of labor.

false p's ineffective pains resembling labor pains but not accompanied by effacement or dilatation of the cervix.

gas p's pains caused by distention of the stomach or intestines by accumulations of air or other gases, occurring as a result of ingestion of gas-forming foods.

girdle p. a painful sensation as of a cord about the waist.

growing p's recurrent quasirheumatic limb pains peculiar to early youth.

heterotopic p. referred p.

homotopic p. pain that is felt at the point of injury.

hunger p. pain coming on at the time for feeling hunger for the next meal; it is a symptom of gastric disorder.

intermenstrual p. pain occurring during the period between the menses, usually about halfway, accompanying extrusion of the oocyte.

jumping p. a peculiar pain in joint diseases when the bone is laid bare by ulceration of the cartilage.

labor p's the rhythmic pains of increasing severity and frequency, caused by contractions of the uterus during childbirth.

lancinating p. a sharp, darting pain.

lightning p's the cutting and intense darting pains of tabes dorsalis.

mechanical p. the most common kind of axial pain, caused when a person puts stress on the lumbar region.

middle p. intermenstrual p.

myofascial p. pain attributed to trigger points in muscles and their fascia, with more specific points of origin than with fibromyalgia.

neurogenic p., neuropathic p. pain, such as that occurring in causalgia or herpetic neuralgia, that results from direct stimulation of nervous tissue of the peripheral or central nervous system (except for sensitized C fibers), generally felt as burning or tingling and often occurring in an area of sensory loss

phantom p., phantom limb p. pain felt as though arising in an absent (amputated) limb; see *phantom limb,* under *limb.*

postprandial p. abdominal pain occurring after eating a meal.

premonitory p's mild uterine contractions before the beginning of true labor.

psychic p. psychalgia (def. 1).

psychogenic p. symptoms of physical pain having psychological origin.

radicular p. root p.

referred p. pain felt in a part other than that in which the cause that produced it is situated.

rest p. a continuous burning pain of the lower leg and foot, beginning or worsening after reclining and being relieved by sitting or standing; it is due to ischemia.

root p. pain caused by disease of a sensory nerve root or roots and felt in the cutaneous areas supplied by the affected roots; some varieties, such as sciatica, may cover extensive areas of a limb. Called also *radicular p.*

somatic p. generally well-localized pain that results from the activation of peripheral nociceptors without injury to the peripheral nerve or central nervous system

starting p's pain and muscular spasm in the early stages of sleep.

stump p. pain arising in the stump in a person with an amputated limb; unlike phantom limb pain, which originates and ends in the brain, it originates from damaged nerve near the site of the amputation.

terebrant p., terebrating p. boring p.

visceral p. pain that results from the activation of nociceptors of the thoracic, pelvic, or abdominal viscera, felt as a poorly localized aching or cramping sensation and often referred to cutaneous sites.

wandering p. pain that repeatedly changes its location.

paint (pānt) 1. a liquid designed for application to the surface, as of the body or a tooth. 2. to apply a liquid to a specific area as a remedial or protective measure.

antiseptic p. a term used to describe immunoglobulin A secreted onto the surfaces of mucous membranes and affording local protection against agents possessing homologous antigens.

Castellani p. carbolfuchsin topical solution.

paint•ing (pānt′ing) 1. application of a liquid, particularly a colored liquid, to a specific area. 2. by extension, covering or labeling a specific area with one or more colors.

chromosome p. a form of fluorescence in situ hybridization in which a variety of different probes, tagged with any of several differently colored fluorochromes, are used simultaneously to uniquely mark individual chromosomes.

pair (pār) 1. a combination of two related, similar, or identical entities or objects. 2. in cardiology, two successive premature beats, particularly two ventricular premature complexes. Called also *couplet.*

base p. a pair of hydrogen-bonded bases, a pyrimidine with a purine base, that bind together two strands, or two parts of a strand, of nucleic acid. In DNA, the pairs are guanine–cytosine and adenine–thymine; in RNA, uracil replaces thymine.

buffer p. a buffer system consisting of an acid and its conjugate base.

ion p. the free electron and the positively charged residual atom that result from the ejection of an orbital electron by ionizing radiation.

pair•ing (pār′ing) the act or process of joining into pairs.

base p. the bonding between purines and pyrimidines in nucleic acids; see under *pair.*

PAIS partial androgen insensitivity syndrome.

pa•ja•ro•e•llo (pah-hah-ro-a′yo) *Ornithodoros coriaceus.*

Pa•jot's law, maneuver (pah-zhōz′) [Charles *Pajot*, French obstetrician, 1816–1896] see under *law* and *maneuver.*

Pal stain (pahl) [Jacob *Pal*, Austrian physician, 1863–1936] see *Stains and Staining Methods,* under *stain.*

palae(o)- for words beginning thus, see those beginning *pale(o)-*.

pa•la•ta (pə-la′tə) [L.] plural of *palatum.*

pal•a•tal (pal′ə-təl) 1. pertaining to the palate. 2. pertaining to the lingual surface of a maxillary tooth. 3. a consonantal speech sound produced with part of the tongue near the hard palate, such as *y, ch,* or *j.*

pal•ate (pal′ət) palatum.

artificial p. speech-aid prosthesis.

bony p., bony hard p. palatum osseum.

cleft p. congenital fissure of the soft palate or both the soft and hard palates, due to faulty fusion of the palatine processes; it typically opens through the roof of the mouth into the nasal cavity and extends anteriorly to the premaxilla, where it deviates to the right or left, following the line of fusion. Called also *palatoschisis, uranoschisis,* and *uranostaphyloschisis* (cleft of both the hard and the soft palate).

hard p. palatum durum.

pendulous p. uvula.

premaxillary p., primitive p. primary p.

primary p., primordial p. the first part of the palate to form in embryonic development, a triangular bony structure formed from the dorsal part of the median palatine process; it represents only a small part of the adult hard palate, that anterior to the incisive fossa.

secondary p. in embryonic development, the part of the palate that forms later than the primary palate, by fusion of the lateral palatine processes; it represents most of the adult hard and soft palates.

smokers' p. nicotine stomatitis.

soft p. palatum molle.

pal•a•tine (pal′ə-tīn) palatal (def. 1).

pal•a•ti•tis (pal″ə-ti′tis) 1. inflammation of the palate. 2. lampas.

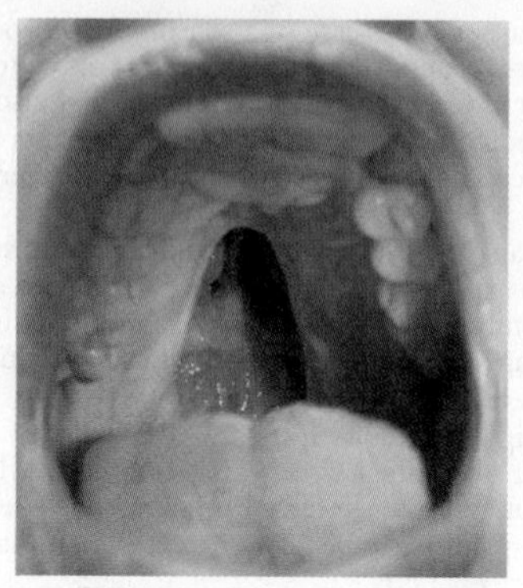

■ Severe cleft palate, the cleft extending from the soft to the hard palate.

palat(o)- [L. *palatum* palate] a combining form denoting relationship to the palate; sometimes used instead of *lingu(o)-* in terms referring to the lingual surface of maxillary teeth.

pal•a•to•glos•sal (pal″ə-to-glos′əl) pertaining to the palate and tongue.

pal•a•tog•na•thous (pal″ə-tog′nə-thəs) [*palato-* + *gnath-* + *-ous*] having a cleft palate.

pal•a•to•graph (pal′ə-to-graf) [*palato-* + *-graph*] an instrument used in palatography.

pal•a•tog•ra•phy (pal″ə-tog′rə-fe) the recording of movements of the palate in speech. See also *palatomyography*.

pal•a•to•max•il•lary (pal″ə-to-mak′sĭ-lar″e) pertaining to the palate and the maxilla.

pal•a•to•my•og•ra•phy (pal″ə-to-mi-og′rə-fe) [*palato-* + *myo-* + *-graphy*] the recording of muscular movements of the palate.

pal•a•to•na•sal (pal″ə-to-na′zəl) [*palato-* + *nasal*] nasopalatine.

pal•a•top•a•gus (pal″ə-top′ə-gəs) [*palato-* + *-pagus*] symmetrical twins conjoined at the palate.

pal•a•to•pha•ryn•ge•al (pal″ə-to-fə-rin′je-əl) pertaining to the palate and pharynx.

pal•a•to•pha•ryn•go•plas•ty (pal″ə-to-fə-ring′go-plas″te) a trimming back of excess palatal and pharyngeal tissue, done in order to widen the airway and relieve obstructive sleep apnea or severe snoring. Called also *uvulopalatoplasty* and *uvulopalatopharyngoplasty*. **palatopharyngoplas′tic** *adj*

pal•a•to•plas•ty (pal′ə-to-plas″te) [*palato-* + *-plasty*] plastic reconstruction of the palate, including cleft palate operations. Called also *uranoplasty*. **palatoplas′tic** *adj*

von Langenbeck p. see *von Langenbeck bipedicle mucoperiosteal flap*, under *flap*.

pal•a•to•ple•gia (pal″ə-to-ple′jə) [*palato-* + *-plegia*] paralysis of the palate.

pal•a•to•prox•i•mal (pal″ə-to-prok′sĭ-məl) pertaining to the palatal (lingual) and proximal surface of a maxillary tooth.

pal•a•tor•rha•phy (pal″ə-tor′ə-fe) surgical correction of a cleft palate, the cleft involving the soft palate and the soft tissues over the hard palate; cf. *palatoplasty*. Called also *staphylorrhaphy* and *uranorrhaphy*.

pal•a•tos•chi•sis (pal″ə-tos′kĭ-sis) cleft palate.

pa•la•tum (pə-la′təm) gen. *pala′ti*, pl. *pala′ta* [L.] [TA] the palate: the partition separating the nasal and oral cavities, consisting anteriorly of a hard bony part and posteriorly of a soft fleshy part.

p. du′rum [TA] hard palate: the anterior part of the palate, characterized by an osseous framework, covered superiorly by mucous membrane of the nasal cavity and, on its oral surface, by mucoperiosteum.

p. mol′le [TA] soft palate: the fleshy part of the roof of the mouth, extending from the posterior edge of the hard palate; from its free inferior border is a projection of variable length, the uvula. Called also *velum palatinum* [TA alternative].

p. os′seum [TA] bony palate: the bony part of the anterior two-thirds of the roof of the mouth, formed by the palatine processes of the maxillae and the horizontal plates of the palatine bones. Called also *bony hard palate*.

pale(o)- [Gr. *palaios* old] a combining form meaning old. Also, *palae(o)-*.

pa•leo•cer•e•bel•lum (pa″le-o-ser″ə-bel′əm) [*paleo-* + *cerebellum*] [TA] the phylogenetically second oldest part of the cerebellum, namely the vermis of the anterior lobe and the pyramis, uvula, and paraflocculus of the posterior lobe. Because this corresponds roughly to the primary site of termination of the major spinocerebellar afferents, the term is sometimes equated with *spinocerebellum*. Cf. *archicerebellum* and *neocerebellum*. **paleocerebel′lar** *adj*

pa•leo•cor•tex (pa″le-o-kor′teks) [*paleo-* + *cortex*] [TA] the portion of the cerebral cortex that, with the archicortex, develops in association with the olfactory system, and which is phylogenetically older and less stratified than the neocortex. It is composed chiefly of the piriform cortex and the parahippocampal gyrus. Spelled also *palaeocortex*.

pa•leo•gen•e•sis (pa″le-o-jen′ə-sis) palingenesis (def. 2).

pa•leo•ge•net•ic (pa″le-o-jə-net′ik) [*paleo-* + *genetic*] originated in the past; said of traits, structures, and other aspects of a species that are not newly acquired.

pa•leo•pa•thol•o•gy (pa″le-o-pə-thol′ə-je) [*paleo-* + *pathology*] the study of disease in bodies preserved from ancient times, such as mummies.

pa•leo•sen•sa•tion (pa″le-o-sən-sa′shən) [*paleo-* + *sensation*] the sensation of severe pain and marked variations of temperature, as compared with phylogenetically newer sensations such as those of light touch and moderate variations of temperature and the epicritic sensations.

pa•leo•stri•a•tum (pa″le-o-stri-a′təm) [*paleo-* + *striatum*] the phylogenetically older part of the corpus striatum represented by the globus pallidus. Cf. *neostriatum*. **paleostria′tal** *adj*

pa•leo•thal•a•mus (pa″le-o-thal′ə-məs) [*paleo-* + *thalamus*] the phylogenetically older part of the thalamus, i.e., the medial portion which lacks reciprocal connections with the neopallium.

pali- [Gr. *palin* backward, or again] a combining form meaning again, often denoting pathologic repetition. Also, *palin-*.

pali•ci•ne•sia (pal″ĭ-sĭ-ne′zhə) palikinesia.

Pali•co•u•rea (pal″ĭ-ko-u′re-ə) a genus of Brazilian plants, some species of which contain fluoroacetates and can cause fatal fluoroacetate poisoning in livestock.

pali•ki•ne•sia (pal″ĭ-kĭ-ne′zhə) [*pali-* + *kinesi-* + *-ia*] a dyskinesia involving pathologic repetition of movements; called also *palicinesia*.

pali•la•lia (pal″ĭ-la′le-ə) palinphrasia.

palin- see *pali-*.

pal•in•drome (pal′in-drōm) [Gr. *palindromos* a running back] in genetics, a DNA or RNA sequence that reads the same in both directions.

pal•in•dro•mia (pal″in-dro′me-ə) [Gr. *palindromia* a running back] the recurrence of a disease. **palindro′mic** *adj*

pal•in•gen•e•sis (pal″in-jen′ə-sis) [*palin-* + *genesis*] the regeneration or restoration of a lost part.

pal•in•graph•ia (pal″in-graf′e-ə) [*palin-* + *graph-* + *-ia*] dysgraphia involving repetition of letters, words, or parts of words.

pa•lin•mne•sis (pal″in-ne′sis) remote memory.

pali•nop•sia (pal″ĭ-nop′se-ə) [*palin-* + *-opsia*] visual perseveration; the pathologic continuance or recurrence of a visual sensation after the stimulus is gone.

pal•in•phra•sia (pal″in-fra′zhə) [*palin-* + Gr. *phrasis* speech + *-ia*] a dysphasia involving repetition of words or phrases; see also *stuttering* (def. 1). Called also *palilalia* and *paliphrasia*.

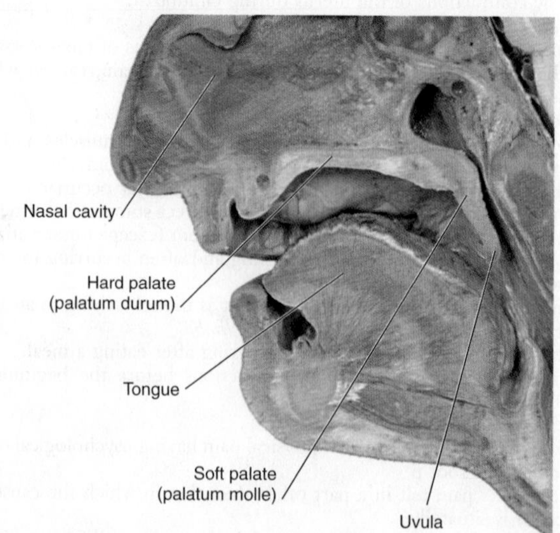

■ Palatum durum (hard palate) and palatum molle (soft palate) in a midline sagittal section.

pali•phra•sia (pal″ĭ-fra′ze-ə) palinphrasia.

pal•i•sade (pal″ĭ-sād′) [Fr. *palissade*, from L. *palus* stake] the arrangement of cells or cellular structures side by side in rows, like pickets in a fence; it is characteristic of some fungi and bacterial cell smears and of cells seen in tissue sections in certain normal and disease states.

p's of Vogt crests of epithelial folds running radially from the sclera to the cornea where corneal epithelial stem cells can be found.

pal•i•viz•u•mab (pal″ĭ-viz′u-mab) a humanized monoclonal antibody produced by recombinant DNA technology and directed against respiratory syncytial virus (RSV); used as a passive immunizing agent in susceptible infants and children, administered intramuscularly.

pal•la•di•um (Pd) (pə-la′de-əm) [L.] a rare, hard, noble metal resembling platinum; specific gravity, 12.16; atomic number, 46; atomic weight, 106.4. It is lighter in weight than platinum and of a neutral color, and is used in alloys for dental and orthodontic appliances.

Pal•la•done (pal′ə-dōn) trademark for a preparation of hydromorphone hydrochloride.

pall•an•es•the•sia (pal″ən-es-the′zhə) [Gr. *pallein* to shake + *anesthesia*] loss or lack of pallesthesia (vibration sense). Called also *apallesthesia.*

pall•es•the•sia (pal″es-the′zhə) [Gr. *pallein* to shake + *esthesia*] the ability to feel mechanical vibrations on or near the body, such as when a vibrating tuning fork is placed over a bony prominence. Called also *vibration sense.* **pallesthet′ic** *adj*

pal•li•al (pal′e-əl) pertaining to the pallium.

pal•li•ate (pal′e-āt) to reduce the severity of; to relieve.

pal•li•a•tive (pal′e-ə-tiv) [L. *palliatus* cloaked] 1. affording relief but not cure. 2. an alleviating medicine.

pal•li•dal (pal′ĭ-dəl) pertaining to the globus pallidus.

pal•li•dec•to•my (pal″ĭ-dek′tə-me) surgical excision of the globus pallidus or extirpation of it by other means (such as chemopallidectomy).

pal•li•do•an•sec•tion (pal″ĭ-do-ən-sek′shən) surgical section of the globus pallidus and ansa lenticularis.

pal•li•do•an•sot•o•my (pal″ĭ-do-ən-sot′ə-me) production of lesions in the globus pallidus and ansa lenticularis.

pal•li•dof•u•gal (pal″ĭ-dof′u-gəl) [*pallidum* + *-fugal*[2]] conducting impulses away from the globus pallidus.

pal•li•do•luy•si•an (pal″ĭ-do-lwe′se-ən) 1. conducting or proceeding from the globus pallidus to the subthalamic nucleus (nucleus of Luys). 2. pertaining to or including the globus pallidus and subthalamic nucleus (nucleus of Luys).

pal•li•dot•o•my (pal″ĭ-dot′ə-me) [*pallidum* + *-tomy*] stereotactic surgery in which lesions are produced in the globus pallidus for treatment of extrapyramidal syndromes.

pal•li•dum (pal′ĭ-dəm) [L. "pale"] globus pallidus.

p. I globus pallidus medialis.

p. II globus pallidus lateralis.

Pal•lis•ter-Kil•li•an syndrome (pal′is-tər kil′e-ən) [Philip David *Pallister*, American geneticist, born 1920; Wolfgang *Killian*, Austrian physician, born 1944] see under *syndrome.*

pal•li•um (pal′e-əm) [L. "cloak"] 1. [TA] cortex cerebri. 2. the cerebral cortex during its period of development.

pal•lor (pal′ər) [L.] paleness; decrease or absence of skin coloration.

palm (pahm, pahlm) [L. *palma*] 1. palma. 2. a tree of the family *Palmae* (q.v.).

betel p. *Areca catechu.*

coconut p. *Cocos nucifera.*

handball p. contusion of the palm of the hand occurring in handball players.

tripe p. a paraneoplastic syndrome in which the palm of the hand is thickened, velvety, and rugose, similar to tripe; often a sign of new or recurrent pulmonary or gastric malignancy.

pal•ma (pahl′mə) gen. and pl. *pal′mae* [L.] [TA] palm: the flexor surface of the hand. Called also *vola* [TA alternative] and *regio palmaris* [TA alternative].

Pal•ma•ceae (pahl-ma′se-e) Palmae.

Pal•mae (pahl′me) the palms, a family of evergreen trees, shrubs, and woody vines, generally found in tropical regions. Genera of medical interest include *Areca, Cocos, Copernicia,* and *Cycas.* Called also *Palmaceae.*

pal•mae (pahl′me) [L.] genitive and plural of *palma.*

pal•mar (pahl′mər) [L. *palmaris; palma* palm] pertaining to the palm.

pal•mar•is (pahl-mar′is) [TA] palmar; a general term designating relationship to the palm of the hand. Called also *volaris* [TA alternative].

pal•mate (pahl′māt) [L. *palma* palm] having a shape resembling that of a hand with the fingers spread.

pal•ma•ture (pahl′mə-chər) [L. *palma* palm] a webbed state of the fingers.

Pal•maz stent (pahl-mahz′) [Julio César *Palmaz*, Argentine-born radiologist in the United States, born 1945] see under *stent.*

pal•mi•tal (pal′mĭ-təl) an aldehyde lipid, the aldehyde form of palmitate; see *plasmalogen.*

pal•mi•tate (pal′mĭ-tāt) the anionic form of palmitic acid.

pal•mit•ic ac•id (pal-mit′ik) [NF] a 16-carbon saturated fatty acid found in most fats and oils, particularly associated with stearic acid. It is one of the most prevalent saturated fatty acids in body lipids. See also table accompanying *fatty acid.*

pal•mi•tin (pal′mĭ-tin) a crystallizable and saponifiable fat from various fats and oils; glyceryl tripalmitate.

pal•mi•to•le•ate (pal″mĭ-to′le-āt) a salt (soap), ester, or anionic form of palmitoleic acid.

pal•mi•to•le•ic ac•id (pal″mĭ-to-le′ik) a monounsaturated 16-carbon fatty acid occurring in many oils, particularly those derived from marine animals. See also table accompanying *fatty acid.*

pal•mi•to•yl (pal″mĭ-to′əl) the acyl radical of palmitic acid. As palmitoyl CoA, a thioester formed with coenzyme A, it can act as a donor of fatty acyl groups in lipid biosynthesis.

palo•no•se•tron hy•dro•chlo•ride (pal-o-no′sə-tron) an antagonist to serotonin receptors, used as an antiemetic; administered by intravenous injection.

palp•a•ble (pal′pə-bəl) perceptible by touch.

pal•pate (pal′pāt) [L. *palpare* to touch] to examine by the hand; to feel.

pal•pa•tion (pal-pa′shən) [L. *palpatio*] the act of feeling with the hand; the application of the fingers with light pressure to the surface of the body for the purpose of determining the consistency of the parts beneath in physical diagnosis.

bimanual p. examination with both hands.

light touch p. light palpation of the surface of the abdomen and thorax with the fingertips for the purpose of finding the outlines of the organs.

pal•pa•to•per•cus•sion (pal″pə-to-pər-kŭ′shən) palpation combined with percussion.

pal•pe•bra (pal′pə-brə) gen. and pl. *pal′pebrae* [L.] [TA] eyelid; either of the two movable folds that protect the anterior surface of the eyeball. **pal′pebral** *adj*

p. infe′rior [TA] lower eyelid: the inferior of the paired movable folds that protect the surface of the eyeball.

p. supe′rior [TA] upper eyelid: the superior of the paired movable folds that protect the surface of the eyeball.

p. ter′tia nictitating membrane.

pal•pe•brae (pal′pə-bre) [L.] genitive and plural of *palpebra.*

pal•pe•bral•is (pal″pə-bra′lis) [L.] palpebral.

pal•pe•brate (pal′pə-brāt) [L. *palpebrare* to wink] 1. to wink. 2. having eyelids.

pal•pe•bra•tion (pal″pə-bra′shən) 1. winking. 2. abnormally frequent winking, as from a tic.

pal•pe•bri•tis (pal″pə-bri′tis) blepharitis.

pal•pi•ta•tion (pal″pĭ-ta′shən) [L. *palpitare* to move frequently and rapidly] a subjective sensation of an unduly rapid or irregular heart beat.

pal•pus (pal′pəs) pl. *pal′pi* [L. *palpare* to touch softly] one of the articulated sensory structures attached to the mouth parts of arthropods.

PALS periarteriolar lymphoid sheath.

pal•sy (pawl′ze) paralysis.

abducens p., abducens nerve p. paralysis of the lateral rectus muscle of the eye due to lesion of the abducens nerve, with internal strabismus and diplopia. Called also *abducens paralysis* and *lateral rectus* or *sixth nerve palsy.*

Bell p. unilateral facial paralysis of sudden onset, due to lesion of the facial nerve and resulting in characteristic distortion of the face.

birth p. see under *paralysis.*

brachial p. see under *paralysis.*

bulbar p. see *progressive bulbar p.*

cerebral p. general name for a large group of persisting, nonprogressive motor disorders appearing in young children and resulting from brain damage caused by birth trauma or intrauterine pathology. The disorders are characterized by delayed or abnormal motor development, such as spastic paraplegia, hemiplegia, or tetraplegia, which is often accompanied by mental retardation, seizures, or ataxia. See also *spastic paraplegia* and *Little disease.*

crossed leg p. palsy of peroneal nerves caused by sitting with one leg crossed over the other.
divers' p. weakness of an area of the body owing to decompression sickness.
Erb p., Erb-Duchenne p. see under *paralysis.*
facial p. Bell p.
fourth nerve p. trochlear nerve p.
ischemic p. see under *paralysis.*
lateral rectus p. abducens p.
long thoracic nerve p. paralysis of the long thoracic nerve with winging of the scapula and inability to raise the arm. Called also *long thoracic neuropathy.*
maternal obstetric p. paralysis affecting some portion of the mother's lower limb due to compression of a nerve during delivery, usually when the fetus is large and the mother is small and has difficult labor. The most common cause is compression of the lumbosacral plexus or its nerves by the fetal head or forceps, resulting in unilateral footdrop.
oculomotor p., oculomotor nerve p. oculomotor paralysis.
oculosympathetic p. Horner syndrome.
printer's p. a condition observed in printers due to chronic antimony poisoning, and marked by neuritis with paralysis, pain in the pelvic region, and papular eruption.
progressive bulbar p. progressive paralysis and atrophy of the muscles of the lips, tongue, mouth, pharynx, and larynx due to lesions of the motor nuclei of the lower brainstem. It is a chronic, generally fatal disease with onset usually in late adulthood; onset may be earlier in patients with amyotrophic lateral sclerosis, syringobulbia, or multiple sclerosis. See also *progressive bulbar p. of childhood* and *Brown-Vialetto-van Laere syndrome.* Called also *bulbar, glossolabial, glossopharyngolabial, labial, labioglossolaryngeal, labioglossopharyngeal,* or *progressive bulbar paralysis;* and *Duchenne paralysis* or *syndrome.*
progressive bulbar p. of childhood, progressive infantile bulbar p. a rare type of progressive bulbar palsy that occurs in young children. Called also *Fazio-Londe atrophy* or *disease.*
progressive supranuclear p. a progressive neurological disorder, having onset during the sixth decade, characterized by supranuclear ophthalmoplegia, especially paralysis of the downward gaze, pseudobulbar paralysis, dysarthria, dystonic rigidity of the neck and trunk, and dementia. Called also *Steele-Richardson-Olszewski syndrome.*
pseudobulbar p. spastic weakness of the muscles innervated by the cranial nerves, i.e., the muscles of the face, pharynx, and tongue, owing to bilateral lesions of the corticospinal tract; symptoms include dysphagia, dysarthria, and spastic facial jerks, sometimes with uncontrolled weeping or laughing and Cheyne-Stokes respiration. Called also *pseudobulbar* or *supranuclear paralysis.*
radial p., radial nerve p., Saturday night p. radial neuropathy.
recurrent laryngeal nerve p. hoarseness or paralysis of structures in and around the larynx owing to damage to the recurrent laryngeal nerve; this may be from compression neuropathy or from disease that affects the nerve.
shaking p. Parkinson disease.
sixth nerve p. abducens p.
spastic bulbar p. pseudobulbar paralysis.
tardy median p. carpal tunnel syndrome.
tardy ulnar p. cubital tunnel syndrome that occurs months to years after injury to the elbow.
third nerve p. oculomotor paralysis.
trochlear p., trochlear nerve p. paralysis of the trochlear nerve, with diplopia and pain at the corner of the orbit; many cases are idiopathic, and a few are complications of herpes zoster ophthalmicus. Called also *fourth nerve p.*
ulnar p., ulnar nerve p. ulnar neuropathy.
wasting p. spinal muscular atrophy.

pal•u•dism (pal'u-diz-əm) malaria.

Pal•u•drine (pal'u-drin) trademark for a preparation of proguanil hydrochloride.

2-PAM pralidoxime.

L-PAM L-phenylalanine mustard; see *melphalan.*

PAM primary amebic meningoencephalitis.

pam•a•brom (pam'ə-brom) [USP] a mild diuretic used in preparations for the relief of premenstrual syndrome.

Pam•e•lor (pam'ə-lor) trademark for a preparation of nortriptyline hydrochloride.

pam•i•dro•nate (APD) (pam″ĭ-dro'nāt) an aminohydroxypropylidene-substituted diphosphonate compound with an affinity for sites of osteoid mineralization; it inhibits bone resorption by adsorbing onto hydroxyapatite crystals in mineralized bone matrix and reducing its solubility, and possibly also by inhibiting osteoclast activity. It is also used in bone imaging complexed with technetium 99m; see table at *technetium.*
p. disodium [USP] the disodium salt of pamidronate; used in the treatment of malignancy-associated hypercalcemia, osteitis deformans, and osteolytic bone metastases associated with breast cancer and myeloma; administered intravenously.

pam•o•ate (pam'o-āt) USAN contraction for 4,4′-methylenebis[3-hydroxy-2-naphthoate].

pam•pin•i•form (pam-pin'ĭ-form) [L. *pampinus* tendril + *form*] shaped like a tendril.

PAN polyarteritis nodosa.

Pan (pan) a genus of primates of the family Pongidae. *P. troglody'tes* is the chimpanzee.

pan- [Gr. *pan* all] prefix signifying all.

pan•a•cea (pan″ə-se'ə) [Gr. *panakeia*] 1. a universal remedy. 2. an ancient name for a healing herb or its juice.

pan•ac•i•nar (pan-as'ĭ-nər) affecting many acini uniformly, including respiratory bronchioles, alveolar ducts, and alveolar sacs.

Pan•a•fil (pan'ə-fil) trademark for a preparation of chlorophyllin copper complex, papain, and urea.

pan•ag•glu•tin•a•ble (pan″ə-gloo'tĭ-nə-bəl) agglutinable with every type of blood serum from the same species, e.g., red blood cells agglutinable with sera of all human blood groups.

pan•ag•glu•ti•na•tion (pan″ə-gloo″tĭ-na'shən) agglutination (e.g., of red blood cells) by the serum of all blood groups of the same species.

pan•ag•glu•ti•nin (pan″ə-gloo'tĭ-nin) [*pan-* + *agglutinin*] an agglutinin which agglutinates the red blood cells of all blood groups in the same species.

pan•an•gi•itis (pan″an-je-i'tis) [*pan-* + *angiitis*] inflammation involving all the coats of the vessel.
diffuse necrotizing p. panangiitis with extensive involvement of the blood vessels.

pan•ar•ter•i•tis (pan″ahr-tə-ri'tis) polyarteritis (def. 1).
p. nodo'sa polyarteritis nodosa.

pan•ar•thri•tis (pan″ahr-thri'tis) [*pan-* + *arthr-* + *-itis*] inflammation of all the joints or of all the structures of a joint.

pan•at•ro•phy (pan-at'rə-fe) [*pan-* + *atrophy*] atrophy affecting several parts; general atrophy.

pan•au•to•nom•ic (pan″aw-tə-nom'ik) pertaining to or affecting the entire autonomic (sympathetic and parasympathetic) nervous system.

Pan•ax (pan'aks) the ginsengs, a genus of perennial herbs of the family Araliaceae, native to parts of Asia and eastern North America. *P. gin'seng* is Chinese ginseng and *P. quinquefo'lius* is American ginseng; both yield the root used in Chinese medicine. See *ginseng* (def. 2).

pan•blas•tic (pan-blas'tik) [*pan-* + *blast-* + *-ic*] pertaining to each of the layers of the blastoderm.

pan•bron•chi•o•li•tis (pan-brong″ke-o-li'tis) a chronic type of infectious inflammation of the airways limited to the bronchioles, seen mainly in East Asia and nearby island countries.

pan•car•di•tis (pan″kahr-di'tis) [*pan-* + *carditis*] diffuse inflammation of the heart, involving the pericardium, myocardium, and endocardium.

pan•cha•kar•ma (pahn″chə-kahr'mə) [Sanskrit "five actions"] a fivefold purification treatment used in ayurveda, consisting of administration of a purgative to eliminate kapha, a laxative of oil or decocted medicines to eliminate pitta, an enema to eliminate vata, inhalation treatment to clear doshas from the head, and bloodletting to purify the blood. There are slight variations on the process, and some of the actions may be omitted in a given case.

pan•chro•mat•ic (pan″kro-mat'ik) [*pan-* + *chromatic*] sensitive to all colors; applied to photographic emulsions.

pan•chro•mia (pan-kro'me-ə) the condition of staining with various dyes.

Pan•coast syndrome, tumor (pan'kōst) [Henry Khunrath *Pancoast,* American radiologist, 1875–1939] see under *syndrome,* and see *pulmonary sulcus tumor,* under *tumor.*

pan•co•lec•to•my (pan″ko-lek'tə-me) excision of the entire colon with creation of an ileostomy.

pan•co•li•tis (pan″ko-li'tis) inflammation of the entire colon.
necrotizing amebic p. a rare but highly fatal complication of amebic dysentery, clinically resembling fulminant ulcerative colitis.

pan•cre•al•gia (pan″kre-al'jə) pancreatalgia.

pan•cre•as (pan'kre-əs) gen. *pancre'atis,* pl. *pancre'ata* [L., from Gr. *pankreas,* from *pan* all + *kreas* flesh] [TA] a large, elongated, racemose gland situated transversely behind the stomach, between the spleen and the duodenum. Its right extremity or *head* (TA, *caput pancreatis*) is larger

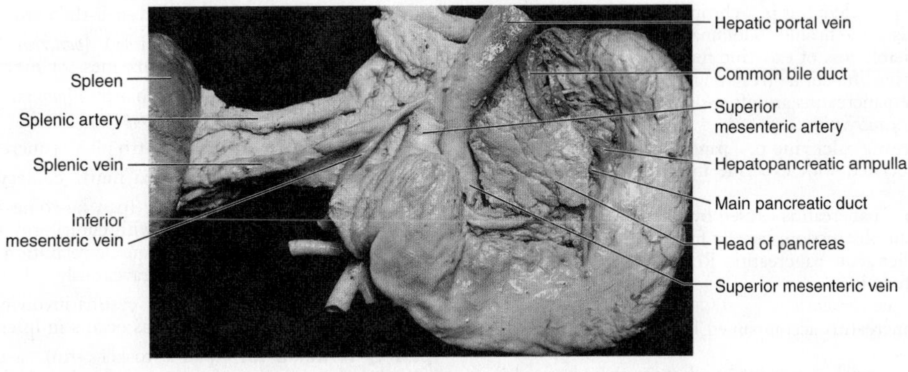

■ Pancreas.

and directed downward; its left extremity or *tail* (TA, *cauda pancreatis*) is transverse and terminates close to the spleen. It is subdivided into lobules by septa that extend into the gland from the thin, areolar tissue that forms an indefinite capsule. The endocrine part *(endocrine pancreas)* consists of the islets of Langerhans, which contain beta cells that produce insulin, alpha cells that produce glucagon, and delta cells that produce somatostatin; all three of these hormones are secreted directly into the bloodstream. Some islets contain PP cells that secrete pancreatic polypeptide. The exocrine part *(exocrine pancreas)* consists of pancreatic acini, secretory units that produce and secrete into the duodenum pancreatic juice, which contains enzymes essential to protein digestion. **pancreat′ic** *adj*

aberrant p. pancreatic rest.

p. accesso′rium [TA], **accessory p.** an inconstant separate part of the head of the pancreas, usually an unattached uncinate process.

annular p. a developmental anomaly in which the pancreas forms a ring around the duodenum.

Aselli p. the mesenteric lymph nodes of certain carnivores. Called also *Aselli glands.*

p. divi′sum a developmental anomaly in which the pancreas is divided into two separate structures, each with its own duct.

dorsal p. an embryonic bud growing out from the endodermal lining of the caudal part of the foregut on the dorsal wall cephalad to the level of the hepatic diverticulum, which forms most of the pancreas and its main duct.

endocrine p. the part of the pancreas that acts as an endocrine gland, consisting of the islets of Langerhans, which secrete insulin, glucagon, somatostatin, and sometimes pancreatic polypeptide directly into the bloodstream. See *pancreas.* Called also *endocrine part of pancreas.*

exocrine p. the part of the pancreas that acts as an exocrine gland, consisting of the pancreatic acini, which produce pancreatic juice and secrete it into the duodenum to aid in protein digestion. See *pancreas.* Called also *exocrine part of pancreas.*

lesser p. processus uncinatus pancreatis.

ventral p. an embryonic bud growing out from the endodermal lining of the caudal part of the foregut on the ventral wall, in the angle between the gut and the hepatic diverticulum, which forms the uncinate process and part of the head of the pancreas and the stem of its main duct.

Willis p., Winslow p. processus uncinatus pancreatis.

pan•cre•a•stat•in (pan″kre-ə-stat′in) a pancreatic peptide derived from a chromogranin, which inhibits secretion of insulin and other endocrine and exocrine pancreatic secretions.

Pan•cre•ase (pan′kre-ās) trademark for preparations of pancrelipase.

pan•cre•a•ta (pan-kre′ə-tə) [L.] plural of *pancreas.*

pan•cre•a•tal•gia (pan″kre-ə-tal′jə) [*pancreat-* + *-algia*] pain in the pancreas.

pan•cre•a•tec•to•my (pan″kre-ə-tek′tə-me) [*pancreat-* + *-ectomy*] surgical removal of all or part of the pancreas.

distal p. removal of the body and tail of the pancreas.

pan•cre•at•ic elas•tase II (pan″kre-at′ik e-las′tās) [EC 3.4.21.71] a serine endopeptidase that catalyzes the cleavage of peptide bonds, preferentially clearing on the carboxyl side of leucine, methionine, and phenylalanine residues. Secreted by the pancreas as the proenzyme proelastase and activated in the duodenum via cleavage by trypsin, it is involved in protein digestion. In a given species, usually either pancreatic elastase or pancreatic elastase II is expressed; in humans it is the latter.

pan•cre•at•ic lip•ase (pan″kre-at′ik li′pās) see under *lipase.*

pancreatic(o)- [L. *pancreaticus* from Gr. *pankreas,* from *pan* all + *kreas* flesh] a combining form denoting relationship to the pancreas, or to the pancreatic duct.

pan•cre•at•i•co•bil•i•ary (pan″kre-at″ĭ-ko-bil′e-ar-e) pertaining to the pancreatic and biliary ducts.

pan•cre•at•i•co•cu•ta•ne•ous (pan″kre-at″ĭ-ko-ku-ta′ne-əs) pertaining to or connecting the pancreas and the skin.

pan•cre•at•i•co•du•o•de•nal (pan″kre-at″ĭ-ko-doo″o-de′nəl) pertaining to or connecting the pancreas and duodenum.

pan•cre•at•i•co•du•od•e•nec•to•my (pan″kre-at″ĭ-ko-doo-od″ə-nek′tə-me) pancreatoduodenectomy.

pan•cre•at•i•co•du•o•de•nos•to•my (pan″kre-at″ĭ-ko-doo″o-də-nos′tə-me) pancreaticoenterostomy with the duct or pancreas anastomosed to the duodenum.

pan•cre•at•i•co•en•ter•ic (pan″kre-at″ĭ-ko-en-ter′ik) pertaining to or connecting the pancreas and the intestine; cf. *enteropancreatic.*

pan•cre•at•i•co•en•ter•os•to•my (pan″kre-at″ĭ-ko-en″tər-os′tə-me) surgical anastomosis of the pancreatic duct, or the divided end of the transected pancreas, with the intestine.

pan•cre•at•i•co•gas•tros•to•my (pan″kre-at″ĭ-ko-gas-tros′tə-me) surgical anastomosis of the pancreatic duct, or the divided end of the transected pancreas, with the stomach.

pan•cre•at•i•co•je•ju•nos•to•my (pan″kre-at″ĭ-ko-jə-joo-nos′tə-me) pancreaticoenterostomy with the duct or pancreas anastomosed to the jejunum.

pan•cre•at•i•co•pleu•ral (pan″kre-at″ĭ-ko-ploor′əl) pertaining to or connecting the pancreas and the pleural cavity.

pan•cre•at•i•co•splen•ic (pan″kre-at″ĭ-ko-splen′ik) splenopancreatic.

pan•cre•a•tin (pan′kre-ə-tin) [USP] a substance from the pancreas of the hog or the ox that contains enzymes such as amylase, trypsin, and lipase; used as a digestive aid in pancreatic insufficiency, and to peptonize milk and other foods.

pan•cre•a•ti•tis (pan″kre-ə-ti′tis) inflammation of the pancreas, which may be acute or chronic, asymptomatic or symptomatic, and is often complicated by autodigestion of pancreatic tissue by its own enzymes. The most common causes are complications from alcoholism and biliary tract conditions such as gallstones; less commonly it may be associated with hyperlipemia, hyperparathyroidism, abdominal trauma from an accident or surgery, vasculitis, or uremia.

acute p. pancreatitis with sudden onset, fever, abdominal pain, nausea, vomiting, tachycardia, and often increased blood levels of pancreatic enzymes. It may be accompanied by complications such as hemorrhaging or necrosis; see *acute hemorrhagic p.* and *acute necrotizing p.*

acute hemorrhagic p. 1. acute pancreatitis in which the autolysis of pancreatic tissue disrupts pancreatic microcirculation, resulting in hemorrhage into the parenchyma and surrounding tissues. Blood staining of the lateral abdominal wall (Turner sign) or periumbilical area (Cullen sign) may result. 2. acute necrotizing p. (def. 2).

acute necrotic p. acute necrotizing p. (def. 2).

acute necrotizing p. 1. a severe type of acute pancreatitis accompanied by necrosis of pancreatic tissue and the surrounding area, often with leakage of pancreatic enzymes to cause chemical imbalances; it often progresses to multiple organ failure and death. 2. in dogs, a condition usually seen in middle-aged obese animals on a high-fat diet; necrosis of the pancreas causes abdominal pain and vomiting. If untreated, it may progress to hyperglycemia, shock, coma, and death. Defs. 1 and 2 called also *acute pancreatic necrosis.*

autoimmune p. chronic pancreatitis in which there are circulating autoantibodies and elevated levels of immunoglobulins; it is often accompanied by other autoimmune disorders and is seen primarily in the elderly.

calcareous p., calcific p., calcifying p. chronic calcifying p.

chronic p. pancreatitis with chronic abdominal pain, progressive fibrosis, and eventually irreversible loss of exocrine function (resulting in steatorrhea) and of endocrine function (resulting in diabetes mellitus). Recurrent attacks of acute pancreatitis are often superimposed, a condition known as *chronic relapsing pancreatitis.*

chronic calcific p., chronic calcifying p. pancreatitis with calcification in the ducts, usually associated with exocrine insufficiency and diabetes mellitus.

chronic obstructive p. pancreatitis caused by dilatation of one of the major ducts proximal to an obstruction, usually from a tumor or scarring; scarring may be from earlier acute pancreatitis. Removal of the obstruction may improve pancreatic function.

chronic relapsing p. see *chronic p.*

gallstone p. acute pancreatitis accompanied by gallstones, one of the most common types.

hereditary p. an autosomal dominant syndrome characterized by recurrent attacks of acute pancreatitis, usually beginning in childhood and resulting from a mutation in chromosome 7q that results in defective production of trypsinogen, so that there is excessive trypsin in the liver, with autodigestion and scarring.

interstitial p. pancreatitis in which pancreatic microcirculation remains intact, with edema, overgrowth of connective tissue, and atrophy of glandular tissue.

tropical p., tropical calcifying p. a type of chronic calcifying pancreatitis observed in India and a few other countries, having an unknown etiology; there may be a hereditary component.

pancreat(o)- [L. *pancreas*, q.v.] a combining form denoting relationship to the pancreas.

pan·cre·a·to·blas·to·ma (pan″kre-ə-to-blas-to′mə) a rare type of malignant pancreatic tumor, having an uncertain origin and usually affecting children.

pan·cre·a·to·du·o·de·nec·to·my (pan″kre-ə-to-doo″o-də-nek′tə-me) excision of the head of the pancreas along with the encircling loop of the duodenum.

pan·cre·a·to·du·o·de·nos·to·my (pan″kre-ə-to-doo″o-də-nos′tə-me) pancreaticoduodenostomy.

pan·cre·a·to·en·ter·os·to·my (pan″kre-ə-to-en″tər-os′tə-me) pancreaticoenterostomy.

pan·cre·a·to·gen·ic (pan″kre-ə-to-jen′ik) arising in or from the pancreas; called also *pancreatogenous.*

pan·cre·a·tog·e·nous (pan″kre-ə-toj′ə-nəs) pancreatogenic.

pan·cre·a·to·gram (pan″kre-at′o-gram) the x-ray film produced by pancreatography.

pan·cre·a·tog·ra·phy (pan″kre-ə-tog′rə-fe) radiography of the pancreas after injection of a contrast medium.

endoscopic retrograde p. pancreatography in which the radiopaque medium is injected into the pancreatic duct at the ampulla of Vater via a cannula introduced through a fiberoptic endoscope. See also *endoscopic retrograde cholangiopancreatography*, under *cholangiopancreatography.*

pan·cre·ato·lith (pan″kre-at′o-lith) pancreatic calculus.

pan·cre·a·to·li·thec·to·my (pan″kre-ə-to-lĭ-thek′tə-me) [*pancreatolith* + *-ectomy*] removal of a calculus from the pancreas.

pan·cre·a·to·li·thi·a·sis (pan″kre-ə-to-lĭ-thi′ə-sis) the presence of calculi in the pancreas or its ductal system, usually associated with pancreatic exocrine (digestive enzymes) and endocrine (insulin) insufficiency, accompanied by steatorrhea, weight loss, and diabetes mellitus. Called also *pancreatic lithiasis* and *pancreolithiasis.*

pan·cre·a·to·li·thot·o·my (pan″kre-ə-to-lĭ-thot′ə-me) [*pancreatolith* + *-tomy*] incision of the pancreas for the removal of a calculus.

pan·cre·a·tol·y·sis (pan″kre-ə-tol′ĭ-sis) pancreolysis.

pan·cre·at·o·my (pan-kre-at′ə-me) pancreatotomy.

pan·cre·a·top·a·thy (pan″kre-ə-top′ə-the) pancreopathy.

pan·cre·a·tos·co·py (pan″kre-ə-tos′cə-pe) [*pancreato-* + *-scopy*] visual examination of the pancreatic duct by means of a small endoscope.

pan·cre·a·tot·o·my (pan″kre-ə-tot′ə-me) [*pancreato-* + *-tomy*] incision of the pancreas.

pan·cre·a·to·tro·pic (pan″kre-ə-to-tro′pik) [*pancreato-* + *-tropic*] having an affinity for or an influence on the pancreas.

pan·cre·a·tro·pic (pan″kre-ə-tro′pik) pancreatotropic.

pan·cre·ec·to·my (pan″kre-ek′tə-me) pancreatectomy.

pan·cre·li·pase (pan″kre-li′pās) [USP] a standardized preparation of hog pancreas, containing enzymes, principally lipase, with amylase and protease, and having the same actions as those of the pancreatic juice; used as a digestive aid in conditions of pancreatic insufficiency.

pan·creo·li·thi·a·sis (pan″kre-o-lĭ-thi′ə-sis) pancreatolithiasis.

pan·cre·ol·y·sis (pan″kre-ol′ĭ-sis) [*pancreas* + *-lysis*] destruction of pancreatic tissue by pancreatic enzymes. **pancreolyt′ic** *adj*

pan·cre·op·a·thy (pan″kre-op′ə-the) [*pancreas* + *-pathy*] any disease of the pancreas. Called also *pancreatopathy.*

pan·creo·tro·pic (pan″kre-o-tro′pik) pancreatotropic.

pan·creo·zy·min (pan′kre-o-zi″min) cholecystokinin.

pan·cu·ro·ni·um bro·mide (pan″ku-ro′ne-əm) a nondepolarizing neuromuscular blocking agent, with curariform action; used as an adjunct to anesthesia to induce skeletal muscle relaxation and to facilitate mechanical ventilation; administered intravenously.

pan·cys·ti·tis (pan″sis-ti′tis) cystitis involving the entire thickness of the wall of the urinary bladder, as occurs in interstitial cystitis.

pan·cy·to·ker·a·tin (pan″si-to-ker′ə-tin) a cocktail of antibodies directed against keratins of various molecular weights, used in immunohistochemical staining to detect cells of epithelial origin.

pan·cy·to·pe·nia (pan″si-to-pe′ne-ə) [*pan-* + *cytopenia*] deficiency of all cellular elements of the blood. See also *erythropenia, leukopenia,* and *thrombocytopenia.*

congenital p., Fanconi p. Fanconi syndrome (def. 1).

tropical canine p. canine ehrlichiosis.

Pan·del (pan-del′) trademark for a preparation of hydrocortisone probutate.

pan·dem·ic (pan-dem′ik) [*pan-* + Gr. *dēmos* people] 1. a widespread epidemic of a disease. 2. widely epidemic; distributed or occurring widely throughout a region, country, or continent or globally.

pan·dem·ic·i·ty (pan″dəm-is′ĭ-te) the state of being pandemic.

Pan·der islands, layer (pahn′der) [Heinrich Christian *Pander*, German anatomist, 1794–1865] see under *island* and *layer.*

pan·dic·u·la·tion (pan″dik-u-la′shən) [L. *pandiculari* to stretch one's self] the act of stretching and yawning.

pan·dys·au·to·no·mia (pan-dis″aw-to-no′me-ə) autonomic neuropathy in both sympathetic and parasympathetic nervous systems, with manifestations that include orthostatic hypotension, anhidrosis, and gastrointestinal involvement.

acute p. acute autonomic neuropathy.

pan·el (pan′əl) 1. a list of names. 2. a group of individuals participating in a specific discussion or activity. 3. a list of names of the medical professionals who are willing to care for insured persons for a stipulated yearly fee under the system of medical insurance carried on by insurance groups under the supervision of the government in Great Britain. 4. the list of the insured persons assigned as clients to a physician under the British National Health Insurance Act. 5. a series of chemical substances, such as drugs or antigens, to which a given animal, tissue, or substance is exposed to test for reactions. 6. a group of related laboratory measurements that reflect the state of function of an organ or system.

pan·en·ceph·a·li·tis (pan″ən-sef″ə-li′tis) a type of encephalitis, probably of viral origin, that produces intranuclear or intracytoplasmic inclusion bodies that cause parenchymatous lesions in both gray and white matter of the brain.

subacute sclerosing p. (SSPE) a rare and devastating form of leukoencephalitis usually affecting children and adolescents. Insidious in onset, it characteristically produces progressive cerebral dysfunction over several weeks or months and death within a year. There is also demyelination with intranuclear inclusion bodies in nerve cells and oligodendroglia. High titers of measles virus in the serum and cerebrospinal fluid have indicated a linkage between this condition and earlier measles infection. Called also *Dawson encephalitis, subacute inclusion body encephalitis, subacute sclerosing leukoencephalopathy, van Bogaert encephalitis,* and *van Bogaert sclerosing leukoencephalitis.*

pan·en·do·scope (pan-en′do-skōp) 1. an endoscope for wide-angle viewing. 2. a cystoscope that permits wide-angle viewing of the urinary bladder and urethra.

oral p. an illuminated tubular device that permits visual observation and audiovisual recording of the larynx and vocal cords during production of speech sounds.

pan·en·dos·co·py (pan″ən-dos′kə-pe) observation by means of a panendoscope.

pan·epi·zo·ot·ic (pan-ep″ĭ-zo-ot′ik) panzootic.

pan·es·the·sia (pan″es-the′zhə) [*pan-* + *esthesia*] the sum of the sensations experienced. **panesthet′ic** *adj*

Pa·neth cells (pah′net) [Josef *Paneth*, Austrian physician, 1857–1890] see under *cell.*

pang (pang) a sudden, piercing pain.

breast p. angina pectoris.

brow p. hemicrania (def. 1).

Pan•glob•u•lin (pan″glob′u-lin) trademark for a preparation of immune globulin intravenous (human).

pan•glos•sia (pan-glos′e-ə) [*pan-* + Gr. *glōssa* tongue] abnormal or pathologic garrulity.

Pan•go•nia (pan-go′ne-ə) the zimbs, a genus of tabanid flies found in Ethiopia that feed on the blood of mammals.

Pan•he•ma•tin (pan-he′mə-tin) trademark for a preparation of hemin.

pan•he•ma•to•pe•nia (pan-he″mə-to-pe′ne-ə) pancytopenia.

pan•hy•po•go•nad•ism (pan-hi″po-go′nad-iz-əm) underdevelopment of all the genital tissues with decreased functional activities of the gonads.

pan•hy•po•pi•tu•i•ta•rism (pan-hi″po-pĭ-too′ĭ-tə-riz-əm) generalized or particularly severe hypopituitarism, which in its complete form leads to absence of gonadal function and insufficiency of thyroid and adrenal cortical function. Dwarfism, regression of secondary sex characters, loss of libido, weight loss, fatigability, bradycardia, hypotension, pallor, depression, and many other manifestations may occur. When cachexia is a prominent feature, it is called *hypophysial* or *pituitary cachexia* or *Simmonds disease.*

prepubertal p. inadequate production of all adenohypophysial hormones that begins before puberty and is associated with subnormal growth. See also *pituitary dwarfism*, under *dwarfism.*

pan•hys•ter•ec•to•my (pan″his-tər-ek′tə-me) [*pan-* + *hysterectomy*] complete removal of the uterus and cervix; total hysterectomy.

pan•hys•tero•ooph•o•rec•to•my (pan-his″tər-o-o″of-ə-rek′tə-me) excision of the body of the uterus, cervix, and ovary.

pan•hys•tero•sal•pin•gec•to•my (pan-his″tər-o-sal″pin-jek′tə-me) excision of the body of the uterus, cervix, and uterine tubes.

pan•hys•tero•sal•pin•go-ooph•o•rec•to•my (pan-his″tər-o-sal″ping-go-o″of-ə-rek′tə-me) excision of the uterus, cervix, uterine tubes, and ovaries.

pan•ic (pan′ik) [from Gr. *Pan* woodland deity who was considered to be the cause of sudden or groundless fear] acute, extreme anxiety with disorganization of personality and function.

homosexual p. an acute, extreme anxiety reaction brought on by circumstances that induce the unconscious fear of being homosexual or of succumbing to homosexual impulses.

Pan•i•cum (pan′ĭ-kum) a genus of grasses used for hay and cereal, including panic grass and millet. Certain species may cause oxalate poisoning and others may cause hepatogenous photosensitization in ruminants.

pan•im•mu•ni•ty (pan″ĭ-mu′nĭ-te) [*pan-* + *immunity*] immunity to several infections caused by bacteria and viruses.

pani•tu•mu•mab (pan″ĭ-too′mə-mab) an antagonist of epidermal growth factor receptors, used in treatment of metastatic colorectal carcinoma; administered by intravenous infusion.

Pan•ix•ine (pan-ik′sēn) trademark for a preparation of cephalexin.

Pan•iz•za plexuses (pah-nēt′sah) [Bartolomeo *Panizza*, Italian anatomist, 1785–1867] see under *plexus.*

pan•leu•ko•pe•nia (pan″loo-ko-pe′ne-ə) a highly contagious and often fatal disease of cats, caused by a parvovirus; characteristics include leukopenia, inactivity, anorexia, diarrhea, and vomiting. Called also *feline* or *infectious feline agranulocytosis, cat* or *feline enteritis, cat* or *feline distemper*, and *cat plague.*

pan•mix•ia (pan-mik′se-ə) random mating.

pan•mix•is (pan-mik′sis) [*pan-* + Gr. *mixis* mixture] random mating.

pan•mu•ral (pan-mu′rəl) [*pan-* + *mural*] pertaining to or affecting the entire wall.

Pan•my•cin (pan-mi′sin) trademark for preparations of tetracycline.

pan•my•eloid (pan-mi′ə-loid) pertaining to all the elements of the bone marrow.

pan•my•elop•a•thy (pan″mi-ə-lop′ə-the) [*pan-* + *myelopathy*] myelopathy involving all the elements of the bone marrow.

Fanconi p. Fanconi syndrome (def. 1).

pan•my•eloph•thi•sis (pan-mi″ə-lof′thĭ-sis) aplastic anemia.

Pan•ner disease (pah′nər) [Hans Jessen *Panner*, Danish radiologist, 1871–1930] see under *disease.*

pan•nic•u•lec•to•my (pə-nik″u-lek′tə-me) surgical excision of the abdominal apron of superficial fat in an obese patient.

pan•nic•u•li (pə-nik′u-li) [L.] genitive and plural of *panniculus.*

pan•nic•u•li•tis (pə-nik″u-li′tis) [*panniculus* + *-itis*] an inflammatory reaction of the subcutaneous adipose tissue; two primary categories are distinguished, depending on the site, called *predominantly lobular p.* and *predominantly septal p.*. Cf. *steatitis.* Called also *adipositis.*

alpha$_1$-antitrypsin deficiency p. a type of relapsing febrile nodular nonsuppurative panniculitis seen in persons with alpha$_1$-antitrypsin deficiency; there are often painful subcutaneous nodules or plaques that may ulcerate.

calcifying p. a type of predominantly lobular panniculitis characterized by calcification of subcutaneous fat, with nodules and induration, usually in cases of renal failure or hyperparathyroidism.

cold p. traumatic panniculitis caused by excessive exposure to cold; children are the most susceptible, but it also occurs in adults who work or otherwise spend long periods outdoors in the winter. Persons who suck excessively on ice or frozen confections may get cold panniculitis around the mouth. Babies and young boys may get it in the scrotum.

connective tissue p. an autoimmune type of panniculitis characterized by inflammatory nodules in the subcutaneous fat progressing to lipoatrophy. Called also *lipoatrophic p.*

cytophagic histiocytic p. a severe variant of relapsing febrile nodular nonsuppurative panniculitis characterized by lobules infiltrated by histiocytes that have phagocytized erythrocytes, leukocytes, and platelets; it is sometimes accompanied by systemic conditions that can be fatal, such as multiorgan failure, coagulopathies with hemorrhaging, and overwhelming infection. In some cases there is an apparent association with T-cell lymphoma.

eosinophilic p. any type in which there are eosinophils in the subcutaneous fat, such as accompanying an insect or arthropod bite or parasitic infection.

factitial p. traumatic panniculitis that is self-induced, such as by blunt trauma (hitting oneself) or by subcutaneous injection of a harmful substance as either self-mutilation or an attempt at self-medication.

gouty p. predominantly lobular panniculitis occurring as a complication of gout, owing to storage of urate crystals in the subcutaneous fat and a resultant granulomatous reaction.

histiocytic cytophagic p. cytophagic histiocytic p.

idiopathic nodular p. relapsing febrile nodular nonsuppurative panniculitis that is idiopathic.

infective p. predominantly lobular panniculitis caused by a bacterial or fungal infection, which may be either by direct inoculation or from infection elsewhere in the body; seen most often in immunocompromised patients.

LE p. lupus erythematosus profundus.

lipoatrophic p. connective tissue p.

lipomembranous p. a type of predominantly lobular panniculitis of the leg, usually in persons with ischemia caused by diabetes mellitus, characterized by degeneration of fat cells and formation of a lipomembrane.

lobular p. 1. any type involving mainly the lobules of adipose tissue; see *predominantly lobular p.* 2. relapsing febrile nodular nonsuppurative p.

lupus p., lupus erythematosus p. lupus erythematosus profundus.

mesenteric p. inflammation with variable fibrosis of mesenteric fat, usually of the small intestine, causing a solid mass that may displace or obstruct the intestine. Some authorities consider this an inflammatory variant of retractile mesenteritis. Called also *mesenteric lipodystrophy.*

nodular nonsuppurative p. relapsing febrile nodular nonsuppurative p.

pancreatic p. a type of predominantly lobular panniculitis occurring secondary to pancreatitis or pancreatic carcinoma.

physical p. panniculitis caused by physical factors, such as cold or a physical trauma.

poststeroid p. a type of predominantly lobular panniculitis seen in children who have been on high-dose corticosteroid therapy that was terminated too rapidly; it is nearly identical to subcutaneous fat necrosis of the newborn, except that affected children are usually two years or older.

predominantly lobular p. one of the two main groups of panniculitides, including those involving mainly the lobules of adipose tissue, such as with necrosis of tissue.

predominantly septal p. one of the two main groups of panniculitides, including those involving primarily the septa and sometimes blood vessels between lobules of adipose tissue; this type is characterized by the development of single or multiple cutaneous nodules.

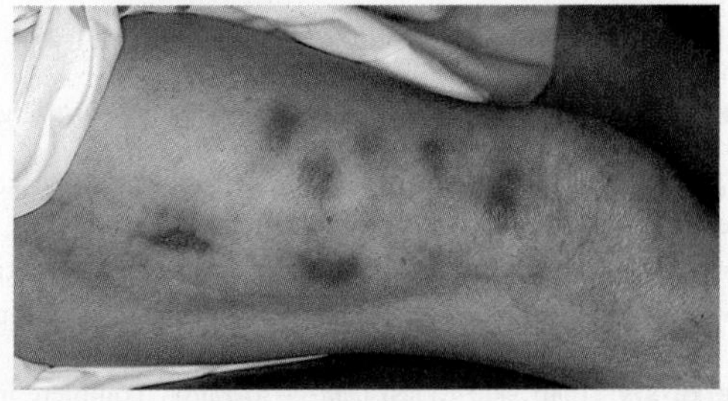

■ Pancreatic panniculitis.

relapsing febrile nodular nonsuppurative p. a type of predominantly lobular panniculitis seen on the lower limbs and trunk, characterized by recurrent fever with single or multiple, erythematous, tender or painless subcutaneous nodules. The nodules resolve and usually leave a depression in the skin. It is most often seen in women and may occur alone or associated with other disorders. Called also *Christian-Weber* or *Weber-Christian disease*, *nodular nonsuppurative p.*, and *Weber-Christian p.*

sclerosing p. lipodermatosclerosis.

septal p. any type involving the septa of subcutaneous tissue; see *predominantly septal p.*

subacute nodular migratory p. a variant of erythema nodosum characterized by discrete nodules with erythematous borders, found asymmetrically on one or both of the lower limbs. The lesions are usually less acute and less numerous than those in classic erythema nodosum; the older central nodules coalesce and clear, and new lesions form nearby, giving the appearance of migration. Called also *chronic erythema nodosum*, *erythema nodosum migrans*, and *Vilanova disease*.

traumatic p. panniculitis, usually of the predominantly lobular type, caused by external trauma. Besides accidental blunt trauma, it may also be caused by cold *(cold p.)* or self-induced trauma *(factitial p.)*.

Weber-Christian p. relapsing febrile nodular nonsuppurative p.

pan•nic•u•lus (pə-nik′u-ləs) gen. and pl. *panni′culi* [L., dim. of *pannus* cloth] a thin layer.

p. adipo′sus [TA] subcutaneous fat: a layer of adipose tissue underlying the dermis. Called also *pannus*.

p. adipo′sus te′lae subcuta′neae abdo′minis [TA] fatty layer of subcutaneous tissue of abdomen: the more superficial layer of the subcutaneous tissue of the abdomen, external to the membranous layer. Called also *Camper fascia*.

p. carno′sus a thin muscular layer within the superficial fascia of animals with a hairy coat; in humans it is represented mainly by the platysma.

pan•nus (pan′əs) [L. "a piece of cloth"] 1. superficial vascularization of the cornea with infiltration of granulation tissue. 2. an inflammatory exudate overlying the lining layer of synovial cells on the inside of a joint, usually occurring in patients with rheumatoid or other inflammatory arthritis and sometimes resulting in fibrous ankylosis of the joint. 3. panniculus adiposus.

degenerative p., p. degenerati′vus 1. growth of connective tissue between the epithelium of the cornea and Bowman membrane. 2. chronic superficial keratitis.

glaucomatous p. degeneration and desquamation of corneal epithelium due to edema in advanced glaucoma.

phlyctenular p. pannus associated with phlyctenular keratitis, the vascularization running all the way around the periphery of the limbus and extending toward the center.

p. sic′cus pannus of the cornea associated with dryness of the cornea and conjunctiva.

p. trachomato′sus pannus occurring secondarily to trachoma, the small fine branching vessels always appearing at the upper limbus and running down under the epithelium into the cornea.

pa•nod•ic (pə-nod′ik) panthodic.

Pa•non•y•chus (pă-non′ĭ-kəs) a genus of mites of the family Tetranychidae.

P. cit′ri the citrus red mite, a species that infests citrus trees and occasionally causes allergic sensitization.

pano•pho•bia (pan″o-fo′be-ə) panphobia.

pan•oph•thal•mia (pan″of-thal′me-ə) panophthalmitis.

pan•oph•thal•mi•tis (pan″of-thəl-mi′tis) [*pan-* + *ophthalmitis*] inflammation of all the structures or tissues of the eye.

pan•op•tic (pan-op′tik) [*pan-* + *opt-* + *-ic*] rendering everything visible; said of a stain which differentiates all the tissues of a specimen. See *Giemsa stain*, at *Stains and Staining Methods* under *stain*.

pan•os•te•itis (pan″os-te-i′tis) [*pan-* + *oste-* + *-itis*] inflammation of every part of a bone.

pan•os•ti•tis (pan″os-ti′tis) panosteitis.

pan•oti•tis (pan″o-ti′tis) [*pan-* + *ot-* + *-itis*] an inflammation of all the parts or structures of the ear.

pan•pho•bia (pan-fo′be-ə) [*pan-* + *-phobia*] fear of everything; a vague and persistent dread of some unknown evil.

pan•proc•to•co•lec•to•my (pan-prok″to-ko-lek′tə-me) excision of the entire rectum and colon, with creation of an ileal stoma.

Pan•ret•in (pan-ret′in) trademark for a preparation of alitretinoin.

pan•ret•i•nal (pan-ret′ĭ-nəl) pertaining to or encompassing the entire retina.

pan•scle•ro•sis (pan″sklə-ro′sis) [*pan-* + *sclerosis*] complete induration of a part or organ.

pan•si•nu•itis (pan″si-nu-i′tis) pansinusitis.

pan•si•nus•ec•to•my (pan″si-nəs-ek′tə-me) excision of the diseased membrane of all of the paranasal sinuses on one side.

pan•si•nus•itis (pan″si-nəs-i′tis) [*pan-* + *sinus* + *-itis*] inflammation involving all of the paranasal sinuses on one side.

pan•sphyg•mo•graph (pan-sfig′mo-graf) [*pan-* + *sphygmo-* + *-graph*] a device for recording cardiac, pulse, and chest movements at the same time.

pan•sporo•blast (pan-spor′o-blast) [*pan-* + *sporo-* + *-blast*] a disporoblastic sporont, i.e., a sporoblast that develops into two or more spores, with or without an enclosing membrane; characteristic of certain protozoa. See *Apansporoblastina* and *Pansporoblastina*.

Pan•sporo•blas•ti•na (pan″spor-o-blas-ti′nə) a suborder of parasitic protozoa (order Microsporida, class Microsporea) in which the sporulation sequence occurs in the host cell within a more or less persistent intracellular sporocyst (with a pansporoblastic membrane); organisms are often dimorphic, with another sporulation sequence not involving such a membrane. The sporoblasts and spores are usually uninucleate when the membrane is present and dinucleate when it is absent. Representative genera include *Amblyospora*, *Pleistophora*, and *Thelohania*.

Pan•stron•gy•lus (pan-stron′jə-ləs) a genus of cone-nose bugs of the family Reduviidae, species of which are vectors of *Trypanosoma*.

P. genicula′tus a vector of *Trypanosoma cruzi* in Panama and Brazil.

P. infes′tans *Triatoma infestans*.

P. megis′tus an important vector of *Trypanosoma cruzi* in Brazil; its local name is *barbeiro* because it frequently bites the face.

pan•sys•tol•ic (pan″sis-tol′ik) [*pan-* + *systole*] pertaining to or affecting all of, or occurring throughout, systole.

pan•ta•chro•mat•ic (pan″tə-kro-mat′ik) [*pant-* + *achromatic*] entirely achromatic.

pan•tal•gia (pan-tal′jə) [*pant-* + *-algis*] pain over the whole body.

pan•ta•mor•phia (pan″tə-mor′fe-ə) [*pant-* + *amorphia*] shapelessness; complete or general deformity.

pan•ta•mor•phic (pan″tə-mor′fik) formless.

pan•tan•en•ceph•a•ly (pan″tan-ən-sef′ə-le) [*pant-* + *anencephaly*] complete absence of the calvaria and brain.

pan•tan•ky•lo•bleph•a•ron (pan-tang″kə-lo-blef′ə-ron) [*pant-* + *ankyloblepharon*] general adhesion of the eyelids to the eyeball and to each other.

Pan•ter•ic (pan-ter′ik) trademark for a preparation of pancreatin.

pan•te•the•ine (pan-tə-the′in) a naturally occurring amide of pantothenic acid and β-mercaptoethanolamine; it is an intermediate in the biosynthesis of coenzyme A, a growth factor for certain bacteria, and a cofactor in certain enzyme complexes (e.g., in fatty acid or polypeptide synthesis).

pan•the•nol (pan′thə-nol) [USP] the alcohol derivative of pantothenic acid; it is converted in the body to pantothenic acid, a member of the B-complex vitamins. Called also *pantothenyl alcohol* and *pantothenol*. The term is sometimes used to refer to the D(+) form of panthenol; see *dexpanthenol*.

pan•thod•ic (pan-thod′ik) [*pan-* + Gr. *hodos* way] radiating in every direction; said of nerve impulses.

Pan•tho•lin (pan′tho-lin) trademark for a preparation of calcium pantothenate.

pant•ing (pant′ing) rapid shallow breathing with a small tidal volume; cf. *tachypnea*.

pant(o)- [Gr. *pas*, gen. *pantos* all] a combining form meaning all, the whole.

pan•to•chro•mism (pan″to-kro′miz-əm) [*panto-* + *chrom-* + *-ism*] the phenomenon of existing in two or more differently colored forms, as a salt.

Pan•toea (pan-te′ə) [Gr. *pantoia* from diverse sources (referring to geographic and ecologic distribution)] a widely distributed genus of gram-negative bacteria of the family Enterobacteriaceae, consisting of nonencapsulated, non–spore-forming straight rods, usually motile with peritrichous flagella. The type species is *P. agglo′merans*.

P. agglo′merans a species found on plants, in water, and in the human intestinal tract. It is a potential pathogen, causing a variety of infections, including those of nosocomial origin. Called also *Enterobacter agglomerans*.

pan•to•graph (pan′to-graf) [*panto-* + *-graph*] an instrument for copying a plane figure to any desired scale.

pan•to•ic ac•id (pan-to′ik) a constituent of pantothenic acid remaining after cleavage of β-alanine.

pan•to•mog•ra•phy (pan″to-mog′rə-fe) a method of tomography for visualization of body curved surfaces at any depth. In dentistry, it may be used for radiography of the maxillary and mandibular dental arches and their associated structures. Called also *panoramic radiography.* **pantomograph′ic** *adj*

pan·to·mor·phia (pan″to-mor′fe-ə) [*panto-* + *morph-* + *-ia*] 1. general or perfect symmetry. 2. ability to assume various shapes, as an ameba.

pan·to·mor·phic (pan″to-mor′fik) able to assume any shape.

Pan·to·paque (pan-to-pāk′) trademark for a preparation of iophendylate.

pan·to·pho·bia (pan″to-fo′be-ə) [*panto-* + *-phobia*] panphobia.

pan·to·pra·zole so·di·um (pan-to′prə-zōl) a proton pump inhibitor with properties similar to those of omeprazole, used in the treatment of erosive esophagitis associated with gastroesophageal reflux disease, administered orally or intravenously, and of pathological hypersecretion associated with Zollinger-Ellison syndrome or other neoplastic conditions, administered intravenously.

pan·to·scop·ic (pan″to-skop′ik) bifocal.

pan·to·then·ate (pan″to-then′āt) a salt of pantothenic acid.

pan·to·then·ic ac·id (pan″to-then′ik) the amide of β-alanine and pantoic acid, a B complex vitamin that is a constituent of coenzyme A; it is distributed ubiquitously in foods, and a deficiency syndrome has not been demonstrated in humans except by experimental administration of the pantothenic acid antagonist ω-methylpantothenic acid.

pan·to·the·nol (pan″to-the′nol) 1. panthenol. 2. dexpanthenol.

pan·to·yl·tau·rine (pan″to-əl-taw′rēn) a competitive inhibitor of pantothenic acid derived by replacement of the carboxyl group by a sulfonyl group; it is the amide of pantoic acid and taurine. Called also *thiopanic acid.*

pan·tro·pic (pan-tro′pik) [*pan-* + *-tropic*] 1. having an affinity for or affecting many tissues or cells. 2. capable of attacking derivatives of any of the three embryonic layers.

pan·tur·bi·nate (pan-tur′bĭ-nāt) the entire structure of a nasal concha, including bone and soft tissue.

Pa·num area (pah′noom) [Peter Ludwig *Panum*, Danish physiologist, 1820–1885] see under *area.*

pan·uve·itis (pan″u-ve-i′tis) inflammation of the entire uveal tract.

pan·zo·ot·ic (pan″zo-ot′ik) [*pan-* + *zootic*] 1. occurring pandemically among animals. 2. a disease that is pandemic among animals. Called also *panepizootic.*

PAO peak acid output.

PAP 1. peroxidase-antiperoxidase; see under *technique.* 2. placental alkaline phosphatase.

pa·pa·in (pə-pa′in, pə-pi′in) 1. [EC 3.4.22.2] an enzyme of the hydrolase class that catalyzes the hydrolysis of proteins and peptides with preferential cleavage at bonds containing arginine, lysine, and glycine residues. It is obtained from the latex of the papaya tree, *Carica papaya.* 2. [USP] a purified preparation of papain used as a protein digestant and as a topical application for enzymatic débridement and promotion of normal healing of surface lesions.

Pap·a·nic·o·laou stain, test (smear) (pap″ə-nik′o-la-oo) [George Nicolas *Papanicolaou*, Greek physician and anatomist in the United States, 1883–1962] see under *test* and see *Stains and Staining Methods*, under *stain.*

Pa·pav·er (pə-pav′ər) a genus of flowering herbs of the family Papaveraceae. *P. somni′ferum*, a pink to purple species, and *P. al′bum*, a silvery white species, are the source of opium (q.v.) and of the poppy seeds (devoid of narcotic alkaloids) that are used as a condiment.

Pa·pav·er·a·ceae (pap″ə-vər-a′se-e) the poppies, a family of plants with often brightly colored flowers. It includes the genera *Argemone*, *Eschscholtzia*, and *Papaver.*

pa·pav·er·ine hy·dro·chlo·ride (pə-pav′ər-in) [USP] the hydrochloride salt of an opium alkaloid, which also may be synthesized; used as a smooth muscle relaxant and vasodilator, especially in the treatment of cerebral and peripheral ischemia associated with arterial spasm and myocardial ischemia complicated by arrhythmias; administered orally, intramuscularly, or intravenously. It is also injected into the corpus cavernosum of the penis in the diagnosis and treatment of erectile dysfunction.

pa·paw (paw′paw) 1. *Carica papaya.* 2. papaya (def. 2). 3. *Asimina triloba.* 4. the fruit of *A. triloba*, which is edible, although ingestion may cause severe skin irritation in sensitive persons; called also *pawpaw.*

pa·pa·ya (pah-pah′yah) [Sp.] 1. *Carica papaya.* 2. the fruit of *Carica papaya*, which contains the enzyme papain. Called also *papaw.*

pa·per (pa′pər) a substance manufactured in thin sheets, prepared from wood, rags, or other fibrous substance which has first been reduced to a pulp.

alkannin p. filter paper dipped in an alcoholic solution of alkannin; alkalis turn it blue, acids red.

articulating p. paper strips coated with ink- or dye-containing wax, used for the marking or locating of occlusal interferences or deflective or interceptive occlusal contacts.

azolitmin p. filter paper saturated with a solution of azolitmin; acids turn it purple to bright red, alkalis turn it blue.

biuret p. filter paper previously dipped in Gies biuret reagent, dried, and cut into strips.

Congo red p. filter paper wet with a 0.2 per cent solution of Congo red in water, dried, and cut in strips.

filter p. a porous, unsized paper used as a filter.

litmus p. bibulous paper impregnated with a solution of litmus, dried, and cut into strips. If slightly alkaline, the paper is blue and is used as a test for acids, which turn it red; if slightly acid, it is red and alkalis turn it blue.

niter p. paper impregnated with potassium nitrate, ignited and used as a moxa or for inhalation in asthma; called also *saltpeter p.*

potassium nitrate p. niter p.

saltpeter p. niter p.

test p. paper that is impregnated with litmus or other indicator.

turmeric p. paper dyed yellow with turmeric; alkalis turn it brown.

Pa·pez circuit (pah-pez′) [James Wenceslas *Papez*, American anatomist, 1883–1958] see under *circuit.*

pa·pil·la (pə-pil′ə) gen. and pl. *papil′lae* [L.] a small nipple-shaped projection, elevation, or structure.

acoustic p. organum spirale.

Bergmeister p. 1. a small mass of neuroglial cells in the center of the embryonic optic disk, surrounding the bulb of the hyaloid artery. 2. a congenital anomaly consisting of a glial veil attached to the anterior aspect of the optic disk, resulting from glial proliferation around the remnants of the posterior part of the hyaloid vessel system.

bile p. p. duodeni major.

circumvallate papillae papillae vallatae.

papil′lae co′nicae conical papillae: sparsely scattered large elevations on the tongue surface, often considered a modified type of filiform papillae.

conoid papillae of tongue papillae conicae.

dental p., dentinal p., p. den′tis [TA] a small mass of condensed mesenchymal tissue in the enamel organ, which differentiates into the dentin and dental pulp.

dermal p., p. der′midis [TA] 1. any of the conical extensions of the collagen fibers, the capillary blood vessels, and sometimes the nerves of the papillary layer of the dermis into corresponding spaces among the downward- or inward-projecting rete ridges on the under surface of the epidermis. On the forehead and ear these are less prominent; on the face, neck, and pubes the relations are reversed and rete ridges extend inward or downward into spaces among a network of dermal ridges. 2. p. pili.

p. duc′tus paroti′dei [TA] papilla of parotid duct: the small papilla marking the orifice of the parotid duct in the mucous membrane of the cheek.

duodenal p., major p. duodeni major.

duodenal p., minor p. duodeni minor.

p. duode′ni ma′jor [TA] major duodenal papilla: a small elevation at the site of the opening of the conjoined common bile duct and pancreatic duct into the lumen of the duodenum. See also *p. duodeni minor.*

p. duode′ni mi′nor [TA] minor duodenal papilla: a small elevation at the site of the opening of the accessory pancreatic duct into the lumen of the duodenum. See also *p. duodeni major.*

papil′lae filifor′mes [TA] filiform papillae: threadlike elevations that cover most of the tongue surface.

papil′lae folia′tae [TA] foliate papillae: parallel mucosal folds on the margins of the tongue at the junction of its body and root.

papil′lae fungifor′mes [TA] fungiform papillae: knoblike projections on the tongue, scattered singly among the filiform papillae.

p. gingiva′lis [TA] gingival papilla: a cone-shaped pad of the interdental gingiva filling the space between two contiguous teeth up to the contact area, as viewed from the labial, buccal, or lingual aspect; called also *interdental p.*, *p. interdentalis* [TA alternative], and *interproximal p.* See also *interdental gingiva*, under *gingiva.*

hair p. p. pili.

ileal p., p. ilea′lis [TA], **ileocecal p.** the conical projection formed by the terminal ileum at its junction with the cecum, with the ileum extending into the large intestine; this structure in the living individual corresponds to the so-called *ileocecal valve* in the cadaver.

p. incisi′va [TA] incisive papilla: a rounded projection at the anterior end of the raphe of the palate.

interdental p. p. gingivalis.

p. interdenta′lis TA alternative for *p. gingivalis.*

interproximal p. p. gingivalis.

p. lacrima′lis [TA] lacrimal papilla: a small elevation on each palpebral margin near the medial angle of the eye; the lacrimal punctum is in its center.

papil′lae lenticula′res lenticular papillae: a series of papillae of the tongue resembling, but less elevated than, the fungiform papillae.

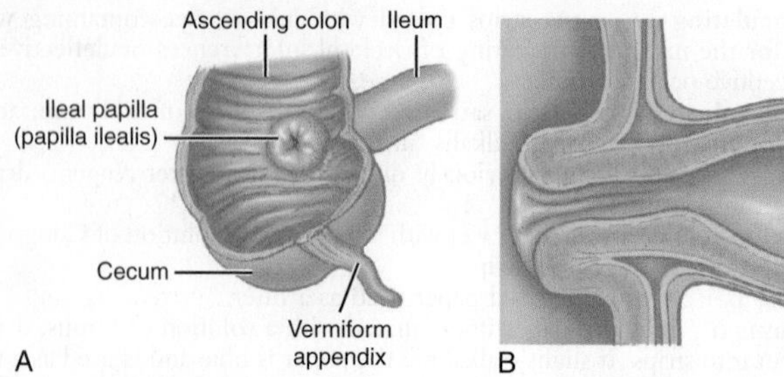

■ Papilla ilealis (ileal papilla). *(A)*, Position within the colon; *(B)*, cross-section of the papilla.

papil′lae lingua′les [TA] lingual papillae: the filiform, fungiform, vallate, foliate, and conical papillae of the tongue.

p. mam′mae, p. mamma′ria [TA], **mammary p.** nipple of the breast: the pigmented projection on the anterior surface of the mammary gland, surrounded by the areola; the lactiferous ducts open onto it. Called also *mammilla, nipple, teat,* and *thelium.*

nerve p., nervous p. neurothele.

p. ner′vi op′tici discus nervi optici.

optic p. discus nervi optici.

palatine p. p. incisiva.

parotid p., p. of parotid duct, p. paroti′dea p. ductus parotidei.

p. pi′li hair papilla: a type of fibrovascular dermal papilla of mesodermal cells that invaginates into the hair bulb.

renal p., p. rena′lis [TA] the blunted apex of a renal pyramid, found in the inner zone of the renal medulla and projecting into a renal sinus.

retromolar p. a small papilla of gingival tissue located at the foot of the ramus of the mandible and attached to the most inferior part of the anterior border of the ramus.

simple papillae of tongue papillae filiformes.

sublingual p. caruncula sublingualis.

papil′lae valla′tae [TA] vallate papillae: the largest papillae of the tongue, 8 to 12 in number, arranged in the form of a V anterior to the sulcus terminalis of the tongue.

p. of Vater p. duodeni major.

pa•pil•lae (pə-pil′e) [L.] genitive and plural of *papilla.*

pap•il•lary (pap′ĭ-lar″e) pertaining to or resembling a papilla, or nipple.

pap•il•late (pap′ĭ-lāt) marked by nipplelike elevations.

pap•il•lec•to•my (pap″ĭ-lek′tə-me) [*papilla* + *-ectomy*] excision of a papilla.

pa•pil•le•de•ma (pap″il-ə-de′mə) edema of the optic disk (papilla), most commonly due to increased intracranial pressure, malignant hypertension, or thrombosis of the central retinal vein; called also *choked disk.*

pap•il•lif•er•ous (pap″ĭ-lif′ər-əs) papillate.

pa•pil•li•form (pə-pil′ĭ-form) [*papilla* + *form*] shaped like a papilla.

pa•pil•li•tis (pap″ĭ-li′tis) [*papilla* + *-itis*] 1. inflammation of a papilla. 2. a form of optic neuritis involving the optic papilla (disk).

necrotizing p., necrotizing renal p. renal papillary necrosis.

pa•pil•lo•ad•e•no•cys•to•ma (pə-pil″o-ad″ə-no-sis-to′mə) papillary cystadenoma (def. 1).

pa•pil•lo•car•ci•no•ma (pə-pil″o-kahr″sĭ-no′mə) papillary carcinoma.

pap•il•lo•ma (pap″ĭ-lo′mə) [*papilla* + *-oma*] a benign epithelial neoplasm producing finger-like or verrucous projections from the epithelial surface. Called also *papillary tumor.* **papillo′matous** *adj*

choroid plexus p. a slow-growing benign tumor of the choroid plexus that often invades the leptomeninges. In children it is usually in a lateral ventricle but in adults it is more often in the fourth ventricle. Hydrocephalus is common, either from obstruction or from tumor secretion of cerebrospinal fluid. If it undergoes malignant transformation it is called a *choroid plexus carcinoma.*

cutaneous p. acrochordon.

fibroepithelial p. a type of papilloma containing extensive fibrous tissue; called also *fibropapilloma.*

intracanalicular p. an arborizing, nonmalignant growth within the ducts of certain glands, especially of the breast.

intracystic p. a papilloma formed within a cyst of a cystadenoma.

intraductal p. a tumor in a lactiferous duct, usually attached to the wall by a stalk; a distinction is often made between the solitary type (tumors found in just one duct and often benign) and the multiple type (tumors found in several or many ducts, often bilaterally, and often premalignant). The solitary type often has a serous or bloody discharge from the nipple, whereas the multiple type does not.

inverted p. papilloma in which the proliferating epithelial cells invaginate into the underlying stroma; it usually occurs in the nasal cavity, urinary bladder, or oral soft tissues *(inverted ductal p.)* of middle-aged males.

inverted ductal p. an intraductal papilloma of the salivary glands, presenting as a nodular submucosal mass in the oral cavity of adults.

inverted schneiderian p. a neoplasm of the nasal wall, having destructive capacity, a tendency to recur, and a potential for malignancy.

rabbit p., Shope p. a viral disease of rabbits marked by the formation of horny warts. These papillomas were the first mammalian tumors shown to be induced by a virus (by Shope in 1933) and the first to be transmitted by purified viral DNA.

squamous p. a papilloma composed of squamous epithelium, such as commonly occurs in the oral cavity.

villous p. papilloma.

pap•il•lo•ma•to•sis (pap″ĭ-lo-mə-to′sis) the development of multiple papillomas.

biliary p. a rare condition of the bile ducts, affecting primarily elderly persons and men more than women, characterized by numerous adenomatous papillomas in the ducts, with cholangitis, abdominal pain, and jaundice; there is a high risk of malignant transformation.

bovine p. an infectious disease of cattle, caused by a papillomavirus and characterized by the development of multiple warts with connective tissue proliferation, occurring mainly on the teats and udder in dairy cattle and the head and neck in beef cattle; calves are affected more often than adults.

canine oral p., canine viral p. a benign viral disease of young dogs, characterized by papillomas on the oral mucous membranes that usually resolve spontaneously in a few weeks; the cause is a papillomavirus.

confluent and reticulate p. a progressive, pruritic skin condition seen primarily in prepubescent girls; it begins on the chest and back as keratotic, pigmented papules that increase in size and spread outward over the body. Centrally located lesions tend to become confluent and peripherally located ones to become reticulate. Called also *Gougerot-Carteaud syndrome.*

equine p. an infectious disease of horses, caused by a papillomavirus and characterized by the development of warts, usually around the face but occasionally around the genitals; it primarily affects animals younger than two years old.

florid p. of nipple nipple adenoma.

juvenile laryngeal p., juvenile laryngotracheobronchial p., recurrent respiratory p. the recurrent growth of benign squamous cell papillomas in the larynx and trachea, caused by the human papillomavirus, and leading to severe narrowing of the airway that may require frequent treatments; onset is in childhood or early adulthood.

subareolar duct p. nipple adenoma.

Pap•il•lo•ma•vi•ri•dae (pap″ĭ-lo″mə-vir′ĭ-de) a family of viruses formerly considered part of the family Papovaviridae, having a nonenveloped icosahedral virion 55 nm in diameter with 72 capsomers in a skew arrangement. The genome consists of a single molecule of double-stranded DNA that has 8,000 base pairs. Replication and assembly take place in the nucleus, and virions are released by cell destruction. Many species cause tumors or other types of cancer. Genera have been named with the word *papillomavirus* preceded by the name of a Greek letter; those of medical or veterinary interest include *Alphapapillomavirus, Betapapillomavirus, Gammapapillomavirus,* and *Mupapillomavirus.*

pap•il•lo•ma•vi•rus (pap″ĭ-lo′mə-vi″rəs) any virus of the family Papillomaviridae. **papillomavi′ral** *adj*

bovine p. (BPV) any of several species of papillomavirus (especially BPV-1, -2, and -4) that cause bovine papillomatosis; there are at least six

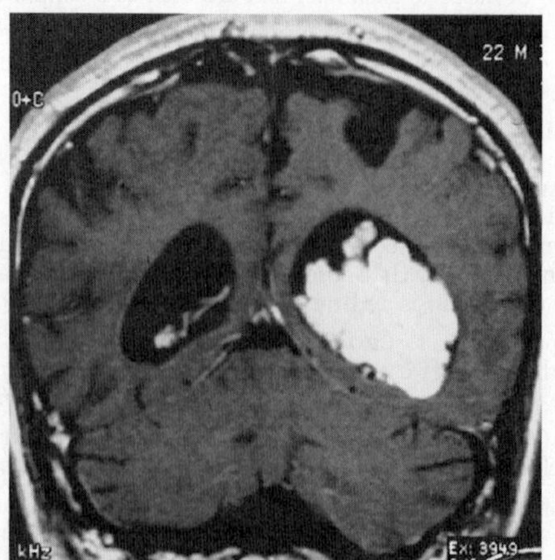

■ Choroid plexus papilloma in the trigone of the left lateral ventricle on a coronal MRI; both lateral ventricles are dilated from hydrocephalus associated with the tumor.

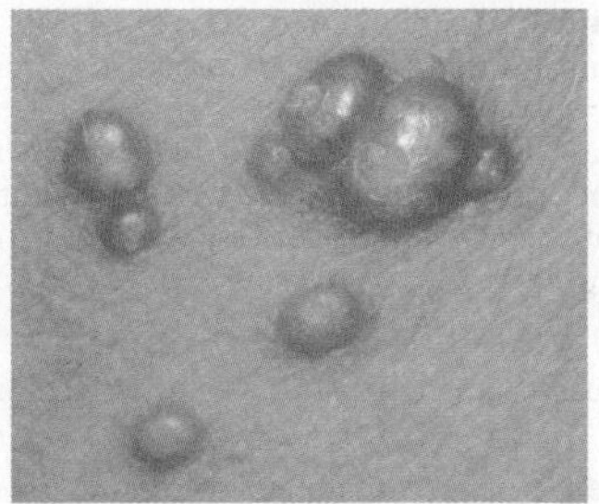

■ Papules.

types with no immunologic cross-reactivity, each type producing a characteristic lesion. Called also *bovine papillomatosis virus.*

cottontail rabbit p. a species of papillomavirus that causes rabbit papilloma.

equine p. a species of papillomavirus that causes equine papillomatosis.

human p. (HPV) any of a number of species of papillomaviruses that cause warts, particularly plantar and genital warts, on the skin and mucous membranes in humans. Dozens of different species and strains have been isolated, now classified in the genera *Alphapapillomavirus*, *Betapapillomavirus*, *Gammapapillomavirus*, and *Mupapillomavirus*. Viruses are transmitted by either direct or indirect contact, and some are associated with malignancies of the genital tract.

rabbit p. cottontail rabbit p.

Pa•pil•lon-Le•fèvre syndrome (pah″pe-yaw′ lə-fev′rə) [M.M. *Papillon*, French dermatologist, 20th century; Paul *Lefèvre*, French dermatologist, 20th century] see under *syndrome.*

pap•il•lo•ret•i•ni•tis (pap″ĭ-lo-ret″ĭ-ni′tis) inflammation of the optic papilla extending to the retina.

pap•il•lo•sphinc•ter•ot•o•my (pap″ĭ-lo-sfingk″tər-ot′ə-me) surgical division of the sphincter of the major duodenal papilla (Oddi sphincter).

pap•il•lo•tome (pap′ĭ-lo-tōm″) a cutting instrument for incising the major duodenal papilla.

pap•il•lot•o•my (pap″ĭ-lot′ə-me) incision of a papilla, as of the duodenal papilla.

Pa•po•va•vi•ri•dae (pə-po″və-vir′ĭ-de) a former family of DNA viruses that included the papillomaviruses and polyomaviruses; see *Papillomaviridae* and *Polyomaviridae.*

pa•po•va•vi•rus (pə-po′və-vi″rəs) [from *pa*pilloma *po*lyoma *va*cuolating agent (SV40) + *virus*] any of the viruses of the former family Papovaviridae. **papovavi′ral** *adj*

lymphotropic p. (LPV) a strain of polyomavirus that was originally isolated from a B-lymphoblastic cell line from an African green monkey; antigenically related viruses occur in many species of primates.

Pap•pen•heim stain (pah′pən-hīm) [Artur *Pappenheim*, German physician, 1870–1916] see *Stains and Staining Methods*, under *stain.*

pap•u•la•tion (pap″u-la′shən) the production of papules.

pap•ule (pap′ūl) [L. *papula*] a small circumscribed, superficial, solid elevation of the skin less than 1 cm (0.5 cm according to some authorities) in diameter. **pap′ular** *adj*

Gottron p's a further development of the Gottron sign in dermatomyositis, consisting of discolored lichenoid flat-topped papules over the knuckles.

moist p., mucous p. condyloma latum.

painful piezogenic pedal p's piezogenic p's.

pearly penile p's numerous tiny white, dome-shaped asymptomatic angiofibromas occurring circumferentially around the penile coronal sulcus.

piezogenic p's transitory, large, soft papules appearing above the heel on the side of one or both feet; they are not inflammatory but are often painful and are elicited by weight bearing with prolonged standing or running. The cause is thought to be temporary herniation of fat tissue and its blood vessels and nerves through connective tissue defects. The papules disappear when pressure is removed. Called also *painful fat herniation* and *painful piezogenic pedal p's.*

prurigo p. the characteristic lesion of prurigo (q.v.).

pruritic urticarial p's and plaques of pregnancy (PUPPP) a common skin condition seen in pregnancy, generally in the third trimester, characterized by eruption of pruritic raised bumps; it usually begins on the abdomen, especially on striae and not near the umbilicus, and often spreads to the thighs.

rheumatoid p's the tender, umbilicated, erythematous papules seen in rheumatoid neutrophilic dermatitis.

split p. a type of fissured papular syphilid sometimes seen at the corners of the mouth.

pap•u•lo•er•y•the•ma•tous (pap″u-lo-er″ə-them′ə-təs) marked by papules on an erythematous surface.

pap•u•lo•eryth•ro•der•ma (pap″u-lo-e-rith″ro-dur′mə) erythroderma with papules.

Ofuji p. a rare type of erythroderma seen primarily in elderly Japanese patients, characterized by papules and pruritus sparing the skinfolds; in some cases it seems to be paraneoplastic.

pap•u•loid (pap′u-loid) resembling a papule.

pap•u•lo•ne•crot•ic (pap″u-lo-nə-krot′ik) characterized by both papules and necrosis.

pap•u•lo•nod•ule (pap″u-lo-nod′ūl) a skin lesion with aspects of both a papule and a nodule.

pap•u•lo•pus•tu•lar (pap″u-lo-pus′tu-lər) both papular and pustular.

pap•u•lo•sis (pap-u-lo′sis) the presence of multiple papules.

bowenoid p. benign reddish brown papules occurring primarily on the genitalia, particularly the penis, in young adults; a viral etiology is suspected and the histologic features are identical to those of Bowen disease.

lymphomatoid p. a usually benign, self-healing, recurrent, asynchronous eruption of hemorrhagic papules, usually on the trunk or limbs, sometimes premalignant. The lesions resemble acute lichenoid pityriasis, and after healing may leave macular scars or crusted scales and a central necrotic mass.

malignant atrophic p. an often fatal disease usually seen in men, characterized by endovasculitis of the skin, gastrointestinal tract, and sometimes other organs, resulting in ischemic infarction of involved tissues. Skin lesions are erythematous papules that become umbilicated and develop porcelain-white centers with telangiectatic borders; these often atrophy and leave white scars. Called also *Degos disease.*

pap•u•lo•squa•mous (pap″u-lo-squa′məs) both papular and scaly.

pap•u•lo•ves•i•cle (pap″u-lo-ves′ĭ-kəl) a papule that changes into a vesicle (blister).

pap•u•lo•ve•sic•u•lar (pap″u-lo-və-sik′u-lər) both papular and vesicular.

pap•y•ra•ceous (pap″ĭ-ra′shəs) [L. *papyraceus*] like paper.

Pa•quin technique (pa′kwin) [Albert J. *Paquin*, Jr., American urologist, 1921–1967] see under *technique.*

para (par′ə) [L. *parere* to bring forth, to bear] a woman who has produced viable young regardless of whether the child was living at birth. Used with Roman numerals to designate the number of pregnancies that have resulted in the birth of viable offspring, as *para 0* (none—nullipara), *para I* (one—primipara), *para II* (two—secundipara), *para III* (three—tripara), *para IV* (four—quadripara), etc. Since the number indicates how many pregnancies, a multiple birth counts as just one in the calculation. Symbol P. Cf. *gravida.*

PAR pseudoautosomal region.

par(a)- [Gr. *para* to, at, or from the side of] a prefix meaning *(a)* beside, near, *(b)* resembling, *(c)* accessory to, *(d)* beyond, *(e)* apart from, *(f)* abnormal.

para- symbol *p-*; in organic chemistry, a prefix indicating a 1,4-substituted benzene ring, e.g., *p*-xylene (1,4-dimethylbenzene) or *p*-nitrophenol (4-nitrophenol).

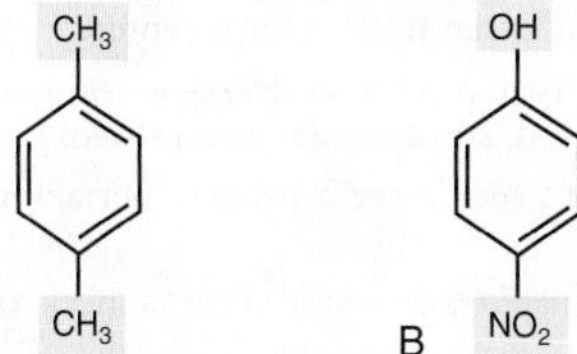

■ Two examples of disubstituted benzene derivatives with substituents in the *para*-position. *(A)*, *p*-xylene (1,4-dimethylbenzene); *(B)*, *p*-nitrophenol.

para-ad•ven•ti•tial (par″ə-ad″vən-tĭ′shəl) near the tunica adventitia.

para-am•i•no•ben•zo•ic ac•id (par″ə-ə-me″no-bən-zo′ik) *p*-aminobenzoic acid.

para-ami•no•hip•pu•ric ac•id (par″ə-ə-me″no-hĭ-pūr′ik) *p*-aminohippuric acid.

para-ami•no•sal•i•cyl•ic ac•id (par″ə-ə-me″no-sal-ĭ-sil′ik) *p*-aminosalicylic acid.

para-an•al•ge•sia (par″ə-an″əl-je′ze-ə) analgesia of the lower part of the body, including the lower limbs. Called also *paranalgesia.*

para-an•es•the•sia (par″ə-an″es-the′zhə) anesthesia of the lower limbs and abdomen; called also *paranesthesia.*

para-aor•tic (par″ə-a-or′tik) near or next to the aorta.

para·ap·pen·di·ci·tis (par″ə-ə-pen″dĭ-si′tis) periappendicitis.

Para·bac·te·roi·des (par″ə-bak″tər-oi′dēz) [*para-* + *Bacteroides*] a genus of gram-negative bacteria of the family Bacteroidaceae, including organisms formerly classified in the genus *Bacteroides*, consisting of anaerobic, non–spore-forming rods that are nonmotile or motile with peritrichous flagella. The type species is *P. distasonis*.

P. distaso′nis a species commonly isolated from human feces; formerly called *Bacteroides distasonis*.

para·ban·ic ac·id (par″ə-ban′ik) the cyclic anhydride of oxaluric acid, an oxidation product of urea.

Par·a·ba·sa·lia (par″ə-bə-sa′le-ə) a phylum of anaerobic, flagellated protozoa, characteristically having at least one parabasal apparatus; orders include Diplomonadida, Retortamonadida, and Trichomonadida.

par·ab·i·on (par-ab′e-on) parabiont.

par·ab·i·ont (par-ab′e-ont) [*para-* + Gr. *bioun* to live] one of two or more organisms living in a condition of parabiosis.

para·bio·sis (par″ə-bi-o′sis) [*para-* + *biosis*] the union of two individuals, as conjoined twins, or of experimental animals by surgical operation. **parabiot′ic** *adj*

vascular p. the crossing of the circulation between two experimental animals by anastomosis of blood vessels.

para·blast (par′ə-blast) [*para-* + *-blast*] the part of the mesoblast from which the blood vessels, lymphatics, etc., are developed. **parablas′tic** *adj*

para·bu·lia (par″ə-bu′le-ə) [*para-* + Gr. *boulē* will + *-ia*] perversion of the will, as when an individual intends to perform a particular action but halts and substitutes either an opposite action or an unrelated alternative; usually seen in schizophrenics.

para·car·di·ac (par″ə-kahr′de-ak) near or beside the heart; called also *juxtacardiac*.

para·car·mine (par″ə-kahr′mēn) a staining medium consisting of carminic acid, calcium chloride, and alcohol.

para·ca·sein (par″ə-ka′sēn) the chemical product of the action of rennin on casein; see *casein*.

par·a·cel·lu·lar (par″ə-sel′u-lər) next to or beside a cell.

Par·a·cel·sus (par″ə-sel′səs) [pseudonym of Philipus Aureolus Theophrastus Bombastus von Hohenheim] the "Luther of Medicine," 1493–1541, a Swiss physician and alchemist who defied the authority of Galen and Avicenna and condemned all medical teaching not based on experience. His alchemical researches led to the introduction of such substances as lead, sulfur, iron, and arsenic into pharmaceutical chemistry. Although he was far ahead of his time in many of his observations (e.g., on metabolic and on occupational diseases), much of his thinking was made obscure by his mysticism.

para·cen·es·the·sia (par″ə-se″nes-the′zhə) [*para-* + *cenesthesia*] any abnormality of the general sense of well-being.

para·cen·te·sis (par″ə-sen-te′sis) [*para-* + *-centesis*] surgical puncture of a cavity with a needle or other hollow instrument for diagnostic or therapeutic aspiration of fluid. **paracentet′ic** *adj*

abdominal p. insertion of a trocar through an incision into the peritoneal cavity to inject a therapeutic agent or remove ascitic fluid. Called also *abdominocentesis* and *peritoneocentesis*.

para·cen·tral (par″ə-sen′trəl) near a center.

para·ceph·a·lus (par″ə-sef′ə-ləs) [*para-* + *-cephalus*] having a rudimentary or misshapen head; see *acephalus paracephalus*.

para·cer·e·bel·lar (par″ə-ser″ə-bel′ər) pertaining to the lateral part of the cerebellum.

para·cer·vi·cal (par″ə-sur′vĭ-kəl) near a neck or cervix, particularly the uterine cervix.

para·cer·vix (par″ə-sur′viks) [*para-* + *cervix*] [TA] the inferior part of the parametrium.

par·ac·et·al·de·hyde (par-as″ət-al′də-hīd) paraldehyde.

par·ac·et·am·ol (par-as″ət-am′ol) acetaminophen.

Para·chla·my·dia (par″ə-klə-mid′e-ə) [*para-* + *Chlamydia* (q.v.)] a genus of bacteria of the family Parachlamydiaceae, consisting of mesophilic cocci with variable Gram staining characteristics; organisms are naturally parasites of free-living amebae and cause respiratory infections in humans. The type species is *P. acanthamoe′bae*.

Para·chla·my·di·a·ceae (par″ə-klə-mid″e-a′se-e) a family of bacteria of the order Chlamydiales that are natural parasites of free-living amebae. It contains the genus *Parachlamydia*.

para·chlo·ro·met·a·xy·le·nol (par″ə-klor″o-met″ə-zi′lə-nol) chloroxylenol.

para·chlo·ro·phe·nol (par″ə-klor″o-fe′nol) [USP] an antibacterial effective against most gram-negative organisms; used as a topical anti-infective.

camphorated p. [USP] a preparation of 33–37 per cent parachlorophenol and 63–67 per cent camphor, used as a dental anti-infective; applied topically to the root canals and the periapical region.

para·chol·era (par″ə-kol′ər-ə) a disease resembling cholera but caused by an organism other than *Vibrio cholerae*.

para·chor·dal (par″ə-kor′dəl) [*para-* + *chordal*] beside or next to the notochord.

Par·a·chor·do·des (par″ə-kor-do′dēz) a genus of the class Nematomorpha. A few cases of human infection with the species *P. pustilo′sus*, *P. tolosa′nus*, and *P. viola′ceus* have been reported from France and Italy.

para·ci·ne·sia (par″ə-si-ne′zhə) parakinesia.

para·ci·ne·sis (par″ə-si-ne′sis) parakinesia.

para·clin·i·cal (par″ə-klin′ĭ-kəl) pertaining to abnormalities (e.g., morphological or biochemical) underlying clinical manifestations (e.g., chest pain or fever).

para·coc·cid·i·oi·dal (par″ə-kok-sid″e-oi′dəl) pertaining to or caused by fungi of the genus *Paracoccidioides*.

Para·coc·cid·i·oi·des (par″ə-kok-sid″e-oi′dēz) a genus of Fungi Imperfecti of the form-family Moniliaceae. *P. brasilien′sis* (called also *Blastomyces brasiliensis*) is the species that causes paracoccidioidomycosis; organisms proliferate by multiple budding yeast cells in the tissues, and produce white aerial mycelia and single or double conidia in media at 25°C or in soil.

para·coc·cid·i·oi·do·my·co·sis (par″ə-kok-sid″e-oi″do-mi-ko′sis) fungal infection by *Paracoccidioides brasiliensis*. The usual form is a chronic condition in adults that begins in the lungs and spreads to the mucocutaneous areas, particularly the buccal mucosa, and may extend to the adjacent skin, tonsils, gastrointestinal lymphatics, liver, and spleen. A less common form is seen in children and is an acute condition with prominent involvement of the reticuloendothelial system that can be fatal. Called also *Almeida* or *Lutz-Splendore-Almeida disease*, *Brazilian* or *South American blastomycosis*, and *paracoccidioidal granuloma*.

para·col·pi·tis (par″ə-kol-pi′tis) [*para-* + *colp-* + *-itis*] paravaginitis.

para·col·pi·um (par″ə-kol′pe-əm) [*para-* + Gr. *kolpos* vagina] the connective and other tissues that surround the vagina.

para·cone (par′ə-kōn) [*para-* + Gr. *kōnos* cone] the mesiobuccal cusp of a maxillary tooth of mammals, which normally occludes between the paraconid and hypoconid of the corresponding lower molar.

para·co·nid (par″ə-ko′nid) [*para-* + *con(o)-* + *-id*] the mesiobuccal cusp of a mandibular molar tooth.

para·cor·tex (par″ə-kor′teks) [*para-* + *cortex*] thymus-dependent area.

par·acou·sis (par″ə-koo′sis) paracusia.

para·cox·al·gia (par″ə-kok-sal′jə) a condition marked by pain simulating that of coxitis.

para·crine (par′ə-krin) [*para-* + Gr. *krinein* to separate] denoting a type of hormone function in which hormone synthesized in and released from endocrine cells binds to its receptor in nearby cells of a different type and affects their function.

par·acu·sia (par″ə-ku′zhə) 1. any deficiency in the sense of hearing; see also *deafness*. Called also *paracusis* and *paracousis*. 2. auditory hallucination.

p. lo′ci inability to locate correctly the origin of sounds.

p. willisia′na paradoxic hearing loss.

par·acu·sis (par″ə-ku′sis) paracusia.

p. of Willis paradoxic hearing loss.

para·cys·tic (par″ə-sis′tik) [*para-* + *cyst-* + *-ic*] perivesical.

para·cys·ti·tis (par″ə-sis-ti′tis) [*para-* + *cyst-* + *-itis*] pericystitis.

para·cys·ti·um (par″ə-sis′te-əm) [*para-* + Gr. *kystis* bladder] the connective and other tissues around the bladder.

para·cyt·ic (par″ə-sit′ik) [*para-* + *cyt-* + *-ic*] denoting cell elements present in the blood or other part of the organism, but enthetic or not normal to it.

para·den·tal (par″ə-den′təl) 1. having some connection with or relation to the science or practice of dentistry. 2. periodontal.

para·den·ti·tis (par″ə-dən-ti′tis) periodontitis.

para·den·ti·um (par″ə-den′she-əm) periodontium (def. 1).

para·den·to·sis (par″ə-dən-to′sis) juvenile periodontitis.

para•des•mose (par″ə-des′mōs) [*para-* + *desmose*] the connection between extranuclear centrioles during mitosis in certain protozoa; see *desmose.*

para•did•y•mal (par″ə-did′ĭ-məl) 1. pertaining to the paradidymis. 2. beside the testis.

para•did•y•mis (par″ə-did′ĭ-mis) [*para-* + Gr. *didymos* testis] [TA] a body made up of a few convoluted tubules in the anterior part of the spermatic cord, considered to be a remnant of the mesonephros; called also *organ of Giraldés, parepididymis,* and *massa innominata.*

para•di•meth•yl•ami•no•benz•al•de•hyde (par″ə-di-meth″əl-ə-me″no-ben-zal′də-hīd) white or pale yellow crystals or crystalline powder, used in the preparation of Ehrlich aldehyde reagent and in the determination of urobilinogen and porphobilinogen.

para•dip•sia (par″ə-dip′se-ə) [*para-* + *dipsia*] an abnormally increased appetite for fluids, which are ingested without relation to bodily need.

para•dox (par′ə-doks) [Gr. *paradoxos* incredible] a statement which seems to be, though it may not be, absurd or self-contradictory.

Opie p. necrotizing local anaphylaxis sometimes acts as a specific protective mechanism.

Simpson p. a form of extreme confounding (q.v.) such that an association between two variables is actually reversed after adjusting for a third.

Weber p. the elongation of a muscle which has been so stretched that it cannot contract.

para•dox•i•cal (par″ə-dok′sĭ-kəl) occurring at variance with the normal rule.

para•du•o•de•nal (par″ə-doo″o-de′nəl, -doo-od′ə-nəl) alongside, near, or around the duodenum.

para•ec•cri•sis (par″ə-ek′rĭ-sis) [*para-* + *-eccrisis*] disordered secretion or excretion.

para•epi•lep•sy (par″ə-ep′ĭ-lep-se) minor focal epilepsy.

para•esoph•a•ge•al (par″ə-e-sof″ə-je′əl) near or beside the esophagus.

para•falx (par″ə-falks′) situated near the falx cerebri or falx cerebelli.

Par. aff. [L.] pars affec′ta (the part affected).

par•af•fin (par′ə-fin) [L. *parum* little + *affinis* akin] 1. [NF] a purified mixture of solid hydrocarbons obtained from petroleum, occurring as an odorless, tasteless, colorless or white, more or less translucent mass; used for embedding histological specimens and as a stiffening agent in pharmaceutical preparations. See also *paraffin bath,* under *bath.* 2. alkane.

hard p. paraffin (def. 1).

light liquid p. light mineral oil.

liquid p. mineral oil.

synthetic p. [NF] paraffin synthesized by catalytic conversion of carbon monoxide and hydrogen to a mixture of paraffin hydrocarbons; used as a stiffening agent in pharmaceutical preparations.

white soft p. white petrolatum.

yellow soft p. petrolatum.

par•af•fin•o•ma (par″ə-fin-o′mə) a chronic granuloma produced by prolonged continuous exposure to the irritation of paraffin.

Par•a•fi•la•ria (par″ə-fĭ-lar′e-ə) a genus of nematodes of the superfamily Filarioides that infect ruminants. *P. bovi′cola* causes dermatorrhagia parasitica (summer bleeding) in cattle. *P. multipapillo′sa* causes the same condition in horses.

Par•a•flex (par′ə-fleks) trademark for preparations containing chlorzoxazone.

para•floc•cu•lus (par″ə-flok′u-ləs) [*para-* + *flocculus*] a small lobe of the cerebellar hemisphere, located immediately cranial to the flocculus. Called also *accessory flocculus.*

dorsal p. pars medialis lobuli biventralis cerebelli.

p. ventra′lis TA alternative for *tonsilla cerebelli.*

ventral p. tonsilla cerebelli.

Para•fon (par′ə-fon) trademark for preparations containing chlorzoxazone.

Para•fos•sar•u•lus (par″ə-fŏ-sar′u-ləs) a genus of fresh water snails of the family Bulimidae.

P. manchou′ricus a species found in eastern Asia and nearby islands. It is the foremost intermediate host of the liver fluke *Opisthorchis sinensis* in Japan and the second most important in China, as well as a carrier of the flukes *O. felineus* and *Echinochasmus perfoliatus.*

para•fre•nal (par″ə-fre′nəl) near a frenum or frenulum.

para•func•tion (par′ə-funk″shən) disordered or abnormal function. parafunc′tional *adj*

para•gam•ma•cism (par″ə-gam′ə-siz-əm) gammacism.

para•gan•glia (par″ə-gang′gle-ə) plural of *paraganglion.*

para•gan•gli•o•ma (par″ə-gang″gle-o′mə) a tumor of the tissue composing the paraganglia.

medullary p. pheochromocytoma.

nonchromaffin p. chemodectoma.

para•gan•gli•on (par″ə-gang′gle-on) pl. *paragan′glia.* A collection of chromaffin cells, derived from neural ectoderm, occurring elsewhere than in the adrenal medulla, usually near the sympathetic ganglia and in relation to the aorta and its branches. Most, if not all, paraganglia secrete epinephrine or norepinephrine. Called also *chromaffin body* and *pheochrome body.*

Para•gard (par′əgahrd) trademark for a type of copper intrauterine device.

para•gen•i•ta•lis (par″ə-gen″ĭ-ta′lis) [*para-* + L. *genitalis* genital] 1. in lower vertebrates, the urinary part of the mesonephros, caudal to the genital part. 2. in higher animals, the paradidymis or paroöphoron.

para•geu•sia (par″ə-goo′zhə) [*para-* + Gr. *geusis* taste + *-ia*] 1. perversion of the sense of taste. 2. a bad taste in the mouth. Called also *dysgeusia.*

para•geu•sic (par″ə-goo′zik) pertaining to or characterized by parageusia.

par•ag•na•thus (pə-rag′nə-thəs) [*para-* + Gr. *gnathos* jaw] 1. a fetus with a supernumerary jaw. 2. in asymmetrical conjoined twins, a parasitic fetus attached laterally to the jaw of the more developed fetus.

par•a•gon•i•mi•a•sis (par″ə-gon″ĭ-mi′ə-sis) infection with flukes of the genus *Paragonimus;* characterized by bronchitis, bronchiectasis, and tuberculoid symptoms. Called also *lung fluke disease* and *paragonimosis.*

par•a•gon•i•mo•sis (par″ə-gon″ĭ-mo′sis) paragonimiasis.

Par•a•gon•i•mus (par″ə-gon′ĭ-məs) [*para-* + Gr. *gonimos* productive; having generative power] a genus of flukes of the family Troglotrematidae; they have two invertebrate hosts, the first a snail, such as *Semisulcospira,* and the second a crab or crayfish, such as *Potamon* or *Eriocheir.*

P. africa′nus a species that parasitizes humans and carnivores in Central Africa.

P. heterotre′ma a species infecting humans in East and Southeast Asia.

P. kellicot′ti a species closely related to *P. westermani,* found in cats, dogs, hogs, minks, and muskrats in the United States.

P. rin′geri *P. westermani.*

P. westerma′ni the lung fluke, a round, pink to brown species found in cysts in the lungs and sometimes in the pleura, liver, abdominal cavity, or elsewhere. It causes parasitic hemoptysis in southern and eastern Asia; infection is acquired through ingestion of infected freshwater crabs or crayfish.

Par•a•gor•di•us (par″ə-gor′de-əs) a genus of sometimes parasitic worms of the class Nematomorpha. Human infections with *P. cinc′tus, P. tricuspida′tus,* and *P. va′rius* have been reported.

para•gram•ma•tism (par″ə-gram′ə-tiz-əm) 1. paraphasia. 2. agrammatism.

para•gran•u•lo•ma (par″ə-gran″u-lo′mə) Hodgkin disease, lymphocyte predominance type.

para•graph•ia (par″ə-graf′e-ə) [*para-* + *graph-* + *-ia*] dysgraphia in which the patient makes mistakes in spelling or writes one word in place of another.

para•he•mo•phil•ia (par″ə-he″mo-fil′e-ə) deficiency of coagulation factor V, an autosomal recessive trait causing a hemorrhagic tendency that is highly variable in intensity.

para•he•pat•ic (par″ə-hə-pat′ik) beside the liver.

para•hip•po•cam•pal (par″ə-hip″o-kam′pəl) near or next to the hippocampus.

para•hor•mone (par″ə-hor′mōn) [*para-* + *hormone*] a substance not conventionally accepted as a true hormone but that exerts hormonelike actions.

para•hyp•no•sis (par″ə-hip-no′sis) [*para-* + *hypnosis*] abnormal sleep, as under hypnosis or during general anesthesia; sometimes characterized by a suggestible state, somnambulism, or an unusual partial awareness of the surroundings.

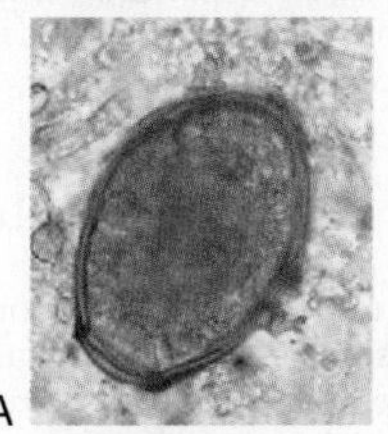

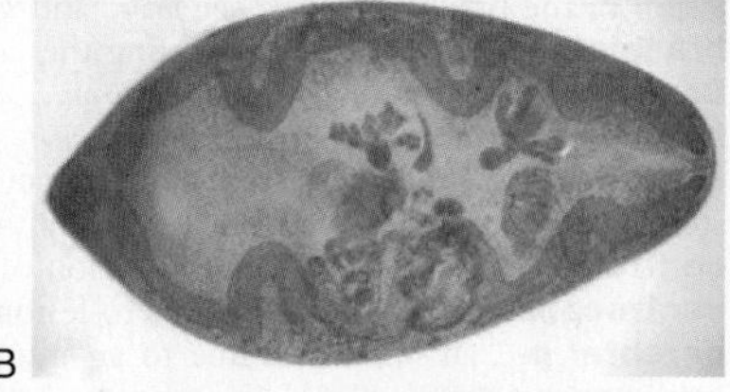

■ *Paragonimus westermani (A),* egg; *(B),* adult, a hermaphrodite having an ovary and two branching testes.

para·hy·poph·y·sis (par″ə-hi-pof′ĭ-sis) an accessory mass of pituitary tissue.

para·in·fec·tious (par″ə-in-fek′shəs) pertaining to manifestations of infectious disease that are caused by the immune response to the infectious agent.

para·ker·a·tin·ized (par″ə-ker′ə-tin-īzd″) pertaining to epithelium in which parakeratosis has occurred.

para·ker·a·to·sis (par″ə-ker″ə-to′sis) persistence of the nuclei of the keratinocytes into the stratum corneum; this is normal only in the epithelium of true mucous membranes of the mouth and vagina.

granular p. a pruritic skin condition usually found in skin furrows, consisting of erythema and hyperkeratotic papules; it was first observed as a reaction to personal hygiene products, but individuals have been found with it who have not been exposed to such substances.

inherited p. an autosomal recessive disease of cattle in Europe and North America in which calves around one month of age develop exanthems and parakeratosis on the legs, head, and neck; growth is stunted and they may die within three months. The cause is deficient uptake of zinc by the intestine, and zinc supplements may be curative. Called also *Adema disease.*

p. pustulo′sa psoriasiform lesions and onycholysis of a fingernail, with erythema, scaling, and blistering of the fingertip, usually seen in children and limited to one digit.

ruminal p. rumenitis with acidosis and hardening and enlargement of the ruminal papillae, most commonly seen in animals fed concentrated, pelleted feed.

p. variega′ta retiform parapsoriasis.

para·ki·ne·sia (par″ə-kĭ-ne′zhə) [*para-* + *kinesi-* + *-ia*] 1. abnormality of motor function resulting in distortion of movements; cf. *dyskinesia.* Called also *paracinesia* and *paracinesis.* 2. in ophthalmology, irregular action of an individual ocular muscle.

para·ki·net·ic (par″ə-kĭ-net′ik) pertaining to or characterized by parakinesia.

para·la·lia (par″ə-la′le-ə) [*para-* + *lal-* + *-ia*] any disturbance of speech, especially the utterance of a vocal sound other than the one desired. Called also *dyslalia.*

p. litera′lis incorrect utterance of certain consonant sounds, often as part of stuttering. Called also *literal paraphasia.*

para·lamb·da·cism (par″ə-lam′də-siz-əm) lambdacism.

par·al·de·hyde (par-al′də-hīd) [USP] a polymerization product of acetaldehyde, having rapid-acting sedative and hypnotic properties; used to control insomnia, excitement, agitation, delirium, and convulsions; administered rectally and intramuscularly and by intravenous infusion.

para·lex·ia (par″ə-lek′se-ə) dyslexia. **paralex′ic** *adj*

par·al·ge·sia (par″əl-je′ze-ə) [*para-* + *algesi-* + *-ia*] any condition marked by abnormal and painful sensations; a painful paresthesia. **paralge′sic** *adj*

par·al·gia (par-al′jə) paralgesia.

par·al·lag·ma (par″ə-lag′mə) [Gr.] displacement of a bone or of the fragments of a broken bone.

par·al·lax (par′ə-laks) [Gr. "change of position"] an apparent displacement of an object due to a change in the observer's position. **parallac′tic** *adj*

binocular p. the seeming difference in position of an object as seen separately by one eye and then by the other, the head remaining stationary. Types include *crossed, direct,* and *vertical p.*

crossed p. binocular parallax occurring in exophoria; when one eye is covered, the object viewed seems to move away from the open eye and toward the covered eye.

direct p. binocular parallax occurring in esophoria; when one eye is covered, the object viewed seems to move toward the open eye and away from the covered eye.

heteronymous p. crossed p.

homonymous p. direct p.

stereoscopic p. binocular p.

uncrossed p. direct p.

vertical p. binocular parallax occurring in vertical diplopia or heterophoria; the object seen seems to move vertically when each eye is closed in turn.

par·al·lel (par′ə-lel) [L. *parallelus*] 1. pertaining to straight lines or planes that do not intersect. 2. pertaining to electric circuit components connected "in parallel" so that the current flow divides, each branch passing through one component, and rejoins; applied by extension to any similar parallel circuit, e.g., the systemic circulation to the various organs. Cf. *series.*

par·al·lel·om·e·ter (par″ə-ləl-om′ə-tər) [*parallel* + *-meter*] an instrument for determining the exact parallel relationships of lines, surfaces, and structures in dental prostheses and casts.

par·al·ler·gy (par-al′ər-je) a condition in which an allergic state, produced by specific sensitization, predisposes the body to react to other allergens with clinical manifestations that differ from the original reaction. **paraller′gic** *adj*

para·lo·gia (par″ə-lo′jə) [*para-* + *log-* + *-ia*] disturbance of the reasoning faculty; marked by delusional or illogical speech.

thematic p. paralogia limited to one subject, on which the mind dwells insistently. Cf. *monomania.*

pa·ral·o·gism (pə-ral′o-jiz-əm) the use of fallacious, meaningless, or illogical thought or language, primarily characteristic of schizophrenia.

pa·ral·o·gous (pə-ral′ə-gəs) [*para-* + *homologous*] related by phylogenetic descent and diverging after duplication within a species; see under *gene.*

pa·ral·o·gy (pə-ral′ə-je) anatomical similarity that has no phylogenetic or functional implication.

pa·ral·y·ses (pə-ral′ĭ-sēz) plural of *paralysis.*

pa·ral·y·sis (pə-ral′ĭ-sis) pl. *paral′yses* [*para-* + *-lysis*] loss or impairment of motor function in a part due to lesion of the neural or muscular mechanism; also, by analogy, impairment of sensory function (sensory paralysis). See also subentries under *hemiplegia, palsy,* and *paraplegia.*

Paralysis

abducens p. see under *palsy.*

p. of accommodation cycloplegia.

p. a′gitans Parkinson disease.

alternate p., alternating p. alternate hemiplegia.

ascending p. spinal paralysis that progresses cephalad.

Avellis p. see under *syndrome.*

Bell p. see under *palsy.*

bilateral p. diplegia.

birth p. obstetric p.

brachial p., brachial plexus p. paralysis of an upper limb from a lesion of the brachial plexus; see *lower* and *upper brachial plexus p.*

brachiofacial p. paralysis affecting the face and an upper limb.

Brown-Séquard p. see under *syndrome.*

bulbar p. progressive bulbar palsy.

cage p. a complex nutritional deficiency resembling osteomalacia, sometimes seen in captive primates.

central p. any paralysis due to a lesion of the brain or spinal cord.

centrocapsular p. paralysis due to lesions of the internal capsule.

cerebral p. any paralysis due to an intracranial lesion; see *cerebral palsy,* under *palsy.*

Chastek p. progressive ataxia and paralysis in silver foxes due to thiamine deficiency following a dietary change from meat to raw fish that contains a thiamine-destroying enzyme.

compression p. paralysis caused by pressure on a nerve, such as crutch paralysis, decubitus paralysis, or severe forms of carpal tunnel syndrome or cubital tunnel syndrome. Cf. *entrapment neuropathy.* Called also *pressure p.*

congenital abducens-facial p., congenital oculofacial p. Möbius syndrome.

conjugate p. loss of ability to perform some of the parallel ocular movements.

coonhound p. acute polyradiculoneuritis.

crossed p., cruciate p. paralysis affecting one side of the face and the opposite side of the body. See also *alternate hemiplegia.*

crural p. paralysis that chiefly affects the thigh or thighs.

crutch p. a type of radial neuropathy caused by pressure of the crutch in the axilla.

Cruveilhier p. spinal muscular atrophy.

curled toe p. a sign of riboflavin deficiency in young chickens; the toes show varying degrees of flexing so that the chick has difficulty walking. Severe deficiency is lethal.

Paralysis *Continued*

decubitus p. paralysis due to pressure on a nerve from lying for a long time in one position.
Dejerine-Klumpke p. Klumpke p.
diaphragmatic p. paralysis of the diaphragm, usually unilateral; called also *phrenoplegia.*
diphtheritic p. a partial paralysis that often follows diphtheria, chiefly affecting the soft palate and throat muscles. Called also *postdiphtheritic p.*
divers' p. decompression sickness.
Duchenne p. 1. progressive bulbar palsy. 2. Erb-Duchenne p.
Duchenne-Erb p. Erb-Duchenne p.
Erb p. 1. Erb-Duchenne p. 2. Erb spastic paraplegia.
Erb-Duchenne p. upper brachial plexus paralysis caused by birth injury; called also *Erb* or *Erb-Duchenne palsy; Duchenne, Duchenne-Erb,* or *Erb p.;* and *Duchenne-Erb syndrome.*
facial p. weakening or paralysis of the facial nerve, as in Bell palsy or Millard-Gubler syndrome.
familial periodic p. any of several autosomal dominant conditions marked by recurring attacks of rapidly progressive flaccid paralysis, further classified on the basis of serum potassium levels; see *hypokalemic periodic p.* and *hyperkalemic periodic p.*
flaccid p. any paralysis accompanied by loss of muscle tone and absence of tendon reflexes in the paralyzed part. Cf. *spastic p.*
fowl p. Marek disease; see under *disease.*
functional p. 1. pseudoparalysis (def. 1). 2. hysterical p.
p. of gaze inability to focus the gaze with either lateral or vertical eye movements, due to pathological processes that usually involve the supranuclear oculomotor centers or pathways. Called also ocular apraxia.
general p. see under *paresis.*
glossolabial p., glossopharyngolabial p. progressive bulbar palsy.
Gubler p. Millard-Gubler syndrome.
hereditary cerebrospinal p. hereditary spastic paraplegia.
hyperkalemic periodic p. an autosomal dominant disorder characterized by recurring attacks of rapidly progressive flaccid paralysis accompanied by high serum potassium levels; due to mutation in the *SCNA4A* gene, (locus 17q13.1-17q13.3), which encodes a subunit of a skeletal muscle sodium channel.
hypoglossal p. paralysis due to a lesion of the hypoglossal nucleus or nerve.
hypokalemic periodic p. an autosomal dominant disorder characterized by recurring attacks of rapidly progressive flaccid paralysis accompanied by low serum potassium levels. Several types have been distinguished: type 1 is due to mutation in the *CACNL1A3* gene (locus: 1q32), which encodes a subunit of a skeletal muscle calcium channel; type 2 is due to mutation in the *SCNA4A* gene, (locus 17q13.1-17q13.3), which encodes a subunit of a skeletal muscle sodium channel.
hysterical p. paralysis in a part owing to a conversion disorder, without any organic neurological cause. Called also *functional p., pseudoparalysis,* and *pseudoparaplegia.*
immune p., immunologic p. immunologic unresponsiveness induced by administration of large doses of antigen; now called *immunologic tolerance.*
infantile p. the major illness of poliomyelitis; see *poliomyelitis.*

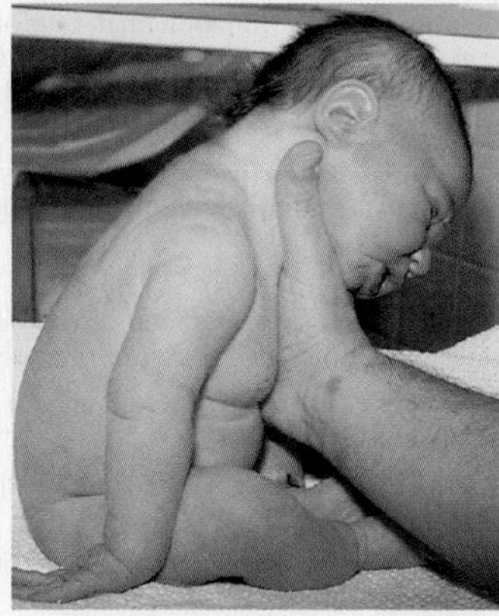

■ Erb-Duchenne paralysis caused by traction injury to C5–C7 spinal cord segments, with characteristic limply adducted and internally rotated arm posture.

infantile cerebral ataxic p. cerebral palsy with ataxia.
infantile cerebrocerebellar diplegic p. cerebral palsy with spastic paraplegia and ataxia.
infantile spinal p. spinal poliomyelitis.
infectious bulbar p. pseudorabies.
ischemic p. local paralysis due to an impairment of the circulation, as by embolism, thrombosis, or trauma; see also *Volkmann contracture,* under *contracture.*
Jamaica ginger p. a form of paralysis of the extremities, especially the legs, that was seen in the 1930s after a type of Jamaican ginger extract ("jake") was accidentally contaminated with the organophosphorus compound tri-*o*-tolyl phosphate and then consumed. Called also *Jamaica ginger polyneuritis.*
juvenile p. general paralysis in young persons.
juvenile p. agitans, juvenile p. agitans (of Hunt) a condition developing in early life, usually familial but occasionally occurring sporadically, marked by increased muscle tonus with the characteristic attitude and facies of paralysis agitans, due to progressive degeneration of the globus pallidus; involvement of the substantia nigra and pyramidal tracts may occur. Called also *paleostriatal syndrome, pallidal atrophy, pallidal syndrome,* and *Ramsay Hunt syndrome.*
Klumpke p., Klumpke-Dejerine p. lower brachial plexus paralysis caused by birth injury, particularly during breech deliveries; called also *Dejerine-Klumpke* or *Klumpke-Dejerine syndrome.*
Kussmaul p., Kussmaul-Landry p. Guillain-Barré syndrome.
labial p., labioglossolaryngeal p., labioglossopharyngeal p. progressive bulbar palsy.
lambing p. pregnancy toxemia in ewes.
Landry p. Guillain-Barré syndrome.
laryngeal p. paralysis of one of the laryngeal muscles, usually because of a lesion of the vagus nerve or the recurrent laryngeal nerve; seen in disorders such as Avellis syndrome, Jackson syndrome, and Vernet syndrome. Called also *laryngoparalysis* and *laryngoplegia.*
lead p. paralysis caused by lead poisoning, with wristdrop due to a peripheral neuritis.
lingual p. paralysis of the tongue.
Lissauer p. an apoplectiform type of general paresis.
local p. paralysis of one muscle or group of muscles.
lower brachial plexus p. atrophic paralysis of the muscles of the forearm and hand due to lesions of the eighth cervical or first dorsal nerve (lower trunk of the brachial plexus). When due to birth trauma it is called *Klumpke-Dejerine p.*
masticatory p. paralysis of the muscles of mastication; see also *trismus* and *trigeminal p.*
maternal obstetric p. see under *palsy.*
medullary tegmental paralyses paralyses due to lesions of the medullary tegmentum, including alternate hemiplegia, Babinski-Nageotte syndrome, Cestan syndrome, and Tapia syndrome.
Millard-Gubler p. see under *syndrome.*
mixed p. combined motor and sensory paralysis.
motor p. paralysis of voluntary muscles.
musculospiral p. radial neuropathy.
nuclear p. any paralysis due to a lesion in a nucleus of origin.
obstetric p. paralysis due to injury received at birth; called also *birth p.*
ocular p. see *amaurosis, cycloplegia,* and *ophthalmoplegia.*
oculomotor p. paralysis of the oculomotor nerve, seen in disorders such as Benedikt syndrome, Claude syndrome, Nothnagel syndrome, and Weber syndrome. Called also *oculomotor* or *third nerve palsy.*
periodic p. any of various diseases characterized by episodic flaccid paralysis or muscular weakness.
peripheral p. loss of power due to some lesion of the nervous mechanism between the nucleus of origin and the muscle.
peroneal p. crossed leg palsy.
phonetic p. vocal fold p.
postdiphtheritic p. diphtheritic p.
postdormital p. sleep paralysis occurring upon waking.
postepileptic p. Todd p.
posthemiplegic p. residual weakness after a stroke.
posticus p. paralysis of the posterior cricothyroid muscle. See also *laryngeal p.*
Pott p. see under *paraplegia.*
predormital p. sleep paralysis occurring prior to falling asleep.
pressure p. compression p.
progressive bulbar p. see under *palsy.*

Paralysis *Continued*

pseudobulbar p. see under *palsy*.
pseudohypertrophic muscular p. see under *dystrophy*.
radial p., radial nerve p. 1. radial neuropathy. 2. in quadrupeds such as horses and dogs, paralysis of elbow and knee muscles owing to injury to the radial nerve. Called also *dropped elbow*.
Ramsay Hunt p. juvenile p. agitans (of Hunt).
range p. Marek disease.
reflex p. paralysis ascribable to peripheral irritation; in some cases secondary changes occur in the spinal cord, and the paralysis ceases to be truly reflex.
rucksack p. a disorder of motor and sensory function of the upper limbs as a result of damage to the brachial plexus caused by the wearing of a backpack (rucksack).
sensory p. loss of sensation resulting from a morbid process.
serum p. peripheral nerve paralysis following administration of serum.
sleep p. paralysis occurring at awakening or sleep onset; it represents extension of the atonia of REM sleep into the waking state and is often seen in those suffering from narcolepsy or sleep apnea. Called also *waking p.* See also *postdormital p.* and *predormital p.*
spastic p. paralysis marked by spasticity of the muscles of the paralyzed part and increased tendon reflexes, due to upper motor neuron lesions. See also *spastic paraplegia*. Cf. *flaccid p.*
spinal p. paralysis due to a lesion of the spinal cord; called also *myeloplegia*.
spinomuscular p. paralysis due to lesion of the gray matter of the spinal cord; see also *spinal muscular atrophy*, under *atrophy*.
supranuclear p. pseudobulbar p.
suprascapular p. paralysis of the suprascapular muscle in a horse due to damage to its nerve. Called also *slipped shoulder, shoulder slip*, and *sweeney* or *sweeny*.
tegmental mesencephalic p. Benedikt syndrome.
thyrotoxic periodic p. recurrent episodes of generalized or local paralysis accompanied by hypokalemia, occurring in association with Graves disease and most often affecting males in the third decade of life; attacks occur especially after exercise or a high-carbohydrate or high-sodium meal and generally last 3 to 12 hours.
tick p. a progressive, ascending type of flaccid paralysis seen in children and domestic animals following the bite of certain ticks. In the northwestern United States and western Canada it is usually caused by *Dermacentor andersoni*, and in other parts of the world numerous other ticks have been implicated, including species of *Amblyomma, Haemaphysalis, Ixodes*, and *Rhipicephalus*. It is usually the result of toxins from the tick's saliva that enter the central nervous system of the host.
Todd p. hemiparesis or monoparesis lasting for a few minutes or hours, or occasionally for several days, after an epileptic seizure; called also *postepileptic p.*
trigeminal p. see under *neuropathy*.
upper brachial plexus p. paralysis of arm muscles due to destruction of the fifth and sixth cervical roots (upper trunk of the brachial plexus); small hand muscles are unaffected. When due to birth trauma it is called *Erb-Duchenne p.*
vasomotor p. paralysis of vasomotor muscles; see also *vasoparesis*. Called also *angioparalysis*.
vocal cord p., vocal fold p. paralysis of one or both or the vocal cords; the voice is weakened but not lost. See also *laryngeal p.* Called also *phonetic p.*
Volkmann ischemic p. see under *contracture*.
waking p. sleep p.
Weber p. see under *syndrome*.
writers' p. writers' cramp.

par•a•lys•or (par′ə-līz″ər) paralyzer.

par•a•lyt•ic (par″ə-lit′ik) [Gr. *paralytikos*] 1. affected with or pertaining to paralysis. 2. a person affected with paralysis.

par•a•lyt•o•gen•ic (par″ə-lit″o-jen′ik) causing paralysis.

par•a•lyz•ant (par′ə-līz″ənt) 1. causing paralysis. 2. an agent that paralyzes.

par•a•lyze (par′ə-līz) to put into a state of paralysis.

par•a•lyz•er (par′ə-līz″ər) a substance which hinders or prevents a chemical reaction; an inhibitor.

para•mag•ne•tism (par″ə-mag′nə-tiz-əm) [*para-* + *magnetism*] the property of being attracted by a magnet and assuming a position parallel to that of a magnetic force without becoming permanently magnetized. **paramagnet′ic** *adj*

para•mas•ti•gote (par″ə-mas′tĭ-gōt) [*para-* + Gr. *mastix* whip] 1. a stage in the life cycle of certain hemoflagellates, in which the kinetoplast is beside the nucleus and the flagellum runs the length of the body before exiting to become free-flowing. 2. having a second, shorter flagellum by the side of a larger one.

para•mas•ti•tis (par″ə-mas-ti′tis) [*para-* + *mastitis*] inflammation of the tissues around the mammary gland.

para•mas•toid (par″ə-mas′toid) near the mastoid process.

para•me•a•tal (par″ə-me-a′təl) near or next to a meatus.

par•a•me•cia (par″ə-me′se-ə) plural of *paramecium*.

Par•a•me•ci•um (par″ə-me′se-əm) [Gr. *paramēkēs* oblong] a genus of ovoid or elongated freshwater protozoa (suborder Peniculina, order Hymenostomatida), some species of which are visible to the naked eye. Certain species have been used as test organisms in cytological, genetic, and other research.

par•a•me•ci•um (par″ə-me′se-əm) pl. *parame′cia*. An organism belonging to the genus *Paramecium*.

para•me•di•an (par″ə-me′de-ən) [*para-* + *median*] near a midline or the median plane.

para•me•di•as•ti•nal (par″ə-me″de-ə-sti′nəl) adjacent to the mediastinum.

para•med•i•cal (par″ə-med′i-kəl) having some connection with or relation to the science or practice of medicine; adjunctive to the practice of medicine in the maintenance or restoration of health and normal functioning. Paramedical workers include physical, occupational, and speech therapists, medical social workers, pharmacists, technicians, and so on.

para•me•nia (par″ə-me′ne-ə) [*para-* + *men-* + *-ia*] dysmenorrhea.

para•me•ni•sci•tis (par″ə-me-nĭ-si′tis) inflammation of the parameniscus.

para•me•nis•cus (par″ə-mə-nis′kəs) the structure or area around the menisci (semilunar fibrocartilages) of the knee.

para•me•si•al (par″ə-me′se-əl) paramedian.

pa•ram•e•ter (pə-ram′ə-tər) [*para-* + *-meter*] 1. a constant in a mathematical expression that distinguishes specific cases, having a definite, fixed value in one case but different values in other cases. For example, in the equation of a straight line, $y = mx + b$, m and b are parameters that specify a particular straight line; changing m changes the slope of the line, while changing b changes the point at which the line crosses the y-axis. 2. in statistics, a value that specifies one of the various members of a family of probability distributions, e.g., the mean or variance of a normal distribution. A parameter is often thought of as the "true value" or "population value" as opposed to the observed value or sample value. 3. a variable whose measure is indicative of a quantity or function that cannot itself be precisely determined by direct methods; e.g., blood pressure and pulse rate are parameters of cardiovascular function, and the level of glucose in blood and urine is a parameter of carbohydrate metabolism.

para•meth•a•sone ac•e•tate (par″ə-meth′ə-sōn) [USP] a glucocorticoid, used chiefly for its antiinflammatory and antiallergic actions; administered orally.

Para•me•tor•chis (par″ə-mə-tor′kis) a genus of trematodes of the family Opisthorchiidae. *P. complex′us* is found in the bile ducts of cats and dogs, sometimes causing jaundice or gastrointestinal disorders.

para•me•tri•al (par″ə-me′tre-əl) 1. pertaining to the parametrium. 2. parametric[1].

para•me•tric[1] (par″ə-me′trik) [*para-* + *metr-* + *-ic*] near the uterus; called also *parametrial*.

para•met•ric[2] (par″ə-met′rik) [*para-* + *metric*] pertaining to or defined in terms of a parameter.

para•me•tri•tis (par″ə-mə-tri′tis) inflammation of the parametrium. **parametri′tic** *adj*

posterior p. inflammation of the cellular tissue around the uterosacral ligaments.

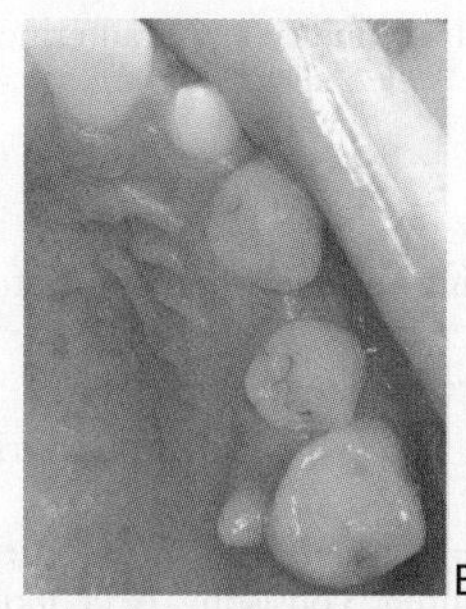

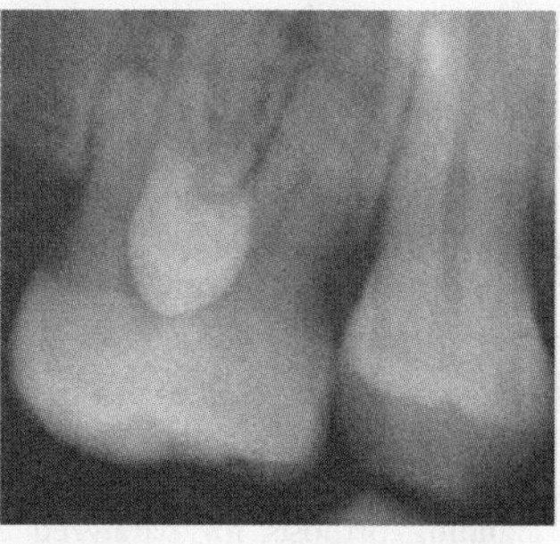

■ Paramolar palatal to a maxillary molar in a patient who also exhibits hypodontia. *(A)*, Clinical appearance; *(B)*, radiograph showing paramolar is rudimentary but fully formed.

para·me·tri·um (par″ə-me′tre-əm) pl. *parame′tria* [*para-* + Gr. *mētra* uterus] [TA] the extension of the subserous coat of the portion of the uterus just above the cervix, out laterally between the layers of the broad ligament.

par·am·ne·sia (par″am-ne′zhə) [*para-* + *amnesia*] a disturbance of memory in which reality and fantasy are confused; cf. *dysmnesia.*

Par·amoe·ba (par″ə-me′bə) [*para-* + *ameba*] a genus of parasitic or free-living ramicristate amebae, protozoa of the order Euamoebida, having both a nucleus and a nucleuslike body; some authorities consider the latter to be a protistan hyperparasite and not a secondary nucleus.

para·mo·lar (par″ə-mo′lər) [*para-* + *molar*] a supernumerary tooth, usually small and rudimentary, sometimes found in the maxilla buccally or lingually to a molar or interproximally between two of the first three molars. Called also *supernumerary molar.*

Par·a·mo·nos·to·mum (par″ə-mo-nos′to-məm) a genus of trematodes. *P. par′vum* infects ducks and chickens in North America.

Par·am·phis·to·ma·ti·dae (par″am-fis″to-mat′ĭ-de) the paramphistomes, a family of parasitic trematodes. Most (such as genera *Calicophoron, Cotylophoron,* and *Paramphistomum*) infest primarily ruminants, but genera *Gastrodiscoides* and *Watsonius* also cause paramphistomiasis in humans.

Par·am·phis·to·ma·toi·dea (par″am-fis-to″mə-toi′de-ə) a superfamily of trematodes that includes the family Paramphistomatidae.

pa·ram·phi·stome (pə-ram′fĭ-stōm) any member of the family Paramphistomatidae, pear-shaped trematodes that have the sucker near the posterior end and infest the intestines of ruminants and occasionally other mammals, causing paramphistomiasis. See also *ruminal fluke.* Called also *amphistome* and *conical fluke.*

par·am·phis·to·mi·a·sis (par″am-fis-to-mi′ə-sis) infestation by intestinal flukes of the family Paramphistomatidae. Most genera are usually found in ruminants; genera *Gastrodiscoides* in Asia and *Watsonius* in Africa may also be found in humans. Adult worms may be present without clinical signs, but immature worms cause more severe manifestations such as enteritis, severe diarrhea, anorexia, and hemorrhaging; heavy infestations can kill cattle and sheep. Called also *amphistomiasis.*

Par·am·phis·to·mum (par″am-fis′to-məm) a genus of trematodes of the family Paramphistomatidae. *P. cer′vi* is found in the rumen and reticulum of ruminants, causing paramphistomiasis.

para·mu·sia (par″ə-mu′ze-ə) [*para-* + Gr. *mousa* music + *-ia*] partial or complete loss of the power of correct musical expression; cf. *amusia.*

par·am·y·loi·do·sis (par-am″ə-loi-do′sis) accumulation of an atypical form of amyloid in tissues.

para·my·oc·lo·nus (par″ə-mi-ok′lə-nəs) [*para-* + *myoclonus*] myoclonus in several unrelated muscles.

p. mul′tiplex term coined by Friedreich to describe a form of myoclonus of unknown etiology starting in the muscles of the upper arms and shoulders and spreading to other parts of the upper body. Called also *Friedreich disease* and *myoclonus multiplex.*

para·myo·to·nia (par″ə-mi″o-to′ne-ə) [*para-* + *myo-* + *ton-* + *-ia*] tonic spasms caused by a disorder of muscular tonicity; cf. *myotonia.*

p. conge′nita an autosomal dominant disorder clinically similar to myotonia congenita, except that the precipitating factor is exposure to cold and the myotonia is aggravated by activity. Like myotonia fluctuans and myotonia permanens and several other disorders, it is due to mutation in the *SCNA4A* gene (locus: 17q23.1-q25.3), which encodes a subunit of a voltage-gated sodium channel. Called also *Eulenburg disease.*

Para·myxo·vi·ri·dae (par″ə-mik″so-vir′ĭ-de) the paramyxoviruses: a family of RNA viruses having a pleomorphic, usually roughly spherical but occasionally filamentous virion 150–300 nm in diameter, consisting of a lipid bilayer membrane with large peplomers surrounding a helical nucleocapsid. The genome consists of a single molecule of negative-sense single-stranded RNA (MW 5–7 × 10^6, size 16 kb). Viruses contain six to ten major polypeptides, including a transcriptase, and are sensitive to lipid solvents, detergents, disinfectants, and extremes of pH; thermostability varies according to genus. Replication occurs in the cytoplasm and assembly is by budding through the plasma membrane. Host range is generally narrow in nature but broad in cultured cells, and transmission is horizontal, chiefly airborne. There are two subfamilies, Paramyxovirinae and Pneumovirinae.

Para·myxo·vi·ri·nae (par″ə-mik″so-vir-i′ne) a subfamily of the family Paramyxoviridae, containing the genera *Avulavirus, Henipavirus, Morbillivirus, Respirovirus,* and *Rubulavirus.*

Para·myxo·vi·rus (par″ə-mik′so-vi″rəs) former name for *Respirovirus.*

para·myxo·vi·rus (par″ə-mik′so-vi″rəs) [*para-* + *myxovirus*] any virus belonging to the family Paramyxoviridae. **paramyxovi′ral** *adj*

avian p. 1 Newcastle disease virus.

par·an·al·ge·sia (par″an-al-je′ze-ə) para-analgesia.

para·na·sal (par″ə-na′zəl) alongside or near the nose.

para·neo·plas·tic (par″ə-ne″o-plas′tik) [*para-* + *neoplastic*] pertaining to changes produced in tissue remote from a tumor or its metastases; see also *paraneoplastic syndrome,* under *syndrome.*

para·neph·ric (par″ə-nef′rik) pertaining to or located in the portion of the retroperitoneum that lies outside the renal fascia; pararenal. Cf *perinephric.*

para·ne·phri·tis (par″ə-nə-fri′tis) [*para-* + *nephritis*] inflammation of the connective tissue around and near the kidney.

para·ne·phro·ma (par″ə-nə-fro′mə) a tumor of the adrenal gland.

par·an·es·the·sia (par″an-es-the′zhə) para-anesthesia.

para·neu·ral (par″ə-noor′əl) [*para-* + *neural*] beside or alongside a nerve.

par·a·noia (par″ə-noi′ah) 1. a term used to describe behavior characterized by well-systematized delusions of persecution, delusions of grandeur, or a combination of the two. There are several disorders in which paranoia may occur: see *delusional disorder, shared psychotic disorder, paranoid personality disorder,* and *paranoid schizophrenia.* 2. former name for the condition now called *delusional disorder.*

par·a·noi·ac (par″ə-noi′ak) paranoid.

par·a·noid (par′ə-noid) 1. pertaining to, characteristic of, or affected with paranoia. 2. a person affected with paranoia.

par·a·no·mia (par″ə-no′me-ə) anomic aphasia.

Para·no·plo·ceph·a·la (par″ə-no″plo-sef′ə-lə) a genus of tapeworms of the family Anoplocephalidae. *P. mamilla′na* infests the stomach and intestines of horses.

para·nor·mal (par″ə-nor′məl) beyond the normal or natural; said of phenomena such as extrasensory perception.

para·nu·cle·ar (par″ə-noo′kle-ər) beside or near a nucleus.

para·op·er·a·tive (par″ə-op′ər-ə-tiv) pertaining to the accessories essential to operative surgery, such as care of instruments and gloves, sterilization, etc.

para·oral (par″ə-or′əl) 1. near or adjacent to the mouth. 2. administered by some route other than by the mouth; said of medication.

par·aor·tic (par″a-or′tik) para-aortic.

para·os·mia (par″ə-os′me-ə) parosmia.

para·ox·on (par″ə-ok′son) the oxygen analog of parathion, of which it is the active metabolite; conversion of parathion to paraoxon occurs primarily in the liver. It also occurs as an environmental degradation product of parathion.

para·ox·o·nase (par″ə-ok′sə-nās) aryldialkylphosphatase.

para·pan·cre·at·ic (par″ə-pan″kre-at′ik) near the pancreas.

para·pa·re·sis (par″ə-pə-re′sis) [*para-* + *paresis*] partial paralysis of the lower limbs.

familial spastic p., hereditary spastic p. see under *paraplegia.*

tropical spastic p. chronic progressive myelopathy.

para·pe·de·sis (par″ə-pə-de′sis) [*para-* + Gr. *pēdēsis* a leaping] passage of body substances into channels not normally conveying them, as of bile pigments into the blood capillaries.

para·peri·to·ne·al (par″ə-per″ĭ-to-ne′əl) near the peritoneum.

para·per·tus·sis (par″ə-pər-tus′is) [*para-* + *pertussis*] an acute respiratory disease clinically indistinguishable from mild or moderate pertussis, caused by *Bordetella parapertussis.* See also *pertussis-like syndrome,* under *syndrome.*

para·pha·ryn·ge·al (par″ə-fə-rin′je-əl) near or beside the pharynx.

para·pha·sia (par″ə-fa′zhə) [*para-* + *-phasia*] a type of dysphasia in which a person uses wrong words or uses words in wrong and senseless combinations; called also *paragrammatism*, *paraphemia*, and *paraphrasia*. **parapha′sic** *adj*

central p. paraphasia due to a brain lesion.

literal p. paralalia literalis.

thematic p. incoherent speech characterized by wandering from the subject.

para·phe·mia (par″ə-fe′me-ə) paraphasia.

para·phen·yl·ene·di·amine (par″ə-fen″əl-ēn-di′ə-mēn) *p*-phenylenediamine.

pa·ra·phia (pə-ra′fe-ə) [*para-* + Gr. *haphē* touch + *-ia*] a disorder of the sense of touch; called also *dysaphia*.

para·phil·ia (par″ə-fil′e-ə) [*para-* + *-philia*] [DSM-IV] a psychosexual disorder characterized by recurrent intense sexual urges, by sexually arousing fantasies, or by behavior involving use of a nonhuman object, the suffering or humiliation of oneself or one's partner, or children or other nonconsenting partners; included are exhibitionism, fetishism, frotteurism, pedophilia, sexual masochism, sexual sadism, transvestic fetishism, and voyeurism.

para·phil·i·ac (par″ə-fil′e-ak) 1. pertaining to paraphilia. 2. an individual exhibiting paraphilia.

para·phi·mo·sis (par″ə-fi-mo′sis) [*para-* + *phimosis*] retraction of phimotic foreskin, causing a painful swelling of the glans; severe cases may cause dry gangrene. See also *phimosis*.

para·pho·nia (par″ə-fo′ne-ə) dysphonia.

para·phra·sia (par″ə-fra′zhə) paraphasia.

para·phre·nia (par″ə-fre′ne-ə) [*para-* + *phren-* + *-ia*] 1. a term which has been used to denote a condition lying midway between paranoia and schizophrenia, in which there are fantastic, absurd, well-systematized delusions without severe personality deterioration. 2. periphrenitis.

para·phren·ic (par″ə-fren′ik) 1. pertaining to or characterized by paraphrenia. 2. an individual exhibiting paraphrenia.

para·phre·ni·tis (par″ə-frə-ni′tis) periphrenitis.

para·phys·e·al (par″ə-fiz′e-əl) paraphysial.

para·phys·i·al (par″ə-fiz′e-əl) pertaining to the paraphysis.

pa·raph·y·sis (pə-raf′ĭ-sis) [Gr. "offshoot"] 1. a thin-walled derivative of the roof plate of the telencephalon, present only temporarily in the human embryo and fetus; called also *paraphysial body*. 2. a sterile thread alongside the spore sac or sexual organs in the hymenial layer of some fungi, especially ascomycetes; also found in mosses and ferns.

para·pin·e·al (par″ə-pin′e-əl) pertaining to the parapineal organ of certain lower vertebrates.

para·plas·tic (par″ə-plas′tik) [*para-* + *plastic*] exhibiting abnormal formative power.

Para·plat·in (par″ə-plat′in) trademark for a preparation of carboplatin.

para·plec·tic (par″ə-plek′tik) [Gr. *paraplēktikos*] paraplegic.

para·ple·gia (par″ə-ple′jə) [*para-* + *-plegia*] paralysis of the lower limbs and lower trunk.

ataxic p. subacute combined degeneration of spinal cord; see under *degeneration*.

Basedow p. muscle weakness accompanying Graves disease, seen most often in the pelvic girdle and thighs, and less often in the upper limbs, around the eyes, or elsewhere.

cerebral p. paraplegia caused by bilateral cerebral lesions.

congenital spastic p. Little disease.

Erb spastic p., Erb syphilitic spastic p. an uncommon form of meningovascular neurosyphilis marked by progressive spasticity and weakness of the legs, paraplegia, muscular atrophy, paresthesia, increased knee and ankle reflexes, and incontinence. Called also *cerebrospinal syphilis*, *Erb paralysis*, *Erb-Charcot disease*, and *syphilitic p.*

familial spastic p. hereditary spastic p.

flaccid p. flaccid paralysis in the lower limbs. Cf. *spastic p.*

hereditary spastic p. any of a group of hereditary disorders consisting of gradually developing paralysis in one, two, or all four limbs, with spasticity. There is degeneration of corticospinal tracts but sensory abnormalities are not present. Called also *hereditary cerebrospinal paralysis*.

infantile spastic p. Little disease.

peripheral p. paraplegia due to a lower motor neuron lesion.

Pott p. paraplegia due to vertebral caries or spinal tuberculosis; called also *Pott paralysis*.

senile p. spastic paraplegia in the elderly, usually caused by transverse lesions of the spinal cord or by anterolateral sclerosis. Called also *tetanoid p.*

spastic p. any of a group of diseases marked by spasticity of the muscles of the paralyzed part and increased tendon reflexes, due to damage to the corticospinal tract. Most varieties are hereditary (see *hereditary spastic p.*), but one variety *(Little disease)* is caused by birth injury or intrauterine conditions. See also *cerebral palsy*, under *palsy*. Called also *spastic diplegia*.

syphilitic p. Erb spastic p.

tetanoid p. senile p.

tropical spastic p. chronic progressive myelopathy.

para·ple·gic (par″ə-ple′jik) 1. pertaining to or of the nature of paraplegia. 2. an individual with paraplegia.

para·ple·gi·form (par″ə-ple′jĭ-form) resembling paraplegia.

para·pneu·mon·ic (par″ə-noo-mon′ik) accompanying or occurring as a complication of pneumonia.

para·po·di·um (pa-rə-po′de-əm) pl. *parapo′dia* [*para-* + Gr. *pous* foot] 1. a standing orthosis for paralyzed children, consisting of a footplate with shoes, bars parallel to the lower limbs, and a padded frame that supports the abdomen and thorax. 2. one of the paired segmented appendages of marine annelids.

par·apoph·y·sis (par″ə-pof′ĭ-sis) [*para-* + *apophysis*] the lower transverse process of a vertebra (processus transversus vertebrae [TA]), or its homologue.

Para·pox·vi·rus (par″ə-poks′vi-rəs) [*para-* + *poxvirus*] a genus of viruses of the subfamily Chordopoxvirinae (family Poxviridae) with serologic cross reactivity, comprising viruses of ungulates, including orf virus, pseudocowpox virus, and bovine papular stomatitis virus.

para·pox·vi·rus (par″ə-poks′vi-rəs) any member of the genus *Parapoxvirus*. **parapoxvi′ral** *adj*

para·prax·ia (par″ə-prak′se-ə) parapraxis.

para·prax·is (par″ə-prak′sis) pl. *paraprax′es* [*para-* + *praxis*] a faulty action, as a slip of the tongue ("freudian slip") or misplacement of an object; attributed by Freud to unconscious motives.

para·proc·ti·tis (par″ə-prok-ti′tis) [*paraproctium* + *-itis*] inflammation of the tissues surrounding the rectum and anus; called also *periproctitis*.

para·proc·ti·um (par″ə-prok′she-əm) [*para-* + Gr. *prōktos* anus] the tissues that surround the rectum and the anus.

para·pro·fes·sion·al (par″ə-pro-fesh′ən-əl) 1. a person who is specially trained in a particular field or occupation to assist a professional such as a physician. 2. allied health professional. 3. pertaining to a paraprofessional.

para·pros·ta·ti·tis (par″ə-pros″tə-ti′tis) periprostatitis.

para·pros·thet·ic (par″ə-pros-thet′ik) adjacent to a prosthesis.

para·pro·tein (par″ə-pro′tēn) M component.

para·pro·tein·emia (par″ə-pro″tēn-e′me-ə) plasma cell dyscrasias.

para·pso·ri·a·sis (par″ə-sə-ri′ə-sis) pl. *parapsori′ases* [*para-* + *psoriasis*] any of a group of slowly evolving erythrodermas, all characterized by scaling, resistance to treatment, and chronicity; it includes the forms of pityriasis lichenoides as well as large plaque and small plaque parapsoriases.

acute p. pityriasis lichenoides et varioliformis acuta.

atrophic p. large plaque p.

chronic p. pityriasis lichenoides chronica.

p. gutta′ta, guttate p. 1. pityriasis lichenoides chronica. 2. small plaque p.

large plaque p. a chronic, asymptomatic to mildly symptomatic eruption consisting of flat, round, red to blue, sometimes large and hardened plaques with superficial scaling; the usual location is on the trunk (especially the hips, buttocks, or female breasts), or the proximal limbs. The retiform type is particularly likely to progress to cutaneous T-cell lymphoma.

p. lichenoi′des retiform p.

p. en plaques see *large plaque p.* and *small plaque p.*

poikilodermatous p. 1. large plaque p. 2. retiform p.

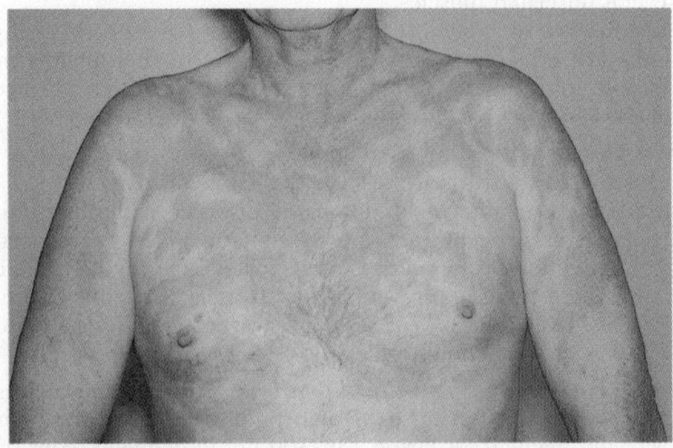

■ Large plaque parapsoriasis.

retiform p. a variant of large plaque parapsoriasis characterized by red to brown, scaly lesions with a netlike distribution, intermixed with deep red plaques, some of which have lichenoid papules. Atrophy and poikiloderma are prominent features of this type, and it is the form most likely to give rise to cutaneous T-cell lymphoma. Called also *p. lichenoides*, *p. variegata*, and *parakeratosis variegata*.

small plaque p. a benign, asymptomatic, chronic eruption consisting of small to moderate sized, red-blue to yellow plaques, found chiefly on the trunk and proximal limbs; plaques have distinct, thin borders and fine, adherent scales, giving the surface a paperlike appearance. Called also *digitate dermatosis*, *p. guttata* and *xanthoerythrodermia perstans*.

p. variega′ta retiform p.

p. variolifor′mis acu′ta pityriasis lichenoides et varioliformis acuta.

p. variolifor′mis chro′nica pityriasis lichenoides chronica.

para•psy•chol•o•gy (par″ə-si-kol′ə-je) [*para-* + *psychology*] the study of psychical effects and experiences which appear to fall outside the scope of physical law, e.g., telepathy and clairvoyance.

para•pul•mo•nary (par″ə-pool′mo-nar-e) near the lung; called also *juxtapulmonary*.

para•pyk•no•mor•phous (par″ə-pik″no-mor′fəs) [*para-* + *pyknomorphous*] neither pyknomorphous nor apyknomorphous, but between the two; staining moderately well. Said of certain nerve cells.

para•py•ram•i•dal (par″ə-pĭ-ram′i-dəl) beside or near a pyramid.

para•quat (par′ə-kwaht) a poisonous dipyridilium compound whose dichloride and dimethylsulfate salts are used as contact herbicides. See *paraquat poisoning*, under *poisoning*.

para•rec•tal (par″ə-rek′təl) beside the rectum.

para•re•flex•ia (par″ə-re-flek′se-ə) dysreflexia.

para•re•nal (par″ə-re′nəl) paranephric.

para•rho•ta•cism (par″ə-ro′tə-siz-əm) rhotacism.

para•ro•san•i•line (par″ə-ro-zan′ĭ-lin) a basic dye occurring as colorless to red crystals, a triphenylmethane derivative; the chief constituent of basic fuchsin (q.v.).

par•ar•rhyth•mia (par″ə-rith′me-ə) parasystole.

para•sa•cral (par″ə-sa′krəl) beside or near the sacrum.

para•sal•pin•ge•al (par″ə-sal-pin′je-əl) beside or in the wall of the uterine tube.

para•sal•pin•gi•tis (par″ə-sal″pin-ji′tis) [*para-* + *salping-* + *-itis*] inflammation of the tissues around a uterine tube.

para•scap•u•lar (par″ə-skap′u-lər) near the scapula.

Par•as•car•is (pər-as′kər-is) a genus of nematodes of the family Ascarididae. *P. equo′rum* is a large parasite that hatches in a horse's intestine and migrates around the body, causing coughing, diarrhea, and other symptoms similar to those of ascariasis.

para•sel•lar (par″ə-sel′ər) near or around the sella turcica.

para•sex•u•al (par″ə-sek′shoo-əl) accomplished by other than sexual means, as by genetic study of in vitro somatic cell hybrids rather than by pedigree studies.

para•sex•u•al•i•ty (par″ə-sek″shoo-al′ĭ-te) abnormal sexuality; usually a paraphilia.

para•sig•ma•tism (par″ə-sig′mə-tiz-əm) sigmatism.

para•si•noi•dal (par″ə-si-noi′dəl) [*para-* + *sino-* + *-oid* + *-al*[1]] situated along the course of a sinus.

para•si•nu•soi•dal (par″ə-si″nə-soi′dəl) sinusoidal (def. 1).

par•a•site (par′ə-sīt) [Gr. *parasitos*] 1. a plant or animal that lives upon or within another living organism at whose expense it obtains some advantage. See *symbiosis*. 2. the smaller, less complete component of asymmetrical conjoined twins, which is attached to and dependent on the autosite.

accidental p. an organism parasitizing an animal other than the usual host, as *Dirofilaria* in humans.

allantoic p. with twins in utero, a weaker twin that takes its blood supply from the stronger through its umbilical circulation.

animal p. any parasite that is a member of the animal kingdom, such as a protozoan, helminth, annelid, or arthropod. Called also *zooparasite*.

coelozoic p. a parasite that lives in a body cavity.

cytozoic p. a parasite that lives in body cells, such as a plasmodium.

diheteroxenic p. a parasite that requires two intermediate hosts.

ectophytic p. a plant ectoparasite.

ectozoic p. an animal ectoparasite.

endophytic p. a plant endoparasite.

entozoic p. a parasite that lives in the lumen of the intestine.

eurytrophic p. an ectoparasite that can feed on various hosts.

facultative p. an organism that may be parasitic upon another but is also capable of independent existence.

hematozoic p. a parasite that lives in the blood.

incidental p. accidental p.

intermittent p. a parasite that lives in its host only part of its life and is free-living at other times. Called also *occasional p.*

karyozoic p. a parasite that lives in cell nuclei.

malarial p. *Plasmodium.*

obligatory p. a parasite that cannot live apart from its host.

occasional p. intermittent p.

periodic p. a parasite that lives in its host for short periods.

permanent p. a parasite that lives in its host from early life until maturity or death of the parasite.

plant p. phytoparasite.

specific p. a parasite that is normal to its current host.

spurious p. an organism that is parasitic on hosts other than humans but may pass through the human body without causing harm.

stenotrophic p. an ectoparasite that can feed on one host only.

temporary p. a parasite that lives free of its host during part of its life cycle.

teratoid p. in asymmetrical conjoined twins, a parasite that appears as a tumorlike mass.

vegetable p. phytoparasite.

par•a•si•te•mia (par″ə-si-te′me-ə) the presence of parasites in the blood, such as malarial parasites or other protozoa.

par•a•sit•ic (par″ə-sit′ik) pertaining to or caused by a parasite.

par•a•sit•i•ci•dal (par″ə-sit″ĭ-si′dəl) antiparasitic (def. 1).

par•a•sit•i•cide (par″ə-sit′ĭ-sīd) [*parasite* + *-cide*] antiparasitic (def. 2).

par•a•sit•ism (par″ə-si′tiz-əm) 1. symbiosis in which one population (or individual) adversely affects the other, but cannot live without it. 2. infection or infestation with parasites.

para•si•tize (par′ah-sĭ-tīz″) to live on or within a host as a parasite.

par•a•si•to•gen•ic (par″ə-si″to-jen′ik) caused by parasites.

par•a•si•toid (par′ə-si″toid) resembling a parasite.

par•a•si•tol•o•gist (par″ə-si-tol′ə-jist) a specialist in parasitology.

par•a•si•tol•o•gy (par″ə-si-tol′ə-je) [*parasite* + *-logy*] the science or study of parasites and parasitism.

par•a•si•to•sis (par″ə-si-to′sis) infection or infestation with parasites.

par•a•si•to•tro•pic (par″ə-si″to-tro′pik) [*parasite* + *-tropic*] having special affinity for parasites.

par•a•si•tot•ro•pism (par″ə-si-tot′rə-piz-əm) parasitotropy.

par•a•si•tot•ro•py (par″ə-si-tot′rə-pe) the affinity of a drug for infective parasites.

para•som•nia (par″ə-som′ne-ə) [*para-* + *somn-* + *-ia*] [DSM-IV] a category of sleep disorders in which abnormal physiological or behavioral events occur during sleep, due to inappropriately timed activation of physiological systems; it includes nightmare disorder, sleep terror disorder, and sleepwalking disorder. Cf. *dyssomnia*.

para•spa•di•as (par″ə-spa′de-əs) [*para-* + Gr. *spadon* a rent] a developmental anomaly in which the urethra opens upon one side of the penis.

para•spe•cif•ic (par″ə-spə-sif′ik) having curative properties in addition to the specific one.

par•a•spi•nal (par″ə-spi′nəl) near the spine; pertaining to a plane along the spine.

para•sple•nic (par″ə-sple′nik) beside the spleen.

para•ster•nal (par″ə-stur′nəl) beside the sternum.

para•sui•cide (par″ə-soo′ĭ-sīd) attempted suicide, emphasizing that in most such attempts death is not the desired outcome.

para•sym•pa•thet•ic (par″ə-sim″pə-thet′ik) of or pertaining to the craniosacral division of the autonomic nervous system; see under *system*.

para•sym•pa•tho•lyt•ic (par″ə-sim″pə-tho-lit′ik) [*parasympathetic* + *-lytic*] 1. producing effects resembling those of interruption of the parasympathetic nerve supply to a part. 2. anticholinergic (def. 2).

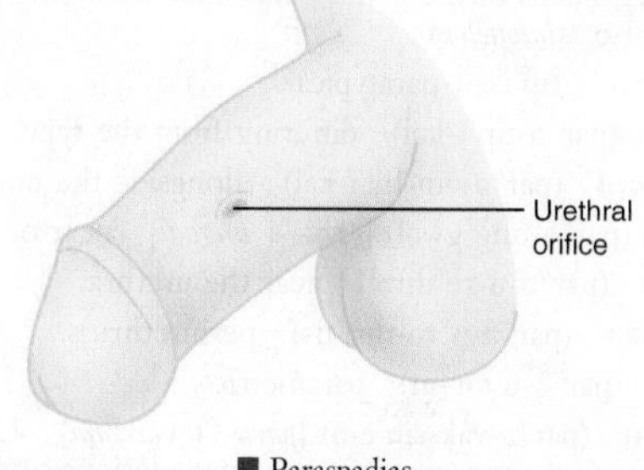

■ Paraspadias.

para·sym·pa·tho·mi·met·ic (par″ə-sim″pə-tho-mĭ-met′ik) [*parasympathetic* + *-mimetic*] 1. producing effects resembling those of stimulation of the parasympathetic nerve supply to a part. 2. cholinergic (def. 2).

para·syno·vi·tis (par″ə-sin″o-vi′tis) [*para-* + *synovitis*] inflammation of the tissues about a synovial sac.

para·sys·to·le (par″ə-sis′tə-le) [*para-* + *systole*] a cardiac irregularity attributed to the interaction of two foci that independently initiate cardiac impulses at different rates; as a rule, one of these foci is the sinoatrial node (the normal pacemaker), and the ectopic focus is usually in the ventricle. Each focus, and thus each rhythm, is protected from the influence of the other.

ventricular p. parasystole in which the ectopic focus is in the ventricle.

para·ten·di·ni·tis (par″ə-ten″dĭ-ni′tis) inflammation of the paratenon, particularly in the knee or ankle.

para·ten·ic (par″ə-ten′ik) denoting an intermediate host, sometimes called transfer host, of a parasite that is not essential to (neither hindering nor hastening) the completion of the parasite's life cycle. See under *host.*

para·ten·on (par″ə-ten′on) [*para-* + Gr. *tenōn* tendon] the fatty areolar tissue filling the interstices of the fascial compartment in which a tendon is situated.

para·thi·on (par″ə-thi′on) an organophosphorus agricultural insecticide that is highly toxic. See *organophosphorus compound poisoning,* under *poisoning.*

para·thor·mone (par″ə-thor′mōn) parathyroid hormone.

para·thy·mia (par″ə-thi′me-ə) [*para-* + *-thymia*] an abnormal, contrary, or inappropriate mood, as seen in schizophrenia.

para·thy·rin (par″ə-thi′rin) parathyroid hormone.

par·a·thy·roid (par″ə-thi′roid) [*para-* + *thyroid*] 1. beside the thyroid gland. 2. *(in the pl.)* parathyroid glands.

para·thy·roid·al (par″ə-thi-roi′dəl) pertaining to the parathyroid glands.

para·thy·roid·ec·to·mize (par″ə-thi″roid-ek′tə-mīz) to excise the parathyroid gland(s).

para·thy·roid·ec·to·my (par″ə-thi″roid-ek′tə-me) [*parathyroid* + *-ectomy*] excision of the parathyroid gland(s).

para·thy·roid·o·ma (par″ə-thi″roid-o′mə) parathyroid adenoma or carcinoma.

para·thy·ro·pri·val (par″ə-thi″ro-pri′vəl) hypoparathyroid.

para·thy·ro·priv·ic (par″ə-thi″ro-priv′ik) hypoparathyroid.

para·thy·ro·tro·phic (par″ə-thi″ro-tro′fik) parathyrotropic.

para·thy·ro·tro·pic (par″ə-thi″ro-tro′pik) having an affinity for or stimulating the growth or hormonal secretion of the parathyroid glands.

para·to·nia (par″ə-to′ne-ə) gegenhalten.

para·tope (par′ə-tōp) [*para-* + *-tope*] an antigen-binding site of an antibody molecule. Cf. *epitope.*

para·tose (par′ə-tōs) an unusual sugar found to be a polysaccharide somatic antigen of *Salmonella* species.

para·tra·cho·ma (par″ə-trə-ko′mə) inclusion conjunctivitis.

para·tro·phic (par″ə-tro′fik) [*para-* + *-trophic*] requiring living material or complex protein matter for food. Cf. *metatrophic.*

para·tu·ber·cu·lo·sis (par″ə-too-bur″ku-lo′sis) 1. a disease resembling tuberculosis but not due to *Mycobacterium tuberculosis.* 2. Johne disease.

para·tu·ber·cu·lous (par″ə-too-bur′ku-ləs) 1. having an indirect relation to tuberculosis. 2. due to conditions produced by tuberculosis. 3. pertaining to paratuberculosis.

para·type (par′ə-tīp) any strain of bacteria, other than the holotype, that is specifically stated to be the one on which the original description of the taxon was based.

para·ty·phoid (par″ə-ti′foid) [*para-* + *typhoid*] 1. see under *fever.* 2. infection due to organisms of the genus *Salmonella* belonging to any serovar but Typhi. See also *salmonellosis.*

para·typ·ic (par″ə-tip′ik) paratypical.

para·typ·i·cal (par″ə-tip′ĭ-kəl) differing from the type.

para·um·bil·i·cal (par″ə-əm-bil′ĭ-kəl) alongside the umbilicus.

para·un·gual (par″ə-ung′gwəl) [*para-* + *ungual*] near or beside a nail.

para·ure·thral (par″ə-u-re′thrəl) near the urethra.

para·ure·thri·tis (par″ə-u″rə-thri′tis) periurethritis.

para·uter·ine (par″ə-u′tər-in) parametric[1].

para·vac·cin·ia (par″ə-vak-sin′e-ə) [*para-* + *vaccinia*] 1. a viral infection of cattle caused by a parapoxvirus, producing lesions similar to those of cowpox and infectious ecthyma on the udders and teats of cows and on the oral mucosa of suckling calves; it begins as small red papules that evolve to vesicles, pustules, and scabbing. It may be transmitted to humans during milking, producing milker's nodules (q.v.); there may then be retransmission to uninfected cows. Called also *pseudocowpox.* 2. milker's nodules.

para·vag·i·nal (par″ə-vaj′ĭ-nəl) beside or next to the vagina.

para·vag·i·ni·tis (par″ə-vaj″ĭ-ni′tis) inflammation of the tissues around the vagina.

para·ve·nous (par″ə-ve′nəs) beside a vein.

para·ver·te·bral (par″ə-vur′tə-brəl) beside the vertebral column.

para·ves·i·cal (par″ə-ves′ĭ-kəl) perivesical.

para·vis·cer·al (par″ə-vis′er-əl) beside a viscus or the visceral branches of the aorta.

par·ax·i·al (par-ak′se-əl) [*para-* + *axial*] situated alongside an axis.

par·ax·on (par-ak′son) [*para-* + *axon*] a collateral branch of an axon.

para·zone (par′ə-zōn) one of the white bands alternating with the dark bands (diazones) in the layers of enamel prisms and seen in cross-section of a tooth.

par·ben·da·zole (par-ben′də-zōl) a veterinary benzimidazole anthelmintic with nematocidal action.

Pa·ré (pah-ra′) Ambroise, 1510–1590. Chief surgeon to three French kings and the greatest surgeon of the 16th century. Paré reformed the treatment of gunshot wounds by abolishing cauterization with boiling oil. He also practiced ligation of arteries after amputation and reintroduced podalic version into obstetrics. His famous aphorism, *Je le pansay, et Dieu le guarit* ("I dressed him and God healed him"), first appeared in 1585, in the fourth edition of his collected works, which he wrote in French to make more accessible.

Par·echo·vi·rus (par-ek′o-vi″rəs) a genus of viruses of the family Picornaviridae; two species, *parechovirus 1* and *parechovirus 2,* infect humans.

par·echo·vi·rus (par-ek′o-vi″rəs) any member of the genus *Parechovirus.* **parechovi′ral** *adj*

p. 1 a species of the genus *Parechovirus,* formerly called *human echovirus* 22, which infects humans but causes few symptoms.

p. 2 a species of the genus *Parechovirus,* formerly called *human echovirus* 23, which infects humans but causes few symptoms.

par·ec·ta·sia (par″ek-ta′zhə) parectasis.

par·ec·ta·sis (par-ek′tə-sis) [*para-* + *ectasis*] excessive stretching or distention of a part or organ.

Par·e·drine (par′ə-drēn) trademark for preparations of hydroxyamphetamine hydrobromide.

par·e·gor·ic (par″ə-gor′ik) [Gr. *parēgorikos* consoling] [USP] a preparation of powdered opium, anise oil, benzoic acid, camphor, diluted alcohol, and glycerin; used as an antiperistaltic, especially in the treatment of diarrhea, and a mild pain reliever; administered orally.

Pa·rel·a·pho·stron·gy·lus (pə-rel″ə-fo-stron′jĭ-lus) a genus of nematodes of the family Protostrongylidae. *P. te′nuis* is normally a harmless parasite of the white-tailed deer, but sometimes it invades the central nervous system of other ruminant species, including sheep and goats, causing fatal neurological disease.

par·en·ce·pha·lia (par″ən-sə-fa′le-ə) [*para-* + *encephal-* + *-ia*] congenital defect of the brain. **parenceph′alous** *adj*

par·en·ceph·a·lo·cele (par″ən-sef′ə-lo-sēl) [*parencephalon* + *-cele*[1]] encephalocele with hernial protrusion of the cerebellum.

pa·ren·chy·ma (pə-reng′kĭ-mə) [Gr. "anything poured in beside"] the essential elements of an organ; in anatomical nomenclature this refers to its functional elements as distinguished from its framework, the stroma. **paren′chymal, parenchym′atous** *adj*

p. pro′statae [TA], **p. of prostate** glandular substance consisting of 30 to 50 small compound tubulosaccular or tubuloalveolar glands, making up the bulk of the prostate; their excretory ducts empty into the prostatic urethra. The parenchyma is surrounded by muscular tissue and permeated by muscular strands.

renal p. the functional tissue of the kidney, consisting of the nephrons.

p. tes′tis [TA], **p. of testis** the functional tissue of the testis, consisting of the seminiferous tubules, Leydig cells, and Sertoli cells.

par·en·chym·a·ti·tis (par″əng-kim″ə-ti′tis) inflammation of a parenchyma.

pa·ren·tal (pə-ren′təl) of, pertaining to, or derived from the parents.

pa·ren·ter·al (pə-ren′tər-əl) [*para-* + *enteral*] not through the alimentary canal, but rather by injection through some other route, such as subcutaneous, intramuscular, intraorbital, intracapsular, intraspinal, intrasternal, or intravenous.

par·epi·did·y·mis (par″ep-ĭ-did′ĭ-mis) paradidymis.

pa•re•sis (pə-re′sis) [Gr. "relaxation"] slight or incomplete paralysis. **paret′ic** *adj*

benign enzootic p. a mild variety of infectious porcine encephalomyelitis.

general p. parenchymatous neurosyphilis in which chronic meningoencephalitis causes gradual loss of cortical function, resulting in progressive dementia and generalized paralysis, which generally occurs 10 to 20 years after the initial infection of syphilis. Called also *Bayle disease, dementia paralytica, paralytic dementia paretic neurosyphilis,* and *syphilitic meningoencephalitis.*

inherited spastic p. a hereditary condition seen in calves during the first year of life, characterized by excessive tonic contractions of the gastrocnemius muscle of first one and later both of the hind legs, with rigidity of the hocks so that the animal is lame and because of lack of exercise fails to gain weight. Called also *Elso heel.*

parturient p. paralysis in a cow near the time of delivery, usually accompanied by hypocalcemia and due to a metabolic disorder. See also *downer cow syndrome,* under *syndrome.* Called also *milk* or *parturient fever.*

par•es•the•sia (par″es-the′zhə) [*para-* + *-esthesia*] an abnormal touch sensation, such as burning, prickling, or formication, often in the absence of an external stimulus. **paresthet′ic** *adj*

Bernhardt p. meralgia paresthetica.

postoperative p. prolonged paresthesia after surgery done with a local anesthetic, especially around the mouth due to injury of the mental nerve or mandibular nerve.

par•fo•cal (pahr-fo′kəl) [L. *par* equal + *focal*] retaining correct focus on changing powers in microscopy.

Par•ham band (pahr′əm) [Frederick William *Parham,* American surgeon, 1856–1927] see under *band.*

par•i•ca (par′ĭ-kə) [Port.] a narcotic snuff prepared from seeds of species of *Piptadenia,* Brazilian trees; the seeds contain dimethyltryptamine and related psychotomimetic indole alkaloids. Called also *cohoba.*

par•i•cal•ci•tol (par″ĭ-kal′sĭ-tol) [USP] a synthetic analogue of vitamin D, used for the prevention and treatment of hyperparathyroidism secondary to chronic renal failure; administered intravenously.

par•i•es (par′e-ēz) pl. *pari′etes* [L.] wall: in anatomy, the structure constituting one side of an organ or body cavity.

p. ante′rior gas′trica [TA] anterior wall of stomach: the part of the stomach wall that is directed toward the anterior surface of the body. Called also *anterior gastric wall* and *anterior stomach wall.*

p. ante′rior vagi′nae [TA] anterior wall of vagina: the wall of the vagina that is intimately associated with the posterior wall of the bladder and urethra.

p. caro′ticus cavita′tis tym′pani [TA] carotid wall of tympanic cavity: the anterior wall of the cavity, related to the carotid canal, in which is lodged the internal carotid artery.

p. exter′nus duc′tus cochlea′ris [TA] external wall of cochlear duct: the part of the ductal wall adjacent to the outer wall of the cochlea.

p. infe′rior or′bitae [TA] inferior wall of orbit: an inner orbital surface formed by surfaces of the maxilla, the zygomatic bone, and the palatine bone; called also *floor of orbit* and *orbital floor.*

p. jugula′ris cavita′tis tym′pani [TA] jugular wall of tympanic cavity: the floor of the tympanic cavity, which is in intimate relation with the jugular fossa, which lodges the bulb of the internal jugular vein.

p. labyrin′thicus cavita′tis tym′pani [TA] labyrinthic wall of tympanic cavity: the wall of the cavity facing medially toward the internal ear; it contains the fenestra vestibuli, the fenestra cochleae, and the promontory. Called also *medial wall of tympanic cavity.*

p. latera′lis or′bitae [TA] lateral wall of orbit: an inner orbital surface formed by the orbital surfaces of the great wing of the sphenoid bone, the zygomatic bone, and the zygomatic process of the frontal bone.

p. mastoi′deus cavita′tis tym′pani [TA] mastoid wall of tympanic cavity: the posterior wall of the cavity, related to the mastoid portion of the temporal bone.

p. media′lis or′bitae [TA] medial wall of orbit: an inner orbital surface formed by parts of the maxillary, lacrimal, ethmoid, and sphenoid bones.

p. membrana′ceus cavita′tis tym′pani [TA] membranous wall of tympanic cavity: the outer wall of the tympanic cavity, formed mainly by the tympanic membrane.

p. membrana′ceus tra′cheae [TA] membranous wall of trachea: the posterior part of the wall of the trachea where the cartilaginous rings are deficient.

p. poste′rior gas′trica [TA] posterior wall of stomach: the part of the stomach wall that is directed toward the posterior surface of the body. Called also *posterior gastric wall* and *posterior stomach wall.*

p. poste′rior vagi′nae [TA] posterior wall of vagina: the vaginal wall intimately associated with the anterior wall of the rectum.

p. supe′rior or′bitae [TA] superior wall of orbit: an inner orbital surface formed chiefly by the orbital plate of the frontal bone and the orbital surface of the lesser wing of the sphenoid bone; called also *roof of orbit.*

p. tegmenta′lis cavita′tis tym′pani [TA] tegmental wall of tympanic cavity: the upper surface of the cavity, formed by part of the petrous portion of the temporal bone. Called also *roof of tympanic cavity* and *roof of tympanum.* See also *tegmen tympani.*

p. tympa′nicus duc′tus cochlea′ris [TA] tympanic wall of cochlear duct: the wall of the cochlear duct that separates it from the scala tympani, composed of the osseous spiral laminae and the basilar membrane. Called also *membrana spiralis ductus cochlearis* [TA alternative] and *spiral membrane of cochlear duct.*

p. vestibula′ris duc′tus cochlea′ris [TA] vestibular wall of cochlear duct: the thin anterior wall of the cochlear duct, which separates it from the scala vestibuli; called also *membrana vestibularis ductus cochlearis* [TA alternative] and *vestibular membrane of cochlear duct.*

pa•ri•e•tal (pə-ri′ə-təl) [L. *parietalis*] 1. of or pertaining to the walls of a cavity. 2. pertaining to or located near the parietal bone, as the parietal lobe.

pa•ri•e•tes (pə-ri′ə-tēz) [L.] plural of *paries.*

pa•ri•e•ti•tis (pə-ri″ə-ti′tis) inflammation of the wall of an organ.

parieto- [L. *paries,* gen. *parietis* wall] a combining form denoting a relation to the parietal bone, the parietal lobe, or a wall of a cavity or organ.

pa•ri•e•to•fron•tal (pə-ri″ə-to-frun′təl) pertaining to the parietal and frontal bones, gyri, or fissures.

pa•ri•e•to•oc•cip•i•tal (pə-ri″ə-to-ok-sip′ĭ-təl) pertaining to the parietal and occipital bones or lobes.

pa•ri•e•to•sphe•noid (pə-ri″ə-to-sfe′noid) pertaining to the parietal and sphenoid bones.

pa•ri•e•to•squa•mo•sal (pə-ri″ə-to-skwah-mo′səl) pertaining to the parietal bone and the squamous portion of the temporal bone.

pa•ri•e•to•tem•po•ral (pə-ri″ə-to-tem′por-əl) pertaining to the parietal and temporal bones or lobes.

pa•ri•e•to•vis•ce•ral (pə-ri″ə-to-vis′ə-rəl) both parietal and visceral; pertaining to the walls of a cavity and the viscera within it.

Pa•ri•naud conjunctivitis, syndrome (pah-re-no′) [Henri *Parinaud,* French ophthalmologist, 1844–1905] see under *syndrome.*

pa•ri pas•su (par′e pas′oo) [L., "at equal pace"] coincidentally with; to the same proportion or degree.

par•i•ty (par′ĭ-te) [L. *parere* to bring forth, produce] para; the condition of a woman with respect to her having borne viable offspring. Cf. *gravidity.*

Park aneurysm (pahrk) [Henry *Park,* English surgeon, 1744–1831] see under *aneurysm.*

Par•ker fluid (pahr′kər) [George Howard *Parker,* American zoologist, 1864–1955] see under *fluid.*

Parkes Web•er syndrome (pahrks-va′bər) [Frederick *Parkes Weber,* English physician, 1863–1962] Sturge-Weber syndrome.

Par•kin•son disease, facies (sign) (pahr′kin-sən) [James *Parkinson,* English physician, 1755–1824] see under *disease* and *facies,* and see also *parkinsonism.*

par•kin•so•ni•an (pahr″kin-so′ne-ən) named for James *Parkinson* or pertaining to parkinsonism.

par•kin•son•ism (pahr′kin-sən-iz″əm) a group of neurological disorders characterized by hypokinesia, tremor, and muscular rigidity. See *Parkinson disease,* under *disease,* and *parkinsonian syndrome,* under *syndrome.*

drug-induced p. a movement disorder seen in reaction to certain medications, such as neuroleptics, tricyclic antidepressants, and calcium channel blockers; characteristics include bradykinesia, masklike facies, tremors, and gait disturbance.

postencephalitic p. parkinsonian syndrome.

Par•lo•del (pahr′lo-del″) trademark for a preparation of bromocriptine mesylate.

Par•nate (pahr′nāt) trademark for a preparation of tranylcypromine sulfate.

par•oc•cip•i•tal (par″ok-sip′ĭ-təl) [*para-* + *occipital*] near the occipital bone.

par•ol•i•vary (par-ol′ĭ-var″e) [*para-* + *olivary*] situated near the olive or olivary nucleus.

par•o•mo•my•cin (par′ə-mo-mi″sin) an aminoglycoside antibiotic derived from *Streptomyces rimosus* var. *paromomycinus,* which is effective against a wide variety of gram-negative, gram-positive, and acid-fast bacteria.

p. sulfate [USP] the sulfate salt of paromomycin, used orally as an antiamebic.

Pa•ro•na space (pah-ro′nah) [Francesco *Parona,* Italian orthopedic surgeon, 1861–1910] see under *space.*

par•onych•ia (par″o-nik′e-ə) [*para-* + *onych-* + *-ia*] inflammation involving the folds of tissue surrounding the nail, with erythema and loss of the cuticle. Called also *perionychia.* See also *onychia.*

Candida **p., candidal p.** paronychia caused by infection with a species of *Candida.*

herpetic p. see under *whitlow.*

par•o•nych•i•al (par″o-nik′e-əl) 1. pertaining to paronychia. 2. pertaining to the nail folds.

par•o•nych•i•um (par″o-nik′e-um) vallum unguis.

par•ooph•o•ri•tis (par″o-of-o-ri′tis) 1. inflammation of the paroöphoron. 2. inflammation of the tissues about the ovary.

par•oöph•o•ron (par″o-of′ə-ron) [*para-* + Gr. *ōon* egg + *pherein* to bear] [TA] an inconstantly present small group of coiled tubules between the layers of the mesosalpinx, being a remnant of the excretory part of the mesonephros. **parooph′oric** *adj*

par•oph•thal•mia (par″of-thal′me-ə) [*para-* + *ophthalmia*] inflammation of the connective tissue around the eye.

par•or•chis (par-or′kis) epididymis.

par•orex•ia (par″o-rek′se-ə) [*para-* + Gr. *orexis* appetite] disordered appetite, with craving for unusual foods; sometimes used synonymously with pica.

par•os•mia (par-oz′me-ə) [*para-* + *osm-*[1] + *-ia*] any disease or perversion of olfaction. Called also *dysosmia* and *paraosmia.* See also *anosmia.*

par•os•te•al (par-os′te-əl) pertaining to the outer surface of the periosteum.

par•os•te•itis (par″os-te-i′tis) [*para-* + *osteitis*] inflammation of the tissues around a bone.

par•os•te•o•sis (par″os-te-o′sis) [*para-* + *osteo-* + *-osis*] ossification of the tissues outside the periosteum.

par•os•ti•tis (par″os-ti′tis) parosteitis.

par•os•to•sis (par″os-to′sis) parosteosis.

pa•rot•ic (pə-rot′ik) parotid (def. 1).

pa•rot•id (pə-rot′id) [*para-* + Gr. *ous* ear] 1. situated or occurring near the ear. 2. pertaining to a parotid gland. 3. glandula parotidea.

pa•rot•i•de•an (pə-rot″ĭ-de′ən) pertaining to the parotid gland.

pa•rot•i•dec•to•my (pə-rot″ĭ-dek′tə-me) [*parotid* + *-ectomy*] excision of the parotid gland.

pa•rot•i•di•tis (pə-rot″ĭ-di′tis) parotitis.

par•o•tin (par′o-tin) an acidic globulin extractable from human parotid gland, which may have some hormonal properties; in rabbits, it promotes mesenchymal growth and calcification of teeth, lowers serum calcium levels, and affects the leukocyte count.

par•oti•tis (par″o-ti′tis) inflammation of the parotid gland; called also *parotiditis.*

bacterial p. infectious parotitis caused by a bacterial infection, most commonly with *Staphylococcus aureus* and less often with *Escherichia coli* or species of *Pseudomonas.*

chronic recurrent p. a rare condition seen in children, characterized by repeated episodes of painful swelling of a parotid gland accompanied by fever; the etiology is unknown.

epidemic p., infectious p. 1. parotitis caused by an infectious agent; see *bacterial p.* and *viral p.* 2. mumps.

postoperative p. infectious, usually suppurative, parotitis following a surgical procedure.

staphylococcal p. the most common type of bacterial parotitis, caused by infection with *Staphylococcus aureus*

suppurative p. bacterial parotitis with suppuration, marked by rapid onset, swelling of the glands, severe pain, and often trismus, low-grade fever, headache, malaise, and leukocytosis. It occurs most often after surgery, in neonates, or in debilitated patients, usually middle-aged or older; patients usually have dehydration and suppression of salivary secretion, and sometimes have been breathing through the mouth or vomiting.

viral p. infectious parotitis caused by a virus; the most common condition is mumps, and less common illnesses are caused by influenza viruses or parainfluenza viruses.

par•ous (par′əs) [L. *parere* to bring forth, produce] having borne one or more viable offspring.

-parous [L. *parere* to bring forth, produce] word termination meaning producing.

par•ovar•i•an (par″o-var′e-ən) 1. situated beside the ovary. 2. pertaining to the parovarium (epoöphoron).

par•ovar•i•ot•o•my (par″o-var″e-ot′ə-me) [*parovarium* + *-tomy*] incision into the parovarium.

par•ova•ri•tis (par″o-və-ri′tis) inflammation of the epoöphoron (parovarium).

par•ova•ri•um (par″o-var′e-əm) [*para-* + *ovarium*] epoöphoron.

par•ox•e•tine hy•dro•chlo•ride (pə-rok′sə-tēn) [USP] a selective serotonin reuptake inhibitor used to treat depressive, obsessive-compulsive, panic, and social anxiety disorders; administered orally.

par•ox•ysm (par′ok-siz-əm) [Gr. *paroxysmos*] 1. a sudden recurrence or intensification of symptoms. 2. a spasm or seizure.

par•ox•ys•mal (par″ok-siz′məl) recurring in paroxysms.

Par•rot atrophy of newborn, pseudoparalysis, etc. (pah-ro′) [Joseph Marie Jules *Parrot*, French physician, 1829–1883] see under *pseudoparalysis* and *sign*, see *marasmus*, and see *ciliospinal reflex*, under *reflex.*

Par•ry disease (par′e) [Caleb Hillier *Parry*, English physician, 1755–1822] toxic nodular goiter.

Par•ry-Rom•berg syndrome (par′e rom′berg) [C.H. *Parry;* Moritz Heinrich *Romberg*, German physician, 1795–1873] facial hemiatrophy.

pars (pahrz) pl. *par′tes* [L. "a portion, piece, share"] part: a particular division or portion of a larger area, organ, or structure.

Pars

Descriptions are given on TA terms, and include anglicized names of specific parts.

p. abdomina′lis aor′tae [TA] abdominal part of aorta: the distal part of the descending aorta, which is the continuation of the thoracic part and gives rise to the inferior phrenic, lumbar, median sacral, superior and inferior mesenteric, middle suprarenal, renal, and testicular or ovarian arteries, and celiac trunk. Called *abdominal aorta* and *aorta abdominalis* [TA alternative].

p. abdomina′lis duc′tus thora′cici [TA] the abdominal part of the thoracic duct; see *ductus thoracicus.*

p. abdomina′lis mus′culi pectora′lis majo′ris [TA] abdominal part of pectoralis major muscle: the portion of the muscle that originates from the aponeurosis of the obliquus externus abdominis.

p. abdomina′lis oeso′phagi [TA] abdominal part of esophagus: the part of the esophagus below the diaphragm, joining the stomach. Called also *abdominal esophagus.*

p. abdomina′lis ure′teris [TA] abdominal part of ureter: that portion of the ureter extending from the kidney to the terminal line of the pelvis.

p. acromia′lis mus′culi deltoi′dei [TA] acromial part of deltoid: the multipennate middle part of the deltoid muscle, arising from the acromion and aiding in abduction of the arm.

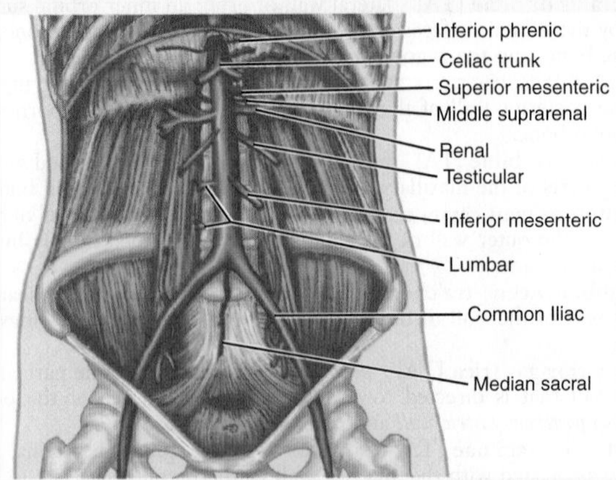

■ Pars abdominalis aortae (abdominal aorta) and its branches.

Pars *Continued*

p. ala′ris mus′culi nasa′lis [TA] alar part of nasalis muscle: the part of the nasalis muscle arising from the maxilla on either side above the lateral incisor tooth and attaching to the alar cartilage of the nose; it assists in opening the nasal aperture. Called also *dilator muscle of naris* and *dilator naris.*

p. alveola′ris mandi′bulae [TA] alveolar part of mandible: the superior portion of the body of the mandible, which contains sockets for the teeth.

p. ante′rior commissu′rae anterio′ris [TA] anterior part of anterior commissure: the smaller anterior part of the commissure, whose fibers interconnect the two olfactory bulbs.

p. ante′rior cul′minis [TA] the anterior part (IV) of the culmen of the cerebellum; it is divided from the posterior part by the intraculminate fissure. Called also *p. ventralis culminis* [TA alternative] and *ventral part of culmen.*

p. ante′rior dor′si lin′guae [TA] anterior part of dorsum of tongue: the part of the dorsum of the tongue anterior to the terminal sulcus. Called also *p. presulcalis dorsi linguae* [TA alternative].

p. ante′rior facie′i diaphragma′ticae he′patis [TA] anterior part of diaphragmatic surface of liver: the part directed toward the anterior surface of the body.

p. ante′rior for′nicis vagi′nae [TA] the anterior part of the fornix of the vagina; called also *anterior fornix.*

p. ante′rior lo′buli centra′lis cerebel′li [TA] the anterior part of the central lobule of the cerebellum (II); called also *p. ventralis lobuli centralis cerebelli* [TA alternative] and *ventral part of central lobule of cerebellum.*

p. ante′rior lo′buli quadrangula′ris anterio′ris [TA] anterior part of anterior quadrangular lobule (HIV): the anterior division of the lobulus quadrangularis anterior cerebelli. Called also *p. ventralis lobuli quadrangularis anterioris* [TA alternative] and *ventral part of anterior quadrangular lobule.*

p. anula′ris vagi′nae fibro′sae digito′rum ma′nus [TA] annular part of fibrous sheaths of fingers: strong transverse bands of fibrous tissue, one in the vagina fibrosa of each finger, crossing the flexor tendons at the level of the upper half of the proximal phalanx.

p. anula′ris vagi′nae fibro′sae digito′rum pe′dis [TA] annular part of fibrous sheaths of toes: fibrous bands in the toes resembling those of similar name in the fingers.

p. aryepiglot′tica mus′culi arytenoi′dei obliq′ui [TA] aryepiglottic part of oblique arytenoid muscle: an inconstant fascicle of the oblique arytenoid muscle, originating from the apex of the arytenoid cartilage and inserting on the lateral margin of the epiglottis. Called also *aryepiglottic muscle* and *musculus aryepiglotticus.*

p. ascen′dens aor′tae [TA] ascending part of aorta: the proximal portion of the aorta, arising from the left ventricle, and giving origin to the right and left coronary arteries before continuing as the arch of the aorta. Called also *aorta ascendens* [TA alternative] and *ascending aorta.*

p. ascen′dens duode′ni [TA] ascending part of duodenum: the terminal part of the duodenum, which goes upwards to end at the duodenojejunal flexure.

p. atlan′tica arte′riae vertebra′lis [TA] atlantic part of vertebral artery: the third part of the artery, which winds behind the lateral mass of the atlas to lie in a groove on the upper surface of the posterior arch of the atlas.

p. autono′mica syste′matis nervo′si periphe′rici TA alternative for *divisio autonomica systematis nervosi peripherici;* see *autonomic nervous system,* under *system.*

p. basa′lis arte′riae pulmona′lis dex′trae [TA] basal part of right pulmonary artery: the part of the pulmonary artery supplying the basal segments of the inferior lobe of the right lung, comprising the anterior, lateral, medial, and basal segmental arteries.

p. basa′lis arte′riae pulmona′lis sinis′trae [TA] basal part of left pulmonary artery: the part of the pulmonary artery supplying the basal segments of the inferior lobe of the left lung, comprising the anterior, lateral, medial, and basal segmental arteries.

p. basila′ris os′sis occipita′lis [TA] basilar part of occipital bone: a quadrilateral plate of the occipital bone that projects superiorly and anteriorly from the foramen magnum.

p. basila′ris pon′tis [TA] basilar part of pons: the part of the pons connecting the cerebrum, cerebellum, and medulla oblongata. It is a broad transverse band that arches across the anterior surface of the superior end of the rhombencephalon; on each side it narrows to enter the cerebellum as the middle cerebellar peduncle. It comprises longitudinal fibers originating at the cerebral cortex, transverse fibers, and the pontine nuclei.

p. buccopharyn′gea mus′culi constricto′ris pharyn′gis supe-rio′ris [TA] buccopharyngeal part of superior constrictor muscle of pharynx: the part of the superior constrictor muscle arising from the pterygomandibular raphe; called also *buccopharyngeal muscle* and *musculus buccopharyngeus.*

p. calcaneocuboi′dea ligamen′ti bifurca′ti calcaneocuboid part of bifurcate ligament: former name for the ligamentum calcaneocuboideum.

p. calcaneonavicula′ris ligamen′ti bifurca′ti calcaneonavicular part of bifurcate ligament: former name for the ligamentum calcaneonaviculare.

p. cana′lis ner′vi op′tici [TA] intracanalicular part of optic nerve: the part of the nerve that runs through the optic canal.

p. cardi′aca gas′trica TA alternative for *cardia.*

p. cartilagi′nea sep′ti na′si [TA] cartilaginous part of nasal septum: the plate of cartilage forming the anterior part of the nasal septum.

p. cartilagi′nea syste′matis skeleta′lis [TA] cartilaginous part of skeletal system: the cartilages of the body.

p. cartilagi′nea tu′bae auditi′vae [TA] cartilaginous part of auditory tube: the part of the tube that is chiefly supported by the tubal cartilage, extending from the pars ossea to the pharyngeal orifice of the auditory tube.

p. caverno′sa arte′riae caro′tidis inter′nae [TA] cavernous part of internal carotid artery: the part located in the cavernous sinus; it has numerous branches, including tentorial basal, tentorial marginal, meningeal, and cavernous branches, branches to trigeminal ganglion, and the inferior hypophysial artery.

p. centra′lis syste′matis nervo′si [TA] the central nervous system, consisting of the brain and spinal cord. Called also *systema nervosum centrale* [TA alternative].

p. centra′lis ventri′culi latera′lis [TA] central part of lateral ventricle: the part of the lateral ventricle found within the parietal lobe; it communicates with the frontal, occipital, and temporal horns. Called also *body of lateral ventricle.*

p. ceratopharyn′gea mus′culi constricto′ris pharyn′gis me′dii [TA] ceratopharyngeal part of middle constrictor muscle of pharynx: the part of the middle constrictor muscle arising from the greater cornu of the hyoid bone; called also *musculus ceratopharyngeus* and *ceratopharyngeal muscle.*

p. cerebra′lis arte′riae caro′tidis inter′nae [TA] cerebral part of internal carotid artery: the terminal part of the artery, which gives off branches comprising the ophthalmic, superior hypophysial, posterior communicating, anterior choroidal, and uncal arteries, and clival and meningeal branches, and then divides into the anterior and middle cerebral arteries in the middle cranial fossa.

p. cervica′lis arte′riae caro′tidis inter′nae [TA] cervical part of internal carotid artery: an unbranched part located in the carotid triangle of the neck.

p. cervica′lis arte′riae vertebra′lis TA alternative for *p. transversaria arteriae vertebralis.*

p. cervica′lis duc′tus thora′cici [TA] the cervical part of the thoracic duct; see *ductus thoracicus.*

p. cervica′lis medul′lae spina′lis [TA] cervical part of spinal cord: the part of the cord that is within the cervical part of the vertebral canal and gives rise to the eight pairs of cervical spinal nerves *(segmenta cervicalia medullae spinalis [1–8]).*

p. cervica′lis oeso′phagi [TA] cervical part of esophagus: the part of the esophagus located in the cervical region, posterior to the trachea and the recurrent laryngeal nerves, anterior to the longus colli muscle and vertebral column, and medial to the lobes of the thyroid gland and the common carotid arteries. Called also *cervical esophagus* and *p. colli oesophagi* [TA alternative].

p. cervica′lis tra′cheae [TA] the part of the trachea located in the cervical region, related anteriorly to the jugular venous arch, sternohyoid and sternothyroid muscles, isthmus of thyroid gland, inferior thyroid veins, thymus, arteria thyroidea ima, posteriorly to the esophagus and recurrent laryngeal nerves, and laterally to the lobes of the thyroid gland and common carotid arteries.

p. chondropharyn′gea mus′culi constricto′ris pharyn′gis me′dii [TA] chondropharyngeal part of middle constrictor muscle of pharynx: the part of the middle constrictor muscle arising from the lesser cornu of the hyoid bone; called also *chondropharyngeal muscle* and *musculus chondropharyngeus.*

p. cilia′ris re′tinae [TA] ciliary part of retina: the two layers of epithelium lining the basal lamina of the ciliary body.

p. clavicula′ris mus′culi deltoi′dei [TA] clavicular part of deltoid muscle: the anterior unipennate portion of the deltoid muscle, originating on the clavicle and assisting pectoralis major in drawing the arm forward and rotating it medially.

p. clavicula′ris mus′culi pectora′lis majo′ris [TA] clavicular part of pectoralis major muscle: the portion of the muscle that originates from the clavicle.

p. coccy′gea medul′lae spina′lis [TA] coccygeal part of spinal cord: the part of the spinal cord that gives rise to the coccygeal spinal nerves *(segmenta coccygea medullae spinalis [1–3]).*

p. coeliacoduodena′lis mus′culi suspenso′rii duode′ni [TA] celiacoduodenal part of suspensory muscle of duodenum: a band of smooth muscle that passes from the terminal duodenum to join the phrenicoceliac part (pars phrenicocoeliaca) and end in connective tissue that attaches to the celiac trunk.

p. col′li oeso′phagi TA alternative for *p. cervicalis oesophagi.*

p. compac′ta substan′tiae ni′grae [TA] compact part of substantia nigra: the posterior part of the substantia nigra, composed of medium-sized cells, many of which are pigmented.

p. convolu′ta lo′buli cortica′lis re′nis convoluted part of cortical lobule of kidney: the part of the renal cortex that surrounds the intracortical prolongations of the pyramids and is composed of convoluted tubules.

p. copula′ris lo′buli paramedia′ni TA alternative for *p. lateralis lobuli biventralis cerebelli.*

p. corneosclera′lis reti′culi trabecula′ris [TA] corneoscleral part of trabecular reticulum: the anterior part of the trabecular reticulum, situated between the venous sinus of the sclera, the scleral spur, and the posterior limiting lamina of the cornea.

par′tes corpo′ris huma′ni [TA] the parts of the human body; a category in official anatomical terminology.

p. costa′lis diaphrag′matis [TA] costal part of diaphragm: the part of the thoracic diaphragm arising from the inner surfaces of the ribs and their cartilages.

p. crania′lis par′tis parasympa′thicae divisio′nis autono′micae syste′matis nervo′si [TA] cranial part of parasympathetic part of autonomic nervous system: the part of the parasympathetic nervous system that includes cranial nerves III, VII, IX, and X and the ciliary, pterygopalatine, otic, submandibular, and sublingual ganglia.

p. cricopharyn′gea mus′culi constricto′ris pharyn′gis inferio′ris [TA] cricopharyngeal part of inferior constrictor muscle of pharynx: the part of the inferior constrictor muscle arising from the cricoid cartilage; called also *cricopharyngeal muscle* or *sphincter* and *musculus cricopharyngeus* [TA alternative].

p. crucifor′mis vagi′nae fibro′sae digito′rum ma′nus [TA] cruciate or cruciform part of fibrous sheaths of fingers: one of the diagonal bundles of the fascia of the fingers that cross each other on the dorsal surface of each digit at the level of the distal end of the proximal phalanx; called also *ligamenta cruciata digitorum manus* and *cruciate ligaments of fingers.*

p. crucifor′mis vagi′nae fibro′sae digito′rum pe′dis [TA] cruciate or cruciform part of fibrous sheaths of toes: one of the bundles of fascial fibers in the toes resembling those of similar name in the fingers; called also *ligamenta cruciata digitorum pedis* and *cruciate ligaments of toes.*

p. cuneifor′mis vo′meris [TA] the wedge-shaped anterior part of the vomer.

p. cupula′ris reces′sus epitympa′nici [TA] cupular space: the part of the epitympanic recess above the head of the malleus.

p. descen′dens aor′tae [TA] the continuation of the aorta from the arch of the aorta, in the thorax, to the point of its division into the common iliac arteries, in the abdomen; divided anatomically into a thoracic part *(pars thoracica aortae)* and an abdominal part *(pars abdominalis aortae).* Called also *aorta descendens* [TA alternative] and *descending aorta.*

p. descen′dens duode′ni [TA] descending part of duodenum: the part between the superior and inferior parts, into which the bile and pancreatic ducts open.

p. dex′tra facie′i diaphragma′ticae he′patis [TA] right part of diaphragmatic surface of liver: the portion that is directed toward the right side of the body, near the ribs on that side.

p. dista′lis adenohypophy′seos [TA] distal part of adenohypophysis: the part that makes up the main body of the gland.

p. dista′lis par′tis prosta′ticae ure′thrae masculi′nae [TA] distal part of prostatic urethra: the portion of the prostatic urethra between the seminal colliculus and where it becomes the intermediate part.

p. dorsa′lis ala′ris lo′buli centra′lis cerebel′li TA alternative for *p. superior alaris lobuli centralis cerebelli.*

p. dorsa′lis cul′minis TA alternative for *p. posterior culminis.*

p. dorsa′lis lo′buli centra′lis cerebel′li TA alternative for *p. posterior lobuli centralis cerebelli.*

p. dorsa′lis lo′buli quadrangula′ris anterio′ris TA alternative for *pars posterior lobuli quadrangularis anterioris.*

p. dura′lis fi′li termina′lis [TA] dural part of filum terminale: the downward prolongation of the spinal dura mater from the lower end of the dural sac, about the level of the second sacral vertebra, to the first coccygeal vertebral segment. Called also *filum terminale externum.*

p. extraocula′ris arte′riae centra′lis re′tinae [TA] extraocular part of central retinal artery: the portion of the artery outside the eyeball, coursing within the dural sheath along with the optic nerve, then piercing the nerve approximately 1.2 cm behind the eyeball, and traveling forward within the center of the nerve to the retina.

p. extraocula′ris ve′nae centra′lis re′tinae [TA] extraocular part of central retinal vein: the short part of the vein outside the eyeball to its junction with the cavernous sinus or superior ophthalmic vein.

p. fibro′sa the dense fibrillar region of nucleolus, where transcription of the ribosomal RNA genes occurs.

p. flac′cida membra′nae tympa′nicae [TA] a small, lax and thin portion of the tympanic membrane between the anterior and posterior malleolar folds. Called also *membrana flaccida* and *Rivinus* or *Shrapnell membrane.*

p. funicula′ris duc′tus deferen′tis [TA] funicular part of ductus deferens: a middle part of the ductus deferens, where it is within the spermatic cord.

p. granulo′sa the granular region of the nucleolus, where ribosomal subunit assembly occurs.

p. glossopharyn′gea mus′culi constricto′ris pharyn′gis superio′ris [TA] glossopharyngeal part of superior constrictor muscle of pharynx: the part of the superior constrictor muscle arising from the side of the root of the tongue. Called also *glossopharyngeal muscle* and *musculus glossopharyngeus.*

p. he′patis dex′tra [TA] right part of liver: the part that receives blood from the right branches of the hepatic portal vein and hepatic artery proper and whose bile flows out through the right hepatic duct. Called also *right liver.*

p. he′patis sinis′tra [TA] left part of liver: the part that receives blood from the left branches of the hepatic portal vein and hepatic artery proper and whose bile flows out through the left hepatic duct. Called also *left liver.*

p. horizonta′lis arte′riae ce′rebri me′diae TA alternative for *p. sphenoidalis arteriae cerebri mediae.*

p. horizonta′lis duode′ni [TA] horizontal part of duodenum: the third, more horizontal or transverse, part of the duodenum, located between the descending and ascending parts, crossing from right to left anterior to the third lumbar vertebra. Called also *p. inferior duodeni* [TA alternative] and *inferior* or *transverse part of duodenum.*

p. ili′aca fas′ciae iliopso′as [TA] ciliac part of iliopsoas fascia: the part of the fascia that invests the iliacus muscle.

p. infe′rior ala′ris lo′buli centra′lis cerebel′li [TA] the inferior part of the wing of the central lobule of the cerebellum (HII); called also *p. ventralis alaris lobuli centralis cerebelli* [TA alternative] and *ventral part of wing of central lobule of cerebellum.*

p. infe′rior duode′ni TA alternative for *p. horizontalis duodeni.*

p. infe′rior ner′vi vestibula′ris [TA] inferior part of vestibular nerve: the inferior branch of the nerve, which has filaments that end in the ampullary crest of the posterior semicircular ducts and the macula of the saccule.

p. infe′rior ve′nae lingula′ris [TA] inferior part of lingular vein: a venous branch that drains the inferior lingular segment of the left lung and drains into the lingular vein. Called also *inferior lingular segmental vein.*

p. infraclavicula′ris plex′us brachia′lis [TA] infraclavicular part of brachial plexus: the part of the brachial plexus that lies in the axilla, below the level of the clavicle. In it arise the medial and lateral pectoral, musculocutaneous, medial brachial cutaneous, medial antebrachial cutaneous, median, ulnar, radial, subscapular, thoracodorsal, and axillary nerves.

p. infraloba′ris ve′nae posterio′ris [TA] infralobar part of posterior vein: a tributary to the posterior branch of the right superior pulmonary vein; called also *infralobar vein.*

p. inguina′lis duc′tus deferen′tis [TA] inguinal part of ductus deferens: a middle part of the ductus deferens, where it is within the inguinal canal.

p. insula′ris arte′riae ce′rebri me′diae [TA] insular part of middle cerebral artery: collectively, the segment of the middle cerebral artery and the branches from it that supply the insula and adjacent areas (M2 segment); the branches comprise the arteriae insulares. See also *segments of middle cerebral artery,* under *segment.*

p. intercartilagi′nea ri′mae glot′tidis [TA] the part of the rima glottidis between the arytenoid cartilages; called also *intercartilaginous glottis, respiratory glottis,* and *interarytenoid space.*

p. interme′dia adenohypophy′seos [TA] intermediate part of adenohypophysis: an ill-defined region between the two lobes of the hypophysis; some systems of nomenclature consider it part of the neurohypophysis. In humans a defined structure develops during embryogenesis, but only scattered cells are retained when the gland matures.

p. interme′dia ure′thrae masculi′nae [TA] intermediate part of male urethra: a short portion of the urethra between the pars prostatica and the pars spongiosa, traversing the deep perineal space. Called also *membranous urethra, membranous part of male urethra* and *p. membranacea urethrae masculinae* [TA alternative].

p. intermembrana′cea ri′mae glot′tidis [TA] the part of the rima glottidis between the vocal folds. Called also *glottis vocalis.*

p. intersegmenta′lis [TA] intersegmental part: any of the veins lying between and draining adjacent bronchopulmonary segments and supplying a main branch of a right or left pulmonary vein; called also *infrasegmental* or *intersegmental vein.*

p. intracrania′lis arte′riae vertebra′lis [TA] intracranial part of vertebral artery: the fourth part of the artery; it pierces the dura and arachnoid mater and ascends anterior to the hypoglossal roots and then medially in front of the medulla oblongata where, at about the lower border of the pons, it joins the opposite artery to form the basilar artery.

p. intracrania′lis ner′vi op′tici [TA] intracranial part of optic nerve: the part of the nerve that lies between the optic canal and the optic chiasm.

p. intralamina′ris ner′vi op′tici intraocula′ris [TA] intralaminar part of intraocular optic nerve: the portion of the intraocular part of the optic nerve that runs through the lamina cribrosa of the sclera.

p. intraloba′ris ve′nae posterio′ris [TA] intralobar part of posterior vein: a tributary of the posterior branch of the right superior pulmonary vein; called also *intersegmental vein.*

p. intramura′lis ure′teris [TA] intramural part of ureter: the short distal portion of the ureter after it bends to run obliquely through the wall of the bladder.

p. intramura′lis ure′thrae masculi′nae [TA] intramural part of male urethra: the short, most proximal, part of the urethra, running almost vertically down from the bladder to where it enters the prostate. Called also *p. preprostatica urethrae masculinae* [TA alternative].

p. intraocula′ris arte′riae centra′lis re′tinae [TA] intraocular part of central retinal artery: the portion of the artery within the eyeball.

p. intraocula′ris ner′vi op′tici [TA] intraocular part of optic nerve: the part of the nerve that is within the eyeball, separated into postlaminar, intralaminar, and prelaminar parts (see *p. postlaminaris nervi optici, p. intralaminaris nervi optici,* and *p. prelaminaris nervi optici*).

p. intraocula′ris ve′nae centra′lis re′tinae [TA] intraocular part of central retinal vein: the portion of the vein that is within the eyeball.

p. intrasegmenta′lis [TA] intrasegmental part: any of the small veins lying within a bronchopulmonary segment and draining into one of the main branches of a right or left pulmonary vein.

p. iri′dica re′tinae [TA] iridial part of retina: the two layers of pigmented epithelium lining the posterior part of the iris.

p. labia′lis mus′culi orbicula′ris o′ris [TA] labial part of orbicularis oris muscle: the part of the muscle whose fibers are restricted to the lips.

p. laryn′gea pharyn′gis [TA] laryngopharynx: the portion of the pharynx that lies below the upper edge of the epiglottis and opens into the larynx and esophagus.

p. latera′lis ar′cus pe′dis longitudina′lis [TA] lateral part of longitudinal arch of foot: the part of the arch formed by the calcaneus, the cuboid bone, and the lateral two metatarsal bones. Called also *lateral longitudinal arch of foot.*

p. latera′lis for′nicis vagi′nae [TA] the lateral part of the fornix of the vagina; called also *lateral fornix.*

p. latera′lis glo′bi pal′lidi media′lis [TA] lateral part of globus pallidus medial segment: the more lateral, or outer, of the two parts into which the medial segment of the globus pallidus is subdivided by the accessory medullary lamina.

p. latera′lis lo′buli biventra′lis cerebel′li [TA] the more lateral part of the biventral lobule of the cerebellum (HVIIIA), separated from the medial part by the intrabiventral fissure and from the lobulus gracilis by the prebiventral fissure. Called also *p. copularis lobuli paramediani* [TA alternative].

p. latera′lis os′sis occipita′lis [TA] lateral part of occipital bone: one of the paired parts of the occipital bone that form the lateral boundaries of the foramen magnum, each being prominently characterized by the presence of one of the occipital condyles.

p. latera′lis os′sis sa′cri [TA] lateral part of sacrum: the part or mass of the sacrum on either side lateral to the dorsal and pelvic sacral foramina; called also *lateral mass of sacrum.*

p. latera′lis ve′nae lo′bi me′dii [TA] lateral part of middle lobe vein: a venous branch draining the lateral segment of the middle lobe of the right lung, emptying into the middle lobe vein. Called also *lateral segmental vein.*

p. li′bera mem′bri inferio′ris [TA] the bones of the thigh, leg, and foot. Called also *skeleton membri inferioris liberi.*

p. li′bera mem′bri superio′ris [TA] the bones of the arm, forearm, and hand. Called also *skeleton membri superioris liberi.*

p. lumba′lis diaphrag′matis [TA] lumbar part of diaphragm: the portion of the thoracic diaphragm that arises from the lumbar vertebrae, comprising the right and left diaphragmatic crura, the right crus arising from the superior three or four vertebrae, and the left from the superior two or three.

p. lumba′lis medul′lae spina′lis [TA], **p. lumba′ris medul′lae spina′lis** lumbar part of spinal cord: the part of the cord that is within the lower thoracic part of the vertebral canal (in adults) and gives rise to the five pairs of lumbar spinal nerves *(segmenta lumbalia medullae spinalis [1–5]).*

p. lumba′lis mus′culi iliocosta′lis lumbo′rum [TA] lumbar part of iliocostalis lumborum: *origin,* iliac crest; *insertion,* angles of lower six or seven ribs; *innervation,* branches of thoracic and lumbar; *action,* extends lumbar spine. Called also *divisio lateralis musculi erectoris spinae lumborum* [TA alternative].

p. lumba′lis mus′culi longis′simus tho′racis [TA] lumbar part of longissimus thoracis: the portion of the longissimus thoracis occurring specifically in the lumbar region; see *musculus longissimus thoracis.* Called also *divisio medialis musculi erectoris spinae lumborum* [TA alternative].

p. magnocellula′ris nu′clei ru′bri [TA] magnocellular part of red nucleus: in humans, the posterior part of the red nucleus, containing a complement of large multipolar cells; the number of these cells is relatively decreased in comparison to the small cells scattered throughout the nucleus; cf. *p. parvocellularis nuclei rubri.*

p. margina′lis mus′culi orbicula′ris o′ris [TA] marginal part of orbicularis oris muscle: the part of the muscle whose fibers blend with those of adjacent muscles.

p. media′lis ar′cus pe′dis longitudina′lis [TA] medial part of longitudinal arch of foot: the part of the longitudinal arch formed by the calcaneus, talus, navicular, cuneiform, and the first three metatarsal bones. Called also *medial longitudinal arch of foot.*

p. media′lis glo′bi pal′lidi media′lis [TA] medial part of globus pallidus medial segment: the more medial, or inner, of the two parts into which the medial segment of the globus pallidus is subdivided by the accessory medullary lamina.

p. media′lis lo′buli biventra′lis cerebel′li [TA] the more medial part of the biventral lobule of the cerebellum (HVIIIB), separated from the lateral part by the intrabiventral fissure and from the tonsilla by the secondary fissure. Called also *lobulus parafloccularis dorsalis* [TA alternative] and *dorsal paraflocculus.*

p. media′lis ve′nae lo′bi me′dii [TA] medial part of middle lobe vein: a venous branch draining the medial segment of the middle lobe of the right lung, emptying into the middle lobe vein. Called also *medial segmental vein.*

Pars *Continued*

p. membrana′cea sep′ti interventricula′ris [TA] membranous part of interventricular septum: the very small, completely membranous area of the interventricular septum of the heart; situated near the root of the aorta, it can be viewed between the opposed margins of the right and posterior semilunar valves of the aorta.
p. membrana′cea sep′ti na′si [TA] membranous part of nasal septum: the anterior inferior part of the nasal septum, beneath the cartilaginous part; it is composed of skin and subcutaneous tissues. Called also *membranous nasal septum* and *membranous septum of nose.*
p. membrana′cea ure′thrae masculi′nae TA alternative for *p. intermedia urethrae masculinae.*
p. mo′bilis sep′ti na′si [TA] mobile part of nasal septum: the part of the nasal septum at the apex of the nose, formed by skin, subcutaneous tissue, the greater alar cartilages, the membranous septum, and the columella; called also *septum mobile nasi.*
p. muscula′ris sep′ti interventricula′ris [TA] muscular part of interventricular septum of heart: the thick muscular partition forming the greater part of the septum between the ventricles of the heart.
p. mylopharyn′gea mus′culi constricto′ris pharyn′gis superio′ris [TA] mylopharyngeal part of superior constrictor muscle of pharynx: the part of the superior constrictor muscle arising from the mylohyoid ridge of the mandible; called also *mylopharyngeal muscle* and *musculus mylopharyngeus.*
p. nasa′lis os′sis fronta′lis [TA] nasal part of frontal bone: the small, irregularly shaped process that projects inferiorly from the medial part of the squama of the frontal bone to articulate with the nasal bones and the frontal processes of the maxillae. Called also *prefrontal bone.*
p. nasa′lis pharyn′gis [TA] nasopharynx: the part of the pharynx that lies above the level of the soft palate.
p. nervo′sa neurohypophy′seos TA alternative for *lobus nervosus neurohypophyseos.*
p. obli′qua mus′culi cricothyroi′dei [TA] the fibers of the cricothyroid muscle that are inserted into the inferior horn, caudal margin, and inner surface of the thyroid cartilage.
p. occlu′sa arte′riae umbilica′lis [TA] the portion of an umbilical artery that atrophies at birth when the placental circulation ceases to become the medial umbilical ligament. Cf. *p. patens arteriae umbilicalis.*
p. olfacto′ria cavita′tis na′si [TA] olfactory region: the superior part of the nasal cavity, the mucosa of which contains most of the receptors for the sense of smell.
p. opercula′ris gy′ri fronta′lis inferio′ris [TA] opercular part of inferior frontal gyrus: the part of the inferior frontal gyrus lying posterior to the ascending ramus of the lateral sulcus and pars triangularis and overlapping the insular lobe (insula). In the hemisphere dominant for speech, it is Broca's motor speech area. See also *operculum frontale* and *operculum frontoparietale.*
p. op′tica re′tinae [TA] optic part of retina: the part of the retina that contains receptors sensitive to light, extending posteriorly from the ora serrata on the inner surface of the choroid and continuous at the optic disk with the optic nerve; it consists of an outer pigmented layer *(stratum pigmentosum retinae)* and an inner, multilayered nervous layer *(stratum nervosum retinae).* See also *retina.*
p. ora′lis pharyn′gis [TA] oropharynx: the division of the pharynx lying between the soft palate and the upper edge of the epiglottis.
p. orbita′lis glan′dulae lacrima′lis [TA] orbital part of lacrimal gland: the main part of the lacrimal gland, limited in front by the orbicularis muscle and the orbital septum.
p. orbita′lis gy′ri fronta′lis inferio′ris [TA] orbital part of inferior frontal gyrus: the part of the inferior frontal gyrus lying below the anterior ramus of the lateral sulcus, which curves around the superciliary border to the orbital surface of the frontal lobe of the cerebral hemisphere anterior to the pars triangularis. See also *operculum frontale* (defs. 1 and 2).
p. orbita′lis mus′culi orbicula′ris oc′uli [TA] orbital part of orbicularis oculi muscle: the part of the orbicularis oculi muscle that arises from the medial margin of the orbit and surrounds it and the palpebral part of the muscle, inserting near the site of origin.
p. orbita′lis ner′vi op′tici [TA] orbital part of optic nerve: the part of the nerve located between the optic canal and the eyeball.
p. orbita′lis os′sis fronta′lis [TA] orbital part of frontal bone: the horizontal part of the bone; it forms the greater part of the roof of the orbit and of the floor of the anterior cranial fossa and is separated from its fellow of the other side by the ethmoid incisure. Called also *orbital plate of frontal bone.*
p. os′sea sep′ti na′si [TA] bony part of nasal septum: the posterior part of the septum, consisting of the perpendicular plate of the ethmoid bone superiorly and of the vomer inferiorly. Called also *bony nasal septum, bony septum of nose,* and *septum nasi osseum* [TA].
p. os′sea syste′matis skeleta′lis [TA] bony part of skeletal system: the bones of the body.
p. os′sea tu′bae auditi′vae [TA] bony part of auditory tube: the part of the tube that lies within the temporal bone, extending from the tympanic orifice to the pars cartilaginea of the auditory tube.
p. palpebra′lis glan′dulae lacrima′lis [TA] palpebral part of lacrimal gland: the part of the gland that projects laterally into the upper eyelid; called also *Rosenmüller gland.*
p. palpebra′lis mus′culi orbicula′ris o′culi [TA] palpebral part of orbicularis oculi muscle: the part of the orbicularis oculi muscle that is contained in the eyelids, originating from the medial palpebral ligament and inserting in the lateral canthus.
p. parasympa′thica divisio′nis autono′micae syste′matis nervo′si [TA] official terminology for *parasympathetic nervous system*; see under *system.*
p. parvocellula′ris nu′clei ru′bri [TA] parvocellular part of red nucleus: the complement of small multipolar cells scattered throughout the red nucleus; in humans, these cells predominate over the large cells in the caudal part of the nucleus; cf. *p. magnocellularis nuclei rubri.*
p. pa′tens arte′riae umbilica′lis [TA] patent part of umbilical artery: the proximal section of the fetal umbilical cord, which remains patent in the adult, although reduced in size. Cf. *p. occlusa arteriae umbilicalis.*
p. pel′vica duc′tus deferen′tis [TA] pelvic part of ductus deferens: the distal part of the ductus deferens, where it is within the pelvic cavity and terminates at the ampulla ductus deferentis.
p. pel′vica par′tis parasympa′thicae divisio′nis autono′micae syste′matis nervo′si [TA] pelvic part of parasympathetic part of autonomic nervous system: the part of the parasympathetic nervous system that includes the second to fourth anterior sacral roots and the sacral splanchnic nerves.
p. pel′vica ure′teris [TA] pelvic part of ureter: the portion of the ureter that extends from the terminal line of the pelvis to the urinary bladder.
p. periphe′rica syste′matis nervo′si [TA] the peripheral part of the nervous system, consisting of the nerves and ganglia outside the brain and spinal cord; called also *peripheral nervous system* and *systema nervosum periphericum* [TA alternative].
p. petro′sa arte′riae caro′tidis inter′nae [TA] petrous part of internal carotid artery: the portion of the artery located in the carotid canal; its branches include the caroticotympanic arteries.
p. petro′sa os′sis tempora′lis [TA] petrous part of temporal bone: a pyramid of dense bone located at the base of the cranium; one of the three parts of the temporal bone, it houses the organ of hearing. Some anatomists divide it into petrous and mastoid subparts and call it the *petromastoid part of temporal bone.* Called also *pyramid of temporal bone.*
p. phrenicocoeli′aca mus′culi suspenso′rii duode′ni [TA] phrenicoceliac part of suspensory muscle of duodenum: a band of skeletal muscle that passes from the right crus of the diaphragm to join the celiacoduodenal part (pars coeliacoduodenalis) and attach to the celiac trunk.
p. pia′lis fi′li termina′lis [TA] pial part of filum terminale: the prolongation of the spinal pia mater from the conus medullaris downward through the lumbar cistern, surrounded by the cauda equina, to attach to the inner aspect of the dural sac about the level of the second sacral vertebra. Called also *filum terminale internum.*
p. pla′na cor′poris cilia′ris orbiculus ciliaris.
p. plica′ta cor′poris cilia′ris corona ciliaris.
p. postcommunica′lis arte′riae ce′rebri anterio′ris [TA] postcommunicating part of anterior cerebral artery: collectively, the branches of the anterior cerebral artery that supply the cortex of the medial parts of the frontal and parietal lobes, comprising the distal medial striate, medial frontobasal, polar frontal, callosomarginal (and its branches), and pericallosal (and its branches) arteries.
p. postcommunica′lis arte′riae ce′rebri posterio′ris [TA] postcommunicating part of posterior cerebral artery: collectively, the branches of the posterior cerebral artery that supply cerebral peduncles, posterior thalamus, colliculi, and pineal and medial geniculate bodies, and choroid plexuses of lateral and third ventricles, comprising the posterolateral central and thalamogeniculate arteries,

and posterior medial choroidal, posterior lateral choroidal, and peduncular branches.

p. poste′rior commissu′rae anterio′ris [TA] posterior part of anterior commissure: the larger posterior portion of the commissure, whose fibers interconnect the middle and inferior temporal gyri, the parahippocampal gyri, and the amygdaloid bodies of the two sides.

p. poste′rior cul′minis [TA] the posterior part (V) of the culmen of the cerebellum; it is divided from the anterior part by the intraculminate fissure. Called also *p. dorsalis culminis* [TA alternative] and *dorsal part of culmen.*

p. poste′rior dor′si lin′guae [TA] posterior part of dorsum of tongue: the part of the dorsum of the tongue posterior to the terminal sulcus. Called also *p. postsulcalis dorsi linguae* [TA alternative].

p. poste′rior facie′i diaphragma′ticae he′patis [TA] posterior part of diaphragmatic surface of liver: the part directed toward the posterior surface of the body.

p. poste′rior for′nicis vagi′nae [TA] the posterior part of the fornix of the vagina; called also *posterior fornix.*

p. poste′rior he′patis [TA] posterior part of liver: term used to refer to the posterior region that is not part of either the left part (TA, *pars hepatis sinistra*) or the right part (TA, *pars hepatis dextra*); this part is coextensive with the caudate lobe. Called also *posterior liver.*

p. poste′rior lo′buli centra′lis cerebel′li [TA] the posterior part of the central lobule of the cerebellum (III); called also *p. dorsalis lobuli centralis cerebelli* [TA alternative] and *dorsal part of central lobule of cerebellum.*

p. poste′rior lo′buli quadrangula′ris anterio′ris [TA] posterior part of anterior quadrangular lobule (HV): the posterior division of the lobulus quadrangularis anterior cerebelli. Called also *p. dorsalis lobuli quadrangularis anterioris* [TA alternative] and *dorsal part of anterior quadrangular lobule.*

p. postlamina′ris ner′vi op′tici intraocula′ris [TA] postlaminar part of intraocular optic nerve: that portion of the intraocular part of the optic nerve that is posterior to the lamina cribrosa of the sclera.

p. postsulca′lis dor′si lin′guae TA alternative for *p. posterior dorsi linguae.*

p. precommunica′lis arte′riae ce′rebri anterio′ris [TA] precommunicating part of anterior cerebral artery: collectively, the branches of the anterior cerebral artery that supply the hypothalamus and lower parts of the corpus striatum, comprising the arteriae centrales anteromediales.

p. precommunica′lis arte′riae ce′rebri posterio′ris [TA] precommunicating part of posterior cerebral artery: collectively, the branches of the posterior cerebral artery anterior to its point of junction with the posterior communicating artery, comprising the posteromedial central arteries, short circumferential arteries, thalamoperforating artery, and collicular artery.

p. prelamina′ris ner′vi op′tici intraocula′ris [TA] prelaminar part of intraocular optic nerve: that portion of the intraocular part of the optic nerve that is anterior to the lamina cribrosa of the sclera.

p. preprosta′tica ure′thrae masculi′nae TA alternative for *p. intramuralis urethrae masculinae.*

p. presulca′lis dor′si lin′guae TA alternative for *p. anterior dorsi linguae.*

p. prevertebra′lis arte′riae vertebra′lis [TA] prevertebral part of vertebral artery: the first part of the artery, from its branching off from the subclavian artery to the point at which it enters the transverse process of the sixth cervical vertebra.

p. profun′da glan′dulae paroti′deae [TA] deep part of parotid gland: that part of the gland located deep to the facial nerve.

p. profun′da mus′culi masse′teris [TA] deep part of masseter muscle: the part whose fibers arise from the medial surface of the zygomatic arch and the fascia over the temporal muscle, and are directed in a vertical inferior direction.

p. profun′da mus′culi sphinc′teris a′ni exter′nus [TA] deep part of external anal sphincter: the part of the sphincter that surrounds the upper part of the anal canal.

p. profun′da par′tis palpebra′lis mus′culi orbicula′ris o′culi [TA] deep part of palpebral part of orbicularis oculi muscle: the part of the orbicularis oculi muscle that arises from the posterior lacrimal ridge of the lacrimal bone, to become continuous with the palpebral portion.

p. prosta′tica ure′thrae masculi′nae [TA] prostatic part of male urethra: the part of the urethra that passes through the prostate; called also *prostatic urethra.*

p. proxima′lis par′tis prosta′ticae ure′thrae masculi′nae [TA] proximal part of prostatic urethra: the first portion of the prostatic urethra, up to and including the seminal colliculus.

p. psoa′tica fas′ciae iliopso′as [TA] psoas part of iliopsoas fascia: the part of the fascia that invests the psoas major muscle.

p. pterygopharyn′gea mus′culi constricto′ris pharyn′gis superio′ris [TA] pterygopharyngeal part of superior constrictor muscle of pharynx: the part of the superior constrictor muscle arising from the caudal part and hamulus of the medial pterygoid plate; called also *pterygopharyngeal muscle* and *musculus pterygopharyngeus.*

p. pylo′rica gas′trica [TA] pyloric part of stomach: the caudal third of the stomach, consisting of the pyloric antrum and canal, and distinguished by the presence of the pyloric glands and by the absence of parietal cells.

p. rec′ta mus′culi cricothyroi′dei [TA] the fibers of the cricothyroid muscle that are inserted into the caudal margin of the thyroid cartilage.

p. rec′ta tu′buli rena′lis straight tubule; see *tubulus rectus proximalis* and *tubulus rectus distalis.*

p. respirato′ria cavita′tis na′si [TA] respiratory region: the part of the nasal cavity inferior to the olfactory region.

p. reticula′ris substan′tiae ni′grae [TA] reticular part of substantia nigra: the anterior part of the substantia nigra, which contains fewer cells than the pars compacta, only some of which contain a small amount of pigment.

p. retrolentifor′mis cap′sulae inter′nae [TA] retrolentiform part of internal capsule: that part of the internal capsule resting on the lateral surface of the thalamus behind the lentiform nucleus, and containing the posterior thalamic radiation. Called also *retrolenticular* or *retrolentiform limb of internal capsule.*

p. sacra′lis medul′lae spina′lis [TA] sacral part of spinal cord: the part of the cord that is within the lumbar part of the vertebral canal and gives rise to the five pairs of sacral spinal nerves *(segmenta sacralia medullae spinalis [1–5]).*

p. scrota′lis duc′tus deferen′tis [TA] scrotal part of ductus deferens: the initial part of the ductus deferens, which is within the scrotum.

p. sphenoida′lis arte′riae ce′rebri me′diae [TA] sphenoid part of middle cerebral artery: collectively, the segment of the middle cerebral artery and the branches from it that supply the internal capsule, thalamus, and corpus striatum (M1 segment); the branches comprise the anterolateral central arteries, anterior temporal artery, and polar temporal artery. Called also *p. horizontalis arteriae cerebri mediae* [TA alternative]. See also *segments of middle cerebral artery,* under *segment.*

p. spina′lis mus′culi deltoi′dei [TA] spinal part of deltoid muscle: the posterior unipennate portion of the deltoid muscle, originating on the lower border of the spine of scapula and acting with latissimus dorsi and teres major in drawing the arm backwards and rotating it laterally.

p. spina′lis ner′vi accesso′rii TA alternative for *radix spinalis nervi accessorii.*

p. spongio′sa ure′thrae masculi′nae [TA] spongy part of male urethra: the portion of the urethra within the corpus spongiosum of the penis. Called also *spongiose* or *spongy urethra.*

p. squamo′sa os′sis tempora′lis [TA] squamous part of temporal bone: the flat, scalelike, anterior and superior portion of the temporal bone; called also *squama temporalis.*

p. sterna′lis diaphrag′matis [TA] sternal part of diaphragm: the portion of the thoracic diaphragm that arises from the inner aspect of the xiphoid process of the sternum.

p. sternocosta′lis mus′culi pectora′lis majo′ris [TA] sternocostal part of pectoralis major muscle: the portion of the muscle that originates from the sternum and the ribs.

p. subcuta′nea mus′culi sphinc′teris a′ni exter′nus [TA] subcutaneous part of external anal sphincter: the part of the sphincter that surrounds the outermost portion of the anal canal.

p. sublentifor′mis cap′sulae inter′nae [TA] sublentiform part of internal capsule: the part of the internal capsule lying inferior to the posterior part of the lentiform nucleus, and containing the temporopontine, geniculocalcarine, and auditory radiation fibers. Called also *sublenticular limb of internal capsule* and *sublentiform limb of internal capsule.*

p. superficia'lis glan'dulae paroti'deae [TA] superficial part of parotid gland: that part of the parotid gland located superficial to the facial nerve.
p. superficia'lis mus'culi masse'teris [TA] superficial part of masseter muscle: the part of the muscle whose fibers arise from the anterior part of the zygomatic arch and are directed inferiorly and posteriorly.
p. superficia'lis mus'culi sphinc'teris a'ni exter'nus [TA] superficial part of external anal sphincter: the part of the sphincter that lies just deep to the subcutaneous part, extending farther toward the rectum.
p. supe'rior ala'ris lo'buli centra'lis cerebel'li [TA] the superior part of the wing of the central lobule of the cerebellum (HIII); called also *p. dorsalis alaris lobuli centralis cerebelli* [TA alternative] and *dorsal part of wing of central lobule of cerebellum.*
p. supe'rior duode'ni [TA] superior part of duodenum: the most proximal part of the duodenum, adjacent to the pylorus; it forms the superior duodenal flexure.
p. supe'rior facie'i diaphragma'ticae he'patis [TA] superior part of diaphragmatic surface of liver: the most superior part of the diaphragmatic surface, projecting convexly upward.
p. supe'rior ner'vi vestibula'ris [TA] superior part of vestibular nerve: the superior branch of the nerve, which has filaments that end in the ampullary crests of the anterior and lateral semicircular ducts and the macula of the utricle.
p. supe'rior ve'nae lingula'ris [TA] superior part of lingular vein: a venous branch that drains the superior lingular segment of the left lung and drains into the lingular vein. Called also *superior lingular segmental vein.*
p. supraclavicula'ris plex'us brachia'lis [TA] supraclavicular part of brachial plexus: the part of the brachial plexus lying in the cervical region above the level of the clavicle, in which arise the dorsal scapular, long thoracic, and suprascapular nerves, and the nerve to the subclavius muscle.
p. sympa'thica divisio'nis autono'micae syste'matis nervo'si [TA] official terminology for *sympathetic nervous system*; see under *system.*
p. tec'ta duode'ni [TA] hidden part of duodenum: a portion of the duodenum that is concealed by the overlying transverse colon, ascending colon, and root of the mesentery.
p. ten'sa membra'nae tympa'nicae [TA] the larger portion of the tympanic membrane; it is tense and firm. Called also *membrana tensa* and *membrana vibrans.*
p. termina'lis i'lei [TA] terminal part of ileum: the part just before the ileum meets the cecum at the ileal orifice and ileal papilla; called also *terminal ileum.*
p. thora'cica aor'tae [TA] thoracic part of aorta: the proximal portion of the descending aorta, which proceeds from the arch of the aorta and gives rise to the bronchial, esophageal, pericardiac, and mediastinal branches, and the superior phrenic, posterior intercostal III to XI, and subcostal arteries; it is continuous through the diaphragm with the abdominal aorta. Called also *thoracic aorta* and *aorta thoracica* [TA alternative].
p. thora'cica duc'tus thora'cici [TA] the thoracic part of the thoracic duct; see *ductus thoracicus.*
p. thora'cica medul'lae spina'lis [TA] thoracic part of spinal cord: the part of the cord that is within the upper three fourths of the thoracic part of the vertebral canal (in the adult) and gives rise to the twelve pairs of thoracic spinal nerves *(segmenta thoracica medullae spinalis [1–12]).*
p. thora'cica mus'culi iliocosta'lis lumbo'rum [TA] thoracic part of iliocostalis lumborum: *origin,* upper borders of angles of six lower ribs; *insertion,* angles of six upper ribs and transverse process of seventh cervical vertebra; *innervation,* branches of thoracic; *action,* keeps thoracic spine erect.
p. thora'cica oeso'phagi [TA] thoracic part of esophagus: the part of the esophagus located in the thoracic region, posterior to the trachea and pericardium and anterior to the vertebral column. Called also *thoracic esophagus.*
p. thora'cica tra'cheae [TA] the part of the trachea that lies posteriorly in the superior mediastinum, separated from the upper four thoracic vertebrae by the esophagus.
p. thyroepiglot'tica mus'culi thyroarytenoi'dei [TA] thyroepiglottic part of thyroarytenoid muscle: fibers of the thyroarytenoid muscle that continue to the margin of the epiglottis; it closes the inlet to the larynx. Called also *thyroepiglottic muscle.*

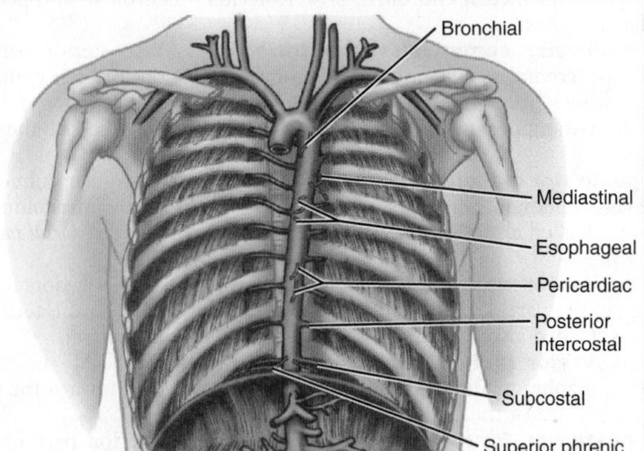

■ Pars thoracica aortae (thoracic aorta) and the arteries and branches to which it gives rise.

p. thyropharyn'gea mus'culi constricto'ris pharyn'gis infe-rio'ris [TA] thyropharyngeal part of inferior constrictor muscle of pharynx: the part of the inferior constrictor muscle arising from the thyroid cartilage; called also *thyropharyngeal muscle* and *musculus thyropharyngeus* [TA alternative].
p. tibiocalca'nea ligamen'ti collatera'lis media'lis [TA] tibiocalcaneal part of medial collateral ligament: the middle portion of the superficial fibers of the medial collateral ligament of the ankle joint, attached superiorly to the medial malleolus of the tibia and inferiorly into nearly the entire length of the sustentaculum tali of the calcaneus. Called also *calcaneotibial ligament, ligamentum calcaneotibiale,* and *tibiocalcaneal* or *tibiocalcanean ligament.*
p. tibionavicula'ris ligamen'ti collatera'lis media'lis [TA] tibionavicular part of medial collateral ligament: the anterior portion of the superficial fibers of the medial collateral ligament of the ankle joint, attached superiorly to the anterior surface of the medial malleolus of the tibia and inferiorly to the navicular bone and the margin of the calcaneonavicular ligament. Called also *ligamentum tibionaviculare* and *tibionavicular ligament.*
p. tibiotala'ris ante'rior ligamen'ti collatera'lis media'lis [TA] anterior tibiotalar part of medial collateral ligament: the deeper portion of the medial collateral ligament of the ankle joint, attached superiorly to the medial malleolus of the tibia and inferiorly to the medial surface of the talus. Called also *ligamentum talotibiale anterius* and *anterior talotibial ligament.*
p. tibiotala'ris poste'rior ligamen'ti collatera'lis media'lis [TA] posterior tibiotalar part of medial collateral ligament: the posterior portion of the superficial fibers of the medial collateral ligament of the ankle joint, attached superiorly to the posterior part of the medial malleolus of the tibia and inferiorly to the medial surface of the talus. Called also *ligamentum talotibiale posterius* and *posterior talotibial ligament.*
p. transver'sa mus'culi nasa'lis [TA] transverse part of nasalis muscle: the part of the nasalis muscle arising from the maxilla on either side just lateral to the nasal notch and inserting on the bridge of the nose; it compresses the nasal opening. Called also *compressor muscle of naris* and *compressor naris.*
p. transver'sa ra'mi sinis'tri ve'nae por'tae he'patis [TA] the transverse part of the left branch of the hepatic portal vein.
p. transversa'ria arte'riae vertebra'lis [TA] cervical part of vertebral artery: the second part of the vertebral artery, ascending through the transverse foramina of the upper six cervical vertebrae; it has spinal and muscular branches. Called also *p. cervicalis arteriae vertebralis* [TA alternative].
p. triangula'ris gy'ri fronta'lis inferio'ris [TA] triangular part of inferior frontal gyrus: the wedge-shaped part of the inferior frontal lobe that lies between the anterior and ascending branches of the lateral sulcus of the cerebral hemisphere bordered by the pars orbitalis anteriorly and the pars opercularis posteriorly. See also *operculum frontale* (defs. 1 and 2).

Pars *Continued*

p. tubera'lis adenohypophy'seos [TA] tuberal part of adenohypophysis: a part consisting of a thin cloak of cells on the anterior and lateral surfaces of the infundibulum. It provides a vascular communication between the hypothalamus and the pituitary gland and secretes some hormones.
p. tympa'nica os'sis tempora'lis [TA] tympanic part of temporal bone: the curved bony plate, developed from the annulus tympanicus of the fetus, forming the anterior and inferior walls and part of the posterior wall of the external auditory meatus in the adult; called also *tympanic plate*.
p. umbilica'lis ra'mi sinis'tri ve'nae por'tae he'patis [TA] umbilical part of left branch: the part of the left branch of the hepatic portal vein that passes from the hilum of the liver to the umbilicus.
p. uteri'na tu'bae uteri'nae [TA] uterine part of uterine tube: the proximal part of the uterine tube, located within the wall of the uterus.
p. uvea'lis reti'culi trabecula'ris [TA] uveal part of trabecular reticulum: the posterior part of the trabecular reticulum, situated between the scleral spur, the ciliary body, and the anterior iris.
p. vaga'lis ner'vi accesso'rii TA alternative for *radix cranialis nervi accessorii*.
p. ventra'lis ala'ris lo'buli centra'lis cerebel'li TA alternative for *p. inferior alaris lobuli centralis cerebelli*.
p. ventra'lis cul'minis TA alternative for *p. anterior culminis*.
p. ventra'lis lo'buli centra'lis cerebel'li TA alternative for *p. anterior lobuli centralis cerebelli*.
p. ventra'lis lo'buli quadrangula'ris anterio'ris TA alternative for *pars anterior lobuli quadrangularis anterioris*.
p. vertebra'lis facie'i costa'lis pulmo'nis [TA] vertebral part of costal surface of lung: the part of the costal surface of each lung related behind to the sides of the vertebral bodies.

Par•son•age-Tur•ner syndrome (pahr'sə-nəj tur'nər) [Maurice John *Parsonage*, British neurologist, 1915–2008; John W. Aldren *Turner*, British neurologist, 1911–1980] neuralgic amyotrophy; see under *amyotrophy*.

pars pla•ni•tis (pahrz pla-ni'tis) a granulomatous uveitis of the pars plana of the ciliary body.

part (pahrt) pars.

Part

For names of parts of various anatomical structures not found here, see under *pars*.

abdominal p. of esophagus pars abdominalis oesophagi.
acromial p. of deltoid muscle pars acromialis musculi deltoidei.
alar p. of nasal muscle pars alaris musculi nasalis.
annular p. of fibrous sheaths of fingers pars anularis vaginae fibrosae digitorum manus.
annular p. of fibrous sheaths of toes pars anularis vaginae fibrosae digitorum pedis.
anterior p. of anterior commissure pars anterior commissurae anterioris cerebri.
anterior p. of anterior quadrangular lobule pars anterior lobuli quadrangularis anterioris.
anterior p. of central lobule of cerebellum pars anterior lobuli centralis cerebelli.
anterior p. of culmen pars anterior culminis.
anterior p. of dorsum of tongue pars anterior dorsi linguae.
atlantic p. of vertebral artery pars atlantica arteriae vertebralis.
autonomic p. of peripheral nervous system autonomic nervous system.
basal p. of left pulmonary artery pars basalis arteriae pulmonis sinistri.
basal p. of right pulmonary artery pars basalis arteriae pulmonis dextri.
basilar p. of occipital bone pars basilaris ossis occipitalis.
basilar p. of pons pars basilaris pontis.
bony p. of auditory tube pars ossea tubae auditivae.
bony p. of nasal septum pars ossea septi nasi.
bony p. of skeletal system pars ossea systematis skeletalis.
cartilaginous p. of auditory tube pars cartilaginea tubae auditivae.
cartilaginous p. of skeletal system pars cartilaginea systematis skeletalis.
cardiac p. of stomach, cardial p. of stomach cardia.
cavernous p. of internal carotid artery pars cavernosa arteriae carotidis internae.
central p. of lateral ventricle pars centralis ventriculi lateralis.
cerebral p. of internal carotid artery pars cerebralis arteriae carotidis internae.
cervical p. of esophagus pars cervicalis oesophagi.
cervical p. of internal carotid artery pars cervicalis arteriae carotidis internae.c
cervical p. of spinal cord pars cervicalis medullae spinalis.
cervical p. of vertebral artery pars transversaria arteriae vertebralis.
clavicular p. of deltoid muscle pars clavicularis musculi deltoidei.
coccygeal p. of spinal cord pars coccygea medullae spinalis.
compact p. of substantia nigra pars compacta substantiae nigrae.
condylar p. of occipital bone pars lateralis ossis occipitalis.
cortical p. of middle cerebral artery the fourth segment of the middle cerebral artery (M4 segment), comprising the inferior and superior terminal branches of the vessel (rami terminales inferiores and rami terminales superiores), which supply the lateral surface of the cerebral hemisphere. See also *segments of middle cerebral artery*, under *segment*.
costal p. of diaphragm pars costalis diaphragmatis.
cranial p. of parasympathetic p. of autonomic nervous system pars cranialis partis parasympathici divisionis autonomicae systematis nervosi.
craniosacral p. of autonomic nervous system pars parasympathica divisionis autonomicae systematis nervosi; see *parasympathetic nervous system*, under *system*.
cruciate p. of fibrous sheaths cruciform part of fibrous sheaths; see entries beginning *pars cruciformis vaginae fibrosae*.
cruciform p. of fibrous sheaths of fingers pars cruciformis vaginae fibrosae digitorum manus.
cruciform p. of fibrous sheaths of toes pars cruciformis vaginae fibrosae digitorum pedis.
dorsal p. of anterior quadrangular lobule pars posterior lobuli quadrangularis anterioris.
dorsal p. of central lobule of cerebellum pars posterior lobuli centralis cerebelli.
dorsal p. of culmen pars posterior culminis.
dorsal p. of lateral geniculate body the part of the lateral geniculate body overlying the dorsal part of the lateral geniculate nucleus.
dorsal p. of medial geniculate body the part of the medial geniculate body overlying the dorsal part of the medial geniculate nucleus. Called also *parvocellular p. of medial geniculate body*.
dorsal p. of wing of central lobule of cerebellum pars superior alaris lobuli centralis cerebelli.
dural p. of filum terminale pars duralis fili terminalis.
endocrine p. of pancreas endocrine pancreas.
exoccipital p. of occipital bone pars lateralis ossis occipitalis.
exocrine p. of pancreas exocrine pancreas.
extraocular p. of central retinal artery pars extraocularis arteriae centralis retinae.
extraocular p. of central retinal vein pars extraocularis venae centralis retinae.
exocrine p. of pancreas exocrine pancreas.

Part *Continued*

fetal p. of placenta the nonmaternal part of the placenta, derived not from the fetus but from the trophoblast that envelops the fetus; from within outward, it consists of amnion, chorionic plate, and chorionic villi. Called also *fetal placenta.*
horizontal p. of duodenum pars horizontalis duodeni.
horizontal p. of middle cerebral artery pars sphenoidalis arteriae cerebri mediae.
inferior p. of duodenum pars horizontalis duodeni.
inferior p. of rhomboid fossa the triangular caudal portion of the rhomboid fossa, extending downward from the rostral part of the taeniae with its apex (the calamus scriptorius) being continuous with the wall of the central canal of the medulla oblongata.
inferior p. of vestibular nerve pars inferior nervi vestibularis.
inferior p. of wing of central lobule of cerebellum pars inferior alaris lobuli centralis cerebelli.
infraclavicular p. of brachial plexus pars infraclavicularis plexus brachialis.
insular p. of middle cerebral artery pars insularis arteriae cerebri mediae.
intermediate p. of male urethra pars intermedia urethrae masculinae.
intermediate p. of rhomboid fossa the wide central portion of the rhomboid fossa, between the superior foveae rostrally and the beginning of the taeniae caudally.
interstitial p. of uterine tube, intramural p. of uterine tube pars uterina tubae uterinae.
intracanalicular p. of optic nerve pars canalis nervi optici.
intracranial p. of optic nerve pars intracranialis nervi optici.
intracranial p. of vertebral artery pars intracranialis arteriae vertebralis.
intralaminar p. of intraocular optic nerve pars intralaminaris nervi optici intraocularis.
intramural p. of male urethra pars intramuralis urethrae masculinae.
intraocular p. of central retinal artery pars intraocularis arteriae centralis retinae.
intraocular p. of central retinal vein pars intraocularis venae centralis retinae.
intraocular p. of optic nerve pars intraocularis nervi optici.
jugular p. of occipital bone pars lateralis ossis occipitalis.
lateral p. of biventral lobe of cerebellum pars lateralis lobuli biventralis cerebelli.
lateral p. of globus pallidus medial segment pars lateralis globi pallidi medialis.
lateral p. of occipital bone pars lateralis ossis occipitalis.
lumbar p. of diaphragm pars lumbalis diaphragmatis.
lumbar p. of iliocostalis lumborum pars lumbalis musculi iliocostalis lumborum.
lumbar p. of longissimus thoracis pars lumbalis musculi longissimus thoracis.
lumbar p. of spinal cord pars lumbalis medullae spinalis.
magnocellular p. of medial geniculate body ventral p. of medial geniculate body.
magnocellular p. of red nucleus pars magnocellularis nuclei rubri.
mastoid p. of temporal bone processus mastoideus ossis temporalis.
maternal p. of placenta the maternally contributed part of the placenta, derived from the decidua basalis; called also *maternal placenta.*
medial p. of biventral lobe of cerebellum pars medialis lobuli biventralis cerebelli.
medial p. of globus pallidus medial segment pars medialis globi pallidi medialis.
membranous p. of male urethra pars intermedia urethrae masculinae.
membranous p. of nasal septum pars membranacea septi nasi.
mobile p. of nasal septum pars mobilis septi nasi.
nasal p. of frontal bone pars nasalis ossis frontalis.
occipital p. of occipital bone squama occipitalis.
opercular p. of middle cerebral artery the third segment of the middle cerebral artery (M3 segment), beginning at the top of the insula as the vessel turns laterally within the lateral cerebral (sylvian) fissure, passing through and supplying the opercula, and ending at the lateral surface of the cerebral hemisphere. See also *segments of middle cerebral artery*, under *segment.*
orbital p. of optic nerve pars orbitalis nervi optici.
parasympathetic p. of autonomic division of nervous system pars parasympathica divisionis autonomicae systematis nervosi; see *parasympathetic nervous system*, under *system.*
parvocellular p. of medial geniculate body dorsal p. of medial geniculate body.
parvocellular p. of red nucleus pars parvocellularis nuclei rubri.
pectineal p. of inguinal ligament ligamentum lacunare.
pelvic p. of parasympathetic p. of autonomic nervous system pars pelvica partis parasympathici divisionis autonomicae systematis nervosi.
petromastoid p. of temporal bone a name given to the pars petrosa ossis temporalis when describing it as having petrous and mastoid parts.
petrous p. of internal carotid artery pars petrosa arteriae carotidis internae.
petrous p. of temporal bone 1. pars petrosa ossis temporalis. 2. sometimes specifically the pars petrosa ossis temporalis excluding the mastoid part (processus mastoideus ossis temporalis).
pial p. of filum terminale pars pialis fili terminalis.
posterior p. of anterior commissure pars posterior commissurae anterioris.
posterior p. of anterior quadrangular lobule pars posterior lobuli quadrangularis anterioris.
posterior p. of central lobule of cerebellum pars posterior lobuli centralis cerebelli.
posterior p. of culmen pars posterior culminis.
posterior p. of dorsum of tongue pars posterior dorsi linguae.
postlaminar p. of intraocular optic nerve pars postlaminaris nervi optici intraocularis.
postsphenoid p. of sphenoid bone, postsphenoidal p. of sphenoid bone the posterior portion of the sphenoid bone; in the fetus it consists of separate basisphenoid, pterygoid, and alisphenoid parts, first cartilaginous and later bony, which fuse to each other and to the presphenoid part before birth. Called also *postsphenoid bone.*
postsulcal p. of dorsum of tongue pars posterior dorsi linguae.
prelaminar p. of intraocular optic nerve pars prelaminaris nervi optici intraocularis.
preprostatic p. of male urethra pars preprostatica urethrae masculinae.
presenting p. 1. the portion of the fetus that is touched by the examining finger through the uterine cervix and, during labor, is bounded by the girdle of resistance. 2. the portion of the body of the fetus that is farthest forward in the birth canal or is closest to it.
presphenoid p. of sphenoid bone, presphenoidal p. of sphenoid bone the anterior portion of the sphenoid bone; it develops separately in the fetus and unites with the postsphenoidal part between the seventh and eighth months of intrauterine life. Called also *presphenoid bone.*
presulcal p. of dorsum of tongue pars anterior dorsi linguae.
prevertebral p. of vertebral artery pars prevertebralis arteriae vertebralis.
pyloric p. of stomach pars pylorica gastrica.
reticular p. of substantia nigra pars reticularis substantiae nigrae.
retrolentiform p. of internal capsule pars retrolentiformis capsulae internae.
sacral p. of spinal cord pars sacralis medullae spinalis.
sphenoid p. of middle cerebral artery pars sphenoidalis arteriae cerebri mediae.
spinal p. of accessory nerve radix spinalis nervi accessorii.
spinal p. of deltoid muscle pars spinalis musculi deltoidei.
spongy p. of male urethra pars spongiosa urethrae masculinae.
squamous p. of frontal bone squama frontalis.
squamous p. of occipital bone squama occipitalis.
squamous p. of temporal bone pars squamosa ossis temporalis.
sternal p. of diaphragm pars sternalis diaphragmatis.
sternocostal p. of diaphragm pars costalis diaphragmatis.
sublentiform p. of internal capsule pars sublentiformis capsulae internae.
subphrenic p. of esophagus pars abdominalis oesophagi.
superior p. of rhomboid fossa the triangular rostral portion of the rhomboid fossa, continuous at its apex with the wall of the cerebral aqueduct and terminating at an imaginary line drawn between the superior foveae.
superior p. of vestibular nerve pars superior nervi vestibularis.

Part *Continued*

superior p. of wing of central lobule of cerebellum pars superior alaris lobuli centralis cerebelli.
supraclavicular p. of brachial plexus pars supraclavicularis plexus brachialis.
sympathetic p. of autonomic division of nervous system pars sympathica divisionis autonomici systematis nervosi; see *sympathetic nervous system*, under *system*.
tabular p. of occipital bone squama occipitalis.
tendinous p. of epicranius muscle galea aponeurotica.
thalamolenticular p. of internal capsule crus posterius capsulae internae.
third p. of quadriceps femoris muscle musculus adductor minimus.
thoracic p. of esophagus pars thoracica oesophagi.
thoracic p. of iliocostalis lumborum pars thoracica musculi iliocostalis lumborum.
thoracic p. of spinal cord pars thoracica medullae spinalis.
thoracolumbar p. of autonomic nervous system pars sympathica divisionis autonomici systematis nervosi; see *sympathetic nervous system*, under *system*.
transverse p. of duodenum pars horizontalis duodeni.
transverse p. of nasal muscle pars transversa musculi nasalis.
tympanic p. of temporal bone pars tympanica ossis temporalis.
vagal p. of accessory nerve radix cranialis nervi accessorii.
vaginal p. of cervix portio vaginalis cervicis.
ventral p. of anterior quadrangular lobule pars anterior lobuli quadrangularis anterioris.
ventral p. of central lobule of cerebellum pars anterior lobuli centralis cerebelli.
ventral p. of culmen pars anterior culminis.
ventral p. of lateral geniculate body the part of the lateral geniculate body overlying the ventral part of the lateral geniculate nucleus.
ventral p. of lateral geniculate nucleus nucleus ventralis corporis geniculati lateralis.
ventral p. of medial geniculate body the part of the medial geniculate body overlying the ventral part of the medial geniculate nucleus; called also *magnocellular p. of medial geniculate body*.
ventral p. of medial geniculate nucleus nucleus ventralis corporis geniculati medialis.
ventral p. of wing of central lobule of cerebellum pars inferior alaris lobuli centralis cerebelli.
vertebral p. of diaphragm pars lumbalis diaphragmatis.

Part. aeq. [L.] par′tes aequa′les (equal parts).

par·tes (pahr′tēz) [L.] plural of *pars*.

Par·the·ni·um (pahr-the′ne-əm) a genus of flowering herbs of the family Compositae. *P. hysterophorus* is wild feverfew, a common cause of airborne contact dermatitis.

par·the·no·gen·e·sis (pahr″thə-no-jen′ə-sis) [Gr. *parthenos* virgin + *-genesis*] a modified form of sexual reproduction with development of a gamete without fertilization, as occurs in some plants and invertebrates, especially arthropods including honey bees and wasps, and in certain lizards. It may occur as a natural phenomenon or be induced by chemical, thermal, or mechanical stimulation *(artificial p.)*.

par·the·no·pho·bia (pahr″thə-no-fo′be-ə) [Gr. *parthenos* virgin + *-phobia*] irrational fear of girls.

par·tho·gen·e·sis (pahr″tho-jen′ə-sis) parthenogenesis.

par·tial·ism (pahr′shəl-iz-əm) a paraphilia characterized by exclusive focus on a body part of the sexual partner.

par·ti·cle (pahr′tĭ-kəl) [L. *particula*, dim. of *pars* part] a tiny mass of material.
 alpha p. a positively charged particle ejected from the nucleus of a radioactive atom, being a high-speed ionized atom of helium. A stream of these particles constitutes alpha rays.
 beta p. an electron emitted from an atomic nucleus during beta decay.
 colloid p's the particles making up the disperse phase of a colloid. See *colloid* (def. 2).
 Dane p. an intact hepatitis B virion.
 disperse p's colloid p's.
 elementary p. any of the subatomic particles, including electrons, protons, neutrons, positrons, neutrinos, muons, etc.
 high-velocity p's subatomic particles, such as electrons, protons, and deuterons, given high speeds in an accelerator.
 nuclear p's Howell-Jolly bodies.
 signal recognition p. a protein-RNA complex that binds to the signal sequence of a nascent protein and a ribosome, arresting the elongation of the polypeptide until the ribosome is associated with the rough endoplasmic reticulum.
 viral p., virus p. virion.

par·tic·u·late (pahr-tik′u-lət) composed of separate particles.

par·ti·tion (pahr-tĭ′shən) something that separates or divides into parts.
 oropharyngeal p. a protective barrier between the oral cavity and the pharynx made of moistened gauze sponges, useful during general anesthesia when a nasal mask is used.

par·ti·tion·ing (pahr-tĭ′shən-ing) dividing into parts.
 gastric p. any of the gastroplasty procedures done for morbid obesity in which a small stomach pouch is walled off for the nutrient flow to pass through; when it is full it signals satiety. See also *gastric stapling*.

par·tu·ri·ent (pahr-tu′re-ənt) [L. *parturiens*] 1. giving birth, or pertaining to childbirth. 2. by extension, a woman in labor.

par·tu·ri·fa·cient (pahr″tu-re-fa′shənt) [L. *parturire* to have the pains of labor + *-facient*] 1. inducing or facilitating childbirth. 2. an agent that induces or facilitates childbirth.

par·tu·ri·om·e·ter (pahr″tu-re-om′ə-tər) [L. *parturitio* childbirth + *-meter*] a device used in measuring the expulsive power of the uterus.

par·tu·ri·tion (pahr″tu-rĭ′shən) [L. *parturitio*] childbirth. **par′tal** *adj*

Part. vic. [L.] parti′tis vi′cibus (in divided doses).

pa·ru·lis (pə-roo′lis) [*para-* + Gr. *oulon* gum] an elevated nodule at the site of a fistula draining a chronic periapical abscess. Called also *gumboil* (or *gum boil*).

par·um·bil·i·cal (par″əm-bil′ĭ-kəl) paraumbilical.

par·vi·cel·lu·lar (pahr″vĭ-sel′u-lər) [L. *parvus* small + *cellular*] composed of small cells, as opposed to *magnicellular*.

par·vo·cel·lu·lar (pahr″vo-sel′u-lər) parvicellular.

Par·vo·vi·ri·dae (pahr″vo-vir′ĭ-de) the parvoviruses: a family of DNA viruses having a nonenveloped virion 18–26 nm in diameter composed of 60 copies of the capsid protein with icosahedral symmetry. The genome consists of a single molecule of linear single-stranded DNA (MW 1.5–2.2 × 10^6, size 4–6 kb). Viruses contain 2–4 major polypeptides, depending on the species, and are resistant to heat, lipid solvents, deoxycholate, and nucleases but sensitive to formalin, β-propiolactone, hydroxylamine, oxidizing agents, and ultraviolet radiation. Replication and assembly occur in the nucleus and require S-phase cellular function in the host cell or the presence of helper virus. Host range is narrow and transmission may be vertical or by mechanical vectors. There are two subclasses: Densovirinae, comprising genera that infect invertebrates, and Parvovirinae, comprising genera that infect vertebrates.

Par·vo·vi·ri·nae (pahr″vo-vir-i′ne) a subfamily of the family Parvoviridae, containing parvoviruses that infect vertebrates; it comprises three genera: *Dependovirus*, *Erythrovirus*, and *Parvovirus*.

Par·vo·vi·rus (pahr′vo-vi″rəs) [*parvo-* + *virus*] parvoviruses; a genus of viruses of the subfamily Parvovirinae (family Parvoviridae) that infect mammals and birds. Viruses multiply in the nucleus and require S-phase cellular

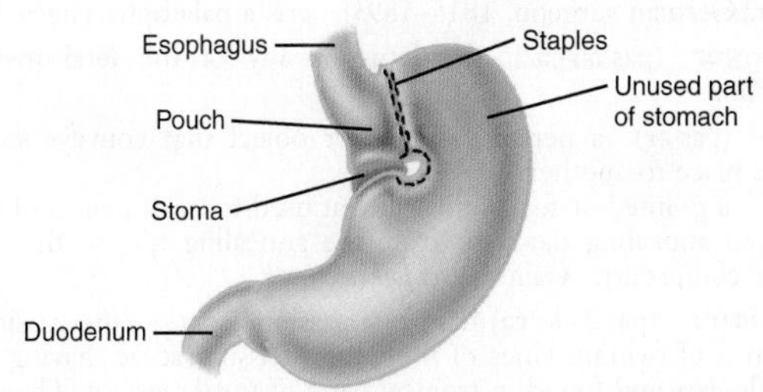

■ Gastric partitioning using a vertical banded gastroplasty.

functions for replication. Transmission is transplacental or by mechanical vector. Human parvoviruses cause transient aplastic crisis, acute arthritis, erythema infectiosum, hydrops fetalis, spontaneous abortion, and fetal death. Animal pathogens include bovine, canine, feline, and goose parvoviruses, feline panleukopenia virus, mink enteritis virus, Aleutian mink disease virus, and various murine parvoviruses.

par•vo•vi•rus (pahr′vo-vi″rəs) [L. *parvus* small + *virus*] any virus of the family Parvoviridae. **parvovi′ral** *adj*

bovine p. a virus of the genus *Parvovirus* infecting cattle that causes diarrhea in calves; infection during the first or second trimesters of gestation may result in abortion. Infection is widespread and antibody to the virus can be found in a high proportion of adult cattle.

canine p. a virus of the genus *Parvovirus* that causes myocarditis in dogs and a type of enteritis called canine parvovirus disease; it is sometimes considered to be a species-specific variant of feline parvovirus.

feline p. a virus of the genus *Parvovirus* that primarily affects cats. Canine parvovirus, feline panleukopenia virus, and mink enteritis virus are sometimes considered to be host-specific variant strains.

goose p. a virus of the genus *Parvovirus* that causes a highly fatal disease of young geese affecting the liver, thyroid, and pancreas.

human p. B19 B19 virus.

human p. RA-1 a species belonging to the genus *Parvovirus* that has been associated with rheumatoid arthritis.

par•vule (pahr′vūl) [L. *parvulus* very small] a very small pill, pellet, or granule.

Par•y•phos•to•mum (par″e-fos′to-məm) a genus of flukes related to *Echinostoma.*

PAS *p*-aminosalicylic acid; periodic acid–Schiff (see under *reaction*).

PASA *p*-aminosalicylic acid.

Pas•cal's law (pahs-kahlz′) [Blaise *Pascal*, French mathematician and physicist, 1623–1662] see under *law.*

pas•cal (Pa) (pas-kal′) [B. *Pascal*] the SI unit of pressure, which corresponds to a force of one newton per square meter.

Pa•schen bodies (pah′shən) [Enrique *Paschen*, German pathologist, 1860–1936] see under *body.*

Pas•er (pās′er) trademark for a preparation of aminosalicylic acid.

PASG pneumatic antishock garment.

Pa•si•ni-Pie•ri•ni atrophoderma (pah-se′ne pya-re′ne) [A. *Pasini*, Argentine physician, early 20th century; L. *Pierini*, Argentine physician, mid-20th century] see under *atrophoderma.*

pas•pal•ism (pas′pəl-iz-əm) poisoning of livestock by ingestion of excessive amounts of *Paspalum commersonii* or *P. scrobiculatum*, grasses containing neurotoxic hydrocarbons; characteristics include tremor, convulsions, and coma. See also *paspalum staggers*, under *staggers.*

Pas•pa•lum (pas′pə-ləm) a genus of grasses commonly eaten by livestock in Asia and Africa. Some species contain a toxic hydrocarbon that can cause paspalism; other species are sometimes contaminated with an ergot and cause paspalum staggers.

pas•pa•lum (pas′pə-ləm) any grass of the genus *Paspalum.*

pas•sage (pas′əj) 1. a channel. 2. the act of moving from one place to another. 3. discharge (def. 3). 4. introduction of infectious material into an experimental animal or culture medium, followed by recovery of the infectious agent. 5. the introduction of a catheter, probe, sound, or bougie through a natural channel such as the urethra.

blind p. successive transfer of infection through experimental animals, chick embryo, or tissue culture, when overt lesions of disease are not apparent, at least in the earlier members of the series.

false p. fistula.

serial p. the successive transfer of a virus or other infectious agent through a series of experimental animals, tissue culture, or synthetic media, with growth occurring in each medium. The process is usually used to attenuate a pathogenic agent.

Pas•sa•vant bar (cushion, pad, ridge) (pahs′ə-vahnt) [Philip Gustav *Passavant*, German surgeon, 1815–1893] crista palatopharyngea.

pas•sen•ger (pas′ən-jər) the fetus or any of the fetal membranes during labor.

pas•ser (pas′ər) a person, animal, or object that conveys something from one place to another.

foil p. a pointed or forked instrument used to carry pellets of gold foil through an annealing flame or from the annealing tray to the prepared cavity for compaction. Called also *foil carrier.*

Pas•si•flo•ra (pas″ĭ-flo′rə) [L. *passio* passion + *flora*] the passion flowers, a genus of twining vines of the family Passifloraceae, having brightly colored flowers and found in tropical parts of the Americas. They contain cyanogenetic glycosides and have caused cyanide poisoning in livestock. *P. incarna′ta* is used medicinally for its sedative and anxiolytic properties.

pas•si•vate (pas′ĭ-vāt) to make the surface of a chemically reactive metal (base metal) less reactive by forming a stable surface reaction compound, usually a metallic oxide.

pas•si•va•tion (pas″ĭ-va′shən) 1. reduction of reactivity of the surface of a chemically reactive metal *(base metal).* 2. the process of making such a surface less reactive.

pas•sive (pas′iv) [L. *passivus*] neither spontaneous nor active; not produced by active efforts.

pas•siv•ism (pas′iv-iz-əm) a submissive attitude or behavior, particularly submission to the will of a sexual partner.

pas•siv•i•ty (pə-siv′ĭ-te) 1. in psychology, an unwillingness, inability, or other failure to take initiative or personal responsibility for routine life events. 2. in dentistry, the condition of rest assumed by the teeth, surrounding tissue, and denture when a removable partial denture is in place but not under masticatory pressure.

paste (pāst) [L. *pasta*] a semisolid preparation containing one or more drug substances, for topical application; the two classes comprise the fatty pastes, thick, stiff ointments that do not flow at body temperature, as well as those made from a single phase aqueous gel.

Ihle p. an ointment containing resorcinol, starch, and zinc oxide in white petrolatum.

Lassar p. zinc oxide and salicylic acid p.

Lassar plain zinc p. zinc oxide p.

zinc oxide p. [USP] a preparation of zinc oxide and starch in white petrolatum, used topically as an astringent and skin protectant; called also *Lassar plain zinc p.*

zinc oxide and salicylic acid p. [USP] a mixture of zinc oxide paste and salicylic acid, used topically as an astringent and local protective. Called also *Lassar p.*

pas•ter (pās′tər) the portion of a bifocal lens ground for near vision.

pas•tern (pas′tərn) the portion of a horse's foot just proximal to the hoof. See also under *bone* and *joint.*

Pas•teur (pahs-toor′) Louis, 1822–1895. French chemist, author of the germ theory of disease, and founder of microbiology, virology, and immunology. Pasteur is famous for disproving spontaneous generation and for his work in stereochemistry, lactic and alcoholic fermentation, microbiology and diseases of wine and beer, diseases of silkworms, anaerobiosis, virulent diseases (anthrax, chicken cholera), and preventive inoculation with attenuated microbes (especially against rabies). Pasteur's work enabled Joseph Lister to develop antiseptic surgery.

Pas•teur effect (reaction) (pahs-toor′) [L. *Pasteur*] see under *effect.*

Pas•teur•el•la (pas″tər-el′ə) [Louis *Pasteur*] a genus of gram-negative, ovoid to rod-shaped bacteria of the family Pasteurellaceae, consisting of nonmotile, fermentative, aerobic to microaerophilic or facultatively anaerobic organisms. Bipolar staining is common. They are parasitic on many species of mammals and birds, causing abscesses and septicemias in humans and respiratory and septic infections in sheep, cattle, and birds. The type species is *P. multoci′da.*

P. aero′genes a species incertae sedis that may cause abortion in pigs and wound infections in humans who have been bitten by infected pigs.

P. anatipes′tifer *Riemerella anatipestifer.*

P. haemoly′tica *Mannheimia haemolytica.*

P. multoci′da a species that is part of the normal flora of the mouth and respiratory tract of many species of mammals and birds; several different biovars and serovars are recognized. In animals it causes hemorrhagic septicemias, pneumonia, local abscesses, and intestinal disease. Human disease is usually from infection of a cat or dog bite or scratch, with localized swelling, abscesses, bronchiectasis, pneumonia, meningitis, and septicemia. See also *P. multocida pneumonia*, under *pneumonia.*

P. pneumotro′pica a species incertae sedis occurring normally and as an occasional pathogen in rodents, and sometimes infecting humans.

P. ure′ae *Actinobacillus ureae.*

Pas•teur•el•la•ceae (pas″tər-el-a′se-e) a family of facultatively anaerobic, nonmotile, gram-negative, coccoid to rod-shaped bacteria of the order Pasteurellales, occurring as parasites in mammals and birds. Organisms of medical interest are contained in the genera *Actinobacillus, Haemophilus, Mannheimia*, and *Pasteurella.*

Pas•teu•rel•la•les (pas″tər-el-a′lēz) an order of bacteria of the class Gammaproteobacteria, phylum Proteobacteria, created on the basis of 16S rRNA sequence analysis; it contains the single family Pasteurellaceae.

pas•teur•el•lo•sis (pas″tər-ə-lo′sis) infection by species of *Pasteurella.*

pneumonic p. infection of the lungs with *Pasteurella* species, usually *P. haemolytica* or *P. multocida.*

septicemic p. hemorrhagic septicemia.

pas•teur•iza•tion (pas″chər-ĭ-za′shən) [Louis *Pasteur*] the process of heating milk or other liquid or solid foods to a particular temperature for

a defined time, to destroy or inactivate microorganisms that would cause spoilage, while retaining the flavor and quality of the food.
cold p., irradiation p. the process of irradiating foods to achieve the effect of traditional pasteurization, but without the use of heat.

Pas•tia lines (sign) (pahs′te-ah) [Constantine Chessec *Pastia*, Romanian physician, 1883–1926] see under *line.*

pas•til (pas′til) pastille.

pas•tille (pas-tēl′) [Fr.] 1. a troche in which the active ingredient is incorporated in a mass of sweetened gum, glycerin, and gelatin base. 2. an aromatic mass to be burnt as a fumigant.

PAT paroxysmal atrial tachycardia; see *paroxysmal tachycardia*, under *tachycardia.*

Pa•tau syndrome (pah-tou′) [Klaus *Patau*, German-born American geneticist, 20th century] trisomy 13 syndrome.

Pat•a•nol (pat′ə-nol) trademark for a preparation of olopatadine hydrochloride.

patch (pach) [L. *pittacium;* Gr. *pittakion*] 1. any area that differs in color or texture from the surrounding surface and is not elevated above it; see also *macule* and *spot.* 2. a small piece of cloth or other material that covers part of another surface. 3. a macule more than 1 cm in diameter.
ash leaf p. see under *macule.*
birth control p. contraceptive p.
Bitot p's see under *spot.*
contraceptive p. a transdermal patch containing an estrogen (usually ethinyl estradiol) and a progestational agent. Called also *birth control p.*
cotton-wool p's see under *spot.*
herald p. the solitary lesion that precedes the general eruption in pityriasis rosea.
Hutchinson p. salmon p. (def. 1).
lance-ovate p. ash leaf macule.
MacCallum p. a sheet of granulation tissue in the myocardium or endocardium, formed by extensive confluence of Aschoff nodules in the myocardium in rheumatic fever.
mucous p. a flat, rounded, gray to white erosion covered by a soft membrane with an erythematous zone, usually on the oral mucosa but sometimes on the anogenital mucosa, in early active secondary syphilis. It contains vast numbers of treponemes and is therefore highly contagious.
Peyer p's noduli lymphoidei aggregati intestini tenuis.
salmon p. 1. a salmon-colored spot seen in the cornea in syphilis; called also *Hutchinson p.* 2. a skin-colored or pink nevus flammeus seen in neonates, usually on either the forehead or the nape of the neck; in most cases it fades completely in time. The one on the neck is popularly known as a stork bite. Called also *nevus simplex.*
shagreen p. a large connective tissue nevus, seen most often in children who have tuberous sclerosis complex; it consists of a skin-colored or pale, elevated, knobby plaque resembling shark or pig skin. The usual location is on the back, especially in the lumbosacral region. Called also *shagreen skin.*
smokers' p's nicotine stomatitis.
soldiers' p's milk spots (def. 1).
transdermal p. a type of transdermal delivery system by which a patch containing medication is placed on the skin so that the medication is gradually absorbed over time.

pa•tel•la (pə-tel′ə) [L., dim of *patera* a shallow dish] [TA] a triangular sesamoid bone, about 5 cm in diameter, situated at the front of the knee in the tendon of insertion of the quadriceps extensor femoris muscle. Called also *knee cap.* **patel′lar** *adj*
p. al′ta an abnormally high patella, the Insall-Salvati ratio being greater than 1.2; called also *high-riding p.*
p. ba′ja (bah′hah) slang term for p. infera.
p. biparti′ta, bipartite p. a patella that is divided into two parts.

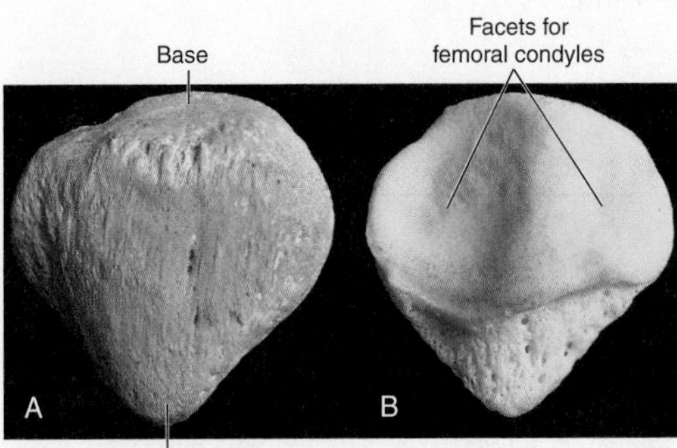

■ Patella. Left patella shown in anterior *(A)* and posterior *(B)* aspects.

p. cu′biti an anomalous sesamoid bone sometimes occurring over the extensor surface of the elbow joint.
floating p. a patella that is separated from the condyles by a large effusion in the knee.
high-riding p. p. alta.
p. in′fera an abnormally low patella, having an Insall-Salvati ratio of less than 1.0; called also *low-riding p.* and *p. baja.*
low-riding p. p. infera.
p. parti′ta a patella that is divided into two or more parts.
slipping p. a patella that is easily movable and readily dislocated.
p. triparti′ta, tripartite p. a patella that is divided into three parts.

pat•el•lal•gia (pat″əl-al′jə) pain in or adjacent to the patella.

pat•el•lec•to•my (pat″ə-lek′tə-me) [*patella* + *-ectomy*] excision or removal of the patella.

pat•el•li•form (pə-tel′ĭ-form) shaped like the patella.

pa•tel•lo•fem•o•ral (pə-tel″o-fem′ə-rəl) pertaining to the patella and the femur.

pat•en•cy (pa′tən-se) [L. *patens* open] the condition of being widely open.
probe p. of foramen ovale incomplete physical closure of the foramen ovale postnatally, although functional closure occurs, so that a probe may be passed between the atria in the adult. It occurs in 20 to 25 per cent of all hearts.

pat•ent (pa′tənt) [L. *patens*] 1. open, unobstructed, or not closed. 2. apparent, evident.

Pat•er•son syndrome (pat′ər-sən) [Donald Ross *Paterson*, Welsh laryngologist, 1863–1939] Plummer-Vinson syndrome.

Pat•er•son–Brown Kel•ly syndrome (pat′ər-sən broun kel′e) [D.R. *Paterson;* A. *Brown Kelly*, Scottish laryngologist, 1865–1941] Plummer-Vinson syndrome.

Pat•er•son-Kel•ly syndrome (pat′ər-sən kel′e) [D.R. *Paterson;* A. Brown *Kelly*] Plummer-Vinson syndrome.

Pa•tey operation (pa′te) [David Howard *Patey*, English surgeon, 1899–1977] see *modified radical mastectomy*, under *mastectomy.*

path (path) 1. a particular course that is followed, or a route that is ordinarily traversed. 2. pathway (defs. 1 and 2).
alvear p. see under *fasciculus.*
condyle p. the course followed by the mandibular condyle in the temporomandibular joint during the various movements of the mandible.
incisor p. the course followed by the incisal edges of the lower anterior teeth in movement of the mandible from the position of normal occlusion to that of edge-to-edge contact with opposing incisors.
p. of insertion the direction or path of a removable partial denture that permits the proper relation of the prosthesis to the hard and soft tissues on insertion, on removal, in function, and at rest. Called also *p. of removal.*
ionization p. the trail of ion pairs produced by ionizing radiation in its passage through matter; called also *ionization track.*
lateral condyle p. the path of the condyle in the glenoid fossa when a lateral mandibular movement is made.
milled-in p's 1. the contours carved by various mandibular movements into the occluding surface of an occlusion rim by teeth or studs placed in the opposing occlusion rim. The curves or contours may be carved into wax, modeling plastic, or plaster of Paris. 2. gliding movements of occlusion rims, which are composed of materials including abrasives.
occlusal p. the course followed by the occlusal surfaces of the lower teeth in movements of the mandible.
occlusal p., generated a registration of the paths of movement of the occlusal surfaces of mandibular teeth on a plastic or abrasive surface attached to the maxillary arch.
p. of removal p. of insertion.

path•er•gia (path-er′je-ə) pathergy.

path•er•gic (path′ər-jik) characterized by pathergy.

path•er•gy (path′ər-je) [*path-* + Gr. *ergon* work] 1. an abnormal reaction to an allergen, either a subnormal reaction or an excessive reaction. 2. the condition of being allergic to numerous antigens; polyvalent allergy.

path•find•er (path′find-ər) 1. an instrument for locating strictures of the urethra. 2. root canal probe.

path(o)- [Gr. *pathos* disease] a combining form denoting relationship to disease.

patho•anat•o•my (path″o-ə-nat′ə-me) anatomic pathology. **patho-anatom′ical** *adj*

patho•bi•ol•o•gy (path″o-bi-ol′ə-je) a branch of pathology that focuses on biological aspects such as structural and functional changes of organs.

path•ob•i•ont (path-ōb′-e-ont) an organism that is normally a harmless symbiont to another, but under certain conditions can become pathogenic.

patho•cli•sis (path″o-klis′is) a specific elemental sensitivity to specific toxins, or a specific affinity of certain toxins for certain systems of organs.

path•odon•tia (path″o-don′shə) dental pathology.

patho•for•mic (path″o-for′mik) [*patho-* + *form* + *-ic*] pertaining to the beginning of disease; said particularly of symptoms at the beginning of mental disorder.

patho•gen (path′o-jən) [*patho-* + *-gen*] any disease-producing agent or microorganism, such as a bacterium, fungus, protozoon, or virus.

patho•gen•e•sis (path″o-jen′ə-sis) [*patho-* + *genesis*] the development of morbid conditions or of disease; more specifically the cellular events and reactions and other pathologic mechanisms occurring in the development of disease. **pathogenet′ic** *adj*

drug p. the production of symptoms of disease by the use of drugs.

path•o•gen•ic (path-o-jen′ik) causing disease or morbid symptoms.

patho•ge•nic•i•ty (path″o-jə-nis′ĭ-te) the quality of producing or the ability to produce pathologic changes or disease.

path•og•e•ny (path-oj′ə-ne) pathogenesis.

pa•thog•no•mon•ic (path″og-no-mon′ik) [*patho-* + Gr. *gnōmonikos* fit to give judgment] specifically distinctive or characteristic of a disease or pathologic condition; a sign or symptom on which a diagnosis can be made.

path•og•no•my (pə-thog′nə-me) [*patho-* + Gr. *gnōmē* a means of knowing] the science of the signs and symptoms of disease.

path•og•nos•tic (path″og-nos′tik) pathognomonic.

pa•thog•ra•phy (pə-thog′rə-fe) [*patho-* + *-graphy*] a history or description of disease.

patho•log•ic (path″o-loj′ik) 1. indicative of or caused by a morbid condition. 2. pertaining to pathology.

patho•log•i•cal (path″o-loj′ĭ-kəl) pathologic.

pa•thol•o•gist (pə-thol′ə-jist) a specialist in pathology.

speech p., speech-language p. a person skilled and certified in speech pathology. Cf. *speech therapist.*

pa•thol•o•gy (pə-thol′ə-je) [*patho-* + *-logy*] 1. the branch of medicine that studies the essential nature of disease, especially the structural, biochemical, and functional changes in the cells, tissues, and organs of the body that cause or are caused by disease. 2. the structural and functional manifestations of disease.

anatomic p. the anatomical study of changes in the function, structure, or appearance of organs or tissues, including postmortem examinations and the study of biopsy specimens. Called also *morbid* or *pathological anatomy* and *pathoanatomy.*

cellular p. cytopathology.

clinical p. pathology applied to the solution of clinical problems, especially the use of laboratory methods in clinical diagnosis.

comparative p. pathology that makes comparisons between diseases of human beings and those of other animals.

dental p. the branch of pathology that treats dental changes in disease. Called also *pathodontia.* See also *oral p.*

experimental p. the study of artificially induced disease processes.

forensic p. a subspecialty of pathology concerned with the medicolegal examination of sudden, unexpected, or violent deaths; duties include the collection of medical evidence, the performance of autopsies to determine the cause and manner of death and, when necessary, the identification of unknown corpses.

functional p. the study of the changes of function due to morbid tissue changes.

general p. the branch of pathology that is concerned with the reactions of cells and tissues to abnormal stimuli and inherited defects that cause disease.

geographical p. the study and comparison of variations in morbidity and mortality in different geographic regions to determine the relationship between these variations and environmental conditions found in each region. Called also *geopathology.*

internal p. medical p.

medical p. the pathology of morbid processes that are not accessible to operative intervention. Cf. *surgical p.*

oral p. the branch of pathology that treats the structural and functional changes in cells, tissues, and organs of the oral cavity that cause or are caused by disease. See also *dental p.*

special p. the study of the pathology of particular diseases or organs.

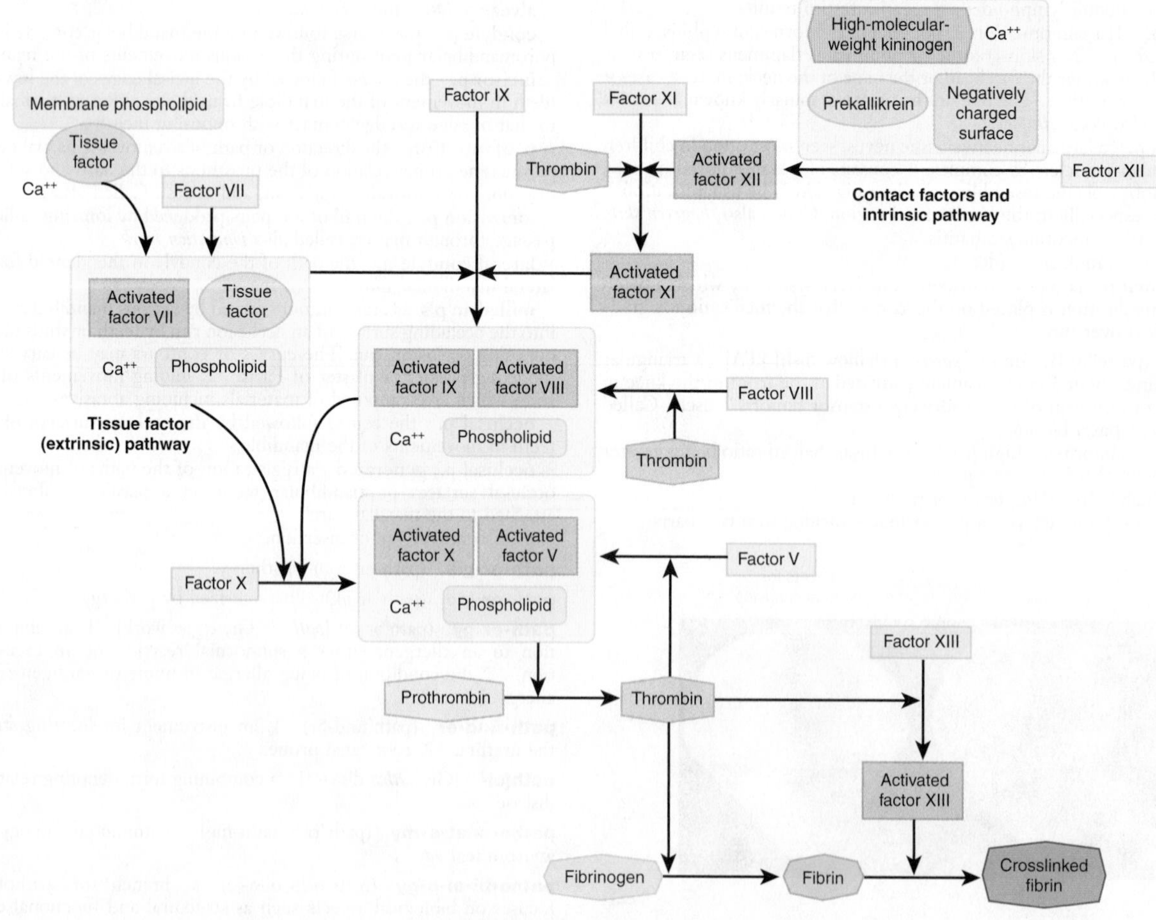

■ Coagulation pathway overview.

speech p., speech-language p. a field of the health sciences dealing with the evaluation of speech, language, and voice disorders and the rehabilitation of patients with such disorders not amenable to medical or surgical treatment.

surgical p. the pathology of disease processes that are surgically accessible for diagnosis or treatment.

systemic p. the branch of pathology that is concerned with the changes in specialized organs and tissues that are responsible for disease.

patho•mi•me•sis (path″o-mi-me′sis) [*patho-* + *mimesis*] mimicry of a disease or disorder, particularly malingering.

patho•mim•ic•ry (path″o-mim′ĭ-kre) pathomimesis.

patho•mor•phism (path″o-mor′fiz-əm) abnormal morphology.

patho•neu•ro•sis (path″o-noo̅-ro′sis) hysterical symptoms due to a chronic disease process.

patho•no•mia (path″o-no′me-ə) [*patho-* + *nom-* + *-ia*] the sum of knowledge regarding the laws of disease.

pa•thon•o•my (pə-thon′ə-me) pathonomia.

patho•pho•bia (path″o-fo′be-ə) [*patho-* + *-phobia*] nosophobia.

patho•phys•i•ol•o•gy (path″o-fiz″e-ol′ə-je) the physiology of disordered function.

patho•poi•e•sis (path″o-poi-e′sis) [*patho-* + *-poiesis*] 1. the causation of disease. 2. the tendency of an individual to become diseased.

patho•psy•chol•o•gy (path″o-si-kol′ə-je) [*patho-* + *psychology*] the psychology of mental disease.

patho•psy•cho•sis (path″o-si-ko′sis) a psychosis arising from organic disease, such as brain tumor, encephalitis, etc.

patho•type (path′o-tīp) pathovar.

patho•var (path′o-vahr, path′o-var) a variant strain of a bacterial species, differentiated by reactions in one or more hosts. Called also *pathotype*.

path•way (path′wa) 1. a course, especially one followed in the attainment of a specific end. Called also *path*. 2. the nerve structures through which an impulse passes between groups of nerve cells or between the central nervous system and an organ or muscle; see also *tract*. 3. metabolic p.

accessory p., accessory conduction p. myocardial fibers that propagate the atrial contraction impulse to the ventricles but are not a part of the normal atrioventricular conducting system; impulses conducted over such a pathway can cause preexcitation (q.v.). See also *Kent bundle*, under *bundle*; *Mahaim fibers*, under *fiber*; and *atriohisian tracts*, under *tract*.

afferent p. the nerve structures through which an impulse, especially a sensory impression, is conducted to the cerebral cortex; see also *ascending tract* and *sensory tract*, under *tract*.

alternative complement p. a pathway of complement activation initiated by a variety of factors other than those initiating the classical complement pathway, including IgA immune complexes, bacterial endotoxins, microbial polysaccharides, and cell walls. It does not include factors C1, C2, and C4 of the classical complement pathway but does include factors B and D and properdin. See illustration at *complement*. The term is sometimes used to denote specifically those steps occurring prior to initiation of formation of the membrane attack complex (C5–C9).

amphibolic p. a group of metabolic reactions with a dual function, providing small metabolites for further catabolism to end products or for use as precursors in synthetic, anabolic reactions. The tricarboxylic acid cycle is an example. See also *anabolism* and *catabolism*.

atrioventricular p. Kent bundle.

auditory p. any of the various sensory pathways for hearing, conducting impulses between the organ of Corti and the cerebral cortex.

biosynthetic p. the sequence of enzymatic steps in the synthesis of a specific end product in a living organism.

central auditory p. the auditory pathway in the central nervous system that runs through the central tract of the auditory nerve.

circus p. the ring or circuit traversed by an excitatory wavefront exhibiting circus movement; see also *reentry*.

classical complement p. the enzymatic cascade containing all the components of complement, C1 through C9, primarily activated by the binding of C1 to antigen-antibody complexes containing IgM, IgG1, IgG2, or IgG3. See illustration at *complement*. The term is sometimes used to denote specifically those steps occurring prior to initiation of formation of the membrane attack complex (C5–C9).

clinical p. a maplike diagram showing the steps a patient should go through for treatment of a given condition.

coagulation p's see *common p. of coagulation*, *extrinsic p. of coagulation*, and *intrinsic p. of coagulation*.

common p. of coagulation the steps in the mechanism of coagulation from the activation of factor X through the conversion of fibrinogen to fibrin. See illustration. See also *intrinsic p. of coagulation* and *extrinsic p. of coagulation*.

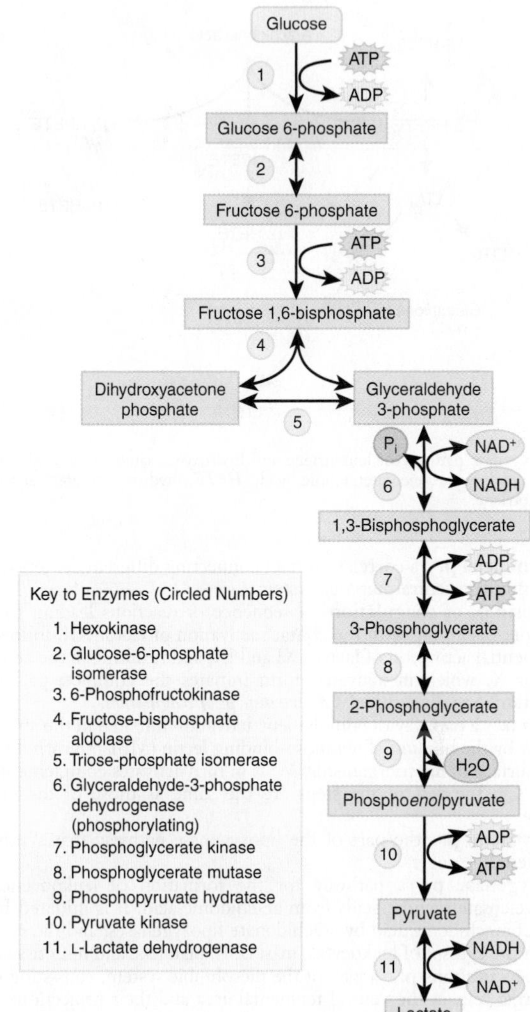

■ Embden-Meyerhof pathway of glucose metabolism, showing also the conversion of pyruvate to lactate.

concealed accessory p. an accessory pathway that conducts impulses unidirectionally from the ventricles to the atria; thus it is not associated with preexcitation but can participate in supraventricular tachycardia.

dentato-rubro-olivary p. Guillain-Mollaret triangle.

efferent p. the nerve structures through which an impulse passes away from the brain, especially for the innervation of muscles, effector organs, or glands; see also *descending tract* and *motor tract*, under *tract*.

Embden-Meyerhof p. (of glucose metabolism), the series of enzymatic reactions in the anaerobic conversion of glucose to lactic acid, resulting in energy in the form of adenosine triphosphate (ATP).

Embden-Meyerhof-Parnas p. Embden-Meyerhof p.

Entner-Doudoroff p. a series of enzymatic reactions in bacteria that convert glucose to pyruvate by way of the intermediate 2-keto-3-deoxy-6-phosphogluconate, forming ATP. It is the major pathway of glucose metabolism in certain strains of *Pseudomonas*.

extrinsic p. of coagulation the mechanism that produces fibrin following tissue injury, beginning with formation of an activated complex between tissue factor and activated factor VII and leading to activation of factor X, which induces the reactions of the common pathway of coagulation. See illustration. Cf. *intrinsic p. of coagulation*.

final common p. a motor pathway consisting of the motor neurons by which nerve impulses from many central sources pass to a muscle or gland in the periphery.

gustatory p. any of the sensory pathways for taste, conducting impulses from the taste buds through the thalamus to the cerebral cortex.

hexosamine p., hexosamine biosynthetic p. a series of enzymatic reactions by which a small amount of glucose is diverted away from the Embden-Meyerhof pathway to form uridine compounds such as uridine-diphosphate-*N*-acetylglucosamine. This is one cause of hyperglycemia-induced and fat-induced insulin resistance and aids formation of compounds such as proteoglycan and *O*-linked glycoproteins.

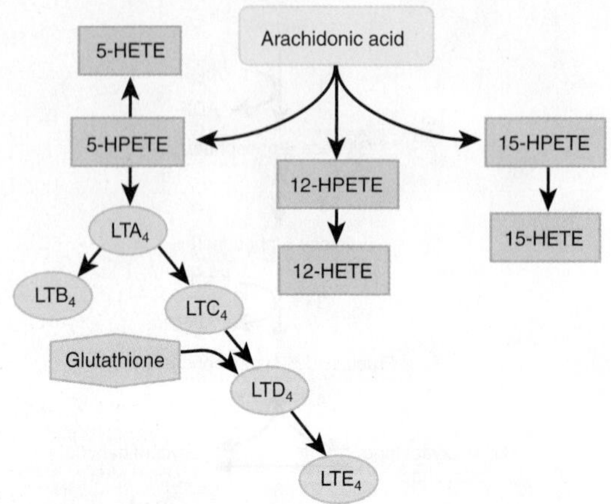

■ Lipoxygenase pathway of leukotriene and hydroxyeicosatetraenoic acid synthesis. *HPETE,* hydroperoxyeicosatetraenoic acid; *HETE,* hydroxyeicosatetraenoic acid; *LT,* leukotriene.

internuncial p. a correlation tract connecting different centers or neurons within the central nervous system.
intrinsic p. of coagulation a sequence of reactions leading to fibrin formation, beginning with the contact activation of factor XII, followed by the sequential activation of factors XI and IX, and resulting in the activation of factor X, which in activated form initiates the common pathway of coagulation. See illustration. Cf. *extrinsic p. of coagulation.*
lectin p. a pathway of complement activation initiated in the absence of antibody by the binding of mannose-binding lectin (MBL) to carbohydrates on the surface of microorganisms. MBL in turn activates complement component C4; the rest of the steps are the same as those of the classical pathway.
leukotriene p. the part of the lipoxygenase pathway that synthesizes leukotriene.
lipoxygenase p. a pathway for the formation of leukotrienes and hydroxyeicosatetraenoic acids from arachidonic acid. It is initiated by oxidation of arachidonic acid by arachidonate lipoxygenases, and the reactions occur in the cytosol of leukocytes, mast cells, platelets, and lung tissue cells.
mesoaccumbens p. a part of the mesolimbic system, consisting of dopaminergic cells in the ventral tegmental area and their projections to the nucleus accumbens; important in reward and motivation.
metabolic p. a series of enzymatic reactions that converts one biological material to another.
motor p. an efferent pathway conducting impulses from the central nervous system to a muscle; see also under *tract.*
olfactory p. the sensory pathway for smell, conducting impulses from the osmoreceptors to the cerebral cortex by way of the olfactory nerves and olfactory tract.
optic p. visual p.
pentose phosphate p. a major branching of the Embden-Meyerhof pathway of carbohydrate metabolism: a pathway of hexose oxidation in which glucose-6-phosphate undergoes two successive oxidations by NADP, the final one being an oxidative decarboxylation to form a pentose phosphate. Called also *phosphogluconate p., hexose monophosphate shunt,* and *pentose shunt.*
perforant p., perforating p. a pathway of fibers originating in the lateral part of the entorhinal area, perforating the subiculum of the hippocampus, and running into the stratum moleculare of the hippocampus, where these fibers synapse with others that go to the dentate gyrus. Called also *perforating fasciculus.*
phosphogluconate p. pentose phosphate p.
properdin p. former name for *alternative complement p.;* see *complement.*
reentrant p. the pathway over which over which an impulse is conducted in reentry (q.v); see also *reentrant mechanism,* under *mechanism.*
sensory p. an afferent pathway that conducts impulses from the receptors in the sense organs to one of the primary receiving areas of the cerebral cortex; see also under *tract.*
visual p. the sensory pathway for sight, conducting impulses from the photoreceptors to the cerebral cortex by way of the optic nerve, optic tract, and optic radiation.

-pathy [Gr. *-patheia,* from *pathos* feeling, disease] a word termination denoting *(a)* a feeling, *(b)* a disease, *(c)* a system of treating disease.

pa•tient (pa′shənt) [L. *patiens*] a person who is ill or who is undergoing treatment for disease.

Pat•rick test (sign) (pat′rik) [Hugh Talbot *Patrick,* American neurologist, 1860–1938] see under *test.*

pat•ri•cli•nous (pat″rĭ-kli′nəs) patroclinous.

pa•tri•lin•e•al (pat″rĭ-lin′e-əl) [L. *pater* father + *linea* line] descended through the male line.

pat•ro•cli•nous (pat″ro-kli′nəs) [Gr. *patēr* father + *klinein* to incline] inheriting or inherited from the father; having characters inherited from the father. Cf. *matroclinous.*

pat•ten (pat′ən) a metallic framework fitted to the base of a shoe to equalize the length of the lower limbs.

pat•tern (pat′ərn) 1. a design to be followed or a device to be used in the construction or fabrication of something. 2. the particular design or arrangement of figures. 3. a characteristic set of traits or actions, as behavior patterns.
action p., fixed action p. a genetically determined sequence of stereotyped acts elicited by specific stimuli and peculiar to a species, such as a courting dance.
full interference p. an interference pattern in which all the motor unit action potentials overlap with others so that none can be measured individually.
interference p. electrical activity in a muscle recorded during maximal voluntary contraction; since a large number of activated motor units are firing asynchronously, some or all of their action potentials overlap (interfere with each other on the recording) and cannot be measured separately. Cf. *full interference p., reduced interference p.,* and *discrete activity.*
occlusal p. the form or design of the occluding surfaces of a tooth or teeth; these forms may be based upon natural or modified anatomic or nonanatomic concepts of teeth.
recruitment p. a description of the sequence of recruitment in a muscle; see also *recruitment frequency* and *recruitment rate.*
reduced interference p. an interference pattern in which only some of the motor unit action potentials overlap each other.
wax p. a reproduction of missing tooth structure or a dental appliance made from casting wax, from which the outline of the mold is made for the casting of a restoration or an appliance.

pat•u•lin (pat′u-lin) a toxic and carcinogenic antibiotic derived from cultures of various fungi, especially *Aspergillus* and *Penicillium;* it causes tremor, paralysis, and death in animals that eat contaminated grain products. Called also *penicidin.*

pat•u•lous (pat′u-ləs) [L. *patulus*] spreading widely apart; open; distended.

Pau•chet procedure (po-sha′) [Victor *Pauchet,* French surgeon, 1869–1936] see under *procedure.*

pauci- [L. *paucus* few] a combining form denoting few. Cf. *olig(o)-.*

pau•ci•ar•thri•tis (paw″se-ahr-thri′tis) oligoarthritis.

pau•ci•ar•tic•u•lar (paw″se-ahr-tik′u-lər) [*pauci-* + *articular*] pertaining to or involving only a few joints.

pau•ci•bac•il•lary (paw″sĭ-bas′ĭ-lar″e) containing just a few bacilli; see *leprosy.*

pau•ci•syn•ap•tic (paw″se-sin-ap′tik) [*pauci-* + *synaptic*] oligosynaptic.

Paul-Bun•nell test (pawl′ bə-nel′) [John Rodman *Paul,* American physician, 1893–1971; Walls Willard *Bunnell,* American physician, 1902–1966] see under *test.*

Paul-Bun•nell-Da•vid•sohn test (pawl′ bə-nel′ da′vid-son) [J.R. *Paul;* W.W. *Bunnell;* Israel *Davidsohn,* American pathologist, 1895–1979] see under *test.*

Paul•li•nia (paw-lin′e-ə) [Simon *Paulli,* Danish botanist, 1603–1680] a genus of woody American vines, occurring chiefly in the tropics and including *P. cupa′na,* or guarana, which is used medicinally.

paunch (pawnch) rumen.

pause (pawz) [Gr. *pauein* to stop] an interruption, or rest.
compensatory p. the pause in impulse generation occurring after an extrasystole, designated as *full* if the sinus node is not reset and the total length of the aberrant plus the following cycle is equivalent to that of two normal cycles, or *incomplete, less than full,* or *noncompensatory* if the sinus node is reset and the normal cycle length disrupted.
noncompensatory p. see *compensatory p.*
sinus p. a transient interruption in the sinus rhythm, of a duration that is not an exact multiple of the normal cardiac cycle. See also *sinus arrest,* under *arrest.*
ventricular p. a momentary delay in rhythmicity in ventricular tachycardia.

Pau•tri•er microabscess (abscess) (po-tre-a′) [Lucien Marius Adolphe *Pautrier,* French dermatologist, 1876–1959] see under *microabscess.*

pave•ment•ing (pāv′mənt-ing) adhesion of leukocytes to the lining endothelium of the blood vessels of an injured part, which occurs as the circulation slows down within the vessels in response to inflammation.

Pa•vet•ta (pə-vet′ə) a genus of shrubs found in southern Africa; various species are poisonous to sheep and cattle, causing gousiekte.

pa•vil•ion (pə-vil′yən) [L. *papilio* butterfly, tent] a dilated or flaring expansion at the end of a passage.

pav•ing (pa′ving) the act or process of laying a hard smooth surface to bear traffic, or the surface so laid.

crazy p. by extension from the masonry term describing paving covered by decorative fine cracks, the appearance of lung tissue on computed tomography in pulmonary alveolar proteinosis or one of several types of pneumonia or pneumonitis.

Pav•lik harness (pahv′lik) [Arnold *Pavlik*, Czech orthopedic surgeon, 1902–1962] see under *harness*.

Pav•lov pouch, stomach (pahv′lof) [Ivan Petrovich *Pavlov*, Russian physiologist, experimental psychologist, and Nobel prize winner, 1849–1936] see under *pouch* and *stomach*.

pav•lov•i•an (pav-lov′e-ən) named for I.P. *Pavlov*.

pa•vor (pa′vor) [L.] terror.

p. diur′nus [L. "day terrors"] attacks of anxiety in children occurring during the afternoon nap.

p. noctur′nus [L. "night terrors"] a sleep disturbance usually occurring in children and characterized by extreme anxiety occurring shortly after sleep onset, with fear and signs of autonomic arousal, inability to be comforted, poor recall of any dream, and later amnesia for the event. Repeated occurrences are called *sleep terror disorder*.

Pav•u•lon (pav′u-lon) trademark for a preparation of pancuronium bromide.

paw (paw) the foot of an animal that is equipped with claws or nails, especially that of a digitigrade or carnivorous animal.

monkey p. see under *hand*.

PAWP pulmonary artery wedge pressure.

paw•paw (paw′paw) 1. papaw (def. 3). 2. papaw (def. 4).

Pax•il (pak′sil) trademark for preparations of paroxetine hydrochloride.

pax•il•lin (pak-sil′in) a cytoskeletal protein, found in focal adhesions and in skeletal and smooth muscle, that links integrins to signaling proteins.

Pax•il•lus (pak-sil′əs) a genus of mushrooms of the family Agaricaceae. *P. involu′tus* is considered edible but can cause gastroenteritis and in some individuals causes systemic reactions including syncope, hemoglobinuria, and decreased haptoglobins in the blood.

Payr clamp, disease (pīr) [Erwin *Payr*, German surgeon, 1871–1946] see under *clamp* and *disease*.

PB *Pharmacopoeia Britannica*.

Pb lead[1] (L. *plum′bum*).

PBB polybrominated biphenyl.

PBG porphobilinogen.

PBI protein-bound iodine.

PBPC peripheral blood progenitor cells.

PBZ trademark for preparations of tripelennamine citrate and tripelennamine hydrochloride.

PC phosphocreatine; sometimes used to designate phosphatidylcholine.

p.c. [L.] post ci′bum (after meals).

PCA passive cutaneous anaphylaxis.

PCB polychlorinated biphenyl.

PcB near point of convergence.

PCC prothrombin complex concentrate.

PCD pterin-4α-carbinolamine dehydratase; see *4a-hydroxytetrahydrobiopterin dehydratase*.

PCE 1. abbreviation for pseudocholinesterase; see *cholinesterase*. 2. trademark for a preparation of erythromycin.

PCEC, PCECV purified chick embryo cell (vaccine).

PCG phonocardiogram.

PCI percutaneous coronary intervention.

pCi picocurie.

Pco_2 the partial pressure of carbon dioxide in the blood; also written P_{co_2}.

PCOS polycystic ovary syndrome.

PCP phencyclidine hydrochloride; pneumocystis pneumonia (formerly *Pneumocystis carinii* pneumonia).

PCR polymerase chain reaction; protein catabolic rate.

PCT porphyria cutanea tarda.

PCV packed-cell volume; pneumococcal 7-valent conjugate vaccine.

PCV7 pneumococcal 7-valent conjugate vaccine.

PCWP pulmonary capillary wedge pressure.

PD prism diopter; interpupillary distance; peritoneal dialysis.

Pd palladium.

PDA patent ductus arteriosus; posterior descending (coronary) artery (ramus interventricularis posterior arteriae coronariae dextrae, q.v.).

PDT photodynamic therapy.

PE phosphatidylethanolamine; phycoerythrin; pulmonary embolism.

PEA pulseless electrical activity.

pea (pe) [Gr. *pisos*] 1. the leguminous vine *Pisum sativum*. 2. the edible seed of *P. sativum*. 3. any of numerous other leguminous vines resembling *P. sativum*. 4. the edible seed of one of these other leguminous vines.

rosary p. 1. *Abrus precatorius*. 2. jequirity bean, so called because it is sometimes used to make rosary beads.

peak (pēk) the top or upper limit of a graphic tracing or of any variable.

Bragg p. a peak in the Bragg curve reflecting a sharp increase in the intensity of ionization produced by an ionizing particle just before its velocity falls to zero.

kilovolts p. (kVp) the highest kilovoltage used in producing a radiograph.

Pé•an clamp (forceps) (pa-ah′) [Jules Émile *Péan*, French surgeon, 1830–1898] see under *clamp*.

pea•nut (pe′nut) 1. *Arachis hypogaea*. 2. the edible tuber of *A. hypogaea*, the source of peanut oil.

pearl (purl) 1. a small rounded mass or body. 2. a rounded mass of tough sputum as seen in the early stages of an attack of bronchial asthma. 3. a small medicated granule, or a glass globule with a single dose of volatile medicine, as amyl nitrite.

Bohn p's see under *nodule*.

Elschnig p's see under *body*.

enamel p. enameloma.

epidermic p's epithelial p's (def. 1).

epithelial p's 1. small cystlike formations along the midline of the hard palate of a newborn, resulting from blockage of ducts from mucous glands; they normally clear up within a few weeks. 2. rounded concentric masses of epithelial cells and keratin found in certain squamous cell carcinomas.

Epstein p's a type of milium sometimes found on the sides of the raphe of the hard palate of the newborn.

gouty p. a sodium urate concretion on the cartilage of the ear in persons with gout.

Laënnec p's soft casts of the smaller bronchial tubes expectorated in bronchial asthma. Cf. *Curschmann spirals*.

PEARS porcine epidemic abortion and respiratory syndrome.

Pear•son correlation coefficient (pēr′sən) [Karl *Pearson*, British statistician, 1857–1936] see under *coefficient*.

Pear•son syndrome (pēr′sən) [H.A. *Pearson*, American physician, 20th century] see under *syndrome*.

peau (po) [Fr.] skin.

p. d'orange (do-rahj′) ["orange skin"] a dimpled condition of the skin, resembling that of an orange, often seen overlying carcinoma of the breast.

peb•ble (peb′əl) colorless, transparent rock crystal from which lenses are sometimes cut.

pé•brine (pa-brēn′) [Fr.] an infectious protozoal disease of silkworms caused by *Nosema bombycis*. Cf. *nosema disease*.

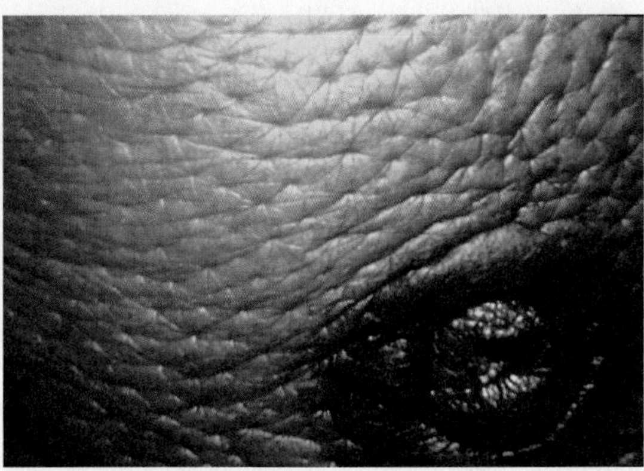

■ Peau d'orange.

pec·ca·ti·pho·bia (pek″ə-tĭ-fo′be-ə) [L. *peccata* sins + *-phobia*] irrational fear of sinning.

pecil(o)- for words beginning thus, see those beginning *poikil(o)-*.

Pec·quet cistern (reservoir), duct (pĕ-ka′) [Jean *Pecquet*, French anatomist, 1622–1674] see *cisterna chyli* and *ductus thoracicus.*

pec·ten (pek′tən) pl. *pec′tines* [L.] 1. a comb; applied to certain anatomical structures because of a fancied resemblance to a comb. 2. p. analis. 3. a pleated projection of choroid into the vitreous in the eye of birds, extending forward from the optic disk.

anal p., p. of anal canal, p. ana′lis [TA] the corrugated epithelium within the anal transitional zone between the pectinate line and the anocutaneous line; called also *pecten.*

p. os′sis pu′bis [TA] the anterior border of the superior ramus of the pubis, beginning at the pubic tubercle and continuing to the iliopubic eminence; called also *pectineal line.*

pec·te·nine (pek′tə-nin) a poisonous alkaloidal compound from a Mexican cactus, *Cereus pecten.*

pec·te·ni·tis (pek″tə-ni′tis) inflammation of the anal pecten.

pec·te·no·sis (pek″tə-no′sis) stenosis of the anal canal caused by a rigid, inelastic ring of tissue of variable width and thickness, between the anal groove and anal crypts, producing bleeding, irritation, and pain on defecation.

pec·te·not·o·my (pek″tə-not′ə-me) [*pecten* + *-tomy*] surgical correction of pectenosis by incision of the ring of tissue causing it.

pec·tic (pek′tik) relating to pectin.

pec·tic ac·id (pek′tik) a complex acid occurring in fruits, containing partially demethylated polymeric galacturonic acids.

pec·tin (pek′tin) [Gr. *pēktos* congealed] 1. a polymer of sugar acids of fruit that forms gels with sugar at the proper pH. 2. [USP] a purified preparation obtained from the acid extract of the inner portion of the rind of citrus fruits or from apple pomace, consisting chiefly of partially methoxylated polygalacturonic acids; used in the treatment of diarrhea, and as a thickening and emulsifying agent in pharmaceutical preparations.

pec·ti·nate (pek′tĭ-nāt) shaped like a comb.

pec·tin·e·al (pek-tin′e-əl, pek″tĭ-ne′əl) pertaining to the os pubis.

pec·ti·nes (pek′tĭ-nēs) [L.] plural of *pecten.*

pec·tin·i·form (pek-tin′ĭ-form) comb-shaped.

pec·ti·za·tion (pek″tĭ-za′shən) [Gr. *pēktikos* curdling] the process of changing to a gel or coagulate.

Pec·to·bac·te·ri·um (pek″to-bak-tēr′e-əm) a genus of gram-negative, facultatively anaerobic, rod-shaped bacteria of the family Enterobacteriaceae, made up of plant pathogens formerly classified in the genus *Erwinia.* The organisms are not human pathogens but have been occasionally isolated from clinical specimens. The type species is *P. caroto′vorum.*

P. caroto′vorum a species that causes soft spots in carrots, potatoes, and other plants; not found in clinical specimens; asparaginase derived from cultures of *P. carotovora* is used as an antineoplastic. Cf *crisantaspase.* Formerly called *Erwinia carotovora.*

pec·to·lyt·ic (pek″to-lit′ik) [*pectin* + *-lytic*] capable of causing the digestion of pectin.

pec·to·ra (pek′tə-rə) [L.] plural of *pectus.*

pec·to·ral (pek′tər-əl) [L. *pectoralis*] thoracic.

pec·to·ral·gia (pek″tə-ral′jə) [*pectoral* + *-algia*] 1. pain in the pectoral muscles; called also *stethalgia, thoracalgia,* and *thoracodynia.* 2. thoracalgia (def. 1).

pec·to·ra·lis (pek″tə-ra′lis, -ral′is) [L., from *pectus,* q.v.] thoracic.

pec·to·ril·o·quy (pek″tə-ril′ə-kwe) [*pectus* + L. *loqui* to speak] voice sounds of increased resonance heard through the chest wall; cf. *egophony* and *bronchophony.* Called also *pectorophony.*

aphonic p. the sound of the whispered voice transmitted through a serous, but not through a purulent, exudate within the pleura. Called also *Baccelli sign.*

whispered p., whispering p. the transmission of the sound of whispered words through the walls of the chest, heard upon auscultation and indicating an area of consolidation. Called also *whispered bronchophony* or *voice.*

pec·to·roph·o·ny (pek″tə-rof′ə-ne) pectoriloquy.

pec·tose (pek′tōs) protopectin.

pec·tous (pek′təs) pertaining to, composed of, or resembling pectin; having a firm, jelly-like consistence.

pec·tun·cu·lus (pek-tung′ku-ləs) [L., dim of *pecten* comb] one of the small longitudinal ridges on the aqueduct of Sylvius.

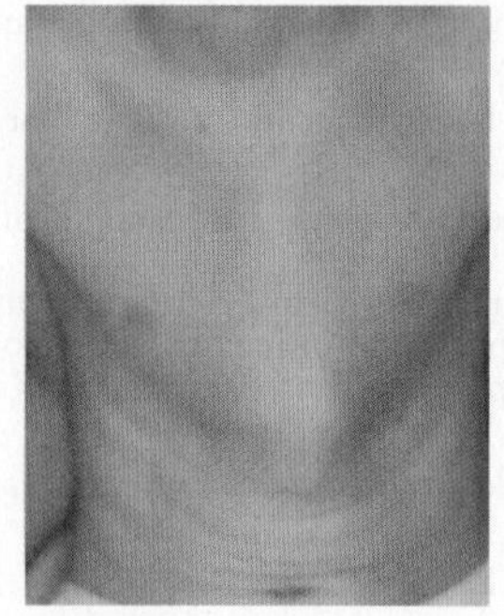

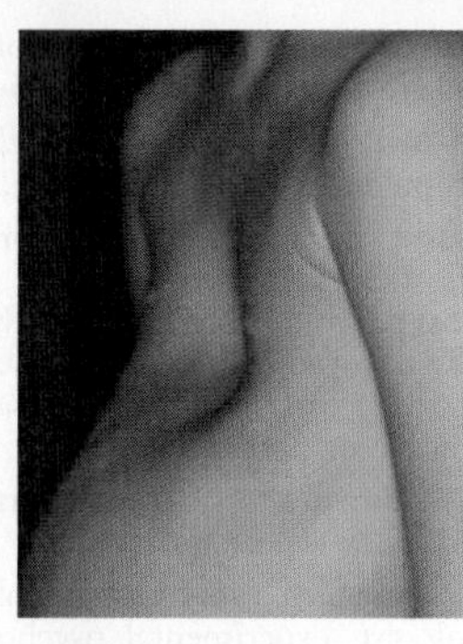

■ *(A),* Pectus carinatum; *(B),* pectus excavatum.

pec·tus (pek′təs) gen. *pec′toris* pl. *pec′tora* [L.] [TA] the front of the chest.

p. carina′tum [L. "keeled breast"] a group of deformities of the anterior chest wall characterized by convex protrusion of the sternum and of the costal cartilages on one or both sides; it is classified by site of greatest prominence as *chondrogladiolar* (sternum and lower costal cartilages) or *chondromanubrial* (sternum and upper costal cartilages). See illustration. Called also *chicken breast, pigeon breast, keeled chest,* and *pigeon chest.*

p. excava′tum [L. "hollowed breast"] a chest in which there is a funnel-shaped depression in the middle of the anterior thoracic wall, with the deepest part in the sternum. Called also *foveated* or *funnel chest, funnel breast, p. recurvatum,* and *koilosternia.* See illustration.

p. gallina′tum p. carinatum.

p. recurva′tum p. excavatum.

ped·al (ped′əl) [L. *pedalis; pes* foot] pertaining to the foot or feet.

pe·dar·throc·a·ce (pe″dahr-throk′ə-se) [*ped-*[1] + *arthrocace*] caries of the joints in children.

pe·da·tro·phia (pe″də-tro′fe-ə) [*ped-*[1] + *atrophia*] marasmus.

ped·er·ast (ped′ər-ast) one who practices pederasty.

ped·er·as·ty (ped′ər-as″te) [*ped-*[1] + Gr. *erastēs* lover] anal intercourse between a man and a boy.

ped·er·in (ped′ər-in) a crystalline toxin isolated from blister beetles of the genus *Paederus.*

pe·des (pe′dēz) [L.] plural of *pes.*

pedi- see *ped(o)-*[2].

pedi·al·gia (ped″e-al′jə) [*pedi-* + *-algia*] podalgia.

Pe·di·a·pred (pēd′e-ə-pred″) trademark for a preparation of prednisolone sodium phosphate.

Pe·di·a·rix (pe′de-ə-riks) trademark for a combination preparation of hepatitis B vaccine (recombinant), diphtheria and tetanus toxoids and acellular pertussis (DTaP) vaccine, and poliovirus vaccine inactivated.

Pe·di·a·zole (pe′de-ə-zōl) trademark for a combination preparation of erythromycin ethylsuccinate and sulfisoxazole acetyl.

pe·di·at·ric (pe″de-at′rik) pertaining to the health of children.

pe·di·a·tri·cian (pe″de-ə-trĭ′shən) a physician who specializes in pediatrics.

pe·di·at·rics (pe″de-at′riks) [*ped-*[1] + *-iatrics*] the branch of medicine that deals with the child, development and care of children, and the nature and treatment of diseases of children.

pe·di·at·rist (pe″de-at′rist) pediatrician.

pe·di·at·ry (pe′de-at″re) pediatrics.

ped·i·cel (ped′ĭ-sel) a footlike part, especially any of the secondary processes of a podocyte that interdigitate with those of other podocytes in a renal corpuscle. Called also *foot process.*

ped·i·cel·la·ria (ped″ĭ-sə-lar′e-ə) pl. *pedicella′riae.* A modified spine with a flexible head, seen in sea urchins and related animals, used in grooming, food getting, and self-defense and the principal site of venom glands.

ped·i·cel·late (ped′ĭ-sə-lāt″) pedunculated.

ped·i·cel·lat·ed (ped′ĭ-sə-lāt″əd) pedunculated.

ped·i·cel·la·tion (ped″ĭ-sə-la′shən) pediculation.

ped·i·cle (ped′ĭ-kəl) [L. *pediculus* little foot] a footlike, stemlike, or narrow basal part or structure, as the stalk by which a nonsessile tumor is attached to normal tissue, or the narrow strip of flap tissue through which it receives its blood supply. Called also *pediculus.*

cone p. the thick triangular or club-shaped ending of a retinal cone cell, which synapses with the bipolar and horizontal cells in the outer plexiform layer.

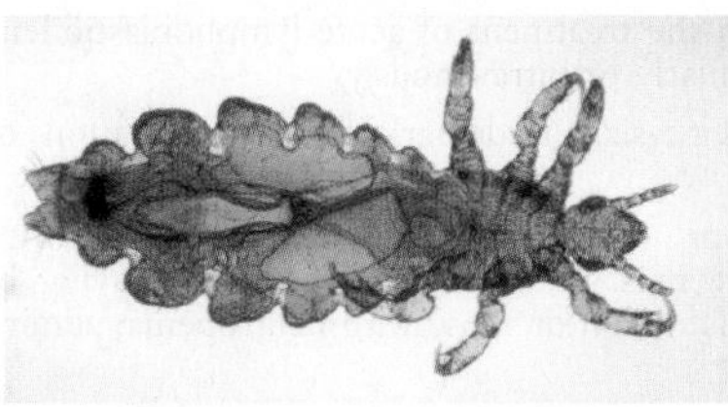

■ *Pediculus humanus capitis;* dorsal view of adult female containing eggs or nits.

p. of lung radix pulmonis.
p. of vertebral arch pediculus arcus vertebrae.

ped•i•cled (ped′ĭ-kəld) having a pedicle.

pe•dic•u•lar (pə-dik′u-lər) pertaining to or caused by lice.

pe•dic•u•late (pə-dik′u-lāt) having a pedicle.

pe•dic•u•la•tion (pə-dik″u-la′shən) the formation of a pedicle; called also *pedicellation.*

pe•dic•u•li (pə-dik′u-li) plural of *pediculus.*

pe•dic•u•li•ci•dal (pə-dik″u-lĭ-si′dəl) destroying lice.

pe•dic•u•li•cide (pə-dik′u-lĭ-sīd) [*pediculus* + *-cide*] an agent that destroys lice.

Ped•i•cu•li•dae (ped″ĭ-ku′lĭ-de) a family of lice (order Anoplura) that includes the genera *Pediculus* and *Phthirus,* which feed on human blood.

pe•dic•u•lo•sis (pə-dik″u-lo′sis) [*pediculus* + *-osis*] infestation with lice of the family Pediculidae, especially infestation with *Pediculus humanus.*
p. ca′pitis infestation of the hair of the head by lice.
p. cor′poris infestation of the body by lice.
p. inguina′lis p. pubis.
p. palpebra′rum infestation of the eyelashes by lice.
p. pu′bis infestation with the pubic louse *Phthirus pubis;* called also *phthiriasis pubis.*

pe•dic•u•lous (pə-dik′u-ləs) infested with lice.

Pe•dic•u•lus (pə-dik′u-ləs) a genus of sucking lice (order Anoplura), of the family Pediculidae.
P. huma′nus a species that feeds on human blood, is a major vector of epidemic typhus, trench fever, and relapsing fever, and causes skin reactions, especially in sensitized persons. It includes two subspecies, *P. humanus capitis* and *P. humanus humanus.*
P. huma′nus cap′itis the head louse, found on the scalp hair.
P. huma′nus cor′poris *P. humanus humanus.*
P. huma′nus huma′nus the body or clothes louse, which lives on the clothing when feeding is not taking place.
P. inguina′lis, **P. pu′bis** *Phthirus pubis.*

pe•dic•u•lus (pə-dik′u-ləs) pl. *pedic′uli* [L.] 1. louse. 2. pedicle: a footlike or stemlike part.
p. ar′cus ver′tebrae [TA] pedicle of vertebral arch: one of the paired parts of the vertebral arch that connect a lamina to the vertebral body; called also *radix arcus vertebrae.*
p. pulmo′nis radix pulmonis.

ped•i•cure (ped′ĭ-kūr) [*pedi-* + *cure*] professional care and treatment of the feet.

Pedi-Dri (ped′ĭ-dri″) trademark for a preparation of nystatin.

ped•i•gree (ped′ĭ-gre) [Fr. *pied de grue,* "crane's foot" (from the appearance of the lines on the pedigree chart)] 1. lineage. 2. a list of ancestors. 3. a chart or diagram of an individual's ancestors used in genetics in the analysis of inheritance of specific traits.

Pe•dio•coc•cus (pe″de-o-kok′əs) a genus of bacteria of the family Lactobacillaceae, consisting of gram-positive, facultatively anaerobic cocci; they are normally found on plants or in dairy products and alcohol-containing beverages, but can produce nosocomial infections.
P. acidilac′tici a species that is a lactic acid bacterium and is normally found on plants, but occasionally causes human infections such as bacteremia or abscesses.
P. pentosa′ceus a species that is a lactic acid bacterium and is normally found on plants, but occasionally causes human infections such as bacteremia or abscesses.

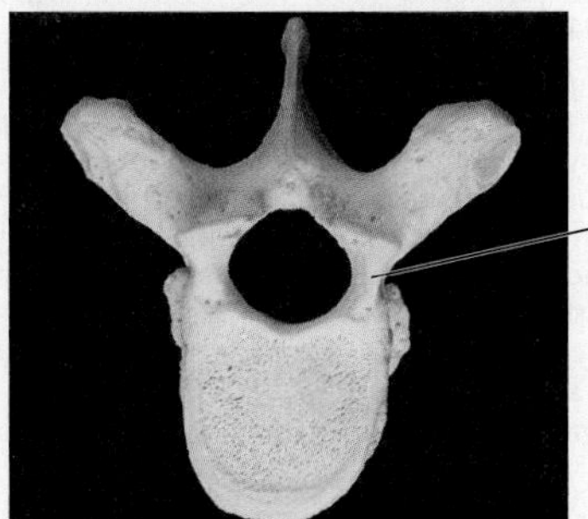

■ Pediculus arcus vertebrae, shown in a superior view of the seventh thoracic vertebra.

pe•dio•don•tia (pe″de-o-don′shə) pediatric dentistry.

Ped•i•pal•pa (ped″ĭ-pal′pə) the whip scorpions, an order of arachnids (not true scorpions) that are nonvenomous but sometimes have irritating secretions; it includes the genus *Mastigoproctus.*

pe•di•tis (pə-di′tis) [*ped-*[2] + *-itis*] pedal osteitis.

ped(o)-[1] [Gr. *pais,* gen. *paidos* child] a combining form denoting relationship to a child. Also, *paed(o)-.*

ped(o)-[2] [L. *pes,* gen. *pedis* foot] a combining form denoting relationship to the foot. Also, *pedi-.*

pe•do•baro•graph (pe″do-bar′o-graf) [*pedo-*[2] + *baro-* + *graph*] an apparatus for recording dynamic variations in downward pressure by different areas of the sole of a foot as a person stands upright or walks. A common type places the subject above a sheet of deformable white film over a glass plate; light reflects differently at different areas on the under side of the plate according to variations in pressure on the plastic sheet, and the differences are recorded.

pe•do•bar•og•ra•phy (pe″do-bə-rog′rə-fe) [*pedo-*[2] + *baro-* + *-graphy*] measurement of dynamic variations in downward pressure by different areas of the sole of a foot, using a pedobarograph.

pe•do•don•tia (pe″do-don′shə) pediatric dentistry.

pe•do•don•tics (pe-do-don′tiks) pediatric dentistry.

pe•do•don•tist (pe-do-don′tist) pediatric dentist.

pe•do•dy•na•mom•e•ter (pe″do-di-nə-mom′ə-tər) [*pedo-*[2] + *dynamometer*] a dynamometer used for the muscles of the lower limb.

pe•do•gen•e•sis (pe″do-jen′ə-sis) [*pedo-*[1] + *-genesis*] the production of offspring by young or larval forms.

pe•do•graph (pe′do-graf) [*pedo-*[2] + *-graph*] an imprint on paper of the weight-bearing surface of the foot, surrounded by a pencil-marked contour of the upper foot.

pe•dol•o•gist (pe-dol′ə-gist) a specialist in pedology.

pe•dol•o•gy (pe-dol′ə-je) [*pedo-*[1] + *-logy*] the systematic study of the life and development of children.

pe•dom•e•ter (pə-dom′ə-tər) [*pedo-*[2] + *-meter*] an instrument for recording the number of steps taken in walking.

pe•do•mor•phism (pe″do-mor′fiz-əm) [*pedo-*[1] + *morph-* + *-ism*] the retention in the adult organism of highly progressive species of bodily characters which at an earlier stage of evolutionary history were actually only infantile. **pedomor′phic** *adj*

pe•dop•a•thy (pə-dop′ə-the) [*pedo-*[2] + *-pathy*] any disease of the foot.

pe•do•phil•ia (pe″do-fil′e-ə) [*pedo-*[1] + *-philia*] [DSM-IV] a paraphilia in which an adult has recurrent, intense sexual urges or sexually arousing fantasies of engaging in or repeatedly engages in sexual activity with a prepubertal child. **pedophil′ic** *adj*

pe•do•pho•bia (pe″de-o-fo′be-ə) [*pedo-*[1] + *-phobia*] irrational fear or dread of children.

pe•dor•thic (pə-dor′thik) pertaining to pedorthics.

pe•dor•thics (pə-dor′thiks) [*pedo-*[2] + *ortho-* + *-ic*] the design, manufacture, fit, and modification of shoes and related foot appliances including ankle and foot orthoses, as prescribed for amelioration of painful or disabling conditions of the lower limb and foot.

pe•dor•thist (pə-dor′thist) an allied health professional trained in pedorthics.

pe•dun•cle (pə-dung′kəl) 1. pedunculus. 2. the stalk by which a nonsessile tumor is attached to normal tissue.
anterior p. of thalamus radiatio thalami anterior.
caudal p. of thalamus radiatio thalami inferior.
central p. of thalamus radiatio thalami centralis.
cerebellar p's pedunculi cerebellares.
cerebellar p., caudal pedunculus cerebellaris inferior.
cerebellar p., cranial pedunculus cerebellaris superior.
cerebellar p., inferior pedunculus cerebellaris inferior.
cerebellar p., middle pedunculus cerebellaris medius.
cerebellar p., pontine pedunculus cerebellaris medius.
cerebellar p., rostral pedunculus cerebellaris superior.
cerebellar p., superior pedunculus cerebellaris superior.
cerebral p. pedunculus cerebri.

p. of flocculus pedunculus flocculi.

inferior p. of thalamus radiatio thalami inferior.

p. of mammillary body a bundle formed by a convergence of afferent fibers in the midbrain tegmentum; it ends in the mammillary body.

olfactory p. in comparative neuroanatomy, the olfactory stalk, especially the region of its attachment to the cerebral hemisphere.

pineal p., p. of pineal body habenula (def. 2).

posterior p. of thalamus radiatio thalami posterior.

superior p. of thalamus radiatio thalami centralis.

thalamic p's, p's of thalamus thalamic radiations.

pe•dun•cu•lar (pə-dung′ku-lər) pertaining to a peduncle.

pe•dun•cu•lat•ed (pə-dung′ku-lāt″əd) provided with a peduncle; opposed to sessile.

pe•dun•cu•lus (pə-dung′ku-ləs) pl. *pedun′culi* [L.] peduncle; a stemlike part, especially a collection of nerve fibers that courses between different areas in the central nervous system.

pedun′culi cerebella′res [TA] cerebellar peduncles: three large bundles of projection fibers on each side of the cerebellum that connect it with other parts of the brain and spinal cord; see *p. cerebellaris inferior, p. cerebellaris medius,* and *p. cerebellaris superior.*

p. cerebella′ris infe′rior [TA] inferior cerebellar peduncle: a composite bundle of nerve fibers in the base of the cerebellum, formed by the union of the restiform body and the juxtarestiform body and connecting the medulla oblongata and spinal cord with the cerebellum. It is located in the lower wall of the fourth ventricle at the caudomedial aspect of the middle cerebellar peduncle. Called also *caudal cerebellar peduncle.*

p. cerebella′ris me′dius [TA] middle cerebellar peduncle: a large bundle of projection fibers originating primarily in the contralateral pontine nuclei and entering the cerebellum, conveying impulses from the cerebral cortex to the cerebellar cortex and nuclei; it is continuous with the pons at the line of attachment of the trigeminal nerve. Called also *brachium pontis* and *pontine cerebellar peduncle.*

p. cerebella′ris supe′rior [TA] superior cerebellar peduncle: a large bundle of projection fibers arising in the cerebellar nuclei, decussating in the caudal mesencephalon; it projects, via the crossed ascending limb, to the red nucleus and thalamus and, via the crossed descending limb, to the reticular and vestibular nuclei and inferior olive. Anterior spinocerebellar tract fibers lie adjacent to each peduncle. Called also *brachium conjunctivum* and *cranial* or *rostral cerebellar peduncle.*

p. ce′rebri [TA] cerebral peduncle: either of the two large paired portions of the midbrain, being separated from each other ventrally by the interpeduncular fossa and continuous dorsally with the mesencephalic tectum. Each peduncle is composed of an anterior portion, the basis pedunculi, consisting of the crus cerebri and the substantia nigra, and a more posterior portion, the tegmentum.

p. floc′culi [TA] peduncle of flocculus: a narrow band of afferent and efferent nerve fibers that connects the nodulus of the cerebellum to the flocculus; its dorsal part is continuous with the anterolateral part of the caudal medullary velum, from which most of its fibers are derived.

Ped•vax•HIB (ped-vaks′hib) trademark for a preparation of *Haemophilus* b conjugate vaccine.

peel (pēl) [L. *pilare* to deprive of hair] 1. the outer covering of something. 2. to remove such an outer covering. 3. a plastic surgery technique involving removal of the outermost layer of skin.

bitter orange p. the dried rind of unripe but fully grown fruit of *Citrus aurantium* Linné, used as a pharmaceutical flavoring agent.

chemical p. chemabrasion.

PEEP positive end-expiratory pressure.

PEF peak expiratory flow.

PEFR peak expiratory flow rate.

PEG percutaneous endoscopic gastrostomy; pneumoencephalography; polyethylene glycol.

peg (peg) a projecting structure.

rete p's rete ridges.

PEG-ADA PEG-adenosine deaminase; see *pegademase.*

peg•ad•e•mase (peg-ad′ə-mās) adenosine deaminase derived from bovine intestine and attached covalently to polyethylene glycol, used in replacement therapy for adenosine deaminase deficiency in patients with severe combined immunodeficiency; administered intramuscularly.

PEG-aden•o•sine de•am•i•nase (PEG-ADA) (ə-den′o-sēn de-am′ĭ-nās) pegademase.

Peg•a•none (peg′ə-nōn) trademark for a preparation of ethotoin.

Peg•a•num (peg′ə-nəm) a genus of herbs of the family Zygophyllaceae. *P. harma′la* L. is African rue, a species whose seeds contain the hallucinogens harmine and harmaline.

peg•as•par•gase (peg-as′pahr-jās) L-asparaginase derived from *Escherichia coli* and covalently linked to polyethylene glycol; used as an antineoplastic in the treatment of acute lymphoblastic leukemia, administered intramuscularly or intravenously.

Peg•a•sys (peg′ə-sis) trademark for a preparation of peginterferon alfa-2a.

peg•fil•gras•tim (peg″fil-gras′tim) a pegylated form of filgrastim, having the same uses as filgrastim for patients having bone marrow or stem cell transplantation or those with neutropenia; administered subcutaneously.

peg•in•ter•fer•on (peg″in″tər-fēr′on) a covalent conjugate of recombinant interferon and polyethylene glycol (PEG); the former moiety acts as a biological response modifier and the latter prolongs the half-life of the compound.

p. alfa-2a a covalent conjugate of recombinant interferon alfa-2a and polyethylene glycol (PEG), used in the treatment of chronic infection by hepatitis C virus or hepatitis B virus; administered subcutaneously.

p. alfa-2b a covalent conjugate of recombinant interferon alfa-2b and polyethylene glycol (PEG), used in the treatment of chronic infection by hepatitis C virus; administered subcutaneously.

PEG-In•tron (peg″in′tron) trademark for a preparation of peginterferon alfa-2b.

pe•gli•col 5 ole•ate (pə-gli′kol) a product obtained by alcoholysis of natural vegetable oils in the presence of polyethylene glycols of molecular weights between 200 and 400, consisting of a mixture of partially mixed esters of glycerin and these polyethylene glycols; the average number of ethylene glycol units is 5. It is used as an emulsifying agent in pharmaceutical preparations. Called also *polyoxyl 5 oleate.*

peg•o•ter•ate (peg″o-ter′āt) a condensation polymer used as a suspending agent in pharmaceutical preparations.

peg•ox•ol 7 ste•a•rate (peg-ok′sōl) a mixture of mono- and distearic esters of ethylene glycol and of polyoxyethylene glycol, the latter having an average molecular weight of 450; the average number of ethylene glycol units is 7. It is used as an emulsifying agent in pharmaceutical preparations.

peg•vis•o•mant (peg-vis′ə-mant) a protein chemically related to human growth hormone that competitively binds to receptors for growth hormone and is used to treat acromegaly.

peg•y•lat•ed (peg′ə-lāt″əd) having polyethylene glycol (PEG) attached; said of certain drugs.

Pel-Eb•stein fever (disease) (pel′ eb′shtīn) [Pieter Klaases *Pel,* Dutch physician, 1852–1919; Wilhelm *Ebstein,* German physician, 1836–1912] see under *fever.*

pe•lade (pə-lahd′) [Fr.] alopecia areata.

pel•age (pel′əj) [Fr.] 1. the hairy coat of mammals. 2. the hairs of the body, limbs, and head collectively.

Pel•a•mis (pel′ə-mis) a genus of sea snakes (family Hydrophiidae). *P. bico′lor* is a venomous species found in the Indian Ocean. *P. platu′rus* is the yellow-bellied sea snake, a venomous species found in many parts of the Indian and Pacific Oceans.

Pel•e•cyp•o•da (pel″e-sip′o-də) [Gr. *pelekys* hatchet + *podos* foot] the bivalves: a class of mollusks which are laterally compressed and have a pair of dorsally hinged lateral shells (valves) and a hatchet-shaped foot for digging; it includes the clams, oysters, and scallops. Called also *Bivalvia.*

Pel•ger-Hu•ët anomaly (pel′gər hu′ət) [Karel *Pelger,* Dutch physician, 1885–1931; G.J. *Huët,* Dutch physician, 1879–1970] see under *anomaly.*

pel•i•o•sis (pel″e-o′sis) [Gr. *peliōsis* extravasation of blood] purpura.

bacillary p. the presence of numerous vasoproliferative, cystic lesions in the liver, spleen, or lymph nodes; it occurs in immunocompromised persons and is caused by *Bartonella henselae.*

p. he′patis, p. of liver the presence of blood-filled lacunae in the parenchyma of the liver, giving it a mottled blue appearance.

Pe•li•zae•us-Merz•ba•cher disease (pa″le-tsa′oos merts′bah-ker) [Friedrich *Pelizaeus,* German physician, 1850–1917; Ludwig *Merzbacher,* German physician, 1875–1942] see under *disease.*

pel•lag•ra (pə-lag′rə) [It. *pelle* skin + *agra* rough] a clinical deficiency syndrome due to deficiency of niacin (or failure to convert tryptophan to niacin) and characterized by dermatitis, inflammation of mucous membranes, diarrhea, and psychic disturbances. The dermatitis occurs on the portions of the body exposed to light or trauma. Mental symptoms include depression, irritability, anxiety, confusion, disorientation, delusions, and hallucinations. **pellag′ral, pellag′rous** *adj*

monkey p. pellagra in caged monkeys, manifested by anorexia, diarrhea, vomiting, emaciation, and finally death.

p. si′ne pella′gra pellagra in which the characteristic dermatitis is not present.

pel•lag•ra•gen•ic (pə-lag″rə-jen′ik) causing pellagra.

pel•lag•roid (pə-lag′roid) a condition resembling pellagra.

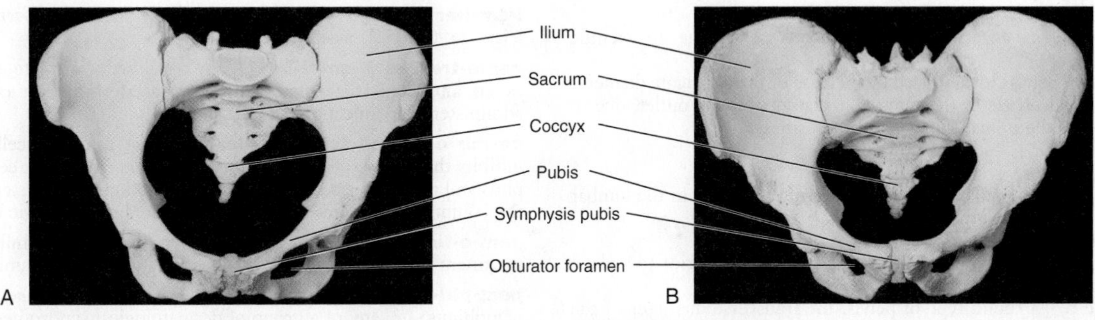

■ Anterior aspect of female *(A)* and male *(B)* pelvis.

Pel·le·gri·ni disease (pel″ə-gre′ne) [Augusto *Pellegrini*, Italian surgeon, 1877–1958] see under *disease*.

Pel·le·gri·ni-Stie·da disease (pel″ə-gre′ne shte′də) [A. *Pellegrini;* Alfred *Stieda*, German surgeon, 1869–1945] Pellegrini disease; see under *disease*.

pel·let (pel′ət) 1. a small pill or granule, such as a small rod- or ovoid-shaped, sterile mass composed of essentially pure steroid hormones, to be implanted under the skin to provide for their slow absorption. 2. a small pill made from sucrose and impregnated with a medicine, used in homeopathy.

pel·li·cle (pel′ĭ-kəl) [L. *pellicula*] 1. a thin skin or film, such as a thin film on the surface of a liquid. 2. in ciliate protozoa, a living outer layer of denser cytoplasm containing the peripheral and surface organelles.

acquired p. a colorless acellular bacteria-free film composed of salivary glycoproteins, deposited on the teeth within minutes after eruption or cleaning.

brown p. a brownish gray to black film formed over a period of time on the surfaces of the teeth, resulting from poor oral hygiene and brushing habits. See also *dental plaque*, under *plaque*.

pel·lic·u·lar (pə-lik′u-lər) pertaining to or characterized by a pellicle.

pel·lic·u·lous (pə-lik′u-ləs) pellicular.

Pel·liz·zi syndrome (pa-lēt′se) [G.B. *Pellizzi*, Italian physician, early 20th century] epiphyseal syndrome.

pel·lu·cid (pə-loo′sid) translucent.

pel(o)- [Gr. *pēlos* mud] a combining form denoting relationship to mud.

Pel·o·de·ra (pel″o-der′ə) *Rhabditis.*

pe·lo·ther·a·py (pe″lo-ther′ə-pe) [*pelo-* + *therapy*] the therapeutic use of earth or mud.

pel·ta (pel′tə) [L. "a shield"] a crescent-shaped membranous structure arising from or covering the axostyle of certain parasitic flagellate protozoa, especially trichomonads.

pel·tate (pel′tāt) [L. *pelta;* Gr. *peltē* shield] scutiform.

pel·ves (pel′vēs) [L.] plural of *pelvis.*

pel·vic (pel′vik) pertaining to the pelvis.

pel·vi·cal·y·ce·al (pel″vĭ-kal″ə-se′əl) pyelocalyceal. Spelled also *pelvicaliceal.*

pel·vi·ceph·a·log·ra·phy (pel″vĭ-sef″ə-log′rə-fe) [*pelvis* + *cephalo-* + *-graphy*] radiographic measurement of the fetal head and of the birth canal.

pel·vi·ceph·a·lom·e·try (pel″vĭ-sef″ə-lom′ə-tre) [*pelvis* + *cephalo-* + *-metry*] measurement of the diameters of the head of the fetus in relation to those of the mother's pelvis.

pel·vi·fem·o·ral (pel″vĭ-fem′ə-rəl) pertaining to or affecting the pelvis and femur.

pel·vi·fix·a·tion (pel″vĭ-fik-sa′shən) surgical fixation of an organ to the pelvic cavity.

pel·vim·e·ter (pel-vim′ə-tər) [*pelvis* + *-meter*] an instrument for measuring the diameters and capacity of the pelvis.

pel·vim·e·try (pel-vim′ə-tre) the measurement of the dimensions and capacity of the pelvis, as by x-ray, computed tomography, or magnetic resonance imaging.

combined p. pelvimetry in which measurements are made both within and outside the body.

pel·vi·og·ra·phy (pel″ve-og′rə-fe) radiography of the organs of the pelvis.

pel·vio·peri·to·ni·tis (pel″ve-o-per″ĭ-to-ni′tis) pelvic peritonitis.

pel·vio·plas·ty (pel′ve-o-plas″te) pyeloplasty.

pel·vi·o·scope (pel′ve-ə-skōp) pelviscope.

pel·vi·os·co·py (pel″ve-os′kə-pe) [*pelvis* + *-scopy*] pelviscopy.

pel·vi·ot·o·my (pel″ve-ot′ə-me) [*pelvis* + *-tomy*] the cutting of the pelvic bones.

pel·vi·peri·to·ni·tis (pel″ve-per″ĭ-to-ni′tis) pelvic peritonitis.

pel·vi·rec·tal (pel″vĭ-rek′təl) pertaining to the pelvis and the rectum.

pel·vis (pel′vis) pl. *pel′ves* [L. "basin"] 1. [TA] the inferior portion of the trunk of the body, bounded anteriorly and laterally by the two hip bones and posteriorly by the sacrum and coccyx; see illustration. The pelvis is divided by a plane passing through the terminal lines into the *p. major* superiorly and the *p. minor* inferiorly. The superior boundary of the pelvic cavity is the *inlet* (*apertura pelvis superior* [TA]), and the inferior boundary of the pelvis minor is the *outlet* (*apertura pelvis inferior* [TA]), which is bounded by the coccyx, the symphysis pubis, and the ischium of either side. The outlet is closed by the coccygeus and levator ani muscles and the perineal fascia, which form the *floor of the pelvis.* The inlet and outlet each have three important diameters: an anteroposterior (conjugate), an oblique, and a transverse, the relations of which determine types variously classified by different authors (see illustration under *diameter*). 2. any basinlike structure.

android p. a pelvis characterized by a wedge-shaped inlet and narrowness of the anterior segment; used as a general designation of a female pelvis showing characters typical of the pelvis in the male.

anthropoid p. a female pelvis characterized by a long anteroposterior diameter of the inlet, which equals or exceeds the transverse diameter.

assimilation p. a pelvis with fusing of the transverse processes in the lumbar or sacral regions; a *high-assimilation pelvis* is one with fusing of the last lumbar vertebra and the sacrum, including six vertebral segments, and a *low-assimilation pelvis* is one with fusing of the last sacral vertebra with the first coccygeal body, including four vertebral segments.

beaked p. one with the pelvic bones laterally compressed and their anterior junction pushed forward, as in osteomalacia.

bony p. p. ossea.

brachypellic p. an oval type of pelvis, the transverse diameter of the inlet exceeding the anteroposterior diameter by 1 to 3 cm.

contracted p. a pelvis in which there is a diminution of 1.5 to 2 cm in any important diameter; when all dimensions are proportionately diminished it is a generally contracted pelvis *(p. justo minor).*

cordate p., cordiform p. a pelvis that is somewhat heart shaped.

coxalgic p. a pelvis that is deformed as a result of hip-joint disease.

dolichopellic p. an elongated pelvis, the anteroposterior diameter of the inlet being greater than the transverse diameter.

dwarf p. a small pelvis seen in several types of dwarfism.

extrarenal p. a renal pelvis that is largely or completely outside the kidney, such as when the kidney has a long shape or when there is obstruction of the ureteropelvic junction.

false p. p. major.

flat p. a pelvis whose anteroposterior dimension is abnormally reduced.

frozen p. a condition, due to infection or carcinoma, in which the adnexa and uterus are fixed in the pelvis.

funnel-shaped p. a female pelvis with a normal inlet, but a greatly narrowed outlet.

giant p. p. justo major.

greater p. p. major.

gynecoid p. a pelvis having a rounded oval shape with a well-rounded anterior and posterior segment; it represents the normal female pelvis.

high-assimilation p. see *assimilation p.*

infantile p. a generally contracted pelvis characterized by an oval shape, a high sacrum, and marked inclination of the walls.

p. jus′to ma′jor a pelvis that is unusually large, with all its dimensions equally increased.

p. jus′to mi′nor a pelvis that is unusually small, with all its dimensions equally reduced; see also *contracted p.*

juvenile p. infantile p.
kyphoscoliotic p. an irregularly contracted pelvis due to rachitic kyphoscoliosis.
kyphotic p. a pelvis characterized by increase of the conjugate diameter at the brim, with decrease of the transverse diameter at the outlet, due to close proximity of the ischial spines and tuberosities.
large p. p. major.
lesser p. p. minor.
lordotic p. a pelvis associated with an anterior curvature in the lumbar region of the vertebral column.
low-assimilation p. see *assimilation p.*
p. ma′jor [TA] greater pelvis: the part of the pelvis superior to a plane passing through the iliopectineal lines.
mesatipellic p. a round type of pelvis, the transverse diameter of the inlet being equal to the anteroposterior diameter or being greater by 1 cm or less.
p. mi′nor [TA] lesser pelvis: the part of the pelvis inferior to a plane passing through the iliopectineal lines; see *pelvis.*
p. na′na dwarf p.
p. obtec′ta a kyphotic pelvis in which the vertebral column extends horizontally across the pelvic inlet.
p. os′sea bony pelvis: the ring of bone forming the skeleton of the pelvis, supporting the vertebral column and resting upon the inferior members, and composed of the two hip bones anteriorly and laterally, and the sacrum and coccyx posteriorly.
osteomalacic p. deformity of the pelvis due to absorption by the bones of their calcium salts, as a result of which the bones become soft and so flexible that they may be stretched or pushed together and cause narrowing of the pelvic inlet.
Otto p. the pelvis with depressed acetabulum seen in protrusio acetabuli.
p. pla′na flat p.
platypellic p., platypelloid p. a pelvis characterized by flattening of the pelvic inlet, with a short anteroposterior and a wide transverse diameter.
Prague p. spondylolisthetic p.
pseudo-osteomalacic p. a deformed pelvis simulating one affected with osteomalacia but resulting from other causes.
rachitic p. a pelvis that is distorted as a result of rickets.
renal p., p. rena′lis [TA] the expanded upper end of the ureter into which the renal calices open, ordinarily lodged within the renal sinus. Under certain conditions a large part of it may be outside the kidney (see *extrarenal p.).*
Rokitansky p. spondylolisthetic p.
round p. a pelvis with an inlet of nearly circular outline.
scoliotic p. a pelvis that is deformed as a result of scoliosis.
simple flat p. a pelvis with a shortened anteroposterior diameter.
small p. p. minor.
p. spino′sa a rachitic pelvis with the crest of the pubis very sharp.
split p. a pelvis with a congenital separation at the pubic symphysis, often associated with exstrophy of the bladder.
spondylolisthetic p. a pelvis in which the pelvic brim is more or less occluded as the result of dislocation of the last, or rarely the fourth or third, lumbar vertebra in front of the sacrum. Called also *Prague* or *Rokitansky p.*
p. spu′ria p. major.
triangular p. a pelvis with a triangular inlet.
true p. p. minor.
p. of ureter p. renalis.

pel·vi·sa·cral (pel′vĭ-sa′krəl) pertaining to the pelvis and the sacrum.

pel·vi·sa·crum (pel″vĭ-sa′krəm) the pelvis and the sacrum together.

pel·vi·scope (pel′vĭ-skōp) an apparatus, usually with a laparoscope, for viewing the pelvis or its contents.

pel·vis·co·py (pel-vis′kə-pe) inspection or visual examination of the pelvis or pelvic viscera, as with a laparoscope or pelviscope. Called also *pelvioscopy.*

pel·vi·sec·tion (pel″vĭ-sek′shən) [*pelvis* + *section*] a cutting of the pelvic bones, such as pubiotomy and symphysiotomy.

pel·vi·ster·num (pel″vĭ-stur′nəm) the cartilage of the symphysis pubis.

pel·vi·tro·chan·te·ri·an (pel″vĭ-tro-kan-tēr′e-ən) relating to the pelvis and the greater trochanter of the femur.

pel·vi·ure·ter·al (pel″ve-u-re′tər-əl) ureteropelvic.

pel·vo·cal·i·ce·al (pel″vo-kal″ĭ-se′əl) pyelocalyceal.

pel·vo·cal·y·ce·al (pel″vo-kal″ə-se′əl) pyelocalyceal.

pel·vos·co·py (pel-vos′kə-pe) pelviscopy.

pel·vo·spon·dy·li·tis (pel″vo-spon″də-li′tis) inflammation of the pelvic portion of the spine.
p. ossi′ficans ankylosing spondylitis.

PEM protein-energy malnutrition.

Pem·ber·ton sign (pem′bər-ton) [Hugh Spear *Pemberton*, British physician, 1890–1956] see under *sign.*

peme·trex·ed di·so·di·um (pem″ə-trek′sed) a folate antagonist used as an antineoplastic agent, acting by interfering with cell replication; administered by injection.

pe·mir·o·last po·tas·sium (pə-mir′o-last″) a mast cell stabilizer that inhibits the release of inflammatory mediators from mast cells and eosinophils and inhibits type I hypersensitivity reactions; administered topically to the conjunctiva to prevent pruritus associated with allergic conjunctivitis.

pem·o·line (pem′o-lēn) a central nervous system stimulant used in the treatment of attention-deficit/hyperactivity disorder; administered orally.

pem·phi·goid (pem′fĭ-goid) [*pemphigus* + *-oid*] 1. like or resembling pemphigus. 2. any of a group of dermatological syndromes similar to but clearly distinguishable from those of the pemphigus group. 3. bullous p.
benign mucosal p., benign mucous membrane p. cicatricial p.
Brunsting-Perry p. see under *syndrome.*
bullous p. a usually mild, self-limited, subepidermal blistering skin disease, sometimes with oral involvement, predominantly affecting the elderly; characteristics include large, tense bullae that rupture to leave denuded areas and have a tendency to heal spontaneously, and cleft formation and deposition of complement, usually with the IgG class of immunoglobulins, at the dermoepidermal junction.
cicatricial p. a benign, chronic, usually bilateral, subepidermal blistering disease chiefly involving the mucous membranes, especially those of the mouth and eye. It chiefly affects the elderly and heals by scarring, which may lead to a slowly progressive shrinkage of the affected mucous membranes and connective tissues. In the eye it is called *ocular pemphigoid.* Called also *benign mucosal* or *benign mucous membrane p.*
dermolytic p. acquired epidermolysis bullosa.
gestational p., p. gestationis herpes gestationis.
localized bullous p. bullous pemphigoid that remains localized, usually at a site on the scalp, trunk, or lower limb.
ocular p., ocular cicatricial p. cicatricial pemphigoid involving the conjunctivae, which eventually may contract and cause blindness. Called also *ocular pemphigus.*

pem·phi·gus (pem′fĭ-gəs) [Gr. *pemphix* blister] 1. any in a group of chronic, relapsing, sometimes fatal autoimmune diseases of the skin, characterized clinically by successive crops of vesicles and bullae, histologically by acantholysis, and immunologically by serum autoantibodies against antigens (see *desmogleins*) in the intracellular zones of the epidermis. Cf. *pemphigoid.* 2. p. vulgaris.
benign familial p. a benign, autosomal dominant dermatitis due to mutation in the *ATP2C1* gene (locus: 3q21-q24), which encodes a Ca^{2+}-ATPase. It is characterized by recurrent bullae and vesicles, usually on the neck, axillae, groin, and other flexural and apposing surfaces. Lesions are in crops and may remain localized or become generalized, rupture, erode, and develop a thick crust. The defect appears to be in keratinocyte cohesion. Called also *Hailey-Hailey disease.*
benign p. vegetans the Hallopeau type of pemphigus vegetans.
Brazilian p. fogo selvagem.
p. erythemato′sus a variant of pemphigus foliaceus, with which it is histologically identical, characterized by a rash resembling lupus erythematosus on the face and lesions resembling seborrhea elsewhere on the body. Immunologically, there is granular deposition of immunoglobulin and complement along the dermoepidermal junction. Called also *Senear-Usher syndrome.*
familial benign p. benign familial p.
p. folia′ceus a superficial, mild, chronic form of pemphigus, usually occurring in the fourth and fifth decades of life, characterized by small flaccid bullae that rupture and crust, as well as localized or generalized exfoliation. It may be limited to the scalp, face, and trunk, or may become generalized.
herpetiform p., p. herpetifor′mis pemphigus with lesions in a herpetiform pattern; some cases are pemphigus foliaceus and others are pemphigus vulgaris.
p. neonato′rum impetigo.
ocular p. see under *pemphigoid.*
paraneoplastic p. a paraneoplastic condition resembling pemphigus vulgaris, characterized by painful erosions of the skin and mucous membranes; the most common underlying malignancies are non-Hodgkin lymphoma and chronic lymphocytic leukemia.
South American p. fogo selvagem.
p. ve′getans a variant of pemphigus vulgaris usually found in intertriginous areas or on the scalp or face, characterized by proliferating warty granulations arising from bullae and having a tendency to coalesce into patches. Two types are distinguished: the more benign *Hallopeau type* is characterized by pustular lesions that resolve without relapsing, and the more severe *Neumann type* is characterized by erosive blisters that evolve into vegetative plaques.

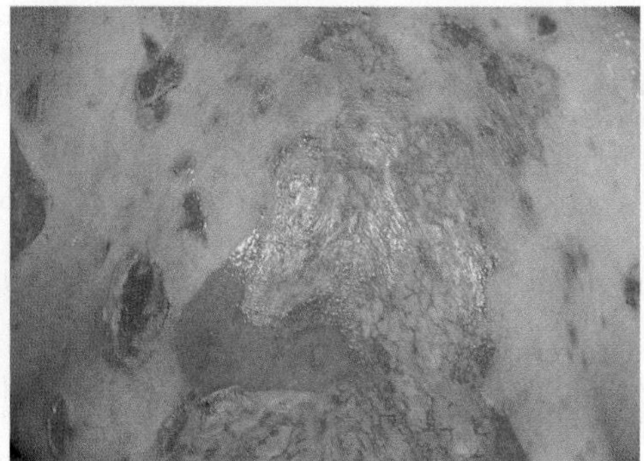

■ Flaccid bullae in pemphigus vulgaris.

p. vulga′ris the most common and severe form of pemphigus, seen usually in persons 40 to 60 years old, characterized by chronic, flaccid, easily ruptured bullae on the skin and mucous membranes. It begins focally but then becomes generalized, leaving large, weeping, denuded surfaces that partially crust over but do not heal and enlarge by confluence. In untreated cases there may be sepsis, cachexia, and electrolyte imbalance that can be fatal.

wildfire p. fogo selvagem.

PEN pharmacy equivalent name.

Pe•ña procedure (pa′nyah) [Alberto *Peña*, Mexican-born American pediatric surgeon, 20th century] posterior sagittal anorectoplasty.

Pen•brit•in (pen-brit′in) trademark for preparations of ampicillin.

pen•bu•to•lol sul•fate (pen-bu′tə-lol) [USP] a nonselective beta-adrenergic blocking agent with intrinsic sympathomimetic activity; administered orally in the treatment of hypertension.

pen•ci•clo•vir (pen-si′klo-vir) an antiviral compound that inhibits viral DNA synthesis and replication in human herpesviruses 1 and 2, used in the treatment of recurrent herpes labialis; applied topically.

pen•del•luft (pen′də-looft″) [Ger. "pendulum breath"] the movement of air back and forth between the lungs, resulting in increased dead space ventilation.

Pen•dred syndrome (pen′dred) [Vaughan *Pendred*, English physician, 1869–1946] see under *syndrome*.

pen•drin (pen′drin) a glycoprotein found on the apical surface of thyroid follicular cells, acting as a transport protein for iodide to leave the cell and aid in formation of thyroxine; mutations in the gene specifying pendrin cause Pendred syndrome (see under *syndrome*).

pen•du•lar (pen′du-lər) having a pendulum-like movement.

pen•du•lous (pen′du-ləs) [L. *pendere* to hang] hanging loosely; dependent.

Pen•e•cort (pen′ə-kort″) trademark for preparations of hydrocortisone.

pe•nec•to•my (pe-nek′tə-me) [*penis* + *-ectomy*] surgical removal of the penis.

pen•e•tra•bil•i•ty (pen″ə-trə-bil′ĭ-te) the ability of x-rays to penetrate matter.

pen•e•trance (pen′ə-trəns) [L. *penetrare* to enter into] in genetics, the frequency of expression of a genotype under defined conditions. If it is less than 100 per cent, the trait is said to exhibit *reduced penetrance* or *lack of penetrance*.

pen•e•trat•ing (pen′ə-trāt-ing) [L. *penetrans*] piercing; entering deeply.

pen•e•tra•tion (pen″ə-tra′shən) [L. *penetratio*] 1. the act of piercing or entering deeply, as by a sharp object, radiation, or a chemical or drug. 2. focal depth.

Pen•e•trex (pen′ə-treks) trademark for a preparation of enoxacin.

pen•e•trom•e•ter (pen″ə-trom′ə-tər) 1. step wedge; a device for measuring the penetrability of x-rays. 2. an apparatus for registering the resistance of semisolid material to penetration.

-penia [Gr. *penia* poverty, need] a word termination indicating an abnormal reduction in number of the element denoted by the root to which it is affixed, as leukopenia.

pen•i•ci•din (pen″ĭ-si′din) patulin.

pen•i•cil•la•mine (pen″ĭ-sil′ə-mēn) [USP] a degradation product of penicillin that chelates certain heavy metals; used orally to reduce the blood copper level in treatment of Wilson disease and to promote excretion of cystine in patients with cystinuria or recurrent cystine calculus formation, by forming a more soluble penicillamine-cystine disulfide. It is also used as a disease-modifying antirheumatic drug in treatment of refractory rheumatoid arthritis.

pen•i•cil•li (pen″ĭ-sil′i) [L.] genitive and plural of *penicillus*.

pen•i•cil•li•ary (pen″ĭ-sil′e-ar″e) [L. *penicillum* brush] resembling a brush or broom.

pen•i•cil•lic ac•id (pen″ĭ-sil′ik) an antibiotic substance produced by several species of *Penicillium* and *Aspergillus;* it has antibacterial activity but is also toxic to animal tissues, causing nephrotoxicity and other damage.

pen•i•cil•lin (pen″ĭ-sil′in) any of a large group of natural or semisynthetic antibacterial antibiotics derived directly or indirectly from strains of fungi of the genus *Penicillium* and other soil-inhabiting fungi grown on special culture media, which exert a bacteriocidal as well as a bacteriostatic effect on susceptible bacteria by interfering with the final stages of the synthesis of peptidoglycan, a substance in the bacterial cell wall. The penicillins, despite their relatively low toxicity for the host, are active against many bacteria, especially gram-positive pathogens (streptococci, staphylococci, pneumococci); clostridia; some gram-negative forms (gonococci, meningococci); some spirochetes *(Treponema pallidum* and *T. pertenue);* and some fungi. Certain strains of some target species, e.g., staphylococci, secrete the enzyme penicillinase, which inactivates penicillin and confers resistance to the antibiotic.

benzathine p. p. G benzathine.

benzyl p. potassium p. G potassium.

benzyl p. sodium p. G sodium.

dimethoxyphenyl p. sodium methicillin sodium.

p. G the most widely used form and the first of the penicillins developed for medicinal use. It is used in the form of the benzathine, potassium, procaine, and sodium salts, principally in the treatment of infections due to penicillin-susceptible gram-positive bacteria, gram-negative cocci, *Treponema pallidum*, and *Actinomyces israelii*. Called also *benzylpenicillin*.

p. G benzathine [USP] a salt having a long-sustained action, obtained by combining penicillin G with *N,N′*-bis(phenylmethyl)-1,2-ethanediamine (2:1); administered orally or intramuscularly.

p. G potassium [USP] the potassium salt of penicillin G; administered orally, intramuscularly, or intravenously.

p. G procaine [USP] a salt having a long-sustained action, obtained by combining penicillin G with procaine (1:1); administered intramuscularly.

p. G sodium [USP] the sodium salt of penicillin G; administered intramuscularly or intravenously.

isoxazolyl p. any of a group of semisynthetic penicillins, including oxacillin and cloxacillin, which combine resistance to penicillinase with acid stability and activity against gram-positive bacteria.

phenoxymethyl p. p. V.

potassium phenoxymethyl p. p. V potassium.

p. V [USP] a semisynthetic oral penicillin prepared from cultures of the mold *Penicillium* in the presence of 2-phenoxyethanol with an autolysate of yeast as the source of nitrogen. It is a broad-spectrum antibiotic having pharmacologic and toxic properties similar to those of other penicillins, and is less potent than penicillin G. Called also *phenoxymethyl p.*

p. V benzathine [USP] the benzathine salt of penicillin V, administered orally.

p. V potassium [USP] the potassium salt of penicillin V; administered orally.

pen•i•cil•lin•ase (pen″ĭ-sil′ĭ-nās) a β-lactamase (q.v.) preferentially cleaving penicillins.

pen•i•cil•lin-fast (pen″ĭ-sĭl′in-fast) resistant to the action of penicillin; said of certain strains of bacteria.

pen•i•cil•li•o•sis (pen′ĭ-sil″e-o′sis) infection with species of *Penicillium*. In humans it is rare, usually a lung infection with fever, coughing, and leukocytosis; in other animals it may cause necrotic rhinitis, mycotoxic nephropathy, or neurological symptoms.

Pen•i•cil•li•um (pen″ĭ-sil′e-əm) [L. *penicillum* brush] a genus of Fungi Imperfecti of the form-class Hyphomycetes, form-family Moniliaceae; they develop fruiting organs resembling a broom or phalanges. Many species are commonly found in the human environment and occasionally cause penicilliosis. When identified, the perfect (sexual) stage is classified in the family Eurotiaceae.

P. chryso′genum a species from which various penicillins are obtained.

P. citreovi′ride a species that sometimes contaminates rice and contains the toxin citreoviridin, which can cause cardiac damage or neurotoxicity.

P. citri′num a species that sometimes contaminates corn and contains the mycotoxin citrinin, which has caused nephropathy and hepatic necrosis in rats and chickens and possibly Balkan nephritis in humans.

P. clavifor′me a toxic species that contains patulin.

P. crusta′ceum *P. glaucum*.

P. cyclo′pium a species that contains mycotoxins such as patulin and penicillic acid.

P. expan′sum a toxic species that contains patulin.

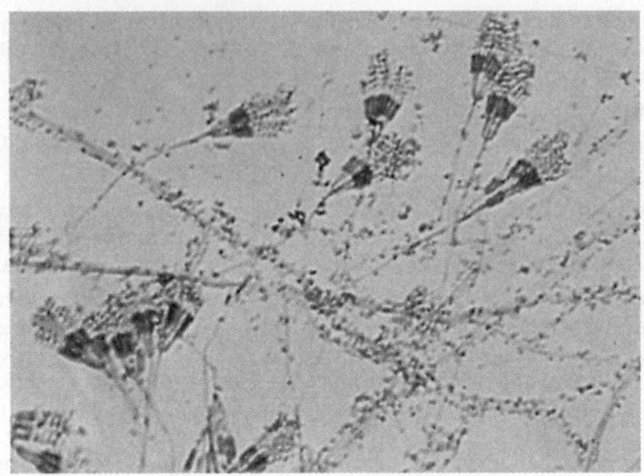

■ *Penicillium*, showing the conidiophores and free conidia.

P. glau'cum a common bluegreen mold; called also *P. crustaceum*.

P. griseoful'vum a species that yields the antibiotic griseofulvin.

P. leu'copus a toxic species that contains patulin.

P. marneffei a species endemic to India, China, Southeast Asia and nearby islands; it causes opportunistic infections that can be fatal in immunocompromised persons.

P. meli'nii a toxic species that contains patulin.

P. nota'tum a species that contains various penicillins and the enzyme glucose oxidase.

P. pa'tulum *P. uticale*.

P. purpuroge'num a species that sometimes contaminates corn and contains the toxin rubratoxin, which causes hepatotoxicity in livestock.

P. ru'brum a species that sometimes contaminates corn and contains the toxin rubratoxin, which causes hepatotoxicity in livestock.

P. utica'le a toxic species that produces patulin; called also *P. patulum*.

P. viridica'tum a species that sometimes contaminates grain and contains the mycotoxins citrinin and ochratoxins; it has caused nephropathy in rats and possibly Balkan nephritis in humans.

pen•i•cil•lo•yl pol•y•ly•sine (pen″ĭ-sil′o-əl pol″e-li′sēn) benzylpenicilloyl polylysine.

pen•i•cil•lus (pen″ĭ-sil′əs) gen. and pl. *penicil'li* [L. "brush"] a structure resembling a brush in appearance.

penicil'li arte'riae sple'nicae [TA] brushlike groups of arterial branches of the lobules of the spleen.

Pe•nic•u•li•na (pə-nik′u-li′nə) a suborder of large, free-living, monomorphic, mainly freshwater protozoa (order Hymenostomatida, subclass Hymenostomatia), characterized by the presence of explosive fusiform trichocysts and three peniculi, often located deep in the buccal cavity; nematodesmata and preoral and postoral sutures and an oral groove occur often. Many species have algal and gram-negative endosymbionts. *Paramecium* is a representative species.

pe•nic•u•lus (pə-nik′u-ləs) pl. *penic'uli* ["little brush"] a modified membrane manifested as a band of fused cilia in the left wall in the buccal cavity of certain ciliate protozoa.

pe•nis (pe′nis) [L.] [TA] the male organ of copulation and of urinary excretion, comprising a root *(radix penis)*, body *corpus penis*, and extremity *glans penis*. The root is attached to the descending portions of the pubic bone by the *crura penis* (see under *crus*), which are the extremities of the corpora cavernosa. The body consists of two parallel cylindrical bodies, the *corpora cavernosa*, and beneath them the *corpus spongiosum*, through which the urethra passes. The glans is covered with mucous membrane and ensheathed by the prepuce, or foreskin. The penis is homologous with the clitoris in the female. **pe'nial, pe'nile** *adj*

buried p. concealed p.

bifid p. diphallus.

clubbed p. penile curvature.

concealed p. a small penis concealed beneath a suprapubic fat pad or the skin of the scrotum, perineum, abdomen, or thigh. It may be congenital or an iatrogenic result of circumcision.

corkscrew p. a defect seen in bulls in which some parts of the penile tunica albuginea stretch more than others during erection, so that a spiral deviation prevents insertion and copulation. Called also *spiral deviation of the penis*.

double p. diphallus.

inconspicuous p. a categorical term denoting a penis that appears to be abnormally small, although the shaft can be abnormal or normal in size; the category includes a variety of anomalies including webbed penis, concealed penis, and micropenis.

p. palma'tus webbed p.

webbed p. a penis that is enclosed by the skin of the scrotum; called also *p. palmatus*.

pe•nis•chi•sis (pe-nis′kĭ-sis) [*penis* + *-schisis*] a fissured state of the penis, such as epispadias, hypospadias, or paraspadias.

pe•ni•tis (pe-ni′tis) inflammation of the penis.

Pen•lac (pen′lak) trademark for a preparation of ciclopirox olamine.

pen•nate (pen′āt) penniform.

pen•ni•form (pen′ĭ-form) [L. *penna* feather + *form*] shaped like a feather; looking like a feather.

pen•ny•ro•yal (pen″e-roi′əl) any of various mint plants, especially *Mentha pulegium*, whose oil was formerly used as a diaphoretic, aromatic, and emmenagogue; use of the leaves or oil as an abortifacient has caused death.

pe•no•plas•ty (pe′no-plas″te) phalloplasty.

pe•no•scro•tal (pe″no-skro′təl) pertaining to the penis and scrotum.

Pen•rose drain (pen′rōz) [Charles Bingham *Penrose*, American gynecologist, 1862–1925] see under *drain*.

pent(a)- [Gr. *pente* five] a combining form meaning five.

pen•ta (pen′tə) pentachlorophenol.

pen•ta•ba•sic (pen″tə-ba′sik) having five replaceable atoms of hydrogen in the molecule.

Pen•ta•car•i•nat (pen″tə-kar′ĭ-nāt) trademark for a preparation of pentamidine isethionate.

Pen•ta•cel (pen′tə-sel) trademark for a combination preparation of diphtheria and tetanus toxoids and acellular pertussis vaccine adsorbed, poliovirus vaccine inactivated, and *Haemophilus* b conjugate (tetanus toxoid conjugate) vaccine.

pen•ta•chlo•ro•phe•nol (pen″tə-klo″ro-fen′ol) a compound used as an insecticide for termite control, an herbicide, and a fungicidal wood preservative; its use has been restricted because it can cause severe toxic reactions such as convulsions, contact dermatitis, and lung, liver, and kidney damage. Called also *penta*.

pen•ta•chro•mic (pen″tə-kro′mik) [*penta-* + *chrom-* + *-ic*] 1. pertaining to or exhibiting five colors. 2. able to distinguish only five of the seven colors of the spectrum.

pen•ta•cyc•lic (pen″tə-sik′lik, -si′klik) containing five fused rings or closed chains in the molecular structure.

pen•tad (pen′tad) 1. any group of five. 2. a pentavalent element or radical.

Reynolds p. biliary colic, jaundice, and fever and chills (i.e., Charcot triad), together with altered mental status and hypotension; it indicates severe cholangitis.

pen•ta•dac•tyl (pen″tə-dak′təl) [*penta-* + *dactyl*] having five fingers or toes on the hand or foot.

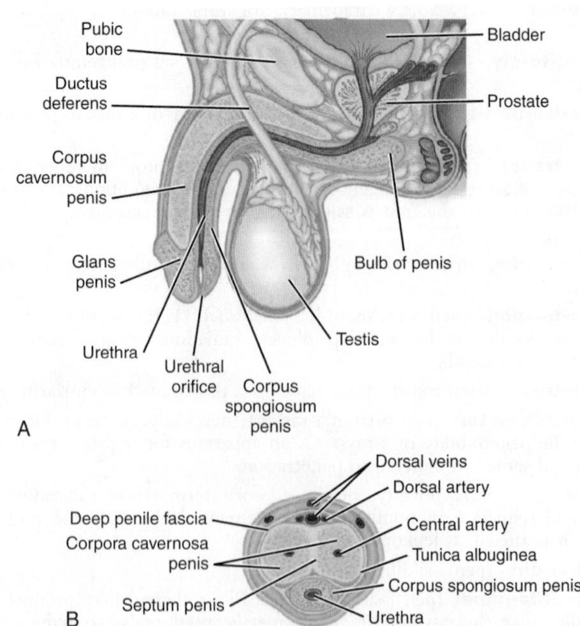

■ Penis. *(A)*, Median sagittal section; *(B)*, transverse section.

pen•ta•ene (pen′tə-ēn) a suffix denoting a chemical compound in which there are five conjugated double bonds.

pen•ta•eryth•ri•tol (pen″tə-ə-rith′rĭ-tol) an alcohol prepared by treating acetaldehyde with formaldehyde in an aqueous solution of calcium hydroxide; used in synthetic resins and in paints and varnishes.

p. tetranitrate (PETN) the nitric acid ester of pentaerythritol, having vasodilator action similar to nitroglycerin, occurring as a white, crystalline powder that may explode on percussion. Called also *niperyt, penthrit.*

pen•ta•eryth•ri•tyl (pen″tə-ə-rith′rĭ-təl) pentaerythritol.

pen•ta•gas•trin (pen″tə-gas′trin) a synthetic pentapeptide consisting of β-alanine and the C-terminal tetrapeptide of gastrin; formerly used in a common gastric function test.

pen•tal•o•gy (pən-tal′ə-je) a combination of five elements or factors, as five concurrent defects or symptoms.

p. of Cantrell a cleft in the inferior part of the sternum associated with midline abdominal defects such as omphalocele, defective pericardium and diaphragm with communication between the pericardial and peritoneal cavities, and cardiac anomalies such as ventricular septal defect or, less often, atrial septal defect, tetralogy of Fallot, or left ventricular diverticulum.

p. of Fallot the four defects of the tetralogy of Fallot accompanied by patent foramen ovale or atrial septal defect.

Pen•tam (pen′tam) trademark for preparations of pentamidine isethionate.

pen•ta•mer (pen′tə-mər) 1. a polymer consisting of five monomers. 2. a viral capsomer having five structural units.

pen•ta•meth•yl•ene•di•amine (pen″tə-meth″əl-ēn-di′ə-mēn) cadaverine.

pen•tam•i•dine is•eth•i•o•nate (pen-tam′ĭ-dēn) an antiinfective administered intravenously or intramuscularly in the treatment of early African trypanosomiasis and leishmaniasis, and intravenously, intramuscularly, or by oral inhalation in the treatment and prophylaxis of pneumocystis pneumonia.

pen•tane (pen′tān) *n*-pentane; an aliphatic hydrocarbon of the methane series, C_5H_{12}, obtained by distillation of petroleum and occurring as a clear, colorless, flammable liquid. It produces anesthesia when inhaled, ingested, or injected.

pen•ta•pep•tide (pen″tə-pep′tīd) a polypeptide containing five amino acids.

pen•ta•pyr•ro•li•din•i•um bi•tar•trate (pen″tə-pĭ-ro″lĭ-din′e-əm) pentolinium tartrate.

Pen•ta•sa (pen-tă′sə) trademark for a preparation of mesalamine.

pen•ta•so•my (pen″tə-so′me) [*penta-* + Gr. *sōma* body] the presence of three additional chromosomes of one type (e.g., 5 X chromosomes) in an otherwise diploid cell (2n + 3).

Pen•ta•span (pen′tə-span″) trademark for a preparation of pentastarch.

pen•ta•starch (pen′tə-stahrch″) an artificial colloid derived from a waxy starch composed of more than 90 per cent amylopectin that has been etherified so that an average of 4 to 5 of the OH groups in every 10 D-glucopyranose units of the starch polymer have been converted to OCH_2CH_2OH groups; used as an adjunct in leukapheresis to increase the erythrocyte sedimentation rate.

pen•ta•stome (pen′tə-stōm) an individual of the phylum Pentastomida; called also *pentastomid* and *tongue worm.*

pen•ta•sto•mi•a•sis (pen″tə-sto-mi′ə-sis) infection with pentastomes.

pen•ta•sto•mid (pen″tə-sto′mid) pentastome.

Pen•ta•sto•mida (pen″tə-sto′mid-ə) the tongue worms, a small phylum that was formerly considered part of Arthropoda, consisting of degenerate wormlike parasites that lack circulatory and respiratory systems. Adults do not have appendages, but have two pairs of hooks near the mouth, and larvae have two or three pairs of rudimentary legs. Adults live in the respiratory passages and body cavities of reptiles, birds, and mammals. Families of importance in human and veterinary medicine include Porocephalidae and Linguatulidae.

pen•ta•tom•ic (pen″tə-tom′ik) [*pent-* + *atom*] 1. containing five atoms. 2. containing five replaceable hydrogen atoms.

Pen•ta•tricho•mo•nas (pen″tə-trik″o-mo′nəs) [*penta-* + *Trichomonas*] a genus of parasitic flagellated protozoa of the order Trichomonadida, phylum Parabasalia, including species formerly in *Trichomonas* that have five anterior flagella.

P. ho′minis one of the most common flagellate species infecting human intestines; it may be present in large numbers but is generally considered to be nonpathogenic. Formerly called *Trichomonas hominis.*

pen•ta•va•lent (pen″tə-va′lənt) having a chemical valence of five; capable of combining with five atoms of hydrogen.

pen•taz•o•cine (pen-taz′o-sēn) a synthetic opioid agonist/antagonist analgesic used for relief of moderate to severe pain.

p. hydrochloride [USP] the hydrochloride salt of pentazocine, administered orally as an analgesic.

p. lactate [USP] the lactate salt of pentazocine, administered intramuscularly, intravenously, or subcutaneously as an analgesic and as an adjunct to anesthesia.

pen•te•tate (pen′tə-tāt) a salt, anion, ester, or complex of pentetic acid.

p. calcium trisodium the calcium trisodium salt of pentetic acid, used as a chelating agent, especially in the treatment of plutonium poisoning. Called also *calcium trisodium pentetate.*

pen•tet•ic ac•id (pen-tet′ik) [USP] diethylenetriamine pentaacetic acid, DTPA; a chelating agent (iron) with the general properties of the edetates. Complexed with radioisotopes it is used as an imaging agent; its uses as a technetium complex (Tc 99m) include renal and brain imaging, renal perfusion studies, assessment of glomerular filtration rate, radionuclide cisternography, and lung imaging; as a complex with indium (In 111) it is used in radionuclide cisternography.

pen•te•tre•o•tide (pen″tə-tre′o-tīd) a conjugate of pentetic acid and the somatostatin analogue octreotide; it binds to somatostatin receptors and is used as the ^{111}In chelate in the imaging of tumors having somatostatin receptors.

Pen•thrane (pen′thrān) trademark for a preparation of methoxyflurane.

pen•thrit (pen′thrit) pentaerythritol tetranitrate.

pen•to•bar•bi•tal (pen″to-bahr′bĭ-təl) [USP] a short- to intermediate-acting barbiturate used as a sedative and hypnotic; administered orally.

p. sodium [USP] the sodium salt of pentobarbital, used as a sedative, particularly as a presurgical adjunct to anesthesia, and as an anticonvulsant for emergency treatment of acute convulsive episodes; administered orally, intramuscularly, intravenously, and rectally.

pen•to•bar•bi•tone (pen″to-bahr′bĭ-tōn) pentobarbital.

pen•to•lin•i•um tar•trate (pen″to-lin′e-əm) a ganglionic blocking agent used as an antihypertensive; administered orally, intramuscularly, and subcutaneously.

pen•to•san (pen′to-san) any member of the class of polysaccharides composed of pentose residues, e.g., arabans or xylans. They occur widely in plants, serving structural and storage functions.

p. polysulfate sodium a polysulfated derivative of a xylose-containing, glucuronate-substituted pentosan, with an average molecular weight between 4000 and 6000 daltons, and having fibrinolytic and anticoagulant actions; used as an antiinflammatory in the treatment of interstitial cystitis; administered orally.

pen•to•sa•zone (pen″tōs′ə-zōn) any osazone formed from a pentose.

pen•tose (pen′tōs) a monosaccharide containing five carbon atoms in a molecule.

pen•tos•emia (pen″to-se′me-ə) the presence of pentose in the blood.

pen•to•side (pen′to-sīd) any glycoside in which the sugar component is a pentose, the most important being the nucleosides.

pen•to•si•dine (pen-to′sĭ-dēn) an advanced glycation end product seen in increased amounts in end-stage renal disease, diabetic nephropathy, and arthritis.

pen•to•stat•in (pen″to-stat′in) an antineoplastic used in the treatment of hairy cell leukemia; administered intravenously.

pen•tos•uria (pen″to-su′re-ə) excretion of pentoses in the urine. **pentosu′ric** *adj*

alimentary p. urinary excretion of pentoses, probably xylose and arabinose, as a normal consequence of excessive ingestion of fruits such as cherries, plums, and grapes, or their juices.

essential p. a benign autosomal recessive deficiency of L-xylulose reductase activity, due to mutation in the *DCXR* gene (locus: 17q25.3), which encodes it, resulting in urinary excretion of high levels of the pentose L-xylulose.

pen•to•syl (pen′tə-səl) a radical of pentose.

pen•to•syl•trans•fer•ase (pen″tə-səl-trans′fər-ās) [EC 2.4.2] any member of a sub-subclass of enzymes of the transferase class that catalyze the transfer of a pentose group from one compound to another.

Pen•to•thal (pen′to-thol) trademark for preparations of thiopental sodium.

pen•tox•ide (pən-tok′sīd) an oxide containing five atoms of oxygen in a molecule.

Pen•tox•il (pen-tok′səl) trademark for a preparation of pentoxifylline.

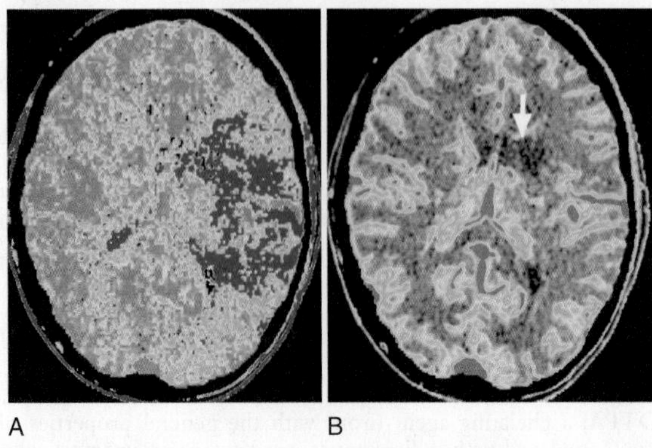

■ Ischemic penumbra on CT perfusion imaging in acute stroke. *(A)*, Mapping of mean transit time (MTT) shows a large deficit corresponding to the entire left middle coronary artery (MCA) territory. *(B)*, Mapping of cerebral blood volume (CBV) shows a small dark-appearing deficit *(arrow)* in the left basal ganglia region, representing the infarcted core. The surrounding area showing a deficit in the MTT map but not the CBV map is the potentially salvageable ischemic penumbra.

pen•tox•if•yl•line (pen″tok-sif′ə-lin) a xanthine derivative that reduces blood viscosity and increases erythrocyte flexibility, microcirculatory flow, and tissue oxygenation; used for the symptomatic treatment of intermittent claudication; administered orally.

pen•tu•lose (pen′tu-lōs) ketopentose.

pen•um•bra (pə-num′brə) [L. *pēne* almost + *umbra*] 1. the area of a shadow where there is partial illumination; it surrounds the umbra. 2. in radiography, an area of blurring around the edges of a structure.
ischemic p. an area of moderately ischemic brain tissue surrounding an area of more severe ischemia; blood flow to this area may be enhanced in order to prevent the spread of a cerebral infarction.

Pen Vee K (pen′ve) trademark for preparations of penicillin V potassium.

PEP phospho*enol*pyruvate; preejection period.

Pep•cid (pep′sid) trademark for preparations of famotidine.

pep•lo•mer (pep′lo-mər) [*peplos* + Gr. *meros* part] one of the knoblike projections, generally composed of glycoproteins, on the surface of the lipoprotein envelope of many enveloped viruses.

pep•los (pep′ləs) [Gr. "robe"] envelope (def. 2).

pep•per (pep′ər) [L. *piper*] 1. any of various plants of the genus *Piper*, or their fruits, particularly the black pepper *(P. nigrum)*, the common spice. 2. any of various plants of the genus *Capsicum*, or their fruits.
cayenne p. capsicum.
Java p. *Piper cubeba.*
red p. capsicum.
tailed p. *Piper cubeba.*

pep•per•mint (pep′ər-mint) 1. *Mentha piperita.* 2. [NF] the dried leaves and flowering tops of *M. piperita*, which have carminative, gastric stimulant, and counterirritant properties; used in flavoring, used internally for gastrointestinal disturbances and liver and gallbladder complaints, used in folk medicine for digestive disturbances, dysmenorrhea, and respiratory infections, and used in homeopathy for colds. See also *peppermint oil*, under *oil.*

pep•sic (pep′sik) peptic.

pep•sin (pep′sin) any of several enzymes of gastric juice that catalyze hydrolysis of proteins to form polypeptides.
p. A [EC 3.4.23.1] an enzyme of the hydrolase class that catalyzes the hydrolysis of proteins with preferential cleavage at phenylalanine, tryptophan, tyrosine, and leucine residues. It is secreted by the gastric mucosa in the form of pepsinogen and has an optimum pH of 1.5 to 2.0.
p. B [EC 3.4.23.2] pepsin similar to pepsin A, formed from pig pepsinogen B. A related enzyme is found in humans.
p. C pepsin similar to pepsin A but highly active with hemoglobin as substrate. In EC nomenclature called *gastricsin.*

pep•sin•o•gen (pep-sin′ə-jən) a proenzyme secreted by chief cells, mucous neck cells, and pyloric gland cells, which is converted into pepsin in the presence of gastric acid or of pepsin itself.

pep•sin•uria (pep″sĭ-nu′re-ə) the presence of pepsin in the urine; it may be associated with duodenal ulcer because of the increased volume of gastric secretion.

pep•stat•in (pep-stat′in) any of the pentapeptide pepsin inhibitors obtained from several species of *Streptomyces*, identified as pepstatins A, B, and C. The A component has been used in the treatment of gastric ulcer.

Pep•tav•lon (pep-tav′lon) trademark for a preparation of pentagastrin.

pep•tic (pep′tik) [Gr. *peptikos*] 1. pertaining to pepsin. 2. pertaining to digestion or to other actions of gastric juice.

pep•ti•dase (pep′tĭ-dās) [EC 3.4] any member of a subclass of enzymes of the hydrolase class that catalyze the hydrolysis of peptide bonds; it comprises the exopeptidases and endopeptidases. Called also *peptide hydrolase.*

pep•tide (pep′tīd) any member of a class of compounds of low molecular weight that yield two or more amino acids on hydrolysis. They are the constituent parts of proteins and are formed by loss of water from the NH_2 and COOH groups of adjacent amino acids. Peptides are known as di-, tri-, tetra- (etc.) peptides depending on the number of amino acids in the molecule. See also *polypeptide.*
agouti-related p. see under *protein.*
amyloid-β p., β-amyloid p. Aβ amyloid.
atrial natriuretic p. (ANP) a hormone involved in natriuresis and the regulation of renal and cardiovascular homeostasis. It is generally 28 amino acids in length but varies somewhat; it is synthesized as a prohormone in the granules of the myocytes of the atrium and is released into the circulation in response to atrial dilatation or increased intravascular fluid volume. Besides causing natriuresis, it also causes diuresis and renal vasodilation and reduces circulating concentrations of renin, aldosterone, and vasopressin, thereby normalizing circulating blood pressure and volume. Called also *atriopeptin* and *atrial natriuretic factor.*
brain natriuretic p., B-type natriuretic p. (BNP) a hormone, originally isolated from porcine brain tissue, having biologic effects similar to those of atrial natriuretic peptide; it is stored mainly in the myocardium of the cardiac ventricles. Blood levels of BNP are elevated in hypervolemic states such as congestive heart failure and hypertension.
C p. the connecting peptide chain that is removed when proinsulin is cleaved to form insulin.
calcitonin gene–related p. a 37–amino acid polypeptide encoded by the calcitonin gene, widely distributed in the central and peripheral nervous systems and also occurring in the adrenal medulla and gastrointestinal tract; it is a potent vasodilator and a neurotransmitter.
corticotropin-like intermediate lobe p. (CLIP) a peptide with a sequence identical to the C-terminal 22 residues of corticotropin, found in the intermediate lobe of the pituitary gland in certain animals; its function, if any, is unknown. It is also produced by human fetuses and may be a regulator of the fetal adrenal glands.
cyclic citrullinated p. (CCP) a synthetic, citrulline-containing peptide with a cyclic structure, used in assays for rheumatoid arthritis; the presence of antibodies to this peptide is highly specific for rheumatoid arthritis.
***N*-formylmethionyl p's** di- and tripeptides in which the N-terminal amino acid residue is *N*-formylmethionine (fMet), which are produced by bacteria in protein synthesis (fMet initiates each polypeptide chain in prokaryotes but is often removed after translation) and which are chemotactic for granulocytes and macrophages but not for lymphocytes.
gastrin-releasing p. a 27–amino acid linear neuropeptide structurally and functionally related to bombesin; it mediates neural release of antral gastrin, causes bronchoconstriction and respiratory tract vasodilation, stimulates growth and mitogenesis of cells in culture, and may act as an excitatory neurotransmitter of enteric interneurons.
glucagon-like p. (GLP) either of two intestinal peptide hormones (GLP-1 and GLP-2) secreted by the L cells in response to ingestion of nutrients, especially carbohydrates and fat-rich meals. GLP-1 inhibits gastric emptying, food intake, and glucagon secretion and stimulates insulin secretion and pancreatic islet proliferation; GLP-2 inhibits antral motility and gastric acid secretion, induces crypt cell proliferation, enhances intestinal epithelial barrier function, stimulates intestinal hexose transport, and inhibits short-term control of food intake.
opioid p. opioid (def. 2).
parathyroid hormone–like p., parathyroid hormone–related p. a peptide somewhat homologous to parathyroid hormone at its amino terminus; it is secreted by certain types of cancer cells and causes hypercalcemia, apparently by acting on the parathyroid receptor, stimulating adenylate cyclase, increasing bone resorption, and inhibiting bone formation. Called also *parathyroid hormone–like protein.*
signal p. see under *sequence.*
vasoactive intestinal p. (VIP) vasoactive intestinal polypeptide.

pep•tide hy•dro•lase (pep′tīd hi′dro-lās) peptidase.

pep•ti•der•gic (pep″tĭ-dur′jik) 1. having an action resembling that of a peptide hormone. 2. activated by, characteristic of, or secreting a peptide hormone or a neuropeptide.

pep•ti•do•gly•can (pep″tĭ-do-gli′kən) a high-molecular-weight polymer that forms the tough, rigid structure of bacterial cell walls. It is made up of three parts: (1) a backbone, composed of alternating *N*-acetylglucosamine and *N*-acetylmuramic acid; (2) a set of identical tetrapeptide side-chains attached to *N*-acetylmuramic acid; and (3) a set of identical peptide cross-bridges. The backbone is the same in all bacterial species;

however, the tetrapeptide side-chains and the peptide cross-bridges vary from species to species.

pep·ti·dyl·ar·gi·nine de·im·i·nase (pep″tĭ-dəl-ahr′jĭ-nēn de-im′ĭ-nās) a family of enzymes of the hydrolase class that catalyze the posttranslational conversion of arginine residues to citrulline residues in the presence of calcium ion. In EC nomenclature, called *protein-arginine deiminase.*

pep·ti·dyl-di·pep·ti·dase (pep″tĭ-dəl″ di-pep′tĭ-dās) [EC 3.4.15] any member of a sub-subclass of enzymes of the hydrolase class that catalyze the cleavage of a dipeptide residue from a free C-terminal end of a peptide or polypeptide.

pep·ti·dyl-di·pep·ti·dase A (pep′tĭ-dəl di-pep′tĭ-dās) [EC 3.4.15.1] an enzyme of the hydrolase class that catalyzes the cleavage of a dipeptide from the C-terminal end of an oligopeptide; it is a zinc protein found on the luminal surface of vascular endothelial cells in the lungs and other tissues. When catalyzing the cleavage of angiotensin I to form the activated angiotensin II, it is also called *angiotensin-converting enzyme;* when catalyzing the cleavage and inactivation of kinins, it is also called *kininase II.* Called also *dipeptidyl carboxypeptidase I.*

pep·ti·za·tion (pep″tĭ-za′shən) increase in the degree of dispersion of a colloid solution; the liquefaction of a colloid gel to form a sol.

Pep·to·coc·ca·ceae (pep″to-kok-a′se-e) [Gr. *pepton* digestion + *kokkos* berry] a family of anaerobic, nonmotile, usually gram-positive bacteria of the order Clostridiales, consisting of spherical cells occurring singly or in pairs, tetrads, chains, or irregular masses. They are found in soil; in the mouth, intestinal tract, and respiratory tract of various animals; and in the human female urogenital tract. Organisms of medical interest are contained in the genera *Peptococcus* and *Ruminococcus.*

Pep·to·coc·cus (pep″to-kok′əs) [Gr. *pepton* digestion + *kokkos* berry] a genus of gram-positive bacteria of the family Peptococcaceae, consisting of anaerobic, chemo-organotrophic cocci, occurring singly or in pairs, tetrads, or irregular masses. Pathogenic species have been assigned to other genera. The type species is *P. ni′ger.*

P. asaccharoly′ticus *Peptoniphilus asaccharolyticus*

P. constella′tus *Streptococcus constellatus.*

P. indo′licus *Peptoniphilus indolicus.*

P. mag′nus *Finegoldia magna.*

pep·to·gen·ic (pep″to-jen′ik) [Gr. *peptein* to digest + *-genic*] 1. producing peptones. 2. promoting digestion; called also *peptogenous.*

pep·tog·e·nous (pep-toj′ə-nəs) peptogenic.

pep·tol·y·sis (pep-tol′ĭ-sis) [*peptone* + *-lysis*] the hydrolysis of peptones. **peptolyt′ic** *adj*

pep·tone (pep′tōn) [Gr. *pepton* digesting] a derived protein, or a mixture of cleavage products produced by the partial hydrolysis of a native protein either by an acid or by an enzyme. Peptones are readily soluble in water and are not precipitatable by heat, by alkalis, or by saturation with ammonium sulfate. **pepton′ic** *adj*

Pep·to·ni·phi·lus (pep″to-nĭ-phil′əs) [*peptone* + Gr. *philos* loving] a genus of gram-positive bacteria of the family Peptostreptococcaceae that do not ferment sugar and use peptone as a major energy source; organisms are non–spore-forming, nonmotile, obligately anaerobic cocci, occurring in pairs, short chains, tetrads, or small clusters. The type species is *P. asaccharoly′ticus.*

P. asaccharoly′ticus an indole-producing species isolated from clinical specimens, including vaginal discharges and ovarian and peritoneal abscesses. Formerly called *Peptococcus asaccharolyticus.*

P. indo′licus an indole-producing species that has been isolated from infections of cows and pigs and is a cause of mastitis in cows. Formerly called *Peptococcus indolicus.*

pep·to·nize (pep′to-nīz) to convert a protein into peptone by the action of an acid or enzyme.

pep·ton·uria (pep″to-nu′re-ə) the presence of peptones in the urine.

Pep·to·strep·to·coc·ca·ceae (pep″to-strep″to-kok-a′se-e) a family of gram-positive, coccoid bacteria of the order Clostridiales; organisms of medical interest are found in the genera *Anaerococcus, Finegoldia, Peptoniphilus, Peptostreptococcus,* and *Tissierella.*

Pep·to·strep·to·coc·cus (pep″to-strep″to-kok′əs) [Gr. *pepton* digestion + *streptos* twisted + *kokkos* berry] a genus of gram-positive bacteria of the family Peptostreptococcaceae, consisting of obligately anaerobic, chemo-organotrophic, nonmotile cocci and coccobacilli. All species except for the type species *P. anaero′bius* have been assigned to other genera.

P. anaero′bius a species that ferments glucose only, isolated in humans from cases of gangrene, infected wounds, puerperal fever, appendicitis, pleurisy, paranasal sinusitis, and osteomyelitis, and from the intestinal tract, oral cavity, and genital secretions.

P. mag′nus *Finegoldia magna.*

P. mi′cros *Micromonas micros.*

per- [L. *per* through] 1. a prefix meaning throughout in space or time, or completely or extremely. 2. a prefix used in chemical terms to denote a large amount or to designate combination of an element in its highest valence.

per·ac·e·tate (per-as′ə-tāt) a salt or derivative of peracetic acid.

per·ace·tic ac·id (per″ə-se′tik) peroxyacetic acid, CH_3COOOH, a strong oxidizing agent sometimes used for sterilization.

per·ac·id (per-as′id) an acid containing more than the usual quantity of oxygen.

per·acid·i·ty (per″ə-sid′ĭ-te) excessive acidity.

per·acute (per″ə-kūt′) [L. *peracutus*] excessively acute or sharp.

Per·a·mel·i·dae (per″ə-mel′ĭ-de) the bandicoots (def. 2), a family of small marsupials that are hosts of a tick that spreads Q fever.

per anum (pər a′nəm) [L.] through the anus.

per·ar·tic·u·la·tion (per″ahr-tik″u-la′shən) [*per-* + *articulation*] diarthrosis.

per·cen·tile (pər-sen′tīl) [*per cent* + *-ile* (by analogy with *quartile, quintile,* etc.)] any one of the 99 values that divide the range of a probability distribution or sample into 100 intervals of equal probability or frequency, e.g., 45 per cent of a population scores below the 45th percentile.

per·cept (pur′sept) 1. something perceived. 2. the mental image of an object in space perceived by the senses.

per·cep·tion (pər-sep′shən) [L. *percipere* to take in completely] the conscious mental registration of a sensory stimulus.

depth p. the proper recognition of depth or the relative distances to different objects in space.

extrasensory p. (ESP) knowledge of, or response to, an external thought or objective event by means other than the senses.

stereognostic p. stereognosis.

per·cep·tive (pər-sep′tiv) 1. pertaining to perception. 2. having keen perception.

per·cep·tiv·i·ty (pur″sep-tiv′ĭ-te) ability to receive sense impressions.

per·chlo·rate (pər-klo′rāt) a salt or ester of perchloric acid.

per·chlor·ic ac·id (pər-klor′ik) a strong mineral acid and oxidizing agent, $HClO_4$.

per·chlo·ride (pər-klor′īd) a chloride that contains more chlorine than the ordinary chloride; an organic compound in which all the hydrogen atoms are substituted by chlorine, as in perchloroethylene (tetrachloroethylene), C_2Cl_4.

per·chlor·meth·ane (pur″klor-meth′ān) carbon tetrachloride.

per·chlor·meth·yl·for·mate (pur″klor-meth″əl-for′māt) diphosgene.

per·chlor·o·eth·y·lene (pər-klor″o-eth′ə-lēn) tetrachloroethylene.

per·cip·i·ent (pər-sip′e-ənt) 1. pertaining to perception. 2. an individual who perceives or is capable of perception.

Per·co·cet (pur′ko-set) trademark for a combination preparation of oxycodone hydrochloride and acetaminophen.

Per·co·dan (pur′ko-dan) trademark for a combination preparation of oxycodone hydrochloride, oxycodone terephthalate, and aspirin.

per·co·late (pur′kə-lāt) [L. *percolare*] 1. to strain; to submit to percolation. 2. to trickle slowly through a substance. 3. a liquid that has been submitted to percolation.

per·co·la·tion (pur″kə-la′shən) [L. *percolatio*] the extraction of the soluble parts of a drug by causing a solvent liquid to flow slowly through it.

per·co·la·tor (pur′kə-la″tər) a vessel used in percolating drugs.

Per·coll (pur′col) trademark for a colloidal suspension of silica used in density gradient centrifugation.

Per·co·lone (pur′kə-lōn) trademark for a preparation of oxycodone hydrochloride.

Per·cor·ten (pər-kor′tən) trademark for preparations of desoxycorticosterone.

per·cuss (pər-kus′) [L. *percutere*] to subject to percussion.

per·cus·si·ble (pər-kus′ĭ-bəl) discoverable on percussion.

per·cus·sion (pər-kush′ən) [L. *percussio*] 1. the act of striking a part with short, sharp blows as an aid in diagnosing the condition of the underlying parts by the sound obtained. 2. a method of massage; see *tapotement.*

auscultatory p. auscultation, usually by stethoscope, of the sound produced by percussion.

bimanual p. the usual manner of percussion in which the middle finger of the left hand is placed against the body wall and is struck a quick blow with the end of the bent right middle finger.

comparative p. percussion of two or more areas in order to compare the sounds obtained.

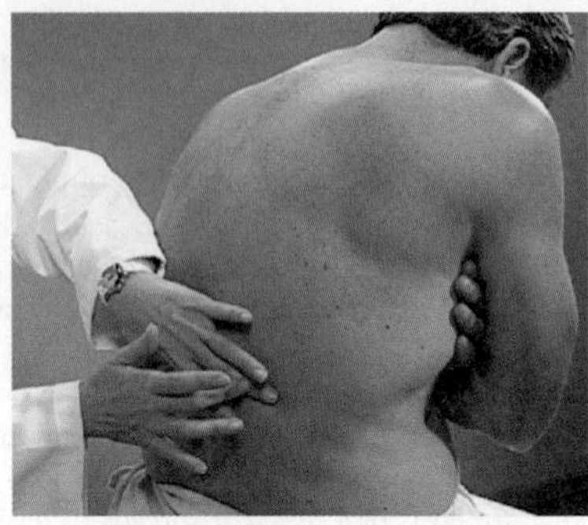

■ Mediate percussion using the middle finger of the nondominant hand as the pleximeter.

deep p. percussion in which a firm blow is struck in order to obtain a note from a deep-seated tissue.
direct p. immediate p.
drop p., drop stroke p. instrumental percussion in which the plexor is allowed to fall by its own weight on to the pleximeter, the elements considered in the examination being the sound heard, the vibrations felt in the handle of the plexor, and the rebound of the plexor seen. Called also *Lerch p.*
finger p. percussion in which the fingers of one hand are used as a plexor, and those of the other as a pleximeter.
fist p. percussion in which the fist is brought down with a moderate thump over the area to be tested.
Goldscheider p. 1. threshold p. 2. orthopercussion.
immediate p. percussion in which no pleximeter is used.
instrumental p. percussion in which a plexor or hammer is used.
Korányi p. see under *auscultation.*
Lerch p. drop p.
mediate p. percussion in which a pleximeter is employed.
Murphy p. piano p.
palpatory p. a combination of palpation and percussion, affording tactile rather than auditory impressions.
paradoxical p. resonance of the chest combined with abundant rales as in acute edema of the lungs.
pencil p. Plesch p.
piano p. percussion by striking the body by the four fingers one after the other, beginning with the little finger; called also *Murphy p.*
Plesch p. percussion within the intercostal spaces to avoid setting the ribs into vibration, the pleximeter finger with the proximal interphalangeal joint flexed at a right angle.
pleximetric p. mediate p.
respiratory p. percussion during respiration so as to bring out the difference in the percussion notes of inhalation and exhalation.
slapping p. percussion made by a slapping blow: used in comparing the resonance.
strip p. percussion which starts from above and progresses downward, thus covering a "strip" of the chest wall.
tangential p. percussion with the pleximeter placed vertically on the body, the strokes being applied to the pleximeter in a direction parallel with the surface of the skin.
threshold p. percussion by tapping lightly with the finger upon a glass rod pleximeter, one end of which, fitted with a rubber cap, rests on an intercostal space; the rod is held at an angle to the body surface, parallel to the borders of the organ to be delimited. This method confines the percussion vibrations to a restricted area. Called also *Goldscheider p.*
topographic p. the demarcation and outlining of a dull area by percussion to determine the boundaries of organs or parts of organs.

per•cus•sor (pər-kus′ər) 1. a vibrator that produces relatively coarse movements. 2. percussion hammer.

per•cu•ta•ne•ous (pur″ku-ta′ne-əs) [*per-* + *cutaneous*] performed through the skin, as injection of radiopaque material in radiological examination, or the removal of tissue for biopsy accomplished by a needle. Cf. *transdermal.*

per•en•ceph•a•ly (per″ən-sef′ə-le) porencephaly.

per•en•ni•al (pə-ren′e-əl) [L. *perennis,* from *per* through + *annus* year] lasting through the year or for several years.

Pe•rey•ra procedure (colposuspension) (pə-ra′rah) [Armand Joseph *Pereyra,* American obstetrician and gynecologist, 1904–1988] see under *procedure.*

Pé•rez sign (pa′rāth) [Jorjen (George) Victor *Pérez,* Spanish physician, 1851–1920] see under *sign.*

per•fect (pur′fəkt) of a fungus, capable of reproducing sexually (with sexual spores). Cf. *imperfect.*

per•fec•tion•ism (pər-fek′shən-iz-əm) the setting for oneself or others of a standard of flawless work or performance, or at least of one that is higher than the situation requires.

per•fil•con A (pər-fil′kon) a hydrophilic contact lens material.

per•fla•tion (pər-fla′shən) [L. *perflatio*] the act of blowing air into a space in order to force out secretions or other substances.

per•flu•bron (pər-floo′bron) [USP] a brominated fluorocarbon used as a contrast medium in magnetic resonance imaging of the gastrointestinal tract; administered orally.

per•flu•or•o•car•bon (pər-floor′o-kahr″bon) any of various substances chemically related to hydrocarbons but with the hydrogen atoms replaced by fluorine atoms. In liquid form, some are used in partial liquid ventilation; in gaseous form they cause environmental damage by collecting in the upper atmosphere.

per•flu•o•ro•chem•i•cal (pər-floor″o-kem′ĭ-kəl) an inert chemical substance with a high oxygen-carrying capacity; some can be emulsified with surfactants and transfused for temporary transport of oxygen in the blood.

per•flu•tren (pər-floo′trən) [USP] a fluorocarbon used as an ultrasound contrast imaging agent in diagnostic cardiology and radiology.

per•fo•rans (pur′fə-ranz) pl. *perforan′tes* [L.] penetrating, perforating; used in reference to muscles, nerves, arteries, and veins that perforate other structures.

per•fo•rat•ed (pur′fə-rāt″əd) [L. *perforatus*] pierced with holes.

per•fo•ra•tion (pur″fə-ra′shən) [L. *perforare* to pierce through] 1. the act of boring or piercing through a part. 2. a hole or break in the containing walls or membranes of an organ or structure of the body.
apical p. root p.
Bezold p. perforation of the inner surface of the mastoid bone; see also *Bezold abscess.*
mechanical p. an artificial opening or hole made by boring, piercing, or cutting through a structure or surface, such as the root of a tooth.
pathologic p. an opening or hole produced in a tissue surface or structure by a pathologic process, such as internal resorption of a tooth.
root p. perforation of the root of a tooth, occurring either iatrogenically during treatment or pathologically from internal resorption.

per•fo•ra•tor (pur′fə-ra″tər) an instrument for piercing bones.

per•for•in (pur′fə-rin) a protein expressed by cytotoxic lymphocytes and forming a transmembrane pore at the site of target cell lysis.

per•for•mance (pər-for′məns) 1. the execution of an action. 2. the act or process of functioning, sometimes measured by a performance scale or a performance test.
ventricular p. the execution of the pumping function of the ventricles, depending on preload, afterload, cardiac contractility, and heart rate; it is measured by cardiac output or work and expressed on a per stroke or per minute basis.

per•fri•ca•tion (pur″frĭ-ka′shən) [L. *perfricare* to rub] rubbing with an ointment or embrocation.

per•frig•er•a•tion (pər-frij″ər-a′shən) frostbite.

per•fu•sate (pər-fu′zāt) a liquid that has been passed over or through the vessels of an organ or tissue.

per•fuse (pər-fūz′) to pour over or through.

per•fu•sion (pər-fu′zhən) 1. the act of pouring over or through, especially the passage of a fluid through the vessels of a specific organ. 2. a liquid poured over or through an organ or tissue.
isolation-p. see under *technique.*
luxury p. abnormally increased flow of blood to an area of the brain, leading to swelling; causes include trauma, nearby cerebral infarction, and epileptogenic focus.
regional p. administration of an agent, particularly a chemotherapeutic agent, directly to a region of the body, commonly done by injecting the agent into a large artery supplying the region.

per•fu•sion•ist (pər-fu′zhən-ist) a technologist who operates the heart-lung machine during cardiopulmonary bypass.

per•go•lide mes•y•late (pur′go-līd″) a long-acting ergot derivative with dopaminergic properties, formerly used as an adjunct in the treatment of parkinsonism, and currently approved only for treatment of equine Cushing syndrome.

Per•go•nal (pur′gə-nəl) trademark for a preparation of menotropins.

peri- [Gr. *peri* around] a prefix meaning near or around.

per•hex•i•line mal•e•ate (pə-hek′sĭ-lēn) a coronary vasodilator, used in the treatment of severe angina pectoris, administered orally.

peri·ac·e·tab·u·lar (per″e-as″ə-tab′u-lər) around the acetabulum.

peri·ac·i·nal (per″e-as′ĭ-nəl) near or around an acinus; called also *periacinous.*

peri·ac·i·nous (per″e-as′ĭ-nəs) periacinal.

Per·i·ac·tin (per″e-ak′tin) trademark for preparations of cyproheptadine hydrochloride.

peri·ad·e·ni·tis (per″e-ad″ə-ni′tis) [*peri-* + *aden-* + *-itis*] inflammation of the tissues around a gland.

p. muco′sa necro′tica recur′rens a recurrent disease of the mucous membranes of unknown etiology, generally considered to be a severe form of recurrent aphthous stomatitis, characterized by deep crateriform ulcers with inflamed borders that leave scars after healing. It usually involves the mucosa of the lips, cheeks, tongue, palate, and anterior tonsillar pillars, but the pharynx, larynx, and genitalia may also be affected. Called also *Mikulicz aphthae, recurring scarring aphthae,* and *Sutton disease.*

peri·ad·ven·ti·tial (per″e-ad″vən-tĭ′shəl) outside the adventitia.

peri·am·pul·lary (per″e-am′pu-lar″e) near or around an ampulla, such as the hepatopancreatic ampulla.

peri·anal (per″e-a′nəl) [*peri-* + *anal*] near or around the anus; cf. *circumanal.*

peri·an·es·the·sia (per″e-an″es-the′zhə) the time from just before anesthesia is administered through the postanesthesia period.

peri·an·gi·itis (per″e-an″je-i′tis) [*peri-* + *angiitis*] perivasculitis.

peri·an·gio·cho·li·tis (per″e-an″je-o-ko-li′tis) pericholangitis.

peri·an·gi·o·ma (per″e-an-je-o′mə) [*peri-* + *angi-* + *-oma*] a tumor that surrounds a blood vessel.

peri·aor·tic (per″e-a-or′tik) near or around the aorta.

peri·aor·ti·tis (per″e-a″or-ti′tis) inflammation of the tissues around the aorta.

peri·apex (per″e-a′peks) the tissue that surrounds the root apex of a tooth (the periodontal ligament and alveolar bone).

peri·ap·i·cal (per″e-ap′ĭ-kəl) [*peri-* + *apic-* + *-al*[1]] at or around the apex of a tooth.

peri·ap·pen·dic·e·al (per″e-ap″ən-dis′e-əl) periappendicular.

peri·ap·pen·di·ci·tis (per″e-ə-pen″dĭ-si′tis) [*peri-* + *appendic-* + *-itis*] inflammation of the tissues around the vermiform appendix.

p. decidua′lis a condition in tubal pregnancy in which, because of adhesions between the appendix and the fallopian tube, decidual cells are present on the peritoneum of the appendix.

peri·ap·pen·dic·u·lar (per″e-ap″ən-dik′u-lər) near or around the vermiform appendix; called also *periappendiceal.*

peri·apt (per′e-apt) [Gr. *periapton* amulet] something worn in the belief that it has power to ward off disease.

peri·aq·ue·duc·tal (per″e-ak″wĭ-duk′təl) near or around an aqueduct.

peri·ar·te·ri·al (per″e-ahr-tēr′e-əl) near or around an artery.

peri·ar·ter·i·tis (per″e-ahr″tə-ri′tis) [*peri-* + *arteritis*] inflammation of the external coats of an artery and of the tissues around the artery.

p. nodo′sa 1. polyarteritis nodosa. 2. a group comprising classic polyarteritis nodosa, allergic granulomatous angiitis, and many systemic necrotizing vasculitides with clinicopathologic characteristics overlapping the two former disorders.

peri·ar·thric (per″e-ahr′thrik) periarticular.

peri·ar·thri·tis (per″e-ahr-thri′tis) inflammation of the tissues around a joint.

calcific p. periarthritis owing to deposition of crystals of basic calcium phosphate.

p. of shoulder periarthritis around the shoulder joint, which may include tendinitis, adhesive capsulitis, and various types of bursitis.

peri·ar·tic·u·lar (per″e-ahr-tik′u-lər) [*peri-* + *articular*] around a joint.

peri·atri·al (per″e-a′tre-əl) near or around the atrium of the heart.

peri·au·ric·u·lar (per″e-aw-rik′u-lər) near or around the auricle of the ear.

peri·ax·i·al (per″e-ak′se-əl) [*peri-* + *axial*] near or around an axis.

peri·ax·il·lary (per″e-ak′sĭ-lar″e) near or around the axilla.

peri·ax·o·nal (per″e-ak′sə-nəl) near or around an axon.

peri·bron·chi·al (per″e-brong′ke-əl) near or around a bronchus.

peri·bron·chi·o·lar (per″e-brong-ki′o-lər) near or around the bronchioles.

peri·bron·chio·li·tis (per″e-brong″ke-o-li′tis) inflammation of the tissues around the bronchioles.

peri·bron·chi·tis (per″e-brong-ki′tis) a form of bronchitis consisting of inflammation and thickening of the peribronchial tissue.

peri·bul·bar (per″e-bul′bər) surrounding the bulb of the eye.

peri·bur·sal (per″e-bur′səl) surrounding a bursa.

peri·cal·i·ce·al (per″e-kal″ĭ-se′əl) pericalyceal.

peri·cal·lo·sal (per″e-kə-lo′səl) near or around the corpus callosum.

peri·ca·lyc·e·al (per″e-kal″ĭ-se′əl) near or around a renal calyx; spelled also *pericaliceal.*

peri·can·a·lic·u·lar (per″e-kan″ə-lik′u-lər) near or around a canaliculus.

peri·cap·il·lary (per″e-kap′ĭ-lar″e) near or around a capillary.

peri·cap·su·lar (per″e-kap′su-lər) surrounding a capsule.

peri·car·dec·to·my (per″e-kahr-dek′tə-me) pericardiectomy.

peri·car·di·ac (per″e-kahr′de-ak) pericardial.

peri·car·di·al (per″e-kahr′de-əl) 1. pertaining to the pericardium. 2. surrounding the heart.

peri·car·di·cen·te·sis (per″e-kahr″de-sen-te′sis) pericardiocentesis.

peri·car·di·ec·to·my (per″e-kahr″de-ek′tə-me) [*pericardium* + *-ectomy*] surgical removal of all or part of the pericardium.

peri·car·dio·cen·te·sis (per″e-kahr″de-o-sen-te′sis) [*pericardium* + *-centesis*] surgical puncture of the pericardial cavity for the aspiration of fluid.

peri·car·di·ol·y·sis (per″e-kahr″de-ol′ĭ-sis) [*pericardium* + *-lysis*] the operation of freeing adhesions between the visceral and parietal pericardium or between the pericardium and surrounding tissues or organs.

peri·car·dio·me·di·as·ti·ni·tis (per″e-kahr″de-o-me″de-as-tĭ-ni′tis) [*pericardium* + *mediastinitis*] pericarditis with mediastinitis; inflammation of the pericardium and mediastinum.

peri·car·dio·phren·ic (per″e-kahr″de-o-fren′ik) pertaining to the pericardium and the diaphragm.

peri·car·dio·pleu·ral (per″e-kahr″de-o-ploor′əl) pertaining to the pericardium and the pleura.

peri·car·di·or·rha·phy (per″e-kahr″de-or′ə-fe) [*pericardium* + *-rrhaphy*] the operation of suturing a wound in the pericardium.

peri·car·di·os·co·py (per″e-kahr″de-os′ko-pe) [*pericardium* + *-scopy*] visualization of the parietal pericardium and epicardium using a flexible fiberoptic bronchoscope or endoscope.

peri·car·di·os·to·my (per″e-kahr″de-os′tə-me) [*pericardium* + *-ostomy*] the creation of an opening into the pericardium, usually for the drainage of effusions.

peri·car·di·ot·o·my (per″e-kahr″de-ot′ə-me) [*pericardium* + *-tomy*] surgical incision of the pericardium.

peri·car·di·tis (per″e-kahr-di′tis) [*pericardium* + *-itis*] inflammation of the pericardium. **pericardit′ic** *adj*

acute benign p., acute idiopathic p. idiopathic p.

adhesive p. a condition resulting from the presence of dense fibrous tissue between the parietal and visceral layers of the pericardium. There may be complete obliteration of the pericardial cavity, or there may be adhesions extending from the pericardium to the mediastinum (mediastinopericarditis), diaphragm, and chest wall (accretio cordis, accretio pericardii).

amebic p. pericardial inflammation occurring as a result of rupture of an amebic abscess of the liver through the diaphragm.

bacterial p. pericardial inflammation produced by bacterial infection, particularly by staphylococci or gram-negative bacilli. See also *purulent p.*

bread-and-butter p. fibrinous pericarditis in which the fibrinous exudate forms a thick shaggy coat over the pericardium, with adhesions between the layers.

carcinomatous p., p. carcinomato′sa pericardial inflammation associated with malignancy of the pericardium.

cholesterol p. pericarditis characterized by cholesterol-laden effusion, resulting from deposition of cholesterol crystals and subsequent inflammatory response including infiltration of the pericardium by lymphocytes, plasma cells, macrophages, and giant cells.

chronic constrictive p., constrictive p. chronic pericarditis in which a fibrotic, thickened, adherent pericardium restricts diastolic filling and cardiac output. It is usually a consequence of a series of events beginning with an acute episode in which fibrin and sometimes calcium are deposited on the pericardial surface, followed by fibrotic scarring and thickening of the pericardium and obliteration of the pericardial space.

dry p. pericardial inflammation not associated with effusion.

p. with effusion pericardial inflammation associated with the collection of a serous or purulent exudate in the pericardial cavity.

effusive constrictive p. pericarditis characterized by pericardial effusion in the presence of visceral pericardial constriction, manifest as continued elevation of right atrial pressure after pericardiocentesis; it often leads to chronic constrictive pericarditis.

fibrinous p., fibrous p. pericarditis characterized by a fibrinous exudate, sometimes accompanied by a small amount of serous effusion; it is usually manifest as a pericardial friction rub. It often progresses to adhesive pericarditis. Cf. *serofibrinous p.*

fungal p. pericardial inflammation due to fungal infection, usually histoplasmosis or coccidioidomycosis.

hemorrhagic p. pericarditis in which the exudate is bloody as well as serous, serofibrinous, or purulent; causes include tuberculosis, uremia, severe acute infections, and neoplasia.

idiopathic p. an acute serofibrinous pericarditis of unknown cause; many patients have recurrent attacks. Called also *acute benign p.*

localized p. chronic inflammation of the pericardium with thickened white or milky epicardial areas.

neoplastic p. pericarditis associated with primary or secondary neoplastic infiltration of the pericardium, often characterized by serous or bloody pericardial effusion, constriction, arrhythmia, or tamponade.

p. obli′terans, obliterating p. an adhesive pericarditis which leads to the obliteration of the pericardial cavity.

postcardiotomy p. pericardial inflammation occurring as a complication following cardiac surgery, characterized by effusion and rarely by constriction.

postinfarction p. acute pericarditis developing within one week after myocardial infarction, manifested as pericardial pain, dyspnea, and a pericardial rub.

postirradiation p. pericardial inflammation, acute or chronic, resulting from high dose radiotherapy, often beginning as exudative effusion with fibrin deposits and sometimes progressing to chronic pericardial effusion or constrictive pericarditis. It may present decades after radiation exposure.

purulent p. pericardial inflammation characterized by pus formation, usually due to bacterial infection, and less often to fungal or viral infection, which may be spread from neighboring tissues, through the blood or lymphatic systems, or via direct implantation in wounds. It is characterized by fibrinopurulent or purulent exudates and often results in constrictive pericarditis and tamponade.

radiation p. postirradiation p.

rheumatic p. pericardial inflammation associated with active rheumatic heart disease, characterized by a fibrinous, serofibrinous, or purulent exudate, sparse to densely shaggy fibrin deposits, chest pain, and pericardial friction rub.

serofibrinous p. pericarditis characterized by a fibrinous exudate accompanied by substantial serous effusion, otherwise resembling fibrinous pericarditis.

serous p. pericarditis characterized by serous effusion, usually produced by a nonbacterial inflammation.

p. sic′ca acute fibrinous pericarditis without effusion.

suppurative p. purulent p.

traumatic p. 1. pericardial inflammation caused by penetrating or nonpenetrating injury to the pericardium; it is characterized by pericardial pain and friction and may lead to hemopericardium or tamponade. 2. in cattle, injury to the pericardium by an ingested hard foreign object such as metallic debris; the object migrates from the reticulum through the diaphragm and lodges against the pericardium, causing inflammation. Exudated fluid collects in the pericardial sac and interferes with the heart's pumping efficiency. Called also *hardware disease* and *traumatic reticulopericarditis.*

tuberculous p. pericarditis secondary to tuberculosis, characterized by effusion of fluid containing fibrin, blood, and sometimes caseous debris, thick shaggy deposits of fibrin, pericardial friction rub, and adhesion of the pericardial layers; it often results in chronic constrictive pericarditis.

uremic p. pericardial inflammation occurring as a complication of uremia; it is characterized by shaggy, vascular, fibrinous exudate on the visceral and parietal pericardial surfaces.

viral p. pericardial inflammation associated with viral infection, usually by coxsackievirus or echovirus, characterized by pericardial friction rub, substantial effusion.

peri•car•di•um (per″ĭ-kahr′de-əm) [L.; *peri-* + Gr. *kardia* heart] 1. [TA] the fibroserous sac that surrounds the heart and the roots of the great vessels, comprising an external layer of fibrous tissue *(p. fibrosum)* and an inner serous layer *(p. serosum).* The base of the pericardium is attached to the central tendon of the diaphragm. 2. pericardial sinus.

adherent p. a pericardium that is abnormally connected with the heart by dense fibrous tissue, as in adhesive pericarditis.

bread-and-butter p. a pericardium having a thick fibrinous deposit on its surfaces; see also *bread-and-butter pericarditis.*

calcified p. a pericardium containing deposits of lime salts.

p. fibro′sum [TA], **fibrous p.** the external layer of the pericardium, consisting of fibrous tissue.

parietal p. lamina parietalis pericardii serosi.

p. sero′sum [TA], **serous p.** the inner serous portion of the pericardium consisting of two layers, the *lamina parietalis pericardii serosi,*

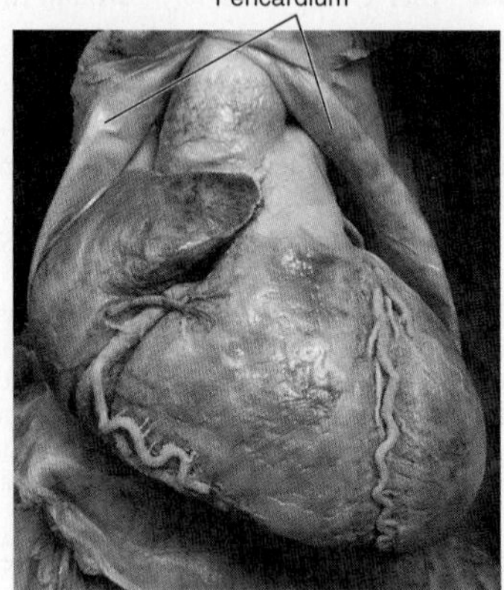

■ Serous pericardium overlying the fibrous pericardium (incised and turned back).

which is apposed to the fibrous pericardium, and the *lamina visceralis pericardii serosi,* or *epicardium,* which is reflected onto the roots of the great vessels and the heart. The space between the two layers is the *cavitas pericardialis.*

shaggy p. bread-and-butter p.

visceral p. lamina visceralis pericardii serosi.

peri•car•dot•o•my (per″e-kahr-dot′ə-me) pericardiotomy.

peri•carp (per′ĭ-kahrp″) [*peri-* + *carp*] the seed vessel or ripened ovary of a flower.

peri•cary•on (per″e-kar′e-on) perikaryon.

peri•ce•cal (per″e-se′kəl) surrounding the cecum.

peri•ce•ci•tis (per″e-se-si′tis) inflammation of the tissues around the cecum.

peri•cel•lu•lar (per″e-sel′u-lər) [*peri-* + *cellular*] surrounding a cell.

peri•ce•men•ti•tis (per″e-se″mən-ti′tis) inflammation of the pericementum (periodontal ligament). See *periodontitis.*

apical p. apical abscess.

chronic suppurative p. marginal periodontitis.

peri•ce•men•tum (per″e-se-men′təm) periodontal ligament. **pericemen′tal** *adj*

peri•cen•tral (per″e-sen′trəl) surrounding a center.

peri•cen•tri•o•lar (per″e-sen″tre-o′lər) around a centriole.

peri•ce•phal•ic (per″e-sə-fal′ik) near or around the head.

peri•cho•lan•gi•tis (per″e-ko″lan-ji′tis) [*peri-* + *cholangi-* + *-itis*] inflammation of the tissues that surround the bile ducts.

peri•cho•le•cys•ti•tis (per″e-ko″lə-sis-ti′tis) inflammation of the tissues around the gallbladder.

gaseous p. emphysematous cholecystitis.

peri•chon•dri•tis (per″e-kon-dri′tis) inflammation of the perichondrium.

peri•chon•dri•um (per″ĭ-kon′dre-əm) [*peri-* + Gr. *chondros* cartilage] [TA] the layer of dense fibrous connective tissue investing all cartilage except the articular cartilage of synovial joints. **perichon′drial** *adj*

peri•chon•dro•ma (per″e-kon-dro′mə) [*perichondrium* + *-oma*] a tumor arising from the perichondrium.

peri•chord (per′ĭ-kord) the investing sheath of the notochord.

peri•chor•dal (per″e-kor′dəl) [*peri-* + *chordal*] around the notochord.

peri•cho•roi•dal (per″e-kor-oi′dəl) surrounding the choroid coat.

peri•chro•ma•tin (per″e-kro′mə-tin) adjacent to a chromatin domain.

peri•co•lic (per″e-kol′ik) around the colon.

peri•co•li•tis (per″e-ko-li′tis) [*peri-* + *colitis*] inflammation around the colon, especially of its peritoneal coat.

peri•co•lon•itis (per″e-ko″lən-i′tis) pericolitis.

peri•col•pi•tis (per″e-kol-pi′tis) perivaginitis.

peri•con•cep•tion•al (per″e-kən-sep′shən-əl) around the time of conception.

peri•con•chal (per″e-kong′kəl) around a concha; cf. *periauricular.*

peri•con•chi•tis (per″e-kong-ki′tis) periorbititis.

peri•cor•ne•al (per″e-kor′ne-əl) surrounding the cornea.

peri•cor•o•nal (per″e-kor′ə-nəl) around the crown of a tooth.

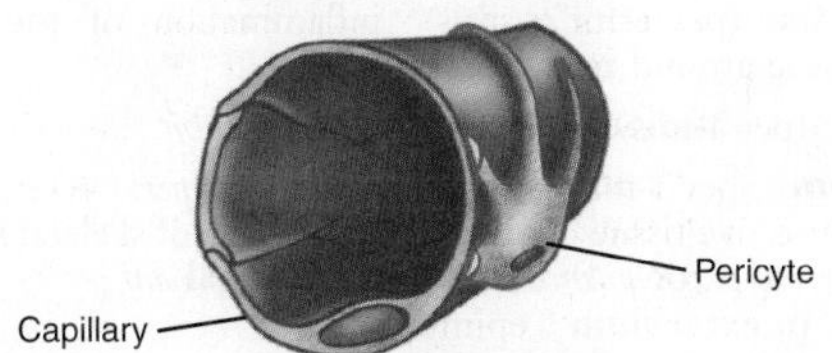

■ Pericyte, its processes wrapped around the capillary epithelium.

peri·cor·o·ni·tis (per″e-kor″o-ni′tis) [*peri-* + *corona* + *-itis*] inflammation of the gingiva surrounding the crown of a tooth. Called also *operculitis.*

peri·cox·itis (per″e-kok-si′tis) inflammation of the tissues about the hip joint.

peri·cra·ni·tis (per″e-kra-ni′tis) inflammation of the external periosteum of the skull.

peri·cra·ni·um (per″e-kra′ne-əm) [*peri-* + *cranium*] [TA] the external periosteum of the skull; called also *periosteum externum cranii* [TA alternative]. **pericra′nial** *adj*

peri·cryp·tal (per″e-krip′təl) around a crypt.

peri·cys·tic (per″e-sis′tik) 1. near or around a cyst. 2. perivesical.

peri·cys·ti·tis (per″e-sis-ti′tis) [*peri-* + *cyst-* + *-itis*] inflammation of the tissues around the bladder.

peri·cys·ti·um (per″ĭ-sis′te-əm) the vascular envelope of certain cysts.

peri·cyte (per′e-sīt) [*peri-* + *-cyte*] a type of elongated cell having the power of contraction; these are found wrapped about the outside of precapillary arterioles, postcapillary venules, and capillaries. Called also *adventitial, pericapillary, perithelial,* or *perivascular cell.*

peri·cy·ti·al (per″e-si′te-əl) around a cell.

peri·cy·to·ma (per″ĭ-si-to′mə) hemangiopericytoma.

peri·dec·to·my (per″ĭ-dek′tə-me) peritectomy.

peri·den·drit·ic (per″e-dən-drit′ik) surrounding the dendrites.

peri·dens (per″ĭ-dens) a supernumerary tooth appearing elsewhere than in the midline of the dental arch.

peri·den·tal (per″e-den′təl) periodontal.

peri·derm (per′ĭ-durm″) [*peri-* + *-derm*] 1. the large-celled outer layer of the two-layered fetal epidermis, which is loosened by hair that grows beneath it and generally disappears before birth. Called also *epitrichium.* 2. the cuticle (eponychium) and hyponychium considered together.

peri·der·mal (per″ĭ-dur′məl) pertaining to the periderm.

peri·des·mic (per″ĭ-dez′mik) 1. pertaining to the peridesmium. 2. periligamentous.

peri·des·mi·tis (per″e-dez-mi′tis) inflammation of the peridesmium.

peri·des·mi·um (per″e-dez′me-əm) [*peri-* + Gr. *desmion* band] the areolar membrane which covers the ligaments.

Peri·dex (per′ĭ-deks) trademark for a preparation of chlorhexidine gluconate.

pe·rid·ia (pə-rid′e-ə) plural of *peridium.*

pe·rid·i·um (pə-rid′e-əm) pl. *perid′ia* [Gr. *pēridion* small leather bag or wallet] the outer coat or limiting membrane enveloping the fruiting body of certain fungi and protozoa.

peri·di·ver·tic·u·lar (per″e-di″vər-tik′u-lər) around a diverticulum.

peri·di·ver·tic·u·li·tis (per″e-di″vər-tik″u-li′tis) inflammation of structures around a diverticulum of the intestine.

peri·don·ti·um (per″ĭ-don′she-əm) periodontium (def. 1).

peri·duc·tal (per″e-duk′təl) surrounding a duct, particularly a duct of the mammary gland.

peri·du·o·de·ni·tis (per″e-doo″o-də-ni′tis) inflammation around the duodenum, which causes deformity of the duodenum as it is surrounded and fixed by peritoneal adhesions.

peri·du·ral (per″e-doo′rəl) around or external to the dura mater.

peri·du·ro·gram (per″e-doo′ro-gram) the film obtained in peridurography.

peri·du·rog·ra·phy (per″e-do͝o-rog′rə-fe) [*peri-* + *dura* + Gr. *graphein* to write] radiography of the spinal canal and interspaces after injection of a contrast medium in the peridural space.

peri·en·ceph·a·li·tis (per″e-en-sef″ə-li′tis) meningoencephalitis.

peri·en·ceph·a·log·ra·phy (per″e-en-sef″ə-log′rə-fe) radiography of the cerebral meninges.

peri·en·ter·ic (per″e-en-ter′ik) near or around the intestine.

peri·en·ter·itis (per″e-en″tər-i′tis) [*peri-* + *enter-* + *-itis*] inflammation of the peritoneal coat of the intestine.

peri·en·ter·on (per″e-en′tər-on) [*peri-* + *enteron*] the primordial embryonic cavity surrounding the viscera.

peri·ep·en·dy·mal (per″e-ep-en′də-məl) near or around the ependyma.

peri·esoph·a·ge·al (per″e-ə-sof′ə-je-əl) around the esophagus.

peri·esoph·a·gi·tis (per″e-ə-sof′ə-ji′tis) inflammation of the tissues around the esophagus.

peri·fas·cic·u·lar (per″e-fə-sik′u-lər) surrounding a fasciculus of nerve or muscle fibers.

peri·fis·tu·lar (per″e-fis′tu-lər) around a fistula.

peri·fo·cal (per″ĭ-fo′kəl) around or surrounding a focus, such as a focus of infection.

peri·fol·lic·u·lar (per″e-fə-lik′u-lər) surrounding a follicle, particularly a hair follicle.

peri·fol·lic·u·li·tis (per″e-fə-lik″u-li′tis) inflammation around the hair follicles.

p. ca′pitis absce′dens et suffo′diens a rare chronic suppurative disease of the scalp, usually seen in young adults, especially men, marked by numerous follicular and perifollicular reactions with formation of nodules that become fluctuant and rupture to produce intercommunicating draining sinuses; upon healing they leave severe scarring and alopecia. Called also *dissecting cellulitis of scalp* and *folliculitis abscedens et suffodiens.*

superficial pustular p. Bockhart impetigo.

peri·for·ni·cal (per″e-for′nĭ-kəl) near a fornix, particularly in the brain.

peri·fu·sate (per″ĭ-fu′zāt) the fluid used in perifusion.

peri·fuse (per″ĭ-fūz′) [*peri-* + L. *fundere* to pour] to pass a bathing fluid around all surfaces of organelles, cells, cell clusters, or tissue held in suspension.

peri·fu·sion (per″ĭ-fu′zhən) the act or process of perifusing.

peri·gan·gli·itis (per″e-gang″gle-i′tis) inflammation of tissues around a ganglion.

peri·gan·gli·on·ic (per″e-gang″gle-on′ik) near or around a ganglion.

peri·gas·tric (per″e-gas′trik) 1. near or around the stomach. 2. pertaining to the peritoneum around the stomach.

peri·gas·tri·tis (per″e-gas-tri′tis) [*peri-* + *gastr-* + *-itis*] inflammation of the peritoneum around the stomach.

peri·gem·mal (per″ĭ-jem′əl) surrounding a taste bud or other bud.

peri·glan·du·lar (per″e-glan′du-lər) surrounding a gland or glands.

peri·glan·du·li·tis (per″e-glan″du-li′tis) inflammation of the tissues around a gland.

peri·gli·al (per″ĭ-gli′əl) surrounding the neuroglial cells.

peri·glos·si·tis (per″e-glos-i′tis) inflammation of the tissues around the tongue.

peri·glot·tic (per″e-glot′ik) near or around the tongue.

peri·graft (per′e-graft) situated or occurring around a graft.

peri·he·pat·ic (per″e-hə-pat′ik) near or around the liver.

peri·hep·a·ti·tis (per″e-hep″ə-ti′tis) [*peri-* + *hepat-* + *-itis*] inflammation of the peritoneal capsule of the liver and of the tissues around the liver.

chlamydial p. perihepatitis due to extension of a chlamydial infection; see also *Fitz-Hugh–Curtis syndrome,* under *syndrome.*

p. chro′nica hyperplas′tica hyaloserositis of the liver; conversion of its peritoneal covering into a white mass resembling the icing of a cake. Called also *frosted* or *icing liver.*

gonococcal p. perihepatitis due to extension of gonorrheal infection; see also *Fitz-Hugh–Curtis syndrome,* under *syndrome.*

peri·her·ni·al (per″e-hur′ne-əl) around a hernia.

peri·hi·lar (per″e-hi′lər) around a hilum.

peri·im·plan·ti·tis (per″e-im-plan-ti′tis) inflammation of the tissue around a dental implant, often with tissue breakdown.

peri·in·su·lar (per″e-in′su-lər) surrounding an island, particularly the insula.

peri·is·let (per″e-i′let) around the islets of Langerhans.

peri·je·ju·ni·tis (per″e-jĕ″joo-ni′tis) inflammation around the jejunum.

peri·kary·on (per″e-kar′e-on) pl. *perikar′ya* [*peri-* + *karyon*] the cell body as distinguished from the nucleus and the processes; applied particularly to neurons.

peri·ke·rat·ic (per″e-kə-rat′ik) surrounding the cornea.

peri·ky·ma·ta (per″e-ki′mə-tə) (pl. of *periky′ma*) [*peri-* + Gr. *kyma* wave] the numerous small transverse ridges on the surface of the enamel of permanent teeth, representing overlapping prism groups; continued abrasion erodes the enamel surface and obliterates them.

peri·lab·y·rinth (per″e-lab′ə-rinth) the tissue surrounding the labyrinth of the ear.

peri·lab·y·rin·thi·tis (per″e-lab″ə-rin-thi′tis) circumscribed labyrinthitis.

peri·la·ryn·ge·al (per″e-lə-rin′je-əl) around the larynx.

peri·len·tic·u·lar (per″e-len-tik′u-lər) surrounding the lens of the eye.

peri·le·sion·al (per″e-le′zhən-əl) near or around a lesion.

peri·lig·a·men·tous (per″e-lig″ə-men′təs) around a ligament.

Pe·ril·la (pə-ril′ə) a genus of herbs found in North America. *P. frutes′cens*, a type of wild mint, contains a poisonous ketone and can cause fatal emphysema in ruminants.

peri·lo·bar (per″e-lo′bər) surrounding a lobe.

peri·lob·u·li·tis (per″e-lob-u-li′tis) inflammation of the tissues surrounding the lobules of the lung.

peri·lymph (per′e-limf) perilympha.

peri·lym·pha (per″e-lim′fə) [*peri-* + *lympha*] [TA] perilymph: the fluid contained within the space separating the membranous labyrinth from the osseous labyrinth; it is entirely separate from the endolymph.

peri·lym·phad·e·ni·tis (per″e-lim-fad″ə-ni′tis) inflammation of the tissues around a lymph gland.

peri·lym·phan·ge·al (per″e-lim-fan′je-əl) near or around a lymphatic vessel.

peri·lym·phan·gi·tis (per″e-lim″fan-ji′tis) inflammation of the tissues around a lymphatic vessel.

peri·lym·phat·ic (per″e-lim-fat′ik) 1. pertaining to the perilymph. 2. around a lymphatic vessel.

peri·man·dib·u·lar (per″e-man-dib′u-lər) near or around the mandible.

peri·mas·ti·tis (per″e-mas-ti′tis) [*peri-* + *mast-* + *-itis*] inflammation of the connective tissue around the mammary gland.

peri·me·a·tal (per″e-me-a′təl) around a meatus.

peri·med·ul·lary (per″e-med′u-lar″e) surrounding a medulla, as the medulla oblongata or the marrow of a bone.

peri·men·in·gi·tis (per″e-men″in-ji′tis) pachymeningitis.

peri·meno·pause (per″e-men′o-pawz) the time just before and after menopause; there are noticeable drops in estrogen levels for three to five years prior to menopause. **perimenopau′sal** *adj*

pe·rim·e·ter (pə-rim′ə-tər) [*peri-* + *-meter*] 1. a line forming the boundary of a plane figure. 2. an apparatus for determining the extent of the peripheral visual field on a curved surface.

  dental p. an instrument for measuring the circumference of a tooth.

peri·met·ric (per″ĭ-met′rik) 1. pertaining to a perimeter. 2. around the uterus. 3. pertaining to the perimetrium.

peri·me·tri·tis (per″ĭ-mə-tri′tis) [*peri-* + *metr-* + *-itis*] inflammation of the perimetrium. **perimetrit′ic** *adj*

peri·me·tri·um (per″ĭ-me′tre-əm) [*peri-* + Gr. *mētra* uterus] TA alternative for *tunica serosa uteri.*

peri·met·ro·sal·pin·gi·tis (per″e-met″ro-sal″pin-ji′tis) inflammation of the uterus and uterine tubes and of surrounding tissues.

  encapsulating p. perimetrosalpingitis with formation of a membrane about the organs involved.

pe·rim·e·try (pə-rim′ə-tre) [*peri-* + *-metry*] determination of the extent of the peripheral visual field by use of a perimeter; cf. *perioptometry.*

peri·mol·y·sis (per″ĭ-mol′ĭ-sis) [shortened from *perimylolysis*, q.v.] erosion of the lingual surfaces of the anterior teeth and the occlusal surfaces of the posterior teeth by acid decalcification; commonly seen in anorexia nervosa and also in other conditions involving chronic regurgitation.

peri·my·eli·tis (per″e-mi″ə-li′tis) 1. endosteitis. 2. spinal meningitis.

peri·my·elog·ra·phy (per″e-mi″ə-log′rə-fe) [*peri-* + *myelo-* + *-graphy*] radiologic examination after injecting iodized oil or other contrast fluid into the subarachnoid space of the spinal cord.

peri·my·lol·y·sis (per″e-mĭ-lol′ĭ-sis) perimolysis.

peri·myo·car·di·tis (per″e-mi″o-kahr-di′tis) [*peri-* + *myocarditis*] combined pericarditis and myocarditis.

peri·myo·en·do·car·di·tis (per″e-mi″o-en″do-kahr-di′tis) pericarditis associated with myocarditis and endocarditis.

peri·myo·si·tis (per″e-mi″o-si′tis) inflammation of the perimysium (connective tissue around muscles).

peri·mys·ia (per″ĭ-mis′e-ə) plural of *perimysium.*

peri·mys·i·um (per″ĭ-mis′e-əm) pl. *perimys′ia* [*peri-* + Gr. *mys* muscle] [TA] the connective tissue demarcating a fascicle of skeletal muscle fibers; called also *internal p.*, or *p. internum.* **perimys′ial** *adj*

  external p., p. exter′num epimysium.

  internal p., p. inter′num perimysium.

peri·na·sal (per″e-na′zəl) perirhinal.

peri·na·tal (per″e-na′təl) [*peri-* + *natal*] pertaining to or occurring in the period shortly before and after birth; variously defined as beginning with completion of the twentieth to twenty-eighth week of gestation and ending 7 to 28 days after birth.

peri·na·tol·o·gist (per″e-na-tol′ə-jist) a specialist in perinatology.

peri·na·tol·o·gy (per″e-na-tol′ə-je) [*perinatal* + *-logy*] the branch of medicine (obstetrics and pediatrics) dealing with the fetus and infant during the perinatal period.

per·in·do·pril er·bu·mine (pə-rin′do-pril) an angiotensin-converting enzyme inhibitor administered orally, alone or in combination with a thiazide diuretic, for treatment of hypertension.

peri·ne·al (per″ĭ-ne′əl) pertaining to the perineum.

peri·neo·cele (per″ĭ-ne′o-sēl) [*perineum* + *-cele*[1]] perineal hernia.

peri·ne·om·e·ter (per″ĭ-ne-om′ə-tər) an instrument for measuring the strength of contractions of the perivaginal muscles.

peri·neo·plas·ty (per″ĭ-ne′o-plas″te) [*perineum* + *-plasty*] plastic surgery of the perineum.

peri·ne·or·rha·phy (per″ĭ-ne-or′ə-fe) [*perineum* + *-rrhaphy*] suture of the perineum, performed for the repair of a laceration.

peri·neo·scro·tal (per″ĭ-ne″o-skro′təl) pertaining to the perineum and scrotum.

peri·ne·ot·o·my (per″ĭ-ne-ot′ə-me) [*perineum* + *-tomy*] surgical incision through the perineum.

peri·neo·vag·i·nal (per″ĭ-ne″o-vaj′ĭ-nəl) pertaining to or communicating between the perineum and the vagina.

peri·neo·vag·i·no·rec·tal (per″ĭ-ne″o-vaj′ĭ-no-rek′təl) pertaining to the perineum, vagina, and rectum.

peri·neo·vul·var (per″ĭ-ne″o-vul′vər) pertaining to the perineum and the vulva.

peri·neph·ric (per″e-nef′rik) immediately adjacent to the kidney, within the renal fascia; perirenal. Cf *paranephric.*

peri·ne·phri·tis (per″e-nə-fri′tis) [*peri-* + *nephr-* + *-itis*] inflammation of perinephric tissue, marked by fever, local pain, and tenderness on pressure. Cf. *perinephric abscess*, under *abscess.* **perinephrit′ic** *adj*

peri·neph·ri·um (per″ĭ-nef′re-əm) [*peri-* + Gr. *nephros* kidney] the peritoneal envelope, renal fascia, and other tissues around the kidney. **perineph′rial** *adj*

peri·ne·um (per″ĭ-ne′əm) [Gr. *perinaion, perineos* the space between the anus and scrotum] 1. [TA] the region and associated structures occupying the pelvic outlet and beneath the pelvic diaphragm; it is bounded anteriorly by the pubic symphysis, anterolaterally by the ischiopubic rami and the ischial tuberosities, posterolaterally by the sacrotuberous ligaments, and posteriorly by the coccyx. The deep limit is the inferior surface of the pelvic diaphragm, and the superficial limit is the skin. 2. the region between the thighs, bounded in the male by the scrotum and anus and in

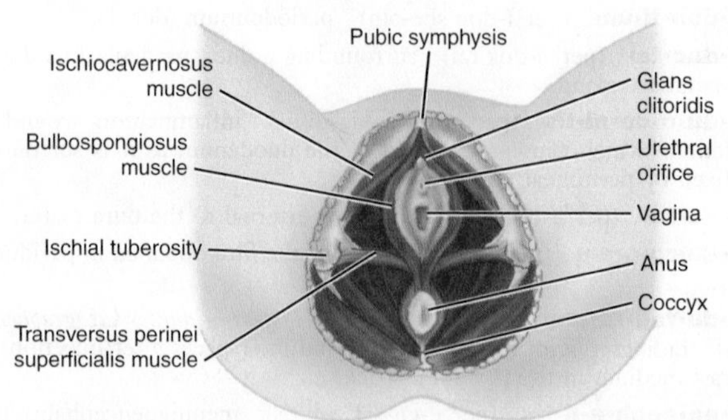

■ Perineum in a female; the diamond-shaped area between the pubic symphysis and coccyx can be divided into anterior urogenital and posterior anal triangles by drawing a line transversely between the ischial tuberosities.

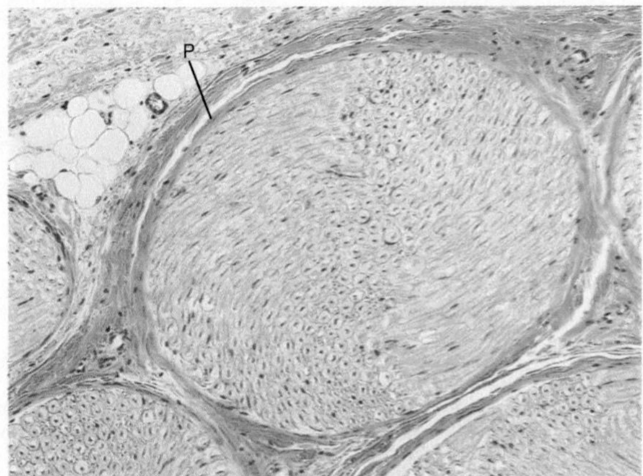

■ Perineurium *(P)* surrounding a bundle of nerve fibers in a cross section of a peripheral nerve.

the female by the vulva and anus, and containing the roots of the external genitalia.

watering can p. a perineum with numerous fistulas leaking urine owing to abscesses or sometimes strictures of the urethra.

peri·neu·ral (per″ĭ-noor′əl) surrounding a nerve or nerves.

peri·neu·ri·tis (per″e-nŏŏ-ri′tis) inflammation of the perineurium. **perineurit′ic** *adj*

peri·neu·ri·um (per″e-noor′e-əm) [*peri-* + Gr. *neuron* nerve] [TA] an intermediate layer of connective tissue in a peripheral nerve, surrounding each bundle (fasciculus) of nerve fibers. See also *epineurium* and *endoneurium*. **perineu′rial** *adj*

peri·nod·al (per″e-no′dəl) near or around a node.

peri·nu·cle·ar (per″e-noo′kle-ər) near or around a nucleus; circumnuclear.

peri·oc·u·lar (per″e-ok′u-lər) near or around the eye.

pe·ri·od (pēr′e-əd) [Gr. *periodos* a going around, circuit, period] an interval or division of time; the time for the regular recurrence of a phenomenon.

absolute refractory p. the portion of the refractory period when a nerve or muscle fiber cannot respond to a stimulus, as contrasted with the relative refractory period. Called also *effective refractory p.*

alveolar p. the period or phase in lung development beginning in utero after the terminal saccular period (about 32 to 36 weeks) and lasting until about eight years of age. The terminal alveolar saccules subdivide several more times and mature alveoli form. Called also *alveolar phase*.

canalicular p. the period or phase of prenatal lung development lasting in different parts of the lungs from the sixteenth or seventeenth week to the twenty-sixth week or later, and followed by the terminal saccular period. Basic structures of the gas-exchanging parts of the lungs form and become vascular, and primordial alveoli called the terminal saccules begin to form, enabling respiration to begin. Fetuses delivered after respiration begins may be viable. Called also *canalicular phase*.

childbearing p. the duration of the reproductive ability in the human female, roughly from puberty to menopause.

effective refractory p. absolute refractory p.

embryonic p. the earliest period or phase of lung development in utero, lasting from the third week after conception to the sixth week; it is sometimes not named as a defined period of lung development, which is instead considered to begin with the following pseudoglandular period. During this period, a ventral respiratory diverticulum (lung bud) arises from the caudal end of the laryngotracheal groove and grows into bronchial buds and the primordial trachea. Called also *embryonic phase*.

ejection p. the second phase of ventricular systole, being the period intervening between the opening and closing of the semilunar valves, during which the blood is being discharged into the aortic and pulmonary arteries. It can be divided into an initial *period of rapid ejection* followed by a *period of reduced ejection* as aortic and ventricular pressures decline from their peaks. Called also *ejection phase* and *sphygmic p.* See illustration at *cardiac cycle*, under *cycle*.

gestation p. the duration of pregnancy, in humans being about 266 days (38 weeks) from the time of fertilization of the oocyte until birth. In obstetrics, the gestation period is instead considered to begin on the first day of the woman's last normal menstrual period prior to fertilization, thus lasting on average 280 days (40 weeks).

half-life p. see *half-life*.

incubation p. 1. the interval of time required for development. 2. the interval between the receipt of infection and the onset of the consequent illness or the first symptoms of the illness (*prodromal stage*). 3. the interval between the entrance into a vector of an infectious agent and the time at which the vector is capable of transmitting the infection. See also *generation time* (def. 1), under *time*. Called also *latent p.*

interdigestive p. a period of relative inactivity in the alimentary tract between two periods of digestive activity.

isoelectric p. on an electrocardiogram, the period between the end of the S wave and the beginning of the T wave, when no potential is recorded because the electrical forces are acting in different directions and neutralize each other.

isometric p. isovolumic p.

isovolumetric p., isovolumic p. in the cardiac cycle, an interval during which the cardiac muscle fibers are contracting or relaxing but the valves are all closed, so that ventricular pressure changes rapidly while volume remains constant; see *p. of isovolumic relaxation* and *p. of isovolumic contraction*.

p. of isovolumic contraction the first phase of ventricular systole, being the short period (0.5 second) lasting from atrioventricular valve closing to semilunar valve opening; as the muscle fibers contract, the ventricular pressure rises rapidly but the ventricular blood volume remains constant. See illustration at *cardiac cycle*, under *cycle*.

p. of isovolumic relaxation a short interval (0.05 second) during ventricular diastole, immediately following the ejection period and lasting from semilunar valve closing to atrioventricular valve opening; as the muscle fibers relax, the ventricular pressure drops and the ventricular blood volume remains constant. See illustration at *cardiac cycle*, under *cycle*.

lag p. the time that elapses between the introduction of a microorganism into a nutrient medium and the initiation of exponential growth.

latency p. 1. latent p. 2. latency stage (def. 1).

latent p. a seemingly inactive period, such as that between exposure to an infection and manifestation of symptoms (*incubation p.*) or between the presentation of a stimulus and the response (*latency*, def. 2).

menstrual p., monthly p. the time of menstruation.

pacemaker refractory p. the interval immediately following either pacemaker sensing or pacing, during which improper inhibition of the pacemaker by inappropriate signals is prevented by temporary inactivation of pacemaker sensing.

preejection p. (PEP) the interval between the onset of ventricular depolarization and the onset of ventricular ejection; it is one of the systolic time intervals (q.v.) used in assessing left ventricular performance and is calculated by subtracting the left ventricular ejection time from the electromechanical systole.

prefunctional p. the time span during morphological and histological development before physiological activity begins.

prodromal p. see under *stage*.

pseudoglandular p. the period or phase of prenatal lung development lasting from about the sixth to the sixteenth week, and followed by the canalicular period. Repeated branching of bronchi and bronchioles takes place to form primordial conductive airways, and the lungs resemble exocrine glands. Fetuses delivered during this phase are not viable because the lungs are not capable of respiration until the twenty-fourth to twenty-sixth week. Called also *pseudoglandular phase*.

quarantine p. 1. the length of time, usually the maximal incubation period of the disease, that must elapse before a person exposed to contagion is regarded as incapable of transmitting or acquiring the disease. See also *quarantine*. 2. a period (originally of 40 days' duration) of detention of vessels, vehicles, or travelers coming from infected or suspected ports or places.

p. of rapid ventricular filling see *p. of ventricular filling*.

reaction p. 1. the stage of rallying from shock after trauma. 2. reaction time.

p. of reduced ventricular filling diastasis; see also *p. of ventricular filling*.

refractory p. the period of depolarization of the cell membrane after excitation, during which the nerve or muscle fiber cannot respond to a second stimulus. See also *absolute refractory p.* and *relative refractory p.*

relative refractory p. the brief period following the absolute refractory period, during which there is repolarization of the cell membrane to the extent that the fiber can respond to a strong stimulus, although the normal resting potential has not been reached.

safe p. the period during the menstrual cycle when conception is considered least likely to occur; it is approximately the ten days after menstruation begins, and the ten days preceding menstruation. See also *rhythm method*, under *method*.

silent p. 1. an interval in the course of a disease in which the symptoms become very mild or disappear for a time. 2. a short period of electrical silence in a muscle, such as is seen just after abrupt unloading.

sphygmic p. ejection p.

terminal saccular p. the period or phase of prenatal lung development lasting, in different parts of the lungs, from the twenty-sixth week or later until near term, and followed by the alveolar period. Walls of the air spaces become thinner and the spaces divide into alveolar saccules with adjacent capillaries; type I and type II alveolar cells begin functioning and surfactant is secreted. Called also *terminal saccular phase.*

p. of ventricular filling in the cardiac cycle, the interval in diastole lasting from atrioventricular valve opening to the start of ventricular contraction and valve closure, during which the ventricular blood volume increases and the pressure drops. The interval is frequently divided into an initial rapid phase of filling and a subsequent slowed phase (diastasis). See also illustration at *cardiac cycle,* under *cycle.*

Wenckebach p. the steadily lengthening P–R interval occurring in successive cardiac cycles in Wenckebach block.

per•io•date (per-i′o-dāt) a salt of periodic acid.

pe•ri•od•ic (pēr′e-od′ik) 1. recurring at regular intervals of time. 2. recurring intermittently or occasionally.

per•iod•ic ac•id (per″i-o′dik) a strong mineral acid and oxidizing agent, HIO_4.

pe•ri•o•dic•i•ty (pēr″e-o-dis′ĭ-te) recurrence at regular intervals of time.

filarial p. the periodic increase of microfilariae in the peripheral blood: nocturnal periodicity occurs in *Wuchereria bancrofti* infection in most endemic areas and in *Brugia malayi* infection; diurnal periodicity occurs in *Loa loa* infection.

lunar p. recurrence synchronized with phases of the moon, such as the reproductive phenomena in certain animals.

malarial p. the more or less regular recurrence of paroxysms at intervals of one, two, or three days in malaria; see under *malaria.*

peri•odon•tal (per″e-o-don′təl) [*peri-* + *odont-* + *-al*[1]] 1. pertaining to the periodontal ligament or periodontium. 2. near or around a tooth; called also *peridental.*

peri•odon•tia (per″e-o-don′shə) 1. plural of *periodontium.* 2. periodontics.

peri•odon•tics (per″e-o-don′tiks) [*peri-* + *odont-* + *-ic*] the branch of dentistry dealing with the study and treatment of diseases of the periodontium.

peri•odon•tist (per″e-o-don′tist) a dentist who specializes in periodontics.

peri•odon•ti•tis (per″e-o-don-ti′tis) [*peri-* + *odont-* + *-itis*] inflammatory reaction of the tissues surrounding a tooth (periodontium), usually resulting from the extension of gingival inflammation (gingivitis) into the periodontium. Periodontitis has been classified in five clinical types: *prepubertal, juvenile, rapidly progressive,* and *adult p.,* and *necrotizing ulcerative gingivoperiodontitis.* Called also *alveolodental osteoperiostitis, cementoperiostitis,* and *paradentitis.*

adult p. the most common form of periodontitis, usually occurring after the age of 35, and usually manifested by slow progression of tissue destruction, which may ultimately result in loss of the teeth.

apical p. inflammatory reaction of the tissues surrounding the root of a tooth.

chronic apical p. periapical granuloma.

juvenile p. a rare form of periodontitis that has an onset at puberty, is more common in females, and is manifested by deep periodontal pockets, usually involving the first molars and incisors. It may be associated with rapidly progressive periodontitis in later life. Called also *paradentosis* and *periodontosis.*

marginal p. a chronic destructive inflammatory periodontal disease that begins as a simple marginal gingivitis and may migrate along the tooth toward the apex, producing periodontal pockets, usually with pus formation, and destruction of the periodontal and alveolar structures, causing the teeth to become loose. Called also *simple p., chronic suppurative pericementitis, Fauchard disease, pyorrhea, pyorrhea alveolaris, Riggs disease,* and *Schmutz pyorrhea.*

prepubertal p. a rare form of periodontitis, probably having an onset soon after eruption of the primary teeth. It occurs in a localized form that involves only some teeth, and in a generalized form that causes rapid destruction of alveolar bone and may or may not affect the permanent teeth.

rapidly progressive p. generalized periodontitis occurring after puberty and before the age of 30 to 35 in those who may or may not have had juvenile periodontitis, characterized by severe and rapid bone destruction, which may progress to abscess formation and tooth loss, or may enter a short or prolonged dormant period.

simple p., p. sim′plex marginal p.

peri•odon•ti•um (per″e-o-don′she-əm) pl. *periodon′tia* [*peri-* + Gr. *odous* tooth] 1. [TA] the tissues that invest or help to invest and support the teeth, including the periodontal ligament, gingivae, cementum, and alveolar and supporting bone. Called also *odontoperiosteum, paradentium,* and *peridontium.* 2. periodontal ligament.

p. insertio′nis [TA] free gingiva: the unattached portion of the gingiva, forming the wall of the gingival crevice. Called also *unattached gingiva* and *free gum.* See also *margo gingivalis.*

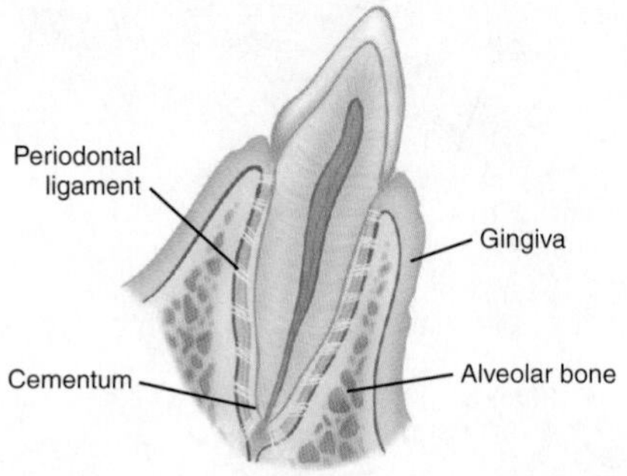

■ Periodontium, showing the periodontal ligament attaching the cementum of the tooth root to the alveolar bone of the socket; the collagen fibers of the ligament are grouped into bundles.

p. protectio′nis [TA] attached gingiva: the part of the gingiva that is firm and resilient and is bound to the underlying cementum and the alveolar bone, thus being immovable.

peri•odon•tol•o•gy (per″e-o-don-tol′ə-je) [*peri-* + *odont-* + *-logy*] the branch of dentistry that deals with the scientific study of the structures and function of the periodontium in health and disease; broader in scope than *periodontics,* which is limited to the diagnosis, prevention, and treatment of periodontal disease, although the two terms are sometimes used interchangeably.

peri•odon•to•sis (per″e-o-don-to′sis) juvenile periodontitis.

Peri•o•gard (per′e-o-gahrd) trademark for a preparation of chlorhexidine gluconate.

peri•om•phal•ic (per″e-om-fal′ik) around the umbilicus.

peri•onych•ia (per″e-o-nik′e-ə) 1. paronychia. 2. plural of *perionychium.*

peri•onych•i•um (per″e-o-nik′e-əm) eponychium.

peri•onyx (per″e-o′niks) [*peri-* + *onyx*] [TA] a relic of the eponychium persisting as a band across the root of the nail, first seen in the eighth month of fetal life.

peri•ooph•o•ri•tis (per″e-o-of″o-ri′tis) [*peri-* + *oophoritis*] inflammation of the tissues around the ovary.

peri•ooph•o•ro•sal•pin•gi•tis (per″e-o-of″o-ro-sal″pin-ji′tis) [*peri-* + *oophoro-* + *salping-* + *-itis*] inflammation of the tissues around an ovary and uterine tube.

peri•oo•the•ci•tis (per-e-o″o-the-si′tis) perioophoritis.

peri•op•er•a•tive (per″e-op′ər-ə-tiv) pertaining to the period extending from the time of hospitalization for surgery to the time of discharge.

peri•oph•thal•mia (per″e-of-thal′me-ə) periophthalmitis.

peri•oph•thal•mic (per″e-of-thal′mik) periocular.

peri•oph•thal•mi•tis (per″e-of″thəl-mi′tis) [*peri-* + *ophthalmitis*] inflammation of the tissues around the eye.

peri•ople (per′e-o″pəl) [*peri-* + Gr. *hoplē* hoof] the layer of soft, light-colored horn covering the outer aspect of the hoof in ungulates.

peri•op•tom•e•try (per″e-op-tom′ə-tre) [*peri-* + *opto-* + *-metry*] the measurement of the peripheral acuity of vision or of the limits of the visual field; cf. *perimetry.*

peri•oral (per″e-or′əl) [*peri-* + *oral*] around or near the mouth; cf. *circumoral.*

peri•or•bit (per″e-or′bit) periorbita.

peri•or•bi•ta (per″e-or′bĭ-tə) [*peri-* + *orbita*] [TA] the periosteal covering of the bones forming the orbit, or eye socket.

peri•or•bi•tal (per″e-or′bĭ-təl) near or around the orbit.

peri•or•bi•ti•tis (per″e-or″bĭ-ti′tis) inflammation of the periorbita.

peri•or•chi•tis (per″e-or-ki′tis) [*peri-* + *orchi-* + *-itis*] inflammation of the tunica vaginalis testis; called also *vaginalitis.*

meconium p. a rare condition seen in infant boys after meconium peritonitis has healed, characterized by a hydrocele of meconium in the scrotum that gradually hardens and often resolves spontaneously in time.

purulent p., p. purulen′ta periorchitis with pus formation.

peri•or•chi•um (per″e-or′ke-əm) lamina parietalis tunicae vaginalis testis.

peri•or•i•fi•cial (per″e-or″ĭ-fish′əl) around an orifice.

peri•ost (per′e-ost) periosteum.

Perio•stat (per′e-o-stat″) trademark for a preparation of doxycycline hyclate.

peri•os•te•itis (per″e-os″te-i′tis) periostitis.

peri•os•teo•ede•ma (per″e-os″te-o-ə-de′mə) edema of the periosteum.

peri•os•te•o•ma (per″e-os-te-o′mə) a morbid bony growth surrounding a bone.

peri•os•teo•med•ul•li•tis (per″e-os″te-o-med″u-li′tis) inflammation of the periosteum and bone marrow.

peri•os•teo•my•eli•tis (per″e-os″te-o-mi″ə-li′tis) [*peri-* + *osteo-* + *myelitis*] inflammation of the entire bone, including periosteum and marrow.

peri•os•teo•phyte (per″e-os′te-o-fīt″) [*periosteum* + *-phyte*] a bony outgrowth on the periosteum.

peri•os•teo•sis (per″e-os″te-o′sis) periostosis.

peri•os•teo•tome (per″e-os′te-o-tōm) an instrument for cutting the periosteum; also an instrument for separating the periosteum from the bone.

peri•os•te•ot•o•my (per″e-os″te-ot′ə-me) [*peri-* + *osteo-* + *-tomy*] surgical incision or slitting of the periosteum.

peri•os•te•ous (per″e-os′te-əs) 1. periosteal. 2. of the nature of periosteum.

peri•os•te•um (per″e-os′te-əm) [*peri-* + Gr. *osteon* bone] [TA] a specialized connective tissue covering all bones of the body, and possessing bone-forming potentialities; in adults, it consists of two layers that are not sharply defined, the external layer being a network of dense connective tissue containing blood vessels, and the deep layer composed of more loosely arranged collagenous bundles with spindle-shaped connective tissue cells and a network of thin elastic fibers. **perios′teal** *adj*

alveolar p. periodontal ligament.

p. exter′num cra′nii TA alternative for pericranium.

peri•os•ti•tis (per″e-os-ti′tis) inflammation of the periosteum. The condition is generally chronic, and is marked by tenderness and swelling of the bone and an aching pain. Acute periostitis is due to infection, is characterized by diffuse suppuration, severe pain, and constitutional symptoms, and usually results in necrosis.

diffuse p. a noncircumscribed periostitis of the long bones.

hemorrhagic p. periostitis in which blood is extravasated beneath the periosteum.

peri•os•to•ma (per″e-os-to′mə) periosteoma.

peri•os•to•med•ul•li•tis (per″e-os″to-med″u-li′tis) periosteomedullitis.

peri•os•to•sis (per″e-os-to′sis) the abnormal deposition of periosteal bone; the condition manifested by development of periosteomas. Called also *periosteosis.*

hyperplastic p. infantile cortical hyperostosis.

peri•os•tos•te•itis (per″e-os-tos″te-i′tis) osteoperiostitis.

peri•os•to•tome (per″e-os′to-tōm) periosteotome.

peri•os•tot•o•my (per″e-os-tot′ə-me) periosteotomy.

peri•otic (per″e-o′tik) [*peri-* + *otic*] 1. near or around the ear, especially the internal ear. 2. pars petrosa ossis temporalis.

peri•ova•ri•tis (per″e-o″və-ri′tis) perioophoritis.

peri•ovu•lar (per″e-ov′u-lər) 1. surrounding an ovum. 2. around the time of ovulation.

peri•pan•cre•at•ic (per″e-pan″kre-at′ik) around or near the pancreas.

peri•pan•cre•a•ti•tis (per″e-pan″kre-ə-ti′tis) [*peri-* + *pancreatitis*] inflammation of tissues around the pancreas.

peri•pap•il•lary (per″e-pap′ĭ-lar″e) around the optic papilla.

peri•par•tum (per″e-pahr′təm) occurring during the last month of gestation or the first few months after delivery, with reference to the mother.

peri•pa•tel•lar (per″e-pə-tel′ər) around the patella.

peri•pa•tet•ic (per″ĭ-pə-tet′ik) ambulatory (def. 1).

peri•pel•vic (per″e-pel′vik) around a renal pelvis.

peri•pe•ni•al (per″e-pe′ne-əl) around the penis.

peri•pha•ryn•ge•al (per″e-fə-rin′je-əl) near or around the pharynx.

pe•riph•er•ad (pə-rif′ər-əd) toward the periphery.

peri•phe•ra•lis (pə-rif″ə-ra′lis) TA alternative for periphericus.

pe•riph•er•aphose (pə-rif′ər-ə-fōs) [*periphery* + *aphose*] a subjective sensation of a dark spot in the line of vision, originating in the peripheral ocular mechanism; cf. *peripherophose.*

peri•phe•ri•cus (per″ĭ-fer′ĭ-kəs) [L., from Gr. *peripherein* to carry around] [TA] peripheral; a general term denoting location away from a center or central structure. Called also *peripheralis* [TA alternative].

pe•riph•er•in (pə-rif′ər-in) 1. a 57-kD protein that polymerizes to form intermediate fibers found in neurons of the peripheral nervous system. 2. a glycoprotein found on the rim region of the membranous disks of the outer segments of the retinal rods, thought to be involved in the assembly, orientation, and stability of the disks; mutations in the gene encoding it can cause retinitis pigmentosa or macular dystrophy.

pe•riph•ero•cen•tral (pə-rif″ər-o-sen′trəl) both peripheral and central.

pe•riph•ero•phose (pə-rif′ə-ro-fōz) [*periphery* + *phose*] any phose or subjective sensation of light originating in the peripheral ocular mechanism; cf. *peripheraphose.*

pe•riph•ery (pə-rif′ə-re) [Gr. *periphereia,* from *peri* around + *pherein* to bear] the outward part or surface or structure; the portion of a system outside the central region. **periph′eral, periph′eric** *adj*

peri•phle•bi•tis (per″e-flə-bi′tis) [*peri-* + *phlebitis*] inflammation of the tissues around a vein or of its external coat. **periphlebit′ic** *adj*

sclerosing p. Mondor disease.

peri•pho•ria (per″ĭ-for′e-ə) cyclophoria.

peri•phre•ni•tis (per″ĭ-frə-ni′tis) [*peri-* + *phrenitis*] inflammation of the diaphragm and structures around it. Called also *paraphrenitis.*

Per•i•pla•ne•ta (per″ĭ-plə-ne′tə) [Gr. *periplanasthai* to wander about] a genus of cockroaches (order Blattaria). *P. america′na* is the American cockroach and *P. australa′siae* is the Australian cockroach.

peri•plasm (per′ĭ-plaz″əm) [*peri-* + *-plasm*] periplasmic space.

peri•plas•mic (per″e-plas′mik) around the plasma membrane; between the plasma membrane and the cell wall of a bacterium.

peri•pleu•ral (per″e-ploor′əl) surrounding the pleura.

peri•pleu•ri•tis (per″e-plo͝o-ri′tis) [*peri-* + *pleur-* + *-itis*] inflammation of the tissues between the pleura and the chest wall.

peri•plo•cin (per″ĭ-plo′sin) a crystallizable glycoside from a woody vine, *Periploca graeca* L. (Asclepiadaceae); it acts like digitalin as a heart tonic and slower of the pulse.

peri•plo•cy•ma•rin (per″ĭ-plo-si′mə-rin) a cardiac glycoside from the bark and wood of *Periploca graeca* L. (Asclepiadaceae).

peri•plog•e•nin (per″ĭ-ploj′ə-nin) an aglycon sterol derivative from periplocin and periplocymarin.

peri•po•lar (per″e-po′lər) near or around a pole or poles.

peri•po•le•sis (per″ĭ-po-le′sis) [Gr. *peripolēsis* a going about] the movement of one cell around another; used to refer to the clustering of lymphocytes around macrophages in lymphoid tissue.

peri•po•ri•tis (per″ĭ-pə-ri′tis) a staphylococcal infection complicating miliaria, with inflammation around the sweat pores, usually affecting infants; called also *periporitis staphylogenes.*

peri•por•tal (per″e-por′təl) near or around the portal vein.

peri•proc•tal (per″e-prok′təl) perirectal.

peri•proc•ti•tis (per″e-prok-ti′tis) paraproctitis.

peri•pros•tat•ic (per″e-pros-tat′ik) near or around the prostate.

peri•pros•ta•ti•tis (per″e-pros″tə-ti′tis) inflammation of the tissues around the prostate; called also *paraprostatitis.*

peri•pros•thet•ic (per″e-pros-thet′ik) near or around a prosthesis.

peri•py•le•phle•bi•tis (per″e-pi″le-flə-bi′tis) [*peri-* + *pylephlebitis*] inflammation of the tissue about the portal vein.

peri•py•lo•ric (per″e-pi-lor′ik) juxtapyloric.

peri•ra•dic•u•lar (per″e-rə-dik′u-lər) around or surrounding a root, especially the root of a tooth.

peri•rec•tal (per″e-rek′təl) around the rectum.

peri•rec•ti•tis (per″e-rek-ti′tis) paraproctitis.

peri•re•nal (per″e-re′nəl) perinephric.

peri•rhi•nal (per″e-ri′nəl) near or around the nose; called also *perinasal.*

peri•sal•pin•gi•tis (per″e-sal″pin-ji′tis) [*peri-* + *salping-* + *-itis*] inflammation of the tissues and peritoneum around a uterine tube.

peri•sal•pin•go•ova•ri•tis (per″e-sal-ping″go-o″və-ri′tis) inflammation involving the ovary and the tissues around the uterine tube.

peri•sal•pinx (per″e-sal′pinks) the peritoneal cover of the upper border of the uterine tube.

peri•scle•ri•um (per″ĭ-skle′re-əm) [*peri-* + Gr. *sklēros* hard] fibrous tissue surrounding ossifying cartilage.

peri•scop•ic (per″ĭ-skop′ik) [*peri-* + Gr. *skopein* to examine] affording a wide range of vision; said of microscopical and meniscus lenses.

peri•sig•moid•itis (per″e-sig″moid-i′tis) inflammation of the peritoneal covering of the sigmoid flexure.

peri•sin•u•ous (per″e-sin′u-əs) near or around a sinus.

peri•si•nus•itis (per″e-si″nəs-i′tis) inflammation of the tissues around a sinus.

peri•sin•u•soi•dal (per″e-si″nə-soi′dəl) surrounding a sinusoid.

peri•splanch•nic (per″ĭ-splank′nik) perivisceral.

peri•splanch•ni•tis (per″e-splank-ni′tis) perivisceritis.

peri•splen•ic (per″e-splen′ik) near or around the spleen.

peri•sple•ni•tis (per″e-splə-ni′tis) [*peri-* + *splen-* + *-itis*] inflammation of the peritoneal coat of the spleen and of the structures around it.

p. cartilagi′nea inflammatory overgrowth of the capsule of the spleen, causing a thickening of cartilaginous hardness.

peri•spon•dyl•ic (per″e-spon-dil′ik) perivertebral.

peri•spon•dy•li•tis (per″e-spon″də-li′tis) [*peri-* + *spondyl-* + *-itis*] inflammation of the parts around a vertebra.

Gibney p. a painful condition of the spinal muscles.

Pe•ris•so•dac•ty•la (pə-ris″o-dak′tə-lə) [Gr. *perissos* odd + *daktylos* finger] an order of mammals, the ungulates with an odd number of toes, including the horse, tapir, and rhinoceros. Cf. *Artiodactyla.*

pe•ris•so•dac•ty•lous (pə-ris″o-dak′tə-ləs) 1. having an odd number of digits on a hand or foot. 2. pertaining to the Perissodactyla.

peri•stal•sis (per″ĭ-stawl′sis) [*peri-* + Gr. *stalsis* contraction] the movement by which the alimentary canal and other tubular organs that have both longitudinal and circular muscle fibers propel their contents; it consists of a wave of contraction passing along the tube for variable distances. **peristal′tic** *adj*

mass p. strong usually brief bursts of peristaltic movements, which propel intestinal contents through long stretches of the intestine or colon, often resulting in defecation.

retrograde p., reversed p. antiperistalsis.

uterine p. rhythmic movements of the myometrium, seen especially druing the follicular phase of the menstrual cycle.

peri•staph•y•line (per″e-staf′ə-līn) [*peri-* + *staphyline*] situated around the uvula.

peri•sto•mal (per″e-sto′məl) 1. adjacent to a stoma. 2. perioral.

peri•stome (per′ĭ-stōm) [*peri-* + Gr. *stoma* mouth] 1. in ciliate protozoa, the buccal area and its encircling adoral zone of membranelles. 2. buccal cavity.

peri•sto•mi•al (per″ĭ-sto′me-əl) pertaining or relating to the peristome or to the area around the cytostome of ciliate protozoa.

peri•stru•mi•tis (per″e-stroo-mi′tis) inflammation extending from an inflamed goiter to the surrounding structures.

peri•stru•mous (per″e-stroo′məs) around or near a goiter.

peri•syl•vi•an (per″e-sil′ve-ən) near the sylvian fissure (sulcus lateralis cerebri).

peri•sy•no•vi•al (per″e-sĭ-no-ve′əl) around a synovial structure.

peri•tec•to•my (per″ĭ-tek′tə-me) [*peri-* + *ectomy*] excision of a ring of conjunctiva behind the limbus, followed by cauterization of the trench thus made.

peri•ten•din•e•um (per″ĭ-tən-din′e-əm) the connective tissue investing larger tendons and extending as septa between the fibers composing them.

peri•ten•di•ni•tis (per″e-ten″dĭ-ni′tis) tenosynovitis.

p. calca′rea a painful condition marked by calcareous deposits in tendons and in peritendinous, capsular, and ligamentous tissues.

p. sero′sa ganglion (def. 3).

peri•ten•di•nous (per″e-ten′dĭ-nəs) around a tendon.

peri•te•non (per″ĭ-te′non) [*peri-* + Gr. *tenōn* tendon] the connective tissue structures associated with a tendon.

peri•ten•o•ne•um (per″ĭ-ten″o-ne′əm) the loose connective tissue covering the surface of tendons and ligaments and penetrating inside to separate the substance into bundles.

peri•ten•o•ni•tis (per″e-ten″ə-ni′tis) tenosynovitis.

peri•ten•on•ti•tis (per″e-ten″on-ti′tis) tenosynovitis.

peri•the•ci•um (per″ĭ-the′se-əm) [*peri-* + Gr. *thēkē* case] the flask-shaped fruiting body of certain molds and ascomycetous fungi (see *ascocarp*) having a pore for the escape of spores.

peri•the•li•o•ma (per″ĭ-the″le-o′mə) hemangiopericytoma.

peri•the•li•um (per″e-the′le-əm) [*peri-* + *thelium*] the layer of connective tissue that surrounds the capillaries and smaller vessels. **perithe′lial** *adj*

Eberth p. a partial layer of cells on the external surface of the capillaries.

peri•tho•rac•ic (per″e-thə-ras′ik) surrounding the thorax.

peri•thy•roi•di•tis (per″e-thi″roi-di′tis) inflammation of the thyroid capsule.

pe•rit•o•my (pə-rit′ə-me) [*peri-* + *-tomy*] surgical incision of the conjunctiva and subconjunctival tissue about the whole circumference of the cornea; usually done as part of enucleation and retinal detachment procedure.

peritone(o)- [L. *peritoneum*, q.v.] a combining form denoting relationship to the peritoneum.

peri•to•ne•al•gia (per″ĭ-to″ne-al′jə) pain in the peritoneum.

peri•to•ne•a•li•za•tion (per″ĭ-tə-ne″əl-ĭ-za′shən) peritonization.

peri•to•ne•al•ize (per″ĭ-to-ne′əl-īz) to cover with peritoneum; called also *peritonize.*

peri•to•nec•to•my (per″ĭ-to-nek′tə-me) surgical removal of part of the peritoneum.

peri•to•neo•cen•te•sis (per″ĭ-to″ne-o-sen-te′sis) [*peritoneo-* + *-centesis*] abdominal paracentesis.

peri•to•ne•og•ra•phy (per″ĭ-to″ne-og′rə-fe) radiography of the peritoneum.

peri•to•neo•mus•cu•lar (per″ĭ-to-ne″o-mus′ku-lər) pertaining to or composed of peritoneum and muscle.

peri•to•ne•op•a•thy (per″ĭ-to-ne-op′ə-the) any disease of the peritoneum.

peri•to•neo•peri•car•di•al (per″ĭ-to-ne″o-per″ĭ-kahr′de-əl) pertaining to the peritoneum and pericardium.

peri•to•neo•pexy (per″ĭ-to′ne-o-pek″se) [*peritoneo-* + *-pexy*] fixation of the uterus by the vaginal route.

peri•to•neo•plas•ty (per″ĭ-to′ne-o-plas″te) peritonization.

peri•to•neo•scope (per″ĭ-to′ne-o-skōp″) laparoscope.

peri•to•ne•os•co•py (per″ĭ-to″ne-os′kə-pe) laparoscopy.

peri•to•ne•ot•o•my (per″ĭ-to″ne-ot′ə-me) laparotomy.

peri•to•neo•ve•nous (per″ĭ-to-ne″o-ve′nəs) communicating with the peritoneal cavity and the venous system.

peri•to•ne•um (per″ĭ-to-ne′əm) [L., from Gr. *peritonaion*, from *per* around + *teinein* to stretch] [TA] the serous membrane lining the abdominopelvic walls *(parietal p.)* and investing the viscera *(visceral p.)*. A strong, colorless membrane with a smooth surface, it forms a double-layered sac that is closed in the male and is continuous with the mucous membrane of the uterine tubes in the female. The potential space between the parietal and visceral peritoneum is called the *peritoneal cavity* (see *cavitas peritonealis* [TA]). **peritone′al** *adj*

abdominal p. p. parietale.

intestinal p. p. viscerale.

parietal p., p. parieta′le [TA] the peritoneum that lines the abdominal and pelvic walls and the inferior surface of the diaphragm.

urogenital p., p. urogenita′le [TA] the peritoneum lining the urogenital structures in the lower pelvis.

visceral p., p. viscera′le [TA] a continuation of the parietal peritoneum reflected at various places over the viscera, forming a complete

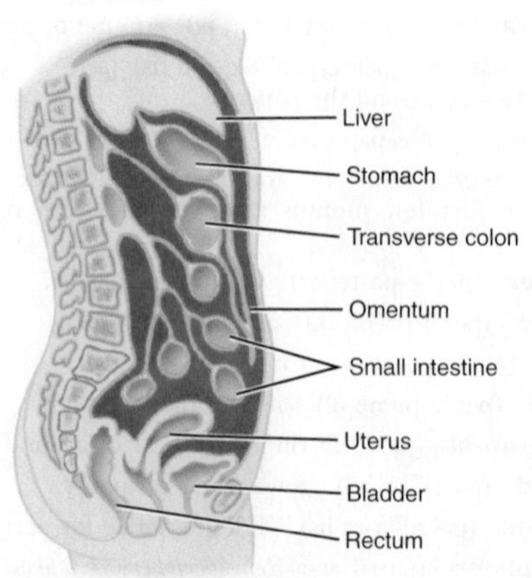

■ Course of the peritoneum *(gray)* in a median sagittal section of a female.

covering for the stomach, spleen, liver, intestines from the distal duodenum to the upper end of the rectum, uterus, and ovaries; it also partially covers some other abdominal organs. It holds the viscera in position by its folds, including the *mesenteries,* the *omenta,* and the *ligaments* of the liver, spleen, stomach, kidneys, bladder, and uterus. The potential space between the visceral and the parietal peritoneum is the *peritoneal cavity* (see *cavitas peritonealis*). The general cavity communicates by the epiploic foramen with the bursa omentalis (or *lesser peritoneal cavity*). Called also *intestinal p.*

peri·to·nism (per″ĭ-to-niz-əm) a condition of shock simulating peritonitis, but without inflammation of the peritoneum.

peri·to·ni·tis (per″ĭ-to-ni′tis) inflammation of the peritoneum, with exudations of serum, fibrin, cells, and pus, usually accompanied by abdominal pain and tenderness, constipation, vomiting, and moderate fever.

adhesive p. peritonitis characterized by adhesions between adjacent serous surfaces.

aseptic p. peritonitis that is not from an infection; the most common cause is an irritating contaminant in fluid used in peritoneal dialysis (see *chemical p.*).

benign paroxysmal p. familial Mediterranean fever.

bile p., biliary p. choleperitoneum.

chemical p. peritonitis due to chemical irritation such as from peritoneal dialysis or from bile leaking out of the intestine.

p. chro′nica fibro′sa encap′sulans chronic peritonitis with formation on the intestine of a white coating of fibrous tissue undergoing hyaline degeneration.

circumscribed p. inflammation limited to a portion of the peritoneum. Called also *localized p.*

diffuse p. inflammation of the greater part of the peritoneum. Called also *general p.*

feline infectious p. a usually fatal contagious viral disease of domestic cats and other felines, caused by a coronavirus; characteristics include slow onset, persistent fever, and varying effects of peritonitis such as pleural or peritoneal effusions and granulomas.

gas p. peritonitis with accumulation of gas in the peritoneum.

general p. diffuse p.

localized p. circumscribed p.

meconium p. peritonitis resulting from perforation of the bowel into the peritoneal cavity in utero or shortly after birth, resulting in escape of meconium into the peritoneal cavity; it occurs most often as a complication of meconium ileus in cystic fibrosis.

pelvic p. 1. perimetritis. 2. peritonitis situated in the pelvis.

perforative p. peritonitis due to a perforation in the digestive tract and escape of its contents.

periodic p. familial Mediterranean fever.

puerperal p. peritonitis following childbirth.

purulent p. peritonitis with pus formation.

sclerosing p. any of several rare complications of long-term peritoneal dialysis; the peritoneum becomes either opaque or tan, wrinkled, and dry. Severe forms, which are often fatal, include formation of a fibrous sac around the small intestine *(sclerosing encapsulating peritonitis),* intestinal obstruction, and calcification of the peritoneum. Called also *peritoneal sclerosis.*

sclerosing encapsulating p. sclerosing peritonitis with formation of a fibrous sac around the intestine; it often progresses to fatal necrosis or obstruction.

septic p. peritonitis caused by a pyogenic microorganism.

spontaneous bacterial p. (SBP) bacterial infection of ascitic fluid without evidence of an intra-abdominal source of infection; seen as a complication of cirrhosis.

traumatic p. acute peritonitis due to trauma.

tuberculous p. peritonitis caused by *Mycobacterium tuberculosis.*

peri·to·ni·za·tion (per″ĭ-to-nĭ-za′shən) the operation of covering a denuded surface of an abdominal organ or the abdominal wall with peritoneum; called also *peritonealization* and *peritoneoplasty.*

peri·to·nize (per′ĭ-to-nīz) peritonealize.

peri·ton·sil·lar (per″e-ton′sĭ-lər) situated around a tonsil.

peri·ton·sil·li·tis (per″e-ton″sĭ-li′tis) inflammation of the peritonsillar tissues.

peri·tra·che·al (per″e-tra′ke-əl) situated around the trachea.

Per·i·trate (per′ĭ-trāt) trademark for preparations of pentaerythritol tetranitrate.

peri·trich (per′ĭ-trik) 1. any ciliate protozoan of the subclass Peritrichia. 2. peritrichous.

Peri·trich·ia (per″ĭ-trik′e-ə) [*peri-* + Gr. *thrix* hair] a subclass of typically cone-shaped, ciliate protozoa (class Oligohymenophorea, phylum Ciliophora), characterized by the presence of a prominent oral ciliary field covering the apical end of the body and spiraling counterclockwise into the infundibulum, a paroral membrane and adoral membranelles that become peniculi, and much reduced somatic ciliature. Many are stalked and sedentary, and others are mobile, all with an aboral scopula. The free-swimming larvae have a locomotory posterior ciliary girdle. It comprises one order: Peritrichida.

Peri·trich·i·da (per″ĭ-trik′ĭ-də) an order of ciliate protozoa (subclass Peritrichia, class Oligohymenophorea) having characters of the subclass. It comprises two suborders: Sessilina and Mobilina.

pe·rit·ri·chous (pə-rit′rĭ-kəs) [*peri-* + *trich-* + *-ous*] 1. having flagella over the entire surface; said of a bacterial cell; see *flagellum.* 2. of flagella, occurring over the entire surface of a bacterial cell. 3. having cilia around the cytostome only; said of Ciliophora. Called also *peritrich.*

peri·tro·chan·ter·ic (per″e-tro″kan-ter′ik) around or near a trochanter.

peri·tu·bu·lar (per″e-too′bu-lər) situated around or near tubules.

peri·um·bil·i·cal (per″e-əm-bil′ĭ-kəl) near or around the umbilicus; called also *periomphalic.*

peri·un·gual (per″e-ung′gwəl) around the nail.

peri·ure·ter·al (per″e-u-re′tər-əl) around the ureter; called also *periureteric.*

peri·ure·ter·ic (per″e-u″rə-ter′ik) periureteral.

peri·ure·ter·itis (per″e-u-re″tər-i′tis) [*peri-* + *ureter-* + *-itis*] inflammation of the tissues around a ureter.

peri·ure·thral (per″e-u-re′thrəl) near or around the urethra.

peri·ure·thri·tis (per″e-u″rə-thri′tis) [*peri-* + *urethr-* + *-itis*] inflammation of the tissues around the urethra; called also *paraurethritis.*

peri·uter·ine (per″e-u′tər-in) around the uterus.

peri·vag·i·nal (per″e-vaj′ĭ-nəl) around the vagina.

peri·vag·i·ni·tis (per″e-vaj″ĭ-ni′tis) inflammation of the tissues around the vagina.

peri·vas·cu·lar (per″e-vas′ku-lər) near or around a vessel.

peri·vas·cu·lar·i·ty (per″ĭ-vas′ku-lar′ĭ-te) an infiltrate of cellular elements of mesodermal origin (including polymorphonuclear leukocytes, lymphocytes, and others) in the perivascular spaces, such as in those of the cerebral parenchyma.

peri·vas·cu·li·tis (per″e-vas″ku-li′tis) inflammation of the tissue surrounding a blood or lymph vessel. Called also *periangiitis.*

peri·ve·nous (per″e-ve′nəs) near or around a vein.

peri·ven·tric·u·lar (per″e-ven-trik′u-lər) around a ventricle; see also under *system.*

peri·ver·te·bral (per″e-vur′tə-brəl) near or around a vertebra.

peri·ves·i·cal (per″e-ves′ĭ-kəl) [*peri-* + *vesic-* + *-al*[1]] near the urinary bladder; called also *paravesical* and *pericystic.*

peri·ve·sic·u·lar (per″e-və-sik′u-lər) near or around a vesicle, such as a seminal vesicle.

peri·ve·sic·u·li·tis (per″e-və-sik″u-li′tis) inflammation of tissue around the seminal vesicle.

peri·vis·cer·al (per″e-vis′ər-əl) near or around a viscus or the viscera.

peri·vis·cer·itis (per″e-vis″ər-i′tis) inflammation around a viscus or around the viscera.

peri·vi·tel·line (per″e-vĭ-tel′ēn) near or around the yolk.

peri·win·kle (per′e-wing″kəl) 1. any of several woody herbs of the genus *Vinca.* 2. *Vinca rosea.*

Madagascar p. *Vinca rosea.*

minor p. *Vinca minor.*

per·le·can (pur′lə-kan) a proteoglycan of the extracellular matrix, consisting of three heparan sulfate chains bound to a 400-kD core and expressed by all cells that make basement membranes, of which it is a major component; it is also a component of cartilage and of the growth plate, where it is essential for long bone growth.

per·lèche (per-lesh′) [Fr.] single or multiple fissures at the corners of the mouth, which may be unilateral or bilateral and may spread to the lips and cheeks. It may be due to a primary or superimposed infection, such as with *Candida albicans,* staphylococci, or streptococci; poor hygiene; drooling of saliva; overclosure of the jaws in edentulous patients or those with ill-fitting dentures; ariboflavinosis; or other causes. Called also *angular cheilitis, cheilosis,* or *stomatitis, migrating cheilitis,* and *intertrigo labialis.*

Per·lia nucleus (per′le-ah) [Richard *Perlia,* German ophthalmologist, late 19th century] see under *nucleus.*

Perl·man syndrome (pərl′mən) [M. *Perlman,* Israeli physician, 20th century] see under *syndrome.*

per·ma·nence (pur′mə-nens) the quality or condition of lasting without essential change.

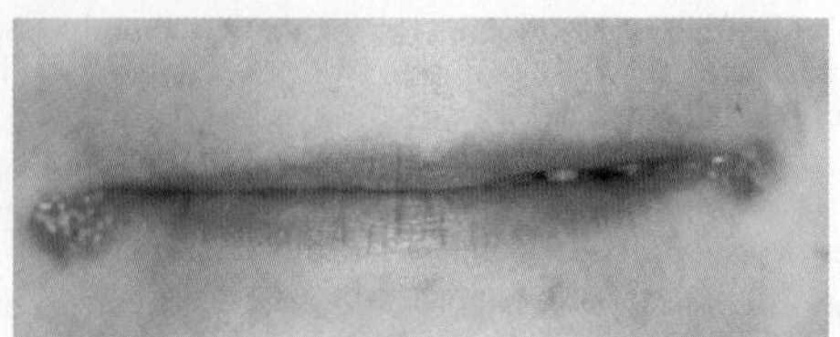

■ Perlèche.

object p. the concept, usually appreciated during the second year of life, that an object continues to exist even when removed from view.

per•man•ga•nate (pər-mang′gə-nāt) the MnO_4^- anion, which has a deep purple color in aqueous solution and is a strong oxidizing agent, or a salt containing this ion.

per•man•gan•ic ac•id (pur″mang-gan′ik) an unstable strong acid and oxidizing agent, $HMnO_4$, existing only in aqueous solution; its salts are permanganates.

Per•ma•pen (pur′mə-pen) trademark for a preparation of penicillin G benzathine.

per•me•a•bil•i•ty (pur″me-ə-bil′ĭ-te) the property or state of being permeable; see also *osmosis.*

per•me•a•bil•i•za•tion (pur″me-ə-bil″ĭ-za′shən) the process of making something permeable, such as a membrane.

per•me•a•ble (pur′me-ə-bəl) [L. *per* through + *meare* to pass] not impassable; allowing passage of a substance. Called also *pervious.*

per•me•ase (pur′me-ās) former term for transport protein.

per•me•ate (pur′me-āt″) 1. to penetrate or pass through, as through a filter. 2. the constituents of a solution or suspension that pass through a filter.

per•me•a•tion (pur″me-a′shən) the act of spreading through or penetrating a substance, tissue, or organ, as by a disease process, such as cancer.

per•meth•rin (pər-meth′rin) a pyrethroid insecticide applied topically in the treatment of infestations by *Pediculus humanus capitis, Sarcoptes scabiei,* and various species of ticks; also applied to objects such as bedding and furniture. In veterinary medicine, used in ear tags for cattle to combat biting flies and in flea collars for cats and dogs.

perm•se•lec•tiv•i•ty (pərm″sə-lek-tiv′ĭ-te) restriction of the permeation of macromolecules across a glomerular capillary wall. A major factor is molecule size relative to the size of the pores through the wall; other important factors include the electrical charge of the molecule versus that of the wall or pore and the physical configuration of the molecule.

per•na (pur′nə) a chlorinated naphthalene, which may cause a serious acne in persons handling it.

per•na•sal (pər-na′səl) [*per-* + *nasal*] performed through the nose.

per•ni•cious (pər-nish′əs) [L. *perniciosus*] harmful; tending toward a fatal outcome.

per•nio (pur′ne-o) pl. *pernio′nes* [L.] chilblain.

per•ni•o•sis (pər-ne-o′sis) chilblain.

pero- [Gr. *pēros* maimed] a combining form meaning deformed.

pe•ro•bra•chi•us (pe″ro-bra′ke-əs) [*pero-* + Gr. *brachiōn* arm] a fetus with deformed upper limbs.

pe•ro•chi•rus (pe″ro-ki′rəs) [*pero-* + Gr. *cheir* hand] a fetus with malformed hands.

pe•ro•cor•mus (pe″ro-kor′məs) [*pero-* + Gr. *kormos* trunk] perosomus.

pe•ro•dac•ty•lus (pe″ro-dak′tə-ləs) [*pero-* + Gr. *daktylos* finger] a fetus with deformity of fingers or toes, or both, especially absence of one or more digits.

pe•ro•me•lia (pe″ro-me′le-ə) severe dysmelia.

pe•rom•e•lus (pe-rom′ə-ləs) [*pero-* + Gr. *melos* limb] a fetus or infant with severe dysmelia.

Pe•ro•mys•cus (pe″ro-mis′kəs) a genus of mice of the family Muridae. *P. leu′copus* is the white-footed mouse, a species that is the primary reservoir in eastern North America for Ixodes scapularis, the tick that spreads Lyme disease. *P. manicula′tus* is the deer mouse, a North American species that is a reservoir for various disease-spreading ticks.

pero•nar•thro•sis (per″o-nahr-thro′sis) [Gr. *peronē* anything pointed for piercing or pinning + *arthrosis*] an articulation in which the surfaces are convex in one direction and concave in the other.

per•o•ne (pər-o′ne) fibula.

per•o•ne•al (per″o-ne′əl) [Gr. *peronē* fibula] pertaining to the fibula or to the lateral aspect of the leg; fibular.

pe•ro•ne•a•lis (pə-ro″ne-a′lis) TA alternative for *fibularis.*

pe•ro•neo•tib•i•al (per″o-ne″o-tib′e-əl) tibiofibular.

Pe•ro•no•spo•ral•es (per″o-no-spə-ra′lēz) [Gr. *peronē* pin + *spora* seed] an order of funguslike organisms of the class Oomycetes, saprobes and plant parasites that reproduce asexually by zoospores and conidia and sexually by oospores. Animal pathogens are included in the family Pythiaceae.

pe•ro•pus (pe′ro-pəs) [*pero-* + Gr. *pous* foot] a fetus with congenital anomalies of one or both feet.

per•oral (pər-or′əl) [*per-* + *oral*] performed through or administered through the mouth.

per os (pər os) [L.] by mouth.

pe•ro•sis (pə-ro′sis) a disease of chicks marked by bone deformities, associated with deficiency of dietary factors such as choline and manganese. **perot′ic** *adj*

pe•ro•so•mus (pe″ro-so′məs) [*pero-* + Gr. *sōma* body] a fetus with greatly deformed body or trunk; called also *perocormus.*

pe•ro•splanch•nia (pe″ro-splank′ne-ə) [*pero-* + *splanchn-* + *-ia*] a developmental anomaly characterized by malformation of the viscera.

per•os•se•ous (pər-os′e-əs) [*per-* + *osseous*] transmitted through bone.

per•ox•i•dase (pər-ok′sĭ-dās) 1. any of a group of enzymes of the oxidoreductase class that catalyze the oxidation of organic substrates by hydrogen peroxide, which is reduced to water [EC 1.11]. These enzymes are heme proteins, found frequently in plants and occasionally in animal tissues. 2. [EC 1.11.1.7] a specific oxidoreductase that catalyzes the reaction of hydrogen peroxide and halide ions to produce cytotoxic acids (such as hypochlorous acid) and other intermediates; these play a role in oxygen-dependent killing of microorganisms and tumor cells. The enzyme is a hemoprotein found in the azurophil granules of neutrophils and the primary lysosomes of monocytes and it has the green color seen in pus. Deficiency of the enzyme, an autosomal recessive or acquired trait, is usually asymptomatic but may predispose affected individuals to severe fungal infections.

per•ox•i•da•tion (pər-ok″sĭ-da′shən) the formation of peroxide radicals.

lipid p. nonenzymatic oxidation of fatty acids to hydroperoxides by strong oxidizing agents such as free radicals.

per•ox•ide (pər-ok′sīd) that oxide of any element which contains more oxygen than any other. More correctly applied to compounds having such linkage as —O—O—; for instance, hydrogen peroxide, H—O—O—H.

per•ox•i•some (pər-ok′sĭ-sōm) a microbody (q.v.), present in all animal cells except erythrocytes and many plant cells, containing over 50 enzymes that participate in a variety of oxidative processes, including reactions involving hydrogen peroxide, purine metabolism, cellular lipid metabolism, and gluconeogenesis. Similar structures *(glyoxysomes),* containing the enzymes of the glyoxylate cycle, are found in certain plants and microorganisms. Defects in peroxisome biosynthesis cause adrenoleukodystrophy and cerebrohepatorenal (Zellweger) syndrome.

peroxy- a prefix indicating the substitution of —O—O— for —O—, as in peroxyacetic acid.

per•oxy•ace•tic ac•id (pər-ok″se-ə-se′tik) peracetic acid.

per•oxy•dol (pər-ok′sĭ-dol) sodium perborate.

per•phen•a•zine (pər-fen′ə-zēn) [USP] a phenothiazine used orally and intramuscularly as an antipsychotic and antiemetic. It is also used in combination with amitriptyline in the treatment of anxiety associated with depression.

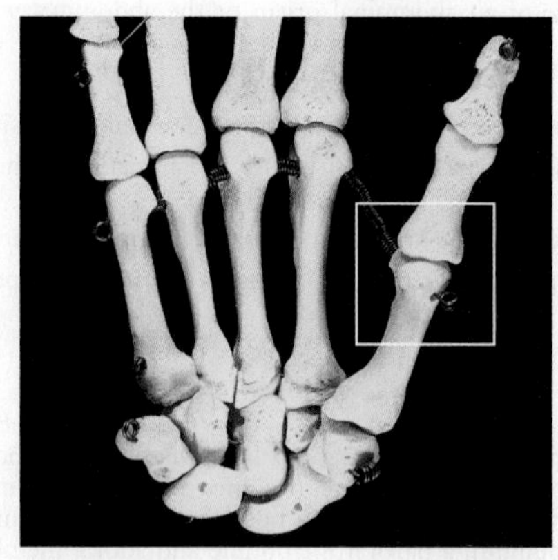

■ Peronarthrosis: metacarpophalangeal joint of the thumb *(box).*

per pri·mam in·ten·ti·o·nem (pər pri′məm in-ten″she-o′nəm) [L.] by first intention; see under *healing.* Written also *per primam.*

per rec·tum (pər rek′təm) [L.] by way of the rectum.

Per·ron·ci·to apparatus (spirals) (per″on-che′to) [Aldo *Perroncito,* Italian histologist, 1882–1929] apparatus of Perroncito; see under *apparatus.*

per·salt (pur′sawlt) a salt of a peracid; a salt whose acid radical has a higher valence than the protosalt.

per sal·tum (pər sawl′təm) [L.] by a leap or bound; denoting a sudden evolutionary development without intermediate stages.

Per·san·tine (pər-san′tēn) trademark for preparations of dipyridamole.

per se·cun·dam in·ten·ti·o·nem (pər se-kun′dəm in-ten″she-o′nəm) [L.] by second intention; see under *healing.* Written also *per secundam.*

per·sev·er·a·tion (pər-sev″ər-a′shən) the inappropriate persistence or repetition of a thought or act after the causative stimulus has ceased or in response to different stimuli, e.g., answering a question correctly and then inappropriately repeating that answer to succeeding questions; most often associated with brain lesions but also seen in schizophrenia.

per·sis·tence (pər-sis′təns) continuation of a behavior or characteristic at a time when it would normally be expected to have disappeared.

hereditary p. of fetal hemoglobin continued production of fetal hemoglobin beyond the point when it is normally replaced by hemoglobin A. Heterozygotes are asymptomatic, while homozygotes have hypochromic microcytic erythrocytes and may have a mild type of thalassemia.

per·sis·ter (pər-sis′tər) [L. *persistere* persist, from *per* through + *sistere* to stand still] in bacteriology, a microorganism that resists a generally toxic level of a drug but is not genetically resistant.

per·so·na (pər-so′nə) [L. "mask"] in jungian psychology, the personality mask or facade presented by a person to the world, as opposed to the *anima,* the inner being.

per·so·nal·i·ty (pur″sə-nal′ĭ-te) the characteristic way that a person thinks, feels, and behaves; the relatively stable and predictable part of a person's thought and behavior; it includes conscious attitudes, values, and styles as well as unconscious conflicts and defense mechanisms. See also under *disorder, trait,* and *type.*

alternating p. dissociative identity disorder.

anancastic p. obsessive-compulsive personality disorder.

as-if p. a personality that is seemingly normal but lacks real, enduring emotion; the person adopts and appears to express ordinary characteristics but is able to summarily discard them and adopt others as situations change.

compulsive p. obsessive-compulsive personality disorder.

cyclothymic p. a temperament characterized by rapid, frequent swings between sad and cheerful moods. See also *cyclothymic disorder,* under *disorder.*

double p., dual p. dissociative identity disorder.

obsessive p. obsessive-compulsive personality disorder.

split p. a colloquial term used for either schizophrenia or dissociative identity disorder.

per·so·nol·o·gy (pur″sə-nol′ə-je) the holistic study of personality, seeking understanding of the aspects of a person through knowledge of the whole. **personolog′ic** *adj*

per·spi·ra·tion (pur″spĭ-ra′shən) [L. *perspirare* to breathe through] 1. sweating. 2. sweat.

insensible p. insensible water loss (see under *loss*).

sensible p. sweating due to secretory activity of sweat glands.

per·sua·sion (pər-swa′zhən) in psychiatry, a therapeutic approach based on direct suggestion and guidance intended to influence favorably attitudes, behavior, and goals.

per·sul·fate (pər-sul′fāt) a salt of persulfuric acid.

per·sul·fide (pər-sul′fīd) a sulfide which contains more sulfur than the ordinary sulfide.

per·sul·fur·ic ac·id (pur″səl-fūr′ik) peroxymonosulfuric acid, H_2SO_5, a strong oxidizing agent.

per·tech·ne·tate (pər-tek′nə-tāt) a salt or ester containing the ion TcO_4^-; see under *technetium* and *uptake.*

Per·thes disease, test (per′təz) [Georg Clemens *Perthes,* German surgeon, 1869–1927] Legg-Calvé-Perthes disease; see under *disease,* and see *tourniquet test,* under *test.*

Per·tik diverticulum (per′tik) [Otto *Pertik,* Hungarian physician, 1852–1913] see under *diverticulum.*

per tu·bam (pər too′bəm) [L.] through a tube.

per·tu·ba·tion (pur″too-ba′shən) perflation or insufflation of the uterine tubes to render them patent.

per·tus·sis (pər-tus′is) [L. *per* intensive + *tussis*] an acute contagious infection of the respiratory tract, usually seen in young children and caused by *Bordetella pertussis.* After an incubation period of about two weeks, there is a *catarrhal stage* for about two weeks, consisting of slight fever, sneezing, runny nose, and dry cough. Then comes the *paroxysmal stage,* lasting three to four weeks, with the characteristic paroxysmal cough that gives the condition its name: the patient has a deep inspiration followed by a series of quick, short coughs that continue until the air is expelled from the lungs to end with a long shrill, whooping inspiration because of spasmodic closure of the glottis. The last stage of disease is the *convalescent stage,* in which paroxysms diminish and finally cease. See also *parapertussis.* Called also *whooping cough.*

per·tus·soid (pər-tus′oid) [*pertussis* + *-oid*] resembling pertussis.

per va·gi·nam (pər və-ji′nəm) through the vagina.

per·ver·sion (pər-vur′zhən) [*per-* + *version*] 1. a turning aside from the normal course; a morbid alteration of function which may occur in emotional, intellectual, or volitional fields. 2. sexual p.; see under *deviation.*

per·vi·ous (pur′ve-əs) [L. *pervius*] permeable.

pes (pes) gen. *pe′dis* pl. *pe′des* [L.] 1. [TA] foot (def. 1). 2. any footlike part.

p. abduc′tus talipes valgus.

p. adduc′tus talipes varus.

p. anseri′nus [L. "goose's foot"] 1. plexus intraparotideus. 2. the combined insertion of the tendinous expansions of the sartorius, gracilis, and semitendinosus muscles.

p. calcaneoca′vus see under *talipes.*

p. cavova′rus see under *talipes.*

p. ca′vus see under *talipes.*

p. equinoval′gus see under *talipes.*

p. equinova′rus see under *talipes.*

p. gi′gas megalopodia.

p. hippocam′pi [TA] a formation of two or three elevations on the rostral end of the ventricular surface of the hippocampus; called also *digitationes hippocampi.*

p. pedun′culi crus cerebri.

p. planoval′gus, p. pla′nus flatfoot.

p. val′gus flatfoot.

p. valgus, congenital convex rocker-bottom foot (def. 1).

p. va′rus see under *talipes.*

pes·sa·ry (pes′ə-re) [L. *pessarium*] 1. an instrument placed in the vagina to support the uterus or rectum or as a contraceptive device. 2. a medicated vaginal suppository.

cup p. a pessary whose top has a cuplike shape to fit the ostium uteri.

diaphragm p. a diaphragm for insertion into the vagina as a barrier contraceptive.

donut p., doughnut p. an inflated soft rubber pessary shaped like a doughnut.

Hodge p. a pessary for use in retrodisplacement of the uterus.

Menge p. a ring pessary with a fixed crossbar holding a detachable stem.

ring p. a round or ring-shaped pessary.

Smith p. a pessary for use in retrodisplacement of the uterus.

stem p. a pessary with a stem for introduction into the cervical canal.

pest (pest) 1. plague. 2. anything, particularly an animal, that is harmful to humans.

avian p., fowl p. 1. Newcastle disease in birds. 2. avian influenza.

p. of small ruminants peste des petits ruminants.

peste (pest) [Fr.] plague.

p. des petits ruminants (PPR) (da pə-te′ ru-me-nah′) ["plague of small ruminants"] a highly fatal viral disease of sheep and goats, prevalent in central and west Africa and the Middle East, caused by a virus of the genus *Morbillivirus* and characterized by fever, necrotic stomatitis, gastroenteritis, and pneumonia. Called also *kata, pest of small ruminants, pseudorinderpest,* and *stomatitis-pneumoenteritis syndrome* or *complex.*

pes·ti·cide (pes′tĭ-sīd) a poison used to destroy pests of any sort, such as a fungicide, herbicide, insecticide, rodenticide, or anthelmintic.

pes·tif·er·ous (pes-tif′ər-əs) [*pestis* + *-ferous*] causing or propagating a pestilence.

pes·ti·lence (pes′tĭ-ləns) [L. *pestilentia*] any virulent contagious or infectious epidemic disease; also an epidemic of such a disease.

pes·ti·len·tial (pes″tĭ-len′shəl) of the nature of a pestilence; producing an epidemic disease.

pes·tis (pes′tis) [L.] plague.

p. equo′rum African horse sickness.

p. ma′jor bubonic plague.

p. mi′nor ambulatory plague.

Pes·ti·vi·rus (pes′tĭ-vi″rəs) [L. *pestis* plague + *virus*] mucosal disease viruses; a genus of viruses of the family Flaviviridae comprising bovine

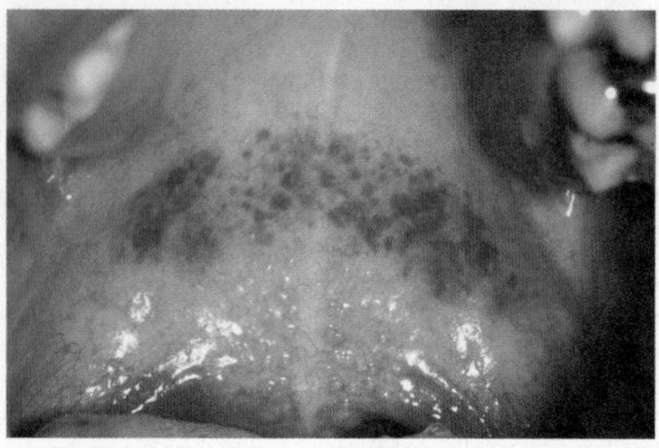

■ Petechiae of the soft palate caused by coughing.

diarrhea virus, hog cholera virus, and border disease virus of sheep. **pestivi′ral** *adj*

pes·tle (pes′əl) [L. *pestillum*] an implement for pounding drugs in a mortar.

PET positron emission tomography.

peta- (P) [Gr. *pente* five, because it is fifth in the series of prefixes for multiples] a combining form used in naming units of measurement to indicate a quantity one quadrillion (10^{15}) times the unit designated by the root with which it is combined.

-petal [L. *petere* to seek] a word termination meaning directed or moving toward, the point of reference being indicated by the word stem to which it is affixed, as centripetal (toward a center), corticipetal (toward the cortex).

pe·te·chia (pə-te′ke-ə) pl. *pete′chiae* [L.] a pinpoint, nonraised, perfectly round, purplish red spot caused by intradermal or submucous hemorrhage. Cf. *ecchymosis*, and see *petechial hemorrhage*, under *hemorrhage*. **pete′chial** *adj*

calcaneal petechiae black heel.

pe·te·chiae (pə-te′ke-e) plural of *petechia*.

Pe·ters anomaly (pa′tərz) [Albert *Peters*, German ophthalmologist, 1862–1938] see under *anomaly*.

peth·i·dine hy·dro·chlo·ride (peth′ĭ-din) meperidine hydrochloride.

pet·i·o·late (pet′e-o-lāt) having a stalk or petiole.

pet·i·o·lat·ed (pet′e-o-lāt-əd) petiolate.

pet·i·ole (pet′e-ōl) a stem, stalk, or pedicle.

epiglottic p. petiolus epiglottidis.

pet·i·oled (pet′e-ōld) petiolate.

pe·ti·o·lus (pə-ti′o-ləs) [L., dim. of *pes* foot] a stem, stalk, or pedicle.

p. epiglot′tidis [TA] epiglottic petiole: the pointed lower end of the epiglottic cartilage, which is attached to the back of the thyroid cartilage.

Pe·tit canal, sinus (pə-te′) [François Pourfour du *Petit*, French anatomist and surgeon, 1664–1741] see *spatia zonularia* and *sinus aortae*.

Pe·tit hernia, ligament, triangle (pə-te′) [Jean Louis *Petit*, French surgeon, 1674–1750] see under *hernia*, see *uterosacral ligament*, under *ligament*, and see *trigonum lumbale inferius*.

Pe·tit's law (pə-tēz′) [Alexis Therese *Petit*, French physicist, 1791–1820] Dulong and Petit's law; see under *law*.

pe·tit mal (pə-te′ mahl) [Fr. "little illness"] see under *epilepsy*.

PETN pentaerythritol tetranitrate.

Pe·tri dish, plate (pe′tre) [Julius Richard *Petri*, German bacteriologist, 1852–1921] see under *dish* and *plate*.

pet·ri·fac·tion (pet″rĭ-fak′shən) [L. *petra* stone + *facere* to make] conversion into a stonelike substance.

pé·tris·sage (pa″trĭ-sahzh′) [Fr.] massage in which the muscles are kneaded and pressed.

pet·roc·cip·i·tal (pet″rok-sip′ĭ-təl) petro-occipital.

pet·ro·la·tum (pet″ro-la′təm) [L.] [USP] a purified mixture of semisolid hydrocarbons obtained from petroleum; used as an ointment base. It is also used as a protective dressing and soothing application to the skin. Called also *mineral* or *petroleum jelly* and *yellow soft paraffin*.

heavy liquid p. mineral oil.

hydrophilic p. [USP] a mixture of cholesterol, stearyl alcohol, and white wax, in white petrolatum; used as an absorbent ointment base and topical skin protectant.

light liquid p. light mineral oil.

liquid p. mineral oil.

white p. [USP] a wholly or nearly decolorized, purified mixture of semisolid hydrocarbons obtained from petroleum; used as an oleaginous ointment base and topical skin protectant.

pe·tro·le·um (pə-tro′le-əm) [L. *petra* stone + *oleum*] a thick natural mixture of solid, liquid, and gaseous hydrocarbons obtained from beneath the surface of the earth. It consists mainly of a mixture of various alkanes, cycloalkanes, and aromatic hydrocarbons as well as small amounts of sulfur, nitrogen, and oxygen compounds.

p. benzin a colorless, volatile, flammable fraction from petroleum distillation, containing largely hydrocarbons of the methane series; it has been variously described as a special grade of ligroin or as a separate but similar fraction with a lower boiling range (35–80°C). It is used chiefly as an extractive solvent.

p. ether a volatile, flammable petroleum distillate, as ligroin or petroleum benzin; sometimes specifically one of these.

pet·rol·iza·tion (pet″rol-ĭ-za′shən) the spreading of petroleum on water for the purpose of destroying mosquito larvae therein.

pet·ro·mas·toid (pet″ro-mas′toid) 1. pertaining to the petrous portion of the temporal bone and its mastoid process. 2. otocranium.

pet·ro·oc·cip·i·tal (pet″ro-ok-sip′ĭ-təl) pertaining to the petrous portion of the temporal bone and to the occipital bone.

pet·ro·pha·ryn·ge·us (pet″ro-fə-rin′je-əs) an occasional muscle arising from the lower surface of the petrous portion of the temporal bone and inserted into the pharynx.

pe·tro·sal (pə-tro′səl) pertaining to the petrous part of the temporal bone.

pet·ro·sec·to·my (pet″ro-sek′tə-me) [*petrous* + *-ectomy*] excision of the air cells of the apex of the petrous part of the temporal bone.

pet·ro·si·tis (pet″ro-si′tis) inflammation of the petrous part of the temporal bone.

pe·tro·so·mas·toid (pĕ-tro″so-mas′toid) petromastoid.

pet·ro·sphe·noid (pet″ro-sfe′noid) pertaining to the sphenoid bone and the petrous part of the temporal bone.

pet·ro·squa·mo·sal (pet″tro-skwə-mo′səl) pertaining to the petrous and squamous parts of the temporal bone.

pet·ro·squa·mous (pet″ro-skwa′məs) petrosquamosal.

pet·rous (pet′rəs) [L. *petrosus*] resembling a rock; hard; stony.

Peu·ced·a·num (pu-sed′ə-nəm) a genus of herbs of the family Umbelliferae, native to Europe and Asia. *P. oreoseli′num* (L.) Munch. is oreoselinum, a medicinal plant.

Peu·ce·tia (pu-se′te-ə) a genus of spiders. *P. vi′ridans* is the lynx spider.

Peutz-Jeg·hers syndrome (pootz′ ja′gerz) [J.L.A. *Peutz*, Dutch physician, 1886–1957; Harold *Jeghers*, American physician, 1904–1990] see under *syndrome*.

pex·ia (pek′se-ə) pexis.

pex·ic (pek′sik) [Gr. *pēxis* fixation] having the power of fixing substances; said of tissues.

pex·in (pek′sin) chymosin.

pex·is (pek′sis) [Gr. *pēxis*] 1. the fixation of matter by a tissue. 2. surgical fixation, usually by suturing.

-pexy [Gr. *pēxis* fixation] a word termination meaning fixation.

Pey·er patches (glands, plaques) (pi′ər) [Johann Conrad *Peyer*, Swiss anatomist, 1653–1712] noduli lymphoidei aggregati intestini tenuis.

pey·o·te (pa-yo′ta) [Sp., from Nahuatl *peyotl*] 1. any of several Mexican cacti of the genus *Lophophora*, especially *L. williamsii* or mescal. 2. a hallucinogenic substance whose active principle is mescaline, found in the flowering heads of *Lophophora williamsii* and consumed in various North American Indian cultures as part of religious ceremonies. Called also *peyotl*.

pey·o·tl (pa-yo′təl) [Nahuatl] peyote.

Pey·ro·nie disease (pa-ro-ne′) [François de la *Peyronie*, French surgeon, 1678–1747] see under *disease*.

Pey·rot thorax (pa-ro′) [Jean Joseph *Peyrot*, French surgeon, 1843–1918] see under *thorax*.

Pez·i·za·les (pez″ĭ-za′lēz) an order of perfect fungi of the subphylum Ascomycotina, series Unitunicatae, usually saprobes, characterized by fleshy ascocarps of various shapes that form as a hymenium, as well as operculate asci. Families of medical significance include Ascobolaceae and Helvellaceae; other families include edible species such as truffles and morels.

Pfan·nen·stiel incision (fahn′ən-shtēl) [Hermann Johann *Pfannenstiel*, German gynecologist, 1862–1909] see under *incision*.

Pfeif·fer phenomenon (reaction) (fi′fər) [Richard Friedrich Johann *Pfeiffer*, German bacteriologist, 1858–1945] see under *phenomenon.*

PFES pelvic floor electrical stimulation.

Pfie·ste·ria (fe-ste′re-ə) [Lois Ann *Pfiester*, American biologist, 1936–1992] a genus of minute, plantlike protozoa of the phylum Dinoflagellata, the cause of red tide in coastal waters of the southeastern United States.

P. piscici′da a species that during one stage of its life cycle produces a neurotoxin that can cause skin lesions and sometimes death in fish, as well as mild neurotoxicity in humans.

Pfi·zer·pen (fi′zər-pen) trademark for a preparation of penicillin G potassium.

PFO patent foramen ovale.

PG prostaglandin; *Pharmacopoeia Germanica.*

pg picogram.

PGAD persistent genital arousal disorder.

PGD preimplantation genetic diagnosis.

PGD_2, PGE_2, $PGF_{2\alpha}$, PGI_2, etc. symbols for various prostaglandins; see *prostaglandin.*

PGL paraganglioma syndrome.

Pgp P-glycoprotein.

Ph Pharmacopeia; phenyl.

pH the symbol relating the hydrogen ion (H^+) concentration or activity of a solution to that of a given standard solution. Numerically the pH is approximately equal to the negative logarithm of H^+ concentration expressed in molarity. pH 7 is neutral; above it alkalinity increases and below it acidity increases.

PHA phytohemagglutinin (def. 2); pseudohypoaldosteronism.

PHA1 pseudohypoaldosteronism type 1.

PHA2 pseudohypoaldosteronism type 2.

pha·ci·tis (fə-si′tis) phakitis.

phac(o)- [Gr. *phakos* lentil, or lentil-shaped object] a combining form denoting relationship *(a)* to a lens, as the crystalline lens, or *(b)* a mole, freckle or nevus, as in phacomatosis. See also words beginning *phak(o)-*.

phaco·ana·phy·lax·is (fak″o-an″ə-fə-lak′sis) [*phaco-* + *anaphylaxis*] hypersensitivity to the protein of the crystalline lens of the eye, induced by escape of material from the lens capsule. See also *lens-induced uveitis.*

phaco·cele (fak′o-sēl) [*phaco-* + *-cele*[1]] the dislocation of the eye lens from its proper place; hernia of the eye lens.

phaco·cyst (fak′o-sist) [*phaco-* + *cyst* (def. 1)] the capsule of the lens (capsula lentis [TA]).

phaco·cys·tec·to·my (fak″o-sis-tek′tə-me) [*phacocyst* + *ectomy*] excision of a portion of the capsule of the lens for cataract.

phaco·cys·ti·tis (fak″o-sis-ti′tis) [*phacocyst* + *-itis*] inflammation about the capsule of the crystalline lens.

phaco·emul·si·fi·ca·tion (fak″o-e-mul″sĭ-fĭ-ka′shən) [*phaco-* + L. *emulgēre* to milk out] a method of cataract extraction in which the lens is fragmented by ultrasonic vibrations and simultaneously irrigated and aspirated.

phaco·ery·sis (fak″o-ə-re′sis) [*phaco-* + Gr. *eryein* to drag away] removal of the lens in cataract by means of suction with an instrument known as an erysiphake; called also *Barraquer method* or *operation.*

phac·oid (fak′oid) [*phaco-* + *-oid*] shaped like a lens or a lentil.

phac·oid·itis (fak″oi-di′tis) phakitis.

pha·col·y·sis (fə-kol′ĭ-sis) [*phaco-* + *lysis*] discission of the crystalline lens, followed by extraction.

phaco·lyt·ic (fak″o-lit′ik) pertaining to or causing dissolution of the crystalline lens.

pha·co·ma (fə-ko′mə) phakoma.

phaco·ma·la·cia (fak″o-mə-la′shə) [*phaco-* + *malacia*] softening of the lens; a soft cataract.

phac·o·ma·to·sis (fak″o-mə-to′sis) phakomatosis.

phaco·meta·cho·re·sis (fak″o-met″ə-ko-re′sis) [*phaco-* + Gr. *metachōrēsis* displacement] displacement of the crystalline lens.

pha·com·e·ter (fə-kom′ə-tər) lensometer.

phaco·pla·ne·sis (fak″o-plə-ne′sis) [*phaco-* + Gr. *planēsis* wandering] abnormal mobility of the crystalline lens.

phaco·scle·ro·sis (fak″o-sklə-ro′sis) [*phaco-* + *sclerosis*] hardening of the crystalline lens, or a cataract that has become hard.

phaco·scope (fak′o-skōp) [*phaco-* + *-scope*] an instrument for viewing accommodative changes of the eye lens.

pha·cos·co·py (fə-kos′kə-pe) the examination of the eye with a phacoscope.

phaco·tox·ic (fak′o-tok″sik) exerting a deleterious effect upon the crystalline lens.

Phae·ni·cia (fe-nish′ə) a genus of greenbottle flies of the family Calliphoridae that are metallic green or blue; some species are important causes of cutaneous myiasis in domestic animals. Called also *Lucilia.*

P. cupri′na a sheep maggot fly of worldwide distribution that causes cutaneous myiasis in sheep and sometimes myiasis in humans. Called also *Lucilia cuprina.*

P. serica′ta a sheep maggot fly of the British Isles that often causes cutaneous myiasis; its larvae (maggots) have also been introduced into infected wounds to facilitate healing. Called also *Lucilia sericata.*

phae(o)- [Gr. *phaios* dun, dusky] a combining form meaning brown or dusky. See also *phe(o)-*.

Phaeo·ac·re·mo·ni·um (fe″o-ak″rə-mo′ne-əm) a genus of Fungi Imperfecti of the form-class Hyphomycetes, form-family Dematiaceae.

P. parasi′ticum a species that causes opportunistic phaeohyphomycosis.

Phaeo·an·nel·lo·my·ces (fe″o-ə-nel″o-mi′sēz) a genus of dematiaceous mitosporic fungi of the group Fungi Imperfecti; *P. wernec′kii* is now called *Hortaea werneckii.*

phaeo·hy·pho·my·co·sis (fe″o-hi″fo-mi-ko′sis) [*phaeo-* + *hyphomycosis*] a hyphomycosis in which the infecting fungus is dark in color, usually of the form-family Dematiaceae. Most are opportunistic infections.

Phae·o·phy·ta (fe″o-fi′tə) in newer systems of classification, a phylum of the kingdom Protista, including brown algae. Called also *Ochrophyta.*

phaeo·spo·ro·tri·cho·sis (fe″o-spor″o-trĭ-ko′sis) phaeohyphomycosis.

phage (fāj) bacteriophage.

-phage [Gr. *phagein* to eat] a word termination denoting one that eats or destroys.

phag·e·de·na (faj″ə-de′nə) [Gr. *phagedaina*; *phagein* to eat] ulceration that spreads rapidly and causes sloughing; see also *phagedenic ulcer*, under *ulcer.* **phagede′nic** *adj*

-phagia [Gr. *phagein* to eat] a word termination denoting relationship to eating or swallowing. Also, *-phagy.*

phag(o)- [Gr. *phagein* to eat] a combining form denoting relationship to eating or consumption by ingestion or engulfing.

phago·cyt·a·ble (fa′go-sīt″ə-bəl) susceptible to phagocytosis.

phago·cyte (fa′go-sīt) [*phago-* + *-cyte*] any cell capable of ingesting particulate matter, such as a *microphage, macrophage,* or *monocyte.* Such cells ingest microorganisms and other particulate antigens that are opsonized (coated with antibody or complement), a process mediated by specific cell-surface receptors (Fc receptors and complement receptors). Other cell types exhibit phagocytosis, but not specific phagocytosis of opsonized particles.

alveolar p. see under *macrophage.*

mononuclear p. any cell of the monocyte-macrophage lineage, including macrophages, monocytes, and their precursors in the monocytic series.

phago·cyt·ic (fa″go-sit′ik) 1. pertaining to or exhibiting phagocytosis. 2. pertaining to phagocytes.

phago·cyt·ize (fa′go-sit″īz) phagocytose.

phago·cy·tol·y·sis (fa″go-si-tol′ĭ-sis) [*phagocyte* + *-lysis*] solution or destruction of phagocytes. **phagocytolyt′ic** *adj*

phago·cy·tose (fa″go-si′tōs) to ingest particles by the process of phagocytosis.

phago·cy·to·sis (fa″go-si-to′sis) endocytosis of particulate material, such as microorganisms or cell fragments. The material is taken into the cell in membrane-bound vesicles (phagosomes) that originate as pinched-off invaginations of the plasma membrane. Phagosomes fuse with lysosomes, forming phagolysosomes in which the engulfed material is killed and digested. See *phagocyte.* **phagocytot′ic** *adj*

induced p. phagocytosis aided by subjecting bacteria to the action of opsonins in the blood.

spontaneous p. phagocytosis of bacteria taking place in an indifferent medium, or phagocytosis of nonantigenic particles.

surface p. enhanced phagocytosis by macrophages and neutrophils of microorganisms or other particulate antigens that are trapped against surfaces, e.g., other leukocytes, fibrin clots, or tissue surfaces; it does not require opsonins.

pha·gol·y·sis (fə-gol′ĭ-sis) phagocytolysis. **phagolyt′ic** *adj*

phago·ly·so·some (fag″o-li′so-sōm) the digestive vacuole formed when the membranes of pre-existent lysosomes within the cytoplasm merge with the phagosome; the lysosomes then discharge their hydrolytic enzymes, resulting in digestion of the phagocytized material.

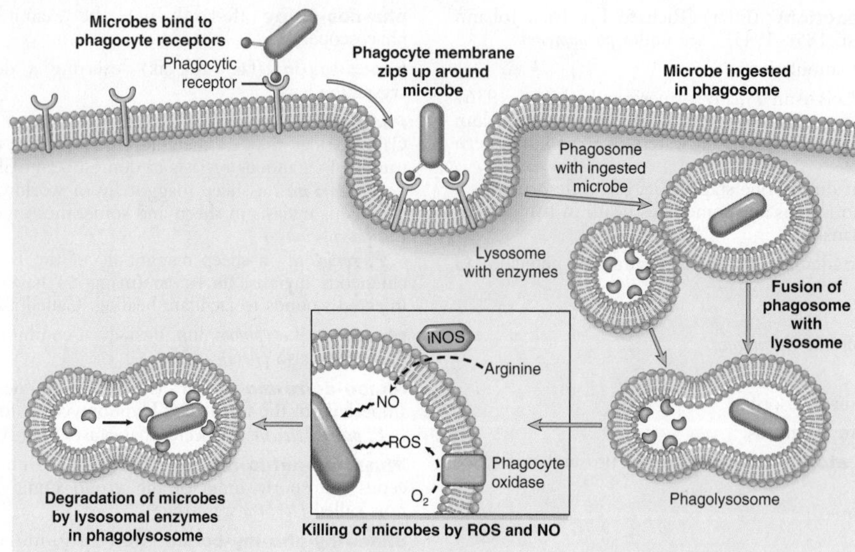

■ Phagocytosis. *iNOS,* Inducible nitric oxide synthase; *NO,* nitric oxide; *ROS,* reactive oxygen species.

phago•ma•nia (fag″o-ma′ne-ə) [*phago-* + *-mania*] an insatiable craving for food, or an obsessive preoccupation with the subject of eating.

phago•pho•bia (fag″o-fo′be-ə) [*phago-* + *-phobia*] irrational fear of eating.

phago•some (fag′o-sōm) [*phago-* + *-some*] the membrane-bounded vesicle in a phagocyte formed by invagination of the cell membrane and the phagocytized material; called also *phagocytotic vesicle.* See also *phagolysosome.*

phago•troph (fag′o-trōf) a holozoic organism.

phago•tro•phic (fag″o-tro′fik) [*phago-* + *-trophic*] holozoic.

phago•type (fag′o-tīp) phage type; see under *type.*

-phagy see *-phagia.*

pha•ki•tis (fa-ki′tis) [*phak-* + *-itis*] inflammation of the crystalline lens.

phak(o)- [Gr. *phakos* a lentil, or lentil-shaped object; a spot on the body, a freckle] for words beginning thus, see also those beginning *phac(o)-.*

pha•ko•ma (fə-ko′mə) [*phak-* + *-oma*] any of the hamartomas found characteristically in the phakomatoses. Written also *phacoma.*

phak•o•ma•to•sis (fak″o-mə-to′sis) pl. *phakomato′ses* [*phakoma* + *-osis*] any of a group of congenital and hereditary developmental anomalies having in common selective involvement of tissues of ectodermal origin (the central nervous system, eye, and skin) and development of hamartomas in these tissues. The group includes neurofibromatosis, tuberous sclerosis complex, Sturge-Weber syndrome, von Hippel-Lindau disease, and ataxia-telangiectasia. Called also *neurocutaneous syndrome.* Written also *phacomatosis.*

pha•lan•ge•al (fə-lan′je-əl) pertaining to a phalanx.

phal•an•gec•to•my (fal″ən-jek′tə-me) excision of a phalanx of a finger or toe.

pha•lan•ges (fə-lan′jēz) plural of *phalanx.*

phal•an•gette (fal″ən-jet′) [Fr.] the distal phalanx of a digit; see *phalanx distalis digitorum manus* and *phalanx distalis digitorum pedis.*

drop p. a condition in which the terminal phalanx of a finger or toe is permanently flexed, as in mallet finger.

phal•an•gi•tis (fal″ən-ji′tis) inflammation of one or more phalanges.

phal•an•gi•za•tion (fal″ən-jĭ-za′shən) surgical separation of the terminal portion of fused digits, without complete extirpation of the connecting web.

phalang(o)- [L. *phalanx,* q.v.] a combining form denoting relationship to a phalanx or to the phalanges.

pha•lan•go•pha•lan•ge•al (fə-lang″go-fə-lan′je-əl) pertaining to two adjoining phalanges of a finger or toe.

phal•an•go•sis (fal″ən-go′sis) [*phalang-* + *-osis*] a condition in which the eyelashes grow in rows.

pha•lanx (fa′lanks) pl. *phalan′ges* [L., from Gr. "a line or array of soldiers"] 1. [TA] any of the bones of the fingers or toes; see *ossa digitorum manus* and *ossa digitorum pedis,* under *os.* 2. any one of a set of plates (made up of supporting cells, q.v.) which are disposed in rows and make up the reticular membrane of the organ of Corti.

Deiters phalanges modified cuticular plates forming the ends of sustentacular epithelial cells of the reticular membrane of the organ of Corti.

phalan′ges digito′rum ma′nus TA alternative for *ossa digitorum manus.*

phalan′ges digito′rum pe′dis TA alternative for *ossa digitorum pedis.*

p. dista′lis digito′rum ma′nus [TA] distal phalanx of fingers: any one of the five terminal bones of the fingers, articulating, except in the thumb, with the phalanx media; called also *p. tertia digitorum manus.*

p. dista′lis digito′rum pe′dis [TA] distal phalanx of toes: any one of the five terminal bones of the toes, articulating, except in the great toe, with the phalanx media; called also *p. tertia digitorum pedis.*

phalanges of fingers ossa digitorum manus.

p. me′dia digito′rum ma′nus [TA] middle phalanx of fingers: any one of the four bones of the fingers (excluding the thumb) situated between the proximal and distal phalanges; called also *p. secunda digitorum manus.*

p. me′dia digito′rum pe′dis [TA] middle phalanx of toes: any one of the four bones of the toes (excluding the great toe) situated between the proximal and distal phalanges; called also *p. secunda digitorum pedis.*

p. pri′ma digito′rum ma′nus p. proximalis digitorum manus.

p. pri′ma digito′rum pe′dis p. proximalis digitorum pedis.

p. proxima′lis digito′rum ma′nus [TA] proximal phalanx of fingers: any one of the five bones of the fingers that articulate with the metacarpal bones and, except in the thumb, with the phalanx media; called also *p. prima digitorum manus.*

p. proxima′lis digito′rum pe′dis [TA] proximal phalanx of toes: any one of the five bones of the toes that articulate with the metatarsal bones and, except in the great toe, with the phalanx media; called also *p. prima digitorum pedis.*

p. secun′da digito′rum ma′nus p. media digitorum manus.

p. secun′da digito′rum pe′dis p. media digitorum pedis.

p. ter′tia digito′rum ma′nus p. distalis digitorum manus.

p. ter′tia digito′rum pe′dis p. distalis digitorum pedis.

phalanges of toes ossa digitorum pedis.

ungual p. of fingers p. distalis digitorum manus.

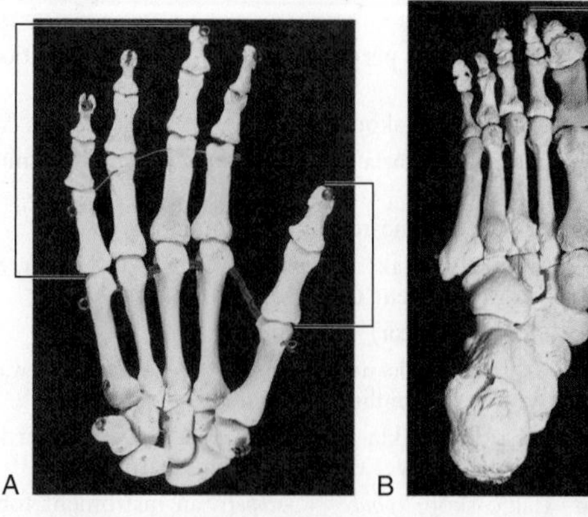

■ Phalanges of the *(A),* hand (palmar view) and *(B),* foot (superior view).

ungual p. of toes p. distalis digitorum pedis.

Pha•lar•is (fə-lar′is) a genus of North American and European grasses commonly found in pastures, certain species of which are called *canary grass.* Various species sometimes cause *Phalaris staggers* and other toxic conditions, including fatal heart failure, in ruminants.

Pha•len sign, test (maneuver) (fa′lən) [George S. *Phalen,* American orthopedic surgeon, 1911–1998] see under *sign* and *test.*

Phal•la•les (fə-la′lēz) the stinkhorns, an order of perfect fungi of the subphylum Basidiomycotina, class Holobasidiomycetes; most species have a fetid mucinous substance around the basidiospores, which are exposed by an internal stalk that grows and breaks out of the basidiocarp.

phal•lal•gia (fə-lal′jə) [*phall-* + *-algia*] pain in the penis.

phal•lec•to•my (fə-lek′tə-me) [*phall-* + *-ectomy*] penectomy.

phal•li (fal′i) genitive and plural of *phallus.*

phal•lic (fal′ik) [Gr. *phallikos*] pertaining or resembling a phallus, or penis.

phal•li•form (fal′ĭ-form) [*phallus* + *form*] phalloid.

phal•lin (fal′in) a poisonous hemolytic glycoside from *Amanita phalloides.*

phal•li•tis (fə-li′tis) [*phall-* + *-itis*] penitis.

phall(o)- [Gr. *phallos* penis] a combining form denoting relationship to the penis.

phal•lo•dyn•ia (fal″o-din′e-ə) [*phallo-* + *-odynia*] phallalgia.

phal•loid (fal′oid) [*phallo-* + *-oid*] shaped like or resembling a penis; called also *phalliform.*

phal•loi•din (fə-loi′din) a heat-stable, bicyclic hexapeptide poison from the mushroom *Amanita phalloides;* see *mushroom poisoning,* under *poisoning.*

phal•loi•dine (fə-loi′dēn) phalloidin.

phal•lon•cus (fə-long′kəs) [*phallo-* + Gr. *onkos* mass] a morbid swelling or tumor of the penis.

phal•lo•plas•ty (fal′o-plas″te) [*phallo-* + *-plasty*] plastic surgery of the penis. **phalloplas′tic** *adj*

phal•lot•o•my (fə-lot′ə-me) [*phallo-* + *-tomy*] incision of the penis.

phal•lo•tox•in (fal′o-tok″sin) any of a group of potent hepatotoxins found in species of *Amanita* mushrooms; because they are not well absorbed in the human gastrointestinal tract, they usually do not do as much damage as the amatoxins do.

phal•lus (fal′əs) gen. and pl. *phal′li* [Gr. *phallos*] 1. penis. 2. a representation of the penis. 3. the primordium of the penis or clitoris that develops from the genital tubercle.

phaner(o)- [Gr. *phaneros* visible] a combining form meaning visible or apparent.

phan•er•o•gam (fan′ər-o-gam) [*phanero-* + Gr. *gamos* marriage] a true seed-bearing plant.

phan•ero•ge•net•ic (fan″ər-o-jə-net′ik) phanerogenic.

phan•er•o•gen•ic (fan″ər-o-jen′ik) [*phanero-* + *-genic*] having a known cause, as opposed to *idiopathic.*

Phan•e•rop•so•lus (fan″ə-rop′sə-ləs) a genus of trematodes found as intestinal parasites in reptiles, birds, and mammals. *P. bon′nei* has been found as a human parasite in Indonesia and Thailand.

phan•tasm (fan′taz-əm) [Gr. *phantasma* appearance] an impression or image not evoked by actual stimuli, and usually recognized as false by the observer; called also *phantom.* Cf. *hallucination.*

phan•ta•sy (fan′tə-se) fantasy.

phan•to•geu•sia (fan″to-goo′zhə) a parageusia consisting of continuous abnormal taste in the mouth, usually metallic or salty, in the absence of any external stimulus.

phan•tom (fan′təm) [Gr. *phantasma* an appearance] 1. phantasm. 2. a model of the body or a body part. 3. in radiology, a device that simulates the conditions encountered when radiation or radioactive material is deposited in tissues, to give a quantitative estimation of its effects.

phan•tos•mia (fant-oz′me-ə) [Gr. *phantasia* imagination + *osm-*[1] + *-ia*] a parosmia consisting of a sensation of smell in the absence of any external stimulus.

phar pharmacy; pharmaceutical; pharmacopeia. Also, *pharm.*

Phar B [L.] Pharma′ciae Baccalau′reus (Bachelor of Pharmacy).

Phar C Pharmaceutical Chemist.

Phar D [L.] Pharma′ciae Doc′tor (Doctor of Pharmacy).

Phar G Graduate in Pharmacy.

Phar M [L.] Pharma′ciae Magis′ter (Master of Pharmacy).

pharm see *phar.*

phar•ma•cal (fahr′mə-kəl) pharmaceutical (def. 1).

phar•ma•ceu•tic (fahr″mə-soo′tik) pharmaceutical (def. 1).

phar•ma•ceu•ti•cal (fahr″mə-soo′tĭ-kəl) [Gr. *pharmakeutikos*] 1. pertaining to pharmacy or to drugs. 2. a medicinal drug.

phar•ma•ceu•tics (fahr″mə-soo′tiks) 1. pharmacy (def. 1). 2. pharmaceutical preparations.

phar•ma•cist (fahr′mə-sist) an individual who is licensed to prepare and sell or dispense drugs and compounds, and to make up prescriptions. Called also *apothecary, druggist,* and *chemist* (British).

pharmaco- [Gr. *pharmakon* medicine] a combining form denoting relationship to a drug or medicine.

phar•ma•co•an•gi•og•ra•phy (fahr″mə-ko-an″je-og′rə-fe) [*pharmaco-* + *angiography*] angiography in which visualization is enhanced by manipulating the flow of blood by the administration of vasodilating and vasoconstricting agents.

phar•ma•co•be•zoar (fahr″mə-ko-be′zor) concretion in the stomach or intestine consisting of undigested parts of medication tablets or capsules; called also *medication bezoar.*

phar•ma•co•chem•is•try (fahr″mə-ko-kem′is-tre) pharmaceutical chemistry.

phar•ma•co•di•ag•no•sis (fahr″mə-ko-di″əg-no′sis) [*pharmaco-* + *diagnosis*] the employment of drugs in the diagnosis of disease.

phar•ma•co•dy•nam•ic (fahr″mə-ko-di-nam′ik) [*pharmaco-* + *dynamic*] pertaining to pharmacodynamics.

phar•ma•co•dy•nam•ics (fahr″mə-ko-di-nam′iks) [*pharmaco-* + *dynamics*] the study of the biochemical and physiological effects of drugs and the mechanisms of their actions, including the correlation of actions and effects of drugs with their chemical structure; also, such effects on the actions of a particular drug or drugs.

phar•ma•co•eco•nom•ics (fahr″mə-ko-ek″ə-nom′iks) the study of economic factors regarding the cost of drug therapy, including their impact on health care systems and society.

phar•ma•co•en•do•cri•nol•o•gy (fahr″mə-ko-en″do-krĭ-nol′ə-je) the study of the influence of drugs on the activity of the endocrine glands, and of the effects of very high levels of hormones on organs and tissues.

phar•ma•co•ep•i•de•mi•ol•o•gy (fahr″mə-ko-ep″ĭ-de″me-ol′ə-je) the study of the factors determining and influencing the frequency and distribution of events related to drug administration in a defined population.

phar•ma•co•ge•net•ics (fahr″mə-ko-jə-net′iks) the clinical study of inherited variation in the nature of responses to drugs, focusing on single genes. In practice, the term is often used interchangeably with *pharmacogenomics.*

phar•ma•co•ge•no•mics (fahr″mə-ko-jə-no′miks) the study of the inherited variations in genes that dictate drug response and the way these can be used to predict individual responses to a drug, using a genome-wide approach. In practice, the term is often used interchangeably with *pharmacogenetics.*

phar•ma•cog•nos•tics (fahr″mə-kog-nos′tiks) pharmacognosy.

phar•ma•cog•no•sy (fahr″mə-kog′nə-se) [*pharmaco-* + Gr. *gnōsis* knowledge] the branch of pharmacology that deals with the biological, biochemical, and economic features of natural drugs and their constituents.

phar•ma•cog•ra•phy (fahr″mə-kog′rə-fe) [*pharmaco-* + *-graphy*] an account or written description of drugs.

phar•ma•co•ki•net•ics (fahr″mə-ko-kĭ-net′iks) the activity or fate of drugs in the body over a period of time, including the processes of absorption, distribution, localization in tissues, biotransformation, and excretion.

phar•ma•col•o•gist (fahr″mə-kol′ə-jist) a specialist in the study of the actions of drugs.

phar•ma•col•o•gy (fahr″mə-kol′ə-je) [*pharmaco-* + *-logy*] the science that deals with the origin, nature, chemistry, effects, and uses of drugs; it includes pharmacognosy, pharmacokinetics, pharmacodynamics, pharmacotherapeutics, and toxicology. **pharmacolog′ic** *adj*

phar•ma•co•ma•nia (fahr″mə-ko-ma′ne-ə) [*pharmaco-* + *-mania*] uncontrollable desire to take or to administer medicines.

phar•ma•co•met•rics (fahr″mə-ko-met′riks) [*pharmaco-* + Gr. *metron* measure] the comparative evaluation of drug activity, distinguished from bioassay in that substances with different chemical constitutions are compared.

phar•ma•co•pe•ia (fahr″mə-ko-pe′ə) [*pharmaco-* + Gr. *poiein* to make] an authoritative treatise on drugs and their preparations; a book containing a list of products used in medicine, with descriptions, chemical tests for determining identity and purity, and formulas for certain mixtures of these substances. It also generally contains a statement of average dosage. The first United States pharmacopeia was published on December 15, 1820, printed in both Latin and English, and its 272 pages included 217 drugs which were considered worthy of recognition. See *USP.* **pharmacopei′al** *adj*

United States P. see under *U.*

phar·ma·co·pho·bia (fahr″mə-ko-fo′be-ə) [*pharmaco-* + *-phobia*] irrational fear of drugs or medicines.

phar·ma·co·phore (fahr′mə-ko-for″) [*pharmaco-* + *-phore*] the group of atoms in a drug molecule which is responsible for the action of the compound.

phar·ma·co·poe·ia (fahr″mə-ko-pe′ə) pharmacopeia.

phar·ma·co·psy·cho·sis (fahr″mə-ko-si-ko′sis) [*pharmaco-* + *psychosis*] any psychosis due to alcohol, drugs, or poisons.

phar·ma·co·ra·di·og·ra·phy (fahr″mə-ko-ra″de-og′rə-fe) radiographic examination of a body organ under the influence of a drug that best facilitates such examination.

phar·ma·co·ther·a·peu·tics (fahr″mə-ko-ther″ə-pu′tiks) [*pharmaco-* + *therapeutics*] study of the uses of drugs in the treatment of disease.

phar·ma·co·ther·a·py (fahr″mə-ko-ther′ə-pe) [*pharmaco-* + *therapy*] the treatment of disease by drugs. Cf. *chemotherapy.* Called also *drug therapy* or *treatment.*

phar·ma·co·vig·i·lance (fahr″mə-ko-vij′ĭ-ləns) the monitoring of the quality and safety of drugs by collection and analysis of data on adverse drug reactions and other safety-related effects of drug administration.

phar·ma·cy (fahr′mə-se) [Gr. *pharmakon* medicine] 1. the branch of the health sciences dealing with the preparation, dispensing, and proper utilization of drugs. 2. a place where drugs are compounded or dispensed.

chemical p. pharmaceutical chemistry.

evidence-based p. the practice of pharmacy in which pharmacists make decisions taking into account the best available, current research evidence, their own expertise, and the needs and preferences of patients. See also under *practice.*

galenic p. the pharmacy of vegetable medicines.

Pharm D [L.] Pharma′ciae Doc′tor (Doctor of Pharmacy).

phar·yn·gal·gia (far″in-gal′jə) [*pharyng-* + *-algia*] pharyngodynia.

phar·yn·gec·ta·sia (far″in-jək-ta′zhə) pharyngoesophageal diverticulum.

phar·yn·gec·to·my (far″in-jek′tə-me) [*pharyng-* + *-ectomy*] surgical removal of a part of the pharynx.

phar·yn·ge·us (far″in-je′əs) [L.] pharyngeal.

phar·yn·gism (far′in-jiz-əm) pharyngospasm.

phar·yn·gis·mus (far″in-jiz′məs) pharyngospasm.

phar·yn·gi·tis (far″in-ji′tis) [*pharyng-* + *-itis*] inflammation of the pharynx. See also *faucitis* and *tonsillitis.* Called also *sore throat.* **pharyngit′ic** *adj*

acute p. inflammation of the throat with dryness and pain, especially on swallowing, followed by moisture of the pharynx, congestion of the mucous membrane, and fever.

aphthous p. herpangina.

atrophic p. a type of chronic pharyngitis involving wasting of the submucous tissue, dryness, and thickened secretions. Called also *p. sicca.*

chronic p. pharyngitis with repeated acute episodes; the most common types are atrophic pharyngitis and hypertrophic pharyngitis.

diphtheritic p. faucial diphtheria.

gangrenous p. pharyngitis characterized by gangrenous patches.

gonococcal p. inflammation of the pharynx from infection with *Neisseria gonorrhoeae*, usually as a result of oral sexual contact.

p. herpe′tica herpangina.

hypertrophic p. a type of chronic pharyngitis with thickening of the mucous membranes, which contain nodules of lymphoid tissue; it is often due to repeated faulty habits of speaking.

membranous p. any type in which there is a fibrous exudate and formation of a false membrane, as seen in Vincent angina, diphtheria, and other conditions.

plague p. pharyngeal plague.

p. sic′ca atrophic p.

streptococcal p. an acute variety caused by infection with *Streptococcus pyogenes;* it occurs in epidemics and is usually spread by droplets or in air, although it can also be spread by direct contact and in food. Characteristics include intense local hyperemia, sometimes with enlargement of cervical lymph nodes and a yellow exudate. Called also *septic sore throat, streptococcal sore throat,* and *streptococcal tonsillitis.*

ulcerative p., p. ulcero′sa pharyngitis with ulceration of the mucous membrane.

vesicular p. herpangina.

pharyng(o)- [Gr. *pharynx* pharynx] a combining form denoting relationship to the pharynx.

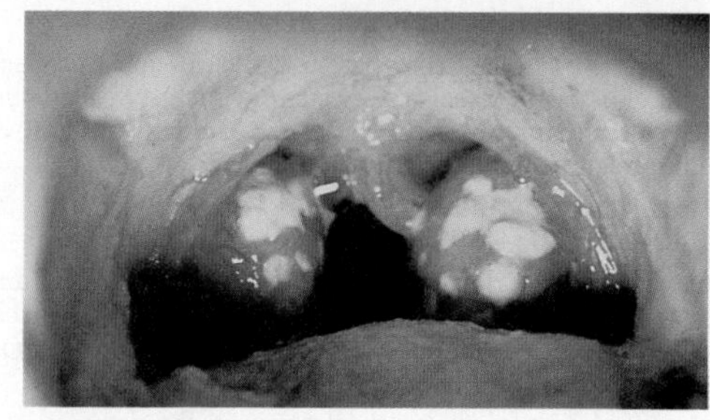

■ Streptococcal pharyngitis, with pus in the tonsillar crypts and palatal petechiae.

pha·ryn·go·cele (fə-ring′go-sēl) [*pharyngo-* + *-cele*[1]] pharyngoesophageal diverticulum.

pha·ryn·go·con·junc·ti·vi·tis (fə-ring″go-kən-junk″tĭ-vi′tis) inflammation involving the pharynx and conjunctiva, the result of a viral infection.

pha·ryn·go·dyn·ia (fə-ring″go-din′e-ə) [*pharyng-* + *-odynia*] pain in the pharynx; called also *pharyngalgia.*

pha·ryn·go·epi·glot·tic (fə-ring″go-ep″ĭ-glot′ik) pertaining to the pharynx and epiglottis.

pha·ryn·go·epi·glot·tid·e·an (fə-ring″go-ep″ĭ-glŏ-tid′e-ən) pharyngoepiglottic.

pha·ryn·go·esoph·a·ge·al (fə-ring″go-ə-sof′ə-je″əl) pertaining to the pharynx and esophagus.

pha·ryn·go·gas·tric (fə-ring″go-gas′trik) pertaining to the pharynx and stomach.

pha·ryn·go·glos·sal (fə-ring″go-glos′əl) glossopharyngeal.

pha·ryn·go·ker·a·to·sis (fə-ring″go-ker″ə-to′sis) keratosis pharyngea.

pha·ryn·go·la·ryn·ge·al (fə-ring″go-lə-ring′je-əl) pertaining to the pharynx and the larynx.

pha·ryn·go·lar·yn·gi·tis (fə-ring″go-lar″in-ji′tis) [*pharyngo-* + *laryngitis*] laryngopharyngitis.

pha·ryn·go·lith (fə-ring′go-lith) [*pharyngo-* + *-lith*] a concretion in the walls of the pharynx.

phar·yn·gol·o·gy (far″ing-gol′ə-je) [*pharyngo-* + *-logy*] the study, diagnosis, and treatment of the pharynx and its diseases.

phar·yn·gol·y·sis (far″ing-gol′ĭ-sis) [*pharyngo-* + *-lysis*] pharyngoparalysis.

pha·ryn·go·max·il·lary (fə-ring″go-mak′sĭ-lar″e) pertaining to the pharynx and the maxillae.

pha·ryn·go·my·co·sis (fə-ring″go-mi-ko′sis) [*pharyngo-* + *mycosis*] any fungal disease of the pharynx.

pha·ryn·go·na·sal (fə-ring″go-na′zəl) nasopharyngeal (def. 1).

pha·ryn·go·oral (fə-ring″go-or′əl) oropharyngeal (def. 1).

pha·ryn·go·pal·a·tine (fə-ring″go-pal′ə-tīn) palatopharyngeal.

pha·ryn·go·pa·ral·y·sis (fə-ring″go-pə-ral′ĭ-sis) [*pharyngo-* + *paralysis*] paralysis of the pharyngeal muscles. Called also *pharyngolysis* and *pharyngoplegia.*

pha·ryn·gop·a·thy (far″ing-gop′ə-the) disease of the pharynx.

pha·ryn·go·plas·ty (fə-ring′go-plas″te) [*pharyngo-* + *-plasty*] plastic operation on the pharynx. **pharyngoplas′tic** *adj*

Hynes p. a technique of pharyngoplasty accomplished by muscle transposition.

pha·ryn·go·ple·gia (fə-ring″go-ple′jə) pharyngoparalysis.

pha·ryn·go·rhi·nos·co·py (fə-ring″go-ri-nos′kə-pe) examination of the nasopharynx and posterior nares with the rhinoscope.

pha·ryn·go·scle·ro·ma (fə-ring″go-sklə-ro′mə) scleroma of the pharynx, usually from extension of rhinoscleroma.

pha·ryn·go·scope (fə-ring′go-skōp) [*pharyngo-* + *-scope*] an instrument for inspecting the pharynx.

phar·yn·gos·co·py (far″ing-gos′kə-pe) direct visual examination of the pharynx.

pha·ryn·go·spasm (fə-ring′go-spaz″əm) [*pharyngo-* + *spasm*] spasm of the pharyngeal muscles. Called also *pharyngism* and *pharyngismus.*

pha·ryn·go·ste·no·sis (fə-ring″go-stə-no′sis) [*pharyngo-* + *stenosis*] narrowing of the lumen of the pharynx.

pha·ryn·gos·to·ma (far″ing-gos′tə-mə) [*pharyngo-* + *stoma*] the opening formed by pharyngostomy.

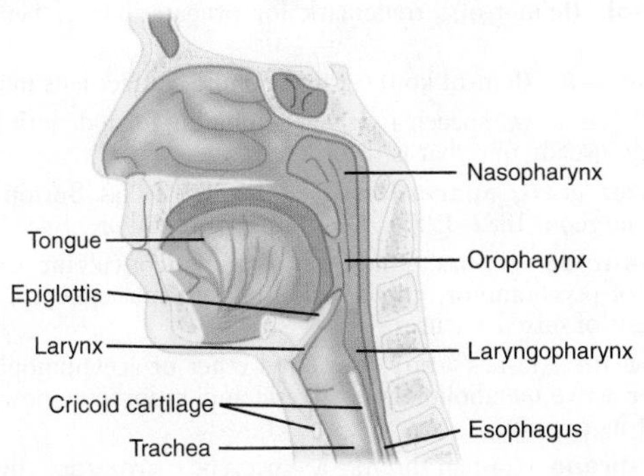

■ Pharynx, divided into the nasopharynx, oropharynx, and laryngopharynx.

pha•ryn•go•stome (fə-ring′go-stōm″) pharyngostoma.

phar•yn•gos•to•my (far″ing-gos′tə-me) [*pharyngo-* + *-stomy*] the surgical creation of an artificial opening into the pharynx.

pha•ryn•go•tome (fə-ring′go-tōm) a cutting instrument used in pharyngeal surgery.

phar•yn•got•o•my (far″ing-got′ə-me) [*pharyngo-* + *-tomy*] surgical incision of the pharynx.

external p. pharyngotomy done through an incision on the external surface of the neck.

internal p. pharyngotomy performed from within the pharynx.

lateral p. the opening of the pharynx from one side.

subhyoid p. external pharyngotomy done through the thyrohyoid membrane.

suprahyoid p. external pharyngotomy in which the suprahyoid muscles are divided and the epiglottic vallecula is entered by following the hyoepiglottic ligament.

pha•ryn•go•ton•sil•li•tis (fə-ring″go-ton″sĭ-li′tis) inflammation of the pharynx and tonsils; called also *tonsillopharyngitis.*

pha•ryn•go•xe•ro•sis (fə-ring″go-ze-ro′sis) [*pharyngo-* + *xerosis*] dryness of the pharynx.

phar•ynx (far′inks) [Gr. "the throat"] [TA] the musculomembranous passage between the mouth and posterior nares and the larynx and esophagus. The part above the level of the soft palate is the *nasopharynx,* which communicates with the auditory tube. The lower portion consists of two sections: the *oropharynx,* which lies between the soft palate and the upper edge of the epiglottis, and the *laryngopharynx,* which lies below the upper edge of the epiglottis and opens into the larynx and esophagus. Called also *throat.* **pharyn′geal** *adj*

phase (fāz) [Gr. *phasis* an appearance] 1. the view that a thing presents to the eye. 2. any one of the varying aspects or stages through which a disease or process may pass. 3. in physical chemistry, any physically or chemically distinct, homogeneous, and mechanically separable part of a system. 4. on an electrodiagnostic recording, that portion of a wave that is between any two consecutive times it crosses the baseline.

p. 0 in cardiac physiology, the phase representing the upstroke of the action potential, in which rapid depolarization occurs after the cell reaches or is driven to threshold potential. It is the result of the opening of fast sodium channels and calcium channels.

p. 1 in cardiac physiology, the initial rapid repolarization phase of the action potential, caused by the closure of the fast sodium channels and an exodus of potassium from the cell.

p. 2 in cardiac physiology, the phase representing the plateau of the action potential, which contributes to the refractory period of the heart; there is a slow entry of calcium into the cell. It is the result of a balance between inward and outward currents and is particularly long in Purkinje and ventricular cells.

p. 3 in cardiac physiology, the terminal rapid repolarization phase of the action potential; it begins with the closing of the slow channels, resulting in an exodus of potassium from the cell and the activation of the sodium-potassium pump. The result is reestablishment of the normal resting potential.

p. 4 in cardiac physiology, the phase representing electrical diastole, i.e. the time between action potentials. It is the resting phase of the electrical cardiac cycle and is steadily maintained in nonpacemaker cells. In pacemaker cells, the membrane potential is normally reduced slowly until threshold potential is reached; if there is an outside stimulus, it may be driven down more rapidly.

alpha p. the estrous stage of the ovarian cycle.

alveolar p. see under *period.*

anagen p. anagen.

anal p. see under *stage.*

beta p. the progestational stage of the ovarian cycle.

canalicular p. see under *period.*

catagen p. catagen.

cholesteric p. a liquid crystal phase that exhibits molecular orientation and arrangement both within and between equispaced planes, being arranged in parallel rows within a layer but twisted slightly between layers so as to form a helix through the layers.

continuous p. a phase that is physically uninterrupted; the continuous portion of a colloid system (see *dispersion medium*).

p. of decline the stage in the growth of a bacterial culture in which the number of live organisms gradually decreases.

disperse p., dispersed p. the internal or discontinuous portion of a colloid system; it is analogous to the solute in a solution. Called also *internal p.* Cf. *dispersion medium.*

double support p. that part of the gait cycle in which both feet are in contact with the floor.

ejection p. see under *period.*

embryonic p. see under *period.*

erythrocytic p. see under *stage.*

estrin p. proliferative stage.

exponential p. logarithmic p.

external p. dispersion medium.

five p's in traditional Chinese medicine, a set of dynamic relations (designated earth, metal, water, wood, and fire) that can be used to categorize relationships among phenomena; sometimes called the five elements because of their superficial resemblance to the elements of alchemy.

follicular p. the first part of the ovarian cycle, lasting from the end of the menstrual phase until ovulation and corresponding to the proliferative phase of the uterine cycle; it is characterized by the development of a dominant ovarian follicle, which reaches maturity by midcycle. At the end of this phase the luteinizing hormone surge and follicle-stimulating hormone surge begin, followed by ovulation.

G_0 p. a special subtype of the G_1 phase, in which cells carry out their normal physiologic functions but do not proliferate. Most of the specialized cells in multicellular organisms enter this phase; they may later return to the cell cycle and enter the S phase.

G_1 p. the part of the cell cycle lasting from the end of cell division (the M phase) until the start of DNA synthesis (the S phase); it is the first part of interphase and is typically the longest cell cycle phase. See also *G_0 p.*

G_2 p. a relatively quiescent part of the cell cycle, the last part of interphase, lasting from the end of DNA synthesis (the S phase) until the start of cell division (the M phase), during which the accuracy of DNA replication is checked and faulty sections repaired.

genital p. see under *stage.*

growth p. one of the stages in the growth of a neoplasm, such as the *radial growth phase* and *vertical growth phase.*

internal p. disperse p.

isovolumetric contraction p., isovolumic contraction p. period of isovolumic contraction.

isovolumetric relaxation p., isovolumic relaxation p. period of isovolumic relaxation.

lag p. the early period following bacterial inoculation into a new medium, a time of stationary population during which the cells adjust to the new environment and synthesize enzymes and intermediates for the subsequent logarithmic phase.

latency p. see under *stage.*

logarithmic p. the stage in the growth of a bacterial culture when a plot of the logarithm of the number of cells against time gives a straight-upward line. Called also *exponential p.*

luteal p. the phase of the ovarian cycle, lasting from ovulation to menstruation, during which the ovarian follicle transforms into the corpus luteum, which secretes progesterone; it corresponds to the secretory phase in the uterus. If fertilization and conception do not take place, the estrogen level falls and the menstrual phase begins.

M p. the part of the cell cycle during which mitosis occurs; subdivided into prophase, metaphase, anaphase, and telophase.

meiotic p. the stage in meiosis in which the reduction of the chromosomes occurs; called also *reduction p.*

menstrual p. the phase of the human menstrual cycle, following the luteal phase and occurring only if fertilization has not taken place. The corpus luteum regresses and is shed through menstruation and growth begins for the ovarian follicle, leading to the follicular phase.

motofacient p. see *motofacient.*

negative p. the initial lowering of the antibody titer following the injection of corresponding antigen.

nematic p. a liquid crystal phase that exhibits molecular orientation without periodicity, having an irregular threadlike surface with little viscosity.

nonmotofacient p. see *motofacient.*

oral p. see under *stage.*

phallic p. see under *stage.*
positive p. the rise in antibody titer that follows the negative phase.
postmeiotic p. the stage following the reduction of the chromosomes in meiosis.
preerythrocytic p. see under *stage.*
premeiotic p., prereduction p. the stage in meiosis preceding reduction of the chromosomes.
proliferative p. the phase of the uterine cycle, corresponding to the follicular phase of the ovarian cycle, during which the functional layer of the endometrium is repaired and proliferates under the influence of estrogen following menstruation .
pseudoglandular p. see under *period.*
radial growth p. an early growth phase of melanoma in which tumor cells are spreading laterally in the epidermis and have not spread into the dermis as in the vertical growth phase.
reduction p. meiotic p.
reversal p. in the process of bone turnover, the period between resorption and formation, during which the resorbed surface is prepared for, in part by depositing the cement subtance to produce the cement line.
S p. the part of the cell cycle between the G_1 and G_2 phases, during which DNA is synthesized and chromosomes are replicated.
secretory p. the phase of the uterine cycle, corresponding to the luteal phase of the ovarian cycle, during which the endometrium, under the influence of progesterone and estrogen from the corpus luteum, thickens and the spiral arteries increase in prominence and become longer and more coiled, with the development of large venous lacunae.
single support p. any part of the gait cycle when just one leg is touching the ground; cf. *double support p.*
smectic p. a liquid crystal phase that exhibits molecular orientation and arrangement in equispaced planes but no periodicity within the planes, having separate layers with little viscosity.
stance p. that part of the gait cycle in which the foot is in contact with the floor and the leg bears the body weight, comprising heel strike, mid stance, and push-off.
stationary p. the stage in the growth of a bacterial culture when the bacteria undergoing division are in equilibrium with those dying, and the number of bacterial cells remains nearly constant.
swing p. that part of the gait cycle in which the foot does not touch the floor and the opposite leg bears the body weight, comprising acceleration, swing through, and deceleration.
synaptic p. synapsis.
telogen p. telogen.
terminal saccular p. see under *period.*
ventricular filling p. see under *period.*
vertical growth p. a growth phase of melanoma more advanced than the radial growth phase; tumor cells are spreading from the epidermis into deeper layers such as the dermis and run the risk of metastasizing.

pha•se•o•lam•in (fə-se″o-lam′in) an α-amylase inhibitor purified from the kidney bean *(Phaseolus vulgaris);* it has been used in preparations alleged to enhance weight control by preventing absorption of ingested carbohydrate.

pha•se•o•lu•na•tin (fa″se-o-loo′nə-tin) linamarin.

Pha•se•o•lus (fa″ze-o′ləs) a large genus of plants of the family Leguminosae, including many edible beans. *P. limen′sis* (the lima bean) and other varieties contain the cyanogen linamarin and can cause cyanide poisoning in animals consuming them in large amounts. *P. vulga′ris* is the kidney bean, a source of phaseolamin and phaseolin.

phase-spe•cif•ic (fāz-spə-sif′ik) having maximum activity during a certain phase of the cell growth cycle; see under *agent.*

-phasia [Gr. *phasis* speech + *-ia*] a combining form denoting a manner of speaking, usually one that is disordered.

pha•sin (fa′sin) any of a group of nitrogenous substances found in seeds, bark, and other plant tissues, which agglutinate red blood corpuscles.

phas•mid (faz′mid) 1. one of a pair of caudal chemoreceptors occurring in certain nematodes. The class Nematoda is sometimes divided into two subclasses, Phasmidia and Aphasmidia, on the basis of the presence or absence of these organs. 2. a nematode belonging to the Phasmidia. Cf. *aphasmid.*

Phas•mid•ia (faz-mid′e-ə) a subclass of Nematoda comprising those organisms possessing phasmids. The following superfamilies are of medical or veterinary importance: Rhabditoidea, Strongyloidea, Oxyuroidea, Ascaridoidea, Spiruroidea, Filarioidea, and Dracunculoidea.

PhB British Pharmacopoeia.

PhD [L.] Philoso′phiae Doc′tor (Doctor of Philosophy).

Phe phenylalanine.

Phelps operation (felps) [Abel Mix *Phelps,* American surgeon, 1851–1902] see under *operation.*

Phe•mer•ol (fe′mər-ol) trademark for preparations of benzethonium chloride.

phem•fil•con A (fem-fil′kon) a hydrophilic contact lens material.

-phemia [Gr. *phēmē* speech + *-ia*] a combining form denoting a manner of speaking, usually one that is disordered.

Phem•is•ter graft, oper•ation (fem′is-tər) [Dallas Burton *Phemister,* American surgeon, 1882–1951] see under *graft* and *operation.*

phe•nac•e•mide (fə-nas′ə-mīd) an oral anticonvulsant used in the treatment of psychomotor, grand mal, and petit mal epilepsy, and in the management of mixed seizures.

phe•nac•e•tin (fə-nas′ə-tin) the ethyl ether of acetaminophen, which is its major active metabolite, an analgesic and antipyretic; now little used because of its toxicity.

phe•nan•threne (fə-nan′thrēn) a tricyclic aromatic hydrocarbon occurring in coal tar and isomeric with anthracene; it is toxic and carcinogenic.

o-phe•nan•thro•line (fə-nan′thrə-lēn) the *ortho* (1,10) isomeric form of phenanthroline, it is a metal chelator often used as an indicator.

phen•ar•sa•zine chlor•ide (fen-ahr′sə-zēn) a toxic compound used as a gas in war and, as a compound with tear gas, in riot control; also used in some wood preserving solutions. It irritates the skin and respiratory tract and also causes nausea, vomiting, depression, and weakness. Called also *adamsite* and *diphenylaminechlorarsine.*

phe•nate (fe′nāt) phenolate.

phen•a•zone (fen′ə-zōn) INN and BAN for *antipyrine.*

phen•a•zo•pyr•i•dine hy•dro•chlo•ride (fen″ə-zo-pir′ĭ-dēn) [USP] a urinary analgesic used orally to relieve symptoms of irritation in cystitis, urethritis, pyelonephritis, prostatitis, and other conditions causing irritation of the lower urinary tract mucosa.

phen•cy•cli•dine hy•dro•chlo•ride (fen-si′klĭ-dēn) a potent veterinary analgesic and anesthetic, sometimes used as a drug of abuse by humans but capable of causing serious psychological disturbances. Abbreviated PCP.

phen•di•met•ra•zine tar•trate (fen″di-met′rə-zēn) [USP] a sympathomimetic amine, related to amphetamine, used as an oral anorectic in the control of exogenous obesity.

phene (fēn) [gr. *phainein* to show] a phenotypic character under control of genetic factors.

phen•el•zine sul•fate (fen′əl-zēn) [USP] a monoamine oxidase inhibitor used as an antidepressant and in the prophylaxis of migraine; administered orally.

Phen•er•gan (fen′ər-gən) trademark for preparations of promethazine hydrochloride.

phen•go•pho•bia (fen″go-fo′be-ə) irrational fear of daylight.

phe•nin•da•mine tar•trate (fə-nin′də-mēn) an antihistamine (H_1 receptor antagonist) with sedative and anticholinergic effects; used in the treatment of allergic rhinitis, allergic conjunctivitis, and cutaneous manifestations of allergic reactions, and as an ingredient in some cough and cold preparations, administered orally.

phen•in•di•one (fen″in-di′ōn) an orally administered indanedione anticoagulant, having a rapid onset and short duration of action; it can cause serious hypersensitivity reactions and is now rarely used

phen•ir•amine mal•e•ate (fĕ-nir′ə-mēn) [USP] an antihistamine with sedative properties, used in the treatment of allergic disorders, including rhinitis, conjunctivitis, and pruritic skin disorders; administered orally, intranasally, or topically to the conjunctiva. It is also used as an ingredient in cough and cold preparations, administered orally.

phen•met•ra•zine hy•dro•chlo•ride (fen-met′rə-zēn) [USP] a central nervous system stimulant formerly used as an anorectic but no longer available because of potential for abuse; see *amphetamine.*

phen(o)- [Gr. *phainein* to show] 1. a combining form denoting a showing or displaying. 2. in chemistry, a prefix denoting a compound derived from benzene.

phe•no•bar•bi•tal (fe″no-bahr′bĭ-təl) [USP] a long-acting barbiturate, used as a sedative, hypnotic, and anticonvulsant, administered orally.
p. sodium [USP] the monosodium salt of phenobarbital, having the actions and uses of the base; administered orally, intravenously, intramuscularly, and subcutaneously.

phe•no•bar•bi•tone (fe″no-bahr′bĭ-tōn) phenobarbital.

phe•no•copy (fe′no-kop″e) [*pheno-* (def. 1) + *copy*] 1. an environmentally induced phenotype mimicking one usually produced by a specific genotype. 2. an individual exhibiting such a phenotype.

phe•nol (fe′nol) 1. [USP] an extremely poisonous, colorless to light pink, crystalline compound, C_6H_5OH, obtained by the distillation of coal tar; it is caustic and disinfectant and is used as a pharmaceutic preservative. Dilute aqueous solutions have been used as topical antiseptics, anesthetics, and antipruritics. Ingestion or absorption through the skin causes phenol poisoning (see under *poisoning*). Called also *carbolic acid*, *hydroxybenzene*, and *oxybenzene*.

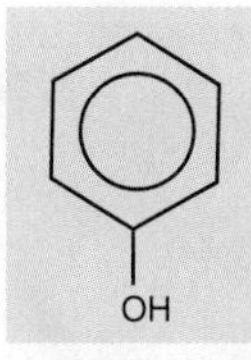

■ Phenol.

2. a generic term for any organic compound containing one or more hydroxyl groups attached to an aromatic carbon ring.
camphorated p. [USP] a mixture of camphor and phenol, applied topically as an antiseptic, anesthetic, and antipruritic.
liquefied p. [USP] an aqueous solution of phenol, containing about 10 per cent of water, having similar actions and uses.

phe•no•late (fe′nə-lāt) 1. to treat with phenol for purposes of sterilization. 2. a salt formed by union of a base with phenol, in which a monovalent metal, such as sodium or potassium, replaces the hydrogen of the hydroxyl group.

phe•no•lat•ed (fe′nə-lāt″əd) charged with phenol.

Phe•no•lax (fe′no-laks) trademark for a preparation of phenolphthalein.

phe•nol•emia (fe″nol-e′me-ə) the presence of phenols in the blood; see *phenol poisoning*, under *poisoning*.

phe•nol•ic (fe-nol′ik) pertaining to or derived from phenol.

phe•nol•iza•tion (fe″nol-ĭ-za′shən) treatment by subjection to the action of phenol.

phe•nol•o•gist (fe-nol′ə-jist) a specialist in phenology.

phe•nol•o•gy (fe-nol′ə-je) [*pheno-* (def. 1) + *-logy*] a study of the effects of climate upon the life and health of living organisms.

phe•nol•phthal•ein (fe″nol-thal′ēn) a cathartic and pH indicator, with a range of 8.5 (colorless) to 9.0 (red).

phe•nol•sul•fon•phthal•ein (PSP) (fe″nol-sul″fon-thal′ēn) a bright to dark red, crystalline powder that has been administered by intramuscular or intravenous injection to test renal function. Called also *phenol red*.

phe•nol•uria (fe″nol-u′re-ə) the presence of phenols in the urine; see *phenol poisoning*, under *poisoning*.

phe•nom•e•nol•o•gy (fə-nom″ə-nol′ə-je) in psychiatry, the study of phenomena in their own right rather than inferring causes, based on the theory that behavior is determined by the way the person perceives reality rather than by objective external reality.

phe•nom•e•non (fə-nom′ə-non) pl. *phenom′ena* [Gr. *phainomenon* that which appears, from *phainesthai* to appear] any observable occurrence or fact; see also *sign* and *symptom*.

Phenomenon

See also under *sign*, *symptom*, and *syndrome*.

Anderson p. clumps of red blood cells in the feces, seen on microscopic examination in amebic dysentery.
arm p. Pool p. (def. 2).
Arthus p. see under *reaction*.
Aschner p. oculocardiac reflex.
Ashman p. aberrant ventricular activation resulting in a short cardiac cycle that follows a normal or long cycle; it is associated with supraventricular premature beats and with atrial fibrillation.
Aubert p. an optical illusion in which a bright vertical line in a dark room tilts to one side when an observer tilts his head to the opposite side.
Austin Flint p. see under *murmur*.
autokinetic visible light p. the apparent spontaneous movement of a pin-point source of light as seen by certain susceptible persons when they gaze steadily at it in a completely blacked-out room.
Babinski p. see under *reflex*.
Becker p. increased pulsation of the retinal arteries, one manifestation of Graves orbitopathy. Called also *Becker sign*.
Bell p. an outward and upward rolling of the eyeball on the attempt to close the eye; it occurs on the affected side in peripheral facial paralysis (Bell palsy).
booster p. on a tuberculin test, an initial false-negative result due to a diminished secondary immune response that becomes positive on subsequent testing.
Bordet-Gengou p. complement fixation.
Bowditch staircase p. treppe.
brake p. the tendency of a muscle to maintain itself in its normal resting position; called also *Rieger p.*
break off p. a state of disconnectedness or unreality experienced by high-altitude pilots. Its symptomatic sensations are apparently indescribable in understandable physical terms, but the condition could be the result of a loss of all the physical sense perceptions.
Chase-Sulzberger p. Sulzberger-Chase p.
clasp-knife p. see under *rigidity*.
cogwheel p. see under *rigidity*.
Cushing p. see under *response*.
Dale p. see under *reaction*.
Danysz p. decrease of the neutralizing influence of an antitoxin when a toxin is added to it in divided portions instead of all at once.
dawn p. the early-morning increase in plasma glucose concentration and thus insulin requirement in a patient with insulin-dependent diabetes mellitus.
Dejerine-Lichtheim p. Lichtheim sign.
d'Herelle p. Twort-d'Herelle p.
doll's head p. an abnormal extraocular muscle manifestation of many ophthalmologic syndromes and conditions: the eyes depress as the head is bent backward.
Erben p. see under *reflex*.
fall-and-rise p. the drop in the number of bacteria that occurs at the beginning of drug treatment and the gradual rise that follows, even while treatment continues.
Felton p. immunologic unresponsiveness or tolerance to pneumococcal polysaccharide induced in mice by administration of large doses of the antigen.
Fick p. a fogging of vision, with the appearance of halos around light, occurring in individuals wearing contact lenses.
finger p. (in hemiplegia), extension of all the fingers or of the thumb and index finger, on pressure against the pisiform bone; called also *Gordon sign*.
first set p. the immune response of the body against a tissue or organ in a host not previously sensitized against the graft antigens. Called also *first set rejection*. See also *second set p.*
flicker p. flicker.
Frégoli p. a form of delusional misidentification in which the subject believes that a stranger, particularly a persecutor, is disguised as various people familiar to the subject. Cf. *Capgras syndrome*.
Friedreich p. the tympanic note of skodaic resonance in pleuritis with effusion varies in pitch during inhalation and exhalation, being higher during inhalation.
Galassi pupillary p. orbicularis pupillary reflex.
Gallavardin p. on auscultation in patients with aortic stenosis and calcified aortic valves, the disappearance of the systolic ejection murmur over the sternum and reappearance at the left ventricular apex, where it mimics that of mitral regurgitation.
Gengou p. complement fixation.
Goldblatt p. see under *hypertension*.
Gowers p. Gowers sign (def. 2).
Grasset p., Grasset-Gaussel p. inability of a patient to raise both lower limbs at the same time, though either can be raised alone; seen in incomplete hemiplegia.
Gunn p. see under *syndrome*.
Gunn pupillary p. Marcus Gunn pupillary p.
Herendeen p. rarely occurring rapid enlargement of a giant cell tumor of bone for several weeks to months after therapeutic irradiation of the lesion.
Hertwig-Magendie p. skew deviation.

Phenomenon *Continued*

hip flexion p. in paraplegia, when the patient attempts to rise from a lying position, the hip flexes on the paralyzed side.
Hoffmann p. increased excitability to electrical stimulation in the sensory nerves; the ulnar nerve is usually tested. Called also *Hoffmann sign.*
Houssay p. hypoglycemia and marked increase in sensitivity to insulin produced in an Houssay animal (an experimental animal deprived of both the pancreas and the pituitary gland).
Hunt paradoxical p. in dystonia musculorum deformans, if the examiner attempts forcible plantar flexion of the foot that is in dorsal spasm there will be increase of the dorsal spasm, but if the patient tries to extend the foot there will be plantar flexion.
iceberg p. cases of clinically apparent disease represent only a small fraction of the total cases of disease, inapparent cases, including preclinical, subclinical, chronic, and latent disease, being even more prevalent.
jaw-winking p. Gunn syndrome.
Kienböck p. paradoxical diaphragm p.
Koch p. if a guinea pig that has been previously infected with tuberculosis organisms is reinjected intracutaneously, the skin over the injected area undergoes necrosis; a superficial ulcer develops and heals quickly, and infection of regional lymph nodes is retarded. The phenomenon demonstrates development of ability to localize tubercle bacilli, which is the principle underlying tuberculin tests.
Koebner p. a cutaneous response seen in certain dermatoses, such as psoriasis, lichen planus, and infectious eczematoid dermatitis, with lesions appearing on uninvolved skin near the site of the skin disease; a similar reaction sometimes occurs on scars or at points where articles of clothing such as belts produce pressure. Called also *isomorphic effect* or *response.*
Kohnstamm p. aftermovement.
Leede-Rumpel p. Rumpel-Leede p.
Liacopoulos p. nonspecific immunosuppression to an antigen induced by administration of large doses of an unrelated antigen.
Liesegang p. the peculiar periodic formation of a precipitate in concentric banded rings, waves, or spirals when two electrolytes diffuse into and meet in a colloid gel.
Lucio p. a local exacerbation reaction occurring in Lucio leprosy. Initially there is ischemic necrosis of the epidermis due to necrotizing vasculitis of small blood vessels of the subpapillary plexus; next, small erythematous lesions erupt and have central necrosis; later, if the eschar is shed, ulceration can be seen, with eventual scar formation. Cf. *erythema nodosum leprosum.*
Marcus Gunn p. Gunn syndrome.
Marcus Gunn pupillary p. with unilateral optic nerve or retinal disease, a difference between the pupillary reflexes of the two eyes when a light is shone alternately into each one with the other eye covered; on the affected side there is abnormally slight contraction or even dilation of the pupil. See also *swinging flashlight test,* under *test.* Called also *Gunn pupillary p.* or *sign* and *Marcus Gunn pupillary sign.*
Meirowsky p. darkening of existing melanin, perhaps by oxidation, beginning within seconds and complete within minutes to a few hours after exposure to ultraviolet radiation of longer wavelengths; it is particularly noticeable in light-skinned individuals (see *tan*).
mucus extravasation p. extravasation of mucus into the surrounding connective tissue from a damaged minor salivary gland excretory duct, followed by an inflammatory reaction leading to the formation of a pool of macrophages and mucin surrounded by a wall of granulation tissue; visible as a small nodule or vesicle on the oral mucosa. Called also *mucocele.* Cf. *mucus retention cyst,* under *cyst.*

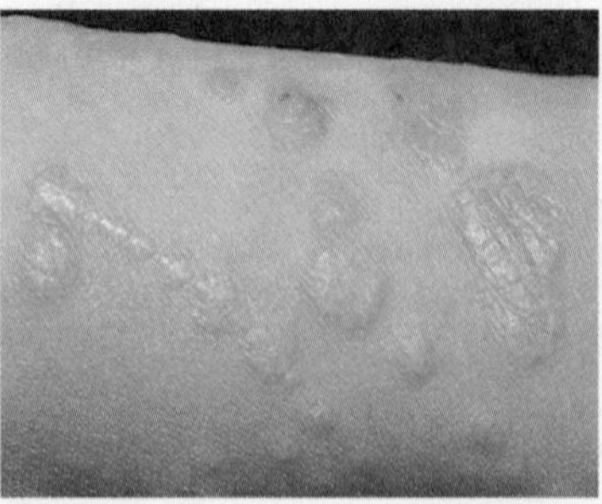

■ Koebner phenomenon in lichen planus.

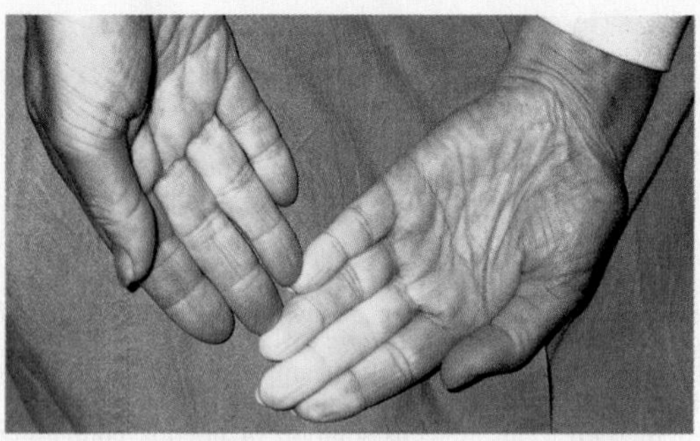

■ Raynaud phenomenon.

Negro p. cogwheel rigidity.
Neisser-Wechsberg p. complement deviation.
no-reflow p. when blood flow is restored to a part following prolonged ischemia, there is initial hyperemia followed by a gradual decline in perfusion until there is almost no blood flow.
nutcracker p. compression of the left renal vein between the aorta and the superior mesenteric artery, causing hypertension in the kidney with flank pain and sometimes fever and gross hematuria. Called also *nutcracker syndrome.*
orbicularis p. orbicularis pupillary reflex.
paradoxical diaphragm p. in phrenic nerve paralysis and diaphragmatic eventration, one hemidiaphragm moves upward on inhalation and downward on exhalation, opposite to the movements on the contralateral side.
paradoxical p. of dystonia Hunt paradoxical p.
paradoxical pupillary p. 1. reversed pupillary reflex. 2. see under *reflex* (def. 2).
Pfeiffer p. the lysis of *Vibrio cholerae* when injected into the peritoneal cavity of an immunized guinea pig; the term is also used to describe the in vitro lysis of cholera vibrios or other bacteria when incubated with specific antibody and complement.
phi p. the perception of the sequential flashing of a stationary row of lights as a moving light.
Piltz-Westphal p. orbicularis pupillary reflex.
pivot shift p. a sign of anterior cruciate ligament disruption: with the knee held at 20° flexion and in neutral rotation and with the muscles relaxed (which lets the femur drop down if the anterior cruciate ligament is torn), a slight valgus or axial force is applied to the knee; subluxation or reduction of the tibia occurs if the anterior cruciate ligament is torn. Called also *pivot shift sign* or *test.*
Pool p. 1. Schlesinger sign. 2. in tetany, the muscles of the upper limb contract when it is raised above the head with the forearm extended, because that causes stretching of the brachial plexus.
psi p. [*psy*che] an experience or effect that appears to be produced without physical agency or intermediation.
Purkinje p. as the intensity of illumination decreases and the eye becomes scotopic, the region of maximum visual acuity shifts from red-yellow to blue-green, the reds becoming less luminous, the blues more luminous. Called also *Purkinje effect* or *shift.*
Queckenstedt p. see under *sign.*
Raynaud p. intermittent bilateral ischemia of the fingers, toes, and sometimes ears and nose, with severe pallor and often paresthesias and pain, usually brought on by cold or emotional stimuli and relieved by heat; it is usually due to an underlying disease or anatomical abnormality. When it is idiopathic or primary it is called *Raynaud disease.*
rebound p. a manifestation of loss of coordination between groups of antagonistic muscles of the limbs in cerebellar dysfunction. It is usually tested by having the patient rest an elbow on a table and try to flex it against the resistance of the examiner; when the resistance is suddenly withdrawn, the affected arm rebounds to the patient's chest, whereas the normal arm flexes only slightly, the flexion being arrested by contraction of antagonistic muscles (the triceps). Called also *Holmes* or *Stewart-Holmes sign.*
reclotting p. thixotropy.

Phenomenon *Continued*

release p. the unhampered activity of a lower center when a higher inhibiting control is removed.
Rieger p. brake p.
R on T p. the occurrence of a premature ventricular complex near the peak of the T wave in electrocardiography; it may lead to ventricular tachycardia or fibrillation.
Rumpel-Leede p. the appearance of minute subcutaneous hemorrhages below the area at which a tourniquet is applied not too tightly for ten minutes upon the upper arm; characteristic of scarlet fever and hemorrhagic diathesis.
satellite p. satellitism, def. 2.
Schellong-Strisower p. fall of systolic blood pressure on assuming an erect posture from the lying down position.
Schlesinger p. see under *sign.*
second set p. the accelerated and intensified rejection by the recipient of a second graft of tissue from the same donor as a consequence of the primary immune response (i.e., antibody production and cell-mediated immunity) induced by the first graft. Called also *second set rejection.*
Sherrington p. the response of the hind limb musculature of an experimental animal on stimulation of a motor nerve that has previously been degenerated.
shot silk p. see under *retina.*
Shwartzman p. see under *reaction.*
Somogyi p. a rebound phenomenon occurring in diabetes mellitus: overtreatment with insulin induces hypoglycemia, which initiates the release of epinephrine, corticotropin, glucagon, and growth hormone, which stimulate lipolysis, gluconeogenesis, and glycogenolysis, which in turn result in hyperglycemia. Called also *rebound hyperglycemia* and *Somogyi effect.*
Splendore-Hoeppli p. the deposition of amorphous, eosinophilic, hyaline material around pathogenic organisms, seen in some fungal and parasitic diseases as the result of a local antigen-antibody reaction.
staircase p. treppe.
Staub-Traugott p. after a glucose load is administered, subsequent loads, given after a short interval, are disposed of at an accelerated rate. See also *Staub-Traugott effect,* under *effect.*
Straus p. see under *reaction.*
Strümpell p. tibialis sign.
Sulzberger-Chase p. abolition of dermal contact hypersensitivity to sensitizing agents, e.g., picryl chloride, produced by prior oral feeding of the agent.
toe p. Babinski reflex.
Trousseau p. spasmodic contractions of muscles provoked by pressure upon the nerves which go to them; seen in tetany.
Tullio p. vertigo induced by high-intensity sounds.
Twort-d'Herelle p. the phenomenon of transmissible bacterial lysis (bacteriophagia). When to a broth culture of typhoid or dysentery bacilli there is added a drop of filtered broth emulsion of the stool from a convalescent typhoid or dysentery patient, complete lysis of the bacterial culture will occur in a few hours. If a drop of this lysed culture is added to another culture of the bacilli, lysis will take place exactly as in the first. A drop of this culture will then dissolve a third culture, and so on through hundreds of transfers. d'Herelle attributed this phenomenon to the action of an ultramicroscopic parasite of bacteria, which he named the *bacteriophage.* See *bacterial virus,* under *virus.*
Tyndall p. see under *effect.*
Wedensky p. on applying a series of rapidly repeated stimuli to a nerve, the muscle contracts quickly in response to the first stimulus and then fails to respond further; but if the stimuli are applied to the nerve at a slower rate, the muscle responds to all of them.
Wenckebach p. see under *block.*
Westphal p. 1. (A.K.O. *Westphal*) orbicularis pupillary reflex. 2. (C.F.O. *Westphal*) see under *sign.*
Westphal-Piltz p. orbicularis pupillary reflex.
Wever-Bray p. cochlear microphonic.

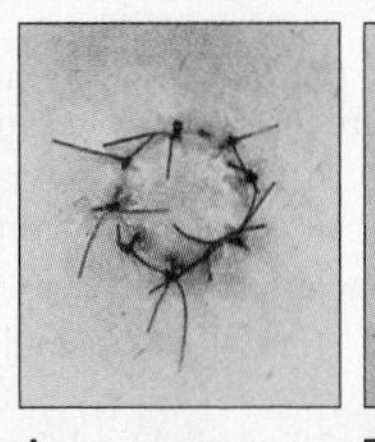

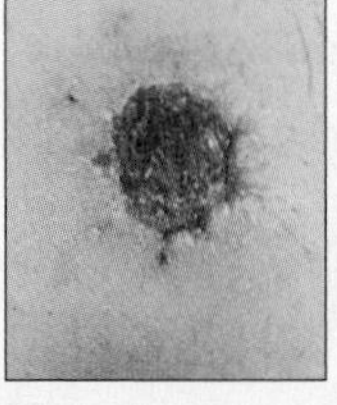

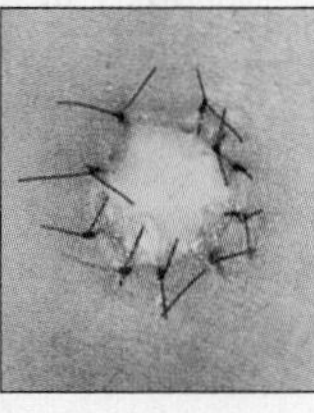

■ Second set phenomenon of a human skin allograft in which the graft has been rejected before it has had time to heal. After a first graft is initially vascularized at day 5 *(A)* and then destroyed by day 12 *(B)*, a second graft from the same donor is not vascularized and is rejected rapidly, by day 7 *(C).*

Phen•op•tic (fen-op′tik) trademark for preparations of phenylephrine hydrochloride.

phe•no•thi•a•zine (fe″no-thi′ə-zēn) 1. a greenish, tasteless, tricyclic organic compound prepared by fusing diphenylamine with sulfur; used as a veterinary anthelmintic. Called also *dibenzothiazine* and *thiodiphenylamine.* 2. any of a group of antipsychotic agents derived from this structure, i.e., all sharing a three-ring structure in which two benzene rings are joined by a sulfur and a nitrogen atom. They are potent alpha-adrenergic and dopaminergic blocking agents, their pharmacologic actions including central nervous system depression, prolongation and potentiation of the effects of narcotic and hypnotic drugs, hypotensive activity, and antispasmodic, antihistaminic, analgesic, sedative, and antiemetic activity.

phe•no•type (fe′no-tīp) [*pheno-* (def. 1) + *type*] the observable morphological, biochemical, and physiological characteristics of an individual, either in whole or with respect to a single or a few traits, as determined by a combination of the genotype and the environment.

Bombay p. a rare blood phenotype produced by the interaction of genes of the ABO blood group and a rare recessive gene at a different locus, resulting in a complete lack of H antigen; cells of individuals with this phenotype lack A, B, and H antigens, and their serum contains anti-A, anti-B, and anti-H antibodies.

McLeod p. a rare blood phenotype with X-linked inheritance in which several antigens of the Kell blood group are weakly expressed; affected individuals sometimes have an anemic condition called *McLeod syndrome.*

phe•no•typ•ic (fe-no-tip′ik) pertaining to or expressive of the phenotype.

phen•ox•ide (fən-ok′sīd) phenolate (def. 2).

phenoxy- a prefix indicating the presence of the group —OC_6H_5, composed of phenyl and an atom of oxygen.

phe•noxy•benz•amine hy•dro•chlo•ride (fə-nok″se-ben′zə-mēn) [USP] an irreversible α-adrenergic blocking agent, chemically related to the nitrogen mustards, with a long duration of action; used to control hypertension and sweating in pheochromocytoma, to treat Raynaud phenomenon, and to treat micturition disorders resulting from neurogenic bladder dysfunction or prostatic obstruction; administered orally.

phe•no•zy•gous (fe″no-zi′gəs) [*pheno-* (def. 1) + *zyg-* + *-ous*] having the cranium much narrower than the face, so that the zygomatic arches are seen when the skull is viewed from above. Cf. *cryptozygous.*

phen•pro•cou•mon (fen-pro′koo-mon) a synthetic coumarin anticoagulant, having a more rapid onset and longer-acting effects than dicumarol and having a marked cumulative effect; administered orally.

phen•pro•pi•o•nate (fen-pro′pe-ə-nāt″) USAN contraction for 3-phenylpropionate.

phen•sux•i•mide (fen-suk′sĭ-mīd) [USP] an anticonvulsant used mainly in the treatment of absence epilepsy, administered orally.

phen•ter•mine (fen′tər-mēn) a sympathomimetic amine related to amphetamine, used as an anorectic; administered orally as a complex with an ion exchange resin to produce a sustained action.

p. hydrochloride [USP] the water-soluble hydrochloride salt of phentermine, used as an anorectic, administered orally.

phen•tol•amine (fen-tol′ə-mēn) an antiadrenergic that blocks the hypertensive action of epinephrine and norepinephrine and most smooth muscle responses involving α-adrenergic receptors.

p. mesylate [USP] the methanesulfonate salt of phentolamine, having the same antiadrenergic actions as the base; administered intramuscularly or intravenously in the prophylaxis and treatment of paroxysmal hypertension associated with surgery for pheochromocytoma and intravenously in the prevention and treatment of cutaneous necrosis and sloughing when extravasation of norepinephrine occurs after intravenous administration.

Phen•u•rone (fen′u-rōn) trademark for a preparation of phenacemide.

phen•yl (Ph) (fen′əl, fe′nəl) the monovalent radical C_6H_5—, derived from benzene by removal of hydrogen. **phenyl′ic** *adj*

p. carbinol benzyl alcohol.

p. hydrate, p. hydroxide phenol (def. 1).

p. mercury acetate phenylmercuric acetate.

p. mercury nitrate phenylmercuric nitrate.

p. salicylate a compound formerly used as an analgesic, antipyretic, intestinal antiseptic, and enteric coating for tablets, and in the prevention of sunburn. In veterinary medicine, it is sometimes used internally as an antipyretic and externally as an antiseptic. Called also *salol.*

phen•yl•a•ce•tic ac•id (fen″əl-ə-se′tik) a catabolite of phenylalanine; it is excessively formed and excreted, sometimes conjugated with glutamine, in phenylketonuria.

phen•yl•ac•e•tyl•urea (fen″əl-as″ə-tēl-u-re′ə) phenacemide.

phen•yl•al•a•nine (Phe, F) (fen″əl-al′ə-nēn) 1. an aromatic essential amino acid, α-amino-β-phenylpropionic acid; most of that ingested is hydroxylated to form tyrosine, which is used for protein synthesis, but small amounts are transaminated to phenylpyruvic acid or decarboxylated. See also table at *amino acid.* 2. [USP] a preparation of phenylalanine used as a dietary supplement.

phen•yl•al•a•nine hy•drox•y•lase (PAH) (fen″əl-al′ə-nēn hi-drok′sə-lās) a monooxygenase that activates molecular oxygen to catalyze the oxidation of phenylalanine to tyrosine, activating oxygen via oxidation of the cofactor tetrahydrobiopterin to dihydrobiopterin. Deficiency of the enzyme results in hyperphenylalaninemia, with the most severe manifestation being phenylketonuria. In official nomenclature, called *phenylalanine 4-monooxygenase* [EC 1.14.16.1].

phen•yl•al•a•nine 4-mono•ox•y•gen•ase (fen″əl-al′ə-nēn mon″o-ok′sə-jən-ās, EC 1.14.16.1) official nomenclature for *phenylalanine hydroxylase.*

phen•yl•al•a•nin•emia (fen″əl-al″ə-nĭ-ne′me-ə) hyperphenylalaninemia.

phen•yl•al•a•nyl (fen″əl-al′ə-nəl) the acyl radical of phenylalanine.

phen•yl•ben•zi•mid•a•zole sul•fon•ic ac•id (fen″əl-ben″zĭ-mid′ə-zōl sul-fon′ik) ensulizole.

***N*-phen•yl•an•thra•nil•ic ac•id** (fen″əl-an″thrə-nil′ik) 2-(phenylamino)benzoic acid: the parent compound of the fenamate analgesics.

phen•yl•bu•ta•zone (fen″əl-bu′tə-zōn) a nonsteroidal antiinflammatory drug of the pyrazolone class; administered orally in the short-term treatment of severe rheumatoid disorders unresponsive to less toxic agents. It is given for periods of less than one week because it can cause aplastic anemia and agranulocytosis.

phen•yl•car•bi•nol (fen″əl-kahr′bĭ-nol) benzyl alcohol.

phe•ny•lene (fen′ə-lēn) a divalent radical, $=C_6H_4$.

***p*-phen•yl•ene•di•amine** (par″ə-fen″əl-ēn-di′ə-mēn) a diamino derivative of benzene used as a dye for hair, garments, and other textiles, as a photographic developing agent, and in a variety of other industrial processes; it is a strong allergen, causing contact dermatitis and bronchial asthma.

phen•yl•eph•rine (fen″əl-ef′rin) a direct-acting sympathomimetic amine that stimulates α-adrenergic receptors and is a powerful vasoconstrictor.

p. hydrochloride [USP] the hydrochloride salt of phenylephrine, used as a vasoconstrictor; used topically to decongest nasal and laryngeal mucous membranes and to produce mydriasis without cycloplegia, and intravenously to maintain blood pressure during spinal and inhalation anesthesia, to treat vascular failure in drug-induced shock, shocklike states, and hypotension, to prolong spinal anesthesia, and to treat paroxysmal supraventricular tachycardia. It is also administered orally as a component of combination antihistaminic-decongestant preparations.

p. tannate the tannate salt of phenylephrine, used as a decongestant in combination antihistaminic-decongestant preparations; administered orally.

phen•yl•hy•dra•zine (fen″əl-hi′drə-zēn) a diazo derivative of aniline, used as a reagent for sugars, ketones, and aldehydes.

phen•yl•in•dane•di•one (fen″əl-in-dān′de-ōn) phenindione.

phen•yl•ke•ton•uria (PKU, PKU1) (fen″əl-ke″to-nu′re-ə) the most severe manifestation of hyperphenylalaninemia (q.v.) that is due to mutation in the *PAH* gene (locus: 12q24.1), which encodes phenylalanine hydroxylase, with virtual absence of enzyme activity and accumulation and excretion of phenylalanine, phenylpyruvic acid, and related compounds. It is an autosomal recessive trait characterized by severe mental retardation, tumors, seizures, hypopigmentation of hair and skin, eczema, and mousy odor, all preventable by early restriction of dietary phenylalanine. Called also *classic p.*

atypical p. non-PKU hyperphenylalaninemia; the term was formerly used to denote tetrahydrobiopterin deficiency disorders.

classic p. phenylketonuria.

maternal p. abnormal fetal development in pregnant women with PKU, probably due to intrauterine exposure of the fetus to high levels of phenylalanine. Miscarriages are frequent and most surviving offspring are severely mentally retarded, often with microcephaly, low birth weight, and congenital anomalies.

variant p. a third category sometimes used in classification of hyperphenylalaninemia due to defects in phenylalanine hydroxylase; it comprises individuals with phenylalanine tolerance intermediate between those with phenylketonuria and those with non-PKU hyperphenylalaninemia, requiring moderate dietary restriction.

phen•yl•lac•tic ac•id (fen″əl-lak′tik) a product of phenylalanine catabolism produced by reduction of phenylpyruvic acid; it is formed and excreted in excess in phenylketonuria.

phen•yl•mer•cu•ric (fen″əl-mər-ku′rik) denoting a compound containing the radical C_6H_5Hg—, forming various antiseptic, antibacterial, and fungicidal salts.

p. acetate [NF] a compound with properties similar to those of phenylmercuric nitrate; used as a bacteriostatic preservative in pharmaceutical preparations. It has also been used as a herbicide. Called also *phenyl mercury acetate.*

p. nitrate [NF] an antibacterial and antifungal compound of phenylmercuric nitrate ($C_6H_5HgNO_3$) and its hydroxide; used as a bacteriostatic preservative in pharmaceuticals. Called also *phenyl mercury nitrate.*

phen•yl•meth•a•nol (fen″əl-meth′ə-nol) benzyl alcohol.

phen•yl•pro•pa•nol•amine (fen″əl-pro″pə-nol′ə-mēn) an adrenergic structurally and pharmacologically related to amphetamine and ephedrine, used as a vasoconstrictor and bronchodilator.

p. bitartrate [USP] the bitartrate salt of phenylpropanolamine, administered orally as a nasal decongestant in combination cold preparations.

p. hydrochloride [USP] the hydrochloride salt of phenylpropanolamine, applied topically as a vasoconstrictor to decongest mucous membranes and administered orally to produce bronchodilation in the symptomatic control of allergic manifestations. It is also used in the treatment of stress incontinence and as an anorexic.

phen•yl•py•ru•vic ac•id (fen″əl-pi-roo′vik) a metabolite of phenylalanine, excessively formed and excreted in phenylketonuria because the major pathway of phenylalanine catabolism, via hydroxylation, is blocked.

phen•yl•thio•car•ba•mide (fen″əl-thi″o-kahr′bə-mīd) phenylthiourea.

phen•yl•thio•urea (fen″əl-thi″o-u-re′ə) a compound used in genetics research; the ability to taste it is inherited as a dominant trait, the compound being intensely bitter to approximately 70 per cent of the population, and nearly tasteless to the rest. Called also *phenylthiocarbamide (PTC).*

phen•yl•tol•ox•amine cit•rate (fen″əl-tol-ok′sə-mēn) an ethanolamine derivative that acts as a sedating antihistamine (H_1 receptor antagonist); administered orally, usually as an ingredient in cough and cold preparations.

phen•y•to•in (fen′ĭ-toin″) [USP] an anticonvulsant used in the treatment of epilepsy other than the petit mal type, the treatment of status epilepticus, and the prevention and treatment of seizures associated with neurosurgery; administered orally. Called also *diphenylhydantoin.*

p. sodium [USP] the monosodium salt of phenytoin, having the same actions and uses as the base; administered orally and intravenously.

phe(o)- [Gr. *phaios* dun, dusky] a combining form meaning brown or dusky. See also *phae(o)-.*

pheo•chrome (fe′o-krōm″) [*pheo-* + *-chrome*] chromaffin.

pheo•chro•mo•blast (fe″o-kro′mo-blast) any of the embryonic structures that develop into chromaffin (pheochrome) cells.

pheo•chro•mo•blas•to•ma (fe″o-kro″mo-blas-to′mə) pheochromocytoma.

pheo•chro•mo•cyte (fe″o-kro′mo-sīt) a chromaffin cell.

pheo•chro•mo•cy•to•ma (fe″o-kro″mo-si-to′mə) [*pheochromocyte* + *-oma*] a usually benign, well-encapsulated, lobular, vascular tumor of chromaffin tissue of the adrenal medulla or sympathetic paraganglia. Because of increased secretion of epinephrine and norepinephrine, hypertension is a cardinal symptom; it may be persistent or intermittent. During severe attacks, there may be headache; sweating; palpitation and tremor; pallor or flushing of the face; nausea and vomiting; pain in the chest and abdomen; and paresthesias of the extremities. Called also *medullary chromaffinoma, medullary paraganglioma, chromaffin cell tumor,* and *pheochromoblastoma.*

pheo•mel•a•nin (fe″o-mel′ə-nin) a sulfur-containing form of melanin found in red hair and oculocutaneous albinism type 3.

phe•re•sis (fə-re′sis) apheresis.

pher•o•mone (fer′ə-mōn) a substance secreted to the outside of the body by an individual and perceived (as by smell) by a second individual of the same species, releasing a specific reaction of behavior in the percipient.

PhG Graduate in Pharmacy; *Pharmacopoeia Germanica.*

phi (fi) [Φ, ϕ] the twenty-first letter of the Greek alphabet.

Phi•al•e•mo•ni•um (fi″əl-ə-mo′ne-əm) a genus of Fungi Imperfecti of the form-class Hyphomycetes, form-family Dematiaceae, closely related to *Acremonium* and *Phialophora. P. obova′tum* has been isolated from hyalohyphomycosis.

phi•a•lide (fi′ə-līd) [Gr. *phialis,* dim. of *phialē* a broad flat vessel] 1. a flask-shaped conidiogenous cell formed in blastic conidiogenesis, projecting from the mycelium and not increasing in length with successive conidium formation. 2. the end cell of a phialophore.

phi•a•lo•co•nid•i•um (fi″ə-lo-kə-nid′e-əm) phialospore.

Phi•a•loph•o•ra (fi″ə-lof′ə-rə) a genus of Fungi Imperfecti of the form-class Hyphomycetes, form-family Dematiaceae. *P. jeansel′mei* and *P. spini′fera* have been reclassified in genus *Exophiala. P. verruco′sa* causes chromoblastomycosis.

phi•a•lo•phore (fi′ə-lə-for″) in certain fungi, the branch of the mycelium that bears at its tip the phialospores.

phi•a•lo•spore (fi′ə-lə-spor) a spore borne at the end of a phialide or a phialophore.

-phil [Gr. *philos* loving, dear] a word termination denoting one having an affinity for something. Also, *-phile.*

-phile see *-phil.*

-philia [Gr. *philein* to love] a word termination denoting *(a)* an abnormal craving or attraction or *(b)* an affinity for an object denoted by the word stem to which it is affixed.

-philic [Gr. *philos* loving] a word termination meaning having an affinity for.

Phi•lippe-Gom•bault tract (fe-lēp′ gom-bo′) [Claudien *Philippe,* French pathologist, 1866–1903; François Alexis Albert *Gombault,* French neurologist, 1844–1904] Gombault-Philippe triangle.

Phil•ly•rea (fĭ-lir′e-ə) a genus of evergreen shrubs of the family Oleaceae, native to the Mediterranean region. *P. latifo′lia* L. has leaves and bark that contain the medicinal substance phillyrin.

phil•ly•rin (fil′ĭ-rin) a crystalline substance that has antimalarial properties, extracted from the leaves and bark of evergreens of the genus *Phillyrea,* especially *P. latifolia* L.

Phi•loph•thal•mus (fi″lof-thal′məs) a genus of trematodes found in many parts of the world, usually in eye infections of birds, and less often in eye infections of mammals.

phil•trum (fil′trəm) [Gr. *philtron* love potion] [TA] the vertical groove in the median portion of the upper lip, a part of the prolabium.

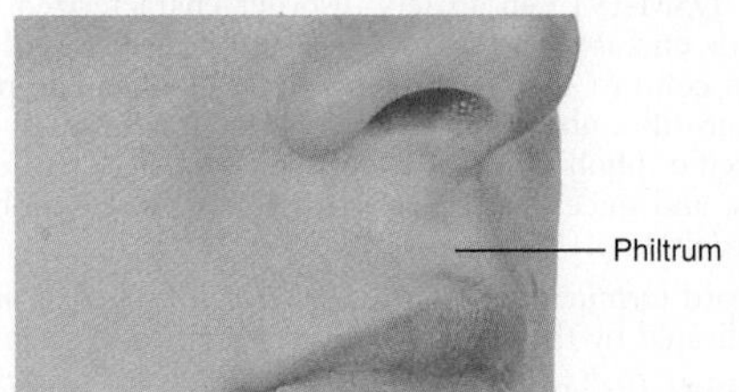

phi•mo•sis (fi-mo′sis) [Gr. *phimōsis* a muzzling or closure] constriction of the preputial orifice so that the prepuce cannot be retracted back over the glans. **phimot′ic** *adj*

pHi•so•Hex (fi′so-heks″) trademark for an emulsion containing hexachlorophene.

phle•bal•gia (flə-bal′jə) [*phleb-* + *-algia*] pain in a vein or varix.

phleb•an•gi•o•ma (fleb″an-je-o′mə) [*phleb-* + *angioma*] venous aneurysm.

phleb•ar•te•ri•ec•ta•sia (fleb″ahr-tēr″e-ek-ta′zhə) [*phleb-* + *arteriectasia*] vasodilation.

phleb•ec•ta•sia (fleb″ek-ta′zhə) [*phleb-* + *-ectasia*] varicosity (def. 1).

p. laryn′gis permanent dilatation of the veins of the larynx, especially those of the vocal cords.

phle•bec•ta•sis (flə-bek′tə-sis) varicosity (def. 1).

phle•bec•to•my (flə-bek′tə-me) [*phleb-* + *-ectomy*] excision of a vein, or of a part of a vein.

phleb•em•phrax•is (fleb″əm-frak′sis) [*phleb-* + *emphraxis*] obstruction of a vein by a plug or clot.

phle•bi•tis (flə-bi′tis) [*phleb-* + *-itis*] inflammation of a vein; when accompanied by thrombus formation it is called *thrombophlebitis.* **phlebit′ic** *adj*

adhesive p. obliterative p.

blue p. phlegmasia cerulea dolens.

enterocolic lymphocytic p. a rare condition of unknown etiology in which there is inflammation of the wall of the intestine and the mesentery without arterial involvement or systemic vasculitis; most patients have acute abdomen and venous thrombi.

p. mi′grans, migrating p. thrombophlebitis migrans.

obliterating p., obliterative p., obstructive p. phlebitis that obstructs a vein.

productive p. phlebosclerosis.

puerperal p. septic inflammation of uterine or other veins following childbirth.

septic p. phlebitis related to a septic process, as in erysipelas, peritonitis, or endometritis. In it the thrombus breaks down and septic emboli are carried to distant parts of the body. Called also *suppurative p.*

sinus p. inflammation of a cerebral sinus.

suppurative p. septic p.

phleb(o)- [Gr. *phleps,* gen. *phlebos* vein] a combining form denoting relationship to a vein or veins. See also words beginning *ven(o)-.*

phle•boc•ly•sis (flə-bok′lĭ-sis) [*phlebo-* + *clysis*] injection of fluid into a vein; called also *venoclysis.*

drip p., slow p. phleboclysis in which the solution is instilled slowly, drop by drop.

phle•bog•e•nous (flə-boj′ə-nəs) originating in a vein.

phlebo•gram (fleb′o-gram) [*phlebo-* + *-gram*] 1. radiograph of a vein taken during phlebography. 2. a tracing of the venous pulse (see illustration under *pulse*) made with a phlebograph or sphygmograph. Called also *venogram.*

phlebo•graph (fleb′o-graf) [*phlebo-* + *-graph*] an instrument for recording the venous pulse.

phle•bog•ra•phy (flə-bog′rə-fe) [*phlebo-* + *-graphy*] 1. angiography of veins. Called also *venography.* 2. the graphic recording of the venous pulse.

ascending p. phlebography in which contrast medium is injected into a vein in the foot and observed as it ascends toward the heart.

descending p. a method for detecting reversed flow of blood: contrast medium is injected into the common femoral vein with the patient in an upright position; since it is heavier than blood the contrast medium may move downward spontaneously or when encouraged by a Valsalva maneuver, thus indicating any incompetent valves or other areas of reversed flow.

phleb•oid (fleb′oid) [*phlebo-* + *-oid*] 1. resembling a vein. 2. venose.

phlebo•lith (fleb′o-lith) [*phlebo-* + *-lith*] a calculus in a vein.

phlebo•li•thi•a•sis (fleb″o-lĭ-thi′ə-sis) [*phlebo-* + *lithiasis*] the presence or development of phleboliths.

phle•bol•o•gy (flə-bol′ə-je) [*phlebo-* + *-logy*] the study of the veins and their diseases.

phlebo•ma•nom•e•ter (fleb″o-mə-nom′ə-tər) a manometer for the direct measurement of venous blood pressure.

phlebo•me•tri•tis (fleb″o-mə-tri′tis) [*phlebo-* + *metr-* + *-itis*] inflammation of the veins of the uterus.

phlebo•phle•bos•to•my (fleb″o-flə-bos′tə-me) operative anastomosis of vein to vein; called also *venovenostomy.*

phlebo•plas•ty (fleb′o-plas″te) [*phlebo-* + *-plasty*] plastic operation for the repair of a vein. **phleboplas′tic** *adj*

phlebo•rhe•og•ra•phy (fleb″o-re-og′rə-fe) [*phlebo-* + *rheography*] a technique for measuring venous volume changes in response to respiration and to compression of the foot or calf, employing a plethysmograph having cuffs applied to the abdomen, thigh, upper, mid, and lower calf, and foot; used in the diagnosis of deep venous thrombosis.

phle•bor•rha•phy (flə-bor′ə-fe) [*phlebo-* + *-rrhaphy*] the suturing of a vein; called also *venorrhaphy, venesuture,* and *venisuture.*

phleb•or•rhex•is (fleb″o-rek′sis) [*phlebo-* + *-rrhexis*] rupture of a vein.

phlebo•scle•ro•sis (fleb″o-sklə-ro′sis) [*phlebo-* + *sclerosis*] fibrous thickening of the walls of the veins; called also *proliferative endophlebitis, venofibrosis, venosclerosis,* and *venous sclerosis.*

phle•bo•sis (flə-bo′sis) abnormal noninflammatory changes in the veins.

phle•bos•ta•sis (flə-bos′tə-sis) [*phlebo-* + *-stasis*] 1. venous stasis. 2. temporary sequestration of a portion of the blood from the general circulation by application of tourniquets on an extremity.

phlebo•ste•no•sis (fleb″o-stə-no′sis) [*phlebo-* + *stenosis*] stenosis or constriction of a vein.

phlebo•throm•bo•sis (fleb″o-throm-bo′sis) [*phlebo-* + *thrombosis*] presence of a clot in a vein, unassociated with inflammation of the wall of the vein. Cf. *thrombophlebitis.* Called also *venous thrombosis.*

phle•bot•o•mist (flə-bot′ə-mist) an individual who practices phlebotomy.

phle•bot•o•mize (flə-bot′ə-mīz) to remove blood by phlebotomy.

Phle•bot•o•mus (flə-bot′ə-məs) [*phlebo-* + Gr. *tomos* a cutting] a genus of small, bloodsucking sandflies of the family Psychodidae; many species are vectors of disease-causing organisms.

P. argen′tipes a vector of *Leishmania donovani* in India.

P. aria′si a vector of *Leishmania infantum* in the Mediterranean region.

P. chinen′sis a vector of *Leishmania infantum* in China.

P. dubosc′qi a vector of *Leishmania major.*

P. lon′gipes the vector of *Leishmania aethiopica* in Ethiopia.

P. ma′jor a vector of *Leishmania infantum* in the Mediterranean region.

P. marti′ni a vector of *Leishmania donovani* in East Africa.

P. nogu′chii a species found in Peru that may transmit *Bartonella bacilliformis,* the etiologic agent of Carrión disease.

P. orienta′lis a vector of *Leishmania infantum* in Sudan.

P. papata′si the vector of the virus of phlebotomus fever; it is also a vector of the protozoa *Leishmania major.*

P. pe′difer the vector of *Leishmania aethiopica* in Kenya.

P. pernicio′sus a vector of *Leishmania infantum* in the Mediterranean region.

P. sergen′ti a vector of *Leishmania tropica* in the Middle East to Indus basin.

P. verruca′rum a vector of *Bartonella bacilliformis,* the etiologic agent of Carrión disease.

phle•bot•o•my (flə-bot′ə-me) [*phlebo-* + *-tomy*] 1. incision of a vein, as for the letting of blood. 2. needle puncture of a vein for the drawing of blood. Called also *venepuncture, venesection, venipuncture, venisection,* and *venotomy.*

bloodless p. phlebostasis (def. 2).

Phleb•o•vi•rus (fleb′o-vi″rəs) [*Phlebotomus* + *virus*] the sandfly fever viruses and uukuviruses; a genus of the family Bunyaviridae. Viruses are classified in two antigenic groups, the sandfly fever group and the Uukuniemi group. The sandfly fever group includes at least 39 species in nine serogroups and ungrouped species; the Uukuniemi group (the uukuviruses), which was previously recognized as a separate genus, contains 12 species in a single serogroup. The sandfly fever group includes the pathogens sandfly fever–Naples, sandfly fever–Sicilian, Toscana, and Rift Valley fever viruses; most sandfly fever viruses are transmitted by sandflies of the genus *Phlebotomus,* but some are mosquito-borne. Uukuviruses are tick-borne and include no known human pathogens. **phlebovi′ral** *adj*

phlegm (flem) [Gr. *phlegma*] 1. abnormally thick mucus secreted by the mucosa of the respiratory tract and expectorated during certain infectious processes. 2. in humoralism, one of the four humors of the body.

phleg•ma•sia (fleg-ma′zhə) [Gr. "heat, inflammation"] inflammation; not currently used except in compound terms (see subentries).

p. al′ba do′lens phlebitis of a femoral vein, occasionally following childbirth or an acute febrile illness; it is characterized by swelling of a lower limb, usually without redness. Called also *galactophlebitis* and *thrombotic p.*

p. ceru′lea do′lens an acute fulminating form of deep venous thrombosis, with reactive arterial spasm and pronounced edema of the extremity and severe cyanosis, purpuric areas, and petechiae; called also *blue phlebitis.*

thrombotic p. p. alba dolens.

phleg•mon (fleg′mon) [Gr. *phlegmonē*] acute subcutaneous inflammation, sometimes with abscess. **phleg′monous** *adj*

pancreatic p. see under *pseudocyst.*

periurethral p. see under *cellulitis.*

pharyngeal p. swelling and necrosis of the wall of the pharynx in cattle, with toxemia and respiratory distress; it may be fatal. Infection with *Fusobacterium necrophorum* is sometimes the cause. Called also *intermandibular cellulitis.*

Phle•um (fle′əm) a genus of grasses (family Gramineae). *P. praten′se* is timothy or timothy grass, a North American species used as fodder for cattle and horses; its pollen causes hay fever in susceptible people. When infested with *Claviceps purpurea,* it can cause ergotism in animals.

phlo•gis•tic (flo-jis′tik) inflammatory.

phlog(o)- [Gr. *phlox,* gen. *phlogos* flame] a combining form denoting relationship to inflammation.

phlo•go•gen•ic (flo″go-jen′ik) [*phlogo-* + *-genic*] causing inflammation.

phlo•gog•e•nous (flo-goj′ə-nəs) phlogogenic.

phlo•rhi•zin (flo-ri′zin) [Gr. *phloios* bark + *rhiza* root] a bitter glycoside from the root bark of apple, cherry, plum, and pear trees; it causes glycosuria *(phlorhizin glycosuria)* by blocking the tubular reabsorption of glucose. Spelled also *phlorizin* and *phlorrhizin.*

phlo•rhi•zin hy•dro•lase (flo-ri′zin hi′dro-lās) glycosylceramidase.

phlo•rhi•zi•nize (flo-ri′zi-nīz) to bring under the influence of phlorhizin.

phlo•rid•zin (flo-rid′zin) phlorhizin.

phlo•rid•zin•ize (flo-rid′zi-nīz) phlorhizinize.

phlo•ri•zin (flo-ri′zin) phlorhizin.

phlo•ro•glu•cin (flor″o-gloo′sin) [*phlorhizin* + Gr. *glykys* sweet] the aglycone of many glycosides, obtained from the bark of apple and other trees, and used as a reagent for pentoses, pentosans, glycuronates, hydrochloric acid in gastric juice, etc. It is an excellent decalcifier of bone specimens.

phlo•ro•glu•ci•nol (flor″o-gloo′sĭ-nol) phloroglucin.

phlor•rhi•zin (flo-ri′zin) phlorhizin.

phlox•ine B (flok′sin) a red acid dye used as a plasma stain in histology and as a component of Mallory phloxine–methylene blue stain.

phlyc•ten (flik′tən) phlyctena.

phlyc•te•na (flik-te′nə) pl. *phlycte′nae* [Gr. *phlyktaina*] 1. a blister made by a burn. 2. a small vesicle containing lymph seen on the conjunctiva in certain conditions. Called also *phlycten.*

phlyc•te•nar (flik′tə-nər) pertaining to or marked by phlyctenae.

phlyc•ten•u•la (flik-ten′u-lə) pl. *phlycten′ulae* [L.] phlyctenule.

phlyc•ten•ule (flik′tən-ūl) [L. *phlyctaenula;* Gr. *phlyktaina* blister] a small phlyctena on the cornea or conjunctiva; called also *phlyctenula.* **phlycten′ular** *adj*

phlyc•ten•u•lo•sis (flik″tən-u-lo′sis) an eye condition characterized by phlyctenules, as phlyctenular keratoconjunctivitis, conjunctivitis, or ophthalmia.

allergic p. phlyctenulosis due to allergy.

tuberculous p. phlyctenulosis due to tuberculous allergy.

PHN postherpetic neuralgia; public health nurse.

pho•bia (fo′be-ə) [Gr. *phobos* fear + *-ia*] a persistent, irrational, intense fear of a specific object, activity, or situation (the phobic stimulus), fear that is recognized as being excessive or unreasonable by the individual having it. When a phobia is a significant source of distress or interferes with social functioning, it is considered a mental disorder (sometimes called a *phobic disorder*); in DSM-IV phobias are classified with the anxiety disorders and are subclassified as agoraphobia, specific phobias, and social phobias. For a list of specific phobias (e.g., *triskaidekaphobia*), see Appendix 4. **pho′bic** *adj*

simple p. specific p.

social p. [DSM-IV] an anxiety disorder characterized by fear and avoidance of social or performance situations in which the individual fears possible embarrassment and humiliation, e.g., fears of speaking, performing, or eating in public. Panic attacks may occur.

specific p. [DSM-IV] an anxiety disorder characterized by persistent and excessive or unreasonable fear of a circumscribed, well-defined object or situation, in contrast to fear of being alone or of public places (agoraphobia) or fear of embarrassment in social situations (social phobia). Common specific phobias involve fear of animals, particularly dogs, snakes, insects, and mice; fear of closed spaces (claustrophobia); and fear of heights (acrophobia).

-phobia a word termination denoting irrational fear of or an aversion to the subject indicated by the stem to which it is affixed.

pho•bo•pho•bia (fo″bo-fo′be-ə) [Gr. *phobos* fear + *-phobia*] irrational fear of one's own fears or of acquiring a phobia.

Pho•ca•ne•ma (fo″kə-ne′mə) *Pseudoterranova.*

pho•co•me•lia (fo″ko-me′le-ə) [Gr. *phōkē* seal + *-melia*] a type of meromelia characterized by absence of the proximal portion of a limb or limbs, the hands or feet being attached to the trunk of the body by a single small, irregularly shaped bone.

pho•com•e•lus (fo-kom′ə-ləs) a person with phocomelia.

Pho•ma (fo′mə) a genus of Fungi Imperfecti of the form-class Coelomycetes, widely found on plants and in the soil. Several species have been occasionally isolated from cases of phaeohyphomycosis.

pho•mop•sin (fo-mop′sin) a mycotoxin found in *Phomopsis leptostromiformis* and *P. rossiana;* it causes mycotoxic lupinosis in grazing animals.

Pho•mop•sis (fo-mop′sis) a genus of Fungi Imperfecti of the form-class Coelomycetes. *P. leptostromifor′mis* and *P. rossia′na* infest plants of the genus *Lupinus* and contain phomopsins, mycotoxins that cause mycotoxic lupinosis in grazing livestock.

phon (fōn) [Gr. *phōnē* voice] a unit of the subjective loudness of a sound.

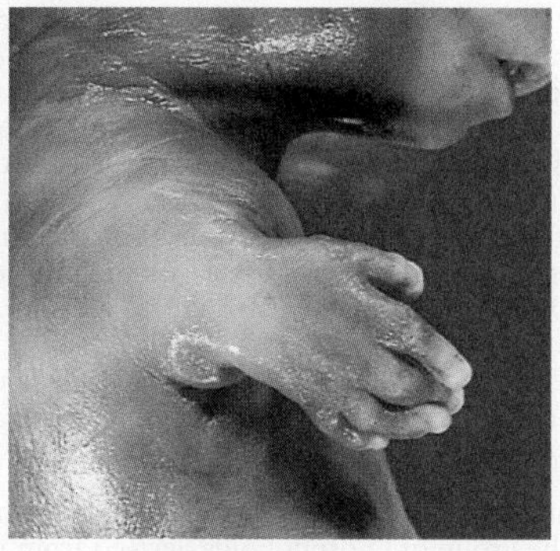

■ Phocomelia.

pho•naco•scope (fo-nak′o-skōp) the apparatus used in phonacoscopy.

pho•na•cos•co•py (fo″nə-kos′kə-pe) [*phon-* + *acou-* + *-scopy*] combined auscultation and percussion by means of a bell-shaped resonating chamber containing a percussion hammer, which is held on the anterior thoracic wall while the examiner listens at the back of the thorax.

pho•nal (fo′nəl) 1. pertaining to sound. 2. vocal.

phon•as•the•nia (fo″nəs-the′ne-ə) [*phon-* + *asthenia*] weakness of voice or difficult phonation from overuse, debilitation, or old age. Called also *myasthenia laryngis* and *vocal fatigue.*

pho•na•tion (fo-na′shən) the utterance of vocal sounds. See also *speech.* pho′natory *adj*

subenergetic p. hypophonia.

superenergetic p. hyperphonia.

pho•neme (fo′nēm) [Gr. *phōnēma* a thing spoken] the smallest speech sound in a language that is distinguishable from others in its class.

phon•en•do•scope (fōn-en′do-skōp) [*phon-* + *endoscope*] a stethoscopic device that intensifies auscultatory sounds, consisting of a shallow metal cup closed by a diaphragm.

pho•net•ic (fə-net′ik) [Gr. *phōnētikos*] pertaining to the articulated sounds of speech; called also *phonic.*

pho•net•ics (fə-net′iks) the science of vocal sounds; called also *phonology.*

pho•ni•at•rics (fo″ne-at′riks) [*phon-* + *-iatrics*] logopedics.

phon•ic (fon′ik, fo′nik) 1. acoustic. 2. phonetic.

pho•nism (fo′niz-əm) a form of synesthesia in which a sensation of hearing is produced by the effect of something seen, felt, tasted, smelled, or thought of.

phon(o)- [Gr. *phōnē* voice] a combining form denoting relationship to sound, often specifically the sound of the voice.

pho•no•an•gi•og•ra•phy (fo″no-an″je-og′rə-fe) the recording and analysis of arterial bruits to estimate the extent of arterial stenosis.

pho•no•aus•cul•ta•tion (fo″no-aws″kəl-ta′shən) auscultation in which a tuning fork is placed over the organ to be examined and its vibrations are listened to through a stethoscope placed over the same organ.

pho•no•car•di•o•gram (fo″no-kahr′de-o-gram) [*phono-* + *cardiogram*] the graphic record produced by phonocardiography.

pho•no•car•dio•graph (fo″no-kahr′de-o-graf) [*phono-* + *cardiograph*] the instrument used in phonocardiography, generally comprising a microphone, amplifier, filters, and a recording device.

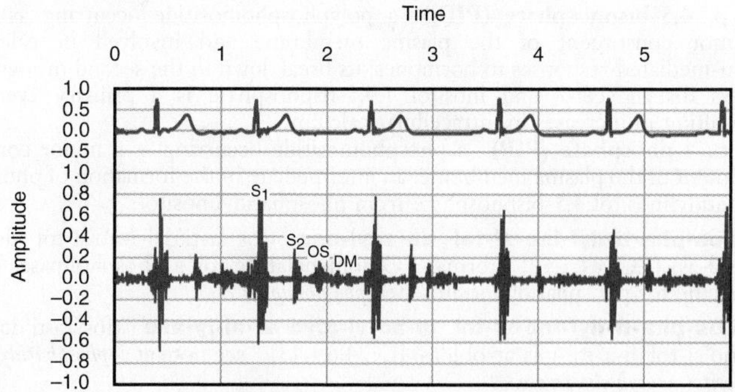

■ Phonocardiogram recorded at the apex in a young adult with rheumatic mitral stenosis. In diastole, there is an opening snap *(OS)* and a diastolic murmur *(DM)* that has presystolic accentuation. *(S_1)*, First heart sound; *(S_2)*, second heart sound.

fetal p. an instrument which provides continuous, instantaneous recording of fetal heart sounds.

pho•no•car•dio•graph•ic (fo″no-kahr″de-o-graf′ik) pertaining to phonocardiography or to a phonocardiogram.

pho•no•car•di•og•ra•phy (fo″no-kahr″de-og′rə-fe) [*phono-* + *cardiography*] the graphic representation of heart sounds, murmurs, or any acoustic phenomena emanating from the heart; in clinical use, the term usually includes recording of the pulse tracings (carotid, apex, and jugular venous) for completeness, and is often combined with other noninvasive methods such as echocardiography.

intracardiac p. the graphic registration of sounds produced by action of the heart by means of a phonocatheter passed into one of the heart chambers.

pho•no•cath•e•ter (fo″no-kath′ə-tər) a device similar in appearance to a conventional catheter, with a microphone at the tip; used in recording the sounds of the heart and great vessels.

pho•no•cath•e•ter•i•za•tion (fo″no-kath″ə-tər-ĭ-za′shən) the use of a phonocatheter for the detection of sounds produced by the circulatory system.

intracardiac p. the passage of a phonocatheter into a chamber of the heart, for the detection of sounds as an aid in diagnosis of cardiac defects.

pho•no•gram (fo′no-gram) [*phono-* + *-gram*] a graphic record of a sound, as of a heart sound.

pho•nol•o•gy (fə-nol′ə-je) [*phono-* + *-logy*] phonetics.

pho•no•mi•cro•sur•gery (fo″no-mi′kro-sur″jər-e) resection of lesions of the vocal folds using an operating microscope introduced through a laryngoscope, done in order to restore or improve the voice.

pho•no•my•oc•lo•nus (fo″no-mi-ok′lə-nəs) myoclonus in which a sound is heard on auscultation of an affected muscle, indicating fibrillar contractions.

pho•no•myo•gram (fo″no-mi′o-gram) [*phono-* + *myo-* + *-gram*] a tracing of the sound produced by muscle action.

pho•no•my•og•ra•phy (fo″no-mi-og′rə-fe) the recording of muscle sounds by an oscillograph to which the sounds are transmitted by a microphone placed over the muscle.

pho•no•pho•bia (fo″no-fo′be-ə) [*phono-* + *-phobia*] irrational fear of sounds or of speaking aloud.

pho•no•pho•re•sis (fo″no-fo-re′sis) the transdermal introduction of a topical agent into the body using mechanical energy supplied by ultrasound.

pho•nop•sia (fo-nop′se-ə) [*phon-* + *-opsia*] a type of photism consisting of a sensation of seeing colors when sounds are heard.

pho•no•scope (fo′no-skōp) [*phono-* + *scope*] an instrument for auscultatory percussion.

pho•nos•co•py (fo-nos′kə-pe) 1. the delimiting of solid and hollow organs (liver, heart, lungs, etc.) by listening with a stethoscope while percussion is made in the vicinity. 2. the use of the phonoscope.

pho•no•se•lec•to•scope (fo″no-sə-lek′tə-skōp) [*phono-* + *select* + *-scope*] an instrument for auscultation by means of which the lower (normal) range of the pulmonary sounds are eliminated, thus emphasizing the higher-pitched pathologic elements.

pho•no•stetho•graph (fo″no-steth′o-graf) an instrument by which the chest sounds are amplified, filtered, and recorded.

pho•no•sur•gery (fo′no-sur″jər-e) a group of surgical procedures whose purpose is to restore, maintain, or enhance the voice.

laryngoplastic p. phonosurgery that restructures the cartilaginous framework of the larynx.

pho•no•trau•ma (fo″no-traw′mə, -trou′mə) damage to the mucosa of the vocal folds caused by abuse or overuse of the voice.

phor•bol (for′bol) a polycyclic alcohol occurring naturally in croton oil; it is the parent compound of the phorbol esters.

p. ester any of several esters of phorbol that are potent cocarcinogens; they are structurally similar to diacylglycerol and can activate protein kinase C. They are used frequently in research to enhance the induction of mutagenesis or tumors by carcinogens.

-phore [Gr. *phoros* carrying] a word termination denoting a carrier of the object designated by the stem to which it is affixed, as a melanophore.

-phoresis [Gr. *phorēsis* a being carried] a word termination indicating transmission, as electrophoresis.

pho•ria (for′e-ə) heterophoria.

pho•ria•scope (for′e-ə-skōp) [*phoria* + *-scope*] a prism-refracting instrument for use in orthoptic training.

Phor•mia (for′me-ə) the blackbottle flies, a genus of blue, black, or green flies of the family Calliphoridae.

P. regi'na a blowfly which causes a cutaneous myiasis of sheep in the United States and Canada. The larvae (maggots) have also been introduced into infected wounds to facilitate healing.

pho•rom•e•ter (fə-rom'ə-tər) [Gr. *phora* movement, range + *-meter*] 1. an instrument to test oculomotor balance. 2. a phoro-optometer.

pho•rom•e•try (fə-rom'ə-tre) use of the phorometer.

pho•ront (for'ont) [Gr. *phora* producing + *ontos* being] the encysted stage or form in the life cycle of certain ciliate protozoa, produced by a tomite and developing into a trophont.

pho•ro-op•tom•e•ter (for″o-op-tom'ə-tər) [Gr. *phora* movement, range + *opto-* + *-meter*] an instrument to test ocular ductions, phorias, refractions, and vergences.

phor•op•ter (for-op'tər) an instrument for evaluation of vision, with lenses placed on dials in a unit that is positioned in front of the patient.

Pho•rop•tor (fo-rop'tor) trademark for a phorometer fitted with a battery of cylindrical lenses.

pho•ro•scope (for'o-skōp) [Gr. *phora* movement, range + *-scope*] a fixed trial frame for eye testing, with a head rest that may be fastened to the table or the wall.

pho•ro•tone (for'o-tōn) [Gr. *phora* movement, range + *tonos* tension] an instrument for exercising the muscles of the eye.

pho•ro•zo•on (for″o-zo'on) [Gr. *phoros* fruitful + *zōon* animal] the asexual stage in the life history of an organism.

phose (fōz) [Gr. *phōs* light] any subjective visual sensation, as of light or color; see *aphose*, *centraphose*, *centrophose*, *chromophose*, *peripheraphose*, *peripherophose*, etc.

phos•gene (fos'jēn) carbonic dichloride, CCl_2O; a highly toxic, colorless gas that causes rapidly fatal pulmonary edema or pneumonia on inhalation; used in the synthesis of a number of organic compounds and formerly used as a war gas.

pho•sis (fo'sis) the production of a phose.

Phos•Lo (foz-lo') trademark for a preparation of calcium acetate.

phos•pha•can (fos'fə-kan) a chondroitin sulfate proteoglycan found in the central nervous system associated with neurons and neural cell adhesion molecules; it is involved in neural-glial interactions associated with nerve differentiation, and the amount increases when there is damage to an axon or spinal cord injury.

phos•pha•gen (fos'fə-jən) any of a group of high energy compounds that are substituted derivatives of phosphoguanidine; they act as reservoirs of phosphate bond energy, donating phosphoryl groups to phosphorylate ADP when ATP levels are low. Phosphocreatine is the phosphagen of vertebrates.

phos•pha•gen•ic (fos″fə-jen'ik) producing or forming phosphate.

phos•pha•tase (fos'fə-tās) a term used in the recommended names of some enzymes of the hydrolase class that are phosphoric monoester hydrolases [EC 3.1.3], catalyzing the release of inorganic phosphate from phosphoric esters. See also *acid phosphatase* and *alkaline phosphatase.*

phos•phate (fos'fāt) [L. *phosphas*] 1. any salt of phosphoric acid or its anions, particularly referring to orthophosphate (inorganic phosphate). 2. any ester of phosphoric acid or of one of its salts or anions; an organic phosphate (q.v.). For specific salts, see entries under the adjectival form, e.g., for *carbamoyl phosphate*, see under *carbamoyl.*

acid p. any phosphate in which only one or two of the three replaceable hydrogen atoms are taken up or replaced.

alkaline p. a phosphate of an alkaline metal, as sodium or potassium.

earthy p. a phosphate of one of the alkaline earth metals.

energy rich p. high-energy p.

high-energy p. an ester, amide, or anhydride of phosphoric acid that contains a high energy phosphate bond (q.v.), e.g., ATP or phosphocreatine.

inorganic p. a salt of phosphoric acid or of any of its anions, usually orthophosphate.

normal p. any phosphate in which all the replaceable hydrogen atoms in phosphoric acid are replaced.

organic p. any ester of phosphoric acid with an organic alcohol, e.g., phospholipids, phosphoproteins, nucleotides, nucleic acids, sugar phosphates, and many small phosphorylated molecules involved in intermediary metabolism.

triple p. a calcium, ammonium, and magnesium phosphate, sometimes found in the urine. See also *struvite.*

phos•phat•ed (fos'fāt-əd) containing phosphates.

phos•pha•te•mia (fos″fə-te'me-ə) hyperphosphatemia.

phos•phates (fos'fāts) any of various combinations of phosphate-containing compounds used as a pharmaceutical source of ionic phosphorous; administered orally or intravenously.

potassium p. 1. [USP] a combination of monobasic and dibasic potassium phosphates used as an electrolyte replenisher. 2. more generally, any potassium-containing source of phosphorus, which includes not only the combination of monobasic and dibasic potassium phosphates but also monobasic potassium phosphate used alone, which is used as an electrolyte replenisher, antiurolithic, and urinary acidifier.

potassium and sodium p. any of various preparations containing both sodium and potassium phosphate in some combination of the monobasic and dibasic salts of each; used as an electrolyte replenisher, urinary acidifier, and antiurolithic.

sodium p. [USP] a combination of monobasic and dibasic sodium phosphates used as an electrolyte replenisher.

phos•phat•ic (fos-fat'ik) pertaining to or containing phosphates.

phos•pha•ti•date (fos″fə-ti'dāt) 1. the anionic form of phosphatidic acid. 2. any of the group of phospholipids derived from phosphatidic acid.

phos•pha•ti•date cy•ti•dyl•yl•trans•fer•ase (fos″fə-ti'dāt si″tĭ-dil″əl-trans'fər-ās) [EC 2.7.7.41] an enzyme of the transferase class that catalyzes the synthesis of CDPdiacylglycerol from CTP and a phosphatidate as a step in the cycle of degradation and resynthesis of phosphoinositides.

phos•pha•ti•date phos•pha•tase (fos″fə-ti'dāt fos'fə-tās) [EC 3.1.3.4] an enzyme of the hydrolase class that catalyzes the cleavage of a phosphate group from a phosphatidate to form a diglyceride; the reaction is a step in the synthesis of triglycerides.

phos•pha•tide (fos'fə-tīd) a phospholipid (q.v.), particularly one derived from phosphatidic acid. The term is sometimes used as a synonym of phosphoglyceride.

phos•pha•ti•dic ac•id (fos″fə-ti'dik) glycerol esterified with long-chain fatty acyl groups at C1 and C2 and phosphorylated at C3; it is the simplest phosphoglyceride (q.v.), the parent compound of most important membrane phospholipids, and a key intermediate in the biosynthesis and degradation of many phosphoglycerides.

phos•pha•ti•dyl (fos″fə-ti'dəl) a term denoting a compound containing a phosphatidic acid group; used also as a prefix to denote such a compound.

phos•pha•ti•dyl•cho•line (PC) (fos″fə-ti″dəl-ko'lēn) a phospholipid in which choline is attached to the phosphate group of phosphatidic acid by an ester linkage; it is a major component of cell membranes and is localized preferentially in the outer surface of the plasma membrane. Called also *lecithin.*

phos•pha•ti•dyl•cho•line–ster•ol *O*-ac•yl•trans•fer•ase (fos″fə-ti″dəl-ko'lēn ster'ol a″səl-trans'fər-ās) [EC 2.3.1.43] an enzyme of the transferase class, secreted by the liver, that catalyzes the formation of cholesteryl esters in high-density lipoproteins by transferring long-chain fatty acid residues from phosphatidylcholine to a sterol. The reaction is a step in the synthesis of lipoproteins. Deficiency of the enzyme, an autosomal recessive trait, is called lecithin–cholesterol acyltransferase (LCAT) deficiency. Called also *lecithin–cholesterol acyltransferase.*

phos•pha•ti•dyl•eth•a•nol•amine (PE) (fos″fə-ti″dəl-eth″ə-nol'ə-mēn) a phospholipid in which ethanolamine is attached to the phosphate group of phosphatidic acid by an ester linkage; it is a major constituent of cell membranes and is localized preferentially in the inner surface of the plasma membrane.

phos•pha•ti•dyl•ino•si•tol (PI) (fos″fə-ti″dəl-ĭ-no'sĭ-tol) a phospholipid in which the sugar inositol is attached to the phosphate group of phosphatidic acid by an ester linkage and the fatty acyl groups are usually arachidonate and stearate; additional phosphates can be attached to the sugar. It is a minor constituent of cell membranes found primarily in the plasma membrane. It is converted by specific kinases to mono- and diphosphorylated forms, phosphoinositides involved in hormonally activated calcium mobilization.

p. 4,5-bisphosphate (PIP_2) a polyphosphoinositide occurring as a minor constituent of the plasma membrane and involved in calcium-mediated responses to hormones; its breakdown to the second messengers diacylglycerol and inositol 1,4,5-triphosphate is a primary event resulting in increases in intracellular calcium.

p. 4-phosphate (PIP) a phosphoinositide occurring as a minor constituent of the plasma membrane; an intermediate in the formation of phosphatidylinositol 4,5-bisphosphate from phosphatidylinositol.

phos•pha•ti•dyl•ino•si•tol de•acyl•ase (fos″fə-ti'dəl-ĭ-no'sĭ-tol de-a'səl-ās) [EC 3.1.1.52] formal EC nomenclature for a phospholipase A_2 specific for phosphatidylinositol. See *phospholipase A_2.*

phos•pha•ti•dyl•ino•si•tol di•ac•yl•glyc•er•ol•ly•ase (fos″fə-ti'dəl-ĭ-no'sĭ-tol di-a″səl-glis'ər-ol li'ās) [EC 4.6.1.13] see note at *1-phosphatidylinositol phosphodiesterase.*

1-phos•pha•ti•dyl•ino•si•tol phos•pho•di•es•ter•ase (fos″fə-ti″dəl-ĭ-no'sĭ-tol fos″fo-di-es'tər-ās) former official nomenclature for a phospholipase C specific for phosphoinositides, catalyzing the cleavage of a diacylglycerol residue from 1-phosphatidylinositol. It is part of a mechanism for mobilization of calcium in response to hormones; it is activated by hormonal binding via a G protein and begins the cycle of phosphoinositide metabolism. It can also play a role in the liberation of arachidonic acid from phosphatidylinositol. NOTE: While this enzyme has officially been renamed *phosphatidylinositol diacylglycerol-lyase* [EC 4.6.1.13], that name and number cover only the bacterial enzyme. The enzyme activity in animals has been determined instead to be part of the activity of the enzyme *phosphoinositide phospholipase C* (q.v.).

phos•pha•ti•dyl•ser•ine (fos″fə-ti″dəl-ser′ēn) a phospholipid in which serine is attached to the phosphate group of phosphatidic acid by an ester linkage; it is an important constituent of cell membranes and is localized preferentially in the inner surface of the plasma membrane. Abbreviated PS.

phos•pha•to•nin (fos″fə-to′nin) any of a group of circulating factors that promote phosphaturia and may play a role in regulating renal tubular phosphate reabsorption. Overexpression results in hyperphosphaturia and hypophosphatemia.

phos•pha•tu•ria (fos″fə-tu′re-ə) 1. excretion of phosphates in the urine; called also *phosphuria.* 2. hyperphosphaturia.

phos•phene (fos′fēn) [Gr. *phōs* light + *phainein* to show] an objective visual sensation that appears with the eyes closed and in the absence of visual light.

accommodation p. the streak of light surrounding the visual field seen in the dark after accommodation.

phos•phide (fos′fīd) any binary compound of phosphorus and another element or radical.

phos•phine (fos′fēn) 1. hydrogen phosphide, PH_3; a toxic malodorous gas and radical. 2. any of a group of organic compounds derived from this; they are similar to amines but are weaker bases. 3. coal tar dye extremely destructive to infusorial life; it is used as a stain. Called also *Philadelphia yellow.*

phos•phite (fos′fīt) any salt of phosphorous acid.

Phos•pho•col P 32 (fos′fo-kol) trademark for a preparation of chromic phosphate P 32.

phos•pho•cre•a•tine (PC) (fos″fo-kre′ə-tin) the phosphagen of vertebrates, a substituted derivative of phosphoguanidine. It is an important storage form of high-energy phosphate, the energy source for muscle contraction; as ATP levels diminish with muscular exertion, the phosphoryl group of phosphocreatine can be donated to ADP to replenish ATP.

phos•pho•di•es•ter (fos″fo-di-es′tər) a diester of phosphoric acid.

phos•pho•di•es•ter•ase (fos″fo-di-es′tər-ās) a term used in the recommended names of some phosphoric diester hydrolases [EC 3.1.4] of the hydrolase class that catalyze the hydrolysis of one of the two ester linkages in a phosphodiester compound.

phos•pho•*enol*•py•ru•vate (fos″fo-e″nol-pi′roo-vāt) a high-energy compound that is a phosphorylated ester of the enol form of pyruvate; it is an intermediate in the Embden-Meyerhof pathway of glucose metabolism, in gluconeogenesis, and in the synthesis of some amino acids. Abbreviated PEP.

phos•pho•*enol*•py•ru•vate car•boxy•ki•nase (GTP) (fos″fo-e″nol-pi′roo-vāt kahr-bok″se-ki′nās) [EC 4.1.1.32] an enzyme of the lyase class that catalyzes the decarboxylation and phosphorylation of oxaloacetate to form phospho*enol*pyruvate, using GTP as a phosphate donor. The enzyme occurs in both the mitochondria and cytosol of mammalian liver, and the reaction is part of the mechanism of gluconeogenesis. Deficiency of the enzyme in mitochondria or cytosol, an autosomal recessive trait, causes infant hypoglycemia. Called also *phosphopyruvate carboxykinase.*

phos•pho•eth•a•nol•amine (fos″fo-eth″ə-nol′ə-mēn) an intermediate in the biosynthesis of phosphatidylethanolamine; elevated levels are excreted in the urine in a number of conditions, including hypophosphatasia, pseudohypophosphatasia, and metabolic bone disease.

phos•pho•fruc•to•al•do•lase (fos″fo-frook″to-al′do-lās) fructose bisphosphate aldolase.

phos•pho•fruc•to•ki•nase 1 (fos″fo-frook″to-ki′nās) 6-phosphofructokinase.

phos•pho•fruc•to•ki•nase 2 (fos″fo-frook″to-ki′nās) 6-phosphofructo-2-kinase.

6-phos•pho•fruc•to•ki•nase (fos″fo-frook″to-ki′nās) [EC 2.7.1.11] an enzyme of the transferase class that catalyzes the phosphorylation of fructose 6-phosphate by ATP to form fructose 1,6-bisphosphate. The reaction is essentially irreversible and is a committed step and a key site of regulation in the Embden-Meyerhof pathway of glucose metabolism. Numerous isozymes occur; deficiency of the muscle isoenzyme, an autosomal recessive trait, is the cause of glycogen storage disease, type VII. Called also *phosphofructokinase 1.*

6-phos•pho•fruc•to-2-ki•nase (fos″fo-frook″to-ki′nās) [EC 2.7.1.105] an enzyme activity that catalyzes the phosphorylation of fructose 6-phosphate by ATP to form fructose 2,6-bisphosphate; it occurs on the same polypeptide as the enzyme activity fructose-2,6-bisphosphate 2-phosphatase (q.v.). In liver, the two activities form part of a mechanism for regulating carbohydrate metabolism. The liver enzyme activity is inhibited via phosphorylation by cyclic-AMP–dependent protein kinase, thus diminishing the rate of formation of fructose 2,6-bisphosphate and slowing glycolysis. Called also *phosphofructokinase 2.*

phos•pho•glob•u•lin (fos″fo-glob′u-lin) a phosphoprotein with globulin as the protein moiety.

phos•pho•glu•co•ki•nase (fos″fo-gloo″ko-ki′nās) [EC 2.7.1.10] an enzyme of the transferase class that catalyzes the phosphorylation of glucose 1-phosphate glucose 1,6-bisphosphate. The reaction product is a necessary intermediate in the phosphoglucomutase reaction.

phos•pho•glu•co•mu•tase (fos″fo-gloo″ko-mu′tās) [EC 5.4.2.2] an enzyme of the isomerase class requiring the presence of the intermediate glucose 1,6-bisphosphate to catalyze the interconversion of glucose 1-phosphate and glucose 6-phosphate, a step in the formation and utilization of glycogen. It also catalyzes the interconversion of the 1-phosphate and 5-phosphate isomers of ribose.

6-phos•pho•glu•co•nate (fos″fo-gloo′kə-nāt) gluconate, the hexonic acid derivative of glucose, phosphorylated at the 6 carbon; it is an intermediate in the pentose phosphate pathway.

phos•pho•glu•co•nate de•hy•dro•gen•ase (de•car•box•y•lat•ing) (fos″fo-gloo′kə-nāt de-hi′dro-jən-ās de″kahr-bok′sə-lāt-ing) [EC 1.1.1.44] an enzyme of the oxidoreductase class that catalyzes the oxidative decarboxylation of 6-phosphogluconate to form ribulose 5-phosphate, reducing $NADP^+$ to NADPH. The reaction is a step in the pentose phosphate pathway of glucose metabolism.

6-phos•pho•glu•co•no•lac•ton•ase (fos″fo-gloo″kə-no-lak′tə-nās) [EC 3.1.1.31] an enzyme of the hydrolase class that catalyzes the formation of 6-phosphogluconate from the corresponding lactone as a step in the pentose phosphate pathway.

phos•pho•glu•cose isom•er•ase (fos″fo-gloo′kōs i-som′ər-ās) glucose-6-phosphate isomerase.

3-phos•pho•glyc•er•al•de•hyde (fos″fo-glis″ər-al′də-hīd) a triose phosphate which results from the splitting of fructose 1,6-diphosphate in muscle metabolism.

phos•pho•glyc•er•ate (fos″fo-glis′ər-āt) an anionic form of phosphoglyceric acid; the 2- and 3-phosphate forms, 2-phosphoglycerate and 3-phosphoglycerate, are enzymatically interconvertible intermediates in the Embden-Meyerhof pathway (q.v.) of glucose metabolism.

phos•pho•glyc•er•ate ki•nase (fos″fo-glis′ər-āt ki′nās) [EC 2.7.2.3] an enzyme of the transferase class that catalyzes the ATP-dependent phosphorylation of 3-phosphoglycerate to form 1,3-bisphosphoglycerate. The reaction is an important energy-transducing step in carbohydrate metabolism. As written, the reaction drives gluconeogenesis; the reverse reaction generates ATP in the catabolism of glucose (see illustration at *Embden-Meyerhof pathway,* under *pathway*). Deficiency of the enzyme, an X-linked trait, causes hemolytic anemia, mental retardation, and behavioral and neurologic abnormalities.

phos•pho•glyc•er•ate mu•tase (fos″fo-glis′ər-āt mu′tās) [EC 5.4.2.1] an enzyme of the isomerase class that catalyzes the interconversion of 3-phosphoglycerate and 2-phosphoglycerate, a step in the Embden-Meyerhof pathway (see illustration under *pathway*). The enzyme requires the presence of a small amount of 2,3-bisphosphoglycerate, which is also an intermediate. Called also *phosphoglyceromutase.*

phos•pho•gly•cer•ic ac•id (fos″fo-glĭ-ser′ik) a phosphate ester of glyceric acid.

phos•pho•glyc•er•ide (fos″fo-glis′ər-īd) a phospholipid in which the phosphate group of a phosphatidic acid is joined in ester linkage to an alcohol moiety, commonly choline, ethanolamine, glycerol, inositol, or serine, forming the corresponding phosphatidyl compound. The phosphoglycerides are a major component of cell membranes.

phos•pho•glyc•ero•mu•tase (fos″fo-glis″ər-o-mu′tās) phosphoglycerate mutase.

phos•pho•gly•co•pro•tein (fos″fo-gli″ko-pro′tēn) a phosphorus-containing glycoprotein.

phos•pho•guan•i•dine (fos″fo-gwahn′ĭ-dēn) 1. phosphorylated guanidine, a high energy compound. 2. a term sometimes used to denote one of the phosphagens because these compounds are substituted derivatives of phosphoguanidine.

phos•pho•hex•ose isom•er•ase (fos″fo-hek″sōs i-som′ər-ās) glucose-6-phosphate isomerase.

phos•pho•ino•si•tide (fos″fo-in-o′sĭ-tīd) any of a number of phosphorylated inositol-containing compounds that play roles in cell activation and calcium mobilization in response to hormones.

phos•pho•ino•si•tide phos•pho•lip•ase C (fos″fo-in-o′sĭ-tīd fos″fo-lip′ās) [EC 3.1.4.11] an enzyme of the hydrolase class that catalyzes the hydrolysis of phosphatidylinositol-4,5-bisphosphate to generate inositol 1,4,5-triphosphate and diacylglycerol, second messengers that initiate a cascade of intracellular responses resulting in cell growth and differentiation and gene expression. The enzyme can also act on phosphatidylinositol, carrying out the reaction formerly ascribed to the enzyme officially called *1-phosphatidylinositol phosphodiesterase* (q.v.). See also *phospholipase C.*

phos•pho•lam•ban (fos″fo-lam′ban) a 22-kilodalton membrane-bound polypeptide of the sarcoplasmic reticulum that stimulates cardiac relaxation; upon phosphorylation by a cyclic AMP–dependent protein kinase, it activates the calcium pump, stimulating the uptake and storage of calcium by the sarcoplasmic reticulum and resulting in relaxation of cardiac muscle.

Phos•pho•line Io•dide (fos′fo-lēn) trademark for a preparation of echothiophate iodide.

phos•pho•lip•ase (fos″fo-lip′ās) any of a number of enzymes that catalyze the hydrolysis of specific ester bonds in phospholipids. Individual enzymes are grouped on the basis of the bond they hydrolyze and are further categorized as carboxylic acid esterases (p. A_1, p. A_2) or phosphodiesterases (p. C, p. D).

p. A_1 [EC 3.1.1.32] any esterase that catalyzes the hydrolysis of the terminal acyl group from a phospholipid, generating a free fatty acid and a lysophospholipid. The enzyme occurs in various forms in all mammalian tissues, particularly the liver and pancreas, and in bee and snake venoms.

p. A_2 [EC 3.1.1.4] any esterase that catalyzes the hydrolysis of the central acyl group from a membrane phospholipid, generating a free fatty acid and a lysophospholipid; this reaction is important in the digestion of dietary phospholipids, and it liberates arachidonic acid for a variety of processes, such as platelet activation. The enzyme occurs in various forms in all mammalian tissues and in snake and bee venoms. EC nomenclature for the enzyme specifically hydrolyzing phosphatidylinositol is *phosphatidylinositol deacylase.*

p. C [EC 3.1.4.3] any esterase that catalyzes the hydrolysis of the phosphoric ester bond of a membrane phospholipid, generating a phosphorylated alcohol and diacylglycerol. Important in the digestion of dietary phospholipids and in various processes dependent on hormonally induced calcium mobilization or arachidonic acid production, they occur in all mammalian tissues and as toxic secretion products of pathogenic bacteria. See also *phosphoinositide phospholipase C.*

p. D [EC 3.1.4.4] any esterase that catalyzes the hydrolysis of the alcohol group from a phospholipid, generating the corresponding phosphatidate. It occurs in various forms, predominantly in plants, but in humans it may be part of a mechanism to generate diacylglycerol for the mobilization of calcium in response to hormones.

phos•pho•lip•id (fos″fo-lip′id) any lipid that contains phosphorus, including those with a glycerol backbone (phosphoglycerides and plasmalogens) or a backbone of sphingosine or related substance (sphingomyelins). Phospholipids are the major form of lipid in all cell membranes.

phos•pho•lip•i•de•mia (fos″fo-lip″ĭ-de′me-ə) the presence of phospholipids in the blood.

phos•pho•lip•i•do•sis (fos″fo-lip″ĭ-do′sis) a type of lipidosis in which phospholipids accumulate in cells and tissues, usually as a result of a reaction with a cationic, amphibolic drug; the precise etiology is unknown.

phos•pho•man•no•mu•tase (fos″fo-man″o-mu′tās) [EC 5.4.2.8] an enzyme of the isomerase class that catalyzes the interconversion of mannose 6-phosphate and mannose 1-phosphate.

phos•pho•man•nose isom•er•ase (fos″fo-man′ōs i-som′ər-ās) mannose-6-phosphate isomerase.

phos•pho•mo•lyb•dic ac•id (fos″fo-mo-lib′dik) a strong acid and oxidizing agent used as a protein precipitant and color reagent; alkaloids, xanthine, uric acid, and other substances reduce phosphomolybdic acid to molybdenum blue. It is also used in histology as a mordant.

phos•pho•mono•es•ter (fos″fo-mon″o-es′tər) a monoester in which phosphate is the ester group.

phos•pho•mono•es•ter•ase (fos″fo-mon″o-es′tər-ās) any of a group of enzymes that act as phosphatases on phosphomonoester substrates; however, the term is usually used to denote acid phosphatase or alkaline phosphatase specifically.

phos•pho•mu•tase (fos″fo-mu′tās) any of the phosphotransferases of the isomerase class, which catalyze the intramolecular transfer of a phosphate group.

phos•pho•nate (fos′fo-nāt) a salt, anion, or ester of phosphonic acid.

phos•pho•ne•cro•sis (fos″fo-nə-kro′sis) phosphorus necrosis.

phos•phon•ic ac•id (fos-fon′ik) the compound $HPO(OH)_2$, or substituted derivatives of the form RPO_3H_2.

phos•pho•ni•um (fos-fo′ne-əm) the univalent radical PH_4^+, forming compounds analogous to those of ammonium.

phos•pho•pe•nia (fos″fo-pe′ne-ə) [*phosphorus* + *-penia*] deficiency of phosphorus in the body; cf. *hypophosphatemia.*

phos•pho•pro•tein (fos″fo-pro′tēn) a protein to which one or more phosphate groups are attached at serine or threonine (rarely tyrosine) residues.

phos•pho•pro•tein phos•pha•tase (fos″fo-pro′tēn fos′fə-tās) [EC 3.1.3.16] an enzyme of the hydrolase class that catalyzes the cleavage of phosphoryl groups from phosphoproteins. Enzymes with this activity are involved in digestion and in the regulation of a variety of enzymes undergoing phosphorylation-dephosphorylation cycles. Called also *protein phosphatase.*

p. p. 1 protein phosphatase 1.

phos•pho•py•ru•vate car•boxy•ki•nase (fos″fo-pi′roo-vāt kahr-bok″se-ki′nās) phospho*enol*pyruvate carboxykinase (GTP).

phos•pho•py•ru•vate hy•dra•tase (fos″fo-pi′roo-vāt hi′drə-tās) [EC 4.2.1.11] an enzyme of the lyase class that catalyzes the dehydration of 2-phosphoglycerate to form phospho*enol*pyruvate, a part of the Embden-Meyerhof pathway of glucose catabolism (see illustration under *pathway*). Called also *enolase.*

phos•pho•rat•ed (fos′fə-rāt″əd) charged or combined with phosphorus.

phos•pho•res•cence (fos″fə-res′əns) the emission of light without appreciable heat; it is characterized by the emission of absorbed light after a delay and at a considerably longer wavelength than that of the absorbed light. Cf. *fluorescence.* **phosphores′cent** *adj*

phos•pho•ri•bo•isom•er•ase (fos″fo-ri″bo-i-som′ər-ās) ribose-5-phosphate isomerase.

phos•pho•ri•bo•syl•amine (fos″fo-ri″bo-sil′ə-mēn) an intermediate product in the synthesis of purines formed from phosphoribosylpyrophosphate and glutamine; excessive production is often a factor in primary gout.

phos•pho•ri•bo•syl•py•ro•phos•phate (PRPP) (fos″fo-ri″bo-səl-pi″ro-fos′fāt) an intermediate in the formation of purines and of purine and pyrimidine nucleotides.

phos•pho•ri•bo•syl•py•ro•phos•phate syn•the•tase (fos″fo-ri″bo-səl-pi″ro-fos′fāt sin′thə-tās) ribose-phosphate pyrophosphokinase.

phos•pho•ri•bo•syl•trans•fer•ase (fos″fo-ri″bo-səl-trans′fər-ās) a term used in the recommended and trivial names of some pentosyltransferases [EC 2.4.2] to denote those that catalyze the transfer of ribose 5-phosphate, usually from phosphoribosylpyrophosphate, to a purine or pyrimidine to form a 5′ nucleotide and inorganic pyrophosphate. These enzymes are important in the biosynthesis of nucleotides.

phos•phor•ic ac•id (fos-for′ik) 1. orthophosphoric acid, the monomeric form H_3PO_4. 2. a general term encompassing the monomeric (orthophosphoric acid), dimeric (pyrophosphoric acid), and polymeric (metaphosphoric acid) forms of the acid. Phosphoric acid is an important metabolite; see *phosphate* and specific acids and salts.

p. a., diluted [NF] a preparation of phosphoric acid in purified water, containing 9.5–10.5 g phosphoric acid per mL; it is used as a solvent in pharmaceutical preparations and orally as a gastric acidifier.

p. a., glacial metaphosphoric acid.

phos•pho•rism (fos′fə-riz″əm) chronic phosphorus poisoning; see under *poisoning.*

phos•pho•rized (fos′fə-rīzd) containing phosphorus.

phos•pho•rol•y•sis (fos″fə-rol′ĭ-sis) cleavage of a chemical bond with simultaneous addition of the elements of phosphoric acid to the residues, as in the splitting of the glycosidic bonds of glycogen catalyzed by the enzyme phosphorylase in carbohydrate metabolism. The reaction is analogous to hydrolysis.

phos•phoro•scope (fos′for-ə-skōp) an instrument for measuring phosphorescence.

phos•pho•rous (fos-for′əs) pertaining to or containing phosphorus.

phos•pho•rous ac•id (fos-for′əs) a reducing inorganic acid, H_3PO_3, which readily absorbs oxygen to form phosphoric acid.

phos•phor•pe•nia (fos″for-pe′ne-ə) phosphopenia.

phos•phor•uria (fos″for-u′re-ə) [*phosphorus* + *-uria*] the presence of free phosphorus in the urine.

phos•pho•rus (P) (fos′fə-rəs) [Gr. *phōs* light + *phorein* to carry] a nonmetallic, allotropic element: poisonous and highly inflammable; atomic number, 15; atomic weight, 30.974. It occurs in three forms—*white* (yellow), *red*, and *black*. It is obtainable from bones, urine, and especially minerals, such as apatite. Phosphorus is an essential element in the diet; it is a major component of the mineral phase of bone and is abundant in all tissues, being involved in some form in almost all metabolic processes. Free phosphorus causes a fatty degeneration of the liver and other viscera, and the inhalation of its vapor often leads to necrosis of the lower jaw. It is used in homeopathic medicine.

p. 32 a radioisotope of phosphorus, atomic mass 32, having a half-life of 14.28 days and emitting only beta particles (1.71 MeV); its therapeutic uses include treatment of polycythemia vera, chronic myelocytic leukemia, chronic lymphocytic leukemia, certain ovarian and prostate carcinomas, palliation of metastatic skeletal disease, and treatment of metastatic intrapleural and intraperitoneal effusions.

phos•pho•ryl (fos′fə-rəl) the trivalent chemical radical ≡P:O.

phos•phor•y•lase (fos-for′ə-lās) 1. any of a group of enzymes catalyzing phosphorolysis of glycosides, transferring the cleaved glycosyl group to inorganic phosphate. The term is usually qualified by adding the name of the substrate acted upon; when used alone it usually denotes glycogen phosphorylase (q.v.) in animals or starch phosphorylase in plants. 2. any of a group of transferases that catalyze the transfer of a phosphate group to an organic acceptor.

phos•phor•y•lase ki•nase (fos-for′ə-lās ki′nās) [EC 2.7.11.19] an enzyme of the transferase class that catalyzes the phosphorylation of (inactive) glycogen phosphorylase *b* to form (active) glycogen phosphorylase *a*, a step in the cascade of reactions regulating glycogenolysis. The enzyme is itself activated via phosphorylation by cyclic-AMP–dependent protein kinase. There are liver and muscle isoforms, each of which comprises four subunits, alpha, beta, gamma, and delta, encoded by multiple genes on multiple chromosomes; the alpha and gamma subunits are differentially encoded and expressed in different tissues while the beta remains constant across the isoforms and the delta is calmodulin. Deficiency of the enzyme causes glycogen storage disease, type IX (q.v.), which is divided into subtypes on the basis of which isoform and specific subunit the mutation affects. Written also *phosphorylase* b *kinase.*

[phos•phor•y•lase] phos•pha•tase (fos-for′ə-lās fos′fə-tās″) [EC 3.1.3.17] an enzyme of the hydrolase class that catalyzes the cleavage of a phosphoryl group from (active) glycogen phosphorylase *a* to form (inactive) phosphorylase *b;* the reaction is part of the mechanism of regulation of glycogenolysis. Recently, this enzyme has been considered to be an activity of the more general enzyme *protein phosphatase 1.*

phos•phor•y•la•tion (fos-for″ə-la′shən) the metabolic process of introducing a phosphate group into an organic molecule. **phosphor′ylated** *adj*

oxidative p. the formation of high energy phosphate bonds by phosphorylation of ADP to ATP coupled to the transfer of electrons from reduced coenzymes (NADH or $FADH_2$) to molecular oxygen via the electron transport chain (see illustration under *chain*). Three molecules of ATP per NADH and two per $FADH_2$ are produced as a result of a proton gradient created across the mitochondrial inner membrane by the electron transport chain.

substrate-level p. the formation of high energy phosphate bonds by phosphorylation of ADP to ATP (or GDP to GTP) coupled to cleavage of a high-energy metabolic intermediate, e.g., succinyl CoA in the tricarboxylic acid cycle.

phos•pho•ryl•y•sis (fos″fə-ril′ĭ-sis) phosphorolysis.

phos•pho•sug•ar (fos′fo-shoog″ər) a sugar in which a hydroxyl group has been esterified with a phosphate group.

Phos•pho•tec (fos′fo-tek) trademark for a kit for the preparation of technetium Tc 99m pyrophosphate.

phos•pho•trans•fer•ase (fos″fo-trans′fər-ās) an enzyme that catalyzes the transfer of a phosphate group, either from one molecule to another [EC 2.7.1–4.2.7.9] or within the same molecule [EC 5.4.2].

phos•pho•tri•ose (fos″fo-tri′ōs) triose phosphate.

phos•pho•tung•state (fos″fo-tung′stāt) a salt of phosphotungstic acid.

phos•pho•tung•stic ac•id (fos″fo-tung′stik) a strong acid and oxidizing agent used as a protein precipitant and color reagent; alkaloids, nitrogenous bases, and other substances reduce phosphotungstic acid to tungsten blue. It is also used in histology as a mordant for hematoxylin and other dyes.

phos•pho•vi•tel•lin (fos″fo-vi-tel′in) phosvitin.

phos•phu•re•sis (fos″fu-re′sis) phosphaturia.

phos•phu•ria (fos-fu′re-ə) phosphaturia.

phos•vi•tin (fos-vi′tin) a phosphoprotein isolated from vitellin in egg yolk; called also *phosphovitellin.*

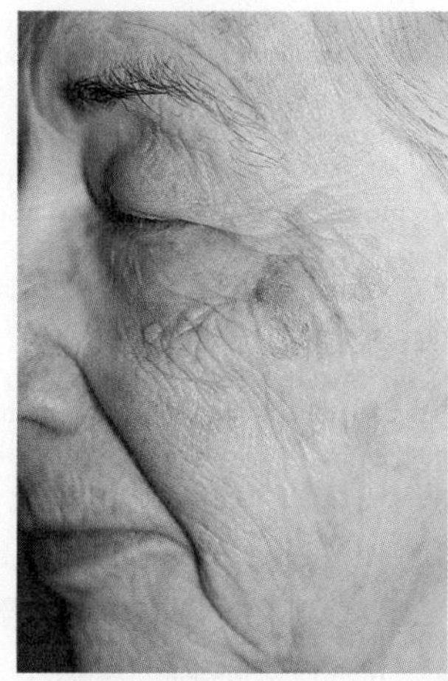

■ Photoaging.

pho•tal•gia (fo-tal′jə) [*phot-* + *-algia*] ocular pain caused by light.

pho•tal•lo•chro•my (fo-tal′ə-kro″me) [*phot-* + *allo-* + *-chrome*] allotropic change with color alteration due to light, as the change of yellow into red phosphorus.

pho•tau•gia•pho•bia (fo-taw″je-ə-fo′be-ə) [Gr. *phōtaugeia* glare + *phobia*] abnormal intolerance of glare.

pho•te•ryth•rous (fo″tə-rith′rəs) deuteranopic.

pho•tes•the•sis (fo″təs-the′sis) [*phot-* + *esthesis*] sensitivity to light.

pho•tic (fo′tik) pertaining to light.

pho•tism (fo′tiz-əm) a synesthesia in which a sensation of color or light is associated with a sensation of hearing, taste, smell, or touch.

phot(o)- [Gr. *phōs*, gen. *phōtos* light] a combining form denoting relationship to light.

pho•to•abla•tion (fo″to-ab-la′shən) volatilization of tissue by ultraviolet rays emitted by a laser.

pho•to•ac•tin•ic (fo″to-ak-tin′ik) giving off both luminous and actinic rays.

pho•to•ac•tive (fo″to-ak′tiv) reacting chemically to sunlight or ultraviolet radiation.

pho•to•ad•ap•ta•tion (fo″to-ad″ap-ta′shən) adaptation by the skin to exposure to ultraviolet radiation, such as erythema or other changes in color; the changes may be either beneficial or harmful.

pho•to•ag•gra•vat•ed (fo″to-ag′rə-vāt″əd) aggravated, though possibly not caused, by exposure to ultraviolet rays, said of skin conditions; see also *photodermatosis.*

pho•to•ag•ing (fo″to-āj′ing) photodamage with premature aging of the skin.

pho•to•al•ler•gen (fo″to-al′ər-jən) an agent that elicits an allergic response to light.

pho•to•al•ler•gy (fo″to-al′ər-je) [*photo-* + *allergy*] a delayed immunologic type of photosensitivity occurring upon exposure to a given chemical substance to which the individual has become previously sensitized. See also *photoallergic contact dermatitis*, under *dermatitis.* Cf. *phototoxicity.* **photoaller′gic** *adj*

pho•to•au•to•troph (fo″to-aw′to-trōf) a photoautotrophic organism.

pho•to•au•to•tro•phic (fo″to-aw″to-tro′fik) requiring for growth only inorganic compounds with carbon dioxide as the sole source of carbon (autotrophic) and deriving energy from photosynthesis; said of algae and certain photosynthetic bacteria.

pho•to•bac•te•ria (fo″to-bak-tēr′e-ə) [*photo-* + *bacteria*] bacteria that derive energy from light by the process of photosynthesis.

Pho•to•bac•te•ri•um (fo″to-bak-tēr′e-əm) [*photo-* + *bacterium*] a genus of halophilic, gram-negative marine bacteria of the family Vibrionaceae, consisting of plump, straight rods that are motile by means of polar flagella; organisms are facultatively anaerobic and chemo-organotrophic, and some are luminescent. The type species is *P. phosphoreum.*

P. dam′selae a nonluminescent species that is a pathogen for marine fish; the subspecies *P. damselae* subsp. *dam′selae* causes wound infections in humans. Formerly called *Vibrio damsela.*

pho•to•bi•ol•o•gy (fo″to-bi-ol′ə-je) [*photo-* + *biology*] a branch of biology that deals with the effect of light on living organisms, including the study of photosynthesis. **photobiolog′ic, photobiolog′ical** *adj*

pho·to·bi·ot·ic (fo″to-bi-ot′ik) [*photo-* + *biotic*] living or thriving only in the light; said of certain organisms such as green plants.

pho·to·ca·tal·y·sis (fo″to-kə-tal′ĭ-sis) the promotion or stimulation of a reaction by light. **photocatalyt′ic** *adj*

pho·to·cat·a·lyst (fo″to-kat′ə-list) a substance by means of which sunlight is utilized, as chlorophyll in the photosynthesis of carbohydrates by green plants.

pho·to·cat·a·lyz·er (fo″to-kat′ə-līz″ər) photocatalyst.

pho·to·cep·tor (fo″to-sep′tər) photoreceptor.

pho·to·chem·i·cal (fo″to-kem′ə-kəl) pertaining to the chemical properties of light; chemically reactive in the presence of light or other radiation.

pho·to·chem·is·try (fo″to-kem′is-tre) [*photo-* + *chemistry*] the branch of chemistry which deals with the chemical properties or effects of light rays or other radiation.

pho·to·che·mo·ther·a·py (fo″to-ke″mo-ther′ə-pe) 1. treatment by means of drugs (such as methoxsalen) that react to ultraviolet radiation or sunlight. 2. photodynamic therapy.

pho·to·chro·mo·gen (fo″to-kro′mə-jən) [*photo-* + *chromo-* + *-gen*] a microorganism whose pigmentation develops as a result of exposure to light, e.g., *Mycobacterium kansasii* (pathogenic for humans), which is yellow-orange if grown in the light, and almost colorless if grown in the dark. See also *nontuberculous mycobacteria*, under *mycobacterium*.

pho·to·chro·mo·ge·nic·i·ty (fo″to-kro″mə-jə-nis′ĭ-te) the property of microorganisms of forming pigment consequent to light exposure; induction occurs within a few minutes in the shorter wavelengths of visible light, pigmentation then occurring within 24 hours if conditions permit continued growth. **photochromogen′ic** *adj*

pho·to·co·ag·u·la·tion (fo″to-ko-ag″u-la′shən) [*photo-* + *coagulation*] condensation of protein material by the controlled use of an intense beam of light (such as from a xenon arc lamp or argon laser); used especially in treatment of retinal detachment and destruction of abnormal retinal vessels, or of intraocular tumor masses.
panretinal p. photocoagulation of almost the entire retina to treat neovascularization, such as in diabetic retinopathy.

pho·to·con·vul·sive (fo″to-kən-vul′siv) photoparoxysmal.

pho·to·cu·ta·ne·ous (fo″to-ku-ta′ne-əs) [*photo-* + *cutaneous*] pertaining to skin conditions in which exposure to light is an important factor, such as photodamage and photodermatosis.

pho·to·dam·age (fo′to-dam″əj) damage to the skin from prolonged exposure to ultraviolet radiation, such as in *actinic dermatitis* and *photoaging*. Called also *dermatoheliosis*.

pho·to·der·ma·ti·tis (fo″to-dur″mə-ti′tis) dermatitis caused by exposure to ultraviolet radiation; see *photoallergic contact dermatitis* and *phototoxic dermatitis*, under *dermatitis*.

pho·to·der·ma·tol·o·gy (fo″to-dur″mə-tol′əje) the study of the effects of light on the skin, including therapeutic effects and pathologic conditions such as photodermatoses.

pho·to·der·ma·to·sis (fo″to-dur″mə-to′sis) any abnormal skin condition caused by a reaction to ultraviolet radiation; cf. *photodamage*.
idiopathic p. any of various types having no known cause, such as chronic actinic dermatitis and polymorphic light eruption.

pho·to·de·tec·tor (fo″to-de-tek′tər) a detector responsive to radiant energy.

pho·to·dis·rup·tion (fo″to-dis-rup′shən) disruption of tissues by laser-produced rapid ionization of molecules.

pho·to·dis·tri·bu·tion (fo″to-dis″trĭ-bu′shən) a pattern of occurrence that corresponds to areas of exposure to the sun or other light, as of skin in photodermatitis.

pho·tod·ro·my (fo-tod′rə-me) [*photo-* + Gr. *dromos* running] the phenomenon of moving toward *(positive p.)* or away from *(negative p.)* light, as in the case of particles in suspension.

pho·to·dy·nam·ic (fo″to-di-nam′ik) [*photo-* + *dynamic*] powerful in the light; used particularly for the action exerted by fluorescent substances in the light.

pho·to·dy·nam·ics (fo″to-di-nam′iks) the science of the activating effects of light on living organisms.

pho·to·dyn·ia (fo″to-din′e-ə) [*photo-* + *-odynia*] photalgia.

pho·to·dys·pho·ria (fo″to-dis-for′e-ə) photophobia.

pho·to·elec·tric (fo″to-e-lek′trik) pertaining to the electric effects of light or other radiation.

pho·to·elec·tron (fo″to-e-lek′tron) an electron emitted from a metallic surface when the latter is illuminated with light, especially with light of short wavelength.

pho·to·er·y·the·ma (fo″to-er″ĭ-the′mə) erythema due to exposure to light.

pho·to·flu·o·ro·gram (fo″to-floor′o-gram) the film produced in photofluorography.

pho·to·flu·o·rog·ra·phy (fo″to-floor-og′rə-fe) the photographic recording of fluoroscopic images on small films, using a fast lens: a procedure used in mass radiography of the chest. Called also *fluororadiography*.

pho·to·flu·o·ro·scope (fo″to-floor′o-skōp) a form of fluoroscope used in making either observations or photographs by means of x-rays.

Pho·to·frin (fo′to-frin) trademark for a preparation of porfimer sodium.

pho·to·gas·tro·scope (fo″to-gas′tro-skōp) [*photo-* + *gastro-* + *-scope*] an apparatus for photographing the interior of the stomach.

pho·to·gen·ic (fo″to-jen′ik) 1. produced by light, as photogenic epilepsy. 2. producing or emitting light; phosphorescent.

pho·to·glot·tog·ra·phy (fo″to-glŏ-tog′rə-fe) glottography using a photoelectric transducer to measure changes in transillumination of the glottis during phonation or respiration.

pho·tog·ra·phy (fo-tog′rə-fe) [*photo-* + *-graphy*] a technique for creating images on sensitized materials by means of light or other radiant energy.
Kirlian p. a photographic technique in which a high-voltage current passed over a subject in contact with photographic film or paper produces an image surrounded by a luminous radiation, or aura, which some claim is a bioenergetic field that can reveal information about the subject's physical health and emotional state.

pho·to·hal·ide (fo″to-hal′īd) any halogen salt that is sensitive to light.

pho·to·he·mo·ta·chom·e·ter (fo″to-he″mo-tə-kom′ə-tər) [*photo-* + *hemo-* + *tacho-* + *-meter*] a device for making a photographic record of the speed of the blood current.

pho·to·het·ero·troph (fo″to-het′ər-o-trōf) a photoheterotrophic organism.

pho·to·het·ero·tro·phic (fo″to-het″ər-o-tro′fik) [*photo-* + *hetero-* + *trophic*] deriving nourishment from organic compounds and energy from visible light.

pho·tohm·ic (fo-to′mik) denoting a change in electric resistance produced by light.

pho·to·in·ac·ti·va·tion (fo″to-in-ak″tĭ-va′shən) inactivation, as of complement, by light.

pho·to·ker·a·tec·to·my (fo″to-ker″ə-tek′tə-me) photorefractive keratectomy.

pho·to·ki·ne·sis (fo″to-kĭ-ne′sis) [*photo-* + *-kinesis*] a change in the rate of motion in response to light, as an increase or decrease in motility of bacteria with a change in illumination. **photokinet′ic** *adj*

pho·to·ky·mo·graph (fo″to-ki′mo-graf) a camera with a moving film for recording movements, as of the string in a string galvanometer; called also a *recording camera*.

pho·to·ky·mog·ra·phy (fo″to-ki-mog′rə-fe) the recording of movements (see *kymography*) with a photokymograph.

pho·tol·o·gy (fo-tol′ə-je) [*photo-* + *-logy*] the branch of physics which treats of light.

pho·to·lu·min·es·cence (fo″to-loo″mĭ-nes′əns) the quality of being luminescent after being exposed to light or other electromagnetic radiation.

pho·tol·y·sis (fo-tol′ĭ-sis) chemical decomposition into simpler units or cleavage of a chemical bond by the action of light or other form of radiant energy. **photolyt′ic** *adj*

pho·to·lyte (fo′to-līt) [*photo-* + Gr. *lyein* to dissolve] any substance decomposable by the action of light.

pho·to·ma (fo-to′mə) a flash of light sparks or color with no objective basis.

pho·to·mag·ne·tism (fo″to-mag′nə-tiz-əm) magnetism induced by the action of light.

pho·to·med·i·cine (fo″to-med′ĭ-sin) the medical specialty dealing with interactions between light and living systems, such as therapeutic uses such as phototherapy and pathologic effects such as photodermatoses.

pho·tom·e·ter (fo-tom′ə-tər) [*photo-* + *-meter*] 1. a device for measuring the intensity of infrared, ultraviolet, or visible light. 2. a device for testing the sensitivity of the eye to light by determining the light minimum.
flame p. a photometer that analyzes the light emitted by a substance in a flame; commonly used for determination of sodium, potassium, lithium, and calcium in biological materials.
flicker p. a photometer in which the frequency of a flickering light can be controlled, formerly used for vision testing. See *flicker*.
Förster p. photoptometer.

pho·tom·e·try (fo-tom′ə-tre) [*photo-* + *-metry*] the measurement of light.

flicker p. see *flicker*.

pho·to·mi·cro·graph (fo″to-mi′kro-graf) [*photo-* + *micro-* + *-graph*] the photograph of a minute object as seen under the light microscope, produced by ordinary photographic methods. Cf. *microphotograph*.

pho·to·mi·crog·ra·phy (fo″to-mi-krog′rə-fe) the production of photomicrographs.

pho·to·mi·cro·scope (fo″to-mi′kro-skōp) a microscope and camera combined for making photomicrographs.

pho·to·mi·cros·co·py (fo″to-mi-kros′kə-pe) photography of enlarged pictures of minute objects with the photomicroscope.

pho·to·mor·pho·gen·e·sis (fo″to-mor″fo-jen′ə-sis) the regulation of form by light, as in the induction of flowering in plants by a minimal period of daylight.

pho·to·myo·clon·ic (fo″to-mi″o-klon′ik) photomyogenic.

pho·to·my·o·gen·ic (fo″to-mi″o-jen′ik) photomyoclonic; denoting an electroencephalographic response to photic stimulation (brief flashes of light) marked by myoclonus of the facial muscles.

pho·ton (fo′ton) [Gr. *phōs*, gen. *phōtos* light] a discrete particle with no mass and no charge, the quantum electromagnetic radiation.

pho·to-onych·ol·y·sis (fo″to-o″nĭ-kol′ĭ-sis) onycholysis resulting from exposure to sunlight or ultraviolet radiation, as after treatment with tetracyclines, methoxsalen, or other photoactive drugs.

pho·to·par·ox·ys·mal (fo″to-par″ok-siz′məl) having an abnormal electroencephalographic response to photic stimulation (brief flashes of light), marked by diffuse paroxysmal discharge recorded as spike-wave complexes; the response may be accompanied by minor seizures. Called also *photoconvulsive*.

pho·top·a·thy (fo-top′ə-the) [*photo-* + *-pathy*] a pathologic effect produced by light.

pho·to·per·cep·tive (fo″to-pər-sep′tiv) [*photo-* + *perceptive*] able to perceive light.

pho·to·pe·ri·od (fo′to-pēr″e-əd) the period of time per day that an organism is exposed to daylight or to artificial light.

pho·to·pe·ri·od·ic (fo″to-pēr″e-od′ik) pertaining to the photoperiod or to photoperiodism.

pho·to·pe·ri·o·dic·i·ty (fo″to-pēr″e-o-dis′ĭ-te) photoperiodism.

pho·to·pe·ri·od·ism (fo″to-pēr′e-əd-iz-əm) the physiologic and behavioral reactions brought about in organisms by changes in the duration of daylight and darkness in a 24-hour period. Called also *photoperiodicity*.

pho·to·phar·ma·col·o·gy (fo″to-fahr″mə-kol′ə-je) [*photo-* + *pharmacology*] the study of the effects of light and other radiations on drugs and on their pharmacological action.

pho·to·phe·re·sis (fo″to-fə-re′sis) [*photo-* + *pheresis*] a technique for treating cutaneous T-cell lymphoma; after administration of a photoactive chemical such as methoxsalen, blood is circulated out of the patient, through a source of ultraviolet radiation, and returned. The therapeutic effect is believed to involve stimulation of the host immune system.

pho·to·phil·ic (fo″to-fil′ik) [*photo-* + *-philic*] thriving in light; said of organisms.

pho·to·pho·bia (fo″to-fo′be-ə) [*photo-* + *-phobia*] abnormal visual intolerance of light. **photopho′bic** *adj*

pho·to·phos·phor·y·la·tion (fo″to-fos″for-ə-la′shən) the formation of ATP occurring in chloroplasts during photosynthesis; it is analogous to oxidative phosphorylation.

cyclic p. the coupling of ATP formation with liberation of the energy arising from a cyclic flow of electrons from the ferredoxin-reducing system back to the chlorophyll.

pho·toph·thal·mia (fo″tof-thal′me-ə) [*phot-* + *ophthalmia*] ophthalmia caused by intense light, such as electric light, rays of a welding arc, or reflection from snow (ophthalmia nivialis).

flash p. ophthalmia produced by exposure to a welding arc.

pho·to·pia (fo-to′pe-ə) day vision; see also *light adaptation*. **photop′ic** *adj*

pho·to·pig·ment (fo″to-pig′mənt) a pigment, such as a retinal pigment, that is unstable in the presence of light.

pho·to·ple·thys·mo·graph (fo″to-plə-thiz′mo-graf) the diode and sensor apparatus used in photoplethysmography.

pho·to·ple·thys·mog·ra·phy (fo″to-pleth″iz-mog′rə-fe) a technique for assessing blood flow by placing a diode that emits infrared light, along with a sensor, on the surface of the skin over a blood vessel; the amount of light reflected back to the sensor is inversely proportional to the number of red blood cells flowing through the vessel.

pho·to·prod·uct (fo′to-prod″əkt) a substance synthesized in the body by the action of light.

pho·to·pro·tec·tion (fo″to-pro-tek′shən) the protection of some cells by exposure to light in the near ultraviolet range prior to exposure to light in the far ultraviolet range.

pho·top·sia (fo-top′se-ə) [*photo-* + *-opsia*] an appearance as of sparks or flashes due to retinal irritation.

pho·top·sin (fo-top′sin) the opsin of the cones of the retina that combines with 11-*cis* retinal to form photochemical pigments (iodopsins). See illustration at *visual cycle*, under *cycle*.

pho·top·sy (fo-top′se) photopsia.

pho·to·ptar·mo·sis (fo″to-tahr-mo′sis) [*photo-* + Gr. *ptarmos* sneezing + *-osis*] sneezing caused by the influence of light.

pho·top·tom·e·ter (fo″top-tom′ə-tər) [*phot-* + *opto-* + *-meter*] a device for testing the acuity of vision by determining the smallest amount of light that will render an object just visible; called also *Förster photometer*

pho·top·tom·e·try (fo″top-tom′ə-tre) [*photo-* + *opto-* + *-metry*] determination of the flicker fusion threshold. See *flicker*.

pho·to·ra·di·a·tion (fo″to-ra″de-a′shən) photodynamic therapy.

pho·to·ra·di·om·e·ter (fo″to-ra″de-om′ə-tər) an apparatus for measuring the quantity of x-rays penetrating any given surface.

pho·to·re·ac·tion (fo″to-re-ak′shən) a chemical reaction initiated or affected by light; called also *photochemical reaction*.

pho·to·re·ac·ti·va·tion (fo″to-re-ak″tĭ-va′shən) reversal of the biological effects of ultraviolet radiation on cells by the action of light-dependent enzymes, as in the repair of DNA by the monomerization of dimerized pyrimidines; such repair can impair the efficacy of ultraviolet disinfection. Called also *photoreversal*.

pho·to·re·cep·tion (fo″to-re-sep′shən) [*photo-* + *re-* + *-ceptor*] the process of detecting radiant energy, usually of wavelengths between 370 and 760 nm, being the range of visible light.

pho·to·re·cep·tive (fo″to-re-sep′tiv) sensitive to stimulation by light.

pho·to·re·cep·tor (fo″to-re-sep′tər) a nerve end-organ or receptor sensitive to light; see also *visual cells*, under *cell*.

pho·to·re·frac·tive (fo″to-re-frak′tiv) pertaining to the refraction of light.

pho·to·res·pi·ra·tion (fo″to-res″pĭ-ra′shən) a process carried out by certain plants, occurring as a result of oxidation of glycolic acid (a product of photosynthesis released by chloroplasts) by glycolic acid oxidase, an enzyme present in the glyoxosomes, ultimately causing an increased output of carbon dioxide.

pho·to·ret·i·ni·tis (fo″to-ret″ĭ-ni′tis) inflammation of the retina due to exposure to intense light, which may result in transient central scotoma.

pho·to·re·ver·sal (fo″to-re-vur′səl) photoreactivation.

Pho·to·rhab·dus (fo″to-rab′dəs) [*photo-* + Gr. *rhabdos* rod] a genus of gram-negative bacteria of the family Enterobacteriaceae, consisting of facultatively anaerobic, non–spore-forming, bioluminescent rods that are motile by peritrichous flagella. Organisms occur as symbionts of nematodes, parasites of insects, and opportunistic pathogens for humans, in whom they cause bacteremia and soft tissue infections. The type species is *P. lumines′cens*.

pho·to·scan (fo′to-skan) a two-dimensional representation (map) of the gamma rays emitted by a radioisotope, revealing its varying concentration in a body tissue, differing from a scintiscan only in that the printout mechanism is a light source exposing a photographic film.

pho·to·scan·ner (fo″to-skan′ər) the system of equipment used in the making of a photoscan.

pho·tos·co·py (fo-tos′kə-pe) [*photo-* + *-scopy*] fluoroscopy.

pho·to·sen·si·tive (fo″to-sen′sĭ-tiv) 1. reacting to light; said of a cell, organ, or organism. 2. having abnormally heightened reactivity of skin or eyes to sunlight.

pho·to·sen·si·tiv·i·ty (fo″to-sen″sĭ-tiv′ĭ-te) [*photo-* + *sensitivity*] 1. ability of a cell, organ, or organism to react to light. 2. an abnormal response of the skin or eyes to sunlight, involving the interaction between photosensitizing substances and sunlight or filtered or artificial light at wavelengths of 280–400 nm. There are two main types: *photoallergy* and *phototoxicity*.

pho·to·sen·si·ti·za·tion (fo″to-sen″sĭ-tĭ-za′shən) 1. the process of photosensitizing. 2. abnormally increased reactivity of the skin or eyes to sunlight.

hepatogenous p. photosensitization caused by accumulation in body tissues of a photosensitizing substance, usually because of inadequate clearance through the liver; it often occurs in ruminants when plants break down in the stomach under anaerobic conditions and form phylloerythrin.

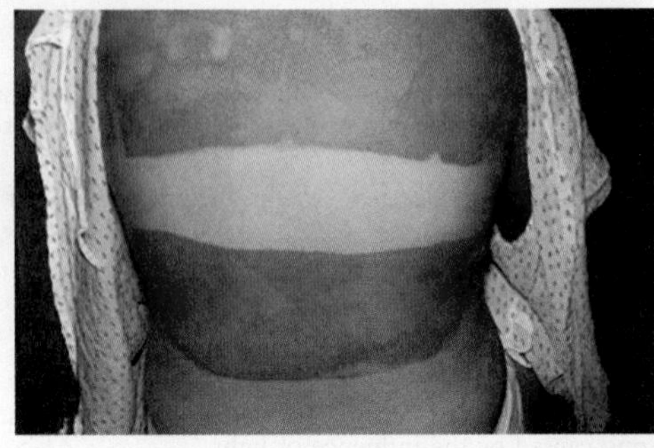

■ Photosensitivity. Severe sunburn in exposed areas after application of a topical photosensitizing cream and exposure to the sun, with sparing of areas under the bathing suit.

pho•to•sen•si•tize (fo″to-sen′sĭ-tīz) [*photo-* + *sensitize*] to sensitize a substance, organism, cell, or tissue to the influence of light. See *photosensitivity*, and see *photodynamic therapy*, under *therapy*.

pho•to•sen•si•ti•zer (fo″to-sen′sĭ-ti″zər) an agent that causes photosensitization.

pho•to•sta•ble (fo′to-sta″bəl) unchanged by the influence of light.

pho•to•syn•the•sis (fo″to-sin′thə-sis) [*photo-* + *synthesis*] a chemical combination caused by the action of light; specifically the formation of carbohydrates (with release of molecular oxygen) from carbon dioxide and water in the chlorophyll tissue of plants and blue-green algae under the influence of light. In bacteria, photosynthesis employs hydrogen sulfide, molecular hydrogen, and other reduced compounds in place of water, so that molecular oxygen is not released. Cf. *chemosynthesis*.

pho•to•tax•is (fo″to-tak′sis) [*photo-* + *taxis*] taxis of an organism elicited in response to the source of light stimulus; called also *heliotaxis*. **phototac′tic** *adj*

pho•to•test•ing (fo″to-test′ing) testing of the reaction of the skin to ultraviolet radiation at various dose levels. Cf. *erythema dose*, under *dose*.

pho•to•ther•a•py (fo″to-ther′ə-pe) [*photo-* + *therapy*] 1. the treatment of disease, e.g., herpes simplex, psoriasis, neonatal hyperbilirubinemia, or seasonal affective disorder, by exposure to light, especially by variously concentrated light rays or specific wavelengths. In complementary medicine, it is used as an adjunct to a wide variety of treatments, such as color therapy. Called also *actinotherapy*. 2. photodynamic therapy.

ultraviolet p. the use of ultraviolet radiation (which may be type A, B, or C, or a combination of types) to treat skin diseases; the radiation is usually generated by an artificial source such as an arc lamp. *Photochemotherapy* is a variant in which photosensitizing drugs are administered beforehand.

pho•to•ther•mol•y•sis (fo″to-thər-mol′ĭ-sis) destruction of tissue by heating it until it vaporizes, such as with a laser for therapeutic purposes.

pho•to•ther•my (fo′to-thur″me) [*photo-* + Gr. *thermē* heat] the heat effects produced by radiant energy. **photother′mal** *adj*

pho•to•tim•er (fo′to-tīm″ər) a device used in radiology and photography to control the exposure interval by terminating the exposure when the amount of incident radiation or light reaches a preset quantity.

pho•tot•o•nus (fo-tot′ə-nəs) [*photo-* + *tonus*] the sensitivity of an organism to light.

pho•to•tox•ic•i•ty (fo″to-tok-sis′ĭ-te) [*photo-* + *toxicity*] a type of photosensitivity that is induced by a toxic substance, in contrast to a photoallergy. See also *phototoxic dermatitis*, under *dermatitis*. **phototox′ic** *adj*

pho•to•trans•duc•tion (fo″to-trans-duk′shən) visual transduction.

pho•to•tro•phic (fo″to-tro′fik) [*photo-* + *-trophic*] capable of deriving energy from light, as in certain green plants and bacteria. Cf. *chemotrophic*.

pho•to•tro•pic (fo″to-tro′pik) exhibiting phototropism.

pho•tot•ro•pism (fo-tot′rə-piz-əm) [*photo-* + *trop-* + *-ism*] 1. tropism of an organism in response to the source of light stimulus. 2. change of color produced in a substance by the action of light.

pho•to•va•por•iza•tion (fo″to-va″por-ĭ-za′shən) laser-produced vaporization of intracellular and extracellular fluids to provide an incision with cauterization of adjacent vessels.

pho•tron•re•flec•tom•e•ter (fo″tron-re″flek-tom′ə-tər) an apparatus for measuring turbidity.

pho•tu•ria (fo-tu′re-ə) [*photo-* + *-uria*] the excretion of urine having a luminous appearance.

PHP pseudohypoparathyroidism.

PHPPA *p*-hydroxyphenylpyruvic acid.

Phrag•mo•ba•sid•io•my•ce•tes (frag″mo-bə-sid″e-o-mi-se′tēz) [Gr. *phragma* fence + *basidium* + Gr. *mykēs* fungus] a class of perfect fungi of the subphylum Basidiomycotina, characterized by having a septate basidium.

Phrag•mo•ba•sid•io•my•ce•ti•dae (frag″mo-bə-sid″e-o-mi-set′ĭ-de) name given to Phragmobasidiomycetes when it is considered a subclass.

phre•nal•gia (fre-nal′jə) [*phren-* + *-algia*] pain in the diaphragm; called also *diaphragmalgia* and *phrenodynia*.

phre•nec•to•my (fre-nek′tə-me) [*phren-* + *-ectomy*] the removal of all or a part of the diaphragm.

phren•em•phrax•is (fren″em-frak′sis) phreniclasia.

phren•ic (fren′ik) 1. pertaining to the diaphragm of the body; called also *diaphragmatic*. 2. mental[1].

phren•i•cec•to•my (fren″ĭ-sek′tə-me) [*phrenic* nerve + *-ectomy*] resection of the phrenic nerve, formerly done to cause paralysis of the diaphragm; called also *phreniconeurectomy*.

phreni•cla•sia (fren″ĭ-kla′zhə) [*phrenic* nerve + Gr. *klasis* crushing] crushing of the phrenic nerve with a clamp, formerly done to cause paralysis of the diaphragm. Called also *phrenemphraxis* and *phrenicotripsy*.

phreni•cla•sis (fren″ĭ-kla′sis) phreniclasia.

phren•i•co•ce•li•ac (fren″ĭ-ko-se′le-ak) pertaining to the diaphragm and the celiac trunk.

phren•i•co•col•ic (fren″ĭ-ko-kol′ik) pertaining to or connecting the diaphragm and colon.

phren•i•co•ex•er•e•sis (fren″ĭ-ko-ek-ser′ə-sis) [*phrenic* nerve + *exeresis*] avulsion of the phrenic nerve; cf. *phrenicectomy* and *phreniclasia*.

phren•i•co•neu•rec•to•my (fren″ĭ-ko-no͝o-rek′tə-me) phrenicectomy.

phren•i•cot•o•my (fren″ĭ-kot′ə-me) [*phrenic* nerve + *-tomy*] surgical division of the phrenic nerve and its accessory, formerly done to cause one-sided paralysis of the diaphragm.

phren•i•co•trip•sy (fren″ĭ-ko-trip′se) [*phrenic* nerve + *-tripsy*] phreniclasia.

Phren•i•lin (fren′ĭ-lin) trademark for a combination preparation of butalbital and acetaminophen.

phre•ni•tis (frə-ni′tis) [*phren-* + *-itis*] inflammation of the diaphragm; called also *diaphragmitis*.

phren(o)- [Gr. *phrēn*, gen. *phrenos* diaphragm, mind] a combining form denoting relationship to the diaphragm, the phrenic nerve, or the mind.

phreno•col•ic (fren″o-kol′ik) phrenicocolic.

phreno•dyn•ia (fren″o-din′e-ə) [*phreno-* + *-odynia*] phrenalgia.

phreno•gas•tric (fren″o-gas′trik) pertaining to the diaphragm and stomach; called also *gastrophrenic*.

phreno•glot•tic (fren″o-glot′ik) pertaining to the diaphragm and the glottis.

phreno•graph (fren′o-graf) [*phreno-* + *-graph*] an apparatus for recording the movements of the diaphragm.

phreno•he•pat•ic (fren″o-hə-pat′ik) [*phreno-* + *hepatic*] pertaining to or connecting the diaphragm and the liver.

phre•nol•o•gist (frə-nol′ə-jist) a person who practices phrenology.

phre•nol•o•gy (frə-nol′ə-je) [*phreno-* + *-logy*] the theory, popular in the 18th and 19th centuries, that mental faculties could be determined by the location of bumps and other topographical features on the skull.

phreno•peri•car•di•tis (fren″o-per″ĭ-kahr-di′tis) [*phreno-* + *pericarditis*] a condition in which the apex of the heart is attached to the diaphragm by adhesions.

phreno•ple•gia (fren″o-ple′jə) diaphragmatic paralysis.

phren•op•to•sis (fren″op-to′sis, fren″o-to′sis) [*phreno-* + *-ptosis*] downward displacement of the diaphragm.

phren•o•sin (fren′o-sin) a cerebroside occurring in the brain and other nervous tissue; it is composed of sphingosine linked to galactose and cerebronic acid.

phren•o•sine (fren′o-sēn) phrenosin.

phreno•spasm (fren′o-spaz″əm) [*phreno-* + *spasm*] spasm of the diaphragm.

phreno•splen•ic (fren″o-splen′ik) pertaining to or connecting the diaphragm and the spleen.

phren•o•tro•pic (fren″o-tro′pik) [*phreno-* + *-tropic*] exerting its principal effect upon the mind.

phric•to•path•ic (frik″to-path′ik) [Gr. *phriktos* producing a shudder + *pathos* disease] causing a shudder; a term applied to a peculiar sensation caused by irritating a hysterical anesthetic area during recovery.

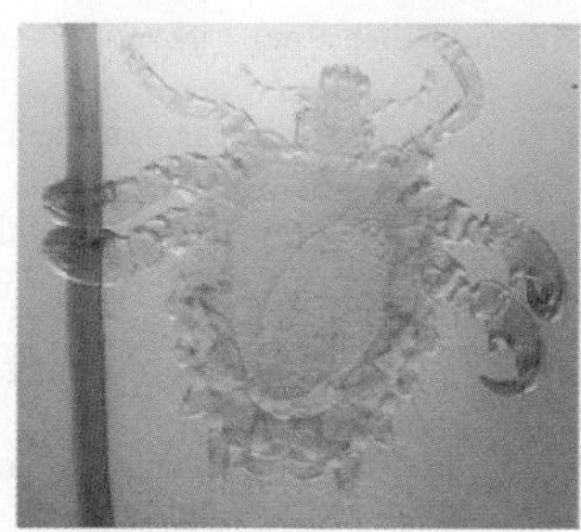

■ *Phthirus pubis* adult female grasping hair shaft, with an egg in her body cavity.

phry•nin (fri′nin) a poisonous substance obtainable from the skin and secretions of various toads; its properties resemble those of digitalin.

phryno•der•ma (frin″o-dur′mə) [Gr. *phrynē* toad + *derma*] follicular hyperkeratosis.

phry•nol•y•sin (fri-nol′ĭ-sin) [Gr. *phrynē* toad + *lysin*] the lysin or toxin from the venom of the fire toad *(Bombinator igneus)*.

phthal•ate (thal′āt) a salt, anion, or ester of phthalic acid.

phthal•ein (thal′ēn) any of a series of coloring matters formed by the condensation of phthalic anhydride with the phenols; some have a cathartic action. See *phenolphthalein.*

alpha-naphthol p. an indicator used in the determination of hydrogen ion concentration; it has a pH range of 9.3–10.5.

orthocresol p. an indicator used in the determination of hydrogen ion concentration; it has a pH range of 8.2–9.8.

phthal•ic ac•id (thal′ik) any of the isomers, but usually the ortho-isomer, of the dicarboxylic acid–substituted benzene ring; the ortho-isomer is used in dye manufacture.

phthal•in (thal′in) any one of a series of colorless compounds formed by reduction of phthalein.

phthir•i•a•sis (thir-i′ə-sis) pediculosis pubis.

p. inguina′lis, pubic p., p. pu′bis pediculosis pubis.

Phthir•us (thir′əs) [Gr. *phtheir* louse] a genus of sucking lice (order Anoplura), of the family Pediculidae, which feed on human blood.

P. pu′bis the pubic or crab louse, a species that infests the hair of the pubic region and which is sometimes found in other hairy areas of the body, such as the eyebrows, eyelashes, and axillae.

phthi•sis (thi′sis, ti′sis) [Gr. *phthisis,* from *phthiein* to decay] a wasting away of the body or a part of the body.

aneurysmal p. the clinical symptoms of chest pain and cough, at first dry and later productive, sometimes with hemoptysis, produced by aneurysm of the ascending aorta and the aortic arch.

p. bul′bi shrinkage and wasting of the eyeball.

p. cor′neae the shriveling and disappearance of the cornea after suppurative keratitis.

phyco- [Gr. *phykos* seaweed] a combining form denoting relationship to seaweed or algae.

phy•co•chrome (fi′ko-krōm) [*phyco-* + *-chrome*] 1. a blue-green pigment from various fresh-water algae of the simplest type. 2. any of the algae that contain both chlorophyll and a blue pigment; the blue-green algae.

phy•co•chro•mo•pro•tein (fi″ko-kro″mo-pro′tēn) a colored, conjugated protein, with respiratory function, found in various seaweeds.

phy•co•eryth•rin (PE) (fi″ko-ə-rith′rin) a red, fluorescent, algal protein that can be coupled to various biological molecules to make them more easily assayed.

Phy•co•my•ce•tes (fi″ko-mi-se′tēz) [*phyco-* + Gr. *mykēs* fungus] in some systems of classification, a class of fungi comprising the common water, leaf, and bread molds, which includes Oomycetes and Zygomycetes as subclasses.

phy•co•my•ce•tous (fi′ko-mi-se′təs) of or pertaining to fungi of the group Phycomycetes.

phy•co•my•co•sis (fi″ko-mi-ko′sis) 1. mucormycosis. 2. zygomycosis.

subcutaneous p. basidiobolomycosis.

phy•la (fi′lə) plural of *phylum.*

phy•lax•is (fə-lak′sis) [Gr. "a guarding"] protection against infection; the bodily defense against infection. **phylac′tic** *adj*

phy•let•ic (fi-let′ik) pertaining to a phylum, or to phylogeny.

-phyll [Gr. *phyllon* leaf] a word termination denoting relationship to leaves, or to chlorophyll.

Phyl•lan•thus (fə-lan′thəs) a genus of herbs, shrubs, and trees of the family Euphorbiaceae, found in tropical and subtropical regions. *P. eng′leri* is a species found in southern Africa; its root and bark contain a potentially deadly toxin, and its local name is suicide plant.

phyl•lid•ea (fə-lid′e-ə) bothridium.

phyll(o)- [Gr. *phyllon* leaf] a combining form denoting relationship to leaves, or to chlorophyll.

phyl•lode (fil′ōd) phyllodes.

phyl•lo•des (fəl-o′dēz) [*phyllo-* + *-oid*] leaflike; term used primarily in reference to tumors that on section show a lobulated, leaflike appearance.

phyl•lo•er•y•thrin (fil″o-er′ĭ-thrin) a derivative of chlorophyll formed in the intestinal canal of ruminant animals and found also in their bile. In cases of hepatic insufficiency it may accumulate in the tissues and cause photosensitization (see *yellows*).

phyl•loid (fil′oid) leaflike. Cf. *phyllodes.*

phyl•lo•quin•one (fil″o-kwin′ōn) phytonadione.

Phyl•lo•sto•mat•i•dae (fil″o-sto-mat′ĭ-de) the leaf-nosed bats, a family of flying mammals of the order Chiroptera found in warm regions of the Americas. Species of medical and veterinary interest are the vampire bats in genera *Desmodus, Diaemus,* and *Diphylla.*

phy•lo•gen•e•sis (fi″lo-jen′ə-sis) phylogeny.

phy•log•e•ny (fi-loj′ə-ne) [Gr. *phylon* tribe + *-geny*] the complete developmental history of a group of organisms. Cf. *ontogeny.* **phylogenet′ic, phylogen′ic** *adj*

phy•lum (fi′ləm) pl. *phy′la* [L., from Gr. *phylon* race] a primary or main division of a kingdom, composed of a group of related classes; in the taxonomy of plants, the term *division* is used instead.

phy•ma (fi′mə) pl. *phy′mata* [Gr. "a growth"] any skin tumor or swelling, especially a circumscribed swelling larger than a tubercle, produced by exudation into the subcutaneous tissue or dermis. **phy′matous** *adj*

phy•ma•ta (fi′mə-tə) [Gr.] plural of *phyma.*

Phy•sa•lia (fi-sa′le-ə) a genus of invertebrates of the phylum Cnidaria, class Hydrozoa, all called Portuguese man-of-war. All species have a large purple air sac that allows them to float on the surface of the water, and from which many long tentacles of stinging polyps hang. The tentacles are equipped with nematocysts that are able to penetrate skin and cause intense pain; paralysis can result from numerous stings.

phy•sal•i•des (fi-sal′ĭ-dēz) plural of *physalis.*

phys•a•lif•er•ous (fis″ə-lif′ər-əs) [*physalis* + *-ferous*] physaliphorous.

phy•sal•i•form (fi-sal′ĭ-form) [*physalis* + *form*] resembling bubbles.

phy•sal•i•phore (fi-sal′ĭ-for) [*physalis* + *-phore*] physaliphorous cell; sometimes used incorrectly for the vacuole within such a cell.

phys•a•liph•o•rous (fis″ə-lif′ə-rəs) [*physalis* + Gr. *phoros* bearing] containing bubbles or vacuoles.

phys•a•lis (fis′ə-lis) pl. *physa′lides* [Gr. *physallis* bubble] a vacuole cavity found in certain cells, such as the giant cells of sarcoma or chordoma.

phys•al•li•za•tion (fis″əl-ĭ-za′shən) [Gr. *physallis* bubble] the formation of a permanent froth when a liquid is shaken together with a gas.

Phys•a•lop•tera (fis″ə-lop′tər-ə) [Gr. *physallis* bubble + *pteron* wing] a genus of nematodes of the family Physalopteridae, superfamily Spiruroidea, found in the stomach and intestine of birds and mammals. *P. cauca′sica* is found in mammals in the Caucasus and parts of Africa. *P. ra′ra* is found in dogs. *P. trunca′ta* is found in chickens and pheasants.

phys•a•lop•ter•i•a•sis (fis″ə-lop-tər-i′ə-sis) infection with *Physaloptera.*

Phys•a•lop•ter•i•dae (fis″əl-op-ter′ĭ-de) a family of nematodes of the superfamily Spiruroidea; they infect birds and mammals. The one genus of veterinary interest is *Physaloptera.*

phys•e•al (fiz′e-əl) pertaining to growth, or to the segment of tubular bone which is concerned mainly with growth (the physis).

phys•iat•rics (fiz″e-at′riks) [*physi-* + *-iatrics*] physiatry.

phys•iat•rist (fiz″e-at′rist) a physician who specializes in physiatry.

phys•iat•ry (fiz″e-at′re) [*physi-* + *-iatry*] the branch of medicine that deals with the prevention, diagnosis, and treatment of disease or injury, and the rehabilitation from resultant impairments and disabilities, using physical agents such as light, heat, cold, water, electricity, therapeutic exercise, and mechanical apparatus, and sometimes pharmaceutical agents. Called also *physiatrics* and *physical medicine.* See also *rehabilitation* (def. 2).

phys•i•cal (fiz′ĭ-kəl) [Gr. *physikos*] pertaining to the body, to material things, or to physics.

phy•si•cian (fĭ-zish′ən) 1. an authorized practitioner of medicine, as one graduated from a college of medicine or osteopathy and licensed by the appropriate board. See also *doctor.* 2. one who practices medicine as distinct from surgery.

p. assistant (PA) a person who has been trained in an accredited program and certified by an appropriate board to perform certain of a physician's duties, including history taking, physical examination, diagnostic tests, treatment, certain minor surgical procedures, etc., all under the responsible supervision of a licensed physician.

attending p. 1. a physician who has admitting privileges at a hospital. 2. the physician with primary responsibility for the care of a patient in a particular case.

emergency p. a specialist in emergency medicine.

family p. a physician engaged in family practice; a medical specialist who plans and provides the comprehensive primary health care of all members of a family, regardless of age or sex, on a continuing basis.

hospital-based p., inpatient p. hospitalist.

resident p. a graduate and licensed physician receiving training in a specialty, usually in a hospital.

Phy•sick pouches (fiz′ik) [Philip Syng *Physick*, American surgeon, 1768–1837] see under *pouch.*

phys•i•co•chem•i•cal (fiz″ĭ-ko-kem′ĭ-kəl) pertaining to physics and chemistry.

phys•ics (fiz′ik) [Gr. *physis* nature] the science of the laws and phenomena of nature, but especially of the forces and general properties of matter and energy.

nuclear p. the study of atomic nuclei and their reactions.

physi(o)- [Gr. *physis* nature] a combining form meaning physical, or denoting relationship to nature or physiology.

phys•io•chem•is•try (fiz″e-o-kem′is-tre) physiologic chemistry, or clinical chemistry. **physiochem′ical** *adj*

phys•i•og•no•my (fiz″e-og′nə-me) [*physio-* + Gr. *gnōmōn* a judge] 1. physiognosis. 2. the attempt to determine temperament and character on the basis of facial features.

phys•i•og•no•sis (fiz″e-og-no′sis) [*physio-* + Gr. *gnōsis* knowledge] diagnosis by means of the facial expression or appearance.

phys•i•o•log•ic (fiz″e-o-loj′ik) normal; not pathologic; characteristic of or conforming to the normal functioning or state of the body or a tissue or organ; physiological.

phys•i•o•log•i•cal (fiz″e-o-loj′ĭ-kəl) pertaining to physiology; physiologic.

phys•i•o•log•i•co•an•a•tom•i•cal (fiz″e-o-loj″ĭ-ko-an″ə-tom′ĭ-kəl) pertaining to physiology and anatomy.

phys•i•ol•o•gist (fiz″e-ol′ə-jist) a specialist in the study of physiology.

phys•i•ol•o•gy (fiz″e-ol′ə-je) [*physio-* + *-logy*] 1. the science of the functions of the living organism and its parts, and of the physical and chemical factors and processes involved. 2. the basic processes underlying the functioning of a species or class of organism, or any of its parts or processes.

animal p. the physiology of animals other than humans; called also *zoophysiology.*

cell p. the scientific study of the phenomena involved in the growth, maintenance, self-regulation, and division of cells; interactions between nucleus and cytoplasm; and the general behavior of protoplasm. Called also cytophysiology.

comparative p. a study of organ functions in various types of animals, vertebrate and invertebrate, in an effort to find fundamental relations in the physiology of members of the entire animal kingdom.

dental p. the study of the function and functional form of the teeth and supporting tissues.

general p. the science of the general laws of life and functional activity.

morbid p., pathologic p. the study of disordered function or of function in diseased tissues.

special p. the physiology of particular organs.

vegetable p. the physiology of plants.

phys•i•ol•y•sis (fiz″e-ol′ĭ-sis) [*physio-* + *-lysis*] natural dissolution and disintegration of tissue.

phys•io•med•i•cal•ism (fiz″e-o-med′ĭ-kəl-iz-əm) [*physio-* + *medicalism*] a system of medical treatment in which only plant remedies are used, excluding those which are poisonous.

phys•i•om•e•try (fiz″e-om′ə-tre) [*physio-* + *-metry*] measurement of the physiologic functions of the body by serologic and physiologic methods.

phys•i•on•o•my (fiz″e-on′ə-me) [*physio-* + Gr. *nomos* law] the science of the laws of nature.

phys•io•patho•log•ic (fiz″e-o-path″ə-loj′ik) pertaining to both the physiologic and pathologic conditions.

phys•io•pa•thol•o•gy (fiz″e-o-pə-thol′ə-je) [*physio-* + *pathology*] the science of functions in disease, or as modified by disease.

phys•i•oph•y•ly (fiz″e-of′ə-le) [*physio-* + Gr. *phylon* tribe] the evolution of bodily functions.

phys•io•ther•a•pist (fiz″e-o-ther′ə-pist) physical therapist.

phys•io•ther•a•py (fiz″e-o-ther′ə-pe) [*physio-* + *therapy*] physical therapy.

phy•sique (fĭ-zēk′) bodily structure, organization, and development.

phy•sis (fi′sis) pl. *phy′ses* [Gr. *phyein* to generate] the segment of tubular bone that is concerned mainly with growth in length of the bone. It consists of four zones: zone of resting cartilage, zone of proliferating cartilage, zone of hypertrophy, and zone of calcification.

phys(o)- [Gr. *physa* air] a combining form denoting relationship to air or gas.

Phy•so•ceph•a•lus (fi″so-sef′ə-ləs) a genus of nematodes of the superfamily Spiruroidea. *P. sexala′tus* is found in the stomach of pigs.

phy•so•hem•a•to•me•tra (fi″so-he″mə-to-me′trə) [*physo-* + *hemato-* + *metra*] the presence of gas and blood within the uterus.

phy•so•hy•dro•me•tra (fi″so-hi″dro-me′trə) [*physo-* + *hydro-* + *metra*] the presence of gas and fluid within the uterus.

phy•so•me•tra (fi″so-me′trə) [*physo-* + *metra*] air or gas in the uterine cavity.

Phy•sop•sis (fi-sop′sis) a subgenus of snails (genus *Bulinus*), several species of which are the intermediate hosts of *Schistosoma haematobium* and other animal schistosomes.

phy•so•pyo•sal•pinx (fi″so-pi″o-sal′pinks) [*physo-* + *pyo-* + *salpinx*] the presence of pus and gas in the uterine tube.

Phy•so•stig•ma (fi″so-stig′mə) [*physo-* + Gr. *stigma* stigma] a genus of tropical plants of the family Leguminosae. *P. veneno′sum* Balf. is the Calabar bean.

phy•so•stig•mine (fi″zo-stig′mēn) [USP] a cholinergic alkaloid having anticholinesterase activity and obtained from the dried ripe seed (Calabar bean) of *Physostigma venenosum;* used topically to produce miosis and decrease of intraocular pressure in glaucoma and parenterally to reverse the central nervous system effects produced by overdosage of anticholinergic drugs (anticholinergic syndrome). Called also *eserine.*

p. salicylate [USP] the salicylate salt of physostigmine with the same properties as the alkaloid.

p. sulfate [USP] the sulfate salt of physostigmine with the same properties as the alkaloid.

phy•so•stig•min•ism (fi″so-stig′min-iz-əm) poisoning by physostigmine.

phy•tag•glu•ti•nin (fi″tə-gloo′tĭ-nin) a phytotoxin which has the power of agglutinating red blood corpuscles.

phy•tal•bu•min (fi″tal-bu′min) [*phyto-* + *albumin*] vegetable albumin.

phy•tan•ate (fi′tən-āt) a salt or anionic form of phytanic acid.

phy•tan•ic ac•id (fi-tan′ik) an unusual 20-carbon branched-chain fatty acid found at high levels in dairy products and fatty tissue of ruminants, and accumulated in tissues of patients with Refsum disease and several peroxisomal disorders.

phy•tan•ic ac•id α-hy•droxy•lase (fi-tan′ik as′id hi-drok′sə-lās) an enzyme that catalyzes the alpha oxidation of phytanic acid, hydroxylating its alpha carbon; the reaction requires molecular oxygen and is stimulated by NADPH and by ferric iron. Deficiency of the enzyme, an autosomal recessive trait, causes Refsum disease.

4-phy•tase (fi′tās) [EC 3.1.3.26] an enzyme of the hydrolase class, present at a low level in ileal mucosa, that hydrolyzes excess dietary phytic acid. Formerly officially called *6-phytase,* based on a different numbering system.

phy•tate (fi′tāt) an anionic form of phytic acid.

-phyte [Gr. *phyton* plant] a combining form denoting a plant or a pathological growth.

phy•tic ac•id (fi′tik) inositol hexaphosphate, a compound occurring in the leaves of plants.

phyt(o)- [Gr. *phyton* plant] a combining form denoting relationship to a plant or plants.

phy•to•a•lex•in (fi″to-ə-lek′sin) any of a group of compounds formed in plants in response to fungal infection, physical damage, chemical injury, or a pathogenic process. Phytoalexins inhibit or destroy the invading agent.

phy•to•an•a•phy•lac•to•gen (fi″to-an″ə-fə-lak′to-jən) [*phyto-* + *anaphylactogen*] an antigen of plant origin that is capable of inducing anaphylaxis; called also *phytosensitinogen.*

phy•to•be•zoar (fi″to-be′zor) [*phyto-* + *bezoar*] a gastric concretion composed of vegetable matter such as skins, seeds, and the fibers of fruit and vegetables.

phy•to•chem•is•try (fi″to-kem′is-tre) [*phyto-* + *chemistry*] the study of plant chemistry, including the chemical processes that take place in plants, the nature of plant chemicals, and the various applications of such chemicals to science and industry.

phy·to·chin·in (fi″to-kin′in) a substance isolated from the leaves of certain grasses, said to have an effect on carbohydrate metabolism resembling that of insulin.

phy·to·dem·ic (fi″to-dem′ik) [*phyto-* + *epidemic*] an epidemic attack of any disease of plants.

phy·to·de·tri·tus (fi″to-de-tri′təs) detritus produced by the disintegration and decomposition of vegetable organisms. Cf. *zoodetritus*.

phy·to·es·tro·gen (fi″to-es′tro-jən) [*phyto-* + *estrogen*] any of a group of weakly estrogenic, nonsteroidal compounds widely occurring in plants; diets containing large amounts of phytoestrogen-containing sources, such as soy, appear to have a preventive effect on cardiovascular disease and osteoporosis.

phy·to·flag·el·late (fi″to-flaj′ə-lāt) [*phyto-* + *flagellate*] any protozoan of a large group exhibiting plantlike behavior, formerly classified in the class Phytomastigophorea.

phy·to·gen·e·sis (fi″to-jen′ə-sis) [*phyto-* + *-genesis*] the origin and development of plants.

phy·tog·e·nous (fi-toj′ə-nəs) [*phyto-* + *-genous*] derived from a plant, or caused by a vegetable growth.

phy·to·he·mag·glu·ti·nin (fi″to-he″mə-gloo′tĭ-nin) a lectin isolated from the red kidney bean *(Phaseolus vulgaris);* it is a hemagglutinin that agglutinates mammalian erythrocytes and a mitogen that stimulates predominantly T lymphocytes. Abbreviated PHA.

phy·toid (fi′toid) [*phyto-* + *-oid*] resembling a plant.

phy·tol (fi′tol) an unsaturated aliphatic alcohol related to xanthophyll, to the carotenoids, and to vitamin A, that exists in chlorophyll as an ester; used in the preparation of vitamin E and phytonadione.

Phy·to·lac·ca (fi″to-lak′ə) a genus of perennial herbs. *P. america′na* is the pokeweed (q.v.) of North America, which contains oxalate and saponins and is medicinal but can be toxic to livestock.

Phy·to·mas·ti·goph·o·ra (fi″to-mas″tĭ-gof′ə-rə) Phytomastigophorea.

Phy·to·mas·ti·goph·o·rea (fi″to-mas″tĭ-go-for′e-ə) [*phyto-* + Gr. *mastix* whip + *phoros* bearing] in older systems of classification, a class of protozoa of the phylum Sarcomastigophora, comprising all of the plantlike (as opposed to animallike) members of the phylum; they are collectively known as phytoflagellates. Members of this group have chromatophores and usually one or two emergent flagella, with ameboid forms occurring in some species. They are mostly free-living and autotrophic. Phytoflagellates are sometimes classified with the algae. Called also *Phytomastigophora*. Cf. *Zoomastigophorea*.

phy·to·mas·ti·goph·o·re·an (fi″to-mas″tĭ-gə-for′e-ən) phytoflagellate.

phy·to·med·i·cine (fi″to-med′ĭ-sin) 1. a preparation of a medicinal herb. 2. herbalism.

phy·to·men·a·di·one (fi″to-men″ə-di′ōn) phytonadione.

phy·to·mi·to·gen (fi″to-mi′to-jən) a substance of plant origin that induces mitosis in human cells.

phy·to·na·di·one (fi-to″nə-di′ōn) 1. a fat-soluble vitamin of the K group (see under *vitamin*) with a phytyl side chain, found in green plants or prepared synthetically and having prothrombinogenic properties. 2. [USP] a preparation of phytonadione used as a prothrombinogenic agent in the treatment of hypoprothrombinemia due to various causes; administered orally or parenterally. Called also *phylloquinone* and *vitamin K_1*.

phy·to·no·sis (fi″to-no′sis) [*phyto-* + *nos-* + *-sis*] any morbid condition due to a plant.

phy·to·par·a·site (fi″to-par′ə-sīt) [*phyto-* + *parasite*] any parasitic plant organism or species.

phy·to·path·o·gen·ic (fi″to-path″o-jen′ik) producing disease in plants.

phy·to·pa·thol·o·gy (fi″to-pə-thol′ə-je) [*phyto-* + *pathology*] 1. the study of plant diseases and their control. 2. the pathology of morbid conditions caused by schizomycetes and other vegetable parasites.

phy·top·a·thy (fi-top′ə-the) [*phyto-* + *-pathy*] any disease of plants.

phy·toph·a·gous (fi-tof′ə-gəs) [*phyto-* + *phag-* + *-ous*] eating vegetable food.

phy·to·pho·to·der·ma·ti·tis (fi″to-fo″to-dur″mə-ti′tis) [*phyto-* + *photo-* + *dermatitis*] phototoxic dermatitis of an area of skin that has been exposed to a plant that contains a psoralen-type photosensitizer; characteristics include burning erythema, then edema with small vesicles that coalesce into large bullae, and later intense residual hyperpigmentation.

phy·to·plank·ton (fi″to-plank′ton) [*phyto-* + *plankton*] the minute plant (vegetable) organisms which, with those of the animal kingdom, make up the plankton of natural waters.

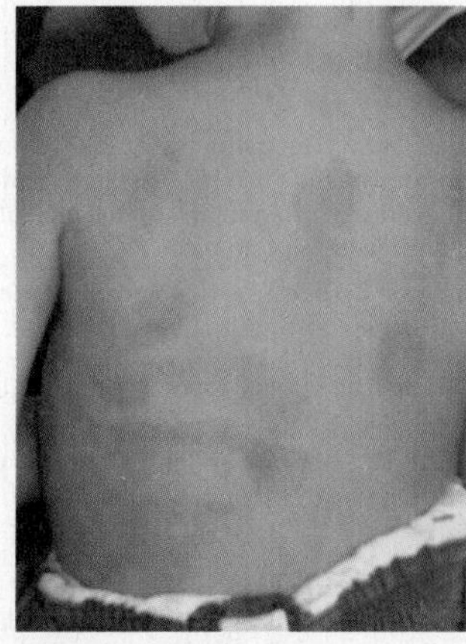

■ Child with phytophotodermatitis, several weeks after contact with his father's hands while they were wet with lime juice immediately before an afternoon at the beach.

phy·to·pre·cip·i·tin (fi″to-pre-sip′ĭ-tin) a precipitin produced by immunization with protein substances of plant origin.

phy·to·sen·si·tin·o·gen (fi″to-sen″sĭ-tin′ə-jən) [*phyto-* + *sensitinogen*] phytoanaphylactogen.

phy·to·sis (fi-to′sis) [*phyto-* + *-osis*] any disease caused by a phytoparasite.

phy·tos·ter·ol (fi-tos′tər-ol″) a plant sterol. See also *sitosterol*.

phy·tos·ter·ol·emia (fi-tos″tər-ol-e′me-ə) sitosterolemia.

phy·to·ther·a·py (fi″to-ther′ə-pe) [*phyto-* + *therapy*] treatment by use of plants.

phy·to·tox·ic (fi′to-tok″sik) 1. pertaining to a phytotoxin, or plant poison. 2. inhibiting the growth of plants.

phy·to·tox·in (fi′to-tok″sin) 1. any toxic substance of plant origin. 2. any of a group of exotoxins produced by certain species of higher plants; they are resistant to proteolytic digestion, and are effective when taken by mouth. Included are abrin, crotin, ricin, and robin.

phy·to·tri·cho·be·zoar (fi″to-tri″ko-be′zor) trichophytobezoar.

phy·to·vi·tel·lin (fi″to-vi-tel′in) vitellin of vegetable origin.

phy·tox·y·lin (fi-tok′sə-lin) [*phyto-* + Gr. *xylon* wood] a substance resembling pyroxylin; used in preparing celloidin sections.

PI phosphatidylinositol; protease inhibitor.

pI the pH of a solution containing a solute at its isoelectric point.

pi (pi) [Π, π] the sixteenth letter of the Greek alphabet.

pia (pi′ə, pe′ə) [L.] 1. tender; soft. 2. pia mater.

pia-ar·ach·ni·tis (pi″ə-ar″ak-ni′tis) leptomeningitis.

pia-arach·noid (pi″ə-ə-rak′noid) [*pia* + *arachnoid*] the pia mater and the arachnoid considered together as one functional unit; the leptomeninges.

pia-glia (pi″ə-gli′ə) a membrane formed by the fusion of the pia mater and the membrana limitans; it constitutes one of the layers of the pia-arachnoid.

pia-in·ti·ma (pi′ə in′tĭ-mə) [*pia* + *intima*] pia-glia.

pia ma·ter (pi′ə ma′tər, pe′ə mah′tər) [L. "tender mother"] [TA] the innermost of the three membranes (meninges) covering the brain and spinal cord, investing them closely and extending into the depths of the fissures and sulci; it consists of reticular, elastic, and collagenous fibers. **pi′al** *adj*

p. m. crania′lis [TA] the pia mater covering the brain, very thin over the cerebral cortex, and thicker over the brainstem; the blood vessels for the brain ramify within it and, as they enter the brain, are accompanied for a short distance by a pial sheath. Called also *p. m. encephali* [TA alternative].

p. m. ence′phali TA alternative for *p. m. cranialis*.

p. m. spina′lis [TA] the pia mater covering the spinal cord and consisting of collagenous fibers, which also form the denticulate ligament and the pial part of the filum terminale, and reticular fibers, which closely invest the cord, form the various septa, and form an investment for the rootlets.

pi·an (pe-ahn′) [Fr.] yaws.

p. bois a form of New World cutaneous leishmaniasis occurring in the forests of the Guianas and northern Brazil, caused by *Leishmania guyanensis*, transmitted chiefly by *Lutzomyia umbratilis*, and characterized by multiple, widespread, deep skin ulcers with nodular lymphatic metastases. Called also *forest yaws*.

hemorrhagic p. verruga peruana.

pi•ar•ach•ni•tis (pi″ar″ak-ni′tis) leptomeningitis.

pi•arach•noid (pi″ə-rak′noid) pia-arachnoid.

pi•blok•to (pĭ-blok′to) [Eskimo] a culture-specific syndrome seen chiefly among Eskimo women, marked by sudden, short-lived attacks of screaming, crying, running naked through the snow, and other dangerous or irrational acts, sometimes with suicidal or homicidal tendencies, often followed by convulsive seizures and coma.

pi•ca (pi′kə) [L. "magpie" (because this bird eats or carries away odd objects)] compulsive eating of nonnutritive substances, such as ice (pagophagia), dirt (geophagia), gravel, flaking paint or plaster, clay, hair (trichophagia), or laundry starch (amylophagia). It also occurs in some patients with iron or zinc deficiencies. In children this syndrome, classified with the eating disorders in DSM-IV, is a rare mental disorder with onset typically in the second year of life; it usually remits in childhood but may persist into adolescence.

PICC peripherally inserted central catheter.

Pich•ia (pich′e-ə) a genus of fungi of the subphylum Ascomycotina, order Endomycetales. It contains the perfect (sexual) stage of a few species of *Candida.*

Pick bodies, disease (pik) [Arnold *Pick*, Czechoslovakian psychiatrist, 1851–1924] see under *body* and *disease* (def. 1).

Pick cells, disease (pik) [Ludwig *Pick*, German physician, 1868–1935] see under *cell*, and see *Niemann-Pick disease*, under *disease*.

pick (pik) any pointed or other sharp device for removing objects from areas that are difficult to access.

apical p. see under *elevator*.

crane p. an elevator for the removal of root fragments of mandibular molar teeth fractured during extraction.

root p. apical elevator.

pick•ling (pik′ling) the process of cleansing newly cast metallic surfaces and removal of oxides and other impurities from metal objects by immersion in an acid solution.

pick•wick•i•an syndrome (pik-wik′e-ən) [from the description of Joe, the fat boy in Dickens' *Pickwick Papers*] see under *syndrome*.

pico- [from It. *piccolo* small] a prefix used in naming units of measurement to indicate one trillionth (10^{-12}) of the unit designated by the root with which it is combined. Symbol p.

pi•co•cu•rie (pCi) (pi″ko-ku′re) a unit of radioactivity, being one trillionth (10^{-12}) of a curie.

pi•co•gram (pg) (pi′ko-gram) one-trillionth (10^{-12}) of a gram.

Pi•cor•na•vi•ri•dae (pĭ-kor″nə-vir′ĭ-de) the picornaviruses: a family of RNA viruses having a nonenveloped icosahedral virion 22–30 nm in diameter without surface features. The genome consists of a single molecule of positive-sense single-stranded RNA (MW approximately 2.5×10^6, size 7.2–8.5 kb). Viruses contain four major polypeptides and are resistant to lipid solvents but sensitive to ultraviolet radiation. Replication and assembly occur in the cytoplasm; virions are released by cell destruction. Host range is narrow and transmission is chiefly mechanical. Genera of medical or veterinary importance include *Aphthovirus*, *Cardiovirus*, *Enterovirus*, *Hepatovirus*, *Parechovirus*, and *Rhinovirus*.

pi•cor•na•vi•rus (pi-kor′nə-vi″rəs) [*pico-* + *r*ibo*n*ucleic *a*cid + *virus*] any virus belonging to the family Picornaviridae. **picornavi′ral** *adj*

pi•co•unit (pi″ko-u′nit) one trillionth (10^{-12}) of a standard unit.

Pi•cras•ma (pi-kraz′mə) a genus of tropical trees of the family Simaroubaceae. *P. excel′sa* (Sw.) Planch. is the bitterwood or Jamaica quassia, source of the medicine quassia.

pic•rate (pik′rāt) any salt of picric acid.

pic•ric ac•id (pik′rik) trinitrophenol.

picr(o)- [Gr. *pikros* bitter] 1. a combining form meaning bitter or denoting relationship to picric acid. 2. denoting relationship to picric acid.

pic•ro•car•mine (pik″ro-kahr′min) a stain prepared from picric acid and carmine and used in microscopy. It consists of a mixture of carmine, ammonia, and distilled water, to which is added an aqueous solution of picric acid.

pic•ro•geu•sia (pik″ro-goo′zhə) [*picro-* + Gr. *geusis* taste + *-ia*] a pathologic bitter taste.

pic•ro•ni•gro•sin (pik″ro-ni-gro′sin) a solution of picric acid and nigrosin in alcohol, used as a stain.

Pic•ror•rhi•za (pik″ro-ri′zə) [*picro-* + Gr. *rhiza* root] a genus of herbs of the family Scrophulariaceae, native to the Himalayas; the rhizome of *P. kurro′a* Royle is tonic and antiperiodic.

pic•ro•sac•cha•rom•e•ter (pik″ro-sak″ə-rom′ə-tər) an instrument used in estimating diabetic sugar.

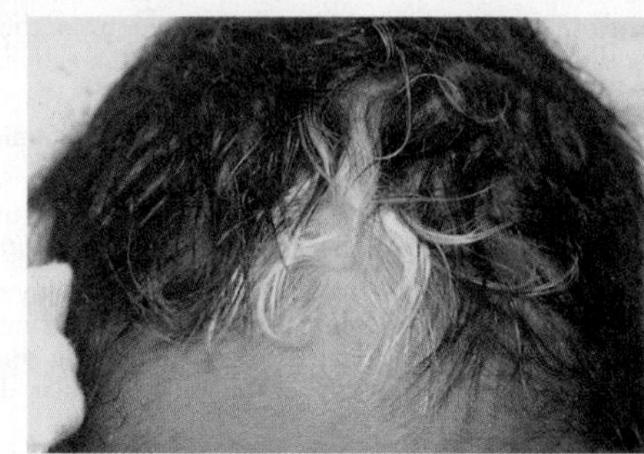

■ Hypopigmented epidermal patches and white forelock characteristic of piebaldism.

pic•ro•scle•ro•tine (pik″ro-skle′ro-tin) a poisonous alkaloid occurring in ergot of rye.

pic•ro•tox•in (pik′ro-tok″sin) an active principle obtained from the seed (cocculus indicus) of *Anamirta cocculus*; it stimulates all portions of the central nervous system by blocking presynaptic inhibition of neural impulses and can cause convulsions. It has been used medicinally as an antidote in the treatment of poisoning by central nervous system depressant drugs, especially the barbiturates, administered intravenously.

pic•ro•tox•in•ism (pik″ro-tok′zin-iz-əm) poisoning by picrotoxin, with hyperactivity of the central nervous system and convulsions.

PID pelvic inflammatory disease.

PIE pulmonary interstitial emphysema; pulmonary infiltration with eosinophilia.

pie•bald (pi′bawld) [L. *pica* magpie + *bald*] exhibiting piebaldism.

pie•bald•ism (pi′bawld-iz-əm) a congenital, autosomal dominant pigmentary disorder in which there are patches of white skin and hair that lack melanocytes, with a characteristic distribution pattern that favors the central anterior trunk, mid-extremities, central forehead, and midfrontal portion of the scalp. There is usually a white forelock. It is often due to mutation in the *KIT* gene (locus: 4q11-q12), a proto-oncogene that encodes a member of the tyrosine kinase family of transmembrane receptors found on the surface of melanocytes.

piece (pēs) a part or portion.

chief p. principal p.

connecting p. 1. neck of spermatozoon. 2. middle p.

end p. the terminal portion of the tail of the spermatozoon; called also *terminal filament*. See illustration at *spermatozoon*.

middle p. an anterior portion of the tail of the spermatozoon, bounded by the neck anteriorly and the anulus posteriorly. Called also *connecting p.* See illustration at *spermatozoon*.

principal p. the main portion of the tail of a spermatozoon, beginning at the anulus and gradually tapering toward the end piece. Called also *chief p.* See illustration at *spermatozoon*.

secretory p. see under *component*.

pie•dra (pya′drə) [Sp. "rock"] a fungal infection of the hair shaft characterized by the presence of dark or pale, firm, irregular nodules composed of fungal elements.

black p. piedra caused by *Piedraia hortae*, characterized by small black or brown gritty nodules on the shafts of the scalp hair; usually seen in tropical regions.

white p. piedra caused by *Trichosporon beigelii*, characterized by white to light brown nodules on the hair of the beard, axilla, or groin, softer than the nodules of the black variety; usually seen in temperate regions. Called also *trichosporosis*.

Pi•e•draia (pi″ə-dri′ə) a genus of fungi of the family Piedraiaceae. *P. hor′tae* is parasitic on hair, causing black piedra.

Pi•e•drai•a•ceae (pi″ə-dri-a′se-e) a family of fungi of the order Dothideales, including the genus *Piedraia*.

pier (pēr) intermediate abutment.

Pi•erre Ro•bin sequence (syndrome) (pyăr-ro-bă′) [*Pierre Robin*, French dentist, 1867–1950] see under *sequence*.

pi•eses•the•sia (pi-e″zes-the′zhə) [Gr. *piesis* pressure + *esthesia*] pressure sense.

pi•esim•e•ter (pi″ə-sim′ə-tər) [Gr. *piesis* pressure + *-meter*] an instrument for testing the sensitiveness of the skin to pressure.

Hales p. a glass tube inserted into an artery for the purpose of ascertaining the blood pressure by the height to which the blood rises in the tube.

-piesis [Gr. *piesis* a pressing or squeezing] a word termination meaning pressure.

pi•ezal•lo•chro•my (pi″ə-zal′ə-kro-me) [*piez-* + *allochromy*] change of color of a substance caused by crushing.

pi•ezes•the•sia (pi″ə-zes-the′zhə) pressure sense.

piez(o)- [Gr. *piezein* to press] a combining form denoting relationship to pressure.

pi•ezo•chem•is•try (pi-e′zo-kem″is-tre) [*piezo-* + *chemistry*] the branch of chemistry that deals with the effect of pressure on chemical phenomena.

pi•ezo•elec•tri•ci•ty (pi-e″zo-e-lek-tris′ĭ-te) [*piezo-* + *electricity*] electrical current generated by mechanical stress in quartz and certain other crystals; analogously, the converse property of expansion or contraction of these materials in response to an applied electric field. **piezoelec′tric** *adj*

pi•ezo•gen•ic (pi-e″zo-jen′ik) caused by pressure.

pi•ezom•e•ter (pi″ə-zom′ə-tər) [*piezo-* + *-meter*] 1. piesimeter. 2. orbitonometer.

PIF prolactin-inhibiting factor; peak inspiratory flow.

pig (pig) 1. a domesticated form of *Sus scrofa*, a farm animal with cloven hoofs that is raised for its meat. 2. something felt to resemble the domesticated pig.
  dancing p. shaker p.
  guinea p. see under G.
  shaker p. a pig suffering from congenital tremor syndrome.

pig•eon•pox (pij′ən-poks) a type of fowlpox seen in pigeons, characterized by pox lesions of the oral mucosa and the eyelids, sometimes resulting in blindness.

pig•ment (pig′mənt) [L. *pigmentum* paint] 1. any normal or abnormal coloring matter of the body. 2. a paintlike medicinal preparation to be applied to the skin.
  anthracotic p. minute carbon particles deposited in lung tissue that give the tissue the black coloration seen in anthracosis.
  bile p. any of the coloring matters of the bile, such as bilirubin, biliverdin, bilicyanin, bilifuscin, bilihumin, biliprasin, and choleprasin.
  blood p. hematogenous p.
  endogenous p. a pigment derived from material normally present in the body.
  exogenous p. a pigment inhaled or ingested and deposited in the lungs and other tissues.
  fatty p. lipid p.
  hematogenous p. any of the pigments derived from hemoglobin, such as hematoidin, hematoporphyrin, hemofuscin, hemosiderin, and methemoglobin.
  hepatogenous p. bile pigment formed in the liver.
  lipid p. any of various pigments having lipid characteristics, some of which also contain protein or iron, the most important one being lipofuscin. Called also *fatty p.*
  lipochrome p. lipochrome.
  malarial p. hemozoin.
  melanotic p. melanin.
  respiratory p's substances, such as hemoglobin, myoglobin, or the cytochromes, which take part in the oxidation processes of the animal body.
  retinal p's the photopigments in retinal rods and cones that respond to certain colors of light and initiate the process of vision.
  visual p's retinal p's.
  wear and tear p. lipochrome.

pig•men•tary (pig′mən-tar″e) pertaining to or of the nature of a pigment.

pig•men•ta•tion (pig″mən-ta′shən) 1. the deposition of pigment. 2. abnormal discoloration of a part by a pigment; see also *dyschromia* and *hyperpigmentation.*
  reticular p., reticulate p., reticulated p. see under *hyperpigmentation.*

pig•ment•ed (pig′mən-təd) colored by deposit of pigment.

pig•men•to•gen•e•sis (pig″mən-to-jen′ə-sis) [*pigment* + *genesis*] the production of pigment.

pig•men•to•gen•ic (pig″mən-to-jen′ik) inducing the formation or deposit of pigment.

pig•men•tol•y•sis (pig″mən-tol′ĭ-sis) [*pigment* + *-lysis*] destruction of pigment.

pig•men•to•phore (pig-men′to-for″) chromatophore.

pi•itis (pi-i′tis) inflammation of the pia mater.

Pil. [L.] pi′lula (pill); pil′ulae (pills).

Pi•la (pi′lə) a genus of freshwater snails of the family Pilidae. *P. co′nica* is the second intermediate host of the fluke *Echinostoma ilocanum* in the Philippines.

pi•la (pi′lə) pl. *pi′lae* [L.] a pillar or pillarlike structure, such as a trabecula of spongy bone.

pi•lae (pi′le) [L.] genitive and plural of *pila.*

pi•lar (pi′lər) [L. *pilaris*] hairy (def. 1).

pil•a•ry (pil′ə-re) hairy (def. 1).

pile[1] (pīl) [L. *pila* pillar] an aggregation of similar elements for generating electricity.
  muscular p. layers of muscular tissue so arranged as to generate an electric current.
  thermoelectric p. a set of slender metallic bars which, on exposure to heat, generates a current of electricity that moves an index and is made to register delicate changes of temperature.
  voltaic p. a battery for current electricity made up of a series of metallic disks.

pile[2] (pīl) [L. *pila* a ball] hemorrhoid.
  sentinel p. a hemorrhoid-like thickening of the mucous membrane at the lower end of a fissure of the anus.

pi•le•us (pi′le-əs) [L. "a close-fitting felt cap"] caul.

pi•li (pi′li) (sing. *pi′lus*) [L.] [TA] the hairs growing out of the skin; see *hair.*

pi•li•al (pi′le-əl) pertaining to a pilus; said of bacteria.

pi•li•ate (pi′le-at) having pili; said of bacteria.

Pil•i•dae (pil′ĭ-de) a family of fresh water snails of the order Mesogastropoda; it includes the genus *Pila.*

pi•lif•er•ous (pi-lif′ər-əs) bearing or producing hair.

pi•li•mic•tion (pi″lĭ-mik′shən) [*pili* + *miction*] passing of urine containing hair or hairlike threads of mucus.

pi•lin (pi′lin) the protein that composes bacterial pili.

pill (pil) [L. *pilula*] tablet.
  radio p. telemetering capsule.

pil•lar (pil′ər) [L. *pila*] a supporting column, usually occurring in pairs.
  anterior p. of fauces arcus palatoglossus.
  anterior p. of fornix columna fornicis.
  articular p's columnlike structures formed by the articulation of the superior and inferior articular processes of the vertebrae; see *processus articularis inferior vertebrarum* and *processus articularis superior vertebrarum.*
  p's of organ of Corti pillar cells.
  p's of diaphragm see *pars lumbalis diaphragmatis.*
  posterior p. of fauces arcus palatopharyngeus.
  posterior p. of fornix crus fornicis.
  Uskow p's two folds of the embryo attached to the dorsolateral portion of the body wall; from these pillars and the septum transversum the diaphragm is formed.

pil•lion (pil′yən) pylon.

pil•low (pil′o) a case or bag stuffed with soft material.
  Frejka p. a type of soft hip abduction orthosis consisting of a pillow wedged between the thighs of an infant to abduct the thighs and correct hip dislocation occurring in developmental dysplasia of the hip. Called also *Frejka pillow splint.*

pill-roll•ing (pil-rōl′ing) see under *tremor.*

pil(o)- [L. *pilus* hair] a combining form denoting relationship to hair, or resembling or composed of hair.

pi•lo•be•zoar (pi″lo-be′zor) trichobezoar.

Pi•lo•car (pi′lo-kahr″) trademark for preparations of pilocarpine hydrochloride.

pi•lo•car•pine (pi″lo-kahr′pēn) [USP] a cholinomimetic alkaloid obtained from leaves of plants of the genus *Pilocarpus*, having predominantly muscarinic effects. When applied to the eye, it produces miosis and a transient rise and persistent fall in intraocular pressure; used in the treatment of glaucoma.
  p. hydrochloride [USP] the monohydrochloride salt of pilocarpine, applied topically to the eye in the treatment of glaucoma or to counteract the effects of cycloplegics and mydriatics following examination or surgery; also administered orally in the treatment of xerostomia resulting from reduced salivary gland function caused by radiotherapy for head and neck cancer or associated with Sjögren syndrome.
  p. nitrate [USP] the nitrate salt of pilocarpine, having the same actions and ophthalmic uses as the hydrochloride salt.

Pi•lo•car•pus (pi″lo-kahr′pəs) [Gr. *pilos* wool or hair wrought into felt + *karpos* fruit] a genus of shrubs of the family Rutaceae, native to tropical regions of the Americas; *P. jaboran′di* and *P. microphyl′lus* have leaves that yield pilocarpine.

pi•lo•cys•tic (pi″lo-sis′tik) [*pilo-* + *cystic*] hollow and containing hairs; said of certain dermoid cysts.

pi•lo•cyt•ic (pi″lo-sit′ik) composed of fiber-shaped cells.

pi•lo•erec•tion (pi″lo-e-rek′shən) horripilation.

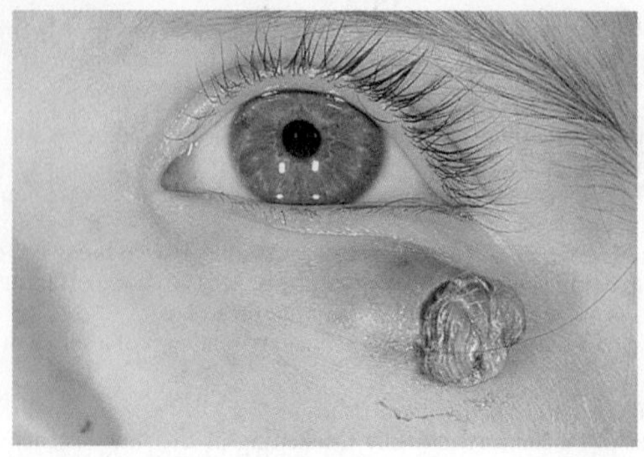

■ Pilomatricoma.

pi•lo•leio•myo•ma (pi″lo-li″o-mi-o′mə) [*pilo-* + *leiomyoma*] a type of leiomyoma cutis, single or multiple, that arises from the arrectores pilorum muscles.

pi•lo•ma•tri•co•ma (pi″lo-ma″trĭ-ko′mə) [*pilo-* + *matrix* + *-oma*] a solitary, benign, calcifying adnexal tumor of hair follicle origin, manifested as a circumscribed, firm, intracutaneous nodule. It usually occurs on the face, neck, or upper limb of a person under age 20. Histological features include a fibrous stroma surrounding nests of basophilic cells and ghost cells. Called also *benign calcified, benign calcifying,* or *Malherbe calcifying epithelioma.*

pi•lo•ma•trix•o•ma (pi″lo-ma″trik-so′mə) pilomatricoma.

pi•lo•mo•tor (pi″lo-mo′tər) [*pilo-* + *motor*] pertaining to the arrector pili muscles; see also *horripilation.*

pi•lo•ni•dal (pi″lo-ni′dəl) [*pilo-* + L. *nidus* nest] pertaining to, characterized by, or having a nidus or tuft of hairs.

Pi•lop•tic (pi-lop′tik) trademark for preparations of pilocarpine hydrochloride.

pi•lose (pi′lōs) [L. *pilosus*] 1. hairy (def. 1). 2. hirsute.

pi•lo•se•ba•ceous (pi″lo-sə-ba′shəs) pertaining to a hair follicle and a sebaceous gland.

Pi•lo•stat (pi′lo-stat″) trademark for preparations of pilocarpine hydrochloride.

Piltz reflex, sign (pilts) [Jan *Piltz,* Polish neurologist, 1870–1931] see *attention reflex of pupil* and *orbicularis pupillary reflex,* under *reflex.*

Piltz-West•phal phenomenon (pilts′ vest′fahl) [J. *Piltz;* Alexander Karl Otto *Westphal,* German neurologist, 1863–1941] orbicularis pupillary reflex.

pi•lu•la (pĭ′lu-lə) pl. *pi′lulae* [L.] pill. **pil′ular** *adj*

pil•ule (pil′ūl) [L. *pilula*] 1. a small pill. 2. pellet.

pi•lus (pi′ləs) gen. and pl. *pi′li* [L.] 1. hair. 2. in microbiology, one of the minute filamentous appendages of certain bacteria; they are considerably smaller and less rigid than flagella and are associated with antigenic properties and sex functions of the cell; called also *fimbria.*

pi′li annula′ti a condition in which hairs appear to have alternating bands of white because air cavities within the shaft reflect light rays back, giving a banded appearance.

pi′li bifurca′ti a rare hair abnormality in which shafts are split in two at various points but back together at other places.

pi′li canali′culi uncombable hair syndrome.

F p. a hollow tubular pilus possessed by (male) F^+ bacterial cells, which carry the F (fertility) plasmid. It forms a connection with a (female) F^- cell in conjugation to allow the transfer of genetic material.

pi′li incarna′ti a condition characterized by ingrown hairs; see under *hair.*

pi′li incarna′ti recur′vi a condition characterized by ingrown hairs that have repenetrated the skin after growing from the hair follicles.

pi′li multige′mini multiple hairs growing from the same follicle, as a result of deep division of its base, producing, in effect, a cluster of separate papillae.

pi′li tor′ti a condition such as Menkes disease that is characterized by twisted hairs (see under *hair*).

pi′li trian′guli et canali′culi uncombable hair syndrome.

Pima (pim′ə) trademark for a preparation of potassium iodide.

pim•e•cro•li•mus (pim″ə-kro-li′məs) a calcineurin inhibitor immunosuppressant produced by a variant of *Streptomyces hygroscopicus;* applied topically to treat moderate to severe atopic dermatitis.

pim•e•li•tis (pim″ə-li′tis) panniculitis.

pimel(o)- [Gr. *pimelē* lard] a combining form denoting relationship to fat.

pim•e•lo•ma (pim″ə-lo′mə) lipoma.

pim•e•lop•ter•yg•i•um (pim″ə-lo-tər-ij′e-əm) [*pimel-* + *pterygium*] a fatty outgrowth on the conjunctiva.

pim•el•or•thop•nea (pim″əl-or″thop-ne′ə) [*pimel-* + *orthopnea*] dyspnea while lying down, due to obesity. Called also *piorthopnea.*

pimo•ben•dan (pim-o-ben′dən) a phosphodiesterase inhibitor with inotropic and vasodilating properties, used to treat mitral valve disease in dogs; administered orally.

pi•mo•zide (pi′mə-zīd) an antipsychotic and antidyskinetic agent, a diphenylbutylpiperidine, used in the treatment of Gilles de la Tourette syndrome; administered orally.

Pim•pi•nel•la (pim″pĭ-nel′ə) [L.] a genus of plants of the family Umbelliferae. *P. ani′sum* L. is anise, a source of anise oil.

pim•ple (pim′pəl) a papule or pustule, usually of the face, neck, or upper trunk, most often due to acne vulgaris.

pin (pin) 1. a long slender metal rod for the fixation of the ends of fractured bones. 2. a peg or dowel by means of which an artificial crown is fixed to the root of a tooth.

friction-locked p., friction-retained p. a metal pin slightly larger than a hole drilled into dentin, forced into the hole and retained in place solely by friction.

Steinmann p. a metal rod for the internal fixation of fractures.

Pi•na•ceae (pi-na′se-e) a large family of evergreen trees and shrubs that have cones and either needles or leaves. It includes the genera *Abies, Pinus,* and *Tsuga.*

pin•a•cy•a•nol (pin″ə-si′ə-nol) an aniline dye used as a tissue stain and for sensitizing photographic plates for red.

Pi•nard maneuver (pe-nahr′) [Adolphe *Pinard,* French obstetrician, 1844–1934] see under *maneuver.*

pince-ci•seaux (pans″se-zo′) [Fr. "forceps-scissors"] a cutting forceps used in iridotomy.

pin•cers (pin′sərz) 1. forceps (def. 1). 2. the median deciduous incisors of the horse; called also *nippers.*

pinch (pinch) 1. to press an object tightly between the thumb and one finger. 2. an act of pinching; used as means of assessing hand dexterity. See also *grip.*

key p. lateral p.

lateral p. the act of pinching an object between the tip of the thumb and the radial side of the forefinger, as when turning a key.

pulp p. the act of pinching an object between the terminal pulp of the thumb and that of one finger.

tip p., tip to tip p. pulp p.

pin•cush•ion•ing (pin′coosh-ən-ing) pincushion deformity.

Pind•borg tumor (pind′borg) [Jens J. *Pindborg,* Danish oral pathologist, born 1921] see *calcifying epithelial odontogenic tumor,* under *tumor.*

pin•do•lol (pin′də-lol) [USP] a nonselective beta-adrenergic blocking agent with intrinsic sympathomimetic activity; administered orally in the treatment of hypertension, angina pectoris, and certain other cardiovascular disorders.

pin•done (pin′dōn) an indanedione anticoagulant used as a rodenticide; it can cause fatal anticoagulant rodenticide poisoning (q.v.) in many mammalian species.

pine[1] (pīn) [L. *pinus*] 1. any tree of the genus *Pinus.* 2. any of numerous other coniferous trees.

longleaf p. *Pinus palustris.*

southern p. *Pinus palustris.*

Swiss mountain p. *Pinus mugo.*

pine[2] (pīn) pining.

pin•e•al (pin′e-əl) [L. *pinealis; pinea* pine cone] 1. pertaining to the pineal body. 2. shaped like a pine cone.

pin•e•al•ec•to•my (pin″e-əl-ek′tə-me) [*pineal* body + *-ectomy*] excision of the pineal body.

pin•e•al•ism (pin′e-əl-iz″əm) any condition due to presumed abnormalities of pineal gland secretion; see also *hyperpinealism* and *hypopinealism.*

pin•e•a•lo•blas•to•ma (pin″e-ə-lo-blas-to′mə) a type of neuroepithelial tumor that is a pinealoma in which the pineal cells are not well differentiated. Called also *pineoblastoma.*

pin•e•a•lo•cyte (pin′e-ə-lo-sīt″) the principal cell of the pineal body, an epithelioid cell with pale-staining cytoplasm, prominent nucleoli, and large nuclei that may be irregularly infolded or lobulated; cords of these cells make up the body of the pineal body. See also *interstitial cells,* under *cell.* Called also *chief cell* and *pineal cell.*

pin•e•a•lo•cy•to•ma (pin″e-ə-lo-si-to′mə) pinealoma.

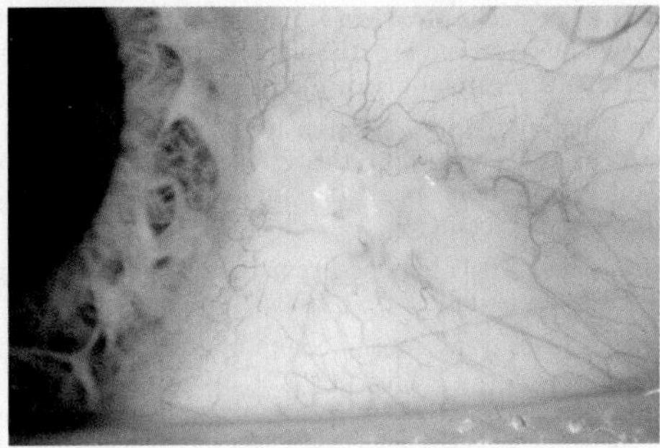
■ Pingueculae.

pin•e•a•lo•ma (pin″e-ə-lo′mə) an uncommon tumor of the pineal body composed of neoplastic nests of large epithelial cells; symptoms include hydrocephalus, conjugate paralysis of upward gaze, disturbances of gait, and precocious puberty, the last possibly due to the suppression of pineal secretion of melatonin. Called also *pinealocytoma* and *pineocytoma.*

ectopic p. pinealoma arising from pineal rests in the midline area, resulting in diabetes insipidus, compression of the optic chiasm, and hypopituitarism.

pin•e•a•lop•a•thy (pin″e-ə-lop′ə-the) any disease of the pineal gland.

pi•nene (pi′nēn) a terpene found in turpentine and many essential oils; used as a solvent and in the manufacture of synthetic camphor, insecticides, and synthetic pine oil.

pin•eo•blas•to•ma (pin″e-o-blas-to′mə) pinealoblastoma.

pin•eo•cy•to•ma (pin″e-o-si-to′mə) pinealoma.

pin•gue•cu•la (ping-gwĕ′ku-lə) gen. and pl. *pingue′culae* [L. "somewhat fatty"] a yellowish spot of proliferation on the bulbar conjunctiva near the sclerocorneal junction, usually on the nasal side; seen in elderly people.

pin•gui•cu•la (ping-gwĭ′ku-lə) pinguecula.

pin•i•form (pin′ĭ-form) [L. *pinea* pine cone + *form*] conical or cone-shaped.

pin•ing (pīn′ing) enzootic marasmus in Scotland due to cobalt deficiency; called also *pine.*

pink•eye (pink′i) 1. acute contagious conjunctivitis. 2. infectious keratoconjunctivitis.

Pin•kus tumor (ping′kəs) [Hermann Karl Benno *Pinkus*, German-born American dermatologist, 1905–1985] premalignant fibroepithelioma.

pin•ledge (pin′lej) a flat floor or shoulder prepared within the tooth structure, into which pin holes are drilled to accommodate pins in a pin-retained cast restoration.

pin•na (pin′ə) [L. "wing"] auricula (def. 1). **pin′nal** *adj*

hairy pinnae hypertrichosis pinnae auris.

pino•cyte (pin′o-, pi′no-sīt) a cell that exhibits pinocytosis.

pino•cyt•ic (pin″o-, pi″no-sit′ik) pertaining to a pinocyte or to pinocytosis.

pino•cy•to•sis (pin″o-, pi″no-si-to′sis) [Gr. *pinein* to drink + *cyto-* + *-osis*] the cellular uptake of extracellular fluid and its contents by enclosing them in vesicles derived from the plasma membrane; it serves as a method of transport for macromolecules. Cf. *macropinocytosis.* **pinocytot′ic** *adj*

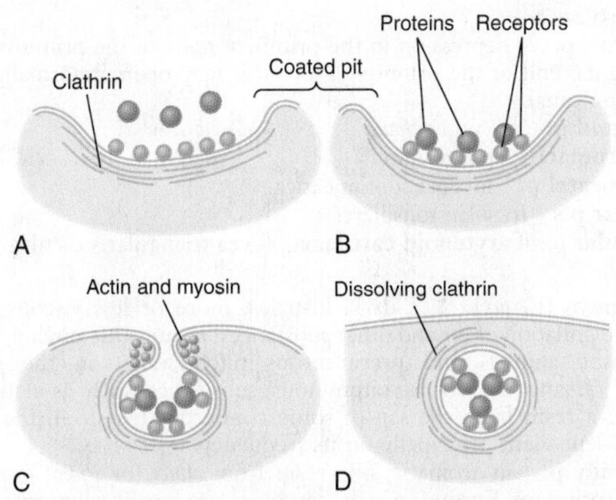

■ Mechanism of pinocytosis of extracellular proteins.

pino•some (pin′o-, pi′no-sōm) [Gr. *pinein* to drink + *-some*] any of the small fluid-filled vesicles found in the cytoplasm during pinocytosis, formed by invaginations of the cell membrane (caveolae) which pinch off and become free. Called also *pinocytotic vesicle.*

Pins sign (pins) [Emil *Pins*, Austrian physician, 1845–1913] Ewart sign.

pint (pt) (pīnt) a unit of liquid measure; in the United States it is 16 fluid ounces, or the equivalent of 0.473 liter. In Great Britain, it is the *imperial pint* and is 20 fluid ounces, or the equivalent of 0.568 liter.

pin•ta (pēn′tah) [Sp. "painted"] a form of treponematosis endemic in certain parts of tropical America, characterized by discolored spots on the skin that may be white, brown, blue, red, or violet; it is caused by *Treponema carateum*, and patients usually have a positive Wassermann reaction. It is believed to be transmitted usually by direct person-to-person contact.

pin•tid (pin′tid) one of the flat erythematous skin lesions constituting the spreading eruption occurring in the second stage of pinta.

Pi•nus (pi′nus) the pines, a large genus of coniferous evergreen trees of the family Pinaceae.

P. mu′go the Swiss mountain pine, a usually low, shrubby pine native to southern Europe; it and its dwarf variant, *P. mu′go* var. *pumi′lio*, are sources of pine needle or dwarf pine needle oil.

P. palus′tris the longleaf or southern pine of the southern United States, a source of pine oil, rosin, turpentine, and other products.

pi•nus (pi′nəs) [L.] glandula pinealis.

pin•worm (pin′wurm″) oxyurid.

pi(o)- [Gr. *piōn* fat] a combining form denoting relationship to fat. See also words beginning *lip(o)-*.

pio•epi•the•li•um (pi″o-ep″ĭ-the′le-əm) [*pio-* + *epithelium*] epithelium in which fatty matter is deposited.

pi•o•glit•a•zone hy•dro•chlo•ride (pi″o-glit′ə-zōn) a thiazolidinedione antidiabetic agent that decreases insulin resistance in the peripheral tissues and liver, used in the treatment of type 2 diabetes mellitus; administered orally.

pi•on (pi′on) [*pi* meso*n*] a subatomic particle, which may be positive, negative, or neutral, with mass intermediate between that of an electron and that of a proton; it carries the force that binds the atomic nucleus together. It is an example of a meson.

Pi•oph•i•la (pi-of′ĭ-lə) a genus of flies. *P. ca′sei* is a fly whose larva is the cheese skipper, a common cause of intestinal myiasis.

pi•or•thop•nea (pi″or-thop′ne-ə, pi″or-thop-ne′ə) pimelorthopnea.

Pi•o•trow•ski sign (reflex) (pe″o-trov′ske) [Alexander *Piotrowski*, German neurologist, 20th century] see under *sign.*

PIP 1. phosphatidylinositol 4-phosphate. 2. proximal interphalangeal; see under *joint.*

PIP_2 phosphatidylinositol 4,5-bisphosphate.

pi•pam•pe•rone (pĭ-pam′pə-rōn) an antipsychotic that has been used in the treatment of schizophrenia.

pip•az•e•thate hy•dro•chlo•ride (pĭ-paz′ə-thāt) a nonnarcotic antitussive; administered orally.

pip•ecol•ic ac•id (pip″ə-kol′ik) a cyclic amino acid occurring as an intermediate in a minor pathway of lysine degradation and at elevated levels in blood in cerebrohepatorenal syndrome and in hyperlysinemia.

pip•e•cu•ro•ni•um bro•mide (pip″ə-ku-ro′ne-əm) a nondepolarizing neuromuscular blocking agent used as an adjunct to anesthesia, inducing skeletal muscle relaxation and facilitating the management of patients on mechanical ventilation; administered intravenously.

Pi•per (pi′pər) [L. "pepper"] a genus of plants of the family Piperaceae, native to southern Asia, Malaysia, and Indonesia. *P. bet′le* is betel, whose leaf is used in the masticatory also called betel. *P. cube′ba* L. f. is the tailed or Java pepper, whose fruit is the cubeb. *P. methys′ticum* is the kava plant (see *kava kava*).

pi•per•a•cil•lin (pi-per′ə-sil″in) [USP] a semisynthetic broad-spectrum penicillin of the ureidopenicillin group, effective against a wide variety of gram-positive and gram-negative aerobic and anaerobic bacteria.

p. sodium [USP] the sodium salt of piperacillin, used in the treatment of infections caused by susceptible organisms and in intra-abdominal surgery for the prevention of infection; administered intramuscularly or intravenously.

pi•per•az•i•dine (pi″pər-az′ĭ-dēn) piperazine.

pi•per•a•zine (pi-per′ə-zēn) [USP] an anthelmintic effective against the parasites *Ascaris lumbricoides* and *Enterobius vermicularis;* it causes a flaccid paralysis of the worm musculature by altering cell membrane permeability and causing hyperpolarization of the membrane. Called also *diethylenediamine* and *piperazidine.*

p. citrate [USP] the citrate salt of piperazine, used in treatment of intestinal roundworm and pinworm infections; administered orally.

p. phosphate the phosphate salt of piperazine, used in treatment of intestinal roundworm and trematode infections.

pi•per•ism (pi′pər-iz-əm) [L. *piper* pepper] poisoning by pepper.

pi•per•o•caine hy•dro•chlo•ride (pi′pər-o-kān″) a local anesthetic used for topical, infiltration, regional, spinal, and caudal anesthesia.

pi•per•o•nyl bu•tox•ide (pi-pur′o-nəl) a synergist used mainly in veterinary medicine in combination with pyrethrins in insecticides and pediculicides.

pi•pet (pi-pet′) pipette.

pi•pette (pi-pet′) [Fr.] 1. a glass or transparent plastic tube used in measuring or transferring small quantities of liquid or gas. 2. to dispense fluid or gas by means of a pipette.

Pi•pi•zan (pi′pĭ-zan) trademark for a preparation of piperazine.

pi•po•bro•man (pĭ″po-bro′mən) an antineoplastic alkylating agent used in the treatment of polycythemia vera, administered orally.

Pip•ra•cil (pip″rə-sil) trademark for a preparation of piperacillin sodium.

pi•pra•drol hy•dro•chlo•ride (pĭ′prə-drol) a central nervous system stimulant, administered orally.

Pip•ta•de•nia (pip″tə-de′ne-ə) a genus of tropical shrubs and trees of the family Leguminosae. Some species from Brazil yield seeds that are made into the narcotic psychotomimetic snuff called *parica.*

Pip•to•ceph•a•lis (pip″to-sef′ə-lis) a genus of fungi of the order Zoopagales; some species contain trichothecenes and can cause alimentary toxic aleukia.

pi•qûre (pe-kūr′) [Fr.] puncture, especially Bernard (diabetic) puncture.

pir•ac•e•tam (pi-ras′ə-tam) a nootropic drug used in treatment of myoclonus of cortical origin; administered orally.

pir•bu•ter•ol (pir-bu′tər-ol) a sympathomimetic agent specific for beta$_2$ receptors, used as a bronchodilator.

p. acetate the acetate ester of pirbuterol, used as a bronchodilator for the treatment of asthma-associated bronchospasm and the treatment and prophylaxis of bronchospasm associated with chronic bronchitis, pulmonary emphysema, or other chronic obstructive airway disease; administered by oral inhalation.

p. hydrochloride the hydrochloride salt of pirbuterol, having actions and uses similar to the acetate ester.

Pi•re•nel•la (pi″rə-nel′ə) a genus of snails of the family Cerithiidae, order Mesogastropoda. *P. co′nica* is a species found in Egypt that is a host of the intestinal fluke *Heterophyes heterophyes.*

pir•en•ze•pine hy•dro•chlo•ride (pir″ən-zĕ′pēn) an antagonist of certain muscarinic receptors that has minimal anticholinergic effects and does not cross the blood-brain barrier, used to inhibit gastric secretion in peptic ulcer.

pir•i•form (pir′ĭ-form) [L. *pirum* a pear + *form*] pear-shaped.

Pi•ro•goff amputation, angle, triangle (pe′ro-gof) [Nikolai Ivanovich *Pirogoff,* Russian surgeon, 1810–1881] see under *amputation,* see *venous angle,* under *angle* and see *hypoglossohyoid triangle,* under *triangle.*

pi•ro•plasm (pi′ro-plaz″əm) any protozoan of the subclass Piroplasmia. Called also *piroplasmid.*

Pi•ro•plas•ma (pi″ro-plaz′mə) former name for *Babesia.*

Pi•ro•plas•mia (pi″ro-plaz-me′ə) [L. *pirum* pear + *plasma*] a subclass of heteroxenous parasitic protozoa (class Sporozoea, subphylum Apicomplexa), occurring as piriform, round, or rod-shaped cells or ameboid cells without a conoid, oocysts, spores, pseudocysts, and flagella, and usually without subpellicular microtubules but with a polar ring and rhoptries. Locomotion is accomplished by flexion, by gliding, or, in sexual stages of certain species, by large axopodium-like organelles *(strahlen).* They are parasitic in the erythrocytes and other circulating and fixed cells of the host, with merogony occurring in vertebrates and sporogony in invertebrates, and producing sporozoites with a single-membraned wall. Ticks are the vectors of most of the piroplasmids. It comprises a single order: Piroplasmida.

pi•ro•plas•mid (pi″ro-plaz′mid) 1. pertaining or relating to protozoa of the subclass Piroplasmia. 2. piroplasm.

Pi•ro•plas•mi•da (pi″ro-plaz′mĭ-də) an order of protozoa (subclass Piroplasmia, class Sporozoea) having the characters of the subclass. Representative genera include *Babesia, Cytauxzoon, Dactylosoma,* and *Theileria.*

pi•ro•plas•mo•sis (pi″ro-plaz-mo′sis) 1. babesiosis. 2. infection by any species of Piroplasmida.

tropical p. see under *theileriasis.*

pir•o•xan•trone hy•dro•chlo•ride (pir″o-zan′trōn) a cytotoxic compound that causes DNA strand breaks and cross-linking; used investigationally in the treatment of carcinoma of the breast.

pir•ox•i•cam (pir-ok′sĭ-kam) a nonsteroidal antiinflammatory drug used for treatment of rheumatoid arthritis, osteoarthritis, ankylosing spondylitis, gout, calcium pyrophosphate deposition disease, and dysmenorrhea; administered orally or rectally.

Pir•quet test (pir-ket′) [Clemens Freiherr von *Pirquet,* Austrian pediatrician, 1874–1929] see under *test.*

pis•ci•cide (pis′ĭ-sīd) any substance poisonous to fish.

Pis•cid•ia (pĭ-sid′e-ə) [L. *piscis* fish + *caedere* to kill] a genus of trees of the family Leguminosae. *P. pisci′pula* (L.) Sarg. (formerly called *P. erythri′na* L.) is Jamaica dogwood, whose bark is a mild anodyne.

pis•ci•din (pĭ-si′din) a neutral principle from *Piscidia piscipula* (L.) Sarg., an anodyne and antispasmodic.

pi•si•form (pi′sĭ-form, piz′ĭ-form) [L. *pisum* pea + *form*] resembling a pea in shape and size.

pi•si•for•mis (pi″sĭ-for′mis) [L.] pisiform.

Pis•ka•cek sign (pis′kə-chek″) [Ludwig *Piskacek,* Austrian obstetrician, 1854–1933] see under *sign.*

Pis•ta•cia (pis-ta′shə) a genus of shrubs and small trees of the family Anacardiaceae, native to various parts of the Northern Hemisphere. *P. lentis′cus* is the mastic tree, source of mastic.

pis•til (pis′til) [L. *pistillus* a pestle] gynecium.

Pi•sum (pi′səm) a genus of vines of the family Leguminosae. *P. sati′vum* is the pea.

PIT plasma iron turnover.

pit (pit) 1. a fovea or indentation, either normal or abnormal. 2. pockmark. 3. to become indented for a short period of time; see *pitting.*

anal p. proctodeum.

arm p. armpit.

auditory p. otic p..

basilar p. a pit in the crown of an incisor tooth above its neck.

coated p's small receptor-bearing pits in the plasma membrane, coated with clathrin on the cytoplasmic surface, that pinch off to form clathrin-coated vesicles enclosing the ligands in receptor-mediated endocytosis.

costal p. fovea costalis inferior.

distal p. fovea distalis dentis.

ear p. preauricular p.

gastric p's foveolae gastricae.

Gaul p's depressions in the corneal epithelium seen in neuroparalytic keratitis.

Herbert p's a characteristic defect left after the healing of a limbal follicle in trachoma.

lens p. a pitlike depression in the ectoderm of the lens placode where the primordial lens is developing.

mesial p. fovea mesialis dentis.

nasal p. olfactory p.

oblong p. of arytenoid cartilage fovea oblonga cartilaginis arytenoideae.

olfactory p. the primordium of a nasal cavity.

otic p. a distinct depression appearing in each otic placode, marking the beginning of embryonic development of the internal ear. Called also *auditory p.* and *otic depression.*

postanal p. foveola coccygea.

preauricular p. a slight depression anterior to the helix and superior to the tragus, sometimes leading to a congenital preauricular cyst or fistula. Called also *ear p.*

primitive p. a depression in the primitive node of the primitive streak at the cranial end of the primitive groove; it may open abnormally into a neurenteric canal.

pterygoid p. see under *fovea.*

p. of stomach epigastrium.

suprameatal p. foveola suprameatica.

tonsillar p's fossulae tonsillares.

triangular p. of arytenoid cartilage fovea triangularis cartilaginis arytenoideae.

pitch (pich) [L. *pix*] 1. a dark, lustrous, more or less viscous residue from the distillation of tar and other substances; it can cause pitch poisoning in domestic animals and precancerous pitch warts on the skin of humans. 2. any of various bituminous substances such as natural asphalt. 3. a resin from the sap of some coniferous trees. 4. the quality of sound dependent principally on its frequency.

Burgundy p. an aromatic, oily resin from *Abies* (or *Picea*) *excelsa,* the Norway spruce of Europe, which has been used as a counterirritant in plasters.

Canada p. a resin from *Tsuga canadensis,* the hemlock tree, used in plasters.

pitch•blende (pich′blend) a black mineral containing uranium oxide; from it are obtained radium, polonium, and uranium.

pith (pith) 1. to pierce the spinal cord or brain; see *pithing.* 2. the soft tissue found in plant stems that often disappears so that the stem becomes hollow. 3. the central core of colorless parenchymatous cells in stems and some roots.

pith•e•coid (pith′ə-koid) [Gr. *pithēkos* ape + *-oid*] apelike.

pith•ing (pith′ing) destruction of the brain and spinal cord by thrusting a blunt needle into the spinal canal and cranium; done on animals to destroy sensibility preparatory to experimenting on their living tissues.

Pith•o•my•ces (pith″o-mi′sēz) a genus of Fungi Imperfecti of the form-family Dematiaceae. *P. charta′rum* contains sporidesmin and causes facial eczema of ruminants.

pith•o•my•co•tox•i•co•sis (pith″o-mi″ko-tok″sĭ-ko′sis) a form of mycotoxicosis in animals from ingestion of fungi of the genus *Pithomyces,* resulting in liver damage and facial eczema of ruminants (see under *eczema*).

Pi•to•cin (pĭ-to′sin) trademark for preparations of oxytocin.

Pi•tres rule, sign (pe′trə) [Jean Albert *Pitres,* French physician, 1848–1927] see under *rule* and *sign.*

Pi•tres•sin (pĭ-tres′in) trademark for a preparation of vasopressin.

pit•ta (pit′ə) [Sanskrit "bile"] according to ayurveda, one of the three doshas, or principles of constitution of the body, condensed from the elements fire and water. Pitta is the principle of transformation energy and governs heat and metabolism in the body, and is concerned with the digestive, enzymatic, and endocrine systems. It is eliminated from the body through sweat.

pit•ting (pit′ing) 1. the formation, usually by scarring, of a small depression. 2. becoming indented with firm pressure and remaining that way when the pressure is removed; see under *edema.* 3. the removal from erythrocytes, by the spleen, of certain structures, such as iron granules, without destruction of the cells.

pi•tu•i•cyte (pĭ-too′ĭ-sīt) [*pituitary* +*-cyte*] any of the dominant and distinctive fusiform cells of the neurohypophysis, which are intermingled with nerve fibers and are regarded as specialized neuroglial cells. According to their morphological appearance on staining with silver, four subtypes are distinguished: adeno-, fibro-, reticulo-, and micropituicytes.

pi•tu•i•ta (pĭ-too′ĭ-tə) [L.] a glutinous mucus.

pi•tu•i•ta•rism (pĭ-too′ĭ-tə-riz″əm) disorder of pituitary function; see *hyperpituitarism* and *hypopituitarism.*

pi•tu•i•tary (pĭ-too′ĭ-tar″e) [L. *pituita* phlegm] 1. hypophysial. 2. hypophysis. 3. a preparation of some part of the pituitary gland of animals (e.g., cattle, pigs, sheep), used therapeutically.

anterior p. 1. adenohypophysis. 2. a preparation of the dried, partially defatted, powdered adenohypophysis of hogs, sheep, or cattle.

pharyngeal p. see under *hypophysis.*

posterior p. 1. neurohypophysis. 2. a powdered preparation of the dried neurohypophysis of certain food animals, having the pharmacological actions of its hormones, *oxytocin* and *vasopressin;* used mainly as an antidiuretic in the treatment of central diabetes insipidus, administered subcutaneously, by nasal inhalation, or by topical application to the nasal mucosa. It may be used to stimulate smooth muscle tissue, especially to produce vasoconstriction in the presence of hemorrhage.

whole p. a preparation of the dried, partially defatted, powdered whole pituitary gland of certain food animals.

pi•tu•i•tec•to•my (pĭ-too″ĭ-tek′tə-me) hypophysectomy.

pit•y•ri•a•sis (pit″ĭ-ri′ə-sis) [Gr. *pityron* bran + *-iasis*] any of various skin diseases characterized by fine, branny scales.

acute lichenoid p. p. lichenoides et varioliformis acuta.

p. al′ba a skin disorder most commonly seen in children or adolescents, usually involving the face, and characterized by round, slightly scaling, hypopigmented patches; it usually involutes spontaneously. Called also *p. maculata, p. simplex,* and *p. streptogenes.*

p. amianta′cea see under *tinea.*

chronic lichenoid p. pityriasis lichenoides chronica.

p. circina′ta p. rotunda.

lichenoid p., p. lichenoi′des a rare, self-limited type of pityriasis with discolored papular lesions, defined as part of the parapsoriasis family; it encompasses a spectrum from pityriasis lichenoides et varioliformis acuta to pityriasis lichenoides chronica.

p. lichenoi′des acu′ta p. lichenoides et varioliformis acuta.

p. lichenoi′des chro′nica a chronic, brown, scaly, macular eruption, usually on the trunk, with epidermal alterations and a perivascular lymphocytic infiltrate. It may either represent progression of pityriasis lichenoides et varioliformis acuta or arise de novo. Called also *chronic p.* and *chronic* or *guttate parapsoriasis.*

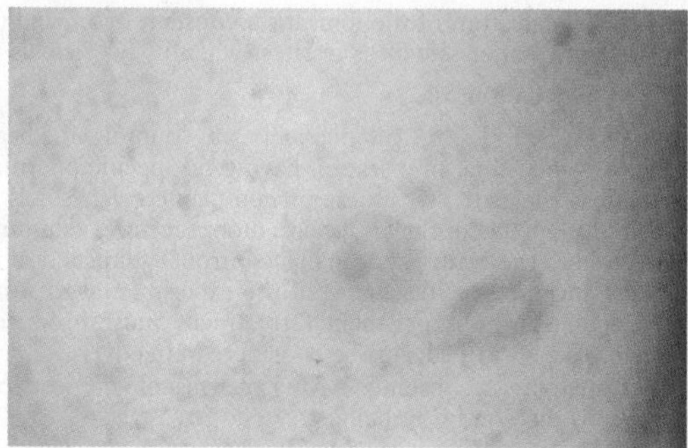

■ Herald patch and surrounding lesions of pityriasis rosea.

p. lichenoi′des et variolifor′mis acu′ta (PLEVA) an acute or subacute, sometimes relapsing, widespread macular, papular, or vesicular eruption that tends to crusting, necrosis, and hemorrhage, which heals to leave pigmented depressed scars, followed by a new crop of lesions. Occasionally, progression to chronic lichenoid pityriasis may occur. Called also *acute lichenoid p., p. lichenoides acuta, acute parapsoriasis,* and *Habermann, Mucha-Habermann,* or *Mucha disease.*

p. lin′guae benign migratory glossitis.

p. macula′ta p. alba.

p. ni′gra tinea nigra.

p. ro′sea a common, acute or subacute, self-limited, exanthematous disease of unknown etiology, whose onset is marked by a solitary pink, reddish, or tan plaque called a herald patch, usually on the trunk, upper limbs, or thighs; subsequent lesions are similar to this but smaller, with vesicular borders, tending to peel and produce a scaly collarette.

p. rotun′da a form of acquired ichthyosis manifested by round, brown, scaly, sharply demarcated patches on the trunk and limbs. The etiology is unknown; some cases may be hereditary, and sometimes it worsens in winter and improves in summer.

p. ru′bra exfoliative dermatitis.

p. ru′bra pila′ris a chronic, inflammatory, cutaneous disease characterized by a patchy rash that begins on the scalp, chest, or face and progresses down the body; there are numerous tiny, red to brown, follicular papules topped by horny plugs that have embedded hairs; there may also be solid confluent hyperkeratosis of the palms and soles with a tendency to fissuring.

p. sic′ca dandruff (def. 2).

p. sim′plex p. alba.

p. sim′plex capilli′tii, p. sim′plex ca′pitis dandruff.

p. steatoi′des an oily variety of dandruff with waxy scales and sometimes an odor.

p. strepto′genes p. alba.

p. versi′color tinea versicolor.

pit•y•roid (pit′ĭ-roid) 1. furfuraceous. 2. branny.

Pit•y•ros•po•ron (pit″ĭ-ros′pə-ron) former name for *Malassezia.*

Pit•y•ros•po•rum (pit″ĭ-ros′pə-rəm) [Gr. *pityron* bran + *sporos* seed] former name for *Malassezia. P. orbicula′re* is *M. furfur* and *P. ova′le* is *M. ovalis.*

piv•a•late (piv′ə-lāt) USAN contraction for trimethylacetate.

piv•am•pi•cil•lin hy•dro•chlo•ride (piv-am″pĭ-sil′in) a derivative of ampicillin, having the same broad spectrum of antibacterial activity and uses as ampicillin.

piv•me•cil•li•nam (piv″mə-sil′ĭ-nəm) INN and BAN for amdinocillin pivoxil.

piv•ot (piv′ət) 1. that on which something turns, such as a dowel or short post. 2. the point of rotation for a removable partial denture.

occlusal p. an elevation contrived on the occlusal surface, usually in the molar region, designed to act as a fulcrum and to induce sagittal mandibular rotation.

pix•el (pik′sel) [contraction of *pix* (short for *pictures*) + *el*ement] a two-dimensional region defining a unit of area on a video display screen.

pi•zo•ty•line (pĭ-zo′tĭ-lēn) an anabolic, antidepressant, and serotonin inhibitor used in treatment of migraine.

piz•zle (piz′əl) popular term used in veterinary medicine for the penis of an animal.

PJRT permanent junctional reciprocating tachycardia.

PJT paroxysmal junctional tachycardia; see *paroxysmal tachycardia,* under *tachycardia.*

PK pyruvate kinase.

pK_a the negative logarithm of the ionization constant of an acid (K_a); the buffering power of a buffer system is greatest when its pK_a equals the pH.

PKU, PKU1 phenylketonuria.

pla•ce•bo (plə-se′bo) [L. "I will please"] any dummy medical treatment; originally, a medicinal preparation having no specific pharmacological activity against the patient's illness or complaint given solely for the psychophysiological effects of the treatment; more recently, a dummy treatment administered to the control group in a controlled clinical trial in order that the specific and nonspecific effects of the experimental treatment can be distinguished—i.e., the experimental treatment must produce better results than the placebo in order to be considered effective.

active p., impure p. a substance having pharmacologic properties that are not relevant to the condition being treated.

place•ment (plās′mənt) position or arrangement, as of the teeth.

lingual p. displacement of a tooth toward the tongue.

pla•cen•ta (plə-sen′tə) pl. *placentas, placen′tae* [L. "a flat cake"] a feto-maternal organ characteristic of true mammals during pregnancy, joining mother and fetus, providing endocrine secretion and selective exchange of soluble, bloodborne substances through an apposition of uterine and trophoblastic vascularized parts. According to species, the area of vascular apposition may be *diffuse, cotyledonary, zonary,* or *discoid;* the nature of apposition may be *labyrinthine* or *villous;* and the intimacy of apposition may vary according to what layers are lost of those originally interposed between maternal and fetal blood (maternal endothelium, uterine connective tissue, uterine epithelium, chorion, extraembryonic mesoderm, and endothelium of villous capillary). The chorion may be joined by and receive blood vessels from either the yolk sac or the allantois, and the uterine lining may be largely shed with the chorion at birth *(deciduate p.)* or may separate from the chorion and remain *(nondeciduate p.).* The human placenta is *discoid, villous, hemochorial, chorioallantoic,* and *deciduate.* After birth, it weighs about 600 g and is about 16 cm in diameter and 2 cm thick, discounting the decidua basalis and the maternal blood in the intervillous space (a principal functional part into which the chorionic villi dip and which leaks out at birth). The villi are grouped into adjoining cotyledons making about 20 velvety bumps on the side of the placenta facing the uterus; the side facing the fetus is smooth and covered with amnion, a thin avascular layer that continues past the edges of the placenta to line the entire hollow sphere of chorion except where it is reflected to cover the umbilical cord. The umbilical cord joins fetus and placenta and usually joins the placenta near the center, although it sometimes inserts at the edge, on the nonplacental chorion, or on an accessory placenta.

accessory p. a placenta that is separate from the main placenta.

p. accre′ta abnormal adherence of part or all of the placenta to the uterine wall, with partial or complete absence of the decidua basalis, especially of the spongiosum layer.

adherent p. a placenta that adheres closely to the wall of the uterus.

annular p. a placenta that extends around the interior of the uterus like a ring or belt.

battledore p. a placenta that has marginal insertion of the umbilical cord.

bidiscoid p. a placenta that has two separate discoid masses, seen in macaques but not humans.

bilobate p., bilobed p. a placenta consisting of two lobes.

p. biparti′ta, bipartite p. bilobate p.

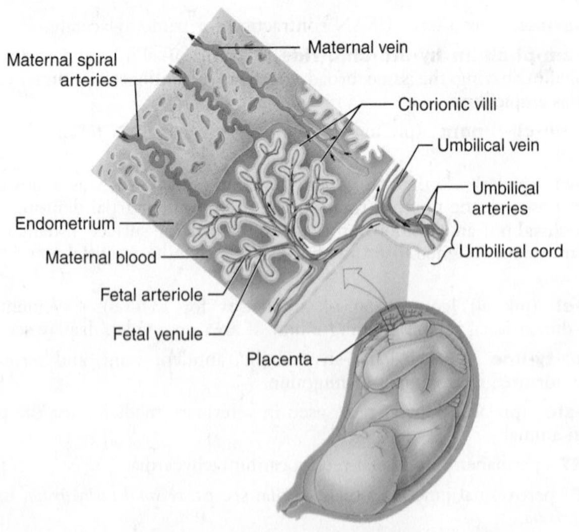

■ Structural features of the placenta.

chorioallantoic p. a placenta in which the allantois joins the chorion or provides its major blood supply.

choriovitelline p. a type of placenta in which the yolk sac becomes an intermediary in the fetal-maternal relationship.

circummarginate p. a placenta that has a smaller ridge of membranous tissue ringing its edge than that seen in a circumvallate placenta.

p. circumvalla′ta, circumvallate p. a placenta in which a dense peripheral ring is raised from the surface and the attached membranes are doubled back over the edge of the placenta.

cirsoid p., p. cirsoi′des a placenta whose vessels appear to be varicose.

complete p. previa placenta previa centralis.

deciduate p., deciduous p. a placenta or type of placentation in which the decidua or maternal parts separate from the uterus and are cast off together with the fetal membranes.

p. diffu′sa 1. a placenta whose tissue is distributed over the chorionic membrane, as in horses and pigs. 2. p. membranacea.

p. dimidia′ta, dimidiate p. bilobate p.

discoid p., p. discoi′dea a disk-shaped placenta.

Duncan p. a placenta that is expelled with the chorionic surface outward; cf. *Schultze p.*

duplex p. bilobate p.

endotheliochorial p. a placenta in which syncytial trophoblast embeds maternal vessels that are bared to their endothelial lining.

epitheliochorial p. a placenta whose uterine epithelial lining is not eroded but merely lies in apposition to the chorion.

p. fenestra′ta a placenta that has spots where tissue is lacking.

fetal p. fetal part of placenta.

fundal p. a placenta that is attached to the fundus of the uterus in the normal manner.

furcate p. lobed p.

hemochorial p. a placenta in which maternal blood comes in direct contact with the chorion; this is the usual type seen in humans.

hemoendothelial p. a placenta in which maternal blood comes in contact with the endothelium of chorionic vessels; this does not occur in humans.

horseshoe p. a type of crescent-shaped placenta sometimes seen in a twin pregnancy.

incarcerated p. retained p.

incomplete p. previa placenta previa partialis.

p. incre′ta placenta accreta with penetration of the myometrium.

labyrinthine p. a placenta in which maternal blood courses in channeled trophoblasts.

lateral p. previa placenta previa marginalis.

lobed p. a placenta that is more or less subdivided into lobes; called also *furcate p.*

maternal p. maternal part of placenta.

p. membrana′cea a placenta that is abnormally thin and spread out over a large area of the uterine wall.

multilobate p., multilobed p., p. multiparti′ta a placenta that has more than three lobes.

p. nappifor′mis p. circumvallata.

nondeciduate p., nondeciduous p. a placenta whose maternal component remains in the uterus instead of being cast off together with the trophoblastic derivatives.

p. percre′ta placenta accreta with invasion of the myometrium all the way to its peritoneal covering, sometimes invading other structures such as the bladder.

p. pre′via a placenta that develops in the lower uterine segment, in the zone of dilatation, so that it covers or adjoins the internal os; painless hemorrhage in the last trimester, particularly during the eighth month, is the most common symptom.

p. pre′via centra′lis central placenta previa; one in which the placenta entirely covers the internal os; called also *complete* or *total placenta previa.*

p. pre′via margina′lis marginal placenta previa; one in which the placenta is just palpable at the margin of the os; called also *lateral placenta previa.*

p. pre′via partia′lis partial placenta previa; one in which the internal os is partially covered; called also *incomplete placenta previa.*

p. reflex′a a placenta whose margin is thickened and appears to turn back on itself.

p. renifor′mis a kidney-shaped placenta.

retained p. a placenta that is either adherent or incarcerated and in consequence fails to be expelled after childbirth.

Schultze p. a placenta that is delivered with the gestation sac inside out, the amnion providing a smooth, glistening surface. Cf. *Duncan p.*

p. spu′ria an accessory placenta that has no blood vessel attachment to the main placenta.

p. succenturia′ta, succenturiate p. an accessory portion attached to the main placenta by an artery and vein.

syndesmochorial p. a type of placenta in which the lining epithelium of the uterus is the only maternal tissue eroded; this type does not occur in humans.

total p. previa placenta previa centralis.

p. tri'loba, trilobate p. a placenta that has three lobes.

p. triparti'ta, tripartite p., p. trip'lex trilobate p.

uterine p. maternal part of placenta.

velamentous p. a placenta in which the umbilical cord is attached to the adjoining membranes, with the umbilical vessels entering the placenta separately.

villous p. a placenta having villi that are outgrowths of the chorion, such as in humans.

yolk-sac p. choriovitelline p.

zonary p., zonular p. 1. annular p. 2. a belt-shaped placenta, as occurs in carnivores.

pla•cen•tal (plə-sen'təl) 1. pertaining to the placenta. 2. a mammal whose young receive nourishment in utero by means of a placenta.

Pla•cen•ta•lia (pla″sən-ta'le-ə) a division of mammals whose embryos are nourished through a placenta; it includes all mammals except marsupials and monotremes.

plac•en•ta•tion (plas″ən-ta'shən) the process of placenta formation and the result, especially with respect to taxonomically relevant aspects of structure. See *placenta.*

plac•en•ti•tis (plas″ən-ti'tis) inflammation of the placenta.

placent(o)- [L. "a flat cake"] a combining form denoting relationship to the placenta.

pla•cen•to•gen•e•sis (plə-sen″to-jen'ə-sis) [*placento-* + *genesis*] the origin and development of the placenta.

pla•cen•to•gram (plə-sen'to-gram″) a film taken in placentography.

plac•en•tog•ra•phy (plas″ən-tog'rə-fe) radiological visualization of the placenta after the injection of a contrast medium.

indirect p. radiographic measurement of the space between the placenta and the presenting head of the fetus, for the recognition of placenta previa.

pla•cen•toid (plə-sen'toid) resembling the placenta.

plac•en•tol•o•gist (plas″ən-tol'ə-jist) a specialist in placentology.

plac•en•tol•o•gy (plas″ən-tol'ə-je) [*placento-* + *-logy*] the scientific study of the development, structure, and functioning of the placenta.

comparative p. the scientific study of the development, structure, and functioning of the placenta in different species of animals.

plac•en•to•ma (plas″ən-to'mə) deciduoma.

plac•en•top•a•thy (plas″ən-top'ə-the) [*placento-* + *-pathy*] any disease of the placenta.

Pla•ci•do disk (plah'se-do) [Antonio *Placido* da Costa, Portuguese ophthalmologist, 1848–1916] see under *disk.*

Plac•i•dyl (plas'ĭ-dəl) trademark for a preparation of ethchlorvynol.

plac•ode (plak'ōd) [Gr. *plax* plate + *eidos* form] a platelike structure, especially a thickened plate of ectoderm in the early embryo, from which a sense organ develops.

auditory p. otic p.

dorsolateral p's a series of placodes giving rise to the acoustic and lateral line organs.

epibranchial p's a series of placodes located dorsal to the pharyngeal (branchial) grooves; they contribute to adjacent cerebral ganglia.

lens p. a thickened area of ectoderm directly overlying the optic vesicle in the early embryo, from which the lens develops.

nasal p., olfactory p. an oval area of thickened ectoderm on the ventrolateral surface of the head of the early embryo, constituting the first indication of the olfactory organ.

otic p. a thickened ectodermal plate located midway alongside the hindbrain in the early embryo, from which the internal ear ultimately develops. Called also *auditory p.*.

plac•oid (plak'oid) platelike or plaquelike.

pla•fond (plah-fon') [Fr. "ceiling"] facies articularis inferior tibiae; so called from its vaulted shape.

pla•gio•ceph•a•ly (pla″je-o-sef'ə-le) [Gr. *plagios* oblique + *-cephaly*] an asymmetric condition of the head, resulting from irregular closure of the cranial sutures. **plagiocephal'ic** *adj*

occipital p., positional p. plagiocephaly with flattening in the occipital region, sometimes related to an infant's continual lying on the back; a unilateral type is seen with torticollis.

plague (plāg) [L. *plaga, pestis;* Gr. *plēgē* stroke] 1. a severe acute or chronic enzootic or epizootic bacterial infection caused by *Yersinia pestis,* which occurs both endemically and epidemically worldwide; it is primarily a disease of urban and sylvatic rodents and is transmitted to humans by the bite of infected fleas, especially species of *Leptopsylla, Nosopsylla,* and *Xenopsylla,* or by contact with or ingestion of infected animals. Human-to-human infection usually occurs by inhalation of plague bacilli–laden droplet aerosols. The most common forms in humans are bubonic plague, pulmonic plague, and septicemic plague. 2. any of various contagious diseases in animals. Called also *pest* and *pestis.*

ambulatory p. a mild form of bubonic plague, usually occurring only in endemic areas, with lymphadenitis, fever, headache, prostration, and a short course. Called also *pestis minor.*

avian p. avian influenza.

bubonic p. the most common form of plague, transmitted by the bite of infected fleas. It is typically characterized by abrupt onset of fever, chills, weakness, and headache, followed by pain, tenderness, and lymphadenopathy (buboes) of the regional lymph nodes, usually inguinal, femoral, axillary, and cervical nodes. There is a marked hemorrhagic tendency with disseminated intravascular coaglation, necrotic purpura, and extensive symmetrical gangrene. Hematogenous dissemination may establish suppurative foci throughout the body. Particularly severe complications include pneumonia (see *pneumonic p.*) and septicemia (see *septicemic p.*).

cat p. panleukopenia.

cattle p. rinderpest.

duck p. an acute contagious herpesvirus infection of ducks, which may also affect geese and swans. It is characterized by vascular damage, with hemorrhage into the tissues and free blood in the body cavities, exanthematous lesions of the mucosa of the digestive tract, lesions of the lymphoid organs, and retrograde changes in the parenchymatous organs. Called also *duck virus enteritis.*

equine p. African horse sickness.

fowl p. avian influenza.

hemorrhagic p. bubonic plague accompanied by hemorrhage.

meningeal p. plague meningitis.

pharyngeal p. a rare form of bubonic plague that may resemble acute tonsillitis, thought to be due to inhalation or ingestion of plague bacilli. Called also *plague pharyngitis.*

pneumonic p., pulmonic p. a rapidly progressive, highly contagious, and often fatal type of plague occurring when the lungs are infected by *Yersinia pestis;* it is accompanied by pneumonia and productive cough with mucoid, blood-stained, foamy, plague bacillus–laden sputum. It may occur as a primary infection, due to inhalation of droplet nuclei expelled during coughing, or as a secondary complication of bubonic plague, due to hematogenous spread of infection from buboes to the lungs; in either case it may subsequently be transmitted to other persons. Called also *plague pneumonia.*

septicemic p. an acute fulminating form of plague with high-density bacteremia and fever, chills, prostration, abdominal pain, shock, and bleeding into skin and other organs. It can occur as a complication of bubonic or pneumonic plague, or can be a primary infection transmitted by fleas that may present and result in death before the appearance of buboes or of pulmonic manifestations. Septicemic plague does not spread from person to person. Called also *plague septicemia.*

swine p. hemorrhagic septicemia of swine.

sylvatic p. bubonic plague occurring in the woods, such as that widely spread among ground squirrels and other wild rodents in the western United States; it is epizootic to humans, such as hunters.

pla•kins (pla'kinz) a group of proteins similar to leukins that can be extracted from platelets.

plako•glo•bin (plak'o-glo″bin) a protein related to the catenins that participates in the linking of cadherins to cytoskeletal filaments in adherens junctions and desmosomes by binding to both the cytoplasmic domain of a cadherin and a cytoskeletal linking protein (catenin or desmoplakin).

pla•na (pla'nə) [L.] plural of *planum.*

pla•nar (pla'nər) 1. flat. 2. of or pertaining to a plane.

pla•nar•i•an (plə-nar'e-ən) any of the free-living flatworms of the class Turbellaria, which are used extensively in biologic studies of regeneration.

Plan B (plan' be') trademark for a preparation of levonorgestrel.

plan•chet (plan'chət) a metal disk on which radioactive samples are mounted and prepared for determination of radioactivity.

Planck constant, theory (plahngk) [Max Karl Ernst Ludwig *Planck,* German physicist, 1858–1947] see under *constant,* and see *quantum theory,* under *theory.*

plane (plān) [L. *planus*] 1. a surface such that a straight line connecting any two of its points lies wholly in the surface. In craniotomy and cephalometry, the term plane is sometimes used interchangeably with line because when viewed from the side (lateral projection), as in a radiograph, it appears as a line. 2. a specified level, as the plane of anesthesia. 3. to rub away or abrade; see *planing.* 4. a superficial incision in the wall of a cavity or between tissue layers, especially in plastic surgery, made so that the precise point of entry into the cavity or between the layers can be determined.

Addison p's a series of planes used as landmarks in the topography of the thorax and abdomen.

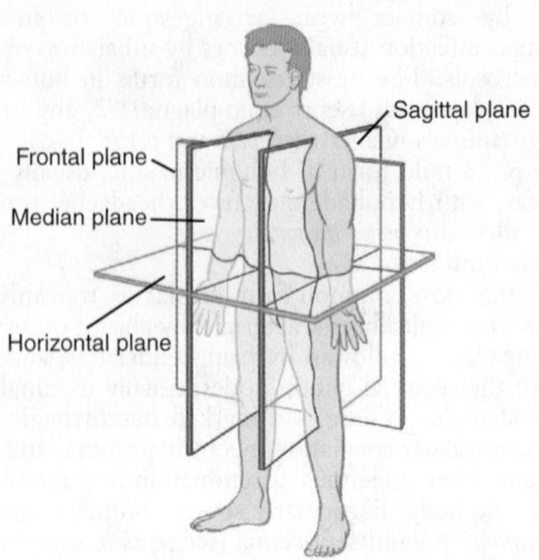

■ Planes of the body, with subject in the anatomical position.

Aeby p. a plane passing through the nasion and basion, perpendicular to the median plane of the cranium.
auricular p. of sacral bone facies auricularis ossis sacri.
auriculoinfraorbital p. Frankfort horizontal p.
axial p. a plane parallel with the long axis of a structure.
axiolabiolingual p. a plane parallel with the long axis of an anterior tooth and passing through its labial and lingual surfaces.
axiomesiodistal p. a plane parallel with the long axis of a tooth and passing through its mesial and distal surfaces.
Baer p. a plane passing through the superior borders of the zygomatic arches.
base p. an imaginary plane upon which is estimated the retention of an artificial denture.
biparietal p. the transverse plane that passes through the two parietal eminences.
bite p. 1. biteplane. 2. occlusal p.
Bolton-nasion p. nasion-postcondylare p.
Broadbent-Bolton p. nasion-postcondylare p.
Broca p. visual p.
buccolingual p. a plane passing through the buccal and lingual surfaces of a posterior tooth.
coronal p's plana frontalia.
cusp p. the small imaginary plane in which buccal cusp tips and lingual cusp tips are located on posterior teeth.
Daubenton p. a plane passing through the opisthion and the inferior edges of the orbits; called also *Daubenton line.*
eye-ear p. Frankfort horizontal p.
facial p. any of several planes passing through craniometric or cephalometric landmarks of the face.
Frankfort horizontal p. a horizontal plane represented in profile by a line between the lowest point on the margin of the orbit and the highest point on the margin of the external acoustic (auditory) meatus.
frontal p's plana frontalia.
frontoparallel p. any plane parallel to the frontal plane.
guide p., guiding p. 1. any plane that guides movement. 2. an orthodontic appliance used to correct crossbite of anterior teeth. 3. two or more vertically parallel surfaces of abutment teeth, so shaped as to direct the path of placement and removal of a partial denture.

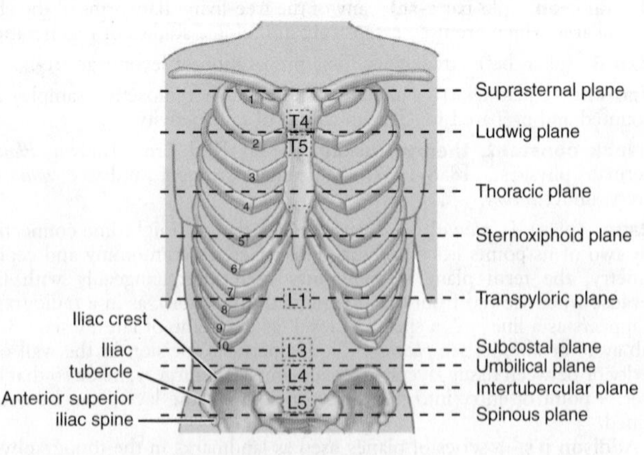

■ Planes of the trunk.

Hensen p. a plane passing through the center of a series of sarcous elements of a muscle fibril.
Hodge p's a series of planes running parallel with the pelvic inlet, the first parallel being in the inlet, the second parallel touching the arch of the pubis and striking the inferior part of the second sacral vertebra, the third cutting the spines of the ischia, and the fourth passing through the tip of the coccyx.
horizontal p. 1. see *plana horizontalia.* 2. in dentistry, a plane passing through a tooth at right angles to its long axis.
interiliac p. planum supracristale.
interparietal p. of occipital bone planum occipitale.
interspinal p., interspinous p. planum interspinale.
intertubercular p. planum intertuberculare.
labiolingual p. a plane passing through the labial and lingual surfaces of an anterior tooth.
Listing p. a transverse vertical plane perpendicular to the anteroposterior axis of the eye, and containing the center of motion of the eyes; in it lie the transverse and vertical axes of ocular rotation.
longitudinal p. any plane parallel to the long axis of the body or of an organ.
Ludwig p. a horizontal plane transecting the trunk at about the level of the joint between the fourth and fifth thoracic vertebrae.
mean foundation p. the mean of the various irregularities in form and inclination of the basal seat (denture-supporting tissues). The ideal condition for denture stability exists when the mean foundation plane is most nearly at right angles to the direction of force.
Meckel p. a plane passing through the auricular and alveolar points.
median p. planum medianum.
median-raphe p. the median plane of the head.
median sagittal p. planum medianum.
mesiodistal p. a plane passing through the mesial and distal surfaces of a tooth.
midclavicular p. linea medioclavicularis.
midpelvic p. pelvic p., narrow.
midsagittal p. planum medianum.
Morton p. a plane passing through the most projecting points of the parietal and occipital protuberances.
nasal p. the flat area between the nostrils on the muzzle of an animal. Called also *planum nasale.*
nasion-postcondylare p. a plane passing at right angles to the median plane, and determined in profile by a line connecting the nasion and postcondylare.
nuchal p. planum nuchale.
occipital p. planum occipitale.
occlusal p., p. of occlusion the hypothetical horizontal plane formed by the contacting surfaces of the upper and lower teeth when the jaws are closed.
orbital p. 1. a plane passing through the two orbital points and perpendicular to the Frankfort horizontal plane; called also *planum orbitale.* 2. visual p.
orbital p. of frontal bone pars orbitalis ossis frontalis.
paramedian p's plana paramediana.
parasagittal p's plana sagittalia.
pelvic p. a plane determined by certain landmarks of the hip bone.
pelvic p., narrow an ovoid plane passing through the apex of the pubic arch, the spines of the ischia, and the end of the sacrum.
pelvic p., wide an irregularly ovoid plane passing from the middle of the pubis to the junction of the second and third sacral vertebrae, at about the center of the excavation of the pelvis.
pelvic p. of outlet a plane passing through the arch of the pubis, the rami of the pubis, the ischial tuberosities, and the tip of the coccyx; see *apertura pelvis inferior.*
principal p. in radiology, the plane which contains the central ray of a radiation beam.
p's of reference planes that are referred to as guides to the locations of specific anatomical sites, or of other planes.
p. of regard a plane passing through the center of rotation and the point of fixation in the eye.
sagittal p's plana sagittalia.
semicircular p. of frontal bone facies temporalis ossis frontalis.
semicircular p. of parietal bone planum temporale.
semicircular p. of squama temporalis facies temporalis partis squamosae.
spinous p. a horizontal plane transecting the trunk at the level of the anterior superior iliac spine.
sternal p. planum sternale.
sternoxiphoid p. a horizontal plane transecting the trunk at about the level of the xiphisternal joint.
subcostal p. planum subcostale.
supracrestal p., supracristal p. planum supracristale.

suprasternal p. a horizontal plane transecting the trunk at the level of the jugular notch.

temporal p. planum temporale.

thoracic p. a horizontal plane transecting the trunk at about the level of the fourth intercostal space.

tooth p. any hypothetical plane passing through a tooth.

transpyloric p. planum transpyloricum.

transtubercular p. planum intertuberculare.

transverse p's plana transversalia.

umbilical p. a horizontal plane transecting the trunk at the level of the umbilicus.

vertical p. any plane of the body perpendicular to a horizontal plane and dividing the body into left and right, or front and back portions, as the sagittal and frontal planes.

visual p. a plane passing through the visual axes of the two eyes; called also *Broca* or *orbital p.*

pla•ni•gram (pla'nĭ-gram) tomogram.

pla•nig•ra•phy (plə-nig'rə-fe) tomography.

pla•nim•e•ter (plə-nim'ə-tər) [L. *planus* plane + *-meter*] an instrument used in measuring the area of surfaces.

plan•ing (plān'ing) 1. the plastic surgery procedure of abrading disfigured skin to promote epithelialization with minimal scarring. It may be done mechanically *(dermabrasion)* or by the application of caustic substances *(chemabrasion)*. 2. see *root p.*

root p. smoothing of the root surface of a tooth after subgingival scaling or curettage.

plank•ton (plank'ton) [Gr. *planktos* wandering] a collective name for the minute free-floating organisms, vegetable and animal, which live in practically all natural waters.

plan•ning (plan'ing) consciously setting forth a scheme to achieve a desired end or goal.

natural family p. rhythm method.

pla•no•cel•lu•lar (pla″no-sel'u-lər) made up of flat cells; cf. *squamous.*

Pla•no•coc•ca•ceae (pla″no-kō-ka'se-e) a family of bacteria of the order Bacillales; medically important organisms are contained in the genus *Kurthia.*

pla•no•con•cave (pla″no-kon-kāv') flat on one side and concave on the other; see under *lens.*

pla•no•con•vex (pla″no-kon-veks') flat on one side and convex on the other; see under *lens.*

pla•nor•bid (plə-nor'bid) 1. a snail of the family Planorbidae. 2. pertaining to snails of the family Planorbidae.

Pla•nor•bi•dae (plə-nor'bĭ-de) [L. *planus* flat + *orbis* ring + *-idae*] a large family of pulmonate fresh-water snails (suborder Basommatophora, order Pulmonata), many species of which are intermediate hosts of pathogenic trematodes; it includes the genera *Biomphalaria, Bulinus, Segmentina,* and *Planorbis* (the type genus).

Pla•nor•bis (plə-nor'bis) a genus of snails of the family Planorbidae. Several species act as intermediate hosts for trematodes such as *Schistosoma mansoni, Fasciolopsis buski,* and species of *Echinostoma.*

plant (plant) any multicellular eukaryotic organism that performs photosynthesis to obtain its nutrition; plants comprise one of the five kingdoms in the most widely used classification of living organisms.

plan•ta (plan'tə) [L.] [TA] sole: the undersurface of the foot. Called also *regio plantaris* [TA alternative]. **plan'tar** *adj*

p. pe'dis former name for *planta.*

plan•tag•i•nis se•men (plan-taj'ĭ-nis se'mən) [L.] plantago seed.

Plan•ta•go (plan-ta'go) the psylliums, a genus of herbs of the family Plantaginaceae whose seeds are used medicinally. There are three important species, *P. in'dica* L., *P. ova'ta* Forskal (blond psyllium), and *P. psyl'lium* L. (Spanish psyllium). See also *plantago seed,* under *seed, psyllium husk,* under *husk,* and *psyllium hydrophilic mucilloid,* under *mucilloid.*

plan•tal•gia (plan-tal'jə) [L. *planta* sole + *-algia*] a painful condition of the sole of the foot.

plan•ta•ris (plan-ta'ris) [L., from *planta* sole of the foot] [TA] plantar; a term designating relationship to the sole of the foot.

plan•ta•tion (plan-ta'shən) [L. *plantare* to plant] the insertion or application of tissue, such as a tooth, or of other material, in or on the human body. Types include *implantation, replantation,* and *transplantation.*

plan•ti•grade (plan'tĭ-grād) [L. *planta* sole + *gradi* to walk] characterized by walking on the full sole of the foot; said of animals such as bears and humans. Cf. *digitigrade* and *unguligrade.*

plan•u•la (plan'u-lə) 1. a larval coelenterate. 2. something resembling such an animal.

invaginate p. gastrula.

pla•num (pla'nəm) pl. *pla'na* [L.] 1. plane. 2. in anatomical nomenclature, a more or less flat surface of a bone or other structure.

pla'na corona'lia TA alternative for *plana frontalia.*

pla'na fronta'lia [TA] frontal planes: planes passing longitudinally through the body from side to side, at right angles to the median plane, and dividing the body into front and back parts. So called because such planes roughly parallel the frontal suture of the skull. Called also *plana coronalia* or *coronal planes* because one of these planes passes through the coronal suture.

pla'na horizonta'lia [TA] horizontal planes: planes at right angles to the long axis of the body.

p. interspina'le [TA] interspinous plane: a horizontal plane transecting the trunk at the level of the anterior superior iliac spines; called also *interspinal line* or *plane.*

p. intertubercula're [TA] intertubercular plane: a horizontal plane transecting the trunk at the level of the iliac tubercles; called also *intertubercular line.*

pla'na, li'neae, et regio'nes planes, lines, and regions: a section of the *Terminologia Anatomica* that contains terms used to describe the surface anatomy of the body.

p. media'num [TA] median plane: the imaginary plane passing longitudinally through the middle of the body from front to back and dividing it into right and left halves. Called also *median sagittal* and *midsagittal plane.*

p. nasa'le nasal plane.

p. nucha'le nuchal plane: the outer surface of the occipital bone between the foramen magnum and the superior nuchal line.

p. occipita'le [TA] occipital plane: the outer surface of the occipital bone superior to the superior nuchal line.

p. orbita'le orbital plane (def. 1).

pla'na paramedia'na [TA] paramedian planes: sagittal planes other than the median plane.

pla'na sagitta'lia [TA] sagittal planes: vertical planes that pass through the body parallel to the median plane (or to the sagittal suture) and divide the body into left and right portions. Included here are the *median* and *paramedian planes.*

p. semiluna'tum the rounded end of a crista ampullaris in a semicircular canal.

p. sterna'le sternal plane: the anterior surface of the sternum.

p. subcosta'le [TA] subcostal plane: a horizontal plane transecting the trunk at the level of the inferior margins of the tenth costal cartilages; called also *infracostal line.*

p. supracrista'le [TA] supracristal plane: a horizontal plane transecting the trunk at the summits of the iliac crests at the level of the fourth lumbar spinous process; called also *supracrestal line* or *plane* and *interiliac plane.*

p. tempora'le [TA] temporal plane: the depressed area on the side of the skull inferior to the inferior temporal line.

p. transpylo'ricum [TA] transpyloric plane: a horizontal plane half way between the superior margins of the manubrium sterni and the pubic symphysis, which usually does not correspond to the level of the pylorus.

pla'na trans'versalia [TA] transverse planes: horizontal planes of the body dividing the body into superior and inferior portions.

pla•nu•ria (pla-nu're-ə) [Gr. *planasthai* to wander + *-uria*] the discharge of urine from an abnormal site.

plaque (plak) [Fr.] 1. any patch or flat area. 2. a superficial, solid, elevated skin lesion equal to or greater than 1.0 cm (0.5 cm according to some authorities) in diameter. Cf. *papule.*

β-amyloid p's, argyrophilic p's neuritic p's.

atheromatous p. fibrous p.

attachment p's small regions of increased density along the sarcolemma of skeletal muscles to which myofilaments seem to attach; cf. *dense bodies,* under *body.*

bacterial p. dental p.

bacteriophage p. a cleared, usually circular, area on a bacterial lawn plate, occurring as a result of lysis of cells by a bacteriophage.

dental p. a soft, thin film of food debris, mucin, and dead epithelial cells deposited on the teeth, providing the medium for the growth of various bacteria. The main inorganic components are calcium and phosphorus, with small amounts of magnesium, potassium, and sodium; the organic matrix consists of polysaccharides, proteins, carbohydrates, lipids, and other components. Plaque plays an important etiologic role in the development of dental caries and periodontal and gingival diseases and provides the base for the development of materia alba; calcified plaque forms dental calculus. Called also *bacterial p.*

ear p. epidermal hyperplasia of the inner surface of the ear in a horse, with raised white plaques resembling papillomas.

eosinophilic p. an ulcerated, circumscribed, raised skin lesion seen in cats, usually on the abdomen or groin, with eosinophilia of the adjacent dermis; it is part of the eosinophilic granuloma complex.

fibrofatty p., fibrolipid p. fibrous p.

fibromyelinic p's areas of overgrowth of medullated fibers and sheaths in areas of incomplete arteriosclerotic necrosis in the cerebral cortex.

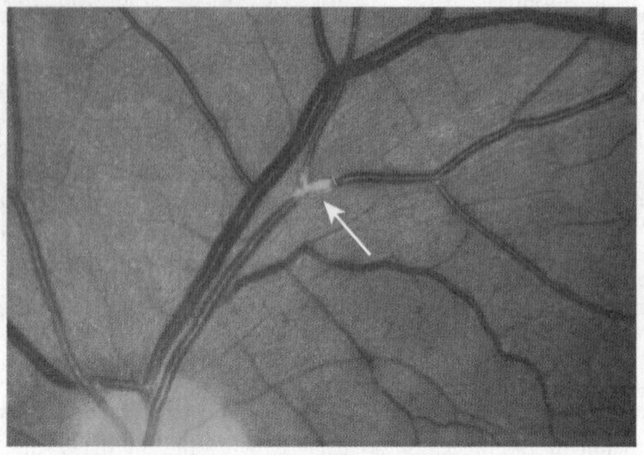

■ Hollenhorst plaque *(arrow).*

fibrous p. the lesion of atherosclerosis, a white to yellow area within an artery that causes the intimal surface to bulge into the lumen; it is composed mainly of collagen and, often, calcium, together with lipid, cell debris, and smooth muscle cells. Called also *atheromatous p.*

Hollenhorst p's atheromatous emboli containing cholesterol crystals in the retinal arterioles, a warning sign of impending serious cardiovascular disease such as stroke, myocardial infarction, aortic aneurysm, or occlusion of the retinal arterioles.

Hutchinson p's a persistent cutaneous manifestation of sarcoidosis consisting of large, flat, slightly elevated plaques, with a predilection for the cheeks, nose, upper limbs, and buttocks; they usually occur bilaterally and symmetrically.

p's jaunes [Fr. "yellow plaques"] old traumatic injuries on the surface of the brain, appearing as depressed, yellowish-brown patches on the crests of the gyri.

Lichtheim p's areas of degeneration in the cerebral white matter that are seen in pernicious anemia.

MacCallum p's irregular thickenings caused by subendocardial lesions, usually in the left atrium, in rheumatic heart disease.

neuritic p's microscopic argyrophilic masses composed of fragmented axon terminals and dendrites surrounding a core of Aβ amyloid; seen in small amounts in the cerebral cortex of normal elderly people and in larger amounts in those with Alzheimer disease. Called also *argyrophil* or *neuritic p's.*

Peyer p's noduli lymphoidei aggregati intestini tenuis.

pleural p's opaque white plaques on the parietal pleura, visible radiographically in cases of asbestosis.

pruritic urticarial papules and p's of pregnancy see under *papule.*

Randall p's small calcium concretions within the tip of the renal papillae; they may project through the surface and serve as foci for the deposition of urinary salts.

Redlich-Fisher miliary p's thickened, dark colored areas in the neuroglia reticulum of the brain, seen in cases of senile psychoses.

senile p's neuritic p's.

talc p's plaques of opaque material on the pleural surfaces of talc miners and processors suffering from talc pneumoconiosis.

Pla·que·nil (pla'kwə-nil) trademark for a preparation of hydroxychloroquine sulfate.

Plas·bu·min (plaz-bu'min) trademark for a preparation of albumin human.

-plasia [Gr. *plasis* molding, from *plassein* to mold] a combining form denoting development or formation.

plasm (plaz'əm) plasma.

-plasm [Gr. *plasma* anything formed or molded] a word termination denoting the constituent substance of cells.

plas·ma (plaz'mə) [Gr. "anything formed or molded"] 1. the fluid portion of the blood in which the particulate components are suspended. *Plasma* is to be distinguished from *serum,* which is the cell-free portion of the blood from which the fibrinogen has been separated in the process of clotting. Called also *blood p.* 2. the lymph deprived of its corpuscles or cells.

antihemophilic human p. normal human plasma that has been processed promptly to preserve the antihemophilic properties of the original blood; used for temporary correction of bleeding tendency in hemophilia.

blood p. plasma (def. 1).

citrated p. blood plasma treated with sodium citrate, which prevents clotting.

fresh frozen p. plasma separated from whole blood and frozen within 8 hours; it contains all coagulation factors including the labile factors V and VIII.

normal human p. sterile plasma obtained by pooling approximately equal amounts of the liquid portion of citrated whole blood from eight or more adult humans, used as a blood volume replenisher.

oxalate p. blood plasma to which ammonium oxalate has been added, formerly used to prevent clotting.

pooled p. a mixture of plasma from several donors.

salt p. blood plasma to which a neutral salt has been added to prevent clotting, such as citrated plasma.

seminal p. the fluid portion of the semen, in which the spermatozoa are suspended.

true p. blood plasma drawn directly from the blood without any change in its gas content.

plas·ma·blast (plaz'mə-blast) [*plasma* + *-blast*] the earliest precursor in the plasmacytic series, which matures to form the proplasmacyte and ultimately the mature plasma cell; it may itself be a derivative of the lymphoblast. **plasmablas'tic** *adj*

plas·ma·cyte (plaz'mə-sīt) plasma cell. **plasmacyt'ic** *adj*

plas·ma·cy·to·ma (plaz″mə-si-to'mə) [*plasmacyte* + *-oma*] 1. plasma cell dyscrasias. 2. solitary myeloma.

multiple p. of bone multiple myeloma.

plas·ma·cy·to·sis (plaz″mə-si-to'sis) the presence of excess plasma cells in the blood.

plas·mal (plaz'məl) a long-chain fatty acid aldehyde produced during hydrolysis of plasmalogens.

plas·ma·lem·ma (plaz″mə-lem'ə) [*plasma* + *-lemma*] 1. plasma membrane. 2. a thin peripheral layer of the ectoplasm in a fertilized oocyte.

plas·ma·lo·gen (plaz-mal'ə-jən) any of various phospholipids in which the group at one C1 of glycerol is an ether-linked alcohol in place of an ester-linked fatty acid, found in myelin sheaths of nerve fibers, cell membranes of muscle, and platelets.

Plas·ma·nate (plaz'mə-nāt) trademark for a commercial preparation of human plasma protein fraction.

plas·ma·phe·re·sis (plaz″mə-fə-re'sis) [*plasma* + *apheresis*] the removal of plasma from withdrawn blood, with retransfusion of the formed elements into the donor; generally, type-specific fresh frozen plasma or albumin is used to replace the withdrawn plasma. The procedure may be done for purposes of collecting plasma components or for therapeutic purposes.

plas·mat·ic (plaz-mat'ik) pertaining to or of the nature of plasma; called also *plasmic.*

plas·ma·tog·a·my (plaz″mə-tog'ə-me) plasmogamy.

plas·mic (plaz'mik) plasmatic.

plas·mid (plaz'mid) [*plasm* + *-id*] an extrachromosomal self-replicating structure found in bacterial cells that carries genes for a variety of functions not essential for cell growth. Plasmids consist of cyclic double-stranded DNA molecules, replicating independently of the chromosomes and transmitting through successive cell divisions genes specifying such functions as antibiotic resistance (R plasmid); conjugation (F plasmid); the production of enzymes, toxins, and antigens; and the metabolism of sugars and other organic compounds. Plasmids can be transferred from one cell to another by conjugation and by transduction. Some plasmids may also become integrated into the bacterial chromosome; these are known as *episomes.*

conjugative p. a plasmid that is transferred from one bacterial cell to another during conjugation.

F p. a conjugative plasmid found in F^+ (male) bacterial cells that leads with high frequency to its transfer and much less often to transfer of the bacterial chromosome. A cell possessing the F plasmid (F^+, male) can form a conjugation bridge (F pilus) to a cell lacking the F plasmid (F^-, female), through which genetic material may pass from one cell to another. Called also *F* or *fertility factor, F element,* and *sex factor.*

F′ p. a hybrid F plasmid that contains also a segment of the host chromosome.

oligomeric p. a plasmid that contains repeating segments of a determinant, formed by recombination between strands during replication and resulting in gene amplification.

R p., resistance p. a conjugative factor in bacterial cells that promotes resistance to agents such as antibiotics, metal ions, ultraviolet radiation, and bacteriophage. R plasmids are large with two functionally distinct parts: a resistance transfer factor (RTF), consisting of genes for autonomous replication and conjugation; and a resistance determinant (R determinant) containing the genes for resistance (R genes); called also *R factor.*

plas·min (plaz'min) [EC 3.4.21.7] a serine endopeptidase that catalyzes the hydrolysis of peptide bonds on the carboxyl side of lysine or arginine residues. The enzyme occurs in plasma as plasminogen, which is activated via cleavage by the plasminogen activators prourokinase, u-plasminogen activator (urokinase), and t-plasminogen (tissue plasminogen activator). Plasmin solubilizes fibrin clots and also degrades various proteins including fibrinogen and coagulation factors V and VII. Plasminogen is activated for therapeutic thrombolysis by recombinant forms of physiologic activators and by streptokinase, a streptococcal enzyme. Bovine plasmin is used for the débridement of wounds. Called also *fibrinolysin.*

plas·min·o·gen (plaz-min′ə-jən) the inactive precursor of plasmin; called also *profibrinolysin.*

plas·min·o·gen ac·ti·va·tor (plaz-min′ə-jən ak′tĭ-va″tər) see under *activator.*

plasm(o)- [Gr. *plasma* anything formed or molded] a combining form denoting relationship to plasma, or to the substance of a cell.

plas·mo·cyte (plaz′mo-sīt) [*plasmo-* + *-cyte*] a plasma cell.

plas·mo·cy·to·ma (plaz″mo-si-to′mə) [*plasmo-* + *-cyte* + *-oma*] 1. plasma cell dyscrasias. 2. solitary myeloma.

plas·mo·dia (plaz-mo′de-ə) plural of *plasmodium.*

plas·mo·di·al (plaz-mo′de-əl) pertaining to plasmodia.

plas·mo·di·ci·dal (plaz″mo-dĭ-si′dəl) [*plasmodia* + L. *caedere* to kill] destructive to plasmodia; cf. *antimalarial.* Called also malariacidal.

plas·mo·di·cide (plaz-mo′dĭ-sīd) an antimalarial agent that destroys the parasites.

plas·mo·di·tropho·blast (plaz-mo″dĭ-tro′fo-blast) syncytiotrophoblast (def. 1).

Plas·mo·di·um (plaz-mo′de-əm) [Gr. *plasma* anything formed or molded] the malarial parasites: a genus of coccidian protozoa of the suborder Haemosporina, order Eucoccidiida. Several species are parasitic in the erythrocytes of mammals; others parasitize birds and reptiles. Protozoal sporozoites concentrate in the salivary glands of female anopheline mosquitoes and are transmitted to the bloodstream of mammals when the mosquito bites them. The first stage inside the mammal's body is the *preerythrocytic* or *exoerythrocytic stage;* the sporozoites migrate through the bloodstream and enter the liver *(intrahepatic stage).* In the liver they develop and multiply within the hepatic cells and become merozoites. Eventually the merozoites burst the hepatic cells and invade erythrocytes to begin the *erythrocytic stage.* Inside the erythrocytes, schizogony takes place and the merozoites are capable of invading other erythrocytes. Some merozoites develop into gametocytes, and when these are ingested by bloodsucking mosquitoes, they begin the *gametocyte stage,* a sexual stage that completes the life cycle, ending with development of new sporozoites inside the mosquito. Malaria in birds is transmitted by culicine mosquitoes.

P. falci′parum the species that causes falciparum malaria; it is characterized by thin "signet-ring" forms of trophozoites and the "crescent" form of the gametes.

P. mala′riae the species that causes quartan malaria; it is characterized by bandlike trophozoites and schizonts with six to twelve merozoites usually arranged in a rosette configuration.

P. ova′le a species found primarily in East and Central Africa that causes ovale malaria and is characterized by oval or fimbriated infected red blood cells.

P. vi′vax the species that causes vivax malaria, characterized by trophozoites having ameboid activity and irregular form, and by Schüffner dots in parasitized red blood cells.

plas·mo·di·um (plaz-mo′de-əm) pl. *plasmo′dia* [*plasmo-* + Gr. *eidos* form] 1. a protozoan of the genus *Plasmodium.* 2. a multinucleate continuous mass of protoplasm formed by aggregation and fusion of myxamebae; also, a protozoan whose body consists of such a mass. Cf. *pseudoplasmodium.*

exoerythrocytic p. a malarial parasite outside a red blood cell; see *preerythrocytic stage,* under *stage.*

plas·mog·a·my (plaz-mog′ə-me) [*plasmo-* + Gr. *gamos* marriage] the union of two or more cells with their nuclei remaining separate; in fertilization, karyogamy follows. Called also *plasmatogamy* and *plastogamy.* Cf. *karyogamy.*

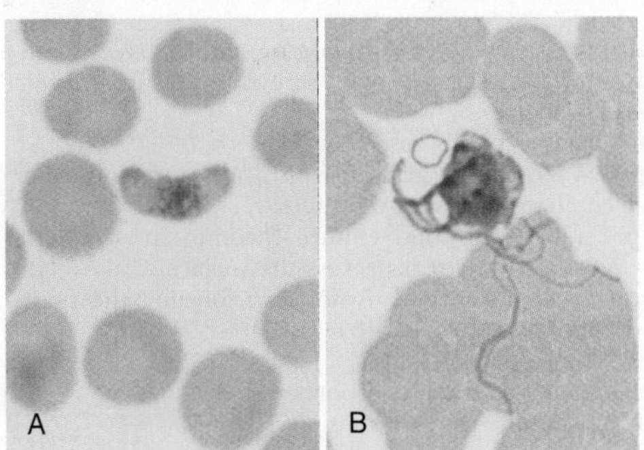

■ *(A), Plasmodium falciparum* female gametocyte; *(B), P. vivax* male gametocytes exflagellating to form microgametes.

plas·moid (plas′moid) an abnormal protein cellular element; see also under *humor.*

plas·mol·y·sis (plaz-mol′ĭ-sis) [*plasmo-* + *-lysis*] contraction or shrinking of the protoplasm of a plant cell or bacterium due to the loss of water by osmotic action. **plasmolyt′ic** *adj*

plas·mo·lyze (plaz′mo-līz) to subject to plasmolysis.

plas·mo·ma (plaz-mo′mə) 1. plasma cell dyscrasias. 2. solitary myeloma.

plas·mon (plaz′mon) [*cytoplasm* + Gr. *-on* neuter ending] the sum total of all nonnuclear genetic material in a cell.

plas·mot·o·my (plaz-mot′ə-me) [*plasmo-* + *-tomy*] reproduction by the separation from the mother cell of smaller masses of protoplasm, each containing several nuclei.

-plast [Gr. *plastos* formed] a word termination denoting any primitive organized unit of living matter, e.g., a granule, an organelle, or a cell.

plas·tein (plas′tēn) the protein synthesized by pepsin from the peptic digestion products of protein.

plas·ter (plas′tər) [L. *emplastrum*] 1. a gypsum material that hardens when mixed with water, used for immobilizing or making impressions of body parts. 2. a pastelike mixture that can be spread over the skin and is adhesive at body temperature, serving purposes such as skin protection and counterirritation.

impression p. a gypsum preparation used for the making of impressions of structures in the mouth.

mustard p. a uniform mixture of powdered black mustard and a solution of suitable adhesive, spread on an appropriate backing material; used as a local irritant.

p. of Paris calcium sulfate hemihydrate reduced to a fine powder; the addition of water produces a porous mass that hardens rapidly. It has been used extensively in making casts and bandages to support or immobilize body parts, and in dentistry for making study models.

salicylic acid p. [USP] a uniform mixture of salicylic acid in a suitable base, spread on paper, cotton cloth, or other backing material; used as a topical keratolytic.

plas·ter of Par·is (par′is) [*Paris,* France, site of gypsum deposits from which it was first made in the early 19th century] see under *plaster.*

plas·tic (plas′tik) [Gr. *plastikos,* from *plassein* to form] 1. tending to build up tissues or to restore a lost part. 2. conformable; capable of being molded. 3. a high-molecular-weight polymeric material, usually organic, capable of being molded, extruded, drawn, or otherwise shaped and then hardened into a form. 4. material that can be molded.

plas·tic·i·ty (plas-tis′ĭ-te) the capability of being molded.

developmental p. the ability, as of a cell, a tissue, or an entire organism, to produce structural, functional, or behavioral alterations in response to changes in the environment.

synaptic p. the ability of synapses to change as circumstances require. They may alter function, such as increasing or decreasing their sensitivity; or they may increase or decrease in actual numbers. This phenomenon is thought to be the main source of the overall plasticity of nervous system pathways.

plas·ti·ci·zer (plas′tĭ-si″zər) any of a group of agents, usually organic, added to other organic or synthetic substances to make them soft and flexible.

plas·tid (plas′tid) any of the specialized organelles in plant cells other than the nucleus and centrosome, such as chloroplasts.

plas·tin (plas′tin) fimbrin.

plas·tog·a·my (plas-tog′ə-me) plasmogamy.

plas·to·gel (plas′to-jel) a gel possessing great plasticity.

plas·tron (plas′tron) [Fr. "breast-plate"] the sternum and costal cartilages.

-plasty [Gr. *plassein* to form] a word termination denoting plastic surgery.

plate (plāt) [Gr. *platē*] 1. a flat structure or layer, such as a thin layer of bone; see also *lamina, layer,* and *stratum.* 2. dental p.; the term is sometimes incorrectly extended to refer to a complete denture. 3. a flat vessel, usually a Petri dish, containing sterile solid medium for the culture of microorganisms. 4. to prepare a culture medium in a Petri dish, or to inoculate such a medium with a bacterial culture.

alar p. lamina alaris.

auditory p. the bony roof of the external acoustic meatus.

axial p. primitive streak.

basal p. 1. lamina basalis. 2. the fused parachordal cartilages, precursors of the occipital bone. 3. the portion of the decidua basalis that becomes the maternal part of the placenta.

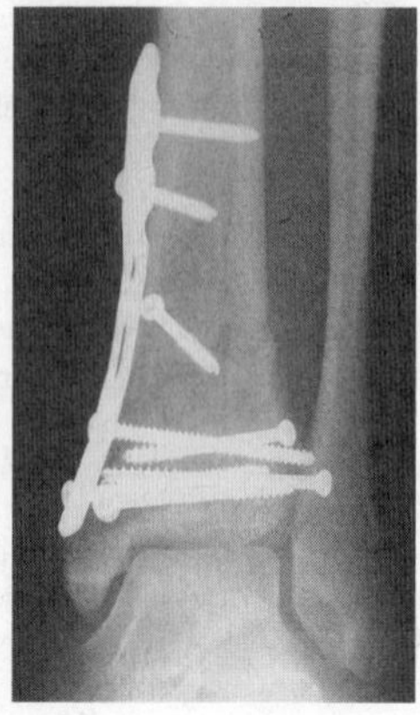

■ Bone plate used for percutaneous fixation of the tibial metaphysis to the diaphysis in the treatment of a pilon fracture.

base p. baseplate (def. 1).

bite p. a removable orthodontic appliance, generally made of acrylic resin, that makes use of adhesion to the palate to provide part of the anchorage needed for the desired tooth movement; used to stimulate eruption of the posterior teeth and to decrease the amount of anterior overbite. Written also *biteplate.*

bone p. a metal bar with perforations for the insertion of screws, used to immobilize fractured segments.

cardiogenic p. an area of splanchnic mesoderm, at first cephalad and later in the pharyngeal region of the embryo, from which the heart arises.

chorionic p. the part of the inner chorionic wall in the area of its uterine attachment, which gives rise to chorionic villi.

compression p. a type of bone plate in which the screws are arranged so that they compress the defect and actively promote closure.

cortical p. a layer of compact bone overlying the spongiosa of the alveolar process on the vestibular and oral aspects of the mandible and maxilla.

cough p. a plate of culture medium on which a patient with a respiratory infection, especially pertussis, coughs.

counting p. in bacteriology, a plate marked off in square centimeters. A Petri dish culture of microorganisms is placed on the plate and colonies per square centimeter are counted. The number of colonies per plate is calculated by multiplying the average count per square centimeter by the area of the Petri dish.

cribriform p. fascia cribrosa.

cribriform p. of ethmoid bone lamina cribrosa ossis ethmoidalis.

cuticular p. a thickened plate that forms the upper surface of the auditory hair cells of the organ of Corti and in which the stereocilia are embedded.

cutis p. dermatome (def. 3).

deck p. roof p.

dental p. a plate of acrylic resin, metal, or other material, which is fitted to the shape of the mouth and serves for the support of artificial teeth.

dermomyotome p. the portion of the embryonic somite remaining after migration of the sclerotomic tissue.

die p. a plate of metal containing dies for forming the cusps in shell crowns.

dorsal p. roof p.

dorsolateral p. lamina alaris.

Eggers p. bone plate used for maintaining apposition of bone segments.

end p. see *end plate,* under *E.*

epiphyseal p. lamina epiphysialis.

equatorial p. the compact group of chromosomes aligned at the equator of the cell during metaphase.

ethmovomerine p. the central part of the ethmoid bone in the fetus.

floor p. the unpaired ventral longitudinal zone of the neural tube, forming the floor of that tube; called also *ventral p.* and *bodenplatte.*

foot p. 1. basis stapedis. 2. a flattened expansion at the end of the limb of the embryo, the precursor of the foot.

force p. force platform.

frontal p. a fetal plate of cartilage between the sides of the ethmoid cartilage and the sphenoid bone.

frontonasal p. a fetal plate from which the external nose is developed.

growth p. lamina epiphysialis.

hand p. a flattened expansion at the end of the limb of the embryo, the precursor of the hand.

horizontal p. of palatine bone lamina horizontalis ossis palatini.

inner p. of calvaria lamina interna calvariae.

Ishihara p's the pseudoisochromatic plates used in the Ishihara test.

jumping-the-bite p., Kingsley p. Kingsley appliance.

Kühne terminal p's the motor end plates of nerves in the muscle spindles.

Lane p's steel plates with holes for screws, used in fixing the fragments of a fractured bone.

lateral mesoblastic p. the thickened portion of either side of the mesoblast.

lateral p. of pterygoid process lamina lateralis processus pterygoidei.

lawn p. a plate of solid culture medium inoculated by swab or with a liquid inoculum so as to produce a uniform confluent growth of microorganisms, used for assay of bacteriophage.

levator p. a small flat structure formed by intertwining of the levator ani muscles in the posterior part of the pelvic region, providing support for the corresponding part of the diaphragm.

lingual p. a major partial denture connector formed as a lingual bar extended to cover the cingula of the lower anterior teeth. When used on the maxillary arch it is often referred to as a *palatal p.*

medial p. of pterygoid process lamina medialis processus pterygoidei.

medullary p. neural p.

mesial p. nephrotome.

metaphase p. equatorial p.

middle p. nephrotome.

Moe p. a stainless steel plate for internal fixation of intertrochanteric fractures of the femur.

motor end p. see under *end plate.*

muscle p. myotome (def. 2).

nail p. unguis.

nephrotome p. nephrotome.

neural p. the thickened plate of ectoderm in the embryo from which the neural tube develops.

notochordal p. head process.

oral p. oropharyngeal membrane.

orbital p. of ethmoid bone lamina orbitalis ossis ethmoidalis.

orbital p. of frontal bone pars orbitalis ossis frontalis.

outer p. of calvaria lamina externa calvariae.

palatal p. see *lingual p.*

paper p. lamina orbitalis ossis ethmoidalis.

parachordal p. basal p. (def. 2).

perpendicular p. of ethmoid bone lamina perpendicularis ossis ethmoidalis.

perpendicular p. of palatine bone lamina perpendicularis ossis palatini.

Petri p. a Petri dish containing a nutrient medium ready for inoculation with the microorganism to be cultured.

pour p. a bacterial culture poured into a Petri dish from a test tube in which the medium has been inoculated.

prechordal p., prochordal p. thickened endoderm, cephalad of the notochord, that combines with ectoderm to become the oropharyngeal membrane.

pseudoisochromatic p. any of a series of charts containing dots of various sizes, brightnesses, and colors, with the dots arranged to form numbers, letters, or other figures that are visible to those with normal color vision but which cannot be discerned by those with color perception defects. See also *Ishihara test,* under *test.*

pterygoid p., lateral lamina lateralis processus pterygoidei.

pterygoid p., medial lamina medialis processus pterygoidei.

quadrigeminal p. lamina tecti mesencephali.

reticular p. a form of nerve ending in the ciliary body consisting of very fine reticulations of granular nerve fiber.

roof p. the unpaired dorsal longitudinal zone of the neural tube, forming its roof; called also *deck p., dorsal p.,* and *deckplatte.*

segmental p. a plate of mesoblast on either side of the notochord at the posterior end of the embryo, from which the mesoblastic segments are formed.

Sherman p. a chrome-cobalt alloy or stainless steel bone plate which can be affixed to a fracture site with screws; often used in open reduction of mandibular fractures.

spiral p. lamina spiralis ossea.

spring p. a dental prosthesis held in place by the elasticity of the base material which abuts against natural teeth.

streak p. a plate of solid culture medium in which the infectious material is inoculated in streaks across the surface.

subgerminal p. a sheet of protoplasm forming the floor of the segmentation cavity of the oocyte.

tarsal p. tarsus (def. 2).

tectal p. lamina tecti mesencephali.

terminal p. lamina terminalis hypothalamus.

tympanic p. pars tympanica ossis temporalis.

urethral p. an endodermal plate that gives rise to the terminal portion of the spongy urethra.

vascular foot p. pericapillary end foot.
ventral p. floor p.
vertical p. of palatine bone lamina perpendicularis ossis palatini.
wing p. lamina alaris.

pla•teau (plă-to′) [Fr.] an elevated and level area.
tibial p. either of the bony surfaces of the tibia, internal and external, closest to the condyles of the femur.
ventricular p. a nearly level part of the intraventricular curve of blood pressure corresponding to the middle of the ejection period of the ventricle.

plate•let (plāt′lət) a disk-shaped structure, 2 to 4 μm in diameter, found in the blood of all mammals and chiefly known for its role in blood coagulation; platelets, which are formed in the megakaryocyte and released from its cytoplasm in clusters, lack a nucleus and DNA but contain active enzymes and mitochondria. See also under *factor*, and see *thrombocytic series*, under *series*. Called also *blood p.* and *thrombocyte*.
blood p. platelet.
giant p. an abnormal large platelet whose membrane lacks glycoprotein Ib so that the platelet cannot bind von Willebrand factor or adhere to the surface of a blood vessel; seen in the Bernard-Soulier syndrome.
gray p. an abnormal platelet with deficient alpha granules, giving it a gray appearance on a Wright stain smear; seen in the bleeding disorder known as *gray platelet syndrome*.

plate•let•phe•re•sis (plāt″lət-fə-re′sis) [*platelet* + *pheresis*] thrombocytapheresis.

plat•form (plat′form) a flat horizontal surface higher than the level of the areas around it.
force p. a small platform that measures variations in downward force between different points on its surface, for assessing stability of stance and posture as a person stands on it; see posturography. Called also *force plate*.

plat•ing (plāt′ing) 1. the act of preparing a bacterial culture on a plate of solid medium in a Petri dish; the preparation of a plate culture. 2. the application of plates to fractured bones for the purpose of holding the fragments in place.

pla•tin•ic (plə-tin′ik) containing platinum in its higher valency.

Pla•ti•nol (plat′ĭ-nol) trademark for preparations of cisplatin.

plat•i•no•sis (plat″ĭ-no′sis) [*platinum* + *-osis*] a morbid condition caused by exposure to soluble platinum salts, with involvement of the upper respiratory tract and allergic skin manifestations.

plat•i•nous (plat′ĭ-nəs) containing platinum in its lower valency.

plat•i•num (Pt) (plat′ĭ-nəm) [L.] a heavy, soft, whitish metal, resembling tin: atomic number, 78; atomic weight, 195.09; specific gravity, 21.37. It also occurs as a black powder *(p. black)* and a spongy substance *(spongy p.)*. Metallic platinum is insoluble except in nitrohydrochloric acid, and is fusible only at very high temperatures; it is therefore used in the manufacture of chemical apparatus. Platinum black and spongy platinum have a strong affinity for oxygen, and act as powerful oxidizing and catalytic agents.
p. chloride platinic tetrachloride, a poisonous substance used as a chemical reagent and formerly in syphilis.

plat•onych•ia (plat″o-nik′e-ə) [Gr. *platys* broad + *onych-* + *-ia*] abnormal flatness and width of the nail.

platy- [Gr. *platys* broad] a combining form meaning broad or flat.

platy•ba•sia (plat″ĭ-ba′se-ə) [*platy-* + *bas-* + *-ia*] bulging upwards of the floor of the posterior cranial fossa adjacent to the foramen magnum due to softening of skull bones or a developmental anomaly; see also *basilar invagination*, under *invagination*. Called also *basilar impression*.

platy•ce•lous (plat″ĭ-se′ləs) [*platy-* + *cel-*[2] + *-ous*] having vertebral centra that are flat in front, or cephalad, and concave caudad.

platy•ceph•a•ly (plat″ĭ-sef′ə-le) [*platy-* + *-cephaly*] the state of being wide headed, or having a breadth-height index of less than 70. **platycephal′ic** *adj*

platy•cne•mia (plat″ik-ne′me-ə) [*platy-* + Gr. *knēmē* leg] compression of the tibia from side to side. **platycne′mic** *adj*

Platy•co•don (plat″ĭ-ko′don) a genus of perennial herbs of the family Campanulaceae having large, blue or white, bell-shaped flowers; *P. grandiflo′rum*, the balloon flower, is a species native to northern Asia that is used in traditional Chinese medicine.

platy•co•ria (plat″ĭ-kor′e-ə) [*platy-* + *cor-* + *-ia*] a dilated condition of the pupil.

platy•cra•nia (plat″ĭ-kra′ne-ə) [*platy-* + *crani-* + *-ia*] artificial flattening of the skull.

platy•glos•sal (plat″ĭ-glos′əl) [*platy-* + *gloss-* + *-al*[1]] having a broad, flat tongue.

platy•hel•minth (plat″ĭ-hel′minth) any member of the phylum Platyhelminthes; called also *flatworm*.

Platy•hel•min•thes (plat″ĭ-həl-min′thēz) [*platy-* + Gr. *helmins* worm] the flatworms, a phylum of acoelomate, dorsoventrally flattened, bilaterally symmetrical invertebrates; classes include Turbellaria, Trematoda, and Cestoidea.

platy•hi•er•ic (plat″e-hi-er′ik) [*platy-* + Gr. *hieron* sacrum + *-ic*] having a wide sacrum with a sacral index of more than 100.

platy•kne•mia (plat″ik-ne′me-ə) platycnemia.

platy•kur•tic (plat″ĭ-kur′tik) [*platy-* + Gr. *kurtos* convex] pertaining to a probability distribution less concentrated about the mean, i.e., having a broader, flatter peak than the normal distribution with the same variance. Cf. *leptokurtic*.

platy•me•ria (plat″ĭ-me′re-ə) a condition in which the femur is excessively compressed from front to back. **platymer′ic** *adj*

platy•mor•phia (plat″ĭ-mor′fe-ə) [*platy-* + *morph-* + *-ia*] having a flat shape; in ophthalmology, a flattened eyeball, resulting in a short anteroposterior axis and hypermetropia. **platymor′phic** *adj*

platy•my•ar•i•an (plat″ĭ-mi-ar′e-ən) [*platy-* + Gr. *mys* muscle] having all muscle cells lying next to the hypodermis, their sarcoplasm being uncovered on three sides next to the body cavity; said of the muscle arrangement in certain nematodes.

platy•my•oid (plat″ĭ-mi′oid) [*platy-* + *myo-* + *-oid*] having the contractile stratum arranged in an even lamina; said of certain muscle cells.

Platy•no•so•mum (plat″ĭ-no-so′mum) a genus of trematodes of the family Dicrocoeliidae. *P. fasto′sum* infests the liver and bile ducts of domestic cats in the southeastern United States and the Caribbean after they eat infested lizards or toads.

platy•pel•lic (plat″ĭ-pel′ik) [*platy-* + Gr. *pella* bowl] having a wide, flat pelvis.

platy•pel•loid (plat″ĭ-pel′oid) platypellic.

platy•phyl•line (plat″ĭ-fil′ēn) an alkaloid from *Senecio platyphyllus* and other species of *Senecio*.

pla•typ•nea (plə-tip′ne-ə) [*platy-* + *-pnea*] dyspnea induced by assumption of the upright position and relieved by assumption of a recumbent position; the opposite of *orthopnea*.

platy•po•dia (plat″ĭ-po′de-ə) flatfoot.

Plat•yr•rhi•na (plat″ĭ-ri′nə) [*platy-* + Gr. *rhis* nose] the New World monkeys, a superfamily of the order Primates (suborder Anthropoidea), characterized by a broad nasal septum and often a prehensile tail.

plat•yr•rhine (plat′ĭ-rīn) [*platy-* + Gr. *rhis* nose] having a broad nose; having a nasal index exceeding 53.

pla•tys•ma (plə-tiz′mə) [Gr.] [TA] a platelike muscle innervated by the cervical branch of the facial nerve; it originates from the fascia of the cervical region and inserts in the mandible and the skin around the mouth. It wrinkles the skin of the neck and depresss the jaw. **platys′mal** *adj*

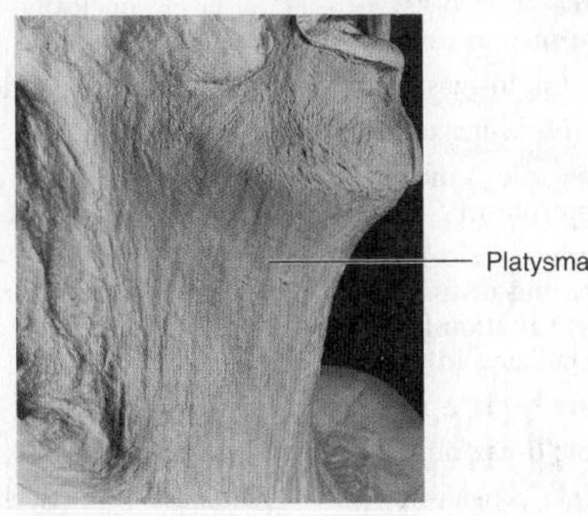

platy•spon•dyl•ia (plat″ĭ-spon-dil′e-ə) platyspondylisis.

platy•spon•dyl•i•sis (plat″ĭ-spon-dil′ĭ-sis) [*platy-* + *spondyl-* + *-sis*] congenital flattening of the vertebral bodies.

Platy•spo•ri•na (plat″ĭ-spə-ri′nə) [*platy-* + *spore*] a suborder of parasitic protozoa (order Bivalvulida, class Myxosporea), usually having bilaterally symmetrical spores with two polar capsules at one pole of the spore in a sutural plane. A representative genus is *Myxosoma*.

platy•staph•y•line (plat″ĭ-staf′ə-lēn) [*platy-* + *staphyline*] having a broad, flat palate.

platy•sten•ce•pha•lia (plat″ĭ-sten″sə-fa′le-ə) platystencephaly.

platy•sten•ceph•a•ly (plat″ĭ-sten-sef′ə-le) [Gr. *platystatos* widest + *enkephalos* brain + *-ia*] a form of dolichocephalism in which the occiput is very wide and pentagonal, the jaws prognathic; observed among South Africans. **platystencephal′ic** *adj*

platy·trope (plat′ĭ-trōp) [*platy-* + Gr. *trepein* to turn] either of two symmetrical parts on opposite sides of the body; a lateral homologue.

Plav·ix (plav′iks) trademark for a preparation of clopidogrel bisulfate.

plec·tin (plek′tin) a 500-kD homodimeric protein chemically related to the plakins, which attaches intermediate filaments to hemidesmosomes and plasma membranes; mutations in the gene for producing plectin causes a type of epidermolysis bullosa simplex.

plec·tron (plek′tron) [Gr. *plēktron* anything to strike with] the hammer form assumed by certain bacilli during sporulation.

PLED periodic lateralized epileptiform discharge.

pledge (plej) a solemn statement of intention.

Nightingale p. a statement of principles for the nursing profession, formulated by a committee in 1893 and subscribed to by student nurses at the time of the capping ceremonies.

pled·get (plej′ət) a small compress or tuft, as of gauze or cotton.

pleg·a·pho·nia (pleg″ə-fo′ne-ə) [Gr. *plēgē* stroke + *aphonia*] auscultation of the chest during percussion over the larynx or trachea in cases in which the patient cannot or is not allowed to speak. The vibrations produced by the percussion take the place of those of the vocal cords.

-plegia [Gr. *plēgē* a blow, stroke] a word termination meaning paralysis, or a stroke.

Pleg·i·sol (ple′jĭ-sol) trademark for a cardioplegic solution containing sodium, potassium, magnesium, calcium, and chloride.

pleio- see *pleo-*.

plei·ot·ro·pism (pli-ot′rə-piz-əm) pleiotropy.

plei·ot·ro·py (pli-ot′rə-pe) [*pleio-* + *-tropy*] the production by a single gene of multiple, apparently unrelated, phenotypic effects. **pleiotrop′ic** *adj*

Pleis·toph·o·ra (plīs-tof′ə-rə) [Gr. *pleistos* most, very many] a genus of parasitic protozoa (suborder Pansporoblastina, order Microsporida), usually found in the muscles of tropical freshwater fish; they have been found in immunocompromised persons, causing microsporidiosis with myositis.

plek·tron (plek′tron) [Gr.] plectron.

Plen·dil (plen′dil) trademark for a preparation of felodipine.

pleo- [Gr. *pleiōn* more] a combining form meaning more, excessive, or multiple. Also, *pleio-*.

pleo·chro·ism (ple′o-kro″iz-əm) pleochromatism. **pleochro′ic** *adj*

pleo·chro·ma·tism (ple″o-kro′mə-tiz-əm) [*pleo-* + *chromat-* + *-ism*] the property possessed by some crystals of transmitting one color in one position and the complementary color in a position at right angles to the first. Called also *pleochroism*. **pleochromat′ic** *adj*

pleo·cy·to·sis (ple″o-si-to′sis) presence of a greater than normal number of cells in the cerebrospinal fluid.

pleo·karyo·cyte (ple″o-kar′e-o-sīt) a large nucleated cell found in cachectic disease such as cancer and tuberculosis.

pleo·mas·tia (ple″o-mas′te-ə) polymastia. **pleomas′tic** *adj*

pleo·ma·zia (ple″o-ma′ze-ə) polymastia.

pleo·mor·phic (ple″o-mor′fik) occurring in various distinct forms; exhibiting pleomorphism.

pleo·mor·phism (ple″o-mor′fiz-əm) [*pleo-* + *morph-* + *-ia*] 1. the assumption of various distinct forms by a single organism or species. 2. in cytomorphology, variation in the size and shape of cells or nuclei. 3. the property of crystallizing in two forms.

pleo·mor·phous (ple″o-mor′fəs) pleomorphic.

pleo·nasm (ple′o-naz″əm) [Gr. *pleonasmos* exaggeration] polymeria.

pleo·nex·ia (ple″o-nek′se-ə) [Gr. "greediness"] a psychiatric disorder characterized by greediness; excessive desire for acquisition of wealth or objects.

ple·on·os·te·o·sis (ple″on-os″te-o′sis) [*pleo-* + *oste-* + *-osis*] abnormally increased ossification; premature and excessive ossification.

Léri p. a hereditary syndrome resulting from premature ossification of epiphyses of the long bones, with broadening and deformity of the digits, flexion contractures of the fingers, broadening and stiffness of the toes and joints, shortening of stature, limitation of movement, and mongolian facies. Inherited as an autosomal dominant trait, the deformities become apparent during the first few years of life.

pleo·no·tia (ple″o-no′she-ə) [*pleo-* + *ot-* + *-ia*] a developmental anomaly characterized by the presence of a supernumerary ear located on the neck.

ple·op·tics (ple-op′tiks) [*pleo-* + *optics*] a technique of eye exercises designed to develop fuller vision of an amblyopic eye and assure proper binocular cooperation.

ple·ro·cer·coid (ple″ro-sur′koid) [Gr. *plēroun* to complete + *cerc-* + *-oid*] the wormlike completed larval stage of certain tapeworms, found in the tissues of vertebrates and invertebrates.

ple·ro·sis (ple-ro′sis) the restoration of lost tissue, as after illness.

Plesch percussion (plesh) [Johann *Plesch*, German physician in England, 20th century] see under *percussion*.

Ple·sio·mo·nas (ple″se-o-mo′nəs) [Gr. *plēsios* near + *monas* unit, from *monos* single] a genus of gram-negative, facultatively anaerobic bacteria of the family Enterobacteriaceae, consisting of motile, rod-shaped organisms with polar flagella, found in the intestinal tracts of mammals. The type species is *P. shigelloi′des*

P. shigelloi′des a species isolated from various animals, associated with diarrhea in humans, especially in tropical and subtropical areas.

ple·sio·mor·phism (ple″se-o-mor′fiz-əm) [Gr. *plesios* near + *morph-* + *-ism*] similarity in form.

ple·sio·mor·phous (ple″se-o-mor′fəs) pertaining to or characterized by plesiomorphism.

ples·ses·the·sia (ples″es-the′zhə) [Gr. *plēssein* to strike + *esthesia*] palpatory percussion; percussion with one hand against a palpating finger of the other hand.

ples·sor (ples′or) percussion hammer.

Ple·tal (pla′tal) trademark for a preparation of cilostazol.

pleth·o·ra (pleth′ə-rə) [L., from Gr. *plēthōrē* fullness, satiety] 1. an excess of blood in a part. 2. by extension, a red florid complexion.

ple·thor·ic (plə-thor′ik) 1. abundant. 2. containing excessive blood; see *plethora* (def. 1).

pleth·ys·mo·gram (plə-thiz′mo-gram) a tracing made by the plethysmograph.

pleth·ys·mo·graph (plə-thiz′mo-graf) [Gr. *plēthysmos* increase + *-graph*] an instrument for determining and registering variations in the volume of an organ, part, or limb and in the amount of blood present or passing through it; also used for recording variations in the size of parts and in the blood supply.

body p. a device for measuring change in body volume, used especially in measuring intrathoracic gas volumes.

digital p. a plethysmograph that registers the change in blood volume taking place in a single finger or toe.

finger p. a digital plethysmograph for a finger.

pleth·ys·mog·ra·phy (pleth″iz-mog′rə-fe) the recording of the changes in the size of a part, particularly as modified by the circulation of the blood in it. Called also *pulse volume recording*.

air p., air-cuff p. a technique for measuring venous hemodynamics, usually in the legs: with the patient supine with lower limbs elevated, a pneumatic cuff attached to a recording device is applied to the limb; volume changes are recorded during a series of exercises.

dynamic venous p. the measurement of changes in limb circumference in response to exercise or passive compression of the limb.

impedance p. a technique for detecting blood volume changes in a part by measuring changes in electrical resistance; used in the diagnosis of deep vein thrombosis. Electrodes are placed around the calf and a pneumatic cuff around the thigh is inflated just enough to cause venous occlusion and then rapidly deflated. The drop in voltage is recorded; it is smaller in a lower limb with deep vein thrombosis than in a normal limb.

respiratory inductive p. a technique that uses elastic bands around the chest and abdomen of the patient to calculate chest and abdominal expansion, respiratory rate, respiratory pattern, and tidal volume.

strain-gauge p. a technique for recording changes in limb circumference employing a rubber tube filled with a conductive fluid; as the tube expands and contracts, the resistance in the fluid changes in proportion to the circumference of the limb; used in the evaluation of deep venous thrombosis and chronic venous insufficiency.

venous occlusion p. the measurement of changes in limb circumference in response to temporary obstruction of venous return.

pleu·ra (ploor′ə) gen. and pl. *pleu′rae* [Gr. "rib, side"] [TA] the serous membrane investing the lungs and lining the thoracic cavity, completely enclosing a potential space known as the pleural cavity. There are two pleurae, right and left, entirely distinct from each other, and they are moistened with a serous secretion that facilitates movements of the lungs in the chest. **pleu′ral** *adj*

cervical p. cupula pleurae.

costal p., p. costa′lis the part of the parietal pleura lining the rib cage.

diaphragmatic p., p. diaphragma′tica the part of the parietal pleura covering the diaphragm.

mediastinal p., p. mediastina′lis the part of the parietal pleura that covers the lateral face of the mediastinum and the structures within it.

parietal p., p. parieta′lis [TA] the portion of the pleura lining the walls of the thoracic cavity.

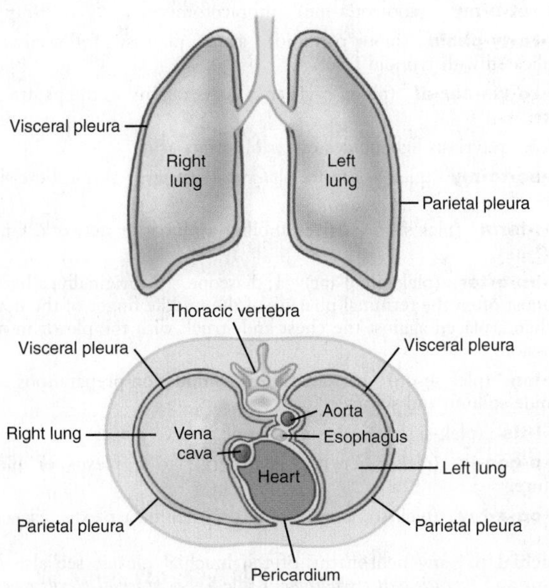

■ Pleura; for purpose of illustration, the pleural cavity is shown as an actual space.

pericardiac p., p. pericardi′aca the portion of the mediastinal pleura covering the pericardium and firmly attached to it.

p. pulmona′lis TA alternative for *p. visceralis.*

pulmonary p. p. visceralis.

visceral p., p. viscera′lis [TA] the portion of the pleura investing the lungs and lining their fissures, completely separating the different lobes; called also *p. pulmonalis* [TA alternative] and *pulmonary p.*

pleu·ra·cen·te·sis (ploor″ə-sen-te′sis) thoracentesis.

pleu·ra·cot·o·my (ploor″ə-kot′ə-me) thoracotomy.

pleu·rae (ploor′e) [L.] genitive and plural of *pleura.*

pleu·ral·gia (plo͞o-ral′jə) [*pleur-* + *-algia*] 1. pleurodynia (def. 1). 2. costalgia (def. 2).

pleu·ram·ni·on (plo͞o-ram′ne-on) an amnion that develops by a process of folding of the somatopleure, a characteristic of many mammals but not humans.

pleu·ra·poph·y·sis (ploor″ə-pof′ĭ-sis) [*pleur-* + *apophysis*] a rib, or its homologue; a rib considered as part of a vertebra.

pleu·rec·to·my (plo͞o-rek′tə-me) [*pleur-* + *-ectomy*] excision of a portion of the pleura.

pleu·ri·sy (ploor′ĭ-se) [Gr. *pleuritis*] inflammation of the pleura, with exudation into its cavity and upon its surface; the two common types are *fibrinous pleurisy* and *pleurisy with effusion.* The inflamed surfaces of the pleura may become permanently united by adhesions. Symptoms include localized chest pain and dry cough; as effusion occurs there is dyspnea but a lessening of pain. Called also *pleuritis.* **pleurit′ic** *adj*

adhesive p. pleurisy in which exudate forms dense adhesions between the visceral and parietal pleurae and partially or totally obliterates the pleural space.

blocked p. encysted p.

cholesterol p. a condition resembling pseudochylothorax, with effusion fluid high in cholesterol.

chylous p. chylothorax.

circumscribed p. encysted p.

costal p. inflammation of the parietal pleura.

diffuse p. pleurisy in which the inflammation involves the entire surface of the pleura.

dry p. fibrinous p.

p. with effusion pleurisy with a pleural effusion (see under *effusion*); types are named according to the type of exudate, such as *chylous p., hemorrhagic p., purulent p.,* and *serous p.* Called also *exudative p.* and *wet p.*

encysted p. pleurisy with adhesions that circumscribe the effused material. Called also *blocked p., circumscribed p.,* and *sacculated p.*

exudative p. p. with effusion.

fibrinous p. pleurisy in which exudate forms fibrinous adhesions between the visceral and parietal pleurae, which partially or totally obliterate the pleural space. Called also *adhesive p.* and *fibrinous* or *fibrosing pleuritis.*

hemorrhagic p. pleurisy with effusion (q.v.) in which the exudate is bloody. See also *hemothorax.*

indurative p. dry pleurisy marked by thickening and hardening of the pleura.

interlobular p. encysted pleurisy enclosed between the lobes of the lung. Called also *interlobitis.*

pulmonary p. inflammation of the pleura that covers the lungs; called also *corticopleuritis* and *visceral p.*

purulent p. empyema (def. 2).

sacculated p. encysted p.

serofibrinous p. pleurisy with effusion (q.v.) with a watery exudate and fibrinous deposits.

serous p. pleurisy with effusion (q.v.) in which the exudate is serous. See also *hydrothorax.*

suppurative p. empyema (def. 2).

visceral p. pulmonary p.

wet p. p. with effusion.

pleu·ri·tis (plo͞o-ri′tis) pleurisy.

fibrinous p., fibrosing p. fibrinous pleurisy.

lupus p. pleurisy, pleural effusion, and fever in patients with systemic lupus erythematosus.

rheumatoid p. pleurisy, pleural effusion, and often empyema in patients with rheumatoid arthritis.

tuberculous p. pleurisy with pleural effusion and multiple tubercles on the pleura in patients with primary tuberculosis.

uremic p. pleurisy, usually of the fibrinous type, with pleural effusion in patients with uremia, often accompanying uremic pericarditis; there are often painful friction rubs and hemothorax.

pleu·ri·tog·e·nous (ploor″ĭ-toj′ə-nəs) causing pleurisy.

pleur(o)- [Gr. *pleura* rib, side] a combining form denoting relationship to the pleura, to the side, or to a rib.

pleu·ro·bron·chi·tis (ploor″o-brong-ki′tis) pleurisy and bronchitis combined.

pleu·ro·cele (ploor′o-sēl) pneumonocele (def. 1).

pleu·ro·cen·te·sis (ploor″o-sen-te′sis) thoracentesis.

Pleu·ro·cer·i·dae (ploor″o-ser′ĭ-de) a family of snails of the order Mesogastropoda that includes the genus *Goniobasis.*

pleu·ro·cho·le·cys·ti·tis (ploor″o-ko″lə-sis-ti′tis) [*pleuro-* + *cholecystitis*] inflammation of the pleura and the gallbladder.

pleu·ro·cu·ta·ne·ous (ploor″o-ku-ta′ne-əs) pertaining to the pleura and the skin.

pleu·rod·e·sis (plo͞o-rod′ə-sis) [*pleuro-* + *-desis*] the artificial production of adhesions between the parietal and the visceral pleura for treatment of persistent pneumothorax or severe pleural effusion; formerly done by physically irritating the pleural surface, it is now usually done with a chemical sclerosing agent.

pleur·odont (ploor′o-dont) [*pleur-* + Gr. *odous* tooth] having teeth attached by one side on the inner surface of the jaw elements, as in certain lizards.

pleu·ro·dyn·ia (ploor″o-din′e-ə) [*pleur-* + *-odynia*] 1. pain in the pleural cavity. 2. costalgia (def. 2). Called also *pleuralgia.*

epidemic p. an acute infectious disease, generally occurring in epidemics among persons under age 20, caused by infection with group A coxsackieviruses or other enteroviruses. The most striking characteristic is sudden sharp paroxysmal pain in the chest over the ribs or in the upper abdomen, which can last for days and is accompanied by fever. There are often relapses after asymptomatic periods. Called also *Bornholm disease* and *epidemic myalgia.*

pleu·ro·esoph·a·ge·al (ploor″o-e-sof″ə-je′əl) pertaining to the pleura and esophagus.

pleu·ro·eso·pha·ge·us (ploor″o-e-so-fa′je-əs) [L.] pleuroesophageal; see under *musculus.*

pleu·ro·gen·ic (ploor″o-jen′ik) pleurogenous.

pleu·rog·e·nous (plo͞o-roj′ə-nəs) [*pleuro-* + *-genous*] originating in the pleura.

pleu·rog·ra·phy (plo͞o-rog′rə-fe) [*pleuro-* + *-graphy*] radiographic examination of the pleural cavity.

pleu·ro·hep·a·ti·tis (ploor″o-hep″ə-ti′tis) [*pleuro-* + *hepat-* + *-itis*] hepatitis with inflammation of a portion of the pleura near the liver.

pleu·ro·lith (ploor′o-lith) [*pleuro-* + *-lith*] a concretion found in the pleura; calcified pleural plaque.

pleu·rol·y·sis (plo͞o-rol′ĭ-sis) [*pleuro-* + *-lysis*] surgical separation of pleural adhesions.

pleu·ro·me·lus (ploor″o-me′ləs) [*pleuro-* + Gr. *melos* limb] an individual with a supernumerary limb arising laterally from the thorax.

pleu·ro·mu·ti·lin (ploor″o-mu′tĭ-lin) any of a class of antibacterial compounds, used in veterinary medicine and now under study for use in humans.

pleu·ro·pa·ri·e·to·pexy (ploor″o-pə-ri′ə-to-pek″se) [*pleuro-* + *parieto-* + *-pexy*] fixation of the visceral pleura to the parietal pleura, thus binding the lung to the chest wall. See also *pleurodesis.*

pleu·ro·peri·car·di·al (ploor″o-per″ĭ-kahr′de-əl) pertaining to both the pleura and the pericardium.

pleu·ro·peri·car·di·tis (ploor″o-per″ĭ-kahr-di′tis) [*pleuro-* + *pericarditis*] inflammation involving both the pleura and the pericardium.

pleu·ro·peri·to·ne·al (ploor″o-per″ĭ-to-ne′əl) pertaining to or communicating between the pleura and the peritoneum, or the pleural and peritoneal cavities.

pleu·ro·pneu·mo·nia (ploor″o-noo͞-mo′ne-ə) 1. pleurisy complicated with pneumonia; called also *pleuritic pneumonia* and *pneumopleuritis.* 2. a contagious disease of cattle and goats caused by infection with *Mycoplasma mycoides;* see *contagious bovine p.* and *contagious caprine p.*

contagious bovine p. pleuropneumonia in cattle, characterized by septicemia, fever, dyspnea, sequestra of infection within the lungs, abnormal lung sounds, and often death.

contagious caprine p. pleuropneumonia in goats, characterized by cough, dyspnea, abnormal lung sounds, and often an early death.

pleu·ro·pneu·mo·nol·y·sis (ploor″o-noo͞″mo-nol′ĭ-sis) [*pleuro-* + *pneumono-* + *lysis*] division of adhesions between the lung and the parietal pleura; see also *pleurolysis.*

pleu·ro·pul·mo·nary (ploor″o-pool′mə-nar″e) pertaining to the pleura and lungs.

pleu·ros·co·py (ploor-os′kə-pe) [*pleuro-* + *-scopy*] thoracoscopy.

pleu·ro·so·ma (ploor″o-so′mə) pleurosomus.

pleu·ro·so·mus (ploor″o-so′məs) [*pleuro-* + Gr. *sōma* body] a fetus with protrusion of the intestine and imperfect development of one upper limb.

pleu·ro·thot·o·nos (ploor″o-thot′ə-nəs) [Gr. *pleurothen* from the side + *tonos* tension] tetanic bending of the body to one side.

pleu·ro·thot·o·nus (ploor″o-thot′ə-nəs) pleurothotonos.

pleu·ro·tome (ploor′o-tōm) an area of the lung supplied with afferent nerve fibers by a single posterior spinal root.

pleu·rot·o·my (ploo͞-rot′ə-me) thoracotomy.

pleu·ro·ty·phoid (ploor″o-ti′foid) acute pleurisy followed by and complicated with typhoid fever.

pleu·ro·vis·cer·al (ploor″o-vis′ər-əl) pertaining to the pleura and the viscera.

PLEVA pityriasis lichenoides et varioliformis acuta.

plex·ec·to·my (plek-sek′tə-me) [*plexus* + *-ectomy*] surgical excision of a plexus.

plex·i·form (plek′sĭ-form) resembling a plexus or network. Cf. *reticular.*

plex·im·e·ter (plek-sim′ə-tər) 1. diascope. 2. originally, a hard plate, now most often the terminal phalanx of the middle finger of the nondominant hand, placed against the chest and struck with the plexor in mediate percussion.

Plex·ion (plek′se-on) trademark for combination preparations of sulfacetamide sodium and sulfur.

plex·i·tis (plek-si′tis) inflammation of a nerve plexus.

plex·o·gen·ic (plek′so-jen″ik) giving rise to a plexus or plexiform structure.

plex·op·a·thy (plek-sop′ə-the) any disorder of a plexus, especially of nerves.

brachial p. any neuropathy of the brachial plexus; see also *brachial paralysis* and *thoracic outlet syndrome.* Called also *brachial plexus neuropathy, brachial syndrome,* and *cervicobrachial syndrome.*

lumbar p. neuropathy of the lumbar plexus.

lumbosacral p. lumbar and sacral plexopathies considered together.

radiation p. injury to a nerve plexus from radiation therapy; the most common site is the brachial plexus after radiation therapy to the axilla in cases of breast cancer.

sacral p. neuropathy of the sacral plexus.

plex·or (plek′sor) percussion hammer, or the index or middle finger of the dominant hand used as a hammer in percussion.

plex·us (plek′səs) pl. *plexus* or *plexuses* [L. "braid"] a network of lymphatic vessels, nerves, or veins. See also *net, network,* and *rete.* **plex′al** *adj*

Plexus

Descriptions are given on TA terms, and include anglicized names of specific plexuses.

annular p. a plexus of nerve fibers encircling the corneal margin.

p. of anterior cerebral artery a thin plexus of sympathetic nerve fibers accompanying the anterior cerebral artery.

aortic p., abdominal p. aorticus abdominalis.

aortic p., thoracic p. aorticus thoracicus.

p. aor′ticus a network of lymphatic vessels about the aorta.

p. aor′ticus abdomina′lis [TA] abdominal aortic plexus: an unpaired nerve plexus composed of interconnecting bundles of fibers that arise from the celiac and superior mesenteric plexuses and descend along the aorta. Receiving branches from the lumbar splanchnic nerves, it becomes the superior hypogastric plexus below the bifurcation of the aorta. Branches of the plexus are distributed along the adjacent branches of the aorta.

p. aor′ticus thoraca′lis, p. aor′ticus thora′cicus [TA] thoracic aortic plexus: a nerve plexus around the thoracic aorta formed by filaments from the sympathetic trunks and vagus nerves, and from which fine twigs accompany branches of the aorta. It is continuous below with the celiac plexus and the abdominal aortic plexus.

p. arte′riae ova′ricae p. ovaricus.

Auerbach p. p. myentericus.

auricular p., posterior a sympathetic nerve plexus on the posterior auricular artery.

p. autono′micus [TA] autonomic plexus: any of the extensive networks of nerve fibers and cell bodies associated with the autonomic nervous system; found particularly in the thorax, abdomen, and pelvis, and containing sympathetic, parasympathetic, and visceral afferent fibers. Called also *visceral p.*

p. basila′ris [TA] basilar plexus: a venous plexus of the dura mater situated over the basilar part of the occipital bone and the posterior portion of the body of the sphenoid, extending from the cavernous sinus to the foramen magnum, and communicating with other dural sinuses.

Batson p. the vertebral plexus (def. 1), considered as a whole system.

p. brachia′lis [TA] brachial plexus: a plexus originating from the anterior branches of the last four cervical spinal nerves and most of the anterior branch of the first thoracic spinal nerves. Situated partly in the neck and partly in the axilla, it is composed successively of anterior branches and trunks (supraclavicular part) which are related to the subclavian artery and which give off the dorsal scapular, long thoracic, subclavius, and suprascapular nerves. The infraclavicular part consists of divisions which lie approximately behind the clavicle and cords and branches in the axilla in relation to the axillary artery. Its branches are medial and lateral pectoral, medial brachial cutaneous, medial antebrachial cutaneous, median, ulnar radial, subscapular, thoracodorsal, and axillary nerves.

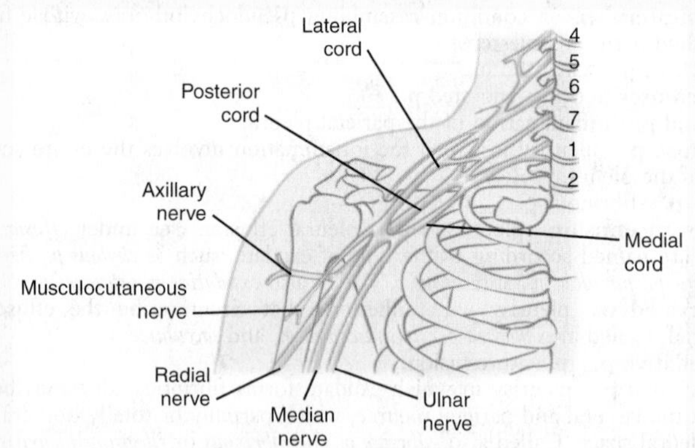

■ Plexus brachialis (brachial plexus). Anterior view, showing the most major branches.

Plexus *Continued*

cardiac p. p. cardiacus.
cardiac p., anterior superficial cardiac p.
cardiac p., deep, cardiac p., great the larger part of the cardiac plexus, situated between the aortic arch and the tracheal bifurcation.
cardiac p., superficial the part of the cardiac plexus that lies beneath the aortic arch to the right of the ligamentum arteriosum.
p. cardi'acus [TA] cardiac plexus: the plexus around the base of the heart, chiefly in the epicardium. It is formed by cardiac branches from the vagus nerves and the sympathetic trunks and ganglia, contains visceral afferent fibers, and shows subdivisions related to the arch of the aorta, right and left atria, and right and left coronary arteries. The cardiac plexus is continuous with the right and left pulmonary plexuses.
p. caro'ticus commu'nis [TA] common carotid plexus: a nerve plexus on the common carotid artery, formed by branches of the internal and external carotid plexuses and the cervical sympathetic ganglia.
p. caro'ticus exter'nus [TA] external carotid plexus: a nerve plexus located around the external carotid artery, formed by the external carotid nerves from the superior cervical ganglion, and supplying sympathetic fibers which accompany the branches of the external carotid artery.
p. caro'ticus inter'nus [TA] internal carotid plexus: a nerve plexus on the internal carotid artery, formed by the internal carotid nerve, which supplies sympathetic fibers to the branches of the internal carotid artery, to the tympanic plexus, to the nerves in the cavernous sinus, and, directly or indirectly, to the cranial parasympathetic ganglia through which they pass.
carotid p. p. caroticus internus.
carotid p., common p. caroticus communis.
carotid p., external p. caroticus externus.
carotid p., internal p. caroticus internus.
p. caverno'sus [TA] a plexus of sympathetic nerve fibers related to the cavernous sinus of the dura mater.
p. caverno'sus con'chae [TA] cavernous plexus of concha: any of the numerous venous plexuses in the thick mucous membrane of the nasal conchae.
cavernous p. p. cavernosus.
cavernous p. of concha p. cavernosus conchae.
celiac p., p. celi'acus p. coeliacus.
cervical p. p. cervicalis.
cervical p., posterior a plexus in the posterior cervical region, formed by posterior rami of the first three or four cervical spinal nerves.
p. cervica'lis [TA] cervical plexus: a nerve plexus formed by the anterior branches of the upper four cervical nerves; arranged as an irregular series of loops, it gives off superficial branches (lesser occipital, greater auricular, transverse cervical, and supraclavicular nerves), and deep branches (phrenic, accessory phrenic, ansa cervicalis, and muscular nerves).
choroid p's infoldings of blood vessels of the pia mater covered by a thin coat of ependymal cells that form tufted projections into the third, fourth, and lateral ventricles of the brain; they are supplied by the choroidal arteries, and they secrete the cerebrospinal fluid. See *p. choroideus ventriculi lateralis, p. choroideus ventriculi tertii,* and *p. choroideus ventriculi quarti.*
choroid p., inferior p. choroideus ventriculi quarti.
p's of choroid artery delicate nerve plexuses accompanying the choroid arteries.
choroid p. of fourth ventricle p. choroideus ventriculi quarti.
choroid p. of lateral ventricle p. choroideus ventriculi lateralis.
choroid p. of third ventricle p. choroideus ventriculi tertii.
p. choroi'deus ventri'culi latera'lis [TA] choroid plexus of lateral ventricle: vascular, fringelike folds of the pia mater in the floor of the pars centralis and the roof of the temporal horn of the lateral ventricle, concerned with production of the cerebrospinal fluid.
p. choroi'deus ventri'culi quar'ti [TA] choroid plexus of fourth ventricle: vascular fringelike folds of the pia mater in the roof of the posterior part of the fourth ventricle and extending into and through the lateral recesses and the foramina of Luschka; concerned with production of the cerebrospinal fluid.
p. choroi'deus ventri'culi ter'tii [TA] choroid plexus of third ventricle: vascular, fringelike folds of the pia mater in the roof of the third ventricle, concerned with production of the cerebrospinal fluid.
ciliary ganglionic p. an autonomic plexus derived from the long and short ciliary nerves, lying on the ciliary muscle, and supplying the dilator and sphincter muscles of the pupil.
p. coccy'geus [TA] coccygeal plexus: a small plexus formed by the anterior branches of the coccygeal and the fifth sacral nerves, and a communication from the fourth sacral nerve, and giving off the anococcygeal nerves.
p. coeli'acus 1. [TA] celiac plexus: a prevertebral plexus that lies on the front and sides of the aorta at the origins of the celiac trunk and superior mesenteric and renal arteries. It contains the paired celiac ganglia, the superior mesenteric ganglion (or ganglia), and small unnamed ganglionic masses. Branches of the plexus extend along all of the adjacent arteries. Called also *solar p.* Also spelled *p. celiacus.* 2. a plexus composed of lymphatic vessels, the superior mesenteric lymph nodes, and the celiac lymph nodes behind the stomach, duodenum, and pancreas. Called also *celiac p.* and *p. celiacus.*
colic p., left the part of the inferior mesenteric plexus that accompanies the left colic artery.
colic p., middle the part of the superior mesenteric plexus that accompanies the middle colic artery.
colic p., right the part of the superior mesenteric plexus that accompanies the right colic artery.
coronary p's, gastric p. gastrici.
coronary p. of heart, anterior a plexus of sympathetic nerve fibers anterior to the heart and related chiefly to the branches of the left coronary artery. Called also *right coronary p. of heart.*
coronary p. of heart, left posterior coronary p. of heart.
coronary p. of heart, posterior a plexus of sympathetic nerve fibers posterior to the heart and related chiefly to the branches of the right coronary artery. Called also *left coronary p. of heart.*
coronary p. of heart, right anterior coronary p. of heart.
coronary p's of stomach, superior p. gastrici.
crural p. p. femoralis.
Cruveilhier p. posterior cervical p.
cystic p. a nerve plexus near the gallbladder, related to the cystic artery.
p. deferentia'lis [TA] deferential plexus: the subdivision of the inferior hypogastric plexus that supplies nerve fibers to the ductus deferens. Called also *p. of ductus deferens.*
p. denta'lis infe'rior [TA] inferior dental plexus: a plexus of nerve fibers from the inferior alveolar nerve, situated around the roots of the lower teeth.
p. denta'lis supe'rior [TA] superior dental plexus: a plexus of fibers from the superior alveolar nerves, situated around the roots of the upper teeth.
diaphragmatic p. phrenic p.
p. of ductus deferens p. deferentialis.
p. ente'ricus [TA] enteric plexus: a plexus of autonomic nerve fibers within the wall of the intestine, and made up of the submucosal, myenteric, and subserosal plexuses; it contains visceral afferent fibers, sympathetic postganglionic fibers, parasympathetic preganglionic and postganglionic fibers, and parasympathetic postganglionic cell bodies.
epigastric p. p. coeliacus.
esophageal p., p. esophagea'lis, p. esopha'geus p. oesophageus.
Exner p. superficial tangential fibers in the molecular layer of the cerebral cortex; called also *molecular p.*
facial p., p. of facial artery a nerve plexus along the facial artery.
p. femora'lis [TA] femoral plexus: a plexus accompanying the femoral artery, derived chiefly from the aortic plexus by way of the common and external iliac plexuses.
gastric p's p. gastrici.
gastric p., inferior the inferior portion of the gastric plexuses, located on the greater curvature of the stomach.
gastric p., left superior gastric p.
gastric p., superior the superior portion of the gastric plexuses, accompanying the left gastric artery on the lesser curvature of the stomach; called also *left gastric p.*
p. gas'trici [TA] gastric plexuses: subdivisions of the celiac portion of the prevertebral plexuses, accompanying the gastric arteries and branches and supplying nerve fibers to the stomach.
gastroepiploic p., left inferior gastric p.
Heller p. an arterial network in the submucosa of the intestine.
hemorrhoidal p. 1. p. venosus rectalis. 2. rectal p. (def. 2).
hemorrhoidal p., external inferior rectal p. (def. 1).
hemorrhoidal p., inferior 1. inferior rectal p. (def. 1). 2. p. rectalis inferior.

hemorrhoidal p., internal superior rectal p. (def. 1).
hemorrhoidal p., middle p. rectalis medius.
hemorrhoidal p., superior 1. superior rectal p. (def. 1). 2. p. rectalis superior.
p. hepa′ticus [TA] hepatic plexus: a subdivision of the celiac plexus accompanying the hepatic artery to the liver.
Hovius p. a venous plexus in the ciliary region connected with the sinus venosus sclerae. Called also *Leber p.*
p. hypogas′tricus hypogastric plexus 1. the hypogastric portion of the prevertebral plexuses; see *p. hypogastricus inferior* and *p. hypogastricus superior.* 2. a plexus of lymphatic vessels in the hypogastric region.
p. hypogas′tricus infe′rior [TA] inferior hypogastric plexus: the plexus formed on each side anterior to the lower part of the sacrum, formed by the junction of the hypogastric and pelvic splanchnic nerves; branches are given off to the pelvic organs. Called also *pelvic p., p. pelvicus* [TA alternative] and *p. pelvina.*
p. hypogas′tricus supe′rior [TA] superior hypogastric plexus: the downward continuation of the abdominal aortic plexus; it lies in front of the upper part of the sacrum, just below the bifurcation of the aorta, receives fibers from the lower lumbar splanchnic nerves, and divides into the right and left hypogastric nerves. Called also *nervus presacralis* [TA alternative] or *presacral nerve.*
ileocolic p. the part of the superior mesenteric plexus that accompanies the ileocolic artery.
p. ili′acus [TA] iliac plexus: any of the plexuses derived chiefly from the aortic plexus and accompanying the common iliac arteries.
p. ili′acus exter′nus a lymphatic plexus situated about the external iliac vessels.
incisive p. a branch of the inferior dental plexus, innervating the canine and incisor teeth of the lower jaw.
infraorbital p. a nerve plexus situated deep to the levator labii superioris muscle, formed by superior labial branches of the infraorbital nerve and branches of the facial nerve.
p. inguina′lis inguinal plexus: a lymphatic plexus situated near the end of the long saphenous vein and along the femoral artery and vein in the iliopectineal fossa.
intercavernous p. a network of venous channels connecting the two cavernous sinuses across both the roof and the floor of the pituitary fossa.
intermesenteric p., lumboaortic p. aorticus abdominalis.
p. intermesente′ricus [TA] intermesenteric plexus: the part of the aortic plexus that is located between the origins of the superior and inferior mesenteric arteries.
interradial p. either of the two striae of Baillarger, external or internal; see *stria laminae granularis internae* and *stria laminae pyramidalis internae.*
intestinal p., submucous p. submucosus.
intramural p. a plexus of autonomous intrinsic nerve cells and fibers that are confined entirely to the intestinal and bladder walls and take part in or regulate local reflexes and activity.
p. intraparoti′deus [TA] parotid plexus: a plexus formed by anastomosis of the terminal branches of the temporal, zygomatic, buccal, marginal mandibular, and cervical rami of the facial nerve, arising in the parotid gland. Called also *p. parotideus.*
intrascleral p. a network of vessels in the sclera, receiving junctional branches from the sinus venosus sclerae.
ischiadic p. p. sacralis.
p. jugula′ris jugular plexus: a plexus of lymphatic vessels along the internal jugular vein.
Leber p. Hovius p.
lienal p. p. splenicus.
p. liena′lis TA alternative for *p. splenicus.*
lingual p. a nerve plexus accompanying the lingual artery.
p. lumba′lis 1. [TA] lumbar plexus: a plexus formed by the anterior branches of the second to fifth lumbar nerves in the psoas major muscle (the branches of the first lumbar nerve often are included). The lower division of the fourth lumbar nerve joins the fifth, and the lumbosacral trunk thus formed becomes part of the sacral plexus. The branches of the first lumbar nerve are the ilioinguinal and iliohypogastric nerves; branches of the plexus proper are the genitofemoral, lateral femoral cutaneous, obturator, and femoral nerves. 2. a lymphatic plexus in the lumbar region.
p. lumba′ris p. lumbalis (def. 1).

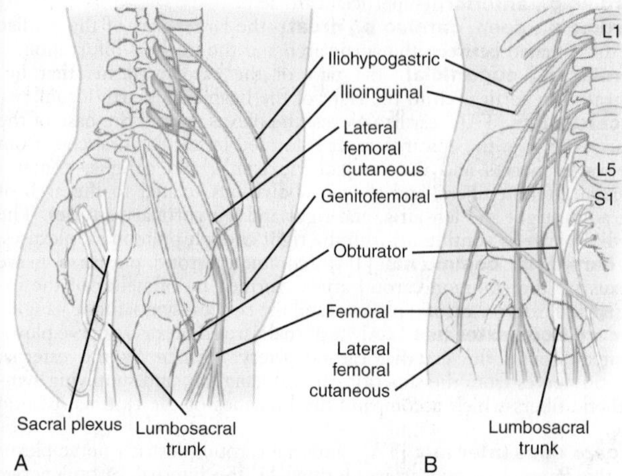

■ Plexus lumbalis (lumbar plexus), in yellow, in lateral *(A)* and anterior *(B)* views, with the divisions forming the lumbosacral trunk shown in white, as is the sacral plexus.

p. lumbosacra′lis [TA] lumbosacral plexus: a term applied to the lumbar and sacral nerve plexuses together, because of their continuous nature.
lymphatic p. an interconnecting network of lymph vessels, i.e., the lymphocapillary vessels, collecting vessels, and trunks, which provides drainage of lymph in a one-way flow.
p. lympha′ticus axilla′ris [TA] axillary lymphatic plexus: a plexus of lymph vessels and nodes in the fossa axillaris.
maxillary p. a nerve plexus that accompanies the maxillary artery.
maxillary p., external p. of facial artery.
p. of medial cerebral artery a thin plexus of sympathetic nerve fibers accompanying the middle cerebral artery.
Meissner p. p. submucosus.
meningeal p. a nerve plexus accompanying the middle meningeal artery.
p. mesente′ricus infe′rior [TA] inferior mesenteric plexus: a subdivision of the aortic plexus accompanying the inferior mesenteric artery.
p. mesente′ricus supe′rior [TA] superior mesenteric plexus: a subdivision of the celiac plexus accompanying the superior mesenteric artery.
molecular p. Exner p.
p. myente′ricus [TA] myenteric plexus: that part of the enteric plexus within the tunica muscularis. Called also *Auerbach p.*
nasopalatine p. a nerve plexus near the incisor foramen.
nerve p. a plexus made up of intermingled nerve fibers.
p. nervo′rum spina′lium [TA] plexus of spinal nerves: a plexus formed by the intermingling of the fibers of two or more spinal nerves, such as the brachial or lumbosacral plexus.
nervous p. nerve p.
occipital p. a nerve plexus accompanying the occipital artery.
p. oesophagea′lis, p. oesopha′geus [TA] esophageal plexus: a plexus surrounding the esophagus formed by branches of the left and right vagi and sympathetic trunks and containing also visceral afferent fibers from the esophagus; it is subdivided into anterior and posterior parts.
ophthalmic p. a nerve plexus accompanying the ophthalmic artery.
p. ova′ricus [TA] ovarian plexus: a subdivision of the aortic plexus, accompanying the ovarian arteries; called also *p. arteriae ovaricae.*
pampiniform p., p. pampinifor′mis [TA] 1. in the male, a plexus of veins from the testicle and the epididymis, constituting part of the spermatic cord. 2. in the female, a plexus of ovarian veins in the broad ligament.
p. pancrea′ticus [TA] pancreatic plexus: a subdivision of the celiac plexus, accompanying pancreatic arteries.
Panizza p's two plexuses of the lymph vessels in the lateral fossae of the frenum of the prepuce.
papillary p. superficial vascular p.

Plexus *Continued*

parotid p., p. paroti′deus p. intraparotideus.
patellar p. a plexus of nerve fibers in front of the knee, formed by communications between branches of the saphenous nerves and the femoral cutaneous nerves.
pelvic p. p. hypogastricus inferior.
p. pel′vicus TA alternative for *p. hypogastricus inferior.*
p. pelvi′na p. hypogastricus inferior.
p. periarteria′lis [TA] periarterial plexus: a network of autonomic and sensory nerve fibers in the adventitia of an artery, some of which follow the course of the artery to reach and innervate other structures and some of which innervate the artery itself.
pericorneal p. anastomosing branches of the anterior conjunctival arteries, arranged in a superficial conjunctival and a deep episcleral layer about the cornea.
peritubular capillary p. a network formed by the peritubular capillaries around the renal tubules.
pharyngeal p. 1. p. pharyngeus. 2. p. pharyngeus nervi vagi.
pharyngeal p. of vagus nerve p. pharyngeus nervi vagi.
p. pharyngea′lis p. pharyngeus.
p. pharyngea′lis ner′vi va′gi p. pharyngeus nervi vagi.
p. pharyn′geus [TA] pharyngeal plexus: a venous plexus posterolateral to the pharynx, formed by the pharyngeal veins, communicating with the pterygoid venous plexus, and draining into the internal jugular vein. Called also *p. pharyngealis.*
p. pharyn′geus ner′vi va′gi [TA] pharyngeal plexus of vagus nerve: a plexus formed chiefly by fibers from branches of the vagus nerves, but also containing fibers from the glossopharyngeal nerves and sympathetic trunks, and supplying motor, general sensory, and sympathetic innervation to the muscles and mucosa of the pharynx and soft palate, except for the tensor veli palatini muscle. Called also *p. pharyngealis nervi vagi.*
phrenic p. a nerve plexus accompanying the inferior phrenic artery to the diaphragm and suprarenal glands.
popliteal p. a plexus of nerve fibers accompanying the popliteal artery.
presacral p. p. venosus sacralis.
prevertebral p′s autonomic nerve plexuses situated in the thorax, abdomen, and pelvis, anterior to the vertebral column; they consist of visceral afferent fibers, preganglionic parasympathetic fibers, preganglionic and postganglionic sympathetic fibers, and ganglia containing sympathetic ganglion cells, and they give rise to postganglionic fibers. The major plexuses are cardiac, pulmonary, esophageal, celiac, mesenteric, and hypogastric. All are closely related to the aorta; those in the abdomen and pelvis supply adjacent viscera by subdivisions which accompany the branches of the aorta and which are named usually after these branches, but sometimes according to the organ supplied.
primary p. a network of capillaries that arise from the superior hypophysial arteries, extend into the median eminence of the hypothalamus, then return to the surface, where they are collected into veins that supply the sinusoids of the adenohypophysis.
prostatic p. 1. p. prostaticus. 2. p. venosus prostaticus.
prostaticovesical p. the plexus venosus vesicalis and the plexus venosus prostaticus considered together; called also *vesicoprostatic plexus.*
p. prosta′ticus [TA] prostatic plexus: a subdivision of the inferior hypogastric plexus that supplies nerve fibers to the prostate and adjacent organs. Called also *Santorini p.*
p. pterygoi′deus [TA] pterygoid plexus: a network of veins corresponding to the second and third parts of the maxillary artery; situated on the lateral surface of the medial pterygoid muscle and on both surfaces of the lateral pterygoid muscle, and draining into the facial vein. Called also *p. venosus pterygoideus.*
pudendal p., p. pudenda′lis p. venosus prostaticus.
p. pulmona′lis [TA] a nerve plexus formed by several strong trunks of the vagus nerve that are joined at the root of the lung by branches from the sympathetic trunk and cardiac plexus. The plexus is often described as having anterior and posterior parts (see *anterior pulmonary p.* and *posterior pulmonary p.*); filaments from each accompany the blood vessels and bronchi into the lungs.
pulmonary p., anterior the smaller portion of the pulmonary plexus, located in front of the root of the lung and interconnected with the posterior pulmonary plexus.
pulmonary p., posterior the larger portion of the pulmonary plexus, located behind the root of the lung and interconnected with the anterior pulmonary plexus.
Quénu hemorrhoidal p. a lymphatic plexus found in the perianal skin.
p. of Raschkow a delicate plexus of nerve fibers beneath the odontoblasts in the dental papilla during the formation of dentin.
rectal p. 1. p. venosus rectalis. 2. see *p. rectalis inferior, p. rectalis medius,* and *p. rectalis superior.*
rectal p., external inferior rectal p. (def. 1).
rectal p., inferior 1. the subcutaneous portion of the rectal venous plexus, below the pectinate line. 2. p. rectalis inferior.
rectal p., internal superior rectal p. (def. 1).
rectal p., middle p. rectalis medius.
rectal p., superior 1. the submucosal portion of the rectal venous plexus, above the pectinate line. 2. p. rectalis superior.
p. recta′lis infe′rior [TA] inferior rectal plexus: a plexus accompanying the inferior rectal artery, derived chiefly from the inferior rectal nerve; called also *inferior hemorrhoidal p.*
p. recta′lis me′dius [TA] middle rectal plexus: a subdivision of the inferior hypogastric plexus, in proximity with and supplying nerve fibers to the rectum; called also *middle hemorrhoidal p.*
p. recta′lis supe′rior [TA] superior rectal plexus: a plexus accompanying the superior rectal artery to the rectum, derived from the inferior mesenteric and hypogastric plexuses. Called also *superior hemorrhoidal p.*
p. rena′lis [TA] renal plexus: a subdivision of the celiac plexus, accompanying the renal artery.
sacral p. 1. p. sacralis. 2. p. venosus sacralis.
sacral p., anterior p. venosus sacralis.
p. sacra′lis [TA] sacral plexus: a plexus that lies in front of the piriform muscle, arising from the anterior branches of the last two lumbar nerves (which form the lumbosacral trunk) and the first four sacral nerves. It has twelve named branches, five supplying pelvic structures (the nerves to the piriformis, to levator ani and coccygeus, and to sphincter ani muscles, the pelvic splanchnic nerves, and the pudendal nerve) and seven helping supply the buttocks and lower limbs (superior and inferior gluteal, posterior femoral cutaneous, perforating cutaneous, and sciatic nerves, and nerves to the quadratus femoris and obturator internus muscles).
sacral lymphatic p. a fine network of lymphatic vessels in the hollow of the sacrum.
Santorini p. 1. p. prostaticus. 2. p. venosus prostaticus.
Sappey subareolar p. a lymphatic plexus situated beneath the areola of the nipple.
solar p. p. coeliacus.
spermatic p. 1. p. testicularis. 2. p. pampiniformis (def. 1).
p. of spinal nerves p. nervorum spinalium.
p. sple′nicus [TA] splenic plexus: a subdivision of the celiac plexus, which accompanies the splenic artery; called also *lienal p.* and *p. lienalis* [TA alternative].
Stensen p. the venous network around the parotid duct.
stroma p. superficial and deep nerve fibrils within the substantia propria of the cornea.
p. subcla′vius [TA] subclavian plexus: a sympathetic nerve plexus on the subclavian artery, arising from the cervicothoracic ganglion, contributing fibers to the phrenic nerve and to the branches of the subclavian artery, and continuing to the axillary artery.
subendocardial terminal p. rami subendocardiales.

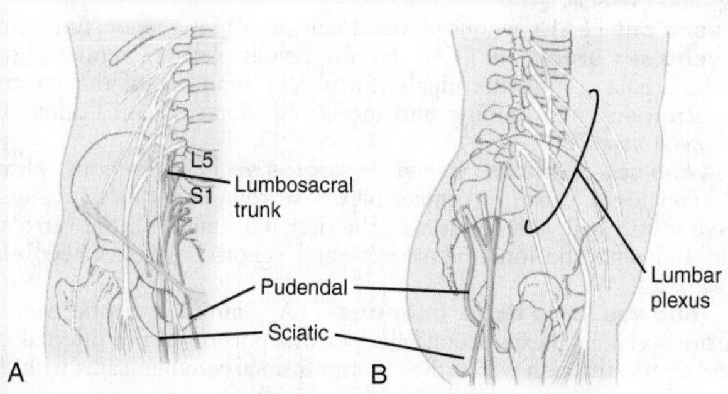

■ Plexus sacralis (sacral plexus), in yellow, in anterior *(A)* and lateral *(B)* views. The lumbar plexus is shown in white.

p. submuco′sus [TA], **submucous p.** submucosal plexus: the part of the enteric plexus that is situated in the submucosa.
subpapillary p. superficial vascular p.
subsartorial p. a nerve plexus deep to the sartorius muscle, formed by communications between branches of the medial femoral cutaneous nerve and the saphenous and obturator nerves.
p. subsero′sus [TA] subserosal plexus: the part of the enteric plexus situated deep to the serosal surface of the tunica serosa.
subtrapezius p. a term sometimes applied to a small plexus situated deep to the trapezius muscle, formed by communications between branches of the accessory nerve and cervical nerves.
supraradial p. Kaes-Bekhterev layer.
p. suprarena′lis [TA] suprarenal plexus: a subdivision of the celiac plexus, in proximity with and supplying nerve fibers to an adrenal (suprarenal) gland.
temporal p., superficial a plexus of nerve fibers accompanying the superficial temporal artery.
p. testicula′ris [TA] testicular plexus: a subdivision of the aortic plexus accompanying the testicular arteries; called also *spermatic p.*
thyroid p., inferior a nerve plexus accompanying the inferior thyroid artery to the larynx, pharynx, and thyroid region.
thyroid p., superior a nerve plexus accompanying the superior thyroid artery to the larynx, pharynx, and thyroid region.
tonsillar p. a plexus around the tonsil, formed by communications between the middle and posterior palatine nerves and the tonsillar branches of the glossopharyngeal nerve; fibers are supplied to the tonsil, soft palate, and region of the fauces.
Trolard p. p. venosus canalis nervi hypoglossi.
tubular capillary p. a vascular network formed by the capillaries around the renal tubules.
p. tympa′nicus [TA] tympanic plexus: a nerve plexus on the promontory of the middle ear, formed by the tympanic and caroticotympanic nerves. It gives off the lesser petrosal nerve and a branch of the greater petrosal nerve and sends sensory fibers to the mucous membrane of the tympanic cavity, the auditory tube, and the mastoid air cells.
p. urete′ricus [TA] ureteric plexus: a plexus supplying the ureter and derived from the renal and hypogastric plexuses.
uterine p. 1. the part of the uterovaginal plexus that supplies nerve fibers to the cervix and lower part of the uterus. 2. p. venosus uterinus.
p. uterovagina′lis 1. [TA] uterovaginal plexus: the subdivision of the inferior hypogastric plexus that supplies nerve fibers to the uterus, ovary, vagina, urethra, and erectile tissue of the vestibule. 2. see *p. venosus uterinus* and *p. venosus vaginalis.*
vaginal p. 1. the part of the uterovaginal plexus that supplies nerve fibers to the walls of the vagina. 2. p. venosus vaginalis.
vascular p. 1. p. vasculosus. 2. p. vascularis.
vascular p., deep a plexus of arterioles and venules found between the dermis and the tela subcutanea, with many interconnections to the superficial vascular plexus; its arterial part is known as the *cutaneous arterial network* or *arterial network of dermis.*
vascular p., superficial a plexus of arterioles and venules found between the papillary and reticular layers of the dermis, with many interconnections to the deep vascular plexus; its arterial part is known as the *subpapillary network* or *rete.* Called also *papillary* or *subpapillary p.*
p. vascula′ris [TA] vascular plexus: a plexus of peripheral nerves through which blood vessels receive innervation.
p. vasculo′sus [TA] vascular plexus: a network of intercommunicating blood vessels.
p. veno′sus [TA] venous plexus: a network of interconnecting veins.
p. veno′sus areola′ris [TA] areolar venous plexus: a venous plexus in the areola around the nipple, formed by branches of the internal thoracic veins and draining into the lateral thoracic vein. Called also *p. venosus mamillae.*
p. veno′sus cana′lis ner′vi hypoglos′si [TA] venous plexus of hypoglossal canal: a venous plexus surrounding the hypoglossal nerve in its canal, and connecting the occipital sinus with the vertebral vein and with the longitudinal vertebral venous sinuses. Called also *Trolard p.*
p. veno′sus caro′ticus inter′nus [TA] internal carotid venous plexus: a venous plexus around the petrosal portion of the internal carotid artery, through which the cavernous sinus communicates with the internal jugular vein.
p. veno′sus fora′minis ova′lis [TA] venous plexus of foramen ovale: a venous plexus that connects the cavernous sinus through the foramen ovale with the pterygoid plexus and the pharyngeal plexus; called also *rete foraminis ovalis.*
p. veno′sus mammil′lae p. venosus areolaris.
p. veno′sus prosta′ticus [TA] prostatic venous plexus: a venous plexus around the prostate gland, receiving the deep dorsal vein of the penis and draining through the vesical plexus and the prostatic veins; called also *p. pudendalis.*
p. veno′sus pterygoi′deus p. pterygoideus.
p. veno′sus recta′lis [TA] rectal venous plexus: a venous plexus that surrounds the lower part of the rectum and drains into the rectal veins; called also *hemorrhoidal p.*
p. veno′sus sacra′lis [TA] sacral venous plexus: the plexus on the pelvic surface of the sacrum that receives the sacral intervertebral veins, anastomoses with neighboring lumbar and pelvic veins, and drains into the middle and lateral sacral veins.
p. veno′sus suboccipita′lis [TA] suboccipital venous plexus: that part of the external vertebral plexus which lies on and in the suboccipital triangle, receives the occipital veins of the scalp, and drains into the vertebral vein.
p. veno′sus uteri′nus [TA] uterine venous plexus: the venous plexus around the uterus, draining into the internal iliac veins by way of the uterine veins.
p. veno′sus vagina′lis [TA] vaginal venous plexus: a venous plexus in the walls of the vagina, which drains into the internal iliac veins by way of the internal pudendal veins.
p. veno′sus vertebra′lis exter′nus ante′rior [TA] anterior external vertebral venous plexus: the venous plexus formed by the anterior external group of veins of the vertebral column that lies on the anterior aspects of the vertebral bodies. See also *venae spinales anteriores.*
p. veno′sus vertebra′lis exter′nus poste′rior [TA] posterior external vertebral venous plexus: the venous plexus formed by the posterior external group of veins of the vertebral column that lie on the posterior aspects of the laminae and around the spinous, articular, and transverse processes of the vertebrae. See also *venae spinales posteriores.*
p. veno′sus vertebra′lis inter′nus ante′rior [TA] anterior internal vertebral venous plexus: the venous plexus formed by the anterior internal group of veins of the vertebral column that lies on the posterior aspects of the vertebral bodies and intervertebral disks, on either side of the posterior longitudinal ligament. See also *venae spinales anteriores.*
p. veno′sus vertebra′lis inter′nus poste′rior [TA] posterior internal vertebral venous plexus: the venous plexus formed by the posterior internal group of veins of the vertebral column that lie on either side of the midline in front of the vertebral arches and ligamenta flava. See also *venae spinales posteriores.*
p. veno′sus vesica′lis [TA] vesical venous plexus: a venous plexus surrounding the upper part of the urethra and the neck of the bladder, communicating with the vaginal plexus in the female and with the prostatic plexus in the male.
venous p. p. venosus.
venous p., areolar p. venosus areolaris.
venous p., hemorrhoidal p. venosus rectalis.
venous p., internal carotid p. venosus caroticus internus.
venous p., prostatic p. venosus prostaticus.
venous p., rectal p. venosus rectalis.
venous p., sacral p. venosus sacralis.
venous p., suboccipital p. venosus suboccipitalis.
venous p., uterine p. venosus uterinus.
venous p., vaginal p. venosus vaginalis.
venous p's, vertebral plexuses of veins related to the vertebral column; see terms beginning *p. venosus vertebralis.*
venous p., vesical p. venosus vesicalis.
venous p. of foot, dorsal rete venosum dorsale pedis.
venous p. of foramen ovale p. venosus foraminis ovalis.
venous p. of hand, dorsal rete venosum dorsale manus.
venous p. of hypoglossal canal p. venosus canalis nervi hypoglossi.
vertebral p. 1. p. vertebralis. 2. (pl.) vertebral venous plexuses.
vertebral p's, external see *p. venosus vertebralis externus anterior* and *p. venosus vertebralis externus posterior.*
vertebral p's, internal see *p. venosus vertebralis internus anterior* and *p. venosus vertebralis internus posterior.*
p. vertebra′lis [TA] vertebral plexus: a nerve plexus accompanying the vertebral artery, formed by fibers from the vertebral and

Plexus *Continued*

cervicothoracic ganglia and carrying sympathetic fibers to the posterior cranial fossa via cranial nerves.
vesical p. 1. p. vesicalis. 2. p. venosus vesicalis.
p. vesica′lis 1. [TA] vesical plexus: the subdivision of the inferior hypogastric plexus that supplies sympathetic nerve fibers to the urinary bladder and parts of the ureter, ductus deferens, and seminal vesicle. 2. p. venosus vesicalis.
vesicoprostatic p. prostaticovesical p.
vidian p. nervus canalis pterygoidei.
visceral p., p. viscera′lis p. autonomicus.

-plexy [Gr. *plēxis* a stroke] a word termination meaning a stroke or seizure.

pli•ca (pli′kə) gen. and pl. *pli′cae* [L.] fold: anatomical nomenclature for a ridge or fold, as of peritoneum or other membrane.

Plica

Descriptions are given on TA terms, and include anglicized names of specific folds.

pli′cae ala′res [TA] alar folds: a pair of folds of the synovial membrane of the knee joint; attached to the medial and lateral margins of the articular surface of the patella, they pass posteriorly, converge, and become continuous with the infrapatellar synovial fold (see *p. synovialis infrapatellaris*).
p. aryepiglot′tica [TA] aryepiglottic fold: a fold of mucous membrane extending on each side between the lateral border of the epiglottis and the summit of the arytenoid cartilage.
p. axilla′ris ante′rior anterior axillary fold.
p. axilla′ris poste′rior posterior axillary fold.
pli′cae caeca′les [TA] cecal folds: the folds of peritoneum on either side of the retrocecal recess, which may connect the cecum to the abdominal wall; written also *plicae cecales.*
p. caeca′lis vascula′ris [TA] vascular cecal fold: the fold of peritoneum that covers the anterior cecal vessels, forming the superior ileocecal recess; written also *p. cecalis vascularis.*
pli′cae ceca′les plicae caecales.
p. ceca′lis vascula′ris p. caecalis vascularis.
p. chor′dae tym′pani [TA] a fold in the mucous membrane of the tympanic cavity overlying the chorda tympani nerve.
pli′cae cilia′res [TA] ciliary folds: low ridges in the furrows between the ciliary processes.
pli′cae circula′res [TA] circular folds: the permanent transverse folds of the luminal surface of the small intestine, involving both the mucosa and submucosa. Called also *Kerckring folds* or *valves.*
p. duodena′lis infe′rior [TA] inferior duodenal fold: a thin fold of peritoneum that bounds the inferior duodenal recess; called also *p. duodenomesocolica* [TA alternative] or *duodenomesocolic fold.*
p. duodena′lis supe′rior [TA] superior duodenal fold: a fold of peritoneum covering the inferior mesenteric vein and the ascending branch of the left colic artery; called also *p. duodenojejunalis* [TA alternative] or *duodenojejunal fold.*
p. duodenojejuna′lis TA alternative for *p. duodenalis superior.*
p. duodenomesoco′lica TA alternative for *p. duodenalis inferior.*
p. epigas′trica TA alternative for *p. umbilicalis lateralis.*
epiglottic p. 1. either of the glossoepiglottic folds; see *p. glossoepiglottica lateralis* and *p. glossoepiglottica mediana.* 2. TA alternative for *p. umbilicalis lateralis.*
p. fimbria′ta [TA] fimbriated fold: the lobulated fold running posteriorly and laterally from the anterior extremity of the frenulum of the tongue.
pli′cae gas′tricae [TA] gastric folds: the series of folds in the mucous membrane of the stomach; they are oriented chiefly longitudinally and partially disappear when the stomach is distended. Called also *gastric rugae* and *rugae of stomach.*
p. gastropancrea′tica [TA] gastropancreatic fold: a crescentic fold of peritoneum formed by the left gastric artery as it runs from the posterior abdominal wall to the lesser curvature of the stomach; called also *left gastropancreatic fold.* Cf. *p. hepatopancreatica.*
p. glossoepiglot′tica latera′lis [TA] lateral glossoepiglottic fold: either of two folds of mucous membrane extending, one on either side, between the base of the tongue and the epiglottis.
p. glossoepiglot′tica media′na [TA] median glossoepiglottic fold: a single fold of mucous membrane between the two lateral glossoepiglottic folds, connecting the base of the tongue and the epiglottis.
p. hepatopancrea′tica [TA] hepatopancreatic fold: a crescentic fold of peritoneum formed by the hepatic artery as it runs forward from the posterior abdominal wall to the lesser omentum; called also *right gastropancreatic fold.* Cf. *p. gastropancreatica.*
p. ileocaeca′lis [TA], **p. ileoceca′lis** ileocecal fold: a fold of peritoneum at the left border of the cecum, extending from the ileum above to the appendix below.
p. incudia′lis [TA], **p. incu′dis** incudal fold: a variable fold in the tunica mucosa of the tympanic cavity, passing from the roof of the cavity to the body and short crus of the incus.
infrapatellar p. p. synovialis infrapatellaris.
p. interarytenoi′dea [TA] interarytenoid fold: a median fold formed by mucous membrane anterior to the transverse arytenoid muscle as it protrudes into the larynx as the muscle approximates the arytenoid cartilages.
p. interurete′rica [TA] interureteric fold: a fold of mucous membrane extending across the fundus of the bladder between the two ureteral orifices, produced by a transverse bundle of muscle fibers; it marks one side of the trigone of the bladder. Called also *p. ureterica* and *interureteric crest* or *ridge.*
pli′cae i′ridis [TA] iridial folds: the numerous minute folds on the posterior surface of the iris.
p. lacrima′lis [TA] lacrimal fold: a fold of mucous membrane at the lower opening of the nasolacrimal duct.
p. longitudina′lis duode′ni [TA] longitudinal fold of duodenum: a mucosal ridge running longitudinally on the inner surface of the medial wall of the descending part of the duodenum.
p. luna′ta p. semilunaris conjunctivae.
p. mallea′ris ante′rior membra′nae tympa′nicae [TA] anterior malleolar fold of tympanic membrane: the line in the tympanic membrane that extends anteriorly from the malleolar prominence and divides the pars tensa from the pars flaccida.
p. mallea′ris ante′rior tu′nicae muco′sae cavita′tis tympa′nicae [TA] anterior malleolar fold of mucous membrane of tympanic cavity: a fold in the tunica mucosa of the tympanic cavity, reflected from the tympanic membrane over the anterior process and ligament of the malleus and part of the chorda tympani nerve.
p. mallea′ris poste′rior membra′nae tympa′nicae [TA] posterior malleolar fold of tympanic membrane: the line in the tympanic membrane that extends posteriorly from the malleolar prominence and divides the pars tensa from the pars flaccida.
p. mallea′ris poste′rior tu′nicae muco′sae cavita′tis tympa′nicae [TA] posterior malleolar fold of mucous membrane of tympanic cavity: a fold of the tunica mucosa of the tympanic cavity, extending from the manubrium of the malleus to the posterior wall of the cavity.
mediopatellar p. p. synovialis mediopatellaris.
p. membra′nae tym′pani exter′na ante′rior p. mallearis anterior membranae tympanicae.
p. membra′nae tym′pani exter′na poste′rior p. mallearis posterior membranae tympanicae.
pli′cae muco′sae vesi′cae bilia′ris [TA] folds of tunica mucosa of gallbladder: the folds in the mucosa that bound the polygonal spaces, giving the interior a honeycombed appearance. Called also *mucosal folds of gallbladder,* and the three TA alternative terms *plicae mucosae vesicae felleae, rugae vesicae biliaris,* and *rugae vesicae felleae.*

Plica *Continued*

pli′cae muco′sae vesi′cae fel′leae TA alternative for *plicae mucosae vesicae biliaris.*

p. ner′vi laryn′gei supe′rior [TA] a fold of mucous membrane in the larynx, overlying the superior laryngeal nerve.

pli′cae palati′nae transver′sae [TA] transverse palatine folds: four to six transverse ridges on the anterior part of the hard palate. Called also *palatine folds, palatine rugae,* and *rugae palatinae.*

pli′cae palma′tae [TA] palmate folds: a system of folds on the anterior and posterior walls of the cervical canal of the uterus, consisting of a median longitudinal ridge and shorter elevations extending laterally and upward. Called also *arbor vitae uteri.*

p. palpebronasa′lis [TA] epicanthus.

p. paraduodena′lis [TA] paraduodenal fold: an inconstant peritoneal fold containing a branch of the left colic artery; see also *Treitz arch,* under *arch.*

p. rectouteri′na [TA] rectouterine fold: a crescentic fold of peritoneum extending from the rectum to the base of the broad ligament on either side, forming the rectouterine pouch.

p. salpingopalati′na [TA] salpingopalatine fold: the mucosal fold passing caudally from the auditory tube to the lateral pharyngeal wall.

p. salpingopharyn′gea [TA] salpingopharyngeal fold: a mucosal fold passing caudally from the posterior lip of the pharyngeal orifice of the auditory tube to the lateral pharyngeal wall.

pli′cae semiluna′res co′li [TA] semilunar folds of colon: crescentic folds in the wall of the colon, projecting into the lumen between the haustra.

p. semiluna′ris conjuncti′vae [TA] semilunar fold of conjunctiva: a fold of mucous membrane at the medial angle of the eye.

p. semiluna′ris fau′cium [TA] semilunar fold of fauces: a curved fold interconnecting the palatoglossal and palatopharyngeal arches and forming the upper boundary of the supratonsillar fossa.

p. spira′lis [TA] spiral fold: a spirally arranged elevation in the mucosa of the first part of the cystic duct; called also *Heister fold* or *valve.*

p. stapedia′lis [TA], **p. stape′dis** stapedial fold: a mucosal fold that passes from the posterior wall of the tympanic cavity along the tympanic membrane and surrounds the stapes.

p. sublingua′lis [TA] sublingual fold: the elevation on the floor of the mouth under the tongue, covering part of the sublingual gland and containing its excretory ducts.

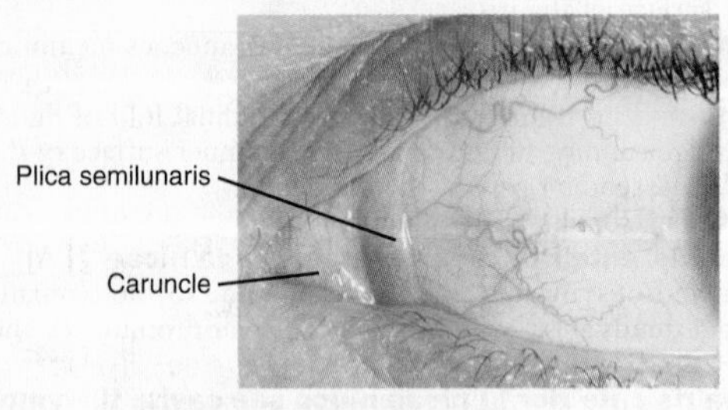

■ Plica semilunaris conjunctivae.

suprapatellar p. p. synovialis suprapatellaris.

p. synovia′lis [TA] synovial fold: an extension of the synovial membrane from its free inner surface into the joint cavity.

p. synovia′lis infrapatella′ris [TA] infrapatellar synovial fold: a large process of synovial membrane, containing some fat, which projects into the knee joint; attached to the infrapatellar adipose body, it passes posteriorly and superiorly to the intercondylar fossa of the femur.

p. synovia′lis mediopatella′ris mediopatellar synovial fold: a fold of synovial membrane in the knee joint, extending obliquely along the medial wall of the joint and inserting on the synovial lining of the infrapatellar fat pad.

p. synovia′lis suprapatella′ris suprapatellar synovial fold: a widely variable fold of synovial membrane in the knee joint, most often occurring as a crescent-shaped medial fold extending from the inferior surface of the quadriceps tendon to the medial edge of the knee joint.

pli′cae transver′sae rec′ti [TA], **pli′cae transversa′les rec′ti** transverse folds of rectum: permanent transverse folds in the rectum, usually three in number (two on the left and one on the right), involving the tunica mucosa and tela submucosa, and the circular layer of the tunica muscularis. Called also *Kohlrausch* or *rectal folds.*

p. triangula′ris [TA] triangular fold: a fold of mucous membrane extending backward from the palatoglossal arch and covering the anteroinferior part of the palatine tonsil.

pli′cae tuba′riae tu′bae uteri′nae [TA] tubal folds of uterine tube: the folds of the mucous lining of the uterine tube, which are high and complex in the ampulla.

p. umbilica′lis latera′lis [TA] lateral umbilical fold: a laterally placed fold of peritoneum on either side of the inferior part of the anterior abdominal wall, overlying the inferior epigastric vessels; called also *p. epigastrica* or *epigastric fold.*

p. umbilica′lis media′lis [TA] medial umbilical fold: a fold of peritoneum on either side of the inferior part of the anterior abdominal wall, covering the obliterated umbilical artery.

p. umbilica′lis media′na [TA] median umbilical fold: the fold of peritoneum that covers the median umbilical ligament; called also *urachal fold.*

p. urete′rica p. interureterica.

p. ve′nae ca′vae sinis′trae [TA] fold of left vena cava: a triangular fold of visceral pericardium occurring between the left superior pulmonary vein and the left pulmonary artery and enclosing the ligament of the left vena cava.

p. ventricula′ris p. vestibularis.

p. vesica′lis transver′sa [TA] transverse vesical fold: a transverse fold of the urogenital peritoneum that extends from the bladder onto the pelvic wall when the bladder is empty.

p. vestibula′ris [TA] vestibular fold: a fold of mucous membrane covering muscle in the larynx, separating the ventricle from the vestibule; called also *false vocal cord* or *fold* and *p. ventricularis.*

pli′cae villo′sae gas′tricae [TA] villous folds of stomach: a fine network of furrows demarcating the gastric areas.

p. voca′lis [TA] vocal fold: a fold of mucous membrane covering the vocalis muscle in the larynx, forming the inferior boundary of the ventricle; called also *chorda vocalis, labium vocale,* and *true vocal cord.*

pli•cae (pli′se) genitive and plural of *plica.*

pli•ca•my•cin (pli″kə-mi′sin) [USP] an antineoplastic antibiotic, produced by *Streptomyces plicatus,* that binds to DNA and inhibits RNA synthesis; it is used for treatment of advanced testicular carcinoma. It also has an inhibiting effect on osteoclasts and is used to treat hypercalcemia and hypercalciuria caused by metastatic malignancy. Administered intravenously. Formerly called mithramycin.

pli•cate (pli′kāt) [L. *plicatus*] plaited or folded.

pli•cat•ic ac•id (plĭ-kat′ik) a water-soluble organic acid found in the wood of *Thuja plicata,* the western red cedar; it causes asthma in susceptible workers.

pli•ca•tion (pli-ka′shən) [L. *plicatus,* past part. of *plicare* to fold] a folding; the taking of tucks in any structure to shorten it, or in the walls of a hollow viscus.

Kelly p. an operation for correction of stress incontinence in women; the connective tissue between the vagina and the urethra and the floor of the bladder are sutured to form a wide shelf of firm tissue supporting the urethra and bladder.

pli•cot•o•my (pli-kot′ə-me) [*plica* + *-tomy*] surgical division of the posterior fold of the tympanic membrane.

pli•ers (pli′ərz) small tong-jawed pincers for bending metals or holding small objects; various forms are much used in dentistry.

plint (plint) plinth.

plinth (plinth) a padded table for a patient to sit or lie on while performing therapeutic exercises.

-ploid [from *diploid* and *haploid*] a word termination denoting (in adjectives) the condition in regard to degree of multiplication of chromosome sets in the karyotype, or (in nouns) an individual or cell having chromosome sets of the particular degree of multiplication in the karyotype indicated by the root to which it is added, as aneuploid, polyploid.

ploi•dy (ploi′de) the status of the chromosome set in the karyotype.

plom•bage (plom-bahzh′) [Fr., "sealing, stopping"] a formerly common method of collapse therapy in which part of the thoracic cavity was surgically filled with inert material.

plop (plop) a dull, faintly explosive sound made on contact by a falling or dropped object.

tumor p. a sound made in early diastole by movement of a pedunculated atrial tumor but easily confused with an opening snap or a third heart sound.

plo•sive (plo′siv) a consonantal speech sound produced by closing off the oral cavity and then releasing with a burst of air, such as an initial *p.* Called also *stop.*

plot (plot) 1. to locate points on a graph. 2. to draw a graph. 3. a graph so produced.

box p. a graphic representation of a frequency distribution of a set of data; for each group is drawn a rectangle with upper and lower limits representing the interquartile range, horizontal line within the rectangle representing the median, and vertical tails ("whiskers") extending above and below the rectangle representing the minimum and maximum values.

bull's-eye p. a polar map of the entire myocardium arranged in multiple concentric circles, representing thallium distribution in the myocardium during exercise testing. Called also *polar p.*

Eadie-Hofstee p. graphic representation of a linear transformation of the Michaelis-Menten equation (q.v.) of enzyme kinetics; *v* is graphed as a function of *v*/[S], resulting in an *x*-intercept of V_{max}/K_M, *y*-intercept of V_{max}, and slope of $-K_M$.

Lineweaver-Burk p. the double reciprocal plot of an enzyme-catalyzed reaction, obtained from the Lineweaver-Burk equation by graphing $1/v$ as a function of 1/[S]. If the reaction obeys Michaelis-Menten kinetics a straight line is obtained with *x*-intercept of $-1/K_M$, *y*-intercept of $1/V_{max}$, and slope of K_M/V_{max}. Although unreliable for large values of $1/v$, the plot is widely used. It is also sometimes used in the classification of enzyme inhibitors, which all cause distinctive alterations in the graph.

polar p. bull's-eye p.

Scatchard p. a graph used in analyzing reversible binding of ligands and receptors, based on the Hill equation where the Hill coefficient is 1.0 (i.e., successive ligands bind independently). The concentration of ligand is varied while that of the receptor is held constant and the ratio of bound to free ligand is plotted as a function of bound ligand.

plo•to•ly•sin (plo″to-li′sin) the hemotoxic fraction of plototoxin.

plo•to•spas•min (plo″to-spaz′min) the neurotoxic fraction of plototoxin.

Plo•to•sus (plo-to′səs) a genus of catfish. *P. linea′tus* is a venomous species of the Indian and Pacific Oceans that has plototoxin on its spines and may be deadly to animals cut or scratched by the spines.

plo•to•tox•in (plo′to-tok″sin) a toxic substance derived from the catfish *Plotosus lineatus,* said to be composed of a hemotoxic fraction *(plotolysin)* and a neurotoxic fraction *(plotospasmin).*

PLP proteolipid protein.

PLT primed lymphocyte typing.

PLTP phospholipid transfer protein.

plug (plug) a lumpy mass that closes or obstructs an opening.

anal p. a mass of epithelial cells that temporarily occludes the anal canal in the embryo.

closing p. a fibrinous coagulum of blood that fills the defect in the endometrial epithelium created by implantation of the blastocyst; within two days it is covered by regenerated uterine epithelium.

copulation p. vaginal p.

Dittrich p's yellow to gray caseous masses of various sizes, consisting of granular debris, fat globules, fatty acid crystals, and bacteria, frequently found in the sputum in cases of bronchiectasis or putrid bronchitis. Called also *Traube p's.*

epithelial p. 1. a mass of ectodermal cells that temporarily closes an opening in the fetus, particularly in the external nares. 2. a mass of epithelium clogging or obstructing an opening.

meconium p. a mass of unusually thick or hard meconium, sometimes found causing intestinal obstruction in an infant; see *meconium plug syndrome,* under *syndrome.*

mucous p. 1. a plug formed by secretions of the mucous glands of the cervix uteri, closing the cervical canal during pregnancy. 2. abnormally thick mucus occluding the bronchi and bronchioles, as in asthma or bronchopulmonary aspergillosis.

Traube p's Dittrich p's.

vaginal p. a plug that forms in the vaginas of animals, especially rodents, after coitus; it consists of a mass of coagulated sperm and mucus; called also *copulation p.*

yolk p. the mass of yolk cells protruding from the blastopore of amphibians at the end of gastrulation.

plug•ger (plug′ər) a dental instrument used for packing, condensing, and compacting filling material into a tooth cavity.

amalgam p. an instrument for packing and condensing plastic amalgam in a prepared tooth cavity.

plum•ba•go (pləm-ba′go) graphite.

plum•bic (plum′bik) [L. *plumbicus* leaden] pertaining to or containing lead.

plum•bism (plum′biz-əm) lead poisoning.

Plum•mer disease, nails, sign (plum′ər) [Henry Stanley *Plummer,* American physician, 1874–1936] see under *disease, nail,* and *sign.*

Plum•mer-Vin•son syndrome (plum′ər vin′s′n) [H.S. *Plummer;* Porter Paisley *Vinson,* American surgeon, 1890–1959] see under *syndrome.*

plu•mose (ploo′mōs) [L. *plumosus,* Fr. *pluma* feather] feathery; resembling a feather.

plum•u•la (plum′u-lə) a set of delicate cross-furrows occasionally found on the upper wall of the aqueduct of Sylvius.

pluri- [L. *plus,* gen. *pluris* more] a combining form meaning several or more.

plu•ri•glan•du•lar (ploor″ĭ-glan′du-lər) [*pluri-* + L. *glandula*] pertaining to, derived from, or affecting several glands. Cf. *polyendocrine.* Called also *multiglandular* and *polyglandular.*

plu•ri•grav•i•da (ploor″ĭ-grav′ĭ-də) [*pluri-* + *gravida*] multigravida.

plu•ri•hor•mo•nal (ploor″ĭ-hor-mo′nəl) [*pluri-* + *hormone*] of or pertaining to several hormones.

plu•ri•loc•u•lar (ploor″ĭ-lok′u-lər) multilocular.

plu•ri•nu•cle•ar (ploor″ĭ-noo′kle-ər) polynuclear.

plu•ri•or•i•fi•cial (ploor″ĭ-or″ĭ-fish′əl) [*pluri-* + *orificial*] pertaining to or affecting several orifices of the body.

plu•rip•a•ra (ploo-rip′ə-rə) [*pluri-* + *para*] multipara.

plu•ri•par•i•ty (ploor″ĭ-par′ĭ-te) multiparity.

plu•ri•po•lar (ploor″ĭ-po′lər) multipolar.

plu•rip•o•tent (plo͝o-rip′ə-tənt) [*pluri-* + *potent*] 1. able to develop (as embryonic cells) or act in any one of several possible ways. 2. able to affect more than one organ or tissue. **pluripo′tency** *n*

plu•ri•po•ten•tial (ploor″ĭ-po-ten′shal) pluripotent.

plu•ri•po•ten•ti•al•i•ty (ploor″ĭ-po-ten″she-al′ĭ-te) pluripotency.

plu•ri•re•sis•tant (ploor″ĭ-re-zis′tənt) resistant to several drugs.

plu•ri•tis•su•lar (ploor″ĭ-tis′u-lər) composed of several tissues.

plu•ri•vis•cer•al (ploor″ĭ-vis′ər-əl) [*pluri-* + *visceral*] pertaining to or affecting several viscera, or organs.

plu•to•ni•um (Pu) (ploo-to′ne-əm) [from the planet *Pluto*] a heavy, metallic, radioactive element of atomic number 94, atomic weight 242, obtained by the addition of neutrons to uranium, thereby changing it into neptunium and then into plutonium.

ply•o•met•rics (pli″o-met′riks) [derivation unknown; possibly a misspelling of *pleiometrics,* from *pleio-* + Gr. *metron* measure] intensive exercises in which muscles are subjected to rapid loading (q.v.) and release, generating a great amount of force in a short period of time. Called also *plyometric exercises.*

Pm promethium.

PMDS persistent müllerian duct syndrome.

PMI point of maximal impulse.

P mi•trale (pe mi-tra′le) in electrocardiography, a pattern of abnormally wide, notched P waves, indicative of prolonged depolarization in a large left atrium; it is commonly associated with mitral valve disease.

PMMA polymethyl methacrylate.

PMN 1. polymorphonuclear. 2. polymorphonuclear neutrophil.

PMR proportionate mortality ratio.

PMS premenstrual syndrome.

-pnea [Gr. *pnoia* breath] a word termination denoting relationship to breathing.

pne(o)- [Gr. *pnein* to breathe] a combining form denoting relationship to the breath.

PNET peripheral neuroectodermal tumor; primitive neuroectodermal tumor.

pneuma- see *pneumat(o)-.*

pneu•mar•thro•gram (noo-mahr′thro-gram) [*pneumo-* + *arthro-* + *-gram*] a radiograph of a joint after it has been injected with air.

pneu•mar•throg•ra•phy (noo″mahr-throg′rə-fe) radiography of a joint after it has been injected with air or gas as a contrast medium; called also *pneumoarthrography.*

pneu•mar•thro•sis (noo″mahr-thro′sis) [*pneumo-* + *arthro-* + *-osis*] 1. the presence of gas or air in a joint. 2. the inflation of a joint with air or gas for the purpose of aiding radiographic examination.

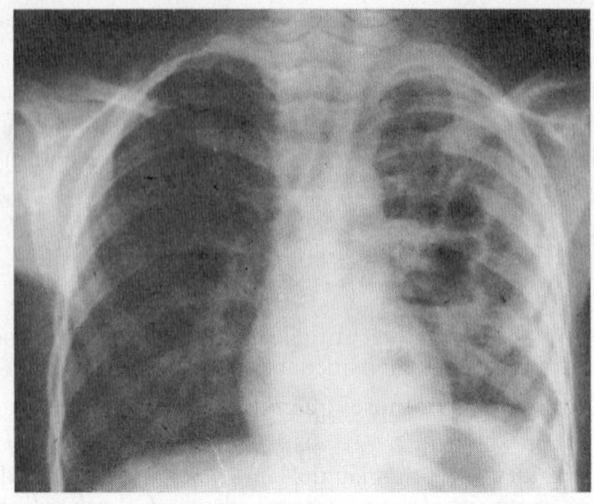

■ Pneumatocele in the upper left lobe of a patient with staphylococcal pneumonia.

pneu•mat•ic (noo-mat′ik) [Gr. *pneuma*, gen. *pneumatos*, air, breath] 1. pertaining to air. 2. respiratory.

pneu•mat•ics (noo-mat′iks) the science which deals with the physical properties of gases.

pneu•ma•tin•u•ria (noo″mə-tĭ-nu′re-ə) pneumaturia.

pneu•ma•ti•za•tion (noo″mə-tĭ-za′shən) the formation of pneumatic cells or cavities in tissue, especially such formation in the temporal bone.

pneu•ma•tized (noo′mə-tīzd) 1. filled with air. 2. containing pneumatic cells.

pneumat(o)- [Gr. *pneuma*, gen. *pneumatos* breath] a combining form denoting relationship to air or gas, or to respiration. Also, *pneuma-*.

pneu•ma•to•car•dia (noo″mə-to-kahr′de-ə) [*pneumato-* + *cardia*] the presence of air in the heart.

pneu•ma•to•cele (noo-mat′o-sēl) [*pneumato-* + *-cele*[1]] 1. a tumor or cyst formed by air or other gas filling an adventitious pouch, such as a laryngocele, tracheocele, or gaseous swelling of the scrotum. Called also *aerocele* and *pneumocele.* 2. a usually benign, thin-walled, air-containing cyst of the lung, as in staphylococcal pneumonia. Called also *pneumocele* and *pneumonocele.*

p. cra′nii, extracranial p. gaseous tumors beneath the scalp after a fracture of the skull that communicates with the paranasal sinuses.

intracranial p. pneumocephalus.

parotid p. enlargement of the parotid glands as a result of blowing air into the parotid ducts. See also *glass-blowers' mouth*, under *mouth*.

pneu•ma•to•ceph•a•lus (noo″mə-to-sef′ə-ləs) pneumocephalus.

pneu•ma•to•gram (noo-mat′o-gram) spirogram.

pneu•ma•to•graph (noo-mat′o-graf″) spirograph.

pneu•ma•to•nom•e•ter (noo″mə-tə-nom′ə-tər) [*pneuma-* + *tonometer*] an applanation tonometer in which air pressure applied through a silicone-rubber membrane in direct contact with the cornea is used to flatten the cornea.

pneu•ma•to•sis (noo″mə-to′sis) [Gr. *pneumatōsis*] the presence of air or gas in an abnormal situation in the body.

p. co′li, p. cystoi′des intestina′lis the presence of thin-walled, gas-containing cysts in the intestinal wall either subserosally or submucosally; the etiology is not known. Called also *intestinal emphysema* and *intestinal p.*

gastric p. air or gas in the wall of the stomach, usually seen in infants secondary to a gastric outlet obstruction or pyloric stenosis.

intestinal p., p. intestina′lis p. cystoides intestinalis.

pneu•ma•tu•ria (noo″mə-tu′re-ə) [*pneumato-* + *-uria*] passage of gas in the urine, usually as a result of a fistula between the bladder and intestine.

pneu•ma•type (noo′mə-tīp) [*pneuma-* + Gr. *typos* type] a breath picture; a deposition of moist breath on a glass surface or mirror, used in the diagnosis of nasal obstructions.

pneu•mec•to•my (noo-mek′tə-me) pneumonectomy.

pneum(o)- [Gr. *pneuma* breath] a combining form denoting relationship to *(a)* respiration, *(b)* the lungs, *(c)* air, *(d)* pneumonia.

pneu•mo•al•veo•log•ra•phy (noo″mo-al″ve-o-log′rə-fe) radiography of the alveoli of the lungs.

pneu•mo•am•ni•os (noo″mo-am′ne-os) the presence of gas in the amniotic fluid.

pneu•mo•an•gi•og•ra•phy (noo″mo-an″je-og′rə-fe) pulmonary angiography.

pneu•mo•ar•throg•ra•phy (noo″mo-ahr-throg′rə-fe) pneumarthrography.

pneu•mo•bil•ia (noo″mo-bil′e-ə) [*pneumo-* + *bile* + *-ia*] the presence of gas in the biliary system.

pneu•mo•bul•bar (noo″mo-bul′bər) pertaining to the lungs and to the respiration center in the medulla oblongata.

pneu•mo•bul•bous (noo″mo-bul′bəs) pneumobulbar.

pneu•mo•car•di•al (noo″mo-kahr′de-əl) cardiopulmonary.

pneu•mo•cele (noo′mo-sēl″) 1. pneumonocele (def. 1). 2. pneumatocele.

pneu•mo•cen•te•sis (noo″mo-sen-te′sis) pneumonocentesis.

pneu•mo•ceph•a•lus (noo″mo-sef′ə-ləs) [*pneumo-* + *-cephalus*] the presence of air in the cranial cavity; called also *intracranial pneumatocele, pneumatocephalus, pneumocrania*, and *pneumoencephalocele.*

pneu•mo•cho•le•cys•ti•tis (noo″mo-ko″lə-sis-ti′tis) emphysematous cholecystitis.

pneu•mo•coc•ce•mia (noo″mo-kok-se′me-ə) the presence of pneumococci in the blood.

pneu•mo•coc•ci (noo″mo-kok′si) plural of *pneumococcus.*

pneu•mo•coc•ci•dal (noo″mo-kok-si′dəl) destroying pneumococci; cf. *antipneumococcal.*

pneu•mo•coc•col•y•sis (noo″mo-kok-ol′ĭ-sis) dissolution of pneumococci.

pneu•mo•coc•co•sis (noo″mo-kok-o′sis) infection with pneumococci; see *pneumococcal pneumonia*, under *pneumonia.*

pneu•mo•coc•co•su•ria (noo″mo-kok″o-su′re-ə) bacteriuria with pneumococci or pneumococcal polysaccharide in the urine.

pneu•mo•coc•cus (noo″mo-kok′əs) pl. *pneumococ′ci* [*pneumo-* + *coccus*] a member of the species *Streptococcus pneumoniae.* **pneumococ′cal, pneumococ′cic** *adj*

pneu•mo•co•lon (noo″mo-ko′lən) [*pneumo-* + *colon*] the presence of air in the colon, either from a penetrating wound or after introduction as an aid to diagnosis.

pneu•mo•co•ni•o•sis (noo″mo-ko″ne-o′sis) [*pneumo-* + *coniosis*] deposition of large amounts of dust or other particulate matter in the lungs, and the subsequent tissue reaction, usually seen in workers in certain occupations and in residents of areas with excessive particulate matter in the air. The definition is usually limited to conditions caused by inorganic dusts, in contrast to those such as byssinosis that are caused by organic dusts. Types range from nearly harmless forms to destructive or fatal conditions and are often named for the implicated substance, such as *aluminosis, anthracosis, asbestosis, graphitosis, siderosis*, or *silicosis.* See table. Called also *pneumokoniosis* and *pneumonoconiosis.*

antimony p. mild pneumoconiosis seen in workers with antimony and its compounds; excessive buildup of antimony in the body may result in antimony poisoning.

bauxite p. a progressive form of pneumoconiosis caused by inhalation of bauxite fumes containing fine particles of alumina and silica. It begins with alveolitis and progresses to emphysema, often with pneumothorax. Called also *bauxite lung, bauxite workers' disease, corundum smelter's lung*, and *Shaver disease.* Cf. *aluminosis.*

coal workers' p. a severe form caused by deposition of large amounts of coal dust in the lungs, usually accompanied by centrilobular emphysema. Different varieties of coal have different risks, and those with certain types of contaminants may cause other types of pneumoconiosis. See also *anthracosis* and *bituminosis.* Called also *black, coal miner's*, or *miner's lung.*

collagenous p. pneumoconiosis in which permanent scarring results, due to fibrogenic dust, such as asbestos or silica, or to altered tissue response to nonfibrogenic dust.

fuller's earth p. a rare type of silicatosis caused by inhalation of the dust of fuller's earth, seen in workers with long-term heavy exposure.

graphite p. silicosis due to inhalation of graphite dust, which often contains up to 10 per cent silica. Called also *graphitosis* and *graphite fibrosis.*

hematite p. mixed dust pneumoconiosis (silicosiderosis) seen in long-term miners of hematite; some patients show diffuse fibrosis throughout a lung while others show nodules primarily in upper lobes.

kaolin p. silicatosis caused by inhaling particles of kaolin. Called also *kaolinosis.*

mica p. silicatosis due to inhalation of and tissue reaction to mica particles; called also *micatosis.*

mixed dust p. pneumoconiosis that is caused by more than one type of dust, such as anthracosilicosis, calcicosilicosis, or silicosiderosis.

noncollagenous p. pneumoconiosis in which the stromal reaction is minimal, consisting chiefly of reticulin fibers.

polyvinyl chloride p. a rare form of pneumoconiosis caused by excessive inhalation of polyvinyl chloride dust.

rheumatoid p. Caplan syndrome.

p. sidero′tica siderosis (def. 1).

Types of Pneumoconiosis

Name	Causative Type of Dust
Aluminosis	Aluminum
Antimony pneumoconiosis	Antimony
Asbestosis	Asbestos
Baritosis	Barium; barite
Bauxite pneumoconiosis	Bauxite
Cadmiosis	Cadmium
Calcicosis	Dusts containing calcium
Chalicosis	Miscellaneous stones
Coal workers' pneumoconiosis	Coal dust
Anthracosis	Anthracite coal
Bituminosis	Bituminous coal
Cobaltosis	Cobalt
Elevator disease	Miscellaneous grains
Hard metal disease	Tungsten carbide, titanium carbide, tantalum carbide
Kaolin pneumoconiosis (kaolinosis)	Kaolin
Mica pneumoconiosis (micatosis)	Mica
Polyvinyl chloride pneumoconiosis	Polyvinyl chloride
Schistosis	Slate
Siderosis	Iron
Silicosis	Silica
Diatomite fibrosis	Diatomaceous earth
Fuller's earth pneumoconiosis	Fuller's earth
Graphite pneumoconiosis (graphitosis)	Graphite
Hematite pneumoconiosis	Hematite
Mixed dust pneumoconioses:	
Anthracosilicosis	Anthracite coal, silica
Calcicosilicosis	Calcium dusts, silica
Labrador lung	Iron, silica, anthophyllite
Siderosilicosis	Iron ore, silica
Stannosis	Tin oxide
Tabacosis	Dried tobacco leaves
Talc pneumoconiosis (talcosis)	Talc
Titanium dioxide pneumoconiosis	Titanium dioxide
Welder's lung	Iron oxide

talc p. a type of silicatosis caused by the inhalation of talc; symptoms include shortness of breath, cough, fatigue, weakness, and weight loss. Prolonged exposure may result in pulmonary fibrosis. Called also *talcosis.*

titanium dioxide p. a mild form of pneumoconiosis seen in workers inhaling excessive amounts of titanium dioxide dust.

pneu•mo•cra•nia (noo″mo-kra′ne-ə) pneumocephalus.

pneu•mo•cra•ni•um (noo″mo-kra′ne-əm) pneumocephalus.

pneu•mo•cys•ti•a•sis (noo″mo-sis-ti′ə-sis) pneumocystis pneumonia.

pneu•mo•cys•tic (noo″mo-sis′tik) pertaining to or caused by *Pneumocystis.*

Pneu•mo•cys•tis (noo″mo-sis′tis) [*pneumo-* + *cyst*] a genus of yeastlike fungi infecting virtually all mammalian species and having a predilection for the lungs, where it is primarily an alveolar pathogen, although disseminated infection may occur in severely immunocompromised hosts. The various species are host-specific, and organisms cannot be grown outside of an infected host.

P. cari′nii a species that formerly included all of the species in the genus, but is now limited to those infecting rats; the agent that infects humans has been reclassified as *P. jiroveci.*

P. jirove′ci a species, formerly included in *P. carinii,* that is the cause of pneumocystis pneumonia (PCP) in humans.

pneu•mo•cys•tis (noo″mo-sis′tis) an individual organism of the genus *Pneumocystis.*

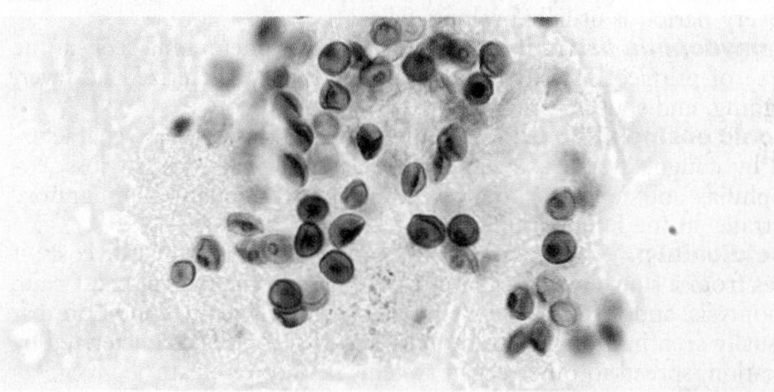

■ *Pneumocystis jiroveci* in bronchoalveolar lavage specimen (methenamine silver stain).

pneu•mo•cys•tog•ra•phy (noo″mo-sis-tog′rə-fe) cystography following injection of air into the bladder.

pneu•mo•cys•to•sis (noo″mo-sis-to′sis) pneumocystis pneumonia.

pneu•mo•cys•to•to•mog•ra•phy (noo″mo-sis″to-to-mog′rə-fe) tomography after inflation of the bladder with air.

pneu•mo•cyte (noo-mo-sīt′) alveolar cell.

pneu•mo•der•ma (noo″mo-dur′mə) [*pneumo-* + *derma*] subcutaneous emphysema.

pneu•mo•dy•nam•ics (noo″mo-di-nam′iks) [*pneumo-* + *dynamics*] 1. the dynamics of the respiratory process. 2. the study of the forces exerted in the process of breathing.

pneu•mo•em•py•e•ma (noo″mo-em″pi-e′mə) pyopneumothorax.

pneu•mo•en•ceph•a•li•tis (noo″mo-ən-sef″ə-li′tis) Newcastle disease in birds.

avian p. Newcastle disease in birds.

pneu•mo•en•ceph•a•lo•cele (noo″mo-en-sef′ə-lo-sēl) pneumocephalus.

pneu•mo•en•ceph•a•lo•gram (noo″mo-ən-sef′ə-lo-gram) the radiograph obtained by pneumoencephalography.

pneu•mo•en•ceph•a•log•ra•phy (PEG) (noo″mo-ən-sef″ə-log′rə-fe) radiographic visualization of the fluid-containing structures of the brain after cerebrospinal fluid is intermittently withdrawn by lumbar puncture and replaced by air, oxygen, or helium; this procedure is no longer performed, having been replaced by metrizamide cisternography.

pneu•mo•en•ceph•a•lo•my•elo•gram (noo″mo-ən-sef″ə-lo-mi-el′o-gram) the radiograph obtained by pneumoencephalomyelography.

pneu•mo•en•ceph•a•lo•my•elog•ra•phy (noo″mo-ən-sef″ə-lo-mi″ə-log′rə-fe) radiographic visualization of the brain and spinal cord after cerebrospinal fluid is removed by lumbar puncture and replaced by gas.

pneu•mo•en•ceph•a•los (noo″mo-ən-sef′ə-los) pneumocephalus.

pneu•mo•en•ter•itis (noo″mo-en″tər-i′tis) [*pneumo-* + *enter-* + *-itis*] inflammation of the lung and intestine.

pneu•mo•fas•cio•gram (noo″mo-fas′e-o-gram) a radiograph of tissue after injection of air into the fascial spaces.

pneu•mo•gas•tric (noo″mo-gas′trik) [*pneumo-* + *gastric*] pertaining to the lungs and stomach; called also *gastropulmonary.*

pneu•mo•gas•trog•ra•phy (noo″mo-gas-trog′rə-fe) [*pneumo-* + *gastrography*] radiography of the stomach after the injection of air.

pneu•mo•gram (noo′mo-gram) 1. a radiogram made after the injection of air into the part. 2. spirogram.

pneu•mo•graph (noo′mo-graf) spirograph.

pneu•mog•ra•phy (noo-mog′rə-fe) 1. radiography of a part after injection of a gas. 2. spirography.

cerebral p. radiography of the brain by pneumoencephalography or ventriculography.

retroperitoneal p. radiography of the abdominal organs after retroperitoneal injection of air or oxygen.

pneu•mo•gy•no•gram (noo″mo-gi′no-gram) a radiograph of the female reproductive organs after injection of air into the uterus.

pneu•mo•he•mo•peri•car•di•um (noo″mo-he″mo-per″ĭ-kahr′de-əm) [*pneumo-* + *hemo-* + *pericardium*] the presence of air or gas and blood in the pericardial cavity.

pneu•mo•he•mo•tho•rax (noo″mo-he″mo-thor′aks) hemopneumothorax.

pneu•mo•hy•dro•me•tra (noo″mo-hi″dro-me′trə) [*pneumo-* + *hydro-* + *metra*] a collection of gas and fluid in the uterine cavity.

pneu•mo•hy•dro•peri•car•di•um (noo″mo-hi″dro-per″ĭ-kahr′de-əm) [*pneumo-* + *hydro-* + *pericardium*] the presence of air or gas and fluid in the pericardial cavity.

pneu•mo•hy•dro•tho•rax (noo″mo-hi″dro-thor′aks) hydropneumothorax.

pneu•mo•ko•ni•o•sis (noo″mo-ko″ne-o′sis) pneumoconiosis.

pneu•mo•lith (noo′mo-lith) [*pneumo-* + *-lith*] a calculus or concretion in the lung, usually composed of calcium salts. Called also *lung calculus* and *pulmolith.*

pneu•mo•li•thi•a•sis (noo″mo-lĭ-thi′ə-sis) the presence of concretions in the lungs.

pneu•mol•o•gy (noo-mol′ə-je) [*pneumo-* + *-logy*] the study of disease of the air passages.

pneu•mol•y•sis (noo-mol′ĭ-sis) pneumonolysis.

pneu•mo•ma•la•cia (noo″mo-mə-la′shə) [*pneumo-* + *-malacia*] morbid softening of lung tissue.

pneu•mo•mas•sage (noo″mo-mə-sahzh′) [*pneumo-* + *massage*] air massage of the tympanum by the alternate compression and rarefaction of the air in the external auditory canal. Called also *pneumatic massage.*

pneu•mo•me•di•as•ti•no•gram (noo″mo-me″de-əs-ti′no-gram) the film produced by pneumomediastinography.

pneu•mo•me•di•as•ti•nog•ra•phy (noo″mo-me″de-as″tĭ-nog′rə-fe) radiography of the mediastinum after injection of nitrous oxide or oxygen through a needle introduced back of the trachea or behind the manubrium.

pneu•mo•me•di•as•ti•num (noo″mo-me″de-əs-ti′nəm) [*pneumo-* + *mediastinum*] the presence of air or gas in the mediastinum, which may interfere with respiration and circulation, and may lead to such conditions as pneumothorax or pneumopericardium. It may occur as a result of trauma or a pathologic process, or it may be induced deliberately as a diagnostic procedure. Called also *Hamman disease* or *syndrome* and *mediastinal emphysema.* See illustration.

pneu•mo•mel•a•no•sis (noo″mo-mel″ə-no′sis) [*pneumo-* + *melanosis*] the blackening of the lung tissue by inhaled coal dust, as in coal workers' pneumoconiosis.

Pneu•mo•mist (noo′mo-mist) trademark for a preparation of guaifenesin.

pneu•mo•my•co•sis (noo″mo-mi-ko′sis) [*pneumo-* + *mycosis*] any fungal disease of the lungs.

pneu•mo•my•elog•ra•phy (noo″mo-mi″ə-log′rə-fe) [*pneumo-* + *myelo-* + *-graphy*] radiographic examination after withdrawal of cerebrospinal fluid and injection of air or gas into the spinal canal.

pneu•mo•nec•ta•sia (noo″mo-nək-ta′zhə) pulmonary emphysema.

pneu•mo•nec•ta•sis (noo″mo-nek′tə-sis) [*pneumon-* + *ectasis*] pulmonary emphysema.

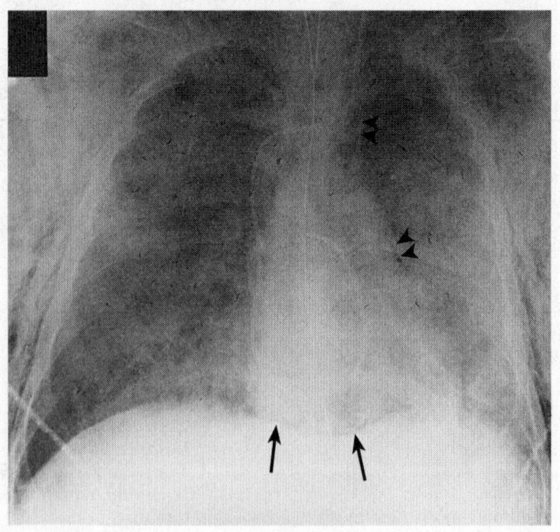

■ Pneumomediastinum, showing characteristic continuous radiolucent line extending from one hemidiaphragm to the other *(arrows)* and air displacing the left mediastinal pleura *(arrowheads).*

pneu•mo•nec•to•my (noo″mo-nek′tə-me) [*pneumon-* + *-ectomy*] surgical removal of lung tissue, especially of an entire lung. Cf. *pneumoresection.* Called also *pulmonectomy.*

pneu•mo•nia (noo-mōn′yə) [Gr. *pneumōnia*] inflammation of the lungs with consolidation. Human pneumonias are most often categorized according to causative organism (such as *amebic p.*, *bacterial p.*, *pneumocystis p.*, *primary atypical p.*, and *viral p.*) or location (such as *apical p.*, *bronchial p.*, and *lobar p.*). See also *pneumonitis.*

Pneumonia

***Acinetobacter* p.** a sometimes fatal type of bacterial pneumonia seen in immunocompromised patients, caused by infection with *Acinetobacter* species. It is usually bronchopneumonia, and characteristics include acute onset of dyspnea with fever, productive cough, chest pain, and abscess formation or empyema.

acute p. severe pneumonia of rapid onset.

acute eosinophilic p. a condition resembling chronic eosinophilic pneumonia but with a more rapid onset and more limited duration, accompanied by acute respiratory failure and diffuse pulmonary infiltrates.

acute interstitial p. the acute form of idiopathic pulmonary fibrosis, now thought to represent a sequel to the acute respiratory distress syndrome. Called also *Hamman-Rich syndrome.*

adenovirus p. viral pneumonia caused by an adenovirus; it is usually mild, but in neonates and the immunocompromised it can be fatal. Characteristics range from interstitial inflammation without necrosis to a necrotizing bronchitis and bronchiolitis with desquamation that may occlude the lumen, and areas of hemorrhagic consolidation alternating with areas of atelectasis.

p. al′ba a fatal desquamative pneumonia of the newborn resulting from congenital syphilis and characterized by white fatty degeneration of the lungs, which appear pale and virtually airless. Called also *white p.* and *white lung.*

alcoholic p. pneumonia associated with alcoholism.

amebic p. pneumonia resulting from amebic abscesses in the lung caused by *Entamoeba histolytica.*

anaerobic p. any pneumonia caused by anaerobic bacteria, usually due to aspiration of contaminated secretions from the mouth, pharynx, or paranasal sinuses, such as with the increased bacterial load of periodontal disease or some other infection. It usually runs a protracted course, progressing to lung cavitation with abscesses and putrid or bloody expectorations.

anthrax p. inhalational anthrax.

apex p., apical p. lobar pneumonia limited to the apex of the lung.

***Aspergillus* p.** a type of fungal pneumonia sometimes seen in pulmonary aspergillosis.

aspiration p. pneumonia due to the entrance of foreign matter, such as food particles or oral secretions, into the respiratory passages or lungs. Called also *deglutition p.* and *inhalation p.*

atypical p., atypical bronchial p. primary atypical p.

atypical interstitial p. fog fever.

bacterial p. pneumonia caused by bacteria, such as *Klebsiella pneumoniae*, *Mycoplasma pneumoniae*, *Staphylococcus aureus*, *Streptococcus pneumoniae*, *Streptococcus pyogenes*, and others.

bronchial p. bronchopneumonia.

brooder p. a lung disease of chicks and other young birds, acquired from moldy grain or straw; it is a form of aspergillosis, usually caused by *Aspergillus fumigatus.*

***Candida* p.** pulmonary candidiasis.

caseous p. tuberculous pneumonia in which necrotic lung tissue is of semisolid consistency and the cut surface resembles cheese. Called also *cheesy p.*

cat p. feline pneumonitis.

central p. lobar pneumonia that begins in the hilum of a lobe of the lung. Called also *core p.*

cheesy p. caseous p.

***Chlamydia trachomatis* p.** a mild type of bacterial pneumonia, usually seen in infants whose mothers are infected with *Chlamydia trachomatis;* characteristics include coughing, tachypnea, and eosinophilia.

chlamydial p. general term for pneumonia caused by members of the phylum Chlamydiae; see *Chlamydophila pneumoniae p.*, *Chlamydiophila psittaci p.*, and *Chlamydia trachomatis p.*

***Chlamydophila pneumoniae* p.** a mild form of primary atypical pneumonia caused by infection with *Chlamydiophila pneumoniae*, characterized by fever, rales, and infiltration of a middle or lower lobe; the recovery period is usually prolonged.

***Chlamydophila psittaci* p.** a severe type of pneumonia seen in the course of psittacosis, lasting several weeks and characterized by fever, coughing, and sputum production.

chronic eosinophilic p. a chronic interstitial lung disease characterized by cough, dyspnea, malaise, fever, night sweats, weight loss, eosinophilia, and a chest film revealing nonsegmental, nonmigratory infiltrates in the lung periphery.

coccidioidal p. pneumonia following primary coccidioidomycosis; it varies from a slowly developing disease with chronic cough, chest pain, hemoptysis, and fever to a more rapidly spreading acute condition that is usually seen in immunocompromised patients and is characterized by cavitation, spread to other organ systems, and often death.

Pneumonia *Continued*

cold agglutinin p. primary atypical p.
contusion p. traumatic p.
core p. central p.
cryptogenic organizing p. bronchiolitis obliterans with organizing pneumonia.
cytomegalovirus p. a type of viral pneumonia seen as an opportunistic infection with a cytomegalovirus in immunocompromised patients; symptoms include fever, a nonproductive cough, dyspnea, and hypoxemia that can be fatal.
deglutition p. aspiration p.
dermal p. a condition produced by injection of virulent pneumococci into the skin of rabbits.
desquamative interstitial p. chronic pneumonia of unknown etiology, characterized by prominence of intra-alveolar macrophages (which were formerly thought to be desquamated large alveolar cells); it is associated with dyspnea and often a nonproductive and harsh cough, and typically occurs in smokers.
p. dis′secans p. interlobularis purulenta.
double p. pneumonia that affects both lungs.
Eaton agent p. mycoplasmal p.
embolic p. 1. pneumonia due to embolism of a blood vessel or vessels of the lungs. 2. in cattle, pneumonia that sometimes follows caudal vena caval thrombosis (q.v.); it often involves abscesses with suppurative pneumonia and aneurysms that may rupture, causing pulmonary hemorrhage that can be either minor, or massive and fatal.
***Enterobacter* p.** a rare type of bacterial pneumonia, usually bronchopneumonia, caused by infection with species of *Enterobacter;* it is usually nosocomial and seen in debilitated patients.
enzootic p. any of several types of mild pneumonias that affect young animals, especially lambs, piglets, and calves, usually caused by viruses or species of *Mycoplasma.*
eosinophilic p. 1. see *acute* and *chronic eosinophilic p.* 2. PIE syndrome (def. 2).
***Escherichia coli* p.** a rare type of bacterial pneumonia caused by infection with *Escherichia coli,* usually in the bronchi or a lower lobe, seen most often in debilitated patients or infants.
fibrous p. pneumonia in which there is an increase in scar tissue during the healing process.
fibrous p., chronic idiopathic pulmonary fibrosis.
Friedländer p. *Klebsiella* p.
fungal p. pneumonia caused by inhaled fungi, usually *Histoplasma capsulatum, Blastomyces dermatitidis,* or *Coccidioides* species; in Central and South America it may be caused by *Paracoccidioides brasiliensis.* Numerous other fungi, such as *Aspergillus* and *Candida,* infect immunocompromised patients. See also *histoplasmosis, North American blastomycosis, coccidioidomycosis,* and *paracoccidioidomycosis.*
gangrenous p. gangrene of the lung.
giant cell p. a rare, often fatal form of interstitial pneumonia caused by the measles virus, affecting children with disease of the reticuloendothelial system (such as leukemia), as well as immunocompromised or otherwise weakened adults; characteristics include multinucleate giant cell inclusion bodies, high fever, tachypnea, hypoxemia, and a harsh dry cough. Called also *Hecht p.*
giant cell interstitial p. a type of pneumonia similar to idiopathic pulmonary fibrosis but with interstitial exudate containing large numbers of irregularly shaped multinucleate giant cells; it is thought to represent the pathologic appearance of hard metal disease.
glanders p. pneumonia associated with glanders, characterized by caseous or calcified granules and pulmonary consolidation; seen in both humans and horses. Called also *p. malleosa.*
***Haemophilus influenzae* p.** bacterial pneumonia caused by infection with *Haemophilus influenzae,* seen mainly in young children and debilitated or immunocompromised adults; it sometimes progresses to life-threatening conditions such as meningitis, pericarditis, endocarditis, and epiglottitis that can cause obstruction of the airway.
Hecht p. giant cell p.
herpes simplex virus p. a type of viral pneumonia seen in neonates or immunocompromised patients, caused by spread of a herpes simplex virus infection into the lungs; characteristics include dyspnea, cough, and hypoxemia in conjunction with other manifestations of the herpesvirus infection.
hypostatic p. pneumonia due to dorsal decubitus in weak or aged persons.
infectious p. of goats contagious caprine pleuropneumonia.
influenzal p., influenza virus p. viral pneumonia caused by an influenza virus, usually the type A virus; some cases are mild, but it can develop into a fulminant condition characterized by high fever, prostration, severe dyspnea, and massive (sometimes rapidly fatal) pulmonary hemorrhagic edema with consolidation. It may be accompanied by a superinfection with bacterial pneumonia.
inhalation p. 1. aspiration p. 2. bronchopneumonia due to the inhalation of irritating substances.
p. interlobula′ris purulen′ta pneumonia with interlobular empyema.
interstitial p. 1. any of various types of pneumonia characterized by thickening of the interstitial tissue. 2. idiopathic pulmonary fibrosis.
interstitial plasma cell p. pneumocystis p.
intrauterine p. pneumonia contracted by the fetus *in utero;* it may result in the death of the fetus or the birth of an infant with fully developed pneumonia.
***Klebsiella* p.** an acute type of bacterial pneumonia caused by infection with *Klebsiella pneumoniae,* usually lobar in type and often limited to the right upper lobe; characteristics include large amounts of inflammatory, sometimes bloody, mucoid exudates in the lung. Called also *Friedländer p.*
***Legionella* p.** pneumonia caused by a species of *Legionella;* see *legionnaire's disease* and *Pittsburgh p.*
lipid p., lipoid p. a rare type of aspiration pneumonia caused by aspiration of oil; mineral oils and vegetable oils usually cause lower grade, chronic inflammation while animal fats tend to cause more acute inflammation and sometimes pulmonary hemorrhage. Called also *oil-aspiration p.*.
lobar p. 1. a type of acute bacterial pneumonia with abundant edema, usually limited to just one lobe of a lung; the most common kind is pneumococcal pneumonia. 2. pneumococcal p.
lobular p. bronchopneumonia.
Löffler p. see under *syndrome.*
lymphocytic interstitial p., interstitial p., lymphoid see under *pneumonitis.*
p. malleo′sa glanders p.
measles virus p. viral pneumonia caused by the measles virus; it ranges from a mild type occurring during a bout of measles to severe, even fatal, giant cell pneumonia.
meningococcal p. a rare type of bacterial pneumonia caused by meningococci *(Neisseria meningitidis);* many cases are subclinical, but some infections become overwhelming, with fever, pleural effusion, and even death. Called also *Neisseria meningitidis p.*
metastatic p. suppurative pneumonia due to bloodborne infection in bacteremia.
migratory p. pneumonia that spreads from one lobe of the lung to others; called also *wandering p.*
***Moraxella* p., *Moraxella catarrhalis* p.** a usually mild type of bacterial pneumonia caused by infection with *Moraxella (Branhamella) catarrhalis,* generally seen in patients with some other debilitating condition, especially smokers with chronic obstructive pulmonary disease. Symptoms include fever and dyspnea.
***Mycoplasma* p., mycoplasmal p.** the most common form of primary atypical pneumonia (q.v.), caused by *Mycoplasma pneumoniae* and occurring most frequently in young adults; called also *Eaton agent p.*
necrotizing p. necrosis of lung tissue in bacterial pneumonia, which may range from small abscesses to massive areas.
***Neisseria meningitidis* p.** meningococcal p.
***Nocardia* p.** the pneumonia seen with severe pulmonary nocardiosis.
obstructive p. pneumonia caused by obstruction of the air passages, as by bronchogenic carcinoma.
oil aspiration p. lipid p.
organizing p. pneumonia characterized by formation of numerous small foci of loose connective tissue called Masson bodies in the bronchioles and alveoli. It may be seen following injury, associated with interstitial lung conditions, or as part of the syndrome called *bronchiolitis obliterans with organizing pneumonia* (or *cryptogenic organizing p.*)
ovine progressive p. a chronic viral disease of sheep caused by a retrovirus, characterized by progressive weight loss and dyspnea that can be fatal. A demyelinating meningoencephalitis may occur, with paresis of the hind limbs progressing to total paralysis and death. The respiratory form is also called *maedi* and the meningoencephalitic form *visna; maedi-visna* is used to describe the entire syndrome.

parainfluenza virus p. viral pneumonia caused by the parainfluenza 3 virus, usually seen in children or immunocompromised adults; characteristics include fever, cough, and dyspnea.
***Pasteurella multocida* p.** a rare type of bacterial pneumonia caused by infection with *Pasteurella multocida,* usually seen in patients with chronic lung disease; characteristics include fever, cough, and dyspnea, sometimes with empyema.
Pittsburgh p. a type of pneumonia resembling legionnaires' disease, caused by *Legionella micdadei,* and occurring as a nosocomial infection especially in immunocompromised patients.
plague p. pneumonic plague.
plasma cell p. pneumocystis p.
pleuritic p. pleuropneumonia (def. 1).
pneumococcal p. a type of acute pneumonia usually caused by *Streptococcus pneumoniae,* with inflammation of one or more lobe(s) of the lung; characteristics include chills followed by sudden fever, dyspnea, tachypnea, pain in the side, and coughing with bloodstained sputum. It usually begins in the lower lobe, which becomes congested *(stage of congestion),* then red and solid *(red hepatization),* and later gray from degeneration of the exudates *(gray hepatization).* In most patients this is followed by the *stage of resolution,* during which the exudates degenerate and are absorbed. Called also *lobar p.*
pneumocystis p. (PCP) a pulmonary disease caused by *Pneumocystis jiroveci,* occurring in premature or malnourished infants and immunocompromised persons. It is characterized by dyspnea, tachypnea, fever, cough, and cyanosis, with cellular detritus containing plasma cells appearing in the lungs; if untreated it leads to pulmonary consolidation, hypoxemia, and death. Called also *pneumocystosis, pneumocystiasis,*interstitial plasma cell p., and, formerly, *Pneumocystis carinii p.*
***Pneumocystis carinii* p.** former name for *pneumocystis p.;* cf. *Pneumocystis jiroveci.*
primary atypical p. a general term applied to any of numerous acute infectious pulmonary diseases, formerly referring to any type other than bacterial pneumonia; causative organisms include *Mycoplasma pneumoniae* (see *mycoplasmal p.*), species of *Rickettsia, Chlamydophila,* and *Chlamydia,* and various viruses (see *viral p.*). All are marked by extensive but tenuous pulmonary infiltration and by fever, malaise, myalgia, sore throat, and a cough that at first is nonproductive but becomes productive and paroxysmal. Called also *atypical, atypical bronchial,* or *cold agglutinin p.*
***Proteus* p.** a rare type of bacterial pneumonia caused by infection with species of *Proteus,* usually *P. mirabilis* or *P. vulgaris;* it usually affects debilitated or immunocompromised patients and is characterized by consolidation with abscesses in the upper lobes.
***Pseudomonas aeruginosa* p.** a form of bacterial pneumonia, usually nosocomial, seen in young children and debilitated or immunocompromised adults, caused by infection with *Pseudomonas aeruginosa;* characteristics include fever and coughing with lung nodules that may be either firm or hemorrhagic and may progress to necrosis of the alveoli with cavitation.
purulent p. suppurative p.
Q fever p. a type of bacterial pneumonia occurring as part of Q fever (infection with *Coxiella burnetii*); it is usually benign and self-limited, with granulomatous infiltrates and linear atelectasis visible radiographically.
respiratory syncytial virus p. viral pneumonia caused by respiratory syncytial virus, seen in infants and young children and occasionally in immunocompromised or otherwise debilitated adults; characteristics include fever, cough, dyspnea, wheezing, and crackles.
rheumatic p. a rare, usually fatal complication of acute rheumatic fever characterized by extensive pulmonary consolidation and rapidly progressive functional deterioration and by alveolar exudate (with the presence of Masson bodies), interstitial infiltrates, and necrotizing arteritis.
***Rhodococcus equi* p.** a type of bacterial pneumonia seen in immunocompromised persons, caused by infection with *Rhodococcus equi,* often after contact with an infected animal; it is often subacute, with consolidation and cavitation visible radiographically.
secondary p. pneumonia seen as a complication of some other disorder, such as influenza or a fungal infection.
***Serratia* p.** a rare type of bacterial pneumonia, usually nosocomial, caused by infection with *Serratia marcescens;* it is often fatal to immunocompromised patients.
staphylococcal p. a common type of bacterial pneumonia, usually bronchopneumonia, caused by infection with *Staphylococcus,* particularly *S. aureus.* Since many strains of *Staphylococcus* are antibiotic-resistant, this type is often seen in hospitals in patients on antibiotic therapy after surgery; it also commonly infects debilitated patients such as those suffering from other respiratory infections or viral infections such as influenza. Characteristics include fever, dyspnea, rales, pleural effusion, and empyema.
streptococcal p. pneumonia caused by a streptococcus other than *S. pneumoniae,* usually *Streptococcus pyogenes;* pleural effusion, with or without empyema, is particularly common.
suppurative p. pneumonia with formation of abscesses in the lungs. Called also *purulent p.*
terminal p. pneumonia that develops during some other disease and often increases the chances of early death of the patient.
traumatic p. pneumonia following an injury to the thorax; called also *contusion p.*
tuberculous p. pneumonia occurring as part of the earliest reaction to infection by *Mycobacterium tuberculosis;* see also *caseous p.* and *exudative tuberculosis.*
tularemic p. pulmonary tularemia.
typhoid p. pneumonia with typhoid symptoms or accompanying typhoid fever; children may develop bronchopneumonia and adults may develop lobar pneumonia, with suppuration and empyema.
unresolved p. pneumonia in which the lung signs fail to clear up within the usual period.
usual interstitial p. idiopathic pulmonary fibrosis.
varicella p., *Varicella zoster* p. viral pneumonia developing as a complication two to six days after the appearance of varicella (chickenpox), seen in adults more often than children. Symptoms may be severe, with violent cough, hemoptysis, and severe chest pains. Radiologically, there are numerous nodular densities, which may coalesce, at the base of each lung, and often enlarged lymph nodes in the hilar region; small nodular calcifications may persist.
ventilator-associated p. the most common nosocomial type of pneumonia, a frequently fatal type seen in patients breathing with a ventilator; it is usually caused by aspiration of contaminated secretions or stomach contents and may be bacterial, viral, or fungal.
verminous p. mild to severe dyspnea and fever in domestic animals due to the presence in the bronchioles or lungs of nematode lungworms, usually of species of *Dictyocaulus, Filaroides, Metastrongylus, Muellerius,* or *Protostrongylus.* Acute episodes may be fatal. In sheep, cattle, goats, and pigs it is called *hoose.* It also occurs in horses, donkeys, dogs, and cats.
viral p. any of numerous pneumonias caused by a virus, such as an adenovirus, influenza virus, parainfluenza virus, or respiratory syncytial virus.
wandering p. migratory p.
white p. p. alba.

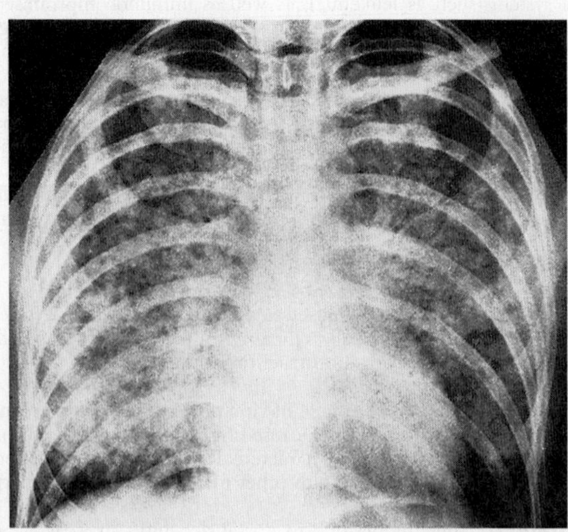

■ Varicella pneumonia. Radiograph taken in the first week, showing widespread soft nodular opacities throughout both lungs, less noticeable at the apices.

Types of Hypersensitivity Pneumonitis

Disease	Source of Antigen	Most Likely Antigen
Bagassosis	Moldy bagasse (pressed sugar cane)	*Thermoactinomyces* spp. and other actinomycetes
Cheese handler's (or washer's) disease or lung	Moldy cheese casings	*Penicillium* spp.
Duck fever	Duck feathers	Duck proteins
Epoxy resin lung	Hot epoxy resin	Phthalic anhydride
Farmer's (harvester's, thresher's) lung	Moldy or contaminated hay	*Aspergillus* spp., *Micropolyspora faeni, Thermoactinomyces vulgaris*, and other actinomycetes
Grain handler's lung	Moldy grain	Miscellaneous fungi
Humidifier lung	Contaminated air conditioners, humidifiers, or dehumidifiers	Amebae, *Cephalosporium* spp., *Penicillium* spp., *Thermoactinomyces*, and other actinomycetes
Malt worker's lung	Moldy barley	*Aspergillus* spp.
Maple bark disease	Moldy maple bark	*Cryptostroma corticale*
Meat wrapper's lung	Meat wrappers or labels	Phthalic anhydride
Miller's lung	Insect-infested wheat	*Sitophilus granarius*
Pigeon breeder's (bird breeder's) lung	Pigeon feces	Pigeon immunoglobulin A
Sequoiosis	Moldy sawdust	*Aureobasidium, Graphium*
Suberosis	Moldy cork dust	*Penicillium* spp.
Turkey handler's disease	Turkey proteins	Turkey products
Wood pulp worker's disease	Moldy wood pulp	*Alternaria* spp.
Wood trimmer's disease	Moldy wood trimmings	*Mucor, Rhizopus*

pneu•mon•ic (noo-mon′ik) [Gr. *pneumonikos*] 1. pertaining to pneumonia. 2. pulmonary (def. 1).

pneu•mo•ni•tis (noo″mo-ni′tis) [*pneumon-* + *-itis*] inflammation of the lungs. See also *pneumonia.*

acute lupus p. a type of pneumonitis that accompanies systemic lupus erythematosus; characteristics include rapid onset, fever, dyspnea, and coughing.

***Ascaris* p.** the most common type of Löffler syndrome, caused by presence in the lungs of the nematode *Ascaris lumbricoides.* Called also *pulmonary ascariasis.*

aspiration p. see under *pneumonia.*

chemical p. pneumonitis caused by the inhalation of chemical irritants; the extent of the injury reflects the concentration of the irritants and the duration of exposure.

cholesterol p. pneumonitis characterized by chronic inflammatory changes and deposition of excessive amounts of cholesterol in the tissues. It is often lobar or segmental in distribution and may resemble primary or metastatic tumor.

feline p. a fatal pneumonitis with conjunctivitis in cats, caused by a strain of *Chlamydophila psittaci.*

granulomatous p. pneumonitis with granulomas, usually resulting from an infection or inhalation of organic dust by a hypersensitive person.

hypersensitivity p. a respiratory hypersensitivity reaction to repeated inhalation of organic particles, usually in an occupational setting, with onset a few hours after exposure to the allergen. Characteristics include fever, fatigue, chills, unproductive cough, tachycardia, and tachypnea; in the chronic form there is interstitial fibrosis with collagenous thickening of the alveolar septa. There are many specific types (see table). Called also *allergic* or *extrinsic allergic alveolitis.*

lupus p. see *acute lupus p.*

lymphocytic interstitial p. an insidious, slowly progressive interstitial lung disease of unknown etiology, marked by diffuse peribronchial and interstitial infiltration of the lungs by lymphocytes, plasma cells, and lymphoblasts; usually seen in immunocompromised patients, especially children, or accompanying Sjögren syndrome. Called also *lymphocytic* or *lymphoid interstitial pneumonia.*

malarial p. pneumonitis caused by *Plasmodium falciparum*, characterized by cough with bloody sputum and coarse rales; in severe cases thromboses may result from the agglutination of parasitized erythrocytes in small blood vessels of the lung.

manganese p. pneumonitis affecting the lower airways and alveoli, caused by inhaling manganese dust or fumes; it may be acute, in which form it is often fatal, or it may be chronic and recurring. See also *manganese poisoning*, under *poisoning.*

mercury p. a sometimes fatal pneumonitis with tracheitis, bronchitis, and bronchiolitis, accompanied by the symptoms of mercury poisoning, caused by the inhalation of mercury fumes.

mouse p. a bronchopneumonia of laboratory mice caused by a strain of *Chlamydia trachomatis.*

pneumocystis p. pneumocystis pneumonia.

radiation p. lung inflammation resulting from radiation exposure, usually radiation therapy, with coughing, dyspnea, and alveolar infiltration, leading to mild to severe or even fatal fibrosis 6 to 9 months after the exposure.

trimellitic anhydride p. hemorrhagic pneumonitis with intra-alveolar hemorrhage and alveolar cell hyperplasia caused by inhalation of trimellitic anhydride fumes.

uremic p. pneumonitis associated with uremia; a butterfly or bat-wing configuration of opacities on the chest radiograph indicates pulmonary edema.

pneumon(o)- [Gr. *pneumon* lung] a combining form denoting relationship to the lungs. For words beginning thus, see also *pneumo-.*

pneu•mo•no•cele (noo-mon′o-sēl) 1. hernial protrusion of lung tissue, as through a fissure in the chest wall. Called also *pleurocele* and *pneumocele.* 2. pneumatocele (def. 2).

pneu•mo•no•cen•te•sis (noo-mo″no-sen-te′sis) [*pneumono-* + *-centesis*] paracentesis of a lung; called also *pneumocentesis.*

pneu•mo•no•coc•cus (noo″mo-no-kok′əs) pneumococcus.

pneu•mo•no•co•ni•o•sis (noo-mo″no-ko″ne-o′sis) pneumoconiosis.

pneu•mo•no•cyte (noo-mon′o-sīt) alveolar cell.

granular p's type II alveolar cells.

membranous p's type I alveolar cells.

pneu•mo•no•en•ter•itis (noo-mo″no-en″tər-i′tis) pneumoenteritis.

pneu•mo•nog•ra•phy (noo″mo-nog′rə-fe) pneumography.

pneu•mo•nol•y•sis (noo″mo-nol′ĭ-sis) [*pneumono-* + *-lysis*] division of the tissues attaching the lung to the wall of the chest cavity so that the lung collapses inward; it was formerly a common method of collapse therapy (q.v.) and is still sometimes done to allow access during thoracic surgery. Called also *pneumolysis.*

pneu•mo•nop•a•thy (noo″mo-nop′ə-the) pneumopathy.

pneu•mo•no•pexy (noo-mo′no-pek″se) [*pneumono-* + *-pexy*] surgical fixation of the lung to the thoracic wall; see also *pleuroparietopexy* and *pleurodesis.* Called also *pneumopexy.*

pneu•mo•nor•rha•gia (noo-mo″no-ra′jə) pulmonary hemorrhage.

pneu•mo•nor•rha•phy (noo″mo-nor′ə-fe) [*pneumono-* + *-rrhaphy*] suture of the lung.

pneu•mo•no•sis (noo″mo-no′sis) pneumopathy.

pneu•mo•no•ther•a•py (noo-mo″no-ther′ə-pe) pneumotherapy.

pneu•mo•not•o•my (noo″mo-not′ə-me) [*pneumono-* + *-tomy*] surgical incision of the lung. Called also *pneumotomy.*

Pneu•mo•nys•soi•des (noo″mo-nis-oi′dēz) a genus of mites of the family Halarachnidae. Its distinction from the genus *Pneumonyssus* has been questioned.

Pneu•mo•nys•sus (noo″mo-nis′əs) a genus of mites of the family Halarachnidae. *P. cani′num* infests the nasal passages of dogs, causing nasal acariasis. *P. simi′cola* is found in the lungs of monkeys.

pneu•mo•par•oti•tis (noo″mo-par″o-ti′tis) pneumatic inflation of the parotid gland.

pneu•mop•a•thy (noo-mop′ə-the) any disease of the lung; called also *pneumonopathy.*

pneu•mo•peri•car•di•um (noo″mo-per″ĭ-kahr′de-əm) [*pneumo-* + *pericardium*] the presence of air or gas in the cavity of the pericardium.

pneu·mo·peri·to·ne·um (noo″mo-per″ĭ-to-ne′əm) [*pneumo-* + *peritoneum*] the presence of gas or air in the peritoneal cavity; it may occur spontaneously, as in subphrenic abscess, or be deliberately introduced as an aid to radiologic examination and diagnosis *(diagnostic p.)* or to achieve exposure during laparoscopy. **pneumoperitone′al** *adj*

pneu·mo·peri·to·ni·tis (noo″mo-per″ĭ-to-ni′tis) [*pneumo-* + *peritonitis*] peritonitis with air or gas in the peritoneal cavity.

pneu·mo·pexy (noo′mo-pek″se) pneumonopexy.

pneu·mo·pha·gia (noo″mo-fa′jə) [*pneumo-* + *-phagia*] aerophagia.

pneu·mo·pho·nia (noo″mo-fo′ne-ə) a form of dysphonia characterized by a breathy voice.

pneu·mo·plas·ty (noo′mo-plas″te) plastic surgery to a lung. **pneumoplas′tic** *adj*

reduction p. surgical removal of nonfunctional lung tissue in cases of advanced emphysema, such as bullectomy in bullous emphysema where giant bullae are compressing the functional lung tissue.

pneu·mo·pleu·ri·tis (noo″mo-ploo̅-ri′tis) pleuropneumonia (def. 1).

pneu·mo·pre·cor·di·um (noo″mo-pre-kor′de-əm) [*pneumo-* + *precordium*] the presence of air in the precordial space.

pneu·mo·pre·peri·to·ne·um (noo″mo-pre-per″ĭ-to-ne′əm) the presence of air or gas in the preperitoneal space; it may occur spontaneously or be deliberately introduced as an aid to radiologic examination and diagnosis.

pneu·mo·py·elog·ra·phy (noo″mo-pi″ə-log′rə-fe) [*pneumo-* + *pyelo-* + *-graphy*] pyelography in which oxygen or air, instead of an opaque solution, is injected into the renal pelvis.

pneu·mo·pyo·peri·car·di·um (noo″mo-pi″o-per″ĭ-kahr′de-əm) pyopneumopericardium.

pneu·mo·pyo·tho·rax (noo″mo-pi″o-thor′aks) pyopneumothorax.

pneu·mo·ra·chi·cen·te·sis (noo″mo-ra″ke-sen-te′sis) pneumorachis (def. 2).

pneu·mo·ra·chis (noo″mo-ra′kis) [*pneumo-* + *rachis*] 1. the presence of a gaseous collection in the spinal canal. 2. the injection of gas into the spinal canal for the facilitation of myelographic examination. See *pneumoencephalomyelography.*

pneu·mo·ra·di·og·ra·phy (noo″mo-ra″de-og′rə-fe) [*pneumo-* + *radiography*] radiography of a part following the injection of air or oxygen, as in pneumoperitoneum.

pneu·mo·re·sec·tion (noo″mo-re-sek′shən) surgical excision of part of a lung; cf. *pneumonectomy.*

pneu·mo·ret·ro·peri·to·ne·um (noo″mo-ret″ro-per″ĭ-to-ne′əm) the presence of air or gas in the retroperitoneal space.

pneu·mor·rha·gia (noo″mo-ra′jə) pulmonary hemorrhage.

pneu·mo·scro·tum (noo″mo-skro′tum) air or gas in the scrotum as a result of trauma or a disease process.

pneu·mo·se·ro·sa (noo″mo-se-ro′sə) injection of air into a joint cavity for fluoroscopy.

pneu·mo·se·ro·tho·rax (noo″mo-se″ro-thor′aks) hydropneumothorax.

pneu·mo·sil·i·co·sis (noo″mo-sil″ĭ-ko′sis) silicosis.

pneu·mo·si·nus di·la·tans (noo″mo-si′nəs di-la′təns) abnormal dilatation of the sphenoidal sinuses with remodeling but without erosion or thinning of the sinus bony walls. The sinuses are well aerated and the mucosa is normal.

pneu·mo·tacho·graph (noo″mo-tak′o-graf) pneumotachygraph.

pneu·mo·ta·chom·e·ter (noo″mo-tə-kom′ə-tər) a transducer used in measuring exhaled air flow.

pneu·mo·tach·y·graph (noo″mo-tak′ĭ-graf) [*pneumo-* + *tachy-* + *-graph*] an instrument for recording the velocity of the respired air.

pneu·mo·tax·ic (noo″mo-tak′sik) [*pneumo-* + Gr. *taxis* arrangement] relating to the regulation of the rate of respiration; see under *center.*

pneu·mo·ther·a·py (noo″mo-ther′ə-pe) the treatment of diseases of the lungs. Called also *pneumonotherapy.*

pneu·mo·ther·mo·mas·sage (noo″mo-thur″mo-mə-sahzh′) [*pneumo-* + *thermo-* + *massage*] the application to the body of hot condensed air to produce an effect resembling massage.

pneu·mo·tho·rax (noo″mo-thor′aks) [*pneumo-* + *thorax*] an accumulation of air or gas in the pleural space; three types are distinguished: *traumatic p., primary spontaneous p.,* and *secondary spontaneous p.* It was formerly sometimes induced for treatment of pulmonary tuberculosis; see *artificial p.*

artificial p. pneumothorax induced intentionally by artificial means; formerly used as a method of collapse therapy (q.v.) in treatment of pulmonary tuberculosis. Called also *induced p.* and *therapeutic p.*

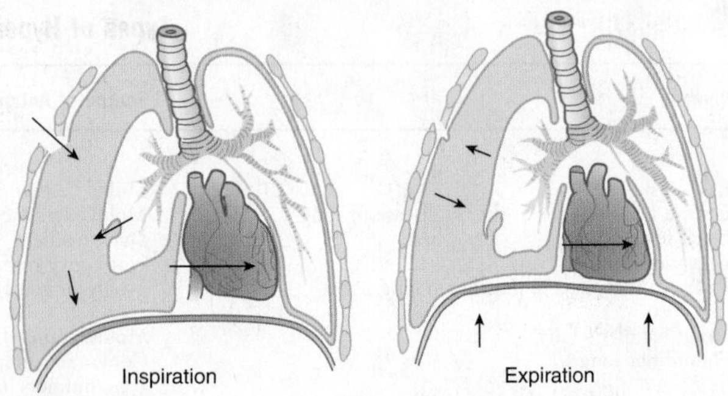

■ Tension pneumothorax with total collapse of the right lung and shift of mediastinal structures to the left. Air is forced into the pleural space during inspiration and cannot escape during expiration.

catamenial p. pneumothorax associated with menstrual periods, believed to represent a consequence of pleural endometriosis.

clicking p. pneumothorax in which there is a clicking sound synchronous with the heartbeat.

closed p. pneumothorax in which pulmonary air leaks into the pleural cavity through a wound in a lung.

diagnostic p. temporary artificial pneumothorax induced in order to demonstrate the parietal or visceral pleura on chest films for detection and localization of tumors of the pleura.

induced p. artificial p.

open p. pneumothorax in which the pleural cavity is exposed to the atmosphere through an open wound in the chest wall. See also *sucking wound.*

pressure p. tension p.

primary spontaneous p. pneumothorax that does not have an obvious external cause, such as that from a ruptured subpleural bleb.

secondary spontaneous p. any type resulting from a known pathologic condition.

tension p. pneumothorax in which the pressure within the pleural space is greater than atmospheric pressure; this may occur when air enters under positive pressure, such as when caused by positive pressure ventilation, or when the tissues around the opening into the pleural cavity act as valves, allowing air to enter but not to escape. The resultant positive pressure in the cavity displaces the mediastinum to the opposite side, with consequent interference with respiration. Called also *pressure p.*

therapeutic p. artificial p.

traumatic p. pneumothorax resulting from chest trauma, such as accompanying a penetrating wound, a fractured rib, or abrupt pressure on a lung.

valvular p. tension p.

pneu·mo·to·mog·ra·phy (noo″mo-to-mog′rə-fe) tomography performed after injection of air or other gas into the region or organ being visualized.

pneu·mot·o·my (noo-mot′ə-me) pneumonotomy.

pneu·mo·tro·pic (noo″mo-tro′pik) 1. having a selective affinity for pulmonary tissue; exerting its principal effect upon the lungs. 2. having a selective affinity for pneumococci.

pneu·mot·ro·pism (noo-mot′rə-piz-əm) the predilection of an agent or organism for lung tissue.

Pneu·mo·tus·sin (noo′mo-tus″in) trademark for combination preparations of hydrocodone bitartrate and guaifenesin.

Pneu·mo·vax 23 (noo′mo-vaks″) trademark for a preparation of pneumococcal vaccine polyvalent.

pneu·mo·ven·tri·cle (noo″mo-ven′trĭ-kəl) [*pneumo-* + *ventricle*] pneumocephalus in one of the cerebral ventricles; called also *pneumoventriculi.*

pneu·mo·ven·tric·u·li (noo″mo-ven-trik′u-li) pneumoventricle.

pneu·mo·ven·tric·u·log·ra·phy (noo″mo-vən-trik″u-log′rə-fe) ventriculography of the cerebral ventricles after the injection of air or gas.

Pneu·mo·vi·ri·nae (noo″mo-vir-i′ne) a subfamily of the Paramyxoviridae containing the genera *Pneumovirus* and *Metapneumovirus.*

Pneu·mo·vi·rus (noo′mo-vi″rəs) [*pneumo-* + *virus*] respiratory syncytial viruses; a genus of viruses of the subfamily Pneumovirinae (family Paramyxoviridae) that includes human and bovine respiratory syncytial viruses and avian pneumovirus.

pneu·mo·vi·rus (noo′mo-vi″rəs) any virus of the genus *Pneumovirus.* **pneumovi′ral** *adj*

avian p. turkey rhinotracheitis virus.

pneu·sis (noo′sis) [Gr. *pneusis* a blowing] ventilation (def. 2).

PNH paroxysmal nocturnal hemoglobinuria.

-pnoea see *-pnea.*

PNS peripheral nervous system.

PO [L.] per os (by mouth, orally).

Po_2, P_{o_2} oxygen partial pressure (oxygen tension).

Po polonium.

pO_2, pO_2 oxygen partial pressure (oxygen tension).

POA pancreatic oncofetal antigen.

Poa (po′ə) a genus of grasses (family Gramineae). *P. praten′sis* is Kentucky bluegrass or June grass, whose pollen causes hay fever.

Pocill. [L.] pocil′lum (a small cup).

pock (pok) a pustule, especially one of the lesions of smallpox.

pock•et (pok′ət) a bag or similar space; see also *cavity, pouch, recess,* and *sac.*

complex p. a spiral type of periodontal pocket involving more than one surface of the tooth, but communicating with the gingival margin only along the surface at which it originates.

compound p. a periodontal pocket involving more than one tooth surface, and communicating with the marginal gingiva along each of the involved surfaces.

endocardial p′s sclerotic thickenings of the mural endocardium, occurring most often on the left ventricular septum below an insufficient aortic valve; called also *regurgitant p′s.*

gingival p. a gingival sulcus deepened by pathological conditions, caused by gingival enlargement with no destruction of the periodontal tissue. Called also *relative p.*

infrabony p., intra-alveolar p. intrabony p.

intrabony p. a periodontal pocket in which the bottom is apical to the level of the adjacent alveolar bone.

pacemaker p. the subcutaneous area in which the pulse generator and pacing leads of an internal pacemaker are implanted, usually developed in the prepectoralis fascia or the retromammary area.

periodontal p. a gingival sulcus that extends abnormally deep into the periodontal ligament apically to the original level of the resorbed alveolar crest.

Rathke p. see under *pouch.*

regurgitant p′s endocardial p′s.

relative p. gingival p.

retraction p. a localized area of atelectasis where the tympanic membrane bulges inward; it may be a precursor of a serious condition such as cholesteatoma or ossicular discontinuity.

Seessel p. see under *pouch.*

simple p. a periodontal pocket involving only one tooth surface.

subcrestal p. intrabony p.

suprabony p., supracrestal p. a periodontal pocket in which the bottom is coronal to the underlying bone.

p′s of Zahn shallow pockets with miniature leaflets, resembling cusps of the semilunar valve, produced in the endocardium of the left ventricle by the regurgitant aortic stream in the presence of insufficiency of the aortic valve.

pock•mark (pok′mahrk) a depressed scar left by a pustule, especially one left by a lesion of smallpox.

Pocul. [L.] po′culum (cup).

po•dag•ra (pə-dag′rə) [*pod-* + *-agra*] gouty pain in the great toe. **podag′ral, podag′ric, podag′rous** *adj*

po•dal•gia (pə-dal′jə) [*pod-* + *-algia*] pain in the foot; cf. *podagra* and *tarsalgia.* Called also *pedialgia* and *pododynia.*

po•dal•ic (pə-dal′ik) [Gr. *pous* foot] pertaining to or accomplished by means of the feet; see under *version.*

pod•ar•thri•tis (pod″ahr-thri′tis) [*pod-* + *arthritis*] inflammation of the joints of the feet.

pod•ede•ma (pod″ə-de′mə) edema of the feet.

pod•en•ceph•a•lus (pod″ən-sef′ə-ləs) [*pod-* + Gr. *enkephalos* brain] a fetus whose brain, without a cranium, hangs by a pedicle.

po•di•a•trist (po-di′ə-trist) a specialist in podiatry; formerly called *chiropodist.*

po•di•a•try (pə-di′ə-tre) [*pod-* + *-iatry*] the specialized field that deals with the study and care of the foot, including its anatomy, pathology, medical and surgical treatment, etc. Formerly called *chiropody.* **podiat′ric** *adj*

pod(o)- [Gr. *pous,* gen. *podos* foot] a combining form denoting relationship to the foot.

Podo•con (pod′o-kon) trademark for a preparation of podophyllum resin.

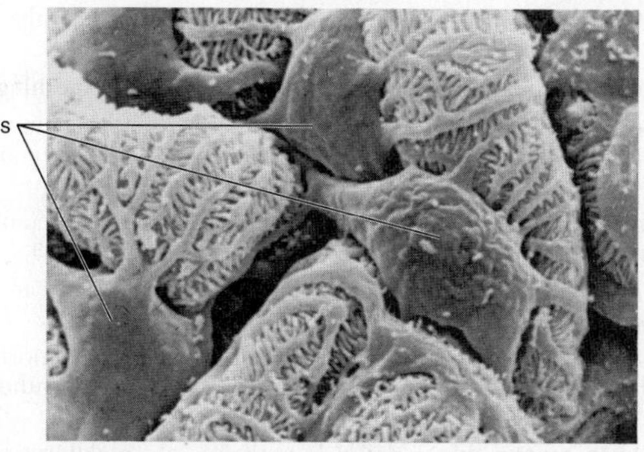

■ Scanning electron micrograph showing podocytes, with their processes (pedicels) interdigitating along the capillary surfaces.

po•do•co•ni•o•sis (po″do-ko″ne-o′sis) lymphedema in the leg and foot caused by absorption of minute particles of silicon; seen primarily in East Africa in persons who work outdoors and do not wear shoes. Called also *mossy foot.*

podo•cyte (pod′o-sīt) [*podo-* + *-cyte*] a modified epithelial cell of the visceral layer of the glomerular capsule in the renal glomerulus; it has a small perikaryon and a number of primary and secondary footlike radiating processes (pedicels) that interdigitate with those of other podocytes and embrace the walls of glomerular capillaries. Called also *visceral epithelial cells.*

po•do•dem•o•di•co•sis (po″do-dem″ə-dĭ-ko′sis) [*podo-* + *demodicosis*] chronic infection of the skin of the feet of dogs or cats by mites of the genus *Demodex,* with pyoderma, alopecia, and scaling.

podo•derm (pod′o-dərm) [*podo-* + *-derm*] on hoofed animals, that portion of the skin that continues downward within the horn capsule of the hoof.

po•do•der•ma•ti•tis (po″do-dur″mə-ti′tis) [*podo-* + *dermatitis*] foot rot of cattle.

podo•dy•na•mom•e•ter (pod″o-di″nə-mom′ə-tər) a dynamometer used for the muscles of the lower limb.

podo•dyn•ia (pod″o-din′e-ə) [*pod-* + *-odynia*] podalgia.

po•dof•i•lox (po-dof′ĭ-loks) a preparation of podophyllotoxin either chemically synthesized or purified from plant extracts; it inhibits cell mitosis and is used topically in the treatment of condyloma acuminatum.

podo•gram (pod′o-gram) [*podo-* + *-gram*] a print of, or an outline tracing of, the sole of the foot.

podo•graph (pod′o-graf) [*podo-* + *-graph*] the instrument used in the making of a podogram.

po•dol•o•gy (po-dol′ə-je) [*podo-* + *-logy*] podiatry.

podo•phyl•lin (pod″o-fil′in) podophyllum resin.

podo•phyl•lo•tox•in (pod″o-fil′o-tok″sin) [*Podophyllum* + *toxin*] a highly toxic compound, the main active component of podophyllum; it has cathartic and antineoplastic properties. Less toxic derivatives such as etoposide and teniposide are used as antineoplastics. See also *podofilox.*

Podo•phyl•lum (pod″o-fil′əm) [*podo-* + Gr. *phyllon* leaf] a genus of perennial North American herbs of the family Berberidaceae. *P. pelta′tum* L. is the source of podophyllotoxin and podophyllum resin.

podo•phyl•lum (pod″o-fil′əm) [USP] the dried rhizome and roots of *Podophyllum peltatum;* called also *Indian apple, mandrake, mandrake root,* and *May apple.* See *podophyllum resin,* under *resin.*

Po•do•stro•ma (po″do-stro′mə) a genus of fungi of the family Hypocreaceae, including the perfect (sexual) stage of some species of *Trichoderma.*

podo•troch•li•tis (pod″o-trok-li′tis) navicular disease.

po•do•troch•lo•sis (po″do-trok-lo′sis) navicular disease.

poe- for words beginning thus, see those beginning *pe-.*

Poe•cil•ia (pe-sil′e-ə) [Gr. *poikilos* spotted, mottled; varied] a genus of minnows; called also *Girardinus.*

P. reticula′ta a species used, especially in tropical America, to control mosquitoes; they eat the larvae of *Anopheles.* Called also *Girardinus poeciloides.*

po•go•ni•a•sis (po″go-ni′ə-sis) [Gr. *pōgōn* beard + *-iasis*] 1. excessive growth of the beard. 2. the growth of a beard on a woman. See also *hirsutism.*

po•go•ni•on (po-go′ne-on) [Gr., dim. of *pōgōn* beard] a craniometric landmark, being the most anterior point in the midline of the chin.

pOH an infrequently used symbol used in expressing the approximate concentration of hydroxide ions in a solution.

-poiesis [Gr. *poiein* to make] a word termination meaning formation.

-poietin [Gr. *poiein* to make] a word termination used in names of hormones to indicate involvement in regulation of the numbers of various cell types in the peripheral blood.

poikil(o)- [Gr. *poikilos* spotted, mottled; varied] a combining form meaning mottled, variable, or irregular.

poi•ki•lo•blast (poi′kĭ-lo-blast″) [*poikilo-* + *-blast*] an abnormally shaped erythroblast.

poi•ki•lo•cyte (poi′kĭ-lo-sīt″) [*poikilo-* + *-cyte*] an abnormally shaped erythrocyte, such as a burr cell, sickle cell, target cell, acanthocyte, elliptocyte, schistocyte, spherocyte, or stomatocyte.

poi•ki•lo•cy•the•mia (poi″kĭ-lo-si-the′me-ə) poikilocytosis.

poi•ki•lo•cy•to•sis (poi″kĭ-lo-si-to′sis) [*poikilocyte* + *-osis*] presence of poikilocytes in the blood; called also *poikilocythemia.*

poi•ki•lo•der•ma (poi″kĭ-lo-dur′mə) pigmentary and atrophic changes in the skin, with both hyperpigmentation and hypopigmentation, so that it has a mottled appearance.

p. atro′phicans vascula′re p. vasculare atrophicans.

bullous acrokeratotic p. Kindler syndrome.

p. of Civatte a skin condition seen on sun-exposed areas, especially the face and back of the neck, usually in middle-aged, fair-skinned persons; characteristics include reticulated, blotchy, red to brown hyperpigmentation, telangiectasias, and interspersed small, pale, atrophic areas. It may be associated with a photosensitivity mechanism.

p. congenita′le Rothmund-Thomson syndrome.

hereditary acrokeratotic p. Kindler syndrome.

p. vascula′re atro′phicans a chronic, localized or generalized skin condition related to large plaque parapsoriasis, characterized by skin discoloration, atrophy, telangiectasias, and sometimes bright red papules; affected skin takes on an erythematous, papery appearance like that of radiodermatitis. The condition may be idiopathic or secondary to other dermatoses, and some cases progress to mycosis fungoides. Called also *p. atrophicans vasculare.*

poi•ki•los•mo•sis (poi″kil-oz-mo′sis) the processes by which a cell or tissue adjusts the osmolarity of its fluid to that of its immediate environment. **poikilosmot′ic** *adj*

poi•ki•lo•sta•sis (poi″kĭ-lo-sta′sis) [*poikilo-* + *-stasis*] the maintenance of stability in the body state (internal environment) by behavioral activities involving movement and selection by the whole organism.

poi•ki•lo•therm (poi-kil′o-thurm″) [*poikilo-* + Gr. *thermē* heat] 1. an animal that exhibits poikilothermy; a so-called cold-blooded animal. 2. ectotherm.

poi•ki•lo•ther•mal (poi″kĭ-lo-thur′məl) poikilothermic.

poi•ki•lo•ther•mia (poi″kĭ-lo-thur′me-ə) poikilothermy.

poi•ki•lo•ther•mic (poi″kĭ-lo-thur′mik) 1. pertaining to or characterized by poikilothermy. 2. ectothermic.

poi•ki•lo•ther•mism (poi″kĭ-lo-thur′miz-əm) poikilothermy.

poi•ki•lo•ther•my (poi″kĭ-lo-thur′me) [*poikilo-* + Gr. *thermē* heat] 1. the exhibition of body temperature which varies with the environmental temperature. 2. the ability of organisms to adapt themselves to variations in the temperature of their environment. Cf. *homeothermy.* 3. ectothermy.

poi•ki•lo•throm•bo•cyte (poi-kil″o-throm′bo-sīt) [*poikilo-* + *thrombocyte*] a platelet of abnormal shape.

poi•ki•lo•thy•mia (poi″kĭ-lo-thi′me-ə) [*poikilo-* + *-thymia*] a mental condition characterized by abnormal variations of mood.

point (point) [L. *punctum*] 1. a small area or spot; the sharp end of an object. 2. to approach the surface, like the pus of an abscess, at a definite spot or place. 3. a tapered, pointed endodontic instrument used for exploring the depth of the root canal in root canal therapy; called also *root canal p.* 4. an anthropometric landmark from which measurements are made. 5. an elongated silver or gutta-percha cone used in root canal obturation.

Point

p. A subspinale.

absorbent p. in root canal therapy, a cone of variable width and taper, usually made of paper or a paper product, used to dry or maintain a liquid disinfectant in the canal. Called also *paper p.*

acupuncture p. acupoint.

Addison p. the midpoint of the epigastric region.

alveolar p. the center of the anterior margin of the alveolar arch.

apophysiary p. subnasal p.

p. Ar articulare.

p. of Arrhigi an electrode site in electrocardiography, 2 to 3 cm to the left of the seventh thoracic vertebra.

p. B supramentale.

p. Ba basion.

Barker p. a point about 3.5 cm above and 3.5 cm behind the middle external auditory meatus, the proper spot to apply the trephine in abscess of the temporosphenoid lobe.

p. Bo Bolton p.

Boas p. a point to the left of the twelfth thoracic vertebra that becomes tender upon pressure in patients with gastric ulcer. Called also *Boas sign.*

boiling p. the temperature at which a liquid will boil (at sea level, or 1 atm, water boils at 100°C, or 212°F); specifically, the temperature at which the equilibrium vapor pressure of a liquid phase equals or slightly exceeds the atmospheric pressure.

Bolton p. a craniometric landmark located at the top of the convex curvature of the retrocondylar fossa, posterior to the condyle and between it and the basal surface of the occipital bone. Called also *p. Bo.*

Broadbent registration p. the midpoint of the perpendicular from the center of the sella turcica to the nasion-postcondylare plane. Called also *p. R.*

Cannon p. see under *ring.*

cardinal p's 1. a group of points on the optic axis, including the nodal points, the principal foci, and the optic center; they may include conjugate focal points of the object and image. Called also *principal p's.* 2. four points within the pelvic inlet: the two sacroiliac articulations and the two iliopectineal eminences.

condenser p. nib.

conjugate p. see under *focus.*

contact p. of tooth area contingens dentis.

convenience p. a small depression at the edge of the floor of the prepared cavity, placed there to retain the first piece of direct filling gold during the process of compaction.

p. of convergence 1. the point at which the lines of sight cross. 2. the point to which rays of light incline.

corresponding p's points upon the two retinae whose impressions unite to produce a single perception. Cf. *disparate p's.*

Cova p. a point at the apex of the costolumbar angle which is tender on pressure in cases of pyelitis of pregnancy.

craniometric p. any one of a set of points of reference assumed for use in craniometry.

critical p. the point of coincidence of the gas and liquid phases, at which the temperature is the critical temperature and the pressure is the critical pressure, and the substance exists as a single phase.

deaf p. one of certain points near the ear where a vibrating tuning fork cannot be heard.

Desjardins p. a point on the abdomen 5 to 7 cm from the umbilicus, on a line joining it to the right axilla; it lies over the head of the pancreas.

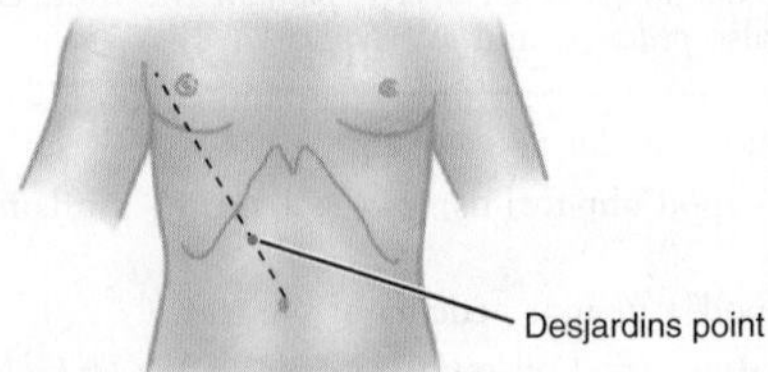

p. of direction see *position* (def. 2).

disparate p's points on the retina which are not paired exactly. Cf. *corresponding p's.*

p. of dispersion in optics, virtual focus.

p. of divergence the conjugate focus from which the light proceeds.

E p. in the apexcardiogram, the peak of the large positive deflection that represents outward motion of the ventricle during systole; it normally coincides with the onset of ejection.

Point *Continued*

p. of election that point at which any particular surgical operation is done by preference.
Erb p. a point 2 to 3 cm above the clavicle and beyond the posterior border of the sternomastoid, at the level of the transverse process of the sixth cervical vertebra; stimulation here contracts various arm muscles.
eye p. the bright circle seen at the crossing point or nearest the approximation of the rays above the microscopical ocular.
far p. the most remote point at which an object is clearly seen when the eye is at rest; called also *punctum remotum.*
p. of fixation 1. the point or object on which the eyes are directed and one's sight is fixed; called also *p. of regard.* 2. the point on the retina, usually the fovea, on which are focused the rays coming from an object directly regarded.
focal p. see *focus* (def. 1), and *cardinal p.* (def. 1).
freezing p. the temperature at which a liquid begins to freeze; that of pure water is 0°C, or 32°F. It is often used interchangeably with *melting p.* but should be reserved for substances being cooled, while melting point is used for substances being heated.
fusion p. melting p.
glenoid p. the center of the glenoid cavity of the scapula.
gutta-percha p. see under *cone.*
Hallé p. a point on the surface of the abdomen overlying the site where the ureter crosses the pelvic brim. It is the point of intersection between a horizontal line connecting the anterior superior iliac spines and a vertical line projected superiorly from the pubic spine.
hinge-axis p. a reference point on the skin corresponding with the terminal hinge axis of the mandible.
hysteroepileptogenous p., hysterogenic p. a point on which, if pressure such as tickling is exerted, a hysteric or hysteroepileptic attack may be produced.
ice p. the true melting point of ice, being the temperature of equilibrium between ice and air-saturated water under one atmosphere pressure.
identical p's corresponding p's.
p. of incidence see *refraction* (def. 2).
isobestic p. the wavelength at which two substances have the same absorptivity, such that if the sum of the concentrations of the compounds in solution is held constant, the absorbance at this point will be invariant as the ratio of the two compounds is varied; existence of one or more such points is indicative of chemical equilibrium between the two compounds.
isoelectric p. the pH of a solution at which a charged molecule does not migrate in an electric field.
isoionic p. the pH of a solution at which a specific ion (usually a protein) contains as many negative charges as positive charges.
J p. the point of intersection between the end of the QRS complex and the onset of the ST segment in electrocardiography.
jugal p. the point of the angle formed by the masseteric and maxillary edges of the malar bone (os zygomaticum).
jugomaxillary p. the point at the anteroinferior angle of the malar bone (os zygomaticum).
Keen p. a point for puncture of the lateral ventricles; 3 cm above and 3 cm behind the external auditory meatus.
Kocher p. a point for puncture of the lateral ventricles; 2.5 cm from the midline, 3.5 cm in front of the bregma.
Krafft p. the temperature above which conjugated bile salts form polymolecular aggregates (micelles) of about 3 to 10 nm in diameter.
lacrimal p. punctum lacrimale.
McBurney p. a point about one third of the distance between the right anterior superior iliac spine and the umbilicus, corresponding with the normal position of the base of the appendix; it is especially tender upon pressure in patients with acute appendicitis.

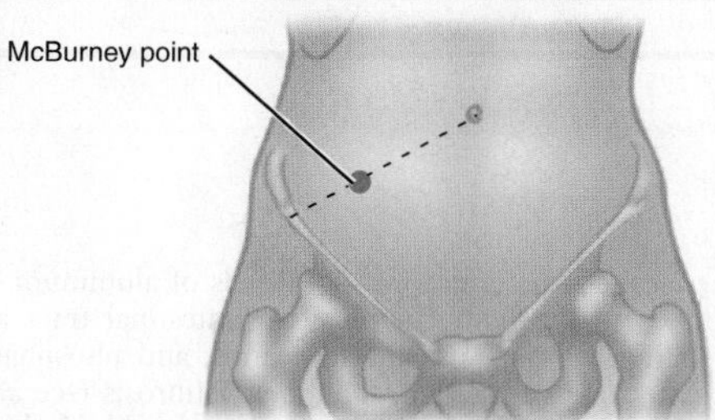

McEwen p. a point above the inner canthus of the eye which is tender in acute frontal sinusitis.
malar p. a point on the external tubercle of the malar bone (os zygomaticum).
p. of maximal impulse (PMI) the point on the chest where the impulse of the left ventricle is felt most strongly, normally in the fifth costal interspace inside the left mammillary line.
maximum occipital p. the point in the occipital bone that is farthest from the glabella.
median mandibular p. a craniometric landmark, being the point at the center of the anterior part of the superior edge of the mandible, at the site of the former mandibular symphysis.
melting p. (mp) the minimum temperature at which a solid begins to liquefy. See also *freezing p.* Cf. *melting temperature* and *fusion temperature.*
mental p. pogonion.
metopic p. metopion.
motor p. 1. the point at which a motor nerve enters a muscle. 2. any point on the skin over a muscle at which the application of galvanic stimulation will cause contraction of a corresponding muscle.
Munro p. a point midway between the umbilicus and the left anterior iliac spine; used for performing abdominal puncture.
nasal p. nasion.
near p. the nearest point at which the eye can distinctly perceive an object; the nearest point of clear vision; called also *punctum proximum.*
near p., absolute the near point for either eye alone with accommodation relaxed.
near p., relative the near point for both eyes with the employment of accommodation.
nodal p's one of two points on the axis of an optical system so situated that a ray falling on one will produce a parallel ray emerging through the other.
normal boiling p. the boiling point at 1 atmosphere pressure.
O p. the nadir of the apexcardiogram, occurring in early diastole at the time of mitral valve opening.
occipital p. the posterior point on the occipital bone.
ossification p. centrum ossificationis.
ossification p., primary centrum ossificationis primarium.
ossification p., secondary centrum ossificationis secundarium.
paper p. absorbent p.
phrenic pressure p. a point along the phrenic nerve between the sternocleidomastoid and the scalenus anticus on the right side; pressure on the point suggests gallbladder disease.
p. Po porion.
pour p. the temperature at which a liquid just begins to flow.
preauricular p. a point on the posterior root of the zygomatic arch just anterior to the auricular point.
pressure p. 1. a point that is particularly sensitive to pressure. 2. one of various locations on the body at which digital pressure may be applied for the control of hemorrhage.
pressure-arresting p. a point at which pressure arrests spasm.
pressure-exciting p. a point at which pressure produces spasm.
principal p's cardinal p's (def. 1).
p. R Broadbent registration p.
reflection p. the point from which a ray of light is reflected.
refraction p. the point at which a ray of light is refracted.
p. of regard p. of fixation (def. 1).
restriction p. a checkpoint late in the G_1 phase of the cell cycle after which the cell is irreversibly committed to entering the S phase; faulty regulation of passage through the restriction point contributes to cell transformation and is a common cause of cancer.
retromandibular tender p. a point behind the superior extremity of the inferior maxilla below the lobule of the ear and in front of the mastoid process. Pressure on this point elicits extreme pain in meningitis.
p. of reversal in retinoscopy, the point at which there is neutralization of movement because the reflex motion is changing to the opposite direction.
root canal p. point (def. 3).
p. SE sphenoethmoidal suture (def. 2).
set p. see under *S.*
silver p. in root canal therapy, a tapered and elongated silver plug that is cemented into the canal as a filling. Called also *silver cone.*
p. SO sphenooccipital synchondrosis (def. 2).

Point *Continued*

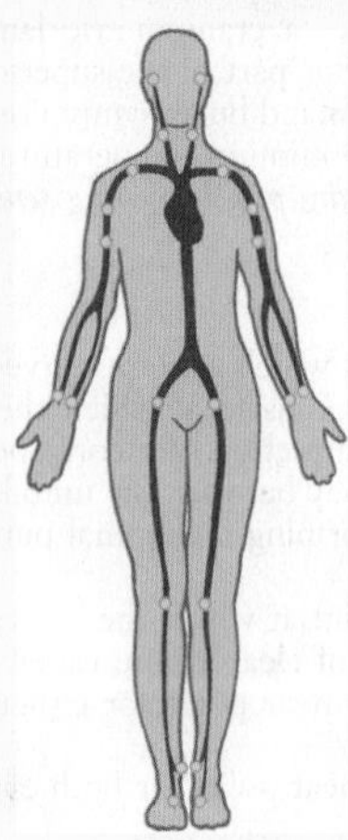

■ Various pressure points used to control hemorrhage.

spinal p. subnasal p.
stereoidentical p's points in space outside of the region within which fusion of double images occurs.
subnasal p. the central point of the root of the anterior nasal spine.
subtemporal p. the point where the sphenotemporal suture and infratemporal crest intersect.
supra-auricular p. a point at the root of the zygomatic process of the temporal bone, directly superior to the auricular point.
supraclavicular p. a point above the clavicle and outside of the sternomastoid where the application of a stimulus causes contraction of the biceps brachii, deltoideus, brachialis, and brachioradialis muscles.
supranasal p. ophryon.
supraorbital p. 1. ophryon. 2. in neuralgia, a tender spot just superior to the supraorbital notch.
sylvian p. a point on the surface of the skull from 29 to 32 mm behind the external angular process of the frontal bone.
tender p. a point on a muscle, ligament, tendon, or area of fascia that causes pain when touched, but without referred pain.
thermal death p. the lowest temperature at which a broth culture of microorganisms can be heat-killed in a 10-minute exposure time.
trigger p. 1. a particular spot on the body on which pressure or other stimulus will give rise to specific sensations or symptoms. 2. a point on a muscle, ligament, tendon, or area of fascia that when touched causes referred pain.
triple p. the temperature and pressure at which three different phases of a substance are in equilibrium. The *triple point of water* (ice, liquid, vapor) is 273.16°K.
vital p. a point in the medulla oblongata, at the respiratory center, puncture of which causes immediate death.
Vogt p., Vogt-Hueter p. a point at the intersection of a horizontal line two fingerbreadths above the zygoma with a vertical line a thumb-breadth behind the ascending sphenofrontal process; here trephination may be performed in traumatic meningeal hemorrhage.
p. Z a point formed by a line perpendicular to the nasion-menton line through the anterior nasal spine.
Ziemssen motor p. motor p.

point•er (point′ər) a contusion at a bony eminence.
hip p. contusion of the bone of the iliac crest or avulsion of muscle attachments of the iliac crest.

Poi•ri•er glands, line (pwah-re-a′) [Paul *Poirier*, French surgeon, 1853–1907] see under *gland* and *line.*

poise (P) (poiz, pwahz) [Jean Leonard Marie *Poiseuille*, French physiologist, 1799–1869] a unit of viscosity of a liquid, equivalent to 10^{-1} pascal•sec. The commonly used unit is the *centipoise*, or one hundredth of a poise.

Poi•seuille's law, space (pwah-swēz′) [J.L.M. *Poiseuille*] see under *law* and *space.*

poi•son (poi′zən) [L. *potio* draft] any substance that, when relatively small amounts are ingested, inhaled, or absorbed, or applied to, injected into, or developed within the body, has chemical action that causes damage to structure or disturbance of function, producing symptoms, illness, or death. See also *toxin* and *venom.* **poi′sonous** *adj*
acrid p. a poison that produces irritation or inflammation, such as the mineral acids, oxalic acid, the caustic alkalis, antimony, arsenic, the salts of copper, some of the compounds of lead, silver nitrate, and the salts of zinc, iodine, cantharides, or phosphorus.
acronarcotic p., acrosedative p. a poison that may produce either irritation, narcotism (or sedation), or both together; most common ones are from plant sources. Stramonium and belladonna are examples of acronarcotics and aconite is an acrosedative.
arrow p. a preparation of plant alkaloids used on arrows in certain primitive societies.
catalyst p. a substance firmly bound to the active areas on the surface of a catalyst, which prevents the adsorption of the reactants for the desired chemical reaction.
corrosive p. any poison which acts by directly destroying tissue.
fatigue p. kenotoxin.
fugu p. tetrodotoxin.
hemotropic p. a poison which has a special affinity for erythrocytes.
irritant p. acrid p.
mitotic p. a toxic principle that interferes with cell division.
muscle p. a poison that interferes with normal action or functioning of muscle.
narcotic p's poisons causing stupor or delirium, such as opium and hyoscyamus.
puffer p. tetrodotoxin.
sedative p's poisons, such as hydrocyanic acid and potassium cyanide, that directly depress the vital centers.
shellfish p. saxitoxin.
toot p. a poison from *Coriaria sarmentosa*, a plant of New Zealand.
vascular p. a poison which acts by affecting the blood vessels.
whelk p. a toxic substance localized in the salivary gland of the whelk; its principal ingredient is tetramethylammonium hydroxide. See also under *poisoning.*

poi•son•ing (poi′zən-ing) the damaging physiologic effects resulting from exposure to poison; see also *intoxication.*

Poisoning

akee p. Jamaican vomiting sickness.
alcohol p. the toxic effects of ingestion of an excess of ethanol, usually from binge drinking (see also *alcoholism*). The most common symptoms are vomiting, stupor, slow or irregular breathing, seizures, blue-tinged or pale skin, and hypothermia. Called also *ethanol p.*
aluminum p. the toxic effects of high levels of aluminum or aluminum compounds in the body. In the gastrointestinal tract aluminum inhibits absorption of calcium, fluorides, iron, and phosphates; inhalation of bauxite fumes may cause pulmonary fibrosis (see *aluminosis*); and aluminum in the bloodstream may lead to neurological symptoms that can be fatal (see *dialysis encephalopathy*, under *encephalopathy*).

Poisoning *Continued*

amnesic shellfish p. a type of shellfish poisoning seen primarily in eastern Canada, caused by ingestion of shellfish that have consumed the diatom *Nitschia pungens,* which contains domoic acid. Symptoms include memory loss, sensorimotor neuropathy, diarrhea, and abdominal cramps.

anticholinergic p. poisoning caused by overdosage with an anticholinergic agent or by ingestion of plants such as jimsonweed that contain belladonna alkaloids. It is characterized by dry mouth, hot, dry, flushed skin, fixed and dilated pupils, sinus tachycardia, urinary retention, disorientation, agitation, impairment of short-term memory, slurred speech, hallucinations, respiratory depression, seizures, and coma; in rare cases death may occur.

anticoagulant rodenticide p. accidental poisoning of domestic animals or livestock, with death from hemorrhaging, after consuming an anticoagulant rodenticide such as an indanedione or warfarin derivative. They may eat the poison itself or may eat rodents that died from such rodenticides.

antimony p. poisoning due to ingestion of antimony compounds, such as from industrial exposure; the symptoms are similar to those of acute arsenic poisoning, with vomiting a prominent symptom. Called also *stibialism.*

arsenic p. poisoning due to systemic exposure to inorganic pentavalent arsenic. *Acute arsenic poisoning,* which may result in shock and death, is marked by erythematous skin eruptions, vomiting, diarrhea, abdominal pain, muscular cramps, and swelling of the eyelids, feet, and hands. *Chronic arsenic poisoning* (called also *arsenicism, arsenism,* or *arsenicosis*), due to ingestion of small amounts over a long period, such as in contaminated drinking water; manifestations include the skin changes known as *arsenical dermatosis;* the fingernail lines known as *Mees lines;* and neurological symptoms such as headache, peripheral neuropathy, and confusion.

barium p. poisoning from excessive ingestion of barium or one of its salts, characterized by gastrointestinal symptoms such as stomach pain, nausea, vomiting, and diarrhea, followed by severe, sometimes fatal hypokalemia with paralysis.

beryllium p. berylliosis.

bismuth p. poisoning from excessive or chronic ingestion of bismuth or its salts; symptoms include anuria, stomatitis, dermatitis, and diarrhea. Called also *bismuthism* and *bismuthosis.*

blister beetle p. cantharidin p.

blood p. septicemia.

bongkrek p. poisoning from bongkrek, a Javanese dish prepared by means of molds from copra press cake. When the fermentation process is faulty, severe poisoning occurs, with vomiting, profuse perspiration, muscle cramps, and coma. Called also *tempeh p.*

boron p. poisoning by ingestion of boron, boric acid, or a borate salt such as sodium borate (borax). Symptoms include weakness, ataxia, tremors, convulsions, and often death.

bracken p. poisoning of animals after eating *Pteridium aquilinum* (bracken). In monogastric animals it consists of severe intoxication due to enzymatic destruction of thiamine by a thiaminase present in the plant; in ruminants it is apparently due to a dialyzable small molecule that causes bone marrow hypoplasia and eventual death. See also *enzootic bovine hematuria,* under *hematuria.*

broom p. poisoning by ingestion of *Cytisus scoparius* or other broom plants, which contain sparteine and cytisine. Characteristics include nausea, vomiting, dizziness, and sometimes clonic convulsions or fatal respiratory paralysis.

buckthorn p. poisoning from ingestion of the fruit of *Karwinskia humboldtiana* (buckthorn), which contains a neurotoxin. Demyelination and axonal degeneration occur in peripheral nerves, slowly progressing to muscle weakness and paralysis that can cause death.

cadmium p. poisoning from excessive ingestion of cadmium or breathing in of its fumes; symptoms include nausea, vomiting, salivation, diarrhea, abdominal pain, and occasionally cardiovascular collapse. Long-term exposure may cause renal disease with tubulopathy and proteinuria.

callistin shellfish p. poisoning caused by ingestion of the shellfish *Callista brevisphonata*; an outbreak in Japan in the 1950s was believed to be due to a choline present in the ovaries of the shellfish.

cantharidin p. poisoning of horses or ruminants by hay contaminated with blister beetles whose bodies contain cantharidin; signs include hyperemia or erosions of the oral and esophageal mucosa, frequent urination, and sometimes shock and death. Called also *blister beetle p.* and *cantharidism.*

carbamate p. poisoning by exposure to excessive amounts of carbamate insecticides; characteristics include salivation, tremors, dyspnea, and occasionally convulsions. See table at *carbamate.*

carbon disulfide p. a condition occurring in workers who excessively inhale fumes of carbon disulfide; characteristics include weakness, sleeplessness, and visual impairment, and sometimes gastric ulcers, encephalopathy, and paralysis.

carbon monoxide p. poisoning due to the inhalation of carbon monoxide and the resulting change of oxyhemoglobin to carboxyhemoglobin (see *carboxyhemoglobinemia*); it may result in tissue hypoxia, cellular anoxia, damage to the central nervous system, and death.

chronic fluoride p., chronic fluorine p. fluorosis.

cobalt p. poisoning from long-term excessive exposure to cobalt, seen in those who work with cobalt and formerly in beer drinkers because for years cobalt was added to beer as a foam stabilizer. Symptoms include nausea, vomiting, tinnitus, nerve deafness, and cardiomyopathy *(beer-drinkers' cardiomyopathy).*

copper p. poisoning by copper or copper salts. In humans it usually follows excessive intake of medicinal cupric sulfate or results from an enzyme deficiency. Characteristics include vomiting, which may be bluegreen, hypotension, jaundice, and coma that may end in death. In animals it is most common in ruminants and pigs after excessive intake of medicinal or fungicidal copper; acute poisoning is characterized by vomiting and convulsions, while chronic poisoning is marked by liver and kidney damage. Chronic buildup of liver copper stores resulting in release of copper into the bloodstream may cause symptoms similar to those of acute poisoning and may be fatal.

corn cockle p. githagism.

cyanide p. poisoning by cyanide compounds, potent rapid-acting substances that cause cellular hypoxia by formation of an inactive complex of cytochrome oxidase and cyanide. Characteristics include nausea without vomiting, dizziness, convulsions, opisthotonos, and death from respiratory paralysis. The usual cause in livestock and other animals is ingestion of plants containing cyanogenetic compounds (see table). In humans it is usually the result of exposure to hydrogen cyanide liquid or gas that is given off by a fungicide, insecticide, or other substance. Cyanide is detoxified by the liver enzyme thiosulfate sulfurtransferase, which catalyzes the reaction of cyanide with thiosulfate to form thiocyanide.

cyanobacteria p. poisoning by cyanobacteria, usually after drinking contaminated water. The most common bacterial genera are *Anabaena, Aphanizomenon, Gloeotrichia, Microcystis (Anacystis), Nodularia,* and *Oscillatoria.* The condition is usually subacute, with liver damage, jaundice, sometimes bloody diarrhea, and photosensitization. Drinking of heavily contaminated water may cause acute symptoms such as muscle tremors, ataxia, dyspnea, cyanosis, and hyperesthesia so that a slight touch may cause convulsions and opisthotonos, which can be fatal.

darnel p. a type of rye grass poisoning caused by ingestion of the seeds of darnel, *Lolium temulentum,* probably only when they are contaminated with a mold such as *Endoconidium temulentum* (see *endoconidiotoxicosis*); in humans this happens when moldy seeds accidentally contaminate flour. Characteristics include giddiness, staggering, vertigo, vomiting, and visual disturbances.

diarrhetic shellfish p. a type of shellfish poisoning caused by ingestion of mussels, scallops, or clams that have fed on algae of either genus *Dinophysis* or *Prorocentrum,* which contain okadaic acid and other toxins. Symptoms include nausea, vomiting, and abdominal cramps.

djenkol bean p. poisoning by the djenkol bean; symptoms vary from lumbar pain, vomiting, and diarrhea to hematuria and proteinuria progressing to anuria and renal failure. Called also *djenkolism.*

elasmobranch p. a form of ichthyosarcotoxism seen after ingestion of certain toxic sharks and skates. One type results from eating the muscle tissue of the shark *Somniosus microcephalus.* Another type is hypervitaminosis A from eating the liver of any of various species.

ergot p. ergotism.

ethanol p. alcohol p.

ethylene glycol p. poisoning from ingestion of ethylene glycol; symptoms include kidney damage, vomiting, hypotension, central nervous system depression, convulsions, coma, and sometimes death.

fish p. ichthyosarcotoxism.

fluoroacetate p. poisoning by fluoroacetate compounds. Carnivores are affected when they eat small animals that have died from fluoroacetate rodenticides, and ruminants are affected when they eat fluoroacetate-containing plants such as *Acacia georginae* or species of *Dichapetalum*, *Gastrolobium*, *Oxylobium*, or *Palicourea*. Poisoning in humans is usually caused by ingestion of rodenticides. Fluoroacetate blocks one of the steps in the tricarboxylic acid cycle, causing neurotoxic effects ranging from ataxia and agitation to convulsions, and cardiac manifestations such as severe tachycardia and cardiomyopathy.

food p. a group of illnesses varying in severity from mild and self-limited to life threatening, caused by ingestion of contaminated food or food that is inherently poisonous. Various microorganisms may cause it, the most common being pathogenic bacteria or their products (bacterial toxins), e.g., *Staphylococcus aureus*, *Bacillus cereus*, *Campylobacter*, *Clostridium botulinum*, *C. perfringens*, *Escherichia coli*, *Vibrio cholerae*, *V. parahaemolyticus*, *Shigella* species, *Salmonella* species, and *Yersinia enterocolitica*. Bacterial food poisoning is usually manifested as bacterial gastroenteritis (q.v.), but it may also be associated with such syndromes as botulism, typhoid fever, and cholera. Neurologic symptoms can also be caused by food poisoning as a result of ingestion of chemically toxic foods, such as certain mushrooms and berries, or ingestion or inhalation of substances such as heavy metals, mercury, or insecticides.

Plants That Can Cause Cyanide Poisoning

Latin Name	Common Name
Acacia leucophloea; A. sieberana	Acacias
Adenia digitata	
Andrachne decaisnei	Andrachne
Anthemis cotula	Mayweed
Aquilegia vulgaris	Columbine
Bahia oppositifolia	
Brachyachne spp.	
Bridelia exaltata	Scrub ironbark tree
Calotis scapigera	
Canthium vaccinifolium	
Cercocarpus spp.	
Chenopodium (certain species)	
Chloris distichophylla	Rhodes grass, windmill grass
Cynodon spp.	Couch grass
Dactyloctenium radulans	
Digitaria sanguinais	A type of crab grass
Dimorphotheca ecklonis	South African daisy
Eleusine indica	Crab grass, crow's foot grass
Eremophila maculata	A type of native fuchsia
Eriobotrya japonica	Loquat
Eschscholtzia spp.	Eschscholtzia, California poppy
Eucalyptus spp.	Eucalyptus
Euphorbia spp.	Spurge
Florestina tripteris	
Glyceria striata	Manna grass
Goodia lotifolia	
Grevillea spp.	Silky oak
Gyrostemon ramulosus	
Hakea spp.	Cushionflower
Haloragis heterophylla	Raspwort, raspweed
Heterodendron oleifolium	(Australian) rosewood
Holcus lanatus	Velvet grass, Yorkshire fog
Hydrangea spp.	Hydrangea
Indigofera australis	Indigo plant
Lambertia spp.	(Australian) honeysuckle
Linum spp.	Flax
Lotonis laxa	
Lotus spp.	Bird's foot trefoil
Loudonia roei	
Macadamia ternifolia	Macadamia
Manihot esculenta	Cassawa, manioc
Nerium oleander	Oleander
Panicum spp.	Coolah grass, klein grass, Guinea grass
Passiflora spp.	Passion flower
Phaseolus limensis	Lima bean
Phyllanthus gasstroemii	
Poranthera microphylla	
Prunus spp.	Apricot, cherry, peach, plum, sloe
Pyrus spp.	Pear
Sambucus nigra	Elder
Sorghum spp.	Johnson grass, sudan grass
Stillingia treculeana	Queen's delight
Suckleya suckleyana	
Trifolium repens	White clover, Landino clover
Triglochin spp.	Arrowgrass
Vicia sativa	Vetch
Xylomelum angustifolium	Sandplain woody pear
Zea mays	Corn
Zieria spp.	

forage p. a type of mycotoxicosis seen in domestic animals, especially horses, resulting from ingestion of food contaminated with a fungus, usually *Fusarium moniliforme*. It causes neurotoxicity, particularly inflammation or softening of the white matter of the brain, with symptoms such as ataxia, tremor, circling, dimmed vision, drowsiness, and sometimes death. See also *moldy corn p.* Called also *leukoencephalitis*, *leukoencephalomalacia*, *mycotoxic leukoencephalomalacia*, and *sleepy staggers*.

fugu p. tetrodotoxism (def. 1).

gossypol p. poisoning from eating cottonseed cake that contains a high proportion of gossypol; most often seen in pigs.

***Gymnothorax* p.** a form of ichthyosarcotoxism produced by ingestion of certain moray eels of the genus *Gymnothorax*.

heavy metal p. poisoning by any of the heavy metals; common conditions include antimony poisoning, arsenic poisoning, cadmium poisoning, cobalt poisoning, lead poisoning, mercury poisoning, thallium poisoning, and zinc poisoning.

hydrogen sulfide p. poisoning by excessive exposure to hydrogen sulfide gas, seen primarily in those who work with petroleum or petrochemicals. The gas is a potent inhibitor of cytochrome-*c* oxidase (q.v.) and poisoning is characterized by metabolic acidosis and anoxia; severe cases may result in coma with death from respiratory paralysis.

iodine p. iodism.

iron p. poisoning from ingestion of excessive iron or iron-containing compounds, such as in children who eat iron supplement tablets like candy; symptoms include ulceration of the gastrointestinal tract, vomiting, vasodilation with shock, metabolic acidosis, liver injury, and coagulation disturbances.

larkspur p. poisoning by the fresh leaves and roots of certain species of *Delphinium* (larkspur), which contain delphinine and other alkaloids. Ingestion may cause immediate death, probably from paralysis of the heart, but more often causes neurological symptoms of less rapid onset that may also end in paralysis and asphyxia.

lead p. poisoning due to the absorption or ingestion of lead or one of its salts. The symptoms include loss of appetite, weight loss, colic, constipation, insomnia, headache, dizziness, irritability, moderate hypertension, albuminuria, anemia, a blue line at the edge of the gums *(lead line)*, encephalopathy (especially in children), and peripheral neuropathy leading to paralysis. Called also *plumbism*.

loco p., locoweed p. locoism.

manganese p. poisoning by manganese, usually caused by inhalation of manganese dust. Symptoms include neurotoxicity with a syndrome resembling parkinsonism, and inflammation throughout the respiratory system; see also *manganese pneumonitis*, under *pneumonitis*. Called also *manganism*.

meat p. acute, often severe gastroenteritis, most often caused by meat contaminated with *Bacillus cereus*, *Clostridium perfringens*, invasive *Escherichia coli*, *Salmonella*, *Staphylococcus aureus*, or *Yersinia enterocolitica*.

mercury p. acute or chronic disease caused by mercury or compounds such as salts that contain it. The *acute* form, due to ingestion, is marked by severe abdominal pain, metallic taste in the mouth, vomiting, bloody diarrhea, oliguria or anuria (usually at onset), and corrosion and ulceration of the entire digestive tract. The *chronic* form, due to absorption by the skin and mucous membranes, inhalation of vapors, or ingestion of mercury salts, is marked by stomatitis, metallic taste in the mouth, a blue line along the border of the gum, sore hypertrophied gums that bleed easily, loosening of teeth, excessive salivation, tremors, incoordination, and psychiatric symptoms such as abnormal excitability, anxiety, and social withdrawal.

methanol p. poisoning from ingestion of methanol (methyl alcohol); symptoms include nerve damage, sometimes seizures and coma, blindness that can be permanent, and sometimes death.

milk p. see under *sickness*.

moldy corn p. forage poisoning occurring when animals eat corn contaminated with the fungus *Fusarium moniliforme*, which contains toxic fumonisins. Called also *cornstalk disease*.

Poisoning *Continued*

molybdenum p. poisoning due to ingestion of large amounts of molybdenum, characterized by weakness, diarrhea, and loss of hair pigmentation; seen primarily in livestock that graze in certain kinds of pastures (see *teart*). Called also *molybdenosis*.
mushroom p. poisoning resulting from ingestion of mushrooms; potentially deadly types result from ingestion of *Amanita phalloides*, *A. verna*, *A. virosa*, and species of *Chlorophyllum*, *Galerina*, and *Lepiota*, which contain neurotoxic amatoxins. The clinical course usually begins with nausea, vomiting, abdominal pain, and diarrhea, followed by a quiescent period of up to 48 hours, and then signs and symptoms of severe liver, kidney, and central nervous system damage that can be fatal.
mussel p. see *shellfish p.*
naphthol p. toxicity caused by the ingestion or absorption through the skin of naphthol, characterized by anemia, jaundice, convulsions, and coma. Called also *naphtholism*.
neurotoxic shellfish p. a relatively mild type of shellfish poisoning caused by the ingestion of mollusks that are contaminated with the protozoan *Karenia brevis*, which contains brevetoxins; characteristics include paresthesias, weakness, abdominal cramps, vomiting, and diarrhea.
nicotine p. poisoning by ingestion of excessive amounts of nicotine, such as in children who eat cigarettes, workers who handle wet tobacco leaves, or persons who overuse nicotine gums or patches. Symptoms include stimulation followed by depression of the central and autonomic nervous systems and occasionally death due to respiratory paralysis. See also *green tobacco sickness*. Called also *nicotinism*.
nicotine sulfate p. poisoning of lambs or calves by nicotine sulfate, formerly used as a component of vermifuges. Symptoms include tremors, rapid respiration, recumbency, and convulsions; severe cases may end in death.
nitrite p. poisoning of ruminants grazing on nitrate-rich plants; the nitrates break down into nitrites in the body. Plants naturally rich in nitrates include *Chenopodium album*, *Salvia reflexa*, and species of *Amaranthus*. Poisoning can also occur in fields heavily dosed with certain fertilizers (see *ammonium nitrate* and *sodium nitrate*). Characteristics include gastroenteritis, diarrhea, potentially fatal methemoglobinemia with anemic anoxia, dyspnea, tremors, and cyanosis.
nitroaniline p. poisoning by nitroaniline, a dye used in paints, inks, and other products, characterized by intense methemoglobinemia.
nutmeg p. severe toxic symptoms produced by ingestion of powdered nutmeg, characterized by narcosis with periods of delirium and excitability.
organophosphorus compound p. poisoning from excessive exposure to an organophosphorus compound (see table at *organophosphorus*); symptoms are usually neurologic and may cause death.
oxalate p. poisoning by oxalic acid or oxalates, usually after ingestion of large quantities of oxalate-containing plants (see table). Characteristics include gastroenteritis, hypotension, hypocalcemia, muscle weakness and twitching, nephrosis, and hyperoxaluria. Called also *oxalism*.
oxygen p. see under *toxicity*.

Plants That Can Cause Oxalate Poisoning

Latin Name	Common Name
Amaranthus retroflexus	Pigweed, prince's feather
Atriplex spp.	Salt bush
Beta spp.	Beet
Calandrinia spp.	Parakeelia
Emex australis	
Enchylaena tomentosa	Barrier salt bush
Halogeton glomeratus	Halogeton
Oxalis spp.	Oxalis
Panicum antidotale	Blue panic grass
Portulaca oleracea	Purslane
Rheum rhaponticum	Rhubarb
Rumex spp.	Dock, sorrel
Salsola kali	Tumbleweed, Russian thistle
Sarcobatus vermiculatus	Greasewood
Setaria sphacelata	
Threlkeldia proceriflora	
Trianthema spp.	Hogweed, pigweed

paralytic shellfish p. a severe type of shellfish poisoning caused by ingestion of bivalve mollusks that are contaminated with dinoflagellates containing saxitoxin, such as species of *Gonyaulax* and related genera. Symptoms include paresthesias of the face and limbs, nausea, vomiting, diarrhea, and sometimes muscle weakness, paralysis, and respiratory failure that can be fatal.
paraquat p. poisoning by paraquat that has been either ingested or absorbed through the skin. Contact with concentrated solutions causes irritation of the skin, cracking and shedding of the nails, and delayed healing of cuts and wounds. After ingestion of large doses, potentially fatal renal and hepatic failure may develop, followed by pulmonary insufficiency.
parathyroid p. the increase in metastatic calcification of organs, particularly the kidneys, when a high calcium diet is given a patient with hyperparathyroidism.
phenol p. poisoning due to ingestion or absorption through the skin of phenol; symptoms include colic, local irritation, corrosion, seizures, cardiac arrhythmias, shock, and respiratory arrest. Called also *carbolism*.
phosphorus p. a condition resulting from ingestion or inhalation of phosphorus, manifested by mandibular necrosis (see *phosphorus necrosis*), toothache, anorexia, weakness, and anemia.
pitch p. an often fatal disorder of domestic animals or livestock, particularly pigs, after they lick or chew on pitch-containing substances such as the tarred walls and floors of pigpens or clay pigeons used in target practice; characteristics include liver damage, anorexia, depression, weakness, jaundice, and anemia.
puffer p., puffer fish p. tetrodotoxism (def. 1).
ragwort p. seneciosis.
ricin p. poisoning by inhalation or ingestion of ricin, characterized by superficial inflammation of the respiratory mucosa, edema of the gastrointestinal tract, and hemorrhages that can be fatal in the lungs and gastrointestinal tract.
rodenticide p. accidental poisoning from the effects of rodenticides after an animal either eats the poison directly or eats a rodent that has died from the poison. See also *fluoroacetate p.* and *anticoagulant rodenticide p.*
rye grass p. poisoning from the eating of rye grass (genus *Lolium*), usually when it is moldy, consisting of mycotoxicosis. Common types are darnel poisoning and rye grass staggers. See also *endoconidiotoxicosis*.
salmon p. poisoning in an animal that has eaten raw fish, especially salmon and trout, that are parasitized by the fluke *Nanophyetus salmincola*, which serves as a vector for rickettsiae. When the etiologic agent is *Neorickettsia helminthoeca*, hemorrhagic enteritis results. A milder form in dogs, caused by an unknown rickettsia, is called *Elokomin fluke fever*.
salt p. poisoning of animals, especially pigs and birds, due to ingestion of too much salt in the absence of available water, marked by excessive thirst, diarrhea, and vomiting, often culminating in death.
saturnine p. lead p.
sausage p. see *allantiasis* and *botulism*.
scombroid p. a form of ichthyosarcotoxism caused by ingestion of a toxic histaminelike substance produced by the action of bacteria on histidine, a normal component of fish flesh; scombroid fish (tuna, bonito, mackerel, etc.) are particularly susceptible to bacterial decomposition. When fish is eaten that is contaminated from being inadequately preserved, the symptoms of the illness develop, including epigastric pain, nausea, vomiting, headache, dysphagia, thirst, urticaria, and pruritus; these usually clear up within 24 hours.
selenium p. poisoning of livestock from grazing on plants that have absorbed excessive selenium from the soil. Areas of selenium-rich soil have been found in the northern Great Plains of North America, Ireland, Israel, China, Russia, and elsewhere. *Chronic selenium poisoning* (called also *alkali disease*) is characterized by cirrhosis of the liver, anemia, loss of hair, erosions of long bones, and emaciation. *Acute selenium poisoning* (called also *blind staggers*) is characterized by impaired vision, an unsteady gait, and increasing incoordination with respiratory failure and often death within 24 hours. Called also *selenosis*.
***Senecio* p.** seneciosis.
shellfish p. acute intoxication caused by ingestion of bivalve mollusks contaminated with neurotoxins. There are four different types: *amnesic*, *diarrhetic*, *neurotoxic*, and *paralytic*.
strychnine p. poisoning by strychnine, which causes excitation of all portions of the central nervous system by blocking postsynaptic inhibition of neural impulses; chronic poisoning is called *strychninism* and can lead to convulsions, respiratory paralysis, and death.

Poisoning *Continued*

tempeh p. bongkrek p.

tetrachloroethane p. a form of poisoning in munition workers caused by inhalation of fumes of tetrachloroethane, and marked by toxic jaundice, headache, anorexia, and gastrointestinal disturbance.

Selenium Accumulators: Plants That Can Cause Selenium Poisoning

Latin Name	Common Name
Acacia cana	Acacia
Aster spp.	Aster
Astragalus (certain species only)*	Andrachne
Atriplex spp.	Salt bush, orache
Castilleja spp.	Paintbrush
Comandra pallida	
Greyia spp.	
Grindelia spp.	Gumweed
Gutierrezia spp.	Broomweed, snakeweed
Machaeranthera spp.	
Morinda reticulata	
Neptunia amplexicaulis	Selenium weed
Oonopsis spp.*	
Penstemon spp.	Penstemon
Sideranthus spp.	
Stanleya spp.	Prince's plume
Xylorrhiza spp.*	

*These plants grow preferentially in selenium-rich soils and are called *selenium indicators*.

tetraodon p. tetrodotoxism (def. 1).

thallium p. poisoning, usually of children or domestic animals, due to ingestion of thallium compounds. It is marked initially by gastrointestinal signs and symptoms such as nausea and abdominal pain. This is followed within a few days by alopecia; neurologic and psychic symptoms such as ataxia, restlessness, delirium, hallucinations, delusions, semicoma, and blindness; and liver and kidney damage. Called also *thallitoxicosis* and *thallotoxicosis*.

TNT p. trinitrotoluene p.

tobacco p. poisoning by tobacco, usually taking the form of nicotine poisoning (q.v.). Called also *tabagism* and *tobaccoism*.

trinitrotoluene p. a form of poisoning in munition workers that work with trinitrotoluene, characterized by dermatitis, gastritis with abdominal pain, vomiting, constipation, flatulence, and blood changes. Called also *TNT p*.

urea p. poisoning of ruminants by excessive consumption of urea, leading to hyperammonemia with tremors, incoordination, dyspnea, convulsions, and sometimes death.

whelk p. poisoning caused by ingestion of whelks that contain whelk poison (q.v.); characterized by intense headache, dizziness, nausea, and vomiting.

zinc p. poisoning from exposure to toxic levels of zinc. Inhalation of freshly oxidized zinc or zinc oxide fumes, as by metal workers, causes metal fume fever (q.v.). Ingestion of high levels of zinc causes gastrointestinal irritation and vomiting, and if chronic can cause hypocupremia, sideroblastic anemia, and neutropenia. Called also *zincalism*.

poi•son ivy (poi′zən i′ve) *Rhus radicans.*
 eastern p. i. name given to *Rhus radicans* to distinguish it from the variant *Rhus rydbergii.*
 western p. i. *Rhus rydbergii.*

Pois•son distribution (pwah-saw′) [Siméon Denis *Poisson*, French mathematician, 1781–1840] see under *distribution.*

poke•root (pōk′root) pokeweed.

poke•weed (pōk′wēd) *Phytolacca americana*, a tall perennial herb of North America; its root has emetic and cathartic properties and has been used in treatment of rheumatic conditions. See also *pokeweed mitogen*, under *mitogen.* Cattle and pigs that eat excessive amounts of it sometimes suffer fatal gastroenteritis and diarrhea because of its content of oxalates and saponins. Called also *pokeroot.*

pol•a•cril•in (pol″ə-kril′in) methacrylic acid ester with divinylbenzene; a synthetic ion exchange resin, supplied in the hydrogen or free acid form; a pharmaceutic aid.
 p. potassium a synthetic ion exchange resin, prepared through polymerization of methacrylic acid and divinylbenzene, and then further neutralized with potassium hydroxide to form the potassium salt of methacrylic acid and divinylbenzene. It is supplied as a pharmaceutical-grade ion exchange resin in a particle size of 100- to 500-mesh; a tablet disintegrant.

Po•land syndrome (anomaly) (po′lənd) [Alfred *Poland*, British physician, 1820–1872] see under *syndrome.*

po•lar (po′lər) [L. *polaris* pertaining to a pole, from *polus* (q.v.)] 1. of or pertaining to a pole; see also under *compound.* 2. being at opposite ends of a spectrum of manifestations, as polar forms of leprosy.

Po•lar•amine (po-lar′ə-mēn) trademark for preparations of dexchlorpheniramine maleate.

po•la•rim•e•ter (po″lə-rim′ə-tər) [*polar* + *-meter*] a device for measuring the rotation of plane polarized light; a polariscope.

po•la•rim•e•try (po″lə-rim′ə-tre) measurement of the rotation of plane polarized light by a liquid or solid.

po•lar•i•scope (po-lar′ĭ-skōp) [*polar* + *-scope*] an instrument for the measurement of polarized light.

po•lar•i•scop•ic (po″lər-ĭ-skop′ik) pertaining to the polariscope or to polariscopy.

po•lar•is•co•py (po″lər-is′kə-pe) the science of polarized light and the use of the polariscope.

po•lar•is•tro•bom•e•ter (po-lar″is-tro-bom′ə-tər) a form of polarimeter used for delicate analyses.

po•lar•i•ty (po-lar′ĭ-te) 1. the fact or condition of having poles. 2. the exhibition of opposite effects at the two extremities. 3. the presence of an axial gradient and exhibition by a nerve of both anelectrotonus and catelectrotonus. 4. the orientation of intracellular structures to the tissue as a whole.
 dynamic p. the specialization of a nerve cell with reference to the flow of impulses.

po•lar•iza•tion (po″lər-ĭ-za′shən) 1. the presence or establishment of polarity. 2. the production of that condition in light by virtue of which its vibrations take place all in one plane or else in circles and ellipses. 3. the accumulation of bubbles of hydrogen gas on the negative plate of a galvanic battery, so that the generation of electricity is impeded. 4. the separation of electric charge so that there is directionality of flow, as between two poles (the anode and the cathode) of an electrolysis cell, or such as that across a biological membrane, which results in a membrane potential. See also *depolarization* and *repolarization.*

po•lar•ize (po′lər-īz) 1. to imbue with polarity. 2. to put into a state of polarization.

po•lar•iz•er (po′lər-īz″ər) an appliance for polarizing light.

po•laro•gram (po-lar′o-gram) the curve of current versus voltage obtained in polarography.

po•lar•og•ra•phy (po″lər-og′rə-fe) an electrochemical technique for identifying and estimating the concentration of reducible elements by means of the dual measurement of the current flowing through an electrochemical cell (which contains the test solution) and the electrical potential between the two electrodes as the potential is increased at a constant rate by an external voltage source. As the voltage reaches the standard electrode potential of the test substance, there is a sharp increase in current flow. The indicator electrode is usually a dropping mercury electrode. **polar-ograph′ic** *adj*

Po•lar•oid (po′lər-oid) trademark for a sheet (film) polarizer utilizing oriented crystals used as a substitute for Nicol prisms and for reducing glare through lenses and windshields.

po•laro•plast (po-lar′o-plast) [*polar* + *plast*] an organelle in microsporidans that imbibes water, swells, and exerts pressure to rupture the polar cap and evert the polar tube through which the sporoplasm escapes to infect the host.

pol•dine meth•yl•sul•fate (pol′dēn) a synthetic quaternary nitrogen anticholinergic used as an adjunct in the treatment of peptic ulcer and gastrointestinal disorders associated with hyperacidity, hypermotility, and spasm, administered orally.

pole (pōl) [L. *polus;* Gr. *polos*] 1. either extremity of an axis, as of the fetal ellipse, or of an organ of the body; called also *polus* or *extremitas.* 2. either of two points that have opposite physical qualities (electric or other).

abembryonic p. the pole of the blastocyst opposite the embryonic pole, that is, further away from the embryoblast; this location is the site of trypsinlike activity that is responsible for the shedding of the zona pellucida.

animal p. 1. the site of an oocyte to which the nucleus is approximated, and from which the polar bodies pinch off. 2. in nonmammalian species, the pole of an egg less heavily laden with yolk than the vegetal pole and therefore exhibiting faster cell division.

anterior p. of eyeball polus anterior bulbi oculi.

anterior p. of lens polus anterior lentis.

antigerminal p. vegetal p.

cephalic p. the end of the fetal ellipse where the head is.

embryonic p. the area of the blastocyst where the embryoblast and the trophoblast are in contact; the embryoblast attaches to the endometrial epithelium at this pole.

frontal p. of cerebral hemisphere, frontal p. of hemisphere of cerebrum polus frontalis hemispherii cerebri.

germinal p. animal p.

inferior p. of kidney extremitas inferior renis.

inferior p. of testis extremitas inferior testis.

lower p. of kidney extremitas inferior renis.

lower p. of testis extremitas inferior testis.

nutritive p. vegetal p.

occipital p. of cerebral hemisphere, occipital p. of hemisphere of cerebrum polus occipitalis hemispherii cerebri.

pelvic p. the end of the fetal ellipse where the breech is.

posterior p. of eyeball polus posterior bulbi oculi.

posterior p. of lens polus posterior lentis.

superior p. of kidney extremitas superior renis.

superior p. of testis extremitas superior testis.

temporal p. of cerebral hemisphere, temporal p. of hemisphere of cerebrum polus temporalis hemispherii cerebri.

tubular p. of renal corpuscle urinary p. of renal corpuscle.

upper p. of kidney extremitas superior renis.

upper p. of testis extremitas superior testis.

urinary p. of renal corpuscle the end of the corpuscle where the proximal tubule exits carrying urine; called also *tubular p.*

vascular p. of renal corpuscle, vascular p. of renal glomerulus the end of the corpuscle and glomerulus where afferent arterioles enter and efferent arterioles exit.

vegetal p., vegetative p., vitelline p. the pole of an oocyte at which the greater amount of food yolk is deposited. Cf. *animal p.*

Pol·e·mo·ni·um (pol″ə-mo′ne-əm) [Gr. *polemōnion*] a widespread genus of annual and perennial herbs. *P. caeru′leum,* is a medicinal species known as Greek valerian or Jacob's ladder.

po·li (po′li) [L.] genitive and plural of *polus.*

pol·i·ca·pram (pol″ĭ-ka′prəm) microcrystals of colloid dimensions used as a tablet binder for pharmaceutical preparations.

po·lice·man (pə-lēs′mən) a glass rod with a piece of rubber tubing on one end, used as a stirring rod and transfer tool in chemical analysis.

poli·clin·ic (pol″e-klin′ik) [Gr. *polis* city + *clinic*] a city hospital, infirmary, or clinic. Cf. *polyclinic.*

pol·i·do·ca·nol (pol″ĭ-do-ka′nol) laureth 9.

pol·i·en·ceph·a·li·tis (pol″e-ən-sef″ə-li′tis) polioencephalitis.

pol·i·fep·ro·san 20 (pol″e-fep′ro-san) a biodegradable polyanhydride copolymer that binds to carmustine so that it does not degrade as fast as usual, thus controlling local delivery of the medication.

po·lio (po′le-o) poliomyelitis.

poli(o)- [Gr. *polios* gray] a combining form denoting relationship to the gray matter of the nervous system.

po·lio·ci·dal (po″le-o-si′dəl) neutralizing the poliomyelitis virus.

po·lio·clas·tic (po″le-o-klas′tik) [*polio-* + Gr. *klastos* breaking] destroying the gray matter of the nervous system; a term applied to the viruses of poliomyelitis, epidemic encephalitis, and rabies.

po·lio·dys·tro·phy (po″le-o-dis′trə-fe) [*polio-* + *dystrophy*] atrophy of the cerebral gray matter.

progressive cerebral p., progressive infantile p. Alpers syndrome.

po·lio·en·ceph·a·li·tis (po″le-o-ən-sef″ə-li′tis) [*polio-* + *encephalitis*] inflammatory disease of the gray substance of the brain.

inferior p. progressive bulbar palsy.

po·lio·en·ceph·a·lo·ma·la·cia (po″le-o-en-sef″ə-lo-mə-la′shə) a highly fatal disease of cattle, sheep, and pigs, caused by a thiamine deficiency; symptoms include edema of the brain with muzzle twitching, opisthotonos, blindness, and inability to stand. Called also *pseudoencephalomalacia* and *cerebrocortical necrosis.*

po·lio·en·ceph·a·lo·me·nin·go·my·eli·tis (po″le-o-ən-sef″ə-lo-mə-ning″go-mi″ə-li′tis) inflammation of the gray matter of the brain and spinal cord and of the meninges covering it.

po·lio·en·ceph·a·lo·my·eli·tis (po″le-o-en-sef″ə-lo-mi″ə-li′tis) inflammation of the gray matter of the brain and spinal cord.

po·lio·en·ceph·a·lop·a·thy (po″le-o-en-sef″ə-lop′ə-the) [*polio-* + *encephalo-* + *-pathy*] disease of the gray matter of the brain.

po·lio·en·ceph·a·lo·tro·pic (po″le-o-ən-sef″ə-lo-tro′pik) having a special affinity for the gray substance of the brain.

po·lio·my·eli·ti·ci·dal (po″le-o-mi″ə-lĭ′tĭ-si″dəl) having the power of destroying poliomyelitis virus.

po·lio·my·eli·tis (po″le-o-mi″ə-li′tis) [*polio-* + *myel-* + *-itis*] an acute infectious disease occurring sporadically or in epidemics and caused by a virus, usually a poliovirus but occasionally a coxsackievirus or echovirus. It is characterized clinically by fever, sore throat, headache, and vomiting, often with stiffness of the neck and back. In the *minor illness (abortive poliomyelitis)* these may be the only symptoms. The *major illness,* which may or may not be preceded by the minor illness, is characterized by involvement of the central nervous system, stiff neck, pleocytosis in the spinal fluid, and sometimes paralysis. (See *nonparalytic p.* and *paralytic p.*) There may be subsequent atrophy of groups of muscles, ending in contraction and permanent deformity. Called also *polio.* The major illness is also called *infantile paralysis* and *acute anterior p.*

abortive p. the minor illness of poliomyelitis; see *poliomyelitis.*

acute anterior p., anterior p. the major illness of poliomyelitis; see *poliomyelitis.*

bulbar p. a serious form of paralytic poliomyelitis in which the medulla oblongata is affected, so that there is often dysfunction of the swallowing mechanism, breathing, and circulation.

endemic p. poliomyelitis occurring sporadically or in a small number of cases, particularly during periods of warm weather.

epidemic p. poliomyelitis occurring in epidemic form.

mouse p., murine p. Theiler disease.

nonparalytic p. the major illness of poliomyelitis when it does not involve paralysis.

paralytic p. the major illness of poliomyelitis when it involves paralysis.

porcine p. infectious porcine encephalomyelitis.

spinal p., spinal paralytic p. the classic form of the major illness, a type of paralytic poliomyelitis affecting the spinal cord and characterized primarily by flaccid paralysis in a limb or limbs.

po·lio·my·elop·a·thy (po″le-o-mi″ə-lop′ə-the) [*polio-* + *myelo-* + *-pathy*] any disease primarily affecting the gray matter of the spinal cord.

po·lio·neu·ro·mere (po″le-o-noor′o-mēr) [*polio-* + *neuro-* + *-mere*] one of the primordial segments of the gray matter of the spinal cord.

po·li·o·sis (po″le-o′sis) [Gr. *polios* gray] circumscribed depigmentation and graying of the hair, particularly of the scalp, in association with a pathologic condition. Cf. *leukotrichia.*

po·lio·vi·rus (po′le-o-vi″rəs) [*poliomyelitis* + *virus*] a species of viruses of the genus *Enterovirus* that cause poliomyelitis. It is separable into three serotypes, designated types 1, 2, and 3. Historically, type 1 has been responsible for about 85 per cent of all paralytic poliomyelitis and for most epidemics, type 3 for about 10 per cent of paralytic poliomyelitis and for occasional epidemics, and type 2 for about 5 per cent of paralytic poliomyelitis. Wild type 2 has now been eliminated worldwide as a result of efforts by the World Health Organization to eradicate poliomyelitis. **poliovi′ral** *adj*

murine p. Theiler virus.

poli·pro·pene (pol″e-pro′pēn) a tablet excipient for pharmaceutical preparations.

pol·ish·ing (pol′ish-ing) creation of a smooth and glossy finish on a surface, as of a tooth or denture.

poli·sog·ra·phy (pol″ĭ-sog′rə-fe) [*poly-* + *iso-* + *-graphy*] radiography in which several exposures are made in the same film.

Po·lis·tes (po-lis′tēz) a genus of wasps of the family Vespidae, having painful stings.

Pol·i·ta·no-Lead·bet·ter technique (pol″ĭ-tah′no led′bet-ər) [Victor A. *Politano,* American urologist, 20th century; Wayland F. *Leadbetter,* American urologist, 20th century] see under *technique.*

Pol·it·zer bag, cone, method (test) (pol′it-zər) [Adam *Politzer,* Hungarian-born otologist in Austria, 1835–1920] see under *bag* and *method;* see *politzerization;* and see *cone of light,* under *cone.*

pol·it·zer·iza·tion (pol″it-zər-ĭ-za′shən) [A. *Politzer*] inflation of the middle ear by means of a Politzer bag. Called also *Politzer method.*

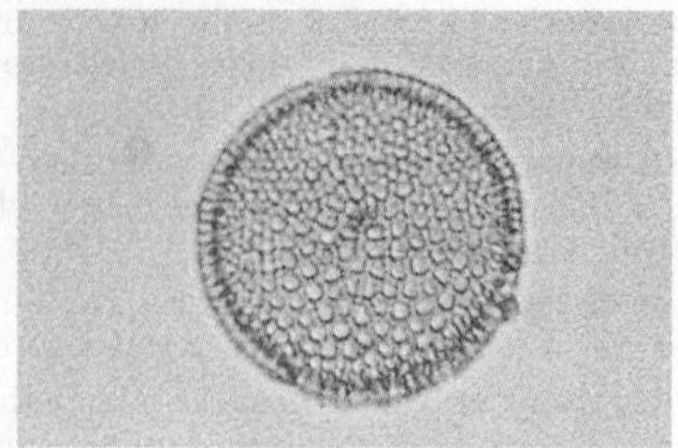

■ Pollen grain.

negative p. displacement of secretion from a cavity through negative pressure produced by means of a Politzer bag.

pol•kis•sen (pōl-kis′ən) [Ger. "pole cushion"] the region of the juxtaglomerular apparatus between the glomerulus and the afferent and efferent arterioles, containing lacelike lacis cells and lying in close contact with the mesangium and the macula densa. Called also *lacis*.

poll (pōl) the back part of the head, especially that of an animal.

pol•la•ki•su•ria (pol″ə-kĭ-su′re-ə) urinary frequency.

pol•la•ki•uria (pol″ə-ke-u′re-ə) [Gr. *pollakis* often + *-uria*] urinary frequency.

polled (pōld) having no horns; said of cattle that have been bred for this inherited trait.

pol•len (pol′ən) the mass of microspores (male fertilizing elements) of flowering plants. Many pollens, especially the airborne pollens, are allergens; i.e., they produce proteinaceous antigens capable of sensitizing susceptible persons and producing allergic symptoms.

pol•le•no•gen•ic (pol″ə-no-jen′ik) [*pollen* + *-genic*] caused by the pollen of plants.

pol•le•no•sis (pol″ə-no′sis) hay fever.

pol•lex (pol′əks) pl. *pol′lices* [L.] [TA] thumb: the first digit of the hand; it is the most preaxial of the five fingers, having only the two phalanges and being opposable to the other four fingers. Called also *digitus primus (I) manus* [TA alternative] and *first finger*. **pol′lical** *adj*

p. exten′sus backward deviation of the thumb.

p. flex′us permanent flexion of the thumb.

p. val′gus deviation of the thumb toward the ulnar side.

p. va′rus deviation of the thumb toward the radial side.

pol•lic•i•za•tion (pol″is-ĭ-za′shən) [L. *pollex* thumb] the replacement or rehabilitation of a thumb, especially surgical construction of a thumb from the index finger or great toe.

pol•li•na•tion (pol″ĭ-na′shən) the transfer of pollen from anther to stigma of a flowering plant.

pol•li•ni•um (po-lin′e-əm) an aggregation of pollen grains held together by a mucilaginous fluid and transported as a whole during pollination.

pol•li•no•sis (pol″ĭ-no′sis) hay fever.

pol•lu•tion (pə-loo′shən) [L. *pollutio*] the act of defiling or making impure.

pol•ly•beak (pol′e-bēk″) [*polly* tame parrot + *beak*] see under *deformity*.

Polo•caine (po′lo-cān) trademark for preparations of mepivacaine hydrochloride.

po•lo•cytes (po′lo-sīts) [Gr. *polos* pole + *-cyte*] polar bodies (def. 1).

po•lo•ni•um (Po) (pə-lo′ne-əm) [L. *Polonia* Poland] a rare metal resembling bismuth, discovered in 1898 in pitchblende; atomic number, 84; atomic weight, 210. It is radioactive, but less so than radium.

pol•ox•a•lene (pol-ok′sə-lēn) [USP] a liquid poloxamer, having a molecular weight of approximately 3000; used as a surfactant in pharmaceutical preparations and in the prevention of bloat in ruminants.

pol•ox•al•kol (pol-ok′sal-kol) poloxamer 188.

pol•ox•a•mer (pol-ok′sə-mər) any of a series of nonionic surfactants of the polyoxypropylene-polyoxyethylene copolymer type, having the general formula $HO(C_2H_4O)_a(C_3H_6O)_b$- $(C_2H_4O)_c$ H, where $a = c$; the molecular weights of the members of the series vary from about 1000 to more than 16,000. The term is used in conjunction with a numerical suffix for individual unique identification of products that may be used as a food, drug, or cosmetic. Poloxamers may be surfactants, emulsifiers, or stabilizers.

p. 182L a liquid poloxamer, having an average molecular weight of 2450; used as a food additive and pharmaceutical aid.

p. 188 a waxy poloxamer, having an average molecular weight of 8350; used as a cathartic, administered orally. Called also *poloxalkol*.

p. 331 a liquid poloxamer, having an average molecular weight of 3800; used as a food additive.

pol•ster (pōl′stər) a small bulge, as on a vessel wall.

po•lus (po′ləs) gen. and pl. *po′li* [L., from Gr. *polos* axis] pole: either extremity of an axis or of an organ.

p. ante′rior bul′bi o′culi [TA] anterior pole of eyeball: the center of the anterior curvature of the eyeball.

p. ante′rior len′tis [TA] anterior pole of lens: the central point of the anterior surface of the lens.

p. fronta′lis hemisphe′rii ce′rebri [TA] frontal pole of cerebral hemisphere: the most prominent part of the anterior end of each hemisphere.

p. infe′rior re′nis TA alternative for *extremitas inferior renis*.

p. infe′rior tes′tis TA alternative for *extremitas inferior testis*.

p. occipita′lis hemisphe′rii ce′rebri [TA] occipital pole of cerebral hemisphere: the most posterior prominence of the occipital lobe of each hemisphere.

p. poste′rior bul′bi o′culi [TA] posterior pole of eyeball: the center of the posterior curvature of the eyeball.

p. poste′rior len′tis [TA] posterior pole of lens: the central point of the posterior surface of the lens.

p. supe′rior re′nis TA alternative for *extremitas superior renis*.

p. supe′rior tes′tis TA alternative for *extremitas superior testis*.

p. tempora′lis hemisphe′rii ce′rebri [TA] temporal pole of cerebral hemisphere: the prominent anterior end of the temporal lobe of each hemisphere.

poly (pol′e) colloquial name for *polymorphonuclear leukocyte*.

poly- [Gr. *polys* many] a combining form meaning many or much.

poly A polyadenylate; polyadenylic acid.

Pol•ya oper•ation (pōl′yah) [Jenö (Eugene) *Polya*, Hungarian surgeon, 1876–1944] see under *operation*.

poly•ac•id (pol″e-as′id) capable of neutralizing several molecules of an acid radical; said of a base or basic radical.

poly•acryl•a•mide (pol″e-ə-kril′ə-mīd) a polymer of acrylamide, having a porosity that is adjustable by changing the composition of the monomer before polymerization; used as an inert support in gel electrophoresis.

poly•ac•rylo•ni•trile (pol″e-ə-kril″o-ni′trīl) a polymer of acrylonitrile used as a hemodialyzer membrane; it is more permeable by diffusion than cuprophane for larger molecules, but fluid removal is rapid and not entirely predictable.

poly•ad•e•ni•tis (pol″e-ad″ə-ni′tis) [*poly-* + *adenitis*] inflammation (adenitis) of several or many glands.

poly•ad•e•no•ma (pol″e-ad″ə-no′mə) adenoma of many glands.

poly•ad•e•no•ma•to•sis (pol″e-ad″ə-no-mə-to′sis) multiple adenomas in a part.

poly•ad•e•nop•a•thy (pol″e-ad″ə-nop′ə-the) 1. polyadenosis. 2. polyendocrinopathy.

poly•ad•e•no•sis (pol″e-ad″ə-no′sis) disorder of several glands, particularly of several endocrine glands. Cf. *polyadenopathy*.

poly•ad•e•nous (pol″e-ad′ə-nəs) [*poly-* + *aden-* + *-ous*] 1. polyendocrine. 2. pluriglandular.

poly•aden•y•late (pol″e-ə-den′ə-lāt) the salt, ester, or anionic form of polyadenylic acid. Abbreviated poly A.

poly•aden•y•lat•ed (pol″e-ə-den′ə-la″təd) having a polyadenylate tail.

poly•aden•y•la•tion (pol″e-ə-den″ə-la′shən) the formation of the polyadenylate tail on eukaryotic RNA molecules or at the 3′ end of viral mRNA, catalyzed by polynucleotide adenylyltransferase.

poly•ad•e•nyl•ic ac•id (pol″e-ad″ə-nil′ik) a homopolymer composed solely of adenylic acid residues; see also *polyadenylate tail*, under *tail*. Abbreviated poly A.

poly•ag•glu•ti•na•tion (pol″e-ə-gloo″tĭ-na′shən) an abnormal condition of erythrocytes in which they agglutinate upon exposure to almost any normal serum due to antigens in their membranes that react to common serum antibodies.

poly•al•co•hol•ism (pol″e-al′kə-hol-iz-əm) intoxication or poisoning by a mixture of different alcohols.

poly•al•ve•o•lar (pol″e-al-ve′ə-lər) having more than the usual number of alveoli, such as a polyalveolar lobe of a lung.

poly•am•ine (pol″e-am′ēn) any compound, e.g., spermine and spermidine, containing two or more amine groups joined by a short hydrocarbon chain. Polyamines are low molecular weight cations and are synthesized within cells to provide intermediates for protein synthesis; they are important in cell growth and proliferation, gene expression, and extracellular matrix synthesis.

poly•an•dry (pol″e-an′dre) [*poly-* + Gr. *aner* man] 1. polygamy in which a woman is concurrently married to more than one man. 2. an animal

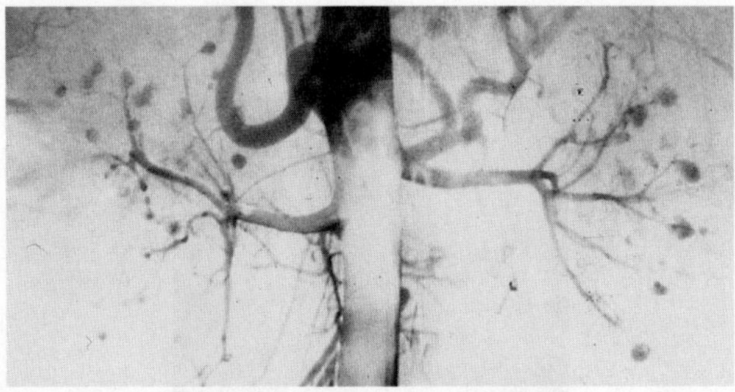

■ Polyarteritis nodosa seen in an arteriogram of a pediatric patient with renovascular hypertension caused by renal artery stenosis, with arterial lesions characterized by multiple thrombi and aneurysms.

mating system seen in polygamous species, in which the female mates with more than one male. 3. union of two or more male pronuclei with one female pronucleus, resulting in polyploidy of the zygote. Cf. *polygyny.*

poly·an·gi·itis (pol″e-an″je-i′tis) inflammation involving multiple blood or lymph vessels.

microscopic p. a type of small vessel vasculitis, usually in the kidneys but sometimes also in the lungs, skin, and nervous system; characteristics are similar to those of polyarteritis nodosa with focal segmental glomerulosclerosis and presence of antineutrophil cytoplasmic autoantibodies.

poly A po·lym·er·ase (pol′e a pə-lim′ər-ās) polynucleotide adenylyltransferase.

poly·ar·cu·ate (pol″e-ahr′ku-ət) characterized by multiple arch-shaped curves.

poly·ar·ter·i·tis (pol″e-ahr″tə-ri′tis) [*poly-* + *arteritis*] 1. multiple inflammatory and destructive arterial lesions; called also *panarteritis.* 2. p. nodosa.

microscopic p. see under *polyangiitis.*

p. nodo′sa (PAN) a form of systemic necrotizing vasculitis involving the small and medium-sized arteries with signs and symptoms resulting from infarction and scarring of the affected organ system. Called also *Kussmaul* or *Kussmaul-Maier disease, necrotizing arteritis, panarteritis nodosa,* and *periarteritis nodosa.*

poly·ar·thral·gia (pol″e-ahr-thral′jə) arthralgia in many different joints.

poly·ar·thric (pol″e-ahr′thrik) [*poly-* + *arthr-* + *-ic*] pertaining to or affecting many joints.

poly·ar·thri·tis (pol″e-ahr-thri′tis) [*poly-* + *arthr-* + *-itis*] an inflammation of several joints together.

acute rheumatic p. see under *arthritis.*

carcinomatous p. asymmetric arthritis of the large and small joints, often in association with malignancy. It has an explosive onset and mimics the appearance of rheumatoid arthritis; it often occurs in older patients and frequently remits upon treatment of the underlying disorder.

chlamydial p. an infectious disease of sheep, and occasionally calves and pigs, in the United States, Australia, and New Zealand, caused by infection with *Chlamydophila psittaci*; characteristics include joint enlargement with edema, fever, and anorexia.

chronic secondary p. Jaccoud arthropathy.

chronic villous p. chronic inflammation of the synovial membrane of several joints.

p. des′truens rheumatoid arthritis.

epidemic p. a disease resembling dengue, caused by the Ross River virus and transmitted by mosquitoes; characteristics include polyarthritis, rash, and fever. It is seen primarily in Australia, New Guinea, and elsewhere in the western Pacific.

infectious p., infectious porcine p. Glasser disease.

migratory p. arthritis that moves from one joint to another in an asymmetric pattern, usually involving large joints such as the ankles, knees, and elbows, seen in conditions such as gonococcal arthritis.

mycoplasmal p. infection in pigs by *Mycoplasma hyorhinis* or *M. hyosynoviae*, often occurring after unusual stresses; characteristics include polyarthritis, swollen joints, and lameness. *M. hyorhinis* infection may be accompanied by polyserositis (see *mycoplasmal polyserositis*).

nonsuppurative p. joint swelling without suppuration in lambs as a result of infection by *Erysipelothrix rhusiopathiae* through a wound. In the acute form, animals have fever and leg pain for two to three weeks; in the chronic form they have permanently swollen joints and are lame.

peripheral p. polyarthritis limited to peripheral joints; asymmetric involvement is common and the number of joints affected tends to be limited. Often the knees and ankles are more involved than the hands or feet.

septic p. septic arthritis in several different joints.

tuberculous p. hypertrophic pulmonary osteoarthropathy.

poly·ar·tic·u·lar (pol″e-ahr-tik′u-lər) [*poly-* + *articular*] affecting many joints.

poly·atom·ic (pol″e-ə-tom′ik) [*poly-* + *atomic*] composed of several atoms.

poly·auxo·troph (pol″e-awk′so-trōf) [*poly-* + *auxo-* + *-trophic*] an organism, especially a mutant, which requires multiple growth factors.

poly·auxo·tro·phic (pol″e-awk″so-tro′fik) requiring multiple growth factors; used especially with reference to a single mutation that causes a multiple requirement.

poly·avi·ta·min·o·sis (pol″e-a-vi″tə-min-o′sis) [*poly-* + *avitaminosis*] a deficiency disease in which more than one vitamin is lacking in the diet.

poly·ax·on·ic (pol″e-ak-son′ik) pertaining to or having several axons.

poly·ba·sic (pol″e-ba′sik) [*poly-* + *basic*] 1. denoting any acid which has several hydrogen atoms replaceable by a base. 2. denoting any salt of a polybasic acid formed by replacing some or all of its hydrogen atoms by a base.

poly·blen·nia (pol″e-blen′e-ə) [*poly-* + *blenn-* + *-ia*] the secretion of an excessive quantity of mucus.

poly·car·bo·phil (pol″e-kahr′bo-fil) [USP] a pharmacologically inert polyacrylic acid cross-linked with divinyl glycol; it is a bulk-forming laxative and also acts as a gastrointestinal absorbent in the treatment of diarrhea.

p. calcium calcium polycarbophil; see under *calcium.*

poly·cel·lu·lar (pol″e-sel′u-lər) multicellular.

poly·cen·tric (pol″e-sen′trik) having many centers.

poly·cen·tric·i·ty (pol″e-sən-tris′ĭ-te) the state or quality of being polycentric.

poly·chei·ria (pol″e-ki′re-ə) [*poly-* + *cheir-* + *-ia*] the condition of having more than two hands.

poly·che·mo·ther·a·py (pol″e-ke″mo-ther′ə-pe) combination chemotherapy.

poly·cho·lia (pol″e-ko′le-ə) hypercholia.

poly·chon·dri·tis (pol″e-kon-dri′tis) inflammation involving many cartilages of the body.

atrophic p., chronic atrophic p., p. chro′nica atro′phicans relapsing p.

relapsing p. a disease of unknown etiology with a chronic course and sometimes recurrence, marked by inflammatory and degenerative lesions of cartilage in the joints, ears, nose, trachea, bronchi, and elsewhere, with deformities such as floppy ear and saddle nose; if the tracheal or bronchial wall collapses, respiratory obstruction may occur. The aorta, sclera, and cornea are also affected. Called also *chronic atrophic p.* and *polychondropathia.*

poly·chon·dro·path·ia (pol″e-kon″dro-path′e-ə) relapsing polychondritis.

poly·chon·drop·a·thy (pol″e-kon-drop′ə-the) relapsing polychondritis.

poly·chrest (pol′e-krest) [*poly-* + Gr. *chrēstos* useful] 1. useful in many conditions. 2. a remedy useful in many diseases.

poly·chro·ma·sia (pol″e-kro-ma′zhə) 1. variation in the hemoglobin content of the erythrocytes of the blood. 2. polychromatophilia.

poly·chro·ma·tia (pol″e-kro-ma′shə) polychromatophilia.

poly·chro·mat·ic (pol″e-kro-mat′ik) [*poly-* + *chromatic*] exhibiting many colors. Cf. *monochromatic.*

poly·chro·mato·cyte (pol″e-kro-mat′o-sīt) polychromatophil.

poly·chro·ma·to·cy·to·sis (pol″e-kro″mə-to-si-to′sis) polychromatophilia.

poly·chro·mato·phil (pol″e-kro-mat′o-fil) [*poly-* + *chromato-* + *-phil*] a cell or other element that is stainable with various stains or colors; called also *polychromatocyte* and *polychromophil.*

poly·chro·ma·to·phil·ia (pol″e-kro″mə-to-fil′e-ə) 1. the quality of being stainable with various different stains or tints. 2. a condition in which the erythrocytes, on staining, show shades of blue tinged with pink; seen in various types of anemia. Called also *polychromasia, polychromatocytosis,* and *polychromophilia.*

poly·chro·ma·to·phil·ic (pol″e-kro″mə-to-fil′ik) pertaining to or characterized by polychromatophilia.

poly·chro·ma·to·sis (pol″e-kro″mə-to′sis) an excess of abnormally staining erythrocytes in the blood; see *polychromatophilia* (def. 2).

poly·chro·me·mia (pol″e-kro-me′me-ə) [*poly-* + *chrom-* + *-emia*] hyperhemoglobinemia.

poly·chro·mic (pol″e-kro′mik) pertaining to or exhibiting many colors.

poly•chro•mo•phil (pol″e-kro′mo-fil) polychromatophil.

poly•chro•mo•phil•ia (pol″e-kro″mo-fil′e-ə) polychromatophilia.

Poly•cil•lin (pol″e-sil′in) trademark for preparations of ampicillin.

poly•cis•tron•ic (pol″e-sis-tron′ik) [*poly-* + *cistron* + *-ic*] spanning or including more than one gene; see *polycistronic messenger RNA*, under *RNA*.

Poly•Cit•ra (pol″e-sit′rə) trademark for preparations containing potassium citrate.

poly•clin•ic (pol″e-klin′ik) [*poly-* + *clinic*] a hospital and school where diseases and injuries of many kinds are studied and treated clinically.

poly•clo•nal (pol″e-klo′nəl) 1. derived from different cells. 2. of or pertaining to multiple clones. Cf. *monoclonal* and *oligoclonal*.

poly•co•ria[1] (pol″e-kor′e-ə) [*poly-* + Gr. *korē* pupil + *-ia*] the existence of more than one pupil in an eye.

p. spu′ria a condition in which the iris contains several openings or holes.

p. ve′ra the existence in the eye of several pupils, each with its own sphincter.

poly•co•ria[2] (pol″e-kor′e-ə) [*poly-* + Gr. *koros* surfeit + *-ia*] the deposit of reserve material in an organ or tissue so as to produce enlargement.

poly•crot•ic (pol″e-krot′ik) [*poly-* + Gr. *krotos* beat] characterized by secondary waves to each beat in the pulse tracing.

pol•yc•ro•tism (pol-ik′rə-tiz-əm) presence of a polycrotic pulse.

poly•cy•clic (pol″e-sik′lik, -si′klik) [*poly-* + *cyclic*] containing more than one ring or cycle (frequency).

poly•cy•e•sis (pol″e-si-e′sis) [*poly-* + *-cyesis*] multiple pregnancy.

poly•cys•tic (pol″e-sis′tik) [*poly-* + *cystic*] containing or made up of many cysts; called also *multicystic*.

poly•cyte (pol′e-sīt) [*poly-* + *-cyte*] an abnormal polymorphonuclear leukocyte of normal size but with more than the usual number of lobes in the nucleus. Cf. *macropolycyte*.

poly•cy•the•mia (pol″e-si-the′me-ə) [*poly-* + *cyt-* + *hem-* + *-ia*] an increase in the total red cell mass of the blood, characterized as either *absolute p.* or *relative p.* Called also *erythrocythemia*, *hypercythemia*, and *hypererythrocythemia*.

absolute p. an increase in red cell mass caused by a sustained overactivity of the erythroid component of the bone marrow, which may occur as a compensatory physiologic response to tissue hypoxia (see *secondary p.*), or as the principal manifestation of polycythemia vera. Cf. *relative p.*

appropriate p. see *secondary p.*

benign p., chronic relative p. stress p.

compensatory p. see *secondary p.*

hypertonic p., p. hyperto′nica stress p.

inappropriate p. see *secondary p.*

myelopathic p., primary p. p. vera.

relative p. a decrease in plasma volume without the change in red blood cell mass of absolute polycythemia, so that the erythrocytes become more concentrated (elevated hematocrit). It occurs in both acute forms (a transient condition due to marked loss of body fluid, lowered fluid intake, or a combination) and chronic forms (see *stress p.*). Called also *spurious p.* and *pseudopolycythemia*.

p. ru′bra, p. ru′bra ve′ra p. vera.

secondary p. any absolute increase in the total red cell mass other than polycythemia vera, usually occurring as a physiologic response to tissue hypoxia. Some types are called *compensatory* or *appropriate*, such as from adjustments for general tissue hypoxia (such as that associated with pulmonary disease, alveolar hypoventilation, cardiovascular disease, or prolonged exposure to high altitude), or from the presence of defective hemoglobin or drugs. Other types are called *inappropriate* and reflect excessive production of erythropoietin due to a disorder of the kidneys or some other organ. Called also *erythrocytosis*.

splenomegalic p. p. vera.

spurious p. 1. relative p. 2. stress p.

stress p. a chronic type of relative polycythemia, seen most often in middle-aged, mildly obese males who are active, anxiety-prone, and hypertensive, occurring without the characteristic symptoms associated with polycythemia vera, i.e., without leukocytosis, splenomegaly, or thrombocytosis. Called also *benign* or *stress erythrocytosis*, *Gaisböck disease*, *pseudopolycythemia*, and *benign*, *chronic relative*, *hypertonic*, or *spurious p.*

p. ve′ra a myeloproliferative disorder of unknown etiology, characterized by abnormal proliferation of all hematopoietic bone marrow elements and an absolute increase in red cell mass and total blood volume. The skin of the face is often ruddy and swollen, and ecchymoses are common. Most patients have splenomegaly, leukocytosis, and thrombocythemia. Hematopoiesis is also reactive in extramedullary sites (liver and spleen), and in time myelofibrosis occurs. Called also *p. rubra* or *p. rubra vera; myelopathic* or *splenomegalic p.;* and *Osler*, *Osler-Vaquez*, *Vaquez*, or *Vaquez-Osler disease*. Cf. *secondary p.*

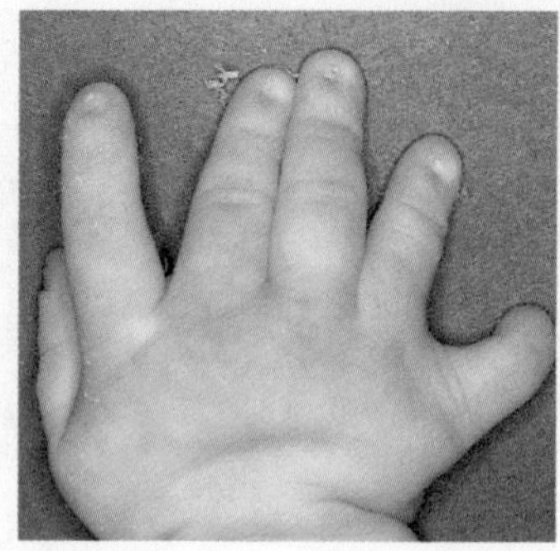

■ Polydactyly.

poly•dac•tyl•ia (pol″e-dak-til′e-ə) polydactyly.

poly•dac•tyl•ism (pol″e-dak′təl-iz-əm) polydactyly.

poly•dac•ty•ly (pol″e-dak′tə-le) [*poly-* + Gr. *daktylos* finger + *-ia*] a developmental anomaly characterized by the presence of more than the usual number of fingers or toes. Called also *polydactylism* and *hyperdactyly*.

poly•de•oxy•ri•bo•nu•cle•o•tide (pol″e-de-ok″se-ri″bo-noo′kle-o-tīd) a polymer of deoxyribonucleotides; deoxyribonucleic acid.

poly•de•oxy•ri•bo•nu•cle•o•tide syn•thase (pol″e-de-ok″se-ri″bo-noo′kle-o-tīd sin′thās) DNA ligase.

poly•dex•trose (pol″e-dek′strōs) a food additive used as a low-calorie replacement for sugar or flour in order to add bulk to breads and pastries that contain artificial sweeteners.

poly•di•meth•yl•si•lox•ane (pol″ī-di-meth″əl-si-lok′sān) a polymeric siloxane in which the substituents are methyl groups; it is the most common form of silicone; see also *dimethicone* and *silicone oil*.

poly•di•ox•an•one (pol″e-di-ok′sə-nōn) a synthetic polymer used as an absorbable suture material.

poly•dip•sia (pol″e-dip′se-ə) [*poly-* + *dipsia*] chronic excessive thirst and intake of fluid; it may have an organic cause, such as the dehydration of diabetes mellitus, diabetes insipidus, or a reaction to medication, or be of psychological origin. Cf. *hyperdipsia*.

psychogenic p. polydipsia without an organic basis, occurring as a result of a mental disorder.

poly•dis•per•soid (pol″e-dis-pur′soid) a colloid in which the disperse phase consists of particles having different degrees of dispersion.

poly•drug (pol′e-drug) more than one drug; used particularly for concurrent abuse of multiple drugs.

poly•dys•pla•sia (pol″e-dis-pla′zhə) [*poly-* + *dysplasia*] faulty development in several types of tissue or several organs or systems.

poly•dys•tro•phy (pol″e-dis′trə-fe) dystrophy of several tissues or structures at the same time. **polydystroph′ic** *adj*

pseudo-Hurler p. mucolipidosis III alpha/beta.

variant pseudo-Hurler p. mucolipidosis III gamma.

poly•elec•tro•lyte (pol″e-e-lek′tro-līt) a large polymer compound of many monomers, each of which carries one or more ionic groups.

poly•em•bry•o•ma (pol″e-em″bre-o′mə) a rare type of germ cell tumor consisting of embryoid bodies and believed to comprise both embryonic and extraembryonic differentiation.

poly•em•bry•o•ny (pol″e-em-bri′o-ne) [*poly-* + *embryo*] the production of two or more embryos from the same oocyte or seed.

poly•en•do•crine (pol″e-en′do-krin) pertaining to or affecting several endocrine glands. Called also *polyadenous*.

poly•en•do•cri•no•ma (pol″e-en″do-krĭ-no′mə) multiple endocrine neoplasia.

poly•en•do•cri•nop•a•thy (pol″e-en″do-krĭ-nop′ə-the) endocrinopathy involving several glands.

pol•y•ene (pol′e-ēn) 1. an aliphatic or alicyclic compound with a carbon chain of four or more atoms and several conjugated double bonds. 2. any of a group of antifungal antibiotics that contain this compound, such as amphotericin, candicidin, and nystatin. They are produced by species of *Streptomyces* and damage cell membranes by forming complexes with sterols.

poly•er•gic (pol″e-ur′jik) able to act in several different ways.

poly•es•the•sia (pol″e-es-the′zhə) [*poly-* + *esthesia*] a dysesthesia in which a single object seems to be felt in several different places, such as may be seen in tabes dorsalis.

poly•es•tra•di•ol phos•phate (pol″e-es″trə-di′ol) a polymer of estradiol phosphate having estrogenic activity similar to that of estradiol; used in the palliative therapy of prostatic carcinoma, administered intramuscularly.

poly·es·trous (pol″e-es′trəs) completing two or more estrous cycles per annual breeding season. Cf. *monestrous.*

poly·ether (pol″e-e′thər) an elastomer made from cyclic ether, used in paste form as an impression material for fixed partial prosthodontic structures, inlays for single quadrants, and dental impressions.

poly·eth·y·lene (pol″e-eth′ə-lēn) polymerized ethylene, (—CH_2—CH_2—)$_n$, a synthetic plastic material, forms of which have been used in reparative surgery.

p. glycol (PEG) [NF] a generic name for mixtures of condensation polymers of ethylene oxide and water, represented by the general formula $H(OCH_2CH_2)_n$ OH, in which *n* is greater than or equal to 4. The term is used in combination with a numeric suffix which indicates the approximate average molecular weight. Those with average molecular weights between 200 and 700 are liquid and those above 1000 are waxlike solids: *p. glycol 3000* (*n* varies from 5 to 5.75) is used as a solvent and dispensing agent in pharmaceutical preparations; *p. glycol 400* (*n* varies from 8.2 to 9.1), *p. glycol 600* (*n* varies from 12.5 to 13.9), and *p. glycol 1500* (*n* varies from 29 to 36) are used as ointment and suppository bases; *p. glycol 1540* (*n* varies from 28 to 36) is used as a vehicle in pharmaceutical preparations; *p. glycol 3350* is used as a laxative; *p. glycol 4000* (*n* varies from 68 to 84) and *p. glycol 6000* (*n* varies from 158 to 204) are used as ointment and suppository bases and as tablet excipients. Called also *macrogol.*

p. glycol monomethyl ether [NF] any of a series of addition polymers of ethylene oxide and methanol, represented by the general formula $CH_3(OHC_2CH_2)_nOH$, in which *n* is the average number of oxyethylene groups. Nominal molecular weights range from 350 to 10,000, the viscosity increasing and the solubility in water and in organic solvents decreasing as the molecular weight increases. Used as an excipient in pharmaceutical preparations.

p. terephthalate any of a group of thermoplastic, fiber-forming polyesters used in textile manufacture; see *Dacron.*

Po·lyg·a·la (po-lig′ə-lə) [*poly-* + Gr. *gala* milk] the milkworts, a genus of plants of the family Polygalaceae, having many species. *P. se′nega* L. is seneca or senega snakeroot, a North American species that yields senega. *P. klotz′chii* is a Brazilian species that causes fatal gastrointestinal and neurological disorders in cattle.

poly·ga·lac·tia (pol″e-gə-lak′she-ə) [*poly-* + *galact-* + *-ia*] excessive secretion of milk.

po·lyg·a·lin (pə-lig′ə-lin) senegenin.

Poly·gam (pol′e-gam) trademark for a preparation of immune globulin intravenous (human).

po·lyg·a·mous (pə-lig′ə-məs) pertaining to polygamy.

po·lyg·a·my (pə-lig′ə-me) [*poly-* + Gr. *gamos* marriage] 1. the concurrent marriage of a woman or man to more than one spouse, as opposed to *monogamy.* 2. animal mating in which the individual mates with more than one partner. See also *polyandry* and *polygyny.*

poly·gan·gli·on·ic (pol″e-gang″gle-on′ik) [*poly-* + *ganglionic*] 1. having or pertaining to several or many ganglia. 2. affecting several lymphatic glands.

poly·gel·ine (pol″e-jel′ēn) a polymer of urea and polypeptides derived from denatured gelatin; used as a plasma expander in hypovolemia.

poly·gene (pol′e-jēn) [*poly-* + *gene*] a member of a group of nonallelic genes whose interaction has an additive effect on a quantitative character, each one having a small effect individually.

poly·gen·ic (pol″e-jen′ik) pertaining to or determined by the action of multiple different genes. Cf. *multifactorial.*

poly·glac·tin 910 (pol″e-glak′tin) a type of multifilament braided material made of purified lactides and glycolides, used in absorbable sutures.

poly·glan·du·lar (pol″e-glan′du-lər) pluriglandular.

poly·glu·cose (pol″e-gloo′kōs) polydextrose that has been made water-soluble by addition of bound molecules of citric acid; used therapeutically in peritoneal dialysis solutions to induce ultrafiltration through the membrane.

poly·glu·co·side (pol″e-gloo′ko-sīd) a polysaccharide composed of glucose residues. Cf. *oligoglucoside.*

poly·glu·ta·mine (pol″e-gloo′tə-mēn) a stretch of glutamine residues in a protein; expanded numbers of such residues are associated with several triplet repeat disorders. See also *polyglutamine disorders,* under *disorder.*

poly·gly·col·ic ac·id (pol″e-gli-kol′ik) a polymer of glycolic acid used for absorbable sutures.

poly·gly·co·nate (pol″e-glik′ə-nāt) a synthetic polymer used as an absorbable suture material.

po·lyg·na·thus (po-lig′nə-thəs, pol″e-nath′əs) [*poly-* + Gr. *gnathos* jaw] asymmetrical conjoined twins with the parasitic twin attached to the jaw of the larger twin. See also *hypognathus.*

pol·y·gon (pol′e-gon) a planar figure bounded by three or more line segments.

frequency p. a graphic method for displaying a frequency distribution, obtained from a histogram by placing a dot at the midpoint of the top of each bar, with a line connecting the dots outlining the polygon.

Poly·go·na·tum (pol″e-go-na′təm) [*poly-* + Gr. *gony* knee] a genus of plants of the family Liliaceae. *P. biflo′rum* (Walt.) Ell. is Solomon seal, a perennial herb of eastern North America used as a tonic, diuretic, emetic, and cathartic; at high doses it is a cardiac poison.

poly·gram (pol′e-gram) a tracing made by a polygraph.

poly·graph (pol′e-graf) [*poly-* + *-graph*] an instrument for simultaneously recording various physiological responses as represented by mechanical or electrical impulses, such as respiratory movements, pulse wave, blood pressure, and galvanic skin responses. Such phenomena reflect emotional reactions which are of use in detecting deception. Popularly known as *lie detector.*

po·lyg·y·ny (pə-lij′ĭ-ne) [*poly-* + Gr. *gynē* woman] 1. polygamy in which a man is married concurrently to more than one woman. 2. an animal mating system seen in polygamous species, in which the male mates with more than one female. 3. union of two or more female pronuclei with one male pronucleus, resulting in polyploidy of the zygote. Cf. *polyandry.*

poly·gy·ria (pol″e-ji′re-ə) polymicrogyria.

poly·he·dral (pol″e-he′drəl) [*poly-* + Gr. *hedra* seat, base] having many faces or sides.

poly·hi·dro·sis (pol″e-hĭ-dro′sis) hyperhidrosis.

poly·his·tio·cy·to·ma (pol″e-his″te-o-si-to′mə) small-cell osteosarcoma.

poly·hy·brid (pol″e-hi′brid) [*poly-* + *hybrid*] a hybrid whose parents differ from each other in more than three characters.

poly·hy·dram·ni·os (pol″e-hi-dram′ne-os) [*poly-* + *hydr-* + *amnion*] excess of amniotic fluid, usually exceeding 2000 mL.

poly·hy·dric (pol″e-hi′drik) containing more than two hydroxyl groups.

poly·hy·per·men·or·rhea (pol″e-hi″pər-men″o-re′ə) [*poly-* + *hyper-* + *menorrhea*] polymenorrhea with abnormally profuse discharge.

poly·hy·po·men·or·rhea (pol″e-hi″po-men″o-re′ə) [*poly-* + *hypo-* + *menorrhea*] polymenorrhea with deficient amount of discharge.

poly·in·fec·tion (pol″e-in-fek′shən) mixed infection.

poly·ion·ic (pol″e-i-on′ik) containing several different ions (e.g., potassium, sodium, etc.), as a polyionic solution.

poly·iso·pre·noid (pol″e-i″so-pre′noid) any isoprenoid that contains multiple isoprene units, such as rubber.

poly·karyo·cyte (pol″e-kar′e-o-sīt) [*poly-* + *karyo-* + *-cyte*] a giant cell containing several nuclei.

poly·ki·ne·ty (pol″e-ki′ne-te) [*poly-* + *kinety*] a row of closely arranged cilia that descends in a counterclockwise spiral into the infundibulum of peritrichous ciliate protozoa.

Poly·kol (pol′ĭ-kol) trademark for preparations of poloxalkol.

poly·lac·tic ac·id (pol″e-lak′tik) a hydrophobic hydroxy acid polymer that is formed into granules and used as a surgical dressing material for dental extraction sites, primarily for prevention of postoperative alveolar osteitis.

poly·lec·i·thal (pol″e-les′ĭ-thəl) macrolecithal.

poly·lep·tic (pol″e-lep′tik) [*poly-* + Gr. *lambanein* to seize] having many remissions and exacerbations.

poly·ly·sine (pol″e-li′sēn) a polypeptide composed of lysine molecules in peptide linkage; used as a carrier for the benzylpenicilloyl moiety in the detection of penicillin sensitivity; see *penicilloyl polylysine.*

poly·ma·con (pol″e-ma′kon) a hydrophilic contact lens material.

poly·mas·tia (pol″e-mas′te-ə) [*poly-* + *mast-* + *-ia*] the presence of more than one pair of mammae, or breasts. Called also *pleomastia.* **polymas′tic** *adj*

Poly·mas·ti·gi·da (pol″e-mas″tĭ-gi′də) in older systems of classification, an order of protozoa of the phylum Sarcomastigophora, subphylum Mastigophora, consisting of small organisms with three to eight or more flagella and usually one or two nuclei; they are found in the digestive tract of various arthropods and vertebrates.

poly·ma·zia (pol″e-ma′ze-ə) polymastia.

poly·me·lia (pol″e-me′le-ə) [*poly-* + *-melia*] a developmental anomaly characterized by the presence of supernumerary limbs.

po·lym·e·lus (pə-lim′ə-ləs) an individual exhibiting polymelia.

poly·me·nia (pol″e-me′ne-ə) polymenorrhea.

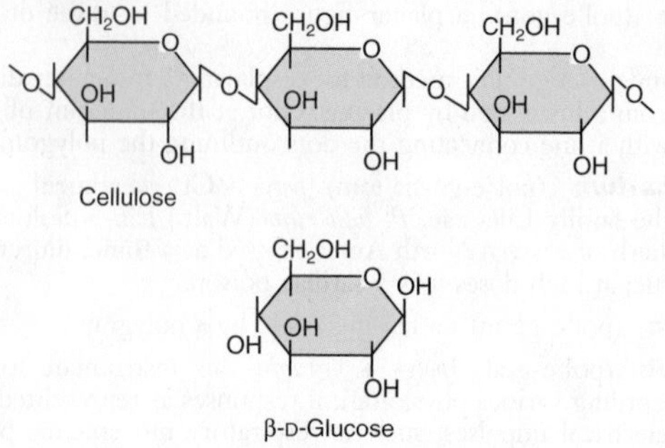

Cellulose

β-D-Glucose

■ The polymer cellulose consists of linked repeating units of the monomer β-D-glucose.

poly·men·or·rhea (pol″e-men″o-re′ə) [*poly-* + *menorrhea*] abnormally frequent menstruation, defined as that occurring at regular intervals of less than 21 days.

poly·mer (pol′ĭ-mər) [*poly-* + Gr. *meros* part] a compound formed by the joining of smaller molecules, referred to as *monomers*. The term is generally used to refer either to a macromolecule made up of a large number of monomers linked by covalent bonds, e.g., polypeptides, nucleic acids, polysaccharides, and plastics, or to a protein made up of several subunits linked by covalent or noncovalent bonds, e.g., hemoglobin or IgM immunoglobulin.
addition p. a compound formed by the repeated combination of smaller molecules (monomers) without the formation of any other products (e.g., polyethylene).
condensation p. a compound formed by the repeated reaction of smaller molecules, involving at the same time the elimination of water or other simple compound (e.g., nylon).
cross-linked p. a polymer that has cross-linking; strength and resistance to solvents make many such polymers suitable for use in dental materials.
polysulfide p. see under *rubber*.

po·lym·er·ase (pə-lim′ər-ās) any enzyme that catalyzes polymerization, especially of nucleotides to polynucleotides.
Taq p. see under *T*.

poly·me·ria (pol″e-mēr′e-ə) [*poly-* + *mer-*[1] + *-ia*] a developmental anomaly characterized by the presence of supernumerary parts or organs of the body.

poly·mer·ic (pol″e-mer′ik) exhibiting the characteristics of a polymer.

po·lym·er·iza·tion (pə-lim″ər-ĭ-za′shən) the act or process of forming a compound (polymer), usually of high molecular weight, by the combination of simpler molecules (monomers).

po·lym·er·ize (pə-lim′ər-īz) to subject to or to undergo polymerization.

poly·meta·car·pia (pol″e-met″ə-kahr′pe-ə) [*poly-* + *metacarpus* + *-ia*] presence of more than the normal number of metacarpal bones.

poly·meta·phos·phate (pol″e-met″ə-fos′fāt) a phosphate polymer that serves as a phosphate reserve in microorganisms, appearing as a metachromatic granule.

poly·meta·tar·sia (pol″e-met″ə-tahr′se-ə) [*poly-* + *metatarsus* + *-ia*] presence of more than the normal number of metatarsal bones.

poly·meth·yl meth·ac·ryl·ate (PMMA) (pol″e-meth″əl meth-ak′rəl-āt) a thermoplastic acrylic resin formed by polymerization of methyl methacrylate; it is used extensively in medicine and dentistry. Written also *polymethylmethacrylate*.

poly·mi·cro·bi·al (pol″e-mi-kro′be-əl) [*poly-* + *microbe*] characterized by the presence of several species of microorganisms.

poly·mi·cro·bic (pol″e-mi-kro′bik) polymicrobial.

poly·mi·cro·gy·ria (pol″e-mi″kro-ji′re-ə) [*poly-* + *micro-* + *gyr-* + *-ia*] a developmental anomaly of the brain characterized by development of numerous small convolutions (microgyri), causing mental retardation. Called also *microgyria* and *polygyria*.

poly·mi·cro·lipo·ma·to·sis (pol″e-mi″kro-lip″o-mə-to′sis) [*poly-* + *micro-* + *lipomatosis*] lipomatosis marked by the presence in the subcutaneous tissues of numerous small lipomas.

poly·mi·cro·tome (pol″e-mi′kro-tōm) [*poly-* + *microtome*] a microtome which cuts several sections at once.

Po·lym·nia (pə-lim′ne-ə) [Gr.; one of the nine Muses] a genus of plants of the family Compositae, having yellow or white flowers. *P. uveda′lia* L., the leafcup or bearsfoot, is anthelmintic, alterative, antispasmodic, and laxative.

poly·morph (pol′e-morf) colloquial term for *polymorphonuclear leukocyte*.

poly·mor·phic (pol″e-mor′fik) [*poly-* + *morph-* + *-ic*] occurring in several or many forms; appearing in different forms at different stages of development. Called also *polymorphous*.

poly·mor·phism (pol″e-mor′fiz-əm) [*poly-* + *morph-* + *-ism*] 1. the existence within a population or species of several different forms of individuals, or the occurrence of different forms or stages in an individual over time. 2. genetic p.
balanced p. a state of equilibrium in which a genetic polymorphism is maintained by a balance between mutation and selection, heterozygotes for the locus having an advantage over either homozygote.
genetic p. the long-term occurrence in a population of multiple alternative alleles at a locus, with the rarest ones being at a frequency greater than could be maintained by recurrent mutation alone.
microsatellite p. the existence of different numbers of tandem repeating units in microsatellites of different individuals; they can be detected by polymerase chain reaction (PCR) and are used extensively as markers, as in genetic linkage and mapping studies, kinship and paternity testing, forensic identification, and analyses of populations. Called also *short tandem repeat p.*
restriction fragment length p. (RFLP) a genetic polymorphism in DNA sequence that can be detected on the basis of differences in DNA fragment lengths produced by digestion with a specific restriction endonuclease.
short tandem repeat p. (STRP) microsatellite p.
single nucleotide p. (SNP) a genetic polymorphism between two genomes that is based on deletion, insertion, or exchange of a single nucleotide.

poly·mor·pho·cel·lu·lar (pol″e-mor″fo-sel′u-lər) [*poly-* + *morpho-* + *cellular*] having cells of many forms.

poly·mor·pho·cyte (pol″e-mor′fo-sīt) polymorphonuclear leukocyte.

poly·mor·pho·nu·cle·ar (pol″e-mor″fo-noo′kle-ər) [*poly-* + *morpho-* + *nuclear*] having a nucleus deeply lobed or so divided that it appears to be multiple.

pol·y·mor·pho·nu·cle·o·cyte (pol″e-mor″fo-nu′kle-o-sīt) polymorphonuclear leukocyte.

poly·mor·phous (pol″e-mor′fəs) polymorphic.

poly·my·al·gia (pol″e-mi-al′jə) myalgia affecting several muscles.
p. arteri′tica, p. rheuma′tica a syndrome in the elderly characterized by proximal joint and muscle pain and a high erythrocyte sedimentation rate; it is sometimes associated with giant cell arteritis.

poly·my·ar·i·an (pol″e-mi-ar′e-ən) [*poly-* + Gr. *mys* muscle] having many muscle cells in each quadrant of a cross section, the cells being coelomyarian in type; said of the muscle arrangement in certain nematodes.

poly·my·oc·lo·nus (pol″e-mi-ok′lə-nəs) myoclonus in several muscles or groups simultaneously or in rapid succession; it occurs in myoclonic epilepsy and in some types of poisoning.

poly·my·op·a·thy (pol″e-mi-op′ə-the) disease affecting several muscles simultaneously.

poly·myo·si·tis (pol″e-mi″o-si′tis) [*poly-* + *myositis*] chronic, progressive myositis with symmetrical weakness of the limb girdles, neck, and pharynx; it can occur in either children or adults. There is usually associated pain and tenderness, and there may be symptoms resembling those of scleroderma, arthritis, systemic lupus erythematosus, or Sjögren syndrome. It is also sometimes associated with malignancy, and may be accompanied by characteristic skin lesions (see *dermatomyositis*).
eosinophilic p. see under *myositis*.

poly·myx·in (pol″e-mik′sin) the generic name for five polypeptide antibiotics (designated A, B, C, D, and E) derived from strains of the soil bacterium *Bacillus polymyxa*, having specific activity against gram-negative bacteria, including *Pseudomonas aeruginosa, Proteus vulgaris, Escherichia coli, Haemophilus influenzae*, and *Klebsiella pneumoniae*. The least toxic members of the group are polymyxins B, usually used in the form of the sulfate salt, and E (see *colistin*).
p. B sulfate [USP] the sulfate salt of the least toxic member of the polymyxin group; used in the treatment of various systemic, urinary tract, ophthalmic, otic, and cutaneous infections due to susceptible gram-negative bacteria, especially *Pseudomonas aeruginosa*, administered orally, parenterally, and topically.

poly·ne·sic (pol″e-ne′sik) [*poly-* + Gr. *nēsos* island] multiple and insular; occurring in many foci.

poly·neu·ral (pol″e-noor′əl) [*poly-* + *neural*] pertaining to or supplied by several nerves.

poly·neu·ral·gia (pol″e-nŏŏ-ral′jə) neuralgia of several nerves.

poly·neu·ric (pol″e-noor′ik) polyneural.

poly·neu·ri·tis (pol″e-nŏŏ-ri′tis) [*poly-* + *neur-* + *-itis*] inflammation of several peripheral nerves at once; called also *multiple neuritis*. **polyneurit′ic** *adj*

acute idiopathic p., acute infectious p., acute infective p., acute postinfectious p. Guillain-Barré syndrome.
anemic p. see under *polyneuropathy.*
cranial p. multiple mononeuropathy involving several cranial nerves, characterized by facial palsy or any of various ocular conditions; sometimes seen as part of sarcoid neuropathy.
endemic p., p. ende′mica beriberi.
Guillain-Barré p. see under *syndrome.*
Jamaica ginger p. see under *paralysis.*
leprous p. sensory or sensorimotor polyneuritis due to inflammation of nerve trunks in association with leprosy.
postinfectious p. Guillain-Barré syndrome.

poly·neu·ro·myo·si·tis (pol″e-noor″o-mi″o-si′tis) polyneuritis with polymyositis.

poly·neu·rop·a·thy (pol″e-noo͞-rop′ə-the) [*poly-* + *neuropathy*] neuropathy of several peripheral nerves simultaneously; called also *multiple* or *peripheral neuropathy.* Some conditions that are actually polyneuropathies are called neuropathies; see under *neuropathy.*
acute postinfectious p. Guillain-Barré syndrome.
amyloid p. polyneuropathy associated with amyloidosis, of either the primary (AL) or familial type; symptoms may include dysfunction of the autonomic nervous system, carpal tunnel syndrome, and sensory disturbances in the extremities such as numbness, hyperesthesia, or paresthesia. See also *familial amyloid p.*
anemic p. polyneuropathy seen in subacute combined degeneration of the spinal cord (see under *degeneration*).
arsenic p., arsenical p. polyneuropathy seen in cases of chronic arsenic poisoning, characterized by sensory disturbances of the extremities and sometimes by a syndrome resembling Guillain-Barré syndrome.
carcinomatous p. paraneoplastic polyneuropathy seen with carcinoma, especially of the lung; it consists of sensory and sensorimotor disturbances such as dysesthesias, paresthesias, and unsteadiness of gait. Cf. *carcinomatous neuromyopathy.*
chronic inflammatory demyelinating p. (CIDP) a slowly progressive, autoimmune type of demyelinating polyneuropathy characterized by progressive weakness and impaired sensory function in the limbs and enlargement of the peripheral nerves, usually with elevated protein in the cerebrospinal fluid. It occurs most commonly in young adults, particularly males, and is related to Guillain-Barré syndrome. Presenting symptoms often include tingling or numbness of the digits, weakness of the limbs, hyporeflexia or areflexia, fatigue, and abnormal sensations.
critical illness p. an idiopathic sensorimotor type of polyneuropathy seen in critically ill patients such as those who are on ventilators or receiving intensive medication.
demyelinating p. any of numerous neurologic conditions in which demyelination of multiple nerves is a primary symptom, such as Charcot-Marie-Tooth disease (type I) and chronic inflammatory demyelinating polyneuropathy.
diabetic p. see under *neuropathy.*
diphtheritic p. Dejerine syndrome (def. 3).
distal symmetric p. the most common type of diabetic neuropathy, with loss of sensation in the feet and sometimes a Charcot joint that deforms the ankle; in some patients this starts with burning or itching in the feet.
erythredema p. acrodynia.
familial amyloid p. autosomal dominant amyloid polyneuropathy, associated with hereditary amyloidosis (q.v.) and involving deposition of amyloid in some combination of the peripheral and autonomic nerves, heart, kidney, and other organs; it was subclassified on the basis of affected kinships, which were found to be associated with specific mutations, but now is usually subclassified on the basis of symptoms and the biochemical composition of the affected fibrils. It most commonly involves one of a variety of point mutations of the *TTR* gene, which encodes transthyretin (see *ATTR amyloidosis,* under *amyloidosis*), but can also be associated with mutations affecting other proteins that can form fibrillar aggregates, such as apolipoprotein A-I.
Guillain-Barré p. see under *syndrome.*
inflammatory demyelinating p. see under *polyradiculoneuropathy.*
motor p. see under *neuropathy.*
nutritional p. polyneuropathy due to nutritional deficits, as seen with beriberi, pellagra, alcoholism, malabsorption syndromes, Strachan syndrome, and other conditions. Cf. *anemic p.*
paraneoplastic p. a paraneoplastic syndrome, sometimes seen with carcinoma, multiple myeloma, or Hodgkin disease, consisting of polyneuropathy with sensory or sensorimotor symptoms. Cf. *carcinomatous pericarditis.* Called also *paraneoplastic neuropathy.*
porphyric p. a severe, often symmetrical type of polyneuropathy that occurs with some varieties of porphyria.
symmetrical sensory p. sensory neuropathy in the limbs, especially their distal parts, seen in diabetes mellitus; it usually develops slowly but occasionally has an acute onset.
uremic p. polyneuropathy caused by the uremia of chronic renal failure, characterized by painless bilateral sensorimotor deficits of the lower limbs and later the upper limbs.

poly·neu·ro·ra·dic·u·li·tis (pol″e-noor″o-rə-dik″u-li′tis) [*poly-* + *neuro-* + *radiculitis*] Guillain-Barré syndrome.

poly·nu·cle·ar (pol″e-noo′kle-ər) 1. of cells, pertaining to or having several nuclei; multinucleated. Cf. *polymorphonuclear.* 2. in organic chemistry, denoting an aromatic compound containing two or more closed rings.

poly·nu·cle·ate (pol″e-noo′kle-āt) polynuclear.

poly·nu·cle·at·ed (pol″e-noo′kle-āt″əd) polynuclear.

poly·nu·cle·o·lar (pol″e-noo-kle′o-lər) having several nucleoli.

poly·nu·cleo·tide (pol″e-noo′kle-o-tīd) a linear polymer of mononucleotides; see *nucleic acid.*

poly·nu·cleo·tide aden·yl·yl·trans·fer·ase (pol″e-noo′kle-o-tīd ə-den″əl-əl-trans′fər-ās) [EC 2.7.7.19] an enzyme of the transferase class that catalyzes the sequential addition of ATP-derived adenylate residues to the 3′ end of a polynucleotide. The enzyme does not require a template. The reaction produces the polyadenylate (poly A) tail characteristic of most eukaryotic messenger RNA molecules. Called also *poly A polymerase.*

poly·nu·cle·o·tide phos·phor·y·lase (pol″e-noo′kle-o-tīd fos-for′ə-lās) polyribonucleotide nucleotidyltransferase.

poly·odon·tia (pol″e-o-don′shə) hyperdontia.

poly·ol (pol′e-ol) an alcohol containing more than two hydroxyl groups, e.g., sugar alcohols, inositol. Called also *polyhydric alcohol.*

poly·ol de·hy·dro·gen·ase (pol′e-ol de-hi′dro-jən-ās) L-iditol 2-dehydrogenase.

poly·o·ma (pol″e-o′mə) a tumor caused by an oncogenic virus of broad host range, originally isolated from parotid gland tumors of mice inoculated with Gross leukemia virus; see also *polyomavirus.*

Poly·o·ma·vi·ri·dae (pol″e-o″mə-vir′ĭ-de) the polyomaviruses, a family of DNA viruses that were formerly grouped together with the papillomaviruses in a family called Papovaviridae; they have a nonenveloped icosahedral virion 40 nm in diameter and a genome of about 5,000 base pairs. The family contains just one genus, *Polyomavirus.*

Poly·o·ma·vi·rus (pol″e-o′mə-vi″rəs) [*poly-* + *-oma* + *virus*] the sole genus of the family Polyomaviridae. Two species, BK polyomavirus and JC polyomavirus, infect humans; others, such as simian virus 40, infect other mammals.

poly·o·ma·vi·rus (pol″e-o′mə-vi″rəs) any virus of the family Polyomaviridae. **polyomavi′ral** *adj*
BK p. a species of the genus *Polyomavirus* that causes widespread infection in childhood (80 per cent of adults being seropositive) and remains latent in the host; it is believed to cause hemorrhagic cystitis and nephritis in immunocompromised patients. Called also *BK virus.*
human p. any of several species of the genus *Polyomavirus* that infect humans.
JC p. a species of the genus *Polyomavirus* that causes widespread infection in childhood (80 per cent of adults being seropositive) and remains latent in the host; it is the cause of progressive multifocal leukoencephalopathy.

poly·onych·ia (pol″e-o-nik′e-ə) [*poly-* + *onych-* + *-ia*] the occurrence of supernumerary nails.

poly·opia (pol″e-o′pe-ə) [*poly-* + *-opia*] the condition in which one object appears as two or more objects.
binocular p. diplopia.
p. monophthal′mica a condition in which an object looked at by one eye appears double.

poly·op·sia (pol″e-op′se-ə) polyopia.

poly·opy (pol′e-o″pe) polyopia.

poly·or·chi·dism (pol″e-or′kĭ-diz-əm) a developmental anomaly characterized by the presence of more than two testes; called also *polyorchism.*

poly·or·chism (pol″e-or′kiz-əm) polyorchidism.

poly·os·tot·ic (pol″e-os-tot′ik) [*poly-* + L. *os* bone] pertaining to or affecting many bones.

poly·otia (pol″e-o′shə) [*poly-* + *ot-* + *-ia*] the condition of having more than two external ears.

poly·ov·u·lar (pol″e-ov′u-lər) pertaining to or produced from more than one oocyte, as in dizygotic twins.

poly·ov·u·la·to·ry (pol″e-ov′u-lə-tor″e) discharging several oocytes in one ovarian cycle.

poly·oxy·eth·y·lene 50 ste·a·rate (pol″e-oks″e-eth′ə-lēn) polyoxyl 50 stearate.

poly·ox·yl (pol″e-oks′əl) any of various mixtures of the mono- and distearate esters of mixed polyoxyethylene diols and the corresponding free diols. The term is used in combination with an identifying number which indicates the average polymer length in oxyethylene units: *p. 8 stearate* and *p. 40 stearate* [USP], in which the average polymer lengths in oxyethylene units are equivalent to about 8 and 40, respectively, are used as surfactants in pharmaceutical preparations.

p. 5 oleate peglicol 5 oleate.

p. 50 stearate a mixture of the mono- and distearate esters of mixed polyoxyethylene diols and the corresponding free diols, the average polymer length being equivalent to about 50 oxyethylene units, occurring as a soft, cream-colored, waxy solid; used as a surfactant and emulsifying agent in pharmaceutical preparations. Called also *polyoxyethylene 50 stearate.*

pol·yp (pol′ip) [Gr. *polypous* a morbid excrescence] an abnormal protruding growth from a mucous membrane; originally applied only to such growths on the mucous membrane of the nose, the term is now applied to ones on any mucous membrane.

adenomatous p. of colon a benign growth in the epithelium of the sigmoid colon or rectum, seen in many persons over age 60 and sometimes preneoplastic; both tubular and villous varieties have been described. It may be sessile or pedunculated and solitary or multiple.

adenomatous p. of stomach a benign growth in the epithelium of the stomach, usually in the antrum, with branching tubules or fingerlike projections and glandular tissue; it may be premalignant or a sign of malignancy nearby. Called also *gastric adenoma.*

aural p. a polyp in the ear; common sites include the external canal, mucosa of middle ear, and eustachian tube.

cardiac p. a ball thrombus or tumor attached by a pedicle to the inside of the heart.

cervical p. a common, relatively innocuous tumor of the uterine cervix, usually in the cervical canal; size varies widely. Such tumors may produce irregular vaginal bleeding.

choanal p's nasal polyps that project posteriorly into the nasopharynx.

cholesterol p's small polypoid excrescences consisting of cholesterol and other lipids, seen projecting into the lumen of the gallbladder in cholesterolosis.

cystic p. a polyp in which the fibrous network is coarse, thus stimulating or producing cysts; called also *hydatid p.*

endocervical p. cervical p.

endometrial p's small, sessile, benign projecting masses on the endometrium, composed of an edematous stroma containing cystically dilated glands.

fibroepithelial p. acrochordon.

gelatinous p. myxoma.

gum p. a small pedunculated growth on the gingiva.

hydatid p. cystic p.

hyperplastic p., inflammatory p. pseudopolyp.

juvenile p's small, benign, hemispheric hamartomas of the large intestine occurring in children; they have an abundant loose fibrovascular stroma containing widely spaced glands. Called also *retention p's.*

laryngeal p's, p's of larynx smooth, rounded, sessile or pedunculated swellings, occurring on the true vocal cords; caused by edema in the lamina propria of the mucous membrane.

lymphoid p's rare, benign tumors of the colon composed of aggregates of lymphoid tissue, usually covered by a fairly regular colonic mucosa.

nasal p's focal accumulations of edema fluid in the mucosa of the nose, with hyperplasia of the associated submucosal connective tissue.

prostatic urethral p's presence of numerous polyps in the prostatic urethra, sometimes causing obstruction, seen in male children as a developmental anomaly and in older males in some inflammatory reactions.

regenerative p. pseudopolyp.

retention p's juvenile p's.

poly·para·si·tism (pol″e-par′ə-si-tiz″əm) infection or infestation by more than one species of parasite.

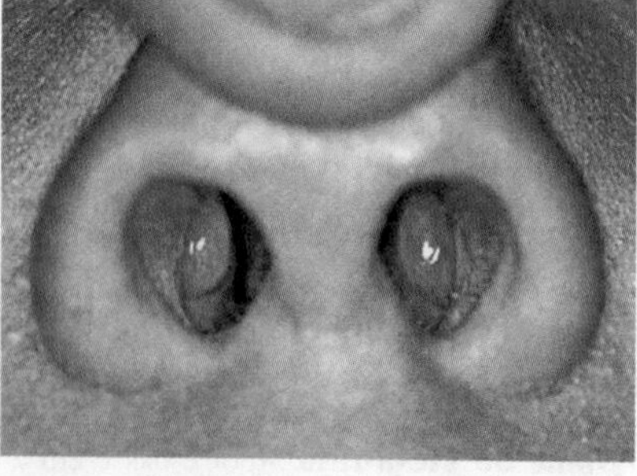

■ Nasal polyps in a patient with cystic fibrosis.

poly·path·ia (pol″e-path′e-ə) [*poly-* + *path-* + *-ia*] the presence of several diseases at once.

pol·yp·ec·to·my (pol″ĭ-pek′tə-me) [*polyp* + *-ectomy*] surgical removal of a polyp.

poly·pep·tide (pol″e-pep′tīd) [*poly-* + *peptide*] a peptide that on hydrolysis yields more than two amino acids; called tripeptides, tetrapeptides, and so on according to the number of amino acids contained. See also *peptide.*

gastric inhibitory p. (GIP), glucose-dependent insulinotropic p. a polypeptide hormone (molecular weight 5165; 43 amino acids) synthesized by K cells in the midzone of the duodenal and jejunal mucosa and released in response to oral glucose, fat, or amino acids; it is a potent insulin stimulant, increases insulin secretion, and inhibits gastric secretion and motility.

islet amyloid p. (IAPP) amylin.

pancreatic p. a hormone (4200 daltons, 36 amino acids) secreted by special endocrine cells in the periphery of some pancreatic islets, the exocrine pancreas, and the intestine; it inhibits pancreatic enzyme secretion and gallbladder contraction, but its physiologic role has not been identified.

parathyroid-like p. a polypeptide with activity like that of parathyroid hormone, causing hypercalcemia; it is produced by tumors of the islet cells and some other organs in multiple endocrine neoplasia type 1.

spasmolytic p. trefoil factor 2.

vasoactive intestinal p. (VIP) a peptide hormone (3326 daltons, 28 amino acids) widely distributed throughout the body but found in highest concentrations in the nervous system and intestines; it is released locally from nerve endings or endocrine cells. Its primary actions are thought to be to serve as a neurotransmitter, to relax smooth muscles of the circulation, intestines, and genitourinary system, to increase secretion of water and electrolytes from the pancreas and intestines, and to release hormones from the pancreatic islets, intestines, and hypothalamus. It is found in excess with VIPomas and the Verner-Morrison syndrome. Called also *vasoactive intestinal peptide.*

poly·pep·ti·de·mia (pol″e-pep″tĭ-de′me-ə) [*polypeptide* + *-emia*] the presence of polypeptides in the blood.

poly·pep·ti·dor·rha·chia (pol″e-pep″tĭ-do-ra′ke-ə) [*polypeptide* + *rhachi-* + *-ia*] the presence of polypeptides in the spinal fluid.

poly·peri·os·ti·tis (pol″e-per″e-os-ti′tis) inflammation of the periosteum of several bones.

p. hyperesthe′tica a chronic disease of the periosteum attended by extreme hyperesthesia of the skin and soft parts.

poly·pha·gia (pol″e-fa′jə) [*poly-* + *-phagia*] excessive eating; gluttony. See also *bulimia.* Called also *hyperphagia.*

poly·pha·lan·gia (pol″e-fə-lan′jə) side-by-side duplication of one or more of the phalanges of a digit.

poly·pha·lan·gism (pol″e-fə-lan′jiz-əm) polyphalangia.

poly·phar·ma·ceu·tic (pol″e-fahr″mə-soo′tik) pertaining to several drugs, especially to the administration of several drugs together.

poly·phar·ma·cy (pol″e-fahr′mə-se) [*poly-* + Gr. *pharmakon* drug] 1. the administration of many drugs together. 2. the administration of excessive medication.

poly·phase (pol′e-fāz) [*poly-* + *phase*] having several phases; containing colloids of several types.

poly·pha·sic (pol″e-fa′zik) having or existing in many phases; having unlike particles in the disperse phase.

poly·phen·ic (pol″e-fen′ik) pleiotropic.

poly·phe·nol ox·i·dase (pol″e-fe′nol ok′sĭ-dās) see *catechol oxidase.*

poly·pho·bia (pol″e-fo′be-ə) [*poly-* + *-phobia*] irrational fear of many things.

poly·phos·pho·ino·si·tide (pol″e-fos″fo-in-o′sĭ-tīd) a multiply phosphorylated phosphoinositide (q.v.), such as phosphatidylinositol 4,5-bisphosphate.

poly·phy·let·ic (pol″e-fi-let′ik) [*poly-* + *phyletic*] arising or descending from more than one cell type; see *polyphyletic theory,* under *theory.*

poly·phy·le·tism (pol″e-fi′lə-tiz-əm) polyphyletic theory; see under *theory.*

poly·phy·le·tist (pol″le-fi′lə-tist) an adherent of the polyphyletic theory; see under *theory.*

poly·phy·odont (pol″e-fi′o-dont) [*poly-* + Gr. *phyein* to produce + *odous* tooth] developing several sets of teeth successively throughout life. Cf. *diphyodont* and *monophyodont.*

poly·pi (pol′ĭ-pi) [L.] plural of *polypus.*

pol·yp·i·form (pə-lip′ĭ-form) polypoid.

poly·plas·tic (pol″e-plas′tik) [*poly-* + *plastic*] 1. containing many structural or constituent elements. 2. undergoing many changes of form.

Poly·plax (pol′e-plaks) a genus of sucking lice (order Anoplura), which parasitize rodents. *P. miacan′tha* is found on rats; *P. serra′ta* infests rabbits and transmits tularemia; and *P. spinulo′sa,* the most common louse of rats, transmits murine typhus.

poly·ploid (pol′e-ploid) [*poly-* + *haploid*] 1. having more than two full sets of homologous chromosomes. There may be three (triploid), four (tetraploid), five (pentaploid), six (hexaploid), seven (heptaploid), eight (octaploid), etc. 2. an individual or cell having more than two full sets of homologous chromosomes. Polyploid organisms, especially plants, are larger than normal and have larger cells. Affected animals are often abnormal in appearance and usually infertile. Cf. *aneuploid.*

poly·ploi·dy (pol′e-ploi″de) the state of being polyploid.

pol·yp·nea (pol″ip-ne′ə) hyperpnea. **polypne′ic** *adj*

poly·po·dia (pol″e-po′de-ə) [*poly-* + *pod-* + *-ia*] the presence of more than two feet.

pol·yp·oid (pol′ĭ-poid) [*polyp* + *-oid*] resembling a polyp.

pol·yp·oi·do·sis (pol″ĭ-poi-do′sis) polyposis.

poly·po·rous (pol′e-por″əs) having many pores.

poly·po·sia (pol″e-po′zhə) [*poly-* + *-posia*] ingestion of abnormally increased amounts of fluids for long periods of time. Cf. *hyperposia.*

pol·yp·osis (pol″ĭ-po′sis) the development of multiple polyps on a part.

attenuated p. coli, attenuated familial adenomatous p. (AFAP) a rare variant form of familial adenomatous polyposis (FAP), characterized by a lower number of polyps, later age of onset, and slightly lower risk of malignancy.

autosomal recessive colorectal adenomatous p. MUTYH-associated p.

cap p. a rare type of polyposis coli in which inflammatory polyps have elongated crypts and caps of purulent, fibrinous exudate.

p. co′li, p. of colon a condition characterized by the occurrence of multiple polyps in the colon, such as familial adenomatous polyposis or juvenile polyposis.

familial adenomatous p. (FAP), familial p. coli, familial intestinal p. an autosomal dominant syndrome in which multiple adenomatous polyps line the mucous membrane of the intestine, particularly the colon, with onset at about puberty; caused by mutation in the *APC* gene (locus: 5q21-q22), a tumor suppressor gene. It is characterized by weight loss, bowel obstruction, and bloody diarrhea; extracolonic signs include pigmented retinal lesions, jaw cysts, sebaceous cysts, and osteomas. If untreated it progresses to malignancy. There is variant form of later onset; see *attenuated familial adenomatous p.*

gastric p. the presence of multiple polyps on the gastric mucosa.

intestinal p. p. coli.

juvenile p., juvenile intestinal p. a disorder characterized by the occurrence of multiple juvenile polyps (q.v.) in the gastrointestinal tract. It can be sporadic or can be an autosomal dominant disorder caused by mutation either in the *SMAD4* gene (locus: 18q21.1), which is a tumor suppressor gene, or in the *BMPR1A* gene (locus: 10q22.3), which encodes a receptor for bone morphogenetic protein. Called also *juvenile polyposis syndrome.*

multiple familial p. familial adenomatous p.

MUTYH-associated p., MYH-associated p. an autosomal recessive disorder closely resembling familial adenomatous polyposis but caused by homozygous mutations in the *MUTYH* gene (locus: 1p34.3-p32.1), which is involved in mismatch repair.

pol·yp·o·tome (pə-lip′ə-tōm) a cutting instrument for removing polyps.

pol·yp·o·trite (pə-lip′ə-trīt) [*polyp* + L. *terere* to crush] an instrument for crushing polyps.

pol·yp·ous (pol′ĭ-pəs) of the nature of a polyp; polyp-like.

poly·prag·ma·sy (pol″e-prag′mə-se) [*poly-* + Gr. *pragma* a doing] polypharmacy.

poly·pro·py·lene (pol″e-pro′pə-lēn″) a widely used synthetic crystalline, thermoplastic polymer with a molecular weight of 40,000 or more, having the general formula $(C_3H_5)_n$. Medical uses include the manufacture of nonabsorbable sutures, surgical casts, and semipermeable membranes for membrane oxygenators.

p. carbonate [NF] a clear, colorless, mobile liquid, $C_4H_6O_3$, used as solvent in oral and topical pharmaceuticals and as a gelling agent.

poly·pty·chi·al (pol″e-ti′ke-əl) [*poly-* + Gr. *ptychē* fold] arranged in several layers; said of glands whose cells are arranged on the basement membrane in several layers. Cf. *monoptychial.*

pol·yp·us (pol′ĭ-pəs) pl. *pol′ypi* [L., from Gr. *polypous,* from *poly-* + *pous* foot] a polyp.

p. cys′ticus cystic polyp.

p. hydatido′sus cystic polyp.

poly·ra·dic·u·li·tis (pol″e-rə-dik″u-li′tis) [*poly-* + *radiculitis*] inflammation of the nerve roots.

poly·ra·dic·u·lo·neu·ri·tis (pol″e-rə-dik″u-lo-nōō-ri′tis) [*poly-* + *radiculoneuritis*] 1. Guillain-Barré syndrome. 2. a disease in dogs similar to human Guillain-Barré syndrome, usually seen in the form of acute polyradiculoneuritis.

acute p. a common type of ascending paralysis in dogs, clinically similar to human Guillain-Barré syndrome; ventral roots of spinal nerves, and other peripheral nerves, undergo segmental demyelination. It was first seen in hunting dogs that had had fights with raccoons. The exact etiology is unclear. Called also *coonhound paralysis.*

poly·ra·dic·u·lo·neu·rop·a·thy (pol″e-rə-dik″u-lo-nōō-rop′ə-the) 1. any disease of the peripheral nerves and spinal nerve roots. 2. Guillain-Barré syndrome.

acute inflammatory demyelinating p. Guillain-Barré syndrome.

chronic inflammatory p., chronic inflammatory demyelinating p. a type of demyelinating polyneuropathy similar to Guillain-Barré syndrome but progressing more slowly or in a fluctuating pattern. The fluctuating variety is sometimes called *chronic relapsing p.*

chronic relapsing p. see *chronic inflammatory demyelinating p.*

inflammatory demyelinating p. see *Guillain-Barré syndrome* and *chronic inflammatory demyelinating p.*

poly·ra·dic·u·lop·a·thy (pol″e-rə-dik″u-lop′ə-the) disease of several spinal nerve roots.

poly·ri·bo·nu·cleo·tide (pol″e-ri″bo-noo′kle-o-tīd) a linear polymer of ribonucleotides; see *ribonucleic acid.*

poly·ri·bo·nu·cleo·tide nu·cleo·ti·dyl·trans·fer·ase (pol″e-ri″bo-noo′kle-o-tīd noo″kle-o-ti′dəl trans′fər-ās) [EC 2.7.7.8] an enzyme of the transferase class that catalyzes the reversible phosphorolysis of RNA molecules or other polyribonucleotides to yield nucleoside diphosphate residues. The bacterial enzyme was used in research elucidating the genetic code. Called also *polynucleotide phosphorylase.*

poly·ri·bo·some (pol″e-ri′bo-sōm) a complex made up of ribosomal subunits assembled among themselves by the filaments of messenger RNA containing the genetic information; they play a role in the synthesis of peptides. Called also *polysome.*

pol·yr·rhea (pol″ĭ-re′ə) [*poly-* + *-rrhea*] a copious fluid discharge.

poly·sac·cha·ride (pol″e-sak′ə-rīd) a carbohydrate that on hydrolysis yields a large number of monosaccharides (variously defined as five or more to eleven or more). Cf. *oligosaccharide.*

bacterial p′s polysaccharides found in bacteria and especially in bacterial capsules.

C p. see under *carbohydrate.*

core p. the constant part of the heteropolysaccharide chain of lipopolysaccharide.

immune p′s polysaccharides which can function as specific antigens, such as capsular substances.

O-specific p. the variable part of the heteropolysaccharide chain of lipopolysaccharide (q.v.); it is responsible for the antigenic specificity.

pneumococcal p., pneumococcus p. any of a large number of polysaccharides derived from the capsule of *Streptococcus pneumoniae;* more than 80 immunologically distinct types have been identified and form the basis of pneumococcal typing. The structure of some is known: *Type 1* is a polymer of trisaccharide units containing galacturonic acids; *Type 2* is a polymer of glucose; *Type 3* is a high molecular weight polymer of glucose and glucuronic acid units (cellobiuronic acid); and *Type 8* consists of glucose and glucuronic acid units alternating with glucosyl-galactose residues.

specific p′s soluble polysaccharides obtained from various microorganisms; in high dilution these specifically precipitate the antisera to the corresponding organisms.

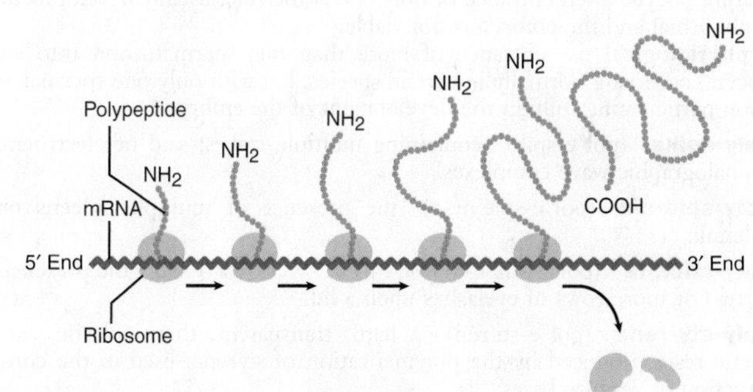

■ Schematic diagram of polyribosomes synthesizing nascent polypeptide chains from a messenger RNA (mRNA) template, the direction proceeding 5′ to 3′.

poly·sce·lia (pol″e-se′le-ə) [*poly-* + Gr. *skelos* leg + *-ia*] a developmental anomaly in which an individual has more than two lower limbs.

po·lys·ce·lus (pə-lis′ə-ləs) an individual with polyscelia.

poly·scope (pol′e-skōp) [*poly-* + *-scope*] diaphanoscope.

poly·sen·si·tiv·i·ty (pol″e-sen″sĭ-tiv′ĭ-te) sensitivity to a number of different stimuli.

poly·sen·so·ry (pol″e-sen′sə-re) multisensory.

poly·se·ro·si·tis (pol″e-sēr″o-si′tis) [*poly-* + *serositis*] general inflammation of serous membranes with serous effusion; see also *Concato disease.*

familial recurrent p. familial Mediterranean fever.

mycoplasmal p. infection of the serous and synovial membranes of pigs by *Mycoplasma hyorhinis,* with acute lameness, fever, and other signs of mild septicemia. It may be accompanied by mycoplasmal polyarthritis. Called also *porcine p.*

periodic p. familial Mediterranean fever.

porcine p. 1. Glasser disease. 2. mycoplasmal p.

recurrent p. familial Mediterranean fever.

poly·si·a·lia (pol″e-si-a′le-ə) ptyalism.

poly·si·a·lic ac·id (pol″si-al′ik) large hydrated polysaccharide similar to K1 of *Escherichia coli.*

poly·si·lox·ane (pol″e-si′lok-sān) any of various polymeric siloxanes, particularly the silicones.

poly·sin·u·itis (pol″e-sin″u-i′tis) polysinusitis.

poly·si·nu·sec·to·my (pol″e-si″nə-sek′tə-me) excision of the diseased membrane of several of the paranasal sinuses.

poly·si·nus·itis (pol″e-si″nəs-i′tis) [*poly-* + *sinusitis*] inflammation of several sinuses at once.

poly·some (pol′e-sōm) polyribosome.

poly·so·mia (pol″e-so′me-ə) [*poly-* + *-somia*] a doubling or tripling of the body of a fetus. See also *conjoined twins,* under *twin.*

poly·so·mic (pol″e-so′mik) 1. pertaining to or exhibiting polysomy. 2. an individual exhibiting polysomy.

poly·som·nog·ra·phy (pol″e-som-nog′rə-fe) [*polygraph* + *somni-* + *-graphy*] the polygraphic recording during sleep of multiple physiologic variables, both directly and indirectly related to the state and stages of sleep, to assess possible biological causes of sleep disorders.

poly·so·mus (pol″e-so′məs) conjoined twins exhibiting polysomia.

poly·so·my (pol″e-so′me) [*poly-* + chromo*some*] an excess of a particular chromosome, resulting from meiotic chromosomal nondisjunction. The chromosome may be duplicated three (trisomy), four (tetrasomy), or more times.

poly·sor·bate (pol″e-sor′bāt) a generic name for esters of sorbitol and its anhydrides condensed with polymers of ethylene oxide, used as surfactant agents: *p. 20,* $C_{58}H_{114}O_{26}$, is polyoxyethylene 20 sorbitan monolaurate; *p. 40,* $C_{62}H_{122}O_{26}$, is polyoxyethylene 20 sorbitan monopalmitate; *p. 60,* $C_{64}H_{126}O_{26}$, is polyethylene 20 sorbitan monostearate; *p. 65,* $C_{100}H_{194}O_{28}$, is polyethylene 20 sorbitan tristearate; *p. 80,* $C_{64}H_{124}O_{26}$, is polyethylene 20 sorbitan monooleate; *p. 85,* $C_{100}H_{188}O_{28}$, is polyethylene 20 sorbitan trioleate. *Polysorbates 20, 40, 60,* and *80* are official in NF.

poly·sper·mia (pol″e-spur′me-ə) [*poly-* + *sperm-* + *-ia*] 1. excessive secretion of semen. 2. polyspermy.

poly·sper·mism (pol″e-spur′miz-əm) 1. polyspermia (def. 1). 2. polyspermy.

poly·sper·my (pol″e-spur′me) fertilization of an oocyte by more than one spermatozoon. Called also *polyspermia.*

pathological p. entrance of more than one spermatozoon into a mature oocyte when entrance of only one is the rule; usually development is abnormal and the embryo is not viable.

physiological p. entrance of more than one spermatozoon into an oocyte, occurring normally in certain species, but with only one spermatozoon participating fully in the development of the embryo.

poly·spike (pol″e-spīk) containing multiple spikes; said of electroencephalographic wave complexes.

poly·sple·nia (pol″e-sple′ne-ə) the presence of multiple spleens or splenuli.

poly·stich·ia (pol″e-stik′e-ə) [*poly-* + Gr. *stichos* row + *-ia*] the presence of two or more rows of eyelashes upon a lid.

poly·sty·rene (pol″e-sti′rēn) a hard, transparent, thermoplastic synthetic resin produced by the polymerization of styrene; used in the construction of denture bases.

poly·sul·fide (pol″e-sul′fīd) 1. a sulfide that has two or more atoms of sulfur. 2. containing polysulfides; see under *rubber.*

poly·sul·fone (pol″e-sul′fōn) a synthetic thermoplastic polymer used as a hemodialyzer membrane.

poly·sus·pen·soid (pol″e-səs-pen′soid) a suspension colloid in which the particles are of different degrees of dispersion.

poly·sy·nap·tic (pol″e-sĭ-nap′tik) involving many synapses in series and therefore a sequence of many neurons; called also *multisynaptic.* Cf. *oligosynaptic.*

poly·syn·dac·ty·ly (pol″e-sin-dak′tə-le) [*poly-* + *syndactyly*] association of polydactyly and syndactyly of varying degrees of the hand and foot.

poly·syn·o·vi·tis (pol″e-sin″o-vi′tis) [*poly-* + *synovitis*] general inflammation of the synovial membranes.

poly·tef (pol′ĭ-tef) a polymer of tetrafluoroethylene, used as a surgical implant material for prostheses, such as artificial vessels and orbital floor implants and for many applications in skeletal augmentation and skeletal fixation. Also used widely in industry, e.g., as an antistick coating for cooking utensils. See also *polymer fume fever,* under *fever.* Called also *polytetrafluoroethylene (PTFE).*

poly·ten·di·ni·tis (pol″e-ten″dĭ-ni′tis) inflammation affecting several tendons.

poly·ten·di·no·bur·si·tis (pol″e-ten″dĭ-no-bər-si′tis) associated bursitis and tendinitis in several parts of the body.

poly·tene (pol′e-tēn) [*poly-* + Gr. *tainia* band] composed of or containing many identical strands of chromatin lying in parallel; see under *chromosome.*

poly·teno·syn·o·vi·tis (pol″e-ten″o-sin″o-vi′tis) inflammation of several or many tendon sheaths at the same time.

poly·te·ny (pol″e-te′ne) successive reduplication of synapsed homologous chromosome pairs without separation into distinct daughter chromosomes or nuclear division.

poly·tet·ra·flu·o·ro·eth·y·lene (PTFE) (pol″e-tet″rə-floor″o-roeth′ə-lēn) polytef.

poly·the·lia (pol″e-the′le-ə) [*poly-* + *thel-* + *-ia*] the presence of more than the usual number of nipples; called also *hyperthelia.*

poly·the·lism (pol″e-the′liz-əm) polythelia.

poly·thene (pol′e-thēn) polyethylene; a formerly used name that is still used in England.

poly·thet·ic (pol″e-thet′ik) [*poly-* + Gr. *thetikos* fit for placing] denoting a taxonomic group classified on the basis of several characters, as opposed to a monothetic group.

poly·thi·a·zide (pol″ĭ-thi′ə-zīd) a thiazide diuretic, used in the treatment of hypertension and edema; administered orally.

po·lyt·o·cous (po-lit′ə-kəs) [*poly-* + *toc-* + *-ous*] giving birth to several offspring at one time.

poly·to·mo·gram (pol″e-to′mo-gram) the record produced by polytomography.

poly·to·mog·ra·phy (pol″e-to-mog′rə-fe) tomography of tissue at several predetermined planes. **polytomograph′ic** *adj*

po·lit·o·mous (po″lit′ə-məs) having more than two parts or sections; cf. *dichotomous.*

poly·trau·ma (pol″e-traw′mə) the occurrence of injuries to more than one body system.

poly·trich·ia (pol″e-trik′e-ə) hypertrichosis.

poly·tri·cho·sis (pol″e-trĭ-ko′sis) hypertrichosis.

Pol·y·trim (pol′e-trim) trademark for a combination preparation of trimethoprim sulfate and polymyxin B sulfate.

poly·tro·phia (pol″e-tro′fe-ə) [*poly-* + *troph-* + *-ia*] excessive nutrition. **polytroph′ic** *adj*

po·lyt·ro·phy (po-lit′rə-fe) polytrophia.

poly·tro·pic (pol″e-tro′pik) [*poly-* + *trop-* + *-ic*] affecting many kinds of bacteria, viruses, or tissues. Cf. *monotropic.*

poly·un·sat·u·rat·ed (pol″e-ən-sach′ər-āt″əd) of a chemical compound, containing two or more double or triple bonds; used particularly of fatty acids, such as linoleic acid.

poly·ure·thane (pol″e-u′rə-thān) any of a group of thermoplastic polymers, artificial rubbers that occur as fibers, coatings, moldable resins, elastomers, and foams; some are used in dentistry, particularly in maxillofacial prostheses.

poly·uria (pol″e-u′re-ə) [*poly-* + *-uria*] the passage of a large volume of urine in a given period, as in diabetes mellitus. Cf. *diuresis.*

poly·va·lent (pol″e-va′lənt) having more than one valence.

poly·vi·nyl (pol″e-vi′nəl) a polymerization product of a monomeric vinyl compound, as polyvinyl chloride.

p. acetate a light- and heat-stable resin formed by the polymerization of vinyl acetate.

p. alcohol see under *alcohol.*

p. chloride a tasteless, odorless, clear hard resin formed by the polymerization of vinyl chloride; its many uses include packaging, clothing, and insulation of pipes and wires. Workers in its manufacture are at risk primarily because of the toxicity of vinyl chloride. Excessive inhalation of its dust can cause polyvinyl chloride pneumoconiosis.

poly·vi·nyl·pyr·rol·i·done (pol″e-vi″nəl-pī-rōl′ĭ-dōn) povidone.

poly·zo·o·sper·mia (pol″e-zo″o-spur′me-ə) a rare condition in which the semen contains excessive numbers of highly motile sperm, with lowered fertility.

po·made (po-mād′) pomatum.

Po·mat·i·op·sis (po-mat″e-op′sis) a genus of amphibious freshwater snails of the family Bulimidae, native to the United States. *P. cincinnatien′sis* and *P. lapida′ria* are intermediate hosts of the lung fluke *Paragonimus kellicotti.*

po·ma·tum (po-ma′təm) [L., from *pomum* apple] a medicated ointment for the hair.

Pom·er·oy technique (operation) (pom′ər-oi) [Ralph Hayward *Pomeroy,* American obstetrician and gynecologist, 1867–1925] see under *technique.*

POMC pro-opiomelanocortin.

POMP a cancer chemotherapy regimen consisting of prednisone, Oncovin (vincristine), methotrexate, and Purinethol (6-mercaptopurine).

Pom·pe disease (pom′pə) [Johann Cassianius *Pompe,* Dutch physician, 20th century] glycogen storage disease (type II).

pom·pho·ly·he·mia (pom″fo-le-he′me-ə) [*pompholyx + hem- + -ia*] the presence of bubbles of gas in the blood, as in decompression sickness.

pom·pho·lyx (pom′fo-liks) [Gr. "bubble"] recurrent eczema with blistering on the palms and soles, particularly along the sides and between the digits, accompanied by pruritus, a burning sensation, and hyperhidrosis. The etiology is unknown, but in some cases it may be an allergic reaction; attacks are self-limited and usually last two to three weeks. Called also *dyshidrotic eczema.*

pon·ceau 3B (pon-so′) scarlet red; see under *red.*

Pon·cet disease (rheumatism) (paw-sa′) [Antonin *Poncet,* French surgeon, 1849–1913] tuberculous arthritis; see under *arthritis.*

Pond. [L.] pon′dere (by weight).

pon·der·al (pon′dər-əl) [L. *pondus,* weight] pertaining to weight.

pon·do·stat·u·ral (pon″do-stat′u-rəl) pertaining to weight and stature.

po·ne·si·a·trics (po-ne″ze-at′triks) [Gr. *ponēsis* toil, exertion + *-iatrics*] a system of therapy in which misdirected neurophysiologic reactions are made perceptible (as by the oscilloscope, electromyograph, etc.) and used as a guide in recognizing and correcting such undesirable responses (dysponesis).

Pon·gi·dae (pon′jĭ-de) the anthropoid apes, a family of primates that includes gibbons, gorillas, orangutans, and chimpanzees. Some are used in laboratory experiments because of their relationship to humans. See also *Anthropoidea* and *Hominoidea.*

Pon·go (pong′go) a genus of primates of the family Pongidae. *P. pyg′maeus* is the orangutan.

po·no·graph (po′no-graf) [Gr. *ponos* toil, suffering, pain + *-graph*] an instrument for estimating and recording sensitiveness of contracting muscles to pain.

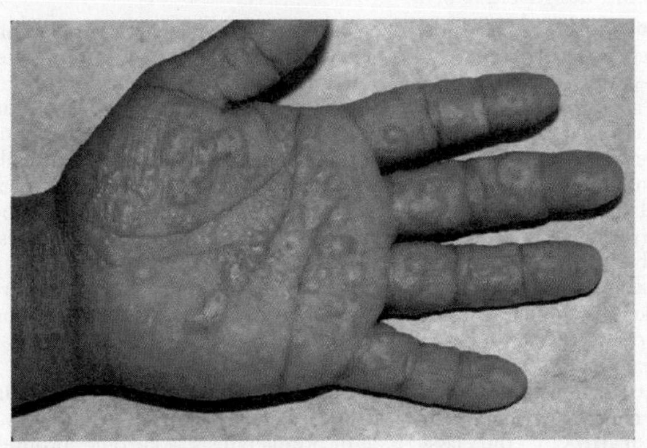

■ Pompholyx.

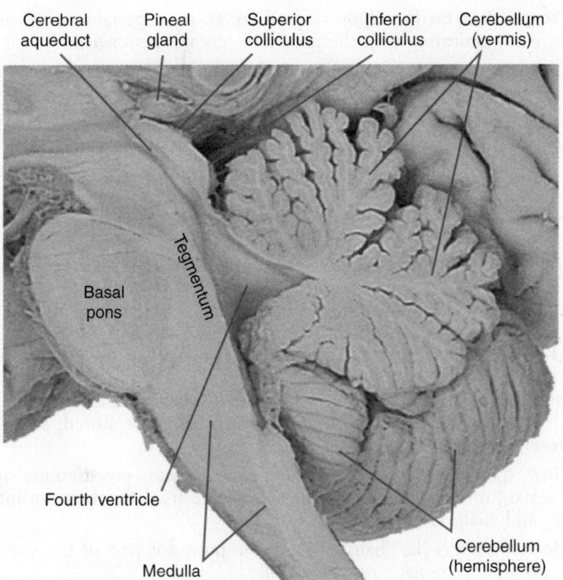

■ Pons and adjacent structures in a midline sagittal section.

pons (ponz) gen. *pon′tis* pl. *pon′tes* [L. "bridge"] 1. bridge: any slip of tissue connecting two parts of an organ. 2. [TA] the part of the central nervous system lying between the medulla oblongata and the mesencephalon, ventral to the cerebellum; it consists of an anterior and a posterior part (see *pars basilaris pontis* and *tegmentum pontis*). See Plate 9. See also *brainstem.*

p. et cerebel′lum TA alternative for *metencephalon* (def. 1).

p. he′patis an occasional projection of fibers partially bridging the longitudinal fissure of the liver.

Pon·se·ti method (pōn-sa′te) [Ignacio *Ponseti,* Spanish-born American orthopedic surgeon, born 1914] see under *method.*

Pon·stel (pon′stel) trademark for a preparation of mefenamic acid.

pon·tes (pon′tēz) [L.] plural of *pons.*

Pon·ti·ac fever (pon′te-ak) [*Pontiac,* Michigan, where an outbreak occurred among occupants of a single building in 1968] see under *fever.*

pon·tic (pon′tik) [L. *pons,* gen. *pontis* bridge] an artificial tooth on a fixed partial denture, which replaces the lost natural tooth, restores its function, and usually occupies the space previously occupied by the natural crown.

pon·tic·u·lar (pon-tik′u-lər) pertaining to a ponticulus.

pon·tic·u·lus (pon-tik′u-ləs) pl. *ponti′culi* [L., dim. of *pons* bridge] 1. a small ridge or bridgelike structure. 2. p. auriculae.

p. auri′culae a ridge of bone running posteriorly from the vestibular fenestra, delineating the superior margin of the tympanic sinus and providing the site of attachment of the posterior auricular muscle.

pon·tile (pon′tīl, pon′tēl) pertaining to the pons; pontine.

pon·tine (pon′tīn, pon′tēn) pertaining to the pons; pontile.

pont(o)- [L. *pons,* gen. *pontis* bridge] a prefix denoting relationship to the pons.

pon·to·bul·bar (pon″to-bul′bər) pertaining to, affecting, or regulated by the pons and the region of the medulla oblongata inferior to it.

pon·to·bul·bia (pon″to-bul′be-ə) syringomyelia extending into the medulla oblongata and pons.

Pon·to·caine (pon′to-kān) trademark for preparations of tetracaine.

pon·to·cer·e·bel·lar (pon″to-ser″ə-bel′ər) 1. pertaining to the pons and the cerebellum. 2. pertaining to the pontocerebellum (neocerebellum [TA]).

pon·to·cer·e·bel·lum (pon″to-ser″ə-bel′um) [*ponto- + cerebellum*] [TA] the portion of the cerebellum whose afferent inflow is predominantly supplied by corticopontocerebellar fibers, roughly corresponding to the cerebellar hemispheres; therefore, the term is sometimes equated with neocerebellum, which is the anatomical division of the cerebellum comprising the lateral parts, including most of the hemispheres and the middle portion of the vermis. Cf. *spinocerebellum* and *vestibulocerebellum.*

pon·to·med·ul·lary (pon″to-med′u-lar″e) pertaining to the pons and the medulla oblongata.

pon·to·mes·en·ce·phal·ic (pon″to-mes″ən-sə-fal′ik) pertaining to or involving the pons and the mesencephalon.

pon•to•pe•dun•cu•lar (pon″to-pə-dung′ku-lər) pertaining to, affecting, or communicating with the pons and cerebral peduncles.

Pool phenomenon (po̅o̅l) [Eugene Hillhouse *Pool*, American surgeon, 1874–1949] 1. see under *phenomenon.* 2. Schlesinger sign.

Pool-Schles•in•ger sign (po̅o̅l′ shla′zing-ər) [E.H. *Pool;* Hermann *Schlesinger*, Austrian physician, 1868–1934] Schlesinger sign.

pool (po̅o̅l) 1. a common reservoir on which to draw; a supply available to be used by a group. 2. to create such a reservoir or supply, such as the mixing of plasma from several donors. 3. an accumulation, as of blood in any part of the body due to retardation of the venous circulation.

gene p. the totality of the genes possessed by all of the members of a population.

metabolic p. the entire mass of labile and reactive substances in the body, to which and from which innumerable substances continuously pass; also used in a restricted sense to mean the extracellular pool or the potassium pool.

storage p. the area of a platelet organelle such as a dense body or an alpha granule where specific chemical constituents are stored; see *storage pool disease*, under *disease.*

pop•lar (pop′lər) any tree of the genus *Populus;* preparations of the bark, leaves, or leaf buds of various species are used for their antiinflammatory and analgesic effects.

pop•les (pop′lez) [L. "ham"] [TA] the posterior part of the knee; see also *regio genus posterior.* **poplit′eal** *adj*

pop•py (pop′e) 1. any plant of the family Papaveraceae. 2. the flower of such a plant.

California p. 1. *Eschscholtzia californica.* 2. a preparation of *E. californica*, used for its sedative, hypnotic, and anxiolytic effects, usually in combination with other herbal sedatives, but sometimes prepared alone as a tea; used also in homeopathy for insomnia.

prickly p. *Argemone mexicana.*

pop•u•la•tion (pop″u-la′shən) [L. *populatio*, from *populus* people] 1. the individuals collectively constituting a certain category or inhabiting a specified geographic area. 2. in statistics, a theoretical concept used to describe an entire group or collection of units, finite or infinite; from it a sample can be drawn.

Pop•u•lus (pop′u-lus) the poplars, a genus of deciduous flowering trees of the family Salicaceae, found in the Northern Hemisphere. *P. can′dicans* Aiton has buds that contain volatile oils and resins and are used medicinally, and the bark, leaves, and leaf buds of a number of species contain salicylic acid derivatives and are used for their antiinflammatory and analgesic effects. See *balm of Gilead* (def. 1).

POR problem-oriented record.

por•ac•tant al•fa (por-ak′tant al′fə) an extract of porcine lung surfactant comprising 99 per cent polar lipids and 1 per cent hydrophobic proteins; administered by instillation via the endotracheal tube in the treatment of neonatal respiratory distress syndrome.

por•ade•nia (por″ə-de′ne-ə) poradenitis.

por•ad•e•ni•tis (por-ad″ə-ni′tis) [*por-*[1] + *adenitis*] a disease of the iliac lymph nodes characterized by formation of small abscesses. Called also *poradenia.*

por•ce•lain (por′sə-lən) 1. a white, translucent, dense ceramic material produced by fusing under high temperature of a mixture of feldspar, kaolin, quartz, whiting, and other substances. 2. dental p.

dental p. a type of porcelain used in dental restorations, either jacket crowns or inlays, artificial teeth, or metal-ceramic crowns. It is essentially a mixture of particles of feldspar and quartz, the feldspar melting first and providing a glass matrix for the quartz.

por•ce•la•ne•ous (por″sə-la′ne-əs) pertaining to or resembling porcelain.

por•cine (por′sīn) [L. *porcus* a pig, hog] pertaining to, characteristic of, or derived from domesticated pigs or other members of the family Suidae. Called also *suid.*

pore (por) [L. *porus*, q.v.] porus; a small opening. **por′al** *adj*

acoustic p., external porus acusticus externus.

acoustic p., internal porus acusticus internus.

alveolar p's openings between adjacent pulmonary alveoli that permit passage of air from one to another; called also *pores of Kohn.*

birth p. metraterm.

dilated p. of Winer a solitary pore on the face, back, or extremities, filled by a keratinous plug that is surrounded by hyperplastic follicular epithelium.

gustatory p. porus gustatorius.

interalveolar p's, p's of Kohn alveolar p's.

nuclear p's small octagonal openings in the nuclear envelope at sites where the two nuclear membranes are in contact and through which transport between the nucleus and the cytoplasm occurs; the pore and the associated structures embedded in its rim form the nuclear pore complex. See also Plate 11.

slit p's small slitlike spaces between the pedicels of the podocytes of the renal glomerulus. Called also *filtration slits.*

sweat p. the opening of a sweat duct on the surface of the skin; called also *porus sudoriferus.*

taste p. porus gustatorius.

por•en•ce•pha•lia (por″en-sə-fal′e-ə) porencephaly.

por•en•ceph•a•li•tis (por″en-sef″ə-li′tis) porencephaly associated with an inflammatory process, such as polioencephalitis.

por•en•ceph•a•ly (por″en-sef′ə-le) the presence of one or more cavities in the brain, which sometimes communicate with the arachnoid space, most often occurring in fetal life or early infancy. Called also *cerebral porosis, perencephaly*, and *porencephalia.* **porencephal′ic, porenceph′alous** *adj*

encephaloclastic p. porencephaly in which the cavities are residues of destructive lesions after birth.

schizencephalic p. porencephaly in which the cavities are the result of maldevelopment of the brain. Called also *schizencephaly.*

por•fi•mer so•di•um (por′fĭ-mər) a hematoporphyrin derivative used as a photosensitizer in photodynamic therapy for esophageal carcinoma and non–small cell lung carcinoma; administered intravenously.

por•fi•ro•my•cin (por″fĭ-ro-mi′sin) the methyl derivative of mitomycin C; an antineoplastic antibiotic derived from *Streptomyces aridus.*

po•ri (po′ri) [L.] genitive and plural of *porus.*

Po•rif•e•ra (pə-rif′ə-rə) [L. *porus* pore + *ferre* to bear] the sponges, a phylum of invertebrates whose bodies are perforated with many pores to admit water from which food is strained.

po•rin (por′in) any of a class of transmembrane matrix proteins found in the outer membranes of mitochondria and some gram-negative bacteria; they form trimers that contain water-filled channels for a variety of small hydrophilic molecules.

po•rio•ma•nia (por″e-o-ma′ne-ə) [Gr. *poreia* walking + *-mania*] an irresistible impulse to travel, run away, or wander off.

po•ri•on (por′e-on) [*por-*[1] + *-on* neuter ending] a craniometric landmark, being the most lateral point on the roof of the bony external acoustic meatus, vertically over the middle of the meatus. Called also *point Po.*

por(o)-[1] [Gr. *poros*, passage] a combining form denoting relationship to a duct, passageway, opening, or pore.

por(o)-[2] [Gr. *pōros* callus, stone] a combining form denoting relationship to a callus or calculus.

po•ro•car•ci•no•ma (por″o-kahr″sĭ-no′mə) [*poro-*[1] + *carcinoma*] an adnexal carcinoma that arises in a sweat pore; cf. *poroma.*

eccrine p. a carcinoma arising from the sweat pore of an eccrine gland, usually occurring as a plaque, ulcer, or pedunculated mass on a limb.

po•ro•ceph•a•li•a•sis (por″o-sef″ə-li′ə-sis) infection with parasitic pentastomes of the order Porocephalida.

Poro•ce•phal•i•da (por″o-sə-fal′ĭ-də) an order of the phylum Pentastomida, including the families Linguatulidae and Porocephalidae.

Poro•ce•phal•i•dae (por″o-sə-fal′ĭ-de) a family of the phylum Pentastomida, having cylindrical bodies. Adults are found in the lungs of reptiles, and larvae are found in various vertebrates. Genera include *Armillifer* and *Porocephalus.*

po•ro•ceph•a•lo•sis (por″o-sef″ə-lo′sis) porocephaliasis.

Po•ro•ceph•a•lus (por″o-sef′ə-ləs) [*poro-*[1] + *-cephalus*] a genus of the phylum Pentastomida, family Porocephalidae. *P. armilla′tus* has been reclassified as *Armillifer armillatus.*

po•ro•fo•con (por″o-fo′kon) either of two hydrophobic contact lens materials, designated A or B.

po•ro•ker•a•to•sis (por″o-ker″ə-to′sis) [*poro-*[2] + *keratosis*] any of several chronic, progressive disorders of keratinization, seen most often in light-skinned persons. The characteristic lesion is round and craterlike with an atrophic center and an elevated, thick, keratotic border formed by a cornoid lamella; lesions may enlarge into circinate, serpiginous, or gyrate forms. Lesions can be premalignant, progressing to basal cell carcinoma or squamous cell carcinoma. It is sometimes inherited as an autosomal dominant disorder, but most cases are sporadic, and a number of factors, including ultraviolet exposure, infection, and immunosuppression, may be involved in its pathogenesis. **porokeratot′ic** *adj*

disseminated superficial actinic p. an autosomal dominant form of porokeratosis, characterized by brown to red, superficial conical papules that occur on sun-exposed skin, usually on the limbs of females over 16 years of age.

linear p. a skin disorder of uncertain heritability, usually appearing in early childhood, characterized by linear papules along Blaschko lines.

p. of Mibelli the classic type of porokeratosis, a chronic, progressive, autosomal dominant type seen most often in males, usually first appearing in early childhood. Lesions are isolated, light brown papules with irregular shapes and a surrounding ridge that is often bifurcated; they may grow to several centimeters in diameter.

p. palma′ris et planta′ris dissemina′ta a variant of punctate porokeratosis characterized by small, superficial, slightly discolored lesions on the soles or palms or both, with gyrate or annular shapes; there may be hundreds of lesions, and they may later appear elsewhere on the body.

p. ptychotro′pica a rare verrucous variant of porokeratosis, affecting the gluteal cleft and characterized by pruritic, confluent plaques in the perianal region that extend symmetrically to the buttocks.

p. puncta′ta palma′ris et planta′ris, punctate p. a skin disorder affecting the palms and soles and occurring during or after adolescence, characterized by tiny keratotic plugs that have elevated margins and do not enlarge; patients often exhibit either linear or Mibelli porokeratosis elsewhere on the body.

po•ro•ma (pə-ro′mə) [Gr. *pōrōma* callus] a type of adnexal adenoma arising within or on the side of a sweat pore.

apocrine p. a poroma arising from the sweat pore of an apocrine sweat gland.

eccrine p. a poroma arising from the sweat pore of an eccrine sweat gland, often on the palm or sole.

po•ro•plas•tic (por″o-plas′tik) both porous and plastic.

po•ro•sis[1] (pə-ro′sis) [Gr. *poros* passage] cavity formation.

cerebral p. porencephaly.

po•ro•sis[2] (pə-ro′sis) [Gr. *pōrōsis*, from *pōros* marble] the formation of the callus in the repair of a fractured bone.

po•ros•i•ty (pə-ros′ĭ-te) 1. the condition of being porous. 2. pore.

po•rot•ic (pə-rot′ik) pertaining to or characterized by porosis favoring the growth of connective tissue.

por•ous (por′əs) penetrated by pores and open spaces.

por•phin (por′fin) a heterocyclic structure composed of four pyrrole rings connected by methylidyne (—CH=) bridges; it is the parent skeleton of the porphyrins.

por•pho•bi•lin•o•gen (por″fo-bĭ-lin′ə-jən) the immediate precursor of the porphyrins, a pyrrole ring with acetyl, propionyl, and aminomethyl side chains; four molecules of porphobilinogen are condensed to form one molecule of uroporphyrinogen III, which is then converted successively to coproporphyrinogen III, protoporphyrin IX, and heme. Porphobilinogen is produced in excess and excreted in the urine in acute intermittent porphyria and several other porphyrias. Abbreviated PBG.

por•pho•bi•lin•o•gen de•am•in•ase (por″fo-bĭ-lin′ə-jən de-am′in-ās) hydroxymethylbilane synthase.

por•pho•bi•lin•o•gen syn•thase (por″fo-bĭ-lin′o-jən sin′thās) [EC 4.2.1.24] an enzyme of the lyase class that catalyzes the condensation of two molecules of δ-aminolevulinate to form porphobilinogen in the synthesis of porphyrins. The enzyme is inhibited by minute quantities of lead poisoning. Genetic deficiency of the enzyme causes a porphyria similar to acute intermittent porphyria but with high urinary levels of δ-aminolevulinic acid, coproporphyrinogen III, and protoporphyrin but not porphobilinogen. Called also *aminolevulinate dehydratase.*

por•pho•bi•lin•o•gen•uria (por″fo-bĭ-lin′o-jə-nu′re-ə) the excretion of urine containing porphobilinogen, as in acute intermittent porphyria.

por•phy•ria (por-fēr′e-ə) [Gr. *porphyra* purple] any of a group of disturbances of porphyrin metabolism, characterized biochemically by marked increase in formation and excretion of porphyrins or their precursors and clinically by various neurologic and cutaneous manifestations. The types are generally classified as hepatic, erythropoietic, and sometimes erythrohepatic, depending on the location of expression of the biochemical defect.

acute p. acute intermittent p.

acute intermittent p. (AIP) an autosomal dominant hepatic porphyria caused by mutation in the *HMBS* gene (locus: 11q23.3), which encodes hydroxymethylbilane synthase; it is manifested by recurrent attacks of abdominal pain, gastrointestinal dysfunction, and neurologic disturbances and by excessive amounts of δ-aminolevulinic acid and porphobilinogen in the urine. Called also *acute p., intermittent acute p., Swedish p.,* and *pyrroloporphyria.*

congenital erythropoietic p. (CEP) an autosomal recessive porphyria due to mutation in the *UROS* gene (locus: 10q25.2-q26.3), which encodes uroporphyrinogen-III synthase, resulting in increased synthesis of uroporphyrinogen I relative to uroporphyrinogen III in bone marrow erythroblasts; it is characterized by cutaneous photosensitivity leading to mutilating skin lesions, by hemolytic anemia and splenomegaly, and by greatly increased urinary excretion of uroporphyrin I and coproporphyrin I. Erythrodontia and hypertrichosis are invariably present. Called also *congenital photosensitive p., Günther disease,* and *erythropoietic uroporphyria.*

congenital photosensitive p. congenital erythropoietic p.

p. cuta′nea tar′da (PCT) the most common form of porphyria, characterized by cutaneous photosensitivity that causes scarring bullae, hyperpigmentation, facial hypertrichosis, and sometimes sclerodermatous thickenings and alopecia; it is frequently associated with alcohol abuse, liver disease, or hepatic siderosis. Urinary levels of uroporphyrin and coproporphyrin are increased and activity of uroporphyrinogen decarboxylase (UROD) is decreased. Three types are generally recognized, all of them heterozygous and clinically apparent beginning in adulthood, precipitated by disease or environmental factors. In types I and III, UROD activity is reduced only in the liver; type I, the most common form, is sporadic but presumed to be genetically determined, while type III is a very rare familial form. Type II is an autosomal dominant form caused by mutation in the *UROD* gene (locus: 1p34); enzyme activity is decreased to approximately 50 per cent systemically. A severe homozygous variant of type II *(hepatoerythropoietic p.)* results in virtual absence of enzyme activity.

cutaneous hepatic p. p. cutanea tarda.

erythrohepatic p. porphyria in which abnormal overproduction of porphyrins and precursors occurs in both liver and bone marrow; when this category is used in classifying porphyrias, it usually includes only erythropoietic protoporphyria. Cf. *erythropoietic p.*

erythropoietic p. porphyria in which excessive formation of porphyrin or its precursors occurs in bone marrow erythroblasts; usually congenital erythropoietic porphyria, but in some classification schemes (those not including a category erythrohepatic porphyria, q.v.) also including erythropoietic protoporphyria.

hepatic p. porphyria in which the excess formation of porphyrin or its precursors is found in the liver; it includes acute intermittent porphyria, variegate porphyria, and hereditary coproporphyria.

hepatoerythropoietic p. (HEP) a severe homozygous form of porphyria cutanea tarda (PCT) type II, believed to result from an autosomal dominant defect in uroporphyrinogen decarboxylase activity; it is clinically identical to PCT but onset is in early childhood and enzyme activity in liver, erythrocytes, and fibroblasts is virtually absent.

intermittent acute p. acute intermittent p.

mixed p., South African genetic p. variegate p.

Swedish p. former name for *acute intermittent p.*

symptomatic p. p. cutanea tarda.

p. variega′ta, variegate p. (VP) an autosomal dominant hepatic porphyria due to mutation in the *PPOX* gene (locus: 1q22), which encodes protoporphyrinogen oxidase, resulting in partial deficiency of enzyme activity. It is characterized by various combinations of chronic cutaneous photosensitivity with lesions and extreme skin fragility, attacks of abdominal pain, neuropathy, and gastrointestinal dysfunction. Fecal protoporphyrin and coproporphyrin are elevated continually and urinary coproporphyrin, δ-aminolevulinic acid, and porphobilinogen are elevated during acute attacks. Called also *mixed p., South African genetic p.,* and *protocoproporphyria.*

por•phy•rin (por′fə-rin) any of a group of compounds containing the porphin structure, four pyrrole rings connected by methylidyne (—CH=) bridges in a cyclic configuration, to which a variety of side chains may be attached. The nature of the side chains is indicated by a prefix, such as *coproporphyrin, etioporphyrin, hematoporphyrin, mesoporphyrin, protoporphyrin,* or *uroporphyrin.* Structural isomers are indicated by roman numerals. Free porphyrins are rarely found in tissues except in disorders of heme biosynthesis *(porphyrias),* but they do occur in the prosthetic groups of hemoglobin, myoglobin, and cytochromes, complexed with metal ions. The term is sometimes used to include porphin or to denote porphin specifically. See also *porphyrinogen* and *chlorophyll.*

por•phy•rin•emia (por″fĭ-rĭ-ne′me-ə) the presence of porphyrin in the plasma or serum.

por•phy•rin•o•gen (por″fə-rin′ə-jən) the reduced form of a porphyrin, containing pyrrole rings linked by methylene (—CH_2—) instead of methylidyne bridges. The porphyrinogen forms are the functional intermediates in the biosynthesis of heme and if oxidized to their corresponding

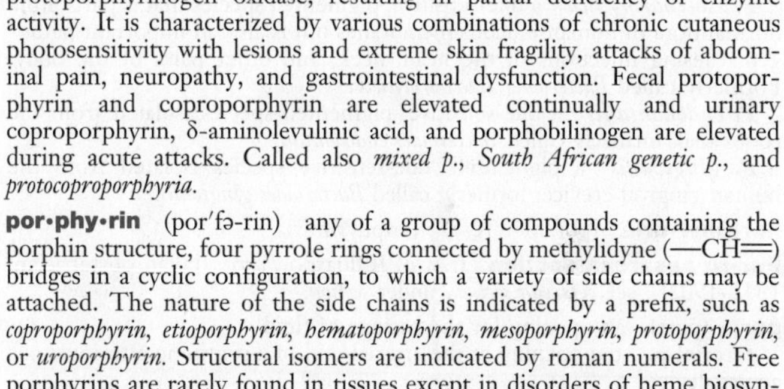

■ Porphyrin. *(A)*, Pyrrole ring; *(B)*, porphin ring; *(C)*, protoporphyrin IX.

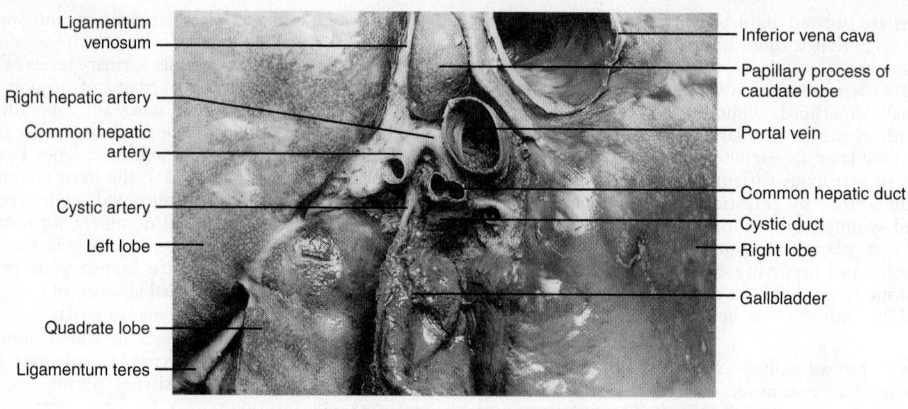

■ Visceral surface of the liver, showing the structures at the porta hepatis.

porphyrins, such as occurs in porphyrias, are irreversibly removed from the biosynthetic pathway and accumulate in tissues. Their nomenclature corresponds to that of the porphyrins.

por·phy·rin·uria (por″fə-rĭ-nu′re-ə) excessive excretion of one or more porphyrins in the urine; see *porphyria.*

Por·phy·ro·mo·na·da·ceae (por″fĭ-ro-mo″nə-da′se-e) a family of gram-negative, rod-shaped bacteria of the phylum Bacteroidetes. It contains the genera *Dysgonomonas* and *Porphyromonas.*

Por·phy·ro·mo·nas (por″fĭ-ro-mo′nəs) [Gr. *porphyra* purple + *monas* unit, from *monos* single] a genus of gram-negative, obligately anaerobic, nonmotile, non–spore-forming, rod-shaped bacteria of the family Porphyromonadaceae that are normal inhabitants of the mucous membranes of the oral cavity; organisms have been isolated from oral infections. Included here are species formerly included in the genus *Bacteroides.* The type species is *P. asaccharoly′tica.*

P. asaccharoly′tica a bile-sensitive, pigmented species that is part of the normal flora of human mucous membranes but is also an important pathogen, causing infections of the head, neck, and other parts of the body. Formerly called *Bacteroides asaccharolyticus.*

P. endodonta′lis a bile-sensitive, pigmented species isolated from the root canal; formerly called *Bacteroides endodontalis.*

P. gingiva′lis a pigmented, bile-sensitive species isolated from the human gingival crevice; formerly called *Bacteroides gingivalis.*

por·phyr·uria (por″fir-u′re-ə) porphyrinuria.

Por·ro cesarean section (por′o) [Edoardo *Porro,* Italian obstetrician, 1842–1902] see *cesarean section,* under *section.*

port (port) an opening for the passage of fluid.

arterial p. the opening at the arterial end of a synthetic arteriovenous access device.

por·ta (por′tə) pl. *por′tae* [L.] anatomical nomenclature for an opening, especially the site of entrance to an organ of the blood vessels and other structures supplying or draining it.

p. he′patis [TA] hepatic portal: the transverse fissure on the visceral surface of the liver where the portal vein and hepatic artery enter the liver and the hepatic ducts leave.

p. lie′nis hilum splenicum.

p. of lung hilum pulmonis.

p. pulmo′nis hilum pulmonis.

p. re′nis hilum renale.

p. of spleen hilum splenicum.

por·ta·ca·val (por″tə-ka′vəl) pertaining to or connecting the portal vein and the vena cava.

por·tal (por′təl) 1. porta. 2. pertaining to a porta, or entrance, especially to the porta hepatis.

hepatic p. porta hepatis.

intestinal p., anterior the region of opening of the embryonic foregut into the yolk sac or unclosed midgut.

intestinal p., posterior the region of opening of the embryonic hindgut into the yolk sac or unclosed midgut.

por·ta·sys·tem·ic (por″tə-sis-tem′ik) portosystemic.

porte-ai·guille (port″a-gwe′) [Fr.] a surgeon's needle holder.

porte·pol·ish·er (port-pol′ish-ər) a hand instrument constructed to hold a wooden point, to be used in a dental engine for applying polishing paste to and burnishing teeth. Written also *porte-polisher.*

Por·ter sign (por′tər) [William Henry *Porter,* Irish physician, 1790–1861] tracheal tugging; see under *tugging.*

Por·ter-Sil·ber chromogens, reaction (por′tər sil′bər) [Curt Culwell *Porter,* American biochemist, 20th century; Robert Howard *Silber,* American biochemist, 20th century] see under *chromogen* and *reaction.*

Por·te·us maze test (por′te-əs) [Stanley David *Porteus,* Australian-born psychologist in United States, 1883–1972] see under *test.*

por·tio (por′she-o) pl. *portio′nes* [L.] portion; a division of a larger anatomical structure. See also *pars* and *part.*

p. mi′nor ner′vi trige′mini radix motoria nervi trigemini.

p. ma′jor ner′vi trige′mini radix sensoria nervi trigemini.

p. supravagina′lis cer′vicis [TA] supravaginal portion of cervix: the part of the cervix uteri that does not protrude into the vagina.

p. vagina′lis cer′vicis [TA] vaginal portion of cervix: the part of the cervix uteri that protrudes into the vagina and is lined with stratified squamous epithelium. Called also *ectocervix* and *exocervix.*

por·tion (por′shən) a part or division of a larger structure; called also *portio* [TA], *part,* and *pars.*

Positions of the Fetus in Various Presentations

Presentation	Point of Direction	Position	Abbreviation
Cephalic Presentation			
Vertex	Occiput	Left occipitoanterior	LOA
		Left occipitoposterior	LOP
		Left occipitotransverse	LOT
		Right occipitoanterior	ROA
		Right occipitoposterior	ROP
		Right occipitotransverse	ROT
Face	Chin	Left mentoanterior	LMA
		Left mentoposterior	LMP
		Left mentotransverse	LMT
		Right mentoanterior	RMA
		Right mentoposterior	RMP
		Right mentotransverse	RMT
Brow	Brow	Left frontoanterior	LFA
		Left frontoposterior	LFP
		Left frontotransverse	LFT
		Right frontoanterior	RFA
		Right frontoposterior	RFP
		Right frontotransverse	RFT
Pelvic Presentation (Breech)			
Complete breech (feet crossed and thighs flexed on abdomen)	Sacrum	Left sacroanterior	LSA
		Left sacroposterior	LSP
		Left sacrotransverse	LST
		Right sacroanterior	RSA
		Right sacroposterior	RSP
		Right sacrotransverse	RST
Incomplete breech	Sacrum	Same designations as above, adding the qualifications footling, knee, etc.	
Shoulder Presentation (Transverse Lie)			
Shoulder	Scapula	Left scapuloanterior	LScA
		Left scapuloposterior	LScP
		Right scapuloanterior	RScA
		Right scapuloposterior	RScP

por·ti·o·nes (por″she-o′nēz) [L.] plural of *portio.*

port·lig·a·ture (port-lig′ə-chər) [Fr. *porte-ligature*] an instrument for applying a ligature in a deep wound.

por·to·en·ter·os·to·my (por″to-en″tər-os′tə-me) surgical anastomosis of the jejunum to an intrahepatic biliary radicle; done to establish a conduit from the intrahepatic bile ducts to the intestine in biliary atresia or stenosis or common duct tumor. Called also *hepatic* or *Kasai p.* and *Kasai operation.*

por·to·gram (por′to-gram) a radiograph of the portal vein.

por·tog·ra·phy (por-tog′rə-fe) radiography of the portal vein after injection of opaque material.

portal p. portography after injection of opaque material into the superior mesenteric vein or one of its branches after laparotomy has been performed.

splenic p. portography after percutaneous injection into the substance of the spleen, usually through the ninth intercostal space in the midaxillary line, of opaque material, which passes immediately into the splenic vein, and then into the portal vein, permitting visualization of those two vessels.

por·to·je·ju·nos·to·my (por″to-je″joo-nos′tə-me) portoenterostomy.

por·to·sys·tem·ic (por″to-sis-tem′ik) connecting the portal and systemic venous circulation. Called also *portasystemic.*

por·to·ve·no·gram (por″to-ve′no-gram) portogram.

por·to·ve·nog·ra·phy (por″to-ve-nog′rə-fe) portography.

Por·tu·guese man-of-war (por′chə-gēs) any cnidarian of the genus *Physalia.*

po·rus (por′əs) gen. and pl. *po′ri* [L., from Gr. *poros* passage] pore; a small opening.

p. acus′ticus exter′nus [TA] the outer end of the external acoustic meatus.

p. acus′ticus inter′nus [TA] the opening of the internal acoustic meatus.

p. gustato′rius [TA] gustatory pore: the small opening of a taste bud onto the surface of the tongue. Called also *taste pore.*

p. op′ticus the opening in the sclera for passage of the optic nerve.

p. sudori′ferus sweat pore.

po·sa·con·a·zole (po″sə-kon′ə-zōl) a triazole antifungal that inhibits synthesis of ergosterol and so disrupts the fungal cell membrane; used in treatment of many different fungal infections, administered orally.

Po·sa·das disease (po-sah′dahs) [Alejandro *Posadas,* Argentine pathologist, 1870–1920] coccidioidomycosis.

Po·sa·das-Wer·ni·cke disease (po-sah′dahs ver′nĭ-ke) [A. *Posadas;* Robert *Wernicke,* Argentine pathologist, 1854–1922] coccidioidomycosis.

-posia [Gr. *posis* a drink + *-ia*] a word termination denoting relationship to drinking, or to intake of fluids.

po·si·tion (pə-zish′ən) [L. *positio*] 1. a bodily posture or attitude assumed by the patient to achieve comfort in certain conditions, or the particular disposition of the body and limbs to facilitate the performance of certain diagnostic or therapeutic procedures. 2. in obstetrics, the situation of the fetus in the pelvis, determined and described by the relation of a given arbitrary point (point of direction) in the presenting part to a given arbitrary point in the coronal plane of the maternal pelvis. For the various possible positions see accompanying table. Cf. *presentation.*

Position

Albert p. a semirecumbent position of the patient for radiography as a means of determining the diameters of the superior strait of the pelvis.

anatomic p., anatomical p. the position of the human body, standing erect, with the face directed anteriorly, the upper limbs at the sides and the palms turned anteriorly (supinated), and the feet pointed anteriorly; used as the position of reference in description of site or direction of various structures or parts as established in official anatomical nomenclature.

batrachian p. a lying position of infants in which the lower limbs are flexed, abducted, and resting on the bed on their outer aspects, somewhat resembling the legs of a frog. Called also *frog leg* or *froglike p.*

Bozeman p. knee-elbow position in which the patient is strapped to supports.

Brickner p. a position for treating shoulder disability, secured by tying the patient's wrist to the head of the bed with the arm supported on a pillow and the head of the bed raised; thus traction with abduction and external rotation is obtained.

Caldwell p. a radiographic position with the forehead and nose against the x-ray plate, used with the Caldwell projection.

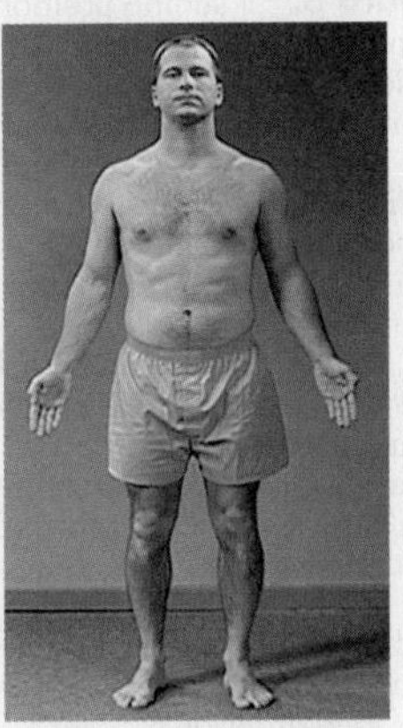

■ Anatomical position.

Casselberry p. a prone position employed after intubation so that the patient may swallow without danger of fluid entering the tube.

centric p. the rest position of the mandible, as it is influenced by the muscle tone, while the patient remains standing or is sitting with jaw open, from which the teeth will come into centric occlusion when the jaw is closed.

***cis* p.** see under *configuration.*

coiled p. the patient lies on one side with hips and knees flexed and thighs drawn up to the body.

decubitus p. the position of an individual lying on a horizontal surface, designated, according to the portion of the body resting on the surface, *dorsal decubitus* (lying on the back), *left lateral decubitus* (on the left side), *right lateral decubitus* (on the right side), or *ventral decubitus* (on the abdomen).

Depage p. a prone position with the pelvis raised to form the apex of an inverted V, while the trunk and lower limbs form the branches of the V.

dorsal p. the posture of a person lying on the back; called also *supine p.*

dorsal elevated p. the patient lies on the back with shoulders and head elevated.

dorsal recumbent p. the patient lies on the back with lower limbs flexed and rotated outward; used in vaginal examination, application of obstetrical forceps, and other procedures.

dorsal rigid p. the patient lies on the back with hips and knees flexed and thighs drawn up to the body.

dorsosacral p. lithotomy p.

Duncan p. the position of the placenta with its margin presenting at the os for delivery.

eccentric p. see under *relation.*

Edebohls p. a dorsal position with knees and thighs drawn up, lower limbs flexed on thighs, and thighs flexed on abdomen; the hips are raised and the thighs abducted. Called also *Simon p.*

Elliot p. a position used for abdominal surgery; the patient lies on the operating table with lower chest elevated by a support under the lower costal margin.

emprosthotonos p. emprosthotonos.

English p. Sims p.

figure four p. the patient lies with one side of the body upwards and the lower limb of that side flexed with its ankle resting on the opposite knee so that the lower limbs are in the shape of a 4.

Position *Continued*

Fowler p. a position in which the patient sits straight upright or leaning back slightly; the legs can be straight or bent at the knees.

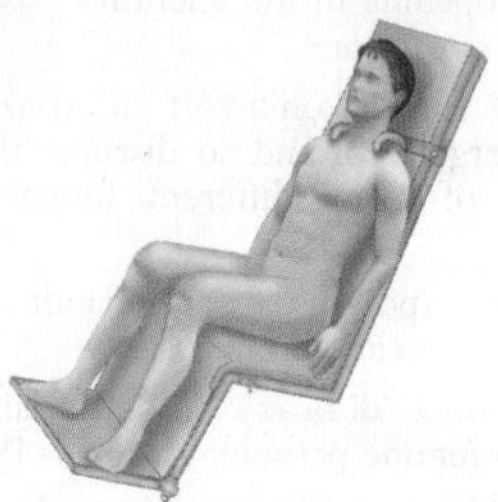

frog leg p., froglike p. batrachian p.
frontal anterior p. frontoanterior p.
frontal posterior p. frontoposterior p.
frontal transverse p. frontotransverse p.
frontoanterior p. a position of the fetus in cephalic presentation in labor, with its brow directed toward the right (RFA) or left (LFA) anterior quadrant of the maternal pelvis.
frontoposterior p. a position of the fetus in cephalic presentation in labor, with its brow directed toward the right (RFP) or left (LFP) posterior quadrant of the maternal pelvis.
frontotransverse p. a position of the fetus in cephalic presentation in labor, with its brow directed toward the right (RFT) or left (LFT) iliac fossa of the maternal pelvis.
Fuchs p. a radiographic position which gives an oblique view of the zygomatic arch projected free of superimposed structures.
genucubital p. knee-elbow p.
genufacial p. a position in which the patient is supported on the knees and face.
genupectoral p. knee-chest p.
hinge p. the position of the condyle in the temporomandibular joint from which an opening by hinge movement is possible beyond the amplitude of rest position.
hinge p., condylar the position of the condyles in the glenoid fossa at which hinge axis movement is possible.
hinge p., mandibular a position of the mandible that allows the condyles to move on the hinge axis during the opening or closing of the jaws.
horizontal p. the patient lies on the back with limbs extended.
jackknife p. a position used for anorectal surgery; the patient lies prone with the buttocks raised. Called also *Kraske p.*
Jones p. acute flexion of the forearm for the treatment of fracture of the internal condyle of the humerus.
knee-chest p. a position in which the patient is supported by knees and chest resting on the table.

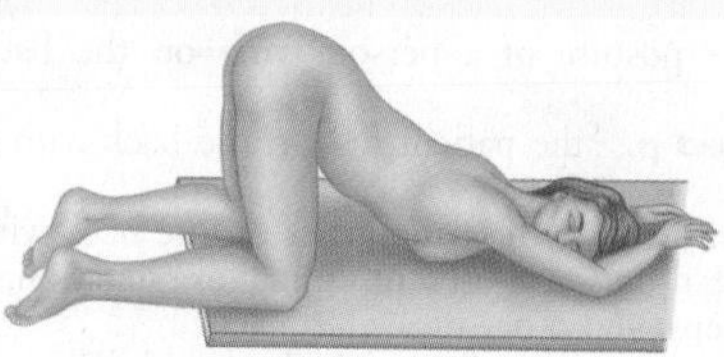

knee-elbow p. a position in which the patient is supported on knees and elbows with the chest elevated from the table.
Kraske p. jackknife p.
lateral recumbent p. Sims p.
lithotomy p. the patient lies in dorsal decubitus with hips and knees flexed and the thighs abducted and externally rotated; called also *dorsosacral p.*

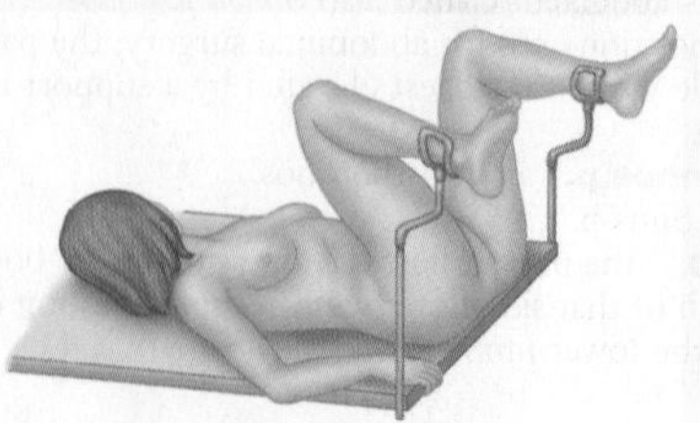

Mayer p. a radiographic position that gives a unilateral superoinferior view of the temporomandibular joint, external auditory canal, and mastoid and petrous processes; helpful in demonstrating fractures and malformations of the temporomandibular joint and in the study of bony atresia of the external auditory canal.
mentoanterior p. a position of the fetus in cephalic presentation in labor, with its chin directed toward the right (RMA) or left (LMA) anterior quadrant of the maternal pelvis.
mentoposterior p. a position of the fetus in cephalic presentation in labor, with its chin directed toward the right (RMP) or left (LMP) posterior quadrant of the maternal pelvis.
mentotransverse p. a position of the fetus in cephalic presentation in labor, with its chin directed toward the right (RMT) or left (LMT) iliac fossa of the maternal pelvis.
mentum anterior p. mentoanterior p.
mentum posterior p. mentoposterior p.
mentum transverse p. mentotransverse p.
occipitoanterior p. a position of the fetus in cephalic presentation in labor, with its occiput directed toward the right (ROA) or left (LOA) anterior quadrant of the maternal pelvis.
occipitoposterior p. a position of the fetus in cephalic presentation in labor, with its occiput directed toward the right (ROP) or left (LOP) posterior quadrant of the maternal pelvis.
occipitosacral p. a position of the fetus in cephalic presentation in labor, with the occiput presenting directly behind, or rotated squarely into the hollow of the sacrum.
occipitotransverse p. a position of the fetus in cephalic presentation in labor, with its occiput directed toward the right (ROT) or left (LOT) iliac fossa of the maternal pelvis.
occiput anterior p. occipitoanterior p.
occiput posterior p. occipitoposterior p.
occiput sacral p. occipitosacral p.
occiput transverse p. occipitotransverse p.
occlusal p. a functional position of the jaws in which contact between some or all of the upper and lower teeth occurs when the mandible is closed, which may or may not coincide with centric occlusion. Called also *occlusal relation.*
opisthotonos p. opisthotonos.
orthopnea p. the patient either sits upright in a chair or assumes an upright or semivertical position by using two or more pillows to support the head and chest from the recumbent position; used for a patient with orthopnea (difficulty breathing except in the upright position).
orthotonos p. orthotonos.
physiologic rest p. rest p.
posterior border p. the most posterior position of the mandible at any specific vertical relation to the maxillae. Called also *posterior border jaw relation.*
prone p. the attitude in which the patient patient lies face down.
rest p. the position of the mandible when its muscles are at rest, the body is in the upright standing or sitting position, and the eyes are focused toward the horizon; the lips are slightly touching and the distance between the upper and lower teeth has a free-way space of about 2 to 5 mm. Called also *physiologic rest p.* and *rest jaw relation.*
reverse Trendelenburg p. a supine position with the patient on a plane inclined with the head higher than the rest of the body and appropriate safety devices such as a footboard.
Robson p. a position for surgery of the biliary tract; the patient lies supine with a sandbag beneath the eleventh and twelfth ribs.
Rose p. the patient is supine with head hanging over the end of the table in full extension so as to enable bleeding to be over the margins of the inverted upper incisors; used to prevent aspiration or swallowing of blood, as from an injured lip.
sacroanterior p. a position of the fetus in breech presentation in labor, with its sacrum directed toward the right (RSA) or left (LSA) anterior quadrant of the maternal pelvis.
sacroposterior p. a position of the fetus in breech presentation in labor, with its sacrum directed toward the right (RSP) or left (LSP) posterior quadrant of the maternal pelvis.
sacrotransverse p. a position of the fetus in breech presentation in labor, with its sacrum directed toward the right (RST) or left (LST) iliac fossa of the maternal pelvis.
sacrum anterior p. sacroanterior p.
sacrum posterior p. sacroposterior p.
sacrum transverse p. sacrotransverse p.

Position *Continued*

scapula anterior p. scapuloanterior p.
scapula posterior p. scapuloposterior p.
scapuloanterior p. a position of the fetus in transverse lie in labor, with its head to the right (RScA) or left (LScA) of the maternal pelvis, and its back anterior.
scapuloposterior p. a position of the fetus in transverse lie in labor, with its head to the right (RScP) or left (LScP) of the maternal pelvis, and its back posterior.
scorbutic p. a pseudoparalytic position characteristic of advanced infantile scurvy; the infant lies quietly with legs flexed at the knees and hips flexed and externally rotated.
semiaxial p. a radiographic position of the head in which the central ray enters at an angle; see *half-axial projection,* under *projection.* Called also *Titterington p.*
semi-Fowler p. a position similar to Fowler position but with the head less elevated.
semiprone p. Sims p.
semireclining p. a partly reclining position seen in heart disease, asthma, and pleural effusion.
Simon p. Edebohls p.
Sims p. the patient lies on the left side with the right knee and thigh flexed and the left upper limb parallel along the back. Called also *English, lateral recumbent,* or *semiprone p.*

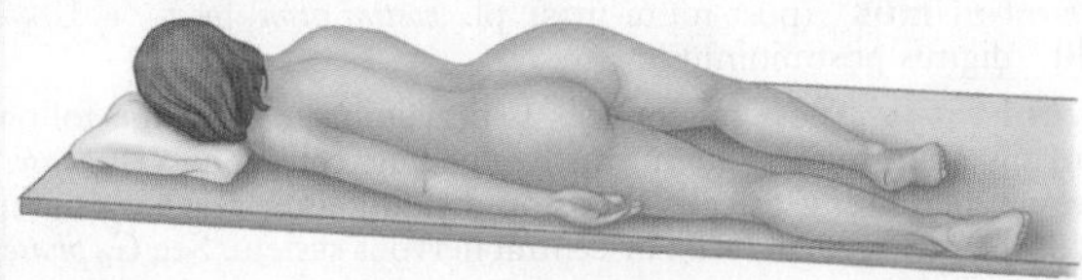

submentovertex p. the position of the head for a submentovertex projection.
supine p. dorsal p.
Titterington p. semiaxial p.
***trans* p.** see under *configuration.*
Trendelenburg p. the patient lies supine on the table or bed, the head of which is tilted downward 30 to 40 degrees, and the table or bed angulated beneath the knees.

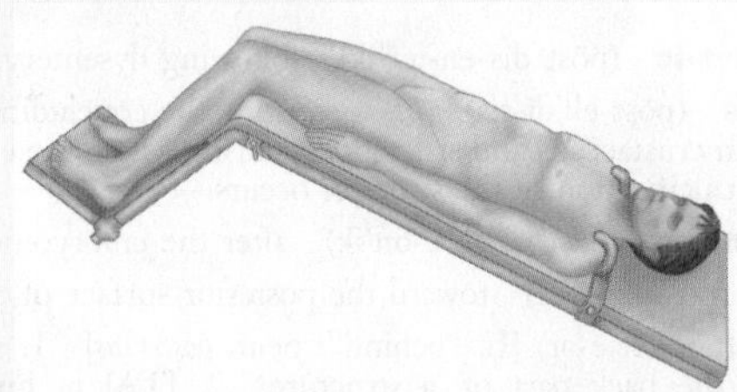

tripod p. 1. a position assumed by the patient with abdominal weakness or meningeal irritation while sitting in bed, supporting the body with the hands in a plane posterior to the pelvis. 2. a sitting position assumed by the patient with respiratory insufficiency, with the hands anterior to the frontal plane. See also *tripoding.*
Valentine p. the patient lies supine with hips flexed by means of a double inclined plane; used in irrigating the urethra.
verticosubmental p. the position of the head for a verticosubmental projection.
Waters p. the position of the head in Waters projection.
Waters p., reverse a radiographic position of the chin and head used to demonstrate the facial bones when the patient cannot be placed in a prone position; it is helpful in demonstrating fractures of the orbits, maxillary sinuses, zygomatic bones, and zygomatic arches.

po•si•tion•er (pə-zish′ən-ər) a resilient elastoplastic removable appliance fitted over the occlusal surfaces of the teeth to obtain limited tooth movement and stabilization, usually at the end of orthodontic treatment. Called also *tooth p.*

pos•i•tive (poz′ĭ-tiv) [L. *positivus*] 1. having a value greater than zero. 2. indicating existence or presence, as chromatin-positive. 3. characterized by affirmation or cooperation.

pos•i•tro•ceph•a•lo•gram (poz″ĭ-tro-sef′ə-lo-gram) [*positron* + *cephalo-* + *-gram*] a record produced by the emission of positrons by isotopes of arsenic administered to facilitate localization of brain tumors.

pos•i•tron (poz′ĭ-tron) [*positive electron*] the antiparticle of the electron, a positive electron; a particle having the mass of the electron but a positive electric charge. Symbol e^+.

po•so•log•ic (po″sə-loj′ik) pertaining to doses.

po•sol•o•gy (po-sol′ə-je) [Gr. *posos* how much + *-logy*] the science of dosage, or a system of dosage.

Pos•sum (pos′əm) [Patient-Operated Selector Mechanism] trademark for a machine designed for the disabled by which, when breathed into in the correct manner, the individual can operate the telephone, ring bells, turn on the television, switch off a light, type a letter, or perform any of a number of other functions by no movement other than that involved in respiration.

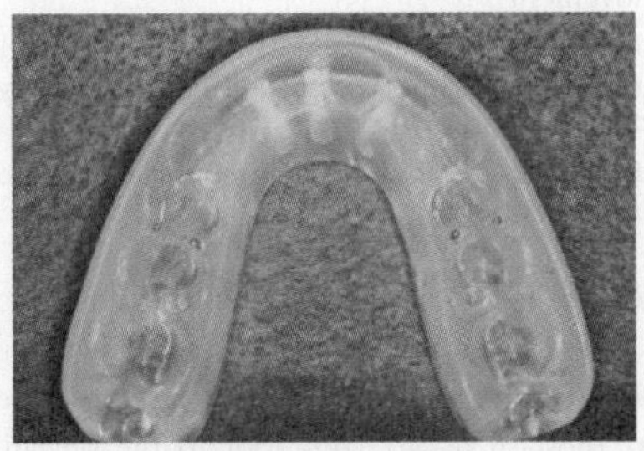

■ Positioner; maxillary occlusal view.

post (pōst) 1. a piece of material firmly secured in an upright position, usually to support something. 2. dowel.
abutment p., implant p. implant abutment.

post- [L. *post* after] a prefix meaning after or behind.

post•al•bu•min (pōst″al-bu′min) a serum protein with an electrophoretic mobility between albumin and alpha-globulin at pH 8.6.

post•anal (pōst-a′nəl) behind or beyond the anus.

post•an•es•the•sia (pōst″an-es-the′zhah) following anesthesia.

post•au•ra•le (pōst″aw-ra′le) a cephalometric landmark, the most posterior point on the helix of the ear.

post•au•ric•u•lar (pōst″aw-rik′u-lər) posterior to the auricle of the ear.

post•ax•i•al (pōst-ak′se-əl) posterior to an axis. In anatomical usage, this refers to the medial (ulnar) aspect of the upper limb, and the lateral (fibular) aspect of the lower limb.

post•bra•chi•al (pōst-bra′ke-əl) on the posterior part of the upper arm.

post•bul•bar (pōst-bul′bər) 1. posterior or distal to a bulb, such as the medulla oblongata. 2. distal to the duodenal bulb.

post•cap•il•lary (pōst-kap′ĭ-lar′e) 1. located just to the venous side of a capillary. 2. venous capillary.

post•car•di•nal (pōst-kahr′dĭ-nəl) pertaining to a pair of embryonic vessels caudal to the heart; see under *vein.*

post•car•di•ot•o•my (pōst″kahr-de-ot′ə-me) occurring after or as a consequence of operating on the heart.

post•cath•e•ter•iza•tion (post-kath″ə-tur″ĭ-za′shən) following catheterization.

post•ca•va (pōst-ka′və) vena cava inferior. **postca′val** *adj*

post•cen•tral (pōst-sen′trəl) posterior to a center, as the postcentral gyrus.

post•ci•bal (pōst-si′bəl) [*post-* + L. *cibum* food] postprandial.

post ci•bum (pōst si′bəm) [L.] after meals (after food).

post•coi•tal (post-koi′təl) after coitus.

post·con·dy·la·re (pōst-kon″də-lar′e) the highest point of the curvature posterior to the occipital condyle.

post·cra·ni·al (pōst-kra′ne-əl) posterior or inferior to the cranium.

post·cu·bi·tal (pōst-ku′bi-təl) on the dorsal side of the forearm.

post·di·as·tol·ic (pōst″di-əs-tol′ik) occurring after diastole.

post·di·crot·ic (pōst″di-krot′ik) occurring after the dicrotic notch and wave of the sphygmogram.

post·diph·ther·it·ic (pōst-dif-thə-rit′ik) after an attack of diphtheria.

post·dor·mi·tum (pōst-dor′mĭ-təm) the period of increasing consciousness interposed between sound sleep and wakening. **post-dor′mital** *adj*

post·dys·en·ter·ic (pōst″dis-en-ter′ik) following dysentery.

post·ec·dy·sis (pōst-ek′dĭ-sis) [*post-* + *ecdysis*] the concluding phase of ecdysis in certain crustaceans and arthropods, during which the endocuticle is secreted and calcification of the skeleton occurs.

post·em·bry·on·ic (pōst″em-bre-on′ik) after the embryonic stage.

pos·te·ri·ad (pos-te′re-ad) toward the posterior surface of the body.

pos·te·ri·or (pos-tēr′e-ər) [L. "behind"; neut. *posterius*] 1. situated in back of, or in the back part of, a structure. 2. [TA] in humans and other bipeds, toward the back surface of the body; called also *dorsal.* 3. in quadruped anatomy, a term sometimes used as a synonym for *caudal.*

postero- [L. *posterus* behind] a combining form denoting relationship to the posterior part.

pos·tero·an·te·ri·or (pos″tər-o-an-tēr′e-ər) from back to front, or from the posterior to the anterior surface, such as the direction of a radiographic projection.

pos·tero·clu·sion (pos″tər-o-kloo′zhən) distoclusion.

pos·tero·ex·ter·nal (pos″tər-o-ek-stur′nəl) situated on the outer side of a posterior aspect.

pos·tero·in·fe·ri·or (pos″tər-o-in-fēr′e-ər) situated posteriorly and inferiorly.

pos·tero·in·ter·nal (pos″tər-o-in-tur′nəl) situated within and toward the posterior surface.

pos·tero·lat·er·al (pos″tər-o-lat′ər-əl) situated posteriorly and to one side.

pos·tero·me·di·al (pos″tər-o-me′de-əl) situated toward the middle of the posterior surface.

pos·tero·me·di·an (pos″tər-o-me′de-ən) situated on the midline of the posterior surface.

pos·tero·pa·ri·e·tal (pos″tər-o-pə-ri′ə-təl) situated at the posterior part of the parietal bone.

pos·tero·su·pe·ri·or (pos″tər-o-soo-pēr′e-ər) situated posteriorly and superiorly.

pos·tero·tem·po·ral (pos″tər-o-tem′po-rəl) situated at the posterior part of the temporal bone.

post·gan·gli·on·ic (pōst″gang-gle-on′ik) situated posterior or distal to a ganglion; said especially of autonomic nerve fibers so located.

post·gle·noid (pōst-gle′noid) behind the glenoid cavity.

post·glo·mer·u·lar (pōst″glo-mer′u-lər) located or occurring distal to a renal glomerulus.

post·he·pat·ic (pōst″hə-pat′ik) 1. posterior to the liver. 2. after the liver has been passed; said of the portal circulation.

post·her·pet·ic (pōst″hər-pet′ik) after an attack of herpes zoster.

pos·thet·o·my (pos-thet′ə-me) [*posth-* + *-tomy*] circumcision.

pos·thio·plas·ty (pos′the-o-plas″te) [*posth-* + *-plasty*] preputioplasty; used chiefly of veterinary procedures.

pos·thi·tis (pos-thi′tis) [*posth-* + *-itis*] inflammation of the prepuce.
enzootic p. see under *balanoposthitis.*

posth(o)- [Gr. *posthē* foreskin] a combining form indicating relationship to foreskin.

pos·tho·lith (pos′tho-lith) [*postho-* + *-lith*] preputial calculus.

post·hu·mous (pos′tu-məs) [L. *postumus* coming after] 1. occurring after death. 2. born after the father's death.

post·hy·oid (pōst-hi′oid) posterior to the hyoid bone.

post·hyp·not·ic (pōst″hip-not′ik) following the hypnotic state.

post·ic·tal (pōst-ik′təl) [*post-* + *-ictal*] occurring after a seizure or sudden attack.

post·ic·ter·ic (pōst-ik-ter′ik) following jaundice.

pos·ti·cus (pos-ti′kəs) [L.] posterior.

post·in·farc·tion (pōst″in-fahrk′shən) following infarction, particularly myocardial infarction.

post·in·fec·tious (pōst″in-fek′shəs) occurring after infection.

post·in·flam·ma·to·ry (pōst″in-flam′ə-tor″e) occurring after or secondary to inflammation.

post·is·chi·al (pōst-is′ke-əl) posterior to the ischium.

post·lin·gual (pōst-ling′gwəl) 1. occurring after the development of language. 2. posterior to the tongue or to a lingula.

post·mas·tec·to·my (pōst″mas-tek′tə-me) following mastectomy.

post·mas·toid (pōst-mas′toid) posterior to the mastoid process.

post·ma·ture (pōst″mə-choor′) overly developed, as a postmature infant. Cf. *postterm pregnancy,* under *pregnancy.*

post·ma·tur·i·ty (pōst″mə-choor′ĭ-te) overdevelopment; the condition of a postmature infant. See also *postmaturity syndrome,* under *syndrome.*

post·me·di·as·ti·nal (pōst″me-de-əs-ti′nəl) 1. posterior to the mediastinum. 2. pertaining to the posterior mediastinum.

post·me·di·as·ti·num (pōst″me-de-əs-ti′nəm) mediastinum posterius.

post·mei·ot·ic (pōst″mi-ot′ik) [*post-* + *meiotic*] occurring after or pertaining to the time following meiosis.

post·meno·pau·sal (pōst″men-o-paw′zəl) occurring after menopause.

post·men·strua (pōst-men′stroo-ə) the period immediately following cessation of a menstrual period.

post·mes·en·ter·ic (pōst″mes-ən-ter′ik) 1. posterior to the mesentery. 2. in the posterior part of the mesentery.

post·mi·ni·mus (pōst-mĭ′nĭ-məs) pl. *postmi′nimi* [*post-* + L. *minimus* small] digitus postminimus.

post·mi·tot·ic (pōst″mi-tot′ik) 1. pertaining to the time following or occurring after mitosis in normally dividing cells. See *G_1 phase,* under *phase.* 2. pertaining to cells that stop dividing after reaching maturity, as cells of the mammalian heart or central nervous system. See *G_0 phase,* under *phase.*

post mor·tem (pōst mor′təm) [L.] after death.

post·mor·tem (pōst-mor′təm) occurring or performed after death; pertaining to the period after death.

post·nar·is (pōst-na′ris) choana (def. 2). **postna′rial** *adj*

post·na·sal (pōst-na′zəl) [*post-* + *nasal*] posterior to the nose.

post·na·tal (pōst-na′təl) occurring after birth, with reference to the newborn. Cf. *postpartum.*

post·op·er·a·tive (pōst-op′ər-ə-tive) occurring after a surgical operation.

post·pal·a·tine (pōst-pal′ə-tīn) posterior to the palate or the palatine bone.

post·par·tal (pōst-pahr′təl) postpartum.

post par·tum (pōst pahr′təm) [L.] after childbirth, or after delivery.

post·par·tum (pōst-pahr′təm) occurring after childbirth, or after delivery, with reference to the mother. Cf. *postnatal.*

post·pran·di·al (pōst-pran′de-əl) after a meal; called also *postcibal.*

post·pu·ber·ty (pōst-pu′bər-te) the period following puberty. **post-pu′beral, postpu′bertal** *adj*

post·pu·bes·cence (pōst″pu-bes′əns) postpuberty. **postpubes′cent** *adj*

post·re·nal (pōst-re′nəl) 1. located behind a kidney. 2. occurring after leaving a kidney, such as renal failure that results from processes impairing normal excretion of urine after it has been formed. Cf. *prerenal.*

post·ro·lan·dic (pōst″ro-lan′dik) posterior to the fissure of Rolando (sulcus centralis).

Post sing. sed. liq. [L.] post sin′gulas se′des liq′uidas (after every watery bowel movement).

post·si·nu·soi·dal (pōst″si-nə-soi′dəl) located beyond a sinusoid or affecting the circulation beyond a sinusoid; used especially to denote the location of vascular resistance in portal hypertension.

post·sphe·noid (pōst-sfe′noid) 1. pertaining to the posterior portion of the body of the sphenoid bone. 2. postsphenoid part of sphenoid bone; see under *part.*

post·sphe·noi·dal (pōst″sfə-noi′dəl) postsphenoid.

post·splen·ic (pōst-splen′ik) posterior to the spleen.

post·ste·not·ic (pōst″stə-not′ik) distal to a stenosed segment.

post·syl·vi·an (pōst-sil′ve-ən) posterior to the sylvian fissure (sulcus lateralis).

post·syn·ap·tic (pōst″sĭ-nap′tik) situated beyond or distal to a synapse, or occurring after the synapse is crossed.

post·term (pōst-tərm′) extending beyond term; said of pregnancy or of an infant.

post·trans·la·tion·al (pōst-trans-la′shən-əl) occurring following translation (def. 2), used of modifications to protein structure that take place after synthesis.

post·trau·mat·ic (pōst″traw-mat′ik) occurring as a result of or after injury.

pos·tu·late (pos′tu-lāt) [L. *postulatum* demanded] a proposition that is assumed or taken for granted.

Koch p's a statement of the kind of experimental evidence required to establish the etiologic relationship of a given microorganism to a given disease. The conditions included are (1) the microorganism must be observed in every case of the disease; (2) it must be isolated and grown in pure culture; (3) the pure culture must, when inoculated into a susceptible animal, reproduce the disease; and (4) the microorganism must be observed in, and recovered from, the experimentally diseased animal.

pos·ture (pos′choor) [L. *postura*] a position of the body. **pos′tural** *adj*

pos·tur·ing (pos′chər-ing) assumption of a pose, particularly one that is exaggerated or unnatural.

catatonic p. assumption of bizarre, fixed poses, sometimes with waxy flexibility, characteristic of catatonic schizophrenia.

decerebrate p. see under *rigidity.*

decorticate p. see under *rigidity.*

extensor p. decerebrate rigidity.

flexor p. decorticate rigidity.

pos·tu·rog·ra·phy (pos″chər-og′rə-fe) testing procedures for upright posture, balance, and sense of equilibrium. The patient stands on a force platform and measurements are taken of head position, hip position, and downward force of the feet; further assessments are done under various conditions of changing visual stimuli and platform position.

post·vac·ci·nal (pōst-vak′sĭ-nəl) occurring after or as a consequence of vaccination for smallpox.

post·vac·cin·i·al (pōst″vak-sin′e-əl) occurring after or as a consequence of vaccinia.

post·ve·ne·re·al (pōst″və-nēr′e-əl) following infection with an organism that causes sexually transmitted disease.

post·vi·tal (pōst-vi′təl) see *postvital staining,* under *staining.*

post·zone (pōst′zōn) see *zone of antigen excess,* under *zone.*

post·zy·got·ic (pōst″zi-got′ik) occurring after the completion of fertilization and formation of the zygote.

Po·ta·ba (po′tə-bə) trademark for preparations of aminobenzoate potassium.

pot·a·ble (po′tə-bəl) [L. *potabilis*] fit to drink; drinkable.

pot AGT potential abnormality of glucose tolerance.

Po·tain sign (po-tă′) [Pierre Carl Edouard *Potain,* French physician, 1825–1901] see under *sign.*

Pot·a·mon (pot′ə-mon) a genus of freshwater crabs (order Decapoda). *P. dentricula′ris, P. dehaa′ni,* and *P. rath′buni* are hosts of the metacercariae of the lung fluke *Paragonimus westermani* in East Asia.

pot·ash (pot′ash) impure potassium carbonate.

sulfurated p. [USP] a mixture of potassium polysulfides and potassium thiosulfate, used as a source of sulfide in pharmaceutical preparations.

pot·as·se·mia (pot″ə-se′me-ə) [*potassium* + *-emia*] kalemia.

po·tas·sic (po-tas′ik) containing potash.

po·tas·si·um (K) (pə-tas′e-əm) a metallic element of the alkali group, many of whose salts are used in medicine. It is a soft, silver-white metal, melting at 58°F; atomic number, 19; atomic weight, 39.102; specific gravity, 0.87. Potassium is the chief cation of muscle and most other cells (intracellular fluid); see also *sodium-potassium pump,* under *pump.*

p. 42 a radioisotope of potassium, atomic mass 42, having a half-life of 12.36 hours and emitting beta particles (3.52 MeV) and gamma rays (0.187 MeV); as the labeled chloride salt it is used as a tracer in studies of potassium interchange in the body.

p. acetate [USP] an electrolyte replenisher and urinary and systemic alkalizer, administered by intravenous infusion and orally.

p. acid phosphate monobasic p. phosphate.

p. acid tartrate p. bitartrate.

p. alum see under *alum.*

p. bicarbonate [USP] a salt, $KHCO_3$, used as a pharmaceutic necessity and as an electrolyte replenisher, antacid, and urinary alkalizer.

p. bitartrate [USP] a compound administered rectally with sodium bicarbonate to produce carbon dioxide, which promotes defecation by distending the rectal ampulla. It is used for the relief of constipation, for the evacuation of the colon before surgical or diagnostic procedures, and for pre- and postpartum bowel emptying. Also used in veterinary medicine as a laxative for small animals and as a diuretic for large animals.

p. carbonate [USP] a compound, K_2CO_3, used in pharmaceutical and chemical manufacturing procedures.

p. chloride [USP] an electrolyte replenisher, KCl, administered orally or by intravenous infusion.

p. citrate [USP] a systemic and urinary alkalizer, electrolyte replenisher, and diuretic; usually administered orally. It is sometimes used in veterinary medicine as a nonirritating diuretic.

p. cyanide an extremely poisonous compound, KCN; formerly used medicinally and now used for various industrial processes and to fumigate fruit trees. See also *cyanide poisoning,* under *poisoning.*

dibasic p. phosphate [USP] the dipotassium salt, K_2HPO_4; used alone or in combination with other phosphate compounds as an electrolyte replenisher, administered orally or intravenously. Called also *dipotassium phosphate.*

p. dichromate $K_2Cr_2O_7$, an oxidizing agent used in Zenker fixative and other histologic fixing solutions.

p. dihydrogen phosphate monobasic p. phosphate.

p. ferricyanide deep-red crystals used in Drabkin solution to test for hemoglobin.

p. gluconate [USP] an electrolyte replenisher used in the prophylaxis and treatment of hypokalemia, administered orally.

p. guaiacolsulfonate $C_7H_7KO_5S$, an expectorant.

p. hydroxide [NF] an alkalizer used in pharmaceutical preparations.

p. iodate a veterinary feed additive used as a source of iodine.

p. iodide [USP] a compound used as an expectorant, as a source of iodine in thyrotoxic crisis and in the preparation of thyrotoxic patients for thyroidectomy, and as an antifungal in the treatment of lymphocutaneous sporotrichosis; administered orally.

p. metaphosphate [NF] a white powder used as a buffering agent in pharmaceutical preparations.

monobasic p. phosphate [NF] the monopotassium salt, KH_2PO_4; used as a buffering agent in pharmaceutical preparations. It is also used, alone or in combination with other phosphate compounds, as an electrolyte replenisher, administered orally or intravenously, and as a urinary acidifier or antiurolithic, administered orally.

p. myronate sinigrin.

p. nitrate [USP] a compound, KNO_3; used as a food preservative.

p. oxalate colorless, odorless crystals used extensively as a reagent.

p. penicillin G penicillin G potassium.

p. perchlorate [USP] a compound, $KClO_4$, that reduces uptake and concentration of iodide, pertechnetate, and other anions by the thyroid and other sites; used in the treatment of iodine-induced hyperthyroidism, as an adjunct to ^{99m}Tc in imaging, and in conjunction with ^{131}I sodium iodide in a test of thyroid function.

p. permanganate [USP] the potassium salt of permanganic acid, having bactericidal, fungicidal, astringent, and oxidizing properties; used in solution as a topical antiinfective. It is also used as an antidote for certain poisons, administered by gastric lavage.

p. phenoxymethyl penicillin penicillin V potassium.

p. phosphate a compound combining potassium and phosphoric acid, in chemistry usually used to denote specifically *dibasic p. phosphate.*

p. phosphates see under *phosphates.*

p. polysulfide any of various compounds having the general formula K_2S_n, for n = 3 to 5; a component of sulfurated potash.

p. sodium tartrate [USP] a compound, $C_4H_4KNaO_6·4H_2O$; used as a cathartic. Called also *Preston salt* and *Rochelle salt.*

p. sorbate [NF] a mold and yeast inhibitor, used as a preservative in pharmaceutical preparations.

p. thiosulfate $K_2S_2O_3$, a component of sulfurated potash.

po·ten·cy (po′tən-se) [L. *potentia* power] 1. the ability of the male to perform coitus. 2. the relationship between the therapeutic effect of a drug and the dose necessary to achieve that effect; a drug with a higher potency will require a smaller dose to produce a given effect. Clinically, potency has little use except as a means to compare the relative activities of pharmaceutic agents. Cf. *efficacy.* 3. the ability of an embryonic part to develop and complete its destiny.

prospective p. the total developmental possibilities of which an embryonic part is capable.

reactive p. see *competence.*

po·ten·tia (po-ten′she-ə) [L.] power.

po·ten·tial (po-ten′shəl) [L. *potentia* power] 1. existing and ready for action but not yet active. 2. the work per unit charge necessary to move a charged body in an electric field from a reference point (usually infinity) to another point, measured in volts. The difference in potential between two points is measured by the work necessary to move a unit positive charge from one to the other.

action p. (AP) the electrical activity developed in a muscle or nerve cell during activity. It may be elicited by electrical, chemical, or mechanical

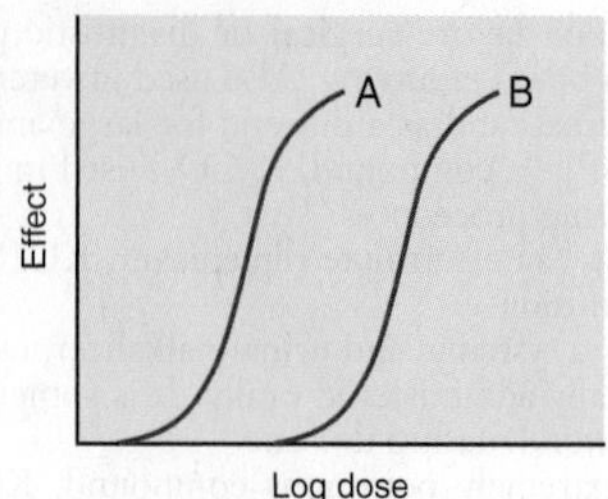

■ Dose-effect curve for two drugs of different potency: Drug A is more potent than drug B.

stimulation, by temperature change, and so on, and results from an influx of sodium ions so that the membrane potential becomes positive. See also *all or none* and *discharge* (def. 4).

after-p. afterpotential.

auditory evoked p. (AEP) in electroencephalography, changes in waves in response to sound; see also *brainstem auditory evoked p.*

bioelectric p. the varying electric potential which accompanies all biochemical processes, as those manifested in the electrocardiogram and the electroencephalogram.

biotic p. the maximum rate at which a population can increase when the age ratio is stable and all environmental conditions are ideal. Called also *reproductive p.*

bizarre high-frequency p. complex repetitive discharge.

brainstem auditory evoked p. (BAEP) that portion of the auditory evoked potential which comes from the brainstem; abnormalities can be analyzed to evaluate comas, to support diagnosis of multiple sclerosis, and to detect early posterior fossa tumors.

cochlear p's see under *microphonic.*

compound action p. see *compound muscle action p.* and *compound nerve action p.*

compound muscle action p. (CMAP) a group of almost simultaneous action potentials from several muscle fibers in the same area; they are usually evoked by stimulation of the supplying motor nerve and are recorded as one multipeaked summated action potential. See also *A wave, F waves, H wave,* and *M wave,* under *wave.*

compound nerve action p. a group of almost synchronous nerve fiber action potentials from the trunk of a motor, sensory, or mixed nerve: they are usually evoked by nerve stimulation and are recorded as a multipeaked summated action potential.

compound sensory nerve action p. sensory nerve action p.

cortical evoked p. an evoked potential recorded from the cerebral cortex. Called also *evoked cortical p.*

demarcation p. injury p.

diastolic p. the transmembrane potential of the cell during electrical diastole.

electric p., electrical p. potential (def. 2).

electrode p. redox p.

end plate p. an action potential that occurs in a stimulated motor end plate, causing initiation of an action potential in the adjacent muscle fiber.

event-related p. a change in waveforms on the electroencephalogram just after a sensory, motor, or cognitive stimulus; cf. *evoked p., readiness p.,* and *contingent negative variation.*

evoked p. (EP) the electrical signal recorded from a sensory receptor, nerve, muscle, or area of the central nervous system that has been

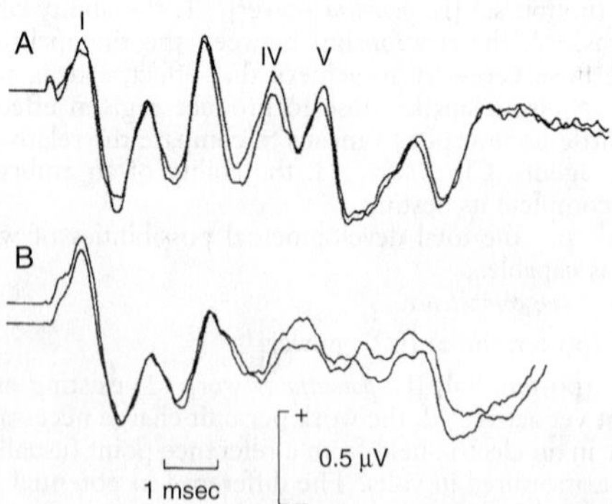

■ Brainstem auditory evoked potential elicited in a normal subject *(A)* and a patient with a structural lesion involving the upper pons *(B);* two trials are superimposed to show replicability.

stimulated, usually by electricity. See also *auditory evoked p., somatosensory evoked p.,* and *visual evoked p.*

evoked cortical p. cortical evoked p.

excitatory postsynaptic p. (EPSP) a transient decrease in membrane polarization induced in a postsynaptic neuron when subjected to a volley of impulses over an excitatory afferent pathway; summation of such potentials may cause discharge by the neuron.

fasciculation p. an electrical potential that occurs with a fasciculation, similar in appearance to a motor unit action potential but occurring spontaneously. These may appear singly or in groups; complex or iterative ones occur in motor unit disorders.

fibrillation p. an abnormal spiked electrical potential associated with fibrillation of a muscle fiber; it occurs spontaneously in some myopathic disorders or may be provoked by movement of a needle electrode.

generator p. the depolarization produced in neural receptors in response to specific kinds of physical stimuli; called also *receptor p.*

inhibitory postsynaptic p. (IPSP) a transient hyperpolarization of membrane potential induced in a postsynaptic neuron when subjected to a volley of impulses over an inhibitory afferent pathway, resulting in a diminished responsiveness of the neuron.

injury p. the difference in recorded electrical potential between the intact longitudinal surface and the injured end of a muscle or nerve; called also *demarcation p.*

membrane p. the electrical potential across a plasma membrane. Cf *action p.* and *resting p.*

morphogenetic p. the degree of strength or ability of an embryonic part to develop into a specific structure.

motor evoked p. the evoked potential of motor nerves, which can be measured to determine the integrity of the motor pathways.

motor unit p. (MUP), motor unit action p. (MUAP) the sum of the recorded action potentials of all the muscle fibers in one motor unit.

muscle action p. compound muscle action p.

muscle fiber action p. the action potential recorded on a muscle fiber spreading in both directions away from the plate region to initiate a contraction; see also *single fiber electromyography.*

myotonic p. see under *discharge.*

negative after-p. see under *afterpotential.*

Nernst p. the voltage produced across a membrane by a concentration gradient of an ion that can diffuse through pores in the membrane while oppositely charged ions cannot pass through the membrane; see *Nernst equation* under *equation.*

nerve p., nerve action p. 1. compound nerve action p. 2. nerve fiber action p.

nerve fiber action p. an action potential recorded from a single nerve fiber; see also *compound nerve action p.*

pacemaker p. the slow diastolic depolarization of cell membranes that normally occurs in the sinoatrial node, atrioventricular node, and His-Purkinje system; under some abnormal conditions it can also occur in atrial and ventricular muscle fibers.

positive after-p. see under *afterpotential.*

postsynaptic p. a change in polarization of a postsynaptic neuron; see *excitatory postsynaptic p.* and *inhibitory postsynaptic p.*

readiness p. a negative potential on the electroencephalogram, which slowly increases and reaches a maximum just before a voluntary movement in a limb; called also *Bereitschaftspotential.*

receptor p. generator p.

redox p. the electrochemical potential of an oxidation-reduction half-reaction under prevailing conditions measured with respect to the standard reduction potential of the hydrogen gas/proton redox couple, which is defined as zero. It is related to its own standard reduction potential by the Nernst equation. Symbol E or E_h.

reproductive p. biotic p.

resting p., resting membrane p. the electrical potential of the inside of a cell at rest relative to the immediate external environment; in nearly all animal cells it is negative (−20 to −100mV) and is maintained mainly by diffusion of potassium ions out of the cell through potassium channels. cf. *action p.*

satellite p. a small abnormal action potential separated from the main motor unit action potential and regularly preceding or following each main action potential on the recording.

sensory p., sensory nerve action p. (SNAP) a compound nerve action potential recorded from a sensory nerve or from the sensory branch of a mixed nerve. Called also *compound sensory nerve action p.*

serrated action p. an action potential whose waveform has several changes in direction without crossing the baseline.

somatosensory evoked p. (SEP) waves recorded from the spinal cord or cerebral hemisphere after electrical stimulation or physiological activation of peripheral sensory fibers; analysis of deviations in latency or amplitude can detect or characterize lesions of the peripheral or sensory conduction pathways.

spike p. the initial very large change in potential of an excitable cell membrane during excitation.

standard electrode p., standard reduction p. the electrochemical potential developed by a half-cell under standard conditions (1 atm pressure; specified temperature, usually 25°C; substances in solution at 1 M concentration) compared to the potential of the hydrogen gas/proton redox couple ($2H^+ + 2e^- \rightleftarrows H_2$) under standard conditions, which by definition has an $E°$ of exactly 0 V. Symbol $E°$.

threshold p. the membrane potential that must be achieved before a membrane channel can open; it differs among the various cardiac membrane channels.

transmembrane p. membrane p.

visual evoked p. (VEP), visual evoked cortical p. in electroencephalography, changes in the evoked cortical potential when the eye is stimulated by light; variations are diagnostic for abnormalities of the visual system and for other disorders, particularly neurological disorders such as multiple sclerosis, that have visual symptoms.

zero p. in electricity, an arbitrary reference point (usually the potential of the earth) used as a zero value in comparison to other electrical potentials.

zeta p. the electric potential across a solid-liquid interface. The zeta potential at the surface of erythrocytes is the net potential produced by both the negative charges on the cell surface and the positive charges in a cloud of cations attracted by the surface charge and forming a layer over the surface; it is responsible for a repelling force between erythrocytes that resists agglutination or rouleau formation.

po•ten•tial•iza•tion (po-ten″shəl-ĭ-za′shən) potentiation (def. 1).

po•ten•ti•a•tion (po-ten″she-a′shən) 1. the increasing of potency; particularly, the synergistic action of two drugs, so that their effect together is greater than the sum of the effects that each one has alone. 2. posttetanic p.

long-term p. a change in efficacy of synapses at monosynaptic junctions lasting from a few days to several weeks, first observed in the hippocampus, dentate gyrus, and nearby areas but now observed elsewhere in the brain. It is thought to be related to long-term information storage and thus to memory.

posttetanic p. an incrementing response, without change of action potential amplitude, that occurs with repetitive nerve stimulation.

po•ten•ti•a•tor (po-ten′she-a-tər) an agent that enhances another agent so that the combined effect is greater than the sum of the effects of each one alone.

po•ten•ti•om•e•ter (po-ten″she-om′ə-tər) an instrument for the accurate measuring of voltage.

po•ten•ti•za•tion (po-ten″tĭ-za′shən) in homeopathy, the process of making a remedy more potent by serial dilution and succussion, or vigorous shaking; the resulting preparation may be so dilute that it is unlikely to contain a single molecule of the original substance.

po•ti•fi•ca•tion (po″tĭ-fĭ-ka′shən) the process of making water fit to drink. Applied to sea water, it is the process of removing sufficient salts to render the remaining fluid safe for drinking.

POTS postural orthostatic tachycardia syndrome.

Pott aneurysm, disease, etc. (pot) [Sir Percivall *Pott*, English surgeon, 1714–1788] see *aneurysmal varix*, under *varix;* see *tuberculosis of spine;* and see under *abscess, curvature, fracture, paraplegia,* and *tumor.*

Pot•ter facies, syndrome (pot′ər) [Edith Louise *Potter*, American physician, 1901–1993] see under *facies* and see *oligohydramnios sequence,* under *sequence.*

Pot•ter version (pot′ər) [Irving W. *Potter*, American obstetrician, 1868–1956] see under *version.*

Potts operation (anastomosis, shunt) (pots) [Willis John *Potts*, American surgeon, 1895–1968] see under *operation.*

pouce (po͞os) [Fr.] the thumb or great toe.

p. flottant (flah-tahn′) ["floating thumb (great toe)"] a thumb or great toe that lacks bones; this may be associated with a number of congenital anomalies or may follow microvascular or plastic surgery.

pouch (pouch) a bag or similar space; see also *cavity, pocket, recess,* and *sac.*

abdominovesical p. the pouch formed by reflection of the peritoneum from the anterior abdominal wall to the distended bladder.

adenohypophysial p. Rathke p.

anal p. the expanded end of the hindgut in certain insects.

anterior p. of Tröltsch recessus anterior membranae tympanicae.

Blake p. a blind pocket of arachnoid connected with the fourth ventricle and the subarachnoid space near the medulla oblongata as a result of abnormal development of the membranous lamina of the auditory tube.

branchial p. pharyngeal p.

craniobuccal p., craniopharyngeal p. Rathke p.

Douglas p., p. of Douglas excavatio rectouterina.

enterocoelic p. a diverticulum of the enteron of the embryo.

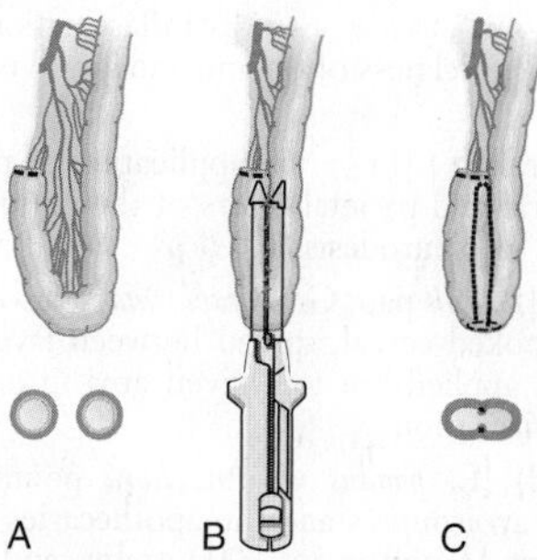

■ Creation of an ileal J pouch using a cutting linear stapler. *(A),* A reservoir is created from the distal ileum; *(B),* the stapler joins two limbs of intestine while dividing the intervening wall; *(C),* the diameter of the resulting pouch is twice the original diameter of the ileum.

guttural p's large mucous sacs in the horse, which are ventral diverticula of the eustachian tube, situated between the base of the cranium and the atlas dorsally and the pharynx ventrally.

Hartmann p. an abnormal sacculation of the neck of the gallbladder.

Heidenhain p. a small pocket of the stomach that has been surgically separated from the body of the stomach, vagally denervated, and made to drain to the exterior; used in the experimental study of gastric physiology. Cf. *Pavlov p.*

hypophysial p. Rathke p.

ileoanal p. see under *reservoir.*

ileocecal p. a type of Mainz pouch that uses intestine from the ileocecal junction.

Indiana p. a type of continent urinary diversion in which part of the ileum and cecum is modified to form a pouch with modification of the ileocecal orifice to maintain continence.

J p. an ileoanal reservoir created by lateral anastomosis of two loops of ileum 15 to 20 cm long.

Kock p. 1. the most common kind of continent ileal reservoir for ileostomy, with a capacity of 500 to 1000 mL and a valve made by intussusception of the terminal ileum. 2. a modification of this pouch, used as a neobladder.

laryngeal p. sacculus laryngis.

Mainz p. any of several continent urinary diversion devices using a section of the rectum and sigmoid colon to create a pouch for maintenance of continence.

Morison p. a pouch of peritoneum inferior to the liver and to the right of the right kidney and extending inferiorly to the transverse mesocolon.

paracystic p. fossa paravesicalis.

pararectal p. fossa pararectalis.

paravesical p. fossa paravesicalis.

Pavlov p. a pocket of stomach that has been surgically separated from the body of the stomach by a mucosal septum, allowed to retain vagal innervation and muscular connection, and made to drain to the exterior; used in the experimental study of gastric physiology. Cf. *Heidenhain p.*

perineal p., deep saccus profundus perinei.

perineal p., subcutaneous saccus subcutaneus perinei.

perineal p., superficial compartimentum superficiale perinei.

pharyngeal p. a lateral diverticulum of the pharynx that meets a corresponding pharyngeal groove in the embryonic ectoderm, forming a closing membrane that may rupture and complete the gill slit as observed in lower vertebrates. Called also *branchial p.* and *visceral p.*

Physick p's inflamed sacculations between the rectal valves, with mucous discharge.

posterior p. of Tröltsch recessus posterior membranae tympanicae.

Prussak p. recessus superior membranae tympanicae.

Rathke p. a diverticulum from the ectodermal roof of the stomodeum of the embryo that lies adjacent to the floor of the diencephalon; from it the adenohypophysis is developed. Its lumen persists in adults as small colloid-filled cysts and clefts at the juncture of the pars distalis and the neurohypophysis. Called also *adenohypophysial,craniobuccal, craniopharyngeal,* or *hypophysial p.*.

rectouterine p., rectovaginal p. excavatio rectouterina.

rectovesical p. excavatio rectovesicalis.

S p. an ileoanal reservoir created by lateral anastomosis of three sections of ileum each 10 to 15 cm long in a configuration resembling the letter S.

Seessel p. a transient outpouching of the embryonic pharynx rostrad of the oropharyngeal membrane and caudal to Rathke pouch.

uterovesical p., vesicouterine p. excavatio vesicouterina.

visceral p. pharyngeal p.

pouch•itis (pouch-i'tis) [*pouch* + *-itis*] inflammation of the mucosa or occasionally of the full thickness of the intestinal wall of an ileal or ileoanal reservoir.

pou•drage (poo-drahzh') [Fr.] the application of powder to a surface, as between the visceral and parietal layers of the pericardium or pleura to promote their fusion in pleurodesis.

poul•tice (pōl'tis) [L. *puls* pap; Gr. *kataplasma*] a soft, moist mass about the consistency of cooked cereal, spread between layers of muslin, linen, gauze, or towels and applied hot to a given area in order to create moist local heat or counterirritation.

pound (lb) (pound) [L. *pondus* weight; *libra* pound] a unit of mass (weight) of both the avoirdupois and the apothecaries' system. The avoirdupois pound contains 16 ounces, or 7000 grains, and is the equivalent of 453.592 gm. The apothecaries' pound contains 12 ounces, or 5760 grains, and is the equivalent of 373.242 gm.

Pou•part ligament, line (poo-pahr') [François *Poupart*, French anatomist, 1661–1708] see *ligamentum inguinale*, and see under *line*.

Po•van (po'van) trademark for a preparation of pyrvinium pamoate.

pov•er•ty (pov'ər-te) the absence or scarcity of requisite substance or elements.

p. of content disordered speech in which quantity is normal but content is altered so that very little or nothing is communicated.

p. of movement the akinesia or bradykinesia seen in subjects with parkinsonism.

po•vi•done (po'vĭ-dōn) [USP] a synthetic polymer principally consisting of linear 1-vinyl-2-pyrrolidone groups, produced as a series of products having mean molecular weights ranging from about 10,000 to about 700,000; used as a dispersing and suspending agent, and has been used as a tablet binder, coating agent, and viscosity-increasing agent in pharmaceutical preparations. Formerly called *polyvinylpyrrolidone (PVP)*. See also *povidone-iodine*.

p.-iodine (PVP-I) [USP] a complex produced by reacting iodine with the polymer povidone; it slowly releases iodine and is used as a topical antiinfective.

Pow•as•san encephalitis, virus (po-wah'sən) [*Powassan*, Ontario, Canada, where the disease was first observed in 1958] see under *encephalitis* and *virus*.

pow•der (pou'dər) [L. *pulvis*] a substance made up of an aggregation of small particles, as that obtained by the grinding or trituration of a solid drug.

absorbable dusting p. an absorbable powder prepared by processing cornstarch, with not more than 2 per cent of magnesium oxide; used for dusting surgeons' rubber gloves and other purposes for which talc is used in the hospital.

bleaching p. chlorinated lime.

dusting p. a fine powder used as a substitute for talc.

impalpable p. a powder so fine that its particles cannot be felt as distinct bodies.

pow•er (pou'ər) [L. *posse* to have power] 1. capability; potency; the ability to act. 2. a measure of magnification, as of a microscope. 3. the rate at which work is done. Symbol *P*. The SI unit of power is the watt. 4. of a statistical test: the probability of correctly rejecting the null hypothesis when a specified alternative holds true; it is equal to 1 minus the probability of a Type II error.

candle p. the numerical expression, in international candles, of the luminous intensity of a light source.

carbon dioxide-combining p., CO_2-combining p. ability of the blood plasma to combine with carbon dioxide, defined as the total CO_2 bound in plasma as bicarbonate at a pCO_2 of 40 mmHg at 25°C. Cf. *alkali reserve*.

defining p. the ability of a lens to make an object clearly visible.

resolving p. the ability of the eye or of a lens to make separately visible small objects that are close together, thus revealing the structure of an object; see also *resolution*.

pox (poks) [variant of *pocks*, from A.S. *pocc* pustule, spot] any of several eruptive or pustular diseases, usually caused by a virus; see specific entries, such as *chickenpox*, *cowpox*, *horsepox*, *rabbitpox*, and *smallpox*.

Pox•vi•ri•dae (poks"vir'ĭ-de) the poxviruses: a family of DNA viruses having a brick-shaped or ovoid virion 220–450 × 140–260 nm consisting of an envelope containing lipid and tubular or globular protein structures surrounding a DNA-containing core and one or two lateral bodies. The genome consists of a single molecule of double-stranded DNA (size 130–375 kbp). Viruses contain over 100 proteins; some are ether-resistant while others are ether-sensitive. Replication and assembly occur in the cytoplasm; virions are released by cell destruction or budding. Host range is narrow and transmission is by fomites, airborne particles, arthropod vectors, or contact. There are two subfamilies: Chordopoxvirinae (poxviruses of vertebrates) and Entomopoxvirinae (poxviruses of insects).

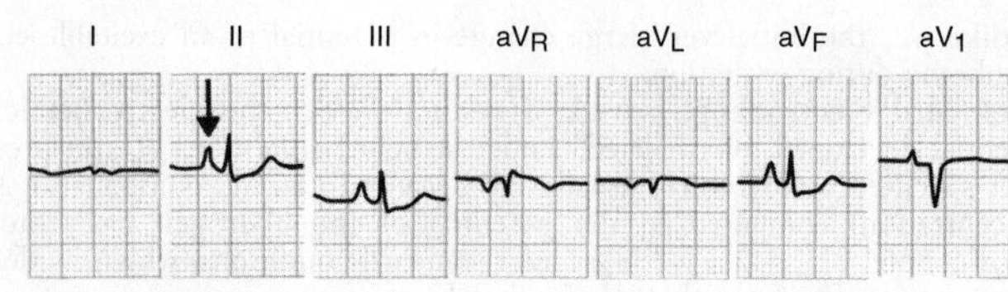

■ P pulmonale. Tall P waves *(arrow)* are seen in leads II, III, aV_F, and V_1 in a patient with chronic lung disease.

pox•vi•rus (poks'vi-rəs) any virus belonging to the family Poxviridae. **poxvi'ral** *adj*

PP [L.] punc'tum prox'imum (near point of accommodation).

PP_i pyrophosphate.

PPD purified protein derivative (tuberculin); see under *tuberculin*.

PPI proton pump inhibitor.

PPLO pleuropneumonialike organisms.

ppm parts per million.

PPoma (pe-pe-o'mə) a rare type of tumor, usually in the head of the pancreas, that secretes pancreatic polypeptide but does not cause endocrine symptoms; many of these grow large and have malignant potential.

PPR peste des petits ruminants.

PPSV pneumococcal vacine polyvalent.

Ppt precipitate; prepared.

P pul•mo•nale (pe pul"mo-na'le) in electrocardiography, a pattern of tall, peaked P waves in leads II, III, and aV_F, indicative of enlargement of the right atrium; it is often associated with pulmonary disease.

PR[1] prosthion; pulmonic regurgitation.

PR[2] [L.] punc'tum remo'tum (far point of accommodation).

Pr praseodymium; presbyopia; prism.

PRA panel-reactive antibody.

prac•tice (prak'tis) [Gr. *praktikē*] the use of one's knowledge in a particular profession, the practice of medicine being the exercise of one's knowledge in the practical recognition and treatment of disease.

contract p. the treatment of the members of a specified group for a lump sum, or at so much per member.

evidence-based p. the practice of health care in which the practitioner systematically finds, appraises, and uses the most current and valid research findings as the basis for clinical decisions. The term is sometimes used to denote evidence-based medicine specifically, but can also include other specialties such as evidence-based nursing, pharmacy, and dentistry.

family p. the medical specialty concerned with the planning and provision of the comprehensive primary health care of all members of a family, regardless of age or sex, on a continuing basis; see also *family physician*. Called also *family medicine*.

general p. the provision of comprehensive medical care regardless of age of the patient or presence of a condition that may temporarily require the services of a specialist; cf. *family p.*

group p. see under *medicine*.

panel p. see *panel* (def. 3).

solo p. the provision of care by a single, self-employed physician or dentist assisted only by auxiliary personnel. Cf. *group medicine*.

prac•ti•tion•er (prak-tish'ən-ər) one who has complied with the requirements of and who is engaged in the practice of medicine, dentistry, or nursing.

general p. a physician in general practice; cf. *family physician.*.

nurse p. see under *nurse*.

prac•to•lol (prak'to-lol) a beta-adrenergic blocking agent having the same actions as propranolol (q.v.). Its use has been found to be associated with an allergic reaction of the eyes, skin, mucous membranes, and ears.

Pra•der stages (prah'dər) [Andrea *Prader*, Swiss pediatrician, 1919–2001] see under *stage*.

Pra•der-Wil•li syndrome (prah'dər vil'e) [A. *Prader;* Heinrich *Willi*, Swiss pediatrician, 1900–1971] see under *syndrome*.

prae- [L. "before"] a prefix meaning before, in front of; for words beginning thus, see also those beginning *pre-*.

prae•cox (pre'koks) [L.] premature, early; see *dementia praecox*.

prag•mat•ag•no•sia (prag"mat-ag-no'zhə) [Gr. *pragma* object + *agnosia*] agnosia.

prag•mat•am•ne•sia (prag"mat-am-ne'zhə) [Gr. *pragma* object + *amnesia*] visual agnosia.

praj•na•pa•ra•dha (pruj″nə-pah-rə-thah′) [Sanskrit] according to ayurveda, deliberate, willful indulgence in unhealthy practices that leads to unbalanced body functions and disease.

pra•kri•ti (prŭ′kre-the) [Sanskrit, from *pra* before + *akriti* creativity] according to ayurveda, a person's underlying characteristic physical and mental constitution and tendencies of expression.

pral•i•dox•ime (pral″ĭ-doks′ēm) a cholinesterase reactivator capable of acting as an antagonist to certain anticholinesterases. Called also *2-PAM.*

p. chloride [USP] the chloride salt of pralidoxime, used as an antidote in the treatment of poisoning due to organophosphates having anticholinesterase activity and to counteract the effects of overdosage by anticholinesterases used in the treatment of myasthenia gravis, administered orally and by intravenous infusion.

pram•i•pex•ole di•hy•dro•chlo•ride (pram″ĭ-pek′sōl) a nonergot dopamine agonist used as an antidyskinetic in the treatment of Parkinson disease; administered orally.

pram•lin•tide ac•e•tate (pram′lin-tīd) a synthetic analogue of amylin that acts as a hypoglycemic, used in treatment of diabetes mellitus; administered by subcutaneous injection.

pram•o•caine hy•dro•chlo•ride (pram′o-kān) INN and BAN for *pramoxine hydrochloride.*

Pra•mo•sone (pră′mo-sōn) trademark for combination preparations of hydrocortisone acetate and pramoxine hydrochloride.

pra•mox•ine hy•dro•chlo•ride (prə-mok′sēn) [USP] a local anesthetic applied topically to the skin and rectal mucous membranes, for temporary relief of pain and pruritus associated with skin and anorectal disorders.

pra•na (prah′nə) [Sanskrit] in ayurvedic tradition, the life force or vital energy, which permeates the body and is especially concentrated along the midline in the chakras. Cf *qi.*

pra•na•ya•ma (prah″nə-yah′mə) [Sanskrit *prana,* q.v.] according to ayurveda, breath control, occurring as one of the eight limbs of raja yoga (see *yoga*); it is used as a means of controlling the energy within the body and the mind and acts as a vitalizing and regenerating force for increasing oxygen exchange that can be used for physical healing.

pran•di•al (pran′de-əl) [L. *prandium* breakfast] pertaining to a meal, especially dinner.

Pran•din (pran′din) trademark for preparations of repaglinide.

pra•seo•dym•i•um (Pr) (pra″ze-o-dim′e-əm) a rare earth element; atomic number, 59; atomic weight, 140.907.

pras•ter•one (pras′tər-ōn) INN for dehydroepiandrosterone.

pra•su•grel (pra′soo-grəl) a platelet inhibitor used as an antithrombotic following angioplasty for acute coronary syndrome; administered orally.

P. rat. aetat. [L.] pro ratio′ne aeta′tis (in proportion to age).

Praus•nitz-Küst•ner reaction (test) (prous′nits kēst′ner) [Otto Carl Willy *Prausnitz,* German hygienist, 1876–1963; Heinz *Küstner,* German gynecologist, 1897–1963] see under *reaction.*

Prav•a•chol (prav′ə-kol) trademark for a preparation of pravastatin sodium.

prav•a•stat•in so•di•um (prav′ə-stat″in) an antihyperlipidemic agent that is an HMG-CoA reductase inhibitor, used to lower blood lipid levels in the treatment of hypercholesterolemia and other forms of dyslipidemia and to reduce the risk of morbidity and mortality associated with atherosclerosis and coronary heart disease; administered orally.

prax•i•ol•o•gy (prak″se-ol′ə-je) [*praxis* + *-logy*] the study of conduct, rather than of thought or consciousness.

prax•is (prak′sis) [Gr. "action"] the doing or performance of action.

pra•ze•pam (praz′ə-pam) a benzodiazepine used as an antianxiety agent in the treatment of anxiety disorders and for short-term relief of anxiety symptoms; administered orally.

pra•zi•quan•tel (pra″zĭ-kwahn′təl) a broad-spectrum anthelmintic used for the treatment of a wide variety of fluke and tapeworm infections; administered orally.

pra•zo•sin hy•dro•chlo•ride (pra′zo-sin) [USP] a quinazoline derivative with vasodilator properties, used as an oral antihypertensive.

pre- [L. *prae-* before] a prefix meaning before, in front of.

pre•adap•ta•tion (pre″a-dap-ta′shən) the acquisition in an ancestral group of certain characters that usually are adaptive to the ancestral mode of life yet at the same time enable a shift in mode of life; for example, lungs in fish ancestral to tetrapods.

pre•ad•i•po•cyte (pre-ad′ĭ-po-sīt″) a precursor to an adipocyte.

pre•ag•o•nal (pre-ag′ə-nəl) preceding the death agony.

pre•al•bu•min (pre″al-bu′min) transthyretin.

pre•an•es•thet•ic (pre″an-əs-thet′ik) occurring before administration of an anesthetic.

pre•an•tral (pre-an′trəl) pertaining to ovarian follicles before they become antral (vesicular) follicles.

pre•aor•tic (pre″a-or′tik) anterior to the aorta.

pre•atax•ic (pre″ə-tak′sik) occurring before or preceding ataxia.

pre•au•ra•le (pre″aw-ra′le) a cephalometric landmark, the point at which a straight line from the postaurale, perpendicular to the long axis of the auricle, meets the base of the auricle.

pre•au•ric•u•lar (pre″aw-rik′u-lər) anterior to the auricle of the ear.

pre•ax•i•al (pre-ak′se-əl) anterior to an axis; in anatomical usage, this refers to the lateral (radial) aspect of the upper limb, and the medial (tibial) aspect of the lower limb.

pre•base (pre′bās) the part of the dorsum of the tongue lying anterior to the base.

pre•be•ta•lipo•pro•tein•emia (pre-ba″tə-lip″o-pro″te-ne′me-ə) hyperprebetalipoproteinemia.

pre•bi•ot•ic (pre″bi-ot′ik) denoting the period before the existence of life on earth.

pre•can•cer (pre′kan-sər) a condition that tends eventually to become malignant. **precan′cerous** *adj*

pre•cap•il•lary (pre-kap′ĭ-lar″e) 1. located just to the arterial side of a capillary. 2. arterial capillary.

pre•car•ci•nom•a•tous (pre-kahr″sĭ-nom′ə-təs) preceding the development of carcinoma.

pre•car•di•ac (pre-kahr′de-ak) anterior to the heart.

pre•car•di•nal (pre-kahr′dĭ-nəl) pertaining to a pair of embryonic vessels cranial to the heart; see under *vein.*

pre•car•di•um (pre-kahr′de-əm) [*pre-* + Gr. *kardia* heart] precordium.

pre•car•ti•lage (pre-kahr′tĭ-ləj) embryonic cartilaginous tissue.

pre•cau•tion (pre-kaw′shən) a protective measure taken in advance.

airborne p's a group of transmission-based precautions used when caring for patients who have diseases that spread through the air, such as tuberculosis, chickenpox, and measles. The patient should be in a private room. Called also respiratory precautions.

contact p's a group of transmission-based precautions used when caring for patients who have diseases that spread through direct skin to skin contact or through indirect contact with contaminated equipment.

droplet p's a group of transmission-based precautions used when caring for patients who have diseases that spread by droplets or dust particles, such as by coughing, sneezing, or talking or during procedures such as suctioning and bronchoscopy. The diseases include rubella, mumps, diphtheria, and influenza.

isolation p's special precautionary measures, practices, and procedures used in the care of patients with contagious or communicable diseases. The Centers for Disease Control and Prevention (CDC) provides explicit and comprehensive guidelines for control of the spread of infectious disease in care of hospitalized patients. The type of infectious disease a patient has dictates the kind of isolation precautions necessary to prevent spread of the disease to others.

respiratory p's airborne precautions.

standard p's a classification of isolation precautions that replaces the former classifications of universal precautions and measures used for isolation of moist body products.

transmission-based p's isolation precautions used when caring for patients with highly transmissible or epidemiologically important pathogens; these constitute additional measures beyond standard precautions. There are three types, depending on the type of disease the patient has: airborne precautions, droplet precautions, and contact precautions.

universal p's a group of measures formerly recommended for protection of noninfected individuals against bloodborne infections such as hepatitis B virus and human immunodeficiency virus, now replaced by the measures called standard precautions.

pre•ca•va (pre-ka′və) vena cava superior. **preca′val** *adj*

Pre•ce•dex (pres′ə-deks) trademark for a preparation of dexmedetomidine hydrochloride.

pre•ce•men•tum (pre″sə-men′təm) cementoid.

pre•cen•tral (pre-sen′trəl) anterior to a center, as the precentral gyrus.

pre•chor•dal (pre-kor′dəl) situated cranial to the notochord; called also *prochordal.*

pre•cip•i•ta•ble (pre-sip′ĭ-tə-bəl) capable of being precipitated.

pre•cip•i•tant (pre-sip′ĭ-tənt) a substance which causes a chemical or mechanical precipitation.

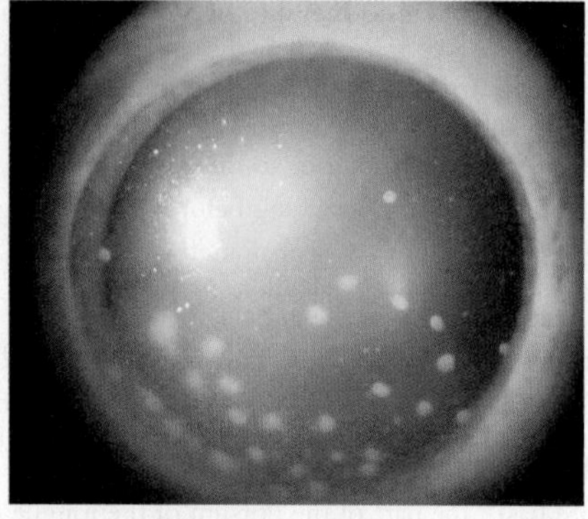

■ Mutton-fat keratic precipitates scattered diffusely on the posterior surface of the cornea.

pre·cip·i·tate (pre-sip′ĭ-tāt) [L. *praecipitare* to cast down] 1. to cause a substance in solution to settle down in solid particles. 2. a deposit made or substance thrown down by precipitation. 3. occurring with undue rapidity, as precipitate labor. 4. in immunology, the product of interaction between soluble macromolecular antigen and the homologous antibody, e.g., the antigen-antibody complex formed as a consequence of the reaction of pneumococcus capsular polysaccharide in solution with specific antiserum.

immune p. see *precipitate.*

keratic p's cellular and fibrinous deposits on the posterior surface of the cornea, occurring after injury or iridocyclitis and giving an appearance of fine drops of dew; see also *keratitis punctata.*

mutton-fat keratic p's coalescent precipitates of inflammatory cells and fibrin that form translucent rings with opaque centers in the anterior chamber of the eye in uveitis.

pre·cip·i·ta·tion (pre-sip″ĭ-ta′shən) [L. *praecipitatio*] the act or process of precipitating.

aluminum p. a technique for production of antibody to specific antigen, using precipitation of antigen by aluminum salts *(aluminum adjuvant);* the absorbed antigen forms a depot at the site of inoculation, from which it is slowly released for a prolonged antibody response.

group p. precipitation by a precipitin in a specific antiserum of an antigen common to a group of closely related microorganisms.

pre·cip·i·tin (pre-sip′ĭ-tin) an antibody to antigen that specifically aggregates the macromolecular antigen in vivo or in vitro to give a visible precipitate.

pre·cip·i·tin·o·gen (pre-sip″ĭ-tin′o-jən) the soluble antigen which stimulates the formation of precipitins and is capable of reacting with them in vitro and in vivo.

pre·cip·i·to·gen (pre-sip′ĭ-to-jən) precipitinogen.

pre·ci·sion (pre-sizh′ən) 1. the quality of being sharply or exactly defined; for example, a measurement with three significant figures is more precise than a measurement with two. Cf. *accuracy.* 2. in statistics, the extent to which a measurement procedure gives the same results when repeated under identical conditions. Under certain conditions, may be called *reliability, repeatability,* or *reproducibility.*

pre·clin·i·cal (pre-klin′ĭ-kəl) before a disease becomes clinically recognizable.

pre·clot·ting (pre-klot′ing) the forcing of a patient's blood through the interstices of a knitted vascular prosthesis prior to implantation to render the graft temporarily impervious to blood by disposition of fibrin and platelets in the interstices; after implantation fibrous ingrowth from the recipient replaces the fibrin-platelet network.

pre·co·cious (pre-ko′shəs) developed more than is usual at a given age.

pre·coc·i·ty (pre-kos′ĭ-te) unusually early development of mental or physical traits.

sexual p. precocious puberty.

pre·cog·ni·tion (pre″kog-nish′ən) [*pre-* + *cognition*] the extrasensory perception of a future event.

pre·col·lag·e·nous (pre″ko-laj′ə-nəs) [*pre-* + *collagenous*] denoting an incomplete stage in the formation of collagen.

pre·co·ma (pre-ko′mə) the neuropsychiatric state preceding coma, as in hepatic encephalopathy.

pre·con·di·tion·ing (pre″kən-dish′ən-ing) the creation of a state in which a stimulus applied later will incur a certain response.

ischemic p. an adaptive response of myocardium injured reversibly by a brief episode of ischemia that increases its resistance to subsequent ischemic episodes.

pre·con·scious (pre-kon′shəs) the part of the mind that is not in immediate awareness but can be consciously recalled with effort, one of the systems of Freud's topographic model of the mind. Cf. *conscious* and *unconscious.*

pre·cor·dia (pre-kor′de-ə) plural of *precordium.*

pre·cor·di·al·gia (pre-kor″de-al′jə) [*precordium* + *-algia*] pain in the precordium.

pre·cor·di·um (pre-kor′de-əm) pl. *precor′dia* [L., from *pre-* + *cor,* gen. *cordis,* heart] the region of the anterior surface of the body covering the heart and stomach; it comprises the epigastric region and the inferior part of the thorax. **precor′dial** *adj*

Pre·cose (pre′kōs) trademark for a preparation of acarbose.

pre·cos·tal (pre-kos′təl) anterior to the ribs.

pre·crit·i·cal (pre-krit′ĭ-kəl) previous to the occurrence of the crisis.

pre·cu·ne·us (pre-ku′ne-əs) [*pre-* + *cuneus*] [TA] a small wedge-shaped convolution on the medial surface of the parietal lobe of the cerebrum, bounded posteriorly by the medial part of the parietooccipital sulcus and anteriorly by the marginal sulcus and posterior paracentral gyrus. **precu′neate** *adj*

pre·cur·sor (pre′kər-sər) [L. *praecursor* a forerunner] 1. something that precedes. 2. in biological processes, a substance from which another, usually more active or mature substance is formed. 3. in clinical medicine, a sign or symptom that heralds another.

Pre·date (pre′dāt) trademark for preparations of prednisolone.

pre·da·tion (pre-da′shən) the derivation by an organism of elements essential for its existence from organisms of other species which it consumes and destroys.

pre·da·tor (prĕ′də-tər) [L. *praedator* a plunderer, pillager] an organism that derives elements essential for its existence from organisms of other species, which it consumes and destroys.

pre·de·cid·u·al (pre″də-sid′u-əl) pertaining to the secretory phase of the uterine cycle.

pre·den·tin (pre-den′tin) the soft fibrillar substance composing the primitive dentin and forming the inner layer of the circumpulpar dentin; called also *dentinoid.*

pre·di·a·be·tes (pre-di″ə-be′tēz) a state of latent impairment of carbohydrate metabolism, in which the criteria for diabetes mellitus are not all satisfied; sometimes controllable by diet alone.

pre·di·as·to·le (pre″di-as′tə-le) the interval immediately preceding diastole in the cardiac cycle.

pre·di·a·stol·ic (pre″di-ə-stol′ik) 1. pertaining to the beginning of diastole. 2. occurring just before diastole.

pre·di·crot·ic (pre″di-krot′ik) occurring before the dicrotic notch and wave of the sphygmogram.

pre·di·ges·tion (pre″di-jes′chən) the partial artificial digestion of food before its ingestion.

pre·dis·pos·ing (pre″dis-pōz′ing) conferring a tendency to disease.

pre·dis·po·si·tion (pre″dis-pə-zish′ən) [*pre-* + *disposition*] a latent susceptibility to disease which may be activated under certain conditions, as by stress.

pre·di·ver·tic·u·lar (pre-di″vər-tik′u-lər) denoting a condition of thickening of the muscular wall of the colon and increased intraluminal pressure but without herniation of the mucosa, i.e., without evidence of diverticulosis.

pred·ni·car·bate (pred″nĭ-kahr′bāt) [USP] a synthetic corticosteroid used topically for the relief of inflammation and pruritus in corticosteroid-responsive dermatoses.

Pred·ni·cen-M (pred′nĭ-sen″) trademark for a preparation of prednisone.

pred·ni·mus·tine (pred″nĭ-mus′tēn) an ester of chlorambucil and prednisone, used as an antineoplastic in treatment of non-Hodgkin lymphoma; administered orally.

pred·nis·o·lone (pred-nis′ə-lōn″) [USP] a synthetic glucocorticoid derived from cortisol, administered orally in replacement therapy for adrenocortical insufficiency and as an antiinflammatory and immunosuppressant in a wide variety of conditions.

p. acetate [USP] the 21-acetate ester of prednisolone, administered by intramuscular injection in replacement therapy for adrenocortical insufficiency and by intra-articular, intralesional, or soft-tissue injection as an antiinflammatory and immunosuppressant in a wide variety of disorders, and applied topically to the conjunctiva in the treatment of allergy and inflammation.

p. hemisuccinate [USP] an ester of hydrocortisone, having actions and uses similar to those of the base.

p. sodium phosphate [USP] a water-soluble ester of prednisolone, having a rapid onset and short duration of action; administered orally or by intramuscular injection in replacement therapy for adrenocortical insufficiency, orally or by intravenous, intramuscular, intra-articular, intralesional, or soft-tissue injection as an antiinflammatory and immunosuppressant in a wide variety of disorders, and applied topically to the conjunctiva in the treatment of allergy and inflammation.

p. sodium succinate [USP] a water-soluble ester of prednisolone, used as a glucocorticoid.

p. tebutate [USP] an ester of prednisolone having a slow onset and long duration of action, used as an antiinflammatory and immunosuppressant; administered by intra-articular, intralesional, or soft-tissue injection.

pred•ni•sone (pred′nĭ-sōn) [USP] a synthetic glucocorticoid derived from cortisone, administered orally as an antiinflammatory and immunosuppressant in a wide variety of disorders.

pre•dor•mi•tum (pre-dor′mĭ-təm) the period of waning consciousness interposed between the waking state and sound slumber. **predor′mital** *adj*

pre•eclamp•sia (pre″ə-klamp′se-ə) a complication of pregnancy characterized by hypertension, edema, and/or proteinuria; when convulsions and coma are associated, it is called *eclampsia.*

pre•ejec•tion (pre″e-jek′shən) occurring prior to ejection.

pre•epi•glot•tic (pre″ep-ĭ-glot′ik) anterior to the epiglottis.

pre•eryth•ro•cyt•ic (pre″ə-rith″ro-sit′ik) before entering an erythrocyte; said of stages in development of species of *Plasmodium.*

pre•ex•ci•ta•tion (pre-ek″si-ta′shən) premature activation of a portion of the ventricles due to transmission of cardiac impulses along an accessory pathway not subject to the physiologic delay of the atrioventricular node. See also *preexcitation syndrome,* under *syndrome.* The term is sometimes used as a synonym for *Wolff-Parkinson-White syndrome.* Called also *ventricular pacemaker*

pre•fron•tal (pre-fron′təl) situated in the anterior part of the frontal lobe or region.

pre•func•tion•al (pre-funk′shən-əl) denoting the period in embryological development during which the organ rudiments are formed but are incapable of performing their specific functions.

pre•gab•a•lin (pre-gab′ə-lin) a derivative of γ-aminobutyric acid (GABA) having anticonvulsant and antinociceptive effects, used in the treatment of neuropathic pain in diabetic neuropathy and postherpetic neuralgia; administered orally.

pre•gan•gli•on•ic (pre″gang-gle-on′ik) situated anterior or proximal to a ganglion; said especially of autonomic nerve fibers so located.

pre•gen•i•tal (pre-jen′ĭ-təl) pertaining to the early stages of psychosexual development (oral and anal), before the genitals have become the dominant influence on sexual behavior.

pre•glo•mer•u•lar (pre″glo-mer′u-lər) located or occurring proximal to a renal glomerulus.

preg•nan•cy (preg′nən-se) [L. *praegnans* with child] 1. the condition of having a developing embryo or fetus in the body, after union of an oocyte and spermatozoon. It is marked by cessation of the menses; nausea on arising in the morning (morning sickness); enlargement of the breasts and pigmentation of the nipples; progressive enlargement of the abdomen. The absolute signs of pregnancy are fetal movements, sounds of the fetal heart, and demonstration of the fetus by x-ray or ultrasound. 2. the period during which a female is pregnant, in humans being about 266 days from the time of fertilization of the oocyte until birth (or 288 days from the last normal menstrual period to birth); see *gestation period,* under *period.*

abdominal p. ectopic pregnancy with development of the embryo in the abdominal cavity.

ampullar p. ectopic pregnancy with development of the embryo in the ampulla of the uterine tube.

bigeminal p. twin p.

broad ligament p. ectopic pregnancy with development of the embryo in the broad ligament.

cervical p. ectopic pregnancy with development of the embryo in the cervical canal.

combined p. simultaneous existence of intrauterine and ectopic pregnancies.

compound p. superimposition of an intrauterine pregnancy on a previously existing ectopic pregnancy, generally a lithopedion.

cornual p. pregnancy in one of the horns of a bicornuate uterus.

ectopic p. development of the embryo outside the uterine cavity; called also *extrauterine p.*

exochorial p. graviditas exochorialis.

extrauterine p. ectopic p.

fallopian p. tubal p.

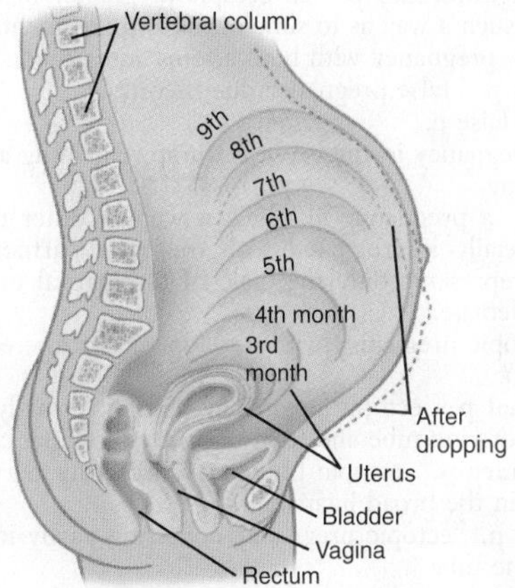

■ Pregnancy—Uterine levels.

false p. absence of the menses and presence of other signs of pregnancy, without occurrence of conception and development of an embryo. It may be due to psychogenic factors, to a tumor or mole, or to endocrine disorders. Called also *pseudocyesis, pseudopregnancy,* and *spurious p.*

gemellary p. twin p.

heterotopic p. combined p.

hydatid p. pregnancy accompanied by formation of a hydatid mole.

hysteric p. phantom p.

interstitial p. ectopic pregnancy with development of the embryo in the part of the uterine tube that is within the wall of the uterus.

intraligamentary p., intraligamentous p. broad ligament p.

intramural p. interstitial p.

intraperitoneal p. ectopic pregnancy within the peritoneal cavity.

membranous p. pregnancy in which the fetus has broken through its membranous envelope and lies in contact with the uterine walls.

mesenteric p. tuboligamentary p.

molar p. conversion of the early embryo into a mole.

multiple p. pregnancy in which two or more fetuses exist simultaneously; it may be *monovular* (resulting from the fertilization of a single oocyte) or *polyovular* (resulting from the fertilization of more than one oocyte). When more than two fetuses coexist, they may come from one zygote or be the result of combined monovular and polyovular twinning. Called also *multiple gestation.*

mural p. interstitial p.

nervous p. phantom p.

ovarian p. ectopic pregnancy with development of the embryo within an ovary.

ovarioabdominal p. ectopic pregnancy that begins ovarian but afterward becomes abdominal.

oviductal p. tubal p.

parietal p. interstitial p.

phantom p. false pregnancy due to psychogenic factors.

plural p. multiple p.

postterm p., prolonged p. pregnancy that has extended beyond 42 completed weeks from the onset of the last menstrual period or 40 completed weeks from conception. See also *postmature infant,* under *infant.*

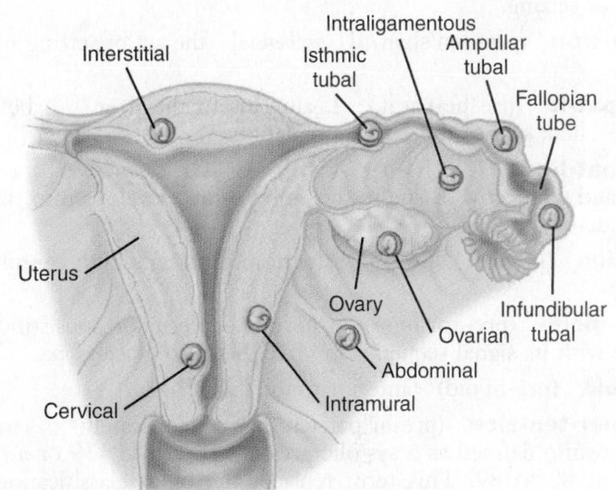

■ Diagram showing locations of ectopic (extrauterine) pregnancy.

pseudointraligamentary p. an ectopic pregnancy in which a sac has been formed in such a way as to simulate an intraligamentary pregnancy.
sarcofetal p. pregnancy with both a fetus and a mole.
sarcohysteric p. false pregnancy due to a mole.
spurious p. false p.
stump p. pregnancy in the cervical stump remaining after a supracervical hysterectomy.
surrogate p. a pregnancy in which a woman other than the female partner is artificially impregnated with the male partner's sperm. The resultant child represents only the male of the marital unit, and may be adopted by the female.
tubal p. ectopic pregnancy with development of the embryo within a uterine tube.
tuboabdominal p. ectopic pregnancy occurring partly in the fimbriated end of the uterine tube and partly in the abdominal cavity.
tuboligamentary p. ectopic pregnancy occurring partly in a uterine tube and partly in the broad ligament.
tubo-ovarian p. ectopic pregnancy occurring partly in the ovary and partly in a uterine tube.
tubouterine p. ectopic pregnancy occurring partly within the uterus and partly in a uterine tube.
twin p. gestation with development of two fetuses.
uteroabdominal p. pregnancy with one fetus in the uterus and another in the abdominal cavity.
uterotubal p. tubouterine p.

preg•nane (preg′nān) a type of saturated 21-carbon steroid hydrocarbon nucleus that is the parent structure of many steroids; two groups of steroids are distinguished as those stemming from 5α-pregnane and those stemming from 5β-pregnane. In the latter group are progesterones, ketones, and several corticosteroids.

preg•nane•di•ol (preg″nān-di′ol) any of several biologically inactive dihydroxy derivatives of progesterone; pregnanediols are metabolic degradation products, found especially in urine of women during pregnancy or the luteal phase of the menstrual cycle.

preg•nane•tri•ol (preg″nān-tri′ol) a metabolite of 17α-hydroxyprogesterone, normally occurring in small amounts in body fluids and urine, but greatly increased in disorders of the adrenal cortex in which 21-hydroxylation of the steroid nucleus is impaired, as in the most common form of congenital adrenocortical hyperplasia with virilism.

preg•nant (preg′nənt) [L. *praegnans*] with child; containing developing young. Called also *gravid.*

preg•nene (preg′nēn) a term used in steroid hormone nomenclature to refer to an unsaturated 21-carbon structure with one double bond and three methyl groups; the δ^4 and δ^5 pregnene steroid nucleus forms the basis of most of the biologically active progestins and corticosteroids.

preg•ne•no•lone (preg-nēn′ə-lōn) 1. an intermediate compound in the synthesis of steroid hormones, formed by cleavage of the side chain of cholesterol between C-20 and C-22. 2. a synthetic preparation of this hormone, used in treatment of rheumatoid arthritis.
p. succinate a nonhormonal sterol derivative that has been used in treatment of rheumatoid arthritis.

Preg•nyl (preg′nil) trademark for a preparation of chorionic gonadotropin.

pre•go•ni•um (pre-go′ne-əm) a recess on the lower edge of the body of the mandible anterior to the angle.

pre•hal•lux (pre-hal′əks) a supernumerary bone of the foot sometimes found growing from the medial border of the scaphoid.

pre•hen•sile (pre-hen′sil) [L. *prehendere* to lay hold of] adapted for grasping or seizing.

pre•hen•sion (pre-hen′shən) [L. *prehensio*] the act of seizing or grasping.

pre•he•pat•ic (pre″he-pat′ik) 1. anterior to the liver. 2. before the liver is reached; said of the portal circulation.

pre•he•pat•i•cus (pre″hə-pat′ĭ-kəs) [*pre-* + Gr. *hēpar* liver] a mass of vascular and connective tissue in the embryo that develops into the interstitial tissue of the liver.

Prehn sign (prān) [D.T. *Prehn*, American physician, 20th century] see under *sign.*

pre•hor•mone (pre-hor′mōn) a hormone precursor consisting of the hormone with its signal sequence in place. See also *prohormone.*

pre•hy•oid (pre-hi′oid) anterior to the hyoid bone.

pre•hy•per•ten•sion (pre-hi″pər-ten′shən) moderately increased blood pressure, defined as a systolic pressure of 120 to 139 or a diastolic pressure of 80 to 89. This term replaces the older classification called *borderline hypertension.*

pre•hy•poph•y•sis (pre″hi-pof′ĭ-sis) adenohypophysis.

pre•ic•tal (pre-ik′təl) [*pre-* + *ictal*] occurring before a stroke or an attack, as before an acute epileptic attack.

pre•in•va•sive (pre″in-va′siv) not yet invading other tissues; see *carcinoma in situ.*

pre•io•ta•tion (pre″i-o-ta′shən) [*pre-* + *iota*] a speech disorder in which an initial *i* sound is converted to *yi.*

Prei•ser disease (pri′zer) [Georg Karl Felix *Preiser*, German orthopedic surgeon, 1879–1913] see under *disease.*

Preisz-No•card bacillus (prīs no-kahr′) [Hugo von *Preisz*, Hungarian bacteriologist, 1860–1940; Edmond Isidore Etienne *Nocard*, French veterinarian, 1850–1903] *Corynebacterium pseudotuberculosis.*

pre•kal•li•kre•in (pre″kal-ĭ-kre′in) a plasma protein that is the proenzyme of plasma kallikrein, being cleaved and activated by activated coagulation factor XII.

pre•lac•te•al (pre-lak′te-əl) preceding the establishment of milk flow; a term applied to the feeding of a newborn baby with carbohydrate-electrolyte solutions to reduce initial weight loss until breast feeding is fully established.

pre•leu•ke•mia (pre-loo-ke′me-ə) myelodysplastic syndrome. **preleuke′mic** *adj*

pre•lim•bic (pre-lim′bik) situated anterior to a limbus; specifically, anterior to the limbus fossae ovalis.

pre•lin•gual (pre-ling′gwəl) occurring before the development of language.

pre-β-lipo•pro•tein (pre″ba-tə-lip″o-pro′tēn) see under *lipoprotein.*

pre•load (pre′lōd) the mechanical state of the heart at the end of diastole, the magnitude of the maximal (end-diastolic) ventricular volume or the end-diastolic pressure stretching the ventricles, calculated as: in isolated cardiac muscle, the force stretching the resting muscle to a given length prior to contraction; in the intact heart, the stress on the ventricular wall at the end of diastole, determined largely by the venous return, total blood volume and its distribution, and atrial activity. It is usually measured as left ventricular end-diastolic volume.

pre•lo•cal•iza•tion (pre″lo-kəl-ĭ-za′shən) the localization in the oocyte or blastomere of materials that will develop into a particular tissue or organ.

pre•lo•co•mo•tion (pre″lo-ko-mo′shən) the movements of a child made with the intention of moving from place to place before motor coordination is sufficiently developed to enable it to walk.

Prel•one (pre′lōn) trademark for a preparation of prednisolone.

PRELP [*p*roline/arginine-*r*ich *e*nd *l*eucine-rich *p*rotein] a leucine-rich repeat protein related to fibromodulin, found in cartilage, sclera, basement membranes, and developing bone; it is thought to play a role in the organization of extracellular matrix.

Pre•lu-2 (pra′loo) trademark for preparations of phendimetrazine tartrate.

pre•ma•lig•nant (pre″mə-lig′nənt) precancerous.

Prem•a•rin (prem′ə-rin) trademark for preparations of conjugated estrogens.

pre•ma•ture (pre-mə-chŏŏr′) [L. *praematurus* early ripe] 1. occurring before the proper time. 2. pertaining to a premature infant; see under *infant.*

pre•ma•tur•i•ty (pre″mə-chŏŏr′ĭ-te) underdevelopment; the condition of a premature infant.

pre•max•il•la (pre″mak-sil′ə) 1. TA alternative for *os incisivum.* 2. the embryonic bone derived from the median nasal prominences that later fuses with the maxilla to form the os incisivum.

pre•max•il•lary (pre-mak′sĭ-lar′e) 1. anterior to the maxilla proper. 2. os incisivum. 3. pertaining to the premaxilla or to the os incisivum.

pre•med•i•cal (pre-med′ĭ-kəl) preceding and preparing for the regular medical course of study, as premedical education.

pre•med•i•cant (pre-med′ĭ-kənt) premedication (def. 2).

pre•med•i•ca•tion (pre″med-ĭ-ka′shən) 1. preliminary administration of a drug preceding a diagnostic, therapeutic, or surgical procedure, as an antibiotic or antianxiety agent. 2. a drug administered for such a purpose.

pre•mei•ot•ic (pre″mi-ot′ik) [*pre-* + *meiotic*] occurring before or pertaining to the time preceding meiosis.

pre•me•nar•che (pre″mə-nahr′ke) the period before menarche (establishment of menstruation). **premenar′chal, premenar′cheal** *adj*

pre•meno•pau•sal (pre″men-o-paw′zəl) preceding menopause.

pre•men•strua (pre-men′stroo-ə) [L.] plural of *premenstruum.*

pre•men•stru•al (pre-men′stroo-əl) occurring before menstruation.

pre·men·stru·um (pre-men′stroo-əm) pl. *premenstrua* [L.] the interval immediately preceding a menstrual period.

pre·mi·tot·ic (pre″mi-tot′ik) occurring before or pertaining to the time preceding mitosis.

pre·mo·lar (P) (pre-mo′lər) [*pre-* + *molar*[2]] 1. see under *tooth.* 2. situated in front of the molar teeth.

pre·mon·i·to·ry (pre-mon′ĭ-tor-e) [L. *praemonitorius*] serving as a warning.

pre·mono·cyte (pre-mon′o-sīt) promonocyte.

pre·mor·bid (pre-mor′bid) occurring before the development of signs or symptoms of disease.

pre·mor·tal (pre-mor′təl) occurring just before death.

Prem·phase (prem′fāz) trademark for a therapeutic regimen of conjugated estrogens and medroxyprogesterone acetate.

Prem·pro (prem′pro) trademark for a combination preparation of conjugated estrogens and medroxyprogesterone acetate.

pre·mu·ni·tion (pre″mu-nish′ən) infection immunity.

pre·mu·ta·tion (pre″mu-ta′shən) increased numbers of triplet repeat sequences in a gene, to the point that although clinical disease is not apparent, the repeats are unstable and prone to undergo further increases during meiosis, crossing the threshold to a level associated with clinical disease.

pre·my·elo·blast (pre-mi′ə-lo-blast″) an early form of a myeloblast.

pre·my·elo·cyte (pre-mi′ə-lo-sīt″) promyelocyte.

pre·na·sa·le (pre″na-sa′le) a cephalometric landmark, the most projecting point, in the median plane, at the tip of the nose.

pre·na·tal (pre-na′təl) [*pre-* + *natal*] existing or occurring before birth, with reference to the fetus. Cf. *antepartal.*

pre·neo·plas·tic (pre″ne-o-plas′tik) preceding the development of a tumor.

pre·op·er·a·tive (pre-op′ər-ə-tiv) preceding an operation.

pre·op·tic (pre-op′tik) anterior to the optic chiasma.

pre·oxy·gen·a·tion (pre-ok″sĭ-jən-a′shən) 1. the prolonged breathing of oxygen to produce denitrogenation before exposure to low atmospheric pressure at high altitudes, as prophylaxis against decompression sickness. 2. the admininistration of 100 percent oxygen before a procedure that produces apnea, such as the induction of anesthesia or tracheal suctioning, in order to increase the oxygen reserve in the lungs and prevent hypoxemia during the period of apnea.

prep·a·ra·tion (prep″ə-ra′shən) [L. *praeparatio*] 1. the act or process of making ready. 2. a medicine made ready for use. 3. an anatomic or pathologic specimen made ready and preserved for study.

biomechanical p. the procedures involved in exposing, enlarging, cleansing, and shaping the pulp chamber and root canal of a tooth by mechanical means.

cavity p. a procedure for establishing in a tooth the biochemically and mechanically acceptable form necessary to receive and retain a restoration. See also *prepared cavity*, under *cavity.*

corrosion p. an anatomic preparation made by injecting the parts to be retained and dissolving the rest of the tissues with some corrosive substance.

heart-lung p. an animal in which only the heart and lungs are kept alive, the blood from the aorta being diverted into an external system of tubes, simulating the systemic circulation, and back via a reservoir to the right atrium; used in studies of heart function.

impression p., touch p. a preparation of bacteria on a slide for examination, made by lightly touching a coverglass to a colony.

pre·par·tal (pre-pahr′təl) [*pre-* + *partal*] antepartum.

pre·pa·tel·lar (pre″pə-tel′ər) in front of the patella.

pre·pa·tent (pre-pa′tənt) before becoming apparent or manifest; in malariology the term is applied to the period elapsing between infection and detection of parasites in the blood.

Pre-Pen (pre′pen) trademark for a preparation of benzylpenicilloyl polylysine.

pre·per·cep·tion (pre″pər-sep′shən) in psychology, anticipation of a perception.

pre·peri·to·ne·al (pre″per-ĭ-to-ne′əl) 1. situated between the parietal peritoneum and the anterior abdominal wall. 2. occurring anterior to the peritoneum.

Prep·i·dil (prep′ĭ-dil) trademark for a preparation of dinoprostone.

pre·pon·der·ance (pre-pon′dər-əns) [*pre-* + L. *pondere* to weigh] the condition of having greater weight, force, or influence.

ventricular p. disproportionate hypertrophy between the ventricles of the heart; diagnosed by the electrocardiograph.

pre·po·ten·tial (pre″po-ten′shəl) the slow diastolic depolarization of the cell membranes of the cardiac pacemaker.

pre·pran·di·al (pre-pran′de-əl) before meals.

pre·pro·hor·mone (pre″pro-hor′mōn) a hormone preproprotein.

pre·pro·in·su·lin (pre″pro-in′sə-lin) the intraglandular precursor of proinsulin, containing a signal sequence at the N-terminal.

pre·pro·pro·tein (pre″pro-pro′tēn) a precursor that is cleaved to form a proprotein.

pre·pros·thet·ic (pre″pros-thet′ik) performed or occurring before insertion of a prosthesis.

pre·pro·tein (pre-pro′tēn) a protein precursor that contains a signal sequence that must be cleaved off to form the protein or proprotein.

pre·pu·ber·ty (pre-pu′bər-te) the period preceding puberty. **prepu′beral, prepu′bertal** *adj*

pre·pu·bes·cence (pre″pu-bes′əns) prepuberty. **prepubes′cent** *adj*

pre·puce (pre′pūs) 1. preputium. 2. preputium penis.

p. of clitoris preputium clitoridis.

p. of penis preputium penis.

redundant p. presence of excessive foreskin that cannot be drawn back over the glans.

pre·pu·tial (pre-pu′shəl) pertaining to the prepuce.

pre·pu·ti·o·plas·ty (pre-pu′she-o-plas″te) plastic surgery of the prepuce.

pre·pu·ti·ot·o·my (pre-pu″she-ot′ə-me) [*preputium* + *-tomy*] incision of the preputium penis on the dorsum or side of the penis, to relieve the constriction in phimosis.

pre·pu·ti·um (pre-pu′she-əm) prepuce: a covering fold of skin.

p. clito′ridis [TA] prepuce of clitoris: a fold formed by the union of the labia minora anterior over the clitoris and united with the glans clitoris.

p. pe′nis [TA] prepuce of penis: the fold of skin covering the glans penis; called also *foreskin.*

pre·py·lor·ic (pre″pi-lor′ik) proximal to the pylorus or pyloric part of the stomach.

pre·re·nal (pre-re′nəl) 1. anterior to a kidney. 2. occurring before the kidney is reached, such as acute renal failure in which the kidney does not receive adequate blood flow. Cf. *postrenal.*

pre·sa·cral (pre-sa′krəl) anterior to or preceding the sacrum.

presby- [Gr. *presbys* old man] a combining form meaning old or denoting relationship to old age.

pres·by·acu·sia (pres″be-ə-ku′zhə) presbycusis.

pres·by·car·dia (pres″be-kahr′de-ə) [*presby-* + *cardia*] impaired cardiac function attributed to the aging process, occurring in association with recognizable changes of senescence in the body and in the absence of convincing evidence of other forms of heart disease.

pres·by·cu·sis (pres″bĭ-ku′sis) [*presby-* + *acou-* + *-sis*] a progressive, bilaterally symmetric sensorineural hearing loss occurring with age.

pres·by·der·ma (pres″be-dur′mə) any of the skin changes associated with aging, such as chronic actinic dermatitis and solar lentigo.

pres·by·esoph·a·gus (pres″be-ə-sof′ə-gəs) alteration in motor function of the esophagus as a result of degenerative changes occurring with advancing age.

pres·by·ope (pres′be-ōp) a person with presbyopia.

pres·by·opia (pres″be-o′pe-ə) [*presby-* + *-opia*] hyperopia and impairment of vision due to advancing years or to old age; it is dependent on diminution of the power of accommodation from loss of elasticity of the crystalline lens, causing the near point of distinct vision to be removed farther from the eye. Abbreviated Pr. **presbyop′ic** *adj*

pre·scap·u·la (pre-skap′u-lə) the suprascapular portion of the scapula.

pre·scap·u·lar (pre-skap′u-lər) 1. anterior to the scapula. 2. pertaining to the prescapula.

pre·scle·rot·ic (pre″sklə-rot′ik) occurring before sclerosis takes place.

pre·scribe (pre-skrīb′) [L. *praescribere* to write before] to designate in writing a remedy for administration.

pre·scrip·tion (prĕ-skrip′shən) [L. *praescriptio*] a written direction for the preparation and administration of a remedy. A prescription consists of the heading or *superscription*—that is, the symbol ℞ or the word Recipe, meaning "take"; the *inscription*, which contains the names and quantities of the ingredients; the *subscription*, or directions for compounding; and the *signature*, usually introduced by the abbreviation S. for *sig′na*, "mark," which gives the directions for the patient which are to be marked on the receptacle.

shotgun p. an irrational prescription that contains a number of ingredients given with the idea that one or more of them may be effective.

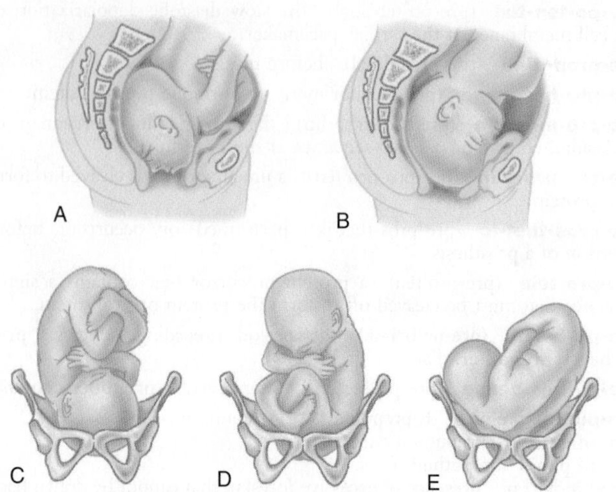

■ Presentations of the fetus. *(A)*, Face presentation; *(B)*, brow presentation; *(C)*, vertex presentation; *(D)*, breech presentation; *(E)*, shoulder presentation.

pre•se•nile (pre-se′nīl) pertaining to a condition resembling senility but occurring in early or middle life.

pre•se•nil•in (pre″sə-nil′in) see under *gene.*

pre•se•nil•i•ty (pre″sə-nil′ĭ-te) premature old age.

pre•se•ni•um (pre-se′ne-əm) the period immediately preceding old age.

pre•sent (pre-zent′) [L. *praesentare* to show] 1. to show or demonstrate. 2. to appear, such as a fetus at the os uteri; see *presenting part,* under *part.* 3. to appear, as for an examination or treatment; said of a patient.

pre•sen•ta•tion (pre″zən-ta′shən) [L. *praesentatio*] 1. the act or process of presenting; see *antigen p.* 2. in obstetrics, that portion of the fetus that is touched by the examining finger through the cervix or, during labor, is bounded by the girdle of resistance.

antigen p. the ingesting and partial digestion of antigens by macrophages, which then present the processed antigen on their surfaces to B and T lymphocytes. (See *antigen-presenting cells,* under *cell.*) The presented antigen is more immunogenic than unprocessed antigen, possibly because it has been broken down into pieces more easily recognized by B and T cells, because it remains on the surface of the presenting cell for a long time, or because it is presented in association with self MHC antigen and thus able to stimulate helper T cells.

breech p. presentation of the buttocks or feet of the fetus in labor.

breech p., complete presentation of the buttocks of the fetus in labor, with the feet alongside the buttocks, the thighs flexed upon the fetal abdomen, and the distal lower limbs flexed upon the thighs; the fetus in essence is in the same attitude as in vertex presentation but with polarity reversed.

breech p., frank presentation of the buttocks of the fetus in labor, with the lower limbs extended against the trunk and the feet lying against the face.

breech p., incomplete presentation of the fetus in labor, with one or both feet or one or both knees of the fetus prolapsed into the maternal vagina.

brow p. presentation of the fetal brow in labor.

cephalic p. presentation of any part of the fetal head in labor, including occiput, brow, or face.

compound p. prolapse of one of the limbs of the fetus alongside the head in cephalic presentation or of one or both arms along with a breech presentation at the beginning of labor.

face p. the presentation of the face of the fetus in labor.

footling p. presentation of the fetus in labor with one (single footling) or both feet (double footling) prolapsed into the maternal vagina.

funic p., funis p. presentation of the umbilical cord in labor.

parietal p. presentation of the parietal portion of the fetal head in labor.

pelvic p. breech p.

placental p. placenta previa.

shoulder p. presentation of the fetal shoulder in labor; see also *oblique lie* and *transverse lie,* under *lie.*

torso p. transverse lie.

transverse p. see under *lie.*

trunk p. transverse lie.

vertex p. the presentation of the vertex of the fetal head in labor.

pre•sep•tal (pre-sep′təl) anterior to a septum.

pre•ser•va•tive (prə-zur′və-tiv) a substance or preparation added to a product to destroy or inhibit the multiplication of microorganisms.

pre•si•nu•soi•dal (pre″si-nə-soi′dəl) anterior to a sinusoid or affecting the circulation before the sinusoids are reached; used especially to denote the location of vascular resistance in portal hypertension.

pre•so•mite (pre-so′mīt) [*pre-* + *somite*] referring to embryos before the appearance of somites; in the human, before 19 days postfertilization.

pre•sper•ma•tid (pre-spur′mə-tid) secondary spermatocyte.

pre•sphe•noid (pre-sfe′noid) 1. pertaining to the anterior part of the body of the sphenoid bone. 2. presphenoid part of sphenoid bone; see under *part.*

pre•sphe•noi•dal (pre″sfə-noi′dəl) presphenoid (def. 1).

pre•spon•dy•lo•lis•the•sis (pre-spon″də-lo-lis-the′sis) a congenital defect in the last lumbar vertebra consisting of a bilateral defect in the neural arches at the pedicles.

pres•som•e•ter (pres-om′ə-tər) manometer.

Jarcho p. an instrument especially designed for measuring pressure during injection of radiopaque material into the uterus in hysterosalpingography.

pres•sor (pres′or) tending to increase blood pressure; said of nerves and chemical substances. Called also *hypertensor.*

pres•so•re•cep•tive (pres″o-re-sep′tiv) sensitive to stimuli due to vasomotor activity, such as blood pressure.

pres•so•re•cep•tor (pres″o-re-sep′tər) baroreceptor.

pres•so•sen•si•tive (pres″o-sen′sĭ-tiv) pressoreceptive.

pres•sure (*P*) (presh′ər) [L. *pressura*] force per unit area; the SI unit is the pascal.

abdominal p. intra-abdominal p.

after p. a sense of pressure that lasts for a short period after removal of the actual pressure.

alveolar p. the pressure exerted by the air in the pulmonary alveoli.

antibiotic p. the amount of an antibiotic in a given environment.

arterial p., arterial blood p. blood p. (def. 2).

atmospheric p. the pressure exerted by the atmosphere, usually considered as the downward pressure of air onto a unit of area of the earth's surface; the unit of pressure at sea level is one *atmosphere.* Pressure decreases with increasing altitude. See also *atmosphere* (def. 2).

back p. the pressure caused by the damming back of the blood in a heart chamber and its tributaries, due to an obstructive heart valve or failing myocardium.

barometric p. atmospheric p.

biting p. occlusal p.

bladder p. intravesical p.

blood p. 1. the pressure of blood against the walls of any blood vessel. 2. the pressure of the blood on the walls of the arteries, dependent on the energy of the heart action, the elasticity of the walls of the arteries, and the volume and viscosity of the blood. The *maximum* or *systolic blood pressure* occurs near the end of the stroke output of the left ventricle of the heart. The *minimum* or *diastolic blood pressure* occurs late in ventricular diastole. *Mean blood pressure* is the average of the blood pressure levels, and *basic blood pressure* is that during quiet rest or basal conditions. See also *hypertension* and *hypotension.*

capillary p. the blood pressure in the capillaries.

central venous p. (CVP) the venous pressure as measured at the right atrium, obtained by means of a central venous catheter whose distal end is attached to a manometer.

cerebral perfusion p. (CPP) the difference between the mean arterial pressure and the intracranial pressure, normally 70–95 mm Hg.

cerebrospinal p. the pressure or tension of the cerebrospinal fluid, normally 100–150 mm Hg as measured by the manometer.

continuous positive airway p. (CPAP) a method of positive pressure ventilation used with patients who are breathing spontaneously, in which pressure in the airway is maintained above the level of atmospheric pressure throughout the respiratory cycle. The purpose is to keep the alveoli open at the end of exhalation and thus increase oxygenation and reduce the work of breathing. Cf. *positive end-expiratory p.*

critical p. the smallest amount of pressure necessary to liquefy a gas at the critical temperature.

detrusor p. the pressure exerted inward by the detrusor urinae muscles of the bladder wall, one of the components of the total intravesical pressure.

detrusor leak point p. as the bladder fills without an increase in abdominal pressure, the level of pressure at which leakage of urine through the urethra occurs; this is a measure of both strength of the urethral sphincters and compliance of the detrusor urinae muscle.

diastolic p., diastolic blood p. see *blood p.*

Donders p. increase of manometric pressure with the instrument placed on the trachea on opening the chest of a dead body; due to collapse of the lung.
end-diastolic p. the pressure in the ventricles of the heart at the end of diastole, usually measured in the left ventricle as an approximation of the end-diastolic volume, or preload.
endocardial p. pressure of blood within the heart.
filling p. see *mean circulatory filling p.*
free hepatic vein p., free hepatic venous p. the venous pressure in a hepatic vein on the vena caval side of a wedged catheter; cf. *wedged hepatic vein p.*
hydrostatic p. the pressure at any level in fluid at rest due solely to the weight of the fluid above it.
intra-abdominal p. the pressure between the viscera within the abdominal cavity. Called also *abdominal p.*
intra-articular p. the pressure within a joint cavity; it is normally subatmospheric at rest, decreased upon flexion, and increased if there is excess fluid in the cavity.
intracranial p. (ICP) the pressure in the space between the skull and the brain, i.e., the pressure of the subarachnoidal fluid.
intraocular p. the pressure of the fluids of the eye against the tunics. It is produced by continual renewal of the fluids within the interior of the eye, and is altered in certain pathological conditions (e.g., glaucoma). It may be roughly estimated by palpation of the eye or measured, directly or indirectly, with specially devised instruments called tonometers. Normal intraocular pressure is symbolized Tn. Called also *intraocular tension.*
intrapleural p. pleural p.
intrathecal p. pressure within a sheath, particularly the pressure of the cerebrospinal fluid within the subarachnoid membrane.
intrathoracic p. pleural p.
intraventricular p. the pressure within one ventricle of the heart.
intravesical p. the pressure exerted on the contents of the urinary bladder, being the sum of the intra-abdominal pressure from outside the bladder and the detrusor pressure exerted by the bladder wall musculature itself. Called also *bladder p.* and *vesical p.*
leak point p. as the bladder fills, the pressure at which leakage occurs through the urethra, used as a measure of strength of the urethral sphincters. See *detrusor leak point p.* and *Valsalva leak point p.*
maximum expiratory p. (MEP) a measure of the strength of respiratory muscles, obtained by having the patient exhale as strongly as possible against a mouthpiece; the maximum value is near total lung capacity.
maximum inspiratory p. (MIP) a measure of the strength of respiratory muscles, obtained by having the patient inhale as strongly as possible with the mouth against a mouthpiece; the maximum value is near the residual volume.
mean arterial p. (MAP) the average pressure within an artery over a complete cycle of one heartbeat; in the brachial artery,

$$\text{MAP} = \text{diastolic pressure} + \frac{\text{systolic pressure} - \text{diastolic pressure}}{3}.$$

mean circulatory filling p. a measure of the average (arterial and venous) pressure necessary to cause filling of the circulation with blood; it varies with blood volume and is directly proportional to the rate of venous return and thus to cardiac output.
negative p. a pressure less than that of the atmosphere.
occlusal p. pressure exerted on the occlusal surfaces of the teeth when the jaws are brought into apposition. Called also *biting p.*
oncotic p. the osmotic pressure due to the presence of colloids in a solution; in the case of plasma–interstitial fluid interaction, it is the force that tends to counterbalance the capillary pressure.
osmotic p. the pressure required to stop osmosis through a semipermeable membrane between a solution and pure solvent; it is proportional to the osmolality of the solution and also to other colligative properties of the solution, including freezing point depression, vapor pressure depression, and boiling point elevation. Symbol π.
osmotic p., effective that part of the total osmotic pressure of a solution which governs the tendency of its solvent to pass through a bordering semipermeable membrane or across another boundary.
partial p. the pressure exerted by each of the components of a gas mixture, such as of gases in the blood.
perfusion p. the difference between the arterial and venous pressures through an organ or capillary bed.
pleural p. the pressure between the visceral pleura and the parietal pleura in the pleural cavity. Called also *intrapleural* or *intrathoracic p.*
positive p. pressure greater than that of the atmosphere.
positive end-expiratory p. (PEEP) a method of positive pressure ventilation used in conjunction with mechanical ventilation; pressure is maintained above the level of atmospheric pressure at the end of exhalation. This is achieved by preventing the complete release of gas during exhalation, usually by means of a valve within the circuit. The purpose is to increase the volume of gas remaining in the lungs at the end of exhalation, thus reducing the shunting of blood through the lungs and improving gas exchange; done in acute respiratory failure to allow reduction of inspired O_2 concentrations. Cf. *continuous positive airway p.*
pulmonary artery wedge p. (PAWP), pulmonary capillary wedge p. (PCWP) blood pressure measured by a catheter wedged into the distal pulmonary artery; it permits indirect measurement of the mean blood pressure in the left atrium.
pulse p. the difference between the systolic and diastolic blood pressures.
resting anal p. the pressure of anal contents against the internal anal sphincter when the colon is at rest.
selection p. an effect produced by a given gene that determines the frequency of a given allele; it may be advantageous for survival *(positive selection pressure)* or disadvantageous *(negative selection pressure).*
solution p. the force that tends to bring into solution the molecules of a solid contained in the solvent.
systolic p., systolic blood p. see *blood p.*
transpulmonary p. the pressure difference between the inner and outer surfaces of the lung, i.e., the pressure tending to inflate or deflate the lungs; equal to the difference between the alveolar pressure and the pleural pressure.
urethral p. the inward pressure exerted by the walls of the urethra, which must be counteracted in order for urine to flow through; see also under *profile.*
Valsalva leak point p. the amount of pressure on the bladder by a Valsalva maneuver at which leakage of urine from the urethra occurs; this is a measure of strength of the urethral sphincters.
venous p. the blood pressure in a vein, such as central venous pressure or wedged hepatic vein pressure.
vesical p. intravesical p.
wedge p. blood pressure measured by a small catheter wedged into a vessel, occluding it; see *pulmonary capillary wedge p.* and *wedged hepatic vein p.*
wedged hepatic vein p., wedged hepatic venous p. the venous pressure measured with a catheter wedged into the hepatic vein. The difference between wedged and free hepatic vein pressures is used to locate the site of obstruction in portal hypertension; it is elevated in that due to cirrhosis but low in cardiac ascites or portal vein thrombosis.

pre·su·bic·u·lum (pre″soo-bik′u-ləm) [TA] a modified six-layered cortex situated between the subiculum and the main part of the parahippocampal gyrus.

pre·sump·tive (pre-zump′tiv) referring to the expected fate of an embryonic part on the basis of an established fate map.

pre·syl·vi·an (pre-sil′ve-ən) pertaining to the anterior or ascending branch of the sylvian fissure (sulcus lateralis).

pre·symp·tom (pre-simp′tom) an indication that is a forerunner of the actual symptoms of a condition.

pre·symp·to·mat·ic (pre″simp-tə-mat′ik) existing before the appearance of symptoms.

pre·syn·ap·tic (pre″sĭ-nap′tik) situated before or proximal to a synapse, or occurring before the synapse is crossed.

pre·sys·to·le (pre-sis′to-le) the interval immediately preceding systole.

pre·sys·tol·ic (pre″sis-tol′ik) 1. pertaining to the beginning of systole. 2. occurring just before systole.

pre·tar·sal (pre-tahr′səl) anterior to the tarsus.

pre·tec·tal (pre-tek′təl) anterior to the tectum mesencephali.

pre·tec·tum (pre-tek′təm) pretectal area.

pre·term (pre-turm′) before completion of the full term; said of pregnancy or of an infant.

pre·throm·bot·ic (pre-throm-bot′ik) preceding the development of thrombosis.

pre·thy·roid (pre-thi′roid) anterior to the thyroid gland or thyroid cartilage.

pre·tib·i·al (pre-tib′e-əl) in front of the tibia.

pre·tu·ber·cu·lo·sis (pre″too-bur″ku-lo′sis) tuberculosis in an incipient and occult stage before any symptoms of the disease have appeared.

Prev·a·cid (prev′ə-sid) trademark for a preparation of lansoprazole.

prev AGT previous abnormality of glucose tolerance.

prev·a·lence (prev′ə-ləns) [L. *praevalēre* to prevail] the number of cases of a disease that are present in a population at a specified time, either at a point in time *(point p.)* or over a period of time *(period p.)*; when the term is unmodified, the former meaning is usually inferred. See *prevalence rate*, under *rate*. Cf. *incidence.*

Prev·a·lite (prev′ə-līt) trademark for a preparation of cholestyramine resin.

Pre•ven (pre-ven′) trademark for a combination preparation of levonorgestrel and ethinyl estradiol.

pre•ven•tive (pre-ven′tiv) 1. serving to avert the occurrence of something. 2. prophylactic (def. 1).

pre•ver•te•bral (pre-vur′tə-brəl) [*pre-* + *vertebral*] anterior to a vertebra or vertebrae.

pre•ves•i•cal (pre-ves′ĭ-kəl) [*pre-* + *vesical*] anterior to the urinary bladder.

pre•vi•a•ble (pre-vi′ə-bəl) not yet viable; said of a fetus incapable of extrauterine existence.

pre•vi•ta•min (pre-vi′tə-min) a precursor of a vitamin.

p. D_3 the immediate precursor to cholecalciferol, produced as a thermally labile intermediate upon irradiation of 7-dehydrocholesterol in the skin; at body temperature, it spontaneously rearranges to form cholecalciferol in approximately three days.

Prev•nar (prev′nahr) trademark for a preparation of pneumococcal 7-valent conjugate vaccine.

Pré•vost law, sign (pra-vo′) [Jean Louis *Prévost*, Swiss physician, 1838–1927] see under *law* and *sign*.

Pre•vo•tel•la (pre″vo-tel′ə) [André Romain *Prévot*, French microbiologist, 1894–1982] a genus of gram-negative, obligately anaerobic, moderately saccharolytic, bile-sensitive bacteria of the family Prevotellaceae, consisting of nonmotile, non–spore-forming, pleomorphic rod-shaped organisms. They are normal inhabitants of the mucous membranes and are found especially in the oral cavity, colon, and vagina; some cause human infections. Included here are a number of species formerly included in the genus *Bacteroides*. The type species is *P. melaninoge′nica*.

P. bi′via a bile-sensitive, nonpigmented species that is moderately fermentative, found in the female genital tract and in the oral cavity, and isolated from infections of the urogenital tract and abdominal region and from breast abscesses. Formerly called *Bacteroides bivius*.

P. buc′cae a nonpigmented species that is a normal inhabitant of the gingival crevice and has been isolated from chest drainage, blood, sinus aspirates, and peritoneal fluid; formerly called *Bacteroides buccae*.

P. cor′poris a pigmented species that has been isolated from various clinical specimens; formerly called *Bacteroides corporis*.

P. denti′cola a pigmented species that is a normal inhabitant of the gingival crevice and has been isolated from various clinical specimens; formerly called *Bacteroides denticola*.

P. di′siens a nonpigmented, weakly fermentative species found in infections of the oral cavity and the female genital tract, and as part of the normal flora of the vagina and mouth; formerly called *Bacteroides disiens*.

P. heparinoly′tica a nonpigmented species that has been isolated from infections of the oral cavity and respiratory tract and from the genital tract; formerly called *Bacteroides heparinolyticus*.

P. interme′dia a weakly fermentative species isolated from the human gingival crevice and various clinical specimens. Formerly called *Bacteroides intermedius* and *B. melaninogenicus* subsp. *intermedius*.

P. melaninoge′nica a coccoid species that produces a black hematin pigment, part of the normal flora of the mucous membranes. It is also an important pathogen in oral, lung, and brain abscesses and occurs in other mixed infections. Formerly called *Bacteroides melaninogenicus* and *B. melaninogenicus* subsp. *melaninogenicus*.

P. ora′lis a nonpigmented, strongly fermentative species found principally in the gingival sulcus, which is occasionally associated with infections of the oral cavity and the respiratory and genital tracts; formerly called *Bacteroides oralis*.

P. o′ris a nonpigmented species that is a normal inhabitant of the gingival crevice and has been isolated from systemic infections; abscesses of the face, neck, and chest; abdominal wound drainage; blood; and peritoneal and spinal fluid. Formerly called *Bacteroides oris*.

P. rumini′cola a nonpigmented, strongly fermentative species isolated from the rumens of cattle, sheep, and elk, and from human abscesses and feces.

Pre•vo•tel•la•ceae (pre″vo-tel-a′se-e) a family of gram-negative, rod-shaped bacteria of the phylum Bacteroidetes. It contains a single genus, *Prevotella*.

Prev•pac (prev′pak) trademark for a therapeutic regimen of lansoprazole, ampicillin, and clarithromycin.

Prey•er reflex (pri′ər) [Thierry Wilhelm *Preyer*, German physiologist, 1841–1897] auricle reflex; see under *reflex*.

pre•zone (pre′zōn) prozone.

pre•zy•ga•poph•y•sis (pre″zi-gə-pof′ĭ-sis) processus articularis superior vertebrarum.

pre•zy•got•ic (pre-zi-got′ik) occurring before the completion of fertilization and formation of the zygote.

PRF prolactin-releasing factor.

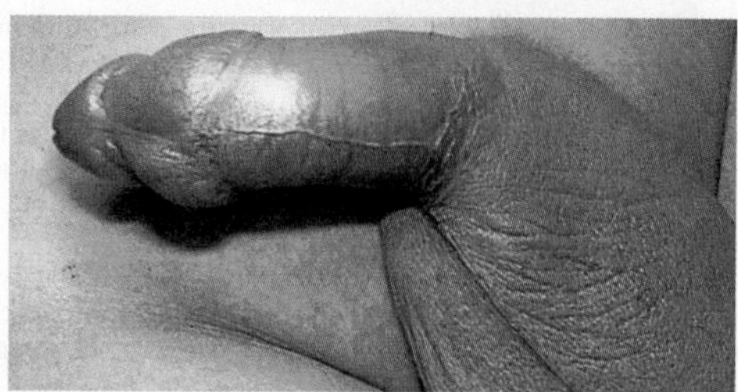

■ Priapism in a youth.

pri•a•pism (pri′ə-piz″əm) [L. *priapismus;* Gr. *priapismos*] persistent abnormal erection of the penis, usually without sexual desire, accompanied by pain and tenderness; causes include diseases and injuries of the spinal cord, vesical calculus, and certain injuries to the penis.

secondary p. priapism caused by obstruction to the outflow of blood through the dorsal vein at the root of the penis.

Price-Jones curve (prīs′-jōnz′) [Cecil *Price-Jones*, English physician, 1863–1943] see under *curve*.

prick (prik) 1. a light puncture. 2. to puncture lightly.

nail p. pricked foot.

prick•le (prik′əl) 1. a small, sharp spine or point. 2. a tingling or smarting sensation.

Prif•tin (prif′tin) trademark for a preparation of rifapentine.

pril•o•caine (pril′o-kān) a local anesthetic used topically, together with lidocaine, to provide dermal analgesia.

p. hydrochloride [USP] the hydrochloride salt of prilocaine; administered parenterally as a local anesthetic in minor surgery and dental procedures.

Pril•o•sec (pril′o-sek) trademark for a preparation of omeprazole.

Prima•cor (prim′ə-kor) trademark for a preparation of milrinone.

pri•map•ter•in (pre-map′tər-in) [from *Primael*, the first patient in whom it was detected + *pterin*] an isomer of biopterin substituted at the 7-position; it accumulates in the urine in patients with a defect in 4a-hydroxytetrahydrobiopterin dehydratase.

pri•map•ter•in•uria (pre-map″tər-ĭ-nu′re-ə) urinary excretion of primapterin, as occurs in tetrahydrobiopterin deficiency that is caused by mutation of the gene encoding 4a-hydroxytetrahydrobiopterin dehydratase.

prim•a•quine phos•phate (prim′ə-kwēn) [USP] an 8-aminoquinoline compound used as an antimalarial against the preerythrocytic stage of *Plasmodium vivax* and *P. ovale* and the gametocyte stage of *P. falciparum*, used especially in the treatment of relapsing vivax malaria; administered orally, sometimes in conjunction with other antimalarials.

pri•mary (pri′mar-e) [L. *primarius* principal; *primus* first] first in order or in time of development; principal.

pri•mase (pri′mās) a DNA-directed RNA polymerase that synthesizes an RNA primer complementary to one of the DNA strands in order to initiate DNA synthesis during DNA replication.

pri•mate (pri′māt) an individual belonging to the order Primates.

Pri•ma•tes (pri-ma′tēz) [L. *primus* first] an order of mammals, including human beings, apes, monkeys, and lemurs. Families include Cercopithecidae, Hominidae, Lemuridae, and Pongidae.

Pri•max•in (pri-mak′sin) trademark for a combination preparation of imipenem and cilastatin sodium.

primed (prīmd) immunologically activated by initial exposure to antigen; said of cells of the immune system.

prim•er (prīm′ər) 1. a substance that prepares for or facilitates the action of another. 2. in genetics, a short piece of DNA or RNA complementary to a given nucleic acid sequence; it acts as the nucleation point from which nucleotides are added to the growing chain, as in DNA replication, sequencing, or the polymerase chain reaction.

cavity p. a substance that enhances adaptation of resin filling materials to cavity walls by inducing wetting between the resinous material and the treated dentin and enamel surfaces.

prim•i•done (prim′ĭ-dōn) [USP] an anticonvulsant used in the treatment of generalized tonic-clonic, nocturnal myoclonic, complex partial, and simple partial epileptic seizures, administered orally.

pri•mi•grav•id (pri″mĭ-grav′id) pregnant for the first time.

pri•mi•grav•i•da (pri″mĭ-grav′ĭ-də) [L. *prima* first + *gravida*] a woman pregnant for the first time; also written gravida I.

pri•mip•a•ra (pri-mip′ə-rə) pl. *primip′arae* [L. *prima* first + *para*] a woman who has had one pregnancy that resulted in a fetus that attained a weight of 500 g or a gestational age of 20 weeks, regardless of whether the infant was living at birth, and regardless of whether it was a single or multiple birth. Also written *para I.*

pri•mi•par•i•ty (pri″mĭ-par′ĭ-te) the condition or fact of being a primipara.

pri•mip•a•rous (pri-mip′ə-rəs) bearing or having borne but one child.

pri•mit•iae (pri-mish′e-e) [L. pl., "first things"] the part of the amniotic fluid discharged before the fetus is extruded.

prim•i•tive (prim′ĭ-tiv) [L. *primitivus*] first in point of time; existing in a simple or early form that shows little complexity.

pri•mor•di•al (pri-mor′de-əl) [L. *primordialis*] original or primitive; of the simplest and most undeveloped character.

pri•mor•di•um (pri-mor′de-əm) pl. *primor′dia* [L. "the beginning"] the earliest discernible indication during embryonic development of an organ or part; called also *anlage* or *rudiment.*

pri•mo•some (pri′mo-sōm) [*primase* + *-some*] a complex of helicase and primase, sometimes with accessory proteins, that moves as a unit along the template DNA during replication, synthesizing RNA primers that initiate the formation of Okazaki fragments.

prim•rose (prim′rōz) 1. a plant of the genus *Primula.* 2. evening p.

evening p. 1. *Oenothera biennis.* 2. a preparation of the oil from the seeds of *O. biennis;* see under *oil.*

Pri•mu•la (pri′mu-lə) a genus of flowering plants of the family Primulaceae. *P. obco′nica* is the cultivated primula or primrose plant, a common cause of allergic contact dermatitis.

prin•ceps (prin′seps) [L.] principal; chief.

Prin•ci•pen (prin′sĭ-pen) trademark for preparations of ampicillin.

prin•ci•ple (prin′sĭ-pəl) [L. *principium*] 1. a chemical component. 2. a substance on which certain of the properties of a drug depend. 3. a law of conduct.

active p. any constituent of a drug that helps to confer upon it a medicinal property.

Doppler p. see under *effect.*

Fick p. a restatement of the law of conservation of mass used in making indirect measurements: the amount of a substance taken up or released by an organ is the product of the blood flow to the organ and the concentration difference of the substance between the arterial and venous systems. It is usually applied as the Fick method (q.v.) or one of the indicator dilution methods (q.v.) to determine cardiac output.

Hardy-Weinberg p. see under *law.*

immediate p. any one of the more or less complex substances of definite chemical constitution into which a heterogeneous substance can be readily resolved.

p. of infinitesimal dose one of the fundamental principles of homeopathy, stating that the more a remedy is diluted (even to the point that none of the medicinal substance is likely to be present) the more powerful and longer lasting will be its effect.

Le Chatelier p. if a biological system is subjected to stress, it will act in such a way as to reduce the stress.

organic p. immediate p.

pleasure p., pleasure-pain p. in psychoanalytic theory, an inborn tendency to avoid pain and seek pleasure through the immediate reduction of tension by either direct or fantasized gratification; cf. *reality p.*

proximate p. immediate p.

reality p. in psychoanalytic theory, the ego functions that modify the demands of the pleasure principle to meet the demands and requirements of the external world.

yin/yang p. in Chinese philosophy, the concept of polar complements existing in dynamic equilibrium and always present simultaneously. In traditional Chinese medicine, a disturbance of the proper balance of yin and yang causes disease, and the goal is to maintain or to restore this balance.

Prin•gle disease (pring′gəl) [John James *Pringle,* British dermatologist, 1855–1922] adenoma sebaceum (def. 2).

Prin•gle maneuver (pring′gəl) [James Hogarth *Pringle,* Scottish surgeon, 1863–1941] see under *maneuver.*

Pri•ni•vil (prin′ĭ-vil) trademark for a preparation of lisinopril.

Prin•zide (prin′zīd) trademark for a combination preparation of lisinopril and hydrochlorothiazide.

Prinz•met•al angina (prints′met-əl) [Myron *Prinzmetal,* American cardiologist, 1908–1994] see under *angina.*

pri•on (pri′on, pre′on) [*protein infectious agent*] any of several protease-resistant, insoluble, transmissible isoforms of the 27–30 kD core of prion protein that cause a group of progressive neurodegenerative diseases (prion diseases). Prions have a pleated sheet conformation rather than the α helix structure that is normal for prion protein, lack detectable nucleic acid, and do not elicit an immune response.

Pris•co•line (pris′ko-lēn) trademark for preparations of tolazoline hydrochloride.

prism (priz′əm) [Gr. *prisma*] a solid of glass, plastic, or a similar substance with a triangular or polygonal cross section, which splits up a ray of light into its constituent colors and turns or deflects light rays toward its base. Prisms are used to correct deviations of the eyes, since they alter the apparent situation of objects. Abbreviated Pr.

adamantine p's, enamel p's prismata adamantina; see under *prisma.*

Maddox p. two prisms with their bases together; used in testing for torsion of the eyeball.

Nicol p. two slabs of Iceland spar cemented together and deflecting a ray of light in such a way that it is split in two, one part (the ordinary ray) being totally reflected and the other (polarized ray) passing through.

Risley p. a prism that rotates in a metal frame marked with a scale; used in testing ocular muscles for imbalance.

pris•ma (priz′mə) pl. *pris′mata* [Gr.] prism.

pris′mata adaman′tina adamantine prisms: the structural units of the tooth enamel, consisting of parallel rods or prisms composed mainly of hydroxyapatite crystals and organic substance and held together with a cement substance, each prism being enveloped in a sheath. Called also *enamel prisms* or *rods.*

pris•ma•ta (priz′mə-tə) [Gr.] plural of *prisma.*

pris•mat•ic (priz-mat′ik) shaped like a prism; produced by a prism.

pris•moid (priz′moid) resembling a prism.

pris•mop•tom•e•ter (priz″mop-tom′ə-tər) [*prism* + *optometer*] an instrument for testing the eye by means of a revolving prism.

pris•mo•sphere (priz′mo-sfēr) [*prism* + *sphere*] a prism combined with a globular lens.

pris•op•tom•e•ter (priz″op-tom′ə-tər) prismoptometer.

Pris•tiq (pris-tēk′) trademark for a preparation of desvenlafaxine succinate.

PRK photorefractive keratectomy.

PRL, Prl prolactin.

p.r.n. [L.] pro re na′ta (according to circumstances).

PRO Professional (or Peer) Review Organization.

Pro proline.

pro- [L. and Gr. "before"] 1. a prefix signifying before or in front of. 2. a prefix denoting a precursor, as of an enzyme or hormone.

pro•ac•cel•er•in (pro″ak-sel′ər-in) factor V; see under *coagulation factors,* at *factor.*

pro•ac•ro•so•mal (pro″ak-ro-so′məl) pertaining to an early stage of development of acrosomes.

pro•ac•ti•va•tor (pro-ak′tĭ-va″tər) the inactive precursor form of an activator, or a factor that requires a chemical change, usually by an enzyme, to become an activator.

C3 p. (C3PA) former name for *factor B.*

pro•al (pro′əl) characterized by forward movement.

Pro•Am•a•tine (pro-am′ə-tēn) trademark for a preparation of midodrine hydrochloride.

pro•am•ni•on (pro-am′ne-on) that part of the embryonal area at the ventral and lateral sides of the head which remains without mesoderm for some time.

pro•an•gio•gen•ic (pro-an″je-o-jen′ik) promoting angiogenesis.

pro•ap•op•tot•ic (pro″ap″op-tot′ic, pro″ap″o-tot′ic) promoting apoptosis.

pro•ar•rhyth•mia (pro″ə-rith′me-ə) cardiac arrhythmia that is either drug-induced or drug-aggravated.

pro•ar•rhyth•mic (pro″ə-rith′mik) inducing or aggravating arrhythmia.

pro•at•las (pro-at′ləs) a rudimentary vertebra that lies in front of the atlas in certain vertebrates and is sometimes seen as an anomaly in humans.

prob•a•bil•i•ty (prob″ə-bil′ĭ-te) [L. *probabilis* probable, from *probare* to test or examine] the likelihood of occurrence of a specified event; it is often represented as a number between 0 (never) and 1 (always) that corresponds to the long-run trial at which an event occurs in a sequence of random independent trials under identical conditions, as the number of trials approaches infinity. Symbol *P.*

significance p. *P* value.

pro•bac•te•rio•phage (pro″bak-te′re-o-fāj″) prophage.

pro•band (pro′band) [Ger., from L. *probandus* "the one to be tested"] an affected person ascertained independently of relatives in a genetic study. Called also *propositus.*

pro·bang (pro′bang) a flexible rod with a ball, tuft, or sponge at one end; used in applying medications to or removing matter from the esophagus or larynx.

Pro-Ban·thine (pro-ban-thīn′) trademark for preparations of propantheline bromide.

probe (prōb) [L. *proba; probare* to test] 1. a slender, flexible instrument designed for introduction into a wound, cavity, or sinus tract for purposes of exploration. 2. a single-stranded DNA or RNA sequence that is labeled, as by radioactivity, and used to detect the presence of a complementary nucleic acid sequence by nucleic acid hybridization (q.v.).

Anel p. a delicate probe for the lacrimal puncta and canals.

blood flow p. an implanted cuff that fits around a surgically exposed artery or vein to detect blood flow.

blunt p. a probe with a blunt end.

Bowman p. one of a set of probes for use on the nasolacrimal ducts.

Brackett p's delicate and flexible probes of silver wire for exploring dental fistulas.

bullet p. a probe used for detecting the presence or location of a bullet.

drum p. a probe with an attachment that emits a sound when it comes in contact with a foreign body.

electric p. a probe that on contact with a foreign body completes an electric circuit, thereby producing a sound.

eyed p. a probe with a slit near one end through which a ligature or tape may be drawn.

fiberoptic p. a flexible probe made up of a bundle of fine glass fibers optically aligned to transmit an image.

heater p. a hollow cylinder with an inner coil for transferring heat to compress tissue and stop bleeding.

imaging p. molecular imaging p.

lacrimal p. a probe designed for use on the lacrimal passages.

molecular imaging p. in molecular imaging, a molecule that can deliver a tracer to a specific organ or tissue to provide a signal on a receptor that can then be picked up by an imaging device. Called also *imaging p.*

periodontal p., pocket p. a probe graduated in millimeters, used to measure the depth and determine the outline of a periodontal pocket and the condition of the crevicular epithelium.

root canal p. in root canal therapy, a hand-operated instrument consisting of a slender, flexible, smooth or edged wire, used for tracing the course of and exploring root canals. Called also *pathfinder, pathfinder broach,* and *smooth broach.*

scissors p. a long, delicate pair of scissors that can be used as a probe.

uterine p. a probe for uterine exploration.

vertebrated p. a flexible probe made up of joined links.

pro·ben·e·cid (pro-ben′ə-sid) [USP] a uricosuric agent that acts by inhibiting the carrier-mediated transport of organic acids in the renal tubule, which increases the excretion of uric acid by blocking its tubular reabsorption and decreases the excretion of penicillins and certain other acidic drugs by blocking their tubular secretion; used in the treatment of hyperuricemia of gout and as an adjunct in antibiotic therapy.

pro·bi·ot·ic (pro″bi-ot′ik) a preparation of nonpathogenic microorganisms introduced into the body for their health benefits, such as *Lactobacillus acidophilus* ingested to modify the intestinal microflora.

pro·bit (pro′bit) [contraction of "*prob*ability un*it*"] a normal variate having mean 5 and standard deviation 1. In quantal biologic assays, the observed responses are often converted to probits (the fraction responding is converted to the probit that cuts off the same fraction of the area under the normal frequency curve) in order to fit a linear log dose–response curve, a procedure based on the assumption that the response thresholds are normally distributed.

pro·bos·cis (pro-bos′is) [*pro-* + Gr. *boskein* to feed, graze] any tubular process or structure of the head or snout of an animal, usually used in feeding.

p. latera′lis a rare congenital deformity marked by absence of the medial and lateral nasal processes and the globular processes; on the affected side, the nasal cavity, choana, and nasal bones are absent and there is a tubular appendage (proboscis) above the medial canthus.

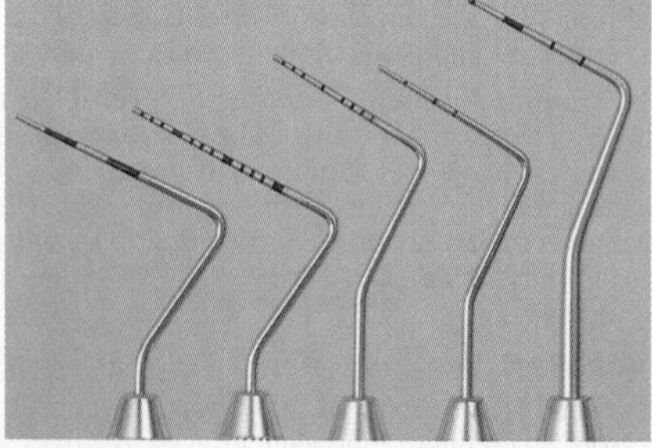

■ Various forms of periodontal probes, with gradations marked on their tips.

pro·bu·col (pro′bu-kōl) an anticholesteremic, used especially as an adjunct to diet for the reduction of elevated serum cholesterol in primary cholesterolemia, administered orally.

pro·cain·a·mide hy·dro·chlo·ride (pro-kān′ə-mīd) [USP] a cardiac depressant used in the treatment of cardiac arrhythmias, administered orally, intramuscularly, or intravenously. Called also *procaine amide hydrochloride.*

pro·caine (pro′kān) a benzoic acid derivative with local anesthetic activity.

p. amide hydrochloride procainamide hydrochloride.

p. hydrochloride [USP] the monohydrochloride salt of procaine; used to produce infiltration anesthesia, peripheral nerve block, and spinal anesthesia.

p. penicillin G see under *penicillin.*

pro·cal·ci·to·nin (pro-kal″sĭ-to′nin) an acute phase protein that is the prohormone of calcitonin. Its serum level is elevated in bacterial infections, but rarely in viral infections, and rises as the severity of the infection increases.

pro·cal·lus (pro-kal′əs) the granulation tissue formed about the site of fracture of a bone; it develops into callus.

Pro·can·bid (pro′kan-bid″) trademark for a preparation of procainamide hydrochloride.

pro·car·ba·zine hy·dro·chlo·ride (pro-kahr′bə-zēn) [USP] an alkylating agent specific for the S phase of the cell cycle used as an antineoplastic, primarily in combination with mechlorethamine, vincristine, and prednisone (MOPP) in the treatment of advanced Hodgkin disease; it is also used in the treatment of non-Hodgkin lymphoma, primary brain tumors, and multiple myeloma; administered orally.

pro·car·boxy·pep·ti·dase (pro″kahr-bok″se-pep′tĭ-dās) a proenzyme of a carboxypeptidase.

pro·car·cin·o·gen (pro″kahr-sin′ə-jən) a chemical substance that becomes carcinogenic only after it is altered by metabolic processes.

Pro·car·dia (pro-kahr′de-ə) trademark for preparations of nifedipine.

Pro·caryo·tae (pro-kar″e-o′te) [*pro-* + Gr. *karyon* nut, kernel] Prokaryotae.

pro·cary·ote (pro-kar′e-ōt) prokaryote. **procaryot′ic** *adj*

pro·cat·er·ol hy·dro·chlo·ride (pro-kat′ər-ol) a β-adrenergic agonist, specific for β_2-adrenergic receptors; administered by inhalation as a bronchodilator for the treatment and prophylaxis of bronchospasm associated with bronchitis, pulmonary emphysema, or other chronic obstructive airway disease, the treatment of asthma-associated bronchospasm, and the prophylaxis of exercise-induced bronchospasm.

Pro·ca·via (pro-ka′ve-ə) a genus of rock hyraxes that live in deserts and hilly regions of Africa and the Middle East; they are common reservoirs for *Leishmania aethiopica.*

pro·ce·dure (pro-se′jər) [L. *procedere,* from *pro* forward + *cedere* move] a series of steps by which a desired result is accomplished. See also under *maneuver, method, operation, surgery,* and *technique.*

Altemeier p. surgical treatment for rectal prolapse or cancer consisting of perineal rectosigmoidectomy and resection of adjacent mesentery.

Anderson p. reconstruction of the hypopharynx and cervical esophagus by the use of bilateral rectangular flaps.

arterial switch p. a one-stage method for anatomical correction of transposition of the great arteries, in which both coronary arteries are transposed to the posterior artery, and the aorta and pulmonary arteries are transected, contraposed, and anastomosed.

Bianchi p. longitudinal division of the bowel and its mesenteric blood supply followed by end-to-end approximation of the bowel segments, used for the treatment of short bowel syndrome.

Bricker p. surgical creation of an ileal conduit with a flat stoma for the collection of urine; the flat contour is achieved by suturing the ileal mucosa to the skin.

Burch p. a type of bladder neck suspension that is a modification of the Marshall-Marchetti-Krantz operation for stress incontinence, consisting of fixation of the lateral vaginal fornices to the iliopectineal ligaments. Called also *Burch colposuspension.*

Camey p. see under *neobladder.*

Csendes p. surgical treatment for gastric ulcers high in the cardia, consisting of subtotal gastrectomy and a large Roux-en-Y anastomosis.

David p. an operative technique for repair of aneurysms of the aortic root with preservation of the aortic valve.

Delorme p. surgical treatment for rectal prolapse consisting of mucosal proctectomy and plication of the muscularis layer.

Dohlman p. an endoscopic technique for repair of a Zenker diverticulum.

endocardial resection p. (ERP) surgical removal of a portion of left ventricular endocardium and underlying myocardium containing an arrhythmogenic area (as determined by intraoperative cardiac mapping) from the base of an aneurysm or infarction; done to relieve ventricular tachycardia in patients with ischemic heart disease.
endorectal pull-through p. ileoanal pull-through anastomosis.
Ertl p. transtibial or transfemoral amputation and myoplasty, with creation of an osteoperiosteal cap to close the medullary canal and, in the transtibial operation, to create a bony bridge between the distal ends of the tibia and fibula, thus increasing stability and weight-bearing ability.
extended endocardial resection p. (EERP) surgical removal of all visible endocardial fibrosis around the base of a left ventricular aneurysm; done to relieve ventricular tachycardia in patients with ischemic heart disease in whom intraoperative cardiac mapping is not possible.
Fick p. see under *method.*
Fontan p. functional correction of tricuspid atresia by anastomosis of, or insertion of a nonvalved prosthesis between, the right atrium and the pulmonary artery with closure of the interatrial communication; it is also used in other selected congenital conditions.
Frey p. an organ-sparing operation for the treatment of chronic pancreatitis, consisting of resection of the head of the pancreas with pancreaticojejunostomy for extended drainage.
Frykman-Goldberg p. surgical treatment for rectal prolapse consisting of resection of the sigmoid colon and rectopexy.
Fulkerson p. a modification of the Maquet procedure, in which the tibial tubercle pedicle is shifted medially as well as elevated and held in place with a screw.
Goldman p. a plastic repair technique for modifying the tip of the nose.
Gomori-Takamatsu p. a method for localizing the alkaline phosphatase enzyme: a tissue secretion is incubated in a buffered solution containing the substrate, glycerophosphate, and calcium ions; hydrolysis of the substrate releases phosphoric acid, and it combines with calcium and precipitates as calcium phosphate. This colorless precipitate is converted to brown cobalt sulfide, which is readily visualized with the microscope.
Hartmann p. resection of a diseased portion of the colon, with the proximal end of the colon brought out as a colostomy and the distal stump or rectum being closed by suture. Colon continuity can later be restored. Called also *Hartmann colostomy* or *operation.*
ileoanal pull-through p. see under *anastomosis.*
Jannetta p. microvascular decompression.
Ladd p. surgical cutting of Ladd bands to correct intestinal malrotation and obstruction.
MAGPI p. [*m*eatal *a*dvancement and *g*lanulo*p*lasty] surgical correction of hypospadias with chordee by meatoplasty and glanuloplasty, creating a neourethra by advancement of the urethral meatus distally.
Maquet p. anterior displacement of the tibial tubercle by creation of a long pedicle of tibial tubercle, which is elevated and held in place by a bone graft taken from the iliac crest; done for relief of severe patellofemoral pain.
Mathieu p. surgical correction of hypospadias of the distal urethra by using perimeatal tissue, making an incision in the glans and suturing the glans together over the defect.
maze p. the surgical division of the normal conduction pathways between the sinoatrial node and the atrioventricular node by a series of incisions in the left atrium to create a maze of conduction pathways; its purpose is to allow a normal impulse to activate the atrium while eliminating macroreentrant circuits; done for the relief of atrial fibrillation.
Mitrofanoff p. appendicovesicostomy.
Nuss p. a minimally invasive technique for correcting pectus excavatum: a convex steel bar is inserted under the sternum through small bilateral thoracic incisions, correcting the deformity and resulting in remodeling of the affected cartilages; the bar is removed once remodeling is complete.
Palomo p. a type of retroperitoneal varicocelectomy done especially in children.
Partington-Rochelle p. a modification of the Puestow procedure, consisting of side-to-side anastomosis between the pancreatic duct and the jejunum, without resection of the tail of the pancreas, done for relief of pain in chronic pancreatitis.
Pauchet p. surgical treatment of a moderately high gastric ulcer by a partial gastrectomy including excision of the ulcer site.
Peña p. posterior sagittal anorectoplasty.
Pereyra p. a type of bladder neck suspension similar to the Burch procedure; a loop of suture or other material is inserted through the paraurethral tissue near the bladder neck and attached to the abdominal fascia.
Puestow p. distal pancreatectomy with side-to-side pancreaticojejunostomy for relief of pain in chronic pancreatitis.
push-back p. see under *technique.*
Ripstein p. a repair procedure for rectal prolapse consisting of mobilization of the rectum, wrapping it with prosthetic mesh, and rectopexy with attachment of the mesh to the presacral fascia.

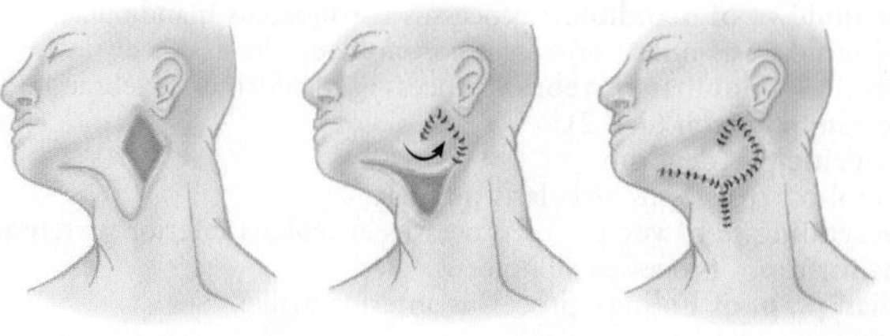
■ V-Y procedure.

Rovsing p. surgical unroofing of renal cysts followed by aspiration of their fluid.
Snodgrass p. surgical correction of hypospadias of the distal urethra by creating a tubular neourethra with a flap of deepithelialized dartos and tunica vaginalis.
Stamey p. a type of bladder neck suspension similar to the Burch procedure, aided by visualization through a cystoscope. Called also *Stamey colposuspension.*
Stoppa p. a tension-free method for treatment of a large or bilateral inguinal hernia, usually done laparoscopically, consisting of placement of nonabsorbable prosthetic plastic mesh across the defect in the inguinal floor. Called also *giant prosthetic reinforcement of visceral sac.*
Sugiura p. esophageal transection with paraesophageal devascularization and devascularization of the abdominal esophagus and proximal stomach; performed for the treatment of bleeding esophageal varices.
Thal p. see under *fundoplication.*
V-Y p. a method of repairing a skin defect in which a V-shaped flap is made proximal to the defect; the flap is transferred to the defect, and the secondary defect thus created is closed to produce a Y-shaped scar.
Wells p. a laparoscopic technique for repair of rectal prolapse, consisting of rectopexy anteriorly and placement of a supportive mesh posteriorly.
Whipple p. radical pancreatoduodenectomy with removal of the distal third of the stomach, the entire duodenum, and the head of the pancreas, with gastrojejunostomy, choledochojejunostomy, and pancreaticojejunostomy; done for cancers or certain other severe disorders of these structures. Called also *Whipple operation.*
Womack p. splenectomy with resection of the superior half of the greater curvature of the stomach, devascularization, and transgastric suturing of the varices; performed for variceal bleeding resulting from portal hypertension.
Young-Dees-Leadbetter p. repositioning of the ureters to a more superior position on the bladder and construction of a new bladder neck sphincter using the trigonal muscle; done for the treatment of urinary incontinence.

pro•ce•lous (pro-se′ləs) [*pro-* + *cel-*[2] + *-ous*] concave on the anterior surface; said of the vertebral centra of certain animals.

pro•ce•phal•ic (pro″sə-fal′ik) [*pro-* + *cephal-* + *-ic*] pertaining to the anterior part of the head.

pro•cer•coid (pro-sur′koid) one of the larval stages of fish tapeworms.

pro•ce•rus (pro-se′rəs) [L.] long; slender.

proc•ess (pros′əs, pro′səs) [L. *processus*] 1. a prominence or projection, as of bone; for names of specific anatomic structures not found here, see official terms under *processus.* 2. a series of operations, events, or steps leading to the achievement of a specific result. 3. to subject to such a series in order to produce desired changes in the original material or achieve some other result.
accessory p. of lumbar vertebra processus accessorius vertebrae lumbalis.
acromial p., acromion p. acromion.
alveolar p. the portion of bone in either the maxilla or the mandible that surrounds and supports the teeth. In the maxilla it is called the *processus alveolaris maxillae*, and in the mandible it is called the *pars alveolaris mandibulae.*
anconeal p. of ulna olecranon.
ascending p. of vertebra processus articularis superior vertebrae.
axillary p. of mammary gland processus axillaris glandulae mammariae.
calcaneal p. of cuboid bone processus calcaneus ossis cuboidei.
caudate p. processus caudatus.
ciliary p's processus ciliares.
Civinini p. processus pterygospinosus.
clinoid p., anterior processus clinoideus anterior.
clinoid p., middle processus clinoideus medius.
clinoid p., posterior processus clinoideus posterior.
cochleariform p. processus cochleariformis.
conoid p. tuberculum conoideum.
coracoid p. processus coracoideus scapulae.

coronoid p. of mandible processus coronoideus mandibulae.
coronoid p. of ulna processus coronoideus ulnae.
costal p. of lumbar vertebra processus costiformis vertebrae lumbalis.
Deiters p. axon (def. 2).
dendritic p. dendrite.
dental p. processus alveolaris maxillae.
descending p. of vertebra processus articularis inferior vertebrae.
ensiform p. processus xiphoideus.
folian p., p. of Folius processus anterior mallei.
foot p. pedicel.
frontonasal p. see under *prominence.*
funicular p. the portion of the tunica vaginalis surrounding the spermatic cord.
hamular p. any hook-shaped process in the body; see *hamulus* and *uncus.*
hamular p. of lacrimal bone hamulus lacrimalis.
hamular p. of sphenoid bone hamulus pterygoideus.
head p. an axial strand of cells in the embryo extending forward from the primitive node; called also *notochordal plate.*
Ingrassia p. ala minor ossis sphenoidalis.
jugular p. processus jugularis ossis occipitalis.
lacrimal p. processus lacrimalis conchae nasalis inferioris.
lateral p. of septal nasal cartilage processus lateralis cartilaginis septi nasi.
long p. of incus crus longum incudis.
long p. of malleus processus anterior mallei.
malar p. processus zygomaticus maxillae.
mammillary p. of lumbar vertebra processus mammillaris vertebrae lumbalis.
mandibular p. see under *prominence.*
mastoid p. processus mastoideus ossis temporalis.
maxillary p. see under *prominence.*
maxillary p. of inferior nasal concha processus maxillaris conchae nasalis inferioris.
mental p. protuberantia mentalis.
nasal p., lateral see under *prominence.*
nasal p., medial see under *prominence.*
odontoblastic p. one of the slender protoplasmic processes in a dentinal tubule, a cytoplasmic extension of the cell body; these processes extend from the dentinoenamel junction and cementodentinal junction to the cell bodies of odontoblasts in the dental pulp. Called also *dentinal fiber* and *Tomes fiber* or *fibril.*
odontoid p. of axis dens axis.
olecranon p. of ulna olecranon.
palatine p., lateral a shelflike projection developing from the medial aspect of each maxillary prominence of the upper jaw in the embryo, later fusing with each other and with the nasal septum to form the palate. Called also *palatal* or *palatine shelf.*
palatine p., median a shelflike projection developing from each median nasal prominence in the embryo, which participates with its fellow in forming the premaxillary portion of the upper jaw. Called also *intermaxillary segment.*
papillary p. processus papillaris.
paramastoid p. of occipital bone, paroccipital p. of occipital bone processus paramastoideus ossis occipitalis.
posterior p. of septal nasal cartilage processus posterior cartilaginis septi nasi.
pterygoid p. processus pterygoideus ossis sphenoidalis.
Rau p., ravian p. processus anterior mallei.
short p. of incus crus breve incudis.
short p. of malleus processus lateralis mallei.
sphenoidal p. of septal nasal cartilage processus posterior cartilaginis septi nasi.
spinous p. spina (def. 1).
spinous p. of vertebra processus spinosus vertebrae.
Stieda p. processus posterior tali.
styloid p. of fibula apex capitis fibulae.
styloid p. of temporal bone processus styloideus ossis temporalis.
styloid p. of radius processus styloideus radii.
styloid p. of ulna processus styloideus ulnae.
sucker p. pericapillary end foot.
synovial p. plica synovialis.
temporal p. of zygomatic bone processus temporalis ossis zygomatici.
Tomes p. 1. a finger-like projection of the ameloblast, occurring during the secretory phase of the cell during amelogenesis, which extends from the point of separation of the adjacent cell membrane to the distal free surface. 2. odontoblastic p.
unciform p. 1. hamulus ossis hamati. 2. uncinate process; see entries beginning *processus uncinatus.*
uncinate p. of cervical vertebra uncus corporis vertebrae cervicalis.
uncinate p. of ethmoid bone processus uncinatus ossis ethmoidalis.
uncinate p. of first thoracic vertebra uncus corporis vertebrae thoracicae primae.
uncinate p. of pancreas processus uncinatus pancreatis.
vermiform p. appendix vermiformis.
xiphoid p. processus xiphoideus.
zygomatic p. of frontal bone processus zygomaticus ossis frontalis.
zygomatic p. of maxilla processus zygomaticus maxillae.
zygomatic p. of temporal bone processus zygomaticus ossis temporalis.

proc·ess·ing (pros′es-ing) the performance of a series of operations in order to produce desired changes in the original material.
central p. the acceptance and interpretation of stimuli by the brain.
protein p. modification of an inactive translation product to a biologically active form, such as a hormone or enzyme, which is then delivered to a target site.
RNA p. modification of a primary transcript to create a functional RNA molecule; alterations vary by type of RNA and between prokaryotes and eukaryotes but include trimming of the ends, addition of a 5′ cap and a polyadenylate tail, removal of introns, and modification of bases.

pro·ces·sus (pro-ses′əs) pl. *proces′sus* [L.] [TA] process: anatomic terminology for a prominence or projection.

Processus

Descriptions are given on TA terms, and include anglicized names of specific processes.

p. accesso′rius ver′tebrae lumba′lis [TA] accessory process of lumbar vertebra: a small nodule on a lumbar vertebra, projecting backward from the posterior surface of the transverse process, lateral and inferior to the mammillary process; a similar process also occurs on the tenth, eleventh, and twelfth thoracic vertebrae.
p. alveola′ris maxil′lae [TA] alveolar process of maxilla: the thick parabolically curved ridge that projects downward and forms the free lower border of the maxilla; it is in front of and lateral to the palatine process and it bears the teeth. Called also *dental process.*
p. ante′rior mal′lei [TA] anterior process of malleus: a slender bony process that arises from the anterior aspect of the neck of the malleus, passes anteriorly and inferiorly to the petrotympanic fissure, and is attached to the petrous portion of the temporal bone by ligamentous fibers. Called also *p. gracilis, folian process, long process of malleus,* and *Rau* or *ravian process.*
p. articula′ris infe′rior ver′tebrae [TA] inferior articular process of vertebra: a process on either side of a vertebra, arising from the inferior surface of the arch near the junction of the lamina and pedicle; it bears a surface that faces anteriorly and inferiorly, articulating with the superior articular process of the vertebra below. Called also *zygapophysis inferior* [TA alternative].
p. articula′ris supe′rior os′sis sa′cri [TA] superior articular process of sacrum: either of two processes projecting posteriorly and medially from the first sacral vertebra at the junctions between the body and the alae; they articulate with the inferior articular processes of the fifth lumbar vertebra.
p. articula′ris supe′rior ver′tebrae [TA] superior articular process of vertebra: a process on either side of a vertebra, arising from the superior surface of the arch near the junction of the lamina and pedicle; it bears a surface that faces posteriorly and superiorly, articulating with the inferior articular process of the vertebra above. Called also *zygapophysis superior* [TA alternative].
p. axilla′ris glan′dulae mamma′riae [TA] axillary process of mammary gland: the superolateral part of the mammary gland that extends toward the axilla; called also *axillary tail* and *p. lateralis glandulae mammariae* [TA alternative].

Processus *Continued*

p. bre′vis mal′lei p. lateralis mallei.
p. calca′neus os′sis cuboi′dei [TA] calcaneal process of cuboid bone: a process projecting posteriorly from the inferomedial angle of the cuboid bone that supports the anterior calcaneus.
p. cauda′tus [TA] caudate process: the right of the two processes seen on the caudate lobe of the liver.
p. cilia′res [TA] ciliary processes: about 70 meridionally arranged ridges or folds projecting from the crown of the ciliary body; they secrete the aqueous humor into the posterior chamber of the eye.
p. clinoi′deus ante′rior [TA] anterior clinoid process: the bony process found on the medial extremity of the posterior border of the lesser wing of the sphenoid bone.
p. clinoi′deus me′dius [TA] middle clinoid process: either of two small inconstant eminences on the internal surface of the sphenoid bone, one on either side of the anterior part of the hypophysial fossa.
p. clinoi′deus poste′rior [TA] posterior clinoid process: either of two tubercles found on the superior angle of either side of the dorsum sellae of the sphenoid bone, giving attachment to the tentorium of the cerebellum.
p. cochlearifor′mis [TA] a small hollow cone of bone at the end of the septum canalis musculotubarii, just anterior to the vestibular window, with an opening through which the tendon of the tensor tympani passes. Called also *cochleariform process.*
p. condyla′ris mandi′bulae [TA] condylar process of mandible: the posterior process on the ramus of the mandible that articulates with the mandibular fossa. Called also *mandibular condyle.*
p. coracoi′deus sca′pulae [TA] coracoid process: a strong curved process that arises from the upper part of the neck of the scapula and overhangs the shoulder joint.
p. coronoi′deus mandi′bulae [TA] coronoid process of mandible: the anterior part of the upper end of the ramus of the mandible, to which the temporal muscle is attached.
p. coronoi′deus ul′nae [TA] coronoid process of ulna: a wide eminence at the proximal end of the ulna, forming the anterior and inferior part of the trochlear incisure.
p. costa′lis ver′tebrae lumba′lis TA alternative for *p. costiformis vertebrae lumbalis.*
p. costifor′mis ver′tebrae lumba′lis [TA] costal process of lumbar vertebra: a process that projects laterally from the transverse process of a lumbar vertebra and resembles a rib. Called also *p. costalis vertebrae lumbalis* [TA alternative].
p. ethmoida′lis con′chae nasa′lis inferio′ris [TA] ethmoidal process of inferior nasal concha: a bony projection above and behind the maxillary process of the inferior nasal concha.
p. falcifor′mis ligamen′ti sacrotubera′lis [TA] falciform process of sacrotuberal ligament: a prolongation of the sacrotuberal ligament, continuing forward along the inner border of the ramus of the ischium from the point of attachment of the ligament on the tuber of the ischium.
p. fronta′lis maxil′lae [TA] frontal process of maxilla: a large, strong, irregular process of bone that projects upward from the body of the maxilla, its medial surface forming part of the lateral wall of the nasal cavity.

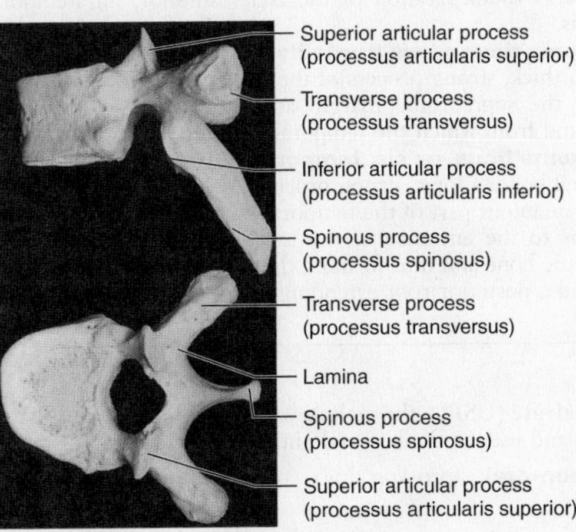

■ Processes of a thoracic vertebra.

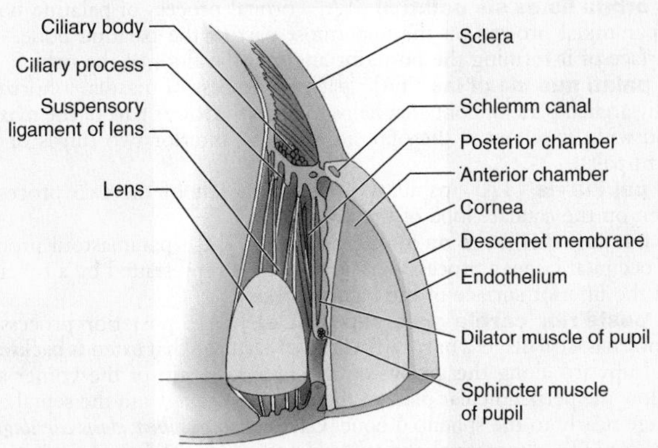

■ Processus ciliares (ciliary processes) and neighboring structures.

p. fronta′lis os′sis zygoma′tici [TA] frontal process of zygomatic bone: the strong, superiorly projecting triangular process of the zygomatic bone lying posterior to the malar surface and between the orbital and temporal surfaces; it unites superiorly with the zygomatic process of the frontal bone and posteriorly with the greater wing of the sphenoid bone.
p. gra′cilis p. anterior mallei.
p. intrajugula′ris os′sis occipita′lis [TA] intrajugular process of occipital bone: a small process that subdivides the jugular notch of the occipital bone into a lateral and a medial part.
p. intrajugula′ris os′sis tempora′lis [TA] intrajugular process of temporal bone: a small ridge on the petrous part of the temporal bone that separates the jugular notch into a medial and a lateral part, corresponding to similar parts of the jugular notch of the facing occipital bone.
p. jugula′ris os′sis occipita′lis [TA] jugular process: either of two processes on the occipital bone that project laterally from the occipital condyles and form the posterior boundary of the jugular foramen.
p. lacrima′lis con′chae nasa′lis inferio′ris [TA] lacrimal process: a process of the inferior nasal concha that articulates with the lacrimal bone.
p. latera′lis cartila′ginis sep′ti na′si [TA] lateral process of septal nasal cartilage: a lateral expansion of the septal cartilage on either side of the nose, fused with the lateral nasal cartilage.
p. latera′lis glan′dulae mamma′riae TA alternative for *p. axillaris glandulae mammariae.*
p. latera′lis mal′lei [TA] lateral process of malleus: a small tapered process that projects laterally from the base of the manubrium mallei and produces the malleolar prominence.
p. latera′lis ta′li [TA] lateral process of talus: a large low process on the lateral surface of the talus, articulating with the lateral malleolus.
p. latera′lis tu′beris calca′nei [TA] lateral process of calcaneal tuberosity: a rough process projecting downward from the lower lateral portion of the tuber calcanei.
p. lenticula′ris incu′dis [TA] lenticular process of incus: a small process on the medial side of the tip of the long limb of the incus, articulating with the head of the stapes.
p. mammilla′ris ver′tebrae lumba′lis [TA] mammillary process of lumbar vertebrae: a tubercle on each superior articular process of the lumbar vertebrae and on the tenth, eleventh, and twelfth thoracic vertebrae.
p. mastoi′deus os′sis tempora′lis [TA] mastoid process: a conical process projecting forward and downward from the external surface of the petrous part of the temporal bone just posterior to the external acoustic meatus. Called also *mastoid bone.*
p. maxilla′ris con′chae nasa′lis inferio′ris [TA] maxillary process of inferior nasal concha: a bony process descending from the ethmoid process of the inferior nasal concha.
p. media′lis tu′beris calca′nei [TA] medial process of calcaneal tuberosity: a rough process projecting downward from the lower medial portion of the tuber calcanei.
p. muscula′ris cartila′ginis arytenoi′deae [TA] muscular process of arytenoid cartilage: the lateral and posterior lower angular projection of the arytenoid cartilage to which the cricoarytenoid muscles are attached.

Processus *Continued*

p. orbita′lis os′sis palati′ni [TA] orbital process of palatine bone: a pyramidal process on the uppermost part of the palatine bone, one surface of it forming the posterior angle of the floor of the orbit.

p. palati′nus maxil′lae [TA] palatine process of maxilla: a horizontally arched plate of bone that helps to form the lower part of the maxilla and with its fellow of the opposite side the anterior two thirds of the hard palate.

p. papilla′ris [TA] papillary process: the left of the two processes seen on the caudate lobe of the liver.

p. paramastoi′deus os′sis occipita′lis [TA] paramastoid process of occipital bone: a process that in humans is represented by a tubercle on the inferior surface of the jugular process.

p. poste′rior cartila′ginis sep′ti na′si [TA] posterior process of septal nasal cartilage: a narrow flat strip of cartilage that extends backward and upward along the groove on the upper margin of the vomer and below the perpendicular plate of the ethmoid bone, from the septal cartilage nearly to the sphenoid bone. Called also *p. sphenoidalis cartilaginis septi nasi* [TA alternative] and *sphenoidal process of septal nasal cartilage.*

p. poste′rior ta′li [TA] posterior process of talus: a backward projection from the posterior portion of the talus, divided into two unequal parts by the sulcus tendinis musculi flexoris hallucis longi tali.

p. pterygoi′deus os′sis sphenoida′lis [TA] pterygoid process of sphenoid bone: either of two processes on the sphenoid bone descending from the points of junction of the greater wings and body of the bone, and each consisting of a lateral and a medial plate (see *lamina lateralis processus pterygoidei* and *lamina medialis processus pterygoidei*).

p. pterygospino′sus [TA] pterygospinous process: a small spine on the posterior edge of the lateral pterygoid plate of the sphenoid bone, giving attachment to the pterygospinous ligament.

p. pyramida′lis os′sis palati′ni [TA] pyramidal process of palatine bone: a strong process projecting downward, backward, and laterally from the lateral part of the posterior margin of the palatine bone and helping to form the pterygoid fossa.

p. sphenoida′lis cartila′ginis sep′ti na′si TA alternative for *p. posterior cartilaginis septi nasi.*

p. sphenoida′lis os′sis palati′ni [TA] sphenoidal process of palatine bone: an irregular mass of bone that projects superiorly and medially from the posterior portion of the superior margin of the perpendicular portion of the palatine bone, and articulates with the body of the sphenoid bone and with the ala vomeris.

p. spino′sus ver′tebrae [TA] spinous process of vertebra: a part of the vertebra projecting backward from the arch, giving attachment to muscles of the back.

p. styloi′deus os′sis metacar′pi ter′tii [TA] styloid process of third metacarpal: a prominent process projecting proximally from the base of the third metacarpal bone.

p. styloi′deus os′sis tempora′lis [TA] styloid process of temporal bone: a long spine projecting inferiorly from the inferior surface of the temporal bone just anterior to the stylomastoid foramen, giving attachment to three muscles and two ligaments.

p. styloi′deus ra′dii [TA] styloid process of radius: a blunt projection from the lateral surface of the distal end of the radius.

p. styloi′deus ul′nae [TA] styloid process of ulna: the medial, non-articular process on the distal extremity of the ulna.

p. supracondyla′ris hu′meri [TA] supracondylar process of humerus: a small inconstant process just proximal to the medial epicondyle of the humerus, giving rise to the ligament of Struthers.

p. tempora′lis os′sis zygoma′tici [TA] temporal process of zygomatic bone: the posterior blunt process of the zygomatic bone that articulates with the zygomatic process of the temporal bone to form the zygomatic arch.

p. transver′sus ver′tebrae [TA] transverse process of vertebra: a process on either side of a vertebra, projecting laterally from the junction between the lamina and the pedicle.

p. tuba′rius an angular process that projects posteriorly from the middle of the posterior edge of the medial pterygoid plate of the sphenoid bone; it provides support for the pharyngeal end of the auditory tube.

p. uncina′tus os′sis ethmoida′lis [TA] uncinate process of ethmoid bone: a curved plate of bone that extends inferiorly and posteriorly from the anterior part of the ethmoid labyrinth.

p. uncina′tus pancre′atis [TA] uncinate process of pancreas: the left and caudal part of the head of the pancreas, which hooks around behind the pancreatic vessels; called also *lesser pancreas.*

p. uncina′tus ver′tebrae cervica′lis TA alternative for *uncus corporis vertebrae cervicalis.*

p. uncina′tus ver′tebrae thora′cicae pri′mae TA alternative for *uncus corporis vertebrae thoracicae primae.*

p. vagina′lis os′sis sphenoida′lis [TA] vaginal process of sphenoid bone: a small plate on the inferior surface of the body of the sphenoid bone on either side, running medially from the medial pterygoid plate to articulate with the ala of the vomer and with the sphenoid process of the palatine bone.

p. vagina′lis peritone′i a diverticulum of the embryonic peritoneal membrane extending into the inguinal canal, accompanying the round ligament in the female, or the testis in its descent into the scrotum in the male (in which case it may be called the *processus vaginalis testis*). It is usually completely obliterated in the female, but a vestige often remains in the male (see *vestigium processus vaginalis*). In females it is often called a *canal of Nuck*, particularly if it persists after birth. Called also *Nuck diverticulum.*

p. vagina′lis tes′tis see *p. vaginalis peritonei.*

p. voca′lis [TA] vocal process: the process of the arytenoid cartilage to which the vocal ligament is attached.

p. xiphoi′deus [TA] xiphoid process: the pointed process of cartilage, supported by a core of bone, connected with the lower end of the body of the sternum. Called also *ensiform* or *xiphoid cartilage; xiphoid bone;* and *xiphisternum.*

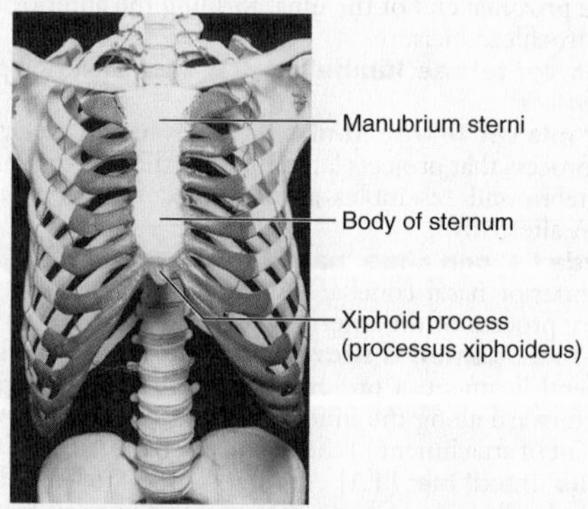

p. zygoma′ticus maxil′lae [TA] zygomatic process of maxilla: the rough triangular eminence that articulates with the zygomatic bone and marks the separation of the facies anterior, infratemporalis, and orbitalis.

p. zygoma′ticus os′sis fronta′lis [TA] zygomatic process of frontal bone: a thick, strong process of the frontal bone, situated at the lateral end of the supraorbital margin and articulating with the zygomatic bone, and from which the temporal line starts.

p. zygoma′ticus os′sis tempora′lis [TA] zygomatic process of temporal bone: a long, strong process arising from the inferior portion of the squamous part of the temporal bone, passing anteriorly from just superior to the entrance of the external acoustic meatus to join the zygomatic bone and thus forming the zygomatic arch. It has an anterior root and a posterior root extending along the temporal bone.

pro•chei•lon (pro-ki′lon) [*pro-* + Gr. *cheilon* lip] tuberculum labii superioris.

pro•chlor•per•a•zine (pro″klor-per′ə-zēn) [USP] a phenothiazine derivative used chiefly as an antiemetic, although it is sometimes used as an antipsychotic or antianxiety agent, administered rectally.

p. edisylate [USP] the ethanedisulfonate salt of prochlorperazine, having the same actions and uses as the base; administered orally, intramuscularly, or intravenously.

p. maleate [USP] the maleate salt of prochlorperazine, having the same actions and uses as the base; administered orally.

pro•chon•dral (pro-kon′drəl) occurring previous to the formation of cartilage.

pro•chor•dal (pro-kor′dəl) prechordal.

pro•chy•mo•sin (pro-ki′mo-sin) the inactive precursor of chymosin (rennin), converted to chymosin by pepsin or autocatalytically.

pro·ci·den·tia (pro″sĭ-den′shə) [L.] 1. prolapse. 2. specifically, prolapse of the uterus to such a degree that the cervix protrudes from the vaginal outlet.

pro·co·ag·u·lant (pro″ko-ag′u-lənt) 1. tending to favor the occurrence of coagulation. 2. a precursor of a natural substance necessary to coagulation of the blood.

pro·cog·ni·tive (pro-kog′nĭ-tiv) reducing disorientation or dementia; said of drugs.

pro·col·la·gen (pro-kol′ə-jən) the precursor molecule of collagen, synthesized in the fibroblast, osteoblast, etc., and cleaved to form collagen extracellularly.

pro·col·la·gen C-en·do·pep·ti·dase (pro-kol′ə-jən en″do-pep′tĭ-dās) [EC 3.4.24.19] an extracellular endopeptidase that catalyzes the cleavage of the C-terminal extension from procollagen, a step in the synthesis of collagen fibers. The enzyme does not require the procollagen substrate to be an intact trimer.

pro·col·la·gen C-pro·tein·ase (pro-kol′ə-jən pro′tēn-ās) procollagen C-endopeptidase.

pro·col·la·gen ga·lac·to·syl·trans·fer·ase (pro-kol′ə-jən gal″ak-tōs″əl-trans′fər-ās) [EC 2.4.1.50] an enzyme of the transferase class that catalyzes the attachment of galactose to hydroxylysine residues in the synthesis of collagen. The donor of the galactose moiety is UDPgalactose, and the enzyme is specific for collagen that is not yet in triple helical form.

pro·col·la·gen glu·co·syl·trans·fer·ase (pro-kol′ə-jən gloo″ko-səl-trans′fər-ās) [EC 2.4.1.66] an enzyme of the transferase class that catalyzes the attachment of glucose to some of the galactose-containing hydroxylysine residues during the synthesis of collagen. The donor of the glucose moiety is UDPglucose, and the enzyme is specific for collagen that is not yet in triple helical form.

pro·col·la·gen-ly·sine 5-di·oxy·gen·ase (pro-kol′ə-jən li′sēn di-ok′sĭ-jən-ās) [EC 1.14.11.4] EC nomenclature for *lysyl hydroxylase.*

pro·col·la·gen N-en·do·pep·ti·dase (pro-kol′ə-jən en″do-pep′tĭ-dās) [EC 3.4.24.14] an extracellular endopeptidase that catalyzes the cleavage of the N-terminal extension from procollagen, a step in the synthesis of collagen. The enzyme requires an intact procollagen trimer as a substrate.

pro·col·la·gen N-pro·tein·ase (pro-kol′ə-jən pro′tēn-ās) procollagen N-endopeptidase.

pro·col·la·gen pep·ti·dase (pro-kol′ə-jən pep′tĭ-dās) an endopeptidase that catalyzes the cleavage of specific terminal segments from procollagen chains, specifically used to denote procollagen N-endopeptidase (q.v.) and procollagen C-endopeptidase (q.v.).

pro·col·la·gen-pro·line di·oxy·gen·ase (pro-kol′ə-jən pro′lēn di-ok′sə-jən-ās) [EC 1.14.11.2] EC nomenclature for *prolyl 4-hydroxylase.*

pro·col·la·gen-pro·line 3-di·oxy·gen·ase (pro-kol′ə-jən pro′lēn di-ok′sə-jən-ās) [EC 1.14.11.7] EC nomenclature for *prolyl 3-hydroxylase.*

pro·con·cep·tive (pro″kən-sep′tiv) 1. aiding or favoring conception. 2. an agent that facilitates or promotes conception.

pro·con·ver·tin (pro″kən-vur′tin) factor VII; see under *coagulation factors,* at *factor.*

pro·cre·a·tion (pro″kre-a′shən) reproduction (def. 2). **pro′creative** *adj*

Pro·crit (pro′krit) trademark for a preparation of epoetin alfa.

proc·tal·gia (prok-tal′jə) [*proct-* + *-algia*] pain in or around the rectum; called also *proctodynia* and *rectalgia.*

p. fu′gax sudden, severe anorectal pain, lasting from a few seconds to a few minutes and then disappearing completely; the patient is symptom-free between episodes, which are generally infrequent. It occurs chiefly in young men, and the etiology is uncertain. The term is often used interchangeably with *levator ani syndrome* (q.v.).

proc·ta·tre·sia (prok″tə-tre′zhə) imperforate anus.

proc·tec·ta·sia (prok″tek-ta′zhə) [*proct-* + *ectasia*] dilatation of the rectum or of the anus.

proc·tec·to·my (prok-tek′tə-me) [*proct-* + *ectomy*] surgical removal of the rectum.

proc·ti·tis (prok-ti′tis) [*proct-* + *-itis*] inflammation of the rectum.

allergic p. in children, allergic gastroenteropathy having its focus in the rectum. In adults, rectal irritation may be caused by chemicals in the rectum, such as after medical procedures or anal intercourse.

eosinophilic p. see under *proctocolitis.*

factitial p. radiation p.

hemorrhagic p. hemorrhage in the rectum caused by radiation damage.

idiopathic p. ulcerative p.

radiation p. radiation colitis in the rectum. Called also *factitial p.*

traumatic p. rectal irritation caused by a foreign body in the rectum, such as during a medical procedure or anal intercourse.

ulcerative p. recurrent ulceration of the mucosa of the rectum, of unknown cause, probably a variant of ulcerative colitis. Called also *idiopathic p.*

proct(o)- [Gr. *prōktos* anus] a combining form designating relationship to the rectum.

proc·to·cele (prok′to-sēl″) rectocele.

proc·to·co·lec·to·my (prok″to-ko-lek′tə-me) surgical removal of the rectum and colon. Called also *coloproctectomy.*

proc·to·co·li·tis (prok″to-ko-li′tis) inflammation of the colon and rectum; called also *coloproctitis* and *rectocolitis.*

eosinophilic p. a manifestion of food allergy, consisting of inflammation of the mucosa of the rectum and colon with eosinophilic infiltration, usually in infants during the first two months of life; it is most often a reaction to cow's milk or soy milk formulas, although it may be provoked in breast-fed infants by food antigens passed in the mother's milk. Most affected infants appear healthy but have rectal edema and blood in the feces.

proc·to·co·lon·os·co·py (prok″to-ko″lən-os′kə-pe) inspection of the interior of the rectum and lower part of the colon.

Proc·to·cort (prok′to-kort) trademark for preparations of hydrocortisone acetate.

Proc·to·Cream (prok′to-crēm) trademark for a preparation of hydrocortisone.

proc·to·cys·to·plas·ty (prok″to-sis′to-plas″te) [*procto-* + *cysto-* + *-plasty*] a plastic operation on the rectum and bladder; operative closure of a rectovesical fistula.

proc·to·cys·tot·o·my (prok″to-sis-tot′ə-me) [*procto-* + *cysto-* + *-tomy*] incision into the bladder from the rectum.

proc·to·dae·um (prok″to-de′əm) proctodeum.

proc·to·de·um (prok″to-de′əm) [*proct-* + Gr. *hodaios* pertaining to a way] an invagination of the surface ectoderm of the embryo at the point where later the anus is formed; called also *anal pit.*

proc·to·dyn·ia (prok″to-din′e-ə) [*proct-* + *-odynia*] proctalgia.

Proc·to·foam-HC (prok′to-fōm) trademark for an aerosol foam containing hydrocortisone acetate and pramoxine hydrochloride; used to relieve anorectal inflammation, pain, swelling, and pruritus.

proc·to·gen·ic (prok″to-jen′ik) [*procto-* + *-genic*] derived from or originating in the rectum.

proc·tog·ra·phy (prok-tog′rə-fe) radiography of the rectum, especially of its movements.

proc·tol·o·gist (prok-tol′ə-jist) a specialist in proctology.

proc·tol·o·gy (prok-tol′ə-je) [*procto-* + *-logy*] the study of the rectum and anus and the nature and treatment of their diseases. **proctolog′ic** *adj*

proc·to·pa·ral·y·sis (prok″to-pə-ral′ĭ-sis) [*procto-* + *paralysis*] paralysis of the muscles of the anus and rectum.

proc·to·pexy (prok′to-pek″se) rectopexy.

proc·to·plas·ty (prok′to-plas″te) [*procto-* + *-plasty*] plastic surgery of the rectum; called also *rectoplasty.*

proc·to·ple·gia (prok″to-ple′jə) [*procto-* + *-plegia*] proctoparalysis.

proc·top·to·sis (prok″top-to′sis, prok″to-to′sis) rectal prolapse.

proc·tor·rha·gia (prok″to-ra′jə) bleeding from the rectum.

proc·tor·rha·phy (prok-tor′ə-fe) [*procto-* + *-rrhaphy*] surgical repair of the rectum.

proc·to·scope (prok′to-skōp) [*procto-* + *-scope*] a speculum or tubular instrument with appropriate illumination for inspecting the rectum. Called also *rectoscope.*

proc·tos·co·py (prok-tos′kə-pe) inspection of the rectum with a proctoscope. Called also *rectoscopy.* **proctoscop′ic** *adj*

proc·to·sig·moid (prok″to-sig′moid) rectosigmoid.

proc·to·sig·moi·dec·to·my (prok″to-sig″moi-dek′tə-me) rectosigmoidectomy.

proc·to·sig·moi·di·tis (prok″to-sig″moi-di′tis) inflammation of the rectum and sigmoid colon.

proc·to·sig·moi·do·scope (prok″to-sig-moid′o-skōp) an instrument for illuminating and viewing the rectum and sigmoid colon.

proc·to·sig·moi·dos·co·py (prok″to-sig″moi-dos′kə-pe) examination of the rectum and sigmoid with the sigmoidoscope.

proc·to·spasm (prok′to-spaz″əm) [*procto-* + *spasm*] spasm of the rectum.

proc·to·ste·no·sis (prok″to-stə-no′sis) [*procto-* + *stenosis*] stricture of the rectum. Called also *rectostenosis.*

proc·tos·to·my (prok-tos′tə-me) [*procto-* + *-stomy*] surgical creation of an artificial opening from the body surface into the rectum.

proc·tot·o·my (prok-tot′ə-me) [*procto-* + *-tomy*] incision into the rectum, as for relief of rectal stricture.

pro·cum·bent (pro-kum′bənt) prone.

pro·cur·sive (pro-kur′siv) [L. *procursivus*] characterized by a tendency to run forward.

pro·cur·va·tion (pro″kər-va′shən) [L. *procurvare* to bend forward] a bending forward, as of the body.

pro·cu·ti·cle (pro-ku′tĭ-kəl) [*pro-* + *cuticle*] the layer of the exoskeleton of certain crustaceans and arthropods beneath the epicuticle, which contains chitin as the principal constituent; it is composed of an endocuticle and an exocuticle.

pro·cy·cli·dine hy·dro·chlo·ride (pro-si′klĭ-dēn) [USP] a synthetic anticholinergic with a direct antispasmodic effect on smooth muscle; used as an antidyskinetic in the treatment of parkinsonism and for the control of drug-induced extrapyramidal reactions (except tardive dyskinesia); administered orally. It is believed to act by partially blocking central cholinergic receptors, which helps balance cholinergic and dopaminergic activity in the basal ganglia.

pro·dro·ma (pro-dro′mə) pl. *prodro′mata* [Gr.] prodrome.

pro·dro·ma·ta (pro-dro′mə-tə) plural of *prodroma*.

pro·drome (pro′drōm) [L. *prodromus;* Gr. *prodromos* forerunning] a premonitory symptom or precursor; a symptom indicating the onset of a disease. **prodro′mal, prodro′mic** *adj*

pro·drug (pro′drug′) [*pro-* + *drug*] a compound that, on administration, must undergo chemical conversion by metabolic processes before becoming an active pharmacological agent; a precursor of a drug.

prod·uct (prod′əkt) something produced.

advanced glycation end p's (AGE) irreversible products of the glycation of proteins, which cause tissue damage; seen when blood glucose concentrations are chronically elevated such as in diabetes mellitus, arthritis, and aging.

Amadori p. a chemically reversible product formed by the combination of Schiff bases.

cleavage p. a substance formed by the splitting of a compound molecule into simpler molecules.

contact activation p. a product of the interaction of blood coagulation factors XII and XI, which functions to activate factor IX.

decay p. a nuclide, which may be stable or radioactive, resulting from the radioactive disintegration of a radionuclide, being formed either directly or as the result of successive transformations in a radioactive series. Called also *daughter*.

end p. the final product resulting from completion of a chain of metabolic reactions.

fibrin degradation p's (FDP), fibrinogen degradation p's, fibrin split p's the protein fragments produced upon enzymatic digestion of fibrin and fibrinogen by plasmin.

fission p. an isotope, usually radioactive, of an element in the middle of the periodic table, produced by fission of a heavy element such as uranium under bombardment by high-energy particles.

ion p. the product of the concentrations of ions in a chemical reaction, each raised to the power of its coefficient in the balanced reaction. The ion product of water, K_W, is a constant equivalent to 10^{-14} at 25°C.

primary gene p. 1. a protein or polypeptide, frequently an enzyme, directly produced by transcription and translation of a gene, rather than by metabolic processing. 2. the unprocessed RNA molecule produced by transcription of a gene.

solubility p. see under *constant*.

spallation p's the many different chemical elements produced in small quantities in nuclear fission.

substitution p. a chemical product obtained by substituting for one element in a molecule an atom or a radical of some other substance.

pro·duc·tive (pro-duk′tiv) producing or forming; said especially of an inflammation that produces new tissue or of a cough that brings forth sputum or mucus.

pro·ec·dy·sis (pro-ek′dĭ-sis) [*pro-* + *ecdysis*] the period of preparation for the process of ecdysis, during which the new cuticle is laid down and the old one ultimately detached from it.

pro·emi·al (pro-e′me-əl) [L. *prooemium* a prelude] prodromal.

pro·en·ceph·a·lon (pro″ən-sef′ə-lon) prosencephalon.

pro·en·zyme (pro-en′zīm) an inactive precursor that can be converted to the active enzyme. Proenzymes, containing extra-long polypeptide chains that block activity, are activated by acid or enzymatic hydrolysis to remove the inhibiting portion.

pro·eryth·ro·blast (pro″ə-rith′ro-blast) the earliest of the immature forms recognizable as a precursor of the mature erythrocyte. It is round, with a large nucleus that occupies most of the cell and is surrounded by a small amount of cytoplasm that is a clear deep blue, often stains unevenly, and shows a pale perinuclear halo. The nucleus is round and red to purple with several nucleoli and consists of a network of fairly uniformly distributed chromatin strands that give it a finely reticular appearance. This term may be used to refer to cells in either normal or abnormal maturation, but some authorities limit it to those involved in normal maturation, in contrast to *promegaloblasts*, in which case it is a synonym of *pronormoblast*. Called also *rubriblast*.

pro·eryth·ro·cyte (pro″ə-rith′ro-sīt) any precursor of an erythrocyte; the term was not adopted by any scheme of red cell morphological development. See *erythrocytic series*, under *series*.

pro·es·tro·gen (pro-es′tro-jən) a substance that has no estrogenic activity itself but can be metabolized in the body to active estrogen.

pro·es·trum (pro-es′trəm) proestrus.

pro·es·trus (pro-es′trəs) [*pro-* + L. *oestrus*] in female mammals that have estrous cycles, the period of heightened follicular activity preceding estrus. Called also *proestrum*.

Proetz test (prōts) [Arthur Walter *Proetz*, American otolaryngologist, 1888–1966] see under *test*.

Pro·fa·si (pro′fə-se) trademark for a preparation of chorionic gonadotropin.

pro·fen·a·mine hydrochloride (pro-fen′ə-mēn) ethopropazine hydrochloride.

pro·fes·sion·al (pro-fesh′ə-nəl) 1. pertaining to one's profession or occupation. 2. a specialist in a particular field or occupation.

allied health p. a person with special training, licensed when necessary, who works under the supervision of a health professional with responsibilities bearing on patient care. Called also *paraprofessional*.

pro·fi·bri·nol·y·sin (pro″fi-brĭ-nol′ĭ-sin) plasminogen.

pro·file (pro′fīl) 1. a simple outline of the shape or form of an object, such as the head or face, viewed from the side. 2. a graph, table, or other summary representing quantitatively a set of characteristics subjected to tests.

antigenic p. the total antigenic content and structure of a tissue or cell.

biophysical p. a numeric scoring system used to assess the well-being of the fetus in high-risk pregnancies, based on the nonstress test combined with sonographic evaluation of fetal breathing, fetal movements, fetal tone, amniotic fluid volume, and, sometimes, the echogenicity of the placenta.

urethral pressure p. (UPP) a record of the resistance of the urethra to fluid flow, measured as variations in urethral pressure (q.v.). A liquid or gas is pumped into the bladder with a catheter in place and the catheter is slowly withdrawn while measurements are taken of the pressure at various points in the urethra. It is usually done from the internal orifice to the external orifice in females and from the internal orifice to the sphincter urethrae muscle in males.

pro·fil·in (pro-fil′in) a 15-kD actin-binding protein that forms a complex with G-actin and prevents it from polymerizing to form F-actin. It also binds to phosphatidylinositol bisphosphate, providing a link between actin organization and signal transduction. See also *gelsolin* and *thymosin β_4*.

Pro·fil·nine SD (pro-fil′nīn) trademark for a preparation of factor IX complex.

pro·fil·om·e·try (pro″fīl-om′ə-tre) the recording of a series of measurements to obtain a profile.

urethral pressure p. the measurement of urethral pressures for a urethral pressure profile.

pro·fon·dom·e·ter (pro″fon-dom′ə-tər) an apparatus for locating a foreign body by the fluoroscope by obtaining three lines of sight that intersect at the foreign body.

pro·fun·da·plas·ty (pro-fun′də-plas″te) reconstruction of the occluded or stenosed deep femoral artery (arteria profunda femoris); called also *profundoplasty*.

pro·fun·do·plas·ty (pro-fun′də-plas″te) profundaplasty.

pro·fun·dus (pro-fun′dəs) [L.] [TA] deep; a term denoting a structure situated deeper than another from the surface of the body.

prog·a·mous (prog′ə-məs) [*pro-* + *gamo-* + *-ous*] previous to fertilization of the oocyte.

pro·gas·ter (pro′gas-tər) [*pro-* + *gaster*] archenteron.

pro·gas·trin (pro-gas′trin) an inactive precursor of gastrin.

pro·ge·nia (pro-je′ne-ə) [*pro-* + *geni-* + *-ia*] prognathism.

pro·gen·i·tal (pro-jen′ĭ-təl) on the external surface of the genitals.

prog·e·ny (proj′ə-ne) [L. *progignere* to bring forth] offspring, or descendants.

pro·ger·ia (pro-jēr′e-ə) [*pro-* + *ger-* + *-ia*] an autosomal dominant syndrome of precocious senility, with affected children developing growth retardation, thinning skin, and fragile bones as young as 18 months, and death from stroke or coronary artery disease usually occurring by 13 years of age. It is caused by mutation in the *LMNA* gene (locus: 1q21.2), which encodes lamin A; the mutation causes partial activation of a cryptic splice site, leading to production of a truncated precursor to lamin A, called progerin, which accumulates at the nuclear envelope, dusrupting the nuclear scaffolding. Cf. *infantilism.* Called also *Hutchinson-Gilford syndrome.*

pro·ger·in (pro-jĕr′in) an abnormal, truncated protein formed during processing of the precursor to lamin A in progeria (q.v.) as a result of mutation of the gene encoding lamins A and C such that a cryptic splice site is activated.

pro·ger·oid (pro-jĕr′oid) resembling progeria, but occurring later in life or affecting only a single organ or tissue.

pro·ges·ta·gen (pro-jes′tə-jən) progestational agent.

pro·ges·ta·tion·al (pro″jəs-ta′shən-əl) 1. a term applied to that phase of the menstrual cycle just before menstruation, when the corpus luteum is active and the endometrium secreting. 2. having effects similar to those of progesterone; see also under *agent.*

pro·ges·te·rone (pro-jes′tə-rōn) 1. the principal progestational hormone of the body, liberated by the corpus luteum, placenta, and in minute amounts by the adrenal cortex; it prepares the uterus for the reception and development of the fertilized oocyte by transforming the endometrium from the proliferative to the secretory stage and maintains an optimal intrauterine environment for sustaining pregnancy. 2. [USP] the same principle isolated from pregnant sows or prepared synthetically; used, usually in the form of synthetic derivatives, as a progestational agent in the treatment of dysfunctional uterine bleeding and abnormalities of the menstrual cycle, as part of postmenopausal hormone replacement therapy, as a test for endogenous estrogen production, and as an adjunct in the treatment of infertility due to partial or complete ovarian failure; administered orally, intramuscularly, or intravaginally. Called also *progestational hormone.*

pro·ges·tin (pro-jes′tin) progestational agent.

pro·ges·to·gen (pro-jes′to-jən) progestational agent.

pro·glos·sis (pro-glos′is) [Gr. *proglōssis*] the tip or apex of the tongue.

pro·glot·tid (pro-glot′id) [*pro-* + *glottis*] one of the segments making up the body of a tapeworm. See *strobila.*

pro·glot·tis (pro-glot′is) pl. *proglot′tides.* Proglottid.

pro·glu·ca·gon (pro-gloo′kə-gon) a prohormone for glucagon, synthesized in alpha cells of the pancreas and L cells of the small intestine.

pro·glu·mide (pro-gloo′mīd) an anticholinergic reported to have a specific inhibitory effect on gastric secretion.

Pro·gly·cem (pro-gli′səm) trademark for a preparation of oral diazoxide.

prog·na·thia (pro-na′the-ə) prognathism.

prog·na·thism (prog′nə-thiz″əm) [*pro-* + *gnath-* + *-ism*] a condition marked by abnormal protrusion of one or both jaws, particularly the mandible, relative to the facial skeleton and soft tissues, so that the person has a gnathic index above 103, with the teeth in mesioclusion. **prognath′ic, prog′nathous** *adj*

prog·na·thom·e·ter (prog′nə-thom′ə-tər) [*prognathous* + *-meter*] an instrument or device for measuring the degree of prognathism.

prog·nose (prog-nōs′) prognosticate.

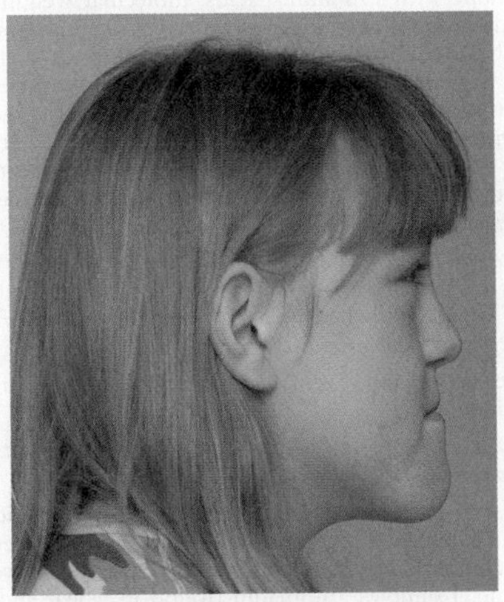

■ Mandibular prognathism.

prog·no·sis (prog-no′sis) [Gr. *prognōsis* foreknowledge] a forecast as to the probable outcome of an attack of disease; the prospect as to recovery from a disease as indicated by the nature and symptoms of the case.

prog·nos·tic (prog-nos′tik) 1. affording an indication as to prognosis. 2. a symptom or sign on which a prognosis may be based.

prog·nos·ti·cate (prog-nos′tĭ-kāt) to forecast the probable outcome of an attack of disease.

prog·nos·ti·cian (prog″nos-tish′ən) one who is skilled in prognosis.

pro·go·no·ma (pro″go-no′mə) [*pro-* + *gon-* + *-oma*] a tumor due to misplacement of tissue as the result of fetal atavism to a stage that does not occur in the life history of the species but does occur in ancestral forms of the species.

melanotic p. melanotic neuroectodermal tumor.

Pro·graf (pro′graf) trademark for preparations of tacrolimus administered orally or intravenously.

pro·gram·ming (pro′gram″ing) the provision of an ordered set of instructions or procedures.

neurolinguistic p. a complementary therapeutic strategy based on the premise that thought is a representation of sensory experience and that behavior can be modified to achieve a desired result by changing the patient's thought patterns and mental strategies in order to give the patient more choices in problem-solving; used for behavior modification and the management of psychosomatic disorders and stress.

pro·gran·u·lo·cyte (pro-gran′u-lo-sīt″) promyelocyte.

pro·grav·id (pro-grav′id) [*pro-* + *gravid*] denoting the phase of the endometrium, under the influence of the corpus luteum, during which it is prepared for pregnancy.

pro·gres·sion (pro-gresh′ən) 1. the act of moving or walking forward; see also *gait.* 2. the process of spreading or becoming more severe.

backward p. retropulsion.

cross-legged p. scissors gait.

saltatory p. saltation (def. 5).

pro·gres·sive (pro-gres′iv) advancing; going forward; going from bad to worse; increasing in scope or severity.

pro·guan·il hy·dro·chlo·ride (pro-gwahn′əl) an antimalarial used in the prophylaxis and treatment of malaria, administered orally. Seldom used in the United States because of the development of resistance by the malarial parasite to proguanil. Called also *chloroguanide hydrochloride.*

pro·hor·mone (pro-hor′mōn) any substance that can be converted into a hormone; see also *prehormone.*

pro·hor·mone con·ver·tase (pro-hor′mōn kən-vur′tās) any of a group of serine endopeptidases of the *trans*-Golgi network and secretory vesicles that catalyze the release of an active hormone from an inactive precursor.

pro·in·flam·ma·to·ry (pro″in-flam′ə-to-re) capable of stimulating inflammation.

pro·in·su·lin (pro-in′sə-lin) a precursor of insulin, with a molecular weight of 8,000 to 10,000; it has minimal hormonal activity and is converted to insulin by removal of the connecting C peptide, leaving the two (A and B)-chain, active insulin molecule.

proj·ect (proj′əkt) [*pro-* + L. *jacĕre* to throw] a task or set of tasks requiring organized effort.

Human Genome P. an international research effort to map and sequence the entire human genome, and to analyze, store, and make available the information obtained.

pro·jec·tion (pro-jek′shən) [*pro-* + L. *jacĕre* to throw] 1. a throwing forward, especially the act of referring impressions made on the sense organs to their proper source, so as to locate correctly the objects producing them. 2. the connection between the cerebral cortex and other parts of the nervous system or organs of special sense. 3. the act of extending or jutting out, or a part that juts out. 4. in psychiatry, an unconscious defense mechanism in which a person attributes to someone else unacknowledged ideas, thoughts, feelings, and impulses felt to be undesirable or unacceptable in himself or herself. 5. the orientation of a radiographic machine in relation to the body or a body part; called also *view.*

anteroposterior (AP) p. a radiographic projection in which the central ray goes from the front to the back of the body or part, with the film at the back.

axial p. a radiographic projection in which the central ray goes from the base to the vertex or from the vertex to the base of a structure.

axillary p. a radiographic projection in which the patient is supine, the upper limb is abducted, and the central ray enters the axilla at an angle; used for visualizing structures in the shoulder region.

brow-down p. a posteroanterior projection of the head with the patient prone.

brow-up p. an anteroposterior projection of the head with the patient supine.

Caldwell p. a posteroanterior projection of the head, used for viewing the frontal and anterior ethmoidal sinuses; the central ray enters the back of the head from a slightly superior angle.

carpal tunnel p. a radiographic projection with the wrist hyperextended and the central ray entering the proximal palm at an angle, for visualization of bones and other structures of the proximal palm and wrist.

cross-table p. a radiographic projection of the spine, pelvis, or lower limb with the patient either prone or supine on a table and the central ray entering laterally.

Didiée p. a rare type of radiographic projection for evaluation of an unstable or repeatedly dislocating shoulder that may have a subtle condition such as the Hill-Sachs lesion; the patient lies prone and the central ray enters the shoulder from a lateral oblique direction.

dorsoplantar p. a radiographic projection of the foot with the central ray passing from the dorsal surface to the plantar surface.

eccentric p. referred sensation.

erroneous p., false p. a misjudging of the position of an object, due to weakness or paralysis of the eye muscles.

frog-leg p. an anteroposterior projection of the abducted hips.

frontal p. a radiographic projection in which the central ray is perpendicular to the frontal plane; it may be either anteroposterior or posteroanterior.

half-axial p. a radiographic projection of the head with the central ray at an angle to the frontal and medial planes; it may be either anteroposterior or posteroanterior. Called also *semiaxial p.*

Heinig p. a radiographic projection for visualization of the sternum and sternoclavicular joint; the upper limb closer to the tube is abducted over the head and the central ray enters the body from an inferior lateral direction, angling toward the opposite shoulder.

Hermodsson p. a rare type of radiographic projection for evaluation of an unstable or repeatedly dislocating shoulder that may have a subtle condition such as the Hill-Sachs lesion; the patient stands with the affected upper limb behind the back and the hand over the lumbar vertebrae, and the central ray enters laterally to the scapula from an inferior posterior direction.

Hughston p. a radiographic projection of the patellofemoral region, with the patient prone, lower limbs at 50 to 60 degrees of flexion, and the central ray at 45 degrees from vertical passing tangentially across the knee.

inferosuperior p. any radiographic projection in which the central ray enters the body or a body part from below.

lateral p. a radiographic projection in which the central ray enters the body or part from the side and is perpendicular to the medial or axial plane.

Laurin p. an axial radiograph of the knees made with the patient seated with the knees flexed at 30 degrees and the lower limbs together; the x-ray tube is placed between the patient's feet and the film is placed against the anterior thighs perpendicular to the beam.

Merchant p. an axial radiograph of the knees made with the patient supine, knees flexed at 45 degrees over the table end, and lower limbs together; the tube is angled 30 degrees below the horizontal and the film is held on the tibia perpendicular to the beam.

mortise p. an anteroposterior projection of the ankle with the foot rotated internally 15 to 20 degrees so that the bases of the tibia and fibula are no longer in front of the talus.

notch p. 1. Stryker notch p. 2. a radiographic projection for visualization of the intercondylar notch of the femur.

oblique p. a radiographic projection in which the central ray enters the body or part at an angle to the frontal and medial or axial planes.

open-mouth p. an anteroposterior projection of the cervical spine, particularly the axis and atlas, done through the open mouth with the patient supine and the central ray pointing vertically downward.

pillar p. a radiographic projection of the articular pillars of the cervical spine, usually with the patient supine and the central ray angled slightly toward the feet from a position above the face; for an unobstructed view, the head may be rotated so that the mandible is not above the spine.

posteroanterior (PA) p. a radiographic projection in which the central ray goes from the back to the front of the body, with the film at the front.

radiographic p. projection (def. 5).

Schüller p. a lateral projection of the head, with the beam originating 30 degrees above horizontal; it allows a view of the antrum, part of the attic, and the head of the malleus.

semiaxial p. half-axial p.

Settegast p. a tangential projection of the patellofemoral region, usually with the patient prone, the knee flexed more than 90 degrees, and the central ray directed vertically downward at the knee. Called also *sunrise p.*

Stenvers p. an oblique projection of the head, done with the head rotated 45 degrees so that the petrous part of the temporal bone is perpendicular to the beam; it allows a view of the petrous apex, the labyrinth, and the internal acoustic meatus.

stress p. a radiographic projection of a movable joint, such as the wrist or knee, while it is under significant stress.

Stryker notch p. a rare type of radiographic projection for evaluation of an unstable or repeatedly dislocating shoulder that may have a subtle condition such as the Hill-Sachs lesion. The patient lies supine with the elbow on the affected side vertical and the hand next to or above the head; the central ray enters anteriorly and angles slightly upwards toward the coracoid process. Called also *notch p.*

submentovertex p. a radiographic projection of the head with the central ray entering under the chin and directed toward the vertex.

sunrise p. Settegast p.

swimmer's p. a radiographic projection of the cervical or thoracic spine with the patient lying supine on a table, the neck hyperextended, the upper limb nearer the camera parallel to the body, and that nearer the film placed above the head; the central ray enters laterally.

tangential p. a radiographic projection with the central ray on a tangent to an organ or part.

thalamocortical p's see under *fiber.*

Towne p. a radiographic projection of the head in which the central ray enters obliquely through the frontal bone, yielding a view of facial structures and the occipital bone; it is an anteroposterior half-axial projection.

tunnel p. a posteroanterior projection in which the knee is flexed 40 to 50 degrees with the patient prone and the foot supported; the central ray is perpendicular to the lower leg for a view of the intercondylar fossa of the femur.

verticosubmental p. a radiographic projection in which the central ray passes from the vertex of the head to the base of the chin, for visualization of the mandible, the base of the skull, and the nasal region.

Waters p. a radiographic projection of the anterior head, used for viewing the maxillary sinuses and sphenoid bone; the central ray enters at an angle through the chin.

West Point p. a rare type of radiographic projection for evaluation of an unstable or repeatedly dislocating shoulder that may have a subtle condition such as the Hill-Sachs lesion. The patient lies prone with the affected upper limb abducted and the forearm hanging off the table; the central ray enters in the scapular region at an angle from the rear to visualize scapular and shoulder structures.

Pro·karyo·tae (pro-kar″e-o′te) the prokaryotes; in some classifications a superkingdom containing the kingdom Monera, in other systems synonymous with Monera. See also *Archaea* and *Bacteria.*

pro·kary·ote (pro-kar′e-ōt) [*pro-* + Gr. *karyon* nut, kernel] any of a group of cellular organisms that lack a true nucleus and nuclear membrane and have nuclear material consisting of a single double-stranded DNA molecule not associated with basic proteins. They lack a cytoskeleton, the cytoplasm is immobile, and organelles are rare. Most have a true cell wall, and all reproduce by cell fission. Organisms are predominantly unicellular but may have filamentous, mycelial, or colonial forms. Prokaryotes are classified into two genetically distinct domains, the Archaea and the Bacteria. Cf. *eukaryote.* **prokaryot′ic** *adj*

pro·ki·net·ic (pro″kĭ-net′ik) stimulating movement or motility, such as drugs that promote gastrointestinal motility.

pro·la·bi·um (pro-la′be-əm) [*pro-* + *labium*] the prominent central part of the upper lip.

pro·lac·tin (PRL, Prl) (pro-lak′tin) [*pro-* + L. *lac* milk] an anterior pituitary hormone with 198 amino acids, molecular weight 23,000, which stimulates and sustains lactation in postpartum mammals after the mammary glands have been prepared by other hormones such as estrogens, progesterone, growth hormone, corticosteroids, and insulin. It also stimulates formation of "milk" in the crop sac of birds such as pigeons and doves (an action formerly used for bioassay), is luteotropic in certain mammals, and has many other effects, including essential roles in the maintenance of immune system functions. Called also *lactogen, luteotropin,* and *lactogenic* or *luteotropic hormone.*

pro·lac·ti·no·ma (pro-lak″tĭ-no′mə) a pituitary adenoma made up of lactotrophs that secretes excessive amounts of prolactin and causes hyperprolactinemia (q.v.). Called also *prolactin cell adenoma, prolactin-secreting adenoma, lactotrope adenoma,* and *lactotroph adenoma.*

pro·lac·to·lib·er·in (pro-lak″to-lib′ər-in) [*prolactin* + *-liberin*] prolactin-releasing hormone.

pro·lac·to·stat·in (pro-lak″to-stat′in) [*prolactin* + *-statin*] prolactin-inhibiting hormone.

pro·lam·in (pro-lam′in, pro′lə-min) any of a group of globular proteins found mainly in cereals; they are soluble in 70–80 per cent alcohol but insoluble in water and absolute alcohol and contain high levels of glutamic acid and proline. Examples are gliadin (found in wheat and rye) and zein (found in corn). Called also *alcohol-soluble protein.*

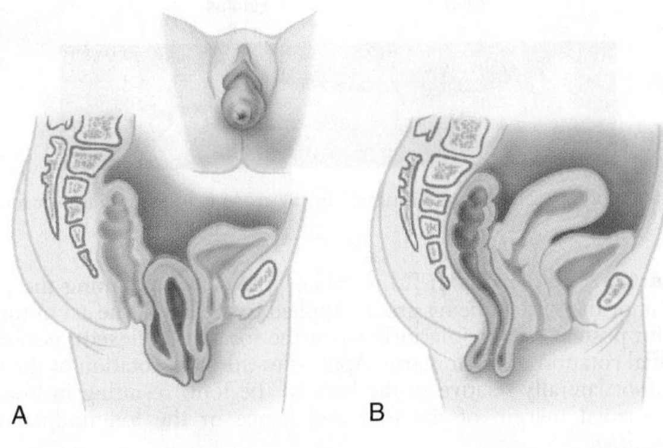

■ *(A)*, Prolapse of uterus; *(B)*, prolapse of rectum.

pro•lapse (pro-laps') [L. *prolapsus; pro* before + *labi* to fall] 1. the falling down, or sinking, of a part or viscus; called also *procidentia* and *ptosis.* 2. to undergo such displacement.

anal p. protrusion of modified anal skin through the anal orifice.

p. of cord premature expulsion of the umbilical cord in labor before the fetus is delivered.

frank p. prolapse of the uterus in which the vagina is inverted and hangs from the vulva.

p. of intervertebral disk herniation of intervertebral disk.

p. of iris protrusion of the iris through a wound in the cornea.

mitral valve p. (MVP) redundancy or hooding of mitral valve leaflets so that they prolapse into the left atrium, often causing mitral regurgitation; see *mitral valve prolapse syndrome*, under *syndrome.* Called also *floppy mitral valve.*

Morgagni p. chronic inflammatory hyperplasia of the mucosa and submucosa of the sacculus laryngis.

mucosal p. prolapse of the mucosa in part of the gastrointestinal tract; in the colon it sometimes occurs with congenital megacolon.

rectal p., p. of rectum protrusion of the rectal mucous membrane through the anus, which can occur to various degrees. *Incomplete* or *partial prolapse* is when there is no displacement of anal sphincter muscle; *complete prolapse* may be either with displacement of anal sphincter muscle or without displacement but with herniation of the colon; and *internal complete* or *concealed prolapse* is when there is intussusception of the rectosigmoid and upper portion of the rectum only as far as the lower rectum. Called also *proctoptosis* and *prolapsus recti.*

uterine p., p. of uterus downward displacement of the uterus so that the cervix is within the vaginal orifice *(first-degree p.)*, the cervix is outside the orifice *(second-degree p.)*, or the entire uterus is outside the orifice *(third-degree p.)*. Called also *descensus uteri* and *hysteroptosis.*

vaginal p. vaginocele (def. 2).

pro•lap•sus (pro-lap'səs) [L.] prolapse.

p. a'ni anal prolapse.

p. rec'ti rectal prolapse.

p. u'teri uterine prolapse.

Pro•las•tin (pro-las'tin) trademark for a preparation of alpha$_1$-proteinase inhibitor (human).

Pro•lene (pro'lēn) trademark for a preparation of polypropylene.

pro•lep•sis (pro-lep'sis) the return of a paroxysm before the expected time. **prolep'tic** *adj*

Pro•leu•kin (pro-loo'kin) trademark for a preparation of aldesleukin.

pro•li•dase (pro'lĭ-dās) X-Pro dipeptidase.

pro•li•dase de•fi•cien•cy (pro'lĭ-dās) an autosomal recessive aminoacidopathy due to mutation in the *PEPD* gene (locus: 19cen-q13.11), which encodes X-Pro dipeptidase; defective cleavage of imidodipeptides results in imidodipeptiduria. Clinical manifestations are variable, but include chronic skin lesions, impaired motor or cognitive development, frequent infections, and skeletal abnormalities.

pro•lif•er•ate (pro-lif'ər-āt) to grow by the reproduction of similar cells.

pro•lif•er•a•tion (pro-lif"ə-ra'shən) [L. *proles* offspring + *ferre* to bear] the reproduction or multiplication of similar forms, especially of cells and morbid cysts. See also *hyperplasia* and *hypertrophy.* **prolif'erative, prolif'erous** *adj*

fibroplastic p. an overgrowth of collagenous connective tissue involving many organs of the body, as occurs in systemic lupus erythematosus, scleroderma, and other collagen diseases.

pro•lif•ic (pro-lif'ik) [L. *prolificus*] fruitful; productive.

pro•lig•er•ous (pro-lij'ər-əs) [L. *proles* offspring + *gerere* to bear] producing offspring.

pro•lin•ase (pro'lĭ-nās) cytosol nonspecific dipeptidase.

pro•line (Pro, P) (pro'lēn) 1. a nonessential amino acid, 2-pyrrolidinecarboxylic acid, a major constituent of collagen (see *tropocollagen*). See also table at *amino acid.* 2. [USP] a preparation of proline used as a dietary supplement.

pro•line de•hy•dro•gen•ase (pro'lēn de-hi'dro-jən-ās) [EC 1.5.99.8] an enzyme of the oxidoreductase class that catalyzes the dehydrogenation of proline to form Δ^1-pyrroline 5-carboxylate, using ubiquinone as an electron acceptor. The enzyme is a flavoprotein (FAD) of the mitochondrial membrane and the reaction is the initial step in the degradation of proline to glutamate. Deficiency of the enzyme, an autosomal recessive trait, is the cause of hyperprolinemia Type I. Called also *proline oxidase.*

pro•line di•pep•ti•dase (pro'lēn di-pep'tĭ-dās) X-Pro dipeptidase.

pro•lin•emia (pro"lĭ-ne'me-ə) hyperprolinemia.

pro•line ox•i•dase (pro'lēn ok'sĭ-dās) proline dehydrogenase.

pro•line ra•ce•mase (pro'lēn ra'sə-mās) [EC 5.1.1.4] an enzyme of the isomerase class that catalyzes the interconversion of L- and D-proline.

Pro•lix•in (pro-lik'sin) trademark for preparations of fluphenazine.

pro•lyl (pro'ləl) the acyl radical of proline.

pro•lyl di•pep•ti•dase (pro'ləl di-pep'tĭ-dās) cytosol nonspecific dipeptidase.

pro•lyl 3-hy•drox•y•lase (pro'ləl hi-drok'sə-lās) an enzyme of the oxidoreductase class that catalyzes the hydroxylation at the 3 position of specific proline residues in nascent procollagen chains. The enzyme requires Fe^{2+}, ascorbate, and α-ketoglutarate for activity. In EC nomenclature, called *procollagen-proline, 3-deoxygenase.*

pro•lyl 4-hy•drox•y•lase (pro'ləl hi-drok'sə-lās) an enzyme of the oxidoreductase class that catalyzes the hydroxylation at the 4 position of specific proline residues in nascent procollagen chains. The enzyme requires Fe^{2+}, ascorbate, and α-ketoglutarate for activity, and the reaction is necessary for thermal stability of the collagen triple helical structure. The enzyme is a tetramer comprising 2α and 2β chains; the β chain in monomeric form is the enzyme protein disulfide-isomerase (q.v.). In EC nomenclature, called *procollagen-proline dioxygenase.*

pro•lym•pho•cyte (pro-lim'fo-sīt) a developmental form in the lymphocytic series (q.v.), intermediate between the lymphoblast and lymphocyte.

PROM premature rupture of membranes.

pro•mas•ti•gote (pro-mas'tĭ-gōt) [*pro-* + Gr. *mastix* whip] a morphological stage in the life cycle of certain trypanosomatid protozoa; the elongate or pear-shaped cell has a central nucleus, anteriorly located kinetoplast and basal body, free-flowing flagellum emerging from the anterior end, and no undulating membrane. Cf. *amastigote, choanomastigote, epimastigote, opisthomastigote,* and *trypomastigote.*

pro•ma•zine hy•dro•chlo•ride (pro'mə-zēn) [USP] a phenothiazine derivative used as an antipsychotic agent; administered orally, intramuscularly, and intravenously.

pro•mega•karyo•cyte (pro-meg"ə-kar'e-o-sīt) a precursor in the thrombocytic series, a large cell intermediate between the megakaryoblast and the megakaryocyte.

pro•meg•a•lo•blast (pro-meg'ə-lo-blast) the earliest developmental form in the abnormal red cell maturation sequence occurring in vitamin B_{12} and folic acid deficiencies; it corresponds to the pronormoblast, but differs from it by its larger size, abundant basophilic cytoplasm, and reticulated, unclumped nuclear chromatin. Several nucleoli are usually present.

pro•meta•phase (pro-met'ə-fās) the phase of cell division that follows prophase; it begins with the disintegration of the nuclear membrane, after which microtubules from each pole of the spindle bind to the kinetochores of the chromosomes, which begin moving toward the cell equator.

pro•meth•a•zine hy•dro•chlo•ride (pro-meth'ə-zēn) [USP] a phenothiazine derivative having marked antihistaminic activity as well as sedative and antiemetic actions; used to provide bedtime, surgical, and obstetrical sedation, to potentiate the action of central depressants, to treat allergic conditions including rhinitis, conjunctivitis, and pruritic skin disorders, to manage nausea, vomiting, and vertigo associated with surgery, pregnancy, and motion sickness, and as an ingredient in cough and cold preparations; administered orally, rectally, intramuscularly, and intravenously.

pro•me•thi•um (Pm) (pro-me'the-əm) the radioactive metallic chemical element of atomic number 61, atomic weight 147.

Pro•me•tri•um (pro-me'tre-um) trademark for a preparation of progesterone.

pro•mine (pro′mēn) a substance widely distributed in animal cells, characterized by its ability to promote cell division and growth. Cf. *retine.*

prom•i•nence (prom′ĭ-nəns) a protrusion or projection; for names of specific anatomical structures, see under *prominentia.*

Ammon scleral p. a prominence on the eyeball of the fetus.

frontonasal p. an expansive facial prominence in the embryo that develops into the forehead and bridge of the nose. Called also *frontonasal process.*

laryngeal p. prominentia laryngea.

mandibular p. the ventral prominence formed by bifurcation of the mandibular (first pharyngeal) arch in the embryo, which unites ventrally with its fellow to form the lower jaw. Called also *mandibular process.*

maxillary p. the dorsal prominence formed by bifurcation of the mandibular (first pharyngeal) arch in the embryo, which joins with the ipsilateral medial nasal prominence in the formation of the upper jaw. Called also *maxillary process.*

nasal p., lateral the more lateral of the two limbs of the horseshoe-shaped elevation bounding a nasal pit in the embryo, which participates in formation of the side and wing of the nose. Called also *lateral nasal process.*

nasal p., medial the more central of the two limbs of the horseshoe-shaped elevation bounding a nasal pit in the embryo, which participates with the ipsilateral maxillary prominence in the formation of half of the upper jaw. Called also *medial nasal process.*

tubal p. torus tubarius.

prom•i•nen•tia (prom″ĭ-nen′shə) gen. and pl. *prominen′tiae* [L.] prominence: a small protrusion on another structure or part.

p. cana′lis facia′lis [TA] prominence of facial canal: an elongated elevation on the medial wall of the tympanic cavity, just inferior to the prominence of the lateral semicircular canal and superior and posterior to the vestibular window.

p. cana′lis semicircula′ris latera′lis [TA] prominence of lateral semicircular canal: a large rounded prominence on the upper portion of the medial wall of the tympanic cavity, between the vestibular window and the mastoid antrum.

p. laryn′gea [TA] laryngeal prominence: a subcutaneous prominence on the front of the neck produced by the thyroid cartilage of the larynx; called also *Adam's apple.*

p. mallea′ris membra′nae tympa′nicae [TA] malleolar prominence of tympanic membrane: a small projection at the upper extremity of the stria mallearis, formed by the lateral process of the malleus. Called also *short process of malleus.*

p. spira′lis [TA] spiral prominence: a prominence on the external wall of the cochlear duct, separating the stria vascularis from the external spiral sulcus.

p. styloi′dea [TA] styloid prominence: an irregular nodule on the posterior portion of the floor of the tympanic cavity, corresponding to the base of the styloid process.

prom•i•nen•tiae (prom″ĭ-nen′she-e) [L.] genitive and plural of *prominentia.*

pro•mono•cyte (pro-mon′o-sīt) a precursor in the monocytic series, being a cell intermediate in development between the monoblast and monocyte.

prom•on•to•ri•um (prom″on-tor′e-əm) pl. *promonto′ria* [L.] promontory: a projecting eminence or process.

p. os′sis sa′cri [TA] promontory of sacrum: the prominent anterior border of the pelvic surface of the body of the first sacral vertebra.

p. tym′pani [TA] promontory of tympanic cavity: the prominence on the medial wall of the tympanic cavity, formed by the first turn of the cochlea; called also *promontory of middle ear.*

prom•on•to•ry (prom′on-tor″e) a projecting eminence or process; for names of specific anatomical structures see under *promontorium.*

p. of middle ear, tympanic p., p. of tympanic cavity promontorium tympani.

pro•mo•ter (prə-mo′tər) 1. a segment of DNA usually occurring upstream from a gene coding region and acting as a controlling element in the expression of that gene; it serves as a recognition signal for an RNA polymerase and marks the site of initiation of transcription. 2. a substance in a catalyst that increases the rate of activity of the catalyst. Cf. *protector.* 3. a type of epigenetic carcinogen that promotes neoplastic growth only after initiation by another substance; called also *cocarcinogen.*

pro•mo•til•i•ty (pro″mo-til′ĭ-te) serving to stimulate motility in the gastrointestinal tract; said of medications.

pro•my•elo•cyte (pro-mi′ə-lo-sīt) a precursor in the granulocytic series, being a cell intermediate in development between a myeloblast and myelocyte and containing a few, as yet undifferentiated, cytoplasmic granules. Called also *premyelocyte* and *progranulocyte.*

pro•nate (pro′nāt) to assume or place in a prone position; see *pronation.*

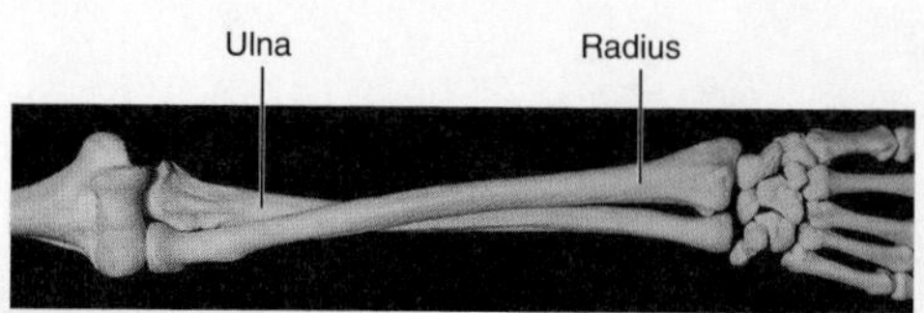

■ Pronation of forearm: the hand is turned by the crossing of the radius over the ulna.

pro•na•tion (pro-na′shən) [L. *pronatio*] the act of assuming the prone position, or the state of being prone. Applied to the hand, the act of turning the palm posteriorly (or inferiorly when the forearm is flexed), performed by medial rotation of the forearm. Applied to the foot, rotation of the front of the foot laterally relative to the back of the foot, resulting in lowering of the medial margin of the foot and hence of the longitudinal arch. Cf. *supination.*

pro•na•to•flex•or (pro-na″to-flek′sər) both pronator and flexor.

pro•na•tor (pro-na′tər) [L.] a muscle that serves to pronate; see *pronation.*

prone (prōn) [L. *pronus* inclined forward] lying face downward; see also *pronation.*

pro•neph•ron (pro-nef′ron) pronephros.

pro•neph•ros (pro-nef′ros) pl. *proneph′roi* [*pro-* + Gr. *nephros* kidney] 1. a vestigial excretory structure that develops in the human embryo at four weeks, before the mesonephros. Although nonfunctional, its duct is later used by the mesonephros, which arises caudal to it. 2. the definitive excretory organ of primitive fishes.

Pro•nes•tyl (pro-nes′təl) trademark for preparations of procainamide hydrochloride.

prong (prong) a conical projection.

nasal p's nasal cannula.

pro•no•grade (pro′no-grād) [L. *pronus* bent downward + *gradi* to walk] characterized by walking with the body approximately horizontal, such as the quadrupeds. Cf. *orthograde.*

pro•nom•e•ter (pro-nom′ə-tər) a goniometer for the forearm.

pro•nor•mo•blast (pro-nor′mo-blast) a term now often considered a synonym of *proerythroblast;* sometimes more specifically one in a course of normal erythrocyte maturation, as opposed to a promegaloblast.

Pron•to•sil (pron′to-sil) trademark for the forerunner of the sulfonamide drugs, first prepared in 1932 and no longer used therapeutically. Called also *P. flavum* and *P. rubrum.*

pro•nu•cle•us (pro-noo′kle-əs) the haploid nucleus occurring after meiosis in the germ cells.

female p. the haploid nucleus of the fully mature oocyte, which loses its nuclear envelope and liberates its chromosomes to meet in synapsis with those similarly derived from the male pronucleus.

male p. the haploid nucleus of the spermatozoon after it has penetrated the oocyte.

pro-opio•mel•a•no•cor•tin (POMC) (pro-o″pe-o-mel″ə-no-kor′tin) [*pro-* + endogenous *opio*ids + *melano*cyte stimulating hormone + *cort*icotropin + *-in*] the 31,000 dalton prohormone that is the precursor of corticotropin, the lipotropins, the melanocyte-stimulating hormones, and the endorphins, all of which are produced by posttranslational proteolytic cleavage in cell types that produce these hormones.

pro•ot•ic (pro-ot′ik) [*pro-* + *otic*] preauricular.

pro•pa•fe•none hy•dro•chlo•ride (pro″pə-fe′nōn) [USP] a sodium channel blocking agent that acts on the Purkinje fibers and myocardium, used in the treatment of life-threatening arrhythmias; administered orally.

prop•a•ga•tion (prop″ə-ga′shən) reproduction (def. 2). **prop′agative** *adj*

pro•pane (pro′pān) a hydrocarbon of the methane series, $CH_3CH_2CH_3$, which is a constituent of natural gas and crude petroleum and occurs as a colorless flammable gas with a characteristic odor.

pro•pan•i•did (pro-pan′ĭ-did) a short-acting anesthetic, derived from eugenol; administered intravenously.

pro•pa•no•ic ac•id (pro″pə-no′ik) systematic name for propionic acid.

pro•pan•the•line bro•mide (pro-pan′thə-lēn) an anticholinergic, which inhibits gastrointestinal hypermotility and hyperacidity; used as adjunctive therapy in the treatment of peptic ulcer and other gastrointestinal disorders, administered orally.

pro•par•a•caine hy•dro•chlo•ride (pro-par′ə-kān) [USP] an anesthetic, applied topically to the conjunctiva.

Pro•pe•cia (pro-pe′shə) trademark for a preparation of finasteride.

pro·pene (pro′pēn) propylene.

2-pro·pene·ni·trile (pro″pēn-ni′trīl) acrylonitrile.

pro·pe·nyl (pro-pe′nəl) a three-carbon radical with one double bond between two of the carbons, $CH_3CH{=}CH{-}$.

pro·per·din (pro′pər-din) a nonimmunoglobulin gamma globulin component of the alternative pathway of complement activation; it complexes with C3b and stabilizes alternative pathway C3 and C5 convertases (C3bBb and $C3b_nBb$). Called also *factor P.*

pro·peri·to·ne·al (pro″pər-ĭ-to-ne′əl) preperitoneal.

prop·er·ty (prop′ər-te) a characteristic quality, ability, capability, or function.

colligative p. any of the properties of solutions that depend only on the concentration of osmotically active particles: boiling point elevation, freezing point depression, osmotic pressure, and vapor pressure lowering.

pro·phage (pro′fāj) [*pro-* + *phage*] the latent stage of a phage in a lysogenic bacterium, in which the viral genome becomes inserted into a specific portion of the host chromosome and is duplicated each cell generation.

pro·phase (pro′fāz) the first stage in cell reduplication. In mitosis, the chromosomes condense, the nucleolus disassembles, and the centrosome separates into two centrioles surrounded by arrays of microtubules (asters), which migrate toward the poles of the cell. In meiosis, the prophase of the first division is highly specialized and consists of five stages: leptotene, zygotene, pachytene, diplotene, and diakinesis (qq.v.). Prophase of the second meiotic division resembles that in mitotic division. See *meiosis* and *mitosis.*

pro·phy·lac·tic (pro″fə-lak′tik) [Gr. *prophylaktikos*] 1. tending to ward off or prevent something, particularly disease. 2. pertaining to prophylaxis. 3. an agent that tends to ward off disease. 4. a device for preventing sexually transmitted disease and/or conception, particularly a condom.

pro·phy·lax·is (pro″fə-lak′sis) [Gr. *prophylassein* to keep guard before] intervention aimed at the prevention of disease; called also *preventive treatment, prophylactic treatment,* and *protective therapy.*

causal p. removal of the cause of a disease.

chemical p. chemoprophylaxis.

collective p. the protection of the community from infection.

dental p. oral p.

drug p. chemoprophylaxis.

individual p. the prevention of infection in an individual.

mechanical p. prevention of the transmission of venereal disease by mechanical means (e.g., a condom).

oral p. cleansing the teeth in the dental office, including removal of plaque, materia alba, calculus, and stains from the exposed and unexposed surfaces of the teeth by scaling and polishing of the teeth, as a preventive measure for the control of local irritational factors. Called also *dental p.*

Pro·phyl·lin (pro-fil′in) trademark for a preparation of chlorophyllin copper complex and sodium propionate.

pro·pid·ium io·dide (pro-pid′e-əm) a fluorescent, intercalating stain for double-stranded nucleic acids, penetrating nonviable cells and fluorescing red; because binding is stoichiometric, it is often used to analyze cellular DNA content.

Pro·pine (pro′pēn) trademark for a preparation of dipivefrin hydrochloride.

pro·pio·lac·tone (pro″pe-o-lak′tōn) a disinfectant effective against gram-positive, gram-negative, and acid-fast bacteria, fungi, and viruses. It is also used to prepare inactivated vaccines because it destroys the nucleic acid core of viruses but does not damage the capsid. Called also *betapropiolactone.*

pro·pi·o·ma·zine hy·dro·chlo·ride (pro″pe-o-ma′zēn) a phenothiazine derivative, used to provide bedtime, perioperative, and obstetrical sedation and as an antiemetic during labor, administered intramuscularly and intravenously.

pro·pi·o·nate (pro′pe-ə-nāt) any salt of propionic acid.

Pro·pi·on·i·bac·te·ri·a·ceae (pro″pe-on″ĭ-bak-tēr″e-a′se-e) a family of bacteria of the suborder Propionibacterineae, order Actinomycetales, consisting of gram-positive, non–spore-forming, anaerobic or aerotolerant, branching or regular rods or filaments. The organisms are inhabitants of the skin and respiratory and intestinal tracts, and are sometimes found in soft tissue infections. Medically important members are contained in the genus *Propionibacterium.*

Pro·pi·o·ni·bac·te·ri·neae (pro″pe-on″ĭ-bak-tə-rin′e-e) a morphologically diverse suborder of aerobic or facultatively anaerobic bacteria of the order Actinomycetales; organisms of medical interest are included in the family Propionibacteriaceae.

Pro·pi·on·i·bac·te·ri·um (pro″pe-on″ĭ-bak-tēr′e-əm) [*pro-* + Gr. *piōn* fat + *baktērion* little rod] a genus of bacteria of the family Propionibacteriaceae, made up of non–spore-forming, anaerobic or aerotolerant, gram-positive rods. The organisms are found as saprophytes in animals and in dairy products, and occasionally cause soft tissue infections.

P. ac′nes a species that is a normal inhabitant of the skin and a frequent contaminant of anaerobic cultures. It is a potential pathogen associated with chronic infections in the blood and bone marrow.

P. granulo′sum a species isolated from the intestinal tract and abscesses. Called also *Corynebacterium granulosum.*

P. jense′nii a species isolated from dairy products and silage, occasionally found in infections.

P. propio′nicum a species that is a normal inhabitant of the body cavities and skin of mammals but can also cause actinomycosis and periodontal disease in humans and infections in cattle.

pro·pi·on·i·bac·te·ri·um (pro″pe-on″ĭ-bak-tēr′e-əm) pl. *propionibacte′ria.* An organism of the genus *Propionibacterium.*

pro·pi·on·ic ac·id (pro″pe-on′ik) a three-carbon saturated fatty acid that can be fermented by several species of bacteria; in mammals it can be converted to the thioester propionyl CoA, a metabolic intermediate.

pro·pi·on·ic·ac·i·de·mia (pro″pe-on″ik-as″ĭ-de′me-ə) 1. an autosomal recessive aminoacidopathy characterized by an excess of propionic acid in the blood and urine, with ketosis, acidosis, hyperglycinemia, hyperglycinuria, and often neurologic complications. The disorder is caused by mutation in either of the genes encoding the two subunits of propionyl-CoA carboxylase (loci: 13q32, 3q21-q22). 2. excess of propionic acid in the blood, such as that characteristic of multiple carboxylase deficiency.

pro·pi·o·nyl (pro′pe-ə-nəl) the acyl radical of propionic acid; the thioester it forms with coenzyme A, propionyl CoA, is an intermediate in the degradation of some amino acids and in the oxidation of odd number chain length fatty acids.

pro·pi·o·nyl-CoA car·boxy·lase (pro′pe-ə-nəl ko-a′ kahr-bok′sə-lās) [EC 6.4.1.3] an enzyme of the ligase class that catalyzes the carboxylation of propionyl CoA to form methylmalonyl CoA; the reaction is part of the route by which three-carbon compounds from some amino acids and from odd-numbered fatty acids are used as fuels. The enzyme is an oligomer comprising 4α and 4β chains and requires a biotin cofactor. Deficiency of enzyme activity due to a defect in either chain, an autosomal recessive trait, causes propionicacidemia; see also *multiple carboxylase deficiency,* under *carboxylase.*

pro·plas·ma·cyte (pro-plaz′mə-sīt) a precursor in the plasmacytic series, being a cell intermediate between the plasmablast and the plasma cell.

pro·plas·min (pro-plaz′min) plasminogen.

Pro·plast (pro′plast) trademark for an alloplastic material that is a porous composite of vitreous carbon fibers and polytef, used for submucosal implantation.

Pro·plex T (pro′pleks) trademark for a preparation of factor IX complex.

pro·po·fol (pro′po-fol) [USP] a short-acting anesthetic and sedative used in induction and maintenance of general anesthesia and also for sedation, as during diagnostic procedures or in patients in intensive care units; administered intravenously.

pro·por·tion (prə-por′shən) [L. *proportio*] the relation of one part to the whole.

pro·pos·i·tus (pro-poz′ĭ-təs) pl. *propo′siti* [L. "the one on display"] 1. proband. 2. more specifically the first proband to be ascertained (index case). Properly, the term is used for a male, with the female counterpart called a *proposita.*

pro·poxy·caine hy·dro·chlo·ride (pro-pok′sĭ-kān) [USP] a local anesthetic, used for infiltration and block anesthesia.

pro·poxy·phene (pro-pok′sĭ-fēn) an opioid analgesic structurally related to methadone. Called also *dextropropoxyphene.*

p. hydrochloride [USP] the hydrochloride salt of propoxyphene, used as an analgesic to provide relief of mild to moderate pain, administered orally.

p. napsylate [USP] the napsylate salt of propoxyphene, having the same actions and uses as the hydrochloride salt.

pro·pran·o·lol (pro-pran′ə-lol) a nonselective beta-adrenergic blocking agent that lacks intrinsic sympathomimetic activity, decreases cardiac rate and output, reduces blood pressure, and is effective in the prophylaxis of migraine.

p. hydrochloride [USP] the hydrochloride salt of propranolol, used as an antiarrhythmic, antianginal, antihypertensive, and antitremor agent, in the management of hypertrophic subaortic stenosis, and in conjunction with an alpha-adrenergic blocking agent in the symptomatic treatment of inoperable pheochromocytoma. It is also used to prevent migraine and to treat myocardial infarction and prevent its recurrence. Administered orally or intravenously.

pro·pri·e·tary (pro-pri′ə-tar-e) protected against free competition by patent, trademark, or other means.

pro·prio·cep·tion (pro″pre-o-sep′shən) perception mediated by proprioceptors or proprioceptive tissues.

pro·prio·cep·tive (pro″pre-o-sep′tiv) 1. pertaining to or characterized by proprioception. 2. pertaining to proprioceptors.

pro·prio·cep·tor (pro″pre-o-sep′tər) sensory nerve terminals found in muscles, tendons, and joint capsules, which give information concerning movements and position of the body; sometimes the receptors in the labyrinth are also considered proprioceptors. See *exteroceptor*, *interoceptor*, and *receptor* (def. 3).

pro·prio·spi·nal (pro″pre-o-spi′nəl) pertaining wholly to the spinal cord; said of ascending and descending nerve fibers that interconnect segments of the spinal cord.

pro·pro·tein (pro-pro′tēn) a precursor of a protein that is converted into the active protein by proteolysis or glycosylation.

prop·tom·e·ter (prop-tom′ə-tər) exophthalmometer.

prop·to·sis (prop-to′sis) exophthalmos.

pro·pul·sion (pro-pul′shən) [*pro-* + *pulsion*] 1. tendency to fall forward in walking. 2. festination.

pro·pyl (pro′pəl) the univalent chemical radical, $CH_3CH_2CH_2$—, from propane.

p. gallate [NF] an alkyl ester of gallic acid, used as an antioxidant in pharmaceutical preparations.

pro·pyl·ene (pro′pə-lēn) chemical name: propene. A gaseous hydrocarbon, $CH_3CH{=}CH_2$, of the olefin series.

p. carbonate [NF] a clear, colorless, mobile liquid used as a solvent in oral and topical pharmaceutical preparations.

p. glycol [USP] a clear, colorless, viscous liquid used as a humectant and solvent in pharmaceutical preparations.

pro·pyl·hex·e·drine (pro″pəl-hek′sə-drēn) [USP] an adrenergic compound used as a vasoconstrictor to decongest nasal mucosa; administered by inhalation.

pro·pyl·io·done (pro″pəl-i′o-dōn) [USP] a radiopaque medium used in bronchography; administered intratracheally.

pro·pyl·par·a·ben (pro″pəl-par′ə-bən) [NF] an antifungal agent, closely related to butylparaben, ethylparaben, and methylparaben; used as a preservative in pharmaceutical preparations.

p. sodium the sodium salt of propylparaben, having the same actions and uses as the base.

pro·pyl·thio·ura·cil (pro″pəl-thi″o-u′rə-sil) [USP] a thyroid inhibitor, used in the treatment of hyperthyroidism; administered orally.

Pro·Quad (pro′kwod) trademark for a preparation of measles, mumps, rubella, and varicella virus vaccine live.

pro re na·ta (p.r.n.) (pro re na′tə) [L.] according to circumstances.

pro·re·nin (pro′re-nin) the inactive precursor of renin, stored in the juxtaglomerular cells of the kidney and activated by cleavage to renin.

pro·ren·nin (pro-ren′in) prochymosin.

Pro·ro·cen·trum (pro″ro-sen′trəm) [*L. prora* prow + *centrum* center] a genus of plantlike, marine and freshwater protozoa of the phylum Dinoflagellata; like other dinoflagellates, when present in vast numbers they can cause red tide. Certain species contain okadaic acid, and if shellfish ingest them, persons eating the contaminated shellfish get diarrhetic shellfish poisoning (see under *poisoning*).

pror·sad (pror′səd) in an anterior direction.

pro·ru·bri·cyte (pro-roo′brĭ-sīt) basophilic erythroblast.

pro·sap·o·sin (pro-sap′ə-sin) a 524–amino acid polypeptide containing four homologous domains of approximately 80 amino acids each; it is processed in the lysosomes to the four active saposins (q.v.).

Pros·car (pros′kahr) trademark for a preparation of finasteride.

pro·scil·lar·i·din (pro-sil-ar′ĭ-din) a cardiac glycoside obtained from squill; it is composed of a molecule of rhamnose linked to a steroid base, and has the same actions and uses as digitalis; administered orally and intravenously.

pro·se·cre·tin (pro″se-kre′tin) a precursor of secretin found in epithelial cells of the duodenum and jejunum.

pro·sec·tion (pro-sek′shən) a carefully prepared dissection for demonstration of anatomic structure.

pro·sec·tor (pro-sek′tər) [L.] one who dissects anatomical subjects for demonstration.

Pro·sed/DS (pro′sed) trademark for a combination preparation of methenamine, phenyl salicylate, methylene blue, benzoic acid, atropine sulfate, and hyoscyamine sulfate.

pros·en·ceph·a·lon (pros″ən-sef′ə-lon) [*pros-* + *encephalon*] 1. [TA] the part of the brain developed from the anterior of the three primary vesicles of the embryonic neural tube; it comprises the diencephalon and telencephalon. 2. the most anterior of the three primary brain vesicles in the embryo, later dividing into the telencephalon and the diencephalon. Called also *forebrain.*

pros(o)- [Gr. *prosō* forward] a prefix meaning forward, or anterior.

Proso·bran·chi·a·ta (pro″so-brang″ke-a′tə) Streptoneura.

proso·cele (pros′o-sēl) prosocoele.

proso·coele (pros′o-sēl) [*proso-* + *-coele*] the foremost cavity of the brain; the ventricular cavity of the prosencephalon.

proso·de·mic (pros″o-dem′ik) [*proso-* + Gr. *dēmos* people] pertaining to or denoting a disease transmitted directly from person to person rather than spread generally (as by a contaminated water supply).

pros·o·dy (pros′o-de) [Gr. *prosodos* a solemn procession] the variation in stress, pitch, and rhythm of speech by which different shades of meaning are conveyed.

proso·gas·ter (pros′o-gas″tər) foregut.

Pro·Som (pro′som) trademark for a preparation of estazolam.

proso·pag·no·sia (pros″o-pag-no′zhə) [*prosop-* + *agnosia*] a form of visual agnosia characterized by an inability to recognize familiar faces, or even one's own face in a mirror, which occurs as a result of bilateral damage to the medioinferior occipital lobes along the medioventral surfaces of the temporal lobes. Called also *face* or *facial agnosia.*

proso·pec·ta·sia (pros″o-pək-ta′zhə) [*prosop-* + *ectasia*] oversized face, as in acromegaly.

Pro·so·pis (pro-so′pis) the mesquites, a genus of shrubs of the family Leguminosae, found in the southwestern United States and other arid regions of the Americas. The beans of *P. juliflo′ra* L. contain a toxin that can cause fatal neurotoxicity in ruminants.

proso·pla·sia (pros″o-pla′zhə) [*proso-* + *-plasia*] 1. abnormal differentiation of tissue. 2. development into a higher level of organization or of function.

prosop(o)- [Gr. *prosōpon* face] a combining form denoting relationship to the face.

pros·o·po·an·os·chi·sis (pros″o-po-ə-nos′kĭ-sis) oblique facial cleft.

pros·o·pop·a·gus (pros″o-pop′ə-gəs) [*prosopo-* + *-pagus*] asymmetrical conjoined twins in which the parasite is attached to the face elsewhere than at the jaw.

pros·o·po·ple·gia (pros″o-po-ple′jə) facial paralysis.

pros·o·pos·chi·sis (pros″o-pos′kĭ-sis) facial cleft (def. 2).

pros·o·po·ster·no·dy·mus (pros″o-po-stur″no-di′məs) [*prosopo-* + *sterno-* + *-didymus*] conjoined twins joined face to face and sternum to sternum.

pros·o·po·tho·ra·cop·a·gus (pros″o-po-thor″ə-cop′ə-gəs) [*prosopo-* + *thoraco-* + *-pagus*] symmetrical conjoined twins united in the frontal plane, the fusion extending from the oral region through the thorax.

pro·spec·tive (prə-spek′tiv) [L. *prospicere* to look forward] 1. looking toward the future. 2. denoting a type of epidemiologic study in which subjects are selected on the basis of factors that are to be examined for their effects on outcomes.

pros·ta·cy·clin (pros″tə-si′klin) a prostaglandin, PGI_2, synthesized by endothelial cells lining the cardiovascular system; it is the most potent known inhibitor of platelet aggregation and a powerful vasodilator and thus is a physiologic antagonist of thromboxane A_2. When used pharmaceutically, it is called *epoprostenol.*

pros·ta·cy·clin syn·thase (pros″tə-si′klin sin′thās) prostaglandin-I synthase.

pros·ta·glan·din (pros″tə-glan′din) [*prostate gland* + *-in* because they were originally thought to originate in the prostate] any of a group of components derived from unsaturated 20-carbon fatty acids, primarily arachidonic acid, via the cyclooxygenase pathway; they are potent mediators of numerous different physiologic processes. The abbreviation for prostaglandin is PG; specific compounds are designated by adding a letter to indicate the type of ring structure and a numerical subscript to indicate the number of double bonds in the hydrocarbon skeleton (e.g., PGE_2, etc.). Most naturally occurring prostaglandins have two double bonds and are synthesized from arachidonic acid (see illustration). The 1 series and 3 series are produced by the same pathway starting with fatty acids that have one fewer or one more double bond than arachidonic acid. The subscript α or β indicates the three-dimensional configuration of alcoholic groups attached to the ring structures (α denotes a substituent below the plane of the ring, β, above the plane). The naturally occurring PGFs all have the α configuration. Prostaglandins act in the cells in which they are synthesized

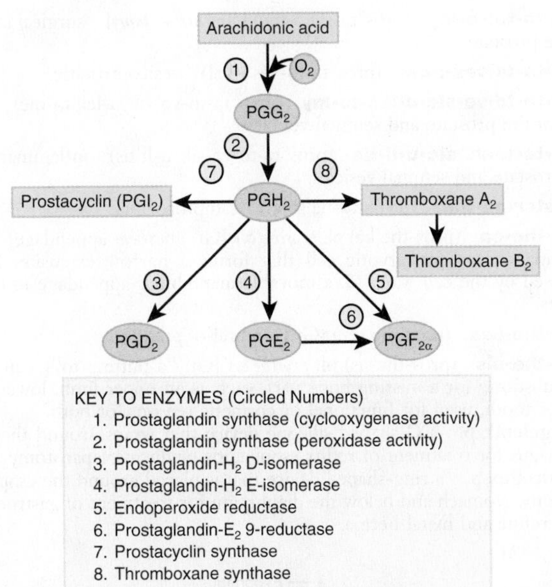

■ Cyclooxygenase pathway of prostaglandin and thromboxane synthesis.

and on surrounding cells, and their actions and effects vary with concentration, hormonal environment, and cell type.

p. D_2 (PGD_2) the major prostaglandin produced by mast cells; it is a mediator of immediate hypersensitivity synthesized and released in response to binding of immunoglobulin E to receptors on the mast cell, and its effects include vasodilation and contraction of nonvascular smooth muscle.

p. E_1 (PGE_1) the analogue of PGE_2 having one double bond; many of its effects, including vasodilation, are similar to those of PGE_2, but unlike PGE_2, it inhibits platelet aggregation. It is used pharmaceutically and called *alprostadil* as a vasodilator in neonates with congenital heart disease and in men with impotence.

p. E_2 (PGE_2) an important prostaglandin produced in the renal medulla, gastrointestinal mucosa, and other tissues; it causes renal vasodilation and inhibition of renal tubular sodium resorption, inhibition of gastric secretion, and either contraction or relaxation of smooth muscle (depending on the tissue). It is also released by macrophages and modulates several inflammatory responses; it increases vascular permeability, increases pain sensitivity, is pyrogenic, and suppresses lymphocyte transformation, release of mediators from mast cells, and cell-mediated cytotoxicity. PGE_2 produced by some tumors causes hypercalcemia by stimulation of bone resorption by osteoclasts. When used pharmaceutically its nonproprietary name is *dinoprostone.*

p. $F_{2\alpha}$ ($PGF_{2\alpha}$) a stable prostaglandin formed from PGH_2 or PGE_2; it stimulates the contraction of uterine and bronchial smooth muscle and produces vasoconstriction in some vessels. As a pharmaceutical, its nonproprietary name is *dinoprost.*

p. $F_{2\alpha}$ tromethamine dinoprost tromethamine.

p. G_2 (PGG_2) a prostaglandin cyclic endoperoxide formed from arachidonic acid by incorporation of two oxygen molecules, catalyzed by the cyclooxygenase activity of prostaglandin-endoperoxide synthase; it is an unstable intermediate and is converted rapidly and spontaneously to PGH_2.

p. H_2 (PGH_2) a prostaglandin cyclic endoperoxide sometimes formed from PGG_2 by the peroxidase reaction of prostaglandin-endoperoxide synthase, although the synthase is not required; it is an unstable intermediate that can be converted to several important prostaglandins and thromboxanes.

p. I_2 (PGI_2) prostacyclin.

pros·ta·glan·din-D syn·thase (pros″tə-glan′din sin′thās) [EC 5.3.99.2] an enzyme of the isomerase class that catalyzes the conversion of the intermediate prostaglandin H_2 (PGH_2) to prostaglandin D_2 (PGD_2). The enzyme requires glutathione. See illustration at *prostaglandin.* Called also *endoperoxide-D-isomerase* and *prostaglandin-H_2 D-isomerase.*

pros·ta·glan·din-en·do·per·ox·ide syn·thase (pros″tə-glan′din en″do-pər-ok′sīd sin′thās) [EC 1.14.99.1] an enzyme of the oxidoreductase class that has both cyclooxygenase and peroxidase activities, which together catalyze the first three reactions in the synthesis of prostaglandins and thromboxanes from arachidonic acid. Its cyclooxygenase activity catalyzes the first two reactions, each of which adds a molecule of oxygen to arachidonic acid, to form the intermediate PGG_2; its peroxidase activity catalyzes the conversion of PGG_2 to the intermediate PGH_2, from which are formed the prostaglandins and thromboxanes. See illustration at *prostaglandin.*

pros·ta·glan·din-E_2 9-re·duc·tase (pros″tə-glan′din re-duk′tās) [EC 1.1.1.189] an enzyme of the oxidoreductase class that catalyzes the reduction of prostaglandin E_2 to prostaglandin $F_{2\alpha}$. It can also act on a variety of similar prostaglandin derivatives with 9-keto or 15-keto groups, reducing them to the corresponding hydroxy compounds. See illustration at *prostaglandin.*

pros·ta·glan·din-E syn·thase (pros″tə-glan′din sin′thās) [EC 5.3.99.3] an enzyme of the isomerase class that catalyzes the conversion of the intermediate prostaglandin H_2 (PGH_2) to prostaglandin E_2 (PGE_2). The enzyme requires glutathione. See illustration at *prostaglandin.* Called also *endoperoxide-E-isomerase* and *prostaglandin-H_2 E-isomerase.*

pros·ta·glan·din-H_2 D-isom·er·ase (pros″tə-glan′din i-som′ər-ās) prostaglandin-D synthase.

pros·ta·glan·din-H_2 E-isom·er·ase (pros″tə-glan′din i-som′ər-ās) prostaglandin-E synthase.

pros·ta·glan·din-I syn·thase (pros″tə-glan′din sin′thās) [EC 5.3.99.4] an enzyme of the isomerase class that catalyzes the conversion of the prostaglandin intermediate prostaglandin H_2 (PGH_2) to prostacyclin (PGI_2). The enzyme acts predominantly in the endothelium of blood vessel walls. See illustration at *prostaglandin.* Called also *prostacyclin synthase.*

pros·ta·glan·din syn·thase (pros″tə-glan′din sin′thās) prostaglandin-endoperoxide synthase.

pros·ta·noid (pros′tə-noid) any of a group of complex fatty acids derived from arachidonic acid, being 20 carbons in length with an internal five- or six-carbon ring; examples are the prostaglandins, prostanoic acid, and the thromboxanes.

pro·sta·ta (pros′tə-tə) [L.] [TA] prostate.

pros·ta·tal·gia (pros″tə-tal′jə) [*prostate* + *-algia*] prostatodynia.

pros·ta·tauxe (pros″tə-tawk′se) prostatomegaly.

pros·tate (pros′tāt) [Gr. *prostates* one who stands before, from *pro* before + *histanai* to stand] a gland in the male that surrounds the bladder neck and urethra. It consists of a median lobe and two lateral lobes, and is made up partly of glandular matter whose ducts empty into the prostatic part of the urethra, and partly of muscular fibers that encircle the urethra. The prostate contributes to the seminal fluid a secretion containing acid phosphatase, citric acid, and proteolytic enzymes that account for the liquefaction of the coagulated semen. Called also *prostata* [TA] and *prostate gland.* **prostat′ic** *adj*

female p. paraurethral glands.

pros·ta·tec·to·my (pros″tə-tek′tə-me) [*prostate* + *-ectomy*] surgical removal of the prostate or of a part of it.

laser p. removal of the prostate after it has been exposed to a laser; there may be either direct contact from the laser with vaporization or an indirect system that causes coagulation necrosis.

perineal p. removal of the prostate through an incision in the perineum.

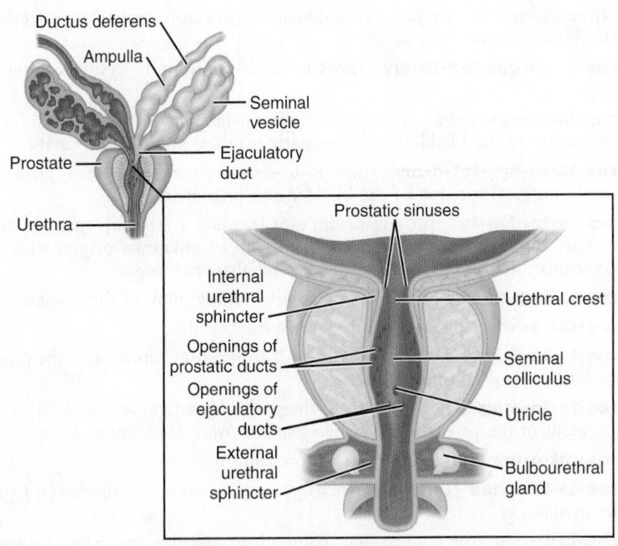

■ Prostate and seminal vesicles.

radical p. removal of the prostate with its capsule, seminal vesicles, ductus deferens, some pelvic fasciae, and sometimes pelvic lymph nodes; performed via either the retropubic or the perineal route.
radical retropubic p. radical prostatectomy through the retropubic space via a suprapubic incision.
retropubic p. see *radical retropubic p.*
retropubic prevesical p. removal of the prostate through a suprapubic incision but without entering the urinary bladder.
suprapubic transvesical p. removal of the prostate through a suprapubic incision and an incision in the urinary bladder.
transurethral p. transurethral resection of the prostate; see under *resection.*
transurethral laser-induced p. (TULIP) a type of laser prostatectomy where only part of the prostate is vaporized so that the rest can move to release pressure on the urethra.
transvesical p. prostatectomy through an incision of the urinary bladder.

pros•ta•tel•co•sis (pros″tə-təl-ko′sis) [*prostate* + *helcosis*] ulceration of the prostate.

pros•tat•i•co•ves•i•cal (pros-tat″ĭ-ko-ves′ĭ-kəl) vesicoprostatic.

pros•ta•tism (pros′tə-tiz″əm) a symptom complex resulting from compression or obstruction of the urethra, usually due to benign prostatic hyperplasia (see under *hyperplasia*). There are both obstructive and neurological symptoms, including diminution in caliber and force of the urinary stream, hesitancy in initiating urination, inability to end it (with subsequent dribbling), a sensation of incomplete bladder emptying, and occasionally urinary retention.
vesical p. urinary retention resembling that in prostatic disease but from other causes.

pros•ta•tisme (pros-tə-tēzm′) prostatism.
p. sans prostate′ the symptoms of prostatic obstruction without enlargement of the prostate.

pros•ta•ti•tis (pros″tə-ti′tis) inflammation of the prostate. **prostatit′ic** *adj*
allergic p. eosinophilic p.
bacterial p. prostatitis caused by bacterial infection, usually from a urinary tract infection, with bacteriuria. *Acute bacterial prostatitis* is a febrile illness with sudden onset; pain in the lumbar and perineal regions, dysuria with frequency, urgency, and nocturia; a tender, swollen prostate; and other symptoms. *Chronic bacterial prostatitis* is a mild condition caused by recurrent urinary tract infections with bacteriuria and variable other symptoms such as pain and dysuria, but only rarely fever.
eosinophilic p. a rare type of granulomatous prostatitis characterized by diffuse infiltration of the prostate by eosinophils, with fever, swelling of the gland, and foci of fibrinoid necrosis; it may superficially resemble carcinoma of the prostate. Since it is usually seen in patients with certain allergies, it is called also *allergic p.*
granulomatous p. prostatitis with granuloma formation, such as from infection with *Mycobacterium tuberculosis,* parasites, or fungi.
nonbacterial p. prostatitis with pain (see *prostatodynia*) and increased numbers of inflammatory cells but without history of urinary tract infection.
nonspecific granulomatous p. granulomatous prostatitis of unknown etiology with focal or diffuse infiltration of the tissues by peculiar, large, pale macrophages.
tuberculous p. a type of granulomatous prostatitis caused by infection with *Mycobacterium tuberculosis.*

pros•ta•to•cys•tec•to•my (pros″tə-to-sis-tek′tə-me) cystoprostatectomy.

pros•ta•to•cys•ti•tis (pros″tə-to-sis-ti′tis) [*prostate* + *cysto-* + *-itis*] inflammation of the bladder neck (prostatic urethra) and bladder cavity.

pros•ta•to•cys•tot•o•my (pros″tə-to-sis-tot′ə-me) [*prostate* + *cysto-* + *-tomy*] surgical incision of the bladder and prostate.

pros•ta•to•dyn•ia (pros″tə-to-din′e-ə) [*prostate* + *-odynia*] pain in the prostate; some authorities limit usage to pain of unknown origin, such as that seen in nonbacterial prostatitis. Called also *prostatalgia.*

pros•ta•tog•ra•phy (pros″tə-tog′rə-fe) radiography of the prostate.

pros•tat•o•lith (pros-tat′o-lith) prostatic calculus.

pros•ta•to•li•thot•o•my (pros″tə-to-lĭ-thot′ə-me) incision of the prostate for the removal of calculus.

pros•ta•to•meg•a•ly (pros″tə-to-meg′ə-le) [*prostate* + *-megaly*] enlargement of the prostate; see *benign prostatic hyperplasia,* under *hyperplasia.*

pros•tat•o•my (pros-tat′ə-me) prostatotomy.

pros•ta•tor•rhea (pros″tə-to-re′ə) [*prostate* + *-rrhea*] a discharge from the prostate.

pros•ta•to•sis (pros″tə-to′sis) congestion of the prostate causing swelling, but without inflammation.

pros•ta•tot•o•my (pros″tə-tot′ə-me) [*prostate* + *-tomy*] surgical incision of the prostate.

pros•ta•to•ves•i•cal (pros″tə-to-ves′ĭ-kəl) vesicoprostatic.

pros•ta•to•ve•sic•u•lec•to•my (pros″tə-to-və-sik″u-lek′tə-me) excision of the prostate and seminal vesicles.

pros•ta•to•ve•sic•u•li•tis (pros″tə-to-və-sik″u-li′tis) inflammation of the prostate and seminal vesicles.

pro•ster•na•tion (pro″stər-na′shən) camptocormia.

pros•the•ca (pros-the′kə) pl. *prosthe′cae* [Gr. *prosthēkē* appendage] 1. an appendage of a prokaryotic cell that forms a narrow extension and is enclosed by the cell wall. 2. a movable mandibular appendage in certain insects.

pros•the•ses (pros-the′sēz) [Gr.] plural of *prosthesis.*

pros•the•sis (pros-the′sis) pl. *prosthe′ses* [Gr. "a putting to"] an artificial substitute for a missing body part, such as an upper limb, lower limb, eye, or tooth, used for functional or cosmetic reasons, or both.
Angelchik p. a C-shaped silicone device that wraps around the distal esophagus for treatment of reflux esophagitis or during laparotomy.
antireflux p. a ring-shaped device that is placed around the esophagus above the stomach and below the diaphragm for treatment of gastroesophageal reflux and hiatal hernia.

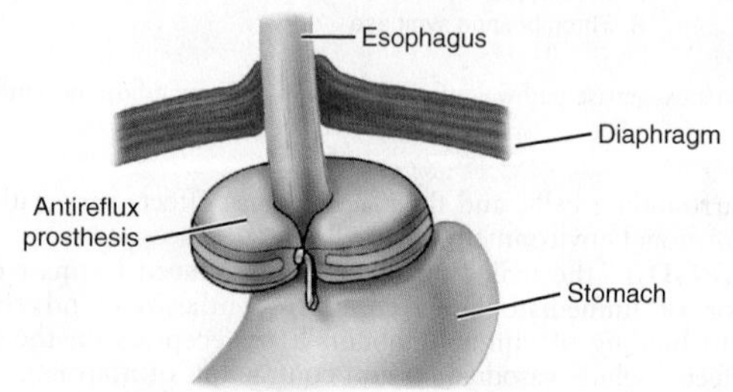

Austin Moore p. a metallic implant used in hip arthroplasty.
body-powered p. a prosthetic upper limb that is controlled by movement of shoulder or pectoral muscles.
Charnley p. an implant for hip arthroplasty consisting of an acetabular cup and a relatively small femoral head component that form a low-friction joint.
cleft palate p. a prosthetic device, such as an obturator, used to correct cleft palate. See also *speech-aid p.,* and *artificial palate,* under *palate.*
definitive p. a prosthesis meant for long-term wear.
dental p. a replacement for one or more of the teeth or other oral structure, ranging from a single tooth to a complete denture. See also *bridge* and *denture.*
endoskeletal p. a limb prosthesis in which support components are primarily internal.
exoskeletal p. a limb prosthesis in which support mechanisms are provided by a rigid external shell.
heart valve p. prosthetic heart valve; see under *valve.*
maxillofacial p. a prosthetic replacement for parts of the maxilla, mandible, or face that are missing or defective because of surgical intervention, trauma, pathology, or developmental malformations. See also under *prosthetics.*
ocular p. 1. artificial eye; see under *eye.* 2. any other aid to vision, e.g., eyeglasses or occluders.
palatal lift p. a type of speech-aid prosthesis sometimes used to aid in closure in cases of velopharyngeal insufficiency.
penile p. a semirigid rod or inflatable device implanted in the penis to provide an erection in men with organic impotence; called also *penile implant.*
Robinson p. a type of stainless steel prosthetic stapes.
speech-aid p. a device designed to close a cleft of the hard or soft palate and to substitute for structures used for normal speech. Called also *artificial palate, obturator,* and *prosthetic speech aid.*
Thompson p. a Vitallium implant used in hip arthroplasty.

pros•thet•ic (pros-thet′ik) 1. pertaining to the use or application of prostheses. 2. serving as a substitute.

pros•thet•ics (pros-thet′iks) the field of knowledge relating to prostheses and their design and use.
dental p., denture p. prosthodontics.
facial p. maxillofacial p.
maxillofacial p. the branch of prosthodontics concerned with anatomic, functional, and cosmetic reconstruction by means of synthetic substitutes of those regions of the maxilla, mandible, and face that have been damaged, absent, or malformed due to illness, injury, congenital defects, or surgical intervention. Called also *facial p.* See also under *prosthesis.*

pros•the•tist (pros′thə-tist) [Gr. *prosthetes* one who adds] an allied health professional trained in prosthetics.

pros•thi•on (PR) (pros′the-on) [Gr. *prosthios* foremost] a craniometric landmark located at the point of the maxillary alveolar process that projects most anteriorly in the midline of the maxilla; used for measuring upper facial height and in determining the gnathic index.

pros•tho•don•tia (pros″tho-don′shə) prosthodontics.

pros•tho•don•tics (pros″tho-don′tiks) [*prosthesis* + Gr. *odous* tooth] the branch of dentistry concerned with the restoration and maintenance of oral function, comfort, appearance, and health of the patient by the replacement of missing teeth and contiguous tissues with artificial substitutes. Called also *dental prosthetics, denture prosthetics, prosthetic dentistry,* and *prosthodontia.*

pros•tho•don•tist (pros″tho-don′tist) a dentist who specializes in prosthodontics.

Pros•tho•gon•i•mus (pros″tho-gon′ĭ-məs) a genus of trematodes. *P. macror′chis* parasitizes chickens, turkeys, and other birds.

pros•tho•ker•a•to•plas•ty (pros″tho-ker′ə-to-plas″te) [*prosthesis* + *kerato-* + *-plasty*] surgical replacement of corneal tissue (as in cataract) by an inert transparent prosthesis.

Pro•stig•min (pro-stig′min) trademark for preparations of neostigmine.

Pros•tin E2 (pros′tin) trademark for preparations of dinoprostone.

Pros•tin F2 Alpha (pros′tin) trademark for preparations of dinoprost tromethamine.

Pros•tin VR (pros′tin) trademark for a preparation of alprostadil.

pros•tra•tion (pros-tra′shən) [L. *prostratio*] extreme exhaustion or powerlessness.

heat p. heat exhaustion.

nervous p. neurasthenia.

pro•tac•tin•i•um (Pa) (pro″tak-tin′e-əm) a radioactive metallic chemical element occurring along with radium in pitchblende, carnotite, and other minerals; atomic weight, 231; atomic number, 91.

Pro•tal•ba (pro-tal′bə) trademark for preparations of protoveratrine A.

pro•tal•bu•mose (pro-tal′bu-mōs) a primary proteose.

pro•ta•mine (pro′tə-mēn) [*prot-* + *amine*] any of a class of basic proteins of low molecular weight, occurring in combination with nucleic acids in the sperm of salmon and certain other fish and having the property of neutralizing heparin.

p. sulfate [USP] a purified mixture of simple protein principles obtained from the sperm or testes of suitable species of fish and able to neutralize heparin; used as an antidote to overdosage with heparin, administered intravenously.

pro•tan (pro′tan) 1. pertaining to protanomaly or protanopia. 2. a person with protanomaly or protanopia.

pro•ta•nom•al (pro″tə-nom′əl) a person with protanomaly.

pro•ta•nom•a•ly (pro″tə-nom′ə-le) [*prot-* + *anomaly*] a type of anomalous trichromasy in which the first, red-sensitive, cones have decreased sensitivity; therefore a greater than normal proportion of lithium red light to thallium green light is required to match a fixed sodium yellow light. **protanom′alous** *adj*

pro•ta•nope (pro′tə-nōp) an individual exhibiting protanopia.

pro•ta•no•pia (pro″tə-no′pe-ə) [*prot-* + *an-*[1] + *-opia*] a dichromasy characterized by retention of the sensory mechanism for two hues only (blue and yellow) of the normal 4-primary quota, and lacking that for red and green and their derivatives, with loss of luminance and shift of brightness and hue curves toward the short-wave end of the spectrum, as in twilight vision. **protanop′ic** *adj*

pro•ta•nop•sia (pro″tə-nop′se-ə) protanopia.

Pro•tea (pro′te-ə) [L.] a genus of trees of the family Proteaceae; many species grow in wet and warm regions and several are medicinal. *P. melli′fera* L. is the sugar protea, which is made into a syrup used for coughs and pulmonary disorders.

pro•te•an (pro′te-ən) [Gr. *Prōteus* an ocean deity able to appear in many different forms] assuming different shapes; changeable in form.

pro•te•ase (pro′te-ās) endopeptidase.

pro•te•a•some (pro′te-ə-sōm) [*protease* + *-some*] a large, cylindrical protease complex occurring in both the nucleoplasm and cytoplasm, consisting of a 20S core that in eukaryotes and Archaea is capped by a regulatory complex at one or both ends; it degrades intracellular proteins that have been marked by the attachment of ubiquitin.

pro•tec•tant (pro-tek′tənt) protective.

pro•tec•tin (pro-tek′tin) a membrane-bound protein, CD59, present in many types of cells; it binds homologous complement factors C8 and C9 and prevents insertion of the membrane attack complex into the membrane, thereby protecting normal bystander cells from lysis after complement activation in nearby bacteria or immune complexes. Called also *membrane inhibitor of reactive lysis.*

pro•tec•tive (pro-tek′tiv) [L. *protegere* to cover over] 1. affording defense or immunity. 2. an agent that provides defense against a deleterious influence, such as a substance applied to the skin *(skin p.)* to avoid the effects of the sun's rays *(solar p.)* or other noxious influences; called also *screen.*

pro•tec•tor (pro-tek′tər) 1. something aimed at preventing damage or other undesirable outcomes; cf. *guard.* 2. a substance in a catalyst that prolongs the rate of activity in the catalyst. Cf. *promoter.*

hip p. a soft pad worn over the hip by a person at risk for falling and breaking a hip.

LATS p. an immunoglobulin found in the serum of patients with Graves disease that neutralizes the capacity of thyroid tissue to bind LATS (long-acting thyroid stimulator); it interferes with the binding of thyrotropin to the human thyroid cell membrane.

pro•tein (pro′tēn) [Gr. *prōtos* first] any of a group of complex organic compounds which contain carbon, hydrogen, oxygen, nitrogen, and usually sulfur, the characteristic element being nitrogen. Proteins, the principal constituents of the protoplasm of all cells, are of high molecular weight and consist essentially of combinations of α-amino acids in peptide linkages. Twenty different amino acids are commonly found in proteins, and each protein has a unique genetically defined amino acid sequence which determines its specific shape and function. Their roles include enzymatic catalysis, transport and storage, coordinated motion, nerve impulse generation and transmission, control of growth and differentiation, immunity, and mechanical support. **protein′ic** *adj*

Protein

p. 4.1 1. an 80-kD protein that helps anchor the cytoskeleton of the erythrocyte to the plasma membrane by binding spectrin to the integral membrane protein glycophorin C; defects of protein 4.1 lead to elliptocytosis, spherocytosis, and pyropoikilocytosis. 2. a superfamily of cytoskeletal proteins, including protein 4.1, ezrin, moesin, radixin, merlin, and talin.

p. A staphylococcal p. A.

AA p. see under *amyloid.*

AAA p's [*A*TPases *a*ssociated with various cellular *a*ctivities] a large family of ATPases that share a highly conserved module of about 230 amino acid residues and serve as molecular chaperones, coupling energy released by ATP hydrolysis to mechanical force. AAA proteins are involved in a variety of intracellular processes, including protein degradation, vesicular transport, microtubule rearrangement, peroxisome assembly, mitochondrial function, signal transduction, cell-cycle control, mitotic spindle formation, and transcription. The family can be extended by the addition of related chaperone proteins to form the superfamily *AAA+ proteins.*

actin-binding p's a large and diverse group of proteins that bind to actin and regulate the dynamics and organization of actin filaments.

acute phase p. any of the non-antibody proteins, produced mainly in the liver, found in increased amounts in serum during the acute phase response; they include C-reactive protein, serum amyloid A protein, fibrinogen, α1-acid glycoprotein, and procalcitonin.

adapter p., adaptor p. a protein that lacks catalytic activity but contains several protein-protein or protein-lipid interaction domains so that it can act as a connector for interactions between molecules and facilitate activation of pathways after receptors have been activated.

agouti-related p. a 132–amino acid protein found in humans and rodents, chemically related to one found in agoutis; it is a powerful appetite stimulant produced primarily in the adrenal gland, hypothalamus, and subthalamic nucleus.

AL p. see under *amyloid.*

alcohol-soluble p. prolamin.

amyloid A p. AA amyloid.

amyloid light chain p. AL amyloid.

Protein *Continued*

amyloid precursor p. (APP) a large transmembrane glycoprotein expressed on the cell surface, of uncertain function; it may be cleaved on the cell surface to a soluble form. Alternatively, cleavage may follow endocytosis, and in some cases then yields abnormal 40 to 43 amino acid peptides that aggregate to form Aβ amyloid associated with Alzheimer disease (q.v.).
bacterial p. a protein formed by bacterial activity.
bacterial cellular p. a protein that forms part of the substance of a bacterium.
bactericidal permeability increasing p. (BPI) a cationic 59-kD antibacterial protein occurring in neutrophil granules; it causes phospholipase activation and phospholipid degradation and increases the permeability of the bacterial cell membrane.
band 3 p. a 90-kD dimeric transmembrane protein occurring in erythrocytes; it is the major anion transport protein and also is the point to which ankyrin binds spectrin to help anchor the erythrocytic cytoskeleton to the plasma membrane.
Bence Jones p. an abnormal plasma or urinary protein, consisting of monoclonal immunoglobulin light chains, excreted in some plasma cell dyscrasias and characterized by its unusual solubility properties: on heating it precipitates at 50°–60°C and redissolves at 90°–100°C, and on cooling it again precipitates and redissolves. See *M component*, under *component*.
binding p. transport p.
bone Gla p. osteocalcin.
bone morphogenetic p. (BMP) any of a group of related proteins involved in induction of bone and cartilage formation and important in embryonic patterning and early skeleton formation. They are metalloproteinases with several highly conserved regions and are members of the transforming growth factor-β superfamily of proteins; binding of BMPs to their corresponding cell-surface receptors begins a signaling cascade that activates transcriptional factors. Recombinant BMPs are used in spine surgery to promote osteogenesis.
p. C a vitamin K–dependent plasma protein that, when activated by thrombin, inhibits the coagulation cascade at the levels of factor V and factor VIII by enzymatic cleavage of the activated forms of these clotting factors; it also enhances fibrinolysis. Deficiency of protein C results in recurrent venous thrombosis.
p. C, activated (APC) protein C that has been activated by thrombin and inhibits the coagulation cascade; see also *drotrecogin alfa*.
CAD p. a protein containing catalytic sites for three enzyme activities: carbamoyl-phosphate synthase (glutamine-hydrolyzing) [EC 6.3.5.5], aspartate carbamoyltransferase [EC 2.1.3.2], and dihydroorotase [EC 3.5.2.3]. The enzyme activities catalyze the first three reactions of pyrimidine biosynthesis.
cAMP receptor p. catabolite activator p.
carrier p. 1. a protein that, when coupled to hapten in vivo or in vitro, renders the hapten capable of eliciting an immune response. See *hapten*. 2. carrier (def. 6).
cartilage oligomeric matrix p. (COMP) a disulfide-linked calcium-binding protein of the cartilage matrix; increased serum levels may be linked to osteoarthritis.
catabolite activator p., catabolite gene activator p. CAP; a bacterial protein, activated by cyclic AMP, that stimulates transcription by binding to certain promoter sites on DNA; called also *cAMP receptor p.* and *cyclic adenosine monophosphate receptor p.*
cationic p's antimicrobial cationic proteins occurring in the primary (azurophilic) granules of neutrophils. They have low molecular weights, are rich in arginine, and appear to inhibit microbial growth. They presumably include the previously characterized substance termed *leukin*.
C4 binding p. a complement system regulatory protein that inhibits activation of the classical pathway; it accelerates decay of the classical pathway C3 convertase by binding to C4b and displacing C2a, and it is also a cofactor for factor I–mediated cleavage of C4b.
channel p. a cell membrane protein containing a transmembrane pore through which ions and small molecules can diffuse; it is most commonly composed of several subunits surrounding the pore. See *channel* (def. 2).
cholesteryl ester transfer p. (CETP) a plasma glycoprotein that plays a role in the movement of cholesterol from the peripheral tissues to the liver by mediating the transfer of cholesteryl esters from HDL cholesterol to apolipoprotein B–containing proteins, which are then metabolized to lipoproteins that are removed from the circulation by receptors in the liver. Deficiency of this protein, an autosomal dominant trait, results in markedly higher plasma levels of HDL cholesterol and apolipoprotein A-I. Called also *lipid transfer p. I.*
citrullinated p. a protein that contains citrulline in place of arginine because an enzyme has interfered with the formation of arginine; see also *cyclic citrullinated peptide*, under *peptide*.
coagulated p. an insoluble form that certain proteins assume when denatured at their isoelectric point by heat, alcohol, ultraviolet rays, or other agents.
coat p. (COP) any of the protein subunits of a coatomer, classified as COPI (involved in transport within the Golgi complex and in retrograde transport from the Golgi complex to the endoplasmic reticulum) and COPII (involved in anterograde protein transport from the Golgi complex to the endoplasmic reticulum).
complement control p. (CCP) any of a superfamily of proteins involved in complement regulation, encoded in a closely linked gene cluster, and having one or more stretches of a common short consensus repeat encoding a 60–amino acid domain. Included are factor H, C4 binding protein, decay accelerating factor, membrane cofactor protein, and several complement receptors. Called also *regulator of complement activation*.
complete p. a protein composed of amino acids in appropriate proportion to each other so that when it is the sole source of protein, the amino acids can all be used by the body; it is therefore more valuable for nutrition than is the partial protein (q.v.).
compound p., conjugated p. a compound in which the protein is linked to a nonprotein (prosthetic) group other than as a salt. Included are nucleoproteins, glycoproteins, lipoproteins, metalloproteins, chromoproteins, hemoproteins, and phosphoproteins. Cf. *simple p.*
constitutive p's proteins produced in fixed amounts, regardless of the organism's need for them.
cord p's the proteins of blood from the umbilical cord.
C-reactive p. (CRP) a globulin that forms a precipitate with the somatic C-polysaccharide of the pneumococcus in vitro; it is the most predominant of the acute phase proteins.
cyclic adenosine monophosphate receptor p. catabolite activator p.
cystic fibrosis transmembrane regulator p. cystic fibrosis transmembrane regulator.
D-bidirectional p. a peroxisomal enzyme with both dehydratase and dehydrogenase activity involved in fatty acid β-oxidation; called also *17β-hydroxysteroid dehydrogenase type 4*. See also *17β-hydroxysteroid dehydrogenase type 4 deficiency*.
denatured p. see *protein denaturation*, under *denaturation*.
derived p. derivatives of the protein molecule formed by hydrolytic changes, including coagulated proteins, proteoses, peptones, and peptides.
encephalitogenic p. myelin basic p.
ERM p's ezrin, radixin, and moesin, three related actin-binding cytoskeletal proteins of the protein 4.1 superfamily; they link the cytoplasmic tails of membrane receptors to actin fibers in the cytoskeleton, as well as playing a role in the formation of microvilli and intercellular junctions and participating in signal transduction pathways.
fibrillar p., fibrous p. a protein that is insoluble in water or dilute salt solution, having extensive secondary structure, such as α-helix or β-pleated sheet structure; included are the principal structural proteins of the body, such as collagens, elastins, keratins, actin, and myosin. Cf. *globular p.*
fusion p. a protein produced by a recombinant DNA construct engineered such that the coding region of one gene is linked distal to the 5′ end of another gene and within its coding region, placing expression of both genes under regulatory control of the second, usually well characterized, gene.
G p. any of a family of similar heterotrimeric proteins of the intracellular portion of the plasma membrane that bind activated receptor complexes and, through conformational changes and cyclic binding and hydrolysis of GTP, directly or indirectly effect alterations in channel gating and so couple cell surface receptors to intracellular responses. Some G proteins are named for their activities, e.g., G_s stimulates and G_I inhibits enzyme activity.
glial fibrillary acidic p. (GFAP) the protein forming the glial filaments of the astrocytes; it is used as an immunohistochemical marker of these cells. It also occurs in radial glia and occasionally in peripheral neuroglia.

Protein *Continued*

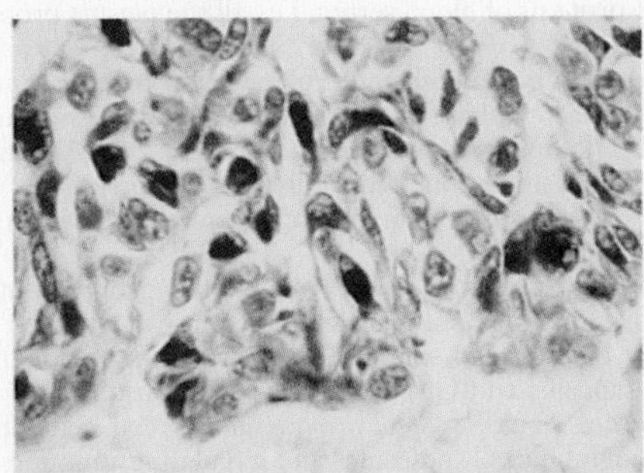

■ Glial fibrillary acidic protein in malignant astrocytoma.

globular p. any of the group of simple proteins soluble in water or dilute salt solution, their polypeptide chains coiled into a globular shape; they constitute most of the proteins in the body, including albumins, globulins, histones, and protamines. Cf. *fibrous p.*

GM_2 activator p. a sphingolipid activator protein that binds GM_2 ganglioside and related glycosphingolipids and presents them to hexosaminidase A for cleavage; it is necessary for enzyme activity. Deficiency results in GM_2 gangliosidosis, AB variant.

green fluorescent p. a fluorescent protein produced by a species of jellyfish; other proteins can be fused to it so that their synthesis and movements can be studied in cell biology research.

GTPase-activating p. a protein that stimulates the GTPase activity of a GTP-binding protein, resulting in the conversion of the protein to its inactive form.

GTP-binding p. any of a number of regulatory proteins, including the G proteins and the monomeric *small GTP-binding proteins,* in which the exchange of GDP for GTP induces a conformational change to produce an active state, while the hydrolysis of GTP to GDP produces an inactive state. GTP-binding proteins act as switches that couple cell-surface receptor activation with intracellular processes such as protein synthesis.

guanyl-nucleotide-binding p. G p.

heat shock p. any of a group of prokaryotic and eukaryotic proteins first identified as being synthesized in response to hyperthermia, hypoxia, or other stresses and believed to enable cells to recover from these stresses, perhaps by enabling recovery of gene expression. Many have been found to be molecular chaperones (q.v.), and these are synthesized abundantly regardless of stress.

high mobility group p's, HMG p's a highly conserved family of small nonhistone nucleoproteins that bind DNA and are involved in controlling transcription. They are important for growth and development, and are regulated by cell cycle–dependent phosphorylation. Those from animals have been classified in three families: HMG-1/2, HMG-14/17 and HMG-I/Y. Members of the HMG-1/2 family contain a conserved motif known as the HMG box (q.v.), which is also found in a variety of other transcription factors.

high-sensitivity C-reactive p. (hs-CRP) see under *test.*

hnRNP p's a diverse group of approximately 30 proteins that associate with nascent heterogeneous nuclear RNA (hnRNA), which is predominantly pre-mRNA, as it is transcribed, forming heterogeneous nuclear ribonucleoprotein particles; they are involved in packaging, splicing, and other posttranscriptional processing of pre-mRNAs, staying bound until the mature mRNAs are transported to the cytoplasm.

immune p. immunoglobulin.

incomplete p. a protein having a ratio of amino acids different from that of the average body protein, and therefore less valuable for nutrition than is the complete protein (q.v.). Called also *partial p.*

inhibitor of apoptosis p. (IAP) any of a class of proteins that play a regulatory role in apoptosis in many species by inhibiting caspase activity, which in turn blocks apoptosis; such proteins are also expressed abnormally in many tumors.

integral membrane p. see *membrane p.*

iron-sulfur p. a group of proteins, including ferredoxins and adrenodoxin, that function in electron transport; they contain iron-sulfur centers of the form $Fe_2S_2Cys_4$ or $Fe_4S_4Cys_4$, where Cys denotes a cysteine residue; the iron atoms undergo reversible transitions between the +2 and +3 oxidation states.

leucine-rich repeat p. any of numerous glycoproteins that contain leucine-rich repeats. Called also *LRR p.*

leukocyte adhesion p. (LAP) β_2 integrin.

link p. an adhesive glycoprotein, existing in three isoforms, that links aggrecan to hyaluronan in cartilage.

lipid transfer p. I cholesteryl ester transfer p.

lipid transfer p. II phospholipid transfer p.

LRR p. leucine-rich repeat p.

M p. 1. see under *component.* 2. a type-specific protein, consisting of two protein chains in a coiled structure, located on the surface of the cell wall of *Streptococcus pyogenes;* it is responsible for adhesion of the bacterium to host epithelial cells and mediates virulence by diminishing activation of the alternative pathway, thereby inhibiting phagocytosis. 3. a permease involved in the transport of β-galactosides across the cell membrane of *Escherichia coli.* 4. matrix p.

maintenance p. the smallest amount of protein upon which the normal conditions of the body can be maintained.

major basic p. (MBP) a cationic 10- to 15-kD protein occurring in eosinophilic granules and having cytotoxic activity against many parasites; it can also induce tissue injury in allergic and inflammatory diseases and, because it induces injury to the bronchial epithelium, is linked to asthma.

matrix p. a nonglycosylated protein occurring between the nucleocapsid and envelope layers of certain viruses, such as orthomyxoviruses, and playing a role in the assembly of the virus particle. Called also *M p.*

membrane p. a protein found in association with the cell membrane, either attached to (peripheral or extrinsic) or inserted in (integral or intrinsic) the membrane; possible roles include enzyme, receptor for a hormone or other molecule, and mediator of active or passive transport of lipid-insoluble substances across the membrane. See Plate 12.

membrane cofactor p. (MCP) a transmembrane protein, CD46, found in most blood cells, endothelial and epithelial cells, and fibroblasts; it restricts the turnover of complement by acting as a cofactor for factor I–mediated catabolism of C3b and C4b.

membrane transport p. a protein that facilitates the transport of one or more specific substances across the plasma membrane; see also *transport p.*

microsomal triglyceride transfer p. (MTP) a protein that occurs in the lumen of the endoplasmic reticulum and is responsible for the transfer of triglycerides and other lipids from the endoplasmic reticulum, where they are synthesized, into the lumen during the assembly of very low density lipoprotein (VLDL). It is believed to act during the translation of apoliporotein B molecules, enabling them to assume the proper conformation.

microtubule-associated p. (MAP) any of a large family of proteins that regulate microtubule assembly and structure; the number and kinds of MAPs vary by cell type and are determined genetically.

mild silver p. see under *silver.*

motor p. a general term encompassing several families of ATP-binding proteins (myosin, kinesin, and dynein) that use the energy from ATP hydrolysis to power movement of subcellular components along a polarized substrate (actin filaments and microtubules).

myelin basic p. (MBP) a basic protein (MW 18,000) that constitutes about 30 per cent of myelin proteins; elevated levels of MBP occur in acute exacerbation of multiple sclerosis and acute cerebral infarction. Immunization of laboratory animals with MBP produces encephalomyelitis by inducing T cell activity that leads to demyelination and lymphoid infiltration. Called also *encephalitogenic p.*

myeloma p. any of the pathological immunoglobulin proteins or fragments, such as M component and Bence Jones protein, secreted by myeloma cells.

native p. unchanged animal or vegetable protein, especially as it occurs in foods.

p53 p. a DNA-binding nuclear protein that regulates transcription of several other genes, playing an essential role in cell-cycle arrest and apoptosis in response to DNA damage or conditions of cellular stress by causing arrest in G_1 phase and inducing transcription of DNA repair genes; it is undetectable or present at very low levels in normal resting cells but present at high levels in a wide variety of transformed cells.

parathyroid hormone–like p., parathyroid hormone–related p. see under *peptide.*

partial p. incomplete p.

Protein *Continued*

penicillin-binding p. any of a group of proteins found in the cell walls of bacteria that are essential to the life of the bacteria and are targeted by penicillin in its bactericidal activity.
peripheral membrane p. see *membrane p.*
phospholipid transfer p. (PLTP) a ubiquitous protein having multiple functions in lipoprotein metabolism; in plasma, it plays an important role in high-density lipoprotein (HDL) metabolism by mediating the transfer of phospholipids from triglyceride-rich lipoproteins to HDL as well as the transfer of phospholipids between HDL molecules.
plasma p's the hundreds of different proteins present in blood plasma, including transport proteins such as albumin, transferrin, and haptoglobin; fibrinogen and other coagulation factors; complement components; immunoglobulins; enzyme inhibitors; precursors of substances such as angiotensin and bradykinin; and many others.
plasma p. fraction see under *fraction.*
prion p. (PrP) a constitutively expressed cell surface glycoprotein, 33–35 kD, of uncertain function; in humans encoded by the *PRNP* gene at locus: 20pter-p12. The 27–30 kD protease-resistant core is the functional, and perhaps only, component of prions; several isoforms have been identified and are responsible for prion disease. Extracellular prion protein aggregates into rod-shaped structures that resemble amyloid.
proteolipid p. (PLP) a hydrophobic protein that is the major constituent of myelin in the central nervous system. Defective synthesis of PLP results in Pelizaeus-Merzbacher disease. Called also *lipophilin.*
R p. any of a group of similar proteins, so named for their rapid electrophoretic mobility relative to intrinsic factor, that avidly bind ingested or circulating cobalamins or analogues and travel with them to the duodenum, where proteolytic digestion frees the vitamin to bind intrinsic factor. Called also *cobalophilin* and *haptocorrin.*
racemized p. protein so changed by chemical or other agents, usually dilute alkali, that its optical activity is lowered and it becomes more resistant to enzymatic hydrolysis. Acid hydrolysis of a racemized protein shows inactivation (racemization) of several of its constituent amino acids.
recombinant p. a protein obtained by introducing recombinant DNA into a heterologous host (microorganism or yeast cell) and causing it to produce the gene product.
retinol binding p. (RBP) an α-globulin synthesized and secreted by the liver. It binds retinol and transthyretin in a 1:1:1 ratio; the complex solubilizes retinol and protects it from glomerular filtration and renal excretion while transporting it to the peripheral tissues.
p. S a vitamin K–dependent plasma protein that inhibits blood clotting by serving as a cofactor for activated protein C. Not to be confused with *S p.*
S p. see *vitronectin.* Not to be confused with *protein S.*
S-100 p. a calcium-binding protein, occurring in three isoforms, that is widely distributed both in normal and neoplastic tissue; it is used as an immunohistochemical marker in initial screening of a number of types of tumors.
SAA p. serum amyloid A p.
serum p's proteins of blood serum, i.e., all the plasma proteins except fibrinogen.
serum amyloid A p. a high-molecular-weight protein synthesized in the liver; it is an acute phase protein and circulates in association with a subclass of HDL lipoproteins. It is the precursor to AA amyloid and accumulates in inflammation. Called also *SAA p.*
simple p. a protein containing only amino acids on complete hydrolysis. Cf. *conjugated p.*
sphingolipid activator p. (SAP) any of a group of nonenzyme lysosomal proteins that stimulate the actions of specific lysosomal hydrolases by binding and solubilizing their sphingolipid substrates; it includes the saposins and GM_2 activator protein (qq.v.).
staphylococcal p. A a *Staphylococcus aureus* cell wall protein that binds immunoglobulin G molecules and circulating immune complexes and is used as a selective immunoadsorbent in biochemical research and in the treatment of idiopathic thrombocytopenic purpura.
strong silver p. see under *silver.*
structural p. a protein whose primary function is to give shape and structure to cells or tissues.
Tamm-Horsfall p. a glycoprotein produced by cells of the ascending limb of the loop of Henle; it is a normal constituent of urine and is the major protein constituent of urinary casts. Called also *uromodulin.*
tau p. [tubulin-associated] any of a family of vertebrate microtubule-associated proteins that promote microtubule assembly and stability; they are found in all cells but are particularly associated with axons of neurons. Abnormally hyperphosphorylated forms are a major component of the paired helical filaments found in neurofibrillary tangles.
transmembrane p. a plasma membrane protein in which the polypeptide chain is exposed on both sides of the membrane.
transport p. a protein that binds to a substance and provides a transport system for it, either in the plasma or across a plasma membrane (see *facilitated diffusion,* under *diffusion*). Some are specific for one substance, such as a hormone, and others bind to several different substances. The term is sometimes used specifically for proteins that bind other proteins. See also *carrier* (def. 6) and *transporter.*
uncoupling p. a protein that occurs in the inner membrane of the mitochondria of brown adipose tissue, important in nonshivering thermogenesis; it dissipates the proton gradient created by the respiratory chain, thus uncoupling oxidation from phosphorylation so that production of heat occurs instead of phosphorylation of ADP to ATP. Called also *thermogenin.*
whole p. protein that has not been split.
Wnt p's a large family of cysteine-rich signaling proteins with a wide variety of functions in embryogenesis, cell fate, self-renewal in normal stem cells, malignant transformation, and organ formation.
zinc finger p. any of a class of nucleic acid–binding proteins that also contain one or more zinc-binding domains (tandemly repeated, highly conserved stretches of 28 nucleotides). The class is named for the fingerlike secondary and tertiary structures formed in the zinc-binding regions of the molecules; individual proteins appear to be involved in transcriptional regulation and in RNA transport.

---

pro·tein·a·ceous (pro″tēn-a′shəs) pertaining to, of the nature of, or consisting of protein.

pro·tein-ar·gi·nine de·im·i·nase (pro′tēn-ahr′jĭ-nēn de-im′ĭ-nās) [EC 3.5.3.15] EC nomenclature for *peptidylarginine deiminase.*

pro·tein·ase (pro′tēn-ās) endopeptidase.

pro·tein di·sul·fide-isom·er·ase (pro′tēn di-sul′fīd-i-som′ə-rās) [EC 5.3.4.1] an enzyme of the isomerase class that catalyzes the rearrangement of disulfide bonds within proteins during folding. It is a monomer identical to one of the subunits of prolyl 4-hydroxylase (q.v.). Called also *disulfide isomerase.*

pro·tein·emia (pro″tēn-e′me-ə) hyperproteinemia.
  Bence Jones p. the presence of Bence Jones protein in serum.

pro·tein-glu·ta·mine γ-glu·ta·myl·trans·fer·ase (pro′tēn gloo′tə-mēn gloo″tə-məl-trans′fər-ās) [EC 2.3.2.13] an enzyme of the transferase class that creates crosslinks within and between fibrin molecules, transferring the glutamyl portion of glutamine side chains to the amino group of lysine side chains: protein-glutamine + lysine-protein = protein-glutamyl lysine-protein + NH_3. The resultant polymerization of fibrin is an important part of blood clotting. It is the activated form of coagulation factor XIII (coagulation factor XIIIa). Called also *transglutaminase.*

pro·tein-his·ti·dine ki·nase (pro′tēn-his′tĭ-dēn ki′nās) [EC 2.7.13] the group of protein kinases comprising those phosphophorylating histidine residues in proteins.

pro·tein ki·nase (pro′tēn ki′nās) [EC 2.7.10–99] any of several groups of enzymes of the transferase class that catalyze the phosphorylation of serine, threonine, tyrosine, or histidine groups in enzymes and other proteins, using ATP as a phosphate donor. Specific protein kinases regulate by phosphorylation enzymes catalyzing key reactions in processes such as glycogen turnover, cholesterol biosynthesis, and amino acid transformations. Further subdivisions include protein-tyrosine kinases [EC 2.7.10], protein-serine/threonine kinases [EC 2.7.11], dual-specificity kinases [EC 2.7.12], and protein-histidine kinases [EC 2.7.13].
  p. k. A cAMP-dependent protein kinase; see under *C.*
  p. k. C [EC 2.7.11.13] any of a family of protein-serine/threonine kinases (q.v.) that are dependent on lipids for activity; they act on a wide variety of proteins and can be activated by calcium but have a requirement for the second messenger diacylglycerol. The enzymes are involved in diverse cellular signaling pathways and have been shown to be a binding site for phorbol esters and other tumor promoters.

pro·tein·o·chrome (pro-tēn′o-krōm) [*protein* + *-chrome*] any one of a series of coloring matters formed by the action of bromine or chlorine on tryptophan.

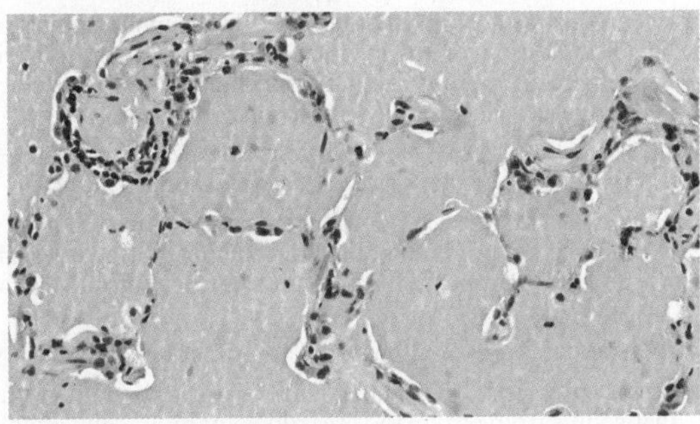

■ Pulmonary alveolar proteinosis. The alveoli are filled with a dense, amorphous, protein-lipid granular precipitate; the alveolar walls are normal.

pro·tein·og·e·nous (pro″tēn-oj′ə-nəs) formed by or from a protein.

pro·tein·ol·o·gy (pro″tēn-ol′ə-je) [*protein* + *-logy*] the scientific study of proteins or of the protein status of the body.

pro·tein·o·sis (pro″tēn-o′sis) the accumulation of excess protein in the tissues.

alveolar p. pulmonary alveolar p.

lipoid p. an autosomal recessive disorder of lipid metabolism due to mutation in the *ECM1* gene (locus: 1q21), which encodes extracellular matrix protein 1; it is characterized by hyaline deposits in the skin and mucosa of the mouth, pharynx, hypopharynx, and larynx, resulting in hoarseness, often from birth, due to infiltration of the vocal cords. Skin lesions begin with recurrent pustules or bullae on the face and distal parts of the limbs, which heal and leave white varioliform scars; later there may be waxy white or yellow papules, nodules, or verrucoid plaques primarily on the face, eyelids, nape, hands, fingers, elbows, and knees. Called also *hyalinosis cutis et mucosae*, *lipoproteinosis*, and *Urbach-Wiethe disease*.

pulmonary alveolar p. a chronic lung disease characterized by dyspnea, productive cough, chest pain, weakness, weight loss, and hemoptysis, and by the filling of the distal alveoli with a bland, eosinophilic, probably endogenous, proteinaceous material that prevents ventilation of affected areas. On computed tomography, the tissue has a characteristic appearance of crazy paving (q.v.).

pro·tein phos·pha·tase (pro′tēn fos′fə-tās) phosphoprotein phosphatase.

p. p. 1 a specific phosphoprotein phosphatase (q.v.) that catalyzes the dephosphorylation of several enzymes involved in the regulation of glycogen metabolism: phosphorylase kinase, glycogen phosphorylase *a*, and glycogen synthase *b*. The enzyme activity encompasses activities formerly assigned to the individual enzymes [phosphorylase] phosphatase and [glycogen-synthase-D] phosphatase.

pro·tein-ser·ine/thre·o·nine ki·nase (pro′tēn sēr′ēn thre′o-nēn ki′nās) [EC 2.7.11] any of the protein kinases that phosphorylate specific serine or threonine residues in proteins. The group is divided into receptor protein serine/threonine kinases (q.v.) and serine/threonine kinases lacking a transmembrane domain; the latter are either separated and named by specificity (see at specific enzyme names) or grouped together as nonspecific serine/threonine protein kinases (q.v.).

pro·tein-ty·ro·sine ki·nase (pro′tēn ti′ro-sēn ki′nās) [EC 2.7.10] a group comprising the protein kinases that catalyze the phosphorylation of tyrosine residues in specific proteins. It is subdivided into the receptor protein-tyrosine kinases and the non-specific protein tyrosine kinases (qq.v.). The enzymes play a variety of roles in the control of cell growth and differentiation. Many of the known oncogenes and proto-oncogenes involved in cancer encode protein-tyrosine kinases, and unregulated activation of these enzymes can lead to oncogenesis as well as to various benign proliferative conditions.

pro·tein-ty·ro·sine-phos·pha·tase (pro′tēn ti′ro-sēn fos′fə-tās) [EC 3.1.3.48] any of a group of enzymes of the hydrolase class that catalyze the removal of phosphate groups from tyrosine residues of proteins. The enzyme activity modulates that of the protein-tyrosine kinases and thus may decrease or inhibit cell growth and tumorigenesis.

pro·tein·uria (pro″te-nu′re-ə) excessive serum proteins in the urine, such as in renal disease, after strenuous exercise, and with dehydration. Called also *albuminuria*. **proteinu′ric** *adj*

accidental p., adventitious p. proteinuria due not to a kidney disease but to some other condition such as hemorrhage in the urinary tract; called also *false p.*

athletic p. effort p.

Bence Jones p. the presence in the urine of Bence Jones protein.

benign p. essential p.

cardiac p. a type of functional proteinuria accompanying congestive heart failure.

colliquative p. proteinuria that is at first mild but then increases suddenly and markedly during convalescence; seen in certain fevers and other conditions.

dietetic p., digestive p. functional proteinuria produced by the eating of certain foods.

effort p. functional proteinuria occurring as a result of vigorous and prolonged exercise of the lower limbs; called also *athletic p.*

essential p. functional proteinuria that is not associated with or followed by renal disease, such as effort proteinuria and the postural proteinurias. Called also *benign p.*

false p. adventitious p.

febrile p. functional proteinuria seen with a fever.

functional p. any proteinuria that is not due to renal disease, such as the transient proteinuria of pregnancy or effort, postural, cardiac, or febrile proteinurias. See also *intermittent p.* and *essential p.* Called also *physiologic p.*

glomerular p. the most common kind of proteinuria, being due to glomerular disease and abnormal permeability of the glomerular capillaries to protein.

intermittent p. functional proteinuria that recurs intermittently; called also *transient p.*

light chain p. overflow proteinuria with increased light chain fragments of immunoglobulins, as in Fanconi syndrome.

lordotic p. postural proteinuria due to lordosis.

nephrogenous p. the usual type of proteinuria, which is caused by renal disease; the two primary types are glomerular proteinuria and tubular proteinuria. Called also *renal p.*

orthostatic p. a form of functional proteinuria, usually seen between the ages of ten and twenty, that occurs on standing erect and disappears on lying down.

overflow p. proteinuria due to hemoglobin, myoglobin, or immunoglobulin loss into the urine due to excessive amounts in the bloodstream, such as in multiple myeloma; it is not usually associated with glomerular or tubular disease.

paroxysmal p. intermittent p.

physiologic p. functional p.

postrenal p. proteinuria that has arisen at some point beyond the renal tubules, such as the renal pelvis, ureter, bladder, prostate, or urethra.

postural p. proteinuria related to body position, such as orthostatic proteinuria or lordotic proteinuria.

prerenal p. proteinuria due primarily to a disease other than one of the kidney, such as heart disease, liver disease, fever, or hyperthyroidism.

pyogenic p. proteinuria due to the absorption of pus cells or exudates, such as in pneumonia or a septic process.

regulatory p. effort p.

renal p. nephrogenous p.

transient p. intermittent p.

tubular p. proteinuria due to excretion of proteins of low molecular weight such as immunoglobulins, which they normally should be reabsorbing.

Pro·teo·bac·te·ria (pro″te-o-bak-tēr′e-ə) [Gr. *Prōteus* an ocean deity able to change shape + *bacteria*] a diverse phylum of gram-negative bacteria, comprising over 1300 species, grouped together on the basis of 16S rRNA sequence analysis; it includes the classes Alphaproteobacteria, Betaproteobacteria, Gammaproteobacteria, Deltaproteobacteria, and Epsilonproteobacteria.

pro·teo·clas·tic (pro″te-o-klas′tik) [*protein* + Gr. *klasis* breakage] splitting up proteins or the protein molecule.

pro·teo·gly·can (pro″te-o-gli′kan) any of a group of polysaccharide-protein conjugates occurring primarily in the matrix of connective tissue and cartilage, composed mainly of polysaccharide chains, particularly glycosaminoglycans, as well as minor protein components. Individual subunits consist of a polypeptide backbone to which many glycosaminoglycan chains are covalently linked; large aggregates resembling bottle brushes are formed when many such subunits are attached via small proteins to long hyaluronan chains.

Pro·te·og·ly·pha (pro″te-og′lĭ-fə) Proteroglypha.

pro·teo·lip·id (pro″te-o-lip′id) 1. a conjugated protein having a lipid component that is soluble in some nonpolar solvents, but insoluble in aqueous solutions. 2. a hydrophobic protein that may or may not have a lipid component and is soluble in some nonpolar solvents.

pro·te·ol·y·sis (pro″te-ol′ĭ-sis) [*protein* + *-lysis*] the splitting of proteins by hydrolysis of the peptide bonds with formation of smaller polypeptides; the process may be catalyzed by proteolytic enzymes, by acids, or by bases.

pro·teo·lyt·ic (pro″te-o-lit′ik) 1. pertaining to, characterized by, or promoting proteolysis. 2. a proteolytic enzyme.

pro·te·ome (pro′te-ōm) [*prot*ein + *-ome*] the complete set of proteins produced from the information encoded in a genome.

pro·teo·me·tab·o·lism (pro″te-o-mə-tab′ə-liz-əm) the metabolism of protein. **proteometabol′ic** *adj*

pro·te·o·mics (pro″te-o′miks) the qualitative and quantitative study of the proteome under various conditions, including protein expression, modification, localization, and function, and protein–protein interactions, as a means of understanding biological processes.

Pro·teo·my·ces (pro″te-o-mi′sēz) Trichosporon.

pro·teo·pep·sis (pro″te-o-pep′sis) [*protein* + Gr. *pepsis* digestion] the digestion of protein. **proteopep′tic** *adj*

pro·teo·pexy (pro′te-o-pek″se) [*protein* + *-pexy*] the fixation of proteins within the organism. **proteopec′tic, proteopex′ic** *adj*

pro·te·ose (pro′te-ōs) [*protein* + *-ose*] a secondary protein derivative or mixture of split products formed by hydrolytic cleavage of the protein molecule that is more complete than the cleavage occurring with primary protein derivatives but less complete than the cleavage forming amino acids. The *primary* proteoses are precipitated by half saturation with ammonium sulfate; the *secondary*, by full saturation.

pro·te·o·some (pro′te-ə-sōm) proteasome.

pro·ter (pro′tər) [Gr. *proteros* front] the anterior daughter organism after transverse division of a ciliate protozoan; cf. *opisthe*.

Pro·ter·og·ly·pha (pro″tər-og′lif-ə) a group of venomous snakes that have small stationary fangs which are grooved rather than hollow and so must be held in the wound if the poison is to reach the deeper tissues. Examples are the Indian cobra and the Sonoran coral snake. Called also *Ankyloproglypha* and *Proteoglypha*.

Pro·te·us (pro′te-əs) [Gr. *Prōteus* an ocean deity able to change shape] a genus of gram-negative, pleomorphic, rod-shaped bacteria of the family Enterobacteriaceae, consisting of facultatively anaerobic, chemo-organotrophic, actively motile organisms. Colonies exhibit swarming. The organisms are found in fecal material, especially in patients treated with oral antibiotics, and are potential pathogens, associated with urinary tract infections, bacteremia, and abdominal and wound infections. The type species is *P. vulga′ris*.

P. incon′stans a former species whose members are now included in the genus *Providencia*.

P. mira′bilis the species most frequently isolated from human clinical material, also found in soil and sewage. It is a leading cause of urinary tract infections and can cause pneumonia in debilitated or immunocompromised patients; see also Proteus *pneumonia*, under *pneumonia*.

P. morga′nii *Morganella morganii*.

P. pen′neri a species that ferments maltose, but is negative for ornithine decarboxylase and indole; it is a cause of urinary tract infections.

P. rett′geri *Providencia rettgeri*.

P. vulga′ris a widespread species found in fecal matter, sewage, and soil. It is a common cause of cystitis and pyelonephritis and is associated with eye and ear infections, pleuritis, peritonitis, and suppurative abscesses. In debilitated or immunocompromised patients it can cause pneumonia (see Proteus *pneumonia*, under *pneumonia*). The species has many serovars. The Ox antigens (Ox-2, Ox-19, Ox-K) react with antibodies formed in rickettsial infections and are used in the Weil-Felix reaction for the diagnosis of typhus, scrub typhus, and Rocky Mountain spotted fever.

Pro·te·us syn·drome (pro′te-əs) [Gr. *Prōteus* an ocean deity able to appear in many different forms] see under *syndrome*.

pro·te·us (pro′te-əs) pl. *pro′tei*. an organism of the genus *Proteus*.

pro·thal·lus (pro-thal′əs) the independent, free-living gametophyte generation of ferns and related lower vascular plants.

pro·throm·bin (pro-throm′bin) [*pro-* + *thrombo-* + *-in* chemical suffix] factor II; see under *coagulation factors*, at *factor*.

pro·throm·bin·ase (pro-throm′bin-āse) 1. the complex formed between activated coagulation factor X and calcium, phospholipid, and modified factor V; it can cleave and activate prothrombin to thrombin. 2. sometimes specifically the active enzyme center of the complex, activated factor X (Xa).

pro·throm·bi·no·gen·ic (pro-throm″bĭ-no-jen′ik) promoting the production of prothrombin (coagulation factor II).

pro·throm·bi·no·pe·nia (pro-throm″bĭ-no-pe′ne-ə) hypoprothrombinemia.

pro·thy·mo·cyte (pro-thi′mo-sīt) a term applied to the lymphoid precursor cell of thymocytes.

pro·tio·dide (pro-ti′o-dīd) in a series of iodides of the same base, the one that contains the smallest amount of iodine.

pro·ti·re·lin (pro-ti′rə-lin) a synthetic preparation of thyrotropin-releasing hormone (q.v.), used diagnostically.

pro·tist (pro′tist) 1. a single-celled eukaryote. 2. any member of the kingdom Protista.

Pro·tis·ta (pro-tis′tə) [Gr. *prōtista* the very first, from *prōtos* first] in the five-kingdom classification of living organisms, a kingdom comprising a diverse group of phylogenically distinct, unicellular eukaryotes, including protozoa, algae, and certain intermediate forms.

pro·ti·um (^{1}H) (pro′te-əm) the mass one isotope of hydrogen; ordinary, or light, hydrogen. See *hydrogen*. Cf. *deuterium* and *tritium*.

prot(o)- [Gr. *prōtos* first] 1. a combining form meaning first or primitive. 2. in chemistry, a prefix denoting the member of a series of compounds with the lowest proportion of the element or radical to which it is affixed.

pro·to·al·bu·mose (pro″to-al′bu-mōs) a primary proteose.

pro·to·anem·o·nin (pro″to-ə-nem′o-nin) a toxic, irritating antibiotic substance that results from enzymatic breakdown of ranunculin after certain plants of the family Ranunculaceae are eaten by an animal; toxic effects include potentially fatal ventricular fibrillation and respiratory failure.

pro·to·bi·ol·o·gy (pro″to-bi-ol′ə-je) [*proto-* + *bio-* + *-logy*] the science that deals with forms of life more minute than bacteria, such as viruses.

pro·to·blast (pro′to-blast) [*proto-* + *-blast*] 1. a cell with no cell wall; an embryonic cell. 2. the nucleus of an oocyte. 3. a blastomere from which a particular organ or part develops.

pro·to·blas·tic (pro″to-blas′tik) pertaining to a protoblast.

pro·to·bro·chal (pro″to-bro′kəl) [*proto-* + Gr. *brochos* mesh] denoting the first stage in the development of an ovary.

Pro·to·cal·liph·o·ra (pro″to-kə-lif′ə-rə) a genus of flies whose larvae feed on nesting birds.

pro·to·cad·he·rin (pro″to-kad-hēr′in) a large family of cadherins, having seven extracellular CAD domains instead of the classic five; they are expressed on neurons and are thought to contribute to the specificity of synaptic connections in the central nervous system.

pro·to·cat·e·chu·ic ac·id (pro″to-kat″ə-choo′ik) 3,4-dihydroxybenzoic acid, a catabolite of epinephrine.

pro·to·chlo·ride (pro″to-klor′id) in a series of chlorides of the same element, the one that contains the least amount of chlorine.

pro·to·chlo·ro·phyll (pro″to-klor′ə-fəl) a substance in plant tissue that is changed by the action of light into chlorophyll.

pro·to·chon·dral (pro″to-kon′drəl) 1. pertaining to the protochondrium. 2. pertaining to a center of chondrification.

pro·to·chon·dri·um (pro″to-kon′dre-əm) [*proto-* + Gr. *chondros* cartilage] a basophil substance developed from precartilage and constituting the intermediate stage in cartilage formation.

Pro·to·coc·ci·di·i·da (pro″to-kok″sĭ-di′ĭ-də) [*proto-* + Gr. *kokkos* berry] an order of parasitic protozoa (subclass Coccidia, class Sporozoea) found in invertebrates, the life cycle of which involves gametogony and sporogony.

pro·to·col (pro′tə-kol) 1. an explicit, detailed plan of an experiment, procedure, or test. 2. the original notes made on a necropsy, experiment, or case of disease.

Balke p., Balke-Ware p. a procedure for assessing cardiovascular health using a graded treadmill exercise test in which the treadmill speed is held constant and its slope increased, with the incremental increases in work so closely spaced as to approach continuity.

Bruce p. a procedure for assessing cardiovascular health using uphill treadmill walking in a graded exercise test; each interval is at a specific load level for three minutes and is followed by another at a prescribed incremental increase in treadmill speed and slope.

Ellestad p. a procedure for assessing cardiovascular health using a graded treadmill exercise test; over six stages the treadmill speed is incrementally raised five times and its slope is raised once.

modified Bruce p. an alteration in the Bruce protocol so that the treadmill is initially horizontal rather than uphill, with the first few intervals increasing the treadmill slope only.

Naughton p. a procedure for assessing cardiovascular health using a graded treadmill exercise test; the selected treadmill speed remains constant through the test but the treadmill slope is raised at the end of each two-minute increment.

pro·to·cone (pro′to-kōn) [*proto-* + Gr. *kōnos* cone] the principal mesiolingual cusp of the upper molar of humans and some other mammals.

pro·to·co·nid (pro″to-ko′nid) [*proto-* + *con(o)-* + *-id*] the mesiobuccal cusp of the lower molars of humans and some other mammals.

pro·to·co·op·er·a·tion (pro″to-ko-op″ər-a′shən) 1. symbiosis in which both populations (or individuals) gain from the association but are able to survive without it. 2. the tendency of animals to cluster in groups and thereby to mutually facilitate the survival of individual organisms.

pro·to·cop·ro·por·phyr·ia (pro″to-kop″ro-por-fir′e-ə) variegate porphyria.

pro•to•di•a•stol•ic (pro″to-di″ə-stol′ik) pertaining to early diastole, i.e., immediately following the second heart sound.

pro•to•du•o•de•num (pro″to-doo″o-de′nəm) the first or proximal portion of the duodenum, extending from the pylorus to the duodenal papilla, and developed embryonically from the foregut.

pro•to•elas•tose (pro″to-e-las′tōs) hemielastin.

pro•to•fi•bril (pro″to-fi′bril) the first elongated unit appearing in the process of formation of any type of fiber.

pro•to•gas•ter (pro′to-gas″tər) archenteron.

pro•to•glob•u•lose (pro″to-glob′u-lōs) a primary product formed in the digestion of globulin.

pro•to•go•no•cyte (pro″to-go′no-sīt) [*proto-* + *gonocyte*] one of the two cells resulting from division of the zygote; in certain lower forms this constitutes the primordial germ cell from which all gametes derive.

pro•to•heme (pro″to-hēm) a heme in which the porphyrin is protoporphyrin; an example is *protoheme IX*, the heme found in hemoglobin.

pro•to•he•min (pro″to-he′min) protoheme in which the iron atom is oxidized to the +3 oxidation state.

pro•to•io•dide (pro″to-i′o-dīd) protiodide.

Pro•to•mas•tig•i•da (pro″to-mas-tij′ĭ-də) Kinetoplastida.

pro•to•mer (pro′to-mər) [*protein* + mono*mer*] one of the identical subunits of which an oligomeric protein is composed.

pro•tom•e•ter (pro-tom′ə-tər) exophthalmometer.

Pro•to•mo•na•di•na (pro″to-mo″nə-di′nə) Kinetoplastida.

pro•ton (pro′ton) [Gr. *prōton*, from *prōtos* first] an elementary particle of positive charge which forms the nucleus of the ordinary hydrogen atom of mass 1; along with neutrons, protons form the nuclei of atoms of all other elements. The proton is the unit of positive electricity; it has one quantum of charge (1.6×10^{-19} coulomb), equivalent to the electron but of opposite polarity, and its mass is 1.67×10^{-27} kilogram, approximately that of the hydrogen ion. Symbol p.

pro•to•neph•ron (pro″to-nef′ron) pronephros.

pro•to•neph•ros (pro″to-nef′ros) pronephros.

pro•to•ni•trate (pro″to-ni′trāt) among several nitrates of the same base, the one that contains the least amount of nitric acid.

Pro•to•nix (pro′tə-niks) trademark for preparations of pantoprazole sodium.

pro•to-on•co•gene (pro″to-ong′ko-jēn) a normal cellular gene that with alteration, such as by mutation, DNA rearrangement, or nearby insertion of viral DNA, becomes an active oncogene; most proto-oncogenes are believed to normally function in cell growth and differentiation. See also *oncogene*.

Pro•to•pam (pro′to-pam) trademark for preparations of pralidoxime.

pro•to•path•ic (pro″to-path′ik) [*proto-* + *path-* + *-ic*] affected first; pertaining to sensing of stimuli in a nonspecific, usually nonlocalized, manner. See *protopathic sensibility*, under *sensibility*.

pro•to•pec•tin (pro″to-pek′tin) any of the precursor polysaccharides from which are derived pectins; they occur in a variety of plants, in the fruits, roots, leaves, and stems.

pro•to•phyl•lin (pro″to-fil′in) a colorless substance that is changed into chlorophyll by the action of air or carbon dioxide.

Pro•to•phy•ta (pro″to-fi′tə) [*proto-* + Gr. *phyton* plant] in former systems of classification, the lowest division of the plant kingdom, consisting of the algae and variously defined to include also the blue-green algae, yeasts, fungi, lichens, bacteria, or viruses.

Pro•top•ic (pro-top′ik) trademark for topical preparations of tacrolimus.

pro•to•pine (pro′to-pin) 1. an alkaloid from *Eschscholtzia californica*, the California poppy, and many other plants; it is an anodyne and hypnotic. 2. a poisonous alkaloid from various species of perennial herbs of the genus *Dicentra*.

pro•to•pla•sia (pro-to-pla′zhah) primary formation of tissue.

pro•to•plasm (pro′to-plaz″əm) [*proto-* + *-plasm*] a general term for the substance of the cell; see *cytoplasm* and *nucleoplasm*. **protoplasmat′ic, protoplas′mic** *adj*

pro•to•plast (pro′to-plast″) [*proto-* + *-plast*] a bacterial, yeast, or fungal cell from which the rigid cell wall has been removed, resulting in a membrane-bound cell that is dependent for its integrity on an isotonic or hypertonic medium. Cf. *spheroplast*.

pro•to•por•phyr•ia (pro″to-por-fir′e-ə) erythropoietic p.

erythrohepatic p. erythropoietic p.

erythropoietic p. (EPP) an autosomal dominant disorder due to mutation in the *FECH* gene (locus: 18q21.3), which encodes ferrochelatase, causing a partial deficiency of the enzyme; it is characterized by increased levels of protoporphyrin in the erythrocytes, plasma, liver, and feces and a wide variety of photosensitive skin changes, ranging from a burning or pruritic sensation to erythema, plaquelike edema, and wheals. The disorder is generally classified as an erythropoietic porphyria, but in classification schemes that include also the category erythrohepatic porphyria, it is classified there.

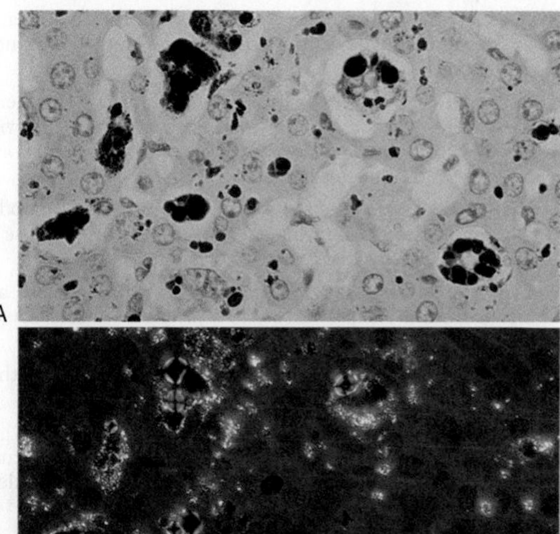

■ Erythropoietic protoporphyria. *(A)*, Brownish-black deposits of protoporphyrin in hepatocytes, canaliculi, Kupffer cells, and ductules (H & E stain). *(B)*, Birefringence of deposits, with a Maltese cross configuration of red birefringence in larger deposits (polarized light).

pro•to•por•phy•rin (pro″to-por′fə-rin) the porphyrin produced by oxidation of the methylene bridge of protoporphyrinogen. Protoporphyrin IX is the only naturally occurring isomer; it is an intermediate in heme biosynthesis, combining with ferrous iron to form protoheme IX, the heme prosthetic group of hemoglobin. It is accumulated and excreted excessively in the feces in erythropoietic protoporphyria and variegate porphyria.

free erythrocyte p. (FEP) protoporphyrin free in the blood rather than incorporated into erythrocytes; in the absence of iron, most is actually bound to zinc as zinc protoporphyrin (q.v.).

zinc p. free erythrocyte protoporphyrin that is bound to zinc. Levels of this chelated form are elevated in iron deficiency and lead poisoning; the nonchelated form is elevated in erythropoietic protoporphyria; and neither is elevated in thalassemia.

pro•to•por•phy•rin•emia (pro″to-por″fə-rĭ-ne′me-ə) the presence of protoporphyrin in the blood; see also *protoporphyria*.

pro•to•por•phy•rin•o•gen (pro″to-por″fə-rin′ə-jən) a porphyrinogen (q.v.) in which two pyrrole rings each have one methyl and one propionate side chain and the other two pyrrole rings each have one methyl and one vinyl side chain. Fifteen isomers are possible but only one, type IX, occurs naturally, produced by oxidative decarboxylation of coproporphyrinogen; it is an intermediate in heme biosynthesis.

pro•to•por•phy•rin•o•gen ox•i•dase (pro″to-por″fə-rin′ə-jən ok′sĭ-dās) [EC 1.3.3.4] an enzyme of the oxidoreductase class that catalyzes the oxidation of protoporphyrinogen IX to protoporphyrin IX, the penultimate step in heme and porphyrin synthesis. Deficiency of the enzyme, an autosomal dominant trait, causes variegate porphyria.

pro•to•pro•te•ose (pro″to-pro′te-ōs) a primary proteose.

pro•to•salt (pro′to-sawlt) in a series of salts of the same base, the one that contains the smallest amount of the substance combining with the base.

Pro•to•spi•ru•ra (pro″to-spi-roo′rə) a genus of nematodes of the family Spiruridae. *P. gra′cilis* is found in the stomachs of cats.

pro•to•spore (pro′to-spor) the first product of progressive cleavage, a multinucleate mass of cytoplasm surrounded by cleavage planes.

Pro•to•stat (pro′to-stat) trademark for a preparation of metronidazole.

pro•to•sto•ma (pro″to-sto′mə) blastopore.

pro•to•stome (pro′to-stōm) [*proto-* + Gr. *stoma* mouth] an individual of the Protostomia.

Pro·to·sto·mia (pro″to-sto′me-ə) a series of the Eucoelomata, including the mollusks, annelids, and arthropods, in all of which the mouth arises from the blastopore.

Pro·to·stron·gy·li·dae (pro″to-stron-jil′ĭ-de) a family of nematodes that includes the genera *Cystocaulus*, *Muellerius*, *Neostrongylus*, *Parelaphostrongylus*, and *Protostrongylus*. Several species are lungworms that infect sheep, goats, and other mammals.

Pro·to·stron·gy·lus (pro″to-stron′jə-ləs) a genus of nematode lungworms of the family Protostrongylidae. *P. rufes′cens* causes hoose or verminous bronchitis in sheep, goats, deer, and rabbits.

pro·to·sty·lid [*proto-* + Gr. *stylis*, gen. *stylidos* little pillar] a dental anomaly ranging from a pit to a furrow to a prominent accessory cusp on the buccal surface of a tooth, particularly a mandibular molar.

pro·to·sul·fate (pro″to-sul′fāt) among several sulfates of the same base, the one containing the smallest proportion of sulfate ion.

Pro·to·the·ca (pro″to-the′kə) [*proto-* + Gr. *thēkē* sheath] a genus of ubiquitous yeastlike organisms thought to be achloric algae, occurring as a spherical, ovoid, or elliptical cells containing several thick-walled autospores. *P. wickerha′mii* and *P. zop′fii* cause protothecosis.

pro·to·the·co·sis (pro″to-the-ko′sis) infection by organisms of the genus *Prototheca*, especially *P. wickerhamii* or *P. zopfii*, varying from cutaneous and subcutaneous lesions to systemic invasion involving internal organs; it may be an opportunistic infection or the result of traumatic implantation of the pathogen into the tissues. In cows it may cause mastitis.

Pro·to·the·ria (pro″to-the′re-ə) [*proto-* + Gr. *thērion* beast, animal] in some systems of classification, a subclass of the Mammalia, including the order Monotremata, the egg-laying mammals.

pro·to·troph (pro′to-trōf) [*proto-* + Gr. *trophē* nourishment] a prototrophic organism.

pro·to·tro·phic (pro″to-tro′fik) having the same growth factor requirements as the ancestral or prototype strain; said of microbial mutants.

pro·tot·ro·py (pro-tot′rə-pe) proton tautomerism. Cf. *anionotropy.*

Pro·to·tu·ni·ca·tae (pro″to-too″nĭ-ka′te) in fungal taxonomy, a series of the subphylum Ascomycotina, consisting of those having a prototunicate ascus. Orders in this series that contain human pathogens are Eurotiales and Onygenales.

pro·to·type (pro′to-tīp) [*proto-* + *type*] 1. the original type or form after which other types or forms are developed. 2. in microbiology, the standard reference strain to which other strains are compared.

pro·to·ver·a·trine (pro″to-ver′ə-trēn) an ester alkaloid obtained from the liliaceous plant *Veratrum album* L. It occurs in two forms, designated A and B, both of which have antihypertensive properties. Protoveratrine A is said to be more active than the B form; the two are usually administered in combination.

pro·to·ver·te·bra (pro″to-vur′tə-brə) 1. somite. 2. the caudal half of a somite that forms most of a vertebra.

pro·tox·ide (pro-tok′sid) in a series of oxides of the same metal, the one containing the smallest amount of oxygen.

Pro·to·zoa (pro″to-zo′ə) [*proto-* + Gr. *zoon* animal] a subkingdom (formerly a phylum) comprising the simplest organisms of the animal kingdom, consisting of unicellular organisms that range in size from submicroscopic to macroscopic; most are free living, but some lead commensalistic, mutualistic, or parasitic existences. According to newer classifications, Protozoa is divided into seven phyla: Sarcomastigophora, Labyrinthomorpha, Apicomplexa, Microspora, Acetospora, Myxozoa, and Ciliophora. Cf. *Metazoa.*

pro·to·zoa (pro″to-zo′ə) plural of *protozoon.*

pro·to·zo·a·ci·dal (pro″to-zo″ə-si′dəl) lethal to protozoa; cf. *antiprotozoal.*

pro·to·zo·a·cide (pro″to-zo′ə-sīd) an agent that kills protozoa; cf. *antiprotozoal.*

pro·to·zo·al (pro″to-zo′əl) protozoan (def. 2).

pro·to·zo·an (pro″to-zo′ən) 1. any individual of the Protozoa; called also *protozoon.* 2. of or pertaining to the Protozoa; called also *protozoal.*

pro·to·zo·ia·sis (pro″to-zo-i′ə-sis) any disease caused by protozoa.

pro·to·zo·ol·o·gy (pro″to-zo-ol′ə-je) the study of protozoa.

pro·to·zo·on (pro″to-zo′on) pl. *protozo′a* [*proto-* + Gr. *zōon* animal] protozoan (def. 1).

pro·to·zo·o·phage (pro″to-zo′o-fāj) [*protozoa* + *-phage*] a cell that has phagocytic action on protozoa.

pro·to·zo·o·sis (pro″to-zo-o′sis) protozoiasis.

pro·trac·tion (pro-trak′shən) [L. *protrahere* to drag forth] 1. drawing out or lengthening. 2. extension or protrusion. 3. a condition in which the teeth or other maxillary or mandibular structures are situated anterior to their normal position.

mandibular p. 1. the protrusive movement of the mandible initiated by the lateral and medial pterygoid muscles acting simultaneously. Cf. *mandibular retraction.* 2. a facial anomaly in which the gnathion lies anterior to the orbital plane.

maxillary p. a facial anomaly in which the subnasion is anterior to the orbital plane.

pro·trac·tor (pro-trak′tər) [*pro-* + L. *trahere* to draw] an instrument for extracting bits of bone, bullets, or other foreign material from wounds.

pro·trans·glu·tam·i·nase (pro-tranz″gloo-tam′ĭ-nās) the proenzyme of protein-glutamine γ-glutamyltransferase (transglutaminase). It is the inactive precursor form of coagulation factor XIII.

pro·trip·ty·line hy·dro·chlo·ride (pro-trip′tə-lēn) [USP] a tricyclic antidepressant of the dibenzocycloheptadiene class; it is also used in the treatment of attention-deficit/hyperactivity disorder and of narcolepsy and associated cataplexy. Administered orally.

Pro·tro·pin (pro-tro′pin) trademark for a preparation of somatrem.

pro·tru·sio (pro-troo′ze-o) [L.] protrusion.

p. aceta′buli a sinking in or subsidence of the floor of the acetabulum with protrusion of the femoral head through it (intrapelvic protrusion) resulting in limitation of movement of the hip joint. Called also *arthrokatadysis* and *Otto disease.*

pro·tru·sion (pro-troo′zhən) [L. *protrudere* to push forward] 1. extension beyond the usual limits, or above a plane surface. 2. the state of being thrust forward or laterally, as in masticatory movements of the mandible; see also subentries under *projection.*

bimaxillary p. the projection of both the maxilla and the mandible beyond normal limits in relation to the cranial base.

bimaxillary dentoalveolar p. the positioning of the entire dentition forward with respect to the facial profile.

disk p. herniation of intervertebral disk.

intrapelvic p. see *protrusio acetabuli.*

pro·tryp·sin (pro-trip′sin) trypsinogen.

pro·tu·ber·ance (pro-too′bər-əns) [*pro-* + L. *tuber* bulge] a projecting part, or prominence; an apophysis, process, or swelling.

p. of chin protuberantia mentalis.

laryngeal p. prominentia laryngea.

mental p. protuberantia mentalis.

occipital p., external protuberantia occipitalis externa.

occipital p., internal protuberantia occipitalis interna.

occipital p., transverse torus occipitalis.

palatine p. torus palatinus.

tubal p. torus tubarius.

pro·tu·ber·an·tia (pro-too″bər-an′shə) gen. and pl. *protuberan′tiae* [L., from *pro-* + *tuber* bulge] protuberance: a projecting part, or prominence.

p. menta′lis [TA] mental protuberance: a more or less distinct and triangular prominence on the anterior surface of the body of the mandible, on or near the median line.

p. occipita′lis exter′na [TA] external occipital protuberance: a prominence at the center of the outer surface of the squama of the occipital bone; it gives attachment to the ligamentum nuchae.

p. occipita′lis inter′na [TA] internal occipital protuberance: the projection of bone at the midpoint of the cruciform eminence, on the internal surface of the squama of the occipital bone, sometimes occurring as a ridge *(crista occipitalis interna).*

pro-UK prourokinase.

pro·uro·ki·nase (pro-UK) (pro″u-ro-ki′nās) the single-chain proenzyme cleaved by plasmin to form u-plasminogen activator (urokinase); it is found circulating in plasma and urine. Although it is inactive in plasma, it is slowly activated in the presence of fibrin clots, which it lyses via fibrin-dependent plasminogen activation. It resembles t-plasminogen activator in having both a higher specific thrombolytic activity and better fibrin specificity than does u-plasminogen activator, and it has been used for therapeutic thrombolysis. Called also *single-chain urokinase-type plasminogen activator.*

Pro·vell (pro-vel′) trademark for a preparation of protoveratrines A and B.

Pro·ven·til (pro-ven′til) trademark for preparations of albuterol.

pro·ven·tric·u·lus (pro″vən-trik′u-ləs) [*pro-* + *ventriculus*] 1. the glandular first portion of the stomach of birds, in which food from the crop is mixed with peptic enzymes and passed to the gizzard. 2. the portion of the foregut in certain invertebrates, e.g., some insects, which may function as a gizzard or as a valve into the stomach.

Pro·vera (pro-ver′ə) trademark for a preparation of medroxyprogesterone acetate.

pro·ver·te·bra (pro-vur′tə-brə) protovertebra.

Pro•vi•den•cia (prov″ĭ-den′shə) [*Providence,* Rhode Island] a genus of gram-negative, facultatively anaerobic, motile, rod-shaped bacteria of the family Enterobacteriaceae, occurring in normal urine and feces. The organisms are potential pathogens associated with urinary tract and secondary tissue infections. The type species is *P. alcalifa′ciens.*

P. alcalifa′ciens a species that does not ferment trehalose or *myo*-inositol; isolated especially from stools of children with diarrhea.

P. rett′geri a species that causes of nosocomial infections, especially of the urinary tract of patients with indwelling catheters. Called also *Proteus rettgeri.*

P. stuar′tii a species that ferments trehalose and *myo*-inositol. It causes nosocomial infections and is a major agent in burn infections.

Pro•vig•il (pro-vij′il) trademark for a preparation of modafinil.

prov•ing (pro͞ov′ing) in homeopathy, the administration of a medicinal substance to healthy persons in doses large enough to elicit a symptomatic response without causing irreversible toxicity in order to determine its therapeutic properties.

pro•vi•rus (pro-vi′rəs) the genome of an animal virus integrated (by crossing over) into the chromosome of the host cell, and thus replicated in all of its daughter cells. It can be activated, spontaneously or by induction, to produce a complete virus; it can also cause transformation of the host cell. **provi′ral** *adj*

pro•vi•sion•al (pro-vizh′ən-əl) formed or performed for temporary purposes; temporary.

pro•vi•ta•min (pro-vi′tə-min) a precursor of a vitamin.

p. A usually β-carotene; however, the term is sometimes used more broadly to denote any of the provitamin A carotenoids.

p. D_2 ergosterol.

p. D_3 7-dehydrocholesterol.

prov•o•ca•tion (prov″ə-ka′shən) challenge (def. 3).

bronchial p. see under *challenge.*

inhalational p. see under *challenge.*

pro•voc•a•tive (pro-vok′ə-tiv) stimulating the appearance of a sign, reflex, reaction, or therapeutic effect.

Pro•vo•cho•line (pro″vo-ko′lēn) trademark for a preparation of methacholine chloride.

Pro•wa•zek bodies (pro-vaht′sək) [Stanislas Joseph Matthias von *Prowazek,* German zoologist, 1875–1915] see under *body.*

Pro•wa•zek-Greeff bodies (pro-vaht′sək grāf′) [S.J.M. von *Prowazek;* Carl Richard *Greeff,* German ophthalmologist, 1862–1938] trachoma bodies, see under *body..*

Pro-X di•pep•ti•dase (di-pep′tĭ-dās″) cytosol nonspecific dipeptidase.

prox•e•mics (prok-se′miks) the study of the effects of spatial distance between persons interacting with each other, and of their orientation toward each other.

prox•i•mad (prok′sĭ-mad) toward the proximal end or in a proximal direction.

prox•i•mal (prok′sĭ-məl) [L. *proximus* next] nearest; closer to any point of reference: opposed to *distal.*

prox•i•ma•lis (prok″sĭ-ma′lis) [L.] [TA] proximal; a term denoting proximity to the point of origin or attachment of an organ or part.

prox•i•mate (prok′sĭ-mət) [L. *proximatus* drawn near] immediate or nearest.

prox•i•mo•atax•ia (prok″sĭ-mo-ə-tak′se-ə) ataxia affecting the proximal part of a limb.

prox•i•mo•buc•cal (prok″sĭ-mo-buk′əl) pertaining to the proximal and buccal surfaces of a posterior tooth.

prox•i•mo•la•bi•al (prok″sĭ-mo-la′be-əl) pertaining to the proximal and labial surfaces of an anterior tooth.

prox•i•mo•lin•gual (prok″sĭ-mo-ling′gwəl) pertaining to the proximal and lingual surfaces of a tooth.

Pro•zac (pro′zak) trademark for preparations of fluoxetine hydrochloride.

pro•zo•nal (pro′zo-nəl) 1. situated before a sclerozone. 2. pertaining to a prozone.

pro•zone (pro′zōn) [*pro-* + *zone*] in an agglutination or precipitin reaction, the zone of higher antibody concentrations within which no reaction occurs. As the antibody concentration is lowered below the prozone, the reaction occurs. This phenomenon may be due simply to antibody excess (such as in the precipitin reaction), or it may be due to blocking antibody or to nonspecific inhibitors in serum. Called also *prezone.*

PrP prion protein.

PRPP phosphoribosylpyrophosphate.

PRU peripheral resistance unit.

Pru•dox•in (proo-dok′sin) trademark for a preparation of doxepin hydrochloride.

pru•i•nate (proo′ĭ-nāt) [L. *pruina* hoarfrost] having the appearance of being covered with hoarfrost.

Pru•let (proo′lət) trademark for a preparation of oxyphenisatin acetate.

Pru•nel•la (proo-nel′ə) a genus of herbs of the family Labiatae, native to Europe and Asia. *P. vulga′ris* L. is called heal-all or self-heal and is astringent and tonic.

Pru•nus (proo′nəs) [L. "plum-tree"] a genus of trees and shrubs of the family Rosaceae, including many that are cultivated for their fruit; the seeds or pits of many varieties contain cyanogenetic compounds such as amygdalin and can cause fatal cyanide poisoning if eaten in large quantities.

P. africa′na the African plum, a tree that yields pygeum.

P. armeni′aca the apricot, whose pit is a source of persic oil.

P. cera′sus the sour cherry, a source of cherry juice.

P. dul′cis the almond, a source of almond oil and bitter almond oil.

P. per′sica the peach, whose pit is a source of persic oil.

P. seroti′na the wild cherry, a large American tree with dark bark and thick oval leaves that yields the flavoring wild cherry (see *wild cherry syrup,* under *syrup*). Both its leaves and its seeds contain cyanogenetic compounds and can cause cyanide poisoning in livestock that consume large amounts.

P. virginia′na the choke cherry, a North American tree whose leaves and seeds contain cyanogenetic compounds and can cause cyanide poisoning in livestock.

pru•ri•go (proo-ri′go) [L. "the itch"] any of various itchy skin eruptions of unknown cause, in which the characteristic lesion (prurigo papule) is dome-shaped and has a small transient vesicle on top; in time this develops crusting or lichenification. **prurig′inous** *adj*

actinic p., p. aestiva′lis a papular type of idiopathic photodermatosis that is a delayed reaction to exposure to sunlight, similar to polymorphous light eruption. It is more common in children and in summer months, and sometimes improving or resolving after puberty. Called also *Hutchinson disease, Hutchinson summer p.,* and *summer p.*

Besnier p., p. of Besnier 1. atopic dermatitis. 2. p. gestationis.

Besnier p. of pregnancy p. gestationis.

p. chro′nica multifor′mis a pruritic condition characterized by prurigo papules, patches of lichenification and eczematization, enlarged regional lymph nodes, and eosinophilia.

p. estiva′lis actinic p.

p. gestatio′nis, p. gestationis of Besnier prurigo occurring in the third trimester of pregnancy, characterized by tiny crust-covered excoriated papules, usually on the extensor surfaces of the limbs but sometimes on the upper trunk or elsewhere; lesions leave postinflammatory residua after they resolve. It usually clears up after delivery but may recur with subsequent pregnancies. Called also *Besnier p. of pregnancy.*

p. gravida′rum p. gestationis.

p. of Hebra p. mitis.

Hutchinson summer p. actinic p.

p. mi′tis a chronic, extremely pruritic type of prurigo that begins in early childhood and is characterized by excoriations, lichenification, and eczematization that become more and more pronounced. It is also accompanied by enlarged glands and other constitutional symptoms. Some authorities consider this to be identical to papular urticaria. Called also *p. of Hebra.*

nodular p., p. nodula′ris a chronic, intensely pruritic form of neurodermatitis, usually in women, on the limbs, especially the anterior thighs and legs. Characteristics include single or multiple, firm nodules that are red, brown, or pink and later become verrucous or fissured; scratching or rubbing of the nodules often makes the condition worse.

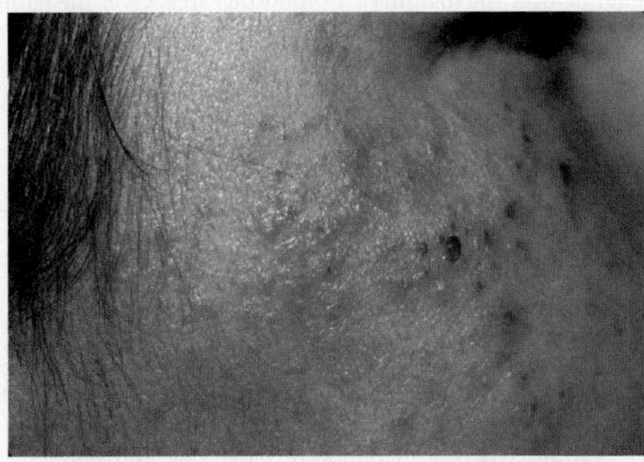

■ Erythematous, excoriated plaques of actinic prurigo.

p. sim′plex a skin condition seen chiefly in middle-aged persons, with prurigo papules at various stages of development, usually in crops, and found most often on the trunk and extensor surfaces of the limbs.

summer p. actinic p..

pru·rit·ic (proo-rit′ik) pertaining to or characterized by pruritus.

pru·rit·o·gen·ic (proo″rit-o-jen′ik) capable of causing or tending to cause pruritus.

pru·ri·tus (proo-ri′təs) [L., from *prurire* to itch] 1. an unpleasant cutaneous sensation that provokes the desire to rub or scratch the skin to obtain relief. Called also *itching.* 2. any of various conditions marked by this sensation; see also *itch.*

p. a′ni intense chronic itching in the anal region.

aquagenic p., bath p. pruritus and other skin sensations, such as burning, lasting for 30 minutes to two hours, after contact with water, without the overt skin changes seen in aquagenic urticaria. The etiology is usually unknown, although sometimes it accompanies polycythemia vera and in other cases it may be familial.

brachioradial p. chronic pruritus of the middle of an arm or the arms, sometimes from damage from ultraviolet radiation (solar pruritus) and sometimes of unknown etiology.

p. hiema′lis asteatotic eczema.

neuropathic p. pruritus caused by a neurologic condition; notalgia paresthetica is one type.

senile p., p. seni′lis itching in the elderly from dryness of the skin; the usual causes are decreased secretion of sweat and sebum and bathing too frequently.

solar p. brachioradial pruritus due to excessive sun exposure, usually in light-skinned persons.

uremic p. generalized itching associated with chronic renal failure and not attributable to other internal or skin disease.

p. vul′vae intense itching of the external genitals of the female, as with lichen sclerosus.

Prus·sak fibers, pouch, space (proo͞′sahk) [Alexander *Prussak,* Russian otologist, 1839–1897] see under *fiber,* and see *recessus superior membranae tympanicae.*

prus·si·ate (prus′e-āt) cyanide.

prus·sic ac·id (prus′ik) hydrogen cyanide.

PS phosphatidylserine; pulmonary stenosis.

ps per second.

pS2 trefoil factor 1.

PSA prostate-specific antigen.

psal·te·ri·al (sal-tēr′e-əl) pertaining to the psalterium.

psal·te·ri·um (sal-tēr′e-əm) [L., from Gr. *psaltērion* harp] 1. commissura fornicis. 2. the omasum.

Psal·y·do·lyt·ta (sal″ĭ-do-lit′ə) a genus of blister beetles (family Meloidae). *P. fus′ca* and *P. substriga′ta* of Africa produce a severe vesicular dermatitis.

psamm(o)- [Gr. *psammos* sand] a combining form meaning sandlike or denoting relationship to sand.

psam·mo·car·ci·no·ma (sam″o-kahr″sĭ-no′mə) [*psammo-* + *carcinoma*] carcinoma containing calcareous matter.

psam·mo·ma (sam-o′mə) [*psamm-* + *-oma*] 1. any tumor that contains psammoma bodies. 2. psammomatous meningioma.

psam·mo·ma·tous (sam-o′mə-təs) characterized by the presence of or containing psammoma bodies.

psam·mous (sam′əs) sandy.

psau·os·co·py (saw-os′kə-pe) [Gr. *psauein* to touch + *-scopy*] a method of physical examination done by passing the ball of the index finger back and forth lightly over the margin of an abnormal area. Over the pathological area the finger seems to encounter greater resistance and the skin seems more tense and less supple.

P_{450}SCC cholesterol monooxygenase (side-chain-cleaving).

PSE portal-systemic or portosystemic encephalopathy.

psel·lism (sel′iz-əm) stuttering (def. 1).

pseud·agraph·ia (soo″də-graf′e-ə) echographia.

pseud·al·bu·mi·nu·ria (so͞od″əl-bu″mĭ-nu′re-ə) adventitious proteinuria.

Pseu·dal·les·che·ria (so͞od″al-əs-kēr′e-ə) a genus of fungi of the family Microascaceae.

P. boy′dii a widely distributed saprobic species commonly isolated from mycetoma and other fungal infections; its perfect (sexual) stage is *Scedosporium apiospermum.* Formerly called *Allescheria boydii.*

pseu·dal·les·che·ri·a·sis (so͞od-al″əs-kə-ri′ə-sis) infection with *Pseudallescheria boydii;* clinical manifestations are highly variable, the most common being eumycotic mycetoma and pulmonary infection. Formerly called *allescheriasis.*

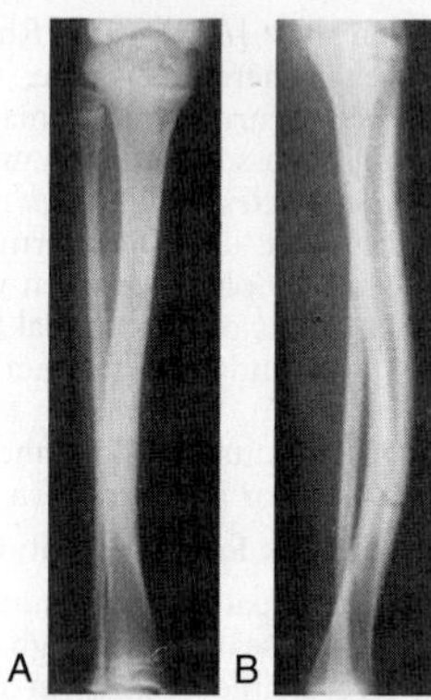

■ Congenital pseudarthrosis of right tibia, anteroposterior view *(A)* and lateral view *(B)*, showing a fracture in the anterior cortex in the distal third.

Pseud·am·phis·to·mum (so͞od″am-fis′to-məm) [*pseud-* + *amphi-* + Gr. *stoma* mouth] a genus of trematodes of the family Opisthorchiidae; called also *Pseudoamphistomum. P. trunca′tum* is found in the bile ducts of various mammals in Europe and India, causing a condition resembling opisthorchiasis.

pseud·an·gi·na (so͞od″ən-ji′nə) pseudoangina.

pseud·an·ky·lo·sis (so͞od″ang-kə-lo′sis) pseudoankylosis.

pseud·aphia (so͞od-a′fe-ə) paraphia.

pseud·ar·thro·sis (so͞od″ahr-thro′sis) [*pseud-* + *arthrosis*] a pathologic entity characterized by deossification of a weight-bearing long bone, followed by bending and pathologic fracture, with inability to form normal callus leading to existence of the "false joint" that gives the condition its name.

Pseud·ech·is (soo-dek′is) [*pseud-* + Gr. *echis* viper] a genus of venomous Australian snakes of the family Elapidae. *P. porphyria′cus* is the Australian blacksnake. See table at *snake.*

pseud·es·the·sia (so͞od″es-the′zhə) [*pseud-* + *esthesia*] 1. synesthesia. 2. a sensation felt without any external stimulus.

pseud(o)- [Gr. *pseudēs* false] a combining form signifying false or spurious.

pseu·do·ac·an·tho·sis (soo″do-ak″an-tho′sis) [*pseudo-* + *acanthosis*] a condition clinically resembling acanthosis.

p. ni′gricans a benign form of acanthosis nigricans associated with obesity that may be associated with endocrine disturbance.

pseu·do·aceph·a·lus (soo″do-a-sef′ə-ləs) [*pseudo-* + *acephalus*] in asymmetrical conjoined twins, a parasitic twin, apparently headless, but with a rudimentary cranium contained in the more developed twin.

pseu·do·ach·a·la·sia (soo″do-ak″ə-la′zhə) lack of motility in the lower esophagus that mimics achalasia but does not involve a muscular problem; the most common cause is a tumor pressing on the exterior surface of the esophagus.

pseu·do·achon·dro·pla·sia (soo″do-a-kon″dro-pla′zhə) [*pseudo-* + *achondroplasia*] an autosomal dominant osteochondrodysplasia caused by mutation in the *COMP* gene (locus: 19p13.1), which encodes cartilage oligomeric protein, important for organization of collagen fibers in the extracellular matrix of chondrocytes. It is a form of dwarfism in which limbs are short but head size and facial features are normal; there are knee and other skeletal deformities and joint hypermobility, and osteoarthritis beginning in early adulthood. The mutation is allelic with that causing one of the forms of multiple epiphyseal dysplasia (q.v.).

pseu·do·ag·glu·ti·na·tion (soo″do-ə-gloo″tĭ-na′shən) rouleau formation.

pseu·do·agraph·ia (soo″do-ə-graf′e-ə) echographia.

pseu·do·ain·hum (soo″do-īn′yoom) a condition resembling ainhum, consisting of annular constrictions around the digits, limbs, or trunk, occurring congenitally (the most severe manifestation being autoamputation in utero) and also seen in a variety of hereditary and nonhereditary disorders.

pseu·do·al·bu·mi·nu·ria (soo″do-al-bu″mĭ-nu′re-ə) adventitious proteinuria.

pseu·do·al·leles (soo″do-ə-lēlz′) [*pseudo-* + *allele*] genes that behave functionally as if they are alleles at the same locus, but that can be shown to be at distinct loci that are separable by recombination. **pseudoallel′ic** *adj*

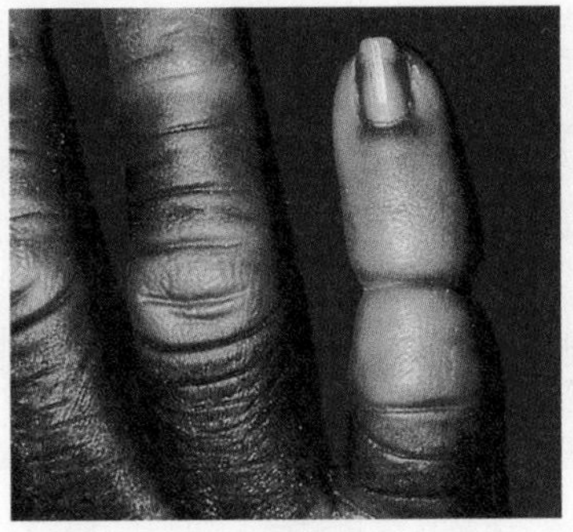

■ Pseudoainhum.

pseu·do·al·ve·o·lar (soo″do-al-ve′ə-lər) simulating an alveolar structure.

Pseu·do·am·phis·to·mum (soo″do-əm-fis′to-məm) *Pseudamphistomum.*

pseu·do·ana·phy·lax·is (soo″do-an″ə-fə-lak′sis) anaphylactoid reaction. **pseudoanaphylac′tic** *adj*

pseu·do·ane·mia (soo″do-ə-ne′me-ə) [*pseudo-* + *anemia*] marked pallor with no clinical or hematological evidence of anemia.

p. angiospas′tica pseudoanemia due to vasoconstriction.

pseu·do·an·eu·rysm (soo″do-an′u-riz″əm) dilatation of a vessel, sometimes with tortuosity, giving the appearance of an aneurysm. Called also *false* or *spurious aneurysm* and *pulsating hematoma.*

pseu·do·an·gi·na (soo″do-an-ji′nə) [*pseudo-* + *angina*] false angina; a syndrome occurring in nervous individuals, marked by precordial pain, fatigue, and lassitude, without evidence of organic disease of the heart.

pseu·do·an·ky·lo·sis (soo″do-ang″kə-lo′sis) fibrous ankylosis.

pseu·do·an·odon·tia (soo″do-an″o-don′shə) [*pseudo-* + *anodontia*] a condition characterized by the presence of multiple unerupted permanent teeth.

pseu·do·an·tag·o·nist (soo″do-an-tag′ə-nist) a muscle that flexes a joint and in so doing enhances the effect of another muscle crossing the joint to act on a more distant one.

pseu·do·ap·o·plexy (soo″do-ap′o-plek″se) [*pseudo-* + *apoplexy*] a condition resembling stroke syndrome (apoplexy), but without cerebral hemorrhage.

pseu·do·ap·pen·di·ci·tis (soo″do-ə-pen″dĭ-si′tis) a condition with symptoms resembling those of appendicitis but not originating in the appendix.

pseu·do·ar·thro·sis (soo″do-ahr-thro′sis) pseudarthrosis.

pseu·do·ath·e·to·sis (soo″do-ath″ə-to′sis) movements of the fingers when the patient closes the eyes and extends the arms, associated with impairment of joint position sense.

pseu·do·at·ro·pho·der·ma col·li (soo″do-at″ro-fo-dur′mə ko′li) a rare skin disease characterized by papillomatous lesions on the neck that resemble vitiligo; it may be a variant of confluent and reticulate papillomatosis.

pseu·do·au·to·so·mal (soo″do-aw″to-so′məl) mimicking the behavior of an autosome; see *pseudoautosomal regions,* under *region.*

pseu·do·ba·cil·lus (soo″do-bə-sil′əs) an exceedingly small, rodlike poikilocyte, resembling a microorganism.

pseu·do·bas·e·dow (soo″do-baz′ə-do) basedoid.

pseu·do·bron·chi·ec·ta·sis (soo″do-brong″ke-ek′tə-sis) a condition in which a bronchiectasis-like pattern appears in the bronchogram of partially atelectatic pulmonary segments when the larger bronchi have become shortened and broadened in outline; these reversible changes do not indicate destruction of the bronchial walls.

pseu·do·bul·bar (soo″do-bul′bər) apparently, but not really, due to a bulbar lesion.

pseu·do·car·ti·lage (soo″do-kahr′tĭ-ləj) chondroid tissue.

pseu·do·car·ti·lag·i·nous (soo″do-kahr″tĭ-laj′ĭ-nəs) composed of a substance resembling cartilage.

pseu·do·cast (soo′do-kast″) a form of urinary sediment resembling a true cast but being accidental in formation, taking the shape of cast by adherence to something else such as a mucous thread or a cotton fiber. Called also *false cast.*

pseu·do·cho·le·cys·ti·tis (soo″do-ko″lə-sis-ti′tis) a syndrome resembling cholecystitis but occurring as an allergic response to eating certain foods.

pseu·do·cho·lin·es·ter·ase (PCE) (soo″do-ko″lin-es′tər-ās) cholinesterase.

pseu·do·chrom·es·the·sia (soo″do-krōm″es-the′zhə) [*pseudo-* + *chrom-* + *esthesia*] a synesthesia in which certain sounds induce sensations of color.

pseu·do·chrom·hi·dro·sis (soo″do-kro″mĭ-dro′sis) [*pseudo-* + *chromhidrosis*] the presence of pigment on the skin caused by the action of pigment-producing bacteria.

pseu·do·chy·lo·tho·rax (soo″do-ki″lo-tho′raks) chyliform effusion.

pseu·do·chy·lous (soo″do-ki′ləs) resembling chyle, but containing no fat. Cf. *chyliform.*

pseu·do·clau·di·ca·tion (soo″do-klaw′dĭ-ka′shən) neurogenic claudication.

pseu·do·clo·nus (soo″do-klo′nəs) a short-lived clonic response.

pseu·do·co·arc·ta·tion (soo″do-ko″ahrk-ta′shən) an imprecise term used to refer to a condition radiographically resembling coarctation, but without compromise of the lumen of the affected structure, such as a "kinked aorta" (which is possibly an aortic arch anomaly).

p. of the aorta a rare congenital anomaly of the arch of the aorta that simulates coarctation radiographically but does not produce occlusion of the vessel.

pseu·do·coe·lom (soo″do-se′lom) in zoology, a body cavity between the mesoderm and endoderm; a persistent blastocoele.

pseu·do·coel·o·mate (soo″do-sēl′o-māt) 1. having a pseudocoelom. 2. an animal having a pseudocoelom, as the aschelminths.

pseu·do·col·loid (soo″do-kol′oid) a mucoid substance sometimes found in ovarian cysts.

pseu·do·col·o·bo·ma (soo″do-kol″o-bo′mə) a line or scar on the iris giving the appearance of a coloboma.

pseu·do·coma (soo′do-co″mə) locked-in syndrome.

pseu·do·cop·u·la·tion (soo″do-cop″u-la′shən) exchange of gametes by close contact between male and female but without intromission, as in frogs.

pseu·do–cor·pus lu·te·um (soo″do-kor′pəs loo-te′əm) a maturing graafian follicle that fails to rupture, retains its oocyte, and then undergoes luteinization.

pseu·do·cow·pox (soo″do-kou′poks) 1. paravaccinia (def. 1). 2. milker's nodules (def. 1).

pseu·do·cox·al·gia (soo″do-kok-sal′jə) Legg-Calvé-Perthes disease.

pseu·do·cri·sis (soo′do-kri″sis) [*pseudo-* + *crisis*] a false crisis; a sudden but temporary abatement of fever.

pseu·do·croup (soo″do-kro͞op′) laryngismus stridulus.

pseu·do·cy·a·nin (soo″do-si′ə-nin) pseudoisocyanin.

pseu·do·cy·e·sis (soo″do-si-e′sis) [*pseudo-* + *-cyesis*] false pregnancy.

pseu·do·cy·lin·droid (soo″do-sə-lin′droid) a shred of mucin in the urine resembling a cylindroid; sometimes of spermatic origin.

pseu·do·cyst (soo′do-sist″) [*pseudo-* + *cyst*] 1. an abnormal or dilated cavity resembling a true cyst but not lined with epithelium. Called also *adventitious* or *false cyst.* 2. a cluster of bradyzoites, small, comma-shaped forms of *Toxoplasma gondii,* enclosed by an irregular wall and sometimes containing thousands of organisms. It represents a resting stage, as opposed to the active, motile stage called the *tachyzoite.* Pseudocysts are found in the tissues, especially muscles and the brain, in chronic (latent) toxoplasmosis. Called also *tissue cyst.*

adrenal p. a cyst of the adrenal gland with no epithelial or endothelial lining, often with thick, irregular walls; it results from adrenal hemorrhage or develops within an adrenal neoplasm. Predisposing factors include trauma to the neck, infection, bleeding diathesis, embolism, aneurysm, or, in infants, anoxia.

p. of auricle, auricular p., endochondral p. a benign, asymptomatic swelling of the auricle of the ear, containing fluid.

p's of lung cystic disease of lung.

pancreatic p. a cystic collection of fluid and necrotic debris whose walls are formed by the pancreas and nearby organs. It occurs as a complication of acute pancreatitis and may subside spontaneously or become secondarily infected and develop into an abscess. Cf. *pancreatic phlegmon,* under *phlegmon.*

paranephric p., pararenal p., perinephric p. urinoma.

pulmonary p's cystic disease of lung.

uriniferous p. urinoma.

pseu·do·de·men·tia (soo″do-də-men′shə) a disorder resembling dementia but that is not due to organic brain disease and is potentially reversible by treatment; usually due to depression or other psychiatric disorder.

depressive p. dementia syndrome of depression; the term is discouraged as technically incorrect because the cognitive deficits are now believed to be real, if reversible.

pseu·do·dex·tro·car·dia (soo″do-dek″stro-kahr′de-ə) a condition in which the heart is displaced to the right, but the ventricles are not inverted nor are the great vessels transposed.

pseu·do·di·a·be·tes (soo″do-di″ə-be′tēz) impaired glucose tolerance due to subclinical diabetes.

uremic p. mellitus impaired glucose tolerance in chronic renal failure.

pseu·do·diph·the·ria (soo″do-dif-thēr′e-ə) any of various infections resembling diphtheria but not caused by *Corynebacterium diphtheriae.* Called also *diphtheroid.*

pseu·do·dis·ease (soo′do-dĭ-zēz″) an occult disease that would never become apparent to a patient during his or her lifetime without the use of diagnostic testing.

pseu·do·di·ver·tic·u·lum (soo″do-di″vər-tik′u-ləm) herniation of the esophageal or intestinal mucosa and submucosa through a tear in the muscular coat. Called also *false diverticulum.*

pseu·do·dom·i·nance (soo″do-dom′ĭ-nəns) [*pseudo-* + *dominance*] 1. appearance of a recessive phenotype in a pedigree, the recessive allele being expressed due to loss of the dominant allele, as by a chromosomal deletion. 2. quasidominance.

pseu·do·dom·i·nant (soo″do-dom′ĭ-nənt) 1. pertaining to pseudodominance (def. 1). 2. quasidominant.

pseu·do·dys·en·tery (soo″do-dis′ən-ter″e) a condition with symptoms of dysentery but due to local irritation rather than to usual causes of dysentery.

pseu·do·ede·ma (soo″do-ə-de′mə) a puffy state resembling edema.

pseu·do·em·bry·on·ic (soo″do-em″bre-on′ik) apparently, but not truly, embryonic.

pseu·do·em·phy·se·ma (soo″do-em″fĭ-ze′mə) a condition resembling emphysema but due to temporary blocking of the bronchial tubes.

pseu·do·en·ceph·a·lo·cele (soo″do-ən-sef′ə-lo-sēl) an encephalocele that is not congenital but caused by disease or injury of the skull.

pseu·do·en·ceph·a·lo·ma·la·cia (soo″do-ən-sef″ə-lo-mə-la′shə) polioencephalomalacia.

pseu·do·en·do·me·tri·tis (soo″do-en″do-mə-tri′tis) a condition simulating endometritis, in which there are changes in the blood vessels, hyperplasia of the stroma and glands, and atrophy.

pseu·do·eo·sin·o·phil (soo″do-e″o-sin′o-fil) a neutrophilic leukocyte with granules showing a predilection for acid dyes.

pseu·do·ephed·rine (soo″do-ə-fed′rin) one of the stereoisomers of ephedrine, having less pressor action and fewer central stimulant effects than ephedrine.

p. hydrochloride [USP] the hydrochloride salt of pseudoephedrine, used as a nasal decongestant, administered orally.

p. sulfate [USP] the sulfate salt of pseudoephedrine, having the same actions and uses as the hydrochloride salt.

pseu·do·epi·lepsy (soo″do-ep′ĭ-lep″se) pseudoseizure.

pseu·do·epiph·y·sis (soo″do-ə-pif′ə-sis) an accessory bone at the distal and the proximal ends of the second metacarpal bone.

pseu·do·es·the·sia (soo″do-es-the′zhə) pseudesthesia.

pseu·do·ex·fo·li·a·tion (soo″do-eks″fo-le-a′shən) exfoliation syndrome.

pseu·do·exo·pho·ria (soo″do-ek″so-for′e-ə) [*pseudo-* + *exophoria*] an outward tendency of the visual axis excited by diminishing the activity of the accommodative centers.

pseu·do·ex·stro·phy (soo″do-eks′trə-fe) a developmental anomaly marked by the characteristic musculoskeletal defects of bladder exstrophy but with no other major defect of the urinary tract.

pseu·do·far·cy (soo′do-fahr″se) lymphangitis epizootica.

pseu·do·fluc·tu·a·tion (soo″do-fluk″choo-a′shən) a movement resembling fluctuation, such as is sometimes seen on tapping lipomas or muscular tissue.

pseu·do·fol·lic·u·li·tis (soo″do-fə-lik″u-li′tis) [*pseudo-* + *folliculitis*] a skin condition resembling folliculitis.

p. bar′bae a condition resembling folliculitis, involving the bearded region, usually seen in men of African descent who have very curly hair and shave their necks. It was formerly thought to be due to a bacterial infection, but that has been disproven; the usual cause is ingrowth of the hair. The primary lesion is a pinhead-sized pustule, pierced by a hair; if neglected, this may lead to impetiginization and crust formation and may become chronic. Popularly known as *razor bumps.*

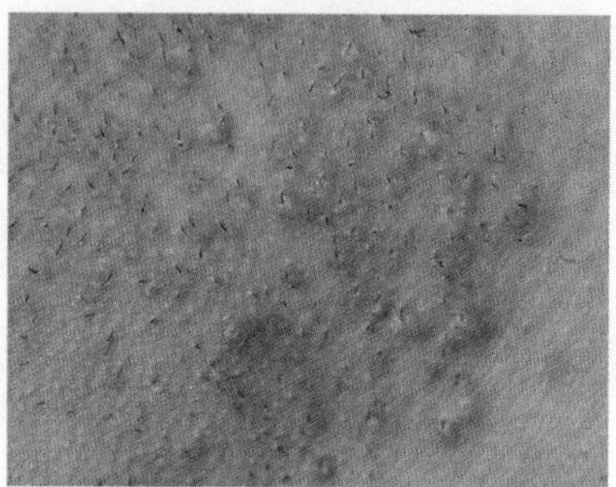

■ Pseudofolliculitis barbae.

pseu·do·frac·ture (soo″do-frak′chər) a condition seen in a radiograph of a bone as a thickening of the periosteum and formation of new bone over what looks like an incomplete fracture.

pseu·do·gan·gli·on (soo″do-gang′gle-on) a thickening of a nerve simulating a ganglion.

Bochdalek p. plexus dentalis superior.

Cloquet p. see under *ganglion.*

Valentin p. intumescentia tympanica.

pseu·do·gene (soo′do-jēn″) [*pseudo-* + *gene*] a DNA sequence that is similar in sequence to an active gene at another locus but that has been inactivated by mutation and is not expressed. Two classes exist: one appears to result from gene duplication and mutation and the other from integration into the genome of DNA copied from processed mRNA molecules.

pseu·do·ges·ta·tion (soo″do-jes-ta′shən) false pregnancy.

pseu·do·geus·es·the·sia (soo″do-gōōs″es-the′zhə) pseudogeusia.

pseu·do·geu·sia (soo″do-goo′zhə) [*pseudo-* + Gr. *geusis* taste + *-ia*] a synesthesia in which taste is experienced in association with a stimulus of a different modality.

pseu·do·glan·ders (soo″do-glan′dərz) 1. epizootic lymphangitis. 2. melioidosis.

pseu·do·glan·du·lar (soo″do-glan′du-lər) resembling some characteristic usually seen in a gland; see *adenoid* (def. 2) and see under *phase.*

pseu·do·gli·o·ma (soo″do-gli-o′mə) a condition resembling glioma, a membrane being produced behind the lens because of failure of the posterior vascular sheath of the lens to atrophy, or because of its replacement by connective tissue.

pseu·do·glob·u·lin (soo″do-glob′u-lin) one of a class of globulins characterized by being soluble in water in the absence of neutral salts and thus not a euglobulin; see also *globulin.*

pseu·do·glot·tic (soo″do-glot′ik) pertaining to the pseudoglottis.

pseu·do·glot·tis (soo″do-glot′is) 1. rima vestibuli. 2. neoglottis.

pseu·do·glu·co·sa·zone (soo″do-gloo-kōs′ə-zōn) a crystalline substance sometimes developed in normal urine in testing for glucose.

pseu·do·gon·or·rhea (soo″do-gon″ə-re′ə) nongonococcal urethritis.

pseu·do·gout (soo′do-gout″) [*pseudo-* + *gout*] calcium pyrophosphate deposition disease, particularly the acute and subacute forms.

pseu·do·graph·ia (soo″do-graf′e-ə) [*pseudo-* + *graph-* + *-ia*] the production of meaningless written symbols imitating letters, the written equivalent of jargon aphasia.

pseu·do·gyn·e·co·mas·tia (soo″do-jin″ə-ko-mas′te-ə) an excess of adipose tissue in the male breast with no increase in glandular tissue. Cf. *gynecomastia.*

pseu·do·hal·lu·ci·na·tion (soo″do-hə-loo″sĭ-na′shən) 1. an image perceived to be occurring externally but that the subject knows is generated within the mind. 2. a hallucination that the subject knows is unreal.

pseu·do·hel·minth (soo″do-hel′minth) [*pseudo-* + *helminth*] something that resembles an endoparasitic worm.

pseu·do·he·mag·glu·ti·na·tion (soo″do-he″mə-gloo″tĭ-na′shən) rouleau formation.

pseu·do·he·ma·tu·ria (soo″do-he″mə-tu′re-ə) the presence in the urine of pigments that give it a pink or red color when hemoglobin and blood cells are not detectable. Called also *false hematuria.*

pseu·do·he·mo·phil·ia (soo″do-he″mo-fil′e-ə) von Willebrand disease.

pseu·do·he·mop·ty·sis (soo″do-he-mop′tĭ-sis) spitting of blood which comes from some source other than the lungs or bronchial tubes.

pseu·do·her·maph·ro·dism (soo″do-hər-maf′ro-diz-əm) pseudohermaphroditism.

pseu·do·her·maph·ro·dite (soo″do-hər-maf′ro-dīt) an individual with pseudohermaphroditism.
female p. an individual with female pseudohermaphroditism. Called also *female intersex.*
male p. an individual with male pseudohermaphroditism. Called also *male intersex.*

pseu·do·her·maph·ro·dit·ism (soo″do-hər-maf′ro-dit-iz″əm) a condition in which an individual is genetically and gonadally of one sex but has significant secondary sex characters of the opposite sex, often with ambiguous external genitalia. Cf. *hermaphroditism.* Called also *androgynism* and *spurious* or *false hermaphroditism.*
female p. a condition in which the affected individual is genetically female and has female gonads (ovaries) but has significant male secondary sex characters. Called also *androgynism* and *gynandrism.*
male p. a condition in which the affected individual is genetically male and has male gonads (testes) but has significant typically female secondary sex characters. Cf. *androgen insensitivity syndrome,* under *syndrome.*

pseu·do·her·nia (soo″do-hur′ne-ə) an inflamed sac or gland simulating strangulated hernia.

pseu·do·het·ero·to·pia (soo″do-het″ər-o-to′pe-ə) displacement of gray or white matter of the brain or cord, produced by unskillful manipulation during autopsy.

pseu·do·hy·dro·ceph·a·lus (soo″do-hi″dro-sef′ə-ləs) abnormally large appearance of a normal-sized head, due to smallness of the face and body, as in Silver syndrome.

pseu·do·hy·dro·ne·phro·sis (soo″do-hi″dro-nə-fro′sis) urinoma.

pseu·do·hypa·cu·sis (soo″do-hīp-ə-ku′sis) [*pseudo-* + *hyp-* + *acusis*] functional hearing loss.

pseu·do·hy·per·ka·le·mia (soo″do-hi″pər-kə-le′me-ə) a laboratory artifact in which serum potassium is elevated when plasma potassium is normal. It occurs in the presence of thrombocytosis or leukocytosis, most commonly in myeloproliferative disorders, because blood clotting causes the release of potassium from platelets and leukocytes.

pseu·do·hy·per·ten·sion (soo″do-hi″pər-ten′shən) a falsely elevated blood pressure reading by sphygmomanometry, occurring particularly in elderly patients, caused by loss of compliance of the arterial walls.

pseu·do·hy·per·tri·cho·sis (soo″do-hi″pər-trĭ-ko′sis) persistence after birth of the fine hair present during fetal life, owing to inability of the skin to throw it off.

pseu·do·hy·per·tri·glyc·er·i·de·mia (soo″do-hi″pər-tri-glis″ə-ri-de′me-ə) false elevation of blood triglyceride levels, usually due to an artifact of testing.

pseu·do·hy·per·tro·phy (soo″do-hi-pur′trə-fe) false hypertrophy; increase of size without true hypertrophy. **pseudohypertro′phic** *adj*
muscular p. increased size of a muscle due not to enlargement of muscle fibers but to infiltration of the muscle with other tissue, such as fat.

pseu·do·hy·pha (soo″do-hi′fə) a string of cells resulting from the building of the blastoconidia, without the cytoplasmic connection of a true hypha; seen in some yeasts.

pseu·do·hy·po·al·dos·ter·on·ism (PHA) (soo″do-hi″po-al-dos′tər-ōn-iz″əm) elevated levels of aldosterone and increased plasma renin activity together with signs and symptoms of mineralocorticoid deficiency, caused by resistance of target tissues to mineralocorticoids.
p. type 1 (PHA1) a hereditary disorder of infancy characterized by severe salt wasting, failure to thrive, and other signs of aldosterone deficiency in association with normal or elevated aldosterone levels, caused by defects in the mineralocorticoid receptor.
p. type 2 (PHA2) an endocrine abnormality of autosomal dominant inheritance, seen primarily in adults, characterized by hyperkalemia without salt wasting and caused by resistance to the mineralocorticoid effects of aldosterone on tubular potassium transport. Called also *Gordon syndrome.*

pseu·do·hy·po·na·tre·mia (soo″do-hi″po-nə-tre′me-ə) a decreased serum sodium concentration that does not correspond to a real hypotonic disorder, i.e., the serum osmolality is normal. It occurs when hyperlipidemia increases the serum non-water volume or hyperproteinemia increases the serum non-sodium solute.

pseu·do·hy·po·para·thy·roi·dism (PHP) (soo″do-hi″po-par″ə-thi′roi-diz″əm) a hereditary condition clinically resembling hypoparathyroidism, but caused by inability to respond to, rather than deficiency of, parathyroid hormone. The major cause is defective G proteins required for signal transduction; in some cases, there is an associated inability to respond to other hormones that require the same G protein types. It is characterized by hypocalcemia and hyperphosphatemia, and is commonly associated with short stature, obesity, short metacarpals, and ectopic calcification.

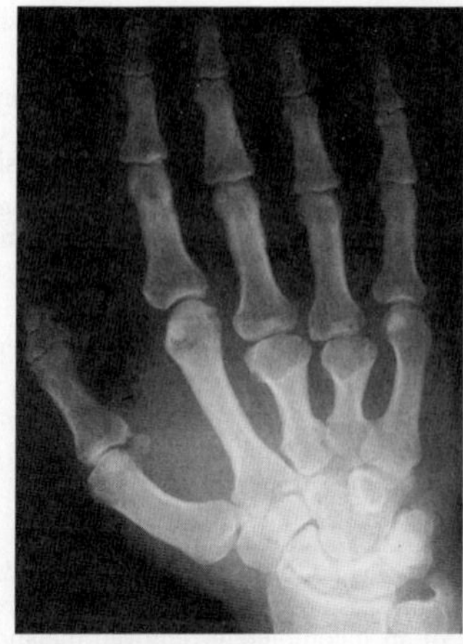
■ Pseudohypoparathyroidism with shortening of the metacarpals of the middle and ring fingers (posteroanterior view).

pseu·do·hy·po·phos·pha·ta·sia (soo″do-hi″po-fos″fə-ta′zhə) a condition resembling hypophosphatasia, characterized by osteopathy of the skull and long bones, muscular hypotonia, hypercalcemia, and increased urinary excretion of phosphoethanolamine. It is distinguished by normal alkaline phosphatase activity.

pseu·do·hy·po·thy·roi·dism (soo″do-hi″po-thi′roi-diz-əm) inability to use thyroxine in tissue cells, despite normal thyroid function, leading to development of symptoms and certain stigmata of hypothyroidism.

pseu·do·ic·ter·us (soo″do-ik′tər-əs) pseudojaundice.

pseu·do·in·farc·tion (soo″do-in-fahrk′shən) the simulation in the electrocardiographic pattern of myocardial infarction, due to disorders other than coronary artery disease.

pseu·do·in·ti·ma (soo″do-in′tĭ-mə) a new layer formed on the intimal surface of a blood vessel graft or vascular prosthesis, consisting of cells other than endothelial cells or proteins such as plasma proteins or collagen. Cf. *neointima.*

pseu·do·iso·chro·mat·ic (soo″do-i″so-kro-mat′ik) seemingly of the same color throughout; in tests for color blindness, this refers to solutions that contain two pigments distinguishable by the normal eye but are seen by a color blind eye as having a single color. Cf. *anisochromatic.*

pseu·do·iso·cy·a·nin (soo″do-i″so-si′ə-nin) an orange metachromatic dye used for the selective demonstration of insulin in pancreatic islet beta cells.

pseu·do·jaun·dice (soo″do-jawn′dis) skin discoloration caused by blood changes and not due to liver disease, as in carotenemia. Called also *pseudoicterus.*

pseu·do·ker·a·tin (soo″do-ker′ə-tin) cytokeratin.

pseu·do·la·mel·lar (soo″do-lə-mel′ər) resembling lamella.

pseu·do·leu·ke·mia (soo″do-loo-ke′me-ə) term formerly used for a group of conditions resembling one another in showing enlarged lymph glands and other characteristics like those seen in leukemia, but without leukemic blood findings. The group included Hodgkin disease, multiple myeloma, agnogenic myeloid metaplasia, and several other conditions.

pseu·do·li·po·ma (soo″do-lĭ-po′mə) a collection of fat within the body that resembles a lipoma; most are the result of tissue separation from trauma with herniation of adipose tissue.

pseu·do·li·thi·a·sis (soo″do-lĭ-thi′ə-sis) any of various conditions with symptoms imitating the presence of calculi when no calculi are present.
biliary p. pain in the bile ducts with symptoms resembling those of cholelithiasis but in the absence of gallstones.

pseu·do·lo·gia (soo″do-lo′jə) [*pseudo-* + *log-* + *-ia*] lying; falsehood.
p. fantas′tica a tendency to tell extravagant and fantastic falsehoods centered about the storyteller, who often comes to believe in and may act on them.

pseu·do·lux·a·tion (soo″do-lək-sa′shən) partial dislocation of a bone.

pseu·do·lym·pho·ma (soo″do-lim-fo′mə) [*pseudo-* + *lymphoma*] any of a group of disorders having a benign course but exhibiting clinical and histologic features suggestive of malignant lymphoma. Called also *lymphocytoma.*
Spiegler-Fendt p. cutaneous lymphoid hyperplasia; see under *hyperplasia.*

Pseu·do·lynch·ia (soo″do-linch′e-ə) a genus of parasitic flies of the family Hippoboscidae. *P. canarien′sis* (called also *P. mari′rah*), parasitizes pigeons and spreads to them a type of malaria, and is also a vector of the protozoon *Haemoproteus columbae.*

pseu·do·mal·func·tion (soo″do-mal-fungk′shən) in cardiac pacing terminology, apparent pacemaker malfunction actually due to an artifact, such as mechanical errors in electrocardiographic analysis.

pseu·do·ma·lig·nan·cy (soo″do-mə-lig′nən-se) [*pseudo-* + *malignancy*] any of several types of tumors exhibiting benign clinical behavior but having a distinctly malignant microscopic appearance; see also *pseudolymphoma* and *pseudomelanoma.*

pseu·do·mam·ma (soo″do-mam′ə) a structure resembling a breast or nipple, such as one found on ovarian dermoid cysts.

pseu·do·ma·nia (soo″do-ma′ne-ə) [*pseudo-* + *-mania*] 1. false or pretended mental disorder. 2. a mental disorder in which the patient admits to crimes actually not committed.

pseu·do·mega·co·lon (soo″do-meg′ə-ko″lən) acquired megacolon.

pseu·do·mel·a·no·ma (soo″do-mel″ə-no′mə) [*pseudo-* + *melanoma*] a benign melanotic lesion resembling a superficial spreading melanoma occurring at the site of an incompletely removed melanocytic nevus.

pseu·do·mel·a·no·sis (soo″do-mel″ə-no′sis) a staining of the tissue after death with pigments from the blood.

pseu·do·me·lia (soo″do-me′le-ə) [*pseudo-* + *-melia*] phantom limb.

pseu·do·mem·brane (soo″do-mem′brān) a layer resembling an organized and living membrane, but made up of coagulated fibrin with bacteria and leukocytes, such as may be formed on mucous membranes in diphtheria or in the colon with *Clostridium difficile* infection. Called also *false membrane* and *neomembrane.* **pseudomem′branous** *adj*

pseu·do·mem·bra·nelle (soo″do-mem′brə-nel) [*pseudo-* + *membranelle*] 1. a membranelle-like organelle, composed of a group of complex kinetofragments, representing a modified frange in certain ciliate protozoa. 2. loosely, any of various membranelle-like ciliary complexes seen in protozoa.

pseu·do·men·in·gi·tis (soo″do-men″in-ji′tis) meningism.

pseu·do·men·stru·a·tion (soo″do-men″stroo-a′shən) uterine discharge unattended with endometrial changes of menstruation, usually occurring in newborn babies.

pseu·do·mo·nad (soo″do-mo′nad) any member of the genus *Pseudomonas.* **pseudomo′nal** *adj*

Pseu·do·mo·na·da·ceae (soo″do-mo″nə-da′se-e) a family of bacteria of the order Pseudomonadales, grouped together on the basis of 16S rRNA sequence analysis and consisting of aerobic, chemo-organotrophic, mostly motile organisms with respiratory metabolism. Medically important organisms are contained in the genus *Pseudomonas.*

Pseu·do·mo·na·da·les (soo″do-mo″nə-da′lēz) an order of bacteria of the class Gammaproteobacteria, phylum Proteobacteria, grouped together by 16S rRNA sequence analysis and consisting of aerobic, chemo-organotrophic organisms with respiratory metabolism; most are motile by means of a polar flagella. It contains the families Pseudomonadaceae and Moraxellaceae.

Pseu·do·mo·nas (soo″do-mo′nəs) [*pseudo-* + Gr. *monas* unit, from *monos* single] a genus of gram-negative bacteria of the family Pseudomonadaceae, consisting of straight or curved rods that are motile by polar flagella. Most species are strict aerobes and some produce pigments; some are fluorescent. The organisms are usually saprophytic, being found in soil, water, and decomposing matter; some are pathogenic for plants and animals. Historically, many unrelated bacteria were classified in the genus. More recently, this genus has been restricted to species related to the type species *P. aerugino′sa.*

P. acido′vorans *Delftia acidovorans.*

P. aerugino′sa the type species of the genus; it produces pyocyanin and fluorescein, which give the color to the "blue pus" observed in certain infections, and it produces a variety of toxins and enzymes. It is a major cause of nosocomial infection, such as *P. aeruginosa* pneumonia or severe infections of the urinary tract, wounds, abscesses, or the bloodstream. It may also cause eye infections in those who use contact lenses.

P. alcali′genes an occasionally opportunistic species found in water reservoirs and recovered from clinical specimens of blood, urine, respiratory tract, and abscesses. It has been associated with empyema and eye infections.

P. cepa′cia *Burkholderia cepacia.*

P. diminu′ta *Brevundimonas diminuta.*

P. fluores′cens a fluorescent species that is an environmental contaminant and occasionally an opportunistic pathogen, causing infections of the urinary tract, wounds, and the bloodstream. It also occurs as a contaminant of blood and blood products used for transfusion, sometimes causing fatal shock.

P. lute′ola a species isolated from nosocomial infections and occasionally other infections such as bacteremia, peritonitis, and appendicitis.

P. mal′lei *Burkholderia mallei.*

P. maltophi′lia *Stenotrophomonas maltophilia.*

P. oryziha′bitans a species that normally inhabits soil and wet environments such as rice paddies, but has been found in nosocomial bacteremia.

P. paucimobi′lis *Sphingomonas paucimobilis.*

P. picket′tii *Ralstonia pickettii.*

P. pseudoalcali′genes a species isolated from water reservoirs and clinical specimens that is sometimes associated with infection.

P. pseudomal′lei *Burkholderia pseudomallei.*

P. pu′tida a fluorescent species that is a common inhabitant of soil, water, and plants, is often isolated from clinical specimens, and can be an opportunistic pathogen.

P. stut′zeri a widespread species often recovered from clinical specimens, which can be an opportunistic pathogen in immunocompromised or debilitated persons.

P. testostero′ni *Comamonas testosteroni.*

P. vesicula′ris *Brevundimonas vesicularis.*

pseu·do·mo·nil·e·thrix (soo″do-mo-nil′ə-thriks) a condition, inherited as an autosomal dominant trait, in which the hairs exhibit irregularly spaced nodal swellings, the internodal areas being normal; cf. *monilethrix.*

pseu·do·mo·sa·i·cism (soo″do-mo-za′ĭ-siz-əm) the presence of two cell lines in only a single sample in amniocentesis or chorionic villus sampling; considered to be due to cell culture artifacts.

pseu·do·mo·tor (soo″do-mo′tər) dyskinetic.

pseu·do·mu·ci·nous (soo″do-mu′sĭ-nəs) resembling mucin; the term has been used for various ovarian neoplasms now known to contain mucin and to be properly denoted mucinous.

pseu·do·my·ce·to·ma (soo″do-mi″sə-to′mə) 1. a rare fungal infection of the dermis and subcutis with *Microsporum canis,* seen in Persian cats. 2. skin lesions in humans caused by infection with *Microsporum canis,* characterized by a tender, pruritic rash; it is seen most often in immunocompromised persons.

pseu·do·my·ia·sis (soo″do-mi-i′ə-sis) the presence of fly maggots in the digestive tract due to ingestion; if present in large numbers, they may cause diarrhea and other symptoms.

pseu·do·my·o·pia (soo″do-mi-o′pe-ə) [*pseudo-* + *myopia*] defective vision resembling myopia, caused by spasm of the ciliary muscle or by failure of relaxation of accommodation.

pseu·do·myo·to·nia (soo″do-mi″o-to′ne-ə) 1. delayed relaxation of a muscle after contraction. 2. former name for complex repetitive discharge.

pseu·do·myx·o·ma (soo″do-mik-so′mə) 1. a gelatinous mass of epithelial mucus resembling a myxoma. 2. p. peritonei.

p. peritone′i the presence in the peritoneal cavity of mucoid matter from a ruptured ovarian cyst or a ruptured mucocele of the appendix; called also *gelatinous ascites* and *hydrops spurius.*

pseu·do·nar·cot·ic (soo″do-nahr-kot′ik) sedative and apparently, but not directly, narcotic.

pseu·do·neo·plasm (soo″do-ne′o-plaz″əm) [*pseudo-* + *neoplasm*] pseudotumor.

pseu·do·neu·ri·tis (soo″do-noo-ri′tis) [*pseudo-* + *neuritis*] a congenital anomaly of the optic papilla in which it becomes hyperemic.

pseu·do·neu·ro·ma (soo″do-noo-ro′mə) false neuroma.

pseu·do·neu·ro·no·pha·gia (soo″do-noo-ro″no-fa′jə) a false appearance of phagocytosis of nerve cells; cf. *satellitosis.*

Pseu·do·no·car·di·a·ceae (soo″do-no-kahr″de-a′se-e) a phenotypically diverse family of gram-positive, aerobic, catalase-positive bacteria of the suborder Pseudonocardineae, order Actinomycetales. Organisms of medical interest are contained in the genera *Amycolatopsis, Saccharomonospora,* and *Saccharopolyspora*

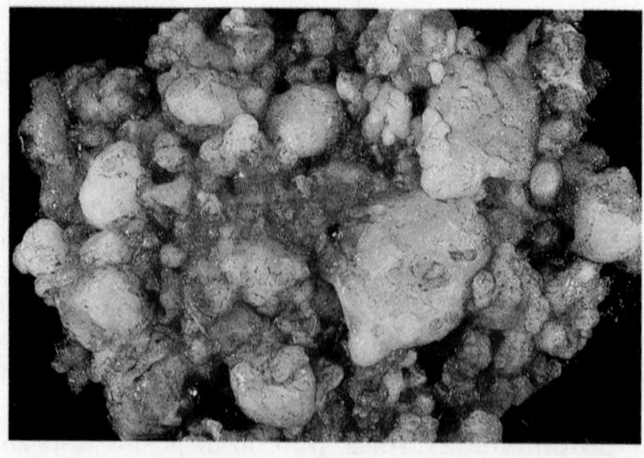

■ Pseudomyxoma peritonei.

Pseu•do•no•car•di•neae (soo″do-no″kahr-din′e-e) a suborder of aerobic bacteria of the order Actinomycetales; medically important organisms are contained in the family Pseudonocardiaceae.

pseu•do•nys•tag•mus (soo″do-nis-tag′məs) end-position nystagmus.

pseu•do•ob•struc•tion (soo″do-ob-struk′shən) a condition simulating obstruction.

intestinal p. a condition characterized by constipation, colicky pain, and vomiting, but without evidence of organic obstruction; it is frequently a motor disorder. See also *Ogilvie syndrome*, under *syndrome*.

pseu•do•ochro•no•sis (soo″do-o-kro′no-sis) a condition resembling ochronosis, but not caused by a disorder of metabolism.

pseu•do•op•to•gram (soo″do-op′to-gram) an optogram in which the rods strip off from the illuminated spot and only the cones remain.

pseu•do•os•teo•ma•la•cia (soo″do-os″te-o-mə-la′shə) rachitic contraction of the pelvis.

pseu•do•pap•il•lary (soo″do-pap′ĭ-lar″e) having a pattern that resembles the growth of papillae but results from necrosis of cells distant from the blood supply, with the preserved cells forming fingerlike projections.

pseu•do•pap•il•le•de•ma (soo″do-pap″ĭ-lə-de′mə) [*pseudo-* + *papilledema*] anomalous elevation of the optic disk.

pseu•do•pa•ral•y•sis (soo″do-pə-ral′ĭ-sis) 1. apparent loss of muscular power because of pain that is not neurologic in origin, marked by defective coordination of movements or by repression of movement. 2. hysterical paralysis.

Parrot p., syphilitic p. apparent paralysis of one or more of the extremities of an infant owing to osteochondritis of an epiphysis in congenital syphilis.

pseu•do•para•ple•gia (soo″do-par″ə-ple′jə) pseudoparalysis of the lower limbs.

pseu•do•par•a•site (soo″do-par′ə-sīt) any object resembling or mistaken for a parasite.

pseu•do•pa•ren•chy•ma (soo″do-pə-reng′kĭ-mə) a mass of hyphae fused together to form a tissuelike structure.

pseu•do•pa•re•sis (soo″do-pə-re′sis) 1. pseudoparalysis (def. 1). 2. hysterical paralysis.

pseu•do•pe•lade (soo″do-pə-lahd′) [*pseudo-* + *pelade*] an uncommon type of cicatricial alopecia, usually seen in women or children, characterized by development of hairless patches and scarring. Some cases may result from earlier conditions such as discoid lupus erythematosus or lichen planus follicularis.

Brocq p. pseudopelade.

pseu•do•pel•lag•ra (soo″do-pə-lag′rə) a condition in alcoholics now recognized as identical to pellagra.

pseu•do•pep•tone (soo″do-pep′tōn) ovomucoid.

pseu•do•peri•car•di•al (soo″do-per″ĭ-kahr′de-əl) seemingly, but not actually, arising from the pericardium.

pseu•do•peri•to•ni•tis (soo″do-per″ĭ-to-ni′tis) peritonism.

pseu•do•per•ox•i•dase (soo-do-pər-ok′sĭ-dās) any of a class of substances, including hemoglobin, that act like peroxidase, catalyzing a reduction-oxidation reaction between hydrogen peroxide and a variety of organic compounds.

pseu•do•pha•kia (soo″do-fa′ke-ə) a condition in which the degenerated crystalline lens is replaced by mesodermal tissue.

p. adipo′sa a condition in which the crystalline lens is replaced by a mass of fatty tissue.

p. fibro′sa replacement of the crystalline lens by a mass of connective tissue that represents hyperplasia of both the anterior and posterior vascular sheaths of the lens.

pseu•do•pha•ko•do•ne•sis (soo″do-fa″ko-do-ne′sis) [*pseudo* + *phakos* + Gr. *donein* to shake] movement of an implanted artificial lens.

pseu•do•pha•kos (soo″do-fa′kəs) [*pseudo-* + Gr. *phakos* lentil-shaped object] an implantable artificial lens used in the treatment of cataracts.

pseu•do•pho•tes•the•sia (soo″do-fo″tes-the′zhə) photism.

Pseu•do•phyl•lid•ea (soo″do-fĭ-lid′e-ə) an order of cestodes in which the scolex typically has two opposing sucking organs. It includes the family Diphyllobothriidae.

pseu•do•phyl•lid•e•an (soo″do-fĭ-lid′e-ən) pertaining to or caused by tapeworms of the order Pseudophyllidea.

pseu•do•plas•mo•di•um (soo″do-plaz-mo′de-əm) [*pseudo-* + *plasmodium*] a multinucleate plasmodium-like body formed by aggregation of myxamebae without fusion of their protoplasm.

pseu•do•pneu•mo•nia (soo″do-noo-mo′ne-ə) a condition marked by the symptoms of pneumonia, but without any lesions in the lungs.

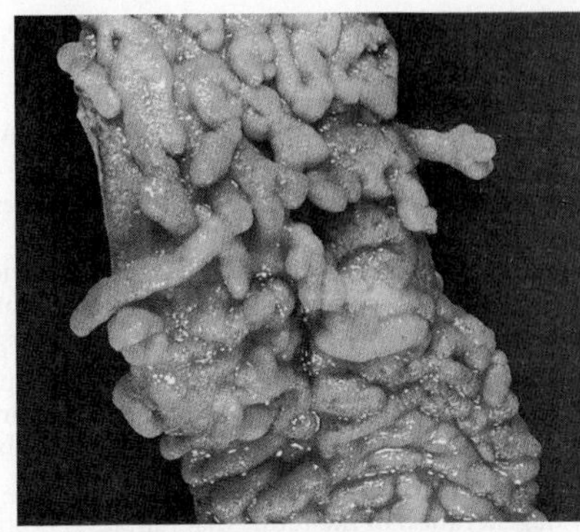

■ Pseudopolyps in ulcerative colitis.

pseu•do•po•dia (soo″do-po′de-ə) [L.] plural of *pseudopodium*.

pseu•do•po•di•o•spore (soo″do-po′de-o-spor) [*pseudopodium* + *spore*] amebula (def. 2).

pseu•do•po•di•um (soo″do-po′de-əm) pl. *pseudopo′dia* [L., from *pseudo-* + Gr. *pous* foot] a temporary cytoplasmic extrusion by means of which an ameba or other ameboid organism or cell moves about or engulfs food. See also *axopodium*, *filopodium*, *lobopodium*, and *reticulopodium*.

pseu•do•poly•cy•the•mia (soo″do-pol″e-si-the′me-ə) 1. stress polycythemia. 2. relative polycythemia.

pseu•do•poly•me•lia (soo″do-pol″e-me′le-ə) an illusory sensation that may be referred to many extreme portions of the body, including the nose, nipples, and glans penis, as well as the hands and feet.

paresthetic p. sensations of pseudopolymelia in the form of paresthesias.

pseu•do•pol•yp (soo″do-pol′ip) a hypertrophied tab of mucous membrane that resembles a polyp but is caused by ulceration surrounding and sometimes undermining a portion of intact mucosa; it is frequently observed in chronic inflammatory diseases such as ulcerative colitis. Called also *hyperplastic*, *inflammatory*, or *regenerative polyp*.

pseu•do•pol•yp•osis (soo″do-pol″ĭ-po′sis) the occurrence of numbers of pseudopolyps in the colon and rectum, as the result of long-standing inflammation.

pseu•do•por•phy•ria (soo″do-por-fēr′e-ə) any of various conditions that are clinically identical to porphyria but not characterized by abnormal excretion of porphyrins; seen most often in patients who are taking certain drugs or are on hemodialysis.

pseu•do•preg•nan•cy (soo″do-preg′nən-se) 1. false pregnancy. 2. the premenstrual stage of the endometrium; so called because it resembles the endometrium just before implantation of the blastocyst.

pseu•do•prog•na•thism (soo″do-prog′nə-thiz-əm) protruding mandible resembling prognathism but due to altered tooth alignment, resulting from malocclusion.

pseu•do•pro•tein•uria (soo″do-pro″te-nu′re-ə) adventitious proteinuria.

pseu•do•pseu•do•hy•po•para•thy•roid•ism (soo″do-soo″do-hi″po-par″ə-thi′roi-diz″əm) an incomplete form of pseudohypoparathyroidism characterized by the same constitutional features but by normal levels of calcium and phosphorus in the serum.

pseu•do•pter•yg•i•um (soo″do-tər-ij′e-əm) a conjunctival scar attached to the cornea, superficially resembling a true pterygium, but usually not firmly adherent to the underlying tissue.

pseu•do•pto•sis (soo″dop-to′sis, soo″do-to′sis) [*pseudo-* + *-ptosis*] decrease in the size of the palpebral aperture.

pseu•do•pu•ber•ty (soo″do-pu′bər-te) development of secondary sex characters and accessory reproductive organs without pubertal levels of gonadotropins and gonadotropin-releasing hormone, most often as a result of the release of steroid hormones by an adrenocortical or gonadal tumor; it may be either isosexual or contrasexual.

precocious p. appearance of some secondary sex characters before the normal age of puberty but without maturation of the gonads. Called also *gonadotropin-independent*, *incomplete*, or *peripheral precocious puberty*.

pseu•do•ra•bies (soo″do-ra′bēz) a highly contagious viral disease caused by a herpesvirus and primarily affecting the central nervous system. It is endemic in pigs; older pigs usually have a mild respiratory infection but piglets often have convulsions and die. It sometimes spreads to cattle, dogs, cats, and other mammals, in which its characteristics include sudden onset, severe pruritus, late paralysis, convulsions, and death within three to four days. Called also *Aujeszky disease* or *itch*, *mad itch*, and *infectious bulbar paralysis*.

Pseu•do•ra•mi•bac•ter (soo″do-ra″mĭ-bak′tər) [*pseudo-* + L. *ramus* branch + *-bacter*] a genus of gram-positive, strictly anaerobic bacteria of the family Eubacteriaceae, consisting of nonmotile non–spore-forming rods that occur in pairs resembling flying birds, clumps, or Chinese characters. The type species is *P. alactoly′ticus*.

P. alactoly′ticus a species isolated from the gingival crevice of persons with periodontal disease and from a variety of soft tissue infections. Formerly called *Eubacterium alactolyticum*.

pseu•do•re•ac•tion (soo″do-re-ak′shən) a false or deceptive reaction; in intradermal tests, a skin reaction due not to the specific protein used in the test but to the protein of the medium used to produce the toxin.

pseu•do•ret•in•i•tis pig•men•to•sa (soo″do-ret″in-i′tis pig″mən-to-sə) pigmentary degeneration of the retina that mimics retinitis pigmentosa but arises from some other cause, such as an intrauterine viral infection or a vascular lesion.

pseu•do•rick•ets (soo″do-rik′əts) renal osteodystrophy.

pseu•do•rin•der•pest (soo″do-rin′dər-pest) peste des petits ruminants.

pseu•do•ro•sette (soo″do-ro-zet′) a radial cluster of tumor cells encircling a small blood vessel; called also *perivascular pseudorosette*.

pseu•do•sar•co•ma (soo″do-sahr-ko′mə) [*pseudo-* + *sarcoma*] sarcomatoid transformation of a carcinoma histologically resembling a sarcoma; cf. *carcinosarcoma*.

pseu•do•sar•co•ma•tous (soo″do-sahr-ko′mə-təs) mimicking sarcoma; used of both benign and malignant lesions that histologically resemble sarcoma.

pseu•do•scle•ro•der•ma (soo″do-sklēr-o-dur′mə) any of various conditions resembling scleroderma or morphea, usually with eosinophilia, deep sclerosis of the skin and subcutaneous tissue, and inflammation. Some types are reactions to drugs or toxins; the Spanish toxic oil syndrome was a deadly type.

pseu•do•scle•ro•sis (soo″do-sklə-ro′sis) [*pseudo-* + *sclerosis*] a condition with the symptoms but not the lesions of multiple sclerosis.

Strümpell-Westphal p., Westphal-Strümpell p. Wilson disease.

pseu•do•scro•tum (soo″do-skro′təm) a solid partition with a median raphe, resembling the scrotum in the male, obliterating the opening into the vagina of a female pseudohermaphrodite.

pseu•do•sei•zure (soo″do-se′zhər) an attack resembling an epileptic seizure but being a type of conversion disorder; it lacks the electroencephalographic characteristics of epilepsy and the patient may be able to stop it by an act of will. Called also *pseudoepilepsy*.

pseud•os•mia (soo-doz′me-ə) [*pseudo-* + *osm-*[1] + *-ia*] a sensation of odor without the appropriate stimulus.

pseu•do•so•lu•tion (soo″do-so-loo′shən) a solution that does not act according to the usual physical laws of solutions; the term is sometimes applied to colloidal systems.

pseu•do•sto•ma (soo″do-sto′mə) [*pseudo-* + *stoma*] an apparent communication between silver-stained endothelial cells.

pseu•do•stra•bis•mus (soo″do-strə-bis′məs) a condition resembling strabismus but caused by an overhanging epicanthus that narrows the visible width of the sclera medial to the iris.

pseu•do•stro•phan•thin (soo″do-stro-fan′thin) a poisonous glycoside from the African shrub *Strophanthus hispidus*.

pseu•do•syn•dac•ty•ly (soo″do-sin-dak′tə-le) fusion of one or more web spaces between the digits secondary to a pathologic process.

pseu•do•ta•bes (soo″do-ta′bēz) [*pseudo-* + *tabes*] any neuropathy with symptoms like those of tabes dorsalis.

diabetic p. a form of diabetic neuropathy with symptoms in the lower limbs such as sensory loss, ataxia, ulceration, and sometimes lancinating pains and joint deformities; sometimes Argyll Robertson pupils occur. Called also *diabetic tabes*.

pupillotonic p. Adie syndrome.

Pseu•do•ter•ra•no•va (psoo″do-ter″ə-no′və) a genus of nematodes of the family Anisakidae; different stages of development are found in marine fishes and sea animals and cause anisakiasis in animals that eat raw or inadequately cooked seafood. Formerly called *Phocanema*.

pseu•do•tet•a•nus (soo″do-tet′ə-nəs) persistent muscular contractions resembling tetanus but not associated with the presence of *Clostridium tetani*.

pseu•do•thrill (soo′do-thril) a condition that simulates a true thrill.

pseu•do•tox•in (soo′do-tok″sin) a poisonous extract from belladonna leaves.

pseu•do•tra•cho•ma (soo″do-trə-ko′mə) a disease of the eye and lids resembling trachoma.

pseu•do•tris•mus (soo″do-tris′məs) a motor disorder of the mouth with symptoms similar to those of trismus.

pseu•do•trun•cus ar•te•ri•o•sus (soo″do-trung′kəs ahr-tēr″e-o′səs) the most severe form of tetralogy of Fallot, accompanied by pulmonary atresia in which outflow is through a single major vessel, the aorta, accompanied by the remnant of the atretic pulmonary artery.

pseu•do•tu•ber•cle (soo″do-too′bər-kəl) a tubercle resembling that of tuberculosis, but not due to the tubercle bacillus.

pseu•do•tu•ber•cu•lo•ma (soo″do-too-bur″ku-lo′mə) a tumor resembling in structure a tuberculoma.

pseu•do•tu•ber•cu•lo•sis (soo″do-too-bur″ku-lo′sis) [*pseudo-* + *tuberculosis*] any of various animal diseases resembling tuberculosis but caused by pathogens other than the tubercle bacillus; caseous swellings resembling tubercular nodules (pseudotubercles) form in organs throughout the body, and there may be fever and diarrhea with a fatal outcome. See *caseous lymphadenitis* and *yersiniosis* (def. 3).

pseu•do•tu•mor (soo″do-too′mər) an enlargement that resembles a tumor; it may result from inflammation, accumulation of fluid, or other causes, and may or may not regress spontaneously. Called also *pseudoneoplasm* and *false tumor*.

p. ce′rebri a condition of raised intracranial pressure with normal cerebrospinal fluid, in the absence of an intracranial mass, hydrocephalus, or other identifiable cause; symptoms include headache, nausea, vomiting, papilledema, and sometimes pulsatile tinnitus. Called also *benign* or *idiopathic intracranial hypertension*.

hepatic p. an inflammatory pseudotumor in the liver.

inflammatory p. a general term for a tumorlike mass representing an inflammatory reaction, occurring in a variety of organs and composed of granulation tissue with leukocyte infiltration. Called also *plasma cell granuloma*.

orbital p. a distinctive, chronic inflammatory reaction in the orbital tissues of the eye, of unknown etiology, that may closely resemble a neoplasm and often becomes bilateral. Symptoms include exophthalmos and congestion of the lids with edema. When limitation of ocular motility also occurs, it is sometimes called *orbital myositis*.

renal p. any mass in the kidney that is normal tissue but mimics something abnormal, such as in Bertin column hypertrophy or a dromedary hump.

pseu•do•ure•mia (soo″do-u-re′me-ə) uremia-like symptoms occurring in acute glomerulonephritis and in hypertensive vascular disease (hypertensive encephalopathy).

pseu•do•ure•tero•cele (soo″do-u-re′tər-o-sēl) a radiographic artifact resembling a ureterocele; it may be due to a cyst, a calcium deposit, or a dilated ureter that is outside the bladder.

pseu•do•uri•dine (soo′do-ūr′ĭ-dēn) 5-ribosyluracil, an unusual nucleotide occurring in transfer RNA; it is produced by posttranscriptional isomerization of uridine and differs from uridine in having the linkage between the 5-carbon of uracil and the 1-carbon of ribose. Symbol ψ.

pseu•do•vac•u•ole (soo″do-vak′u-ōl) a round space within certain red blood cells that contains an animal microorganism.

pseu•do•ven•tri•cle (soo″do-ven′trĭ-kəl) cavum septi pellucidi.

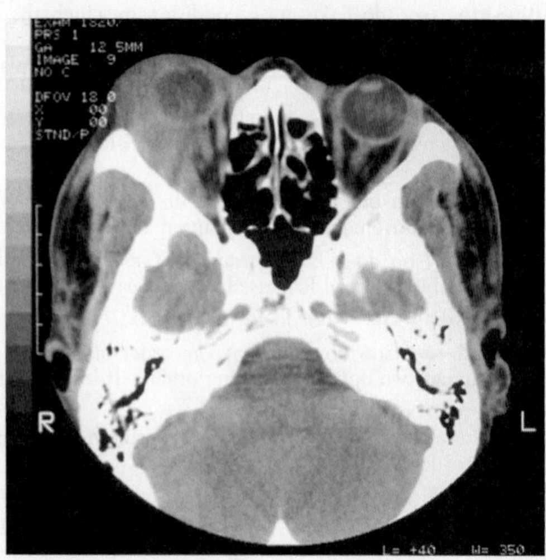

■ Orbital pseudotumor. Axial CT scan showing diffuse orbital inflammation of the right side.

pseu•do•ver•ti•go (soo″do-vur′tĭ-go) any dizziness or other form of lightheadedness that resembles vertigo but does not involve a sense of rotation. Among many possible causes are hyperventilation, orthostatic hypotension, and panic disorder.

pseu•do•voice (soo′do-vois) the vocal sounds produced under proper training after laryngectomy; see also *esophageal speech.*

pseu•do•vom•it•ing (soo″do-vom′it-ing) regurgitation of matter from the stomach without expulsive effort.

pseu•do•xan•thine (soo″do-zan′thēn) 1. a compound from muscle tissue or nucleic acids. 2. a compound from uric acid.

pseu•do•xan•tho•ma elas•ti•cum (soo″do-zan-tho′mə e-las′tĭ-kəm) an inherited disorder usually appearing after puberty with skin, eye, and cardiovascular manifestations, most of which result from basophilic degeneration of elastic tissue; it is usually an autosomal recessive disorder caused by mutation in the *ABCC6* gene (locus: 16p13.1), which encodes a transmembrane transporter important in elastic fiber assembly; some pseudodominance may also occur. Symptoms include small yellow cutaneous macules and papules that merge to form plaques, mainly in flexural areas; lax, inelastic, redundant skin; angioid streaks in the retina; arterial insufficiency in the lower limbs; premature calcification of peripheral arteries; reduced arterial pulses; symptoms of coronary insufficiency, hypertension, and mitral valve prolapse; and gastrointestinal and other hemorrhages. Called also *nevus elasticus.*

psi pounds per square inch.

psi•co•fur•a•nine (si″ko-fūr′ə-nēn) a nucleoside antibiotic produced by *Streptomyces hygroscopicus* that has antibacterial and antitumor activity.

psi•lo•cin (si′lo-sin) a hallucinogenic compound found in some species of *Psilocybe;* its chemical structure and activity are similar to those of psilocybin.

Psi•lo•cy•be (si″lo-si′be) a genus of mushrooms of the family Strophariaceae, native to the southern United States and Mexico; several species are sources of psilocybin and psilocin and are consumed in some North American Indian cultures as part of religious ceremonies.

psi•lo•cy•bin (si″lo-si′bin) a hallucinogenic crystalline compound with indole characteristics, isolated from mushrooms of the genus *Psilocybe,* especially *P. mexicana* Heim.

psit•ta•cine (sit′ə-sīn) [Gr. *psittakos* parrot] of or relating to parrots, parakeets, and related birds. See also *psittacosis.*

psit•ta•co•sis (sit″ə-ko′sis) [Gr. *psittakos* parrot + *-osis*] 1. an acute or chronic respiratory and systemic disease of wild and domestic birds, caused by infection with *Chlamydophila psittaci;* it was originally seen in psittacine birds and is transmissible to other animals. Called also *chlamydiosis.* 2. human infection by *C. psittaci,* generally acquired by inhalation of dried bird excreta containing the pathogen; it may also be acquired by handling feathers or tissues of infected birds, through an open skin lesion, or from the bite of an infected bird. It may be asymptomatic, have mild influenzalike symptoms, or manifest as severe pneumonia that lasts several weeks (see Chlamydophila psittaci *pneumonia,* under *pneumonia*). Called also *parrot disease* or *fever* and *ornithosis.*

PSM presystolic murmur.

PSMA prostate-specific membrane antigen.

pso•as (so′as) [Gr. genitive of *psoa* muscles of lower back] see *musculus psoas major* and *musculus psoas minor,* under *musculus.*

pso•dy•mus (sŏ′dĭ-məs) [*psoas* + *-didymus*] conjoined twins with two heads and trunks, but single at and below the loins.

pso•itis (so-i′tis) [*psoas* + *-itis*] inflammation of a psoas muscle or of its sheath.

Pso•ra•lea (so-ra′le-ə) a genus of plants of the family Leguminosae, many of which contain psoralens. The fruit of *P. coralifolia* is used in traditional Chinese medicine in topical preparations for alopecia and vitiligo.

psor•a•len (sor′ə-lən) 1. any of a group of photosensitizing constituents of plants such as *Ammi majus* or *Psoralea corylifolia;* examples are methoxsalen and trioxsalen. They are used in various perfumes or drugs and can cause phototoxic dermatitis. 2. any of the plants that contain one of these substances.

Psor•con (sor′kon) trademark for a preparation of diflorasone diacetate.

Pso•rer•ga•tes (sor″ər-ga′tēz) a genus of parasitic mites; *P. o′vis* causes pruritus and dermatitis in sheep. Called also *Psorobia.*

pso•ri•as•i•form (so″re-as′ĭ-form) resembling psoriasis.

pso•ri•a•sis (sə-ri′ə-sis) [Gr. *psōriasis*] any of a group of common chronic, squamous dermatoses with variable symptoms and courses; some are inherited. Principal histological findings are Munro microabscesses and spongiform pustules; also seen are rounded, circumscribed, erythematous, dry, scaling patches of various sizes, covered by gray, silvery, or white, umbilicated, lamellar scales. The most common sites are extensor surfaces, nails, scalp, genitalia, and the lumbosacral region. **psoriat′ic** *adj*

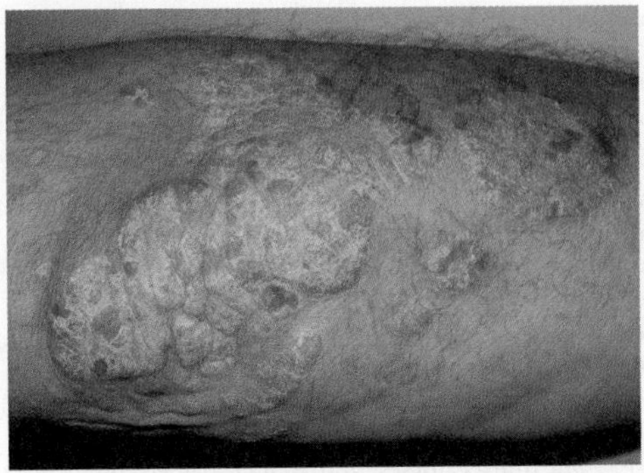

■ Psoriasis.

annular p., p. annula′ris, p. annula′ta psoriasis characterized by ring-shaped lesions with central healing; called also *circinate p.*

arthritic p., p. arthropa′thica psoriatic arthritis.

Barber p. localized pustular p.

p. bucca′lis a rare form of psoriasis that affects the oral mucosa.

p. circina′ta, circinate p. annular p.

discoid p. psoriasis characterized by round lesions with distinct borders; lesions may coalesce to form plaques, resulting in *plaque psoriasis.* Called also *nummular p.*

erythrodermic p., exfoliative p. a severe generalized erythrodermic condition usually developing chronically, such as in a reaction to topical therapy or ultraviolet exposure. Occasionally it occurs as the initial manifestation of psoriasis and has severe characteristics such as massive skin exfoliation associated with serious systemic illness and abnormalities of temperature and cardiovascular regulation that may even be fatal. Called also *psoriatic erythroderma.*

flexural p. inverse p.

follicular p. a rare form of psoriasis in which papules form around hair follicles; in adults it is mainly on the thighs, and in children it is more often on the trunk and tending to form large plaques.

generalized pustular p. severe and generalized pustular psoriasis, usually in patients with psoriatic arthritis or erythrodermic psoriasis. Characteristics include high fever, leukocytosis, hypocalcemia, arthralgia, malaise, and other systemic symptoms, sometimes resulting in death. Called also *von Zumbusch* or *Zumbusch p.*

p. gutta′ta, guttate p. psoriasis characterized by the abrupt appearance of small droplike lesions over much of the skin surface, especially on the trunk and proximal limbs; seen primarily in children and young adults, especially following streptococcal infections.

inverse p. a condition resembling seborrheic dermatitis. Lesions are moist and erythematous; have a few soft, greasy scales; and are found in flexures such as the axillae and the inguinal region, or in skinfolds such as in the inframammary, intergluteal, and perianal areas and on the palms, soles, and nails. Called also *flexural* or *volar p.* See also *seborrheic p.*

p. invetera′ta psoriasis characterized by confluent lesions and thickening and hardening of the skin.

p. lin′guae a rare form of psoriasis that affects the mucosa of the tongue.

localized pustular p. pustular psoriasis localized to the skin of the palms or the soles of the feet; there may also be psoriasis at other sites. It is accompanied by swelling, erythema, and local tenderness. Called also *Barber p., pustulosis palmaris et plantaris,* and *palmoplantar pustulosis.*

nummular p., p. nummula′ris discoid p.

p. ostra′cea, ostraceous p. rupioid p.

palmar p. a variant of palmoplantar psoriasis occurring only on the palms of the hands.

palmoplantar p., p. of palms and soles 1. localized pustular p. 2. inverse psoriasis limited to the palms and soles. Called also *volar p.*

plantar p. a variant of palmoplantar psoriasis occurring only on the soles of the feet.

plaque p. the most common type of psoriasis, in which lesions are in round plaques with distinct borders.

pustular p. chronic, relapsing psoriasis characterized by vesicles or pustules, generally occurring in association with a focal infection elsewhere in the body. Two types are recognized: a more severe *generalized pustular p.* and a less severe *localized pustular p.*

rupioid p., p. rupioi′des psoriasis in which the lesions form thick, tough patches covered with scales, somewhat resembling the outside of an oyster shell. Called also *p. ostracea.*

seborrheic p. inverse psoriasis of the scalp and adjacent facial areas.

volar p. 1. palmoplantar p. 2. localized pustular p.

von Zumbusch p. generalized pustular p.
p. vulga′ris psoriasis.
Zumbusch p. generalized pustular p.

Pso·ri·at·ec (sor″e-at′ek) trademark for a preparation of anthralin.

Pso·ro·bia (so-ro′be-ə) *Psorergates.*

Pso·roph·o·ra (sə-rof′o-rə) a genus of large, annoying mosquitoes of the tribe Aedini, subfamily Culicinae; their larvae prey on the larvae of other mosquitoes. Some species, particularly *P. ferox′* and *P. lut′zii,* act as carrier hosts of the eggs of *Dermatobia hominis.*

psor·oph·thal·mia (sor″of-thal′me-ə) [Gr. *psōrophthalmia*] a form of ulcerative marginal blepharitis.

Pso·rop·tes (sə-rop′tēz) a genus of mites of the family Psoroptidae, the cause of psoroptic mange (q.v.). *P. cuni′culi* infests the ears of rabbits and goats; *P. e′qui* infests horses; and *P. o′vis* (called also *P. bo′vis*) causes sheep scab in sheep and scabies in cattle and horses.

pso·rop·tic (sə-rop′tik) pertaining to or caused by *Psoroptes.*

Pso·rop·ti·dae (so-rop′tĭ-de) a family of parasitic long-legged mites, many of which cause mange in various animal species. Genera include *Chorioptes, Otodectes,* and *Psoroptes.*

PSP phenolsulfonphthalein.

PSRO Professional Standards Review Organization.

PSTI pancreatic secretory trypsin inhibitor.

PSVT paroxysmal supraventricular tachycardia.

psy·chal·ga·lia (si″kəl-ga′le-ə) psychalgia.

psy·chal·gia (si-kal′jə) [*psych-* + *-algia*] 1. pain, usually in the head and perceived as being of emotional origin, that may accompany intolerable ideas, obsessions, or hallucinations; called also *psychic pain.* 2. psychogenic pain; see also *pain disorder,* under *disorder.*

psy·chal·gic (si-kal′jik) pertaining to or characterized by psychalgia.

psy·cha·tax·ia (si″kə-tak′se-ə) a disordered mental condition marked by confusion and inability to concentrate.

psy·che (si′ke) [Gr. *psychē* the organ of thought and judgment] 1. the human faculty for thought, judgment, and emotion; the mental life, including both conscious and unconscious processes; the mind in its totality, as distinguished from the body. 2. the soul or self.

psy·che·del·ic (si″kə-del′ik) [*psyche* + Gr. *dēlos* manifest, evident] 1. pertaining to or characterized by hallucinations, distortions of perception and awareness, and sometimes psychotic-like behavior. 2. a drug that produces such effects.

psy·chi·a·trist (si-ki′ə-trist) a physician who specializes in psychiatry.

psy·chi·a·try (si-ki′ə-tre) [*psych-* + *-iatry*] the branch of medicine that deals with the study, treatment, and prevention of mental disorders. **psychiat′ric** *adj*

addiction p. a subspecialty concerned with the diagnosis and treatment of addiction and other problems related to substance use.
administrative p. the branch of psychiatry concerned with the organization and management of mental health programs and facilities, including public and private hospitals, clinics, and centers.
biological p. the subspecialty that emphasizes biochemical, neurological, and pharmacological causes and treatment approaches.
community p. the branch of psychiatry concerned with the detection, prevention, and treatment of mental disorders as they develop within psychosocial, cultural, or geographical areas, with emphasis given to environmental factors.
consultation liaison p. the subspecialty that connects psychiatry with other areas of medicine, bringing a psychosocial approach to the biological treatment of organic illness. Called also *liaison p.*
cross-cultural p., cultural p. the study of mental illness and mental health among different societies, nations, and cultures; called also *transcultural p.*
descriptive p. psychiatry based on the study of observable symptoms and behavioral phenomena, rather than underlying psychodynamic processes; cf. *dynamic p.*
dynamic p. psychiatry based on the study of the unconscious mechanisms, conflicts, and other emotional processes that motivate and underlie human behavior, rather than the more observable behaviors themselves; cf. *descriptive p.*
existential p. psychiatry based on the existential philosophy of Kierkegaard, Heidegger, Jaspers, and others, holding the view that persons must take responsibility for their own existence.
forensic p. psychiatry that deals with the legal aspects of mental disorders.
geriatric p. geropsychiatry.
industrial p. the branch of psychiatry concerned with the diagnosis and prevention of mental illness in the work setting, including aspects of absenteeism, accident proneness, personnel policies, occupational fatigue, substance abuse, vocational adjustment, retirement, interpersonal relations, and related phenomena.
liaison p. consultation liaison p.
military p. the study and treatment of psychiatric problems done under the auspices of military organizations such as induction centers, training facilities, and military hospitals; it includes emergency and nonemergency treatment for active-duty and retired military personnel and their dependents.
occupational p. industrial p.
orthomolecular p. psychiatry based on the theory that psychiatric illnesses are due to disturbances in the molecular environment of the brain and can be cured by restoration of optimal concentrations of substances normally present in the body, such as vitamins *(orthomolecular therapy).* Cf. *orthomolecular medicine.*
preventive p. the branch of psychiatry broadly concerned with the amelioration, control, and limitation of psychiatric disability. It is often categorized as *primary*—measures to prevent a disorder; *secondary*—therapeutic measures to limit a disorder; and *tertiary*—measures and intervention to reduce impairment or disability following a disorder.
social p. the branch of psychiatry concerned with the cultural, ecologic, and sociologic facts that engender, precipitate, intensify, prolong, or otherwise complicate maladaptive patterns of behavior and their treatment.
transcultural p. cross-cultural p.

psy·chic (si′kik) pertaining to the psyche or to the mind; mental.

psych(o)- [Gr. *psychē* the mind, reason] a combining form denoting relationship to the psyche, or to the mind.

psy·cho·acous·tics (si″ko-ə-ko͞os′tiks) a branch of psychophysics involving the study of the relationship between acoustic stimuli and behavior.

psy·cho·ac·tive (si″ko-ak′tiv) psychotropic.

psy·cho·an·a·lep·tic (si″ko-an″ə-lep′tik) [*psycho-* + *analeptic*] exerting a stimulating effect upon the mind.

psy·cho·anal·y·sis (si″ko-ə-nal′ĭ-sis) 1. a theory of human mental phenomena and behavior (Freud). 2. a method of investigation into the contents of the mind. 3. a therapeutic technique based on Freud's theory, focusing on the influence that unconscious forces such as repressed impulses, internal conflicts, and childhood trauma have on the mental state. The therapist elicits from patients past emotional experiences and their influence on current mental life, so as to delineate the conflicts and mechanisms by which a pathologic mental state has been produced to furnish hints for psychotherapeutic procedures. The method employs free association, recall and interpretation of dreams, and interpretation of transference and resistance phenomena.

psy·cho·an·a·lyst (si″ko-an′ə-list) a practitioner of psychoanalysis.

psy·cho·an·a·lyt·ic (si″ko-an″ə-lit′ik) pertaining to psychoanalysis.

psy·cho·au·di·to·ry (si″ko-aw′dĭ-tor″e) pertaining to the conscious and intelligent perception of sound.

psy·cho·bi·o·log·i·cal (si″ko-bi″o-loj′ĭ-kəl) pertaining to psychobiology.

psy·cho·bi·ol·o·gist (si″ko-bi-ol′ə-jist) a specialist in psychobiology.

psy·cho·bi·ol·o·gy (si″ko-bi-ol′ə-je) 1. a field of study examining the relationship between brain and mind, studying the effect of biological influences, including biochemical, neurological, and pharmacological factors, on psychological functioning or mental processes. Called also *biopsychology.* 2. Adolf Meyer's school of psychiatric thought, in which the human being is viewed as an integrated unit, incorporating psychological, social, and biological functions, with behavior a function of the total organism.

psy·cho·ca·thar·sis (si″ko-kə-thahr′sis) [*psycho-* + *catharsis*] catharsis (def. 2).

psy·cho·chem·is·try (si″ko-kem′is-tre) the science that deals with the relationship between chemistry and psychologic processes.

psy·cho·chrome (si′ko-krōm) [*psycho-* + *-chrome*] a subjective mental association between any bodily sensation and some particular color.

psy·cho·chrom·es·the·sia (si″ko-krōm″es-the′zhə) chromesthesia.

psy·cho·cor·ti·cal (si″ko-kor′tĭ-kəl) [*psycho-* + *cortical*] pertaining to the mind and to the cortex of the brain as the site of mental functions.

psy·cho·cu·ta·ne·ous (si″ko-ku-ta′ne-əs) pertaining to the relations between mental or emotional factors and skin disorders; see *psychodermatology.*

psy·cho·der·ma·tol·o·gy (si″ko-dur″mə-tol′ə-je) the study of the relations between mental or emotional factors and skin disorders; called also *psychocutaneous medicine.*

psy·cho·di·ag·no·sis (si″ko-di″əg-no′sis) the use of psychological methods of assessment in the diagnosis of psychiatric disorders.

psy·cho·di·ag·nos·tics (si″ko-di″əg-nos′tiks) psychodiagnosis.

Psy·cho·di·dae (si-ko′dĭ-de) a family of flies, the owl flies or sandflies, of the order Diptera, characterized by small size, long legs, and abundant hair on both wings and body. It includes the genera *Lutzomyia* and *Phlebotomus.*

psy·cho·dom·e·ter (si″ko-dom′ə-tər) an instrument for measuring the rate of mental processes.

psy·cho·dom·e·try (si″ko-dom′ə-tre) [*psycho-* + Gr. *hodos* way + *-metry*] measurement of the rate of mental processes.

psy·cho·dra·ma (si′ko-drah″mə) a form of group psychotherapy in which patients dramatize their own or assigned life situations in order to achieve insight into personalities, relationships, conflicts, and emotional problems, and to alter faulty behavior patterns.

psy·cho·dy·nam·ics (si″ko-di-nam′iks) [*psycho-* + *dynamics*] the interplay of conscious and unconscious motivational forces, such as wishes, drives, emotions, conflict, and defense mechanisms, that gives rise to the expression of mental processes, as in attitudes, behavior, or symptoms.

psy·cho·dys·lep·tic (si″ko-dis-lep′tik) [*psycho-* + Gr. *dys-* bad + *lēpsis* a taking hold] inducing a dreamlike or delusional state of mind.

psy·cho·en·do·crine (si-ko-en′do-krin) psychoneuroendocrine.

psy·cho·en·do·cri·nol·o·gy (si-ko-en″do-krĭ-nol′ə-je) psychoneuroendocrinology.

psy·cho·gal·van·ic (si″ko-gal-van′ik) pertaining to certain changes in the electrical properties of the skin that are presumed to have a psychologic component, such as in galvanic skin responses.

psy·cho·gal·va·nom·e·ter (si″ko-gal″və-nom′ə-tər) an instrument similar to a polygraph, able to detect changes in skin resistance to electric current.

psy·cho·gen·e·sis (si″ko-jen′ə-sis) [*psycho-* + *-genesis*] 1. mental development. 2. production of a symptom or illness by psychic factors.

psy·cho·gen·ic (si″ko-jen′ik) [*psycho-* + *-genic*] produced or caused by psychological factors. See also *psychosomatic.*

psy·cho·ger·i·at·rics (si″ko-jer″e-at′riks) geropsychiatry.

psy·cho·gram (si′ko-gram) [*psycho-* + *-gram*] 1. psychograph. 2. a visual sensation associated with a mental idea, as of a certain number that appears visualized when it is thought of.

psy·cho·graph (si′ko-graf) [*psycho-* + *-graph*] 1. a chart for recording graphically the personality traits of an individual. 2. a written description of the mental functioning of an individual.

psy·cho·ki·ne·sis (si″ko-kĭ-ne′sis) [*psycho-* + *-kinesis*] the postulated direct influence of volitional action on a physical object, or the influence of mind on matter without the intermediation of physical force.

psy·cho·lag·ny (si′ko-lag″ne) [*psycho-* + Gr. *lagneia* lust] the experiencing of sexual enjoyment from imagining or thinking of sexual acts.

psy·cho·lep·sy (si′ko-lep″se) [*psycho-* + Gr. *lēpsis* a taking hold, a seizure] a sudden, intense lowering of mood level, usually of short duration, in individuals with unstable psychic tension.

psy·cho·lin·guis·tics (si″ko-ling-gwis′tiks) the study of psychological aspects of language acquisition, processing, and production, on the part of both the producer and the receiver.

psy·chol·o·gist (si-kol′ə-jist) a qualified specialist in psychology.

psy·chol·o·gy (si-kol′ə-je) [*psycho-* + *-logy*] the branch of science that deals with the mind and mental processes, especially in relation to human and animal behavior. **psycholog′ic, psycholog′ical** *adj*

abnormal p. the study of mental disorders and behavior disturbances.

analytic p., analytical p. the system of psychology founded by Carl G. Jung, based on the concepts of the collective unconscious and the complex.

animal p. the study of the mental activity of animals.

behavioristic p. see *behaviorism.*

child p. the study of the development of the mind of the child.

clinical p. the use of psychologic knowledge and techniques in the treatment of persons with mental, emotional, behavior, and developmental disorders.

cognitive p. the branch of psychology that deals with how the human mind receives and interprets impressions and ideas.

community p. the application of psychological principles to the study and support of the mental health of individuals in their social context.

comparative p. the study of behavior using a comparison of species as a source of knowledge.

criminal p. the study of the mentality, the motivation, and the social behavior of criminals.

depth p. the study of unconscious mental processes.

developmental p. the study of changes in behavior that occur through the life span.

dynamic p. psychology that stresses the causes of and motivations for behavior.

environmental p. study of the effects of the physical and social environment on behavior.

experimental p. the study of mental operations and behaviors by the employment of controlled laboratory procedures.

gestalt p. see *gestaltism.*

individual p. Alfred Adler's psychological theory that stresses the role of compensation for feelings of inferiority as the source of psychological and interpersonal problems.

physiologic p., physiological p. the branch of psychology that studies the relationship between physiologic and psychologic processes.

social p. psychology that focuses on social interaction, on the ways in which actions of others influence the behavior of an individual.

psy·chom·e·ter (si-kom′ə-tər) an instrument used in psychometry.

psy·cho·me·tri·cian (si″ko-mə-trish′ən) a person skilled in psychometry.

psy·cho·met·rics (si″ko-met′riks) psychometry.

psy·chom·e·try (si-kom′ə-tre) [*psycho-* + *-metry*] systematic measurement of mental processes and behavioral acts.

psy·cho·mo·tor (si″ko-mo′tər) pertaining to motor effects of cerebral or psychic activity.

psy·cho·neu·ral (si″ko-noor′əl) relating to the totality of neural events initiated by a sensory input and leading to storage, to discrimination, or to an output of any kind.

psy·cho·neu·ro·en·do·crine (si-ko-noor″o-en′do-krin) pertaining to the interaction between the endocrine system, the central nervous system, and a person's mental or emotional state; see also *psychoneuroendocrinology.*

psy·cho·neu·ro·en·do·cri·nol·o·gy (si″ko-noor″o-en″do-krĭ-nol′ə-je) [*psycho-* + *neuroendocrinology*] the study of the effects of the nervous and endocrine system on emotional processes.

psy·cho·neu·ro·im·mu·nol·o·gy (si″ko-noor″o-im″u-nol′ə-je) the study of the interactions between psychological factors (such as stress or conditioned reaction), the central nervous system, and immune function as modulated by the neuroendocrine system.

psy·cho·neu·ro·sis (si″ko-nŏŏ-ro′sis) neurosis.

psy·cho·path (si′ko-path″) former term for a person with antisocial personality disorder.

psy·cho·pa·thol·o·gy (si″ko-pə-thol′ə-je) [*psycho-* + *pathology*] 1. the pathology of mental disorders; the branch of medicine that deals with the causes and nature of mental disease. 2. abnormal, maladaptive behavior or mental activity.

psy·chop·a·thy (si-kop′ə-the) [*psycho-* + *-pathy*] broadly, a mental disorder; sometimes used specifically for *antisocial personality disorder.* **psychopath′ic** *adj*

psy·cho·phar·ma·col·o·gy (si″ko-fahr″mə-kol′ə-je) 1. the study of the action of drugs on psychological functions and mental states. 2. the use of drugs to modify psychological functions and mental states.

psy·cho·phys·i·cal (si″ko-fiz′ĭ-kəl) pertaining to the mind and its relation to physical manifestations.

psy·cho·phys·ics (si″ko-fiz′iks) [*psycho-* + *physics*] the science dealing with the quantitative relationships between the characteristics or patterns of physical stimuli and the resultant sensations.

psy·cho·phys·io·log·ic (si″ko-fiz″e-o-loj′ik) [*psycho-* + *physiologic*] 1. psychosomatic. 2. pertaining to psychophysiology (physiologic psychology).

psy·cho·phys·i·ol·o·gy (si″ko-fiz″e-ol′ə-je) physiologic psychology.

psy·cho·ple·gic (si″ko-ple′jik) an agent that lessens cerebral activity or excitability.

psy·cho·pro·phy·lax·is (si″ko-pro″fĭ-lak′sis) a technique of natural childbirth using mental and physical training aimed at the suppression of painful sensations associated with labor and delivery; see also *Lamaze method,* under *method.* **psychoprophylac′tic** *adj*

psy·cho·sen·so·ri·al (si″ko-sən-sor′e-əl) psychosensory.

psy·cho·sen·so·ry (si″ko-sen′sə-re) pertaining to the conscious perception of sensory impulses to the mind and to sensation.

psy·cho·ses (si-ko′sēz) plural of *psychosis.*

psy·cho·sex·u·al (si″ko-sek′shoo-əl) pertaining to the mental or emotional aspects of sex or sexuality.

psy·cho·sine (si′ko-sēn) a cerebroside derivative lacking its fatty acyl chain; it is sphingosine linked via its 1-hydroxyl group to a monosaccharide group.

psy·cho·sis (si-ko'sis) pl. *psycho'ses* [*psych-* + *-osis*] 1. a mental disorder characterized by gross impairment in reality testing as evidenced by delusions, hallucinations, markedly incoherent speech, or disorganized and agitated behavior, usually without apparent awareness on the part of the patient of the incomprehensibility of this behavior; called *psychotic disorder* in DSM-IV. 2. the term is also used in a more general sense to refer to mental disorders in which mental functioning is so impaired that it interferes grossly with the patient's capacity to meet the ordinary demands of life. Historically, the term has been applied to many conditions, e.g., manic-depressive psychosis, that were first described in psychotic patients, although many patients with the disorder are not judged psychotic.

acute delusional p. bouffée délirante.

affective p. a psychosis in which a disturbance in mood is the prominent characteristic; see *mood disorders*, under *disorder*.

alcoholic p's psychoses associated with alcohol use and involving organic brain damage; the category includes alcohol withdrawal delirium, Korsakoff syndrome, and hallucinosis and paranoia accompanying alcoholism.

bipolar p. see under *disorder*.

brief reactive p. a brief psychotic disorder (q.v.) occurring in response to a stressful life event.

depressive p. a psychosis characterized by severe depression; now more commonly described as a form of major depressive disorder (q.v.) with psychotic features.

drug p. any psychosis associated with drug use.

functional p. a psychosis for which organic disease or dysfunction cannot be found to play a causative role.

Korsakoff p. see under *syndrome*.

interictal p. psychotic symptoms occurring between attacks of epilepsy, especially temporal lobe epilepsy.

manic p. the manic phase of bipolar disorder.

manic-depressive p. former name for bipolar disorder; see *bipolar disorders* (def. 2), under *disorder*.

organic p. psychosis that has a known or presumed organic etiology.

postictal p. psychotic symptoms occurring after a seizure, most often when there is a cluster of seizures that may have been followed by a lucid period of one to three days. Some patients have hallucinations or delusions, with danger of suicide or other violence in response to an imaginary command; others have anxiety or panic disorders.

postpartum p. psychosis in a woman who has recently given birth.

prison p. any psychosis for which a prison environment has been a precipitating factor.

reactive p. brief reactive p.

schizoaffective p. see under *disorder*.

senile p. depressive or paranoid delusions or hallucinations or other mental disorders due primarily to degeneration of the brain in old age, as in senile dementia.

toxic p. a psychosis due to the ingestion of toxic agents (e.g., alcohol, opium) or to the presence of toxins within the body.

psy·cho·so·cial (si"ko-so'shəl) pertaining to or involving both psychic and social aspects.

psy·cho·so·mat·ic (si"ko-so-mat'ik) [*psycho-* + *somat-* + *-ic*] pertaining to the mind-body relationship; having bodily symptoms of psychic, emotional, or mental origin; called also *psychophysiologic.* See also under *disorder.*

psy·cho·stim·u·lant (si"ko-stim'u-lənt) 1. producing a transient increase in psychomotor activity. 2. a drug that produces such effects, such as caffeine, methylphenidate, or the amphetamines.

psy·cho·sur·gery (si"ko-sur'jər-e) brain surgery performed for treatment of psychiatric disorders; called also *psychiatric surgery* and *functional neurosurgery.* **psychosur'gical** *adj*

psy·cho·tech·nics (si"ko-tek'niks) [*psycho-* + Gr. *technē* art] the employment of psychological methods in studying sociological and other problems.

psy·cho·ther·a·peu·tics (si"ko-ther"ə-pu'tiks) psychotherapy.

psy·cho·ther·a·py (si"ko-ther'ə-pe) [*psycho-* + *therapy*] treatment of mental disorders and behavioral disturbances using verbal and nonverbal communication, including such psychological techniques as support, suggestion, persuasion, reeducation, reassurance, and insight, in order to alter maladaptive patterns of coping, relieve emotional disturbance, and encourage personality growth. It is usually contrasted with therapies involving physical interventions, such as drug or convulsive therapies. See also under *therapy.*

brief p. any of numerous forms of psychotherapy limited to a preagreed number of sessions, generally 10 to 20, or having a termination date; most types are active and directive, and many are oriented toward a specific problem or symptom. See table.

existential p. psychotherapy based on the existential philosophy of Kierkegaard, Heidegger, Jaspers, etc., in which the emphasis is on present interactions and feeling experiences rather than on rational thinking.

Selected Brief Psychotherapy Methods

Brief dynamic psychotherapy (BDP)
Brief psychotherapy for stress-response syndromes (BPSRS)
Cognitive-behavioral therapy (CBT)
Dialectical behavior therapy (DBT)
Interpersonal psychotherapy (IPT)
Short-term anxiety-provoking psychotherapy (STAPP)
Short-term dynamic psychotherapy (STDP)
Supportive-expressive (SE) psychotherapy
Time-limited psychotherapy (TLP)
Time-limited dynamic psychotherapy (TLDP)

group p. see under *therapy.*

interpersonal p. a form of brief psychotherapy that treats mood disorders by addressing interpersonal problems, emphasizing that the mood disorder is a medical illness and focusing on healing current relationships in a specific problem area in the here and now.

psychoanalytic p. psychoanalysis (def. 3).

supportive p. psychotherapy aimed at reinforcing a patient's defenses, relieving immediate crises or acute disequilibria, reducing symptoms to a premorbid level, and promoting the healthy aspects of the patient, without probing emotional conflicts or trying to alter the basic personality. Specific methods include advice; guidance; reassurance; desensitization; art, music, or dance therapy; and occupational therapy.

psy·chot·ic (si-kot'ik) 1. pertaining to, characterized by, or caused by psychosis. 2. a person exhibiting psychosis.

psy·chot·o·gen·ic (si-kot"o-jen'ik) psychotomimetic.

psy·chot·o·mi·met·ic (si-kot"o-mĭ-met'ik) [*psychosis* + *-mimetic*] 1. pertaining to, characterized by, or producing manifestations like those of a psychosis, such as visual hallucinations, distortion of perception, and schizophrenia-like behavior. 2. a drug or other agent that has such effects; called also *psychotogenic.*

psy·cho·tro·pic (si"ko-tro'pik) [*psycho-* + *-tropic*] exerting an effect upon the mind; capable of modifying mental activity; usually applied to drugs that affect the mental state. Called also *psychoactive.*

psychr(o)- [Gr. *psychros* cold] a combining form denoting relationship to cold.

psy·chro·al·gia (si"kro-al'jə) a painful feeling of cold. Cf. *cryesthesia.*

psy·chro·es·the·sia (si"kro-es-the'zhə) [*psychro-* + *esthsia*] a state in which a part of the body, though objectively warm when touched, is experienced as being cold.

psy·chrom·e·ter (si-krom'ə-tər) [*psychro-* + *-meter*] an apparatus for measuring atmospheric moisture by the difference in reading of two thermometers, one with a dry bulb and one with a wet bulb.

sling p. an instrument in which the thermometers are swung through the air to facilitate evaporation from the wet bulb.

psy·chro·phile (si'kro-fīl) an organism that grows best at low temperatures.

psy·chro·phil·ic (si"kro-fil'ik) [*psychro-* + *-philic*] fond of cold; said of bacteria that grow in the cold, often growing best between 15° and 20° C. See also *mesophilic* and *thermophilic.*

psyl·li·um (sil'e-əm) 1. a plant of the genus *Plantago. Blond p.* is *P. ovata* and *Spanish p.* is *P. psyllium.* 2. the husk *(psyllium husk)* or seed *(plantago* or *psyllium seed)* of various species of *Plantago*; used as a bulk-forming laxative.

PT prothrombin time.

Pt platinum.

pt pint.

PTA plasma thromboplastin antecedent (factor XI; see under *coagulation factors*, at *factor*).

ptar·mus (tahr'məs) [Gr. *ptarmos*] spasmodic sneezing. **ptar'mic** *adj*

PTC plasma thromboplastin component (factor IX; see under *coagulation factors*, at *factor*); phenylthiocarbamide.

PTCA percutaneous transluminal coronary angioplasty.

PteGlu pteroylglutamate or pteroylglutamic acid; see *folic acid.*

pter the end of the short arm of a chromosome.

pter·i·dine (ter'ĭ-dēn) a bicyclic aromatic nitrogenous compound or the class of compounds containing such a ring structure. Most naturally occurring pteridine derivatives are pterins.

Pte·ri·di·um (tə-rid'e-əm) a genus of ferns. *P. aquili'num* L. Kuhn (Polypodia'ceae) is the bracken. See also *bracken poisoning*, under *poisoning.*

pter·in (ter'in) [Gr. *pteron* wing] the 2-amino, 4-hydroxy derivative of pteridine; the term is also used to denote the class of compounds containing

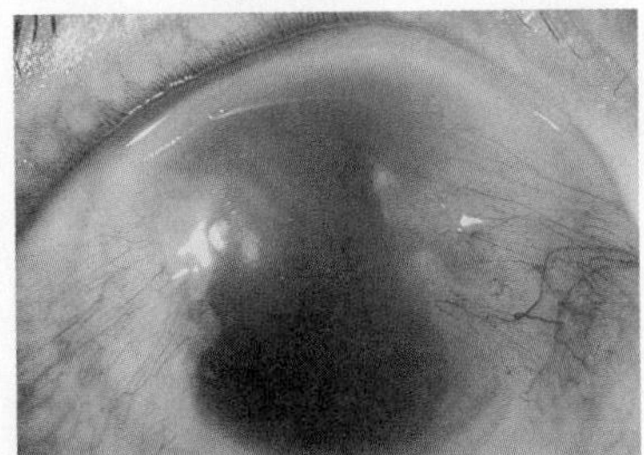

■ Pterygia of both the lateral and medial canthi.

such a ring structure, such as tetrahydrobiopterin or folic acid. Pterins are so named because they were first identified in the wings of butterflies.

pter·in-4α-car·bin·ol·amine de·hy·dra·tase (PCD) (ter′in kahr″bin-ol′ə-mēn de-hi′drə-tās) 4a-hydroxytetrahydrobiopterin dehydratase.

pte·ri·on (tēr′e-on) [Gr. *pteron* wing] [TA] a point at the junction of the frontal, parietal, temporal, and greater wing of the sphenoid bone; about 3 cm posterior to the external angular process of the orbit.

pte·ro·ic ac·id (tə-ro′ik) a constituent of folic acid consisting of *p*-aminobenzoic acid linked to a substituted pteridine by a methylene bridge.

pter·o·yl·glu·ta·mate (PteGlu) (ter″o-əl-gloo′tə-māt) an anionic form of pteroylglutamic (folic) acid. See *folic acid.*

pter·o·yl·glu·tam·ic ac·id (PteGlu) (ter″o-əl-gloo-tam′ik) folic acid.

pter·o·yl·poly·glu·ta·mate (ter″o-əl-pol″e-gloo′tə-māt) any of the folate compounds having more than one glutamate residue; it is the usual form in which folates are stored in foods and in body tissues.

pte·ryg·i·um (tə-rij′e-əm) pl. *ptery′gia* [Gr. *pterygion* wing] 1. a winglike structure. 2. especially, an abnormal triangular fold of membrane in the interpalpebral fissure, extending from the conjunctiva to the cornea; it is immovably united to the cornea at its apex, firmly attached to the sclera in its middle portion, and merged with the conjunctiva at its base.

p. col′li a congenital condition in which there is a thick fold of skin on the side of the neck from the mastoid region to the acromion; it occurs in association with genetic syndromes such as Turner syndrome and Noonan syndrome. Called also *webbed neck.*

congenital p. epitarsus.

pter·y·goid (ter′ĭ-goid) [Gr. *pterygōdēs* like a wing] shaped like a wing.

pter·y·go·man·dib·u·lar (ter″ĭ-go-man-dib′u-lər) pertaining to the pterygoid process and the mandible.

pter·y·go·max·il·lary (ter″ĭ-go-mak′sĭ-lar-e) pertaining to a pterygoid process and the maxilla.

pter·y·go·pal·a·tine (ter″ĭ-go-pal′ə-tīn) pertaining to a pterygoid process and to the palate bone; in anatomy it is sometimes interchangeable with the term *sphenopalatine.*

PTFE polytetrafluoroethylene; see *polytef.*

PTH parathyroid hormone.

Pthir·us (thir′əs) *Phthirus.*

pto·maine (to′mān, to-mān′) [Gr. *ptōma* carcass] any of several toxic bases formed by decarboxylation of an amino acid, often by bacterial action, such as cadaverine, muscarine, neurine, ptomatropine, or putrescine.

pto·mat·ro·pine (to-mat′ro-pēn) [*ptomaine* + *atropine*] a poison from putrid sausages and the viscera of corpses of those dead from typhoid fever; it has effects somewhat like those of atropine.

ptosed (tōst) affected with ptosis; prolapsed.

pto·sis (to′sis) [Gr. *ptōsis* fall] 1. prolapse. 2. drooping of the upper eyelid; called also *blepharoptosis.*

p. adipo′sa, false p. an apparent ptosis caused by a fold of skin and fat hanging down below the border of the eyelid.

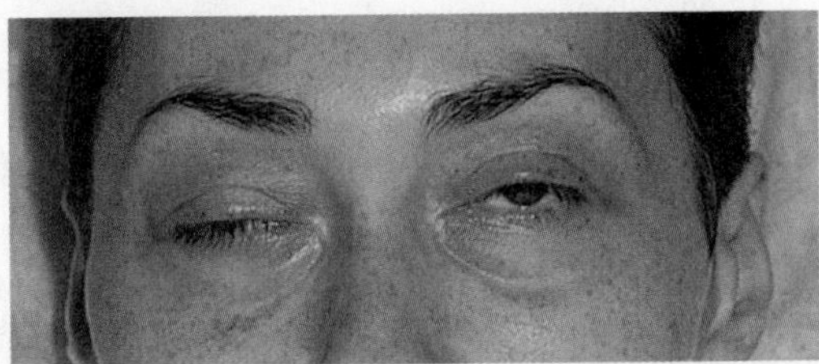

■ Bilateral ptosis.

aponeurogenic p., aponeurotic p. the most common acquired ptosis, caused by a defect in the aponeurosis of the levator palpebrae superioris muscle. Cf. *involutional p.*

congenital p. ptosis present at birth and resulting from maldevelopment of the levator palpebrae superioris muscle.

Horner p. moderate ptosis with retraction of the eyeball, miosis, and flushing of the affected side of the face, due to lesions of the cervical sympathetic nerves, part of the symptom complex called *Horner syndrome.* Called also *p. sympathetica.*

involutional p. ptosis resulting from degeneration of the attachment of the levator palpebrae superioris muscle to the eyelid; it is usually caused by a defect in the aponeurosis *(aponeurotic p.)*, but it can have other causes, such as fatty degeneration of the muscle. The term is often used synonymously with *aponeurotic p.*

p. lipomato′sis ptosis produced by lipoma of the eyelid.

mechanical p. acquired ptosis due blepharochalasis or to the presence of a mass, such as a tumor of the eyelid or scar tissue, that weighs down the lid or interferes with movement.

morning p. waking p.

myogenic p. acquired ptosis occurring as a manifestation of myopathy involving the levator palpebrae superioris muscle or the myoneural junction.

neurogenic p. ptosis due to dysfunction of the of the third cranial nerve or of the sympathetic innervation of the superior tarsal muscle (Müller muscle).

renal p. nephroptosis.

p. sympathe′tica Horner p.

waking p. temporary paralysis of the upper lid on awakening from sleep.

-ptosis [Gr. *ptōsis* fall] a word termination indicating downward displacement.

ptot·ic (tot′ik) pertaining to or affected with ptosis.

PTPS 6-pyruvoyltetrahydropterin synthase.

PTRA percutaneous transluminal renal angioplasty.

PTS 6-pyruvoyltetrahydropterin synthase.

PTSD posttraumatic stress disorder.

PTT partial thromboplastin time.

pty·al·a·gogue (ti-al′ə-gog) sialagogue.

pty·a·lec·ta·sis (ti″ə-lek′tə-sis) [*ptyalo-* + *ectasis*] 1. operative dilatation of a salivary duct. 2. dilatation of one of the ducts of the salivary glands.

pty·a·lin (ti′ə-lin) [Gr. *ptyalon* spittle] α-amylase occurring in saliva.

pty·a·lism (ti′ə-liz″əm) [Gr. *ptyalismos*] excessive salivation. Called also *hyperptyalism, hypersalivation, ptyalorrhea, salivation, sialism,* and *sialorrhea.*

pty·a·lize (ti′ə-līz) to increase or stimulate the secretion of saliva.

ptyal(o)- [Gr. *ptyalon* saliva] a combining form denoting relationship to saliva. See also words beginning *sial(o)-.*

pty·alo·cele (ti-al′o-sēl) [*ptyalo-* + *-cele*[1]] a cystic tumor containing saliva.

sublingual p. ranula.

pty·al·o·gen·ic (ti″ə-lo-jen′ik) [*ptyalo-* + *-genic*] formed from or by the action of saliva.

pty·a·log·ra·phy (ti″ə-log′rə-fe) [*ptyalo-* + *-graphy*] sialography.

pty·a·lo·li·thi·a·sis (ti″ə-lo-lĭ-thi′ə-sis) [*ptyalo-* + *lith-* + *-iasis*] sialolithiasis.

pty·a·lo·li·thot·o·my (ti″ə-lo-lĭ-thot′ə-me) sialolithotomy.

pty·a·lor·rhea (ti″ə-lo-re′ə) [*ptyalo-* + *-rrhea*] ptyalism.

pty·oc·ri·nous (ti-ok′rĭ-nəs) [Gr. *ptyon* a winnowing shovel, or fan + *krinein* to separate] elaborating secretion in the form of granules that are eventually extruded; said of unicellular glands such as goblet cells that secrete in this way. Cf. *diacrinous.*

Pu plutonium.

pu·bar·che (pu-bahr′ke) the beginning of puberty, signaled by growth of the pubic hair.

pu·ber·tas (pu-bur′təs) [L.] puberty.

p. prae′cox precocious puberty.

pu·ber·ty (pu′bər-te) [L. *pubertas*] the period during which the secondary sex characters begin to develop and the capability of sexual reproduction is attained. **pu′beral, pu′bertal** *adj*

central precocious p. precocious puberty caused by premature hypothalamic-pituitary-gonadal maturation; it is always isosexual and involves not only development of secondary sex characters but also development of the gonads. Increases in height and weight and osseous maturation are accelerated, and early closing of the epiphyses leads to short stature. Cf.

precocious pseudopuberty, under *pseudopuberty*. Called also *complete*, *gonadotropin-dependent*, or *true precocious p.*

complete precocious p. central precocious p.

constitutional precocious p. precocious puberty occurring in otherwise normal children generally with a family history of early onset of puberty. The age range for such individuals overlaps the upper range for those with idiopathic precocious puberty.

contrasexual precocious p. precocious puberty in which secondary sex characters of the opposite sex are developed; called also *heterosexual precocious p.*

delayed p. delayed onset of secondary sex characters significantly beyond the average; a common definition for girls is lack of breast enlargement by age 13 or menses by age 15, and for boys lack of testicular enlargement by age 14.

gonadotropin-dependent precocious p. central precocious p.

gonadotropin-independent precocious p. precocious pseudopuberty.

heterosexual precocious p. contrasexual precocious p.

idiopathic precocious p. central precocious puberty in which no underlying causative lesion can be found; it affects mainly girls and is usually sporadic, although there is a hereditary form whose occurrence is confined largely to boys.

incomplete precocious p. precocious pseudopuberty.

isosexual precocious p. precocious puberty in which sex characters are consistent with the sex of the individual.

neurogenic precocious p. central precocious puberty that is caused by a lesion of the central nervous system, such as tumor, congenital defect, or trauma.

peripheral precocious p. precocious pseudopuberty.

precocious p. onset of sexual maturation at an earlier age than normal, defined as two standard deviations below the mean, or before age 8 in girls and 9 in boys. It is usually hormonal *(central precocious p.)*, but occasionally it occurs in otherwise normal children *(constitutional precocious p.)* Called also *sexual precocity* and *pubertas praecox*.

true precocious p. central precocious p.

pu•bes (pu′bēz) gen. *pu′bis* [L.] 1. [TA] pubic hairs; the hairs covering the pubic region. 2. hypogastrium.

pu•bes•cence (pu-bes′əns) the state of being pubescent.

pu•bes•cent (pu-bes′ənt) [L. *pubescens* becoming hairy] 1. reaching sexual maturation; see *puberty*. 2. covered with down or lanugo.

pu•bic (pu′bik) pertaining to or situated near the pubes, the os pubis, or the pubic region.

pu•bio•plas•ty (pu′be-o-plas″te) a plastic operation on the pubes.

pu•bi•ot•o•my (pu″be-ot′ə-me) [*pubis* + *-tomy*] surgical separation of the pubic bone lateral to the median line.

pu•bis (pu′bis) [L., gen. of *pubes*] TA alternative for *os pubis*.

pu•bo•coc•cyg•e•al (pu″bo-kok-sij′e-əl) pertaining to the pubis and coccyx or to the musculus pubococcygeus.

pu•bo•coc•cy•ge•us (pu″bo-kok-sij′e-əs) pertaining to the pubis and coccyx; see under *musculus*.

pu•bo•fem•o•ral (pu″bo-fem′ə-rəl) pertaining to the os pubis and femur.

pu•bo•pros•tat•ic (pu″bo-pros-tat′ik) pertaining to the os pubis and prostate.

pu•bo•rec•tal (pu″bo-rek′təl) pertaining to the pubis and rectum or to the musculus puborectalis.

pu•bo•rec•ta•lis (pu″bo-rek-ta′lis) pertaining to the pubis and rectum; see under *musculus*.

pu•bo•tib•i•al (pu″bo-tib′e-əl) pertaining to the pubes and tibia.

pu•bo•ves•i•cal (pu″bo-ves′ĭ-kəl) vesicopubic.

PUBS percutaneous umbilical blood sampling; see *cordocentesis*.

pu•den•da (pu-den′də) [L.] plural of *pudendum*.

pu•den•dum (pu-den′dəm) pl. *puden′da* [L., from *pudere* to be ashamed] the external genitalia, especially of the female; see also *p. femininum*. **puden′dal, pu′dic** *adj*

p. femini′num [TA] female pudendum: that portion of the female genitalia comprising the mons pubis, labia majora, labia minora, vestibule of the vagina, bulb of the vestibule, greater and lesser vestibular glands, and vaginal orifice. Commonly used to denote the entire external female genitalia (i.e., to include the clitoris and urethra as well). Cf. *vulva*.

pu•er•ile (pu′ər-il) [L. *puerilis*; *puer* child] pertaining to childhood or to children; childish.

pu•er•pera (pu-ur′pər-ə) [L. *puer* child + *parere* to bring forth, to bear] a woman who has just given birth to an infant.

pu•er•per•ant (pu-ur′pər-ənt) puerpera.

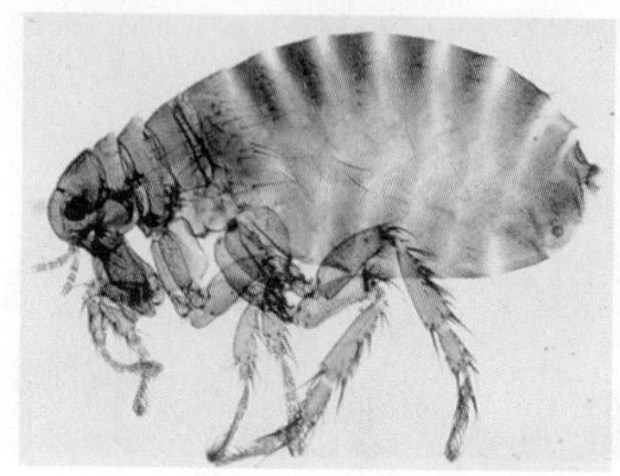

■ *Pulex irritans.*

pu•er•pe•ri•um (pu″ər-pēr′e-əm) [L.] the period from the end of the third stage of labor until involution of the uterus is complete, usually lasting 3 to 6 weeks. **puer′peral** *adj*

Pue•stow procedure (pu′sto) [Charles Bernard *Puestow*, American surgeon, 1902–1973] see under *procedure*.

PUFA polyunsaturated fatty acid.

puff (puf) [A.S. *pyffan*] 1. a short, blowing, auscultation sound. 2. chromosome p.

chromosome p. in genetics, one of the temporarily swollen regions of the polytene chromosome, constituting a diffuse, uncoiled region of the chromosome and resulting from localized synthesis of DNA or RNA.

puff•er (puf′ər) puffer fish.

puff•ing (puf′ing) localized enlargement in giant polytene chromosomes; see *chromosome puff*, under *puff*.

Pu•lex (pu′leks) [L. "flea"] a genus of fleas that are parasitic on various mammals.

P. cheo′pis *Xenopsylla cheopis*.

P. duge′si *P. irritans*.

P. ir′ritans the common flea, which is parasitic on the skin of humans and domestic animals; its bite produces itching.

P. pe′netrans *Tunga penetrans*; see *chigoe*.

pu•lex (pu′leks) pl. *pu′lices* [L.] a flea of the genus *Pulex*.

Pul•heems (pul′hēmz) a system of medical classification for recording the physical and mental status of recruits in the British armed services, representing: P, physical capacity; U, upper limbs; L, lower limbs; H, hearing (acuity); EE, eyesight (visual acuity); M, mental capacity; S, stability (emotional).

pu•lic•i•cide (pu-lis′ĭ-sīd) [*pulex* + *-cide*] an agent destructive to fleas.

Pu•lic•i•dae (pu-lis′ĭ-de) a family of fleas of the order Siphonaptera; four genera are important to humans: *Ctenocephalides*, *Hoplopsyllus*, *Pulex*, and *Xenopsylla*.

pull (po͝ol) 1. to strain a muscle. 2. the injury sustained in a muscle strain.

pull-through (pool′throo) the surgical pulling of one segment of intestine through a segment distal to it. See under *operation*, and see *ileoanal pull-through anastomosis*, under *anastomosis*.

pul•lu•late (pul′u-lāt) to germinate.

pul•lu•la•tion (pul″u-la′shən) [L. *pullulare* to sprout] the act or process of budding, as in yeast, or of sprouting; germination.

Pul•mi•cort (pul′mĭ-kort) trademark for preparations of budesonide.

pul•mo (pool′mo) gen. *pulmo′nis* pl. *pulmo′nes* [L.] [TA] lung.

p. dex′ter [TA] right lung; see *lung*.

p. sinis′ter [TA] left lung; see *lung*.

pulm(o)- [L. *pulmo* lung] a combining form denoting relationship to the lungs; see also words beginning *pulmon(o)-*.

pul•mo•aor•tic (pool″mo-a-or′tik) aorticopulmonary.

pul•mo•gram (pool′mo-gram) a radiograph of the lungs.

Pul•mo•lite (pul′mo-līt″) trademark for a kit for the preparation of technetium Tc 99m albumin aggregated.

pul•mo•lith (pool′mo-lith) [*pulmo-* + *-lith*] pneumolith.

pul•mo•nal (pool′mo-nəl) pulmonary (def. 1).

pul•mo•nary (pool′mo-nar″e) [L. *pulmonarius*] 1. pertaining to the lungs. Called also *pneumonic* and *pulmonic*. 2. pulmonic (def. 2).

Pul•mo•nata (pul″mə-na′tə) an order of snails and slugs of the subclass Euthyneura, including genera with lungs or respiratory sacs. Many are intermediate hosts of trematodes and other pathogens. Its suborders include Basommatophora and Stylommatophora.

pul•mo•nec•to•my (pool″mo-nek′tə-me) pneumonectomy.

pul•mo•nes (pəl-mo′nes) [L.] plural of *pulmo.*

pul•mon•ic (pool-mon′ik) 1. pulmonary. 2. pertaining to the pulmonary artery.

pul•mo•ni•tis (pool″mo-ni′tis) pneumonitis.

pulmon(o)- [L. *pulmo*, gen. *pulmonis* lung] a combining form denoting relationship to the lungs; see also words beginning *pulmo-*.

pul•mo•nol•o•gist (pool″mə-nol′ə-jist) a specialist in pulmonology.

pul•mo•nol•o•gy (pool″mo-nol′ə-je) the medical specialty concerned with the anatomy, physiology, and pathology of the lungs.

pul•mo•no•per•i•to•ne•al (pool″mə-no-per″ĭ-to-ne′əl) pertaining to or communicating with the lungs and the peritoneum.

Pul•mo•zyme (pul′mo-zīm) trademark for a preparation of dornase alfa.

pulp (pulp) [L. *pulpa* flesh] any soft, juicy animal or vegetable tissue, such as the dental pulp or splenic pulp. **pul′pal** *adj*

coronal p. pulpa coronalis.

dead p. necrotic p.

dental p. pulpa dentis.

devitalized p. necrotic p.

digital p. the mass of tissue forming the soft cushion on the palmar or plantar surface of the distal phalanx of a finger or toe.

enamel p. stellate reticulum.

exposed p. dental pulp that has become exposed to the external environment because of trauma or disease.

mummified p. the dry, shriveled pulp seen in dry gangrene.

necrotic p., nonvital p. dental pulp that has been deprived of its blood and nerve supply and is no longer composed of living tissue; there may or may not be bacterial invasion. Necrosis is evidenced by insensitivity to stimulation by electricity, heat, cold, or trauma. Called also *dead p.* and *devitalized p.* See also *gangrenous pulp necrosis*, under *necrosis.*

putrescent p. necrotic pulp that has been invaded by putrefactive microorganisms and has a foul odor.

radicular p. pulpa radicularis.

red p. pulpa rubra.

splenic p. pulpa splenica.

tooth p. pulpa dentis.

vertebral p. nucleus pulposus disci intervertebralis.

vital p. dental pulp that has both vascularity and sensation, i.e is not necrotic.

white p. pulpa alba.

pul•pa (pul′pə) gen. and pl. *pul′pae* [L. "flesh"] pulp: any soft, juicy tissue.

p. al′ba [TA] white pulp: the portion of the spleen involved in the immune response, appearing as gray specks on the cut surface of the organ. It comprises the T lymphocyte–rich periarteriolar lymphoid sheaths in which are interspersed the B lymphocyte–containing splenic lymphoid nodules.

p. corona′lis [TA] coronal pulp; the portion of the dental pulp in the crown portion of the pulp cavity.

p. den′tis [TA] dental pulp: the richly vascularized and innervated connective tissue of mesodermal origin contained in the central cavity of a tooth and delimited by the dentin; it has formative, nutritive, sensory, and protective functions. The portion within the tooth chamber proper is the *p. coronalis*, and that within the root is the *p. radicularis.* Called also *endodontium* and *tooth pulp.*

p. liena′lis TA alternative for *p. splenica.*

p. radicula′ris [TA] radicular pulp; the portion of the dental pulp in the root canal of a tooth.

p. ru′bra [TA] red pulp: the dark, reddish-brown substance that fills up the interspaces of the sinuses of the spleen as the splenic cords and forms the bulk of the splenic parenchyma, acting as a filter for the blood.

p. sple′nica [TA] splenic pulp: the parenchyma of the spleen, composed of red *(p. rubra)* and white pulp *(p. alba)*; called also *p. lienalis* [TA alternative].

pul•pal•gia (pəl-pal′je-ə) pain in the pulp of a tooth.

pul•pec•to•my (pəl-pek′tə-me) [*pulp* + *-ectomy*] root canal therapy consisting of complete extirpation of the dental pulp. Called also *dental pulp extirpation.*

pul•pi•tis (pəl-pi′tis) pl. *pulpi′tides* [*pulp* + *-itis*] inflammation of the dental pulp, usually due to bacterial infection in dental caries, tooth fracture, or other conditions causing exposure of the pulp to bacterial invasion. Chemical irritants, thermal factors, hyperemic changes, and other factors may also cause pulpitis.

anachoretic p. pulpitis caused by bacteria that circulate in the bloodstream and settle at sites of pulpal inflammation; it is usually the result of a chemical or mechanical injury.

closed p. pulpitis characterized by the absence of a direct communication between the dental pulp and the oral environment.

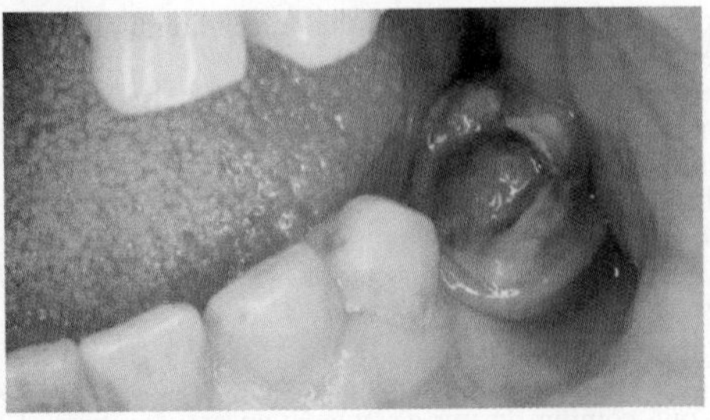

■ Chronic hyperplastic pulpitis with erythematous granulation tissue extruding from the pulp chamber of the mandibular first molar.

hyperplastic p. a chronic productive type of pulpitis usually occurring in teeth with large carious lesions; it is characterized by proliferation of the dental pulp tissue, filling the cavity with a pedunculated or sessile, pinkish red, fleshy mass.

open p. pulpitis characterized by the presence of a direct communication between the dental pulp and the oral environment.

reversible p. pulpitis in which the pulp may recover spontaneously; it is usually asymptomatic until pain is caused by some external stimulus.

pulp•less (pulp′ləs) without pulp; having the pulp removed.

pul•pot•o•my (pəl-pot′ə-me) [*pulp* + *-tomy*] root canal therapy consisting of partial excision of the dental pulp. Called also *pulp amputation.*

pul•py (pul′pe) soft or pultaceous.

pul•sate (pul′sāt) to beat rhythmically, as the heart.

pul•sa•tile (pul′sə-tīl) characterized by a rhythmical pulsation.

pul•sa•tion (pəl-sa′shən) [L. *pulsatio*] a throb or rhythmical beat, as of the heart.

expansile p. a pulsation that expands with each beat of the pulse; it reflects an increase in volume of a mass, usually an aneurysm.

suprasternal p. arterial pulsation in the region of the suprasternal notch, due to dilatation and/or elongation of the aortic arch or to aneurysm.

pul•sa•tor (pul′sa-tər) an apparatus for maintaining respiration.

Bragg-Paul p. a pulsator consisting of an air bag placed around the patient's chest and abdomen and rhythmically inflated and deflated by an electric pump.

pulse (puls) [L. *pulsus* stroke] 1. the rhythmic expansion of an artery, palpable with the finger. See also *pulse rate*, under *rate*, and *beat.* 2. any rhythmic expansion, such as a venous pulse. 3. a brief surge, as of current or voltage.

abdominal p. the pulse over the abdominal aorta.

abrupt p. quick p. (def. 1).

allorhythmic p. irregular p.

alternating p. pulsus alternans.

anacrotic p. a pulse in which the ascending limb of the tracing shows a transient drop in amplitude, or a notch.

anadicrotic p. a pulse in which the ascending limb of the tracing has two waveforms separated by a notch, signifying a transient drop in amplitude.

anatricrotic p. a pulse in which the ascending limb of the tracing shows three small additional waves or notches.

apical p. the pulse over the apex of the heart, as heard through a stethoscope or palpated.

arterial pressure p. pressure p.

atrial liver p. a presystolic pulse corresponding to the atrial venous pulse, sometimes occurring in tricuspid stenosis.

atrial venous p., atriovenous p. a venous pulse in the neck having an accentuated a wave during atrial systole, owing to increased force of contraction of the right atrium; a characteristic of tricuspid stenosis.

biferious p. pulsus bisferiens.

bigeminal p. a pulse in which beats occur as two in rapid succession separated from the following pair by a longer interval; it is usually related to regularly occurring ventricular premature beats.

bisferious p. pulsus bisferiens.

bounding p. strong p.

brachial p. a pulse felt over the brachial artery at the inner aspect of the elbow.

cannonball p. Corrigan p.

capillary p. Quincke p.

carotid p. the pulse in the carotid artery; tracings of it can be used in timing the phases of the cardiac cycle.

catacrotic p. a pulse in which the descending limb of the tracing has a notch.

catadicrotic p. a pulse in which the descending limb of the tracing has a notch between two small additional waveforms.

catatricrotic p. a pulse in which the descending limb of the tracing has two notches between three small waveforms.

centripetal venous p. an abnormal venous pulse caused by a systolic volume expansion that passes from the arteries through the capillaries and venules into the larger veins.

collapsing p. Corrigan p.

Corrigan p. a jerky pulse with a full expansion, followed by a sudden collapse, occurring in aortic regurgitation. Called also *cannonball, collapsing, pistol-shot, trip-hammer,* or *water-hammer p.*

coupled p. bigeminal p.

dicrotic p. a pulse whose tracing has two peaks instead of the usual one, the second one coming during diastole as an exaggeration of the dicrotic wave. See also *anacrotic p.* and *catadicrotic p.*

dorsalis pedis p. a pulse felt on the dorsum of the foot between the first and second metatarsal bones; in 8 to 10 per cent of the population it cannot be detected.

dropped-beat p. intermittent p.

entoptic p. the subjective sensation of seeing in the dark a flash of light at each heart beat.

epigastric p. abdominal p.

febrile p. a type of pulse that is both strong and quick, seen in fever.

femoral p. a pulse felt over the femoral artery in the femoral triangle.

filiform p. thready p.

formicant p. low-tension p.

frequent p. a pulse with a rate faster than normal; called also *pulsus frequens* and *quick p.*

full p. strong p.

funic p. the pulse through the umbilical artery.

gate p. an electrical pulse that serves as a control signal for a gate (q.v.).

hard p. high-tension p.

high-tension p. a pulse characterized by a gradual impulse, long duration, slow subsidence, and a firm, cordy state of the artery between the beats.

infrequent p. slow p.

intermittent p. a pulse in which various beats are dropped. Called also *dropped-beat p.*

irregular p. a pulse in which the beats occur at irregular intervals; called also *allorhythmic p.*

jerky p. a type of pulse that is both quick and strong; called also *sharp p.* and *vibrating p.*

jugular p. a venous pulse seen or felt over the internal jugular vein.

Kussmaul p. paradoxical p.

labile p. a pulse that is normal when the patient is resting but increased by sitting, standing, or exercise.

low-tension p. a pulse with sudden onset, short duration, low amplitude, and quick decline, easily obliterated by pressure. Called also *formicant* or *soft p.* and *pulsus formicans, mollis, parvus,* or *vacuus.*

monocrotic p. a pulse in which the tracing has just one waveform per beat of the artery.

nail p. the pulsation of blood under the nails; sometimes demonstrated by the onychograph.

paradoxical p. a pulse that markedly decreases in size during inhalation, such as the one often seen in constrictive pericarditis. Called also *Kussmaul p.* or *sign* and *pulsus paradoxus.*

paradoxical p., reversed a rise in arterial pressure during inhalation, seen in hypertrophic obstructive cardiomyopathy and some cases of tricuspid insufficiency and atrioventricular dissociation.

pistol-shot p. Corrigan p.

plateau p. a pulse that is slowly rising and sustained.

polycrotic p. a pulse whose tracing shows secondary pulse waves; see *dicrotic p.* and *tricrotic p.*

popliteal p. a pulse palpated in the popliteal fossa, most easily detected when the patient is lying prone with the knee flexed about 45 degrees.

posterior tibial p. a pulse felt over the posterior tibial artery just posterior to the medial malleolus on the inner aspect of the ankle.

pressure p. the arterial pulse caused directly by systole; see also *blood pressure,* under *pressure.* Called also *arterial pressure p.*

quadrigeminal p. a pulse with a pause after every fourth beat.

quick p. 1. a pulse that strikes the finger smartly and leaves it quickly; called also *pulsus celer* and *abrupt* or *short p.* 2. frequent p.

Quincke p. alternate blanching and flushing of the skin. This may be elicited in several ways, such as by observing the nail bed or skin at the root of the nail while pressing on the end of the nail. Caused by pulsation of subpapillary arteriolar and venous plexuses, it is sometimes seen in aortic insufficiency and other disorders, but may occur in normal persons under certain conditions. It was originally thought to be due to pulsation of the capillaries, hence the name *capillary p.* Called also *Quincke sign.*

radial p. a pulse felt over the radial artery.

radiofrequency p. a short burst of electrical energy at a given radio frequency.

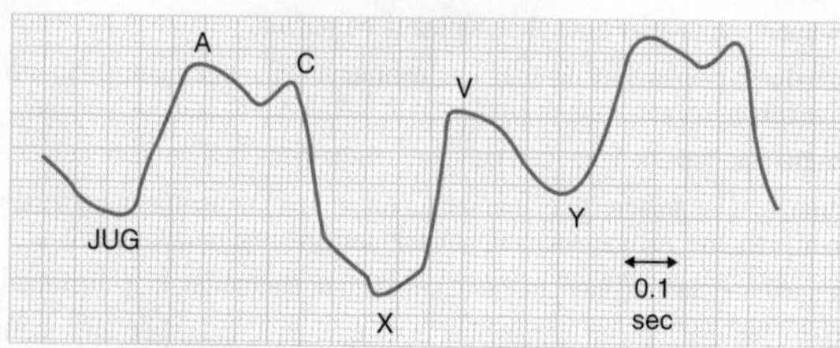

■ Normal jugular venous pulse: *A,* a positive wave due to contraction of the right atrium; *C,* a positive deflection due to bulging of the tricuspid valve toward the atria at the onset of ventricular contraction; *X,* a negative deflection due to atrial relaxation; *V,* a positive deflection due to filling of the right atrium against the closed tricuspid valve during ventricular contraction; *Y,* a negative deflection due to emptying of the right atrium upon ventricular relaxation.

respiratory p. a pulse observed normally in the superficial cervical veins after rapid exercise or at other times of increased respiration.

retrosternal p. a venous pulse perceptible just above the suprasternal notch.

Riegel p. a pulse that is diminished in size during exhalation.

running p. a pulse with small irregular excursions.

sharp p. jerky p.

short p. quick p. (def. 1).

slow p. a pulse with less than the usual number of pulsations per minute. Called also *infrequent* or *vagus p.* and *pulsus tardus.*

soft p. low-tension p.

strong p. a forcible pulse of high amplitude; see also *high-tension p.* Called also *bounding, full,* or *tense p.* and *pulsus fortis, magnus,* or *plenus.*

tense p. strong p.

thready p. a pulse that is very fine and scarcely perceptible. Called also *filiform p.* and *pulsus filiformis.*

tricrotic p. a pulse in which the tracing shows three expansions of the artery in one beat. See also *anatricrotic p.* and *catatricrotic p.*

trigeminal p. a pulse with a pause after every third beat.

trip-hammer p. Corrigan p.

unequal p. a pulse in which some of the beats are strong and others weak.

vagus p. slow p.

venous p. the pulsation that occurs in a vein, usually observed at the right jugular vein just above the sternoclavicular junction.

vermicular p. a small rapid pulse giving to the finger a sensation of wormlike movement.

vibrating p. jerky p.

water-hammer p. Corrigan p.

wiry p. a small, tense pulse.

pulse•less (puls′ləs) lacking a pulse.

pul•sion (pul′shən) a pushing forward, or outward, or to either side.

pul•sus (pul′səs) pl. *pul′sus* [L., from *pellere* to beat] pulse.

p. abdomina′lis abdominal pulse.

p. alter′nans alternating pulse: a pulse in which there is regular alternation of weak and strong beats without changes in cycle length, usually indicative of serious myocardial disease.

p. bife′riens p. bisferiens.

p. bige′minus bigeminal pulse.

p. bisfe′riens a pulse with two strong systolic peaks separated by a midsystolic dip, usually seen in pure aortic regurgitation and aortic regurgitation with stenosis. Called also *biferious* or *bisferious pulse.*

p. ce′ler quick pulse (def. 1).

p. dif′ferens inequality of the pulse observable at corresponding sites on either side of the body.

p. filifor′mis thready pulse.

p. for′micans low-tension pulse.

p. for′tis strong pulse.

p. fre′quens frequent pulse.

p. irregula′ris perpe′tuus irregular pulse.

p. mag′nus strong pulse.

p. mag′nus et ce′ler a pulse that is both strong and quick; see *febrile pulse* and *jerky pulse.*

p. mol′lis low-tension pulse.

p. paradox′us paradoxical pulse.

p. par′vus low-tension pulse.

p. par′vus et tar′dus a slow pulse that is also low-tension.

p. ple′nus strong pulse.

p. tar′dus slow pulse.

p. trige′minus trigeminal pulse.

p. va′cuus low-tension pulse.

p. veno′sus venous pulse.

pul•ta•ceous (pəl-ta′shəs) [L. *pultaceus*] like a pulp or poultice.

pulv. [L.] pul′vis (powder).

pul·ver·iza·tion (pul″vər-ĭ-za′shən) [L. *pulvis* powder] the reduction of any substance to powder.

pul·ver·u·lent (pəl-ver′u-lənt) [L. *pulverulentus*] powdery; dustlike.

pul·vi·nar (pəl-vi′nər) [L. "a cushioned seat"] the prominent, cushion-like mass of nuclei that forms the posterior extremity of the thalamus, which overhangs the medial and lateral geniculate bodies and is separated inferiorly from the medial geniculate body by the brachium of the superior colliculus; it receives fibers from other thalamic nuclei and gives off widespread cortical projections. In official terminology, called *pulvinar thalami.*

p. tha′lami [TA] official terminology for *pulvinar.*

p. tu′nicae inter′nae segmen′ti arteria′lis anastomo′sis arteriove′nae glomerifor′mis the wall of the internal coat of the arterial segment of the anastomosis arteriovenosa glomeriformis, consisting of three to six layers of contractile glomus cells. Called also *p. tunicae intimae segmenti arterialis anastomosis arteriovenae glomeriformis.*

pul·vi·nate (pul′vĭ-nāt) [L. *pulvinus* cushion] shaped like a cushion.

pu·mex (pu′məks) [L.] pumice.

pum·ice (pum′is) [USP] a substance of volcanic origin, consisting chiefly of complex silicates of aluminum, potassium, and sodium, occurring as a very light, hard, rough, porous, grayish powder; used in dentistry as an abrasive or polishing agent, the effect achieved depending on the particle size.

pump (pump) 1. an apparatus for drawing or forcing fluids or gases. 2. to draw or force fluids or gases.

acid p. proton p.

air p. a pump for exhausting or forcing in air.

bile salt export p. a canalicular transport protein for carrying bile salts out of hepatocytes, coded for by a gene on chromosome 2q24; deficiency of this protein causes a type of progressive familial intrahepatic cholestasis.

blood p. a machine used to propel blood through the tubing of extracorporeal circulation devices, designed to do so without damaging blood constituents, particularly the erythrocytes. See also *centrifugal p.* and *roller p.*

breast p. a manual or electric pump for abstracting milk from the breast.

calcium p. the mechanism of active transport of calcium (Ca^{2+}) across a membrane, as of the sarcoplasmic reticulum of muscle cells, against a concentration gradient; the mechanism is driven by the hydrolysis of ATP by the membrane-bound enzyme Ca^{2+}-ATPase.

cardiac balloon p. intra-aortic balloon p.

centrifugal p. a blood pump in which centrifugal force generated by cones or impellers rotating in a closed unit returns the blood to the patient.

efflux p. a transmembrane protein that can expel substances such as drugs from inside the cell.

electrogenic p. a protein channel pump in which the ion exchange is not one-to-one and hyperpolarization results on one side of the membrane. Cf. *sodium p.*

hydrogen p. proton p.

infusion p. a device for injecting a measured amount of fluid during a specific interval of time.

infusion-withdrawal p. a pump for the simultaneous injection and withdrawal of fluid at the same rate.

insulin p. an externally worn pump that can supply insulin to subcutaneous tissues through a plastic tube; a large bolus is infused before every meal and a continuous basal rate of insulin is maintained at other times. Called also *continuous subcutaneous insulin infusion.*

intra-aortic balloon p. (IABP) a pump used in intra-aortic balloon counterpulsation (q.v.).

Lindbergh p. a perfusion apparatus by means of which an organ removed from the body may be kept alive indefinitely.

muscle p. compression of veins by the contraction of skeletal muscles, forcing blood towards the heart against the flow of gravity; seen particularly in the deep veins of the lower limbs. Called also *venous p.*

Na^+-K^+ p. Na^+,K^+-ATPase.

peristaltic p. a pump that moves liquid through tubing by alternate contractions and relaxations on the tubing.

proton p. a system for transporting protons (hydrogen ions) across cell membranes, often exchanging them for other positively charged ions; it may be driven by energy supplied by ATP metabolism, light, or a flow of electrons. See also *H^+,K^+-ATPase.* Called also *hydrogen p.*

roller p. a blood pump in which flow is maintained by the compression of the tubing containing the blood between a continuously moving roller and a curved back plate.

sodium p., sodium-potassium p. Na^+,K^+-ATPase.

stomach p. a pump for removing the contents from the stomach.

venous p. muscle p.

pump·kin (pump′kin) an annual vine *Cucurbita pepo,* that produces large, orange fruits with a thick rind and many seeds; the seeds are used for symptomatic relief of benign prostatic hyperplasia; it is also used for a variety of indications in folk medicine.

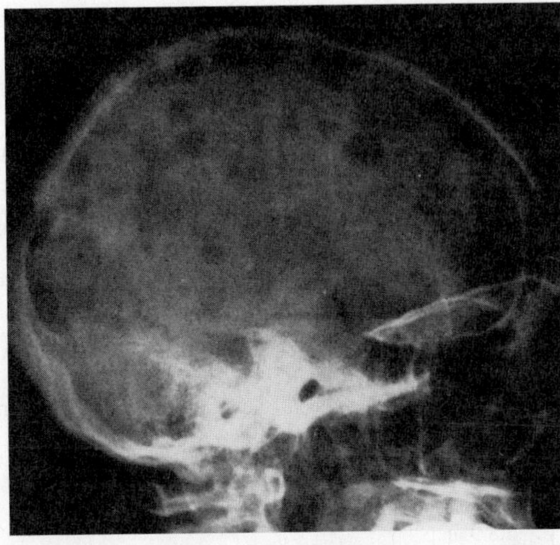

■ Punched-out lesions, most visible in the calvarium, in a lateral view of the skull in multiple myeloma.

pump-oxy·gen·a·tor (pump′ ok″sĭ-jə-na′tər) an apparatus, usually extracorporeal, comprising an arterial pump and blood oxygenator plus filters and traps, for saturating blood with oxygen and perfusing the body tissue; used for cardiopulmonary bypass during cardiac surgery.

punch (punch) an instrument for indenting, perforating, or excising a disk or segment of tissue or other material.

biopsy p. a round knife used to remove a small amount of skin or other tissue; see also *punch biopsy,* under *biopsy.*

pin p. an instrument for perforating a metal backing to receive the pins for fastening artificial teeth.

plate p. a punch for cutting out parts of an artificial dental plate.

rubber dam p. an instrument for punching holes in a rubber dam in order to permit passage of the dam over the crowns of teeth.

punch drunk (punch′drunk″) showing symptoms of chronic traumatic encephalopathy (see under *encephalopathy*).

punched-out (puncht′out″) having the appearance of substance or tissue having been removed with a punch.

punc·ta (pungk′tə) [L.] plural of *punctum.*

punc·tal (pungk′təl) pertaining to the punctum lacrimale.

punc·tate (pungk′tāt) resembling or marked with points or dots.

punc·ti·form (pungk′tĭ-form) 1. like a point; located in a point. 2. in bacteriology, denoting very minute colonies.

punc·to·graph (pungk′to-graf) [*punctum* + *-graph*] an instrument for the radiographic localization of foreign bodies in the tissues.

punc·tum (pungk′təm) pl. *punc′ta* [L.] 1. a tiny spot or point. 2. anatomical nomenclature for a point or other tiny area.

p. cae′cum blind spot.

imperforate p. congenital atresia of the punctum lacrimale, resulting in epiphora; it is particularly common in small breeds of dogs and in pigs.

p. lacrima′le [TA] lacrimal point: the opening on the lacrimal papilla of an eyelid, near the medial angle of the eye, into which tears from the lacrimal lake drain to enter the lacrimal canaliculi.

p. lu′teum macula lutea.

p. ossificatio′nis centrum ossificationis.

p. ossificatio′nis prima′rium centrum ossificationis primarium.

p. ossificatio′nis secunda′rium centrum ossificationis secundarium.

p. prox′imum near point.

p. remo′tum far point.

punc′ta vasculo′sa tiny red spots marking the cut surface of the white substance of the brain, produced by blood from divided vessels.

punc·tum·e·ter (pəngk-tum′ə-tər) [*punctum* + *-meter*] an instrument for measuring the range of accommodation.

punc·ture (pungk′chər) [L. *punctura*] 1. the act of piercing or penetrating with a pointed object or instrument. 2. a wound so made.

Bernard p. puncture of the brain of an experimental animal at a specific point of the floor of the fourth ventricle to cause diabetes *(puncture diabetes)* and glycosuria. Called also *diabetic p.*

Blom-Singer p. tracheoesophageal p.

cisternal p. puncture of the cisterna cerebellomedullaris through the posterior atlanto-occipital membrane for the purpose of withdrawing cerebrospinal fluid; called also *intracisternal p.* and *suboccipital p.*

cranial p. cisternal p.
diabetic p. Bernard p.
dural p. lumbar p.
exploratory p. puncture of a cavity or tumor and removal of some portion of the contents for examination.
heat p. elevation of the temperature of the animal body produced by puncturing the base of the brain.
intracisternal p. cisternal p.
Kronecker p. in experimental medicine, puncture of the inhibitory nerve center of the heart by means of a long fine needle.
lumbar p. the withdrawal of fluid from the subarachnoid space in the lumbar region, usually between the third and fourth lumbar vertebrae, for diagnostic or therapeutic purposes. Called also *dural, spinal,* or *thecal p., rachiocentesis,* and *spinal tap.*
spinal p. lumbar p.
splenic p. puncture of the spleen to obtain a specimen of splenic tissue for examination or to measure portal pressure.
sternal p. removal of bone marrow from the manubrium of the sternum through an appropriate needle.
suboccipital p. cisternal p.
thecal p. lumbar p.
tracheoesophageal p. a one-way plastic valve placed in a surgically created tracheoesophageal fistula to restore speech after laryngectomy. Called also *Blom-Singer p.*
transethmoidal p. a technique for obtaining postmortem biopsy specimens of the brain, using a trocar inserted through the nostril.
ventricular p. puncture of a cerebral ventricle for the purpose of withdrawing fluid.

pun·gent (pun′jənt) [L. *pungens* pricking] sharp or biting; somewhat acrid.

Pun·nett square (pun′ət) [Reginald Crundall *Punnett,* English geneticist, 1875–1967] see under *square.*

Pun·ti·us (pun′te-əs) a genus of fresh-water fish.
P. java′nicus a species placed in fresh-water ponds in certain areas of the world, because it eliminates the weeds necessary for the propagation of mosquitoes.

PUO pyrexia of unknown origin.

pu·pa (pu′pə) [L. "a doll"] the second stage in the development of an insect, between the larva and the imago. **pu′pal** *adj*

pu·pil (pu′pil) [L. *pupilla* girl] the opening at the center of the iris of the eye, through which light enters the eye; in official terminology, called *pupilla.* See also *iris.* **pu′pillary** *adj*

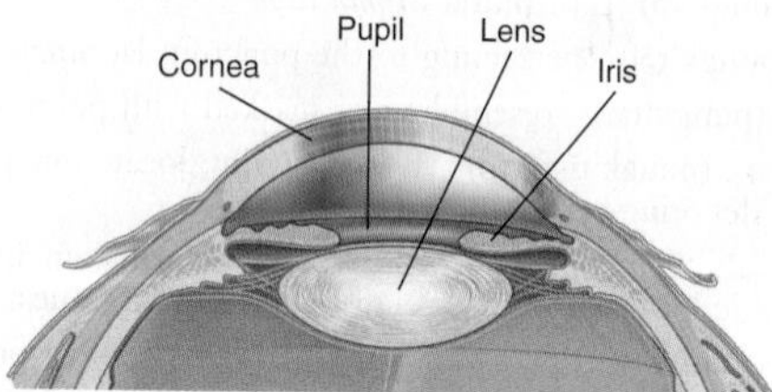

Adie p. tonic p.
Argyll Robertson p. a pupil that is miotic and responds to accommodation effort, but not to light; it is most commonly seen in cases of neurosyphilis.
artificial p. a pupil made by iridectomy.
Behr p. contralateral dilatation of the pupil in lesions of the optic tract.
bounding p. a pupil that shows alternating dilatation and contraction; see *hippus.*
Bumke p. dilation of the pupil after a psychic stimulus.
cat's-eye p. a pupil whose aperture is narrow and vertical.
cornpicker's p's dilated pupils resulting from exposure to dust from jimsonweed (which contains stramonium) in the cornfield.
fixed p. a pupil that does not react either to light or on convergence, or in accommodation.
Hutchinson p. a condition of the pupils in which one is dilated and the other not.
keyhole p. a pupil with a coloboma or a sector iridectomy on one side of the margin.
Marcus Gunn p. the defect of pupillary movement seen in the Marcus Gunn pupillary phenomenon.
myotonic p. tonic p.
pinhole p. a pupil that is extremely contracted.
skew p's a condition in which one of the ocular axes deviates upward and the other downward.
stiff p. Argyll Robertson p.
tonic p. a usually unilateral condition of the eye in which the affected pupil is larger than the other and has light-near dissociation, responding slowly to accommodation and convergence and reacting to light only after prolonged exposure to dark or light. Called also *Adie p., myotonic p.,* and *pupillotonia.* See also *Adie syndrome,* under *syndrome.*

pu·pil·la (pu-pil′ə) pl. *pupil′lae* [L. "girl"] [TA] pupil.

pu·pil·la·to·nia (pu″pil-ə-to′ne-ə) tonic pupil.

Pu·pil·li·dae (pu-pil′ĭ-de) a family of small to minute terrestrial snails and slugs of the suborder Stylommatophora, commonly found in moist wooded regions in North America; it includes the genus *Chondrina.*

pupill(o)- [L. *pupilla,* q.v.] a combining form denoting relationship to the pupil.

pu·pil·lo·graph (pu-pil′o-graf) [*pupillo-* + *-graph*] an instrument that detects responses of the pupil of the eye.

pu·pil·lom·e·ter (pu″pĭ-lom′ə-tər) [*pupillo-* + *-meter*] an instrument for measuring the width or diameter of the pupil; called also *coreometer.*

pu·pil·lom·e·try (pu″pĭ-lom′ə-tre) measurement of the diameter or width of the pupil of the eye; called also *coreometry.*

pu·pil·lo·mo·tor (pu″pĭ-lo-mo′tər) pertaining to the movement of the pupil.

pu·pil·lo·ple·gia (pu″pĭ-lo-ple′jə) [*pupillo-* + *-plegia*] tonic pupil.

pu·pil·lo·scope (pu-pil′o-skōp) 1. an instrument for observing the pupil and its reactions. 2. retinoscope.

pu·pil·lo·sta·tom·e·ter (pu-pil″o-stə-tom′ə-tər) [*pupillo-* + Gr. *statos* placed + *-meter*] an instrument for measuring the distance between the pupils.

pu·pil·lo·to·nia (pu″pĭ-lo-to′ne-ə) tonic pupil.

PUPPP pruritic urticarial papules and plaques of pregnancy.

pure (pūr) [L. *purus*] free from mixture with or contamination by other materials; a reagent is *chemically pure* when it contains no other chemicals that might interfere with its action.

pur·ga·tion (pər-ga′shən) [L. *purgatio*] evacuation (def. 2). **pur′gative** *adj*

purge (purj) [L. *purgare* to cleanse, to purify] 1. to cleanse or purify, to remove undesirable substances from something, such as from marrow in an autologous bone marrow transplant or food from the stomach or intestines. 2. to remove fecal matter from the intestines; see *evacuation* (def. 2). 3. a cathartic.

pu·ric (pu′rik) pertaining to purine.

pu·ri·fi·ca·tion (pūr″ĭ-fĭ-ka′shən) the separating of foreign or contaminating elements from a substance of interest.
affinity p. the removal of contaminating elements by means of affinity chromatography.

pu·ri·form (pu′rĭ-form) [L. *pus,* gen. *puris* pus + *form*] resembling pus; called also *puruloid* and *pyoid.*

pu·rine (pu′rēn) [L. *purum* pure + *urine*] a heterocyclic compound, $C_5H_4N_4$, which is not found free in nature, but is variously substituted to produce a group of compounds known as *purines* or *purine bases* (see illustration under *base*), of which uric acid is a metabolic end product. The purine bases include adenine and guanine, which are constituents of nucleic acids, and hypoxanthine and xanthine.
amino p. aminopurine.
methyl p's alkaloids formed from purines by substituting methyl groups, usually in positions 1, 3, 7. The principal ones are caffeine, theobromine, and theophylline.

pu·rin·emia (pu″rĭ-ne′me-ə) the presence of purine bases in the blood. **purine′mic** *adj*

pu·rine-nu·cleo·side phos·phor·y·lase (pu′rēn noo′kle-o-sīd fos-for′ə-lās) [EC 2.4.2.1] an enzyme of the transferase class that catalyzes the cleavage of purine nucleosides to form purines and ribose 1-phosphates in the degradation of nucleotides and nucleic acids. Absence of activity, an autosomal recessive trait, results in defective cell-mediated immunity.

pu·ri·ner·gic (pu″rin-ur′jik) stimulated or activated by purine bases or nucleotides.

Pu·rine·thol (pu′rēn-thol) trademark for a preparation of mercaptopurine.

pu·rino·lyt·ic (pu″rin-o-lit′ik) [*purine* + *-lytic*] splitting up purines.

pu·rin·om·e·ter (pu″rin-om′ə-tər) [*purine* + *-meter*] an apparatus for estimating the quantity of purine bodies in the urine.

Pur·kin·je cells, fibers, etc. (pər-kin′je) [Jan Evangelista *Purkinje,* Czech physiologist, 1787–1869] see under *cell, fiber, figure, network, phenomenon, system,* and *vesicle* and see *stratum purkinjense corticis cerebelli.*

Pur•kin•je-San•son mirror images (pər-kin′je sah-saw′) [J.E. *Purkinje;* Louis Joseph *Sanson,* French physician, 1790–1841] see under *image.*

pu•ro•mu•cous (pu″ro-mu′kəs) mucopurulent.

pu•ro•my•cin (pūr″o-mi′sin) an antibiotic produced by *Streptomyces alboniger,* which has been used experimentally as an antineoplastic because of its ability to inhibit protein synthesis; it also has trypanosomicidal and amebicidal activity and was formerly used in the treatment of African trypanosomiasis and amebic dysentery.

pur•ple (pur′pəl) 1. a color between blue and red. 2. a substance of this color used as a dye or indicator.

bromcresol p. an indicator, dibromo-*o*-cresolsulfonphthalein, used in the determination of hydrogen ion concentration, being yellow at pH 5.2 and purple at pH 6.8. Written also *bromocresol p.*

visual p. rhodopsin.

Pur•pu•ra (pur′pu-rə) a genus of marine snails of the family Muricidae. Some species furnish a purple dye and others contain the neurotoxin purpurine or murine.

pur•pu•ra (pur′pu-rə) [L. "purple"] 1. any of a group of conditions characterized by ecchymoses or other small hemorrhages in the skin, mucous membranes, or serosal surfaces; causes include blood disorders, vascular abnormalities, and trauma. 2. any of several conditions similar to the traditional purpura group, which may be caused by decreased platelet counts, platelet abnormalities, vascular defects, or reactions to drugs.

actinic p. benign sun-induced damage to the dermis, usually on sun-exposed parts of the arms and hands of elderly persons, with darkened macules and patches; sometimes it is caused by minor trauma or shearing movements. Called also *solar p.*

allergic p., anaphylactoid p. Henoch-Schönlein p.

p. annula′ris telangiecto′des a rare type of chronic pigmented purpura that usually begins on the lower limbs and becomes more generalized; the original punctate erythematous lesions coalesce to form annular or serpiginous patterns. Involution is slow and may be followed by atrophy and loss of hair in the area. Called also *Majocchi p.* or *disease.*

brain p. a hemorrhagic encephalopathy resembling acute necrotizing hemorrhagic encephalomyelitis, but without the inflammatory or necrotic changes of that disorder. It is marked by small pericapillary hemorrhages in the white matter of the brain, with adjacent demyelination and destruction of the axons; clinical manifestations include stupor and coma. The etiology is uncertain, but it is sometimes secondary to viral pneumonia or arsenical intoxication. Called also *pericapillary encephalorrhagia.*

chronic pigmented p. any of a group of benign dermatoses of unknown etiology, not associated with underlying systemic disease, consisting of minimal inflammation with cayenne pepper spots on the skin; included are lichen aureus, pigmented purpuric lichenoid dermatitis, purpura annularis telangiectodes, and Schamberg disease. Called also *pigmented purpuric dermatitis* or *dermatosis* and *p. pigmentosa chronica.*

fibrinolytic p., p. fibrinoly′tica purpura secondary to and accompanied by increased breakdown of fibrin in the blood.

p. ful′minans a form of nonthrombocytopenic purpura seen mainly in children, usually following an infectious disease such as scarlet fever or varicella; characteristics include fever, shock, anemia, and sudden and rapidly spreading symmetrical skin hemorrhages of the lower limbs, often with extensive intravascular thromboses and gangrene.

p. hemorrha′gica 1. idiopathic thrombocytopenic p. 2. an acute, usually fatal disease of horses that may occur after a respiratory tract infection; characteristics include subcutaneous edema and petechiae around the head with tachycardia.

Henoch p. a variety of Henoch-Schönlein purpura characterized by acute visceral symptoms such as vomiting, diarrhea, abdominal distention, hematuria, and renal colic, and without articular symptoms. Called also *p. nervosa.*

Henoch-Schönlein p. a form of nonthrombocytopenic purpura, sometimes a type of hypersensitivity vasculitis and sometimes of unknown cause, usually seen in children and associated with symptoms including urticaria, erythema, arthropathy, arthritis, gastrointestinal symptoms, and renal involvement. Called also *allergic* or *anaphylactoid p., Schönlein-Henoch p.,* and *Schönlein-Henoch syndrome.*

hypergammaglobulinemic p. Waldenström p.

idiopathic p., idiopathic thrombocytopenic p., immune thrombocytopenic p. a type of thrombocytopenic purpura that is not directly associated with any definable systemic disease but often follows a systemic infection; it has been found to be an autoimmune condition, caused by antigens against platelets, resulting in ecchymoses, petechiae, and other bleeding. There are both acute and chronic forms: the *acute form* has a sudden onset, is more common in children, and usually resolves spontaneously within a few months; the *chronic form* has a slower onset, is more common in adults, and may be recurrent.

inflammatory p. palpable p.

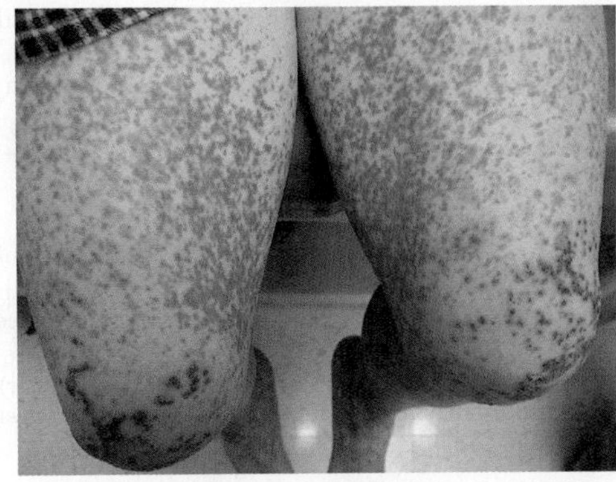

■ Rash of Henoch-Schönlein purpura.

itching p. a recurrent, pruritic, eruptive hemorrhagic dermatosis, usually seen in males, manifested as erythematous macules with punctate purpura beginning on the lower limbs and spreading to the trunk, upper limbs, and in severe cases the large flexural areas.

Majocchi p. p. annularis telangiectodes.

p. nervo′sa Henoch p.

nonthrombocytopenic p. purpura without any decrease in the platelet count of the blood. Called also *p. simplex.*

palpable p. firm, hemorrhagic papules or plaques up to several centimeters in diameter that do not blanch when the skin is pressed, typically resulting from inflammatory vascular injury or infectious microemboli.

p. pigmento′sa chro′nica, p. pigmento′sa progressi′va chronic pigmented p.

primary thrombocytopenic p. idiopathic thrombocytopenic p.

psychogenic p. painful bruising syndrome; the term is sometimes used more narrowly to denote only those cases without evidence of sensitivity to erythrocytes.

retiform p. purpura with lesions in a reticular pattern; it may be either inflammatory (see *palpable purpura*) or noninflammatory.

p. rheuma′tica Schönlein p.

Schamberg p. see under *disease.*

Schönlein p. Henoch-Schönlein purpura with articular and dermatological symptoms but without gastrointestinal symptoms. Called also *p. rheumatica* and *Schönlein disease.*

Schönlein-Henoch p. Henoch-Schönlein p.

secondary thrombocytopenic p. thrombocytopenic purpura occurring as a consequence of a primary hematologic disease such as leukemia, or an underlying systemic nonhematologic entity.

p. seni′lis a type of purple to red, irregularly shaped hemorrhages beneath the skin of the upper and lower limbs of elderly persons. See also *steroid p.*

p. sim′plex nonthrombocytopenic p.

solar p. actinic p.

steroid p. hemorrhages found beneath the skin of the upper and lower limbs owing to attrition of dermal and vascular connective tissue from long-term treatment with adrenocortical steroid hormones; it is identical in appearance to purpura senilis.

thrombocytopenic p., thrombopenic p. 1. any form of purpura in which the platelet count is decreased; it may be either *primary (idiopathic)* or *secondary.* See also *thrombotic thrombocytopenic p.* 2. primary thrombocytopenic p.

thrombotic thrombocytopenic p. a form of thrombotic microangiopathy usually seen in adults, characterized by thrombocytopenia with thromboses in terminal arterioles and capillaries; other symptoms include hemolytic anemia, azotemia, fever, and bizarre neurological manifestations. Some authorities consider it identical to the hemolytic uremic syndrome. Called also *microangiopathic* or *microangiopathic hemolytic anemia* and *Moschcowitz disease.*

Waldenström p., Waldenström hypergammaglobulinemic p. a syndrome of increased circulating immunoglobulin G with vasculitis and purpuric lesions on the lower legs, seen primarily in women, often with an underlying immunologic disorder. Called also *hypergammaglobulinemic p.*

pur•pu•ric (pər-pu′rik) of the nature of, pertaining to, or affected with purpura.

pur•pu•rin (pur′pu-rin) 1. a glycoside from madder root that has been used as a nuclear stain; called also *alizarin No. 6* and *alizarinopurpurin.* 2. uroerythrin. 3. purpurine.

pur•pu•rine (pur′pu-rēn) 1. a neurotoxic substance derived from the median zone of the hypobranchial or purple gland of gastropods of the genus *Purpura,* thought to be an ester or a mixture of esters of choline;

the substance is called *murexine* when derived from snails of the genus *Murex*. 2. purpurin (def. 1).

pur·pu·rin·uria (pur″pu-rĭ-nu′re-ə) the presence of uroerythrin in the urine.

pur·pu·rog·e·nous (pur″pu-roj′ə-nəs) [L. *purpura* purple + *-genous*] producing visual purple (rhodopsin).

purr (pur) a low vibratory murmur.

purr·ing (pur′ing) having a tremulous quality, like the purr of a cat.

Pur·ti·lo syndrome (pər-te′lo) [David T. *Purtilo*, American physician, 20th century] X-linked lymphoproliferative syndrome; see under *syndrome*.

Purt·scher disease (angiopathic retinopathy) (poor′cher) [Otmar *Purtscher*, German ophthalmologist, 1852–1927] see under *disease*.

pu·ru·lence (pu′roo-ləns) [L. *purulentia*] the condition of being purulent.

pu·ru·len·cy (pu′roo-len″se) purulence.

pu·ru·lent (pu′roo-lənt) [L. *purulentus*] 1. pertaining to or consisting of pus. 2. containing pus. 3. suppurative. 4. caused by pus; called also *pyogenous*.

pu·ru·loid (pu′roo-loid) puriform.

pus (pus) gen. *pu′ris* pl. *pu′ra* [L.] a liquid inflammation product made up of leukocytes, cellular debris, and a thin protein-rich fluid called liquor puris.

blue p. pus with a bluish tint, seen in certain suppurative infections, the color comes from a bacterial pigment called pyocyanin, produced by *Pseudomonas aeruginosa*.

burrowing p. pus that is not walled off but extends between fascial planes, sometimes for long distances.

chocolate p. the dark brown pus seen in amebic liver abscess.

green p. pus having a greenish tint.

laudable p., p. laudan′dum a term once applied to a creamy yellow, odorless pus, secreted by a healthy granulating surface and regarded as indicative of less danger than other varieties.

sanious p. bloody pus, often ichorous and ill smelling.

pus·tu·la (pus′tu-lə) pl. *pus′tulae* [L.] pustule.

pus·tu·la·tion (pus″tu-la′shən) the formation of pustules; see also *pustulosis*.

pus·tule (pus′tūl) [L. *pustula*] a visible collection of pus within or beneath the epidermis. **pus′tular** *adj*

Kogoj spongiform p. spongiform p.

malignant p. the initial skin lesion of cutaneous anthrax; called also *malignant carbuncle*.

multilocular p. a pustule with several compartments, indicating origin from a spongiotic vesicle within the epidermis rather than from infection in a follicle, a sweat pore, or subepidermal tissues.

simple p. unilocular p.

spongiform p., spongiform p. of Kogoj a focal area of spongiosis beneath the stratum corneum of the epidermis, lined with edematous cells and containing neutrophils in the intercellular spaces; it is a cardinal sign of active psoriasis and is also found in other dermatoses such as seborrheic dermatitis. Cf. *Munro microabscess*.

unilocular p. a pustule having a single cavity, suggesting origin in a follicle, sweat pore, or subepidermal tissue; called also *simple p.*

pus·tu·lo·der·ma (pus″tu-lo-dur′mə) [*pustule* + *derma*] pustulosis.

toxic p. acute generalized exanthematous pustulosis.

pus·tu·lo·sis (pus″tu-lo′sis) a skin condition marked by an outbreak of pustules.

acute generalized exanthematous p. (AGEP) a type of acute, febrile drug eruption consisting of many small pustules within large areas of edematous erythema. Called also *pustular eruption, pustular drug eruption*, and *toxic pustuloderma*.

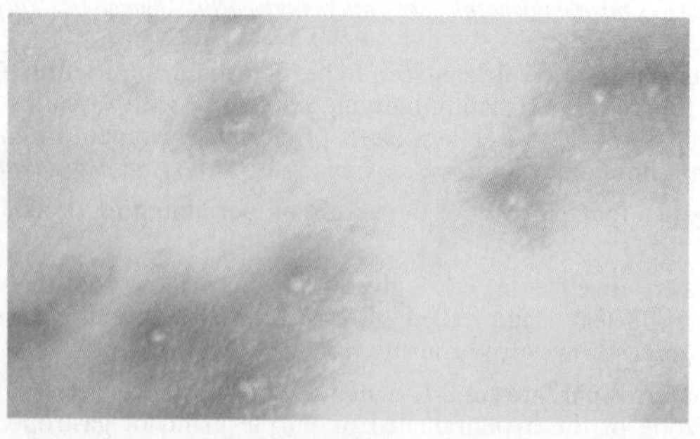

■ Pustules.

p. palma′ris et planta′ris, palmoplantar p. 1. localized pustular psoriasis. 2. a pustular eruption similar to localized pustular psoriasis except without psoriasis.

pu·ta·men (pu-ta′mən) [L. "shell"] [TA] the larger, darker (in unstained brain slices) and more lateral part of the lentiform nucleus, separated from the lateral globus pallidus by the lateral medullary lamina. **puta′minal** *adj*

Put·nam-Da·na syndrome (put′nəm da′nə) [James Jackson *Putnam*, American neurologist, 1846–1918; Charles Loomis *Dana*, American neurologist, 1852–1935] see *subacute combined degeneration of spinal cord*, under *degeneration*.

pu·tre·fac·tion (pu″trə-fak′shən) [L. *putrefactio*] enzymic decomposition, especially of proteins, with the production of foul-smelling compounds, such as hydrogen sulfide, ammonia, and mercaptans. Cf. *fermentation*. **putrefac′tive, pu′trid** *adj*

pu·tre·fy (pu′trə-fi) to decompose, with the production of foul-smelling compounds; a term applied especially to the decomposition of proteins and organic matter.

pu·tres·cence (pu-tres′əns) partial or complete rottenness. **putres′cent** *adj*

pu·tres·cine (pu-tres′ēn) chemical name: tetra-methylene-diamine. A polyamine first found in decaying animal tissues but now known to occur in almost all tissues and in cultures of certain bacteria. It is formed by decarboxylation of ornithine and is itself a precursor of spermidine.

Puus·epp reflex (pu′sep) [Lyudvig Martinovich *Puusepp*, Estonian neurosurgeon, 1875–1942] see under *reflex*.

PUVA psoralen plus ultraviolet A; see under *therapy*.

PVB a cancer chemotherapy regimen consisting of Platinol (cisplatin), vinblastine, and bleomycin.

PVC polyvinyl chloride.

PVL periventricular leukomalacia.

PVP polyvinylpyrrolidone, former name for *povidone*.

PVP-I povidone-iodine.

PVS permanent vegetative state; persistent vegetative state.

PWA person with AIDS.

PWM pokeweed mitogen.

py·ar·thro·sis (pi″ahr-thro′sis) [*pyo-* + *arthr-* + *-osis*] acute suppurative arthritis.

Pyc·nan·the·mum (pik-nan′thə-məm) [Gr. *pyknos* dense + *anthemon* bloom] the mountain mints, a genus of American herbs of the family Labiatae; they are aromatic and carminative and resemble pennyroyal or spearmint in taste and smell.

pyc·nid·ium (pik-nid′e-əm) a flask-shaped or spherical fruiting body whose inner wall is lined with conidiogenous cells.

pycn(o)- for words thus beginning, see those beginning *pykn(o)-*.

py·elec·ta·sia (pi″ə-lək-ta′zhə) pyelectasis.

py·elec·ta·sis (pi″ə-lek′tə-sis) [*pyel-* + *ectasis*] dilatation of the renal pelvis.

py·el·ic (pi-el′ik) pertaining to the renal pelvis; called also *renipelvic*.

py·eli·tis (pi″ə-li′tis) [*pyel-* + *-itis*] inflammation of the renal pelvis, often accompanied by symptoms such as pain and tenderness in the loins, irritability of the bladder, bloody or purulent urine, and a peculiar pain on flexion of the thigh. See also *pyelonephritis*. **pyelit′ic** *adj*

cystic p., p. cys′tica pyelitis with formation of submucosal cysts.

emphysematous p. pyelitis with air or gas only in the collecting system; see also *emphysematous pyelonephritis*, under *pyelonephritis*.

encrusted p. pyelitis with ulcers encrusted with urinary salts.

p. glandula′ris pyelitis with conversion of transitional mucosal into cylindrical epithelium, with formation of glandular acini.

p. granulo′sa pyelitis with exuberant granulations.

p. gravida′rum pyelonephritis of pregnancy.

hematogenous p. pyelitis in which the infection comes from the blood.

hemorrhagic p. pyelitis with hemorrhage.

suppurative p. pyelitis with abscesses and pyonephrosis.

pyel(o)- [Gr. *pyelos* pelvis] a combining form denoting relationship to the renal pelvis.

py·elo·cal·i·ce·al (pi″ə-lo-kal″ĭ-se′əl) pyelocalyceal.

py·elo·cali·ec·ta·sis (pi″ə-lo-kal″e-ek′tə-sis) [*pyelo-* + *caliectasis*] hydronephrosis.

py·elo·cal·y·ce·al (pi″ə-lo-kal″ĭ-se′əl) pertaining to the renal pelvis and calices; spelled also *pyelocaliceal*. Called also *pelvicalyceal* and *pelvocalyceal*.

py·elo·cu·ta·ne·ous (p″ə-lo-ku-ta′ne-əs) pertaining to or communicating between the renal pelvis and the skin.

py·elo·cys·ti·tis (pi″ə-lo-sis-ti′tis) [*pyelo-* + *cyst-* + *-itis*] inflammation of the renal pelvis and the bladder; called also *cystopyelitis.*

py·elo·du·o·de·nal (pi″ə-lo-doo″ə-de′nəl) pertaining to or connecting the renal pelvis and the duodenum.

py·elo·gram (pi′ə-lo-gram) [*pyelo-* + *-gram*] a radiograph of the kidney and ureter, especially one showing the renal pelvis.

dragon p. bizarre forms in the pyelogram seen in cases of polycystic kidneys.

py·elo·graph (pi′ə-lo-graf) pyelogram.

py·elog·ra·phy (pi″ə-log′rə-fe) [*pyelo-* + *-graphy*] radiography of the renal pelvis and ureter after the structures have been filled with a contrast solution.

air p. pneumopyelography.

antegrade p. pyelography in which the contrast medium is introduced by percutaneous needle puncture into the renal pelvis.

ascending p. retrograde p.

p. by elimination, excretion p. intravenous p.

intravenous p. pyelography with intravenous injection of a contrast medium that passes quickly into the urine.

lateral p. pyelography in which the patient lies in lateral position with the side to be examined next to the film.

respiration p. pyelography with a diphasic film showing the kidney under several phases of the respiratory cycle.

retrograde p. pyelography in which the contrast fluid is injected into the renal pelvis through the ureter.

wash-out p. pyelography in which the radiograph is taken after the kidneys have been filled with a contrast solution and then "washed out" by water diuresis, increasing the contrast between a normal and a malfunctioning kidney.

py·elo·il·eo·cu·ta·ne·ous (pi″ə-lo-il″e-o-ku-ta′ne-əs) pertaining to the renal pelvis, ileum, and skin; see under *anastomosis.*

py·elo·in·ter·sti·tial (pi″ə-lo-in″tər-stish′əl) pertaining to the interstitial tissue of the renal pelvis.

py·elo·li·thot·o·my (pi″ə-lo-lĭ-thot′ə-me) [*pyelo-* + *lithotomy*] the operation of excising a renal calculus from the renal pelvis.

py·elo·ne·phri·tis (pi″ə-lo-nə-fri′tis) [*pyelo-* + *nephr-* + *-itis*] inflammation of the kidney and renal pelvis because of bacterial infection; it begins in the interstitial tissues *(interstitial nephritis)* and rapidly extends to involve the tubules *(tubulointerstitial nephritis)*, glomeruli *(glomerulonephritis)*, and then the renal blood vessels.

acute p., acute bacterial p., acute suppurative p. pyelonephritis of sudden onset characterized by fever, chills, pain in the costovertebral region or flanks, and symptoms of bladder inflammation. Called also *acute focal bacterial nephritis.*

ascending p. pyelonephritis caused by a urinary tract infection that has spread up the ureter into the kidney.

calculous p. pyelonephritis caused by urinary calculi.

chronic p. pyelonephritis attributed to cicatricial effects of a previous infection or to recurring or progressive infection. It is usually of insidious onset and occasionally may lead to chronic renal insufficiency.

contagious bovine p. an inflammatory condition of cattle due to infection of the kidneys and urinary tract with *Corynebacterium renale*; characteristics include painful, swollen kidneys and thickened, inflamed walls throughout the urinary tract, with hematuria and pyuria. Other domestic animals occasionally suffer from a similar condition.

emphysematous p. a rare, life-threatening complication of acute pyelonephritis, in which gas collects in the renal collecting system and parenchyma and may cause necrosis; seen in diabetics with gas produced by lactose-fermenting bacteria, in ureteral obstruction, and in certain other conditions.

p. gravida′rum, p. of pregnancy a renal infection during pregnancy characterized by dilatation of the renal pelvis and the ureters; some degree of ureteric obstruction may be caused by the gravid uterus.

xanthogranulomatous p. a form of chronic pyelonephritis characterized by enlargement of the kidney with loss of function, thickening and adhesion of the perirenal tissue and capsule, and destruction of parenchymal tissue; calculi, foam cells, granulomas, and medullary abscesses may also be seen. It is frequently associated with infection by *Proteus* spp.

py·elo·ne·phro·sis (pi″ə-lo-nə-fro′sis) [*pyelo-* + *nephr-* + *-osis*] disease of the kidney and renal pelvis; see *pyelonephritis.*

py·elop·a·thy (pi″ə-lop′ə-the) [*pyelo-* + *-pathy*] any disease of the renal pelvis.

py·elo·phle·bi·tis (pi″ə-lo-flə-bi′tis) [*pyelo-* + *phlebitis*] inflammation of the veins of the renal pelvis.

py·elo·plas·ty (pi′ə-lo-plas″te) [*pyelo-* + *-plasty*] a plastic operation on the renal pelvis, especially the ureteropelvic junction. **pyeloplas′tic** *adj*

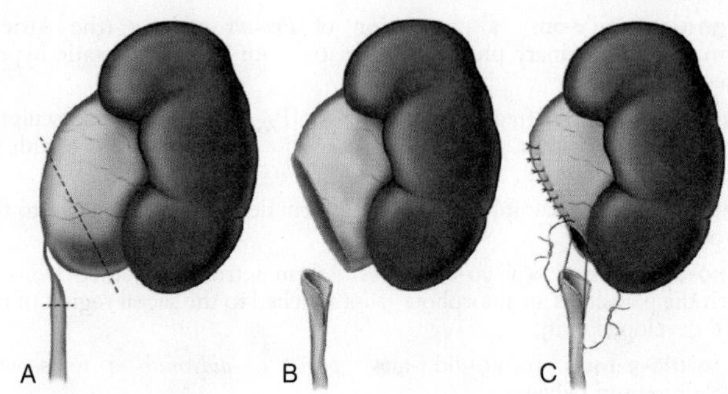

■ Dismembered pyeloplasty used for reduction of redundant renal pelvis. *(A)*, Excision of redundant portion between traction sutures; *(B)*, closure of cephalad aspect of pelvis down to the dependent portion; *(C)*, anastomosis of dependent aspect of pelvis to proximal ureter.

Anderson-Hynes p. dismembered p.

Culp-DeWeerd p. pyeloplasty in which a spiral flap is turned down and incorporated into the adjacent ureter.

dismembered p. a pyeloplasty procedure for redundancy of the renal pelvis, consisting of excision of the ureteropelvic junction and part of the pelvis and reattachment of the spatulated end of the ureter to the remaining pelvis. Called also *Anderson-Hynes p.*

Foley Y-V p. pyeloplasty for repair of an obstructed and high ureteropelvic junction; a V-shaped flap is made from part of the renal pelvis and inserted into a Y-shaped incision whose angle is at the junction.

py·elos·co·py (pi″ə-los′kə-pe) [*pyelo-* + *-scopy*] observation of the renal pelvis under the fluoroscope after intravenous or retrograde injection of a contrast medium.

py·elo·si·nus (pi″ə-lo-si′nus) pertaining to a renal pelvis and renal sinus.

py·elos·to·my (pi″ə-los′tə-me) [*pyelo-* + *-stomy*] a rare procedure in which an opening is surgically created directly into the renal pelvis for temporary urinary diversion, in contrast to the more common nephrostomy.

py·elot·o·my (pi″ə-lot′ə-me) [*pyelo-* + *-tomy*] incision of the renal pelvis.

py·elo·ure·ter·ec·ta·sis (pi″ə-lo-u-re″tər-ek′tə-sis) dilatation of a renal pelvis and ureter.

py·elo·ure·ter·i·tis (pi″ə-lo-u-re″tər-i′tis) [*pyelo-* + *ureteritis*] inflammation of a ureter and renal pelvis.

p. cys′tica pyeloureteritis in which subendothelial cysts project into the lumen of the ureter and renal pelvis; see also *ureteritis cystica.*

py·elo·ure·ter·og·ra·phy (pi″ə-lo-u-re″tər-og′rə-fe) pyelography.

py·elo·ure·ter·ol·y·sis (pi″ə-lo-u-re″tər-ol′ə-sis) [*pyelo-* + *uretero-* + *-lysis*] the surgical freeing of fibrous bands or adhesions near the junction of the renal pelvis and ureter.

py·elo·ure·tero·plas·ty (pi″ə-lo-u-re′tər-o-plas″te) ureteropyelostomy.

py·elo·ve·nous (pi″ə-lo-ve′nəs) pertaining to the renal pelvis and renal veins.

py·em·e·sis (pi-em′ə-sis) [*pyo-* + *-emesis*] vomiting of pus or purulent matter.

py·e·mia (pi-e′me-ə) [*py-* + *-emia*] a general septicemia in which secondary foci of suppuration occur and multiple abscesses are formed. The condition is marked by fever, chills, sweating, jaundice, and abscesses in various parts of the body. Called also *metastatic infection.* **pye′mic** *adj*

arterial p. pyemia due to the dissemination of septic emboli from the heart.

cryptogenic p. pyemia in which the source of infection is unidentified.

otogenous p. pyemia originating from inflammation in the ear.

portal p. suppurative pylephlebitis.

tick p. a condition seen in lambs in the British Isles up to the age of three months, in which the bite of the tick *Ixodes ricinus* becomes infected by *Staphylococcus aureus*, sometimes with septicemia or bacteremia that can be fatal.

Py·e·mo·tes (pi″ə-mo′tēz) a genus of parasitic mites. *P. tri′tici* and *P. ventrico′sus* are called *straw itch mites;* both species parasitize the larvae of insects, are found in the straw of cereals, and cause the dermatitis known as *grain itch.*

py·en·ceph·a·lus (pi″en-səf′ə-ləs) brain abscess.

py·e·sis (pi-e′sis) suppuration.

py·gal (pi′gəl) gluteal.

py·gal·gia (pi-gal′jə) [*pygo-* + *-algia*] pain in the buttocks.

py·ge·um (pij′e-əm) a preparation of *Prunus africana* (the African plum), used for urinary problems associated with benign prostatic hyperplasia.

pyg·ma·li·on·ism (pig-ma′le-on-iz″əm) [*Pygmalion*, a Greek sculptor who fell in love with a statue he had carved] the falling in love with an object made by oneself.

pyg(o)- [Gr. *pygē* rump] a combining form denoting relationship to the buttocks.

py·go·amor·phus (pi″go-ə-mor′fəs) asymmetrical conjoined twins in which the parasite is an amorphous mass attached to the sacral region of the more developed twin.

py·go·did·y·mus (pi″go-did′ĭ-məs) [*pygo-* + *-didymus*] a fetus with double hips and pelvis.

py·gom·e·lus (pi-gom′ə-ləs) [*pygo-* + Gr. *melos* limb] a fetus with a supernumerary limb or limbs attached to or near the buttock.

py·gop·a·gus (pi-gop′ə-gəs) [*pygo-* + *-pagus*] conjoined twins consisting of two nearly complete individuals joined at the sacrum so that the two components are back to back.

p. parasi′ticus asymmetrical conjoined twins in which the parasitic twin is attached to the sacral region of the more developed twin.

py·gop·a·gy (pi-gop′ə-je) the condition of being a pygopagus.

py·go·style (pi′go-stīl) a flat bone at the end of the vertebral column of birds, representing the union of several vertebrae and serving as a site of attachment for the tail feathers. Called also *plowshare bone*.

pykn(o)- [Gr. *pyknos* thick, frequent] a combining form meaning thick, compact, or frequent. Also *pycn(o)-*.

pyk·no·cyte (pik′no-sīt″) a distorted, contracted, occasionally spiculed erythrocyte; these occur normally in small numbers in full-term infants but are seen in greater numbers in hemolytic disorders.

pyk·no·cy·to·sis (pik″no-si-to′sis) conspicuous increases in the numbers of pyknocytes in the blood.

pyk·no·dys·os·to·sis (pik″no-dis″os-to′sis) an autosomal recessive disorder caused by mutation in the *CTSK* gene (locus: 1q21), which encodes cathepsin K, resulting in osteoclast dysfunction. It is characterized by short stature, osteosclerosis, fragility of bone, partial agenesis of terminal digits of hands and feet, cranial anomalies, frontal and occipital bossing, and hypoplasia of the angle of the mandible.

pyk·nom·e·ter (pik-nom′ə-tər) [*pykno-* + *-meter*] an instrument for determining the specific gravity of fluids.

pyk·nom·e·try (pik-nom′ə-tre) measurement by the pyknometer.

pyk·no·mor·phic (pik″no-mor′fik) pyknomorphous.

pyk·no·mor·phous (pik″no-mor′fəs) [*pykno-* + *morph-* + *-ous*] having the stainable elements compactly arranged; a term applied to certain nerve cells.

pyk·no·sis (pik-no′sis) [Gr. *pyknōsis* condensation] a thickening, especially degeneration of a cell in which the nucleus shrinks in size and the chromatin condenses to a solid, structureless, basophilic mass or masses.

pyk·not·ic (pik-not′ik) [Gr. *pyknōtikos*] 1. serving to close the pores. 2. pertaining to pyknosis.

Pyle disease (pīl) [Edwin *Pyle*, American physician, 1891–1961] metaphyseal dysplasia; see under *dysplasia*.

pyle- [Gr. *pylē* gate] a combining form denoting relationship to the portal vein.

py·le·phle·bi·tis (pi″le-flə-bi′tis) [*pyle-* + *phlebitis*] inflammation of the portal vein; it usually results from intestinal disease.

adhesive p. pylethrombophlebitis.

suppurative p. pylephlebitis with pyemia; called also *portal pyemia*.

py·le·throm·bo·phle·bi·tis (pi″le-throm″bo-flə-bi′tis) [*pyle-* + *thrombophlebitis*] thrombosis and inflammation of the portal vein.

py·le·throm·bo·sis (pi″le-throm-bo′sis) thrombosis of the portal vein.

py·lic (pi′lik) [Gr. *pylē* gate] portal (def. 2).

py·lon (pi′lon) a tube, often adjustable, that connects the socket of a prosthetic lower limb to the prosthetic foot.

py·lo·rec·to·my (pi″lo-rek′tə-me) [*pylor-* + *-ectomy*] excision of the pylorus; called also *gastropylorectomy*.

py·lo·ri·ste·no·sis (pi-lor″ĭ-stə-no′sis) pyloric stenosis.

py·lo·ri·tis (pi″lor-i′tis) inflammation of the pylorus.

pylor(o)- [L. *pylorus*, q.v.] a combining form denoting relationship to the pylorus.

py·lo·ro·du·od·e·ni·tis (pi-lor″o-doo-od″ə-ni′tis) inflammation of the pyloric and duodenal mucosa.

py·lo·ro·gas·trec·to·my (pi-lor″o-gas-trek′tə-me) pylorectomy.

py·lo·ro·my·ot·o·my (pi-lor″o-mi-ot′ə-me) a type of pyloroplasty done for congenital pyloric stenosis, consisting of longitudinally incising thickened serosa and muscularis down to the mucosa. Called also *Ramstedt* or *Fredet-Ramstedt operation*.

py·lo·ro·plas·ty (pi-lor′o-plas″te) [*pyloro-* + *-plasty*] incision of the pylorus and reconstruction of the channel through it, such as to relieve obstruction or accelerate gastric emptying after a vagotomy for peptic ulcers. See also *pyloromyotomy* and *pylorotomy*. **pyloroplas′tic** *adj*

double p. posterior pyloromyotomy combined with the Heineke-Mikulicz pyloroplasty.

Finney p. reconstruction of the pylorus and pyloric outlet by means of a longitudinal incision through the pylorus and adjacent walls of the stomach and duodenum and the establishment of a new anastomosis between the stomach and duodenum.

Heineke-Mikulicz p. reconstruction of the pyloric channel by incising the pylorus longitudinally and suturing the incision transversely.

py·lo·ros·co·py (pi″lor-os′kə-pe) [*pyloro-* + *-scopy*] inspection of the pylorus with an endoscope.

py·lo·ro·spasm (pi-lor′o-spaz″əm) [*pyloro-* + *spasm*] spasm of the pylorus or of the pyloric portion of the stomach.

congenital p. spasm of the pylorus in infants due to prenatal conditions.

reflex p. pylorospasm due to extragastric conditions.

py·lo·ro·ste·no·sis (pi-lor″o-stə-no′sis) pyloric stenosis.

py·lo·ros·to·my (pi″lor-os′tə-me) [*pyloro-* + *-stomy*] surgical formation of an opening through the abdominal wall into the stomach near the pylorus.

py·lo·rot·o·my (pi″lor-ot′ə-me) [*pyloro-* + *-tomy*] a type of pyloroplasty involving incision of the pylorus.

py·lo·rus (pi-lor′əs) [Gr. *pyloros*, from *pylē* gate + *ouros* guard] [TA] the most distal part of the stomach, surrounded by a strong band of circular muscle; the stomach contents are emptied through it into the duodenum. Usage is variable, with the term referring sometimes to the entire pyloric part of the stomach and at others to just a section of it, such as the pyloric antrum, canal, or opening. **pylor′ic** *adj*

py(o)- [Gr. *pyon* pus] a combining form denoting relationship to pus.

pyo·ar·thro·sis (pi″o-ahr-thro′sis) acute suppurative arthritis.

pyo·blen·nor·rhea (pi″o-blen″o-re′ə) suppurative blennorrhea.

pyo·cele (pi′o-sēl″) [*pyo-* + *-cele*[1]] 1. distention of a cavity or tube due to retention of pus. 2. specifically, such a condition of pus in the scrotum.

pyo·ce·lia (pi″o-se′le-ə) [*pyo-* + *celi-* + *-ia*] pus in the abdominal cavity.

pyo·ceph·a·lus (pi″o-sef′ə-ləs) brain abscess.

pyo·cin (pi′o-sin) [*pyo-* + *-cin*, from L. *caedere* to kill] a protein bacteriocin produced by certain strains of *Pseudomonas aeruginosa*.

pyo·coc·cus (pi″o-kok′əs) any pus-forming coccus. **pyococ′cic** *adj*

pyo·col·pos (pi″o-kol′pos) [*pyo-* + Gr. *kolpos* vagina] a collection of pus within the vagina.

pyo·cy·an·ic (pi″o-si-an′ik) pertaining to or characterized by blue pus.

pyo·cy·a·nin (pi″o-si′ə-nin) [*pyo-* + *cyan-* + *-in* chemical suffix] a blue-green pigment produced by *Pseudomonas aeruginosa;* it gives the color to blue pus.

pyo·cyst (pi′o-sist) [*pyo-* + *cyst*] a cyst containing pus.

pyo·cys·tis (pi″o-sis′tis) pus in the urinary bladder.

pyo·der·ma (pi″o-dur′mə) [*pyo-* + *derma*] any purulent skin disease. Called also *pyodermia*.

blastomycosis-like p. pyoderma with verrucous plaques and purulent sinuses; it is usually from a bacterial infection and is seen most often in immunocompromised persons.

chancriform p., p. chancrifor′me facie′i an eroded, ulcerated, nodular, solitary lesion with a rolled edge, usually on the face but sometimes elsewhere; it closely resembles a syphilitic chancre, and generally occurs in association with regional lymphadenopathy. The lesion usually involutes and heals with scarring.

p. facia′le an acute, localized skin disease of the face, seen almost exclusively in girls and young women; it is usually in the absence of acne and is characterized by intense erythema, abscesses, cysts, and sinus tracts between deep-seated lesions. If untreated, it may heal to leave severe scarring.

p. fis′tulans sini′fica hidradenitis suppurativa.

p. gangreno′sum a rapidly evolving, idiopathic, chronic, debilitating type of neutrophilic dermatosis that usually accompanies a systemic disease such as ulcerative colitis or certain forms of arthritis; characteristics include irregular, boggy, blue-red ulcers with undermined borders surrounding purulent necrotic bases.

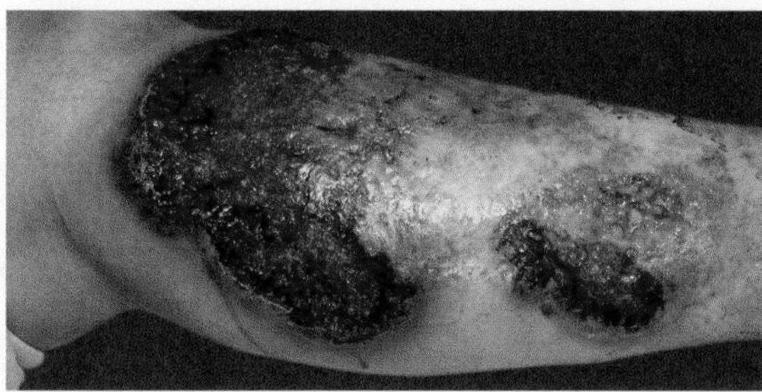

■ Pyoderma gangrenosum in a patient with chronic ulcerative colitis.

juvenile p. a skin disease of unknown etiology seen in puppies, particularly shorthaired breeds; characteristics include pustular lesions of the skin of the face, head, and sometimes other parts of the body with fever and lymphadenopathy. The commonly seen submandibular lymphadenopathy gives the disease its nickname *puppy strangles.* Called also *juvenile cellulitis.*

malignant p. a destructive, progressive, ulcerative, suppurative skin disease resembling pyoderma gangrenosum, usually found on the head, neck, or trunk; it may develop spontaneously or at the site of trauma and then enlarge peripherally.

p. ve′getans see under *dermatitis.*

pyo•der•mia (pi″o-dur′me-ə) pyoderma.

pyo•gen•e•sis (pi″o-jen′ə-sis) [*pyo-* + *-genesis*] the formation of pus; cf. *suppuration.* Called also *pyopoiesis.*

pyo•gen•ic (pi″o-jen′ik) producing pus; called also *pyopoietic.*

py•og•e•nous (pi-oj′ə-nəs) purulent (def. 4).

pyo•he•mo•tho•rax (pi″o-he″mo-thor′aks) [*pyo-* + *hemothorax*] a collection of pus and blood in the pleural space.

pyo•hy•dro•ne•phro•sis (pi″o-hi″dro-nə-fro′sis) hydropyonephrosis.

py•oid (pi′oid) puriform.

pyo•me•tra (pi″o-me′trə) [*pyo-* + *metra*] an accumulation of pus within the uterus.

pyo•me•tri•tis (pi″o-mə-tri′tis) purulent inflammation of the uterus.

pyo•me•tri•um (pi″o-me′tre-əm) pyometra.

pyo•my•o•ma (pi″o-mi-o′mə) a leiomyoma that has undergone suppuration.

pyo•myo•si•tis (pi″o-mi″o-si′tis) [*pyo-* + *myositis*] an acute bacterial infection of skeletal muscle, usually seen in the tropics; in temperate regions it may be seen in immunocompromised or debilitated individuals. It occurs spontaneously without other foci of infection and is most commonly caused by *Staphylococcus aureus.* The primary characteristic is suppuration followed by abscess formation within the fascial covering of the affected muscle or muscles. Called also *spontaneous bacterial myositis* and *tropical p.*

tropical p. pyomyositis.

pyo•ne•phri•tis (pi″o-nə-fri′tis) purulent inflammation of the kidney.

pyo•neph•ro•li•thi•a•sis (pi″o-nef″ro-lĭ-thi′ə-sis) [*pyo-* + *nephrolithiasis*] calculous pyonephrosis.

pyo•neph•ro•sis (pi″o-nə-fro′sis) [*pyo-* + *nephrosis*] infected hydronephrosis that has progressed to suppurative destruction of the renal parenchyma, with extensive or complete loss of renal function. **pyonephrot′ic** *adj*

calculous p. the presence of stones and pus in the kidney.

pyo•ova•ri•um (pi″o-o-var′e-əm) abscess of an ovary.

pyo•peri•car•di•tis (pi″o-per″ĭ-kahr-di′tis) purulent pericarditis.

pyo•peri•car•di•um (pi″o-per″ĭ-kahr′de-əm) [*pyo-* + *pericardium*] the presence of pus in the pericardial cavity.

pyo•peri•to•ne•um (pi″o-per″ĭ-to-ne′əm) [*pyo-* + *peritoneum*] pus in the peritoneal cavity.

pyo•peri•to•ni•tis (pi″o-per″ĭ-to-ni′tis) purulent peritonitis.

pyo•pha•gia (pi″o-fa′jə) [*pyo-* + *-phagia*] the swallowing of pus.

py•oph•thal•mia (pi″of-thal′me-ə) [*py-* + *ophthalmia*] a suppurative condition of the eye; called also *pyophthalmitis.*

py•oph•thal•mi•tis (pi″of-thəl-mi′tis) pyophthalmia.

pyo•phy•lac•tic (pi″o-fi-lak′tik) [*pyo-* + *phylactic*] serving as a defense against purulent infection.

pyo•phy•so•me•tra (pi″o-fi″so-me′trə) [*pyo-* + *physo-* + *metra*] a collection of pus and gas in the uterus.

pyo•pneu•mo•cho•le•cys•ti•tis (pi″o-noo″mo-ko″lə-sis-ti′tis) [*pyo-* + *pneumo-* + *cholecystitis*] emphysematous cholecystitis with pus.

pyo•pneu•mo•cyst (pi″o-noo′mo-sist) [*pyo-* + *pneumo-* + *cyst*] a cyst containing pus and gas.

pyo•pneu•mo•hep•a•ti•tis (pi″o-noo″mo-hep″ə-ti′tis) abscess of the liver with pus and gas in the abscess cavity.

pyo•pneu•mo•peri•car•di•um (pi″o-noo″mo-per″ĭ-kahr′de-əm) [*pyo-* + *pneumo-* + *pericardium*] the presence of pus and gas or air in the pericardial cavity.

pyo•pneu•mo•peri•to•ne•um (pi″o-noo″mo-per″ĭ-to-ne′əm) pus and gas in the peritoneal cavity.

pyo•pneu•mo•peri•to•ni•tis (pi″o-noo″mo-per″ĭ-to-ni′tis) [*pyo-* + *pneumo-* + *peritonitis*] peritonitis with pus and gas in the peritoneal cavity.

pyo•pneu•mo•tho•rax (pi″o-noo″mo-thor′aks) [*pyo-* + *pneumothorax*] a collection of pus and air or gas in the pleural cavity. Called also *pneumoempyema* and *pneumopyothorax.*

pyo•poi•e•sis (pi″o-poi-e′sis) pyogenesis. **pyopoiet′ic** *adj*

pyo•py•elec•ta•sis (pi″o-pi″ə-lek′tə-sis) pyonephrosis.

py•or•rhea (pi″o-re′ə) [*pyo-* + *-rrhea*] 1. periodontitis (def. 1). 2. marginal periodontitis.

p. alveola′ris marginal periodontitis.

Schmutz p. marginal periodontitis.

py•or•rhe•al (pi″o-re′əl) pertaining to or characterized by periodontitis or marginal periodontitis.

pyo•ru•bin (pi″o-roo′bin) a bright-red, water-soluble, nonfluorescent pigment produced by some strains of *Pseudomonas aeruginosa.*

pyo•sal•pin•gi•tis (pi″o-sal″pin-ji′tis) [*pyo-* + *salping-* + *-itis*] purulent salpingitis.

pyo•sal•pin•go-ooph•o•ri•tis (pi″o-sal-ping″go-o″of-ə-ri′tis) inflammation of an ovary and uterine tube, with accumulation of pus.

pyo•sal•pin•go-oo•the•ci•tis (pi″o-sal-ping″go-o″o-the-si′tis) pyosalpingo-oophoritis.

pyo•sal•pinx (pi″o-sal′pinks) [*pyo-* + *salpinx*] a collection of pus in a uterine tube.

pyo•scle•ro•sis (pi″o-sklə-ro′sis) an inflammatory, purulent sclerosis.

pyo•se•mia (pi″o-se′me-ə) pyospermia.

pyo•sep•ti•ce•mia (pi″o-sep″tĭ-se′me-ə) pyemia combined with septicemia.

pyo•sper•mia (pi″o-spur′me-ə) [*pyo-* + *sperm-* + *-ia*] pus in the semen.

pyo•stat•ic (pi″o-stat′ik) [*pyo-* + *-static*] 1. stopping or hindering the process of suppuration; called also *antipyogenic.* 2. an agent that has this effect.

pyo•sto•ma•ti•tis (pi″o-sto″mə-ti′tis) [*pyo-* + *stomatitis*] a suppurative inflammation of the mouth.

p. ve′getans a variant of dermatitis vegetans involving the oral mucosa, sometimes seen in association with ulcerative colitis or some other gastrointestinal disturbance. The primary lesions are miliary abscesses that tend to form groups and become proliferative, soft, red, folded, and verrucous, sometimes spreading over the entire oral cavity. They may remain confined to the mouth or may coexist with typical dermatitis vegetans.

pyo•tho•rax (pi″o-tho′raks) [*pyo-* + *thorax*] empyema (def. 2).

pyo•um•bil•i•cus (pi″o-əm-bil′ĭ-kəs) infection of the umbilicus.

pyo•ura•chus (pi″o-u′rə-kəs) the presence of pus in the urachus.

pyo•ure•ter (pi″o-u-re′tər) [*pyo-* + *ureter*] an accumulation of pus in a ureter.

pyo•ve•sic•u•lo•sis (pi″o-və-sik″u-lo′sis) an accumulation of pus in the seminal vesicles.

pyo•xan•thine (pi″o-zan′thin) a brownish red pigment derivable by oxidation from pyocyanin.

pyo•xan•those (pi″o-zan′thōs) [*pyo-* + Gr. *xanthos* yellow] a yellow pigment produced by the oxidation of pyocyanin in blue pus when exposed to air.

Pyr•a•lis (pir′ə-lis) a genus of widely distributed small moths. *P. farina′lis* is a meal moth that acts as a host for parasites such as tapeworms of the genus *Hymenolepis.*

pyr•a•mid (pir′ə-mid) [Gr. *pyramis*] a pointed or cone-shaped structure or part; called also *pyramis* [TA]. The term is often used alone to indicate the pyramid of the medulla oblongata.

p. of cerebellum pyramis vermis.

p's of Ferrein radii medullares.

p's of kidney pyramides renales; see under *pyramis.*

Lalouette p. lobus pyramidalis glandulae thyroideae.

p. of light see under *cone.*

Malacarne p. the posterior end of the pyramid of the vermis.

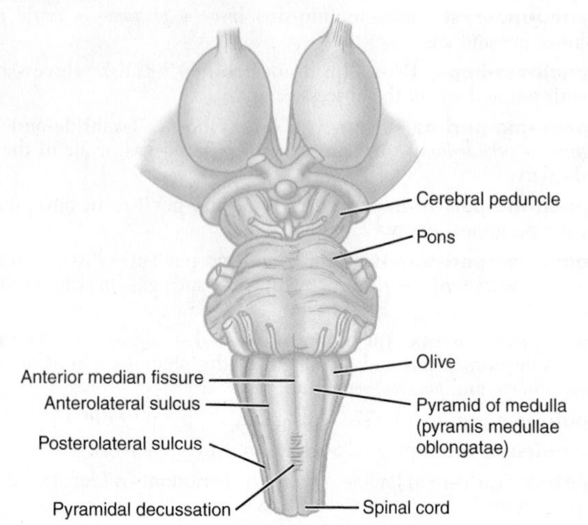

■ Pyramis medullae oblongatae (pyramid of medulla) in an anterior (inferior) view of the brainstem.

p's of Malpighi pyramides renales; see under *pyramis*.
p. of medulla oblongata pyramis medullae oblongatae.
petrous p. pars petrosa ossis temporalis.
renal p's pyramides renales; see under *pyramis*.
p. of temporal bone pars petrosa ossis temporalis.
p. of thyroid lobus pyramidalis glandulae thyroideae.
p. of tympanum eminentia pyramidalis.
p. of vermis pyramis vermis.
p. of vestibule pyramis vestibuli.

py•ram•i•dal (pĭ-ram′ĭ-dəl) [L. *pyramidalis*] 1. shaped like a pyramid. 2. pertaining to the pyramidal tract.

py•ram•i•da•le (pĭ-ram″ĭ-da′le) [L.] os triquetrum.

py•ram•i•da•lis (pĭ-ram″ĭ-da′lis) [L.] pyramidal; see under *musculus*.

py•ram•i•des (pĭ-ram′ĭ-dēz) [Gr.] plural of *pyramis*.

py•ram•i•dot•o•my (pĭ″ram-ĭ-dot′ə-me) section of the pyramidal tract.

pyr•a•mis (pir′ə-mis) pl. *pyra′mides* [Gr.] pyramid: a part or structure with a pointed or conical shape.

p. bul′bi TA alternative for *p. medullae oblongatae*.

p. medul′lae oblonga′tae [TA] pyramid of medulla oblongata: either of two rounded masses, one on either side of the anterior median fissure of the medulla oblongata, composed of motor fibers from the cerebral cortex to the spinal cord and medulla oblongata. Called also *p. bulbi* [TA alternative].

pyra′mides rena′les [TA] renal pyramids: the conical masses that make up the substance of the renal medulla; they contain the loops of Henle, the collecting ducts, and the straight arterioles of the kidney.

p. ver′mis [TA] pyramid of vermis (VIII): the part of the vermis of the cerebellum between the tuber vermis and the uvula, continuous with the lobulus biventer of the cerebellar hemisphere.

p. vesti′buli [TA] pyramid of vestibule: the triangular-shaped anterior end of the vestibular crest.

py•ran (pi′ran) a heterocyclic compound:

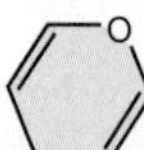

It is the ring structure that forms the basis of the pyranoses.

pyr•a•nose (pir′ə-nōs) any sugar containing a pyran ring structure, a cyclic form that ketoses and aldoses may take in solution. See also individual sugars, e.g., *glucopyranose*.

py•ran•o•side (pĭ-ran′o-sīd) a glycoside in which the sugar is in pyranose configuration.

py•ran•tel (pĭ-ran′təl) a broad-spectrum anthelmintic, effective against pinworms and roundworms; it acts as a depolarizing neuromuscular blocking agent, producing spastic paralysis of the parasite. Usually seen as the pamoate salt.

p. pamoate [USP] the pamoate salt of pyrantel, used for treatment of ascariasis and enterobiasis, administered orally.

p. tartrate the tartrate salt of pyrantel, having the same actions as the pamoate salt.

py•ran•yl (pi′ran-əl) the radical C_5H_5O-, derived from pyran by removal of hydrogen.

pyr•a•zin•a•mide (PZA) (pir″ə-zin′ə-mīd) [USP] an antibacterial derived from nicotinic acid, used as a tuberculostatic, administered orally.

py•ra•zine (pĭ′rə-zēn) an aromatic compound comprising a six-membered ring with nitrogen atoms at positions 1 and 4; it is a component of the folates and of the isoalloxazine ring system of flavins.

pyr•az•o•lone (pir-az′o-lōn) any of a class of nonsteroidal antiinflammatory drugs that have been used in the treatment of arthritis and other musculoskeletal and joint disorders; because of toxicity, few are still used.

pyra•zo•lo•py•rim•i•dine (pir″ə-zo-lo-pi-rim′ĭ-dēn) any in a class of sedative hypnotics that have effects similar to those of the benzodeazepines.

py•rec•tic (pi-rek′tik) [Gr. *pyrektikos* feverish] 1. febrile. 2. pyrogenic. 3. pyrogen.

py•rene (pi′rēn) a carcinogenic polycyclic hydrocarbon, $C_{16}H_{10}$, used in biochemical research.

Py•re•no•chae•ta (pi″rə-no-ke′tə) a genus of Fungi Imperfecti of the form-class Coelomycetes, widely found on plants and in the soil. *P. ro′meroi* has been isolated from cases of eumycotic mycetoma.

py•re•noid (pi′rə-noid) [Gr. *pyrēn* fruit stone + *-oid*] one of the proteinaceous refringent bodies found closely associated with the chloroplasts of most phytoflagellates; involved in the synthesis and storage of polysaccharide.

py•re•ther•a•py (pi″rə-ther′ə-pe) [Gr. *pyr* fever + *therapy*] pyretotherapy.

py•reth•rin (pi-reth′rin) either of two esters, *pyrethrin I* and *pyrethrin II*, found in the flowers of certain species of *Chrysanthemum*, used alone or in combination with piperonyl butoxide as an insecticide and topical pediculicide. See also *pyrethrum extract*, under *extract*.

py•reth•roid (pi-reth′roid) any of a group of growth regulators, analogous to insect juvenile hormones, that interfere with the development of insect larvae; used in the control of insects that are harmful in the adult stage.

Py•re•thrum (pi-re′thrəm) former genus name applied to certain plants of genus *Chrysanthemum* that are sources of pyrethrins.

py•re•thrum (pi-re′thrəm) [Gr. *pyrethron*] the species of *Chrysanthemum* that contain pyrethrins.

py•ret•ic (pi-ret′ik) [Gr. *pyretos* fever] 1. febrile. 2. pyrogenic. 3. pyrogen.

pyret(o)- [Gr. *pyretos* fever] a combining form denoting relationship to fever.

py•ret•o•gen (pi-ret′o-jən) pyrogen.

py•re•to•gen•e•sis (pi″rə-to-jen′ə-sis) [*pyreto-* + *-genesis*] the origin and causation of fever.

py•re•to•gen•ic (pi″rə-to-jen′ik) pyrogenic.

py•re•tog•e•nous (pi″rə-toj′ə-nəs) 1. caused by high body temperature. 2. pyrogenic.

py•re•tog•ra•phy (pi″rə-tog′rə-fe) [*pyreto-* + *-graphy*] a description of fever.

py•re•tol•o•gy (pi″rə-tol′ə-je) [*pyreto-* + *-logy*] the sum of what is known regarding fevers; the science of fevers.

py•re•tol•y•sis (pi″rə-tol′ĭ-sis) [*pyreto-* + *-lysis*] 1. reduction of fever. 2. lysis that is hastened by fever.

py•re•to•ther•a•py (pi″rə-to-ther′ə-pe) [*pyreto-* + *therapy*] 1. treatment of a disease by raising the patient's temperature, such as by physical means or injection of fever-producing vaccines. Called also *fever therapy*, *therapeutic fever*, and *pyretherapy*. 2. the treatment of fever.

py•rex•ia (pi-rek′se-ə) fever. **pyrex′ial** *adj*

Pyr•i•ben•za•mine (pir″ĭ-ben′zə-mēn) trademark for preparations of tripelennamine.

pyr•i•dine (pir′ĭ-dēn) a toxic, colorless, liquid hydrocarbon comprising a substituted benzene ring, C_5H_5N, usually derived from coal tar; it is used as a laboratory and industrial intermediate.

Py•rid•i•um (pĭ-rid′e-əm) trademark for preparations of phenazopyridine hydrochloride.

pyr•i•do•stig•mine bro•mide (pir″ĭ-do-stig′mēn) [USP] a cholinesterase inhibitor, which acts by inhibiting destruction of acetylcholine and so facilitating transmission of impulses across the neuromuscular junction; used as a cholinergic in the symptomatic treatment of myasthenia gravis and for reversal of the effects of nondepolarizing neuromuscular blocking agents such as tubocurarine after surgery; administered orally, intravenously, or intramuscularly.

pyr•i•dox•al (pir″ĭ-dok′səl) one of the forms of vitamin B_6 (q.v.).

p. phosphate pyridoxal phosphorylated at the hydroxymethyl group of C-5; it is the prosthetic group of many enzymes involved in amino acid transformations.

pyr•i•dox•amine (pir″ĭ-dok′sə-mēn) one of the three active forms of vitamin B_6.

pyr•i•dox•ic ac•id (pir″ĭ-dok′sik) oxidation product of pyridoxal, the principal urinary excretion product of vitamin B_6.

pyr•i•dox•ine (pēr″ĭ-dok′sēn) one of the forms of vitamin B_6 (q.v.).

p. hydrochloride [USP] the hydrochloride salt of pyridoxine, used in the prophylaxis and treatment of vitamin B_6 deficiency and as an antidote in the treatment of cycloserine and isoniazid poisoning.

pyr•i•form (pir′ĭ-form) piriform.

py•ril•amine (pə-ril′ə-mēn) an ethylenediamine derivative with antihistaminic, sedative, and hypnotic actions.

p. maleate [USP] the maleate salt of pyrilamine, used as an antihistamine in the treatment of hypersensitivity reactions and pruritic skin disorders, and as an ingredient in cough and cold preparations; administered orally.

p. tannate the tannate salt of pyrilamine, having the same actions and uses as the maleate salt.

pyr•i•meth•amine (pir″ĭ-meth′ə-mēn) [USP] a folic acid antagonist, used as an antimalarial, especially for suppressive prophylaxis, and also used concomitantly with a sulfonamide in the treatment of toxoplasmosis, administered orally.

py•rim•i•dine (pə-rim′ĭ-dēn) an organic compound, a metadiazine, $C_4H_4N_2$, which is the fundamental form of the pyrimidine bases. These are mostly oxy or amino derivatives, for example, 2,4-dioxypyrimidine is uracil, 2-oxy-4-aminopyrimidine is cytosine, and 2,4-dioxy-5-methylpyrimidine is thymine, all of which are constituents of nucleic acid. See illustration of *purine and pyrimidine bases*, under *base*.

py•rim•i•dine-nu•cleo•side phos•phor•y•lase (pə-rim′ĭ-dēn noo′kle-o-sīd″ fos-for′ə-lās) [EC 2.4.2.2] an enzyme of the transferase class that catalyzes the cleavage of pyrimidine nucleosides to form pyrimidines and ribose 1-phosphates in the degradation of nucleotides and nucleic acids.

py•rin (pi′rin) a 781–amino acid protein (MW 86,000) expressed primarily in the cytoplasm of neutrophils and monocytes and believed to regulate neutrophil-mediated inflammation; mutations of the gene that codes for this protein cause familial Mediterranean fever. Called also *marenostrin*.

pyr•i•thi•amine (pir″ĭ-thi′ə-mēn) a synthetic compound that by metabolic competition can cause symptoms of thiamine deficiency.

pyr(o)- [Gr. *pyr* fire] 1. a combining form denoting relationship to fire or heat. 2. in chemistry, a prefix meaning produced by heating. 3. in inorganic chemistry, a prefix indicating a dimeric acid anhydride, e.g., pyrophosphoric acid.

py•ro•bo•rate (pi-ro-bor′āt) any salt of pyroboric acid.

py•ro•bo•ric ac•id (pi″ro-bor′ik) a dimer of boric acid, $H_2B_4O_7$, produced by heating boric acid. Called also *tetraboric acid*.

py•ro•cat•e•chin (pi″ro-kat′ə-kin) pyrocatechol.

py•ro•cat•e•chol (pi″ro-kat′ə-kol) a compound comprising the aromatic portion in the synthesis of endogenous catecholamines, obtained by distilling catechu or a related substance or produced synthetically. It is a reagent and was formerly used as a topical antiseptic. Called also *catechol* and *pyrocatechin*.

py•ro•dex•trin (pi″ro-dek′strin) dextrin.

py•ro•gal•lic ac•id (pi″ro-gal′ik) pyrogallol.

py•ro•gal•lol (pi″ro-gal′ol) a poisonous acid derived from gallic acid, used as a reagent, photographic developer, mordant for wool, and dye constituent. Called also *pyrogallic acid*.

py•ro•gen (pi′ro-jən) [*pyro-* + *-gen*] a fever-producing substance.

bacterial p. a fever-producing agent of bacterial origin; endotoxin.

endogenous p. fever-producing subtances produced by the macrophages or other cells in response to infection or to events inducing cell-mediated immunity; included are interleukin-1 and tumor necrosis factor.

exogenous p. a fever-producing agent of external origin; types include bacterial endotoxins and other microbial products, certain types of antigen-antibody complexes, viruses, synthetic polynucleotides, incompatible blood and blood products, and androgen breakdown products such as etiocholanone. The action is mediated by an endogenous pyrogen.

leukocytic p. interleukin-1.

py•ro•ge•net•ic (pi″ro-jə-net′ik) pyrogenic.

py•ro•gen•ic (pi″ro-jen′ik) [*pyro-* + *-genic*] causing fever. Called also *febrifacient* and *pyretic*.

py•rog•e•nous (pi-roj′ə-nəs) pyrogenic.

py•ro•glob•u•lin (pi″ro-glob′u-lin) [*pyro-* + *globulin*] a monoclonal immunoglobulin that precipitates irreversibly upon heating to 56°C (as opposed to Bence Jones proteins, which precipitate but redissolve on cooling).

py•ro•glob•u•lin•emia (pi″ro-glob″u-lin-e′me-ə) the presence of pyroglobulin in the blood, occurring most frequently in multiple myeloma, Waldenström macroglobulinemia, and other lymphoproliferative disorders, although it occasionally is seen without known associated disease.

py•ro•glu•ta•mate (pi″ro-gloo′tə-māt) 5-oxoproline.

py•ro•glu•tam•ic ac•id (pi″ro-gloo-tam′ik) 5-oxoproline.

py•ro•glu•tam•ic•ac•id•uria (pi″ro-gloo-tam″ik-as″ĭ-du′re-ə) generalized deficiency of glutathione synthetase; see *glutathione synthetase deficiency*.

py•ro•lag•nia (pi″ro-lag′ne-ə) [*pyro-* + Gr. *lagneia* lust] sexual gratification from witnessing or making fires.

py•ro•lig•ne•ous (pi″ro-lig′ne-əs) [*pyro-* + *ligneous*] pertaining to the destructive distillation of wood.

Py•ro•lite (pi′ro-līt) trademark for a kit for the preparation of technetium Tc 99m (pyro- and trimeta-) phosphates.

py•rol•y•sis (pi-rol′ĭ-sis) [*pyro-* + *-lysis*] decomposition of organic substances under the influence of a rise in temperature.

Py•ro•lyte (pi′ro-līt) trademark for a type of pyrolytic carbon.

py•ro•ma•nia (pi″ro-ma′ne-ə) [*pyro-* + *-mania*] [DSM-IV] an impulse control disorder characterized by the compulsion to set or watch fires in the absence of monetary or other gain, the act being preceded by tension or arousal and resulting in pleasure or relief.

erotic p. pyrolagnia.

py•rom•e•ter (pi-rom′ə-tər) [*pyro-* + *-meter*] an instrument for measuring the intensity of heat, especially for very high temperatures that cannot be measured with a mercury thermometer.

py•ro•nin (pi′ro-nin) any of several basic xanthene dyes ranging from pink-red to purple-red in color, used as histological stains and as specific stains for RNA. Spelled also *pyronine*.

p. B a basic xanthene dye used as a stain for bacteria, molds, and RNA.

p. G p. Y.

p. Y a basic xanthene dye used as a bacterial stain and as the RNA-staining component of methyl green–pyronin stain.

py•ro•nine (pi′ro-nēn) pyronin.

py•ro•nin•o•phil•ia (pi″ro-nin″o-fil′e-ə) increased affinity for pyronin dyes, characteristic of cells with high levels of cytoplasmic RNA.

py•ro•nino•phil•ic (pi″ro-nin″o-fil′ik) 1. pertaining to or exhibiting pyroninophilia. 2. staining selectively with pyronin dyes.

py•ro•pho•bia (pi″ro-fo′be-ə) [*pyro-* + *-phobia*] abnormal fear of fire.

py•ro•phos•pha•tase (pi″ro-fos′fə-tās) any enzyme that catalyzes the hydrolysis of a pyrophosphate bond, cleaving between the two phosphate groups. See also *inorganic pyrophosphatase*.

py•ro•phos•phate (pi″ro-fos′fāt) any salt, anion, or ester of pyrophosphoric acid. Formed during many metabolic reactions, it is an important intermediate because its large free energy of hydrolysis makes the reactions essentially irreversible. The symbol PP_i denotes the uncombined form.

py•ro•phos•pho•ki•nase (pi″ro-fos″fo-ki′nās) a term used in the recommended names of the diphosphotransferases.

py•ro•phos•pho•ric ac•id (pi″ro-fos-for′ik) the ester-linked dimeric form of phosphoric acid, $H_4P_2O_7$. See also *phosphoric acid*.

py•ro•phos•pho•trans•fer•ase (pi″ro-fos″fo-trans′fər-ās) diphosphotransferase.

py•ro•poi•ki•lo•cyt•ic (pi″ro-poi″kĭ-lo-sit′ik) characterized by or of the nature of the heat-sensitive poikilocytes that occur in pyropoikilocytosis.

py•ro•poi•ki•lo•cy•to•sis (pi″ro-poi″kĭ-lo-si-to′sis) presence in the blood of numerous bizarre-shaped heat-sensitive poikilocytes.

hereditary p. an autosomal recessive blood disorder in which there are many different types of heat-sensitive poikilocytes and erythrocyte fragments, with severe hemolytic anemia. It resembles severe hereditary elliptocytosis, but there are few if any elliptocytes.

py•ro•sis (pi-ro′sis) [Gr. *pyrōsis* burning] heartburn.

py•rot•ic (pi-rot′ik) [Gr. *pyrōtikos* fit for burning] 1. caustic; burning. 2. pertaining to heartburn (pyrosis).

py•roxy•lin (pir-ok′sə-lin) [*pyr-* + Gr. *xylon* wood] [USP] a product of the action of a mixture of nitric and sulfuric acids on cotton, consisting chiefly of cellulose tetranitrate; a necessary ingredient of collodion. Called also *guncotton* and *nitrocellulose*.

pyr·ro·caine hy·dro·chlo·ride (pir'o-kān) a local anesthetic used in dentistry to produce infiltration and nerve block anesthesia.

pyr·role (pir-ōl') 1. a toxic, basic heterocyclic compound:

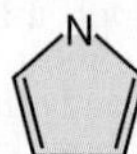

It is used in the manufacture of pharmaceuticals. 2. a substituted derivative of this structure.

pyr·rol·i·dine (pir-ol'ĭ-dēn) a simple base, tetramethylene imine, obtained from tobacco or prepared from pyrrole.

pyr·ro·line (pir'o-lēn) pyrrole in which one of the two double bonds has been hydrogenated.

Δ^1-p. 5-carboxylate a carboxy derivative of pyrroline that acts as an intermediate in the degradation and synthesis of proline.

1-pyr·ro·line-5-car·box·y·late de·hy·dro·gen·ase (pir'o-lēn kahr-bok'sə-lāt de-hi'dro-jən-ās) [EC 1.5.1.12] an enzyme of the oxidoreductase class that catalyzes the dehydrogenation of Δ^1-pyrroline 5-carboxylate to glutamate, using NAD^+ as an electron acceptor; the reaction is a step in the degradation of proline and excess ornithine. The enzyme can also oxidize the 3-hydroxy derivative of Δ^1-pyrroline 5-carboxylate to form 4-hydroxyglutamate. Deficiency of the enzyme, an autosomal recessive trait, is the cause of hyperprolinemia, type II.

pyr·ro·line-5-car·box·y·late re·duc·tase (pir'o-lēn kahr-bok'sə-lāt re-duk'tās) [EC 1.5.1.2] an enzyme of the oxidoreductase class that catalyzes the irreversible reduction of Δ^1-pyrroline 5-carboxylate to proline, using NADPH (or NADH) as an electron donor; the reaction is the final step in the biosynthesis of proline from glutamate or ornithine. The enzyme may also reduce the 3-hydroxy analog of pyrroline 5-carboxylate to form hydroxyproline.

pyr·ro·line 5-car·box·y·late syn·thase (pir'o-lēn kahr-bok'sə-lāt sin'thās) a mitochondrial enzyme activity that catalyzes the conversion of glutamate to Δ^1-pyrroline 5-carboxylate, an intermediate in the synthesis of proline. ATP is hydrolyzed in the reaction and NADPH is the electron donor.

pyr·ro·liz·i·dine (pĭ-ro-liz'ĭ-dēn) any of a group of alkaloids found in various plants, causing hepatotoxic syndromes in ruminants. Included are jacobine, monocrotaline, retrorsine, senecifoline, and senecine.

pyr·ro·lo·por·phyr·ia (pir"ə-lo-por-fir'e-ə) acute intermittent porphyria.

py·ru·vate (pi'roo-vāt) a salt, ester, or anionic form of pyruvic acid. In biochemistry, the term is used interchangeably with pyruvic acid, even though pyruvate technically refers to the negatively charged ion. Pyruvate is the end product of glycolysis, and it in turn may be converted to lactate or acetyl CoA or to ethanol (as in yeasts).

py·ru·vate car·box·y·lase (pi'roo-vāt kahr-bok'sə-lās) [EC 6.4.1.1] an enzyme of the ligase class that catalyzes the irreversible carboxylation of pyruvate to form oxaloacetate. The enzyme is a mitochondrial protein containing a biotin prosthetic group, requiring Mg^{2+} or Mn^{2+} and acetyl CoA, and occurs in liver but not in muscle. The reaction is necessary for gluconeogenesis from lactate or amino acids forming pyruvate and also provides four-carbon compounds for the tricarboxylic acid cycle. Deficiency of the enzyme, an autosomal recessive trait, causes severe psychomotor retardation and lactic acidosis in infants; there is a particularly severe, rapidly fatal form, in which hyperammonemia, hypercitrullinemia, and hyperlysinemia are also present.

py·ru·vate de·car·box·y·lase (pi'roo-vāt de"kahr-bok'sə-lās) [EC 4.1.1.1] an enzyme of the lyase class that catalyzes the decarboxylation of 2-keto acids to form aldehydes, part of the anaerobic fermentation pathway that produces ethanol and CO_2 from glucose. The enzyme occurs in yeast and requires thiamine pyrophosphate as a cofactor.

py·ru·vate de·hy·dro·gen·ase (ac·e·tyl-trans·fer·ring) (pi'roo-vāt de-hi'dro-jən-ās as'ə-təl trans'fər-ing) [EC 1.2.4.1] an enzyme of the oxidoreductase class that is a component of the multienzyme pyruvate dehydrogenase complex (q.v.). The enzyme catalyzes the oxidative decarboxylation of pyruvate, forming acetyl bound to the cofactor thiamine pyrophosphate; the acetyl is subsequently transferred to the lipoamide linked to the side chain of a lysine residue of the enzyme dihydrolipoyllysine-residue acetyltransferase, which is also part of the complex. Deficiency of the enzyme causes lacticacidemia, ataxia, psychomotor retardation, and sometimes lactic acidosis.

[py·ru·vate de·hy·dro·gen·ase (ac·e·tyl-trans·fer·ring)] ki·nase (pi'roo-vāt de-hi'dro-jən-ās as'ə-təl trans'fər-ing ki'nās) [EC 2.7.11.2] an enzyme of the transferase class that catalyzes the phosphorylation of the decarboxylase component of the pyruvate dehydrogenase complex, inactivating the complex. It is inhibited by pyruvate and ADP.

[py·ru·vate de·hy·dro·gen·ase (ac·e·tyl-trans·fer·ring)]-phos·pha·tase (pi'roo-vāt de-hi'dro-jən-ās as'ə-təl trans'fər-ing fos'fə-tās) [EC 3.1.3.43] an enzyme of the hydrolase class that catalyzes the dephosphorylation of the pyruvate dehydrogenase complex, which activates the complex. Deficiency of the enzyme causes metabolic acidosis with high levels of lactic, pyruvic, and free fatty acids in serum.

py·ru·vate de·hy·dro·gen·ase com·plex (pi'roo-vāt de-hi'dro-jən-ās kom'pleks) see under *complex*.

py·ru·vate ki·nase (PK) (pi'roo-vāt ki'nās) [EC 2.7.1.40] an enzyme of the transferase class that catalyzes the transfer of high energy phosphate from phospho*enol*pyruvate to ADP to yield ATP and pyruvate. It is one of two reactions generating ATP in the Embden-Meyerhof pathway (see illustration under *pathway*) and a key regulatory site in this pathway. The enzyme has three distinct isozymes. Deficiency of pyruvate kinase activity in erythrocytes, an autosomal recessive trait, results in hemolytic anemia.

py·ru·vate ki·nase (PK) de·fi·cien·cy (pi'roo-vāt ki'nās) an autosomal recessive disorder caused by mutation in the *PKLR* gene (locus: 1q21), which encodes the liver and erythrocyte isozymes of pyruvate kinase. It is the most common glycolytic enzyme defect in the Embden-Meyerhof pathway and is characterized by chronic hemolytic anemia of widely variable severity.

py·ru·ve·mia (pi"roo-ve'me-ə) increased pyruvic acid in the blood.

py·ru·vic ac·id (pi-roo'vik) α-ketopropionic acid, $CH_3COCOOH$, the end product of the Embden-Meyerhof pathway of glucose metabolism, also produced by the catabolism of several amino acids. Pyruvate can be converted to acetyl coenzyme A, which can enter the tricarboxylic acid cycle for aerobic production of energy or be used for fatty acid synthesis. Energy can be obtained anaerobically by conversion of pyruvate to lactate (which occurs in mammalian muscle tissue) or to ethanol, small organic acids, and many other compounds (microbial fermentations). Pyruvate can also be converted to oxaloacetate, the first step in gluconeogenesis.

6-py·ru·voyl-tet·ra·hy·drop·ter·in syn·thase (PTPS, PTS) (pi-roo"vo-əl-tet"rə-hi-drop'tər-in sin'thās) an enzyme catalyzing the rate-limiting reaction in the synthesis of tetrahydrobiopterin from guanosine triphosphate. Deficiency of the enzyme, an autosomal recessive trait caused by mutation of the *PTS* gene, which encodes the enzyme, is a form of tetrahydrobiopterin deficiency (q.v.).

pyr·vin·i·um pam·o·ate (pir-vin'e-əm) [USP] an anthelmintic that acts by preventing the uptake of exogenous glucose and is administered orally in the treatment of enterobiasis.

Py·thi·a·ceae (pith"e-a'se-e) a family of aquatic, moldlike chromists of the order Pythiales, consisting mainly of plant parasites with some saprobes, having an intracellular mycelium and sporangia borne singly on branching sporangiophores; it includes a genus pathogenic for animals, *Pythium*.

Py·thi·a·les (pith"e-a'lēs) an order of chromists of the subclass Saprolegniomycetidae; organisms pathogenic for animals are included in the family Pythiaceae.

pyth·i·o·sis (pith"e-o'sis) infection by *Pythium insidiosum*, primarily affecting horses and mules but also seen in dogs and cattle, in India, Indonesia, Europe, and the southern United States; characteristics include formation of subcutaneous abscesses that enlarge until the overlying skin is destroyed, leaving large raw surfaces. It is often confused with cutaneous habronemiasis because of the close clinical similarity between the two conditions. Human infection occurs rarely, with manifestations that may be primarily subcutaneous, ocular, vascular, or systemic; disease is often rapidly progressive, severe, and resistant to treatment. Called also *bursati*, *hyphomycosis destruens equi*, *leeches*, and *swamp cancer*.

Py·thi·um (pith'e-əm) [Gr. *pythein* to make rot] a genus of root-parasitic, moldlike chromists of the family Pythiaceae, having filamentous sporangia and smooth-walled spherical oogonia. Most members are plant parasites.

P. insidio'sum a species that causes pythiosis in animals and occasionally infects humans.

py·tho·gen·e·sis (pi"tho-jen'ə-sis) [Gr. *pythein* to rot + *-genesis*] the origination of a process of decay or decomposition.

py·tho·gen·ic (pi"tho-jen'ik) [Gr. *pythein* to rot + *-genic*] causing decay or decomposition.

py·thog·e·nous (pi-thoj'ə-nəs) caused by putrefaction or filth.

py·u·ria (pi-u're-ə) [*pyo-* + *-uria*] the presence of pus in the urine.

miliary p. the presence in the urine of small miliary inclusions consisting of pus cells, blood cells, and epithelium.

PZA pyrazinamide.

PZD partial zona dissection.

PZI protamine zinc insulin.

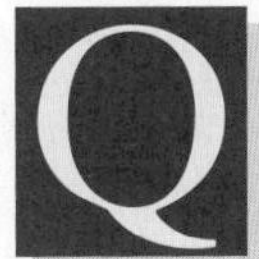

Q ubiquinone.

Q electric charge; heat; reaction quotient.

Q_{10} temperature coefficient; ubiquinone.

Q rate of blood flow.

q the long arm of a chromosome.

q. [L.] qua′que (each, every).

q electric charge; ubiquinone; (in statistics) the probability of an alternative event occurring where *p* is the probability of the specified event and $q = 1 - p$. Cf. *p*.

Q an•gle [Q for *quadriceps*] see under *angle*.

q.d. [L.] qua′que di′e (every day) *(on the JCAHO "Do Not Use" List).*

Q fe•ver (ku′ fe′vər) [Q for *query;* so called because the etiologic agent was unknown when it was first reported in Queensland, Australia, in 1935] see under *fever*.

q.h. [L.] qua′que ho′ra (every hour).

qi (che) [Mandarin Chinese "life energy"] one of the basic substances that according to traditional Chinese medicine pervade the body; a subtle influence or vital energy that is the cause of most physiologic processes and whose proper balance is necessary for maintaining health. Several types of qi are present in the body; disturbances, such as blockage in the flow of qi along the meridians (q.v.), cause disease. Spelled also *chi* and *ch'i*.

q.i.d. [L.] qua′ter in di′e (four times a day).

qi gong (che′ kung′) [Chinese] qi cultivation, a broad range of practices, incorporating meditation, movement exercises, and breath control, whose purpose is to manipulate and develop qi, and ranging in application from the meditative systems of spiritual practitioners to medical practice to the martial arts; in traditional Chinese medicine, it is used both for self-therapy and by practitioners to correct imbalances of qi in others.

q.l. [L.] quan′tum li′bet (as much as desired).

QNS Queen's Nursing Sister (of Queen's Institute of District Nursing).

qns quantity not sufficient.

q.p. [L.] quan′tum pla′ceat (as much as desired).

q.q.h. [L.] qua′que quar′ta ho′ra (every four hours).

Qq.hor. [L.] qua′que ho′ra (every hour).

QS_2 electromechanical systole.

q.s. [L.] quan′tum sa′tis (sufficient quantity).

q-sort (ku′sort) a technique of personality assessment in which the subject (or an observer) indicates the degree to which a standardized set of descriptive statements applies to the subject.

q.suff. [L.] quan′tum suf′ficit (as much as suffices).

qt quart.

qter the end of the long arm of a chromosome.

quack (kwak) [from *quacksalver*, q.v.] one who fraudulently claims to have ability and experience in the diagnosis and treatment of disease or the effects to be achieved by the treatment.

quack•ery (kwak′ər-e) the fraudulent misrepresentation of one's ability and experience in the diagnosis and treatment of disease or of the effects to be achieved by the treatment offered.

quack•sal•ver (kwak-sal′vər) [Dutch "salve peddler"] one claiming special merit for treatment with medications and salves.

Quad•ra•moid (kwod′rə-moid) trademark for an oral suspension of trisulfapyrimidines.

quad•ran•gle (kwod′rang-gəl) 1. quadrilateral. 2. a dental instrument having four angulations in the shank connecting the handle, or shaft, with the working portion of the instrument, known as the blade, or nib. Cf. *binangle*, *monangle*, and *triple-angle*.

quad•ran•gu•lar (kwod-rang′gu-lər) [*quadri-* + *angular*] having four angles.

quad•rant (kwod′rənt) [L. *quadrans* quarter] 1. one quarter of a circle; that portion of the circumference of a circle that subtends an angle of 90 degrees. 2. any one of four corresponding parts or quarters, as of the abdominal surface, the field of vision, the dentition, or the tympanic membrane.

quad•ran•tal (kwod-ran′təl) resembling or affecting a quadrant.

quad•rant•an•o•pia (kwod″rənt-ə-no′pe-ə) [*quadrant* + *an-*[1] + *-opia*] hemianopia in one fourth of the visual field, bounded by a vertical and a horizontal radius. Called also *tetartanopia* and *quadrant hemianopia*.

quad•rant•an•op•sia (kwod″rənt-ə-nop′se-ə) quadrantanopia.

quad•ran•tec•to•my (kwod″rən-tek′tə-me) a form of partial mastectomy involving en bloc excision of tumor in one quadrant of breast tissue, as well as the pectoralis major muscle fascia and overlying skin.

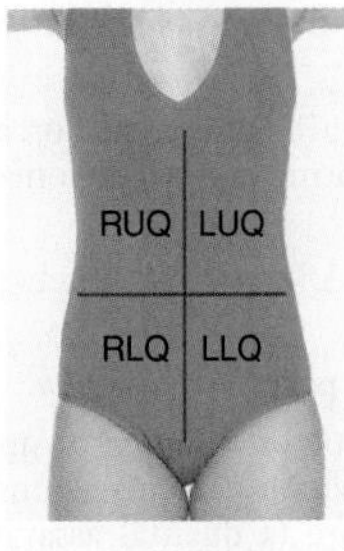

■ Quadrants of the abdomen. *RUQ,* Right upper quadrant; *LUQ,* left upper quadrant; *RLQ,* right lower quadrant; *LLQ,* left lower quadrant.

quad•rate (kwod′rāt) [L. *quadratus* squared] square or squared; four sided.

quad•ra•ti•pro•na•tor (kwod-ra″tĭ-pro-na′tər) musculus pronator quadratus.

quad•ra•tus (kwod-ra′təs) [L.] squared; four sided.

quadr(i)- [L. *quattuor* four] a prefix signifying four, or fourfold.

quad•ri•ba•sic (kwod″rĭ-ba′sik) having four replaceable atoms of hydrogen.

quad•ri•ceps (kwod′rĭ-seps) [*quadri-* + L. *caput* head] four headed; possessing four heads.

q. fe′moris musculus quadriceps femoris.

quad•ri•ceps•plas•ty (kwod′rĭ-seps-plas″te) plastic repair of a ruptured quadriceps femoris muscle.

quad•ri•cus•pid (kwod″rĭ-kus′pid) [*quadri-* + *cuspid*] 1. having four cusps; said of a tooth, or of a semilunar (aortic or pulmonary) valve with four cusps. 2. a tooth with four cusps.

quad•ri•den•tate (kwod″rĭ-den′tāt) forming four coordinate covalent bonds in a chelate.

quad•ri•dig•i•tate (kwod″rĭ-dij′ĭ-tāt) tetradactylous.

quad•ri•gem•i•nal (kwod″rĭ-jem′ĭ-nəl) [L. *quadrigeminus*] 1. fourfold, or in four parts; forming a group of four. 2. pertaining to the corpora quadrigemina.

quad•ri•gem•i•nus (kwod″rĭ-jem′ĭ-nəs) [L.] quadrigeminal.

quad•ri•gem•i•ny (kwod″rĭ-jem′ĭ-ne) [*quadri-* + L. *geminus* twin] 1. occurrence in fours. 2. the occurrence of a quadrigeminal pulse.

quad•ri•lat•er•al (kwod″rĭ-lat′ər-əl) [*quadri-* + *lateral*] 1. having four sides. 2. a figure that has four sides; called also *quadrangle*. 3. a postulate with four parts.

Celsus q. "Notae vero inflammationis sunt quattuor, rubor et tumor, cum calore et dolore." There are in fact four signs of inflammation—redness, swelling, heat, and pain.

quad•ri•loc•u•lar (kwod″ri-lok′u-lər) [*quadri-* + *locular*] having four cells, cavities, or chambers.

quad•rip•a•ra (kwod-rip′ə-rə) [*quadri-* + *para*] a woman who has had four pregnancies which resulted in viable offspring; also written *para IV*.

quad•ri•pa•re•sis (kwod″rĭ-pə-re′sis) tetraparesis.

quad•ri•par•tite (kwod″rĭ-pahr′tīt) having four parts or divisions.

quad•ri•ple•gia (kwod″rĭ-ple′jə) [*quadri-* + *-plegia*] paralysis of all four limbs; called also *tetraplegia*.

quad•ri•ple•gic (kwod″rĭ-ple′jik) 1. of, pertaining to, or characterized by quadriplegia. 2. an individual with quadriplegia.

quad•ri•po•lar (kwod″rĭ-po′lər) having four poles, as a cell.

quad•ri•sect (kwod′rĭ-sekt) [*quadri-* + L. *secare* to cut] to cut into four parts.

quad•ri•sec•tion (kwod″rĭ-sek′shən) [*quadri-* + *section*] division into four parts.

quad•ri•tu•ber•cu•lar (kwod″rĭ-too-bur′ku-lər) having four tubercles or cusps; said of teeth.

quad•ri•va•lent (kwod″rĭ-va′lənt) 1. effective against four different entities, as diseases or strains of a pathogen. 2. tetravalent.

quad•ru•ped (kwod′roo-ped″) [*quadri-* + L. *pes* foot] 1. four-footed. 2. an animal having four feet.

quadrupl. [L.] quadruplica′to (four times as much).

quad•rup•let (kwod-ro͞op′lət) [L. *quadrupulus* fourfold] one of four offspring produced in one gestation period.

qua•le (kwa′le) the quality of a thing; especially the quality of a sensation or other conscious process.

qual•i•ta•tive (kwahl′ĭ-ta″tiv) [L. *qualitativus*] pertaining to quality. Cf. *quantitative.*

qual•i•ty (kwahl′ĭ-te) 1. a characteristic or attribute. 2. in radiology, the ability of a particular form or type of ionizing radiation to penetrate matter.

Quant sign (kwahnt) [C.A.J. *Quant,* Dutch physician, early 20th century] see under *sign.*

quan•ta (kwahn′tə) [L.] plural of *quantum.*

quan•tal (kwahn′təl) 1. of or relating to quanta. 2. denoting an all-or-none response, one for which partial responses are undetectable or are not measured, or a procedure (a quantal assay) in which such a response is measured.

quan•tile (kwahn′tīl) [*quantity* + *-ile* (by analogy with *quartile, percentile,* etc.)] any of the values that divide the range of an observed or theoretical probability distribution into a given number of equal, ordered parts; examples are the median, quartiles, and percentiles. Each value divides the range into two specified parts, with the part below the value corresponding to a prescribed fraction p and the part above to $1 - p$.

quan•tim•e•ter (kwahn-tim′ə-tər) [L. *quantus* how much + *-meter*] an apparatus for measuring the quantity of x-rays generated by a tube.

quan•ti•ta•tive (kwahn′tĭ-ta″tiv) [L. *quantitativus*] 1. denoting or expressing a quantity. 2. relating to the proportionate quantities or to the amount of the constituents of a compound.

quan•ti•ty (kwahn′tĭ-te) 1. a characteristic, as of energy or mass, susceptible of precise physical measurement. 2. a measurable amount.

quan•tum (kwahn′təm) pl. *quan′ta* [L. "as much as"] a unit of energy under the quantum theory. It is hν, in which h is Planck constant, 6.626×10^{-34} joule second, and ν is the frequency of vibration with which the energy is associated. See *quantum theory,* under *theory.*

q. of light a quantity of light (radiant energy) equivalent to the frequency of the light times 6.626×10^{-34} joule second.

quan•tum li•bet (kwahn′təm li′bət) [L.] as much as desired.

quan•tum sat•is (kwahn′təm sat′is) [L.] a sufficient quantity.

quan•tum suf•fi•cit (kwahn′təm suf′ĭ-sit) [L.] as much as suffices.

quar•an•tine (kwor′ən-tēn, kwahr′ən-tēn) [Ital. *quarantina,* from L. *quadraginta* forty] 1. restriction of freedom of movement of apparently well individuals who have been exposed to infectious disease, imposed for the usual maximal incubation period of the disease *(quarantine period).* Cf. *surveillance* (def. 2). 2. quarantine period; see under *period.* 3. the place where persons are detained for inspection. 4. to detain or isolate on account of suspected contagion.

quart (qt) (kwort) [L. *quartus* fourth] one fourth of a gallon; in the United States it is equal to 0.946 liter and in Great Britain it is an *imperial quart* and is equal to 1.14 liters.

quar•tan (kwor′tən) [L. *quartanus,* pertaining to the fourth] recurring every 72 hours (fourth day, counting the day of the previous paroxysm). See *malaria.*

quar•ter (kwor′tər) the part of a horse's hoof lying between the heel and the toe.

false q. a cleft from top to bottom of the quarter of a horse's hoof.

quar•tile (kwor′tīl) [L. *quartilis* pertaining to a fourth, from *quartus* fourth] any of the three values that divide the range of a probability distribution into four parts of equal probability; i.e., the 1st, 2nd, and 3rd quartiles are the 25th, 50th, and 75th percentiles.

quar•tip•a•ra (kwor-tip′ə-rə) quadripara.

quar•ti•sect (kwor′tĭ-səkt) [L. *quartus* fourth + *secare* to cut] to cut into four parts.

quar•ti•ster•nal (kwor″tĭ-stur′nəl) [L. *quartus* fourth + *sternum* sternum] pertaining to the fourth sternebra, or the bony segment of the sternum opposite the fourth intercostal space.

quartz (kworts) a crystalline form of silica; workers inhaling excessive amounts of its dust may suffer from silicosis. Called also *rock crystal.*

Quar•zan (kwahr′zan) trademark for a preparation of clidinium bromide.

quasi- [L. *quasi* as if, as though] a prefix meaning almost, seemingly, or resembling.

qua•si•dip•loid (kwah″ze-dip′loid) [*quasi-* + *diploid*] 1. having two sets of chromosomes but with an abnormal distribution. In tissue cell cultures, a chromosome of one pair may be missing and may be replaced by an extra chromosome from another pair. 2. an organism or cell that is quasidiploid.

qua•si•dom•i•nance (kwah″ze-dom′ĭ-nəns) [*quasi-* + *dominance*] the mimicking of dominance in inheritance, with roughly half of the offspring expressing a phenotype, but actually caused by mating of a carrier of a recessive gene with an individual homozygous for the gene; it can be distinguished from dominance by examination of an extended pedigree. **quasidom′inant** *adj*

qua•si•spe•cies (quah″ze-spe′sēz) one of a population of closely related genotypes coexisting as a result of mutations of the original genotype, with selective pressures causing the genotypes to assume a distribution in the center of which is the most frequent, and often fittest, genotype. The heterogeneous mixture of closely related viruses within an individual host are quasispecies.

quas•sa•tion (kwah-sa′shən) [L. *quassatio*] the crushing of drugs, or their reduction to small pieces.

Quas•sia (kwosh′ə) [*Quassi,* 18th century slave of Surinam, who used it] a genus of tropical trees of the family Simaroubaceae whose wood is used as an antipyretic. *Q. ama′ra* L. is Surinam quassia, a source of medicinal quassia.

quas•sia (kwosh′ə) 1. any of various tropical trees of the genera *Picrasma* and *Quassia.* 2. the dried, bitter heartwood of *Picrasma excelsa* (Jamaica quassia) or *Quassia amara* (Surinam quassia); it has been used as an enema for pinworms.

Quat., quat. [L.] quat′tuor (four).

qua•ter in die (kwah′ter in de′a) [L.] four times a day.

qua•ter•nary (kwah′tər-nar″e, kwah-tur′nər-e) [L. *quaternarius,* from *quattuor* four] 1. fourth in order. 2. containing four elements or groups.

Qua•tre•fages angle (kah″trə-fahzh′) [Jean Louis Armand de *Quatrefages* de Bréau, French naturalist, 1810–1892] parietal angle.

qua•ze•pam (kwah′zə-pam) [USP] a benzodiazepine used as a sedative and hypnotic in the treatment of insomnia; administered orally.

Queck•en•stedt sign (phenomenon, test) (kwek′ən-shtet″) [Hans Heinrich Georg *Queckenstedt,* German physician, 1876–1918] see under *sign.*

Quel•i•cin (kwel′ĭ-sin) trademark for a preparation of succinylcholine chloride.

quench•ing (kwench′ing) 1. extinguishing, suppressing, or diminishing a physical property, as the rapid chilling of a hot metal by plunging it into cold liquid. 2. in biochemistry, decrease of fluorescence from an excited molecule by interference that reduces the fluorescence intensity, such as deexcitation of the fluorescent molecule by collision with other molecules, absorption of fluorescent emission by the surrounding medium, or a decrease or shift in wavelength of fluorescence due to chemical interaction of the fluorescent molecule with other molecules. 3. in liquid scintillation counting, interference with generation or propagation of light energy from the sample, decreasing the counting efficiency of the detector. 4. the termination of secondary and subsequent ionizations in a detector to give it time to become sensitive again.

fluorescence q. a technique for measuring the primary interaction of antigen and antibody by determination of the amount of light absorbed by bound antigen from fluorescent-labeled antibody exposed to ultraviolet radiation.

Quénu hemorrhoidal plexus (ka-nu′) [Eduard André Victor Alfred *Quénu,* French surgeon, 1852–1933] see under *plexus.*

Qué•nu-Mu•ret sign (ka-nu′ mu-ra′) [E.A.V.A. *Quénu;* Paul Louis *Muret,* French surgeon, early 20th century] see under *sign.*

Quer•cus (kwur′kəs) [L.] the oaks, a genus of large, leaf-bearing, hardwood trees of the family Fagaceae. *Q. al′ba* (the white oak) and other species make the excrescence called the nutgall (q.v.). Oaks have gallic and tannic acids in their leaves and acorns, making those parts poisonous to livestock.

Quer•vain (kār-vă′) see *de Quervain.*

ques•tion•naire (kwes″chə-nār′) a set of questions used to obtain personal information or to gather statistically useful data.

CAGE q. a simple, four-question screening instrument for alcoholism; patients are asked if they feel that they should *cut down* on alcohol intake, are *annoyed* at criticism, feel *guilt* about alcohol use, or use an alcoholic "*eye opener*" in the morning.

Ques•tran (kwes′tran) trademark for preparations of cholestyramine resin.

que•ti•a•pine fu•ma•rate (quĕ-ti′ə-pēn) a dibenzothiazepine derivative that is an antagonist to multiple neurotransmitter receptors in the brain, used as an antipsychotic in the treatment of schizophrenia and other psychotic disorders; administered orally.

Quey•rat erythroplasia (ka-rah′) [Louis Auguste *Queyrat,* French dermatologist, 1856–1933] penile intraepithelial neoplasia; see under *neoplasia.*

Quick test (kwik) [Armand James *Quick,* American physician, 1894–1978] see under *test.*

quick (kwik) 1. rapid. 2. alive. 3. pregnant and able to feel the fetal movements.

quick•en•ing (kwik′ən-ing) the first recognizable movements of the fetus, appearing usually from the sixteenth to the twentieth week of pregnancy.

quick•lime (kwik′līm) calcium oxide.

quid•ding (kwid′ing) a condition in horses in which food is taken into the mouth, repeatedly chewed, and then expelled; it may be caused by injuries to the mouth, disorders of the teeth or gums, paralysis of the muscles of mastication, or some other condition causing inability to swallow.

quil•la•ia (kwĭ-la′yə) the dried inner bark of *Quillaja saponaria*, formerly used in medicine for its local irritant action. Its chief constituent is quillaic acid, and it is used as an emulsifier and surfactant. Called also *soap bark*, *soap tree bark*, and *quillay bark*.

Quil•la•ja (kwĭ-la′yə) [Sp. Am. *quillai*] a genus of trees of the family Rosaceae. *Q. sapona′ria* Molina is a species native to South America that is a source of quillaia.

quin•a•crine hy•dro•chlo•ride (kwin′ə-krin) an antimalarial, antiprotozoal, and anthelmintic, used especially for suppressive therapy of malaria and in the treatment of giardiasis and tapeworm infestations, administered orally. Called also *chinacrine hydrochloride* and *mepacrine hydrochloride*.

Quin•a•glute (kwin′ə-glo͞ot) trademark for a preparation of quinidine gluconate.

quin•ag•o•lide hy•dro•chlo•ride (kwin-ag′o-līd) a non-ergot dopamine D_2 antagonist with actions and uses similar to those of bromocriptine mesylate, used in treatment of hyperprolactinemia, such as with a prolactinoma; it can also be used as a growth hormone suppressant in the treatment of acromegaly. Administered orally.

quin•al•bar•bi•tone (kwin″əl-bahr′bĭ-tōn) secobarbital.

quin•al•dic ac•id (kwin-al′dik) a catabolite of tryptophan that is excreted in the urine. Called also *quinaldinic acid*.

quin•al•din•ic ac•id (kwin″əl-din′ik) quinaldic acid.

quin•a•pril hy•dro•chlo•ride (kwin′ə-pril″) [USP] an angiotensin-converting enzyme inhibitor used in the treatment of hypertension, alone or in combination with a thiazide diuretic, and congestive heart failure; administered orally.

quin•azo•line (kwin-az′o-lēn) a bicyclic aromatic ring structure comprising a benzene ring linked to a pyridine derivative having nitrogen substituents at positions 1 and 3; the parent compound of prazosin and related drugs.

Quin•cke edema (disease), pulse (sign) (kwing′kə) [Heinrich Irenaeus *Quincke*, German physician, 1842–1922] see *angioedema* and see under *pulse*.

quin•eth•a•zone (kwin-eth′ə-zōn) a sulfonamide derivative that has a different chemical structure from but the same pharmacologic actions as the thiazide diuretics, used in the treatment of hypertension and edema; administered orally.

quin•ic ac•id (kwin′ik) a compound found in cinchona bark and in many plants. Called also *kinic acid*.

Quin•i•dex (kwin′ĭ-deks) trademark for a preparation of quinidine sulfate.

quin•i•dine (kwin′ĭ-dēn) the dextrorotatory isomer of quinine obtained from various species of *Cinchona* and their hybrids, and from *Remijia peduncluata*, or prepared from quinine. It has cardiac depressant activity, and is as potent an antimalarial as quinine but is rarely used for the latter effect except when quinine is not immediately available.

q. gluconate [USP] the gluconate salt of quinidine, having the same actions as the base; used in the treatment of certain cardiac arrhythmias, administered orally or intravenously, and in the treatment of life-threatening falciparum malaria, administered intravenously.

q. polygalacturonate a salt of quinidine, having the same actions and uses as the base; administered orally in the treatment of certain cardiac arrhythmias.

q. sulfate [USP] the sulfate salt of quinidine, having the same actions and uses as the base; administered orally in the treatment of certain cardiac arrhythmias.

■ Quinazoline.

qui•nine (kwin′in, kwin-ēn′, kwi′nīn) [L. *quinina*] an alkaloid of cinchona, which suppresses the asexual forms of all malarial parasites during the erythrocytic stage and has a slight effect on *Plasmodium vivax* and *P. malariae* during the gametocyte stage. Once widely used to prevent and control malaria, it has been largely replaced by less toxic and more effective synthetic antimalarials, and is now used chiefly (usually in the form of one of its soluble salts) in the treatment of falciparum malaria resistant to other antimalarials. Quinine also has analgesic, antipyretic, mild oxytocic, cardiac depressant, and sclerosing properties, and it decreases the excitability of the motor end plate.

q. dihydrochloride the dihydrochloride salt of quinine, having the same actions and uses as the base; administered orally or parenterally.

q. hydrochloride the hydrochloride salt of quinine, having the same actions and uses as the base; administered orally.

q. sulfate [USP] the dihydrate sulfate salt of quinine, having the same actions and uses as the base, and also used to prevent nocturnal cramps in the legs and feet; administered orally.

q. and urea hydrochloride a double salt of quinine and urea hydrochloride, which has been used to produce sclerosing, thrombosis, and obliteration of internal hemorrhoids and varicose veins.

qui•nin•ism (kwin′ĭ-niz″əm) cinchonism.

quin•o•line (kwin′o-lēn) a heterocyclic nitrogenous compound comprising a benzene ring linked to one of pyridine, derivable from quinine, coal tar, and various other sources, or synthesized; used as a preservative for anatomical specimens.

quin•o•lin•ic ac•id (kwin″o-lin′ik) a cyclic, nitrogen-containing, dicarboxylic compound for which a class of glutamate receptors has an affinity; it may play a role in neurodegenerative disorders.

quin•o•lone (kwin′o-lōn) any of a group of synthetic antibacterial agents that includes nalidixic acid, cinoxacin, rosoxacin, and the fluoroquinolones.

fluorinated 4-q. fluoroquinolone.

qui•none (kwi′nōn, kwin′ōn) any of a group of highly conjugated aromatic diketones, usually in the *ortho* or *para* configuration, derived from benzene or from multiple ring hydrocarbons such as anthracene or naphthalene; they are subclassified on the basis of ring structure (e.g., anthraquinone or benzoquinone), are mild oxidizing agents, and are usually colored yellow, red, or orange. The term is often used specifically to denote benzoquinone (q.v.), particularly 1,4-benzoquinone.

quin•o•noid (kwin′o-noid) resembling a quinone or containing a quinone (particularly a benzoquinone) ring structure.

Quinq. [L.] quin′que (five).

quin•que•cus•pid (kwing″kwə-kus′pid) [L. *quinque* five + *cuspid*] 1. having five cusps. 2. a tooth with five cusps.

quin•que•tu•ber•cu•lar (kwing″kwə-too-bur′ku-lər) having five tubercles or cusps.

quin•que•va•lent (kwing″kwə-va′lənt) pentavalent.

quin•qui•na (kin-ke′nə) cinchona (def. 2).

quin•sy (kwin′ze) [Gr. *kynanche* sore throat] peritonsillar abscess.

quint- [L. *quintus* fifth] a prefix signifying five or fifth.

Quint. [L.] quin′tus (fifth).

quin•tan (kwin′tən) [L. *quintanus* of the fifth] recurring every fifth day, as a fever.

quin•tes•sence (kwin-tes′əns) [*quint-* + *essence*] the highly concentrated extract of any substance.

quin•tile (kwin′tīl) [L. *quintilis* pertaining to a fifth, from *quintus* fifth] any of the four values that divide the range of a probability distribution into five parts of equal probability, i.e., the 1st, 2nd, 3rd, and 4th quintiles are the 20th, 40th, 60th, and 80th percentiles.

quin•tip•a•ra (kwin-tip′ə-rə) [*quint-* + *para*] a woman who has had five pregnancies which resulted in viable offspring; also written *para V*.

quin•ti•ster•nal (kwin″tĭ-stur′nəl) [*quint-* + *sternal*] denoting the fifth bony portion of the sternum, or the part above the xiphoid process and adjacent to the fifth intercostal space.

Quin•ton-Scrib•ner shunt (kwin′tən skrib′nər) [Wayne E. *Quinton*, American nephrologist, 20th century: Belding H. *Scribner*, American nephrologist, born 1921] see under *shunt*.

quin•tup•let (kwin-tup′lət) [L. *quintuplex* five-fold] one of five offspring produced in one gestation period.

quin•u•pris•tin (kwin-u′pris-tin) a semisynthetic streptogramin antibacterial effective against a variety of gram-positive organisms, inhibiting the late phase of protein synthesis in the bacterial ribosome. It is used in conjunction with dalfopristin in the treatment of serious bacteremia caused by vancomycin-resistant *Enterococcus faecium* and complicated skin and skin structure infections caused by *Streptococcus pyogenes* or methicillin-sensitive *Staphylococcus aureus;* administered intravenously.

quis·qual·ic ac·id (kwis-kwah′lik) an excitotoxin found in the *Quisqualus* nut; it has actions and experimental uses similar to those of kainic acid.

quit·tor (kwit′or) a fistulous sore on the quarters or the coronet of a horse's foot.

simple q. local inflammation resulting in a slough, with formation of pus immediately above the hoof.

skin q. a painful ulcer of the skin above the hoof.

subhorny q. inflammation from the coronary band to beneath the hoof, with pus formation in the sensitive tissue.

tendinous q. quittor in which inflammation extends into the tendons of the leg and the ligaments of the joint.

Quix·in (kwik′sin) trademark for a preparation of levofloxacin.

quo·ad vi·tam (kwo′ad vi′tam) [L.] so far as life is concerned.

Quotid. [L.] quotid′ie (daily).

quo·tid·i·an (kwo-tid′e-ən) [L. *quotidianus* daily] recurring every day; applied to the type of fever caused by certain forms of malarial parasites.

quo·tient (kwo′shənt) a number obtained as the result of division; a number indicating how many times one number is contained in another.

achievement q. a percentage statement of the extent to which a child has progressed in learning in proportion to his or her ability. Abbreviated AQ.

albumin q. the amount of albumin in the blood plasma divided by the amount of albumin present in the blood.

caloric q. the quotient obtained by dividing the heat evolved (expressed in calories) by the oxygen consumed (expressed in milligrams) in a metabolic process.

D q. the ratio of glucose to nitrogen in the urine.

growth q. that part of the entire food energy which is used for growth.

intelligence q. the measure of intelligence obtained by dividing the patient's mental age, as ascertained by the Binet test, by chronological age and multiplying the result by 100. Abbreviated IQ.

protein q. the number obtained by dividing the quantity of globulin in the blood plasma by the quantity of albumin.

reaction q. for a balanced chemical equation, the product of the concentrations of the reaction products, each raised to the power equal to the coefficient of the product in the equation, divided by the concentrations of the reactants, each raised to the power equal to its coefficient. For the equation $aA + bB + \ldots = rR + sS + \ldots$,

$$Q = \frac{[R]^r[S]^s}{[A]^a[B]^b}.$$

At equilibrium the reaction quotient equals the equilibrium constant.

respiratory q. (RQ) the ratio of the volume of carbon dioxide given off by the body tissues to the volume of oxygen absorbed by them; usually equal to the corresponding volumes given off and taken up by the lungs.

q.v. [L.] quan′tum vis (as much as you please); quod vi′de (which see).

Qvar (ku′vār) trademark for preparations of beclomethasone dipropionate.

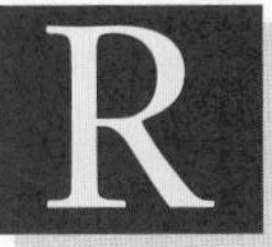

R arginine; organic radical; Rankine (see under *scale*); rate; expiratory exchange ratio; Réaumur (see under *scale*); resistance (def. 3); respiration; rhythm; right; roentgen; rough (colony).

R. [L.] remo'tum (far).

R resistance (def. 3); gas constant.

***R*-** [L. *rectus* right] a stereodescriptor used to specify the absolute configuration of compounds having asymmetric carbon atoms. The four different substituents at the asymmetric carbon atom are ranked according to the Cahn-Ingold-Prelog sequence rules; then, looking at the molecule with the lowest ranking substituent pointing directly away from the viewer, if the other three substituents are in clockwise order going from highest to lowest ranked, the configuration is *R;* otherwise *S.* Example: L-threonine is (2*S*:3*R*)-2-amino-3-hydroxybutanoic acid.

R_A, R_{AW} airway resistance.

R_e Reynolds number.

R_f in paper or thin-layer chromatography, the distance moved by a solute spot from the origin expressed as a fraction of the distance moved by the solvent front.

℞ [L.] re'cipe (take). See *prescription.*

r ring chromosome; drug resistance.

r correlation coefficient; distance; radius; drug resistance.

r_s Spearman rank correlation coefficient.

ρ rho, the seventeenth letter of the Greek alphabet; symbol for *correlation coefficient* (of a population).

RA rheumatoid arthritis.

Ra radium.

RAAS renin-angiotensin-aldosterone system.

Rab•A•vert (rāb'ə-vert") trademark for a preparation of rabies vaccine (purified chick embryo cell vaccine).

rab•bet•ting (rab'ət-ing) impaction of the denticulated broken surfaces of a fractured bone.

rab•bit (rab'it) any of various species of short-tailed lagomorphs, long-eared burrowing mammals of the family Leporidae, originally from Europe and Asia but later introduced into the Americas, Australia, and elsewhere, becoming pests and sometimes reservoirs for disease such as tularemia. Rabbits are often used in laboratory medicine.

Watanabe heritable hyperlipidemic (WHHL) r. a mutant strain of rabbits that have a genetic deficiency of LDL (low-density lipoprotein) receptors similar to that occurring in human familial hypercholesterolemia; they are used in studies of lipoprotein metabolism and atherogenesis.

rab•bit•pox (rab'it-poks) an acute eruptive skin disease of rabbits, caused by a virus closely related to the vaccinia virus; it is often fatal.

ra•bep•ra•zole so•di•um (rə-bep'ra-zōl) a proton pump inhibitor used to limit gastric acid secretion in treatment of erosive or ulcerative gastroesophageal reflux disease and other conditions marked by excessive secretion of gastric acid; administered orally.

rab•id (rab'id) [L. *rabidus*] infected with rabies.

ra•bies (ra'bēz, ra'be-ēz) [L. *rabere* to rage] an acute infectious disease of the central nervous system that can affect almost any mammal, caused by a virus of the genus *Lyssavirus.* It is usually spread by contamination with virus-laden saliva of bites from infected animals, although aerosol infection can occur via the respiratory route, transplantation, or ingestion of infected tissues. Many different mammals can be vectors. The incubation period is highly variable, depending on the size of the inoculum and the site of the bite, being shorter after a bite near the brain than after one farther away. Symptoms usually include paresthesia, pain, or a burning sensation at the site of inoculation; periods of hyperexcitability, hallucinations, delirium, and bizarre behavior alternating with periods of calmness and lucidity; painful spasms of pharyngeal and laryngeal muscles, hypersalivation, and fearfulness provoked by attempts to drink or even by the sight of fluids (hydrophobia); convulsions; meningismus; paralysis; and coma. Recovery is rare, with death usually associated with respiratory depression and cardiorespiratory failure. Formerly the term *hydrophobia* was used as a synonym for rabies in general rather than for just the symptom of the paralytic phase.

dumb r. paralytic r.

furious r. a stage or form of rabies in which excessive motor activity is prominent.

paralytic r. a stage or form of rabies in which the most prominent symptom is ascending paralysis. Called also *dumb r.*

ra•bi•form (ra'bĭ-form) resembling rabies.

Rab•son-Men•den•hall syndrome (rab'sən men'dən-hawl) [S.M. *Rabson,* American physician, 20th century; E.N. *Mendenhall,* American physician, 20th century] see under *syndrome.*

ra•ce•mase (ra'sə-mās) a term used in the names of some enzymes of the subclass racemases and epimerases [EC 5.1] to denote those that catalyze inversion of the configuration around the asymmetric carbon atom in a substrate having only one center of asymmetry; thus, racemers are interconverted. Cf. *epimerase.*

ra•ce•mate (ra'sə-māt) an equimolecular mixture of two enantiomorphic isomers, being optically inactive in solution because of the presence of the same number of dextro- and levorotatory molecules. In the solid state it may have the properties of a loosely bound molecular compound. Called also *racemic form, racemic mixture,* or *racemic modification.*

ra•ce•me•thi•o•nine (rās"ə-mə-thi'o-nēn) a racemic mixture of D- and L-methionine, administered orally as a urinary acidifier to reduce skin irritation in incontinence and diaper rash in infants and to reduce urine odor.

ra•ce•mic (ra-se'mik) made up of two enantiomorphic isomers and therefore optically inactive.

ra•ce•mi•za•tion (ra"sə-mĭ-za'shən) the transformation of one half of the molecules of an optically active compound into molecules which possess exactly the opposite (mirror-image) configuration, with complete loss of rotatory power because of the statistical balance between equal numbers of dextro- and levorotatory molecules. Cf. *mutarotation.*

rac•e•mose (ras'ə-mōs) [L. *racemosus*] resembling a bunch of grapes on its stalk.

ra•ceph•e•drine hy•dro•chlo•ride (ra-sef'ə-drēn) the racemic form of ephedrine hydrochloride, having the same actions and uses.

rac•er (ra'sər) any of several species of fast-moving colubrid snakes.

black r. blacksnake (def. 2).

ra•chi•al (ra'ke-əl) spinal (def. 2).

ra•chi•al•gia (ra"ke-al'jə) rachiodynia.

ra•chi•cen•te•sis (ra"ke-sen-te'sis) [*rachi-* + *-centesis*] lumbar puncture.

ra•chid•i•al (ra-kid'e-əl) spinal (def. 2).

ra•chid•i•an (ra-kid'e-ən) spinal (def. 2).

ra•chi•graph (ra'ke-graf) [*rachi-* + *-graph*] an instrument for recording the outlines of the spine and back.

ra•chil•y•sis (ra-kil'ĭ-sis) [*rachi-* + *-lysis*] mechanical treatment of a curved vertebral column by combined traction and pressure.

rachi(o)- [Gr. *rhachis* spine] a combining form denoting relation to the spine.

ra•chio•camp•sis (ra"ke-o-kamp'sis) [*rachio-* + Gr. *kampsis* curve] curvature of the vertebral column.

ra•chio•cen•te•sis (ra"ke-o-sen-te'sis) [*rachio-* + *-centesis*] lumbar puncture.

ra•chio•chy•sis (ra"ke-ok'ĭ-sis) [*rachio-* + Gr. *chysis* a pouring] the effusion of a fluid within the vertebral canal.

ra•chi•odyn•ia (ra"ke-o-din'e-ə) [*rachio-* + *-odynia*] pain in the vertebral column. Called also *rachialgia.* Cf. *spondylodynia.*

ra•chio•ky•pho•sis (ra"ke-o-ki-fo'sis) kyphosis.

ra•chi•om•e•ter (ra"ke-om'ə-tər) [*rachio-* + *-meter*] an instrument for measuring curvatures of the vertebral column.

ra•chio•my•eli•tis (ra"ke-o-mi"ə-li'tis) [*rachio-* + *myelitis*] myelitis (def. 1).

ra•chi•op•a•gus (ra"ke-op'ə-gəs) [*rachio-* + *pagus*] symmetrical conjoined twins united back to back in the sagittal plane, fusion being limited to the upper trunk and cervical region.

ra•chi•op•a•thy (ra"ke-op'ə-the) [*rachio-* + *-pathy*] spondylopathy.

ra•chio•sco•li•o•sis (ra"ke-o-sko"le-o'sis) lateral curvature of the spine.

ra•chio•tome (ra'ke-o-tōm) an instrument for cutting the vertebrae.

ra•chi•ot•o•my (ra"ke-ot'ə-me) [*rachio-* + *-tomy*] incision of a vertebra or of the vertebral column.

ra•chip•a•gus (ra-kip'ə-gəs) [*rachi-* + *-pagus*] vertebrodidymus.

ra•chis (ra'kis) [Gr. *rhachis* spine] columna vertebralis.

ra•chis•chi•sis (ra-kis'kĭ-sis) [*rachi-* + *-schisis*] congenital fissure of the vertebral column; see also *spina bifida.*

r. partia'lis merorachischisis.

r. poste'rior spina bifida.

r. tota'lis fissure of the entire vertebral column; called also *holorachischisis.* See also *spina bifida.*

ra•chit•ic (ra-kit'ik) pertaining to or affected with rickets.

ra•chi•tis (ra-ki'tis) [Gr. *rachitis*] 1. rickets. 2. spondylitis.

r. feta'lis anula'ris the formation before birth of anular thickenings on the long bones.

r. feta'lis microme'lica deficient longitudinal growth of the bones of the fetus.

rach•i•tism (rak'ĭ-tiz"əm) a tendency to rickets.

ra•chit•o•gen•ic (rə-kit"o-jen'ik) causing rickets.

rach•i•tome (ra'kĭ-tōm) rachiotome.

ra•chit•o•my (rə-kit'ə-me) rachiotomy.

rac•lo•pride (rak'lo-prīd) an antipsychotic compound related to sulpiride; used investigationally.

r. C 11 [USP] raclopride in which a portion of the molecules have been labeled at the *o*-methyl position with ^{11}C, used as a tracer in tomographic studies of neurological disorders associated with D_2 dopaminergic receptor dysfunction; administered intravenously.

RAD right axis deviation.

rad[1] (rad) [acronym for *r*adiation *a*bsorbed *d*ose] a unit of measurement of the absorbed dose of ionizing radiation; it corresponds to an energy transfer of 100 ergs per gram of any absorbing material (including tissues). The biological effect of 1 rad varies with the kind of radiation the tissue is exposed to.

rad[2] abbreviation for *radian.*

rad. [L.] ra'dix (root).

ra•dec•to•my (ra-dek'tə-me) [*radix* + *-ectomy*] root amputation.

Rad•for•dia (rad-for'de-ə) a genus of mites of the family Myobiidae; *R. ensi'fera* is found on laboratory rats and sometimes causes severe pruritus with alopecia.

ra•di•a•bil•i•ty (ra"de-ə-bil'ĭ-te) the property of being radiable.

ra•di•a•ble (ra'de-ə-bəl) capable of being penetrated by radiation, especially by x-rays.

ra•di•ad (ra'de-ad) toward the radius or radial side of the forearm.

ra•di•al (ra'de-əl) [L. *radialis*] 1. pertaining to a radius. 2. pertaining to the lateral aspect of the forearm as opposed to the medial (ulnar) aspect. 3. radiating; spreading outward from a common center.

ra•di•a•lis (ra"de-a'lis) [L., from *radius,* q.v.] [TA] radial; a general term denoting relationship to the radius or to the radial aspect of the forearm.

ra•di•an (rad) (ra'de-ən) [from *radius*] the SI unit of measurement of plane angles, equal to the angle subtended to the center of a circle by an arc whose length is equal to the radius of the circle. One radian equals $360°/2\pi$ or approximately 57.296°.

ra•di•ant (ra'de-ənt) [L. *radians*] 1. diverging from a common center. 2. emitting radiation or heat. 3. transmitted by radiation.

ra•di•ate (ra'de-āt) [L. *radiare, radiatus*] 1. to diverge or spread from a common point. 2. arranged in a radiating manner.

ra•di•a•tio (ra-de-a'she-o) pl. *radiatio'nes* [L., from *radiare* to furnish with spokes] a radiation or radiating structure; used in anatomical nomenclature to designate a collection of nerve fibers connecting different portions of the brain.

r. acus'tica [TA] acoustic radiation: a fiber tract arising in the medial geniculate nucleus and passing laterally in the sublenticular portion of the internal capsule to terminate in the transverse temporal gyri; the radiation provides reciprocal connections and forms part of the inferior thalamic peduncle.

r. cor'poris callo'si [TA] radiation of corpus callosum: the projection of fibers from the corpus callosum to all parts of the neopallium.

r. op'tica [TA] optic radiation: a fiber tract that begins at the lateral geniculate body, passes laterally through the pars retrolentiformis of the internal capsule, follows the lateral wall of the lateral ventricle, immediately internal to the tapetum, and ends in the striate area on the medial surface of the occipital lobe on either side of the calcarine sulcus; the radiation provides reciprocal connections and forms part of the posterior thalamic peduncle. Called also *geniculocalcarine tract, occipitothalamic radiation,* and *radiation of Gratiolet.*

r. tha'lami ante'rior [TA] anterior thalamic radiation: the group of thalamocortical fibers of the anterior limb of the internal capsule connecting the medial and anterior thalamic nuclei and the cortex of the frontal lobe.

r. tha'lami centra'lis [TA] central thalamic radiation: the group of thalamocortical fibers of the posterior limb of the internal capsule, presumably carrying general sensory impulses from the ventral thalamic nuclei to the postcentral gyrus. Called also *superior thalamic radiation.*

r. tha'lami infe'rior [TA] inferior thalamic radiation: the smallest of the four thalamic peduncles; it connects the medial geniculate body with certain areas of the cortex of the temporal lobe, forming one of the principal components of the ansa peduncularis. Called also *inferior peduncle of thalamus.*

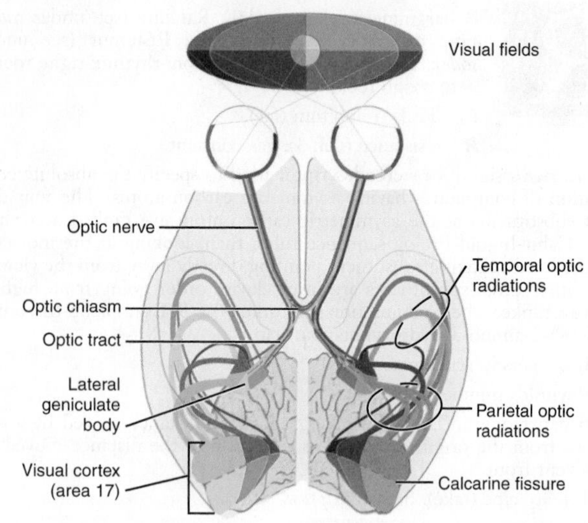

■ Optic radiations (radiationes opticae); the extent of their spread is exaggerated for clarity.

r. tha'lami poste'rior [TA] posterior thalamic radiation: the group of thalamocortical fibers of the retrolentiform part of the internal capsule connecting the cortices of the occipital and parietal lobes and the caudal parts of the thalamus.

ra•di•a•tion (ra"de-a'shən) [L. *radiatio,* q.v.] 1. divergence from a common center. 2. a structure made up of divergent elements, as one of the fiber tracts in the brain; for official names of specific structures, see under *radiatio.* 3. energy transmitted by waves through space or through some medium; usually referring to electromagnetic radiation when used without a modifier. By extension, a stream of particles, such as electrons, neutrons, protons, or alpha particles.

α-r. see under *ray.*

acoustic r. radiatio acustica.

actinic r. see under *ray.*

adaptive r. evolution from a generalized, primitive species to diverse, specialized species, each adapted to a distinct mode of life.

alpha r. see under *ray.*

annihilation r. radiation produced by the collision and annihilation of a particle and its antiparticle, especially the two 0.511 MeV gamma ray photons produced by the annihilation of a positron and an electron.

auditory r. radiatio acustica.

β-r. see under *ray.*

background r. radiation arising from radioactive material other than that directly under consideration or study. Background radiation due to cosmic rays and natural radioactivity in the environment is always present; additional background radiation may be due to the presence of other radioactive material in the vicinity, to radioactive components of building materials, etc.

beta r. see under *ray.*

braking r. bremsstrahlung.

Cerenkov r. visible light emitted by a high-speed charged particle moving through a transparent medium at a speed greater than the speed of light in that medium.

r. of corpus callosum radiatio corporis callosi.

corpuscular r. radiation consisting of streams of subatomic particles, such as protons, deuterons, electrons, positrons, and neutrons.

direct r. primary r.

electromagnetic r. see under *wave.*

γ-r., gamma r. see under *ray.*

r. of Gratiolet radiatio optica.

heterogeneous r. radiation consisting of a beam of particles of various energies, or having different frequencies, or containing different types of particles.

homogeneous r. radiation consisting of an extremely narrow band of frequencies or a beam of monoenergetic particles of a single type.

infrared r. see *infrared.*

interstitial r. energy emitted by radium, radon, or some other radiopharmaceutical inserted directly into the tissue; see *interstitial radiotherapy,* under *radiotherapy.*

ionizing r. corpuscular or electromagnetic radiation capable of producing ionization, directly or indirectly, in its passage through matter.

monochromatic r. radiation having a single wavelength.

monoenergetic r. radiation of a given type, as of alpha, beta, or gamma rays, in which all particles or photons originate with and have the same energy.

occipitothalamic r., optic r. radiatio optica.

photochemical r. the part of the radiant spectrum that produces chemical changes.

primary r. radiation coming directly from a source, such as a radioactive substance or an x-ray tube, without interactions with matter.

pyramidal r. the projection of fibers from the cerebral cortex to the pyramidal tract of the medulla oblongata.

scattered r., secondary r. radiation whose direction has been changed by interaction with matter in its passage through a substance. See also *scattering.*

tegmental r. fibers radiating laterally from the red nucleus.

thalamic r's the four two-way radiations of thalamocortical fibers that connect the dorsal thalamus with many parts of the cerebral cortex; they form a major portion of the internal capsule and the corona radiata. See terms beginning *radiatio thalami,* under *radiatio.* Called also *thalamic peduncles.*

thalamic r., anterior radiatio thalami anterior.

thalamic r., central radiatio thalami centralis.

thalamic r., inferior radiatio thalami inferior.

thalamic r., posterior radiatio thalami posterior.

thalamic r., superior radiatio thalami centralis.

thalamostriate r. the extension of fibers from the thalamus and hypothalamus to the corpus striatum.

thalamotemporal r. radiatio acustica.

r's of thalamus thalamic r's.

ultraviolet r. see under *ray.*

ra•di•a•ti•o•nes (ra-de-a″she-o′nēz) [L.] plural of *radiatio.*

rad•i•cal (rad′ĭ-kəl) [L. *radicalis*] 1. directed to the cause; directed to the root or source of a morbid process, as radical surgery. 2. a group of atoms which enters into and goes out of chemical combination without change, and which forms one of the fundamental constituents of a molecule. Organic radicals are symbolized R.

acid r. 1. the electronegative element which combines with hydrogen to form an acid. 2. all of an acid except the hydroxyl group.

alcohol r. all of the alcohol molecule except the hydrogen atom of the —OH group; an alkoxy radical.

color r. chromophore.

free r. a radical that carries an unpaired electron; such radicals are extremely reactive, with a very short half-life (10^{-5} second or less in an aqueous solution).

oxygen r. a toxic metabolite of oxygen, such as superoxide or singlet oxygen, capable of damaging microorganisms and normal tissues.

rad•i•ces (rad′ĭ-sēz) [L.] plural of *radix.*

ra•dic•i•form (ra-dis′ĭ-form) [*radix* + *form*] shaped like a root; shaped like the root of a tooth.

rad•i•cle (rad′ĭ-kəl) [L. *radicula*] any one of the smallest branches of a vessel or nerve. Called also *radicula* and *ramulus.*

rad•i•cot•o•my (rad″ĭ-kot′ə-me) rhizotomy.

ra•dic•u•la (rə-dik′u-lə) [L.] radicle.

ra•dic•u•lal•gia (rə-dik″u-lal′jə) pain due to disease of the spinal nerve roots.

ra•dic•u•lar (rə-dik′u-lər) of or pertaining to a root (radix) or radicle.

ra•dic•u•lec•to•my (rə-dik″u-lek′tə-me) [*radicula* + *-ectomy*] excision of a rootlet, especially resection of spinal nerve roots.

ra•dic•u•li•tis (rə-dik″u-li′tis) [*radicula* + *-itis*] inflammation of the root of a spinal nerve, especially of that portion of the root which lies between the spinal cord and the intervertebral canal. Called also *radicular neuritis.*

ra•dic•u•lo•gan•gli•o•ni•tis (rə-dik″u-lo-gang″gle-o-ni′tis) inflammation of the posterior spinal nerve roots and their ganglia.

ra•dic•u•log•ra•phy (rə-dik″u-log′rə-fe) radiography of nerve roots.

ra•dic•u•lo•med•ul•lary (rə-dik″u-lo-med′u-lar″e) pertaining to or affecting the nerve roots and the spinal cord.

ra•dic•u•lo•me•nin•go•my•eli•tis (rə-dik″u-lo-mə-ning″go-mi″ə-li′tis) meningomyeloradiculitis.

ra•dic•u•lo•my•elop•a•thy (rə-dik″u-lo-mi″ə-lop′ə-the) myeloradiculopathy.

ra•dic•u•lo•neu•rop•a•thy (rə-dik″u-lo-nōō-rop′ə-the) disease of the nerve roots and nerves.

ra•dic•u•lop•a•thy (rə-dik″u-lop′ə-the) disease of the nerve roots, such as from inflammation or impingement by a tumor or a bony spur.

cervical r. radiculopathy of cervical nerve roots, often with neck or shoulder pain; compression of nerve roots is a common cause in this area.

diabetic r. radiculopathy, most commonly involving the thoracic and upper lumbar roots, that accompanies diabetes mellitus; it is often associated with significant weight loss.

lumbar r. any disease of lumbar nerve roots, such as from disk herniation or compression by a tumor or bony spur, with lower back pain and often paresthesias. One type is sciatica.

lumbosacral r. disease of nerve roots of the lumbar and sacral segments of the spinal cord.

spondylotic caudal r. compression of the cauda equina due to encroachment upon a congenitally small spinal canal by spondylosis, resulting in pseudoclaudication or more profound neural disorders of the lower limbs.

thoracic r. a rare type of radiculopathy involving the thoracic nerve roots, with pain in a bandlike distribution around the chest.

thoracoabdominal r. radiculopathy involving the thoracic and lumbar nerve roots, the most common form of diabetic radiculopathy; symptoms are pain and dysesthesias in the chest and abdomen.

ra•dic•u•lo•plex•op•a•thy (rə-dik″u-lo-pleks-op′ə-the) disease of nerve roots and plexuses.

lumbosacral r. lumbosacral radiculoplexus neuropathy.

ra•dic•u•lo•plex•us (rə-dik″u-lo-plek′səs) a plexus of spinal nerves with its nerve roots, considered as a unit.

lumbosacral r. the lumbosacral plexus and its nerve roots considered together.

ra•di•ec•to•my (ra″de-ek′tə-me) [*radix* + *-ectomy*] root amputation.

ra•dii (ra′de-i) [L.] genitive and plural of *radius.*

radi(o)- [L. *radius,* q.v.] 1. a combining form denoting relationship *(a)* to the radius (def. 2) or *(b)* to radiant energy, rays, or ionizing radiation. 2. in chemistry, a combining form denoting a radioactive isotope of the element to which it is affixed, e.g., radiocarbon, radiogold.

ra•dio•ac•tin•i•um (ra″de-o-ak-tin′e-əm) a substance formed by the disintegration of actinium.

ra•dio•ac•tive (ra″de-o-ak′tiv) having the property of radioactivity.

ra•dio•ac•tiv•i•ty (ra″de-o-ak-tiv′ĭ-te) 1. emission of corpuscular or electromagnetic radiations consequent to nuclear disintegration, a natural property of all chemical elements of atomic number above 83; this can also be induced in all other known elements. 2. the quality of having such emissions.

artificial r., induced r. radioactivity produced by bombarding an element with high velocity particles, as the radioactivity of synthetic nuclides.

ra•dio•al•ler•go•sor•bent (ra″de-o-al″ər-go-sor′bənt) denoting a radioimmunoassay technique for the measurement of specific IgE antibody to a variety of allergens; see under *tests.*

ra•dio•au•to•gram (ra″de-o-aw′to-gram) autoradiograph.

ra•dio•au•to•graph (ra″de-o-aw′to-graf) autoradiograph.

ra•dio•bi•cip•i•tal (ra″de-o-bi-sip′ĭ-təl) pertaining to the radius and the biceps muscle of the arm.

ra•dio•bi•ol•o•gist (ra″de-o-bi-ol′ə-jist) a specialist in radiobiology.

ra•dio•bi•ol•o•gy (ra″de-o-bi-ol′ə-je) a branch of biology concerned with the effect of light, ultraviolet radiation, and ionizing radiation upon living tissue or organisms. **radiobiolog′ical** *adj*

ra•dio•cal•ci•um (ra″de-o-kal′se-əm) any of several radioactive isotopes of calcium. The isotopes ^{45}Ca, with a half-life of 163 days and emitting beta particles of energy 0.255 MeV, and ^{47}Ca, with a half-life of 4.54 days and emitting beta particles of energy 1.98 and 0.67 MeV and gamma rays of energy 1.30, 0.81, and 0.49 MeV, have been used as tracers in the study of calcium metabolism.

ra•dio•cap•i•tel•lar (ra″de-o-kap″ĭ-tel′ər) pertaining to the radius and the capitulum humeri (capitellum).

ra•dio•car•bon (ra″de-o-kahr′bon) a radioactive isotope of carbon, such as ^{11}C or ^{14}C.

ra•dio•car•ci•no•gen•e•sis (ra″de-o-kahr″sĭ-no-jen′ə-sis) cancer formation caused by exposure to radiation.

ra•dio•car•dio•gram (ra″de-o-kahr′de-o-gram) the graphic record obtained by radiocardiography.

ra•dio•car•di•og•ra•phy (ra″de-o-kahr″de-og′rə-fe) 1. the graphic recording of the variation with time of the concentration, in a selected chamber of the heart, of a radioactive isotope, usually injected intravenously. 2. radioelectrocardiography.

ra•dio•car•pal (ra″de-o-kahr′pəl) pertaining to the radius and carpus.

ra•dio•car•pus (ra″de-o-kahr′pəs) musculus flexor carpi radialis.

ra•dio•chem•is•try (ra″de-o-kem′is-tre) the branch of chemistry which treats of radioactive materials.

ra·dio·che·mo·ther·a·py (ra″de-o-ke-mo-ther′ə-pe) chemoradiotherapy.

ra·dio·chro·ism (ra″de-o-kro′iz-əm) [*radio-* + Gr. *chroa* color] the capacity of a substance to absorb certain radioactive and x-rays.

ra·dio·col·loids (ra″de-o-kol′oids) radioisotopes in pure form in solution, which tend to behave more like colloids than solutes.

ra·dio·con·trast (ra″de-o-kon′trast) contrast (def. 2).

ra·dio·cur·a·ble (ra″de-o-kūr′ə-bəl) curable by radiation therapy.

ra·dio·cys·ti·tis (ra″de-o-sis-ti′tis) radiation cystitis.

ra·di·ode (ra′de-ōd) an instrument for the therapeutic application of a radioactive source.

ra·dio·dense (ra′de-o-dens″) radiopaque.

ra·dio·den·si·ty (ra″de-o-den′sĭ-te) radiopacity.

ra·dio·der·ma·ti·tis (ra″de-o-dur″mə-ti′tis) radiation dermatitis.

ra·dio·di·ag·no·sis (ra″de-o-di″əg-no′sis) diagnosis by means of x-rays and radiographs.

ra·dio·di·ag·nos·tics (ra″de-o-di″əg-nos′tiks) the art of x-ray diagnosis.

ra·dio·dig·i·tal (ra″de-o-dij′ĭ-təl) pertaining to the radius and fingers.

ra·di·odon·tics (ra″de-o-don′tiks) dental radiology.

ra·di·odon·tist (ra″de-o-don′tist) dental radiologist.

ra·dio·ecol·o·gy (ra″de-o-e-kol′ə-je) the science dealing with the effects of radiation on species of plants and animals in natural communities or ecosystems.

ra·dio·elec·tro·car·dio·gram (ra″de-o-e-lek″tro-kahr′de-o-gram″) the graphic recording obtained by radioelectrocardiography.

ra·dio·elec·tro·car·di·o·graph (ra″de-o–əlek″tro-kahr′de-o-graf″) a device for transmission of electrocardiographic signals in radioelectrocardiography.

ra·dio·elec·tro·car·di·og·ra·phy (ra″de-o-e-lek″tro-kahr″de-og′rə-fe) an electrocardiography technique done by radiotelemetry.

ra·dio·el·e·ment (ra″de-o-el′ə-mənt) any chemical element having radioactive properties.

ra·dio·en·ceph·a·lo·gram (ra″de-o-ən-sef′ə-lo-gram″) the graphic record obtained by radioencephalography.

ra·dio·en·ceph·a·log·ra·phy (ra″de-o-ən-sef″ə-log′rə-fe) 1. REG; the study of the passage of an injected tracer through the cerebral blood vessels as revealed by an external scintillation counter. 2. the recording of changes in the electric potential of the brain without direct attachment between the recording apparatus and the subject, the impulses being beamed by radio waves from the subject to the receiver.

ra·dio·fre·quen·cy (ra″de-o-fre′kwən-se) radio frequency.

Ra·dio·gard·ase (ra″de-o-gahr′dās) trademark for a preparation of Prussian blue.

ra·dio·gen·e·sis (ra″de-o-jen′ə-sis) the production of rays or radioactivity.

ra·di·o·gen·ic (ra″de-o-jen′ik) [*radio-* + *-genic*] produced by irradiation.

ra·dio·gold (ra′de-o-gōld″) one of the radioactive isotopes of gold, particularly ^{198}Au. See *gold Au 198,* under *gold.*

ra·dio·gram (ra′de-o-gram″) radiograph.

ra·dio·graph (ra′de-o-graf″) a film produced by radiography.

bite-wing r. a type of dental radiograph that reveals the crowns, necks, coronal thirds of the roots of both the upper and lower teeth, and the dental arches, produced on dental x-ray film that has a central protruding tab or wing on which the teeth close to hold the film in position (bite-wing film).

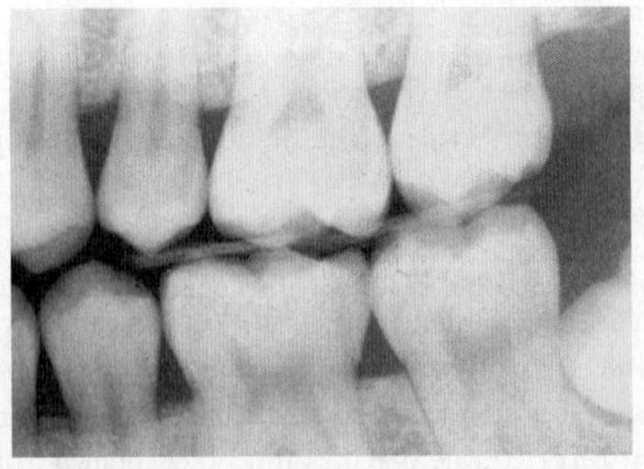

■ Bite-wing radiograph of normal teeth, free from caries.

cephalometric r. a radiograph of the head, including the mandible, in full lateral view; used for making cranial measurements. Called also *cephalogram.*

lateral oblique jaw r. a radiograph of the mandible that unilaterally reveals the mandible from symphysis to condyle.

lateral ramus r. a radiograph of the mandibular ramus and condyle.

lateral skull r. a radiograph of the sinuses and lateral aspects of the skeletal structures of the cranium.

maxillary sinus r. Waters view r.

panoramic r. a type of extraoral body-section radiograph on which the maxilla and the mandible are depicted on a single film. Called also *orthopantograph.*

submental vertex r., submentovertex r. the radiograph made from a submentovertex projection.

Waters projection r., Waters view r. the radiograph made from a Waters projection.

ra·di·og·ra·phy (ra″de-og′rə-fe) [*radio-* + *-graphy*] the making of film records (radiographs) of internal structures of the body by passage of x-rays or gamma rays through the body to act on specially sensitized film. Formerly called *roentgenography.* **radiograph′ic** *adj*

body section r. tomography.

digital r. a technique in which x-ray absorption is quantified by the assignment of a number to the amount of x-rays reaching the detector; the information is entered into a computer and manipulated to produce an optimal image.

digital subtraction r. use of digital subtraction to monitor the flow of contrast medium on radiographs over time; the most common application is digital subtraction angiography.

double-contrast r. mucosal relief r.

electron r. a technique in which a latent electron image is produced on clear plastic by passing x-ray photons through a gas with a high atomic number; this image is then developed into a black-and-white picture.

mass r. examination by x-rays of the general population or of large groups of the population.

miniature r., mass the use of miniature x-ray film in mass radiography.

mucosal relief r. radiography of the mucosa of the gastrointestinal tract in two stages: first a high concentration of contrast medium is injected; then when most of that has been evacuated, air or an effervescent substance is injected to inflate the organ; the light coating of contrast medium on the mucosal surface clearly reveals any abnormalities. Called also *double-contrast r.*

panoramic r. pantomography.

selective r. radiography of certain segments of the population, chosen on some specific basis such as symptoms.

serial r. the taking of several exposures of a selected area at arbitrary intervals.

spot-film r. the making of localized instantaneous radiographs during the course of a fluoroscopic examination. See also *spot film,* under *film.*

ra·dio·hu·mer·al (ra″de-o-hu′mər-əl) pertaining to the radius and humerus.

ra·dio·im·mu·ni·ty (ra″de-o-ĭ-mu′nĭ-te) a condition of decreased sensitivity to radiation sometimes produced by repeated irradiation.

ra·dio·im·mu·no·as·say (ra″de-o-im″u-no-as′a) a highly sensitive and specific assay method that uses the competition between radiolabeled and unlabeled substances in an antigen-antibody reaction to determine the concentration of the unlabeled substance; it can be used to determine antibody concentrations or to determine the concentration of any substance against which specific antibody can be produced. Abbreviated RIA.

ra·dio·im·mu·no·de·tec·tion (ra″de-o-im″u-no-de-tek′shən) immunodetection by means of the specific interaction of radiolabeled antibody with antigen, as the use of labeled antibody to detect elevated levels of a specific antigen in the diagnosis of certain cancers.

ra·dio·im·mu·no·dif·fu·sion (ra″de-o-im″u-no-dĭ-fu′zhən) immunodiffusion conducted with radioisotope-labeled antibodies or antigens.

ra·dio·im·mu·no·elec·tro·pho·re·sis (ra″de-o-im″u-no-e-lek″tro-fə-re′sis) immunoelectrophoresis in which a radiolabeled antigen or antibody is located within a specific precipitin arc using autoradiography.

ra·dio·im·mu·no·im·ag·ing (ra″de-o-im″u-no-im′ə-jing) imaging in which a radiolabled antibody is introduced into the body to react specifically with its appropriate antigen and thus enable a structure or system of interest to be visualized, as by scintigraphy (immunoscintigraphy).

ra·dio·im·mu·no·pre·cip·i·ta·tion (ra″de-o-im″u-no-pre-sip″ĭ-ta′shən) see under *assay.*

ra·dio·im·mu·no·scin·tig·ra·phy (ra″de-o-im″u-no-sin-tig′rə-fe) immunoscintigraphy.

ra·dio·im·mu·no·sor·bent (ra″de-o-im″u-no-sor′bənt) denoting a radioimmunoassay technique for measuring IgE in samples of serum; see under *tests.*

ra·dio·io·dine (ra″de-o-i′o-dīn) any of the nine radioactive isotopes of iodine; ^{131}I, ^{125}I, and ^{123}I are the most commonly used in the diagnosis and treatment of both benign and malignant disease of the thyroid gland and in the scintiscanning of such organs as the lung, liver, and kidney.

ra·dio·iron (ra″de-o-i′ərn) any radioactive isotope of iron; see *iron 55* and *iron 59*.

ra·dio·iso·tope (ra″de-o-i′sə-tōp) an isotope which is radioactive; one having an unstable nucleus and emitting characteristic radiation during its decay to a stable form. Radioisotopes have important diagnostic and therapeutic uses in clinical medicine and research. See also *radiopharmaceutical* and *radiotherapy*.

carrier-free r. see *carrier-free*.

ra·dio·la·bel (ra′de-o-la″bəl) 1. radioactive label. 2. to incorporate such a radioactive label into a compound.

ra·dio·lab·eled (ra″de-o-la′bəld) marked by incorporation of a radioisotope. See also *radioactive tracer*, under *tracer*.

ra·dio·le·sion (ra″de-o-le′zhən) a lesion caused by exposure to radiation.

ra·dio·li·gand (ra″de-o-li′gand, rad″e-o-lig′ənd) a radiolabeled substance, e.g., an antigen, used in the quantitative measurement of an unlabeled substance by its binding reaction to a specific antibody or other receptor site.

ra·di·ol·o·gist (ra″de-ol′ə-jist) a physician who specializes in the use of x-rays and other forms of radiation in the diagnosis and treatment of disease.

dental r. a dentist who specializes in dental radiology. Called also *radiodontist*.

ra·di·ol·o·gy (ra″de-ol′ə-je) [*radio-* + *-logy*] the branch of the health sciences concerned with radioactive substances and radiant energy and with the diagnosis and treatment of disease by means of both ionizing (e.g., x-rays) and nonionizing (e.g., ultrasound) radiation. **radiolog′ic, radiolog′ical** *adj*

dental r. the branch of radiology dealing primarily with orofacial structures. Called also *radiodontics*.

interventional r. the branch of radiology concerned with providing diagnosis and treatment of disease by a variety of percutaneous procedures performed under the guidance of radiologic imaging.

nuclear r. radionuclide scanning.

oral r. dental radiology.

ra·dio·lu·cen·cy (ra″de-o-loo′sən-se) the property of being radiolucent.

ra·dio·lu·cent (ra″de-o-loo′sənt) [*radio-* + L. *lucēre* to shine] permitting the passage of x-rays or other forms of radiant energy with little attenuation; radiolucent areas appear dark on the exposed film.

ra·di·o·lus (ra-de′o-ləs) [L., dim. of *radius* ray] a probe, staff, or sound.

ra·di·om·e·ter (ra″de-om′ə-tər) an instrument for detecting and measuring radiant energy.

ra·dio·mi·crom·e·ter (ra″de-o-mi-krom′ə-tər) [*radio-* + *micro-* + *-meter*] a sensitive radiometer for detecting minute amounts of radiant energy.

ra·dio·mi·met·ic (ra″de-o-mi-met′ik) [*radio-* + *-mimetic*] exerting effects similar to those of ionizing radiation.

ra·dio·mus·cu·lar (ra″de-o-mus′ku-lər) going from the radial artery or nerve to the muscles.

ra·dio·ne·cro·sis (ra″de-o-nə-kro′sis) destruction of tissue caused by radiation; called also *radiation necrosis*.

ra·dio·neu·ri·tis (ra″de-o-nŏŏ-ri′tis) neuritis resulting from excessive exposure to ionizing radiation.

ra·di·o·ni·tro·gen (ra″de-o-ni′trə-jən) any radioactive isotope of nitrogen; see also *nitrogen 13*.

ra·dio·nu·clide (ra″de-o-noo′klīd) a nuclide that disintegrates with the emission of corpuscular or electromagnetic radiations. Called also *radioactive nuclide*.

ra·dio·opac·i·ty (ra″de-o-o-pas′ĭ-te) radiopacity.

ra·di·opac·i·ty (ra″de-o-pas′ĭ-te) the property of being radiopaque.

ra·di·opaque (ra″de-o-pāk′) [*radio-* + *opaque*] not penetrable by x-rays or other forms of radiant energy; radiopaque areas appear light or white on the exposed film.

ra·dio·pa·thol·o·gy (ra″de-o-pə-thol′ə-je) pathology having to do with the effects of radiation on tissues.

ra·dio·phar·ma·ceu·ti·cal (ra″de-o-fahr″mə-soo′tĭ-kəl) a radioactive pharmaceutical, nuclide, or other chemical used for diagnostic or therapeutic purposes.

ra·dio·phar·ma·cy (ra″de-o-fahr′mə-se) the preparation of radioactive pharmaceuticals and radionuclides.

ra·dio·pho·bia (ra″de-o-fo′be-ə) [*radio-* + *-phobia*_] irrational anxiety about the damaging effects of x-rays and sources of radiation.

ra·dio·phos·pho·rus (ra″de-o-fos′fə-rəs) either of two radioactive isotopes of phosphorus, ^{32}P and ^{33}P. See *phosphorus 32; chromic phosphate P 32*, and *sodium phosphate P 32*.

ra·dio·pho·tog·ra·phy (ra″de-o-fo-tog′rə-fe) photography of the fluorescent image produced by an x-ray beam.

ra·dio·phy·lax·is (ra″de-o-fə-lak′sis) the modifying effect of a small dose of radiation on the reaction to a large subsequent radiation.

ra·dio·phys·ics (ra″de-o-fiz′iks) the physics of radiology.

ra·dio·po·tas·si·um (ra″de-o-po-tas′e-əm) a radioactive isotope of potassium; see *potassium 42*.

ra·dio·po·ten·ti·a·tion (ra″de-o-po-ten″she-a′shən) the action of a drug in enhancing the effect of irradiation.

ra·dio·prax·is (ra″de-o-prak′sis) [*radio-* + *praxis*] use of rays of light, electricity, etc., in treatment of disease.

ra·dio·pro·tec·tant (ra″de-o-pro-tek′tənt) 1. providing protection against the toxic effects of ionizing radiation. 2. radioprotector.

ra·dio·pro·tec·tor (ra″de-o-pro-tek′tər) an agent that provides protection against the toxic effects of ionizing radiation.

ra·dio·pul·mo·nog·ra·phy (ra″de-o-pul″mə-nog′rə-fe) a rapid method for estimation of ventilation of localized lung areas, based on measurement of variation in intensity of low-voltage x-rays passed through the lungs during breathing.

ra·dio·re·ac·tion (ra″de-o-re-ak′shən) a bodily reaction, especially a skin reaction, to radiation.

ra·dio·re·cep·tor (ra″de-o-re-sep′tər) 1. a receptor for the stimuli that are excited by radiant energy, such as light or heat. 2. a receptor to which a radioligand can bind; see also *radioreceptor assay*, under *assay*.

ra·dio·re·sis·tance (ra″de-o-re-zis′təns) resistance, as of tissue or cells, to the injurious effects of radiation. **radioresist′ant** *adj*

ra·dio·re·spon·sive (ra″de-o-re-spon′siv) reacting to irradiation.

ra·di·os·co·py (ra″de-os′kə-pe) [*radio-* + *-scopy*] fluoroscopy.

ra·dio·sen·si·bil·i·ty (ra″de-o-sen″sĭ-bil′ĭ-te) radiosensitivity.

ra·dio·sen·si·tive (ra″de-o-sen′sĭ-tiv) sensitive to radiant energy, such as x-ray or other radiation; said of skin, tumor tissue, etc.

ra·dio·sen·si·tive·ness (ra″de-o-sen′sĭ-tiv-nis) radiosensitivity.

ra·dio·sen·si·tiv·i·ty (ra″de-o-sen″sĭ-tiv′ĭ-te) sensitivity, as of the skin or other tissue, to radiant energy, such as x-ray or other radiation.

ra·dio·sen·si·ti·zer (ra″de-o-sen′sĭ-ti″zər) a chemotherapeutic agent used to enhance the effect of radiation therapy.

ra·dio·so·di·um (ra″de-o-so′de-əm) a radioactive isotope of sodium; see *sodium 22* and *sodium 24*.

ra·dio·ste·re·os·co·py (ra″de-o-ster″e-os′kə-pe) [*radio-* + *stereo-* + *-scopy*] the inspection of the interior organs by means of x-rays.

ra·dio·stron·ti·um (ra″de-o-stron′she-əm) a radioactive isotope of strontium, four of medical importance being the isotopes ^{85}Sr, ^{87m}Sr, ^{89}Sr, and ^{90}Sr. See also individual isotopes under *strontium*.

ra·dio·sul·fur (ra″de-o-sul′fər) a radioactive isotope of sulfur. See *sulfur 35*.

ra·dio·sur·gery (ra″de-o-sur′jər-e) surgery in which tissue destruction is by means of ionizing radiation rather than surgical incision; the radiation may be from an implant or an external source.

stereotactic r., stereotaxic r. stereotactic surgery in which lesions are produced by ionizing radiation.

ra·dio·tel·em·e·try (ra″de-o-tə-lem′ə-tre) telemetry in which the data is transmitted by radio waves from the object of measurement to the recording apparatus.

ra·dio·ther·a·peu·tics (ra″de-o-ther″ə-pu′tiks) 1. the body of knowledge comprising the available information regarding the therapeutic use of ionizing radiation. 2. radiotherapy.

ra·dio·ther·a·pist (ra″de-o-ther′ə-pist) a specialist in radiotherapy.

ra·dio·ther·a·py (ra″de-o-ther′ə-pe) [*radio-* + *therapy*] the treatment of disease by ionizing radiation. Called also *irradiation* and *radiation therapy*.

adjuvant r. radiotherapy used in addition to surgical resection in the treatment of cancer.

conformal r. external beam radiotherapy in which multiple beams are focused by computer-controlled collimators so that the distribution of the radiation dose matches the shape of tumor and the dose received by uninvolved tissues is minimized.

extended field r. see under *irradiation*.

external beam r. treatment by radiation emitted from a source located at a distance from the body; called also *beam therapy, external beam therapy,* and *teleradiotherapy.*
hemibody r. see under *irradiation.*
high-voltage r. radiotherapy in which the radiation has a voltage greater than 300 kV. See *orthovoltage r., supervoltage r.,* and *megavoltage r.*
hyperfractionated r. hyperfractionation.
intraoperative r. (IORT) the use of a single high dose of radiation at the time of surgery as adjuvant therapy in tumor resection.
interstitial r. that administered with the radioactive element contained in devices (e.g., needles or wire) inserted directly into the tissues.
intracavitary r. that in which the radioactive element is introduced into a natural body cavity.
inverted Y field r. see under *irradiation.*
involved field r. see under *irradiation.*
mantle field r. see under *irradiation.*
megavoltage r. radiotherapy in which the radiation has voltage of 1000 kV or more.
neoadjuvant r. radiotherapy used as neoadjuvant therapy (q.v.) for cancer. Called also *preoperative r.*
orthovoltage r. radiotherapy in which the radiation has voltage between 140 and 400 kV.
preoperative r. neoadjuvant r.
supervoltage r. radiotherapy in which the radiation has voltage between 400 and 1000 kV.

ra•di•ot•o•my (ra″de-ot′ə-me) [*radio-* + *-tomy*] tomography.

ra•dio•tox•emia (ra″de-o-tok-se′me-ə) toxemia produced by radiation or a radioactive substance.

ra•dio•tox•ic•ity (ra″de-o-tok-sis′ĭ-te) radiation toxicity.

ra•dio•tra•cer (ra″de-o-tra′sər) radioactive tracer.

ra•dio•trans•par•en•cy (ra″de-o-trans-par′ən-se) radiolucency. radiotranspar′ent *adj*

ra•di•o•tro•pic (ra″de-o-tro′pik) influenced by radiation.

ra•di•ot•ro•pism (ra″de-ot′ro-piz-əm) a tropism with regard to radiation.

ra•dio•ul•nar (ra″de-o-ul′nər) pertaining to the radius and ulna.

ra•di•sec•to•my (ra″de-sek′tə-me) [*radix* + *-ectomy*] root amputation.

rad•ish (rad′ish) 1. any of various plants of the genus *Raphanus.* 2. the edible root of *Raphanus sativus,* used for bronchitis and dyspepsia.

ra•di•um (ra′de-əm) [from its radiant quality] a rare radioactive element in the uranium decay series. It has an atomic weight of 226, an atomic number of 88, and a half-life of 1600 years. It is found mainly in pitchblende and undergoes spontaneous disintegration with formation of a gas called radon (half-life = 3.85 days). In this process it emits alpha particles. Radon (alpha emitter) on deposit in solid form disintegrates into a series of decay products: radium A (half-life = 3 minutes), radium B (half-life = 26.7 minutes), and radium C (half-life = 19.5 minutes). The beta particles and gamma radiation used in clinical therapy originate from radium B and C. With radium in a sealed container and the same number of atoms of each decay product disintegrating per second, radium and its decay products are in equilibrium. In this state, the formation of beta particles and gamma rays reaches its maximum. In clinical gamma-ray therapy, shielding off of the beta particles can be accomplished by a metallic container, e.g., of gold or platinum. A glass-walled container permits irradiation with beta particles as well as gamma rays.

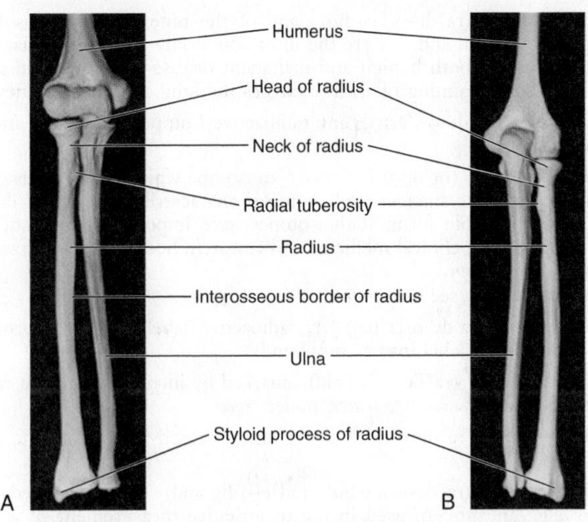

■ Radius and ulna. *(A),* Anterior view; *(B),* posterior view.

ra•di•us (ra′de-əs) gen. and pl. *ra′dii* [L. "spoke" (of a wheel)] 1. a line segment from the center to the circumference of a circle or the surface of a sphere; the length of such a segment. Symbol *r.* 2. [TA] the bone on the outer or thumb side of the forearm, articulating proximally with the humerus and ulna and distally with the ulna and carpus. See illustration and Plate 40.
r. cur′vus Madelung deformity.
r. fix′us a straight line from the hormion to the inion.
ra′dii len′tis [TA] radii of lens: imaginary lines extending from the midpoint of the axis of the lens of the eye to the capsule of the lens.
ra′dii medulla′res [TA] medullary rays: cortical extensions of bundles of tubules from the renal pyramids.
van der Waals r. the distance at which there is a balance between van der Waals attractive and repulsive forces in the formation of chemical bonds.

ra•dix (ra′diks) gen. *ra′dicis* pl. *ra′dices* [L.] root: the most inferior part, or a part by which a structure is anchored, as the portion of a hair, nail, or tooth that is buried in the tissues, or the part of a nerve adjacent to the center to which it is connected.

Radix

Descriptions are given on TA terms and include anglicized names of specific roots.

r. ante′rior an′sae cervica′lis r. superior ansae cervicalis.
r. ante′rior ner′vi spina′lis [TA] anterior root of spinal nerve: the motor division of each spinal nerve, attached centrally to the spinal cord and joining peripherally with the corresponding posterior (sensory) root to form the nerve before it emerges through the intervertebral foramen. It conveys motor fibers to skeletal muscle and contains preganglionic autonomic fibers at thoracolumbar and sacral levels. There are 31 anterior and 31 posterior roots: 8 cervical, 12 thoracic, 5 lumbar, 5 sacral, and 1 coccygeal. Called also *ventral* or *motor root of spinal nerve, r. ventralis nervi spinalis,* and *r. motoria nervi spinalis* [TA alternative].
r. ar′cus ver′tebrae pediculus arcus vertebralis.
r. basa′lis ante′rior ve′nae basa′lis commu′nis anterior basal root of common basal vein: a venous root draining the anterior basal segment of the right lung and emptying into the common basal vein.
r. cli′nica [TA] clinical root: that portion of a tooth below the clinical crown, being attached to the gingiva or alveolus.
r. cochlea′ris ner′vi vestibulocochlea′ris the central continuation of the cochlear nerve from the spiral ganglion, passing dorsal to the inferior cerebellar peduncle to enter the brain; called also *r. inferior nervi vestibulocochlearis.*
r. crania′lis ner′vi accesso′rii [TA] cranial root of accessory nerve: the nerve rootlets originating from the nucleus ambiguus and emerging from the side of the medulla oblongata; although they are part of the vagus nerve, they are so named because they were originally considered to be part of the accessory nerve. They join briefly with the spinal root of the accessory nerve to form the trunk of accessory nerve; upon exiting the jugular foramen, they split from the spinal part, immediately unite with the vagus nerve, and are distributed to the soft palate, constrictors of the pharynx, and the larynx. Called also *pars vagalis nervi accessorii* [TA alternative].
r. den′tis [TA] root of tooth: the portion of a tooth which is covered by cementum, proximal to the neck of the tooth and ordinarily embedded in the dental alveolus; called also *anatomical root.*

Radix *Continued*

r. dorsa'lis ner'vi spina'lis r. posterior nervi spinalis.
r. facia'lis nervus canalis pterygoidei.
r. infe'rior an'sae cervica'lis [TA] inferior root of ansa cervicalis: a strand of filaments connecting the ansa cervicalis with branches of the second and third cervical nerves; called also *r. posterior ansae cervicalis* and *posterior root of ansa cervicalis.*
r. infe'rior ner'vi vestibulocochlea'ris r. cochlearis nervi vestibulocochlearis.
r. interme'dia gan'glii pterygopala'tini TA alternative for *nervus petrosus major.*
r. latera'lis ner'vi media'ni [TA] lateral root of median nerve: the fibers contributed to the median nerve by the lateral cord of the brachial plexus.
r. latera'lis trac'tus op'tici [TA] lateral root of optic tract: fibers from the optic tract that enter the lateral geniculate body.
r. lin'guae [TA] root of tongue: the portion of the tongue posterior to the sulcus terminalis, being attached inferiorly to the hyoid bone, and directed posteriorly and superiorly.
r. media'lis ner'vi media'ni [TA] medial root of median nerve: the fibers contributed to the median nerve by the medial cord of the brachial plexus.
r. media'lis trac'tus op'tici [TA] medial root of optic tract: fibers from the optic tract that enter the superior colliculus and the pretectal region.
r. mesente'rii [TA] root of mesentery: the line of attachment of the mesentery to the posterior abdominal wall, extending from the duodenojejunal flexure near the second lumbar vertebra diagonally downward to the upper border of the right sacroiliac joint.
r. moto'ria ner'vi spina'lis TA alternative for *r. anterior nervi spinalis.*
r. moto'ria ner'vi trige'mini [TA] motor root of trigeminal nerve: the smaller of the two roots by which the trigeminal nerve is attached to the side of the pons; it contains proprioceptive as well as motor fibers, and continues deep to the trigeminal ganglion to join the mandibular nerve. Called also *portio minor nervi trigemini.*
r. nasa'lis TA alternative for *r. nasi.*
r. na'si [TA] root of nose: the upper portion of the nose, which is attached to the frontal bone. Called also *r. nasalis* [TA alternative].
r. nasocilia'ris gan'glii cilia'ris TA alternative for *r. sensoria ganglii ciliaris.*
r. oculomoto'ria gan'glii cilia'ris TA alternative for *r. parasympathica ganglii ciliaris.*
r. parasympa'thica gan'glii cilia'ris [TA] parasympathetic root of ciliary ganglion: a short collection of fibers passing from the inferior branch of the oculomotor nerve to the posterior inferior portion of the ciliary ganglion; it contains preganglionic parasympathetic fibers for the sphincter papillae and the ciliary muscle. Called also *r. oculomotoria ganglii ciliaris* [TA alternative], *ramus nervi oculomotorii ad ganglion ciliare* [TA alternative], and *motor, short,* or *oculomotor root of ciliary ganglion.*
r. parasympa'thica gan'glii o'tici TA alternative for *nervus petrosus minor.* NOTE: when considering the ganglia of the pars parasympathica, this is the preferred term in the official nomenclature.

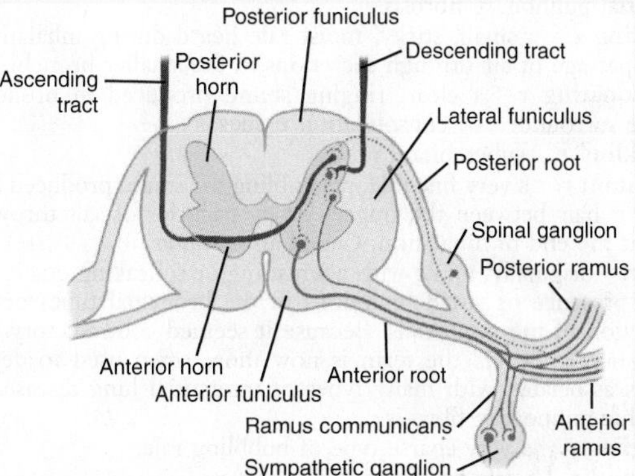

■ Diagram of a horizontal section of the spinal cord, with posterior and anterior roots and a spinal nerve.

r. parasympa'thica ganglio'rum pelvico'rum [TA] parasympathetic root of pelvic ganglia: *origin,* sacral plexus—S3–S4; *distribution,* leaving the sacral plexus, they enter the inferior hypogastric plexus and supply the pelvic organs; *modality,* preganglionic parasympathetic and visceral afferent. Called also *nervi splanchnici pelvici* [TA alternative] and *pelvic splanchnic nerves.*
r. parasympa'thica gan'glii pterygopalati'ni TA alternative for *nervus petrosus major.* NOTE: when considering the ganglia of the pars parasympathica, this is the preferred term in the official nomenclature.
r. parasympa'thica gan'glii sublingua'lis, r. parasympa'thica gan'glii submandibula'ris TA alternative for *chorda tympani.* NOTE: when considering the ganglia of the pars parasympathica, this is the preferred term in the official nomenclature.
r. pe'nis [TA] root of penis: the proximal, attached portion of the penis, consisting of the diverging crura of the corpora cavernosa and the bulb.
r. pi'li root of hair.
ra'dices plex'us brachia'lis [TA] roots of brachial plexus: the anterior branches of the four lower cervical spinal nerves and the first thoracic nerve, which combine to form the trunks of the brachial plexus; see *rami ventrales nervorum cervicalium* and *rami ventrales nervorum thoracicorum,* under *ramus.*
r. poste'rior an'sae cervica'lis r. inferior ansae cervicalis.
r. poste'rior ner'vi spina'lis [TA] posterior root of spinal nerve: the sensory division of each spinal nerve, attached centrally to the spinal cord and joining peripherally with the anterior (motor) root to form the nerve before it emerges through the intervertebral foramen: each posterior root bears a spinal ganglion and conveys sensory fibers to the spinal cord. There are 31 anterior and 31 posterior nerve roots: 8 cervical, 12 thoracic, 5 lumbar, 5 sacral, and 1 coccygeal. Called also *dorsal* or *sensory root of spinal nerves, r. dorsalis nervi spinalis,* and *r. sensoria nervi spinalis* [TA alternative].
r. pulmo'nis [TA] root of lung: the attachment of either lung, comprising the structures entering and emerging at the hilum; called also *pedicle of lung.*
r. senso'ria gan'glii cilia'ris [TA] sensory root of ciliary ganglion: sensory fibers from the cornea, iris, ciliary body, and choroid that pass through the ciliary ganglion to the nasociliary nerve. Called also *r. nasociliaris ganglii ciliaris* [TA alternative], *ramus communicans nervi nasociliaris cum ganglio ciliari,* [TA alternative], and *long* or *nasociliary root of ciliary ganglion.*
r. senso'ria gan'glii o'tici TA alternative for *rami ganglionares nervi mandibularis ad ganglion oticum.*
r. senso'ria gan'glii pterygopalati'ni TA alternative for *rami ganglionares nervi maxillaris ad ganglion pterygopalatinum.*
r. senso'ria gan'glii submandibula'ris TA alternative for *rami ganglionares nervi lingualis ad ganglion submandibulare.*
r. senso'ria ner'vi spina'lis TA alternative for *r. posterior nervi spinalis.*
r. senso'ria ner'vi trige'mini [TA] sensory root of trigeminal nerve: the larger of the two roots by which the trigeminal nerve is attached to the side of the pons. It contains sensory fibers and expands into a large flat ganglion (the trigeminal ganglion) which gives rise to the ophthalmic, maxillary, and mandibular nerves. Called also *portio major nervi trigemini.*
r. spina'lis ner'vi accesso'rii [TA] spinal root of accessory nerve: the nerve rootlets originating from the gray matter of the spinal cord and emerging from the side of the cord as far down as the fifth or sixth cervical vertebrae; they ascend in the vertebral canal, pass through the foramen magnum, briefly join with the part of the vagus nerve that is often called the cranial root of accessory nerve to form the trunk of the accessory nerve, and exit the jugular foramen; there the spinal root fibers split from the cranial and supply the sternocleidomastoid and trapezius muscles. Called also *pars spinalis nervi accessorii* [TA alternative].
r. supe'rior an'sae cervica'lis [TA] superior root of ansa cervicalis: fibers of the first or second cervical nerve, descending in company with the hypoglossal nerve, connecting it with the ansa cervicalis and helping supply the infrahyoid muscles. Called also *r. anterior ansae cervicalis* and *anterior root of ansa cervicalis.*
r. supe'rior ner'vi vestibulocochlea'ris r. vestibularis nervi vestibulocochlearis.

Radix *Continued*

r. sympa′thica gan′glii cilia′ris [TA] sympathetic root of ciliary ganglion: postganglionic fibers from the superior cervical ganglion, derived from the internal carotid plexus, to the ciliary ganglion, for distribution by the short ciliary nerves to the dilator muscle of the pupil, orbital muscle and tarsal muscles, and blood vessels of the eyeball.

r. sympa′thica gang′lii pterygopalati′ni TA alternative for *nervus petrosus profundus.* NOTE: when considering the ganglia of the pars parasympathica, this is the preferred term in the official nomenclature.

r. un′guis root of nail: the proximal portion of the nail, situated in the sulcus of the matrix of the nail.

r. ventra′lis ner′vi spina′lis r. anterior nervi spinalis.

r. vestibula′ris ner′vi vestibulocochlea′ris vestibular root of vestibulocochlear nerve: the central continuation of the vestibular nerve from the vestibular ganglion, entering the brain, just lateral to the intermediate nerve and immediately superior to the restiform body. Called also *r. superior nervi vestibulocochlearis* and *superior root of vestibulocochlear nerve.*

ra•dix•in (rə-dik′sin) an actin-binding protein, related to ezrin and moesin, see *ERM proteins*, under *protein.*

ra•don (Rn) (ra′don) a heavy, colorless, gaseous, radioactive element; atomic weight, 222; atomic number, 86; obtained by the breaking up of radium, and used in radiotherapy. ^{219}Rn is a radioactive isotope of the actinium radioactive series. ^{220}Rn is a radioactive isotope of the thorium radioactive series.

Ra•do•vi•ci sign (rah-do-ve′che) [André *Radovici*, French physician, 20th century] see *palm-chin reflex*, under *reflex.*

RAE right atrial enlargement; see *atrial enlargement*, under *enlargement.*

Rae•der syndrome, paratrigeminal syndrome (ra′dər) [Johan Georg *Raeder*, Norwegian ophthalmologist, 1889–1956] see under *syndrome.*

raf•fi•nose (raf′ĭ-nōs) a nonreducing trisaccharide occurring abundantly in sugar beets and other plants; it is composed of galactose linked α-(1,6) to glucose, which is linked β-(1,2) to fructose. Formerly called *melitose.*

ra•fox•a•nide (rə-fok′sə-nīd) a salicylanilide anthelmintic used in cattle and sheep.

raft (raft) a floating platform or similar structure composed of an aggregate of buoyant materials.

lipid r. a region of the plasma membrane rich in cholesterol and sphingolipids; such regions are responsible for functions such as signal transduction and vesicle formation. Cf. *caveola.*

rage (rāj) a state of violent anger.

sham r. an outburst of behavior in a decorticated animal, resembling fear or anger; a similar phenomenon may be observed in humans with insulin-induced hypoglycemia or carbon monoxide poisoning.

rag•o•cyte (rag′o-sīt) [*Ragg* (*r*heumatoid serum *agg*lutinator) + *-cyte*] a polymorphonuclear leukocyte with cytoplasmic inclusions of ingested aggregated IgG, rheumatoid factor, fibrin, and complement, found in the joints in rheumatoid arthritis. Called also *RA cell.*

rag•weed (rag′wēd) any of various species of plants of the genus *Ambrosia* whose pollen can cause hay fever.

rag•wort (rag′wərt) any of various poisonous plants of the genus *Senecio.*

Rah•nel•la (rə-nel′ə) [Otto *Rahn*, German-American microbiologist, 1881–1957] a genus of gram-negative, facultatively anaerobic, rod-shaped bacteria of the family Enterobacteriaceae, occurring in fresh water and occasionally isolated from human clinical specimens. The type species is *R. aqua′tilis.*

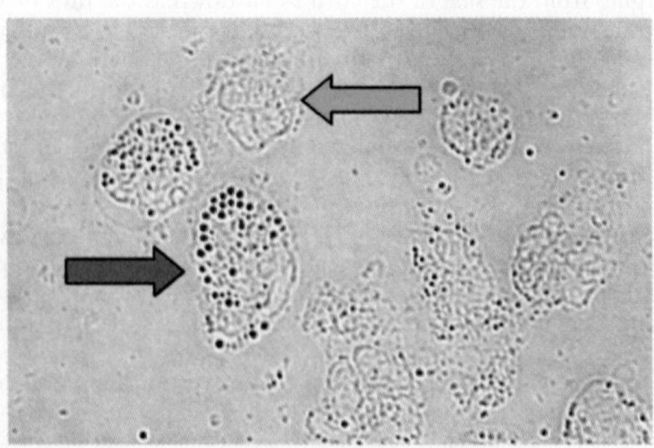

■ Ragocyte *(blue arrow)* from a patient with rheumatoid arthritis, showing the typical granules; an adjacent cell lacks ragocyte granules *(green arrow).*

ra•i•gan (ra′ĭ-gan) [Chinese] dried mushrooms of the species *Omphalia lapidescens*, an anthelmintic used in Chinese medicine.

Rail•li•e•tia (ri″le-e′she-ə) [Louis-Joseph Alcide *Railliet*, French biologist, 1852–1930] a genus of parasitic mites; *R. au′ris* is found in the ears of cattle and sometimes causes ulceration.

Rail•li•e•ti•na (ri″le-ə-ti′nə) [L.-J.A. *Railliet*] a genus of tapeworms of the family Davaineidae, many species of which infect birds, domestic fowl, and mammals. *R. asia′tica, R. celeben′sis, R. demararien′sis, R. formosa′na, R. loechesa′lavezi*, and *R. madagascarien′sis* have been reported from human infections.

rail•li•e•ti•ni•a•sis (ri″le-ə-tĭ-ni′ə-sis) infection with tapeworms of the genus *Raillietina.*

Rai•ney corpuscle (ra′ne) [George *Rainey*, British anatomist, 1801–1884] see under *corpuscle.*

RAIU radioactive iodine uptake.

ra•jas (rah-jus′) [Sanskrit] according to ayurveda, one of the three gunas, characterized by activity, stimulation, and movement, in contrast to inertia (tamas) and equilibrium (sattva). All movement and activity of the mind and body is due to rajas.

rak•ing (ra′king) gathering, moving, scraping, or loosening, as with a rake.

back r. extraction of impacted feces from the rectum of an animal.

rale (rahl) a discontinuous sound (q.v.) consisting of a series of short nonmusical noises, heard primarily during inhalation; called also *crackle.*

amphoric r. a coarse, musical, and tinkling rale caused by the splashing of fluid in a cavity connected with a bronchus. Called also *bottle sound.*

atelectatic r. a nonpathologic rale that is dissipated by deep breathing or coughing and is best observed at the margin of a lung. This type is frequently heard in those who breathe feebly and superficially, when on deep inhalation the moist walls of the unexpanded alveoli are suddenly forced apart by the entering air; after a few deep inhalations these rales are lost. Called also *marginal* or *border r.*

border r. atelectatic r.

bubbling r. a moist rale heard when air passes through areas of bronchi that contain mucus.

cavernous r. a hollow and metallic rale caused by the alternate expansion and contraction of a pulmonary cavity during respiration.

cellophane r. a rale resembling the rustling of cellophane, heard in interstitial pulmonary fibrosis.

clicking r. a small, sticky, moist rale heard during inhalation, caused by the passage of air through secretions in the smaller bronchi.

consonating r. a clear, ringing sound produced in bronchial tubes that are surrounded by consolidation tissues.

crackling r. subcrepitant r.

crepitant r. a very fine rale, resembling the sound produced by rubbing a lock of hair between the fingers or by particles of salt thrown on fire; heard at the end of inhalation. Called also *crepitus.*

dry r. originally, a rale with a whistling or squeaking quality produced by the presence of viscid secretions in the bronchial tubes or by spastic contraction of the tube walls. Because it seemed contradictory to refer to such a rale as "dry," the term is now more often used to describe fine crackles associated with many types of interstitial lung disease, including idiopathic pulmonary fibrosis.

gurgling r. a very coarse type of bubbling rale.

guttural r. a rale produced in the throat.

marginal r. atelectatic r.

metallic r. consonating r.

moist r. any of numerous rales produced by the presence of liquid in the bronchial tubes.

mucous r. bubbling r.

subcrepitant r. a fine, moist rale heard in conditions associated with liquid in the smaller tubes; called also *crackling r.*

tracheal r. a rale produced in the trachea.

vesicular r. crepitant r.

Ral•gro (ral′gro) trademark for a preparation of zeranol.

ral•ox•i•fene hy•dro•chlo•ride (ral-ok′sĭ-fēn) a selective estrogen receptor modulator that has estrogenlike effects on bone, increasing bone mineral density, and on lipid metabolism, decreasing total and LDL cholesterol, but not on breast and uterine tissue; used for the prevention of postmenopausal osteoporosis; administered orally.

Ral•sto•nia (rawl-sto′ne-ə) [Ericka *Ralston*, American bacteriologist, 20th century] a genus of aerobic, nonfermentative gram-negative bacteria of the family Burkholderiaceae, consisting of motile and nonmotile, non–spore-forming, catalase- and oxidase-positive rods. Several species are associated with human infections. The type species is *R. picket′tii.*

R. picket′tii a species of low virulence, isolated from numerous clinical and environmental sources; human infection occurs in immunocompromised patients and as a result of the use of contaminated infusates. Formerly called *Pseudomonas pickettii.*

ral•teg•ra•vir (ral-teg′rə-vir) an antiretroviral agent used in treatment of human immunodeficiency virus infection, usually in combination with other agents; administered orally.

ral•ti•trex•ed di•so•di•um (ral″tĭ-trek′səd) a quinazoline folate analogue that inhibits thymidylate synthase; used as an antineoplastic in the treatment of advanced colorectal carcinoma, administered intravenously.

Ra•man effect (rah′mahn) [Sir Chandrasekhara Venkata *Raman*, Indian physicist, 1888–1970; winner of the Nobel prize for physics in 1930] see under *effect.*

ra•mel•te•on (rə-mel′te-ən) a melatonin receptor agonist used as a hypnotic in the treatment of insomnia characterized by difficulty with sleep onset; administered orally.

RAMC Royal Army Medical Corps.

ra•mi (ra′mi) [L.] genitive and plural of *ramus.*

Ra•mi•klor•rid•i•um (ra″mĭ-klor-id′e-əm) a genus of fungi of the form-family Dematiaceae.

R. macken′ziei a species seen most often from the Middle East to India, causing brain abscesses and sometimes meningitis.

ram•i•cot•o•my (ram″ĭ-kot′ə-me) [*ramus* + *-tomy*] ramisection.

ra•mi•cris•tate (ra″me-kris′tāt) having branching mitochondrial cristae; said of amebae.

ram•i•fi•ca•tion (ram″ĭ-fĭ-ka′shən) [*ramus* + L. *facere* to make] 1. distribution in branches. 2. a branch or set of branches. 3. the manner of branching.

ram•i•fy (ram′ĭ-fi) [*ramus* + L. *facere* to make] 1. to branch; to diverge in various directions. 2. to traverse in branches.

ra•mi•pril (rə-mi′pril) an angiotensin-converting enzyme inhibitor used in the treatment of hypertension and post–myocardial infarction congestive heart failure; administered orally. It is also used to reduce the risk of myocardial infarction, stroke, and death in patients considered at high risk for a major cardiovascular event.

Ra•mi•rez ashy dermatosis (rah-me′rās) [Oswaldo *Ramirez* C., Salvadoran dermatologist, mid-20th century] erythema dyschromicum perstans.

rami•sec•tion (ram″ĭ-sek′shən) [*ramus* + *section*] the operation of cutting one or more of the rami communicantes of the sympathetic nervous system; called also *ramicotomy, ramisectomy,* and *sympathetic ramisection.*

ram•i•sec•to•my (ram″ĭ-sek′tə-me) ramisection.

ram•itis (ram-i′tis) [*ramus* + *-itis*] inflammation of a ramus.

Ramm•stedt see *Ramstedt.*

ra•mol•lisse•ment (rah″mo-lēs-maw′) [Fr.] softening.

Ra•mon flocculation test (rah-maw′) [Gaston *Ramon*, French bacteriologist 1886–1963] see under *test.*

Ra•mond sign (rah-maw′) [Louis *Ramond*, French internist, 1879–1952] see under *sign.*

ra•mose (ra′mōs) [L. *ramus* branch] branching; having many branches.

ram•part (ram′pahrt) a broad, encircling embankment.

maxillary r. a ridge or mound of epithelial cells seen in that portion of the jaw of the embryo which is to become the alveolar border.

Ram•say Hunt paralysis, syndrome (ram′ze hunt′) [James *Ramsay Hunt*, American neurologist, 1872–1937] see *dyssynergia cerebellaris progressiva;* see *juvenile paralysis agitans (of Hunt),* under *paralysis;* and see under *syndrome.*

Rams•den eyepiece (ramz′dən) [Jesse *Ramsden*, English instrument maker and optician, 1735–1800] see under *eyepiece.*

Ram•stedt operation (rahm′shtet) [Conrad *Ramstedt*, German surgeon, 1867–1963] see *Fredet-Ramstedt operation,* under *operation.*

ra•mu•lus (ra′mu-ləs) pl. *ra′muli* [L., dim. of *ramus*] radicle.

ra•mus (ra′məs) gen. and pl. *ra′mi* [L.] branch: anatomic terminology for a smaller structure given off by a larger one, or into which the larger structure, such as a blood vessel or nerve, divides. **ra′mal** *adj*

Ramus

Descriptions are given on TA terms and include anglicized names of specific branches.

r. accesso′rius arte′riae menin′geae me′diae [TA] accessory branch of middle meningeal artery: a branch arising from the middle meningeal artery, or directly from the maxillary artery, and entering the middle cranial fossa through the foramen ovale to supply the trigeminal ganglion, walls of the cavernous sinus, and neighboring dura mater.

r. acetabula′ris arte′riae circumflex′ae fe′moris media′lis [TA] acetabular branch of medial circumflex femoral artery: a branch of the medial circumflex artery of the thigh, distributed to the head of the femur and to the acetabulum. Called also *acetabular artery.*

r. acetabula′ris arte′riae obturato′riae [TA] acetabular branch of obturator artery: a branch distributed to the hip joint; called also *acetabular artery.*

r. acromia′lis arte′riae suprascapula′ris [TA] acromial branch of suprascapular artery: a branch distributed to the acromion process.

r. acromia′lis arte′riae thoracoacromia′lis [TA] acromial branch of thoracoacromial artery: a branch distributed to the deltoid muscle and acromion process.

ra′mi alveola′res superio′res anterio′res ner′vi maxilla′ris [TA] anterior superior alveolar branches of maxillary nerve: branches from the infraorbital nerve that innervate the incisor and canine teeth of the upper jaw, help form the superior dental plexus, and give terminal twigs to the floor of the nose; *modality,* general sensory.

r. alveola′ris supe′rior me′dius ner′vi maxilla′ris [TA] middle superior alveolar branch of maxillary nerve: a branch from the infraorbital nerve that innervates the premolar teeth of the upper jaw by way of the superior dental plexus; *modality,* general sensory.

ra′mi alveola′res superio′res posterio′res ner′vi maxilla′ris [TA] posterior superior alveolar branches of maxillary nerve: branches that innervate the maxillary sinus, cheek, gums, and molar and premolar teeth of the upper jaw; they form part of the superior dental plexus; *modality,* general sensory.

rami anastomo′tici rami communicantes (def. 2).

r. anastomo′ticus arte′riae lacrima′lis cum arte′ria menin′gea me′dia [TA] anastomotic branch of lacrimal artery with middle meningeal artery: a recurrent meningeal branch of the lacrimal artery that passes back via the lateral part of the orbital fissure and anastomoses with the anastomotic branch of the middle meningeal artery.

r. anastomo′ticus arte′riae menin′geae me′diae cum arte′ria lacrima′li [TA] anastomotic branch of middle meningeal artery with lacrimal artery: a branch of the middle meningeal artery that is distributed to the orbit and anastomoses with the anastomotic branch of the lacrimal artery.

r. ante′rior arte′riae obturato′riae [TA] anterior branch of obturator artery: a branch that passes forward around the medial margin of the obturator foramen, on the obturator membrane, and is distributed to the obturator and adductor muscles.

r. ante′rior arte′riae pancreaticoduodena′lis inferio′ris [TA] anterior branch of inferior pancreaticoduodenal artery: a branch that passes in front of the head of the pancreas and then ascends to

Ramus *Continued*

anastomose with the anterior superior pancreaticoduodenal artery; it supplies the head of the pancreas and adjoining parts of the duodenum.

r. ante′rior arte′riae recurren′tis ulna′ris [TA] anterior branch of ulnar recurrent artery: a branch that helps supply the pronator teres and brachialis muscles and runs to the front of the medial epicondyle, supplying the elbow joint and adjacent structures.

r. ante′rior arte′riae rena′lis [TA] anterior branch of renal artery: a branch supplying the anterior, superior, and inferior segments of the kidney.

r. ante′rior duc′tus hepa′tici dex′tri [TA] the anterior branch of the right hepatic duct, draining anterior segments of the right liver.

r. ante′rior ner′vi auricula′ris mag′ni [TA] anterior branch of great auricular nerve; a branch distributed to the skin of the face over the parotid gland; *modality*, general sensory.

ra′mi anterio′res nervo′rum cervica′lium [TA] anterior branches of cervical nerves: eight nerve branches of which the upper four form the cervical plexus and the lower four form most of the brachial plexus; see also *r. anterior nervi spinalis.* See illustration at *ramus posterior nervi spinalis.* Called also *rami ventrales nervorum cervicalium* [TA alternative].

r. ante′rior ner′vi coccy′gei [TA] anterior branch of coccygeal nerve: a branch of the last spinal nerve, emerging from the sacral hiatus and contributing to the coccygeal plexus; called also *r. ventralis nervi coccygei* [TA alternative].

r. ante′rior ner′vi cuta′nei antebra′chii media′lis [TA] anterior branch of medial cutaneous nerve of forearm: a branch that innervates the skin of the front and medial aspect of the forearm; *modality*, general sensory.

ra′mi anterio′res nervo′rum lumba′lium [TA] anterior branches of lumbar nerves: the anterior branches of the five lumbar spinal nerves; the upper four form the lumbar plexus, and the fifth and a part of the fourth form part of the sacral plexus. Called also *rami ventrales nervorum lumbalium* [TA alternative].

r. ante′rior ner′vi obturato′rii [TA] anterior branch of obturator nerve: a branch that supplies the gracilis and the adductor longus and brevis muscles and the pectineus, and occasionally gives off a branch to the skin of the medial side of the thigh and leg; *modality*, motor and general sensory.

ra′mi anterio′res nervo′rum sacra′lium [TA] anterior branches of sacral nerves: branches of the five sacral spinal nerves; the upper four emerge from the sacrum through the anterior foramina and contribute to the sacral plexus, and the fifth emerges through the sacral hiatus and, with a communication from the fourth, contributes to the coccygeal plexus. Called also *rami ventrales nervorum sacralium* [TA alternative].

r. ante′rior ner′vi spina′lis [TA] anterior branch of spinal nerve: the anterior and usually larger of the two branches into which each spinal nerve divides almost as soon as it emerges from the intervertebral foramen; the anterior branches supply anterior and lateral parts of the trunk and all parts of the limbs.

ra′mi anterio′res nervo′rum thoracico′rum TA alternative for *nervi intercostales.* NOTE: Although the term is official alternative terminology for the nervi intercostales, it encompasses both the 11 nervi intercostales and also the nervus subcostalis, which is the anterior ramus from the twelfth thoracic nerve.

r. ante′rior sul′ci latera′lis ce′rebri [TA] anterior branch of lateral cerebral sulcus: a branch that runs forward a short distance into the inferior frontal gyrus.

anterior rami of thoracic nerves rami anteriores nervorum thoracicorum.

r. ante′rior ve′nae pulmona′lis dex′trae superio′ris TA alternative for *vena anterior lobi superioris pulmonis dextri.*

r. ante′rior ve′nae pulmona′lis sinis′trae superio′ris TA alternative for *vena anterior lobi superioris pulmonis sinistri.*

r. apica′lis ve′nae pulmona′lis dex′trae superio′ris TA alternative for *vena apicalis.*

r. apicoposte′rior ve′nae pulmona′lis sinis′trae superio′ris TA alternative for *vena apicoposterior.*

r. articula′ris [TA] articular branch: any of the branches of a mixed (afferent or efferent) peripheral nerve supplying a joint and its associated structures.

ra′mi articula′res arte′riae descenden′tis genicula′ris [TA] articular branches of descending genicular artery: branches that pass downward in the vastus medialis muscle and help supply the knee joint.

r. ascen′dens arte′riae circumflex′ae fe′moris latera′lis [TA] ascending branch of lateral circumflex femoral artery: a branch that runs upward along the trochanteric line of the femur and between the gluteus medius and minimus muscles, and anastomoses with branches of the superior gluteal artery. It helps supply the upper thigh muscles.

r. ascen′dens arte′riae circumflex′ae fe′moris media′lis [TA] ascending branch of medial circumflex femoral artery: a branch that ascends in front of the quadratus femoris muscle to the trochanteric fossa, and there anastomoses with gluteal arteries.

r. ascen′dens arte′riae circumflex′ae i′lium profun′dae [TA] ascending branch of deep circumflex iliac artery: a branch leaving the deep circumflex iliac artery near the anterior superior iliac spine, rising between and distributing to the transversus abdominis and internal oblique muscles.

r. ascen′dens arte′riae segmenta′lis anterio′ris pulmo′nis dex′tri [TA] ascending branch of anterior segmental artery of right lung: one of the branches of the anterior segmental artery that supply the anterior segment of the superior lobe of the right lung.

r. ascen′dens arte′riae segmenta′lis ante′rioris pulmo′nis sinis′tri [TA] ascending branch of anterior segmental artery of left lung: one of the branches of the anterior segmental artery that supply the anterior segment of the superior lobe of the left lung.

r. ascen′dens arte′riae segmenta′lis posterio′ris pulmo′nis dex′tri [TA] ascending branch of posterior segmental artery of right lung: one of the branches of the posterior segmental artery that supply the posterior segment of the superior lobe of the right lung.

r. ascen′dens arte′riae segmenta′lis posterio′ris pulmo′nis sinis′tri [TA] ascending branch of posterior segmental artery of left lung: one of the branches of the posterior segmental artery that supply the posterior segment of the superior lobe of the left lung.

r. ascen′dens ra′mi superficia′lis arte′riae transver′sae col′li [TA] the ascending branch of the superficial branch of the transverse cervical artery.

r. ascen′dens sul′ci latera′lis ce′rebri [TA] ascending branch of lateral cerebral sulcus: a branch that runs superiorly a short distance into the inferior frontal gyrus.

r. atria′lis anastomo′ticus ra′mi circumflex′i arte′riae corona′riae sinis′trae [TA] atrial anastomotic branch of circumflex branch of left coronary artery: a branch of the circumflex branch of the left coronary artery that passes the interatrial septum to anastomose with the right coronary artery; called also *atrial anastomotic artery* and *anastomotic atrial artery.*

ra′mi atria′les arte′riae corona′riae dex′trae [TA] atrial branches of right coronary artery: branches of the right coronary artery, consisting of anterior and lateral branches chiefly distributed to the right atrium, and usually a single posterior branch distributed to the right and left atria.

ra′mi atria′les ra′mi circumflex′i arte′riae corona′riae sinis′trae [TA] atrial branches of circumflex branch of left coronary artery: branches distributed to the left atrium, consisting of anterior, lateral, and posterior groups.

r. atria′lis interme′dius arte′riae corona′riae dex′trae [TA] intermediate atrial branch of right coronary artery: a branch of the right coronary artery arising opposite to the marginal branch and ascending to over the right atrium; called also *right intermediate atrial artery.*

r. atria′lis interme′dius ra′mi circumflex′i arte′riae corona′riae sinis′tri [TA] intermediate atrial branch of circumflex branch of left coronary artery: a branch that distributes along the left atrium above the coronary sulcus; called also *left intermediate atrial artery.*

ra′mi atrioventricula′res ra′mi circumflex′i arte′riae corona′riae sinis′trae [TA] atrioventricular branches of circumflex branch of left coronary artery: small recurrent branches distributed to the atria and ventricles.

ra′mi auricula′res anterio′res arte′riae tempora′lis superficia′lis [TA] anterior auricular branches of superficial temporal artery: branches that supply the lateral aspect of the pinna and the external acoustic meatus. Called also *anterior auricular arteries.*

r. auricula′ris arte′riae auricula′ris posterio′ris [TA] auricular branch of posterior auricular artery: a branch supplying the pinna and adjacent skin.

r. auricula′ris arte′riae occipita′lis [TA] auricular branch of occipital artery: an inconstant branch of the occipital artery that helps supply the medial aspect of the pinna.

r. auricula′ris ner′vi va′gi [TA] auricular branch of vagus nerve: a branch arising from the superior ganglion of the vagus, innervating the cranial surface of the auricle, the floor of the external acoustic meatus, and the adjacent part of the tympanic membrane; *modality*, general sensory.

r. autono′micus [TA] autonomic branch: any of the branches of the parasympathetic or sympathetic nerves of the autonomic nervous system.

r. basa′lis ante′rior ve′nae basa′lis commu′nis TA alternative for *vena basalis anterior*.

r. basa′lis tento′rii arte′riae caro′tidis inter′nae [TA] tentorial basal branch of internal carotid artery: a twig from the cavernous part of the internal carotid artery that supplies the base of the tentorium.

ra′mi bronchia′les arte′riae thora′cicae inter′nae [TA] bronchial branches of internal thoracic artery: small, variable branches of the internal thoracic artery, with distribution to the bronchi and trachea. Called also *anterior bronchial arteries*.

ra′mi bronchia′les ner′vi va′gi [TA] branches of the vagus that supply the bronchi and the pulmonary vessels, both directly and by way of the anterior and posterior parts of the pulmonary plexus; there are two or three short anterior branches and numerous longer posterior branches; *modality*, parasympathetic and visceral afferent.

ra′mi bronchia′les par′tis thora′cicae aor′tae [TA] bronchial branches of thoracic part of aorta: branches arising from the thoracic aorta to supply the bronchi and lower trachea, and passing along the posterior sides of the bronchi to ramify about the respiratory bronchioles; distributed also to adjacent lymph nodes, pulmonary vessels, and pericardium, and to part of the esophagus. Called also *bronchial arteries*.

ra′mi bucca′les ner′vi facia′lis [TA] buccal branches of facial nerve: branches that innervate the zygomatic, levator labii superioris, buccinator, and orbicularis oris muscles; *modality*, motor and general sensory.

ra′mi calca′nei arte′riae tibia′lis posterio′ris [TA] calcaneal branches of posterior tibial artery: branches that arise from the posterior tibial artery and are distributed to the medial aspect and back of the heel.

ra′mi calca′nei latera′les ner′vi sura′lis [TA] lateral calcaneal branches of sural nerve: branches that innervate the skin on the back of the leg and the lateral side of the foot and heel; *modality*, general sensory.

ra′mi calca′nei media′les ner′vi tibia′lis [TA] medial calcaneal branches of tibial nerve: branches supplying the medial side of the heel and of the posterior part of the sole; *modality*, general sensory.

ra′mi calca′nei ramo′rum malleola′rium latera′lium arte′riae fibula′ris [TA] calcaneal branches of lateral malleolar branches of peroneal artery: branches distributed to the lateral aspect and back of the heel.

r. calcari′nus arte′riae occipita′lis media′lis [TA] calcarine branch of medial occipital artery: a branch that supplies the calcarine fissure.

ra′mi capsula′res arteria′rum intrarena′lium [TA] capsular branches of intrarenal arteries: branches that supply the renal capsule.

ra′mi capsula′res arte′riae rena′lis [TA] capsular branches of renal artery: branches that supply the renal capsule. Called also *capsular arteries* and *perirenal arteries*.

ra′mi cardi′aci cervica′les inferio′res ner′vi va′gi [TA] inferior cardiac branches of the vagus nerve: branches (sometimes called cervicothoracic) arising from the vagi and from the recurrent laryngeal nerves at the thoracic inlet, and joining cervicothoracic sympathetic cardiac nerves, the combined nerves passing to the cardiac plexus; *modality*, parasympathetic and visceral afferent.

ra′mi cardi′aci cervica′les superio′res ner′vi va′gi [TA] superior cervical cardiac branches of vagus nerve: variable branches arising from the vagus in the cervical region and usually joining the cervical sympathetic cardiac nerves. The conjoined nerves then descend in front of, or behind, the arch of the aorta to the cardiac plexus; *modality*, parasympathetic and visceral afferent.

ra′mi cardi′aci thora′cici [TA] thoracic cardiac branches: branches of the second through fourth or fifth thoracic ganglia of the sympathetic trunk, supplying the heart and having a sympathetic (accelerator) modality as well as a visceral afferent one (chiefly for pain). Called also *thoracic cardiac nerves* and *nervi cardiaci thoracici*.

ra′mi cardi′aci thora′cici ner′vi va′gi [TA] thoracic cardiac branches of the vagus nerve: branches which arise in the thorax from the right and left vagus and left recurrent laryngeal nerves. They go directly to the posterior walls of the atria, to the coronary plexuses, and to the anterior pulmonary plexuses.

r. carpa′lis dorsa′lis arte′riae radia′lis [TA] dorsal carpal branch of radial artery: a branch running medially deep to the extensor tendons and helping form the dorsal carpal rete.

r. carpa′lis dorsa′lis arte′riae ulna′ris [TA] dorsal carpal branch of ulnar artery: a variable branch of the ulnar artery that runs laterally deep to the tendons of the ulnar muscles of the wrist, helping to form the dorsal carpal rete.

r. carpa′lis palma′ris arte′riae radia′lis [TA] palmar carpal branch of radial artery: a branch that passes medially behind the flexor tendons on the palmar aspect of the wrist and forms a network with a corresponding branch of the ulnar artery.

r. carpa′lis palma′ris arte′riae ulna′ris [TA] palmar carpal branch of ulnar artery: a branch that passes laterally behind the flexor tendons on the palmar aspect of the wrist and forms a network with a corresponding branch of the radial artery.

ra′mi cau′dae nu′clei cauda′ti arte′riae choroi′deae anterio′ris [TA] branches of anterior choroidal artery to tail of caudate nucleus: small branches that supply the tail of the caudate nucleus.

r. cervica′lis ner′vi facia′lis TA alternative for *r. colli nervi facialis*.

ra′mi chiasma′tici arte′riae choroi′deae anterio′ris [TA] branches of anterior choroidal artery to optic chiasm: small branches that supply the optic chiasm.

r. chiasma′ticus arte′riae communican′tis posterio′ris [TA] chiasmatic branch of posterior communicating artery: a branch that supplies the optic chiasm.

ra′mi choroi′dei posterio′res latera′les arte′riae ce′rebri posterio′ris [TA] lateral choroidal branches of the posterior cerebral artery: branches that supply the choroid plexus of the lateral ventricle and the thalamus.

ra′mi choroi′dei posterio′res media′les arte′riae ce′rebri posterio′ris [TA] medial choroidal branches of posterior cerebral artery: branches that supply the choroid plexus of the third ventricle.

ra′mi choroi′dei ventri′culi latera′lis arte′riae choroi′deae anterio′ris [TA] choroidal branches to lateral ventricle: small branches of the anterior choroidal artery that supply the choroid plexus of the lateral ventricle.

r. choroi′deus ventri′culi quar′ti arte′riae inferio′ris posterio′ris cerebel′li [TA] choroidal branch to fourth ventricle: a branch of the posterior inferior cerebellar artery that supplies the choroid plexus of the fourth ventricle.

ra′mi choroi′dei ventri′culi ter′tii arte′riae choroi′deae anterio′ris [TA] choroidal branches to third ventricle: small branches of the anterior choroidal artery that supply the third ventricle.

r. cingula′ris arte′riae callosomargina′lis [TA] the cingular branch of the callosomarginal artery, supplying the cingulate gyrus.

r. circumflex′us arte′riae corona′riae sinis′trae [TA] circumflex branch of left coronary artery: a branch that curves around to the back of the left ventricle in the coronary sulcus, supplying the left ventricle and left atrium. Called also *circumflex artery*.

r. circumflex′us fibula′ris arte′riae tibia′lis posterio′ris [TA] fibular circumflex branch of posterior tibial artery: a branch that winds laterally around the neck of the fibula, helping supply the soleus muscle and contributing to the anastomosis around the knee joint; called also *r. circumflexus peronealis arteriae tibialis posterioris* [TA alternative]. and *fibular circumflex artery*.

r. circumflex′us peronea′lis arte′riae tibia′lis posterio′ris TA alternative for *r. circumflexus fibularis arteriae tibialis posterioris*.

r. clavicula′ris arte′riae thoracoacromia′lis [TA] clavicular branch of thoracoacromial artery: a vessel that passes medially to supply the subclavius muscle.

ra′mi cliva′les par′tes cerebra′lis arte′riae caro′tidis inter′nae [TA] clival branches of cerebral part of internal carotid artery: twigs from the cerebral part of the internal carotid artery that supply the clivus.

r. cochlea′ris arte′riae vestibulocochlea′ris [TA] cochlear branch of vestibulocochlear artery: a branch that supplies the cochlea.

ra′mi coeli′aci ner′vi va′gi [TA] celiac branches of vagus nerve: branches that arise from both the anterior and posterior vagal trunks and join the celiac plexus; *modality*, parasympathetic and visceral afferent. Called also *celiac nerves*.

r. co′licus arte′riae ileoco′licae [TA] colic branch of ileocolic artery: a branch that passes upward on the ascending colon and anastomoses with the right colic artery; called also *ascending ileocolic artery*.

r. collatera′lis arte′riae intercosta′lis posterio′ris [TA] collateral branch of posterior intercostal artery: a branch helping supply the thoracic wall, arising from a posterior intercostal artery near the angle of the rib and running forward in the lower part of the corresponding intercostal space.

r. col′li ner′vi facia′lis [TA] cervical branch of facial nerve: a branch lying deep to and innervating the platysma muscle; *modality*, motor. Called also *r. cervicalis nervi facialis* [TA alternative].

ra′mi communican′tes 1. communicating branches between two nerves; in official terminology called *rami communicantes nervorum spinalium*. 2. branches connecting two arteries. Called also *rami anastomotici*.

r. commu′nicans al′bus ner′vi spina′lis [TA] white communicating branch of spinal nerve: one of the two types of communicating nerve branches between a sympathetic ganglion and a spinal nerve; the white type are mostly myelinated, send impulses from the spinal nerves to and through the ganglia, and are located mainly in the thoracic and upper lumbar region. Cf. *r. communicans griseus nervi spinalis*.

r. commu′nicans arte′riae fibula′ris [TA] communicating branch of peroneal artery: a communicating branch between the peroneal and the posterior tibial arteries, distributed to the interosseous membrane and supramalleolar region.

r. commu′nicans cochlea′ris ner′vi vestibula′ris [TA] cochlear communicating branch of vestibular nerve: a branch of the vestibular nerve that unites with the cochlear nerve.

r. commu′nicans fibula′ris ner′vi fibula′ris commu′nis [TA] sural communicating branch of common peroneal nerve: a small branch arising from the common peroneal nerve, either with the lateral cutaneous sural nerve or separately; distally it joins the medial sural cutaneous nerve to form the sural nerve. Called also *r. communicans peroneus nervi peronei communis* [TA alternative].

r. commu′nicans gri′seus ner′vi spina′lis [TA] gray communicating branch of spinal nerve: one of the two types of communicating nerve branches between a sympathetic ganglion and a spinal nerve; these branches are gray (unmyelinated) and carry postganglionic impulses back to the spinal nerves and then to the periphery, supplying blood vessels, sweat glands, and smooth muscles. Cf. *r. communicans albus nervi spinalis*.

ra′mi communican′tes ner′vi auriculotempora′lis cum ner′vo facia′li [TA] communicating branches of auriculotemporal nerve with facial nerve: branches containing sensory fibers from the auriculotemporal nerve that join the facial nerve within the parotid gland, to be distributed with branches of the latter.

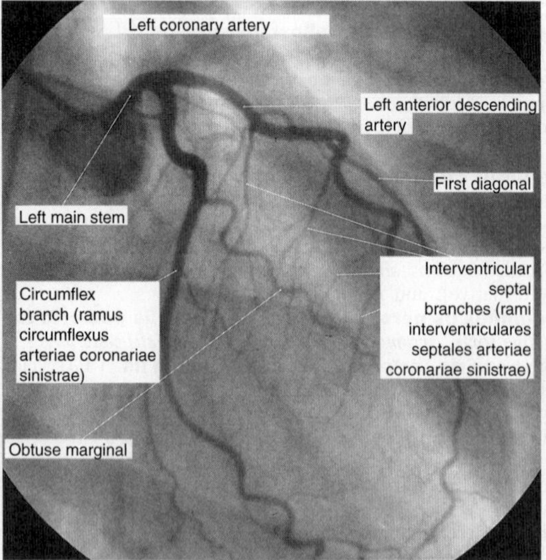

■ Left coronary artery with circumflex branch (ramus circumflexus arteriae coronariae sinistrae) and interventricular septal branches (rami interventriculares septales arteriae coronariae sinistrae), shown in anterior oblique view in a left coronary arteriogram.

r. commu′nicans ner′vi facia′lis cum ner′vo glossopharyn′geo [TA] communicating branch of facial nerve with glossopharyngeal nerve: a branch that interconnects the glossopharyngeal nerve and the facial nerve after emergence of the latter from the stylomastoid foramen.

r. commu′nicans ner′vi glossopharyn′gei cum chor′da tym′pani [TA] communicating branch of glossopharyngeal nerve with chorda tympani: a small branch that interconnects the glossopharyngeal nerve and the chorda tympani.

r. commu′nicans ner′vi glossopharyn′gei cum ner′vo auriculo-tempora′li [TA] communicating branch of glossopharyngeal nerve with auriculotemporal nerve: a branch carrying postganglionic parasympathetic fibers from the glossopharyngeal nerve to the auriculotemporal nerve for distribution to the parotid gland.

r. commu′nicans ner′vi glossopharyn′gei cum ra′mo auricula′ri ner′vi va′gi [TA] communicating branch of glossopharyngeal nerve with auricular branch of vagus nerve: a small branch connecting the glossopharyngeal nerve with the auricular branch of the vagus nerve.

r. commu′nicans ner′vi glossopharyn′gei cum ra′mo menin′geo ner′vi va′gi [TA] communicating branch of glossopharyngeal nerve with meningeal branch of vagal nerve: a branch that carries autonomic fibers destined for the meninges from the glossopharyngeal nerve to the meningeal branch of the vagal nerve.

r. commu′nicans ner′vi interme′dii cum ner′vo va′go [TA] communicating branch of intermediate nerve with vagus nerve: a branch of the intermediate nerve that communicates with the vagus nerve.

r. commu′nicans ner′vi interme′dii cum plex′u tympa′nico [TA] communicating branch of intermediate nerve with tympanic plexus: a branch of the intermediate nerve that communicates with the tympanic plexus.

r. commu′nicans ner′vi lacrima′lis cum ner′vo zygoma′tico [TA] communicating branch of lacrimal nerve with zygomatic nerve: a branch that carries parasympathetic postganglionic fibers originating in the pterygopalatine ganglion and destined for the lacrimal gland.

r. commu′nicans ner′vi laryn′gei superio′ris cum ner′vo la-ryn′geo recurren′te [TA] communicating branch of superior laryngeal nerve with recurrent laryngeal nerve: a small branch interconnecting the internal branch of the superior laryngeal nerve with the recurrent laryngeal nerve, behind or in the posterior cricoarytenoid muscle. Called also *Galen nerve*.

ra′mi communican′tes ner′vi lingua′lis cum ner′vo hypoglos′so [TA] communicating branches of lingual nerve with hypoglossal nerve: plexiform terminal branches interconnecting the lingual and hypoglossal nerves just in front of the hyoglossus muscle.

r. commu′nicans ner′vi media′ni cum ner′vo ulna′ri [TA] communicating branch of median nerve with ulnar nerve: a small branch across the flexor digitorum profundus muscle, connecting the median with the ulnar nerve.

r. commu′nicans ner′vi nasocilia′ris cum gan′glio cilia′ri TA alternative for *radix sensoria ganglii ciliaris*.

ra′mi communican′tes nervo′rum spina′lium [TA] communicating branches of spinal nerves: branches connecting spinal nerves with sympathetic ganglia, each spinal nerve receiving a gray communicating ramus, and the thoracic and upper lumbar spinal nerves having in addition a white communicating ramus. Called also *rami communicantes*.

r. commu′nicans ner′vi va′gi cum ner′vo glossopharyn′geo [TA] communicating branch of vagus nerve with glossopharyngeal nerve; see *r. communicans nervi glossopharyngei cum ramo auriculari nervi vagi*.

r. commu′nicans perone′us ner′vi perone′i commu′nis TA alternative for *r. communicans fibularis nervi fibularis communis*.

r. commu′nicans ulna′ris ner′vi radia′lis [TA] ulnar communicating branch of radial nerve: a small branch in the hand that interconnects the most medial dorsal digital nerve from the superficial branch of the radial nerve with the adjacent most lateral dorsal digital nerve from the dorsal branch of the ulnar nerve.

r. co′ni arterio′si arte′riae corona′riae dex′trae [TA] conus arteriosus branch of right coronary artery: the first ventricular branch of the right coronary artery, which supplies the conus arteriosus, and anastomoses with the left conus artery (branch) of the anterior interventricular branch of the left coronary artery; called also *conal* or *conus artery*, *right conus artery*, and *third conus artery*.

r. co′ni arterio′si arte′riae corona′riae sinis′trae [TA] conus arteriosus branch of left coronary artery: a small branch of the anterior interventricular branch of the left coronary artery, which supplies the conus arteriosus, and anastomoses with the right conus artery (branch) of the right coronary artery; called also *conal* or *conus artery* and *left conus artery*.
ra′mi cor′poris amygdaloi′dei arte′riae choroi′deae anterio′ris [TA] branches of anterior choroidal artery to amygdaloid body: small branches that supply the amygdaloid body.
r. cor′poris callo′si dorsa′lis arte′riae occipita′lis media′lis [TA] dorsal branch to corpus callosum: a branch of the medial occipital artery that supplies the dorsum of the corpus callosum.
ra′mi cor′poris genicula′ti latera′lis arte′riae choroi′deae anterio′ris [TA] branches of anterior choroidal artery to lateral geniculate body: small branches that supply the lateral geniculate body.
ra′mi cortica′les inferio′res arte′riae ce′rebri me′diae TA alternative for *rami terminales inferiores arteriae cerebri mediae.*
ra′mi cortica′les superio′res arte′riae ce′rebri me′diae TA alternative for *rami terminales superiores arteriae cerebri mediae.*
r. costa′lis latera′lis arte′riae thora′cicae inter′nae [TA] lateral costal branch of internal thoracic artery: an occasional branch passing inferolaterally behind the ribs, supplying ribs and costal cartilages, and anastomosing with the posterior intercostal arteries.
r. cricothyroi′deus arte′riae thyroi′deae superio′ris [TA] cricothyroid branch of superior thyroid artery: a vessel running medially over the cricothyroid muscle, toward the cricothyroid ligament, and anastomosing with its fellow of the opposite side. Called also *cricothyroid artery*.
ra′mi cru′ris ce′rebri arte′riae choroi′deae anterio′ris [TA] branches of anterior choroidal artery to crus cerebri: small branches that supply the crus cerebri.
ra′mi cru′ris posterio′ris cap′sulae inter′nae arte′riae choroi′deae anterio′ris [TA] branches of anterior choroidal artery to posterior limb of internal capsule: small branches that supply the posterior limb of the internal capsule of the cerebrum.
r. cuta′neus [TA] cutaneous branch: a branch of a mixed (afferent or efferent) peripheral nerve innervating a region of the skin.
r. cuta′neus ante′rior abdomina′lis ner′vi intercosta′lis [TA] anterior abdominal cutaneous branch of intercostal nerve: a branch from the intercostal nerve that contributes to innervation of the skin in the anteromedial abdominal region. Its modality is general sensory.
ra′mi cuta′nei anterio′res ner′vi femora′lis [TA] anterior cutaneous branches of femoral nerve: branches that innervate the skin on the front and medial aspect of the thigh and patella and contribute to the subsartorial and patellar plexuses; *modality*, general sensory.
r. cuta′neus ante′rior ner′vi iliohypogas′trici [TA] anterior cutaneous branch of iliohypogastric nerve: a branch that runs forward between the internal and external oblique muscles and innervates the skin over the pubis; *modality*, general sensory.
r. cuta′neus ante′rior pectora′lis ner′vi intercosta′lis [TA] anterior pectoral cutaneous branch of intercostal nerve: a branch from the intercostal nerve that contributes to innervation of the skin in the anteromedial thoracic region; in the breast region it sends further branches (see *rami mammarii mediales rami cutanei anterioris pectoralis nervi intercostalis*). Its modality is general sensory.
ra′mi cuta′nei cru′ris media′les ner′vi saphe′ni [TA] medial crural cutaneous branches of saphenous nerve: branches distributed by the saphenous nerve to the skin of the medial aspect of the leg; *modality*, general sensory.
r. cuta′neus latera′lis abdomina′lis ner′vi intercosta′lis [TA] lateral abdominal cutaneous branch of intercostal nerve: a branch from the intercostal nerve that, through its anterior and posterior subdivisions, innervates the skin of the lateral and posterior body wall; it has a general sensory modality.
r. cuta′neus latera′lis arte′riae intercosta′lis posterio′ris [TA] lateral cutaneous branch of posterior intercostal artery: a branch arising from a posterior intercostal artery, supplying the anterolateral thoracic wall. The branches of the third through fifth posterior intercostal arteries give off small mammary branches.
r. cuta′neus latera′lis ner′vi iliohypogas′trici [TA] lateral cutaneous branch of iliohypogastric nerve: a nerve branch distributed to the skin over the side of the buttock; *modality*, general sensory.
r. cuta′neus latera′lis pectora′lis ner′vi intercosta′lis [TA] lateral pectoral cutaneous branch of intercostal nerve: a branch from the intercostal that, through its anterior and posterior subdivisions, innervates the skin of the lateral and posterior body wall; it has a general sensory modality. Those of the fourth through sixth anterior thoracic branches send further branches (see *rami mammarii laterales rami cutanei lateralis pectoralis nervi intercostalis*).
r. cuta′neus latera′lis ra′mi dorsa′lis arte′riae intercosta′lis posterio′ris [TA] lateral cutaneous branch of dorsal branch of posterior intercostal artery: a branch from the dorsal branch of each posterior intercostal artery that supplies the posterolateral aspect of the thorax.
r. cuta′neus media′lis ra′mi dorsa′lis arte′riae intercosta′lis posterio′ris [TA] medial cutaneous branch of dorsal branch of posterior intercostal artery: a branch of the dorsal branch of each posterior intercostal artery that supplies the skin adjacent to the vertebral column.
r. cuta′neus ner′vi obturato′rii [TA] cutaneous branch of obturator nerve: a variable branch arising from the anterior branch of the obturator nerve, forming part of the subsartorial plexus, and supplying the skin of the medial aspect of the thigh and leg; *modality*, general sensory.
r. cuta′neus poste′rior ra′mi posterio′ris ner′vi thora′cici [TA] posterior cutaneous branch of posterior branch of thoracic nerve: cutaneous branches of either of the two divisions of a dorsal branch; see *r. lateralis rami posterior nervi thoracici* and *r. medialis rami posterior nervi thoracici*.
r. deltoi′deus arte′riae profun′dae bra′chii [TA] deltoid branch of profunda brachii artery: a branch distributed to the brachialis and deltoid muscles, and anastomosing with the posterior circumflex humeral artery.
r. deltoi′deus arte′riae thoracoacromia′lis [TA] deltoid branch of thoracoacromial artery: a branch of the thoracoacromial artery descending with the cephalic vein and helping to supply the deltoid and pectoralis major muscles.
ra′mi denta′les arte′riae alveola′ris inferio′ris [TA] dental branches of inferior alveolar artery: branches arising from the inferior alveolar artery in the mandibular canal and supplying the inferior teeth.
ra′mi denta′les arteria′rum alveola′rium superio′rum anterio′rum [TA] dental branches of anterior superior alveolar arteries: branches that supply the incisor and canine teeth.
ra′mi denta′les arte′riae alveola′ris superio′ris posterio′ris [TA] dental branches of posterior superior alveolar artery: branches that supply the molar and premolar teeth.
ra′mi denta′les inferio′res plex′us denta′lis inferio′ris [TA] inferior dental branches of inferior dental plexus: branches that innervate the lower teeth; *modality*, general sensory.
ra′mi denta′les superio′res plex′us denta′lis superio′ris [TA] superior dental branches of superior dental plexus: branches that innervate the teeth of the upper jaw; *modality*, general sensory.
r. descen′dens arte′riae circumflex′ae fe′moris latera′lis [TA] descending branch of lateral circumflex femoral artery: a branch passing from the lateral circumflex artery (sometimes directly from the deep femoral) to the knee, and supplying the thigh muscles.
r. descen′dens arte′riae occipita′lis [TA] descending branch of occipital artery: a branch that arises from the occipital artery on the obliquus capitis superior muscle and divides into superficial and deep branches, supplying the trapezius and deep neck muscles.
r. descen′dens arte′riae segmenta′lis anterio′ris pulmo′nis dex′tri [TA] descending branch of anterior segmental artery of right lung: one of the branches of the anterior segmental artery that supply the anterior segment of the superior lobe of the right lung.
r. descen′dens arte′riae segmenta′lis anterio′ris pulmo′nis sinis′tri [TA] descending branch of anterior segmental artery of left lung: one of the branches of the anterior segmental artery that supply the anterior segment of the superior lobe of the left lung.
r. descen′dens arte′riae segmenta′lis posterio′ris pulmo′nis dex′tri [TA] ascending branch of posterior segmental artery of right lung: one of the branches of the posterior segmental artery that supply the posterior segment of the superior lobe of the right lung.
r. descen′dens arte′riae segmenta′lis posterio′ris pulmo′nis sinis′tri [TA] descending branch of posterior segmental artery of left lung: one of the branches of the posterior segmental artery that supply the posterior segment of the superior lobe of the left lung.
r. descen′dens ra′mi superficia′lis arte′riae transver′sae col′li [TA] descending branch of the superficial branch of the transverse cervical artery.

r. dex′ter arte′riae hepa′ticae pro′priae [TA] right branch of hepatic artery proper: the right of the two branches into which the hepatic artery proper normally divides; it supplies the right liver, and a branch, the cystic artery, supplies the gallbladder.
r. dex′ter ve′nae por′tae he′patis [TA] right branch of hepatic portal vein: a branch distributed to the right liver.
r. digas′tricus ner′vi facia′lis [TA] digastric branch of facial nerve: a branch that innervates the posterior belly of the digastric muscle; *modality*, motor; called also *digastric nerve.*
r. diplo′icus arte′riae supraorbita′lis [TA] diploic branch of supraorbital artery: a small branch arising as the artery passes through the supraorbital notch and supplying the diploë of the frontal bone and the lining of the frontal sinus.
ra′mi dista′les latera′les stria′ti arteria′rum centra′lium anterolatera′lium [TA] distal lateral striate branches of anterolateral central arteries: branches supplied by the middle cerebral artery, supplying the basal nuclei of the brain and its internal capsule.
r. dorsa′lis arte′riae intercosta′lis posterio′ris [TA] dorsal branch of posterior intercostal artery: a branch arising from a posterior intercostal artery, passing backward with the dorsal branch of the corresponding intercostal nerve to supply the posterior thoracic wall; it has several spinal branches and a medial and a lateral cutaneous branch.
r. dorsa′lis arte′riae intercosta′lis posterio′ris pri′mae [TA] dorsal branch of first intercostal artery: the dorsal branch arising from the first posterior intercostal artery. Its distribution is similar to that of the other posterior intercostals; see *r. dorsalis arteriae intercostalis posterioris.*
r. dorsa′lis arte′riae intercosta′lis posterio′ris secun′dae [TA] dorsal branch of second intercostal artery: the dorsal branch arising from the second posterior intercostal artery. Its distribution is similar to that of the other posterior intercostals; see *r. dorsalis arteriae intercostalis posterioris.*
r. dorsa′lis arte′riae lumba′lis [TA] dorsal branch of lumbar artery: the larger of the two branches into which each lumbar artery (four or five) divides; it supplies lumbar back muscles, joints, and skin, and gives off a spinal branch.
r. dorsa′lis arte′riae subcosta′lis [TA] dorsal branch of subcostal artery: a branch supplying back muscles, its distribution being similar to that of the dorsal branches of the posterior intercostal arteries.
ra′mi dorsa′les lin′guae arte′riae lingua′lis [TA] dorsal lingual branches of lingual artery: branches of the lingual artery arising beneath the hyoglossus muscle and supplying the tonsil and the back of the tongue.
ra′mi dorsa′les nervo′rum cervica′lium TA alternative for *rami posteriores nervorum cervicalium.*
r. dorsa′lis ner′vi coccy′gei TA alternative for *r. posterior nervi coccygei.*
ra′mi dorsa′les nervo′rum lumba′lium TA alternative for *rami posteriores nervorum lumbalium.*
ra′mi dorsa′les nervo′rum sacra′lium TA alternative for *rami posteriores nervorum sacralium.*
ra′mi dorsa′les nervo′rum thoracico′rum TA alternative for *rami posteriores nervorum thoracicorum.*
r. dorsa′lis ner′vi ulna′ris [TA] dorsal branch of ulnar nerve: a large cutaneous branch that arises from the ulnar nerve and passes down the distal portion of the forearm to the medial side of the back of the hand, where it divides usually into three, sometimes four, dorsal digital nerves; *modality*, general sensory.
r. dorsa′lis ve′nae intercosta′lis posterio′ris TA alternative for *vena dorsalis venae intercostalis posterioris.*
ra′mi duodena′les arte′riae pancreaticoduodena′lis superio′ris anterio′ris [TA] duodenal branches of anterior superior pancreaticoduodenal artery: vessels that supply the duodenum.
ra′mi duodena′les arte′riae pancreaticoduodena′lis superio′ris posterio′ris [TA] duodenal branches of posterior superior pancreaticoduodenal artery: vessels supplying the duodenum.
ra′mi epididyma′les arte′riae testicula′ris [TA] epididymal branches of testicular artery: they are distributed to the epididymis.
r. exter′nus ner′vi accesso′rii [TA] external branch of accessory nerve: the branch of the accessory nerve that originates from the spinal roots of the nerve; it sends muscular branches to supply the sternocleidomastoid and trapezius muscles.
r. exter′nus ner′vi laryn′gei superio′ris [TA] external branch of superior laryngeal nerve: the smaller of the two branches into which the superior laryngeal nerve divides, descending under cover of the sternothyroid muscle and innervating the cricothyroid and the inferior constrictor of the pharynx; *modality*, motor.
r. femora′lis ner′vi genitofemora′lis [TA] femoral branch of genitofemoral nerve: a branch arising by division of the genitofemoral nerve above the inguinal ligament; entering the femoral sheath, it turns forward and supplies the skin of the femoral triangle; *modality*, general sensory. Called also *nervus lumboinguinalis.*
r. fronta′lis anteromedia′lis arte′riae callosomargina′lis [TA] the anteromedial frontal branch of the callosomarginal artery.
r. fronta′lis arte′riae menin′geae me′diae [TA] frontal branch of middle meningeal artery: a branch lodged in grooves on the sphenoid and parietal bones and supplying the dura mater of the front of the brain. A part of it is sometimes enclosed in a bony canal.
r. fronta′lis arte′riae tempora′lis superficia′lis [TA] frontal branch of superficial temporal artery: a tortuous terminal branch that supplies the forehead and frontal scalp.
r. fronta′lis intermediomedia′lis arte′riae callosomargina′lis [TA] the intermediomedial frontal branch of the callosomarginal artery.
r. fronta′lis posteromedia′lis arte′riae callosomargina′lis [TA] the posteromedial frontal branch of the callosomarginal artery.
ra′mi gangliona′res ner′vi lingua′lis ad gan′glion submandibula′re [TA] ganglionic branches of lingual nerve to submandibular ganglion: branches which interconnect the lingual nerve and the submandibular ganglion, and by which the ganglion is suspended from the nerve; they carry preganglionic fibers that derive from the chorda tympani and synapse in the submandibular ganglion and postganglionic fibers. Called also *radix sensoria ganglii submandibularis* [TA alternative] and *motor* or *sensory root of submandibular ganglion.*
ra′mi gangliona′res ner′vi mandibula′ris ad gan′glion o′ticum [TA] ganglionic branches of mandibular nerve to otic ganglion: branches of the mandibular nerve that communicate with the otic ganglion. Called also *radix sensoria ganglii otici* [TA alternative].
ra′mi gangliona′res ner′vi maxilla′ris ad gan′glion pterygopalati′num [TA] ganglionic branches of maxillary nerve to pterygopalatine ganglion: fibers connecting the maxillary nerve to the pterygopalatine ganglion. Called also *radix sensoria ganglii pterygopalatini* [TA alternative] and *sensory root of pterygopalatine ganglion.*
ra′mi gangliona′res trigemina′les arte′riae caro′tidis inter′nae [TA] branches of internal carotid artery to trigeminal ganglion: short branches from the cavernous part of the internal carotid artery that supply the trigeminal ganglion.
ra′mi gas′trici anterio′res trun′ci vaga′lis anterio′ris [TA] anterior gastric branches of anterior vagal trunk: branches arising from the anterior trunk of the vagus near the cardiac end of the stomach, innervating the anterior aspect of the lesser curvature and the anterior surface of the stomach almost to the pylorus; *modality*, parasympathetic and visceral afferent.
ra′mi gas′trici arte′riae gastroomenta′lis dex′trae [TA] gastric branches of right gastroomental artery: vessels that supply both surfaces of the stomach.
ra′mi gas′trici arte′riae gastroomenta′lis sinis′trae [TA] gastric branches of left gastroomental artery: vessels that supply both surfaces of the stomach.
ra′mi gas′trici posterio′res trun′ci vaga′lis posterio′ris [TA] posterior gastric branches of posterior vagal trunk: branches arising from the posterior vagal trunk near the cardiac end of the stomach and innervating the cardiac orifice and fundus, the posterior aspect of the lesser curvature, and the posterior surface of the stomach to the pyloric antrum; *modality*, parasympathetic and visceral afferent.
r. genita′lis ner′vi genitofemora′lis [TA] genital branch of genitofemoral nerve: a branch arising from the genitofemoral nerve above the inguinal ligament; entering the inguinal canal through the deep ring, it supplies the cremaster and continues to the skin of the scrotum or of the labium majus, and that of the adjacent area of the thigh; *modality*, general sensory and motor.
ra′mi ge′nus cap′sulae inter′nae arte′riae choroi′deae anterio′ris [TA] branches of anterior choroidal artery to genu of internal capsule: small branches that supply the genu of the internal capsule of the cerebrum.
ra′mi gingiva′les inferio′res plex′us denta′lis inferio′ris [TA] inferior gingival branches of inferior dental plexus: branches

originating from the inferior dental plexus and innervating the gingivae of the lower jaw; *modality,* general sensory.
ra′mi gingiva′les ner′vi menta′lis [TA] gingival branches of mental nerve: branches that innervate the gums; *modality,* general sensory.
ra′mi gingiva′les superio′res plex′us denta′lis superio′ris [TA] superior gingival branches of superior dental plexus: branches arising from the superior dental plexus and innervating the gingivae of the upper jaw; *modality,* general sensory.
r. glandula′ris ante′rior arte′riae thyroi′deae superio′ris [TA] anterior glandular branch of superior thyroid artery: a branch principally supplying the anterior surface of the thyroid gland, and anastomosing with the artery of the opposite side.
ra′mi glandula′res arte′riae facia′lis [TA] glandular branches of facial artery: branches given off to the submandibular gland by the facial artery as it passes over the lateral surface of the gland.
ra′mi glandula′res arte′riae thyroi′deae inferio′ris [TA] glandular branches of the inferior thyroid artery: branches distributed to the inferior surface of the thyroid gland.
r. glandula′ris latera′lis arte′riae thyroi′deae superio′ris [TA] lateral glandular branch of superior thyroid artery: a branch distributed to the lateral surface of the thyroid gland.
r. glandula′ris poste′rior arte′riae thyroi′deae superio′ris [TA] posterior glandular branch of superior thyroid artery: a branch distributed mainly to the medial and lateral surfaces of the thyroid gland; it anastomoses with the inferior thyroid artery.
ra′mi glo′bi pal′lidi arte′riae choroi′deae anterio′ris [TA] branches of anterior choroidal artery to globus pallidus: small branches that supply the globus pallidus.
r. gy′ri angula′ris arte′riae ce′rebri me′diae [TA] branch of middle cerebral artery to angular gyrus: a branch originating in the inferior terminal branch of middle cerebral artery and supplying the angular gyrus.
ra′mi helici′ni arte′riae uteri′nae [TA] helicine branches of uterine artery: the exceedingly tortuous terminal branches of the uterine artery in the uterine muscle. Called also *helicine arteries.*
ra′mi hepa′tici trun′ci vaga′lis anterio′ris [TA] hepatic branches of anterior vagal trunk: branches (sometimes only one) arising from the anterior vagal trunk, contributing to the hepatic plexus, and helping innervate the liver, gallbladder, pancreas, pylorus, and duodenum; *modality,* parasympathetic and visceral afferent.
ra′mi hippocam′pi arte′riae choroi′deae anterio′ris [TA] branches of anterior choroidal artery to hippocampus: small branches that supply the hippocampus.
r. hypothala′micus arte′riae communican′tis posterio′ris [TA] hypothalamic branch of posterior communicating artery: a branch that supplies the hypothalamus.
r. ilea′lis arte′riae ileoco′licae [TA] ileal branch of ileocolic artery: a branch that passes upward and to the left of the lower ileum and anastomoses with the end of the superior mesenteric artery.
r. ili′acus arte′riae iliolumba′lis [TA] iliac branch of iliolumbar artery: one of the two branches into which the iliolumbar artery divides in the iliac fossa; it supplies the iliacus muscle and sends a large nutrient branch to the ilium.
r. infe′rior ner′vi oculomoto′rii [TA] inferior branch of oculomotor nerve: the branch of the oculomotor nerve that innervates the medial and inferior rectus and inferior oblique muscles of the eyeball and, via the motor root of the ciliary ganglion and then the short ciliary nerves, supplies the sphincter pupillae and ciliary muscles; *modality,* motor and parasympathetic.
ra′mi inferio′res ner′vi transver′si col′li [TA] inferior branches of transverse nerve of neck: the more inferior of the branches that arise from the transverse cervical nerve near the anterior border of the sternocleidomastoid muscle, innervating skin and subcutaneous tissue in the anterior cervical region; *modality,* general sensory.
r. infe′rior os′sis pu′bis [TA] inferior ramus of pubic bone: the short flattened bar of bone that projects from the body of the pubic bone in a posteroinferolateral direction to meet the ramus of the ischium. See illustration at *ramus ossis ischii.*
r. infe′rior ra′mi profun′di arte′riae glu′teae superio′ris [TA] inferior branch of deep branch of superior gluteal artery: the lower division of the deep branch of the superior gluteal artery, accompanied by the superior gluteal nerve and helping supply the gluteus medius, gluteus minimus, and tensor fasciae latae muscles and the hip joint and ilium.
r. infrahyoi′deus arte′riae thyroi′deae superio′ris [TA] infrahyoid branch of superior thyroid artery: a vessel running along the inferior border of the hyoid bone, supplying the infrahyoid region, and anastomosing with its fellow of the opposite side.
r. infrapatella′ris ner′vi saphe′ni [TA] infrapatellar branch of saphenous nerve: a branch running inferolaterally from the saphenous nerve to the patellar plexus; *modality,* general sensory.
ra′mi inguina′les arte′riae puden′dae exter′nae profun′dae [TA] inguinal branches of deep external pudendal artery: branches arising from the deep external pudendal arteries and supplying the inguinal region.
ra′mi intercosta′les anterio′res arte′riae thora′cicae inter′nae [TA] anterior intercostal branches of internal thoracic artery: twelve branches, two in each of the upper six intercostal spaces, that supply the intercostal spaces and the pectoralis major muscle. Within each space both branches run laterally, the upper anastomosing with the posterior intercostal artery, the lower with the collateral branch of that artery.
ra′mi interganglion′res trun′ci sympa′thici [TA] interganglionic branches of sympathetic trunk: the branches that interconnect the ganglia of the sympathetic trunk.
r. inter′nus ner′vi accesso′rii [TA] internal branch of accessory nerve: the branch of the trunk of accessory nerve that begins as what has been called cranial root of the accessory nerve (now identiified as part of the vagus nerve), and joins the vagus nerve immediately upon branching off the trunk; it carries motor fibers that are distributed to the soft palate, pharyngeal constrictors, and larynx.
r. inter′nus ner′vi laryn′gei superio′ris [TA] internal branch of superior laryngeal nerve: the larger of the two branches of the superior laryngeal nerve, which innervates the mucosa of the epiglottis, base of the tongue, and larynx; *modality,* general sensory.
r. interventricula′ris ante′rior arte′riae corona′riae sinis′trae [TA] anterior interventricular branch of left coronary artery: the branch of the left coronary artery that runs to the apex of the heart in the anterior interventricular sulcus, supplying the ventricles and most of the interventricular septum. See illustration at *ramus marginalis dexter arteriae coronariae dextrae.* Called also *anterior interventricular artery.*
r. interventricula′ris poste′rior arte′riae corona′riae dex′trae [TA] posterior interventricular branch of right coronary artery: a branch running toward the apex of the heart in the posterior interventricular sulcus, supplying the diaphragmatic surface of the ventricles and part of the interventricular septum.
ra′mi interventricula′res septa′les arte′riae corona′riae dex′trae [TA] interventricular septal branches of right coronary artery: numerous relatively small branches of the posterior interventricular branch of the right coronary artery that supply about the posterior one-third of the interventricular septum. Called also *posterior interventricular septal arteries* and *posterior septal arteries.*
ra′mi interventricula′res septa′les arte′riae corona′riae sinis′trae [TA] interventricular septal branches of left coronary artery: branches of the anterior interventricular branch of the left coronary artery that supply about the anterior two-thirds of the interventricular septum. See illustration at *ramus circumflexus arteriae coronariae sinistrae.* Called also *anterior interventricular septal arteries* and *anterior septal arteries.*
ischial r. r. ossis ischii.
ischiopubic r., r. ischiopu′bicus [TA] the inferior ramus of the pubis and the adjacent part of the ramus of the ischium, considered as a unit.
r. of ischium r. ossis ischii.
ra′mi isth′mi fau′cium ner′vi lingua′lis [TA] branches from the lingual nerve to the isthmus of the fauces; *modality,* general sensory.
r. of jaw r. mandibulae.
ra′mi labia′les anterio′res arte′riae puden′dae exter′nae profun′dae [TA] anterior labial branches of deep external pudendal artery: branches that arise from the deep external pudendal artery and supply the labium majus; called also *anterior labial arteries of vulva.*
ra′mi labia′les ner′vi menta′lis [TA] labial branches of mental nerve: branches of the mental nerve that innervate the lower lip; *modality,* general sensory.
ra′mi labia′les posterio′res arte′riae puden′dae inter′nae [TA] posterior labial branches of internal pudendal artery: two branches arising from the internal pudendal artery in the anterior part of the ischiorectal fossa, helping to supply the ischiocavernosus and bulbospongiosus

muscles, and supplying the labium majus and labium minus. Called also *posterior labial arteries of vulva.*
ra′mi labia′les superio′res ner′vi infraorbita′lis [TA] superior labial branches of infraorbital nerve: branches of the infraorbital nerve that are distributed to mucous membranes of the mouth and skin of the upper lip; *modality,* general sensory.
ra′mi laryngopharyn′gei gan′glii cervica′lis superio′ris [TA] laryngopharyngeal branches of superior cervical ganglion: branches from the superior cervical ganglion to the larynx and walls of the pharynx; *modality,* sympathetic.
r. latera′lis arte′riae superio′ris cerebel′li [TA] the lateral branch of the superior cerebellar artery.
r. latera′lis duc′tus hepa′tici sinis′tri [TA] the lateral branch of the left hepatic duct, draining lateral segments of the left liver.
r. latera′lis interventricula′ris anterio′ris arte′riae corona′riae sinis′trae [TA] lateral branch of the anterior interventricular branch of the left coronary artery.
r. latera′lis na′si arte′riae facia′lis [TA] lateral nasal branch of the facial artery: a branch supplying the ala and dorsum of the nose.
r. latera′lis ner′vi supraorbita′lis [TA] lateral branch of supraorbital nerve: a branch of the supraorbital nerve that supplies the frontal sinus, upper eyelid, and skin and subcutaneous tissue of the forehead and scalp laterally as far as the temporal region; *modality,* general sensory.
ra′mi latera′les pon′tis [TA] lateral pontine branches: the longer pontine arteries, which arise from the posterolateral and lateral aspects of the basilar artery and course circumferentially around the brainstem, sending penetrating vessels into the pons. Called also *circumferential pontine branches;* they are often subdivided into short and long circumferential pontine branches.
r. latera′lis ra′mi posterio′ris ner′vi cervica′lis [TA] lateral branch of posterior branch of cervical nerve: the lateral branch that arises from the posterior branch of a cervical nerve and supplies adjacent muscles.
r. latera′lis ra′mi posterio′ris ner′vi lumba′lis [TA] lateral branch of posterior branch of lumbar nerve: a branch that runs inferolaterally from the posterior branch of each lumbar nerve and innervates adjacent muscle; these branches have upper terminal branches that constitute the superior cluneal nerves and innervate the skin of the buttock.
r. latera′lis ra′mi posterio′ris ner′vi sacra′lis [TA] lateral branch of posterior branch of sacral nerve: a branch that arises from the posterior branch of one of the three upper sacral nerves and supplies the posterior gluteal skin.
r. latera′lis ra′mi posterio′ris ner′vi thora′cici [TA] lateral branch of posterior branch of thoracic nerve: the lateral of the terminal divisions of the posterior branch; it supplies first its corresponding levator costae muscle and then the longissimus thoracis and iliocostalis thoracis muscles. The lower branches pierce the latissimus dorsi and supply the skin of the back.
ra′mi liena′les arte′riae liena′lis TA alternative for *rami splenici arteriae splenicae.*
r. lingua′lis ner′vi facia′lis [TA] lingual branch of facial nerve: an inconstant branch of the facial nerve sometimes arising together with the stylohyoid branch, and helping to supply the styloglossal and glossopalatine muscles; *modality,* motor.
ra′mi lingua′les ner′vi glossopharyn′gei [TA] lingual branches of glossopharyngeal nerve: branches of the glossopharyngeal nerve that innervate the posterior third of the tongue; *modality,* general and special sensory.
ra′mi lingua′les ner′vi hypoglos′si [TA] lingual branches of hypoglossal nerve: branches of the hypoglossal nerve that innervate the intrinsic and extrinsic muscles of the tongue; *modality,* motor.
ra′mi lingua′les ner′vi lingua′lis [TA] lingual branches of lingual nerve: branches that innervate the anterior two-thirds of the tongue, adjacent areas of the mouth, and the gums; *modality,* general and special sensory.
r. lingula′ris ve′nae pulmona′lis sinis′trae superio′ris TA alternative for *vena lingularis.*
ra′mi lo′bi cauda′ti par′tis transver′sae ve′nae por′tae he′patis [TA] caudate branches of transverse part of hepatic portal vein: the branches of the left branch of the portal vein that drain the caudate lobe (pars posterior hepatis).
r. lo′bi me′dii ve′nae pulmona′lis dex′trae superio′ris TA alternative for *vena lobi medii.*
r. lumba′lis arte′riae iliolumba′lis [TA] lumbar branch of iliolumbar artery: a branch that arises from the iliolumbar artery in the iliac fossa and ascends to supply the psoas and quadratus lumborum muscles, sending a spinal branch through the intervertebral foramen just above the sacrum.
ra′mi malleola′res latera′les arte′riae fibula′ris [TA] lateral malleolar branches of peroneal artery: branches that supply the lateral aspect of the ankle and give off calcaneal branches to the lateral aspect and back of the heel.
ra′mi malleola′res media′les arte′riae tibia′les posterio′ris [TA] medial malleolar branches of posterior tibial artery: vessels supplying the area of the medial malleolus and giving off calcaneal branches to the medial aspect and back of the heel.
ra′mi mamma′rii latera′les arte′riae thora′cicae latera′lis [TA] lateral mammary branches of lateral thoracic artery: branches that supply the mammary gland.
ra′mi mamma′rii latera′les ra′mi cuta′nei latera′lis arte′riae intercosta′lis posterio′ris [TA] lateral mammary branches of lateral cutaneous branch of posterior intercostal artery: branches that arise from each of the third, fourth, and fifth posterior intercostal arteries to supply the pectoral muscles, skin, and mammary tissue.
ra′mi mamma′rii latera′les ra′mi cuta′nei latera′lis pectora′lis ner′vi intercosta′lis [TA] the lateral mammary branches of the lateral pectoral cutaneous branch of the intercostal nerve: *modality,* general sensory.
ra′mi mamma′rii media′les ra′mi cuta′nei anterio′ris pectora′lis ner′vi intercosta′lis [TA] the medial mammary branches of the anterior pectoral cutaneous branch of the intercostal nerve; *modality,* general sensory.
ra′mi mamma′rii media′les ra′mi perforan′tium arte′riae thora′cicae inter′nae [TA] medial mammary branches of perforating branch of internal thoracic artery: branches that arise from the second, third, and fourth perforating branches of the internal thoracic artery and help supply the mammary gland.
r. mandi′bulae [TA] ramus of mandible: a quadrilateral process projecting superiorly from the posterior part of either side of the mandible. Called also *r. of jaw.*
r. margina′lis dex′ter arte′riae corona′riae dex′trae [TA] right marginal branch of right coronary artery: a branch that passes toward the apex of the heart along the acute margin of the heart and ramifies over the right ventricle; called also *right marginal artery.* See illustration.
r. margina′lis mandibula′ris ner′vi facia′lis [TA] marginal mandibular branch of facial nerve: a branch of the facial nerve that runs forward from the front of the parotid gland along the border of the mandible, deep to the platysma and depressor anguli oris muscles, supplying the latter and the risorius, depressor labii inferioris, and mentalis muscles; *modality,* motor.
r. margina′lis sinis′ter ra′mi circumflex′i arte′riae corona′riae sinis′trae [TA] left marginal branch of circumflex branch of left coronary artery: a branch that follows the left margin of the heart and supplies the left ventricle. Called also *left marginal artery.*

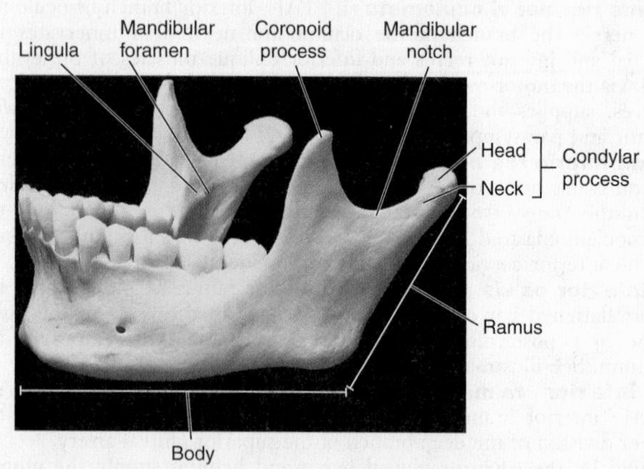

■ Ramus mandibulae (ramus of mandible), which together with the corpus mandibulae (body of the mandible) composes the mandible.

r. margina′lis sul′ci cin′guli [TA] marginal branch of cingulate sulcus: the posterior portion of the cingulate sulcus that turns off at a right angle and is directed toward the dorsal margin of the cerebral hemisphere, separating the precuneus and the paracentral lobule. Called also *sulcus marginalis* [TA alternative] and *marginal sulcus.*
r. margina′lis tento′rii arter′iae caro′tidis inter′nae [TA] tentorial marginal branch of internal carotid artery: a twig from the cavernous part of the internal carotid artery that supplies the margin of the tentorium.
ra′mi mastoi′dei arte′riae auricula′ris posterio′ris [TA] mastoid branches of posterior auricular artery: branches that supply the mastoid cells.
r. mastoi′deus arte′riae occipita′lis [TA] mastoid branch of occipital artery: a branch that enters the cranial cavity through the mastoid foramen and supplies the dura mater, diploe, and mastoid cells. Called also *mastoid artery.*
r. media′lis arte′riae superio′ris cerebel′li [TA] the medial branch of the superior cerebellar artery.
r. media′lis duc′tus hepa′tici sinis′tri [TA] the medial branch of the left hepatic duct, draining medial segments of the left liver.
r. media′lis ner′vi supraorbita′lis [TA] medial branch of supraorbital nerve: a nerve branch that supplies the frontal sinus, upper eyelid, and skin and subcutaneous tissue of the forehead and adjacent scalp as far back as the parietal bone; *modality,* general sensory.
ra′mi media′les pon′tis [TA] medial pontine branches: the shorter pontine arteries, which arise from the posterior aspect of the basilar artery and enter the pons along its anterior median groove. Called also *paramedian pontine branches.*
r. media′lis ra′mi posterio′ris ner′vi cervica′lis [TA] medial branch of posterior branch of cervical nerve: the medial branch that arises from the posterior branch of a cervical nerve and supplies muscle, periosteum, ligaments, and joints; all except the first and sometimes the sixth through eighth have an eventual cutaneous distribution.
r. media′lis ra′mi posterio′ris ner′vi lumba′lis [TA] medial branch of posterior branch of lumbar nerve: a branch of the posterior branch of each lumbar nerve, mainly innervating deep muscle but also helping supply ligaments, periosteum, and joints.
r. media′lis ra′mi posterio′ris ner′vi sacra′lis [TA] medial branch of posterior branch of sacral nerve: a branch arising from the posterior branch of one of the three upper sacral nerves and innervating the multifidus muscle.
r. media′lis ra′mi posterio′ris ner′vi thora′cici [TA] medial branch of posterior branch of thoracic nerve: one of the terminal divisions of the posterior branch of the thoracic nerve, supplying periosteum, ligaments, and joints. Those of the upper thoracic nerves supply the skin of the back, and those of the lower nerves supply primarily the erector spinae muscle.
ra′mi mediastina′les arte′riae thora′cicae inter′nae [TA] mediastinal branches of internal thoracic artery: branches that supply areolar tissue, pericardium, lymph nodes, and the thymus in the anterior and superior mediastina. Called also *anterior mediastinal arteries.*

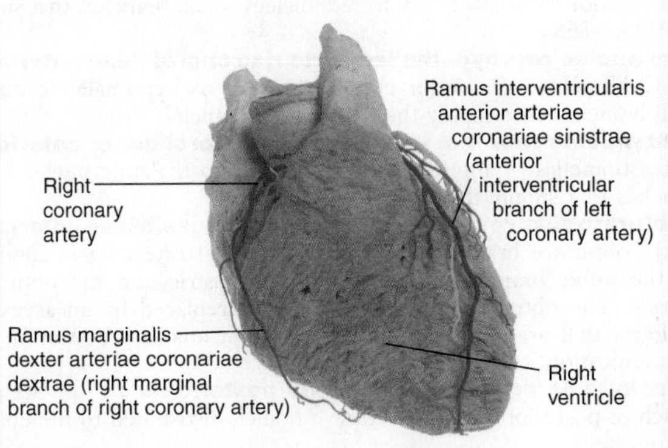

■ Anterior view of the heart showing several rami of the coronary arteries.

ra′mi mediastina′les par′tis thora′cicae aor′tae [TA] mediastinal branches of thoracic part of aorta: small vessels supplying connective tissue and lymph nodes in the posterior mediastinum.
ra′mi medulla′res latera′les arte′riae vertebra′lis [TA] lateral medullary branches of posterior inferior cerebellar artery: branches supplying the undersurface of the hemisphere of the cerebellum and anastomosing with the anterior inferior cerebellar and superior cerebellar branches of the basilar artery.
ra′mi medulla′res media′les arte′riae vertebra′lis [TA] medial medullary branches of posterior inferior cerebellar artery, ramifying on the cerebellar vermis between the hemispheres.
r. membra′nae tym′pani ner′vi auriculotempora′lis [TA] branch to tympanic membrane of auriculotemporal nerve: a branch given to the tympanic membrane by the nerve of the external acoustic meatus, a branch of the auriculotemporal nerve; *modality,* general sensory.
r. menin′geus ante′rior arte′riae ethmoida′lis anterio′ris [TA] anterior meningeal branch of anterior ethmoidal artery; a branch that supplies the dura mater. Called also *anterior meningeal artery.*
r. menin′geus arte′riae occipita′lis [TA] meningeal branch of occipital artery: one or more variable branches of the occipital artery that enter the posterior fossa and supply the dura mater.
ra′mi menin′gei arte′riae vertebra′lis [TA] meningeal branches of vertebral artery: branches, anterior and posterior, arising from the vertebral artery in the foramen magnum and ramifying in the posterior cranial fossa to supply the dura mater, including the falx cerebelli and bone.
r. menin′geus ner′vi mandibula′ris [TA] meningeal branch of mandibular nerve: a branch that arises from the trunk of the mandibular nerve, re-enters the cranium through the foramen spinosum, accompanies the middle meningeal artery to supply the dura mater, and also helps innervate the mucous membrane of the mastoid air cells. Called also *nervus spinosus* [TA alternative].
r. menin′geus ner′vi maxilla′ris [TA] meningeal branch of maxillary nerve: a branch arising from the maxillary nerve in the middle cranial fossa, accompanying the middle meningeal artery, and supplying the dura mater; *modality,* general sensory. Called also *meningeal nerve* and *nervus meningeus medius.*
r. menin′geus ner′vi spina′lis [TA] meningeal branch of spinal nerve: the small branch of each spinal nerve that re-enters the intervertebral foramen to supply the dura mater, vertebral column, and associated ligaments. Called also *r. recurrens nervi spinalis* [TA alternative].
r. menin′geus ner′vi va′gi [TA] meningeal branch of vagus nerve: a branch that arises in the jugular foramen from the superior ganglion of the vagus nerve, innervating dura mater of the posterior cranial fossa.
r. menin′geus par′tis caverno′sae arte′riae caro′tidis inter′nae [TA] meningeal branch of cavernous part of internal carotid artery: a twig from the cavernous part of the internal carotid artery that supplies the meninges of the anterior cranial fossa.
r. menin′geus par′tis cerebra′lis arte′riae caro′tidis inter′nae [TA] meningeal branch of cerebral part of internal carotid artery: a twig from the cerebral part of the internal carotid artery that supplies the meninges of the anterior cranial fossa.
r. menin′geus recur′rens arte′riae ophthal′micae [TA] recurrent meningeal branch of ophthalmic artery: a branch that passes back through the superior orbital fissure and anastomoses with a branch of the meningeal artery between the internal and external carotid arteries.
r. menin′geus recur′rens ner′vi ophthal′mici [TA] tentorial branch of ophthalmic nerve: a branch that arises from the ophthalmic nerve close to its origin from the trigeminal ganglion, turning back to innervate the dura mater of the tentorium cerebelli and falx cerebri; *modality,* general sensory. Called also *r. tentorius nervi ophthalmici* [TA alternative].
r. menta′lis arte′riae alveola′ris inferio′ris [TA] mental branch of inferior alveolar artery: a branch arising from the inferior alveolar artery in the mandibular canal, which leaves the canal at the mental foramen, supplies the chin, and anastomoses with its fellow of the opposite side and with the submental and inferior labial arteries. Called also *mental artery.*
ra′mi menta′les ner′vi menta′lis [TA] mental branches of mental nerve: branches that innervate the skin of the chin; *modality,* general sensory.
r. muscula′ris [TA] muscular branch: a branch of a peripheral nerve or vessel that supplies muscle.

Ramus *Continued*

ra′mi muscula′res arte′riae vertebra′lis [TA] muscular branches of vertebral artery: branches of the transverse part of the vertebral artery that supply the deep muscles of the neck and anastomose with the descending branch of the occipital artery and the deep cervical artery.

ra′mi muscula′res ner′vi axilla′ris [TA] muscular branches of axillary nerve: branches that innervate the deltoid and teres minor muscles; *modality*, motor.

ra′mi muscula′res ner′vi femora′lis [TA] muscular branches of femoral nerve: branches that innervate the anterior thigh muscles; *modality*, motor.

ra′mi muscula′res ner′vi fibula′ris profun′di [TA] muscular branches of deep peroneal nerve: branches that innervate the tibialis anterior, extensor hallucis longus, extensor digitorum longus, and peroneus tertius muscles; *modality*, motor.

ra′mi muscula′res ner′vi fibula′ris superficia′lis [TA] muscular branches of superficial peroneal nerve: branches that innervate the peroneus longus and peroneus brevis muscles; *modality*, motor.

ra′mi muscula′res nervo′rum intercosta′lium [TA] muscular branches of intercostal nerves: branches that supply numerous muscles of the lateral and ventral regions of the thorax and abdomen.

ra′mi muscula′res ner′vi media′ni [TA] muscular branches of median nerve: branches that innervate most of the flexor muscles on the front of the forearm and most of the short muscles of the thumb; *modality*, motor.

ra′mi muscula′res ner′vi musculocuta′nei [TA] muscular branches of musculocutaneous nerve: branches that innervate muscles of the upper arm; *modality*, motor and general sensory. See *branch to biceps brachii*, *branch to brachialis*, and *branch to coracobrachialis*, under *branch*.

ra′mi muscula′res ner′vi radia′lis [TA] muscular branches of radial nerve: branches that innervate the triceps, anconeus, brachioradialis, and extensor carpi radialis muscles; a branch to the brachialis muscle is probably sensory; *modality*, motor and sensory.

ra′mi muscula′res ner′vi tibia′lis [TA] muscular branches of tibial nerve: branches that supply muscles of the back of the leg; *modality*, motor.

ra′mi muscula′res ner′vi ulna′ris [TA] muscular branches of ulnar nerve: branches that innervate the flexor carpi ulnaris muscle and the ulnar half of the flexor digitorum profundus; *modality*, motor.

ra′mi muscula′res ra′mi anterio′ris ner′vi obturato′rii [TA] muscular branches of anterior branch of obturator nerve: branches arising from the anterior ramus of the obturator nerve and innervating the gracilis and adductor longus muscles, usually the adductor brevis, and often the pectineus; *modality*, motor.

ra′mi muscula′res ra′mi exter′ni ner′vi accesso′rii [TA] muscular branches of external branch of accessory nerve: the branches of the external branch of the accessory nerve that supply the sternocleidomastoid and trapezius muscles.

ra′mi muscula′res ra′mi posterio′ris ner′vi obturato′rii [TA] muscular branches of posterior branch of obturator nerve: branches arising from the posterior ramus of the obturator nerve and innervating the obturator externus and adductor brevis muscles, and sometimes the adductor magnus; *modality*, motor.

r. mus′culi stylopharyn′gei ner′vi glossopharyn′gei [TA] stylopharyngeal branch of glossopharyngeal nerve: a branch that supplies the stylopharyngeal muscle; *modality*, motor.

r. mylohyoi′deus arte′riae alveola′ris inferio′ris [TA] mylohyoid branch of inferior alveolar artery: a branch that descends with the mylohyoid nerve in the mylohyoid sulcus to supply the floor of the mouth.

ra′mi nasa′les anterio′res latera′les arte′riae ethmoida′lis anterio′ris [TA] anterior lateral nasal branches of anterior ethmoidal artery; twigs of the anterior ethmoidal artery that descend into the nasal cavity with the anterior ethmoidal nerve and supply the lateral nasal wall.

r. nasa′lis exter′nus ner′vi ethmoida′lis anterio′ris [TA] external nasal branch of anterior ethmoidal nerve: a branch that is essentially a continuation, or terminal branch, of the anterior ethmoidal nerve, innervating the skin of the dorsal part of the nose; *modality*, general sensory.

ra′mi nasa′les exter′ni ner′vi infraorbita′lis [TA] external nasal branches of infraorbital nerve: they innervate the skin of the side of the nose; *modality*, general sensory.

ra′mi nasa′les inter′ni latera′les ner′vi ethmoida′lis anterio′ris [TA] lateral internal nasal branches of anterior ethmoidal nerve: branches arising from the internal nasal branches of the anterior ethmoidal nerve and innervating the mucosa of the lateral wall of the nasal cavity; *modality*, general sensory.

ra′mi nasa′les inter′ni media′les ner′vi ethmoida′lis anterio′ris [TA] medial internal nasal branches of anterior ethmoidal nerve: branches arising from the internal nasal branches of the anterior ethmoidal nerve and supplying the nasal septum; *modality*, general sensory.

ra′mi nasa′les inter′ni ner′vi ethmoida′lis anterio′ris [TA] internal nasal branches of anterior ethmoidal nerve: the medial and lateral branches that innervate the nasal septum and the mucous membrane of the lateral wall of the nasal cavity; *modality*, general sensory.

ra′mi nasa′les inter′ni ner′vi infraorbita′lis [TA] internal nasal branches of infraorbital nerve: branches that innervate the mobile septum of the nose; *modality*, general sensory.

ra′mi nasa′les posterio′res inferio′res ner′vi palati′ni majo′ris [TA] inferior posterior nasal branches of greater palatine nerve: nerve branches of the maxillary nerve, usually branches of the greater palatine nerve, that supply the middle and inferior nasal meatus and inferior conchae; *modality*, general sensory.

ra′mi nasa′les posterio′res superio′res latera′les ner′vi maxilla′ris [TA] lateral superior posterior nasal branches of maxillary nerve: branches that supply the superior and middle nasal conchae and the posterior ethmoidal sinuses; *modality*, general sensory.

ra′mi nasa′les posterio′res superio′res media′les ner′vi maxilla′ris [TA] medial superior posterior nasal branches of maxillary nerve: nerve branches, usually branches of the nasopalatine nerve, that supply the nasal septum; *modality*, general sensory.

ra′mi nervo′rum arte′riae caro′tidis inter′nae [TA] twigs from the cavernous part of the internal carotid artery that supply the nerves of the walls of the cavernous and inferior petrosal sinuses.

r. ner′vi oculomoto′rii arte′riae communican′tis posterio′ris [TA] oculomotor nerve branch of posterior communicating artery: the branch that supplies the oculomotor nerve.

r. ner′vi oculomoto′rii ad gan′glii cilia′re TA alternative for *r. parasympathica ganglii ciliaris.*

r. no′di atrioventricula′ris arte′riae corona′riae dex′trae [TA] atrioventricular nodal branch of right coronary artery: a branch of the right coronary artery usually arising opposite the origin of the posterior interventricular artery and inserting into the atrioventricular node. Called also *atrioventricular nodal artery.*

r. no′di atrioventricula′ris ra′mi circumflex′i arte′riae corona′riae sinis′trae [TA] atrioventricular nodal branch of circumflex branch of left coronary artery: a branch of the left coronary artery occasionally found supplying the atrioventricular node.

r. no′di sinuatria′lis arte′riae corona′riae dex′trae [TA] sinoatrial nodal branch of right coronary artery: a branch of the right coronary artery that supplies the right atrium, encircles the base of the superior vena cava, and inserts into the sinoatrial node. Called also *nodal artery*, *sinoatrial* or *sinuatrial nodal artery*, and *sinus node artery.*

r. no′di sinuatria′lis ra′mi circumflex′i arte′riae corona′riae sinis′trae [TA] sinoatrial nodal branch of circumflex branch of left coronary artery: a branch of the left coronary artery occasionally found supplying the sinoatrial node.

ra′mi nu′clei ru′bri arte′riae choroi′deae anterio′ris [TA] branches of anterior choroidal artery to red nucleus: small branches that supply the red nucleus.

ra′mi nucleo′rum hypotha′lami arte′riae choroi′deae anterio′ris [TA] branches of anterior choroidal artery to hypothalamic nuclei: small branches that supply the hypothalamic nuclei.

ra′mi nucleo′rum tha′lami arte′riae choroi′deae anterio′ris [TA] branches of anterior choroidal artery to thalamic nuclei: small branches that supply the thalamic nuclei.

r. obturato′rius ra′mi pu′bici arte′riae epigas′tricae inferio′ris [TA] obturator branch of inferior epigastric artery: a vessel connecting the pubic branches of the inferior epigastric and the obturator arteries. The obturator artery is sometimes replaced by an accessory obturator that arises from the inferior epigastric artery by way of this communication.

r. occipita′lis arte′riae auricula′ris posterio′ris [TA] occipital branch of posterior auricular artery: a branch distributed to the epicranial muscle.

ra′mi occipita′les arte′riae occipita′lis [TA] occipital branches of occipital artery: a medial and a lateral branch of the occipital artery, distributed to the scalp and, through the meningeal branch, to the dura mater.

r. occipita′lis ner′vi auricula′ris posterio′ris [TA] occipital branch of posterior auricular nerve: a branch supplying the occipital belly of the occipitofrontalis muscle; *modality,* motor.

r. occipitotempora′lis arte′riae occipita′lis media′lis [TA] occipitotemporal branch of medial occipital artery: a branch that supplies the occipital and temporal areas of the cerebral cortex.

ra′mi oesophagea′les arte′riae gas′tricae sinis′trae [TA] esophageal branches of left gastric artery: branches that supply the esophagus; called also *inferior esophageal arteries.* Spelled also *rami esophageales arteriae gastricae sinistrae.*

ra′mi oesophagea′les arte′riae thyroi′deae inferio′ris [TA] esophageal branches of inferior thyroid artery: branches that supply the esophagus; spelled also *rami esophageales arteriae thyroideae inferioris.*

ra′mi oesophagea′les ganglio′rum thora′cicorum [TA] esophageal branches of thoracic ganglia: sympathetic nerve branches from the thoracic ganglia, helping to innervate the thoracic and abdominal esophagus. Spelled also *rami esophageales gangliorum thoracicorum.*

ra′mi oesophagea′les par′tis thora′cicae aor′tae [TA] esophageal branches of thoracic part of aorta: branches, usually two, that arise from the front of the aorta to supply the esophagus; spelled also *rami esophageales partis thoracicae aortae.*

ra′mi oesopha′gei ner′vi laryn′gei recurren′tis [TA] esophageal branches of recurrent laryngeal nerve: branches that help innervate the esophagus; *modality,* visceral afferent and general sensory; spelled also *rami esophagei nervi laryngei recurrentis.*

ra′mi omenta′les arte′riae gastroomenta′lis dex′trae [TA] omental branches of right gastro-omental artery: branches that supply the greater omentum.

ra′mi omenta′les arte′riae gastroomenta′lis sinis′trae [TA] omental branches of left gastro-omental artery; branches that supply the stomach and greater omentum.

r. orbita′lis arte′riae menin′geae me′diae [TA] the orbital branch of the middle meningeal artery.

ra′mi orbita′les ner′vi maxilla′ris [TA] orbital branches of pterygopalatine ganglion: branches passing from the pterygopalatine ganglion through the inferior orbital fissure to supply the orbital periosteum and the ethmoidal and sphenoidal sinuses; *modality,* general sensory and parasympathetic.

r. os′sis is′chii [TA] ramus of ischium: the flattened bar of bone that projects from the inferior end of the body of the ischium in an anterosuperomedial direction to meet the inferior ramus of the pubis. It forms part of the border of the obturator foramen. See illustration.

r. ova′ricus arte′riae uteri′nae [TA] ovarian branch of uterine artery: the terminal branch of the uterine artery, which supplies the ovary and anastomoses with the ovarian artery.

r. palma′ris ner′vi media′ni [TA] palmar branch of median nerve: a branch arising from the median nerve in the lower part of the forearm and supplying the skin of the central palm and of the thenar eminence; *modality,* general sensory.

r. palma′ris ner′vi ulna′ris [TA] palmar branch of ulnar nerve: a branch arising from the ulnar nerve in the lower part of the forearm, supplying the cutaneous structures of the medial part of the palm; *modality,* general sensory.

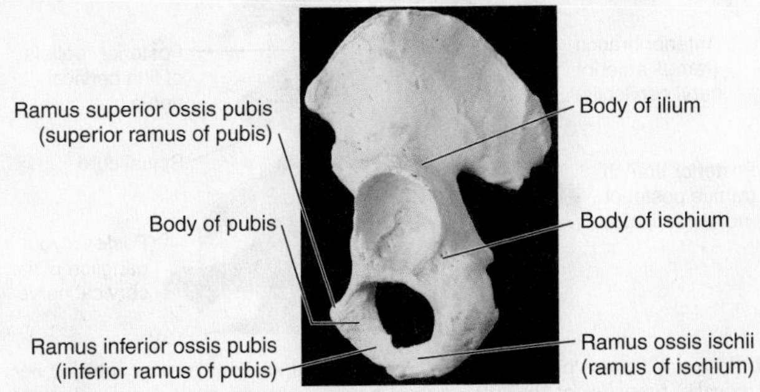

■ Lateral surface of left hip bone, showing the ramus ossis ischii, ramus superior ossis pubis, and ramus inferior ossis pubis.

r. palma′ris profun′dus arte′riae ulna′ris [TA] deep palmar branch of ulnar artery: a branch that accompanies the deep palmar branch of the ulnar nerve and joins the radial artery to form the deep palmar arch.

r. palma′ris superficia′lis arte′riae radia′lis [TA] superficial palmar branch of radial artery: a branch arising from the radial artery in the lower part of the forearm and supplying the thenar eminence.

ra′mi palpebra′les inferio′res ner′vi infraorbita′lis [TA] inferior palpebral branches of infraorbital nerve: branches that supply the skin and conjunctiva of the lower eyelid; *modality,* general sensory.

ra′mi palpebra′les ner′vi infratrochlea′ris [TA] palpebral branches of infratrochlear nerve: branches that help supply the eyelids; *modality,* general sensory.

ra′mi pancrea′tici arte′riae pancreaticoduodena′lis superio′ris anterio′ris [TA] pancreatic branches of the anterior superior pancreaticoduodenal artery: vessels that supply the pancreas.

ra′mi pancrea′tici arte′riae pancreaticoduodena′lis superio′ris posterio′ris [TA] pancreatic branches of posterior superior pancreaticoduodenal artery: vessels that supply the pancreas.

ra′mi pancrea′tici arte′riae sple′nicae [TA] pancreatic branches of splenic artery: branches that supply the pancreas, arising from the splenic artery during its tortuous course along the superior border of the body of the pancreas.

ra′mi paracentra′les arte′riae callosomargina′lis [TA] paracentral branches of callosomarginal artery: branches arising from the postcommunicating part of the anterior cerebral artery and supplying the cerebral cortex and medial central sulcus. Called also *paracentral artery.*

r. parieta′lis arte′riae menin′geae me′diae [TA] parietal branch of middle meningeal artery: a vessel that arises in the middle cranial fossa, grooves the temporal and parietal bones, and supplies the posterior dura mater.

r. parieta′lis arte′riae occipita′lis media′lis [TA] parietal branch of medial occipital artery: the branch of the medial occipital artery that supplies the parietal lobe.

r. parieta′lis arte′riae tempora′lis superficia′lis [TA] parietal branch of superficial temporal artery: the posterior terminal branch of the superficial temporal artery, supplying the scalp in the parietal region.

ra′mi parietooccipita′les arte′riae pericallo′sae [TA] parietooccipital branches of anterior cerebral artery: branches arising from the postcommunicating part of the anterior cerebral artery and supplying the parietal lobe and sometimes the occipital lobe.

r. parietooccipita′lis arte′riae occipita′lis media′lis [TA] parietooccipital branch of medial occipital artery: a vessel that supplies the cortex of the medial surface of the hemisphere up to the area of the parietooccipital sulcus.

r. paroti′deus arte′riae auricula′ris posterio′ris [TA] parotid branch of the posterior auricular artery: a branch supplying the parotid gland.

r. paroti′deus arte′riae tempora′lis superficia′lis [TA] parotid branch of superficial temporal artery: a branch supplying the parotid gland and the temporomandibular joint.

ra′mi paroti′dei ner′vi auriculotempora′lis [TA] parotid branches of auriculotemporal nerve: branches that bear postganglionic fibers from the otic ganglion to the parotid gland; *modality,* parasympathetic.

ra′mi paroti′dei ve′nae facia′lis parotid branches of facial vein: TA alternative for the parotid veins opening into the facial vein; see *venae parotideae.*

ra′mi par′tis retrolentifor′mis cap′sulae inter′nae arte′riae choroi′deae anterio′ris [TA] branches of anterior choroidal artery to retrolentiform limb of internal capsule: small branches that supply the retrolentiform limb of the internal capsule of the cerebrum.

ra′mi pectora′les arte′riae thoracoacromia′lis [TA] pectoral branches of thoracoacromial artery: branches that descend between the pectoralis major and minor muscles, supplying these muscles and the mammary gland.

ra′mi peduncula′res arte′riae ce′rebri poste′rioris [TA] peduncular branches of posterior cerebral artery: branches that supply the cerebral peduncles.

ra′mi perforan′tes ar′cus palma′ris profun′dus [TA] perforating branches of deep palmar arch: vessels connecting the palmar metacarpal arteries and deep palmar arch with the dorsal metacarpal arteries, between the bases of the metacarpal bones and in the interosseous spaces.

r. per′forans arte′riae fibula′ris [TA] perforating branch of peroneal artery: a branch passing forward from the peroneal artery where the interosseous membrane and the tibiofibular syndesmosis are continuous and descending to supply the syndesmosis and the ankle joint.

ra′mi perforan′tes arteria′rum metatarsea′rum planta′rium [TA] perforating branches of plantar metatarsal arteries: vessels connecting the plantar metatarsal arteries with the dorsal metatarsal arteries through the interosseous spaces.

ra′mi perforan′tes arte′riae thora′cicae inter′nae [TA] perforating branches of internal thoracic artery: six branches, one in each of the upper six intercostal spaces, supplying the pectoralis major muscle and adjacent skin; the second, third, and fourth branches give off mammary branches.

r. pericardi′acus ner′vi phre′nici [TA] pericardiac branch of phrenic nerve: a branch arising from the phrenic or accessory phrenic nerve and supplying the pericardium; *modality*, general sensory.

ra′mi pericardi′aci par′tis thora′cicae aor′tae [TA] pericardial branches of thoracic part of aorta: small branches from the aorta distributed to the surface of the pericardium.

ra′mi peridenta′les arte′riae alveola′ris inferio′ris [TA] peridental branches of inferior alveolar artery: branches arising from the inferior alveolar artery in the mandibular canal and supplying the roots and pulp of the teeth.

ra′mi peridenta′les arteria′rum alveola′rum superio′rum anterio′rum [TA] peridental branches of anterior superior alveolar arteries: branches supplying the gingivae of the upper teeth.

ra′mi peridenta′les arte′riae alveola′ris superio′ris posterio′ris [TA] peridental branches of posterior superior alveolar artery: branches arising from the posterior superior alveolar artery and supplying the maxillary gingivae.

ra′mi perinea′les ner′vi cuta′nei fe′moris posterio′ris [TA] perineal branches of posterior femoral cutaneous nerve: branches arising from the posterior femoral cutaneous nerve at the lower margin of the gluteus maximus muscle and innervating the skin of the external genitalia; *modality*, general sensory.

r. petro′sus arte′riae menin′geae me′diae [TA] petrosal branch of middle meningeal artery: a branch that arises in the region of the petrous part of the temporal bone, entering the hiatus for the greater petrosal nerve and anastomosing with the stylomastoid artery.

ra′mi pharyngea′les arte′riae pharyn′geae ascenden′tis [TA] pharyngeal branches of ascending pharyngeal artery: irregular vessels supplying the pharynx.

ra′mi pharyngea′les arte′riae thyroi′deae inferio′ris [TA] pharyngeal branches of inferior thyroid artery: vessels that supply the pharynx.

r. pharyn′geus arte′riae cana′lis pterygoi′dei [TA] pharyngeal branch of artery of pterygoid canal: a branch lying medial to the pterygopalatine ganglion.

ra′mi pharyn′gei ner′vi glossopharyn′gei [TA] pharyngeal branches of glossopharyngeal nerve: branches innervating the mucous membrane of the oropharynx, with a general sensory modality.

ra′mi pharyn′gei ner′vi laryn′gei recurren′tis [TA] pharyngeal branches of recurrent laryngeal nerve: small nerve branches that innervate the inferior constrictor muscle of the pharynx.

r. pharyn′geus ner′vi va′gi [TA] pharyngeal branch of vagus nerve: any of several branches that innervate the pharyngeal muscles and mucosa and have motor and general sensory modalities.

ra′mi phrenicoabdomina′les ner′vi phre′nici [TA] phrenicoabdominal branches of phrenic nerve: branches of the phrenic or accessory phrenic nerve that supply the diaphragm; *modality*, general sensory and motor.

r. postcentra′lis ra′mi dorsa′lis arte′riae intercosta′lis posterio′ris [TA] postcentral branch of dorsal branch of posterior intercostal artery: one of the spinal branches of the dorsal branch of a posterior intercostal artery; it is the branch that tracks behind the vertebral body.

r. poste′rior arte′riae obturato′riae [TA] posterior branch of obturator artery: a branch passing backward around the lateral margin of the obturator foramen, on the obturator membrane, supplying muscles around the ischial tuberosity and giving off an acetabular branch.

r. poste′rior arte′riae pancreaticoduodena′lis inferio′ris [TA] posterior branch of inferior pancreaticoduodenal artery: a branch that ascends behind the head of the pancreas, which it sometimes pierces, and anastomoses with the posterior superior pancreaticoduodenal artery; it supplies the head of the pancreas and adjoining parts of the duodenum.

r. poste′rior arte′riae recurren′tis ulna′ris [TA] posterior branch of ulnar recurrent artery: a branch running to the back of the medial epicondyle, supplying the elbow joint and neighboring muscles.

r. poste′rior arte′riae rena′lis [TA] posterior branch of renal artery: a branch supplying the posterior segment of the kidney.

r. poste′rior duc′tus hepa′tici dex′tri [TA] the posterior branch of the right hepatic duct, draining posterior segments of the right liver.

r. poste′rior ner′vi auricula′ris mag′ni [TA] posterior branch of great auricular nerve: a branch, formed by division of the great auricular nerve, that innervates the skin over the mastoid process and the back of the external ear; *modality*, general sensory.

ra′mi posterio′res nervo′rum cervica′lium [TA] posterior branches of cervical nerves: branches of the eight cervical spinal nerves, further subdividing into lateral and medial branches (see *r. lateralis rami posterior nervi cervicalis* and *r. medialis rami posterior nervi cervicalis*). See illustration at *ramus posterior nervi spinalis.* Called also *rami dorsales nervorum cervicalium* [TA alternative].

r. poste′rior ner′vi coccy′gei [TA] posterior branch of coccygeal nerve: a branch of the last spinal nerve, helping to innervate the skin over the coccyx. Called also *r. dorsalis nervi coccygei* [TA alternative].

r. poste′rior ner′vi cuta′nei antebra′chii media′lis [TA] posterior branch of medial antebrachial cutaneous nerve: a branch that innervates the skin of the posteromedial and medial aspects of the forearm; *modality*, general sensory.

ra′mi posterio′res nervo′rum lumba′lium [TA] posterior branches of the five lumbar spinal nerves; they subdivide into lateral and medial branches (see *r. lateralis rami posterioris nervi lumbalis* and *r. medialis rami posterioris nervi lumbalis*). Called also *rami dorsales nervorum lumbalium* [TA alternative].

r. poste′rior ner′vi obturato′rii [TA] posterior branch of obturator nerve: a branch that descends to innervate the knee joint, giving muscular branches to the obturator externus, adductor magnus, and sometimes the adductor brevis muscle; *modality*, general sensory and motor.

ra′mi posterio′res nervo′rum sacra′lium [TA] posterior branches of sacral nerves: branches of the five sacral spinal nerves, emerging from the sacrum through the posterior foramina; they subdivide into medial and lateral branches (see *r. medialis rami posterioris nervi sacralis* and *r. lateralis rami posterioris nervi sacralis*). Called also *rami dorsales nervorum sacralium* [TA alternative].

r. poste′rior ner′vi spina′lis [TA] posterior branch of spinal nerve: the posterior and usually smaller of the two branches into which each spinal nerve divides almost as soon as it emerges from the intervertebral foramen; the posterior branches supply the skin, muscles, joints, and bone of the posterior part of the neck and trunk. Most of these branches further subdivide into a medial and a lateral portion.

ra′mi posterio′res nervo′rum thoracico′rum [TA] posterior branches of thoracic nerves: branches of the twelve thoracic spinal nerves; they subdivide into lateral and medial and posterior cutaneous branches; see *r. lateralis rami posterioris nervi thoracici*, *r. medialis rami posterioris nervi thoracici*, and *r. cutaneus posterior rami posterioris*

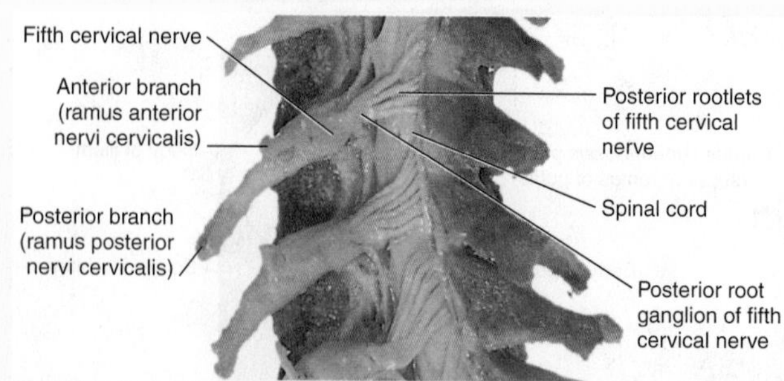

■ Posterior (ramus posterior nervi cervicalis) and anterior (ramus anterior nervi cervicalis) branches of the fifth cervical nerve, the nerve itself forming from the union of ventral and dorsal nerve roots, just distal to the ganglion on the dorsal root, within the intervertebral foramen.

nervi thoracici. Called also *rami dorsales nervorum thoracicorum* [TA alternative].

r. poste′rior sul′ci latera′lis ce′rebri [TA] posterior branch of lateral cerebral sulcus: the part of the lateral cerebral sulcus that runs obliquely posteriorly between the temporal and the parietal lobes.

r. poste′rior ve′nae pulmona′lis dex′trae superio′ris TA alternative for *vena posterior lobi superioris pulmonis dextri.*

r. poste′rior ventri′culi sinis′tri ra′mi circumflex′i arte′riae corona′riae sinis′trae [TA] posterior left ventricular branch of circumflex branch of left coronary artery: an interventricular continuation of the circumflex branch; there may be two or three vessels.

r. posterolatera′lis dex′ter arte′riae corona′riae dex′trae [TA] an inconstant branch of the right coronary artery.

ra′mi precunea′les arte′riae pericallo′sae [TA] precuneal branches of pericallosal artery: vessels originating in the postcommunicating part of the anterior cerebral artery and supplying the inferior precuneus. Called also *precuneal arteries.*

r. prelamina′ris ra′mi dorsa′lis arte′riae intercosta′lis posterio′ris [TA] prelaminar branch of dorsal branch of posterior intercostal artery: one of the spinal branches of the dorsal branch of a posterior intercostal artery; it is the branch that tracks in front of the lamina of the vertebral arch.

r. profun′dus arte′riae circumflex′ae fe′moris media′lis [TA] deep branch of medial circumflex femoral artery: a branch ascending toward the trochanteric fossa, and anastomosing with gluteal branches.

r. profun′dus arte′riae glu′teae superio′ris [TA] deep branch of superior gluteal artery: a branch passing forward between the gluteus medius and minimus muscles, and dividing into superior and inferior branches.

r. profun′dus arte′riae planta′ris media′lis [TA] deep branch of medial plantar artery: a branch that supplies the anteromedial aspect of the sole, anastomosing with the medial three plantar metatarsal arteries.

r. profun′dus arte′riae transver′sae col′li [TA] official terminology for the dorsal scapular artery when it is the deep branch of the transverse cervical artery; see *arteria dorsalis scapulae.*

r. profun′dus ner′vi planta′ris latera′lis [TA] deep branch of lateral plantar nerve: a branch that accompanies the lateral plantar artery on its medial side and the plantar arch, innervating the interossei, the second, third, and fourth lumbrical, and the adductor hallucis muscles, and some articulations; *modality,* general sensory.

r. profun′dus ner′vi radia′lis [TA] deep branch of radial nerve: a branch arising from the radial nerve and winding laterally around the radius to the back of the forearm, supplying the supinator, extensor digitorum, extensor digiti minimi, and extensor carpi ulnaris muscles, and often the extensor carpi radialis brevis muscle. Its continuation, the posterior interosseous nerve, supplies distal forearm muscles and the carpal and intercarpal joints; *modality,* motor.

r. profun′dus ner′vi ulna′ris [TA] deep branch of ulnar nerve: the deep branch that is accompanied by the deep palmar branch of the ulnar artery, rounds the hook of the hamate bone, and follows the deep palmar arch beneath the flexor tendons, supplying the wrist joint, the interossei, third and fourth lumbrical, and adductor pollicis muscles, and usually the deep head of the flexor pollicis brevis muscle; *modality,* general sensory and motor.

ra′mi prosta′tici arte′riae vesica′lis inferio′ris [TA] prostatic branches of inferior vesical artery: branches that supply the prostate and communicate with corresponding vessels on the opposite side.

ra′mi proxima′les latera′les stria′ti arteria′rum centra′lium anterolatera′lium [TA] proximal lateral striate branches of anterolateral central arteries: branches supplied by the middle cerebral artery, supplying the basal nuclei of the brain and its internal capsule.

ra′mi pterygoi′dei arte′riae maxilla′ris [TA] pterygoid branches of maxillary artery: branches that supply the pterygoid muscles.

pubic r., inferior r. inferior ossis pubis.

pubic r., superior r. superior ossis pubis.

r. pu′bicus arte′riae epigas′tricae inferio′ris [TA] pubic branch of inferior epigastric artery: a branch that arises from the inferior epigastric artery near the deep inguinal ring and descends on the back of the pubis, anastomosing through an obturator branch with the pubic branch of the obturator artery.

r. pu′bicus arte′riae obturato′riae [TA] pubic branch of obturator artery: a branch that ascends on the pelvic surface of the ilium, anastomosing with its fellow of the other side and with the pubic branch of the inferior epigastric artery.

r. pu′bicus ve′nae epigas′tricae inferio′ris TA alternative for *vena pubica.*

r. of pubis see *r. inferior ossis pubis* and *r. superior ossis pubis.*

r. of pubis, ascending r. superior ossis pubis.

r. of pubis, descending r. inferior ossis pubis.

ra′mi pulmona′les plex′us pulmona′lis [TA] pulmonary branches of pulmonary plexus: branches of the anterior and posterior pulmonary plexuses that accompany the blood vessels and bronchi into the lungs; *modality,* sympathetic and visceral afferent.

ra′mi pulmona′les thora′cici ganglio′rum thoracico′rum [TA] pulmonary thoracic branches of thoracic ganglia: branches from the second to the fourth, fifth, or sixth thoracic ganglia to the posterior pulmonary plexus, sometimes going on to follow intercostal arteries to the hilum of the lung.

ra′mi radicula′res arte′riae vertebra′lis [TA] radicular branches of vertebral artery: one type of spinal branch of the cervical part of the vertebral artery; the radicular branches enter the vertebral foramina and follow and supply the roots of individual spinal nerves.

r. recur′rens ner′vi spina′lis TA alternative for *r. meningeus nervi spinalis.*

r. rena′lis ner′vi splanch′nici mino′ris [TA] renal branch of lesser splanchnic nerve: a branch from the lesser splanchnic nerve to the aorticorenal ganglion; *modality,* sympathetic preganglionic fibers and visceral afferent.

ra′mi rena′les ner′vi va′gi [TA], **ra′mi rena′les plex′us coeli′aci** renal branches of vagus nerve: branches passing from the vagal trunks via the celiac plexus to the kidney; *modality,* parasympathetic and visceral afferent.

ra′mi sacra′les latera′les arte′riae sacra′lis media′nae [TA] lateral sacral branches of median sacral artery: branches that anastomose with the lateral sacral arteries laterally.

r. saphe′nus arte′riae descenden′tis ge′nus [TA] saphenous branch of descending genicular artery: a vessel that accompanies the saphenous nerve between the sartorius and gracilis muscles on the medial side of the knee, supplying the skin and anastomosing with the medial inferior genicular artery.

ra′mi scrota′les anterio′res arte′riae puden′dae exter′nae profun′dae [TA] anterior scrotal branches of deep external pudendal artery: branches arising from the deep external pudendal artery and supplying the anterior scrotal region in the male; called also *anterior scrotal arteries.*

ra′mi scrota′les posterio′res arte′riae puden′dae inter′nae [TA] posterior scrotal branches of internal pudendal artery; two branches arising from the internal pudendal artery in the anterior part of the ischiorectal fossa, helping to supply the ischiocavernosus and bulbospongiosus muscles, and distributed to the scrotum. Called also *posterior scrotal arteries.*

ra′mi septa′les anterio′res arte′riae ethmoida′lis anterio′ris [TA] anterior septal branches of anterior ethmoidal artery; twigs of the anterior ethmoidal artery that descend into the nasal cavity with the anterior ethmoidal nerve and supply the nasal septum.

ra′mi septa′les posterio′res arte′riae sphenopalati′nae [TA] posterior septal branches of sphenopalatine artery: branches that anastomose with the ethmoidal arteries.

r. sep′ti na′si arte′riae labia′lis superio′ris [TA] nasal septum branch of superior labial artery: a branch that ramifies on the lower and front part of the nasal septum.

r. sinis′ter arte′riae hepa′ticae pro′priae [TA] left branch of hepatic artery proper: a branch that supplies the left liver.

r. sinis′ter ve′nae por′tae he′patis [TA] left branch of hepatic portal vein: a branch distributed to the left liver.

r. si′nus caro′tici ner′vi glossopharyn′gei [TA] branch of glossopharyngeal nerve to carotid sinus: a branch that supplies the pressoreceptors and chemoreceptors of the carotid sinus and carotid body with visceral afferent fibers.

r. si′nus caverno′si arte′riae caro′tidis inter′nae [TA] a twig from the cavernous part of the internal carotid artery that supplies the walls of the cavernous sinus.

ra′mi spina′les arte′riae cervica′lis ascenden′tis [TA] spinal branches of ascending cervical artery: branches that help supply the vertebral canal.
r. spina′lis arte′riae iliolumba′lis [TA] spinal branch of iliolumbar artery; a branch that passes through the intervertebral foramen between the fifth lumbar vertebra and the sacrum to help supply the contents of the vertebral canal.
r. spina′lis arte′riae intercosta′lis posterio′ris pri′mae [TA] spinal branch of first posterior intercostal artery: a vessel arising from the dorsal branch of the first posterior intercostal artery, entering the intervertebral foramen to help supply the contents of the vertebral canal.
r. spina′lis arte′riae intercosta′lis posterio′ris secun′dae [TA] spinal branch of second posterior intercostal artery: a vessel arising from the dorsal branch of the second posterior intercostal artery, entering the intervertebral foramen to help supply the contents of the vertebral canal.
r. spina′lis arte′riae lumba′lis [TA] spinal branch of lumbar artery: a branch arising from the dorsal branch of a lumbar artery and entering an intervertebral foramen with the spinal nerve to help supply the contents of the vertebral canal.
r. spina′lis arte′riae sacra′lis latera′lis [TA] spinal branch of lateral sacral artery: a vessel arising from a lateral sacral artery and entering the pelvic sacral foramen to help supply the contents of the vertebral canal.
r. spina′lis arte′riae subcosta′lis [TA] spinal branch of subcostal artery: a spinal branch corresponding to those arising from the dorsal branches of the posterior intercostal arteries; it enters the vertebral canal to help supply the contents of the canal.
ra′mi spina′les arte′riae vertebra′lis [TA] spinal branches of vertebral artery: branches of the cervical part of the vertebral artery; they supply the spinal cord and its meninges, the vertebral bodies, and the intervertebral disks.
ra′mi spina′les ra′mi dorsa′lis arte′riae intercosta′lis posterio′ris [TA] spinal branches of dorsal branch of posterior intercostal artery: branches that arise from the dorsal branch of each posterior intercostal artery and enter the vertebral canal through the vertebral foramen to supply the vertebrae, spinal cord, and meninges. They may arise as a single spinal branch, enter the foramen, and then divide into individual spinal branches, or may arise from the dorsal branch as a number of independent spinal branches.
r. spina′lis ve′nae intercosta′lis posterio′ris TA alternative for *vena spinalis venae intercostalis posterioris.*
ra′mi sple′nici arte′riae sple′nicae [TA] splenic branches of splenic artery: the terminal branches of the splenic artery, which follow the trabeculae; called also *rami lienales arteriae lienalis* [TA alternative].
r. stape′dius arte′riae auricula′ris posterio′ris [TA] stapedial branch of posterior auricular artery: a variable branch supplying the stapedius muscle and tendon.
ra′mi sterna′les arte′riae thora′cicae inter′nae [TA] sternal branches of internal thoracic artery: branches that supply the sternum and the transversus thoracis muscle.
ra′mi sternocleidomastoi′dei arte′riae occipita′lis [TA] sternocleidomastoid branches of occipital artery: branches of the occipital artery, usually an upper and a lower, that supply the sternocleidomastoid and adjacent muscles. Called also *sternocleidomastoid arteries.*
r. sternocleidomastoi′deus arte′riae thyroi′deae superio′ris [TA] sternocleidomastoid branch of superior thyroid artery: a branch that arises from the superior thyroid artery, but sometimes directly from the external carotid artery, passing across the carotid sheath to supply the middle portion of the sternocleidomastoid muscle.
r. stylohyoi′deus ner′vi facia′lis [TA] stylohyoid branch of facial nerve: a branch that arises from the facial nerve just below the base of the skull to innervate the stylohyoid muscle; *modality,* motor.
ra′mi subendocardia′les [TA] subendocardial branches: small ramifications of the conducting system of the heart (Purkinje fibers), which form a plexus in the papillary muscles and ventricles. Called also *Purkinje network* and *subendocardial terminal network.*
ra′mi subscapula′res arte′riae axilla′ris [TA] subscapular branches of axillary artery: branches that supply the subscapularis muscle.
ra′mi substan′tiae ni′grae arte′riae choroi′deae anterio′ris [TA] branches of anterior choroidal artery to substantia nigra: small branches that supply the substantia nigra.
ra′mi substan′tiae perfora′tae anterio′ris arte′riae choroi′deae anterio′ris [TA] branches to anterior perforated substance: small branches of the anterior choroidal artery that supply the anterior perforated substance.
r. superficia′lis arte′riae circumflex′ae fe′moris media′lis [TA] superficial branch of medial circumflex femoral artery: a branch passing between the quadratus femoris and the proximal border of the adductor magnus and anastomosing with the inferior gluteal, lateral circumflex femoral, and first perforating arteries.
r. superficia′lis arte′riae glu′teae superio′ris [TA] superficial branch of superior gluteal artery: a branch that ramifies to supply the gluteus maximus muscle.
r. superficia′lis arte′riae planta′ris media′lis [TA] superficial branch of medial plantar artery: a branch that supplies the medial side of the great toe.
r. superficia′lis arte′riae transver′sae col′li [TA] superficial branch of transverse cervical artery: a branch that arises from the transverse cervical artery at the anterior border of the levator scapulae muscle; it has ascending and descending branches that supply the levator scapulae, trapezius, and splenius muscles.
r. superficia′lis ner′vi planta′ris latera′lis [TA] superficial branch of lateral plantar nerve: a branch that arises from the lateral plantar nerve at the lateral border of the quadratus plantae muscle and passes forward, dividing into a lateral part that innervates skin of the lateral side of the sole and little toe, joints of the toe, and the flexor digiti minimi brevis muscle, and a medial part, a common plantar digital nerve, that gives two proper plantar digital nerves to the adjacent sides of the fourth and fifth toes; *modality,* general sensory.
r. superficia′lis ner′vi radia′lis [TA] superficial branch of radial nerve: the continuation of the radial nerve that accompanies the radial artery in the forearm, winds dorsalward, supplies the lateral side of the back of the hand, and divides into dorsal digital nerves that supply the skin of the dorsal surface and adjacent surfaces of the thumb, index, and middle fingers, and sometimes the radial side of the ring finger; *modality,* general sensory.
r. superficia′lis ner′vi ulna′ris [TA] superficial branch of ulnar nerve: the branch of the ulnar nerve in the hand that supplies the palmaris brevis muscle and divides into a proper palmar digital nerve for the medial side of the little finger, a common palmar digital nerve giving off two proper nerves to supply adjacent sides of the little and fourth fingers, and sometimes palmar digital nerves also for the adjacent sides of the third and fourth fingers; *modality,* general sensory and motor.
r. supe′rior ner′vi oculomoto′rii [TA] superior branch of oculomotor nerve: the upper and smaller of the two branches of the oculomotor nerve, which supplies the superior rectus muscle and, terminally, the levator palpebrae superioris; *modality,* motor.
ra′mi superio′res ner′vi transver′si col′li [TA] superior branches of transverse cervical nerve: the upper of the branches that arise from the transverse cervical nerve near the anterior border of the sternocleidomastoid muscle, innervating skin and subcutaneous tissue in the anterior cervical region; *modality,* general sensory.
r. supe′rior os′sis pu′bis [TA] superior ramus of pubic bone: the bar of bone projecting from the body of the pubic bone in a posterosuperolateral direction to the iliopubic eminence and forming part of the acetabulum. See illustration at *ramus ossis ischii.* Called also *superior pubic r.*
r. supe′rior ra′mi profun′di arte′riae glu′teae superio′ris [TA] superior branch of deep branch of superior gluteal artery: the upper division of the deep branch of the superior gluteal artery, extending as far as the anterior superior iliac spine and helping supply the gluteus medius, gluteus minimus, and tensor fasciae latae muscles.
r. supe′rior ve′nae pulmona′lis dex′trae inferio′ris TA alternative for *vena superior lobi inferioris pulmonis dextri.*
r. supe′rior ve′nae pulmona′lis sinis′trae inferio′ris TA alternative for *vena superior lobi inferioris pulmonis sinistri.*
r. suprahyoi′deus arte′riae lingua′lis [TA] suprahyoid branch of lingual artery: a branch passing along the upper border of the hyoid bone, supplying suprahyoid muscles and anastomosing with its fellow of the other side.

Ramus *Continued*

r. tempora'lis ante'rior arte'riae ce'rebri me'diae [TA] anterior temporal branch of middle cerebral artery: a branch arising from the inferior terminal branch of the middle cerebral artery and supplying the lateral surface of the anterior temporal lobe. Called also *anterior temporal artery.*

ra'mi tempora'les anterio'res arte'riae occipita'lis latera'lis [TA] anterior temporal branches of lateral occipital artery: branches that supply the cortex of the anterior part of the temporal lobe.

ra'mi tempora'les interme'dii arte'riae occipita'lis latera'lis [TA] intermediate temporal branches of lateral occipital artery: branches that supply the cortex of the middle part of the temporal lobe. Called also *rami temporales medii arteriae occipitalis lateralis* [TA alternative].

ra'mi tempora'les me'dii arte'riae occipita'lis latera'lis TA alternative for *rami temporales intermedii arteriae occipitalis lateralis.*

r. tempora'lis me'dius arte'riae ce'rebri me'diae [TA] middle temporal branch of middle cerebral artery: a branch arising from the inferior terminal branch of the middle cerebral artery and supplying the lateral surface of the temporal lobe between the anterior and posterior rami. Called also *middle temporal artery.*

ra'mi tempora'les ner'vi facia'lis [TA] temporal branches of facial nerve: terminal branches of the facial nerve that innervate the anterior and superior auricular muscles, the frontal belly of the occipitofrontal muscle, and the orbicularis oculi and corrugator muscles; *modality,* motor.

r. tempora'lis poste'rior arte'riae ce'rebri me'diae [TA] posterior temporal branch of middle cerebral artery: a branch arising from the inferior terminal branch of the middle cerebral artery and supplying the lateral surface of the posterior temporal lobe. Called also *posterior temporal artery.*

ra'mi tempora'les posterio'res arte'riae occipita'lis latera'lis [TA] posterior temporal branches of lateral occipital artery: branches that supply the cortex of the posterior part of the temporal lobe.

ra'mi tempora'les superficia'les ner'vi auriculotempora'lis [TA] superficial temporal branches of auriculotemporal nerve: branches to the skin of the scalp in the temporal region; *modality,* general sensory.

r. temporooccipita'lis arte'riae ce'rebri me'diae [TA] temporooccipital branch of middle cerebral artery: a branch arising from the inferior terminal branch of the middle cerebral artery and supplying the lateral surface of the posterior temporal and occipital lobes.

r. tento'rii ner'vi ophthal'mici TA alternative for *r. meningeus recurrens nervi ophthalmici.*

ra'mi termina'les inferio'res arte'riae ce'rebri me'diae [TA] inferior terminal branches of middle cerebral artery: branches arising from the middle cerebral artery and including the anterior temporal, middle temporal, posterior temporal, and temporooccipital branches, and branch to angular gyrus; they supply the temporal and occipital lobes. Called also *rami corticales inferiores arteriae cerebri mediae* [TA alternative].

ra'mi termina'les superio'res arte'riae ce'rebri me'diae [TA] superior terminal branches of middle cerebral artery: branches arising from the middle cerebral artery and including the lateral frontobasal, prefrontal, anterior parietal, and posterior parietal arteries, and the arteries of precentral sulcus, of central sulcus, and of postcentral sulcus; they supply the frontal and parietal lobes. Called also *rami corticales superiores arteriae cerebri mediae* [TA alternative].

ra'mi thy'mici arte'riae thora'cicae inter'nae [TA] thymic branches of internal thoracic artery: branches distributed to the thymus gland in the anterior mediastinum; called also *thymic arteries.*

r. thyrohyoi'deus an'sae cervica'lis [TA] thyrohyoid branch of ansa cervicalis: a branch from the superior root of the ansa cervicalis, innervating the thyrohyoid muscle; *modality,* motor.

r. tonsil'lae cerebel'li arte'riae inferio'ris posterio'ris cerebel'li [TA] tonsillar branch of posterior inferior cerebellar artery: a branch that ascends upward from the posterior inferior cerebellar artery to the tonsil of the cerebellum to supply the dentate nucleus of the cerebellum.

r. tonsilla'ris arte'riae facia'lis [TA] tonsillar branch of facial artery: a vessel ascending from the facial artery on the pharynx to supply the tonsil and the root of the tongue.

ra'mi tonsilla'res ner'vi glossopharyn'gei [TA] tonsillar branches of glossopharyngeal nerve: branches that supply the mucosa over the palatine tonsil and the adjacent portion of the soft palate; *modality,* general sensory.

ra'mi tonsilla'res nervo'rum palatino'rum mino'rum [TA] tonsillar branches of lesser palatine nerves: branches that innervate the palatine tonsils.

ra'mi trachea'les arte'riae thora'cicae inter'nae [TA] the tracheal branches of the internal thoracic artery.

ra'mi trachea'les arte'riae thyroi'deae inferio'ris [TA] tracheal branches of inferior thyroid artery: vessels supplying the trachea.

ra'mi trachea'les ner'vi laryn'gei recurren'tis [TA] tracheal branches of recurrent laryngeal nerve: branches distributed to the tracheal mucosa; *modality,* general sensory.

ra'mi trac'tus op'tici arte'riae choroi'deae anterio'ris [TA] branches of anterior choroidal artery to optic tract: small branches that supply the optic tract.

r. transver'sus arte'riae circumflex'ae fe'moris latera'lis [TA] transverse branch of lateral circumflex femoral artery: a branch that pierces the vastus lateralis muscle, turning around the femur to anastomose with the transverse branch of the medial circumflex femoral artery and with other arteries, deep to the gluteus maximus muscle.

r. transver'sus arte'riae circumflex'ae fe'moris media'lis transverse branch of medial circumflex femoral artery: a branch that passes between the quadratus femoris and adductor magnus muscles, supplying them, and then turning around the femur to anastomose with the transverse branch of the lateral circumflex femoral artery and with other arteries, deep to the gluteus maximus muscle.

ra'mi tuba'rii arte'riae ova'ricae [TA] tubal branches of ovarian artery: branches distributed to the uterine tubes.

r. tuba'rius arte'riae uteri'nae [TA] tubal branch of uterine artery: a branch that supplies the uterine tube and the round ligament.

r. tuba'rius plex'us tympa'nici [TA] tubal branch of tympanic plexus: a branch given to the auditory tube from the tympanic plexus; *modality,* general sensory.

ra'mi tu'beris cine'rei arte'riae choroi'deae anterio'ris [TA] branches of anterior choroidal artery to tuber cinereum: small branches that supply the tuber cinereum.

ra'mi urete'rici arte'riae duc'tus deferen'tis [TA] ureteral branches of artery of ductus deferens: branches that supply the lower portion of the ureter.

ra'mi urete'rici arte'riae ova'ricae [TA] ureteral branches of ovarian artery: branches distributed to the ureter.

ra'mi urete'rici arte'riae rena'lis [TA] ureteral branches of renal artery: branches that supply the upper portion of the ureter.

ra'mi urete'rici arte'riae testicula'ris [TA] ureteral branches of testicular artery: branches distributed to the ureter.

ra'mi vagina'les arte'riae recta'lis me'diae [TA] a branch of the middle rectal artery that supplies the vagina.

ra'mi vagina'les arte'riae uteri'nae [TA] vaginal branches of uterine artery: two median longitudinal vessels formed by anastomosis of branches of the uterine and vaginal arteries, one of which descends in front of and the other behind the vagina. Called also *azygos arteries of vagina.*

ra'mi ventra'les nervo'rum cervica'lium TA alternative for *rami anteriores nervorum cervicalium.*

r. ventra'lis ner'vi coccy'gei TA alternative for *r. anterior nervi coccygei.*

ra'mi ventra'les nervo'rum lumba'lium TA alternative for *rami anteriores nervorum lumbalium.*

ra'mi ventra'les nervo'rum sacra'lium TA alternative for *rami anteriores nervorum sacralium.*

ra'mi ventra'les nervo'rum thoracico'rum, ventral rami of thoracic nerves rami anteriores nervorum thoracicorum.

r. ver'mis supe'rior arte'riae supe'rioris cerebel'li arteria vermis superior.

r. vestibula'ris poste'rior arte'riae vestibulocochlea'ris [TA] posterior vestibular branch of vestibulocochlear artery: a branch that supplies the saccule, basal end of the cochlea, and most of the semicircular canals.

r. viscera'lis r. autonomicus.

Ramus *Continued*

ra′mi zygoma′tici ner′vi facia′lis [TA] zygomatic branches of facial nerve: branches that cross the zygomatic bone and innervate the orbicularis oculi muscle; *modality*, motor.

r. zygomaticofacia′lis ner′vi zygoma′tici [TA] zygomaticofacial branch of zygomatic nerve: a branch that passes from the lateral wall of the orbit, piercing the zygomatic bone to supply overlying skin; *modality*, general sensory.

r. zygomaticotempora′lis ner′vi zygoma′tici [TA] zygomaticotemporal branch of zygomatic nerve: a branch that passes from the lateral wall of the orbit, piercing the zygomatic bone to innervate skin of the anterior temporal region; *modality*, general sensory.

ran•cid (ran′sid) [L. *rancidus*] having a musty, rank taste or smell; applied to fats that have undergone decomposition, with the liberation of fatty acids.

ran•cid•i•fy (ran-sid′ĭ-fi) to decompose, with the liberation of fatty acids; a term applied especially to the decomposition of fats.

ran•cid•i•ty (ran-sid′ĭ-te) the quality of being rancid.

Ran•dall plaques (ran′dəl) [Alexander *Randall*, American urologist, 1883–1951] see under *plaque.*

ran•dom (ran′dəm) [Old French *randon* violence] pertaining to a chance-dependent process, particularly one that occurs according to a known probability distribution.

ran•dom•iza•tion (ran″dəm-ĭ-za′shən) assignment of experimental subjects to treatment groups according to some known probability distribution governed by chance, so that the distribution of subjects within each group should vary only by chance.

ran•dom•ized (ran′dəm-īzd) having subjects who are chosen through randomization; said of clinical trials.

Ra•nex•a (rā-nek′sə) trademark for a preparation of ranolazine hydrochloride.

range (rānj) 1. the difference between the upper and lower limits of a variable or of a series of values. 2. an interval in which values sampled from a population, or the values in the population itself, are known to lie. 3. the geographic region in which a given species is found.

r. of accommodation the alteration in the refractive state of the eye produced by accommodation. It is the difference in diopters between the refraction by the eye adjusted for its far point and that when adjusted for its near point. Called also *amplitude of accommodation.*

r. of audibility see under *limit.*

interquartile r. the difference between the data values at the 75th and 25th percentiles, encompassing the middle 50 per cent of the data.

r. of motion the range, measured in degrees of a circle, through which a joint can be extended and flexed. See also under *exercise.*

normal r., r. of normal see *reference values*, under *value.*

ran•i•my•cin (ran-ĭ-mi′sin) an antibacterial antibiotic derived from a variant of *Streptomyces lincolnensis.*

ra•nine (ra′nīn) [L. *raninus*, from *rana* frog] 1. pertaining to a frog. 2. ranular. 3. sublingual.

ra•ni•ti•dine (rə-nĭ′tĭ-dēn) a histamine H_2 receptor antagonist, which inhibits gastric acid secretion.

r. hydrochloride [USP] the hydrochloride salt of ranitidine, used to inhibit gastric acid secretion in the prophylaxis and treatment of gastric and duodenal ulcer, gastroesophageal reflux disease, and conditions that cause gastric hypersecretion; administered orally, intravenously, or intramuscularly.

rank (rangk) 1. in statistics, the position of a sample observation (or population value) in the sequence of sample values (or population values) arranged in order, usually from lowest to highest. 2. to place in such an order.

Ran•ke angle (rahng′kə) [Hans Rudolph *Ranke*, Dutch anatomist, 1849–1887] see under *angle.*

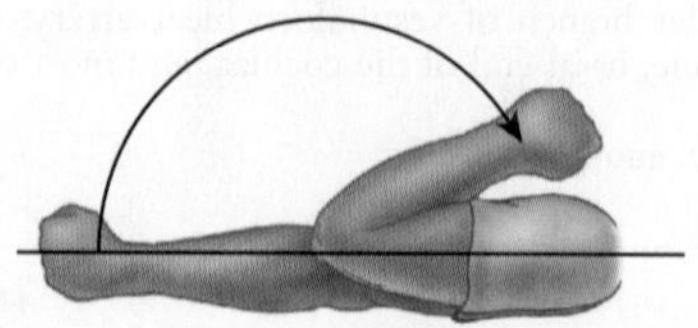

■ Range of motion of the elbow joint.

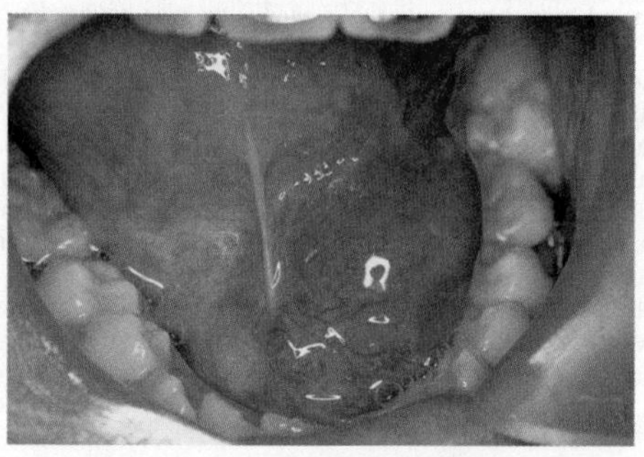

■ Ranula.

Ran•ke complex (rahng′kə) [Karl Ernst von *Ranke*, German internist, 1870–1926] primary complex; see under *complex.*

Ran•kine scale (rang′kin) [William John Macquorn *Rankine*, Scottish engineer and physicist, 1820–1872] see under *scale.*

ra•no•la•zine hy•dro•chlo•ride (rə-no′lə-zēn) an anti-ischemic and antianginal drug used for the treatment of chronic angina pectoris; administered orally.

Ran•son criteria (ran′sən) [John H.C. *Ranson*, American physician, 1938–1995] see under *criterion.*

ran•u•la (ran′u-lə) [L., dim. of *rana* frog] a form of retention cyst of the floor of the mouth, usually due to obstruction of the ducts of the submaxillary or sublingual glands, presenting a slowly enlarging painless deep burrowing mucocele of one side of the mouth. Called also *sublingual cyst* and *sublingual ptyalocele.* **ran′ular** *adj*

plunging r. a rare type of ranula that has become invasive and penetrates into the mylohyoid muscle, the submental region, or the submandibular region.

Ra•nun•cu•la•ceae (rə-nung″ku-la′se-e) a family of flowering plants, most of which contain the glycoside ranunculin; when the plants are eaten, the ranunculin breaks down to form the lethal toxin protoanemonin. Genera include *Aconitum*, *Actaea*, *Anemone*, *Cimicifuga*, *Clematis*, *Delphinium*, *Helleborus*, *Hydrastis*, and *Ranunculus.*

ra•nun•cu•lin (rə-nung′ku-lin) a glycoside found in most plants of the family Ranunculaceae; when the plants are eaten, enzymes in animals convert ranunculin to protoanemonin, a toxin that can be lethal.

Ra•nun•cu•lus (rə-nung′ku-ləs) the crowfoots and buttercups, a genus of plants of the family Ranunculaceae. Some species are poisonous, because they contain the glycoside ranunculin, which when ingested is enzymatically broken down into highly toxic protoanemonin.

Ran•vier crosses, nodes, segment (internode), tactile disks (rahn-vya′) [Louis Antoine *Ranvier*, French pathologist, 1835–1922] see under *cross*, *disk*, and *node*, and see *internodal segment* under *segment.*

RAO right anterior oblique.

Ra•oult's law (rah-o͞olz′) [François Marie *Raoult*, French physical chemist, 1830–1901] see under *law.*

Rap•a•mune (rap′ə-mūn) trademark for a preparation of sirolimus.

rap•a•my•cin (rap-ə-mi′sin) sirolimus.

rape[1] (rāp) [L. *rapere* to seize] nonconsensual sexual penetration of an individual, obtained by force or threat, or in cases in which the victim is not capable of consent.

rape[2] (rāp) [L. *rapum*] *Brassica napus*, an edible plant whose seeds are the source of rapeseed oil.

ra•pha•nia (rə-fa′ne-ə) [Gr. *raphanos* radish] poisoning by seeds of the wild radish, *Raphanus raphanistrum.*

ra•phae (ra′fe) plural of *raphe.*

Ra•phan•us (rə-fan′əs) [L., from Gr. *raphanos* radish] the radishes, a genus of plants of the family Cruciferae native to Europe and Asia. *R. raphanis′trum* is the wild radish, whose seeds contain a poisonous mustard oil glycoside (see *raphania*). *R. sati′vus* is cultivated for food.

ra•phe (ra′fe) gen. *raphēs* pl. *ra′phae* [Gr. *rhaphē*] a seam; in anatomy, the line of union of the halves of any of various symmetrical parts.

abdominal r. linea alba.

amniotic r. the line of junction of the amniotic folds in the amnion of those vertebrates in which it is formed by folding.

r. anococcy′gea, anococcygeal r. corpus anococcygeum.

r. cor′poris callo′si, r. of corpus callosum see *stria longitudinalis medialis corporis callosi* and *stria longitudinalis lateralis corporis callosi.*

lateral palpebral r. r. palpebralis lateralis.

median r. of medulla oblongata, r. media′na medul′lae oblonga′tae r. medullae oblongatae.

median r. of neck, posterior ligamentum nuchae.

median r. of perineum r. perinei.

median r. of pons, r. media′na ponti′na r. pontis.

r. medul′lae oblonga′tae [TA] raphe of medulla oblongata: a median line at the union of the two lateral halves of the medulla oblongata, continuing into the pontine tegmentum; called also *median r. of medulla oblongata* and *r. mediana medullae oblongatae.*

midpalatine r. r. palati.

r. pala′ti [TA] palatine raphe: a narrow whitish streak at the midline of the roof of the mouth (both the hard and soft palates), extending from the incisive papilla to the tip of the uvula; it may occur as a ridge in front and as a groove posteriorly. Called also *midpalatine r.*

palatine r., median r. palati.

r. palpebra′lis latera′lis a thin horizontal band of connective tissue extending from the external angle of the rima palpebralis to the lateral margin of the orbit.

r. pe′nis [TA], **r. of penis** a narrow dark streak or ridge continuous posteriorly with the raphe scroti and extending forward for a variable distance along the midline of the urethral surface of the penis; in the newborn it may extend to the tip of the glans.

perineal r., r. perinea′lis, r. perine′i [TA] a ridge along the median line of the perineum that runs forward from the anus; in the male, it is continuous with the raphe of the scrotum and the raphe of the penis. Called also *median r. of perineum.*

pharyngeal r., r. pharyn′gis [TA] a more or less distinct band of connective tissue extending downward from the base of the skull along the posterior wall of the pharynx in the median plane, and giving attachment to the constrictor muscles of the pharynx.

r. pon′tis [TA] raphe of pons: a median line at the union of the two lateral halves of the pons, which is a continuation of the raphe of the medulla oblongata into the pontine tegmentum; called also *median r. of pons* and *r. mediana pontina.*

r. pterygomandibula′ris [TA] pterygomandibular raphe: a tendinous line between the buccinator and the constrictor pharyngis superior muscles, from which the middle portions of both muscles originate.

scrotal r., r. scrota′lis r. scroti.

r. scro′ti [TA], **r. of scrotum** a ridge along the surface of the scrotum in the median line, dividing it into nearly equal lateral parts; it is continuous with the perineal raphe and the raphe of the penis.

ra•phes (ra′fēz) genitive singular of *raphe.*

Rap•pa•port classification (rap′ə-port) [Henry *Rappaport,* American pathologist, 1913–2003] see under *classification.*

rap•port (rah-por′) [Fr.] a relation of harmony and accord between two persons, as between patient and physician.

rap•ture of the deep popular name for *nitrogen narcosis.*

rar•e•fac•tion (rar″ə-fak′shən) [L. *rarefactio*] the condition of being or becoming less dense; diminution in density and weight, but not in volume.

RAS[1] renal artery stenosis; renin-angiotensin system.

RAS[2] [*ra*t *s*arcoma; the transforming gene was obtained during passage of the Harvey murine sarcoma virus through a rat] any of a family of human proto-oncogenes related to oncogenes first identified in Harvey murine sarcoma virus (H-*ras*) and Kirsten murine sarcoma virus (K-*ras*). Mammalian cells contain three 21 kDa Ras proteins (H- K- and N-Ras) that act as GTP-binding proteins with GTPase activity, and are important in the cell cycle; specific point mutations can lead to oncogenesis.

ra•sa•ji•line mes•y•late (rə-saj′ĭ-lēn) a monoamine oxidase inhibitor used as an antiparkinsonian agent; administered orally.

ra•sa•ya•na (rah″sah-yah′nə) any of a group of herbal remedies with antioxidant properties used in ayurveda to promote health, provide defense against disease, and promote longevity.

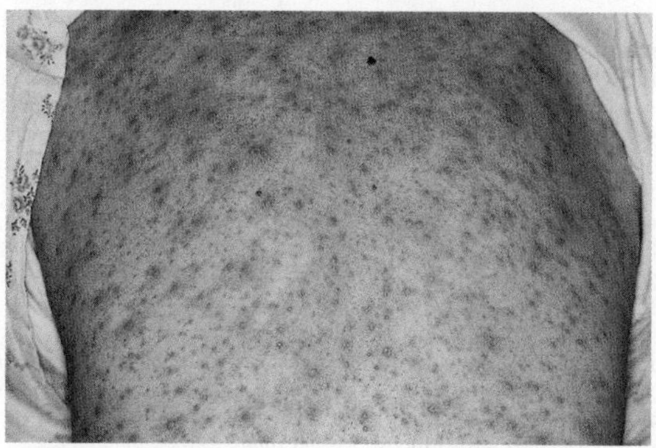

■ Pleomorphic rash of varicella.

ras•bur•i•case (ras-būr′ĭ-kās) a recombinant form of urate oxidase, used in treatment of hyperuricemia in children who have leukemia, lymphoma, or solid tumors; administered by intravenous infusion.

rash (rash) a temporary eruption on the skin, such as in urticaria, a drug eruption, or an exanthem.

brown-tail r. see under *dermatitis.*

butterfly r. a rash formed by a skin eruption across the nose and adjacent areas of the cheeks, as in systemic lupus erythematosus, seborrheic dermatitis, and rosacea. Called also *butterfly.*

caterpillar r. see under *dermatitis.*

diaper r. popular term for *diaper dermatitis.*

drug r. see under *eruption.*

heat r. miliaria rubra.

heliotrope r. a pink to purple rash seen most often around the eyes of persons with dermatomyositis.

napkin r., nappy r. popular terms for *diaper dermatitis.*

nettle r. urticaria in domestic animals as an allergic reaction to nettles.

sun r. popular term for *solar dermatitis.*

wandering r. benign migratory glossitis.

Rash•kind balloon atrial septostomy (rash′kind) [W.J. *Rashkind,* American surgeon, 20th century] see under *septostomy.*

ra•sion (ra′zhən) [L. *rasio*] the grating of drugs with a file.

Ras•mus•sen aneurysm (rahs′mo͝o-sən) [Fritz Waldemar *Rasmussen,* Danish physician, 1834–1877] see under *aneurysm.*

Ras•mus•sen encephalitis (syndrome) (rahs′mo͝o-sən) [Theodore Brown *Rasmussen,* American neurologist in Canada, 1910–2002] see under *encephalitis.*

rasp (rasp) 1. a coarse file used in surgery. Called also *raspatory* and *xyster.* 2. to file with this instrument.

ras•pa•to•ry (ras′pə-to-re) [L. *raspatorium*] rasp (def. 1).

rasp•ber•ry (raz′ber-e) 1. either *Rubus iridaeus* or *R. strigosus.* 2. the fruit of either *R. iridaeus* or *R. strigosus,* used as a flavoring agent. See also under *juice* and *syrup.*

RAST radioallergosorbent test.

Ras•tel•li operation (rahs-tel′e) [Gian Carlo *Rastelli,* Italian cardiovascular surgeon, 1933–1970] see under *operation.*

rat (rat) any of numerous small rodents of the genus *Rattus* and related genera of the family Muridae; many are aggressive and omnivorous pests found around human dwellings. Rats not only cause great economic loss but also are vectors of disease; they harbor at least eleven species of intestinal parasites that are transmissible to humans, such as tapeworms, roundworms, and trichinae; and they are reservoirs for the infective agents of plague,

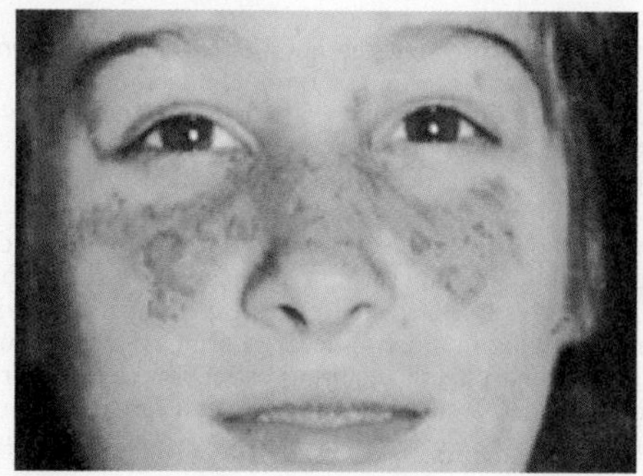

■ Butterfly rash in systemic lupus erythematosus.

typhus, Weil disease, and rat-bite fever. Albino mutants of some species are used as laboratory animals.

albino r. white r.

BB r. a strain that serves as a model of type 1 diabetes mellitus.

black r. *Rattus rattus,* the European black rat and the one most commonly responsible for transmitting plague to humans by means of its flea *Xenopsylla cheopis.*

brown r. *Rattus norvegicus,* a brownish-gray species that is larger than the black rat, and has short ears and tail. Called also *barn rat, gray rat, Norway rat, sewer rat,* and *wharf rat.*

bush r. wood r.

cotton r. any member of the genus *Sigmodon.*

fa/fa r. a rat homozygous for the *fa* gene; such rats are genetically obese, hyperphagic, and hyperinsulinemic, with normal intravenous but abnormal oral glucose tolerance. Used as an experimental model of insulin resistance associated with glucose intolerance.

Fischer 344 r. an inbred strain of albino laboratory rats developed in 1920; used particularly in cancer research.

Holtzman r. a strain of albino rat descended originally from the S–D strain, which originated from Wistar Institute sometime before 1929.

Long-Evans r. a strain of rat, developed at the University of Rochester, characterized by a brown to black head and shoulders.

multimammate r. see under *mouse.*

Munich-Wistar r. an inbred strain of rat much used in experimental medicine.

pack r. wood r.

rice r. any member of the genus *Oryzomys.*

Sprague-Dawley r. a strain of albino rat developed by the Sprague-Dawley Animal Company, widely used in experimental work because of its calmness and ease of handling.

trade r. wood r.

white r. an albino form of *Rattus rattus* or of *R. norvegicus* which is much used as a laboratory animal.

Wistar r. a strain of albino rat developed at the Wistar Institute but which has spread so widely to other institutions that there is probably marked dilution of the strain.

wood r. a rat of the genus *Neotoma,* also known as *bush rat, pack rat,* and *trade rat.* These rats are hosts of fleas and ticks.

Zucker r. a mutant strain of laboratory rats existing as a lean phenotype (genotype Fa/Fa or Fa/fa) and a genetically obese phenotype (genotype fa/fa); the obese Zucker rat is used as an experimental model of juvenile-onset obesity.

rate (rāt) [L. *rata,* from *rates* calculated] 1. the amount of change of a physical quantity or number of occurrences of an event per unit time. 2. in epidemiology and demography, the frequency of an event in a specified population; correctly applied only to fractions for which all of the cases contributing to the numerator are also counted in the denominator and for which the denominator is the entire population at risk. Rates are often multiplied by a factor to give the number of events per 1000, 10,000, or 100,000 population. 3. more generally, a term sometimes used to denote some measured quantity with respect to another. Symbol R.

Rate

adjusted r. a fictitious summary rate statistically adjusted to remove the effect of a demographic or other influential variable such as age or sex, thus permitting unbiased comparison between groups having different underlying compositions with respect to these variables. Called also *standardized r.* Cf. *crude r.* and *specific r.*

attack r. in the analysis of acute outbreaks of disease, the proportion of persons who are exposed to the disease during the outbreak who do become ill.

basal metabolic r. an expression of the rate at which oxygen is utilized by the body cells, or the calculated equivalent heat production by the body, in a fasting subject at complete rest. Abbreviated BMR. See also *basal metabolism,* under *metabolism.*

birth r. a rate in which the numerator is the number of live births in a geographic area in a defined period, usually one year. The denominator of the *crude birth rate* is the average total population or the midyear population in the area during the period. Specific birth rates for subsets of the population may also be calculated, e.g., an *age-specific birth rate,* limited to the population of females of a defined age range.

case r. attack r.

case fatality r. the proportion of persons contracting a disease who die of that disease: the numerator is the number of deaths caused by a disease and the denominator is the number of diagnosed cases of the disease. Called also *case fatality ratio, fatality r.,* and *lethality r.*

circulation r. the amount of blood pumped through the body by the heart per unit time; usually expressed in milliliters or liters per minute.

crude r. the total number of events occurring in an entire population over a period of time, without reference to any of the individuals or subgroups within the population. Cf. *adjusted r.* and *specific r.*

cumulative incidence r. the proportion of an initially disease-free population developing a disease over a fixed interval, calculated by cumulating the proportions developing the disease within short subintervals.

death r. a rate expressing the number of deaths in a population at risk. The *crude death rate* is the ratio of the number of deaths in a geographic area in one year divided by the average or midyear population in the area during the year. An *age-specific death rate* is the ratio of the number of deaths occurring in a specified age group in one year to the average or midyear population of that group. A *cause-specific death rate* is the ratio of the number of deaths due to a specified cause in one year to the average or midyear total population. Called also *mortality r.*

DEF r. an expression of dental caries experience in deciduous teeth: calculated by adding number of decayed primary teeth requiring filling *(D),* decayed primary teeth requiring extraction *(E),* and primary teeth successfully filled *(F);* missing primary teeth are not included in the calculation.

DMF r. an expression of the condition of the teeth based on the number of teeth decayed, missing, indicated for removal and of those filled or bearing restorations: calculated by adding the number of carious permanent teeth requiring filling *(D),* carious permanent teeth requiring extraction *(Mr),* permanent teeth previously extracted because of caries *(Mp),* and permanent teeth filled *(F)* Number of DMF teeth per child of a specific age or age group is calculated by the formula:

$$\frac{D + Mr + Mp + F}{\text{number of children examined}} = \text{DMF}.$$

dose r. the amount of any agent administered per unit of time.

erythrocyte sedimentation r. (ESR) the rate at which erythrocytes precipitate out from a well-mixed specimen of venous blood, measured by the distance the top of the column of erythrocytes falls in a given time interval under specified conditions; an increase in rate is usually due to elevated levels of plasma proteins, especially fibrinogen and immunoglobulins, which decrease the zeta potential on erythrocytes by dielectric shielding and thus promote rouleau formation. It is increased in monoclonal gammopathy, hypergammaglobulinemia due to inflammatory disease, hyperfibrinogenemia, active inflammatory disease, and anemia. The traditional methods of calculating ESR are the *Westergren method* and the *Wintrobe method.* See also *zeta sedimentation ratio* under *ratio.*

fatality r. 1. the death rate in a specific group of persons simultaneously affected by some event, such as a natural disaster. 2. case fatality r.

fertility r. a measure of fertility in a defined population over a specified period of time, usually one year; particularly the *general fertility r.,* but also including more specific rates such as those for females of a given parity or a particular decade in age or that describing the completed rate for females who have finished childbearing.

fetal death r., fetal mortality r. the ratio of the number of fetal deaths in one year to the total number of both live births and fetal deaths in that year. Cf. *fetal death ratio.*

first incidence r. incidence r.

five-year survival r. an expression of the number of survivors with no trace of disease five years after each has been diagnosed or treated for the same disease.

flow r. flow (def. 2).

general fertility r. the most widely used measure of fertility; the number of live births in a geographic area in a year per 1000 women of childbearing age, which is usually defined as age 15 to 44 years.

glomerular filtration r. (GFR) the quantity of glomerular filtrate formed per unit time in all nephrons of both kidneys, equal to the

Rate *Continued*

inulin clearance; usually measured clinically by the endogenous creatinine clearance.

growth r. an expression of the increase in size of an organic object per unit time, calculations usually being made as to both the absolute and the relative increment.

heart r. the number of contractions of the ventricles of the heart per unit of time (usually a minute). It usually corresponds to the pulse rate, but occasionally some of the contractions of the left ventricle fail to produce peripheral pulse waves, so that the rate of the pulse at the wrist is less than that of the heart.

incidence r. the probability of developing a particular disease during a given period of time; the numerator of the rate is the number of new cases during the specified time period and the denominator is the population at risk during the period. Cf. *prevalence r.*

infant death r., infant mortality r. the ratio of the number of deaths in one year of children less than one year of age to the number of live births in that year.

lethality r. case fatality r.

maternal death r., maternal mortality r. a rate in which the numerator is the number of maternal deaths ascribed to puerperal causes in one year; the number of live births in that year is often used as the denominator, although to make a true rate the denominator should be the number of pregnancies (live births and fetal deaths). Called also *puerperal death* or *mortality r.*

maximal midexpiratory flow r., maximum midexpiratory flow r. maximum midexpiratory flow.

monthly fecundity r. (MFR) a measure of the number of pregnancies occurring in a single menstrual cycle for a specified group of women.

morbidity r. a rate in which the numerator is a number of cases of a disease and the denominator is the number of people at risk for the disease; it can denote either of the more precise terms *incidence r.* and *prevalence r.*

mortality r. death r.

mutation r. the number of new mutations at a given locus per unit of time, generally per generation or per cell division.

neonatal death r., neonatal mortality r. the ratio of the number of deaths in one year of children less than 28 days of age to the number of live births in that year.

oocyst r. the percentage of wild female mosquitoes found to contain oocysts in the midgut.

output exposure r. in radiology, the exposure to radiation at a specified point per unit of time, usually expressed in roentgens per minute.

parasite r. the percentage of persons in a particular age group or area that are found to be infected with parasites, such as malarial parasites.

peak expiratory flow r. (PEFR) see under *flow.*

peak inspiratory flow r. see under *flow.*

perinatal death r., perinatal mortality r. the ratio of the number of the sum of fetal deaths after 28 or more weeks of gestation (stillbirths) and deaths of infants less than 7 days of age in one time period and population to the sum of the number of live births and fetal deaths after 28 or more weeks of gestation (stillbirths) in that same time period and population.

plasma refilling r. in hemodialysis, the rate at which plasma that has been withdrawn and dialyzed flows back into the patient's circulatory system.

postneonatal death r., postneonatal mortality r. the ratio of the number of deaths in a given year of children between the 28th day of life and the first birthday relative to the difference between the number of the live births and neonatal deaths in that year; the denominator is sometimes simplified, less correctly, to the number of live births. The ratio is sometimes approximated as the difference between the infant mortality rate and the neonatal mortality rate.

prevalence r. the number of people in a population who have a disease or other condition at a given time: the numerator of the rate is the number of existing cases of the condition at a specified time and the denominator is the total population. Time may be a point or a defined interval; if unspecified it is traditionally the former. Cf. *incidence r.*

protein catabolic r. (PCR) a calculation derived by multiplying 6.25 times the amount of nitrogen in grams excreted in the urine over a given time period; this represents the amount of protein catabolized by the body in excess of protein synthesis. In a healthy steady state of nitrogen balance it approximates the amount of protein in the diet.

puerperal death r., puerperal mortality r. maternal mortality r.

pulse r. the rate of pulsation noted in a peripheral artery per minute, normally from 50 to 100.

relative survival r. a statistical comparison between the rate of patients in a cohort surviving for a certain length of time and the survival rate of a comparable group in the general population.

respiration r. the number of breaths per minute, usually measured by movements of the chest.

secondary attack r. the attack rate in a closed exposed group, such as a household. The index case, which brings the group to the attention of the investigator, and also other initial cases occurring too early to be related to the index case are excluded from both the numerator and the denominator when possible.

sedimentation r. the rate at which a sediment is deposited in a given volume of solution, especially when subjected to the action of a centrifuge; see also *erythrocyte sedimentation r.*

sickness r. morbidity r.

single nephron glomerular filtration r. (SNGFR) the estimated glomerular filtration rate for a single nephron, the product of the surface area for filtration and the average of values along the length of a glomerular capillary.

slew r. the rate of change of the voltage between the positive and negative peaks on the electrogram, or the rate of change in the steepest portion if the electrogram is monophasic.

specific r. a rate that applies to a specific demographic subgroup, e.g., individuals of a specific age, sex, or race, giving the total number of events in relation only to that subgroup. Cf. *adjusted r.* and *crude r.*

sporozoite r. the percentage of wild female mosquitoes found to contain sporozoites in the glands.

standardized r. adjusted r.

stillbirth r. fetal death r.

Westergren sedimentation r. Westergren method.

Rath·ke column, cysts, duct, etc. (raht′kə) [Martin Heinrich *Rathke*, German anatomist, 1793–1860] see under *column, cyst, duct, fold,* and *pouch,* see *craniopharyngioma,* and see *trabeculae cranii,* under *trabecula.*

rat·i·cide (rat′ĭ-sīd) an agent destructive to rats.

ra·tio (ra′she-o) [L.] an expression of the quantity of one substance or entity in relation to that of another; the relationship between two quantities expressed as the quotient of one divided by the other.

AC/A r. the amount of convergence in prism diopters divided by the amount of accommodation in diopters that is required for both eyes to be directed at an object. If it is too high, the person has esotropia; if it is too low, the person has exotropia. Called also *AC/A r.*

A-G r. albumin-globulin r.

albumin/creatinine r. the ratio of albumin to creatinine in the urine, calculated as a measure of albuminuria.

albumin-globulin r. the ratio of albumin to globulin in blood serum, plasma, or urine in various types of renal or liver disease, a formerly widely used assessment of protein composition that is now being replaced by quantitiative measurement of specific serum proteins.

aldosterone-renin r. the ratio between plasma aldosterone concentration and plasma renin activity, a test for primary aldosteronism.

arm r. a figure expressing the relation of the length of the longer arm of a mitotic chromosome to that of the shorter arm.

Blackburne-Peel r. the ratio of the perpendicular distance between the tibial and patellar articular surfaces to the length of the patellar articular surface with the knee in 30° of flexion; it is equal to 0.8 in the normal knee.

body-weight r. body weight in grams divided by stature in centimeters.

cardiothoracic r. the ratio of the transverse diameter of the heart to the internal diameter of the chest at its widest point just above the level of the dome of the diaphragm, such as on radiographic examination; it is a rough guide to cardiac enlargement, being normally less than 0.5. Called also *cardiothoracic index.*

case fatality r. see under *rate.*

concentration r. the ratio of the average concentration of a solid in the urine to its concentration in the blood.

conduction r. in cardiac physiology, the ratio of atrial to ventricular depolarizations, measured as the ratio of P waves to QRS complexes in the electrocardiogram; it is normally 1:1.

critical r. any of a class of tests of statistical significance in which a parameter is divided by its standard error; e.g., in the *t*-test, the critical ratio is the difference between two means divided by the standard error of that difference. The larger the ratio, the more likely the difference is significant.

cross-product r. odds r.

curative r. therapeutic r.

expiratory exchange r. respiratory exchange r.

extraction r. the extent to which the plasma concentration of a substance is reduced as the blood flows through a clearing organ; calculated by the formula

$$E = \frac{C_A - C_V}{C_A},$$

where E is the extraction rate, C_A is the inflow plasma concentration, and C_V is the outflow plasma concentration.

***F*-r.** the variance between the means of several groups relative to the variance within the groups; used in the *F*-test (q.v.) in the analysis of variance (ANOVA).

fetal death r. the ratio of fetal deaths in one year to the number of live births in that year. Cf. *fetal death rate.*

grid r. in radiology, the ratio of the height of the lead strips to the width of the interspacing of a grid.

hand r. the ratio of the length of the hand to its width.

holdaway r. a means of expressing the relationship of the pogonion and the lower incisor to the nasion-basion plane; used in radiographic cephalometric diagnosis.

Insall-Salvati r. the ratio of the length of the ligamentum patellae to the height of the patella, equal to approximately 1 in the normal knee.

inspiratory-expiratory r. the ratio of the inspiratory time to the expiratory time during the breathing cycle. Normally, expiratory time is longer than inspiratory time; if the inspiratory time is longer than the expiratory time, gas trapping may result.

karyoplasmic r. nucleocytoplasmic r.

ketogenic-antiketogenic r. the proportion between substances that form glucose in the body and those that form fatty acids.

lecithin/sphingomyelin r. the ratio of lecithin to sphingomyelin concentration in the amniotic fluid, used to predict the degree of pulmonary maturity of the fetus and thus the risk of respiratory difficulties for the newborn. Called also *L/S ratio.*

likelihood r. 1. an index of diagnostic marker tests, the odds of a disease given a specified test value relative to the odds of the disease in the study population. It can be calculated for either a positive or a negative test, the former (LR+) being the ratio of the sensitivity to the false-positive error rate and the latter (LR−) being the ratio of the false-negative error rate to the specificity. Depending on how it is written, it can be viewed either as a risk ratio or an odds ratio. 2. see under *test.*

L/S r. lecithin/sphingomyelin r.

mendelian r. the ratio of offspring having particular phenotypes or genotypes expected on the basis of Mendel's laws from the mating of two individuals with specific phenotypes or genotypes.

nucleocytoplasmic r., nucleoplasmic r. the ratio of nuclear to cytoplasmic volume.

nutritive r. the ratio between the digestible protein and the digestible fats and carbohydrates in a ration in stock feeding.

odds r. the ratio of the probability of occurrence of one event to that of its alternative; it is often used in epidemiological analysis as it closely approximates relative risk.

proportionate mortality r. (PMR) 1. the ratio of the number of deaths from a particular cause to the total number of deaths in the same time period. 2. in occupational epidemiology, the ratio of observed deaths due to a specific cause in an occupational cohort to the expected deaths due to that cause, as determined by the proportion of deaths from the cause in the general population or comparison population, multiplied by 100. Cf. *standardized mortality r.*

protein/creatinine r. the ratio of protein to creatinine in the urine, calculated as a measure of proteinuria.

relative risk r. relative risk.

respiratory exchange r. the ratio of carbon dioxide output to oxygen uptake in respiration. Symbol R. Called also *expiratory exchange r.*

risk r. relative risk.

sex r. the proportion of one sex to the other; by tradition the number of males in a population to the number of females, usually stated as the number of males per 100 females.

signal-to-noise r. the ratio between the amplitude of a signal being measured and that of the noise (q.v.).

standardized morbidity r. (SMR) a ratio like a standardized mortality ratio except that cases of disease rather than deaths are the observed data.

standardized mortality r. (SMR) the ratio of the number of observed deaths in a study population to the number of expected deaths in that population. The expected deaths are calculated by classifying the study group by demographic variables such as age, sex, or race; computing the expected deaths for each class by multiplying the number of individuals in the study group in that class by the class-specific death rate in a standard reference population; and adding the expected deaths in all classes. Cf. *proportionate mortality r.* (def. 2).

stimulation r. (SR) see *lymphocyte proliferation test,* under *test.*

therapeutic r. the fraction of the minimal lethal dose of a drug that is therapeutically effective; called also *curative r.*

urea excretion r. the ratio of the number of milligrams of urea in the urine excreted in one hour to the number of milligrams in 100 mL of blood; the normal ratio is 50.

urea reduction r. (URR) the fractional reduction in blood urea nitrogen during a single hemodialysis session, expressed as a percentage, measured to assess adequacy of hemodialysis.

ventilation-perfusion r. the ratio of oxygen received in the pulmonary alveoli to the flow of blood through the corresponding alveolar capillaries.

zeta sedimentation r. (ZSR) a measurement comparable to the erythrocyte sedimentation rate, except that it is unaffected by anemia. The packed-cell volume *(zetacrit)* of a blood specimen is calculated by centrifuging the specimen in a *Zetafuge,* a specially designed instrument that produces controlled cycles of compaction and dispersion and allows rouleaux to form and sediment rapidly. The zetacrit divided into the true hematocrit gives the zeta sedimentation ratio.

ra·tion (ră′shən, ra′shən) [L. *ratio* proportion] a fixed allowance of food or drink per day or other unit of time.

basal r. a ration giving the required energy, but lacking in one or more vitamins.

ra·tion·al (ră′shən-əl) [L. *rationalis* reasonable] based upon reason; characterized by possession of one's reason.

ra·tio·nale (ră″shən-al′) [L.] a rational exposition of principles; the logical basis of a procedure.

ra·tion·al·iza·tion (ră″shən-əl-ĭ-za′shən) a type of defense mechanism in which one justifies, by an incorrect application of reason, attitudes and behavior that would otherwise be unacceptable.

rat-tails (rat′tālz) a swollen condition of the hair papillae over the flexor tendons of a horse's legs, due to filth and bacteria.

rat·tle·snake (rat′əl-snāk) any of the New World pit vipers of the genera *Crotalus* and *Sistrurus,* having a series of cornified interlocking segments at the tip of the tail; when disturbed they vibrate the tail to produce the characteristic rattling or buzzing sound. See table at *snake.*

eastern diamondback r. *Crotalus adamanteus,* a large venomous snake found along the East and Gulf Coasts of the United States.

ground r. 1. massasauga. 2. pygmy r.

Massasauga r. massasauga.

Mojave r. *Crotalus scutulatus scutulatus,* a poisonous species found in the southwestern United States.

prairie r. *Crotalus viridis viridis,* a venomous snake found in the prairies and plains of the midwestern United States.

pygmy r. *Sistrurus miliarius,* a small venomous species found in the southeastern United States.

timber r. *Crotalus horridus,* a venomous yellowish-brown snake found from the East Coast of the United States west into Texas.

western diamondback r. *Crotalus atrox,* a venomous snake found in the southwestern United States and northern Mexico.

Rat·tus (rat′əs) a genus of small rodents, including several common species of rats (q.v.). *R. norve′gicus* is the brown rat and *R. rat′tus* is the black rat.

Rau process (rou) [Johann J. *Rau* (L. *Ravius*), Dutch anatomist, 1668–1719] see *processus anterior mallei.*

Rau·ber layer (rou′bər) [August Antinous *Rauber,* German-born anatomist in Estonia, 1841–1917] see under *layer.*

Rau·wi·loid (rou′wĭ-loid) trademark for preparations of alseroxylon.

Rau·wol·fia (rou-wool′fe-ə) [Leonhard *Rauwolf,* 16th century German botanist] a large genus of tropical trees and shrubs of the family Apocyanaceae. Many species provide alkaloids of medical interest, such as reserpine, and have long been used medicinally in South America, Africa, and Asia.

R. serpenti′na a small shrub native to India and elsewhere in Asia, containing many alkaloids, particularly reserpine and rescinnamine; its dried root is the medicinal substance called *rauwolfia serpentina.*

rau·wol·fia (rou-wool′fe-ə) 1. any member of the genus *Rauwolfia.* 2. the medicinal dried root or an extract of the dried root of *Rauwolfia.*

r. serpenti′na [USP] the dried root of *Rauwolfia serpentina,* sometimes with fragments of rhizome and aerial stem bases attached; used as an antihypertensive and to treat nervousness and insomnia; also used in folk medicine for various uses and in Indian medicine for poisonous bites and other uses.

Rau•zide (rou′zīd) trademark for preparations of rauwolfia serpentina with bendroflumethiazide.

RAV Rous-associated virus.

Ra•vitch technique (ra′vich) [Mark M. *Ravitch*, American surgeon, 1910–1989] see under *technique.*

Ra•vi•us (ra′ve-əs) see *Rau.*

ray (ra) [L. *radius* spoke] 1. a line emanating from a center. 2. a distinct portion of electromagnetic radiation that proceeds in a specific direction. 3. any of various marine elasmobranch fishes with flattened bodies and narrow tails. See also *stingray.*

α-r's alpha r's.

actinic r's light rays that produce chemical changes. In general, light rays have more of this property the farther they are from the center of the visible spectrum, so that infrared, red, violet, and ultraviolet are the most actinic.

alpha r's high-speed helium nuclei that have been ejected from radioactive substances. Owing to their high velocity (one tenth that of light) their kinetic energy is so great that a single alpha particle produces a microscopic flash of light when it hits a spinthariscope; when it hits another atom (as of nitrogen) it may cause it to disintegrate.

anode r's positive r's.

β-r's, beta r's electrons ejected from radioactive substances with velocities that may be as high as 0.98 of the velocity of light.

cathode r's negative particles of electricity streaming out in a vacuum tube at right angles to the surface of the cathode and away from it irrespective of the position of the anode. They move in a straight line unless deflected by a magnet. By striking on solids they generate x-rays. See also *electron stream.*

central r. the straight line passing through the center of the radiation source and the center of the final beam-limiting diaphragm.

characteristic r's x-rays emitted as a result of the rearrangement of electrons in the inner shells of atoms, as when electrons are ejected from the inner shells by high-speed bombarding electrons or when an orbital electron is captured by the nucleus during radioactive decay; the wavelengths of the rays produced depend on the element and the energy levels involved. Cf. *characteristic fluorescent r's.*

characteristic fluorescent r's secondary rays emitted as a result of the rearrangement of electrons in the inner shells of atoms; identical with characteristic rays (q.v.) except that characteristic rays are caused by the bombardment of the x-ray tube target by electrons, whereas characteristic fluorescent rays are caused by primary ray photon bombardment of an absorbing material.

chemical r. actinic r.

convergent r. a ray that is approaching a focus; it may be produced by passage through a convex lens or by reflection from a concave mirror.

δ-r's, delta r's secondary beta rays produced in a gas by the passage of alpha particles.

digital r. 1. a digit of the hand or foot and the corresponding portion of the metacarpus or metatarsus, considered as a continuous structural unit. 2. in the embryo, a mesenchymal condensation of the hand or foot plate that outlines the pattern of a future digit.

divergent r's rays coming from a source nearer than infinity, or a pencil or bundle of light rays directed away from a focus after passing through a concave lens or after being reflected from a convex mirror.

dynamic r's rays that are active physically or therapeutically.

fluorescent r's characteristic fluorescent r's.

γ-r's, gamma r's electromagnetic radiation of short wavelengths emitted by the nucleus of an atom during a nuclear reaction. They consist of high energy photons, have no mass and no electric charge, and travel with the speed of light and are usually associated with beta rays.

glass r's the rays formed in an x-ray tube by the cathode rays striking the glass wall of the tube, so called to distinguish them from the x-rays originating at the anticathode.

grenz r's very soft x-rays with a wavelength of about 20 nm, lying between x-rays and ultraviolet rays in the electromagnetic spectrum.

hard r's, hard x-r's x-rays of short wavelength, high energy, and great penetrative power.

heat r's see *radiant heat,* under *heat.*

incident r. see *reflection* (def. 2), and *refraction* (def. 2).

indirect r's rays formed at the surface of the glass of the cathode ray tube.

infrared r's invisible rays just below the red end of the visible spectrum; their wavelengths range between 0.75 and 1000 μm; see *infrared.*

infra roentgen r's grenz r's.

intermediate r's electromagnetic waves whose wavelengths lie between those of ultraviolet rays and x-rays.

luminous r's rays of the visible spectrum (see under *spectrum*).

medullary r's radii medullares.

parallel r's rays that come from a source at an infinite distance; divergent rays may be made parallel by means of a convex lens or a concave mirror.

positive r's streams of positively charged atoms traveling at high speed from the anode of a partially evacuated tube under the influence of an applied voltage.

reflected r. see *reflection* (def. 2).

refracted r. see *refraction* (def. 2).

roentgen r's x-r's.

Sagnac r's secondary beta rays formed when gamma rays are reflected from a metal surface.

soft r's, soft x-r's x-rays that have a long wavelength, low energy, and little penetrative power.

ultraviolet r's invisible rays that are just beyond the violet end of the visible spectrum; their wavelengths range between 4 and 400 nm; see *ultraviolet.*

W r's intermediate r's.

x-r's electromagnetic waves of short wavelengths (approximately 0.01 to 10 nm) or corresponding quanta (wave mechanics), produced when electrons moving at high velocity impinge on various substances, especially heavy metals. They are commonly generated by passing a current of high voltage (10,000 volts or more) through a Coolidge tube. They can penetrate most substances to some extent, some more readily than others, and transform a photographic plate, which enables their use for *radiography.* They can also cause certain substances to fluoresce, making *fluoroscopy* possible. Because of the high energy of their quanta, they strongly ionize tissue through which they pass by means of the photoelectrons (both primary and secondary) that they liberate. This makes them useful in treatment of various pathological conditions (see *radiotherapy*). Formerly called *roentgen r's.*

Ray•mond-Ces•tan syndrome (ra-maw′ ses-tah′) [F. *Raymond;* Raymond *Cestan,* French neurologist, 1872–1934] see under *syndrome.*

Ray•naud disease (gangrene), phenomenon, sign (ra-no′) [Maurice *Raynaud,* French physician, 1834–1881] see under *disease* and *phenomenon,* and see *acrocyanosis.*

Raz•a•dyne (raz′ə-dīn) trademark for a preparation of galantamine hydrobromide.

ra•zox•ane (ra-zok′sān) an antineoplastic that may reduce the cardiac toxicity of doxorubicin and related antitumor anthracyclines when given in conjunction with those drugs.

Rb rubidium.

RBBB right bundle branch block; see *bundle branch block,* under *block.*

RBC red blood cell; red blood cell count.

RBC IT red blood cell iron turnover.

RBD REM sleep behavior disorder.

RBE relative biological effectiveness.

RBP retinol binding protein.

RCA regulator of complement activation; right coronary artery.

R-CHOP a cancer chemotherapy regimen consisting of rituximab, cyclophosphamide, hydroxydaunomycin (doxorubicin), Oncovin (vincristine), and prednisone.

rCBF regional cerebral blood flow.

RCM Royal College of Midwives.

RCN Royal College of Nursing.

RCOG Royal College of Obstetricians and Gynaecologists.

RCP Royal College of Physicians.

rcp reciprocal translocation.

RCS Royal College of Surgeons.

RCSEd Royal College of Surgeons of Edinburgh.

RCSI Royal College of Physicians in Ireland.

RCT randomized controlled trial.

RCU red cell utilization.

RCVS Royal College of Veterinary Surgeons.

RD reaction of degeneration; Registered Dietitian.

rd rutherford.

RDA recommended dietary allowance; right displacement of the abomasum.

RDE receptor-destroying enzyme.

RE radium emanation (see *radon*); right eye; retinol equivalent.

Re rhenium.

re- [L.] a prefix meaning back or again.

re•ab•sorb (re″əb-sorb′) 1. to absorb again; to undergo or to subject to reabsorption. 2. resorb.

re·ab·sorp·tion (re″ab-sorp′shən) 1. the act or process of absorbing again. 2. resorption.

tubular r. selective reabsorption by the kidneys of substances such as glucose, proteins, or sodium that were previously secreted into the renal tubules, after which they are returned to the circulating blood.

re·act (re-akt′) 1. to respond to a stimulus. 2. to enter into chemical action.

re·ac·tance (re-ak′təns) the part of electric impedance that arises from inductors and capacitors. It is a part of the impedance of electric current flow in an alternating current electric circuit. Symbol *X*.

re·ac·tant (re-ak′tənt) an original substance entering into a chemical reaction.

acute phase r. see under *protein.*

re·ac·tion (re-ak′shən) [*re-* + L. *agere* to act] 1. opposite action, or counteraction. 2. response. 3. the phenomena caused by the action of chemical agents; a chemical process in which one substance is transformed into another substance or substances. For named reactions not defined here, see under *test.* 4. in psychology, the mental and/or emotional state elicited in response to any particular situation.

Reaction

acetic acid r. Rivalta r.

acid r. 1. a reaction in which an acid participates. 2. a surplus of hydrogen ions in a solution or a pH below 7.0. 3. any test by which a surplus of hydrogen ions is recognized, such as the reddening of blue litmus.

acrosome r. a sequence of structural changes seen in spermatozoa in the vicinity of an oocyte in the uterine tube, believed to facilitate their entry into the oocyte: the outer membrane of the acrosome fuses at multiple points with the overlying plasma membrane of the head of the spermatozoon, creating openings through which enzymes of the acrosome are liberated.

acute situational r., acute stress r. a transient, self-limiting acute emotional reaction to severe psychological stress; it is variably defined as comprising one or more of the following DSM-IV categories: *adjustment disorder*, *brief reactive psychosis*, *acute stress disorder*, and *posttraumatic stress disorder.* Called also *transient situational disturbance.*

adjustment r. see under *disorder.*

agglutination r. a positive result on an agglutination test: formation of an aggregate upon mixing soluble antibody with particulate antigen molecules in an aqueous medium; the visible aggregates are formed when specific antibody crosslinks the antigens.

alarm r. the physiologic effects in response to acute stress, fright, or rage (increased blood pressure and cardiac output, increased blood flow to skeletal muscles, decreased flow to the viscera, increased rate of glycolysis and blood glucose concentration), mediated by sympathetic nervous system discharge and release of adrenal medullary hormones; called also *fight-or-flight r.* See also *stress r.*

alkaline r. 1. the presence in a solution of more hydroxyl ions than hydrogen ions, i.e., a pH greater than 7.0. 2. any test by which such a solution is recognized, such as the bluing of red litmus.

allergic r. hypersensitivity r.; used particularly to denote a type I hypersensitivity r.

allograft r. the rejection of an allogeneic graft by a normal host; called also *homograft r.*

alpha-naphthol r. Molisch test (defs. 2, 3).

anamnestic r. see under *response.*

anaphylactic r. anaphylaxis.

anaphylactoid r. a reaction resembling generalized anaphylaxis but not caused by IgE-mediated allergic reaction, instead being due to nonimmunologic degranulation of mast cells with release of the pharmacological mediators involved in anaphylaxis. Called also *anaphylactoid shock.*

anaplerotic r. a reaction that restores the concentration of crucial intermediates that have been depleted in cellular function; called also *anaplerosis.*

anniversary r. abnormal behavior, symptoms, illness, or dreams occurring on the anniversary of a disturbing event.

antibody-mediated cytotoxic hypersensitivity r. type II hypersensitivity r.

antibody-mediated hypersensitivity r. 1. type II hypersensitivity r. 2. occasionally, any hypersensitivity reaction in which antibodies are the primary mediators, as contrasted with those mediated by T lymphocytes; included are *types I, II,* and *III hypersensitivity r's.*

antigen-antibody r. the reversible binding of antigen to homologous antibody brought about by the formation of weak bonds between antigenic determinants on antigen molecules and antigen binding sites on immunoglobulin molecules. Certain effects, e.g., precipitation and agglutination reactions and viral neutralization, result from the binding itself; other effects, e.g., complement activation and opsonization, result from conformational changes that occur in immunoglobulin molecules with antigen binding and enable them to interact with complement proteins and Fc receptors on phagocytes.

antiglobulin r. the agglutination of particles (usually erythrocytes) that have been (1) sensitized by the adsorption of soluble antigen, (2) treated with antibody to that antigen, and (3) treated with antiserum to the serum globulin of the animal species that produced the antibody.

anxiety r. a reaction characterized by abnormal apprehension or uneasiness; see also *anxiety disorders*, under *disorder.*

Arias-Stella r. changes in cells of the endometrial epithelium consisting chiefly of bizarre-shaped hyperchromatic enlarged nuclei and loss of cellular polarity; cytoplasmic vacuolation is occasionally present. It is thought to be associated with presence of chorionic tissue in an intrauterine or extrauterine site and is sometimes seen in ectopic pregnancy.

Arthus r. the development of an inflammatory lesion, with induration, erythema, edema, hemorrhage, and necrosis, a few hours after intradermal injection of antigen into a previously sensitized animal producing precipitating antibody; it is classed as a type III hypersensitivity reaction in the Gell and Coombs classification of immune responses. The lesion results from the precipitation of antigen-antibody complexes, which causes complement activation and the release of complement fragments that are chemotactic for neutrophils; large numbers of neutrophils infiltrate the site and cause tissue destruction by release of lysosomal enzymes. Called also *Arthus phenomenon.*

Arthus-type r. any pathologic process involving the same mechanism as the Arthus reaction, i.e., deposition of immune complexes and complement activation, as in immune complex disease.

associative r. a reaction in which the response is withheld until the idea presented has suggested an associated idea.

axon r., axonal r. the neurodegeneration seen in a neuron following the severing of its axon, including central chromatolysis with displacement of the nucleus; called also *axonal*, *Nissl*, or *retrograde degeneration.*

Bekhterev (Bechterew) r. in cases of tetany, the minimum of electric current needed to arouse muscular contraction needs to be diminished at every interruption or change of density in order to prevent tetanic contraction.

Bence Jones r. the precipitation of protein by heat followed by its redissolving on boiling and being precipitated again on cooling.

Berthelot r. the reaction of ammonia with Berthelot reagent to form phenol-indophenol, a stable, deep blue product; used in colorimetric methods for ammonia and urea.

Bittorf r. in renal colic, the pain produced by squeezing the testicle or pressing the ovary radiates to the kidney.

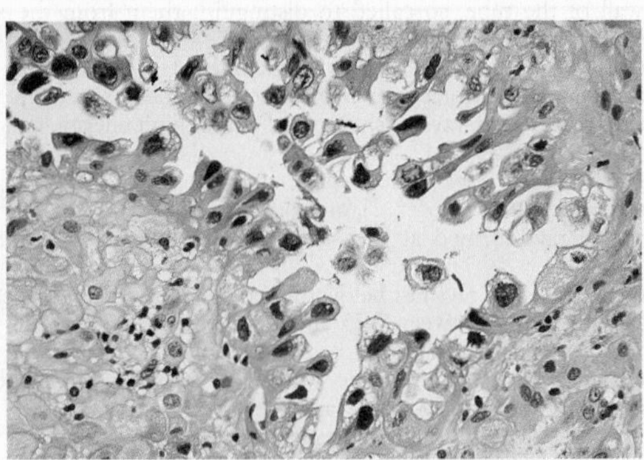

■ Arias-Stella reaction in endometrial mucosa.

biuret r. formation of a chelate having an intense violet-red color when biuret or compounds having two or more adjacent peptide bonds (e.g., proteins) are reacted with copper sulfate in alkaline solution; the reaction forms the basis for a colorimetric method for detection of protein (biuret test).
Bordet-Gengou r. complement fixation.
cadaveric r. total loss of electrical response in the affected muscles in familial periodic paralysis.
Cannizzaro r. the reaction which certain aldehydes may undergo in concentrated alkali; one molecule of the aldehyde is reduced to the corresponding alcohol and another molecule is simultaneously oxidized to the salt of a carboxylic acid.
capsular r. the reaction of the capsular substance of bacteria with a homologous antibody.
carbamino r. alpha-amino acids unite with CO_2 in the presence of alkalis or alkaline earths to form salts of carbamino-carboxylic acids. This reaction is used in studying the course of protein digestion.
Casoni r. see *Casoni intradermal test,* under *test.*
cell-mediated hypersensitivity r. type IV hypersensitivity r.
chromaffin r. the taking on of a deep brown color by tissue of the adrenal medulla or other types that contain the catecholamines epinephrine and norepinephrine, within 12 hours after it is placed in a dichromate solution; this can be used to detect pheochromocytomas and other tumors that produce catecholamines. See also *chromaffin cells,* under *cell.*
cockade r. the reaction of a sensitized guinea pig to intradermal injection of tuberculin; it consists of a large papule with a necrotic, hemorrhagic center.
complement fixation r. see under *fixation.*
congenital leukemoid r. transient myeloproliferative disorder.
conglutination r. a characteristic agglutination reaction obtained by a mixture of conglutinin, cells (e.g., bacteria or red cells), fresh complement, and a cell-specific immune serum from which the agglutinins have been removed by absorption. See *conglutinin.*
consensual r. 1. crossed reflex. 2. an involuntary action that accompanies a voluntary action.
conversion r. see under *disorder.*
cross r. the interaction of an antigen with an antibody formed against a different antigen with which the first antigen shares identical or closely related antigenic determinants.
cutaneous r. a positive reaction indicating immunity or hypersensitivity in a skin test. Called also *skin r., cutireaction,* and *dermoreaction.*
cytotoxic hypersensitivity r. type II hypersensitivity r.
Dale r. an in vitro test for anaphylactic sensitization in the guinea pig: a small amount of the antigen added to a tissue bath in which is immersed the excised uterine horn (smooth muscle) of an anaphylactically sensitized guinea pig causes contraction of the sensitized uterine muscle. Called also *Schultz-Dale r.* NOTE: Schultz employed intestinal muscle; Dale used uterine muscle from virgin guinea pigs.
defense r. see under *mechanism.*
r. of degeneration the reaction to electric stimulation of muscles whose nerves have degenerated. It consists of a loss of response to a faradic stimulus in a muscle and to galvanic and faradic stimulus in a nerve. Galvanic irritability of the muscle is increased. Abbreviated Ea. R. (Ger. *Entartungs-Reaktion*) and RD.
delayed hypersensitivity r. a reaction of cell-mediated immunity, named in contrast to immediate hypersensitivity reactions because its onset is 24 to 72 hours after the antigenic challenge; the term is usually used to denote the subset of type IV hypersensitivity reactions (Gell and Coombs classification) involving cytokine release and macrophage activation, as opposed to direct cytolysis, but can be used more broadly, even sometimes being used synonymously with *type IV hypersensitivity r.* The classic delayed hypersensitivity reaction is the tuberculin reaction observed in skin testing.
depressive r. depression; the term is sometimes used to denote specific types of depression, such as reactive depression, or any of various mood disorders in which depression plays the predominant role.
desmoplastic r. see *desmoplastic.*
diazo r. Ehrlich diazo r.
Dick r. see under *test.*
digitonin r. the formation of a precipitate on treating a sterol, such as cholesterol or ergosterol, with digitonin; employed to define cholesterol esters which do not precipitate in total serum cholesterol determinations.
displacement r. a chemical reaction in which a reactant displaces a functional group from a substrate and becomes bound in the position formerly occupied by the leaving group; see also *displacement.*
dissociative r. see under *disorder.*
dopa r. the reaction by which dopa is changed into melanin under the influence of monophenol monooxygenase.
downgrading r. a type 1 lepra reaction, similar in appearance to the reversal reaction (upgrading reaction), but representing a deterioration in the immune response to *Mycobacterium leprae,* worsening of clinical symptoms, and an increased index of *M. leprae* in the tissues. It may be seen during antileprosy treatment if the strain of *M. leprae* has become drug resistant or the patient has had poor compliance with the drug regimen.
egg yellow r. the appearance of a yellow foam in an Ehrlich diazo reaction before the addition of ammonia, thought to indicate acute pneumonia.
Ehrlich aldehyde r. the reaction of urobilinogen with *p*-dimethylaminobenzene to form a red-colored substance; used for semiquantitative determination of urobilinogen in urine and feces.
Ehrlich diazo r. a reaction of a pure pink or red color resulting from the action of diazotized sulfanilic acid and ammonia upon certain aromatic substances, e.g., urobilinogen, found in the urine in some conditions. This reaction has diagnostic value in hepatic disease, typhoid fever, and measles and prognostic value in tuberculosis.
erythrocyte sedimentation r. see under *rate.*
r. of exhaustion reaction to electric stimulation seen in conditions of exhaustion. In it the reaction normally produced by a certain current can be reproduced only by an increase in the current.
Fernandez r. a delayed hypersensitivity reaction in the lepromin test.
Feulgen r. a specific histochemical reaction for DNA: after acid hydrolysis at 60°C, tissue sections are stained in Schiff reagent; DNA stains magenta.
fight-or-flight r. alarm r.
foreign body r. a granulomatous inflammatory reaction evoked by the presence of an exogenous material in the tissues, a characteristic feature of which is the formation of foreign body giant cells.
fuchsinophil r. a reaction seen when certain substances that have been stained with fuchsin retain the stain on being treated with picric acid alcohol.
graft-versus-host r. see under *disease.*
Grignard r. see under *reagent.*
group r. see under *agglutination.*
hemagglutination-inhibition r. the inhibition by antibodies of viral agglutination of red cells.
hemianopic pupillary r. reaction in certain cases of hemianopia in which the stimulus of light thrown upon one side of the retina causes the iris to contract, while light thrown on the other side arouses no response. Called also *Wernicke r.*
Henle r. a staining dark brown of the cells of the adrenal medulla on treatment with chromium salts.
Herxheimer r. Jarisch-Herxheimer r.
homograft r. allograft r.
hunting r. periods of vasoconstriction alternating with periods of vasodilatation in a finger or other part exposed to temperatures below 15°C, as if the body were hunting for an equilibrium point of skin temperature.
hypersensitivity r. a reaction in which the body mounts an exaggerated or inappropriate immune response to a substance either foreign or perceived as foreign, resulting in local or general tissue damage. Such reactions are usually classified as types I–IV on the basis of the Gell and Coombs classification (q.v.).

type I a hypersensitivity reaction that occurs within minutes when a sensitized individual is reexposed to antigen, resulting from interaction of IgE and the antigen; clinical manifestations can range from localized dermatitis, urticaria, or angioedema to allergic rhinitis or asthma to systemic anaphylaxis. The first exposure to the antigen induces the production of IgE antibodies that bind to receptors on mast cells and basophils. Upon subsequent exposure the antigen cross-links receptor-bound IgE molecules, triggering production and release of a diverse array of mediators that act on other cells, producing symptoms such as bronchospasm, edema, mucous secretion, and inflammation. Called also *immediate hypersensitivity r.*

type II tissue or cell damage resulting from the interaction of antibodies and antigens on cell surfaces; specific IgG or IgM against cell surface or extracellular matrix antigens or cell surface receptors binds and causes damage at the site

Reaction *Continued*

of binding by any of several mechanisms involving either complement activation and lysis or opsonization mediated by receptors for Fc or C3b, leading to phagocytosis and destruction by macrophages and neutrophils. Examples of disorders caused by such tissue damage include myasthenia gravis, hemolytic anemia, Goodpasture syndrome, and Rh incompatibility and transfusion reactions. Called also *antibody-mediated hypersensitivity r.* and *cytotoxic hypersensitivity r.*

type III local or general inflammatory response due to formation of circulating antigen-antibody complexes and their deposition in tissues; the complexes activate complement and other inflammatory mediators, initiating processes including increased vascular permeability, stimulation of mast cell degranulation and neutrophil chemotaxis and accumulation, and aggregation of platelets, and resulting in tissue damage. Ensuing diseases, called also *immune complex diseases,* can be roughly classified as being due to persistent infection, to autoimmunity, or to inhalation of antigenic material; examples include serum sickness, Arthus reaction, subacute bacterial endocarditis, systemic lupus erythematosus, and farmer's lung. Called also *immune complex–mediated hypersensitivity r.*

type IV a reaction of cell-mediated immunity, the immune response being initiated by antigen-specific T lymphocytes; in contrast to the reactions of immediate hypersensitivity, reactions take one or more days to develop and can be transferred by lymphocytes but not by serum. Reactions are mediated by T lymphocytes both through release of cytokines and through direct cytolysis. In the former mechanism, release of vasoactive and chemotactic cytokines is triggered by contact between the T cells and specific antigens on antigen-presenting cells; the cytokines attract and activate non–antigen-specific monocytes and macrophages, resulting in local erythema and induration, and leading to granuloma formation and necrosis if the eliciting stimulus cannot be eliminated. A common example is the tuberculin reaction elicited in skin testing for tuberculosis. In direct cytolysis, sometimes called *cell-mediated cytotoxicity,* cytotoxic T lymphocytes interact with foreign antigens presented by class I MHC molecules on cell surfaces, causing lysis of these foreign cells, as in allograft rejection. Type IV reactions can be induced by intracellular parasites, such as certain viruses, mycobacteria, and fungi, foreign tissue, tumor cells, soluble proteins, and haptens. The term is often equated with *delayed hypersensitivity reaction,* although the latter term is sometimes restricted to cytokine-mediated reactions (as contrasted with direct cytolysis). Called also *cell-mediated* or *T cell–mediated hypersensitivity r.*

id r. a sterile secondary skin eruption occurring in sensitized patients as a result of circulation of allergenic products from a primary site of infection; the morphology and site of the lesion vary.

r. of identity a reaction pattern seen in double diffusion in two dimensions: the precipitin lines between the antigen wells and the antiserum well stop at their point of intersection, indicating that the antigen samples are identical. See also *r. of nonidentity* and *r. of partial identity.* See illustration.

immediate hypersensitivity r. 1. type I hypersensitivity r. 2. occasionally, any hypersensitivity reaction mediated by antibodies and developing rapidly, generally in minutes to hours (i.e., *type I, II,* or *III hypersensitivity r.*), as distinguished from those mediated by T lymphocytes and macrophages and generally requiring 24 to 72 hours to develop (*type IV hypersensitivity r's,* sometimes called *delayed hypersensitivity r's*).

immune r. see under *response.*

immune complex–mediated hypersensitivity r. type III hypersensitivity r.

intracutaneous r., intradermal r. the reaction to an intracutaneous injection of antigen in a skin test.

Jaffe r. creatinine when treated with picric acid in strongly alkaline solution gives an intense red color.

Jarisch-Herxheimer r. a transient, short-term immunologic reaction commonly seen following antibiotic treatment of syphilis and less often in other diseases, such as borreliosis, brucellosis, typhoid fever, and trichinellosis. Manifestations include fever, chills, headache, myalgias, and exacerbation of cutaneous lesions. The reaction has been attributed to liberation of endotoxin-like substances or antigens from the killed or dying microorganisms, but its exact pathogenesis is unclear. Called also *Herxheimer r.*

johnin r. a skin reaction like the tuberculin reaction, produced by filtrates of cultures of *Mycobacterium avium* subsp. *paratuberculosis* (see *johnin*); used in the diagnosis of Johne disease in cattle.

Jolly r. failure of response to faradic stimulation in a muscle, the power of voluntary contraction as well as the response to galvanic stimulation being retained.

Jones-Mote r. a weak type IV hypersensitivity reaction to protein antigens associated with basophil infiltration, occurring on challenge a few days after priming with a protein antigen in aqueous solution or in Freund incomplete adjuvant. Called also *cutaneous basophil hypersensitivity.*

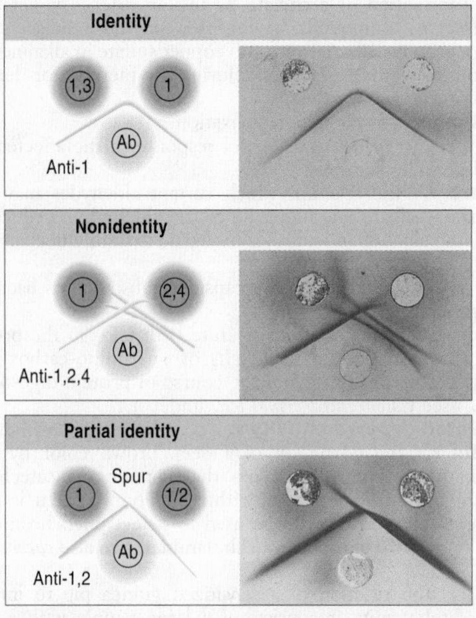

■ Double diffusion used to indicate the relationship between antigens *(blue, with numerals indicating epitopes present)* and a particular test antibody *(yellow). (Top),* Reaction of identity; the antibody is precipitating identical epitopes in each preparation. *(Middle),* Reaction of nonidentity; the antibody preparation distinguishes the three different antigens, each of which forms an arc. *(Bottom),* Reaction of partial identity; the antibody preparation reacts with both epitopes, forming a line of identity (anti–epitope 1) with the addition of a spur of nonidentity (anti–epitope 2).

late phase r. an IgE-mediated immune reaction occurring 5 to 8 hours after exposure to antigen, after the wheal and flare reactions of immediate hypersensitivity have diminished; it is characterized by inflammation, with accumulation of neutrophils, basophils, eosinophils, and $CD4^+$ T lymphocytes, pruritus, and minor cellular infiltration. Prostaglandins are not formed. Inflammation subsides after reaching a maximum around 24 hours after exposure.

lengthening r. the elongation of the extensor muscles which permits flexion of a limb.

lepra r. an acute or subacute hypersensitivity reaction occurring either during the course of antileprosy treatment or in untreated cases of leprosy. There are two types, now often called *type 1* and *type 2.* Type 1 includes the *reversal* or *upgrading reaction* and the *downgrading reaction,* which are delayed hypersensitivity reactions. Type 2 is *erythema nodosum leprosum,* a type III hypersensitivity reaction.

lepromin r. either of the results of a lepromin test; see *Fernandez r.* and *Mitsuda r.*

leukemic r., leukemoid r. a peripheral blood picture resembling that of leukemia or indistinguishable from it on the basis of morphologic appearance alone, with leukocytosis of varying degrees and increased numbers of immature cells in circulation. It may be seen with infections such as tuberculosis, brucellosis, toxoplasmosis, staphylococcal infections, and streptococcal infections; with inflammatory disorders such as glomerulonephritis, rheumatoid arthritis, liver failure, and diabetic acidosis; with tumors and granulomatous infiltration of bone marrow; and with intoxications such as eclampsia, severe burns, and mercury poisoning.

Liebermann-Burchard r. see under *test.*

ligase chain r. a type of DNA amplification technique that uses DNA ligase to link adjacent pairs of synthetic oligonucleotides that have been hybridized to complementary regions on each strand of the double-stranded target DNA, with the product used as a template for subsequent cycles of amplification of the sequence in question. Because the ligation reaction requires perfect base pairing, sequence variation at the ligation site can be demonstrated.

Loeb decidual r. the presence of a glass bead or other irritant causes the formation of a small deciduoma in the uterine mucosa when corpora lutea are developing normally.
Lohmann r. an easily reversible reaction occurring in muscle, in which the high-energy phosphate bond of ATP is transferred to creatine, forming creatine phosphate; the reaction is catalyzed by creatine kinase.
Machado-Guerreiro r., Machado-Guerreiro r. see under *test.*
manic-depressive r. former name for bipolar disorder; see *bipolar disorders* (def. 2), under *disorder.*
Mantoux r. see under *test.*
Marchi r. failure of the degenerated myelin sheath of a nerve to become discolored when treated with osmic acid.
Mazzotti r. the set of adverse reactions, which may be severe or rarely life-threatening, that accompany the administration of diethylcarbamazine in onchocerciasis, most commonly an intensely pruritic rash, but sometimes also systemic manifestations such as fever, malaise, lymph node swelling, eosinophilia, arthralgias, tachycardia, and hypotension; if numerous microfilariae are present in the eyes, blindness may occur. See also *Mazzotti test*, under *test.*
Mitsuda r. the appearance of a wheal after three or four weeks in the *lepromin test.*
mixed agglutination r. agglutination of a mixture of different cell types by antibody directed against an antigenic determinant present on all of the cells.
mixed leukocyte r., mixed lymphocyte r. see under *culture.*
Molisch r. see under *test.*
Moloney r. see under *test.*
Montenegro r. see *leishmanin test*, under *test.*
myasthenic r. progressively diminished response of a muscle to repeated electric stimuli.
Nagler r. the formation of an opaque zone around colonies of *Clostridium perfringens* on egg yolk agar, produced by the action of a diffusible lecithinase.
near-point r. constriction of the pupil when the gaze is fixed on a near point.
Neufeld r. when pneumococci and other capsulated microorganisms are mixed with specific immune serum there occurs in addition to agglutination a swelling (Ger. *quellung*) of the capsules of the organisms, owing to the binding of antibody with the capsular polysaccharide; called also *capsular swelling* and *quellung r.*
neurotonic r. muscular contraction persisting after the stimulus which produced it has ceased.
neutral r. the presence of an equal number of H^{+} and OH^{-} ions in a solution, i.e., a pH of 7.0.
Ninhydrin r. see *triketohydrindene hydrate test*, under *test.*
r. of nonidentity a reaction pattern seen in double diffusion in two dimensions: the precipitin lines between the antigen wells and the antiserum well cross, indicating that the antigen samples have no antigenic determinants in common. See also *r. of identity* and *r. of partial identity.*
obsessive-compulsive r. see under *disorder.*
Oestreicher r. xanthydrol r.
orbicularis r. orbicularis pupillary reflex.
oxidation-reduction r. redox r.
pain r. dilatation of the pupil on a feeling of pain.
parallergic r. see *parallergy.*
r. of partial identity a reaction pattern seen in double diffusion in two dimensions: one of the precipitin lines between the antigen wells and the antiserum well stops at the point of intersection, whereas the other continues past it, indicating that the antigen samples have some, but not all, antigenic determinants in common. See also *r. of identity* and *r. of nonidentity.*
PAS r. periodic acid–Schiff r.
passive cutaneous anaphylaxis r. passive cutaneous anaphylaxis.
passive cutaneous Arthus r. a variation of the Arthus reaction in which a nonimmune host is inoculated with large quantities of precipitating antibody intravenously, followed by local cutaneous inoculation of antigen.
Pasteur r. see under *effect.*
Paul-Bunnell r. see under *test.*
periodic acid–Schiff r. a tissue section is exposed to periodic acid, which oxidizes hydroxyl groups on adjacent carbon atoms or adjacent hydroxyl groups and amino groups to aldehydes, and then is stained with Schiff reagent, which forms an additional product with aldehydes to produce a red or magenta reaction product; used to test for glycogen, epithelial mucins, neutral polysaccharides, and glycoproteins. Called also *PAS r.*
peroxidase r. the appearance of deep-blue granules in leukocytes of marrow origin when stained with Goodpasture stain, distinguishing them from cells of lymphatic origin.
Pfeiffer r. see under *phenomenon.*
phobic r. phobic disorder; see *phobia.*
photochemical r. photoreaction.
P-K r. Prausnitz-Küstner r.
polymerase chain r. (PCR) a type of rapid nucleic acid amplification of specific DNA or RNA sequences, allowing small quantities of short sequences to be analyzed without cloning: oligonucleotide primers are annealed to single-stranded nucleotide sequences, which are copied by polymerase; the number of copies is geometrically amplified by repeated cycles of annealing and copying.
Porter-Silber r. the reaction of the dihydroxyacetone side chain of certain 17-hydroxycorticosteroids (Porter-Silber chromogens) with phenylhydrazine in acid, which produces a yellow color; an index of adrenocortical function now largely supplanted by immunoassay techniques.
Prausnitz-Küstner r. a type I hypersensitivity reaction produced in a nonatopic subject by intradermal injection of serum from an atopic subject, followed 12 or more hours later by an injection of antigen into the same site; the presence of specific IgE antibody in the transferred serum results in a classic wheal and flare reaction to the antigen. Once the standard method of demonstrating IgE, this test is no longer used because of the risk of transmitting hepatitis and because serum IgE can now be measured by in vitro assays, e.g., RAST and RIST. Called also *P-K r.* or *test* and *Prausnitz-Küstner test.*
precipitin r. the formation of an insoluble precipitate by reaction of antigen and antibody; it occurs only with multivalent antigens and is dependent on electrolyte concentration, pH, temperature, and the relative concentrations of antigen and antibody, the amount of precipitate formed increasing to a maximum and then decreasing as the relative antigen concentration is increased.
prozone r. see *prozone.*
pseudoallergic r. a clinical state exhibiting what appear to be the signs and symptoms of an immediate hypersensitivity reaction but with no evidence for an immunologic mechanism.
psychotic depressive r. psychosis characterized by depressed mood resulting from a specific event, usually in a patient without prior history of severe depression; the condition has been incorporated into major depressive disorder.
quellung r. [Ger. "swelling"] Neufeld r.
redox r. a reaction in which there is transfer of electrons from an electron donor (the reducing agent) to an electron acceptor (the oxidizing agent).
reversal r. a type 1 lepra reaction usually occurring during chemotherapy in borderline leprosy. It is a type of delayed hypersensitivity

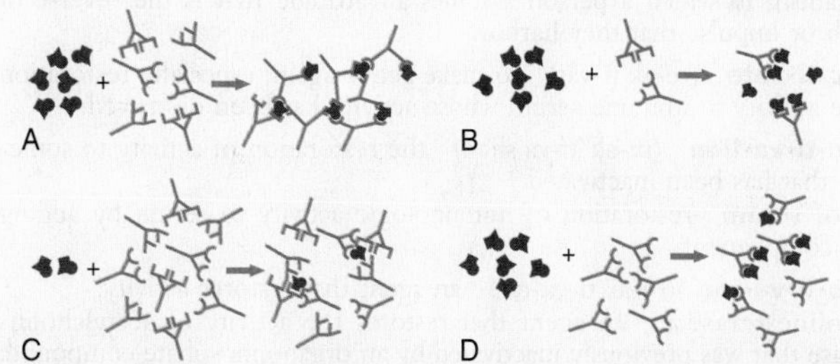

■ Schematic of precipitin reactions with different proportions of antigen and antibody. Antigenic proteins that elicit antibody responses are depicted as having three different antibody-binding sites on their surface. Polyclonal antibodies with three different specificities (box, triangle, circle) are also depicted. *(A)*, Under conditions of antigen–antibody equivalence, there is maximum cross-linking and visible precipitin formation. *(B)*, With antigen excess, the resulting small soluble immune complexes do not form a visible precipitate. *(C)*, With antibody excess, small soluble complexes are also formed; lattice formation is insufficient to cause visible precipitation. *(D)*, Under conditions of equivalence but in the presence of monoclonal, rather than polyclonal, antibodies, each antigen binds only at a single site; there is no cross-linking and no visible precipitate.

Reaction *Continued*

reaction with "upgrading" of cell-mediated immunity to *Mycobacterium leprae;* this process tends to move the disease toward the tuberculoid pole. The reaction is chiefly characterized by erythema, edema, tenderness of preexisting quiescent lesions, appearance of new lesions, neuritis with nerve damage, fever, adenopathy, and an elevated leukocyte count. Called also *upgrading r.* See also *downgrading r.*

reverse passive Arthus r. the reaction produced when precipitating antibody is inoculated into a skin site in an experimental animal, followed in 30 minutes to 2 hours by inoculation of the homologous antigen, either intravenously or intracutaneously at the same site. Thus the usual anatomical locations of precipitating antibody and antigen in an Arthus reaction are reversed.

reversible r. a chemical reaction that may occur in either direction, depending on conditions; the products may react to re-form the reactants.

righting r's responses of the head and eyes that occur as the body processes sensory input from the visual and vestibular systems; they maintain the orientation of the head and body with respect to the vertical.

Rivalta r. a reaction for distinguishing fluids of transudation and exudation, utilizing acetic acid.

Schick r. see under *test.*

Schultz-Dale r. see *Dale r.*

second set r. see under *phenomenon.*

Selivanoff r. see under *test.*

serological r., serum r. seroreaction.

serum sickness–like r. see *serum sickness,* under *sickness.*

shortening r. the shortening that succeeds the lengthening reaction when a limb is brought back into the extended position.

Shwartzman r., generalized a generalized reaction following two intravenous injections of endotoxin separated by 24 hours; it is characterized by widespread hemorrhages, bilateral cortical necrosis of the kidneys, and a marked fall in leukocyte and platelet counts and usually results in death of the animal.

Shwartzman r., localized a localized cutaneous reaction consisting of vascular necrosis, petechial hemorrhages, and leukocyte infiltration that occurs at the site of an original subcutaneous injection of endotoxin approximately 24 hours after an intravenous injection of the same or another endotoxin given at a site other than the original injection site.

skin r. cutaneous r.

startle r. the various psychophysiological phenomena, including involuntary motor and autonomic reactions, evidenced by an individual in reaction to a sudden, unexpected stimulus, as a loud noise.

Straus r. when material containing virulent glanders bacilli is inoculated into the peritoneal cavity of male guinea pigs, scrotal lesions develop; called also *Straus phenomenon.*

stress r. any of the biological reactions to adverse stimuli, physical, mental, or emotional, internal or external, that tend to disturb the organism's homeostasis; should these compensating reactions, physiological or psychological, be inadequate or inappropriate, they may lead to disorders. See *alarm r.* and *acute stress r.;* see *general adaptation syndrome,* under *syndrome;* and see *acute stress disorder, adjustment disorder,* and *posttraumatic stress disorder,* under *disorder.*

substitution r. a chemical reaction in which one atom or functional group replaces another in a molecule.

sympathetic stress r. alarm r.

T cell–mediated hypersensitivity r. type IV hypersensitivity r.

tendon r. see under *reflex.*

toxin-antitoxin r. the antigen-antibody reaction between a toxin and antitoxin.

transfusion r. any symptoms due to agglutination or hemolysis of the recipient's blood cells when blood for transfusion is incorrectly matched (see *crossmatching*), or when the recipient has a hypersensitivity reaction to some element of the donor blood.

trigger r. see under *action.*

tuberculin r. induration or vesiculation as a delayed reaction at the site of a tuberculin test (q.v.), a positive result.

Turnbull blue r. blue-black coloration produced when tissue containing chemically active iron is treated with potassium ferrocyanide and hydrochloric acid.

upgrading r. reversal r.

vasovagal r. see under *syncope.*

vestibular pupillary r. dilatation of the pupils arising from stimulation of the external auditory canal.

Voges-Proskauer r. see under *test.*

Wassermann r. see under *test.*

Weil-Felix r. see under *test.*

Wernicke r. hemianopic pupillary r.

wheal and erythema r., wheal and flare r. the characteristic local cutaneous reaction consisting of an elevated, blanched wheal surrounded by a spreading "flare" of erythema that occurs within a few minutes at the site of a minor nonpenetrating skin injury and also in response to administration of allergen to an atopic individual; it is caused by release of histamine from mast cells.

white-graft r. an immune reaction to a tissue graft, e.g., a skin graft, as a result of which the grafted tissue does not become vascularized due to rapid rejection.

Widal r. see under *test.*

xanthydrol r. when tissue from a uremic patient is fixed in a solution of xanthydrol in glacial acetic acid, a large deposit of xanthydrol occurs in the tissue.

zed r. a reaction that appears in infants in cases of starvation after the starvation is relieved; it consists of a slight gain in weight, elevation of temperature, and the appearance of watery feces containing a large number of cells.

---

re•ac•tion-for•ma•tion (re-ak′shən for-ma′shən) a type of defense mechanism in which a person assumes an attitude that is the reverse of a wish or impulse that they harbor.

re•ac•ti•vate (re-ak′tĭ-vāt) to make active again; especially restoration of the activity to immune serum whose activity has been destroyed.

re•ac•ti•va•tion (re-ak″tĭ-va′shən) the restoration of activity to something that has been inactivated.

r. of serum restoration of immunologic activity to serum by adding fresh complement.

re•ac•ti•va•tor (re-ak′tĭ-va-tər) an agent that restores activity.

cholinesterase r. an agent that restores the activity of acetylcholinesterase that was previously inactivated by an organophosphate compound; see *pralidoxime.*

re•ac•tive (re-ak′tiv) characterized by reaction; readily responsive to a stimulus.

re•ac•tiv•i•ty (re″ak-tiv′ĭ-te) 1. the process or property of being reactive. 2. in electroencephalography, the capability of alternation of a given pattern of electrical activity upon sensory stimulation or other physiological change.

persistent light r. chronic actinic dermatitis.

re•ac•to•gen•ic (re-ak″to-jen′ik) [*reaction* + *-genic*] causing an excessive local or systemic reaction; said of vaccine.

read•ing (rēd′ing) understanding of written or printed symbols representing words.

lip r., speech r. the understanding of speech through observation of the movement of the lips of the speaker. Called also *visual hearing.*

re•a•gent (re-a′jənt) [*re-* + *agent*] a substance employed to produce a chemical reaction so as to detect, measure, produce, etc., other substances.

amino-acid r. a 0.5 per cent solution of sodium β-naphthoquinone-4-sulfonate freshly prepared.

arsenic–sulfuric acid r. Rosenthaler r.

Benedict r. any of several alkaline copper sulfate solutions used for Benedict test for glucose.

Berthelot r. an alkaline solution of phenol and hypochlorite, used in the Berthelot reaction.

Bial r. orcinol 1.5 g, fuming hydrochloric acid 500 g, ferric chloride (10 per cent) 20–30 drops.

biuret r. any of various alkaline copper sulfate solutions containing a variety of stabilizers, used in the biuret reaction (q.v.).

Bogg r. dissolve 25 g of phosphotungstic acid in 125 mL of water. Dilute 25 mL of concentrated hydrochloric acid to 100 mL. Mix the two solutions.

diazo r. a reagent consisting of two solutions which are mixed just prior to the test in the proportion of 25 mL of solution *A* to 0.75 mL of *B.* Solution *A:* sulfanilic acid, 1 g; distilled water, 1000 mL. Solution *B:* sodium nitrite, 0.5 g: distilled water, 100 mL.

Ehrlich aldehyde r. 4 g of paradimethylaminobenzaldehyde in a mixture of 80 mL of concentrated hydrochloric acid and 380 mL of ethyl alcohol.

Ehrlich diazo r. Solution *A:* dissolve 5 g of sodium nitrite in 1 L of distilled water. Solution *B:* dissolve 5 g of sulfanilic acid and 50 mL of hydrochloric acid in 1 L of distilled water. For use mix 1 part of *A* with 50 to 100 parts of *B.*

Fouchet r. 1.0 g ferric chloride and 25.0 g trichloroacetic acid dissolved in water to make 100 mL; see *Fouchet test,* under *test.*

general r. a reagent that indicates the general class of bodies to which a substance belongs.

Grignard r. any of several compounds of magnesium with an organic radical and a halogen; these reagents undergo reactions with many substances, producing important products.

Lloyd r. an especially fine preparation of fuller's earth obtained by elutriation; used to absorb alkaloids from solutions.

Millon r. see under *test.*

Nessler r. an aqueous solution of 5 per cent potassium iodide, 2.5 per cent mercury bichloride, and 16 per cent potassium hydroxide; used as a test for ammonia.

Ninhydrin r. trademark for a preparation of triketohydrindene hydrate.

Rosenthaler r. *(for alkaloids),* 1 part of potassium arsenate in 100 parts of concentrated sulfuric acid.

Schiff r. a reagent for testing for the presence of aldehydes, prepared by dissolving 0.25 g of fuchsin in 1 liter of water and decolorizing by passing sulfur dioxide into it. In the presence of aldehyde the blue color is restored.

Scott-Wilson r. add 90 g sodium hydroxide in solution to 5 g mercuric cyanide in solution, then add 1.45 g silver nitrate solution with constant stirring.

splenic r. any drug or stimulus which causes the spleen to contract.

re•a•gin (re′ə-jin) [*reagent* + *-in*] 1. the antibody that mediates type I hypersensitivity reactions; in humans, IgE. 2. former name for the serum antibody detected by the Wassermann test.

re•a•gin•ic (re″ə-jin′ik) pertaining to reagin.

re•al•gar (re′al-gahr″) [Ar. *rahj al-ghar* powder of the mine] arsenic disulfide, As_2S_2: a pigment.

real-time (rēl′tīm) capable of updating information as quickly as it is received, so that the data can be used to create continuously updated output, such as a moving video display; see under *ultrasonography.*

ream•er (rēm′ər) in root canal therapy, an engine-driven or hand-operated instrument for canal enlargement, consisting of a serrated triangular shaft twisted into a loosely spiraled form.

re•an•i•ma•tion (re-an″ĭ-ma′shən) the process of restoring life or liveliness.

eye r. microsurgical restoration of function of a paralyzed eye sphincter.

facial r. the use of surgical procedures to improve facial appearance and motion in facial paralysis.

re•at•tach•ment (re″ə-tach′mənt) 1. joining together parts that have been separated. 2. the recementing of a dental crown or other prosthesis. 3. embedding of new periodontal ligament fibers into new cementum and the attachment of gingival epithelium to tooth surface previously denuded by disease.

Ré•au•mur scale, thermometer (ra″o-mūr′) [René Antoine Feschault de *Réaumur,* French naturalist, 1683–1757] see under *scale* and *thermometer.*

re•base (re-bās′) to refit a denture by means of the replacement of the denture base material without changing the occlusal relations of the teeth.

Reb•e•tol (reb′ə-tol) trademark for a preparation of ribavirin.

Reb•e•tron (reb′ə-tron) trademark for a packaged combination of Rebetol (ribavirin) and Intron A (interferon alfa-2b).

re•bound (re′bound) a reversed response on the withdrawal of a stimulus; see also under *phenomenon* and *tenderness.*

acid r. an increased rate of gastric acid secretion occurring 30 to 60 minutes after eating.

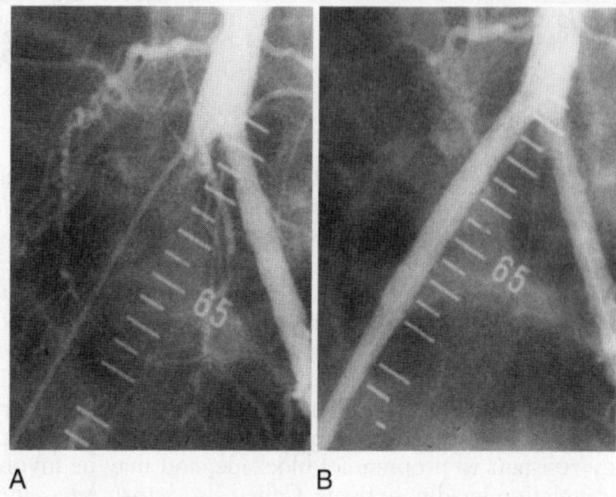

■ Recanalization. Occlusion of right common iliac artery *(A)* treated by recanalization and stent placement *(B).*

adiposity r. an increase in body mass index that normally occurs at about age six following a steady decline during early childhood.

heparin r. the return of anticoagulant activity following neutralization of heparin in a patient's blood by protamine.

REM r. the phenomenon in which a subject deprived of REM (rapid eye movement) sleep for a prolonged period will, on being permitted to sleep undisturbed, compensate by having increased REM sleep.

urea r. a sudden increase in release of urea into the bloodstream by cells and organs that normally store it, seen in the first 15 minutes to an hour after urea has been removed by dialysis; this is caused by flow-volume dysequilibrium.

re•cal•ci•fi•ca•tion (re-kal″sĭ-fĭ-ka′shən) the restoration of calcium salts to the bodily tissues.

re•call[1] (re-kawl′) to remember or recollect.

re•call[2] (re′kawl) the process of bringing information back into consciousness.

re•can•a•li•za•tion (re-kan″ə-lĭ-za′shən) formation of new canals or paths, especially blood vessels, through an obstruction such as a clot. Called also *canalization.*

re•ca•pit•u•la•tion (re″kə-pit″u-la′shən) see under *theory.*

re•cei•ver (re-sēv′ər) 1. a vessel for collecting a gas or a distillate. 2. the portion of an apparatus by which electric energy is converted into signals which may be seen or heard.

re•cep•tac•u•lum (re″səp-tak′u-ləm) pl. *receptac′ula* [L., from *recipere* to receive] a receptacle or container; that which serves for receiving or containing something.

r. chy′li cisterna chyli.

r. gan′glii petro′si fossula petrosa.

r. Pecquet′i cisterna chyli.

re•cep•tive (re-cep′tiv) capable of receiving or of responding to a stimulus.

re•cep•tor (re-sep′tər) [L. *recipere* to receive, accept] 1. a molecular structure within a cell or on the cell surface and characterized by (1) selective binding of a specific substance and (2) a specific physiologic effect that accompanies the binding, e.g., membrane receptors for peptide hormones, neurotransmitters, antigens, complement fragments, and immunoglobulins, and nuclear receptors for steroid hormones. 2. a sensory nerve terminal that responds to stimuli of various kinds; classified in various ways including by the type of stimulus (see *chemoreceptor, mechanoreceptor, photoreceptor,* and *thermoreceptor*) and by the location in the body (see *exteroceptor, interoceptor,* and *proprioceptor*).

Receptor

α-adrenergic r's adrenergic receptors that respond to norepinephrine and to such blocking agents as phenoxybenzamine and phentolamine. They are subdivided into two types: α_1, found in smooth muscle, heart, and liver, with effects including vasoconstriction, intestinal relaxation, uterine contraction and pupillary dilation, and α_2, found in platelets, vascular smooth muscle, nerve termini, and pancreatic islets, with effects including platelet aggregation, vasoconstriction, and inhibition of norepinephrine release and of insulin secretion. Called also *alpha* or *alpha-adrenergic receptors.*

adrenergic r. a site on an effector organ innervated by postganglionic adrenergic fibers of the sympathetic nervous system, classified as either α-adrenergic or β-adrenergic according to its reaction to

norepinephrine and epinephrine, as well as to certain blocking and stimulating agents. Called also *adrenoceptor* and *adrenoreceptor.*
alpha r's, alpha-adrenergic r's α-adrenergic r's.
β-adrenergic r's adrenergic receptors that respond particularly to epinephrine and to such blocking agents as propranolol. They are subdivided into two basic types: β_1, found in the myocardium and causing lipolysis and cardiac stimulation, and β_2, found in smooth and skeletal muscle and liver and causing bronchodilation, vasodilation, and increased presynaptic release of norepinephrine. A third type, β_3, is atypical; it is more sensitive to norepinephrine than to epinephrine, is relatively resistant to propranolol blockade, and may be involved in lipolysis regulation in adipose tissue. Called also *beta* or *beta-adrenergic r's.*
B cell antigen r's monomeric IgM, IgD, and (on memory cells only) IgG that is attached to the cell membrane of B lymphocytes and which, in conjunction with T cell help, triggers B cell activation on contact with antigen.
beta r's, beta-adrenergic r's β-adrenergic r's.
cell-surface r. membrane r.
cholinergic r. a type of cell-surface receptor that binds the neurotransmitter acetylcholine and mediates its action on postjunctional cells. Types include parasympathetic autonomic effector cells, sympathetic and parasympathetic autonomic ganglion cells, striated muscle, and certain central neurons. Two classes are often distinguished: *muscarinic r's* and *nicotinic r's.* Called also *cholinoceptor.*
cold r. a cutaneous thermoreceptor particularly sensitive to temperatures between 15°and 35°C. See also *paradoxical cold response,* under *response.*
complement r's cell-surface receptors for products of complement reactions, with roles including recognition of pathogens, phagocytosis, adhesion, and clearance of immune complexes. At least nine types exist, with the best characterized being CR1–4, which bind C3 fragments already bound to a surface. Other complement receptors are named according to ligand (e.g., C5a receptor).

CR1 CD35 or C3b receptor; a membrane glycoprotein specific for C3b and C4b and expressed on erythrocytes and many other cell types including neutrophils, monocytes, T and B lymphocytes, and eosinophils; its roles include inhibition of C3 convertases, stimulation of phagocytosis of complement-coated particles and microorganisms, and clearance of immune complexes from the circulation.

CR2 CD21 or C3d receptor; a single-chain membrane glycoprotein present on B lymphocytes, follicular dendritic cells, and certain epithelial cells; it is specific for complement fragments iC3b and C3dg, produced by cleavage of bound C3b by factor I and is involved in B lymphocyte activation. CR2 is the Epstein-Barr virus receptor and also binds interferon-α.

CR3 glycoprotein Mac-1.

CR4 a β_2 integrin (CD11c/CD18) expressed on monocytes, macrophages, neutrophils, and NK cells that binds to inactivated C3b (iC3b) and to the fragment C3dg and also mediates leukocyte adhesion. It is involved in both Fc receptor–mediated and Fc-independent phagocytosis. It comprises an α and a β chain; the latter is common also to CR3. Called also *glycoprotein p150,95* and *p150,95.*

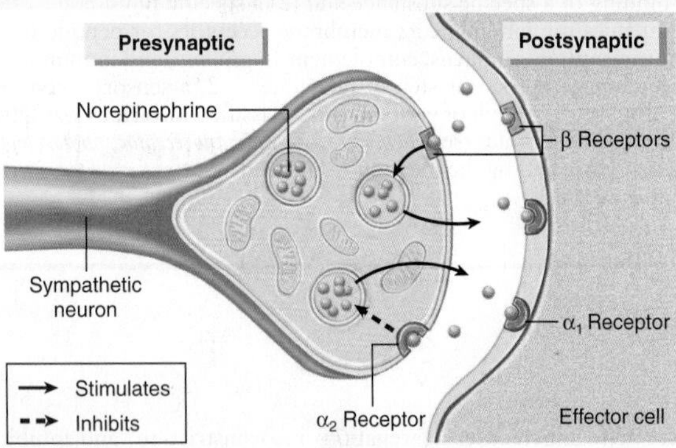

■ Adrenergic receptor; simplified schematic view of adrenergic nerve ending and the effector cell with its receptors. When norepinephrine is released, it enters the synaptic cleft to bind to α_1- and β-adrenergic receptors on the effector cell; there is also a short feedback loop in which norepinephrine binds to α_2- and β-adrenergic receptors on the neuron to inhibit or stimulate further release, respectively.

contact r. mechanoreceptor.
cutaneous r. any of the various types of sense organs found in the dermis or epidermis, usually a mechanoreceptor, thermoreceptor, or nociceptor; see also *exteroceptor.*
cytokine r's transmembrane proteins that bind cytokines via extracellular domains, acting to convert an extracellular signal to an intracellular one; they are divided into families on the basis of sequence homologies and folding motifs.
distance r. teleceptor.
dopaminergic r's receptors that are stimulated by the neurotransmitter dopamine and mediate the activation (by D_1 receptors) and inactivation (by D_2 receptors) of adenylate cyclase.
estrogen r. (ER) a type of nuclear receptor consisting of a cellular regulatory protein that binds estrogens, found on nearly all cell types, but particularly in estrogen-sensitive tissues such as the uterus and breast. Cytoplasmic levels are measured in surgically removed breast carcinoma; high levels indicate that a positive response to endocrine therapy is likely.
Fc r's specific cell-surface receptors for antigen-antibody complexes or aggregated immunoglobulins that bind a site in the Fc portion of the immunoglobulin molecule and may exhibit specificity for particular immunoglobulin classes. Fc receptors are found on B cells, K cells, macrophages, neutrophils, and eosinophils, and, during some developmental stages, on T cells; those on K cells, macrophages, and neutrophils bind to opsonizing antibodies bound to antigens and trigger phagocytosis of the antigen.
GABA r's, γ-aminobutyric acid r's membrane receptors that bind the neurotransmitter γ-aminobutyric acid to facilitate its inhibitory effect on postsynaptic cells. There are two types: the more common *GABA A receptors* are ligand-gated chloride channels that attenuate postsynaptic potentials on neuron bodies and dendrites and inhibit the release of neurotransmitters at nerve terminals; the less common *GABA B receptors* include G proteins and activate cellular coupling systems to either open potassium channels, prevent the opening of calcium channels, or inhibit the production of cyclic adenosine monophosphate.
G protein–coupled r's (GPCR) a large superfamily of membrane receptors whose intracellular effects are mediated by G proteins; they are expressed in all eukaryotes and comprise seven transmembrane domains. Specific GCPRs recognize a wide range of signals, including photons, cations, odorants, eicosanoids, lipids, neurotransmitters, and hormones.
gustatory r. a receptor for taste, located in the taste cell of a taste bud.
H_1 r's, H_2 r's see *histamine.*
hair follicle r's rapidly adapting receptors that surround the roots of hair follicles.
histamine r's see *histamine.*
homing r. a cell-surface molecule that directs tissue- or organ-specific attachment of that cell; specifically, one of the surface proteins of lymphocytes that mediate their attachment to a particular type of vascular endothelium.
IgE r's membrane receptors for immunoglobulin E (IgE) on mast cells and basophils; the IgE molecules are bound by a site in the Fc region, leaving their antigen-binding sites exposed; binding of a multivalent antigen that cross-links the receptors triggers release of mediators of immediate hypersensitivity.
insulin r's specific membrane receptors for insulin found on target cells. When insulin binds to a receptor, either the receptor protein kinase is activated, leading to the activation of other protein kinases within the cell, or the occupied receptors move to coated pits and are endocytosed; in the latter case, in addition to the effects mediated by kinases, a few effects may depend on degradation products.
itch r. a hypothetical receptor that is particularly sensitive to itching sensations, thought to be located in free nerve endings in the epidermis and dermis.
J-r's mechanoreceptors in the walls of pulmonary alveoli, in close contact with capillaries; they respond to interstitial fluid in the lungs to induce a response of rapid, shallow breathing or dyspnea. Called also *juxtacapillary r's.*
joint r. any of several mechanoreceptors that occur in joint capsules and respond to deep pressure and to other stimuli such as stress or change in position.
juxtacapillary r's J-r's.

Receptor *Continued*

LDL r's, low-density lipoprotein r's specific receptors for low-density lipoprotein (LDL) found in coated pits on the surface of mammalian cells. The coated pits are internalized, forming coated vesicles from which LDL receptors are recycled back to the plasma membrane while LDL particles are transferred to lysosomes, where they are degraded, releasing free cholesterol, phospholipids, and amino acids. Genetic defects in LDL receptors are responsible for familial hypercholesterolemia.
membrane r. a receptor located on or in the plasma membrane; called also *cell-surface r.*
muscarinic r. a type of cholinergic receptor that is stimulated by the alkaloid muscarine and blocked by atropine; it is found on autonomic effector cells as well as central neurons in the thalamus and cerebral cortex. Three types may be distinguished on the basis of pharmacologic specificity and five types on the basis of molecular structure; a number of differing nomenclatures have been applied to these types.
muscle r. a mechanoreceptor found in a muscle or tendon; see *muscle spindle* under *spindle* and *Golgi tendon organ* under *organ.*
N_1-r's nicotinic receptors that are preferentially blocked by hexamethonium; they occur on autonomic ganglion cells.
N_2-r's nicotinic receptors that are preferentially blocked by decamethonium; they occur on striated muscle.
nicotinic r. a type of cholinergic receptor that is stimulated initially and blocked at high doses by the alkaloid nicotine and blocked by tubocurarine. These receptors are acetylcholine-gated ion channels and are found on autonomic ganglion cells, striated muscle, and spinal central neurons. See *N_1-r's* and *N_2-r's.*
nonadapting r. a mechanoreceptor, such as a nociceptor, that responds to stimulation with a continual steady discharge and little or no accommodation over time.
nuclear r. any of various receptors that are located in the nucleus of a cell and respond to substances that cross the cell membrane without passing through the transducing systems of the membrane; steroid hormones, thyroid hormones, and vitamin metabolites such as retinoids and calcitriol bind to nuclear receptors.
olfactory r. a chemoreceptor in the nasal epithelium that is sensitive to stimulation, giving rise to the sensation of odors.
opiate r., opioid r. any of a number of types of receptors for opiates and opioids; at least seven different types are postulated at different locations in the body, grouped into three major classes (δ, κ, and μ) according to the specific substances they bind and to the specific physiological effect(s) (e.g., analgesia, respiratory depression, or a psychotomimetic effect) that binding causes or inhibits. See accompanying table.
orphan r. a protein identified as a putative receptor on the basis of structural homology with a known class of receptors but without identification of possible ligands or evidence of function.
paciniform r's see under *corpuscle.*
pain r. nociceptor.
pressure r. slowly adapting r.
P2X r's ATP-gated channels.
purinergic r's membrane receptors widely expressed in the brain, peripheral tissues, and circulating blood cells, that bind purine bases or nucleotides. They are grouped by ligand as P1 (adenosine), P2X (ATP-gated channels, q.v.), and P2Y, (GTP). Most mediate their responses by G proteins.
rapidly adapting r. a mechanoreceptor that responds quickly to stimulation but that rapidly accommodates and stops firing if the stimulus remains constant, such as Meissner corpuscles or pacinian corpuscles.
ryanodine r. [from its sensitivity to the plant alkaloid *ryanodine*] a tetrameric receptor containing a calcium ion channel, located in the sarcoplasmic reticulum of muscle cells and the endoplasmic reticulum of nerve cells; it exists in three isoforms, each opening in response to a different activator to release stored calcium into the cytosol. Point mutations in the gene encoding this receptor are one cause of malignant hypothermia.

Opioid Receptor Classes

Class and Subclass	Endogenous Ligand	Action
delta (δ)	leu-enkephalin	*Increase in:* feeding, growth hormone release; *Decrease in:* dopamine release
δ_1		Supraspinal analgesia
δ_2		Supraspinal and spinal analgesia
kappa (κ)		*Increase in:* feeding, psychotomimesis, sedation; *Decrease in:* gastrointestinal motility
κ_1	dynorphin A; dynorphin B; α-neoendorphin	Supraspinal analgesia; *Increase in:* diuresis
κ_2		
κ_3		Supraspinal analgesia
mu (μ)	met-enkephalin; β-endorphin	*Increase in:* feeding, sedation
μ_1		Supraspinal analgesia; *Decrease in:* acetylcholine release
μ_2		Spinal analgesia; *Increase in:* growth hormone release; *Decrease in:* dopamine release, gastrointestinal motility, respiratory function

sensory r. receptor (def. 2).
slowly adapting r. a mechanoreceptor that responds slowly to stimulation and continues firing as long as the stimulus continues, such as Merkel disks or Ruffini endings.
steroid r., steroid hormone r. a type of nuclear receptor consisting of a protein of high molecular weight, found in the target tissue of a given steroid hormone.
stretch r. a sense organ in a muscle or tendon that responds to elongation; see *Golgi tendon organ* under *organ* and *muscle spindle* under *spindle.*
tactile r. a mechanoreceptor for the sense of touch; called also *touch r.*
T cell antigen r. (TCR) the characteristic marker of T lymphocytes, consisting of two polypeptide chains linked by a disulfide bridge. Two forms exist: TCR-1, composed of α and β chains and occurring on helper and cytotoxic T cells, and the much less common TCR-2, composed of γ and δ chains and occurring on certain T cells of the gut and epidermis; both forms are associated with the CD3 molecule. The T cell antigen receptor has a constant and a variable (antibody-binding) portion and recognizes both specific foreign antigens and self MHC antigens; both must be seen simultaneously to trigger T cell activation.
thermal r. thermoreceptor.
touch r. tactile r.
vibration r. a rapidly adapting receptor sensitive to vibrations.
visual r. photoreceptor.
volume r's postulated receptors that respond to increased plasma extracellular fluid volume and stimulate corrective measures.
warmth r. a cutaneous thermoreceptor particularly sensitive to temperature between 30° and 45°C.

re·cep·tor pro·tein ser·ine/thre·o·nine ki·nase (re-sep′tər pro′tēn sēr′ēn thre′o-nēn ki′nās) [EC 2.7.11.30] a group comprising those protein-serine/threonine kinases with a transmembrane domain. Each occurs as a pair of different subunits, with each subunit having a cytoplasmic kinase domain. When brought together by binding their dimeric protein ligands (e.g., transforming growth factorβ, activins, inhibins, bone morphogenetic proteins), the subunits act together to initiate signaling cascades by activating cytoplasmic transcription factors that regulate genes required for control of cellular proliferation and differentiation. Cf. *non-specific serine/threonine protein kinase.*

re•cep•tor pro•tein-ty•ro•sine ki•nase (re-sep′tər pro′tēn ti′ro-sēn ki′nās) [EC 2.7.10.1] a group comprising those protein-tyrosine kinases with a transmembrane domain and cytoplasmic tyrosine kinase activity. They are involved in cellular signaling pathways; binding of extracellular growth factor ligands (e.g., epidermal growth factor, fibroblast growth factors, transforming growth factor-α, platelet-derived growth factor, insulin) leads to dimerization and activation of receptors, autophosphorylation, and then binding and activation of effector proteins that control cellular proliferation and differentiation. Cf. *non-specific protein-tyrosine kinase.*

re•cess (re′ses) a small empty space or hollow; for specific anatomic structures not found here, see under *recessus.* See also *cavity, pocket,* and *pouch.*

accessory r. of elbow recessus sacciformis articulationis cubiti.

acetabular r. fossa acetabuli.

anterior r. of interpeduncular fossa the portion of the interpeduncular fossa located on the midline immediately caudal to and between the corpora mammillaria; called also *Tarin r.* or *space.*

anterior r. of tympanic membrane recessus anterior membranae tympanicae.

aorticomediastinal r. a small space between the ramifications of the left pulmonary artery and descending thoracic aorta, into which tissue of the left lung intrudes.

azygoesophageal r. a small space between the azygos vein and the esophagus, into which tissue of the lower lobe of the right lung intrudes.

azygomediastinal r. a small space between the azygos vein and mediastinum, into which tissue of the right lung intrudes.

chiasmatic r. recessus supraopticus.

facial r. a roughly triangular depression on the surface of the temporal bone, bounded on two sides by the facial nerve and with an apex at the external genu of the facial nerve. Called also *suprapyramidal r.*

Hyrtl r. recessus epitympanicus.

infundibular r. recessus infundibuli.

infundibuliform r. recessus pharyngeus.

laryngopharyngeal r. recessus piriformis.

lateral r. of fourth ventricle recessus lateralis ventriculi quarti.

lateral r. of nasopharynx recessus pharyngeus.

middle pharyngeal r. bursa pharyngealis.

optic r. recessus supraopticus.

paracolic r's sulci paracolici.

pineal r. recessus pinealis.

pleural r's recessus pleurales.

posterior r. of interpeduncular fossa the portion of the interpeduncular fossa that slightly undermines the anterior margin of the pons.

posterior r. of tympanic membrane recessus posterior membranae tympanicae.

Reichert r. recessus cochlearis vestibuli.

retroannular r. a deep groove formed by the cell membrane immediately behind the annulus of spermatozoa of some species.

r. of Rosenmüller recessus pharyngeus.

sacciform r. of articulation of elbow recessus sacciformis articulationis cubiti.

saccular r. recessus sphericus vestibuli.

sphenoethmoidal r. recessus sphenoethmoidalis.

subhepatic r. recessus subhepaticus.

subphrenic r. recessus subphrenicus.

superior r. of tympanic membrane recessus superior membranae tympanicae.

supraoptic r. recessus supraopticus.

suprapineal r. recessus suprapinealis.

suprapyramidal r. facial r.

supratonsillar r. fossa supratonsillaris.

Tarin r. anterior r. of interpeduncular fossa.

triangular r. a small triangular recess sometimes found on the anterior wall of the third ventricle of the brain, with its base below the anterior commissure and its sides formed by the converging columns of the fornix.

r's of Tröltsch see *recessus membranae tympani anterior* and *recessus membranae tympani posterior.*

tubotympanic r. the elongate recess derived from the first pharyngeal pouch; its distal part contributes to the formation of the tympanic membrane, its proximal part elongates to form the pharyngotympanic tube, and its cavity gives rise to the tympanic cavity and mastoid antrum.

utricular r. recessus ellipticus vestibuli.

r's of vestibule see *recessus cochlearis vestibuli, recessus ellipticus vestibuli,* and *recessus sphericus vestibuli.*

re•ces•sion (re-sesh′ən) [L. *recedere* to draw back or away] the drawing away of a tissue or part from its normal position.

angle r. recession of the angle of the anterior chamber of the eye; see also under *glaucoma.*

gingival r. the drawing back of the gingivae from the necks of the teeth with exposure of root surfaces.

r. of ocular muscle surgical displacement of the insertion of an ocular muscle posteriorly; done to weaken the stronger muscle in strabismus.

re•ces•sive (re-ses′iv) 1. tending to recede; not exerting a ruling or controlling influence. 2. in genetics, pertaining to phenotypic expression of an allele only in homozygotes, i.e., when the allele is carried by both members of a pair of homologous chromosomes (or hemizygotes, for X-linked traits).

re•ces•siv•i•ty (re″ses-iv′ĭ-te) the phenotypic expression of a gene only in a homozygote, not in a heterozygote also possessing a dominant allele for that locus.

re•ces•sus (re-ses′əs) pl. *reces′sus* [L.] recess: a cavity, pocket, or pouch.

r. ante′rior membra′nae tympa′nicae [TA] anterior recess of tympanic membrane: a pocket in the tympanic membrane formed by the tunica mucosa between the anterior malleolar fold and the anterior superior part of the pars tensa of the membrane, ending blindly above.

r. cochlea′ris vesti′buli [TA] cochlear recess of vestibule: a small depressed area on the medial wall of the vestibule of the ear, situated just below the posterior end of the crista vestibuli, and perforated with foramina through which nerve fibers pass to the posterior portion of the ductus cochlearis. Called also *Reichert recess.*

r. costodiaphragma′ticus pleura′lis [TA] costodiaphragmatic recess of pleura: the pleural recess situated at the junction of the costal and diaphragmatic pleurae; called also *sinus phrenicocostalis.*

r. costomediastina′lis pleura′lis [TA] costomediastinal recess of pleura: a wedge-shaped space, not completely filled with lung tissue, along the line at which the costal pleura meets the mediastinal pleura in front; called also *sinus costomediastinalis pleurae.*

r. duodena′lis infe′rior [TA] inferior duodenal recess: a pocket in the peritoneum on the left side of the ascending part of the duodenum, bounded by the inferior duodenal fold.

r. duodena′lis supe′rior [TA], **r. duodenojejuna′lis** superior duodenal recess: a peritoneal pocket behind the superior duodenal fold.

r. ellip′ticus vesti′buli [TA] elliptical recess of the vestibule: an oval depressed area in the roof and medial wall of the vestibule of the internal ear, situated above and behind the crista and pierced by 25 to 30 small foramina through which nerves come from the internal acoustic meatus to the utricle, which occupies the depression. Called also *r. utricularis vestibuli* [TA alternative].

r. epitympa′nicus [TA] epitympanic recess: the portion of the tympanic cavity above the level of the tympanic membrane, containing the greater part of the incus and the upper half of the malleus. Called also *attic, epitympanum, epitympanic space,* and *Hyrtl recess.*

r. hepatorena′lis [TA] hepatorenal recess: a pocket of the subhepatic space that lies between the liver and the kidney.

r. ileocaeca′lis infe′rior [TA] inferior ileocecal recess: a peritoneal pocket situated behind the ileocecal fold, above the vermiform appendix below the ileum, and medial to the cecum; also spelled *r. ileocecalis inferior.*

r. ileocaeca′lis supe′rior [TA] superior ileocecal recess: a peritoneal pocket situated behind and below the vascular cecal fold, above the ileum and medial to the lower end of the ascending colon; also spelled *r. ileocecalis superior.*

r. ileoceca′lis infe′rior r. ileocaecalis inferior.

r. ileoceca′lis supe′rior r. ileocaecalis superior.

r. infe′rior bur′sae omenta′lis [TA] inferior omental recess: the lower portion of the omental bursa, including its extension down into the great omentum. It is bounded in front by the posterior wall of the stomach, and behind by the pancreas, the transverse colon and its mesocolon, the left suprarenal gland, and part of the left kidney.

r. infundibula′ris TA alternative for *r. infundibuli.*

r. infundi′buli [TA] infundibular recess: a funnel-shaped depression in the floor of the third ventricle of the brain, immediately caudal to the optic chiasm and within the infundibulum of the hypophysis. Called also *r. infundibularis* [TA alternative].

r. intersigmoi′deus [TA] intersigmoidal recess: a shallow peritoneal pocket running downward and to the left at the base of the sigmoid mesocolon.

r. latera′lis ventri′culi quar′ti [TA] lateral recess of fourth ventricle: a narrow, curved prolongation of the cavity of the fourth ventricle of the brain, extending laterally onto the dorsal surface of the restiform body; it contains a lateral prolongation of the choroid plexus and provides for the passage of cerebrospinal fluid into the subarachnoid space.

r. liena′lis TA alternative for *r. splenicus.*

r. membra′nae tym′pani ante′rior r. anterior membranae tympanicae.

r. membra′nae tym′pani poste′rior r. posterior membranae tympanicae.

r. membra′nae tym′pani supe′rior r. superior membranae tympanicae.

r. op′ticus recessus supraopticus.

r. paraduodena′lis [TA] paraduodenal recess: a pocket occasionally found in the peritoneum behind a fold containing a branch of the left colic artery.

r. pharyn′geus [TA] pharyngeal recess: a wide, slitlike lateral extension in the wall of the nasopharynx, superior and posterior to the pharyngeal orifice of the auditory tube; called also *Rosenmüller cavity* or *fossa*.

r. phrenicomediastina′lis pleura′lis [TA] phrenicomediastinal recess of pleura: the pleural recess situated at the line of junction of the diaphragmatic and mediastinal pleurae.

r. pinea′lis [TA] pineal recess: an extension of the third ventricle into the stalk of the pineal body.

r. pirifor′mis [TA] piriform recess: a pear-shaped fossa in the wall of the laryngeal pharynx lateral to the arytenoid cartilage and medial to the lamina of the thyroid cartilage. Called also *piriform fossa* or *sinus*.

r. pleura′les [TA] pleural recesses: the spaces where the different portions of the pleura join at an angle and which are never completely filled by lung tissue; see *r. costodiaphragmaticus pleuralis*, *r. costomediastinalis pleuralis*, and *r. phrenicomediastinalis pleuralis*. Called also *sinus pleurae*.

r. pneumatoente′ricus either of the paired embryonic excavations alongside the dorsal mesogastrium, the right one sometimes persisting as the infracardiac bursa.

r. poste′rior membra′nae tympa′nicae [TA] posterior recess of tympanic membrane: a pocket in the tympanic membrane formed by the tunica mucosa between the posterior malleolar fold and the posterior superior part of the pars tensa of the membrane, ending blindly above.

r. retrocaeca′lis [TA] retrocecal recess: a peritoneal pocket extending upward behind the cecum and sometimes behind the colon; also spelled *r. retrocecalis*.

r. retroceca′lis r. retrocaecalis.

r. retroduodena′lis [TA] retroduodenal recess: an occasional peritoneal pocket extending behind the horizontal and ascending parts of the duodenum.

r. saccifor′mis articulatio′nis cu′biti [TA] sacciform recess of articulation of elbow: the distal bulging of the articular capsule of the elbow joint, situated between the incisura radialis ulnae and the circumferentia articularis radii.

r. saccifor′mis articulatio′nis radioulna′ris dista′lis [TA] sacciform recess of distal radioulnar articulation: a bulging of the synovial membrane of the articular capsule of the distal radioulnar joint, which extends proximally between the radius and ulna beyond the point of their articular surfaces.

r. saccula′ris vesti′buli TA alternative for *r. sphericus vestibuli*.

r. sphenoethmoida′lis [TA] sphenoethmoidal recess: the most superior and posterior part of the nasal cavity, above the superior nasal concha, into which the sphenoidal sinus opens.

r. sphe′ricus vesti′buli [TA] spherical recess of vestibule: a circular depressed area in the anteroinferior portion of the medial wall of the vestibule of the internal ear. It is pierced by 12 to 15 small foramina through which nerves come from the internal acoustic meatus to the saccule, which occupies the depression. Called also *r. saccularis vestibuli* [TA alternative].

r. sple′nicus [TA] splenic recess: an extension of the omental bursa to the left behind the gastrosplenic ligament almost to the spleen; called also *r. lienalis* [TA alternative].

r. subhepa′ticus [TA] subhepatic space: the peritoneal pocket just inferior to the liver, with a surface next to the kidney.

r. subphre′nicus [TA] subphrenic space: the space between the diaphragm and subjacent abdominal organs.

r. subpopli′teus [TA] subpopliteal recess: a prolongation of the synovial tendon sheath of the popliteus muscle outside the knee joint into the popliteal space.

r. supe′rior membra′nae tympa′nicae [TA] superior recess of tympanic membrane: a recess in the tympanic membrane formed by the tunica mucosa between the neck of the malleus and the pars flaccida of the membrane and ending blindly below. Called also *Prussak pouch* or *space*.

r. supe′rior bur′sae omenta′lis [TA] superior omental recess: a long, narrow peritoneal pocket leading from the vestibule upward toward the liver, between the inferior vena cava on the right, the esophagus on the left, the gastrohepatic ligament in front, and the diaphragm behind.

r. supraop′ticus [TA] supraoptic recess: a depression in the floor of the third ventricle of the brain, between the chiasma behind and the lamina terminalis in front. Called also *r. opticus* and *optic recess*.

r. suprapinea′lis [TA] suprapineal recess: the posterior extension of the third ventricle of the brain above and around the pineal body.

r. utricula′ris vesti′buli, r. utri′culi vestibula′ris TA alternative for *r. ellipticus vestibuli*.

re•cid•i•va•tion (re-sid″ĭ-va′shən) relapse, recurrence, or repetition, as of a disease or condition or of a pattern of behavior, particularly a criminal act.

re•cid•i•vism (re-sid′ĭ-viz-əm) a tendency to relapse into a previous condition, disease, or pattern of behavior, particularly a return to criminal behavior.

re•cid•i•vist (re-sid′ĭ-vist) [Fr. *récidiviste*, from L. *recidere* to fall back] one who tends to relapse, especially a person who tends to return to criminal habits after treatment or punishment.

rec•i•pe (res′ĭ-pe) 1. [L.] take; used at the head of a physician's prescription, and usually indicated by the symbol ℞. See *prescription*. 2. a formula for the preparation of a specific combination of ingredients.

re•cip•i•ent (re-sip′e-ənt) one who receives, as blood in transfusion, or a tissue or organ graft.

universal r. a person thought to be able to receive blood of any group without agglutination of the donor cells.

re•cip•ro•cal (re-sip′rə-kəl″) 1. being equivalent or complementary. 2. inversely related; opposing.

re•cip•ro•ca•tion (re-sip″ro-ka′shən) [L. *reciprocare* to move backward and forward] 1. the act of giving and receiving in exchange; the complementary interaction of two distinct entities. 2. an alternating back-and-forth movement. 3. in dentistry, the means by which one part of a removable partial denture framework is made to counter the effect created by another part of the framework.

re•cir•cu•la•tion (re-sur″ku-la′shən) in hemodialysis, circulation of part of the blood from the venous line to the arterial line, thus reducing concentration gradients across the hemodialyzer membranes and reducing the efficiency of the procedure.

Reck•ling•hau•sen canals, disease, disease of bone (rek′ling-hou″zen) [Friedrich Daniel von *Recklinghausen*, German pathologist, 1833–1910] see under *canal*, and see *neurofibromatosis 1*, under *neurofibromatosis*, and *osteitis fibrosa cystica*.

Reck•ling•hau•sen-Ap•ple•baum disease (rek′ling-hou-zen ahp′əl-boum) [F.D. von *Recklinghausen;* L. *Applebaum*, German physician, 20th century] hemochromatosis.

Re•clast (re′klast) trademark for a preparation of zoledronic acid.

re•cog•ni•tion (rek″əg-nĭ′shən) 1. the act of recognizing (seeing something as familiar). 2. the state of being seen as familiar. 3. the interaction of immunologically competent cells with antigen; it begins with binding of the antigen to specific antigen receptors on B and T lymphocytes then proceeds to an immune response directed against the antigen. Called also *antigen r.*

re•coil (re′koil) the act or state of pulling back quickly, as towards a resting position upon removal of a strong opposing force.

elastic r. the ability of a stretched elastic object or organ, such as the lung or bladder, to return to its resting position. See also *elastance*.

re•com•bi•nant (re-kom′bĭ-nənt) 1. the new entity (e.g., gene, protein, cell, individual) that results from genetic recombination. 2. pertaining or relating to such an entity. See also under *DNA*.

Re•com•bi•nate (re-kom′bĭ-nāt) trademark for a preparation of antihemophilic factor (recombinant).

re•com•bi•na•tion (re″kom-bĭ-na′shən) 1. the reunion, in the same or a different arrangement, of formerly united elements which have become separated. 2. in genetics, the process that creates new combinations of genes by shuffling the linear order of the DNA, such as occurs naturally by crossing over of homologous chromosomes during meiosis or of homologous DNA sequences in somatic cells during mitosis, or occurs in vitro when DNA or RNA is manipulated for genetic engineering.

bacterial r. in bacterial genetics, the process of producing a new gene by any of several processes, e.g., the sexual union of two parents, molecular crossing over between two DNA strands, or transformation.

somatic r. the rearrangement of genetic material by bringing together a set of inherited, initially separated, DNA sequences by deletion of the intervening DNA; in immature B and T lymphocytes, it is the method by which the variety of genes encoding the diverse repertoire of antigen receptors is generated.

Re•com•bi•vax HB (re-kom′bĭ-vaks″) trademark for a preparation of hepatitis B vaccine (recombinant).

re•com•pres•sion (re″kəm-presh′ən) the restoration of pressure, especially the return to conditions of normal pressure after exposure to greatly diminished atmospheric pressure.

re•con•sti•tu•tion (re″kon-stĭ-too′shən) 1. a type of regeneration in which a new organ forms by the rearrangement of tissues rather than from new formation at an injured surface. 2. the restoration to original form of a substance previously altered for preservation and storage, as the restoration to a liquid state of blood serum or plasma that has been dried and stored.

re•con•struc•tion (re″kən-struk′shən) 1. the act or process of reassembling or re-forming from constituent parts. 2. surgical restoration of function of a part, such as with a bypass or plastic surgery.

aortic r. restoration of function to a damaged aorta, as by bypass or aortoplasty.

arterial r. restoration of arterial blood supply to a part, as by a bypass, arterioplasty, or endarterectomy.

image r. from projections radiography in which two- or three-dimensional images of an object are reconstructed from a set of mathematical projections, as in transverse axial tomography.

venous r. restoration of venous drainage of a part, as by a graft or phleboplasty.

re·con·tour (re-kon′to͞or) 1. to give new shape or contour to. 2. in dentistry, to change the contour of a crown or a complete or partial denture.

rec·ord (rek′ord) a permanent or long-lasting account of something (as on film, in writing, etc). See also under *registration.*

chew-in r., functional 1. a record of the natural chewing movements of the mandible made on the occlusion rim by the teeth or scribing studs. 2. a record of movements of the mandible made on the occluding surface of the opposing occlusion rim by the teeth or scribing studs; produced by simulated chewing movements. 3. a record of lateral and protrusive movements of the mandible made on the occlusal surface of the occlusion rim by the teeth or scribing studs on an opposing rim; produced during simulated movements of bruxism.

face-bow r. a registration by means of a face-bow of the position of the hinge axis and/or the condyles; used to orient the maxillary cast to the opening and closing axis of the articulator.

interocclusal r. bite registration.

interocclusal r., centric a record of the centric jaw position (relation).

interocclusal r., eccentric a record of a jaw relation other than the centric relation.

interocclusal r., lateral a record of a lateral eccentric jaw position.

interocclusal r., protrusive a record of a protruded eccentric jaw position.

jaw relation r. a registration of any positional relationship of the mandible in reference to the maxillae; these records may be of any of the many vertical, horizontal, or orientation relations.

maxillomandibular r. a record of the relation of the mandible to the maxilla.

occluding centric relation r. a registration of centric relation made at the established occlusal vertical dimension.

problem-oriented r. (POR) an approach to patient care record keeping that focuses on those specific health problems of the patient that require immediate attention and on the structuring of a cooperative health care plan designed to cope with the identified problems. The components basic to the POR are: *the data base*, which provides information obtained from the variety of sources required for each patient regardless of diagnosis or presenting problems; *the problem list*, which contains those major problems currently needing attention and serves as the basis of a plan of care; *the plan*, which specifies what is to be done with regard to each problem; *the progress notes*, which document the observations, assessments, nursing care plans, physician's orders, etc., of all health care personnel directly involved in the care of the patient. See also *SOAP*.

profile r. a record showing the sagittal outline form or profile of the face.

protrusive r. a registration of a forward position of the mandible with reference to the maxilla.

terminal jaw relation r. a record of the relationship of the mandible to the maxilla made at the vertical relation of occlusion and at the centric position.

re·cord·ing (re-kōrd′ing) the making of a record.

pulse volume r. plethysmography.

re·cru·des·cence (re″kroo-des′əns) [L. *recrudescere* to become sore again] the recurrence of symptoms after a temporary abatement. Cf. *relapse.* **recrudes′cent** *adj*

re·cruit·ment (re-kro͞ot′mənt) 1. the gradual increase to a maximum in a reflex when a stimulus of unaltered intensity is prolonged. 2. in audiology, an abnormally large increase in the perceived loudness of a sound caused by a slight increase in its intensity. 3. in muscle physiology, the orderly increase in number of activated motor units with increasing strength of voluntary muscle contractions. See also *recruitment pattern.*

follicle r. the process by which certain primordial ovarian follicles begin growing in a given menstrual cycle.

Rect. [L.] rectifica′tus (rectified).

rec·tal·gia (rek-tal′jə) proctalgia.

rec·tec·to·my (rek-tek′tə-me) proctectomy.

rec·ti·fi·ca·tion (rek″tĭ-fĭ-ka′shən) [L. *rectificatio*] 1. the act of making straight, pure, or correct. 2. redistillation of a liquid to purify it. 3. conversion of alternating current to direct current.

spontaneous r. a transverse lie which rectifies itself before labor begins.

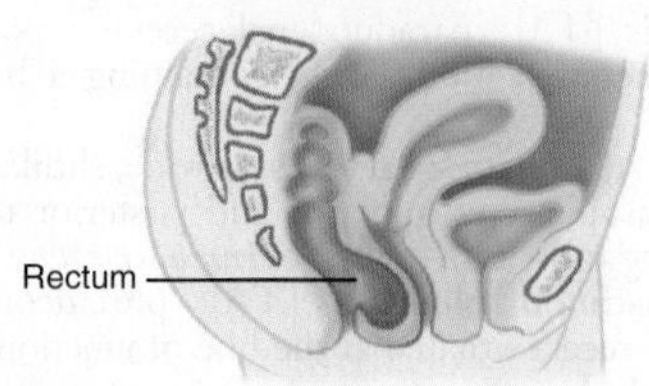

■ Rectocele.

rec·ti·fied (rek″tĭ-fīd) refined; made straight; converted to direct current (DC).

rec·ti·fi·er (rek′tĭ-fi″ər) a device for obtaining a direct (unidirectional) current from an alternating current.

thermionic r. a rectifier consisting of an electric valve in which the electrons are supplied by a heated electrode.

rec·tis·chi·ac (rek-tis′ke-ak) pertaining to the rectum and the ischium.

rec·ti·tis (rek-ti′tis) proctitis.

rect(o)- [L. *rectum*] a combining form designating relationship to the rectum. See also words beginning *proct(o)-*.

rec·to·ab·dom·i·nal (rek″to-ab-dom′ĭ-nəl) pertaining to the rectum and abdomen.

rec·to·cele (rek′to-sēl) [*recto-* + *-cele*[1]] hernial protrusion of part of the rectum into the vagina; called also *proctocele* and *rectovaginal hernia.*

rec·to·coc·cy·ge·al (rek″to-kok-sij′e-əl) pertaining to the rectum and the coccyx.

rec·to·coc·cy·ge·us (rek″to-kok-sij′e-əs) [L.] rectococcygeal; see under *musculus.*

rec·to·co·li·tis (rek″to-ko-li′tis) proctocolitis.

rec·to·cu·ta·ne·ous (rek″to-ku-ta′ne-əs) pertaining to or communicating between the rectum and the skin.

rec·to·cys·tot·o·my (rek″to-sis-tot′ə-me) proctocystotomy.

rec·to·la·bi·al (rek″to-la′be-əl) pertaining to or communicating between the rectum and a labium majus.

rec·to·pexy (rek′to-pek″se) [*recto-* + *-pexy*] fixation of the rectum to some adjacent tissue or organ by suture; called also *proctopexy.*

rec·to·plas·ty (rek′to-plas″te) proctoplasty.

rec·to·ro·mano·scope (rek″to-ro-man′ə-skōp) proctosigmoidoscope.

rec·to·ro·ma·nos·co·py (rek″to-ro-mə-nos′kə-pe) [*recto-* + L. *romanum* sigmoid + *-scopy*] proctosigmoidoscopy.

rec·to·scope (rek′to-skōp) proctoscope.

rec·tos·co·py (rek-tos′kə-pe) proctoscopy.

rec·to·sig·moid (rek″to-sig′moid) 1. pertaining to the rectum and sigmoid colon. 2. the rectum and the sigmoid colon considered together.

rec·to·sig·moi·dec·to·my (rek″to-sig″moi-dek′tə-me) excision of the rectum and sigmoid; called also *proctosigmoidectomy.*

perineal r. rectosigmoidectomy through a perineal incision; see also *Altemeier procedure*, under *procedure.*

rec·to·sig·moi·dos·to·my (rek″to-sig″moi-dos′tə-me) 1. creation of an artificial opening between the sigmoid colon and the rectum; called also *sigmoidorectostomy.* 2. the opening so created.

rec·to·sig·moi·dos·co·py (rek″to-sig″moi-dos′kə-pe) proctosigmoidoscopy.

rec·to·ste·no·sis (rek″to-stə-no′sis) proctostenosis.

rec·tos·to·my (rek-tos′tə-me) proctostomy.

rec·tot·o·my (rek-tot′ə-me) proctotomy.

rec·to·ure·ter·al (rek″to-u-re′tər-əl) ureterorectal.

rec·to·ure·thral (rek″to-u-re′thrəl) pertaining to or communicating between the rectum and the urethra. Called also *urethrorectal.*

rec·to·uter·ine (rek″to-u′tər-in) pertaining to or connecting the rectum and the uterus; called also *uterorectal.*

rec·to·vag·i·nal (rek″to-vaj′ĭ-nəl) pertaining to or communicating between the rectum and vagina.

rec·to·ves·i·cal (rek″to-ves′ĭ-kəl) pertaining to or communicating between the rectum and urinary bladder. Called also *vesicorectal.*

rec·to·ves·i·co·vag·i·nal (rek″to-ves″ĭ-ko-vaj′ĭnəl) vesicovaginorectal.

rec·to·ves·tib·u·lar (rek″to-vəs-tib′u-lər) pertaining to or communicating between the rectum and the vestibule of the vagina.

rec•to•vul•var (rek″to-vul′vər) pertaining to or communicating between the rectum and vulva.

rec•tum (rek′təm) [L. "straight"] [TA] the distal portion of the large intestine, beginning anterior to the third sacral vertebra as a continuation of the sigmoid and ending at the anal canal. **rec′tal** *adj*

rec•tus (rek′təs) [L.] straight; anatomical terminology for a straight structure, such as a muscle (see entries beginning *musculus rectus*).

re•cum•bent (re-kum′bənt) lying down.

re•cu•per•a•tion (re-koo″pər-a′shən) [L. *recuperatio*] the recovery of health and strength.

re•cur•rence (re-kur′əns) [L. *re-* again + *currere* to run] the return of symptoms after a remission; see also *relapse* and *recrudescence.*

re•cur•rent (re-kur′ənt) [L. *recurrens* returning] 1. running back, or toward the source. 2. returning after remissions.

re•cur•va•tion (re″kər-va′shən) [L. *recurvatio*] a backward bending or curvature.

red (red) [L. *rubrum*] 1. the color produced by the longest waves of the visible spectrum, approximately 630 to 750 nm. 2. a dye or stain with this color.

alizarin r. S, alizarin water-soluble r. sodium alizarinsulfonate.

aniline r. basic fuchsin.

basic r. 2 safranin O.

basic r. 9 rosaniline.

bromphenol r. an indicator, dibromphenolsulfonphthalein, used in determining hydrogen ion concentration, being yellow at pH 5.2 and red at pH 6.8. Written also *bromophenol r.*

carmine r. a stain derived from carmine.

cerasine r. Sudan III.

chlorophenol r. a pH indicator with a range of 5.2 (yellow) to 6.8 (red).

Congo r. an odorless, dark red or reddish brown powder that decomposes on exposure to acid fumes; used as a biological stain, as an indicator with a pH range of 3.0 (blue-violet) to 5.2 (red), and as a diagnostic aid in amyloidosis See also under *tests.*

cotton r. safranin O.

cotton r. B, cotton r. C Congo r.

cotton r. 4 B benzopurpurine 4 B.

cresol r. an indicator, ortho-cresol-sulfonphthalein, used in the determination of the hydrogen ion concentration. It has a pH range of 7.2 to 8.8, being yellow at 7.2 and red at 8.8.

dianil r. 4 C, dianin r. 4 B benzopurpurine 4 B.

direct r. Congo r.

direct r. 4 B benzopurpurine 4 B.

indigo r., indoxyl r. a coloring matter produced by heating an aqueous solution of indoxyl to 130°C.

magdala r. a basic dye used for staining connective tissue. It is a mixture of monoamino- and diamino-naphthosafranins.

methyl r. a dye, used as an indicator in the determination of hydrogen ion concentration, with a pH range of 4.4 (red) to 6 (yellow).

naphthaline r. magdala r.

neutral r. a basic red fluorochrome dye used as a pH indicator with a range of 6.8 (red) to 8 (yellow) and as a stain, particularly for supravital staining of granules and vacuoles.

oil r. Sudan III.

oil r. IV scarlet r.

oil r. O a red diazo dye that is more soluble in fat than in water or alcohols; used as a stain for neutral fats.

phenol r. phenolsulfonphthalein.

provisional r. a colored lipin obtained from rhodopsin.

scarlet r. a red fat-soluble azo dye, used as a biological stain for fats. Called also *oil r. IV, ponceau 3B, scarlet R, scharlach R,* and *Sudan IV.*

Sudan r. magdala r.

toluylene r. neutral r.

tony r. Sudan III.

trypan r. an acid azo dye used as a vital stain and which possesses some trypanocidal activity.

re•de•cus•sate (re″de-kus′āt) to form a secondary decussation.

red•foot (red′foot) a fatal condition of unknown etiology affecting newborn lambs, in which the sensitive lamina of the feet become exposed owing to detachment of the overlying horn.

re•dia (re′de-ə) pl. *re′diae* [F. *Redi,* Italian naturalist, 1626–1698] a larval stage of certain trematode parasites, which develops in the body of a snail host and gives rise to daughter rediae or to the cercariae.

re•dif•fer•en•ti•a•tion (re″dif-ər-en″she-a′shən) the return of a dedifferentiated tissue or part to its original or another more or less similar condition.

Redig. in pulv. [L.] rediga′tur in pul′verem (let it be reduced to powder).

Red. in pulv. [L.] reduc′tus in pul′verem (reduced to powder).

red•in•te•gra•tion (red-in″tə-gra′shən) [L. *redintegrare* to make whole again] 1. the restoration or repair of a lost or damaged part. 2. a psychic process in which a part of a complex stimulus revokes the complete reaction that was previously made to the complex stimulus as a whole. 3. reintegration (def. 2).

re•dis•lo•ca•tion (re″dis-lo-ka′shən) dislocation recurring after reduction.

re•dox (re′doks) oxidation-reduction.

re•dresse•ment (rə-dres-maw′) [Fr.] 1. a second or repeated dressing. 2. correction of a deformity.

re•duce (re-do͞os′) [*re-* + L. *ducere* to lead] 1. to restore to the normal place or relation of parts, as to *reduce* a fracture. 2. in chemistry, to submit to reduction. 3. to decrease in weight.

re•duced (re-do͞ost′) 1. returned to the proper place or position, as a *reduced* fracture. 2. restored to a metallic form, as *reduced* iron. 3. altered by a chemical change involving a gain of electrons.

re•du•ci•ble (re-doo′sĭ-bəl) capable of being reduced.

re•duc•tant (re-duk′tənt) the electron donor in an oxidation-reduction (redox) reaction.

re•duc•tase (re-duk′tās) a term used in the recommended names of some enzymes of the oxidoreductase class [EC 1], usually denoting those catalyzing reactions physiologically important solely for reduction of a metabolite.

5α-r. an enzyme that catalyzes the irreversible reduction of testosterone to dihydrotestosterone with NADPH as the hydrogen donor. Deficiency of the enzyme, with resultant deficiency in dihydrotestosterone, is an autosomal recessive condition characterized by male pseudohermaphroditism, prepubertal ambiguous or female-type external genitalia (usually some form of perineal hypospadias), and some masculinization at puberty without gynecomastia.

re•duc•tion (re-duk′shən) [L. *reductio*] 1. the correction of a fracture, dislocation, or hernia. 2. in chemistry, the addition of hydrogen to a substance, or more generally, the gain of electrons.

breast r. popular name for reduction mammaplasty.

r. of chromosomes the passing of the members of a chromosome pair to the daughter cells during meiosis, each daughter cell receiving half the diploid number.

closed r. the manipulative reduction of a fracture or dislocation without incision.

r. en masse reduction of a strangulated hernia included within its sac, so that the strangulation is not relieved.

lung volume r. see under *surgery.*

open r. reduction of a fracture or dislocation after incision into the site.

weight r. the lessening of one's body weight by a regimen designed for that purpose.

re•dun•dan•cy (re-dun′dən-se) [L. *redundare* to overflow] the presence of multiple copies of a gene in a genome, or of the same or similar DNA sequences.

re•du•pli•ca•tion (re″doo-plĭ-ka′shən) [L. *reduplicatio*] 1. a doubling back. 2. the recurrence of paroxysms of a double type. 3. duplication (def. 3).

ureteral r. double ureter.

re•du•vi•id (re-du′vĭ-id) 1. belonging to the family Reduviidae. 2. an insect of the family Reduviidae.

Re•du•vi•i•dae (re″du-vi′ĭ-de) a family of winged hemipterous insects of the suborder Heteroptera, including various biting species called cone-nose bugs, kissing bugs, and assassin bugs. Many have painful bites, and some species transmit Chagas disease. Genera include *Eratyrus, Eutriatoma, Melanolestes, Panstrongylus, Reduvius* (type genus), *Rhodnius,* and *Triatoma.*

Re•du•vi•us (re-du′ve-us) a genus of hemipterous blood-sucking insects. *R. persona′tus* has a painful bite that may cause nausea, urticaria, or other allergic symptoms.

red•wa•ter (red′waw-tər) 1. bovine babesiosis. 2. bacillary hemoglobinuria.

Reed cells (rēd) [Dorothy *Reed,* American pathologist, 1874–1964] Reed-Sternberg cells.

Reed-Hodg•kin disease (rēd′ hoj′kin) [D. *Reed;* Thomas *Hodgkin,* English physician, 1798–1866] Hodgkin disease.

Reed-Stern•berg cells (rēd′ stərn′bərg) [D. *Reed;* Carl von *Sternberg,* Austrian pathologist, 1872–1935] see under *cell.*

reef (rēf) an infolding or tuck of tissue, as a tuck made in plication.

re•en•try (re-en′tre) reexcitation of a region of cardiac tissue by a single impulse, continuing for one or more cycles and sometimes resulting in ectopic beats or tachyarrhythmias. It can exist over either an anatomical or a functional area of slowed impulse conduction and requires also refractoriness of tissue to stimulation and an area of unidirectional block to conduction. See also *reflection* and *reentrant mechanism,* under *mechanism.* **reen′trant** *adj*

anatomical r. reentry in which the block to conduction is an anatomical obstacle; it is usually described by the ring model.

anisotropic r. reentry that is functional in not occurring around an anatomical obstacle but whose functional properties are conferred by the inherent structural anisotropy of the cardiac muscle fibers; thus it has qualities of both functional and anatomical reentry.

atrial r. reentry in which the entire reentrant circuit lies within one or both atria, excluding the sinus node.

atrioventricular nodal r., AV nodal r. an arrhythmia-causing mechanism in which two opposing pathways are established within the atrioventricular node (longitudinal dissociation); the anterograde pathway, which is usually slower, activates the ventricles and the retrograde pathway, which is usually faster, activaties the atria. This mechanism is responsible for approximately half of symptomatic paroxysmal supraventricular tachycardias.

functional r. reentry in which the block to conduction is due to functional heterogeneity of the electrophysiological properties of regions of cardiac tissue; it is usually described by the leading circle model.

intra-atrial r. atrial r.

reflected r. reflection (def. 4).

sinus nodal r. reentry in which impulses traverse a reentrant circuit within or near the sinus node before being conducted to the rest of the heart.

Re•Fac•to (re-fak′to) trademark for a preparation of antihemophilic factor (recombinant).

re•fect (re-fekt′) to induce refection.

re•fec•tion (re-fek′shən) [L. *reficere* to restore] recovery; repair: applied specifically to the ability of the flora of the cecum of rats to synthesize vitamins of the B group from deficient diets and supply them to the host animal. **refec′tious** *adj*

re•feed•ing (re-fēd′ing) restoration of normal nutrition after a period of fasting or starvation; see also *refeeding syndrome,* under *syndrome.*

re•ferred (re-furd′) of sensory phenomena, perceived at a site other than the one being stimulated; see under *pain* and *sensation.*

re•fill•ing (re-fil′ing) flowing back in, such as of a liquid into a container.

plasma r. plasma refilling rate.

re•fine (re-fīn′) to purify or free from foreign matter.

re•flect•ed (re-flek′təd) turned or bent back; mirrored.

re•flec•tion (re-flek′shən) [L. *reflexus,* past part. of *reflectere* to bend back] 1. a turning or bending back; a bending back upon its course. 2. in physics, the turning back of a ray of light, sound, or heat when it strikes against a surface that it does not penetrate. The ray before reflection is known as the *incident ray;* after reflection, it is the *reflected ray.* 3. an image produced by this process. 4. a special form of reentry in which an impulse crosses a narrow area of diminished responsiveness to excite distal tissue, pauses long enough for repolarization of proximal tissue, and returns, retracing its pathway and reexciting the same fibers in reverse rather than traversing a circuit. If the returning impulse is strong enough, a seesaw movement of current can result, causing tachyarrhythmias.

pericardial r. a point or line of folding along which the lamina visceralis pericardii serosi (visceral pericardium) becomes the lamina parietalis pericardii serosi (parietal pericardium).

re•flec•tor (re-flek′tər) a device for reflecting light or sound.

dental r. a mouth mirror used to reflect light on the field of action during a dental operation or examination.

re•flex (re′fleks) [L. *reflexus,* past part. of *reflectere* to bend back] 1. reflected. 2. a reflected action or movement; the sum total of any particular involuntary activity. See *reflex arc* and *reflex action.* 3. a reflection or a reflected image of an object.

Reflex

abdominal r's, abdominal skin r's contractions of abdominal muscles on scratching of the skin of the abdominal wall.

abdominocardiac r. any reflex in the heart produced by stimulating the abdominal sympathetic nerves. See also *Livierato sign,* under *sign.*

Abrams heart r. contraction of the myocardium, with reduction in the area of cardiac dullness, which results when the skin of the precordial region is irritated. It is observed with the fluoroscope.

accommodation r. the coordinated changes that occur when the eye adapts itself for near vision; they are constriction of the pupil, convergence of the eyes, and increased convexity of the lens.

Achilles r., Achilles tendon r. triceps surae r.

acoustic r. contraction of the stapedius muscle in response to intense sound. Called also *cochleostapedial r.* and *stapedial r.*

acquired r. conditioned response.

adductor r. of foot Hirschberg sign.

adductor r. of thigh on tapping the tendon of the adductor magnus with the thigh in abduction, contraction of the adductors results.

allied r's reflexes in which two afferent stimuli use the same common pathway or produce effects on two synergistic muscles.

anal r., anal wink r. contraction of the anal sphincter on scratching or other irritation of the skin of the anus.

ankle r. triceps surae r.

antagonistic r's reflex movements occurring not in the muscle which has been stretched but in its antagonist.

anticus r. Piotrowski sign.

antigravity r's reflexes that keep the antigravity muscles in extension to hold the body upright.

ascending excitatory r. the component of the peristaltic reflex in which muscles proximal to a bolus contract and actively push the bolus along.

Aschner r. oculocardiac r.

atavistic r. primitive r.

atriopressor r. rise in arterial blood pressure (vasoconstriction) attributed to a change of pressure in the right atrium and great veins.

attention r. of pupil alteration of size in the pupil when the attention is suddenly fixed; called also *Piltz r.*

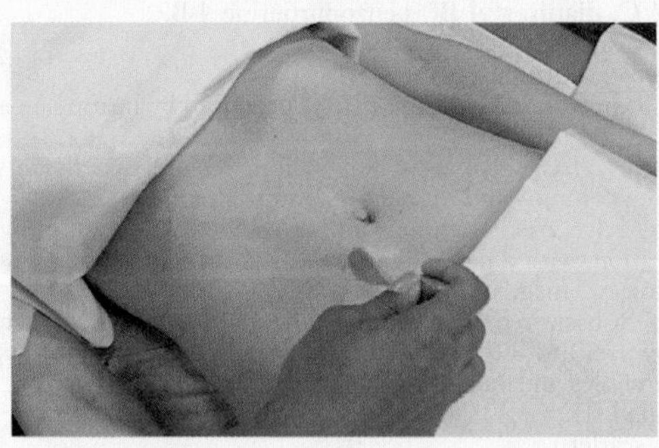

■ Examination of abdominal reflexes.

attitudinal r's reflexes having to do with the position of the body, primarily controlled by input from receptors in the utriculus; called also *statotonic r's.*

audito-oculogyric r. a turning of both eyes in the direction of a sudden sound.

auditory r. any reflex caused by stimulation of the auditory (vestibulocochlear) nerve, especially momentary closure of both eyes produced by a sudden sound.

auricle r. involuntary movement of the auricle of the ear produced by auditory stimuli (more pronounced in some other animals than in humans).

auriculocervical nerve r. Snellen r.

auriculopalpebral r. Kisch r.

autonomic r. a response of smooth muscle, glands, and conducting tissue of the heart, which alters the functional state of the innervated organ.

axon r. a reflex resulting from a stimulus applied to one branch of a nerve, which sets up an impulse that moves centrally to the point of division of the nerve, where it is reflected down the other branch to the effector organ.

Babinski r. dorsiflexion of the big toe on stimulating the sole of the foot; normal in infants but in others a sign of a lesion in the central nervous system, particularly in the pyramidal tract. Called also *Babinski phenomenon* or *sign* and *toe phenomenon* or *sign.*

Babkin r. pressure by the examiner's thumbs on the palms of both hands of the infant results in opening of the infant's mouth; it is elicited in many newborn infants, normal and abnormal, except when lethargic or comatose.

Bainbridge r. rise in pressure in, or increased distention of, the large somatic veins or the right atrium results in acceleration of the heartbeat.

bar r. a pathological reflex in which movement of one lower limb is followed by similar movements of the other when the patient is recumbent; indicative of a lesion, often a tumor, in the prefrontal area.

Barkman r. contraction of the rectus abdominis muscle on the same side after stimulation of the skin just below one of the nipples.

baroreceptor r. the reflex responses to stimulation of baroreceptors of the carotid sinus and aortic arch, regulating blood pressure by controlling heart rate, strength of heart contractions, and diameter of blood vessels.

basal joint r. finger-thumb r.

Bechterew r. Bekhterev r.

behavior r. conditioned response.

Bekhterev r. 1. Bekhterev deep r. 2. hypogastric r. 3. nasal r. 4. paradoxical pupillary r.

Bekhterev deep r. with corticospinal tract lesions, if the toes and foot are passively flexed in a plantar direction and then released, they will flex in a dorsal direction and the knees and hip will also flex.

Bekhterev-Mendel r. Mendel-Bekhterev r.

Bezold r., Bezold-Jarisch r. a cardiovascular reflex occurring upon stimulation of chemoreceptors, primarily in the left ventricle, by certain antihypertensive alkaloids and similar substances; afferent vagal fibers carry the impulses to the medulla oblongata, after which impulses carried back by efferent vagal fibers cause reflex bradycardia and hypotension.

biceps r. contraction of the biceps muscle of the arm when its tendon is tapped.

bladder r. the reflex contracting and emptying of the urinary bladder in response to filling, the first step in the micturition reflex; it can be voluntarily inhibited by impulses from the brain in patients with normal neurological function.

blink r. 1. corneal r. (def. 1). 2. blink responses considered together.

brachioradialis r. tapping on the lower end of the radius produces flexion of the forearm.

Brain r. an extension of the hemiplegic flexed upper limb when the patient assumes a quadrupedal posture; called also *quadrupedal extensor r.*

brainstem r's reflexes regulated at the level of the brainstem, such as pupillary, pharyngeal, and cough reflexes and the control of respiration. Their prolonged absence is one criterion of brain death.

bregmocardiac r. pressure upon the bregmatic fontanelle slows the action of the heart.

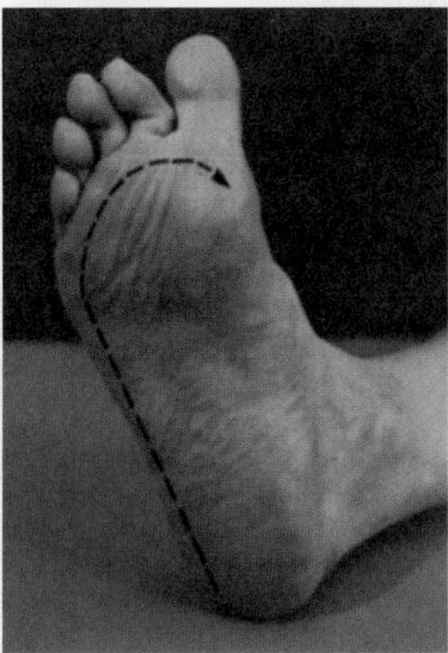

■ Babinski reflex.

Brissaud r. contraction of the tensor muscle of fascia lata on tickling the sole.

Brudzinski r. see under *sign.*

bulbocavernosus r. bulbospongiosus r.

bulbomimic r. in coma from stroke syndrome, pressure on the eyeball causes contraction of facial muscles on the side opposite the lesion; in coma from toxic causes, the reflex occurs on both sides. Called also *facial r.* and *Mondonesi r.*

bulbospongiosus r. contraction of the bulbospongiosus muscle in response to a tap on the dorsum of the penis; called also *bulbocavernous, penile,* or *virile r.*

carotid sinus r. pressure on, or in, the carotid artery at the level of its bifurcation, causing reflex slowing of the heart rate; this reflex originates in the wall of the sinus of the internal carotid artery. See *carotid sinus syndrome,* under *syndrome.*

cat's eye r. leukokoria.

cerebral cortex r. Haab r.

Chaddock r. stimulation below the external malleolus produces extension of the great toe; it occurs in lesions of the pyramidal tract.

chain r. a series of reflexes, each serving as a stimulus to the next one, representing a complete activity.

chin r. jaw r.

choked r. in fluoroscopy, absence of movement of the retinal illumination on reaching the point of reversal.

ciliary r. the movement of the pupil in accommodation.

ciliospinal r. painful stimulation of the skin of the neck, face, or another body part dilates the ipsilateral pupil. Called also *Parrot sign.*

clasp-knife r. see under *rigidity.*

closed loop r. a reflex, such as a stretch reflex, in which the stimulus (such as muscle stretch) decreases when it receives feedback from the response mechanism.

cochleo-orbicular r., cochleopalpebral r. contraction of the orbicularis palpebrarum muscle when a sharp, sudden noise is made close to the ear; it does not occur in total deafness from labyrinthine disease.

cochleopupillary r. a reaction of the iris to a loud sound, consisting of contraction of the pupil followed by dilatation.

cochleostapedial r. acoustic r.

cold pressor r. immersion of the hand in ice water for several minutes causes vasoconstriction, tachycardia, and transient hypertension due to activation of the sympathetic nervous system.

concealed r. a reflex elicited by a stimulus but concealed by a more dominant reflex elicited by the same stimulus.

conditioned r. see under *response.*

conjunctival r. closure of the eyelid when the conjunctiva is touched.

consensual r. crossed r.

consensual light r. stimulation of one eye by light produces a reflex response in the opposite pupil.

convergency r. convergence of the visual axes with fixation on a near point.

convulsive r. a reflex in which several muscles contract convulsively without coordination.

coordinated r. a reflex in which several muscles react so as to produce an orderly and useful movement.

corneal r. 1. irritation of the cornea results in reflex closure of the lids; called also *blink r., eyelid closure r.,* and *lid r.* 2. reflection of light from the cornea.

corneomandibular r. movement of the lower jaw toward the side opposite the eye whose cornea is lightly touched, the mouth being open.

corneomental r. wrinkling of the muscles on one side of the chin when pressure is applied to the cornea.

corneopterygoid r. corneomandibular r.

coronary r. the reflex that controls the caliber of the coronary blood vessels.

cough r. the sequence of events initiated by the sensitivity of the lining of the airways and mediated by the medulla as a consequence of impulses transmitted by the vagus nerve, resulting in coughing, i.e., the clearing of the passageways of foreign matter.

cranial r. any reflex whose paths are connected directly with the brain.

cremasteric r. stimulation of the skin on the front and inner side of the thigh retracts the testis on the same side. The presence of this reflex indicates integrity of the first lumbar nerve segment of the spinal cord or its root; absence indicates damage of the first lumbar nerve

segment or its root or lesion of the corticospinal tract. Cf. *Geigel r.* and *hypogastric r.*
crossed r. a response on the side of the body opposite to the side being stimulated, such as the consensual light reflex or the crossed adductor reflex.
crossed adductor r. adduction of one lower limb when an attempt is made to elicit the quadriceps jerk on the opposite side.
crossed extension r. reflex extension of a limb or body part in response to a flexion reflex in the contralateral part.
cuboidodigital r. Mendel-Bekhterev r.
Cushing r. see under *response.*
cutaneous pupillary r. ciliospinal r.
dartos r. vermicular contractions of the dartos muscle when a cold or stroking stimulus is applied to the perineum; called also *scrotal r.*
dazzle r. a reflex by which a strong light shining on the eyes causes an immediate closing of the eyelids which lasts as long as the stimulus.
deep r., deep tendon r. tendon r.
defecation r. rectal r.
delayed r. a reflex that occurs some time after the stimulus provoking it has been received.
depressor r. a response to stimulation resulting in decreased motor activity.
descending inhibitory r. the component of the peristaltic reflex in which muscles distal to a bolus relax so that the bolus can move along.
digital r. Hoffmann sign (def. 2).
direct light r. contraction of the sphincter iridis and reduction of the size of the pupillary aperture immediately after a ray of light is thrown upon the retina through the pupil.
diving r. a reflex involving cardiovascular and metabolic adaptations to conserve oxygen while diving into water; seen in reptiles, birds, and mammals, including humans.
doll's eye r. oculocephalic r.
dorsal r. contraction of the back muscles in response to stimulation of the skin over the erector spinae muscle; called also *erector spinae r.*
dorsocuboidal r. Mendel-Bekhterev r.
elbow r. triceps r.
embrace r. Moro r.
emergency light r. contraction of the pupils, closure of the eyelids, and lowering of the eyebrows.upon excessive stimulation of the retina by light.
enterogastric r. inhibition of gastric motility when something enters the duodenum, such as when chyme proceeds downward from the stomach.
epigastric r. contraction of the abdominal muscles caused by stimulating the skin of the epigastrium or over the fifth and sixth intercostal spaces near the axilla.
Erben r. slowing down of the pulse upon bending the head and trunk strongly forward, due to vagal excitability; called also *Erben phenomenon* or *sign.*
erector spinae r. dorsal r.
esophagosalivary r. excessive salivation due to irritation of the esophagus, as by a tumor or gastroesophageal reflux; called also *Roger r.*
external auditory meatus r. Kisch r.
eyeball compression r., eyeball-heart r. oculocardiac r.
eyelid closure r. 1. corneal r. (def. 1). 2. conjunctival r.
facial r. bulbomimic r.
faucial r. reflex vomiting caused by irritation of the fauces, cf. *pharyngeal r.*
femoral r. Remak r.
finger-thumb r. passive flexion of the metacarpophalangeal joint of one of the fingers causes flexion of the basal joint and extension of the terminal joint of the thumb; called also *basal joint r.* and *Mayer r.*
flexion r., flexor r. a reflex that results in movement of a limb or part toward the body, often in response to a painful stimulus; it may cause a crossed extension reflex in the contralateral body part.
fontanelle r. Grünfelder r.
foveal r. the dotlike reflex of light caused by the foveola retinae, seen during ophthalmoscopy.
front-tap r. in spinal irritability, a tap on the skin muscles of the extended leg causes contraction of the gastrocnemius muscle.
fundus r. red r.
fusion r. the reflex that tends to merge the images on the two retinas into a single impression.
gag r. pharyngeal r.
galvanic skin r. see under *response.*
gastrocolic r. an increase in intestinal and colonic peristaltic activity following entrance of food into the empty stomach.
gastroileal r. an increase in ileal motility and opening of the ileocecal valve when food enters the empty stomach.
gastropancreatic r. an increase in pancreatic secretion induced by distention of the corpus of the stomach; it is mediated by the vagus nerve.
Gault cochleopalpebral r. cochleopalpebral r.
Geigel r. a reflex in the female corresponding to the cremasteric reflex in the male: when the inner anterior aspect of the upper thigh is stroked, there is a contraction of the muscular fibers at the upper edge of the Poupart ligament. Cf. *hypogastric r.* Called also *inguinal r.*
Gifford r., Gifford-Galassi r. orbicularis pupillary r.
glabellar r., glabella tap r. reflex blinking of the eyes when the glabella is tapped; normally the patient stops blinking after the second or third tap, but in Parkinson disease and certain kinds of cerebral degeneration the blinking continues even when many taps are done.
gluteal r. contraction of the gluteal muscles when the skin of the buttock is stroked.
Gordon r. flexor r., paradoxical.
grasp r., grasping r. a grasping motion of the fingers or toes in response to stimulation; it is normal in infants, but pathologic in older persons.
Grünfelder r. dorsal flexion of the great toe with a fanwise spreading of the other toes elicited by continued pressure at the corner of the posterior lateral fontanelle; normal in infants but a sign of middle ear disease in older children.
gustolacrimal r. syndrome of crocodile tears.
H-r. a monosynaptic reflex elicited by stimulating a nerve, particularly the tibial nerve, with an electric shock. See also *H wave.*
Haab r. bilateral pupillary contraction when the patient sits in a darkened room, and without accommodation or convergence directs attention to a bright object already within the field of vision. Called also *cerebral cortex r.*
heart r. Abrams heart r.
heel-tap r. a reflex occurring in disease of the pyramidal tract, consisting of fanning and plantar flexion of the toes produced by a tap on the patient's heel.
hepatojugular r. incorrect term for *hepatojugular reflux.*
Hering-Breuer r. the neurologic mechanism that tends to limit respiratory excursions. Stimuli from the sensory endings in the lungs and perhaps in other parts passing up the vagus nerves tend to limit both inhalation and exhalation in ordinary breathing.
Hirschberg r. see under *sign.*
Hoffmann r. Hoffmann sign (def. 2).
Hughes r. virile r. (def. 2).
hypochondrial r. sudden inhalation caused by quick pressure beneath the lower border of the ribs.
hypogastric r. contraction of the muscles of the lower abdomen on stroking the skin of the inner surface of the thigh; cf. *cremasteric r.* and *Geigel r.* Called also *Bekhterev r.*
ileogastric r. inhibition of gastric motility by distention of the ileum.
inborn r. unconditioned response.
indirect r. crossed r.
infraspinatus r. outward rotation of the upper limb and straightening of the elbow upon tapping of a point over the scapula on a line bisecting the angle formed by its spine and its inner border.
inguinal r. Geigel r.
interscapular r. contraction of the scapular muscles when a stimulus is applied between the scapulae. Called also *scapular r.*
intestinointestinal r. inhibition of activity elsewhere in the intestine when one part of it has become overdistended or its mucosa has become irritated.
inverted radial r. a flexion of the fingers without movement of the forearm, produced by tapping the lower end of the radius; it indicates disease of the fifth cervical segment of the spinal cord associated with damage of the pyramidal tract below that level.
iris contraction r. pupillary r.
ischemic r. the elevation of arterial pressure in response to cerebral ischemia.
jaw r., jaw jerk r. closure of the mouth caused by a downward blow on the lower jaw while it hangs passively open; this is most obvious

with lesions of the corticospinal tract and is seen less often in healthy individuals. Called also *jaw jerk*, *chin r.*, and *mandibular r.*
Joffroy r. twitching of the gluteal muscles on pressure against the buttocks, seen in spastic paralysis.
Juster r. extension of the fingers instead of flexion on stimulation of the palm.
juvenile r. a glistening white reflection from the smooth surface of the retina in young people.
Kehrer r., Kisch r. closure of the eye as a result of tactile or thermal stimulation of the deepest part of the external auditory meatus and tympanum.
knee jerk r. patellar r.
Kocher r. contraction of the abdominal muscle on compression of the testicle; called also *testicular compression r.*
labyrinthine r's vestibular r's.
lacrimal r. secretion of tears elicited by touching or otherwise irritating the conjunctiva or the cornea.
Landau r. when an infant is held in the prone position, the entire body forms a convex upward arc; gentle pressure on the head or gravity flexes the neck and hip, reversing the arc.
laryngeal r. a type of cough reflex in which irritation of the fauces and larynx causes cough.
laughter r. laughter brought on by tickling.
let-down r. the ejection or release of milk from the alveoli of the breast into the ducts, caused by a combination of neurogenic and hormonal reflexes involving the hormone oxytocin and, to a lesser extent, vasopressin; called also *milk ejection r.* and *milk let-down r.*
lid r. corneal r. (def. 1).
Liddell and Sherrington r. stretch r.
light r. 1. cone of light. 2. a circular spot of light seen reflected from the retina with the retinoscopic mirror. 3. pupillary r. (def. 1).
lip r. a reflex movement of the lips of sleeping babies, which occurs on tapping near the angle of the mouth.
local r. a reflex whose arc does not pass through the spinal cord, such as occurs in the enteric nervous system. See also *intramural plexus*, under *plexus*.
Lovén r. general vasodilatation of an organ when its afferent nerve is stimulated; this secures a maximal supply of blood to the organ, together with a general rise of blood pressure.
lumbar r. dorsal r.
McCarthy r. supraorbital r.
McCormac r. patelloadductor r.
McDowall r. a decrease in systemic blood pressure following vagotomy, due to abolishment of the afferent impulses from the atria, which normally induce vasoconstriction.
macular r. in ophthalmoscopy, a ring-shaped reflection of light surrounding the macula lutea.
Magnus and de Kleijn neck r's extension of both ipsilateral limbs, or one, or part of a limb, and increase of tonus on the side to which the chin is turned when the head is rotated to the side, and flexion with loss of tonus on the side to which the occiput points; a sign of decerebrate rigidity except in infants. See also *tonic neck r.*
mandibular r. jaw r.
Marinesco-Radovici r. palm-chin r.
mass r. in severe injury of the spinal cord, stimulation below the level of the lesion produces flexion reflexes of the lower extremity, evacuation of the bowels and bladder, and sweating of the skin below the level of the lesion. Called also *Riddoch mass r.*
Mayer r. finger-thumb r.
Mendel r., Mendel dorsal r. of foot Mendel-Bekhterev r.
Mendel-Bekhterev r. percussion of the dorsum of the foot normally causes dorsal flexion of the second to fifth toes; in certain organic nervous conditions it causes plantar flexion of the toes. Called also *Bekhterev-Mendel*, *cuboidodigital*, *dorsocuboidal*, *Mendel*, or *tarsophalangeal r.*
micturition r. any of the reflexes necessary for effortless evacuation of urine and subconscious maintenance of continence: vesical contraction following distention of the bladder, vesical contraction evoked by urethral flow, vesical contraction evoked by proximal urethral distention, relaxation of the urethra resulting from running liquid in the urethra, distention of the bladder resulting in relaxation of the external sphincter, relaxation of the proximal urethral smooth muscle by distention of the bladder, and vesical contraction related to running liquid through the urethra.
milk ejection r., milk let-down r. let-down r.
Mondonesi r. bulbomimic r.
Morley peritoneocutaneous r. when any of the cerebrospinal nerve endings in the peritoneum or subperitoneal tissues are irritated, pain will be referred to the corresponding segmental skin area.
Moro r., Moro embrace r. flexion of an infant's thighs and knees, fanning and then clenching of the fingers, with arms first thrown outward then brought together as if in an embrace, produced by a sudden stimulus such as the table being struck next to the child, or by sudden extension of the neck when the head is allowed to fall backward or the child is pulled up by both hands from a lying position and then let go. It is seen normally in infants up to 3 to 4 months of age but is abnormal if it persists beyond that time. Called also *embrace r.* and *startle r.*
muscular r. stretch r.
myenteric r. peristaltic r.
myopic r. Weiss r.
myotatic r. stretch r.
nasal r. tickling of the mucosa of the nasal cavity produces contraction of the facial muscles on the same side of the face; called also *Bekhterev r.*
nasolabial r. sudden retroversion of the head, stretching of the back, retroversion of the arms at the shoulder, extension and pronation of the forearms, and extension and adduction of the legs, elicited by a slight vertical sweeping motion touching the tip of the nose; it frequently occurs in healthy infants, and disappears around the fifth month of age.
nasomental r. contraction of the mentalis muscle on tapping the side of the nose with a percussion hammer.
neck r's reflex adjustments in trunk posture and limb position caused by stimulation of proprioceptors in the neck joints and muscles when the head is turned; this tends to maintain a constant orientation between the head and the body.
neck righting r. rotation of the trunk in the direction in which the head of the supine infant is turned; this reflex is absent or decreased in infants with spasticity.
nociceptive r's reflexes initiated by painful stimuli.
obliquus r. stimulation of the skin below Poupart ligament contracts a part of the external oblique muscle.
oculoauricular r. slight flattening of the pinna of one ear against the skull when the eyes deviate strongly to the opposite side. Absence on

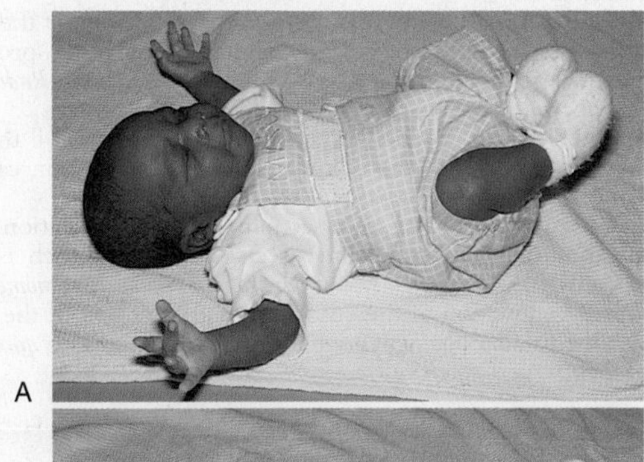

A

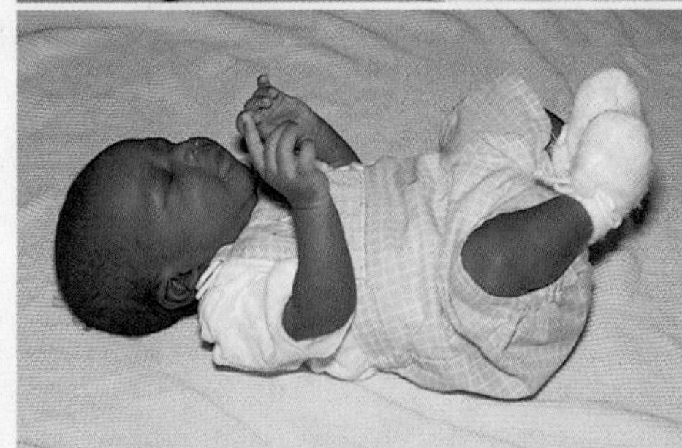

B

■ Moro reflex. After a loud noise or an abrupt change in the infant's head position, there is first symmetrical abduction and extension of the extremities *(A)* followed by symmetrical adduction and flexion *(B)*.

one side indicates facial nerve palsy at or proximal to the stylomastoid foramen.

oculocardiac r. a slowing of the rhythm of the heart following compression of the eyes. A slowing of from 5 to 13 beats per minute is normal; one of from 13 to 50 or more is exaggerated; one of from 1 to 5 is diminished. If ocular compression produces acceleration of the heart, the reflex is called *inverted.* Called also *Aschner r.* or *phenomenon.*

oculocephalic r., oculocephalogyric r. when the head is rotated laterally, the eyes deviate synergistically in the opposite direction; assessed in premature infants and the comatose to test for integrity of function of the oculomotor nerves and brainstem. Called also *doll's eye r.* or *sign* and *Cantelli sign.*

oculopharyngeal r. rapid deglutition together with spontaneous closing of the eyes in response to irritation of the conjunctiva.

oculopupillary r. stimulation of the cornea or of the eyelid results in dilation and then contraction of both pupils; called also *oculosensory r.* and *trigeminus r.*

oculosensory r. oculopupillary r.

oculovagal r. pressure on the eyeball induces ectopic atrioventricular beats or rhythm.

open loop r. a reflex, such as a flexion reflex, in which the stimulus causes activity that it does not further control and that does not give it feedback.

Oppenheim r. dorsiflexion of the big toe on stroking downward along the medial side of the tibia, seen in pyramidal tract disease.

opticofacial winking r. closure of the eyelids when an object is brought suddenly into the field of vision.

orbicularis r. orbicularis pupillary r.

orbicularis oculi r. normal contraction of the orbicularis oculi muscle, with resultant closing of the eye, on percussion at the outer aspect of the supraorbital ridge, over the glabella, or around the margin of the orbit.

orbicularis pupillary r. unilateral contraction of the pupil, followed by dilatation after closure or attempted closure of eyelids that are forcibly held apart. Called also *Galassi pupillary, orbicularis,* or *Westphal-Piltz phenomenon* and *Gifford, Gifford-Galassi,* or *Westphal pupillary r.*

orienting r. the response of an animal to an unexpected or novel stimulus or alteration of a stimulus; it involves adjustments of head, body, or sensory organs to pay close attention to the stimulus. In higher vertebrates including humans it is mediated at the brainstem level. Called also *orienting response.*

palatal r., palatine r. swallowing when the palate is stimulated; called also *swallowing r.*

palmar r. flexion of the fingers in response to scratching of the palm.

palm-chin r., palmomental r. twitching of the chin produced by stimulating (scratching) the palm; called also *Marinesco-Radovici r.* and *Radovici sign.*

paradoxical flexor r. dorsiflexion of the great toe or of all the toes when the deep muscles of the calf are pressed upon, seen in cases of pyramidal tract disease; called also *Gordon r.*

paradoxical pupillary r. 1. reversed pupillary r. 2. dilatation of the pupil on exposure to light; sometimes seen in conditions such as tabes dorsalis. Called also *Bekhterev r.* and *paradoxical pupillary phenomenon.*

patellar r. contraction of the quadriceps and extension of the lower limb when the patellar ligament is tapped; called also *knee jerk, quadriceps jerk, knee jerk r.,* and *quadriceps r.*

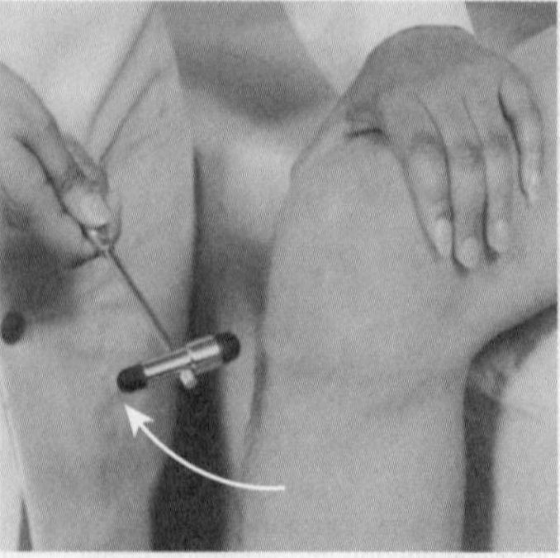

■ Eliciting the patellar reflex.

patelloadductor r. crossed adduction of the thigh produced by tapping the quadriceps tendon as in the patellar reflex; called also *McCormac r.*

pathologic r. a reflex that is not normal, but is the result of a pathologic condition, and may serve as a sign of disease.

pectoral r. with the subject's upper limb placed halfway between adduction and abduction and the examiner's finger in the muscle tendon near the humerus, adduction and slight internal rotation are normally produced by a sharp blow of the finger.

penile r., penis r. bulbospongiosus r.

perianal r. anal r.

periosteal r. contraction of a muscle after tapping of a nearby bone that lies just below the surface of the skin; see *radial r., tibioadductor r.,* and *ulnar r.*

peristaltic r. when a portion of the intestine is irritated or distended, the area just proximal contracts (see *ascending excitatory r.*) and the area just distal relaxes (see *descending inhibitory r.*).

peritoneointestinal r. inhibition of motility of the stomach and intestine resulting from retroperitoneal irritation or hemorrhage.

pharyngeal r. contraction of the constrictor muscle of the pharynx elicited by touching the back of the pharynx; called also *gag r.*

phasic r. coordinated r.

Philippson r. excitation of the knee extensor on one side induced by inhibition in the extensor of the other.

pilomotor r. horripilation (production of goose flesh) when the skin is stroked.

Piltz r. attention r. of pupil.

placing r. flexion followed by extension of the lower limb when the infant is held erect and the dorsum of the foot is drawn along the under edge of a table top, seen in the normal infant up to the age of six weeks.

plantar r. contraction of the toes when the sole of the foot is irritated; cf. *Babinski r.*

platysmal r. contraction of the pupil when the platysma is nipped.

pollicomental r. palm-chin r.

postural r. a reflex consisting of some change of posture.

pressor r. a reflex that increases the blood pressure.

Preyer r. auricle r.

primitive r. any of a group of stereotypic reflexes, such as the Moro and rooting reflexes, that are directed by centers in the brainstem and are normal in newborns but disappear in infancy in most individuals; their reappearance later in life indicates cerebral, subcortical, or diffuse frontal lobe pathology. Called also *atavistic r.*

proprioceptive r. a reflex that is initiated by a stimulus to a proprioceptor.

psychic r. a reflex aroused by a stored-up impression of memory, such as the secretion of saliva at the sight or thought of good-tasting food.

psychocardiac r. increase in the pulse rate on recalling an individual emotional experience.

psychogalvanic r. galvanic skin response.

pulmonocoronary r. reflex vasoconstriction of the coronary arteries, mediated by the vagus nerves, such as with a pulmonary embolism.

pupillary r. 1. contraction of the pupil on exposure of the retina to light. Called also *light r.* and *pupillary light r.* 2. any reflex involving the iris, changing the size of the pupil in response to a stimulus, e.g., change in illumination, change in point of fixation, sudden loud noise, or emotional stimulus.

pupillary light r. pupillary r. (def. 1).

Puusepp r. abduction of the little toe on stimulating the posterior external part of the sole of the foot; indicative of lesions of the extrapyramidal and pyramidal tracts.

quadriceps r. patellar r.

quadrupedal extensor r. Brain r.

radial r. flexion of the forearm, following tapping on the lower end of the radius; when the fingers flex as well, it indicates hyperreflexia.

rectal r. the process by which the accumulation of feces in the rectum excites defecation; called also *defecation r.*

rectoanal inhibitory r. relaxation of the internal anal sphincter in response to increased pressure in the rectum; it can be tested by inflating a balloon in the lumen. It is absent in cases of congenital megacolon.

red r. a luminous red appearance seen upon the retina during retinoscopy; called also *fundus r.*

regional r. segmental r.

Reflex *Continued*

Remak r. plantar flexion of the first three toes and sometimes of the foot, with extension of the knee on stroking of the upper anterior surface of the thigh, a sign of a spinal cord lesion; called also *femoral r.*
renointestinal r. inhibition of motility of the intestine resulting from renal irritation.
renorenal r. a reflex pain or anuria in a sound kidney in cases in which the other kidney is diseased.
retrobulbar pupillary r. slight dilation of the pupil, which contracts under light stimulation and then dilates while the light stimulation is still present.
reversed pupillary r. any abnormal pupillary reflex opposite to one that occurs normally, such as dilation of the pupil when the retina is stimulated by light. Called also *paradoxical pupillary r.* or *phenomenon.*
Riddoch mass r. mass r.
righting r. the ability to assume optimal position when there has been a departure from it.
Roger r. esophagosalivary r.
rooting r. a reflex seen normally in newborns, in which stimulation of the side of the cheek or the upper or lower lip causes the infant to turn the mouth and face to the stimulus. In older persons it indicates pathology.
Rossolimo r. when the plantar surface of the toes is tapped, if there is plantar flexion of the toes, this indicates lesions of the pyramidal tract.
Ruggeri r. acceleration of the pulse following strong convergence of the eyeballs toward something very close to the eyes; it indicates sympathetic excitability.
Saenger r. see under *sign.*
scapular r. interscapular r.
scapulohumeral r. adduction with outward rotation of the humerus produced by percussing along the inner edge of the scapula.
Schäffer r. dorsiflexion of the great toe on pinching the Achilles tendon at its middle third; seen in organic hemiplegia.
scratch r. a spinal reflex by which an itch or other irritation of the skin causes a nearby body part to move over and briskly rub the affected area.
scrotal r. dartos r.
segmental r. a reflex controlled by a single segment or region of the spinal cord.
senile r. a gray reflection from the pupil of aged people due to hardening of the lens.
sexual r. the reflex of erection and ejaculation produced by stimulation of the genitals.
shot-silk r. shot-silk retina.
simple r. a reflex involving a single muscle.
skin r. a reflex occurring on stimulation of the skin.
skin pupillary r. ciliospinal r.
Snellen r. unilateral congestion of the ear upon stimulation of the distal end of the divided great auricular nerve; called also *auriculocervical nerve r.*
snout r. pursing of the lips into a snout shape when there is a light tap near the midline of the lips, occurring normally during infancy; although its appearance later in life may indicate neurologic disease, it is also seen in healthy individuals.
sole r. plantar r.
somatointestinal r. inhibition of intestinal motility when the skin over the abdomen is stimulated.

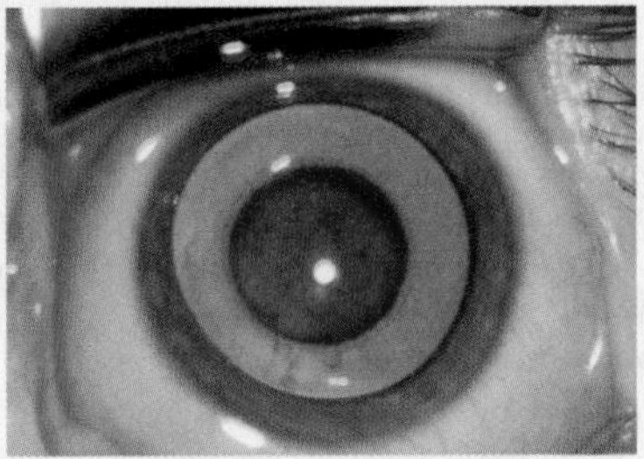

■ Red reflex partially blocked by cataract (direct ophthalmoscopy).

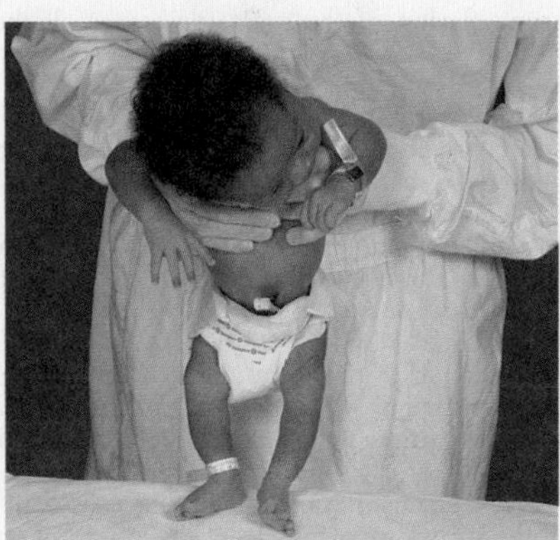

■ Stepping reflex.

spinal r. any reflex whose arc is connected with a center in the spinal cord.
stapedial r. acoustic r.
startle r. 1. Moro r. 2. see under *reaction.*
static r. any of the reflexes for maintenance of position and righting of the body, such as the *postural reflex, righting reflex,* or *vestibular reflexes.*
statotonic r's attitudinal r's.
stepping r. 1. movements of progression elicited when the infant is held upright and inclined forward with the soles of the feet touching a flat surface; it is obtainable in the normal infant up to the age of six weeks. 2. extension of the hind leg of a dog when the plantar surface of the foot is pressed.
Stookey r. with the lower limb semiflexed at the knee, flexion of the limb when the tendons of the semimembranosus and the semitendinosus muscles are tapped.
stretch r. reflex contraction of a muscle in response to passive longitudinal stretching; called also *Liddell and Sherrington r.* and *myotatic r.* See also *muscle spindle,* under *spindle.*
Strümpell r. movement of the lower limb with adduction of the foot produced by stroking the thigh or abdomen.
sucking r. sucking movements of the mouth elicited by the touching of an object to an infant's lips; this is sometimes seen in adults, particularly the elderly, with certain neurologic or degenerative conditions.
suck-swallow r. rhythmical sucking and swallowing movements in an infant when a finger or nipple is placed in the mouth.
superficial r. any withdrawal reflex elicited by noxious or tactile stimulation of the skin, cornea, or mucous membrane, including the corneal reflex, pharyngeal reflex, cremasteric reflex, and others.
supinator longus r. brachioradialis r.
supraorbital r. contraction of the orbicularis oculi muscle when the supraorbital nerve is tapped; called also *McCarthy r.*
suprapatellar r. with the subject's lower limb extended, a kicking back of the patella when it is struck by the examiner's curved index finger.
suprapubic r. stroking the abdomen above Poupart ligament causes deviation of the linea alba toward the side that is stroked.
supraumbilical r. epigastric r.
swallowing r. palatal r.
tapetal light r. the glowing of eyes in the dark, as occurs in some carnivorous animals.
tarsophalangeal r. Mendel-Bekhterev r.
tendon r. involuntary contraction of a muscle after brief stretching caused by percussion of its tendon; tendon reflexes include the biceps reflex, triceps reflex, quadriceps reflex, and others. Called also *deep* or *deep tendon r.* and *tendon jerk* or *reaction.*
testicular compression r. Kocher r.
threat r. sudden closure of the eyes at a sign of danger.
Throckmorton r. a variation of the Babinski reflex elicited by percussion of the metatarsophalangeal region in the dorsum of the foot.
tibioadductor r. tapping of the tibia on the medial side results either in homolateral adduction of the lower limb or crossed adduction from side to side.

Reflex *Continued*

toe r. if strong flexion of the great toe causes all the muscles of the lower limb to flex, this is a sign of a pathologic state that involves hyperreflexia.
tonic r. 1. a reflex in which an appreciable period of time passes between muscle contraction and relaxation. 2. a reflex that maintains the reflex contractions that are the basis of posture.
tonic neck r. a reflex in the newborn consisting of extension of the upper limb and sometimes the lower limb on the side to which the head is forcibly turned, with flexion of the contralateral limbs; cf. *Magnus and de Kleijn neck r's.*
trained r. conditioned response.
triceps r. contraction of the belly of the triceps muscle and slight extension of the upper limb when the tendon of the muscle is tapped directly, with the limb flexed and fully supported and relaxed. Called also *elbow r.* or *jerk.*
triceps surae r. plantar flexion of the foot caused by a twitchlike contraction of the triceps surae muscle, elicited by a tap on the Achilles tendon preferably while the patient kneels on a bed or chair, the feet hanging free over the edge; called also *Achilles jerk, ankle jerk, triceps surae jerk,* and *Achilles, Achilles tendon,* or *ankle r.*
trigeminus r. oculopupillary r.
ulnar r. tapping of the styloid process of the ulna results in pronation of the hand.
unconditioned r. see under *response.*
urinary r. micturition r.
vagus r. abnormal sensitiveness to pressure over the course of the vagus nerve.

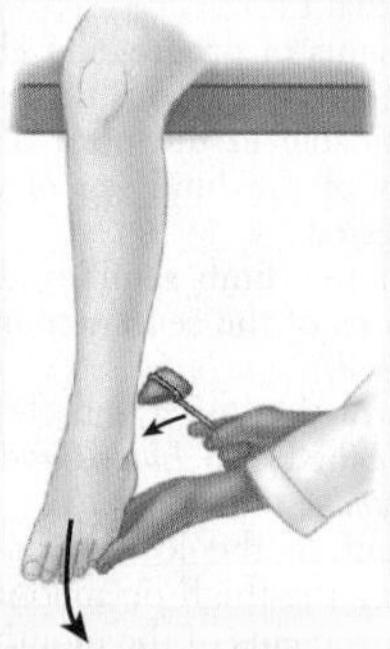

■ Triceps surae reflex.

vascular r., vasopressor r. vasoconstriction with a rise in blood pressure caused by neural stimulation.
vertebra prominens r. pressure upon the last cervical vertebra of an animal reduces the tone of all four limbs.
vesical r. bladder r.
vesicointestinal r. inhibition of intestinal motility due to irritation of the bladder.
vestibular r's the reflexes for maintaining the position of the eyes and body in relation to changes in orientation of the head; the neural pathways are complex, traveling from the vestibular nerve to the vestibular nuclei and thence to the involved muscles of the eye and body; cf. *static r.*
vestibuloocular r. nystagmus or deviation of the eyes in response to stimulation of the vestibular system by angular acceleration or deceleration or when the caloric test is performed (irrigation of the ears with warm or cool water or air). See *caloric test* and *harmonic acceleration test,* under *test.*
virile r. 1. bulbospongiosus r. 2. in the flaccid penis, a sudden reflexive downward jerk elicited by pulling upward the foreskin or glans penis. Called also *Hughes r.*
visceral r. a reflex in which the stimulus is set up by some state of an internal organ.
viscerocardiac r. reflex alteration in cardiac rhythm or contractility caused by visceral excitation.
visceromotor r. contraction of abdominal muscles (abdominal rigidity) over a diseased viscus.
viscerosensory r. a response or reaction to pressure on some part of the body due to disease of some internal organ.
viscerotrophic r. degeneration of any peripheral tissue as a result of chronic inflammation of any of the viscera.
vomiting r. vomiting due to reflexive stimulation of muscles of the gastrointestinal tract and throat, allowing their contents to be forcibly expelled; it is mediated by centers in the medulla oblongata and can be set in motion by many different stimuli such as touching the back of the pharynx. See also *pharyngeal r.*
water-silk r. shot-silk retina.
Weiss r. a curved reflection seen with the ophthalmoscope on the fundus of the eye to the nasal side of the disk; believed to be indicative of myopia.
Westphal pupillary r., Westphal-Piltz r. orbicularis pupillary r.
withdrawal r. a nociceptive reflex in which a body part is quickly moved away from a painful stimulus.
zygomatic r. lateral motion of the lower jaw to the percussed side on percussion over the zygoma.

re•flex•o•gen•ic (re-flek″so-jen′ik) [*reflex* + *-genic*] 1. producing or increasing reflex action. 2. resulting from a reflex action.

re•flex•og•e•nous (re″flek-soj′ə-nəs) reflexogenic.

re•flexo•graph (re-flek′so-graf) [*reflex* + *-graph*] an instrument for graphically recording a reflex.

re•flex•ol•o•gy (re″flek-sol′ə-je) 1. the science or study of reflexes. 2. a therapeutic technique based on the premise that areas exist in the hands or feet that correspond to the organs and systems of the body and that stimulation of these areas by pressure can affect the corresponding organ or system.

re•flex•om•e•ter (re″flek-som′ə-tər) [*reflex* + *-meter*] an instrument for measuring the force necessary to produce myotatic contraction.

re•flexo•phil (re-flek′so-fil) [*reflex* + *-phil*] characterized by exaggerated activity of reflexes.

re•flexo•ther•a•py (re-flek″so-ther′ə-pe) reflex therapy.

Re•flu•dan (rə-floo′dan) trademark for a preparation of lepirudin.

re•flux (re′fləks) [*re-* + *flux*] a backward or return flow. Cf. *backflow* and *regurgitation* (def. 1).

duodenogastric r. reflux of the contents of the duodenum into the stomach; it may occur normally, especially during fasting.
alkaline r. reflux of alkaline contents of the duodenum into the stomach or esophagus; see *alkaline reflux gastritis* and *alkaline reflux esophagitis.*
duodenogastroesophageal r. gastroesophageal r.
enterogastric r. duodenogastric r.
esophageal r. gastroesophageal r.
gastroesophageal r. reflux of the stomach and duodenal contents into the esophagus, which sometimes occurs normally, particularly in the distended stomach postprandially, or as a chronic pathological condition that leads to the conditions known as *gastroesophageal reflux disease* and *reflux esophagitis.*
hepatojugular r. distention of the jugular vein induced by pressure over the liver; it suggests insufficiency of the right heart; sometimes incorrectly called *hepatojugular reflex.*
intrarenal r. reflux of urine into the renal parenchyma.
laryngopharyngeal r. (LPR) a complication of gastroesophageal reflux caused by reflux from the esophagus into the pharynx, characterized by a variety of intermittent chronic symptoms, including hoarseness, cough, throat clearing, globus pharyngeus, and dysphagia.
valvular r. backflow of blood past a venous valve in the lower limb due to venous insufficiency.
venous r. any reflux of blood in the veins, usually of the lower limbs, due to venous insufficiency.
vesicoureteral r., vesicoureteric r. the passage of urine from the bladder back into a ureter; called also *vesicoureteral regurgitation.*

re•fract (re-frakt′) [L. *refringere* to break apart] 1. to cause to deviate. 2. to ascertain errors of ocular refraction.

re•frac•ta do•si (re-frak′tə do′si) [L.] in repeated and divided doses.

re•frac•tile (re-frak′til) capable of refracting.

re•frac•tion (re-frak′shən) 1. the act or process of refracting; specifically the determination of the refractive errors of the eye and their correction by glasses. 2. the deviation of light in passing obliquely from one medium to another of different density. The deviation occurs at the surface

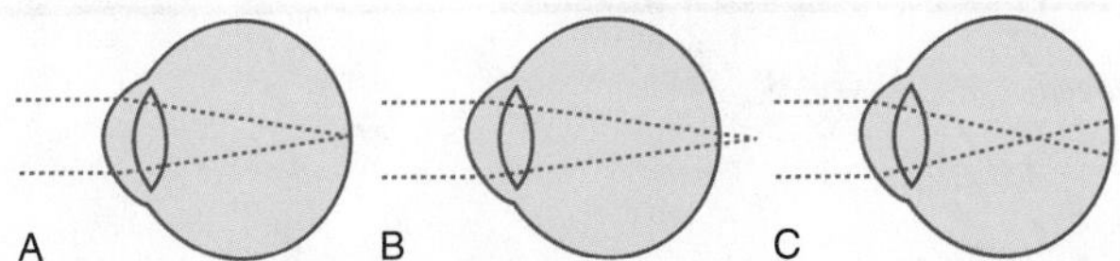

■ Refraction by the eye in *(A)* emmetropia; *(B)* hyperopia; and *(C)* myopia.

of junction of the two mediums, which is known as the refracting surface. The ray before refraction is called the *incident ray;* after refraction it is the *refracted ray.* The point of junction of the incident and the refracted ray is known as the *point of incidence.* The angle between the incident ray and a line perpendicular to the refracting surface at the point of incidence is known as the *angle of incidence;* that between the refracted ray and this perpendicular is called the *angle of refraction.* The sine of the angle of incidence divided by the sine of the angle of refraction gives the *relative index of refraction.*

cycloplegic r. a type of static refraction, measured after lens accommodation is paralyzed by administration of cycloplegic eye drops.

double r. birefringence.

dynamic r. the normal accommodation of the eye, which is being continually exerted without conscious effort.

ocular r. the refraction of light produced by the mediums of the normal eye and resulting in the focusing of images upon the retina.

static r. the refraction of the eye when its accommodation is paralyzed.

re·frac·tion·ist (re-frak′shən-ist) an individual skilled in determining the refracting power of the eyes and correcting refractive defects.

re·frac·tive (re-frak′tiv) pertaining to or subserving a process of refraction; having the power to refract.

re·frac·tiv·i·ty (re″frak-tiv′ĭ-te) the quality of being refractive; the power or ability to refract.

re·frac·tom·e·ter (re″frak-tom′ə-tər) [*refraction* + *-meter*] 1. an instrument for measuring the refractive power of the eye. 2. an instrument for determining the indexes of refraction of various substances, particularly for determining the strength of lenses of spectacles.

re·frac·tom·e·try (re″frak-tom′ə-tre) the measurement of refractive power with the refractometer.

re·frac·tor (re-frak′tər) a device for retinoscopic examination of the eye to determine its refractive power.

re·frac·to·ri·ness (re-frak′tə-re″nes) the state of being refractory.

postrepolarization r. refractoriness to stimuli that exists even after a fiber has completely repolarized; see also *absolute refractory period,* under *period.*

re·frac·to·ry (re-frak′tə-re) [L. *refractorius*] 1. resistant to treatment. See also *resistance.* 2. not responding to a stimulus; see under *period.*

re·frac·ture (re-frak′chər) the operation of breaking over again a bone which has been fractured and has united with a deformity; called also *anaclasis.*

re·fran·gi·bil·i·ty (re-fran″jĭ-bil′ĭ-te) susceptibility to being refracted; the quality of being refrangible. refran′gible *adj*

re·fresh (re-fresh′) 1. to freshen. 2. to denude a wound of epithelium to enhance tissue repair.

re·frig·er·a·tion (re-frij″ər-a′shən) cooling.

re·frin·gent (re-frin′jənt) refractive.

Ref·sum disease (syndrome) (ref′soom) [Sigvald Bernhard *Refsum,* Norwegian physician, 1907–1991] see under *disease.*

re·fu·sion (re-fu′zhən) [L. *refusio*] the return of blood to the circulation after temporary removal or stoppage of flow.

REG radioencephalography.

re·gain·er (re-gān′ər) space regainer; a space maintainer that pushes back teeth that have crowded the edentulous area. See also under *maintainer* and *retainer.*

r.-maintainer an orthodontic appliance combining the characteristics of a space regainer and a maintainer.

space r. regainer.

Re·gaud residual body (rə-go′) [Claude *Regaud,* French radiologist, 1870–1940] see *residual body of Regaud,* under *body.*

re·gen·er·a·tion (re-jen″ər-a′shən) [*re-* + *generation*] the natural renewal of a structure, as of a lost tissue or part.

epimorphic r. epimorphosis.

guided tissue r. treatment of the tissue of an accidental or surgical wound using microporous membranes as barriers to undesirable types of cells so that only the desired types of cells can enter the wound and regenerate.

morphallactic r. morphallaxis.

reg·i·men (rej′ĭ-mən) [L. "guidance"] a strictly regulated scheme of medication, diet, exercise, or other activity designed to achieve certain ends. See also *method, technique, therapy,* and *treatment.*

re·gio (re′je-o) pl. *regio′nes* [L. "a space enclosed by lines"] region: general anatomical nomenclature for an area on the surface of the body within defined boundaries.

Regio

Descriptions are given on TA terms and include anglicized names of specific regions.

regio′nes abdomina′les [TA] abdominal regions: the various anatomical regions of the abdomen including the right and left hypochondriac, flank (lateral), and groin (inguinal) regions, and the epigastric, umbilical, and pubic regions. See illustration at *abdomen.*

r. ana′lis [TA] anal region: the portion of the perineal region surrounding the anus; called also *anal triangle.*

r. antebrachia′lis [TA] antebrachial region; see *r. antebrachii anterior* and *r. antebrachii posterior.*

r. antebrachia′lis ante′rior TA alternative for *r. antebrachii anterior.*

r. antebrachia′lis poste′rior TA alternative for *r. antebrachii posterior.*

r. antebra′chii ante′rior [TA] anterior region of forearm: the anterior, or palmar, region of the forearm; called also *r. antebrachialis anterior* [TA alternative].

r. antebra′chii poste′rior [TA] posterior region of forearm: the posterior, or dorsal, region of the forearm; called also *r. antebrachialis posterior* [TA alternative].

r. auricula′ris [TA] auricular region: the surface region of the head about the ear.

r. axilla′ris [TA] axillary region: the region of the thorax around the fossa axillaris.

r. brachia′lis [TA] brachial region: see *r. brachii anterior* and *r. brachii posterior.*

r. brachia′lis ante′rior TA alternative for *r. brachii anterior.*

r. brachia′lis poste′rior TA alternative for *r. brachii posterior.*

r. bra′chii ante′rior [TA] anterior region of arm: the anterior region of the arm; called also *r. brachialis anterior* [TA alternative].

r. bra′chii poste′rior [TA] posterior region of arm: the posterior region of the arm; called also *r. brachialis posterior* [TA alternative].

r. bucca′lis [TA] buccal region: the region of the cheek.

r. calca′nea [TA] heel region: the region of the foot overlying the calcaneus.

regio′nes ca′pitis [TA] the various anatomical regions of the head, including the frontal, parietal, occipital, temporal, auricular, mastoid, and facial regions.

r. carpa′lis [TA] carpal region: see *r. carpalis anterior* and *r. carpalis posterior.*

r. carpa′lis ante′rior [TA] anterior region of wrist: the anterior aspect of the wrist.

r. carpa′lis poste′rior [TA] posterior region of wrist: the posterior aspect of the wrist.

regio′nes cervica′les [TA] the various anatomical regions of the neck, including the anterior, lateral, and posterior cervical regions and the sternocleidomastoid region; called also *cervical regions.*

r. cervica′lis ante′rior [TA] anterior cervical region: the region of the neck anterior to the sternocleidomastoid muscle, subdivided into the submandibular, carotid, muscular, and submental triangles. Called also *trigonum cervicale anterius* [TA alternative], *trigonum colli anterius* [TA alternative], and *anterior cervical triangle.*

Regio *Continued*

r. cervica′lis latera′lis [TA] lateral cervical region: the region of the neck lateral to the sternocleidomastoid region (posterior to the sternocleidomastoid muscle); called also *trigonum cervicale posterius* [TA alternative], *trigonum colli laterale* [TA alternative], and *posterior cervical triangle.*
r. cervica′lis poste′rior [TA] posterior cervical region: the region of the neck posterior to the regio cervicalis lateralis. Called also *nuchal region* and *r. colli posterior* [TA alternative].
r. col′li poste′rior TA alternative for *r. cervicalis posterior.*
r. cox′ae [TA] hip region: the region of the lower limb overlying the hip joint.
r. cru′ris [TA] leg region: the lower leg, including the regio cruris anterior, the regio cruris posterior, the regio talocruralis anterior, and the regio talocruralis posterior.
r. cru′ris ante′rior [TA] the anterior region of the leg.
r. cru′ris poste′rior [TA] the posterior region of the leg.
r. cubita′lis [TA] cubital region: the area of the upper limb about the elbow.
r. cubita′lis ante′rior [TA] the anterior region around the elbow.
r. cubita′lis poste′rior [TA] the posterior or dorsal region around the elbow.
r. deltoi′dea [TA] deltoid region: the surface region overlying the deltoid muscle.
regio′nes dorsa′les [TA] regions of back: the various anatomical regions of the back, including the vertebral, sacral, scapular, infrascapular, and lumbar regions. Called also *regiones dorsi* [TA alternative]. See illustration.
r. dorsa′lis ma′nus [TA] back or dorsum of hand: the hand surface opposite the palm.
r. dorsa′lis pe′dis TA alternative for *dorsum pedis.*
regio′nes dor′si TA alternative for *regiones dorsales.*
r. epigas′trica TA alternative for *epigastrium.*
r. facia′lis [TA] the facial region, which includes the various anatomical regions of the face: the orbital, nasal, parotid, oral, mental, infraorbital, buccal, and zygomatic regions.
r. fe′moris [TA] femoral region: the region overlying the femur.
r. fe′moris ante′rior [TA] the anterior region of the thigh.
r. fe′moris poste′rior [TA] the posterior region of the thigh.
r. fronta′lis [TA] frontal region: the surface region of the head overlying the frontal bone.
r. ge′nus [TA] knee region: the region of the lower limb overlying the knee joint, comprising the *regio genus anterior* and the *regio genus posterior.*
r. ge′nus ante′rior [TA] the anterior region about the knee.
r. ge′nus poste′rior [TA] the posterior region about the knee, including the popliteal fossa.
r. glutea′lis [TA] gluteal region: the region overlying the gluteal muscles.
r. hypochondri′aca [TA] TA alternative for *hypochondrium.*
r. inframamma′ria [TA] inframammary region: the region of the anterior aspect of the thorax situated inferior to either mamma and superior to the inferior border of the twelfth rib.
r. infraorbita′lis [TA] infraorbital region: the region inferior to the eye, adjacent to the regio nasalis.

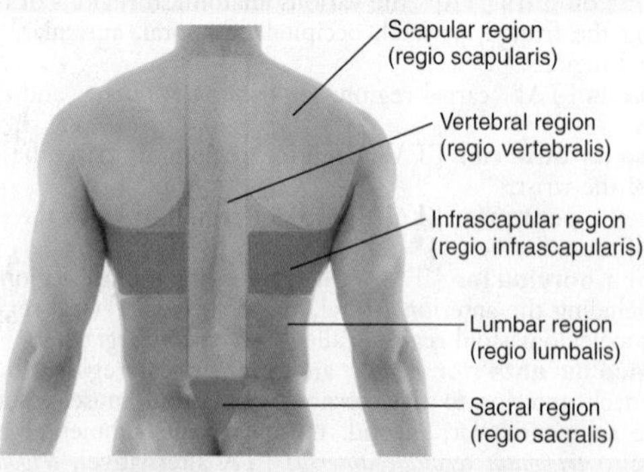

■ Regiones dorsales (regions of back).

r. infrascapula′ris [TA] infrascapular region: the region of the back inferior to the scapula and lateral to the inferior thoracic vertebrae. See illustration at *regiones dorsales.*
r. inguina′lis TA alternative for *inguen.*
r. latera′lis TA alternative for *latus*[2].
r. lumba′lis [TA] lumbar region: that part of each side of the back between the thorax and pelvis. See illustration at *regiones dorsales.*
r. mamma′ria [TA] mammary region: the region of the anterior aspect of the thorax, around the mammary gland.
r. ma′nus [TA] hand region: the region of the upper limb distal to the antebrachial region and comprising the various regions of the hand and wrist.
r. mastoi′dea [TA] mastoid region: the region of the head on either side roughly corresponding to the outline of the mastoid process of the temporal bone.
regio′nes mem′bri inferio′ris [TA] the various anatomical regions of the lower limb, including the gluteal, hip, femoral, knee, leg, and foot regions.
regio′nes mem′bri superio′ris [TA] the various anatomical regions of the upper limb, including the deltoid, brachial, cubital, antebrachial, and hand regions.
r. menta′lis [TA] mental region: the region of the chin.
r. metacarpa′lis [TA] metacarpal region: the region of the surface of the hand overlying the metacarpals.
r. metatarsa′lis [TA] metatarsal region: the region of the foot overlying the metatarsals.
r. nasa′lis [TA] nasal region: the region of the face about the nose.
r. occipita′lis [TA] occipital region: the surface region of the head overlying the occipital bone.
r. ora′lis [TA] oral region: the region of the face about the mouth.
r. orbita′lis [TA] orbital region: the region of the face about the eye; called also *ocular region.*
r. palma′ris TA alternative for *palma.*
r. parieta′lis [TA] parietal region: the surface region of the head on either side roughly corresponding to the outline of the parietal bone.
r. parotideomasseter′ica [TA] parotid region: the region of the face on either side, about the parotid gland and masseter muscle.
r. pectora′lis [TA] pectoral region: the aspect of the thorax, or chest, bounded by the pectoralis major muscle and including the lateral pectoral, mammary, and inframammary regions.
r. pectora′lis latera′lis [TA] lateral pectoral region: the region of the anterior thorax lateral to the pectoral region, bounded by the axillary region and the hypochondrium.
r. pe′dis [TA] foot region: the region of the lower limb distal to the leg region *(regio cruris),* comprising the various regions of the ankle and foot.
r. perinea′lis [TA] perineal region: the region overlying the pelvic outlet, including the anal and urogenital regions.
r. planta′ris TA alternative for *planta.*
r. presterna′lis [TA] presternal region: the region of the chest superficial to the sternum.
r. pu′bica TA alternative for *hypogastrium.*
r. retromalleola′ris latera′lis [TA] lateral retromalleolar region: the region posterior to the lateral malleolus of the fibula.
r. retromalleola′ris media′lis [TA] medial retromalleolar region: the region posterior to the medial malleolus of the tibia.
r. sacra′lis [TA] sacral region: the region of the back overlying the sacrum. See illustration at *regiones dorsales.*
r. scapula′ris [TA] scapular region: the region of the back overlying the scapula. See illustration at *regiones dorsales.*
r. sternocleidomastoi′dea [TA] sternocleidomastoid region: the region of the neck overlying the sternocleidomastoid muscle.
r. su′rae [TA] sural region: the region on the posterior aspect of the leg around the calf; see *sura.*
r. talocrura′lis ante′rior [TA] anterior talocrural region: the anterior aspect of the lower limb between the leg and foot; called also *anterior ankle region.*
r. talocrura′lis poste′rior [TA] posterior talocrural region: the posterior aspect of the lower limb between the leg and foot; called also *posterior ankle region.*
r. tarsa′lis [TA] ankle region: the region overlying the tarsal bones.
r. tempora′lis [TA] temporal region: the surface region of the head on either side roughly corresponding to the outline of the temporal bone.

Regio *Continued*

regio′nes thora′cicae anterio′res et latera′les [TA] anterior and lateral thoracic regions: the various regions of the chest, including the presternal, pectoralis, mammary, inframammary, and axillary regions, infraclavicular and axillary fossae, and clavipectoral trigone.
r. umbilica′lis TA alternative for *umbilicus* (def. 2).
r. urogenita′lis [TA] urogenital region: the portion of the perineal region surrounding the urogenital organs. Called also *genitourinary region* and *urogenital triangle.*
r. vertebra′lis [TA] vertebral region: the middle region of the back, overlying the vertebral column. See illustration at *regiones dorsales.*
r. zygoma′tica [TA] zygomatic region: the region of the face on either side, about the zygomatic bone.

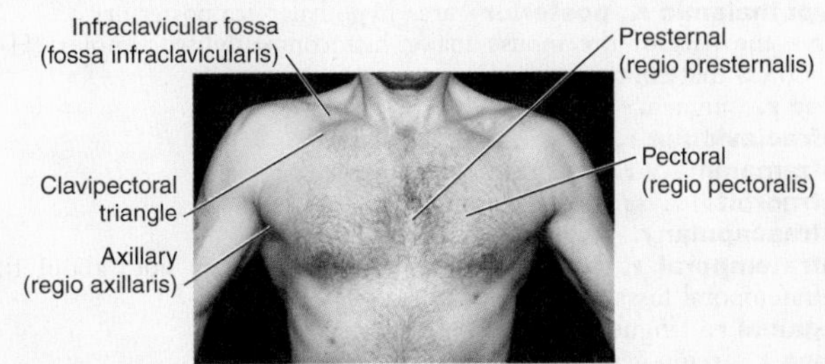

■ Shoulder and chest with regiones thoracicae anteriores et laterales (anterior and lateral thoracic regions) indicated.

re•gion (re′jən) a plane area with more or less definite boundaries; for names of specific regions not listed here, see under *regio.* **re′gional** *adj*

Region

abdominal r's regiones abdominales.
r. of accommodation the space including all points to which the eye can be adjusted by accommodation.
AN r. see *nodus atrioventricularis.*
anal r. regio analis.
ankle r. regio tarsalis.
ankle r., anterior regio talocruralis anterior.
ankle r., posterior regio talocruralis posterior.
antebrachial r. regio antebrachialis.
anterior r. of arm regio brachii anterior.
anterior r. of elbow regio cubitalis anterior.
anterior r. of forearm regio antebrachii anterior.
anterior r. of knee regio genus anterior.
anterior r. of leg regio cruris anterior.
anterior r. of neck regio cervicalis anterior.
anterior r. of thigh regio femoris anterior.
anterior r. of wrist regio carpalis anterior.
auricular r. regio auricularis.
axillary r. regio axillaris.
r's of back regiones dorsales.
basilar r. the base of the skull.
brachial r. regio brachialis.
Broca r. see under *convolution.*
buccal r. regio buccalis.
C r. constant r.
calcaneal r. regio calcanea.
carpal r. regio carpalis.
cervical r's regiones cervicales.
cervical r., anterior regio cervicalis anterior.
cervical r., lateral regio cervicalis lateralis.
cervical r., posterior regio cervicalis posterior.
chiasmatic r. area hypothalamica rostralis.
ciliary r. the part of the eye occupied by the ciliary body and its adjuncts.
complementarity determining r. (CDR) the hypervariable regions of an immunoglobulin or T cell receptor variable region that interact with complementary amino acids on an antigen or major histocompatibility complex molecule and form the antigen-binding site.
constant r. the C-terminal portion of an immunoglobulin heavy chain (C_H) or light chain (C_L), comprising one homology region in light chains and three or four in heavy chains; it has a constant amino acid sequence for chains of a single type produced by one individual. Constant regions vary among the heavy chain classes and subclasses (isotypic variation) and among individuals (allotypic variation). Called also *C r.* See illustration at *immunoglobulin.*
cubital r. regio cubitalis.
deltoid r. regio deltoidea.
dorsal r. of foot dorsum pedis.
dorsal lip r. 1. the mesodermal tissue around the dorsal lip of the blastopore of an amphibian. 2. an analogous region in the human embryo that serves as the organizer which by induction initiates and controls early development.
encephalic r. lamina alaris.
epigastric r. epigastrium.
extrapolar r. the region of the body that lies outside the influence of the poles in electrotherapy.
Fab r. see *Fab.*
facial r. regio facialis.
Fc r. see *Fc.*
femoral r. regio femoris.
foot r. regio pedis.
frontal r. regio facialis.
genitourinary r. regio urogenitalis.
gluteal r. regio glutealis.
hand r. regio manus.
heel r. regio calcanea.
hinge r. a short flexible region between the C_H1 and C_H2 domains of immunoglobulin heavy chains which allows each of the Fab regions (the "arms" of the Y-shaped immunoglobulin molecule) to move independently as necessary to bind to antigens. See illustration at *immunoglobulin.*
hip r. regio coxae.
homogeneously staining r's (HSR) long unbanded regions on chromosomes created by gene amplification; they are tumor markers indicative of solid neoplasms with poor prognosis.
homology r's regions of immunoglobulin heavy and light chains containing about 110 amino acid residues and forming compact globular domains stabilized by one intrachain disulfide bond; they have a high degree of sequence homology and similar three-dimensional structure. Each variable region (V_H and V_L) of heavy and light chains and the light chain constant region (C_L) are coextensive with a single homology region. Heavy chain constant regions are composed of three (in γ, δ, and α chains) or four (in μ and ε chains) homology regions, C_H1, C_H2, C_H3, and C_H4, and a hinge region separating C_H1 and C_H2.
hypervariable r's regions a few amino acids in length within immunoglobulin heavy and light chain variable regions at which the amino acid sequence is extremely variable; there are three in light chains and four in heavy chains. They contain most of the amino acid residues forming the antigen-binding site.
hypogastric r. hypogastrium.
hypothalamic r., anterior area hypothalamica rostralis.
hypothalamic r., dorsal area hypothalamica dorsalis.
hypothalamic r., intermediate area hypothalamica intermedia.
hypothalamic r., lateral area hypothalamica lateralis.

Region *Continued*

hypothalamic r., posterior area hypothalamica posterior.
I r. the part of the mouse major histocompatibility complex (H-2 complex) that contains the immune response genes.
iliac r. inguen.
infraclavicular r. fossa infraclavicularis.
inframammary r. regio inframammaria.
infraorbital r. regio infraorbitalis.
infrascapular r. regio infrascapularis.
infratemporal r. the area of the head on either side, about the infratemporal fossa.
inguinal r. inguen.
knee r. regio genus.
lateral r. latus[2].
lateral r. of neck regio cervicalis lateralis.
leg r. regio cruris.
locus control r. (LCR) a segment of DNA situated apart from a structural gene or cluster of genes but acting in *cis* to increase the transcriptional activity of the gene or cluster, probably by opening and remodeling chromatin structure.
lumbar r. regio lumbalis.
mammary r. regio mammaria.
mammillary r. area hypothalamica posterior.
mastoid r. regio mastoidea.
mental r. regio mentalis.
metacarpal r. regio metacarpalis.
metatarsal r. regio metatarsalis.
motor r. see under *area.*
mylohyoid r. the region on the lingual surface of the mandible to which the mylohyoid muscle is attached.
N r. see *nodus atrioventricularis.*
nasal r. regio nasalis.
NH r. see *nodus atrioventricularis.*
nuchal r. regio cervicalis posterior.
nucleolar organizing r. (NOR), nucleolus organizing r. a chromosomal region, morphologically distinguishable as a secondary constriction, that encodes ribosomal RNA; it is surrounded by a fibrillar center of a nucleolus. In humans there are five, located on the short arms of the acrocentric chromosomes. Called also nucleolar or nucleolus organizer.
occipital r. regio occipitalis.
ocular r. regio orbitalis.
olfactory r. pars olfactoria cavitatis nasi.
opticostriate r. nuclei basales; see under *nucleus.*
oral r. regio oralis.
orbital r. regio orbitalis.
palmar r. palma.
parietal r. regio parietalis.
parotid r. regio parotideomasseterica.
pectoral r. regio pectoralis.
pectoral r., lateral regio pectoralis lateralis.
perichromatin r. the boundary zone between the chromatin domains and the interchromosomal domain of the cell nucleus, forming a compartment in which RNA processing and replication and DNA replication occur.
perineal r. regio perinealis.
plantar r. planta.
posterior r. of arm regio brachii posterior.
posterior r. of elbow regio cubitalis posterior.
posterior r. of forearm regio antebrachii posterior.
posterior r. of knee regio genus posterior.
posterior r. of leg crural region, posterior.
posterior r. of neck regio cervicalis posterior.
posterior r. of thigh regio femoris posterior.
posterior r. of wrist regio carpalis posterior.
precordial r. an area of the anterior surface of the body covering the heart and part of the epigastrium down to the level of the twelfth ribs.

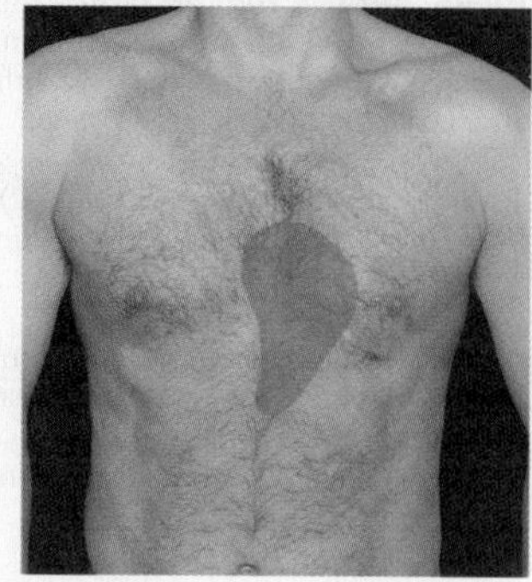

■ Precordial region.

prefrontal r. see under *area.*
preoptic r. 1. area hypothalamica rostralis. 2. area preoptica.
presternal r. regio presternalis.
presumptive r. an area of the blastula which has been proved under normal conditions to develop into a specific organ or type of tissue.
pretectal r. area pretectalis.
pseudoautosomal r's (PAR) short regions of homology on the sex chromosomes that pair and recombine during meiosis. PAR1 is located at the tip of the short arm; PAR2 is smaller and located at the tip of the long arm.
pubic r. hypogastrium.
respiratory r. pars respiratoria cavitatis nasi.
retromalleolar r., lateral regio retromalleolaris lateralis.
retromalleolar r., medial regio retromalleolaris medialis.
rolandic r. primary somatomotor area.
sacral r. regio sacralis.
scapular r. regio scapularis.
sensory r's primary receiving areas.
sternocleidomastoid r. regio sternocleidomastoidea.
supraclavicular r. the region superior to the clavicle.
supraoptic r. the part of the anterior hypothalamic region dorsal to the optic chiasm, containing the paraventricular, supraoptic, and anterior hypothalamic nuclei.
sural r. regio surae.
talocrural r., anterior regio talocruralis anterior.
talocrural r., posterior regio talocruralis posterior.
temporal r. regio temporalis.
trabecular r. the region of the embryonic cranium from which the sphenoid bone is developed.
trochanteric r. regio coxae.
tuberal r. area hypothalamica intermedia.
umbilical r. umbilicus (def. 2).
urogenital r. regio urogenitalis.
V r., variable r. the N-terminal portion, composing one homology region, of an immunoglobulin heavy chain (V_H) or light chain (V_L); it varies in amino acid sequence among chains of a single type. The antigen binding sites of immunoglobulin molecules are formed by parts of the V_H and V_L regions; thus the V_H and V_L amino acid sequences determine the antigenic specificity of the antibody molecule. Although variable regions vary among antibodies of different specificity (idiotype variation), all of the immunoglobulins produced by a single clone of plasma cells (a clonotype) have the same variable regions but may have different constant regions. See illustration at *immunoglobulin.*
vertebral r. regio vertebralis.
vestibular r. the lowest and the movable portion of the nose; see *vestibulum nasi.*
zygomatic r. regio zygomatica.

re·gi·o·nes (re″je-o′nēz) [L.] plural of *regio.*

reg·is·trant (rej′is-trənt) a nurse who is listed on the books of a registry as available for duty.

reg·is·trar (rej′is-trahr) 1. an official keeper of records. 2. in British hospitals, a resident specialist who acts as assistant to the chief or attending specialist.

reg·is·tra·tion (rej″is-tra′shən) 1. in dentistry, the making of a record of the jaw relations present, or of those desired. 2. the record so produced. See also under *record.*

bite r., interocclusal r. a record of the positional relation of the teeth or jaws to each other, made on occlusal surfaces of occlusion rims or teeth in a plastic material which hardens, such as plaster of Paris or wax.

occlusal r. bite r.

reg•is•try (rej′is-tre) 1. an office where a nurse may have his or her name listed as being available for duty. 2. a central agency for the collection of pathologic material and related clinical, laboratory, x-ray, and other data in a specified field of pathology, so organized that the data can be properly processed and made available for study.

Reg•lan (reg′lan) trademark for preparations of metoclopramide hydrochloride.

Reg•o•nol (reg′o-nol) trademark for preparations of pyridostigmine bromide.

Reg•ra•nex (reg′rə-neks) trademark for a preparation of becaplermin.

re•gres•sion (re-gresh′ən) [L. *regressio* a return] 1. a return to a former or earlier state. 2. a subsidence of symptoms or of a disease process. 3. a return to earlier, especially to infantile, patterns of thought or behavior, a characteristic of many mental disorders also exhibited by normal persons in many situations, e.g., feelings of helplessness and dependency in a patient with a serious physical illness. 4. a functional relationship between the mean value of a random variable and the corresponding values of one or more variables identified by the experimenter (the independent variables).

linear r. the statistical procedure for fitting a straight regression line to observed data, usually by minimizing the sum of the squared deviations of the observed values of the dependent variable from the regression line *(least-squares regression)*.

logistic r. a multivariate statistical method used for modeling the probability of occurrence of a dichotomous outcome as a function of multiple independent variables; it always yields a probability between 0 and 1.

multiple r. a form of linear regression or other regression method analyzing the effects of multiple independent variables simultaneously.

r. toward the mean the statistical tendency in successive generations to exhibit values closer and closer to the mean; see *Galton's law of regression*, under *law*.

re•gres•sive (re-gres′iv) going back; subsiding; characterized by regression.

Reg•ro•ton (reg′ro-ton) trademark for a combination preparation of chlorthalidone and reserpine.

reg•u•lar (reg′u-lər) [L. *regularis; regula* rule] normal or conforming to rule; occurring at proper or fixed intervals.

Reg•u•lar Il•e•tin (reg′u-lər il′ə-tin) see under *Iletin*.

reg•u•la•tion (reg″u-la′shən) [L. *regula* rule] 1. the act of adjusting or state of being adjusted to a certain standard. 2. in biology, the adaptation of form or behavior of an organism to changed conditions. 3. the power to form a whole embryo from stages before the gastrula.

reg•u•la•tor (reg′u-lə-tər) a mechanism or process that controls another mechanism or process.

r. of complement activation (RCA) complement control protein.

cystic fibrosis transmembrane r. (CFTR), cystic fibrosis transmembrane conductance r. a transmembrane protein produced by the *CFTR* gene, primarily functioning as a cAMP-regulated chloride channel that also regulates other ion channels, and found in cell membranes of the respiratory epithelium, pancreas, salivary glands, sweat glands, intestines, and reproductive tract. Numerous mutations, particularly a deletion causing omission of a phenylalanine residue from the protein, have been associated with cystic fibrosis.

reg•u•la•to•ry (reg′u-lə-tor″e) pertaining to or effecting regulation.

re•gur•gi•tant (re-gur′jĭ-tənt) [*re-* + L. *gurgitare* to flood] flowing back or in the opposite direction from normal.

re•gur•gi•ta•tion (re-gur″jĭ-ta′shən) [*re-* + L. *gurgitare* to flood] 1. flow in the opposite direction from normal, as the backward flowing of blood into the heart or between heart chambers. See also *reflux*. 2. movement of undigested or partially digested food upward through the esophagus; see also *vomiting* and *rumination*.

aortic r. (AR) the backflow of blood from the aorta into the left ventricle, owing to aortic valve insufficiency; it may be chronic or acute.

mitral r. (MR) the backflow of blood from the left ventricle into the left atrium, owing to mitral valve insufficiency; it may be acute or chronic, and is usually due to mitral valve prolapse, rheumatic heart disease, or a complication of cardiac dilatation.

pulmonic r. (PR) the backflow of blood from the pulmonary artery into the right ventricle, owing to pulmonary valve insufficiency.

tricuspid r. (TR) the backflow of blood from the right ventricle into the right atrium, owing to tricuspid valve insufficiency.

valvular r. regurgitation of the blood through the orifices of the heart valves owing to imperfect closing of the valves; see *aortic, mitral, pulmonic,* and *tricuspid r.*

vesicoureteral r. see under *reflux*.

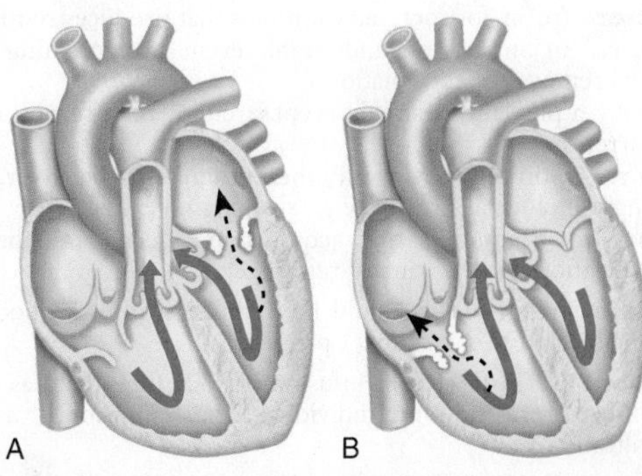

■ *(A)*, Mitral regurgitation (systole); valve incompetence allows backflow from the left ventricle into the left atrium. *(B)*, Tricuspid regurgitation (systole); valve incompetence allows backflow of blood from the right ventricle into the right atrium.

re•ha•bil•i•ta•tion (re″hə-bil″ĭ-ta′shən) [L. *rehabilitare* to rehabilitate] 1. the restoration of normal form and function after injury or illness. 2. the restoration of the ill or injured patient to optimal functional level in the home and community in relation to physical, psychosocial, vocational, and recreational activity.

neuromuscular r. rehabilitation of damaged nerves and muscles to a level at which they can do relatively complex movements.

vocational r. programs designed to help persons with disabilities acquire gainful employment either for the first time or after an illness or accident.

re•ha•bil•i•tee (re″hə-bil′ĭ-te) a person undergoing rehabilitation.

Reh•man•nia (ra-man′e-ə) [Joseph *Rehmann*, Russian physician, died 1831] a genus of tender perennial herbs native to China, Korea, and Japan, including *R. glutino′sa* (di huang), whose roots are used in traditional Chinese medicine.

re•hy•dra•tion (re″hi-dra′shən) the restoration of water or of fluid content to a patient or to a substance that has become dehydrated; see also *oral rehydration therapy*, under *therapy*.

Rei•chert cartilage, etc. (ri′kərt) [Karl Bogislaus *Reichert*, German anatomist, 1811–1883] see under *cartilage, recess,* and *scar*.

Reid's base line (rēd) [Robert William *Reid*, Scottish anatomist, 1851–1939] see *base line*, under *line*.

Reif•en•stein syndrome (ri′fən-stīn) [Edward Conrad *Reifenstein* Jr., American endocrinologist, 1908–1975] see under *syndrome*.

rei•ki (ra′ke) [Japanese, from *rei* spirit-guided + *ki* vital energy] a healing tradition of Eastern origin whose purpose is to rebalance the complex energy systems that compose the body when they have become out of balance. This unbalancing may have physical manifestations, which can be relieved by the channeling of energy from an unlimited universal energy source through the hands of the practitioner.

Reil band, etc. (rīl) [Johann Christian *Reil*, German anatomist, 1759–1813] see under *ribbon*, and see *lobus insularis* and *trigonum lemnisci*.

re•im•plan•ta•tion (re″im-plan-ta′shən) the planting back of tissue or a structure, such as a tooth, in or near the site from which it was previously lost or removed.

ureteral r. ureteroneocystostomy.

re•in•fec•tion (re″in-fek′shən) a second infection by the same pathogenic agent, or a second infection of the same person or organ by a different pathogenic agent.

re•in•force•ment (re″in-fors′mənt) in behavioral science, the presentation of a stimulus following a response that increases the frequency of subsequent responses; see *positive r.* and *negative r.*

continuous r. a schedule of reinforcement in which each response results in a reward.

covert r. the use of an imagined rather than a physical reward to increase behavioral frequency.

giant prosthetic r. of visceral sac Stoppa procedure.

negative r. presentation of an unpleasant, undesirable event that strengthens responses leading to its removal or termination.

partial r. any of several schedules of reinforcement (q.v.) in which a response yields a reward only at certain times or after certain numbers of responses.

positive r. presentation of a desirable event that strengthens future occurrences of the behavior that preceded it.

r. of reflex the increasing of a reflex response by causing the patient to perform some mental or physical concentration while the reflex is being elicited.

re•in•forc•er (re″in-for′sər) any stimulus that produces reinforcement.

negative r. an unpleasant, undesirable event strengthening responses leading to its removal or termination.

positive r. a pleasant, desirable event strengthening responses preceding its occurrence.

primary r. a stimulus having an inherent effect on behavior, generally one affecting a biological process, e.g., sleeping or eating.

secondary r. a stimulus that acquires its effects on behavior only through association with a primary reinforcer.

re•in•fu•sate (re″in-fu′zāt) fluid for reinfusion into the body, usually after being subjected to a treatment process.

re•in•fu•sion (re″in-fu′zhən) infusion of body fluid that has previously been withdrawn from the same individual, e.g., reinfusion of ascitic fluid after ultrafiltration.

Rein•ke crystalloids (crystals), edema, space (rīn′kə) [Friedrich Berthold *Reinke*, German anatomist, 1862–1919] see under *crystalloid*, *edema*, and *space*.

re•in•ner•va•tion (re″in-ər-va′shən) restoration of nerve function to a part from which it was lost; it may occur spontaneously or be achieved by nerve grafting.

re•in•oc•u•la•tion (re″in-ok″u-la′shən) an inoculation that follows a previous one with the same virus.

re•in•te•gra•tion (re″in-tə-gra′shən) 1. biological integration after a state of disruption. 2. restoration of harmonious mental function after disintegration of the personality in mental illness. Called also *redintegration*.

re•in•tu•ba•tion (re″in-too-ba′shən) intubation performed after extubation.

re•in•ver•sion (re″in-vur′zhən) restoration to its normal place of an inverted organ, especially restoration of an inverted uterus.

re•in•vo•ca•tion (re″in-vo-ka′shən) reactivation.

Reis•sei•sen muscles (rīs′i-sen) [Franz Daniel *Reisseisen*, German anatomist, 1773–1828] see under *muscle*.

Reiss•ner fiber, membrane (rīs′nər) [Ernst *Reissner*, German anatomist, 1824–1878] see under *fiber*, and see *paries vestibularis ductus cochlearis*.

Rei•ter syndrome (ri′tər) [Hans *Reiter*, German physician, 1881–1969] see under *syndrome*.

re•it•er•a•ture (re-it″ər-ə-tu′re) [L.] repeat or renew, as a prescription.

re•jec•tion (re-jek′shən) an immune response against grafted tissue that may result in failure of the graft to survive; called also *graft r.*

acute r., acute cellular r. the classic type of graft rejection, occurring 1 to 3 weeks after transplantation or following a cessation of immunosuppressive therapy and resulting primarily from the cell-mediated immune response of the recipient against incompatible human leukocyte antigens; it is manifested histologically as extensive infiltration of the graft by mononuclear cells, primarily small lymphocytes, accompanied by edema and interstitial hemorrhage.

cellular r. acute r.

chronic r. a gradual progressive loss of function of the transplanted organ occurring months or years after transplantation.

first set r. see under *phenomenon*.

graft r. see *rejection*.

hyperacute r. graft rejection occurring immediately after transplantation and resulting from the presence of preformed, circulating cytotoxic antibodies against antigens (often non-HLA antigens) on the graft. Antigen-antibody complexes on vascular endothelium initiate an Arthus-type reaction (type III reaction) in which complement activation results in infiltration by neutrophils, endothelial injury, and occlusion of capillaries with fibrin-platelet thrombi; adequate blood flow to the graft is never established.

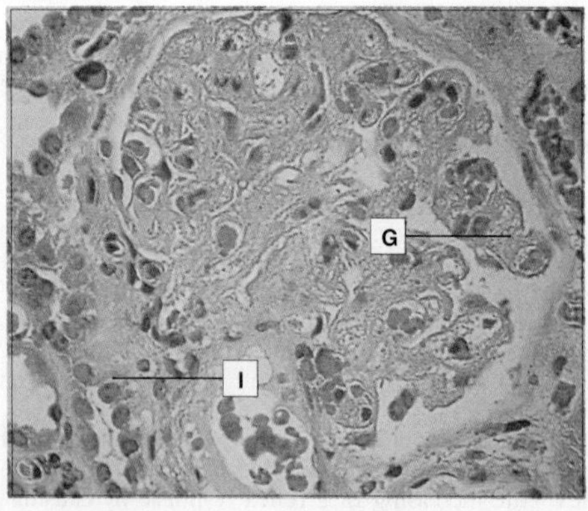

■ Renal histology showing acute rejection. Small lymphocytes and other cells are infiltrating *(I)* the interstitium of the graft. *(G)*, glomerulus.

second set r. see under *phenomenon*.

re•ju•ve•nes•cence (re-joo″və-nes′əns) [*re-* + L. *juvenescere* to become young] a renewal of youth or of strength and vigor.

Rel•a•fen (rel′ə-fen) trademark for a preparation of nabumetone.

re•lapse (re′laps, rə-laps′) [L. *relapsus*, past part. of *relabi* to fall back] the return of a disease after its apparent cessation. Cf. *recrudescence*.

intercurrent r. a relapse occurring before the temperature has reached a normal level.

rebound r. return of some of the symptoms of a disease on cessation of treatment, applied especially to the relapse of patients with rheumatoid arthritis on withdrawal of cortisone or ACTH (Hench).

re•laps•ing (rə-lap′sing, re′lap-sing) recurrent; denoting an illness that is characterized by periods of remission alternating with attacks of symptomatic disease.

re•la•tion (re-la′shən) [L. *relatio* a carrying back] the condition or state of one object or entity when considered in connection with another.

acentric r. eccentric jaw r.

buccolingual r. the position of a tooth or space in the dental arch in relation to the tongue and the cheek.

centric r. the position of the mandible, obtained principally by operator guidance, in which the condyles are in the rearmost uppermost position in the fossae of the temporomandibular joint. Called also *median retruded jaw r.* and *true centric*.

dynamic r's the relations existing between two objects or entities when one or both of them are moving or constantly changing, as the relation between the mandible and the maxilla.

eccentric r., eccentric jaw r. any relation of the mandible to the maxilla other than the centric relation; called also *acentric r.* and *eccentric position*.

eccentric jaw r., acquired an eccentric relation of the mandible to the maxilla that is assumed in order to bring the teeth into centric occlusion.

Frank-Starling r. Starling's law of the heart.

jaw r. any relation of the mandible to the maxilla, variously designated as centric, eccentric, median, occlusal, protrusive, and the like. Called also *maxillomandibular r.*

lateral occlusal r. the relation of the mandible to the maxilla when the lower jaw is in a position to either side of centric relation.

length-tension r. the relationship between the tension placed on a resting muscle, or preload, and the length of that muscle; see *Starling's law of the heart*, under *law*.

maxillomandibular r. jaw r.

median jaw r. the relation between the maxilla and the mandible when the lower jaw is in the median sagittal plane, without being displaced to either side; ideally, median and centric relations should coincide.

median retruded jaw r. centric r.

object r's the emotional bonds formed between one person and another, as contrasted with interest in and love for oneself and usually described as the capacity for love for and appropriate reaction to others.

occlusal r. see under *position*.

posterior border jaw r. see under *position*.

protrusive jaw r. an occlusal position in which the mandible is protruded. See also *prognathism*.

rest jaw r. rest position.

ridge r. the positional relation of the mandibular ridge to the maxillary ridge.

static r's the relations existing between two objects or entities when neither one of them is moving or changing in any way.

unstrained jaw r. the relation between the mandible and the maxilla that exists when a state of balanced tonus exists among all the muscles involved, being achieved without undue or unnatural force and causing no distortion of the tissues of the temporomandibular joints.

re•lax•ant (re-lak′sənt) [L. *relaxare* to loosen] 1. lessening or reducing tension. 2. an agent that lessens tension.

muscle r. an agent that specifically aids in reducing muscle tension, as those acting at the polysynaptic neurons of motor nerves (e.g., meprobamate) or at the neuromuscular junction (curare and related compounds); see also *neuromuscular blocking agent*, under *agent*.

re•lax•a•tion (re″lak-sa′shən) 1. a lessening of tension. 2. a mitigation of pain.

isometric r. relaxation of a muscle without shortening.

isovolumetric r., isovolumic r. see under *period*.

re•lax•in (re-lak′sin) a water-soluble polypeptide (molecular weight approx. 8000) extractable from the corpus luteum of pregnancy; it produces relaxation of the pubic symphysis and dilation of the uterine cervix in certain animal species. Its role in the pregnant human female is uncertain.

re·lease (re-lēs′) 1. the act of removing from restraint. 2. surgical incision or cutting of soft tissue to bring about relaxation.

lateral r. surgical division of the lateral patellar retinaculum, sometimes done in cases of chondromalacia patellae caused by patella alta.

tendon r. tenotomy.

Re·len·za (rə-len′zə) trademark for a preparation of zanamivir.

re·li·a·bil·i·ty (re-li″ə-bil′ĭ-te) 1. the tendency of a system to be resistant to failure. 2. precision (def. 2).

re·lief (re-lēf′) [L. *relevatio*] 1. the mitigation or removal of pain or distress. 2. the reduction or elimination of undesirable pressure or force from a specific area under a denture base. See also under *chamber* and *space.* 3. a thin lining of adhesive or hard baseplate wax in the master cast beneath lingual bar connectors or bar portions of the lingual plates, areas where major connectors will contact thin tissue, and beneath framework extension onto bridge areas for attachment of resin bases, which correspond accurately to the tissue topography. See also *blockout.*

re·lieve (re-lēv′) [L. *relevare* to lighten] to mitigate or remove pain or distress.

re·line (re-līn′) to resurface the tissue side of a denture with new base material in order to achieve a more accurate fit.

Rel·pax (rel′paks) trademark for a preparation of eletriptan hydrobromide.

re·lux·a·tion (re″lək-sa′shən) redislocation.

REM rapid eye movements (see also under *sleep*); reticular erythematous mucinosis.

rem (rem) [*r*oentgen-*e*quivalent–*m*an] the quantity of any ionizing radiation which has the same biological effectiveness as 1 rad of x-rays; 1 rem = 1 rad × RBE (relative biological effectiveness).

Re·mak ganglion (ra′mahk) [Robert *Remak*, German neurologist, 1815–1865] see under *ganglion.*

Re·mak reflex, sign (ra′mahk) [Ernst Julius *Remak*, German neurologist, 1848–1911] see under *reflex* and *sign.*

rem·e·dy (rem′ə-de) [L. *remedium*] anything that cures, palliates, or prevents disease. **reme′dial** *adj*

Bach r's, Bach flower r's a set of 38 flower essences, developed as a milder alternative to homeopathic remedies, that produce mental or emotional but not physical symptoms upon proving; they are used to treat mental and emotional complaints and have no direct effect on physical symptoms.

concordant r's in homeopathy, remedies of similar action but of dissimilar origin.

inimic r's in homeopathy, remedies whose actions are antagonistic.

Rescue R. trademark for a Bach remedy composed of the essences of five flowers (cherry plum, clematis, impatiens, rock rose, and star of Bethlehem) used for the acute treatment of stress.

tissue r's the twelve remedies which, according to the biochemical school of homeopathy, form the mineral bases of the body.

Re·mer·on (re′mer-on) trademark for a preparation of mirtazapine.

Rem·i·cade (rem′ĭ-kād) trademark for a preparation of infliximab.

rem·i·fen·ta·nil hy·dro·chlo·ride (rem″ĭ-fen′tə-nil) an ultra–short-acting opioid analgesic, used as an anesthesia adjunct.

Re·mij·ia (re-mij′e-ə) a genus of shrubs of the family Rubiaceae. *R. peduncula′ta* Flueck. is a source of cuprea bark, which contains cinchona alkaloids.

re·min·er·al·i·za·tion (re-min″ər-əl-ĭ-za′shən) the restoration of mineral elements, as of calcium salts to bones or teeth.

Rem·i·nyl (rem′ə-nəl) trademark for a preparation of galantamine hydrobromide.

re·mis·sion (re-mish′ən) [L. *remissio*] a diminution or abatement of the symptoms of a disease; also the period during which such diminution occurs.

re·mit·tence (re-mit′əns) temporary abatement, without actual cessation, of symptoms. **remit′tent** *adj*

rem·nant (rem′nənt) something remaining; a residue; a vestige.

chylomicron r's partially metabolized chylomicrons that have lost most of their triglycerides via degradation in muscle and adipose tissue but retain their cholesteryl esters; they reenter the bloodstream and are taken up into hepatic cells via receptor-mediated endocytosis. Within the liver, they are digested and their cholesteryl esters cleaved to generate free cholesterol.

re·mod·el·ing (re-mod′əl-ing) reorganization or renovation of an old structure.

bone r. absorption of bone tissue and simultaneous deposition of new bone; in normal bone the two processes are in dynamic equilibrium.

cardiac r. geometric and structural changes in heart chambers, usually ventricles, with decline in function that can lead to heart failure; the most common cause is cardiomyopathy, such as from the strain of hypertension or following myocardial infarction. Called also *myocardial r.* See also *ventricular r.*

cerebral vascular r. dysplastic changes in cerebral arteries with thickening of the tunica media and narrowing of the lumen; this may occur in hypertension and make the brain more susceptible to an infarct.

chromatin r. alterations in chromatin structure that affect the behavior of the chromosomes, often specifically changes in nucleosome structure causing regions adjacent to actively transcribed genes to become hypersensitive to cleavage by nucleases, as by disruption of DNA–histone contacts, releasing the histones, or by sliding of nucleosomes along the DNA.

myocardial r. cardiac r.

reverse r. in a heart that has undergone cardiac remodeling, the return to a more normal state, such as after medical treatment.

ventricular r. the most common type of cardiac remodeling, usually in the left ventricle.

Re·mod·u·lin (rĕ-mod′u-lin) trademark for a preparation of treprostinil sodium.

re·mo·ti·va·tion (re-mo″tĭ-va′shən) any of various group therapy techniques used with long-term, withdrawn patients in mental hospitals to stimulate their communication, vocational, and social skills and interest in their environment.

re·my·elin·a·tion (re-mi″ə-lĭn-a′shən) restoration of a myelin sheath after demyelination has taken place from a disease or injury.

ren (ren) gen. *re′nis* pl. *re′nes* [L.] [TA] kidney (q.v.): either of the two organs in the lumbar region that excrete the urine.

Re·nac·i·din (re-nas′ĭ-din) trademark for a preparation of citric acid, gluconolactone, and magnesium carbonate.

Re·na·gel (re′nə-jel) trademark for a preparation of sevelamer hydrochloride.

re·nal (re′nəl) [L. *renalis*] pertaining to the kidney; called also *nephric.*

Re·naut bodies (rə-no′) [Joseph Louis *Renaut*, French physician, 1844–1917] see under *body.*

Ren·du-Os·ler-Web·er syndrome (ron-du′ ōs′lər va′bər) [Henri Jules Louis Marie *Rendu*, French physician, 1844–1902; Sir William *Osler*, Canadian physician, 1849–1919; Frederick Parkes *Weber*, British physician, 1863–1962] hereditary hemorrhagic telangiectasia.

re·nes (re′nēz) [L.] plural of *ren.*

Ren·ese (rə-nēs′) trademark for preparations of polythiazide.

Ren·ese-R (rə-nēs′) trademark for a combination preparation of polythiazide and reserpine.

ren·i·form (ren′ĭ-form) [*ren-* + *form*] shaped like a kidney.

re·nin (re′nin) [EC 3.4.23.15] an enzyme of the hydrolase class that catalyzes cleavage of the leucine-leucine bond in angiotensinogen to generate angiotensin I. The enzyme is synthesized as inactive prorenin in the kidney and released into the blood in the active form in response to various metabolic stimuli. See also *renin-angiotensin-aldosterone system*, under *system.* Not to be confused with *rennin* (chymosin).

big r. prorenin.

re·nin·ism (re′nin-iz″əm) a condition marked by overproduction of renin; see also *hyperreninemia.*.

primary r. a syndrome of hypertension, hypokalemia, hyperaldosteronism, and elevated plasma renin activity, due to proliferation of juxtaglomerular cells.

re·nin·o·ma (ren″ĭ-no′mə) juxtaglomerular cell tumor.

reni·pel·vic (ren″ĭ-pel′vik) pyelic.

ren·net (ren′ət) a commercial preparation of chymosin (rennin), used to make cheeses and rennet custards.

ren·nin (ren′in) chymosin.

ren(o)- [L. *ren* kidney] a combining form denoting relationship to a kidney.

re·no·col·ic (re″no-kol′ik) pertaining to or communicating between the kidney and the colon. Called also *nephrocolic.*

re·no·co·lon·ic (re″no-kə-lon′ik) renocolic.

re·no·cor·ti·cal (re″no-kor′tĭ-kəl) pertaining to the renal cortex.

re·no·cu·ta·ne·ous (re″no-ku-ta′ne-əs) nephrocutaneous.

re·no·cys·to·gram (re″no-sis′to-gram) renogram.

re·no·du·o·de·nal (re″no-doo-ə-de′nəl) pertaining to or communicating between the kidney and the duodenum.

re·no·gas·tric (re″no-gas′trik) gastrorenal.

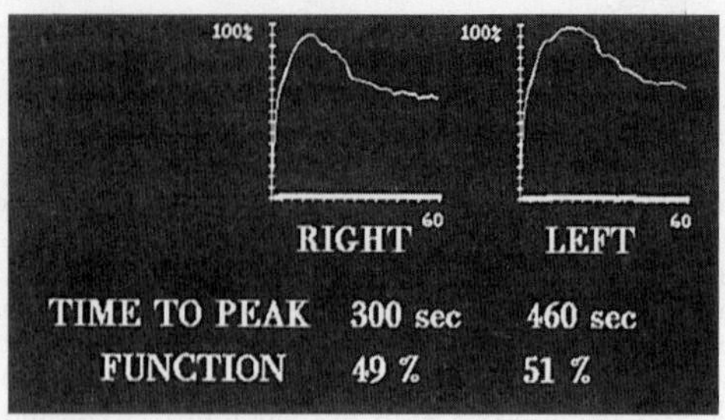

■ Renogram, showing background-corrected activity versus time to assess the relative renal function.

Re•no•graf•in (re″no-graf′in) trademark for preparations of diatrizoate sodium and diatrizoate meglumine.

re•no•gram (re′no-gram) a graphic record of kidney function produced by externally monitoring the level of radioactivity in the bladder as a radiopharmaceutical agent enters it from the kidney via the ureters; called also *nephrogram* and *renocystogram.*

re•nog•ra•phy (re-nog′rə-fe) [*reno-* + *-graphy*] radiography of the kidney; called also *nephrography.*

diuresis r. a well-hydrated patient with an empty bladder is administered a radiopharmaceutical agent and 20 minutes later a diuretic such as furosemide; the pattern of washout of the radiopharmaceutical is monitored to assess first the functioning of the collecting system and then the transport capacity of the upper urinary tract.

re•no•in•tes•ti•nal (re″no-in-tes′tĭ-nəl) enterorenal.

re•no•med•ul•lary (re″no-med′u-lar″e) [*reno-* + *medullary*] pertaining to the medulla of the kidney.

re•no•pri•val (re″no-pri′vəl) pertaining to, characterized by, or resulting from deprivation of kidney function.

re•no•pro•tec•tion (re″no-prə-tek′shən) protection of the kidney against harmful effects such as of a drug or other chemical. **renoprotec′tive** *adj*

Re•no•quid (re′no-kwid) trademark for a preparation of sulfacytine.

re•nos•co•py (re-nos′kə-pe) nephroscopy.

re•no•tro•phic (re″no-tro′fik) renotropic.

re•no•tro•pic (re″no-tro′pik) 1. having a special affinity for kidney tissue. 2. having the ability to increase kidney size; called also *renotrophic.*

Re•no•va (re-no′və) trademark for preparations of tretinoin.

re•no•vas•cu•lar (re″no-vas′ku-lər) [*reno-* + *vascular*] pertaining to or affecting the blood vessels of the kidney.

Ren•shaw cells (ren′shaw) [Birdsey *Renshaw*, American neurophysiologist, 1911–1948] see under *cell.*

re•nun•cu•lus (re-nung′ku-ləs) renal lobe; see *lobi renales*, under *lobus.*

Reo•Pro (re′o-pro″) trademark for a preparation of abciximab.

Reo•vi•ri•dae (re″o-vir′ĭ-de) the reoviruses: a family of RNA viruses having a nonenveloped icosahedral virion 60–80 nm in diameter; virions have two protein shells, the particle with the outer shell removed being referred to as the core. The genome consists of 10 to 12 structural segments of linear double-stranded RNA (total MW 12–20 × 10^6, 10–27 kbp depending on the genus). Virions contain 10–12 structural proteins, including a transcriptase, and are resistant to heat but sensitive to lipid solvents. Replication and assembly occur in the cytoplasm. Transmission is by the fecal-oral route, by fomites, or by arthropod vectors. Vertebrate pathogens are included in the genera *Orthoreovirus, Orbivirus, Rotavirus, Coltivirus,* and *Aquareovirus.* Other genera contain arthropod and plant pathogens.

reo•vi•rus (re′o-vi″rəs) [*r*espiratory and *e*nteric *o*rphan + *virus*] 1. any virus belonging to the family Reoviridae. 2. any virus belonging to the genus *Orthoreovirus.* **reovi′ral** *adj*

re•ox•i•da•tion (re-ok″sĭ-da′shən) the act of taking up oxygen again, as by hemoglobin.

re•oxy•gen•a•tion (re-ok″sĭ-jə-na′shən) in radiobiology, the phenomenon in which hypoxic (and thus radioresistant) tumor cells become more exposed to oxygen (and thus more radiosensitive) by coming into closer proximity to capillaries after death and loss of other tumor cells due to previous irradiation.

Rep. [L.] repeta′tur (let it be repeated).

rep (rep) [*r*oentgen *e*quivalent *p*hysical] an unofficial unit of the amount of radiation of any kind which yields an amount of energy transferred to the tissue equal to that transferred by 1 roentgen of hard x- or γ-radiation (200 V or greater); it is approximately 93 ergs per gram of water or soft tissue.

re•pag•li•nide (rə-pag′lĭ-nīd) an oral hypoglycemic agent that acts by stimulating the release of insulin from functioning beta cells in the pancreatic islet tissue; used, often in combination with metformin, in the treatment of type 2 diabetes mellitus.

re•pair (re-pār′) 1. restoration to sound condition after damage or injury. 2. physical or mechanical restoration of damaged or diseased tissues by the growth of healthy new cells or by surgical apposition.

Canadian r. Shouldice r.

Bassini r. repair of inguinal hernia, with high ligation of the sac, reinforcement of the floor of the canal, and placement of the spermatic cord under the external oblique anastomosis. Called also *Bassini operation.*

Cooper ligament r. McVay r.

global genome r. (GGR) the form of nucleotide excision repair (q.v.) occurring throughout the genome; a complex of proteins identifies DNA damage by detection of distortions in the DNA helix. A variety of mutations affecting this pathway have been associated with xeroderma pigmentosum. Cf. *transcription-coupled r.*

hymen r. hymenoplasty.

Lichtenstein r. tension-free hernioplasty in which the inguinal floor is reinforced by a sheet of mesh placed between the fascia transversalis and the aponeurosis of the external oblique muscle.

McVay r. repair of an inguinal hernia by suturing the conjoined tendon (inguinal falx) first to the pectineal ligament (Cooper ligament) from the pubic tubercle laterally to the femoral canal and then to the inguinal ligament beyond the femoral canal, with recreation of the internal inguinal ring.

mismatch r. correction of unpaired or mispaired bases in DNA strands, resulting from errors introduced during DNA replication, by excision of defective single-strand segments and synthesis of new ones; the process is directed by mismatch repair genes.

nucleotide excision r. (NER) repair of bulky lesions introduced into DNA by damage, such as that induced by ultraviolet light; at least 30 proteins are involved and the process consists of recognition of the lesion, strand separation at the site, single strand incision on both sides of the lesion with excision of the lesion-containing single-stranded fragment, and DNA synthesis and ligation to fill and close the gap. It comprises two subpathways that differ in their recognition of DNA damage: global genome repair and transcription-coupled repair (qq.v.).

postreplication r. a damage tolerance mechanism that allows DNA synthesis to continue across damaged regions of DNA when the lesions have not been repaired prior to replication; the gaps resulting in the daughter strands are filled in by recombination with intact undamaged parental strands.

Shouldice r. a modification of the Bassini repair, with a continuous suture being used instead of an interrupted suture.

transcription-coupled r. (TCR) the form of nucleotide excision repair (q.v.) acting on the transcribed strand of genes; blocking of RNA polymerase progression by DNA damage initiates the repair process. Mutations affecting this pathway have been associated with Cockayne syndrome. Cf. *global genome r.*

re•par•a•tive (re-par′ə-tiv) pertaining to or effecting repair.

re•pa•ten•cy (re-pa′tən-se) [*re-* + *patency*] reestablishment of the opening in a part or vessel which has been closed.

re•peat (re-pēt′) something done or occurring more than once, particularly over and over.

long terminal r's (LTR) identical DNA sequences occurring at each end of an integrated retrovirus and essential for integration of the molecule into host DNA; each is several hundred nucleotides long and contains a short, inverted, repeated sequence at each of its own ends. Many also contain elements regulating the expression of the DNA they surround.

leucine-rich r. (LRR) a type of short motif of a protein that has about 24 residues and 5 leucines, which makes a hydrophobic region that participates in protein-protein interactions. See *leucine-rich repeat protein*, under *protein.*

short tandem r. (STR), simple sequence r. (SSR) microsatellite.

tandem r. 1. arrangement of two or more copies of a nucleotide sequence adjacent to each other within a segment of DNA. 2. arrangement of two or more copies of a gene or two or more copies of a segment of a chromosome adjacent to each other on a chromosome.

trinucleotide r., triplet r. an unstable DNA sequence of three nucleotides, occurring in some human genes and normally repeated in tandem 5 to 50 times; expansion above that number has been linked to certain genetic disorders. The triplet sequences always begin with C and end with G (see *genetic code*, under *code*). See also *triplet repeat disorders*, under *disorder.*

variable number tandem r's (VNTR) different numbers of tandemly repeated oligonucleotide sequences in the alleles of a gene; such polymorphism can be useful in genetic mapping. See also *minisatellite.*

re•peat•a•bil•i•ty (re-pēt″ə-bil′ĭ-te) precision (def. 2).

re·pel·lent (re-pel′ənt) [L. *repellere* to drive back] able to repel or drive off; also an agent so acting, as *insect repellent.*

re·pel·ler (re-pel′ər) an instrument used in labor of animals to push back the fetus until the head and limbs can be properly placed for normal delivery.

re·per·co·la·tion (re″pər-ko-la′shən) [*re-* + *percolation*] a second or repeated percolation with the same materials.

re·per·fu·sion (re″pər-fu′zhən) restoration of blood flow to an area or part that was temporarily ischemic.

re·pe·ta·tur (re″pe-ta′tūr) [L.] let it be repeated.

re·pig·men·ta·tion (re-pig″men-ta′shən) restoration of pigmentation to skin that has lost it.

re·place·ment (re-plās′ment) 1. substitution; see also *replacement therapy*, under *therapy*. 2. arthroplasty.
  articular r., joint r. arthroplasty.
  total joint r. see under *arthroplasty.*

re·plan·ta·tion (re″plan-ta′shən) the replacement of an organ or other structure, such as a digit, limb, or tooth, to the site from which it was previously lost or removed; called also *reimplantation.*

re·plen·ish·er (re-plen′ish-ər) an agent that restores what has been lost, used up, or is lacking.

re·ple·tion (re-ple′shən) [L. *repletio*] the condition of being full.

rep·li·case (rep′lĭ-kās) 1. an RNA-directed RNA polymerase. 2. more generically, any enzyme that replicates nucleic acids, i.e., a DNA or RNA polymerase.

rep·li·ca·tion (rep″lĭ-ka′shən) [L. *replicatio* a fold backwards] 1. a turning back of a part so as to form a duplication. 2. repetition of an experiment to ensure accuracy. 3. the process of duplicating or reproducing, as the replication of an exact copy of a strand of DNA or RNA.
  DNA r. the production of multiple identical copies of a DNA molecule by unwinding the two strands of the double helix and forming a new complementary strand to each.
  semiconservative r. the mode in which DNA is replicated, each daughter molecule having one newly synthesized strand and one strand from the parent molecule.

rep·li·ca·tion er·ror-pos·i·tive (rep″lĭ-ka′shən er′ər poz′ĭ-tiv) a term sometimes used to denote the phenotype associated with microsatellite instability (q.v.).

rep·li·ca·tive (rep′lĭ-ka″tiv) pertaining to replication.

rep·li·con (rep′lĭ-kon) a unit of DNA that contains an initiation point and a termination point and is capable of self-replication. In bacteria, plasmids, and viruses, there is a single replicon, while a eukaryotic chromosome contains many.

rep·li·some (rep′lĭ-sōm) [*replication* + *-some*] a complex consisting of a primosome and other proteins involved in DNA replication that moves along as the complementary strand is synthesized.

re·po·lar·iza·tion (re-po″lər-ĭ-za′shən) the reestablishment of polarity, especially the return of cell membrane potential to resting potential after depolarization. See also *potassium channel* and *sodium channel*, under *channel.*
  early r. a normal variant of the usually isoelectric ST segment in which the segment is elevated at its J point; it is seen mostly in children, young adults, and black men.

re·po·si·tion·ing (re″pə-zish′ən-ing) 1. changing the position of something. 2. the replacing of a structure or part to its normal site.
  jaw r. the changing of any relative position of the mandible to the maxilla, usually by altering the occlusion of the natural or artificial teeth.
  muscle r. surgical replacement of a muscle attachment into a more acceptable functional position.

re·pos·i·tor (re-poz′ĭ-tər) an instrument used in returning a displaced organ or tissue to the normal position.

re·pos·i·to·ry (re-poz′ĭ-tor-e) a place where something is stored; used in pharmacology to refer to the injection, usually intramuscularly, of a long-acting drug, which is slowly absorbed and is therefore prolonged in its action.

re·pres·si·ble (re-pres′ĭ-bəl) capable of undergoing repression.

re·pres·sion (re-presh′ən) 1. the act of restraining, inhibiting, or suppressing. 2. in psychiatry, an unconscious defense mechanism in which unacceptable ideas, fears, and impulses are thrust out or kept out of consciousness. 3. gene r.
  coordinate r. parallel diminution of the concentrations of the several enzymes of a metabolic pathway, resulting from increases in the level of repressor.
  endproduct r. enzyme r.

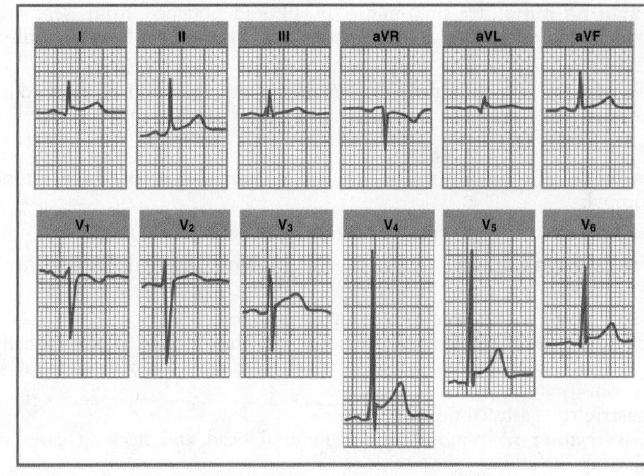

■ Early repolarization. The benign ST segment elevations are usually most marked in the midprecordial leads (V_4 here)

  enzyme r. interference, usually by the endproduct of a pathway, with synthesis of the enzymes of that pathway.
  gene r. the inhibition of gene transcription of an operon; in prokaryotes the mechanism involves binding of the operon by a repressor, sometimes also requiring the binding of a corepressor or absence of an inducer. The end result is frequently a decrease in the level of an enzyme.

re·pres·sor (re-pres′ər) [L. "a restrainer"] in genetics, a protein produced by a regulator gene that binds to the operator region of a structural gene to block initiation of transcription of the gene or operon.

re·pro·duc·i·bil·i·ty (re″pro-doo″sĭ-bil′ĭ-te) precision (def. 2).

re·pro·duc·tion (re″pro-duk′shən) [*re-* + L. *productio* production] 1. the production of offspring by organized bodies; called also *procreation* and *propagation.* 2. the creation of a similar object or situation; duplication; replication.
  asexual r. reproduction without the fusion of gametes, as by fission or budding.
  bisexual r. see *sexual r.*
  cytogenic r. reproduction in which the new individual proceeds from a single germ cell or zygote.
  sexual r. reproduction by the fusion of a female gamete and a male gamete (called also *bisexual r.*, *amphigony*, *gamogenesis*, and *syngamy*) or by development of an unfertilized egg (called also *unisexual r.*). See also *parthenogenesis.*
  somatic r. reproduction in which the new individual proceeds from a multicellular fragment produced by fission or budding.
  unisexual r. see *sexual r.*
  vegetative r. asexual r.

re·pro·duc·tive (re″pro-duk′tiv) pertaining to or characterized by reproduction.

Re·pro·nex (re′pro-neks) trademark for a preparation of menotropins.

rep·til·ase (rep′til-ās) an enzyme from Russell's viper venom that clots fibrinogen and can be used to determine blood coagulation time.

rep·tile (rep′tīl) any member of the class Reptilia.

Rep·til·ia (rep-til′e-ə) a class of aquatic or terrestrial, cold-blooded vertebrates, including snakes, lizards, turtles, alligators, and crocodiles, as well as the extinct dinosaurs, which have bodies covered with horny scales or plates and breathe by means of lungs; most lay eggs outside of the body.

re·pul·lu·la·tion (re-pul″u-la′shən) [*re-* + *pullulation*] renewed growth by sprouting.

re·pul·sion (re-pul′shən) [L. *re-* back + *pellere* to drive] 1. the act of driving apart or away; a force which tends to drive two bodies apart. It is the opposite of attraction. 2. in genetics, the occurrence on opposite chromosomes in a double heterozygote of the two mutant alleles of interest. Cf. *coupling.*

Re·quip (re′kwip) trademark for a preparation of ropinirole hydrochloride.

RES reticuloendothelial system.

re·sa·zu·rin (re-sa′zu-rin) a quinone-imine compound used as a pH indicator with a pH range of 3.8 (orange) to 6.5 (violet). It is also used as an indicator of redox potential, turning from blue (oxidized) to pink (partially reduced) to colorless (fully reduced).

re·scin·na·mine (re-sin′ə-min) an alkaloid obtained from *Rauwolfia serpentina* and other species of *Rauwolfia;* administered orally as an antihypertensive.

Re·scrip·tor (re-skrip′tor) trademark for a preparation of delavirdine mesylate.

res·cue (res′ku) salvage.

Res·cu·la (res′ku-lə) trademark for a preparation of unoprostone isopropyl.

re·sect (re-sekt′) to remove part or all of an organ or tissue.

re·sec·ta·ble (re-sek′tə-bəl) capable of being resected; lending itself to resection.

re·sec·tion (re-sek′shən) [L. *resectio*] excision.

bladder neck r. surgical removal of the bladder neck, usually done by the transurethral route to treat obstruction or neurogenic dysfunction.

gastric r. gastrectomy.

Girdlestone r. removal of the femoral head and neck in cases of severe hip infection.

root r., root-end r. apicoectomy.

sleeve r. see under *lobectomy.*

submucous r. a formerly common technique for correction of a deviated nasal septum: the mucous membrane is opened and a portion of the underlying tissue is excised and repositioned or replaced.

transurethral r. (TUR) endoscopic removal of tissue through the urethra in the treatment of genitourinary disorders, such as bladder tumor, prostate hyperplasia, or ejaculatory duct obstruction; see also *transurethral r. of bladder tumor* and *transurethral r. of the prostate.*c

transurethral r. of bladder tumor (TURBT) removal of a tumor of the urinary bladder by means of a cystoscope passed through the urethra.

transurethral r. of the prostate (TURP) prostatectomy done with a cystoscope passed through the urethra.

wedge r. removal of a triangular-shaped segment of tissue.

re·sec·to·scope (re-sek′to-skōp) an instrument with a wide-angle telescope and an electrically activated wire loop for transurethral removal or biopsy of lesions of the bladder, prostate, or urethra.

re·sec·tos·co·py (re″sək-tos′kə-pe) resection or biopsy of lesions by means of the resectoscope.

re·ser·pine (rə-sur′pēn) [USP] an alkaloid isolated from the root of *Rauwolfia serpentina* and other species of *Rauwolfia;* used as an antihypertensive, administered orally.

re·serve (re-zurv′) 1. to hold back for future use. 2. a supply, beyond that ordinarily used, which may be utilized in an emergency.

adrenal r. the amounts of adrenal hormones available for bodily purposes; when it is low, a person has adrenal insufficiency.

alkali r., alkaline r. the amount of conjugate base components of the blood buffers; since bicarbonate is the most important of these conjugate bases, the blood bicarbonate is often considered to be equivalent.

bone marrow r. a storage pool of mature neutrophils in the bone marrow, which can be released as needed.

cardiac r. the potential ability of the heart to perform a wide range of work beyond that required under basal conditions, depending on changing demands of various physiological or pathological states; usually expressed as a percentage increase above normal.

contractile r. the additional amount of contractility that can be elicited from abnormally contracting ventricular wall segments by application of a suitable stimulus.

ovarian r. the number and quality of oocytes in the ovaries of a woman of childbearing age.

renal r. the increase in glomerular filtration rate that is seen for 2 to 4 hours after intake of a high-protein meal.

re·ser·voir (rez′ər-vwahr) [Fr. *réservoir,* from *réserver* to reserve] 1. a place or cavity for storage. 2. cisterna. 3. an alternate or passive host or carrier that harbors pathogenic organisms or parasites, without injury to itself, and serves as a source from which other individuals can be infected. Called also *reservoir host* or *r. of infection.*

cardiotomy r. in cardiopulmonary bypass, a collection chamber for blood suctioned from the heart chambers and pericardium.

continent ileal r. 1. an intra-abdominal pouch having a volume of at least 500 mL and a valve; it maintains continence of feces and is emptied by a catheter when full. See also *Kock pouch.* 2. ileal neobladder.

continent urinary r. neobladder.

ileoanal r. a pouch for the retention of feces, formed by suturing together multiple limbs of ileum and connected to the anus by a short conduit of ileum; done in conjunction with colectomy and ileoanal anastomosis to provide for continent elimination of feces in the management of ulcerative colitis.

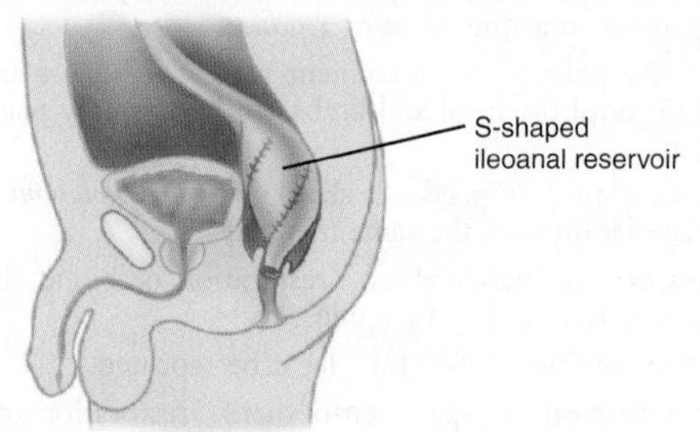

r. of infection reservoir (def. 3).

Ommaya r. a device implanted beneath the galea aponeurotica for instillation of medication or removal of fluid through a catheter in a lateral ventricle of the brain.

Pecquet r. cisterna chyli.

re·shap·ing (re-shāp′ing) a restoration or change of shape, as of a crown, bridge, or denture.

res·i·dent (rez′ĭ-dənt) 1. a graduate and licensed physician receiving training in a specialty, usually in a hospital. 2. resident physician. 3. being or pertaining to such a physician.

re·sid·ua (re-zid′u-ə) [L.] plural of *residuum.*

re·sid·u·al (re-zid′u-əl) [L. *residuus*] remaining or left behind.

res·i·due (rez′ĭ-doo) [L. *residuum,* from *re-* back + *sidere* to sit] 1. a remainder; that which remains after the removal of other substances. 2. in biochemistry, the portion of a molecule that remains after it has lost some of its components, such as an amino acid residue.

amino acid r. an amino acid molecule that has lost a water molecule by becoming joined to a molecule of another amino acid.

day r. the thoughts, feelings, and ideas related to the events of the day that appear in or shape the contents of the dreams that night.

re·sid·u·um (re-zid′u-əm) pl. *resid′ua* [L.] 1. a residue or remainder. 2. in coccidian protozoa, the material remaining after completion of different stages in the life cycle of the parasite. Called also *residual body.*

gastric r. the contents of the stomach during the interdigestive period, such as in the morning before eating.

re·sil·ience (rə-zil′yəns) [L. *resilire* to leap back] 1. the property of being able to return to the original form after distortion, as by bending, compressing, or stretching. 2. the ability to recover readily from an illness. 3. resiliency.

re·sil·ien·cy (rə-zil′yən-se) 1. resilience. 2. a measure of the energy required to stress an object to the proportional limit (see under *limit*).

re·sil·i·ent (re-zil′yənt) [L. *resiliens*] elastic; returning to its former shape or size after distortion.

res·in (rez′in) [L. *resina*] 1. any of various highly combustible semisolids or amorphous solids that are insoluble in water, mostly soluble in alcohol or ether, and generally soft and sticky but hardening after exposure to cold. Chemically diverse, they occur naturally as exudations from plants or from insects feeding on plants, and they can also be produced synthetically. 2. a compound made by condensation or polymerization of low-molecular-weight organic compounds.

acrylic r's a class of thermoplastic resins, ethylene derivatives containing a vinyl group, produced by polymerization of acrylic or methacrylic acid or their derivatives; used in a variety of medical and dental applications, including medical prostheses and instruments and dental restorations, prostheses, and appliances. They are also used as adsorbents in chromatography and as ion exchange resins.

activated r. self-curing r.

anion exchange r. an ion exchange resin (q.v.) that exchanges anions; pharmacologic uses include treatment of familial hypercholesterolemia and of pruritus associated with partial biliary obstruction.

A-stage r. resole.

autopolymer r. self-curing r.

cation exchange r. an ion exchange resin (q.v.) that exchanges cations; pharmacologic uses include treatment of hyperkalemia and prevention of formation of calcium-containing renal calculi.

cholestyramine r. [USP] a strongly basic anion exchange resin in the chloride form, consisting of styrene-divinylbenzene copolymer with quaternary ammonium functional groups, having an affinity for bile acids, which it binds into an insoluble complex that is excreted in the feces, resulting in elimination of bile acids from the enterohepatic circulation and in increased oxidation of cholesterol to bile acids; administered orally as adjunctive therapy to diet in the management of patients with elevated cholesterol due to familial hyperlipoproteinemia, type IIa (patients with pure hypercholesterolemia), for the relief of pruritus associated with cholestasis occurring in partial biliary obstruction, and to treat diarrhea due to excess bile acids in the colon.

cold-curing r. self-curing r.

composite r. resin matrix composite.

copolymer r. a resin produced by the concurrent and joint polymerization of two or more different monomers or polymers.

C-stage r. resite.

cyanoacrylate r. a resin based on alkyl 2-cyanoacrylates, used in surgical sutures and periodontal dressings.

direct filling r. a resin or a composite, usually an acrylic, that is inserted directly into the prepared cavity and allowed to polymerize at the temperature in the mouth.

epoxy r. a thermosetting resin based on reactivity of the epoxide group, which is characterized by toughness, adhesibility, chemical resistance, dielectric properties, and dimensional stability; several modified types are used as denture base material. Inhalation of its vapors can cause *epoxy resin lung*, a form of hypersensitivity pneumonitis.

heat-curing r. a resin that requires the use of heat to effect its polymerization.

ion exchange r. a high molecular weight, insoluble polymer of simple organic compounds with the ability to exchange its attached ions for other ions in the surrounding solution. They are classified as *(a) cation* or *anion exchange resins*, depending on which ions the resin exchanges, and *(b) carboxylic, sulfonic*, etc., depending on the nature of the active groups.

ionomer r. a copolymer of ethylene and a vinyl monomer with an acid group to form a transparent resilient thermoplastic material; used in flasks, bottles, and tubing.

light-activated r., light-cured r. a resin whose polymerization is activated by exposure to light; dental resins are usually activated by blue light (wavelength 400–500 nm).

podophyllum r. [USP] a powdered mixture of resins removed from podophyllum by percolation with alcohol and subsequent precipitation upon addition of acidified water; used as a topical caustic in the treatment of laryngeal papillomas, condylomata acuminata, keratoses, and other epitheliomas; available as a 25 per cent solution in alcohol, which may be diluted for use. Called also *podophyllin.* See also *podophyllotoxin.*

quick-cure r., self-curing r. any resin that can be polymerized by the addition of an activator and a catalyst without the use of external heat; used in dental restorations and repairs. Called also *activated r., autopolymer r.*, and *cold-curing r.*

styrene r. polystyrene.

synthetic r. an amorphous, organic, semisolid or solid material produced from low-molecular-weight organic compounds by polymerization or condensation.

thermoset r., thermosetting r. a resin that after its initial hardening reaction remains rigid or solid when cooled and reheated; several are used in dentistry, e.g, epoxy resin.

vinyl r. a thermoplastic resin, an ethylene derivative containing the vinyl radical, $CH_2{=\!=}CH{-\!-}$.

res•i•noid (rez′ĭ-noid) 1. resembling a resin. 2. a substance resembling a resin. 3. a dry therapeutic precipitate prepared from a vegetable tincture.

res•i•nous (rez′ĭ-nəs) [L. *resinosus*] of the nature of a resin.

re•sis•tance (re-zis′təns) [L. *resistere* to stand back] 1. opposition, or counteracting force. 2. the natural ability of an organism to resist microorganisms or toxins produced in disease. 3. the opposition to the flow of electrical current between two points of a circuit; it is the voltage drop between the two points divided by the current flow, in SI units expressed in ohms. Symbol R or *R.* 4. in psychiatry, conscious or unconscious defenses that prevent material in the unconscious, as repressed thoughts, from coming into awareness.

airway r. the opposition of the tracheobronchial tree to air flow: the mouth-to-alveoli pressure difference divided by the air flow. Symbol R_A or R_{AW}.

androgen r. androgen insensitivity.

complete androgen r. complete androgen insensitivity syndrome.

drug r. 1. the ability of a microorganism or virus to withstand the effects of a drug that are lethal to most members of its species. *Primary drug resistance* refers to initial infection by a resistant organism; *secondary drug resistance* is resistance that develops during the course of therapy. See also *multidrug r.* Microbial resistance to a drug can be symbolized by the superscript R, *R*, r, or *r* attached to the name of the drug. 2. resistance by a tumor cell line to a cytotoxic compound or compounds.

electrical r. resistance (def. 3).

environmental r. the sum of the physical and biologic factors that prevent a species from reproducing at its maximum rate.

glucocorticoid r. decreased sensitivity target tissues and a consequent elevation in circulating adrenocortical hormone levels, without the clinical features of Cushing syndrome; manifestations range from asymptomatic hyperadrenocorticism to syndromes of mineralocorticoid or adrenocortical androgen excess. It may be secondary to infectious, allergic, or inflammatory processes or result from sporadic or familial mutations in the glucorticoid receptor.

incomplete androgen r. partial androgen insensitivity syndrome.

insulin r. impairment of normal biologic responses to insulin, which may result from abnormalities in the beta-cell products, binding of insulin to antagonists such as anti-insulin antibodies, defects in receptors, reduced numbers of receptors, or defects in the insulin action cascade in the target cell. It can also be caused by excessive quantities of growth hormone, adrenocortical steroids, or some other regulators, or by chronic hyperinsulinemia secondary to hyperphagia. Incidence is increased with conditions such as obesity, diabetes mellitus, acromegaly, uremia, and certain rare, possibly genetic, autoimmune disorders.

internal r. the electrical resistance within a voltage source, e.g., a battery, power supply, or generator.

mineralocorticoid r. pseudohypoaldosteronism.

multidrug r., multiple drug r. 1. drug resistance to multiple drugs. 2. a phenomenon seen in some malignant cell lines: cells that have developed natural resistance to a single cytotoxic compound are also resistant to structurally unrelated chemotherapy agents.

partial androgen r. partial androgen insensitivity syndrome.

peripheral vascular r. total peripheral r.

pleiotropic drug r. multidrug r.

pulmonary vascular r. the vascular resistance of the pulmonary circulation, equal to the difference between the mean pulmonary arterial pressure and the left atrial filling pressure divided by the cardiac output.

total peripheral r. the vascular resistance of the systemic circulation: the difference between the mean arterial pressure and central venous pressure divided by the cardiac output. Called also *peripheral vascular r.*

total pulmonary r. pulmonary vascular r.

vascular r. the opposition to blood flow in a vascular bed; it is the pressure drop across the bed divided by the blood flow, conventionally expressed in peripheral resistance units or in dyne•sec•cm^{-5}. Symbol RR or *R.*

venous r. resistance to blood flow by a vein; under normal conditions it depends largely on extrinsic factors such as compression by surrounding structures. Thrombi often but not always cause an increase in resistance.

re•sis•tin (re-zis′tin) a 114 amino acid adipocytokine that has been implicated in the development of insulin resistance; it has been suggested that it may be the link between obesity and insulin resistance, but its role remains unclear. It has also been found in the synovial fluid of patients with inflammatory joint disease.

re•sis•tive (re-zis′tiv) pertaining to or characterized by resistance.

res•ite (res′īt) an insoluble, infusible cross-linked form produced by further reaction of resole under heat.

res•ole (res′ōl) a thermosetting resin in the uncured, unformed state, consisting primarily of partially condensed phenol alcohols.

res•o•lu•tion (rez″o-loo′shən) [L. *resolutum*, from *resolvere* to unbind] 1. the subsidence of a pathologic state, as the subsidence of an inflammation, or the softening and disappearance of a swelling. 2. the perception as separate of two adjacent objects or points. In microscopy, it is the minimal distance at which two adjacent objects can be distinguished as separate. The resolving power of an instrument depends on the wavelength of the radiation used and the numerical aperture of the system; it is expressed in microns distance or lines per millimeter. 3. a measure of the fineness of detail that can be discerned in an image.

re•solve (re-zolv′) [L. *resolvere*] 1. to restore to the normal state after some pathologic process. 2. to separate a thing into its component parts.

re•sol•vent (re-zol′vənt) [L. *resolvens* dissolving] 1. promoting resolution or the dissipation of a pathologic growth. 2. an agent that promotes resolution.

res•o•nance (rez′o-nəns) [L. *resonare* to echo] 1. the prolongation and intensification of sound produced by transmission of its vibrations to a cavity, especially a sound elicited by percussion. See also *dullness* and *flatness.* 2. a vocal sound as heard in auscultation. 3. mesomerism.

amphoric r. a sound heard upon percussion or auscultation, resembling that produced by blowing over the mouth of an empty bottle, as in amphoric respiration. See also *cavernous voice*, under *voice.* Called also *amphoric murmur.*

bandbox r. the extremely resonant sound elicited by percussion in cases of emphysema of the lungs. Called also *bandbox sound.*

cough r. a peculiar auscultatory sound elicited by coughing.

cracked-pot r. a peculiar sound elicited by percussion over a pulmonary cavity that communicates with a bronchus. Called also *cracked-pot sound.*

electron paramagnetic r., electron spin r. in spectrometry, a measure of electron spin as an indication of the presence and extent of activity of free radicals in an organic reaction. Abbreviated EPR or ESR.

hydatid r. a peculiar sound heard in the combined auscultation and percussion of a hydatid cyst.

nuclear magnetic r. a measure, by means of applying an external magnetic field to a solution in a constant radiofrequency field, of the magnetic moment of atomic nuclei to determine the structure of organic compounds. This technique is used in magnetic resonance imaging (q.v.).

osteal r. the sound elicited by percussion over a bony structure.

skodaic r. increased percussion resonance at the upper part of the chest, with flatness below it; heard above a large pleural effusion or area of consolidation. Called also *Skoda sign* or *tympany* and *skodaic tympany.*

tympanic r. tympanitic r. (def. 2).

tympanitic r. 1. the peculiar sound elicited by percussing a tympanitic abdomen. 2. the drumlike reverberation of a cavity full of air; called also *tympanic r.*

vesicular r. vesicular breath sounds; see under *sound.*

vesiculotympanitic r. a resonance, heard upon auscultation, that is partly vesicular and partly tympanitic. Called also *wooden r.*

vocal r. (VR) the sound of ordinary speech as heard through the chest wall.

whispering r. whispered pectoriloquy.

wooden r. vesiculotympanitic r.

res·o·nant (rez′o-nənt) giving a vibrant sound on percussion.

res·o·na·tor (rez′o-na″tər) an instrument used to intensify sounds. In electricity, an electrical circuit in which oscillations of a certain frequency are set up by oscillations of the same frequency in another circuit.

re·sorb (re-sorb′, re-zorb′) to take up or absorb again; to undergo resorption.

re·sor·cin (rə-sor′sin) resorcinol.

re·sor·ci·nism (rə-sor′sĭ-niz″əm) chronic poisoning by resorcinol, resulting in methemoglobinemia, paralysis, and damage to the capillaries, kidneys, heart, and nervous system.

re·sor·ci·nol (rə-sor′sĭ-nol) [USP] a bactericidal, fungicidal, keratolytic, exfoliative, and antipruritic agent, used especially as a topical keratolytic in the treatment of acne and other dermatoses, such as seborrheic dermatitis. Called also *resorcin.*

r. monoacetate [USP] the monoacetate salt of resorcinol, used topically as an antiseborrheic and keratolytic.

re·sorp·tion (re-sorp′shən) [L. *resorbere* to swallow again] 1. the loss of substance through physiologic or pathologic means, such as loss of dentin and cementum of a tooth, or of the alveolar process of the mandible or maxilla. 2. reabsorption of fluid.

bone r. a type of bone loss (resorption) due to osteoclastic activity.

idiopathic r. resorption of calcified tissues without apparent cause.

root r. resorption in which cementum or dentin is lost from the root of a tooth owing to cementoclastic or osteoclastic activity in conditions such as trauma of occlusion or neoplasms.

tooth r., external resorption of calcified dental tissue, beginning on the external surface of the root and extending to the cementum, dentin, and eventually into the root canal. See also *internal tooth r.* (def. 1).

tooth r., internal 1. an unusual form of tooth resorption beginning centrally in a tooth, and apparently initiated by inflammatory hyperplasia of the pulp, characterized by a pink hued area on the crown showing the hyperplastic vascular pulp tissue filling the resorbed area. Called also *chronic perforating hyperplasia* and *pink tooth of Mummery.* 2. external tooth resorption that ramifies into the dentin.

tubular r. see under *reabsorption.*

Res·pi·Gam (res′pĭ-gam) trademark for a preparation of respiratory syncytial virus immune globulin intravenous.

res·pir·a·ble (res′spər-ə-bəl) 1. suitable for respiration. 2. small enough to be inhaled, such as an irritating particle.

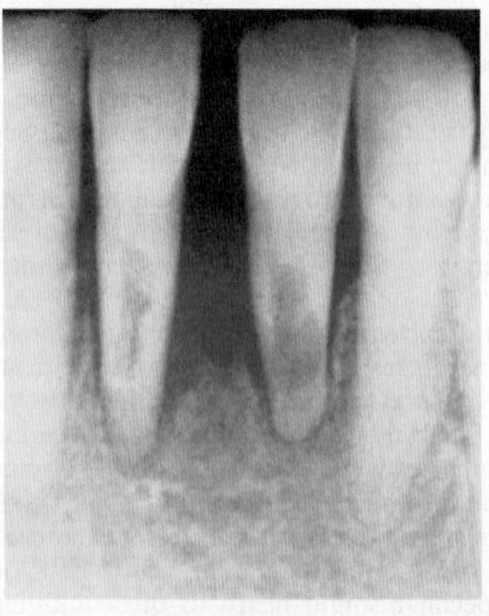

■ Internal tooth resorption, showing a fusiform enlargement of the pulpal chamber.

res·pi·ra·tion (res″pĭ-ra′shən) [L. *respiratio*] 1. the exchange of oxygen and carbon dioxide between the atmosphere and the cells of the body. The process includes *ventilation* (inhalation and exhalation), the diffusion of oxygen from pulmonary alveoli to the blood and of carbon dioxide from the blood to the alveoli, and the transport of oxygen to and carbon dioxide from the body cells. Symbol R. 2. ventilation (def. 2). 3. the metabolic processes by which cells generate energy, chiefly in the form of ATP, by the oxidation of organic molecules such as glucose, with the release of carbon dioxide, water, and other oxidized products; called also *cell* or *cellular r.*

abdominal r. respiration maintained by contribution of the diaphragm and respiratory muscles. Cf. *thoracic r.*

aerobic r. the oxidative transformation of certain substrates into secretory products, the released energy being used in the process of assimilation.

amphoric r. respiration characterized by amphoric resonance, heard over pulmonary cavities or pneumothorax.

anaerobic r. a form of respiration in which energy is released from chemical reactions in which free oxygen takes no part.

artificial r. any artificial method of ventilation in which air is forced into and out of the lungs of a person who has stopped breathing. It may be either mechanical (see *mechanical ventilation*) or done as an emergency procedure with no mechanical equipment. The most effective nonmechanical emergency technique is the *mouth-to-mouth method;* other less used techniques are the *Holger Nielsen method, Schafer method,* and *Silvester method* (see under *method*). Called also *artificial* or *assisted ventilation.*

asthmoid r. wheezing respiration like that of bronchial asthma.

Biot r. breathing characterized by irregular periods of apnea alternating with periods in which four or five breaths of identical depth are taken; seen in patients with increased intracranial pressure. Called also *Biot breathing* or *sign.*

bronchial r. bronchial breath sounds; see under *sound.*

bronchocavernous r. breath sounds intermediate in character between bronchial and cavernous, heard over a lung cavity with solidified lung tissue adjacent to it.

bronchovesicular r. bronchovesicular breath sounds; see under *sound.*

cavernous r. cavernous breath sounds; see under *sound.*

cell r., cellular r. respiration (def. 3).

Cheyne-Stokes r. breathing characterized by rhythmic waxing and waning of the rate and depth of respiration, with regularly recurring periods of apnea; seen especially in coma resulting from affection of the nervous centers.

cogwheel r. breathing characterized by peculiar jerky inhalations; the sounds of inhalation and exhalation are not continuous but are split into two or more separate sounds. Called also *interrupted* or *jerky r.*

collateral r. see under *ventilation.*

controlled diaphragmatic r. the intentional use of abdominal respiration in order to limit the motion of the apices of the lung.

costal r. thoracic r.

diaphragmatic r. respiration that is mainly performed by the diaphragm.

divided r. respiration marked by a pause between the sounds of inhalation and those of exhalation.

electrophrenic r. (EPR) artificial respiration induced by electric stimulation of the phrenic nerve to produce rhythmic contractions of the diaphragm, done to provide ventilatory support in patients with diaphragmatic paralysis. Called also *diaphragmatic* or *phrenic pacing.*

external r. the exchange of gases between the lungs and the blood. Cf. *internal r.*

fetal r. gaseous interchange through the placenta.

forced r. deliberate hyperventilation.

internal r. the exchange of gases between the body cells and the blood; cf. *external r.* Called also *tissue r.*

interrupted r., jerky r. cogwheel r.

Kussmaul r., Kussmaul-Kien r. a pattern of deep and rapid respiration, seen particularly in metabolic acidosis. Called also *air hunger.*

paradoxical r. respiration in which all or part of a lung is deflated during inhalation and inflated during exhalation, as with flail chest or paralysis of the diaphragm.

periodic r. Cheyne-Stokes r.

puerile r. respiration in which the breathing sounds are more intense than those of normal adult respiration and resemble those of childhood.

suppressed r. respiration without any appreciable sound, as may occur in extensive consolidation of the lung or in pleuritic effusion.

thoracic r. respiration performed by the intercostal and other thoracic muscles. Cf. *abdominal r.* Called also *costal r.*

tissue r. internal r.

tubular r. bronchial breath sounds; see under *sound.*

vesicular r. vesicular breath sounds; see under *sound.*

vesiculocavernous r. cavernous breath sounds with a vesicular quality, indicating a cavity surrounded by healthy lung tissue.

vicarious r. increased action in one lung when that of the other lung is diminished.

res·pi·ra·tor (res′pĭ-ra″tər) ventilator (def. 2).

cuirass r. see under *ventilator.*

Drinker r. a type of negative-pressure ventilator consisting of a metal tank enclosing the body of the patient with the head outside. It was formerly in wide use, but its use has now decreased in favor of less cumbersome cuirass and jacket ventilators. Called also *tank ventilator* and, popularly, *iron lung.*

Engström r. a volume-controlled, piston-operated respirator with a sine wave airflow pattern.

res·pi·ra·to·ry (res′pər-ə-tor″e) [*re-* + L. *spirare* to breathe] pertaining to respiration. Called also *pneumatic.*

res·pi·rol·o·gist (res″pĭ-rol′ə-jist) respiratory therapist.

res·pi·rol·o·gy (res″pĭ-rol′ə-je) respiratory care.

res·pi·rom·e·ter (res″pĭ-rom′ə-tər) an instrument for determining the character of the respiratory movements.

res·pi·ro·pha·sic (res″pĭ-ro-fa′zik) pertaining to or varying between different phases of respiration.

Res·pi·ro·vi·rus (res′pĭ-ro-vi″rəs) a genus of viruses of the family Paramyxoviridae, subfamily Paramyxovirinae, that cause chiefly respiratory infections in a variety of vertebrate hosts. Species include human parainfluenza viruses 1 and 3 and Sendai virus. Formerly called *Paramyxovirus.*

re·sponse (re-spons′) [L. *respondere* to answer, reply] an action or movement due to the application of a stimulus. Called also *reaction.*

acute phase r. a group of physiologic processes occurring soon after the onset of infection, trauma, inflammatory processes, and some malignant conditions. The most prominent change is a dramatic increase of acute phase proteins, especially C-reactive protein, in the serum. Also seen are fever, increased vascular permeability, and a variety of metabolic and pathologic changes.

anamnestic r. secondary immune r.

antiviral r. virologic r.

auditory brainstem r. (ABR) *for sensorineural hearing loss:* a test that tracks nerve signals arising in the internal ear as they travel along the auditory nerve to the brain region responsible for hearing. A small speaker placed near the ear makes a clicking sound, and electrodes record the nerve signal as it travels. The test can determine where along the nerve there is a lesion responsible for sensorineural hearing loss, often due to a benign tumor.

autoimmune r. an immune response against an autoantigen.

blink r's compound muscle action potentials evoked in the orbicularis oculi muscles by stimulation of the skin innervated by the supraorbital nerve. An early response (the R_1 wave) occurs on the same side as the stimulation and a later response (the R_2 wave) occurs on both sides along with a twitch of both orbicularis oculi muscles. Called also *blink reflexes.*

booster r. secondary immune r.

conditioned r. a response evoked by a conditioned stimulus; one occurring to a stimulus that was incapable of evoking it before conditioning.

Cushing r. tachycardia, increased systemic blood pressure, and slow, irregular breathing in response to an increase in intracranial pressure. Called also *Cushing phenomenon* or *reflex.*

decremental r., decrementing r. a progressive decrease in amplitude of successive M waves upon repetitive nerve stimulation (q.v.); it may indicate impaired neuromuscular transmission, neuropathy, myopathy, or motor neuron disease. Cf. *incremental r.*

electrodermal r. galvanic skin r.

F r. F waves (def. 2); see under *wave.*

galvanic skin r. the alteration in electrical resistance of the skin associated with sympathetic nerve discharge. Called also *electrodermal, psychogalvanic,* or *sympathetic skin r.* and *psychogalvanic reflex.*

hepatic arterial buffer r. a compensation mechanism of the hepatic circulation; when blood flow in eiher the hepatic artery or the portal vein is diminished, that in the other increases in an effort to maintain perfusion of the liver.

immune r. any response of the immune system to an antigenic stimulus, including antibody production, cell-mediated immunity, and immunologic tolerance. The responses causing tissue injury are generally classified into the types described by the Gell and Coombs classification (see under *classification*). See also *hypersensitivity reaction,* under *reaction.*

immune r., primary the immune response occurring on the first exposure to an antigen. After a lag or latent period of from 3 to 14 days depending on the antigen, specific antibodies appear in the blood. There is a peak of IgM production lasting several days followed immediately by a peak of IgG production. Antibody production ceases after several weeks, but memory cells remain in circulation.

immune r., secondary the immune response occurring on the second and subsequent exposures to an antigen; compared to a primary immune response, the lag period is shorter, the peak antibody titer is higher and lasts longer, IgG production predominates, the antibodies produced have a higher affinity for the antigen, and a much smaller dose of the antigen is required to initiate the response. Called also *anamnestic r.* and *booster r.*

incremental r. the progressive increase in amplitude of successive M waves upon repetitive nerve stimulation (q.v.); excessive increase is pathologic. Cf. *decrementing r.*

inflammatory r. the various changes that tissue undergoes when it becomes inflamed; see *inflammation.*

isomorphic r. Koebner phenomenon.

M r. see under *wave.*

orienting r. see under *reflex.*

paradoxical cold r. an inappropriate sensation of cold due to response of some cold receptors to contact with an object having a temperature above 45°C.

psychogalvanic r., psychogalvanic skin r. galvanic skin r.

relaxation r. a group of physiologic changes that cause decreased activity of the sympathetic nervous system and consequent relaxation after stimulation of certain regions of the hypothalamus. They are the opposite of the alarm reaction and may be self-induced through techniques such as meditation and biofeedback.

reticulocyte r. increase in the formation of reticulocytes in response to a bone marrow stimulus, such as that provided by administration of a hematinic.

sympathetic skin r. galvanic skin r.

triple r., triple r. of Lewis a physiologic reaction of the skin to stroking with a blunt instrument: first a red line develops at the site of stroking, owing to the release of histamine or a histaminelike substance, then a flare develops around the red line due to vasodilation, and finally a wheal is formed as a result of local edema.

unconditioned r. a response elicited spontaneously by an unconditioned stimulus; an unlearned response, i.e., one that occurs naturally. Called also *inborn* or *unconditioned reflex.*

virologic r. response to therapy with an antiviral agent; called also *antiviral r.*

rest (rest) 1. repose after exertion. 2. a fragment of embryonic tissue that has been retained within the adult organism; called also *embryonic, epithelial,* and *fetal r.* 3. the part of a removable partial denture that rests on the abutment tooth, and thus prevents movement of the denture and helps in providing occlusal support.

aberrant r. choristoma.

adrenal r's glandulae suprarenales accessoriae.

bed r. confinement of a patient to bed.

carbon r. the amount of carbon in the deproteinized blood.

cingulum r. lingual r.

embryonic r., epithelial r., fetal r. see *rest* (def. 2).

incisal r. a metallic part or extension of a removable partial denture that rests on the prepared incisal edge of an anterior abutment tooth.

lingual r. a metallic part or extension of a removable partial denture that rests on the prepared lingual surface of an anterior abutment tooth and thus provides support or indirect retention. Called also *cingulum r.*

Malassez r. the remaining cells of the root sheath in the periodontal ligament, which persist and sometimes form an epithelial network and occasionally develop into a dental cyst.

nephrogenic r's remnants of renal blastema tissue found in or around the kidney, sometimes precursors of Wilms tumor.

occlusal r. a rest placed on the occlusal surface of a posterior tooth for transmitting occlusal stresses parallel to its long axis and holding the clasp in its predetermined position; a component of removable partial dentures. Called also *occlusal stop.*

pancreatic r. ectopic pancreatic tissue, usually in the stomach or small intestine, forming a polyplike lesion.

precision r. a prefabricated, rigid, metallic extension of a fixed or removable partial denture, consisting of two closely fitted interlocking parts, the insert of which fits into a box-type rest or keyway (female) portion of the attachment in the cast restoration of a tooth.

recessed r. a rigid extension of a partial denture, which contacts a definite seat prepared in the surface of a tooth.

semiprecision r. a denture rest, sometimes supplemented by a spring-loaded plunger or clip, which fits into a seat in an abutment tooth that has been specially deepened to provide added retention. See also under *attachment.*

suprarenal r's glandulae suprarenales accessoriae.

surface r. a rigid extension of a partial denture, which contacts the unaltered extracoronal surface of a tooth.

Walthard cell r's see under *islet.*

Re·sta·sis (rə-sta′sis) trademark for a preparation of cyclosporine.

rest·bite (rest′bīt) the relation of the teeth when the jaw is at rest.

re·ste·no·sis (re″stə-no′sis) recurrent stenosis, especially of a cardiac valve, after surgical correction of the primary condition. **restenot′ic** *adj*

false r. stenosis recurring after failure to divide either commissure of the cardiac valve beyond the area of incision of the papillary muscles.

true r. restenosis occurring after complete opening of one or both of the commissures of the cardiac valve involved.

res•ti•form (res′tĭ-form) [L. *restis* rope + *form*] shaped like a rope.

res•ti•tu•tion (res″tĭ-too′shən) [L. *restitutio*] 1. an active process of restoration. 2. the spontaneous realignment of the fetal head with the fetal body, after delivery of the head.

res•to•ra•tion (res″tə-ra′shən) [L. *restaurare* to review, rebuild] 1. the act of renewing, rebuilding, or reconstructing. 2. the return to a previous state or condition, as of health. 3. the process of replacing by artificial means a missing, damaged, or diseased tooth or teeth or any part thereof. See also *filling* and *prosthetic r.*, and see *restorative dentistry*, under *dentistry*. 4. the act of re-forming the contours of parts of teeth destroyed by lesions or injury, thereby restoring their functional properties.

buccal r. the replacement, usually with silver alloy, gold, or plastic, of the buccal portion of a posterior tooth lost through caries or injury.

cast r. a dental restoration that is created outside the mouth from impressions of the prepared tooth, then bonded and cemented into place; included are inlays and onlays. Called also *indirect r.* Cf. *direct r.*

cusp r. restoration of the summit of a cusp or the incisal edge of a tooth, done for functional or cosmetic reasons.

direct r. a dental restoration created directly in the area being restored, using soft materials that are shaped to fit the tooth, such as amalgam or composite. Cf. *cast r.*

facial r. the replacement, usually with silver alloy, gold, or acrylic resin, of the facial portion of a posterior tooth lost through caries or injury.

indirect r. cast r.

prosthetic r. 1. the replacement of a lost or absent body part with an artificial structure, such as the use of an inlay, crown, bridge, or partial or complete denture, or other appliance to replace lost tooth structure, teeth, or oral tissue or structure. 2. any appliance, such as an inlay, crown, bridge, or partial or complete denture, used to replace lost tooth structure, teeth, or oral tissue or structure.

Res•tor•il (res′tə-ril″) trademark for a preparation of temazepam.

re•straint (re-strānt′) the forcible confinement or control of a subject, as of a violently psychotic or irrational person.

re•stric•tion (re-strik′shən) 1. a limitation. 2. a thing or process that limits.

fetal growth r. see under *retardation.*

gastric r. any of various surgical treatments for morbid obesity in which part of the stomach is closed off from the flow of nutrients through the alimentary canal, such as gastric banding, gastric bypass, and gastric partitioning.

intrauterine growth r. fetal growth retardation.

MHC r. the phenomenon of certain cell–cell interactions in the immune response occurring only between cells haploidentical for a major histocompatibility complex (MHC). Helper T cells are activated by antigen only when the antigen is "seen" in conjunction with self class II MHC antigens (Ia antigens in mice, HLA-DR antigens in humans) as is the case when antigen is presented by macrophages. Cytotoxic T cells are activated by and kill only cells displaying foreign antigens (e.g., viral antigens or tumor antigens) plus self class I MHC antigens (K or D antigens in mice, HLA-A, -B, or -C antigens in humans).

re•sub•limed (re″səb-līmd′) subjected to repeated processes of sublimation.

re•su•pi•na•tion (re″soo-pĭ-na′shən) [L. *resupinare* to turn on the back] 1. the act of turning upon the back or dorsum. 2. the position of one lying upon the back.

re•sus•ci•ta•tion (re-sus″ĭ-ta′shən) [L. *resuscitare* to revive] the restoration to life or consciousness of one apparently dead; it includes such measures as artificial respiration and cardiac massage.

active compression-decompression r. a type of cardiopulmonary resuscitation done with a device for closed chest cardiac massage that allows not only compression of the chest but also actively assisted expansion of the chest by means of a suction bellows.

brain r. cerebral r.

cardiocerebral r. an intervention for cardiac arrest, consisting of continual chest compressions that are not interrupted by mouth-to-mouth resuscitation.

cardiopulmonary r. (CPR) the artificial substitution of heart and lung action as indicated for cardiac arrest or apparent sudden death resulting from electric shock, drowning, respiratory arrest, and other causes. The two major components of CPR are rescue breathing and closed chest cardiac massage.

cerebral r. restoration of function to the brain after an insult such as a stroke, hypoxia, or coma. Called also *brain r.*

expired air r. (EAR) rescue breathing.

mouth-to-mouth r. a rescue breathing technique: with the victim supine, the rescuer places a hand under the nape of the victim's neck and a hand on the victim's forehead, also pressing victim's nostrils closed; the rescuer takes a deep breath and exhales between the victim's lips (two pairs of lips forming an airtight seal). This is repeated quickly four times to inflate the victim's lungs before allowing the first exhalation.

re•sus•ci•ta•tor (re-sus′ĭ-ta″tər) an apparatus for initiating respiration in cases of asphyxia.

cardiopulmonary r. an apparatus that simultaneously assists the patient's breathing and applies external cardiac massage.

re•su•ture (re-soo′chər) secondary suture.

re•syn•chro•ni•za•tion (re-sing″krə-nĭ-za′shən) restoration of synchrony between two or more signals (such as waves) that were originally synchronized but had been in desynchronization.

re•tain•er (re-ta′nər) 1. a device for retaining or keeping something in position. 2. the part of a denture that unites the abutment tooth with the suspended portion of the bridge, such as an inlay, partial crown, or complete crown. 3. an orthodontic device for maintaining in position the teeth and jaws. 4. any form of clasp, attachment, or other device used for the fixation or stabilization of a prosthetic appliance. 5. the portion of a fixed prosthesis attaching a pontic to the abutment teeth.

continuous bar r. continuous clasp.

direct r. a clasp or attachment applied to an abutment tooth, by which a removable partial denture is maintained in position.

Hawley r. an orthodontic appliance consisting of a removable palatal wire and an acrylic bite plate resting against the palate, used to stabilize teeth after their movement or as a basis for tooth movement by providing anchorage for other attachments. Called also *Hawley appliance.*

indirect r. a part of a removable partial denture that assists the direct retainers in preventing displacement of distal-extension denture bases by functioning through lever action on the opposite side of the fulcrum line.

matrix r. a mechanical device designed to engage the ends of a matrix band or strip and to tighten the matrix around the tooth.

space r. an orthodontic appliance that retains the space created by premature loss of a tooth or the space to be filled by an erupting tooth. See also under *maintainer* and *regainer.*

re•tar•da•tion (re″tahr-da′shən) [L. *retardare* to slow down, impede] delay; hindrance; delayed development.

borderline mental r. [DSM-IV] borderline intellectual functioning.

fetal growth r., intrauterine growth r. birth weight below the tenth percentile for gestational age for infants in a given population; classified as *symmetric* or *proportionate* (both weight and length below normal) and *asymmetric* or *disproportionate* (weight below normal, length normal). Called also *fetal* or *intrauterine growth restriction.*

mental r. [DSM-IV] a mental disorder characterized by significantly subaverage general intellectual functioning associated with impairments in adaptive behavior and manifested during the developmental period. It is classified on the basis of severity as *mild, moderate, severe,* and *profound;* a fifth subgroup, *borderline intellectual functioning,* is sometimes included.

mild mental r. [DSM-IV] mental retardation in which IQ is between 50–55 and 70; the person can develop social and communication skills during the preschool period, has minimal sensorimotor impairment, by the late teens can acquire academic skills up to the sixth grade level, and usually achieves social and vocational skills adequate for minimal self-support.

moderate mental r. [DSM-IV] mental retardation in which IQ is between 35–40 and 50–55; the person may talk or learn to communicate but has poor social awareness and only fair motor development, is unlikely to progress to the second grade level in academic skills, but can profit from vocational training and with moderate supervision can perform personal care.

motor r. abnormal slowness of movements of muscles, as seen with congenital or other orthopedic or neurologic disorders and psychiatric conditions such as depression.

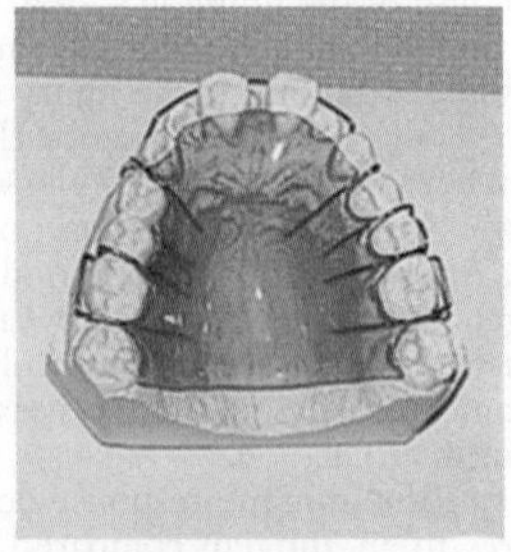

■ Hawley retainer.

profound mental r. [DSM-IV] mental retardation in which IQ is less than 20–25; the person has limited sensorimotor development, may achieve very limited self-care, and requires a highly structured environment with constant supervision.

psychomotor r. generalized slowing of mental and physical activity, as is common in depression and in catatonic schizophrenia.

severe mental r. [DSM-IV] mental retardation in which IQ is between 20–25 and 35–40; the person has poor motor development and minimal speech in the preschool period, may learn to talk by the late teens, can be trained in elementary hygiene skills, and as an adult may learn to perform simple work under close supervision.

Ret•a•vase (ret′ə-vās) trademark for a preparation of reteplase.

retch (rech) to try to vomit; called also *gag.*

retch•ing (rech′ing) a strong involuntary effort to vomit.

re•te (re′te) pl. *re′tia* [L. "net"] anatomical nomenclature for a network, especially of arteries or veins. See also *net, network,* and *plexus.* **re′tial** *adj*

r. acromia′le [TA] acromial rete or network: a network formed by ramification of the acromial branch of the thoracoacromial artery on the acromion process.

r. arterio′sum [TA] arterial network: an anastomotic network formed by arteries just before they become arterioles or capillaries.

r. arterio′sum der′midis arterial network of dermis: the arterial portion of the deep vascular plexus, found in the skin at the boundary between the dermis and the tela subcutanea. Called also *r. cutaneum* and *cutaneous arterial network.*

r. arterio′sum subpapilla′re subpapillary network: the arterial portion of the superficial vascular plexus, found in the skin at the boundary between the papillary and reticular layers. Called also *r. subpapillare.*

articular r. r. vasculosum articulare.

articular cubital r., articular r. of elbow r. articulare cubiti.

articular r. of knee r. articulare genus.

r. articula′re cu′biti [TA] articular network of elbow: an arterial network formed on the posterior aspect of the elbow by the posterior ulnar recurrent, inferior and superior ulnar collateral, and interosseous recurrent arteries.

r. articula′re ge′nus [TA] articular network of knee: an extensive arterial network on the capsule of the knee joint, supplying branches to the contiguous bones and joints. It is formed by the genicular arteries, the termination of the deep femoral artery, the descending branch of the lateral circumflex artery, and the tibial recurrent artery.

r. calca′neum [TA] calcaneal rete or network: an arterial network on the posterior and lower surfaces of the calcaneus, receiving branches from the calcaneal branches of the peroneal artery and the lateral malleolar branches of the peroneal artery.

carpal r., dorsal r. carpale dorsale.

r. carpa′le dorsa′le [TA] dorsal carpal network: an arterial rete formed by the dorsal radial carpal and dorsal ulnar carpal arteries and giving off the second, third, and fourth dorsal metacarpal arteries to the dorsum of the hand and the second, third, and fourth fingers. Called also *dorsal* or *posterior carpal arch.*

r. cuta′neum r. arteriosum dermidis.

dorsal venous r. of foot r. venosum dorsale pedis.

dorsal venous r. of hand r. venosum dorsale manus.

r. fora′minis ova′lis plexus venosus foraminis ovalis.

r. of Haller, r. halle′ri r. testis.

r. lymphocapilla′re [TA] lymphocapillary network: any of the closed, freely communicating networks formed by the lymphocapillary vessels.

malleolar r., lateral r. malleolare laterale.

malleolar r., medial r. malleolare mediale.

r. malleola′re latera′le [TA] lateral malleolar rete or network: a small arterial network on the lateral malleolus, formed by the lateral anterior malleolar artery, the perforating branch of the peroneal artery, and the lateral tarsal artery.

r. malleola′re media′le [TA] medial malleolar rete or network: a small arterial network on the medial malleolus, formed by the medial anterior malleolar artery and branches from the posterior tibial artery.

r. mira′bile 1. [TA] a vascular network formed by division of an artery or a vein into a large number of smaller vessels that subsequently reunite into a single vessel; in the human this occurs only in the arterioles that supply the glomeruli of the kidney. 2. arterial anastomosis of the brain occurring between the external and internal carotid arteries as a result of longstanding thrombosis of the internal carotid arteries.

r. ole′crani r. articulare cubiti.

r. ova′rii a homologue of the rete testis, developed in the early female fetus but vestigial in the adult.

patellar r. r. patellare.

r. patella′re [TA] patellar rete or network: a network of arterial branches surrounding the patella and derived from the various arteries of the knee.

plantar r., plantar venous r. r. venosum plantare.

r. subpapilla′re, subpapillary r. r. arteriosum subpapillare.

r. tes′tis [TA] a network of channels formed by the straight seminiferous tubules, traversing the mediastinum testis and draining into the efferent ductules; called also *r. of Haller.*

r. vasculo′sum articula′re [TA] articular vascular network: an anastomotic network of blood vessels in or around a joint; called also *articular r.*

r. veno′sum [TA] venous network: an anastomotic network of small veins.

r. veno′sum dorsa′le ma′nus [TA] dorsal venous network of hand: a venous network on the back of the hand, formed by the dorsal metacarpal veins.

r. veno′sum dorsa′le pe′dis [TA] dorsal venous network of foot: a superficial network of anastomosing veins on the dorsum of the foot proximal to the transverse venous arch, draining into the great and the small saphenous veins.

r. veno′sum planta′re [TA] plantar venous network: a thick venous network in the subcutaneous tissue of the sole of the foot. Called also *plantar venous rete* and *plantar cutaneous venous network.*

re•ten•tate (re-ten′tāt) in a filtration process, the part of a solution that does not cross the membrane, as opposed to the diffusate.

re•ten•tion (re-ten′shən) [L. *retentio,* from *retentare* to hold firmly back] 1. the act or process of keeping in possession, or of holding in place or position. 2. the persistent keeping within the body of matter normally excreted. 3. in cavity preparation, the prevention of displacement of a restoration. 4. in orthodontic therapy, the period during which the patient is wearing an appliance(s) to maintain and stabilize the teeth in the position into which they were moved.

denture r. the holding in proper position in the mouth of a removable denture. See *direct r.* and *indirect r.*

direct r. denture retention through the use of attachments or clasps that resist removal from the abutment teeth. See under *retainer.*

indirect r. retention in the mouth of a removable partial denture by means of an indirect retainer.

surgical r. retention in the mouth of a dental prosthesis by means of attachments embedded in the oral tissues.

urinary r. accumulation of urine within the bladder because of inability to urinate.

ret•e•plase (ret′ə-plās) a deletion mutant of alteplase (recombinant tissue plasminogen activator) produced by recombinant DNA technology and having a longer half-life than the parent compound; used as a thrombolytic agent in the treatment of myocardial infarction, administered intravenously.

re•tia (re′te-ə) [L.] plural of *rete.*

re•tic•u•la (rə-tik′u-lə) [L.] plural of *reticulum.*

re•tic•u•lar (rə-tik′u-lər) [L. *reticularis*] 1. pertaining to or resembling a net, network, or reticulum. Cf. *plexiform.* 2. pertaining to the reticulum of a ruminant.

re•tic•u•lat•ed (rə-tik′u-lāt″əd) reticular (def. 1).

re•tic•u•la•tion (rə-tik″u-la′shən) [L. *reticulum* a net] in radiology, a network of wrinkles or corrugations in the emulsion of an x-ray film resulting from sharp temperature differences between processing solutions.

re•tic•u•lin (rə-tik′u-lin) the constituent protein of the reticular fibers; it has been shown to be type III collagen.

re•tic•u•li•tis (rə-tik″u-li′tis) [*reticul-* + *-itis*] inflammation of the reticulum of a ruminant animal.

reticul(o)- [L. *reticulum* dim. of *rete* net] a combining form denoting a relationship to a reticulum or to a reticular structure.

re•tic•u•lo•cyte (rə-tik′u-lo-sīt″) [*reticulo-* + *-cyte*] an immature erythrocyte showing a basophilic reticulum under vital staining.

re•tic•u•lo•cy•to•gen•ic (rə-tik″u-lo-si″to-jen′ik) causing the formation of reticulocytes.

re•tic•u•lo•cy•to•pe•nia (rə-tik″u-lo-si″to-pe′ne-ə) [*reticulocyte* + *-penia*] a decrease in the number of reticulocytes in the blood.

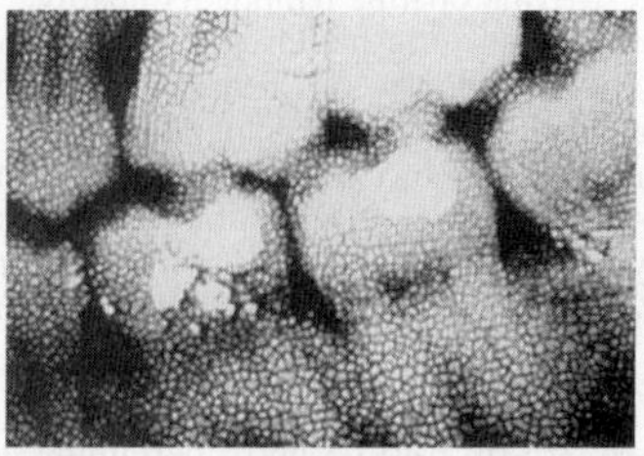

■ Reticulation.

re·tic·u·lo·cy·to·sis (rə-tik″u-lo-si-to′sis) an increase in the number of reticulocytes in the peripheral blood.

re·tic·u·lo·en·do·the·li·al (rə-tik″u-lo-en″do-the′le-əl) pertaining to tissues having both reticular and endothelial attributes; see under *system.*

re·tic·u·lo·en·do·the·li·o·sis (rə-tik″u-lo-en″do-the-le-o′sis) [*reticuloendothelium* + *-osis*] hyperplasia of reticuloendothelial tissue.

leukemic r. hairy cell leukemia.

re·tic·u·lo·en·do·the·li·um (rə-tik″u-lo-en″do-the′le-əm) the tissue of the reticuloendothelial system.

re·tic·u·lo·his·tio·cy·tary (rə-tik″u-lo-his″te-o-si′tər-e) reticulohistiocytic (def. 1).

re·tic·u·lo·his·tio·cyt·ic (rə-tik″u-lo-his″te-o-sit′ik) 1. pertaining to or composed of histiocytes (macrophages) in the reticuloendothelial system; see also *reticulohistiocytoma.* 2. pertaining to or of the nature of a reticulohistiocytoma; see under *granuloma.*

re·tic·u·lo·his·tio·cy·to·ma (re-tik″u-lo-his″te-o-si-to′mə) [*reticulo-* + *histiocytoma*] a granulomatous proliferation of lipid-laden macrophages and multinucleated giant cells whose pale eosinophilic cytoplasm has a ground-glass appearance. It occurs in two clinically different but histologically indistinguishable forms, *reticulohistiocytic granuloma* and *multicentric reticulohistiocytosis.*

re·tic·u·lo·his·tio·cy·to·sis (rə-tik″u-lo-his″te-o-si-to′sis) [*reticulo-* + *histiocytosis*] the formation of multiple reticulohistiocytomas.

multicentric r. one of the two types of reticulohistiocytoma, a rare systemic disease seen mainly in women, characterized by polyarthritis of the hands and large joints with nodular swellings in the skin, bone, and mucous and synovial membranes and sometimes swellings on the wrists; there may be evidence of internal malignancy. It may become quiescent, leaving only crippling arthropathy and disfigured skin, or it may progress to multiple organ involvement and eventual death. Called also *lipid* or *lipoid dermatoarthritis.*

re·tic·u·loid (rə-tik′u-loid) 1. resembling reticulosis. 2. a condition resembling reticulosis.

actinic r. chronic actinic dermatitis.

re·tic·u·lo·nod·u·lar (rə-tik″u-lo-nod′u-lər) having a pattern that is reticular and contains nodules, such as a lung with asbestosis or any of various kinds of pneumonia.

re·tic·u·lo·pe·nia (rə-tik″u-lo-pe′ne-ə) reticulocytopenia.

re·tic·u·lo·peri·car·di·tis (rə-tik″u-lo-per″ĭ-kahr-di′tis) inflammation of the reticulum and pericardium of a ruminant.

traumatic r. traumatic pericarditis (def. 2).

re·tic·u·lo·peri·the·li·um (rə-tik″u-lo-per″ĭ-the′le-əm) retoperithelium.

re·tic·u·lo·peri·to·ni·tis (rə-tik″u-lo-per″ĭ-tə-ni′tis) inflammation of the reticulum and peritoneal cavity of a ruminant.

traumatic r. inflammation following perforation of the wall of the reticulum by an ingested foreign object such as metallic debris; it is often benign, but if the object pierces another organ, serious complications may arise. See also *traumatic pericarditis* (def. 2). Called also *hardware disease.*

re·tic·u·lo·pi·tu·i·cyte (rə-tik″u-lo-pĭ-too′ĭ-sīt) see *pituicyte.*

re·tic·u·lo·po·di·um (rə-tik″u-lo-po′de-əm) reticulopo′dia [*reticulo-* + Gr. *pous* foot] a filamentous pseudopodium with interconnected branches. Cf. *axopodium, filopodium,* and *lobopodium.* Called also *rhizopodium.*

re·tic·u·lo·ru·men (rə-tik″u-lo-ru′mən) the reticulum and rumen considered as a unit; called also *ruminoreticulum.*

re·tic·u·lo·ru·mi·nal (rə-tik″u-lo-roo′mĭ-nəl) pertaining to the rumen and reticulum. Called also *ruminoreticular.*

re·tic·u·lo·sis (rə-tik″u-lo′sis) [*reticul-* + *-osis*] an abnormal increase in cells derived from or related to reticuloendothelial cells, such as that seen in leukemia and lymphoma.

familial hemophagocytic r., familial histiocytic r. familial hemophagocytic lymphohistiocytosis.

histiocytic medullary r. hemophagocytic lymphohistiocytosis.

inflammatory r. granulomatous meningoencephalitis.

lipomelanotic r. dermatopathic lymphadenopathy.

malignant midline r., midline malignant r. polymorphic r.

pagetoid r. a usually solitary skin lesion of long duration and slow growth characterized by large numbers of abnormal mononuclear cells infiltrating the epidermis and an underlying, reactive, mixed dermal infiltrate. Some authorities consider it an indolent, epidermotropic form of cutaneous T-cell lymphoma. Called also *Woringer-Kolopp disease.*

polymorphic r. a type of angiocentric immunoproliferative lesion involving midline structures of the nose and face; called also *malignant midline* or *midline malignant reticulosis.*

re·tic·u·lo·spi·nal (rə-tik″u-lo-spi′nəl) pertaining to a reticular formation and the spinal cord.

re·tic·u·lo·the·li·um (rə-tik″u-lo-the′le-əm) the retothelium.

re·tic·u·lum (rə-tik′u-ləm) pl. *retic′ula* [L., dim. of *rete* net] 1. a small network, especially one within a cell. 2. reticular tissue. 3. the second stomach of a ruminant; its mucous membranes are covered with many small pockets. Called also *honeycomb.*

agranular endoplasmic r. smooth endoplasmic r.

Chiari r. Chiari network.

Ebner r. a network of cells in the seminiferous tubules.

endoplasmic r. (ER) an organelle of all eukaryotic cells, consisting of an interconnecting network of tubules, flat saccules (cisternae), and vesicles extending from the nuclear envelope to the cell surface, and specialized for protein processing and lipid synthesis; there are three specialized regions: the *rough endoplasmic reticulum, smooth endoplasmic reticulum,* and *transitional endoplasmic reticulum,* (qq.v.). See Plate 12.

granular endoplasmic r. rough endoplasmic r.

reti′cula lie′nis trabeculae splenicae.

rough endoplasmic r. a region of the endoplasmic reticulum that bears large numbers of ribosomes on the outer surface of its membrane and is specialized for protein synthesis and folding.

sarcoplasmic r. a special form of smooth endoplasmic reticulum found in association with the T tubules in the sarcoplasm of striated muscle and comprising a system of cisternae and tubules forming a plexus around each myofibril. It contains large numbers of calcium pumps and ryanodine receptors and is a storage compartment for calcium ions, which it releases in response to an action potential in the adjacent T tubule to cause muscular contraction.

smooth endoplasmic r. a region of the endoplasmic reticulum composed of tubular elements lacking ribosomes and associated with many metabolic processes, including carbohydrate metabolism, the synthesis of lipids, cholesterol, and carbohydrates, and drug metabolism.

stellate r. the soft, middle part of the enamel organ of a developing tooth, the cells being separated by an increase in the gelatinous intercellular substance that forces the cells apart without breaking the intercellular connections, giving them a stellate appearance and providing protection later for the enamel-forming cells.

r. trabecula′re [TA] a trabecula of loose fibers found at the iridocorneal angle between the anterior chamber of the eye and the venous sinus of the sclera; the aqueous humor filters through the spaces between the fibers into the sinus and passes into the bloodstream. The reticulum is divided into a corneoscleral part and a uveal part. Called also *Hueck ligament, ligamentum pectinatum anguli iridocornealis, pectinate ligament, pectinate ligament of iris,* and *trabecular meshwork.*

transitional endoplasmic r. the final cisterna of the endoplasmic reticulum, from which vesicles bud during the transport of proteins to the Golgi complex for further processing.

re·ti·form (re′tĭ-form, ret′ĭ-form) plexiform.

Ret·in-A (ret″in-a′) trademark for preparations of tretinoin.

ret·i·na (ret′ĭ-nə) [L.] [TA] the innermost of the three tunics of the eyeball, surrounding the vitreous body and continuous posteriorly with the optic nerve. It is divided into the *pars optica,* which rests upon the choroid, the *pars ciliaris,* which rests upon the ciliary body, and the *pars iridica,* which rests upon the posterior surface of the iris. The pars optica is subdivided into an outer, pigmented layer *(stratum pigmentosum)* and an inner, transparent layer *(stratum nervosum).* The stratum nervosum is divided into nine layers, as follows (see illustration): (1) the internal limiting membrane; (2) the nerve fiber layer; (3) the layer of ganglion cells; (4) the inner plexiform layer; (5) the inner nuclear layer; (6) the outer plexiform layer; (7) the outer nuclear layer; (8) the external limiting membrane; (9) the layer of rods and cones. The layer of rods and cones is the percipient part of the retina, responding to visual stimuli by a photochemical reaction; it is connected with the nerve fiber layer by nerve fibers that join to form the optic nerve. In the center of the posterior part of the retina is the *macula lutea,* the most sensitive portion of the retina, with the fovea centralis at its center. About 0.25 cm inside the fovea is the point of entrance of the optic nerve and the central artery of the retina; at this point the retina is incomplete and forms the blind spot.

detached r. a retina whose inner layers are separated from the pigment epithelial layer; see *retinal detachment,* under *detachment.*

leopard r. see under *fundus.*

shot-silk r. an opalescent effect, as of changeable silk, sometimes seen in the retinas of young persons. Called also *shot-silk phenomenon* or *reflex* and *watered-silk r.*

tessellated r., tigroid r. see under *fundus.*

watered-silk r. shot-silk r.

ret·i·nac·u·lum (ret″ĭ-nak′u-ləm) pl. *retina′cula* [L. "a rope, cable"] a structure that retains an organ or tissue in place.

r. cauda′le [TA] caudal retinaculum: a fibrous band that extends from the tip of the coccyx to the adjacent skin and thus forms the foveola coccygea.

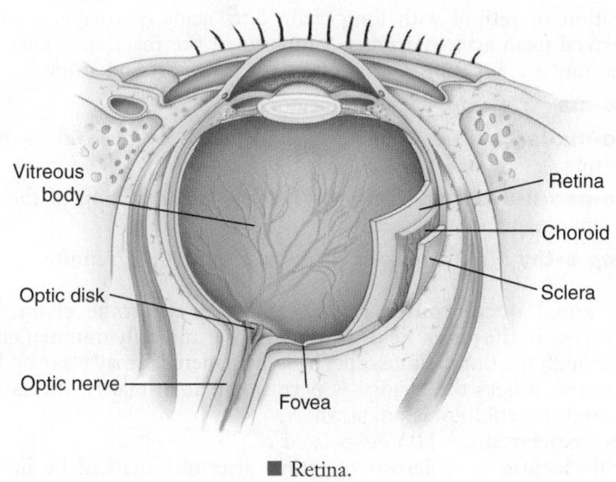

■ Retina.

retina′cula cu′tis [TA] skin ligaments: bands of connective tissue attaching the dermis to the subcutaneous tissue.

extensor r. of hand r. musculorum extensorum manus.

flexor r. of foot r. musculorum flexorum pedis.

flexor r. of hand r. musculorum flexorum manus.

inferior extensor r. of foot r. musculorum extensorum inferius pedis.

inferior fibular r., inferior peroneal r. r. musculorum fibularium inferius.

lateral patellar r. r. patellae laterale.

medial patellar r. r. patellae mediale.

r. musculo′rum extenso′rum infe′rius pe′dis [TA] inferior extensor retinaculum of foot: a Y-shaped band of fascia passing from the lateral side of the upper surface of the calcaneus across the foot to attach by one arm to the medial malleolus and by the other to the medial side of the plantar aponeurosis.

r. musculo′rum extenso′rum ma′nus [TA] extensor retinaculum of hand: the distal part of the antebrachial fascia, overlying the extensor tendons.

r. musculo′rum extenso′rum supe′rius pe′dis [TA] superior extensor retinaculum of foot: the thickened lower portion of the fascia on the front of the leg, attached to the tibia on one side and the fibula on the other, and serving to hold in place the extensor tendons that pass beneath it.

r. musculo′rum fibula′rium infe′rius [TA] inferior peroneal retinaculum: a fibrous band that arches over the tendons of the peroneal muscles and holds them in position on the lateral side of the calcaneus; called also *r. musculorum peroneorum inferius* [TA alternative] and *inferior fibular r.*

r. musculo′rum fibula′rium supe′rius [TA] superior peroneal retinaculum: a fibrous band that arches over the tendons of the peroneal muscles and helps to hold them in place below and behind the lateral malleolus; it extends from the malleolus downward and backward to the calcaneus. Called also *r. musculorum peroneorum superius* [TA alternative] and *superior fibular r.*

r. musculo′rum flexo′rum ma′nus [TA] flexor retinaculum of hand: a heavy fibrous band continuous with the distal part of the antebrachial fascia, completing the carpal canal through which pass the tendons of the flexor muscles of the hand and fingers.

r. musculo′rum flexo′rum pe′dis [TA] flexor retinaculum of foot: a strong band of fascia that extends from the medial malleolus down onto the calcaneus. It holds in place the tendons of the tibialis posterior, flexor digitorum, and flexor hallucis muscles as they pass to the sole of the foot, and gives protection to the posterior tibial vessels and tibial nerve. Called also *ligamentum laciniatum.*

r. musculo′rum peroneo′rum infe′rius [TA] TA alternative for *r. musculorum fibularium inferius.*

r. musculo′rum peroneo′rum supe′rius [TA] TA alternative for *r. musculorum fibularium superius.*

r. patel′lae latera′le [TA] lateral patellar retinaculum: a fibrous membrane from the tendon of the vastus lateralis muscle, attached to the lateral margin of the patella and then along the side of the patellar ligament, and inserted into the tibia as far distal as the fibular collateral ligament; it also blends with the iliotibial tract of the fascia lata. Called also *lateral patellar ligament.*

r. patel′lae media′le [TA] medial patellar retinaculum: a fibrous membrane from the tendon of the vastus medialis muscle, attached to the medial margin of the patella and then along the side of the patellar ligament, and inserted into the tibia as far distal as the tibial collateral ligament.

superior extensor r. of foot r. musculorum extensorum superius pedis.

superior fibular r., superior peroneal r. r. musculorum fibularium superius.

Weitbrecht r. retinacular fibers attached to the neck of the femur.

ret•i•nal (ret′ĭ-nəl) 1. pertaining to the retina. 2. the aldehyde of retinol, derived from absorbed dietary carotenoids or esters of retinol and having vitamin A activity. In the retina, retinal combines with opsins of rods (scotopsins) and cones (photopsins), functioning as the prosthetic group in the resulting visual pigments rhodopsin and the iodopsins.

11-*cis* r. a retinal isomer that combines with opsins to form photoreceptive molecules, in the rods combining with scotopsin to form rhodopsin and in the cones combining with photopsins to form several iodopsins. In the presence of light, it is converted to the all-*trans* isomer.

all-*trans* r. a retinal isomer formed from the 11-*cis* isomer upon bleaching of the photoreceptor proteins of the retina by light; the isomer dissociates from the opsins and is reconverted to the 11-*cis* isomer in the dark to renew the visual cycle.

ret•i•nal isom•er•ase (ret′ĭ-nəl i-som′ər-ās) [EC 5.2.1.3] an enzyme of the isomerase class that catalyzes the interconversion of the all-*trans* and 11-*cis* isomers of retinal. The reaction regenerates 11-*cis* retinal in the visual cycle.

ret•i•nal re•duc•tase (ret′ĭ-nəl re-duk′tās) alcohol dehydrogenase (NAD(P)$^+$).

ret•ine (ret′ēn) a substance stated to be widely distributed in animal cells, which is characterized by its ability to retard cell division and growth. Cf. *promine.*

ret•i•ni•tis (ret″ĭ-ni′tis) inflammation of the retina; used in the older ophthalmologic literature to denote impairment of sight, perversion of vision, edema, and exudation into the retina, and occasionally by hemorrhages into the retina.

actinic r. inflammation of the retina due to exposure to actinic light rays.

r. albuminu′rica retinitis associated with kidney disease. Cf. *arteriosclerotic retinopathy* and *hypertensive retinopathy.*

r. circina′ta, circinate r. circinate retinopathy.

Coats r. see under *disease.*

cytomegalovirus r. one of the most common types of opportunistic infection with cytomegalovirus in immunocompromised patients, beginning with visual field limitations and progressing to retinal necrosis and hemorrhage that often causes blindness.

diabetic r. see under *retinopathy.*

disciform r. disciform macular degeneration.

exudative r. Coats disease.

gravidic r. retinitis that accompanies the albuminuria of pregnancy.

hypertensive r. see under *retinopathy.*

Jacobson r. syphilitic r.

Jensen r. retinochoroiditis juxtapapillaris.

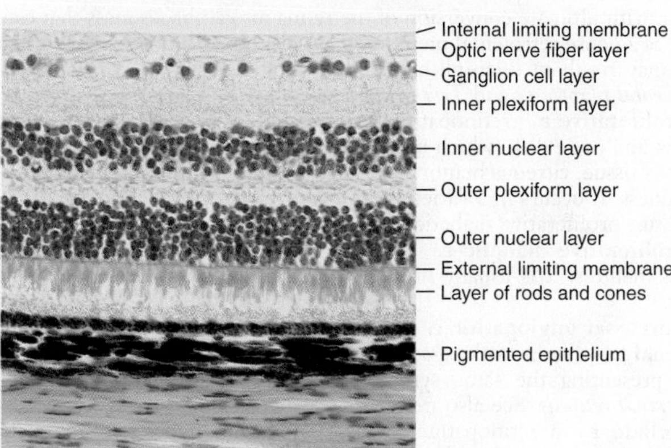

■ Layers of the optic part of the retina.

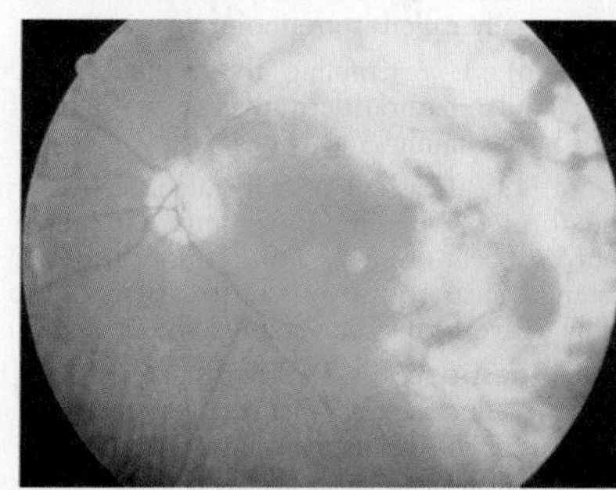
■ Cytomegalovirus retinitis involving the posterior pole and threatening the fovea.

leukemic r. see under *retinopathy.*
metastatic r. retinitis caused by septic emboli in the retinal vessels.
nephritic r. renal retinopathy.
r. pigmento'sa a group of diseases, frequently hereditary, marked by progressive loss of retinal response (as elicited by the electroretinogram), retinal atrophy, attenuation of the retinal vessels, and clumping of the pigment, with contraction of the field of vision. It may be transmitted as a dominant, recessive, or X-linked trait and is sometimes associated with other genetic defects.
r. pigmento'sa si'ne pigmen'to retinitis pigmentosa without clumping of pigment.
r. proli'ferans, proliferating r. retinitis caused by intraocular hemorrhage, with neovascularization and formation of fibrous tissue bands that extend into the vitreous from the surface of the retina; retinal detachment is sometimes a sequela.
r. puncta'ta albes'cens retinitis characterized by a diffusion of white spots on the retina.
renal r. see under *retinopathy.*
r. sclopeta'ria a severe traumatic retinal lesion, as from the impact of a bullet.
serous r., simple r. simple inflammation of the superficial layers of the retina.
solar r. retinitis due to excessive exposure to sunlight.
r. stella'ta stellate retinopathy.
striate r. retinitis characterized by gray or yellowish streaks just behind the retinal vessels.
suppurative r. retinitis due to pyemic infection.
syphilitic r., r. syphili'tica retinitis complicating syphilitic iritis.
uremic r. retinitis accompanying uremia.

ret•i•no•blas•to•ma (ret″ĭ-no-blas-to′mə) [*retina* + *blastoma*] a malignant, often congenital blastoma, occurring in both hereditary and sporadic forms, composed of tumor cells arising from embryonic retinal cells. it appears in one or both eyes in children under 5 years of age, and is usually diagnosed initially by a bright white or yellow pupillary reflex (leukokoria). It is caused by germline or somatic mutations, or both, in both alleles of the retinoblastoma *(RB1)* gene. Called also *glioma retinae.*
endophytic r., r. endo'phytum a retinoblastoma that begins in the inner layers of the retina and spreads toward the center of the globe; called also *glioma endophytum.*
exophytic r., r. exo'phytum a retinoblastoma that begins in the outer layers of the retina and spreads away from the center of the globe; called also *glioma exophytum.*

ret•i•no•cer•e•bral (ret″ĭ-no-sə-re′brəl, -ser′ə-brəl) affecting both the retina and cerebrum; see *von Hippel-Lindau disease,* under *disease.*

ret•i•no•cho•roid (ret″ĭ-no-kor′oid) pertaining to the retina and the choroid.

ret•i•no•cho•roi•di•tis (ret″ĭ-no-kor-oi-di′tis) chorioretinitis.
r. juxtapapilla'ris a condition seen in young healthy subjects, marked by a small inflammatory area on the fundus close to the papilla; called also *Jensen retinitis* or *retinochoroiditis.*
toxoplasmic r. see under *chorioretinitis.*

ret•i•no•cy•to•ma (ret″ĭ-no-si-to′mə) a rare benign variant of retinoblastoma composed of viable cells with substantial photoreceptor differentiation and often fleurettes; vision is often normal. Called also *retinoma.*

ret•i•no•di•al•y•sis (ret″ĭ-no-di-al′ĭ-sis) [*retina* + *dialysis*] disinsertion of the retina; detachment of the retina at its peripheral insertion.

ret•i•no•graph (ret′ĭ-no-graf) a photograph of the retina.

ret•i•nog•ra•phy (ret″ĭ-nog′rə-fe) photography of the retina.

ret•i•no•ic ac•id (ret″ĭ-no′ik) an oxidized derivative of retinol, formed by carboxylation of the aldehyde group of retinal (q.v.). It is believed to be the form of vitamin A that plays a role in the development and growth of bone and in the maintenance of normal epithelial structures. In pharmacology, the term is often used alone to mean the all-*trans* isomer *(tretinoin)*; the 13-*cis* isomer is usually called isotretinoin.

ret•i•noid (ret′ĭ-noid) 1. resembling the retina. 2. retinol, retinal, or any structurally similar natural derivative or synthetic compound; the latter need any not have vitamin A activity.

ret•i•nol (ret′ĭ-nol) a 20-carbon primary alcohol occurring as several isomers; it is the form of vitamin A (vitamin A_1) found in mammals. Most dietary sources occur as esters of retinol, also the predominant forms for storage and transport; the de-esterified alcohol can be converted to the metabolically active forms retinal and retinoic acid.

ret•i•nol de•hy•dro•gen•ase (ret′ĭ-nol de-hi′dro-jən-ās) [EC 1.1.1.105] an enzyme of the oxidoreductase class that catalyzes the reversible oxidation of retinol to retinal, using NAD^+ as an electron acceptor.

ret•i•nol *O*-fat•ty-ac•yl•trans•fer•ase (ret′ĭ-nol fat′e a″səl-trans′fər-ās) [EC 2.3.1.76] an enzyme of the transferase class that catalyzes the esterification of retinol with long chain fatty acids (particularly palmitic acid) derived from acyl coenzyme A molecules; the reaction occurs in the intestinal mucosa, creating retinyl esters for transport and storage.

ret•i•no•ma (ret″ĭ-no′mə) retinocytoma.

ret•i•no•ma•la•cia (ret″ĭ-no-mə-la′shə) [*retina* + *malacia*] softening of the retina.

ret•i•no•pap•il•li•tis (ret″ĭ-no-pap″ĭ-li′tis) inflammation of the retina and the optic papilla.

ret•i•nop•a•thy (ret″ĭ-nop′ə-the) [*retina* + *-pathy*] 1. retinitis. 2. retinosis.
acute zonal occult outer r. (AZOOR) a syndrome characterized by blind spots in the visual fields with photopsia and only minimal changes visible through the ophthalmoscope; in some patients it may clear up within a year, but in others the change is permanent. It primarily affects young women, and the etiology is unknown.
AIDS-associated r. HIV-associated r.
arteriosclerotic r. sclerosis of retinal arterioles marked by increased tortuosity, attenuation, copper-wire appearance, perivascular sheathing, nipping at arteriovenous crossings, small, scattered hemorrhaging, and small, white, well-defined exudates with no surrounding edema.
background r., background diabetic r. nonproliferative diabetic r.
bull's eye r. see under *maculopathy.*
cancer-associated r. (CAR) retinal changes as part of a paraneoplastic syndrome, with dysfunction of the rods and cones and progressive loss of vision.
central angiospastic r. central serous r.
central serous r. a usually self-limiting condition marked by acute localized detachment of the neural layer or the pigmented layer of the retina in the region of the macula, causing farsightedness.
circinate r. a condition marked by a circle of white spots enclosing the macular area, leading to complete foveal blindness; called also *retinitis circinata* or *circinate retinitis.*
diabetic r. the retinal changes associated with diabetes mellitus; see *proliferative diabetic r.* and *nonproliferative diabetic r.*
exudative r. Coats disease.
hemorrhagic r. retinopathy marked by profuse hemorrhaging in the retina, occurring in diabetes, occlusion of the central vein, and hypertension.
HIV-associated r. a usually asymptomatic microangiopathy affecting the retina, seen in human immunodeficiency virus infection; it is manifested by transient cotton-wool spots, and occasionally hemorrhages, microaneurysms, and other lesions of the microvasculature. Called also *retinal microvasculopathy* and *AIDS-associated r.*
hypertensive r. retinopathy associated with essential or malignant hypertension; changes may include irregular narrowing of the retinal arterioles, hemorrhages in the nerve fiber layers and the outer plexiform layer, exudates and cotton-wool patches, a lipid star in the macula, arteriosclerotic changes, and, in malignant hypertension, papilledema. Called also *hypertensive retinitis.* See also *renal r.* and *stellate r.*
leukemic r. a condition occurring in leukemia, with paleness of the fundus resulting from infiltration of the retina and choroid with leukocytes, and swelling of the disk with blurring of its margin.
nonproliferative diabetic r. a type of diabetic retinopathy usually seen in the early stages of the condition, characterized by progression of microaneurysms, punctate hemorrhages within the retina, yellow exudates, cotton-wool spots, and sometimes macular edema that can compromise vision. Called also background diabetic r.
pigmentary r. see *retinitis pigmentosa.*
r. of prematurity a bilateral retinopathy typically occurring in premature infants treated with high concentrations of oxygen, characterized by vascular dilatation, proliferation, and tortuosity, edema, and retinal detachment, with ultimate conversion of the retina into a fibrous mass that can be seen as a dense retrolental membrane; usually, growth of the eye is arrested and may result in microphthalmia, and blindness may occur. Called also *retrolental fibroplasia* and *Terry syndrome.*
proliferative r. retinopathy characterized by neovascularization of the retina and optic disk (which may project into the vitreous), proliferation of fibrous tissue, vitreous hemorrhage, and eventually retinal detachment with blindness. It occurs in a variety of inflammatory conditions and in diabetes mellitus; proliferative diabetic retinopathy is the most common type.
proliferative diabetic r. proliferative retinopathy accompanying diabetes mellitus; it is usually preceded by nonproliferative diabetic retinopathy.
Purtscher angiopathic r. Purtscher disease.
renal r. a retinopathy associated with renal and hypertensive disorders, and presenting the same symptoms as hypertensive retinopathy; called also *renal retinitis.* See also *stellate r.*
stellate r. a retinopathy not associated with hypertensive, renal, or arteriosclerotic disorders, but presenting the same symptoms as hypertensive retinopathy; called also *stellate retinitis.* See also *renal r.*

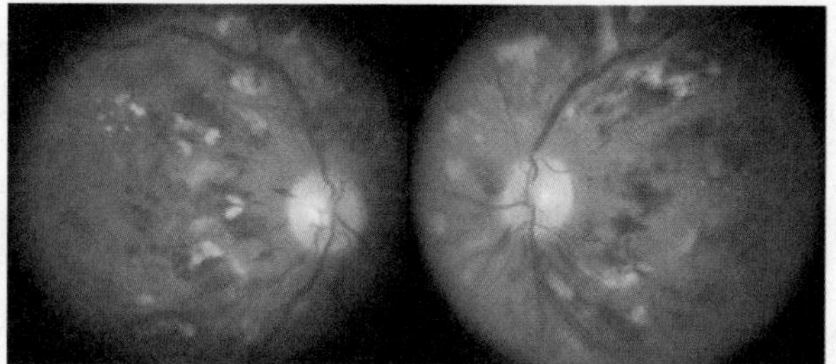

■ Ophthalmoscopy of severe proliferative diabetic retinopathy showing diffuse retinal hemorrhages in all quadrants and neovascularization.

ret•i•no•pexy (ret′ĭ-no-pek″se) restoring of the retina to its proper anatomical location.

pneumatic r. a treatment for retinal detachment involving injection of gas into the posterior vitreous cavity in such a way that the gas bubble presses against the area of torn retina, forcing it back into place.

ret•i•nos•chi•sis (ret″ĭ-nos′kĭ-sis) [*retina* + *-schisis*] splitting of the retina: in the *juvenile form* the splitting occurs in the nerve fiber layer, and in the *adult form* in the external plexiform layer. The disorder is usually more benign and slowly progressive than retinal detachment.

ret•i•no•scope (ret′ĭ-no-skōp″) an instrument for performing retinoscopy; called also *skiascope.*

ret•i•nos•co•py (ret″ĭ-nos′kə-pe) [*retina* + *-scopy*] an objective method for investigating, diagnosing, and evaluating refractive errors of the eye, by projection of a beam of light into the eye and observation of the movement of the illuminated area on the retina surface and of the refraction by the eye of the emergent rays. Called also *skiascopy* and *skiametry.*

book r. dynamic retinoscopy in which the patient focuses on reading a book; commonly used with children.

dynamic r., near point r. retinoscopy in which the patient fixes the gaze on a target at a near distance; accommodation is active.

static r. retinoscopy in which the patient fixes the gaze on a target at a long distance in order to relax accommodation.

ret•i•no•sis (ret″ĭ-no′sis) [*retina* + *-osis*] any of various degenerative, noninflammatory conditions of the retina.

ret•i•no•top•ic (ret″ĭ-no-top′ik) relating to the organization of the visual pathways and visual area of the brain.

ret•i•no•tox•ic (ret′ĭ-no-tok″sik) exerting a toxic or deleterious effect upon the retina.

ret•i•nyl (ret′ĭ-nəl) pertaining to or derived from retinol.

ret•i•nyl-pal•mi•tate es•ter•ase (ret′ĭ-nəl pal′mĭ-tāt es′tər-ās) [EC 3.1.1.21] an enzyme of the hydrolase class that catalyzes the cleavage of palmitic acid from the corresponding retinyl ester to form the free alcohol retinol. The reaction occurs in the intestinal lumen and in the liver in the metabolism of vitamin A.

re•to•peri•the•li•um (re″to-per″ĭ-the′le-əm) [*rete* + *peri-* + *thelium*] the layer of cells covering a reticular framework.

Re•tor•ta•mo•nad•i•da (re-tor″tə-mo-nad′ĭ-də) an order of parasitic, flagellate, intestinal protozoa of the phylum Sarcomastigophora, having two to four flagella, one of which is turned posteriorly and associated with a ventral cytosomal region; Golgi apparatus and mitochondria are absent. Representative genera include *Chilomastix* and *Retortamonas.*

Re•tor•tam•o•nas (re″tor-tam′o-nas) [L. *retortus* bent back + Gr. *monas* unit, from *monos* single] a genus of biflagellate, nonpathogenic, parasitic, intestinal protozoa of the order Retortamonadida, phylum Sarcomastigophorea, found in various insects, amphibians, reptiles, and mammals; they have two anterior flagella, one of which extends posteriorly and trails from the body.

re•to•thel (re′to-thel) reticuloendothelial.

re•to•the•li•um (re″to-the′le-əm) [*rete* + *thelium*] the layer of cells covering a reticular tissue. **retothe′lial** *adj*

re•trac•tile (re-trak′təl) [L. *retractilis*] susceptible of being drawn back.

re•trac•tion (re-trak′shən) [L. *retrahere* to draw back] 1. the act of drawing back; the condition of being drawn back. 2. distal movement of teeth, usually accomplished with an orthodontic appliance.

clot r. the drawing away of a blood clot from the wall of a vessel, a stage of wound healing caused by contraction of platelets.

gingival r. the displacement of the marginal gingiva away from a tooth.

mandibular r. 1. drawing back or retracting the mandible, accomplished by contraction of the middle and posterior parts of the temporal muscles and the suprahyoid muscle. 2. the condition of the mandible in which it lies posterior to the orbital plane. Cf. *mandibular protraction.*

Selected Surgical Retractors

Adson retractor	Hibbs retractor
Alm retractor	Hohmann retractor
Army-Navy retractor	Jansen retractor
Aufricht retractor	Leyla-Yasargil retractor
Balfour retractor	Lowsley retractor
Beckman retractor	Martin retractor
Bennett retractor	Masson-Judd retractor
Budde retractor	Miller-Senn retractor
Burford retractor	Millin retractor
Converse alar retractor	Miltex retractor
Davidson retractor	Mollison retractor
Deaver retractor	Morris retractor
DeBakey-Cooley retractor	Ollier retractor
Denis Brown retractor	O'Sullivan-O'Connor retractor
Doane retractor	Parker retractor
Doyen retractor	Ragnell retractor
Finochietto retractor	Richardson retractor
Fomon retractor	Rigby retractor
Frazier retractor	Roux retractor
Glenner retractor	Senn retractor
Greenberg retractor	Senn-Kanavel retractor
Harrington retractor	USA retractor
Heaney retractor	Weitlaner retractor

re•trac•tor (re-trak′tər) 1. an instrument for maintaining operative exposure by separating the edges of a wound and holding back underlying organs and tissues; many shapes, sizes, and styles are available. See accompanying table. 2. any retractile muscle.

Emmet r. a self-retaining vaginal speculum.

Moorehead r. an instrument for retracting the lips, cheeks, or margins of a surgical wound. It fits over the crown of the head and is provided with metal buttons, to which shields (or retractors) of desired shapes or sizes may be attached.

re•trad (re′trad) [L. *retro* backward] toward a posterior or dorsal part.

re•triev•al (re-tre′vəl) in psychology, the process of obtaining memory information from wherever it has been stored.

retr(o)- [L. *retro* backward] a prefix meaning backward, or located behind.

ret•ro•ac•e•tab•u•lar (ret″ro-as″ə-tab′u-lər) posterior to the acetabulum.

ret•ro•ac•tion (ret″ro-ak′shən) action in a reversed direction; cf. *reaction.*

ret•ro•au•ric•u•lar (ret″ro-aw-rik′u-lər) postauricular.

ret•ro•buc•cal (ret″ro-buk′əl) pertaining to the posterior part of the mouth near the cheek.

ret•ro•bul•bar (ret″ro-bul′bər) [*retro-* + *bulbar*] 1. posterior or inferior to the medulla oblongata. 2. posterior to the eyeball.

ret•ro•cal•ca•ne•al (ret″ro-kal-ka′ne-əl) posterior to the calcaneus.

ret•ro•cal•ca•neo•bur•si•tis (ret″ro-kal-ka″ne-o-bər-si′tis) retrocalcaneal bursitis.

ret•ro•cer•vi•cal (ret″ro-sur′vĭ-kəl) posterior to the cervix uteri.

ret•ro•ces•sion (ret″ro-sesh′ən) [L. *retrocessio*] 1. a going backward or backward displacement; cf. *retrodeviation.* 2. backward displacement of the uterus.

ret•ro•chi•as•mat•ic (ret″ro-ki-as-mat′ik) located posterior to the optic chiasm, such as a tumor.

ret•ro•coch•le•ar (ret″ro-kok′le-ər) 1. posterior to the cochlea. 2. denoting the eighth cranial nerve and cerebellopontine angle as opposed to the cochlea.

ret•ro•col•lic (ret″ro-kol′ik) 1. nuchal. 2. torticollar.

ret•ro•col•lis (ret″ro-kol′is) [*retro-* + *collum*] spasmodic torticollis in which the head is drawn directly backward.

ret•ro•cru•ral (ret″ro-kroo′rəl) 1. posterior to the lower limb. 2. posterior to any crus.

ret•ro•cur•sive (ret″ro-kur′siv) [*retro-* + L. *currere* to run] marked by stepping backward.

ret•ro•de•vi•a•tion (ret″ro-de″ve-a′shən) any displacement backward; a general term that includes retroversion, retroflexion, and other deviations. Called also *retrodisplacement* and *retroposition.*

ret•ro•dis•place•ment (ret″ro-dis-plās′mənt) retrodeviation.

ret•ro•fill•ing (ret″ro-fil′ing) a method of root canal therapy in which the canal is filled from the apex, which has been surgically exposed;

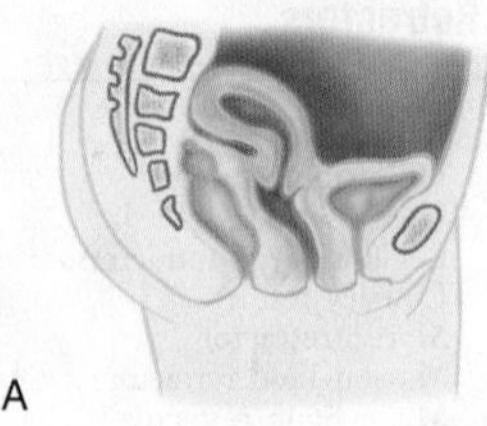

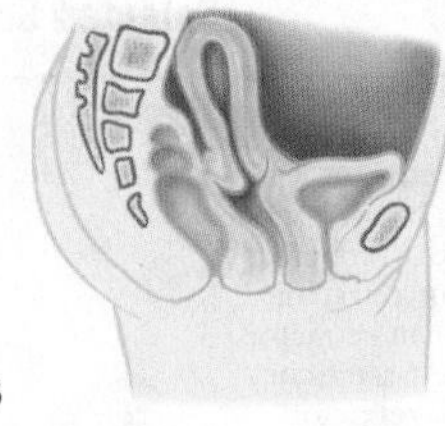

■ Retroflexion *(A)* and retroversion *(B)* of uterus.

zinc-free silver alloy is the most commonly used filling material. Called also *reverse filling* and *root-end filling*.

ret·ro·flexed (ret′ro-flekst) bent posteriorly; cf. *retroflexion*.

ret·ro·flex·ion (ret″ro-flek′shən) [*retro-* + *flexion*] the bending of an organ or part so that its top is turned posteriorly; particularly, the bending posteriorly of the body of the uterus toward the cervix, resulting in a sharp angle at the point of bending.

ret·ro·gas·se·ri·an (ret″ro-gə-sēr′e-ən) pertaining to the sensory (posterior) root of the trigeminal (gasserian) ganglion.

ret·ro·gna·thia (ret″ro-nath′e-ə) retrognathism.

ret·ro·gnath·ism (ret″ro-nath′iz-əm) [*retro-* + *gnath-* + *-ism*] abnormal posterior positioning of one or both jaws, particularly the mandible, relative to the facial skeleton and soft tissues. Called also *retrognathia*. retrognath′ic *adj*

ret·ro·grade (ret′ro-grād) [*retro-* + L. *gradi* to step] 1. moving backward or against the usual direction of flow. 2. degenerating, deteriorating, or catabolic.

ret·ro·gres·sion (ret″ro-gresh′ən) [*retro-* + L. *gressus* course] degeneration; deterioration; regression; return to an earlier, less complex condition.

ret·ro·in·fec·tion (ret″ro-in-fek′shən) migration of newly hatched larval pinworms *(Enterobius vermicularis)* from the perianal region back into the anus and intestine.

ret·ro·jec·tion (ret″ro-jek′shən) [*retro-* + L. *jacere* to throw] irrigation of a cavity by injection of fluid.

ret·ro·lab·y·rin·thine (ret″ro-lab″ə-rin′thēn) posterior to a labyrinth.

ret·ro·len·tal (ret″ro-len′təl) behind the lens of the eye.

ret·ro·lis·the·sis (ret″ro-lis′thə-sis) retrospondylolisthesis.

ret·ro·mo·lar (ret″ro-mo′lər) behind a molar.

ret·ro·mor·pho·sis (ret″ro-mor-fo′sis) retrograde metamorphosis.

ret·ro·pa·rot·id (ret″ro-pə-rot′id) behind a parotid gland.

ret·ro·per·i·stal·sis (ret″ro-per″ĭ-stawl′sis) reversed peristalsis.

ret·ro·peri·to·ne·al (ret″ro-per″ĭ-to-ne′əl) external to or posterior to the peritoneum.

ret·ro·peri·to·ne·um (ret″ro-per″ĭ-to-ne′əm) spatium retroperitoneale.

ret·ro·peri·to·ni·tis (ret″ro-per″ĭ-to-ni′tis) inflammation in the retroperitoneal space.

fibrous r. retroperitoneal fibrosis.

ret·ro·pha·ryn·ge·al (ret″ro-fə-rin′je-əl) 1. pertaining to the posterior part of the pharaynx. 2. posterior to the pharynx.

ret·ro·phar·yn·gi·tis (ret″ro-far″in-ji′tis) inflammation of the posterior part of the pharynx.

ret·ro·phar·ynx (ret″ro-far′inks) the posterior part of the pharynx.

ret·ro·pla·cen·tal (ret″ro-plə-sen′təl) posterior to the placenta.

ret·ro·pla·sia (ret″ro-pla′zhə) [*retro-* + *-plasia*] retrograde metaplasia; degeneration of a tissue or cell into a more primitive type.

ret·ro·posed (ret′ro-pōzd″) [*retro-* + L. *positus* placed] displaced backward or posteriorly.

ret·ro·po·si·tion (ret″ro-pə-zish′ən) retrodeviation.

ret·ro·po·son (ret″ro-po′zon) retrotransposon.

ret·ro·pu·bic (ret″ro-pu′bik) posterior to the pubic arch.

ret·ro·pul·sion (ret″ro-pul′shən) [*retro-* + *pulsion*] 1. a driving back. 2. a tendency to walk backward involuntarily, seen in some varieties of parkinsonism; called also *backward progression*. 3. an abnormal gait in which the body is bent backward.

ret·ro·re·nal (ret″ro-re′nəl) postrenal (def. 1).

ret·ror·sine (ret′ror-sin) a poisonous pyrrolizidine alkaloid found in various species of *Senecio*, causing seneciosis in ruminants.

ret·ro·sig·moid·al (ret″ro-sig-moi′dəl) posterior to the sigmoid sinus.

ret·ro·spec·tive (ret″ro-spek′tiv) [L. *retrospicere* to look back at] 1. looking backward, or directed toward the past. 2. denoting a type of epidemiologic study in which patients are selected on the basis of an outcome (or lack thereof) and examined for factors that might be associated with the outcome.

ret·ro·spon·dy·lo·lis·the·sis (ret″ro-spon″də-lo-lis-the′sis) posterior displacement of one vertebral body on the subjacent body.

ret·ro·ster·nal (ret″ro-stur′nəl) [*retro-* + *sternal*] situated or occurring posterior to the sternum.

ret·ro·sym·phys·i·al (ret″ro-sim-fiz′e-əl) posterior to the symphysis pubis.

ret·ro·tor·sion (ret″ro-tor′shən) a decrease in the torsion angle of the femur, resulting in external deviation of the thigh.

ret·ro·trans·po·son (ret″ro-tranz-po′zon) a transposable element that generates a RNA intermediate, from which a new element is created by reverse transcription and inserted at a new site. Called also *retroposon*.

ret·ro·uter·ine (ret″ro-u′tər-in) posterior to the uterus.

ret·ro·ver·sio·flex·ion (ret″ro-vur″se-o-flek′shən) retroversion combined with retroflexion.

ret·ro·ver·sion (ret″ro-vur′zhən) the tipping of an entire organ or part in a posterior direction, such as the tipping back of the entire uterus in relation to the pelvic axis.

ret·ro·vert·ed (ret″ro-vur′təd) in a condition of retroversion.

ret·ro·ves·i·cal (ret″ro-ves′ĭ-kəl) posterior to the urinary bladder.

Ret·ro·vir (ret′ro-vir) trademark for preparations of zidovudine.

Ret·ro·vi·ri·dae (ret″ro-vir′ĭ-de) the retroviruses: a family of RNA viruses having a virion 80–100 nm in diameter consisting of a lipid-containing envelope with peplomers, surrounding an icosahedral capsid. The genome consists of two identical molecules of polyadenylated positive-sense single-stranded RNA; the monomers are connected at the 5′ end by hydrogen bonds and each has a molecular weight of approximately 3×10^6 and a size of 3.5–9 kb, depending on the genus. Viruses contain seven major polypeptides, including a reverse transcriptase, and are resistant to ultraviolet light but sensitive to lipid solvents and detergents. Replication is unique: genomic RNA serves as a template for DNA synthesis via reverse transcriptase; complementary DNA is synthesized from viral DNA and integrated into the host cell DNA, where it is used for transcription. Assembly occurs by budding through the plasma membrane. Most retroviruses are oncogenic. Genera of medical or veterinary importance are *Alpharetrovirus*, *Betaretrovirus*, *Gammaretrovirus*, *Deltaretrovirus*, *Lentivirus*, and *Spumavirus*.

ret·ro·vi·rol·o·gy (ret″ro-vi-rol′ə-je) the branch of microbiology that is concerned with retroviruses and the diseases they cause.

ret·ro·vi·rus (ret′ro-vi″rəs) any virus of the family Retroviridae. retrovi′ral *adj*

BLV-HTLV r's former name for the genus *Deltaretrovirus*.

human endogenous r's (HERV) retroviruslike sequences found in the human genome, thought to constitute the remains of true retroviruses that were absorbed through evolution; at least one is thought to be linked to expression of tumor cells.

mammalian type B r's former name for the genus *Betaretrovirus*.

mammalian type C r's a group of viruses in the genus *Gammaretrovirus* that infect mammals; it includes the feline and murine leukemia viruses. They have a dense, centrally located core within a lipoprotein envelope covered with barely visible spikes; replication occurs at the inner surface of the plasma membrane at the same time as budding.

re·tru·sion (re-troo′zhən) [L. *re-* back + *trudere* to shove] 1. the state of being located posterior to the normal position, such as the mandible or a tooth displaced in the line of occlusion. 2. the backward movement of the mandible. 3. the pressing backward of the teeth.

Rett syndrome (ret) [Andreas *Rett*, Austrian physician, 20th century] see under *syndrome*.

re·turn (re-turn′) a coming back.

venous r. the flow of blood into the heart from the peripheral vessels.

Ret·zi·us fibers, space (cavity), veins (ret′ze-oos) [Anders Adolf *Retzius*, Swedish anatomist, 1796–1860] see under *fiber* and *vein*, and see *spatium retropubicum*.

Ret·zi·us foramen, lines (striae, stripes) (ret′ze-oos) [Magnus Gustav *Retzius*, Swedish anatomist, 1842–1919] see *apertura lateralis ventriculi quarti*, and see *incremental lines*, under *line*.

re·up·take (re-up′tāk) reabsorption of a previously secreted substance.

re·vac·ci·na·tion (re″vak-sĭ-na′shən) a second vaccination.

re·vas·cu·lar·iza·tion (re-vas″ku-lər-ĭ-za′shən) 1. the restoration of blood supply, as after a wound. 2. the restoration of an adequate blood supply to a part, such as with a bypass or angioplasty procedure.

renal r. surgical correction of occlusion of a renal artery through a technique such as renal artery endarterectomy or one of the bypass procedures.

re•ve•hent (rə-ve′hənt) carrying back; said of veins and arteries.

re•ver•ber•a•tion (re-vur″bə-ra′shən) [L. *reverberare* to cause to rebound] duration of neuronal activity well beyond an initial stimulus due to transmission of impulses along branches of nerves arranged in a circle, permitting positive feedback; it occurs in the brain and perhaps elsewhere and is thought to be related to processes such as learning, memory, and habituation. See also *reverberating circuit*, under *circuit*.

Re•ver•din graft, needle (rĕ-ver-dă′) [Jacques Louis *Reverdin*, Swiss surgeon, 1842–1929] see *pinch graft*, under *graft*, and see under *needle*.

re•ver•sal (re-vur′səl) a turning or change to go in the opposite direction.

sex r. a change in characteristics from those typical of one sex to those typical of the other. *Primary sex reversal* is that resulting from errors in sex determination, the initial development of testes or ovaries; *secondary sex reversal* is that resulting from errors in the consequent differentiation of the male or female phenotype.

vasectomy r. surgical restoration of connection between ducts or vessels in a man who has previously had a vasectomy. Types include vasoepididymostomy and vasovasostomy.

re•verse tran•scrip•tase (re-vurs′ tran-skrip′tās) RNA-directed DNA polymerase.

re•ver•si•ble (re-vur′sĭ-bəl) capable of going through a series of changes in either direction, forward or backward, as a reversible chemical reaction.

re•ver•sion (re-vur′zhən) [*re-* + *version*] 1. regression (def. 1). 2. in genetics, the mutation of a mutant phenotype so that the original function is restored; the term can be used specifically to denote mutation of the DNA such that the parental base sequence is regained (reverse mutation), but can be also be used more broadly to describe production of an altered base sequence that nevertheless encodes the original amino acid or masking of the first alteration by a second via suppression (q.v.).

antigenic r. a change in the antigenic structure of adult cells to that of immature cells, as in certain tumors.

true r. reversion occurring via reverse mutation, restoring the parental nucleotide sequence.

Re•ver•sol (re-vur′sol) trademark for a preparation of edrophonium chloride.

Rev•ex (rev′eks) trademark for a preparation of nalmefene hydrochloride.

Rev-Eyes (rev′īz) trademark for a preparation of dapiprazole hydrochloride.

Re•Via (re-vi′ə) trademark for a preparation of naltrexone hydrochloride.

Re•vil•liod sign (rĕ-ve-yo′) [Jean Léonard Adolphe *Revilliod*, Swiss physician, 1835–1919] see under *sign*.

re•vi•ves•cence (re″vi-ves′əns) [L. *revivescere* to revive] the renewal of vital activities.

re•viv•i•fi•ca•tion (re-viv″ĭ-fĭ-ka′shən) [*re-* + *vivi-* + *facere* to make] 1. restoration to life or consciousness. 2. refreshing of diseased surfaces to promote their union.

Rev•lim•id (rev-lim′id) trademark for a preparation of lenalidomide.

rev•o•lute (rev′o-lo͞ot) turned back or curled back.

re•vul•sion (re-vul′shən) [L. *revulsio;* from *re-* back + *vellere* to draw] the drawing of blood from one part to another, as occurs in counterirritation.

Rex•ed laminae (rek″sed) [B. *Rexed*, 20th century] see under *lamina*.

Rey•a•taz (ra′ə-taz) trademark for a preparation of atanazavir sulfate.

Reye syndrome (ri) [Ralph Douglas Kenneth *Reye*, Australian physician, 20th century] see under *syndrome*.

Reye-John•son syndrome (ri′ jon′sən) [R.D.K. *Reye;* George Magnus *Johnson*, American physician, born 1935] Reye syndrome.

Rey•nals (ra-nahlz′) see *Duran-Reynals*.

Rey•nolds number (ren′əldz) [Osborne *Reynolds*, Irish physicist, 1842–1912] see under *number*.

Rey•nolds Risk Score (ren′əldz) [*Reynolds* Center, Harvard Medical School, named for Donald W. *Reynolds*, American philanthropist, 1906–1993] see under *score*.

Rez•i•pas (rez′ĭ-pas) trademark for a preparation of para-aminosalicylic acid.

RF radio frequency; rheumatoid factor.

RFA right frontoanterior; see *frontoanterior position*, under *position*.

RfD reference dose.

RFI renal failure index.

RFLP restriction fragment length polymorphism.

RFP right frontoposterior; see *frontoposterior position*, under *position*.

RFPSG Royal Faculty of Physicians and Surgeons of Glasgow.

RFT right frontotransverse; see *frontotransverse position*, under *position*.

RGN Registered General Nurse (Scotland).

RGO reciprocating gait orthosis.

Rh rhodium.

Rh_{null} symbol for a rare blood type in which all Rh factors are lacking; see also *Rh-null syndrome*, under *syndrome*.

Rh antibody, blood group, factor [from *Rhesus* monkeys, whose blood was found to contain the factor in 1940] see under *antibody*, *blood group*, and *factor*.

Rhab•di•a•soi•dea (rab″de-ə-soi′de-ə) in some classifications, a superfamily of phasmids, including the genus *Strongyloides*.

rhab•dit•ic (rab-dit′ik) pertaining or belonging to *Rhabditis*, or to the Rhabditoidea.

Rhab•di•ti•dae (rab-dit′ĭ-de) a family of nematodes that contains both free-living and parasitic species. Genera of medical or veterinary interest include *Rhabditis* and *Strongyloides*.

rhab•dit•i•form (rab-dit′ĭ-form) rhabdoid.

Rhab•di•tis (rab-di′tis) [Gr. *rhabdos* rod] a genus of minute phasmid nematodes of the superfamily Rhabditoidea, family Rhabditidae, living mostly in damp earth, and as an accidental parasite in animals.

R. ho′minis a species found in human feces.

R. intestina′lis a species found in human feces.

R. niel′lyi a species found as an accidental parasite on human skin.

R. pel′lio a species found in the human genitourinary tract.

R. strongyloi′des a species that usually lives in decaying vegetable matter but may invade broken skin and cause rhabditic dermatitis.

rhab•di•toid (rab′dĭ-toid) rhabdoid.

Rhab•di•toi•dea (rab″dĭ-toi′de-ə) a superfamily of phasmids, some members of which are free-living and others parasitic to plants and animals; it includes the genera *Rhabditis* and *Strongyloides*.

rhabd(o)- [Gr. *rhabdos* rod] a combining form meaning rod-shaped or denoting relationship to a rod.

rhab•doid (rab′doid) [*rhabdo-* + *-oid*] resembling a rod; rod-shaped.

rhab•do•myo•blast (rab″do-mi′o-blast″) [*rhabdo-* + *myoblast*] the prototypic cell of rhabdomyosarcoma, containing an eccentric nucleus, eosinophilic cytoplasm, and sometimes cross striations resembling those of striated muscle; it may be round, spindle-shaped, or racquet-shaped (strap or tadpole cell). **rhabdomyoblas′tic** *adj*

rhab•do•myo•blas•to•ma (rab″do-mi″o-blas-to′mə) [*rhabdo-* + *myo-* + *blastoma*] rhabdomyosarcoma.

rhab•do•myo•chon•dro•ma (rab″do-mi″o-kon-dro′mə) [*rhabdo-* + *myo-* + *chondroma*] a benign mesenchymoma containing striated muscle and cartilaginous elements.

rhab•do•my•ol•y•sis (rab″do-mi-ol′ĭ-sis) [*rhabdo-* + *myo-* + *-lysis*] disintegration or dissolution of muscle, associated with excretion of myoglobin in the urine.

exertional r. 1. rhabdomyolysis due to intense, prolonged physical exertion, with symptoms often resembling those elicited by exercise in persons with occlusive arterial disease. 2. severe muscular soreness and recumbency in an animal during exercise, either after it does unusually strenuous exercise or when it returns to heavy exercise after a prolonged rest; symptoms include heavy sweating, rapid pulse, and stiffness of gait, sometimes with myoglobinuria. See also *azoturia* (def. 2) and *capture myopathy*.

rhab•do•my•o•ma (rab″do-mi-o′mə) [*rhabdo-* + *myoma*] a benign tumor derived from striated muscle. The cardiac form is considered to be a hamartoma and is often associated with tuberous sclerosis; the extracardiac form is a true neoplasm and is often divided into fetal and adult forms on the basis of the degree of cellular differentiation, distribution, patient age, and other factors.

rhab•do•myo•myx•o•ma (rab″do-mi″o-mik-so′mə) [*rhabdo-* + *myo-* + *myxoma*] a benign mesenchymoma containing striated muscle cell and myxoid elements.

rhab•do•myo•sar•co•ma (rab″do-mi″o-sahr-ko′mə) [*rhabdo-* + *myo-* + *sarcoma*] a highly malignant tumor of striated muscle derived from primitive mesenchymal cells and exhibiting differentiation along rhabdomyoblastic lines, including but not limited to the presence of cells with recognizable cross striations. It occurs in three forms: *pleomorphic r.*,

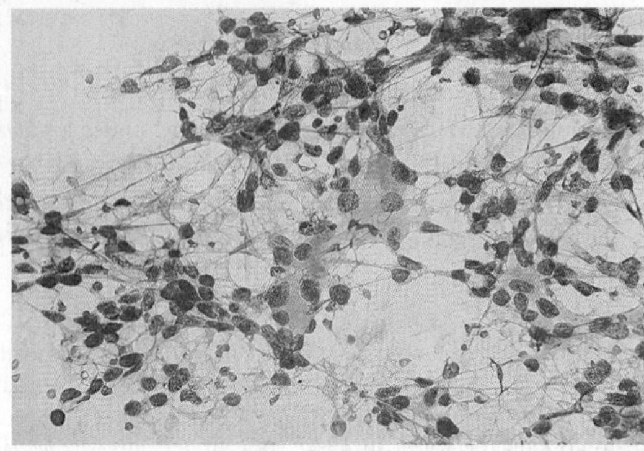

■ Alveolar rhabdomyosarcoma in the forearm of a six-year-old child, showing characteristic round, spindled, and plumper rhabdoid cells (Papanicolaou stain).

alveolar r., and *embryonal r.* Called also *rhabdomyoblastoma* and *rhabdosarcoma*.

alveolar r. a rhabdomyosarcoma containing dense proliferations of small round cells among fibrous septa that form alveoli; it occurs mainly in adolescents and young adults and affects muscles of the extremities, trunk, orbit, and elsewhere.

botryoid r. see under *sarcoma*.

embryonal r. the most common form of rhabdomyosarcoma, containing alternating loosely cellular areas having myxoid stroma and densely cellular areas having spindle cells; it occurs mainly in infants and young children and affects the head and neck, lower genitourinary tract, pelvis, and extremities. Sarcoma botryoides is a subtype.

orbital r. rhabdomyosarcoma in the orbit and surrounding structures, usually superior to the globe; the most common types are embryonal and alveolar. It may affect patients of any age and is the most common primary malignant orbital tumor in children.

paratesticular r. a tumor of the spermatic cord, usually seen in boys under age 15, presenting as a scrotal mass that may grow rapidly; most cases are embryonal rhabdomyosarcomas.

pleomorphic r. a rhabdomyosarcoma seen in skeletal muscles, usually in the limbs of adults, possibly representing dedifferentiation of skeletal muscle cells; the cells are large and have bizarre hyperchromatic nuclei.

r. of prostate a variety of embryonal rhabdomyosarcoma seen mainly in the prostates of young men; it is large and fleshy and may grow fast, filling the pelvis.

Rhab•do•ne•ma (rab″do-ne′mə) *Rhabditis.*

rhab•dos (rab′dos) [Gr. "rod"] a straight cytopharyngeal apparatus with walls supported by nematodesmata and sometimes containing toxicysts; it is characteristic of the lower ciliate protozoa.

rhab•do•sar•co•ma (rab″do-sahr-ko′mə) rhabdomyosarcoma.

rhab•do•sphinc•ter (rab″do-sfingk′tər) [*rhabdo-* + *sphincter*] 1. musculus sphincter urethrae externus urethrae femininae. 2. musculus sphincter urethrae externus urethrae masculinae.

Rhab•do•vi•ri•dae (rab″do-vir′ĭ-de) the rhabdoviruses: a family of RNA viruses having a bullet- or rod-shaped virion 130–430 × 45–100 nm consisting of a lipid-containing envelope, with large G-protein peplomers, surrounding a helical nucleocapsid. The genome consists of a single molecule of negative-sense single-stranded RNA (MW 3.5–4.6 × 10^6, size 11–15 kb). Viruses contain four or five major polypeptides, including a transcriptase, and are sensitive to lipid solvents, detergents, and proteolytic enzymes. Replication occurs in the cytoplasm and assembly is by budding on the plasma membrane or intracytoplasmic membranes. Transmission is by biologic or mechanical vectors. Vertebrate pathogens are included in the genera *Vesiculovirus*, *Lyssavirus*, and *Ephemerovirus*; at least six serogroups of viruses that infect animals and a large number of ungrouped viruses have not yet been assigned to genera.

rhab•do•vi•rus (rab′do-vi″rəs) [*rhabdo-* + *virus*] any virus of the family Rhabdoviridae. **rhabdovi′ral** *adj*

rhachi- for words beginning thus, see those beginning *rachi-*.

Rhad•in•o•vi•rus (rad′ĭ-no-vi″rus) a genus of viruses of the subfamily Gammaherpesvirinae (family Herpesviridae) containing both human and animal pathogens; species include human herpesvirus 8 and several that infect farm animals or other mammals.

rhag•a•des (rag′ə-dēz) [pl. of Gr. *rhagas* rent] fissures, cracks, or fine linear scars in the skin, such as around the mouth or in other regions where the skin moves frequently.

rha•gad•i•form (rə-gad′ĭ-form) [*rhagades* + *form*] resembling rhagades.

rhag•i•on•id (raj″e-on′id) a fly of the family Rhagionidae.

Rhag•i•on•i•dae (raj″e-on′ĭ-de) the snipe flies, a family of biting flies; the genera *Spaniopsis*, *Suragina*, and *Symphoromyia* contain species that are vicious biters.

rham•nose (ram′nōs) a methylpentose structurally derived from mannose (6-deoxymannose); the L- isomer occurs naturally as a component of many plant glycosides and of lipopolysaccharides of some gram-negative bacteria.

rham•no•side (ram′no-sīd) a glycoside that on hydrolysis yields rhamnose.

Rham•nus (ram′nəs) [L., from Gr. *rhamnos* a kind of prickly shrub] a genus of trees and shrubs of the family Rhamnaceae, often with a cathartic bark and fruit. Among them are *R. cathar′tica*, or common buckthorn, *R. purshia′na* D.C., or cascara buckthorn, the source of cascara sagrada, and *R. fran′gula*, or alder buckthorn.

rha•pha•nia (rə-fa′ne-ə) raphania.

rha•phe (ra′fe) [Gr. *rhaphē*] raphe.

rheg•ma (reg′mə) [Gr. *rhēgma*] 1. tear. 2. fracture.

rheg•ma•tog•e•nous (reg″mə-toj′ə-nəs) arising from or caused by a rhegma or tear.

rhe•ni•um (Re) (re′ne-əm) a chemical element; atomic number, 75; atomic weight, 186.2.

r. 186 a radioactive isotope of rhenium, atomic mass 186, having a half-life of 3.78 days and emitting beta particles (1.077, 0.933 MeV) and gamma rays (0.137, 0.632, 0.768 MeV); in the form of a colloid suspension it has been injected into joints for synoviorthesis.

r. 188 a radioactive isotope of rhenium. atomic mass 188, having a half-life of 16.9 hours and emitting beta particles (2.12, 1.96 MeV) and gamma rays (0.155 MeV).

rhe(o)- [Gr. *rheos* current] a combining form denoting relationship to an electric current, or to a flow, as of fluids.

rheo•base (re′o-bās) [*rheo-* + *base*] the minimal electric current of infinite duration necessary to produce a twitch in a muscle.

rhe•og•ra•phy (re-og′rə-fe) the recording of flow of a fluid.

light reflection r. a type of photoplethysmography used to assess deep venous thrombosis; the diode and sensor are placed on the medial surface of the calf over the vein to be tested.

rhe•ol•o•gy (re-ol′ə-je) the science of the deformation and flow of matter, such as the flow of blood through the heart and blood vessels.

Rheo•mac•ro•dex (re″o-mak′ro-deks) trademark for a preparation of dextran 40.

rhe•om•e•ter (re-om′ə-tər) [*rheo-* + *-meter*] galvanometer.

rheo•nome (re′o-nōm) [*rheo-* + Gr. *nemein* to distribute] an apparatus for determining the effect of irritation on a nerve.

rheo•scope (re′o-skōp) [*rheo-* + *-scope*] an instrument for detecting the presence of an electric current.

rheo•stat (re′o-stat) [*rheo-* + *-stat*] an appliance for regulating the resistance and thus controlling the amount of current entering an electric circuit.

rhe•os•to•sis (re″os-to′sis) [*rheo-* + *ostosis*] a condition of hyperostosis marked by the presence of streaks in the bones; see also *melorheostosis*.

rheo•ta•chyg•ra•phy (re″o-tə-kig′rə-fe) [*rheo-* + *tachy-* + *-graphy*] the recording of the variation in the electromotive action of muscles.

rheo•tax•is (re″o-tak′sis) [*rheo-* + *-taxis*] the orientation of an organism in a stream of liquid, with its long axis parallel with the direction of fluid flow.

negative r. rheotaxis with movement of the organism in the same direction as that of the liquid.

positive r. rheotaxis with movement of the organism in the opposite direction to that of the liquid.

rhe•ot•ro•pism (re-ot′ro-piz-əm) rheotaxis.

rhe•sus (re′səs) rhesus monkey.

Rhe•um (re′əm) the rhubarbs, a genus of plants of the family Polygonaceae, some species of which are cathartic.

R. officina′le Baill., a species whose dried roots and rhizomes are used as a laxative.

R. palma′tum Chinese rhubarb; a widely cultivated species native to western and northwestern China, similar to *R. rhaponticum*, whose dried rhizome is used medicinally

R. rhapon′ticum L., the common edible garden rhubarb; its leaves are rich in oxalates and can cause oxalate poisoning (q.v.).

rheum (rōōm) [Gr. *rheuma* flux] a watery discharge.

rheu•ma•tal•gia (roo″mə-tal′jə) chronic rheumatic pain.

rheu•ma•tid (roo′mə-tid) any skin lesion or eruption etiologically associated with rheumatism.

rheu·ma·tism (roo'mə-tiz-əm) [L. *rheumatismus;* Gr. *rheumatismos*] popular name for any of a variety of disorders marked by inflammation, degeneration, or metabolic derangement of connective tissue structures of the body, especially the joints and related structures, including muscles, bursae, tendons, and fibrous tissue, with pain, stiffness, or limitation of motion. Rheumatism confined to the joints is more precisely called *arthritis.* **rheumat'ic** *adj*

desert r. primary coccidioidomycosis.

fibroblastic r. a rare joint disease, usually in the hands, characterized by polyarthralgia and painless subcutaneous nodules, sometimes progressing to contractures; the etiology is unknown.

muscular r. fibrositis.

nonarticular r. any of several syndromes characterized by nonarthritic pain in and around a joint; one type is fibromyalgia.

palindromic r. a condition in which there are repeated episodes of arthritis and periarthritis without fever and without producing irreversible changes in the joints.

Poncet r., tuberculous r. tuberculous arthritis.

rheu·ma·to·gen·ic (roo″mə-to-jen'ik) [*rheumatism* + *-genic*] producing or causing rheumatism.

rheu·ma·toid (roo'mə-toid) [*rheumatism* + *-oid*] 1. resembling rheumatism. 2. associated with rheumatoid arthritis.

rheu·ma·tol·o·gist (roo″mə-tol'ə-jist) a specialist in rheumatic conditions.

rheu·ma·tol·o·gy (roo″mə-tol'ə-je) the branch of medicine dealing with rheumatic disorders, their causes, pathology, diagnosis, treatment, etc.

rheu·ma·to·sis (roo″mə-to'sis) any disorder attributed to rheumatic origin.

Rheu·ma·trex (roo'mə-treks″) trademark for preparations of methotrexate.

rhex·is (rek'sis) [Gr. *rhēxis* a breaking forth, bursting] the rupture of an organ or vessel.

rhi·go·sis (rĭ-go'sis) [Gr. *rhigōsis* a shivering] the ability to feel cold; see *temperature sense,* under *sense.* **rhigot'ic** *adj*

rhi·nal (ri'nəl) [*rhin-* + *-al*[1]] nasal (def. 1).

rhi·nal·gia (ri-nal'jə) [*rhin-* + *-algia*] pain in the nose. Called also *rhinodynia.*

rhi·nal·ler·go·sis (ri″nal-ər-go'sis) [*rhin-* + *allergy* + *-osis*] allergic rhinitis.

rhi·nede·ma (ri″nə-de'mə) [*rhin-* + *edema*] edema of the nose.

rhi·nen·ce·pha·lia (ri″nən-sə-fa'le-ə) rhinocephaly.

rhi·nen·ceph·a·lon (ri″nən-sef'ə-lon) [*rhin-* + *encephalon*] 1. a term generally applied to certain parts of the brain previously thought to be concerned entirely with olfactory mechanisms, including the olfactory nerves, bulbs, tracts, and subsequent connections (all olfactory in function) and the limbic system (not primarily olfactory in function); it is homologous with the olfactory portions of the brain in certain other animals. Called also *olfactory brain* and *smell brain.* 2. a term formerly used in official terminology to designate the area of the brain comprising the substantia perforata anterior, stria diagonalis (Broca), area subcallosa, and gyrus paraterminalis. 3. one of the portions of the telencephalon in the embryo.

rhi·nen·ceph·a·lus (ri″nən-sef'ə-ləs) rhinocephalus.

rhin·i·on (rin'e-on) [Gr., dim. of *rhis*] a cephalometric landmark located at the lower end of the suture between the nasal bones.

rhi·nism (ri'niz-əm) rhinolalia.

rhi·ni·tis (ri-ni'tis) [*rhin-* + *-itis*] inflammation of the mucous membrane of the nose.

acute r., acute catarrhal r. an acute congestion of the mucous membrane of the nose, marked by dryness, followed by increased mucous secretion from the membrane, impeded respiration through the nose, and pain. Called also *coryza.*

allergic r. a general term used to denote any allergic reaction of the nasal mucosa; it may occur perennially *(nonseasonal allergic r.)* or seasonally *(hay fever).*

anaphylactic r. allergic r.

atopic r. nonseasonal allergic r.

atrophic r. a chronic form of rhinitis that is nonallergic and noninfectious, marked by wasting of the mucous membrane and the glands. In the early stages there are small dry areas with crusting, either with viscid secretions or without secretions (see *r. sicca*). In later stages the nasal passages become enlarged and have a foul smell, progressing to ozena (q.v.). It is sometimes the result of trauma, and vascular damage by radiation therapy, environmental irritants, and disease has also been implicated.

atrophic r. of swine a disease of young swine caused by severe persistent inflammation of the nasal mucosa; severe cases may result in marked atrophy of the turbinate bones and lateral displacement of the snout. The primary inflammatory reaction may be caused by a variety of agents, including a virus. See also *inclusion body r.*

r. caseo'sa rhinitis with a caseous, gelatinous, fetid discharge.

chronic r. long-term inflammation of nasal mucous membranes, manifested as either *hypertrophic rhinitis* or *atrophic rhinitis.*

fibrinous r. membranous r.

gangrenous r. a gangrenelike inflammation of the nasal mucosa. See also *cancrum nasi.*

hypertrophic r. a form of rhinitis that is nonallergic and noninfectious, and in which the mucous membrane thickens and swells. See also *vasomotor r.*

inclusion body r. mucopurulent rhinitis and sinusitis of young pigs due to infection with a cytomegalovirus; severe cases may be marked by atrophy of the turbinate bones (see *atrophic r. of swine*) and distortion of the snout, sneezing, stunting of growth, and, histologically, by the presence of inclusion bodies in scrapings of the nasal mucous membranes.

r. medicamento'sa rhinitis that is nonallergic and noninfectious and is caused by rebound vasodilation after prolonged or excessive use of vasoconstricting nasal sprays or drops.

membranous r. chronic rhinitis with the formation of a false membrane, as in nasal diphtheria. Called also *fibrinous r.* and *pseudomembranous r.*

necrotic r. suppuration, necrosis, and swelling of the nose of a pig due to infection by *Fusobacterium necrophorum* that enters through a wound. Called also *bullnose.*

nonseasonal allergic r., perennial r. allergic rhinitis that may occur continuously or intermittently all year round; it is caused by an allergen to which the individual is more or less always exposed, such as house dust, danders, and food, and is characterized by sudden attacks of sneezing, swelling of the nasal mucosa with a profuse watery discharge, itching of the eyes, and lacrimation. Called also *atopic r.* Cf. *hay fever.*

porcine inclusion body r. inclusion body r.

pseudomembranous r. membranous r.

seasonal allergic r. hay fever.

r. sic'ca atrophic rhinitis without secretions.

syphilitic r. rhinitis caused by syphilis, characterized by ulceration, caries of the nasal bone, and a fetid discharge.

tuberculous r. rhinitis due to tuberculosis, characterized by ulceration, caries of the nasal bone, and ozena.

vasomotor r. 1. a form of hypertrophic rhinitis with symptoms similar to those of allergic rhinitis; transient changes in vascular tone and permeability are brought on by such stimuli as chilling, fatigue, anger, and anxiety. 2. any type of allergic or nonallergic rhinitis not caused by an infectious agent.

rhin(o)- [Gr. *rhis,* gen. *rhinos* nose] a combining form denoting relationship to the nose, or a noselike structure.

rhi·no·an·tri·tis (ri″no-ən-tri'tis) [*rhino-* + *antritis*] inflammation of the nasal cavity and the antrum of Highmore. Called also *nasoantritis.*

rhi·no·can·thec·to·my (ri″no-kan-thek'tə-me) rhinommectomy.

rhi·no·cele (ri'no-sēl) rhinocoele.

rhi·no·ceph·a·lus (ri″no-sef'ə-ləs) a fetus exhibiting rhinocephaly.

rhi·no·ceph·a·ly (ri″no-sef'ə-le) [*rhino-* + *-cephaly*] a developmental anomaly characterized by the presence of a proboscis-like nose superior to eyes that are partially or completely fused into one.

rhi·no·chei·lo·plas·ty (ri″no-ki'lo-plas″te) [*rhino-* + *cheiloplasty*] plastic surgery of the nose and lip.

Rhi·no·clad·i·el·la (ri″no-klad″e-el'ə) a genus of imperfect fungi of the form-class Hyphomycetes, form-family Dematiaceae. *R. aquasper'sa* causes chromoblastomycosis.

rhi·no·coele (ri'no-sēl) [*rhino-* + *-coele*] the ventricle of the olfactory lobe of the brain.

Rhi·no·cort (ri'no-kort) trademark for preparations of budesonide.

rhi·no·dyn·ia (ri″no-din'e-ə) [*rhin-* + *-odynia*] rhinalgia.

rhi·no·en·to·moph·tho·ro·my·co·sis (ri″no-en″to-mof″thə-ro-mi-ko'sis) the usual form of conidiobolomycosis, marked by development of large polyps in the subcutaneous tissues of the nose and paranasal sinuses; orbital involvement with unilateral blindness may follow. Sometimes, especially in weak or immunocompromised patients, it can spread to the central nervous system and cause fatal rhinocerebral zygomycosis. Called also *rhinofacial zygomycosis.*

Rhi·noes·trus (ri-nes'trəs) a genus of flies of the family Oestridae whose larvae occur in the nasal passages of horses in Europe, Asia, and Africa; they may deposit larvae in the human eye.

rhi·nog·e·nous (ri-noj'ə-nəs) [*rhino-* + *-genous*] arising in the nose.

rhi·no·ky·pho·sis (ri″no-ki-fo'sis) [*rhino-* + *kyphosis*] the presence of an abnormal hump in the ridge of the nose.

rhi•no•la•lia (ri″no-la′le-ə) [*rhino-* + *lal-* + *-ia*] altered speech due to abnormality of nasal structures; see *hypernasality* and *hyponasality.* Called also *rhinism* and *rhinophonia.*
 r. aper′ta hypernasality.
 r. clau′sa hyponasality.
 open r. hypernasality.

rhi•no•lar•yn•gi•tis (ri″no-lar″in-ji′tis) inflammation of the mucous membrane of the nose and larynx.

rhi•no•lar•yn•gol•o•gy (ri″no-lar″in-gol′ə-je) [*rhino-* + *laryngology*] a branch of otorhinolaryngology that focuses on the nose and larynx and their diseases.

rhi•no•lith (ri′no-lith) [*rhino-* + *-lith*] a nasal stone or concretion. Called also *nasal calculus.*

rhi•no•li•thi•a•sis (ri″no-lĭ-thi′ə-sis) the presence of rhinoliths in the nose.

rhi•nol•o•gist (ri-nol′ə-jist) a specialist in rhinology.

rhi•nol•o•gy (ri-nol′ə-je) [*rhino-* + *-logy*] the medical specialty that deals with the nose and its diseases.

rhi•no•ma•nom•e•ter (ri″no-mə-nom′ə-tər) [*rhino-* + *manometer*] a manometer used in rhinomanometry; called also *nasomanometer.*

rhi•no•ma•nom•e•try (ri″no-mə-nom′ə-tre) measurement of the airflow and pressure within the nose during respiration; nasal resistance or obstruction can be calculated from the data obtained.

rhi•nom•e•ter (ri-nom′ə-tər) [*rhino-* + *-meter*] an instrument for measuring the nose and nasal cavities.
 acoustic r. an apparatus that measures the dimensions of the nasal cavity by transmitting small sound waves and charting their reflections off various parts of the cavity.

rhi•nom•mec•to•my (ri″no-mek′tə-me) [*rhin-* + Gr. *omma* eye + *ectomy*] excision of the inner canthus of the eye.

rhi•no•my•co•sis (ri″no-mi-ko′sis) fungal infection of the nasal mucosa.

rhi•no•ne•cro•sis (ri″no-nə-kro′sis) necrosis of the nasal bones.

rhi•no•nem•me•ter (ri″no-nem′ə-tər) a device for measuring nasal air flow rates. Cf. *pneumotachometer.*

rhi•no•path•ia (ri″no-path′e-ə) rhinopathy.
 r. vasomoto′ria vasomotor rhinitis.

rhi•nop•a•thy (ri-nop′ə-the) [*rhino-* + *-pathy*] any disease of the nose.

rhi•no•pha•ryn•ge•al (ri″no-fə-rin′je-əl) nasopharyngeal.

rhi•no•phar•yn•gi•tis (ri″no-far″in-ji′tis) nasopharyngitis.

rhi•no•pha•ryn•go•lith (ri″no-fə-ring′go-lith) [*rhino-* + *pharyngo-* + *-lith*] calculus of the nasal pharynx.

rhi•no•phar•ynx (ri″no-far′inks) pars nasalis pharyngis.

rhi•no•pho•nia (ri″no-fo′ne-ə) rhinolalia.

rhi•no•phy•co•my•co•sis (ri″no-fi″ko-mi-ko′sis) rhinoentomophthoromycosis.

rhi•no•phy•ma (ri″no-fi′mə) [*rhino-* + *phyma*] the most common type of phymatous rosacea, a severe facial condition with sebaceous hyperplasia, seen most often in men, involving the lower half of the nose and sometimes adjacent cheek areas.

rhi•no•plas•ty (ri′no-plas″te) [*rhino-* + *-plasty*] a plastic surgical operation on the nose, either reconstructive, restorative, or cosmetic. **rhinoplas′tic** *adj*
 Carpue r. Indian r.
 English r. reconstruction of the nose using flaps from the cheeks.

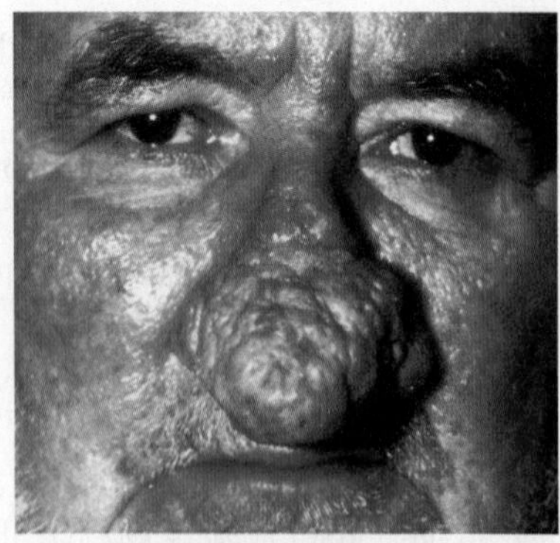

■ Rhinophyma.

 Indian r. reconstruction of the nose by a flap of skin taken from the forehead, with its pedicle at the root of the nose; called also *Carpue operation.*
 Italian r. tagliacotian r.
 Joseph r. an operation for modification of the shape of the nose by resection of the dorsal osteocartilaginous hump with a saw.
 tagliacotian r. reconstruction of the nose by a flap of skin taken from the arm, the flap remaining attached to the arm until union has taken place; called also *Italian* or *tagliacotian operation.*

rhi•no•pneu•mo•ni•tis (ri″no-noo″mo-ni′tis) [*rhino-* + *pneumonitis*] inflammation of the nasal and pulmonary mucous membranes.
 equine viral r. a highly contagious disease of horses caused by a herpesvirus; characteristics include mild respiratory infection in young animals and abortion in mares exposed for the first time; in the latter it is called *equine virus abortion.*

rhi•nor•rha•gia (ri″no-ra′jə) [*rhino-* + *-rrhagia*] epistaxis.

rhi•nor•rha•phy (ri-nor′ə-fe) [*rhino-* + *-rrhaphy*] an operation for epicanthus performed by excising a fold of skin from the nose and closing the opening with sutures.

rhi•nor•rhea (ri″no-re′ə) [*rhino-* + *-rrhea*] the free discharge of a thin nasal mucus.
 cerebrospinal fluid r. discharge of cerebrospinal fluid through the nose; see also *cerebrospinal fluid fistula.*

rhi•no•sal•pin•gi•tis (ri″no-sal-pin-ji′tis) [*rhino-* + *salpingitis*] inflammation of the nasal mucosa and the eustachian tube.

rhi•no•scle•ro•ma (ri″no-sklə-ro′mə) [*rhino-* + *scleroma*] a granulomatous disease in which hard patches or nodules form on the nose and nasopharynx, thought to be due to *Klebsiella rhinoscleromatis*; it occurs in Egypt, Eastern Europe, and Central and South America.

rhi•no•scope (ri′no-skōp) [*rhino-* + *-scope*] an instrument used in nasal examinations; various types of specula and endoscopes may be used. Called also *nasoscope.*

rhi•nos•co•py (ri-nos′kə-pe) examination of the nasal passages with a rhinoscope. **rhinoscop′ic** *adj*
 anterior r. rhinoscopy of anterior nasal structures through the nares.
 median r. examination of superior structures in the nasal cavity, such as the openings of the ethmoid cells, by means of a long nasal speculum.
 posterior r. rhinoscopy of posterior nasal structures through the nasopharynx.

rhi•no•si•nu•si•tis (ri″no-si″nəs-itis) [*rhino-* + *sinus* + *-itis*] inflammation of the paranasal sinuses; called also *nasosinusitis.*

rhi•no•spo•rid•i•o•sis (ri″no-spor-id″e-o′sis) [*rhino-* + Gr. *sporidion* dim. of *sporos* seed] a chronic, localized granulomatous fungal infection with *Rhinosporidium seeberi*, affecting mucocutaneous tissues, usually of the nose but sometimes elsewhere in the body; characterized by polyps, papillomas, and other wartlike lesions.

Rhi•no•spo•rid•i•um see•beri (ri″no-spor-id′e-əm se′bər-i) the as yet unisolated organism, presumably a fungus, that causes rhinosporidiosis.

rhi•no•ste•no•sis (ri′no-stə-no′sis) narrowing of a nasal passage.

rhi•not•o•my (ri-not′ə-me) [*rhino-* + *-tomy*] incision into the nose.

rhi•no•tra•che•itis (ri″no-tra″ke-i′tis) [*rhino-* + *tracheitis*] inflammation of the nasal mucous membranes and trachea.
 feline r., feline viral r. the feline respiratory disease complex when it is caused by feline herpesvirus 1, usually manifesting as an acute febrile infection of the upper respiratory tract and conjunctivae in kittens, with a mucopurulent discharge from the eyes and nose, photophobia, coughing, and sneezing.
 infectious r., infectious bovine r. an acute, infectious, febrile disease of cattle, caused by bovine herpesvirus 1 and marked by inflammation and ulceration of the upper respiratory tract, which may be followed by pneumonia, coughing, profuse discharge from the eyes and nose, excessive salivation, anorexia, and, in pregnant cows, abortion.

Rhi•no•vi•rus (ri′no-vi″rəs) [*rhino-* + *virus*] a genus of viruses of the family Picornaviridae that infect the upper respiratory tract and cause the common cold. Over 100 antigenically distinct types infect humans; bovine and equine rhinoviruses have also been isolated.

rhi•no•vi•rus (ri′no-vi″rəs) any virus belonging to the genus *Rhinovirus.* **rhinovi′ral** *adj*

Rhi•pi•ceph•a•lus (ri″pĭ-sef′ə-ləs) [Gr. *rhipis* fan + *-cephalus*] a genus of ticks of the family Ixodidae, parasitic on many different mammals and serving as vectors for bacteria, protozoa, viruses, and other disease-producing organisms.
 R. appendicula′tus the brown ear tick, a species that parasitizes cattle and other ungulates from Sudan south through East Africa to South Africa; it is the usual vector for *Theileria parva*, which causes East Coast fever, and can also transmit other protozoa and viruses.

R. bur'sa a species found from the Mediterranean basin across into Central Asia, usually parasitizing sheep and goats; it is a vector for the protozoa *Babesia* and *Theileria* in domestic animals and for viruses causing Crimean-Congo hemorrhagic fever and other conditions in humans.

R. capen'sis a species found on cattle and horses in East Africa and southern Africa and serving as a vector for East Coast fever.

R. evert'si a species found on horses, cattle, and other herbivores in eastern and southern Africa; it may serve as a vector for *Theileria parva*, the cause of East Coast fever, as well as *Rickettsia conorii* or various other protozoa, bacteria, or viruses.

R. pulchel'lus a species that parasitizes herbivores in East Africa and is a vector for Nairobi sheep disease and East Coast fever.

R. sangui'neus the brown dog tick, a common species found on domestic animals around the world, serving as a vector for disease-causing bacteria and viruses. Pathogens that it spreads include *Rickettsia rickettsii* and species of *Ehrlichia* and *Babesia*.

R. si'mus the black pitted tick, a species that parasitizes mammals in central and southern Africa and serves as a vector for East Coast fever, tick paralysis, and other diseases.

R. tura'nicus a species that attacks cattle and horses in Europe, Asia, and Africa and serves as a vector for *Rickettsia conorii* and species of *Babesia*.

rhitid(o)- for words beginning thus, see those beginning *rhytid(o)-*.

rhiz(o)- [Gr. *rhiza* root] a combining form denoting relationship to a root.

Rhi·zo·bi·a·ceae (ri-zo″be-a′se-e) a phenotypically diverse family of bacteria of the order Rhizobiales, grouped together on the basis of 16S rRNA sequence analysis. Organisms of medical interest are contained in the genus *Rhizobium*.

Rhi·zo·bi·a·les (ri-zo″be-a′lēz) an order of bacteria of the class Alphaproteobacteria, phylum Proteobacteria, comprising a heterogeneous group of gram-negative bacteria based on 16S rRNA sequence analysis. Pathogenic organisms are included in the families Bartonellaceae, Bradyrhizobiaceae, and Brucellaceae.

Rhi·zo·bi·um (ri-zo′be-əm) [*rhizo-* + Gr. *bios* life] a genus of gram-negative, non–spore-forming, motile, aerobic, rod-shaped bacteria of the family Rhizobiaceae. Organisms produce nodules on the roots of leguminous plants and fix free nitrogen symbiotically. The type species is *R. leguminosa'rum*.

R. radiobac'ter a species that is an occasional opportunistic human pathogen, usually associated with infection of devices such as intravascular catheters and nephrostomy tubes. Formerly called *Agrobacterium radiobacter*.

rhi·zo·blast (ri′zo-blast) [*rhizo-* + *-blast*] flagellar rootlet.

Rhi·zoc·to·nia (ri-zok-to′ne-ə) a genus of imperfect fungi of the form-class Hyphomycetes. *R. legumini'cola* contains the mycotoxin slaframine and sometimes contaminates clover hay, causing slobbers (q.v.) in farm animals.

rhi·zo·don·tro·py (ri″zo-don′trə-pe) [*rhizo-* + *odont-* + *-tropy*] 1. the act of rotating a tooth root. 2. the act of attaching an artificial crown to a tooth root by means of a pivot.

rhi·zo·don·try·py (ri″zo-don′trĭ-pe) [*rhizo-* + *odont-* + Gr. *trephination*] surgical perforation of a tooth root to provide a channel of egress for a confined fluid.

rhi·zoid (ri′zoid) [*rhiz-* + *-oid*] 1. rootlike; resembling a root. 2. a filamentous rootlike structure of fungi and certain algae that extends into the substrate. See illustration at *mold*.

rhi·zoi·dal (ri-zoi′dəl) rhizoid (def. 1).

rhi·zol·y·sis (ri-zol′ə-sis) percutaneous radiofrequency rhizotomy.

Rhi·zo·mas·tig·i·da (ri″zo-mas-tij′ĭ-də) [*rhizo-* + Gr. *mastix* whip] in former systems of classification, an order of zooflagellates characterized by the presence of one to many flagella and pseudopodia occurring simultaneously or at different times in the trophozoite.

rhi·zome (ri′zōm) [Gr. *rhizōma* root stem] the subterraneous root stock of a plant.

rhi·zo·mel·ic (ri-zo-mel′ik) [*rhizo-* + *mel-* + *-ic*] pertaining to or involving the hip joint and shoulder joint.

rhi·zo·me·nin·go·my·eli·tis (ri″zo-mə-ning″go-mi″ə-li′tis) meningomyeloradiculitis.

Rhi·zo·mu·cor (ri″zo-mu′kor) [*rhizo-* + L. *mucor* bread mold] a genus of saprobic fungi of the family Mucoraceae, having few, poorly developed rhizoids. *R. pusil'lus* sometimes causes mucormycosis or opportunistic infections in humans; in other animals it is a more common pathogen and is a major cause of bovine mycotic infection.

rhi·zo·plast (ri′zo-plast) [*rhizo-* + *-plast*] flagellar rootlet.

Rhi·zop·o·da (ri-zop′ə-də) [*rhizo-* + Gr. *pous* foot] 1. a superclass of protozoa of the phylum Sarcomastigophora, comprising the amebae; the majority are free-living in soil and water, but some are parasitic or pathogenic. 2. Sarcodina.

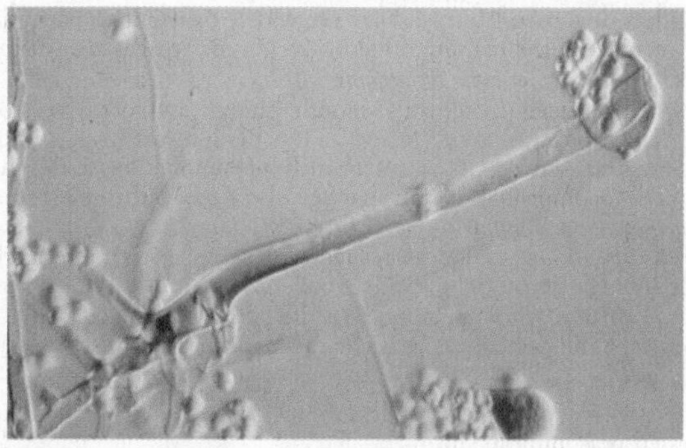

■ *Rhizopus.*

rhi·zo·po·di·um (ri″zo-po′de-əm) pl. *rhizopo'dia* [*rhizo-* + Gr. *pous* foot] reticulopodium.

Rhi·zo·pus (ri′zo-pəs) [*rhizo-* + Gr. *pous* foot] a genus of fungi of the family Mucoraceae, characterized by sporangiophores that arise from nodes at the point where the rhizoids are formed and by a hemispherical columella; it is widespread as a saprobe and a facultative parasite of fruits and vegetables.

R. arrhi'zus *R. oryzae*.

R. microspo'rus a species that causes mucormycosis.

R. ory'zae the most common cause of mucormycosis in humans; it occasionally infects other animals. Called also *R. arrhizus*.

R. rhizopodifor'mis a species that causes human mucormycosis and is an important cause of bovine mycotic abortion and of gastritis in cattle and pigs. Called also *Mucor rhizopodiformis*.

rhi·zot·o·my (ri-zot′ə-me) [*rhizo-* + *-tomy*] interruption of a cranial or spinal nerve root; see also *neurolysis* (def. 4).

anterior r. division of the anterior or motor spinal nerve roots.

chemical r. rhizotomy by injection of a neurolytic chemical such as glycerol or phenol adjacent to the nerve root; see also *glycerol r.* and *chemical neurolysis*.

dorsal r. posterior r.

glycerol r. chemical rhizotomy of the trigeminal or spinal nerves by injection of glycerol; see also *chemical neurolysis*.

percutaneous r. trigeminal rhizotomy not involving brain surgery, such as glycerol rhizotomy or percutaneous radiofrequency rhizotomy.

percutaneous radiofrequency r. trigeminal rhizotomy in which radio waves are used to destroy part of the trigeminal ganglion.

posterior r. division of the posterior or sensory spinal nerve roots; done for relief of intractable pain. Called also *dorsal r.*

retrogasserian r. trigeminal r.

trigeminal r. destruction of part of the sensory root of the trigeminal nerve above the trigeminal ganglion, or of the ganglion itself, for the relief of trigeminal neuralgia. The most common surgical techniques used are the Dandy and Frazier-Spiller operations; nonsurgical techniques include percutaneous radiofrequency rhizotomy and glycerol rhizotomy. Called also *retrogasserian r.*

rho (ro) [Ρ, ρ] the seventeenth letter of the Greek alphabet.

Spearman r. Spearman rank correlation coefficient.

rho·da·mine (ro′də-mēn) [*rhod-* + *amine*] any of a group of red fluorescent dyes used to label proteins in immunofluorescence techniques.

r. B a basic red fluorescent dye used in dyeing paper, as a reagent for heavy metals, and as a stain in immunofluorescence techniques; used as a component of the Truant auramine-rhodamine stain.

rho·da·nate (ro′də-nāt) a salt of rhodanic acid.

rho·dan·ic ac·id (ro-dan′ik) 1. thiocyanic acid. 2. rhodanine.

rho·da·nine (ro′də-nēn) a reagent that gives colored products with aldehydes and ketones.

rho·di·um (ro′de-əm) [Gr. *rhodon* rose] a hard and rare metal of the platinum group; atomic number, 45; atomic weight, 102.905.

Rhod·ni·us (rod′ne-əs) a genus of South American insects of the family Reduviidae. *R. prolix'us* is a species that transmits *Trypanosoma cruzi*, the etiologic agent of Chagas disease.

rhod(o)- [Gr. *rhodon* rose] a combining form meaning red.

Rho·do·coc·cus (ro″do-kok′əs) [*rhodo-* + *coccus*] a genus of bacteria of the family Nocardiaceae, consisting of nonmotile, gram-positive, aerobic, chemo-organotrophic organisms that form a mycelium that breaks up into bacillary and coccal forms. They are widely distributed, occurring especially in soil and the manure of herbivores; some species are pathogenic.

R. bronchia'lis *Gordonia bronchialis.*

R. e'qui a species that forms smooth, shiny, orange to red colonies with elemental hyphae, found in soil and in the intestinal tracts and feces of numerous mammals; it causes bronchopneumonia in foals and can infect immunocompromised humans. See also *Rhodococcus equi pneumonia,* under *pneumonia.* Called also *Corynebacterium equi.*

R. erythropo'lis a species associated with various infections including peritonitis, pneumonia, and eye infections.

R. rhodo'chrous the type species of the genus, associated with various infections including pneumonia, bacteremia, and pericarditis.

Rho•do•den•dron (ro″də-den′drən) a genus of shrubs and trees found in the Northern Hemisphere; they contain andromedotoxin and have caused poisoning in sheep.

rho•do•gen•e•sis (ro″do-jen′ə-sis) [*rhodo-* + *-genesis*] the restoration of the purple tint to rhodopsin after it has become bleached by the action of light.

rho•do•phy•lax•is (ro″do-fə-lak′sis) [*rhodo-* + *phylaxis*] the ability of the retinal epithelium to regenerate rhodopsin. **rhodophylac′tic** *adj*

rho•dop•sin (ro-dop′sin) [*rhodo-* + *opsin*] visual purple: a photosensitive purple-red chromoprotein in the retinal rods that is bleached and activated by light, producing stimulation of the retinal sensory endings as it is formed and degraded in the visual cycle (see illustration under *cycle*). It is a conjugated protein containing an 11-*cis* retinal prosthetic group linked to opsin.

rho•dop•sin ki•nase (ro-dop′sin ki′nās) [EC 2.7.11.14] an enzyme that phosphorylates activated rhodopsin, enabling it to bind arrestin and thus inhibiting its binding to transducin; the reaction occurs in the deactivation of activated rhodopsin during the visual cycle.

Rho•do•spi•ril•la•les (ro″do-spi″rĭ-la′lēz) [Gr. *rhodon* rose + *Spirillum*] a morphologically, metabolically, and ecologically diverse order of bacteria of the class Alphaproteobacteria, phylum Proteobacteria, grouped together on the basis of 16S rRNA sequence analysis. Medically important organisms are contained in the family Acetobacteraceae.

Rho•do•tor•u•la (ro″do-tor′u-lə) a genus of yeastlike imperfect fungi of the form-family Cryptococcaceae. *R. glu'tinis* is a nonpathogenic species from the air, potatoes, and the skin in seborrhea. *R. ru'bra* is a skin contaminant that occasionally causes opportunistic infections.

rho•do•tox•in (ro′do-tok″sin) a poisonous compound from the flowers and leaves of various shrubs and trees, such as *Rhododendron;* it is also found in honey from *Rhododendron* flowers.

RhoGAM (ro′gam) trademark for a preparation of Rh_0(D) immune globulin.

rhomb•en•ceph•a•li•tis (rom″ben-sef″ə-li′tis) inflammation of the rhombencephalon; a combination of brainstem encephalitis and cerebellitis.

rhomb•en•ceph•a•lon (rom″ben-sef′ə-lon) [Gr. *rhombos* rhombus + *enkephalos* brain] 1. the part of the brain developed from the posterior of the three primary brain vesicles of the embryonic neural tube; it comprises the metencephalon (cerebellum and pons) and myelencephalon (medulla oblongata). 2. the most caudal of the three primary brain vesicles in the embryo, later dividing into the metencephalon and myelencephalon. 3. the most caudal of the three primary brain vesicles in the embryo, later dividing into the metencephalon and myelencephalon. Called also *hindbrain.*

rhom•bo•coele (rom′bo-sēl) ventriculus terminalis medullae spinalis.

rhom•boid (rom′boid) [Gr. *rhombos* rhombus + *-oid*] 1. having a shape similar to a rectangle that has been skewed to one side so that the angles are oblique. 2. a plane figure having such a shape.

Michaelis r. a diamond-shaped area over the posterior aspect of the pelvis formed by the dimples of the posterior superior spines of the ilia, the lines formed by the gluteal muscles, and the groove at the distal end of the vertebral column.

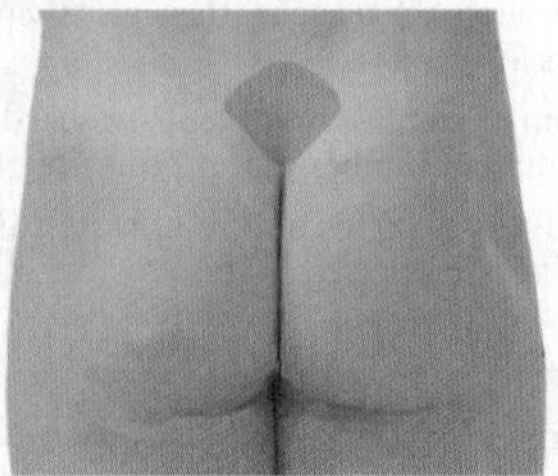

■ Michaelis rhomboid.

rhom•bo•mere (rom′bo-mēr) one of a series of segmental elevations (neuromeres) dividing the developing rhombencephalon.

Rhom•bo•mys (rom′bo-mis) a genus of large rodents of the family Muridae. *R. opi'mus* is the great gerbil, a species that lives in colonies in deserts from the Middle East and Central Asia to northwestern India; it is a common reservoir for *Leishmania major,* which causes cutaneous leishmaniasis.

rhon•chus (rong′kəs) pl. *rhon′chi* [L., from Gr. *rhonchos* a snoring sound] a continuous sound (q.v.) consisting of a dry, low-pitched, snore-like noise, produced in the throat or bronchial tube due to a partial obstruction such as by secretions. Sometimes called *sonorous r.* (q.v.). **rhon′chal, rhon′chial** *adj*

sibilant r. wheeze (def. 1).

sonorous r. a term sometimes used in place of *rhonchus* to distinguish it from a *wheeze* or *sibilant rhonchus.*

whistling r. wheeze (def. 1).

Rho•pa•lo•psyl•lus (ro″pə-lo-sil′əs) a genus of fleas. *R. cavi'cola* is the South American cavy flea, which transmits *Yersinia pestis.*

rhop•try (rōp′tre) [Gr. *rhopalon* club] in apicomplexan protozoa, either of two electron-dense, paired, tubular, saccular, or club-shaped organelles that arise anteriorly, extend toward the posterior end of the body of the organism, and form part of the apical complex. Called also *toxoneme.*

rho•ta•cism (ro′tə-sizm) a speech disorder consisting of imperfect pronunciation of the *r* sound. Called also *pararhotacism.*

rhu•barb (roo′bahrb) 1. any of various members of the genus *Rheum.* 2. the dried rhizome and root of *Rheum officinale,* used as a laxative.

Chinese r. 1. *Rheum palmatum.* 2. a preparation of the dried rhizome of *R. palmatum,* used as a laxative; it is also used for a variety of indications in traditional Chinese medicine and in homeopathy for diarrhea and teething.

r-HuEPO recombinant human erythropoietin; see *epoetin.*

Rhus (rus) [L., gen. *rhois*] the sumacs, a genus of vines, shrubs, and trees of the family Anacardiaceae; most species are native to North America. Some species contain urushiol, a highly allergenic oleoresin mixture, and contact with them produces a severe dermatitis *(rhus dermatitis)* in sensitive persons. Extracts of the leaves and twigs of some species (see *poison ivy extract* and *poison oak extract,* under *extract*) have been used in the prophylaxis and treatment of dermatitis associated with these species. See also *Toxicodendron.*

R. diversilo'ba western poison oak, a species of tree found in western North America that causes rhus dermatitis.

R. quercifo'lia *R. toxicodendron.*

R. ra'dicans poison ivy, a North American species that causes rhus dermatitis; it is usually a climbing vine, but a variant called *Rhus rydbergii* is free-standing. Called also *Toxicodendron radicans.*

R. rydber'gii a variant of *Rhus radicans* that is freestanding, found in the western United States and Canada. Called also *Toxicodendron rydbergii.*

***R. toxica'rium,* R. toxicoden′dron** eastern poison oak, a species found in eastern North America that causes rhus dermatitis. Called also *R. quercifolia, Toxicodendron toxicarium,* and *T. toxicodendron.*

R. ver'nix poison sumac, a North American species that causes rhus dermatitis; called also *Toxicodendron vernix.*

rhus (rus) any member of the genus *Rhus.* See also *rhus dermatitis,* under *dermatitis.*

rhythm (rith′əm) [L. *rhythmus;* Gr. *rhythmos*] a measured movement; the recurrence of an action or function at regular intervals. **rhyth′mic, rhyth′mical** *adj*

accelerated atrioventricular (AV) junctional r. a cardiac rhythm in which increased rhythmicity of the atrioventricular junction causes it to initiate a series of ectopic impulses, usually occurring at a rate of 70 to 130 beats per minute.

accelerated idioventricular r. a rapid ventricular rhythm, approximately 60 to 110 beats per minute; it usually results from premature beats or an escape rhythm generated by slowing of the sinus pacemaker or acceleration of a ventricular pacemaker.

alpha r. a uniform rhythm of waves in the normal electroencephalogram, showing an average frequency of 10 per second; see *alpha waves* under *wave.* Called also *Berger r.* and *alpha activity.*

atrial escape r. a cardiac dysrhythmia occurring when sustained suppression of sinus impulse formation causes other atrial foci to act as cardiac pacemakers.

atrioventricular (AV) junctional r. the heart rhythm that results when the atrioventricular junction acts as pacemaker.

atrioventricular (AV) junctional escape r. a cardiac rhythm of four or more AV junctional escape beats at a rate below 60 beats per minute, the impulses originating in the AV junction due to absence of normal impulse generation by or conduction from the sinus node or atria.

atrioventricular (AV) nodal r. atrioventricular (AV) junctional r.

Berger r. alpha r.
beta r. a rhythm in the electroencephalogram consisting of waves smaller than those of the alpha rhythm, having an average frequency of 25 per second; see *beta waves* under *wave.* Called also *beta activity.*
biologic r. biorhythm.
circadian r. the regular recurrence in cycles of approximately 24 hours from one point to another, such as with certain biological activities that recur regardless of long periods of darkness or other changes in environmental conditions.
circamensual r. recurrence in cycles of about one month (30 days).
circannual r. recurrence of a phenomenon in cycles of about one year.
circaseptan r. regular recurrence in cycles of about seven days (one week).
circus r. circus movement (def. 2).
coupled r. heart beats occurring in pairs, the second beat of the pair usually being a ventricular premature beat; see also *bigeminal pulse* and *bigeminy.*
delta r. rhythm on the electroencephalogram consisting of delta waves. Called also *delta activity.*
ectopic r. a heart rhythm initiated by a focus outside the sinoatrial node.
escape r. a heart rhythm initiated by lower centers when the sinoatrial node fails to initiate impulses, its rhythmicity is depressed, or its impulses are completely blocked.
gallop r. an auscultatory finding of three *(triple r.)* or four *(quadruple r.)* heart sounds; the extra sounds occur in diastole and are related either to atrial contraction (S_4 gallop), to early rapid filling of a ventricle (S_3 gallop), or to concurrence of both events (summation gallop).
gamma r. a rhythm of waves in the electroencephalogram having a frequency of 50 per second.
idioventricular r. a sustained series of impulses propagated by an independent pacemaker within the ventricles, with a rate of 20 to 50 beats per minute. See also *accelerated idioventricular r.*
infradian r. the regular recurrence in cycles of more than 24 hours from one stated point to another, such as certain biologic activities that occur at such intervals, regardless of conditions of illumination.
junctional r. atrioventricular junctional r.
junctional escape r. atrioventricular junctional escape r.
mu r. a pattern of rapid activity sometimes seen on an electroencephalogram over the central regions during wakefulness; waves have rounded electropositive and pointed electronegative components and are of little diagnostic significance.
nodal r. atrioventricular junctional r.
nyctohemeral r. a day and night rhythm.
pendulum r. alternation in the rhythm of the heart sounds in which the diastolic sound is equal in time, character, and loudness to the systolic sound, the beat of the heart resembling the tick of a watch.
quadruple r. the gallop rhythm cadence produced when all four heart sounds, S_1 to S_4, recur in successive cardiac cycles. Cf. *triple r.* and *summation gallop.*
reciprocal r. a cardiac dysrhythmia established by a sustained reentrant mechanism in which impulses traveling back toward the atria through the atrioventricular junction also travel forward to reexcite the ventricles; thus each cycle contains a reciprocal beat, with two ventricular contractions.
reciprocating r. a cardiac dysrhythmia in which an impulse initiated in the atrioventricular node travels both up toward the atria and down toward the ventricles, followed by cycles of bidirectional propagation of the impulse that alternately initiate from the impulses traveling up toward the atria and those traveling down toward the ventricles.
reentrant r. an abnormal cardiac rhythm resulting from a reentry circuit.
sinoatrial r. sinus r.
sinus r. normal heart rhythm originating in the sinoatrial node.
supraventricular r. any cardiac rhythm originating above the ventricles, either normally in the sinoatrial node or abnormally elsewhere in the atria or in the atrioventricular node. Cf. *supraventricular arrhythmia.*
theta r. rhythm on the electroencephalogram consisting of theta waves (q.v.). Called also *theta activity.*
triple r. the gallop rhythm cadence produced when three heart sounds recur in successive cardiac cycles, due to the presence of either a third or a fourth heart sound. Cf. *quadruple r.*
ultradian r. the regular recurrence in cycles of less than 24 hours from one stated point to another, such as certain biologic activities that occur at such intervals, regardless of conditions of illumination.
ventricular escape r. idioventricular r.
ventricular r. 1. idioventricular r. 2. any cardiac rhythm controlled by a focus within the ventricles.

rhyth·mic·i·ty (rith-mis′ĭ-te) 1. the state of being rhythmical. 2. automaticity (def. 2).

rhy·tid (ri′tid) pl. *rhy′tides.* A wrinkle in the skin.

rhyt·i·dec·to·my (rit″ĭ-dek′tə-me) [*rhytid-* + *-ectomy*] plastic surgery to eliminate wrinkles from the facial skin by excising loose or redundant tissue; popularly called *face-lift.* Called also *rhytidoplasty.*

rhytid(o)- [Gr. *rhytis,* gen. *rhytidos* wrinkle] a combining form denoting relationship to wrinkles. Also *rhitid(o)-.*

rhyt·i·do·plas·ty (rit′ĭ-do-plas″te) rhytidectomy. **rhytidoplas′tic** *adj*

rhyt·i·do·sis (rit″ĭ-do′sis) [Gr. *rhytidōsis; rhytis* wrinkle] a wrinkling of the cornea.

RIA radioimmunoassay.

rib (rib) 1. costa (def. 1). 2. something resembling this bone.
abdominal r's, asternal r's costae spuriae.
bicipital r. an anomalous rib resulting from fusion of the anterior part of the seventh cervical vertebra with the first thoracic rib.
cervical r. costa cervicalis.
false r's costae spuriae.
floating r's costae fluitantes.
slipping r. a rib whose attaching cartilage is repeatedly dislocated.
spurious r's costae spuriae.
sternal r's costae verae.
Stiller r. an abnormally movable tenth rib.
true r's costae verae.
vertebral r's costae fluitantes.
vertebrocostal r's the upper three false ribs of either side, articulating with the vertebrae and connected by cartilage to the costal cartilage of the ipsilateral seventh rib.
vertebrosternal r's costae verae.

ri·ba·vi·rin (ri″bə-vi′rin) [USP] a nucleoside analogue resembling guanosine; it is a broad-spectrum antiviral active against a wide variety of DNA and RNA viruses; used in the treatment of severe viral pneumonia caused by respiratory syncytial virus, particularly in high-risk infants with underlying conditions such as cardiopulmonary disease, administered by oral inhalation. It is also used in conjunction with interferon alfa-2b in the treatment of chronic hepatitis C, administered orally.

Rib·bert's theory (rib′ərts) [Moritz Wilhelm Hugo *Ribbert,* German pathologist, 1855–1920] see under *theory.*

rib·bon (rib′ən) a bandlike structure.
r. of Reil the rostral part of the lemniscus medialis.
synaptic r. 1. in the eye, a dense lamella surrounded by a halo of synaptic vesicles, found at a right angle to the apex of the synaptic ridge in the outer plexiform layer of the retina. 2. in the internal ear, a structure similar to that found in the eye, occurring in varying numbers in the cytoplasm of the hair cells.

Ribes ganglion (rēb) [François *Ribes,* French surgeon, 1765–1845] see under *ganglion.*

ri·bi·tol (ri′bĭ-tol) a sugar alcohol formed by reduction of the carbonyl group of ribose; it is a constituent of a class of teichoic acids.

ri·bo·fla·vin (ri′bo-fla″vin) 1. vitamin B_2, a heat-stable, water-soluble flavin comprising a substituted isoalloxazine ring system linked to ribitol. It serves as a component of two coenzymes, FAD and FMN, of flavoproteins, which function as electron carriers in oxidation-reduction processes. It occurs in milk, organ meats, eggs, leafy green vegetables, whole grains and enriched cereals and breads, and various algae, and is an essential nutrient for humans, the requirement being related to body size, metabolic rate, and growth rate. Deficiency of the vitamin is known as ariboflavinosis (q.v.). 2. [USP] an official preparation of riboflavin, used in the treatment and prophylaxis of riboflavin deficiency; administered orally and parenterally.
r. 5′-phosphate flavin mononucleotide.
r. 5′-phosphate sodium [USP] a preparation of the sodium salt of riboflavin 5′-phosphate, administered orally or parenterally in the treatment of dietary riboflavin deficiency.

ri·bo·fla·vin ki·nase (ri″bo-fla′vin ki′nās) [EC 2.7.1.26] an enzyme of the transferase class that catalyzes the phosphorylation of riboflavin to form flavin mononucleotide (FMN), a cofactor for electron transfer reactions.

ri·bo·nu·cle·ase (ri″bo-noo′kle-ās) any nuclease (q.v.) specifically catalyzing the cleavage of phosphate ester linkages in ribonucleic acids; the ribonucleases are grouped as those cleaving internal bonds (endoribonucleases) and those cleaving at termini (exoribonucleases).
r. I pancreatic r.
pancreatic r. [EC 3.1.27.5] an endoribonuclease isolated from the pancreas of ruminants and used extensively in studies of enzyme mechanics and in molecular biology research; it catalyzes cleavage specifically of terminal pyrimidine nucleoside 3′-phosphate residues. Called also *r. I, RNase, RNase I,* and *RNase A.*

ri·bo·nu·cle·ic ac·id (RNA) (ri″bo-noo-kle′ik) the nucleic acid in which the sugar is ribose, constituting the genetic material in the RNA viruses and playing a role in the flow of genetic information in all cells. Ribosyl moieties are linked via phosphate groups attached to their 5′ and 3′ hydroxyl groups to form the backbone of a linear polymer, with purine and pyrimidine bases attached to the sugars as side chains. The characteristic bases adenine (A), uracil (U), cytosine (C), and guanine (G) are specified by the presence of thymine (T), A, G, and C, respectively, in the gene being transcribed. Many RNA molecules contain bases modified by posttranscriptional processing (methylation, deamination, isomerization), and although mainly single-stranded, some contain regions of secondary structure such as base pairing between self-complementary sequences, which stabilizes specific conformations. In most viruses with an RNA genome, the RNA is single-stranded, but several families have a double-stranded RNA genome. For specific types of RNA, see under *RNA.*

ri·bo·nu·cleo·pro·tein (RNP) (ri″bo-noo″kle-o-pro′tēn) a complex of protein and ribonucleic acid.

heterogeneous nuclear r. (hnRNP) a complex of what has historically been called heterogeneous nuclear RNA (hnRNA), but is predominantly pre-mRNA, and approximately 30 different proteins, the proteins being called *hnRNP proteins* (q.v.).

small nuclear r. (snRNP) any of a group of ribonucleoproteins, each composed of a small nuclear RNA (snRNA) associated with approximately 10 to 20 polypeptides; five snRNP's form key components of the spliceosome, being thus involved in processing of pre-mRNA's.

small nucleolar r. any of a group of ribonucleoproteins, each composed of a small nucleolar RNA (snoRNA) and specific proteins; see *small nucleolar RNA,* under *RNA.*

ri·bo·nu·cleo·side (ri″bo-noo′kle-o-sīd) a nucleoside in which the purine or pyrimidine base is combined with ribose.

ri·bo·nu·cleo·side di·phos·phate re·duc·tase (ri″bo-noo′kle-o-sīd″ di-fos′fāt re-duk′tās) [EC 1.17.4.1] an enzyme of the oxidoreductase class that catalyzes the formation of 2′-deoxyribonucleotides from the corresponding ribonucleoside diphosphates using NADPH as the ultimate electron donor. The deoxyribonucleoside diphosphates are used in DNA synthesis. Called also *ribonucleotide reductase.*

ri·bo·nu·cleo·tide (ri″bo-noo′kle-o-tīd) a nucleotide in which the purine or pyrimidine base is combined with ribose.

ri·bo·nu·cleo·tide re·duc·tase (ri″bo-noo′kle-o-tīd″ re-duk′tās) ribonucleoside diphosphate reductase.

ri·bo·pho·rin (ri′bo-for″in) either of two abundant transmembrane glycoproteins (designated I and II) of the rough endoplasmic reticulum that bind to the large subunits of ribosomes during translocation; they are also subunits of oligosaccharyltransferase, anchoring a third subunit that carries out the transfer reaction in *N-linked glycosylation.*

ri·bo·py·ra·nose (ri″bo-pir′ə-nōs) ribose occurring in the cyclic pyranose configuration; it is the usual form in solution although not in ribonucleic acids.

ri·bose (ri′bōs) an aldopentose found in riboflavin and ribonucleic acid (RNA) as well as in free ribonucleosides and ribonucleotides.

r. 5-phosphate a phosphorylated form of ribose occurring as an intermediate in the pentose phosphate pathway and in the synthesis of nucleotides.

ri·bose-5-phos·phate isom·er·ase (ri′bōs fos′fāt i-som′ər-ās) [EC 5.3.1.6] an enzyme of the isomerase class that catalyzes the interconversion of ribulose 5-phosphate and ribose 5-phosphate. The reaction is part of the pentose phosphate pathway and is important in ribose metabolism.

ri·bose-phos·phate py·ro·phos·pho·ki·nase (ri′bōs fos′fāt pi″ro-fos″fo-ki′nās) [EC 2.7.6.1] an enzyme of the transferase class that catalyzes the phosphorylation of ribose 5-phosphate to form 5-phosphoribosyl-1-pyrophosphate, the initial reactant in purine and pyrimidine nucleotide biosynthesis. Enhanced enzyme activity, an X-linked recessive trait, leads to increased purine synthesis and causes primary gout. Called also *phosphoribosylpyrophosphate synthetase.* In official nomenclature, the preferred name is now *ribose-phosphate diphosphokinase.*

ri·bo·some (ri′bo-sōm) [*ribo*nucleic acid + *-some*] a large molecular structure, approximately 12 nm wide and 25 nm long, having two dissociable subunits, that is the site of protein synthesis (see *translation*). Ribosomes found in the cytosol of eukaryotes have a sedimentation coefficient of 80S; the subunits have coefficients of 60S and 40S and together contain four different ribosomal RNA (rRNA) chains and about 80 different proteins. Ribosomes found in prokaryotes and mitochondria are smaller (70S, with 50S and 30S subunits containing a total of three rRNAs and 55 proteins) and also differ from eukaryotic ribosomes in their sensitivity to certain antibiotics. **riboso′mal** *adj*

ri·bo·syl (ri′bo-səl) a glycosyl radical formed from ribose by removal of the anomeric hydroxyl group.

5-ri·bo·syl·ura·cil (ri″bo-səl-ūr′ĭ-sil) pseudouridine.

Ri·bot's law (re-bōz′) [T. *Ribot,* French neurologist, 19th century] see under *law.*

ri·bo·thy·mi·dine (ri″bo-thi′mĭ-dēn) the ribosyl analogue of thymidine, a rare base found in small amounts in transfer RNA.

ri·bo·vi·rus (ri′bo-vi″rəs) RNA virus.

ri·bo·zyme (ri′bo-zīm″) [*ribo*nucleic acid + *-zyme*] an RNA molecule with catalytic activity; different classes exist, and the reactions they catalyze may be intramolecular, e.g., self-splicing, or intermolecular, e.g., maturation of tRNA molecules. Secondary and tertiary structure is important to activity.

ri·bu·lose (ri′bu-lōs) a ketopentose isomeric with ribose and occurring in phosphorylated form *(ribose 5-phosphate)* as an intermediate in the pentose phosphate pathway.

ri·bu·lose-phos·phate 3-epim·er·ase (ri′bu-lōs fos′fāt ə-pim′ər-ās) [EC 5.1.3.1] an enzyme of the isomerase class that catalyzes the interconversion of ribulose 5-phosphate and xylulose 5-phosphate. The reaction is a part of the pentose phosphate pathway.

RIC Royal Institute of Chemistry.

rice (rīs) 1. *Oryza sativa.* 2. the seed or grain of *O. sativa,* which consists mainly of starch and is used as a food and a dusting powder.

r. polishings the pericarp and germ layers of rice; they are a rich source of thiamine but are removed in the production of white rice.

Ri·chards-Run·dle syndrome (rich′ərdz run′dəl) [B.W. *Richards,* British physician, 20th century; A.T. *Rundle,* British physician, 20th century] see under *syndrome.*

Ri·chet aneurysm (re-sha′) [Didier Dominique Alfred *Richet,* French surgeon, 1816–1891] see *fusiform aneurysm,* under *aneurysm.*

Rich·ner-Han·hart syndrome (rik′nər hahn′hahrt) [Hermann *Richner,* Swiss physician, 20th century; Ernst *Hanhart,* Swiss physician, 1891–1973] type II tyrosinemia.

Rich·ter hernia (rik′tər) [August Gottlieb *Richter,* German surgeon, 1742–1812] see under *hernia.*

Rich·ter syndrome (rik′tər) [Maurice Nathaniel *Richter,* American pathologist, 20th century] see under *syndrome.*

Rich·ter-Mon·ro line (rik′tər mən-ro′) [A.G. *Richter;* Alexander *Monro* (Secundus), Scottish anatomist and surgeon, 1733–1817] Monro-Richter line.

ri·cin (ri′sin) a phytotoxin found in the seeds of the castor oil plant *(Ricinus communis),* used in synthesis of immunotoxins; ingestion causes ricin poisoning.

ri·cin·ism (ri′sĭ-niz-əm) ricin poisoning.

ri·cin·ole·ic ac·id (ri″sin-o-le′ik) 1. an unsaturated 18-carbon fatty acid constituting 80 per cent of the fatty acid content of castor oil. 2. a mixture of fatty acids obtained by hydrolysis of castor oil and used intravaginally to restore or maintain normal vaginal acidity.

Ric·i·nus (ris′ĭ-nəs) [L.] a genus of plants of the family Euphorbiaceae. *R. commu′nis* is the castor bean or castor oil plant, which yields castor oil but whose seed (the castor bean) contains the phytotoxin ricin and causes ricin poisoning.

rick·ets (rik′əts) [thought to be a corruption of Gr. *rhachitis* a spinal complaint] an interruption in the development and mineralization of the growth plate of bone, with radiographic abnormalities, osteomalacia, bone pain, fatigability, growth retardation, and often hypotonia, convulsions, and tetany. Biochemical abnormalities include hypocalcemia, elevated serum alkaline phosphatase, hypophosphatemia, and decreased intestinal absorption of calcium and phosphorus. It is caused by a variety of defects in vitamin D, calcium, and phosphorus homeostasis, including dietary deficiencies or malabsorption, primary disorders of bone matrix, and acquired or inherited metabolic and hormonal abnormalities. See also *osteomalacia.*

adult r. osteomalacia.

anticonvulsant r. rickets occurring in children receiving long-term anticonvulsant therapy; the drugs induce vitamin D deficiency (frequently compounded by dietary insufficiency of the vitamin) and hypocalcemia, hypophosphatemia, and secondary hyperparathyroidism by increasing the rate of conversion of the vitamin to inactive metabolites.

autosomal dominant hypophosphatemic r. (ADHR), autosomal dominant vitamin D–resistant r. a form of familial hypophosphatemic rickets with autosomal dominant inheritance and caused by mutation in the *FGF23* gene (locus: 12p13.3), which encodes a member of the fibroblast growth factor family. Clinically it is similar to X-linked hypophosphatemia but shows incomplete penetrance and variable age at onset.

familial hypophosphatemic r. any of several inherited disorders of proximal renal tubular function causing phosphate loss, hypophosphatemia, and skeletal deformities, including rickets and osteomalacia. The group is genetically heterogeneous and clinically variable. See *X-linked*

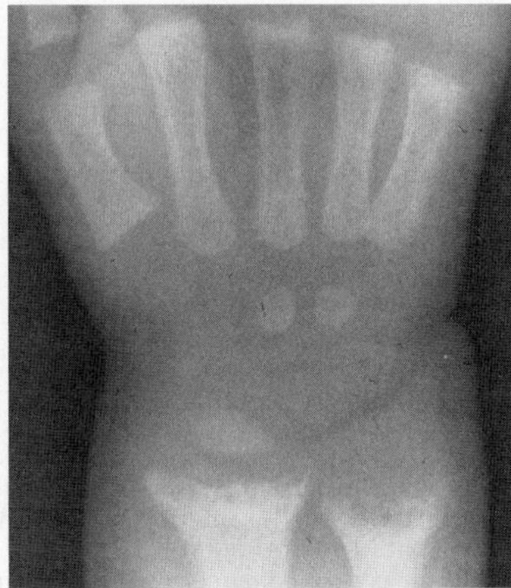

■ Rickets, with characteristic cupping and fraying of the metaphyseal ends of the radius and ulna.

hypophosphatemia, autosomal dominant hypophosphatemic r., and *hereditary hypophosphatemic r. with hypercalciuria*.

fetal r. achondroplasia.

hepatic r. rickets associated with hepatic disease, believed to result from inadequate absorption of vitamin D.

hereditary hypophosphatemic r. with hypercalciuria a form of familial hypophosphatemic rickets caused by mutation in the *SLC34A3* gene (locus: 9q34), which encodes a cotransporter important in maintenance of inorganic phosphate concentration at the kidney; hypophosphatemia is accompanied by elevated levels of serum 1,25-dihydroxyvitamin D, increased intestinal absorption of calcium and phosphate, and hypercalciuria.

hypophosphatemic r. any of a group of disorders characterized by rickets associated with hypophosphatemia, resulting from dietary phosphorus deficiency *(antacid-induced osteomalacia)* or due to defects in renal tubular function that may be either hereditary *(familial hypophosphatemic rickets)* or acquired. While skeletal deformities such as genu varum and short stature are present, neither hypocalcemia, myopathy, nor tetany occur, and serum parathyroid hormone is normal.

oncogenous r. oncogenous osteomalacia occurring in children.

pseudodeficiency r. vitamin D–dependent r. type I and type II.

pseudovitamin D–deficiency r. vitamin D–dependent r., type I; the term is sometimes used to denote types I and II collectively.

refractory r. vitamin D–resistant r.

renal r. rickets occurring in children and secondary to renal dysfunction asociated with hyperphosphatemia; the term is also used more loosely as a synonym of *renal osteodystrophy*.

scurvy r. rachitic changes in the skeleton associated with infantile scurvy.

vitamin D–dependent r., type I an autosomal recessive disorder characterized by rickets with myopathy, hypocalcemia, moderate hypophosphatemia, secondary hyperparathyroidism, and subnormal serum concentrations of 1,25-dihydroxyvitamin D. The disorder can be overcome by high doses of vitamin D or physiologic doses of calcitriol and is caused by any of several enzyme defects in the pathway by which vitamin D is converted to its active form 1,25-dihydroxyvitamin D.

vitamin D–dependent r., type II an autosomal recessive disorder similar to type I but with elevated serum concentrations of 1,25-dihydroxyvitamin D. The disorder cannot be overcome by high levels of vitamin D or its metabolites and is caused by end organ refractoriness to the active metabolite, owing to defective receptor binding, absence of the receptors, or post-receptor defects. Multiple variants exist, subdivided as those with or without alopecia.

vitamin D–refractory r. vitamin D–resistant r.

vitamin D–resistant r. 1. X-linked hypophosphatemia. 2. any of a group of disorders characterized by rickets but not responding to high doses of vitamin D; most are forms of familial hypophosphatemic rickets.

X-linked hypophosphatemic r. X-linked hypophosphatemia.

rick•ett•se•mia (rik″ət-se′me-ə) the presence of rickettsiae in the blood.

Rick•ett•sia (rĭ-ket′se-ə) [Howard Taylor *Ricketts*, American pathologist, 1871–1910] a genus of bacteria of the family Rickettsiaceae, made up of small rod-shaped to coccoid, often pleomorphic microorganisms. The cells have typical cell walls, possess no flagella, are gram-negative, and multiply only inside host cells. They occur in the cytoplasm of cells or free in the lumen of the gut in lice, fleas, ticks, and mites, by which they are transmitted to mammals. Various species contain organisms that cause typhus fevers and spotted fevers. The type species is *R. prowaze′kii*.

R. aeschliman′nii a rare species found in Morocco that causes rash and sloughing of the skin.

R. afri′cae a species seen in southern Africa, spread by the ticks *Amblyomma hebraeum* and *A. variegatum*, the cause of African tick-bite fever.

R. a′kari the etiologic agent of rickettsialpox, transmitted by the mite *Liponyssoides sanguineus* from the reservoir of infection in house mice.

R. austra′lis the etiologic agent of Queensland tick typhus, transmitted from infected marsupials by ixodid ticks.

R. cono′rii the etiologic agent of boutonneuse fever, transmitted by the bites of various species of ixodid ticks, including those of the genera *Amblyomma, Haemaphysalis, Hyalomma*, and *Rhipicephalus*. The principal animal reservoirs are dogs and rodents.

R. fe′lis the etiologic agent of cat flea typhus, transmitted by the cat flea *(Ctenocephalides felis)* and having the opossum as reservoir.

R. heilongjiangen′sis a species seen in China that causes a macular rash with sloughing of the skin.

R. ho′nei the etiologic agent of Flinders Island spotted fever, transmitted by the reptile tick *Aponomma hydrosauri*.

R. japo′nica the etiologic agent of Japanese spotted fever, transmitted by ixodid ticks.

R. par′keri a species found in the southern United States, spread by the tick *Amblyomma maculatum;* it causes mild rickettsiosis in domestic animals and may occasionally infect humans.

R. prowaze′kii the etiologic agent of epidemic typhus and the recrudescent infection Brill-Zinsser disease. The organisms are transmitted between humans via the louse *Pediculus humanus* var. *corporis* and from flying squirrels to humans by fleas and lice.

R. quinta′na *Bartonella quintana*.

R. rickett′sii the usual etiologic agent of Rocky Mountain spotted fever, transmitted by ticks of the genera *Dermacentor, Rhipicephalus, Haemaphysalis, Amblyomma* and *Ixodes*, which have their natural reservoirs in rodents, dogs, and foxes.

R. sennet′su *Neorickettsia sennetsu*.

R. sibi′rica the etiologic agent of North Asian or Siberian tick typhus, which is transmitted from infected rodents by ticks of the genera *Dermacentor* and *Haemaphysalis*.

R. slova′ca a species first isolated in Slovakia that causes fever, a macular rash, and sloughing of the skin.

R. tsutsugamu′shi *Orientia tsutsugamushi*.

R. ty′phi the etiologic agent of murine typhus, transmitted from infected rats to humans chiefly by rat fleas. Called also *R. typhi (mooseri)*.

R. ty′phi (moo′seri) *R. typhi*.

rick•ett•sia (rĭ-ket′se-ə) pl. *rickett′siae*. Any scotobacterium of the order Rickettsiales.

Rick•ett•si•a•ceae (rĭ-ket″se-a′se-e) a family of bacteria of the order Rickettsiales, made up of small rod-shaped, ellipsoidal, coccoid, or diplococcus-shaped, obligately intracellular, often pleomorphic microorganisms occurring in arthropods, by which they are transmitted to vertebrates, causing disease. Medically important organisms are contained in the genera *Rickettsia* and *Orientia*.

rick•ett•siae (rĭ-ket′se-e) plural of *rickettsia*.

rick•ett•si•al (rĭ-ket′se-əl) caused by rickettsiae.

Rick•ett•si•a•les (rĭ-ket″se-a′lēz) an order of bacteria of the class Alphaproteobacteria, phylum Proteobacteria, comprising small, gram-negative, nonflagellated, rod-shaped or coccoid, often pleomorphic microorganisms that multiply only inside the cells of the host. Bacteria are found as parasites in arthropods (which may serve as vectors), helminths, and vertebrates; some species are pathogenic. The order includes the families Anaplasmataceae and Rickettsiaceae.

rick•ett•si•al•pox (rĭ-ket′se-əl-poks″) a mild self-limited febrile disease caused by *Rickettsia akari*, transmitted to humans by the mite *Liponyssoides sanguineus*, an ectoparasite of the house mouse. Characteristics include an escharlike primary cutaneous lesion, generalized papulovesicular rash, headache, and backache. Called also *Kew Gardens spotted fever*.

rick•ett•si•ci•dal (rĭ-ket″sĭ-si′dəl) lethal to rickettsiae; cf. antirickettsial.

rick•ett•si•o•sis (rĭ-ket″se-o′sis) infection with rickettsiae.

canine r. see under *ehrlichiosis*.

rick•ett•sio•stat•ic (rĭ-ket″se-o-stat′ik) inhibiting growth of rickettsiae; cf. antirickettsial.

ric•tal (rik′təl) pertaining to a fissure.

ric•tus (rik′təs) [L.] 1. a fissure or cleft. 2. a gaping, as of the mouth.

RID radial immunodiffusion.

Rid•au•ra (rid-aw′rə) trademark for a preparation of auranofin.

Rid•doch mass reflex (rid′ok) [George *Riddoch*, British neurologist, 1888–1947] see under *reflex*.

Rid•e•al-Walk•er coefficient, method (test) (rid′e-əl wawk′ər) [Samuel *Rideal*, English chemist, 1863–1929; J.T. Ainslie *Walker*, English chemist, 1868–1930] see *phenol coefficient*, under *coefficient*, and see under *method*.

ridge (rij) a projection or projecting structure; see also *carina*, *crest*, and *crista*.

alveolar r. the bony ridge of the maxilla or mandible, which contains the alveoli.

alveolar r., residual the bony ridge remaining after disappearance of the alveoli from the alveolar process following removal or loss of the teeth. Called also *edentulous r.* and *residual r.*

basal r. cingulum (def. 3).

bicipital r., anterior crista tuberculi minoris.

bicipital r., external crista tuberculi majoris.

bicipital r., internal crista tuberculi minoris.

bicipital r., outer, bicipital r., posterior crista tuberculi majoris.

buccocervical r., buccogingival r. a ridge or prominence on the buccal surface above the cementoenamel junction of posterior teeth.

bulbar r's spiral endocardial thickenings in the bulbus cordis that fuse to form the aorticopulmonary septum, separating the bulbus cordis into aortic and pulmonary trunks.

cerebral r's of cranial bones variable ridges on the inner surface of the cranium, corresponding to the sulci of the brain.

deltoid r. tuberositas deltoidea.

dental r. any linear elevation on the crown of a tooth named according to the surface or cusp on which it is located or in recognition of some other characteristic.

dermal r's cristae cutis.

edentulous r. alveolar r., residual.

epipericardial r. a ventral ridge separating the ventral ends of the pharyngeal (branchial) arches in the embryo from the pericardial swelling.

fingerprint r's cristae cutis.

gastrocnemial r. a ridge on the posterior surface of the femur, giving attachment to the gastrocnemius muscle.

genital r. gonadal r.

gluteal r. tuberositas glutea.

gonadal r. an elevation of thickened mesothelium and underlying mesenchyme on the ventromedial border of the embryonic mesonephros; the primordial germ cells become embedded in it, establishing it as the primordium of the ovary or testis. Called also *genital r.* or *fold*.

healing r. an indurated ridge that normally forms deep to the skin along the length of a healing wound and extends about 1 cm on each side of the wound.

incisal r. the part of the crown of an anterior tooth that makes up the actual incisal portion; see *incisal surface*, under *surface*.

intertrochanteric r. crista intertrochanterica.

interureteric r. plica interureterica.

linguocervical r., linguogingival r. cingulum (def. 3).

longitudinal r. of hard palate the part of the palatine raphe that is on the hard palate.

mammary r. a ridge of thickened epithelium from axilla to groin on each side in the mammalian embryo, along which nipples and mammary glands develop, all but one pair usually disappearing in the human. Called also *mammary crest* and *mammary* or *milk line*.

r. of mandibular neck a blunt, smooth ridge passing obliquely downward and forward from the mandibular condyle on the medial surface of the mandibular neck and ramus, serving as their buttress.

marginal r. crista marginalis.

mesonephric r. the more lateral portion of the urogenital ridge, which gives rise to the mesonephros.

middle r. of femur linea pectinea.

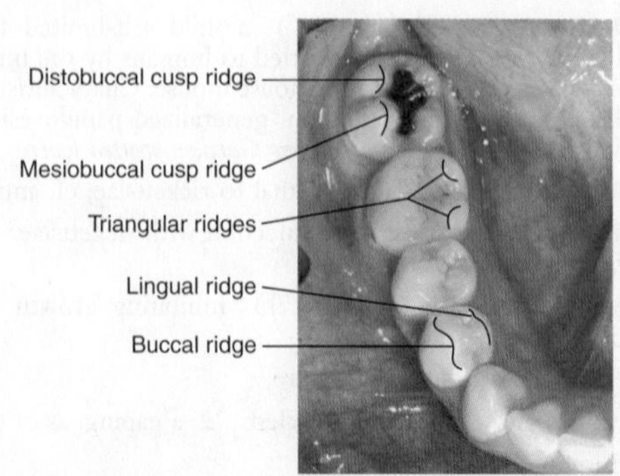

■ Dental ridges, in a superior view of the mandible.

milk r. mammary r.

mylohyoid r. linea mylohyoidea mandibulae.

r. of neck of rib crista colli costae.

r. of nose agger nasi.

oblique r. crista obliqua.

oblique r's of scapula lineae musculares scapulae.

palatine r's, transverse plicae palatinae transversae.

palatopharyngeal r., Passavant r. crista palatopharyngea.

pectoral r. crista tuberculi majoris.

pharyngeal r. crista palatopharyngea.

pterygoid r. crista infratemporalis.

residual r. alveolar r., residual.

rete r's the inward projections of the epidermis into the dermis at the dermal-epidermal junction, as seen histologically in vertical sections. Called also *rete pegs*.

rough r. of femur linea aspera.

semicircular r. of parietal bone, inferior linea temporalis inferior ossis parietalis.

semicircular r. of parietal bone, superior linea temporalis superior ossis parietalis.

skin r's cristae cutis.

sphenoid r. crista sphenoidalis.

sublingual r. frenulum linguae.

superciliary r. arcus superciliaris.

supinator r. crista musculi supinatoris.

supplemental r. an abnormal ridge on the surface of a tooth.

supracondylar r. of humerus, lateral crista supraepicondylaris lateralis humeri.

supracondylar r. of humerus, medial crista supraepicondylaris medialis humeri.

supraepicondylar r. of humerus, lateral crista supraepicondylaris lateralis humeri.

supraepicondylar r. of humerus, medial crista supraepicondylaris medialis humeri.

supraorbital r. arcus superciliaris.

suprarenal r. a caudal projection of the dorsal portion of the pleuroperitoneal membrane of the embryo, in which the adrenal cortex develops.

supravalvular r. of aorta crista supravalvularis aortae.

supravalvular r. of pulmonary trunk crista supravalvularis trunci pulmonalis.

synaptic r. a wedge-shaped projection in the retina of a cone pedicle or of a rod spherule, on either side of which lie the horizontal cells whose dendrites are inserted into the ridge.

taste r's papillae foliatae.

tentorial r. a ridge on the inner surface of the cranium just superior to the groove for the transverse sinus, to which the tentorium is attached.

transverse r. crista transversalis.

transverse r's of sacrum lineae transversae ossis sacri.

transverse r's of vaginal wall rugae vaginales.

trapezoid r. linea trapezoidea.

triangular r. crista triangularis.

urethral r. carina urethralis vaginae.

urogenital r. a longitudinal ridge or fold in the embryo, lateral to the root of the dorsal mesentery, which later subdivides longitudinally into the mesonephric and gonadal ridges.

wolffian r. mesonephric r.

rid•gel (rid′jəl) ridgling.

ridg•ing (rij′ing) in plastic surgery, a visible line or ridge at the margin of an area that has been surgically planed; occasionally encountered when beveling at the junction of treated and untreated areas has not been performed.

ridg•ling (rij′ling) an animal, especially a horse, with one or both testes undescended.

Rid•ley sinus (rid′le) [Humphrey *Ridley*, English anatomist, 1653–1708] sinus circularis.

Rie•chert-Mun•din•ger apparatus, technique (re′kərt moon′ding-ər) [T. *Riechert*, German neurosurgeon, 20th century; F. *Mundinger*, German neurosurgeon, born 1924] see under *apparatus* and *technique*.

Rie•del lobe, thyroiditis (disease, struma) (re′del) [Bernhard Moritz Carl Ludwig *Riedel*, German surgeon, 1846–1916] see under *lobe* and *thyroiditis*.

Rie•der cell leukemia, lymphocyte (cell) (re′dər) [Hermann *Rieder*, German roentgenologist, 1858–1932] see under *leukemia* and *lymphocyte*.

Rie•gel pulse (re′gəl) [Franz *Riegel*, German physician, 1843–1904] see under *pulse*.

Rie•ger anomaly, syndrome (re′gər) [Herwigh *Rieger*, German ophthalmologist, 1898–1986] see under *anomaly* and *syndrome*.

Riehl melanosis (rēl) [Gustav *Riehl*, Austrian dermatologist, 1855–1943] see under *melanosis*.

Rie•me•rel•la (re″mər-el′ə) a genus of gram-negative bacteria of the family Flavobacteriaceae, consisting of aerobic, nonmotile, non-spore-forming rods occurring in pairs or short chains; organisms are oxidase- and catalase-positive. The type species is *R. anatipes′tifer*.

R. anatipes′tifer a species that causes infectious avian serositis. Formerly called *Moraxella anatipestifer* and *Pasteurella anatipestifer*.

Ries•man sign (rēs′mən) [David *Riesman*, American physician, 1867–1940] see under *sign*.

RIF resistance-inducing factor; right iliac fossa; rifampin.

rif•a•bu•tin (rif″ə-bu′tin) [USP] an antibacterial derived from rifamycin S, used for the prevention of disseminated *Mycobacterium avium* complex (MAC) disease in patients with advanced human immunodeficiency virus infection; administered orally.

Rif•a•din (rif′ə-din) trademark for preparations of rifampin.

Rif•a•mate (rif′ə-māt) trademark for a combination preparation of rifampin and isoniazid.

rif•am•pi•cin (rif′am-pĭ-sin) INN for *rifampin*.

rif•am•pin (RIF) (rif-am′pin) [USP] a semisynthetic derivative of rifamycin SV, having the antibacterial actions and uses of the rifamycin (q.v.) group of antibiotics; administered orally or intravenously. Called also *rifampicin*.

rif•a•my•cin (rif″ə-mi′sin) any of a family of antibiotics biosynthesized by a strain of *Amycolatopsis rifamycinica*, effective against a broad spectrum of bacteria, including gram-positive cocci, some gram-negative bacilli, and *Mycobacterium tuberculosis* and certain other mycobacteria. The five components are designated A, B, C, D, and E; rifamycins O, S, and SV are derivatives of the B component, and AG and X are derivatives of the O component. In the United States the rifamycins are used only for the initial treatment and retreatment of pulmonary tuberculosis and for prophylaxis of meningococcal infections in close contacts of patients with *Neisseria meningitidis* infection; they have been used in other countries to treat various infectious diseases due to susceptible organisms, such as leprosy, gonorrhea, and biliary tract and respiratory infections.

rif•a•pen•tine (rif″ə-pen′tēn) a synthetic rifamycin antibiotic used in conjunction with other antituberculosis medications in the treatment of pulmonary tuberculosis; administered orally.

Rif•a•ter (rif′ə-tər) trademark for a combination preparation of rifampin, isoniazid, and pyrazinamide.

rif•ax•i•min (rif-ak′sĭ-min) a semisynthetic antibacterial compound, derived from rifamycin, that inhibits bacterial RNA synthesis, used for the treatment of traveler's diarrhea caused by noninvasive strains of *Escherichia coli;* administered orally.

Rift Val•ley fever (rift′ val′e) [*Rift Valley*, Kenya, where it was first described in 1931] see under *fever*.

Riga-Fede disease (re′gah fa′da) [Antonio *Riga*, Italian physician, 1832–1919; Francesco *Fede*, Italian pediatrician, 1832–1913] see under *disease*.

Riggs disease (rigz) [John Mankey *Riggs*, American dentist, 1810–1885] marginal periodontitis.

right-hand•ed (rīt han′dəd) using the right hand preferentially, or more skillfully than the left, in voluntary motor acts. See also *handedness* and *laterality*.

ri•gid•i•ty (rĭ-jid′ĭ-te) [L. *rigiditas; rigidus* stiff] stiffness or inflexibility, chiefly that which is abnormal or morbid; called also *rigor*.

cadaveric r. rigor mortis.

catatonic r. maintenance of a rigid posture in spite of attempts to be moved, characteristic of catatonic schizophrenia.

clasp-knife r. an exaggerated stretch reflex of skeletal muscles seen in spasticity and decerebrate rigidity, resembling the opening of a penknife or clasp knife; there is increased resistance to the extensors (induced by passive flexion of a joint), which suddenly gives way on exertion of further pressure. Called also *clasp-knife effect, phenomenon, reflex*, or *spasticity*.

cogwheel r. rigidity of a muscle that gives way in a series of little jerks upon being passively stretched, analogous to the ratcheting movement when a spring-loaded rod drops into the successive notches of a cog. Called also *cogwheel phenomenon* or *sign* and *Negro phenomenon* or *sign*.

congenital articular r. rigid or deformed joints in newborn calves or lambs; a hereditary variety is seen among Charolais cattle, and a type acquired in utero is part of the Akabane virus disease. Called also *congenital arthrogryposis*.

decerebrate r. an abnormal body posture produced by decerebration. In experimental animals it is marked by rigid extension of the lower limbs (hindlimbs in a quadruped). In humans it is manifested by the person lying in rigid extension with the upper limbs internally rotated at the shoulders and pronated; elbows, knees, and hips rigidly extended; and fingers, ankles, and toes flexed. Called also *decerebrate* or *extensor posturing*.

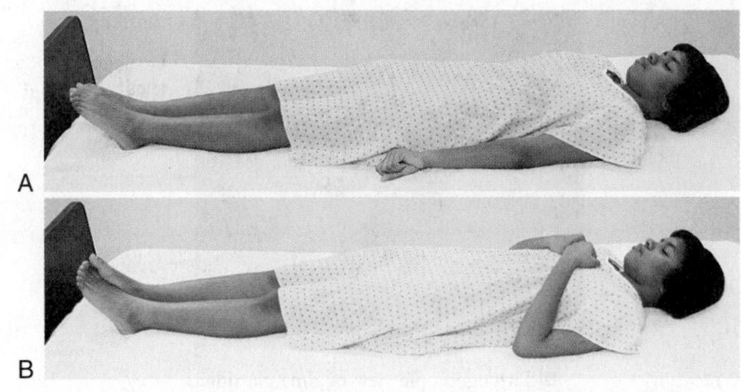

■ *(A)*, Decerebrate rigidity; *(B)*, decorticate rigidity.

decorticate r. an abnormal body posture indicative of a lesion in the cerebral hemispheres or disruption of the corticospinal tracts; the patient has bilateral adduction of the shoulders, pronation and flexion of the elbows and wrists, and extension, internal rotation, and plantar flexion of the lower limbs. Called also *decorticate* or *flexor posturing*.

hemiplegic r. rigidity of the paralyzed limbs in hemiplegia.

lead pipe r. diffuse muscular rigidity resembling the resistance to bending of a thin-walled metal pipe; seen in parkinsonism.

mydriatic r. orbicularis pupillary reflex.

nuchal r. stiffness of or inability to move the neck, often a sign of some underlying condition such as cerebral hemorrhage, a tumor in the area, or bacterial meningitis.

paratonic r. an intermittent abnormal increase in resistance to passive movement in a comatose patient.

postmortem r. rigor mortis.

rig•or (rig′or, ri′gor) [L.] 1. a chill. 2. rigidity.

acid r. coagulation of the protein of muscle produced by acids.

calcium r. arrest of cardiac muscle in full contraction, caused by an excess of calcium.

heat r. rigidity of muscles induced by heat.

r. mor′tis the stiffening of a dead body, accompanying the depletion of adenosine triphosphate in the muscle fibers.

water r. a condition of rigor in a muscle caused by immersing it in water.

Ri•ley-Day syndrome (ri′le da′) [Conrad Milton *Riley*, American pediatrician, 1913–2005; Richard Lawrence *Day*, American pediatrician, 1905–1989] dysautonomia.

Ri•ley-Smith syndrome (ri′le smith′) [Harris Dewitt *Riley*, Jr., American pediatrician, born 1925; William Robert *Smith*, American physician, born 1931] see under *syndrome*.

Ril•u•tek (ril′u-tək) trademark for a preparation of riluzole.

ril•u•zole (ril′u-zōl) a compound used in the treatment of amyotrophic lateral sclerosis; it prolongs survival time but does not improve muscular strength or neurologic function.

rim (rim) a border or edge.

acetabular r. limbus acetabuli.

bite r. occlusion r.

occlusion r., record r. a border constructed on temporary or permanent denture bases for the purpose of recording the maxillomandibular relation and for positioning the teeth. Called also *bite-block, bitelock*, and *bite r.*

ri•ma (ri′mə) gen. and pl. *ri′mae* [L.] a cleft, crack, or similar opening. **ri′mal** *adj*

r. a′ni crena analis.

r. glot′tidis [TA] fissure of glottis: the elongated opening between the true vocal cords and between the arytenoid cartilages. It consists of an intercartilaginous part and an intermembranous part; see *pars intercartilaginea rimae glottidis* and *pars intermembranacea rimae glottidis*.

intercartilaginous r. pars intercartilaginea rimae glottidis.

intermembranous r. pars intermembranacea rimae glottidis.

r. o′ris [TA] oral fissure: the longitudinal opening of the mouth, between the lips.

r. palpebra′rum [TA] palpebral fissure: the longitudinal opening between the eyelids.

r. puden′di [TA] pudendal cleft: the cleft between the labia majora in which the urethra and vagina open.

r. vesti′buli [TA] fissure of vestibule: the space between the right and left vestibular folds of the larynx.

Rim•ac•tane (rim-ak′tān) trademark for a preparation of rifampin.

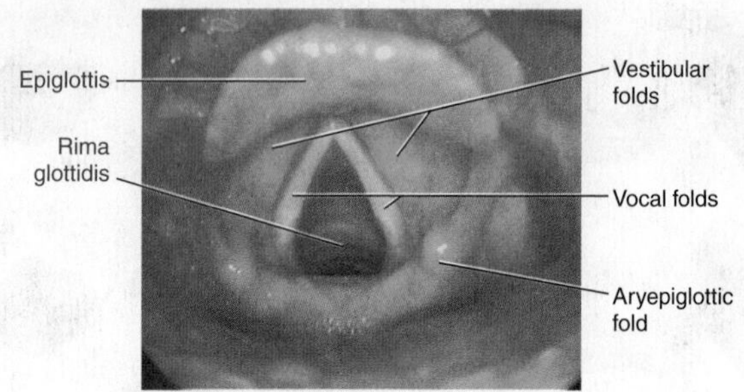

■ Laryngoscopic view of rima glottidis.

ri•mae (ri′me) [L.] genitive and plural of *rima.*

ri•man•ta•dine hy•dro•chlo•ride (ri-man′tə-dēn) [USP] an antiviral agent of the adamantane group, used in treatment and prophylaxis of influenza A.

ri•mex•o•lone (rĭ-mek′sə-lōn″) [USP] a corticosteroid used as a topical antiinflammatory in the treatment of inflammation following eye surgery and of anterior uveitis.

Rim•i•fon (rim′ĭ-fon) trademark for a preparation of isoniazid.

rim•i•ter•ol hy•dro•bro•mide (rim″ĭ-ter′ōl) an adrenergic used as a bronchodilator.

rim•ose (rim′ōs) [L. *rima* crack] marked by cracks and fissures.

Rim•so-50 (rim′so) trademark for a preparation of dimethyl sulfoxide.

rim•u•la (rim′u-lə) pl. *ri′mulae* [L.] a minute fissure, especially of the spinal cord or brain.

RIND reversible ischemic neurologic deficit.

rin•der•pest (rin′dər-pest) [Ger. *Rinder* cattle + *pest* plague] a disease of cattle, which sometimes affects sheep and swine and is caused by a paramyxovirus; symptoms are fever and croupous, ulcerative diphtheritic lesions of the gastrointestinal tract. Called also *cattle plague.*

Rind•fleisch folds (rint′flīsh) [Georg Eduard *Rindfleisch*, German physician, 1836–1908] see under *fold.*

ring (ring) [from A.S. *hring*;] 1. any annular or circular organ or area; for names of specific anatomical structures, see under *anulus.* See also *circle* and *circulus.* 2. in chemistry, a collection of atoms united in a continuous or closed chain.

abdominal r. anulus inguinalis profundus.

Albl r. a circular shadow observed in a radiograph of the skull, caused by an aneurysm of a cerebral artery.

amnion r. the attached margin of the amnion about the umbilicus of the fetus.

annular r's round or oval opacities surrounding a translucent area in a radiograph of the lung, indicative of cavitation in pulmonary tuberculosis. Called also *pleural rings.*

anorectal r. musculus sphincter ani internus.

apical r. polar r.

atrial r. the ring surrounding the opening between the atrium and ventricle of the primitive vertebrate heart; represented in the mammalian heart by the atrioventricular node.

atrioventricular r's, atrioventricular valve r's see *anulus fibrosus dexter/sinister cordis.*

Balbiani r. a large chromosome puff on a polytene chromosome where RNA synthesis is taking place.

Bandl r. pathologic retraction r.; see *retraction r.*

benzene r. the closed hexagon of carbon atoms in benzene (C_6H_6), from which the different benzene compounds are derived by replacement of the hydrogen atoms.

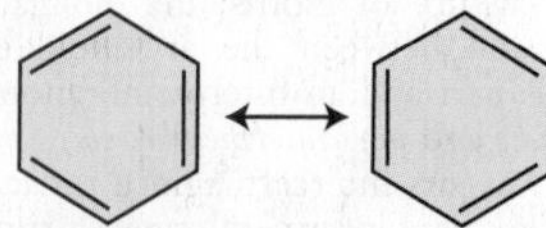

■ Benzene ring structure represented as a hybrid of two possible ring structures; sometimes called a resonance hybrid.

Bickel r. Waldeyer tonsillar r.

Cabot r's Cabot ring bodies; see under *body.*

Cannon r. in the radiograph after a barium meal, a narrow area or focal contraction at the middle third of the transverse colon, representing the junction of the primitive midgut and hindgut and marking an area of overlap between the superior and inferior nerve plexuses.

capsular tension r. in cataract surgery, a small ring that is inserted into the lens capsule for support when the supportive structure of the lens is particularly weak.

carbocyclic r. a chemical ring that includes only carbon atoms.

cardiac lymphatic r. anulus lymphaticus cardiae.

Carpentier r. a semi-rigid prosthetic ring used in annuloplasty to restore competence to a regurgitant cardiac valve.

casting r. 1. a cylinder used as a container for the investment and mold during the process of casting. 2. refractory flask.

ciliary r. orbiculus ciliaris.

circumaortic venous r. see under *collar.*

common tendinous r. anulus tendineus communis.

conjunctival r. anulus conjunctivae.

constriction r. 1. a contracted area of the uterus, allegedly possible at any level, occurring where the resistance of the uterine contents is slight, as over a depression in the contour of the fetal body, or below the presenting part. Cf. *retraction r.* 2. contractile r.

contact r. a patterned injury or powder burn on the body surface at the site of a wound caused by a gunshot fired close to the point of entry.

contraceptive r., contraceptive vaginal r. a vaginal ring that contains a combination of progestins and estrogens, for slow release as a contraceptive device.

contractile r. a narrow band of actin filaments and myosin II, encircling the equator of a dividing cell, that pinches in to separate the daughter cells from one another. Called also *constriction r.*

contraction r. see *constriction r.* and *retraction r.*

coronary r. see under *band.*

crural r. anulus femoralis.

cytoplasmic r. an octagonal array of protein subunits located on the cytoplasmic side of the nuclear pore, each unit having a filament that extends into the cytoplasm; the filaments may mediate transport into the nucleus through the nuclear pore complex.

distal r. terminal r.

Duran r. a flexible prosthetic ring used in annuloplasty to restore competence to a regurgitant cardiac valve.

esophageal r., esophagogastric r. Schatzki r.

femoral r. anulus femoralis.

fibrocartilaginous r. of tympanic membrane anulus fibrocartilagineus membranae tympani.

fibrous r's of heart see anulus fibrosus dexter/sinister cordis.

fibrous r. of intervertebral disk anulus fibrosus disci intervertebralis.

Fleischer r. an incomplete annular pigmented line at the base of the cone in keratoconus.

Fleischer-Strümpell r. Kayser-Fleischer r.

germ r. the proliferating marginal zone of the early blastoderm that is about to become the lips of the blastopore.

glaucomatous r. a light yellowish ring around the optic disk in glaucoma, indicating atrophy of the choroid.

halo r. see under *device.*

hernial r. a ring through which a hernia protrudes, such as a dilated internal inguinal ring.

heterocyclic r. a chemical ring that includes atoms of different elements.

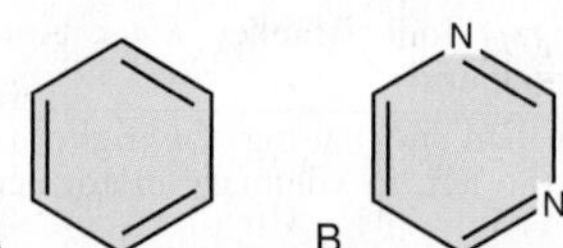

■ *(A)*, Benzene, having a homocyclic ring structure; *(B)*, pyrimidine, having a heterocyclic ring structure.

homocyclic r. a chemical ring in which all the members are atoms of the same element.

inguinal r., deep anulus inguinalis profundus.

inguinal r., external anulus inguinalis superficialis.

inguinal r., internal anulus inguinalis profundus.

inguinal r., superficial anulus inguinalis superficialis.

interpubic fibrous r. discus interpubicus.

intravaginal r. vaginal r.

r. of iris, greater anulus iridis major.

r. of iris, lesser anulus iridis minor.

isocyclic r. homocyclic r.

Kayser-Fleischer r. a golden brown or green discoloration at the level of the Descemet membrane in the limbic region of the cornea, due to the deposition of copper in Wilson disease and other liver disorders.

Landolt r's broken rings used in testing of visual acuity, the width of the ring and the break in its continuity each being one-fifth of its overall diameter; the observer is to identify the orientation of the break,

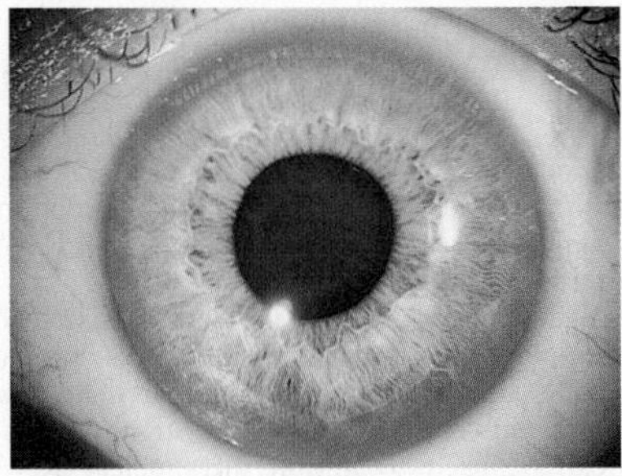

■ Kayser-Fleischer ring in Wilson disease.

with the ability to identify a break subtending 1 minute of arc corresponding to 20/20 vision.

Liesegang r's 1. see under *phenomenon.* 2. concentric laminations due to deposition of calcium, such as occur within some tumors or other lesions.

Löwe r. a ring in the visual field caused by the macula lutea.

Lower r's see anulus fibrosus dexter/sinister cordis.

lower esophageal r. Schatzki r.

lymphoid r. Waldeyer tonsillar r.

Maxwell r. a ring resembling the Löwe ring but smaller and fainter.

middle r. a barrel-shaped structure of the nuclear pore complex, consisting of eight transmembrane proteins in a spokelike arrangement and lying between the cytoplasmic and nucleoplasmic rings. Called also *central framework* and *spoke r.*

mitral r., mitral valve r. see *anulus fibrosus dexter/sinister cordis.*

neonatal r. see *neonatal line,* under *line.*

nuclear r., nucleoplasmic r. an octagonal array of protein subunits located on the nucleoplasmic side of the nuclear pore, each unit having a filament that extends into the nucleoplasm; the filaments are joined together at the ends by a terminal ring to form a basketlike structure (nuclear basket), which may mediate transport out the nucleus through the nuclear pore complex.

pathologic retraction r. see *retraction r.*

periosteal bone r. see under *collar.*

pelvic r. pelvis ossea.

physiologic retraction r. see *retraction r.*.

pleural r's annular r's.

polar r. an electron-dense, annular, anterior thickening of the pellicle of apicocomplexan protozoa, occurring at some stage in the life cycle, and forming part of the apical complex. Called also *apical r.*

retraction r. a circular thickening and indentation occurring in normal labor going around the junction of the isthmus and corpus uteri. It is often normal *(physiologic retraction ring),* delineating the upper contracting portion and the lower dilating portion. Sometimes it is abnormally persistent *(pathologic retraction ring),* such as in prolonged labor or certain other labor conditions, when it may obstruct expulsion of the fetus. Cf. *constriction r.*

right/left fibrous r. of heart see *anulus fibrosus dexter/sinister cordis.*

Schatzki r. a fibrous, annular constriction of the lower esophagus, usually at the junction of the esophageal and gastric mucosa; in some persons it is congenital and in others it results from scar tissue. Called also *esophageal* or *lower esophageal r.*

Schwalbe r., Schwalbe anterior border r. a circular ridge composed of collagenous fibers surrounding the outer margin of the Descemet membrane.

scleral r. a white ring seen adjacent to the optic disk in ophthalmoscopy when the retinal pigment epithelium and choroid do not extend to the disk.

sewing r. a cloth-covered ring that surrounds a prosthetic heart valve and holds it in position.

signet r. 1. a ring that has a much thicker portion; see under *cell.* 2. ring form.

Soemmering r. 1. a doughnut-shaped remnant of lens behind the pupil, occurring after cataract surgery or secondary to trauma as a result of contact between the anterior capsule and the posterior capsule, which traps varying amounts of lens substance peripherally; called also *Soemmering ring cataract.* 2. a developmental cataract in which the primary lens cells fail to develop or are absorbed during intrauterine disease. Later developing subcapsular cells, having no fetal nucleus around which to grow, form doughnut-shaped ring cataracts.

spoke r. middle r.

terminal r. a round structure at the end of the nuclear basket of a nuclear pore complex, able to adapt to the size of proteins and mRNA that are moving between the nucleus and the cytoplasm. Called also *distal r.*

tracheal r's cartilagines tracheales.

tricuspid r., tricuspid valve r. see *anulus fibrosus dexter/sinister cordis.*

tympanic r. anulus tympanicus.

umbilical r. anulus umbilicalis.

vaginal r. a thin plastic ring containing one or more drugs; it is placed inside the vagina for controlled drug release over an extended period, as for delivery of hormones. Called also *intravaginal r.*

vaginal contraceptive r. contraceptive vaginal r.

vascular r. any of various developmental anomalies in which the aortic arches encircle the trachea and esophagus, sometimes compressing them.

r. of Vieussens limbus fossae ovalis.

Vossius r. a ring of pigment on the lens caused by pressure of the pupillary margin against the lens following a contusion.

Waldeyer tonsillar r. the circular series of lymphoid tissue formed by the lingual, pharyngeal, and faucial tonsils. Called also *Bickel* or *lymphoid r.*

Zinn r. anulus tendineus communis.

ring-bone (ring′bōn) exostosis involving the first or second phalanx of the horse, resulting in lameness if the articular surfaces are affected.

low r.-b. buttress foot.

Ring·er injection, irrigation (mixture, solution) (ring′ər) [Sydney *Ringer,* English physiologist, 1835–1910] see under *injection* and *irrigation.*

ring·womb (ring′wo͞om) failure of the cervix of a ewe to dilate during parturition, usually resulting in the death of the lamb in utero.

ring·worm (ring′wərm) popular name for tinea (in humans) or dermatophytosis (in other animals); so called because of the ring-shaped configuration of the lesions.

r. of the beard tinea barbae.

black dot r. one of two common types of tinea capitis; this type is caused most often by *Trichophyton tonsurans* and occasionally by *T. violaceum.* There are multiple areas of alopecia studded with black dots representing infected hairs broken off at or below the surface of the scalp. See also *gray patch r.*

r. of the body tinea corporis.

r. of the face tinea faciei.

r. of the foot tinea pedis.

gray patch r. one of two common types of tinea capitis; this type is caused most often by *Microsporum audouinii* and sometimes by *M. canis, M. ferrugineum,* or *M. gypseum.* There are multiple gray scaly lesions and stubs of broken hairs, and the inflammatory response is minimal. The condition is benign and resolves spontaneously. See also *black-dot r.*

r. of the groin tinea cruris.

r. of the hand tinea manuum.

honeycomb r. favus.

r. of the nails onychomycosis.

Oriental r. tinea imbricata.

r. of the scalp tinea capitis.

Tokelau r. tinea imbricata.

Rin·ne test (rin′ə) [Heinrich Adolf *Rinne,* German otologist, 1819–1868] see under *test.*

Ri·o·lan anastomosis, arch, etc. (re″o-lah′) [Jean *Riolan,* French physician and physiologist, 1580–1657] see under *anastomosis, arch, bone, muscle, nosegay,* and *ossicle.*

RIPA radioimmunoprecipitation assay.

RIPHH Royal Institute of Public Health and Hygiene.

Rip·stein procedure (rip′stēn) [Charles B. *Ripstein,* American surgeon, 1913–2003] see under *procedure.*

RISC RNA-induced silencing complex.

Ris·don approach (riz′don) [E. Fulton *Risdon,* Canadian plastic surgeon, 1880–1968] see under *approach.*

ris·ed·ro·nate so·di·um (ris-ed′rə-nāt″) a diphosphonate inhibitor of bone resorption, used for the prevention and treatment of osteoporosis and for the treatment of osteitis deformans; administered orally.

risk (risk) [Fr. *risque,* from L. *resecare* to cut off] a danger or hazard, the probability of suffering harm or other unfavorable outcome.

attributable r. the amount or proportion of incidence of disease or death (or risk of disease or death) in individuals exposed to a specific risk factor that can be attributed to exposure to that factor; the difference in the risk for unexposed versus exposed individuals. The term is sometimes incorrectly used to denote *population attributable r.*

competing r. an event that removes a subject from being at risk for the outcome under study; e.g., death from automobile accident is a competing risk that removes a subject from the risk of heart disease.

empiric r. the probability that a trait will occur or recur in a family, based solely on experience rather than on knowledge of the causative mechanism. Cf. *genetic r.*

genetic r. the probability that a trait will occur or recur in a family, based on knowledge of its pattern of genetic transmission. Cf. *empiric r.*

population attributable r. in a total population, the proportion of a disease incidence, or risk of the disease, that can be attributed to exposure to a specific risk factor; the difference between the risk in the total population and the risk in the unexposed group.

relative r. for a disease, death, or other outcome, the ratio of the incidence rate among individuals with a given risk factor to the incidence rate among those without it.

Ris·ley prism (riz′le) [Samuel Doty *Risley*, American ophthalmologist, 1845–1920] see under *prism.*

Ris·per·dal (ris′pər-dal) trademark for preparations of risperidone.

ris·per·i·done (ris-per′ĭ-dōn) a benzisoxazole derivative used as an antipsychotic agent, administered orally. Its mechanism of action is unknown, but its activity may result from a combination of dopamine and serotonin antagonism.

Ris·ser jacket (ris′ər) [Joseph C. *Risser*, American orthopedic surgeon, 1892–1942] see under *jacket.*

RIST radioimmunosorbent test.

ris·to·ce·tin (ris″to-se′tin) an antibiotic substance produced by the fermentation of *Nocardia lurida;* formerly used in treatment of severe staphylococcal infections resistant to other antibiotics.

ri·sus (ri′səs) [L.] laughter.

r. sardo′nicus a grinning expression produced by spasm of the facial muscles, seen in tetanus and certain types of poisoning.

Rit·a·lin (rit′ə-lin) trademark for preparations of methylphenidate hydrochloride.

Rit·gen maneuver (method) (rit′gen) [Ferdinand August Marie Franz von *Ritgen*, German gynecologist, 1787–1867] see under *maneuver.*

rit·o·drine hy·dro·chlor·ide (rit′o-drēn) [USP] a beta$_2$-adrenergic agent used as a smooth muscle (uterine muscle) relaxant to delay uncomplicated premature labor; administered orally and intravenously.

ri·to·na·vir (ri-to′nə-vir) [USP] an HIV protease inhibitor that causes formation of immature, noninfectious viral particles; used in the treatment of human immunodeficiency virus infection and acquired immunodeficiency syndrome; administered orally.

Rit·ter disease (rit′ər) [Gottfried *Ritter* von Rittershain, German physician, 1820–1883] staphylococcal scalded skin syndrome.

rit·u·al (rich′u-əl) in psychiatry, behavior performed compulsively to relieve anxiety, as in obsessive-compulsive disorder.

Ri·tux·an (rĭ-tuk′sən) trademark for a preparation of rituximab.

ri·tux·i·mab (rĭ-tuk′sĭ-mab) a chimeric murine/human monoclonal antibody that binds the CD 20 antigen; used as an antineoplastic in the treatment of CD20-positive, B-cell non-Hodgkin lymphoma; administered intravenously.

ri·val·ry (ri′vəl-re) a state of competition or antagonism.

binocular r., retinal r. the apparent alternate displacement of two figures when viewed together, there being no fusion into a continuous picture of the images of the two eyes.

sibling r. competition between siblings for the love, affection, and attention of one or both parents or for other recognition or gain.

Ri·val·ta reaction (test) (re-vahl′tah) [Fabio *Rivalta*, Italian pathologist, late 19th century] see under *reaction.*

riv·a·stig·mine tar·trate (riv″ə-stig′mēn) a reversible cholinesterase inhibitor, believed to increase the level of acetylcholine available in the central nervous system; administered orally as an adjunct in the treatment of mild to moderate dementia of the Alzheimer type.

ri·vi·ni·an (rĭ-vin′e-ən) named for Augustus Quirinus *Rivinus.*

Ri·vi·nus ducts, gland, membrane, notch (rĭ-ve′nəs) [Augustus Quirinus *Rivinus*, German anatomist and botanist, 1652–1723] see *ductus sublinguales minores, glandula sublingualis, pars flaccida membranae tympanicae,* and *incisura tympanica.*

ri·vus (ri′vəs) pl. *ri′vi* [L.] a brook, or little stream.

r. lacrima′lis [TA] the pathway by which the tears reach the lacrimal lake from the excretory ductules of the lacrimal gland.

ri·za·trip·tan ben·zo·ate (ri″zə-trip′tan) a selective serotonin receptor agonist used in the acute treatment of migraine; administered orally.

riz·i·form (riz′ĭ-form) resembling grains of rice.

RLF retrolental fibroplasia; see *retinopathy of prematurity,* under *retinopathy.*

RLL right lower lobe; see *lobus inferior pulmonis dextri.*

RMA right mentoanterior; see *mentoanterior position,* under *position.*

RML right middle lobe; see *lobus medius pulmonis dextri.*

RMP right mentoposterior; see *mentoposterior position,* under *position.*

RMS trademark for a preparation of morphine sulfate.

RMT right mentotransverse; see *mentotransverse position,* under *position.*

RN registered nurse.

Rn radon.

RNA ribonucleic acid.

ambisense RNA negative-sense RNA that functions not only as a template for the transcription of complementary RNA but also as a template for protein synthesis.

antisense RNA (asRNA) an RNA molecule transcribed off the coding, rather than the template, strand of DNA, and thus complementary to the sense (messenger) RNA; hybridization between the sense and antisense RNA molecules prevents translation of the mRNA in bacteria. In vitro, antisense RNA can be used to inhibit intranuclear RNA processing in eukaryotic cells.

complementary RNA (cRNA) viral RNA that is transcribed from negative-sense RNA and serves as a template for protein synthesis.

heterogeneous nuclear RNA (hnRNA) in eukaryotes, a diverse group of long primary transcripts formed in the nucleus, mostly comprising pre-mRNA.

messenger RNA (mRNA) RNA molecules, usually 400 to 10,000 bases long, that serve as templates for protein synthesis (translation); in eukaryotes they have characteristic posttranscriptional modifications, the 5′-cap and poly A tail. The base sequence of an mRNA transcript completely specifies the corresponding polypeptide amino acid sequence.

negative-sense RNA viral RNA that has a base sequence complementary to that of mRNA; during replication it serves as a template for the transcription of viral complementary RNA, which in turn serves as a template for protein synthesis.

polycistronic messenger RNA a messenger RNA that contains more than one initiation site and encodes more than one gene product; usually denoting the single transcript transcribed from a prokaryotic operon and ultimately translated into multiple polypeptides.

positive-sense RNA viral RNA that has the same base sequence as mRNA; during replication, it functions as mRNA and serves as a template for protein synthesis.

precursor RNA any of the unprocessed RNA primary transcripts in the eukaryotic nucleus; see *pre-mRNA, pre-rRNA,* and *pre-tRNA.*

pre-mRNA, pre-messenger RNA any of the large RNA molecules constituting a primary transcript of a structural gene in eukaryotes, containing introns and exons and constituting the majority of the heterogeneous nuclear RNA; it must be processed by polyadenylation, capping, and splicing to become mature messenger RNA (mRNA).

pre-rRNA, pre-ribosomal RNA the large primary transcript that is synthesized and processed in the nucleolus to yield three of the mature rRNA molecules found in eukaryotic ribosomes (18S, 5.8S, and 28S in higher eukaryotes). Small nucleolar RNA's (snoRNA's) assist in processing.

pre-tRNA, pre-transfer RNA any of the primary transcripts of eukaryotic transfer RNA (tRNA) genes, synthesized in the nucleoplasm, and cleaved, modified, and sometimes spliced before transport through nuclear pore complexes to the cytoplasm, as mature tRNA.

ribosomal RNA (rRNA) the most abundant form of RNA; together with proteins it forms the ribosomes, playing a structural role and also a role in ribosomal binding of mRNA and tRNAs. Individual chains are conventionally designated by their sedimentation coefficients. Eukaryotic ribosomes contain four different rRNA chains (5S, 5.8S, 18S, and 28S), synthesized in the nucleolus and constituting the bulk of the ribosome; prokaryotic ribosomes contain three (5S, 16S, and 23S).

small interfering RNA (siRNA) any of a number of small (about 22 nucleotides), double-stranded RNA molecules that are incorporated (with one strand being discarded) into RNA-induced silencing complexes, which they guide to complementary messenger RNA sequences where they induce degradation during the process of RNA interference.

small nuclear RNA (snRNA) any of an abundant class of small RNA molecules found in the nucleus in eukaryotes; five uracil-rich snRNA's (U1, U2, U4, U5, U6) occur complexed with proteins as small nuclear ribonucleoproteins (snRNP's) and play a role in posttranscriptional RNA processing.

small nucleolar RNA (snoRNA) any of a class of small RNA's localized to the eukaryotic nucleolus and, as small nucleolar ribonucleoproteins (snoRNP's), involved in processing and modification of rRNA molecules and assembly of ribosomes. At least some are encoded within the introns of other genes.

transfer RNA (tRNA) small RNA molecules, 73–93 nucleotides, occurring in cells in 20 or more varieties and functioning in translation; each variety carries a specific amino acid to a site specified by an RNA codon, binding to amino acid and ribosome, and to the codon via an anticodon region. All have numerous modified bases and extensive secondary structure; see illustration.

RNA-di·rect·ed DNA po·lym·er·ase (dĭ-rek′təd pə-lim′ər-ās) [EC 2.7.7.49] an enzyme of the transferase class that catalyzes the

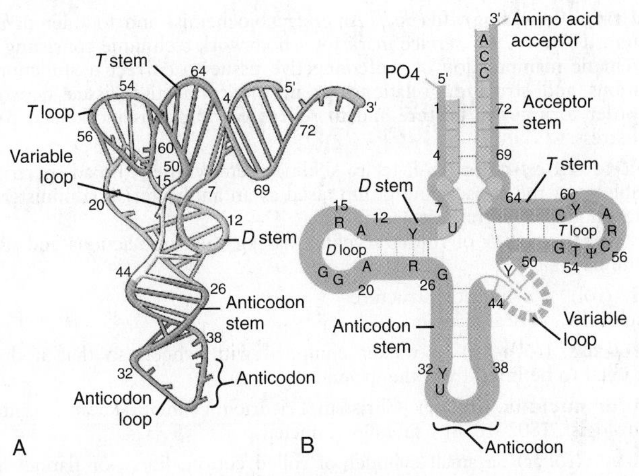

■ Schematic diagram of features common to transfer RNA (tRNA) molecules, depicting the anticodon and amino acid attachment regions. Lines between chains represent hydrogen-bonded base pairs. *(A)*, Backbone model; *(B)*, planar model. The characteristic cloverleaf is formed by the hairpin and loop structures that result from intrachain hydrogen bonding. Single letter code for bases: *A*, adenine; *C*, cytosine; *G*, guanine; *R*, any purine; *T*, thymine; *U*, uracil; *A*, adenine; *Y*, any pyrimidine; *ψ*, pseudouridine.

template-directed, step-by-step addition of deoxyribonucleotides to the 3′ end of a DNA or RNA primer or growing DNA chain, using a single-stranded RNA template. The enzyme occurs in retroviruses and the DNA is an intermediate in the formation of progeny RNA from the original virion RNA. See also *retrovirus.* Called also *reverse transcriptase.*

RNA-di•rect•ed RNA po•lym•er•ase (dĭ-rek′təd pə-lim′ər-ās) [EC 2.7.7.48] an enzyme of the transferase class that catalyzes the template-directed step-by-step addition of ribonucleotides to the 3′ end of a growing RNA chain, using a single-stranded RNA template. The reaction is important for transcription, and in some cases replication, of RNA in most RNA viruses except retroviruses.

RNAi RNA interference.

RNA po•lym•er•ase (pə-lim′ər-ās) 1. a general term denoting any enzyme catalyzing the template-directed incorporation of ribonucleotides into an RNA chain; see *DNA-directed RNA polymerase* and *RNA-directed RNA polymerase.* 2. DNA-directed RNA polymerase.

RNA rep•li•case (rep′lĭ-kās) RNA-directed RNA polymerase.

RNase ribonuclease, sometimes used specifically to denote pancreatic ribonuclease.

R. I, R. A pancreatic ribonuclease.

RNP ribonucleoprotein.

ROA right occipitoanterior; see *occipitoanterior position,* under *position.*

roach (rōch) cockroach.

roar•ing (ror′ing) a rough sound on inhalation and sometimes on exhalation by a horse, usually due to obstruction in the respiratory tract or laryngeal hemiplegia.

rob robertsonian translocation.

Ro•bax•in (ro-bak′sin) trademark for preparations of methocarbamol.

Ro•bax•i•sal (ro-bak′sĭ-sal) trademark for a combination preparation of methocarbamol and aspirin.

ro•ben•i•dine hy•dro•chlo•ride (ro-ben′ĭ-dĕn) a compound related to guanidine, formerly used as a coccidiostat for poultry.

Ro•bert ligament (ro-bār′) [César Alphonse *Robert,* French surgeon, 1801–1862] see under *ligament.*

Rob•erts syndrome (rob′ərts) [John Bingham *Roberts,* American surgeon, 1852–1924] see under *syndrome.*

Rob•ert•shaw tube (rob′ərt-shaw) [Frank L. *Robertshaw,* British anesthesiologist, 20th century] see under *tube.*

Rob•ert•son sign (rob′ərt-sən) [William Egbert *Robertson,* American physician, 1869–1956] see under *sign.*

ro•bin (ro′bin) a phytotoxin found in the bark of the tree *Robinia pseudacacia,* which has caused poisoning of livestock.

Ro•bin•ia (ro-bin′e-ə) a genus of North American shrubs and trees of the family Leguminosae. *R. pseudaca′cia* is the black locust or black acacia tree, whose bark contains the phytotoxin robin and has caused poisoning in livestock.

Rob•i•now syndrome (dwarfism) (rob′ĭ-nou) [Meinhard *Robinow,* German-born American physician, 1909–1997] see under *syndrome.*

Rob•in•son circle (rob′in-sən) [Frederick Byron *Robinson,* American anatomist, 1857–1910] see under *circle.*

Ro•bi•nul (ro′bĭ-nəl) trademark for preparations of glycopyrrolate.

Ro•bi•son ester (ro′bĭ-sən) [Robert *Robison,* British chemist, 1884–1941] glucose 6-phosphate.

Ro•bi•tus•sin (ro″bĭ-tus′in) trademark for preparations of guaifenesin.

Rob•son line, position (rob′sən) [Sir Arthur William Mayo *Robson,* London surgeon, 1853–1933] see under *line* and *position.*

ro•bust (ro-bust′) in statistics, a somewhat imprecise term that is applied to a procedure that is relatively insensitive to violations of the assumptions on which it is based or to procedures that are based on weaker (more easily satisfied) assumptions, e.g., nonparametric tests.

Ro•cal•trol (ro′kal-trōl) trademark for preparations of calcitriol.

Ro•ceph•in (ro-sef′in) trademark for a preparation of ceftriaxone sodium.

Ro•cha•li•maea (ro″kə-li-me′ə) [Henrique da *Rocha-Lima,* French physician in Germany, 1879–1956] a former genus of bacteria, now included in the genus *Bartonella.*

Ro•chon-Du•vi•gneaud syndrome (ro-shaw′doo-ve-nyo′) [André *Rochon-Duvigneaud,* French ophthalmologist, late 19th century] superior orbital fissure syndrome.

rock•ing (rok′ing) moving back and forth repetitively and rhythmically.

body r. a rhythmic backward and forward motion in a sitting position.

Rocky Moun•tain spotted fever (rok′e moun′tən) [*Rocky Mountains* of western United States, where it was first observed in 1899] see under *fever.*

ro•cu•ro•ni•um bro•mide (ro″ku-ro′ne-əm) a nondepolarizing neuromuscular blocking agent, structurally related to and less potent than vecuronium, used as an adjunct in general anesthesia to facilitate endotracheal intubation and as a skeletal muscle relaxant during surgery or mechanical ventilation; administered intravenously.

rod (rod) 1. a straight, slim mass of substance. 2. retinal r.

Auer r's see under *body.*

Corti r's, r's of Corti pillar cells.

Cotrel-Dubousset r. a rigid contoured rod used in Cotrel-Dubousset instrumentation.

enamel r's the approximately parallel rods or prisms forming the enamel of teeth. They are enclosed in a sheath of organic matter (the enamel rod sheath, or prism sheath) and are embedded in the interprismatic or cement substance.

Harrington r. a rigid, contoured metal rod used in Harrington instrumentation.

Knodt r. a rigid, contoured rod used in Knodt instrumentation.

König r's a series of steel bars each of which gives a note of certain pitch when struck.

Luque r. a rigid, contoured stainless steel rod used in Luque instrumentation.

Maddox r's a set of parallel cylindrical glass rods used in testing for heterophoria. The rods, placed before the eye, distort the image of a point source of light into a long streak perpendicular to the axis of the rods, interfere with fusion, and break up binocular vision.

Meckel r. see under *cartilage.*

muscle r. myofibril.

olfactory r. the slender apical portion of an olfactory bipolar neuron, a modified dendrite, extending as a cylindrical process from the nucleus to surface of the epithelium.

retinal r. one of the two types of visual cells, along with retinal cones, having synapses internally with bipolar retinal cells. Rods serve night vision and detection of motion. Their synaptic terminals are spherical, and their dendritic inner and outer segments are long and cylindrical. Rods have membranous disks, free saccules that contain rhodopsin and are completely enclosed by the outer cell membrane. There are about 120 million rods in the retina. None are in the foveola; the greatest concentration is about 20 degrees away from the fovea centralis, and the density gradually decreases approaching the periphery of the retina. Called also *rod* and *rod cell.*

ro•dent (ro′dənt) [L. *rodere* to gnaw] 1. any mammal of the order *Rodentia.* 2. gnawing; corroding.

Ro•den•tia (ro-den′shə) the rodents, an order of mammals characterized by large chisel-shaped incisors in the upper and lower jaws; common animals in this group include rats, mice, and squirrels. Numerous species serve as reservoirs for infectious diseases.

ro•den•ti•cide (ro-den′tĭ-sīd) 1. destructive to rodents. 2. any agent for destroying rodents.

anticoagulant r. an anticoagulant that kills rodents by causing massive hemorrhaging; some of these substances can also kill other mammals that

Anticoagulant Rodenticides

Brodifacoum	Difenacoum
Bromadiolone	Diphenadione (diphaenone)
Chlorophacinone	Pindone
Coumachlor	Valone
Coumafuryl	Warfarin
Coumatetralyl	

accidentally ingest them. Most are derivatives of indanedione or warfarin. See table.

ro·den·tine (ro-den′tīn) pertaining to a rodent.

Roent·gen (rent′gən) see *Röntgen*.

roent·gen (rent′gən) [Wilhelm Konrad *Röntgen*, German physicist and Nobel prize winner, 1845–1923] the international unit of x- or γ-radiation. It is the quantity of x- or γ-radiation such that the associated corpuscular emission per 0.001293 gram of dry air (1 cm^3 at 0°C and 760 mm Hg) produces in air ions carrying 1 electrostatic unit of electrical charge of either sign. Symbol R.

roent·gen rays (rent′gen) [W.K. *Röntgen*] x-rays; see under *ray*.

roent·geno·graph (rent′gən-o-graf) radiograph.

roent·gen·og·ra·phy (rent″gən-og′rə-fe) radiography. **roentgenograph′ic** *adj*

roent·gen·ol·o·gist (rent″gən-ol′ə-jist) radiologist.

roent·gen·ol·o·gy (rent″gən-ol′ə-je) radiology.

roent·geno·scope (rent-gen′o-skōp) fluoroscope.

roent·gen·os·co·py (rent″gən-os′kə-pe) fluoroscopy.

ro·fe·cox·ib (ro″fə-cok′sib) a nonsteroidal antiinflammatory drug of the COX-2 inhibitors group, used in treatment of osteoarthritis, acute pain, and dysmenorrhea; administered orally.

Ro·fer·on-A (ro-fēr′on) trademark for a preparation of interferon alfa-2a.

Ro·gaine (ro′gān) trademark for preparations of minoxidil.

Ro·ger disease, symptom (ro-zha′) [Henri Louis *Roger*, French physician, 1809–1891] see under *disease* and *symptom*.

Ro·ger reflex (ro-zha′) [Georges Henri *Roger*, French physiologist, 1860–1946] esophagosalivary reflex.

Röhl marginal corpuscles (rərl) [Wilhelm *Röhl*, German physician, 1881–1929] see under *corpuscle*.

Ro·hyp·nol (ro-hip′nəl) trademark for a preparation of flunitrazepam.

Ro·ki·tan·sky diverticulum, hernia, pelvis (ro″kĭ-tahn′ske) [Karl Freiherr von *Rokitansky*, Czech pathologist in Austria, 1804–1878] see *traction diverticulum*, under *diverticulum*, see *massive hepatic necrosis*, under *necrosis*, and see *spondylolisthetic pelvis*, under *pelvis*.

Ro·ki·tan·sky-Asch·off sinuses (ro″kĭ-tahn′ske ahsh′of) [K.F. von *Rokitansky;* Karl Albert Ludwig *Aschoff*, German pathologist, 1866–1942] see under *sinus*.

Ro·ki·tan·sky-Cush·ing ulcers (ro″kĭ-tahn′ske koosh′ing) [K.F. von *Rokitansky;* Harvey Williams *Cushing*, American surgeon, 1869–1939] see under *ulcer*.

Ro·ki·tan·sky-Kü·ster-Hau·ser syndrome (ro″kĭ-tahn′ske ke′stər hou′zer) [K.F. von *Rokitansky;* Hermann *Küster*, German gynecologist, early 20th century; G.A. *Hauser*, Swiss physician, 20th century] Mayer-Rokitansky-Küster-Hauser syndrome.

ro·lan·dic (ro-lan′dik) described by or named for Luigi *Rolando*, Italian anatomist, 1773–1831.

Ro·lan·do angle, cells, etc. (ro-lahn′do) [L. *Rolando*] see under *angle*, *cell*, and *line;* see *motor area*, under *area;* and see *sulcus centralis cerebri* and *tuberculum trigeminale*.

role (rōl) the behavior pattern that an individual presents to others.
 gender r. the public expression of gender; the image projected by a person that identifies their maleness or femaleness, which need not correspond to their gender identity (q.v.).
 sick r. the role played by a person who has defined himself or herself as ill, with or without validation of the role by health care providers or family members. Adoption of the sick role changes the behavioral expectations of others toward sick persons. They are exempted from normal social responsibilities and not held responsible for the condition; they are obliged to "want to get well" and to seek competent medical help. The sick role also involves behavioral changes, including increased attention to the body and bodily functions, regression (increase in dependent behavior), narrowing of interests, and emotional overreactions.

Rol·fing (rawl′fing) [Ida *Rolf*, American biochemist and founder of the system, 1896–1979] service mark for a bodywork technique consisting of systematic manipulation of the connective tissue to correct dysfunctional fixations and structural relationships in the connective tissue network in order to improve posture and to relieve chronic musculoskeletal pain and stress.

ro·li·tet·ra·cy·cline (ro-lĭ-tet″rə-si′klin) a semisynthetic broad-spectrum antibiotic of the tetracycline group, used as an antibacterial, administered intravenously or intramuscularly.
 r. nitrate a salt of rolitetracycline, having the same actions and uses as the base.

roll (rōl) a cylindrical structure.
 scleral r. calcar sclerae.

roll·a·tor (rōl′a-tər) a walker equipped with wheels so that it does not need to be lifted from the ground.

Rol·ler nucleus (rol′ər) [Christian Friedrich Wilhelm *Roller*, German neurologist, 1802–1878] sublingual nucleus.

roll·er (rōl′ər) a small cylinder of rolled cotton, linen, or flannel for surgical use.

Rol·le·ston rule (rol′əs-tən) [Sir Humphrey Davy *Rolleston*, English physician, 1862–1944] see under *rule*.

Rol·let stroma (rol′et) [Alexander *Rollet*, Austrian physiologist, 1834–1903] see under *stroma*.

Rol·let syndrome (ro-la′) [J. *Rollet*, French physician, 20th century] orbital apex syndrome; see under *syndrome*.

Ro·ma·ña sign (ro-mah′nyah) [Cecilio *Romaña*, Argentine physician in Brazil, 20th century] see under *sign*.

Ro·mano-Ward syndrome (ro-mah′no word′) [C. *Romano*, Italian physician, born 1923; O.C. *Ward*, Irish physician, 20th century] see under *syndrome*.

Ro·ma·now·sky (Ro·ma·nov·sky) stain (method) (ro″mə-nou′ske, ro″mə-nof′ske) [Dimitri Leonidovich *Romanowsky* (or *Romanovsky*), Russian physician, 1861–1921] see *Stains and Staining Methods*, under *stain*.

Ro·maz·i·con (ro-maz′ĭ-kon) trademark for a preparation of flumazenil.

Rom·berg disease (trophoneurosis), sign (test), spasm (rom′bərg) [Moritz Heinrich *Romberg*, German physician, 1795–1873] see *facial hemiatrophy*, under *hemiatrophy*, and see under *sign* and *spasm*.

rom·berg·ism (rom′bərg-iz-əm) [M.H. *Romberg*] Romberg sign.

ro·mi·plo·stim (ro″mĭ-plo′stim) a thrombopoietin receptor agonist used for treatment of immune thrombocytopenic purpura; administered by subcutaneous injection.

Rom·me·laere sign (rom-ə-lār′) [Guillaume *Rommelaere*, Belgian physician, 1836–1916] see under *sign*.

Rom·ney Marsh disease (rom′ne mahrsh) [*Romney Marsh*, England, where it was first reported] struck.

ron·geur (raw-zhur′) [Fr. "gnawing, biting"] a forcepslike instrument for cutting tough tissue, particularly bone. See table.

Ro·ni·a·col (ro-ni′ə-kol) trademark for preparations of nicotinyl alcohol.

ro·nid·a·zole (ro-nid′ə-zōl) a veterinary antiprotozoal and antimicrobial used to treat histomoniasis and swine dysentery.

Rön·ne nasal step (rur′nə) [Henning Kristian Trappaud *Rönne*, Danish ophthalmologist, 1878–1947] see under *step*.

ron·nel (ron′əl) an organophosphorus insecticide, effective against flies, roaches, screw worms, and cattle grub.

Rönt·gen (rent′gen) Wilhelm Konrad, 1845–1923. German physicist. For his discovery of x-rays in 1895, while experimenting with a cathode ray tube, he received the first Nobel prize in physics in 1901.

Rood method (rōōd) [Margaret *Rood*, American physical therapist, 20th century] see under *method*.

roof (rōōf) a covering structure; see also *tectum* and *tegmen*.

Selected Rongeurs

Bacon rongeur	Lempert and Carroll rongeur
Cloward rongeur	Sauerbruch rongeur
Fulton rongeur	Stille rongeur
Kerrison rongeur	Stille-Luer rongeur
Leksell rongeur	Stookey rongeur
Lempert rongeur	Zaufal-Jansen rongeur

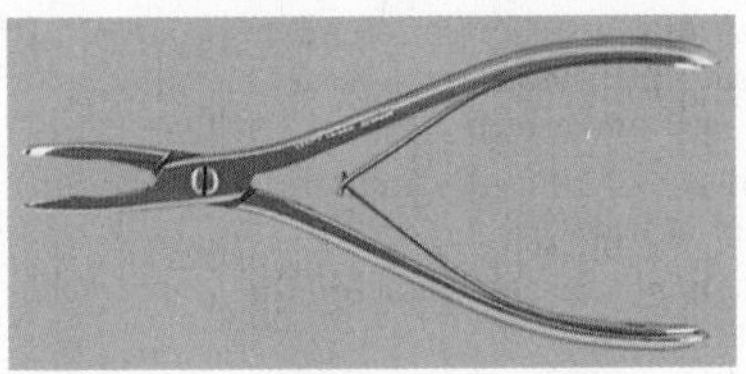

■ Rongeur.

r. of fourth ventricle tegmen ventriculi quarti.
r. of lateral ventricle the superior covering of a lateral ventricle, formed by parts of the corpus callosum and its tapetum as well as the tail of the caudate nucleus and the stria terminalis.
r. of mouth palatum.
r. of nasal cavity the superior surface of the cavity, formed by portions of the sphenoid, ethmoid, frontal, and nasal bones; it is narrow anteriorly and wider posteriorly.
nasopharyngeal r., r. of nasopharynx fornix pharyngis.
r. of orbit paries superior orbitae.
r. of skull calvaria.
r. of third ventricle the tela choroidea ventriculi tertii and the ependyma, which form the superior covering structures of the third ventricle.
r. of tympanic cavity paries tegmentalis cavitatis tympani.
r. of tympanum 1. tegmen tympani. 2. paries tegmentalis cavitatis tympani.

room (rōōm) an enclosed place in a building, set apart for specific purposes such as the performance of procedures.
anechoic r. see under *chamber.*
delivery r. a hospital room to which an obstetrical patient is taken for delivery.
emergency r. popular name for *emergency department.*
labor r. predelivery r.
operating r. a room in a hospital equipped and used for surgical operations.
postdelivery r. a recovery room for the care of obstetric patients immediately after delivery.
predelivery r. a hospital room where an obstetric patient remains during the first stage of labor, i.e., from the time the pains begin until she is ready for delivery; called also *labor r.*
recovery r. postanesthesia care unit.

room·ing-in (rōōm′ing-in) the practice of keeping a newly born infant in a crib near the mother's bed, instead of in a nursery, during the hospital stay.

Roos test (rōōs) [David B. *Roos*, American surgeon, late 20th century] see under *test.*

root (rōōt) 1. radix. 2. the lowermost part of a plant or other structure.
anatomical r. the portion of a tooth that is covered by cementum; see *radix dentis.*
r's of ansa cervicalis see *radix superior ansae cervicalis* and *radix inferior ansae cervicalis.*
anterior r. of ansa cervicalis radix superior ansae cervicalis.
anterior r. of spinal nerve radix anterior nervi spinalis.
anterior r. of zygomatic process of temporal bone a short thick continuation of the inferior border of the zygomatic process, extending medially to the articular tubercle.
r. of aorta, aortic r. the dense fibrous area that encircles the aortic valve and constitutes the junction between the aortic vestibule of the left ventricle and the aorta.
r. of arch of vertebra pediculus arcus vertebrae.
bitter r. gentian.
r's of brachial plexus radices plexus brachialis.
clinical r. radix clinica.
r. of clitoris crus clitoridis.
cochlear r. of vestibulocochlear nerve radix cochlearis nervi vestibulocochlearis.
cranial r. of accessory nerve radix cranialis nervi accessorii.
dorsal r. of spinal nerve radix posterior nervi spinalis.
facial r., r. of facial nerve a motor nerve root consisting of fibers passing from the nucleus of the facial nerve to the facial colliculus, and from there through the ventral surface of the lower part of the pons, where the sensory root (the nervus intermedius) joins it to form the facial nerve.
r. of hair the proximal portion of a hair embedded in the hair follicle; called also *radix pili.*
inferior r. of ansa cervicalis radix inferior ansae cervicalis.
inferior r. of vestibulocochlear nerve radix cochlearis nervi vestibulocochlearis.
lateral r. of median nerve radix lateralis nervi mediani.
lateral r. of optic tract radix lateralis tractus optici.
licorice r. licorice (def. 2).
lingual r. the root of a posterior tooth nearest to the tongue, especially on a maxillary molar.
long r. of ciliary ganglion radix sensoria ganglii ciliaris.
r. of lung radix pulmonis.
mandrake r. podophyllum.
medial r. of median nerve radix medialis nervi mediani.
medial r. of optic tract radix medialis tractus optici.
r. of mesentery radix mesenterii.
motor r. of ciliary ganglion radix parasympathica ganglii ciliaris.
motor r. of mandibular nerve a small root that emerges from the trigeminal ganglion and combines with the corresponding sensory root to form the mandibular nerve.
motor r. of spinal nerve radix anterior nervi spinalis.
motor r. of submandibular ganglion rami ganglionares nervi lingualis ad ganglion submandibulare.
motor r. of trigeminal nerve radix motoria nervi trigemini.
r. of nail radix unguis.
nasociliary r. of ciliary ganglion radix sensoria ganglii ciliaris.
nerve r's the anterior and posterior roots of the spinal nerves; see *radix anterior nervi spinalis* and *radix posterior nervi spinalis.* Called also *spinal r's.*
nerve r., motor radix posterior nervi spinalis.
nerve r., sensory radix anterior nervi spinalis.
r. of nose radix nasi.
oculomotor r. of ciliary ganglion radix parasympathica ganglii ciliaris.
orizaba jalap r. ipomea.
r. of otic ganglion the preganglionic fibers of the lesser petrosal nerve.
palatine r. the root of a maxillary molar tooth located nearest to the palate.
parasympathetic r. of ciliary ganglion radix parasympathica ganglii ciliaris.
parasympathetic r. of otic ganglion nervus petrosus minor.
parasympathetic r. of pterygopalatine ganglion nervus petrosus major.
parasympathetic r. of sublingual ganglion, parasympathetic r. of submandibular ganglion chorda tympani.
physiological r. the portion of a tooth proximal to the gingival crevice, or embedded in the dental alveolus.
posterior r. of ansa cervicalis radix inferior ansae cervicalis.
posterior r. of spinal nerve radix posterior nervi spinalis.
posterior r. of zygomatic process of temporal bone a continuation of the superior border of the zygomatic process, extending above the external acoustic meatus and ending continuous with the supramastoid crest.
retained r. 1. a tooth root, or part of a root, remaining in the soft tissue or in bone following trauma, extensive tooth decay, or incomplete extraction. 2. a tooth root intentionally retained to prevent resorption of the alveolar process.
sensory r. of ciliary ganglion radix sensoria ganglii ciliaris.
sensory r. of mandibular nerve a large root that emerges from the trigeminal ganglion and combines with the corresponding motor root to form the mandibular nerve.
sensory r. of otic ganglion rami ganglionares nervi mandibularis ad ganglion oticum.
sensory r. of pterygopalatine ganglion rami ganglionares nervi maxillaris ad ganglion pterygopalatinum.
sensory r. of spinal nerve radix posterior nervi spinalis.
sensory r. of submandibular ganglion rami ganglionares nervi lingualis ad ganglion submandibulare.
sensory r. of trigeminal nerve radix sensoria nervi trigemini.
short r. of ciliary ganglion radix parasympathica ganglii ciliaris.
spinal r's nerve r's.
spinal r. of accessory nerve radix spinalis nervi accessorii.
r's of spinal nerves nerve r's.
superior r. of ansa cervicalis radix superior ansae cervicalis.
superior r. of vestibulocochlear nerve radix vestibularis nervi vestibulocochlearis.
sympathetic r. of ciliary ganglion radix sympathica ganglii ciliaris.
sympathetic r. of pterygopalatine ganglion nervus petrosus profundus.
r. of tongue radix linguae.
r. of tooth radix dentis.
ventral r. of spinal nerve radix anterior nervi spinalis.
vestibular r. of vestibulocochlear nerve radix vestibularis nervi vestibulocochlearis.

root·let (rōōt′lət) 1. a small root or rootlike structure or a division of such a structure. 2. radicle.

flagellar r. one of the delicate striated fibrils of the flagellar root system that arise from the basal body and run deep into the cytoplasm, perhaps serving as anchoring organelles or having a skeletal function. They occur most commonly in phytoflagellate protozoa, and were formerly thought to connect the basal body to the nucleus of the cell. Called also *rhizoblast* and *rhizoplast.*

r's of spinal nerve fila radicularia nervi spinalis.

ROP right occipitoposterior; see *occipitoposterior position,* under *position.*

ro•pin•i•role hy•dro•chlo•ride (ro-pin′ĭ-rōl″) a dopamine agonist used as an antidyskinetic in the treatment of Parkinson disease; administered orally.

ro•pi•va•caine hy•dro•chlo•ride (ro-piv′ə-kān) a local anesthetic of the amide type, used for percutaneous infiltration anesthesia, peripheral nerve block, and epidural block.

ro•ri•din (ro′rĭ-din) any of several trichothecene mycotoxins found in species of *Stachybotrys,* especially *S. alternans,* causing stachybotryotoxicosis.

Ror•schach test (ror′shahk) [Hermann *Rorschach,* Swiss psychiatrist, 1884–1922] see under *test.*

Ro•sa (ro′zə) the roses, a genus of flowering, usually prickly, plants of the family Rosaceae. *R. al′ba* L., *R. centifo′lia* L., *R. damasce′na* Mill., and *R. gal′lica* L. have flowers that yield rose oil.

ro•sa•cea (ro-za′she-ə) [L. feminine of *rosaceus* rose-colored, shortened from *acne rosacea*] a chronic skin disease, usually involving the middle third of the face, characterized by persistent erythema and often by telangiectasia with acute episodes of edema, papules, and pustules; it affects both men and women, but is often more severe in men. It is associated with an excess of cathelicidin and stratum corneum tryptic enzyme, which results in the formation of an abnormal inflammatory peptide that is responsible for the lesions. Complications include rosacea keratitis and rhinophyma. Called also *acne rosacea.*

erythematotelangiectatic r. rosacea characterized by facial flushing and erythema, often with telangiectasia; some patients also have edema, burning sensations, and roughness or scaling of the skin.

r. ful′minans pyoderma faciale.

granulomatous r. rosacea characterized by hard yellow to brown papules or nodules that occur on the medial and lateral areas of the face as well as around the mouth. Called also *lupoid* or *papular r.*

inflammatory r. papulopustular r.

lupoid r. granulomatous r.

ocular r. bloodshot, burning eyes with symptoms of rosacea, sometimes accompanied by blepharitis and conjunctivitis.

papular r. granulomatous r.

papulopustular r. rosacea characterized by central facial erythema with papules and pustules around the face; it resembles acne vulgaris but does not include comedones.

phymatous r. rosacea involving the lower part of the nose, characterized by sebaceous hyperplasia and swelling; the most common type is rhinophyma.

steroid r. rosacea developing as a reaction to administration of topical steroids, causing periorificial dermatitis on the face.

vascular r. erythematotelangiectatic r.

ro•sa•ce•i•form (ro-za′she-ĭ-form″) resembling rosacea.

Ro•sai-Dorf•man disease (ro′zi dorf′mən) [Juan *Rosai,* American pathologist, 20th century; Ronald F. *Dorfman,* American pathologist, 20th century] see under *disease.*

ro•san•i•line (ro-zan′ĭ-lin) a basic dye derived from triphenylmethane, occurring as reddish brown crystals, which is soluble in acids and alcohol and slightly soluble in water. It is used, usually as the hydrochloride, in the preparation of other dyes and as a component of basic fuchsin.

ro•sa•ra•mi•cin (ro″zə-rə-mi′sin) a macrolide antibiotic, derived from *Micromonospora rosaria,* having a broad spectrum of antibacterial activity against gram-positive bacteria and some activity against gram-negative bacteria; the butyrate, propionate, sodium phosphate, and stearate salts have antibacterial activity similar to that of the base.

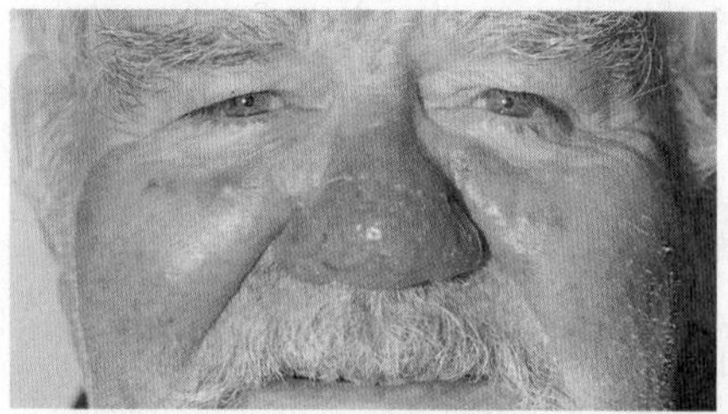

■ Rosacea.

ro•sa•ry (ro′zə-re) a structure resembling a string of beads.

rachitic r. see under *bead.*

scorbutic r. see under *bead.*

Rose position (rōz) [Frank Atcherly *Rose,* British surgeon, 1873–1935] see under *position.*

rose (rōz) [L. *rosa*] 1. any plant of the genus *Rosa.* 2. a dark pink or light red color.

r. bengal a dye, the dichlor- or tetrachlorerythrosin, $NaO{\bullet}(C_6HI_2{\bullet}O)_2C{\bullet}C_6H_2Cl_2{\bullet}COONa$.

r. bengal sodium I 131 [USP] rose bengal in which a portion of the molecules contain radioiodine (^{131}I), used as a radioactive tracer in the liver function test called the rose bengal test.

ro•se•in (ro′ze-in) fuchsin.

rose•mary (rōz′mar-e) *Rosmarinus officinalis.*

Ro•sen method (ro′zən) [Marion *Rosen,* German-born American physical therapist and body worker, born 1914] see under *method.*

Ro•sen•bach sign (ro′zən-bahk) [Ottomar *Rosenbach,* German physician, 1851–1907] see under *sign.*

Ro•sen•berg-Berg•strom syndrome (ro′zən-bərg burg′strəm) [Alan L. *Rosenberg,* American physician, 20th century; Lavonne *Bergstrom,* American physician, 20th century] see under *syndrome.*

Ro•sen•berg-Chu•tor•i•an syndrome (ro′zən-bərg choo-tor′e-ən) [Roger N. *Rosenberg,* American physician, 20th century; Abe Milton *Chutorian,* American physician, born 1929] see under *syndrome.*

Ro•sen•mül•ler organ, etc. (ro′zən-me″lər) [Johann Christian *Rosenmüller,* German anatomist, 1771–1820] see *epoöphoron, nodus lymphoideus inguinalis profundus proximalis,* and *recessus pharyngeus.*

Ro•sen•thal canal (ro′zən-tahl) [Isidor *Rosenthal,* German physiologist, 1836–1915] canalis spiralis modioli.

Ro•sen•thal syndrome (ro′zen-thawl) [Robert Louis *Rosenthal,* American hematologist, born 1923] factor XI deficiency; see under *deficiency.*

Ro•sen•thal vein (ro′zən-tahl) [Friedrich Christian *Rosenthal,* German anatomist, 1779–1829] vena basalis.

ro•se•o•la (ro-ze′o-lə, ro″ze-o′lə) [L.] 1. a type of rose-colored rash seen most often in an infectious disease such as measles or other exanthematous diseases. 2. exanthema subitum.

r. infan′tum exanthema subitum.

Ro•se•o•lo•vi•rus (ro″ze-o′lo-vi″rəs) [*roseola* + *virus*] a genus of viruses of the subfamily Betaherpesvirinae (family Herpesviridae), containing species human herpesviruses 6 (the etiologic agent of exanthema subitum) and human herpesvirus 7.

Ro•seo•mo•nas (ro″ze-o-mo′nəs) [L. *roseus* rose-colored + Gr. *monas* unit, from *monos* single] a genus of gram-negative bacteria of the family Acetobacteraceae, consisting of plump cocci, coccobacilli, or short rods, occurring singly and in pairs or short chains. Organisms are aerobic, catalase- and urease-positive, and oxidase-variable and produce a pale pink pigment; motility is variable.

R. gilar′dii the type species of the genus, which can cause bacteremia in weak or immunocompromised persons.

ro•sette (ro-zet′) [Fr. "little rose"] a structure, formation, or part occurring in a loosely attached cluster resembling a rose, such as *(a)* the clusters of polymorphonuclear leukocytes around a globule of lysed nuclear material, observed in a test for systemic lupus erythematosus; *(b)* a unique glandular complex near the oral area of certain ciliate protozoa, of unknown function; or *(c)* the symmetrical segmenter stage of certain malarial parasites, especially *Plasmodium malariae.*

E r. see under *assay.*

EAC r. see under *assay.*

ependymal r. glandlike structures consisting of tumor cells with epithelial features and having long, slender processes extending into a lumen; seen in ependymoma.

Flexner-Wintersteiner r. a cell formation found in retinoblastoma and certain other ophthalmic tumors, with columnar cells radiating out from a clear central core and separated from it by a membrane; spokes like those of a wheel may also be seen, representing rods and cones.

Homer Wright r. a circular or spherical grouping of dark tumor cells around a pale, eosinophilic, central area that contains neurofibrils but lacks a lumen; seen in some medulloblastomas, neuroblastomas, and retinoblastomas or other ophthalmic tumors.

ro•sig•lit•a•zone mal•e•ate (ro-sig-lit′ə-zōn) a thiazolidinedione antidiabetic agent that increases insulin sensitivity, used in the treatment of type 2 diabetes mellitus; administered orally.

ro•sin (roz′in) the solid resin obtained from *Pinus palustris* and other species of pine, occurring as angular, translucent, amber-colored fragments, often covered with yellow dust; it contains about 90 per cent resin. It has been widely used in the preparation of plasters and ointments, as well as chewing gums, varnishes, and polishes, but its use has declined because it is a common cause of allergic contact dermatitis.

Ros•ma•ri•nus (ros″mə-ri′nəs) [L. "sea-dew"] a genus of plants of the family Labiatae. *R. officina′lis* L. is rosemary, a species native to southern Europe and Turkey that is the source of rosemary oil.

ro•sox•a•cin (ro-soks′ə-sin) a broad-spectrum quinolone antibacterial agent, administered orally.

Ros•so•li•mo reflex (sign) (ros″o-le′mo) [Gregorij Ivanovich *Rossolimo*, Russian neurologist, 1860–1928] see under *reflex*.

Ros•tan asthma (ros-tah′) [Louis Léon *Rostan*, French physician, 1790–1866] cardiac asthma.

ros•tel•lum (ros-tel′əm) pl. *rostel′la* [L. "little beak"] a small protuberance or beak, especially the fleshy protuberance of the scolex of a tapeworm, which may or may not bear hooks.

ros•tra (ros′trə) plural of *rostrum*.

ros•trad (ros′trad) 1. toward a rostrum; situated nearer the rostrum in relation to a specific point of reference. 2. cephalad.

ros•tral (ros′trəl) [L. *rostralis*, q.v.] 1. pertaining to or resembling a rostrum; having a rostrum or beak. 2. toward a rostrum or beak. 3. in human anatomy, toward the oral and nasal region, which may mean superior (for areas of the spinal cord) or anterior (for brain areas).

ros•tra•lis (ros-tra′lis) [L., from *rostrum* beak] [TA] rostral.

ros•trate (ros′trāt) [L. *rostratus* beaked] having a beaklike process.

ros•tri•form (ros′trĭ-form) [*rostrum* + *form*] shaped like a beak.

ros•tro•cau•dal (ros″tro-kaw′dəl) cephalocaudal.

ros•trum (ros′trəm) pl. *ros′trums* or *ros′tra* [L. "beak"] a beaklike appendage or part.

r. cor′poris callo′si [TA] rostrum of corpus callosum: the anterior and lower end of the corpus callosum, passing from the genu caudally toward the anterior commissure.

r. sphenoida′le [TA] sphenoidal rostrum: the prominent ridge on the inferior surface of the sphenoid bone that articulates with a deep depression between the wings of the vomer.

ro•su•va•stat•in cal•ci•um (rə-soo′və-stat″in) a synthetic HMG-CoA reductase inhibitor that acts as an antihyperlipidemic by inhibiting cholesterol synthesis; used in treatment of hypercholesterolemia and other forms of dyslipidemia, administered orally.

ROT right occipitotransverse; see *occipitotransverse position*, under *position*.

Rot see *Roth*.

rot (rot) 1. decay (def. 1). 2. liver r.

benign foot r. foot rot of sheep that is mainly confined to the skin between the digits; lameness is less severe than with virulent foot rot. Called also *scald* and *foot scald*.

bovine foot r. foot r. of cattle.

contagious foot r. virulent foot r.

fleece r. dermatitis in sheep resulting from prolonged skin wetness, accompanied by matted wool and exudation; it is often a precursor of cutaneous myiasis.

foot r. inflammation with interdigital dermatitis and mild to severe necrosis of the hoof of an animal, caused by a bacterial infection; in cattle and sheep it is exacerbated in wet or cold weather or soggy pastures, and in pigs it usually follows trauma. See *foot r. of cattle*, *foot r. of pigs*, and *foot r. of sheep*.

foot r. of cattle inflammation of the foot of a cow or bull, with dermatitis between the digits, lameness, fever, swelling of the coronet, and necrotic foul-smelling material around the lesion. It is thought to be caused by infection with *Fusobacterium necrophorum*. Called also *bovine foot r.*, *foul in the foot*, *interdigital necrobacillosis*, and *pododermatitis*.

foot r. of pigs a noncontagious foot infection of pigs, usually caused by *Fusobacterium necrophorum* or *Corynebacterium pyogenes* that invades through lesions on lateral digits of the hind legs, often after trauma such as from living in a pen with a hard or abrasive floor. Abscess formation is followed by lameness and sometimes permanent foot deformity. Called also *porcine foot r.*

foot r. of sheep infection of the hooves of sheep with *Fusobacterium necrophorum* or *Bacteroides nodosus*. There are two varieties, *benign foot r.* and *contagious* or *virulent foot r.*

jungle r. warm water immersion foot.

liver r. a form of fascioliasis seen in cattle and sheep, and occasionally humans, characterized by fibrosis of the liver with anemia and weight loss; severe cases can be fatal. The infecting fluke is *Fasciola hepatica*.

ovine foot r. foot r. of sheep.

pizzle r., sheath r. enzootic balanoposthitis.

porcine foot r. foot r. of pigs.

strawberry foot r. dermatophilosis in sheep.

virulent foot r. foot rot of sheep with chronic necrosis of the hoof and underlying dermis, destruction and eventual detachment of the hoof, lameness, and recumbency. The cause is usually a combined infection with *Fusobacterium necrophorum* and *Bacteroides nodosus*, and it is worse in wet or cold weather or in a soggy pasture. Called also *contagious foot r.*

ro•tab•la•tion (ro″tab-la′shən) an atherectomy technique in which a rotating bur is inserted through a catheter into an artery; the burr rotates and debulks atherosclerotic plaque. Called also *rotational ablation* or *atherectomy*.

Ro•ta•hal•er (ro′tə-hāl″ər) trademark for a type of dry powder inhaler that delivers single doses of medication.

ro•tam•e•ter (ro-tam′ə-tər) a flow-rate meter of variable area with a rotating float in a tapered tube, used for measuring the flow of gases in administering an anesthetic.

Ro•ta•rix (ro′tə-riks) trademark for a preparation of rotavirus vaccine, live, oral.

ro•ta•ry (ro′tə-re) marked by or produced by rotation.

ro•tate (ro′tāt) to turn around an axis; to twist.

Ro•ta•Teq (ro′tə-tek) trademark for a preparation of rotavirus vaccine, live, oral, pentavalent.

ro•ta•tion (ro-ta′shən) [L. *rotare* to turn] 1. the process of turning around an axis; movement of a body about its axis, called the *axis of rotation*. 2. the turning of the fetal head through 90 degrees during labor so that the long diameter of the head corresponds with the long diameter of the pelvic outlet. It should occur naturally, but if it does not the rotation may be accomplished manually or instrumentally by the obstetrician. See also *maneuver*. 3. a turning around a central axis without undergoing any displacement from the axis. See also *hinge movement*, under *movement*. 4. a procedure whereby a malturned tooth is turned into its normal position. 5. malposition due to an abnormal turning of a tooth around its longitudinal axis.

molecular r. the figure obtained by multiplying the specific rotation by the molecular weight and dividing by 100.

optical r. the quality of certain optically active substances whereby the plane of polarized light is changed, so that it is rotated in an arc the length of which is characteristic of the substance.

specific r. the arc through which a substance of specified concentration rotates the plane of polarization in a specified light path, as observed in a polarimeter.

torsional r. torsion.

van Ness r. fusion of the knee joint and rotation of the ankle to function as the knee; done to correct a congenitally missing femur.

wheel r. torsion (def. 3).

ro•ta•tion•plas•ty (ro-ta′shən-plas″te) the moving of a rotation flap over a defect.

ro•ta•tor (ro′ta-tər) 1. causing rotation. 2. a muscle that rotates a body part; see *musculi rotatores*.

ro•ta•to•ry (ro″tə-tor′e) occurring in or caused by rotation.

Ro•ta•vi•rus (ro′tə-vi″rəs) [L. *rota* wheel + *virus*] the rotaviruses, a genus of viruses of the family Reoviridae that have a wheellike appearance; they are transmitted by the fecal-oral route and cause acute infantile gastroenteritis and diarrhea in young children and many animal species. There are six antigenic groups (A–F). See Plate 49.

ro•ta•vi•rus (ro′tə-vi″rəs) [L. *rota* wheel + *virus*] any member of the genus *Rotavirus*. **ro′taviral** *adj*

Rotch sign (roch) [Thomas Morgan *Rotch*, American physician, 1849–1914] see under *sign*.

ro•te•none (ro′tə-nōn) a poisonous compound from the dried roots and other parts of plants of the genera *Derris* and *Lonchocarpus;* used as an insecticide.

ro•texed (ro′tekst) rotated and bent to one side.

ro•tex•ion (ro-tek′shən) act of rotating and flexing; also the state of being rotated and flexed.

Roth disease (rōt) [Vladimir Karlovich *Roth* (or *Rot*), Russian neurologist, 1848–1916] meralgia paresthetica.

Roth spots, vas aberrans (rōt) [Moritz *Roth*, Swiss physician, 1839–1915] see under *spot*, and see *ductuli aberrantes*.

Roth-Bern•hardt disease (rōt′ bern′hahrt) [V.K. *Roth;* Martin *Bernhardt*, German neurologist, 1844–1915] meralgia paraesthetica.

Ro•the•ra test (roth′ər-ah) [Arthur Cecil Hamel *Rothera*, Australian biochemist, 1880–1915] see under *test*.

Roth•ia (roth′e-ə) [Genevieve D. *Roth*, American bacteriologist, 20th century] a genus of bacteria of the family Micrococcaceae, consisting of aerobic, gram-positive, non–acid-fast, non–spore-forming organisms occurring in coccoid, diphtheroid, and branched filament forms. The type species is *R. dentocario'sa*.

R. dentocario'sa a species found in the oral cavities of primates, particularly in plaque and calculus deposits on the teeth and in carious material. It is a cause of infective endocarditis, bacteremia, pneumonia, and peritonitis.

R. mucilagino'sa a species that is a normal inhabitant of the oral cavity and pharynx and can cause infective endocarditis.

Roth·mann-Ma·kai syndrome (rot'mahn maw'koi) [Max *Rothmann*, German pathologist, 1868–1915; Endre *Makai*, Hungarian surgeon, 20th century] see under *syndrome*.

Roth·mund-Thom·son syndrome (rot'moond tom'son) [August von *Rothmund*, Jr., German physician, 1830–1906; Mathew Sidney *Thomson*, English dermatologist, 1894–1969] see under *syndrome*.

Ro·tor syndrome (ro-tōr') [Arturo B. *Rotor*, Filipino physician, 20th century] see under *syndrome*.

ro·tox·amine (ro-toks'ə-mēn) the *l*-isomer of carbinoxamine, having antihistaminic potency about twice that of the racemic form.

r. tartrate the tartrate salt of rotoxamine, having the same actions as the base; used in the treatment of allergic disorders, administered orally.

rott·le·ra (rot'lər-ə) kamala (def. 2).

rouge (ro͞ozh) a fine red powder composed of iron oxide (Fe_2O_3), usually in cake form but sometimes impregnated on paper or cloth; used in dentistry as a polishing agent for restorations of gold and precious metal alloys.

Rou·get bulb (roo-zha') [Antoine D. *Rouget*, French physiologist, 19th century] bulb of ovary.

Rou·get cell, muscle (roo-zha') [Charles Marie Benjamin *Rouget*, French physiologist and anatomist, 1824–1904] see *pericyte*, and see under *muscle*.

rough (ruf) not smooth; having an irregular surface.

rough·age (ruf'əj) indigestible material such as fibers, cellulose, etc., in the diet.

Roug·non-Heb·er·den disease (ro͞on-yaw' heb'ər-dən) [Nicholas François *Rougnon* de Magny, French physician, 1727–1799; William *Heberden*, Sr., English physician, 1710–1801] angina pectoris.

rou·leau (roo-lo') pl. *rouleaux'* [Fr. "roll"] an abnormal group of red blood cells adhering together like a roll of coins.

round·worm (round'wərm) nematode.

Rous sarcoma (rous) [Francis Peyton *Rous*, American pathologist and Nobel prize winner, 1879–1970] see under *sarcoma*.

Rous·sy-De·je·rine syndrome (roo-se' dĕ-zhĕ-rēn') [Gustave *Roussy*, French pathologist, 1874–1948; Joseph Jules *Dejerine*, French neurologist, 1849–1917] thalamic syndrome.

Rous·sy-Lé·vy syndrome (hereditary areflexic dystasia) (roo-se' la-ve') [G. *Roussy;* Gabrielle *Lévy*, French neurologist, 1886–1935] see under *syndrome*.

Rou·vière node (roo-vyār') [Henri *Rouvière*, French anatomist and embryologist, 1875–1952] see under *node*.

Roux-en-Y anastomosis (operation) (roo-en-wi, Fr. roo″ahn-e-grek') [César *Roux*, Swiss surgeon, 1857–1926] see under *anastomosis*.

Rov·sing procedure, sign, syndrome (rov'sing) [Niels Thorkild *Rovsing*, Danish surgeon, 1862–1927] see under *procedure*, *sign*, and *syndrome*.

Ro·wa·sa (row-a'sə) trademark for preparations of mesalamine.

Rox·a·nol (rok'sə-nol) trademark for preparations of morphine sulfate.

rox·ar·sone (rok-sahr'sōn) [USP] an arsenical used in veterinary practice for the treatment of coccidiosis and necrotic enteritis in poultry and for the treatment of swine dysentery.

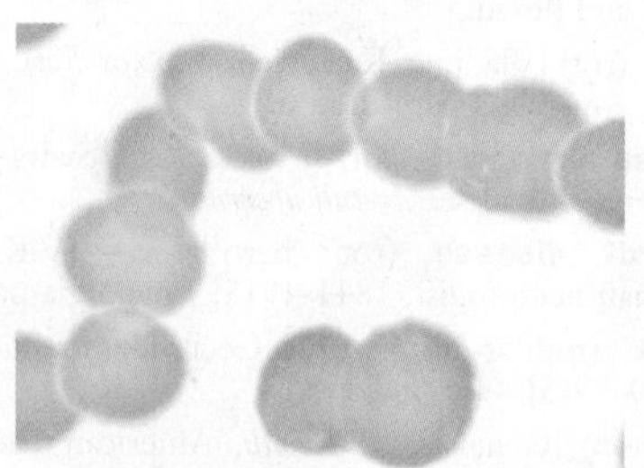

■ Human red blood cells arranged in rouleaux.

Rox·i·cet (rok'sĭ-set″) trademark for combination preparations of oxycodone hydrochloride and acetaminophen.

Rox·i·co·done (rok-se-ko'dōn) trademark for preparations of oxycodone hydrochloride.

Ro·ze·rem (ro-zēr'em) trademark for a preparation of ramelteon.

RPC reactive perforating collagenosis.

RPE retinal pigment epithelium; see *stratum pigmentosum retinae*.

RPF renal plasma flow.

R Ph Registered Pharmacist.

RPLND retroperitoneal lymph node dissection; see under *lymphadenectomy*.

rpm revolutions per minute.

RQ respiratory quotient.

RRA Registered Record Administrator.

-rrhage [Gr. *rhegnynai* to burst forth] a word termination denoting abnormal or excessive flow. Also, *-rrhagia*.

-rrhagia see *-rrhage*.

-rrhaphy [Gr. *rhaphē* suture] a word termination denoting suture or operative repair.

-rrhea [Gr. *rhoia* flow] a word termination denoting flow or discharge.

-rrhexis [Gr. *rhēxis*, from *rhēgnynai* to burst] a word termination denoting the action or process of breaking, rupturing, or splitting.

-rrhoea see *-rrhea*.

rRNA ribosomal RNA.

16S r. one of the component RNA molecules of the prokaryotic ribosome (see *ribosomal RNA*, under *RNA*); phylogenetic analysis of the nucleotide sequence of the gene encoding it is widely used in the taxonomic classification of prokaryotes.

RSA right sacroanterior; see *sacroanterior position*, under *position*.

RScA right scapuloanterior; see *scapuloanterior position*, under *position*.

RSCN Registered Sick Children's Nurse.

RScP right scapuloposterior; see *scapuloposterior position*, under *position*.

RSM Royal Society of Medicine.

RSNA Radiological Society of North America.

RSP right sacroposterior; see *sacroposterior position*, under *position*.

RST right sacrotransverse; see *sacrotransverse position*, under *position*.

RSTMH Royal Society of Tropical Medicine and Hygiene.

RSV respiratory syncytial virus; Rous sarcoma virus.

RTA renal tubular acidosis.

RTF resistance transfer factor.

Ru ruthenium.

RU-486 mifepristone.

rub (rub) 1. to move something over a surface with friction. 2. the action of such movement. 3. friction r.

friction r. an auscultatory sound caused by the rubbing together of two serous surfaces, as in a pericardial rub or pleural friction rub; called also *rub*.

pericardial r., pericardial friction r. a scraping or grating noise heard with the heart beat, usually a to-and-fro sound, associated with pericarditis or other pathological condition of the pericardium.

pleural r., pleural friction r., pleuritic r. a rub produced by friction between the visceral and costal pleurae.

Ru·barth disease (roo'bahrt) [Sven *Rubarth*, Swedish veterinarian, 20th century] hepatitis contagiosa canis; see under *hepatitis*.

rub·ber (rub'ər) 1. an elastic material made from the milky latex of any of various trees of the genera *Hevea* and *Ficus*. 2. a synthetic product resembling this material.

polysulfide r. an elastomeric synthetic rubber used in dentistry as an impression material for fixed partial prosthodontic structures, inlays for single quadrants, and dental impressions.

rub·bing (rub'ing) moving something over a surface with friction.

coin r. firm rubbing of the edge of a coin or similar object in lines or circles along the skin of the trunk or back, often producing ecchymoses or welts; in Asian cultures, it is used to eliminate blood stagnation and promote normal circulation and metabolism in the treatment of conditions such as pain, fever, stiffness, nausea, and respiratory illnesses. Called also *gua sha* and *cao gio*.

ru·be·fa·cient (roo″bə-fa'shənt) [*ruber* + *-facient*] 1. causing reddening of the skin. 2. an agent that reddens the skin by producing active or passive hyperemia.

ru•bel•la (roo-bel′ə) [L., from *rubellus* reddish, from *ruber* red] an acute, usually benign, infectious disease caused by viruses of genus Rubivirus, a togavirus, affecting most often children and nonimmune young adults. The virus enters the respiratory tract via droplet nuclei and spreads to the lymphatic system. The first symptoms are a slight cold, sore throat, and fever, followed by enlargement of the postauricular, suboccipital, and cervical lymph nodes, and later appearance of a fine pink rash that begins on the head and spreads to become generalized. Transplacental infection of the fetus as a result of maternal infection in the first trimester can cause death of the conceptus or developmental anomalies in the newborn infant (see *congenital rubella syndrome*, under *syndrome*). Called also *German measles* and *three-day measles.* In French and Spanish the word *rubeola* is used for this disease.

Ru•bens flap (roo′bənz) [Peter Paul *Rubens*, Flemish painter, 1577–1640] see under *flap.*

ru•be•o•la (roo-be′o-lə, roo-be-o′lə) [dim. of L. *rubeus* red] 1. measles. 2. French and Spanish term for *rubella.*

ru•be•o•sis (roo″be-o′sis) redness, usually referring to the eyes.

r. i′ridis a condition characterized by formation of new blood vessels and connective tissue on the surface of the iris, frequently seen in diabetics *(r. i′ridis diabe′tica)* and following occlusion of the central retinal vein or artery. If untreated, it can develop into severe, intractable glaucoma.

r. re′tinae a condition characterized by formation of new blood vessels in front of the optic papilla in retinitis proliferans; this may be seen in either nondiabetics or diabetics *(r. re′tinae diabe′tica)*, and if untreated can lead to retinal detachment.

ru•ber (roo′bər) [L.] red.

ru•bes•cent (roo-bes′ənt) [L. *rubescere* to become red] reddish; becoming red.

Ru•bex (roo′beks) trademark for a preparation of doxorubicin hydrochloride.

ru•bid•i•um (Rb) (roo-bid′e-əm) [L. *rubidus* red] a rare metallic alkaline element; atomic number, 37; atomic weight, 85.47.

r. 82 a radioactive isotope of rubidium, atomic mass 82, having a half-life of 1.273 minutes; it decays by positron emission (3.15 MeV) and is used as a tracer in positron emission tomography.

r. chloride Rb 82 [USP] the chloride salt of ^{82}Rb, used for positron emission tomography in the diagnosis of cardiac disease; administered intravenously.

ru•bid•o•my•cin (roo-bid′o-mi″sin) daunorubicin.

ru•big•i•nose (roo-bij′ĭ-nōs) [L. *rubigo* rust] having a rusty, brownish color; said of sputum.

ru•big•i•nous (roo-bij′ĭ-nəs) rubiginose.

ru•bin (roo′bin) fuchsin.

Ru•bin•stein syndrome (roo′bin-stīn) [Jack Herbert *Rubinstein*, American pediatrician, born 1925] see under *syndrome.*

Ru•bin•stein-Tay•bi syndrome (roo′bin-stīn ta′be) [J.H. *Rubinstein;* Hooshang *Taybi*, Iranian-born American radiologist, 1919–2006] see under *syndrome.*

Ru•bi•vi•rus (roo′bĭ-vi″rəs) [L. *rubeus* red + *virus*] rubella virus; a genus of viruses of the family Togaviridae containing the cause of rubella.

Rub•ner's law (roob′nərz) [Max *Rubner*, German physiologist, 1854–1932] see under *law.*

ru•bor (roo′bor) [L.] redness, one of the cardinal signs of inflammation.

Ru•bra•tope-57 (roo′brə-tōp) trademark for a preparation of cyanocobalamin Co 57.

ru•bra•tox•in (roo′brətok″sin) a mycotoxin found in *Penicillium purpurogenum* and *P. rubrum*, which contaminate corn and can cause hepatotoxicity in livestock.

ru•bri•blast (roo′brĭ-blast) proerythroblast.

ru•bric (roo′brik) red; specifically, pertaining to the red nucleus.

ru•bri•cyte (roo′brĭ-sīt) [L. *rubrum* red + *-cyte*] polychromatophilic erythroblast.

ru•bro•spi•nal (roo″bro-spi′nəl) pertaining to the red nucleus and the spinal cord.

ru•bro•tha•lam•ic (roo″bro-thə-lam′ik) pertaining to the red nucleus and the thalamus.

Ru•bu•la•vi•rus (roo′bu-lə-vi″rəs) [L. *rubula inflans* mumps] a genus of viruses of the subfamily Paramyxovirinae (family Paramyxoviridae); species that cause human disease include human parainfluenza viruses 2 and 4 and mumps virus.

Ru•bus (roo′bəs) [L.] a genus of prickly plants of the family Rosaceae, including brambles, raspberries, and blackberries. The root barks of several species of blackberry are tonic and astringent and have been used to treat diarrhea. *R. idae′us* L. and *R. strigo′sus* Michx. are varieties of raspberry (q.v.).

ruc•tus (ruk′təs) [L.] eructation.

Rud syndrome (rood) [Einar *Rud*, Danish physician, 20th century] see under *syndrome.*

ru•di•ment (roo′dĭ-mənt) 1. a structure that has remained undeveloped, or one with little or no function at present but which was functionally developed earlier either in the individual or in its phylogenetic ancestors. 2. primordium.

lens r. see under *placode.*

ru•di•men•ta•ry (roo″dĭ-men′tə-re) 1. imperfectly developed. 2. vestigial.

ru•di•men•tum (roo″dĭ-men′təm) pl. *rudimen′ta* [L. "a first beginning"] 1. primordium. 2. rudiment (def. 1).

Ru•di•mi•cro•spo•rea (roo″dĭ-mi″kro-spor′e-ə) [*rudi*ment + *micro-* + *spore*] a class of protozoa (phylum Microspora) found as hyperparasites of gregarines in annelids, the spores of which have a simple extrusion apparatus consisting of a polar cap and a thick polar tube extending backward from the cap, bending laterally and terminating in an infundibulum; a polaroplast and posterior vacuole are absent. It comprises one order: Metchnikovellida.

rue (roo) [L. *Ruta*] 1. *Ruta graveolens.* 2. any of various plants that resemble *R. graveolens.*

African r. *Peganum harmala.*

Ru•fen (roo′fən) trademark for preparations of ibuprofen.

Ruf•fi•ni ending (brush, corpuscle, cylinder, end-organ) (roo-fe′ne) [Angelo *Ruffini*, Italian anatomist, 1864–1929] see under *ending.*

ru•fous (roo′fəs) erythristic.

ru•ga (roo′gə) pl. *ru′gae* [L.] a ridge, wrinkle, or fold, as of mucous membrane.

gastric rugae, rugae gas′tricae plicae gastricae.

ru′gae palati′nae, palatine rugae plicae palatinae transversae.

rugae of stomach plicae gastricae.

rugae of vagina, ru′gae vagina′les [TA] small transverse folds of the mucous membrane of the vagina extending outward from the columns.

ru′gae vesi′cae bilia′ris, ru′gae vesi′cae fel′leae TA alternatives for *plicae mucosae vesicae biliaris.*

ru•gae (roo′je) [L.] plural of *ruga.*

Rug•ge•ri reflex (sign) (roo-ja′re) [Ruggero *Ruggeri*, Italian physician, 1823–1905] see under *reflex.*

ru•gine (roo-zhēn′) a raspatory.

ru•gose (roo′gōs) [L. *rugosus*] characterized by wrinkles.

ru•gos•i•ty (roo-gos′ĭ-te) [L. *rugositas*] 1. the condition of being wrinkled. 2. a fold, wrinkle, or ruga.

ru•gous (roo′gəs) [L. *rugosus*] rugose.

RUL right upper lobe; see *lobus superior pulmonis dextri.*

rule (rōōl) [L. *regula*] a statement of conditions commonly observed in a given situation, or a statement of a prescribed course of action to obtain a result. Cf. *law.*

Allen r. the extended body parts of warm-blooded species (tail, ears, and limbs) are relatively shorter in the colder regions of a species range than in the warmer.

Arey r. the total length of an embryo or fetus in inches, for the first five months, equals the numerical sum of the number of the previous lunar months since conception; for the last five lunar months, it equals the product of the number of the month multiplied by 2.

Bartholomews r. of fourths if the uterine fundus is one-fourth of the way from the pubic symphysis to the umbilicus, the pregnancy is of two months' duration; one-half of the way, three months' duration; three-quarters of the way, four months' duration; at the umbilicus, five months' duration. The fundus then rises one-quarter of the way to the ensiform process each month until the ninth, when it sinks to the level it occupied at eight months.

Bergmann r. for geographically dispersed races of warm-blooded species of animals, body size is smaller in warmer parts of the species range than in colder parts of the range.

r. of bigeminy bigeminy tends to be self-perpetuating because the premature complexes both precipitate and are caused by long cardiac cycles.

Budin r. a bottle-fed baby should not take more than 10 per cent of its own weight of cow's milk per day.

Cahn-Ingold-Prelog sequence r's in chemistry, a set of rules used to determine the absolute configuration of chiral molecules by assigning priority rankings to the atoms attached to a chiral center. Atoms directly attached to the chiral center are ranked in order of decreasing atomic number; if these are alike then the groups incorporating the atoms are ranked using the site of difference nearest the chiral center, with identical groups ranked on the basis of their nearest neighbors. Multiple bonds are treated as if the atoms of the bond are replicated once for each extra bond. Isotopes are ranked by descending atomic mass. See also *E-*, *Z-*, *R-*, and *S-*.

delivery date r. Nägele r.

dermatomal r. the theory that visceral pain is referred to the dermatomes supplied by the posterior roots through which the visceral afferent impulses reach the spinal cord.

Durham r. a definition of criminal responsibility from a 1954 federal court of appeals case, Durham vs. United States; the court held that "an accused is not criminally responsible if his unlawful act was the product of mental disease or mental defect." In 1972 the same court reversed itself and adopted the American Law Institute formulation (see under *formulation*).

Goodsall r. a guide to classification of anal fistulas; those with external openings in the posterior half of the perianal area usually originate in the posterior half of the anus and those with external openings in the anterior perineum usually originate in the anterior quadrant of the anus.

Haase r. the total length of an embryo or fetus in centimeters, for the first five months, equals the square of the number of lunar months since conception; for the last five months it equals the product of the number of the month multiplied by 5.

Hardy-Weinberg r. see under *law*.

Hudson lactone r. molecular optical rotation of a carbohydrate or its derivatives is given as the sum of the rotation contributions at each asymmetric center. Certain other empirical conclusions may also be drawn from existing data.

Jackson r. see under *law*.

Liebermeister r. in febrile tachycardia, the pulse beats increase at the rate of about eight per minute to every degree centigrade of temperature.

McDonald r. the length in centimeters of the abdominal contour from the upper margin of the pubic symphysis to the fundus of the uterus, divided by 3.5, gives the duration of pregnancy in lunar months; applicable only after the sixth month of pregnancy.

M'Naghten r. a definition of criminal responsibility formulated in 1843 by English judges questioned by the House of Lords as a result of the acquittal of Daniel M'Naghten on grounds of insanity. It holds that "to establish a defense on the ground of insanity, it must be clearly proved that, at the time of committing the act, the party accused was laboring under such a defect of reason, from disease of the mind, as not to know the nature and quality of the act he was doing, or, if he did know it, he did not know he was doing what was wrong" and further that a defendant who "labors under partial delusions only and is not in other respects insane ... must be considered in the same situation as to responsibility as if the facts with respect to which the delusion exists were real." These rules are still used in many American jurisdictions.

Nägele r. to predict the first day of labor and confinement, subtract three months from one year after the first day of the last menstruation and add seven days.

r. of nines a method of estimating the extent of body surface that has been burned in an adult; the body surface is divided into sections of 9 per cent or multiples of 9 per cent. See accompanying table. For children the Lund-Browder classification provides a more accurate estimate.

octet r. when atoms combine to form molecules, they tend to share or transfer electrons until eight (four pairs) are in the valence shell of each atom.

phase r. a heterogeneous chemical system of p coexistent phases and c variable components has $c - p + 2$ degrees of freedom or variations of phase, i.e., the sum of its coexistent phases and its possible changes of phase exceeds the number of its components by 2.

Pitres' r. see under *law*.

Rule of Nines

Region	Percentage of Body Surface
Head and neck	9%
Anterior trunk	18%
Posterior trunk	18%
Left arm	9%
Right arm	9%
Left leg	18%
Right leg	18%
Genitalia and perineum	1%

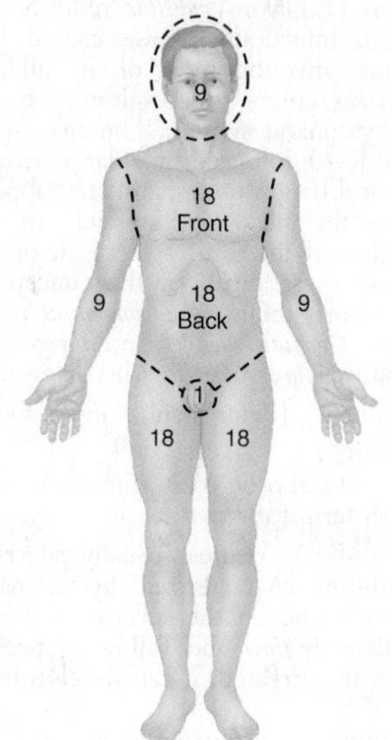

■ Rule of nines.

Rolleston r. the ideal systolic pressure for an adult is the figure represented by 100 plus half the age in years.

van't Hoff r. the velocity of chemical reactions is increased twofold or more for each rise of 10°C in temperature; it is generally true when temperatures approximate those under which the reaction normally occurs. Called also *van't Hoff's law*. See also *temperature coefficient*, under *coefficient*.

Weigert-Meyer r. in cases of double ureter, the ureter from the upper pole of the kidney usually opens below and medial to the one from the lower pole. Called also *Weigert-Meyer law*.

Weinberg r. the total number of dizygotic twins in any population is twice the number of twins of different sex, and the sum of these subtracted from the total number of all twins gives the number of monozygotic twins.

ru•men (roo′mən) [L. "throat"] the first stomach of a ruminant, consisting of a huge sac lined by a mucous membrane, with several subdivisions, where partially chewed food is stored prior to rumination. Called also *paunch*. **ru′minal** *adj*

ru•men•i•tis (roo″mə-ni′tis) inflammation of the rumen.

ru•men•ot•o•my (roo″mə-not′ə-me) [*rumen* + *-tomy*] surgical incision of the rumen of an animal to remove a foreign body or impacted food or to evacuate gases.

ru•mi•nant (roo′mĭ-nənt) 1. any of the suborder Ruminantia (order Artiodactyla), hoofed mammals that have four stomachs (the *rumen, reticulum, omasum,* and *abomasum*), through which the food passes in digestion. It includes cattle, sheep, goats, deer, and antelopes. 2. chewing the cud.

Ru•mi•nan•tia (roo″mĭ-nan′she-ə) the ruminants, a suborder of mammals of the order Artiodactyla.

ru•mi•na•tion (roo″mĭ-na′shən) [L. *ruminare* to think over] 1. in ruminants, the casting up of food (called *cud*) out of the rumen and chewing of it a second time; called also *cudding*. 2. in humans, the regurgitation of food after almost every meal, part of it being vomited and the rest swallowed; sometimes seen in infants *(rumination disorder)* or in mentally retarded individuals. 3. repeated, excessive thinking about an event or situation.

ru•mi•na•tive (roo′mĭ-nə″tiv) characterized by rumination; constantly dwelling on certain topics or ideas.

Ru•mi•no•coc•cus (roo″mĭ-no-kok′əs) [*rumen* + Gr. *kokkos* berry] a genus of anaerobic, gram-positive bacteria of the family Lachnospiraceae, occurring as spherical to elongated cocci, which are involved in the fermentation of cellulose in the rumens of cattle and sheep. The type species is *R. flavefa′ciens*.

ru•mi•no•re•tic•u•lar (roo″mĭ-no-rə-tik′u-lər) reticuloruminal.

ru•mi•no•re•ti•cu•lum (roo″mĭ-no-rə-tik′u-ləm) reticulorumen.

Rum-K (rum′kay) trademark for a preparation of potassium chloride.

rump (rump) the buttock or gluteal region.

Rum•pel-Leede phenomenon (sign, test) (room′pəl lēd′) [Theodor *Rumpel*, German physician, 1862–1923; Carl Stockbridge *Leede*, American physician, 1882–1964] see under *phenomenon*.

Run•dles-Falls syndrome (run'dəlz fawlz') [Ralph Wayne *Rundles*, American internist, 1911–1991; Harold Francis *Falls*, American ophthalmologist and geneticist, 1909–2006] hereditary sideroblastic anemia.

runt (runt) a young animal with growth retardation.

Run•yon classification, group (run'yən) [Ernest H. *Runyon*, American microbiologist, 20th century] see under *classification.*

ru•pia (roo'pe-ə) [Gr. *rhypos* filth] thick, dark, raised, lamellated, adherent crusts on the skin, such as those seen in late secondary syphilis. ru'pial *adj*

ru•pi•oid (roo'pe-oid) resembling rupia.

rup•ture (rup'chər) 1. forcible tearing or disruption of tissue. 2. to forcibly disrupt tissue. 3. hernia.

premature membrane r. (PROM), premature r. of membranes rupture of the fetal membranes before the onset of labor, with leakage of amniotic fluid from the vagina.

Ru•sco•ni anus (roo-sko'ne) [Mauro *Rusconi*, Italian biologist, 1776–1849] see *blastopore.*

Rus•cus (rus'kəs) a genus of European evergreen herbs of the family Liliaceae, having erect woody stems, small scalelike leaves, small greenish flowers, and red berries; *R. aculea'tus* (butcher's broom) is used medicinally.

Rush (rush) Benjamin, 1745–1813. American physician and statesman, born in Philadelphia; he was the first professor of chemistry at the College of Philadelphia and wrote the first American book on chemistry. Rush was a Surgeon General in the Continental Army and physician to Pennsylvania Hospital, where he introduced clinical instruction; he was the founder of the Philadelphia Dispensary (the first in America), founder of the Philadelphia College of Physicians, and professor of the Institutes of Medicine (i.e., physiology and pathology) and Clinical Medicine at the University of Pennsylvania. Rush was the first American to investigate mental illness, to write on cholera infantum, and to notice focal infection in teeth; he was a founder of experimental physiology; and he also wrote on alcoholism, personal hygiene, and public health and on the great yellow fever epidemic in Philadelphia (1793). Rush's views on that epidemic (that it originated locally and was not imported) and his treatment of the sufferers (excessive purging and blood letting) caused controversy and lawsuits.

rush (rush) 1. to move fast. 2. fast movement.

peristaltic r. a powerful wave of contractile activity that travels long distances down the small intestine; it is caused by intense irritation or unusual distention. Called also *peristaltic reflex.*

Rus•sell bodies (rus'əl) [William *Russell*, Scottish physician, 1852–1940] see under *body.*

Rus•sell dwarf, syndrome (dwarfism) (rus'əl) [Alexander *Russell*, British pediatrician, 1914–2003] see under *dwarf* and see *Silver-Russell syndrome*, under *syndrome.*

Rus•sell effect (rus'əl) [William James *Russell*, English chemist, 1830–1909] see under *effect.*

Rus•sell traction (rus'əl) [R. Hamilton *Russell*, Australian surgeon, 1860–1933] see under *traction.*

Rus•sell's viper, viper venom (rus'əl) [Patrick *Russell*, English physician in Syria, 1727–1805] see under *viper* and *venom.*

Rus•sell-Sil•ver syndrome (dwarfism) (rus'əl sil'vər) [A. *Russell;* Henry K. *Silver*, American pediatrician, 20th century] Silver-Russell syndrome.

Rust disease, syndrome (roost) [Johann Nepomuk *Rust*, Austrian surgeon, 1775–1840] see under *disease* and *syndrome.*

rust (rust) 1. iron oxide or hydroxide, forming a reddish deposit on metallic iron where the latter has been exposed to moisture; also a similar deposit on other metals that have been exposed to dampness. 2. a fungus of the order Uredinales, members of which cause the plant disease also called rust. 3. a fungal disease of plants, caused by members of the class Uredinales and characterized by the formation of spots on their skin that resemble the rust of metals.

rut (rut) [L. *rugitus* roaring] 1. the period or season of heightened sexual activity in some male mammals that coincides with the season of estrus in the females. 2. estrus.

Ru•ta (roo'tə) a genus of strong-scented flowering herbs of the family Rutaceae, native to Europe and Asia. *R. graveo'lens* is rue, a species whose leaves contain oil that is an irritant poison.

ru•the•ni•um (Ru) (roo-the'ne-əm) a rare, very hard metallic element; atomic weight, 101.07; atomic number, 44.

Ruth•er•ford's theory (ruth'ər-fordz) [William *Rutherford*, Scottish physiologist, 1839–1899] frequency theory.

ruth•er•ford (rd) (ruth'ər-fərd) [Sir Ernest *Rutherford*, British physicist, 1871–1937] the unit representing one million disintegrations of radioactive matter per second.

ru•ti•do•sis (roo″tĭ-do'sis) rhytidosis.

ru•tin (roo'tin) a bioflavonoid (q.v.) obtained from buckwheat and other plants.

Ru•val•ca•ba syndrome (roo″vahl-ka'bə) [R.H. *Ruvalcaba*, American physician, born 1934] see under *syndrome.*

Ruysch glomerulus, membrane, etc. (roish) [Frederic *Ruysch*, Dutch anatomist, 1638–1731] see *glomerulus renis* and *lamina choroidocapillaris*, and see under *muscle* and *tube.*

ruysch•ian (roi'she-an) named for Frederic *Ruysch.*

RV residual volume; Rotavirus (or rotavirus); rotavirus vaccine.

RVAD right ventricular assist device.

RVH right ventricular hypertrophy; see *ventricular hypertrophy*, under *hypertrophy.*

Rye classification (ri) [*Rye*, New York, where a conference in 1965 adopted the classification] see under *classification.*

rye (ri) 1. *Secale cereale.* 2. the seed of *S. cereale*, which is used as food and can grow a fungus that is the source of ergot.

spurred r. see *ergot* (def. 1).

Ryle tube (rīl) [John Alfred *Ryle*, British physician, 1889–1950] see under *tube.*

Ryth•mol (rith'mol) trademark for a preparation of propafenone hydrochloride.

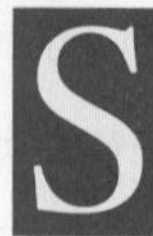

S spherical lens; serine; siemens; smooth (see under *colony*); substrate; sulfur; Svedberg unit; sacral vertebrae (S1 through S5).

S. [L.] sig′na (mark); see *prescription* and *signature* (def. 1).

S entropy.

S- [L. *sinister* left] a stereodescriptor used to specify the absolute configuration of compounds having asymmetric carbon atoms. See *R-*.

S_1 first heart sound; see under *sound*.

S_2 second heart sound; see under *sound*.

S_3 third heart sound; see under *sound* and see *gallop rhythm* under *rhythm*.

S_4 fourth heart sound; see under *sound* and see *gallop rhythm* under *rhythm*.

S_f Svedberg flotation unit.

s second.

s. [L.] se′mis (half); sinis′ter (left).

s sample standard deviation.

s^{-1} reciprocal second; ms^{-1} is equivalent to m/s.

$\bar{s}$ [L.] si′ne (without).

Σ the Greek capital letter sigma; used in mathematics to indicate a sum:

$$\sum_{i=1}^{n} x_i = x_1 + x_2 + x_3 + \ldots + x_n.$$

σ sigma, the eighteenth letter of the Greek alphabet; symbol for *standard deviation*.

σ^2 variance.

SA sinoatrial.

S.A. [L.] secun′dum ar′tem (according to art).

SAAG serum-ascites albumin gradient.

Sa•bin vaccine (sa′bin) [Albert Bruce *Sabin*, Polish-born American virologist, 1906–1993] poliovirus vaccine live oral.

Sa•bin-Feld•man syndrome (sa′bin feld′mən) [A.B. *Sabin*; Harry Alfred *Feldman*, American epidemiologist, 1914–1985] see under *syndrome*.

sab•i•nism (sab′ĭ-niz-əm) poisoning by savin.

sab•i•nol (sab′ĭ-nol) a terpene alcohol from the evergreen shrub *Juniperus sabina* which is the chief constituent of savin oil.

Sa•bou•raud dextrose agar (sah-boo-ro′) [Raymond Jacques Adrien *Sabouraud*, French dermatologist, 1864–1938] see under *culture medium*.

Sab•ou•rau•di•tes (sab″oo-ro-di′tēz) *Microsporum*.

Sa•bril (sa′bril) trademark for a preparation of vigabatrin.

sab•u•lous (sab′u-ləs) [L. *sabulosus; sabulum* sand] gritty or sandy.

sa•bur•ra (sə-bur′ə) [L.] foulness of the stomach, mouth, or teeth. **sabur′ral** *adj*

sac (sak) [L. *saccus;* Gr. *sakkos*] a pouch or bag.

abdominal s. the part of the embryonic coelom that develops into the abdominal cavity.

air s. 1. in birds, one of the air-filled cavities connected with the air passages of the lungs and usually with cavities in the bones; they assist in respiration and lower the body's specific gravity. Domestic fowl have one or two unpaired sacs and three symmetrically arranged pairs including cranial, thoracic, and abdominal pairs. 2. *(in the pl.)* sacculi alveolares.

allantoic s. the dilated portion of the allantois which becomes a part of the placenta in many mammals; in humans it becomes the urachus.

alveolar s′s sacculi alveolares.

amniotic s. the sac formed by the amnion, containing the amniotic fluid; popularly known as the *bag of waters*.

anal s. in carnivores, either of two sacs found between the internal and external anal sphincters, lined with sebaceous glands and in some species with apocrine glands.

aneurysmal s. the chamber of a sacculated aneurysm.

aortic s. the homologue in mammalian embryos of the ventral aorta, from which arise the arteries of the pharyngeal arches.

chorionic s. the sac formed by the vertebrate chorion, surrounding the embryo, amniotic cavity, and amniotic sac and contributing to the fetal part of the placenta.

conjunctival s. saccus conjunctivalis.

dental s. a concentric layer of connective tissue in which the enamel organ and dental papilla are embedded, which completely surrounds the developing tooth after the epithelial attachment that connects the enamel organ with the dental lamina disintegrates.

dural s. 1. the portion of the spinal dura mater extending caudally from the level of the first or second lumbar vertebra to the attachment at the filum terminale externum, about the first or second sacral vertebra, and containing the lumbar cistern, cauda equina, cerebrospinal fluid, and filum terminale internum. 2. more broadly, the entire length of the spinal dura mater from the foramen magnum to the attachment at the filum terminale externum; located in the vertebral canal and containing the spinal cord, spinal roots, and the contents of the lumbar cistern.

embryonic s. blastocyst.

enamel s. the enamel organ during the stage in which its outer layer forms a sac enclosing the whole dental germ.

endolymphatic s. saccus endolymphaticus.

gestation s., gestational s. a sac comprising the extraembryonic membranes that envelop the embryo or fetus; in humans, it is formed by the fused amnion and chorion.

greater peritoneal s. the peritoneum of the peritoneal cavity proper.

heart s. pericardium.

hernial s. the pouch of peritoneum enclosing a hernia.

Hilton s. sacculus laryngis.

lacrimal s. saccus lacrimalis.

lesser s., lesser peritoneal s. bursa omentalis.

Lower s′s the bulbus inferior venae jugularis and bulbus superior venae jugularis.

omental s. bursa omentalis.

pericardial s. pericardium.

pleural s. cavitas pleuralis.

serous s. the sac made up of the pleura, pericardium, and peritoneum.

tear s. saccus lacrimalis.

terminal s′s thin-walled dilatations that develop at the ends of the respiratory bronchioles during fetal development; they develop a close relationship with the capillaries and their appearance marks the point at which limited respiration becomes possible. Called also *primitive* or *primordial alveoli* and *terminal saccules*.

vitelline s. yolk s.

yolk s. the extraembryonic membrane that connects with the midgut; formed during the development of higher vertebrates. In human embryos, the yolk sac is formed in the second week of development from the exocoelomic membrane and exocoelomic cavity as the primary yolk sac. As the extraembryonic coelom forms, extraembryonic endodermal cells migrate from the hypoblast inside the primary yolk sac and form a smaller secondary yolk sac, pinching off a large portion of the primary yolk sac, which decreases in size and eventually disappears. In human embryos, the yolk sac contains no yolk and does not serve a primary nutritive function; it is often called the umbilical vesicle. However, it does serve several functions; it is the first hematopoietic organ of the embryo and its vitelline circulation plays an important role in the early embryonic circulation. It is also the site of origin of the primordial germ cells. During organogenesis, the yolk sac provides endodermal cells that form the primordial midgut; lateral folding of the embryo reduces the connection between the midgut and yolk sac to a yolk stalk. The yolk sac shrinks and by 20 weeks is usually undetectable. In marsupial and placental mammals, the yolk sac produces a complete vitelline circulation in the early embryo and then undergoes regression; in oviparous vertebrates, it encloses the yolk mass, breaks down yolk, and makes it available to the developing organism.

sac•brood (sak′brōōd) an infectious disease of the larvae of bees, caused by a virus.

sac•cade (sə-kād′) [Fr. "jerking"] the series of involuntary, abrupt, rapid, small movements or jerks of both eyes simultaneously in changing the point of fixation on a visualized object, such as the series of jumps the

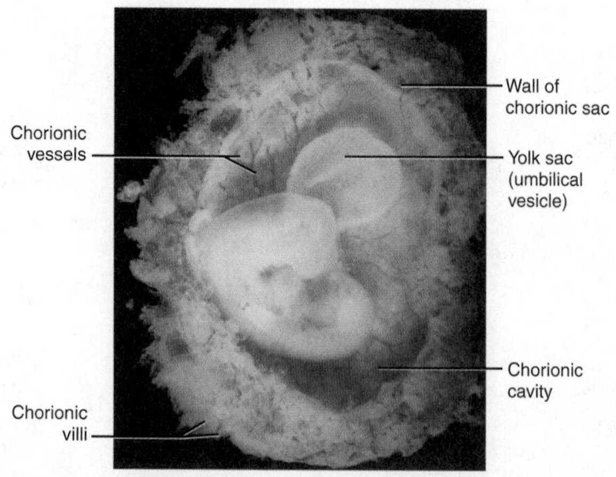

■ Yolk sac of an embryo at Carnegie stage 14, about 32 days.

eyes make in scanning a line of print. See also *saccadic movement* under *movement*. saccad′ic *adj*

sac·cate (sak′āt) [L. *saccatus*] 1. saccular. 2. contained in a sac.

sac·cha·rate (sak′ə-rāt) a salt of a saccharide.

sac·cha·reph·i·dro·sis (sak″ə-ref″ĭ-dro′sis) [*sacchar-* + Gr. *ephidrōsis* sweating] the discharge of sugar in the sweat.

sac·char·ic ac·id (sə-kar′ik) 1. glucaric acid. 2. more generally, any dicarboxylic sugar acid.

sac·cha·ride (sak′ə-rīd) one of a series of carbohydrates, including the sugars. The saccharides are divided into monosaccharides, oligosaccharides, and polysaccharides, according to the number of monosaccharide groups ($C_nH_{2n}O_{n-1}$) composing them.

sac·char·i·fi·ca·tion (sə-kar″ĭ-fĭ-ka′shən) [*sacchar-* + L. + *facere* to make] conversion of starch into sugar.

sac·cha·rim·e·ter (sak″ə-rim′ə-tər) [*sacchar-* + *-meter*] a device for estimating the proportion of sugar in a solution. It may be either a polarimeter, a hydrometer, or a closed container in which the volume of CO_2 produced by fermentation may be assayed.

sac·cha·rin (sak′ə-rin) [NF] a white crystalline compound, several hundred times sweeter than sucrose; used as a sweetening agent in pharmaceutical preparations.

s. calcium [USP] the calcium salt of saccharin, used as a nonnutritive sweetener when sugar is contraindicated.

s. sodium [USP] the sodium salt of saccharin, used like the calcium salt.

sac·cha·rine (sak′ə-rīn) [Gr. *sakcharon* sugar] sugary; having a sweet taste.

sac·char·i·nol (sə-kar′ĭ-nol) saccharin.

sacchar(o)- [Gr. *sakcharon* sugar] a combining form denoting relationship to sugar.

sac·cha·ro·lyt·ic (sak″ə-ro-lit′ik) [*saccharo-* + *-lytic*] capable of breaking the glycosidic bonds in saccharides.

sac·cha·ro·me·tab·o·lism (sak″ə-ro-mə-tab′o-liz-əm) [*saccharo-* + *metabolism*] the metabolism of sugar. **saccharometabol′ic** *adj*

sac·cha·rom·e·ter (sak″ə-rom′ə-tər) saccharimeter.

Sac·cha·ro·mo·no·spo·ra (sak″ə-ro-mon″o-spor′ə) [L. *Saccharum* generic name of sugarcane + *mono-* + Gr. *sporos* seed] a genus of gram-positive bacteria of the family Pseudonocardiaceae, consisting of thermophilic and mesophilic organisms that form a nonfragmenting, branched mycelium and produce aerial hyphae bearing single spores. The type species is *S. vi′ridis*.

S. vi′ridis a thermophilic species occurring in high-temperature habitats such as leaf litter, manure, and compost; it is a significant cause of hypersensitivity pneumonitis.

Sac·cha·ro·my·ces (sak″ə-ro-mi′sēz) [*saccharo-* + Gr. *mykēs* fungus] a genus of yeasts, fungi of the family Saccharomycetaceae. Many species formerly put in this genus have now been classified elsewhere.

S. baya′nus *S. pastorianus.*

S. boular′dii a species that is used as a probiotic in treatment of diarrhea.

S. carlsbergen′sis a species used in microbiological assay in measuring vitamin B_6 in the urine, and in the brewing of beer; it has been implicated in a few cases of mycosis of the stomach.

S. cerevi′siae brewers' yeast or bakers' yeast, a species with oval or spherical cells, used for alcoholic fermentation and leavening in bread; it occasionally causes lung disease.

S. dairen′sis a species with oval or elliptical cells that produces a fermentation in milk; called also *S. galacticolus.*

S. ellipsoi′deus a species that forms elliptical cells that are solitary or in branching chains; it causes alcoholic fermentation in wines.

S. fra′gilis a species that is sometimes part of the normal flora of the human throat and gastrointestinal tract but can also cause opportunistic infection.

S. galacti′colus *S. dairensis.*

S. glu′tinis *Rhodotorula glutinis.*

S. granulomato′sus *Cryptococcus neoformans.*

S. guttula′tus *Saccharomycopsis guttulatus.*

S. mesente′ricus *Candida mesenterica.*

S. mycoder′ma *Candida vini.*

S. neofor′mans *Cryptococcus neoformans.*

S. pastoria′nus a species from fermenting wine and beer; it has been implicated in a few cases of mycosis of the stomach. Called also *S. bayanus.*

sac·cha·ro·my·ces (sak″ə-ro-mi′sēz) pl. *saccharomyce′tes*. An organism of the genus *Saccharomyces.*

Sac·cha·ro·my·ce·ta·ceae (sak″ə-ro-mi″sə-ta′se-e) a family of fungi of the order Endomycetales, including unicellular yeasts that reproduce sexually by formation of ascospores; it includes the genera *Hansenula, Saccharomyces,* and *Saccharomycopsis.*

sac·cha·ro·my·ce·tes (sak″ə-ro-mi-se′tēz) plural of *saccharomyces.*

sac·cha·ro·my·cet·ic (sak″ə-ro-mi-set′ik) pertaining to or due to the presence of saccharomycetes.

sac·cha·ro·my·ce·tol·y·sis (sak″ə-ro-mi″sə-tol′ĭ-sis) [*saccharomycetes* + *-lysis*] the splitting up of saccharomycetes.

Sac·cha·ro·my·cop·sis (sak″ə-ro-mi-kop′sis) a genus of perfect yeasts of the family Saccharomycetaceae. *S. guttula′tus* is found in the intestines of herbivores and can cause enteritis.

sac·cha·ro·pine (sak′ə-ro-pēn″) an intermediate in the metabolism of lysine, formed by condensation of lysine and α-ketoglutarate; it accumulates abnormally in some disorders of lysine degradation.

sac·cha·ro·pine de·hy·dro·gen·ase (sak′ə-ro-pēn″ de-hi′dro-jən-ās) an enzyme activity that catalyzes oxidative cleavage of saccharopine to form α-aminoadipate semialdehyde and glutamate, using NAD^+ as an electron acceptor. The reaction is the second step in the major route of lysine degradation; the enzyme activity is part of the bifunctional enzyme α-aminoadipic semialdehyde synthase (q.v.). Enzyme activity is absent in hyperlysinemia and the variant saccharopinuria. In official nomenclature called *saccharopine dehydrogenase (NAD⁺, L-glutamate-forming).*

sac·cha·ro·pine de·hy·dro·gen·ase (NAD⁺, L-glu·ta·mate-form·ing) (sak′ə-ro-pēn″ de-hi′dro-jən-ās gloo′tə-māt form′ing) [EC 1.5.1.9] official nomenclature for *saccharopine dehydrogenase.*

sac·cha·ro·pine de·hy·dro·gen·ase (NADP⁺, L-ly·sine-form·ing) (sak′ə-ro-pēn″ de-hi′dro-jən-ās li′sēn form′ing) [EC 1.5.1.8] official nomenclature for *lysine-ketoglutarate reductase.*

sac·cha·ro·pin·emia (sak″ə-ro-pĭ-ne′me-ə) an excess of saccharopine in the blood, as in hyperlysinemia or saccharopinuria.

sac·cha·ro·pin·uria (sak″ə-ro-pĭ-nu′re-ə) 1. excretion of saccharopine in the urine. 2. a variant form of hyperlysinemia; it is similarly due to mutation in the *AASS* gene (locus: 7q31.3), which encodes α-aminoadipic semialdehyde synthase, but while the activity of saccharopine dehydrogenase is absent, substantial lysine-ketoglutarate reductase activity is retained. It is clinically similar to hyperlysinemia but with higher urinary saccharopine and lower lysine.

Sac·cha·ro·po·ly·spo·ra (sak″ə-ro-pol″e-spor′ə) [L. *Saccharum* generic name of sugarcane + Gr. *poly* many + *sporos* seed] a genus of bacteria of the family Pseudonocardiaceae, consisting of branching filaments that fragment into rod-shaped elements; organisms are gram-positive, aerobic, and non–acid-fast. The type species is *S. hirsu′ta.*

S. erythrae′a a species that is the source of the antibiotic erythromycin. Formerly called *Streptomyces erythreus.*

S. rectivir′gula a thermophilic species isolated from compost, hay, and grain that is the principal cause of farmer's lung. Formerly called *Micropolyspora faeni.*

Sac·cha·rum (sak′ə-rəm) a genus of plants of the family Gramineae. *S. officina′rum* L. is sugar cane, a major commercial source of sucrose.

sac·ci (sak′si) genitive and plural of *saccus.*

sac·ci·form (sak′sĭ-form) [*saccus* + *form*] saccular.

sac·cu·lar (sak′u-lər) shaped like a bag or sac; called also *saccate* and *sacciform.*

sac·cu·lat·ed (sak′u-lāt″əd) [L. *sacculatus*] having saccules.

sac·cu·la·tion (sak″u-la′shən) 1. the quality of being sacculated, or pursed out with little pouches. 2. sacculus.

s's of colon haustra coli.

sac·cule (sak′ūl) [L. *sacculus*] 1. sacculus. 2. sacculus vestibularis.

air s's, alveolar s's sacculi alveolares.

laryngeal s., s. of larynx sacculus laryngis.

terminal s's see under *sac.*

vestibular s. sacculus vestibularis.

sac·cu·li (sak′u-li) [L.] genitive and plural of *sacculus.*

sac·cu·li·tis (sak″u-li′tis) inflammation of a small sac or saccule.

anal s. inflammation of the anal sacs, usually accompanied by an infection.

sac·cu·lo·coch·le·ar (sak″u-lo-kok′le-ər) pertaining to the sacculus and cochlea.

sac·cu·lus (sak′u-ləs) gen. and pl. *sac′culi* [L., dim. of *saccus*] a little pouch or sac.

sac′culi alveola′res alveolar saccules: the spaces into which the alveolar ducts open distally, and with which the alveoli communicate; called also *alveolar sacs.*

sacculi of Beale tiny pits in the mucous membrane of the common bile duct.

s. laryn′gis [TA] laryngeal saccule: a diverticulum extending upward from the front of the laryngeal ventricle, between the vestibular fold medially and the thyroarytenoid muscle and thyroid cartilage laterally; called also *appendage* or *appendix of ventricle of larynx*, *Hilton sac*, and *laryngeal pouch*.

s. vestibula′ris [TA] saccule: the smaller of the two divisions of the membranous labyrinth within the vestibule; it communicates with the cochlear duct by way of the ductus reuniens.

sac•cus (sak′əs) gen. and pl. *sac′ci* [L., from Gr. *sakkos*] a pouch or bag, or a baglike structure.

s. an′ticus one of the four pouches in the fetal middle ear, later developing into the anterior recess of the tympanic membrane.

s. conjunctiva′lis [TA] conjunctival sac: the potential space, lined by conjunctiva, between the eyelids and the eyeball.

s. endolympha′ticus [TA] endolymphatic sac: the blind, flattened cerebral end of the endolymphatic duct.

s. lacrima′lis [TA] lacrimal sac: the dilated upper end of the nasolacrimal duct.

s. me′dius one of the four pouches in the fetal middle ear, later subdividing to form the epitympanum and the region of the petrous part of the temporal bone.

s. pos′ticus one of the four pouches in the fetal middle ear, later developing into the round window, oval window, and sinus tympani.

s. profun′dus perine′i [TA] deep perineal pouch: the region superior (deep) to the perineal membrane and extending to the pelvic diaphragm; called also *spatium profundum perinei* [TA alternative] and *deep perineal space*.

s. subcuta′neus perine′i [TA] subcutaneous perineal pouch: a potential space between the membranous layer of the perineal subcutaneous tissue and the superficial layer of the fascia of the perineal muscles.

s. supe′rior one of the four pouches in the fetal middle ear, later developing into the posterior recess of the tympanic membrane, part of the mastoid process, and the space below the incus.

SACH solid ankle cushion heel; see under *foot*.

Sachs disease (saks) [Bernard Parney *Sachs*, American neurologist, 1858–1944] see *Tay-Sachs disease*, under *disease*.

sa•crad (sa′krad) toward the sacrum, or sacral aspect.

sa•cral•gia (sa-kral′jə) [*sacr-* + *-algia*] pain in the sacrum.

sa•cral•iza•tion (sa″krəl-ĭ-za′shən) anomalous fusion of the fifth lumbar vertebra to the first segment of the sacrum, so that the sacrum consists of six segments.

sa•crar•thro•gen•ic (sa″krahr-thro-jen′ik) [*sacr-* + *arthro-* + *-genic*] resulting from disease of a sacral joint.

sa•crec•to•my (sa-krek′tə-me) [*sacr-* + *-ectomy*] excision or resection of the sacrum.

sac•ri•fice (sak′rĭ-fīs) to kill an experimental animal.

sacr(o)- [L. *sacrum*, q.v.] a combining form denoting relationship to the sacrum.

sa•cro•an•te•ri•or (sa″kro-an-tēr′e-ər) having the sacrum directed forward; see under *position*.

sa•cro•coc•cy•ge•al (sa″kro-kok-sij′e-əl) pertaining to or located in the region of the sacrum and coccyx.

sa•cro•coc•cyx (sa″kro-kok′siks) the sacrum and coccyx together.

sa•cro•col•po•pexy (sa″kro-kol′po-pek″se) [*sacro-* + *colpopexy*] a surgical procedure, performed transabdominally or laparoscopically, for correction of prolapse of the vaginal vault by securing it to the anterior surface of the sacrum.

sa•cro•cox•al•gia (sa″kro-kok-sal′jə) pain in the sacroiliac joint.

sa•cro•cox•itis (sa″kro-kok-si′tis) [*sacro-* + *coxa* + *-itis*] inflammation of the sacroiliac joint.

sa•cro•dyn•ia (sa″kro-din′e-ə) [*sacro-* + *-odynia*] pain in the sacral region.

sa•cro•il•i•ac (sa″kro-il′e-ak) pertaining to the sacrum and ilium; denoting the joint or articulation between the sacrum and ilium and the ligaments associated therewith.

sa•cro•il•i•itis (sa″kro-il″e-i′tis) inflammation (arthritis) in the sacroiliac joint.

pyogenic s. septic arthritis in the sacroiliac joint.

sa•cro•lis•the•sis (sa″kro-lis-the′sis) the condition in which the sacrum lies anterior to the fifth lumbar vertebra.

sa•cro•lum•bar (sa″kro-lum′bər, -bahr) [*sacro-* + *lumbar*] pertaining to the sacrum and the loin.

sa•cro•peri•ne•al (sa″kro-per″ĭ-ne′əl) pertaining to the sacrum and the perineum.

sa•cro•pos•te•ri•or (sa″kro-pos-tēr′e-ər) having the sacrum directed backward; see under *position*.

sa•cro•prom•on•to•ry (sa″kro-prom′ən-tor-e) the promontory of the sacrum.

sa•cro•sci•at•ic (sa″kro-si-at′ik) pertaining to the sacrum and the ischium.

sac•ro•sid•ase (sak-ro′sĭ-dās) an enzyme derived from yeast that catalyzes the hydrolysis of terminal fructose residues of disaccharides, including sucrose; used as a substitute to replace the sucrase activity lacking in sucrase-isomaltase deficiency, administered orally.

sa•cro•spi•nal (sa″kro-spi′nəl) [*sacro-* + *spinal*] pertaining to the sacrum and the spine, or vertebral column.

sac•ro•spi•nous (sa″kro-spi′nəs) sacrospinal.

sa•crot•o•my (sa-krot′ə-me) [*sacro-* + *-tomy*] the operation of cutting into the lower end of the sacrum.

sa•cro•trans•verse (sa″kro-trans-vərs′) relating to the direction of the fetal sacrum in breech presentation; see under *position*.

sa•cro•uter•ine (sa″kro-u′tər-in) pertaining to the sacrum and the uterus.

sa•cro•ver•te•bral (sa″kro-vur′tə-brəl) pertaining to the sacrum and the vertebral column.

sa•crum (sa′krəm) [L. "sacred"] the triangular bone just below the lumbar vertebrae; see *os sacrum* [TA]. See illustration. **sa′cral** *adj*

assimilation s. see *assimilation pelvis*, under *pelvis*.

scimitar s. a congenitally deformed sacrum shaped like a scimitar, usually accompanied by other defects such as anorectal or neural anomalies.

tilted s. a condition marked by separation of the sacroiliac joint and forward displacement of the sacrum.

sac•to•sal•pinx (sak″to-sal′pinks) [Gr. *saktos* stuffed + *salpinx*] dilatation of the inflamed uterine tube by retained secretions.

SAD seasonal affective disorder.

sad•dle (sad′əl) 1. a support whose shape fits the contour of the object resting upon it. 2. a saddle-shaped structure or part. 3. denture base s.

denture base s. the part of a complete or partial denture that rests on the basal seat and to which the teeth are attached. Called also *saddle*. See also *denture base*, under *base*.

sa•dism (sa′diz-əm, sad′iz-əm) [Comte Donatien Alphonse François, Marquis de *Sade*, French novelist, 1740–1814] the act or instance of gaining pleasure from inflicting physical or psychological pain on another; the term is usually used to denote *sexual s.* **sa′dist** *n* **sadis′tic** *adj*

anal s. in freudian theory, the destructive and aggressive manifestations of anal erotism, such as aggressiveness, selfishness, and stinginess.

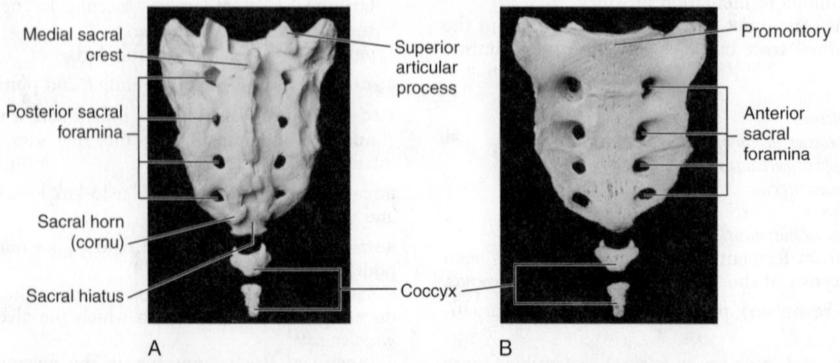

■ Dorsal *(A)* and pelvic *(B)* surfaces of the sacrum and coccyx.

oral s. in freudian theory, a sadistic form of oral erotism manifested by fantasies of chewing, biting, or otherwise using the mouth, lips, or teeth aggressively or destructively.

phallic s. in freudian theory, the aggressive and destructive tendencies associated with the childhood phallic stage of development, stemming from the child's interpretation of sexual intercourse as aggressive and violent.

sexual s. [DSM-IV] a paraphilia in which sexual gratification is derived from hurting, humiliating, or otherwise inflicting physical or psychological suffering on another.

sa•do•ma•so•chism (sa″do-mas′ə-kiz-əm) a state characterized by both sadistic and masochistic tendencies. **sadomas′ochist** *n* **sadomaso-chis′tic** *adj*

SADS Schedule for Affective Disorders and Schizophrenia; sudden adult, arrhythmia, or arrhythmic death syndrome.

Sae•misch operation, ulcer (za′mish) [Edwin Theodor *Saemisch*, German ophthalmologist, 1833–1909] see under *operation*, and see *ulcus serpens corneae.*

Saeng•er sign (reflex) (zāng′er) [Alfred *Saenger*, German neurologist, 1861–1921] see under *sign.*

Saethre-Chot•zen syndrome (sa′trə kot′zən) [Haakon *Saethre*, Norwegian psychiatrist, 1891–1945; Fritz *Chotzen*, German psychiatrist, 1871–1937] Chotzen syndrome.

saf•flow•er (saf′low-ər) *Carthamus tinctorius.*

saf•ra•nin O (saf′rə-nin) a basic red aniline dye used as a nuclear stain and as a counterstain in the Gram method. Spelled also *safranine O.*

saf•role (saf′rol) a methylene ether obtained from sassafras oil, formerly used as an anodyne and flavoring but now restricted because it is carcinogenic.

saf•ro•sin (saf′ro-sin) eosin I bluish.

sage (sāj) *Salvia officinalis*, an herb whose leaves contain a volatile oil and are sudorific, carminative, and astringent; the dried leaves are used as an antisecretory agent in hyperhidrosis, sialorrhea, pharyngitis, and bronchitis.

sag•it•tal (saj′ĭ-təl) [L. *sagittalis; sagitta* arrow] 1. shaped like or resembling an arrow; straight. 2. situated in the plane of the sagittal suture or parallel to it; said of an anteroposterior plane or section parallel to the median plane of the body.

sag•it•ta•lis (saj″ĭ-ta′lis) [TA] sagittal: a general term denoting a structure situated in the plane of or parallel to the sagittal suture.

sa•go (sa′go) a starch mainly derived from the pith of various species of palm, chiefly of the genus *Sagus.*

Sah•li method (zah′le) [Herman *Sahli*, Swiss physician, 1856–1933] acid hematin method.

St. John's wort (sānt jonz wort) [NF] any of various species of the genus *Hypericum; H. perforatum* is the medicinal herb, which is used as a mild antidepressant, sedative, and anxiolytic; it is also used topically for inflammation of the skin, contusions, myalgia, and first-degree burns.

Saint triad (sānt) [Charles Frederick Morris *Saint*, South African radiologist, 20th century] see under *triad.*

Sai•zen (si′zen) trademark for a preparation of somatropin.

Sa•ka•ti-Ny•han syndrome (sah′kah-te ni′han) [Nadia *Sakati*, American pediatrician, 20th century; William Leo *Nyhan*, American pediatrician, born 1926] see under *syndrome.*

Sak•se•naea (sak″sə-ne′ə) a genus of fungi of the family Saksenaeaceae, characterized by coenocytic hyphae and flask-shaped sporangia. *S. vasifor′mis* is a soil saprobe that occasionally causes mucormycosis in immunocompromised or debilitated patients.

Sak•se•naea•ceae (sak″sən-e-a′se-e) a family of fungi of the order Mucorales, having sporangia that may be either lageniform and columellate or lobate and acolumellate; it includes one pathogenic genus, *Saksenaea.*

S.A.L. [L.] secun′dum ar′tis le′ges (according to the rules of art).

sal (sal) [L.] salt.

s. ammoniac ammonium chloride.

s. so′da sodium carbonate.

s. vola′tile ammonium carbonate.

Sala cells (sah′lah) [Luigi *Sala*, Italian zoologist, 1863–1930] see under *cell.*

Sal•a•gen (sal′ə-jən) trademark for a preparation of pilocarpine hydrochloride.

sal•a•man•der (sal″ə-man′dər) [Gr. *salamandra* a kind of lizard] any member of the order Caudata, tailed amphibians often used in experiments.

sal•a•man•drine (sal″ə-man′drēn) a poisonous base from the skin of a species of salamander.

sal•an•tel (sal′ən-təl) a veterinary anthelmintic.

sal•a•zo•sul•fa•pyr•i•dine (sal″ə-zo-sul″fə-pir′ĭ-dēn) sulfasalazine.

sal•bu•ta•mol (sal-bu′tə-mol) INN and BAN for *albuterol.*

Sal•flex (sal′fleks) trademark for preparations of salsalate.

sal•i•cin (sal′ĭ-sin) a precursor of salicylic acid, contained in the bark of the willow (*Salix* spp.) and poplar (*Populus* spp.), that is responsible for the antiinflammatory and antipyretic effects of willow bark.

sal•i•cyl•am•ide (sal″ĭ-səl-am′īd) an amide of salicylic acid used as an analgesic and antipyretic, administered orally.

sal•i•cyl•an•i•lide (sal″ĭ-səl-an′ĭ-līd) any of several compounds usually prepared by the interaction of salicylic acid and aniline; some are anthelmintics and others are topical antifungal agents. See *closantel, niclosamide, oxyclozanide*, and *rafoxanide.*

sal•i•cyl•ate (sal″ĭ-sil′āt, sə-lis′ə-lāt) 1. a salt, anion, or ester of salicylic acid. 2. any of a group of related compounds derived from salicylic acid, such as acetylsalicylic acid (aspirin); such compounds inhibit prostaglandin synthesis and have analgesic, antipyretic, and antiinflammatory activity.

choline s. the choline salt of salicylic acid, used as an analgesic, antipyretic, antiinflammatory, and antirheumatic; administered orally.

choline and magnesium s's choline magnesium trisalicylate; see under *trisalicylate.*

magnesium s. [USP] the magnesium salt of salicylic acid, used as an analgesic, antipyretic, antiinflammatory, and antirheumatic; administered orally.

methyl s. see under *methyl.*

sodium s. [USP] the monosodium salt of salicylic acid, used as an analgesic, antiinflammatory, antipyretic, and antirheumatic; administered orally.

sal•i•cyl•at•ed (sal′ĭ-sil″āt-əd) containing or impregnated with salicylic acid.

sal•i•cyl•azo•sul•fa•pyr•i•dine (sal″ĭ-sil-az″o-sul″fə-pir′ĭ-dēn) sulfasalazine.

sal•i•cyl•emia (sal″ĭ-sə-le′me-ə) [*salicylate* + *-emia*] the presence of salicylate in the blood.

sal•i•cyl•ic ac•id (sal′ĭ-sil′ik) [USP] a substituted benzoic acid derivative, obtained from the bark of the white willow and wintergreen leaves, and also prepared synthetically; it is used as a topical keratolytic and caustic to treat a variety of skin disorders including acne, seborrheic dermatitis of the scalp, plantar warts, and corns; see also *benzoic and salicylic acids ointment*, under *ointment.*

sal•i•cyl•ism (sal′ĭ-sil″iz-əm) the commonly occurring toxic effects of excessive dosage with salicylic acid or its salts, usually marked by tinnitus, nausea, and vomiting.

sal•i•cyl•sul•fon•ic ac•id (sal″ĭ-səl-sul-fon′ik) sulfosalicylic acid.

sal•i•cyl•ur•ic ac•id (sal″ĭ-səl-ūr′ik) the glycine conjugate of salicylic acid, a form in which salicylates are excreted in the urine.

sal•i•fi•a•ble (sal′ĭ-fi″ə-bəl) [*sal* + L. *fieri* to become] capable of combining with acids so as to form salts.

sal•i•fy (sal′ĭ-fi) to convert into a salt.

sa•lim•e•ter (sə-lim′ə-tər) [*sal* + *-meter*] a hydrometer for ascertaining the concentration of saline solutions.

sa•line (sa′lēn, sa′līn) [L. *salinus; sal* salt] salty; of the nature of a salt; containing a salt or salts.

normal s. (NS), physiological s. physiologic saline solution.

sal•i•nom•e•ter (sal″ĭ-nom′ə-tər) an instrument (hydrometer) for direct reading of the salt content of a liquid.

sal•i•no•my•cin (sal″in-o-mi′sin) an antibiotic produced by *Streptomyces albus*; used as a coccidiostat in poultry.

sa•li•va (sə-li′və) [L.] the clear, alkaline, somewhat viscid secretion from the parotid, submaxillary, sublingual, and smaller mucous glands of the mouth. It serves to moisten and soften the food, keeps the mouth moist, and contains α-amylase, a digestive enzyme which converts starch into maltose. The saliva also contains mucin, serum albumin, globulin, leukocytes, epithelial debris, and potassium thiocyanate. Certain toxins frequently occur in it. **sal′ivary** *adj*

artificial s. saliva substitute.

chorda s. submaxillary saliva produced in response to stimulation of the chorda tympani nerve, less viscid and turbid than that of the unstimulated gland.

ganglionic s. saliva obtained by irritating the submaxillary gland.

lingual s. the secretion of Ebner glands and other serous glands of the tongue.

parotid s. saliva produced by the parotid gland; thinner and less viscid than the other varieties.

ropy s. saliva which is highly viscid.

sublingual s. saliva produced by the sublingual gland, the most viscid of all.

submaxillary s. saliva produced by the submaxillary gland.

sympathetic s. submaxillary saliva produced in response to stimulation of its sympathetic nerve supply; more viscid and turbid than that of the unstimulated gland.

sal•i•vant (sal′ĭ-vənt) salivatory.

sa•li•va•ria (sal″ĭ-var′e-ə) in some systems of classification, a subgroup of the genus *Trypanosoma* comprising species whose developmental cycle is completed in the salivary glands (anterior station) of the vector, with transmission by inoculation when the vector bites the definitive host. The group includes the subgenera *Duttonella*, *Nannomonas*, and *Trypanozoon*. Cf. *stercoraria*.

sal•i•var•i•an (sal″ĭ-var′e-ən) pertaining to or caused by trypanosomes of the salivaria group.

sal•i•vate (sal′ĭ-vāt) to produce an excessive flow of saliva.

sal•i•va•tion (sal″ĭ-va′shən) [L. *salivatio*] 1. the secretion of saliva. 2. ptyalism.

sal•i•va•tor (sal′ĭ-va″tər) an agent that causes salivation.

sal•i•va•to•ry (sal′ĭ-və-tor″e) causing salivation.

Sa•lix (sa′liks) [L.] a genus of deciduous shrubs and trees of the family Salicaceae, widespread in temperate and cold regions, having unisexual flowers, usually narrow leaves, and strong, lightweight wood; some species (white willow) are used medicinally.

Salk vaccine (sawk) [Jonas Edward *Salk*, American physician and virologist, 1914–1995] see *poliovirus vaccine inactivated*, under *vaccine*.

Sal•kow•ski test (sahl-kof′ske) [Ernst Leopold *Salkowski*, German physiologic chemist, 1844–1923] see under *test*.

sal•met•er•ol xin•a•fo•ate (sal-met′ər-ol) a β-adrenergic agonist, specific for β_2-adrenergic receptors; administered by inhalation as a bronchodilator for the treatment and prophylaxis of bronchospasm associated with asthma, bronchitis, pulmonary emphysema, or other chronic obstructive airway disease, and the prophylaxis of exercise-induced bronchospasm.

sal•min (sal′min) a toxic substance derived from the sperm of salmon.

Sal•mo•nel•la (sal″mo-nel′ə) [Daniel Elmer *Salmon*, American pathologist, 1850–1914] a genus of gram-negative bacteria of the family Enterobacteriaceae, consisting of non–spore-forming, facultatively anaerobic rods, usually motile with peritrichous flagella. The genus comprises two species, *S. bongori* and *S. enterica*, the latter containing six subspecies, and is separable into over 2400 serovars on the basis of O (somatic), Vi (capsular), and H (flagellar) antigens; O antigens are grouped into serogroups, of which six (A, B, C_1, C_2, D, and E) cause nearly all infections of warm-blooded animals. Pathogenic members are widely distributed in the animal kingdom and cause enteric fevers (typhoid and paratyphoid), septicemia, and gastroenteritis. In reporting *Salmonella* infections, the full taxonomic designation may be abbreviated, so that *S. enterica* subs. *enterica* serovar Typhi can become *Salmonella* serovar Typhi or *Salmonella* Typhi. The type species is *S. ente′rica*.

S. abor′tus e′qui *S. enterica* subsp. *enterica* serovar Abortusequi.

S. abor′tus o′vis *S. enterica* subsp. *enterica* serovar Abortusovis.

S. ago′na *S. enterica* subsp. *enterica* serovar Agona.

S. arizo′nae *S. enterica* subsp. *arizonae*.

S. bon′gori a species isolated mainly from cold-blooded animals and the environment.

S. choleraesu′is *S. enterica* subsp. *enterica* serovar Choleraesuis.

S. dub′lin *S. enterica* subsp. *enterica* serovar Dublin.

S. ente′rica a species containing most of the serovars of *Salmonella*, divided into six subspecies; most infections of warm-blooded animals are caused by the subspecies *S. enterica* subsp. *enterica*.

S. ente′rica **subsp.** *arizo′nae* a subspecies found in reptiles, birds, and domestic animals, and also isolated from dried egg powder and other food sources. Ingestion of contaminated food produces gastroenteritis and salmonellosis, and less often bacteremias and local infections. The organisms may ferment lactose rapidly. Formerly called *S. arizonae*.

S. ente′rica **subsp.** *diarizo′nae* a subspecies biphasic for the H antigen, found in cold-blooded animals and occasionally in persons having contact with such animals; there are more than 300 serovars.

S. ente′rica **subsp.** *ente′rica* a subspecies found mainly in warm-blooded animals, containing multiple biovars, many of which cause diseases such as paratyphoid fever, septicemia, and gastroenteritis.

S. ente′rica **subsp.** *ente′rica* **serovar Abortuse′qui** a group B serovar that causes infectious abortion in mares; not found in other animals. Formerly called *S. abortus equi*.

S. ente′rica **subsp.** *ente′rica* **serovar Abortuso′vis** a group B serovar that causes abortion in sheep; formerly called *S. abortus ovis*.

S. ente′rica **subsp.** *ente′rica* **serovar Ago′na** a group B serovar first isolated in West Africa and later found around the world; formerly called *S. agona*.

S. ente′rica **subsp.** *ente′rica* **serovar Choleraesu′is** a strain pathogenic for many different animals, associated with hog cholera in pigs and paratyphoid fever, gastroenteritis, and septicemia in humans. Formerly called *S. choleraesuis* and *S. suipestifer*.

S. ente′rica **subsp.** *ente′rica* **serovar Dub′lin** a group D serovar frequently isolated from cattle, sheep, and pigs in the United States and northern Europe; it causes septicemia, enteritis, and abortion. Formerly called *S. dublin*.

S. ente′rica **subsp.** *ente′rica* **serovar Enteri′tidis** a group B serovar that frequently causes enteritis in humans; see Salmonella *enteritis*. Formerly called *S. enteritidis*.

S. ente′rica **subsp.** *ente′rica* **serovar Gallina′rum** a group B serovar that causes fowl typhoid; it has little or no pathogenicity for humans. It is nonmotile and contains O antigen but no H antigen. Formerly called *S. gallinarum-pullorum*.

S. ente′rica **subsp.** *ente′rica* **serovar Hei′delberg** a group B serovar frequently isolated from poultry and humans; formerly called *S. heidelberg*.

S. ente′rica **subsp.** *ente′rica* **serovar Litch′field** a group C serovar originally isolated in North America and later found in other parts of the world.

S. ente′rica **subsp.** *ente′rica* **serovar Montevide′o** a group C serovar originally isolated in South America but later found in other parts of the world.

S. ente′rica **subsp.** *ente′rica* **serovar New′port** a group C serovar, one of the most common ones isolated in the United States; formerly called *S. newport*.

S. ente′rica **subsp.** *ente′rica* **serovar Paraty′phi A** a group A serovar that causes mild paratyphoid fever; formerly called *S. paratyphi* and *S. paratyphi A*.

S. ente′rica **subsp.** *ente′rica* **serovar Paraty′phi B** a group B serovar, the most common cause of paratyphoid fever in northern parts of North America and Europe; formerly called *S. paratyphi B* and *S. schottmuelleri*.

S. ente′rica **subsp.** *ente′rica* **serovar Paraty′phi C** a group C serovar that is the most frequent cause of paratyphoid fever in parts of Asia, Africa, and northeastern Europe, and causes other serious diseases in northern South America. Formerly called *S. hirschfeldii* and *S. paratyphi C*.

S. ente′rica **subsp.** *ente′rica* **serovar Saintpaul′** a group B serovar originally isolated in Europe but now found around the world.

S. ente′rica **subsp.** *ente′rica* **serovar Schwar′zengrund** a group B serovar first isolated in Southeast Asia but now found around the world.

S. ente′rica **subsp.** *ente′rica* **serovar Sen′dai** a group D serovar originally isolated in Japan; it causes septicemia and typhoid fever.

S. ente′rica **subsp.** *ente′rica* **serovar Ty′phi** a group D serovar that is a strict parasite of humans, is transmitted by water or food contaminated by human feces, and causes typhoid fever. Strains containing the Vi antigen are designated V strains; those that have partially lost Vi antigen, V-W strains; and those that do not contain Vi antigen, W strains. The species is sometimes subdivided into phage types on the basis of susceptibility to empirically numbered bacteriophages. Formerly called *S. typhi*.

S. ente′rica **subsp.** *ente′rica* **serovar Typhimu′rium** a group B serovar normally found in rats and mice, frequently causing food poisoning and paratyphoid fever in humans in North America and northern Europe. In immunocompromised persons it can cause recurrent fevers and diarrhea. Formerly called *S. typhimurium*.

S. ente′rica **subsp.** *hou′tenae* a subspecies monophasic for the H antigen, found in cold-blooded animals and sometimes in persons having contact with such animals; formerly called *houtenae*.

S. ente′rica **subsp.** *sala′mae* a group D serovar originally isolated in East Africa and now found around the world; formerly called *S. salamae*.

S. enteri′tidis *S. enterica* subsp. *enterica* serovar Enteritidis.

S. gallina′rum-pullo′rum *S. enterica* subsp. *enterica* serovar Gallinarum.

S. hei′delberg *S. enterica* subsp. *enterica* serovar Heidelberg.

S. hirschfel′dii *S. enterica* subsp. *enterica* serovar Paratyphi C.

S. hou′tenae *S. enterica* subsp. *houtenae*.

S. new′port *S. enterica* subsp. *enterica* serovar Newport.

S. paraty′phi *S. enterica* subsp. *enterica* serovar Paratyphi A.

S. paraty′phi A *S. enterica* subsp. *enterica* serovar Paratyphi A.

S. paraty′phi B *S. enterica* subsp. *enterica* serovar Paratyphi B.

S. paraty′phi C *S. enterica* subsp. *enterica* serovar Paratyphi C.

S. pullo′rum *S. enterica* subsp. *enterica* serovar Gallinarum.

S. sala′mae *S. enterica* subsp. *salamae*.

S. schottmuel′leri *S. enterica* subsp. *enterica* serovar Paratyphi B.

S. suipes′tifer *S. enterica* subsp. *enterica* serovar Choleraesuis.

S. ty′phi *S. enterica* subsp. *enterica* serovar Typhi.

S. typhimu′rium *S. enterica* subsp. *enterica* serovar Typhimurium.

sal•mo•nel•la (sal″mo-nel′ə) pl. *salmonel′lae*. A bacterium of the genus *Salmonella*.

sal•mo•nel•lal (sal″mo-nel′əl) caused by salmonellae.

sal•mo•nel•lo•sis (sal″mo-nəl-o′sis) infection with a species of *Salmonella;* in humans it is most often manifested as food poisoning with acute gastroenteritis, vomiting, diarrhea, and occasionally septicemia; typhoid fever and paratyphoid fever are also *Salmonella* infections.

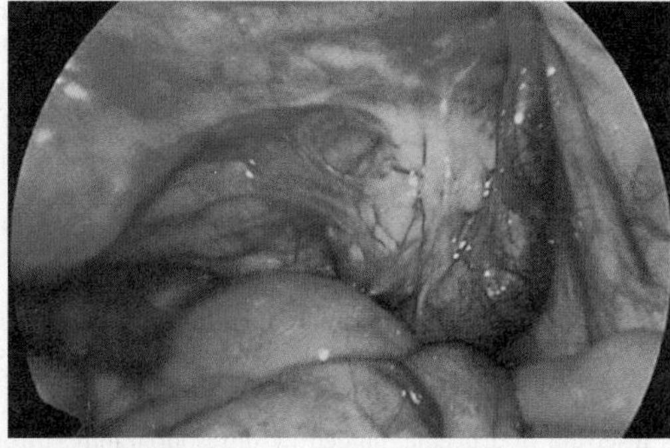

■ Acute salpingitis with dense adhesions that obscure the ovary. Dye has been instilled into the swollen uterine tube on the right *(blue)*.

Recurrent fevers and diarrhea with more serious gastrointestinal symptoms are seen in immunocompromised patients. *Salmonella* infections also cause abortions in horses and sheep and diarrhea and typhus in chickens.

sa·lol (sa′lol) phenyl salicylate.

sal·pin·gec·to·my (sal″pin-jek′tə-me) [*salping-* + *-ectomy*] surgical removal of a uterine tube; called also *tubectomy*.
  abdominal s. salpingectomy done through an incision in the abdomen.

sal·pin·gem·phrax·is (sal″pin-jəm-frak′sis) [*salping-* + *emphraxis*] obstruction of the auditory tube.

sal·pin·gi·an (sal-pin′je-ən) tubal.

sal·pin·gi·on (sal-pin′je-on) a point at the apex of the petrous bone on its lower surface.

sal·pin·git·ic (sal″pin-jit′ik) pertaining to or characterized by salpingitis.

sal·pin·gi·tis (sal″pin-ji′tis) [*salping-* + *-itis*] 1. inflammation of the uterine tube. 2. inflammation of the auditory tube.
  chronic interstitial s. inflammation of the uterine tube associated with infiltration of mucosa, connective tissue, and muscle with lymphocytes and plasma cells.
  eustachian s. salpingitis (def. 2).
  hemorrhagic s. inflammation of the uterine tube associated with rupture of a blood vessel and effusion of blood.
  hypertrophic s. pachysalpingitis.
  s. isth′mica nodo′sa inflammation and nodular thickening of parts of both uterine tubes, usually of the isthmic and proximal ampullary portions; tubal epithelium is found within the myosalpinx or beneath the serosa, resulting from diverticula from the tubal lumen. Called also *nodular s.*
  mural s. pachysalpingitis.
  nodular s. s. isthmica nodosa.
  parenchymatous s. pachysalpingitis.
  s. pro′fluens inflammation of the uterine tube, with accumulation in its lumen of fluid that ultimately escapes.
  pseudofollicular s. inflammation of the uterine tube characterized by agglutination of its walls, causing a formation of saccules.
  purulent s., suppurative s. inflammation of the uterine tube with suppuration; called also *pyosalpingitis*.
  tuberculous s. infection of the uterine tube by the tubercle bacillus, *Mycobacterium tuberculosis*.

salping(o)- [Gr. *salpinx* tube] a combining form denoting relationship to a tube, specifically to the uterine or to the auditory tube.

sal·pin·go·cele (sal-ping′go-sēl) [*salpingo-* + *-cele*[1]] hernial protrusion of a uterine tube.

sal·pin·gog·ra·phy (sal″ping-gog′rə-fe) [*salpingo-* + *-graphy*] radiography of the uterine tubes after the injection of an opaque medium.

sal·pin·gol·y·sis (sal″ping-gol′ĭ-sis) surgical lysis of adhesions involving the uterine tubes.

sal·pin·go-ooph·o·rec·to·my (sal-ping″go-o-of″ə-rek′tə-me) surgical removal of a uterine tube and ovary. Called also *ovariosalpingectomy*, *oophorosalpingectomy*, and *tubo-ovariotomy*.

sal·pin·go-ooph·o·ri·tis (sal-ping″go-o-of″ə-ri′tis) inflammation of a uterine tube and ovary.

sal·pin·go-ooph·oro·cele (sal-ping″go-o-of′ə-ro-sēl) hernia containing a uterine tube and ovary.

sal·pin·go-oo·the·ci·tis (sal-ping″go-o″o-the-si′tis) [*salpingo-* + *oothec-* + *-itis*] salpingo-oophoritis.

sal·pin·go-ovar·i·ec·to·my (sal-ping″go-o-var″e-ek′tə-me) salpingo-oophorectomy.

sal·pin·go-ovar·i·ot·o·my (sal-ping″go-o-var″e-ot′o-me) salpingo-oophorectomy.

sal·pin·go·peri·to·ni·tis (sal-ping″go-per″ĭ-to-ni′tis) inflammation of the peritoneum covering the uterine tube.

sal·pin·go·pexy (sal-ping′go-pek″se) [*salpingo-* + *-pexy*] operative fixation of a uterine tube.

sal·pin·go·pha·ryn·ge·al (sal-ping″go-fə-rin′je-əl) pertaining to the auditory tube and the pharynx.

sal·pin·go·plas·ty (sal-ping′go-plas″te) [*salpingo-* + *-plasty*] plastic repair of a uterine tube; called also *tuboplasty*. **salpingoplas′tic** *adj*

sal·pin·gor·rha·phy (sal″ping-gor′ə-fe) [*salpingo-* + *-rrhaphy*] suture of the uterine tube.

sal·pin·gos·co·py (sal″ping-gos′kə-pe) endoscopic visualization of the uterine tubes via the fimbrial ends of the tubes, the endoscope being inserted into the peritoneal cavity via an incision made for laparoscopy or laparotomy.

sal·pin·go·sto·mat·o·my (sal-ping″go-sto-mat′ə-me) [*salpingo-* + *stoma* + *-tomy*] surgical resection of a portion of the uterine tube, with creation of a new abdominal ostium.

sal·pin·go·sto·mato·plas·ty (sal-ping″go-sto-mat′o-plas″te) salpingostomatomy.

sal·pin·gos·to·my (sal″ping-gos′tə-me) [*salpingo-* + *-stomy*] 1. formation of an opening or fistula into a uterine tube. 2. surgical restoration of the patency of a uterine tube.

sal·pin·got·o·my (sal″ping-got′ə-me) [*salpingo-* + *-tomy*] surgical incision of a uterine tube.
  abdominal s. salpingotomy done through an incision in the abdominal wall.

sal·pin·go·u·re·ter·al (sal-ping″go-u-re′tər-əl) pertaining to or connecting a uterine tube and a ureter.

sal·pinx (sal′pinks) [Gr.] 1. a tube. 2. TA alternative for *tuba uterina*.
  s. auditi′va tuba auditiva.

sal·sa·late (sal′sə-lāt) [USP] a dimer of salicylic acid, which hydrolyzes in vivo to form salicylate; used for treatment of osteoarthritis, rheumatoid arthritis, and related rheumatic disorders, administered orally.

salt (sawlt) [A.S. *sealt*] 1. sodium chloride; common, or table, salt. 2. any compound of a base and an acid; any compound of an acid some of whose replaceable hydrogen atoms have been substituted. 3. *(in the pl.)* saline cathartic.
  acid s. any salt in which the combining power of the acid is not completely exhausted. Cf. *persalt*.
  basic s. any salt with more than the normal proportion of the basic elements.
  bile s's conjugates of glycine or taurine with bile acids, formed in the liver and excreted in the bile; they are powerful detergents that disperse fat globules in the intestine, enabling fats to be digested and absorbed.
  bone s's the crystalline salts deposited in the organic matrix (principally collagen fibers) of bone, composed chiefly of calcium and phosphate.
  buffer s. a salt, such as sodium bicarbonate or sodium phosphate, the anion of which functions as a conjugate base in a buffer system.
  double s. any salt in which the two hydrogen atoms of a dibasic acid have been replaced by two separate metals or basic radicals, as in potassium sodium tartrate.
  Epsom s. magnesium sulfate.
  Glauber s. sodium sulfate.
  halide s., haloid s. any binary compound of a metal or basic radical with a halogen (chlorine, iodine, bromine, or fluorine).
  neutral s., normal s. any salt which is neither acidic nor basic in reaction.
  oral rehydration s's (ORS) [USP] a dry mixture of sodium chloride, potassium chloride, dextrose, and either sodium citrate or sodium bicarbonate; dissolved in water for use in oral rehydration therapy (q.v.).
  Preston s., Rochelle s., Seignette s. potassium sodium tartrate.
  smelling s's aromatized ammonium carbonate: stimulant and restorative.
  Wurster s's the univalent oxidation products of the aromatic *p*-diamines. They are free radicals which may polymerize in a sufficiently concentrated solution and at low temperatures or in the solid state.

sal·ta·tion (sal-ta′shən) [L. *saltatio*, from *saltare* to jump] 1. the action of leaping. 2. the jerky dancing or leaping that sometimes occurs in chorea. 3. saltatory conduction. 4. in genetics, a dramatic and abrupt inherited change in the phenotype of an organism due to a mutation. 5. sudden increases or changes in the course of an illness; called also *saltatory progression*.

sal·ta·to·ri·al (sal″tə-tor′e-əl) saltatory.

sal·ta·to·ry (sal′tə-tor″e) pertaining to or characterized by saltation; see also under *evolution* and *spasm.*

Sal·ter lines (sawl′tər) [Sir Samuel James A. *Salter*, English dentist, 1825–1897] Owen lines; see under *line.*

Sal·ter-Har·ris fracture (sawl′tər har′is) [Robert Bruce *Salter*, Canadian surgeon, born 1924; W. Robert *Harris*, Canadian surgeon, born 1922] see under *fracture.*

salt·ing in (sawl′ting in) dissolving proteins by raising the salt concentration; certain proteins that are insoluble in pure water dissolve when small amounts of neutral salt are added.

salt·ing out (sawl′ting out) precipitation of proteins by raising the salt concentration; any soluble protein will precipitate out of solution if enough neutral salt is added.

sa·lu·bri·ous (sə-loo′bre-əs) [L. *salubris*] conducive to health; wholesome.

sal·ure·sis (sal″u-re′sis) [*sal* + *-uresis*] the excretion of sodium and chloride ions in the urine.

sal·uret·ic (sal″u-ret′ik) 1. pertaining to, characterized by, or promoting saluresis. 2. an agent that promotes saluresis.

sal·u·tary (sal′u-tar″e) [L. *salutaris*] favorable to the preservation or restoration of health.

Sal·u·ten·sin (sal″u-ten′sin) trademark for a combination preparation of hydroflumethiazide and reserpine.

sal·vage (sal′vəj) [Fr.] pertaining to therapeutic measures taken late in the treatment process after other measures have failed. Called also *rescue.*

sal·var·san (sal′vər-sən) arsphenamine.

salve (sav) ointment.

Sal·via (sal′ve-ə) [L.] a genus of plants of the family Labiatae. *S. offici-na′lis* L. is the medicinal herb sage (q.v.). *S. reflex′a* L. is mintweed, an Australian plant rich in nitrates, which can cause fatal nitrite poisoning in ruminants.

Salz·mann nodular corneal dystrophy (zahlts′mahn) [Maximilian *Salzmann*, Austrian-born ophthalmologist in Germany, 1862–1954] see under *dystrophy.*

sam·an·da·rine (sə-man′də-rin) a poisonous alkaloid from the skin of various salamanders.

sa·mar·i·um (Sm) (sə-mar′e-əm) a very rare, metallic element; atomic number, 62; atomic weight, 150.35.

s. 153 a radioactive isotope of samarium, atomic mass 153, having a half life of 46.70 hours and emitting beta particles (0.81, 0.71, 0.64 MeV) and gamma rays (0.103, 0.070 MeV); it has been used in synoviorthesis.

s. Sm 153 lexidronam (Sm 153-EDTMP) [USP] samarium 153 complexed with ethylenediaminetetramethylenephosphonic acid, a bone-seeking diphosphonate complex that concentrates in areas of bone turnover; used in the palliative treatment of patients with osteoblastic metastatic bone lesions, administered intravenously.

Sam·bu·cus (sam-boo′kus) the elders, a genus of flowering berry-producing trees of Europe and North America. The most common species are *S. canaden′sis* L. of North America and *S. ni′gra* L. (Caprifoliaceae). Their berries (elderberries) contain a volatile oil that has been used to treat wounds, burns, and ulcers and as a laxative and diuretic; animals eating large amounts may have toxic reactions and diarrhea.

SAMHSA Substance Abuse and Mental Health Services Agency.

Sam·pao·le·si line (sahm″pah-o-la′se) [Roberto *Sampaolesi*, Argentine ophthalmologist, late 20th century] see under *line.*

sam·ple (sam′pəl) [L. *exemplum* example] 1. a representative part taken to typify the whole. 2. a subset of a population that is selected for inclusion in a research study.

accidental s. convenience s.

cluster s. a variation of a random sample in which the population is divided into groups on the basis of some shared characteristic (such as hospitals grouped by geographic region) and a random sample is drawn from each group.

convenience s. a type of nonprobability sample in which the population selected is easily accessible to the researcher; available subjects are simply entered into the study without any attempt at randomization. Called also *accidental s.*

nonprobability s. a sample in which not every element of the population has an equal chance of being selected, so that the sample is not representative and generalizations cannot be made to the entire population.

probability s. random s.

purposive s. a type of nonprobability sample in which the researcher consciously selects specific elements or subjects for inclusion in order to ensure inclusion of certain characteristics relevant to the study.

quota s. a convenience sample that is adjusted to ensure that certain subgroups are not underrepresented.

random s. a sample chosen from a population in such a way that each choice is independent of the other choices and every member of the population has an equal probability of being chosen.

stratified s. a sample in which the population has been divided into multiple mutually exclusive groups or strata before the sample was chosen; the most common form uses random samples, so that the term is often used to denote a *stratified random s.*

stratified random s. a stratified sample in which random samples are chosen within each stratum. Sometimes called *stratified s.*

sam·pling (sam′pling) the selection or making of a sample.

chorionic villus s. (CVS) a procedure used for prenatal diagnosis at 9 to 12 weeks′ gestation (7 to 10 weeks after fertilization). One method is aspiration of fetal tissue for analysis by catheter through the cervix from the villous chorion (chorion frondosum), under ultrasonic guidance. Another method is insertion of a needle, guided by ultrasonography, through the mother′s abdominal and uterine walls into the uterine cavity. Spelled also *chorionic villous sampling.* Called also *chorionic villus biopsy.*

inferior petrosal sinus s. (IPSS) a test for the cause of Cushing syndrome: catheters are inserted into the inferior petrosal sinuses and venous blood is withdrawn and analyzed for its levels of corticotropin; this is then compared with corticotropin levels in the patient′s peripheral blood. If the ratio of central to peripheral corticotropin is above 3.0, the Cushing syndrome is of central origin *(Cushing disease)*, usually from a pituitary adenoma.

percutaneous umbilical blood s. (PUBS), percutaneous umbilical cord s. cordocentesis.

systematic s. selection of study objects conducted when an ordered list of all members of the population is available; subjects are chosen from the list at a given uniform interval from each other, using a starting point that is selected randomly.

Sam·sca (sam′skə) trademark for a preparation of tolvaptan.

san·a·tive (san′ə-tiv) [L. *sanare* to heal] having a tendency to heal; curative.

san·a·to·ry (san′ə-tor″e) [L. *sanatorius*] salubrious.

Sanc·to·ri·us (sank-to′re-əs) [It. Santorio Santorio, 1561–1636] an Italian physician, professor of medicine at Padua, who devised several instruments of precision (e.g., a clinical thermometer and a pulse clock), and made quantitative experiments on basal metabolism or "insensible perspiration."

sanc·tu·ary (sangk′choo̅-ar″e) an area in the body where a drug tends to collect and to escape metabolic breakdown.

sand (sand) small, gritty particles, usually of some mineral such as silica.

brain s. corpora arenacea.

hydatid s. sediment that floats freely in the fluid of a hydatid cyst after rupture of brood capsules, consisting of scolices and cellular debris.

sand·crack (sand′krak) see under *crack.*

San·ders disease (san′dərz) [Murray *Sanders*, American bacteriologist, 20th century] epidemic keratoconjunctivitis.

sand·fly (sand′fli) 1. any of various two-winged flies of the families Heleidae, Simuliidae, and Psychodidae. 2. more specifically, any fly of the genus *Phlebotomus.*

Sand·hoff disease (zahnd′hof) [K. *Sandhoff*, German biochemist, 20th century] see under *disease.*

San·di·fer syndrome (san′dĭ-fər) [Paul *Sandifer*, British radiologist, 20th century] see under *syndrome.*

Sand·im·mune (san′dim-ūn) trademark for preparations of cyclosporine.

San·do·glob·u·lin (san″do-glob′u-lin) trademark for a preparation of immune globulin intravenous (human).

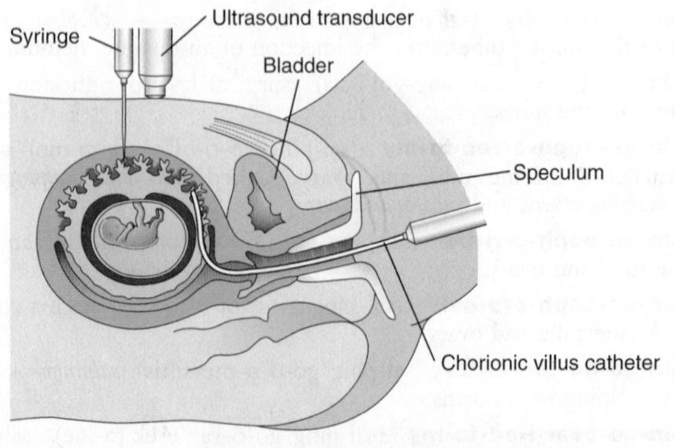

■ Chorionic villus sampling.

San•do•sta•tin (san′do-stat″in) trademark for preparations of octreotide acetate.

Sand•with bald tongue (sand′with) [Fleming Mant *Sandwith*, British physician, 1853–1918] see under *tongue.*

sane (sān) [L. *sanus*] of sound mind; compos mentis.

San•fi•lip•po syndrome (san-fĭ-lip′o) [Sylvester J. *Sanfilippo*, American pediatrician, 20th century] see under *syndrome.*

Sän•ger see *Saenger.*

sangui- [L. *sanguis* blood] a combining form denoting relationship to blood; see also terms beginning with *hemat(o)-* and *hem(o)-*.

san•guic•o•lous (sang-gwik′ə-ləs) [*sangui-* + L. *colere* to dwell] inhabiting or living in the blood.

san•guif•er•ous (sang-gwif′ər-əs) [*sangui-* + *-ferous*] 1. containing blood. 2. circulatory (def. 3).

san•gui•na•rine (sang″gwĭ-na′rēn) an alkaloid obtained from *Argemone mexicana* and related species; see also *epidemic dropsy*, under *dropsy.*

san•guin•e•ous (sang-gwin′e-əs) pertaining to or containing blood; bloody.

san•guin•o•lent (sang-gwin′ə-lənt) [L. *sanguinolentus*] of a bloody tinge.

san•gui•no•pu•ru•lent (sang″gwĭ-no-pu′roo-lənt) containing both blood and pus.

san•gui•nous (sang′gwi-nəs) sanguineous.

san•guis (sang′gwis) [L.] TA alternative for *haema;* see *blood.*

san•guiv•o•rous (sang-gwiv′ə-rəs) hematophagous.

sa•ni•es (sa′ne-ēz) [L.] a fetid discharge from a wound or ulcer, containing serum, pus, and blood. **sa′nious** *adj*

san•i•tar•i•an (san″ĭ-tar′e-ən) a person who is expert in matters of sanitation and public health.

san•i•tar•i•um (san″ĭ-tar′e-əm) [L.] an institution for the promotion of health. The word was originally coined to designate the institution established by the Seventh Day Adventists at Battle Creek, Michigan, to distinguish it from institutions providing care for mental or tuberculous patients.

san•i•tary (san′ĭ-tar″e) [L. *sanitarius*] pertaining to health or promoting or conducive to health; usually used in reference to an environment that is clean, i.e., without an agent that is deleterious to health.

san•i•ta•tion (san″ĭ-ta′shən) [L. *sanitas* health] the establishment of environmental conditions favorable to health.

san•i•ti•za•tion (san″ĭ-tĭ-za′shən) the process of making or the quality of being made sanitary; see *sanitize.*

san•i•tize (san′ĭ-tīz) to clean and sterilize, as eating or drinking utensils.

san•i•ty (san′ĭ-te) [L. *sanitas* soundness] soundness, especially soundness of mind.

San Joa•quin Val•ley fever (disease) (san′ wah-kēn′ val′e) [*San Joaquin Valley*, California, where the disease is particularly prominent] primary coccidioidomycosis.

San•o•rex (san′ə-reks) trademark for a preparation of mazindol.

San•sert (san′sərt) trademark for a preparation of methysergide maleate.

San•som sign (san′səm) [Arthur Ernest *Sansom*, English physician, 1838–1907] see under *sign.*

San•son images (sah-saw′) [Louis Joseph *Sanson*, French physician, 1790–1841] Purkinje-Sanson mirror images; see under *image.*

San•ta•vuo•ri disease (syndrome) (sahn″tah-vwo′re) [Pirkko *Santavuori*, Finnish physician, 20th century] Haltia-Santavuori disease; see under *disease.*

San•ta•vuo•ri-Hal•tia disease (syndrome) (sahn″tah-vwo′re hahl′te-ah) [P. *Santavuori;* M. *Haltia*, Finnish physician, 20th century] Haltia-Santavuori disease; see under *disease.*

San•to•ri•ni cartilage, etc. (sahn″to-re′ne) [Giovanni Domenico *Santorini*, Italian anatomist, 1681–1737] see *cartilago corniculata, ductus pancreaticus accessorius, ligamentum cricopharyngeum, musculus risorius, papilla duodeni major, plexus prostaticus*, and *tuberculum corniculatum.*

SAP sphingolipid activator protein (or saposin).

sap (sap) the natural juice of a living organism or tissue.
cell s. cytosol.

sa•phe•na (sə-fe′nə) [L., from Gr. *saphēnēs* manifest] any of the three venae saphenae; see entries beginning *vena saphena.* **saphe′nous** *adj*

saph•e•nec•to•my (saf″ə-nek′tə-me) [*saphena* + *-ectomy*] excision of a saphenous vein.

saph•en•og•ra•phy (saf″ən-og′rə-fe) phlebography of the great saphenous vein after injection of contrast medium at the ankle.

sap•id (sap′id) [L. *sapidus*] having or imparting an agreeable taste.

sa•po (sa′po) [L. "soap"] soap.

sa•pog•e•nin (sə-poj′ə-nin) a compound resulting from the decomposition of saponin.

sa•po•na•ceous (sap″o-na′shəs) [L. *sapo* soap] of a soapy quality or nature.

Sa•po•na•ria (sa″po-nar′e-ə) a genus of plants of the family Caryophyllaceae. *S. officina′lis* is soapwort, whose root contains saponin and sapotoxin and was formerly used in skin diseases; livestock eating the plant may get enteritis with diarrhea.

sa•pon•i•fi•a•ble (sə-pon″ĭ-fi′ə-bəl) capable of being hydrolyzed to give a fatty acid salt and an alcohol; said of lipids.

sa•pon•i•fi•ca•tion (sə-pon″ĭ-fĭ-ka′shən) [L. *sapo* soap + *facere* to make] hydrolysis of an ester by an alkali, resulting in the production of a free alcohol and an alkali salt of the ester acid; originally, the act or process of converting fats into soaps and glycerol by heating with alkalis.

sa•pon•i•fy (sə-pon′ĭ-fi) 1. to produce saponification. 2. to undergo saponification.

sap•o•nin (sap′o-nin) any of a group of glycosides found in plants such as *Quillaja saponaria* and *Saponaria officinalis;* they form a durable foam when their watery solutions are shaken and even in high dilutions can dissolve red blood cells. Their aglycon is sapogenin.
cholan s's a group of saponins that on hydrolysis yield sterol-like compounds.
triterpenoid s's a group of saponins that on hydrolysis yield 1,2,7-trimethyl naphthalene.

sap•o•phore (sap′o-for) [L. *sapor* taste + *-phore*] the group of atoms in the molecule of a compound that gives the substance its characteristic taste.

sap•o•sin (SAP) (sap′ə-sin) any of four homologous glycoproteins, designated A through D, cleaved from the precursor prosaposin and belonging to the group of sphingolipid activator proteins; each stimulates lysosomal hydrolysis of specific glycosphingolipids by one or more acid hydrolases. Deficiency of SAP-B causes a variant form of metachromatic leukodystrophy, and deficiency of SAP-C is a cause of Gaucher disease.

sa•po•tox•in (sa′po-tok″sin) any of various toxic saponins found in such plants as *Agave lechuguilla, Phytolacca americana, Quillaja saponaria*, and *Saponaria officinalis.* Livestock consuming these plants may suffer from enteritis or gastroenteritis with diarrhea that can be fatal.

Sapo•vi•rus (sap′o-vi″rəs) a genus of viruses of the family Caliciviridae that cause self-limited, acute foodborne gastroenteritis; called also *Sapporo-like virus.*

Sap•pey fibers, ligament, veins (sah-pa′) [Marie Philibert Constant *Sappey*, French anatomist, 1810–1896] see under *fiber* and *ligament*, and see *venae paraumbilicales.*

sap•phism (saf′iz-əm) [*Sappho*, Greek poetess, about 600 B.C.] homosexuality between women; lesbianism.

Sap•pin•ia (să-pin′e-ə) a genus of free-living amebae that usually live in the soil, but have occasionally been found in cases of granulomatous amebic encephalitis; the most common species is *S. diploi′dea.*

sapr(o)- [Gr. *sapros* rotten] a combining form meaning rotten or putrid, or designating relationship to decay or to decaying material.

sap•robe (sap′rōb) [*sapro-* + Gr. *bios* life] an organism, usually referring to a fungus, that feeds on dead or decaying organic matter. Cf. *saprophyte.* **sapro′bic** *adj*

Sap•ro•leg•nia (sap″ro-leg′ne-ə) [*sapro-* + Gr. *legnon* border] a genus of partially saprobic aquatic chromists of the order Saprolegniales; they can cause parasitic disease in fish and amphibians.

Sap•ro•leg•ni•a•les (sap″ro-leg″ne-a′lēz) an order of mostly saprobic funguslike chromists of the subclass Saprolegniomycetidae (class Oomycetes), having an extensive mycelial thallus without cross walls. Genera include *Saprolegnia* and *Achlya.*

Sap•ro•leg•nio•my•ce•ti•dae (sap″ro-leg″ne-o-mi-set′ĭ-de) a subclass of the class Oomycetes; it includes the orders Salprolegniales and Pythiales.

sap•ro•no•sis (sap″ro-no′sis) a disease caused by organisms of the environment.

sa•proph•i•lous (sə-prof′ĭ-ləs) [*sapro-* + *-phil* + *-ous*] saprophytic.

sap•ro•phyte (sap′ro-fīt) [*sapro-* + *-phyte*] an organism that lives on dead or decaying plant or animal material; said especially of plants or so-called plantlike organisms, such as certain protozoa and bacteria. Fungi with this characteristic are called *saprobes.* See also *autophyte* and *saprozoic.*

sap·ro·phyt·ic (sap″ro-fit′ik) 1. pertaining to or of the nature of a saprophyte. 2. saprozoic.

sap·ro·zo·ic (sap″ro-zo′ik) [*sapro-* + *zoic*] having a type of nutrition involving uptake of organic materials in dissolved form obtained from dead or decaying plant or animal matter; said of animals or so-called animal-like organisms (e.g., certain protozoa). Called also *saprophytic*. Cf. *holozoic* and *saprophytic*.

sa·quin·a·vir (sə-kwin′ə-vir) [USP] an HIV protease inhibitor that causes formation of immature, noninfectious viral particles; used in the treatment of human immunodeficiency virus infection and acquired immunodeficiency syndrome; administered orally.

s. mesylate [USP] the mesylate salt of saquinavir, having the same actions and uses as the base; administered orally.

Sar·a·fem (sār′ə-fem) trademark for preparations of fluoxetine hydrochloride.

sar·al·a·sin ac·e·tate (sə-ral′ə-sin) an angiotensin II receptor antagonist, which has been used as an antihypertensive in the treatment of severe hypertension and in the diagnosis of renin-dependent hypertension.

Sar·ci·na (sahr′sĭ-nə) [L. "package," "bundle"] a genus of spherical, gram-positive bacteria of the family Clostridiaceae, occurring in cubical packets of eight or more cells, formed by division in three perpendicular planes; organisms are nonmotile, strictly anaerobic, and chemo-organotrophic, with a fermentative metabolism. They are common soil inhabitants and are found on cereal grains and in the digestive tracts of animals and occasionally in clinical specimens. The type species is *S. ventri′culi*.

sar·ci·na (sahr′sĭ-nə) pl. *sar′cinae*. 1. A spherical bacterium occurring predominantly in cubical packets of eight cells as a consequence of failure of daughter cells to separate following cell division in three planes. 2. an organism of the genus *Sarcina*.

sarc(o)- [Gr. *sarx, sarkos* flesh] a combining form denoting relationship to flesh.

sar·co·blast (sahr′ko-blast) [*sarco-* + *-blast*] myoblast.

sar·co·car·ci·no·ma (sahr″ko-kahr″sĭ-no′mə) carcinosarcoma.

sar·co·cele (sahr′ko-sēl) [*sarco-* + *-cele*[1]] any fleshy swelling or tumor of the testis.

sar·co·cyst (sahr′ko-sist) [*sarco-* + *cyst*] 1. a protozoan of the genus *Sarcocystis*. 2. one of the elongated, cylindrical, membrane-bound hyaline bodies of the protozoan *Sarcocystis*, containing the trophozoites known as Rainey corpuscles; they are found in the muscles of individuals with sarcocystosis.

sar·co·cys·tin (sahr″ko-sis′tin) a toxin obtained from species of *Sarcocystis*.

Sar·co·cys·tis (sahr″ko-sis′tis) [*sarco-* + Gr. *kystis* bladder] a genus of coccidian protozoa (suborder Eimeriina, order Eucoccidiida) that are parasitic in birds, reptiles, and mammals and occur as elongated cylindrical bodies called sarcocysts in the host's muscles. They have an obligatory two-host life cycle, with sexual reproduction in the definitive host (a carnivore) and asexual reproduction, including schizogony and sarcocyst formation. Infection of the definitive host is usually the result of eating meat of an infected animal; infection of the intermediate host occurs when these animals accidentally ingest sarcocysts from feces contaminating their food supply. See also *sarcocystosis*.

S. boviho′minis a species for which cattle are the specific intermediate hosts and humans the definitive hosts; it causes intestinal sarcocystosis in humans. Together with *S. suihominis*, formerly considered to be a single species, *S. hominis*.

S. ho′minis see *S. bovihominis* and *S. suihominis*.

S. lindeman′ni former name for a species causing human infection, which was found to be a combination of other species.

S. suiho′minis a species for which pigs are the specific intermediate hosts and humans the definitive hosts; it causes intestinal sarcocystosis in humans. Together with *S. bovihominis*, formerly considered to be a single genus, *S. hominis*.

sar·co·cys·to·sis (sahr″ko-sis-to′sis) infection with protozoa of the genus *Sarcocystis*, which in humans is usually asymptomatic or manifested either by muscle cysts associated with myositis or myocarditis or by intestinal infection. It is usually transmitted by the eating of raw or undercooked beef or pork containing sporocysts of the parasites or by ingestion of sporocysts from the feces of an infected animal, usually in contaminated soil. Heavy infections in cattle and other animals may be associated with anorexia, emaciation, fever, nervousness, lameness, hypersalivation, anemia, and abortion. Called also *sarcosporidiasis* and *sarcosporidiosis*.

Sar·co·di·na (sahr″ko-di′nə) [Gr. *sarkōdēs* fleshlike] in older classifications of protozoa, a subphylum of the phylum Sarcomastigophora, including those organisms that alter their body shape and move about and acquire food by extension of pseudopodia (cytoplasmic organelles of various types), or by protoplasmic flow without discrete pseudopodia. Some have flagella during certain stages. The body of some sarcodines is naked, while in others an external or internal test or skeleton is present.

sar·co·dine (sahr′ko-dīn) 1. pertaining to the subphylum Sarcodina. 2. any individual protozoan of the subphylum Sarcodina. Called also *sarcodinian*.

sar·co·din·i·an (sahr″ko-din′e-ən) sarcodine.

sar·co·gen·ic (sahr″ko-jen′ik) [*sarco-* + *-genic*] forming muscle.

sar·co·gly·can (sahr″ko-gli′kan) any of a family of transmembrane glycoproteins of the sarcolemma, constituting a subcomplex of the dystrophin-glycoprotein complex that associates with dystrophin and mediates muscle membrane stability. It includes α-, β-, γ-, δ-, ε-, and ζ-sarcoglycans, with the α- form being the most common. Mutations in sarcoglycans have been linked to various types of muscular dystrophy and cardiomyopathy.

sar·co·gly·ca·nop·a·thy (sahr″ko-gli″kə-nop′ə-the) a general term encompassing the types of limb-girdle muscular dystrophy that are caused by mutations in the genes coding for sarcoglycans α, β, γ, and δ.

sar·coid (sahr′koid) [*sarc-* + *-oid*] 1. sarcoidosis. 2. a sarcomalike tumor. 3. fleshlike.

Boeck s. sarcoidosis.

Darier-Roussy s. a form of sarcoidosis characterized by large nodules in a subcutaneous location.

equine s. a common wartlike benign cutaneous tumor of horses, caused by an unidentified virus.

Schaumann s. sarcoidosis.

Spiegler-Fendt s. cutaneous lymphoid hyperplasia; see under *hyperplasia*.

sar·coi·do·sis (sahr″koi-do′sis) [*sarcoid* + *-osis*] a chronic, progressive, systemic granulomatous reticulosis of unknown etiology, characterized by hard tubercles (q.v.). It can affect almost any organ or tissue, including the skin, lungs, lymph nodes, liver, spleen, eyes, and small bones of the hands and feet. Laboratory findings may include hypercalcemia and hypergammaglobulinemia. There is usually low or absent reactivity to tuberculin, and in active cases the Kveim test is positive. Called also *sarcoid*, *Besnier-Boeck disease*, *Boeck disease* or *sarcoid*, and *Schaumann disease*, *sarcoid*, or *syndrome*.

acute s. types having an abrupt onset and a high rate of spontaneous remission.

cardiac s. involvement of the heart in sarcoidosis, with lesions ranging from a few asymptomatic, microscopic granulomas to widespread infiltration of the myocardium by large masses of sarcoid tissue, often leading to arrhythmias, heart block, mitral regurgitation, or sudden death.

chronic s. types having an insidious onset and slow development.

muscular s. sarcoidosis involving the skeletal muscles, with sarcoid tubercles, interstitial inflammation with fibrosis, and disruption and atrophy of the muscle fibers.

sar·co·lem·ma (sahr″ko-lem′ə) [*sarco-* + *-lemma*] the delicate plasma membrane which invests every striated muscle fiber. **sarcolem′mic**, **sarcolem′mous** *adj*

L-sar·co·ly·sin (sahr″ko-li′sin) melphalan.

sar·co·ma (sahr-ko′mə) pl. *sarcomas, sarco′mata* [*sarc-* + *-oma*] any of a group of tumors usually arising from connective tissue, although the term now includes some of epithelial origin; most are malignant. Many types have prefixes denoting the type of tissue or structure involved; see *chondrosarcoma, fibrosarcoma, lymphosarcoma, myxosarcoma, osteosarcoma, rhabdomyosarcoma*, and so on. **sarco′matous** *adj*

adipose s. liposarcoma.

alveolar soft part s. a well-circumscribed, slow growing, painless, highly metastatic malignant neoplasm of unknown cell origin, characterized

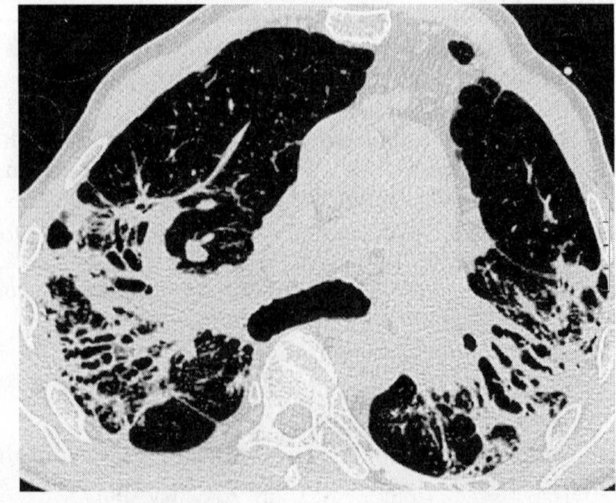

■ Sarcoidosis. High resolution CT scan shows areas of conglomerate fibrosis in a perihilar distribution with associated bronchial distortion and volume loss.

by a distinctive alveolar pattern, usually seen on the limbs, head, or neck of young adults.

ameloblastic s. see under *fibrosarcoma.*

avian s. any of a group of rare sarcomas of fowls, transmitted by retroviruses related to avian leukosis virus; the earliest known one was the Rous sarcoma. Called also *chicken s.*

botryoid s., s. botryoi′des a variety of embryonal rhabdomyosarcoma, arising in submucosal tissue, presenting grossly as a polypoid grapelike structure, and found most often in young children or infants in the upper vagina, cervix uteri, or neck of the urinary bladder.

chicken s. avian s.

chloromatous s. chloroma.

chondroblastic s. the chondroblastic form of osteosarcoma.

clear cell s. of kidney a malignant kidney tumor similar to Wilms tumor but with a poorer prognosis; its cells have pale or clear cytoplasm and are arranged uniformly in vascularized nests. It often metastasizes to bone.

embryonal s. Wilms tumor.

endometrial stromal s. a pale, polypoid, fleshy, malignant tumor of the endometrial stroma, usually arising from the uterine fundus.

epithelioid s. a rare, frequently metastatic tumor consisting of lobulated masses of spindle cells and epithelioid cells surrounding a necrotic center; it usually arises in the deep soft tissues of the distal limbs of young adults, particularly males.

Ewing s. a highly malignant, metastatic, primary tumor of bone, closely related to a primitive neuroectodermal tumor; it is usually found in the diaphyses of long bones, ribs, or flat bones of children or adolescents. Characteristics include saucerization of the cortex, patchy, permeative destruction, and often a large soft tissue mass; the most common symptoms include pain, swelling, leukocytosis, and fever. Called also *Ewing tumor.*

fascial s. a sarcoma arising in the fasciae about the joints, especially in the lower limbs.

fibroblastic s. the fibroblastic form of osteosarcoma.

fowl s. chicken s.

giant cell s. 1. a form of giant cell tumor of bone (q.v.) that arises malignant de novo, rather than transforming to malignancy. 2. sarcoma characterized by large anaplastic (giant) cells.

granulocytic s. chloroma.

hemangioendothelial s. hemangiosarcoma.

Hodgkin s. Hodgkin disease, lymphocyte depletion type.

idiopathic multiple pigmented hemorrhagic s. Kaposi s.

immunoblastic s. of B cells large cell, immunoblastic lymphoma composed predominantly of B cells.

immunoblastic s. of T cells large cell, immunoblastic lymphoma made up predominantly of T cells.

Jensen s. a malignant tumor in mice transmissible to healthy mice by transplanting a small portion of the tumor. Called also *Jensen tumor.*

Kaposi s. a multicentric, malignant neoplastic vascular proliferation characterized by bluish-red cutaneous nodules, usually on the lower limbs, that slowly increase in size and number and spread to more proximal sites. The tumors have endothelium-lined channels and vascular spaces mixed with aggregates of spindle-shaped cells; they may remain confined to skin and subcutaneous tissue, but widespread visceral involvement may occur. The condition is endemic in certain parts of Central Africa and Central and Eastern Europe, and a virulent and disseminated form occurs in immunocompromised patients. It is caused by human herpesvirus 8. Called also *multiple idiopathic hemorrhagic s.* and *idiopathic multiple pigmented hemorrhagic s.*

Kupffer cell s. hepatic angiosarcoma.

lymphatic s. diffuse lymphoma.

melanotic s. malignant melanoma.

mixed cell s. malignant mesenchymoma.

multiple idiopathic hemorrhagic s. Kaposi s.

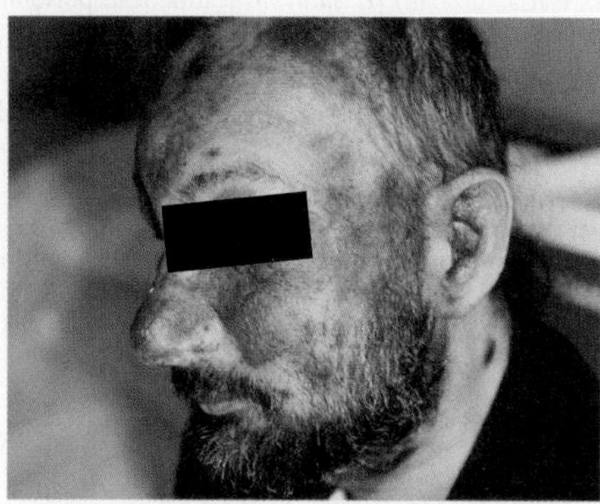

■ Kaposi sarcoma.

multipotential primary s. of bone small-cell osteosarcoma.

neurogenic s. malignant peripheral nerve sheath tumor.

osteoblastic s. the osteoblastic form of osteosarcoma.

osteogenic s. osteosarcoma.

parosteal s. see under *osteosarcoma.*

polymorphous s. malignant mesenchymoma.

pseudo–Kaposi s. unilateral subacute to chronic dermatitis, often with postinflammatory hyperpigmentation, occurring in association with underlying arteriovenous fistula, which closely resembles Kaposi sarcoma both clinically and histologically.

reticulum cell s. histiocytic lymphoma.

reticulum cell s. of the brain former name for *primary central nervous system lymphoma.*

Rous s. a type of avian sarcoma transmitted by a retrovirus; it metastasizes freely and is sometimes highly lethal. Experimental inoculation into other fowl produces similar growths. This was the first sarcoma known to be caused by a virus.

soft tissue s. a general term for a malignant tumor derived from extraskeletal connective tissue, including fibrous, fat, smooth muscle, nerve, vascular, histiocytic, and synovial tissue, with almost all lesions originating from primitive mesoderm. Tumors arising in Schwann cells are also included.

spindle cell s. 1. any sarcoma composed of spindle-shaped cells; cf. *rhabdomyosarcoma.* 2. a type of soft tissue sarcoma whose cells are spindle-shaped; it is usually resistant to radiation therapy and may be of either high or low grade malignancy.

synovial s. synoviosarcoma.

telangiectatic s. a sarcoma that develops a rich vascular network; the endothelial cells may be mistaken for the neoplastic element.

sar·co·ma·gen·ic (sahr″ko-mə-jen′ik) causing sarcoma. See also *cancerigenic.*

Sar·co·mas·ti·goph·o·ra (sahr″ko-mas″tĭ-gof′ə-rə) [*sarco-* + Gr. *mastix* whip + *phoros* bearing] a phylum comprising protozoa that typically possess an endosome nucleus characterized by a ring of nuclear chromatin around a central chromatin-free region, and are motile by means of flagella, pseudopodia, or both types of locomotor organs. The phylum is sometimes divided into subphyla Mastigophora (the flagellates), Sarcodina (the amebae), and Opalinata (the opalinids).

sar·co·ma·ta (sahr-ko′mə-tə) plural of *sarcoma.*

sar·co·ma·toid (sahr-ko′mə-toid) resembling sarcoma.

sar·co·ma·to·sis (sahr″ko-mə-to′sis) a condition characterized by the formation of sarcomas.

sar·co·mere (sahr′ko-mēr) [*sarco-* + *-mere*] the contractile unit of myofibrils; sarcomeres are repeating units, delimited by the Z bands along the length of the myofibril. See Plate 32.

sar·co·neme (sahr′ko-nēm) [*sarco-* + Gr. *nēma* thread] microneme.

sar·co·pe·nia (sahr″ko-pe′ne-ə) [*sarco-* + *-penia*] age-related reduction in skeletal muscle mass in the elderly.

Sar·coph·a·ga (sahr-kof′ə-gə) [*sarco-* + Gr. *phagein* to eat] a genus of gray flesh flies of the family Sarcophagidae. The larvae of several species have been found in wounds, ulcers, and nasal passages of animals. The most important species is *S. haemorrhoida′lis.* Other species are *S. carna′ria, S. dux, S. fuscicau′da, S. nificor′nis,* and *S. rubicor′nis.*

Sar·co·phag·i·dae (sahr″ko-faj′ĭ-de) the flesh flies, a family of insects of the order Diptera; genera *Sarcophaga* (type genus) and *Wohlfahrtia* cause myiasis. **sarcoph′agid** *adj*

sar·co·plasm (sahr′ko-plaz″əm) [*sarco-* + *-plasm*] the interfibrillary matter of the striated muscles; the substance in which the fibrillae of the muscle fiber are embedded. **sarcoplas′mic** *adj*

sar·co·plast (sahr′ko-plast) [*sarco-* + *-plast*] an interstitial cell of a muscle, itself capable of being transformed into a muscle.

sar·co·poi·et·ic (sahr″ko-poi-et′ik) [*sarco-* + Gr. *poiein* to make] producing flesh or muscle.

Sar·cop·syl·la (sahr″kop-sil′ə) *Tunga.*

Sar·cop·tes (sahr-kop′tēz) [*sarco-* + Gr. *koptein* to cut] a genus of mites of the family Sarcoptidae. *S. scabie′i* is the scabies or itch mite of humans, which causes scabies. Varieties of the same species cause mange in other animals.

sar·cop·tic (sahr-kop′tik) of, relating to, or caused by *Sarcoptes.*

Sar·cop·ti·dae (sahr-kop′tĭ-de) a family of acarid mites; genera of medical and veterinary interest include *Notoedres* and *Sarcoptes.*

sar·cop·ti·do·sis (sahr-kop″tĭ-do′sis) infestation with *Sarcoptes.*

sar·co·sine (sahr′ko-sēn) an amino acid occurring as an intermediate in the metabolism of choline in the kidney and liver; it is normally not detectable in human blood or urine.

sar·co·sine de·hy·dro·gen·ase (sahr′ko-sēn de-hi′dro-jən-ās) [EC 1.5.99.1] a mitochondrial enzyme of the oxidoreductase class that catalyzes the oxidative demethylation of sarcosine to form glycine; electrons are transferred via its flavin (FAD) cofactor to electron transfer flavoprotein. Folate is also a cofactor. The reaction occurs in the inner mitochondrial membrane in liver and kidney; deficiency of the enzyme, an autosomal recessive trait, results in sarcosinemia.

sar·co·si·ne·mia (sahr″ko-sĭ-ne′me-ə) accumulation of sarcosine in the blood along with elevated excretion in the urine, caused by deficiency of activity of the enzyme sarcosine dehydrogenase. The enzyme deficiency can be an autosomal recessive disorder caused by mutation in the *SARDH* gene (locus: 9q33-q34), which encodes the apoenzyme, or it can be caused by a defect in electron transfer flavoprotein (q.v.) or by severe folate deficiency.

sar·co·si·nu·ria (sahr″ko-sĭ-nu′re-ə) excretion of sarcosine in the urine.

sar·co·sis (sahr-ko′sis) [*sarco-* + *-osis*] abnormal increase of flesh.

sar·co·span (sahr′ko-span) an integral membrane protein with four transmembrane domains, expressed in cardiac and skeletal muscle as well as many other tissues; it is believed to play a role anchoring other proteins to the lipid bilayer. In skeletal muscle, it is part of the dystrophin-glycoprotein complex.

Sar·co·spo·rid·ia (sahr″ko-spor-id′e-ə) in former systems of classification, an order of sporozoan protozoa that included the genus *Sarcocystis.*

sar·co·spo·rid·i·an (sahr″ko-spor-id′e-ən) similar to or caused by protozoa of the genus *Sarcocystis.*

sar·co·spo·rid·i·a·sis (sahr″ko-spor″ĭ-di′ə-sis) sarcocystosis.

sar·co·spo·rid·i·o·sis (sahr″ko-spor-id″e-o′sis) sarcocystosis.

sar·cos·to·sis (sahr″kos-to′sis) [*sarco-* + *ostosis*] ossification of fleshy tissues.

sar·co·style (sahr′ko-stīl) [*sarco-* + Gr. *stylos* column] 1. a myofibril. 2. a bundle of myofibrils; called also *Kölliker* or *muscle column.*

sar·cot·ic (sahr-kot′ik) [Gr. *sarkōtikos*] 1. promoting the growth of flesh. 2. pertaining to sarcosis.

sar·co·tu·bules (sahr″ko-too′būlz) membrane-limited structures that extend throughout the sarcoplasm and form a closely meshed canalicular network around each myofibril.

sar·cous (sahr′kəs) pertaining to flesh or to muscular tissues.

sar·gram·os·tim (sahr-gram′o-stim) [USP] granulocyte-macrophage colony-stimulating factor developed by recombinant technology that acts to stimulate hematopoiesis and decrease neutropenia, used as an adjuvant to myelosuppressive cancer chemotherapy, to promote myeloid engraftment in bone marrow transplantation or hematopoietic stem cell transplantation, and to enhance peripheral progenitor cell yield in autologous hematopoietic stem cell transplantation; administered intravenously or subcutaneously.

sa·rin (zah-rēn′) an organophosphorus compound that is a potent cholinesterase inhibitor and is used as a nerve gas; symptoms of poisoning include bronchial constriction, convulsions, and often death. See also *organophosphorus compound poisoning*, under *poisoning.*

Sa·ro·tham·nus (sa″ro-tham′nəs) [Gr. *saron* broom + *thamnos* shrub] *Cytisus.*

Sar·ra·ce·nia (sar″ə-se′ne-ə) [Michel *Sarrazin*, Canadian physician and naturalist, 1659–1734] a genus of plants of the family Sarraceniaceae. *S. purpu′rea* L. is the most common pitcher plant of North America; the secretion of its pitcher contains digestant enzymes and is a stimulant, diuretic, and laxative.

SARS severe acute respiratory syndrome.

SARS-CoV SARS-associated coronavirus.

sar·sa (sahr′sə) gen. *sar′sae.* Sarsaparilla.

sar·sa·pa·ril·la (sahr″sə-pə-ril′ə, sas″pə-ril′ə) [Sp. *zarzaparrilla*, fr. *zarza* briar + *parrilla* vine] 1. any of various plants of the genus *Smilax.* 2. the dried root of any of various species of *Smilax*, used as a flavoring agent in beverages, and in the treatment of psoriasis and other skin conditions and in homeopathy. It contains sarsasapogenin, a precursor in the manufacture of compounds in the pregnane series.

sar·sa·sapo·gen·in (sahr″sə-sap″o-jen′in) a steroid sapogenin from sarsaparilla.

Sas·sa·fras (sas′ə-fras) [L.] a genus of trees of the family Lauraceae. *S. albi′dum* Nutt. (called also *S. varifo′lia* and *S. officina′le*) is a North American tree whose root contains the toxic and carcinogenic sassafras oil.

sat·el·lite (sat′ə-līt) [L. *satelles* companion] 1. a subservient smaller body that is under the influence of a larger one. 2. a vein that closely accompanies an artery, such as the brachial. 3. a minor, or attendant, lesion situated near a larger one. 4. a globoid mass of chromatin attached at the secondary constriction to the ends of the short arms of acrocentric autosomes. It may occur ectopically on other chromosomes through translocation; such heteromorphisms can be heritable and are sometimes associated with clinical conditions. 5. exhibiting satellitism. 6. the posterior of a pair of gregarines undergoing syzygy.

bacterial s. satellite colony.

centriolar s. one of the small dense, amorphous bodies associated with the centrioles, which serve as nucleation sites for polymerization of tubulin to form microtubules.

chromosomal s. satellite (def. 4).

sat·el·li·tism (sat′ə-li-tiz-əm) 1. the presence or formation of satellites. 2. the phenomenon in which certain bacterial species grow more vigorously in the immediate vicinity of colonies of other unrelated species (e.g., *Haemophilus influenzae* near a colony of staphylococci), owing to the production of an essential metabolite by the latter species.

platelet s. a phenomenon sometimes seen in blood that has been anticoagulated with ethylenediaminetetraacetic acid (EDTA), in which platelets surround or adhere to leukocytes.

sat·el·li·to·sis (sat″ə-li-to′sis) accumulation of neuroglial cells about neurons; seen whenever neurons are damaged.

sa·ti·e·ty (sə-ti′ə-te) [L. *satietas*] 1. sufficiency. 2. full gratification of appetite or thirst, with abolition of the desire to eat or drink.

early s. a sensation of the stomach being full after just part of an average meal has been consumed; this is sometimes a precursor of nausea.

sa·tra·tox·in (sa′trə-tok″sin) any of several trichothecene mycotoxins found in species of *Stachybotrys*, especially *S. alternans*, causing stachybotryotoxicosis.

Sat·tler layer (zaht′lər) [Hubert *Sattler*, Austrian ophthalmologist, 1844–1928] see under *layer.*

satt·va (sahth′və) [Sanskrit] according to ayurveda, the purest aspect of the three gunas, characterized by equilibrium; it is responsible for health and contentment of the mind and body and is associated with the mind, consciousness, or intelligence that maintains health.

sa·tu·mo·mab (sə-too′mo-mab) a monoclonal antibody specific to colorectal and ovarian adenocarcinomas; see *indium In 111 satumomab pendetide.*

sat·u·rat·ed (sach′ə-rāt-əd) 1. of a chemical compound, having all the chemical affinities satisfied; i.e., no double or triple bonds are present. The term is most commonly used for carbon-carbon bonds, as in saturated fatty acids. 2. of a solution, containing as much solute as may be dissolved under stated conditions.

sat·u·ra·tion (sach″ə-ra′shən) [L. *saturatio*] 1. the act of saturating or condition of being saturated. 2. in radiotherapy, the delivery of a maximum tolerable tissue dose within a short time period and then maintenance of this biologic effect for an extended period of time by additional smaller fractional doses.

oxygen s. a measure of the degree to which oxygen is bound to hemoglobin, usually measured by a pulse oximeter, given as a percentage calculated by dividing the maximum oxygen capacity into the actual oxygen content and multiplying by 100.

transferrin s. the percentage of transferrin bound to iron in a serum sample, calculated by the formula

$$\frac{\text{serum iron}}{\text{total iron} - \text{binding capacity (TIBC)}} \times 100;$$

used in evaluation of patients with iron deficiency or overload.

sat·ur·nine (sat′ər-nīn) [L. *saturninus*, from *saturnus* lead] 1. pertaining to or caused by lead. 2. having the dull, heavy properties associated with lead.

sat·ur·nism (sat′ər-niz-əm) [L. *saturnus* lead] lead poisoning.

sat·y·ri·a·sis (sat″ĭ-ri′ə-sis) [Gr. *satyros* satyr + *-iasis*] hypersexuality in a male; cf. *nymphomania.*

sat·y·ro·ma·nia (sat″ĭ-ro-ma′ne-ə) hypersexuality in a male.

sau·cer (saw′sər) a rounded, shallow depression.

auditory s. otic placode.

sau·cer·iza·tion (saw″sər-ĭ-za′shən) 1. the excavation of tissue to form a shallow shelving depression usually performed to facilitate drainage from infected areas of bone. 2. the shallow, saucer-like depression on the upper surface of a vertebra which has suffered a compression fracture.

```
    H   H   H   H   H   H   H   H   H   H   H   H   H   H   H   O
    |   |   |   |   |   |   |   |   |   |   |   |   |   |   |   //
H—C—C—C—C—C—C—C—C—C—C—C—C—C—C—C—C—O—H
    |   |   |   |   |   |   |   |   |   |   |   |   |   |   |
    H   H   H   H   H   H   H   H   H   H   H   H   H   H   H
```

■ Palmitic acid, a common saturated fatty acid.

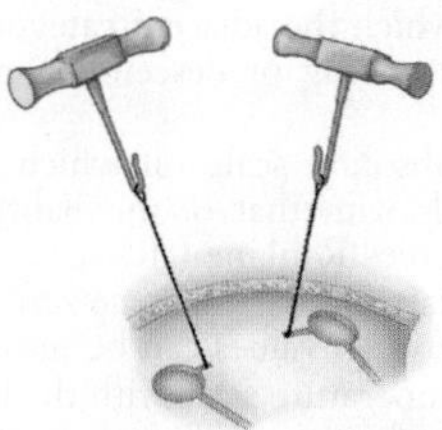

■ Gigli wire saw as used in removing segment of the skull.

Saun•ders disease, sign (sawn′dərz) [Edward Watt *Saunders*, American physician, 1854–1927] see under *disease* and *sign.*

Saus•sure hygrometer (so-sūr′) [Horace Bénédict de *Saussure*, Swiss physicist, 1740–1799] see under *hygrometer.*

sav•in (sav′in) [L. *sabina*] *Juniperus sabina*, whose fresh tops are the source of savin oil; it is also used in homeopathy.

saw (saw) a cutting instrument with a cutting or serrated edge.

bayonet s. a surgical bone saw used for the excision of the nasal dorsal hump.

crown s. a form of trephine.

Gigli wire s. a flexible wire with saw teeth.

hole s. a trephine.

separating s. a saw for separating teeth.

saw pal•met•to (saw pal-met′o) 1. *Serenoa repens*, a small creeping palm of the southeastern United States. 2. [NF] the partially dried, ripe fruit of *S. repens*, used for urinary problems associated with benign prostatic hyperplasia.

saxi•tox•in (sak′sĭ-tok″sin) a powerful, heat-stable, low molecular weight neurotoxin synthesized and secreted by certain dinoflagellates, such as species of *Gonyaulax;* it accumulates in the tissues of bivalve mollusks feeding on the dinoflagellates, and persons eating such mollusks can get either neurotoxic or paralytic shellfish poisoning (see under *poisoning*). Called also *shellfish poison.*

Sayre apparatus (sa′ər) [Lewis Albert *Sayre*, American surgeon, 1820–1900] see under *apparatus.*

SB sinus bradycardia.

Sb antimony (L. *sti′bium*).

SBE subacute bacterial endocarditis; see *infective endocarditis*, under *endocarditis.*

SBFT small bowel follow-through.

SBMA spinobulbar muscular atrophy.

SBP spontaneous bacterial peritonitis.

SC secretory component; closure of semilunar valves; subcutaneous.

Sc scandium.

scab (skab) 1. a crust formed on the surface of a wound. 2. to become covered with such a crust. 3. scabies in domestic animals.

foot s. sheep s.

head s. acariasis on the head of an animal, most commonly a sheep.

sheep s. psoroptic mange in sheep, the most common type of mange in that species, caused by the mite *Psoroptes ovis*, which infests the skin at the base of the hairs. A scab forms, which later detaches along with the wool; open sores may lead to infection, emaciation, and even death.

sca•bet•ic (skə-bet′ik) scabietic.

sca•bi•cide (ska′bĭ-sīd) 1. destructive to *Sarcoptes scabiei;* used in the treatment of scabies. 2. an agent for destroying *Sarcoptes scabiei.*

sca•bies (ska′bēz) [L., from *scabere* scratch] 1. a contagious dermatitis of various different animals, caused by the mite *Sarcoptes scabiei;* the egg-laying female mite digs into the upper layer of the epidermis and makes raised sinuous burrows (cuniculi), which then cause a papular eruption accompanied by intense pruritus sometimes associated with eczema from scratching and secondary bacterial infection. Called also *seven-year itch* (in humans) and *sarcoptic mange* (in other animals). 2. psoroptic mange in cattle and horses caused by *Psoroptes ovis.*

crusted s., Norwegian s. a rare, severe form of scabies caused by an unusually heavy mite infestation, seen especially in senile, mentally retarded, or immunocompromised patients, those with poor sensation, or those with severe systemic disease; it is thought to represent an abnormal host immune response to the mites and is characterized by crusting dermatitis of the hands and feet; horny debris under the nails; erythematous, scaling plaques on the neck, scalp, and trunk; and usually lymphadenopathy and eosinophilia.

s. incognito scabies whose symptoms are masked but not eradicated because it has been treated with corticosteroids.

sca•bi•et•ic (ska″be-et′ik) pertaining to or affected with scabies.

SCAD de•fi•cien•cy short-chain acyl-CoA dehydrogenase deficiency; see under *acyl-CoA dehydrogenase.*

scaf•fold (skaf′əld) an artificial network of synthetic or biological tissue that supports ingrowth of fibrous tissue to strengthen a graft.

sca•la (ska′lə) pl. *sca′lae* [L. "staircase"] a stairlike structure; applied especially to various passages of the cochlea.

s. of Löwenberg, s. me′dia ductus cochlearis.

s. tym′pani [TA] the perilymph-filled part of the cochlea that is continuous with the scala vestibuli at the helicotrema, is separated from other cochlear structures by the spiral lamina and the basilar membrane of the cochlear duct, and ends blindly near the fenestra cochleae. Called also *tympanic canal of cochlea.*

s. vesti′buli [TA] the perilymph-filled part of the cochlea that begins in the vestibule, is separated from other cochlear structures by the spiral lamina and Reissner membrane of the cochlear duct, and becomes continuous with the scala tympani at the helicotrema. Called also *vestibular canal.*

sca•lar (ska′lər) [L. *scalaris* pertaining to a ladder or staircase] 1. a quantity that has magnitude only (as opposed to also having direction), such as mass or temperature. Cf. *vector*. 2. pertaining to such a quantity.

sca•lar•i•form (skə-lar′ĭ-form) [*scalar* + *form*] resembling the rungs of a ladder.

scald (skawld) 1. a burn caused by hot liquid or hot, moist vapor. 2. to burn with hot liquid or steam. 3. interdigital dermatitis. 4. benign foot rot.

foot s. 1. interdigital dermatitis. 2. benign foot rot.

scale[1] (skāl) [L. *scala*, usually pl. *scalae*, a series of steps] a scheme or device by which some property may be evaluated or measured, such as a linear surface bearing marks at regular intervals, representing certain predetermined units.

absolute s., absolute temperature s. 1. a temperature scale with its zero at absolute zero (−273.15°C, −459.67°F). 2. Kelvin s.

Apgar s. see under *score.*

Arthritis Impact Measurement S. a questionnaire for assessing the health and functioning over the past month of a person with a rheumatic disease; it asks a long series of questions and assigns numbers from 1 for almost always impaired to 5 for never impaired.

Ashworth S. a scale to assess the severity of spasticity of a part, now modified and used most commonly as the *Modified Ashworth Scale;* it measures the increase in tone as the muscle is stretched and assigns numbers from 0 (no increase in tone) to 4 (complete rigidity of the part on flexion or extension).

ASIA s. Frankel classification.

Baumé s. a scale for expressing the specific gravity of liquids, based on the extent to which the liquid is lighter or heavier than water.

Bayley S's of Infant Development a psychological test for assessing development of infants, using motor, mental, and behavioral development scales.

binary s. dichotomous s.

Blessed Dementia Rating S. a tool for assessing the severity of dementia. It contains 22 items and measures changes over the preceding six months in everyday activities; in self-care habits; and in personality, interests, and drives. Ratings are based on information gathered from relatives or friends of the patient.

Borg s. a numerical scale for assessing dyspnea, from 0 representing no dyspnea to 10 as maximal dyspnea.

Brazelton behavioral s. a method for assessing infant behavior by its responses to environmental stimuli.

Brief Psychiatric Rating S. (BPRS) a rating scale for assessing psychopathology on the basis of a small number of items, usually 16 to 24, encompassing psychosis, depression, and anxiety symptoms.

Cattell Infant Intelligence S. a test of general motor and cognitive development, assessed by performance of tasks, in the first 18 months of life.

Celsius s. (C) a temperature scale on which 0° is officially 273.15 kelvins and 100° is 373.15 kelvins. Before 1948 (and still, unofficially) the degree Celsius (°C) was called the degree centigrade (°C) with 0° at the freezing point of fresh water and 100° at the boiling point, at normal atmospheric pressure (760 mm Hg). See also *kelvin* and Appendix 6 for Celsius-Fahrenheit, Fahrenheit-Celsius equivalents.

centigrade s. a scale in which the interval between two fixed points is divided into 100 equal units, as the Celsius scale.

Charrière s. French s.

Columbia Mental Maturity S. a test of specific kinds of mental function and general abilities, suitable for children (ages 3 to 12) with no speech or with limited physical capabilities, such as those with cerebral palsy.

Coma Recovery S.-Revised (CRS-R) an assessment instrument for differentiating the minimally conscious state from the vegetative state, similar in structure to the Glasgow Coma Scale but with more detailed subscales designed to detect subtle signs of recovery of awareness.

continuous s. an interval scale in which the intervals can be broken into finer and finer gradations, e.g., blood glucose or weight scales.

Defensive Functioning S. a scale comprising defense mechanisms used to prevent or allay anxiety.

dichotomous s. a nominal scale that has two categories.

dimensional s. interval s.

Dunfermline s. a scale for assessing the nutritional status of children: 1, superior condition; 2, passable condition; 3, requiring supervision; 4, requiring medical treatment.

Epworth Sleepiness S. a tool for measuring how sleepy a person is during daytime or working hours, using a scale of 1 to 5 for whether the person is unlikely or likely to fall asleep in a series of situations such as watching television, having a quiet conversation, or being stalled in traffic.

Fahrenheit s. (F) a temperature scale, obsolescent but still commonly used in the United States, in which the lowest temperature attainable by a freezing mixture of ice and salt is denoted as 0° and the normal temperature of the human body was originally denoted as 96°. Fresh water freezes at about 32° and boils at about 212° under average atmospheric pressure. See also *Celsius s.* and Appendix 6 for Celsius-Fahrenheit, Fahrenheit-Celsius equivalents.

Fitzpatrick s. a rating of skin types according to degree of reactivity to or absorption of ultraviolet radiation, assigning Roman numerals from I (least reactive, usually dark skin) to VI (most reactive, usually pale skin).

French s. a scale for denoting the size of catheters, sounds, and other tubular instruments; one French unit (symbol F) is 0.33 mm in diameter, so that an 18 French or 18F needle has a diameter of 6 mm.

GAF s. Global Assessment of Functioning s.

Gaffky s. a scale formerly used widely in denoting the prognosis in tuberculosis, based on the number of tubercle bacilli in the sputum.

Glasgow Coma S. a standardized system for assessing response to stimuli in a neurologically impaired patient; reactions are given a numerical value in three categories (eye opening, verbal responsiveness, and motor responsiveness), and the three scores are then added together. The lowest values are the worst clinical scores.

Glasgow Outcome S. a scale used to describe outcome after serious head injury, based on the general level of social functioning regained. Patients are assigned to one of five categories: good recovery, moderately disabled, severely disabled, vegetative, or dead.

Global Assessment of Functioning s. a rating of psychiatric status from 1 (lowest level of functioning) to 100 (highest level), assessing psychological, social, and occupational functioning; widely used in studies of treatment effectiveness. Called also *GAF s.*

gray s. 1. the range of different shades of gray that can be displayed for use in a CT scan display. 2. see under *ultrasonography*.

Hamilton Depression Rating S. a scale that scores the severity of depression on the basis of a semistructured interview eliciting depression-related symptoms.

homigrade s. a temperature scale in which 0° is the melting point of ice (0°C, 32°F), 100° is the normal human body temperature (37°C, 98.6°F), and 270° is the boiling point of water.

hydrometer s. a scale used for expressing the specific gravity of liquids.

interval s. a scale for classifying data, in which the values have intrinsic order and all intervals have an inherent and equal distance between, e.g., age or temperature scales. Called also *dimensional s.* Cf. *ratio s.*

Karnofsky s., Karnofsky performance s. a widely used performance scale, assigning scores ranging from 0 for a nonfunctional or dead patient to 100 for one with completely normal functioning.

Kelvin s. an absolute temperature scale in which the unit of measurement, the kelvin, is equivalent to the degree Celsius, so that the ice point is 273.15 kelvins and the boiling point of water is 373.15 kelvins.

nominal s. the weakest qualitative, not quantitative or ordered, classification of the samples into separate categories so that each possible result belongs to only one category, with the categories not able to be ordered relative to each other, e.g., one dealing with religion or sex and not size, weight, or temperature. Cf. *ordinal s.*

nonlinear s. a scale in which the divisions corresponding to the steps are unequal, such as one with divisions that show logarithmic or exponential growth or change.

ordinal s. a scale used to classify data into qualitative ordered categories, e.g., defining socioeconomic status as low, medium, or high; the values have a distinct order but intervals are created arbitrarily and lack an intrinsic numerical equality.

Penn Spasm Frequency S. a scale that measures the frequency of spasms and assigns numbers from 0 for no spasms to 4 for more than 10 per hour.

performance s. a scale that measures a patient's ability to function, serving as a prognostic indicator of seriousness of disease or disability. The most widely used scale is the Karnofsky scale.

ranked s. a scale in which the adjacent categories are arranged according to a progressively ascending or descending magnitude, as an ordinal scale or interval scale.

Rankine s. (R) an absolute scale on which the incremental unit of measurement corresponds with that of the Fahrenheit scale, so that the ice point is at 491.67 degrees Rankine (°R).

ratio s. an interval scale (q.v.) with a true zero point, e.g., mass, length, or income; thus ratios between values can be meaningfully defined.

Réaumur s. (R) a temperature scale with the ice point at 0 degrees and the normal boiling point of water at 80 degrees Réaumur (°R).

Social and Occupational Functioning Assessment S. (SOFAS) a scale that describes the level of an individual's social and occupational functioning, either present or past; unlike the GAF scale, it is not directly influenced by the severity of the individual's psychological symptoms.

temperature s. a scale used for expressing the degree of heat, based on absolute zero as a reference point (absolute scale), or with a certain value arbitrarily assigned to such temperatures as the ice point and boiling point of water under certain stipulated conditions, the range between and beyond them being divided into a designated number of identical units.

visual analog s. a scale that enables a patient to indicate the perceived level of intensity of a symptom (such as pain) by locating its position on a line representing a range from least intensity to greatest intensity.

Wechsler Adult Intelligence S. (WAIS) a group of tests for assessment of intellectual functioning in adults.

Wechsler Intelligence S. for Children (WISC) a group of tests for assessment of intellectual functioning in children ages 5 to 15.

scale[2] (skāl) [Old Fr. *escale* shell, husk] 1. a thin, compacted, flaky fragment, such as of bone or enamel. 2. a bit of dry, horny epidermis, usually ready to be sloughed; called also *squama* and *squame.* 3. a thin fragment of tartar or other concretion on the surface of a tooth. 4. to remove such fragments and concretions from the tooth surface and beneath the gingival margin with a scaler.

adhesive s. a scale of epidermis that is not readily sloughed, as in lupus erythematosus.

sca•lene (ska′lēn) [Gr. *skalēnos* uneven] 1. uneven; unequally three-sided. 2. pertaining to one of the scalene muscles (see terms beginning *musculus scalenus*).

sca•le•nec•to•my (ska″lə-nek′tə-me) [*scalenus* + *-ectomy*] the surgical resecting of a scalenus muscle.

sca•le•not•o•my (ska″lə-not′ə-me) [*scalenus* + *-tomy*] sectioning of the scalene muscles to restrict respiratory activity of the upper thorax and thus induce apical rest; formerly used in treatment of pulmonary tuberculosis.

sca•le•nus (ska-le′nəs) [L., from Gr. *skalēnos*] uneven (scalene); see under *musculus.*

scal•er (ska′lər) 1. a dental instrument used in removing scale (plaque and calculus) from tooth surfaces. 2. an electronic instrument for rapid counting of radiation-induced pulses emitted from a Geiger counter or other radiation detectors.

chisel s. periodontal chisel.

deep s. one of several types of scalers designed for removal of subgingival deposits from the teeth.

double-ended s. a scaler with blades on both sides of the handle, one blade for the right side, the other for the left.

hoe s. a scaler made with different angular relationships of shank and handle, but with the blade bent at a 99° angle, and the flattened termination surface beveled at an angle of 45°, used for planing and smoothing root surfaces.

sickle s. a scaler that removes tenacious supragingival or subgingival deposits; it has a sickle-like blade with flattened sides and a trapezoidal cross section.

superficial s. one of several types of scalers designed for removal of supragingival deposits from the teeth.

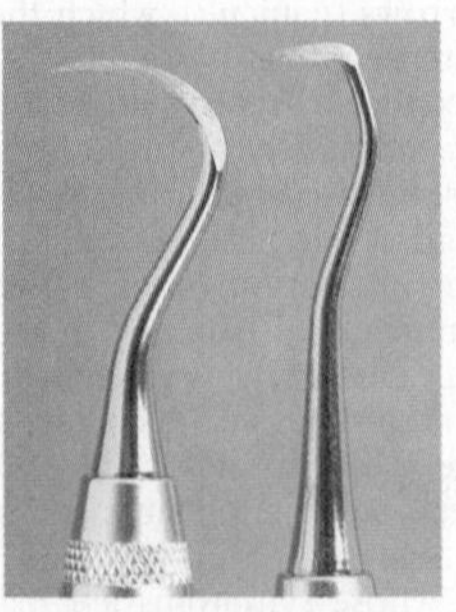

■ Sickle scalers.

ultrasonic s. an ultrasonic instrument with a tip for supplying high-frequency vibrations, used to remove adherent deposits from the teeth and bits of inflamed tissue from the walls of the gingival crevice.

scal•ing (ska′ling) removal of scale (plaque and calculus) from a tooth.
deep s. removal of plaque and calculus from the surface of a tooth apical to the gingival margin, usually accumulated in periodontal pockets. Called also *subgingival s.* and *root s.*
root s. deep s.
subgingival s. deep s.
ultrasonic s. removal of debris, plaque, and calculus from the surface of the teeth with an ultrasonic scaler.

scalp (skalp) that part of the skin of the head, exclusive of the face and ears, that is normally covered with hair.
double s. thinning of the bones of the scalp in young sheep, usually because of an inadequate diet; called also *cappie.*

scal•pel (skal′pəl) [L. *scalpellum*] a small surgical knife with a straight handle and, usually, a blade with a convex edge.

sca•ly (ska′le) [L. *squamosus*] pertaining to or characterized by scales.

scam•mo•ny (skam′ə-ne) [L. *scammonium, scammonia*] 1. *Convolvulus scammonia.* 2. the dried root of *C. scammonia* or the resin derived from it; formerly used as a cathartic. 3. any of various other plants of the family Convolvulaceae, or the root or resin derived therefrom.
Mexican s. ipomea.

scan (skan) 1. to examine or map the body, or one or more organs or regions of it, by gathering information with a sensing device. 2. the data or image so obtained, often designated according to the organ under examination, as *brain scan, kidney scan, thyroid scan,* etc. 3. shortened form of *scintiscan.*
A-s. display on a cathode ray tube of ultrasonic echoes, in which one axis represents the time required for return of the echo and the other corresponds to the strength of the echo.
B-s. display on a cathode ray tube of ultrasonic echoes, in which the position of a bright dot on the tube corresponds to the time elapsed and the brightness of the spot to the strength of the echo; movement of the transducer across the skin surface yields a two-dimensional cross-sectional display.
CAT s., CT s. computerized axial tomography, or the image obtained from it.
Meckel s. a technetium-99m pertechnetate gastric-mucosa scan used to demonstrate ectopic gastric mucosa, particularly in Meckel diverticulum.
M-mode s. the image obtained using M-mode echocardiography, showing the motion (M) over time of a monodimensional ("icepick") section of the heart.
PET s. positron emission tomography, or the image obtained from it.
ventilation-perfusion s., V/Q s. a scintigraphic technique for demonstrating perfusion defects in normally ventilated areas of the lung in the diagnosis of pulmonary embolism, consisting of the imaging of the distribution of an inhaled radionuclide followed by the imaging of the perfusion of the lungs by an injected radionuclide.

scan•di•um (Sc) (skan′de-əm) a very rare metallic element; atomic number, 21; atomic weight, 44.956.

scan•ner (skan′ər) equipment used for making scans or scanning.
EMI s. an instrument for reconstructing tomographic images for display; see *computed tomography,* under *tomography.*
scintillation s. scintiscanner.

scan•ning (skan′ing) 1. the act of examining visually, as a small area or different isolated areas, in detail. 2. the act of examining with a sensing device, as to perform a scan. 3. scanning speech.
infarct avid s. see under *scintigraphy.*
MUGA s., multiple gated acquisition s. equilibrium radionuclide angiocardiography.
radioisotope s., radionuclide s. production of a two-dimensional record or image representing the gamma rays emitted by a radioactive isotope (radionuclide) concentrated in a specific tissue of the body, such as the brain or thyroid gland.
thallium s. see *thallium-201 myocardial perfusion scintigraphy,* under *scintigraphy,* and *thallium stress test,* under *test.*

sca•nog•ra•phy (skan-og′rə-fe) a method of making radiographs by the use of a narrow slit beneath the tube in such a manner that only a line or sheet of x-rays is employed and the x-ray tube moves over the object so that all the rays of the central beam pass through the part being radiographed at the same angle.

scan•sion (skan′shən) scanning speech.

Scan•zo•ni maneuver (operation) (skahn-tso′ne) [Friedrich Wilhelm *Scanzoni,* German obstetrician, 1821–1891] see under *maneuver.*

sca•pha (ska′fə) [L. "a skiff"] [TA] the long curved depression that separates the helix of the ear from the antihelix; called also *scaphoid fossa* and *fossa helicis.*

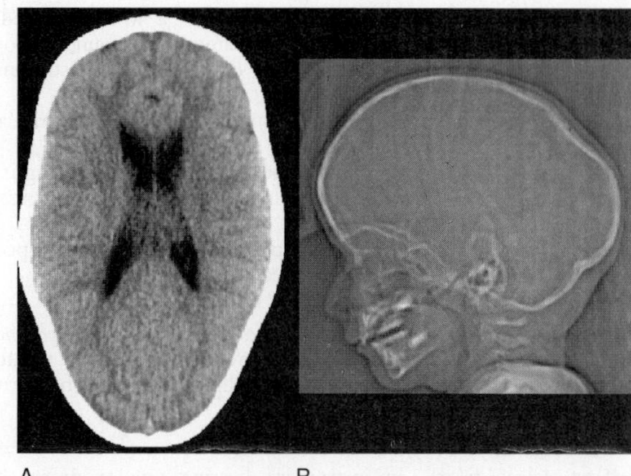

■ Scaphocephaly in a brain CT scan *(A)* and lateral radiograph *(B).*

sca•phi•on (ska′fe-on) [Gr. *skaphion* a small bowl or basin] basis cranii externa.

scaph(o)- [Gr. *skaphē* skiff or light boat] a combining form meaning boat-shaped.

scapho•ce•pha•lia (skaf″o-sə-fa′le-ə) scaphocephaly.

scapho•ceph•a•ly (skaf″o-sef′ə-le) [*scapho-* + *-cephaly*] anteroposterior elongation of the skull, with bitemporal narrowing. Because it is usually caused by sagittal synostosis (premature closure of the sagittal suture), the two terms are often used synonymously. **scaphocephal′ic, scaphoceph′alous** *adj*

scaph•oid (skaf′oid) [*scaph-* + *-oid*] shaped like a boat; called also *navicular.* Used especially in reference to the most lateral bone in the proximal row of carpal bones; see *os scaphoideum.*

scaph•oid•itis (skaf″oi-di′tis) inflammation of the scaphoid bone.
tarsal s. 1. inflammation involving the navicular (scaphoid) bone of the tarsus. 2. Köhler bone disease (def. 1).

scapho•lu•nate (skaf″ə-loo′nāt) pertaining to the scaphoid and lunate bones.

Scap•to•co•sa (skap″to-ko′sə) a genus of wolf spiders (family Lycosidae). *S. rapto′ria* is a Brazilian species whose powerful hemolytic venom causes necrotic arachnidism.

scap•u•la (skap′u-lə) pl. *scap′ulae* [L.] [TA] the flat, triangular bone in the back of the shoulder, articulating with the ipsilateral clavicle and humerus; called also *shoulder blade.* See Plate 40. **scap′ular** *adj*
alar s., s. ala′ta winged s.
elevated s. Sprengel deformity.
Graves s. scaphoid s.
scaphoid s. a scapula in which the vertebral border is more or less concave.
winged s. a scapula having a prominent vertebral border.

scap•u•lal•gia (skap″u-lal′jə) pain in the scapular region.

scap•u•lary (skap″u-lar′e) a shoulder bandage, with the appearance of a pair of suspenders or braces, to hold in place a body bandage or girdle.

scap•u•lec•to•my (skap″u-lek′tə-me) surgical removal of the scapula.

scap•u•lo•an•te•ri•or (skap″u-lo-an-tēr′e-ər) denoting a position of the fetus in transverse lie, with the scapula directed anteriorly.

scap•u•lo•cla•vic•u•lar (skap″u-lo-klə-vik′u-lər) pertaining to the scapula and the clavicle.

scap•u•lo•dyn•ia (skap″u-lo-din′e-ə) [*scapula* + *-odynia*] pain in the region of the shoulder.

scap•u•lo•hu•mer•al (skap″u-lo-hu′mər-əl) pertaining to the scapula and the humerus.

scap•u•lo•per•o•ne•al (skap″u-lo-per-o-ne′əl) pertaining to or involving both the scapula and the fibula or outer calf.

scap•u•lo•pexy (skap′u-lo-pek″se) [*scapula* + *-pexy*] surgical fixation of the scapula.

scap•u•lo•pos•te•ri•or (skap″u-lo-pos-tēr′e-ər) denoting a position of the fetus in transverse lie, with the scapula directed posteriorly.

scap•u•lo•tho•rac•ic (skap″u-lo-thə-ras′ik) pertaining to the scapula and thorax.

sca•pus (ska′pəs) pl. *sca′pi* [L.] anatomical nomenclature for a shaft or shaftlike structure.
s. pi′li hair shaft.

scar (skahr) [Gr. *eschara* the scab or eschar on a wound caused by burning] 1. a mark remaining after the healing of a wound or other morbid process; called also *cicatrix*. 2. any of various manifestations of an earlier event.

apical s. a translucent area of bone commonly found around the apex of a tooth after root canal therapy or other endodontic treatment.

hypertrophic s. a scar formed by exuberant cicatrization, giving it the appearance of a keloid but without the latter's tendency to progressive extension or to recurrence after excision.

Reichert s. an area over the implanting blastocyst of some species, consisting of a fibrinous membrane in place of the decidual tissue.

white s. of ovary corpus albicans (def. 1).

scar·i·fi·ca·tion (skar″ĭ-fĭ-ka′shən) [L. *scarificatio*, Gr. *skariphismos* a scratching up] production in the skin of many small, superficial scratches or punctures, as for the introduction of smallpox vaccine. The term is sometimes used erroneously for scarring.

scar·i·fi·ca·tor (skar′ĭ-fĭ-ka″tər) scarifier.

scar·i·fi·er (skar′ĭ-fi″ər) an instrument bearing one or more sharp points, used in scarification.

scar·la·ti·na (skahr″lə-te′nə) [L. "scarlet"] scarlet fever. **scarlat′inal** *adj*

scar·la·tin·i·form (skahr″lə-tin′ĭ-form) resembling scarlet fever, especially its skin eruption.

scar·lat·i·noid (skahr-lat′ĭ-noid) scarlatiniform.

scar·let (skahr′lət) 1. bright red tinged with orange or yellow. 2. a dye or stain with this color.

Biebrich s. an azo dye used as a plasma stain.

s. G Sudan III.

s. R scarlet red; see under *red*.

Scar·pa fascia, etc. (skahr′pah) [Antonio *Scarpa*, Italian anatomist and surgeon, 1747–1832] see under *fascia* and *foramen;* see *posterior staphyloma* under *staphyloma;* and see *cornu superius marginis falciformis*, *ganglion vestibulare*, *membrana tympanica secundaria*, *nervus nasopalatinus*, and *trigonum femorale*.

scar·ring (skahr′ing) cicatrization.

renal s. focal areas of thinning of the renal cortex with indentations on the surface of the kidney, resulting from destruction of tubules and nephrons by reflux nephropathy or pyelonephritis.

SCAT sheep cell agglutination test.

Scat·chard plot (skach′ərd) [George *Scatchard*, American chemist, 1892–1973] see under *plot*.

scat(o)- [Gr. *skōr*, gen. *skatos* dung] a combining form denoting relation to dung, or fecal matter; see also words beginning *skat(o)-*.

sca·tol (ska′tōl) skatole.

scato·lo·gia (skat″ah-lo′jə) scatology (def. 2).

telephone s. a paraphilia in which sexual arousal or activity is linked to the placing of obscene phone calls.

scato·log·ic (skat″o-loj′ik) pertaining to or characterized by scatology.

sca·tol·o·gy (skah-tol′ə-je) [*scato-* + *-logy*] 1. the study and analysis of feces, as for diagnostic purposes. 2. a preoccupation with feces, filth, or obscenities.

sca·to·ma (skə-to′mə) fecaloma.

sca·toph·a·gy (skə-tof′ə-je) coprophagy.

sca·tos·co·py (skə-tos′kə-pe) [*scato-* + *-scopy*] inspection of the feces.

scat·ter (skat′ər) the change in energy or momentum of radiation or particles (e.g., photons or x-rays) produced by interaction with the medium through which the rays or particles pass. See also *backscatter*.

scat·ter·gram (skat′ər-gram) scatterplot.

scat·ter·ing (skat′ər-ing) a change in direction of a photon or subatomic particle as the result of a collision or interaction.

Compton s. modified scattering; the deflection of an incident photon by interaction with a free electron or an orbital electron of much lower energy than the photon; the photon is deflected from its original path and gives up part of its energy to displace the electron.

Thomson s. unmodified scattering; deflection of a photon by interaction with an atom with no loss of energy by the photon.

scat·ter·plot (skat′ər-plot) a plot in rectangular coordinates of paired observations of two random variables, each observation plotted as one point on the graph; the scatter or clustering of points provides an indication of the relationship between the two variables. Called also *scatter diagram* or *scattergram*.

scav·en·ger (skav′ən-jər) a substance that influences the course of a chemical reaction by ready combination with free radicals.

ScD [L.] Scien′tiae Doc′tor (Doctor of Science).

ScDA [L.] scapulo-dextra anterior (right scapuloanterior, a position of the fetus; see *position*).

scDNA single copy DNA.

ScDP [L.] scapulo-dextra posterior (right scapuloposterior, a position of the fetus; see *position*).

sce·do·spo·ri·o·sis (se″do-spor″e-o′sis) pseudallescheriasis.

Sce·do·spo·ri·um (se-do-spor′e-əm) a genus of Fungi Imperfecti of the form-class Hyphomycetes, form-family Moniliaceae; its perfect (sexual) stage is *Pseudallescheria*. *S. apiosper′mum* is the anamorph of *P. boydii*, a major cause of eumycotic mycetoma. *S. proli′ficans*, formerly called *S. infla′tum*, has been isolated from several cases of osteomyelitis. Formerly called *Monosporium*.

SCFA short-chain fatty acids.

Scha·fer method (sha′fər) [Sir Edward Albert Sharpey-*Schafer*, English physiologist, 1850–1935] artificial respiration; see under *respiration*.

Schä·fer syndrome (sha′fər) [Erich *Schäfer*, German physician, 20th century] see under *syndrome*.

Schäf·fer reflex (shāf′ər) [Max *Schäffer*, German neurologist, 1852–1923] see under *reflex*.

Scham·berg disease (dermatosis, purpura) (shahm′bərg) [Jay Frank *Schamberg*, American dermatologist, 1870–1934] see under *disease*.

Scham·roth test (sign) (sham′roth) [Leo *Schamroth*, South African cardiologist in the United States, 1924–1988] see under *test*.

Schanz disease, syndrome (shahnts) [Alfred *Schanz*, German orthopedist, 1868–1931] see under *disease* and *syndrome*.

schar·lach R (shahr′lak) scarlet red.

Schat·zki ring (shaht′ske) [Richard *Schatzki;* German-born American radiologist, 1901–1992] see *esophageal ring*, under *ring*.

Schau·dinn fluid (shou′din) [Fritz Richard *Schaudinn*, German bacteriologist, 1871–1906] see under *fluid*.

Schau·mann bodies, disease, sarcoid, syndrome (shou′mahn) [Jörgen *Schaumann*, Swedish dermatologist, 1879–1953] see under *body*, and see *sarcoidosis*.

Schau·ta operation (shou′tah) [Friedrich *Schauta*, Austrian gynecologist, 1849–1919] see under *operation*.

SChE serum cholinesterase.

Sche·de operation (sha′də) [Max *Schede*, German surgeon, 1844–1902] see under *operation*.

sched·ule (sked′ūl) a formal list, plan of procedure, or timetable.

S. for Affective Disorders and Schizophrenia (SADS) a semistructured interview administered by a professional and designed to yield diagnostic information about current and lifetime incidences of affective disorders and schizophrenia.

Diagnostic Interview S. (DIS) a structured interview, administered by trained nonclinicians, assessing lifetime as well as current occurrence of symptoms of a variety of mental disorders; diagnoses are aided by computer algorithms.

Gesell developmental s. a test of the developmental status of infants that includes assessment of motor development, adaptive behavior, language development, and personal-social behavior.

s. of reinforcement a series of rules governing the delivery or nondelivery of reinforcement; it may occur after every response (continuous reinforcement) or not (partial reinforcement). In partial reinforcement, delivery may occur after predetermined amounts of time (*intervals*) or numbers of responses (*ratios*), either of these being unvarying (*fixed*) or changing (*variable*), e.g., a *fixed-interval s.* or a *variable ratio s.*

Scheibe aplasia, deafness (shi′bə) [A. *Scheibe*, American physician, early 20th century] see under *aplasia* and *deafness*.

Scheie operation, syndrome (sha) [Harold Glendon *Scheie*, American ophthalmologist, 1909–1990] see under *operation* and *syndrome*.

Schei·ner experiment (shi′nər) [Christoph *Scheiner*, German astronomer, 1575–1650] see under *experiment*.

sche·ma (ske′mə) [Gr. *schēma* form, shape] a plan, outline, or arrangement.

sche·mat·ic (ske-mat′ik) serving as a diagram or model.

scheme (skēm) 1. a plan or plot. 2. a diagram or chart detailing a system or plan.

decay s. a diagram detailing the disintegration pattern for an atom, showing transitions between various energy states.

Sche·pel·mann sign (sha′pəl-mahn) [Emil *Schepelmann*, German physician, 20th century] see under *sign*.

sche·ro·ma (ske-ro′mə) xerophthalmia.

-schesis [Gr. *schesis* holding back or suppression] word element signifying suppression of a process.

Scheu·er·mann disease, kyphosis (shoi′ər-mahn) [Holger Werfel *Scheuermann*, Danish surgeon, 1877–1960] osteochondrosis of the vertebrae; see *osteochondrosis*.

Schick sign, test (reaction) (shik) [Béla *Schick*, Hungarian pediatrician in the United States, 1877–1967] see under *sign* and *test*.

Schiff reagent (shif) [Hugo (Ugo) *Schiff*, German chemist in Italy, 1834–1915] see under *reagent*.

Schil·der disease (encephalitis) (shil′dər) [Paul Ferdinand *Schilder*, Austrian-born neurologist in the United States, 1886–1940] see under *disease*.

Schil·ler test (shil′ər) [Walter *Schiller*, Austrian pathologist in the United States, 1887–1960] see under *test*.

Schil·ling leukemia (shil′ing) [Victor Theodor Adolf Georg *Schilling*, German hematologist, 1883–1960] acute monocytic leukemia.

Schil·ling test (shil′ing) [Robert Frederick *Schilling*, American hematologist, born 1919] see under *test*.

Schim·mel·busch disease (shim′əl-boosh″) [Curt *Schimmelbusch*, German surgeon, 1860–1895] cystic disease of the breast; see under *disease*.

Schim·mel·pen·ning syndrome (shim′əl-pen″ing) [Gustav W. *Schimmelpenning*, German dermatologist, born 1928] sebaceous nevus syndrome.

schin·dy·le·sis (skin″də-le′sis) [Gr. *schindylēsis* a splintering] [TA] a form of articulation in which a thin plate of one bone is received into a cleft in another, as in the articulation of the perpendicular plate of the ethmoid bone with the vomer. Called also *wedge-and-groove joint*.

Schi·nus (shi′nəs) a genus of flowering trees of the family Anacardiaceae. *S. terebinthifolius* is the Brazilian pepper tree or Florida holly tree; its sap and crushed berries are common causes of urushiol dermatitis in southern Florida.

Schin·zel-Gie·di·on syndrome (shin′tsel ge′de-on) [Albert A.G.L. *Schinzel*, Austrian geneticist, born 1944; Andres *Giedion*, Swiss radiologist, born 1925] see under *syndrome*.

Schi·øtz tonometer (she-ets′) [Hjalmar *Schiøtz*, Norwegian physician, 1850–1927] see under *tonometer*.

Schir·mer syndrome (shir′mər) [Rudolf *Schirmer*, German ophthalmologist, 1831–1896] see under *syndrome*.

-schisis [Gr. *schisis* cleft] a combining form denoting a cleft or cleavage.

schis·ta·sis (skis′tə-sis) cleft (def. 2).

schist(o)- [Gr. *schistos* split] a combining form meaning split, cleft, or divided.

schis·to·cor·mia (shis″-, skis″to-kor′me-ə) [*schisto-* + Gr. *kormos* trunk + *-ia*] a developmental anomaly characterized by a fissure of the abdomen, with lower limbs rudimentary or lacking. Called also *schistosomia*.

schis·to·cor·mus (shis″-, skis″to-kor′məs) a fetus exhibiting schistocormia.

schis·to·cyte (shis′-, skis′to-sīt) a fragment of an erythrocyte, commonly observed in the blood in hemolytic anemias; called also *helmet cell* and *schizocyte*.

schis·to·cy·to·sis (shis″-, skis″to-si-to′sis) the accumulation of schistocytes in the blood; called also *schizocytosis*.

schis·to·me·lia (shis″-, skis″to-me′le-ə) [*schisto-* + *-melia*] a developmental anomaly characterized by a cleft condition of a limb.

schis·tom·e·lus (shis-, skis-tom′ə-ləs) a fetus exhibiting schistomelia.

schis·to·sis (shis-, skis-to′sis) [*schist* a form of slate + *-osis*] pneumoconiosis in slate workers.

Schis·to·so·ma (shis″-, skis″to-so′mə) [*schisto-* + Gr. *sōma* body] a genus of blood flukes, parasitic trematodes of the family Schistosomatidae; called also *Bilharzia*.

S. bo′vis a species found in the portal system of sheep and cattle in Iraq, Africa, and certain islands in the Mediterranean.

S. haemato′bium a common parasite that causes schistosomiasis in humans in North Africa, other Mediterranean coastal regions, and the Arabian Peninsula. The adult worms are found in the veins, especially those of the vesical plexus, producing irritability of the bladder, hematuria, and dysentery. The parasites enter the body through the skin of persons coming in contact with infested waters, the invertebrate hosts being small snails of the genus *Bulinus*, including the subgenus *Physopsis*. Called also *Bilharzia haematobia*.

S. in′dicum a species occurring in cattle, sheep, goats, and other ruminants in India and southern Africa.

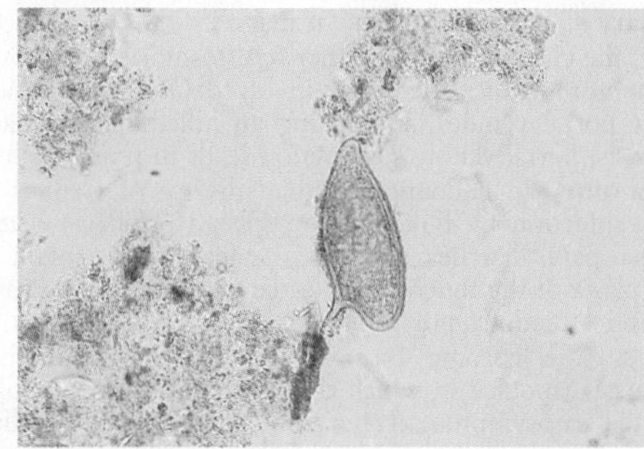

■ *Schistosoma mansoni* egg, showing prominent lateral spine.

S. intercala′tum a species found in the veins of humans, horses, and ruminants in Central and West Africa; it causes schistosomiasis intercalatum by penetrating the skin of persons coming in contact with infested water. The transmitting hosts are snails of the genus *Bulinus*.

S. japo′nicum a species found in the veins of animals in Japan, China, the Philippines, Taiwan, and Indonesia; it causes schistosomiasis japonica by penetrating the skin of persons coming in contact with infested waters. The usual transmitting hosts are small snails of the genus *Oncomelania*.

S. manso′ni a species found in the veins of animals in Egypt and elsewhere in Africa as well as in South America and the West Indies; it causes schistosomiasis mansoni by penetrating the skin of persons coming in contact with infested waters. The transmitting hosts are planorbid snails, especially those of the genus *Biomphalaria*.

S. mat′theei a species found in the portal mesenteric vein of various species of mammals in southern Africa.

S. mekon′gi a species found in Laos and Cambodia that differs from *S. japonicum* chiefly in requiring a different intermediate host.

S. spinda′le a species parasitic in ruminants in India, Malaysia, Indonesia, and southern Africa, and sometimes causing cercarial dermatitis in humans.

schis·to·so·ma·ci·dal (shis″-, skis″to-so″mə-si′dəl) schistosomicidal.

schis·to·so·ma·cide (shis″-, skis″to-so′mə-sīd) schistosomicide.

schis·to·so·mal (shis″-, skis″to-so′məl) pertaining to or caused by *Schistosoma*. Called also *bilharzial*.

Schis·to·so·ma·ti·dae (shis″-, skis″tə-so-mat′ĭ-de) a family of trematodes, including the genera *Heterobilharzia*, *Schistosoma*, *Schistosomatium*, and *Trichobilharzia*.

Schis·to·so·ma·ti·um (shis″-, skis″to-so-ma′she-əm) a genus of blood flukes of the family Schistosomatidae. *S. douthit′ti* is usually found in the hepatic portal veins of the meadow mouse but sometimes causes cercarial dermatitis in humans.

schis·to·some (shis′-, skis′to-sōm) 1. an individual fluke of the genus *Schistosoma*. 2. sometimes extended to refer to any fluke of the family Schistosomatidae.

schis·to·so·mia (shis″-, skis″to-so′me-ə) [*schisto-* + *soma* + *-ia*] a developmental anomaly characterized by a fissure of the abdomen, with lower limbs (in humans) or hind limbs (in quadrupeds) rudimentary or lacking.

schis·to·so·mi·a·sis (shis″-, skis″to-so-mi′ə-sis) infection with flukes of the genus *Schistosoma;* called also *bilharziasis* and *bilharziosis*.

cutaneous s. cercarial dermatitis.

eastern s. s. japonica.

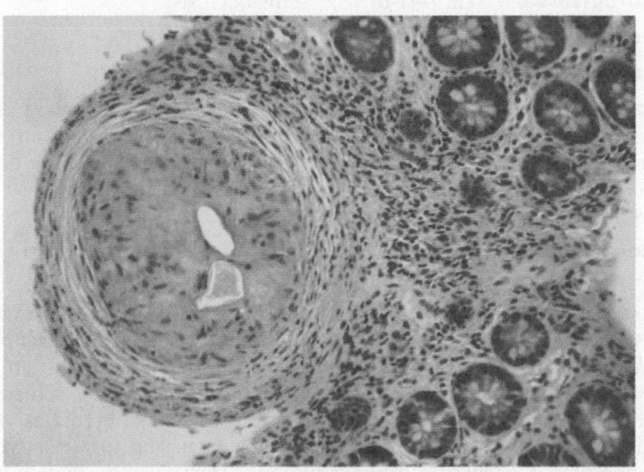

■ Schistosomiasis. Colon biopsy specimen showing a schistosome egg granuloma.

genitourinary s., s. haemato′bia urinary s.

hepatic s. the chronic form of either schistosomiasis mansoni or schistosomiasis japonica in which the liver is involved. Ova of the parasites lodge in the hepatic portal venules, stimulating an inflammatory reaction with pipestem fibrosis; portal venous destruction leads to portal hypertension.

s. intercala′tum an endemic intestinal disease of Central and West Africa due to infection by flukes of the species *Schistosoma intercalatum*, with abdominal pain, diarrhea in which the feces may contain blood and mucus, hyperplasia of the mucosa of the rectal valves, inflammation of the rectal walls, and sometimes polyposis.

intestinal s. the chronic form of either schistosomiasis mansoni or schistosomiasis japonica in which the intestinal tract is involved. Most of those infected are asymptomatic but some have intermittent diarrhea and blood and mucus in the feces.

s. japo′nica infection by *Schistosoma japonicum*. Acute infection in the early stages produces a condition called Katayama fever, which resembles serum sickness. Chronic effects of infection, which may be severe, are caused by fibrosis around the eggs deposited by the parasite in the liver, lungs, and central nervous system.

Manson s., s. manso′ni infection with *Schistosoma mansoni*, which lives mainly in the inferior and superior mesenteric veins but migrates to deposit eggs in venules, primarily of the large intestine. Eggs lodging in the liver may lead to peripheral fibrosis, hepatosplenomegaly, and ascites. Called also *Manson disease*.

Oriental s. s. japonica.

pulmonary s. schistosomiasis in which migrating parasites cause a type of pneumonia, and the ova, and sometimes the adult worms, cause embolization of pulmonary arterioles. Allergic pneumonia, allergic asthma, and emphysema may occur.

urinary s., vesical s. infection with *Schistosoma haematobium*, involving the urinary tract and causing cystitis and hematuria; called also *endemic hematuria*, *genitourinary s.*, and *s. haematobia*.

visceral s. infection with either *Schistosoma mansoni* or *S. japonicum*, as opposed to urinary schistosomiasis.

schis•to•so•mi•ci•dal (shis″-, skis″to-so″mĭ-si′dəl) killing schistosomes; cf. *antischistosomal*.

schis•to•so•mi•cide (shis″-, skis″to-so′mĭ-sīd) an agent that kills schistosomes; cf. *antischistosomal*.

schis•to•so•mu•lum (shis″-, skis″to-som′u-ləm) pl. *schistoso′mula*. A stage in the life cycle of a schistosome occurring just after it has penetrated human skin as a cercaria; it loses its tail and becomes physiologically modified in order to be capable of anaerobic metabolism in the bloodstream.

Schis•to•so•mum (shis″-, skis″to-so′məm) *Schistosoma*.

schis•to•so•mus (shis″-, skis″to-so′məs) a fetus with schistosomia.

schiz•am•ni•on (skiz-am′ne-ən) [*schiz-* + *amnion*] an amnion formed by cavitation over or in the embryoblast, as in human development.

schiz•ax•on (skiz-ak′son) an axon which is divided into two equal, or nearly equal, branches.

schiz•en•ce•phal•ic (skiz″ən-sə-fal′ik) having abnormal clefts in the brain substance; see under *porencephaly*.

schiz•en•ceph•a•ly (skiz″ən-sef′ə-le) [*schiz-* + Gr. *enkephalos* brain] schizencephalic porencephaly.

schiz(o)- [Gr. *schizein* to divide] a combining form meaning split, cleft, or divided.

schizo•af•fec•tive (skit′so-ə-fek′tiv) pertaining to or exhibiting features of both schizophrenic and mood disorders.

schizo•cyte (skiz′o-sīt) schistocyte.

schizo•cy•to•sis (skiz″o-si-to′sis) schistocytosis.

schizo•gen•e•sis (skiz″o-jen′ə-sis) fission (def. 2).

schi•zog•e•nous (skĭ-zog′ə-nəs) reproducing by fission.

schi•zog•o•ny (skĭ-zog′ə-ne) [*schizo-* + Gr. *gonē* seed] a form of asexual reproduction characteristic of certain sarcodines and sporozoa in which daughter cells are produced by multiple fission of the nucleus of the parasite (schizont) followed by segmentation of the cytoplasm to form separate masses around each smaller nucleus.

schizo•gy•ria (skiz″o-ji′re-ə) a condition in which the cerebral convolutions are marked by wedge-shaped cracks.

schiz•oid (skit′soid) 1. characterized by or resulting from excessive shyness, sensitivity, social withdrawal, and introversion; see *schizoid personality disorder*, under *disorder*. 2. a term used loosely to refer to any of a variety of characteristics related to schizophrenia, including schizophrenia-like traits said to indicate a predisposition to schizophrenia as well as any disorder other than schizophrenia either occurring in a relative of a schizophrenic or occurring more commonly than average in families of schizophrenics.

schizo•ki•ne•sis (skit″so-kĭ-ne′sis) the condition in which, when an overt specific conditioned response has been extinguished, concomitant nonspecific responses continue to be elicited by the stimulus.

schiz•ont (skiz′ont) [*schizo-* + Gr. *ōn*, *ontos* being] the multinucleate stage or form in the development of certain sporozoa and sarcodine protozoa during schizogony. See also *meront* and *segmenter*.

schi•zon•ti•cide (skĭ-zon′tĭ-sīd) an agent that destroys schizonts.

schizo•nych•ia (skiz″o-nik′e-ə) onychoschizia.

schizo•pha•sia (skit″so-fa′zhə) word salad; see under *W*.

schizo•phre•nia (skit″so-fre′ne-ə) [*schizo-* + *phren* + *-ia*] [DSM-IV] a mental disorder or heterogeneous group of disorders (the schizophrenias or schizophrenic disorders) comprising most major psychotic disorders and characterized by disturbances in form and content of thought (loosening of associations, delusions, and hallucinations), mood (blunted, flattened, or inappropriate affect), sense of self and relationship to the external world (loss of ego boundaries, dereistic thinking, and autistic withdrawal), and behavior (bizarre, apparently purposeless, and stereotyped activity or inactivity). The definition and clinical application of the concept of schizophrenia have varied greatly. The DSM-IV criteria emphasize marked disorder of thought (delusions, hallucinations, or other thought disorder accompanied by disordered affect or behavior), deterioration from a previous level of functioning, and chronicity (duration of more than 6 months), thus excluding from this classification conditions referred to by others as acute, borderline, simple, or latent schizophrenia.

acute s. acute schizophrenic episode; a condition characterized by acute onset of schizophrenic symptoms; since DSM-IV defines schizophrenia as a chronic disorder, such conditions must now be classified in another psychotic syndrome, such as schizophreniform disorder, brief psychotic disorder, or schizoaffective disorder.

ambulatory s. mild schizophrenia that is compensated well enough that patients can maintain themselves in the community without hospitalization.

borderline s. latent s.

catatonic s. [DSM-IV] a type of schizophrenia characterized by marked psychomotor disturbance, including some combination of motoric immobility (stupor, catalepsy), excessive motor activity, extreme negativism, mutism, echolalia, echopraxia, and peculiarities of voluntary movement such as posturing, mannerisms, grimacing, or stereotyped behaviors.

childhood s. schizophrenia-like symptoms with onset before puberty, characterized by autistic, withdrawn behavior, failure to develop an identity separate from the mother's, and gross developmental immaturity, a category that formerly included all types of childhood "psychosis" including symbiotic psychosis and infantile autism. DSM-IV, taking the position that there is no clear relationship between these disorders and adolescent and adult schizophrenia and other psychotic disorders, calls them pervasive developmental disorders.

disorganized s. [DSM-IV] a type of schizophrenia characterized by frequent incoherence, marked loosening of associations, or grossly disorganized behavior and flat or grossly inappropriate affect and that does not meet the criteria for the catatonic type; associated features include extreme social withdrawal, grimacing, mannerisms, mirror gazing, inappropriate giggling, and other unusual behavior.

hebephrenic s. disorganized s.

latent s. a type of schizophrenia characterized by clear symptoms of schizophrenia but no history of a psychotic schizophrenic episode; it includes conditions that have been called ambulatory, borderline, prepsychotic, pseudoneurotic, and pseudopsychopathic schizophrenia in which has there has been no acute psychotic episode. Patients described by these terms do not fit the DSM-IV definition of schizophrenia; most would be classified as having schizotypal personality disorder (q.v.).

paranoid s. [DSM-IV] a type of schizophrenia characterized by preoccupation with one or more systematized delusions or with frequent auditory hallucinations but without disorganized speech, disorganized or catatonic behavior, or flat or inappropriate affect.

prepsychotic s. latent s.

process s. schizophrenia having a particularly debilitating course and poor prognosis.

residual s. [DSM-IV] a type of schizophrenia characterized by a history of one or more episodes of schizophrenia with prominent psychotic symptoms, current lack of such symptoms, but continuing presence of other schizophrenic symptoms, such as blunted or inappropriate affect, social withdrawal, eccentric behavior, illogical thinking, or loosening of associations.

schizoaffective s. see under *disorder*.

simple s. a type of schizophrenia characterized by gradual, insidious loss of drive, social withdrawal, and emotional apathy, but without prominent psychotic features. It is often considered to be a form of personality disorder; see *schizotypal personality disorder*, under *disorder*.

undifferentiated s. [DSM-IV] a type of schizophrenia characterized by the presence of prominent psychotic symptoms but not classifiable as catatonic, disorganized, or paranoid.

schizo•phren•ic (skit″so-fren′ik) 1. pertaining to or characterized by schizophrenia. 2. a person affected with schizophrenia.

schizo•phren•i•form (skit″so-fren′ĭ-form) resembling schizophrenia.

Schiz•oph•yl•lum (skiz-of′ĭ-ləm) a genus of fungi of the subphylum Basidiomycotina, order Aphyllophorales. *S. commu′ne* has been isolated from human infections, including maxillary sinusitis.

schizo•pro•so•pia (skiz″o-pro-so′pe-ə) facial cleft (def. 2).

Schizo•py•ren•i•da (skiz″o-pĭ-ren′ĭ-də) [*schizo-* + Gr. *pyrēn* fruit stone] an order of ameboid protozoa of the class Lobosa, phylum Sarcomastigophora; they are typically cylindrical, and monopodial. Some species have temporary flagellate stages during their life cycle. Representative genera include *Naegleria* and *Vahlkampfia.*

schizo•tax•ia (skit″so-tak′se-ə) a genetic predisposition to schizophrenia.

schizo•tho•rax (skiz″o-thor′aks) thoracoschisis.

schizo•to•nia (skiz″o-to′ne-ə) [*schizo-* + *ton-* + *-ia*] division of the influx of tone to the muscles, so that, for instance, in the upper limbs the flexors become hypertonic, while in the lower limbs the extensors become hypertonic.

schizo•trich•ia (skiz″o-trik′e-ə) trichoschisis.

Schizo•tryp•a•num (skiz″o-trip′ə-nəm) [*schizo-* + Gr. *trypanon* borer] 1. in some systems of protozoa classification, a stercorarian subgenus of the genus *Trypanosoma,* including *T. cruzi.* 2. in some systems of classification, this is considered a genus genetically distinct from *Trypanosoma,* and the species causing Chagas disease is called *S. cruzi.*

schizo•ty•pal (skit″so-ti′pəl) exhibiting eccentricities in behavior and communication style, and decreased ability to form social relationships, similar to those of schizophrenia but less severe. See *schizotypal personality disorder,* under *disorder.*

schizo•zo•ite (skiz″o-zo′īt) merozoite.

Schlat•ter disease (sprain) (shlah′tər) [Carl *Schlatter,* Swiss surgeon, 1864–1934] see *Osgood-Schlatter disease,* under *disease.*

Schlat•ter-Os•good disease (shlah′tər oz′good) [C. *Schlatter;* Robert Bayley *Osgood,* American orthopedist, 1873–1956] see *Osgood-Schlatter disease,* under *disease.*

Schlemm canal, ligaments (shlem) [Friedrich S. *Schlemm,* German anatomist, 1795–1858] see *sinus venosus sclerae,* and under *ligament.*

Schlep•per (shlep′ər) [Ger. *Schlepper,* hauler, tractor, tugboat] carrier (def. 7).

Schle•sin•ger sign (phenomenon) (shla′sing-ər) [Hermann *Schlesinger,* Austrian physician, 1866–1934] see under *sign.*

Schlich•ter test (shlik′tər) [Jakub G. *Schlichter,* American internist, 20th century] see *serum bactericidal activity test,* under *test.*

Schmidt syndrome[1] (shmit) [Adolf *Schmidt,* German physician, 1865–1918] see under *syndrome.*

Schmidt syndrome[2] (shmit) [Martin Benno *Schmidt,* German pathologist, 1863–1949] see under *syndrome.*

Schmidt-Lan•ter•man incisures (clefts), segment (shmit′ lan′tər-mən) [Henry D. *Schmidt,* American anatomist, 1823–1888; A.J. *Lanterman,* American anatomist in Germany, late 19th century] see under *incisure,* and see *medullary segment,* under *segment.*

Schmin•cke tumor (shming′kə) [Alexander *Schmincke,* German pathologist, 1877–1953] lymphoepithelioma.

Schmorl body, disease, nodule (shmorl) [Christian Georg *Schmorl,* German pathologist, 1861–1932] see under *body, disease,* and *nodule.*

Schna•bel caverns (shnah′bəl) [Isidor *Schnabel,* Austrian ophthalmologist, 1842–1908] see under *cavern.*

Schnei•der carmine (shni′dər) [Franz Coelestin *Schneider,* German chemist, 1813–1897] see under *carmine.*

schnei•de•ri•an (shni-de′re-ən) named for Conrad Victor *Schneider,* German physician, 1614–1680.

Schnitz•ler syndrome (shnits′lər) [L. *Schnitzler,* French dermatologist, 20th century] see under *syndrome.*

Schoe•ma•ker line (shoo′mah-kər) [Jan *Schoemaker,* Dutch surgeon, 1871–1940] see under *line.*

Schön's theory (shurnz) [Wilhelm *Schön,* German ophthalmologist, 1848–1917] see under *theory.*

Schön•lein purpura (disease) (shurn′līn) [Johann Lukas *Schönlein,* German physician, 1793–1864] purpura rheumatica.

Schön•lein-Hen•och purpura (disease) (shurn′līn hen′ŏk) [J.L. *Schönlein;* Eduard Heinrich *Henoch,* German pediatrician, 1820–1910] Henoch-Schönlein purpura.

schra•dan (shra′dan) octamethyl pyrophosphoramide.

Schre•ger bands (shra′gər) [Christian Heinrich Theodor *Schreger,* Danish anatomist, 1768–1833] Hunter-Schreger bands; see under *band.*

Schrei•ber maneuver (shri′bər) [Julius *Schreiber,* German physician, 1849–1932] see under *maneuver.*

Schroe•der disease (shrur′dər) [Robert *Schroeder,* German gynecologist, 1884–1959] see under *disease.*

Schroe•der van der Kolk's law (shrur′dər vahn dār kolks) [Jacob Ludwig Conrad *Schroeder van der Kolk,* Dutch physiologist, 1797–1862] see under *law.*

Schu•chardt incision (shoo′kahrt) [Karl August *Schuchardt,* German surgeon, 1856–1901] paravaginal incision.

Schüff•ner dots, stippling (shēf′nər) [Wilhelm August Paul *Schüffner,* German pathologist, 1867–1949] see under *dot* and *stippling.*

Schül•ler disease (syndrome) (she′lər) [Artur *Schüller,* Austrian neurologist, 1874–1958] see *Hand-Schüller-Christian disease,* under *disease,* and see *osteoporosis circumscripta cranii.*

Schül•ler-Chris•tian disease (syndrome) (she′lər kris′chən) [A. *Schüller;* Henry A. *Christian,* American physician, 1876–1951] Hand-Schüller-Christian disease; see under *disease.*

Schultz syndrome (angina) (shoolts) [Werner *Schultz,* German internist, 1878–1947] agranulocytosis.

Schultz-Dale reaction (shoolts′ dāl′) [W. *Schultz;* Sir Henry Hallett *Dale,* English physiologist and pharmacologist, 1875–1968] see under *reaction.*

Schult•ze cells, tract (shoolt′sə) [Max Johann Sigismund *Schultze,* German biologist, 1825–1874] see *olfactory cells,* under *cell,* and *fasciculus interfascicularis.*

Schult•ze fold (shoolt′sə) [Bernhard Sigismund *Schultze,* German gynecologist, 1827–1919] see under *fold.*

Schult•ze sign (shoolt′sə) [Friedrich *Schultze,* German physician, 1848–1934] Chvostek sign; see under *sign.*

Schult•ze-Chvos•tek sign (shoolt′sə kvos′tek) [F. *Schultze;* Franz *Chvostek,* Austrian surgeon, 1835–1884] Chvostek sign.

Schumm test (shoom) [Otto *Schumm,* German chemist, early 20th century] see under *test.*

Schütz fasciculus (bundle, tract) (shēts) [Hugo *Schütz,* German neurologist, early 20th century] see *fasciculus longitudinalis dorsalis.*

Schwa•bach test (shvah′bahk) [Dagobert *Schwabach,* German otologist, 1846–1920] see under *test.*

Schwal•be corpuscles, etc. (shvahl′bə) [Gustav Albert *Schwalbe,* German anatomist, 1844–1917] see under *corpuscle, fissure, nucleus, ring, sheath,* and *space.*

Schwann cell, membrane (sheath), nucleus, substance (shvahn) [Theodor *Schwann,* German anatomist and physiologist, 1810–1882] see under *cell* and *nucleus,* and see *neurilemma.*

schwan•ni•tis (shwah-ni′tis) schwannosis.

schwan•no•gli•o•ma (shwah″no-gli-o′mə) schwannoma.

schwan•no•ma (shwah-no′mə) 1. a neoplasm originating from Schwann cells (of the myelin sheath) of neurons; the two types are neurilemomas and neurofibromas. Called also *schwannoglioma* and *Schwann cell tumor.* 2. neurilemoma.

acoustic s. see under *neuroma.*

cellular s. a type of schwannoma that contains compact, hypercellular fascicles and is found most often adjacent to the vertebral column.

granular cell s. see under *tumor.*

malignant s. malignant peripheral nerve sheath tumor.

plexiform s. a rare type of schwannoma characterized by an interconnecting multinodular pattern of intraneural growth, arising most often in soft tissues of the head and neck.

vestibular s. acoustic neuroma.

schwan•no•ma•to•sis (shwah″no-mə-to′sis) the occurrence of multiple schwannomas, usually indicating that a person has a genetic predisposition to them; this is sometimes an autosomal dominant condition, such as neurofibromatosis type 2.

schwan•no•min (shwah-no′min) merlin.

schwan•no•sis (shwah-no′sis) hypertrophy of the neurilemma (sheath of Schwann).

Schwartz-Jam•pel syndrome (shworts′ jam′pəl) [Oscar *Schwartz,* American pediatrician, born 1919; Robert Steven *Jampel,* American ophthalmologist, born 1926] see under *syndrome.*

Schwartz-Jam•pel-Aber•feld syndrome (shworts′ jam′pəl a′bər-feld) [O. *Schwartz;* R.S. *Jampel;* D.C. *Aberfeld,* British physician, 20th century] see under *syndrome.*

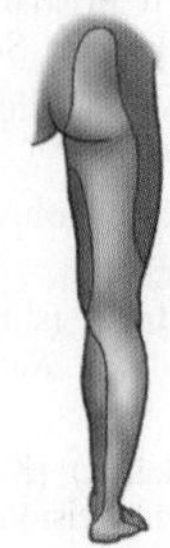

■ Distribution of pain in sciatica.

Schwart•ze sign (shvahrt′zə) [Hermann Hugo Rudolf *Schwartze*, German otologist, 1837–1910] see under *sign*.

Schwarz activator, appliance (shvahrtz) [Arthur Martin *Schwarz*, Austrian orthodontist, 20th century] see *bow activator*, under *activator*, and see under *appliance*.

Schwe•di•au•er (shva′de-ou″ər) see *Swediaur*.

Schweig•ger-Sei•del sheath (shvi′gər-si′dəl) [Franz *Schweigger-Seidel*, German physiologist, 1834–1871] see under *sheath*.

Schwen•in•ger-Buz•zi anetoderma (shven′in-gər boot′se) [Ernst *Schweninger*, German physician, 1850–1924; Fausto *Buzzi*, Swiss dermatologist, 1858–1907] see under *anetoderma*.

SCI spinal cord injury.

sci•age (se-ahzh′) [Fr.] a sawing movement in massage.

Sci•an•na blood group (se-ah′nah) [*Scianna*, surname of the propositus first reported on in the 1960s] see under *blood group*.

sci•at•ic (si-at′ik) [L. *sciaticus;* Gr. *ischiadikos*] 1. ischial. 2. pertaining to or located near the sciatic nerve; called also *ischiadic* and *ischiatic*.

sci•at•i•ca (si-at′ĭ-kə) [L.] a syndrome characterized by pain radiating from the back into the buttock and along the posterior or lateral aspect of the lower limb; it is most often caused by protrusion of a low lumbar intervertebral disk. The term is also used to refer to pain anywhere along the course of the sciatic nerve. Called also *Cotugno disease* and *sciatic neuralgia* or *neuropathy*.

SCID severe combined immunodeficiency.

sci•ence (si′əns) [L. *scientia* knowledge] 1. the systematic observation of natural phenomena for the purpose of discovering laws governing those phenomena. 2. the body of knowledge accumulated by such means.

applied s. science that is concerned with the application of discovered laws to the matters of everyday living.

behavioral s. the interdisciplinary study of behavior for the purpose of understanding persons as individual and social beings; it involves principally psychology, sociology, and anthropology, but also political science and other social sciences.

pure s. science that is concerned solely with the discovery of unknown laws relating to particular facts.

sci•en•tist (si′ən-tist) an individual learned in science, especially one active in some particular field of investigation.

sci•er•opia (si-ər-o′pe-ə) [Gr. *skieros* shady + *-opia*] visual defect in which objects appear in a shadow.

scil•la (sil′ə) [L.] squill.

scil•la•bi•ose (sil″ə-bi′ōs) a disaccharide obtained by acid hydrolysis of scillaren A.

scil•la•ren (sil′ə-rən) a mixture of cardioactive glycosides, scillaren A and B, from fresh squill.

scil•lir•o•side (sil′ir-o-sīd) a cardiac glycoside that is the active principle in red squill (q.v.); in small amounts it causes convulsions and in larger amounts cardiac arrest.

scim•i•tar (sim′ĭ-tahr) [Persian *shimshir*] 1. a sword used in the Middle East that curves to one side. 2. shaped like such a sword.

scin•ti•an•gi•og•ra•phy (sin″tĭ-an″je-og′rə-fe) angioscintigraphy.

scin•ti•gram (sin′tĭ-gram) the graphic record obtained by scintigraphy.

scin•tig•ra•phy (sin-tig′rə-fe) the production of two-dimensional images of the distribution of radioactivity in tissues after the internal administration of radionuclide, the images being obtained by a scintillation camera. **scintigraph′ic** *adj*

acute infarct s. infarct avid s.

exercise thallium s. thallium-201 scintigraphy performed in conjunction with an exercise stress test; see *thallium stress test*, under *test*.

gated blood pool s. equilibrium radionuclide angiocardiography.

infarct avid s. scintigraphy performed following myocardial infarction to confirm infarction as well as detect, localize, and quantify regions of myocardial necrosis. A radiotracer that concentrates in these regions, usually technetium ^{99m}Tc pyrophosphate, is administered intravenously and images are obtained with a gamma camera. For maximal sensitivity, the study is performed between 24 and 72 hours after infarction.

myocardial perfusion s. scintigraphy performed using a radiotracer that traverses the myocardial capillary system and enters myocardial cells; after the radionuclide, usually thallium 201, is introduced into the bloodstream, regional myocardial blood flow and cell viability are assessed using immediate and delayed images. Scintigraphy is frequently combined with an exercise stress test in the diagnosis of coronary artery disease. See also *thallium-201 myocardial perfusion s.* and *thallium stress test*, under *test*.

technetium Tc 99m pyrophosphate s. infarct avid s.

thallium-201 myocardial perfusion s. the most common type of myocardial perfusion scintigraphy; the radionuclide used is thallium 201 in the form of thallous chloride. It is most frequently performed in conjunction with exercise stress tests in the diagnosis of coronary artery disease, but is sometimes performed on resting patients to detect transient ischemia or myocardial infarction. See also *thallium stress test*, under *test*.

scin•til•la•tion (sin″tĭ-la′shən) [L. *scintilla* spark] 1. an emission of sparks. 2. a subjective visual sensation, as of seeing sparks. 3. a particle emitted in disintegration of a radioactive element.

scin•ti•pho•to•graph (sin″tĭ-fo′to-graf) scintigram.

scin•ti•pho•tog•ra•phy (sin″tĭ-fo-tog′rə-fe) scintigraphy.

scin•ti•re•nog•ra•phy (sin″tĭ-re-nog′rə-fe) scintigraphy of the kidney.

scin•ti•scan (sin′tĭ-skan) a two-dimensional representation (map) of the radiation emitted by a radioisotope, revealing its varying concentration in specific tissues of the body, such as the brain, kidney, or thyroid gland.

scin•ti•scan•ner (sin″tĭ-skan′ər) the system of equipment used in the making of a scintiscan.

scirrh(o)- [Gr. *skirrhos* hard] a combining form meaning hard, or denoting relationship to a hard cancer or scirrhous carcinoma.

scir•rhoid (skir′oid) [*scirrho-* + *-oid*] resembling scirrhous carcinoma.

scir•rhous (skir′əs) [L. *scirrhosus*] pertaining to or of the nature of a hard cancer; see also under *carcinoma*.

scir•rhus (skir′əs) [Gr. *skirrhos*] scirrhous carcinoma.

scis•sion (sizh′ən) [L. *scindere* to split] fission; splitting. In chemistry, the splitting of a molecule into two or more simpler molecules.

scis•sors (siz′ərz) a cutting instrument with two opposed shearing blades. See accompanying table.

canalicular s. delicate scissors with one of the blades probe pointed; used in slitting the lacrimal canal.

cannula s. scissors used in slitting a canal lengthwise.

craniotomy s. strong F-shaped shears for use in opening the fetal head.

Fox s. delicate, fine-pointed scissors designed to gain access to interproximal areas for the removal of small tissue tabs or slight soft tissue deformities during gingivoplasty or gingivectomy.

Liston s. scissors for cutting plaster-of-Paris bandages.

Smellie s. short, strong-bladed scissors with external cutting edges, used in craniotomy.

scis•sors-bite (siz′erz-bīt′) see under *bite*.

Sciu•ri•dae (syoo′rĭ-de) the squirrel family, a family of rodents usually having long bushy tails and strong hind legs; there are both tree-dwelling and ground-dwelling genera. Genera of public health interest include *Ammospermophilus*, *Cynomys*, *Marmota*, and *Spermophilus*.

ScLA [L.] scapulo-laeva anterior (left scapuloanterior, a position of the fetus; see *position*).

SCLC small cell lung carcinoma.

scle•ra (sklēr′ə) gen. and pl. *scle′rae* [L., from Gr. *skleros* hard] [TA] the tough white outer coat of the eyeball, covering approximately the posterior

Selected Scissors

Barraquer scissors	Mayo scissors
Castroviejo scissors	Metzenbaum scissors
curved Mayo scissors	Nelson scissors
DeWecker scissors	Potts-Smith scissors
Jako scissors	Thorek scissors
Knapp scissors	Vannas scissors
Littler scissors	Westcott scissors
McGuire scissors	

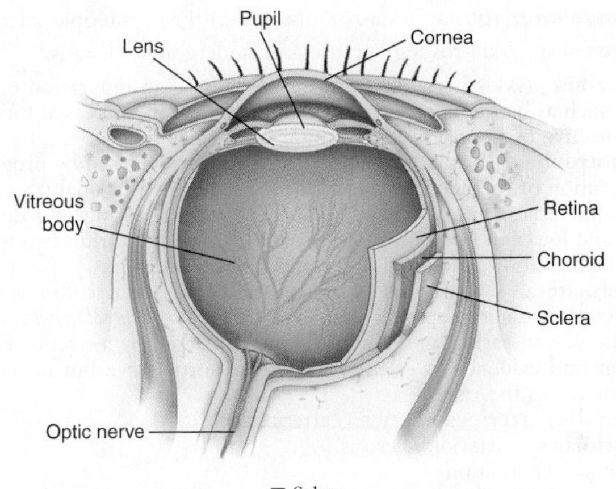

■ Sclera.

five-sixths of its surface, and continuous anteriorly with the cornea and posteriorly with the external sheath of the optic nerve. **scler'al** *adj*

blue s. a condition of unusual blueness of the sclera; it is normal in infants, but is also a prominent feature of osteogenesis imperfecta, and is seen in certain other abnormalities.

scle•rad•e•ni•tis (sklēr″ad-ə-ni′tis) [*sclero-* + *aden-* + *-itis*] inflammation and hardening of a gland.

scle•ra•ti•tis (sklēr″ə-ti′tis) scleritis.

scle•ra•tog•e•nous (sklēr″ə-toj′ə-nəs) sclerogenous.

scle•rec•ta•sia (sklēr″ək-ta′zhə) [*scler-* + *ectasia*] a bulging out of the sclera.

scle•rec•ta•sis (sklə-rek′tə-sis) sclerectasia.

scle•rec•to•iri•dec•to•my (sklə-rek″to-ir″ĭ-dek′tə-me) [*sclerectomy* + *iridectomy*] the operation of excision of a portion of the sclera and of the iris for glaucoma; called also *Lagrange operation.*

scle•rec•to•iri•do•di•al•y•sis (sklə-rek″to-ir″ĭ-do-di-al′ĭ-sis) [*sclera* + *-ectomy* + *irido-* + *dialysis*] sclerectomy and iridodialysis.

scle•rec•tome (sklə-rek′tōm) an instrument for performing sclerectomy.

scle•rec•to•my (sklə-rek′tə-me) [*sclero-* + *ectomy*] excision of the sclera by scissors (Lagrange operation), by punch (Holth operation), or by trephining (Elliot operation).

scle•re•de•ma (sklēr″ə-de′mə) [*scler-* + *edema*] diffuse, symmetrical, woodlike, nonpitting induration of the skin of unknown etiology, typically beginning on the head or neck and spreading progressively to involve the upper limbs, thorax, and sometimes extracutaneous sites. It is usually preceded by an infectious process, especially with a staphylococcus, and usually occurs in association with diabetes mellitus. Women are affected much more often than men, and the condition resolves spontaneously in a few months. Called also *Buschke s.* Although it is not restricted to adults, it is called also *s. adultorum.*

s. adulto′rum, Buschke s. scleredema.

diabetic s., s. diabetico′rum scleredema associated with diabetes mellitus.

s. neonato′rum misnomer for *sclerema.*

scle•re•ma (sklə-re′mə) [*scler-* + (ed)*ema*] a severe, sometimes fatal type of predominantly lobular panniculitis seen chiefly in preterm, sick, or debilitated infants suffering from a serious underlying illness. Characteristics include diffuse, rapidly progressive, nonpitting induration of the adipose tissue, so that the skin becomes cold, pale, and inflexible or boardlike. Called also *s. adiposum, s. neonatorum,* and *Underwood disease.*

s. adipo′sum, s. neonato′rum sclerema.

scle•ren•ce•pha•lia (sklēr″ən-sə-fa′le-ə) sclerencephaly.

scle•ren•ceph•a•ly (sklēr″ən-sef′ə-le) [*sclero* + Gr. *enkephalos*] sclerosis of the brain.

scle•ri•a•sis (sklə-ri′ə-sis) [Gr. *sklēriasis*] a hardened state of an eyelid.

scle•ri•rit•o•my (sklēr″ĭ-rit′ə-me) [*scler-* + *iritomy*] incision of the sclera and iris in anterior staphyloma.

scle•ri•tis (sklə-ri′tis) [*scler-* + *-itis*] inflammation of the sclera, with dilation of the scleral, episcleral, and bulbar conjunctival vessels. It may be confined to a sector or diffuse, and presents with severe, boring pain, photophobia, tearing, and decreased visual acuity. It is often associated with systemic disease, particulary rheumatoid arthritis. Cf. *episcleritis.*

anterior s. inflammation of the sclera adjoining the limbus of the cornea; often subclassified as diffuse, nodular, necrotizing, or necrotizing without inflammation (scleromalacia perforans).

brawny s. a virulent, usually bilateral scleritis involving a thickening of the periphery of the cornea.

diffuse s. the most benign form of anterior scleritis, characterized by widespread injection of the conjunctival and episcleral vessels.

necrotizing s. a severe form of anterior scleritis characterized by progressive necrosis, with thinning of the sclera, through which the underlying uvea can be seen to varying degrees, by painful avascular patches, and potentially resulting in perforation of the globe; usually associated with a serious systemic disease and involvement of multiple organs.

necrotizing s. without inflammation scleromalacia perforans.

nodular s. a form of anterior scleritis characterized by the presence of an immobile, injected nodule in the inflamed area; it may progress to necrotizing scleritis.

posterior s. scleritis involving the posterior sclera, the vagina bulbi, and the underlying retina and choroid.

scler(o)- [Gr. *sklēros* hard] a combining form meaning hard, often used especially to denote relationship to the sclera.

scle•ro•ad•i•pose (sklēr″o-ad′ĭ-pōs) composed of fibrous and fatty tissue.

scle•ro•blas•te•ma (sklēr″o-blas-te′mə) [*sclero-* + *blastema*] the embryonic tissue that takes part in the formation of bone. **scleroblaste′mic** *adj*

scle•ro•cho•roi•di•tis (sklēr″o-ko″roi-di′tis) inflammation of the sclera and the choroid coat, resulting in atrophy of both coats and protrusion of the former.

s. ante′rior inflammation involving the choroid and anterior portions of the sclera and causing anterior staphyloma.

s. poste′rior a condition seen in progressive myopia in which posterior staphyloma occurs in the region of the optic disk.

scle•ro•con•junc•ti•val (sklēr″o-kon″jənk-ti′vəl) pertaining to the sclera and conjunctiva.

scle•ro•con•junc•ti•vi•tis (sklēr″o-kən-junk″tĭ-vi′tis) inflammation of the sclera and the conjunctiva.

scle•ro•cor•nea (sklēr″o-kor′ne-ə) the sclera and the cornea considered as forming a single coat or layer.

scle•ro•cor•ne•al (sklēr″o-kor′ne-əl) pertaining to the sclera and the cornea.

scle•ro•dac•tyl•ia (sklēr″o-dak-til′e-ə) sclerodactyly.

scle•ro•dac•ty•ly (sklēr″o-dak′tə-le) [*sclero-* + Gr. *daktylos* finger] localized scleroderma of the digits, as in acrosclerosis.

scle•ro•der•ma (sklēr″o-dur′mə) [*sclero-* + *derma*] 1. chronic hardening and thickening of the skin, a finding in various different diseases; there are two primary forms: *localized scleroderma* and *systemic scleroderma.* Called also *dermatosclerosis.* 2. systemic s.

circumscribed s. 1. localized s. 2. morphea.

diffuse s., generalized s. systemic s.

linear s. localized scleroderma in which the induration is in bandlike formations, with hyperpigmentation, hypopigmentation, and atrophy of the skin, subcutaneous tissue, muscle, and bone. When it involves the frontal or frontoparietal area of the forehead and the scalp, it is called *coup de sabre.* Called also *linear morphea.*

localized s. 1. scleroderma confined to the skin and subcutaneous tissue or secondarily involving the musculoskeletal system. It occurs in three forms: morphea, linear scleroderma, and coup de sabre. Called also *circumscribed s.* Cf. *systemic s.* 2. morphea.

systemic s. a systemic disorder of the connective tissue characterized by fibrosis with hardening and thickening of the skin, as well as abnormalities of both microvasculature (telangiectasias) and larger vessels (Raynaud phenomenon); there are also fibrotic degenerative changes in body organs such as the heart, lungs, kidneys, and gastrointestinal tract. It may be confined to the face and hands for long periods or may progress, spread

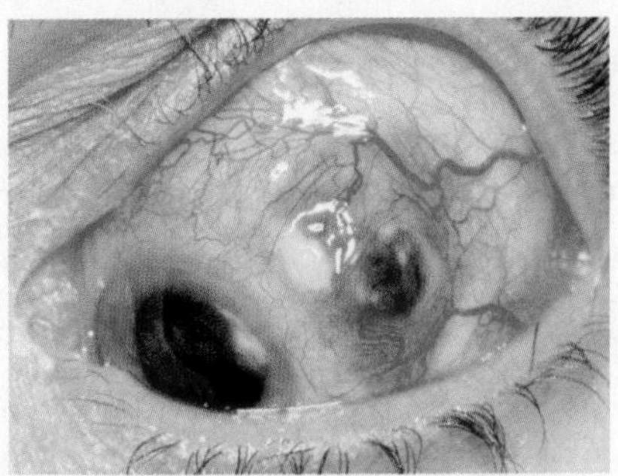

■ Necrotizing scleritis in rheumatoid arthritis. Active scleral inflammation surrounds an area of tissue loss, with uveal tissue visible in the areas of scleral loss.

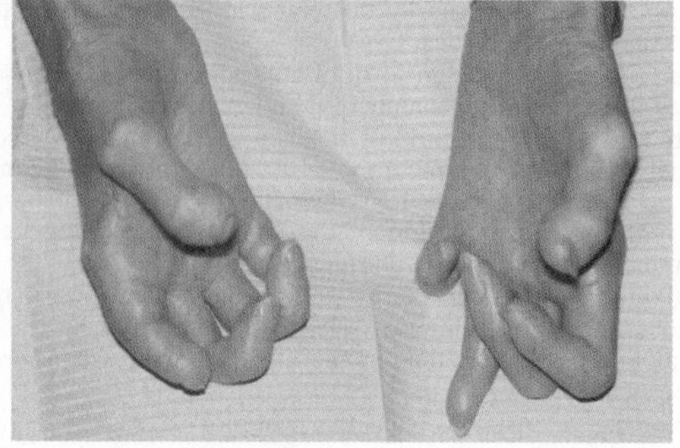

■ Systemic scleroderma with characteristic tense shiny skin and fixed clawlike position of the fingers caused by acro-osteolysis and flexion contractures.

diffusely, and become generalized. Called also *diffuse s.* and *systemic sclerosis.* See also *CREST syndrome.*

scle•ro•der•ma•tous (sklēr″o-dur′mə-təs) pertaining to or characterized by scleroderma.

scle•ro•der•moid (scle″ro-dur′moid) resembling scleroderma.

scle•ro•des•mia (sklēr″o-des′me-ə) [*sclero-* + *desm-* + *-ia*] hardening of ligaments.

scle•ro•em•bo•li•za•tion (sklēr″o-em″bə-lĭ-za′shən) sclerotherapy accompanied by embolization, used most often for varicoceles.

scle•ro•gen•ic (sklēr″o-jen′ik) sclerogenous.

scle•rog•e•nous (sklə-roj′ə-nəs) [*sclero-* + *-genous*] producing sclerosis or sclerous tissue.

scle•ro•gum•ma•tous (sklēr″o-gum′ə-təs) composed of fibrous and gummatous tissue.

scle•roid (sklēr′oid) [*sclero-* + *-oid*] having a hard texture.

scle•ro•iri•tis (sklēr″o-i-ri′tis) inflammation of the sclera and of the iris.

scle•ro•ker•a•ti•tis (sklēr″o-ker″ə-ti′tis) inflammation of the sclera and of the cornea.

scle•ro•ker•a•to•iri•tis (sklēr″o-ker″ə-to-i-ri′tis) inflammation of the sclera, cornea, and iris.

scle•ro•ker•a•to•sis (sklēr″o-ker″ə-to′sis) sclerokeratitis.

scle•ro•ma (sklə-ro′mə) [Gr. *sklērōma* induration] a hardened patch or induration, especially of the nasal or laryngeal tissues. See also *laryngoscleroma, pharyngoscleroma,* and *rhinoscleroma.*

scle•ro•ma•la•cia (sklēr″o-mə-la′shə) [*sclero-* + *malacia*] degeneration and thinning (softening) of the sclera.

s. per′forans a form of nodular scleritis in which necrosis and atrophy occur without inflammation and usually without pain. Marked thinning of the sclera exposes the dark underlying uvea, the nodules may coalesce, and perforation of the globe readily occurs. It is most often associated with rheumatoid arthritis.

scle•ro•mere (sklēr′o-mēr) [*sclero-* + *-mere*] 1. any segment or metamere of the skeletal system. 2. the caudal half of a sclerotome (def. 3).

scle•ro•myx•ede•ma (sklēr″o-mik″sə-de′mə) [*sclero-* + *myxedema*] the most serious form of lichen myxedematosus, accompanied by scleroderma, producing exaggerated furrowing of the skin, especially on the face; it sometimes proves fatal.

scle•ro•nych•ia (sklēr″o-nik′e-ə) [*sclero-* + *onych-* + *-ia*] a simultaneous thickening and dryness of the nails.

scle•ro•nyx•is (sklēr″o-nik′sis) [*sclero-* + *nyxis*] surgical puncture of the sclera.

scle•ro-ooph•o•ri•tis (sklēr″o-o-of″ə-ri′tis) sclerosing inflammation of an ovary.

scle•ro-oo•the•ci•tis (sklēr″o-o″o-the-si′tis) sclero-oophoritis.

scle•roph•thal•mia (sklēr″of-thal′me-ə) [*sclero-* + *-ophthalmia*] the condition in which, from imperfect differentiation of the sclera and cornea, the periphery of the cornea is opaque and only the central part remains clear.

scle•ro•pro•tein (sklēr″o-pro′tēn) [*sclero-* + *protein*] a simple protein characterized by its insolubility and fibrous structure, usually serving a supportive or protective function in the body; called also *albuminoid.*

scle•ro•sal (sklə-ro′səl) indurated.

scle•ro•sant (sklə-ro′sənt) sclerosing agent.

scle•rose (sklə-rōs′) to undergo sclerosis; to harden.

sclé•rose en plaques (skla-rōz′ ahn plahk) [Fr.] multiple sclerosis.

scle•ros•ing (sklə-rōs′ing) causing or undergoing sclerosis.

scle•ro•sis (sklə-ro′sis) [Gr. *sklērōsis* hardness] an induration or hardening, such as hardening of a part from inflammation, increased formation of connective tissue, or disease of the interstitial substance.

amyotrophic lateral s. a motor neuron disease marked by progressive degeneration of the neurons that give rise to the corticospinal tract and of the motor cells of the brainstem and spinal cord, resulting in a deficit of upper and lower motor neurons; it usually ends fatally within two to three years. Called also *Lou Gehrig disease* and *Charcot syndrome.*

anterolateral s. sclerosis of the ventral and lateral columns of the spinal cord, leading to spastic paraplegia; called also *ventrolateral s.*

aortic s. an early stage of aortic stenosis marked by a systolic ejection murmur and evidence of calcification of the aortic valve but no pressure gradient across the valve.

arterial s., arteriocapillary s. arteriosclerosis.

arteriolar s. arteriolosclerosis.

bone s. eburnation.

combined s. subacute combined degeneration of spinal cord; see under *degeneration.*

concentric s. Baló disease.

dentinal s. regressive alteration in tooth substance with calcification of the dentinal tubules, usually caused by trauma, abrasion, or normal aging processes, and producing translucent zones (transparent dentin).

diaphyseal s. diaphyseal dysplasia.

diffuse s. sclerosis that affects large areas of the brain and spinal cord.

diffuse cerebral s. the infantile form of metachromatic leukodystrophy; see under *leukodystrophy.*

diffuse systemic s. systemic s.

endocardial s. see under *fibroelastosis.*

Erb s. primary lateral s.

focal glomerular s. focal segmental glomerulosclerosis.

gastric s. linitis plastica.

glomerular s. glomerulosclerosis.

hippocampal s. loss of neurons in the hippocampal region with gliosis, sometimes seen with epilepsy. Called also *mesial temporal s.*

hyperplastic s. a form of arteriosclerosis seen in small arteries and arterioles as a subintimal thickening of the wall of the vessel.

lateral s. a motor neuron disease consisting of degeneration of the lateral columns of the spinal cord, leading to spastic paraplegia. See *amyotrophic lateral s.* and *primary lateral s.*

lobar s. presence of narrow, scar-distorted convolutions over a large area (lobe) of the surface of the cerebral hemispheres; seen frequently in cerebral palsy.

medial calcific s. Mönckeberg arteriosclerosis.

mesial temporal s. hippocampal s.

miliary s. sclerosis occurring in minute spots with miliary lesions.

Mönckeberg s. see under *arteriosclerosis.*

multiple s. (MS) a disease in which there are foci of demyelination throughout the white matter of the central nervous system, sometimes extending into the gray matter; symptoms usually include weakness, incoordination, paresthesias, speech disturbances, and visual complaints. The course of the disease is usually prolonged, so that the term *multiple* also refers to remissions and relapses that occur over a period of many years. Four types are recognized, based on the course of the disease: *relapsing remitting, secondary progressive, primary progressive,* and *progressive relapsing.* The etiology is unknown.

Pelizaeus-Merzbacher s. see under *disease.*

peritoneal s. sclerosing peritonitis.

posterolateral s. subacute combined degeneration of spinal cord; see under *degeneration.*

primary lateral s. a form of motor neuron disease in which the degenerative process is limited to the corticospinal pathways. Called also *Erb s.*

progressive systemic s. systemic scleroderma that has spread to involve wide areas of skin, especially on the trunk.

subendocardial s. endocardial fibroelastosis.

systemic s. see under *scleroderma.*

tuberous s. (TSC) see under *complex.*

valvular s. fibrous thickening of a cardiac valve, especially the mitral valve.

vascular s. arteriosclerosis.

venous s. phlebosclerosis.

ventrolateral s. anterolateral s.

scle•ro•skel•e•ton (sklēr″o-skel′ə-ton) [*sclero-* + *skeleton*] those parts of the bony skeleton that are formed by the ossification of ligaments, tendons, or fasciae.

scle•ro•ste•no•sis (sklēr″o-stə-no′sis) [*sclero-* + *stenosis*] induration or hardening combined with contraction.

Scle•ros•to•ma (sklə-ros′to-mə) *Strongylus.*

S. duodena′le *Ancylostoma duodenale.*

S. syn'gamus *Syngamus trachea.*

scle•ros•to•my (sklə-ros'tə-me) [*sclero-* + *-stomy*] the surgical creation of an opening through the sclera; it is usually performed in the treatment of glaucoma.

scle•ro•ther•a•py (sklēr″o-ther'ə-pe) the injection of a chemical irritant (see *sclerosing agent,* under *agent*) into a vein to produce inflammation and eventual fibrosis and obliteration of the lumen, as for the treatment of hemorrhoids, varicose veins, varicocele, or esophageal varices.

scle•ro•tia (sklə-ro'she-ə) plural of *sclerotium.*

scle•rot•ic (sklə-rot'ik) 1. hard, or hardening; affected with sclerosis. 2. scleral.

scle•rot•i•ca (sklə-rot'ĭ-kə) [L. *scleroticus;* Gr. *sklēros* hard] sclera.

scle•rot•ic ac•id (sklə-rot'ik) an acid found in ergot, of which it is one of the active principles.

scle•rot•i•co•cho•roid•itis (sklə-rot″ĭ-ko-kor″oid-i'tis) sclerochoroiditis.

Scle•ro•tin•ia (sklēr″o-tin'e-ə) a genus of fungi of the family Sclerotiniaceae, which includes many pathogens of plants. Its imperfect (sexual) stage is *Monilia.*

Scle•ro•tin•i•a•ceae (sklēr″o-tin-e-a'se-e) a family of fungi of the order Helotiales; it includes the genus *Sclerotinia.*

scle•ro•ti•tis (sklēr″o-ti'tis) scleritis.

scle•ro•ti•um (sklə-ro'she-əm) [L. *sclerotica* hard] 1. in fungi, a hard mass of intertwined mycelia, usually with pigmented walls resistant to adverse environmental conditions; it will germinate to produce new hyphae under favorable conditions or in response to a chemical stimulus from a prospective host. 2. in certain protozoa, a multinucleate hard cyst into which the plasmodium divides in response to adverse environmental conditions, such as desiccation; sclerotia will germinate and fuse together to produce a new plasmodium under favorable conditions.

scle•ro•tome (sklēr'o-tōm) [*sclero-* + *-tome*] 1. an instrument used in the incision of the sclera. 2. the area of a bone innervated from a single spinal segment. 3. one of the paired masses of mesenchymal tissue, separated from the ventromedial part of a somite, which develop into vertebrae and ribs.

scle•rot•o•my (sklə-rot'ə-me) [*sclero-* + *-tomy*] surgical incision of the sclera.

anterior s. the surgical opening of the anterior chamber of the eye, chiefly done for the relief of glaucoma.

posterior s. an opening made into the vitreous through the sclera, as for detached retina or the removal of a foreign body.

scle•rous (sklēr'əs) indurated.

ScLP [L.] scapulo-laeva posterior (left scapuloposterior, a position of the fetus; see *position*).

SCM State Certified Midwife.

sco•le•ces (sko'lə-sēz) [L.] plural of *scolex.*

sco•le•coid (sko'lə-koid) [Gr. *skōlekoeidēs* vermiform] 1. resembling a worm. 2. resembling a scolex; hydatid.

sco•lex (sko'leks) pl. *sco'leces, sco'lices* [Gr. *skōlēx* worm] the attachment organ (holdfast) of a tapeworm, generally considered the anterior, or cephalic, end.

sco•li•ces (sko'lĭ-sēz) plural of *scolex.*

sco•li•ci•dal (sco″lĭ-si'dəl) lethal to scolices of tapeworms.

sco•li•cide (sco'lĭ-sīd) an agent lethal to scolices of tapeworms.

scoli(o)- [Gr. *skolios* twisted] a combining form meaning twisted or crooked.

sco•lio•ky•pho•sis (sko″le-o-ki-fo'sis) [*scolio-* + *kyphosis*] combined lateral (scoliosis) and posterior (kyphosis) curvature of the spine.

sco•lio•ra•chit•ic (sko″le-o-rə-kit'ik) affected with scoliosis and rickets.

sco•li•o•si•om•e•try (sko″le-o-se-om'ə-tre) [*scoliosis* + *-metry*] measurement of curvatures, especially those of the vertebral column.

sco•li•o•sis (sko″le-o'sis) [Gr. *skoliōsis* curvation] an appreciable lateral deviation in the normally straight vertical line of the spine. Cf. *kyphosis* and *lordosis.* **scoliot'ic** *adj*

cicatricial s. scoliosis due to a cicatricial contraction following caries or necrosis.

coxitic s. scoliosis in the lumbar region caused by hip disease.

empyematic s., empyemic s. scoliosis caused by empyema.

habit s. scoliosis due to improper posture.

inflammatory s. scoliosis caused by vertebral disease; called also *osteopathic s.*

myopathic s. paralytic s.

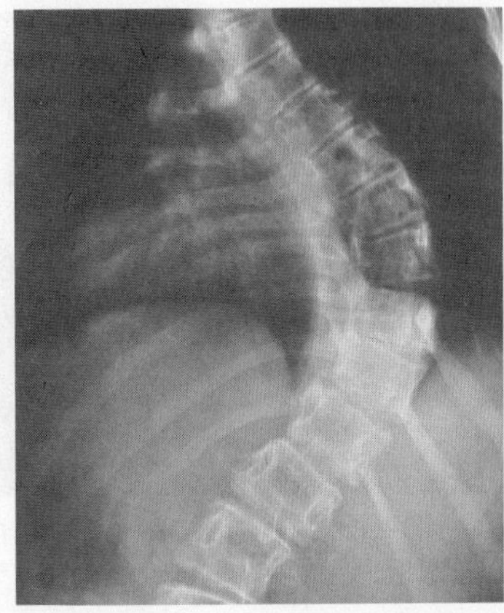

■ Severe thoracic scoliosis (posteroanterior projection).

ocular s., ophthalmic s. scoliosis attributed to excessive tilting of the head by a person suffering from astigmatism or muscle imbalance.

osteopathic s. inflammatory s.

paralytic s. scoliosis resulting from muscle paralysis; called also *myopathic s.*

rachitic s. spinal curvature due to rickets.

rheumatic s. scoliosis due to rheumatism of the dorsal muscles.

sciatic s. listing of the lumbar part of the spine away from the affected side in sciatica.

static s. scoliosis due to difference in the length of the lower limbs.

sco•li•o•som•e•ter (sko″le-o-som'ə-tər) an apparatus for measuring curves, especially those of the vertebral column.

sco•lio•tone (sko'le-o-tōn) an apparatus for the forcible correction of scoliosis.

Sco•lo•pen•dra (sko″lo-pen'drə) [Gr. *skolops* anything pointed] a genus of venomous centipedes (class Chilopoda). The bite of some large species may produce a severe local inflammation attended with pain, glandular enlargement, vomiting, headache, vertigo, and fever. *S. he'ros* and *S. mor'sitans* are American species; *S. gigan'tea* is a tropical species.

sco•lop•sia (sko-lop'se-ə) [Gr. *skolops* anything pointed] a suture between two bones that allows motion of one on the other.

scom•broid (skom'broid) 1. of or pertaining to the suborder Scombroidea. 2. a fish of the suborder Scombroidea. See also under *poisoning.*

Scom•broi•dea (skom-broi'de-ə) a suborder of larger, bony, marine fish having oily flesh, including tunas, bonitos, mackerels, albacores, and skipjacks. The flesh of these fish may contain a toxic histaminelike substance and, if ingested, can cause scombroid poisoning.

scom•bro•tox•ic (skom'bro-tok″sik) pertaining to or caused by scombrotoxin.

scom•bro•tox•in (skom'bro-tok″sin) the histaminelike toxin formed in scombroid fish by bacterial action; it causes scombroid poisoning.

scoop (sko͞op) a spoonlike instrument for evacuating cavities.

Mules s. a form of curet used in eye operations.

sco•pa•rin (sko-pa'rin) a diuretic principle found in scoparius.

sco•pa•ri•us (sko-pa're-əs) the tops of *Cytisus scoparius,* or broom; they contain the alkaloid sparteine and the principle scoparin, and are diuretic, cathartic, and emetic. Scoparius is abused by being smoked for its euphoric properties. Called also *spartium.*

-scope [Gr. *skopein* to view, examine] a word termination denoting an instrument for examining or observing.

sco•po•la (sko-po'lə) the dried rhizome and larger roots of *Scopolia carniolica,* which contains the same constituents as belladonna and is used as an anticholinergic.

sco•po•lag•nia (sko″po-lag'ne-ə) scopophilia.

sco•pol•a•mine (sko-pol'ə-mēn) an anticholinergic alkaloid, derived from several solanaceous plants, including *Atropa belladonna, Hyoscyamus niger, Datura* species, and *Scopolia* species. It has effects on the autonomic nervous system similar to those of atropine. It is used as an antiemetic, particularly in motion sickness; administered transdermally. Called also *hyoscine.*

s. hydrobromide [USP] the trihydrate salt of scopolamine, used as an antisialagogue preanesthetic medication and as an adjunct to general anesthesia, administered parenterally; as an antiemetic, administered orally or parenterally; and as a cycloplegic and mydriatic, applied topically to the conjunctiva.

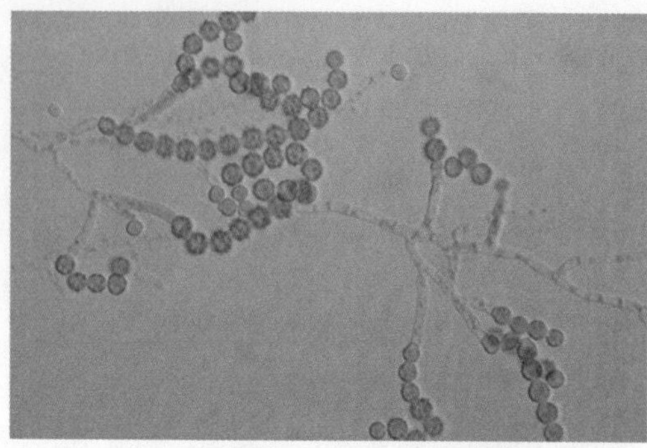

■ *Scopulariopsis.* The clusters of conidiophores are annellides that increase in length as conidia are formed; the conidia tend to remain in chains on the annellides.

Sco·po·lia (sko-po′le-ə) [Johann-Antoni *Scopoli,* Italian physician, 1723–1788] a genus of plants of the family Solanaceae. *S. carnio′lica atropoi′des* Jacq., a European species, and *S. japo′nica* and *S. lu′rida,* Asian species, contain scopolamine and their rhizomes and roots have properties like those of hyoscyamus and belladonna.

sco·pom·e·ter (sko-pom′ə-tər) [Gr. *skopein* to examine + *-meter*] an instrument for measuring the turbidity of solutions, i.e., the density of a precipitate.

sco·pom·e·try (sko-pom′ə-tre) measurement of the optical density of a precipitate to determine the amount of a substance in suspension.

sco·po·phil·ia (sko-po-fil′e-ə) [Gr. *skopein* to view + *-philia*] usually, voyeurism, but the disorder is sometimes divided into active and passive forms, *active scopophilia* being voyeurism and *passive scopophilia* being exhibitionism.

sco·po·pho·bia (sko″po-fo′be-ə) [Gr. *skopein* to view + *-phobia*] irrational fear of being seen.

scop·to·phil·ia (skop″to-fil′e-ə) scopophilia.

scop·to·pho·bia (skop″to-fo′be-ə) scopophobia.

scop·u·la (skop′u-lə) [L. "small brush"] an aboral organelle of peritrichous protozoa comprising a field of kinetosomes and immobile cilia, which may function as a holdfast organ or may be the origin of the stalk.

Scop·u·lar·i·op·sis (skop″u-lar″e-op′sis) a genus of Fungi Imperfecti of the family Moniliaceae. *S. brevicau′lis* can cause onychomycosis and other forms of scopulariopsosis.

scop·u·lar·i·op·so·sis (skop″u-lar″e-op-so′sis) infection with a fungus of the genus *Scopulariopsis,* usually in the form of onychomycosis caused by *S. brevicaulis.*

-scopy [Gr. *skopein* to examine] a word termination denoting the act of examining.

scor·bu·tic (skor-bu′tik) [L. *scorbuticus*] pertaining to or affected with scurvy.

scor·bu·ti·gen·ic (skor-bu″tĭ-jen′ik) causing scurvy.

scor·bu·tus (skor-bu′təs) [L.] scurvy.

score (skor) a rating, usually expressed numerically, based on achievement or the degree to which certain qualities or conditions are present.

APACHE s. [*a*cute *p*hysiological *a*ssessment and *c*hronic *h*ealth *e*valuation] a widely used method for assessing severity of illness in acutely ill patients in intensive care units, taking into account a variety of routine physiological parameters. A variation called the *APACHE II score* has been developed that assesses 12 physiologic variables along with age and chronic health status. Benign or normal findings get low numbers, and a total score of more than 8 raises concern.

Apgar s. a numerical expression of the condition of a newborn infant, usually determined at 60 seconds after birth, being the sum of points gained on assessment of the heart rate, respiratory effort, muscle tone, reflex irritability, and color. Cf. *recovery s.*

Ballard s. either of two assessment systems for the gestational age of a neonate, assigning whole numbers from -1 for premature to +5 for postmature, considering several different parameters; one score assesses neuromuscular maturity and a second one assesses various aspects of the body surface for gestational age.

Bishop s. a score for estimating the prospects of induction of labor in a primigravida, arrived at by evaluating the extent of cervical dilatation, effacement, the station of the fetal head, consistency of the cervix, and the cervical position in relation to the vaginal axis.

Child-Pugh s., Child-Turcotte-Pugh s. see under *classification.*

DeMeester s. a composite score derived from six parameters measured during 24-hour gastroesophageal pH monitoring, used for rating the severity of gastroesophageal reflux disease.

disease activity s. a calculation of the degree of impairment of the joints in a person with rheumatoid arthritis, assessing significant limitations of movement, tenderness, and swelling of a number of joints; it is usually done for either 28 or 44 joints.

Gleason s. see under *grade.*

lod s. [*lo*garithm of the *od*ds favoring linkage] a score that measures the likelihood of two genes showing a specified recombination value, indicating linkage.

propensity s. an assessment of the effect that factors in a person's background have on the probability that they will be chosen for a treatment group in a clinical trial that is less than completely randomized.

recovery s. a number expressing the condition of an infant at various stipulated intervals more than one minute after birth; it is based on the same features assessed by the Apgar score at 60 seconds after birth.

Reynolds Risk S. an algorithm for stratification of risk of cardiovascular disease in healthy persons. It is based on age; smoking status; systolic blood pressure; total cholesterol, high-density lipoprotein, and high-sensitivity C-reactive protein levels; and family history of cardiovascular disease.

standard s. *z* value.

stroke s. any of various scoring systems that seek to characterize a patient's clinical state following a stroke.

***z* s.** see under *value.*

scor·ings (skor′ings) small transverse lines caused by increased density of bone, seen in radiographs at the metaphysis of growing bones, and due to temporary cessation of growth.

scor·pi·on (skor′pe-ən) any arthropod of the order Scorpionida.

bark s. any of various species of *Centruroides.*

black s. *Euscorpius italicus.*

fat-tailed s. any of various members of the genus *Androctonus.*

whip s. any arachnid of the order Pedipalpa.

Scor·pi·o·nes (skor-pe-o′nēz) Scorpionida.

Scor·pi·on·ida (skor-pe-on′ĭ-də) the scorpions, an order of arachnids with elongated bodies, usually found in tropical or subtropical climates. Numerous genera of the families Buthidae and Hemiscorpiidae are stinging or venomous, usually with venomous stings on their erectile tails. Called also *Scorpiones.*

scor·pi·on·ism (skor′pe-ən-iz″əm) poisoning by scorpion stings.

scot(o)- [Gr. *skotos* darkness] a combining form denoting relationship to darkness.

sco·to·chro·mo·gen (sko″to-kro′mo-jən) [*scoto-* + *chromo-* + *-gen*] a microorganism whose pigmentation develops in the dark as well as in the light; specifically, a member of Runyon Group II of the nontuberculous mycobacteria, but applicable also to many other organisms. See also *nontuberculous mycobacteria,* under *mycobacterium.*

sco·to·chro·mo·ge·nic·i·ty (sko″to-kro″mo-jə-nis′ĭ-te) the property of forming pigment in the dark, the coloration occurring irrespective of exposure to light. **scotochromogen′ic** *adj*

sco·to·din·ia (sko″to-din′e-ə) [*scoto-* + Gr. *dinos* whirl] dizziness with blurring of vision and headache. Called also *apoplectic vertigo* and *tenebric vertigo.*

sco·to·ma (sko-to′mə) pl. *scoto′mata* [Gr. *skotōma*] 1. an area of lost or depressed vision within the visual field, surrounded by an area of less depressed or of normal vision. 2. mental s.

absolute s. a scotoma in which perception of light is entirely lost.

annular s. a circular scotoma surrounding the point of fixation; called also *ring s.*

arcuate s. a scotoma arising at or near the blind spot and arching inferiorly or superiorly toward the nasal field, following the paths of the retinal nerve fibers.

aural s., s. au′ris loss of ability to perceive auditory stimuli coming from a certain direction.

Bjerrum s. a further development of a Seidel scotoma in which the sickle-shaped defect contiguous to the blind spot extends above and below the fixation point and encircles it more or less completely.

cecocentral s. centrocecal s.

central s. a scotoma that corresponds with the point of fixation and interferes with or entirely abolishes central vision.

centrocecal s. a horizontal oval scotoma that extends from the point of fixation to the blind spot.

color s. an isolated area of defective color vision.

flittering s. teichopsia.

hemianopic s. a scotoma that affects half of the central visual field. Cf. *hemianopia.*

mental s. in psychiatry, a figurative blind spot in a person's psychological awareness, the patient being unable to gain insight into and to understand his mental problems; lack of insight.

motile s's floating opacities, not true scotomata, occurring in the vitreous, muscae volitantes being an example of such a defect.

negative s. a scotoma appearing as a blank spot in the visual field; the patient is unaware of it, and it is detected only by examination.

paracentral s. a scotoma found near the point of fixation.

peripapillary s. a scotoma near the one corresponding to the optic disk.

peripheral s. a scotoma distant from the point of fixation, toward the periphery of the visual field.

physiologic s. the area of the visual field corresponding with the optic disk, in which the photosensitive receptors are absent.

positive s. a scotoma subjectively perceived as a black spot in the visual field, and of which the patient is aware.

relative s. a scotoma in which perception of light is only diminished, or the loss is restricted to light of certain wavelengths.

ring s. annular s.

scintillating s. teichopsia.

Seidel s. a further development of an arcuate scotoma, extending out at one end or both ends; the concavity of the prolongation is always directed toward the fixation point.

sco•to•ma•graph (sko-to′mə-graf) [*scotoma* + *-graph*] an instrument for recording a scotoma.

sco•to•ma•ta (sko-to′mə-tə) plural of *scotoma.*

sco•tom•a•tous (sko-tom′ə-təs) pertaining to or affected with scotoma.

sco•tom•e•ter (sko-tom′ə-tər) [*scotoma* + *-meter*] an instrument for diagnosing and measuring scotomata.

Bjerrum s. campimeter.

sco•tom•e•try (sko-tom′ə-tre) the measurement of isolated areas of depressed vision (scotomata) within the visual field.

sco•to•phil•ia (sko″to-fil′e-ə) nyctophilia.

sco•to•pho•bia (sko″to-fo′be-ə) [*scoto-* + *-phobia*] irrational fear of darkness.

sco•to•pia (sko-to′pe-ə) night vision. **scotop′ic** *adj*

sco•top•sin (sko-top′sin) the opsin of the rods of the retina that combines with 11-*cis* retinal to form rhodopsin. See illustration at *visual cycle,* under *cycle.*

sco•tos•co•py (sko-tos′kə-pe) retinoscopy.

scours (skourz) diarrhea in animals other than humans.

black s. acute dysentery in cattle, accompanied by intestinal hemorrhage producing a dark color of the feces; the etiology is unknown. See also *bloody s.* and *winter dysentery.*

bloody s. swine dysentery.

calf s. see under *diarrhea.*

peat s. molybdenum poisoning in grazing cattle.

weanling pig s. 1. postweaning diarrhea. 2. coliform gastroenteritis.

white s. neonatal diarrhea in calves, lambs, and foals during the first few days after birth, usually caused by enteropathogenic strains of *Escherichia coli* and less often by other bacteria or viruses; marked by fever, dehydration, and depression, with fetid light-colored feces that may be bloodstained late in the disease.

winter s. see under *dysentery.*

scr scruple.

scra•pie (skra′pe) the first of the prion diseases to be recognized, occurring in sheep and goats and characterized by severe pruritus, muscular incoordination, and increasing debility, ending in death.

scratch (skrach) 1. to scrape or rub a surface lightly with the nails or with a sharp or jagged instrument, particularly to relieve itching. Called also *excoriate.* 2. to make shallow cuts on a surface. 3. a slight wound; called also *excoriation.* 4. to make a thin grating sound.

Means-Lerman s. a systolic grating sound heard in the second left intercostal space during exhalation in hypertension, caused by friction between the pleural and pericardial surfaces.

scratch•es (skrach′əz) greasy heel.

screen (skrēn) 1. a structure resembling a curtain or partition, used as a protection or shield, e.g., against excessive radiation exposure; see also *shield.* 2. a large flat surface upon which light rays are projected. 3. protective (def. 2). 4. to examine by fluoroscopy (Great Britain). 5. to separate well individuals in a population from those who have an undiagnosed disease, defect, or other pathologic condition or who are at high risk, by means of tests, examinations, or other procedures. See also *screening.*

Bjerrum s. tangent s.

fluorescent s. a sheet of cardboard, paper, or glass coated with suitable material, which fluoresces visibly, as calcium tungstate, used as an intensifying screen in radiography; as the chief part of a fluoroscope; as a substitute for a fluoroscope in a darkened room.

intensifying s. a thin sheet of celluloid or other substance coated with a finely divided substance which fluoresces under the influence of x-rays and intended to be used in close contact with the emulsion of a photographic plate or film for the purpose of reinforcing the image.

oral s. vestibular s.

skin s. a substance applied to the skin to protect it from the effects of the sun's rays or other noxious agents.

solar s., sun s. sunscreen.

tangent s. a large square of black cloth, stretched on a frame, hung from a roller, and having a central mark for fixation; used with a campimeter to map the field of vision. Called also *Bjerrum s.*

vestibular s. an acrylic resin removable orthodontic appliance that covers the labial or buccal surface of one or both dental arches, fitting between the oral mucosa and the teeth; used to treat oral habits and to stimulate tooth movement. Called also *oral s.* and *oral shield.*

screen•ing (skrēn′ing) 1. examination or testing of a group of individuals to separate those who are well from those who have an undiagnosed disease or defect or who are at high risk. 2. fluoroscopy (Great Britain).

antibody s. a method of determining the presence and amount of anti-HLA antibodies in the serum of a potential allograft recipient: aliquots of the recipient's serum are mixed with a panel of leukocytes from well-characterized cell donors and complement is added. Reaction between the recipient's pre-existing antibody and specific antigen in the donor cells leads to cell lysis; the percentage of different cells lysed provides a rough measure of the sensitization of the recipient (referred to as the *panel reactive antibody*).

mass s. screening performed on or made available to an entire population.

multiphasic s., multiple s. screening in which various diagnostic procedures are employed during the same screening program.

prescriptive s. screening performed for the early detection of disease or disease precursors in apparently well individuals so that health care can be provided early in the course of the disease or before the disease becomes manifest.

screw (skroo) a solid cylinder with a helical thread on its exterior surface, used to hold two objects together.

pedicle s. a screw that goes into the pedicle of a vertebral arch, often in the lumbar region, used in various types of instrumentation.

screw•worm (skroo′wərm) the larva of *Cochliomyia hominivorax.*

Scrib•ner shunt (skrib′nər) [Belding H. *Scribner,* American nephrologist, born 1921] Quinton-Scribner shunt.

scro•bic•u•late (skro-bik′u-lāt) [L. *scrobiculatus*] marked with pits or cavities.

scrof•u•la (skrof′u-lə) former name for *tuberculous cervical lymphadenitis.*

scrof•u•lo•der•ma (skrof″u-lo-dur′mə) [*scrofula* + *derma*] a type of cutaneous tuberculosis affecting children and young adults, representing either direct extension of tuberculosis into the skin from underlying structures such as cervical lymph nodes, bone, or a lung, or contact exposure to tuberculosis. It is manifested by painless subcutaneous swellings that evolve into cold abscesses, ulcers, and draining sinus tracts. Called also *tuberculosis colliquativa.*

scro•tec•to•my (skro-tek′tə-me) [*scrotum* + *-ectomy*] partial or complete excision of the scrotum.

scro•ti•tis (skro-ti′tis) inflammation of the scrotum.

scro•to•plasty (skro′to-plas″te) [*scrotum* + *-plasty*] plastic surgery of the scrotum.

scro•tum (skro′təm) [L. "bag"] [TA] the pouch that contains the testes and their accessory organs. It is composed of skin, the tunica dartos, the

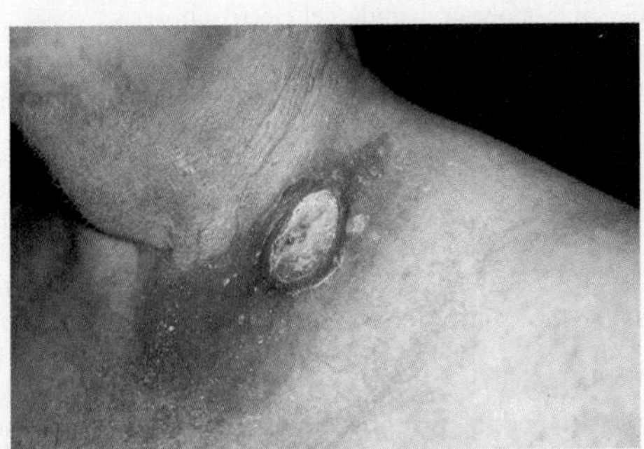

■ Scrofuloderma; the lesion is an extension from an underlying lymph node.

spermatic, cremasteric, and infundibuliform fasciae, and the tunica vaginalis testis. **scro'tal** *adj*

bifid s. separation of the two halves of the scrotum, as in penoscrotal transposition.

lymph s. elephantiasis scroti.

watering-can s. a condition in which the undersurface of the scrotum and the perineum have multiple sinuses discharging urine, owing to neglected stricture of the nearby urethra.

scru•ple (℈, scr) (skroo'pəl) [L. *scrupulus*, dim. of *scrupus* a sharp stone, a worry or anxiety] a unit of mass (weight) of the apothecaries' system, being 20 grains, or the equivalent of 1.296 g.

scru•pu•los•i•ty (skroo″pu-los'ĭ-te) excessive meticulousness or punctiliousness, usually related to moral or religious questions.

Scul•te•tus bandage (skəl-te'təs) [Johannes *Schultes* (L. *Scultetus*), German surgeon, 1595–1645] see under *bandage.*

scul•te•tus (skəl-te'təs) [J. *Schultes* (*Scultetus*)] Scultetus bandage.

scu-PA single-chain urokinase-type plasminogen activator; see *prourokinase.*

scur•vy (skur've) [L. *scorbutus*] a condition due to deficiency of ascorbic acid (vitamin C) in the diet and marked by weakness, anemia, spongy gums, a tendency to mucocutaneous hemorrhages and a brawny induration of the muscles of the lower limbs.

hemorrhagic s. infantile s.

infantile s. a nutritional disease of infants characterized by the same symptoms as scurvy in adults; called also *Barlow disease.*

scute (skūt) [L. *scutum* shield] 1. any squama or scalelike structure. 2. tympanic s.

tympanic s. the bony plate which divides the upper part of the tympanic cavity from the mastoid cells.

scu•tel•lum (sku-tel'əm) pl. *scutel'la* [L. "little shield," dim. of *scutum* shield] the third of the four chitinous plates making up the dorsum of the thorax of an insect.

scu•ti•form (sku'tĭ-form) [*scutum* + *form*] shaped like a shield; called also *thyroid.*

scu•tu•la (sku'tu-lə) plural of *scutulum.*

scu•tu•lum (sku'tu-ləm) pl. *scu'tula* [L. "little shield"] a yellow, perifollicular, saucerlike or cup-shaped crust with a cheesy odor, composed of dense mats of mycelia and epithelial debris, characteristic of favus. **scu'tular** *adj*

scu•tum (sku'təm) [L. "shield"] 1. tympanic scute. 2. cartilago thyroidea. 3. a hard chitinous plate on the anterior portion of the dorsal surface of hard-bodied ticks.

s. pec'toris sternum.

scyb•a•la (sib'ə-lə) plural of *scybalum.*

scy•ba•lum (sib'ə-ləm) pl. *scy'bala* [Gr. *skybalon*] a dry, hard mass of fecal matter in the intestine. **scy'balous** *adj*

Scy•pho•zoa (si″fo-zo'ə) a class of the phylum Cnidaria, including forms that have a medusa stage, such as jellyfish; numerous species have toxic stings.

Scy•ta•lid•ium (si″tə-lid'e-əm) a genus of Fungi Imperfecti of the form-class Coelomycetes, usually found in soil or wood. *S. hyali'num* is a synanamorph of *Hendersonula toruloides* and has been isolated from cases of phaeohyphomycosis.

SD skin dose; standard deviation.

SDA [L.] sacro-dextra anterior (right sacroanterior, a position of the fetus; see *position*).

SDP [L.] sacro-dextra posterior (right sacroposterior, a position of the fetus; see *position*).

SDS sodium dodecyl sulfate.

SDS-PAGE SDS–polyacrylamide gel electrophoresis.

SDT [L.] sacro-dextra transversa (right sacrotransverse, a position of the fetus; see *position*).

SE standard error; sphenoethmoidal suture (def. 2).

Se selenium.

Sea•bright ban•tam syndrome (se'brīt ban'təm) [from *Seabright bantam* chickens, a breed in which the rooster has this condition] pseudohypoparathyroidism.

Sea•dor•na•vi•rus (se-ə-dor'nə-vi″rəs) [*S*outh *E*ast *A*sia *do*deca *RNA virus*] a genus of viruses of the family Reoviridae; a species pathogenic to humans is Banna virus.

seal (sēl) 1. something that effects a firm closure. 2. to secure or close tightly. 3. in dentistry, a material, usually plastic, that hardens in the mouth; used to close the coronal opening in a tooth during endodontic treatment. See also *sealant.* 4. a die with a raised emblem used to mark something.

border s. the contact of the denture border with the underlying or adjacent tissues to prevent the passage of air or other substances.

double s. a seal consisting of gutta-percha underneath another material (e.g., temporary cement); used to close the coronal opening in a tooth during endodontic treatment.

posterior palatal s. the seal at the posterior border of a denture produced by displacing some of the soft tissue covering the palate by extra pressure developed in the impression or by scraping a depression in the cast.

Solomon s. *Polygonatum biflorum.*

velopharyngeal s. see under *closure.*

seal•ant (se'lənt) an agent that protects against access from the outside or leakage from the inside; sealer.

dental s. a coating material capable of mechanically bonding to the surface of a tooth and offering protection against decay-causing external chemical or physical agents.

fibrin s. see under *glue.*

fissure s. see *pit and fissure s.*

pit and fissure s. a dental sealant used to occlude noncarious pits and fissures on occlusal tooth surfaces, thereby preventing caries-producing microorganisms and debris from entering.

seal•er (se'lər) an agent that protects against access from the outside or leakage from the inside; sealant.

endodontic s. root canal s.

root canal s. in root canal therapy, a substance used for cementing silver and gutta-percha cones to the tooth structure. Called also *endodontic s.* and *root canal cement.*

seam (sēm) a line of union.

osteoid s. on the surface of a bone, the narrow region of newly formed organic matrix not yet mineralized.

pigment s. the portion of the pigmented epithelium of the iris which bends forward around the pupillary border.

search•er (surch'ər) a type of sound used to search for calculi in the bladder. Called also *stone-searcher.*

sea•sick•ness (se'sik-nis) nausea and malaise caused by the motion of a ship. Written also *sea sickness.*

sea•son•al (se'zən-əl) of, depending on, or occurring in a particular season of the year.

seat (sēt) a part on which the base of something rests or sits.

basal s. oral tissues which support a complete or partial denture.

rest s. see under *area.*

seat•worm (sēt'wərm) oxyurid.

sea ur•chin (se' ur'chin) any of various marine animals of the class Echinoidea, having round bodies enclosed in a shell with spiny processes and pedicellariae protruding from it. Genera such as *Diadema* and *Echinothrix* may secrete venom from glands on the pedicellariae.

sea•weed (se'wēd) a plant growing in the sea, especially one of the algae.

se•ba•ce•o•ma (sə-ba″se-o'mə) term proposed for the subset of sebaceous hyperplasia in which tumors are poorly differentiated.

se•ba•ceous (sə-ba'shəs) [L. *sebaceus*] 1. pertaining to or containing sebum. 2. secreting sebum.

Sé•bi•leau hollow, muscle (sa″be-lo') [Pierre *Sebileau*, French surgeon, 1860–1953] see under *hollow* and *muscle.*

se•bo•cyte (se'bo-sīt″) a sebum-producing cell within a sebaceous gland.

se•bo•gen•e•sis (se″bo-jen'ə-sis) the production of sebum.

se•bo•pso•ri•a•sis (se″bo-sə-ri'ə-sis) a variant of seborrheic dermatitis that has fewer dry scales and more yellow, greasy scales.

seb•or•rhea (seb″o-re'ə) [*sebum* + *-rrhea*] 1. excessive secretion of sebum; called also *hypersteatosis.* 2. seborrheic dermatitis.

s. adipo'sa, s. oleo'sa seborrhea in which the secretion is oily, seen especially on the nose and forehead.

s. sic'ca dry, scaly seborrheic dermatitis.

seb•or•rhe•al (seb″o-re'əl) seborrheic (def. 1).

seb•or•rhe•ic (seb″o-re'ik) 1. characterized by or pertaining to seborrhea. 2. pertaining to those areas of the body in which sebaceous glands are abundant, including the scalp, face, chest, back, axilla, and groin.

seb•or•rhi•a•sis (seb″o-ri'ə-sis) seborrheic psoriasis.

se•bos•ta•sis (se-bos'tə-sis) cessation of sebum production, with resultant dry skin.

sebo•tro•pic (seb″o-tro'pik) having an affinity for sebaceous glands.

se•bum (se′bəm) [L. "suet"] the secretion of the sebaceous glands, a thick, semifluid substance composed of fat and epithelial debris from the cells of the malpighian layer. Called also *cutaneous s.*

cutaneous s., s. cuta′neum sebum.

s. palpebra′le the secretion of the tarsal glands.

Se•ca•le (se-ka′le) [L. "rye"] a genus of plants of the grass family (Gramineae). *S. cerea′le* L. is rye.

Sec•kel bird-headed dwarf, syndrome (dwarfism) (sek′əl) [Helmut Paul George *Seckel*, American physician, 1900–1960] see *bird-headed dwarf*, under *dwarf*, and see under *syndrome*.

seco•bar•bi•tal (sek″o-bahr′bĭ-təl) [USP] a short-acting barbiturate with hypnotic and sedative effects. Called also *quinalbarbitone*.

s. sodium [USP] the monosodium salt of secobarbital, having the same actions as the base; administered orally, intravenously, or intramuscularly as a sedative and hypnotic, particularly a presurgical adjunct to anesthesia, and intravenously or intramuscularly as an anticonvulsant in the treatment of tetanus.

se•co•dont (se′ko-dont) [L. *secare* to cut + Gr. *odous* tooth] having teeth in which the tubercles of the molars are provided with cutting edges, as in many carnivorous mammals.

Sec•o•nal (sek′o-nahl) trademark for preparations of secobarbital sodium.

sec•ond (s) (sek′ənd) the SI unit of time, equal to the duration of 9,192,631,770 periods of the radiation corresponding to the transition between the two hyperfine levels of the ground state of cesium 133.

sec•on•dary (sek′ən-dar″e) [L. *secundarius*, from *secundus* second] 1. second or inferior in order of time, place, or importance. 2. derived from or consequent to a primary event or thing.

sec•ond in•ten•tion (sek′ənd in-ten′shən) see under *healing*.

se•cre•ta (se-kre′tə) [L. pl.] secretion (def. 2).

se•cret•a•gogue (se-krēt′ə-gog) [*secretion* + *-agogue*] 1. stimulating secretion. 2. an agent that stimulates secretion.

se•crete (se-krēt′) [L. *secernere*, *secretum* to separate] to separate or elaborate cell products.

se•cre•tin (se-kre′tin) a strongly basic polypeptide hormone secreted by the mucosa of the duodenum and upper jejunum when acid chyme enters the intestine. It stimulates the release of pancreatic juice by the pancreas and to a lesser extent bile by the liver, both of which contain bicarbonate and change the pH of the duodenum from acid to alkaline, thereby facilitating the action of intestinal digestive enzymes. Secretin is used in pancreatic function tests and tests for gastrinoma; see *secretin test*, under *test*.

se•cre•tion (se-kre′shən) [L. *secretio*, from *secernere* to secrete] 1. the process of elaborating a specific product as a result of the activity of a gland; this activity may range from separating a specific substance of the blood to the elaboration of a new chemical substance. 2. material that is secreted.

antilytic s. saliva secreted by the submaxillary gland with nerves intact, as distinguished from that secreted when the nerve is divided.

external s. a secretion discharged by an exocrine gland (q.v.) to an external or internal surface of the body. Cf. *internal s.*

internal s. a hormone; a substance secreted by an organ or structure of the endocrine system (q.v.). Cf. *external s.*

paralytic s. secretion from a gland after paralysis or division of its nerve.

se•cre•to•gogue (se-kre′tə-gog) secretagogue.

se•cre•to•in•hib•i•to•ry (se-kre″to-in-hib′ĭ-tor″e) antisecretory (def. 1).

se•cre•to•mo•tor (se-kre″to-mo′tər) exciting or stimulating secretion; said of nerves.

se•cre•to•mo•tory (se-kre″to-mo′tor-e) secretomotor.

se•cre•tor (se-kre′tər) 1. an individual expressing the autosomal dominant phenotype of secreting the ABH antigens of the ABO blood group in the saliva and other body fluids. See also *nonsecretor*. 2. the gene that determines this phenotype.

se•cre•to•ry (se-kre′tə-re, se′krə-tor″e) pertaining to secretion or affecting the secretions.

sec•tile (sek′tīl) [L. *sectilis*, from *secare* to cut] 1. susceptible of being cut. 2. one of several parts into which a whole is divided.

sec•tio (sek′she-o) pl. *sectio′nes* [L., from *secare* to cut] 1. an act of cutting. 2. section: anatomic terminology for a segment or subdivision of an organ.

sec•tion (sek′shən) [L. *sectio*] 1. an act of cutting. 2. a cut surface. 3. a segment or subdivision of an organ; called also *sectio* [TA]. 4. a supplemental taxonomic category subordinate to a subgenus but superior to a species or series.

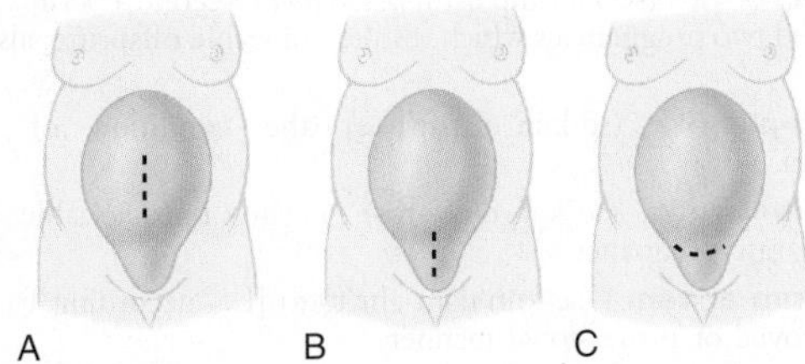

■ Cesarean section. *(A)*, Classic; *(B)*, low vertical; *(C)*, transverse incisions.

abdominal s. laparotomy.

celloidin s. a section cut by a microtome from tissue that has been embedded in celloidin.

cervical cesarean s. lower segment cesarean s.

cesarean s. incision through the abdominal and uterine walls for delivery of a fetus. Called also *abdominal delivery*.

classic cesarean s. cesarean section in which the upper segment, or corpus, of the uterus is incised.

coronal s. frontal s.

corporeal cesarean s. classic cesarean s.

extraperitoneal cesarean s. cesarean section performed without incision of the peritoneum, the peritoneal fold being displaced upward and the bladder being displaced downward or to the midline, the uterus then being opened by an incision in its lower segment.

frontal s. a longitudinal section parallel with the long axis of the body and at right angles to a sagittal section; it divides the body into a dorsal and a ventral part. Called also *coronal s.*

frozen s. a section cut by a microtome from tissue that has been frozen.

Latzko cesarean s. extraperitoneal cesarean section with the uterine incision made through one side of the lower segment of the uterus.

lower segment cesarean s. cesarean section in which the lower uterine segment is incised, either transperitoneally or extraperitoneally.

low vertical cesarean s. cesarean section done transperitoneally with a low vertical uterine incision that is usually made after downward reflection of the bladder.

Munro Kerr cesarean s. cesarean section in which the lower uterine segment is opened transversely through the uterovesical fold, without displacement of the bladder.

paraffin s. a section cut by a microtome from tissue which has been embedded in paraffin.

perineal s. external urethrotomy.

Porro cesarean s. cesarean section with extirpation of the uterine corpus and ovaries; of historical interest.

sagittal s. a longitudinal section that follows the sagittal suture and runs the entire length of the body, thus dividing the latter into more or less equal right and left halves, or a section parallel to it.

serial s. histologic section made in a consecutive order and so arranged for the purpose of microscopic examination.

step s's multiple sequential levels prepared for histopathologic diagnosis of small biopsies; step sectioning consumes less material than serial sectioning.

transperitoneal cesarean s. cesarean section performed with an incision through the uterovesical fold of peritoneum.

transverse s. a section made at right angles to the long axis of a body or structure.

transverse cesarean s. cesarean section done transperitoneally with incision of the enterovesical peritoneum and downward displacement of the bladder followed by a low transverse version of the uterus.

sec•ti•o•nes (sek″she-o′nēz) [L.] plural of *sectio*.

sec•tor (sek′tər) [L. "cutter"] 1. the area of a circle included between an arc and the radii bounding it. 2. an area, zone, or part of something. 3. to divide into sectors.

sec•to•ri•al (sek-tor′e-əl) [L. *sector* cutter] 1. pertaining or relating to a sector. 2. in genetics, pertaining to the presence of a sector of tissue which carries a somatic mutation and which is therefore different phenotypically from the tissues of the rest of the body. 3. cutting or adapted for cutting, as the molar teeth of carnivores.

Sec•tral (sek′tral) trademark for a preparation of acebutolol hydrochloride.

se•cun•di•grav•i•da (sə-kun″dĭ-grav′ĭ-də) [L. *secundus* second + *gravida*] a woman pregnant for the second time; also written *gravida II*.

se•cun•di•na (sek″ən-di′nə) pl. *secundi′nae* [L., from *secundus* following] afterbirth.

se•cun•di•nae (sek″ən-di′ne) [L.] afterbirth.

se•cun•dines (sek′ən-dēnz, se-kun′dēnz) [L. *secundinae*] afterbirth.

se•cun•dip•a•ra (se″kən-dip′ə-rə) [L. *secundus* second + *para*] a woman who has had two pregnancies which resulted in viable offspring; also written *para II.*

se•cun•di•par•i•ty (se-kun″dĭ-par′ĭ-te) the condition of being a secundipara.

se•cun•dip•a•rous (se″kən-dip′ə-rəs) having borne viable offspring in two separate pregnancies.

se•cun•dum ar•tem (se-kun′dəm ahr′təm) [L. "according to the art"] in an approved or professional manner.

se•cu•rin (sə-kūr′in) a protease inhibitor that binds separase; its degradation releases separase to cleave cohesin and initiate chromatid separation in anaphase. Securin is overexpressed in some pituitary tumors and can act as an oncogene in cultured cells.

SED skin erythema dose; see *erythema dose,* under *dose.*

Sed•a•pap (sed′ə-pap) trademark for a combination preparation of butalbital and acetaminophen.

se•da•tion (sə-da′shən) [L. *sedatio*] the production of a sedative effect; the act or process of calming.

conscious s. a state of sedation in which the conscious patient is rendered free of fear, apprehension, and anxiety through the use of pharmacologic agents.

sed•a•tive (sed′ə-tiv) [L. *sedativus*] 1. allaying activity and excitement. 2. an agent that allays excitement; see also *tranquilizer.* Called also *calmative.*

sed•en•tary (sed′ən-tar″e) [L. *sedentarius*] 1. sitting habitually; of inactive habits. 2. pertaining to a sitting posture.

Sé•dil•lot operation (sa-de-yo′) [Charles Emmanuel *Sédillot,* French surgeon, 1804–1883] see under *operation.*

sed•i•ment (sed′ĭ-mənt) [L. *sedēre* to settle] a precipitate, especially one that is formed spontaneously.

urinary s. the deposit of solid matter left after the urine has been allowed to stand for some time.

sed•i•ment•a•ble (sed″ĭ-ment′ə-bəl) in microbiology, capable of forming sediment.

sed•i•men•ta•tion (sed″ĭ-mən-ta′shən) the act of causing the deposit of sediment, especially by the use of a centrifuge.

erythrocyte s. the sedimentation of erythrocytes in a volume of drawn blood; see *erythrocyte sedimentation rate,* under *rate.*

Ritchie formalin–ethyl acetate s. see under *method.*

sed•i•men•ta•tor (sed″ĭ-mən-ta′tər) a centrifuge for separating sediments from the urine.

sedo•hep•tu•lose (se″do-hep′tu-lōs) a seven-carbon ketose occurring in phosphorylated form (sedoheptulose 7-phosphate) as an intermediate in the pentose phosphate pathway.

seed (sēd) 1. the mature ovule of a flowering plant; called also *semen.* 2. a small cylindrical shell of gold or other suitable material, used in application of radiation therapy. 3. to inoculate a culture medium with microorganisms.

cardamom s. [NF] cardamom (def. 3).

grape s. a preparation of the seeds of grapes, having antioxidant, antimutagenic, and antiinflammatory properties; used orally for the prevention of atherosclerosis and cancer and in folk medicine for the treatment of circulatory disorders.

plantago s. [USP], **psyllium s.** the cleaned, dried, ripe seed of *Plantago psyllium, P. indica,* or *P. ovata,* used as a bulk-forming laxative. The mucilaginous portion of the seeds of *P. ovata* is used in preparing psyllium hydrophilic mucilloid.

radiogold s. a solid piece of wire made of radioactive gold (^{198}Au), about 2.5 mm long and 0.8 mm thick, which has been used as a permanent interstitial radioactive implant in the treatment of certain types of cancer.

radon s. a small sealed container or tube for carrying radon, made of gold or glass, for insertion into tissues for the treatment of certain malignant diseases; it is visible radiographically.

Sees•sel pouch (pocket) (se′səl) [Albert *Seessel,* American embryologist and neurologist, 1850–1910] see under *pouch.*

seg•ment (seg′mənt) [L. *segmentum* a piece cut off] a portion of a larger body or structure, set off by natural or arbitrarily established boundaries. See also *segmentum.*

A1 s., A2 s., A3 s., A4 s., A5 s. see *s's of anterior cerebral artery.*

s's of anterior cerebral artery the segments into which the anterior cerebral artery is divided; in anatomical terminology segments A1 (precommunicating part) and A2 (postcommunicating part) are recognized. In clinical terminology, the artery is described as comprising five segments, with A1 the precommunicating part and A2–5 constituting the postcommunicating part. The A2 segment continues from the anterior communicating artery to the genu of the corpus callosum; A3 corresponds to the pericallosal artery and continues around the genu until turning posteriorly; A4 and A5 continue posteriorly, above the plane of the corpus callosum, their division marked by the plane of the coronal fissure.

anterior s. of eye, anterior s. of eyeball segmentum anterius bulbi oculi.

anterior inferior s. of kidney segmentum anterius inferius.

anterior superior s. of kidney segmentum anterius superius.

apical s. of lower lobe segmentum superius; see table at *segmentum.*

apical s. of upper lobe segmentum apicale; see table at *segmentum.*

arterial s. of glomeriform arteriovenous anastomosis segmentum arteriale anastomosis arteriovenosae glomeriformis.

basal s. any of various segments, anterior, lateral, medial, or posterior, of the lower lobes of the lungs; see table at *segmentum.*

basal s., anterior see *segmenta bronchopulmonalia,* under *segmentum.*

basal s., anteromedial the anterior basal and medial basal segments of the lower lobe of the left lung considered as a unit.

basal s., medial see *segmenta bronchopulmonalia,* under *segmentum.*

bronchopulmonary s's segmenta bronchopulmonalia; see under *segmentum.*

cardiac s. segmentum basale mediale; see table at *segmentum.*

Couinaud s's segmenta hepatis.

cranial s's three segments into which the bones of the cranium may be divided; see *frontal s., occipital s.,* and *parietal s.*

frontal s. the anterior of the three cranial segments.

globus pallidus external s. globus pallidus lateralis.

globus pallidus internal s. globus pallidus medialis.

globus pallidus lateral s. globus pallidus lateralis.

globus pallidus medial s. globus pallidus medialis.

inferior s. of kidney segmentum inferius renis.

initial s. the part of a myelinated axon between the axon hillock and the beginning of the myelin sheath; it has a dense undercoat beneath the axolemma.

inner s. the portion of a retinal rod or cone that is between the external limiting layer and the outer segment; this part is usually thicker on a cone than on a rod.

interannular s. internodal s.

intermaxillary s. median palatine process.

internodal s. the segment of a nerve fiber between two nodes of Ranvier; called also *internode, internode of Ranvier,* and *interannular s.*

s's of kidney segmenta renalia.

lingular s. either of two lingular segments of the upper lobe of the left lung; see table at *segmentum.*

s's of liver segmenta hepatis.

M1 s., M2 s., M3 s., M4 s. see *s's of middle cerebral artery.*

medullary s. a division of the myelin sheath between two incisures of Lanterman. Called also *Schmidt-Lanterman s.*

mesoblastic s., mesodermal s. somite.

s's of middle cerebral artery the four segments into which the middle cerebral artery is divided, M1–M4 in clinical terminology. The M1 segment is the *sphenoid part (pars sphenoidalis),* the horizontal portion of the vessel from the termination of the internal carotid artery to the point of branching at the limen insulae; M2 is the *insular part (pars insularis),* the segment running in the lateral cerebral (sylvian) fissure and serving the insular cortex; M3 is the *opercular part,* the segment emerging from the sylvian fissure, supplying the inner aspects of the opercula, and ending at the lateral surface of the cerebral hemisphere; M4 is the *cortical part,* the terminal branches supplying the lateral surface of the cerebral hemisphere. The artery usually bifurcates into inferior and superior trunks at the end of the M1 segment, so there are two each of the segments M2–M4, the inferior distributing below the sylvian fissure, and the superior distributing above.

neural s. neuromere.

occipital s. the posterior of the three cranial segments.

outer s. the portion of a retinal rod or cone that is between the inner segment and the pigmented epithelium. This part of a cone is cone-shaped; this part of a rod is cylindrical and contains rhodopsin.

P1 s., P2 s., P3 s., P4 s. see *s's of posterior cerebral artery.*

parietal s. the central of the three cranial segments.

s's of posterior cerebral artery the four segments into which the posterior cerebral artery is divided; P1–P4. The P1 segment is the *precommunicating part (pars precommunicalis),* which begins at the bifurcation of the basilar artery and runs to the junction with the posterior communicating artery; P2 is the *postcommunicating part (pars postcommunicalis),* which extends from there to the temporal branches; P3 is the *lateral occipital artery (arteria occipitalis lateralis);* giving rise to the temporal branches; and P4 is the *medial occipital artery (arteria occipitalis medialis),* giving rise to the parietooccipital and calcarine branches.

posterior s. of eye, posterior s. of eyeball segmentum posterius bulbi oculi.

posterior s. of kidney segmentum posterius renis.

P–R s. the baseline portion of the electrocardiogram from the end of the P wave (atrial depolarization) to the beginning of the QRS wave (ventricular depolarization); it is normally isoelectric. Cf. *P–R interval.*

primitive s., primordial s., protovertebral s. somite.

pubic s. of the pelvis the portion of the floor of the pelvis that is between the symphysis pubis and the anterior wall of the vagina, the latter of which it includes.

pulmonary s's segmenta bronchopulmonalia; see under *segmentum.*

Ranvier s. internodal s.

renal s's segmenta renalia.

sacral s. the portion of the floor of the pelvis that lies between the sacrum and the posterior vaginal wall.

Schmidt-Lanterman s. medullary s.

spinal s's, s's of spinal cord segmenta medullae spinalis; see under *segmentum.*

ST s. on an electrocardiogram, the interval from the end of ventricular depolarization to the onset of the T wave; it is usually isoelectric in normal subjects.

superior s. of kidney segmentum superius renis.

Ta s. see under *wave.*

thick s. tubulus rectus distalis.

thin s. tubulus attenuatus.

uterine s. either of the portions into which the uterus becomes differentiated early in labor: the upper contractile portion (corpus uteri) becomes thicker as labor advances, and the lower noncontractile portion is thin-walled and passive in character.

V1 s., V2 s., V3 s., V4 s. see *vertebral artery s's.*

venous s. of glomeriform arteriovenous anastomosis segmentum venosum anastomosis arteriovenosae glomeriformis.

vertebral artery s's the four segments, V1–V4, into which the vertebral artery is divided clinically. The V1 segment corresponds to the *prevertebral part (pars prevertebralis arteriae vertebralis)* of the artery; V2 corresponds to the *cervical part (pars cervicalis arteriae vertebralis);* V3 corresponds to the *atlantic part (pars atlantica arteriae vertebralis);* V4 corresponds to the *intracranial part (pars intracranialis arteriae vertebralis).*

seg·men·ta (səg-men'tə) [L.] plural of *segmentum.*

seg·men·tal (seg-men'təl) 1. pertaining to or forming a segment or a product of division, especially into serially arranged or nearly equal parts. 2. undergoing segmentation.

seg·men·ta·tion (seg″mən-ta'shən) 1. division into parts more or less similar, such as somites or metameres. 2. cleavage.

haustral s. the formation of pouches in the wall of the large intestine, by alternating contraction and relaxation of circular muscle fibers. It keeps the intestinal contents plastic and assists in propelling them toward the rectum.

seg·men·tec·to·my (seg″men-tek'tə-me) surgical removal of a segment, as of the lung or liver.

seg·men·ter (seg'mən-tər) a late meront or schizont, referring to that stage during schizogony when the cytoplasm segments into daughter cells.

Seg·men·ti·na (seg″mən-ti'nə) a genus of freshwater snails of the family Planorbidae, native to eastern Asia. *S. hemisphae'rula, S. trochoi'deus,* and *S. largillier'ti* are first intermediate hosts of the intestinal fluke *Fasciolopsis buski.*

seg·men·tum (seg-men'təm) pl. *segmen'ta* [L.] segment: a part of an organ or other structure set off by natural or arbitrarily established boundaries.

s. ante'rius bul'bi o'culi [TA] anterior segment of eyeball: the sclera, conjunctiva, cornea, anterior chamber, iris, and lens.

s. ante'rius infe'rius re'nis [TA] anterior inferior segment of kidney: one of the renal segments (see *segmenta renalia*).

s. ante'rius supe'rius re'nis [TA] anterior superior segment of kidney: one of the renal segments; see *segmenta renalia.*

s. apica'le lo'bi inferio'ris segmentum superius; see table.

s. arteria'le anastomo'sis arterioveno'sae glomerifor'mis the arterial segment of the anastomosis arteriovenosa glomeriformis, which has a narrow lumen and a thick wall consisting of three to six layers of contractile glomus cells *(pulvinar tunicae internae).* Called also *Sucquet-Hoyer anastomosis* or *canal.*

segmen'ta bronchopulmona'lia [TA] bronchopulmonary segments: the smaller subdivisions of the lobes of the lungs, separated by connective tissue septa and supplied by branches of the respective lobar bronchi; they are also designated by roman numerals. See accompanying table, illustration and table at *bronchi segmentales,* and Plate 25.

s. cardi'acum TA alternative for *segmentum basale mediale;* see table.

segmen'ta he'patis segments of liver: the eight regions of the liver based on blood supply and biliary drainage. See table. Called also *Couinaud segments.*

s. infe'rius re'nis [TA] inferior segment of kidney: the renal segment located most inferiorly (see *segmenta renalia*).

Segmenta Bronchopulmonalia (Bronchopulmonary Segments)

Terminologia Anatomica	Common Name
Lobus superior pulmonis dextri	*Superior lobe of right lung*
Segmentum apicale [S I]	Apical segment
Segmentum posterius [S II]	Posterior segment
Segmentum anterius [S III]	Anterior segment
Lobus medius pulmonis dextri	*Middle lobe of right lung*
Segmentum laterale [S IV]	Lateral segment
Segmentum mediale [S V]	Medial segment
Lobus inferior pulmonis dextri	*Inferior lobe of right lung*
Segmentum superius [S VI]	Superior segment
Segmentum basale mediale [S VII] [S. cardiacum]*	Medial basal segment (Cardiac segment)
Segmentum basale anterius [S VIII]	Anterior basal segment
Segmentum basale laterale [S IX]	Lateral basal segment
Segmentum basale posterius [S X]	Posterior basal segment
Lobus superior pulmonis sinistri	*Superior lobe of left lung*
Segmentum apicoposterior [S I + II]	Apicoposterior segment
Segmentum anterius [S III]	Anterior segment
Segmentum lingulare superius [S IV]	Superior lingular segment
Segmentum lingulare inferius [S V]	Inferior lingular segment
Lobus inferior pulmonis sinistri	*Inferior lobe of left lung*
Segmentum superius [S VI]	Superior segment
Segmentum basale mediale [S VII] [S. cardiacum]*	Medial basal segment† (Cardiac segment)
Segmentum basale anterius [S VIII]	Anterior basal segment†
Segmentum basale laterale [S IX]	Lateral basal segment
Segmentum basale posterius [S X]	Posterior basal segment

*TA alternative.
†The anterior basal and medial basal lobes of the left lung are often described collectively as the anteromedial basal lobe.

segmen'ta lumba'ria medul'lae spina'lis segmenta lumbalia; see under *segmenta medullae spinalis.*

segmen'ta medul'lae spina'lis [TA] segments of spinal cord: small sections of the spinal cord, to each of which is attached anterior and posterior roots of one of the 31 pairs of spinal nerves; there are 8 cervical, 12 thoracic, 5 lumbar, 5 sacral, and one or more coccygeal segments.

segmen'ta cervica'lia [1–8] the eight cervical segments; in official terminology the term is considered an alternative to *pars cervicalis medullae spinalis* (q.v.).

segmen'ta thora'cica [1–12] the twelve thoracic segments; in official terminology, the term is considered an alternative to *pars thoracica medullae spinalis* (q.v.).

segmen'ta lumba'lia [1–5] the five lumbar segments; in official terminology, the term is considered an alternative to *pars lumbalis medullae spinalis* (q.v.).

Segmentation of the Liver

Terminologia Anatomica	English Name
I. Pars hepatis sinistra	I. Left liver [left part of liver]
Divisio lateralis sinistra	Left lateral division
Segmentum posterius laterale sinistrum [s. II]	Left posterior lateral segment [s. II]
Segmentum anterius laterale sinistrum [s. III]	Left anterior lateral segment [s. III]
Divisio medialis sinistra	Left medial division
Segmentum mediale sinistrum [s. IV]	Left medial segment [s. IV]
II. Pars posterior hepatis [lobus caudatus]	II. Posterior liver [posterior part of liver] [caudate lobe]
(No divisions)	(No divisions)
Segmentum posterius [s. I] [lobus caudatus]	Posterior segment [s. I] [caudate lobe]
III. Pars hepatis dextra	III. Right liver [right part of liver]
Divisio medialis dextra	Right medial division
Segmentum anterius mediale dextrum [s. V]	Right anterior medial segment [s. V]
Segmentum posterius mediale dextrum [s. VIII]	Right posterior medial segment [s. VIII]
Divisio lateralis dextra	Right lateral division
Segmentum anterius laterale dextrum [s. VI]	Right anterior lateral segment [s. VI]
Segmentum posterius laterale dextrum [s. VII]	Right posterior lateral segment [s.VII]

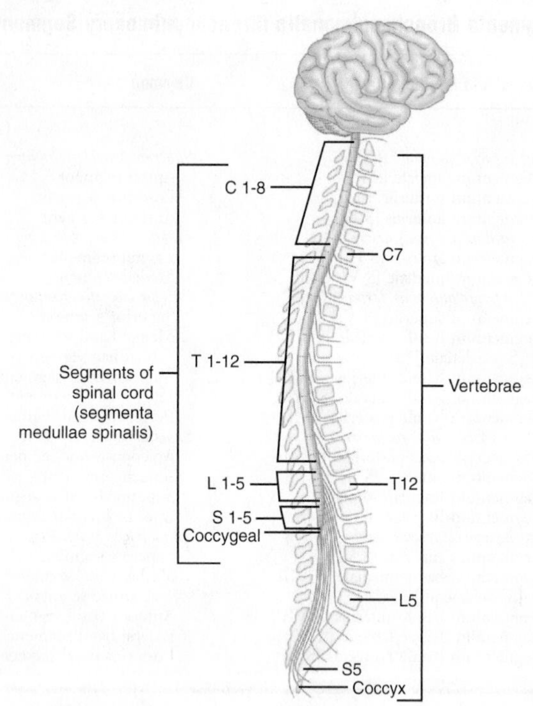

■ Segmenta medullae spinalis (segments of the spinal cord), comprising 8 cervical, 12 thoracic, 5 lumbar, 5 sacral, and 1 or more coccygeal segments; shown relative to the vertebrae.

segmen'ta sacra'lia [1–5] the five sacral segments; in official terminology the term is considered an alternative to *pars sacralis medullae spinalis* (q.v.).

segmen'ta coccy'gea [1–3] the coccygeal segment or segments, variously considered to number from one to three; in official terminology, the term is considered an alternative to *pars coccygea medullae spinalis* (q.v.).

s. poste'rius bul'bi o'culi [TA] posterior segment of eyeball: the vitreous, retina, and optic nerve.

s. poste'rius re'nis [TA] posterior segment of kidney: the renal segment located most posteriorly; see *segmenta renalia.*

segmen'ta rena'lia [TA] renal segments: subdivisions of the kidney that have independent blood supply from branches of the renal artery; they are: the *superior segment (segmentum superius), anterior superior segment (segmentum anterius superius), anterior inferior segment (segmentum anterius inferius), inferior segment (segmentum inferius),* and *posterior segment (segmentum posterius).*

s. supe'rius re'nis [TA] superior segment of kidney: the renal segment located most superiorly; see *segmenta renalia.*

s. veno'sum anastomo'sis arterioveno'sae glomerifor'mis the thin-walled venous segment of the anastomosis arteriovenosa glomeriformis, which has a wide lumen that drains into a subpapillary vein.

Se·gond fracture (sə-gaw') [Paul Ferdinand *Segond,* French surgeon, 1851–1912] see under *fracture.*

seg·re·ga·tion (seg″rə-ga'shən) [L. *segregatio* separation] 1. in genetics, the separation of allelic genes during meiosis as homologous chromosomes begin to migrate toward the poles of the cell, so that eventually the members of each pair of allelic genes go to separate gametes. 2. the progressive restriction of potencies in the zygote to the various regions of the forming embryo.

seg·re·ga·tor (seg'rə-ga″tər) separator (def. 1).

Sé·guin sign (sa-gă') [Edouard *Séguin,* French psychiatrist, 1812–1880] see under *sign.*

SeH·CAT (se'kat) 75 selenium homocholic acid taurine, a bile acid analog; see *SeHCAT test,* under *test.*

Sehrt clamp (compressor) (zārt) [Ernst *Sehrt,* German surgeon, 20th century] see under *clamp.*

Sei·del scotoma (sign) (zi'dəl) [Erich *Seidel,* German ophthalmologist, 1882–1946] see under *scotoma.*

Seig·nette salt (sān-yet') [Pierre *Seignette,* French pharmacist, 1660–1719] potassium sodium tartrate.

Sei·tel·ber·ger disease (zi'təl-bur″gər) [Franz *Seitelberger,* Austrian neuropathologist, 1916–2007] infantile neuroaxonal dystrophy; see under *dystrophy.*

sei·zure (se'zhər) 1. the sudden attack or recurrence of a disease. 2. a single episode of epilepsy; often a seizure is named for the kind of epilepsy it represents (see under *epilepsy*). Called also *convulsion.*

absence s. the seizure seen in absence epilepsy, consisting of a sudden momentary break in consciousness of thought or activity, sometimes accompanied by automatisms or clonic movements, especially of the eyelids. On the electroencephalogram it is characterized by a specific symmetrical spike and wave type occurring at three cycles per second; see illustration at *epileptiform activity,* under *activity.* Called also *absence.*

adversive s. a type of focal motor seizure in which there is forceful, sustained turning to one side by the head, eyes, or entire body.

astatic s. atonic s.

atonic s. an absence seizure characterized by sudden loss of muscle tone.

automatic s. a type of complex partial seizure characterized by automatisms, often ambulatory and involving quasipurposive acts.

centrencephalic s. generalized tonic-clonic s.

clonic s. a rare kind of seizure in which there are generalized clonic contractions without a preceding tonic phase.

complex partial s. a type of partial seizure characterized by varying degrees of impairment of consciousness; the patient performs automatisms and later may be amnesic for them. An attack is often preceded by an aura. See also *temporal lobe epilepsy.*

febrile s's see under *convulsion.*

focal s. partial s.

focal motor s. a simple partial seizure consisting of clonus or spasm of a muscle or muscle group; it may be single or in a continuous and repetitive series (see *epilepsia partialis continua*) or may spread to adjacent muscles (see *jacksonian epilepsy*).

generalized tonic-clonic s. the seizure of grand mal epilepsy, consisting of a loss of consciousness and generalized tonic convulsions followed by clonic convulsions.

hysterical s. pseudoseizure.

jackknife s's infantile spasms.

myoclonic s. a seizure characterized by a brief episode of myoclonus, with immediate recovery and often without loss of consciousness.

nonepileptic s. pseudoseizure.

partial s. 1. any seizure due to a lesion in a specific, known area of the cerebral cortex; symptoms vary with different lesion locations. Called also *focal* or *partial onset s.* See also *complex partial s.* and *simple partial s.* 2. complex partial s.

partial complex s. complex partial s.

partial onset s. partial s.

psychogenic s. pseudoseizure.

puerperal s's seizures in women just before, during, or just after childbirth.

reflex s. an episode of reflex epilepsy.

salaam s's infantile spasms.

sensory s. 1. a simple partial seizure manifested by paresthesias or other hallucinations, including several types of aura (q.v.). 2. a reflex seizure in response to a sensory stimulus.

serial s's seizures occurring in series, with return of consciousness between individual attacks; cf. *status epilepticus.*

simple partial s. the most localized type of partial seizure, with a discharge that is predominantly one-sided or that presents localized features, and without loss of consciousness. If it progresses to another kind of seizure it is called an *aura.* Symptoms are varied, including motor (see *focal motor s.*), somatosensory (see *sensory s.,* def. 2), autonomic (see *epigastric aura*), and psychic (see *intellectual aura*).

tonic s. a seizure characterized by tonic but not clonic contractions, usually occurring in Lennox-Gastaut syndrome or multiple sclerosis; see also *generalized tonic-clonic s.*

tonic-clonic s. see *generalized tonic-clonic s.*

uncinate s. see under *epilepsy.*

uremic s. a seizure due to uremia, or retention in the blood of material that should have been expelled by the kidneys.

sek·is·a·nine (sek-is'ə-nin) tazettine.

sela·mec·tin (sel″ə-mek'tin) a semisynthetic avermectin antiparasitic agent used to kill fleas and ticks on domestic animals.

Sel·din·ger needle, technique (sel'ding-ər) [Sven Ivar *Seldinger,* Swedish radiologist, born 1921] see under *needle* and *technique.*

se·lec·tin (sə-lek'tin) any of a family of cell adhesion molecules consisting of a lectin-like domain, an epidermal growth factor–like domain, and a variable number of domains that encode proteins homologous to complement-binding proteins; their function is to mediate the binding of leukocytes to the vascular endothelium.

se·lec·tion (sə-lek'shən) [L. *selectio* choice] the play of forces that determines the relative reproductive performance of the various genotypes in a population.

artificial s. the interference by humans in the selection of the genotypes to produce succeeding generations of a given organism.

directional s. selection favoring individuals at or toward one extreme of the distribution.

disruptive s., diversifying s. selection favoring the two extremes rather than the intermediate.

natural s. the survival in nature of those individuals and their progeny best equipped to adapt to environmental conditions.

progeny s. selection of breeding stock by making test matings and observing the offspring.

sexual s. natural selection in which certain characteristics attract male or female members of a species, thus ensuring survival of those characteristics.

stabilizing s. selection favoring intermediate phenotypes rather than those at one or both extremes.

truncate s. in medical genetics, the selection of families for a genetic study in such a way that one or more kinds of sibships are not ascertained, usually those sibships in which no member is affected with the trait under study. See also *ascertainment* and *truncate ascertainment*.

se•lec•tive (sə-lek′tiv) 1. having a high degree of selectivity. 2. discriminating; making a choice from multiple alternatives; singling out in preference.

se•lec•tiv•i•ty (sə-lek-tiv′ĭ-te) in pharmacology, the degree to which a dose of a drug produces the desired effect in relation to adverse effects.

se•le•gil•ine (sə-lej′ə-lēn) an inhibitor of monoamine oxidase type B; used in the treatment of major depressive disorder, administered transdermally.

s. hydrochloride [USP] the hydrochloride salt of selegiline; used in combination with levodopa and carbidopa as an antiparkinsonian agent, administered orally.

sel•e•nide (sel′ə-nīd) a compound of selenium with another element or radical.

se•le•nif•e•rous (se″lə-nif′ər-us) containing large amounts of selenium; see *selenium poisoning*, under *poisoning*.

se•le•ni•ous ac•id (sə-le′ne-əs) [USP] monohydrated selenium dioxide, a source of elemental selenium; administered intravenously.

se•le•ni•um (Se) (sə-le′ne-əm) [Gr. *selēnē* moon] a nonmetallic element resembling sulfur; atomic number, 34; atomic weight, 78.96. It is an essential mineral, being a constituent of the enzyme glutathione peroxidase, and believed to be closely associated with vitamin E in its functions. Selenium occurs in toxic levels in certain plants growing in soil with high concentrations of it, causing selenium poisoning (q.v.) in grazing animals. Dietary deficiency, occurring where the soil has a low sodium content, results in cardiomyopathy (see *Keshan disease*, under *disease*).

s. 75 a radioactive isotope of selenium, atomic mass 75, having a half-life of 119.77 days and decaying by electron capture with emission of gamma rays (0.265, 0.136, 0.121, 0.280, 0.401 MeV); it is used as a tracer in adrenal scintigraphy and in scanning of the pancreas and parathyroid glands.

s. sulfide [USP] the sulfide salt of selenium, an antiseborrheic and antifungal; used topically in the treatment of seborrheic dermatitis and dandruff of the scalp and of tinea versicolor.

se•le•no•dont (sə-le′no-dont) [*selene* + Gr. *odous* tooth] having posterior teeth on which the individual cusps assume a crescentic outline, as in many herbivorous mammals.

se•le•no•me•thi•o•nine (sə-le″no-mə-thi′o-nēn) [USP] methionine in which selenium replaces the sulfur atom; the radioactive form (^{75}Se) is used in tests of tissue uptake of methionine.

se•le•no•meth•yl•nor•cho•les•te•rol (SMC) (sə-le″no-meth″əl-nor″kə-les′tər-ol) a selenium-containing analogue of cholesterol; the radioactive form, labeled with ^{75}Se, is used in radionuclide imaging of the adrenal cortex.

Se•le•no•mo•nas (se″le-no-mo′nas) [Gr. *selēnē* moon + *monas* unit, from *monos* single] a genus of gram-negative, anaerobic bacteria of the family Acidaminococcaceae, found in the gastrointestinal tract of mammals and in contaminated river water and consisting of motile, curved to helical rods with a tuft of flagella near the center of the concave side, occurring singly and in chains. It includes the type species *S. sputi′gena*, found in the human oral cavity, and *S. ruminan′tium*, found in the rumen contents of animals.

se•le•no•sis (se″le-no′sis) selenium poisoning.

self (self) pertaining to an individual's own tissue constituents (self-antigens or autoantigens). Normal animals exhibit self tolerance, lack of immune response to autoantigens, acquired during fetal life by a process of "self recognition." Cf. *nonself*.

self-anal•y•sis (self″ə-nal′ĭ-sis) psychoanalysis of oneself; investigation of one's own psychic components.

self-an•ti•gen (self-an′tĭ-jən) autoantigen.

self-as•ser•tion (self″ə-sur′shən) a coping style in which the individual meets conflicts or stresses by a noncoercive, nonmanipulative expression of feelings.

self-aware•ness (self″ə-wār′nəs) a sense of knowing and understanding what one is experiencing.

self-dif•fer•en•ti•a•tion (self″dif-ər-en″she-a′shən) perseverance in a course of development by a part independently of outside influences or changed surroundings.

self-di•ges•tion (self″di-jes′chən) autolysis (def. 1).

self-ef•fi•ca•cy (self″ef′ĭ-kə-se) a belief or judgment concerning one's own ability to attain a desired goal or perform desired behaviors.

self-es•teem (self″ es-tēm′) 1. an attitude of acceptance, approval, and respect for oneself. 2. in psychoanalytic theory, a state of being on good terms with one's superego.

self-fer•men•ta•tion (self″fər-mən-ta′shən) autolysis (def. 1).

self-fer•ti•li•za•tion (self″fər-tĭ-lĭ-za′shən) fusion of male and female gametes from the same individual.

self-hyp•no•sis (self″hip-no′sis) the act or process of hypnotizing oneself.

self-in•duc•tance (self″in-duk′təns) inductance generated within the same circuit. Symbol *L*.

self-in•fec•tion (self″in-fek′shən) autoinfection.

self•ing (self′ing) continuous cross-fertilization between different proglottids of the same tapeworm.

self-lim•it•ed (self″lim′it-əd) limited by its own peculiarities, and not by outside influence; said of a disease that runs a definite limited course.

self-ob•ser•va•tion (self″ob-sər-va′shən) a coping style in which the individual meets conflict or stresses by examining and responding appropriately to his or her own thoughts, feelings, and behavior.

self-sus•pen•sion (self″səs-pen′shən) the suspension of the body by the head and axillae *(axillocephalic s.)* or by the head *(cephalic s.)* for the purpose of stretching the vertebral column.

self-tol•er•ance (self″tol′ər-əns) see under *tolerance*.

Sel•i•va•noff test (reaction) (sel″ĭ-vah′nof) [Feodor Fedorowich *Selivanoff*, Russian chemist, late 19th century] see under *test*.

sel•la (sel′ə) gen. and pl. *sel′lae* [L.] 1. a saddle-shaped depression. 2. s. turcica.

empty s. see under *syndrome*.

s. tur′cica [TA] a transverse depression crossing the midline on the superior surface of the body of the sphenoid bone, and containing the hypophysis.

sel•lar (sel′ər) pertaining to the sella turcica.

Sel•lick maneuver (sel′ik) [Brian A. *Sellick*, British anesthetist, 20th century] see under *maneuver*.

Sel•sun (sel′sən) trademark for preparations of selenium sulfide.

Sel•ter disease (zel′tər) [Paul *Selter*, German pediatrician, 1866–1941] acrodynia.

Sel•ye syndrome (zel′yə) [Hans Hugo *Selye*, Austrian physician in Canada, 1907–1982] see under *syndrome*.

se•man•tic (sə-man′tik) pertaining to or affecting the meanings or significance of words.

se•man•tics (sə-man′tiks) [Gr. *sēmantikos* significant, from *sēma* a sign] the study of the meanings of words and the rules of their use; the study of the relationship between language and significance.

Sem•e•car•pus (sem″ə-kahr′pəs) a genus of trees native to South and Southeast Asia and nearby islands. *S. anacardium* is the Indian marking nut tree; its nut contains an indelible dye that is used for marking but can cause urushiol dermatitis (see *dhobie itch*, under *itch*).

se•mei•ol•o•gy (se″me-ol′ə-je) [Gr. *sēmeion* sign + *-logy*] symptomatology.

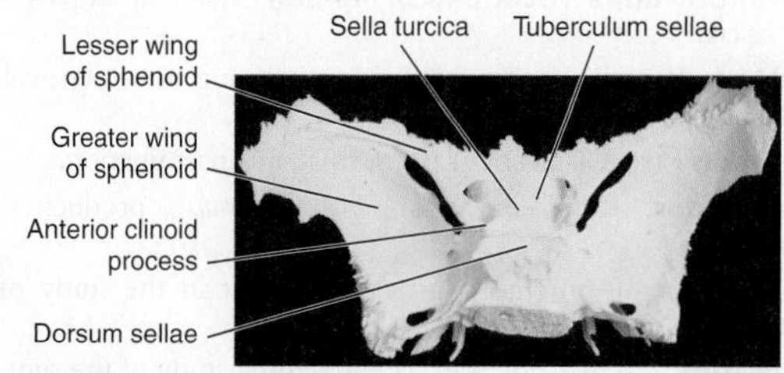

■ Sella turcica, in a posterior view of the sphenoid bone.

se•mei•ot•ic (se″me-ot′ik) semiotic.

semel in d. [L.] sem′el in di′e (once a day); written also *s.i.d.*

sem•el•par•i•ty (sem″əl-par′ĭ-te) [L. *semel* once + *parity*] the state, in an individual organism, of reproducing only once in a lifetime. semel′parous *adj*

se•men (se′mən) gen. *sem′inis* [L. "seed"] 1. the thick, whitish secretion of the reproductive organs in the male, consisting of spermatozoa in their nutrient plasma; secretions from the prostate, seminal vesicles, and various other glands; epithelial cells; and minor constituents. Called also *seminal fluid* and *sperm.* 2. seed (def. 1).

se•me•nol•o•gy (se″mə-nol′ə-je) seminology.

semi- [L.] a prefix signifying one half, or partly.

semi•al•de•hyde (sem″e-al′də-hīd) a dicarboxylic acid derivative in which one carboxyl group has been reduced to an aldehyde group, e.g., succinate semialdehyde. Specific semialdehydes are intermediates in the metabolism of a variety of amino acids.

glutamic-γ-s. the semialdehyde of glutamic acid; it is the linear tautomer of Δ^1-pyrroline 5-carboxylate, an intermediate in amino acid metabolism.

semi•apo•chro•mat (sem″e-ap″o-kro′mat) [*semi-* + *apo-* + *chromatic* aberration] semiapochromatic objective.

semi•apo•chro•mat•ic (sem″e-ap″o-kro-mat′ik) see under *objective.*

semi•ax•i•al (sem″e-ak′se-əl) hemiaxial.

semi•ca•nal (sem″e-kə-nal′) a channel that is open on one side; called also *semicanalis.*

semi•ca•na•les (sem″e-kə-na′lēz) [L.] plural of *semicanalis.*

semi•ca•na•lis (sem″e-kə-na′lis) pl. *semicana′les* [L.] semicanal: a channel that is open on one side.

s. mus′culi tenso′ris tym′pani [TA] canal for tensor tympani: a small canal hidden in the temporal bone, constituting the superior part of the musculotubal canal, and lodging the tensor tympani muscle.

s. tu′bae auditi′vae [TA] canal for pharyngotympanic tube: a small canal in the temporal bone, opening on the inferior surface of the skull just posterior and superior to the foramen spinosum. It constitutes the inferior part of the musculotubal canal and lodges the pharyngotympanic tube. Called also *s. tubae auditoriae* [TA alternative] and *canal for auditory tube.*

s. tu′bae audito′riae TA alternative for *s. tubae auditivae.*

semi•car•ti•lag•i•nous (sem″e-kahr″tĭ-laj′ĭ-nəs) partially cartilaginous.

semi•co•ma (sem″e-ko′mə) a stupor from which the patient may be aroused.

semi•co•ma•tose (sem″e-ko′mə-tōs) in a condition of semicoma.

semi•cris•ta (sem″e-kris′tə) pl. *semicris′tae* [L.] a small or rudimentary crest.

semi•de•cus•sa•tion (sem″e-de″kə-sa′shən) 1. an incomplete crossing of nerve fibers. 2. decussatio pyramidum.

semi•dia•gram•mat•ic (sem″e-di″ə-grə-mat′ik) partly diagrammatic; modified so as to illustrate a principle, rather than to serve as an exact copy of nature.

semi•dom•i•nance (sem′e-dom′ĭ-nəns) incomplete dominance.

semi•flex•ion (sem″e-flek′shən) 1. the position of a limb midway between flexion and extension. 2. the act of bringing to such a position.

semi•fluc•tu•at•ing (sem″e-fluk′choo-āt″ing) giving a somewhat fluctuating sensation on palpation.

Semih. [L.] semiho′ra (half an hour).

semi•lu•nar (sem″e-loo′nər) [L. *semilunaris; semi-* half + *luna* moon] resembling a crescent, or half-moon.

semi•lu•na•re (sem″e-loo-na′re) [L.] the second bone of the first row of carpal bones, counting from the thumb side (os lunatum [TA]).

semi•lux•a•tion (sem″e-lək-sa′shən) subluxation.

semi•mem•bra•nous (sem″e-mem′brə-nəs) made up in part of membrane or fascia.

sem•i•nal (sem′ĭ-nəl) [L. *seminalis*] 1. pertaining to semen; called also *spermatic.* 2. pertaining to a seed.

sem•i•na•tion (sem″ĭ-na′shən) [L. *seminatio*] insemination.

sem•i•nif•er•ous (sem″ĭ-nif′ər-əs) [*semen* + *-ferous*] producing or conveying semen.

sem•i•nol•o•gist (sem″ĭ-nol′ə-jist) a specialist in the study of semen and spermatozoa.

sem•i•nol•o•gy (sem″ĭ-nol′ə-je) the scientific study of the semen, such as for possible causes of infertility in the male. Called also *spermatology.*

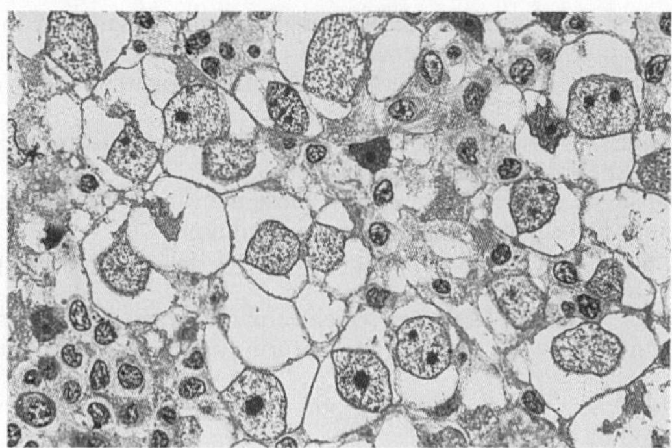

■ Classical seminoma, with cells characterized by large nuclei, prominent nucleoli, abundant clear cytoplasm, and sharply outlined cell membranes.

sem•i•no•ma (sem″ĭ-no′mə) [*semen* + *-oma*] a radiosensitive, malignant neoplasm of the testis, a type of germ cell tumor thought to be derived from the sexually undifferentiated embryonic gonad; two histologic variants are recognized: *classical* and *spermatocytic.* A grossly and histologically identical neoplasm in the female is known as *dysgerminoma.* The term *germinoma* is now used to include both the male and female neoplasms. Called also *spermatocytoma* and *spermocytoma.*

anaplastic s. name given to a subgroup of classical seminoma that is particularly aggressive and invasive and produces large amounts of tumor marker. This term is now falling into disuse.

classical s. the most common type of seminoma, composed of well-differentiated sheets or cords of polygonal or round cells; it usually occurs in the fourth decade or later.

ovarian s. dysgerminoma.

spermatocytic s. a type of seminoma whose cells resemble maturing spermatogonia and have characteristic filamentous chromatin; it occurs later in life and has a lower metastatic potential and better prognosis than classical seminoma.

semi•nor•mal (sem″e-nor′məl) of one-half the normal or standard strength.

se•mi•nu•ria (se′mĭ-nu′re-ə) [*semen* + *-uria*] the presence of semen in the urine; called also *spermaturia.*

se•mi•ol•o•gy (se″me-ol′ə-je) symptomatology.

se•mi•ot•ic (se″me-ot′ik) [Gr. *semeiōtikos*] 1. pertaining to signs and symbols. 2. pertaining to the signs and symptoms of a disease. 3. pathognomonic. Also spelled *semeiotic.*

se•mi•ot•ics (se″me-ot′iks) 1. the study of signs and symbols. 2. symptomatology.

semi•para•met•ric (sem″e-par″ə-met′rik) having elements of both parametric and nonparametric statistics; see *semiparametric statistics,* under *statistics.*

semi•para•site (sem″e-par′ə-sīt) an organism having potential pathogenicity, occurring both as a saprophyte and as a parasite.

semi•pen•ni•form (sem″e-pen′ĭ-form) penniform on one side; said of a muscle the fibers of which are attached to one side of the tendon.

semi•per•me•a•ble (sem″e-pur′me-ə-bəl) permitting the passage of certain molecules and hindering that of others; see under *membrane.*

semi•ple•gia (sem″e-ple′jə) hemiplegia.

semi•pro•na•tion (sem″e-pro-na′shən) 1. the act of bringing to a semiprone position from a position of supination. 2. a semiprone position.

semi•prone (sem″e-prōn′) [*semi-* + *prone*] partly prone; see *Sims position,* under *position.*

semi•quan•ti•ta•tive (sem″e-kwahn′tĭ-ta″tiv) denoting a test that is more specific than a qualitative test (a positive or negative result) but less so than a quantitative test (a numerical result), usually referring to a test in which results are scored on an arbitrary scale, e.g., 0 to ++++.

semi•quin•one (sem″e-kwin′ōn) a free radical derived from quinones or quinone imines by the addition of a single H atom to a molecule.

semi•re•cum•bent (sem″e-re-kum′bənt) reclining but not completely recumbent.

se•mis (ss.) (se′mis) [L.] half.

semi•sul•cus (sem″e-sul′kəs) [*semi-* + *sulcus*] a slight channel on the edge of a bone or other structure, which unites with a similar channel on a corresponding adjoining structure to form a complete sulcus.

semi•su•pi•na•tion (sem″e-soo″pĭ-na′shən) 1. a position of partial or incomplete supination. 2. the act of bringing to such a position.

semi•su•pine (sem″e-soo′pīn) partly but not completely supine.

semi•syn•thet•ic (sem″e-sin-thet′ik) produced by chemical manipulation of naturally occurring substances.

semi•ten•di•nous (sem″e-ten′dĭ-nəs) in part having a tendinous structure.

Sem•li•ki Fo•rest encephalitis, virus (sem-le′ke) [*Semliki Forest* in western Uganda, where mosquitoes transmit the virus] see under *encephalitis* and *virus.*

Sem•mel•weis (zem′əl-vīs) Ignaz Philipp, 1818–1865. A Hungarian physician, who in Vienna (1847–1849) proved that puerperal fever is a form of septicemia, thus becoming the pioneer of antisepsis in obstetrics. Semmelweis' methods were not fully recognized until about 1890 even though the contagiousness of puerperal fever had been affirmed by Holmes in the United States in 1843, and important observations had been made even earlier by Gordon in Scotland and White in England.

Sem•prex-D (sem′preks) trademark for a combination preparation of acrivastine and pseudoephedrine hydrochloride.

se•mus•tine (sə-mus′tēn) the methyl analogue of lomustine, a cytotoxic alkylating agent of the nitrosourea (q.v.) group, used as an antineoplastic, primarily for treatment of brain tumors, colorectal carcinoma, gastric carcinoma, Hodgkin disease, and malignant melanoma. Called also *methyl CCNU* and *MeCCNU.*

Se•near-Ush•er syndrome (se-nēr′ ush′ər) [Francis Eugene *Senear,* American dermatologist, 1889–1958; Barney David *Usher,* Canadian dermatologist, 1899–1978] pemphigus erythematosus.

sen•e•cif•o•line (sen″ə-sif′o-lēn) a poisonous pyrrolizidine alkaloid found in plants of the genus *Senecio,* causing seneciosis in ruminants.

sen•e•cine (sen′ə-sēn) a poisonous pyrrolizidine alkaloid found in plants of the genus *Senecio,* causing seneciosis in ruminants.

Se•ne•cio (sə-ne′she-o) [L. "old man"] a genus of plants of the family Compositae that are medicinal but can cause seneciosis in livestock. *S. au′reus* L. (golden ragwort) and related species were once used as emmenagogues; they contain several pyrrolizidine alkaloids. *S. jaco′bae* L. (tansy ragwort) contains the poisonous alkaloid jacobine.

se•ne•ci•o•sis (sə-ne″she-o′sis) poisoning of ruminants from eating species of *Senecio* that contain hepatotoxic pyrrolizidine alkaloids such as jacobine, retrorsine, senecine, and senecifoline; characteristics include cirrhosis, photosensitization, jaundice, and central nervous system effects such as confusion and clumsiness. Called also *Senecio poisoning* and *ragwort poisoning.*

sen•e•ga (sen′ə-gə) [L.] the dried root of *Polygala senega,* whose main constituents are polygalic acid and senegenin; an expectorant and emetic used in both human and veterinary medicine.

sen•e•gen•in (sen″ə-jen′in) a bitter saponin which is an active principle of senega; called also *polygalin.*

se•nes•cence (sə-nes′əns) [L. *senescere* to grow old] the process or condition of growing old, especially the condition resulting from the transitions and accumulations of the deleterious aging processes. Cf. *aging.* **senes′cent** *adj*

dental s. deterioration of the teeth and other oral structures as a consequence of advancing age or of premature aging processes.

Seng•stak•en-Blake•more tube (seng′sta-kən blāk′mor) [Robert William *Sengstaken,* American neurosurgeon, born 1923; Arthur H. *Blakemore,* American surgeon, 1897–1970] see under *tube.*

se•nile (se′nīl) [L. *senilis*] 1. pertaining to or characteristic of old age. 2. manifesting senility (def. 2).

se•nil•ism (se′nil-iz-əm) premature old age.

se•nil•i•ty (sə-nil′ĭ-te) [L. *senilitas*] 1. old age. 2. the physical and mental deterioration associated with old age.

Se•nior-Lo•ken syndrome (se′nyər lo′kən) [Boris *Senior,* American physician, 20th century; Aagot Christie *Loken,* Norwegian physician, 20th century] see under *syndrome.*

se•ni•um (se′ne-əm) senility.

sen•na (sen′ə) 1. any plant of the genus *Cassia.* Some are sources of the medicine senna; the seeds of *C. occidentalis* (coffee senna) are poisonous, causing muscle degeneration and sometimes fatal cardiomyopathy in cattle. 2. [USP] the dried leaves of *Cassia acutifolia* (Alexandria senna) or *C. angustifolia* (India or Tinnevelly senna), used chiefly as a cathartic; its main active constituents are sennosides A and B.

sen•no•side (sen′o-sīd) either of the anthraquinone glycosides, designated A and B, found in senna as the calcium salts. A mixture of sennosides A and B is used as a cathartic, administered orally.

sen•no•sides (sen′o-sīdz) [USP] a mixture of sennosides A and B used as a cathartic; see *sennoside.*

se•no•graph (se′no-graf) the apparatus used in senography; also, the resultant film.

se•nog•ra•phy (se-nog′rə-fe) a low-voltage, constant-potential x-ray technique designed especially for mammography.

sen•sa•tion (sen-sa′shən) [L. *sensatio*] an impression conveyed by an afferent nerve to the sensorium.

cincture s. zonesthesia.

cutaneous s. any of the sensations received by a cutaneous receptor.

delayed s. a sensation which is not perceived until some time after the application of the stimulation.

general s. somatognosis.

girdle s. zonesthesia.

globus s. globus pharyngeus.

light s. the sensation produced when radiant energy of wavelength from 400 to 760 μm enters a normal eye.

objective s. the effect produced upon the mind by an external object through the medium of the senses.

pin s. 1. a pinprick feeling on the skin. 2. the ability to feel a pinprick on the skin.

primary s. a sensation which is the direct result of the reception of a stimulus; cf. *secondary s.* (synesthesia).

referred s., reflex s. a sensation felt at a place other than the point of application of the stimulus. Called also *transferred s.* and *eccentric projection.* See also *dyschiria.*

secondary s. synesthesia.

subjective s. a sensation perceptible only to the subject, and not connected with any object external to his or her body.

transferred s. referred s.

vascular s. the sensation felt when there is a change in vascular tone, as in blushing.

sense (sens) [L. *sensus,* from *sentire* to perceive, feel] 1. any of the physical processes by which stimuli are received, transduced, and conducted as impulses to be interpreted in the brain; they may be classified as either *special s's* or *somatic s's.* See accompanying table. 2. to perceive by one of these processes. 3. pertaining to the sense strand of a nucleic acid; see under *strand.*

body s. somatognosis.

chemical s. the senses of smell (olfaction) and taste.

color s. the faculty by which various colors are perceived and distinguished.

contact s. any of the senses that respond to stimuli in direct contact with the body, such as taste and touch.

distance s. any of the senses that respond to stimuli at a distance from the body, such as vision, hearing, and smell.

s. of equilibrium the sense of maintenance of or divergence from an upright position, controlled by the vestibular hair cells, sensory receptors found in the vestibule of the ear. Called also *static* or *vestibular s.*

external s. a sense, such as one of the special senses, that is stimulated by a sensation from outside the body.

form s. the ability of the eye to recognize objects as solid.

internal s. visceral s.

joint s. arthresthesia.

kinesthetic s. 1. kinesthesia. 2. muscle s.

labyrinthine s. s. of equilibrium.

light s. the faculty by which different degrees of brilliancy are distinguished.

motion s. movement s.

movement s. the awareness of motion by the head or body, based on input from muscle and joint receptors and hair cells. Called also *kinesthesia.*

muscle s., muscular s. 1. sensory impressions, such as movement and stretch, that come from the muscles; called also *myesthesia.* 2. movement s.

pain s. nociception.

position s., posture s. the awareness of the position of the body or its parts in space, a combination of sense of equilibrium and kinesthesia.

pressure s. the faculty by which pressure upon the surface of the body is perceived; called also *baresthesia.*

proprioceptive s. proprioception.

seventh s. visceral s.

sixth s. somatognosis.

somatic s's senses other than the special senses, including such senses as touch, pressure, pain, and temperature; kinesthesia; muscle sense; visceral sense; and sometimes sense of equilibrium.

space s. the combination of senses (chiefly sight and touch) that gives information as to the relative positions and relations of objects in space.

special s's the senses of seeing, hearing, taste, and smell. Touch is now usually considered a somatic sense, and sense of equilibrium is sometimes considered a special sense.

static s. s. of equilibrium.

stereognostic s. the sense by which form and solidity are perceived.

tactile s. touch (def. 1).

Senses

Common Name	Other Names	Absence of Sense	Selected Disorders of Sense
Special Senses			
Vision	Sight	Blindness (amaurosis)	Diplopia, myopia, presbyopia
Hearing	Audition	Deafness (anakusis)	Dysacusis, hearing loss, hyperacusis, hypoacusis
Olfaction	Smell, osmesthesia, osphresis	Anosmia (anophresia, olfactory anesthesia)	Parosmias (dysosmias) Cacosmia, heterosmia, hyperosmia, hyposmia
Taste	Gustation	Ageusia (gustatory anesthesia)	Parageusias (dysgeusias) Hypergeusia, hypogeusia
Somatic Senses			
Touch	Tactile sense, taction	Anaphia (tactile anesthesia)	Paraphias (dysaphias) Tactile hyperesthesia (hyperaphia), tactile hypoesthesia
Pain sense	Algesia, agesthesia, nociception	Analgesia	Hypalgesia, hyperalgesia
Pallesthesia	Vibration sense, palmesthesia	Pallanesthesia (apallesthesia)	Hyperpallesthesia, hypopallesthesia
Pressure sense	Baresthesia, barognosis, piesesthesia, piezesthesia	Baragnosis (abarognosis)	—
Temperature sense	Thermesthesia, thermoesthesia	Thermoanesthesia (thermoanalgesia)	Cryanesthesia, cryesthesia, crymodynia, hypercryesthesia, hyperthermalgesia, isothermognosis, thermohyperesthesia, thermohypoesthesia
Tickling	Gargalesthesia	Gargalanesthesia	—
Bathyesthesia	Deep sensibility	Bathyanesthesia	Bathyhyperesthesia, bathyhypesthesia
Movement sense	Kinesthesia, motion sense	Akinesthesia	—
Muscle sense	Myesthesia, kinesthetic sense	Muscle anesthesia (amyoesthesia)	Muscular hyperesthesia
Posture sense	Position sense	Autotopagnosia (somatotopagnosia)	—
Somatognosis	Body sense, sixth sense	Asomatognosia, anosognosia	—
Stereognosis	Stereocognosy	Astereognosis (astereocognosy, stereoagnosis)	—
Topesthesia	—	Atopagnosia (topoanesthesia)	—
Trichesthesia	Hair sensibility	—	—
Visceral sense	Internal sense, seventh sense, splanchnesthesia	Visceral anesthesia	—
Classification Unclear			
Sense of equilibrium	Equilibrium, static sense, vestibular sense, labyrinthine sense	—	Disequilibria (dizziness, dysstasia, vertigo)

temperature s. the faculty by which differences in temperature are distinguished by the thermoreceptors; called also *thermesthesia* and *thermoesthesia.*

time s. the ability to distinguish time intervals.

vestibular s. s. of equilibrium.

vibration s. pallesthesia.

visceral s. the awareness of sensations that arise from the viscera and stimulate the interoceptors; sensations include pain, pressure or fullness, and organ movement. Called also *splanchnesthesia.*

sensi- [L. *sensus,* from *sentire* to perceive, feel] a combining form denoting relationship to perception or feeling.

sen·si·bil·i·ty (sen″sĭ-bil′ĭ-te) [L. *sensibilitas*] susceptibility of feeling; ability to feel or perceive.

bone s. pallesthesia.

common s. somatognosis.

deep s. sensibility to stimuli such as pain, movement, and pressure that activate receptors below the body surface but not in the viscera. It includes joint sensibility (arthresthesia) and muscle sense (myesthesia). Called also *bathyesthesia.*

electromuscular s. sensibility of muscles to electric stimulation.

epicritic s. the sensibility of the skin to precise stimulations which furnishes the means for making fine discriminations of touch and temperature. Cf. *protopathic s.*

joint s. arthresthesia.

mesoblastic s. deep s.

pallesthetic s., palmesthetic s. pallesthesia.

proprioceptive s. proprioception.

protopathic s. sensibility to crude stimulations such as pain, temperature, and some forms of touch, which acts as a defensive agency against pathologic changes in the tissues. Cf. *epicritic s.*

splanchnesthetic s. visceral sense.

vibratory s. pallesthesia.

sen·si·bil·i·za·tion (sen″sĭ-bil-ĭ-za′shən) 1. the act of making more sensitive. 2. sensitization.

sen·si·ble (sen′sĭ-bəl) [L. *sensibilis*] 1. capable of sensation. 2. perceptible to the senses.

sen·sif·er·ous (sen-sif′ər-əs) [*sensi-* + *-ferous*] transmitting sensations.

sen·sim·e·ter (sen-sim′ə-tər) [*sensi-* + *-meter*] an instrument for measuring the degree of sensitiveness of anesthetic and hyperesthetic areas on the body.

Sen·si·par (sen′sĭ-pahr) trademark for a preparation of cinacalcet hydrochloride.

sen·si·tive (sen′sĭ-tiv) [L. *sensitivus*] 1. able to receive or respond to stimuli. 2. sometimes used to mean having too quick, too acute, or some other abnormal response to stimulation.

sen·si·tiv·i·ty (sen″sĭ-tiv′ĭ-te) 1. the state or quality of being sensitive. 2. the smallest concentration of a substance that can be reliably measured by a particular analytical method. 3. the conditional probability that a person having a disease will be correctly identified by a clinical test, i.e., the number of true positive results divided by the total number with the disease (which is the sum of the numbers of true positive plus false negative results). Cf. *specificity* and *predictive value.*

analytical s. sensitivity (def. 2).

antibiotic s., antimicrobial s. see under *susceptibility.*

diagnostic s. sensitivity (def. 3).

insulin s. the body's response to insulin; it is reduced in states of insulin resistance (q.v.), such as diabetes mellitus.

multiple chemical s. a variable group of symptoms, sometimes disabling, attributed to exposure to chemicals in the environment that are not considered harmful to the average person at the levels they are encountered. Some authorities consider this diagnosis controversial.

proportional s. the relationship in which a response bears some quantitative algebraic relationship to the intensity of the stimulus.

sen·si·ti·za·tion (sen″sĭ-tĭ-za′shən) 1. immunization. 2. sensibilization (def. 1). 3. exposure to allergen that results in the development of hypersensitivity. 4. the coating of erythrocytes with antibody so that they are subject to lysis by complement in the presence of homologous antigen, the first stage of a complement fixation test.

autoerythrocyte s. an abnormal reaction in which intradermal injection of a patient's own erythrocytes produces a painful ecchymosis; see *painful bruising syndrome,* under *syndrome.*

central s. a proposed mechanism for the cause of chronic pain conditions and migraine, by which nociceptors in the central nervous system become hypersensitive to stimuli as a result of tissue damage or inflammation.

covert s. a form of aversive conditioning in which the frequency of undesirable behavior is lessened by mentally associating it with unpleasant mental images.

photodynamic s. the increased lethal effects of light on microorganisms when certain dyes are present in the solution.

Rh s. see under *isoimmunization.*

spinal s. alteration of neural pathways through the spinal cord to make them more sensitive, especially to pain.

sen·si·tized (sen′sĭ-tīzd) rendered sensitive.

sen·si·tiz·er (sen′sĭ-ti″zər) an allergen or irritant that, after an initial sensitizing exposure, produces atopic or contact dermatitis in secondary exposures.

sens(o)- see *sensi-*.

sen·so·mo·tor (sen″so-mo′tər) sensorimotor.

sen·sor (sen′sər) something that senses; a natural system or synthetic device specifically designed to respond to a physical stimulus (light, heat, pressure, etc.) by generating an impulse that can be measured or otherwise interpreted, or used as a control.

Sen·sor·caine (sen′sər-kān″) trademark for preparations of bupivacaine hydrochloride.

sen·so·ri·al (sen-sor′e-əl) [L. *sensorialis*] pertaining to the sensorium.

sen·so·ri·glan·du·lar (sen″sə-re-glan′du-lər) producing glandular activity as one of the consequences of stimulation of the sensory nerves.

sen·so·ri·mo·tor (sen″sə-re-mo′tər) both sensory and motor.

sen·so·ri·mus·cu·lar (sen″sə-re-mus′ku-lər) producing reflex muscular action in response to a sensory impression.

sen·so·ri·neu·ral (sen″sə-re-noor′əl) 1. of or pertaining to a sensory nerve. 2. pertaining to or affecting a sensory nerve or mechanism.

sen·so·ri·um (sən-sor′e-əm) [L. *sentire* to experience, to feel the force of] 1. any of the primary receptive areas. 2. the condition of a subject relative to the subject's consciousness or mental clarity.

sen·so·ri·vas·cu·lar (sen″sə-re-vas′ku-lər) producing vascular changes as a result of stimulation applied through the sensory nerves.

sen·so·ri·vaso·mo·tor (sen″sə-re-vas″o-mo′tər) sensorivascular.

sen·so·ry (sen′sə-re) [L. *sensorius*] pertaining to or subserving sensation.

sen·ti·ent (sen′she-ənt) [L. *sentiens*] able to feel; sensitive; having sensation or feeling.

sen·ti·nel (sen′tĭ-nəl) an individual or object that gives a warning or indicates danger.

SEP somatosensory evoked potential.

sep·a·rase (sep′ə-rās) [EC 3.4.22.49] a protease that cleaves a subunit of cohesin to initiate the separation of sister chromatids in anaphase.

sep·a·ra·tion (sep″ə-ra′shən) 1. the process of taking apart or the state of having been taken apart. 2. the forcing apart of adjacent teeth having tight contact, as with a separating wire prior to banding in orthodontic therapy.

s.-individuation the process usually seen in infants by which the child identifies itself as different from the primary caretaker while maintaining an emotional attachment.

shoulder s. separation or dislocation of the shoulder at the acromioclavicular joint occurring in athletes.

sep·a·ra·tor (sep′ə-ra″tər) 1. a device for keeping two or more things apart. 2. a device or instrument for wedging teeth apart, especially proximal teeth having a tight contact, as for the examination of proximal surfaces, finishing a restoration, or before banding in orthodontic therapy. Called also *space maintainer.*

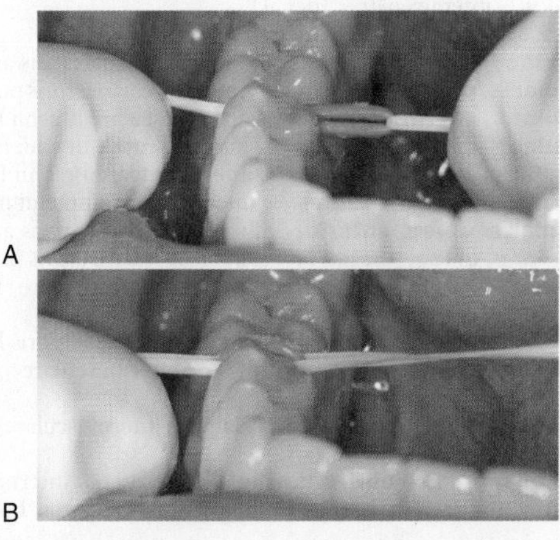

■ Placing an elastomeric ring separator between two molars.

Seph·a·dex (sef′ə-deks) trademark for cross-linked dextran beads, a medium for molecular sieve chromatography.

se·pia (se′pe-ə) [L., from Gr. *sēpia* cuttlefish] 1. a dark brown, inspissated inky juice secreted by the cuttlefish *(Sepia),* a squidlike cephalopod marine mollusk. 2. a dark brown–colored pigment.

se·pi·ap·ter·in re·duc·tase (se″pe-ap′tər-in re-duk′tās) [EC 1.1.1.153] an enzyme of the oxidoreductase class that catalyzes the final two-step, NADPH-dependent, reduction reaction in the biosynthesis of tetrahydrobiopterin (BH4), acting on the 6-pyruvoyltetrahydropterin intermediate formed by 6-pyruvoyltetrahydropterin synthase. It also catalyzes a step in the alternative salvage pathway of BH4 synthesis, and the reduction of various other carbonyl substances. Deficiency of the enzyme, an autosomal recessive trait, leads to BH4 and neurotransmitter deficiencies without hyperphenylalaninemia, manifesting as dopa-responsive dystonia.

se·pi·um (se′pe-əm) [L., from Gr. *sēpia* cuttlefish] the bone or internal shell of the cuttlefish, used in preparing polishing agents and tooth powder, and hung in bird cages to supply a supplementary source of lime. Called also *cuttlebone.*

sep·sin (sep′sin) [Gr. *sēpsis* decay] a poisonous crystallizable substance from decaying yeast and from animal matter.

Sep·sis (sep′sis) a genus of flies. *S. viola′cea* is the common dung fly, which can spread various diseases.

sep·sis (sep′sis) [Gr. *sēpsis* decay] 1. the presence in the blood or other tissues of pathogenic microorganisms or their toxins. 2. septicemia.

catheter s. sepsis occurring as a complication of intravenous catheterization.

incarcerated s. an infection that is latent after the primary lesion has apparently healed but may be activated by a slight trauma.

mouse s., murine s. an infectious disease of mice, due to *Erysipelothrix rhusiopathiae;* called also *mouse* or *murine septicemia.*

oral s. a disease condition in the mouth or adjacent parts which may affect the general health through the dissemination of toxins.

postanginal s. Lemierre syndrome.

puerperal s. see under *fever.*

Sept. [L.] sep′tem (seven).

sep·ta (sep′tə) [L.] plural of *septum.*

sep·tal (sep′təl) pertaining to a septum; see also under *area.*

sep·ta·nose (sep′tə-nōs) a monosaccharide having a seven-numbered ring structure.

sep·tate (sep′tāt) divided by a septum or septa.

sep·ta·tion (sep-ta′shən) division into parts by a septum or septa.

sep·ta·tome (sep′tə-tōm) septotome.

sep·tec·to·my (sep-tek′tə-me) [*sept-* + *-ectomy*] excision of part or all of a septum, particularly the nasal septum.

atrial s. surgical creation of a defect in the interatrial septum; performed to allow interatrial blood mixing in transposition of great vessels.

sep·te·mia (sep-te′me-ə) septicemia.

sep·ti (sep′ti) [L.] genitive of *septum.*

sep·tic (sep′tik) [L. *septicus;* Gr. *sēptikos*] produced by or due to decomposition by microorganisms; putrefactive.

sep·ti·ce·mia (sep″tĭ-se′me-ə) [*septic* + *-emia*] systemic disease associated with the presence and persistence of pathogenic microorganisms or their toxins in the blood. Called also *blood poisoning* and *sepsis.* **septice′mic** *adj*

coliform s. *Escherichia coli* s.

cryptogenic s. septicemia in which the focus of infection is not evident during life.

***Escherichia coli* s.** septicemia caused by *Escherichia coli* in the systemic circulation, seen most often in children or domestic animals; characteristics include shock, hypothermia, and coma that can be fatal. Called also *coliform s.* and *colisepticemia.*

***Haemophilus* s. of cattle** former name for *histophilosis.*

hemorrhagic s. any of a group of animal diseases caused by infection with *Pasteurella multocida* or *Mannheimia haemolytica;* called also *septicemic pasteurellosis.*

hemorrhagic s. of cattle infection of cattle with *Pasteurella multocida,* characterized by sudden fever, salivation, nervous prostration, pneumonia, subcutaneous petechiae or hemorrhages, and often death within a few days.

hemorrhagic s. of sheep a septicemic infection of young sheep by *Mannheimia haemolytica* or *P. multocida,* usually characterized by coughing with a discharge from the nose and eyes; a more severe form with pneumonia can be fatal.

hemorrhagic s. of swine infection of swine with *Pasteurella multocida,* characterized by bronchopneumonia, occasionally with pleuritis and pericarditis. Called also *swine plague.*

mouse s., murine s. see under *sepsis.*

plague s. septicemic plague.

puerperal s. see under *fever*.

rabbit s. pasteurellosis in rabbits, a common contagious disease caused by infection with *Pasteurella multocida*, characterized by inflammation of mucous membranes in the respiratory tract, sometimes with otitis media, conjunctivitis, abscesses, or pneumonia that can be fatal. Called also *snuffles*.

sep·ti·co·py·emia (sep″tĭ-ko-pi-e′me-ə) septicemia and pyemia combined. **septicopye′mic** *adj*

sep·ti·grav·i·da (sep″tĭ-grav′ĭ-də) [L. *septem* seven + *gravida*] a woman pregnant for the seventh time; also written *gravida VII*.

sep·ti·me·tri·tis (sep″tĭ-me-tri′tis) [*septic* + *metritis*] septic inflammation of the uterus.

sep·ti·neu·ri·tis (sep″tĭ-noo͝-ri′tis) neuritis due to sepsis.

Nicolau s. a generalized, diffuse neuritis of the entire nervous system due to the multiplication and migration of viruses in nervous tissue, as occurs in rabies.

sep·tip·a·ra (sep-tip′ə-rə) [L. *septem* seven + *para*] a woman who has had seven pregnancies which resulted in viable offspring; also written *para VII* or *VII-para*.

sep·ti·va·lent (sep″tĭ-va′lənt) [L. *septem* seven + *valens* able] able to combine with or to replace seven hydrogen atoms.

sept(o)- [L. *septum*, q.v.] a combining form denoting relationship to a septum.

Sep·to·caine (sep′to-kān) trademark for a combination preparation of articaine hydrochloride and epinephrine, used as a dental anesthetic.

sep·to·mar·gi·nal (sep″to-mahr′jĭ-nəl) pertaining to the margin of a septum.

sep·to·na·sal (sep″to-na′zəl) pertaining to the nasal septum.

sep·to·plas·ty (sep′to-plas″te) [*septo-* + *-plasty*] surgical reconstruction of the nasal septum. **septoplas′tic** *adj*

sep·to·rhi·no·plas·ty (sep″to-ri′no-plas″te) [*septo-* + *rhino-* + *-plasty*] a plastic operation combining reconstruction of the nasal septum and correction of deformities of the external nose. **septorhinoplas′tic** *adj*

sep·tos·to·my (sep-tos′tə-me) [*septo-* + *-stomy*] surgical creation of an opening in a septum.

balloon atrial s., Rashkind balloon atrial s. surgical creation of an opening in the interatrial septum of the heart by passage of a balloon catheter from the right atrium through the septum to the left atrium, at which point the balloon is inflated and the catheter is then withdrawn to create an interatrial septal defect; performed in transposition of the great vessels with an intact septum.

sep·to·tome (sep′to-tōm) an instrument for operating on the nasal septum.

sep·tot·o·my (sep-tot′ə-me) [*septo-* + *-tomy*] incision of the nasal septum.

Sep·tra (sep′trə) trademark for combination preparations of trimethoprim and sulfamethoxazole.

sep·tu·la (sep′tu-lə) [L.] plural of *septulum*.

sep·tu·lum (sep′tu-ləm) pl. *sep′tula* [L., dim. of *septum*] a small separating wall or partition.

sep′tula tes′tis [TA] septa of testis: connective tissue lamellae from the inner surface of the tunica albuginea, uniting to form the mediastinum testis.

sep·tum (sep′təm) gen. *sep′ti* pl. *sep′ta* [L. *saeptum* past part. of *saepire* to fence or wall off] 1. a dividing wall or partition. 2. septal area. 3. s. pellucidum.

Septum

Descriptions are given on TA terms and include anglicized names of specific anatomic structures.

alveolar s., s. alve′oli 1. interalveolar s. 2. interradicular s.

aorticopulmonary s. a septum, formed by fusion of the bulbar ridges, that divides the bulbus cordis into aortic and pulmonary trunks.

atrial s. s. interatriale cordis.

atrioventricular s. of heart, s. atrioventricula′re cor′dis [TA] the portion of the membranous part of the interventricular septum between the right atrium and left ventricle.

s. of auditory tube s. canalis musculotubarii.

Bertin septa columnae renales.

bony s. of eustachian canal s. canalis musculotubarii.

bony nasal s., bony s. of nose pars ossea septi nasi.

s. bul′bi ure′thrae the fibrous septum dividing the interior of the bulb of the urethra into two approximately equal parts.

s. cana′lis musculotuba′rii [TA] septum of musculotubal canal: the thin lamella of bone that divides the musculotubal canal into the semicanals for the tensor tympani muscle and the auditory tube.

cartilaginous s. of nose pars cartilaginea septi nasi.

cervical s., intermediate, s. cervica′le interme′dium [TA] a glial–pia mater septum which dips into the dorsal intermediate sulcus of the dorsal funiculus of the cervical and upper thoracic parts of the spinal cord; it separates the fasciculus gracilis and fasciculus cuneatus.

cloacal s. urorectal s.

Cloquet s. s. femorale.

s. corpo′rum cavernoso′rum clito′ridis [TA] septum of corpora cavernosa of clitoris: an incomplete fibrous septum between the two lateral halves of the clitoris.

crural s. s. femorale.

deviated s. lateral malposition of the nasal septum owing to injury or a congenital malformation, so that one part of the nasal cavity is smaller than the other; it seldom causes complications, but occasionally may handicap breathing, block the normal flow of mucus from the sinuses during a cold, or prevent proper drainage of infected sinuses.

Douglas s. the septum formed by the union of Rathke folds, forming the rectum of the fetus.

enamel s. see under *cord*.

femoral s., s. femora′le [TA] the thin fibrous membrane that helps to close the anulus femoralis; it is derived from the fascia transversalis, is perforated for the passage of lymphatic vessels, and is embedded in fat.

s. of frontal sinuses s. sinuum frontalium.

gingival s. the part of the gingiva interposed between adjoining teeth.

s. glan′dis pe′nis [TA], **s. of glans penis** an incomplete fibrous septum in the median plane of the glans penis, especially below the urethra.

interalveolar s. 1. any of the septa interalveolaria mandibulae or septa interalveolaria maxillae. 2. one of the thin septa that separate adjacent pulmonary alveoli, containing connective tissue constituents of the respiratory tissue and the capillary network of the blood supply of the lung. Called also *alveolar s.*

sep′ta interalveola′ria mandi′bulae [TA] interalveolar septa of mandible: the partitions between the tooth sockets in the alveolar part of the mandible.

sep′ta interalveola′ria maxil′lae [TA] interalveolar septa of maxilla: the partitions between the tooth sockets in the alveolar process of the maxilla.

interatrial s. of heart, s. interatria′le cor′dis [TA] the wall that separates the atria of the heart.

interdental s. interalveolar s. (def. 1).

interlobular s. interalveolar s. (def. 2).

intermuscular s., anterior crural s. intermusculare cruris anterius.

intermuscular s., posterior crural s. intermusculare cruris posterius.

intermuscular s. of arm, external s. intermusculare brachii laterale.

intermuscular s. of arm, internal s. intermusculare brachii mediale.

intermuscular s. of arm, lateral s. intermusculare brachii laterale.

intermuscular s. of arm, medial s. intermusculare brachii mediale.

intermuscular s. of leg, anterior s. intermusculare cruris anterius.

intermuscular s. of leg, posterior s. intermusculare cruris posterius.

intermuscular s. of thigh, external s. intermusculare femoris laterale.

intermuscular s. of thigh, lateral s. intermusculare femoris laterale.

intermuscular s. of thigh, medial s. intermusculare femoris mediale.

s. intermuscula′re ante′rius cru′ris s. intermusculare cruris anterius.

s. intermuscula′re bra′chii latera′le [TA] lateral intermuscular septum of arm: the fascial sheet extending from the lateral border of

Septum *Continued*

the humerus to the under surface of the fascia investing the arm; called also *s. intermusculare humeri laterale.*
s. intermuscula′re bra′chii media′le [TA] medial intermuscular septum of arm: the fascial sheet extending from the medial border of the humerus to the under surface of the fascia investing the arm; called also *s. intermusculare humeri mediale.*
s. intermuscula′re cru′ris ante′rius [TA] anterior crural intermuscular septum: a fascial sheet extending between the extensor digitorum longus and the peroneal muscles to the anterior fibular crest. Called also *anterior intermuscular s. of leg* and *s. intermusculare anterius cruris.*
s. intermuscula′re cru′ris poste′rius [TA] posterior crural intermuscular septum: a fascial sheet extending between the peroneal and soleus muscles to the lateral fibular crest. Called also *posterior intermuscular s. of leg* and *s. intermusculare posterius cruris.*
s. intermuscula′re fe′moris latera′le [TA] lateral intermuscular septum of thigh: the fascial sheet in the thigh separating the vastus lateralis muscle from the biceps femoris.
s. intermuscula′re fe′moris media′le [TA] medial intermuscular septum of thigh: the fascial sheet in the thigh separating the vastus medialis from the adductor and the pectineus muscles.
s. intermuscula′re hu′meri latera′le s. intermusculare brachii laterale.
s. intermuscula′re hu′meri media′le s. intermusculare brachii mediale.
s. intermuscula′re poste′rius cru′ris s. intermusculare cruris posterius.
interradicular s. any of the septa interradicularia mandibulae or septa interradicularia maxillae; called also *alveolar s.* and *interalveolar s.*
sep′ta interradicula′ria mandi′bulae [TA] interradicular septa of mandible: the thin bony partitions separating the crypts of a mandibular dental alveolus occupied by the separate roots of a multirooted tooth.
sep′ta interradicula′ria maxil′lae [TA] interradicular septa of maxilla: the thin bony partitions separating the crypts of a maxillary alveolus occupied by the separate roots of a multirooted tooth.
s. intersinua′le fronta′le s. sinuum frontalium.
s. intersinua′le sphenoida′le septum sinuum sphenoidalium.
interventricular s. of heart, s. interventricula′re cor′dis [TA] the partition that separates the left ventricle from the right ventricle, consisting of a muscular and a membranous part; called also *ventricular s.* See illustration.
Körner s. a bony plate sometimes found dividing the interior part of the mastoid into medial and lateral portions; it results from fusion of the squamous and petrous parts of the bone.
s. lin′guae [TA], **s. lingua′le** lingual septum: the median vertical fibrous part of the tongue.
s. lu′cidum s. pellucidum.
median s. of spinal cord, dorsal, median s. of spinal cord, posterior s. medianum posterius medullae spinalis.
s. media′num dorsa′le medul′lae spina′lis s. medianum posterius medullae spinalis.
s. media′num poste′rius medul′lae spina′lis [TA] posterior median septum of spinal cord: a neuroglial septum that is a continuation of the posterior median sulcus of the spinal cord, penetrating the substance of the cord and extending almost to the central canal. Called also *dorsal median s. of spinal cord* and *s. medianum dorsale medullae spinalis.*

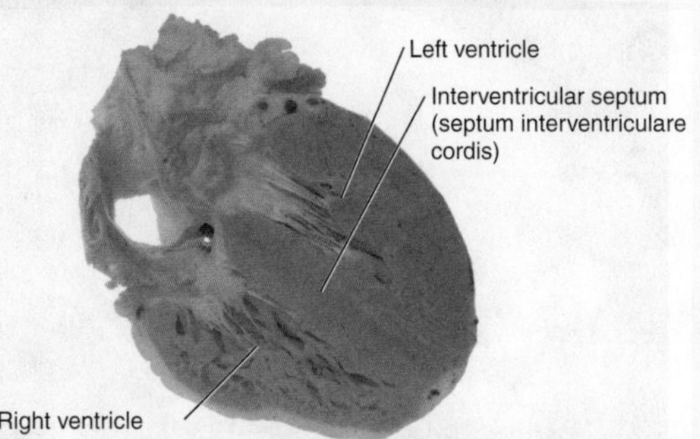

■ Septum interventriculare cordis (interventricular septum) between the cardiac ventricles.

mediastinal s., s. mediastina′le mediastinum (def. 2).
membranous nasal s., membranous s. of nose pars membranacea septi nasi.
s. mo′bile na′si, mobile s. of nose pars mobilis septi nasi.
s. of musculotubal canal s. canalis musculotubarii.
nasal s. s. nasi.
nasal s., bony pars ossea septi nasi.
nasal s., cartilaginous pars cartilaginea septi nasi.
nasal s., membranous pars membranacea septi nasi.
s. nasa′le TA alternative for *s. nasi.*
s. na′si [TA] septum of nose: the partition separating the two nasal cavities in the midplane, composed of cartilaginous, membranous, and bony parts. Called also *nasal s.* and *s. nasale* [TA alternative].
s. na′si os′seum [TA] pars ossea septi nasi.
neural s. a prolongation, chiefly in the lower vertebrates, of the general investing fascia, extending medially from the surface toward the skeleton; represented in humans by the ligamentum nuchae and the supraspinous and interspinous ligaments.
s. of nose s. nasi.
orbital s., s. orbita′le [TA] a fibrous membrane anchored to the periorbita along the entire margin of the orbit, extending to the levator palpebrae superioris muscle in the upper lid and to the tarsal plate in the lower lid; called also *tarsal membrane.*
s. pectinifor′me s. penis.
s. pellu′cidum [TA] pellucid septum: a double membrane separating the anterior horns of the lateral ventricles of the brain; situated in the median plane, it is bounded superiorly and rostrally by the corpus callosum and inferiorly by the body and columns of the fornix. Called also *s. lucidum.*
s. pe′nis [TA], **s. of penis** the fibrous sheet between the two corpora cavernosa of the penis, formed by union of the tunicae albugineae of the two sides.
pharyngeal s. oropharyngeal membrane.
placental septa decidual tissue that forms incomplete partitions between placental cotyledons; the septa are covered with trophoblast and contain a core of maternal tissue.
precommissural s., s. precommissura′le a septum situated anterior to the rostral commissure of the cerebrum, corresponding in part to the paraterminal gyrus, which consists of dorsal, ventral, medial, and caudal nuclear groups; called also *s. verum.*
s. pri′mum the first septum in the embryonic heart, dividing the primordial atrium into right and left chambers.
rectovaginal s. fascia rectovaginalis.
s. rectovagina′le TA alternative for fascia rectovaginalis.
rectovesical s. fascia rectoprostatica.
s. rectovesica′le TA alternative for fascia rectoprostatica.
scrotal s., s. scro′ti [TA], **s. of scrotum** a fibromuscular partition in the median plane, dividing the scrotum into two nearly equal parts.
s. secun′dum the second septum in the embryonic heart, to the right of the septum primum; after birth it fuses with the septum primum to close the foramen ovale and form the interatrial septum.
s. si′nuum fronta′lium [TA] septum of frontal sinuses: a thin lamina of bone in the lower part of the frontal bone, lying more or less in the median plane, that separates the frontal sinuses. Called also *s. intersinuale frontale.*
s. si′nuum sphenoida′lium [TA], **sphenoidal s., s. of sphenoidal sinuses** a usually asymmetric, thin lamina of bone in the body of the sphenoid bone, lying more or less in the median plane and separating the sphenoidal sinuses. Called also *s. intersinuale sphenoidale.*
spurious s., s. spu′rium a structure formed by union of the two folds, one on either side, guarding the opening of the sinus venosus into the dorsal wall of the right atrium of the heart in the early embryo. It disappears early in the fetal period, taking no part in atrial separation.
subarachnoidal s. an incomplete fibrous sheath which lies in the median plane and which connects the arachnoid to the pia mater along the posterior median sulcus of the cervical and upper thoracic parts of the spinal cord.
septa of testis septula testis.
s. of tongue s. linguae.
tracheoesophageal s. the septum that, during the fourth week of embryonic development, separates the trachea from the ventral surface of the primordial esophagus; it forms by fusion of the tracheoesophageal folds.

Septum *Continued*

transverse s. of ampulla crista ampullaris.
s. transver′sum a thick plate of mesodermal tissue that occupies the space between the thoracic cavity and yolk stalk in the early embryo, forming a transverse partition partially separating the coelomic cavity into thoracic and abdominal portions. It gives rise to the central tendon of the diaphragm.
urorectal s. the caudally and outwardly growing wedge of endoderm-covered mesoderm that divides the cloaca into the urogenital sinus and rectum, and the cloacal outlet into the urogenital orifice and anus; called also *urorectal fold* and *cloacal s.*
s. of ventricles of heart, ventricular s. s. interventriculare cordis.
s. ve′rum s. precommissurale.

sep•tup•let (sep-tup′lət) [L. *septuplum* a group of seven] one of seven offspring produced in one gestation period.

seq. luce [L.] sequen′ti lu′ce (the following day).

se•quel (se′kwəl) sequela.

se•que•la (sə-kwel′ə) pl. *seque′lae* [L.] any lesion or affection following or caused by an attack of disease.
postpolio sequelae, postpoliomyelitis sequelae see under *syndrome.*

se•quence (se′kwəns) [L. *sequi* to follow] 1. a connected series of events or things. 2. in dysmorphology, a pattern of multiple anomalies derived from a single known or presumed prior anomaly or mechanical factor. Called also *anomalad* and *complex.* 3. the order of arrangement of residues or constituents in a biological polymer, as the order of nucleotides in DNA or RNA, or of amino acids in a protein. 4. a specific fragment or segment of a biological polymer, with a known arrangement of its residues. 5. to ascertain the order of the residues of a biological polymer.
adenoma-carcinoma s. the evolutionary progression of a colorectal adenoma to a carcinoma.
***Alu* repeat s.** any of a family of related, repetitive, dimeric DNA sequences, named for their cleavage by the restriction endonuclease *Alu I.* The sequences are approximately 300 base pairs long and are interspersed throughout the primate genome in up to a million copies per haploid genome; some can generate copies of themselves, which can insert elsewhere into the genome.
amniotic band s. see under *syndrome.*
consensus s. a sequence of nucleotides that is common to different genes or genomes, usually with some variations but showing substantial similarity; frequently, the prototype sequence that most others approach.
flanking s. in a nucleic acid, a short stretch of nucleotides immediately adjacent to either end of the region under consideration.
gene s. the ordered arrangement of nucleotides into codons in a gene.
insertion s. (IS) a small bacterial transposable element containing only genes that encode transposition functions and having a short run of inverted repeated sequences at each of its termini, it causes duplication of the recipient DNA site into which it inserts, one copy of the recipient DNA flanking it on each side. It may act as an individual transposable element, or it may occur in pairs as the termini of more complex transposons.
intervening s. intron.
leader s. signal s.
nearest neighbor s. the sequence determined by nearest neighbor sequence analysis.
oligohydramnios s. a group of anomalies, usually causing death shortly after birth, caused by compression of the fetus secondary to oligohydramnios, which may result from renal agenesis or other fetal urinary tract defects or from leakage of amniotic fluid; infants have characteristic flattened facies *(Potter facies)* and skeletal abnormalities such as clubbed feet and contracted joints, often with hypoplasia of the lungs.
Pierre Robin s. the triad of micrognathia, cleft palate, and glossoptosis, with backward and upward displacement of the larynx and angulation of the manubrium sterni; cleft palate makes sucking and swallowing difficult, permitting easy access of fluids into the larynx. Respiratory failure secondary to upper airway obstruction can be fatal. It evolves due to abnormally hypoplastic development of the mandible between gestational weeks 7 to 11, and may appear in association with other syndromes or as an isolated entity. Called also *Pierre Robin syndrome.*
pulse s. in magnetic resonance imaging, the order, spacing, and type of radio frequency pulses that produce magnetic resonance images according to changes in the gradients of the magnetic field.
signal s., targeting s. a sequence of 15 to 30 amino acids occurring at the N-terminal end of the precursors of secretory proteins; it is required for transport of the protein across the membrane of the rough endoplasmic reticulum into the cisternae, where it is immediately cleaved off by an endopeptidase. Called also *leader s.* and *signal peptide.*

se•ques•ter (sə-kwes′tər) [L.; Fr. *sequestrer* to shut up illegally] 1. to detach or separate abnormally a small portion from the whole; see *sequestration* and *sequestrum.* 2. to isolate a constituent of a chemical system by chelation or other means; cf. *sequestrant.*

se•ques•tra (se-kwes′trə) [L.] plural of *sequestrum.*

se•ques•tral (se-kwes′trəl) pertaining to or of the nature of a sequestrum.

se•ques•trant (sə-kwes′trənt) a sequestering agent, as, for example, cholestyramine resin, which binds bile acids in the intestine, thus preventing their absorption.

se•ques•tra•tion (se″kwəs-tra′shən) [L. *sequestratio*] 1. the formation of a sequestrum. 2. the isolation of a patient. 3. a net increase in the quantity of blood within a limited vascular area, occurring physiologically, with or without forward flow persisting, or produced artificially by the application of tourniquets.
bronchopulmonary s. pulmonary s.
corneal s. see under *sequestrum.*
disk s. see *sequestered disk*, under *disk.*
extralobar s. extralobar pulmonary sequestration; see *pulmonary s.*
intralobar s. intralobar pulmonary sequestration; see *pulmonary s.*
pulmonary s. loss of connection of lung tissue, and sometimes bronchi, with the bronchial tree and with the pulmonary veins, the tissue receiving its arterial supply from the systemic circulation. The mass may be completely separated anatomically and physiologically from normally connected lung *(extralobar pulmonary s.)* or be in anatomical contiguity with and partly surrounded by normal lung *(intralobar pulmonary s.).* Called also *accessory lung* and *bronchopulmonary s.*

se•ques•trec•to•my (se″kwəs-trek′tə-me) [*sequestrum* + *-ectomy*] the surgical removal of a sequestrum.

se•ques•trot•o•my (se″kwəs-trot′ə-me) [*sequestrum* + *-tomy*] sequestrectomy.

se•ques•trum (sə-kwes′trəm) pl. *seques′tra* [L.] 1. any tissue that has become sequestered. 2. a piece of dead bone that has become separated during the process of necrosis from the sound bone.
corneal s. a condition in cats in which a section of corneal stroma becomes dark colored and sometimes detached; it may be due to a herpesvirus infection or to tissue irritation from a disease process. Called also *corneal sequestration.*
primary s. a sequestrum that is entirely detached.
secondary s. a sequestrum that is partially detached and may be pushed into place.
tertiary s. a sequestrum that is separated by only a slight dividing line and remains in its place.

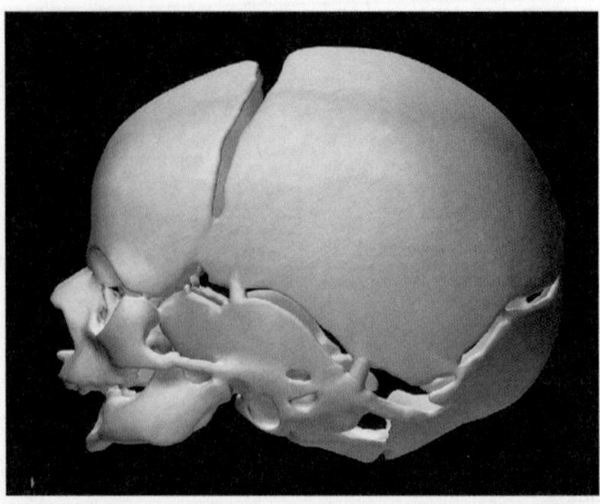

■ Pierre Robin sequence; lateral view of the craniofacial skeleton showing a small retruded mandible.

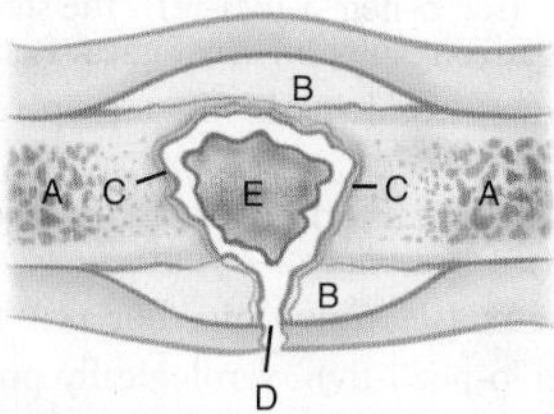

■ Formation of a sequestrum: *(A)*, sound bone; *(B)*, new bone; *(C)*, granulations lining involucrum; *(D)*, cloaca; *(E)*, sequestrum.

se•quoi•o•sis (se″kwoi-o′sis) a type of hypersensitivity pneumonitis seen in logging and sawmill workers, caused by inhalation of sawdust of *Sequoia* and similar trees that contains fungal spores of *Aureobasidium* or *Graphium*.

Ser serine.

se•ra (se′rə) [L.] plural of *serum*.

Ser-A-Gen (ser′ə-jən) trademark for combination preparations of reserpine, hydralazine hydrochloride, and hydrochlorothiazide.

se•ral•bu•min (sēr″al-bu′min) albumin (def. 2).

Ser-Ap-Es (sər-ap′əs) trademark for combination preparations of reserpine, hydralazine hydrochloride, and hydrochlorothiazide.

Ser•ax (ser′aks) trademark for preparations of oxazepam.

Se•re•noa (sə-re′o-ə) a genus of nearly stemless palms of the southeastern United States, having nearly round leaves and ovoid fruits, including *S. re′pens*, the *saw palmetto*.

Ser•e•vent (ser′ə-vent) trademark for a preparation of salmeterol xinafoate.

Ser•gent white adrenal line (sār-zhaw′) [Emile *Sergent*, French physician, 1867–1943] see under *line*.

ser•gly•cin (ser-gli′sin) an intracellular proteoglycan, consisting of a 12-kD core with 24 serine-glycine repeats that are the attachment sites for about 15 glycosaminoglycans; it is expressed by leukocytes and binds histamine in secretory granules.

se•ri•al (se′re-əl) arranged in or forming a series.

se•ri•al•o•graph (se″re-al′o-graf) an apparatus for making series of x-ray pictures.

ser•i•cin (ser′ĭ-sin) silk glue or silk gelatin; a protein derivable from silk.

Ser•i•co•pel•ma (ser″ĭ-ko-pel′mə) a genus of huge hairy spiders of the family Theraphosidae. *S. commu′nis* is the black tarantula.

se•ries (sēr′ēz) [L. "row"] 1. a group or succession of objects or substances arranged in regular order or forming a kind of chain. 2. a group of related tests leading up to either a diagnosis or the ruling out of a given diagnosis. 3. pertaining to electric circuit components connected "in series" so that the current flow goes through each component without branching; applied by extension to any similar series circuit, e.g., the pulmonary and systemic circulations. Cf. *parallel*. 4. a taxonomic category of fungi falling between a subphylum and an order and based on the type of ascus the organism possesses.

basophil s., basophilic s. see *granulocytic s.*

eosinophil s., eosinophilic s. see *granulocytic s.*

erythrocyte s., erythrocytic s. the succession of morphologically distinguishable cells that are stages in erythrocyte development; the precursor cells detected in vitro are the *burst-forming unit–erythroid* and *colony-forming unit–erythroid*, which are followed in order of maturity by the *proerythroblast*, *basophilic erythroblast* or *normoblast*, *polychromatophilic erythroblast* or *normoblast*, *orthochromatic erythroblast* or *normoblast*, *reticulocyte*, and *erythrocyte*.

gastrointestinal s. upper gastrointestinal s.

granulocyte s., granulocytic s. the succession of morphologically distinguishable cells that are stages in granulocyte development; after the *colony-forming unit–granulocyte-macrophage*, the stages in order of maturity are the *myeloblast*, *promyelocyte*, *myelocyte*, and *metamyelocyte*, followed by the *band* or *stab cell*, which is the least mature form normally found in the peripheral blood, and the mature segmented (polymorphonuclear) *granulocyte*. Commitment to one of the granulocyte lines occurs in stem cells before the myeloblast stage, so that there are distinct basophilic, eosinophilic, and neutrophilic series, although all three include the same morphologic stages. Formerly called the *myelocytic*, *myeloid*, or *leukocytic s.*

Hofmeister s. the sequence of ions arranged with respect to their effects on the solubility of proteins, e.g., on their salting-out effects; called also *lyotropic s.*

homologous s. a series of organic compounds each member of which differs from the one preceding it by having one more CH_2 group.

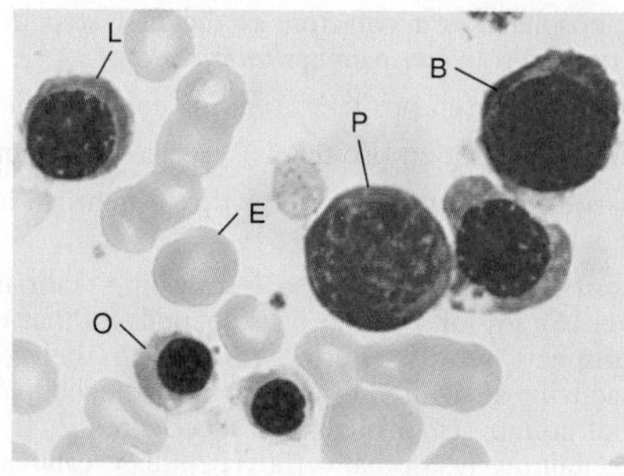

■ Stages in the erythropoietic series: *P*, proerythroblast; *B*, basophilic erythroblast; *L*, polychromatophilic erythroblast; *O*, orthochromatic erythroblast; *E*, erythrocyte.

leukocytic s. granulocytic s.

lymphocyte s., lymphocytic s. a series of morphologically distinguishable cells once thought to represent stages in lymphocyte development: in order of maturity, the lymphoblast, "prolymphocyte," and lymphocyte. It is now known that lymphocyte precursors are morphologically indistinguishable from small lymphocytes and that lymphoblasts are not precursors but activated lymphocytes that have been transformed in response to antigenic stimulation.

lyotropic s. Hofmeister s.

monocyte s., monocytic s. the succession of developing cells that ultimately culminates in the monocyte; after the *colony-forming unit-granulocyte-macrophage*, the stages in order of maturity are the *monoblast*, *promonocyte*, and the mature *monocyte*.

myelocytic s., myeloid s. granulocytic s.

neutrophil s., neutrophilic s. see *granulocytic s.*

plasmacyte s., plasmacytic s. a series of morphologically distinguishable cells that are stages in plasma cell development: in order of maturity, the plasmablast (an activated B cell usually referred to as a large lymphocyte or lymphoblast), proplasmacyte, and plasmacyte.

thrombocyte s., thrombocytic s. the succession of morphologically distinguishable cells that are stages in platelet (thrombocyte) development: in order of maturity, the megakaryoblast, promegakaryocyte, and megakaryocyte, which fragments to form platelets.

upper gastrointestinal s. a barium study of the upper gastrointestinal tract using a series of radiographs. Called also *barium meal*.

ser•ine (Ser, S) (sēr′ēn) 1. a naturally occurring, nonessential amino acid, 2-amino-3-hydroxypropionic acid; it may be synthesized from glycine. See also table at *amino acid*. 2. [USP] a preparation of serine used as a dietary supplement.

L-ser•ine am•mo•nia-ly•ase (sēr′ēn ə-mo′ne-ə li′ās) [EC 4.3.1.17] an enzyme of the lyase class that catalyzes the elimination of ammonia from L-serine, with formation of a double bond to yield pyruvate. The enzyme contains a pyridoxal phosphate prosthetic group.

L-ser•ine de•hy•dra•tase (sēr′ēn de-hi′drə-tās) former official name for *L-serine ammonia-lyase*.

ser•ine en•do•pep•ti•dase (sēr′ēn en″do-pep′tĭ-dās) [EC 3.4.21] any member of the group of endopeptidases containing at the active site a triad of serine, aspartate, and histidine residues involved in catalysis. Included are enzymes active in digestion, blood coagulation, immune reactions, and fertilization of the oocyte. Called also *serine protease* or *proteinase*.

ser•ine hy•droxy•meth•yl•trans•fer•ase (sēr′ēn hi-drok″se-meth″əl-trans′fər-ās) glycine hydroxymethyltransferase.

ser•ine C-pal•mi•to•yl•trans•fer•ase (sēr′ēn pahl″mĭ-to″əl-trans′fər-ās) [EC 2.3.1.50] an enzyme of the transferase class that catalyzes the condensation of palmitoyl CoA and L-serine to yield 3-dehydrosphinganine,

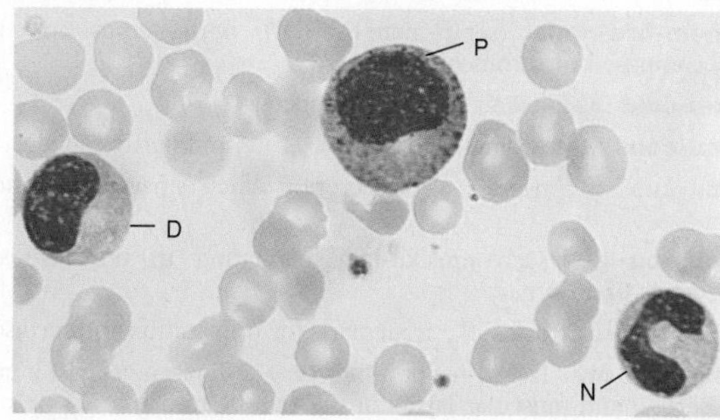

■ Several stages of the granulocytic series. *D*, Neutrophilic metamyelocyte; *P*, promyelocyte; *N*, neutrophilic band cell.

with pyridoxal phosphate as a cofactor, as the first step in sphingolipid biosynthesis. Written also *serine palmitoyltransferase.*

ser•ine pro•te•ase (sēr′ēn pro′te-ās) serine endopeptidase.

ser•ine pro•tein•ase (sēr′ēn pro′tēn-ās) serine endopeptidase.

ser•ine/thre•o•nine ki•nase (sēr′ēn thre′o-nēn ki′nās) protein-serine/threonine kinase.

ser•ine-type car•boxy•pep•ti•dase (sēr′ēn-tīp″ kahr-bok″se-pep′tĭ-dās) 1. [EC 3.4.16] any of a group of exopeptidases that contain diisopropyl fluorophosphate–sensitive serine residues in their catalytic sites, have optimum activity at acid pH, and catalyze the hydrolytic cleavage of the C-terminal amino acid from a peptide chain. 2. [EC 3.4.16.1] a specific serine-containing lysosomal carboxypeptidase catalyzing this reaction and acting on a variety of peptides.

SERM selective estrogen receptor modulator.

ser•mo•rel•in ac•e•tate (sur″mo-rel′in) the acetate salt of a synthetic peptide corresponding to a portion of growth hormone–releasing hormone; used in the treatment of idiopathic growth hormone deficiency in prepubertal children; administered subcutaneously.

ser(o)- [L. *serum* whey, watery substance] a combining form denoting relationship to serum.

se•ro•al•bu•min•ous (sēr″o-al-bu′min-əs) 1. containing serum and albumin. 2. pertaining to or containing serum albumin.

se•ro•con•ver•sion (sēr″o-kən-vur′zhən) [*sero-* + *conversion*] the change of a patient's serologic test results from negative to positive, indicating development of antibodies in response to infection or immunization.

se•ro•con•vert (sēr″o-kən-vert′) to undergo seroconversion.

se•ro•cul•ture (sēr′o-kul″chər) [*sero-* + *culture*] a bacterial culture on blood serum.

se•ro•cys•tic (sēr″o-sis′tik) made up of serous cysts.

se•ro•di•ag•no•sis (sēr″o-di″əg-no′sis) [*sero-* + *diagnosis*] diagnosis made by using serologic tests. **serodiagnos′tic** *adj*

se•ro•en•te•ri•tis (sēr″o-en″tə-ri′tis) perienteritis.

se•ro•epi•de•mi•ol•o•gy (se″ro-ep″ĭ-de″me-ol′ə-je) [*sero-* + *epidemiology*] epidemiology in which serologic studies of individuals and populations are used to monitor or study infectious diseases.

se•ro-fast (sēr″o-fast′) serum-fast.

se•ro•fib•rin•ous (sēr″o-fi′brin-əs) both serous and fibrinous.

se•ro•fi•brous (sēr″o-fi′brəs) pertaining to serous and fibrous surfaces, as, serofibrous apposition.

se•ro•floc•cu•la•tion (sēr″o-flok″u-la′shən) [*sero-* + *flocculation*] flocculation produced in blood serum by an antigen.

se•ro•group (sēr′o-groo͞p) [*sero-* + *group*] 1. a group of bacteria containing a common antigen, possibly including more than one serovar (q.v.), species, or genus. A serogroup is a tentative and unofficial designation, used in the classification of certain genera of bacteria, e.g., *Leptospira, Salmonella, Shigella,* and *Streptococcus.* 2. a group of viral species that are closely related antigenically.

se•rol•o•gist (sēr-ol′ə-jist) a specialist in serology.

se•rol•o•gy (sēr-ol′ə-je) [*sero-* + *-logy*] originally, the study of the in vitro reactions of immune sera, e.g., precipitin, agglutination, and complement fixation reactions. The term is now used to refer to the use of such reactions to measure serum antibody titers in infectious disease (serologic tests), to the clinical correlations of the antibody titer (the "serology" of a disease), and to the use of serologic reactions to detect antigens (e.g., "serologically defined" human leukocyte antigens). **serolog′ic, serolog′ical** *adj*
diagnostic s. serodiagnosis.

se•ro•ma (sēr-o′mə) [*ser-* + *-oma*] a tumorlike collection of serum in the tissues.

se•ro•mem•bra•nous (sēr″o-mem′brə-nəs) both serous and membranous; composed of serous membrane.

se•ro•mu•coid (sēr″o-mu′koid) seromucous.

se•ro•mu•cous (sēr″o-mu′kəs) partly serous and partly mucous.

se•ro•mu•cus (sēr″o-mu′kəs) a secretion which is part serum and part mucus.

se•ro•mus•cu•lar (sēr″o-mus′ku-lər) pertaining to the serous and muscular coats of an organ.

Sero•my•cin (ser″o-mi′sin) trademark for preparations of cycloserine.

se•ro•my•ot•o•my (se″ro-mi-ot′ə-me) [*sero-* + *myo-* + *-tomy*] a cutting into the serosal and muscular layers of the wall of an organ.

se•ro•neg•a•tive (sēr″o-neg′ə-tiv) serologically negative; showing negative results on serological examination; showing a lack of antibody.

se•ro•neg•a•tiv•i•ty (sēr″o-neg″ə-tiv′ĭ-te) the state of being seronegative, or of showing negative results on serological examination.

Se•ro•phene (se′ro-fēn) trademark for a preparation of clomiphene citrate.

se•ro•phil•ic (sēr″o-fil′ik) a term used to describe a bacterium whose growth is enhanced in the presence of serum.

se•ro•pneu•mo•tho•rax (sēr″o-noo″mo-thor′aks) hydropneumothorax.

se•ro•pos•i•tive (sēr″o-poz′ĭ-tiv) serologically positive; showing positive results on serological examination; showing a high level of antibody.

se•ro•pos•i•tiv•i•ty (sēr″o-poz″ĭ-tiv′ĭ-te) the state of being seropositive, or of showing positive results on serologic examination.

se•ro•prev•a•lence (se″ro-prev′ə-ləns) the proportion of a population seropositive for a specific antibody.

se•ro•prog•no•sis (sēr″o-prog-no′sis) the prognosis of a disease based on the results of serologic tests.

se•ro•pu•ru•lent (sēr″o-pu′roo-lənt) both serous and purulent.

se•ro•pus (sēr′o-pus″) serum mingled with pus.

Ser•o•quel (ser′o-kwel) trademark for a preparation of quetiapine fumarate.

se•ro•re•ac•tion (sēr″o-re-ak′shən) serological reaction; a reaction demonstrating a specific antibody or antigen in serum.

se•ro•re•lapse (sēr″o-re′laps) a definite rise in serological titer occurring after treatment.

se•ro•re•sis•tance (sēr″o-re-zis′təns) failure of the serological titer to fall satisfactorily after treatment. **seroresis′tant** *adj*

se•ro•re•ver•sal (sēr″o-re-ver′səl) a fall in serological titer after treatment.

se•ro•re•ver•sion (sēr″o-re-ver′zhən) [*sero-* + *reversion*] spontaneous or induced conversion from a seropositive to a seronegative state.

se•ro•sa (sēr-o′sə, sēr-o′zə) 1. tunica serosa. 2. chorion.
s. of bladder tunica serosa vesicae urinariae.
s. of esophagus tunica serosa oesophagi.
s. of gallbladder tunica serosa vesicae biliaris.
s. of large intestine tunica serosa intestini crassi.
s. of liver tunica serosa hepatis.
s. of parietal pleura tunica serosa pleurae parietalis.
s. of pericardium tunica serosa pericardii.
s. of peritoneum tunica serosa peritonei.
s. of small intestine tunica serosa intestini tenuis.
s. of spleen tunica serosa splenica.
s. of stomach tunica serosa gastrica.
s. of testis tunica serosa testis.
s. of urinary bladder tunica serosa vesicae urinariae.
s. of uterine tube tunica serosa tubae uterinae.
s. of uterus tunica serosa uteri.
s. of visceral pleura tuncia serosa pleurae visceralis.

se•ro•sal (sēr-o′səl) pertaining to or composed of serosa.

se•ro•sa•mu•cin (sēr-o″sə-mu′sin) a protein resembling mucin, found in inflammatory ascitic exudates.

se•ro•san•guin•e•ous (sēr″o-sang-gwin′e-əs) pertaining to or containing both serum and blood.

se•ro•se•rous (sēr″o-sēr′əs) pertaining to two or more serous membranes.

se•ro•si•tis (sēr″o-si′tis) pl. *serosi′tides* [*serous membrane* + *-itis*] inflammation of a serous membrane.
infectious avian s. a septicemic disease of ducklings and geese, characterized by fibrinous peritonitis, pericarditis, and airsacculitis, and caused by *Riemerell anatipestifer.* Called also *new duck disease* in ducklings and *goose influenza* in geese.
multiple s. polyserositis.

se•ros•i•ty (sēr-os′ĭ-te) the quality possessed by serous fluids.

se•ro•stat•us (sēr″o-stat′əs) status in relation to presence or absence of a given antibody; see *seropositivity* and *seronegativity.*

Sero•stim (ser′o-stim) trademark for a preparation of somatropin.

se•ro•sur•vey (sēr″o-sur′va) a population survey using a serologic test to screen for exposure and immunity to an infectious disease.

se•ro•sy•no•vi•al (sēr″o-sĭ-no′ve-əl) both serous and synovial.

se•ro•syn•o•vi•tis (sēr″o-sin″o-vi′tis) [*sero-* + *synovitis*] synovitis with effusion of serum.

se•ro•ther•a•py (sēr″o-ther′ə-pe) [*sero-* + *therapy*] treatment of disease by injection of immune serum or antitoxin.

se•ro•tho•rax (sēr″o-thor′aks) hydrothorax.

ser•o•ton•er•gic (ser″o-tōn-ur′jik) serotoninergic.

se•ro•to•nin (ser″o-to′nin) a monoamine vasoconstrictor, synthesized in the intestinal chromaffin cells or in central or peripheral neurons and found in high concentrations in many body tissues, including the intestinal mucosa, pineal body, and central nervous system. Produced enzymatically from tryptophan by hydroxylation and decarboxylation, it has many physiologic properties, such as inhibition of gastric secretion, stimulation of smooth muscle, serving as a central neurotransmitter, and being a precursor of melatonin. It is also found in animal species from coelenterates to vertebrates, in bacteria, and in many plants. Called also *5-hydroxytryptamine*.

sero•to•nin•er•gic (ser″o-to″nin-ur′jik) 1. containing or activated by serotonin, as the neurons of the raphe nuclei of the brainstem. 2. of or pertaining to neurons that secrete serotonin, which, in turn, stimulates release of pituitary hormones. Called also *serotonergic*.

se•ro•type (sēr′o-tīp″) 1. the type of a microorganism as determined by the kinds and combinations of constituent antigens present in the cell. 2. serovar. 3. to distinguish organisms on the basis of their constituent antigens.

heterologous s. a related but not identical serotype.

homologous s. an identical serotype.

se•rous (sēr′əs) [L. *serosus*] 1. pertaining to or resembling serum. 2. producing or containing serum, as a serous gland or cyst.

se•ro•vac•ci•na•tion (sēr″o-vak″sĭ-na′shən) injection of serum combined with bacterial vaccination to produce passive immunity by the former and active immunity by the latter.

se•ro•var (sēr′o-var) a taxonomic subdivision of bacteria based on the kinds and combinations of constituent antigens present in the cell, or a formula expressing the antigenic analysis on which such a subdivision is based. Called also *serotype*. See also *serogroup*.

Ser•pa•zide (ser′pə-zīd) trademark for combination preparations of reserpine, hydralazine hydrochloride, and hydrochlorothiazide.

Ser•pen•tes (ser′pen-tēz) *Ophidia*.

ser•pig•i•nous (sər-pij′ĭ-nəs) [L. *serpere* to creep] having a wavy or much indented margin.

ser•pin (sur′pin) [*ser*ine protease *in*hibitor] any of a superfamily of high-molecular-weight, structurally related glycoproteins that act as serine protease (serine endopeptidase) inhibitors. They have a specific, highly ordered tertiary structure with a mobile reaction center, although individual serpins are highly specific for particular endopeptidases. Among their targets are serine endopeptidases involved in coagulation, complement activation, fibrinolysis, inflammation, and tissue remodeling.

Ser•pu•li•na•ceae (sur″pu-lĭ-na′se-e) [L. *serpulina* little snake] a family of gram-negative, helical bacteria of the order Spirochaetales; organisms of medical interest are contained in the genus *Brachyspira*.

ser•rat•ed (ser′āt-ed) [L. *serratus*, from *serra* saw] having a sawlike edge.

Ser•ra•tia (sə-ra′she-ə) [Serafino *Serrati*, Italian physicist, 18th century] a genus of gram-negative, facultatively anaerobic bacteria of the family Enterobacteriaceae, consisting of motile, peritrichously flagellated rods, sometimes capsulated. Most strains produce white, pink, or red pigments. The organisms occur widely on plants, in soil, and in water. Many species are opportunistic pathogens, causing infections of the endocardium, blood, wounds, and urinary and respiratory tracts in immunocompromised patients. The type species is *S. marces′cens*.

S. liquefa′ciens the species most commonly found in the natural environment, consisting of nonpigmented, ornithine decarboxylase–positive organisms; it sometimes occurs as an opportunistic pathogen.

S. marces′cens the species most frequently isolated from human infections, divided into a number of biogroups on the basis of pigmentation and physiological and nutritional characteristics; it is an opportunistic pathogen, causing nosocomial bacteremia, endocarditis, and pneumonia in immunocompromised patients. See also *Serratia pneumonia*, under *pneumonia*.

S. odori′fera a species with a characteristic musty, potato-like odor, occasionally isolated from plants or food and rarely found as an opportunistic pathogen.

S. rubidae′a a species with pigmented strains that is ornithine decarboxylase negative, found in ripe coconuts; strains have been isolated rarely from human patients.

ser•ra•tion (sə-ra′shən) [L. *serratio*] 1. a structure or formation with teeth like those of a saw. 2. the condition of being serrated. 3. on an electrodiagnostic recording, part of an abnormal wave that has several changes in direction without crossing the baseline.

ser•ra•tus (sə-ra′təs) [L.] serrated.

serre•fine (sār-fēn′) [Fr.] a small spring forceps for compressing bleeding vessels.

Serres angle, glands (sār) [Antoine Etienne Reynaud Augustin *Serres*, French physiologist, 1786–1868] see *metafacial angle*, under *angle*, and *Epstein pearls*, under *pearl*.

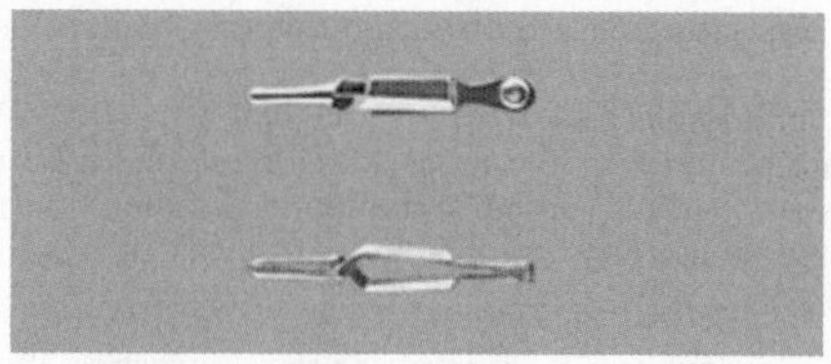

■ Serrefines.

Ser•to•li cell (ser-to′le) [Enrico *Sertoli*, Italian histologist, 1842–1910] see under *cell*.

ser•tra•line hy•dro•chlo•ride (sur′trə-lēn) a selective serotonin reuptake inhibitor, used to treat depressive, obsessive-compulsive, and panic disorders; administered orally.

se•rum (sēr′əm) pl. *serums, se′ra* [L. "whey"] 1. the clear portion of any body fluid; the clear fluid moistening serous membranes. 2. blood s. 3. antiserum.

active s. a serum that contains complement.

anticomplementary s. a serum which interferes with or destroys the activity of complement.

antilymphocyte s. (ALS) antiserum derived from animals that have been immunized against human lymphocytes, a powerful nonspecific immunosuppressive agent that causes destruction of circulating lymphocytes.

antirabies s. [USP] antiserum obtained from the blood serum or plasma of animals (generally horses) immunized with rabies vaccine; used for postexposure prophylaxis against rabies. Rabies immune globulin is used instead (because of its lower incidence of adverse reactions), if available.

antitetanic s. (ATS) tetanus antitoxin.

antitoxic s. antitoxin.

articular s. synovia.

bacteriolytic s. serum containing a bacteriolysin capable of inducing complement-dependent lysis of a bacterium.

blood s. the clear liquid that separates from the blood when it is allowed to clot completely. It is therefore blood plasma from which fibrinogen has been removed in the process of clotting.

blood s., glycerin blood serum containing glycerin.

blood grouping s's [USP] preparations containing particular antibodies against red cell antigens, used for blood typing. Those most commonly used are the anti-A and anti-B blood grouping serums, used to determine ABO blood types, and the anti-Rh blood grouping serums (anti-D, anti-C, anti-E, anti-c, and anti-e), used to determine Rh blood types.

convalescence s., convalescent s., convalescents′ s. blood serum from a patient convalescing from an infectious disease, formerly used as a prophylactic injection in such diseases as measles, scarlet fever, or whooping cough.

despeciated s. a heterologous antiserum treated to remove some of the species-specific proteins so that it is less likely to cause anaphylaxis.

foreign s. heterologous s. (def. 1).

heterologous s. 1. serum obtained from an animal belonging to a species different from that of the recipient. 2. serum prepared from an animal immunized by an organism differing from that against which it is to be used.

homologous s. 1. serum obtained from an animal belonging to the same species as the recipient. 2. serum prepared from an animal immunized by the same organism against which it is to be used.

hyperimmune s. antiserum with an especially high antibody titer produced by repeated antigen injections.

immune s. antiserum.

inactivated s. serum which has been heated, usually at 56°C for 30 minutes, to destroy the lytic activity of contained complement components.

leukocyte typing s. [USP] a preparation of serum derived from blood or plasma obtained from animals or from human donors and containing antibody for the identification of human leukocyte antigens; used for in vitro histocompatibility testing.

Loeffler blood s., Löffler blood s. see *Loeffler coagulated serum medium* under *culture medium*.

lymphatolytic s. serum which destroys lymphatic tissues, such as the spleen and lymph glands.

monovalent s. antiserum containing antibodies against only one of several strains or species of microorganisms or only one of a group of antigens.

normal s. serum from a normal untreated animal.

pericardial s. pericardial fluid.

polyvalent s. antiserum containing antibodies to a group of two or more strains or species of microorganism or to a group of two or more antigens.

pooled s. the mixed serum from a number of individuals.

pregnancy s. blood serum taken from pregnant women.

Sclavo s. a specific anti-anthrax serum that may be used against human anthrax.

specific s. monovalent s.

truth s. a misnomer for the drugs sometimes employed in narcoanalysis, especially amobarbital sodium and thiopental sodium; the agent used is not a serum and its use does not guarantee truthfulness.

se·ru·mal (sēr-oo′məl) pertaining to or formed from serum.

se·rum-fast (sēr′əm-fast″) resistant to the destructive effect of serum; said of bacteria.

Serv. [L.] ser′va (keep, preserve).

ser·vo·mech·a·nism (ser″vo-mek′ə-niz-əm) a control system in which feedback is used to control errors in another system. The term is also applied to biological systems, such as the mechanism that controls the diameter of the pupil of the eye according to the amount of incident light.

ser·yl (sēr′əl, ser′əl) the acyl radical of serine.

ses·a·me (ses′ə-me) [L. *sesamum;* Gr. *sēsamon*] 1. *Sesamum indicum.* 2. the seeds of *S. indicum,* which yield sesame oil.

ses·a·moid (ses′ə-moid) [L. *sesamoides;* Gr. *sēsamon* sesame + *eidos* form] 1. denoting a small nodular bone embedded in a tendon or joint capsule. 2. a sesamoid bone. See under *bone.*

ses·a·moi·di·tis (ses″ə-moi-di′tis) inflammation of the sesamoid bones and surrounding structures of a horse's foot.

Ses·a·mum (ses′ə-məm) [L.] a genus of herbs of the family Pedaliaceae, native to hot regions of Africa and Asia. *S. in′dicum* L. is sesame, the source of sesame oil.

sesqui- [L. *sesqui* a half more] a prefix meaning one and a half.

ses·qui·ox·ide (ses″kwe-ok′sid) a compound of three parts of oxygen with two of another element.

ses·qui·sul·fate (ses″kwe-sul′fāt) a sulfate containing three parts of sulfuric acid united with two of another element.

ses·qui·sul·fide (ses″kwe-sul′fīd) a sulfide containing three parts of sulfur united with two of another element.

ses·sile (ses′il) [L. *sessilis*] attached by a base; not pedunculated or stalked.

Ses·sin·ia (sə-sin′e-ə) the coconut beetles, a genus of blister beetles (family Meloidae), found on various Pacific islands.

ses·ta·mibi (ses″tə-mib′e) a compound comprising six substituted isocyanide (isonitrile) chains; as a complex with radiolabeled technetium (Tc 99m) it is used in studies of myocardial perfusion and thyroid and parathyroid imaging. See table at *technetium.*

set (set) 1. to align bones or bone fragments, as in reducing a fracture. 2. in psychology, a readiness to perceive or respond in a certain way because of past experience, requirements of a task, etc.

phalangeal s. a surgical office procedure for correction of deformities of the lesser toes, involving incision to reach the bony joint and manipulation for proper positioning.

se·ta (se′tə) pl. *se′tae* [L.] 1. bristle. 2. any bristlelike structure, such as the multicellular stalk of certain plants.

se·ta·ceous (se-ta′shəs) [L. *setaceus,* from *seta* bristle] slender and rigid, like a bristle.

Se·ta·ria (se-tar′e-ə) 1. a large genus of grasses found in Europe and North America, often used for forage or hay. *S. sphacela′ta* and other species contain oxalates and can cause oxalate poisoning in livestock that eat large amounts of them. 2. a genus of nematodes of the superfamily Filarioides. *S. equi′na* is found in the abdominal cavities of various mammals. *S. labiatopapillo′sa* (or *S. cer′vi*) is an African species found in the peritoneal cavities of cattle, game animals, and occasionally humans.

set-fast (set′fast) azoturia (def. 2).

se·tif·er·ous (se-tif′ər-əs) setigerous.

se·tig·er·ous (se-tij′ər-əs) [*seta* + L. *gerere* to carry] bearing bristles (setae); called also *setiferous.*

se·ton (se′ton) [Fr. *seton;* L. *seta* bristle] a thread of silk, linen, or other finely drawn material for passage through a sinus, fistula, or epithelial tract, often to serve as a guide for subsequent dilatation with instruments of larger diameter.

set-point (set′point) the target value of a controlled variable that is maintained physiologically by bodily control mechanisms for homeostasis, e.g., the point at which body temperature is controlled by the hypothalamic thermostat. Written also *set point.*

Set·te·gast projection (set′ə-gahst) [H. *Settegast,* German radiologist, 20th century] see under *projection.*

set·up (set′əp) 1. organization or arrangement. 2. the arrangement of teeth on a trial denture base.

diagnostic s. a procedure involving dissection of teeth from a plaster model and repositioning of the teeth in desired positions to aid in case analysis preliminary to constructing an orthodontic appliance.

Se·ver disease (se′vər) [James Warren *Sever,* American orthopedic surgeon, 1878–1964] see under *disease.*

se·vel·a·mer hy·dro·chlo·ride (sə-vel′ə-mər) a phosphate binder administered orally to reduce serum phosphorus concentrations in treatment of hyperphosphatemia and ectopic calcification in patients with end-stage renal disease.

Sev·in (sev′in) trademark for a preparation of carbaril.

se·vo·flu·rane (se″vo-floo′rān) an inhalation anesthetic used for the induction and maintenance of general anesthesia.

sew·age (soo′əj) the used water supply of a community, consisting of an aqueous suspension of feces and other waste materials; the contents of sewers.

SEWHO shoulder-elbow-wrist-hand orthosis.

sex (seks) [L. *sexus*] 1. the distinction between male and female, found in most species of animals and plants, based on the type of gametes produced by the individual or the category into which the individual fits on the basis of that criterion. Ova are produced by the female and spermatozoa by the male; the union of these distinctive germ cells being the prerequisite for the production of a new individual in sexual reproduction. 2. see *gender identity,* under *identity.* 3. sexual intercourse. 4. to determine whether an individual is male or female.

chromosomal s. sex as determined by the sex chromosome constitution in somatic cells, in humans being the XX (female) or the XY (male) genotype, without regard to phenotypic manifestations; called also *genetic s.*

endocrinologic s. sex determined by gender-specific hormonal patterns. See also *phenotypic s.*

genetic s. chromosomal s.

genital s. phenotypic s.

gonadal s. that part of the phenotypic sex that is determined by the gonadal tissue present, whether ovarian or testicular.

morphological s. that part of the phenotypic sex that is determined by the morphology of the external genitals.

nuclear s. the sex as determined on the basis of the presence or absence of sex chromatin in somatic cells, its presence normally indicating the XX (female) genotype, and its absence the XY (male) genotype.

phenotypic s., somatic s. the phenotypic manifestations of sex such as presence of genital organs and secondary sex characters, under endocrine influences; see also *endocrinologic s., gonadal s.,* and *morphological s.*

sex-[1] [L. *sex* six] a combining form meaning six.

sex-[2] [L. *sexus* sex] a combining form denoting relationship to sex or sexuality.

sex·dig·i·tate (seks-dij′ĭ-tāt) [*sex-*[1] + *digitate*] having six digits; see *hexadactyly.*

sex·duc·tion (seks-duk′shən) F-duction.

sex-in·flu·enced (seks-in′floo-ənst) pertaining to something differing between the sexes; see under *trait.*

sex·iv·a·lent (sek-siv′ə-lənt) hexavalent.

sex-lim·it·ed (seks-lim′it-əd) affecting individuals of one sex only; see under *trait.*

sex-linked (seks′linkt) 1. carried on one of the sex chromosomes, as a gene; see under *gene.* 2. by extension, sexually determined, as an inherited trait determined by such a gene; see under *trait.*

sex·ol·o·gy (sek-sol′ə-je) [*sex-*[2] + *-logy*] the study of sex and sexual relations and their evolutionary, physiological, developmental, and sociological aspects.

sex·tant (seks′tənt) one of the six equal parts into which the dental arch may be divided: maxillary right, left, and anterior and mandibular right, left, and anterior.

sex·ti·grav·i·da (seks″tĭ-grav′ĭ-də) [L. *sextus* sixth + *gravida*] a woman pregnant for the sixth time; also written *gravida VI.*

sex·tip·a·ra (seks-tip′ə-rə) [L. *sextus* sixth + *para*] a woman who has had six pregnancies which resulted in viable offspring; also written *para VI* or *VI-para.*

sex·tup·let (seks-tup′lət) [L. *sextus* sixth] one of six offspring produced in one gestation period.

sex·u·al (sek′shoo-əl) [L. *sexualis*] 1. pertaining to, characterized by, involving, or endowed with sex, sexuality, the sexes, or the sex organs and their functions. 2. characterized by the property of maleness or femaleness. 3. pertaining to reproduction involving both male and female gametes. 4. implying or symbolizing erotic desires or activity.

sex•u•al•i•ty (sek″shoo-al′ĭ-te) 1. the characteristic quality of the male and female reproductive elements. 2. the constitution of an individual in relation to sexual attitudes or activity.

infantile s. in freudian theory, the erotic life of infants and children, encompassing the oral, anal, and phallic stages of psychosexual development.

sex•u•al•iza•tion (sek″shoo-al-ĭ-za′shən) the endowing of an object or function with sexual significance or instinct, as occurs with various body parts during development; it may also occur indirectly and unconsciously for seemingly unrelated events or objects.

Sé•za•ry cell, syndrome (erythroderma) (sa-zah-re′) [Albert *Sézary*, French dermatologist, 1880–1956] see under *cell* and *syndrome.*

SF-1 steroidogenic factor 1.

SFEMG single fiber electromyography.

SGA 1. Subjective Global Assessment. 2. small for gestational age; see under *infant.*

SGOT serum glutamic-oxaloacetic transaminase; see *aspartate transaminase.*

SGPT serum glutamic-pyruvic transaminase; see *alanine transaminase.*

shad•ow (shad′o) 1. an attenuated image of an actual object, as a faded or colorless erythrocyte. 2. a figure or image created by the interruption of light or other rays, such as the representation on a radiograph of radiopaque structures.

bat's wing s. a radiographic shadow that radiates through both lungs from the hilar region toward the periphery, leaving a clear zone at the apices, periphery, and bases.

heart s. cardiac silhouette.

Purkinje s's see under *figure.*

shad•ow-cast•ing (shad′o-kast′ing) a technique for increasing the visibility of ultramicroscopic specimens under the microscope by applying a coating of chromium, gold, or other metal.

shaft (shaft) a long slender part, such as the diaphysis of a long bone. Called also *scapus* [TA].

s. of femur corpus ossis femoris.

s. of fibula corpus fibulae.

hair s. the long cylindrical part that is the major portion of a hair, sometimes referring to only the portion that extends beyond the surface of the skin. Called also *scapus pili.*

s. of humerus corpus humeri.

s. of metacarpal bone corpus ossis metacarpi.

s. of metatarsal bone corpus ossis metatarsi.

s. of penis corpus penis.

s. of phalanx of hand corpus phalangis manus.

s. of phalanx of foot corpus phalangis pedis.

s. of radius corpus radii.

s. of rib corpus costae.

s. of tibia corpus tibiae.

s. of ulna corpus ulnae.

shag•gy (shag′e) 1. covered with, having, or resembling rough long hair or wool. 2. having a rough texture or surface or hairlike processes.

sha•green (shə-grēn′) 1. a type of untanned leather covered with granulations. 2. the rough skin of various types of sharks. 3. having a rough, nevoid surface and a resemblance to shark skin; see *shagreen patch,* under *patch.*

Shah-Waar•den•burg syndrome (shah′ vahr′den-boorg) [Krishnakumar N. *Shah*, Indian physician, late 20th century; Petrus Johannes *Waardenburg*, Dutch ophthalmologist, 1886–1979] Waardenburg syndrome type 4; see under *syndrome.*

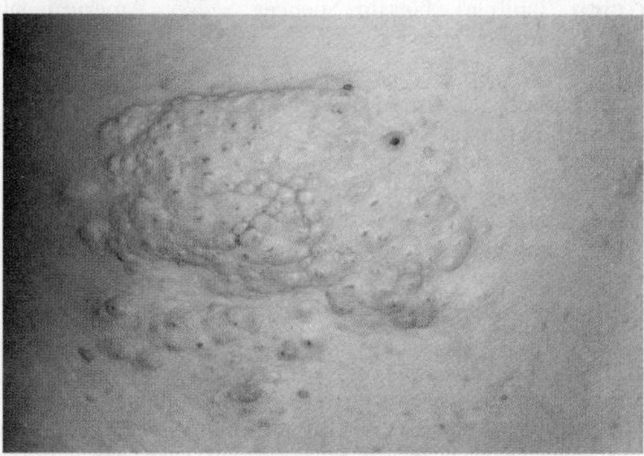

■ Shagreen patch in tuberous sclerosis.

sham (sham) 1. a hoax; a fraudulent imitation. 2. not genuine; fraudulent; marked by falseness.

sha•man•ism (shah′-, sha′mə-niz″əm) a traditional system, occurring in tribal societies, in which certain individuals, or shamans, are believed to be gifted with access to an invisible spiritual world and, through the use of specific rituals, ceremonies, and physical objects, are able to mediate between the spiritual and physical worlds for the purpose of healing, divination, and affecting events in the physical world.

shank (shangk) 1. leg (def. 1). 2. crus (def. 2).

shap•ing (shāp′ing) an operant conditioning technique used in behavior therapy in which new behavior is produced by providing reinforcement for progressively closer approximations of the final desired behavior. Called also *successive approximation.*

shark (shahrk) any of numerous elasmobranch fishes, usually found in the ocean; some are carnivorous and predatory and may attack humans. See also *elasmobranch poisoning.*

Greenland s. *Somniosus microcephalus.*

Shar•pey fibers (shahr′pe) [William *Sharpey*, Scottish anatomist and physiologist, 1802–1880] see under *fiber.*

shave (shāv) 1. to cut at or parallel to the surface of the skin. 2. to remove the beard or other body hair by such a process. 3. to cut thin slices from or to cut into thin slices.

Sha•ver disease (sha′vər) [Cecil Gordon *Shaver*, Canadian physician, 20th century] bauxite pneumoconiosis.

SHBG sex hormone–binding globulin.

shear (shēr) 1. an applied force that tends to cause an opposite but parallel sliding motion of the planes of an object. 2. the strain resulting from such force.

sheath (shēth) [L. *vagina;* Gr. *thēkē*] a tubular structure enclosing or surrounding some organ or part.

anterior tarsal tendon s's vaginae tendinum tarsales anteriores.

arachnoid s. the continuation of the arachnoidea mater around the optic nerve, forming part of the internal sheath of the optic nerve.

bulbar s. vagina bulbi.

carotid s., carotid s. of cervical fascia vagina carotica fasciae cervicalis.

caudal s. a tubular cytoplasmic structure at the base of the nucleus in the early spermatid.

chordal s. notochordal s.

common flexor s. vagina communis tendinum musculorum flexorum.

common tendon s. of peronei vagina communis tendinum musculorum fibularium.

crural s. femoral s.

dentinal s. Neumann s.

dermal s. the layer of dermis adjacent to a hair follicle.

dorsal carpal tendon s's vaginae tendinum carpales dorsales.

dural s. vagina externa nervi optici.

enamel prism s., enamel rod s. a sheath of organic tissue completely or partially surrounding each enamel prism. Called also *prism s.* and *rod s.*

external s. of optic nerve vagina externa nervi optici.

s. of eyeball vagina bulbi.

femoral s. the fascial covering of the proximal portion of the femoral vessels, derived from the intra-abdominal fascia; the most medial portion of the sheath, separated by a septum, forms the canalis femoralis. Called also *crural s.*

fibrous s's of fingers vaginae fibrosae digitorum manus.

fibrous s. of optic nerve vagina externa nervi optici.

fibrous s. of spermatozoon the fibrous sheath surrounding the principal piece of the tail of a spermatozoon.

fibrous tendon s. stratum fibrosum vaginae tendinis.

fibrous s's of toes vaginae fibrosae digitorum pedis.

fibular tarsal tendon s's vaginae tendinum tarsales fibulares.

Henle s. endoneurium.

Hertwig s., s. of Hertwig root s. (def. 1).

inner s. of optic nerve, internal s. of optic nerve vagina interna nervi optici.

intertubercular tendon s. vagina tendinis intertubercularis.

s. of Key and Retzius endoneurium.

lamellar s. perineurium.

Mauthner s. axolemma.

medullary s. myelin s.

mitochondrial s. a sheath of circumferentially oriented mitochondria, arranged end to end, that surrounds the middle piece of a spermatozoon and is thought to control the movements of the tail.

muscle s. fascia propria musculi.

myelin s. the cylindrical covering on the axons of some neurons; it consists of concentric layers of myelin, formed in the peripheral nervous system by the plasma membrane of Schwann cells, and in the central nervous system by oligodendrocytes. It is interrupted at intervals along its length by gaps known as nodes of Ranvier. Myelin is an electrical insulator that serves to speed the conduction of nerve impulses. See also *myelinated nerve fibers*, under *fiber*. Called also *medullary s.*

nerve s. myelin s.

Neumann s., s. of Neumann an area of interface between peritubular and intertubular dental structures. Called also *dentinal s.*

neurilemmal s. neurilemma.

notochordal s. an elastic sheath surrounding the notochord.

s's of optic nerve the internal and external meningeal sheaths of the optic nerve within the orbit, continuous with the meninges of the brain. See *vagina externa nervi optici* and *vagina interna nervi optici*.

outer s. of optic nerve vagina externa nervi optici.

palmar carpal tendon s's vaginae tendinum carpales palmares.

periarterial lymphatic s., periarteriolar lymphatic s., periarteriolar lymphoid s. (PALS) any of the sheaths of lymphatic tissue surrounding the arteries that have left the splenic trabeculae; the sheaths are mainly composed of T lymphocytes, at intervals expanding to form the B lymphocyte–containing splenic lymphoid nodules, and together composing the white pulp of the spleen.

perinephric s. fascia renalis.

perivascular s. a pia glial membrane which accompanies blood vessels into the brain.

pial s. the continuation of the pia mater around the optic nerve, forming part of the internal sheath of the optic nerve.

plantar tendon s. of peroneus longus vagina plantaris tendinis musculi fibularis longi.

prism s. enamel prism s.

rectus s., s. of rectus abdominis muscle vagina musculi recti abdominis.

rod s. enamel prism s.

root s. 1. an epithelial extension of the cervical loop of the enamel organ, consisting of the inner and outer enamel epithelium, and directing the number and morphological growth of the roots. It is bordered externally by the dental sac and internally by developing cementum and root dentin, and ultimately becomes the epithelial diaphragm. Called also *Hertwig s.* and *s. of Hertwig*. 2. the epithelial portion of the hair follicle, divided into the *inner root sheath* and the *outer root sheath*. The inner root sheath has three layers: *Huxley layer*, *Henle layer*, and the *cuticle of the root sheath*. The outer root sheath does not have distinct layers and merges with the epidermis near the skin surface.

Scarpa s. fascia cremasterica.

Schwalbe s. the thin envelope of an elastic fiber.

s. of Schwann neurilemma.

Schweigger-Seidel s. a spindle-shaped thickening in the walls of the second portion of the arterial branches forming the penicilli in the spleen; see *sheathed artery*, under *artery*. Called also *ellipsoid*.

s. of styloid process vagina processus styloidei.

synovial s. vagina synovialis.

synovial s's of fingers vaginae synoviales digitorum manus.

synovial tendon s. stratum synoviale vaginae tendinis.

synovial s's of toes vaginae synoviales digitorum pedis.

tendon s. vagina tendinis.

tendon s. of abductor pollicis longus and extensor pollicis brevis vagina tendinum musculorum abductoris longi et extensoris pollicis brevis.

tendon s. of extensores carpi radiales vagina tendinum musculorum extensorum carpi radialium.

tendon s. of extensor carpi ulnaris vagina tendinis musculi extensoris carpi ulnaris.

tendon s. of extensor digitorum and extensor indicis vagina tendinum musculorum extensoris digitorum et extensoris indicis.

tendon s. of extensor digitorum longus vagina tendinum musculi extensoris digitorum longi.

tendon s. of extensor digiti minimi vagina tendinis musculi extensoris digiti minimi.

tendon s. of extensor hallucis longus vagina tendinis musculi extensoris hallucis longi.

tendon s. of extensor pollicis longus vagina tendinis musculi extensoris pollicis longi.

tendon s. of flexor carpi radialis vagina tendinis musculi flexoris carpi radialis.

tendon s. of flexor digitorum longus vagina tendinum musculi flexoris digitorum longi.

tendon s. of flexor hallucis longus vagina tendinis musculi flexoris hallucis longi.

tendon s. of flexor pollicis longus vagina tendinis musculi flexoris pollicis longi.

tendon s. of tibialis anterior vagina tendinis musculi tibialis anterioris.

tendon s. of tibialis posterior vagina tendinis musculi tibialis posterioris.

tendon s's of toes vaginae tendinum digitorum pedis.

tibial tarsal tendon s's vaginae tendinum tarsales tibiales.

Shee•han syndrome (she′ən) [Harold Leeming *Sheehan*, English pathologist, 1900–1988] see *postpartum pituitary necrosis*, under *necrosis*.

sheep-pox (shēp-poks) a contagious disease of sheep caused by a poxvirus, which is characterized by fever, systemic disturbances, and widespread skin lesions on non-woolbearing areas or where the hair is not long; it is usually more severe, often fatal, in younger animals. Called also *ovine smallpox* and *variola ovina*.

sheet (shēt) 1. a rectangular piece of cotton, linen, etc., for a bed covering. 2. any structure resembling such a covering.

β s., beta s., β pleated s., beta pleated s. pleated s.

draw s. a folded sheet placed under a patient in bed so that it may be withdrawn without lifting the patient.

pleated s. a secondary structure occurring in many proteins, consisting of several polypeptide chains running in the same direction (a parallel pleated sheet) or in alternating directions (an antiparallel pleated sheet) and joined by hydrogen bonds between the imino hydrogen of each peptide bond and the carbonyl oxygen of a peptide bond in the next chain over. Called also *β structure*, *β s.*, and *β pleated s.*

secretory s. the simplest form of multicellular gland, consisting of secreting cells alone, e.g., the surface epithelium of the mammalian gastric mucosa.

shelf (shelf) a broad, flat surface, normal or abnormal, in the body.

buccal s. the surface of the mandible from the residual alveolar ridge or the alveolar ridge to the external oblique line in the region of the lower buccal vestibule; it is covered with cortical bone.

dental s. the shelflike epithelial invagination formed by the dental ridge, beneath which the dental papillae are formed.

palatal s., palatine s. lateral palatine process.

shel•lac (shə-lak′) a product of lac from India, produced on various plants by an insect, *Laccifer lacca* Kerr (Coccidae); sometimes used in dentistry and surgery, and in coating confections and medicinal tablets.

shen (shen) one of the basic substances that according to traditional Chinese medicine pervade the body, usually translated "spirit," encompassing both the mind of the individual and healthy mental and physical function.

Shen•ton line (arch) (shen′tən) [Edward Warren Hine *Shenton*, English radiologist, 1872–1955] see under *line*.

Shep•herd fracture (shep′ərd) [Francis John *Shepherd*, Canadian surgeon, 1851–1929] see under *fracture*.

Sher•man plate (shur′mən) [Harry Mitchell O'Neill *Sherman*, American surgeon, 1854–1921] see under *plate*.

Sher•ring•ton's law (sher′ing-tənz) [Sir Charles Scott *Sherrington*, British physiologist and Nobel prize winner, 1857–1952] see under *law*.

Shew•a•nel•la (shoo″ə-nel′ə) [James M. *Shewan*, Scottish microbiologist, 20th century] a genus of gram-negative bacteria of the family Alteromonadaceae, consisting of straight or curved rods that are motile by a single polar flagellum; organisms are facultatively anaerobic, chemoheterotrophic, and oxidase- and catalase-positive. Some species have been isolated from polymicrobial human infections. The type species is *S. putrefa′ciens*.

S. al′gae the species most commonly associated with human infection.

S. putrefa′ciens a ubiquitous, genetically heterogeneous species that is a cause of food spoilage and is infrequently associated with human disease.

SHH Sonic Hedgehog; see *SHH gene*, under *gene*.

shi•at•su (she-ot′soo) [Japanese "finger pressure"] a Japanese form of acupressure, in which pressure is applied by the practitioner, using the thumb, elbow, or knee, perpendicularly to the skin at acupoints, combined with passive stretching and rotation of the joints.

Shib•ley sign (shib′le) [Gerald Spencer *Shibley*, American physician, 1890–1981] see under *sign*.

shield (shēld) any protecting structure.

Buller s. a watch glass fitted over the unaffected eye to guard it from infection from the affected eye.

embryonic s. the double-layered disc from which the embryo proper develops; see *embryonic disc*, under *disc*.

eye s. a covering for the eyes to protect them from light or injury.

lead s. in radiology, a lead barrier for protecting personnel from radiation.

nipple s. a cover to protect the nipple of a nursing woman.

oral s. see under *screen*.

shift (shift) a change, as of position or status.

antigenic s. a sudden, major change in the antigenicity of a virus, seen especially in influenza viruses, resulting from the recombination of the genomes of two virus strains; it is associated with pandemics because hosts do not have immunity to the new strain. Cf. *antigenic drift*, under *drift*.

chloride s. the exchange of chloride (Cl^-) and bicarbonate (HCO_3^-) between the plasma and the red blood cells; it takes place whenever HCO_3^- is generated or decomposed within the red cells.

Doppler s. the magnitude of the change in frequency caused by the Doppler effect.

s. to the left an increase in the percentage of neutrophils that have only one or two lobes, seen in some bacterial infections. See *Arneth count*, under *count.*

Purkinje s. see under *phenomenon.*

s. to the right an increase in the percentage of neutrophils with 5 or more lobes, seen most often in cobalamine and folate deficiencies. See *Arneth count*, under *count.*

stage s. a change in stage of a case of cancer, usually referring to improvement (change to a lower stage); it may be due to treatment or to any of various other causes.

Shi·ga bacillus, toxin (she′gah) [K. *Shiga*, Japanese bacteriologist, 1871–1957] see *Shigella dysenteriae* type 1, and see under *toxin.*

Shi·gel·la (shĭ-gel′ə) [K. *Shiga*] a genus of gram-negative, facultatively anaerobic, rod-shaped bacteria of the family Enterobacteriaceae, consisting of nonmotile bacilli that cannot utilize citrate as a sole carbon source and that ferment carbohydrates with acid but no gas production. The genus consists of four species, differentiated by biochemical reactions: *S. dysenteriae* (subgroup A), *S. flexneri* (subgroup B), *S. boydii* (subgroup C), and *S. sonnei* (subgroup D). Their normal habitat is the intestinal tract of humans and other primates; all species cause bacillary dysentery and shigellosis. Phylogenetically, *Shigella* is a pathovar of *Escherichia coli*, but because of long use its treatment as a separate genus has been preserved. The type species is *S. dysente′riae.*

S. boy′dii a species that causes acute diarrhea, especially in tropical regions. It has 19 serovars, all of which ferment mannitol but not lactose.

S. dysente′riae a highly pathogenic species that causes severe bacillary dysentery; there are 15 serovars, none of which ferment lactose or mannitol. *S. dysenteriae* 1 is the classic Shiga bacillus and produces a potent neurotoxin.

S. flexne′ri a species that causes severe bacillary dysentery. It has six serovars and two variants (X and Y); type 2 produces an enterotoxin. The organisms ferment mannitol but not lactose. Called also *Flexner bacillus.*

S. son′nei a species that causes a mild but frequently encountered form of bacillary dysentery; there is a single serovar but two forms or phases, I (smooth colonies) and II (rough colonies), each with its own specific antigen.

shi·gel·la (shĭ-gel′ə) pl. *shigel′lae.* A bacterium of the genus *Shigella.*

shi·gel·lo·sis (shĭ′gə-lo′sis) any of the intestinal conditions produced by infection with species of *Shigella*, such as bacillary dysentery (see under *dysentery*).

shim (shim) in magnetic resonance imaging, adjustment of the magnetic field to correct lack of homogeneity.

shin (shin) 1. the crest or anterior edge of the tibia. 2. the anterior aspect of the lower limb below the knee.

bucked s's sore s's.

cucumber s. a tibia which is curved with the concavity forward.

saber s. a tibia with a marked anterior convexity as seen in congenital syphilis, yaws, and osteitis deformans.

sore s's periostitis of the large metacarpal or metatarsal bone of the horse.

shin·gles (shing′gəlz) [L. *cingulus*] herpes zoster.

shiv·er (shiv′ər) 1. a slight chill or tremor. 2. to tremble, as from a chill.

shiv·er·ing (shiv′ər-ing) involuntary trembling or quivering of the body caused by contraction or twitching of the muscles, a physiologic method of heat production in mammals.

SHML sinus histiocytosis with massive lymphadenopathy; see *Rosai-Dorfman disease*, under *disease.*

shock (shok) 1. a sudden disturbance of mental or physical equilibrium. 2. a condition of profound hemodynamic and metabolic disturbance characterized by failure of the circulatory system to maintain adequate perfusion of vital organs. It may result from inadequate blood volume (hypovolemic shock), inadequate cardiac function (cardiogenic shock), or inadequate vasomotor tone (neurogenic shock and septic shock). Called also *circulatory collapse.*

anaphylactic s. shock due to an allergic reaction; see *anaphylaxis.*

anaphylactoid s. see under *reaction.*

burn s. shock resulting from the loss of plasma into a burn wound.

cardiac s., cardiogenic s. shock resulting from primary failure of the heart in its pumping function, as in myocardial infarction, severe cardiomyopathy, or mechanical obstruction or compression of the heart; clinical characteristics are similar to those of hypovolemic shock.

circulatory s. shock (def. 2).

deferred s., delayed s. shock occurring a considerable time after the injury is received.

diastolic s. the cardiac impulse that strikes the palpating hand in early diastole.

electric s. the immediate effects produced by the passage of an electric current through any part of the body, e.g., painful stimulation of nerves or tetanic contractions of muscles.

endotoxic s., endotoxin s. septic shock due to release of endotoxins by gram-negative bacteria.

hematogenic s. hypovolemic s.

hemorrhagic s. hypovolemic shock resulting from hemorrhage.

histamine s. a reaction resembling anaphylactic shock produced in experimental animals by histamine injection.

hypoglycemic s. 1. insulin s. 2. a hypoglycemic reaction resulting from severe adrenocortical insufficiency, especially during fasting.

hypovolemic s. shock resulting from insufficient blood volume for the maintenance of adequate cardiac output, blood pressure, and tissue perfusion. Without modification the term refers to absolute hypovolemic shock caused by acute hemorrhage or excessive fluid loss. Relative hypovolemic shock refers to a situation in which the blood volume is normal but insufficient because of widespread vasodilation as in neurogenic shock or septic shock. Clinical characteristics include hypotension; hyperventilation; cold, clammy, cyanotic skin; a weak and rapid pulse; oliguria; and mental confusion, combativeness, or anxiety. Called also *hematogenic* or *oligemic s.*

insulin s. a hypoglycemic reaction to overdosage of insulin, a skipped meal, or strenuous exercise in an insulin-dependent diabetic; early symptoms are tremor, irritability, dizziness, cool moist skin, hunger, and tachycardia; if untreated it can progress to coma (see *diabetic coma*) and convulsions. Called also *hypoglycemic s.*

irreversible s. a condition in which the changes produced cannot be corrected by treatment, and death is inevitable.

neurogenic s. shock resulting from neurogenic vasodilation, which can be produced by cerebral trauma or hemorrhage, spinal cord injury, deep general or spinal anesthesia, or toxic central nervous system depression.

oligemic s. hypovolemic s.

osmotic s. exposure of membrane-bound stuctures to an extremely hypotonic environment, which results in rupture of the membrane and loss of contents; used to lyse cells and organelles.

pleural s. a hypotensive condition sometimes following thoracentesis, characterized by cyanosis, pallor, dilated pupils, and disturbance of pulse and respiration.

secondary s. shock appearing one or more hours after injury; delayed shock.

septic s. shock associated with overwhelming infection, usually infection with gram-negative bacteria, although it may be produced by other bacteria, viruses, fungi, or protozoa. It is thought to result from the action of endotoxins or other products of the infectious agent on the vascular system causing large volumes of blood to be sequestered in capillaries and veins; activation of the complement and kinin systems and the release of histamine, cytokines, prostaglandins, and other mediators may be involved. Clinical characteristics include initial chills and fever, warm flushed skin, increased cardiac output, and a lesser degree of hypotension than with hypovolemic shock; if therapy is ineffective, it may progress to the clinical picture associated with hypovolemic shock.

serum s. anaphylactic shock resulting from administration of foreign serum to a sensitized individual.

shell s. former term for combat-related posttraumatic stress disorder; now used colloquially.

spinal s. the loss of spinal reflexes after injury of the spinal cord, which affects the muscles innervated by the cord segments situated below the site of the lesion.

surgical s. shock that occurs during or after surgical operation.

testicular s. the effect of a sharp blow upon the testes.

traumatic s. any shock produced by trauma.

vasogenic s. shock caused by marked vasodilation.

Shope fibroma, papilloma (shōp) [Richard Edwin *Shope*, American pathologist, 1902–1966] see *rabbit fibroma*, under *fibroma*, and *rabbit papilloma*, under *papilloma.*

short·sight·ed·ness (short′sīt-əd-nis) myopia.

shot-com·pres·sor (shot-kəm-pres′ər) see under *compressor.*

shot·ty (shot′e) like shot; resembling the pellets used in shotgun cartridges; usually applied to mildly to moderately enlarged collections of lymph nodes.

shoul·der (shōl′dər) the junction of the upper limb and trunk; also that part of the trunk that is bounded at the back by the scapula. See also *regio deltoidea.*

drop s. depression of one shoulder below the level of the other.

frozen s. popular but misleading term for *adhesive capsulitis.*

loose s. a condition seen in progressive muscular atrophy in which, when attempts are made to lift the patient by grasping the upper arms, the arms move up but the trunk remains behind.

slipped s. suprascapular paralysis.

shoul•der-blade (shōl′dər-blād) scapula.

shoul•der slip (shōl′dər slip) suprascapular paralysis.

Shoul•dice repair (shōl′dīs) [Edward Earl *Shouldice*, Canadian surgeon, 1890–1965] see under *repair.*

show (sho) 1. a tiny amount or appearance of something. 2. bloody s.

bloody s. vaginal discharge of blood-tinged mucus, usually meaning that the cervix has begun to dilate and the onset of labor is imminent.

Shprint•zen's syndrome (shprint′sən) [Robert J. *Shprintzen*, American geneticist, 20th century] velocardiofacial syndrome.

Shprint•zen-Gold•berg syndrome (shprint′sən gōld′bərg) [Robert J. *Shprintzen;* Rosalie B. *Goldberg*, American geneticist, 20th century] velocardiofacial syndrome.

Shrap•nell membrane (shrap′nəl) [Henry Jones *Shrapnell*, English anatomist and Army surgeon, 1761–1841] pars flaccida membranae tympanicae.

shrink•age (shring′kəj) a reduction in size, extent, or quantity.

casting s. the decrease in volume of a metal dental cast as it cools and hardens.

polymerization s. the decrease in volume of dental resin as polymerization occurs.

shud•der (shud′ər) 1. an involuntary or convulsive quiver or shake. 2. in a pulse tracing, the graphic representation of a thrill.

carotid s. vibrations seen at the crest of the carotid pulse tracing in aortic stenosis; used also of the underlying thrill felt on palpation of the carotid artery.

Shul•man syndrome (shool′mən) [Lawrence Edward *Shulman*, American rheumatologist, born 1919] eosinophilic fasciitis.

shunt (shunt) 1. to turn to one side; to divert or bypass. 2. a passage or anastomosis between two natural channels, especially between blood vessels; it may be formed either physiologically (e.g., to bypass a thrombosis), or by a structural anomaly. 3. a surgically created anastomosis. 4. the operation of forming such an anastomosis.

arteriovenous s. 1. anastomosis arteriolovenularis. 2. a U-shaped plastic tube inserted between an artery and a vein (usually between the radial artery and cephalic vein), bypassing the capillary network, a formerly common means of arteriovenous access.

Blalock-Taussig s. see under *operation.*

Buselmeier s. a modification of the Quinton-Scribner shunt in which the Silastic tube is implanted under the skin, with two ports projecting through the skin.

cardiovascular s. an abnormality of blood flow between the sides of the heart or between the systemic and pulmonary circulation; see *left-to-right s.* and *right-to-left s.*

cerebrospinal fluid s. a shunt for draining off cerebrospinal fluid in cases of hydrocephalus, such as a ventricular shunt.

Denver s. a modification of the LeVeen peritoneovenous shunt that includes a manual pump mechanism for ascitic fluid.

gastrorenal s. an abnormal anastomosis between gastric varices and the left renal vein.

Glenn s. see under *operation.*

hexose monophosphate s. pentose phosphate pathway.

left-to-right s. diversion of blood from the left side of the heart to the right side or from the systemic to the pulmonary circulation through an anomalous opening such as a septal defect or patent ductus arteriosus.

LeVeen s. peritoneovenous s.

Linton s. splenorenal s.

lumboperitoneal s. a communication between the lumbar subarachnoid space and the peritoneum by means of a plastic tube with an in-line pressure-flow regulator; created to permit drainage of cerebrospinal fluid for relief of communicating hydrocephalus.

mesocaval s. a portosystemic shunt between the superior mesenteric vein and the inferior vena cava, done for the treatment of esophageal varices in portal hypertension.

pentose s. pentose phosphate pathway.

peritoneovenous s. a surgically implanted subcutaneous plastic tube for continuous shunting of ascites fluid from the peritoneal cavity to the jugular vein; a pressure-activated valve buried in the abdominal wall ensures one-way flow.

portacaval s. a portosystemic shunt between the portal vein and vena cava, done for treatment of portal hypertension.

portosystemic s. a surgically created shunt that connects the portal and systemic circulations, such as a mesocaval, portacaval, or splenorenal shunt, for treatment of portal hypertension. Called also *portosystemic anastomosis.*

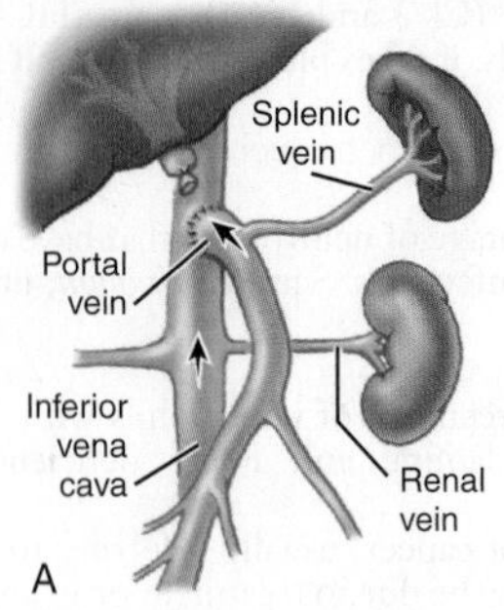

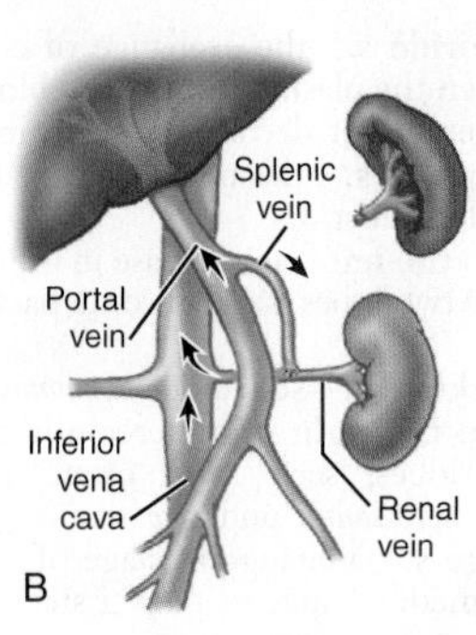

■ Shunts diverting portal venous blood flow from the liver. *(A)*, Portacaval shunt; *(B)*, splenorenal shunt.

postcaval s. portacaval s.

Potts s. see under *operation.*

pulmonary s. movement of blood from the venous circulation to the arterial circulation without participating in gas exchange, resulting in hypoxemia.

Quinton-Scribner s. an arteriovenous shunt formerly widely used for hemodialysis, consisting of an external cannula composed of a U-shaped Silastic tube with Teflon tips, connecting the radial artery and the cephalic vein.

reversed s., right-to-left s. diversion of blood from the right side of the heart to the left side or from the pulmonary to the systemic circulation through an anomalous opening one as a septal defect or patent ductus arteriosus.

Scribner s. Quinton-Scribner s.

splenorenal s. after removal of the spleen, anastomosis of the splenic vein to the left renal vein; done for the treatment of esophageal varices in portal hypertension. Called also *Linton s.*

splenorenal s., distal anastomosis of the distal splenic vein to the inferior vena cava with preservation of the spleen; done for the treatment of esophageal varices in portal hypertension. Called also *Warren s.*

Thomas s. an arteriovenous shunt for hemodialysis, consisting of a Silastic cannula with Dacron cuffs inserted between the femoral artery and femoral vein.

Torkildsen s. ventriculocisternal s.

transjugular intrahepatic portosystemic s. (TIPS) an artificial percutaneous shunt between the hepatic and portal veins within the liver with placement of an expandable stent in the tract created; it is done by a transjugular route under radiologic guidance for treatment of bleeding esophageal varices.

ventricular s. any of the shunts that drain cerebral ventricles to relieve hydrocephalus.

ventriculoatrial s. an artificial communication between a cerebral ventricle and a cardiac atrium, done with a plastic tube with an in-line pressure-flow regulator, to permit drainage of cerebrospinal fluid for relief of hydrocephalus.

ventriculocisternal s. a formerly common procedure in which a communication was surgically established between a lateral ventricle and the cisterna magna for drainage of cerebrospinal fluid in hydrocephalus. Called also *Torkildsen s.* or *operation* and *ventriculocisternostomy.*

ventriculoperitoneal s. the most common shunt for relief of hydrocephalus, consisting of an artificial channel between a cerebral ventricle and the peritoneum made with plastic tubing.

ventriculopleural s. a communication between a cerebral ventricle and the pleural cavity by means of a plastic tube with an in-line pressure-flow regulator, done for the relief of hydrocephalus.

ventriculovenous s. an artificially created communication between a cerebral ventricle and the internal jugular vein by means of a plastic tube

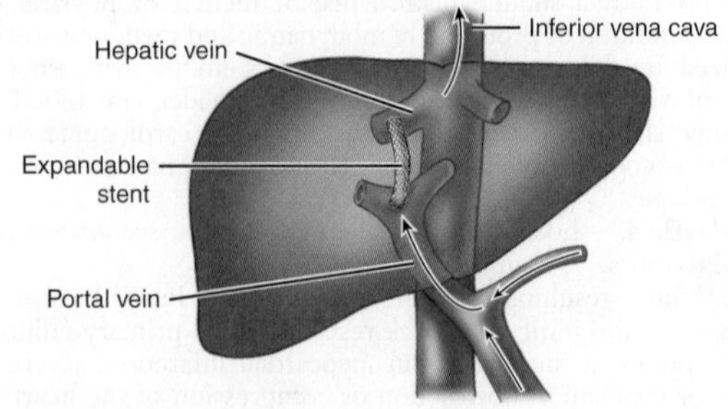

■ Transjugular intrahepatic portosystemic shunt.

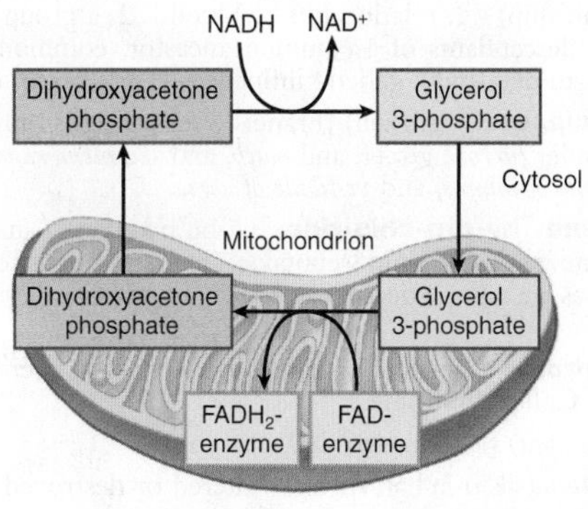

■ Glycerol phosphate shuttle.

with an in-line pressure-flow regulator, permitting drainage of cerebrospinal fluid for relief of hydrocephalus.

Warren s. distal splenorenal s.

Waterston s. see under *operation.*

shut·tle (shut′əl) [A.S. *scytel* a dart] in biochemistry, a mechanism for the transport of electrons or an organic group, or both, across a membrane.

glycerol phosphate s. a cyclic mechanism for transferring electrons from cytosolic NADH to the mitochondrial electron transport chain and thus to oxygen, acting by means of enzyme-catalyzed redox reactions that interconvert glycerol 3-phosphate and dihydroxyacetone phosphate. It occurs primarily in white fibers of striated muscle and nervous tissue. See illustration.

malate-aspartate s. a mechanism for transferring electrons into mitochondria from the cytosol of red fibers of skeletal muscle, heart, and the brain, involving cytosolic and mitochondrial forms of the enzymes malate dehydrogenase and aspartate transaminase, and two transmembrane carriers. Electrons from cytosolic NADH are used to reduce oxaloacetate to malate, which enters the mitochondrial matrix and donates electrons to NAD^+, becoming reoxidized to oxaloacetate. To return to the cytosol, oxaloacetate is first transaminated to form aspartate, which can traverse the membrane; once in the cytosol it is deaminated to oxaloacetate.

Shwach·man syndrome (shwahk′mən) [Harry *Shwachman*, American pediatrician, 1910–1986] see under *syndrome.*

Shwach·man-Di·a·mond syndrome (shwahk′mən di′ə-mond) [H. *Shwachman;* Louis Klein *Diamond*, American pediatrician, 1902–1999] see under *syndrome.*

Shwartz·man reaction (phenomenon) (shwahrts′mən) [Gregory *Shwartzman*, Russian bacteriologist in the United States, 1896–1965] see under *reaction.*

Shy-Dra·ger syndrome (shi′ dra′gər) [George Milton *Shy*, American neurologist, 1919–1967; Glenn A. *Drager*, American neurologist, 1917–1967] see under *syndrome.*

Shy-Ma·gee syndrome (shi′ mə-gee′) [G.M. *Shy;* Kenneth Raymond *Magee*, American physician, born 1926] central core disease.

SI 1. Système International d'Unités, or International System of Units. See under *unit.* 2. stimulation index; see *lymphocyte proliferation test*, under *test.*

Si silicon.

SIAD syndrome of inappropriate antidiuresis.

SIADH syndrome of inappropriate antidiuretic hormone.

si·al·a·den (si-al′ə-dən) a salivary gland.

si·al·ad·e·nec·to·my (si″əl-ad″ə-nek′tə-me) sialoadenectomy.

si·al·ad·e·ni·tis (si″əl-ad″ə-ni′tis) inflammation of a salivary gland.

chronic nonspecific s. an inflammatory disease of the major salivary glands, characterized by intermittent swelling that may lead to fibrous degeneration, resulting from obstruction of the salivary ducts by calculi, foreign bodies, tumors, or scar formation, with subsequent bacterial invasion.

si·al·ad·e·nog·ra·phy (si″əl-ad″ə-nog′rə-fe) radiography of the salivary glands and ducts.

si·al·ad·e·no·ma (si″əl-ad″ə-no′mə) a benign tumor of the salivary glands.

s. papilli′ferum a benign exophytic papillomatous lesion of the salivary glands, usually occurring in the hard palate or buccal mucosa of male adults; it appears to originate from the superficial portion of the salivary gland excretory duct.

si·al·ad·e·nop·athy (si″əl-ad″ən-op′ə-the) [*sial-* + *adeno-* + *-pathy*] sialadenosis.

benign lymphoepithelial s. see under *lesion.*

si·al·ad·e·no·sis (si″əl-ad″ə-no′sis) [*sial-* + *adenosis*] a disease of a salivary gland; see also *sialadenitis.* Called also *sialadenopathy.*

si·al·ad·e·not·o·my (si″əl-ad″ə-not′ə-me) sialoadenotomy.

si·a·la·gog·ic (si″ə-lə-goj′ik) promoting the flow of saliva.

si·al·a·gogue (si-al′ə-gog) [*sial-* + *-agogue*] an agent that promotes the flow of saliva. Called also *ptyalagogue.*

si·a·late (si′ə-lāt) any salt of a sialic acid.

si·al·ec·ta·sia (si″əl-ek-ta′zhə) dilatation of a salivary duct.

si·al·en·dos·co·py (si″əl-en-dos′kə-pe) endoscopic examination of the salivary ducts and glands.

si·al·ic (si-al′ik) [Gr. *sialikos*] 1. pertaining to the saliva. 2. pertaining to sialic acid.

si·al·ic ac·id (si-al′ik) an *N*-acyl derivative of neuraminic acid, e.g., *N*-acetylneuraminic acid; sialic acids occur in many polysaccharides, glycoproteins, and glycolipids in animals and bacteria.

si·al·i·dase (si-al′ĭ-dās) neuraminidase.

si·al·i·do·sis (si-al″ĭ-do′sis) an autosomal recessive lysosomal storage disorder caused by mutation in the *NEU1* gene (locus: 6p21.3), which encodes neuraminidase. It is often subclassified on the basis of clinical manifestations.

s. type I the milder form of sialidosis, lacking dysmorphic features and having onset usually in the second decade; it is characterized by myoclonus, ocular cherry red spot with progressive loss of visual acuity, and storage of sialyloligosaccharides.

s. type II the more severe form of sialidosis, having the characteristics of the milder form and additionally characterized by somatic abnormalities, coarse facies, and dysostosis multiplex. It occurs as several variants of increasing severity with earlier age of onset; that of infantile onset is characterized also by visceromegaly and mental retardation, and the congenital form is additionally characterized by ascites, hydrops fetalis, facial edema, inguinal hernias, and early death.

si·a·line (si′ə-lin) [L. *sialinus*] salivary.

si·al·ism (si′əl-iz-əm) [Gr. *sialismos*] ptyalism.

si·al·is·mus (si″əl-iz′məs) ptyalism.

si·a·li·tis (si″ə-li′tis) 1. sialadenitis. 2 inflammation of a salivary duct.

sial(o)- [Gr. *sialon* saliva] a combining form denoting relationship to *(a)* saliva or the salivary glands or *(b)* sialic acid.

si·a·lo·ad·e·nec·to·my (si″ə-lo-ad″ə-nek′tə-me) [*sialo-* + *aden-* + *-ectomy*] excision of a salivary gland.

si·a·lo·ad·e·ni·tis (si″ə-lo-ad″ə-ni′tis) sialadenitis.

si·a·lo·ad·e·not·o·my (si″ə-lo-ad″ə-not′ə-me) [*sialo-* + *adeno-* + *-tomy*] incision and drainage of a salivary gland.

si·alo·aer·oph·a·gy (si″ə-lo-ār-of′ə-je) [*sialo-* + *aero-* + *-phagy*] excessive swallowing of saliva and air.

si·alo·an·gi·ec·ta·sis (si″ə-lo-an″je-ek′tə-sis) [*sialo-* + *angi-* + *ectasis*] dilatation of the salivary ducts.

si·alo·an·gi·itis (si″ə-lo-an″je-i′tis) inflammation of the salivary ducts. Called also *sialodochitis* and *sialoductitis.*

si·alo·an·gi·og·ra·phy (si″ə-lo-an″je-og′rə-fe) radiography of the ducts of the salivary glands after injection of radiopaque material.

si·alo·an·gi·tis (si″ə-lo-an-ji′tis) sialoangiitis.

si·alo·cele (si′ə-lo-sēl″) [*sialo-* + *-cele*[1]] a salivary cyst or tumor.

si·a·lo·da·cry·o·ad·e·ni·tis (si″ə-lo-dak″re-o-ad″ə-ni′tis) severe inflammation of the salivary and lacrimal glands in rats, caused by a coronavirus. Characteristics include exophthalmos, facial swelling, and redness around the eyes. It is usually self-limiting, but severe forms can lead to blindness.

si·alo·do·chi·tis (si″ə-lo-do-ki′tis) sialoangiitis.

si·alo·do·cho·plas·ty (si″ə-lo-do′ko-plas″te) [*sialo-* + Gr. *dochos* receptacle + *-plasty*] plastic operation on the salivary ducts.

si·alo·duc·ti·tis (si″ə-lo-dək-ti′tis) sialoangiitis.

si·a·lo·en·dos·co·py (si″ə-lo-en-dos′kə-pe) sialendoscopy.

si·a·log·e·nous (si″ə-loj′ə-nəs) [*sialo-* + *-genous*] producing saliva.

si·alo·gly·co·con·ju·gate (si-al″o-gli″ko-kon-ju′gət) a compound comprising a sialic acid residue in glycosidic linkage with a glycoconjugate; most of the sialic acid in body fluids and tissues is so complexed.

si·alo·gly·co·pro·tein (si″ə-lo-gli″ko-pro′tēn) sialoprotein.

si·alo·gog·ic (si″ə-lo-goj′ik) sialagogic.

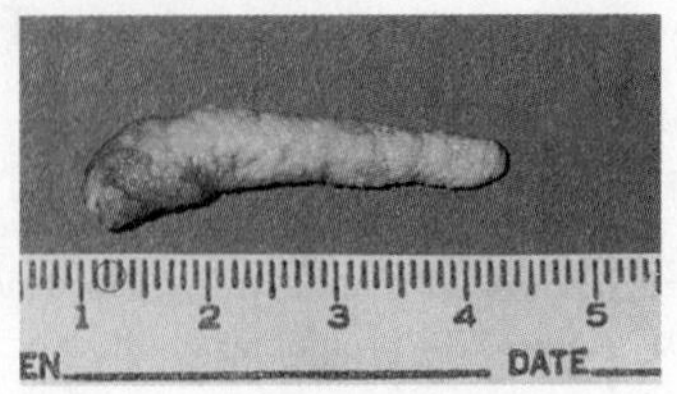

■ Sialolith.

si•alo•gogue (si-al′o-gog) sialagogue.

si•alo•gram (si-al′o-gram) [*sialo-* + *-gram*] a radiograph produced by sialography.

si•alo•graph (si-al′o-graf) sialogram.

si•a•log•ra•phy (si″ə-log′rə-fe) [*sialo-* + *-graphy*] radiographic demonstration of the salivary ducts by means of the injection of substances opaque to x-radiation.

si•alo•lith (si-al′o-lith) [*sialo-* + *-lith*] a calcareous concretion or calculus in the salivary ducts or glands, involving most commonly the submaxillary gland and its duct, less frequently the parotid and sublingual glands and their ducts, and seldom the minor salivary glands. Called also *salivary calculus* and *salivary stone.*

si•alo•li•thi•a•sis (si″ə-lo-lĭ-thi′ə-sis) [*sialo-* + *lithiasis*] a condition characterized by the presence of sialoliths. Called also *ptyalolithiasis.*

si•alo•li•thot•o•my (si″ə-lo-lĭ-thot′ə-me) [*sialolith* + *-tomy*] incision of a salivary gland or duct for the removal of a calculus.

si•al•o•ma (si″ə-lo′mə) a salivary tumor.

si•alo•meta•pla•sia (si″ə-lo-met″ə-pla′zhə) metaplasia of the salivary glands.

necrotizing s. a benign inflammatory condition of the minor salivary glands, simulating mucoepidermoid and squamous cell carcinoma. Histological findings usually show lobular necrosis and ductal and glandular metaplasia.

si•alo•mu•cin (si″ə-lo-mu′sin) a mucin whose carbohydrate groups contain a sialic acid.

si•alo•pha•gia (si′ə-lo-fa′jə) [*sialo-* + *-phagia*] excessive swallowing of saliva.

si•alo•pro•tein (si″ə-lo-pro′tēn) a glycoprotein that contains sialic acid as one of the carbohydrates. Called also *sialoglycoprotein.*

bone s. an acidic glycoprotein of the bone matrix, synthesized by a number of cells associated with the skeleton, that binds osteocyte integrins to the bone.

si•a•lor•rhea (si″ə-lo-re′ə) [*sialo-* + *-rrhea*] ptyalism.

si•a•los•che•sis (si″ə-los′kə-sis) [*sialo-* + *-schesis*] suppression of the salivary secretion.

si•a•lo•se•mei•ol•o•gy (si″ə-lo-se″mi-ol′ə-je) [*sialo-* + *semeiology*] analysis of the saliva as a means of determining the physiologic status of the patient, especially in regard to metabolic processes.

si•alo•sis (si″ə-lo′sis) [*sial-* + *-osis*] 1. the flow of saliva. 2. ptyalism.

si•alo•ste•no•sis (si″ə-lo-stə-no′sis) [*sialo-* + *stenosis*] stenosis, or narrowing, of a salivary duct.

si•alo•sy•rinx (si″ə-lo-sir′inks) [*sialo-* + *syrinx*] 1. a salivary fistula. 2. a syringe for washing out the salivary ducts, or a drainage tube for the salivary ducts.

si•al•yl•ol•i•go•sac•cha•ride (si-al″əl-ol″ĭ-go-sak′ə-rīd) any of the oligosaccharides to which are attached one or more sialic acid residues; they accumulate when neuraminidase (sialidase) activity is deficient, as in sialidosis and galactosialidosis.

si•al•yl•trans•fer•ase (si-al″əl-trans′fər-ās) a term used in the recommended names of some enzymes of the transferase class that catalyze the formation of sialylglycoconjugates via transfer of the sialic acid group from CMP to one of several glycoconjugate acceptors.

sib (sib) [A.S. *sib* kin] 1. a blood relative; one of a group of persons, all of whom are descendants of a common ancestor. 2. sibling.

sib•i•lant (sib′ĭ-lənt) [L. *sibilans* hissing] 1. having a shrill, hissing, or whistling character. 2. a consonant sound produced with a hiss, such as *s, sh, z,* or *zh.*

sib•ling (sib′ling) [A.S. *sib* kin + *ling* a diminutive] any of two or more offspring of the same parents; a brother or sister. Called also *sib.*

si•bor•ox•ime (si″bo-rok′sēm) a compound which, complexed with technetium 99m, constitutes a BATO that has been used in brain imaging; see table at *technetium.*

sib•ship (sib′ship) 1. relationship by blood. 2. a group of persons, all of whom are descendants of a common ancestor, commonly used as the basis of study to determine genetic influences. 3. a group of siblings.

Sib•son fascia, etc. (sib′sən) [Francis *Sibson,* English physician, 1814–1876] see under *furrow, groove,* and *notch,* and see *membrana suprapleuralis, musculus scalenus minimus,* and *vestibule of aorta.*

si•bu•tra•mine hy•dro•chlo•ride (sĭ-bu′trə-mēn) an inhibitor of norepinephrine and serotonin reuptake, structurally related to amphetamine, used as an anorectic in the management of obesity; withdrawn from market.

Si•card syndrome (se-kahr′) [Jean Athanase *Sicard,* French neurologist, 1872–1929] Collet syndrome.

sic•cant (sik′ənt) [L. *siccare* to dry] drying.

sic•co•la•bile (sik″o-la′bəl, -la′bīl) altered or destroyed by drying.

sic•co•sta•bile (sik″o-sta′bəl, -sta′bīl) not altered by drying.

sic•cus (sik′əs) [L.] dry.

sick (sik) 1. not in good health; afflicted by disease; ill. 2. affected with nausea.

sick bay (sik ba) hospital and dispensary quarters on a naval vessel or station.

sick•le•mia (sik-le′me-ə) sickle cell anemia.

sick•ling (sik′ling) the development of sickle cells in the blood, as in sickle cell anemia.

sick•ness (sik′nis) disease.

acute mountain s. mountain sickness that appears a few hours after exposure to high altitude, characterized by fatigue, dizziness, breathlessness, headache, nausea, vomiting, insomnia, impairment of mental capacity, and prostration. Called also *Acosta disease.*

aerial s. altitude s.

African horse s. an infectious disease of horses and mules caused by orbivirus; it is endemic in most of sub-Saharan Africa but has also been found in Europe and the Middle East. Four types are distinguished: the *respiratory type* (fever, dyspnea, copious fluid discharge, and usually a fatal inhalation pneumonia), the *cardiac type* (edema of the head with widespread petechiae, often but not always fatal), the *mixed cardiac and respiratory type,* and a mild type called *horse sickness fever.* Called also *pestis equorum* and *equine plague.*

African sleeping s. African trypanosomiasis.

air s. airsickness.

altitude s. the condition resulting from difficulty in adjusting to diminished oxygen pressure at high altitudes. It may take the form of mountain sickness (q.v.), high-altitude pulmonary edema, or cerebral edema. Called also *high-altitude s.*

athletes' s. weakness, blurred vision, nausea, and headache, following a short period of intense physical exercise.

aviation s. airsickness.

balloon s. altitude sickness occurring during balloon ascents.

bay s. Haff disease.

bush s. enzootic marasmus in New Zealand due to cobalt deficiency.

caisson s. decompression s.

car s. carsickness.

chronic mountain s. mountain sickness characterized by loss of tolerance to hypoxia in a previously acclimatized person, with secondary polycythemia. It occurs in two types: an *emphysematous* type in which dyspnea is the dominant symptom and bronchitis, laryngitis, and cyanosis are often present; and an *erythremic* type in which there is an erythremic color that becomes cyanotic on mild exertion, with fatigue, headache, episodic stupor, paresthesias, anorexia, nausea, vomiting, and decreased visual acuity. Called also *Andes disease* and *Monge disease.*

compressed-air s. decompression s.

decompression s. joint pains, respiratory manifestations, skin lesions, and neurologic signs occurring in aviators who ascend too quickly to high altitudes or in persons who have been breathing compressed air in caissons or diving apparatus if air pressure is reduced too rapidly, because gases that were dissolved in the blood under the high pressure suddenly go out of solution and form bubbles that go into the capillaries and interfere with blood flow. Called also *caisson s.* or *disease, compressed-air s., divers' palsy,* and *divers' paralysis.*

East African sleeping s. see under *trypanosomiasis.*

gall s. anaplasmosis.

Gambian horse s. a fatal type of nagana seen in horses throughout central Africa, caused by *Trypanosoma congolense.*

Gambian sleeping s. West African trypanosomiasis.

grass s. a usually fatal disease of horses occurring after they have been put to graze on grass, usually between May and July; characteristics include dysphagia, severe diarrhea, dehydration, interrupted peristalsis, and priapism. It was first observed in Scotland but has now spread across northern Europe and elsewhere. Called also *grass disease.*

green tobacco s. a transient, recurrent form of nicotine poisoning seen in tobacco harvesters, caused by absorption of dissolved nicotine from wet tobacco leaves through unprotected skin; symptoms include headache, dizziness, vomiting, and prostration.
high-altitude s. altitude s.
horse s. see *African horse s.* and *Gambian horse s.*
Jamaican vomiting s. a type of poisoning seen in Jamaica and nearby areas of the West Indies, due to ingestion of damaged or unripe fruit of the akee tree *(Blighia sapida)*, which contains the toxins hypoglycine A and B; characteristics include vomiting of acute onset followed by convulsions, coma, and often death. Called also *akee poisoning.*
lambing s. a condition of ewes almost identical with milk fever of cows.
laughing s. pseudobulbar paralysis.
milk s. acute, often fatal poisoning in humans who drink milk, or eat milk products or meat, from cattle or sheep that were poisoned by eating plants containing tremetol (see *trembles*); the human disease is marked by weakness, anorexia, vomiting, constipation, and sometimes muscular tremors. Called also *milk poisoning.*
morning s. a type of nausea seen in women early in pregnancy; called also *emesis gravidarum, nausea gravidarum,* and *vomiting of pregnancy.*
motion s. sickness caused by motion experienced in any kind of travel, such as sea sickness, train sickness, car sickness, and air sickness.
mountain s. high altitude sickness caused by exposure to altitude high enough to cause hypoxia, occurring as a result of decreased atmospheric pressure with consequent lowering of arterial oxygen content. It occurs as acute, subacute, and chronic forms. The subacute and chronic forms can be cured by descent to a lower altitude. Called also *mountain disease.*
radiation s. a condition resulting from exposure to a whole-body dose of over 1 gray of ionizing radiation, characterized by the symptoms of the acute radiation syndrome (see under *syndrome*). Its severity varies with the dose level.
railroad s. transit tetany.
Rhodesian sleeping s. East African trypanosomiasis.
salt s. enzootic marasmus in Florida.
sea s. seasickness.
serum s. a hypersensitivity reaction to the administration of foreign serum or serum proteins characterized by fever, urticaria, arthralgia, edema, and lymphadenopathy. It is caused by the formation of circulating antigen-antibody complexes that are deposited in tissues and trigger tissue injury mediated by complement and polymorphonuclear leukocytes. Serum sickness is classed with the Arthus reaction and other immune complex diseases as a type III hypersensitivity reaction (Gell and Coombs classification). Although serum sickness is now rare because of the replacement of most animal-derived antisera with human immune globulins, an identical illness *(serum sickness–like reaction* or *syndrome)* can be produced by hypersensitivity reactions to penicillin and other drugs.
sleeping s. 1. African trypanosomiasis. 2. any disease characterized by increasing drowsiness and lethargy. Some are caused by protozoa, such as African trypanosomiasis; others are viral infections, such as St. Louis encephalitis and eastern, western, and Venezuelan equine encephalomyelitis.
space s. space adaptation syndrome.
stiff s. bovine ephemeral fever.
subacute mountain s. a type of mountain sickness that is milder than the chronic form and similar clinically to the acute form except for being persistent and amenable to cure by a descent in altitude.
sweating s. a febrile, tickborne illness affecting African cattle, especially calves, due to a toxin produced by *Hyalomma truncatum,* and characterized by the presence of moist eczematous lesions of the mucous membranes. Called also *tick toxicosis.*
three-day s. bovine ephemeral fever.
turning s. an unusual form of bovine theileriasis in which *Theileria parva* invades the central nervous system, causing either acute attacks of spinning followed by unconsciousness or chronic circling and incoordination.
veld s., veldt s. heartwater.
vomiting s. Jamaican vomiting s.
West African sleeping s. see under *trypanosomiasis.*
x-ray s. radiation s.

Sid blood group (sid) [from part of the name of the English propositus first reported on in the 1960's] see under *blood group.*

s.i.d. [L.] sem'el in di'e (once a day); written also *semel in d.*

side (sīd) the lateral (right or left) portion or aspect of the body, a part, or a structure. See also *latus* (2).
balancing s. the segment of a denture or dental arch on the side opposite to that toward which the mandible is moved. The term pertains to occlusion and bears no relation to masticatory activity. Called also *nonfunctioning s.*
dominant s. the half of the body in which a person is stronger; writing and eating are usually done with the hand on the dominant side. See also *handedness* and *laterality.*

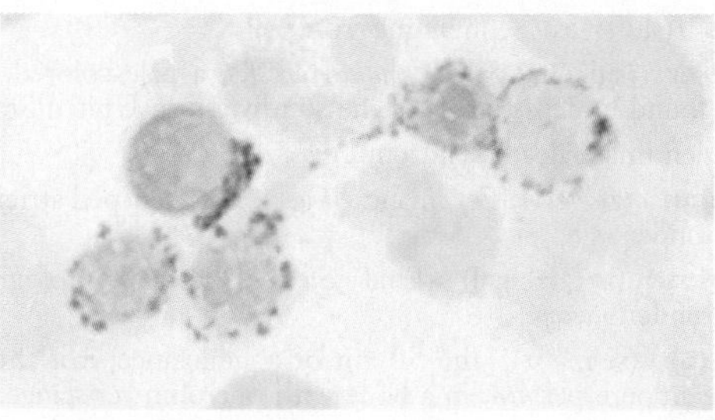

■ Ringed sideroblasts (iron stain, bone marrow).

functioning s. working s.
nonfunctioning s. balancing s.
working s. the segment of a denture or dental arch on the same side as that toward which the mandible is moved. The term pertains to occlusion and bears no relation to masticatory activity. Called also *functioning s.*

side•bone (sīd'bōn) a condition of horses marked by ossification of the lateral cartilages of the third phalanx of the foot.

sid•er•in•uria (sid″ər-ĭ-nu're-ə) [*sidero-* + *-uria*] excretion of iron in the urine, such as in hemosiderinuria.

sider(o)- [Gr. *sidēros* iron] a combining form denoting relationship to iron.

sid•ero•blast (sid'ər-o-blast″) a normoblast that contains granules of iron in the form of ferritin in its cytoplasm and stains with Prussian blue.
ringed s. an abnormal sideroblast containing many iron granules in its mitochondria in a ring shape around the periphery of the nucleus, as seen in sideroblastic anemia.

sid•ero•cyte (sid'ər-o-sīt″) an erythrocyte containing granules of ferritin in its cytoplasm.

sid•ero•der•ma (sid″ər-o-dur'mə) bronzed coloration of the skin from the deposition of iron derived from degenerated hemoglobin.

sid•ero•fi•bro•sis (sid″ər-o-fi-bro'sis) fibrosis of the spleen marked by iron-containing deposits.

sid•ero•my•cin (sid″ər-o-mi'sin) any of a class of antibiotics structurally related to hydroxamic acid that inhibit bacterial growth by interfering with iron uptake. Sideromycins are synthesized by certain species of actinomycetes.

sid•ero•pe•nia (sid″ər-o-pe'ne-ə) [*sidero-* + *-penia*] iron deficiency.
siderope'nic *adj*

sid•ero•phage (sid'ər-o-fāj″) a macrophage laden with phagocytosed iron-containing particles.

sid•ero•phil (sid'ər-o-fil″) 1. siderophilous. 2. a siderophilous tissue or structure.

sid•er•oph•il•in (sid″ər-of'ĭ-lin) transferrin.

sid•er•oph•i•lous (sid″ər-of'ĭ-ləs) [*sidero-* + Gr. *philein* to love] having a tendency to absorb iron.

sid•ero•phore (sid'ər-o-for″) [*sidero-* + *-phore*] 1. a substance that binds iron. 2. a macrophage containing hemosiderin. 3. a compound produced by certain species of mycobacteria and enterobacteria that chelates iron and facilitates its uptake by the cell.

sid•ero•scope (sid'ər-o-skōp) [*sidero-* + *-scope*] a magnet or other appliance for determining the presence of metallic iron as a foreign body in the eye.

sid•er•o•sil•i•co•sis (sid″ər-o-sil″ĭ-ko'sis) a type of mixed dust pneumoconiosis consisting of siderosis with silicosis, due to the inhalation of dust containing particles of iron ore and silica. Called also *silicosiderosis.*

sid•er•o•sis (sid″ər-o'sis) 1. a benign type of pneumoconiosis caused by the inhalation of iron particles; it usually becomes serious only when combined with silicosis (see *siderosilicosis*). Called also *pneumoconiosis siderotica* and *pulmonary s.* 2. hyperferremia. 3. hemosiderosis.
Bantu s. African iron overload.
s. bul'bi the deposit of an iron pigment within the eyeball.
s. conjuncti'vae a rust brown or yellowish discoloration of the conjunctiva due to the presence of an iron foreign body; the condition may also be seen in hemochromatosis.
hepatic s. see under *hemosiderosis.*
nutritional s. excessive iron in the blood due to a diet very high in iron and low in protein and calories.
pulmonary s. siderosis (def. 1).
urinary s. hemosiderinuria.

sid•er•ot•ic (sid″ər-ot'ik) pertaining to or characterized by siderosis.

sid•er•ous (sid′ər-əs) containing iron.

side•wind•er (sīd′wīnd-ər) *Crotalus cerastes*, a pale-colored venomous rattlesnake found in desert areas of the southwestern United States.

SIDS sudden infant death syndrome.

Sie•gert sign (ze′gert) [Ferdinand *Siegert*, German pediatrician, 1865–1946] see under *sign.*

Sie•gle otoscope (ze′gəl) [Emil *Siegle*, German otologist, 1833–1900] see under *otoscope.*

sie•mens (S) (se′mənz) the SI unit of conductance; it is the conductance of one ampere per volt in a body with one ohm resistance.

Sie•mer•ling nucleus (ze′mer-ling) [Ernst *Siemerling*, German neurologist and psychiatrist, 1857–1931] see under *nucleus.*

sieve (siv) a device having pores or perforations of uniform size used for separating objects or particles of different sizes.

molecular s. a crystalline substance having uniform pores of molecular size that adsorbs smaller but not larger molecules; used in chemical separation.

sie•vert (Sv) (se′vərt) the SI unit of radiation absorbed dose equivalent, defined as that producing the same biologic effect in a specified tissue as 1 gray of high-energy x-rays; 1 sievert equals 100 rem.

sig. [L.] sig′na (mark).

sigh (si) [L. *suspirium*] an audible and prolonged inhalation, followed by an audible exhalation.

sight (sīt) [A.S. *sihth*] vision (defs. 1, 2).

day s. nyctalopia.
far s., long s. hyperopia.
near s. myopia.
night s. hemeralopia.
old s. presbyopia.
short s. myopia.

sig•ma•tism (sig′mə-tiz-əm) a speech disorder consisting of incorrect, difficult, or too frequent use of the *s* sound. See also *lisping.* Called also *parasigmatism.*

Sig•mo•don (sig′mə-don) the cotton rats, a genus of rodents of the family Muridae found in warm regions of the Americas. *S. his′pidus* of Florida and the Caribbean is a vector for hantavirus pulmonary syndrome.

sig•moid (sig′moid) [Gr. *sigmoeidēs*, from the letter *sigma* + *eidos* form] 1. shaped like the letter S or the letter C. 2. colon sigmoideum.

sig•moid•ec•to•my (sig″moi-dek′tə-me) excision of the sigmoid colon; called also *sigmoid colectomy.*

sig•moid•itis (sig″moi-di′tis) inflammation of the sigmoid colon.

sig•moido•cys•to•plas•ty (sig-moi″do-sis′to-plas″te) sigmoid cystoplasty.

sig•moido•pexy (sig-moi′do-pek″se) [*sigmoid* + *-pexy*] suspension of the sigmoid colon, usually performed for treatment of rectal prolapse.

sig•moido•proc•tos•to•my (sig-moi″do-prok-tos′tə-me) rectosigmoidostomy.

sig•moido•rec•tos•to•my (sig-moi″do-rək-tos′tə-me) rectosigmoidostomy.

sig•moido•scope (sig-moi′do-skōp) a rigid or flexible endoscope with appropriate illumination for examining the sigmoid colon.

sig•moid•os•co•py (sig″moi-dos′kə-pe) inspection of the sigmoid colon through a sigmoidoscope. **sigmoidoscop′ic** *adj*

sig•moido•sig•moi•dos•to•my (sig-moi″do-sig-moi-dos′tə-me) 1. surgical creation of an anastomosis between two portions of the sigmoid colon. 2. the opening so created.

sig•moid•os•to•my (sig″moi-dos′tə-me) [*sigmoid* + *-stomy*] 1. formation of an artificial opening from the body surface into the sigmoid colon. 2. the opening so created.

sig•moid•ot•o•my (sig″moi-dot′ə-me) operative incision into the sigmoid colon.

sig•moido•ves•i•cal (sig-moi″do-ves′ĭ-kəl) pertaining to or communicating between the sigmoid colon and the urinary bladder. Called also *vesicosigmoid.*

sign (sīn) [L. *signum*] an indication of the existence of something; any objective evidence of a disease, i.e., such evidence as is perceptible to the examining physician, as opposed to the subjective sensations (symptoms) of the patient.

Sign

For terms not found here, see also under *phenomenon, reflex, symptom,* and *syndrome.*

Aaron s. a sensation of pain or distress in the epigastric or precordial region on pressure over the McBurney point in appendicitis.

Abadie s. 1. [Charles *Abadie*] spasm of the levator palpebrae superioris muscle; a sign of Graves disease. 2. [Jean *Abadie*] insensibility of the Achilles tendon to pressure; seen in tabes dorsalis.

accessory s. any nonpathognomonic sign of disease.

accordion s. alternating bands of high and low attenuation, resembling the bellows of an accordion, on computed tomography of the colon, resulting from entrapment of contrast material between edematous haustral folds; a sign of pseudomembranous colitis.

air crescent s. on a CT scan of the lung, the appearance of an intracavitary mass partly surrounded by air that has entered the cavity secondary to necrosis; it is usually a late finding in pulmonary aspergillosis but may occur in other conditions.

air-cushion s. Klemm s.

Allis s. relaxation of the fascia between the iliac crest and the greater trochanter, so that leg length is unequal, a sign of fracture of the neck of the femur.

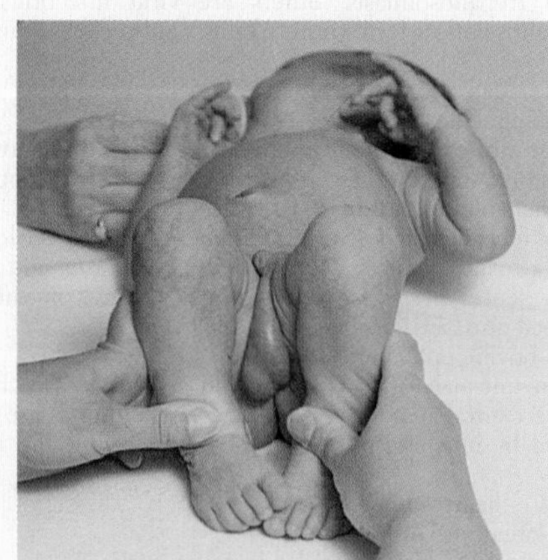

■ Examination for Allis sign: checking for unequal upper leg length.

Amoss s. in painful flexure of the spine, patients, when rising to a sitting posture from lying in bed, do so by supporting themselves with the hands placed far back in the bed.

Anghelescu s. inability to bend the spine while lying on the back so as to rest on the head and heels alone, seen in tuberculosis of the vertebrae.

antecedent s. any precursory indication of an attack of disease.

anterior drawer s. see under *test.*

anterior tibial s. tibialis s.

anticus s. Piotrowski s.

Argyll Robertson pupil s. see under *pupil.*

Arroyo s. asthenocoria.

assident s. accessory s.

Auenbrugger s. a bulging of the epigastrium, due to extensive pericardial effusion.

Auspitz s. the appearance of multiple fine bleeding points when a scale is removed from a psoriatic plaque, caused by thinning of the epidermis over the dermal papillae.

Babinski s. 1. loss or lessening of the Achilles tendon reflex in sciatica: this distinguishes it from hysterical sciatica. 2. a misnomer for Babinski reflex. 3. in hemiplegia, the contraction of the platysma muscle in the healthy side is more vigorous than on the affected side, as seen in opening the mouth, whistling, blowing, etc. 4. when a hemiplegic patient is lying with arms crossed upon the chest, and makes an effort to sit up, the thigh on the paralyzed side is flexed upon the pelvis and the heel is lifted from the ground, while on the healthy side the limb does not move. 5. when the paralyzed forearm is placed in supination, it turns over to pronation: seen in organic paralysis. Called also *pronation s.*

Babinski toe s. Babinski reflex.

Baccelli s. aphonic pectoriloquy.

Baillarger s. inequality of the pupils in general paresis.

Ballance s. resonance of right flank when the patient lies on the left side; said to be present in splenic rupture.

Ballet s. external ophthalmoplegia, with loss of all voluntary eye movements, the pupillary movements and reflex eye movements persisting; seen in Graves disease and conversion disorders.

Bamberger s. 1. allochiria. 2. presence of signs of consolidation at the angle of the scapula, which disappear when the patient leans forward; a sign of pericardial effusion.

banana s. a flattened and curved, bananalike shape of the cerebellar hemispheres seen in axial section in sonography of the fetal skull; a sign of the Arnold-Chiari deformity.

Bárány s. caloric test.

Bard s. in organic nystagmus the oscillations of the eye increase as the patient's attention follows the finger moved alternately from one side to the other; but in congenital nystagmus the oscillations disappear under similar conditions.

Barré s. contraction of the iris is slower in mental deterioration.

Barré pyramidal s. the patient lies face down and the lower limbs are flexed at the knee; if there is disease of the pyramidal tracts, the patient will be unable to maintain this position.

Bastian-Bruns s. see under *law*.

Battle s. discoloration over the skin of the mastoid region of the skull, in the line of the posterior auricular artery, the ecchymosis first appearing near the tip of the mastoid process; seen in fracture of the base of the skull.

Becker s. see under *phenomenon*.

Béclard s. a sign of the maturity of the fetus consisting of a center of ossification in the lower epiphysis of the femur.

Beevor s. 1. a sign of functional paralysis consisting of inability of the patient to inhibit the antagonistic muscles. 2. upward deviation of the umbilicus on attempting to lift the head, caused by contraction of the upper but not the lower abdominal muscles and indicative of a spinal cord lesion in the region of the lower thoracic vertebrae.

Bekhterev s. 1. Bekhterev deep reflex. 2. paralysis of the facial muscles for automatic movements.

Bell s. see under *phenomenon*.

Berger s. an irregularly shaped or elliptical pupil in the early stages of tabes dorsalis, paralytic dementia, and certain paralyses.

Bergman s. in urologic radiography, when there is a neoplasm in the ureter a dilation is seen immediately below it, and a catheter tends to coil in this dilated portion; when there is an obstructing stone, the ureter below it is collapsed rather than dilated.

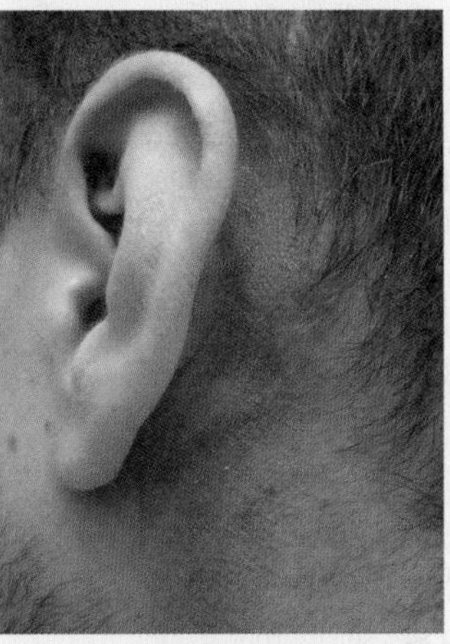

■ Battle sign.

Bethea s. the examiner stands beside the patient and places fingertips on upper surfaces of corresponding ribs high in the patient's axillae; if the patient has less respiratory movement of ribs on one side, this indicates impairment of chest expansion. Called also *Bethea method.*

Bezold s. an inflammatory swelling below the apex of the mastoid process; evidence of mastoiditis.

Biernacki s. analgesia of the ulnar nerve in general paresis and tabes dorsalis.

Biot s. see under *respiration.*

Bjerrum s. see under *scotoma.*

Blumberg s. pain on abrupt release of steady pressure (rebound tenderness) over the site of a suspected abdominal lesion; seen in peritonitis.

Boas s. see under *point.*

bonbon s. a sign of tardive dyskinesia in which a person presses the tip of the tongue against the inside of the cheek.

Bonnet s. pain on thigh adduction in sciatica.

Bordier-Fränkel s. Bell phenomenon.

Boston s. Graefe s.

Bouillaud s. permanent retraction of the chest in the precordial region; a sign of adherent pericardium.

bowler hat s. on a radiograph of the colon, a shadow resembling a bowler hat, representing the filling defect of either a sessile polyp on the inferior wall or a diverticulum.

bowstring s. after a straight-leg raising test is performed, the knee is flexed to reduce radicular pain; return of the pain when pressure is applied to the popliteal fossa is a positive sign of lumbar radiculopathy.

Boyce s. a gurgling sound heard on pressure by the hand on the side of the neck; seen in diverticulum of the esophagus.

Bozzolo s. a visible pulsation of the arteries within the nostrils; said to indicate aneurysm of the thoracic aorta.

Bragard s. with the knee stiff, the lower limb is flexed at the hip until the patient experiences pain; the foot is then dorsiflexed. Increase of pain points to disease of the nerve root.

Branham s. bradycardia produced by digital closure of an artery proximal to an arteriovenous fistula.

Braunwald s. occurrence of a weak pulse instead of a strong one immediately after a premature ventricular contraction.

Broadbent s. a retraction seen on the left side of the back, near the eleventh and twelfth ribs, related to pericardial adhesion.

Broadbent inverted s. pulsations synchronizing with ventricular systole on the posterior lateral wall of the chest in gross dilatation of the left atrium.

Brockenbrough s. occurrence of a weak pulse instead of a strong one immediately after a premature ventricular contraction; indicative of idiopathic hypertrophic subaortic stenosis.

broken straw s. a sharply angulated spindle cell resembling a broken straw; characteristic of the spindle cell form of embryonal rhabdomyosarcoma.

Brown s. blanching of the tympanic membrane and of the area behind it, seen with pneumatic pressure on the membrane; it indicates presence of a vascular tumor or other lesion in the middle ear.

Brown-Séquard s. see under *syndrome.*

Brudzinski s. 1. in meningitis, flexion of the neck usually results in flexion of the hip and knee; called also *neck s.* 2. in meningitis, when passive flexion of the lower limb on one side is made, a similar movement will be seen in the opposite limb; called also *contralateral s.*

Brunati s. the appearance of opacities in the cornea during the course of pneumonia or typhoid fever.

Bruns s. see under *syndrome.*

Bryant s. lowering of the axillary folds in dislocation of the shoulder.

bulbar s's dysfunction of muscles in the lower face and throat that are supplied by motor nerves coming off the brainstem, which causes difficulties in breathing, swallowing, talking, and other functions of the throat; these are seen with conditions such as spinobulbar muscular atrophy and amyotrophic lateral sclerosis.

Burton s. lead line.

buttonhole s. invagination of a nodule when pressed with a finger, a characteristic of neurofibromatosis.

calcium s. on a chest radiograph, the calcified intima of the aorta is separated more than 1 cm from the outer border of the aorta; a rare finding suggestive of aortic dissection.

Cantelli s. oculocephalic reflex.

cardinal s's (of inflammation), dolor, calor, rubor, tumor, and functio laesa; see *inflammation.*
cardiorespiratory s. a change in the normal pulse-respiration ratio from 4:1 to 2:1; seen in infantile scurvy.
Carman s., Carman-Kirklin s., Carman-Kirklin meniscus s. meniscus s.
Carnett s. a test for parietal tenderness: the abdomen is palpated while the patient holds the anterior abdominal muscles tense; the tense muscles prevent the examiner's fingers from coming in contact with the underlying viscera and any tenderness elicited over them will be parietal in location. Tenderness elicited over relaxed muscles may be either parietal or intra-abdominal in origin; that present with relaxed muscles and absent with tense muscles is due to a subparietal lesion and its cause is inside the abdomen; that found with both relaxed and tensed muscles is due to an anterior parietal lesion and its cause is outside the abdominal cavity.
Carvallo s. in tricuspid regurgitation, augmentation of the pansystolic murmur by inspiration.
Cegka s. invariability of the cardiac dullness during the different phases of respiration; a sign of adherent pericardium.
Chaddock s. see under *reflex.*
Chadwick s. a dark bluish or purplish-red and congested appearance of the vaginal and cervical mucosa, an indication of pregnancy.
chandelier s. an informal term for the raising of the arms toward the ceiling (that is, toward the chandelier) in response to intense pain, or the apprehension of intense pain; used especially of pain caused by movement of the cervix during pelvic examination in women with pelvic inflammatory disease.
Charcot s. the raising of the eyebrow in peripheral facial paralysis, and the lowering of the same part in facial contraction.
Cheyne-Stokes s. see under *respiration.*
Chilaiditi s. positioning of the colon between the liver and the diaphragm on x-ray; called also *hepatoptosis.*
Chvostek s., Chvostek-Weiss s. spasm of the facial muscles elicited by tapping the facial nerve in the region of the parotid gland; seen in tetany. Called also *Schultze* or *Schultze-Chvostek s.*
Claude hyperkinesis s. reflex movements of paretic muscles elicited by painful stimuli.
Cleeman s. creasing of the skin just above the patella, indicative of fracture of the femur with overriding of fragments.
Codman s. in rupture of the supraspinatus tendon, the upper limb can be passively abducted without pain, but when support for it is removed and the deltoid muscle contracts suddenly, pain occurs again.
cogwheel s. see under *rigidity.*
coiled spring s. a concentric ring pattern of the mucosa of the intestine, seen on barium enema examination in a variety of diseases, including posttraumatic hematoma of the duodenum, acute appendicitis, intussusception of the appendix, mucocele, endometriosis of the appendix, and carcinoma.
Cole s. deformity of the duodenal contour as seen in the radiograph, a sign of the presence of duodenal ulcer.
colon cutoff s. a radiographic sign of appendiceal perforation or colonic spasm, consisting of absence of gas and feces in the right lower quadrant, reflex dilatation of the transverse colon, and sharp cutoff of gas at the hepatic flexure.
commemorative s. any sign of a previous disease.
Comolli s. a sign of scapular fracture consisting of the appearance in the scapular region, shortly after the accident, of a triangular swelling reproducing the shape of the body of the scapula.
complementary opposition s. Hoover s. (def. 1).
contralateral s. Brudzinski s. (def. 2).
Coopernail s. ecchymosis on the perineum and scrotum or labia: a sign of fracture of the pelvis.
Cope s. psoas s.
Corrigan s. 1. see under *line.* 2. see under *pulse.*
cortical rim s. in computed tomography of the kidney, a thin rim of peripheral cortex that is perfused and visible when other parts of the cortex are not, because of capsular collateral arteries; it indicates cortical necrosis, renal vein thrombosis, or infarction of the nonperfused parts. Called also *rim s.*
cortical ring s. ring-shaped appearance of the cortex of the scaphoid bone on radiography of the wrist, caused by abnormal orientation of the scaphoid following disruption of the scaphoid ligament; a sign of scapholunate dislocation. Called also *signet ring s.*

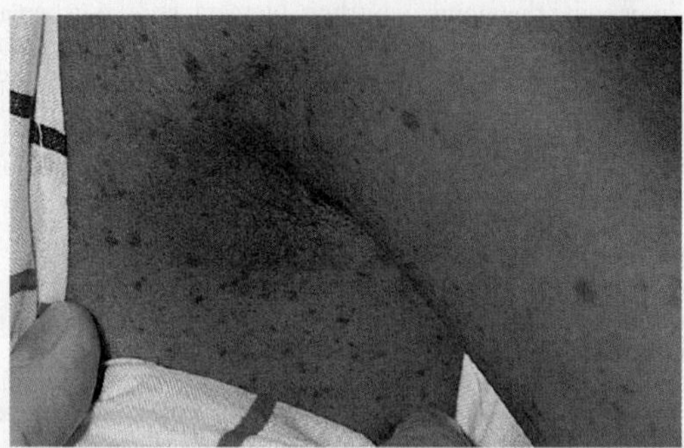

■ Crowe sign.

coughing s. Huntington s.
Courvoisier s. severe jaundice with a palpable, nontender gallbladder, indicating obstruction of biliary passages from something other than a gallstone, possibly a tumor; see *Courvoisier's law,* under *law.*
Cowen s. when light is shone into one pupil, there is jerky constriction of the contralateral pupil in Graves disease.
crescent s. meniscus s.
Crichton-Browne s. tremor of the outer angles of the eyes and of the labial commissures in the earlier stages of general paresis.
Crowe s. appearance of freckles in the axillae, a sign of neurofibromatosis. Called also *axillary freckling.*
CT angiogram s. enhanced pulmonary vessels against a background of low attenuation material seen on computed tomography of the lung; first described in bronchioloalveolar carcinoma but also seen in a variety of other pulmonary conditions.
Cullen s. a bluish discoloration of the skin around the umbilicus, indicative of intraperitoneal hemorrhage; seen most often with acute hemorrhagic pancreatitis or a fallopian tube ruptured from an ectopic pregnancy.
Dalrymple s. one manifestation of Graves orbitopathy, consisting of retraction of the eyelids so that the palpebral opening is abnormally wide. See also *Stellwag s.*
D'Amato s. in pleural effusion, the location of dullness is altered from the vertebral area in the sitting position to the heart region when the patient assumes a lateral position on the side opposite the effusion.
Darier s. urtication and itching occurring on rubbing the lesions of urticaria pigmentosa.
Dawbarn s. in acute subacromial bursitis, when the upper limb hangs by the side palpation over the bursa causes pain, but when it is abducted this pain disappears.
Dejerine s. aggravation of symptoms of radiculitis produced by coughing, sneezing, and straining at stool.
Delbet s. in aneurysm of the main artery of a limb, if the nutrition of the part distal to the aneurysm is maintained, although the pulse may have disappeared, the collateral circulation is sufficient.
Demarquay s. fixation or lowering of the larynx during phonation and deglutition; a sign of syphilis of the trachea.
Demianoff s. with the patient in dorsal decubitus position, extreme pain when the attempt is made to lift an extended lower limb above ten degrees, a sign of a lesion in the erector spinae muscles of the lumbar region. Cf. *Lasègue s.*
de Musset s. Musset s.
Dennie s. Morgan fold.
Desault s. a sign of intracapsular fracture of the femur, consisting of alteration of the arc described by rotation of the greater trochanter, which normally describes the segment of a circle, but in this fracture rotates only as the apex of the femur as it rotates about its own axis.
d'Espine s. in the normal person, on auscultation over the spinous processes, pectoriloquy ceases at the bifurcation of the trachea, and in infants opposite the seventh cervical vertebra. If pectoriloquy is heard lower than this, it indicates enlargement of bronchial lymph nodes.
dip and plateau s. square root s.
Dixon Mann s. Mann s.

doll's eye s. oculocephalic reflex.
Dorendorf s. fullness of a supraclavicular fossa on one side in aneurysm of the aortic arch.
double bubble s. on a radiograph of the abdomen, appearance of two foci of gas, one in the stomach and the other in the duodenum, signifying duodenal obstruction. The same sign, but consisting of the stomach and duodenum distended by fluid, may be observed in the fetus by ultrasonography.
double duct s. simultaneous dilatation of the common bile duct and the pancreatic duct with contiguous narrowing, as seen with cholangiopancreatography, indicating possible carcinoma of the head of the pancreas or the ampulla of Vater.
drawer s's see under *test.*
drooping lily s. a deformity seen on excretory urography of a duplex kidney, with the forcing of the lower collecting system and ureter outward and downward to resemble the shape of a drooping lily; it is caused by obstruction and dilation of the upper collecting system.
Drummond s. a whiff heard at the open mouth during respiration in cases of aortic aneurysm.
DTP s. [*d*istal *t*ingling on *p*ercussion] Tinel s.
Dubois s. shortness of the little finger in congenital syphilis.
Duchenne s. the sinking in of the epigastrium on inhalation in paralysis of the diaphragm or in certain cases of hydropericardium.
Dugas s. see under *test.*
Dunphy s. increased abdominal pain on coughing, a sign of acute appendicitis.
Dupuytren s. 1. a crackling sensation on pressure over a sarcomatous bone. 2. in congenital dislocation of the head of the femur, there is a free up-and-down movement of the head of the bone.
Duroziez s. see under *murmur.*
E s. reversed three s.
echo s. echolalia.
Elliot s. 1. induration of the edge of a syphilitic skin lesion. 2. a scotoma extending from the blind spot and made up of numerous points or spots.
Ely s. see under *test.*
Enroth s. abnormal fullness of the eyelids, a manifestation of Graves orbitopathy.
Erben s. see under *reflex.*
Erichsen s. when the iliac bones are sharply pressed toward each other pain is felt in sacroiliac disease but not in hip disease.
Eustace Smith s. Smith s.
Ewart s. bronchial breathing and dullness on percussion at the lower angle of the left scapula, a sign of pericardial effusion.
Ewing s. tenderness at the upper inner angle of the orbit: a sign of obstruction of the outlet of the frontal sinus.
external malleolar s. Chaddock reflex.
fabere s. Patrick test; see under *test.*
facial s. Chvostek s.
Fajersztajn crossed sciatic s. in sciatica, the hip on the affected side can be flexed only when the knee is flexed, not when the limb is held straight; flexing the sound thigh with the limb on that side held straight causes pain on the affected side.
fallen lung s. a radiographic sign of rupture of the trachea or a mainstem bronchus, in which the collapsed lung sags posteriorly and laterally away from the hilum.
fan s. spreading apart of the toes following the stroking of the sole of the foot; it forms part of the Babinski reflex.
fat pad s. distention and displacement of the fat adjacent to a joint capsule, usually in the elbow or knee, visible on a radiograph when the joint is flexed; a sign of a fracture within the joint that involves little or no bone displacement.
figure three s. a pair of bulges in the wall of the aortic arch, one above and one below the aortic knuckle, seen on a radiograph and signifying coarctation of the aorta. See also *reversed three s.* Called also *three s.*
finger-escape s. the hand is held with the fingers extended and adducted; in cervical myelopathy the fourth and fifth (and sometimes the middle) fingers flex and abduct. See also *myelopathy hand*, under *hand.*
finger-in-glove s. a radiographic sign seen in conditions that cause central bronchiectasis, in which mucus-filled, dilated bronchi appear as V- or Y-shaped opacities resembling gloved fingers.
flag s. a band of light hair seen in children who have recovered from kwashiorkor.
floating tooth s. on radiographic examination of the mandible, erosion of the bony alveoli around the teeth so that they seem to be floating in space; it occurs in some forms of histiocytosis X.
forearm s. Léri s.
formication s. Tinel s.
Fothergill s. an abdominal wall mass that does not cross the midline and remains palpable when the rectus abdominis muscle is contracted indicates presence of a hematoma in the rectus abdominis.
Fränkel s. excessive range of passive movement of the hip joint, indicating diminished tone of the surrounding musculature in tabes dorsalis.
Friedreich s. diastolic collapse of the cervical veins due to adherent pericardium.
Froment paper s. abnormal flexion of the distal phalanx of the thumb when a sheet of paper is held between the thumb and the radial surface of the index finger; a sign of a lesion of the ulnar nerve.
frontal release s's a group of primitive reflexes seen normally in infants and suppressed in adults, but released in adults with brain lesions, especially of the frontal lobe. These include the grasping, rooting, snout, and sucking reflexes.
Gaenslen s. with the patient in the supine position, the knee and hip on one side are held in flexed position by the patient, while the other lower limb, hanging over the edge of the table, is pressed down by the examiner to produce hyperextension of the hip: pain occurs on the affected side in lumbosacral disease.
Galeazzi s. in development dysplasia of the hip, apparent shortening of the femur, as shown by the difference of knee levels with the knees and hips flexed at right angles with the patient lying on a flat table.
Gauss s. an increase in uterine mobility seen early in pregnancy.
Gianelli s. Tournay s.
Glasgow s. a systolic sound in the brachial artery in latent aneurysm of the aorta.
Goggia s. in health, the fibrillary contraction produced by striking and then pinching the brachial biceps extends throughout the whole muscle; in debilitating disease, such as typhoid fever, the contraction is local.
Golden S s. a radiographic sign seen when a hilar mass, usually a tumor, causes peripheral atelectasis, most often of the right upper lobe. The central convexity caused by the mass and the distal concavity resulting from atelectasis together give the affected fissure an S shape.
Goldstein s. wide space between the great toe and the adjoining toe, seen in Down syndrome.
Goldthwait s. with the patient supine, one lower limb is raised by the examiner with one hand, the other hand being placed under the patient's lower back; leverage is then applied to the side of the pelvis. If the patient feels pain before the lumbar spine is moved, the lesion is a sprain of the sacroiliac joint. If pain does not appear until after the lumbar spine moves, the lesion is in the sacroiliac or lumbosacral articulation.
Goodell s. softening of the cervix uteri as a sign of pregnancy.
Gordon s. finger phenomenon (def. 1).
Gorlin s. the ability to touch the tip of the nose with the tongue, frequently a sign of Ehlers-Danlos syndrome.
Gottron s. a cutaneous sign pathognomonic of dermatomyositis, consisting of symmetrical macular violaceous erythema, with or without edema, over extensor surfaces such as the knuckles, elbows, or knees.
Gowers s. 1. abrupt intermittent oscillation of the iris under the influence of light; seen in certain stages of tabes dorsalis. 2. a sign of pseudohypertrophic muscular dystrophy; to stand from the supine position, the patient rolls to the prone position, kneels, and pushes up to a

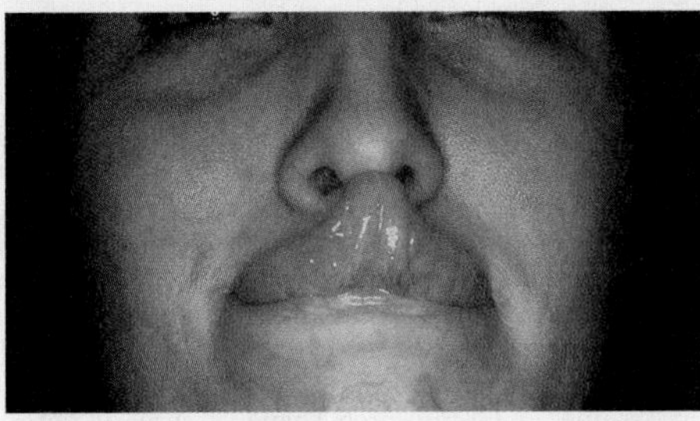

■ Gorlin sign.

standing position with hands against shins, knees, and thighs. Called also *Gowers maneuver* or *phenomenon.*
Graefe s. failure of the upper lid to move downward promptly and evenly with the eyeball in looking downward; instead it moves tardily and jerkingly, a manifestation of Graves orbitopathy. Called also *lid lag* and *Boston* or *von Graefe s.*
Grancher s. equality of pitch of exhalations and inhalations, a sign of obstruction to exhalation.
Granger s. if in the radiograph of an infant two years old or less, the anterior wall of the lateral sinus is visible, extensive destruction of the mastoid is indicated.
Grasset s., Grasset-Bychowski s. Grasset phenomenon.
Grasset-Gaussel-Hoover s. Hoover s. (def. 1).
Grey Turner s. Turner s.
Griesinger s. edematous swelling behind the mastoid process; seen in thrombosis of the transverse sinus.
Griffith s. lower lid lag on upward gaze, a manifestation of Graves orbitopathy.
Grocco s. 1. see under *triangle.* 2. extension of the liver dullness to the left of the midspinal line, indicating enlargement of the organ.
Guilland s. brisk flexion at the hip and knee joint when the contralateral quadriceps muscle is pinched; a sign of meningeal irritation.
Gunn s. 1. Gunn crossing s. 2. Marcus Gunn pupillary phenomenon. 3. see under *syndrome.*
Gunn crossing s. a crossing of an artery over a vein in the fundus of the eye, indicative of essential hypertension.
Gunn pupillary s. Marcus Gunn pupillary phenomenon.
Hahn s. persistent rotation of the head from side to side in cerebellar disease of childhood.
hair collar s. the presence of a tuft of long, dark hair surrounding a ring of alopecia on a baby's scalp; this is sometimes indicative of an underlying dysraphism.
Hall s. a tracheal diastolic shock felt in aneurysm of the aorta.
halo s. 1. a halo effect produced in the radiograph of the fetal head between the subcutaneous fat and the cranium; said to be indicative of intrauterine death of the fetus. 2. a sign of cerebrospinal fluid in rhinorrhea: a drop of bloody nasal discharge is placed on a cloth; if it contains cerebrospinal fluid, there will be a light-colored ring radiating out farther than the blood. 3. an early computed tomographic finding in pulmonary aspergillosis, consisting of a ring of ground-glass opacity surrounding a primary nodule; it is occasionally seen in other pulmonary conditions, including mycoses, carcinoma, and pneumonia.
Hamman s. a precordial crunching, clicking, or knocking sound, synchronous with each heart beat, heard on auscultation in such conditions as acute mediastinitis, pneumomediastinum, and pneumothorax. Called also *Hamman murmur.*
hard s's obvious objective findings on the basis of which a specific diagnosis can be made; cf *soft s's.*
harlequin s. reddening of the lower half of the laterally recumbent body and blanching of the upper half, due to temporary vasomotor disturbance in newborn infants.
Haudek s. a projecting shadow in radiographs of penetrating gastric ulcer, due to settlement of bismuth in pathologic niches of the stomach wall; called also *Haudek niche.*
Hawkins s. in fractures of the talar neck, a radiolucent zone beneath the subchondral plate of the head of the talus, indicative of disuse osteoporosis; its absence reflects increased risk of talar avascular necrosis.
Heberden s. see under *node.*
Hegar s. softening of the lower segment of the uterus, an indication of pregnancy.
Heilbronner s. see under *thigh.*
Heim-Kreysig s. a depression of the spaces between the ribs, seen along with the cardiac systole in adhesive pericarditis.
Helbing s. medialward curving of the Achilles tendon as viewed from behind; seen in flatfoot.
Hennebert s. rotatory nystagmus when positive or negative pressure is applied to the tympanic membrane, indicative of labyrinthitis with leakage of perilymph; positive pressure (air compression) causes nystagmus toward the affected side, and negative pressure (air rarefaction) causes nystagmus away from the affected side.
Hennings s. an angular deformity of the angulus of the stomach, in which it assumes a Gothic arch shape; a sign of chronic gastric ulcer. Called also *Gothic arch formation.*
Hill s. disproportionate femoral systolic hypertension, seen in aortic regurgitation and certain other conditions involving increased stroke volume.
Hirschberg s. adduction, inversion, and slight plantar flexion of the foot on stroking the inner aspect (not the sole) of the foot from the great toe to the heel; called also *adductor reflex of foot.*
Hitzelberger s. anesthesia of medial, posterior, or superior areas of the external auditory canal caused by an acoustic neuroma that is pressing against the facial nerve.
Hoehne s. absence of uterine contractions during delivery despite repeated injections of oxytocics, regarded as a sign of rupture of the uterus.
Hoffmann s. 1. see under *phenomenon.* 2. in hemiplegia, a sudden nipping of the nail of the index, middle, or ring finger will produce flexion of the terminal phalanx of the thumb and of the second and third phalanges of some other finger; called also *digital* or *Hoffmann reflex.*
Holmes s. rebound phenomenon.
Homans s. pain on passive dorsiflexion of the foot; a sign of thrombosis of deep calf veins.
Hoover s. 1. in the normal state or in genuine paralysis, if the supine patient is directed to press the whole lower limb against the surface, there will be a lifting movement in the opposite limb; this phenomenon is absent in hysteria and malingering. Called also *Grasset-Gaussel-Hoover s.* 2. movement of the costal margins toward the midline during inhalation, occurring bilaterally in pulmonary emphysema and unilaterally in conditions causing flattening of the diaphragm, such as pleural effusion and pneumothorax.
Hope s. double heart beat in aortic aneurysm.
Horner s. Spalding s.
Horsley s. if there is a difference in the temperature in the two axillae, the higher temperature will be on the paralyzed side.
Howship-Romberg s. pain passing down the inner side of the thigh to the knee due to pressure on the obturator nerve by an obturator hernia.
Hueter s. the absence of the transmission of osseous vibration in cases of fracture with fibrous material interposed between the fragments.
Huntington s. the patient lies supine, with lower limbs hanging over the edge of a table, and is told to cough. If the coughing produces flexion of the thigh and extension of a paralyzed lower limb, it indicates that the paralysis is due to an upper motor neuron lesion.
Hutchinson s. 1. interstitial keratitis and a dull-red discoloration of the cornea in congenital syphilis. 2. see under *tooth.* 3. see under *triad.*
hyperkinesis s. Claude hyperkinesis s.
iliopsoas s. with the patient lying supine, the leg is elevated and extended against resistance; if this causes pain, it indicates appendicitis with a retrocecal abscess.
impingement s. when the shoulder is flexed forward with the humerus internally rotated and its greater tubercle against the surface of the acromion, pain indicates an overuse injury to the arm muscles, as in the impingement syndrome (q.v.).
Jendrassik s. paralysis of the extraocular muscles, one manifestation of Graves orbitopathy.
jugular s. Queckenstedt s.
Kanavel s. a point of maximum tenderness in the palm 2.5 cm proximal to the base of the little finger in infection of tendon sheath.
Kantor s. string s.
Karplus s. a modification of the vocal resonance, in which, on auscultation over a pleural effusion, the vowel *u* spoken by the patient is heard as *a.*
Keen s. increased diameter of the lower limb at the malleoli in Pott fracture of the fibula.
Kehr s. severe pain in the left shoulder in some cases of rupture of the spleen.
Kellock s. increase of the vibration of the ribs on sharp percussion with one hand, the other hand being placed firmly on the thorax under the nipple; a sign of pleural effusion.
Kerandel s. deep hyperesthesia accompanied by pain, often retarded, after some slight blow upon a bony projection of the body; seen in African trypanosomiasis.
Kergaradec s. uterine souffle.
Kernig s. a sign of meningitis: the patient can easily and completely extend the lower limb when in dorsal decubitus position but not when

in the sitting posture or when lying with the thigh flexed upon the abdomen.
Kerr s. alteration of the texture of the skin below the somatic level in lesions of the spinal cord.
Kestenbaum s. a decrease in number of arterioles traversing the optic disk margin as a criterion for optic atrophy.
Kleist s. the fingers of the patient when gently elevated by the fingers of the examiner will hook into the examiner's fingers; indicative of frontal and thalamic lesions.
Klemm s. in the radiograph in chronic appendicitis, there is often an indication of tympanites in the right lower quadrant.
Klippel-Weil s. flexion and adduction of the thumb when the patient's flexed fingers are quickly extended by the examiner; indicative of pyramidal tract disease.
Knies s. unequal dilatation of the pupils, one manifestation of Graves orbitopathy.
Kocher s. a sign of Graves' orbitopathy: the examiner places one hand on a level with the patient's eyes and then lifts it higher; the patient's upper lid springs up more quickly than the eyeball does.
Koplik s. see under *spot.*
Kreysig s. Heim-Kreysig s.
Krisovski (Krisowski) s. cicatricial lines radiating from the mouth in congenital syphilis.
Kussmaul s. 1. distention of the jugular veins during inhalation, seen in constrictive pericarditis and mediastinal tumor. 2. paradoxical pulse.
Küstner s. a cystic tumor on the median line anterior to the uterus in cases of ovarian dermoids.
Lafora s. picking of the nose regarded as an early sign of cerebrospinal meningitis.
Langoria s. relaxation of the extensor muscles of the thigh; a symptom of intracapsular fracture of the femur.
Lasègue s. 1. in sciatica, flexion of the hip is painful when the knee is extended, but painless when the knee is flexed. This distinguishes the disorder from disease of the hip joint. Cf. *Demianoff s.* 2. dorsiflexion of the foot during the straight-leg lift test exacerbates the pain in S1 radiculopathy.
Laugier s. a condition in which the styloid process of the radius and of the ulna are on the same level; seen in fracture of the lower part of the radius.
leg s. 1. Schlesinger s. 2. Neri s.
lemon s. scalloping of the frontal bones giving the skull a lemon-shaped configuration in axial section in sonography of the fetal skull during the second trimester of pregnancy; a sign of the Arnold-Chiari deformity.
Léri s. passive flexion of the hand and wrist of the affected side in hemiplegia shows no normal flexion at the elbow.
Leser-Trélat s. sudden appearance and rapid increase in size and number of seborrheic keratoses, which may be a sign of internal malignancy, especially of the gastrointestinal tract.
Lhermitte s. the development of sudden, transient, electric-like shocks spreading down the body when the patient flexes the head forward; seen mainly in multiple sclerosis but also in compression and other disorders of the cervical cord.
Lichtheim s. in some types of motor aphasia the patient cannot speak but can indicate with fingers the number of syllables in a word being thought of. Called also *Dejerine-Lichtheim phenomenon.*
Linder s. with the patient either lying down or sitting with lower limbs outstretched, passive flexion of the head will cause pain in the lower limb or the lumbar region in sciatica.
Livierato s. vasoconstriction when the abdominal sympathetic nerve is irritated by striking the anterior abdomen along the xiphoumbilical line.
Lucas s. distention of the abdomen in the early stages of rickets.
Ludloff s. swelling and ecchymosis at the base of Scarpa triangle together with inability to raise the thigh when in a sitting posture, a sign of traumatic separation of the epiphysis of the greater trochanter.
Luftsichel s. [Ger. "air sickle"] a sickle-shaped paramediastinal radiolucency seen on the chest radiograph in upper pulmonary lobe collapse and caused by hyperinflation of the superior segment of the ipsilateral lower lobe.
McBurney s. tenderness upon pressure at the McBurney point (two thirds of the way from the umbilicus to the anterior superior spine), indicative of acute appendicitis.
Macewen s. on percussion of the skull behind the junction of the frontal, temporal, and parietal bones, there is a more resonant note than normal in internal hydrocephalus and cerebral abscess. Called also *cracked-pot sound* and *cranial cracked-pot sound.*
McGinn-White s. a Q wave and late inversion of the T wave in lead III, low ST intervals and T waves in lead II, and inverted T waves in chest leads V_2 and V_3, the electrocardiographic evidence of right ventricular dilatation due to massive pulmonary embolism, plus the clinical signs of acute cor pulmonale.
McMurray s. see under *test.*
Magendie s., Magendie-Hertwig s. skew deviation.
Magnan s. formication.
Mahler s. a steady increase of pulse rate without corresponding elevation of temperature; seen in thrombosis.
Maisonneuve s. marked hyperextensibility of the hand, a symptom of Colles fracture.
Mann s. with Graves orbitopathy, the two eyes appear not to be on the same level. Called also *Dixon Mann s.*
Mannkopf s. increase in the frequency of the pulse on pressure over a painful spot; not present in simulated pain.
Marcus Gunn pupillary s. see under *phenomenon.*
Marie s. tremor of the body or extremities in Graves disease and other types of hyperthyroidism.
Marie-Foix s. withdrawal of lower leg on transverse pressure of tarsus or forced flexion of toes even though the lower limb as a whole is incapable of voluntary movement.
Marinesco s. Marinesco succulent hand.
Mean s. Kocher s.
Mendel-Bekhterev s. see under *reflex.*
meniscus s. the radioscopic appearance of a crescentic shadow made by the crater of a gastric ulcer: when the convexity of the crescent points outward the ulcer is on the lesser curvature; when the convexity points downward the ulcer is distal to the angular incisure. Called also *Carman, Carman-Kirklin,* or *crescent s.*
Mennell s. an examining thumb is placed over the posterosuperior spine of the sacrum and then made to slide, first outward and then inward. If on pressure over the former point tenderness is detected, it is due to a sensitive deposit in the structures of the gluteal aspect of the posterosuperior spine. If the tenderness is over the inner point, it is probable that the superior ligaments of the sacroiliac joint are strained and sensitive. If the tenderness is increased by pressure backward on the anterosuperior aspect of the ilium and decreased by pulling forward the crest from behind, this is positive proof that it is caused by the sensitive ligaments.
Mercedes-Benz s. shadows shaped like the logo of the Mercedes-Benz automobile, seen on radiographs of the gallbladder; they indicate the presence of gas-filled fissures within gallstones, although the gallstones themselves may not be visible.
Mexican hat s. a shadow resembling a large-brimmed Mexican hat, seen on a radiograph of the colon; it represents the filling defect caused by a pedunculated polyp on the inferior wall.
Minor s. the method of rising from a sitting position characteristic of the patient with sciatica; the patient leans on the healthy side, balancing on that leg, placing one hand on the back and taking weight off the affected leg.
Möbius s., Moebius s. inability to keep the eyeballs converged due to insufficiency of the internal rectus muscles; a manifestation of Graves orbitopathy.
Mosler s. sternal tenderness in acute myeloblastic leukemia.
moulage s. a waxy cast appearance of bowel segments, a radiographic sign of celiac disease.
Mulder s. when the foot is compressed from the sides and the involved distal metatarsal space is digitally compressed, if a Morton neuroma is present the involved nerve will snap below the metatarsal heads, sometimes making an audible click. Called also *Mulder click.*
Müller s. a sign of aortic insufficiency consisting of pulsation of the uvula and redness of the tonsils and velum palati, occurring synchronously with the action of the heart.
Munson s. abnormal bulging of the lower lid when the patient rolls the eyes downward, caused by keratoconus (abnormal curvature of the cornea).
Murphy s. a sign of gallbladder disease consisting of interruption of the patient's deep inhalation when the physician's fingers are pressed deeply beneath the right costal arch, below the hepatic margin.

Musset s. rhythmical jerking movement of the head; seen in cases of aortic aneurysm and aortic insufficiency.
Myerson s. a sign of Parkinson disease: ready induction of blepharospasm when the frontalis muscle is tapped.
neck s. Brudzinski s. (def. 1).
Negro s. cogwheel rigidity.
Neri s. 1. a sign of organic hemiplegia, consisting in the spontaneous bending of the knee of the affected side as the leg is passively lifted, the patient being in the dorsal position. 2. with the patient standing, forward bending of the trunk will cause flexion of the knee on the affected side in lumbosacral and iliosacral lesions.
niche s. Haudek s.
Nicoladoni s. Branham s.
Nikolsky s. ready separation of the outer layer of the epidermis from the basal layer with sloughing of the skin produced by minor trauma such as a sliding or rubbing pressure on the skin; this may occur in pemphigus, certain hereditary blistering skin diseases, staphylococcal scalded skin syndrome, toxic epidermal necrolysis, and thermal burns.
Ober s. see under *test.*
objective s. a sign that can be seen, heard, or felt by the diagnostician; called also *physical s.*
obturator s. a sign of appendicitis: hypogastric or adductor pain elicited by passive internal rotation of the flexed thigh, due to contact between an inflammatory process and the internal obturator muscle.
Oliver s. tracheal tugging; see under *tugging.*
Oppenheim s. see under *reflex.*
orbicularis s. in hemiplegia, inability to close the eye on the paralyzed side without closing the other eye.
Ortolani s. the presence of a palpable click in and out as the hip is reduced by abduction and dislocated by adduction in developmental dysplasia of the hip; called also *Ortolani click.*
Osler s. the presence of Osler nodes on the hands and feet, pathognomonic of subacute bacterial endocarditis.
Pace s. with the patient seated, the examiner abducts the thigh and rotates it externally; pain indicates the presence of levator ani syndrome.
Parkinson s. see under *facies.*
Parrot s. 1. ciliospinal reflex. 2. bony nodes on the outer table of the skull of infants with congenital syphilis, so that it has a hot cross bun or buttock shape; called also *Parrot nodes, hot cross bun skull,* and *natiform skull.*
Pastia s. see under *line.*
patent bronchus s. the radiologic finding of an unobstructed bronchus supplying a collapsed lung, lobe, or segment.
Patrick s. see under *test.*
Pemberton s. a sign of thoracic inlet narrowing, such as by a goiter or tumor; when the patient raises the arms above the head, there is venous congestion of the face and often respiratory distress.
Pérez s. a friction sound heard over the sternum when the patient raises and drops the upper limbs; a sign of mediastinal tumor or of aneurysm of the arch of the aorta.
Phalen s. appearance of numbness or paresthesias within 30 to 60 seconds during the Phalen test, a positive sign for carpal tunnel syndrome.

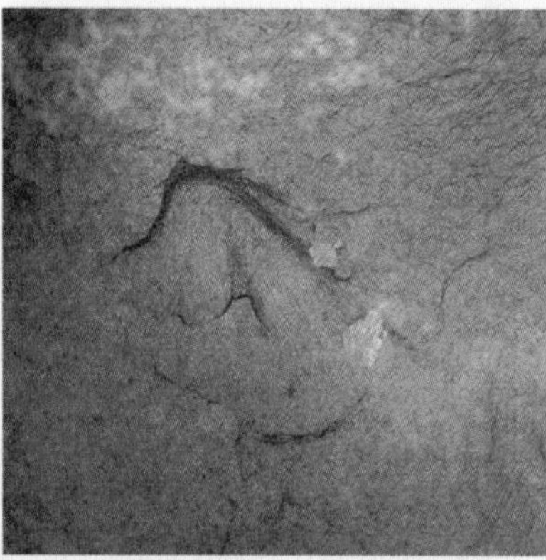

■ Positive Nikolsky sign: epidermal detachment caused by mechanical pressure on an area of erythematous skin in toxic epidermal necrolysis.

physical s. objective s.
Piltz s. 1. attention reflex of pupil; see under *reflex.* 2. orbicularis pupillary reflex.
Pins s. Ewart s.
Piotrowski s. percussion of the anterior tibialis muscle produces dorsal flexion and supination of the foot. When this reflex is excessive it indicates organic disease of the central nervous system. Called also *anticus s.* or *reflex.*
Piskacek s. asymmetrical enlargement of the corpus uteri due to enlargement of the pregnant uterus in the cornual region, usually over the site of implantation.
Pitres s. hypoesthesia of the scrotum and testes in tabes dorsalis.
pivot shift s. see under *phenomenon.*
placental s. implantation bleeding.
Plummer s. inability to step up onto a chair or to walk up steps, seen in Graves disease and other forms of hyperthyroidism.
Pool-Schlesinger s. Schlesinger s.
Porter s. tracheal tugging.
posterior drawer s. see under *test.*
Potain s. 1. extension of percussion dullness over the arch of the aorta, in dilatation of the aorta, from the manubrium to the third costal cartilage on the right-hand side. 2. timbre métallique.
prayer s. digital contractures in the hand, a sign of diabetes mellitus, seen when the patient holds the palms of the hands together as if praying.
Prehn s. elevation and support of the scrotum will relieve the pain in epididymo-orchitis, but not in torsion of the testicle.
Prévost s. a sign of hemiplegia, such as with middle cerebral artery stroke: conjugate deviation of the head and eyes, the eyes looking toward the affected hemisphere and away from the paralyzed limbs.
pronation s. 1. Babinski s. (def. 5). 2. pronation of the forearm caused by passive flexion, seen in hemiplegia; called also *Strümpell s.*
pseudo-Babinski s. in poliomyelitis, the Babinski reflex is modified so that only the big toe is extended, because all the foot muscles except the dorsiflexors of the big toe are paralyzed.
pseudo-Graefe s. slow descent of the upper lid on looking down, and quick ascent on looking up; seen in conditions other than Graves disease.
psoas s. flexion of or pain on hyperextension of the hip due to contact between an inflammatory process and the psoas muscle; the inflammation may indicate appendicitis. Called also *Cope s.*
puddle s. a method for detecting ascites in the abdominal cavity: the patient lies prone for five minutes, then rises to hands and knees; the part of the ventral abdomen containing the fluid "puddle" shows a loss of high-frequency vibration that can be detected and measured by flicking a finger against the flank and abdomen and listening through a stethoscope.
pulvinar s. bilateral hyperintensity of the pulvinar seen on magnetic resonance imaging, a sign of new variant Creutzfeldt-Jakob disease.
pyramid s., pyramidal s. any sign pointing to disease of the pyramidal tract.
Quant s. a T-shaped depression in the occipital bone, sometimes seen in rickets.
Queckenstedt s. when the veins in the neck are compressed on one or both sides, in healthy persons there is a rapid rise in the pressure of the cerebrospinal fluid, which returns quickly to normal when pressure is taken off the neck. When there is a block in the vertebral canal the pressure of the cerebrospinal fluid is affected little or not at all by this maneuver. Called also *Queckenstedt phenomenon* or *test.*
Quénu-Muret s. in aneurysm, the main artery of the limb is compressed and then a puncture is made at the periphery; if blood flows, the collateral circulation is probably established.
Quincke s. see under *pulse.*
raccoon s. raccoon eyes; see under *eye.*
radialis s. inability to close the fist without marked dorsal extension of the wrist, seen in hemiplegia; called also *Strümpell s.*
Radovici s. palm-chin reflex.
Ramond s. rigidity of the erector spinae muscle indicative of pleurisy with effusion; the rigidity relaxes when the effusion becomes purulent.
Raynaud s. acrocyanosis.
Remak s. either polyesthesia or a prolongation of the lapse of time before a painful impression is perceived, seen in tabes dorsalis.

Sign *Continued*

reservoir s. the ability of a patient to produce cerebrospinal fluid rhinorrhea at will by moving the head, indicating presence of a fistula with pooling in a paranasal sinus.
reversed three s. a pair of indentations, one on either side of the aortic knuckle, seen on barium contrast imaging of the esophagus and representing mirror images of a figure three sign; it signifies coarctation of the aorta. Called also *E s.*
Revilliod s. orbicularis s.
Riesman s. 1. Snellen s. 2. softening of the eyeball in diabetic coma.
rim s. cortical rim s.
Robertson s. 1. fibrillary contraction of the pectoralis muscle over the cardiac area in approaching death from heart disease. 2. absence of pupillary dilatation on pressure over alleged painful areas in malingering. 3. in ascites, fullness and tension in the patient's flanks, felt by the examiner with the patient supine.
Romaña s. unilateral ophthalmia with palpebral edema, conjunctivitis, and swelling of regional lymph glands as a sign of Chagas disease.
Romberg s. swaying of the body or falling when standing with the feet close together and the eyes closed; the result of loss of joint position sense, seen in tabes dorsalis and other diseases affecting the posterior columns. Called also *rombergism* and *Romberg test.*
Rommelaere s. an abnormally small proportion of normal phosphates and of sodium chloride in the urine in cancerous cachexia.
rope s. the presence of skin-colored to slightly erythematous linear indurations extending from the upper back to the axilla; pathognomonic for interstitial granulomatous dermatitis.
Rosenbach s. absence of the abdominal skin reflex, indicative of inflammatory disease of the intestines or of hemiplegia on the side where the sign is present.
Rossolimo s. see under *reflex.*
Rotch s. dullness on percussion of the right fifth intercostal space, a sign of pericardial effusion.
Rovsing s. pressure over the point on the left side corresponding to the McBurney point on the right will elicit the typical pain at the McBurney point in appendicitis.
Ruggeri s. see under *reflex.*
Rumpel-Leede s. see under *phenomenon.*
Saenger s. a light reflex of the pupil that has ceased returns after a short stay in the dark; observed in cerebral syphilis but not in tabes dorsalis.
Sansom s. 1. marked increase of the area of dullness in the second and third intercostal spaces, due to pericardial effusion. 2. a rhythmical murmur heard with a stethoscope applied to the lips in aneurysm of the thoracic aorta.
Saunders s. on wide opening of the mouth there take place in children associated movements of the hand consisting of opening of the hand and extension and separation of the fingers; called also *mouth-and-hand synkinesia.*
Schamroth s. see under *test.*
Schepelmann s. in dry pleurisy, the pain is increased when the patient bends his body toward the normal side, whereas in intercostal neuralgia it is increased by bending toward the affected side.
Schick s. stridor heard on exhalation in an infant with tuberculosis involving the bronchial glands.
Schlesinger s. in tetany, if the patient's lower limb is held at the knee joint and flexed strongly at the hip joint, there will soon be an extensor spasm at the knee joint, with extreme supination of the foot. Called also *Pool* or *Schlesinger phenomenon.*
Schultze s., Schultze-Chvostek s. Chvostek s.
Schwartze s. a pink blush behind the tympanic membrane, sometimes seen in otosclerosis because of hyperemia of the mucous membrane around the promontory.
scimitar s. on a radiograph of the chest, a scimitar-shaped shadow to the right of the lower border of the heart, representing the anomalous vein of the scimitar syndrome.
Séguin s. the involuntary contraction of the muscles just before an epileptic attack.
Seidel s. see under *scotoma.*
setting sun s. downward deviation of the eyes, so that each iris resembles a sun setting beneath the lower lid, with white sclera exposed between it and the upper lid; this indicates increased intracranial pressure (such as from hemorrhage or ependymitis), hydrocephalus, or a pineal gland tumor.

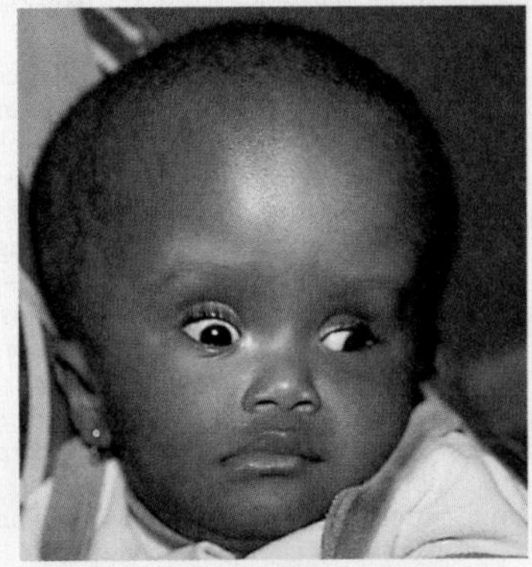

■ Setting sun sign in infant with hydrocephalus.

shawl s. poikiloderma on the shoulders and upper trunk in the area often covered by a shawl, a sign of dermatomyositis.
Shibley s. in the presence of consolidation of the lung or a collection of fluid in the pleural cavity, all spoken vowels are heard through the stethoscope as "ah."
Siegert s. in Down syndrome, the little fingers are short and curved inward.
signet ring s. in diagnostic imaging, a ring-shaped appearance caused by a pathologic process, such as that seen on radiographs of the wrist in scapholunate dislocation or that caused by a dilated bronchus on computed tomography of the lung. See also *cortical ring s.*
Silex s. furrows radiating from the mouth in congenital syphilis.
Simon s. 1. [C.E. *Simon*] retraction or fixation of the umbilicus during inhalation. 2. [J. *Simon*] absence of the usual correlation between the movements of the diaphragm and thorax; seen in beginning meningitis.
Skoda s. skodaic resonance.
Smith s. a murmur heard in cases of enlarged bronchial glands on auscultation over the manubrium with the patient's head thrown back.
Snellen s. the bruit heard with a stethoscope over the closed eye in Graves disease; see also *Graves orbitopathy,* under *orbitopathy.*
soft s's minor objective findings that are often associated with a morbid condition, although they are not pathognomonic for it; cf. *hard s's.*
sonographic Murphy s. evidence of gallstones on an ultrasound examination combined with pain over the gallbladder indicates presence of acute cholelithiasis.
Soto-Hall s. with the patient lying supine, on flexion of the spine beginning at the neck and going downward, pain will be felt at the site of the lesion in back abnormalities.
Spalding s. on an x-ray of a fetus in utero, overriding of the bones of the vault of the skull indicates that the fetus is dead.
spinal s. a sign of pleurisy consisting of tonic contraction of the spinal muscles on the diseased side.
spine s. reluctance to flex the spine anteriorly, owing to pain, a sign of poliomyelitis or meningitis.
split pleura s. a rim of thickened and enhanced parietal and visceral pleura surrounding a loculated pleural fluid collection on contrast-enhanced computed tomography; a sign of empyema.
square root s. in constrictive pericarditis, the diastolic level of the right ventricular pressure curve is initially normal but rapidly rises abnormally.
stairs s. difficulty in descending a stairway in tabes dorsalis.
steeple s. on a radiograph of the airway, an area of narrowing or obstruction above a wider area, sometimes seen in children with croup or epiglottitis.
Stellwag s. a sign of Graves orbitopathy: infrequent and incomplete blinking accompanied by Dalrymple sign.
Sternberg s. a sign of pleurisy consisting of sensitiveness to palpation of the muscles of the shoulder girdle.
Stewart-Holmes s. rebound phenomenon.
Stierlin s. absence of the normal shadow on a radiographic image of the colon after a barium enema, due to an indurating or ulcerating process such as tuberculosis of the cecum or colon.

Sign *Continued*

Strauss s. increase of fat following the use of fatty foods in chylous ascites.
string s. in radiography of the colon, a stringlike configuration of contrast material through a filling defect; called also *Kantor s.*
string of beads s. 1. a series of round shadows resembling a string of beads or pearls, seen on a radiograph of the small intestine, indicating bubbles of trapped gas surrounded by the fluid of an obstructed and distended bowel. 2. the appearance on an angiogram of an artery affected by fibromuscular dysplasia, with areas of protruding aneurysms alternating with areas of thinning and stenosis.
Strümpell s. 1. tibialis s. 2. radialis s. 3. pronation s. (def. 2).
Strunsky s. a sign for detecting lesions of the anterior arch of the foot. The examiner grasps the toes and flexes them suddenly. This procedure is painless in the normal foot, but causes pain if there is inflammation of the anterior arch.
Suker s. a manifestation of Graves orbitopathy, consisting of deficient complementary fixation in lateral eye rotation.
Sumner s. on gentle palpation of the iliac fossa, a slight increase in tonus of the abdominal muscles may indicate appendicitis, stone in the ureter or kidney, or a twisted pedicle of an ovarian cyst.
swinging flashlight s. Marcus Gunn pupillary phenomenon.
Tay s. cherry-red spot.
Theimich lip s. a protrusion or pouting of the lips elicited by tapping the orbicularis oris muscle.
Thomas s. the flexion deformity seen in a hip in the Thomas test.
three s. figure three s.
Throckmorton s. see under *reflex.*
thumb s. 1. the thumblike appearance of the swollen epiglottis on a lateral radiograph of the neck in epiglottitis. 2. in Marfan syndrome, the entire nail of the thumb projects beyond the ulnar border of the hand when the thumb is crossed over the palm without assistance. Cf. *wrist s.*
thumbprint s. thumb s. (def. 1).
tibialis s. dorsal flexion of the foot when the thigh is drawn up toward the body; seen in spastic paralysis of the lower limb. Called also *Strümpell s.* or *phenomenon* and *anterior tibial s.*
Tinel s. a tingling sensation in the distal end of a limb when percussion is made over the site of a divided nerve. It indicates a partial lesion or the beginning regeneration of the nerve. Called also *DTP s.*, *formication s.*, and *distal tingling on percussion.*

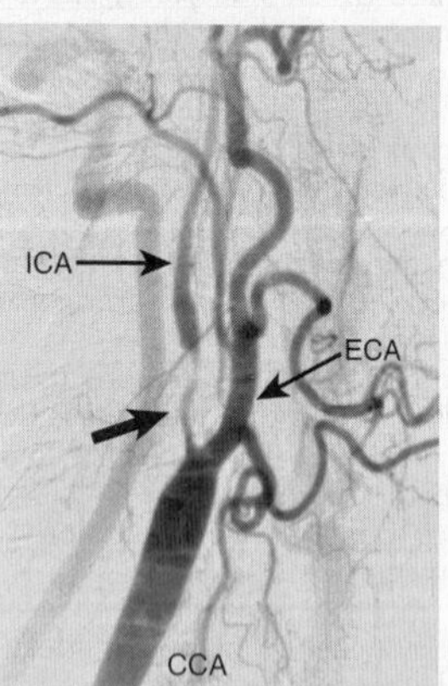

■ String sign *(short arrow)* in angiography, reflecting severe form of near occlusion of internal carotid artery beyond a point of critical stenosis. *CCA*, Common carotid artery; *ECA*, external carotid artery; *ICA*, internal carotid artery.

toe s. Babinski reflex.
Tournay s. unilateral dilatation of the pupil of the abducting eye on extreme lateral fixation.
Traube s. a loud sound like a pistol shot heard in auscultation over the femoral arteries in aortic regurgitation. Called also *pistol-shot sound.*
Trendelenburg s. 1. see under *test.* 2. see under *gait.*
trepidation s. patellar clonus.
Tresilian s. a reddish appearance of the parotid duct in mumps.
Troisier s. signal node.
Trousseau s. 1. see under *phenomenon.* 2. tache cérébrale.
Turner s. discoloration (bruising) and induration of the skin of the costovertebral angle caused by extravasation of blood in acute hemorrhagic pancreatitis. Called also *Grey Turner s.*
Turyn s. in sciatica, if the patient's great toe is bent dorsally, pain will be felt in the gluteal region.
twin peak s. a sonographic sign of dichorionic twinning consisting of a triangular zone whose echotexture is similar to that of the placenta, wider at the chorionic surface of the placenta and tapering to a point within the intertwin membrane.
Unschuld s. a nonspecific early sign of diabetes mellitus: a tendency to cramping in the calves.
Vanzetti s. in sciatica the pelvis is always horizontal in spite of scoliosis, but in other lesions with scoliosis the pelvis is inclined.
vein s. a bluish cord along the midaxillary line formed by the swollen junction of the thoracic and superficial epigastric vein; seen in tuberculosis involving the bronchial glands and in superior vena cava obstruction.
vital s's the pulse, respiration, and (body) temperature.
von Graefe s. Graefe s.
Waddell s's five signs indicating that a patient's low back pain is being intensified by psychological factors: tenderness that is not localized but spread over a wide area; production of pain by rotation of the pelvis or shoulders; decrease in pain behavior when the patient is distracted by the examiner; weakness or sensory disturbance that is not limited in a normal anatomic distribution; and overreaction, i.e. excessive body language or verbalization during the examination.
Wartenberg s. 1. a sign of ulnar palsy, consisting of a position of abduction assumed by the little finger. 2. reduction or absence of the pendulum movements of the upper limb in walking; seen in patients with cerebellar disease.
Weber s. see under *syndrome.*
Weill s. absence of expansion in the subclavicular region of the affected side in infantile pneumonia.
Wernicke s. hemiopic pupillary reaction.
Westermark s. transient clearing (avascularity) of the normal radiologic shadow of pulmonary tissue distal to a pulmonary embolism.
Westphal s. loss of the knee jerk in tabes dorsalis.
Wilder s. an early sign of Graves orbitopathy, consisting of a slight twitch of the eyeball when it changes its movement from adduction to abduction or vice versa.
Williamson s. markedly diminished blood pressure in the lower limb as compared with that in the upper limb on the same side, seen in pneumothorax and pleural effusion.
Wimberger s. symmetrical erosions of the proximal tibia seen radiographically in infants with congenital syphilis.
Winterbottom s. enlargement of posterior cervical lymph nodes in African trypanosomiasis.
Wood s. relaxation of the orbicularis muscle, fixation of the eyeball, and divergent strabismus, indicative of profound anesthesia.
wrist s. in Marfan syndrome, the thumb overlaps the distal phalanx of the fifth finger when grasping the opposite wrist.

sig•na (sig′nə) [L.] mark, or write; abbreviated S.S. or sig. on prescriptions. See *prescription.*

sig•nal•ing (sig′nəl-ing) the sending of information.
adrenergic s. the transmission of a chemical stimulus that activates adrenergic receptors.
cell s. synthesis and release by a cell of a substance, such as a hormone, that binds to receptors on and effects a specific response in a target cell.
retrograde s. the sending of information back across a synapse from a target organ or muscle to a nerve ending, causing modification of the signal intensity from the nerve.

sig•nal•ment (sig′nəl-mənt) [Fr. *signaler* to describe, from L. *signum* mark] in veterinary practice, a description consisting of the species, breed, age, and sex of an animal.

sig•na•ture (sig′nə-chər) [L. *signatura*] 1. the part of a prescription that gives directions to the patient for taking of medicine; abbreviated S. or sig. See *prescription.* 2. a characteristic feature of a substance that in folk medicine may be regarded as an indicator of its medicinal virtues: the eyelike mark on the flower of the euphrasia was considered to show its usefulness in eye diseases; the liverlike shape of the leaf of liverwort pointed to its use in hepatic diseases; and the yellow color of saffron indicated its use in jaundice.

sig•nif•i•cant (sig-nif′ĭ-kənt) in statistics, probably resulting from something other than chance.

sign•ing (sīn′ing) communication between individuals, especially the deaf, using signs made with the hands and fingers. Called also *dactylology*.

Sig. n. pro. [L.] sig′na nom′ine pro′prio (label with the proper name).

sig•ua•te•ra (sig″wə-ta′rə) [Sp.] ciguatera.

si•ki•mi (se′ke-me) [Japanese] *Illicium religiosum*.

sik•im•i•tox•in (sik-im′ĭ-tok″sin) a poisonous substance found in *Illicium religiosum* (sikimi).

sil•a•fil•con A (sil″ə-fil′kon) a hydrophilic contact lens material.

sil•a•fo•con A (sil″ə-fo′kon) a hydrophobic contact lens material.

Si•las•tic (sĭ-las′tik) trademark for polymeric silicone substances that have the properties of rubber but are biologically inert; used in surgical prostheses.

sil•den•a•fil cit•rate (sil-den′ə-fil″) a phosphodiesterase inhibitor that relaxes the smooth muscle of the penis, thereby facilitating blood flow to the corpus cavernosum; used to treat erectile dysfunction in impotence therapy.

si•lence (si′ləns) [L. *silēre* to be quiet] a state of being silent.

electrical s. in electroencephalography and electromyography, absence of measurable electrical activity in tissue.

electrocerebral s. (ECS) electrical silence in the cerebral cortex. Temporary silence may occur with overdoses of depressant drugs such as barbiturates and benzodiazepines, with hypothermia, or with cardiogenic shock. Permanent silence is one of the criteria for a diagnosis of brain death. Called also *electrocerebral inactivity*.

si•len•cer (si′lən-sər) in molecular genetics, any of a class of nucleotide sequences that function as *cis*-acting negative regulators of transcription.

si•len•cing (si′lən-sing) the process of making or keeping something silent.

gene s. negative regulation of gene expression; it includes processes that inhibit transcription of genes, such as DNA methylation, and posttranscriptional processes, such as the degradation of messenger RNA by RNA interference.

si•lent (si′lənt) 1. noiseless. 2. producing no detectable signs or symptoms.

Si•lex sign (se′leks) [Paul *Silex*, German ophthalmologist, 1858–1929] see under *sign*.

si•lex (si′leks) [L. "flint"] a refined form of silica powder, which may be mixed with water or a mouthwash solution to form a fine abrasive paste for polishing metal castings.

Silf•ver•skiöld syndrome (sil′vər-shərld) [Nils G. *Silfverskiöld*, Swedish orthopedist, 1888–1957] see under *syndrome*.

sil•hou•ette (sil″ə-wet′) [Fr.] the outline or contour of a thing.

cardiac s. the contour of the heart appearing on radiographs of the chest.

cardiopericardial s. the contour of the heart and pericardium appearing on radiographs of the chest.

cardiovascular s. the contour of the heart and great vessels appearing on radiographs of the chest.

sil•i•ca (sil′ĭ-kə) [L. *silex* flint] SiO_2, silicon dioxide or silicic anhydride, occurring in nature as agate, sand, amethyst, chalcedony, cristobalite, flint, quartz, and tridymite. It is one of the major constituents of dental porcelain and a common filler in resin composites; in granular form it serves as a dental abrasive and polishing agent. See also *silicosis*.

sil•i•cate (sil′ĭ-kāt) [L. *silicus*] a salt of any of the silicic acids.

sil•i•ca•to•sis (sil″ĭ-kə-to′sis) pneumoconiosis caused by the inhalation of the dust of silicates, particularly aluminum silicate and magnesium silicate (e.g., asbestos, fuller's earth, kaolin, mica, or talc). See *asbestosis*, and see other types under *pneumoconiosis*.

si•lic•ea (sĭ-lis′e-ə) a homeopathic preparation of silica.

si•li•ceous (sĭ-lish′əs) containing silica or a compound of silicon.

si•lic•ic ac•id (sĭ-lik′ik) the molecular species $Si(OH)_4$ occurring in hydrated forms of silica, e.g., silica gel.

si•li•cious (sĭ-lish′əs) siliceous.

sil•i•co•an•thra•co•sis (sil″ĭ-ko-an″thrə-ko′sis) anthracosilicosis.

sil•i•co•flu•o•ride (sil″ĭ-ko-floor′īd) fluorosilicate.

sil•i•con (Si) (sil′ĭ-kon) [L. *silex* flint] a nonmetallic element occurring in nature as silicon dioxide, usually called silica; atomic number, 14; atomic weight, 28.086.

s. carbide a compound produced by the reaction of silicon and carbon at extremely high temperature; it ranks next to diamond in hardness and is used in dentistry as an abrasive and refractory.

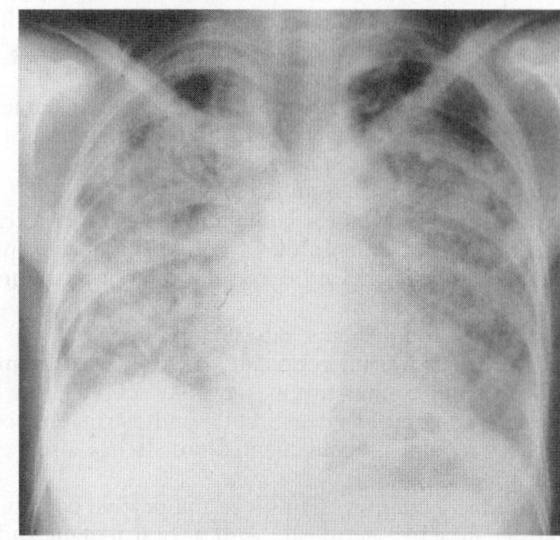

■ Acute silicosis showing alveolar filling in a 28-year-old woman who inhaled fine particles of silica from abrasive powder.

colloidal s. dioxide [NF] a submicroscopic fumed silica prepared by the vapor-phase hydrolysis of a silicon compound; used as a tablet diluent and as a suspending and thickening agent.

s. dioxide 1. silica. 2. [NF] a preparation of purified silica, used as a pharmaceutical dispersing and suspending agent.

s. fluoride SiF_4, a colorless gas sometimes fatal to workers in superphosphate factories.

sil•i•cone (sil′ĭ-kōn) a polymeric organic siloxane; any of a large group of organic compounds comprising alternating silicon and oxygen atoms linked to organic radicals, $(R_2SiO)_n$, the most common substituent being a methyl group. They occur as liquids, semisolids, or solids as a function of molecular weight and degree of polymerization, and range in viscosity from less than one to greater than one million centistokes. Functionally, silicones are usually divided into fluids (or oils), greases, waxes, resins, gums, and elastomers (silicone rubber), and uses have included wetting agents and surfactants, lubricants, defoaming agents, sealants, coolants, surgical membranes, contact lenses, implants, and dental impression materials. See also under *oil*.

sil•i•co•pro•tein•o•sis (sil″ĭ-ko-pro″tēn-o′sis) a rapidly fatal pneumoconiosis occurring several weeks to months after massive exposure to silica dust, characterized by the presence of proteinaceous fluid in the air spaces.

sil•i•co•sid•er•o•sis (sil″ĭ-ko-sid″ər-o′sis) siderosilicosis.

sil•i•co•sis (sil″ĭ-ko′sis) [*silica* + *-osis*] pneumoconiosis due to the inhalation of the dust of stone, sand, or flint containing silica, with formation of generalized nodular fibrotic changes in both lungs. Since many common minerals contain silica, there are numerous different types of silicosis. Called also *pneumosilicosis*. **silicot′ic** *adj*

infective s. silicotuberculosis.

sil•i•co•tu•ber•cu•lo•sis (sil″ĭ-ko-too-ber″ku-lo′sis) tuberculous infection of the silicotic lung; called also *infective silicosis* and *tuberculosilicosis*.

sil•i•qua (sil′ĭ-kwə) [L.] a pod, or husk.

s. oli′vae amiculum olivare.

sil•i•quose (sil′ĭ-kwōs) pertaining to or resembling a pod or husk.

silk (silk) the protein filament produced by the larvae of various insects; braided, degummed silk obtained from the cocoons of the silkworm *Bombyx mori* is used as a nonabsorbable suture material.

virgin s. silk from which the adhesive protein sericin has not been removed; used as a suture material in ophthalmic microsurgery.

silk•worm (silk′wərm) the larva of *Bombyx mori*.

si•lox•ane (si-lok′sān) any of various compounds based on a substituted backbone of alternating silica and oxygen molecules; in polymeric form they are also called *polysiloxanes*, and those in which the side chain substituents are organic radicals, i.e., organic siloxanes, are silicones (q.v.). The most common are the polydimethylsiloxanes, having methyl substituents.

Sil•va•dene (sil′və-dēn) trademark for a preparation of silver sulfadiazine.

Sil•ver syndrome (sil′vər) [Henry K. *Silver*, American pediatrician, born 1918] Silver-Russell syndrome; see under *syndrome*.

sil•ver (Ag) (sil′vər) a white, soft, malleable, and ductile metallic element; atomic number, 47; atomic weight, 107.870. Its compounds are extensively used in medicine and in x-ray and photographic films; metallic silver is used in surgery and in the manufacture of instruments. In dentistry, it is used chiefly in prostheses, in alloys such as amalgam, in soldering, to neutralize the color imparted by copper in alloys, and as points to obliterate the root canal.

s. chloride an insoluble white salt, AgCl, that darkens in light.

colloidal s. a silver preparation in which the silver exists as free ions to only a small extent. See *strong s. protein* and *mild s. protein.*

colloidal s. iodide silver iodide in solution rendered stable by gelatin, an antiseptic for treating inflammations of mucous membranes.

fused s. nitrate toughened s. nitrate.

methenamine s. see under *methenamine.*

mild s. protein a preparation containing 19–23 per cent of silver, rendered colloidal by the presence of, or combination with, protein; it is used as a topical antiinfective in various rectal, ocular, vaginal, urethral, otic, nasal, and pharyngeal infections.

molded s. nitrate toughened s. nitrate.

s. nitrate [USP] a powerful germicide, $AgNO_3$, used as an antiseptic, applied topically to the conjunctiva as a prophylactic against ophthalmia neonatorum, and also used as an antiseptic and astringent, especially in infections of the skin and mucous membranes. It has also been used to purify drinking water.

strong s. protein a compound of silver and protein containing 7.5–8.5 per cent of silver; an active germicide with a local irritant and astringent effect. It may cause argyria.

s. sulfadiazine [USP] the silver derivative of sulfadiazine, having bactericidal activity against many gram-positive and gram-negative organisms, as well as being effective against yeasts; used as a topical antiinfective for the prevention and treatment of wound sepsis in patients with second and third degree burns.

toughened s. nitrate [USP] a compound prepared by fusing silver nitrate with hydrochloric acid, sodium chloride, or potassium nitrate, occurring as white crystalline masses molded into pencils or cones, and containing 94.5 per cent of silver nitrate; used as a caustic and applied topically after being dipped in water. Called also *lunar caustic, fused silver nitrate,* and *molded silver nitrate.*

Sil·ver-Rus·sell syndrome (dwarfism) (sil′vər rus′əl) [H.K. *Silver;* Alexander *Russell,* British pediatrician, 1914–2003] see under *syndrome.*

Sil·ver·man needle (sil′vər-mən) [Irving *Silverman,* American surgeon, 20th century] see under *needle.*

Sil·ver·man syndrome (sil′vər-mən) [Frederic Noah *Silverman,* American pediatrician, 1914–2006] Currarino-Silverman syndrome.

Sil·ves·tri·ni-Cor·da syndrome (sil-vəs-tre′ne kor′dah) [R. *Silvestrini,* Italian physician, 20th century; L. *Corda,* Italian physician, 20th century] see under *syndrome.*

Sil·vi·us (sil′ve-əs) a genus of Australian biting flies of the family Tabanidae.

Si·ly·bum (sil′ĭ-bəm) a genus of thistles, including *S. maria′num,* the milk thistle.

sil·y·mar·in (sil″ĭ-mar′in) an extract from the seeds of the milk thistle *(Silybum marianum),* used for the treatment of chronic liver disease.

Sim·a·ru·ba (sim″ə-roo′bə) a genus of tropical American trees of the family Simaroubaceae; several species are medicinal. The root bark of *S. ama′ra* Aubl. is a bitter tonic and astringent, and has been used in amebiasis; its active principle is simarubidin.

si·ma·zine (si′mə-zēn) an herbicide used in gardens; it is toxic to ruminants, causing liver and kidney damage and neurotoxicity that can be fatal.

Sim·dax (sim′daks) trademark for a preparation of levosimendan.

si·meth·i·cone (sĭ-meth′ĭ-kōn) [USP] a mixture of dimethicones and silicon dioxide, with a molecular weight between 14,000 and 21,000, occurring as a translucent, gray, viscous fluid. It is administered orally as an antifoaming agent in gastroscopy, and is also used as an antiflatulent and as a releasing agent in pharmaceutical preparations. Called also *dimethicone* or *activated dimethicone.* It is used in veterinary medicine in the treatment and prevention of bloat in cattle.

sim·i·an (sim′e-ən) [L. *simia* ape] of, pertaining to, or resembling an ape or a monkey.

si·mi·lia si·mi·li·bus cu·ran·tur (sĭ-mĭ′le-ə sĭ-mĭ′lĭ-bəs ku-ran′tər) [L. "likes are cured by likes"] the doctrine, which lies at the foundation of homeopathy, that a disease is cured by those remedies that produce effects resembling the disease itself.

si·mil·li·mum (sĭ-mil′ĭ-məm) [L. "likest"] the homeopathic remedy that most exactly reproduces the symptoms of any disease.

Sim·ka·nia (sim-ka′ne-ə) [*Simona Kahane,* Israeli microbiologist, b. 1945] a genus of bacteria of the family Simkaniaceae, consisting of small coccoid organisms that multiply only within the cytoplasm of host cells by a unique developmental cycle (see Chlamydiales); organisms are naturally parasites of free-living amebae. The type species is *S. negevensis.*

S. negeven′sis a species that is associated with human respiratory disease.

Sim·ka·ni·a·ceae (sim-ka″ne-a′se-e) a family of bacteria of the order Chlamydiales, consisting of small coccoid microorganisms incapable of synthesizing ATP that multiply only within the cytoplasm of host cells by the unique developmental cycle common to the Chlamydiales (q.v.). It contains the genus *Simkania.*

Sim·monds disease (syndrome) (zim′əndz) [Morris *Simmonds,* German physician, 1855–1925] panhypopituitarism.

Si·mon sign[1] (si′mən) [Charles Edmund *Simon,* American physician, 1866–1927] see under *sign.*

Si·mon sign[2] (si′mən) [Sir John *Simon,* English surgeon, 1816–1904] see under *sign.*

Si·mo·nart thread (band) (se″mo-nahr′) [Pierre Joseph Cécilien *Simonart,* Belgian obstetrician, 1817–1847] see under *thread.*

Si·mons disease (ze′monz) [Arthur *Simons,* German physician, 20th century] partial lipodystrophy.

sim·ple (sim′pəl) [L. *simplex*] 1. neither compound nor complex; single. 2. an old term for any herb with real or supposed medicinal virtues.

Sim·plex·vi·rus (sim′pleks-vi″rəs) [herpes *simplex* + *virus*] the herpes simplex virus group, a genus of ubiquitous viruses of the subfamily Alphaherpesvirinae (family Herpesviridae) that infect various animals; included are human herpesviruses 1 and 2, bovine herpesvirus 2, and herpesvirus B.

Simp·son forceps (simp′sən) [Sir James Young *Simpson,* Scottish obstetrician, 1811–1870] see under *forceps.*

Sims position, speculum (simz) [James Marion *Sims,* American gynecologist, 1813–1883] see under *position* and *speculum.*

sim·ul (sim′əl) [L.] at the same time as.

sim·u·la·tion (sim″u-la′shən) [L. *simulatio*] 1. an imitation or pretense. 2. the act of counterfeiting a disease; malingering. 3. the mimicking of one disease by another.

Monte Carlo s. see under *method.*

sim·u·la·tor (sim″u-la′tər) something that simulates, such as an apparatus that simulates conditions that will be encountered in real life.

Sim·u·lect (sim′u-lekt) trademark for a preparation of basiliximab.

Si·mu·li·i·dae (si″mu-le′ĭ-de) a family of small flies of the suborder Nematocera, characterized by a humped back and short stubbed antennae of 10 or 11 segments. It contains approximately 600 species, known variously as black flies, buffalo gnats, or turkey gnats. The females of several species are vicious biters.

Si·mu·li·um (si-mu′le-əm) a genus of flies of the family Simuliidae; many species bite animals and spread disease.

S. amazo′nicum a species that is a vector of *Mansonella ozzardi* in Brazil and Guyana.

S. arc′ticum a species found in Alaska.

S. columbaczen′se a species found in southern Europe that causes fatal anemia in domestic animals.

S. damno′sum a species that is an intermediate host of *Onchocerca volvulus* in Africa.

S. metal′licum a Mexican species that transmits *Onchocerca volvulus.*

S. ochra′ceum a Mexican species that transmits *Onchocerca volvulus.*

S. pecua′rium the buffalo gnat, which attacks horses and cattle.

S. venus′tum a species found in Denmark and many parts of North America.

si·mul·tag·no·sia (si″məl-tag-no′zhah) simultanagnosia.

si·mul·tan·ag·no·sia (si″məl-tān″əg-no′zhah) impaired purposeful search of a complex visual display, reflecting a difficulty in integrating the parts as a whole; called also *simultagnosia.*

SIMV synchronized intermittent mandatory ventilation.

sim·va·stat·in (sim′və-stat″in) [USP] an antihyperlipidemic agent that is an HMG-CoA reductase inhibitor, used to lower blood lipid levels in the treatment of hypercholesterolemia and other forms of dyslipidemia and to reduce the risk of morbidity and mortality associated with atherosclerosis and coronary heart disease; administered orally.

si·nal (si′nəl) pertaining to a sinus; sinusal.

sin·al·bin (sin-al′bin) a glycoside found in white (or yellow) mustard; animals eating large quantities of these plants, especially the seeds, may develop fatal gastroenteritis.

Sin·a·pis (sin′ə-pis) former genus name for the mustards, plants now classified in genus *Brassica.*

sin·ca·lide (sin′kə-līd) [USP] the synthetic C-terminal octapeptide of cholecystokinin, used to stimulate gallbladder contraction in gallbladder function testing and cholecystography; administered intravenously.

sin·ci·put (sin′sĭ-pət) [L.] [TA] official name for *forehead,* considered as a part of the body; cf. *frons.* **sincip′ital** *adj*

Sind·bis fever, virus (sind′bis) [*Sindbis,* Egypt, village where the fever was observed in the 1950s] see under *fever* and *virus.*

Sin·ding-Lar·sen disease (sin′ding-lahr′sən) [Christian Magnus Falsen *Sinding-Larsen*, Norwegian physician, 1866–1930] Larsen disease; see under *disease*.

Sin·ding-Lar·sen–Jo·hans·son disease (sin′ding-lahr′sən yo-hahn′sən) [C.M.F. *Sinding-Larsen;* Sven Christian *Johansson*, Swedish surgeon, 1880–1959] Larsen disease; see under *disease*.

Sin·e·met (sin′ĕ-met) trademark for a combination of carbidopa and levodopa.

Sin·e·quan (sin′ə-kwahn) trademark for a preparation of doxepin hydrochloride.

sin·ew (sin′u) the tendon of a muscle.
weeping s. an encysted ganglion, chiefly on the back of the hand, containing synovial fluid.

sing. [L.] singulo′rum (of each).

sin·gle blind (sing′gəl blīnd) pertaining to a clinical trial or other experiment in which subjects do not know which treatment they are receiving.

Sin·gu·lair (sing′gu-lăr″) trademark for a preparation of montelukast sodium.

sin·gul·ta·tion (sing″gəl-ta′shən) a hiccup.

sin·gul·tous (sing-gul′təs) affected with hiccup.

sin·gul·tus (sing-gul′təs) [L.] hiccup.

sin·i·grin (sin′ĭ-grin) potassium myronate, a glycoside found in black or brown mustard *(Brassica nigra)* and horseradish *(Armoracia lapathifolia)*, from which allyl isothiocyanate is derived. Animals eating large quantities of these plants, especially their seeds, can develop fatal gastroenteritis.

si·nis·ter (sĭ-nis′tər) [L.] [TA] left: a term denoting the left-hand one of two similar structures, or the one situated on the left side of the body.

si·nis·trad (sĭ-nis′trad) to or toward the left.

sin·is·tral (sin′is-trəl) [L. *sinistralis*] 1. pertaining to the left side. 2. left-handed.

sin·is·tral·i·ty (sin″is-tral′ĭ-te) the preferential use, in voluntary motor acts, of the left member of the major paired organs of the body, as the left ear, eye, hand, and foot. See also *laterality* and *handedness*.

sinistr(o)- [L. *sinister* left] a combining form meaning left, or denoting relationship to the left side.

sin·is·tro·car·dia (sin″is-tro-kahr′de-ə) [*sinistro-* + Gr. *kardia* heart] displacement of the heart leftward in the thorax.

sin·is·tro·cer·e·bral (sin″is-tro-ser′ə-brəl) pertaining to or situated in the left cerebral hemisphere.

sin·is·troc·u·lar (sin″is-trok′u-lər) [*sinistro-* + *ocular*] left-eyed; having the left eye the dominant eye.

sin·is·troc·u·lar·i·ty (sin″is-trok″u-lar′ĭ-te) the state of having the left eye the dominant eye.

sin·is·tro·gy·ra·tion (sin″is-tro-ji-ra′shən) [*sinistro-* + *gyration*] a turning to the left, as a movement of the eye or the plane of polarization.

sin·is·tro·man·u·al (sin″is-tro-man′u-əl) [*sinistro-* + *manual*] left-handed.

sin·is·trop·e·dal (sin″is-trop′ə-dəl) [*sinistro-* + *pedal*] using the left foot in preference to the right.

sin·is·tro·tor·sion (sin″is-tro-tor′shən) levoclination.

sin(o)- [L. *sinus*, q.v.] a combining form denoting relationship to a sinus.

si·no·a·or·tic (si″no-a-or′tik) pertaining to a sinus and the aorta.

si·no·atri·al (si″no-a′tre-əl) pertaining to the sinus venosus (sinus of venae cavae) and the atrium of the heart; called also *sinuatrial.*

si·no·bron·chi·tis (si″no-brong-ki′tis) [*sino-* + *bronchitis*] chronic paranasal sinusitis with recurrent bronchitis.

si·nog·ra·phy (si-nog′rə-fe) [*sino-* + *-graphy*] radiography of the sinuses or of a pathologic sinus.

si·nom·e·nine (si-nom′ə-nin) a toxic crystalline alkaloid from the root of *Sinomenium acutum*, structurally related to thebaine.

Si·no·me·ni·um (si″no-me′ne-əm) a genus of plants of the family Menispermaceae. *S. acu′tum* (Thumb.) Rehd. Wils. is a species native to eastern Asia whose root is a source of the toxic alkaloid sinomenine.

Si non val. [L.] si non va′leat (if it is not enough).

si·no·pul·mo·nary (si″no-pool′mə-nar″e) involving the paranasal sinuses and the lungs.

si·nos·co·py (si-nos′kə-pe) [*sino-* + *-scopy*] endoscopic examination of a paranasal sinus; called also *sinusoscopy.*

si·no·spi·ral (si″no-spi′rəl) pertaining to the sinus venosus (sinus of venae cavae) and having a spiral course; said of certain bundles of cardiac muscle fibers. See also under *fiber*.

si·no·ven·tric·u·lar (si″no-vən-trik′u-lər) pertaining to the sinus venosus (sinus of venae cavae) and the ventricle of the heart.

sin·ter (sin′tər) [Ger.] 1. a chemical sedimentary rock deposited by mineral springs, especially one containing silica or calcium carbonate. 2. to transform a powder into a solid mass by heating below the melting point under specific conditions of pressure and decreased surface area.

sin·u·ate (sin″u-āt) having a wavy margin.

sinu·at·ri·al (sin″u-a′tre-əl) sinoatrial.

Si·nu·mist-SR (si′nu-mist) trademark for a preparation of guaifenesin.

sin·u·ous (sin′u-əs) [L. *sinuosus*] bending in and out; winding.

si·nus (si′nəs) pl. *si′nus* or *sinuses* [L. "a hollow"] 1. a cavity, channel, or space, such as a venous sinus or paranasal sinus. 2. an abnormal channel or fistula permitting the escape of pus.

Sinus

Descriptions are given on TA terms, and include anglicized names of specific sinuses.

accessory s's of the nose s. paranasales.
air s. an air-containing space within the substance of a bone.
anal s's, s. ana′les [TA] furrows, with pouchlike recesses at the lower end, separating the anal columns; called also *anal crypts, sinuses of Morgagni*, and *s. rectales.*
anterior s's, s. anterio′res cellulae ethmoidales anteriores.
s. of anterior chamber the narrow space at the edge of the anterior chamber of the eye, between the border of the cornea and the root of the iris.
s. aor′tae [TA] aortic sinus: a dilatation between the aortic wall and each of the semilunar cusps of the aortic valve; from two of these sinuses the coronary arteries take origin. Called also *Petit s., s. of Morgagni*, and *s. of Valsalva.*
Arlt s. s. of Maier.
basilar s. plexus basilaris.
s. of Bochdalek hiatus pleuroperitonealis.
branchial s. an abnormal cavity or space that opens externally on the inferior third of the neck, anterior to the sternocleidomastoid muscle; it usually results from persistence of the second pharyngeal groove and cervical sinus.
Breschet s. s. sphenoparietalis.
s. caro′ticus [TA], **carotid s.** the dilated portion of the internal carotid artery, situated above the division of the common carotid artery into its two main branches, or sometimes on the terminal portion of the common carotid artery, containing in its wall pressoreceptors that are stimulated by changes in blood pressure.
s. caverno′sus [TA], **cavernous s.** either of two sinuses of the dura mater, irregularly shaped and located at either side of the body of the sphenoid bone, extending from the medial end of the superior orbital fissure in front to the apex of the petrous temporal bone behind. Each sinus receives the corresponding superior ophthalmic vein, superficial middle cerebral vein, and the sphenoparietal sinus, and communicates with the opposite cavernous sinus by the anterior and posterior cavernous sinuses and with the transverse sinuses and internal jugular vein by way of the superior and inferior petrosal sinuses, respectively. Each cavernous sinus commonly comprises one or more main venous channels and contains the internal carotid artery and abducent nerve and, in the lateral wall of the sinus, the oculomotor, trochlear, ophthalmic, and maxillary nerves.
cervical s. a temporary depression caudal to the second pharyngeal (hyoid) arch, containing the succeeding pharyngeal arches; it is overgrown by the second pharyngeal arch and closes off as the cervical vesicle.

Sinus *Continued*

circular s., s. circula′ris the venous ring around the hypophysis formed by the two cavernous and the anterior and posterior intercavernous sinuses; called also *Ridley s.*
s. circula′ris i′ridis s. venosus sclerae.
coccygeal s. a pilonidal sinus just over or close to the tip of the coccyx. Called also *sacrococcygeal s.*
s. corona′rius [TA], **coronary s.** the terminal portion of the great cardiac vein, which lies in the coronary sulcus between the left atrium and ventricle, and empties into the right atrium between the orifice of the inferior vena cava and the atrioventricular orifice.
cortical s′s lymph sinuses in the cortex of a lymph node, which arise from the marginal sinuses and continue into the medullary sinuses; called also *intermediate s′s.*
costodiaphragmatic s. recessus costodiaphragmaticus pleuralis.
costomediastinal s. of pleura, s. costomediastina′lis pleu′rae recessus costomediastinalis pleuralis.
costophrenic s. recessus costodiaphragmaticus pleuralis.
cranial s′s s. durae matris.
dermal s. a congenital sinus tract extending from the surface of the body, between the bodies of two adjacent lumbar vertebrae, to the spinal canal.
s′s of dura mater, s. du′rae ma′tris [TA] large venous channels forming an anastomosing system between the layers of the cranial dura mater. They are devoid of valves, do not collapse when drained, and in some parts contain trabeculae. They drain the cerebral veins and some diploic and meningeal veins into the veins of the neck. Those at the base of the skull also drain most of the blood from the orbit. In some places they communicate with superficial veins by small emissary vessels. Called also *cranial s′s, s. venosi durales,* and *venous s′s of dura mater.*
dural s′s, dural venous s′s s. durae matris.
s. epididy′midis [TA], **s. of epididymis** a long, slitlike serous pocket between the upper part of the testis and the overlying epididymis.
Eternod s. a loop of vessels connecting the vessels of the chorion with those in the underside of the yolk sac.
ethmoid s′s, ethmoidal s′s cellulae ethmoidales.
ethmoidal s′s, anterior cellulae ethmoidales anteriores.
ethmoidal s′s, middle cellulae ethmoidales mediae.
ethmoidal s′s, posterior s. ethmoidales posteriores.
s. ethmoida′les cellulae ethmoidales.
s. ethmoida′les anterio′res cellulae ethmoidales anteriores.
s. ethmoida′les me′dii cellulae ethmoidales mediae.
s. ethmoida′les posterio′res cellulae ethmoidales posteriores.
Forssell s. a smooth space in the wall of the stomach surrounded by folds of the mucosa; seen on radiographic examination.
frontal s., s. fronta′lis [TA] one of the paired irregular shaped paranasal sinuses located in the frontal bone deep to the superciliary arch, separated from its fellow of the opposite side by a bony septum; it communicates by way of the nasofrontal duct with the middle meatus of the nasal cavity on the same side.
Guérin s. lacuna magna.
Huguier s. a depression in the tympanum between the fenestra ovalis and the fenestra rotunda.
s. intercaverno′sus ante′rior [TA] the anterior of the two sinuses of the dura mater connecting the two cavernous sinuses, passing anterior to the infundibulum of the hypophysis.

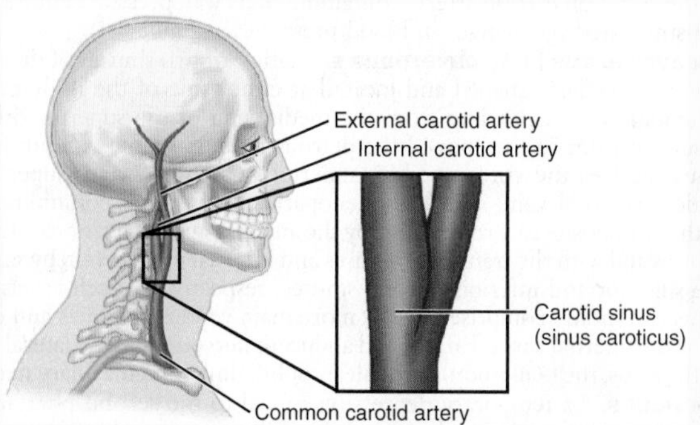

■ Sinus caroticus (carotid sinus) and carotid arteries in a deep dissection of the right side of the neck.

s. intercaverno′sus poste′rior [TA] the posterior of the two sinuses of the dura mater connecting the two cavernous sinuses, passing posterior to the infundibulum of the hypophysis.
intercavernous s., anterior s. intercavernosus anterior.
intercavernous s., posterior s. intercavernosus posterior.
intermediate s′s cortical s′s.
s. of kidney s. renalis.
lacteal s′s, s. lacti′feri [TA], **lactiferous s′s** enlargements in the lactiferous ducts just before they open onto the mammary papilla.
laryngeal s., s. of larynx ventriculus laryngis.
lateral s. s. transversus durae matris.
s. liena′lis TA alternative for *s. splenicus.*
longitudinal s., inferior s. sagittalis inferior.
longitudinal s., superior s. sagittalis superior.
lymph s′s, lymphatic s′s irregular tortuous spaces within lymph nodes through which a continuous stream of lymph passes to enter the efferent lymphatic vessels. See also *cortical s′s, marginal s′s,* and *medullary s′s.*
s. of Maier a slight diverticulum from the upper part of the lacrimal sac, into which the lacrimal canaliculi open, either together or separately; called also *Arlt s.*
marginal s′s 1. discontinuous venous lacunae, relatively free of villi, near the edge of the placenta. They were originally thought to be circumferentially continuous and important for placental drainage; their existence has not been confirmed. 2. bowl-shaped lymph sinuses separating the capsule from the cortical parenchyma of a lymph node, and from which lymph flows into the cortical sinuses; called also *subcapsular s′s.* 3. see *s. marginalis.*
s. margina′lis [TA] marginal sinus: any of the variably developed veins that connect the occipital sinus with the vertebral venous plexuses.
mastoid s′s cellulae mastoideae.
s. maxilla′ris [TA], **maxillary s.** one of the paired paranasal sinuses located in the body of the maxilla on either side and communicating with the middle meatus of the nasal cavity on the same side. Called also *antrum of Highmore.*
s. me′dii cellulae ethmoidales mediae.
medullary s′s lymph sinuses in the medulla of a lymph node, which divide the lymphoid tissue into a number of medullary cords.
Meyer s., s. Mey′eri a small depression in the floor of the external auditory canal just in front of the tympanic membrane.
middle s′s cellulae ethmoidales mediae.
s. of Morgagni 1. *(in the pl.)* s. anales. 2. sinus aortae. 3. ventriculus laryngis.
mucous s′s of male urethra lacunae urethrales urethrae masculinae.
nail s. the space underlying the advancing free edge of the fingernail or toenail; called also *s. unguis.*
oblique s. of pericardium, s. obli′quus pericar′dii [TA] a recess of serous pericardium that passes upward behind the left atrium and between the left and right pulmonary veins.
occipital s., s. occipita′lis [TA] one of the sinuses of the dura mater; it begins in right and left branches called the marginal sinuses, and then passes upward along the attached margin of the cerebellar falx to end in the confluence of the sinuses.
oral s. stomodeum.
paranasal s′s, s. paranasa′les [TA] the mucosa-lined air cavities in the cranial bones that communicate with the nasal cavity, including the ethmoidal, frontal, maxillary, and sphenoid sinuses.
parasinoidal s′s lacunae laterales.
pericardial s. an enlarged blood-filled portion of the hemocoelom surrounding the heart in many invertebrates with open circulatory systems, such as arthropods. Called also *pericardium.*
s. pericar′dii s. transversus pericardii.
Petit s. sinus aortae.
petrosal s., inferior s. petrosus inferior.
petrosal s., superior s. petrosus superior.
s. petrosquamo′sus [TA], **petrosquamous s.** an inconstant sinus, one of the sinuses of the dura mater; it runs along the petrosquamous fissure, connecting posteriorly with the transverse sinus and anteriorly with the retromandibular vein.
s. petro′sus infe′rior [TA] inferior petrosal sinus: one of the sinuses of the dura mater, arising from the cavernous sinus and running along the line of the petrooccipital synchondrosis to the superior bulb of the internal jugular vein.

Sinus *Continued*

s. petro′sus supe′rior [TA] superior petrosal sinus: one of the sinuses of the dura mater, arising at the cavernous sinus, passing along the attached margin of the cerebellar tentorium, and draining into the transverse sinus.
phrenicocostal s., s. phrenicocosta′lis recessus costodiaphragmaticus pleuralis.
pilonidal s. a suppurating fistulous tract, most often in the coccygeal region *(coccygeal sinus)* and containing a tuft of hair; occasionally these are found in other regions of the body. It is usually the result of repeated friction that has caused hairs to penetrate the skin. Called also *piliferous cyst, pilonidal cyst,* and *pilonidal fistula.*
piriform s. recessus piriformis.
s. pleu′rae, pleural s's recessus pleurales.
pleuroperitoneal s. hiatus pleuroperitonealis.
s. pocula′ris utriculus prostaticus.
posterior s's, s. posterio′res s. ethmoidales posteriores.
s. poste′rior cavita′tis tympa′nicae [TA] posterior sinus of tympanic cavity: a groove in the posterior wall of the tympanic cavity inferior to the pyramidal eminence.
prostatic s., s. prosta′ticus [TA] the posterolateral recess between the seminal colliculus and the wall of the urethra, where the prostatic ductules empty into the urethra.
s. of pulmonary trunk s. trunci pulmonalis.
pyriform s. recessus piriformis.
rectal s's, s. recta′les s. anales.
s. rec′tus [TA] straight sinus: one of the sinuses of the dura mater, situated in the line of union of the cerebral falx and the cerebellar tentorium, formed by the junction of the great cerebral vein and the inferior sagittal sinus, and ending in a transverse sinus, usually the left, at the confluence of the sinuses.
renal s., s. rena′lis [TA] a cavity within the substance of the kidney, occupied by the renal pelvis, calices, vessels, nerves, and fat.
s. reu′niens the sinus venosus of the embryonic heart into which empty all the veins that go to the heart.
rhomboid s. ventriculus terminalis medullae spinalis.
Ridley s. s. circularis.
Rokitansky-Aschoff s's small outpouchings of the mucosa of the gallbladder extending through the lamina propria and the muscular layer.
sacrococcygeal s. coccygeal s.
sagittal s., inferior s. sagittalis inferior.
sagittal s., superior s. sagittalis superior.
s. sagitta′lis infe′rior [TA] inferior sagittal sinus: one of the sinuses of the dura mater; it is small and situated in the posterior half of the lower concave border of the falx cerebri, and it opens into the upper end of the straight sinus. Called also *inferior longitudinal s.*
s. sagitta′lis supe′rior [TA] superior sagittal sinus: one of the sinuses of the dura mater; it begins in front of the crista galli and extends backward in the convex border of the falx cerebri. Near the internal occipital protuberance it ends in a variable way in the confluence of the sinuses, usually ending in the right transverse sinus. It receives the superior cerebral veins, communicates with the lateral lacunae, and is partially invaginated by arachnoidal granulations. Called also *superior longitudinal s.*
sigmoid s., s. sigmoi′deus [TA] either of two sinuses of the dura mater, continuations of the transverse sinuses; each curves downward from the tentorium cerebelli to become continuous with the superior bulb of the internal jugular vein.
soleal s's widened areas of the veins of the legs near the soleus muscle, which may expand in cases of venous stasis.

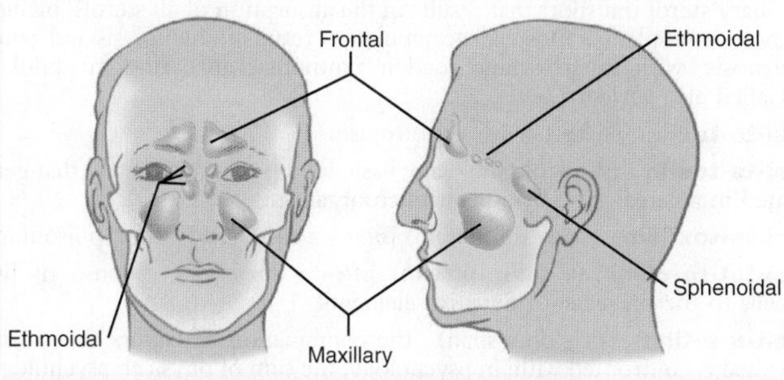

■ Sinus paranasales (paranasal sinuses).

sphenoid s., sphenoidal s., s. sphenoida′lis [TA] one of the paired paranasal sinuses in the anterior part of the body of the sphenoid bone, communicating with the superior meatus of the nasal cavity on the same side; the two are separated from each other by a septum.
sphenoparietal s., s. sphenoparieta′lis [TA] either of two sinuses of the dura mater, each beginning at a meningeal vein next to the apex of the small wing of the sphenoid bone and draining into the anterior part of the cavernous sinus. Called also *Breschet s.*
s. of spleen, splenic s., s. sple′nicus [TA] a dilated venous sinus not lined by ordinary endothelial cells, found in the splenic pulp; called also *s. lienalis* [TA alternative].
straight s. s. rectus.
subcapsular s's marginal s's (def. 2.)
tarsal s., s. tar′si [TA] the space between the calcaneus and talus, containing the interosseous ligament; called also *tarsal canal.*
tentorial s. s. rectus.
terminal s. a vein which encircles the vascular area in the blastoderm.
tonsillar s. fossa tonsillaris.
s. tonsilla′ris TA alternative for *fossa tonsillaris.*
transverse s. of dura mater s. transversus durae matris.
transverse s. of pericardium s. transversus pericardii.
s. transver′sus du′rae ma′tris [TA] transverse sinus of dura mater: either of two large sinuses of the dura mater that begin in a variable fashion at the confluence of the sinuses near the internal occipital protuberance. Each follows the attached margin of the tentorium cerebelli to the petrous temporal bone, where it becomes the sigmoid sinus. At their origin in the confluence, one sinus, usually the right, is continuous with the superior sagittal sinus and the other, usually the left, is continuous with the straight sinus.
s. transver′sus pericar′dii [TA] transverse sinus of pericardium: a passage behind the aorta and pulmonary trunk and in front of the atria; it is lined by serous pericardium.
traumatic s. a sinus due to trauma.
s. trun′ci pulmona′lis [TA] sinus of pulmonary trunk: a slight dilatation between the wall of the pulmonary trunk and each of the semilunar cusps of the pulmonary trunk valve.
s. tym′pani [TA] tympanic sinus: a deep fossa in the posterior part of the tympanic cavity; it is bounded superiorly by the eminentia pyramidalis and inferiorly by the subiculum promontorii, and it opens anteriorly into the fossula fenestrae cochleae.
s. of tympanic cavity, posterior s. posterior cavi tympani.
s. un′guis nail s.
unroofed coronary s. congenital complete or partial absence of the partition dividing the coronary sinus from the left atrium, allowing the shunting of blood from the left atrium through the coronary sinus into the right atrium.
urachal s. dilatation of part of the urachus at the umbilical end, either congenitally or as a result of a urachal cyst that has begun to drain to the surface.
urogenital s., s. urogenita′lis an elongated sac formed by division of the cloaca in the early embryo, communicating with the mesonephric ducts and primordial urinary bladder; it forms most of the bladder in both sexes, the vestibule, urethra, and vagina in the female, and most of the urethra in the male.
uterine s's venous channels in the wall of the uterus in pregnancy.
s. of Valsalva sinus aortae.
s. of venae cavae, s. vena′rum cava′rum [TA] the portion of the right atrium bounded medially by the interatrial septum and laterally by the crista terminalis, and into which the superior and inferior venae cavae empty; it is often called the sinus venosus because it develops from that embryonic structure.
s. veno′sus 1. [TA] venous sinus: the common venous receptacle in the embryonic heart, attached to the posterior wall of the primordial atrium; it receives the umbilical and vitelline veins and the common cardinal veins. 2. venous s. (def. 1). 3. s. venarum cavarum.
s. veno′si dura′les s. durae matris.
s. veno′sus scle′rae [TA] venous sinus of sclera: a circular channel at the junction of the sclera and cornea, which is the main pathway for elimination of aqueous humor from the eye. Called also *Schlemm canal.*
venous s. 1. a large vein or channel for the circulation of venous blood, such as one of the sinuses of the dura mater. 2. s. venosus (def. 1).
venous s's of dura mater s. durae matris.
venous s. of sclera s. venosus sclerae.
s. ventri′culi Forssell s.

si·nus·al (si'nə-səl) pertaining to a sinus.

si·nus·itis (si″nəs-i'tis) inflammation of a sinus, usually a paranasal sinus; it may be purulent or nonpurulent, acute or chronic. Types are named for the sinus involved.

ethmoid s. inflammation of an ethmoid sinus; called also *ethmoiditis.*

frontal s. inflammation of a frontal sinus.

infectious s. of turkeys a common, sometimes highly fatal respiratory disease of turkeys and game birds, caused by pleuropneumonialike organisms (q.v.) and marked by swelling below the eyes and sneezing; called also *airsac disease.*

maxillary s. inflammation of a maxillary sinus; called also *antritis.*

sphenoid s. inflammation of a sphenoid sinus; called also *sphenoiditis.*

si·nus·oid (si'nə-soid) [*sinus* + *-oid*] 1. resembling a sinus. 2. vas sinusoideum.

discontinuous s. see *vas sinusoideum.*

fenestrated s. see *vas sinusoideum.*

si·nus·oi·dal (si″nə-soi'dəl) 1. located in a sinusoid or affecting the circulation in the region of a sinusoid; used especially to denote the location of vascular resistance in portal hypertension. 2. shaped like or pertaining to a sine wave.

si·nus·os·co·py (si″nəs-os'ko-pe) sinoscopy.

si·nus·ot·o·my (si″nə-sot'ə-me) [*sinus* + *-tomy*] incision into a sinus.

si·nu·spi·ral (si″nu-spi'rəl) sinospiral.

si·nu·ven·tric·u·lar (si″nu-vən-trik'u-lər) sinoventricular.

Si op. sit [L.] si o'pus sit (if it is necessary).

si·phon (si'fən) [Gr. *siphōn* tube] a bent tube with two arms of unequal length, used to transfer liquids from a higher to a lower level by the force of atmospheric pressure.

s. caro'ticum [TA], **carotid s.** the innermost section of the petrosal part of the internal carotid artery just before the artery enters the cranial cavity.

si·phon·age (si'fon-əj) the use of the siphon, as in gastric lavage or in draining the bladder.

Si·pho·na ir·ri·tans (si-fo'nə ir'ĭ-təns) *Haematobia irritans.*

Si·pho·nap·tera (si″fo-nap'tər-ə) [Gr. *siphon* tube + *apteros* wingless] the fleas, an order of insects whose bodies are laterally compressed, highly chitinized and sclerotized, and wingless; they are blood-sucking ectoparasites of mammals and birds. More than 800 species have been described, grouped in six or more families.

Si·phun·cu·la·ta (si-fun″ku-la'tə) Anoplura.

Si·phun·cu·li·na (si-fun″ku-li'nə) a genus of dipterous insects of the family Chloropidae. *S. funi'cola* is the common eye fly of India, where it spreads conjunctivitis and trachoma.

Sip·ple syndrome (sip'əl) [John H. *Sipple*, American physician, born 1930] multiple endocrine neoplasia, type 2A; see under *neoplasia.*

Sip·py diet (sip'e) [Bertram Welton *Sippy*, American physician, 1866–1924] see under *diet.*

si·reno·me·lia (si″rən-o-me'le-ə) apodal symmelia.

si·ren·om·e·lus (si″rən-om'ə-ləs) a fetus with apodal symmelia; called also *apus, sympus apus,* and *sireniform fetus.*

sir·i·a·sis (sir-i'ə-sis) sunstroke.

siRNA small interfering RNA.

si·ro·li·mus (sĭ-ro'lĭ-məs) a macrolide antibiotic obtained from a variant of *Streptomyces hygroscopicus,* having immunosuppressant properties; administered orally to prevent rejection of kidney transplants.

-sis [Gr. suffix of action] a word termination denoting an action, process, or condition. Appears most commonly in the suffixes *-asis, -esis, -iasis,* and *-osis.*

SISI short increment sensitivity index.

siso·mi·cin (sis″o-mi'sin) an aminoglycoside antibiotic derived from *Micromonospora inyoensis,* closely related to the C_{1a} component of the gentamicin complex; it is bactericidal for many gram-negative and some gram-positive organisms, having a range of activity similar to that of gentamicin.

s. sulfate [USP] the sulfate salt of sisomicin, used in the treatment of infections caused by susceptible gram-negative organisms; administered intravenously or intramuscularly.

sis·ter (sis'tər) the nurse in charge of a hospital ward (Great Britain).

Sis·ter Mary Jo·seph nodule (sis'tər mār'e jo'səf) [*Sister Mary Joseph* Dempsey, American Roman Catholic nun and medical worker, 1856–1929] see under *nodule.*

Sis·trunk operation (sis'trənk) [Walter *Sistrunk*, American surgeon, 1880–1933] see under *operation.*

Sis·tru·rus (sis-troo'rəs) a genus of small rattlesnakes of the family Crotalidae; they are widely distributed throughout the United States and have symmetrical plates covering their heads. *S. catena'tus* is the massasauga and *S. milia'rius* is the *pygmy rattlesnake.* See table at *snake.*

si·ta·glip·tin phos·phate (si″tə-glip'tin) a dipeptidyl-peptidase-4 inhibitor that acts in response to elevated blood sugar to slow the inactivation of incretins, thereby increasing insulin release and decreasing circulating glucagon levels, used in the treatment of type 2 diabetes mellitus; administered orally.

site (sīt) a place, position, or locus.

active s. the part of an enzyme or other catalyst at which the reaction occurs; it is the three-dimensional region of the molecule that binds the substrate and facilitates its conversion to a reaction product. See also *binding s.* and *catalytic s.*

allosteric s. a specific site on a multi-subunit enzyme that is not the substrate binding site but that when reversibly bound by an effector induces a conformational change in the enzyme, altering its catalytic properties.

antigen-binding s., antigen-combining s. the region of the immunoglobulin molecule that binds to antigens; there is one such site on each of the two Fab regions of each immunoglobulin monomer.

binding s. in an enzyme or other protein, the three-dimensional configuration of specific groups on specific amino acids that binds particular compounds such as substrates or effectors, with high affinity and specificity. Cf. *catalytic s.*

catalytic s. in an enzyme, the portion of the active site that converts the substrate to a reaction product or otherwise interacts with it. Cf. *binding s.*

combining s. antigen-binding s.

cryptic splice s. an unusual splice site with a sequence similar to that of the consensus splice site; it is usually unused but can become competitive with the normal site if either is mutated.

fragile s. a nonstaining gap in the chromatin of a metaphase chromosome, usually in both chromatids, and inherited in a mendelian fashion; the chromosome is easily breakable at this site. In cultured human cells, fragile sites are expressed under conditions of folate or thymidine deprivation or in the presence of methotrexate.

immunologically privileged s's regions of the body that are not normally accessible to effector cells of the immune system and thus sites where allograft rejection does not occur and tumors escape immune surveillance, e.g., the meninges of the brain and the anterior chamber of the eye.

restriction s. a base sequence in a DNA segment recognized by a particular restriction endonuclease.

sequence-tagged s. (STS) a short length (200–500 base pairs) of DNA that has a single occurrence in the genome and can be detected and amplified by the polymerase chain reaction; useful in physical mapping of the genome.

splice s. the nucleotides that span the intron–exon junction in a eukaryotic primary transcript of a split gene and function in excision and splicing reactions; those at the 5′ end form the splice donor site, while those at the 3′ end constitute the splice acceptor site.

sit(o)- [Gr. *sitos* food] a combining form denoting relationship to food.

Si·to·phi·lus (si-tof'ĭ-lus) a genus of weevils. *S. grana'rius* is the wheat weevil, which feeds on and lays eggs in kernels of grain; hypersensitivity to it causes miller's lung.

si·to·pho·bia (si″to-fo'be-ə) [*sito-* + *-phobia*] irrational fear of eating or of food.

si·tos·ter·ol (si-tos'tər-ol) 1. a generic term for a group of closely related natural plant sterols, the individual compounds being designated by Greek letters, and sometimes subscript numerals, as α_1, α_2, α_3, β, and γ, on the basis of differing characteristics. 2. a pharmaceutical preparation consisting of β-sitosterol and related plant sterols, used as an anticholesterolemic agent.

si·tos·ter·ol·emia (si-tos″tər-ol-e'me-ə) excessive levels of sitosterols in the blood and tissues, caused by a hereditary defect in intestinal and biliary sterol transport that results in the absorption of all sterols, including those from plants. Sitosterol accumulation results in hemolysis and xanthomatosis, with tuberous and tendon xanthomas appearing in childhood. Called also *phytosterolemia.*

si·to·tax·is (si″to-tak'sis) sitotropism.

si·to·tox·in (si'to-tok″sin) any basic food poison, especially that generated in a cereal food by a plant microorganism.

si·to·tox·ism (si″to-tok'siz-əm) [*sito-* + *tox-* + *-ism*] food poisoning.

si·tot·ro·pism (si-tot'ro-piz-əm) [*sito-* + *tropism*] response of living cells to the presence of nutritive elements.

sit·u·a·tion (sich″o͞o-a'shən) the combination of factors that an individual is confronted with; in psychology, the sum of physical, psychological, and sociocultural factors that act on persons and influence their behavior.

si·tus (si'təs) pl. *si'tus* [L.] site, or position.

s. ambi'guus heterotaxy syndrome.

s. inver′sus, s. inver′sus vis′cerum lateral transposition of the viscera of the thorax and abdomen; a familial pattern and consanguineous parents have been reported. Complete transposition of the viscera in the absence of other defects is structurally sound, but see *dextrocardia, levocardia,* and *Kartagener syndrome.*
s. perver′sus dislocation of any viscus.
s. so′litus the normal position of the viscera.
s. transver′sus s. inversus.

SIV simian immunodeficiency virus.

Si vir. perm. [L.] si vi′res permit′tant (if the strength will permit).

Sjö•gren syndrome (shur′gren) [Henrik Samuel Conrad *Sjögren,* Swedish ophthalmologist, 1899–1986] see under *syndrome.*

Sjö•gren-Lars•son syndrome (shur′gren lahr′sən) [Karl Gustaf Torsten *Sjögren,* Swedish physician, 1896–1974; Tage Konrad Leopold *Larsson,* Swedish physician, 1905–1998] see under *syndrome.*

SK streptokinase.

skat•ole (skat′ōl) [Gr. *skōr,* gen. *skatos* dung] a crystalline amine, with a strong characteristic odor, from human feces. It is produced by the decomposition of proteins in the intestine and directly from the amino acid tryptophan by decarboxylation.

ska•tox•yl (skə-tok′sil) an oxidation product of skatole, found in the urine in certain cases of disease of the large intestine.

ske•las•the•nia (ske″ləs-the′ne-ə) [Gr. *skelos* leg + *asthenia*] weakness of the lower limbs.

Ske•lax•in (skə-laks′in) trademark for a preparation of metaxalone.

skel•e•tin (skel′ə-tin) any of a number of gelatinous substances occurring in invertebrate tissue, and including chitin, sericin, spongin, etc.

skel•e•ti•za•tion (skel″ə-tĭ-za′shən) 1. extreme emaciation. 2. the removal of the soft parts from the skeleton.

skel•e•tog•e•nous (skel″ə-toj′ə-nəs) producing skeletal or bony structures.

skel•e•tog•e•ny (skel″ə-toj′ə-ne) the formation of the skeleton; the origin and development of the skeleton.

skel•e•ton (skel′ə-tən) [Gr. "a dried body, mummy"] the hard framework of the animal body, especially the bony framework of the body of higher vertebrate animals; the bones of the body collectively. See Plate 40. See also *endoskeleton, exoskeleton,* and *visceral skeleton.* **skel′etal** *adj*
appendicular s., s. appendicula′re [TA] the bones of the upper and lower limbs.
axial s., s. axia′le [TA] the bones of the cranium, vertebral column, ribs, and sternum.
cardiac s. the fibrous or fibrocartilaginous framework that supports and gives attachment to the cardiac muscle fibers and valves, and the roots of the aorta and pulmonary trunk; it includes the anuli fibrosi cordis, left and right fibrous trigones, membranous part of the interventricular septum, and the infundibular tendon. Called also *fibrous s. of heart.*
fibrous s. of heart cardiac s.
s. of heart cardiac s.
s. mem′bri inferio′ris li′beri pars libera membri inferioris.
s. mem′bri superio′ris li′beri pars libera membri superioris.
thoracic s., s. thora′cicus s. thoracis.
s. thora′cis [TA] skeleton of thorax: the skeletal framework enclosing the thorax, consisting of the thoracic vertebrae and intervertebral disks, the ribs and costal cartilages, and the sternum; called also *rib cage* and *thoracic cage.*
visceral s. the portion of the skeleton that protects the viscera, including the sternum, ribs, pelvis, and os coxae.

skel•e•to•ni•za•tion (skel″ə-tə-nĭ-za′shən) 1. the process of reducing to a skeletal form or of eliminating excess elements. 2. the application of an algorithm to a digital image in order to eliminate data obscuring the structure of interest. 3. abnormal prominence of the orbital rim due to thinning or drooping of the underlying soft tissues. 4. in rhinoplasty, the elevation of the soft tissues from the underlying framework of the nose.

skel•e•to•pia (skel″ə-to′pe-ə) [*skeleton* + Gr. *topos* place] the position of an organ in relation to the skeleton.

skel•e•to•py (skel′ə-to″pe) skeletopia.

Skel•id (skel′id) trademark for a preparation of tiludronate disodium.

Skene ducts (tubules), glands (skēn) [Alexander Johnston Chalmers *Skene,* American gynecologist, 1838–1900] see *ductus paraurethrales urethrae femininae,* and see *paraurethral glands,* under *gland.*

ske•ni•tis (ske-ni′tis) inflammation of the paraurethral glands (Skene glands).

skew (sku) 1. deviating from a straight line; slanting. 2. asymmetric or antisymmetric. 3. of a probability distribution, not symmetric about the mean.

skew•foot (sku′foot) any deformity of the foot in which its forepart deviates toward the midline; see *metatarsus varus* and *talipes varus.*

skew•ness (sku′nis) of a probability distribution, lack of symmetry about the mean, or any measure of the lack of symmetry.

skia- [Gr. *skia* shadow] a combining form denoting reference to shadows, especially of internal structures as produced by x-rays.

skia•gram (ski′ə-gram) radiograph.

ski•am•e•try (ski-am′ə-tre) retinoscopy.

skia•scope (ski′ə-skōp) retinoscope.

ski•as•co•py (ski-as′kə-pe) retinoscopy.

skill (skil) an ability acquired through training or experience.
fine motor s's see under *function.*
gross motor s's see under *function.*

Skil•lern fracture (skil′ərn) [Penn Gaskell *Skillern,* American surgeon, 20th century] see under *fracture.*

skim•ming (skim′ing) the removing of floating matter from a liquid.
plasma s. the action of red cells in flowing blood which leaves a zone near the wall of a vessel that is relatively free of cells.

skin (skin) the outer integument or covering of the body, consisting of the dermis and epidermis, and resting upon the subcutaneous tissue; called also *cutis* [TA]. See illustration.
alligator s. see *ichthyosis.*
bronzed s. bronze-colored skin, as seen in Addison disease and hemochromatosis.
collodion s. skin resembling collodion, as in some forms of ichthyosis; see also *collodion baby,* under *baby.*
crocodile s. see *ichthyosis.*
deciduous s. keratolysis exfoliativa.
elastic s. Ehlers-Danlos syndrome.
farmers' s. actinic elastosis.
fish s. see *ichthyosis.*
glossy s. atrophoderma neuriticum.
granulomatous slack s. a rare variant of cutaneous T-cell lymphoma characterized by folds of lax, pendulous skin, usually in the groin or axilla, with a granulomatous infiltrate and clonal T cells.
India rubber s. Ehlers-Danlos syndrome.
lax s. cutis laxa.
leopard s. a manifestation of onchodermatitis consisting of depigmented areas surrounding darkened areas that are adjacent to hair follicles, It is usually located on the shins, with epidermal thinning with breakdown of dermal collagen, which can interfere with mobility of the part.
loose s. cutis laxa.
marble s. cutis marmorata.
piebald s. piebaldism.
porcupine s. skin having sharp points resembling the quills of a porcupine, as in ichthyosis hystrix.
sailors' s. actinic elastosis.
shagreen s. see under *patch.*
tissue-engineered s. a skin equivalent (q.v.) created by culturing skin cells.
toad s. follicular hyperkeratosis.

skin•fold (skin′fōld) the layer of skin and subcutaneous fat raised by pinching the skin and letting the underlying muscle fall back to the bone; measurements of skinfold thickness (most often taken over the biceps or triceps muscles, above the iliac crest, or below the scapula) are used to estimate the percentage of body fat. See also *triceps skinfold thickness,* under *thickness.*
triceps s. (TSF) the skinfold on the arm over the triceps muscle; see *triceps skinfold thickness,* under *thickness.*

Skin•ner box (skin′ər) [Burrhus Frederic *Skinner,* American psychologist, 1904–1990] see under *box.*

Skin•ner classification (skin′ər) [C.N. *Skinner,* American dentist, early 20th century] see under *classification.*

skler(o)- for words beginning thus, see those beginning *scler(o)-.*

Sko•da sign (tympany) (sko′dah) [Josef *Skoda,* Czech-born physician in Austria, 1805–1881] skodaic resonance.

sko•da•ic (sko-da′ik) named for Josef *Skoda.*

skole- for words beginning thus, see those beginning *scole-.*

sko•pom•e•ter (sko-pom′ə-tər) an instrument for measuring color, cloudiness, and other optical phenomena of liquids without using standards for comparison.

SKSD streptokinase-streptodornase.

skull (skul) the skeleton of the head, including the cranium and the mandible. See illustration.
cloverleaf s. kleeblattschädel.
hot cross bun s. 1. Parrot sign (def. 2). 2. caput quadratum.

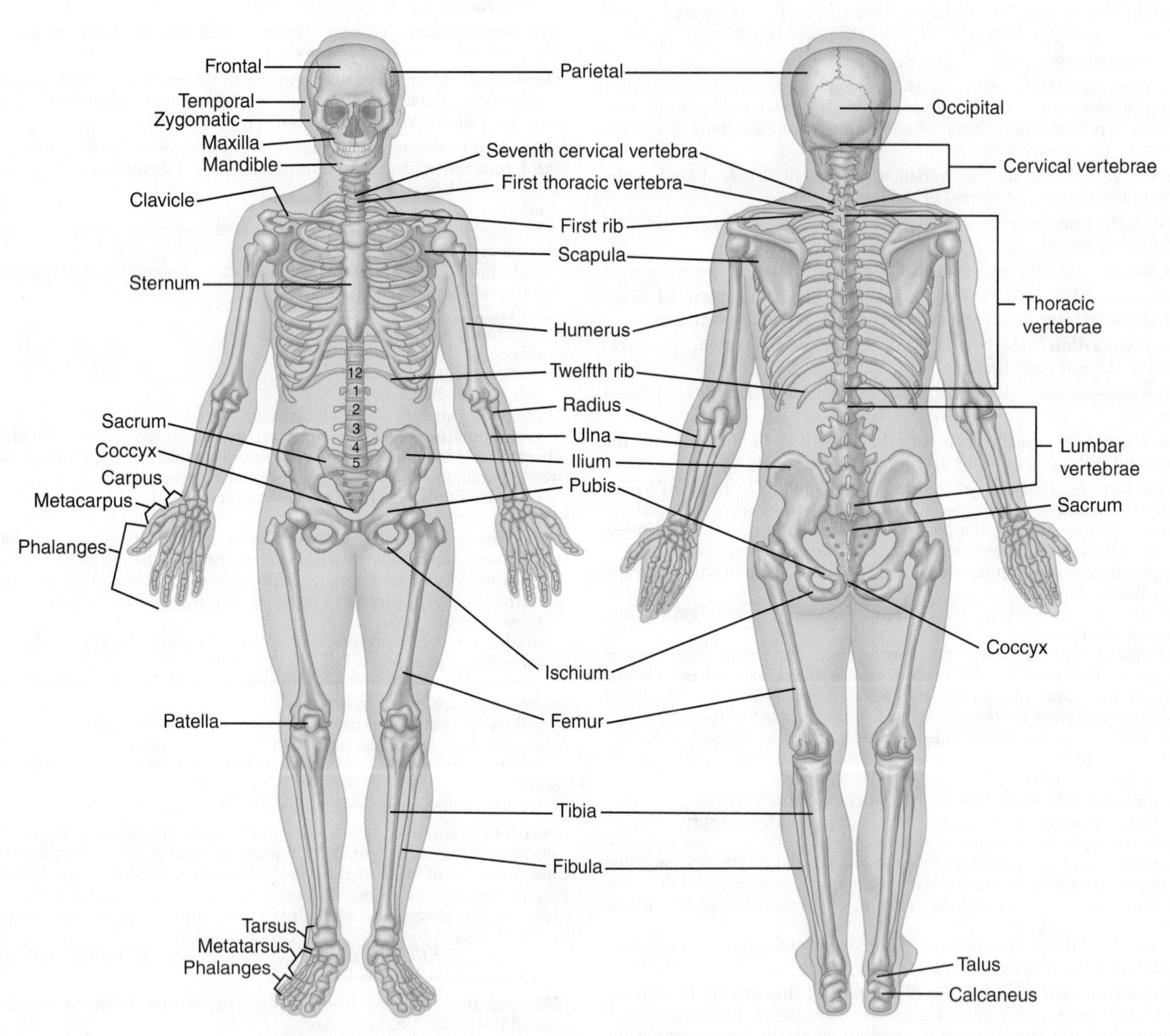

■ **PLATE 40**—ANTERIOR AND POSTERIOR VIEWS OF THE HUMAN SKELETON

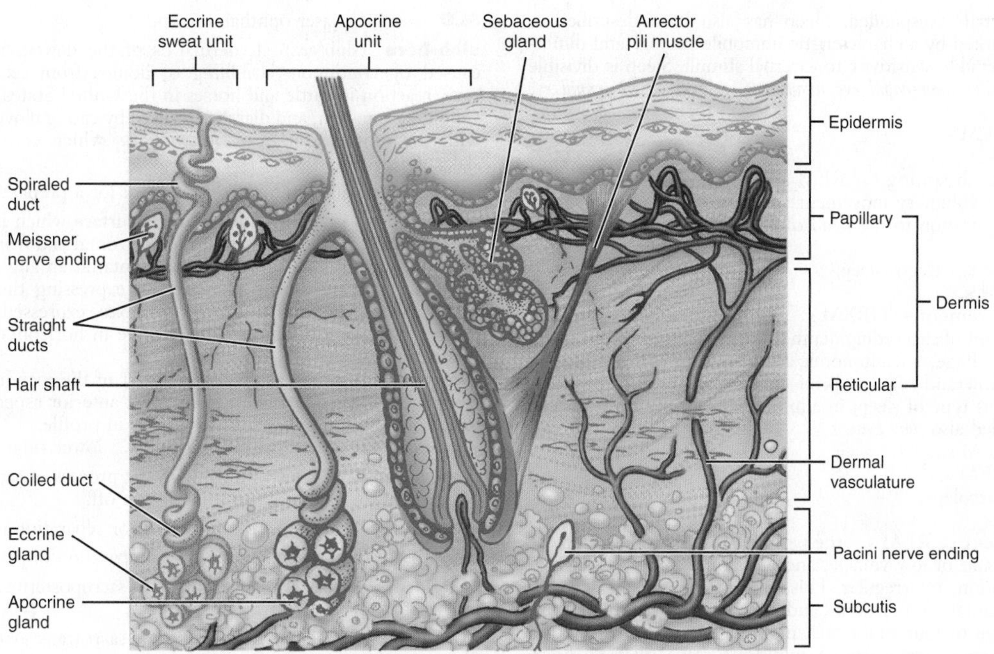

■ Diagram of a cross section of the skin.

lacuna s. craniolacunia.
maplike s. a skull marked by irregular tracings resembling outlines on a map; seen in x-ray films of the cranial bones in Hand-Schüller-Christian disease.
natiform s. 1. Parrot sign (def. 2). 2. caput quadratum.
steeple s., tower s. oxycephaly.
West lacuna s., West-Engstler s. a honeycomb appearance of the skull in radiographs, associated with spina bifida or meningocele and occasionally with encephalocele.

SKY spectral karyotype.

sl slyke.

SLA [L.] sacro-laeva anterior (left sacroanterior, a position of the fetus; see *position*).

SLAC scapholunate advanced collapse.

slaf•ra•mine (slaf′rə-mēn) a sialogogic mycotoxin found in *Rhizoctonia leguminicola*, which causes slobbers (q.v.) in livestock.

slant (slant) 1. a sloping surface of agar in a test tube. 2. slant culture.

SLE systemic lupus erythematosus.

SLED sustained low-efficiency dialysis.

sleep (slēp) a period of rest for the body and mind, during which volition and consciousness are in partial or complete abeyance and the

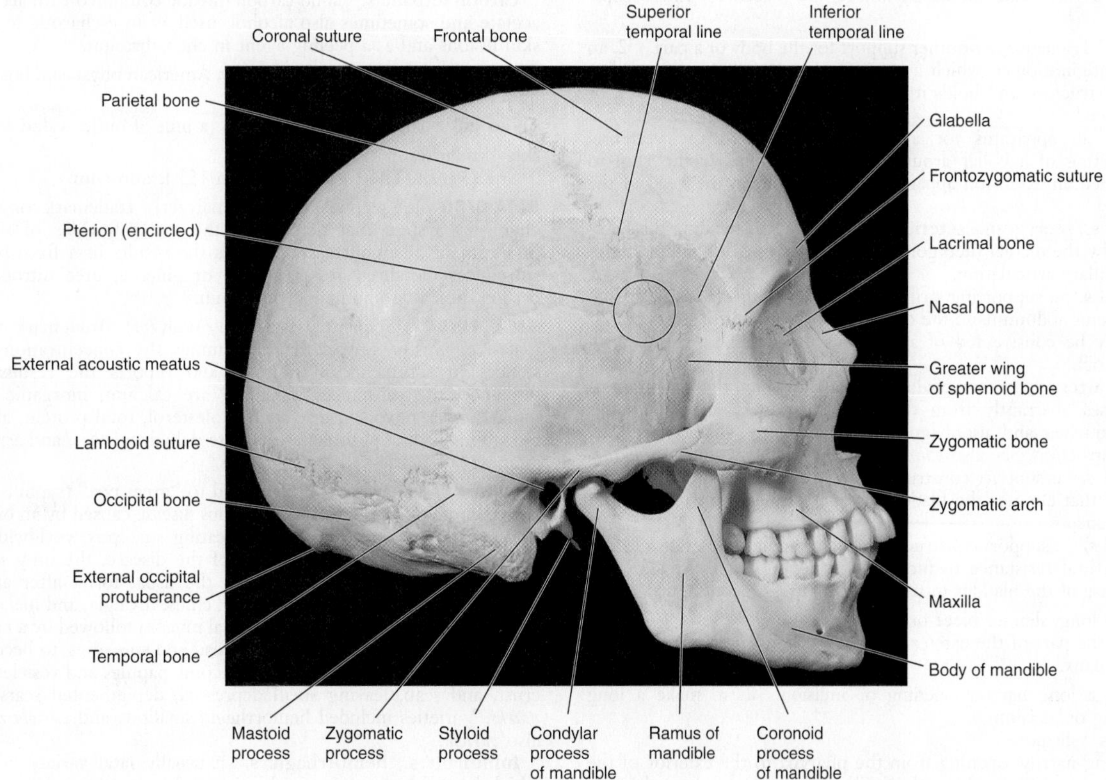

■ Lateral view of the skull.

bodily functions partially suspended. Sleep has also been described as a behavioral state marked by a characteristic immobile posture and diminished but readily reversible sensitivity to external stimuli. Sleep is divisible into two types: *NREM (non–rapid eye movement) s.* and *REM (rapid eye movement) s.*

active s., D s. REM s.

deep s. NREM s.

desynchronized s., dreaming s. REM s.

electric s. loss of voluntary movement and presence of general anesthesia induced by application to the head of a rapidly interrupted electric current.

electrotherapeutic s. electrosleep.

fast wave s. REM s.

non–rapid eye movement s., NREM s. the dreamless period of sleep, consisting of four stages of succeeding depth, during which the brain waves are slow and of high voltage, and autonomic activities, such as heart rate and blood pressure, are low and regular. Brief episodes of REM sleep occur at intervals during this type of sleep; in adults, about 80 per cent of sleep is NREM sleep. Called also *slow wave s.*

orthodox s. NREM s.

paradoxical s. REM s.

paroxysmal s. narcolepsy.

quiet s. NREM s.

rapid eye movement s., REM s. the period of sleep during which the brain waves are fast and of low voltage, and autonomic activities, such as heart rate and respiration, are irregular. This type of sleep is associated with dreaming, mild involuntary muscle jerks, and rapid eye movements (REM). It usually occurs three to four times each night at intervals of 80 to 120 minutes, each occurrence lasting from 5 minutes to more than an hour. In adults, about 20 per cent of sleep is REM sleep and 80 per cent is NREM (non–rapid eye movement) sleep. Called also *desynchronized, dreaming,* or *paradoxical s.* See also *REM rebound,* under *rebound.*

S s., slow wave s., synchronized s. NREM s.

twilight s. a condition of analgesia and amnesia, produced by hypodermic administration of morphine and scopolamine. In this state the patient, although responding to pain, does not retain it in memory. Formerly widely used in obstetrics.

sleep·talk·ing (slēp′tawk-ing) somniloquism.

sleep·walk·ing (slēp′wawk-ing) somnambulism.

slee·py·grass (sle′pe-gras) *Stipa viridula.*

Slen·trol (slen′trōl) trademark for a preparation of dirlotapide.

slice (slīs) in tomography, a cross-sectional plane of the body selected for imaging.

slide (slīd) a glass plate on which objects are placed for microscopic examination.

sling (sling) 1. a bandage or other support for the body or a part. 2. an anatomical configuration in which a long narrow structure passes underneath another structure and holds it up; it may be normal, anomalous, or surgically induced.

Glisson s. an apparatus for applying extension to the vertebral column, consisting of a collar around the neck and under the chin to which is attached an extension apparatus over a pulley at the head of the patient's bed.

mandibular s., pterygomasseteric s. a structure suspending the mandible, formed by the medial pterygoid and masseter muscles and aiding in mandibulomaxillary articulation.

pubovaginal s. a supporting strip placed underneath the bladder from one edge of rectus abdominis to the other in the treatment of stress incontinence; it may be constructed of autologous or allogeneic tissue or of synthetic material.

pulmonary artery s. a rare cardiac anomaly in which the left pulmonary artery arises aberrantly from the right pulmonary artery and lies between the trachea and esophagus; it is frequently characterized by respiratory obstruction. See also *pulmonary sling syndrome,* under *syndrome.*

suburethral s. a support constructed from muscle, ligament, or synthetic material that elevates the bladder from underneath in treatment of stress incontinence.

vaginal wall s. a support constructed using a vaginal wall graft in order to provide urethral resistance to increased intra-abdominal pressure and stabilize the base of the bladder in treatment of stress incontinence.

slip (slip) a long, slender piece or strip.

central s. the part of the extensor tendon of a finger that inserts into the middle phalanx.

slit (slit) 1. a long narrow opening or incision. 2. to make a long narrow opening or incision.

filtration s's slit pores.

gill s. a long narrow opening from the pharynx to the exterior of the body of many aquatic animals, such as fishes and salamanders, through which water is drawn to bathe the gills.

SLO scanning laser ophthalmoscope.

slob·bers (slob′ərz) 1. dermatitis of the dewlap in domestic rabbits, caused by continuous dribbling of liquids from feeding devices. 2. a toxic reaction in cattle and horses in the United States, with excessive salivation, lacrimation, and diarrhea, caused by eating clover hay contaminated with the fungus *Rhizoctonia leguminicola,* which contains the mycotoxin slaframine.

Slo-Ni·a·cin (slo-ni′ə-sin) trademark for a preparation of niacin.

slope (slōp) 1. an inclined plane; a surface which is neither horizontal nor vertical. 2. to deviate from the horizontal and from the vertical plane; said of a surface intersecting the horizontal at an angle between 1 and 90 degrees. 3. a mathematical means of expressing the position of a line relative to the horizontal and vertical axes, expressed as the ratio of the change in vertical distance to the change in horizontal distance when the line is traversed.

lower ridge s. the slope of the crest of the mandibular residual ridge from the third molar region to its most anterior aspect in relation to the lower border of the mandible as viewed in profile.

mandibular anteroposterior ridge s. lower ridge s.

slough (sluf) 1. necrotic tissue in the process of separating from viable portions of the body. 2. to shed or cast off.

slough·ing (sluf′ing) the formation or separation of a slough.

Slow-K (slo′ka′) trademark for a preparation of potassium chloride.

SLP [L.] sacro-laeva posterior (left sacroposterior, a position of the fetus; see *position*).

SLT [L.] sacro-laeva transversa (left sacrotransverse, a position of the fetus; see *position*).

Slu·der method, neuralgia (syndrome) (sloo′dər) [Greenfield *Sluder,* American laryngologist, 1865–1925] see under *method* and *neuralgia.*

sludge semisolid particles, sometimes partially suspended in a liquid.

biliary s. semisolid particles in the bile, containing calcium bilirubinate and sometimes tiny stones (see *microlithiasis*), seen in early stages of cholestasis.

sludg·ing (sluj′ing) the settling out of solid particles from solution.

s. of blood intravascular agglutination.

slug (slug) any of numerous terrestrial gastropods closely related to the snails but having a rudimentary or absent shell; they are divided between the subclasses Euthyneura and Streptoneura. Some are intermediate hosts of parasitic trematodes.

slur·ry (slur′e) a watery mixture or suspension of insoluble matter.

slush (slush) partially melted snow or a substance resembling it.

carbon dioxide s. solid carbon dioxide combined with acetone or ethyl acetate and sometimes also alcohol; used as an escharotic to treat various skin lesions and as a peeling agent in chemabrasion.

Sly syndrome (sli) [William S. *Sly,* American physician, born 1932] see under *syndrome.*

slyke (sl) (slīk) [D.D. Van Slyke] a unit of buffer value.

Sm samarium.

Sm 153-EDTMP samarium Sm 153 lexidronam.

SMA 6/60 [Sequential Multiple Analyzer] trademark for an automated chemistry system that determines the concentrations of six substances in serum in 60 minutes and reports the results in a fixed sequence; the substances measured are creatinine or glucose, urea nitrogen, chloride, carbon dioxide, sodium, and potassium.

SMA 12/60 [Sequential Multiple Analyzer] trademark for an automated chemistry system that determines the concentrations of 12 substances in serum in 60 minutes and reports the results in a fixed sequence; the substances measured are calcium, inorganic phosphorus, glucose, urea nitrogen, uric acid, cholesterol, total protein, albumin, total bilirubin, alkaline phosphatase, lactate dehydrogenase, and aspartate transaminase.

small·pox (smawl′poks) [compared to "great pox" (syphilis)] an acute, highly contagious, often fatal infectious disease caused by an orthopoxvirus. Vaccination has succeeded in eradicating smallpox worldwide; therefore, since there are no animal vectors of the disease, the only source of the virus is in medical laboratories. In the usual form, after an incubation period and a prodrome of high fever, chills, myalgia, and malaise, petechial reddish spots would appear on the oral mucosa followed by a raised macular cutaneous rash starting on the forehead and spreading to become generalized. The lesions would evolve to become papules and vesicles, umbilicate, crust, and scab, leaving small depressed, depigmented scars called *pockmarks.* Varieties included hemorrhagic smallpox and *variola minor.* Called also *variola.*

fulminant s., hemorrhagic s. a usually fatal variety of smallpox in which hemorrhages occur in the skin and mucous membranes.

ovine s. sheep-pox.

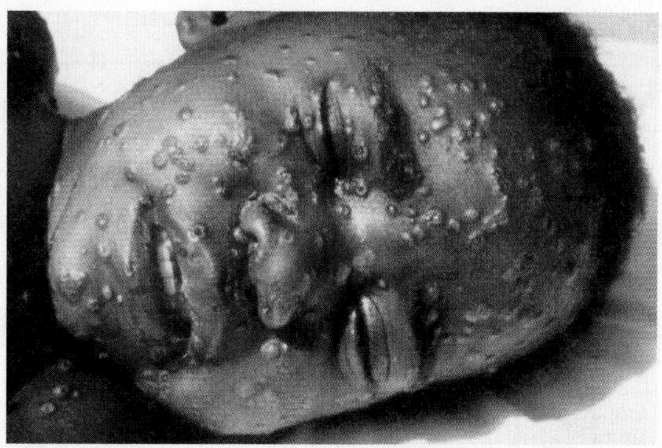

■ Smallpox.

SMC selenomethylnorcholesterol.

smear (smēr) a specimen for microscopic study prepared by spreading the material across the glass slide.

buccal s. a specimen obtained by gently scraping the inside of the cheek with a small spatula; used to examine the DNA or chromosomal complement of the individual, as in paternity testing or the sex chromatin test.

Pap s., Papanicolaou s. see under *test.*

smeg•ma (smeg′mə) [Gr. *smēgma* soap] a type of secretion of sebaceous glands, found chiefly beneath the prepuce; it consists principally of desquamated epithelial cells and sometimes has a cheesy consistency. smegmat′ic *adj*

smeg•ma•lith (smeg′mə-lith) a calcareous concretion in the smegma.

smell (smel) 1. olfaction. 2. odor.

smell-brain (smel′brān) rhinencephalon (def. 1).

Smel•lie method, scissors (smel′e) [William *Smellie*, British obstetrician, 1697–1763] see under *scissors* and see *Mauriceau maneuver*, under *maneuver*.

smi•la•cin (smi′lə-sin) [Gr. *smilakinos* pertaining to smilax] a poisonous glycoside, from sarsaparilla.

Smi•lax (smi′laks) [L., Gr. "bindweed"] a genus of climbing plants of the family Liliaceae. Several species are called sarsaparilla and are sources of the flavoring sarsaparilla; some have a starchy root that was formerly used as food and is used medicinally.

Smith dislocation, fracture (smith) [Robert William *Smith*, Irish surgeon, 1807–1873] see under *dislocation* and *fracture*.

Smith sign (smith) [Eustace *Smith*, English physician, 1835–1914] see under *sign*.

Smith-Lem•li-Opitz syndrome (smith′ lem′le o′pits) [David W. *Smith*, American pediatrician, 1926–1981; Luc *Lemli*, American physician, 20th century; John Marius *Opitz*, American pediatrician, born 1935] see under *syndrome*.

Smith-Pe•ter•sen nail (smith′-pa′tər-sen) [Marius Nygaard *Smith-Petersen*, American orthopedic surgeon, 1886–1953] see under *nail*.

Smith-Strang disease (smith′ strang′) [Allan J. *Smith*, British physician, 20th century; Leonard Birnie *Strang*, British physician, born 1925] see under *disease*.

SMO supramalleolar orthosis.

smog (smog) a mixture of smoke and fog; a colloid system in which the disperse phase consists of a mixture of gas and moisture and the dispersion medium is air.

smoke (smōk) a colloid system in which one or more solids is dispersed in a gas or vapor.

SMON subacute myelo-opticoneuropathy.

SMR standardized morbidity ratio; standardized mortality ratio.

smut (smut) 1. any fungus of the order Ustilaginales. 2. contamination of cereal grass (wheat, oats, rye, corn) by one of these fungi, particularly of the genera *Tilletia*, *Ustilago*, and *Urocystis*. Ingestion of contaminated seeds can cause poisoning; see *ergotism* and *ustilaginism*.

corn s. a smut of *Zea mays* caused by *Ustilago maydis;* ingestion of the infected seeds causes ustilaginism.

rye s. ergot (def. 1).

wheat s. smut on wheat caused by *Tilletia tritici*; ingestion causes glomerulonephritis in livestock.

S.N. [L.] secun′dum natu′ram (according to nature).

Sn tin (L. *stan′num*).

sn- [for *s*tereospecific *n*umbering] a chemical prefix used to indicate stereoisomers of glycerol derivatives: the glycerol chain is numbered as if it were derived from L-glyceraldehyde. This provides an unambiguous numbering. The enantiomer is obtained by reversing the numbering. For example *sn*-glycerol 1-phosphate is the same as L-glycerol 1-phosphate; the enantiomer D-glycerol 1-phosphate is the same as L-glycerol 3-phosphate or *sn*-glycerol 3-phosphate. See D-.

snail (snāl) any of numerous gastropods that have external spiral shells; they are divided between the subclasses Euthyneura and Streptoneura. Many snails in tropical countries are intermediate hosts of parasitic trematodes; the miracidium of the parasite develops into a cercaria in the body of the snail. Cf. *slug*.

snake (snāk) 1. a limbless reptile of the suborder Ophidia, some of which are poisonous. See table. 2. any of various worms that resemble members of Ophidia.

black s. blacksnake.

brown s. a venomous elapid snake of Australia and New Guinea belonging to the genus *Demansia*.

cabbage s. see *Mermithidae*.

colubrid s. colubrid (def. 1).

coral s. any of various venomous snakes of the genera *Micrurus* and *Micruroides;* called also *harlequin s.*

coral s., Arizona *Micruroides euryxanthus*.

coral s., Eastern a subspecies of *Micrurus fulvius* found in the Southeastern United States.

coral s., Sonoran *Micruroides euryxanthus*.

coral s., Texas a subspecies of *Micrurus fulvius* found in Texas and nearby areas.

crotalid s. crotalid (def. 1).

elapid s. elapid (def. 1).

hair s. see *Gordius*.

harlequin s. coral s.

poisonous s′s 1. venomous s′s. 2. snakes that contain poison, either in venom glands or in other organs or tissues.

sea s. a snake of the family Hydrophiidae.

tiger s. *Notechis scutatus*.

venomous s′s snakes that secrete substances (venoms) capable of producing a deleterious effect on either the blood (see *hemotoxin*) or the nervous system (see *neurotoxin*); the venom is injected into the body of the victim by the snake's bite. Called also *poisonous s′s*, *thanatophidia*, and *toxicophidia*.

viperine s. true viper.

snake•root (snāk′ro͞ot) 1. any plant of the genus *Asarum*. 2. any of certain other plants, such as *Polygala senega*, formerly used as remedies for snakebite.

seneca s., senega s. *Polygala senega*.

SNAP sensory nerve action potential.

snap (snap) a short sharp sound.

mitral opening s. an opening snap caused by abnormal movement of the mitral valve, usually due to mitral stenosis.

opening s. a short, sharp sound occurring in early diastole, caused by abrupt halting at its maximal opening of an abnormal atrioventricular valve; usually indicative of a stenotic valve that is still pliable.

tricuspid opening s. an opening snap caused by abnormal movement of the tricuspid valve, usually due to valvular stenosis.

snap•per (snap′ər) any of various carnivorous marine fish of the family Lutjanidae, found in tropical waters; they are often eaten, but sometimes contain ciguatoxin and cause ciguatera.

snare (snār) a wire loop or noose for removing polyps and tumors by encircling them at the base and closing the loop.

Sned•don syndrome (sned′ən) [Ian Bruce *Sneddon*, English dermatologist, 1915–1987] see under *syndrome*.

Sned•don-Wil•kin•son disease (sned′ən wil′kin-sən) [I.B. *Sneddon;* Darrell Sheldon *Wilkinson*, English dermatologist, 20th century] see *subcorneal pustular dermatosis*, under *dermatosis*.

sneeze (snēz) 1. to expel air forcibly and spasmodically through the nose and mouth. 2. an involuntary, sudden, violent, and audible expulsion of air through the mouth and nose. Called also *sternutation*.

sneeze•weed (snēz′wēd) *Helenium*.

Snell's law (snelz) [Willebrord van Roijen *Snell*, Dutch astronomer and mathematician, 1591–1626] see under *law*.

Snel•len chart, etc. (snel′ən) [Hermann *Snellen*, Dutch ophthalmologist, 1834–1908] see under *chart*, *eye*, *sign*, *test*, and *test type*.

SNGFR single nephron glomerular filtration rate.

SNM Society of Nuclear Medicine.

Snod•grass procedure (snod′gras) [Warren *Snodgrass*, American physician, late 20th century] see under *procedure*.

Important Venomous Snakes

Family	Type of Fangs	Common Names	Type of Venom	Distribution	Remarks
Colubridae	Rear, immovable, grooved	Colubrids	Mostly mild	Warm parts of both hemispheres	Over 1000 species, the few poisonous ones not dangerous
		Boomslang	Hemorrhagin	South Africa	Arboreal, timid
Elapidae	Front, immovable, grooved	Elapids	Predominantly neurotoxin	Mostly in Old World	Over 150 species, very poisonous
		Cobras	Mostly neurotoxin	Africa, India, Asia, Philippines, Celebes	Spitting cobra in Africa aims at eyes
		Kraits	Strong neurotoxin	India, Southeast Asia, Indonesia	Sluggish, often buried in dust
		Mambas	Neurotoxin	Tropical West Africa	Arboreal
		Blacksnake	Neurotoxin	Australia	Large snake, wet terrain
		Copperhead	Neurotoxin	Australia, Tasmania, Solomons	Damp environment
		Brown snake	Neurotoxin	Australia, New Guinea	Slender
		Tiger snake	Strong neurotoxin	Australia	Dry environment, aggressive, very dangerous
		Death adder	Neurotoxin	Australia, New Guinea	Sandy terrain
		Coral snakes	Neurotoxin	United States, tropical America	About 26 species, 2 in southern United States
Hydrophiidae	Front, immovable, hollow	Sea snakes	Some mild, others very toxic	Tropical, Indian and Pacific Oceans	Rudder-like tail, gentle, over 50 species
Viperidae	Front, movable, hollow	True vipers; viperines; viperids	Predominantly hemotoxin	Entirely in Old World	About 50 species
		European viper	Hemotoxin	Europe (rare), North Africa, Near East	Dry rocky country
		Russell's viper	Hemotoxin	Southeast Asia, Java, Sumatra	Mostly open terrain, deadly
		Sand vipers	Hemotoxin	Northern Sahara	Buried in sand
		Puff adder	Hemotoxin	Arabia, Africa	Open terrain, sluggish
		Gaboon viper	Neurotoxin and hemotoxin	Tropical West Africa	Forests, deadly
		Rhinoceros viper	Hemotoxin	Tropical Africa	Wet forests
Crotalidae	Front, movable, hollow	Pit vipers; crotalids; crotalines	Predominantly hemotoxin	Old and New Worlds; none in Africa	Over 80 species, pit between eye and nostril
		Habu viper	Neurotoxin	Warmer parts of East Asia, Ryukyu Islands	Caves and dry rocky country
		Rattlesnakes	Predominantly hemotoxin	North, Central, and South America	South American form neurotoxic
		Bushmaster	Hemotoxin	Central and South America	Wet forests, large
		Fer-de-lance	Hemotoxin	Central America, northern South America, few West Indies	Common on plantations
		Palm vipers	Hemotoxin	Southern Mexico, Central and South America	Arboreal, small, greenish, bites face
		Copperhead	Hemotoxin	United States	Dry stony terrain
		Water moccasin	Hemotoxin	Southeast United States to Texas	Swamps
		Asiatic pit vipers	Hemotoxin	Southeast Asia, Taiwan	Most arboreal

snore (snor) 1. rough, noisy breathing during sleep, due to vibration of the uvula and soft palate; called also *stertor.* 2. to produce such sounds during sleep.

snoRNA small nucleolar RNA.

snoRNP small nucleolar ribonucleoprotein.

snout (snout) the long, specialized upper lip and apex of the nose seen in pigs and certain other animals.

snow (sno) a freezing or frozen mixture consisting of discrete particles or crystals.

carbon dioxide s. solid carbon dioxide, formed by rapid evaporation of liquid carbon dioxide; it gives a temperature of about −79°C (−110°F). It has been used in cryotherapy to freeze the skin and produce local anesthesia with arrest of blood flow. In the form of carbon dioxide slush, it is used as an escharotic to destroy skin lesions such as warts or moles and as a peeling agent for chemabrasion.

snow•blind•ness (sno′blīnd-nis) temporary loss of sight due to injury to superficial cells of the cornea caused by ultraviolet rays of the sun reinforced by those reflected by snow.

SNP (snip) single nucleotide polymorphism.

SNRI serotonin-norepinephrine reuptake inhibitor; see also *selective norepinephrine reuptake inhibitor*, under *inhibitor*.

snRNA small nuclear RNA.

snRNP (snurp) small nuclear ribonucleoprotein.

SNS sympathetic nervous system.

snuff (snuf) a medicinal or errhine powder to be inhaled through the nose.

snuf•fles (snuf′əlz) 1. a catarrhal discharge from the nasal mucous membrane in infants, generally in congenital syphilis. 2. rabbit septicemia.

SO sphenooccipital synchondrosis (def. 2).

SOAP (sōp) [*s*ubjective data; *o*bjective data; *a*ssessment; *p*lan] a device for conceptualizing the process of recording the progress notes in the *problem-oriented record* (see under *record*): *S* indicates subjective data obtained from the patient and others close to him; *O* designates objective data obtained by observation, physical examination, diagnostic studies, etc.; *A* refers to assessment of the patient's status through analysis of the problem, possible interaction of the problems, and changes in the status of the problems; *P* designates the plan for patient care.

soap (sōp) [L. *sapo*] any compound of one or more fatty acids, or their equivalents, with an alkali. Soap is detergent and is used as a cleanser.

green s. [USP] a soap made by the saponification of vegetable oils, excluding coconut oil and palm kernel oil, without the removal of glycerin, the alkali being potassium hydroxide. It is the chief ingredient of green soap tincture (q.v.). Called also *medicinal soft s.* and *soft s.*

hexachlorophene liquid s. [USP] a solution of hexachlorophene in a 10 to 13 per cent solution of a potassium soap, used as a topical antiinfective and detergent.

medicinal soft s., potash s., soft s. green s.

superfatted s. a soap having an excess of fat over that necessary to neutralize all the alkali.

soap•stone (sōp′stōn) the solid stony form in which talc (q.v.) is found in nature. Called also *steatite*.

So•ave operation (so-ah′va) [F. *Soave*, Italian pediatric surgeon, 20th century] see under *operation*.

SOB shortness of breath.

so•cial•iza•tion (so″shəl-ĭ-za′shən) the process by which society integrates the individual, and the individual learns to behave in socially acceptable ways.

so•cio•acu•sis (so″se-o-ə-ku′sis) noise-induced hearing loss due to prolonged exposure to high levels of noise.

so•cio•bi•ol•o•gist (so″se-o-bi-ol′ə-jist) a specialist in sociobiology.

so•cio•bi•ol•o•gy (so″se-o-bi-ol′ə-je) the branch of theoretical biology that proposes that animal (including human) behavior has a biological basis controlled by the genes; the study of the biological basis of behavior. **sociobiolog′ic, sociobiolog′ical** *adj*

so•ci•o•gen•ic (so″se-o-jen′ik) arising from or imposed by society.

so•ci•om•e•try (so″se-om′ə-tre) [L. *socius* fellow + *-metry*] the branch of sociology concerned with the measurement of human social behavior.

so•cio•path•ic (so″se-o-path′ik) pertaining to antisocial behavior or to antisocial personality disorder.

so•cio•ther•a•py (so″se-o-ther′ə-pe) any treatment emphasizing socioenvironmental and interpersonal rather than intrapsychic factors.

sock•et (sok′ət) 1. a hollow or depression, into which a corresponding part fits. 2. gomphosis.

dry s. a condition sometimes occurring after tooth extraction, particularly after traumatic extraction, resulting in a dry appearance of the exposed bone in the socket, due to disintegration or loss of the blood clot. It is basically a focal osteomyelitis without suppuration and is accompanied by severe pain (alveolalgia) and foul odor. Called also *alveolar osteitis* and *alveolitis sicca dolorosa*.

eye s. orbita.

tooth s. alveolus dentalis.

so•da (so′də) a term loosely applied to sodium bicarbonate (baking s.), sodium hydroxide (caustic s.), or sodium carbonate (washing s.).

baking s., bicarbonate of s. sodium bicarbonate.

caustic s. sodium hydroxide.

s. lime [NF] a mixture of calcium oxide and sodium or potassium hydroxide or both; a reagent used to absorb carbon dioxide in anesthesia machines, in oxygen therapy, and in the determination of the basal metabolic rate.

so•di•um (Na) (so′de-əm) a soft, silver white, alkaline metallic element; atomic number, 11; atomic weight, 22.990; specific gravity, 0.971. With a valence of 1, it has a strong affinity for oxygen and other nonmetallic elements. Sodium provides the chief cation of the extracellular body fluids. See also *sodium pump*, under *pump*. The salts of sodium are the most widely used salts in medicine. NOTE: For sodium salts not listed below, see the name of the active ingredient.

Sodium

s. 22 a radioactive isotope of sodium, atomic mass 22, having a half-life of 2.60 years and decaying by positron emission (0.545, 1.83 MeV) with electron capture and emission of gamma rays (1.275 MeV). It has been used in the determination of body sodium space and total exchangeable sodium.

s. 24 a radioactive isotope of sodium, atomic mass 24, having a half-life of 14.66 hours and emitting beta particles (1.389, 4.17 MeV) and gamma rays (1.369, 2.754 MeV); it has been used in the determination of sodium space and total exchangeable sodium.

s. acetate [USP] the trihydrate sodium salt of acetic acid, used as a source of sodium ions in solutions for hemodialysis and peritoneal dialysis. It has also been used as a systemic and urinary alkalizer, diuretic, and expectorant.

s. acetate C 11 [USP] sodium acetate in which a portion of the molecules have been labeled with carbon 11, used as a tracer in positron emission tomography in the study of cardiac metabolism; administered intravenously.

s. acid phosphate monobasic s. phosphate.

s. alginate [NF] a purified carbohydrate product extracted from brown seaweeds with dilute alkali; used as a suspending agent. It is also used for its emulsifying, stabilizing, thickening, and water-binding qualities in foods, medicines, and cosmetics.

s. alizarinsulfonate a yellow-brown or orange-yellow powder used as a stain in microscopy, as a reagent for aluminum, as an acid-base indicator, and in the determination of fluorine. Called also *alizarin red S* and *alizarin water-soluble red*.

s. ascorbate [USP] the monosodium salt of ascorbic acid, administered parenterally as an antiscorbutic and nutritional supplement, as an adjunct to improve absorption in the treatment of iron deficiency anemia and to improve chelation during deferoxamine therapy for chronic iron toxicity; also used as an antioxidant in pharmaceuticals and food.

s. aurothiomalate INN for *gold sodium thiomalate;* see under *gold*.

s. benzoate [NF] the sodium salt of benzoic acid, $C_7H_5NaO_2$, used as an antifungal preservative in pharmaceutical preparations and foods. It may also be used as a test for liver function, administered orally or intravenously.

s. bicarbonate [USP] the monosodium salt of carbonic acid, $NaHCO_3$, used as an electrolyte replenisher and systemic alkalizer, administered by intravenous injection or infusion. It is also administered orally as a gastric antacid and urinary alkalizer, and is applied topically in solution to wash the nose, mouth, or vagina, and as a cleansing enema; sometimes used in solution as a dressing for minor burns. Called also *baking soda* and *bicarbonate of soda*.

s. biphosphate monobasic s. phosphate.

s. bisulfite the monosodium salt of sulfurous acid, $HNaO_3S$, used as an antioxidant and stabilizing agent in pharmaceutical preparations.

s. borate [NF] the sodium salt of boric acid, $Na_2B_4O_7$, used as an alkalizing agent in pharmaceutical preparations. It has also been used for its weak antibacterial and mild astringent properties in lotions and ear and eye preparations. Called also *borax*, *s. pyroborate*, and *s. tetraborate*.

s. calcium edetate, s. calciumedetate edetate calcium disodium.

s. carbonate [NF] the disodium salt of carbonic acid, used as an alkalizing agent in pharmaceutical preparations. Called also *sal soda*.

s. chloride common table salt: a mineral soluble in water and found widely distributed over the earth, such as in sea water. It is a necessary constituent of the body and consequently of the diet, making up over 90 per cent of the inorganic constituents of the blood serum, and is the principal salt involved in maintaining osmotic tension of blood and tissues. It is used in medicine [USP] for many purposes, such as in the preparation of isotonic and physiologic saline solutions; as a fluid and electrolyte replenisher; as an isotonic vehicle for drugs; as an antihypercalcemic; as an antidote to silver nitrate poisoning, administered by intravenous infusion; as a topical antiinflammatory; to irrigate wounds and body cavities; as an enema to flush the colon and promote evacuation; as a mucolytic, administered by inhalation; and as a topical osmotic agent in ophthalmology. Also used widely as a food preservative and seasoning.

s. chromate the disodium salt of chromic acid; it is toxic and has a variety of industrial uses. See also *s. chromate Cr 51*.

s. chromate Cr 51 sodium chromate prepared using the radioactive isotope chromium 51; used as a biological tracer to tag erythrocytes and estimate red cell or whole blood volume as well as for red cell survival time demonstrations and sequestration studies, and for the diagnosis of gastrointestinal bleeding. Labeled platelets are used for platelet survival studies.

s. citrate [USP] the trisodium salt of citric acid, used as an anticoagulant for blood or plasma that is to be fractionated or for blood that is to be stored. It is also administered orally as a urinary alkalizer.

s. cyanide an extremely poisonous compound, NaCN, used for various industrial processes and to fumigate fruit trees. See also *cyanide poisoning*, under *poisoning*.

dibasic s. phosphate [USP] the heptahydrate disodium salt of phosphoric acid; used alone or in combination with other phosphate compounds, it is given intravenously as an electrolyte replenisher, orally or rectally as a laxative, and orally as a urinary acidifier and as an antiurolithic.

s. dodecyl sulfate (SDS) the more usual name for sodium lauryl sulfate when used as an anionic detergent to solubilize proteins.

s. ferric gluconate a ferric oxide hydrate directly bonded to sucrose chelated with gluconate, used as a hematinic, especially in treatment of hemodialysis patients with iron deficiency anemia who are also receiving erythropoietin therapy. Administered by intravenous injection.

Sodium *Continued*

s. fluoride [USP] a dental caries prophylactic, NaF; used in the fluoridation of water and applied topically to the teeth.
s. fluoroacetamide a sodium salt related chemically to sodium fluoroacetate, also used as a rodenticide and causing poisoning similar to fluoroacetate poisoning in many mammals.
s. fluoroacetate the sodium salt of fluoroacetic acid, a toxin found in the South African tree *Dichapetalum cymosum*; it is used as a rodenticide, but is also poisonous to mammals other than rodents. See *fluoroacetate poisoning*, under *poisoning*.
s. fluosilicate s. silicofluoride.
s. folate a water-soluble compound used in treatment of various anemias and sprue. See also *folic acid*.
s. glutamate 1. the monosodium salt of L-glutamic acid, used as a pharmaceutic necessity, and also used to enhance the flavor of foods. See also *Chinese restaurant syndrome*, under *syndrome*. 2. monosodium glutamate.
s. hyaluronate hyaluronan.
s. hydroxide [NF] a caustic alkali, NaOH, used as an alkalizing agent in pharmaceutical preparations. Called also *caustic soda*.
s. hypochlorite the sodium salt of hypochlorous acid, NaClO, having germicidal and disinfectant properties. See also under *solution*.
s. hyposulfite s. thiosulfate.
s. iodide [USP] a binary haloid, NaI, used in various conditions as a source of iodine. It is also used as an expectorant.
s. iodide I 123 [USP] sodium iodide labeled with ^{123}I; administered orally or intravenously in thyroid uptake tests and thyroid imaging.
s. iodide I 125 sodium iodide labeled with ^{125}I; administered orally or intravenously as a tracer in tests of thyroid functioning and in thyroid imaging.
s. iodide I 131 [USP] sodium iodide labeled with ^{131}I; used as a tracer in thyroid uptake tests and thyroid imaging and used in the treatment of hyperthyroidism and thyroid carcinoma; administered orally or intravenously.
s. ipodate ipodate sodium.
s. lactate [USP] the sodium salt of racemic or inactive lactic acid, used intravenously in one-sixth molar solution as a fluid and electrolyte replenisher to combat acidosis.
s. lauryl sulfate [NF] an anionic surfactant, used as a wetting agent, emulsifying aid, and detergent in various cosmetic and dermatologic preparations. See also *s. dodecyl sulfate*.
s. metabisulfite [NF] an antioxidant, $Na_2S_2O_5$, used in pharmaceutical preparations.
monobasic s. phosphate [USP] the monohydrate, dihydrate, or anhydrous monosodium salt of phosphoric acid; used in buffer solutions. Used alone or in combination with other phosphate compounds, it is given intravenously as an electrolyte replenisher, orally or rectally as a laxative, and orally as a urinary acidifier and as an antiurolithic.
s. monofluorophosphate [USP] a dental caries prophylactic, applied topically to the teeth.
s. morrhuate morrhuate sodium.
s. nitrate a compound, $NaNO_3$, used as a reagent, in fertilizers, and in certain industrial processes; it is sometimes responsible for nitrite poisoning in livestock.
s. nitrite [USP] an antidote for cyanide poisoning, $NaNO_2$; it reduces hemoglobin to methemoglobin, which has a greater affinity for cyanide than does cytochrome oxidase. It is also used as a preservative in cured meats and other foods.
s. nitroferricyanide, s. nitroprusside [USP] an antihypertensive used in the treatment of acute congestive heart failure and of hypertensive crisis and to produce controlled hypotension during surgery, administered by intravenous infusion. It is also used as a reagent and testing solution.
s. para-aminosalicylate aminosalicylate sodium.
s. perborate a compound, $NaBO_3 \cdot 4H_2O$, prepared by interaction of boric acid or sodium borate with sodium or hydrogen peroxide. It is an antiseptic, used in 2 per cent solution as a mouthwash and in a 10–20 per cent powder in dentifrices.
s. permanganate a strongly oxidizing substance used as a disinfectant.
s. pertechnetate Tc 99m [USP] official nomenclature for *technetium 99m pertechnetate*.
s. phenylbutyrate an agent used as adjunctive treatment to control the hyperammonemia of urea cycle enzyme disorders; administered orally.
s. phosphate any of various compounds of sodium and phosphoric acid; usually used to denote specifically *dibasic s. phosphate*.
s. phosphate P 32 [USP] sodium phosphate labeled with radiophosphorus (^{32}P); used in the treatment of polycythemia vera, chronic myelocytic leukemia, and chronic lymphocytic leukemia, in the localization of certain tumors, and in the palliation of metastatic skeletal disease; administered orally or intravenously.
s. phosphates see under *phosphates*.
s. polyphosphate disodium salt of polyphosphoric acid; a pharmaceutic aid, $(NaPO_3)_n$, where $n = 12$ to 20.
s. polystyrene sulfonate [USP] a cation exchange resin prepared in the sodium form, each gram of which exchanges 110–135 mg of potassium, calculated on the anhydrous basis; used as an antihyperkalemic, administered orally or rectally.
potassium s. tartrate see under *potassium*.
s. propionate [NF] the sodium salt of propionic acid, having antifungal properties; used alone or in combination with calcium propionate or other agents as a preservative to inhibit mold production in bakery and dairy products and other foods and in pharmaceuticals. It is also used as a topical antifungal to treat mycoses.
s. pyroborate s. borate.
s. salicylate see under *salicylate*.
s. silicofluoride a compound added to water to produce 0.7 to 1 part per million of fluorine, to prevent dental caries, and also used in insecticides. Called also *s. fluosilicate*.
s. stearate [NF] a mixture of sodium stearate, sodium palmitate, and small amounts of the sodium salts of other fatty acids; used as a stiffening and emulsifying agent in pharmaceutical preparations.
s. stibocaptate a trivalent antimony compound, used as an antischistosomal, administered intramuscularly. Called also *antimony sodium dimercaptosuccinate* and *stibocaptate*.
s. sulfate [USP] the decahydrate disodium salt of sulfuric acid, used orally as a cathartic or laxative and also administered by gastric lavage in the treatment of barium poisoning. Called also *Glauber salt*.
s. sulfite Na_2SO_3, fairly stable in the anhydrous form; used as a reagent and as a preservative and antioxidant.
s. tetraborate s. borate.
s. tetradecyl sulfate an anionic surfactant with sclerosing properties; used as a wetting agent, as a detergent, and as a sclerosing agent in sclerotherapy for varicose veins.
s. thiamylal thiamylal sodium.
s. thiosulfate [USP] a compound used intravenously as an antidote to cyanide poisoning; also used in solution as a foot bath to prevent ringworm infection at swimming pools and public showers, topically in tinea versicolor, and in measuring the volume of extracellular body fluid and the renal glomerular filtration rate.
s. trimetaphosphate the trisodium salt of metaphosphoric acid, used as a pharmaceutic aid.
s. urate see under *urate*.

so·di·um-po·tas·si·um ATP·ase (so′de-əm-po-tas′e-əm a-te-pe′ās) Na^+,K^+-ATPase.

so·do·ku (so′do-koo) [Japanese *so* rat + *doku* poison] Japanese name for the spirillary form of rat-bite fever.

sod·o·my (sod′ə-me) [*Sodom*, biblical city near the Dead Sea] 1. anal intercourse. 2. any of various nonreproductive sexual acts, particularly anal intercourse.

Soem·mer·ing ring (ring cataract) (sur′mər-ing) [Samuel Thomas von *Soemmering*, German anatomist, 1755–1830] see under *ring*.

SOFAS Social and Occupational Functioning Assessment Scale.

sof·ten·ing (sof′en-ing) malacia.
colliquative s. see under *necrosis*.

Soh·val-Sof·fer syndrome (so′vahl sof′ər) [Arthur R. *Sohval*, American internist, 1904–1985; Louis J. *Soffer*, American endocrinologist, 1904–1995] see under *syndrome*.

Sol. [L.] solution.

sol (sol) [*sol*ution] a colloid system in which the dispersion medium is liquid or gas; the latter is usually called an *aerosol*.

metal s. a colloidal dispersion of a metal in a liquid. Such dispersions often have catalytic properties similar to those of enzymes, and are therefore sometimes called inorganic enzymes.

So•la•na•ceae (so″lə-na′se-e) a large family of widely distributed herbs, shrubs, and trees, having great economic importance, and including many poisonous and medicinal species. *Atropa, Capsicum, Datura, Duboisia, Hyoscyamus, Nicotiana, Scopolia,* and *Solanum* are important genera.

so•la•na•ceous (so″lə-na′shəs) of or pertaining to the family Solanaceae.

so•la•nine (so′lə-nēn) a steroidal glycoalkaloid found in several species of *Solanum,* such as the nightshades and the green spots on potatoes; if ingested, it can cause erythrolysis, central nervous system depression, and often fatal respiratory failure.

so•la•noid (so′lə-noid) [*solanum* + *-oid*] resembling a raw potato in texture.

So•la•num (so-la′nəm) [L. "nightshade"] a large genus of plants of the family Solanaceae. It includes the potato, tomato, eggplant, several of the nightshades, and many poisonous and medicinal species. *S. carolinen′se* L. is a poisonous North American species. *S. dimidia′tum, S. fastigia′tum,* and *S. kweben′se* cause crazy cow syndrome respectively in the United States, Brazil, and South Africa. *S. malacox′ylon* is a South American species that causes enzootic calcinosis in ruminants.

so•lap•sone (so-lap′sōn) an antibacterial derivative of dapsone, having actions similar to those of the parent compound but less toxic; used as a leprostatic, administered orally and intramuscularly. Called also *solasulfone.*

So•la•quin (so′lə-kwin) trademark for preparations of hydroquinone.

so•lar (so′lər) [L. *solaris*] 1. pertaining to the sun. 2. denoting the great sympathetic plexus and its principal ganglia (especially the celiac); so called because of their radiating nerves.

So•lar•aze (so′lər-āz) trademark for a preparation of diclofenac sodium.

so•la•ri•um (so-lar′e-əm) [L.] a room especially designed to allow exposure to light of the sun or to artificial light.

so•la•sul•fone (so″lə-sul′fōn) solapsone.

sol•a•tion (sol-a′shən) the conversion of a gel into a sol.

sold•er (sod′ər) [L. *solidatio* making solid, fastening] 1. a fusible metal or alloy of metals used to unite pieces of metals with higher fusion temperatures. 2. to fasten together pieces of metal through the use of this material.

sole (sōl) [L. *solea; planta*] 1. planta. 2. the inferior surface of a horse's hoof.

so•le•al (so′le-əl) [L. *solea* a sandal with straps] pertaining to the calf or to the musculus soleus.

solen(o)- [Gr. *sōlēn* a channel, gutter, pipe] a combining form denoting relationship to a pipe or gutter; tubular or grooved.

So•le•nog•ly•pha (so″lə-nog′lĭ-fə) [*soleno-* + Gr. *glyphein* to cut out with a knife] a group of venomous snakes with fangs that are hollow like a hypodermic needle and that normally fold back against the roof of the mouth but can be erected for striking and piercing. Examples are the massasauga and the rattlesnakes.

so•le•noid (so′lə-noid) [Gr. *sōlēnoeidēs* pipe-shaped, from *sōlēn* pipe] 1. a coil of insulated wire in which a magnetic field is produced by a flow of electric current. 2. a coil surrounding a movable iron core that is pulled in when the coil is energized. It can be used to perform some mechanical work, such as opening a valve, or as a switch. 3. a model for the higher order structure of eukaryotic DNA, formed by supercoiling of nucleosomes, each turn containing approximately six nucleosomes, and constituting the characteristic 30-nm chromatin fiber; the solenoids in turn make up the chromatin loops of the condensed chromosome.

so•le•no•nych•ia (so″lə-no-nik′e-ə) median nail dystrophy.

So•le•no•po•tes (so″lə-no-po′tēz) [*soleno-* + Gr. *pōtēs* a drinker] a genus of sucking lice (order Anoplura); *S. capilla′tus* is found on cattle.

So•le•nop•sis (so″lə-nop′sis) the fire ants, a genus of stinging ants of the family Formicidae; they inflict painful, burning stings that cause local or systemic reactions. *S. gemina′ta* is indigenous to the United States. *S. saevis′sima rich′teri* is an aggressive species native to South America that has now been seen in North America.

so•le•us (so′le-əs) [L. *solea* a sandal with straps] see *musculus soleus.*

sol•fer•i•no (sol″fər-e′no) fuchsin.

Sol•ga•nal (sol′gə-nal″) trademark for a preparation of aurothioglucose.

sol•id (sol′id) [L. *solidus*] 1. not fluid or gaseous. 2. not hollow. 3. a substance or tissue not fluid or gaseous.

color s. a three-dimensional geometrical body, devised to show the relation of all hues and brightnesses, including black, white, and grays, in their various modes.

Sol•i•da•go (sol″ĭ-da′go) [L.] the goldenrods, a genus of composite-flowered plants (family Compositae). *S. virgau′rea* L., of Europe and North America, is aromatic and diuretic. Certain other species are toxic or deadly to livestock.

so•li•fen•a•cin suc•ci•nate (so″lĭ-fen′ə-sin) an antimuscarinic used in treatment of irritable bladder; administered orally.

sol•ip•sism (sōl′ip-siz-əm) [L. *solus* alone + *ipse* self] the belief that the world exists only in the mind of the individual, or that it consists solely of an individual person and their own experiences. **solipsis′tic** *adj*

So•lir•is (sə-lir′is) trademark for a preparation of eculizumab.

sol•i•tary (sol′ĭ-tar″e) 1. alone; separated from others. 2. living alone or in pairs only.

Sol•o•mon syndrome (sol′ə-mən) [Lawrence M. *Solomon,* American pediatric dermatologist, late 20th century] sebaceous nevus syndrome.

sol•pu•gid (sol-pu′jid) an individual of the order Solpugida.

Sol•pu•gida (sol″pu-jid′ə) the jointed spiders, a family of hairy spiders that are differentiated from other spiders by having a segmented abdomen more broadly joined to the cephalothorax; solpugids can inflict deep painful bites and are found mainly in desert, tropical, and subtropical areas.

sol•u•bil•i•ty (sol″u-bil′ĭ-te) the quality or fact of being soluble; susceptibility of being dissolved.

sol•u•ble (sol′u-bəl) [L. *solubilis*] susceptible of being dissolved.

Solu-Cor•tef (sol″u-kor′tef) trademark for a preparation of hydrocortisone sodium succinate.

Sol•u-Med•rol (sol″u-med′rol) trademark for a preparation of methylprednisolone sodium succinate.

Sol•u•rex (sol′u-reks″) trademark for a preparation of dexamethasone sodium phosphate.

Sol•u•rex LA (sol′u-reks″) trademark for a preparation of dexamethasone acetate.

so•lute (sol′ūt) a substance dissolved in a solvent; a solution consists of a solute and a solvent.

so•lu•tio (so-loo′she-o) [L., from *solvĕre* to dissolve] solution.

so•lu•tion (sə-loo′shən) [L. *solutio*] 1. a homogeneous mixture of one or more substances (solutes) dispersed molecularly in a sufficient quantity of dissolving medium (solvent). The solute may be gas, liquid, or solid; the solvent is usually liquid, but may be solid, as in a solid solution of copper in silver (sterling silver). 2. in pharmacology, a term used to denote a liquid preparation containing one or several soluble chemical substances usually dissolved in water and not, for various reasons, falling into another category (e.g., syrup, elixir). 3. the process of dissolving. 4. a loosening or separation.

Solution

ACD s. anticoagulant citrate dextrose s.

acetic acid otic s. [USP] a solution of glacial acetic acid in a nonaqueous solvent; used topically to treat otitis externa caused by *Pseudomonas, Candida,* and *Aspergillus.*

acid citrate dextrose s. anticoagulant citrate dextrose s.

acidulated phosphate fluoride s. sodium fluoride and acidulated phosphate topical s.

Albright s. a solution consisting of 75 g of sodium citrate, 25 g of potassium citrate, 140 g of citric acid, and 1000 mL of water; used in the treatment of renal tubular acidosis.

alcoholic s. a solution in which alcohol is used as the solvent.

aluminum acetate topical s. [USP] an astringent solution prepared from aluminum subacetate topical solution by the addition of glacial acetic acid and water; used as a gargle or mouthwash and applied

to the skin as a wet dressing, diluted with 10 to 40 parts water. Called also *Burow s.*
aluminum subacetate topical s. [USP] a solution containing aluminum sulfate, acetic acid, precipitated calcium carbonate, and water, used topically on the skin and mucous membranes as an astringent. It is also used as a topical antiseptic and as a wet dressing in various skin diseases.
ammonia s. see *dilute ammonia s.* and *strong ammonia s.*
anisotonic s. a solution having tonicity differing from that of the standard of reference.
anticoagulant citrate dextrose s. [USP] a solution of citric acid, sodium citrate, and dextrose in water for injection, used as an anticoagulant in the preservation of whole blood.
anticoagulant citrate phosphate dextrose s. [USP] a solution containing citric acid, sodium citrate, monobasic sodium phosphate, and dextrose in water for injection; used for preservation of whole blood or red cells for up to 21 days. Called also *citrate phosphate dextrose s.* and *CPD s.*
anticoagulant citrate phosphate dextrose adenine s. [USP] a solution consisting of anticoagulant citrate phosphate dextrose solution and adenine; used for the preservation of whole blood or red cells for up to 35 days. Called also *CPDA-1 s.*, *CPD-adenine s.*, and *citrate phosphate dextrose adenine s.*
anticoagulant heparin s. [USP] a sterile solution of heparin sodium in sodium chloride injection, used as an anticoagulant in the preservation of whole blood.
anticoagulant sodium citrate s. [USP] a solution of sodium citrate in water for injection, used for the storage of whole blood, the preparation of blood for fractionation, and the preparation of citrated human plasma.
antipyrine and benzocaine otic s. [USP] a solution of antipyrine and benzocaine in glycerin instilled into the ear canal for relief of pain and inflammation in acute otitis media and as an adjunct in cerumen removal.
antipyrine, benzocaine, and phenylephrine hydrochloride otic s. [USP] a solution of antipyrine, benzocaine, and phenylephrine hydrochloride in a suitable nonaqueous solvent; instilled into the ear canal for relief of pain and inflammation in acute otitis media.
APF s. sodium fluoride and acidulated phosphate topical s.
aqueous s. a solution in which water is used as the solvent.
Benedict s. an aqueous solution of sodium citrate, sodium carbonate, and copper sulfate. Its normal blue color changes to yellow, orange, or red in the presence of a reducing sugar such as glucose. It is used in urinalysis.
Bouin s. see under *fluid.*
buffer s. a solution which resists appreciable change in its hydrogen ion concentration when acid or alkali is added to it.
Burow s. aluminum acetate topical s.
calcium hydroxide topical s. [USP] a clear, colorless liquid with an alkaline reaction, containing at least 140 mg of calcium hydroxide per 100 mL at 25°C; used in preparing various astringent formulations for topical application to the skin and mucous membranes. Called also *lime water.*
carbamide peroxide topical s. [USP] a solution of carbamide peroxide in anhydrous glycerin, used as a cerumen-softening agent and as a dental cleanser and antiinflammatory.
carbolfuchsin s. see *carbolfuchsin.*
carbolfuchsin topical s. [USP] a dark purple solution containing basic fuchsin, phenol, resorcinol, acetone, alcohol, and purified water; used as a topical antifungal in the treatment of dermatophytosis, tinea, and other skin infections. Called also *Castellani paint.*
cardioplegic s. a cold solution injected into the aortic root or coronary ostia to induce cardiac arrest and protect the heart from damage during open heart surgery; it is usually potassium in either a buffered electrolyte solution or blood.
carmine s. a deep red, rather viscous liquid, compounded of carmine, dilute ammonia solution, glycerin, and water; used as a coloring agent.
Carnoy s. an acid fixative used for studying animal and plant tissue, particularly the cell nucleus and chromosomes; composed of: dehydrated alcohol and glacial acetic acid, and sometimes also chloroform. Called also *Carnoy fluid.*
centinormal s. hundredth-normal s.
citrated Locke s. a solution of sodium chloride, potassium chloride, calcium chloride, and sodium citrate in distilled water, with pH adjusted to 7.4.
citrate phosphate dextrose s. anticoagulant citrate phosphate dextrose s.
citrate phosphate dextrose adenine s. anticoagulant citrate phosphate dextrose adenine solution.
colloid s., colloidal s. imprecise terms for a *colloidal system;* see *colloid* (def. 2).
compound iodine s. strong iodine s.
contrast s. a solution of a substance opaque to the x-ray, used to facilitate radiographic visualization of some organ or structure in the body.
CPD s. anticoagulant citrate phosphate dextrose s.
CPDA-1 s., CPD-adenine s. anticoagulant citrate phosphate dextrose adenine s.
crystal violet s. gentian violet topical s.
Czapek-Dox s. Czapek-Dox agar; see under *culture medium.*
Dakin s. a diluted sodium hypochlorite solution, often specified as containing 0.5 per cent available chlorine; it has been used as a topical antiinfective for skin and wounds.
decimolar s. a solution having one-tenth the concentration of a molar solution.
decinormal s. tenth-normal s.
desonide and acetic acid otic s. a solution of desonide and acetic acid used topically for the treatment of superficial external auditory canal infections accompanied by inflammation.
dexamethasone sodium phosphate ophthalmic s. [USP] a sterile aqueous solution of dexamethasone sodium phosphate, instilled into the conjunctival sac in the treatment of inflammatory and allergic conditions and into the otic canal for the treatment of superficial external auditory canal infections accompanied by inflammation.
dilute ammonia s., diluted ammonium hydroxide s. a colorless, transparent, alkaline liquid, containing 9 to 10 percent of ammonia; used as a pharmaceutic necessity. Called also *ammonia water.*
disclosing s. a solution used for the purpose of making something apparent, such as one to be painted on the surface of a tooth in order to stain, and thus render visible, foreign matter or bacterial plaque.
double-normal s. a solution having double the strength of a normal solution; designated 2 N.
Drabkin s. an aqueous solution containing 1.0 g sodium bicarbonate, 0.05 g potassium cyanide, and 0.20 g potassium ferricyanide per liter; used to lyse red cells and convert hemoglobin to cyanmethemoglobin in hemoglobinometry.
Fehling s. an alkaline cupric sulfate solution similar to Benedict reagent.
ferric subsulfate s. [USP] a reddish-brown aqueous solution of basic ferric sulfate, prepared from ferrous sulfate, sulfuric acid, and nitric acid; used as an astringent and hemostatic.
fiftieth-normal s. a solution having one-fiftieth the strength of a normal solution: designated N/50 or 0.02 N.
fixative s. see *fixative.*
Flemming s. a solution for hardening histological specimens, consisting of chromium trioxide, osmium tetroxide, glacial acetic acid, and water.
formaldehyde s. [USP] a solution of formaldehyde in water, containing not less than 37 per cent of formaldehyde; used as a disinfectant and as a preservative and fixative for pathologic specimens. Called also *formalin* and *formol.*
formol-Zenker s. Zenker-formol fixative.
gentian violet topical s. [USP] a purple liquid with a slight odor of alcohol, containing gentian violet, alcohol, and purified water, applied topically to the skin and mucous membranes in infections associated with gram-positive bacteria and molds. Called also *crystal violet s.* and *methylrosaniline chloride s.*
Gilson s. a fixative solution consisting of mercury bichloride, nitric acid, glacial acetic acid, 70 per cent alcohol, and water.
Gowers s. a solution of sodium sulfate, glacial acetic acid, and water, used for the dilution of blood prior to counting red blood cells with a hemocytometer.
Gram s. see under *stain.*
gram molecular s. molar s.
half-normal s. a solution having half the strength of a normal solution; designated N/2.
Hayem s. a solution of mercury bichloride, sodium chloride, and sodium sulfate, used in diluting blood prior to counting red blood cells with a hemocytometer.

heparin lock flush s. [USP] a sterile preparation of heparin sodium injection with sufficient sodium chloride to make it isotonic with blood, used to maintain patency of indwelling intravascular devices designed for intermittent injection or infusion therapy or blood sampling.
hundredth-normal s. a solution having one-hundredth the strength of a normal solution; designated N/100 or 0.01 N.
hydrogen peroxide topical s. [USP] a solution containing 2.5–3.5 g hydrogen peroxide per 100 mL; used as a topical antiinfective to the skin and mucous membranes.
hydroxypropyl methylcellulose ophthalmic s. [USP] a sterile solution containing 85–115 per cent hydroxypropyl methylcellulose; applied topically to the conjunctiva to protect the cornea during certain ophthalmic procedures and to lubricate the cornea.
hyperbaric s. a solution having a greater specific gravity than a standard of reference, such as one used for spinal anesthesia having a specific gravity greater than that of the spinal fluid, causing it to migrate downward and produce anesthesia below the level of injection.
hypobaric s. a solution having a specific gravity less than that of a standard of reference, such as one used for spinal anesthesia having a specific gravity less than that of the spinal fluid, causing it to migrate upward and produce anesthesia above the level of injection.
iodine topical s. [USP] transparent, reddish brown liquid, with the odor of iodine, consisting of iodine and sodium iodide in purified water, each 100 mL of which contains 1.8 to 2.2 g of iodine and 2.1 to 2.6 g of sodium iodide; used as a topical antiinfective.
isobaric s. a solution having the same specific gravity as a standard of reference, such as one used for spinal anesthesia having a specific gravity the same as that of the spinal fluid, causing it to remain and produce anesthesia at the level of injection.
Kinyoun carbolfuchsin s. Kinyoun carbolfuchsin. See also *Kinyoun staining method*, at *Table of Stains and Staining Methods*, under *stain.*
Labarraque s. sodium hypochlorite solution, diluted with an equal volume of water.
lactated Ringer s. see under *injection.*
lactulose s. [USP] an aqueous solution prepared from lactulose concentrate, consisting principally of lactulose, with small quantities of lactose and galactose and traces of other related sugars; used to reduce blood ammonia levels in the treatment of hepatic encephalopathy, administered orally.
Lang s. a hardening fluid containing corrosive mercury bichloride, sodium chloride, and acetic acid, in water.
Locke s. a solution of sodium chloride, calcium chloride, potassium chloride, sodium bicarbonate, and dextrose; used in physiological experiments to keep the mammalian heart beating.
Locke-Ringer s. a test solution containing sodium chloride, potassium chloride, calcium chloride, magnesium chloride, sodium bicarbonate, dextrose, and water.
Lugol s. strong iodine s.
magnesium citrate oral s. [USP] a colorless to slightly yellow, clear, effervescent liquid, with a sweet, acidulous taste and a lemon flavor, prepared using magnesium carbonate, anhydrous citric acid, syrup, talc, lemon oil, potassium bicarbonate, and purified water; used as a cathartic.
methoxsalen topical s. [USP] a preparation containing 9.2 to 10.8 mg of methoxsalen per mL; used in conjunction with exposure to ultraviolet light to facilitate repigmentation in idiopathic vitiligo.
methylcellulose ophthalmic s. [USP] a sterile solution of methylcellulose, applied topically to protect the cornea during certain ophthalmic procedures and to lubricate the cornea.
methylrosaniline chloride s. gentian violet topical s.
molal s. a solution containing 1 mole of solute dissolved in 1000 g of solvent.
molar s. a solution each liter of which contains 1 mole of solute per liter of solution: designated M/1 or 1 M. The concentration of other solutions may be expressed in relation to that of molar solutions as tenth-molar (M/10 or 0.1 M), etc.
molecular disperse s. a solution in which the dispersed particles have a diameter of about 0.1 picometer.
Monsel s. ferric subsulfate s.
Nessler s. see under *reagent.*
normal s. a solution in which each liter contains 1 equivalent weight of the dissolved substance: designated N/1 or 1 N.
normal saline s., normal salt s. physiologic saline s.
ophthalmic s. a sterile solution, essentially free from foreign particles and suitably compounded and dispensed, for instillation into the eye.
oral sodium phosphate s. a solution of mixed phosphate salts of sodium, to be taken orally as a laxative prior to colonoscopy.
Perenyi s. an embryological fixing solution, consisting of 10 per cent solution of nitric acid, alcohol, and 0.5 per cent solution of chromic acid.
physiologic saline s., physiologic salt s., physiologic sodium chloride s. a 0.9 per cent aqueous solution of sodium chloride, which is isotonic with blood serum.
potassium citrate and citric acid oral s. [USP] a solution of potassium citrate and citric acid monohydrate in an aqueous medium, providing approximately 2 mmol potassium per mL and used as an electrolyte replenisher.
Ringer s. see under *injection* and *irrigation.*
saline s., salt s. a solution of sodium chloride in purified water.
saturated s. a solution in which the solvent has taken up all of the dissolved substance that it can hold in solution.
sclerosing s. a solution of a sclerosing agent, for use in sclerotherapy.
seminormal s. half-normal s.
Shohl s. a solution containing 140 g citric acid and 98 g hydrated crystalline salt of sodium citrate in distilled water to make 1000 mL; used to correct electrolyte imbalance in the treatment of renal tubular acidosis.
sodium chloride s. see under *injection* and *irrigation.*
sodium fluoride and acidulated phosphate topical s. [USP] a fluoride-containing preparation, consisting of sodium fluoride, hydrofluoric acid, and phosphoric acid, with concentrations of 1.23 per cent fluoride ion and 0.98 per cent phosphoric acid, pH of 3.0 to 3.5; applied topically to the teeth as a dental caries prophylactic.
sodium hypochlorite s. [USP] a clear, pale, greenish yellow liquid with the odor of chlorine, containing 4–6 per cent sodium hypochlorite; used as a disinfectant for utensils, etc., but not suitable for application to wounds. It has also been used as a deodorant and bleaching agent. In diluted form, usually at a strength of approximately 0.5 per cent available chlorine, it has been used as a local anti-infective and wound irrigant. See also *Dakin s.*
sodium hypochlorite topical s. [USP] a colorless to light yellow liquid containing between 0.20 and 0.32 g of sodium hypochlorite in a topical solution; used as a local anti-infective.
sodium phosphates rectal s. [USP] a solution of dibasic sodium phosphate and monobasic sodium phosphate, or dibasic sodium phosphate and phosphoric acid, in purified water; used as a cathartic; called also sodium phosphate and biphosphate enema and sodium phosphates enema.
solid s. a crystalline phase of solution that is homogeneous but has several different chemical components, whose molecules are randomly distributed on the points of the space lattice. See also under *alloy.*
standard s. a solution that contains in each liter a definitely stated amount of reagent; usually expressed in terms of normality (equivalent weights of solute per liter of solution) or molarity (moles of solute per liter of solution).
strong ammonia s. [NF], **stronger ammonium hydroxide s.** a colorless, transparent, strongly alkaline liquid containing 27–31 per cent ammonia; used as a solvent and as a source of ammonia in pharmaceutical preparations. Called also *stronger ammonia water.*
strong iodine s. [USP] a transparent, deep brown liquid, with the odor of iodine, containing in purified water 4.5–5.5 g of iodine and 9.5–10.5 g of potassium iodide in 100 mL; used as a source of iodine in preparation for thyroid surgery, administered orally, and in Gram method and other staining methods. Called also *Lugol s.*
supersaturated s. an unstable solution that contains more of the solute than it can permanently hold.
susa s. a decalcifying solution used for fixing animal tissue, composed of mercury bichloride, sodium chloride, trichloroacetic acid, formaldehyde solution, and water.
TAC s. a solution of tetracaine, epinephrine (adrenaline), and cocaine, used as a local anesthetic in the emergency treatment of uncomplicated lacerations.
tenth-normal s. a solution having one-tenth the strength of a normal solution: designated N/10 or 0.1 N.
test s's standard solutions (in purity and concentration) of specified chemical substances used in performing certain test procedures.

Solution *Continued*

thousandth-normal s. a solution having one-thousandth the strength of a normal solution: designated N/1000 or 0.001 N.
Toison s. a fluid used in diluting blood for the counting of the erythrocytes, consisting of gentian violet, sodium chloride, sodium sulfate, glycerin, and water. Called also *Toison fluid.*
Tyrode s. a modified Locke solution containing magnesium.
University of Wisconsin s. a preservation solution used to flush organs before cold storage prior to transplantation to prevent cold-induced cell injury.
volumetric s. a solution that contains a specific quantity of solute per stated unit of volume; see also *standard s.*
xanthan gum s. [NF] a solution of xanthan gum, methylparaben, and propylparaben in purified water; used as a suspending, stabilizing, emulsifying, and thickening agent.
Zenker s. see under *fixative.*
Ziehl-Neelsen carbolfuchsin s. Ziehl-Neelsen carbolfuchsin. See also *Ziehl-Neelsen staining method,* at *Table of Stains and Staining Methods,* under *stain.*

solv. [L.] sol've (dissolve).

sol•vate (sol'vāt) a compound of one or more molecules of a solvent with the ions or with the molecules of a dissolved substance.

sol•va•tion (sol-va'shən) chemical combination of a solvent with the solute.

sol•vent (sol'vənt) [L. *solvere* to dissolve] 1. dissolving; effecting a solution. 2. a substance, usually a liquid, that dissolves or that is capable of dissolving; the component of a solution that is present in greater amount. Cf. *solute.*

sol•vol•y•sis (sol-vol'ĭ-sis) a general term for double decomposition reactions of the type of hydrolysis, ammonolysis, and sulfolysis.

So•ma (so'mə) trademark for combination preparations of carisoprodol and aspirin.

so•ma (so'mə) [Gr. *sōma* body] 1. the body as distinguished from the mind. 2. the body tissue as distinguished from the germ cells. 3. the cell body of a neuron.

so•mal (so'məl) somatic.

som•a•lin (som'ə-lin) a cardioactive glycoside from plants of the genus *Adenium.*

so•man (so'man) an organophosphorus compound that is a potent cholinesterase inhibitor and is used as a nerve gas; symptoms of poisoning include bronchial constriction, convulsions, and often death. See also *organophosphorus compound poisoning,* under *poisoning.*

so•ma•tal•gia (so″mə-tal'jə) [*somato-* + *-algia*] generalized bodily pain.

so•mat•es•the•sia (so″mat-es-the'zhə) [*somato-* + *esthesia*] 1. somatic sense. 2. somatognosis.

so•mat•es•thet•ic (so″mat-əs-thet'ik) pertaining to somatesthesia (somatognosis).

so•mat•ic (so-mat'ik) [Gr. *sōmatikos*] 1. pertaining to or characteristic of the soma or body. 2. pertaining to the body wall in contrast to the viscera.

so•mat•i•co•visc•er•al (so-mat″ĭ-ko-vis'ər-əl) pertaining to the body proper and viscera.

so•ma•tist (so'mə-tist) an individual who believes that mental disorders are of physical origin and are based on bodily lesions.

so•ma•ti•za•tion (so″mə-tĭ-za'shən) in psychiatry, the conversion of mental experiences or states into bodily symptoms.

somat(o)- [Gr. *sōma,* gen. *sōmatos* body] a combining form denoting relationship to the body.

so•mato•chrome (so-mat'o-krōm) [*somato-* + *-chrome*] any neuron that has cytoplasm completely surrounding the nucleus and easily stainable Nissl bodies.

so•ma•to•cri•nin (so″mə-to-kri'nin) growth hormone–releasing hormone.

so•mato•derm (so-mat'o-dərm) [*somato-* + *-derm*] somatic layer.

so•mato•form (so-mat'o-form) [*somato-* + L. *forma* form] denoting physical symptoms that cannot be attributed to organic disease and appear to be of psychic origin.

so•ma•to•gen•e•sis (so″mə-to-jen'ə-sis) [*somato-* + *-genesis*] the formation or emergence of bodily structure out of hereditary sources; the formation of somatoplasm out of germ plasm.

so•ma•to•ge•net•ic (so-mat″o-jə-net'ik) 1. pertaining to somatogenesis. 2. somatogenic.

so•ma•to•gen•ic (so″mə-to-jen'ik) [*somato-* + *-genic*] originating in the cells of the body, as a disease process; opposed to psychogenic.

so•ma•tog•no•sis (so″mə-tog-no'sis) [*somato-* + Gr. *gnōsis* recognition] the general feeling of the existence of one's body and of the functioning of the organs. Called also *cenesthesia, somatesthesia, somesthesia,* and *body* or *sixth sense.*

so•mato•gram (so-mat'o-gram) [*somato-* + *-gram*] a radiograph of the body.

so•ma•to•lib•er•in (so″mə-to-lib'ər-in) growth hormone–releasing hormone.

so•ma•tol•o•gy (so″mə-tol'ə-je) [*somato-* + *-logy*] the study of the body, including both anatomy and physiology.

so•ma•to•mam•mo•tro•pin (so″mə-to-mam'o-tro″pin) a family of hormones, including growth hormone and prolactin, produced by the anterior pituitary, and human placental lactogen, produced by the placenta.
chorionic s. human placental lactogen.

so•ma•to•me•din (so″mə-to-me'din) any of several peptides formed in the liver and other tissues and found in plasma, complexed with transport proteins; they stimulate cellular growth and replication, particularly in bone and muscle, as second messengers in the somatotropic actions of growth hormone and also have insulin-like biological activities. Two such peptides have been isolated, insulinlike growth factors I and II (see under *factor*).
s. A former name for *insulinlike growth factor II.*
s. C former name for *insulinlike growth factor I.*

so•ma•to•meg•a•ly (so″mə-to-meg'ə-le) gigantism.

so•ma•tom•e•try (so″mə-tom'ə-tre) [*somato-* + *-metry*] measurement of the body.

so•ma•to•mo•tor (so″mə-to-mo'tər) pertaining to movements of the body.

so•mato•pleure (so-mat'o-ploor) [*somato-* + Gr. *pleura* side] the embryonic body wall, formed by ectoderm and somatic mesoderm. **somatopleur'al** *adj*

so•ma•to•psy•chic (so″mə-to-si'kik) [*somato-* + *psychic*] pertaining to both body and mind; relating to the effects of the body on the mind.

so•ma•tos•chi•sis (so″mə-tos'kĭ-sis) [*somato-* + *-schisis*] a developmental anomaly characterized by a fissure of the trunk.

so•ma•tos•co•py (so″mə-tos'kə-pe) [*somato-* + *-scopy*] viewing or examination of the body.

so•ma•to•sen•sory (so″mə-to-sen'sə-re) pertaining to sensations received in the skin and deep tissues.

so•ma•to•sex•u•al (so″mə-to-sek'shoo-əl) [*somato-* + *sexual*] pertaining to the physical manifestations of sexual development.

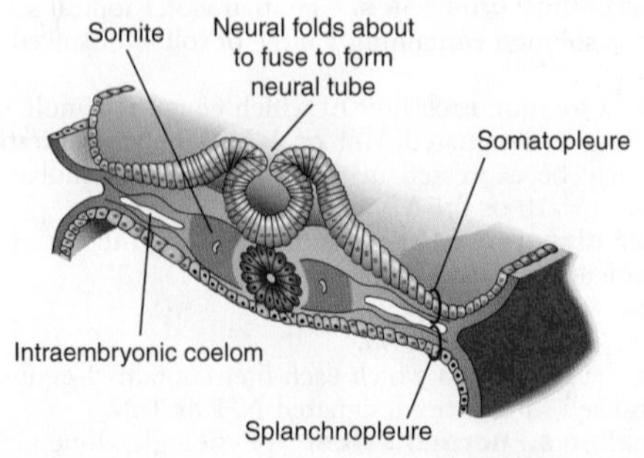

■ Somatopleure and splanchnopleure on transverse section through embryonic disc of a 21-day embryo.

so•ma•to•splanch•no•pleur•ic (so″mə-to-splank″no-ploor′ik) pertaining to the somatopleure and the splanchnopleure.

so•ma•to•stat•in (SS) (so″mə-to-stat′in) [*somato*tropin + *-statin*] any of several cyclic tetradecapeptides elaborated primarily by the median eminence of the hypothalamus and by the delta cells of the pancreatic islets; they inhibit release of growth hormone, thyrotropin, and corticotropin by the adenohypophysis, of insulin and glucagon by the pancreas, of gastrin by the gastric mucosa, of secretin by the intestinal mucosa, and of renin by the kidney. Called also *growth hormone release–inhibiting hormone* and *somatotropin release–inhibiting hormone.*

so•ma•to•stat•i•no•ma (som″ə-to-stat″ĭ-no′mə) a rare type of tumor that secretes somatostatin; most are islet cell tumors associated with diabetes mellitus or abnormal glucose tolerance, but some are found in the duodenum.

so•ma•to•ther•a•py (so″mə-to-ther′ə-pe) [*somato-* + *therapy*] biological treatment of mental disorders, such as by electric shock or drug therapy.

so•ma•to•to•nia (so″mə-to-to′ne-ə) [*somato-* + *ton-* + *-ia*] a temperament type characterized by love of physical adventure, boundless energy, boldness, aggressiveness, and need for exercise and activity; the behavioral counterpart of mesomorphy.

so•ma•to•top•ag•no•sia (so″mə-to-tōp″ag-no′zhə) [*somato-* + *top-* + *agnosia*] autotopagnosia.

so•ma•to•top•ic (so″mə-to-top′ik) related to particular areas of the body; describing the organization of the motor area of the brain, control of the movement of different parts of the body being centered in specific regions of the cortex.

so•mato•trope (so-mat′o-trōp) somatotroph.

so•mato•troph (so-mat′o-trōf) an acidophil of the adenohypophysis that stains preferentially with orange G and secretes growth hormone. Called also *somatotrope cell, somatotroph cell,* and *alpha acidophil.*

so•ma•to•tro•phic (so″mə-to-tro′fik) somatotropic.

so•ma•to•tro•phin (so′mə-to-tro″fin) growth hormone.

so•ma•to•tro•pic (so″mə-to-tro′pik) [*somato-* + *-tropic*] 1. having an affinity for or stimulating the body or the body cells; also having an influence on the body. 2. having a stimulating effect on body nutrition and growth. 3. having the properties of a growth hormone (somatotropin).

so•ma•to•tro•pin (so′mə-to-tro″pin) growth hormone.

so•ma•to•tro•pi•no•ma (so″mə-to-tro″pĭ-no′mə) growth hormone–secreting adenoma.

so•mato•type (so-mat′o-tīp) [*somato-* + *type*] a particular category of body build, determined on the basis of certain physical characteristics. See *ectomorph, endomorph,* and *mesomorph.*

so•mato•typ•ing (so-mat′o-tīp″ing) a method of studying objectively the physical types of individuals.

so•ma•trem (so′mə-trem) a biosynthetic pharmaceutical preparation of human growth hormone, prepared by recombinant technology, using *Escherichia coli,* and differing from the natural human hormone in containing an additional methionine residue at the terminus. It is used to treat growth failure and AIDS-associated cachexia or weight loss, administered intramuscularly or subcutaneously.

so•mat•ro•pin (so-mat′ro-pin) [USP] a pharmaceutical preparation of growth hormone, having the same amino acid sequence as the natural hormone. Originally derived from cadaver pituitary glands, the human form is now biosynthetic, prepared by recombinant means from *Escherichia coli.* It is used to treat growth failure and AIDS-associated cachexia or weight loss, administered intramuscularly or subcutaneously.

So•mat•u•line (so-mat′u-lēn) trademark for a preparation of lanreotide acetate.

Som•a•vert (som′ə-vərt) trademark for a preparation of pegvisomant.

-some [Gr. *soma* body] a word termination denoting a body.

so•mes•the•sia (so″mes-the′zhə) somatognosis. **somesthet′ic** *adj*

SOMI sternal-occipital-mandibular immobilizer.

-somia [Gr. *sōma* body + *-ia*] a word termination denoting a condition of the body.

so•mite (so′mīt) one of the paired, blocklike masses of mesoderm, arranged segmentally alongside the neural tube of the embryo, forming the vertebral column and segmental musculature; called also *mesoblastic, mesodermic, primitive, primordial,* or *protovertebral segment.*

som•nam•bu•lance (som-nam′bu-ləns) somnambulism.

som•nam•bu•la•tion (som-nam″bu-la′shən) somnambulism.

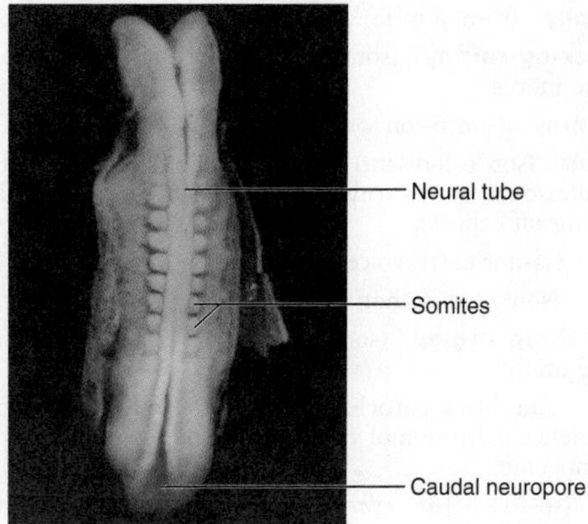

■ Somites in a 22-day embryo.

som•nam•bu•lism (som-nam′bu-liz-əm) [L. *somn-* + *ambulare* to walk] rising out of bed and walking about or performing other complex motor behavior during an apparent state of sleep, usually occurring in the first third of the night and lasting a few minutes to a half hour. The individual is relatively unresponsive, not alert, not easily awakened, and usually amnesic for the episode later. Called also *noctambulation, sleepwalking,* and *somnambulance.* See also *sleepwalking disorder,* under *disorder.*

som•nam•bu•list (som-nam′bu-list) an individual who walks while asleep.

somn(i)- [L. *somnus* sleep] a combining form denoting relationship to sleep.

som•ni•fa•cient (som″nĭ-fa′shənt) hypnotic (defs. 1 and 2).

som•nif•er•ous (som-nif′ər-əs) hypnotic (def. 1).

som•nif•ic (som-nif′ik) hypnotic (def. 1).

som•nil•o•quence (som-nil′o-kwəns) somniloquism.

som•nil•o•quism (som-nil′o-kwiz-əm) [*somni-* + L. *loqui* to speak] talking during sleep.

som•nil•o•quist (som-nil′o-kwist) an individual who talks while sleeping.

som•nil•o•quy (som-nil′o-kwe) somniloquism.

Som•ni•o•sus (som″ne-o′səs) a genus of sharks. *S. microce′phalus* is the Greenland shark, a species with a small head, weak jaws, and small teeth whose muscle tissue is poisonous, causing elasmobranch poisoning.

som•no•cin•e•ma•to•graph (som″no-sin″ə-mat′o-graf) [*somnus* + *cinematograph*] an apparatus for recording movements made during sleep.

som•no•lence (som′nə-ləns) [L. *somnolentia* sleepiness] drowsiness or sleepiness, particularly in excess. **som′nolent** *adj*

som•no•len•tia (som″nə-len′shə) [L.] 1. drowsiness, or somnolence. 2. sleep drunkenness.

som•nol•o•gy (som-nol′ə-je) the study of sleep.

So•mo•gyi phenomenon (effect), unit (so′mo-je) [Michael *Somogyi,* American biochemist, 1883–1971] see under *phenomenon* and *unit.*

son•ant (so′nənt) voiced.

so•nar•og•ra•phy (so″nər-og′rə-fe) ultrasonic scanning that provides a two-dimensional image corresponding to clear sections of acoustic interfaces in tissues.

So•na•ta (so-nah′tə) trademark for a preparation of zaleplon.

sonde (sond) [Fr.] sound (def. 4).

s. coudé (koo-da′) ["bent sound"] a catheter with an elbow, or sharp, beaklike bend, near the end.

sone (sōn) a unit of loudness, being the loudness of a simple tone of 1,000 cycles per second, 40 decibels above a listener's threshold.

son•i•cate (son′ĭ-kāt) 1. to expose to sound waves. 2. to disrupt bacteria by exposure to high-frequency sound waves. 3. the products of such disruption.

son•i•ca•tion (son″ĭ-ka′shən) exposure to sound waves; see *sonicate.*

Son•ne dysentery (son′ə) [Carl Olaf *Sonne,* Danish bacteriologist, 1882–1948] see under *dysentery.*

sono•gram (son′o-gram) a record or display obtained by ultrasonic scanning.

sono•graph•ic (son″o-graf′ik) ultrasonographic.

so·nog·ra·phy (sə-nog′rə-fe) ultrasonography.

sono·hys·ter·og·ra·phy (son″o-his″tər-og′rə-fe) sonographic examination of the uterus.

sono·lu·cen·cy (son″o-loo′sən-se) the property of being sonolucent.

sono·lu·cent (son″o-loo′sənt) in ultrasonography, permitting the passage of ultrasound waves without reflecting them back to their source (without giving off echoes).

so·nor·ant (sə-nor′ənt) voiced.

so·no·rous (son′ə-rəs, sə-nor′əs) [L. *sonorus*] resonant; sounding.

son·o·u·re·throg·ra·phy (son″o-u″rə-throg′rə-fe) sonographic examination of the urethra.

soot (soot) fine black particles, composed mainly of carbon, resulting from incomplete combustion of various fuels; long-term skin exposure to it can be carcinogenic.

So·pho·ra (so-fo′rə) [Ar. *sofara*] a genus of trees and shrubs of the family Leguminosae. The root and seed of *S. tomento′sa* are used in India to arrest choleraic vomiting. *S. secundiflo′ra* is the mescal bean, one of the North American plants called *locoweed.*

so·por (so′por) [L.] unnaturally deep or profound sleep. **so′porous** *adj*

so·po·rif·er·ous (so″por-if′ər-əs) [*sopor* + *-ferous*] inducing deep or profound slumber.

sop·o·rif·ic (sop″o-rif′ik, so″po-rif′ik) [*sopor* + L. *facere* to make] 1. causing or inducing profound sleep. 2. hypnotic (def. 2).

S. op. s. [L.] si o′pus sit (if it is necessary).

sor·af·e·nib (sor-af′ə-nib) an inhibitor of multiple kinases, prescribed in treatment of unresectable hepatocellular carcinoma and advanced renal cell carcinoma; administered orally.

sorb (sorb) to attract and retain substances by absorption or adsorption.

sor·be·fa·cient (sor″bə-fa′shənt) [*sorb* + *-facient*] absorbefacient.

sor·bent (sor′bənt) an agent that sorbs; see *absorbent* and *adsorbent.*

sor·bic ac·id (sor′bik) 2,4-hexadienoic acid, a compound found in berries of the mountain ash *Sorbus aucuparia* and in many other plants; it inhibits the growth of yeasts and molds and is used as an antimicrobial preservative.

sor·bi·tan (sor′bĭ-tən) a generic name for an anhydride of sorbitol, whose fatty acids are surfactants (*s. monolaurate* [NF], *s. monooleate* [NF], *s. monopalmitate* [NF], *s. monostearate* [NF], *s. sesquioleate* [NF], *s. trioleate* [NF], *s. tristearate*) used as emulsifiers in pharmaceutical preparations. See also *polysorbate.* Called also *sorbitol anhydride.*

sor·bi·tol (sor′bĭ-tol) 1. a six-carbon sugar alcohol formed by reduction of the carbonyl group of glucose and occurring naturally in a variety of fruits. It is a precursor of the fructose in seminal plasma and is also found in lens deposits in diabetes mellitus. 2. [NF] an official preparation used in pharmaceutical preparations as a sweetening agent, tablet excipient, humectant, and stabilizer, in foods as a bulk sweetening agent, and as an osmotic laxative. Called also *glucitol.*

sor·bi·tol de·hy·dro·gen·ase (sor′bĭ-tol de-hi′dro-jən-ās) L-iditol 2-dehydrogenase.

Sor·bi·trate (sor′bĭ-trāt) trademark for preparations of isosorbide dinitrate.

Sor·da·ri·a·ceae (sor″də-re-a′se-e) a family of fungi of the order Sordariales; it includes the genera *Neurospora* and *Chaetomium.*

Sor·da·ri·a·les (sor-da″re-a′lēz) an order of perfect fungi of the subphylum Ascomycotina, series Unitunicatae, characterized by inoperculate asci; most are saprobes. It includes the family Sordariaceae.

sor·des (sor′dēz) [L. "filth"] dirt; debris; especially the encrustations and accumulations of food, epithelial matter, and bacteria collected on the teeth and lips during a prolonged fever.

sore (sor) 1. a popular term for almost any lesion of the skin or mucous membranes. 2. painful.
  bay s. chiclero ulcer.
  bed s. decubitus ulcer.
  canker s. recurrent aphthous stomatitis.
  chrome s. chrome ulcer.
  cold s. herpes febrilis.
  desert s. a type of phagedenic ulcer seen in South Africa and Australia, with initial papulovesicular lesions on the limbs, which later rupture and form painful ulcers; it probably represents an infected ulcer from some previously neglected lesion.
  pressure s. decubitus ulcer.
  saddle s. see under *gall.*
  soft s. chancroid.
  summer s's cutaneous habronemiasis.
  veldt s. desert s.
  venereal s. any sore that accompanies or manifests a venereal disease.

sore·head (sor′hed) elaeophoriasis.

So·ret band, effect (phenomenon) (so-ra′) [Charles *Soret,* French physicist, 1854–1904] see under *band* and *effect.*

sore throat (sor thrōt) 1. pharyngitis. 2. faucitis.
  clergyman's s. t. hypertrophic pharyngitis after speaking at length, as in a clergyman or other public speaker. Called also *dysphonia clericorum.*
  epidemic streptococcal s. t. streptococcal pharyngitis.
  septic s. t. streptococcal pharyngitis.
  spotted s. t. follicular tonsillitis.
  streptococcal s. t. see under *pharyngitis.*
  ulcerated s. t. gangrenous pharyngitis.

Sor·ghum (sōr′gum) a genus of grasses (family Gramineae); several species are sources of the syrup called sorghum. Three species, *S. halepen′se* (Johnson grass), *S. sudanen′se* (Sudan grass), and *S. vulga′re* (also called *S. bi′color*), are commonly used as fodder for cattle and horses but contain cyanogenetic compounds and when eaten fresh can cause cyanide poisoning. Johnson grass and Sudan grass can cause hay fever.

so·ri (so′ri) plural of *sorus.*

So·ria·tane (so′re-ə-tān) trademark for a preparation of acitretin.

Sor·ine (sor′in) trademark for preparations of sotalol hydrochloride.

sorp·tion (sorp′shən) [L. *sorbere* to suck in] the process or state of being sorbed; absorption or adsorption.

Sors·by syndrome (sorz′be) [Arnold *Sorsby,* British ophthalmologist, 1900–1980] see under *syndrome.*

sort·er (sor′tər) a device for sorting.
  fluorescence-activated cell s. (FACS) an automated instrument that separates cell populations labeled with fluorescent antibodies or other fluorescent labels. The sample stream is broken up into droplets which are electrostatically charged and deflected into different collecting tubes depending on the measured fluorescence of the droplets.

so·rus (so′rəs) pl. *so′ri* [Gr. *sōros* heap] a mass, group, or cluster of spores, sporangia, or reproductive bodies occurring in certain plants, fungi, and protozoa.

S.O.S. [L.] si o′pus sit (if it is necessary).

So·ta·cor (so′tə-kor″) trademark for a preparation of sotalol hydrochloride.

so·ta·lol hy·dro·chlo·ride (so′tə-lol) a non-cardioselective beta-adrenergic blocking agent used in the treatment of life-threatening cardiac arrhythmias; administered orally.

So·to-Hall sign (so″to-hawl′) [Ralph *Soto-Hall,* American surgeon, 20th century] see under *sign.*

So·tos syndrome (so′tōs) [Juan Fernandez *Sotos,* American pediatrician, born 1927] cerebral gigantism; see under *gigantism.*

souf·fle (soo′fəl) [Fr. "a puff"; L. *sufflare* to blow] a soft, blowing, auscultatory sound; called also *bruit de soufflet.*
  cardiac s. any cardiac or vascular murmur of a blowing quality.
  funic s., funicular s. a hissing souffle synchronous with the fetal heart sounds, and supposed to be produced in the umbilical cord.
  mammary s. a functional cardiac murmur with a blowing sound, heard over the breasts in late pregnancy and during lactation; it may be either restricted to systole or continuous.
  placental s. a souffle supposed to be produced by the blood current in the placenta.
  splenic s. a sound said to be sometimes audible over a diseased spleen.
  umbilical s. funic s.
  uterine s. a sound made by the blood within the arteries of the gravid uterus.

sound (sound) [L. *sonus*] 1. a pressure wave that propagates through an elastic medium, which may be a gas, liquid, or solid; waves with a frequency between 20 and 20,000 Hz provide the stimulus for the subjective sensation of hearing. 2. the effect produced on the organ of hearing and its central connections by the vibrations of air or some other medium. 3. a noise, normal or abnormal, heard within the body; for other sounds see under *bruit, fremitus, murmur,* and *rale.* 4. an instrument to be introduced into a cavity to detect a foreign body or to dilate a stricture.
  adventitious s's abnormal auscultatory sounds heard over the lungs, such as rales, rhonchi, or any of the abnormal types of resonance; they are usually characterized as either *continuous s's* or *discontinuous s's.* Cf. *breath s's.*
  aortic ejection s. an ejection sound due to abnormality of structure or function of the aortic valve or aorta.
  aortic second s. (A_2) the audible vibrations related to the closure of the aortic valve. See also *second heart s.*
  atrial s. fourth heart s.

auscultatory s's sounds heard on auscultation, such as heart sounds, Korotkoff sounds, breath sounds, or adventitious sounds.
bandbox s. see under *resonance.*
bellows s. to-and-fro murmur.
bottle s. amphoric rale.
bowel s's relatively high-pitched abdominal sounds caused by propulsion of contents through the lower part of the colon.
breath s's auscultatory sounds heard in relation to the patient's breathing; they are usually listened for over a lung or a bronchus. Types include *bronchial, bronchovesicular, vesicular,* and *cavernous breath sounds.* Cf. *adventitious sounds.*
bronchial breath s's breath sounds with a high pitch like that of blowing through a tube. In healthy persons they are heard over the normal manubrium sterni on auscultation during respiration. When heard elsewhere they are pathologic and may indicate areas of adjacent consolidated or compressed lung. Called also *bronchial breathing* and *bronchial* or *tubular respiration.*
bronchovesicular breath s's breath sounds intermediate between bronchial and vesicular, with inhalation and exhalation being of similar duration and quality. They are heard normally near the anterior part of the first two intercostal spaces and on the back between the scapulae. When heard over the lung they usually indicate an area of partial consolidation. Called also *bronchovesicular respiration.*
cardiac s's heart s's.
cavernous breath s's abnormal breath sounds marked by a peculiar prolonged hollow resonance, usually due to an underlying cavity in the lung. Called also *cavernous respiration.*
continuous s's adventitious sounds that last longer than 0.2 sec; they include wheezes and rhonchi.
cracked-pot s. 1. see under *resonance.* 2. Macewen sign.
cranial, cracked-pot s. Macewen sign.
discontinuous s's adventitious sounds that last less than 0.2 sec and come in a series; the most common kind are rales (crackles).
ejection s's high-pitched clicking sounds occurring shortly after the first heart sound, at the time of maximal opening of the semilunar valves; seen in patients with abnormalities of these valves or dilatations of the aortic or pulmonary arteries. The sounds may be described as aortic or pulmonic and vascular or valvular. Called also *ejection clicks.*
entotic s's sounds that originate within the ear, such as tinnitus.
esophageal s. a long, flexible sound for exploring the esophagus.
first heart s. (S_1) the heart sound occurring during closure of the mitral and tricuspid valves; it is dull, firm, prolonged, and is heard as a "lubb" sound. It begins with an inaudible, low-frequency vibration (M) occurring at the onset of ventricular systole, followed by two intense, high-frequency vibratory bursts associated with mitral and tricuspid valve closure (M_1 and T_1, respectively), and ending with several variable low-intensity vibrations. Splitting of M_1 and T_1 is not usually discernible in normal adults.
flapping s. the peculiar sound made by the closure of the heart valves.
fourth heart s. (S_4) the heart sound associated with atrial contraction, occurring during the presystolic phase of diastole. It is rarely audible in normal hearts but when accentuated is usually called an *S_4 gallop.* See also *gallop rhythm,* under *rhythm.*
friction s. see under *rub.*
heart s's the sounds heard over the cardiac region in auscultation, which are produced by the functioning of the heart. The first and second are normally audible as the "lubb-dupp"sound, the third is normally audible only in youth, and the fourth is normally inaudible. See also individual sounds and see entries under *gallop* and *gallop rhythm,* under *rhythm.*
hippocratic s's succussion s's.
Korotkoff s's sounds heard during auscultatory determination of blood pressure, heard in an artery that was previously relaxed but becomes suddenly distended beyond the point where the pneumatic cuff is placed.
lacrimal s. a sound of small caliber for use in the lacrimal canal.
Le Fort s. a urethral sound with a screw tip for attachment of a filiform, used to pass through tight strictures.
metallic s. a sound having a metallic quality heard especially over cavities in the chest.
muscle s. the sound heard over a muscle when in a condition of contraction.
nonejection systolic s. midsystolic click.
percussion s. any sound obtained by percussion.
pericardial friction s. see under *rub.*
physiological s's sounds heard when the auditory canals are plugged, caused by the rush of blood through blood vessels in or near the internal ear and by adjacent muscles in continuous low frequency vibration.
pistol-shot s. Traube sign.
pulmonic ejection s. an ejection sound due to abnormality of structure or function of the pulmonary valve or artery.

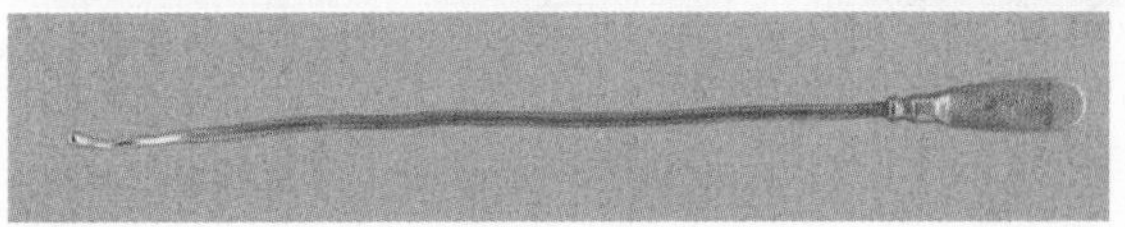

■ Uterine sound.

pulmonic second s. the audible vibrations related to the closure of the pulmonary valve; abbreviated P_2. See also *second heart s.*
respiratory s's breath s's.
second heart s. (S_2) the heart sound occurring during closure of the two semilunar valves at the beginning of diastole, and heard as a "dupp"sound. It consists of two sharp, high frequency vibrations representing closure of the aortic (A_2) then pulmonary (P_2) valves; the sounds are generally merged on expiration but split on inspiration in normal adults.
S_3 gallop s. see under *gallop.*
S_4 gallop s. see under *gallop.*
shaking s's succussion s's.
speech s. one of the minimal elements of a spoken language, such as a consonant or vowel. See also *phoneme.*
subjective s. phonism.
succussion s's splashing sounds heard over a distended stomach or in hydropneumothorax during succussion. Called also *hippocratic s's.*
systolic ejection s's ejection s's.
third heart s. (S_3) the heart sound associated with low frequency vibrations of the ventricular walls during rapid ventricular filling in early diastole. It is normally detected only in youthful patients unless accentuated due to cardiac disease; it is then usually called an *S_3 gallop.* See also *gallop rhythm,* under *rhythm.*
tick-tack s's heart sounds that have a pendulum rhythm.
to-and-fro s. see under *murmur.*
urethral s. a long, thin, slightly conical steel sound for exploring and dilating the urethra.
uterine s. a long, flexible sound for exploring the uterus.
valvular ejection s. an ejection sound resulting from abnormality of one or both semilunar valves. Cf. *vascular ejection s.*
vascular ejection s. an ejection sound resulting from abnormality of the pulmonary artery or aorta without abnormality of either semilunar valve. Cf. *valvular ejection s.*
vesicular breath s's low-pitched sounds heard on auscultation over the normal lung during ventilation. Called also *vesicular resonance.*
voice s's auscultatory sounds heard over the lungs or airways when the patient speaks; increased resonance indicates consolidation or an airless lung underlying an effusion. Types include *bronchophony, egophony, laryngophony, pectoriloquy, tracheophony,* and *cavernous voice.*
water-wheel s. bruit de moulin.
white s. a mixture of all frequencies of mechanical vibration perceptible as sound.
Winternitz s. a type of double-lumen catheter.
xiphisternal crunching s. a peculiar sound, of unknown origin, frequently heard (20 per cent of healthy men) over the lower sternum and xiphoid process.

sour·cil (soor-sēl′) [Fr. "eyebrow"] a curvilinear area of increased bone density in the roof of the acetabulum, caused by the pressure of the femoral head in weight bearing.

South·ern blot (blot analysis, blot hybridization) (suth′ərn) [E.M. *Southern,* British biologist, born 1938] see under *blot.*

sow·dah (sou′dah) [Ar. "black"] a type of onchodermatitis seen in Yemen and Saudi Arabia, usually on one or both lower limbs, characterized by black pigmentation, thickening, and roughness of the skin, edema, intense pruritus, papules, and regional lymphadenopathy. Similar cases have been reported in the Sudan and West Africa.

Soxh·let apparatus (soks′let) [Franz Ritter von *Soxhlet,* German chemist, 1848–1926] see under *apparatus.*

soy (soi) soybean.

soya (soi′yə) soybean.

soy·bean (soi′bēn) the bean of the leguminous plant, *Glycine max.* It contains little starch, is rich in protein, and also contains high levels of phytoestrogens.

sp. [L.] spir′itus (spirit).

SP-40,40 clusterin.

SPA sperm penetration assay.

space (spās) 1. a delimited area. 2. an actual or potential cavity of the body; called also *spatium* [TA]. 3. the expanse of the universe beyond the earth and its atmosphere.

Space

For descriptions of specific anatomic structures not listed here, see under *spatium.*

alveolar dead s. the difference between physiologic dead space and anatomic dead space, representing the space in alveoli occupied by air that does not participate in oxygen–carbon dioxide exchange (see *alveolar ventilation,* under *ventilation*). It varies in different parts of the lungs and under different conditions.
anatomic dead s. the portions of the airway, from the nose and mouth to the terminal bronchioles, in which exchange of oxygen and carbon dioxide does not occur. Cf. *physiologic dead s.*
anterior paranephric s., anterior pararenal s. a compartment of the retroperitoneal space bounded posteriorly by the renal fascia and anteriorly by the posterior parietal peritoneum, containing the retroperitoneal portions of the colon, duodenum, and pancreas.
apical s. the region between the wall of the alveolus and the apex of the root of a tooth.
axillary s. axilla.
Bogros s. spatium retroinguinale.
Bowman s. urinary s.
bregmatic s. fonticulus anterior.
buccal s. a tissue space lateral to the buccopharyngeal fascia, between the buccinator and masseter muscles; it contains the buccal fat pad, Stensen duct, and the facial artery.
Burns s. spatium suprasternale.
capsular s. urinary s.
carotid s., carotid bundle s. the potential space within the carotid sheath, extending from the base of the skull to the superior mediastinum.
cartilage s's the spaces in hyaline cartilage which contain the cartilage cells.
cavernous s's of corpora cavernosa of penis cavernae corporum cavernosorum penis.
cavernous s's of corpus spongiosum of penis cavernae corporis spongiosi penis.
cell s's the spaces in the ground substance of connective tissue enclosing the connective tissue corpuscles.
circumlental s. see *spatia zonularia,* under *spatium.*
Colles s. a space under the perineal fascia containing the transversus perinei, ischiocavernosus, and bulbocavernosus muscles, the posterior scrotal or labial vessels and nerves, and the bulbous portion of the urethra.
complemental s. portions of the pleural cavity that are not occupied by lung tissue, such as the triangular spaces below the lower borders of the lungs and irregular spaces about the heart.
corneal s's the spaces between the lamellae of the substantia propria of the cornea which contain corneal cells and tissue fluid; called also *interlamellar s's.*
cupular s. pars cupularis recessus epitympanici.
Czermak s's spatia interglobularia; see under *spatium.*
danger s. a subdivision of the spatium retropharyngeum, lying in the midline between the alar fascia and the prevertebral fascia and extending from the base of the skull to the level of the diaphragm; so called because it provides a route by which infection of the pharynx can spread to the mediastinum. Called also *prevertebral s.*
dead s. 1. space remaining after closure of surgical or other wounds, permitting the accumulation of blood or serum and resultant delay in healing. 2. see *anatomic dead s.* and *physiologic dead s.*
Disse s's, s's of Disse perisinusoidal s's.
Douglas s. excavatio rectouterina.
epicerebral s. the potential space between the brain and the pia mater.
epidural s. 1. spatium epidurale. 2. an artifactual space created between the dura mater and the inner table of the skull as a result of trauma or a pathologic process.
episcleral s. spatium episclerale.
epispinal s. the potential space between the substance of the spinal cord and the pia mater.
epitympanic s. recessus epitympanicus.
escapement s's spaces which permit the escape of material being comminuted between the occlusal surfaces of the teeth, provided by the cusps and ridges, sulci and developmental ridges of the teeth, and the embrasures between the teeth.
extradural s. spatium epidurale.
extraperitoneal s. spatium extraperitoneale.
s's of Fontana spatia anguli iridocornealis; see under *spatium.*
freeway s. interocclusal distance.
globular s's of Czermak spatia interglobularia.
H. s. Holzknecht s.
haversian s. canalis nutricius.
Henke s. a space containing connective tissue between the vertebral column and the pharynx and esophagus.
His perivascular s's perivascular s's.
Holzknecht s. the middle one of the three clear lung fields in the radiograph of the chest in oblique projection when the rays pass from the left posteriorly to the right anteriorly; called also *H. s., prevertebral s.,* and *retrocardiac s.*
iliocostal s. the area between the twelfth rib and the crest of the ilium.
infrahyoid s's the potential spaces in the neck just inferior to the hyoid bone, including the anterior visceral and retropharyngeal spaces.
interarytenoid s. pars intercartilaginea rimae glottidis.
intercostal s. spatium intercostale.
intercristal s. the space within the inner membrane of a mitochondrion, occupied by the mitochondrial matrix. Called also *matrix space.*
interdental s. interproximal s.
interfascial s. spatium episclerale.
interglobular s's spatia interglobularia.
interlamellar s's corneal s's.
intermembrane s., intermembranous s. a narrow space between the inner and outer membranes of a mitochondrion, including its inward projections between the cristae.
interocclusal s. see under *distance.*
interosseous s's of metacarpus spatia interossea metacarpi.
interosseous s's of metatarsus spatia interossea metatarsi.
interpeduncular s. fossa interpeduncularis.
interpleural s. mediastinum (def. 2).
interproximal s., interproximate s. the space between the proximal surfaces of adjoining teeth; sometimes used to designate especially the space between the proximal surfaces of adjoining teeth that is gingival to the area of contact *(septal s.).* Cf. *embrasure.*
interradicular s. 1. the space between roots. 2. in dentistry, the entire extent of the space between the roots of a tooth, from apex to base.
interseptal s. a space between the two folds guarding the opening of the sinus venosus; the space disappears as the folds unite to form the spurious septum in the heart of the early embryo.
intervaginal s. spatium episclerale.
intervaginal s's of optic nerve spatia intervaginalia nervi optici.
intervillous s. the space of the placenta into which the chorionic villi project and through which maternal blood circulates.
s's of iridocorneal angle spatia anguli iridocornealis.
Kiernan s's the triangular spaces bounded by the invaginated Glisson capsule between the liver lobules, containing the larger interlobular branches of the portal vein, hepatic artery, and hepatic duct.
Kiesselbach s. see under *area.*
Kretschmann s. a depressed area in the recessus epitympanicus, below Prussak space.
Larrey s's intervals between those parts of the diaphragm which are attached to the ribs and that which is attached to the sternum.
leeway s. see *Nance leeway s.*

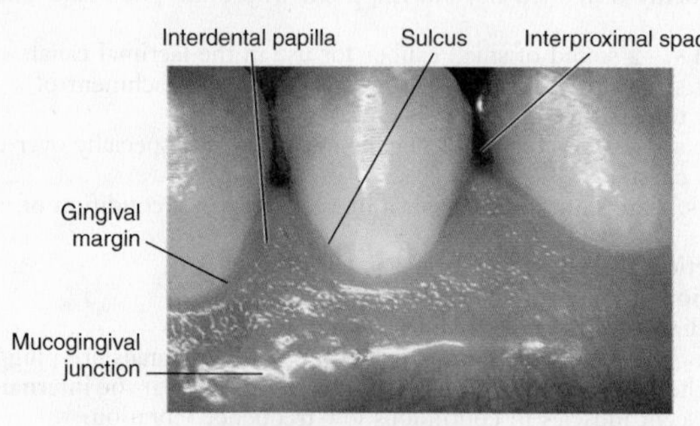

■ Interproximal space.

Space *Continued*

Lesshaft s. see under *triangle.*
lymph s. any space in tissue occupied by lymph.
Magendie s's subarachnoid spaces between the pia and arachnoid, corresponding to the principal sulci of the brain.
mandibular s. a tissue space formed by splitting of the superficial layer of the cervical fascia at the inferior border of the mandible, containing the anterior part of the ramus of the mandible and adjacent structures.
marrow s. cavitas medullaris.
masticator s. a potential space of the neck anterior and lateral to the pharyngomaxillary space, formed by splitting of the superficial layer of the deep cervical fascia and containing the muscles of mastication, the ramus and posterior part of the mandible, branches of the mandibular nerve, and the maxillary artery and its branches.
matrix s. intercristal s.
Meckel s. cavum trigeminale.
mediastinal s. mediastinum (def. 2).
medullary s. cavitas medullaris.
midpalmar s. the palmar space lying between the middle metacarpal bone and the radial side of the hypothenar eminence.
Mohrenheim s. a groove on the deltoid muscle for the cephalic vein and a branch of the acromiothoracic artery.
Nance leeway s. the amount by which the space occupied by the deciduous canine and first and second deciduous molars exceeds that occupied by the canine and premolar teeth of the permanent dentition, usually averaging 1.7 mm on each side of the dental arch.
Nuel s's fluid-filled spaces in the organ of Corti, between the outer pillar cells and outer hair cells.
palmar s. a large fascial space in the hand, divided by a fibrous septum into the midpalmar space and the thenar space.
paraglottic s. a laryngeal space bounded inferiorly by the conus elasticus, medially by the quadrangular membrane, posteriorly by the mucosa of the piriform fossa, and anterolaterally by the thyroid cartilage.
parapharyngeal s. pharyngomaxillary s.
parasinoidal s's lacunae laterales.
paravertebral s. prevertebral s. (def. 1).
paravesical s's a pair of subdivisions of the extraperitoneal space found lateral to the prevesical space.
Parona s. a space between the pronator quadratus muscle and the deep flexor tendons in the forearm, about 5 cm above the wrist, in direct continuity with the tendon sheaths and the midpalmar space.
parotid s. a potential space within the parotid fascia, containing the parotid gland.
perforated s., anterior substantia perforata rostralis.
perforated s., posterior substantia perforata posterior.
periaxial s. a fluid-filled cavity surrounding the nuclear bag and myotubule regions of a muscle spindle.
perichoroidal s. spatium perichoroideum.
perilymphatic s. spatium perilymphaticum.
perineal s., deep saccus profundus perinei.
perineal s., superficial compartimentum superficiale perinei.
perinephric s. perirenal s.
perineuronal s. the extracellular compartment surrounding nerve cells of the central nervous system; its histologic appearance as a space is an artifact.
perinuclear s. a space, approximately 30 nm wide and continuous with the lumen of the endoplasmic reticulum, separating the inner and outer membranes of the nuclear envelope. Called also *perinuclear cistern* or *cisterna.*
peripharyngeal s. spatium peripharyngeum.
periplasmic s. a zone between the plasma membrane and the outer membrane of the cell wall of gram-negative bacteria.
perirenal s. the compartment of the retroperitoneal space that lies within the renal fascia and contains the kidney, perirenal fat, adrenal gland, and proximal ureter. Called also *perinephric s.*
perisinusoidal s's small spaces that separate the sinusoids of the liver from the cells of its parenchyma and that store the lymph of the liver. Called also *Disse s's.*
peritonsillar s. a potential space of the neck bounded by the palatine tonsil, the superior constrictor muscle of the pharynx, and the anterior and posterior faucial arches.
perivascular s's spaces, often only potential, that surround blood vessels for a short distance as they enter the brain; their inner wall is formed by a prolongation of a membrane like the arachnoid, and the outer wall by a continuation of the pia; the intervening channel communicates with the subarachnoid space. Called also *His perivascular s's* and *Virchow-Robin s's.*
perivesical s's subdivisions of the extraperitoneal space found anterior to the urinary bladder.
perivesical s., anterior spatium retropubicum.
perivitelline s. in mammals, a fluid-filled space between the plasma membrane of the oocyte and the zona pellucida; in many other animals, one separating the plasma membrane of the egg from the fertilization membrane (e.g., amphibians) or chorion (e.g., fish).
pharyngeal s., lateral spatium lateropharyngeum.
pharyngeal mucosal s. a potential space of the neck on the airway side of the buccopharyngeal fascia, extending from the base of the skull to the level of the cricoid cartilage and containing muscles, the torus tubarius, salivary glands, and mucosal and lymphoid tissue.
pharyngomaxillary s. a potential space of the neck bounded by the buccopharyngeal fascia, the internal pterygoid muscle, and the prevertebral fascia, forming a cone with its base at the sphenoid bone and its apex at the hyoid bone; it is divided by the styloid process into anterior and posterior compartments, the latter containing the carotid sheath and cranial nerves IX–XII. Called also *parapharyngeal s.* and *lateral pharyngeal s.*
phrenocostal s. the space between the outer edge of the diaphragm and the costal surface.
physiologic dead s. the anatomic dead space plus the alveolar dead space; it reflects nonuniformity of ventilation and perfusion in different parts of the lung.
pleural s. cavitas pleuralis.
pneumatic s. a portion of bone occupied by air-containing cells; applied especially to spaces in the bones of the head constituting the paranasal sinuses.
Poiseuille s. the part of the lumen of a tube where no flow of liquid occurs, as next to the wall of a blood vessel, where the red cells are virtually motionless and constitute a layer over which the inner layers of liquid slide.
popliteal s. fossa poplitea.
posterior paranephric s., posterior pararenal s. a compartment of the retroperitoneal space lying between the posterior renal fascia and the transversalis fascia, containing mainly adipose tissue.
preepiglottic s. a fat-filled laryngeal space bounded superiorly by the vallecula and hyoepiglottic ligament, posteriorly by the epiglottis and quadrangular membrane, and anteriorly by the thyrohyoid membrane and thyroid cartilage.
preperitoneal s. spatium retropubicum.
preputial s. the space between the prepuce and the glans penis.
presacral s. a subdivision of the extraperitoneal space found between the urinary bladder and the sacrum. Called also *retrorectal s.*
pretracheal s. anterior visceral s.
prevertebral s. 1. a potential space between the prevertebral fascia and the bodies of the vertebrae, attached to the transverse process of the vertebrae, and extending from the base of the skull to the coccyx; it contains muscles, nerves, the vertebral artery and vein, and the vertebral bodies. Called also *paravertebral s.* 2. danger s. 3. Holzknecht s.
prevesical s. spatium retropubicum.
prezonular s. portion of the eyeball anterior to the zonula ciliaris, occupied by the aqueous humor.
proximal s., proximate s. interproximal s.
Prussak s. recessus superior membranae tympanicae.
quadrangular s., quadrilateral s. a potential space in the shoulder region, bounded by the long head of the triceps brachii muscle, the teres minor muscle, the surgical neck of the humerus, and the teres major muscle; the axillary nerve, posterior circumflex humeral artery, and adjacent veins pass through it.
Reinke s. a potential space between the vocal ligament and the overlying mucosa; inflammation results in Reinke edema.
relief s. a space between the slightly elevated lingual bar type of the major connector and the underlying soft tissue; it allows for a minor degree of settling of a removable partial denture without impinging on the structure over which the bar passes.
respiratory dead s. the part of either the anatomic or the physiologic dead space that represents a volume of air that does not take part in alveolar ventilation.
retrobulbar s. the space lying behind the fascia of the bulb of the eye, containing the eye muscles and the ocular vessels and nerves.

Space *Continued*

retrocalcaneal s. the space between the posterior calcaneus and the calcaneal tendon, occupied by the calcaneal bursa.
retrocardiac s. Holzknecht s.
retroesophageal s. spatium retropharyngeum.
retroinguinal s. spatium retroinguinale.
retromylohyoid s. the part of the alveololingual sulcus just lingual to the retromolar pad, and posterior to the lingual tuberosity.
retro-ocular s. retrobulbar s.
retroperitoneal s. spatium retroperitoneale.
retropharyngeal s. 1. spatium retropharyngeum. 2. retrovisceral s.
retropubic s. spatium retropubicum.
retrorectal s. presacral s.
retrovisceral s. a subdivision of the spatium retropharyngeum lying between the pretracheal and prevertebral layers of the deep cervical fascia. Called also *retropharyngeal s.*
Retzius s. 1. spatium perilymphaticum. 2. spatium retropubicum.
Schwalbe s's spatia intervaginalia nervi optici.
semilunar s. Traube s.
septal s. that portion of the interproximal space gingival to the contact area of adjacent teeth in a dental arch.
subarachnoid s. spatium subarachnoideum.
subcapsular s. the potential space between the renal parenchyma and the renal capsules.
subdural s. spatium subdurale.
subepicranial s. the potential space between the epicranius muscle and the pericranium; it is traversed by small arteries which supply the pericranium and by the emissary veins connecting the intracranial venous sinuses with the superficial veins of the scalp.
subgingival s. gingival crevice.
subhepatic s. recessus subhepaticus.
sublingual s. the superior part of the submandibular space, containing the sublingual gland and loose connective tissue surrounding the tongue.
submandibular s. a potential space of the neck bounded by the oral mucosa and tongue anteriorly and medially; the superficial layer of the deep cervical fascia laterally, and the hyoid bone inferiorly; it comprises two spaces, the sublingual and submaxillary spaces, divided by the mylohyoid muscle.
submaxillary s. the inferior part of the submandibular space; see *trigonum submandibulare.*
submental s. the medial part of the submaxillary space; see *trigonum submentale.*
subphrenic s. recessus subphrenicus.
subumbilical s. the somewhat triangular space within the body cavity just inferior to the umbilicus.
suprahyoid s's the potential spaces of the neck and pharyngeal region superior to the hyoid bone, including the pharyngomaxillary and submandibular spaces.
suprasternal s. spatium suprasternale.
Tarin s. anterior recess of interpeduncular fossa.
Tenon s. spatium episclerale.
thenar s. the palmar space lying between the middle metacarpal bone and the tendon of the flexor pollicis longus.
thiocyanate s. a quantitative expression of the space occupied by the extracellular fluid in the body, computed after intravenous injection of sodium thiocyanate.
thyrohyal s. the depressed space between the thyroid cartilage and hyoid bone in front.
Traube s. an area on the left anterior inferior part of the thorax, over which the air in the stomach produces a vesiculotympanitic sound.
Tröltsch s's see *recessus membranae tympani anterior* and *recessus membranae tympani posterior.*
urinary s. a narrow chalice-shaped cavity in the renal glomerulus between the visceral layer and the parietal layer of the glomerular capsule, continuous with the lumen of the proximal convoluted tubule. Called also *Bowman* or *capsular s.*
Virchow-Robin s's perivascular s's.
visceral s. a potential space between the pretracheal fascia and the prevertebral fascia, extending from the hyoid bone to the mediastinum and containing the lower pharynx, larynx, trachea, esophagus, thyroid, great vessels, and areolar tissue. It is subdivided into the *anterior visceral, posterior visceral (retrovisceral),* and *visceral vascular or carotid spaces.*
visceral s., anterior a potential space in the neck surrounded by the pretracheal layer of the deep cervical fascia; it contains the thyroid gland, the esophagus, and the trachea. Called also *pretracheal s.*
visceral s., posterior spatium retropharyngeum.
visceral vascular s. carotid s.
Westberg s. the space between the pericardium and the beginning of the aorta.
yolk s. the space formed by retraction of the yolk from the zona pellucida.
zonular s's spatia zonularia.

spac·er (spās′ər) 1. something that separates or keeps other things apart; see *spacer DNA,* under *DNA.* 2. on a metered dose inhaler, a chamber between the inhaler canister and the patient's mouth where droplets of medication can slow down and evaporate so that there is less direct impact on the oropharynx.

spac·ing (spās′ing) the creation or arranging of spaces.
third s. the shift of fluid from the intravascular compartment into other compartments, as by extravasation into the interstitial space or accumulation in the intestinal lumen, where it is not available to support circulation.

Spal·ding sign (spawl′ding) [Alfred Baker *Spalding,* American obstetrician and gynecologist, 1874–1942] see under *sign.*

Spal·lan·za·ni's law (spahl″ahn-tsah′nēz) [Lazaro *Spallanzani,* Italian anatomist, 1729–1799] see under *law.*

spal·la·tion (spaw-la′shən) splintering; the process of breaking into small bits; see *spallation products,* under *product.*

span (span) 1. a measurement of reach or extent. 2. the distance in a fully extended hand between the tips of the thumb and little finger. 3. the distance between the tips of the fingers with the upper limbs extended.

Span·i·op·sis (span″e-op′sis) a genus of blood-sucking flies of the family Rhagionidae found in Australia.

spar (spahr) a nonmetallic, rather lustrous mineral.
Iceland s. a crystalline form of calcium carbonate, usually found in Iceland, and used in making Nicol prisms.

spar·flox·a·cin (spahr-flok′sə-sin) a synthetic, broad-spectrum fluoroquinolone antimicrobial agent administered orally.

spar·ga·no·sis (spahr″gə-no′sis) infection with migrating spargana (tapeworm larvae of the genera *Diphyllobothrium* and *Spirometra*), which invade the subcutaneous tissues, causing inflammation and fibrosis that resembles cellulitis.

spar·ga·num (spahr′gə-nəm) pl. *spar′gana* [Gr. *sparganon* swaddling clothes] the larval stage (plerocercoid) of certain cestodes, especially of the genera *Diphyllobothrium* and *Spirometra,* which may migrate in the subcutaneous tissues of animals and cause sparganosis.

spar·te·ine (spahr′tēn) [L. *spartium* broom] a poisonous alkaloid obtained from the legumes *Cytisus scoparius* (broom), *Lupinus luteus* (yellow lupin bean), *L. niger* (black lupin bean), and *Anagyris foetida* (Mediterranean stinkbush). See *lupinosis* and *broom poisoning.*

spar·ti·um (spahr′she-əm) [Gr. *spartos* broom plant] scoparius.

spasm (spaz′əm) [L. *spasmus;* Gr. *spasmos*] 1. a sudden, violent, involuntary contraction of a muscle or a group of muscles, attended by pain and interference with function, producing involuntary movement and distortion. 2. a sudden but transitory constriction of a passage, canal, or orifice.
s. of accommodation spasm of the ciliary muscles, producing excess of accommodation for near objects.
athetoid s. a spasm in which the affected member makes movements like those of athetosis.
Bell s. facial s.
bronchial s. bronchospasm.
cadaveric s. rigor mortis causing movements of the limbs.
carpopedal s. spasm of the hand or foot, or of the thumbs or great toes, seen in tetany.
clonic s. a spasm consisting of clonic contractions; see also *clonus.*
dancing s. saltatory s.
diffuse esophageal s. strong, uncoordinated, nonpropulsive contractions of the esophagus evoked by swallowing, with chest pain, seen especially in the elderly. Sometimes the esophageal lumen appears coiled on the

radiograph (*corkscrew* or *curling esophagus*). Called also *esophageal s.* or *dysrhythmia, esophagism, esophagospasm,* and *neurogenic* or *spastic dysphagia.*

esophageal s. diffuse esophageal s.

facial s. tonic spasm of the muscles supplied by the facial nerve, either involving the entire side of the face or confined to a limited region around the eye. Called also *Bell s.* and *convulsive* or *facial tic.*

fixed s. permanent rigidity of a muscle or set of muscles.

glottal s., glottic s. laryngospasm.

habit s. see under *tic.*

hemifacial s. facial spasm confined to one side.

histrionic s. facial s.

infantile s's, infantile massive s's a syndrome of severe myoclonus appearing in the first 18 months of life and associated with general cerebral deterioration; it is marked by severe flexion spasms of the head, neck, and trunk and extension of the limbs. Called also *jackknife seizures* or *spasms; salaam convulsions, seizures,* or *spasms;* and *West syndrome.*

inspiratory s. spasmodic contraction of the muscles of inhalation.

intention s. muscular spasm occurring on attempting voluntary movement.

jackknife s's infantile s's.

laryngeal s. laryngospasm.

levator s. levator ani syndrome.

lock s. a firm tonic spasm that seems to lock the fingers together, as in writers' cramp and in similar affections.

massive s. a spasm characterized by contraction of most of the body musculature. Cf. *seizure* and *infantile massive s.*

mixed s. a spasm in which there are both extensor and flexor movements.

mobile s. athetosis.

myopathic s. a spasm that accompanies a disease of the muscles.

nictitating s. winking s.

nodding s. spasmus nutans.

phonatory s. spasm of the tensors of the vocal cords, which interferes with speech. See also *dysphonia spastica.*

progressive torsion s. dystonia musculorum deformans.

respiratory s. spasm of the muscles of respiration.

retrocollic s's retrocollis.

Romberg s. trismus.

rotatory s. intermittent spasm of the splenius muscle causing rotation of the head; cf. *retrocollis* and *torticollis.*

salaam s's infantile s's.

saltatory s. clonic spasm of the muscles of the lower limbs, producing a peculiar jumping or springing motion, seen in conditions such as Gilles de la Tourette syndrome, saltatory chorea, and the jumping diseases. Called also *Bamberger disease, dancing spasm,* and *saltatory tic.*

sphincter s. spasm of a sphincter muscle, particularly an anal sphincter.

tetanic s., tonic s. tetanus (def. 2).

tonoclonic s. a convulsive twitching of the muscles.

torsion s. spasm marked by a twisting or turning of the body, especially of the pelvis, as in dystonia musculorum deformans.

toxic s. a spasm that is due to a poison.

winking s. spasmodic twitching of the orbicularis palpebrarum muscle and of the eyelid.

writers' s. writers' cramp.

spasm(o)- [Gr. *spasmos* spasm] a combining form denoting relationship to a spasm.

spas·mod·ic (spaz-mod′ik) [Gr. *spasmōdēs*] of the nature of a spasm.

spas·mo·gen (spaz′mo-jən) [*spasmo-* + *-gen*] a substance that produces or causes spasms.

spas·mo·gen·ic (spaz″mo-jen′ik) relating to the production of or causing spasms.

spas·mol·y·sis (spaz-mol′ĭ-sis) the elimination or checking of spasm.

spas·mol·y·sin (spaz-mol′ĭ-sin) trefoil factor 2.

spas·mo·lyt·ic (spaz″mo-lit′ik) antispasmodic.

spas·mo·phil·ic (spaz″mo-fil′ik) marked by a tendency to spasms.

spas·mus (spaz′məs) [L.] spasm.

s. nu′tans nodding of the head accompanied by nystagmus, seen in infants and young children; called also *nodding spasm.*

spas·tic (spas′tik) [Gr. *spastikos*] 1. of the nature of or characterized by spasms. 2. hypertonic, so that the muscles are stiff and the movements awkward; see *cerebral palsy,* under *palsy,* and *spastic paraplegia,* under *paraplegia.*

spas·tic·i·ty (spas-tis′ĭ-te) the state of being spastic; see *spastic* (def. 2).

clasp-knife s. see under *rigidity.*

inherited periodic s. an autosomal recessive muscle disorder seen in adult cattle; upon arising, for a few seconds to 30 minutes the animal is unable to flex the hindlimbs or walk and may have limb tremors. Called also *stretches.*

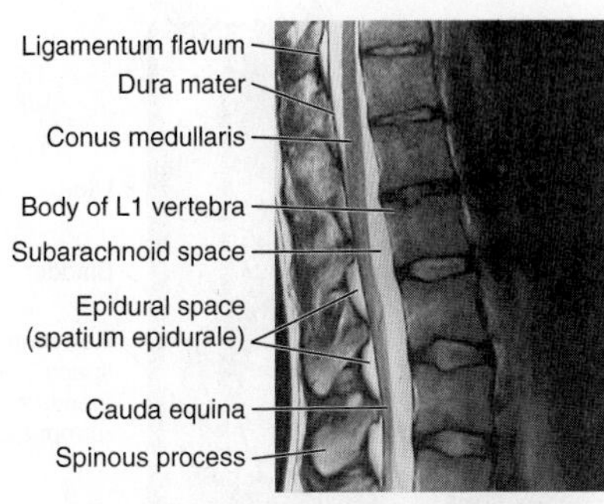

■ Lumbar spine showing spinous processes and epidural spaces (spatia epiduralia).

spa·tia (spa′she-ə) [L.] plural of *spatium.*

spa·tial (spa′shəl) pertaining to space.

spa·ti·um (spa′she-əm) pl. *spa′tia* [L.] space: an actual or potential delimited area or open region.

spa′tia an′guli i′ridis, spa′tia an′guli iridocornea′lis [TA] spaces of iridocorneal angle: the spaces between the fibers of the pectinate ligament through which communication is effected between the anterior chamber and the canal of Schlemm. Called also *spaces of Fontana.*

s. epidura′le [TA] epidural space: the space between the dura mater and the walls of the vertebral canal, containing venous plexuses and fibrous and alveolar tissue. Called also *epidural cavity, s. extradurale* [TA alternative], *extradural space,* and *s. peridurale* [TA alternative].

s. episclera′le [TA] episcleral space: the space between the bulbar fascia and the eyeball; called also *s. intervaginale* and *intervaginal* or *Tenon space.*

s. extradura′le TA alternative for *s. epidurale.*

s. extraperitonea′le [TA] extraperitoneal space: the space between the parietal peritoneum and the transversalis fascia, containing the extraperitoneal fascia around various organs; it is subdivided into the spatium retroperitoneale, the spatium retropubicum, and the spatium retroinguinale.

s. intercosta′le [TA] intercostal space: the space intervening between two adjacent ribs.

s. interfascia′le s. episclerale.

spa′tia interglobula′ria interglobular spaces: numerous small irregular spaces on the outer surface of the dentin in the root of a tooth. Called also *Czermak spaces* and *globular spaces of Czermak.*

spa′tia interos′sea metacar′pi [TA] interosseous spaces of metacarpus: the four spaces between the metacarpal bones.

spa′tia interos′sea metatar′si [TA] interosseous spaces of metatarsus: the four spaces between the metatarsal bones.

s. intervagina′le s. episclerale.

spa′tia intervagina′lia ner′vi op′tici intervaginal spaces of optic nerve: the subdural or subarachnoid spaces between the internal and external sheaths of the optic nerve; called also *Schwalbe space.*

s. lateropharyn′geum [TA] lateral pharyngeal space: the part of the spatium peripharyngeum that is lateral to the pharynx.

s. leptomenin′geum TA alternative for *s. subarachnoideum.*

s. perichoroidea′le, s. perichoroi′deum [TA] perichoroidal space: any of the spaces between the laminae of the nonvascular layer of the choroid nearest the sclera.

s. peridura′le TA alternative for *s. epidurale.*

s. perilympha′ticum [TA] perilymphatic space: the fluid-filled space separating the membranous from the osseous labyrinth; called also *Retzius space.*

s. peripharyn′geum [TA] peripharyngeal space: the space around the pharynx, which is filled with areolar tissue; it is subdivided into the *s. lateropharyngeum* and the *s. retropharyngeum.*

s. profun′dum perine′i TA alternative for *saccus profundus perinei.*

s. retroinguina′le [TA] retroinguinal space: the subdivision of the extraperitoneal space bounded by the peritoneum above and the fascia transversalis below. Called also *Bogros space.*

s. retroperitonea′le [TA] retroperitoneal space: the subdivision of the extraperitoneal space between the posterior parietal peritoneum and the posterior abdominal wall, containing the kidneys, suprarenal glands, ureters, duodenum, ascending and descending colon, pancreas, and the large vessels and nerves. Called also *retroperitoneum.*

s. retropharyn′geum [TA] retropharyngeal space: the part of the spatium peripharyngeum that lies just behind the prevertebral layer of the deep cervical fascia, extending from the base of the skull to the level of the second thoracic vertebra. It is subdivided into the *retrovisceral space* (also called the *retropharyngeal space*) and the *prevertebral* or *danger space.* Called also *retroesophageal space* and *posterior visceral s.*

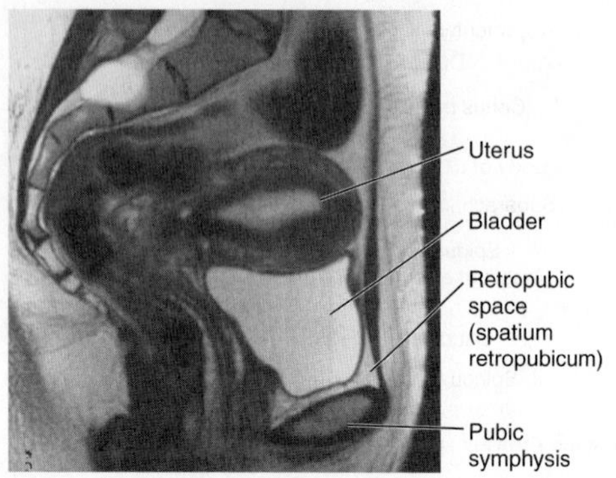

■ Sagittal MRI during menstruation, showing the spatium retropubicum (retropubic space).

s. retropu′bicum [TA] retropubic space: the part of the extraperitoneal space between the inferior aspect of the apex of the bladder, the fascia transversalis, and the posterosuperior aspect of the pubic symphysis, extending along the sides of the bladder to the lateral ligaments and limited inferiorly by the puboprostatic ligaments. Called also *prevesical* or *Retzius space.*

s. subarachnoi′deum [TA] subarachnoid space: the space between the arachnoidea mater and the pia mater, containing cerebrospinal fluid and bridged by delicate trabeculae; called also *s. leptomeningeum* [TA alternative].

s. subdura′le [TA] subdural space: an artifactual space between the dura mater and the arachnoid, formerly believed to be a narrow fluid-containing space; in the normal brain the arachnoid is attached to the dura, and space occurs only as the result of trauma or a pathologic process.

s. superficia′le perine′i TA alternative for *compartimentum superficiale perinei.*

s. suprasterna′le [TA] suprasternal space: a slitlike interval between the deep and superficial layers of the cervical fascia, above the manubrium of the sternum; it contains the lower parts of the anterior jugular veins and the jugular venous arch, the sternal heads of the sternocleidomastoid muscle, and sometimes a lymph node.

spa′tia zonula′ria [TA] zonular spaces: the lymph-filled interstices between the fibers of the zonula ciliaris, communicating with the posterior chamber of the eye; called also *Petit canal.*

spat•u•la (spach′ə-lə) [L.] 1. a flat, blunt, usually flexible instrument, used for spreading plasters and for mixing ointments and masses. 2. a spatulate structure.

s. mal′lei umbo membranae tympanicae.

spat•u•lar (spach′ə-lər) spatulate (def. 1).

spat•u•late (spach′ə-lāt) 1. having a flat blunt end. 2. to mix or manipulate with a spatula. 3. to make a longitudinal incision in the cut end of a tubular structure and spread it open in order to increase the size of the opening for anastomosis.

spat•u•la•tion (spach″ə-la′shən) 1. the mixing of combined materials to a homogeneous mass by repeatedly scraping them up and smoothing out the mass on a flat surface with a spatula. 2. the process of spatulating the end of a tube; see *spatulate* (def. 3).

spav•in (spav′in) 1. any of various enlargements of the tarsus of equines, usually medially and distal to the tibiotarsal articulation and involving the metatarsals. 2. bone s.

blood s. dilatation of either or both of the medial metatarsal veins or the saphenous veins, forming a soft enlargement on the dorsomedial surface of the tarsus.

bog s. distention of the synovial capsule of the tibiotarsal joint.

bone s. osteoperiostitis or arthritis of the intertarsal or tarsometatarsal joints, often leading to exostosis and ankylosis; locations include anterior, posterior, and high. See also *occult s.* Called also *spavin.*

occult s. a bone spavin without visible radiographic exostoses, confined to the joint surfaces between two bones.

spav•ined (spav′ind) affected with spavin.

spay (spa) to castrate a female animal, usually by oophorohysterectomy.

SPCA serum prothrombin conversion accelerator (factor VII; see *coagulation factors,* under *factor*).

Spear•man rank correlation coefficient (rho) (spēr′mən) [Charles Edward *Spearman,* British psychologist, 1863–1945] see under *coefficient.*

spear•mint (spēr′mint) 1. any of various species of mint. *Mentha spicata* is common spearmint and *M. cardiaca* is Scotch spearmint. 2. the dried leaves and flowering tops of *M. spicata* or *M. cardiaca,* used as a flavoring agent and source of spearmint oil.

spe•cial•ism (spesh′əl-iz″əm) limitation of practice or study to a particular branch of medicine or surgery.

spe•cial•ist (spesh′əl-ist) a physician whose practice is limited to a particular branch of medicine or surgery, especially one who, by virtue of advanced training, is certified by a specialty board as being qualified to so limit his practice.

clinical nurse s., nurse s. see under *nurse.*

spe•cial•iza•tion (spesh″əl-ĭ-za′shən) in medicine, medical practice limited to some special branch of medicine or surgery.

spe•cial•ty (spesh′əl-te) the field of practice of a specialist.

spe•ci•a•tion (spe″se-a′shən) the evolutionary formation of new species, or the process of such formation.

spe•cies (spe′shēz, spe′sēz) [L.] 1. a taxonomic category subordinate to a genus (or subgenus), and superior to a subspecies or variety, composed of individuals possessing common characters distinguishing them from other categories of individuals of the same taxonomic level. In taxonomic nomenclature, species are designated by the genus name followed by a Latin or latinized adjective or noun. 2. a group of objects having common attributes.

concordant s. see under *xenograft.*

diovulatory s. any of the species of animals in which females ordinarily discharge two oocytes in one ovarian cycle.

discordant s. see under *xenograft.*

fugative s. a species of plant or animal that inhabits or grows in a region for only a short period of time.

monovulatory s. any of the species of animals in which females usually discharge only one oocyte in any ovarian cycle.

polyovulatory s. any of the species of animals in which the females normally discharge several oocytes (3–16) at each ovarian cycle.

reactive oxygen s. biologically active, partially reduced derivatives of molecular oxygen (O_2), including the superoxide radical, hydrogen peroxide, and the hydroxyl radical. They are produced by normal metabolic processes and may also be produced by the absorption of energy, such as ultraviolet or ionizing radiation, and can damage biological systems.

type s. in bacteriology, the species that characterizes a genus, usually the first species validly described in the genus, but it may be one arbitrarily designated as such for classification purposes.

spe•cies-spe•cif•ic (spe″sēz-spə-sif′ik) 1. characteristic of a particular species. 2. having a characteristic effect on, or interaction with, cells or tissues of members of a particular species; said of an antigen, drug, or infective agent.

spe•cif•ic (spə-sif′ik) [L. *specificus*] 1. pertaining to a species. 2. produced by a single kind of microorganism. 3. restricted in application, effect, etc., to a particular structure, function, etc. 4. a remedy specially indicated for a particular disease. 5. in immunology, pertaining to the special affinity of antigen for the corresponding antibody.

spec•i•fic•i•ty (spes″ĭ-fis′ĭ-te) 1. the quality or state of being specific. 2. the conditional probability that a person not having a disease will be correctly identified by a clinical test, i.e., the number of true negative results divided by the total number of those without the disease (which is the sum of the numbers of true negative plus false positive results). Cf. *sensitivity* and *predictive value.*

diagnostic s. specificity (def. 2).

neuronal s. the invariance of the locations, trajectories, and spatial arrangement of neurons in all members of the same species.

spec•i•men (spes′ĭ-mən) 1. a sample or part of a thing, or of several things, taken to show or to determine the character of the whole, as a specimen of urine. 2. a preparation of tissue for pathological examination or of a normal tissue, organ, or organism for study of its structure.

corrosion s. a preparation of an organ, such as the liver, by injection of certain of its structures, as the arteries and veins, and chemical digestion of surrounding substance.

speck•les (spek′əlz) concentrations of components involved in RNA processing, scattered throughout the cell nucleus; it is uncertain whether they are storage areas for inactive factors or play a more active role in messenger RNA metabolism.

SPECT single-photon emission computed tomography.

spec•ta•cles (spek′tə-kəlz) glasses.

Spec•ta•zole (spek′tə-zōl) trademark for a preparation of econazole nitrate.

spec•ti•no•my•cin (spek″tĭ-no-mi′sin) an antibiotic, derived from *Streptomyces spectabilis,* that has moderate antibacterial activity against many gram-positive and gram-negative organisms, but is especially effective against *Neisseria gonorrhoeae.* It is also used in veterinary medicine in bacterial enteritis and coccidiosis of dogs.

s. hydrochloride [USP] a salt of spectinomycin used in the treatment of acute gonorrheal urethritis and proctitis in the male and acute gonorrheal cervicitis and proctitis in the female.

spec·tra (spek′trə) plural of *spectrum.*

spec·tral (spek′trəl) 1. pertaining to a spectrum. 2. performed by means of a spectrum.

spec·trin (spek′trin) a dimeric contractile protein that with ankyrin, actin, glycophorin, and other cytoskeleton proteins forms a fibrous network beneath the plasma membrane of erythrocytes that maintains cell shape and flexibility; defects of spectrin lead to elliptocytosis, spherocytosis, and pyropoikilocytosis.

spectr(o)- [L. *spectrum* image] a combining form denoting relationship to a spectrum or to an image.

Spec·tro·bid (spek′tro-bid″) trademark for a preparation of bacampicillin hydrochloride.

spec·tro·col·or·im·e·ter (spek″tro-kul″ər-im′ə-tər) [*spectro-* + *colorimeter*] an ophthalmospectroscope using a source of light from a selected wavelength of the spectrum to detect color blindness for one color.

spec·tro·flu·o·rom·e·ter (spek″tro-floo͝-rom′ə-tər) an optical instrument for analysis of fluorescence spectra.

spec·tro·graph (spek′tro-graf) [*spectro-* + *-graph*] an instrument for photographing spectra on a sensitive photographic plate.

mass s. mass spectrometer.

spec·trom·e·ter (spek-trom′ə-tər) [*spectro-* + *-meter*] 1. an instrument for measuring the index of refraction by measuring the external angle of a prism of the substance. 2. a spectroscope for measuring the wavelengths of rays of a spectrum.

infrared s. a device that analyzes the chemical composition of a substance either by passing infrared light through a specimen and characterizing its absorption spectrum or by measuring the amount of infrared light emitted by excited atoms or molecules in a specimen; infrared light is emitted or absorbed in a given band in proportion to the concentration of the molecule characterized by the band.

mass s. an analytical instrument which identifies a substance by sorting a stream of electrified particles (ions) according to their mass; the sorting is most commonly done as follows: when the stream of charged particles enters a magnetic field, the particles are deflected into semicircular paths varying with their mass and charge components, ultimately striking a photographic plate or photomultiplier tube sensor. Called also *mass spectrograph.*

Mossbauer s. an instrument that detects small changes in interaction between an atomic nucleus and its environment caused by changes in temperature, pressure, and chemical state; used in chemical-physical research with applications in medicine.

spec·trom·e·try (spek-trom′ə-tre) the determination of the wavelengths or frequencies of the lines in a spectrum.

tandem mass s. (MS/MS) a two-step technique used to analyze a sample for a predetermined set of substances, either by using a separate mass spectroscope for each step or by performing the steps sequentially using the same spectroscope. In the first stage, a predetermined set of ions is selected for fragmentation; in the second, mass spectra are produced for the fragments. Used in screening newborns for multiple metabolic disorders from a single blood sample.

spec·tro·pho·to·flu·o·rom·e·ter (spek″tro-fo″to-floo͝-rom′ə-tər) an analytical instrument combining the techniques of spectrophotometry and fluorescence analysis.

spec·tro·pho·tom·e·ter (spek″tro-fo-tom′ə-tər) [*spectro-* + *photometer*] an apparatus for estimating the quantity of coloring matter in solution by the quantity of light absorbed (as indicated by the spectrum) in passing through the solution. Cf. *colorimeter.*

absorption s. an analytical instrument for comparing the absorption of radiation of a given wavelength with a standard to identify a sample material.

spec·tro·pho·tom·e·try (spek″tro-fo-tom′ə-tre) the use of the spectrophotometer.

spec·tro·po·lar·im·e·ter (spek″tro-po″lər-im′ə-tər) a combined spectroscope and polariscope for determining optical rotation.

spec·tro·scope (spek′trə-skōp) [*spectro-* + *-scope*] an instrument for developing and analyzing spectra.

spec·tros·co·py (spek-tros′kə-pe) [*spectro-* + *-scopy*] the propagation and analysis of spectra; examination by means of a spectroscope. **spectroscop′ic** *adj*

infrared s. examination by means of an infrared spectrometer, to study systems or molecules by examining their interactions with infrared radiation.

spec·trum (spek′trəm) pl. *spec′tra* [L. "image"] 1. a charted band of wavelengths of electromagnetic vibrations obtained by refraction and diffraction. See *invisible s.* and *visible s.* 2. by extension, any measurable range of activity, such as an antibacterial spectrum or the range of manifestations of a disease.

absorption s. the spectrum afforded by light that has passed through various gaseous media, each gas absorbing those rays of which its own spectrum is composed.

action s. 1. the range of wavelength of incident light producing a response in some material under study, such as an enzyme to be inactivated by radiation. 2. a graph plotting the magnitude of this response as a function of the wavelength of the incident light.

antibacterial s. the range of bacteria affected by an antibiotic.

broad-s. effective against a wide range of microorganisms; said of an antibiotic. Called also *wide-spectrum.*

chemical s. the part of the spectrum that includes actinic rays (ultraviolet rays).

chromatic s., color s. the portion of the range of wavelengths of electromagnetic waves (from 770 to 390 nm) that gives rise to the sensation of color (red to violet) to the normally perceptive eye; it is coincident with the *visible spectrum.*

continuous s. a spectrum in which absorption lines are not developed.

continuous x-ray s. bremsstrahlung (def. 1).

electromagnetic s. the continuous range of electromagnetic energy from cosmic rays to electric waves, including gamma rays, x-rays, ultraviolet rays, visible light, infrared waves, and radio waves.

fortification s. a form of migraine aura characterized by scintillating or zigzag bands of colored light forming the edge of an area of teichopsia. Called also *fortification figures.*

invisible s. the part of the electromagnetic spectrum whose wavelengths are less than 390 nm (ultraviolet, grenz rays, x-rays, and gamma rays) and between 770 and 12,000 nm (infrared).

narrow-s. effective against only one group or a few groups of microorganisms; said of an antibiotic.

ocular s. afterimage.

oculoauriculovertebral s. (OAVS) the association of hemifacial microsomia with vertebral and ocular defects, often in combination with anomalies of the cardiovascular, respiratory, genitourinary, and central nervous systems; its manifestations are highly variable. Most cases are sporadic, but instances of autosomal dominant or recessive inheritance have been reported. Cf. *oculoauriculovertebral dysplasia,* under *dysplasia.*

solar s. the portion of the electromagnetic spectrum that emanates from the sun, including the visible spectrum and small portions of the infrared radiations and ultraviolet radiations just beyond the visible spectrum.

visible s. the part of the electromagnetic spectrum, with wavelengths between 770 and 390 nm, that is capable of stimulating specialized sense organs and is perceptible as light.

wide-s. broad-s.

x-ray s. the spectrum of a heterogeneous beam of x-rays produced by a suitable grating, generally a crystal.

spec·u·lum (spek′u-ləm) pl. *spec′ula* [L. "mirror"] an instrument that exposes the interior of a passage or cavity of the body by enlarging the opening.

bivalve s. a speculum with two adjustable blades.

Cook s. a three-pronged rectal speculum.

duck-billed s. a type of bivalve vaginal speculum.

eye s., eyelid s. lid s.

Graves s. a type of two-valved vaginal speculum.

Kelly s. a tubular rectal speculum fitted with an obturator; called also *Kelly sphincteroscope.*

lid s. an appliance for keeping the eyelids apart. Called also *eye* or *eyelid s.* and *blepharostat.*

Martin s. a rectal speculum consisting of a conical cylinder with an obturator.

rectal s. a speculum that enlarges the diameter of the rectum for an examination.

Sims s. a double duck-billed vaginal speculum.

stop s. an eye speculum with an appliance for controlling the degree to which its branches spread.

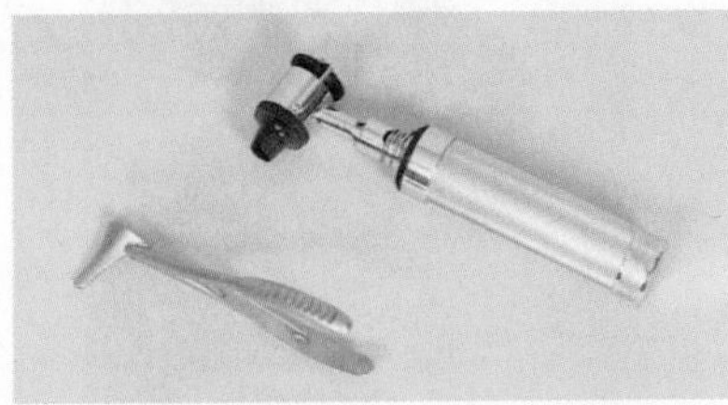

■ Nasal specula.

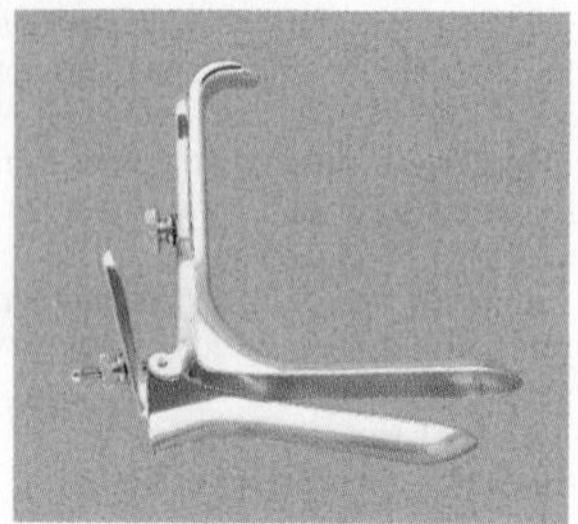
■ Graves speculum.

vaginal s. a speculum that enlarges the vaginal opening for use in a vaginal examination.

Spee curve (curvature) (shpa) [Ferdinand Graf von *Spee*, German embryologist, 1855–1937] see under *curve.*

speech (spēch) the utterance of vocal sounds conveying ideas. Cf. *phonation.*

alaryngeal s. esophageal s.

cerebellar s. speech seen with cerebellar lesions, varying from jerky or scanning to explosive. See also *scanning s.* and *explosive s.*

cleft palate s. dysphasia due to a cleft palate, often characterized by hypernasality, difficulty with fricatives, and other problems due to velopharyngeal insufficiency.

clipped s. speech in which the words are slurred over and uncompleted; called also *scamping s.* and *slurred s.*

echo s. echolalia.

esophageal s. a method of speech used after laryngectomy, with sound produced by vibration of the column of air in the esophagus against the contracting cricopharyngeal sphincter.

explosive s. speech uttered with more force than necessary; see also *cerebellar s.*

mirror s. a speech abnormality in which the order of syllables in a sentence is reversed.

plateau s. speech which is characterized by a level, monotonous, unvaried pitch.

pressured s. logorrhea.

scamping s. clipped s.

scanning s. 1. slurring, monotonous speech sometimes seen in multiple sclerosis. 2. staccato s.

slurred s. clipped s.

staccato s. speech in which each syllable is uttered separately; seen in multiple sclerosis.

telegraphic s. speech consisting of only certain prominent words and lacking modifiers, articles, and other ancillary words. It is typical of children around age two but in older persons it is a form of agrammatism.

spell (spel′) a short period of time, of indefinite length.

breath-holding s. sudden cessation of breathing with loss of consciousness, usually in a young child, often in reaction to an emotional trauma such as scolding or startle. The most common kind is the *cyanotic breath-holding spell* in which the child becomes cyanotic and may have clonic jerks and opisthotonos. A less common type is the *pallid breath-holding spell,* in which the child becomes pale and hypotonic and may have a tonic seizure.

Spe•mann induction (shpa′mahn) [Hans *Spemann*, German zoologist and Nobel prize winner, 1869–1941] see under *induction.*

Spence tail (spens) [James *Spence*, Scottish surgeon, 19th century] see under *tail.*

Spens syndrome (spenz) [Thomas *Spens*, Scottish physician, 1769–1842] Adams-Stokes syndrome; see under *syndrome.*

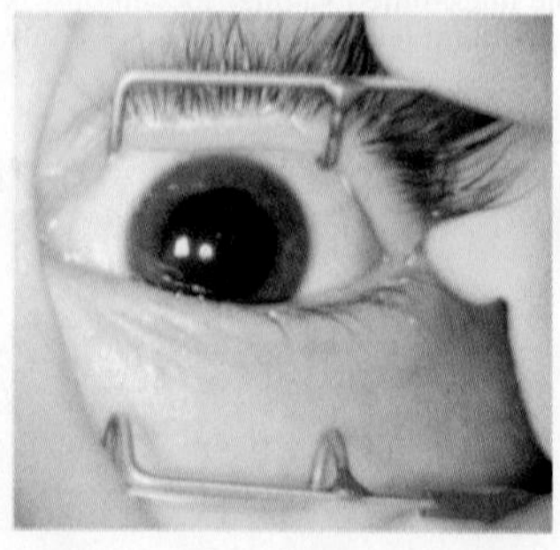
■ Lid speculum.

sperm (spurm) [Gr. *sperma* seed] 1. spermatozoon. 2. semen (def. 1).

muzzled s. a spermatozoon that cannot adhere to the oocyte, as when the acrosome is deficient.

washed s. sperm from a sample that has undergone sperm washing in preparation for artificial insemination; see under *washing.*

sper•ma•ceti (spur″mə-set′e) [Gr. *sperma* seed + *kētos* whale] a waxy substance obtained from the head of the sperm whale, *Physeter macrocephalus,* occurring as white, somewhat translucent, slightly unctuous masses, having a crystalline fracture and a pearly luster; used in the preparation of ointment bases.

synthetic s. cetyl esters wax.

sper•mag•glu•ti•na•tion (spur″mə-gloo″tĭ-na′shən) the agglutination of spermatozoa.

sper•mat•ic (spər-mat′ik) [L. *spermaticus;* Gr. *spermatikos*] 1. seminal. 2. spermatozoal.

sper•ma•tid (spur′mə-tid) a cell derived from a secondary spermatocyte by fission, and capable of undergoing spermiogenesis to develop into a spermatozoon; called also *spermatoblast.*

sper•ma•ti•tis (spur″mə-ti′tis) deferentitis.

spermat(o)- [Gr. *sperma,* gen. *spermatos* seed] a combining form denoting a relationship to sperm or to the male aspect of reproduction; also *sperm(o)-.*

sper•ma•to•blast (spur′mə-to-blast″) [*spermato-* + *-blast*] a term originally applied to Sertoli cells, but now having the same meaning as *spermatid.*

sper•ma•to•cele (spur′mə-to-sēl″) [*spermato-* + *-cele*[1]] a cystic distention of the epididymis or the rete testis containing spermatozoa.

sper•ma•to•ce•lec•to•my (spər-mat″o-sə-lek′tə-me) [*spermatocele* + *-ectomy*] excision of a spermatocele.

sper•ma•to•ci•dal (spur″mə-to-si′dəl) spermicidal.

sper•ma•to•cide (spər-mat′o-sīd″) spermicide.

sper•ma•to•cyst (spur′mə-to-sist″) [*spermato-* + *cyst*] spermatocele.

sper•ma•to•cy•tal (spur″mə-to-si′təl) pertaining to spermatocytes.

sper•ma•to•cyte (spər-mat′o-sīt) [*spermato-* + *-cyte*] either of two intermediate stages in the development of spermatids.

primary s. a diploid cell that has derived from a spermatogonium and can subsequently begin meiosis and divide into two haploid secondary spermatocytes.

secondary s. one of the two haploid cells into which a primary spermatocyte divides, and which in turn gives origin to spermatids.

sper•ma•to•cy•to•gen•e•sis (spur″mə-to-si″to-jen′ə-sis) the first stage of formation of spermatozoa, in which the spermatogonia develop into spermatocytes and then into spermatids.

sper•ma•to•cy•to•ma (spur″mə-to-si-to′mə) seminoma.

sper•ma•to•gen•e•sis (spur″mə-to-jen′ə-sis) [*spermato-* + *-genesis*] the process of formation of spermatozoa, including both spermatocytogenesis and spermiogenesis.

sper•ma•to•ge•net•ic (spur″mə-to-jə-net′ik) 1. pertaining to spermatogenesis. 2. spermatogenic.

sper•ma•to•gen•ic (spur″mə-to-jen′ik) [*spermato-* + *-genic*] producing semen or spermatozoa.

sper•ma•tog•e•nous (spur″mə-toj′ə-nəs) spermatogenic.

sper•ma•tog•e•ny (spur″mə-toj′ə-ne) spermatogenesis.

sper•ma•to•gone (spur′mə-to-gōn″) spermatogonium.

sper•ma•to•go•nia (spur″mə-to-go′ne-ə) plural of *spermatogonium.*

sper•ma•to•go•ni•um (spur″mə-to-go′ne-əm) pl. *spermatogo′nia* [*spermato-* + Gr. *gonē* generation] an undifferentiated germ cell of a male, originating in a seminiferous tubule and dividing into two primary spermatocytes; called also *spermatogonial cell* and *spermatophore.*

sper•ma•toid (spur′mə-toid) [*spermato-* + *-oid*] resembling a spermatozoon.

sper•ma•tol•o•gy (spur′mə-tol′ə-je) [*spermato-* + *-logy*] seminology.

sper•ma•tol•y•sin (spur″mə-tol′ĭ-sin) a lysin that destroys spermatozoa; cf. *spermicide.*

sper•ma•tol•y•sis (spur′mə-tol′ĭ-sis) [*spermato-* + *-lysis*] destruction or dissolution of spermatozoa. **spermatolyt′ic** *adj*

sper•ma•to•phore (spur′mə-to-for″) [*spermato-* + *-phore*] 1. a capsule containing several spermatozoa, extruded by certain invertebrates. 2. spermatogonium.

sper•ma•to•poi•et•ic (spur″mə-to-poi-et′ik) spermatogenic.

sper•ma•to•tox•ic (spur′mə-to-tok″sik) 1. spermicidal. 2. having a destructive or toxic effect on spermatozoa.

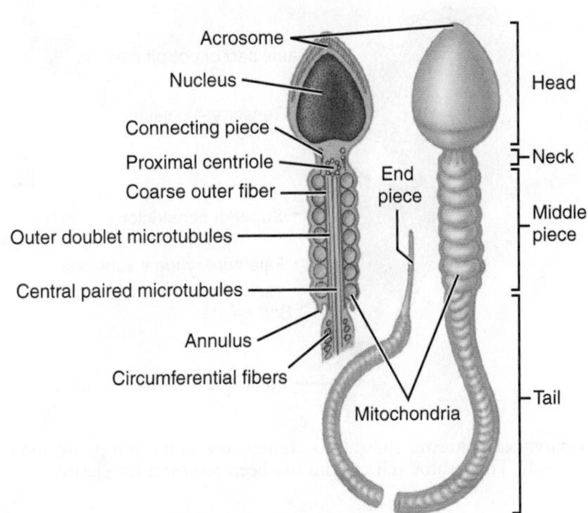

■ Human spermatozoon: side view (in cross-section) and flat view.

sper•ma•tox•in (spur′mə-tok″sin) spermotoxin.

sper•ma•to•zoa (spur″mə-to-zo′ə) [Gr.] plural of *spermatozoon.*

sper•ma•to•zoid (spur″mə-to-zoid) [*spermatozoon* + *-oid*] 1. spermatozoon. 2. the male germ cell in plants.

sper•ma•to•zo•on (spur″mə-to-zo′on) pl. *spermatozo′a* [*spermato-* + Gr. *zōon* animal] a mature male germ cell, the specific output of the testes. It is the generative element of the semen which serves to fertilize the oocyte, and contains the genetic information to be transmitted to the zygote by the male. It consists of a head (or nucleus), a neck, a middle piece, and a tail with an end piece. Spermatozoa, formed in the seminiferous tubules, are derived from spermatogonia, which first develop into spermatocytes, which, in turn, undergo meiosis to produce spermatids; the spermatids then differentiate into spermatozoa. Called also *sperm.* spermatozo′al *adj*

sper•ma•tu•ria (spur″mə-tu′re-ə) [*spermato-* + *-uria*] seminuria.

sper•mi•a•tion (spur″me-a′shən) the release of mature spermatozoa from the Sertoli cells.

sper•mi•ci•dal (spur″mĭ-si′dəl) [*sperm* + L. *caedere* to kill] destructive to spermatozoa; called also *spermatocidal* and *spermatotoxic.*

sper•mi•cide (spur′mĭ-sīd) an agent that destroys spermatozoa; called also *spermatocide.*

sper•mid (spur′mid) spermatid.

sper•mi•dine (spur′mĭ-dēn) a polyamine, first found in human semen but now known to occur in almost all tissues, in association with nucleic acids; it is formed from putrescine and is itself a precursor of spermine.

sper•mi•duct (spur′mĭ-dukt″) [*sperm* + *duct*] the ejaculatory duct and ductus deferens together.

sper•mine (spur′mēn) a polyamine, first found in human semen but now known to occur in almost all tissues in association with nucleic acids, being formed from spermidine.

spermi(o)- see *spermat(o)-.*

sper•mio•gen•e•sis (spur″me-o-jen′ə-sis) the second stage in the formation of spermatozoa, when spermatids transform into spermatozoa.

sper•mio•gram (spur′me-o-gram) laboratory examination and analysis of a semen sample, including such factors as pH, ejaculate volume, total sperm count, and sperm morphology, motility, density, and vitality.

sperm(o)- see *spermat(o)-.*

sper•mo•blast (spur′mo-blast) [*spermo-* + *-blast*] spermatid.

sper•mo•cy•to•ma (spur″mo-si-to′mə) seminoma.

sper•mo•lith (spur′mo-lith) [*spermo-* + *-lith*] seminal vesicle calculus.

sper•mol•y•sis (spər-mol′ĭ-sis) spermatolysis.

Sper•moph•i•lus (spər-mof′ĭ-ləs) a genus of ground squirrels (family Sciuridae) that harbor organisms transmissible to humans. *S. bee′cheyi* is a species of California that is often infected with plague; also, it and the species *S. mol′lis* of Utah and *S. orego′nus* of Oregon are natural reservoirs of *Francisella tularensis.*

sper•mo•plasm (spur′mo-plaz″əm) [*spermo-* + *-plasm*] the protoplasm of a spermatid.

sper•mo•tox•ic (spur′mo-tok″sik) 1. spermicidal. 2. spermatotoxic (def. 2).

sper•mo•tox•in (spur′mo-tok″sin) a toxin destructive to spermatozoa, especially a cytotoxic antibody produced by injecting an animal with spermatozoa; cf. *spermicide.* Called also *spermatoxin.*

SPF sun protection factor; specific-pathogen free, a term applied to animals reared for laboratory experiments and known to be free of specific pathogens.

sp gr specific gravity.

sph spherical or spherical lens.

Sphae•ri•a•les (sfe″re-a′lēz) an order of perfect fungi of the subphylum Ascomycotina, series Unitunicatae, characterized by inoperculate asci. Many fungi formerly in this order have now been assigned elsewhere, such as in the order Sordariales.

sphaer(o)- for words beginning thus, see also those beginning *spher(o)-.*

Sphae•roi•des (sfe-roi′dēz) a genus of marine puffer fish of the family Tetraodontidae. Their flesh contains tetrodotoxin, and consumption without special cooking can cause fatal tetrodotoxism.

Sphe•ci•dae (sfe′sĭ-de) the solitary wasps, a family of flying insects of the order Hymenoptera that have a long thin body and delicate wings; many species can sting. Members of this family live in comparative isolation.

sphen•eth•moid (sfən-eth′moid) sphenoethmoid.

sphe•ni•on (sfe′ne-on) pl. *sphe′nia* [Gr. *sphēn* wedge + *on* neuter ending] the cranial point at the sphenoid angle of the parietal bone.

sphen(o)- [Gr. *sphēn* wedge] a combining form denoting relationship to the sphenoid bone or to a wedge, or meaning wedge-shaped.

sphe•no•bas•i•lar (sfe″no-bas′ĭ-lər) pertaining to the sphenoid bone and the basilar part of the occipital bone. Cf. *sphenooccipital.*

sphe•noc•cip•i•tal (sfe″nok-sip′ĭ-təl) sphenooccipital.

sphe•no•ceph•a•ly (sfe″no-sef′ə-le) [*spheno-* + *-cephaly*] a developmental anomaly characterized by a wedge-shaped appearance of the head.

sphe•no•eth•moid (sfe″no-eth′moid) sphenoethmoidal.

sphe•no•eth•moi•dal (sfe″no-eth-moi′dəl) pertaining to the sphenoid and ethmoid bones.

sphe•no•fron•tal (sfe″no-fron′tal) pertaining to the sphenoid and frontal bones.

sphe•noid (sfe′noid) [*sphen-* + *-oid*] 1. wedge-shaped; see os sphenoidale. 2. sphenoidal.

sphe•noi•dal (sfe-noi′dəl) pertaining to the sphenoid bone; sphenoid.

sphe•noi•di•tis (sfe″noi-di′tis) sphenoid sinusitis.

sphe•noi•dos•to•my (sfe″noi-dos′tə-me) [*sphenoid* + *-ostomy*] operative removal of the anterior wall of the sphenoidal sinus.

sphe•noi•dot•o•my (sfe″noi-dot′ə-me) incision into the sphenoidal sinus.

sphe•no•ma•lar (sfe″no-ma′lər) sphenozygomatic.

sphe•no•max•il•lary (sfe″no-mak′sĭ-lar″e) pertaining to the sphenoid bone and the maxilla.

sphe•no•oc•cip•i•tal (sfe″no-ok-sip′ĭ-təl) pertaining to the sphenoid and occipital bones.

sphe•no•or•bi•tal (sfe″no-or′bĭ-təl) pertaining to the sphenoid bone and the orbits.

sphe•no•pal•a•tine (sfe″no-pal′ə-tīn) pertaining to or in relation with the sphenoid and palatine bones; in anatomy it is sometimes interchangeable with the term *pterygopalatine.*

sphe•no•pa•ri•e•tal (sfe″no-pə-ri′ə-təl) pertaining to the sphenoid and parietal bones.

sphe•no•pe•tro•sal (sfe″no-pə-tro′səl) pertaining to the sphenoid bone and the petrous part of the temporal bone.

sphe•nor•bi•tal (sfe-nor′bĭ-təl) sphenoorbital.

sphe•no•squa•mo•sal (sfe″no-skwə-mo′səl) pertaining to the sphenoid bone and the squamous part of the temporal bone.

sphe•no•tem•po•ral (sfe″no-tem′pə-rəl) pertaining to the sphenoid and temporal bones.

sphe•not•ic (sfe-not′ik) [*spheno-* + *otic*] denoting a fetal bone which becomes that part of the sphenoid bone adjacent to the carotid groove.

sphe•no•tur•bi•nal (sfe″no-tur′bĭ-nəl) both sphenoid and turbinate, or pertaining to the sphenoid and turbinate bones.

sphe•no•vo•mer•ine (sfe″no-vo′mər-in) pertaining to the sphenoid and the vomer.

sphe•no•zy•go•mat•ic (sfe″no-zi″go-mat′ik) pertaining to the sphenoid and zygomatic bones.

sphere (sfēr) [Gr. *sphaira* sphere] a three-dimensional round body; called also *globe*. **spher′ical** *adj*
embryotic s. morula.
segmentation s. morula.
vitelline s., yolk s. morula.

spher(o)- [Gr. *sphaira* a ball or globe] a combining form meaning round, or denoting relationship to a sphere.

sphe•ro•cyl•in•der (sfēr-o-sil′in-dər) a combined spherical and cylindrical lens.

sphe•ro•cyte (sfēr′o-sīt) [*sphero-* + *-cyte*] a small, globular, completely hemoglobinated erythrocyte without the usual central pallor, found characteristically in hereditary spherocytosis but also observed in acquired hemolytic anemia.

sphe•ro•cyt•ic (sfēr″o-sit′ik) characterized by the presence of spherocytes.

sphe•ro•cy•to•sis (sfēr″o-si-to′sis) the presence of spherocytes in the blood; called also *microspherocytosis*.
hereditary s. a group of clinically and genetically heterogeneous hereditary disorders characterized by the presence of spherocytes, hemolytic anemia, abnormal fragility of erythrocytes, jaundice, and splenomegaly; molecular defects affect various proteins important to the erythrocyte cytoskeleton. Called also *congenital hemolytic* or *spherocytic anemia*, and *Minkowski-Chauffard syndrome*.

sphe•roid (sfēr′oid) [*sphero-* + *-oid*] a globular body, or one resembling a sphere.

sphe•roi•dal (sfēr-oi′dəl) having the form or shape of a sphere.

sphe•roi•din (sfēr-oi′din) [*Sphaeroides* a genus of puffer fish] a toxic fraction from tetrodotoxin.

sphe•rom•e•ter (sfēr-om′ə-tər) [*sphero-* + *-meter*] an instrument for measuring the curvature of a surface.

sphe•ro•pha•kia (sfēr″o-fa′ke-ə) [*sphero* + *phak-* + *ia*] a developmental defect in which a smaller, more spherical optic lens than normal is formed, with partial or complete aplasia of the zonule.

sphe•ro•plast (sfēr′o-plast) a membrane-bound, spherical cell that results after partial or complete removal of the cell wall from a bacterial, yeast, or fungal cell; it is dependent for its integrity on an isotonic or hypertonic medium. Cf. *protoplast* (def. 3).

sphe•rule (sfēr′ūl) [L. *sphaerula* little ball] 1. a small sphere. 2. a type of spherical, multinucleate cell seen in the parasitic stage of *Coccidioides immitis*, in which endospores are developed.
rod s. the pear-shaped ending of a retinal rod cell, which synapses with the bipolar and horizontal cells in the outer plexiform layer.

sphe•ru•lin (sfēr′u-lin) a skin test antigen prepared from spherule-endospore phase *Coccidioides immitis* organisms; it detects almost all persons who are coccidioidin-positive, as well as a group of coccidioidin-negative persons with previous *C. immitis* exposure. Cf. *coccidioidin*.

sphinc•ter (sfingk′tər) [L., from Gr. *sphinktēr* that which binds tight] a ringlike band of muscle fibers that constricts a passage or closes a natural orifice; called also *musculus sphincter* [TA]. **sphinc′teral, sphincter′ic** *adj*
anal s., external musculus sphincter ani externus.
anal s., internal musculus sphincter ani internus.
s. a′ni see *musculus sphincter ani externus* and *musculus sphincter ani internus*.
artificial genitourinary s. an implantable prosthetic device for treating urinary incontinence due to an incompetent or absent sphincter; an artificial sphincter is created with an inflatable cuff around the bladder neck or bulbar urethra.
s. of bile duct, Boyden s., s. of Boyden musculus sphincter ductus choledochi.
cardiac s., cardioesophageal s. lower esophageal s.
cloacal s. the developing muscle surrounding the caudal end of the cloaca in the embryo; its posterior part will become the external anal sphincter and its anterior part becomes the superficial transverse perineal, bulbospongiosus, and ischiocavernosus muscles.
cornual s. tubal s.
cricopharyngeal s. pars cricopharyngea musculi constrictoris pharyngis inferioris.
esophageal s., lower (LES) the terminal few centimeters of the esophagus, near the esophagogastric junction, which prevents reflux of gastric contents into the esophagus. Called also *cardiac*, *cardioesophageal*, or *gastroesophageal s.*
esophageal s., upper (UES) the upper 3 to 5 cm of the esophagus, including the cricopharyngeal muscle, which prevents the aspiration of air from the pharynx into the esophagus.
external s. of female urethra musculus sphincter urethrae externus urethrae femininae.

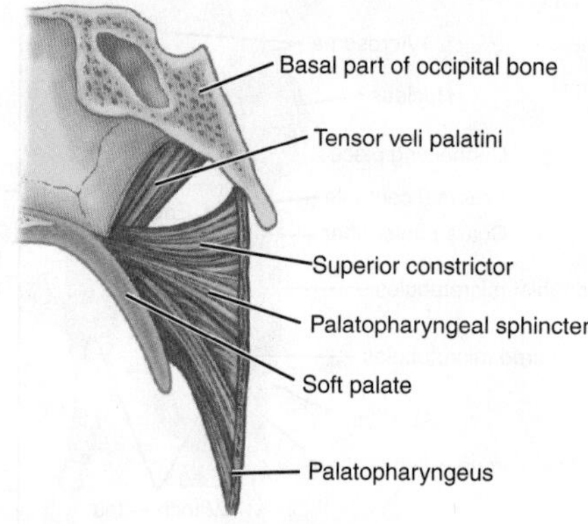

■ Palatopharyngeal sphincter shown in a sagittal view of the soft palate and adjoining pharyngeal wall. The levator veli palatini has been removed for clarity.

external s. of male urethra musculus sphincter urethrae externus urethrae masculinae.
gastroesophageal s. lower esophageal s.
Glisson s. musculus sphincter ampullae hepatopancreaticae.
hepatic s. a thickened portion of the muscular coat of the hepatic veins near their entrance into the inferior vena cava.
s. of hepatopancreatic ampulla musculus sphincter ampullae hepatopancreaticae.
Hyrtl s. an incomplete band or thickening of the muscle fibers in the rectum about 10 cm above the anus in the upper part of the rectal ampulla; called also *rectal s.*
internal s. of urethra musculus sphincter urethrae internus.
s. i′ridis musculus sphincter pupillae.
Nélaton s. see under *fold*.
O'Beirne s. rectosigmoid s.
s. o′culi musculus orbicularis oculi.
s. of Oddi musculus sphincter ampullae hepatopancreaticae.
s. o′ris musculus orbicularis oris.
palatopharyngeal s. a transverse band of muscle fibers in the posterior wall of the pharynx, derived from the superior constrictor or palatopharyngeus muscle, which contracts during swallowing to form the crista palatopharyngea; it also contracts during speech in persons with cleft palate.
pancreatic s., s. of pancreatic duct musculus sphincter ductus pancreatici.
pharyngoesophageal s. upper esophageal s.
precapillary s. a smooth muscle fiber encircling a true capillary where it originates from the arterial capillary, which can open and close the capillary entrance.
preprostatic s. musculus sphincter urethrae internus.
prepyloric s. a band of muscle fibers in the wall of the stomach proximal to the pyloric sphincter.
s. pupil′lae musculus sphincter pupillae.
pyloric s. musculus sphincter pyloricus.
rectal s. Hyrtl s.
rectosigmoid s. circular muscle fibers in the wall of the large intestine at the junction of the sigmoid colon and rectum; called also *O'Beirne s.*
smooth s. musculus sphincter urethrae internus.
striated s. 1. musculus sphincter urethrae externus urethrae femininae. 2. musculus sphincter urethrae externus urethrae masculinae.
supracollicular s. musculus sphincter urethrae internus.
tubal s. an encircling band of muscle fibers at the junction of the uterine tube and the uterus.
s. ure′thrae, urethral s. see *musculus sphincter urethrae internus*, *musculus sphincter urethrae externus urethrae femininae*, and *musculus sphincter urethrae externus urethrae masculinae*.
urethral s., external see *musculus sphincter urethrae externus urethrae femininae* and *musculus sphincter urethrae externus urethrae masculinae*.
urethral s., internal musculus sphincter urethrae internus.
urethral s. of female urethra, external musculus sphincter urethrae externus urethrae femininae.
urethral s. of male urethra, external musculus sphincter urethrae externus urethrae masculinae.
s. vagi′nae compressor vaginae.
s. vesi′cae, vesical s. musculus sphincter urethrae internus.

sphinc•ter•al•gia (sfingk″tər-al′jə) [*sphincter* + *-algia*] pain in a sphincter muscle, such as an anal sphincter.

sphinc•ter•ec•to•my (sfingk″tər-ek′tə-me) [*sphincter* + *-ectomy*] excision of any sphincter, such as the sphincter iridis.

sphinc•ter•is•mus (sfingk″tər-iz′məs) sphincter spasm.

sphinc·ter·itis (sfingk″tər-i′tis) inflammation of a sphincter, particularly of the sphincter of Oddi.

sphinc·ter·ol·y·sis (sfingk″tər-ol′ĭ-sis) [*sphincter* + *lysis*] the operation of separating the iris from the cornea in anterior synechia.

sphinc·ter·om·et·ry (sfingk″tər-om′ə-tre) measurement of the opening of the sphincter vesicae; called also *cystosphincterometry.*

sphinc·tero·plas·ty (sfingk′tər-o-plas″te) [*sphincter* + *-plasty*] surgical repair of a defective sphincter. **sphincteroplas′tic** *adj*

sphinc·tero·scope (sfingk′tər-o-skōp″) an instrument, such as a speculum, for inspecting the anal sphincter.

Kelly s. see under *speculum.*

sphinc·ter·os·co·py (sfingk″tər-os′kə-pe) inspection of a sphincter.

sphinc·tero·tome (sfingk′tər-o-tōm″) an instrument for cutting a sphincter.

sphinc·ter·ot·o·my (sfingk″tər-ot′ə-me) [*sphincter* + *-tomy*] incision of a sphincter.

internal s. incision of the internal anal sphincter in treatment of an anal fissure.

precut s. in cannulation and sphincterotomy for procedures in the common bile duct, initial cutting of the papilla of Vater when the opening is particularly blocked or stenosed.

sphin·ga·nine (sfing′gə-nēn) a dihydroxy derivative of sphingosine and similarly a common component of sphingolipids in mammals.

sphingo- [Gr. *sphingein* to bind fast] a combining form denoting relationship to sphingosine or a sphingolipid.

Sphin·go·bac·te·ri·um (sfing″go-bak-tēr′e-əm) a genus of gram-negative, aerobic or facultatively anaerobic, rod-shaped bacteria of the family Flavobacteriaceae, characterized by production of a yellow pigment. They were formerly considered part of the genus *Flavobacterium* and are opportunistic pathogens in humans.

S. multivo′rum a species isolated from cases of bacteremia and peritonitis.

S. spiritivo′rum a species occasionally recovered from the blood of patients with bacteremia.

sphin·go·ga·lac·to·side (sfing″go-gə-lak′to-sīd) a substance composing part of the material characteristic of the spleen in Gaucher disease.

sphin·go·in (sfing′go-in) a leukomaine from the substance of the brain.

sphin·go·lip·id (sfing″go-lip′id) a lipid in which the backbone is sphingosine or a related base; the basic unit is a ceramide (q.v.) which is attached via its 1-hydroxyl group to a polar head group. The sphingolipids include sphingomyelins, cerebrosides, and gangliosides.

sphin·go·lip·i·do·sis (sfing″go-lip″ĭ-do′sis) [*sphingolipid* + *-osis*] any of various lysosomal storage diseases characterized by abnormal storage of sphingolipids.

cerebral s. neuronal ceroid lipofuscinosis.

sphin·go·lipo·dys·tro·phy (sfing″go-lip″o-dis′trə-fe) sphingolipidosis.

Sphin·go·mo·na·da·ceae (sfing″go-mo″nə-da′se-e) a family of gram-negative bacteria of the order Sphingomonadales. Organisms of medical interest are contained in the genus *Sphingomonas.*

Sphin·go·mo·na·da·les (sfing″go-mo″nə-da′lēz) an order of bacteria of the class Alphaproteobacteria, phylum Proteobacteria, consisting of gram-negative, non–spore-forming, chemoheterotrophic rod-shaped, ovoid, or pleomorphic cells; most species are aerobic with respiratory metabolism. It contains the single family Sphingomonadaceae.

Sphin·go·mo·nas (sfing″go-mo′nəs) [*sphingo-* + Gr. *monas* unit, from *monos* single] a genus of free-living, gram-negative bacteria of the family Sphingomonadaceae, consisting of non–spore-forming, motile or nonmotile straight or slightly curved rods or ovoid cells; organisms are aerobic, catalase-positive, and oxidase-positive or -negative. Organisms of medical interest are contained in the type species *S. paucimo′bilis.*

S. paucimo′bilis a genus found widely distributed in soil and water that is an opportunistic pathogen in immunocompromised persons; nosocomial infections are associated with contaminated water, ventilators, and catheters. Formerly called *Pseudomonas paucimobilis.*

sphin·go·my·elin (sfing″go-mi′ə-lin) any of the group of sphingolipids in which the head group is phosphorylated choline, making them sphingophospholipids; they are the only phospholipids not derived from glycerol in humans. They occur in membranes, primarily in nervous tissue, and are accumulated abnormally in Niemann-Pick disease.

sphin·go·my·elin·ase (sfing″go-mi′ə-lin-ās) sphingomyelin phosphodiesterase.

sphin·go·my·eli·no·sis (sfing″go-mi″ə-lin-o′sis) Niemann-Pick disease.

sphin·go·my·elin phos·pho·di·es·ter·ase (sfing″go-mi′ə-lin fos″fo-di-es′tər-ās) [EC 3.1.4.12] an enzyme of the hydrolase class that catalyzes the cleavage of sphingomyelin to ceramide and phosphorylated choline in the major pathway for sphingomyelin degradation. Deficiency of the enzyme, an autosomal recessive trait, causes Niemann-Pick disease. Called also *sphingomyelinase.*

sphin·go·phos·pho·lip·id (sfing″go-fos″fo-lip′id) a phospholipid derived from sphingosine or a related base; in higher animals, the most abundant are the sphingomyelins.

sphin·go·sine (sfing′go-sēn) an amino alcohol with a long unsaturated hydrocarbon chain; sphingosine and its derivative sphinganine are the major bases of the sphingolipids in mammals.

sphin·go·sine *N*-ac·yl·trans·fer·ase (sfing′go-sēn a″səl-trans′fər-ās) [EC 2.3.1.24] an enzyme of the transferase class that catalyzes the transfer of a fatty acyl group from an acyl (usually stearoyl) coenzyme A to sphingosine to form a ceramide. The reaction occurs in microsomes as a step in the synthesis of sphingolipids.

sphyg·mic (sfig′mik) [Gr. *sphygmikos*] pertaining to the pulse.

sphygm(o)- [Gr. *sphygmos* pulse] a combining form denoting relationship to the pulse.

sphyg·mo·chro·no·graph (sfig″mo-kro′no-graf) [*sphygmo-* + *chronograph*] a form of self-registering sphygmograph.

sphyg·mo·dy·na·mom·e·ter (sfig″mo-di″nə-mom′ə-tər) [*sphygmo-* + *dynamometer*] an instrument for determining the force of the pulse.

sphyg·mo·gram (sfig′mo-gram) [*sphygmo-* + *gram*] the record or tracing made by a sphygmograph; it consists of a curve having a sudden rise *(primary elevation),* followed by a sudden fall, after which there is a gradual descent marked by a number of secondary elevations. Called also *pulse curve.*

sphyg·mo·graph (sfig′mo-graf) [*sphygmo-* + *graph*] an instrument for registering the movements, form, and force of the arterial pulse. **sphygmograph′ic** *adj*

sphyg·mog·ra·phy (sfig-mog′rə-fe) the production of pulse tracings with the sphygmograph.

sphyg·moid (sfig′moid) [*sphygm-* + *-oid*] resembling a pulse.

sphyg·mol·o·gy (sfig-mol′ə-je) [*sphygmo-* + *-logy*] the sum of what is known regarding the pulse.

sphyg·mo·ma·nom·e·ter (sfig″mo-mə-nom′ə-tər) an instrument for measuring blood pressure in the arteries. There are many forms of the instrument, often named for the person who devised them, such as *Riva-Rocci s., Faught s., Erlanger s., Janeway s., Mosso s., Rogers s., Stanton s., Tycos s.*

sphyg·mom·e·ter (sfig-mom′ə-tər) [*sphygmo-* + *-meter*] an instrument for measuring the force and frequency of the pulse.

sphyg·mo·met·ro·graph (sfig″mo-met′ro-graf) an apparatus for recording the maximal and minimal arterial blood pressures.

sphyg·mo·met·ro·scope (sfig″mo-met′ro-skōp) an instrument for taking the blood pressure by the auscultatory method.

sphyg·mo·os·cil·lom·e·ter (sfig″mo-os″ĭ-lom′ə-tər) a form of sphygmomanometer in which the disappearance and reappearance of the pulse are indicated by an oscillating needle.

sphyg·mo·pal·pa·tion (sfig″mo-pal-pa′shən) the act of palpating or feeling the pulse.

sphyg·mo·phone (sfig′mo-fōn) [*sphygmo-* + Gr. *phōnē* sound] an apparatus for rendering audible the vibrations of the pulse.

sphyg·mo·ple·thys·mo·graph (sfig″mo-plə-thiz′mo-graf) a plethysmograph which traces a record of the pulse, together with the curve of fluctuation of volume.

sphyg·mo·scope (sfig′mo-skōp) [*sphygmo-* + *-scope*] a device formerly used to make the pulse beat visible.

sphyg·mos·co·py (sfig-mos′kə-pe) examination of the pulse.

sphyg·mo·sys·to·le (sfig″mo-sis′tə-le) [*sphygmo-* + *systole*] the part of the sphygmogram that corresponds to the systole of the heart.

sphyg·mo·to·nom·e·ter (sfig″mo-to-nom′ə-tər) [*sphygmo-* + *tonometer*] an instrument for measuring the elasticity of the arterial walls.

sphyg·mo·vis·co·sim·e·try (sfig″mo-vis″ko-sim′ə-tre) [*sphygmo-* + *viscosimetry*] measurement of the blood pressure and the viscosity of the blood.

spi·ca (spi′kə) [L. "ear of wheat"] spica bandage.

spic·u·lat·ed (spik′u-lāt″əd) having spicules; spiny.

spic·ule (spik′ūl) [L. *spiculum*] a sharp, needle-like body. **spic′ular** *adj*

spic·u·lum (spik′u-ləm) pl. *spic′ula* [L.] spicule.

spi·der (spi′dər) 1. any arachnid of the order Araneae, usually characterized by a body in two parts: the cephalothorax, which has eight legs attached, and the abdomen. Some species have venomous bites. Cf. *arachnidism.* 2. spider angioma.

arterial s. spider angioma.

banana s. *Heteropoda venatoria*, a large tropical spider, sometimes found outside the tropics in shipments of fruit such as bananas; its bite is painful but not serious.

bird s. any of various members of the family Theraphosidae, large hairy tropical spiders reputed to sometimes catch and eat small birds.

black widow s. *Latrodectus mactans*, a species found in the United States, whose bite causes pain and sometimes death.

brown s. *Loxosceles laeta*, the species whose bite causes loxoscelism in South America.

brown recluse s. *Loxosceles reclusa*, the species whose bite causes loxoscelism in North America.

cat-headed s. *Mastophora gasteracanthoides*, a venomous spider of Peru, Chile, and Argentina whose bite causes necrotic spots on vineyard workers.

comb-footed s. any member of the family Theridiidae.

European wolf s. European tarantula.

funnel-web s. any spider of the Australian genus *Atrax*. Six species have venomous bites, and the bite of *A. robustus* has caused human deaths.

hobo s. *Tegenaria agrestis*.

jointed s. any member of the family Solpugida.

lynx s. *Peucetia viridans*, a species that squirts a corrosive spray that produces painful burns in the eye of its prey.

tree funnel-web s. *Atrax formidabilis*, an Australian spider with a venomous bite.

vascular s. spider angioma.

wandering s. *Ctenus ferus*, a South American species with a painful bite. Severe reactions may involve weakness, irregular heartbeat, breathing difficulties, and temporary blindness; in young children deaths have occurred.

wolf s. any spider of the family Lycosidae.

Spie·ghel line (shpe′gəl) [Adriaan van der *Spieghel* (L. *Spigelius*), Flemish anatomist, 1578–1625] linea semilunaris.

Spie·gler-Fendt pseudolymphoma (sarcoid) (shpe′gler fent′) [Eduard *Spiegler*, Austrian dermatologist, 1860–1908; Heinrich *Fendt*, Austrian dermatologist, 19th century] cutaneous lymphoid hyperplasia; see under *hyperplasia*.

Spiel·mey·er-Vogt disease (shpēl′mi-ər fōkt′) [Walter *Spielmeyer*, German physician, 1879–1935; Heinrich *Vogt*, German physician, early 20th century] Vogt-Spielmeyer disease; see under *disease*.

spi·ge·li·an (spi-je′le-ən) named for Adriaan van der *Spieghel*.

spike (spīk) a sharp upward deflection in a curve, such as the main deflection of the oscillographic tracing of the action potential wave, the following smaller wave being called the *after-potential*. See also under *potential*.

end-plate s's the biphasic type of end-plate activity.

Spi·lan·thes (spi-lan′thēz) [Gr. *spilos* spot + Gr. *anthos* flower] a genus of composite-flowered plants (family Compositae). *S. acmel′la* Murr., the Para cress of tropical America and Asia, is a mosquito larvicide and was formerly used as a remedy for toothache.

spill·way (spil′wa) embrasure.

spin (spin) the angular momentum of a nucleus or electron.

spi·na (spi′nə) gen. and pl. *spi′nae* [L.] 1. spine: a thornlike process or projection. 2. columna vertebralis.

s. bi′fida a neural tube defect characterized by defective closure of the vertebral arch, through which the spinal cord and meninges may protrude *(s. bifida cystica)* or may not *(s. bifida occulta)*. Cf. *rachischisis*. Called also *hydrocele spinalis* and *cleft spine*.

s. bi′fida ante′rior a defect of closure on the anterior surface of the vertebral canal, often associated with defective development of the abdominal and thoracic viscera.

s. bi′fida aper′ta s. bifida manifesta.

s. bi′fida cys′tica spina bifida in which there is protrusion through the defective vertebral arch of a cystic swelling involving the meninges (meningocele), spinal cord (myelocele), or both (meningomyelocele).

s. bi′fida manifes′ta spina bifida with detectable external manifestations; it includes all types of spina bifida cystica and a few types of spina bifida occulta. Called also *s. bifida aperta*.

s. bi′fida occul′ta spina bifida in which there is a defect of the vertebral arch without protrusion of the spinal cord or meninges.

s. bi′fida poste′rior a defect of closure on the posterior surface of the vertebral canal.

s. fronta′lis s. nasalis ossis frontalis.

s. he′licis [TA] spine of helix: a small, forward-projecting cartilaginous process on the anterior portion of the helix at about the junction of the helix and its crus, just above the tragus.

s. ili′aca ante′rior infe′rior [TA] anterior inferior iliac spine: a blunt bony process projecting forward from the lower part of the anterior margin of the ilium, just above the acetabulum.

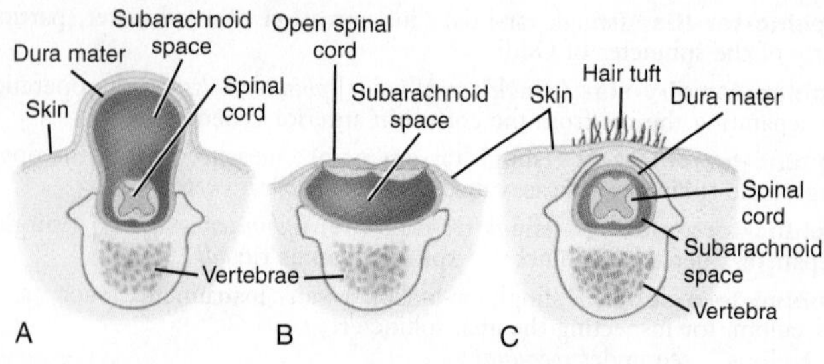

■ *(A)*, Spina bifida cystica with meningocele resulting from absence of the laminae of the vertebral arch; characterized by protrusion of the meninges. *(B)*, Spina bifida cystica with myelocele resulting from absence of the vertebral arch; characterized by myeloschisis and protrusion of the defective spinal cord. *(C)*, Spina bifida occulta; characterized by failure of fusion of the laminae of the vertebral arch.

s. ili′aca ante′rior supe′rior [TA] anterior superior iliac spine: a blunt bony projection on the anterior border of the ilium, forming the anterior end of the iliac crest.

s. ili′aca poste′rior infe′rior [TA] posterior inferior iliac spine: a blunt bony projection from the posterior border of the ilium, corresponding to the posterior lower extremity of the facies auricularis and the posterior upper extremity of the incisura ischiadica major.

s. ili′aca poste′rior supe′rior [TA] posterior superior iliac spine: a blunt bony projection on the posterior border of the ilium, forming the posterior end of the iliac crest.

s. ischia′dica [TA], s. ischia′lis spine of ischium: a strong process of bone projecting backward and medialward from the posterior border of the ischium, on a level with the lower border of the acetabulum and serving to separate the major and minor ischiadic notches. Called also *ischial spine*.

s. mea′tus s. suprameatica.

s. menta′lis infe′rior [TA] inferior mental spine: the lower part of a small bony projection located on the internal surface of the mandible, near the lower end of the midline and above the anterior end of the mylohyoid line, serving for attachment of the geniohyoid muscle. Called also *inferior genial tubercle*.

s. menta′lis supe′rior [TA] superior mental spine: the upper part of a small bony projection located on the internal surface of the mandible, near the lower end of the midline and above the anterior end of the mylohyoid line, serving for attachment of the genioglossus muscle. Called also *superior genial tubercle*.

s. nasa′lis ante′rior maxil′lae [TA] anterior nasal spine of maxilla: the sharp anterosuperior projection at the anterior extremity of the nasal crest of the maxilla.

s. nasa′lis os′sis fronta′lis [TA] nasal spine of frontal bone: a rough and somewhat irregular process of bone projecting downward and forward from the front part of the inferior surface of the pars nasalis of the frontal bone and fitting between the nasal bones and the ethmoid bone; called also *s. frontalis*.

s. nasa′lis poste′rior os′sis palati′ni [TA] posterior nasal spine of palatine bone: a small, sharp, backward-projecting bony spine forming the medial posterior angle of the horizontal plate of the palatine bone; called also *nasal spine of palatine bone*.

s. os′sis sphenoida′lis [TA] spine of sphenoid bone: a small bony process projecting inferiorly from the inferior aspect of the greater wing of the sphenoid bone where the wing projects into the angle between the petrous and squamous portions of the temporal bone; it is just posterior to the foramen spinosum and serves for attachment of the sphenomandibular and pterygospinous ligaments.

spi′nae palati′nae [TA] palatine spines: ridges which are laterally placed on the inferior surface of the maxillary part of the hard palate, separating the palatine sulci.

s. sca′pulae [TA] spine of scapula: a triangular plate of bone attached by one edge to the back of the scapula, its tip being at the vertebral border of the scapula; it passes laterally toward the shoulder joint and at its base bears the acromion.

s. suprameata′lis TA alternative for *s. suprameatica*.

s. suprамea′tica [TA] suprameatal spine: a pointed process that sometimes projects from the temporal bone, just above and at the back of the external acoustic meatus. Called also *Henle spine* and *s. suprameatalis* [TA alternative].

s. trochlea′ris [TA] trochlear spine: a spicule of bone on the anteromedial part of the orbital surface of the frontal bone for attachment of the trochlea of the superior oblique muscle; when absent, it is represented by the trochlear fovea.

s. tympa′nica ma′jor [TA] greater tympanic spine: a spine of the temporal bone forming the anterior edge of the tympanic notch (deficient part of tympanic sulcus).

s. tympa′nica mi′nor [TA] lesser tympanic spine: a spine of the temporal bone forming the posterior edge of the tympanic notch.

s. vento′sa a true dactylitis occurring mostly in infants and young children, characterized by enlargement of the fingers or toes, with caseation, sequestration, and sinus formation.

spi•nae (spi′ne) [L.] genitive and plural of *spina.*

spi•nal (spi′nəl) [L. *spinalis*] 1. pertaining to a spine. 2. pertaining to the vertebral column; called also *rachial, rachidial,* and *rachidian.* 3. pertaining to the spinal cord's functioning independently from the brain; see under *animal* and *reflex.*

spi•na•lis (spi-na′lis) [L.] spinal.

spi•nate (spi′nāt) [L. *spinatus*] having thorns; shaped like a thorn.

spin•dle (spin′dəl) 1. a rod or pin that tapers at one end or both ends, or something having this shape. 2. the fusiform figure occurring in the cell nucleus during the metaphase of mitosis, composed of microtubules radiating from the centrioles and connecting the centrally located chromosomes at their centromeres. Called also *mitotic s.* and *nuclear s.* 3. a type of fusiform brain wave occurring on the electroencephalogram in groups at a frequency of about 14 per second, usually while the patient is falling asleep. 4. muscle s.

aortic s. the dilated part of the aorta just below the isthmus; called also *His s.*

Axenfeld-Krukenberg s. Krukenberg s.

cleavage s. any spindle formed during cleavage of the zygote.

enamel s's clublike structures in the inner third of the dental enamel, believed to be terminals of protoplasmic processes of the odontoblasts that have passed across the dentinoenamel junction.

His s. aortic s.

Krukenberg s. a vertical spindle-shaped, brownish-red opacity on the posterior surface of the cornea.

mitotic s. spindle (def. 2).

muscle s. a fusiform end organ found between skeletal muscle fibers and acting as a mechanoreceptor; the muscle spindles are arranged in parallel with muscle fibers, and respond to passive stretch of the muscle but cease to discharge if the muscle contracts isotonically, thus signaling muscle length. The muscle spindle is the receptor responsible for the stretch or myotatic reflex. Called also *neuromuscular s.*

neuromuscular s. muscle s.

neurotendinous s. Golgi tendon organ.

nuclear s. spindle (def. 2).

sleep s's bursts of activity at frequencies of about 14 per second, seen on the electroencephalogram in light or early sleep.

tendon s. Golgi tendon organ.

urine s's spindle-shaped, urine-filled segments of the ureter due to occlusion.

spine (spīn) 1. spina (def. 1). 2. columna vertebralis. 3. bar (def. 6).

alar s., angular s. spina ossis sphenoidalis.

bamboo s. the rigid spine produced by ankylosing spondylitis; so called because of the radiographic appearance caused by lipping of the vertebral margins.

cervical s. the part of the spine comprising the cervical vertebrae.

cleft s. spina bifida.

dendritic s. gemmule (def. 2).

frontal s. spina nasalis ossis frontalis.

s. of helix spina helicis.

hemal s. a ventral projection from the hemal arch, which is attached to the underside of certain vertebral centra in lower vertebrates.

Henle s., s. of Henle spina suprameatica.

iliac s. any of four bony projections on the ilium; see terms beginning *spina iliaca.*

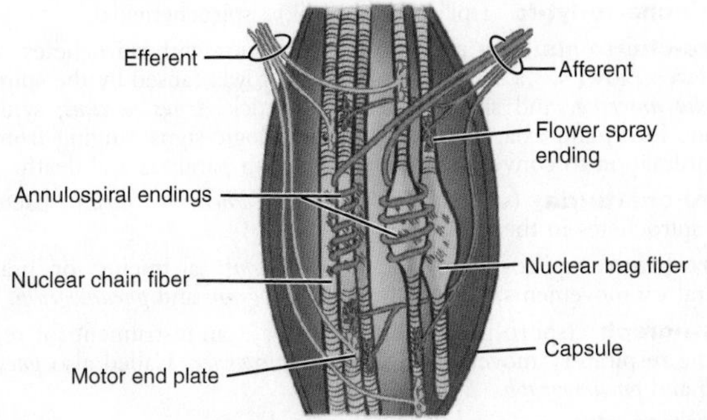

■ Diagrammatic cross-section of a muscle spindle showing the intrafusal fibers and afferent and efferent endings.

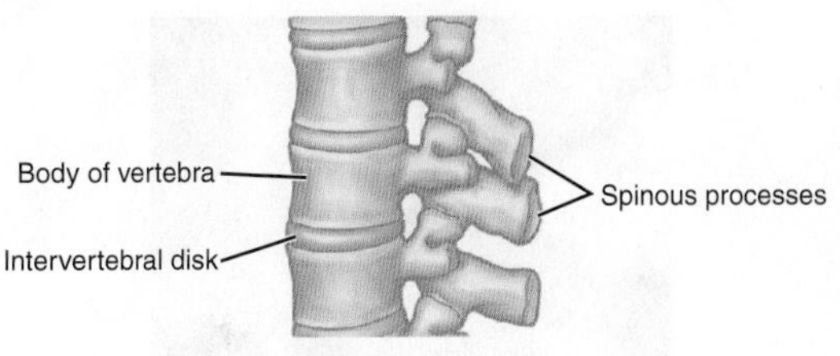

■ Kissing spines.

iliac s., anterior inferior spina iliaca anterior inferior.

iliac s., anterior superior spina iliaca anterior superior.

iliac s., posterior inferior spina iliaca posterior inferior.

iliac s., posterior superior spina iliaca posterior superior.

ischial s., s. of ischium spina ischiadica.

kissing s's a condition in which the spinous processes of adjacent vertebrae are in contact; called also *Baastrup disease* or *syndrome.*

lumbar s. the part of the spine comprising the lumbar vertebrae.

s. of maxilla spina nasalis anterior maxillae.

meatal s. spina suprameatica.

mental s., inferior spina mentalis inferior.

mental s., superior spina mentalis superior.

nasal s., anterior 1. spina nasalis anterior maxillae. 2. a cephalometric landmark: the tip of this spine as seen on the x-ray film in norma lateralis.

nasal s., posterior spina nasalis posterior ossis palatini.

nasal s. of frontal bone spina nasalis ossis frontalis.

nasal s. of palatine bone spina nasalis posterior ossis palatini.

nasal s. of palatine bone, posterior spina nasalis posterior ossis palatini.

neural s. processus spinosus vertebrae.

peroneal s. of calcaneus trochlea fibularis calcanei.

pharyngeal s. tuberculum pharyngeum.

poker s. the ankylosed spine produced by rheumatoid spondylitis; so called because of its rigidity.

pubic s., s. of pubis tuberculum pubicum.

rigid s. poker s.

s. of scapula spina scapulae.

sciatic s. spina ischiadica.

s. of sphenoid bone, sphenoidal s. spina ossis sphenoidalis.

suprameatal s. spina suprameatica.

thoracic s. the part of the spine comprising the thoracic vertebrae.

thoracolumbar s. see under *junction.*

tympanic s., anterior, tympanic s., greater spina tympanica major.

tympanic s., lesser, tympanic s., posterior spina tympanica minor.

typhoid s. a painful condition of the spine due to osteomyelitis of the vertebrae following typhoid fever.

Spi•nel•li operation (spe-nel′e) [Pier Giuseppe *Spinelli,* Italian gynecologist, 1862–1929] see under *operation.*

Spin•hal•er (spin′hāl-ər) trademark for a type of dry powder inhaler that delivers single doses of medication.

spi•nif•u•gal (spi-nif′u-gəl) [*spin-* + *-fugal*[2]] going, conducting, or moving away from the spinal cord.

spi•nip•e•tal (spi-nip′ə-təl) [*spin-* + *-petal*] tending, conducting, or moving toward the spinal cord.

spinn•bar•keit (spin′bahr-kīt) [Ger.] the formation of an elastic thread by mucus of the uterine cervix when it is drawn out; the time of maximum elasticity usually precedes or coincides with ovulation.

spin(o)- [L. *spina* spine] a combining form denoting relationship to the spine. See also words beginning spondyl(o)- and vertebr(o)-.

spi•no•bul•bar (spi″no-bul′bər) 1. pertaining to the spinal cord and the medulla oblongata. 2. extending from the spinal cord to the medulla oblongata.

spi•no•cel•lu•lar (spi″no-sel′u-lər) containing, made up of, or marked by prickle cells.

spi•no•cer•e•bel•lar (spi″no-ser″ə-bel′ər) pertaining to the spinal cord and the cerebellum.

spi•no•cer•e•bel•lum (spi″no-ser″ə-bel′əm) [*spino-* + *cerebellum*] [TA] the portion of the cerebellum serving as the primary site of termination of the major spinocerebellar afferents, roughly corresponding to the vermis of the cerebellum, the anterior lobe, the paramedian lobule (in which the body is represented), and the paraflocculus; this term is sometimes equated with paleocerebellum. Cf. *vestibulocerebellum* and *pontocerebellum.*

spi•no•cor•ti•cal (spi″no-kor′tĭ-kəl) pertaining to or extending between the spinal cord and the cerebral cortex.

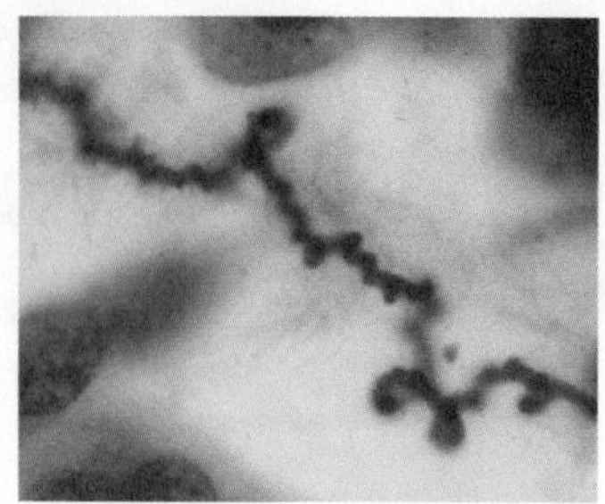

■ Curschmann spiral.

spi•no•cos•tal•is (spi″no-kos-ta′lis) the serratus posterior superior and inferior muscles together.

spi•no•gle•noid (spi″no-gle′noid) pertaining to the spine of the scapula and the glenoid cavity.

spi•no•gram (spi′no-gram) a radiograph of the spine or of the spinal cord.

spi•no•pel•vic (spi″no-pel′vik) pertaining to or affecting the spine and the pelvis.

spi•nop•e•tal (spi-nop′ə-təl) spinipetal.

spi•nose (spi′nōs) spinous.

spi•no•tec•tal (spi″no-tek′təl) tectospinal.

spi•no•tha•lam•ic (spi″no-thə-lam′ik) pertaining to or extending between the spinal cord and the thalamus.

spi•nous (spi′nəs) [L. *spinosus*] 1. like a spine; acanthoid. 2. pertaining to a spine or to a spinelike process.

spir. [L.] spir′itus (spirit).

spir•a•cle (spir′ə-kəl) [L. *spirare* to breathe] a breathing orifice of arthropods; an accessory opening for the intake of water in the respiratory system of cartilaginous fish.

spir•ad•e•no•car•ci•no•ma (spīr-ad″ə-no-kahr″sĭ-no′mə) [*spir-*[1] + *adenocarcinoma*] a type of adnexal carcinoma of a sweat gland, representing a spiradenoma that has undergone malignant transformation.

spir•ad•e•no•ma (spīr″ad-ə-no′mə) [*spir-*[1] + *adenoma*] a type of adnexal adenoma that is poorly differentiated; it may tend towards either eccrine or apocrine gland tissue.

eccrine s. a benign, solitary, deep-seated nodule arising from the coil portion of an eccrine sweat gland.

spi•ral (spi′rəl) [L. *spiralis*, from *spira*; Gr. *speira*] 1. winding about a center like a coil or the thread of a screw; called also *helical.* 2. a winding structure. See also *coil*, *helix*, *vortex*, and *whorl.*

Curschmann s's coiled mucinous fibrils sometimes found in the sputum in bronchial asthma. Cf. *Laënnec pearls.*

Perroncito s's apparatus of Perroncito.

spir•a•my•cin (spir″ə-mi′sin) a macrolide antibiotic produced by *Streptomyces ambofaciens;* effective against many gram-positive and some gram-negative organisms, as well as *Toxoplasma gondii*; used as an alternative agent in the treatment of toxoplasmosis during pregnancy. It is occasionally used to treat bacterial infections. Administered orally, intravenously, or rectally.

spi•ril•la (spi-ril′ə) [L., dim. of *spira* coil] plural of *spirillum.*

Spi•ril•la•ceae (spi″ril-a′se-e) a family of gram-negative, microaerophilic, motile, helical bacteria of the order Nitrosomonadales, occurring in stagnant freshwater environments. It contains a single genus, *Spirillum.*

spi•ril•lary (spi′rĭ-lar″e) pertaining to or caused by spirilla.

spi•ril•lo•sis (spi″rĭ-lo′sis) any disease condition caused by spirilla within the body.

Spi•ril•lum (spi-ril′əm) [L., dim. of *spira* coil] a genus of gram-negative bacteria of the family Spirillaceae, consisting of short, rigid, helical cells with bipolar flagella; organisms are motile, and microaerophilic or aerobic, with a respiratory metabolism, and are found in stagnant freshwater environments. The type species is *S. vo′lutans.*

S. mi′nus a species of gram-negative bacteria incertae sedis of the family Spirillaceae, consisting of rigid, tightly coiled, spiral rods that are motile by bipolar flagella. It is a normal parasite of the nasopharynx of rats and mice and is the etiologic agent of the spirillary form of rat-bite fever.

spi•ril•lum (spi-ril′əm) pl. *spiril′la* [L., dim. of *spira* coil] 1. a bacterium of the genus *Spirillum.* 2. more generally, any spiral-shaped bacterium.

spir•it (spir′it) [L. *spiritus*] 1. any volatile or distilled liquid. 2. an alcoholic or hydroalcoholic solution of a volatile material. 3. in traditional Chinese medicine, shen (q.v.).

aromatic ammonia s. [USP], **aromatic s. of ammonia** a preparation compounded of ammonium carbonate, strong ammonia solution, lemon oil, lavender oil, nutmeg oil, alcohol, and purified water; used as a respiratory stimulant in syncope, weakness, or threatened faint. In veterinary medicine, it is used as a respiratory and circulatory stimulant, and sometimes as a carminative and antacid.

benzaldehyde s. a mixture of benzaldehyde, alcohol, and distilled water; used as a flavoring agent.

camphor s. [USP] a solution of camphor and alcohol, used topically as a local counterirritant.

compound orange s. an alcoholic preparation containing orange, lemon, coriander, and anise oils; used as a flavoring agent.

peppermint s. [USP] a preparation of peppermint, peppermint oil, and alcohol, containing in 100 mL between 9.0 and 11.0 mL of peppermint oil; used as a digestive aid and flavor. Called also *essence of peppermint.*

s's of turpentine turpentine oil.

Spi•ri•va (spi-re′və) trademark for a preparation of tiotropium bromide.

spir(o)-[1] [Gr. *speira* coil] a combining form denoting relationship to a coil or spiral.

spir(o)-[2] [L. *spirare* to breathe] a combining form denoting relationship to the breath or to breathing.

Spi•ro•cer•ca (spi″ro-ser′kə) a genus of nematodes of the superfamily Spiruroidea. *S. lu′pi* (called also *S. sanguinolen′ta*) infests the walls of the aorta, esophagus, and stomach of canines and felines, forming large nodules; see *spirocercosis.*

Spi•ro•cer•ci•dae (spi″ro-sur′kĭ-de) a family of nematodes of the superfamily Spiruroidea, many species of which infect the digestive tracts of mammals. Genera of veterinary interest include *Ascarops*, *Physocephalus*, and *Spirocerca.*

spi•ro•cer•co•sis (spi″ro-sər-ko′sis) infestation of the esophagus or aorta of a canine or feline with *Spirocerca lupi*, which forms large nodules that sometimes obstruct the lumen and sometimes undergo transformation into a sarcoma.

Spi•ro•chae•ta•ceae (spi″ro-ke-ta′se-e) [*spiro-*[1] + Gr. *chaitē* hair] a family of bacteria of the order Spirochaetales consisting of slender, undulating, motile organisms, 6 to 500 μm in length, occurring in the form of spirals with one or more complete turns in the helix. Organisms of medical interest are contained in the genera *Borrelia* and *Treponema.*

Spi•ro•chae•ta•les (spi″ro-ke-ta′lēz) an order of bacteria of the class Spirochaetes comprising free-living, commensal, and parasitic organisms, with some being pathogenic; organisms of medical interest are contained in the families Spirochaetaceae, Leptospiraceae, and Serpulinaceae.

Spi•ro•chae•tes (spi″ro-ke′tēz) 1. a phylum of bacteria consisting of gram-negative, highly flexible, helical cells that are motile by protoplasmic flagella; organisms are chemo-organotrophic and may be anaerobic, microaerophilic, facultatively anaerobic, or aerobic. Members are free-living or associated with animal hosts; some are pathogenic. It contains the single class Spirochaetes. 2. the sole class of the order Spirochaetes. It contains the single order Spirochaetales.

spi•ro•che•tal (spi″ro-ke′təl) pertaining to or caused by spirochetes.

spi•ro•chete (spi′ro-kēt) [*spiro-*[1] + Gr. *chaitē* hair] a spiral bacterium; a general term for any microorganism of the order Spirochaetales; it includes the common pathogenic genera *Borrelia*, *Leptospira*, and *Treponema.*

spi•ro•che•te•mia (spi″ro-ke-te′me-ə) [*spirochete* + *-emia*] the presence of spirochetes in the blood.

spi•ro•che•ti•ci•dal (spi″ro-ke″tĭ-si′dəl) [*spirochete* + L. *caedere* to kill] destructive to spirochetes.

spi•ro•che•tol•y•sin (spi″ro-ke-tol′ĭ-sin) a substance that causes lysis of spirochetes.

spi•ro•che•to•lyt•ic (spi″ro-ke″to-lit′ik) spirocheticidal.

spi•ro•che•to•sis (spi″ro-ke-to′sis) infection with spirochetes.

avian s., fowl s. a septicemic disease of fowls caused by the spirochete *Borrelia anserina*, and spread by the fowl tick *Argas persicus;* symptoms include fever, anorexia, diarrhea, and neurologic signs ranging from mild incoordination to convulsions, sometimes with paralysis and death.

spi•ro•che•tu•ria (spi″ro-ke-tu′re-ə) [*spirochete* + *-uria*] bacteriuria with spirochetes in the urine.

spi•ro•gram (spi′ro-gram) [*spiro-*[2] + *-gram*] a tracing or graph of respiratory movements. Called also *pneumatogram* and *pneumogram.*

spi•ro•graph (spi′ro-graf) [*spiro-*[2] + *-graph*] an instrument for registering the respiratory movements. See also *spirometer.* Called also *pneumatograph* and *pneumograph.*

spi•rog•ra•phy (spi-rog′rə-fe) the graphic measurement of breathing, including breathing movements and breathing capacity. See also *spirometry.* Called also *pneumography.*

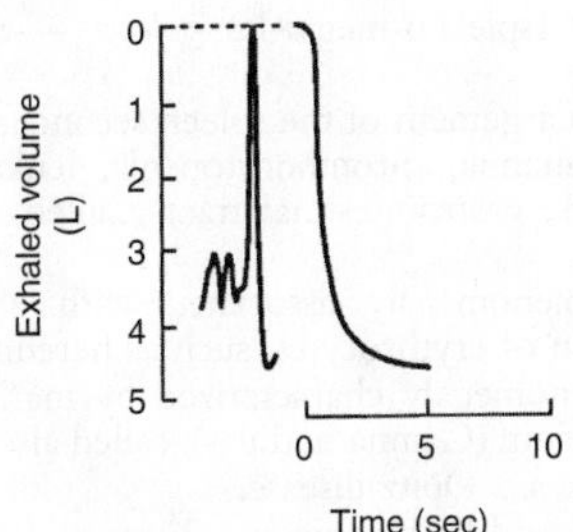

■ Normal spirogram, showing first quiet breathing then a maximal inspiration and expiration without concern for timing, followed by a timed maximal inspiration and as complete, forceful, and rapid an exhalation as possible.

spi•roid (spi′roid) resembling a spiral; cf. *helicoid.*

spi•ro•in•dex (spi″ro-in′deks) [*spiro-*[2] + *index*] the value obtained by dividing the vital capacity by the height of the individual.

spi•ro•lac•tone (spi″ro-lak′tōn) any of a group of compounds bearing 17α-propionic acid as gamma-lactone with 17β-hydroxyl, capable of opposing the action of sodium-retaining steroids on renal transport of sodium and potassium. Three such compounds have been studied. The first contains angular methyl groups at C_{13} and C_{10}, and is 3-(3-keto-17β-hydroxy-4-androsten-17α-yl)-propionic acid-γ-lactone; the second, without the angular methyl group at C_{10}, is more potent; and the third (spironolactone), with a thioacetyl group at C_7, is highly active orally.

spi•ro•ma (spi-ro′mə) spiradenoma.

spi•rom•e•ter (spi-rom′ə-tər) [*spiro-*[2] + *-meter*] an instrument for measuring the air inhaled into and exhaled from the lungs, such as in pulmonary function tests.

Spi•ro•me•tra (spi″ro-me′trə) [*spiro-*[1] + Gr. *metra* womb, uterus] a genus of tapeworms of the family Diphyllobothriidae, parasites of fish-eating cats, dogs, and birds. Infection in humans is caused by eating inadequately cooked fish.

S. erinaceieuropae′i a species parasitic in humans, dogs, and cats.

S. mansonoi′des a species parasitic in dogs and cats, especially bobcats, which may cause diarrhea and anemia; infection with the larvae may cause sparganosis in humans.

spi•ro•met•ric (spi″ro-met′rik) pertaining to spirometry or the spirometer.

spi•rom•e•try (spi-rom′ə-tre) the measurement of the breathing capacity of the lungs, such as in pulmonary function tests. See also *spirography.*

bronchoscopic s. bronchospirometry.

incentive s. a maneuver in which maximum inhalations are done by the patient and sustained with the encouragement of visual feedback until predicted inspiratory reserve volume is achieved.

spir•o•no•lac•tone (spi″rə-no-lak′tōn) [USP] a synthetic 17-spirolactone steroid and aldosterone antagonist that is a potassium-sparing diuretic; it blocks the aldosterone-dependent exchange of sodium and potassium in the distal renal tubule, which increases excretion of sodium and water and decreases excretion of potassium. Used in the treatment of edema, hypokalemia, primary aldosteronism, and, usually in combination with other drugs, hypertension.

Spi•rop•tera (spi-rop′tər-ə) a genus of nematodes of the family Habronematidae. *S. neoplas′tica* causes gastric carcinoma in rats.

spi•ro•scope (spi′ro-skōp) [*spiro-*[2] + *-scope*] an apparatus for respiration exercises by which the patient can see the amount of water displaced in a given time and thus gauge his respiratory capacity.

spi•ros•co•py (spi-ros′kə-pe) the use of the spiroscope.

Spi•ru•roi•dea (spi″roo-roi′de-ə) a superfamily of phasmid nematodes, including the families Gnathostomatidae, Physalopteridae, Spirocercidae, and Thelaziidae.

Spitz nevus (spits) [Sophie *Spitz,* American pathologist, 1910–1956] see under *nevus.*

Spitz•ka nucleus, tract (spits′kə) [Edward Charles *Spitzka,* New York neurologist, 1852–1914] see *Perlia nucleus,* under *nucleus,* and see *tractus posterolateralis.*

Spitz•ka-Lis•sau•er tract (column) (spits′kə lis′ou-ər) [E.C. *Spitzka;* Heinrich *Lissauer,* German neurologist, 1861–1891] tractus posterolateralis.

splanch•nes•the•sia (splank″nes-the′zhə) visceral sense. **splanchnesthet′ic** *adj*

splanch•nic (splank′nik) 1. visceral. 2. pertaining to one of the splanchnic nerves.

splanch•ni•cec•to•my (splank″nĭ-sek′tə-me) [*splanchnic* + *-ectomy*] resection of one or more of the splanchnic nerves for the treatment of hypertension or intractable pain.

splanch•ni•cot•o•my (splank″nĭ-kot′ə-me) [*splanchnic* + *-otomy*] splanchnicectomy.

splanchn(o)- [Gr. *splanchnos* viscus] a combining form denoting relationship to a viscus, now used primarily in embryology. For terms not found here, see those beginning *enter(o)-* or *viscer(o)-*.

splanch•no•coele (splank′no-sēl) [*splanchno-* + *-coele*] the portion of the embryonic body cavity, or coelom, from which are developed the abdominal, pericardial, and pleural cavities; called also *pleuroperitoneal cavity.*

splanch•no•cra•ni•um (splank″no-kra′ne-əm) viscerocranium.

splanch•no•derm (splank′no-dərm) splanchnopleure.

splanch•nol•o•gy (splank-nol′ə-je) [*splanchno-* + *-logy*] 1. the scientific study of the viscera of the body. 2. the body of knowledge about the viscera.

splanch•no•meg•a•ly (splank″no-meg′ə-le) organomegaly.

splanch•no•pleure (splank′no-ploor) [*splanchno-* + Gr. *pleura* side] the layer formed by the union of the splanchnic mesoderm with endoderm; from it are developed the muscles, as well as the connective tissue of the digestive tube. Called also *splanchnoderm.* **splanchnopleu′ral** *adj*

splanch•not•o•my (splank-not′o-me) viscerotomy.

S-plasty (es′plas″te) in plastic surgery, a technique for distributing the contractile forces of wound healing in more than one direction by making an S-shaped incision, instead of a straight line, in areas where skin is loose.

splay•foot (spla′foot) flatfoot.

splay•leg (spla′leg) myofibrillar hypoplasia.

spleen (splēn) [Gr. *splēn;* L. *splen*] a large glandlike but ductless organ in the upper part of the abdominal cavity on the left side lateral to the cardiac end of the stomach; it has a flattened oblong shape and is about 125 mm long, the largest structure in the lymphoid system. It has a purple color and a pliable consistency, and is distinguished by two types of tissue: red pulp and white pulp, named for their appearance on the cut surface of the organ. The spleen disintegrates red blood cells and sets free hemoglobin, which the liver converts into bilirubin; it serves as a reservoir of blood; and it produces lymphocytes and plasma cells. During fetal life and in the newborn it gives rise to new red blood cells. It has other important functions whose full scope has not been entirely determined. Called also *splen* [TA] and *lien* [TA alternative]. **splen′ic** *adj*

accessory s. splen accessorius.

bacon s. a spleen with areas of amyloid degeneration, giving its cut surfaces the appearance of fried bacon.

cyanotic s. a contracted form of spleen due to passive congestion.

diffuse waxy s. amyloid degeneration of the spleen involving especially the coats of the venous sinuses and the reticulum of the organ.

enlarged s. splenomegaly.

flecked s. of Feitis multiple necroses of the spleen, characterized by nonembolic multiple areas of anemic necrosis.

floating s. a spleen displaced and abnormally movable; called also *wandering s.*

Gandy-Gamna s. siderotic splenomegaly.

lardaceous s. waxy s.

movable s. floating s.

porphyry s. a spleen which is the seat of nodular infiltration.

sago s. a spleen having on its cut surface the appearance of grains of sago; due to amyloid infiltration.

speckled s. flecked s. of Feitis.

wandering s. floating s.

waxy s. a spleen affected with amyloid degeneration; called also *lardaceous s.*

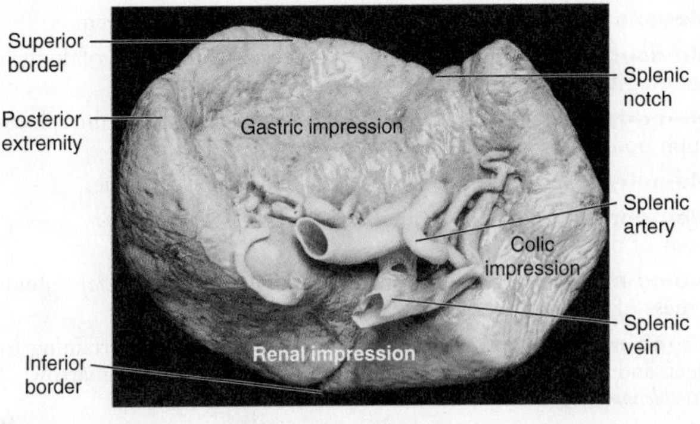

■ Spleen; visceral surface.

splen (splen) [Gr. *splēn*] [TA] a large glandlike but ductless organ in the upper part of the abdominal cavity; see *spleen*. Called also *lien* [TA alternative].

s. accesso′rius [TA] accessory spleen: a connected or detached outlying portion, or exclave, of the spleen; called also *lien accessorius* [TA alternative], *splenulus*, and *splenunculus*.

sple•nal•gia (sple-nal′jə) [*splen-* + *-algia*] pain in the spleen; called also *splenodynia*.

sple•nat•ro•phy (sple-nat′rə-fe) atrophy of the spleen.

Splen•do•re-Hoep•pli phenomenon (splen-dor′ra hur′ple) [Alphonso *Splendore*, Italian physician in Brazil, 1871–1953; Reinhard J. C. *Hoeppli*, Swiss parasitologist, 1893–1973] see under *phenomenon*.

sple•nec•ta•sis (sple-nek′tə-sis) splenomegaly.

sple•nec•to•mize (sple-nek′tə-mīz) to remove the spleen.

sple•nec•to•my (sple-nek′tə-me) [*splen-* + *-ectomy*] excision or extirpation of the spleen.

sple•nec•to•pia (sple″nek-to′pe-ə) [*splen-* + *ectopia*] displacement of the spleen; wandering or floating spleen.

sple•nel•co•sis (sple″nəl-ko′sis) [*splen-* + *elcosis*] ulceration of the spleen.

sple•ne•mia (sple-ne′me-ə) [*splen-* + *-emia*] congestion of the spleen with blood.

sple•nem•phrax•is (sple″nəm-frak′sis) [*splen-* + *emphraxis*] congestion of the spleen.

sple•ni•al (sple′ne-əl) pertaining to the splenium corporis callosi or to the splenius muscle.

splen•ic•ter•us (splen-ik′tər-əs) [*splen-* + *icterus*] inflammation of the spleen associated with jaundice.

splen•i•form (splen′ĭ-form) resembling the spleen.

splen•i•ser•rate (splen″ĭ-ser′āt) pertaining to the splenius and the serratus muscles.

sple•ni•tis (sple-ni′tis) [*splen-* + *-itis*] inflammation of the spleen, a condition usually produced by pyemia. It is attended by enlargement of the organ with pus, and is marked by much local pain.

sple•ni•um (sple′ne-um) [L., from Gr. *splēnion* bandage] 1. a bandlike structure. 2. a bandage or compress. 3. s. corporis callosi.

s. cor′poris callo′si [TA] the posterior rounded end of the corpus callosum; it conveys visual information between the two cerebral hemispheres.

splen(o)- [Gr. *splēn* spleen] a combining form denoting relationship to the spleen.

sple•no•blast (sple′no-blast) the cell from which a splenocyte develops.

sple•no•cele (sple′no-sēl) [*spleno-* + *-cele*[1]] hernia of the spleen.

sple•no•col•ic (sple″no-kol′ik) [*spleno-* + *colic* (def. 1)] pertaining to the spleen and colon.

sple•no•cyte (sple′no-sīt) the monocyte characteristic of the spleen.

sple•no•dyn•ia (sple″no-din′e-ə) splenalgia.

sple•nog•e•nous (sple-noj′ə-nəs) arising in or formed by the spleen.

sple•no•gram (sple′no-gram) 1. a radiograph of the spleen. 2. a differential count of the cells found in a stained preparation of material obtained by splenic puncture.

sple•nog•ra•phy (sple-nog′rə-fe) [*spleno-* + *-graphy*] 1. radiography of the spleen. 2. a description of the spleen.

sple•no•hep•a•to•meg•a•ly (sple″no-hep″ə-to-meg′ə-le) hepatosplenomegaly.

sple•noid (sple′noid) [*spleno-* + *-oid*] resembling the spleen.

sple•nol•o•gy (sple-nol′ə-je) [*spleno-* + *-logy*] the sum of knowledge regarding the spleen, its functions and diseases.

sple•no•lym•phat•ic (sple″no-lim-fat′ik) pertaining to the spleen and lymph nodes.

sple•nol•y•sis (sple-nol′ĭ-sis) destruction of spleen tissue.

sple•no•ma (sple-no′mə) pl. *splenomas*, *spleno′mata* [*spleno-* + *-oma*] a tumor of the spleen.

sple•no•ma•la•cia (sple″no-mə-la′shə) [*spleno-* + *-malacia*] abnormal softness of the spleen; softening of the spleen.

sple•no•med•ul•lary (sple″no-med′u-lar″e) 1. of or pertaining to the spleen and bone marrow. 2. formed in the spleen and bone marrow; called also *splenomyelogenous*.

sple•no•me•ga•lia (sple″no-mə-ga′le-ə) splenomegaly.

sple•no•meg•a•ly (sple″no-meg′ə-le) [*spleno-* + *-megaly*] enlargement of the spleen.

congestive s. enlargement of the spleen secondary to portal hypertension, with ascites, anemia, thrombocytopenia, leukopenia, and episodic hemorrhage from the gastrointestinal tract. Called also *Banti disease* and *splenic anemia*.

hemolytic s. splenomegaly associated with any disorder causing increased degradation of erythrocytes, such as hereditary spherocytosis.

siderotic s. splenomegaly characterized by marked fibrosis with deposit of iron and calcium (Gamna nodules); called also *Gandy-Nanta disease*.

thrombophlebitic s. Opitz disease.

tropical s. 1. visceral leishmaniasis. 2. see under *syndrome*.

sple•nom•e•try (sple-nom′ə-tre) determination of the size of the spleen.

sple•no•my•elog•e•nous (sple″no-mi″ə-loj′ə-nəs) splenomedullary (def. 2).

sple•no•my•elo•ma•la•cia (sple″no-mi″ə-lo-mə-la′shə) [*spleno-* + *myelo-* + *-malacia*] softening of the spleen and bone marrow.

sple•no•neph•ric (sple″no-nef′rik) pertaining to the spleen and the kidney.

sple•no•neph•rop•to•sis (sple″no-nef″rop-to′sis, sple″no-nef″ro-to′sis) [*spleno-* + *nephro-* + *-ptosis*] downward displacement of the spleen and kidney on the same side.

sple•no•pan•cre•at•ic (sple″no-pan″kre-at′ik) pertaining to the spleen and the pancreas.

sple•nop•a•thy (sple-nop′ə-the) [*spleno-* + *-pathy*] any disease of the spleen.

sple•no•pexy (sple′no-pek″se) [*spleno-* + *-pexy*] surgical fixation of a mobile spleen.

sple•no•phren•ic (splen″o-fren′ik) [*spleno-* + *-phren-* + *-ic*] pertaining to the spleen and diaphragm.

sple•no•por•tog•ra•phy (sple″no-por-tog′rə-fe) splenic portography.

sple•nop•to•sis (sple″nop-to′sis, sple″no-to′sis) [*spleno-* + *-ptosis*] prolapse or downward displacement of the spleen.

sple•no•re•nal (sple″no-re′nəl) pertaining to the spleen and kidney, or to splenic and renal veins.

sple•nor•rha•gia (sple″no-ra′jə) [*spleno-* + *-rrhagia*] hemorrhage from the spleen.

sple•nor•rha•phy (sple-nor′ə-fe) [*spleno-* + *-rrhaphy*] surgical repair of the spleen.

sple•no•sis (sple-no′sis) a condition in which multiple implants of splenic tissue are present throughout the peritoneal cavity.

sple•not•o•my (sple-not′ə-me) [*spleno-* + *-tomy*] surgical incision of the spleen.

sple•no•tox•in (sple′no-tok″sin) a toxin produced by or acting on the spleen.

sple•nu•lus (splĕ′nu-ləs) pl. *sple′nuli* [L.] splen accessorius.

sple•nun•cu•lus (sple-nung′ku-ləs) splen accessorius.

splice•o•some (spli′so-sōm) [Middle Dutch *splissen* + *-some*] a large ribonucleoprotein complex, composed of various small nuclear ribonucleoproteins (snRNP) as well as other protein factors, that attaches to specific sites on pre-mRNA and catalyzes splicing out of their introns in the formation of mature mRNA.

splic•ing (spli′sing) [Middle Dutch *splissen*] the joining together of two nucleic acid segments so as to form a new genetic combination; see *DNA s.* and *RNA s.*

alternative s. the splicing of RNA at variable positions on the primary transcript as a function of the type of tissue or of the developmental stage, removing varying introns to yield distinct mRNA's that encode specific proteins; it is a mechanism for developmental regulation and for tissue specificity.

DNA s. the attachment of individual DNA molecules to each other, as occurs in vivo in the assembly of functional vertebrate immunoglobulin genes, or in vitro in various techniques of recombinant DNA technology.

RNA s. the removal (splicing out) of introns from a primary transcript and the subsequent joining (splicing together) of exons in the production of a mature RNA molecule.

splint (splint) 1. an appliance, either rigid or flexible, used to hold in position a displaced or movable part or to keep in place and protect an injured part. See also *orthosis*. 2. the act of fastening or confining with such an appliance. 3. to fasten or confine with such an appliance. 4. see *splinting* (def. 2). 5. an exostosis on the splint bone of a horse; see also *splints*.

abutment s. adjacent tooth restorations that have been rigidly united at their proximal contact areas to form a single abutment with multiple roots.

air s. a temporary splint consisting of an inflated tube that wraps around a limb for immobilization in emergency situations. Called also *inflatable s.*

airplane s. a static orthosis that holds the upper limb in abduction at the level of the shoulder; used following burns in the axillary region and for short periods following surgery to the shoulder or brachial plexus.

anchor s. a splint for fracture of the jaw, with metal loops fitting over the teeth and held together by a rod.

Anderson s. a splint for external-internal fixation of fractures: two or more long screws, Kirschner wire, or nails are inserted through the tissues into the bone above and below the fracture; each group of screws, wires or nails is attached to an external plate and the plates are joined by an adjustable screw.

Angle s. a splint for fracture of the mandible.

Asch s. a splint used in operations on the nose.

Balkan s. see under *frame.*

banjo traction s. a dynamic orthosis to aid extension of the fingers using a banjo-shaped steel bar attached to the fingers with rubber bands and plastic rings.

bite s. occlusal s.

boutonnière s. a dynamic orthosis designed to limit or correct boutonnière deformities; it encourages palmar displacement of the lateral tendons of the fingers, causing them to act as flexors and stabilize the proximal interphalangeal joints.

cap s. a plastic or metallic fracture or stabilization appliance designed to cover the crowns of the teeth and usually cemented in place.

carpal tunnel s. see under *brace.*

coaptation s's small splints adjusted about a fractured limb for the purpose of producing coaptation of fragments.

Denis Browne s. a type of ankle-foot orthosis consisting of a pair of metal foot splints joined by a cross bar; used in talipes equinovarus.

dynamic s. see under *orthosis.*

Essig-type s. a stainless steel wire passed labially and lingually around a segment of the dental arch and held in position by individual ligature wires around the contact areas of the teeth; used to stabilize fractured or re-positioned teeth.

flexor hinge s. a dynamic type of wrist-hand orthosis for a weak or paralyzed hand, activated by movements of the wrist; metacarpophalangeal flexion is accomplished via a spring and hinge mechanism when the wrist extends. Called also *flexor hinge orthosis.*

fracture s. 1. a device fabricated of metal or plastic and used to fix segments in the treatment of fractures or facial deformities. 2. a plastic material contoured to the lingual and buccal-labial aspects of the teeth and fixed with wire or cement.

Frejka pillow s. Frejka pillow.

functional s. dynamic orthosis.

Gilmer s. a stainless steel wire fastening for holding the lower teeth to the upper ones in fracture of the mandible.

Gunning s. a type of interdental splint used in treating fractures of the mandible or maxilla.

hand s. a splint that supports weakened hand muscles, with or without a wrist component; called also *hand orthosis.*

Hodgen s. a formerly common leg splint resembling a Thomas splint but with only half a ring.

inflatable s. air s.

interdental s. a splint for jaw fractures, held in place by wires passed around the teeth.

Keller-Blake s. a hinged half-ring modification of the Thomas splint for fracture of the femur.

Kingsley s. a splint for jaw fractures, consisting of a baseplate adapted to the upper dental arch, with stout metal arms extending out through the mouth and curving backward along the sides of the cheeks to provide fixation to the head cap.

Kirschner wire s. see under *wire.*

Kirschner-Eimer s. an external splint used in veterinary medicine for fixation of a long bone fracture, consisting of transverse pins driven into the bone above and below the fracture and an external clamp to hold the pins (and thus the bone fragments) in position.

knuckle bender s. a dynamic type of hand splint used to release extension contractures of the metacarpophalangeal joints. It maintains the knuckles in a flexion angle just smaller than where pain begins; over time, the joint tissues yield and stretch and the splint is readjusted.

labial s. an appliance of plastic or metal, or both, made to conform to the outer aspect of the dental arch; used in the management of jaw and facial injuries.

lingual s. a splint similar to the labial splint, but conforming to the inner aspect of the dental arch.

Liston s. a fracture splint for the femur, usually made of straight strips of wood with padding, adapted to the side of the body and thigh.

lively s. dynamic orthosis.

occlusal s. a removable dental appliance, usually plastic, covering one or both dental arches in an effort to minimize the damaging effect of bruxism and other occlusal habits; it is usually worn at night. Called also *bite, night* or *occlusal guard* and *bite s.*

opponens s. see under *orthosis.*

plaster s. a splint composed of gauze impregnated with plaster of Paris.

plastic s. pneumatic orthosis.

resting s. static orthosis.

shin s's an overuse injury characterized by strain of the flexor digitorum longus muscle occurring in athletes, with pain along the shin.

Stader s. a splint used in veterinary medicine for external-internal fixation of fractures, consisting of a metal bar that bridges the fracture and has steel pins at each end for insertion into the bone; the ends of the fractured bone are drawn together by adjusting screws.

static s. see under *orthosis.*

swan neck s. a dynamic type of hand splint designed to limit or correct swan neck deformity by restricting extension of the proximal interphalangeal joints while permitting full flexion.

Taylor s. see under *brace.*

tenodesis s. see under *orthosis.*

therapeutic s. dynamic orthosis.

Thomas s. a knee-ankle-foot orthosis consisting of two rigid rods attached to an ovoid ring that fits around the thigh; used in emergencies or for transporting patients, or combined with other apparatus to provide traction.

ulnar deviation s. a dynamic type of hand splint designed to restrict or correct ulnar deviation; metacarpophalangeal flexion is reduced but otherwise hand function is possible.

wrist s. a splint that supports or protects weakened wrist muscles; it may or may not have forearm or hand components. Called also *wrist orthosis.*

wrist cock-up s. a dynamic type of wrist splint that stabilizes and immobilizes a subluxated wrist to alleviate pain in normal hand functions.

wrist-hand s. see under *orthosis.*

splin•ter (splin′tər) 1. a small slender fragment, as a piece of fractured bone. 2. to break into small fragments.

splint•ing (splin′ting) 1. treatment by use of a splint. 2. in dentistry, the application of a fixed restoration to join two or more teeth into a single rigid unit. 3. rigidity of muscles in an effort to avoid pain caused by movement of a part.

splints (splints) development of exostoses, sometimes with inflammation, of the splint bones of horses.

split•ting (split′ing) 1. the division of a single object into two or more objects or parts. 2. in psychoanalytic theory, a primitive defense mechanism in which "objects" (persons) possessing a natural mix of positive and negative attributes are perceived as being either "all good" or "all bad." Characteristic of very young children, it is also seen in patients with borderline personality disorder and sometimes in those with other personality disorders or psychoses.

fixed s. of S_2 abnormal splitting of the second heart sound in which the gap between the aortic and pulmonic components does not vary with the phases of respiration. It is heard in patients with atrial septal defects.

s. of heart sounds the presence of two components in the first or second heart sound complexes; used chiefly to denote the separation of the elements of the second sound, with the first component heard normally corresponding to aortic valve closure (aortic second sound) and the second to pulmonic valve closure (pulmonic second sound). The gap between the two components normally varies with the phases of respiration.

reversed s. of S_2 altered splitting of the second heart sound such that the order of the components is reversed; pulmonic valve closure precedes aortic valve closure. It occurs when left-sided ejection is delayed or left-sided systole is prolonged.

sagittal s. of mandible intraoral osteotomy of the ascending mandibular ramus and posterior body of the mandible in the sagittal plane for correction of prognathism, retrognathism, or open bite; an alternative procedure confines the split to the body of the mandible.

wide s. of S_2 altered splitting of the second heart sound in which the gap between the aortic and pulmonic valve closures is increased, usually due to hemodynamic or electrical abnormalities that cause delay of the pulmonic second sound.

spol•i•go•typ•ing (spol′ĭ-go-tīp″ing) [*spacer* + *oligotyping*] an oligotyping technique for distinguishing strains of *Mycobacterium tuberculosis* by the presence or absence of certain spacer DNA sequences.

spon•dee (spon′de) [L. *spondeum* of a libation] any word of two syllables having equal stress on each syllable (e.g., pancake); used in tests of speech reception threshold.

spon•dy•lal•gia (spon″də-lal′jə) spondylodynia.

spon•dyl•ar•thri•tis (spon″dəl-ahr-thri′tis) [*spondyl-* + *arthritis*] arthritis of the spine.

s. ankylopoie′tica ankylosing spondylitis.
seronegative s. an arthritis of the seronegative spondyloarthropathies group.

spon·dyl·ar·throc·a·ce (spon″dəl-ahr-throk′ə-se) [*spondyl-* + *arthr-* + Gr. *kakē* badness] tuberculosis of the vertebrae.

spon·dyl·ar·throp·a·thy (spon″dəl-ahr-throp′ə-the) spondyloarthropathy.

spon·dyl·ex·ar·thro·sis (spon″dəl-eks″ahr-thro′sis) [*spondyl-* + Gr. *exarthrōsis* dislocation] dislocation of a vertebra.

spon·dy·li·tis (spon″də-li′tis) inflammation of the vertebrae; called also *rachitis.* **spondylit′ic** *adj*

s. ankylopoie′tica, s. ankylo′sans ankylosing s.

ankylosing s. a form of degenerative joint disease that affects the spine. It is a systemic illness of unknown etiology, affecting young persons predominantly, and producing pain and stiffness as a result of inflammation of the sacroiliac, intervertebral, and costovertebral joints; paraspinal calcification, with ossification and ankylosis of the spinal joints, may cause complete rigidity of the spine and thorax. Called also *Bekhterev arthritis* or *disease, Bekhterev s.; Marie-Strümpell s.* or *disease; Strümpell-Marie disease; rheumatoid* or *rhizomelic s.; s. deformans;* and *rhizomelic spondylosis.*

Bekhterev (Bechterew) s., s. defor′mans ankylosing s.

hypertrophic s. spondylitis with evidence of hypertrophic changes in the vertebrae.

s. infectio′sa inflammation of the vertebrae caused by a specific pathogen.

Marie-Strümpell s. ankylosing s.

muscular s. a morbid condition of the spine resulting from muscular weakness and not a true inflammation.

posttraumatic s. Kümmell disease.

rheumatoid s., rhizomelic s. ankylosing s.

traumatic s. spondylitis occurring as a result of injury to the vertebrae.

s. tuberculo′sa, tuberculous s. spinal tuberculosis.

s. typho′sa inflammation of the vertebrae following typhoid fever.

spon·dy·li·ze·ma (spon″də-li-ze′mə) [*spondyl-* + Gr. *izēmia* depression] downward displacement of a vertebra in consequence of the destruction or softening of the one below it.

spondyl(o)- [Gr. *spondylos* vertebra] a combining form denoting relationship to a vertebra, or to the vertebral column.

spon·dy·lo·ar·thri·tis (spon″də-lo-ahr-thri′tis) spondylarthritis.

spon·dy·lo·ar·throp·a·thy (spon″də-lo-ahr-throp′ə-the) disease of the joints of the spine.

seronegative s's a general term comprising a number of degenerative joint diseases having common clinical, immunologic, pathologic, and radiographic features, including synovitis of the peripheral joints, enthesopathy, bony ankylosis of the large peripheral joints, lack of rheumatoid factor, and, in many cases, a positive status for the human leukocyte antigen HLA-B27. Included in this group are *enteropathic arthritis, psoriatic arthritis, ankylosing spondylitis,* and *Reiter syndrome.*

spon·dy·loc·a·ce (spon″də-lok′ə-se) [*spondylo-* + Gr. *kakē* badness] tuberculosis of the vertebrae.

spon·dy·lo·dyn·ia (spon″də-lo-din′e-ə) [*spondyl-* + *-odynia*] pain in a vertebra. Called also *spondylalgia.* Cf. *rachiodynia.*

spon·dy·lo·epi·phys·e·al (spon″də-lo-ep″ĭ-fiz′e-əl) pertaining to the vertebrae and the epiphyses.

spon·dy·lo·lis·the·sis (spon″də-lo-lis-the′sis) [*spondyl-* + *olisthe* + *-sis*] forward displacement (olisthy) of one vertebra over another, usually of the fifth lumbar over the body of the sacrum, or of the fourth lumbar over the fifth, usually due to a developmental defect in the pars interarticularis. **spondylolisthet′ic** *adj*

congenital s. dysplastic s.

degenerative s. spondylolisthesis caused by long-standing instability due to progressive degeneration of the spinal joints, usually accompanied by rotation of the affected disk.

dysplastic s. spondylolisthesis resulting from congenital anomalies of the lumbosacral junction, allowing the fifth lumbar vertebra to slip forward on the first sacral vertebra. Called also *congenital s.*

isthmic s. spondylolisthesis accompanied by a lesion of the pars interarticularis, divided into three subtypes on the basis of the type of lesion: *lytic* (stress fracture of the pars interarticularis), *elongated* (elongation of the pars interarticularis due to continuous cracking and healing), and *acute fracture.*

pathological s. spondylolisthesis due to alterations in the structure of the pedicle, the pars articularis, or the articular processes caused by bone disease.

traumatic s. spondylolisthesis due to acute fracture of the facets, pedicle, or lamina, rather than of the pars interarticularis.

spon·dy·lol·y·sis (spon″də-lol′ĭ-sis) [*spondylo-* + *-lysis*] dissolution of a vertebra; a condition marked by platyspondylia, aplasia of the vertebral arch, and separation of the pars interarticularis.

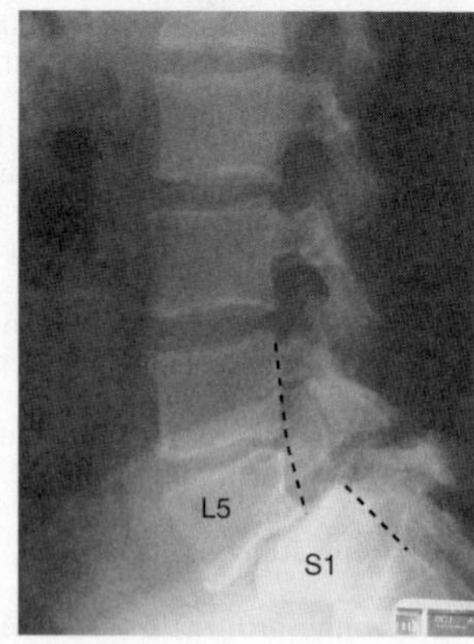

■ Spondylolisthesis due to spondylolysis; discontinuity of the posterior elements of L5 allowed forward slippage of L5 on S1.

spon·dy·lo·ma·la·cia (spon″də-lo-mə-la′shə) softening of vertebrae.

spon·dy·lop·a·thy (spon″də-lop′ə-the) [*spondylo-* + *-pathy*] any disorder of the vertebrae; called also *rachiopathy.*

traumatic s. Kümmell disease.

spon·dy·lop·to·sis (spon″də-lop-to′sis, spon″də-lo-to′sis) spondylolisthesis.

spon·dy·lo·py·o·sis (spon″də-lo-pi-o′sis) [*spondylo-* + *pyo-* + *-sis*] suppuration of a vertebra or of vertebrae.

spon·dy·los·chi·sis (spon″dĭ-los′kĭ-sis) rachischisis.

spon·dy·lo·sis (spon″də-lo′sis) 1. ankylosis of a vertebral joint. 2. degenerative spinal changes due to osteoarthritis.

cervical s. degenerative joint disease affecting the cervical vertebrae, intervertebral disks, and surrounding ligaments and connective tissue, sometimes with pain or paresthesia radiating along the upper limbs as a result of pressure on the nerve roots.

s. chro′nica ankylopoie′tica ankylosing spondylitis.

lumbar s. degenerative joint disease affecting the lumbar vertebrae and intervertebral disks, causing pain and stiffness, sometimes with sciatic radiation due to nerve root pressure by associated protruding disks or osteophytes.

rhizomelic s. ankylosing spondylitis.

s. uncovertebra′lis cervical spondylosis affecting the uncinate process of a vertebra.

spon·dy·lo·syn·de·sis (spon″də-lo-sin-de′sis) spinal fusion.

spon·dy·lot·ic (spon″də-lot′ik) pertaining to or due to spondylosis.

spon·dy·lot·o·my (spon″də-lot′ə-me) rachitomy.

spon·dy·lous (spon′də-ləs) vertebral.

sponge (spunj) [Gr. *spongia*] 1. a member of the invertebrate phylum Porifera. 2. the elastic fibrous skeleton of such an animal, used mainly as an absorbent. 3. an absorbent pad of gauze or other material.

absorbable gelatin s. [USP] a sterile, absorbable, water-insoluble gelatin-base sponge; used as a local hemostatic.

Bernays s. compressed disks of cotton that expand under moisture, used in treatment of epistaxis.

contraceptive s. a sponge impregnated with spermacide, inserted into the vagina before sexual intercourse to prevent pregnancy.

fibrin s. a spongy form of fibrin, used as a hemostatic.

gelatin s. a spongy form of denatured gelatin used as a hemostatic, especially when wet with thrombin.

spon·gi·form (spun′jĭ-form) resembling a sponge.

spongi(o)- [L., *spongia* sponge] a combining form meaning like a sponge, or denoting relationship to a sponge.

spon·gio·blast (spun′je-o-blast) [*spongio-* + *-blast*] 1. any of the embryonic epithelial cells that develop near the neural tube and later become transformed, some into neuroglial and some into ependymal cells. 2. amacrine cell.

spon·gio·blas·to·ma (spun″je-o-blas-to′mə) any tumor containing spongioblasts; considered to be one of the neuroepithelial tumors. See *gliosarcoma, glioblastoma,* and *polar s.*

s. multifor′me glioblastoma.

polar s., s. pola′re a rare malignant brain tumor seen from childhood to young adulthood, characterized by palisades of unipolar spongioblasts; sites may be either cerebral or cerebellar. Called also *piloid astrocytoma* and *unipolar s.*

unipolar s., s. unipola′re polar s.

spon•gio•cyte (spun′je-o-sīt″) 1. neuroglial cell. 2. a type of cell with spongy vacuolated protoplasm found in the adrenal cortex.

spon•gio•cy•to•ma (spun″je-o-si-to′mə) spongioblastoma.

spon•gi•oid (spun′je-oid) spongiform.

spon•gio•sa (spun″je-o′sə) [L.] 1. spongy. 2. substantia spongiosa ossium.

spon•gio•sa•plas•ty (spun″je-o′sə-plas″te) autoplasty of the substantia spongiosa ossium to potentiate formation of new bone or to cover bone defects.

spon•gi•o•sis (spun″je-o′sis) intercellular edema of the epidermis, giving the tissue a spongelike appearance due to the formation of microvesicles. **spongiot′ic** *adj*

eosinophilic s. spongiosis accompanied by infiltration of the epidermis by eosinophils.

spon•gio•si•tis (spun″je-o-si′tis) periurethritis.

spon•gy (spun′je) of a spongelike appearance or texture.

spon•ta•ne•ous (spon-ta′ne-əs) [L. *spontaneus*] 1. voluntary; instinctive. 2. occurring without external influence.

Spon•tin (spon′tin) trademark for a lyophilized preparation of ristocetins A and B.

spoon (spōōn) 1. a metallic instrument with an oval bowl to which a handle is attached. 2. spoon excavator.

Daviel s. an instrument used in removing the crystalline lens from the eye.

sharp s. a surgical instrument consisting of a spoon with sharp edges for scraping away granulations.

Volkmann s. sharp s.

spo•rad•ic (spə-rad′ik) [from Gr. *sperein* to sow seed] neither endemic nor epidemic; occurring occasionally in a random or isolated manner.

spo•ran•gia (spə-ran′je-ə) plural of *sporangium.*

spo•ran•gio•phore (spə-ran′je-o-for) [*sporangium* + *-phore*] a specialized hypha that gives rise to a sporangium.

spo•ran•gio•spore (spə-ran′je-o-spor) a spore contained in a sporangium.

spo•ran•gi•um (spə-ran′je-əm) pl. *sporan′gia* [*spore* + Gr. *angeion* vessel] a fungal or protozoal cell that produces spores internally (sporangiospores) by the process called *progressive cleavage.* See also illustration at *mold.* **sporan′gial** *adj*

Spo•ra•nox (spor′ə-noks) trademark for preparations of itraconazole.

spo•ra•tion (spo-ra′shən) sporulation.

spore (spor) [L. *spora*, Gr. *spora* seed] 1. a refractile, oval body formed within bacteria, especially genera of the family Bacillaceae *(Bacillus, Clostridium, Desulfotomaculum, Sporolactobacillus, Sporosarcina)*, which is regarded as a resting stage during the life history of the cell, and is characterized by its resistance to environmental changes. Called also *bacterial s.* 2. the reproductive element, produced sexually or asexually, of one of the lower organisms, such as protozoa, fungi, or algae. See *asexual s.*, *sexual s.*, and *sporulation.*

asexual s. a spore produced without a sexual process, such as in an imperfect fungus; see *aleuriospore*, *chlamydospore*, *conidium*, *endospore*, and *zoospore.*

bacterial s. see *spore* (def. 1).

resting s. a spore that has thick walls and remains dormant for a long period, usually to survive adverse conditions, after which it can germinate.

sexual s. a spore produced by a sexual process, such as in a perfect fungus; see *ascospore*, *basidiospore*, *oospore*, and *zygospore.*

swarm s. zoospore.

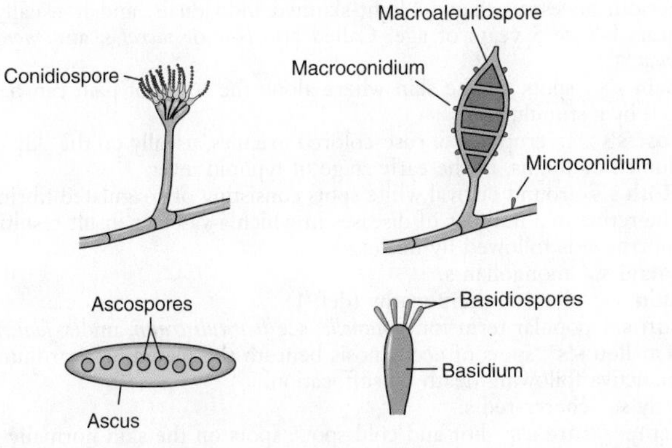

■ Various types of fungal spores.

spo•ri•ci•dal (spor″ĭ-si′dəl) [*spore* + L. *caedere* to kill] destroying spores.

spo•ri•cide (spor′ĭ-sīd) an agent that destroys spores.

spo•ri•des•min (spor″ĭ-des′min) a poison isolated from the fungus *Pithomyces chartarum;* it causes facial eczema and liver damage in sheep and cattle in New Zealand and Australia.

Spo•rid•i•a•les (spə-rid″e-a′lēz) in some systems of classification, an order of perfect fungi of the subphylum Basidiomycotina, including part of what others call order Ustilaginales. It contains the genera *Filobasidiella* and *Filobasidium.*

spo•rif•er•ous (spə-rif′ər-əs) [*spore* + *-ferous*] producing or bearing spores; called also *sporiparous.*

spo•rip•a•rous (spə-rip′ə-rəs) sporiferous.

spor(o)- [Gr. *sporos* seed] a combining form denoting relationship to a spore.

spo•ro•blast (spor′o-blast) [*sporo-* + *-blast*] 1. an immature coccidian sporocyst. 2. a mass of spore-forming cells within a pansporoblastic membrane.

Spo•rob•o•lo•my•ces (spə-rob″ə-lo-mi′sēz) a genus of Fungi Imperfecti of the form-class Hyphomycetes; several species have been isolated from human infections.

spo•ro•cyst (spor′o-sist) [*sporo-* + *cyst*] 1. any cyst, envelope, or sac containing spores or reproductive cells. 2. a germinal saclike stage in the life cycle of digenetic trematodes produced by metamorphosis of a miracidium and giving rise to rediae. 3. a stage in the life cycle of certain coccidian protozoa contained within an oocyst, produced by a sporoblast, and giving rise to sporozoites.

spo•ro•do•chi•um (spor″o-do′ke-əm) a cushion-shaped mass of hyphae covered with conidiophores.

spo•ro•duct (spor′o-dəkt) [*sporo-* + *duct*] a tubelike structure through which spores of certain sporozoans and some fungi pass to the outside of the cell.

spo•ro•gen•e•sis (spor″o-jen′ə-sis) [*sporo-* + *genesis*] sporulation (def. 1).

spo•ro•gen•ic (spor″o-jen′ik) pertaining to or characterized by sporulation. Called also *sporogenous.*

spo•rog•e•nous (spə-roj′ə-nəs) sporogenic.

spo•rog•e•ny (spə-roj′ə-ne) [*sporo-* + *-geny*] sporulation (def. 1).

spo•rog•o•ny (spə-rog′ə-ne) [*sporo-* + Gr. *goneia* generation] 1. sporulation (def. 1). 2. in protozoa, sporulation involving multiple fission of a sporont (schizogony), resulting in the production of sporocysts (if present in the life cycle) and sporozoites.

spo•ront (spor′ont) [*sporo-* + Gr. *ōn*, *ontos* being] a zygote of coccidian protozoa enclosed within an oocyst, which undergoes sporogony to produce sporoblasts, each of which forms a sporocyst containing sporozoites.

spo•ro•phore (spor′o-for) [*sporo-* + *-phore*] the part of a spore-producing organism that supports the spores.

spo•ro•phyte (spor′o-fīt) [*sporo-* + *-phyte*] the diploid or asexual stage in the alternation of generations (metagenesis) in plants.

spo•ro•plasm (spor′o-plaz″əm) [*sporo-* + *-plasm*] 1. the protoplasm of spores. 2. the central dinucleate mass of cytoplasm of certain protozoa that leaves the spore through the polar tube as an amebula to infect the host.

spo•ro•plas•mic (spor″o-plaz′mik) pertaining to or of the nature of sporoplasm.

Spo•ro•thrix (spor′o-thriks) a genus of Fungi Imperfecti of the form-class Hyphomycetes, form-family Moniliaceae. *S. schen′ckii* (formerly called *Sporotrichum schenckii*) causes sporotrichosis. Many other species, including *S. car′nis*, cause the formation of white mold on meat in cold storage.

spo•rot•ri•chin (spə-rot′rĭ-kin) a derivative of *Sporothrix schenckii* used as a skin test in the diagnosis of sporotrichosis.

spo•ro•tri•cho•sis (spor″o-trĭ-ko′sis) [*sporo-* + *trich-* + *-osis*] chronic fungal infection with *Sporothrix schenckii;* in most species it is characterized by nodular lesions of the cutaneous and subcutaneous tissues and adjacent lymphatics that suppurate and ulcerate. It is acquired by fungal implantation into the skin by trauma or through an abrasion, or by inhalation into the lungs. The infection may remain localized or may be disseminated by the bloodstream to involve the osteoarticular and musculoskeletal tissues, viscera, mucous membranes, central nervous system, eye, or genitourinary system.

spo•ro•tri•chot•ic (spor″o-tri-kot′ik) 1. pertaining to or caused by fungi of the genus *Sporothrix.* 2. pertaining to sporotrichosis.

Spo•rot•ri•chum (spə-rot′rĭ-kəm) [*sporo-* + Gr. *thrix* hair] a genus of soil-inhabiting Fungi Imperfecti of the form-class Hyphomycetes,

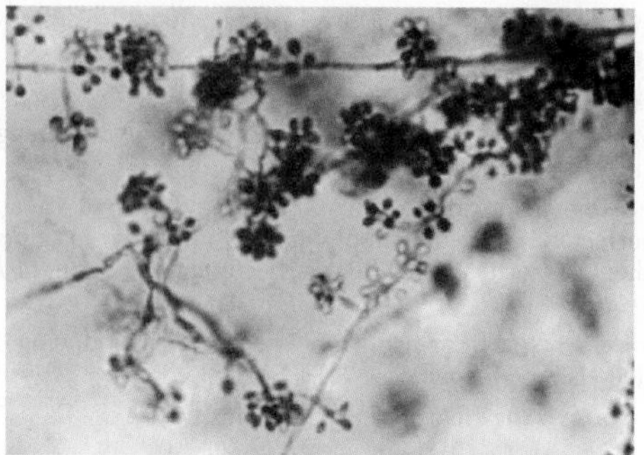
■ Mold phase of *Sporothrix schenckii,* showing sympodial conidia borne in clusters at the ends of lateral conidiophores.

form-family Moniliaceae; it formerly also included those now in the genus *Sporothrix.*

Spo•ro•zoa (spor″o-zo′ə) [*sporo-* + Gr. *zōon* animal] 1. Sporozoea. 2. in some former systems of classification, a subphylum and in others a class of protozoa, the members of which have been assigned to four phyla: Apicomplexa, Acetospora, Microspora, and Myxozoa. The organisms in the last three phyla form spores; many of the Apicomplexa do not. 3. Apicomplexa.

spo•ro•zoa (spor″o-zo′ə) plural of *sporozoon.*

spo•ro•zo•an (spor″o-zo′ən) [*sporo-* + Gr. *zōon* animal] 1. any protozoon of the class Sporozoea. 2. any of a large group of protozoa that form spores; phyla of medical or veterinary significance include Apicomplexa, Microspora, and Myxozoa. Called also *sporozoon.* 3. pertaining or relating to the protozoa in these groups.

Spo•ro•zoea (spor″o-ze′ə) a class of homoxenous or heteroxenous parasitic protozoa (phylum Apicomplexa) having a conoid (if present) forming a complete cone; both sexual and asexual phases; oocysts generally containing infective sporozoites that result from sporogeny; flagella in microgametes of some groups; and pseudopods (if present) used for feeding only. Locomotion of mature organisms is by means of body flexion, gliding, or undulation of longitudinal ridges on the body surface. Subclasses of medical interest are Coccidia and Piroplasmia. Called also *Sporozoa.*

spo•ro•zo•ite (spor″o-zo′īt) [*sporo-* + *zo-* + *-ite*] the elongate, nucleated, motile infective stage resulting from sporogony in certain protozoa. In malaria, the sporozoites of *Plasmodium* spp. are liberated from the oocysts in the mosquito, accumulate in the vector's salivary glands, and are transferred to the definitive host by the bite of the infected mosquito.

spo•ro•zo•on (spor″o-zo′on) pl. *sporozo′a.* Sporozoan (defs. 1 and 2).

spor•u•lar (spor′u-lər) pertaining to a spore.

spor•u•la•tion (spor″u-la′shən) 1. the formation of spores. Called also *sporogenesis, sporogeny,* and *sporogony.* 2. the liberation of spores.

spor•ule (spor′ūl) 1. a small spore. 2. spore.

spot (spot) a circumscribed area distinguished by its color, such as on the skin; see also *dot, macule,* and *patch.*

acoustic s's the maculae sacculi and maculae utriculi.

age s. solar lentigo.

ash leaf s. see under *macule.*

Bitot s's superficial, foamy gray, triangular spots on the conjunctiva, consisting of keratinized epithelium; they are associated with vitamin A deficiency. See also *xerosis conjunctivae.*

blind s. 1. discus nervi optici. 2. mental scotoma.

blue s. 1. *(in the pl.)* maculae ceruleae. 2. mongolian s.

Brushfield s's small white spots on the periphery of the iris, usually crescentic, with the concavity outward, frequently but not exclusively seen in children with Down syndrome.

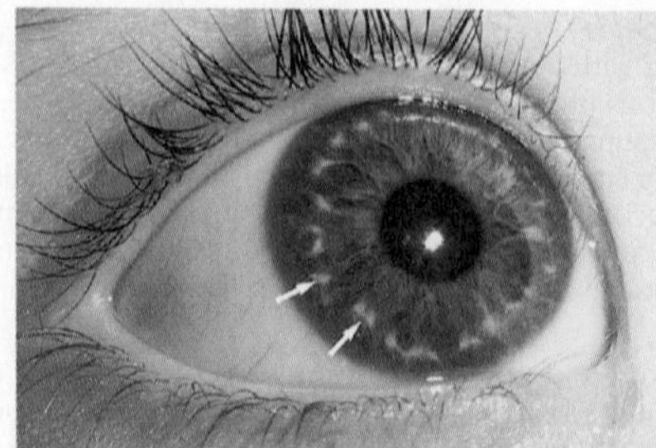
■ Brushfield spots *(arrows)* in a child with Down syndrome.

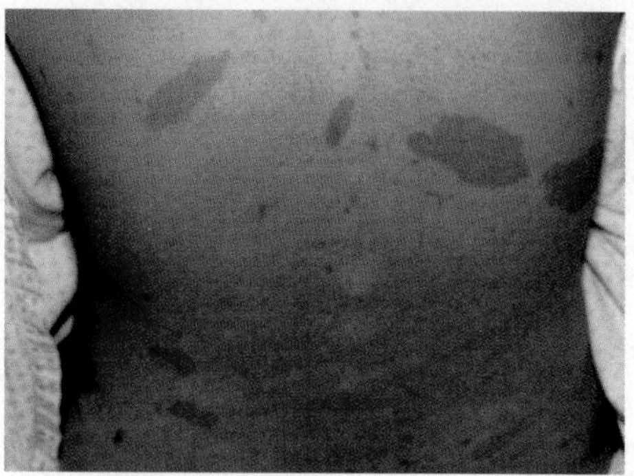
■ Café au lait spots on the back of a 9-year-old girl.

café au lait s's (kă-fa′o la′) [Fr. "coffee with milk"] pigmented macules of a distinctive light brown color, as in neurofibromatosis and Albright syndrome. Called also *café au lait macules.*

cayenne pepper s's tiny red dots on the skin, caused by tiny hemorrhages from capillaries in the upper dermis within or on the border of lesions of chronic pigmented purpura.

cherry-red s. a red circular area (the choroid) surrounded by gray-white retina, seen through the fovea centralis of the eye in Tay-Sachs disease and several other neurodegenerative storage diseases. It is caused by accumulation of sphingolipids in retinal ganglion cells, giving a whitish appearance to areas with such cells; the parafoveal area has many, while the fovea has none. Called also *Tay s.* or *sign.* See illustration at *Tay-Sachs disease,* under *disease.*

cold s. see *temperature s's.*

cotton-wool s's white or gray soft-edged opacities in the retina composed of cytoid bodies; seen in hypertensive retinopathy, lupus erythematosus, and other conditions. Called also *cotton-wool exudates* or *patches.*

deaf s. see under *point.*

De Morgan s. cherry angioma.

eye s. 1. the rudiment of an eye in the embryo. 2. eyespot.

flame s's flame-shaped hemorrhages in the nerve fiber layer of the retina.

focal s. the part of the target of an x-ray tube which is bombarded by the focused electron stream when the tube is energized.

Fordyce s's see under *granule.*

germinal s. the nucleolus of an oocyte.

hot s. 1. see *temperature s's.* 2. the sensitive area of a neuroma. 3. an area of increased density on an x-ray or thermographic film. 4. a region of a genome that has a particularly high tendency for recombination or mutation.

Koplik s's small, irregular, bright red spots on the buccal and lingual mucosa, with a minute bluish white speck in the center of each; seen in the prodromal stage of measles. Called also *Koplik sign.*

lance-ovate s. ash leaf macule.

light s. cone of light.

liver s. 1. solar lentigo. 2. *(in the pl.)* tinea versicolor.

Mariotte s. discus nervi optici.

Maurer s's see under *dot.*

mental blind s. mental scotoma.

milk s's, milky s's 1. whitish spots of fibrous thickening seen on the visceral layer of the pericardium. 2. aggregations of macrophages in the omentum or the subserous layer of the pleura and peritoneum.

mongolian s. a congenital melanocytic nevus that is flat, smooth, and blue-gray to brown; the usual location is in the lumbosacral area. It occurs far more in dark-skinned people (especially those of East Asian or Native American ancestry) than in light-skinned individuals, and it usually disappears before 5 years of age. Called also *blue* or *sacral s.* and *mongolian macula.*

pain s's spots on the skin where alone the sense of pain can be produced by a stimulus.

rose s's an eruption of rose-colored macules, usually on the skin of the abdomen or thighs, in the early stage of typhoid fever.

Roth s's round or oval white spots consisting of coagulated fibrin seen in the retina in a number of diseases in which a vascular insult resulting in hemorrhage is followed by healing.

sacral s. mongolian s.

shin s's diabetic dermopathy (def. 1).

soft s. popular term for *fontanelle;* see *fonticuli cranii,* under *fonticulus.*

Tardieu s's spots of ecchymosis beneath the pleura, pericardium, and conjunctiva following death by suffocation.

Tay s. cherry-red s.

temperature s's hot and cold spots: spots on the skin normally anesthetic to pain and pressure and sensitive respectively to heat and cold; they

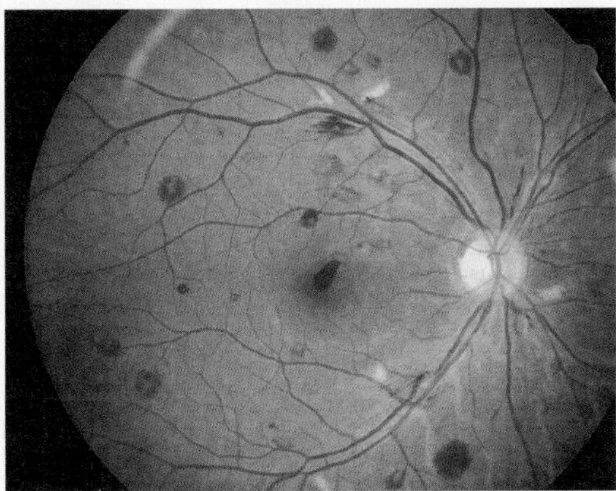

■ Roth spots, multiple hemorrhages, and perivascular infiltrates in a patient with leukemia.

are arranged in lines, often somewhat curved, and show the peculiar arrangement of the end-organ with respect to the temperature sense.

warm s's minute areas in the skin that are peculiarly sensitive to temperatures above body temperature; see *temperature s's.*

yellow s. macula lutea.

sprain (sprān) a joint injury in which some of the fibers of a supporting ligament are ruptured but the continuity of the ligament remains intact.

eversion s. an uncommon type of sprain to the ankle, in which the foot twists laterally and medial ankle ligaments are injured.

inversion s. the most common type of sprain to the ankle, in which the foot twists medially and lateral ankle ligaments are injured.

rider's s. sprain of the adductor longus muscle of the thigh, resulting from strain in riding horseback.

Schlatter s. Osgood-Schlatter disease.

spray (spra) a liquid minutely divided or nebulized as by a jet of air or steam.

needle s. a water spray administered through a device having needle-sized jets.

pepper s. an aerosolized form of oleoresins from capsicum, highly irritant to the skin and mucous membranes; used similarly to tear gas.

spread•er (spred′ər) an instrument for distributing something over a broad area.

root canal filling s. in root canal therapy, a hand-operated, smooth, pointed, tapered metal instrument used to compress filling material laterally against the walls of the canal to make room for insertion of additional cones.

spread•ing (spred′ing) a stretching out or expanding.

antigen s. the expansion of antigen-producing capabilities within a cell or from one cell to another, thought to be an important mechanism for the development of certain autoimmune conditions.

Spren•gel deformity (shpreng′gəl) [Otto Gerhard Karl *Sprengel*, German surgeon, 1852–1915] see under *deformity.*

spring (spring) 1. a piece of resilient metal, such as a hardened coiled steel wire, that will return to its original shape after bending. 2. a resilient wire attached to a denture or other appliance.

auxiliary s. a short piece of wire attached to an orthodontic appliance to serve as a lever to apply force to a tooth or teeth.

bow s. a loop spring with the shape of a labial bow; used in a removable orthodontic appliance to move teeth.

closed s. 1. a spring that has both ends attached. 2. in orthodontic appliances, a spring that has only one end anchored in the active plate.

coil s. a spiral winding of fine resilient wire; attached to orthodontic appliances to open or to close spaces between teeth.

finger s. a finger-shaped stainless steel wire spring; used interproximally as an open spring in removable orthodontic appliances.

Kesling s. a tooth-spacing spring used to gain separation between the teeth to facilitate band placement in fitting orthodontic appliances.

loop s. a closed orthodontic spring having a variety of different shapes, from that of a hairpin to that of a bow.

open s. a spring whose ends are free.

paddle s. a paddle-shaped wire spring used in removable orthodontic appliances; it is activated by bending it toward the tooth.

separating s. a spring placed between the teeth to obtain separation.

uprighting s. a coiled spring used for uprighting teeth in orthodontic therapy.

Z s. a spring bent in the form of a Z with a coil loop at each end, used to move an individual tooth or groups of teeth buccally or labially.

Sprinz-Du•bin syndrome (sprints′ doo′bin) [Helmuth *Sprinz*, German-born American pathologist, 1911–1990; Isidore Nathan *Dubin*, American pathologist, 1913–1981] Dubin-Johnson syndrome.

Sprinz-Nel•son syndrome (sprints′ nel′sun) [H. *Sprinz;* R.S. *Nelson*, American physician, 20th century] Dubin-Johnson syndrome.

sprue (sproo) [Dutch *spruw*] 1. a chronic form of malabsorption syndrome occurring in tropical and nontropical forms. 2. in a dental casting, an opening in the investment through which the molten alloy or metal can reach the mold space after the wax has been eliminated.

celiac s. see under *disease.*

collagenous s. a rare, often fatal condition resembling celiac disease but not responsive to dietary gluten withdrawal, characterized by extensive deposition of collagen in the lamina propria of the colon.

nontropical s. celiac disease.

refractory s. 1. malabsorption and flat jejunal mucosa, signs of celiac disease that do not respond to withdrawal of dietary gluten. 2. celiac disease in which initial responsiveness to gluten withdrawal deteriorates with time; it is often characterized by persistent absence of villi in the proximal mucosa and malabsorption even during the initial period of clinical responsiveness. Called also *unclassified s.*

tropical s. a malabsorption syndrome occurring in the tropics and subtropics; the malabsorption usually leads to protein-energy malnutrition and often folic acid deficiency anemia and stomatitis. It is relatively uncommon in children, and the cause is unknown.

unclassified s. refractory s.

Spry•cel (spri′sel) trademark for a preparation of dasatinib.

SPS trademark for a preparation of sodium polystyrene sulfonate.

Spt. [L.] spir′itus (spirit).

Spu•ma•vi•ri•nae (spu″mə-vir-i′ne) the foamy viruses: a former subfamily of the Retroviridae, containing the genus *Spumavirus.*

Spu•ma•vi•rus (spu′mə-vi″rəs) [L. *spuma* foam + *virus*] the foamy viruses, a genus of nonpathogenic viruses of the family Retroviridae, having characteristic virion morphology with a central condensed core and prominent surface spikes. They are named for the foamy appearance of infected cells in cultures, caused by extensive vacuolation. Capsid assembly occurs in the cytoplasm prior to budding through the plasma membrane. Organisms can induce persistent, asymptomatic infection in numerous different mammals.

spu•ma•vi•rus (spu′mə-vi″rəs) any virus of the genus *Spumavirus.*

spur (spur) 1. a pointed projection; called also *calcar.* 2. in dentistry, a piece of metal projecting from a plate, band, or other dental appliance.

calcaneal s. an abnormal bony projection on the calcaneus, most often its posterior or plantar surface; some are benign, but others cause severe pain when a person walks. Called also *heel s.*

calcarine s. calcar avis.

heel s. calcaneal s.

s. of malleus on the head of the malleus, a projection on the inferior margin of the facet for the incus; called also *cog tooth of malleus.*

occipital s. an abnormal process of bone on the occipital bone behind the posterior process of the atlas.

olecranon s. an abnormal process of bone at the insertion of the triceps muscle.

plantar s. a calcaneal spur on the plantar surface, causing pain that may be severe when a person walks.

scleral s. calcar sclerae.

spu•ri•ous (spu′re-əs) [L. *spurius*] simulated; not genuine; false.

Spur•ling test (spur′ling) [Roy Glenwood *Spurling*, American neurosurgeon, 1894–1968] see under *test.*

spu•tum (spu′təm) [L.] matter ejected from the respiratory tract through the mouth. Called also *expectoration.*

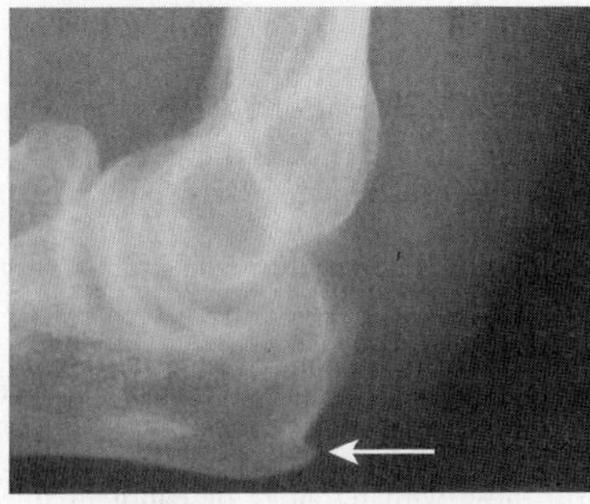

■ Olecranon spur *(arrow).*

albuminoid s. a yellowish, frothy sputum of persons from whom large amounts of pleural fluid have been withdrawn; believed to be due to pulmonary edema.

globular s. nummular s.

green s. sputum with a greenish tint due to a bile pigment (as in certain types of jaundice) or presence of *Pseudomonas aeruginosa*.

nummular s. sputum in rounded disks, shaped somewhat like coins.

prune juice s. dark reddish brown, bloody sputum, seen in lung conditions such as certain forms of pneumonia, cancer, or gangrene.

rusty s. sputum stained with blood or blood pigments, as in pneumococcal pneumonia.

SQ subcutaneous.

squa•lane (skwah′lān) [NF] a saturated hydrocarbon obtained by hydrogenation of squalene from fish oil and used as an oleaginous vehicle in pharmaceuticals.

squa•lene (skwa′lēn) [first isolated from *Squalus*, a genus of sharks] an unsaturated, symmetrical, 30-carbon triterpene intermediate formed in the biosynthesis of cholesterol and all other cyclic triterpenes. It can be isolated from shark and other fish oils and some plants.

squa•ma (skwa′mə) pl. *squa′mae* [L.] 1. in anatomy, a flat, platelike structure. 2. scale (def. 2).

s. alveola′ris type I alveolar cell.

external mental s. protuberantia mentalis.

s. of frontal bone, s. fronta′lis [TA] frontal squama: the broad, curved portion of the frontal bone, situated superior to the supraorbital margin and forming the forehead.

occipital s. squama occipitalis.

s. occipita′lis [TA] squamous part of occipital bone: the largest of the four parts of the occipital bone, extending from the posterior edge of the foramen magnum to the lambdoid suture, its external surface bearing the external occipital protuberance and nuchal lines.

perpendicular s. s. frontalis.

superior occipital s. os interparietale.

temporal s., s. of temporal bone, s. tempora′lis pars squamosa ossis temporalis.

squa•mate (skwa′māt) 1. scaly. 2. squamous (def. 2).

squa•ma•ti•za•tion (skwa″mə-tĭ-za′shən) squamous metaplasia.

squame (skwām) [L. *squama*] 1. squama (def. 1). 2. scale (def. 2).

squam(o)- [L. *squama* scale] a combining form denoting relationship to a scale or a squama (q.v.).

squa•mo•cel•lu•lar (skwa″mo-sel′u-lər) [*squamo-* + *cellular*] having squamous cells.

squa•mo•fron•tal (skwa″mo-fron′təl) pertaining to the squama frontalis.

squa•mo•mas•toid (skwa″mo-mas′toid) [*squamo-* + *mastoid*] pertaining to the squamous and mastoid portions of the temporal bone.

squa•mo•oc•cip•i•tal (skwa″mo-ok-sip′ĭ-təl) pertaining to the squama occipitalis.

squa•mo•pa•ri•e•tal (skwa″mo-pə-ri′ə-təl) [*squamo-* + *parietal*] pertaining to the pars squamosa ossis temporalis and the parietal bone.

squa•mo•pe•tro•sal (skwa″mo-pə-tro′səl) [*squamo-* + *petrosal*] pertaining to the squamous and petrous parts of the temporal bone.

squa•mo•sa (skwa-mo′sə) [L.] 1. squamous (def. 2). 2. scaly.

squa•mo•sal (skwa-mo′səl) 1. squamous (def. 2). 2. scaly.

squa•mo•so•pa•ri•e•tal (skwa-mo″so-pə-ri′ə-təl) squamoparietal.

squa•mo•sphe•noid (skwa″mo-sfe′noid) sphenosquamosal.

squa•mo•tem•po•ral (skwa″mo-tem′pə-rəl) pertaining to the squamous portion of the temporal bone.

squa•mous (skwa′məs) [L. *squamosus* scaly] 1. scaly. 2. resembling a squama; flattened or platelike.

squa•mo•zy•go•mat•ic (skwa″mo-zi″go-mat′ik) [*squamo-* + *zygomatic*] pertaining to the squamous portions of the temporal bone and the zygomatic bone.

square (skwār) a plane figure with four equal sides and four right angles.

Punnett s. in genetics, a grid with margins that shows the genotypes of the gametes of each parent (in the margins) and their possible progeny (in the squares).

squat•ting (skwaht′ing) a position of flexion of the knees and hips, the buttocks being lowered to the level of the heels. It is sometimes adopted by the parturient at delivery. Children with certain types of cyanotic cardiac defects, particularly those with tetralogy of Fallot, frequently adopt the position.

		Affected parent A/a	
	Gametes	A	a
Normal parent a/a	a	A/a Affected	a/a normal
	a	A/a Affected	a/a normal

■ Punnett square diagramming the probabilities for inheritance of a hypothetical dominant trait upon crossing a heterozygote with a homozygote lacking the trait (normal).

squill (skwil) [Gr. *skilla*] 1. any of various plants of the genus *Urginea*, particularly *U. maritima* or *U. indica*. 2. the fleshy inner scales of the bulb of *U. maritima* or *U. indica;* a distinction is made between those with white bulbs *(white squill)* and those with red bulbs *(red squill)*. Called also *scilla*.

red s. 1. a variety of *Urginea maritima* that has red bulbs. 2. the fleshy inner scales of the bulb of this plant, a source of the cardiac glycoside scilliroside; it can cause convulsions or cardiac arrest and is used as a rodenticide.

white s. 1. a variety of *Urginea maritima* that has white bulbs. 2. the fleshy inner scales of the bulb of this plant, a source of the cardiac glycosides glucoscillaren A, scillaren A, and proscillaridin A, as well as other principles; it is used as a cardiotonic, and also has a variety of uses in folk medicine.

squil•lit•ic (skwĭ-lit′ik) pertaining to or containing squill.

squint (skwint) strabismus; for types of squint not entered here, see under *strabismus*.

accommodative s. esotropia.

comitant s., concomitant s. concomitant strabismus.

convergent s. esotropia.

divergent s. exotropia.

upward and downward s. hypertropia.

squir•rel (skwur′əl) any of numerous species of rodents of the family Sciuridae; several are reservoirs of plague and other diseases.

antelope s. any squirrel of the genus *Ammospermophilus*.

ground s. any of several ground-dwelling members of the genus *Spermophilus*, found in many northern regions of the world, sometimes reservoirs of plague.

Russian ground s. *Spermophilus citellus* and other species found in northern Europe and Siberia, which are sometimes reservoirs of plague.

SR stimulation ratio; see *lymphocyte proliferation test* under *test*.

Sr strontium.

sr steradian.

SRBC sheep red blood cell.

SRC (sahrk) a human proto-oncogene homologous to the v-*src* oncogene first identified as the transforming determinant in Rous sarcoma virus; it encodes Src tyrosine kinase and mutations have been associated with various forms of cancer. In nonhuman species, it is usually written as *Src* or *src*.

Src ty•ro•sine ki•nase (sahrk ti′ro-sēn ki′nās) a family of related non-specific protein-tyrosine kinases, the prototype of which is the protein encoded by the *SRC* proto-oncogene; they are highly conserved, act as cellular switches for growth and differentiation, and are themselves controlled by phosphorylation. They are normally kept in the inactive state by regulatory segments that cover the active site of the protein; mutations that alter protein activity have been associated with various forms of cancer, including small-cell lung, colon, and breast carcinomas, neuroblastoma, and rhabdomyosarcoma.

SRF skin reactive factor.

SRH somatotropin-releasing hormone.

SRIF somatotropin release–inhibiting factor; see *somatostatin*.

SRN State Registered Nurse (England and Wales).

sro•ta (sro′tə) [Sanskrit] according to ayurveda, channels in the body through which nutrients and waste flow for body function. Srotas range from the gross, such as the digestive tract, urinary tract, respiratory cavity, spleen, and blood vessels, to the imperceptible, such as the meridians, bone marrow, and sarcolemma, and are classified by their origin and by the substances that they carry.

SRS-A slow-reacting substance of anaphylaxis.

SRT speech reception (or recognition) threshold.

SS somatostatin.

ss. [L.] se′mis (half).

SSD[1] source-skin distance.

SSD[2] trademark for preparations of silver sulfadiazine.
ssDNA single-stranded DNA.
SSKI trademark for a preparation of potassium iodide.
SSPE subacute sclerosing panencephalitis.
SSR simple sequence repeat.
SSRI selective serotonin reuptake inhibitor.
ssRNA single-stranded RNA.
SSS sick sinus syndrome; specific soluble substance.
s.s.s. [L.] stra′tum su′per stra′tum (layer upon layer).
S.S.V. [L.] sub sig′no vene′ni (under a poison label).
ST sinus tachycardia.
S.T. 37 trademark for a solution of hexylresorcinol.
St stoke.
St. [L.] stet (let it stand); stent (let them stand).

stab[1] (stab) [A.S. *stabben* stab] 1. to pierce or wound with a pointed instrument. 2. to thrust a pointed instrument into something. 3. stab culture.

stab[2] (stab) [Ger. *stab* staff] shaped like or resembling a staff or rod.

sta·bi·late (sta′bĭ-lāt) a population of microorganisms preserved in a genetically stable and viable condition (as by freeze-drying or low temperature); distinguished from a strain that may be maintained by subculture.

sta·bile (sta′bəl, sta′bīl) [L. *stabilis* stable, abiding] not moving; stationary; resistant to chemical change; opposed to *labile*.
heat s. thermostabile.

sta·bi·lim·e·try (sta″bĭ-lim′ə-tre) stabilometry.

sta·bil·i·ty (stə-bil′ĭ-te) the quality of maintaining a stable character in the presence of forces threatening to disturb it; resistance to change.
dimensional s. the resistance of a material to change in its shape or measurements.

sta·bil·iza·tion (sta″bil-ĭ-za′shən) the creation of a stable state.

sta·bi·liz·er something that promotes stabilization.
mood s. any of various drugs that lessen the mood swings of bipolar disorder.

sta·bi·lom·e·try (sta″bĭ-lom′ə-tre) assessment of a person's postural stability and equilibrium by recording oscillations in the center of gravity as electrical signals.

sta·ble (sta′bəl) 1. not moving, fixed, firm. 2. constant (def. 1).

stac·ca·to (stə-kah′to) [Ital. "detached"] delivered in a quick, jerky manner, with an interval between each two syllables. See also *staccato speech*, under *speech*.

stachy·bot·ry·o·tox·i·co·sis (stak″e-bot″re-o-tok″sĭ-ko′sis) mycotoxicosis in livestock caused either by eating contaminated feed or by sleeping on contaminated bedding containing fungi of the genera *Stachybotrys* or *Myrothecium*, especially *S. alternans*, or *M. verrucaria*, which contain roridins, satrotoxins, and verrucarins. It has been seen in France, southeastern Europe, Brazil, and Russia. Initial symptoms include fever, diarrhea, and incoordination; continued exposure can lead to hemorrhaging in various organs, sometimes followed by coma and death. Humans working in contaminated areas have occasionally also been affected.

Stachy·bot·rys (stak″e-bot′ris) a genus of Fungi Imperfecti of the order Moniliales. *S. alter′nans* (called also *S. at′ra* or *S. charta′rum*), which has been found contaminating animal feed and bedding, contains roridins, satratoxins, and verrucarins, which cause stachybotryotoxicosis.

stack·ing (stak′ing) piling something together in an orderly way.
insulin s. the taking of an additional dose of insulin too soon after the previous dose, thus causing hypoglycemia.

stac·tom·e·ter (stak-tom′ə-tər) [Gr. *staktos* oozing out in drops + *-meter*] an instrument for measuring drops.

Sta·der splint (sta′dər) [Otto *Stader*, American veterinary surgeon, 20th century] see under *splint*.

Sta·de·ri·ni nucleus (stah′də-re″ne) [Rutilio *Staderini*, Italian anatomist, late 19th century] nucleus intercalatus.

sta·di·om·e·ter (sta″de-om′ə-tər) [*stadium* + *-meter*] a device for measuring height; the usual type is a calibrated bar with a movable headpiece.

Sta·dol (sta′dol) trademark for preparations of butorphanol tartrate.

staff (staf) 1. a wooden rod or rodlike structure. 2. a grooved director used as a guide for the knife in surgery. 3. the professional personnel of a hospital. 4. band cell.
s. of Aesculapius a rod or staff with a snake entwined around it, commonly appearing in the ancient representations of Aesculapius, the god of medicine. It is the symbol of medicine and is the official emblem of the American Medical Association. See illustration.

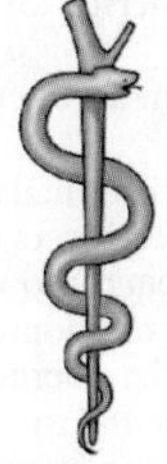
■ Staff of Aesculapius.

attending s. the corps of attending physicians and surgeons of a hospital.
consulting s. the corps of physicians and surgeons attached to a hospital who do not visit regularly, but may be consulted by members of the attending staff.
house s. the resident physicians and surgeons of a hospital.

stage (stāj) 1. a period or distinct phase in the course of a disease, the life history of an organism, or any biological process. See also *staging*. 2. the platform of a microscope on which a slide is placed for viewing of the specimen.
amphibolic s. the stage of an infectious disease between the acme and the decline, in which the diagnosis is uncertain.
anal s. in psychoanalytic theory, the second stage of psychosexual development, occurring between the ages of 1 and 3 years, during which the infant's activities, interests, and concerns are on the anal zone; it is preceded by the oral stage and followed by the phallic stage.
asexual s. anamorph.
bell s. the third stage of odontogenesis, a time of morphodifferentiation and histodifferentiation in which the enamel organ changes in shape from a cap to a bell that has four distinct layers.
cap s. the second stage of odontogenesis, a time of proliferation characterized by formation of the enamel cap in the tooth germ and organization of the dental cells into three layers.
Carnegie s's 23 numbered stages of human embryonic development defined by anatomical characteristics such as the appearance of the developing limbs.
cold s. the chill or rigor period of an intermittent fever such as malaria.
eruptive s. 1. the period during the course of an eruptive fever or exanthem when the rash is present. 2. the period in tooth development when the tooth is erupting.
erythrocytic s. in the life cycle of malarial parasites (protozoa of genus *Plasmodium*), the stage where they are inside erythrocytes of its mammalian host, developing from a sporozoite into a merozoite.
exoerythrocytic s. preerythrocytic s.
expulsive s. second stage of labor.
first s. of labor the earliest stage of labor, ending with dilatation of the os uteri.
fourth s. of labor a name sometimes applied to the immediate postpartum period.
gametocyte s., gametocytic s. in the life cycle of malarial parasites (protozoa of genus *Plasmodium*), the stage after the erythrocytic stage; the merozoites have become gametocytes, are ingested by mosquitoes, and develop into sporozoites within the mosquito's body.
genital s. in psychoanalytic theory, the last stage in psychosexual development, occurring during puberty, during which the person can achieve sexual gratification from genital-to-genital contact and is capable

Erickson's Eight Stages of Man

Psychosexual Stage	Approximate Age	Crisis
Oral-sensory	Birth to 18 mo.	Trust/mistrust
Anal-muscular	18 mo. to 3 years	Antonomy/shame, self-doubt
Genital-locomotor control	3 to 5 years	Initiative/guilt
Latency	5 to 13 years	Industry, competence/ inferiority, failure
Puberty	13 to 21 years	Identity/role confusion
Genitality (young adulthood)	21 to 40 years	Intimacy/isolation
Productivity (adulthood)	40 to 60 years	Generativity/self-absorption, stagnation
Maturity	60 years to death	Integrity, self-worth/despair

of a mature relationship with a person of the opposite sex; it follows the latency stage.

hot s. the period of pyrexia in an intermittent fever such as malaria.

imperfect s. anamorph.

intrahepatic s. in the life cycle of malarial parasites (protozoa of genus *Plasmodium*), the part of the preerythrocytic stage when sporozoites have invaded the liver and are developing into merozoites.

lamina-bud s. the first stage of odontogenesis, characterized by initial formation of the tooth bud and development of dental lamina.

latency s. 1. in psychoanalytic theory, the period of relative quiescence in psychosexual development, lasting from age 5 or 6 years to adolescence, during which interest in persons of the opposite sex ceases and children tend to associate mainly with persons of their own sex; it is preceded by the phallic stage and followed by the genital stage. 2. latent period.

mechanical s. a platform of a microscope by which the specimen being viewed can be moved in either of two mutually perpendicular directions.

oral s. in psychoanalytic theory, the earliest stage of psychosexual development, lasting from birth to about 18 months, during which the oral zone is the center of the infant's needs, expression, and pleasurable erotic experiences; it is followed by the anal stage.

perfect s. teleomorph.

phallic s. in psychoanalytic theory, the third stage in psychosexual development, lasting from age 2 or 3 years to 5 or 6 years, during which sexual interest, curiosity, and pleasurable experiences are centered on the penis in boys and the clitoris in girls; it is preceded by the anal stage and followed by the latency stage.

placental s. third s. of labor.

Prader s's a classification system for genetic females with excessive androgens that cause disorders of sexual development, ranging from stage I (phenotypically female) through three stages of ambiguous genitalia to stage V (phenotypically male).

preeruptive s. 1. the stage before the eruptive stage of a fever; cf. *prodromal s.* 2. the period of tooth development, before tooth eruption, characterized by growth of the coronal portion of the tooth, prior to the beginning of the growth of the root.

preerythrocytic s. in the life cycle of malarial parasites (protozoa of genus *Plasmodium*), the period after parasites are inside the mammal, bird, or reptile host but have not yet invaded the erythrocytes for the erythrocytic stage; they first swim freely in the bloodstream and then invade the liver for the intrahepatic stage. Called also *exoerythrocytic s.*

premenstrual s. the condition of the uterine mucosa after ovulation and formation of a corpus luteum.

prodromal s. the period of early symptoms of a disease; see *prodrome.* In an infectious disease process, this is after the incubation period and just before the appearance of characteristic symptoms. Called also *prodromal period.*

progestational s. the secretory stage of the menstrual cycle immediately preceding menstruation or implantation of the blastocyst.

proliferative s. the phase of the uterine mucosa following the first rest stage; the mucosa shows hypertrophy of glands and increase of lining epithelium.

pyretogenic s. the stage of invasion of a febrile attack.

rest s. the stage of the uterine mucosa immediately following the completion of menstruation.

ring s. see under *form.*

second s. of labor the period during which the infant is expelled from the uterus and vagina. Called also *expulsive s.*

sexual s. teleomorph.

s's of sleep see *NREM sleep*, under *sleep.*

sweating s. the final stage of a malarial paroxysm, marked by sweating.

Tanner s's a series of stages of physical maturity of adolescents, taking into account the development of pubic hair, external genitals in boys, and breasts in girls.

third s. of labor the period following expulsion of the infant and ending with expulsion of the placenta and membranes from the uterus. Called also *placental s.*

transitional pulp s. a condition of the dental pulp in which chronic inflammatory cells are present but not in sufficient quantities to constitute a typical inflammatory exudate, usually resulting from abrasion, attrition, caries, periodontal disease, or a reaction to a restorative procedure.

ugly duckling s. a development stage in the mixed dentition before the maxillary canine teeth erupt; the crowns of upper central and lateral incisors flare distally, with a diastema between the incisors.

stag•gers (stag′ərz) 1. incoordination in animals. 2. a form of vertigo occurring in decompression sickness.

blind s. 1. any of various syndromes in animals characterized by wandering, unsteady gait, and lack of awareness of the surroundings. 2. acute selenium poisoning; see under *poisoning.* 3. gid.

grass s. 1. locoism. 2. lactation tetany.

paspalum s. a temporary type of paspalism seen in livestock that eat seeds of paspalum grasses contaminated with an ergot; characteristics include tremors and ataxia.

***Phalaris* s.** head nodding, incoordination, and sometimes convulsions in ruminants grazing on certain species of *Phalaris* (canary grass). The etiology is unknown, but it occurs more often in cool weather when the grass is growing rapidly.

rye grass s. 1. a neurotoxic disease seen in ruminants in North America, Europe, Australia, and New Zealand after they eat the rye grass *Lolium perenne* when it is contaminated by an endophytic fungus; characteristics include head nodding, incoordination, limb stiffness, and opisthotonos, all of which soon subside if the animals stop eating the grass. 2. a neurotoxic disease resembling the mycotoxic disease, seen in sheep in Australia and South Africa after they eat the rye grass *Lolium rigidum* when its seed galls are carrying a nematode infected with species of *Corynebacterium.* Characteristics include tremor, ataxia, seizures, nystagmus, and opisthotonos, often ending fatally.

sleepy s., stomach s. forage poisoning.

***Zamia* s., zamia s.** the neurotoxic effects seen in ruminants after they eat seeds or leaves of zamias or other cycads; characteristics include ataxia of the hind limbs that may progress to paralysis.

stag•ing (stāj′ing) 1. the determination of distinct phases or periods in the course of a disease, the life history of an organism, or any biological process. 2. the classification of neoplasms according to the extent of the tumor; see *TNM s.*

TNM s. staging of tumors according to three basic components: primary tumor (T), regional nodes (N), and metastasis (M). Adscripts are used to denote size and degree of involvement; for example, 0 indicates undetectable, and 1, 2, 3, and 4 a progressive increase in size or involvement. Thus a tumor may be described as T1N2M0.

stag•nant (stag′nənt) 1. motionless; not flowing or moving. 2. inactive; not developing or progressing.

Stahr gland (shtahr) [Hermann *Stahr*, German anatomist and pathologist, 1868–1947] see under *gland.*

stain (stān) 1. any dye, reagent, or other material used in producing coloration, such as a substance used in coloring tissues or microorganisms for microscopical study. For specific stains, see *Stains and Staining Methods* below. 2. a superficial discoloration, or an artificially colored spot in the skin.

acid s. a stain that is acid in reaction and more readily colors the protoplasm of cells.

acid-fast s. a staining procedure for demonstrating acid-fast microorganisms; see *auramine-rhodamine s., Fite method, Kinyoun staining method* and *Ziehl-Neelsen staining method* at *Stains and Staining Methods.*

basic s. a stain that is basic in reaction and shows an affinity for the nuclei of cells.

contrast s. material used to color an unstained portion of a tissue after another portion has been stained with another dye.

counter s. counterstain.

differential s. a stain that aids differentiation of various elements in a specimen.

electron s's substances containing heavy atoms, such as osmic tetroxide, uranyl, and lead ions, which, under certain conditions, act as "electron stains," comparable to histologic stains, by combining selectively with certain regions of the specimen; used in the visualization of the ultrastructure.

extrinsic s. a stain that can be removed from a tooth surface by polishing.

heavy metal s. any of the elements of high atomic weight often used as stains in electron microscopy.

intrinsic s. a stain that is within the enamel of a tooth and cannot be removed by polishing.

lipoid s. a stain made from a lipid or fatlike substance, such as Sudan III.

metachromatic s. a stain that colors certain cell constituents a color different from that of the stain itself.

neutral s. a compound that combines an acid dye and a basic dye, the cation and anion of the resulting salt each having a different color.

nuclear s. a stain that has a special affinity for the nuclei of cells.

plasmatic s., plasmic s. a stain that colors the tissue uniformly throughout.

port-wine s. a persistent dark red to purple nevus flammeus, usually on the face, growing proportionately with the affected child. At first it is

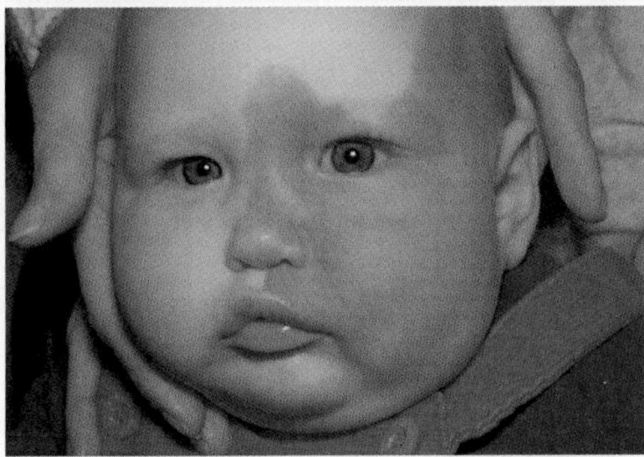

■ Port-wine stain.

macular, but it may later develop angiomatous overgrowths. Port-wine stains often occur in association with other congenital abnormalities, such as the Klippel-Trénaunay and Sturge-Weber syndromes. Called also *port-wine mark* or *nevus*.

protoplasmic s. a stain that has a special affinity for the protoplasm of cells.

selective s. a stain that has a special affinity for a certain tissue element, staining it more vividly than, or to the exclusion of, other elements of the same specimen.

thiazine-eosinate s. any of a group of neutral stains used in hematology and histology that combine an eosin dye, usually eosin Y, as the anionic component and one or more thiazine dyes as the cationic component. The prototype is the Romanowsky stain.

tumor s. an area of increased density in a radiograph due to collection of contrast material in distorted and abnormal vessels, prominent in the capillary and venous phases of arteriography, and presumed to indicate neoplasm.

Stains and Staining Methods

Listing some of the preparations and methods commonly employed in histologic and pathologic technique *(arranged alphabetically)*. For other stains, see under *blue*, *red*, etc.

acid fuchsin s. a diffuse stain containing acid fuchsin and diluted hydrochloric acid in purified water, for demonstrating axons and as a component of connective tissue stains.

Albert diphtheria s. a stain containing toluidine blue and methyl (or malachite) green. Following treatment with iodine solution, the metachromatic granules appear black, the bars dark green to black, and the remainder of the diphtheria bacillus a light green.

alum-carmine s. a preparation of ordinary alum and carmine.

Alzheimer s. a methylene blue and eosin polychrome stain for demonstrating Negri bodies.

Anthony capsule s. a method of demonstrating the capsules of bacteria. A smear of a milk culture is air dried, or a smear is mixed with milk and dried. The slide is stained with crystal violet and washed with copper sulfate. The capsule appears unstained against a purple background; the cells are deeply stained.

auramine-rhodamine s. Truant auramine-rhodamine s.

azan s. Heidenhain's modification of Mallory triple stain.

Benda s. a method for demonstrating nerve tissue.

Best carmine s. a stain for demonstrating glycogen.

Bethe method a method of fixing methylene blue stains of nerve fibers.

Bielschowsky method a method for demonstrating axons and neurofibrils using an ammoniacal silver stain.

Bodian method a method of staining nerve fibers and nerve endings with colloidal silver.

Bowie s. a stain used to demonstrate the slightly basophilic cytoplasm and the specific granules of juxtaglomerular cells.

Cajal method a method of staining astrocytes by a gold chloride–mercuric chloride compound.

Cajal double method a method of demonstrating ganglion cells.

carbolfuchsin s. carbolfuchsin used in a stain, particularly for detection of acid-fast bacteria; see *Kinyoun staining method*, *Ziehl-Neelsen staining method*, and *Fite method*. It is also used as a counterstain for *Legionella pneumophila* following other routine stains. Stained cells appear pink to red.

carbol–gentian violet s. a solution containing gentian violet and phenol (carbolic acid).

Castaneda s. a method of demonstrating rickettsiae. A smear is air dried and treated with methylene blue, then counterstained with safranin O, washed, and air dried. Rickettsiae appear blue against red cellular elements.

Ciaccio s. a stain for demonstrating lipids.

Davenport s. a stain for demonstrating various elements of nerve tissue, dependent upon the special affinity of nerve cells and their processes for silver.

Delafield hematoxylin s. a preparation of hematoxylin, alcohol, ammonia alum, water, glycerin, and methanol, used as a nuclear stain.

Dieterle s. a silver impregnation method for staining *Legionella* and other organisms. Slides are sensitized in uranyl nitrate, treated with gum mastic, incubated in silver nitrate, and developed in a solution of hydroquinone, sodium sulfite, acetone, formaldehyde, pyridine, and gum mastic. Cells stain black on a yellow-tan background.

Ehrlich acid hematoxylin s. a preparation of hematoxylin, used as a nuclear stain.

Ehrlich triacid s. a stain containing acid fuchsin, orange G, and methyl green; used for demonstrating various formed elements in the blood.

F method chromosomes are treated with phosphate buffer, rinsed and stored for 60–72 hours in saline citrate solution, then fixed in methanol-acetic acid, and stained by the Feulgen method.

Feulgen method a method of demonstrating chromatin and deoxyribonucleic acid (DNA).

Fite method a staining method used for acid-fast microorganisms. Tissue sections are deparaffinized in 2:1 xylene and peanut oil, then stained with Ziehl-Neelsen carbolfuchsin, decolorized with acid alcohol, and counterstained with methylene blue.

Fontana s. a method of staining spirochetes by silver impregnation, using ammoniacal silver nitrate solution.

Fontana-Masson s. an ammoniacal silver nitrate stain for melanin and argentaffin material; used in the diagnosis of melanoma, pheochromocytoma, and carcinoid tumors.

F-staining method F m.

Giemsa s. a solution containing azure II-eosin, azure II, glycerin, and methanol; used for staining protozoan parasites such as *Plasmodium* and *Trypanosoma*, for chlamydiae, for differential staining of blood smears, and for viral inclusion bodies. Stained elements appear pink to purple to blue.

Gimenez s. a method for staining chlamydiae, rickettsiae, and *Legionella*. Smears are stained with carbol–basic fuchsin solution, washed, and counterstained with malachite green. Cells appear red against a greenish background.

Golgi s. any of several stains that were widely used for staining nerve cells and their processes.

Golgi-Cox s. a modification of one of Golgi's original methods, used for staining ganglion cells.

Gomori s's stains used for histological demonstration of enzymes, especially phosphatases and lipases in sections; also methods for demonstration of connective tissue fibers and secretion granules.

Gomori methenamine silver (GMS) s. methenamine silver s.

Gomori trichrome s. a one-step mixture of stains used to identify an increase in collagenous connective tissue fibers or to differentiate between collagen and smooth muscle fibers; it combines a plasma stain (chromotrope 2R) and a connective tissue fiber stain (fast green FCF, light green, or aniline blue), with phosphotungstic acid, and acetic acid. The mixture differentially stains a variety of cytoplasmic inclusions associated with various disease states, such as ragged red fibers.

Gomori-Wheatley s. a rapid type of trichrome stain for demonstrating structural details of intestinal protozoa. The solution is as follows: chromotrope 2R 0.6 g, light green SF 0.3 g, phosphotungstic acid 0.7 g, acetic acid 1.00 mL, and distilled water 100.00 mL.

Stains and Staining Methods *Continued*

Goodpasture s. a method for demonstrating the peroxidase reaction.
Gram method, Gram s. an empirical staining procedure in which microorganisms are stained with crystal violet, treated with 1:15 dilution of strong iodine solution, decolorized with ethanol or ethanol-acetone, and counterstained with a contrasting dye, usually safranin O. Those microorganisms that retain the crystal violet stain are said to be gram-positive, and those that lose the crystal violet stain by decolorization but stain with the counterstain are said to be gram-negative. Gram-positive organisms that lose the stain easily, so that samples appear to be a mixture of gram-positive and gram-negative organisms, are said to be gram-variable.
Grimelius argyrophil method a method for demonstrating granule-containing cells such as APUD cells. Incubation in a buffered silver nitrate solution is followed by reduction in a hydroquinone and sodium sulfite solution; reactive cell granules appear black.
Grocott-Gomori methenamine–silver nitrate s. a method for demonstrating actinomycetes and fungi in tissue. Sections are treated with chromic acid, stained with methenamine-silver nitrate solution, and counterstained with light green solution. Cells appear brown against a green background.
Hale iron s. a stain used on substances with a high acid polysaccharide content because of the ability of polyanionic polysaccharides to bind polyvalent cations. Its main component is colloidal iron (Fe^{3+}).
Hansel s. a stain used to detect eosinophils in urine or other body fluids, the eosinophils staining red against a background of blue.
Harris hematoxylin s. a nuclear stain containing hematoxylin, aluminum sulfate, mercuric oxide, and alcohol in water; modified preparations lacking the mercuric oxide also exist.
Heidenhain iron hematoxylin s. an important cytological method for the demonstration of most cellular structures: nuclei, chromosomes, centrioles, fibrils, mitochondria, cilia, etc.
hemalum s. a nuclear stain containing hematoxylin and alum, widely used, especially in combination with eosin.
hematoxylin-eosin s. a mixture of hematoxylin in distilled water and aqueous eosin, usually eosin Y, solution, widely employed for routine examination of tissues; numerous variations are employed in execution of the stain.
hematoxylin-eosin-azure II s. a method for the staining of blood-forming organs; called also *Maximow method.*
Hiss capsule s. a method of demonstrating bacterial capsules. Smears are treated with crystal violet, heated, and rinsed with copper sulfate solution. Capsules appear as pale blue halos around deep blue to purple cells.
Hortega method a method of demonstrating microglia, employing ammoniacal silver carbonate.
India ink capsule s. a method of demonstrating cell capsules, especially of *Cryptococcus neoformans.* The smear is mixed with India ink, covered with a coverglass, and examined microscopically. Capsules appear as a clear halo around the cells against a black background.
iron hematoxylin method a staining procedure in which the sections are treated with an iron salt, stained with hematoxylin, and differentiated with the same iron salt.
Jenner method a method for demonstrating blood corpuscles.
Kinyoun staining method a stain for acid-fast organisms that does not require heating the stained slides. A heat-fixed smear is treated with Kinyoun carbolfuchsin. The slide is washed with water, decolorized with acid alcohol, and counterstained with methylene blue. Acid-fast organisms appear red against a blue background. Cf. *Ziehl-Neelsen staining method.*

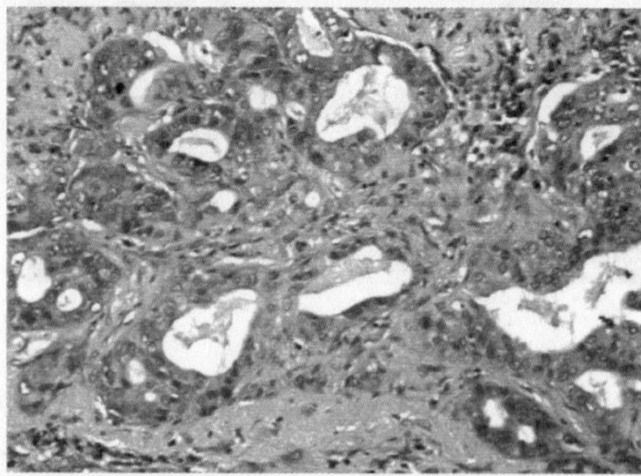

■ Hematoxylin-eosin stain showing a glandular pattern of cell growth in an adenocarcinoma specimen.

Leifson flagella s. a method for demonstrating bacterial flagella. Smears are air dried, treated with alcoholic pararosaniline–tannic acid solution, and washed. Flagella are visible against a clear background.
Leishman s. a mixture of alkaline methylene blue and eosin in methanol for staining blood cells and certain parasites; also used for G banding of chromosomes.
Levaditi method a method for demonstrating *Treponema pallidum* in sections, employing reduced silver.
lithium-carmine s. a diffuse stain used intravitally for the demonstration of macrophages.
Löffler alkaline methylene blue s. a simple stain used especially for demonstrating granules in *Corynebacterium diphtheriae.* Methylene blue made alkaline with potassium hydroxide is applied to a smear briefly and the slide washed. Granules appear deep blue in lighter blue cells.
Lugol iodine s. strong iodine solution.
Luxol fast blue s. trademark for a group of dyes used in histology as stains for complex lipids, particularly myelin; they have a marked affinity for phospholipids, lecithin, and cephalin.
Macchiavello s. a stain used for chlamydiae. The heat-fixed smear is stained with basic fuchsin, decolorized in citric acid, and counterstained with methylene blue. Organisms stain red against a blue background.
Mallory acid fuchsin, orange G, and aniline blue s. a stain for demonstrating connective tissue and secretion granules. Called also *Mallory triple s.*
Mallory phloxine–methylene blue s. a stain used in histology to demonstrate connective tissue.
Mallory phosphotungstic acid–hematoxylin s. a stain used for demonstrating nuclear and cytoplasmic detail and connective tissue fibers.
Mallory triple s. Mallory acid fuchsin, orange G, and aniline blue s.
Marchi method a method of demonstrating degenerated nerve fibers, the tissue first being fixed in a solution containing potassium bichromate, which prevents the normal myelinated fibers from staining with osmic acid.

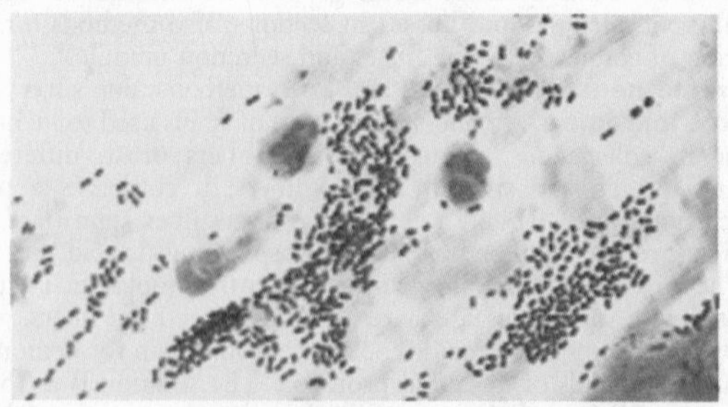

■ Gram stain demonstrating gram-positive diplococci in sputum smear.

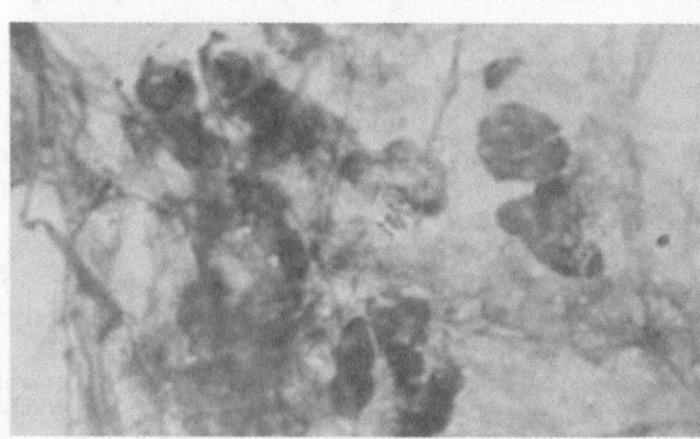

■ Kinyoun staining method used to demonstrate acid-fast bacilli *(Mycobacterium tuberculosis)* in sputum smear.

Stains and Staining Methods *Continued*

Masson s., Masson trichrome s. a trichrome stain for tissue including pituitary, thyroid, nerve, epithelial, and connective tissue.

Maximow method hematoxylin-eosin-azure II.

May-Grünwald s. an alcoholic neutral mixture of methylene blue and eosin.

Mayer hemalum s. an aqueous solution of hematein, alum, thymol, and 90 per cent alcohol.

Mayer mucihematein s. a specific stain for mucin.

methenamine silver s. 1. *(for argentaffin cells)* a methenamine silver solution used together with gold chloride, sodium thiosulfate, and a safranin O counterstain; argentaffin granules are black while granules of mast cells remain red. 2. *(for fungi)* Grocott-Gomori methenamine–silver nitrate s.

methyl green–pyronin s. a solution of methyl green and pyronin (usually pyronin Y) used as a differential stain for DNA and RNA: DNA is stained blue-green by methyl green and RNA is stained red by pyronin.

Milligan trichrome s. a differential stain for connective tissue and smooth muscle. Nuclei and muscle appear magenta; collagen appears green or blue, depending on whether fast green or aniline blue is used as a counterstain; and red blood cells appear orange to orange red.

Nissl method a method employed in the study of nerve cell bodies.

Pal-Weigert method a modification of the Weigert myelin sheath method used in the study of myelinated nerves; the specimen being treated is immersed for several weeks in a solution containing potassium bichromate.

Papanicolaou s. a method of staining smears of secretions from the respiratory, digestive, or genitourinary tract for examination of exfoliated cells, to detect the presence of a malignant process; used in the Papanicolaou test (see under *test*).

Pappenheim s. the original methyl green–pyronin staining method, used to differentiate between basophilic granules of erythrocytes and nuclear fragments.

PAS s., periodic acid–Schiff s. see under *reaction.*

phosphotungstic acid–hematoxylin s. see *Mallory phosphotungstic acid–hematoxylin s.*

Q method, Q banding method, quinacrine fluorescent method see under *banding.*

R method see under *banding.*

Ranson pyridine silver s. a stain used for demonstrating nerve cells and their processes.

R banding method see under *banding.*

resorcin-fuchsin s. Weigert resorcin-fuchsin s.

reverse Giemsa method R banding.

Romanowsky (Romanovsky) s. the prototype of the many eosin–polychrome methylene blue stains for blood smears and malarial parasites, including Giemsa stain, Leishman stain, and Wright stain.

Seller s. a combination of alcoholic solutions of methylene blue and basic fuchsin which stains Negri bodies a bright red against a purplish-pink background; used in rapid diagnosis of rabies.

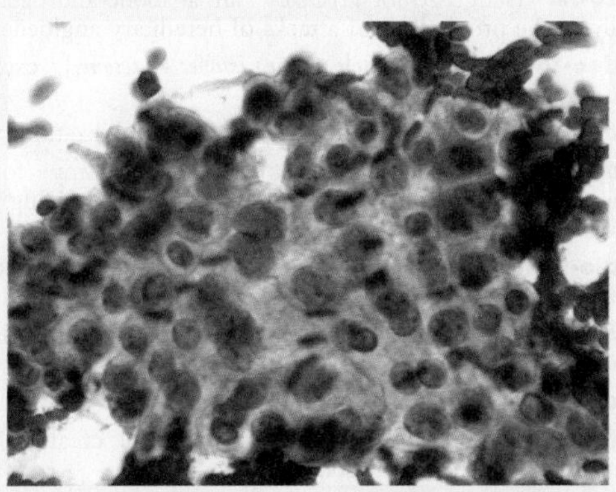

■ Papanicolaou stain showing clusters of cells with foamy or vacuolated cytoplasm in a fine-needle aspiration biopsy specimen of adenocarcinoma.

Steiner s. a staining method for detecting spirochetes and nonfilamentous bacteria in paraffin-embedded tissue by first sensitizing it to silver and then exposing it to silver nitrate.

Sternheimer-Malbin s. a stain used in urinalysis which has ready affinity for hyaline casts, epithelial casts, red cells, bladder epithelial nuclei, nuclei of vaginal epithelium, and trichomonads, staining each a different color.

Sudan black B fat s. a stain used to demonstrate *Legionella* and fat vacuoles in bacterial cells. A heat-fixed smear is treated with Sudan black B, cleared with xylol, and counterstained with safranin. Fat vacuoles stain blue-black; bacterial cells stain pink.

T method a method for staining only the terminal ends of chromosomes by means of either Giemsa stain or acridine orange; it results in bands (T bands) of dark violet (Giemsa) or fiery orange (acridine orange).

tetrachrome s. a stain combining eosin Y, methylene blue, azur A, and methylene violet, in methyl alcohol.

trichrome s. any staining method having three dyes of different colors, usually with the sample being exposed sequentially, such as the Gomori or Masson trichrome stains.

Truant auramine-rhodamine s. a method for demonstrating mycobacteria. A smear is heat fixed, stained with auramine-rhodamine solution, decolorized, counterstained with potassium permanganate, and examined under ultraviolet light; acid-fast organisms glow with a yellow-orange color.

T-staining method T m.

Unna-Pappenheim s. a variation of methyl green–pyronin stain, used to detect plasma cells and demonstrate nucleoproteins.

van Gieson s. any of several staining solutions formerly widely used for connective tissue samples.

Verhoeff s. a type of iron hematoxylin staining method for demonstrating elastic tissue.

Verhoeff-van Gieson s. a histopathological stain for demonstrating elastic fibers.

von Kossa s. a silver nitrate stain for bone mineral.

Warthin-Starry silver s. a method for staining *Bartonella* and spirochetes. A smear is air-dried, immersed in absolute ethanol, washed in distilled water, and incubated in 2 per cent silver nitrate. The cover glass is then developed in a mixture of silver nitrate, gelatin, glycerol, agar, and hydroquinone. Organisms appear black on a light background.

Wayson s. a method used to demonstrate polar staining. A smear is treated with a mixture of basic fuchsin and methylene blue with phenol, washed with water, and dried. It is used especially to demonstrate *Yersinia pestis* in specimens from tissues and lymph nodes.

Weigert fibrin s. a method, many variations of which have been used in both fixation and staining; stains gram-positive bacteria as well as fibrin.

Weigert iron hematoxylin s. a simple method for staining most nuclear and cytoplasmic constituents.

Weigert myelin sheath method a method of demonstrating the myelin sheath of nerve cell processes.

Weigert neuroglia fiber s. a complicated method for demonstrating fibrous glia, which works best on human material.

Weigert resorcin-fuchsin s. a method for the demonstration of elastic fibers.

Weil s. a method for staining myelin sheaths.

Wirtz-Conklin spore s. a smear is heated with malachite green, rinsed, then counterstained with safranin. Spores appear green in red-stained cells.

Wright s. a mixture of eosin Y and polychrome methylene blue, used for staining blood smears and for detection of malarial parasites in the blood.

Ziehl-Neelsen staining method a stain for acid-fast organisms. A heat-fixed smear is flooded with Ziehl-Neelsen carbolfuchsin, heated for 5 minutes, cooled, and washed. The slide is decolorized with acid alcohol, washed, and counterstained with methylene blue. Acid-fast organisms appear red against a blue background. Cf. *Kinyoun staining method.*

stain•ing (stān′ing) 1. the artificial coloration of a substance, such as the introduction or application of material to facilitate examination of tissues, microorganisms, or other cells under the microscope. For various staining methods, see *Stains and Staining Methods*, under *stain*. 2. modification of the color of the teeth or denture base to achieve a more lifelike appearance.

bipolar s. staining at the two poles only, or staining differently at the two poles.

differential s. staining with a substance for which different bacteria or different elements of the bacteria or specimen being stained show varying affinities, resulting in their differentiation.

double s. staining with two different dyes which have an affinity for different tissue elements.

fluorescent s. a technique for visualizing specific cellular or tissue components by treating a specimen with a fluorochrome that binds specifically to the component of interest and observing the specimen by fluorescence microscopy.

intravital s. vital s.

multiple s. staining with several different dyes to facilitate identification of different tissue elements.

negative s. staining of the background and not the organism, to facilitate the microscopical study of bacteria.

polar s. staining in which the ends of the rod stain deeply while the central portion of the organism is nearly or quite unstained, as in the pasteurellas.

postvital s. staining occurring after death of a tissue previously stained by vital methods.

preagonal s. vital s.

relief s. a method of staining that colors the background and leaves the cells uncolored.

simple s. staining with a single substance, such as the staining of microorganisms with a single dye.

substantive s. the coloration of tissues by direct absorption of dyes in which they are immersed.

supravital s. staining of living tissue removed from the body, but before cessation of the chemical life of the cells.

telomeric s., terminal s. differential staining of chromosomes to stain chromosome telomeric regions, consisting of pretreatment with a heated salt solution before treatment with buffered Giemsa stain or acridine orange; only the telomeric regions of the chromosomes retain the stain.

triple s. staining with three different dyes to facilitate identification of the different elements.

vital s. staining of a tissue by a dye which is introduced into a living organism and which, by virtue of affinity for certain tissues, will stain those tissues; called also *intravital s.*

stal•ag•mom•e•ter (stal″əg-mom′ə-tər) [Gr. *stalagmos* dropping + *-meter*] an instrument for measuring surface tension by determining the exact number of drops in a given quantity of a liquid.

stalk (stawk) an elongated, more or less slender anatomical structure resembling the stem of a plant; see also *peduncle* and *pedunculus*.

allantoic s. the slender tube interposed between the urogenital sinus and allantoic sac in the embryo; its intraembryonic part is the precursor of the urachus.

body s. connecting s.

cerebellar s. any of the cerebellar peduncles.

connecting s. a bridge of mesoderm connecting the caudal end of the early embryo with the trophoblastic tissues and eventually giving passage to embryonic blood vessels connecting with the placenta; it is the precursor of part of the umbilical cord. Called also *body s.*

hypophysial s. infundibulum neurohypophyseos.

infundibular s. 1. infundibulum neurohypophyseos. 2. see under *stem*.

neural s. infundibulum neurohypophyseos.

optic s. a slender structure attaching the optic vesicle, and later the optic cup, to the brain wall in the embryo.

pineal s. habenula (def. 2).

pituitary s. infundibulum neurohypophyseos.

rectal s. ligamentum recti laterale.

s's of thalamus thalamic peduncles.

yolk s. the narrow duct connecting the yolk sac with the midgut of the early embryo; it becomes partly incorporated into the embryo and usually undergoes complete obliteration, although part may persist as a diverticulum from the small intestine *(ileal* or *Meckel diverticulum)*. Called also *omphaloenteric, umbilical*, or *vitelline duct*.

stal•li•my•cin hy•dro•chlo•ride (stal″ĭ-mi′sin) an antibacterial administered in the form of a topical ointment.

sta•men (sta′mən) the structure of a flower which bears the male gamete, or pollen.

Sta•mey procedure (colposuspension) (sta′me) [Thomas Alexander *Stamey*, American urologist, born 1928] see under *procedure*.

stam•i•na (stam′ĭ-nə) [L.] vigor or endurance.

Stamm gastrostomy (shtahm) [M. *Stamm*, German surgeon, late 19th century] see under *gastrostomy*.

stam•mer•ing (stam′ər-ing) a speech disorder marked by involuntary pauses; sometimes used synonymously with *stuttering*, especially in Great Britain.

Stam•no•so•ma (stam″no-so′mə) [Gr. *stamnos* jar + *sōma* body] a genus of flukes. *S. arma′tum* and *S. formosa′num* are parasites of birds, but experimental human infections have been reported.

stance (stans) the posture and general bodily orientation of a person standing. Cf. *gait*.

stan•dard (stan′dərd) something established as a measure or model to which other similar things should conform.

stan•dard•iza•tion (stan″dərd-ĭ-za′shən) 1. the bringing of any preparation to a specified standard as to quality or ingredients. 2. the formulation of standards for a substance or for a procedure.

stan•dard•ize (stan′dərd-īz) to compare with or conform to a standard; to establish standards.

stand•still (stand′stil) suspension of activity or movement.

atrial s. cardiac arrhythmia in which there is a pause in atrial contraction, as occurs secondary to sinus arrest or sinoatrial block, the ventricle continuing to respond to its own pacemaker.

cardiac s. cessation of contraction of the myocardium.

sinus s. see under *arrest*.

ventricular s. cardiac arrhythmia in which there is an absence of ventricular contraction.

Stan•ford-Bi•net test (stan′fərd be-na′) [*Stanford* University, where test was revised for use in the U.S.; Alfred *Binet*, French physiologist and psychologist, 1857–1911] see under *test*.

Stan•ley bacillus (stan′le) [*Stanley*, England, where it was first isolated] see under *bacillus*.

Stan•ley Kent see *Kent*.

stan•nic (stan′ik) containing tin as a quadrivalent element.

s. chloride a caustic liquid used as a mordant in dyemaking and for various other purposes; it is toxic and corrosive if inhaled or spilled on the skin.

s. oxide a compound found in nature as the mineral cassiterite, or produced through a reaction between tin and concentrated nitric acid at high temperatures. Used as a polishing agent for glass, metals, and especially to produce a high polish on metallic dental restorations. Called also *tin oxide*.

stan•nif•er•ous (stan-if′ər-əs) [L. *stannum* tin + *-ferous*] containing tin.

stan•no•sis (stan-o′sis) benign pneumoconiosis due to the inhalation of tin oxide; it is symptomless unless accompanied by silicosis.

stan•nous (stan′əs) containing tin as a bivalent element.

s. chloride tin chloride, $SnCl_2$, used in the anhydrous and dihydrated forms as a reagent and, as the dihydrate, as a pharmaceutic aid.

s. fluoride [USP] a compound, SnF_2, applied topically to the teeth as a dental caries prophylactic.

s. pyrophosphate $Sn_2P_2O_7$, a diagnostic aid used in bone imaging.

stan•o•lone (stan′o-lōn) an anabolic-androgenic steroid that is a semisynthetic form of dihydrotestosterone.

stan•o•zo•lol (stan′o-zo-lol″) [USP] an anabolic-androgenic steroid, used orally in the prophylaxis of attacks of hereditary angioedema.

sta•pe•dec•to•my (sta″pə-dek′tə-me) [*stapes* + *-ectomy*] excision of the stapes.

sta•pe•di•ol•y•sis (stə-pe″de-ol′ĭ-sis) stapes mobilization.

sta•pe•dio•plas•ty (stə-pe′de-o-plas″te) stapedectomy followed by replacement with a prosthetic stapes, done to correct hearing loss due to otosclerosis. **stapedioplas′tic** *adj*

sta•pe•dio•te•not•o•my (stə-pe″de-o-tə-not′ə-me) the cutting of the tendon of the stapedius muscle.

sta•pe•dio•ves•tib•u•lar (stə-pe″de-o-vəs-tib′u-lər) pertaining to the stapes and vestibule.

sta•pe•di•us (stə-pe′de-əs) musculus stapedius.

sta•pe•dot•o•my (sta″pə-dot′ə-me) the surgical creation of a small opening in the footplate of the stapes.

sta•pes (sta′pēz) gen. *stape′dis* [L. "stirrup"] [TA] the innermost of the auditory ossicles, shaped somewhat like the stirrup used in horse riding; it articulates by its head with the incus, and its base is inserted into the oval window (fenestra vestibuli). Called also *stirrup*. See illustration at *ossicula auditus*, under *ossiculum*. **stape′dial** *adj*

staph•i•sa•gria (staf″ĭ-sa′gre-ə) [Gr. *staphis* raisin + *agrios* wild] the seeds of *Delphinium staphisagria*, which were formerly used as a topical parasiticide; the plant and its seeds are poisonous and narcotic, containing numerous alkaloids such as delphinine, delphinoidine, delphisine, and staphisagrine.

staph·i·sa·grine (staf″ĭ-sa′grin) a poisonous alkaloid found in the seeds of *Delphinium staphisagria.*

staph·y·line (staf′ə-līn) 1. botryoid. 2. uvular.

staph·y·lin·id (staf″ə-lin′id) 1. pertaining to or due to beetles of the family Staphylinidae. 2. a beetle of the family Staphylinidae.

Staph·y·lin·i·dae (staf″ə-lin′ĭ-de) the rove beetles, a family of beetles that feed on decaying animal or vegetable matter; some species produce an irritating substance that causes blistering.

sta·phyl·i·on (stə-fil′e-on) [Gr. "little grape"] an encephalometric landmark on the posterior edge of the hard palate at the median line.

staph·y·li·tis (staf″ə-li′tis) uvulitis.

staphyl(o)- [Gr. *staphylē* a bunch of grapes] a combining form denoting resemblance to a bunch of grapes, used especially to denote relationship to the uvula or to staphylococci.

Sta·phy·lo·coc·ca·ceae (staf″ə-lo-kŏ-ka′se-e) a family of gram-positive, facultatively anaerobic bacteria of the order Bacillales; medically important organisms are included in the genera *Gemella* and *Staphylococcus.*

staph·y·lo·coc·cal (staf″ə-lo-kok′əl) pertaining to or caused by staphylococci.

staph·y·lo·coc·ce·mia (staf″ə-lo-kok-se′me-ə) [*staphylococcus* + *-emia*] the presence of staphylococci in the blood, causing septicemia.

staph·y·lo·coc·ci (staf″ə-lo-kok′si) plural of *staphylococcus.*

staph·y·lo·coc·cic (staf″ə-lo-kok′sik) staphylococcal.

staph·y·lo·coc·cin (staf″ə-lo-kok′sin) a bacteriocin produced by certain strains of *Staphylococcus aureus.*

staph·y·lo·coc·co·sis (staf″ə-lo-kok-o′sis) infection caused by staphylococci; see *staphylococcal endocarditis, impetigo, parotitis,* and *pneumonia,* and see *staphylococcal scalded skin syndrome,* under *syndrome.*

Sta·phy·lo·coc·cus (staf″ə-lo-kok′əs) [Gr. *staphylē* bunch of grapes + *kokkos* berry] a ubiquitous genus of gram-positive, mainly facultatively anaerobic bacteria of the family Staphylococcaceae consisting of cocci, usually unencapsulated, 0.5 to 1.5 µm in diameter, occurring singly or in pairs, tetrads, short chains, or irregular clusters; organisms are chemo-organotrophic, non–spore-forming, nonmotile, and usually catalase-positive. Staphylococci are important inhabitants of the skin, cutaneous glands, and mucous membranes; several species are important pathogens, causing a wide variety of infections, as well as producing a number of toxins. The type species is *S. au′reus.*

S. au′reus a species comprising the yellow-pigmented, coagulase-positive pathogenic forms of the genus; it causes serious suppurative infections and systemic disease, including impetigo bullosa, staphylococcal pneumonia, and staphylococcal scalded skin syndrome, and has developed resistance to nearly all classes of antibiotics. This species also produces toxins that cause food poisoning and toxic shock syndrome.

S. ca′pitis a coagulase-negative species that can cause bacteremia or infective endocarditis.

S. epider′midis the most common coagulase-negative species inhabiting the skin and mucous membranes; many strains are pathogens or secondary invaders and cause mainly nosocomial diseases, including wound infection, urinary tract infection, bacteremia, subacute bacterial endocarditis, infection of catheters and other indwelling devices, and postoperative endophthalmitis.

S. haemoly′ticus a coagulase-negative species sometimes occurring on the skin and mucous membranes; it is associated with infections of wounds, the urinary tract, and the conjunctiva, and with septicemia.

S. ho′minis a coagulase-negative species that is a common inhabitant of the skin; it is associated with infections of wounds, the urinary tract, and the conjunctiva, and with septicemia.

S. hy′icus a species that infects pigs through wounds in the skin and causes greasy pig disease.

S. interme′dius a coagulase-negative species found most often in dogs, such as in skin or eye infections; it infects the wounds of persons who are bitten by infected dogs.

S. lugdunen′sis a coagulase-negative species that is a transient inhabitant of the skin; it is a potential pathogen, associated with a wide variety of infections, including skin and soft tissue infections, bacteremia, and endocarditis.

S. saccharoly′ticus a coagulase-negative species that can cause bacteremia or endocarditis in susceptible persons.

S. saprophy′ticus a coagulase-negative species that is an inhabitant of the genitourinary skin; organisms are usually harmless commensals but can cause community-acquired urinary tract infections.

S. sciu′ri a coagulase-negative species usually found in nonhuman mammals such as squirrels, cattle, and pigs; it occasionally causes opportunistic skin infections in humans.

S. si′mulans a coagulase-negative species that is a common animal pathogen and a rare cause of human infection, most often of the urinary tract or wounds.

S. war′neri a coagulase-negative species that is a cause of nosocomial infections and of bacteremia in premature neonates.

staph·y·lo·coc·cus (staf″ə-lo-kok′əs) pl. *staphylococ′ci.* An organism of the genus *Staphylococcus.*

coagulase-negative staphylococci *Staphylococcus* species that do not produce coagulase; included here are all species associated with humans except for *S. aureus.* Some are normal inhabitants of the skin and mucous membranes and potential pathogens, causing mainly nosocomial infections of the skin, soft tissues, and respiratory and genitourinary tracts; infections of implanted devices and vascular grafts; bacteremia; endocarditis; endophthalmitis; osteomyelitis; and peritonitis.

staph·y·lo·der·ma (staf″ə-lo-dur′mə) cutaneous pyogenic infection by staphylococci.

staph·y·lo·ki·nase (staf″ə-lo-ki′nās) a bacterial kinase produced by certain strains of staphylococci, which can activate plasminogen in the blood of various species of animals.

staph·y·lol·y·sin (staf″ə-lol′ə-sin) a principle with hemolytic activity produced by staphylococci.

α s., alpha s. a hemolysin produced by pathogenic staphylococci which lyses both sheep and rabbit erythrocytes at 37°C and has leukocidin activity.

β s., beta s. a hot-cold hemolysin produced by staphylococci which lyses sheep but not rabbit erythrocytes in the cold following preliminary incubation at 37°C.

δ s., delta s. a hemolysin produced by pyogenic staphylococci which lyses red cells from humans and several other species; it differs immunologically from the α and β staphylolysins, and is both dermonecrotic and lethal.

ε s., epsilon s. a hemolysin formed almost exclusively by nonpathogenic, coagulase-negative strains of staphylococci.

γ s., gamma s. a hemolysin produced by staphylococci which is similar to, but serologically distinguishable from, the α staphylolysin.

staph·y·lo·ma (staf″ə-lo′mə) [Gr. *staphylōma* a defect in the eye inside the cornea] protrusion of the cornea or sclera lined with uveal tissue, resulting from inflammation. **staphylom′atous** *adj*

annular s. staphyloma of the sclera in the ciliary region, extending around the margin of the cornea.

anterior s. scleral or corneal staphyloma in the anterior part of the eye.

ciliary s. scleral staphyloma in the part covered by the ciliary body.

s. cor′neae, corneal s. 1. ectasia of the cornea with adherent uveal tissue; called also *projecting s.* 2. staphyloma formed by an iris which has protruded through a wound in the cornea.

s. cor′neae racemo′sum staphyloma corneae (def. 2) in which there are a number of perforations from which small portions of iris protrude.

equatorial s. scleral staphyloma occurring in the equatorial region of the eye.

intercalary s. staphyloma that occurs in the rim of sclera anterior to the insertion of the ciliary body.

posterior s., s. posti′cum backward bulging of the sclera at the posterior pole of the eye; called also *Scarpa s.*

projecting s. s. corneae.

retinal s. a forward bulging of the retina.

Scarpa s. posterior s.

scleral s. protrusion of the contents of the eyeball at a point where the sclera has become too thin.

uveal s. protrusion of the uvea through a ruptured sclera.

staph·yl·op·to·sis (staf″əl-op-to′sis) uvuloptosis.

staph·y·lor·rha·phy (staf″ə-lor′ə-fe) palatorrhaphy.

staph·y·los·chi·sis (staf″ə-los′kĭ-sis) bifid uvula.

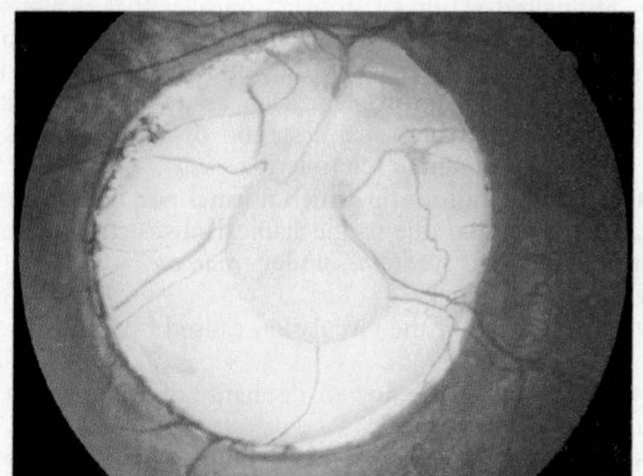

■ Posterior staphyloma.

staph·y·lo·tox·in (staf′ə-lo-tok″sin) any of the several toxins produced by *Staphylococcus aureus;* see *staphylococcal toxin,* under *toxin.*

sta·ple (sta′pəl) 1. a stainless steel wound closure device. 2. to close a wound with such a device.

stap·ling (sta′pling) the act or process of fastening with staples.

gastric s., stomach s. gastric partitioning in which the stomach is divided by a wall of staples.

star (stahr) 1. a symmetrical, round geometrical figure with five or more points radiating out from a center. 2. any structure resembling such a figure.

dental s. a marking on the incisor teeth of horses, first appearing in the lower central incisors at about the age of eight years; used in judging a horse's age.

lens s's starlike lines formed within the lens of the eye by fibers which pass from the anterior to the posterior surface.

s's of Verheyen venae stellatae renis.

Winslow s's whorls of capillary vessels from which arise the vorticose veins of the choroid coat of the eyeball.

starch (stahrch) [A.S. *stercan* to stiffen] 1. any of a group of polysaccharides of the general formula $(C_6H_{10}O_5)_n$, composed of a long-chain polymer of glucose in the form of amylose and amylopectin; it is the chief storage form of energy reserve (carbohydrates) in plants. 2. [NF] a preparation consisting of the granules separated from the mature grain of corn or wheat, or from potato tubers, occurring as irregular, angular, white masses or fine powder; used as a dusting powder and as a filler, binder, and disintegrant in pharmaceutical preparations.

pregelatinized s. [NF] starch processed to rupture all or part of the granules in the presence of water, and subsequently dried; used as a tablet excipient in pharmaceutical preparations.

resistant s. dietary starch that is not digested in the small intestine and continues on into the large intestine, where it has qualities similar to those of dietary fiber; high levels of resistant starch are thought to benefit intestinal physiology in ways similar to high fiber diets.

soluble s. starch partially hydrolyzed with hydrochloric acid so that it is water soluble; usually amylodextrin.

starch phos·phor·y·lase (stahrch fos-for′ə-lās) see *phosphorylase.*

Star·gardt disease (macular degeneration) (shtahr′gahrt) [Karl Bruno *Stargardt,* German ophthalmologist, 1875–1927] see under *disease.*

Star·ling curve, hypothesis, law (stahr′ling) [Ernest Henry *Starling,* English physiologist, 1866–1927] see under *curve, hypothesis,* and *law.*

Star·lix (stahr′liks) trademark for a preparation of nateglinide.

Starr-Ed·wards valve (stahr′ ed′wərdz) [Albert *Starr,* American surgeon, born 1926; Miles Lowell *Edwards,* American electrical engineer, 1898–1982] see under *valve.*

start·er (stahr′tər) a culture of microorganisms used to initiate fermentation, as in dairy products.

star·tle (stahr′təl) [A.S. *stertlen* to run about] 1. to make a quick involuntary movement as in alarm, surprise, or fright. 2. to become alarmed, surprised, or frightened.

star·va·tion (stahr-va′shən) [A.S. *sterven* to die] long-continued and extreme deprivation of food and resulting morbid effects.

stas·i·mor·phia (stas″ĭ-mor′fe-ə) stasimorphy.

stas·i·mor·phy (stas′ĭ-mor″fe) [Gr. *stasis* standing + *morphē* form] deformity or abnormality of shape in any organ, due to arrest of development.

sta·sis (sta′sis) [Gr. "a standing still"] 1. a stoppage or diminution of the flow of blood or other body fluid in any part. 2. a state of equilibrium among opposing forces.

bile s., biliary s. cholestasis.

gastric s. impaired action of stomach muscles that is less severe than gastroparesis; symptoms include weight loss, nausea, and vomiting. It may follow gastric surgery, such as when the vagus nerve has been damaged; be part of a neuromuscular problem such as autonomic neuropathy or peripheral neuropathy; or be a manifestation of a systemic disorder such as diabetes mellitus or systemic scleroderma.

intestinal s. any condition in which normal passage of intestinal content is impaired; it may be due to mechanical obstruction or impaired intestinal motility. See *stasis syndrome,* under *syndrome.*

papillary s. papilledema.

pressure s. stoppage of the circulation caused by undue pressure on a part.

urinary s. stoppage of the flow or discharge of urine, which may occur at any level of the urinary tract.

venous s. cessation or impairment of venous flow, such as with venous insufficiency; see also *stasis ulcer,* under *ulcer.* Called also *phlebostasis* and *venostasis.*

-stasis [Gr. "a standing still"] a word termination indicating the maintenance of (or maintaining) a constant level; preventing increase or multiplication.

STAT [*s*ignal *t*ransducer and *a*ctivator of *t*ranscription] any of a family of mobile transcription factors that are part of the pathway that leads from cytokines to cytokine receptors to Janus kinases to STAT's, which upon phosphorylation form activated dimers that enter the nucleus and activate expression of various genes.

stat. [L.] sta′tim (at once, immediately).

-stat [Gr. *-states* one who causes to stand, from *histanai* to cause to stand] a word termination denoting an agent that inhibits growth without killing, or a device that maintains something in a steady state.

state (stāt) [L. *status*] 1. condition or situation; see also *status.* 2. the crisis, or the turning point of an attack of disease.

acute confusional s. delirium.

alpha s. the state of relaxation and peaceful wakefulness, associated with prominent alpha brain wave activity.

anelectrotonic s. the condition which occurs in a nerve near the anode during the passage of a continuous current.

asexual s. anamorph.

borderline s. a diagnostic term used when it is difficult to determine which of two states are indicated by the presenting symptoms, generally for a state that has some characteristics of psychosis but in which the patient has some contact with reality.

carrier s. the state of being a carrier (q.v.) of a disease.

catelectrotonic s. the condition of a nerve near the cathode during the passage of an electric current.

central excitatory s. a condition in which there is stored up in a reflex center of the spinal cord a number of stimuli which do not reveal themselves in reflex response.

correlated s. dynamic equilibrium.

de-efferented s. locked-in syndrome.

dreamy s. a state of altered consciousness lasting for a few minutes and accompanied by hallucinations; associated with temporal lobe lesions. See also *temporal lobe epilepsy,* under *epilepsy,* and *petit mal status,* under *status.*

excited s. the condition of a nucleus, atom, or molecule produced by the addition of energy to the system as the result of absorption of photons or of inelastic collisions with other particles or systems.

ground s. the condition of lowest energy of a nucleus, atom, or molecule, as opposed to the excited state.

hypercoagulable s. a pathologic condition of hypercoagulability of the blood.

hyperglycemic hyperosmolar s., hyperglycemic hyperosmolar nonketotic s., hyperosmolar hyperglycemic s. a metabolic derangement in which there is an abnormally high serum glucose level without ketoacidosis, causing fluid loss from cells to extracellular fluid. The cells become dehydrated, blood volume decreases, polyuria ensues, and some patients lapse into a coma *(hyperglycemic hyperosmolar coma)* that can be fatal. The condition occurs as a complication of borderline and unrecognized diabetes mellitus, in pancreatic disorders that interfere with production of insulin, as a complication of extensive burns, in conditions marked by an excess of steroids, or in acute stress conditions including infections. It also may develop during total parenteral nutrition, hemodialysis, or peritoneal dialysis.

hypnagogic s. the state of semiconsciousness that immediately precedes falling asleep.

hypnopompic s. the state of semiconsciousness that immediately precedes complete awakening from sleep.

imperfect s. anamorph.

indifferent s. the earliest period of genital development, during which the gonads are sexually undifferentiated *(indifferent gonads).*

inotropic s. cardiac contractility.

local excitatory s. the condition of a nerve produced by an ineffectual stimulus.

metastable s. 1. an excited state with an unusually long lifetime, ranging from 10^{-6} second to several minutes. 2. an intermediate state between the ground and excited states, requiring additional energy before decay to the ground state can occur.

minimally conscious s. a level of consciousness higher than the vegetative state, characterized by limited but discernible evidence of awareness of self or the environment.

oxidation s. see under *number.*

perfect s. teleomorph.

permanent vegetative s. (PVS) the presence of a vegetative state three months after nontraumatic brain damage or 12 months after traumatic brain damage.

persistent vegetative s. (PVS) the presence of a vegetative state one month after acute brain damage.

plastic s., pluripotent s. the state of parts of the zygote or very early embryo in which they may develop into any adult tissue or part.

refractory s. a condition of subnormal excitability of muscle and nerve following excitation.

resting s. the physiological condition achieved by complete bed rest for a period of at least one hour, a condition required in a number of different tests of various body functions.

sexual s. teleomorph.

singlet s. the excited state occurring when one electron of a pair is excited to a higher energy level without changing its spin; it is unstable and can decay to either a ground state or a triplet state.

steady s. dynamic equilibrium.

triplet s. the excited state resulting when an electron is activated by absorbing a photon, moves to an outer orbital of higher energy, with the electron spin parallel to that of the other unpaired electron; it is a long-lived state that cannot decay to a ground state unless the spin changes again.

twilight s. a temporary absence of consciousness in which the patient may perform certain acts involuntarily and without remembrance of them afterward. Examples are complex partial seizures, absence seizures, and dreamy states.

vegetative s. a condition of profound nonresponsiveness in a state of apparent wakefulness, usually due to widespread lesions of the cerebral cortex and thalamus. Awareness of the self or of the environment is completely absent and there is no evidence of purposeful behavior; sleep/wake cycles occur, hypothalamic and brainstem autonomic functions are at least partially preserved, and stereotypic responses such as yawning and chewing are present.

stath•mo•ki•ne•sis (stath″mo-ki-ne′sis) a state of arrested mitosis, or pseudometaphase, as that induced by subjecting cells to the action of an agent such as colchicine, which destroys the fibrillar structure of cell spindles and thus permits the calculation of mitosis time.

stat•ic (stat′ik) [Gr. *statikos* causing to stand, from *histanai* to cause to stand] 1. at rest; in equilibrium; not in motion. 2. not dynamic.

-static a word termination meaning inhibiting, or denoting an agent that inhibits, or pertaining to the maintenance of a constant level.

Stat•icin (stat′ĭ-sin) trademark for a preparation of erythromycin.

stat•ics (stat′iks) the phase of mechanics that deals with the action of forces and systems of forces on bodies at rest.

sta•tim (sta′tim) [L.] immediately, at once. Abbreviated *stat.*

-statin [Gr. *stasis* a standing still] a word termination denoting cessation or inhibition; used in names of hormones.

stat•ins (stat′inz) [from the ending *-statin* that occurs in the names of drugs of this class] HMG-CoA reductase inhibitors.

sta•tion (sta′shən) [L. *statio*, from *stare* to stand still] 1. a position or location. 2. the location of the presenting part of the fetus in the birth canal in relation to an imaginary plane passing through the ischial spines, which is designated as zero. In one system, the location is given in whole centimeters, ranging from −5 (above the plane) to +5 (below the plane). In an older alternative system, the long axis of the birth canal is divided into thirds above and below the plane and the location is given by thirds, from −3 (above the plane) to +3 (below the plane). 3. a specified site to which the sick and wounded are brought.

anterior s. the part of the digestive system of a vector where salivarian species of *Trypanosoma* develop.

posterior s. the part of the digestive system of a vector where stercorarian species of *Trypanosoma* develop.

sta•tion•ary (sta′shən-ar″e) [L. *stationarius*] not subject to variations or to changes of place.

sta•tis•tic (stə-tis′tik) [back formation from *statistics*, q.v.] 1. an item of numerical data. 2. a value summarizing, representing, or characterizing some aspect of a sample or the population from which the sample was drawn.

sta•tis•tics (stə-tis′tiks) [Ger. *Statistik* originally "political science of state affairs," from L. *status* state] 1. a collection of numerical data. 2. a discipline devoted to the collection, analysis, and interpretation of numerical data using the theory of probability, concerned particularly with methods for drawing inferences about characteristics of a population from examination of a random sample.

bayesian s. a somewhat controversial statistical methodology that, unlike conventional statistics, which treats population parameters as fixed (though unknown) values, treats parameters as random variables with a specified probability distribution, termed the prior (or *a priori*) distribution. Bayes theorem is then used to convert the probability distribution of an observable statistic (treated as a conditional probability for a given parameter value) to a conditional probability distribution of the parameter values for a given value of the observable statistic. This distribution is termed the posterior (or *a posteriori*) distribution because it assigns a probability to each parameter value that depends on the observed data. The controversial point is the prior distribution, which represents a subjective opinion of the experimenter as to the *a priori* credibility of the various parameter values; for example, in estimating the probability of the presence of a particular disease given a positive test result, the prior distribution represents the experimenter's judgment of the prevalence of the disease in the population under study.

descriptive s. the use of statistical methods to measure and describe characteristics of groups, without drawing inferences about the population in general.

inferential s. the use of statistical methods to generalize conclusions from sample data, using theories of probability to estimate population parameters.

nonparametric s. a statistical methodology that can be used on data without making the assumption that the data are drawn from a population with a normal or other specified distribution. See also under *test*.

parametric s. statistical methodology that depends upon assumptions about the distribution of the data, e.g., that the data approximate a normal distribution and are homoscedastic.

semiparametric s. statistical methodology that combines both parametric and nonparametric elements; used for estimating population parameters when a function is unknown, such as the distribution function of a random variable that has not been observed.

vital s. the data, usually collected by governmental bodies, detailing the rates of birth, death, disease, marriage, and divorce in a population.

stato•acous•tic (stat″o-ə-ko͞os′tik) pertaining to balance and hearing.

stato•co•nia (stat″o-ko′ne-ə) [Gr. *statos* standing + *konos* dust] plural of *statoconium*.

stato•co•ni•um (stat″o-ko′ne-əm) [TA] one of the minute calciferous granules within the gelatinous statoconic membrane surmounting the acoustic maculae *(membrana statoconiorum macularum)*. Called also *otolith*, *otolite*, *otoconium*, and *ear crystal*.

stato•lith (stat′o-lith) 1. statoconium. 2. a solid or semisolid body occurring in the statocyst of animals.

sta•tom•e•ter (stə-tom′ə-tər) exophthalmometer.

sta•ture (stach′oor) [L. *statura*] the height or tallness of a person standing. **stat′ural** *adj*

familial short s., genetic short s. a syndrome of short stature (q.v.) with normal growth velocity, normal onset and progression of puberty, normal skeletal age, and short stature in close relatives such as parents.

psychosocial short s. deprivation dwarfism.

short s. in pediatric growth assessment, reduced length or height, defined variously as being below the third or the fifth percentile for age when plotted on a growth chart. Cf. *dwarfism*.

tall s. term sometimes used in pediatrics for height that is more than 2 standard deviations above the norm for a child's age; in a minority of cases it may be a sign of a disorder. Cf. *gigantism*.

sta•tus (sta′təs) [L.] state; particularly used in reference to a morbid condition.

absence s. a type of petit mal status that lasts for several hours and has few stereotyped or abnormal movements.

s. asthma′ticus a particularly severe episode of asthma that does not respond adequately to ordinary therapeutic measures and may require hospitalization.

s. calci′fames calcium hunger.

s. chore′icus a severe and persistent form of chorea.

complex partial s. status epilepticus consisting of a series of complex partial seizures without return to full consciousness in between. Called also *psychomotor s.*

s. convulsi′vus s. epilepticus (def. 1).

s. criba′lis, s. cribro′sus a sievelike condition of the brain due to dilatation of the perivascular lymph spaces.

s. cri′ticus a severe and persistent form of tabetic crises.

s. dysmyelina′tus, s. dysmyelinisa′tus Hallervorden-Spatz disease.

s. dysra′phicus any faulty closure of the embryonic neural tube, with faulty formation of midline adult structures that may include the vertebral column, sternum, breasts, or palate. Cf. *neural tube defect*, under *defect*.

s. epilep′ticus 1. a continuous series of generalized tonic-clonic seizures without return to consciousness, a life-threatening emergency. Called also *convulsive s. epilepticus*. 2. any prolonged series of similar seizures without return to full consciousness between them; the two major types are *convulsive s. epilepticus*, which is life-threatening, and *nonconvulsive s. epilepticus*, which is serious but not usually life-threatening.

s. epilepticus, convulsive s. epilepticus (def. 1).

s. epilepticus, nonconvulsive status epilepticus that does not include generalized tonic-clonic seizures; see *complex partial s.*, *petit mal s.*, and *epilepsia partialis continua*.

s. epilepticus, tonic-clonic s. epilepticus (def. 1).

s. hemicra′nicus s. migrainosus.

s. lacuna′ris, s. lacuno′sus a condition of the brain marked by numerous small infarcts *(lacunar infarcts)* or losses of substance.

s. lympha′ticus developmentally normal hyperplasia of lymphoid tissue and the thymus, formerly thought to be an important cause of sudden death (by airway obstruction) in infants; called also *s. thymicolymphaticus*, and *s. thymicus*.

s. marmora′tus a usually congenital condition marked by excessive myelinization of the nerve fibers of the corpus striatum, as in Vogt syndrome; called also *état marbré*.

s. migraino′sus a state marked by constantly recurring attacks of migraine; called also *s. hemicranicus*.

performance s. ability of a patient to function as measured by a performance scale.

petit mal s. any of a variety of clinical disorders with symptoms ranging from momentary interruption of consciousness to longer-lasting spells of loss of motor control. They have a distinctive pattern on the electroencephalogram, with spike and wave discharges at three cycles per second. See also *absence epilepsy*, under *epilepsy*.

s. prae′sens the condition of a patient at the time of observation.

psychomotor s. complex partial s.

simple partial s. epilepsia partialis continua.

s. thymicolympha′ticus, s. thy′micus s. lymphaticus.

s. verruco′sus a wartlike appearance of the cerebral cortex, produced by disorderly arrangement of the neuroblasts so that the formation of fissures and sulci is irregular and unpredictable.

s. vertigino′sus prolonged vertigo.

Staub-Trau•gott effect (test), phenomenon (shtoub′ trou′got) [Hans *Staub*, Swiss internist, 1890–1967; Carl *Traugott*, German internist, 20th century] see under *effect* and *phenomenon*.

Stauf•fer syndrome (staw′fər) [Maurice H. *Stauffer*, American gastroenterologist, 20th century] see under *syndrome*.

stau•ri•on (staw′re-on) [Gr., dim. of *stauros* cross] a point at the crossing of the median and transverse palatine sutures.

stau•ro•ple•gia (staw″ro-ple′jə) [Gr. *stauros* cross + *-plegia*] alternate hemiplegia.

staves•acre (stāvz-a′kər) 1. *Delphinium staphisagria*. 2. staphisagria.

stav•u•dine (stav′u-dēn) [USP] a nucleoside analogue of thymidine that inhibits human immunodeficiency virus (HIV) replication, used in the treatment of HIV infection; administered orally.

stax•is (stak′sis) [Gr. "a dripping"] hemorrhage.

stay (sta) 1. a narrow structure that gives support. 2. bar (def. 6).

frog s. bar (def. 6).

s. of white line adminiculum lineae albae.

STD sexually transmitted disease.

STE subperiosteal tissue expander.

steal (stēl) diversion of something from its normal course, usually refering to blood flow in occlusive arterial disease.

cerebral s., subclavian s. in occlusive disease of the subclavian artery, a reversal of blood flow in the ipsilateral vertebral artery from the basilar artery to the subclavian artery beyond the point of occlusion; this may deprive the brain of blood and cause the subclavian steal syndrome.

ste•a•ral•de•hyde (ste″ə-ral′də-hīd) a long-chain, aliphatic free aldehyde found in plasmalogens, giving the so-called plasmal reaction upon direct treatment of the tissue with Schiff reagent.

ste•a•rate (ste′ə-rāt) any salt (soap), ester, or anionic form of stearic acid.

ste•a•ric ac•id (ste-ar′ik) [*stear-* + *-ic*] 1. a saturated 18-carbon fatty acid occurring in most fats and oils, particularly the oils of land animals and fats of tropical plants; stearic and palmitic acids are the two most common saturated fatty acids in body fluids. See also table at *fatty acid*. 2. [NF] a preparation containing a mixture of stearic and palmitic acids, prepared by hydrogenation of fats and oils that are derived from edible sources unless the preparation is for external use only; used as a tablet and capsule lubricant and as an emulsifying and solubilizing agent.

ste•ar•i•form (ste-ar′ĭ-form) fatlike.

ste•a•rin (ste′ə-rin) tristearin.

stear(o)- [Gr. *stear*, gen. *steatos* fat] a combining form denoting relationship to fat.

ste•a•rop•tene (ste″ə-rop′tən) [*stearo-* + Gr. *ptēnos* volatile] the more solid component of a volatile oil, cf. *eleoptene*.

ste•a•ro•yl (stēr′o-əl) the acyl radical of stearic acid.

ste•a•ro•yl-CoA 9-de•sat•u•rase (ste-ar′o-əl ko-a′ de-sach′u-rās) [EC 1.14.19.5] an enzyme activity of the oxidoreductase class that catalyzes the desaturation of stearoyl coenzyme A to form oleoyl coenzyme A. It is part of a complex in the endoplasmic reticulum that also includes a flavoprotein (FAD), cytochrome b_5, and cytochrome-b_5 reductase. Called also *acyl-CoA desaturase*.

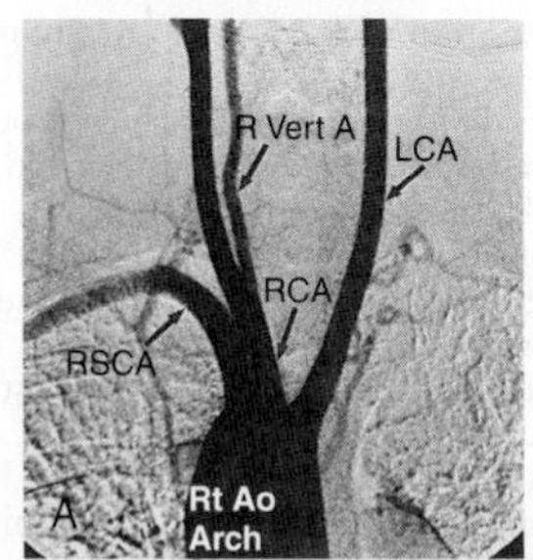

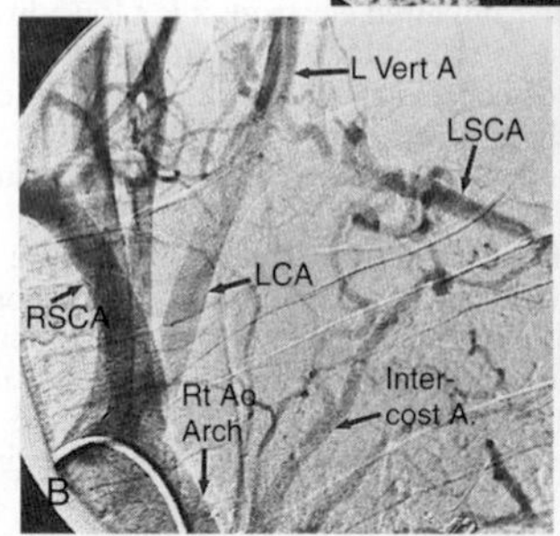

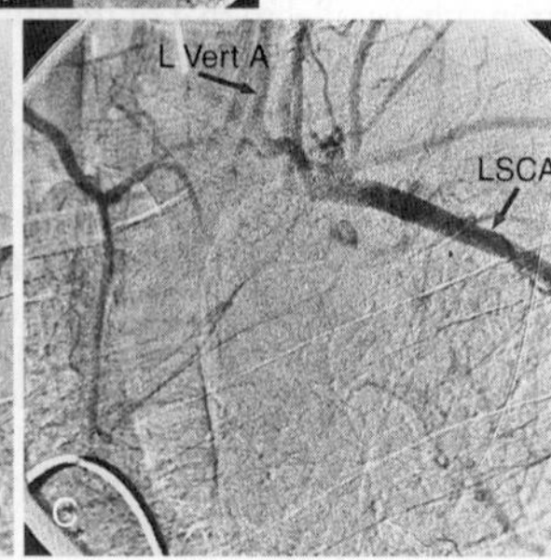

■ Symptomatic congenital subclavian steal in a 21-year-old man. *(A)*, Arteriogram of early phase shows right aortic arch *(Rt Ao Arch)* from which arise a right subclavian artery *(RSCA)*, right carotid artery *(RCA)*, right vertebral artery *(R Vert A)*, and left carotid artery *(LCA)*. The left subclavian artery *(LSCA)* is conspicuously absent. *(B)*, Subsequent phase shows LSCA filling from the left vertebral artery *(L Vert A)*. *Intercost A*, Intercostal artery. *(C)*, Later phase shows further filling of LSCA from L Vert A.

ste•ar•rhea (ste″ə-re′ə) steatorrhea.

ste•a•tite (ste′ə-tīt) soapstone.

ste•a•ti•tis (ste″ə-ti′tis) [*steato-* + *-itis*] 1. inflammation of adipose tissue. See also *panniculitis*. 2. yellow fat disease.

nutritional s. yellow fat disease.

steat(o)- stear(o)-.

ste•a•to•crit (ste′ə-to-krit″) [*steato-* + Gr. *krinein* to separate] a semiquantitative method for assessing the amount of fat in feces.

acid s. a screening test for fat malabsorption: an acidified stool sample is centrifuged to yield solid, liquid, and fatty layers and the proportion of fat is expressed as a volumetric percentage (lipid phase/solid phase), with normal being less than 10 percent.

ste•a•to•cys•to•ma (ste″ə-to-sis-to′mə) a pale to flesh-colored epidermal cyst, typically with an intricately infolded thin epidermal lining, without a granular layer, incorporating abortive hair follicles and at times sebaceous, eccrine, or apocrine structures, and containing lanugo and an oily material. These lesions are clinically similar and may be related to eruptive vellus hair cysts (see under *cyst*).

s. mul′tiplex development of numerous steatocystomas, especially involving the skin over the sternum, proximal limbs, or the scrotum in males; it is often an autosomal dominant disorder chiefly affecting males at birth or presenting around the time of puberty.

ste•a•tog•e•nous (ste″ə-toj′ə-nəs) lipogenic.

ste•a•to•hep•a•ti•tis (ste″ə-to-hep″ə-ti′tis) fatty liver with inflammation. **steatohepatit′ic** *adj*

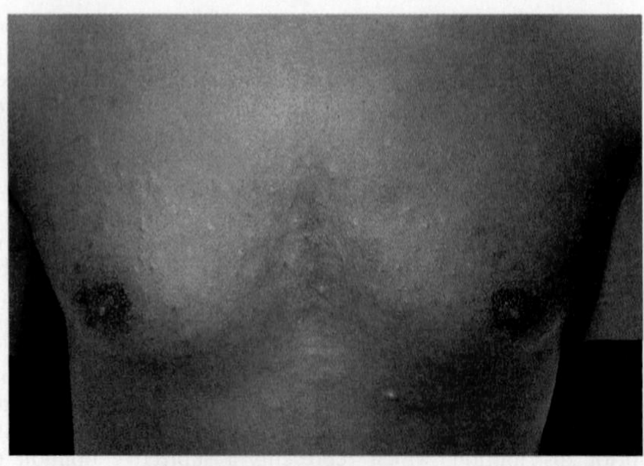

■ Steatocystoma multiplex.

nonalcoholic s. (NASH) an inflammatory disease of the liver of uncertain pathogenesis, histologically resembling alcoholic hepatitis but occurring in nonalcoholic patients, most often obese women with type 2 diabetes mellitus; clinically it is generally asymptomatic or mild, but fibrosis or cirrhosis may result.

ste·a·tol·y·sis (ste″ə-tol′ĭ-sis) lipolysis.

ste·a·to·lyt·ic (ste″ə-to-lit′ik) lipolytic.

ste·a·to·ma (ste″ə-to′mə) pl. *steato′mata, steatomas* [*steat-* + *-oma*] a fatty mass retained within a sebaceous gland.

ste·a·to·ma·to·sis (ste″ə-to-mə-to′sis) 1. lipomatosis. 2. steatocystoma multiplex.

ste·a·tom·ery (ste″ə-tom′ər-e) [*steato-* + Gr. *mēros* thigh] a deposit of fat on the outer aspects of the thighs and buttocks.

ste·a·to·ne·cro·sis (ste″ə-to-nə-kro′sis) fat necrosis.

ste·a·to·pyg·ia (ste″ə-to-pij′e-ə) [*steato-* + *pyg-* + *-ia*] excessive fatness of the buttocks, usually seen in women. **steatop′ygous** *adj*

ste·a·tor·rhea (ste″ə-to-re′ə) [*steato-* + *-rrhea*] excessive amounts of fats in the feces, as in malabsorption syndromes.

idiopathic s. celiac disease.

ste·a·to·sis (ste″ə-to′sis) fatty change.

s. cardi′aca cardiomyoliposis.

hepatic s., liver s. fatty liver.

macrovesicular s. fatty change in which a single large droplet occupies most of the cell, displacing the cytoplasm and nucleus to a ring around the droplet. Called also *macrosteatosis.* Cf. *microvesicular s.*

microvesicular s. fatty change in which numerous small lipid droplets are present in the cytoplasm. Called also *microsteatosis.* Cf. *macrovesicular s.*

STEC Shiga toxin–producing *Escherichia coli.*

stech·i·ol·o·gy (stek″e-ol′ə-je) stoichiology.

stech·i·om·e·try (stek″e-om′ə-tre) stoichiometry.

Steele-Ri·chard·son-Ol·szew·ski syndrome (stēl′ rich′ərd-sən ol-shev′ske) [John C. *Steele*, Canadian neurologist, born 1934; John Clifford *Richardson*, Canadian neurologist, 1909–1986; Jerzy *Olszewski*, Polish-born Canadian neurologist, 1913–1966] progressive supranuclear palsy; see under *palsy.*

Steell murmur (stēl) [Graham *Steell*, English physician, 1851–1942] Graham Steell murmur; see under *murmur.*

steg·no·sis (steg-no′sis) [Gr. *stegnōsis* obstruction] constriction; stenosis.

steg·not·ic (steg-not′ik) 1. pertaining to, characterized by, or promoting stegnosis. 2. astringent.

Steg·o·my·ia (steg″o-mi′yə) [Gr. *stegos* roof + *myia* fly] a subgenus of mosquitoes of the genus *Aedes*, native to various Pacific islands.

Stein-Lev·en·thal syndrome (stīn′ lev′ən-thahl) [Irving Freiler *Stein*, Sr., American gynecologist, 1887–1976; Michael Leo *Leventhal*, American obstetrician and gynecologist, 1901–1971] polycystic ovary syndrome; see under *syndrome.*

Stein·brock·er syndrome (stīn′brok-ər) [Otto *Steinbrocker*, American physician, 20th century] shoulder-hand syndrome.

Steind·ler operation (stīnd′lər) [Arthur *Steindler*, American orthopedic surgeon, 1878–1959] see under *operation.*

Stei·ner syndrome (shti′nər) [L. *Steiner*, German physician, early 20th century] Curtius syndrome.

Stei·nert disease (shti′nərt) [Hans *Steinert*, German physician, early 20th century] myotonic dystrophy; see under *dystrophy.*

Stein·mann pin (shtīn′mahn) [Fritz *Steinmann*, Swiss surgeon, 1872–1932] see under *pin.*

Stein·stras·se (shtīn′shtrah-sə) [Ger. "stone street"] urinary tract obstruction due to fragments of calculi that become lodged in the ureter after extracorporeal shock wave lithotripsy.

Stel·a·zine (stel′ə-zēn) trademark for preparations of trifluoperazine hydrochloride.

stel·la (stel′ə) pl. *stel′lae* [L.] star.

s. len′tis hyaloi′dea the posterior pole of the crystalline lens.

s. len′tis iri′dica the anterior pole of the crystalline lens.

stel·late (stel′āt) [L. *stellatus*] shaped like a star; arranged in a roset, or in rosets.

stel·lec·to·my (stə-lek′tə-me) removal of the stellate ganglion; done for the relief of pain.

Stel·lite (stel′it, stel′īt) trademark for any of a group of nonferrous, very hard, noncorrosive alloys composed chiefly of cobalt and chromium, with or without small amounts of other metals added. Used especially in the manufacture of cutting tools such as surgical instruments.

stel·lu·la (stel′u-lə) pl. *stel′lulae* [L., dim. of *stella*] little star.

stellulae of Verheyen, stel′lulae verhey′enii venae stellatae renis.

Stell·wag sign (shtel′vahk) [Carl von Carion *Stellwag*, Austrian ophthalmologist, 1823–1904] see under *sign.*

stem (stem) a stalklike supporting structure; see also *peduncle.*

brain s. brainstem; see under *B.*

femoral s. in arthroplasty of the hip or knee, the part of the prosthesis that inserts into the end of the trimmed and prepared femur.

s. of hair follicle name sometimes given to the segment of the hair follicle between the bulb and the isthmus.

humeral s. in arthroplasty of the shoulder or elbow, the part of the prosthesis that inserts into the end of the trimmed and prepared humerus.

infundibular s. the inferior part of the infundibulum hypothalami; it contains the neural connections of the pituitary gland and is continuous with the tuber cinereum.

stem bro·me·lain (stem bro′mə-lān) [EC 3.4.22.32] see *bromelain.*

STEMI ST elevation myocardial infarction.

Sten·der dishes (shten′dər) [Wilhelm P. *Stender*, German manufacturer, 19th century] see under *dish.*

sten·i·on (sten′e-on) pl. *sten′ia* [Gr. *stenos* narrow + *-on* neuter ending] an encephalometric landmark, the craniometrical point situated at each end of the smallest transverse diameter of the head in the temporal region.

Ste·no (ste′no) see *Stensen.*

sten(o)- [Gr. *stenos* narrow] a combining form meaning contracted or narrow.

steno·breg·mat·ic (sten″o-breg-mat′ik) [*steno-* + *bregmatic*] having the superior and anterior portions of the head narrowed.

steno·ce·pha·lia (sten″o-sə-fa′le-ə) stenocephaly.

steno·ceph·a·ly (sten″o-sef′ə-le) [*steno-* + *-cephaly*] excessive narrowness of the head. **stenoceph′alous** *adj*

steno·cho·ria (sten″o-kor′e-ə) [*steno-* + Gr. *chōros* space] stenosis, or narrowing.

steno·cro·ta·phia (sten″o-kro-ta′fe-ə) [*steno-* + *crotaphion* + *-ia*] narrowness of the temporal region.

steno·crot·a·phy (sten″o-krot′ə-fe) stenocrotaphia.

steno·pe·ic (sten″o-pe′ik) [*sten-* + Gr. *opē* opening] having a narrow slit or opening.

ste·nosed (stə-nōzd′) narrowed or constricted.

ste·no·sis (stə-no′sis) pl. *steno′ses* [Gr. *stenōsis*] an abnormal narrowing of a duct or canal; called also *arctation, coarctation,* and *stricture.* **stenot′ic** *adj*

aortic s. (AS) narrowing of the aortic orifice or of the supravalvular or subvalvular regions; see also *supravalvular aortic s.* and *subvalvular aortic s.*

buttonhole mitral s. mitral stenosis in which adhesion and shortening of the mitral cusps produces a diaphragmatic slit resembling a buttonhole; called also *fishmouth mitral s.*

calcific aortic s. the most common type of aortic stenosis, characterized by calcific nodules around the cusps of the aortic valve.

caroticovertebral s. atherosclerotic stenosis of the cervical portions of the vertebral arteries, resulting in cerebral ischemia.

cicatricial s. stenosis caused by the contraction of a cicatrix.

fishmouth mitral s. buttonhole mitral s.

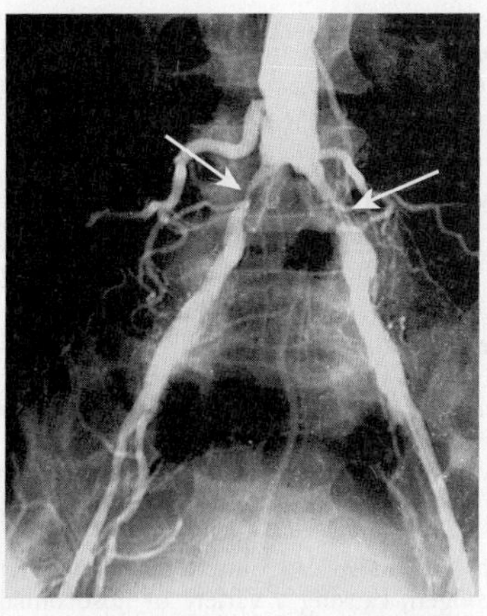

■ Bilateral severe stenosis of the common iliac arteries *(arrows);* seen in a standard contrast angiogram.

granulation s. stenosis or narrowing caused by the deposit of granulations or by their contraction.

hypertrophic pyloric s. pyloric stenosis caused by muscular hypertrophy and mucosal edema, occurring chiefly in infants; symptoms include nausea, vomiting, epigastric pain, anorexia, weight loss, dehydration, and hypochloremic alkalosis; affected infants have a palpable pyloric mass and visible peristalsis.

hypertrophic subaortic s., idiopathic hypertrophic subaortic s. (IHSS) a form of hypertrophic cardiomyopathy in which the left ventricle is hypertrophied (commonly with disproportionate involvement of the interventricular septum) and the cavity is small; it is marked by obstruction to left ventricular outflow. Called also *muscular subaortic s.*

infantile hypertrophic gastric s. congenital hypertrophy and hyperplasia of the musculature of the pyloric sphincter, occurring within the first few weeks of life and leading to partial obstruction of the gastric outlet.

infundibular s. stenosis below the pulmonary valve, within the infundibulum (conus arteriosus) of the right ventricle of the heart. Called also *subpulmonic infundibular s.*

lumbar spinal s. spinal s.

meatal s. stenosis of the urinary meatus, seen most often in boys or men as a complication of circumcision and meatitis.

mitral s. a narrowing of the left atrioventricular orifice (mitral orifice); see also *buttonhole mitral s.*

muscular subaortic s. idiopathic hypertrophic subaortic s.

papillary s. sphincter of Oddi dysfunction.

postdiphtheritic s. stenosis of the larynx or trachea following diphtheria.

pulmonary s. (PS) narrowing of the opening between the pulmonary artery and the right ventricle, usually at the level of the valve leaflets.

pyloric s. obstruction of the pyloric orifice of the stomach; it may be congenital as in hypertrophic pyloric stenosis (q.v.), or acquired due to peptic ulcers or prepyloric carcinoma.

rectal s. stenosis or stricture of the rectum. Called also *proctostenosis* and *rectostenosis.*

renal artery s. (RAS) narrowing of one or both renal arteries, caused by atherosclerosis or fibromuscular dysplasia, so that renal function is impaired (see also *ischemic nephropathy*, under *nephropathy*). The resultant increase in renin release by the affected kidney causes renovascular hypertension, and bilateral stenosis may result in chronic renal failure.

spinal s. narrowing of the vertebral canal, nerve root canals, or intervertebral foramina of the lumbar spine caused by encroachment of bone upon the space; symptoms are caused by compression of the cauda equina and include pain, paresthesias, and neurogenic claudication. The condition may be either congenital or due to spinal degeneration. Called also *lumbar spinal s.* See also *spinal compression* under *compression.*

subaortic s. aortic stenosis due to an obstructive lesion in the left ventricle below the aortic valve, causing a pressure gradient across the obstruction within the ventricle. See also *idiopathic hypertrophic subaortic s.*

subglottic s. stenosis of the trachea below the glottis. A congenital form results in neonatal stridor or laryngotracheitis, often requiring tracheotomy but resolving with age. An acquired form is caused by repeated intubations.

subpulmonic infundibular s. infundibular s.

subvalvular aortic s. subaortic s.

supravalvular aortic s. a rare form of aortic stenosis occurring above the aortic valve, usually caused by a complete circumferential fibrous ring of constricting tissue at the level of the sinus of Valsalva. See also *Williams syndrome*, under *syndrome.*

tricuspid s. (TS) narrowing or stricture of the tricuspid orifice of the heart.

valvular s. stenosis affecting any of the valves of the heart; see *aortic s.*, *mitral s.*, *pulmonary s.*, and *tricuspid s.*

steno·ther·mal (sten″o-thur′məl) stenothermic.

steno·ther·mic (sten″o-thur′mik) [*steno-* + *therm-* + *-ic*] capable of development only within a narrow range of temperature, e.g., a bacterial culture.

steno·tho·rax (sten″o-thor′aks) [*steno-* + *thorax*] abnormal narrowness of the chest.

Steno·tro·pho·mo·nas (sten″o-tro″fo-mo′nəs) [*steno-* + *tropho-* + Gr. *monas* unit, from *monos* single] a genus of gram-negative, β-lactamase–producing bacteria of the family Xanthomonadaceae, consisting of aerobic, nonfermentative, chemo-organotrophic, straight or curved rods that are motile by two or more flagella and occur singly or in pairs; organisms are typically soil and water inhabitants. The type species is *S. maltophi′lia.*

S. maltophi′lia a widespread, antibiotic-resistant species that is an opportunistic pathogen, causing a variety of nosocomial infections, most commonly bacteremia and pneumonia. Formerly called *Pseudomonas maltophilia* and *Xanthomonas maltophilia.*

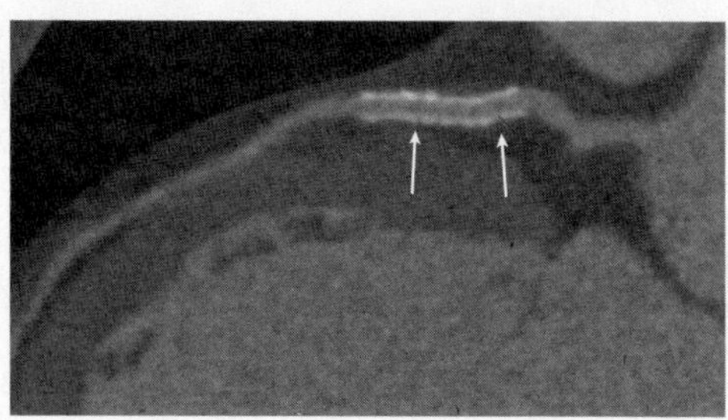

■ Patent stent *(arrows)* in the proximal anterior interventricular branch of the left coronary artery.

Sten·sen canal, duct, etc. (sten′sən) [Niels *Stensen* (Nicolaus *Steno*), Danish physician, anatomist in Italy, 1638–1686] see under *experiment* and *plexus*, and see *canales incisivi*, *ductus parotideus*, and *foramina incisiva.*

Stent graft, mass (stent) [Charles R. *Stent*, English dentist, 1845–1901] see under *mass* and see *inlay graft* under *graft.*

stent (stent) [from Charles R. *Stent*] 1. a mold for keeping a skin graft in place, made of Stent mass or some acrylic or dental compound. 2. a slender rodlike or threadlike device used to provide support for tubular structures that are being anastomosed, or to induce or maintain their patency. See also *endoprosthesis.* 3. to apply or insert a stent.

drug-eluting s. a coronary artery stent coated with a pharmaceutic agent that is slowly released to resist restenosis of the vessel.

intravascular s. a metal wire or tube introduced into a stenotic blood vessel to create and maintain luminal patency; it may be self-expanding or balloon-expandable.

Palmaz s. an intravascular stent made of rigid wire mesh; it is introduced by a guidewire and then expanded into place by a balloon.

pigtail s. a ureteral stent with a curl near the end like that of a pig's tail to maintain it in place.

T-Y s. a stent with both T-shaped and Y-shaped sections, used for keeping an airway patent after trauma or a burn.

ureteral s. a stent inserted into the ureter to maintain patency in stenosis or in healing after trauma or surgery.

step (step) one of a series of foot rests on different levels, or a structure resembling it.

Rönne nasal s. a steplike defect in the nasal side of the visual field; seen in glaucoma.

ste·pha·ni·al (stə-fa′ne-əl) pertaining to the stephanion.

ste·pha·ni·on (stə-fa′ne-ən) [Gr. *stephanos* crown + *-on* neuter ending] the point on the side of the cranium at which the coronal suture meets the superior temporal line.

Ste·phano·fi·la·ria (stef″ə-no-fī-lar′e-ə) a genus of nematodes of the superfamily Filarioidea. *S. stile′si* causes stephanofilariasis in cattle in the United States.

steph·a·no·fi·la·ri·a·sis (stef″ə-no-fil″ə-ri′ə-sis) a chronic skin disease of cattle in certain parts of the United States, due to infestation with the nematode *Stephanofilaria stilesi;* called also *filarial* or *verminous dermatitis* and *stephanofilarosis.*

steph·a·no·fil·a·ro·sis (stef″ə-no-fil″ə-ro′sis) stephanofilariasis.

Steph·a·nu·ri·dae (stef″ə-nu′rĭ-de) a family of nematodes that includes the genus *Stephanurus.*

Steph·a·nu·rus (stef″ə-nu′rəs) a genus of nematode parasites of the family Stephanuridae. *S. denta′tus* is parasitic in the urinary tract and occasionally other organs in pigs.

ste·ra·di·an (sr) (stə-ra′de-ən) [Gr. *ster-* solid + *radian*] the SI unit of measurement of solid angles, equivalent to the angle subtended at the center of a sphere by an area on its surface equal to the square of its radius. A full sphere subtends 4π steradians.

Ster·a·pred (ster′ə-pred″) trademark for a preparation of prednisone.

sterc(o)- [L. *stercus* dung] a combining form denoting relationship to feces.

ster·co·bi·lin (stur″ko-bi′lin) [*sterco-* + *bilin*] a bile pigment derivative, formed by air oxidation of stercobilinogen, which is in turn derived by reduction of bilirubin; it is a brown-orange-red pigmentation contributing to the color of feces and urine.

ster·co·bi·lin·o·gen (stur″ko-bi-lin′o-jən) a bilirubin metabolite and precursor of stercobilin, formed by reduction of urobilinogen.

ster·co·lith (stur′ko-lith) [*sterco-* + *-lith*] fecalith.

ster·co·ra·ceous (stur″kə-ra′shəs) [L. *stercoraceus*] fecal.

ster·co·ral (stur′kə-rəl) fecal.

ster·co·ra·ria (stur″kə-rar′e-ə) in some systems of classification, a subgroup of the genus *Trypanosoma* comprising species whose developmental cycle is completed in the hindgut (posterior station) of the vector, with transmission by fecal contamination during biting of the host by the vector. The group includes the subgenera *Megatrypanum, Herpetosoma,* and *Schizotrypanum.* Cf. *salivaria.*

ster·co·rar·i·an (stur″kə-rar′e-ən) pertaining to or caused by trypanosomes of the stercoraria group.

ster·co·ro·ma (stur″kə-ro′mə) fecaloma.

ster·co·rous (stur′kə-rəs) [L. *stercorosus*] fecal.

Ster·cu·lia (stər-ku′le-ə) a large genus of mostly tropical trees and shrubs of the family Sterculiaceae, named for the stercorous (manurelike) odor of certain species. Some species have edible seeds and others are medicinal. *S. u′rens* and other species yield the gummy exudate called *karaya gum.*

ster·cu·lia (stər-ku′le-ə) 1. any plant of the genus *Sterculia.* 2. karaya gum.

stereo- [Gr. *stereos* solid] a combining form meaning solid, having three dimensions, or firmly established.

ster·eo·acu·i·ty (ster″e-o-ə-ku′ĭ-te) [*stereo-* + *acuity*] visual acuity with stereoscopic vision.

ster·eo·ag·no·sis (ster″e-o-ag-no′sis) astereognosis.

ster·eo·an·es·the·sia (ster″e-o-an″es-the′zhə) [*stereo-* + *anesthesia*] inability to identify by touch the form, size, weight, and texture of objects, owing to cortical disease or an interruption of nerve tracts. Cf. *astereognosis.*

ster·eo·ar·throl·y·sis (ster″e-o-ahr-throl′ĭ-sis) [*stereo-* + *arthro-* + *-lysis*] operative formation of a movable new joint in cases of bony ankylosis.

ster·eo·aus·cul·ta·tion (ster″e-o-aws″kəl-ta′shən) auscultation by means of two phonendoscopes each on different parts of the chest. One tube of each instrument is placed in the ears, the other tube of each being closed with the fingers.

ster·eo·blas·tu·la (ster″e-o-blas′tu-lə) a solid blastula, all of whose cells reach the external surface.

ster·eo·blind (ster″e-o-blīnd′) [*stereo-* + *blind*] lacking in stereopsis.

ster·eo·cam·pim·e·ter (ster″e-o-kam-pim′ə-tər) [*stereo-* + *campimeter*] an instrument for studying unilateral central scotomas and defects in the central retinal area.

ster·eo·chem·i·cal (ster″e-o-kem′ĭ-kəl) pertaining to stereochemistry, or to the space relations of the atoms of a molecule.

ster·eo·chem·is·try (ster″e-o-kem′is-tre) 1. the chemical theory that supposes an arrangement of the atoms of certain molecules in three-dimensional spaces. 2. the branch of chemistry concerned with the space relations between atoms.

ster·eo·cil·i·a (ster″e-o-sil′e-ə) (sing. *stereocil′ium*) [*stereo-* + *cilium*] long, nonmotile microvilli found on the free surface of hair cells of the internal ear and on pseudostratified epithelial cells of the male epididymis; they have cores of cross-linked actin filaments but, unlike true cilia, do not have axonemes. Cf. *kinocilium.*

ster·eo·cine·flu·o·rog·ra·phy (ster″e-o-sin″ə-flo͝o-rog′rə-fe) photographic recording by motion picture camera of x-ray images produced by stereofluoroscopy, affording three-dimensional visualization.

ster·eo·cog·no·sy (ster″e-o-kog′no-se) stereognosis.

ster·eo·flu·o·ros·co·py (ster″e-o-flo͝o-ros′kə-pe) stereoscopic fluoroscopy.

ster·e·og·no·sis (ster″e-og-no′sis) [*stereo-* + Gr. *gnōsis* knowledge] 1. the faculty of perceiving and understanding the form and nature of objects by the sense of touch. 2. perception by the senses of the solidity of objects.

ster·e·og·nos·tic (ster″e-og-nos′tik) pertaining to stereognosis.

ster·eo·gram (ster′e-o-gram) 1. a stereoscopic radiograph. 2. a stereoscopic drawing.

ster·eo·graph (ster′e-o-graf) stereogram.

ster·eo·iso·mer (ster″e-o-i′so-mər) one of a group of compounds having a stereoisomeric relationship.

ster·eo·isom·er·ism (ster″e-o-i-som′ər-iz-əm) [*stereo-* + *isomerism*] the relationship between two or more isomers that have the same structure (the same linkages between atoms) but different configurations (spatial arrangements) in contrast to constitutional isomerism in which the isomers have different structures. Stereoisomers are further classified into *enantiomers,* those having molecules that are mirror images of each other, and *diastereomers,* those that do not. An older classification used the subdivisions optical and geometric isomerism (q.v.), which did not include all forms of stereoisomerism. Called also *configurational, stereochemical,* or *spatial isomerism.* **stereoisomer′ic** *adj*

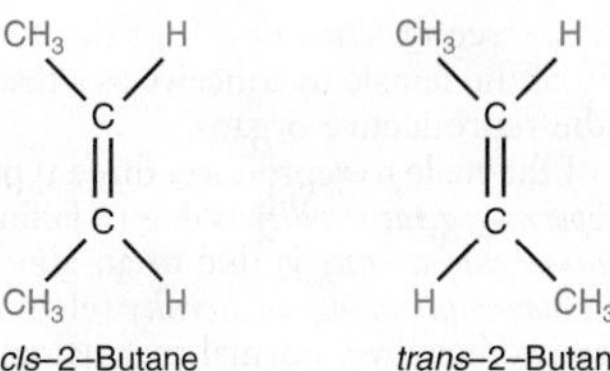

■ Stereoisomerism, exemplified by a pair of *cis-trans* diastereomers.

ster·e·ol·o·gy (ster″e-ol′ə-je) the study of the three-dimensional properties of objects usually seen in two dimensions.

ster·e·om·e·ter (ster″e-om′ə-tər) [*stereo-* + *-meter*] an instrument for performing stereometry.

ster·e·om·e·try (ster″e-om′ə-tre) the measurement of the cubic or solid contents of a solid body, or of the capacity of a hollow space.

ster·eo·oph·thal·mo·scope (ster″e-o-of-thal′mo-skōp) binocular ophthalmoscope.

Ster·eo·or·thop·ter (ster″e-o-or-thop′tər) trademark for a mirror-reflecting instrument used to correct strabismus.

ster·eo·pho·rom·e·ter (ster″e-o-fo-rom′ə-tər) [*stereo-* + *phorometer*] a phorometer with a stereoscopic attachment.

ster·eo·pho·to·mi·cro·graph (ster″e-o-fo″to-mi′kro-graf) a stereoscopic photograph of a microscopical subject.

ster·e·op·sis (ster″e-op′sis) [*stereo-* + Gr. *opsis* vision] stereoscopic vision.

ster·eo·ra·di·og·ra·phy (ster″e-o-ra″de-og′rə-fe) the making of a radiograph giving an impression of depth as well as of width and height.

ster·eo·ra·di·om·e·try (ster″e-o-ra″di-om′ə-tre) measurement of the solid dimensions of a radiopaque object from its stereoscopic radiographs.

ster·eo·sal·pin·gog·ra·phy (ster″e-o-sal″ping-gog′rə-fe) salpingography in which an impression of depth is achieved.

ster·eo·scope (ster′e-o-skōp″) [*stereo-* + *-scope*] an instrument for producing the appearance of solidity and relief by combining the images of two pictures of an object seen from slightly dissimilar viewpoints.

ster·eo·scop·ic (ster″e-o-skop′ik) having the effect of a stereoscope; giving to objects seen a solid or three-dimensional appearance.

ster·eo·spe·cif·ic (ster″e-o-spə-sif′ik) exhibiting marked specificity for one of several stereoisomers of a substrate or reactant; said of enzymes or of synthetic organic reactions.

ster·eo·tac·tic (ster″e-o-tak′tik) [*stereo-* + L. *tactus* touch] 1. characterized by precise positioning in space; said especially of discrete areas of the brain that control specific functions. 2. pertaining to types of surgery or radiotherapy that use a system of three-dimensional coordinates to locate the site to be operated on or irradiated. 3. thigmotactic.

ster·eo·tax·ic (ster″e-o-tak′sik) 1. stereotactic. 2. thigmotactic.

ster·eo·tax·is (ster″e-o-tak′sis) 1. stereotactic surgery. 2. thigmotaxis.

ster·eo·taxy (ster″e-o-tak′se) stereotactic surgery.

ster·e·ot·ro·pism (ster″e-ot′rə-piz-əm) [*stereo-* + *tropism*] thigmotropism. **stereotrop′ic** *adj*

ster·eo·typ·ic (ster″e-o-tip′ik) having a fixed, unvarying form.

ster·eo·ty·py (ster′e-o-ti″pe) [*stereo-* + Gr. *typos* type] the persistent repetition or sameness of acts, ideas, or words, frequently occurring in disorders such as autistic disorder and schizophrenia.

Ste·re·um (ste′re-əm) a genus of bracken fungi of the order Aphyllophorales, including some species causing tree and wood rot.

ste·ric (ste′rik) pertaining to the arrangement of atoms in space; pertaining to stereochemistry.

ste·rig·ma (ste-rig′mə) pl. *sterig′mata* [Gr. *stērigma* support] 1. the narrow stalk at the end of a basidium that gives rise to basidiospores. 2. metula.

ste·rig·ma·to·cys·tin (stə-rig″mə-to-sis′tin) a mycotoxin produced by *Aspergillus versicolor,* which sometimes contaminates corn; it is hepatotoxic and carcinogenic.

ster·i·lant (ster′ĭ-lənt) a sterilizing agent; see *antibiotic* and *disinfectant.*

ster·ile (ster′il) [L. *sterilis*] 1. unable to produce offspring; in females, called also *barren.* 2. aseptic.

ste·ril·i·ty (stə-ril′ĭ-te) [L. *sterilitas*] 1. inability to produce offspring, i.e., either to conceive *(female s.)* or to induce conception *(male s.)* Cf. *infertility.* 2. asepsis.

absolute s. complete and irremediable inability to produce offspring.

aspermatogenic s. see *male s.*

dysspermatogenic s. see *male s.*
female s. inability of the female to conceive as a result of a structural or functional defect in the reproductive organs.
male s. inability of the male to reproduce; three types are distinguished according to cause: *aspermatogenic sterility* is due to failure to produce living spermatozoa; *dysspermatogenic sterility* is due to an abnormality in spermatozoa production; and *normospermatogenic sterility* refers to those with causes other than inability to produce live, normal spermatozoa.
normospermatogenic s. see *male s.*
primary s. 1. sterility caused by absence of some factor essential for reproduction. 2. sterility in which no offspring has ever been produced.
relative s. infertility.
secondary s. 1. inability to produce further offspring after having conceived or induced conception. 2. sterility resulting from a noncongenital defect.

ster•i•li•za•tion (ster″ĭ-lĭ-za′shən) 1. the complete destruction or elimination of all living microorganisms, accomplished by physical methods (dry or moist heat), chemical agents (ethylene oxide, formaldehyde, alcohol), radiation (ultraviolet, cathode), or mechanical methods (filtration). 2. any procedure by which an individual is made incapable of reproduction, as by castration, vasectomy, or salpingectomy.
culdoscopic s. an older method of sterilization of a female using an endoscope to visualize the fallopian tubes and ovaries; the endoscope is inserted through an incision in the posterovaginal cervix to locate the fallopian tubes, which are then drawn out through the vaginal incision and severed.
fractional s., intermittent s. destruction of microbial viability by successive application of the procedure at intervals, to allow spores to develop into vegetative forms, which are more easily destroyed.
laparoscopic s. sterilization of a female using an endoscope to visualize the fallopian tubes and surrounding structures; the endoscope is guided into the abdominal cavity through a small puncture made by a trocar inserted immediately below the umbilicus. A second small puncture is made in the lower abdomen so that cautery forceps can be inserted for electrocoagulation and severing of the tubes.

ster•i•lize (ster′ĭ-līz) 1. to render sterile; to free from microorganisms. 2. to render incapable of reproduction.

ster•i•liz•er (ster′ĭ-līz″ər) an apparatus used for the destruction of microorganisms; see *sterilization* (def. 1).

Ster•i•sil (ster′ĭ-sil) trademark for a preparation of hexetidine.

ster•nad (ster′nad) toward the sternum, or sternal aspect.

ster•nal•gia (stər-nal′jə) [*stern-* + *-algia*] pain in the sternum; called also *sternodynia.*

Stern•berg giant cells, sign (shtərn′bərg) [Carl von *Sternberg,* Austrian pathologist, 1872–1935] see *Reed-Sternberg cells,* under *cell,* and see under *sign.*

Stern•berg-Reed cells (shtərn′bərg rēd′) [C. von *Sternberg;* Dorothy *Reed,* American pathologist, 1874–1964] see *Reed-Sternberg cells,* under *cell.*

ster•ne•bra (stur′nə-brə) pl. *ster′nebrae* [*sternum* + *vertebrae*] any of the segments of the developing sternum in the embryo, which later fuse to form the corpus sterni.

ster•nen (stur′nən) pertaining to the sternum alone.

stern(o)- [L. *sternum,* q.v.] a combining form denoting relationship to the sternum.

ster•no•cla•vic•u•lar (stur″no-klə-vik′u-lər) pertaining to the sternum and clavicle.

ster•no•cla•vic•u•la•ris (stur″no-klə-vik″u-lar′is) [L.] sternoclavicular.

ster•no•clei•dal (stur″no-kli′dəl) [*sterno-* + *cleid-* + *-al*[1]] sternoclavicular.

ster•no•clei•do•mas•toid (stur″no-kli″do-mas′toid) pertaining to the sternum, clavicle, and mastoid process.

ster•no•cos•tal (stur″no-kos′təl) [*sterno-* + *costal*] pertaining to the sternum and ribs.

ster•nod•y•mus (stər-nod′ĭ-məs) thoracopagus.

ster•no•dyn•ia (ster″no-din′e-ə) sternalgia.

ster•no•go•ni•om•e•ter (stur″no-go″ne-om′ə-tər) an instrument for measuring the sternal angle.

ster•no•hy•oid (stur″no-hi′oid) pertaining to the sternum and to the hyoid bone.

ster•noid (stur′noid) resembling the sternum.

ster•no•mas•toid (stur″no-mas′toid) pertaining to the sternum and the mastoid process.

ster•nop•a•gus (stər-nop′ə-gəs) thoracopagus.

ster•no•peri•car•di•al (stur″no-per″ĭ-kahr′de-əl) pertaining to the sternum and the pericardium.

ster•no•scap•u•lar (stur″no-skap′u-lər) pertaining to the sternum and the scapula.

ster•nos•chi•sis (stər-nos′kĭ-sis) cleft sternum.

Ster•no•sto•ma (stur″no-sto′mə) a genus of mites that infest the trachea and bronchi of wild and domestic birds and cause respiratory difficulty.

ster•no•thy•roid (stur″no-thi′roid) pertaining to the sternum and to the thyroid cartilage or gland.

ster•not•o•my (stər-not′ə-me) [*sterno-* + *-tomy*] the operation of cutting through the sternum.
median s. incision through the midline of the sternum, done to gain access to thoracic organs and other structures.

ster•no•tra•che•al (stur″no-tra′ke-əl) [*sterno-* + *tracheal*] pertaining to the sternum and to the trachea.

ster•no•try•pe•sis (stur″no-tri-pe′sis) [*sterno-* + *trypesis*] surgical perforation of the sternum.

ster•no•ver•te•bral (stur″no-vur′tə-brəl) pertaining to the sternum and vertebrae.

ster•no•xi•phop•a•gus (stur″no-zi-fop′ə-gəs) [*sterno-* + *xipho-* + *-pagus*] a type of thoracopagus in which conjoined twins are united in the region of the xiphoid process of the sternum.

ster•num (stur′nəm) [L., from Gr. *sternon*] [TA] a longitudinal unpaired plate of bone forming the middle of the anterior wall of the thorax; it articulates above with the clavicles and along its sides with the cartilages of the first seven ribs. Its three parts are the manubrium, the body (corpus sterni), and the xiphoid process (processus xiphoideus). **ster′nal** *adj*
cleft s. a developmental defect in which the sternum is longitudinally fissured as a result of incomplete fusion of the cartilaginous sternal bars. Called also *sternal cleft.*

ster•nu•ta•tion (stur″nu-ta′shən) [L. *sternutatio*] sneeze (def. 2).

ster•nu•ta•tor (stur′nu-ta″tər) a gas or other substance that causes sneezing.

ster•nu•ta•to•ry (stər-nu′tə-tor″e) [L. *sternutatorius*] 1. producing or causing sneezing. 2. an agent that causes sneezing.

stern•zel•len (shtern′tsel-en) [Ger.] hepatic stellate cells.

ster•oid (ster′oid) any of a group of lipids that contain a hydrogenated cyclopentanoperhydrophenanthrene ring system. Substances included in this group include progesterone, adrenocortical hormones, sex hormones, cardiac aglycones, bile acids, sterols (such as cholesterol), saponins, toad poisons, and some carcinogenic hydrocarbons.
adrenal cortical s., adrenocortical s. corticosteroid.
anabolic s., anabolic-androgenic s's (AAS) any of a group of synthetic derivatives of testosterone having pronounced anabolic properties and relatively weak androgenic properties; they are used clinically mainly to promote growth and repair of body tissues in diseases or states promoting catabolism or tissue wasting.
gonadal s. sex s.
ovarian s. a gonadal steroid produced by the ovary, such as an estrogen or a progestational agent.
sex s. a steroid hormone produced by a gonad, such as an estrogen, androgen, or progestational agent. Called also *gonadal s.*

ster•oid 11β-mono•oxy•gen•ase (ster′oid mon″o-ok′sə-jən-ās) [EC 1.14.15.4] an enzyme of the oxidoreductase class that catalyzes the NADPH-dependent hydroxylation of steroids at the 11 position as a step in the synthesis of steroid hormones. The enzyme is a mitochondrial cytochrome P-450 acting as a terminal oxidase in an electron transport chain

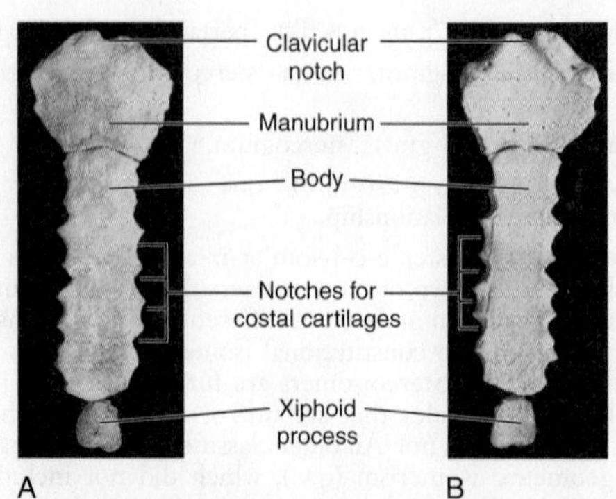

■ Sternum. *(A),* Anterior view; *(B),* posterior view.

that also includes adrenodoxin and a flavoprotein. Deficiency of the enzyme, an autosomal recessive trait, is called 11β-hydroxylase deficiency and causes congenital adrenal hyperplasia (type IV). The enzyme may include the enzyme activities of corticosterone 18-monooxygenase (q.v.). Called also *11β-hydroxylase.*

ster·oid 17α-mono·oxy·gen·ase (ster′oid mon″o-ok′sə-jən-ās) [EC 1.14.99.9] an enzyme of the oxidoreductase class that catalyzes the hydroxylation of steroids at the 17 position. The enzyme is a microsomal cytochrome P-450 that accepts electrons from NADPH via a flavoprotein. The reactions catalyzed are steps in the synthesis of steroid hormones, including cortisol, androgens, and estrogens. Deficiency of the enzyme, an autosomal recessive trait, is called 17α-hydroxylase deficiency and causes congenital adrenal hyperplasia (type V). The enzyme also possesses 17α-hydroxyprogesterone aldolase activity. Called also *17α-hydroxylase.*

ster·oid 21-mono·oxy·gen·ase (ster′oid mon″o-ok′sə-jən-ās) [EC 1.14.99.10] an enzyme of the oxidoreductase class that catalyzes the NADPH-dependent hydroxylation of steroids at the 21 position. The enzyme is a microsomal cytochrome P-450, requires a flavoprotein for reducing equivalents, and is part of the steroid hormone synthesis system. Deficiency of the enzyme, an autosomal recessive trait, inhibits conversion of 17-hydroxyprogesterone to 11-deoxycortisol; it is called 21-hydroxylase deficiency (q.v.) and causes congenital adrenal hyperplasia (type III). Called also *21-hydroxylase.*

ste·roi·do·gen·e·sis (stə-roi″do-jen′ə-sis) the biosynthesis of steroids, as by the adrenal glands and gonads.

ste·roi·do·gen·ic (stə-roi′do-jen′ik) producing or giving rise to steroids.

ster·oid sul·fa·tase (ster′oid sul′fə-tās) steryl-sulfatase.

ster·ol (ster′ol) [*stereo-* + *-ol*] any of a group of steroids with a long (8–10 carbons) aliphatic side-chain at position 17 and at least one alcoholic hydroxyl group, usually at position 3; sterols have lipidlike solubility. Examples are cholesterol and ergosterol.

ster·ol *O*-ac·yl·trans·fer·ase (ster′ol a″səl-trans′fər-ās) [EC 2.3.1.26] an enzyme of the transferase class that catalyzes the transfer of acyl groups from acyl coenzyme A to cholesterol to form cholesteryl esters, a step in the metabolism of cholesterol. Called also *acyl CoA:cholesterol acyltransferase* and *cholesterol acyltransferase.*

ster·ol es·ter·ase (ster′ol es′tər-ās) [EC 3.1.1.13] an enzyme of the hydrolase class that catalyzes the cleavage of cholesterol and other sterol esters and triglycerides. Deficiency of the lysosomal enzyme causes the allelic autosomal recessive disorders Wolman disease and cholesteryl ester storage disease. Called also *acid lipase* and *cholesterol esterase.*

ster·tor (stur′tor) [L.] snore (def. 1).

hen-cluck s. a respiration sound like a hen's cluck in cases of postpharyngeal abscess.

ster·to·rous (stur′tə-rəs) characterized by snoring (stertor).

ster·yl-sul·fa·tase (ster′əl sul′fə-tās) [EC 3.1.6.2] a microsomal enzyme of the hydrolase class that catalyzes the cleavage of the sulfate group from sulfated sterols. Deficiency of the enzyme, an X-linked trait, causes X-linked ichthyosis. Called also *steroid sulfatase.*

steth·acous·tic (steth″ə-koos′tik) heard with the stethoscope.

steth·al·gia (steth-al′jə) 1. thoracalgia (def. 1). 2. pectoralgia (def. 1).

steth(o)- [Gr. *stēthos* chest] a combining form denoting relationship to the chest.

stetho·cyr·to·graph (steth″o-sir′to-graf) [*stetho-* + *cyrto-* + *-graph*] an instrument for measuring and recording the curves of the chest. Called also *stethokyrtograph.*

stetho·go·ni·om·e·ter (steth″o-go″ne-om′ə-tər) [*stetho-* + *goniometer*] an apparatus for measuring the curvature of the chest.

stetho·graph (steth′o-graf) [*stetho-* + *-graph*] an instrument for recording movements of the chest.

steth·og·ra·phy (steth-og′rə-fe) [*stetho-* + *-graphy*] use of the stethograph to record movements of the chest.

stetho·kyr·to·graph (steth″o-kir′to-graf) stethocyrtograph.

steth·om·e·ter (steth-om′ə-tər) [*stetho-* + *-meter*] an instrument for measuring the circular dimension or expansion of the chest. Called also *thoracometer.*

stetho·my·itis (steth″o-mi-i′tis) stethomyositis.

stetho·my·o·si·tis (steth″o-mi″o-si′tis) [*stetho* + *myo-* + *-itis*] inflammation of the muscles of the chest.

stetho·pa·ral·y·sis (steth″o-pə-ral′ĭ-sis) paralysis of the chest muscles.

stetho·phone (steth′o-fōn) [*stetho-* + Gr. *phōnē* voice] 1. an instrument designed to transmit stethoscopic sounds so that many persons can hear them simultaneously. 2. a term proposed as a more accurate name for stethoscope.

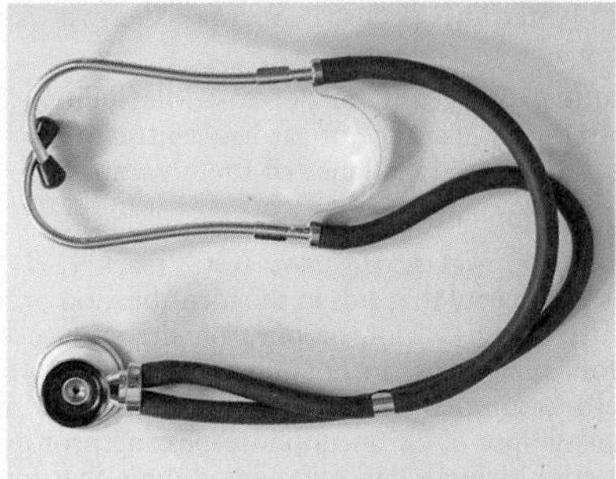

■ Stethoscope.

stetho·pho·nom·e·ter (steth″o-fo-nom′ə-tər) [*stetho-* + *phono-* + *-meter*] an instrument for measuring the intensity of auscultatory sounds.

stetho·poly·scope (steth″o-pol′ĭ-skōp) [*stetho-* + *poly-* + *-scope*] a stethoscope for the simultaneous use of several persons.

stetho·scope (steth′o-skōp) [*stetho-* + *-scope*] an instrument for performing mediate auscultation, through which respiratory, cardiac, pleural, arterial, venous, uterine, fetal, intestinal, and other internal body sounds are conveyed to the ear of the examiner; numerous different forms and sizes are available. **stethoscop′ic** *adj*

binaural s. a stethoscope with two adjustable branches, designed for use with both ears.

DeLee-Hillis s. a type of fetal stethoscope worn on the head of the examiner, used for listening to the fetal heart.

differential s. a stethoscope by means of which sounds at two different portions of the body may be compared.

electronic s. an electronic amplifier of sounds within the body; selective controls permit tuning for low or high frequency tones. An auxiliary output permits the recording or viewing of audio patterns.

esophageal s. a stethoscope that is positioned within the esophagus to transmit heart and respiratory sounds.

steth·os·co·py (steth-os′kə-pe) examination by means of the stethoscope.

stetho·spasm (steth′o-spaz″əm) spasm of the chest muscles.

Ste·vens-John·son syndrome (ste′vənz jon′sən) [Albert Mason *Stevens,* American pediatrician, 1884–1945; Frank Chambliss *Johnson,* American pediatrician, 1894–1934] see under *syndrome.*

Ste·wart-Holmes sign (stoo′ərt hōmz′) [Purves *Stewart,* English physician, 1869–1949; Eric Gordon *Holmes,* English neurologist, 1876–1965] rebound phenomenon.

Ste·wart-Treves syndrome (stoo′ərt trēvz) [Fred Waldorf *Stewart,* American oncologist, 1894–1991; Norman *Treves,* American physician, 20th century] see under *syndrome.*

sthe·nia (sthe′ne-ə) [*sthen-* + *-ia*] a condition of strength and activity.

sthen·ic (sthen′ik) active; strong.

sthen(o)- [Gr. *sthenos* strength] a combining form denoting relationship to strength.

sthen·om·e·try (sthen-om′ə-tre) [*stheno-* + *-metry*] the measurement of bodily strength.

STI sexually transmitted infection; systolic time intervals.

stib·i·al·ism (stib′e-əl-iz-əm) [L. *stibium* antimony] antimony poisoning.

stib·i·at·ed (stib′e-āt″əd) [L. *stibium* antimony] containing antimony.

stibo·cap·tate (stib″o-kap′tāt) BAN for *sodium stibocaptate.*

stibo·phen (stib′o-fən) a trivalent antimony compound, formerly used as an anthelmintic, chiefly in the treatment of schistosomiasis, but superseded by less toxic agents.

Stick·er disease (shtik′ər) [Georg *Sticker,* German hygienist, 1860–1960] erythema infectiosum.

Stick·ler syndrome (stik′lər) [Gunnar B. *Stickler,* German-born American pediatrician, born 1925] hereditary progressive arthro-ophthalmopathy.

Stie·da disease, fracture (shte′dah) [Alfred *Stieda,* German surgeon, 1869–1945] see *Pellegrini disease,* under *disease,* and see under *fracture.*

Stie·da process (shte′dah) [Ludwig *Stieda,* German anatomist, 1837–1918] see *processus posterior tali.*

Stier•lin sign (shtēr′lin) [Eduard *Stierlin*, German surgeon, 1878–1919] see under *sign*.

stiff•ness (stif′nis) 1. rigidity or decreased flexibility. 2. ankylosis.
chamber s. reduced elastance of cardiac ventricles.
myocardial s. decreased elastance of the myocardium.

sti•fle (sti′fəl) stifle joint.

stig•ma (stig′mə) pl. *stigmas, stig′mata* [Gr. "mark"] 1. any mental or physical mark or peculiarity that aids in the identification or in the diagnosis of a condition. 2. a mark, spot, or pore on the surface of an organ or organism. 3. follicular s. 4. in botany, the uppermost part of a pistil, which secretes a moist, sticky substance to trap and hold the pollen that reaches it. 5. an eyespot of chromatophore-bearing protozoa, such as certain euglenoids, comprising a dark pigmented mass that functions in light detection by shielding the photoreceptor cells from specific wavelengths. 6. a distinguishing personal trait that is perceived as or actually is physically, socially, or psychologically disadvantageous. 7. *(in the pl.)* gill slits around the pharynx in urochordates, through which pass respiratory and feeding currents. 8. *(in the pl.)* purpuric or hemorrhagic lesions of the hands and/or feet, which resemble crucifixion wounds.
follicular s. a spot on the surface of an ovary where the vesicular ovarian follicle will rupture and permit passage of the secondary oocyte during ovulation.
Giuffrida-Ruggieri s. abnormal shallowness of the glenoid fossa.
malpighian s's the points where the smaller veins enter into the larger veins of the spleen.

stig•mal (stig′məl) stigmatic.

stig•mas•te•rol (stig-mas′tə-rol) an unsaturated plant sterol initially isolated from the Calabar bean *(Physostigma)* and also found in other plant fats such as soybean oil, rapeseed oil, and cocoa butter; it is used as a starting material in the manufacture of synthetic progesterone.

stig•ma•ta (stig′mə-tə) [Gr.] plural of *stigma*.

stig•mat•ic (stig-mat′ik) pertaining to a stigma.

stig•ma•tism (stig′mə-tiz-əm) 1. the condition due to or marked by stigmata. 2. the accurate rendition of points by a lens system.

stig•ma•ti•za•tion (stig″mə-tĭ-za′shən) 1. the act or process of developing or being identified as possessing one or more stigmata. 2. the act or process of negatively labeling or characterizing another. 3. stigmatism (def. 1).

stig•ma•tom•e•ter (stig″mə-tom′ə-tər) [*stigma* + *-meter*] an instrument for testing the refraction of the eye by retinoscopy and for direct ophthalmoscopy.

stig•ma•to•phil•ia (stig-mə-to-fil′e-ə) [Gr. *stigma* mark made by a pointed instrument + *-philia*] a paraphilia in which sexual excitement depends on piercing or tattooing the body.

Stil•bel•la•ceae (stil-bə-la′se-e) a family of Fungi Imperfecti of the form-order Moniliales, including the genus *Dendrodochium*.

stil•bene (stil′bēn) an unsaturated hydrocarbon that is the nucleus of diethylstilbestrol and related compounds; it is used in the manufacture of dyes and optical bleaches.

stil•bes•trol (stil-bes′trol) diethylstilbestrol.

Sti•le•sia (sti-le′zhə) a genus of cestodes of the family Anoplocephalidae. *S. globipuncta′ta* is found in the small intestines of ruminants; heavy infestations can be fatal.

sti•let (sti-let′) [Fr. *stilette*] stylet.

sti•lette (sti-let′) [Fr.] stylet.

Still disease (stil) [Sir George Frederick *Still*, English physician, 1868–1941] systemic onset juvenile rheumatoid arthritis; see under *arthritis*.

still•birth (stil′burth″) the delivery of a dead child; see *fetal death*, under *death*.

still•born (stil′born″) born dead.

Stil•ler rib (stil′ər) [Berthold *Stiller*, Hungarian physician, 1837–1922] see under *rib*.

Stil•ling canal, etc. (shtil′ing) [Benedict *Stilling*, German anatomist, 1810–1879] see *canalis hyaloideus* and *nucleus thoracicus posterior* and see under *fiber* and *fleece*.

Stil•ling syndrome (shtil′ing) [Jakob *Stilling*, German ophthalmologist, 1842–1915] Duane syndrome; see under *syndrome*.

Stil•ling-Türk-Du•ane syndrome (shtil′ing tērk dwān) [J. *Stilling*; Siegmund *Türk*, Swiss ophthalmologist, late 19th century; Alexander *Duane*, American ophthalmologist, 1858–1926] Duane syndrome; see under *syndrome*.

Stil•phos•trol (stil-fos′trōl) trademark for preparations of diethylstilbestrol diphosphate.

sti•lus (sti′ləs) pl. *sti′li* [L.] stylus.

Stim•ate (stim′āt) trademark for a preparation of desmopressin acetate.

Stim•son meth•od (stim′sən) [Lewis A. *Stimson*, American surgeon, 1844–1917] see under *method*.

stim•u•lant (stim′u-lənt) [L. *stimulans*] 1. producing stimulation; especially producing stimulation by causing tension on muscle fiber through the nervous tissue. 2. an agent or remedy that produces stimulation.
central s. a stimulant of the central nervous system.
cerebral s. a stimulant that increases the functional activities of the brain.
diffusible s. a stimulant that acts quickly and strongly, but transiently.
general s. a stimulant that acts upon the whole body.
local s. a stimulant that affects only, or mainly, the part to which it is applied.
nervous s. central s.
spinal s. a stimulant that acts upon and through the spinal cord.
topical s. local s.
uterine s. an agent that stimulates uterine contractions or menstruation.
vascular s., vasomotor s. a stimulant that affects the vasomotor centers.

stim•u•late (stim′u-lāt) to excite to functional activity.

stim•u•la•tion (stim″u-la′shən) [L. *stimulatio*, from *stimulare* to goad] the act or process of stimulating; the condition of being stimulated.
areal s. stimulation of an extended portion of a sense organ.
audio-visual-tactile s. the simultaneous rhythmic excitation of the receptors for the senses of hearing, sight, and touch.
controlled ovarian s. see under *hyperstimulation*.
deep brain s. (DBS) mild high frequency electrical stimulation of a specific area of the thalamus, globus pallidus, or subthalamic nucleus by means of an electrode implanted in the brain, controlled by a battery implanted just below the clavicle, which the patient can turn off and on. The electrical signals block those signals from the brain that cause tremor and some other related dysfunctions; the procedure is used in the treatment of movement disorders including Parkinson disease, essential tremor, and dystonia.
functional electrical s. (FES), functional neuromuscular s. (FNS) the application of an electrical current by means of a prosthesis, some parts of which may be implanted, to stimulate and restore partial function to muscle disabled by neurological lesions.
gastric electrical s. (GES) a treatment for severe gastroparesis, consisting of implantation of electrodes on the proximal antral wall and delivery of mild, high frequency electrical stimulation.
nonspecific s. stimulation of a sense organ by a modality other than the usual one, such as when pressure or an electric current stimulates the retina.
paradoxical s. application of a warm object to one of the cold spots of the body produces a sensation of cold.
paraspecific s. nonspecific s.
pelvic floor electrical s. (PFES) functional electrical stimulation of the muscles of the pelvic floor, delivered through a vaginal or rectal probe, used in the treatment of stress incontinence.
punctual s. excitation of a sense organ by stimulation at a single point.
repetitive nerve s. repeated supramaximal stimulation of a motor nerve while recording the M wave of its muscle to note any changes in the wave. Types of responses include the *decrementing response, incrementing response, postactivation exhaustion*, and *postactivation facilitation*.
transcranial direct current s. application of a weak direct current to the brain, which alters the firing rate of neurons; its use as a treatment for major depression, some types of stroke syndrome, and other conditions is being explored.
transcranial magnetic s. electrical stimulation of a relatively superficial area of the brain by a current generated by an electromagnet placed against the skull; used in testing of function of different areas.
transcutaneous electrical nerve s. (TENS), transcutaneous nerve s. (TNS) electrical stimulation of nerves for relief of pain, either by electrodes attached to the skin or by an apparatus manually held against the skin; the stimulus interferes with neural transmission of pain signals and thus has an analgesic effect.
vagal nerve s. (VNS), vagus nerve s. delivery of electrical current to the left vagus nerve in the neck by means of an electronic pulse generator implanted in the chest, just under the clavicle; used in the treatment of epilepsy and intractable depression.

stim•u•la•tor (stim′u-la″tər) 1. any agent that excites functional activity. 2. in electrodiagnosis, an instrument that applies pulses of current to stimulate a nerve, muscle, or area of the central nervous system.
Bimler s. see under *appliance*.
electronic s. stimulator (def. 2).
human thyroid adenylate cyclase s's (HTACS) thyroid-stimulating immunoglobulins.

long-acting thyroid s. (LATS) the original name given to thyroid-stimulating immunoglobulins, referring to a mouse bioassay in which thyroid stimulation by this substance peaks later than that induced by thyroid-stimulating hormone.

stim•u•la•to•ry (stim′u-lə-tor″e) capable of stimulating or causing stimulation.

stim•u•li (stim′u-li) plural of *stimulus.*

stim•u•lon (stim′u-lon) a viral antigen postulated to have anti-interferon activity and which therefore promotes the multiplication of other viruses.

stim•u•lus (stim′u-ləs) pl. *stim′uli* [L. "goad"] any agent, act, or influence that produces functional or trophic reaction in a receptor or in an irritable tissue.

adequate s. a stimulus of the specific form of energy to which the receptor is most sensitive; called also *homologous s.*

aversive s. a stimulus that, when applied following the occurrence of a response, decreases the strength of that response on later occurrences.

chemical s. a chemical substance capable of exciting a response in an organism mediated through specialized nerve endings.

conditioned s. a stimulus that acquires the capacity to evoke a particular response by repeated pairing with another stimulus that is naturally capable of eliciting the response (*unconditioned s.*).

discriminative s. a stimulus, associated with reinforcement, which exerts control over a particular form of behavior; the subject discriminates between closely related stimuli and responds positively only in the presence of that stimulus.

electric s. a galvanic, induced, or other electric current or shock as applied to a responsive tissue.

eliciting s. any stimulus, conditioned or unconditioned, which elicits a response.

heterologous s. a stimulus that produces an effect or sensation when applied to part of a nerve tract.

heterotopic s. a stimulus to heart contraction arising elsewhere than in the sinoatrial node, the normal pacemaker of the heart.

homologous s. adequate s.

liminal s. threshold s.

maximal s. a stimulus of just sufficient intensity to cause the maximal amplitude of the evoked potential; see also *supramaximal s.*

mechanical s. a stimulant application of mechanical force, as in friction or pinching.

patterned s. a photic stimulus consisting of a checkerboard or other pattern of alternating light and dark areas, used to elicit visual evoked potentials.

reinforcing s. reinforcer.

subliminal s., subthreshold s. a stimulus too weak to produce a perceivable response.

supraliminal s. suprathreshold s.

supramaximal s. a stimulus more intense than a maximal one; used in electrodiagnostic studies to ensure that the evoked potential stays at its maximum level.

suprathreshold s. a stimulus whose strength is greater than the minimum required to just elicit a response.

threshold s. a stimulus that is just strong enough to elicit a response; see also *threshold* (defs. 1 and 2).

unconditioned s. any stimulus naturally capable of eliciting a specific response.

sting (sting) 1. an injury caused by the venom of a plant or animal (biotoxin) introduced into or contacted by the individual, often exacerbated by mechanical trauma caused by the organ responsible for its introduction. 2. the organ used to inflict such injury.

Irukandji s. see under *syndrome.*

sting•er (sting′er) colloquial term for pain, paresthesia, and transient weakness and numbness of the upper extremity caused by neurapraxia of the brachial plexus or a cervical nerve root.

sting•ray (sting′ra) any of various rays having sharp barbed venomous spines near the base of the tail; different species vary from a few centimeters to several meters in length. Stinging causes cardiovascular symptoms such as vasoconstriction and bradycardia.

Sti•pa (sti′pə) a genus of grasses (family Gramineae). *S. viri′dula* is sleepygrass, a species found in the southwestern United States that is poisonous to cattle and horses and is said to be a powerful narcotic, diuretic, sudorific, and cardiac poison.

stipe (stīp) [L. *stipes* tree trunk] in botany, a stalk, especially that of a mushroom or seaweed or the stem of a fern frond.

stip•pled (stip′əld) [Dutch *stippelen* to keep spotting] marked by small spots or flecks.

stip•pling (stip′ling) [Dutch *stippelen* to keep spotting] 1. the appearance of fine light or dark dots, or a spotted appearance. 2. the appearance of the retina as if dotted with light and dark points. 3. gingival s.

epiphyseal s. the radiographic appearance of punctate opacities in the epiphyses, representing foci of calcification; seen in chondrodysplasia punctata.

basophilic s. the presence of basophilic granules, consisting of precipitated ribosomal RNA, in the cytoplasm of erythrocytes, seen in conditions of defective heme synthesis (such as β-thalassemia) and in lead poisoning. Called also *punctate basophilia.*

gingival s. a condition in which the gingiva presents a minutely lobulated surface, like that of an orange peel, which is a normal adaptive process of the gingiva and its absence or reduction indicates gingival disease.

malarial s. the finely granular appearance often seen in stained erythrocytes that harbor parasites of tertian malaria; see *Maurer dots* and *Schüffner dots.*

Maurer s. malarial stippling with Maurer dots.

Schüffner s. malarial stippling with Schüffner dots.

sti•ro•fos (sti′ro-fos) a veterinary insecticide.

stir•rup (stur′əp) 1. a structure or device resembling the stirrup of a saddle, or the portion of an apparatus on which to rest the feet. 2. the stapes.

Finochietto s. an apparatus for exerting skeletal traction in fractures of the lower limb, with a U-shaped steel band passed over the posterior process of the calcaneus and fixed by a cross bar, from which traction is applied.

stitch (stich) 1. suture (def. 2). 2. suture (def. 4). 3. popular term for a severe, sudden pain, generally at the costal margin on one side.

sto•chas•tic (sto-kas′tik) [Gr. *stochastikos* conjecturing] pertaining to a random process, used particularly to refer to a time series of random variables.

stoe•chi•ol•o•gy (stek″e-ol′ə-je) stoichiology.

Stoerk blennorrhea (shturk) [Carl *Stoerk*, Austrian laryngologist, 1832–1899] see under *blennorrhea.*

stoi•chi•ol•o•gy (stoi″ke-ol′ə-je) [Gr. *stoicheion* element + *-logy*] the science of elements, especially the physiology of the cellular elements of tissues.

stoi•chi•om•e•try (stoi″ke-om′ə-tre) [Gr. *stoicheion* element + *-metry*] the study of the numerical relationships of chemical elements and compounds and the mathematical laws of chemical changes; the mathematics of chemistry.

stoke (St) (stōk) a unit of kinematic viscosity, being that of fluid with a viscosity of 1 poise and a density of 1 gram per cubic centimeter; it is equal to 10^{-4} meter squared per second.

Stokes amputation (operation) (stōks) [Sir William *Stokes*, Irish surgeon, 1839–1900] Gritti-Stokes amputation.

Stokes collar, law, syndrome (stōks) [William *Stokes*, Irish physician, 1804–1878] see under *collar* and *law* and see *Adams-Stokes syndrome*, under *syndrome.*

Stokes-Ad•ams attack, syndrome (syncope) (stōks′ ad′əmz) [W. *Stokes;* Robert *Adams*, Irish physician, 1791–1875] see *Adams-Stokes attack*, under *attack* and *Adams-Stokes syndrome*, under *syndrome.*

Stok•vis-Tal•ma syndrome (stok′vis tahl′mah) [Barend Joseph E. *Stokvis*, Dutch physician, 1834–1902; Sape *Talma*, Dutch physician, 1847–1918] enterogenous cyanosis.

sto•lon (sto′lon) [L. *stolo*, gen. *stolonis* shoot] a runner that can develop roots and a stem; in fungi an aerial hypha that forms rhizoids and an aerial mycelium when it contacts the surface of the substrate. See illustration at *mold.*

sto•ma (sto′mə) pl. *stomas, sto′mata* [Gr. "mouth"] 1. any minute pore, orifice, or opening on a free surface. 2. the opening established in the abdominal wall by colostomy, ileostomy, or a similar operation. 3. the opening between two portions of the intestine in an anastomosis.

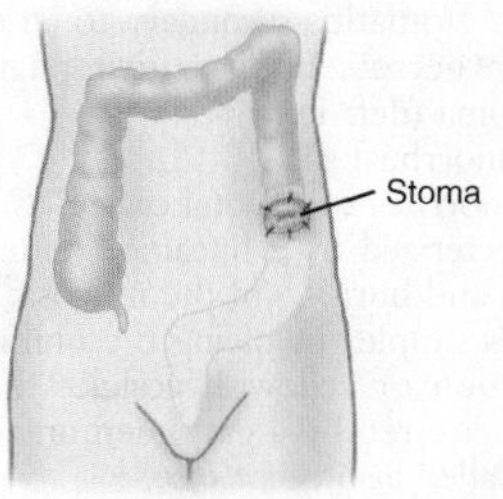

■ Stoma resulting from a descending colostomy.

defunctioning s., loop s. the stoma of a defunctioning or loop ileostomy.

stom·ach (stum′ək) [L. *stomachus;* Gr. *stomachos*] 1. gaster. 2. in ruminants, any of four expansions of the alimentary canal between the esophagus and the duodenum; the first three, the *rumen, reticulum,* and *omasum,* are called *forestomachs,* and the fourth, the *abomasum,* is analogous to the stomach of a nonruminant. 3. the midgut of an invertebrate.
bilocular s. hourglass s.
cardiac s. cardia.
cascade s. an atypical form of hourglass stomach; on a radiograph the posterior wall is seen to be drawn up, and contrast medium first fills the upper sac and then cascades into the lower sac.
cup-and-spill s. a radiographic finding in which the barium remains for a time in the gastric fundus, before spilling over into the main cavity of the stomach, as a result of pressure by a distended colon.
dumping s. the stomach complication seen in dumping syndrome (see under *syndrome*).
hourglass s. a stomach more or less completely and permanently divided into two parts, resembling an hourglass in shape; the deformity is due to scarring that complicates chronic gastric ulcer.
leather bottle s. linitis plastica.
miniature s. Pavlov s.
Pavlov s. a portion of the stomach of a dog isolated from communication with the rest of the stomach and opening on to the abdominal wall through a fistula; used in studying gastric secretion.
thoracic s. a stomach that has moved up above the diaphragm in a hiatal hernia.
upside-down s. thoracic s.
waterfall s. cascade s.
watermelon s. gastric antral vascular ectasia.

stom·a·chal (stum′ə-kəl) gastric.

sto·mach·ic (sto-mak′ik) 1. gastric. 2. a medicine that promotes the functional activity of the stomach.

sto·ma·de·um (sto″mə-de′əm) stomodeum.

sto·mal (sto′məl) pertaining to a stoma; called also *stomatal.*

sto·mal·gia (sto-mal′jə) stomatalgia.

sto·ma·ta (sto′mə-tə) [Gr.] plural of *stoma.*

sto·ma·tal (sto′mə-təl) stomal.

sto·ma·tal·gia (sto″mə-tal′jə) pain in the mouth; called also *stomatodynia.*

sto·mat·ic (sto-mat′ik) pertaining to the mouth.

sto·ma·ti·tis (sto″mə-ti′tis) pl. *stomati′tides* [*stomat-* + *-itis*] inflammation of the oral mucosa, due to local or systemic factors, which may involve the buccal and labial mucosa, palate, tongue, floor of the mouth, and the gingivae.
allergic s. stomatitis caused by exposure to allergens or as a manifestation of an allergic condition. See also *s. venenata.*
angular s. perlèche.
s. aphtho′sa, aphthous s. recurrent aphthous s.
s. area′ta mi′grans benign migratory glossitis.
s. arsenica′lis stomatitis due to arsenic poisoning.
bismuth s. stomatitis due to bismuth poisoning, characterized by a thin blue-black line in the marginal gingivae *(bismuth line),* pigmentation of the buccal mucosa, sore tongue, metallic taste, and a burning sensation of the mouth. Called also *bismuth gingivitis.*
bovine papular s. a mild disease of young cattle, caused by a poxvirus, with oral lesions resembling those of foot-and-mouth disease.
catarrhal s. transitory inflammation of the oral mucosa, sometimes with gingivitis, erythema, swelling, and occasionally epithelial desquamation; believed to be caused by the oral bacterial flora.
contact s. s. venenata.
denture s. inflammation of the oral mucosa seen in some patients with new dentures or with old, ill-fitting ones, caused by *Candida albicans*; characterized by redness, swelling, and pain of mucosa that is in contact with the denture. Called also *chronic atrophic candidiasis* and *denture sore mouth.*
s. exanthema′tica stomatitis secondary to an exanthematous disease.
fusospirochetal s. necrotizing ulcerative gingivostomatitis.
gangrenous s. noma (def. 1).
gonococcal s. gonorrheal s.
gonorrheal s. gonorrhea of the oral cavity, usually transmitted by orogenital contact, characterized by a linear or flattened eruption associated with redness, itching, and burning of the mucosa. Called also *gonococcal s.*
herpetic s. herpes simplex involving the oral mucosa and lips, characterized by the formation of yellowish vesicles that rupture and produce ragged painful ulcers covered by a gray membrane and surrounded by an erythematous halo. Called also *vesicular s.*
infectious s. a general term for a usually mild infection of the oral mucosa, beginning with a circumscribed red, itchy area.

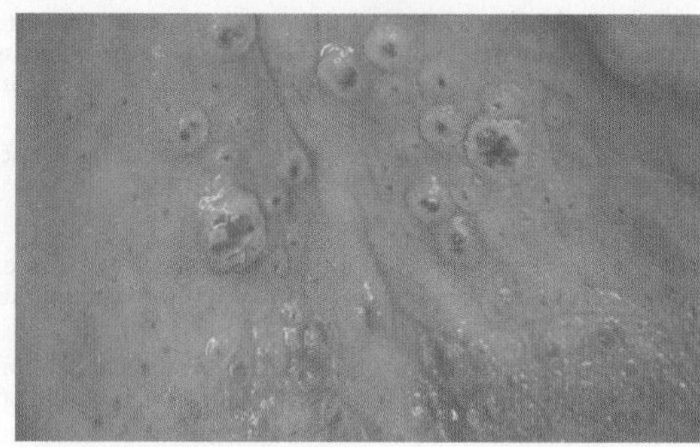

■ Nicotine stomatitis on the hard palate of a pipe smoker.

s. intertro′pica tropical s.
lead s. the oral manifestations of lead poisoning, including the *lead line,* a bluish line along the free gingival margin, pigmentation of the mucosa in contact with the teeth, metallic taste, excessive salivation, and swelling of the salivary glands.
s. medicamento′sa stomatitis due to an allergic reaction to drugs, ingested, absorbed through the skin or mucosa, or given by hypodermic injection. Principal symptoms include vesicles, erosion, ulcers, erythema, purpura, angioedema, burning, and itching. See also *s. venenata.*
membranous s. infection of the oral mucosa, accompanied by the formation of a false membrane.
mercurial s., mercury s. stomatitis due to mercury poisoning; symptoms include necrotic and ulcerative lesions and discoloration similar to lead lines of the gingivae, soreness of gums, strong metallic taste, foul breath, ptyalism, and necrosis of the alveolar process.
mycotic s. thrush (def. 1).
necrotic s. calf diphtheria in the oral cavity.
s. nicoti′na, nicotine s. a condition believed to be a variant of oral leukoplakia, seen in smokers of tobacco, particularly heavy pipe smokers. Characteristics include grayish white nodules or papules on the palate with a red spot in the center of each, representing dilated orifices of accessory palatal salivary glands; thickening, keratinization, and epithelial wrinkling with development of fissures and cracks may occur in later stages. Called also *smokers' palate* or *patches.*
nonspecific s. inflammation of the oral mucosa occurring in association with other conditions, such as menstruation, diabetes, or uremia.
recurrent aphthous s. a recurrent disease of unknown etiology, characterized by the appearance on the oral mucosa of one or more small round or oval ulcers that are covered by a grayish fibrinous exudate and surrounded by a bright red halo. The lesions usually persist for 7 to 14 days and then heal without scarring. A severe form is known as *periadenitis mucosa necrotica recurrens.* Called also *aphthae, aphthous s.,* and *canker sore.*
s. scarlati′na a condition of the oral mucosa seen in scarlatina (scarlet fever), characterized in the early stages by fiery red coloration, congestion, and exudate of the throat, and by strawberry tongue and raspberry tongue in the later stages.
s. scorbu′tica stomatitis associated with vitamin C deficiency, characterized by red swollen gums, gingival ulcers and gangrene, periodontal destruction, loose teeth, hemorrhage from the dental pulp, hypoplasia of the dental enamel, arrest of dentin formation, and exaggerated sensitivity of the oral mucosa to irritants. See also *scurvy.*
syphilitic s. stomatitis due to systemic syphilis.
tropical s. the stomatitis associated with tropical sprue.
ulcerative s. stomatitis characterized by the appearance of shallow ulcers on the cheeks, tongue, and lips.
ulcerative s. of sheep contagious ecthyma.
uremic s. the oral manifestation of uremia, consisting of a peculiar odor of the breath, erythema, exudation, ulcerations, pseudomembrane formation, and burning sensations.
s. venena′ta an allergic condition of the oral mucosa resulting from contact with a substance to which the patient is sensitized, including cosmetics, dentifrices, mouthwashes, and dental materials, as well as drugs applied topically; inflammation and edema of the mucosa accompanied by burning and sometimes itching are the principal symptoms. Called also *contact s.* See also *s. medicamentosa.*
vesicular s. 1. herpetic s. 2. a viral infection in swine, cattle, and horses, caused by a rhabdovirus and characterized by vesicular eruptions on the oral mucosa. There may also be vesicles in swine on the snout and interdigital spaces, in cattle on the udder and teats, and in horses on the coronary band. It must be distinguished from foot-and-mouth disease.
Vincent s. necrotizing ulcerative gingivitis.

stomat(o)- [Gr. *stoma,* gen. *stomatos* mouth] a combining form denoting relationship to the mouth or to the ostium uteri. Also, *stom(o)-.*

sto·ma·to·cyte (sto′mə-to-sīt) an abnormal erythrocyte in which a slit or mouthlike area replaces the normal circle of pallor, usually due to edema. See also *stomatocytosis.* **stomatocyt′ic** *adj*

sto·ma·to·cy·to·sis (sto″mə-to-si-to′sis) the presence of stomatocytes in the blood, as seen in liver disease, Rh null syndrome, a rare congenital type of hemolytic anemia, and a few other conditions. Called also *hydrocytosis.*

dehydrated hereditary s. (DHS) a rare, autosomal dominant, well-compensated hemolytic anemia characterized by erythrocyte (RBC) dehydration and caused by a defect in membrane cation permeability, with excessive efflux of potassium ions relative to sodium; dehydration appears as elevated MCHC and MCV, with decreased osmotic fragility but increased sensitivity to shear stress. RBC morphology can include stomatocytes, target cells, spiculated erythrocytes, and macrocytes. Called also *hereditary xerocytosis.*

sto·ma·to·dyn·ia (sto″mə-to-din′e-ə) stomatalgia.

sto·ma·to·dys·o·dia (sto″mə-to-dis-o′de-ə) halitosis.

sto·ma·to·gen·e·sis (sto″mə-to-jen′ə-sis) [*stomato-* + *genesis*] a morphologic process seen in ciliate protozoa in which all oral structures and associated organelles are formed or existing ones are replaced.

sto·ma·to·glos·si·tis (sto″mə-to-glos-i′tis) inflammation involving the oral mucous membranes and the tongue, occurring in nutritional disorders such as pellagra, beriberi, vitamin B complex deficiency, and in infections, etc.

sto·ma·tog·nath·ic (sto″mə-tog-nath′ik) [*stomato-* + *gnathic*] denoting the mouth and jaws collectively.

sto·ma·tog·ra·phy (sto″mə-tog′rə-fe) [*stomato-* + *-graphy*] a description of the mouth.

sto·ma·to·la·lia (sto″mə-to-la′le-ə) [*stomato-* + *lal-* + *-ia*] hyponasality.

sto·ma·tol·o·gist (sto″mə-tol′ə-jist) a specialist in stomatology.

sto·ma·tol·o·gy (sto″mə-tol′ə-je) [*stomato-* + *-logy*] the branch of medical science concerning the mouth and its diseases, functions, and structure; called also *oralogy.* See also *dentistry.* **stomatolog′ic** *adj*

sto·ma·to·ma·la·cia (sto″mə-to-mə-la′she-ə) [*stomato-* + *malacia*] excessive or abnormal softness of the oral structures.

sto·ma·to·me·nia (sto″mə-to-me′ne-ə) [*stomato-* + *men-*+ *-ia*] bleeding from the mucous membrane of the mouth at the time of menstruation.

sto·mat·o·my (sto-mat′ə-me) [*stoma-* + *-tomy*] surgical incision of the ostium uteri.

sto·ma·to·my·co·sis (sto″mə-to-mi-ko′sis) [*stomato-* + *mycosis*] any oral disease due to a fungus.

sto·ma·top·a·thy (sto″mə-top′ə-the) [*stomato-* + *-pathy*] any pathological condition of the mouth.

sto·ma·to·plas·ty (sto′mə-to-plas″te) [*stomato-* + *-plasty*] plastic repair of defects of or reconstruction of the mouth. **stomatoplas′tic** *adj*

sto·ma·tor·rha·gia (sto″mə-to-ra′jə) [*stomato-* + *-rrhagia*] hemorrhage from the mouth.

s. gingiva′rum hemorrhage from the gingivae.

sto·ma·tos·chi·sis (sto″mə-tos′kĭ-sis) cleft lip.

sto·ma·to·scope (sto-mat′o-skōp) [*stomato-* + *-scope*] an instrument used in inspecting the mouth.

sto·ma·tot·o·my (sto″mə-tot′ə-me) stomatomy.

sto·mi·on (sto′me-ən) [Gr. *stomion,* dim. of *stoma* mouth] a cephalometric landmark, being the midpoint in the oral fissure when the lips are closed.

stom(o)- see *stomat(o)-.*

sto·mo·de·um (sto″mo-de′əm) [*stomo-* + Gr. *hodaios* pertaining to a way] an invagination of the surface ectoderm of the embryo during the fourth week, at the point where later the mouth is formed. **stomode′al** *adj*

sto·mos·chi·sis (sto-mos′kĭ-sis) cleft lip.

Sto·mox·ys (sto-mok′sis) a genus of flies of the family Muscidae. *S. bouffar′di* transmits trypanosomes to goats in South America. *S. cal′citrans* is the stable fly, a common biting pest that transmits many diseases, such as anthrax, infectious anemia, surra, and tetanus.

-stomy [Gr. *stoma* mouth] a word termination denoting the surgical creation of an artificial opening into a hollow organ (colostomy, tracheostomy) or a new opening between two such structures (gastroenterostomy); also denoting the opening so created.

stone (stōn) 1. calculus. 2. a unit of weight in Great Britain, the equivalent of 14 pounds (avoirdupois), or about 6.34 kg. 3. an abrading instrument or tool, such as one used for sharpening instruments.

bladder s. vesical calculus.

chalk s. articular calculus.

dental s. a very strong dental plaster composed chiefly of the α-hemihydrate of gypsum, used for construction of casts of the oral structures.

infection s. struvite calculus.

kidney s. renal calculus.

pulp s. denticle (def. 2).

salivary s. sialolith.

stone-search·er (stōn′sər-chər) searcher.

Stook·ey reflex (stook′e) [Byron Polk *Stookey,* American neurosurgeon, 1887–1966] see under *reflex.*

stool (stōōl) feces.

fatty s. feces containing fat; see *steatorrhea.*

pipestem s., ribbon s. long flattened feces seen in lower rectal stricture.

rice-water s's the characteristic and diagnostic watery, light gray to clear diarrhea of cholera, containing flecks of mucous material, epithelial cells, and many cholera vibrios.

silver s. silver-colored feces due to a mixture of melena and fat, sometimes seen in persons with tropical sprue or biliary tract obstruction, or in children with diarrhea who are given sufonamides.

spinach s. a type of dark green feces, the color of cooked spinach, formerly seen in infants who had been given calomel.

stop (stop) 1. to come to a halt. 2. to cease, discontinue, or arrest. 3. any device that serves to prevent further progression or advancement. 4. plosive.

centric s. facies approximalis dentis.

glottal s. a speech sound made by closure of the glottis and then an explosive release.

occlusal s. see under *rest.*

Stop·pa procedure (stop′ə) [René E. *Stoppa,* French surgeon, 1921–2006] see under *procedure.*

sto·rax (stor′aks) [L. *storax, styrax,* from Gr. *styrax*] [USP] a balsam from the trunk of *Liquidambar orientalis* Mill (Levant s.), a tree of western Asia, or of *L. styraciflua* L. (American s.) of North America, used as an ingredient of compound benzoin tincture (see under *tincture*). It has been used as an expectorant and topical parasiticide. Called also *styrax.*

stor·i·form (stor′ĭ-form) [L. *storea, storia* a rush mat + *form*] having an irregularly whorled pattern somewhat like that of a straw mat; said of the microscopic appearance of dermatofibrosarcomas.

storm (storm) crisis (def. 2).

sympathetic s. severe sympathetic hyperactivity (see under *hyperactivity*), seen most often after head injury or as a reaction to certain drugs.

thyroid s., thyrotoxic s. see under *crisis.*

Storm van Leeu·wen chamber (storm vahn la′vən) [William *Storm van Leeuwen,* Dutch pharmacologist, 1882–1933] see under *chamber.*

Stox·il (stok′sil) trademark for a preparation of idoxuridine.

STP standard temperature and pressure: 0°C and 760 mm Hg.

STPD standard temperature and pressure, dry; denoting a volume of dry gas at 0° C and a pressure of 760 mm Hg.

STR short tandem repeat.

stra·bis·mol·o·gy (strə″biz-mol′ə-je) the study of strabismus.

stra·bis·mom·e·ter (stra″biz-mom′ə-tər) [*strabismus* + *-meter*] an apparatus for measuring strabismus; called also *ophthalmotropometer* and *strabometer.*

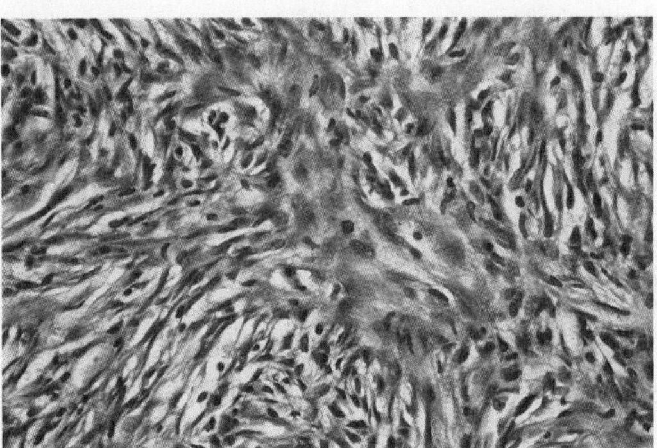

■ Storiform pattern in dermatofibrosarcoma protuberans.

stra•bis•mom•e•try (strə″biz-mom′ə-tre) [*strabismus* + *-metry*] measurement of the amount of strabismus; called also *ophthalmotropometry* and *strabometry.*

stra•bis•mus (strə-biz′məs) [Gr. *strabismos* a squinting] an eye condition in which the visual axes cannot be directed at the same point of fixation under normal conditions of seeing. The various forms of strabismus are spoken of as *tropias,* with their direction indicated by the appropriate prefix, such as cyclotropia, esotropia, exotropia, hypertropia, and hypotropia. Called also *cast, heterotropia, manifest deviation,* and *squint.* **strabis′mal, strabis′mic** *adj*

absolute s. strabismus that occurs at all distances of the fixation point; called also *constant s.*

accommodative s. strabismus caused by excessive or deficient effort at accommodation.

alternating s., bilateral s., binocular s. strabismus that affects each eye alternately.

comitant s., concomitant s. strabismus caused by faulty insertion of the eye muscles, resulting in the same amount of deviation in whatever direction the eyes are looking, because the squinting eye follows the movements of the other eye; called also *muscular s.* and *concomitant squint.*

constant s. absolute s.

convergent s. esotropia.

cyclic s. intermittent strabismus that recurs at regular intervals.

s. deor′sum ver′gens strabismus in which the visual axis of the squinting eye falls below the fixation point.

divergent s. exotropia.

external s. exotropia.

incomitant s. nonconcomitant s.

intermittent s. strabismus that occurs only at intervals.

internal s. esotropia.

kinetic s. strabismus due to spasm of the muscles controlling ocular movements.

latent s. strabismus that occurs only when one eye is occluded.

manifest s. strabismus that is evident in binocular vision.

mechanical s. strabismus caused by pressure or traction on the eye, as by a tumor, producing deflection.

monocular s., monolateral s. unilateral s.

muscular s. concomitant s.

noncomitant s., nonconcomitant s. strabismus in which the amount of deviation of the squinting eye varies according to the direction in which the eyes are turned; called also *incomitant s.*

nonparalytic s. concomitant strabismus that is not due to paralysis of the extraocular muscles.

paralytic s. strabismus that is due to paralysis of an eye muscle.

s. sur′sum ver′gens strabismus in which the visual axis of the squinting eye lies above the fixation point.

unilateral s., uniocular s. strabismus affecting only one eye.

vertical s. strabismus in which the deviation of the visual axis is in the vertical plane; see *hypertropia* and *hypotropia.*

stra•bom•e•ter (strə-bom′ə-tər) strabismometer.

stra•bom•e•try (strə-bom′ə-tre) strabismometry.

strabo•tome (strab′o-tōm) a knife for performing strabotomy.

stra•bot•o•my (strə-bot′ə-me) [Gr. *strabos* squinting + *-tomy*] cutting of the tendon of an eye muscle for treatment of strabismus.

Stra•chan syndrome (strawn) [William Henry Williams *Strachan,* British physician, 1857–1921] see under *syndrome.*

Stra•chan-Scott syndrome (strawn′ skot′) [W.H.W. *Strachan;* Sir Henry Harold *Scott,* British physician, 1874–1956] Strachan syndrome.

strad•dle (strad′əl) 1. to extend over or across, to be on both sides. 2. to have one leg on each opposite side of something.

strah•len (strah′lən) [Ger. "streaming," "ray"] a large locomotor organelle resembling an axopodium; seen in protozoa of the subclass Piroplasmia.

strain (strān) 1. to exercise or use to an extreme, potentially harmful, degree. 2. excessive effort or undue exercise. 3. an overstretching or overexertion of some part of the musculature. 4. to filter something or subject it to colation. 5. change in the size or shape of a body as the result of an externally applied force; expressed as the fractional or percentage change in dimension resulting from the application of stress (q.v.). 6. a group of organisms within a species or variety, characterized by some particular quality, such as rough or smooth strains of bacteria.

cell s. cells derived from a primary culture by the selection and cloning of cells with specific properties; cells are adapted to culture but do not have the potential for infinite division. Cf. *cell line.*

heterologous s. a strain of microorganisms different from the strain originally isolated, tested, etc.

high-jumper's s. strain of the rotator muscles of the thigh occurring in high jumpers.

homologous s. a strain of microorganisms similar to the strain originally isolated, tested, etc.

R s., rough s. a type of strain that results from bacterial dissociation; rough or R colonies have a dull, uneven surface and irregular border, the growth in fluid media tends to flake out, no capsules are seen, and the culture tends to be less virulent.

reference s. a strain of bacteria or other microorganisms used as a standard of reference, which appears to meet the criteria of the type strain but is not officially accepted as a neotype.

resistant s. a strain of organisms that is resistant to the effects of the agents, such as antibiotics or insecticides, used to control them.

S s., smooth s. a type of strain that results from bacterial dissociation; smooth or S colonies have a smooth surface and an unbroken border, growth in fluid media tends to be diffuse; capsules, if present at all, are found in this strain, and the culture tends to be more virulent.

Vi s. a strain of bacteria, especially *Salmonella typhi,* that contains the Vi (virulence) antigen of Felix.

wild-type s. the strain used as a standard for a given species or variety of organism, usually presumed to be the type found in nature. See also *wild type,* under *type.*

strain•er (strān′ər) an apparatus for straining.

strait (strāt) a narrow passageway.

inferior pelvic s. apertura pelvis inferior.

superior pelvic s. apertura pelvis superior.

strait•jack•et (strāt′jak″ət) a device for restraining the limbs, especially the arms, of a violently disturbed person; it consists of a canvas jacket with long sleeves that can be fastened behind the back of the patient.

stra•mo•ni•um (strə-mo′ne-əm) 1. *Datura stramonium.* 2. the dried leaf and flowering or fruiting tops of *D. stramonium,* a source of hyoscyamine and scopolamine and having anticholinergic and parasympatholytic effects. It is used in folk medicine for various respiratory problems, in Chinese medicine for pain and respiratory problems, and in homeopathy for infection, cramps, and ocular inflammation. Called also *jimson weed* and *thorn apple.*

strand (strand) a thread or fiber or a structure resembling one.

antisense s. the strand of a double-stranded nucleic acid that is complementary to the sense strand, in DNA being thus the template on which the mRNA is synthesized. Cf. *sense s.* See also *antisense RNA,* under *RNA.*

coding s. sense s.

lagging s. in DNA replication, the strand that is synthesized in the direction opposite that in which the replication fork moves; because it must be synthesized in the 5′ to 3′ direction and the replication fork moves along the strand in the 3′ to 5′ direction, it is replicated in short fragments (Okazaki fragments), which are later joined. Cf. *leading strand.* See illustration at *replication fork,* under *fork.*

lateral enamel s. lateral dental lamina.

leading s. in DNA replication, the strand that is synthesized in the same direction as the replication fork moves, i.e., in the 5′ to 3′ direction; it is synthesized as a continuous strand. Cf. *lagging strand.* See illustration at *replication fork,* under *fork.*

sense s. the strand of a double-stranded nucleic acid that encodes the product; in DNA it is the strand that encodes the RNA, having thus the same base sequence except changing T for U in the RNA. Called also *coding s.* Cf. *antisense s.*

template s. antisense s.

stran•gal•es•the•sia (strang″gəl-es-the′zhə) [Gr. *strangalizein* to choke + *esthesia*] zonesthesia.

stran•gle (strang′gəl) [L. *strangulare*] choke (def. 1).

stran•gles (strang′gəlz) 1. in horses, an infectious disease characterized by a mucopurulent inflammation of the respiratory mucous membrane, with lymph node abscesses, and caused by *Streptococcus equi.* Called also *equine* or *horse distemper.* 2. in pigs, infection of the lymph nodes of the neck and pharynx with heavily encapsulated abscesses.

bastard s. a usually fatal complication of strangles in horses involving spread of abscesses to organs such as the lungs, brain, or lymph nodes of the trunk.

puppy s. juvenile pyoderma.

stran•gu•lat•ed (strang′gu-lāt″əd) [L. *strangulatus*] congested by reason of constriction or hernial stricture, with compromise of the blood supply; see *hernia.*

stran·gu·la·tion (strang″gu-la′shən) [L. *strangulatio*] 1. choke (def. 2). 2. arrest of the circulation in a part, due to compression. See *hemostasis* (def. 2).

stran·gu·ria (strang-gu′re-ə) strangury.

stran·gu·ry (strang′gu-re) [Gr. *stranx* drop + *ouron* urine] slow and painful discharge of the urine, due to spasm of the urethra and bladder.

strap (strap) 1. a band or strip, such as a strap muscle. 2. a band of adhesive tape used in attaching parts to each other; see also *strapping*. 3. to bind down tightly.

Montgomery s's straps made of lengths of adhesive tape, used to secure dressings that must be changed frequently. Called also *Montgomery tapes*.

strap·ping (strap′ing) the application of strips of adhesive tape, one overlapping the other, to cover and exert pressure upon an extremity or other area of the body; see illustration and see also *bandage*.

Gibney s. see under *bandage*.

stra·ta (stra′tə) [L.] plural of *stratum*.

strat·i·fi·ca·tion (strat″ĭ-fĭ-ka′shən) [L. *stratum* layer + *facere* to make] 1. disposal in layers. 2. in statistical analysis, separation of a sample into subsamples on the basis of specified criteria, in order to control for the effects of confounding variables.

strat·i·fied (strat′ĭ-fīd) formed or arranged in layers.

strat·i·form (strat′ĭ-form) [*stratum* + *-form*] having a layered structure.

stra·tig·ra·phy (strə-tig′rə-fe) [*stratum* + *-graphy*] tomography.

Strat·tera (strə-ter′ə) trademark for a preparation of atomoxetine hydrochloride.

stra·tum (strat′əm, stra′təm) pl. *stra′ta* [L.] in anatomy, a sheetlike mass of substance; see also *layer* and *lamina*.

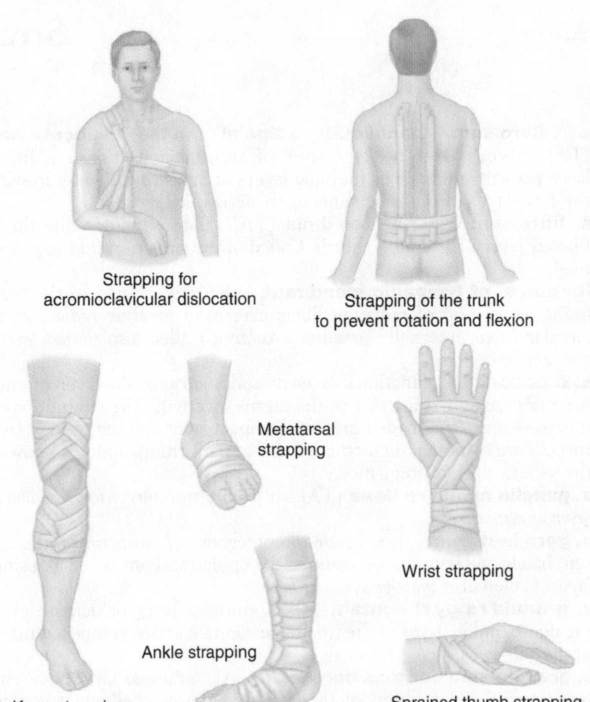

■ Various types of strapping.

Stratum

Descriptions are given on TA terms, and include anglicized names of specific terms.

s. adamanti′num dental enamel.

s. basale of endometrium basal layer of endometrium: the deepest layer of the endometrium, which contains the blind ends of the uterine glands; the cells of this layer undergo minimal change during the sexual cycle.

s. basale of epidermis basal layer of epidermis: the deepest stratum of the epidermis, beneath the stratum spinosum, composed of a single layer of deeply basophilic cells. See figure at *epidermis* and see also *s. germinativum*.

s. cine′reum s. griseum superficiale colliculi superioris.

s. circula′re mus′culi detruso′ris vesi′cae [TA] circular layer of detrusor: the substantial middle layer of three ill-defined interlacing layers composing the detrusor muscle of the bladder, forming a circular course between two layers of longitudinally arranged smooth muscle cell bundles.

s. circula′re tu′nicae muscula′ris co′li [TA] circular layer of muscular coat of colon: the inner layer of circularly coursing fibers in the muscular coat (tunica muscularis) of the colon.

s. circula′re tu′nicae muscula′ris gas′tricae [TA] circular layer of muscular coat of stomach: the layer of circularly coursing fibers in the muscular coat (tunica muscularis) of the stomach.

s. circula′re tu′nicae muscula′ris intesti′ni ten′uis [TA] circular layer of muscular coat of small intestine: the inner layer of circularly coursing fibers in the muscular coat (tunica muscularis) of the small intestine.

s. circula′re tu′nicae muscula′ris par′tis prosta′ticae ure′thrae [TA] circular layer of muscular coat of prostatic urethra: circularly arranged smooth muscle fibers in the outer aspect of the nonstriated muscle layer of the prostatic urethra.

s. circula′re tu′nicae muscula′ris rec′ti [TA] circular layer of muscular coat of rectum: the inner layer of circularly coursing fibers in the muscular coat (tunica muscularis) of the rectum.

s. circula′re tu′nicae muscula′ris ure′thrae femini′nae [TA] circular layer of muscular coat of female urethra: circularly arranged smooth muscle fibers in the outer aspect of the nonstriated muscle layer of the female urethra, mingling with the skeletal muscle fibers forming the inner part of the external urethral sphincter.

s. circulare of tympanic membrane circular layer of tympanic membrane: the inner part of the fibrous stratum of the membrane, consisting of circularly coursing fibers deep to the mucous layer of the tympanic membrane; it is best developed near the periphery.

s. cor′neum horny layer: the outermost layer of the epidermis, consisting of cells that are dead and desquamating. See figure at *epidermis*.

stra′ta cor′nus ammo′nis TA alternative for *strata hippocampi*.

s. cuta′neum of tympanic membrane cutaneous layer of tympanic membrane: a very thin form of skin that constitutes the lateral layer of the tympanic membrane.

s. exter′num longitudina′le mus′culi detruso′ris vesi′cae [TA] external longitudinal layer of detrusor: the outer layer of smooth muscle fibers of three ill-defined interlacing layers composing the detrusor muscle of the bladder, arranged in longitudinally oriented bundles.

s. fibro′sum cap′sulae articula′ris TA alternative for *membrana fibrosa capsulae articularis*.

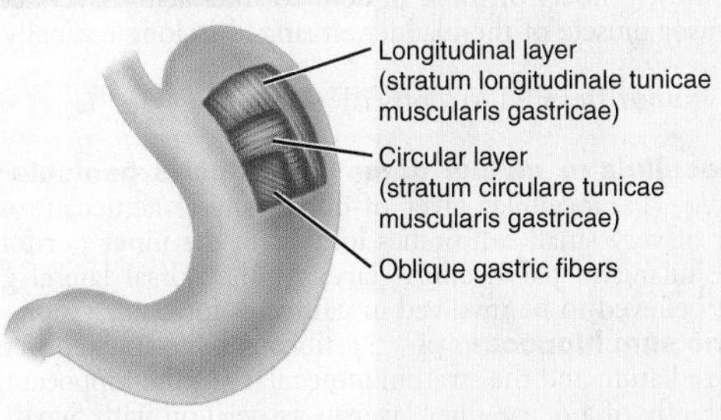

■ Layers (strata) of the muscular coat of the stomach (stratum circulare tunicae muscularis gastricae).

Stratum *Continued*

s. fibro′sum panni′culi adipo′si te′lae subcuta′neae [TA] fibrous layer of fatty layer of subcutaneous tissue: a fibrous layer present singly or in multiple layers in areas of the body in which the fatty layer of the subcutaneous tissue is thick.

s. fibro′sum vagi′nae ten′dinis [TA] fibrous tendon sheath: the fibrous layer of a tendon sheath. Called also *vagina fibrosa* [TA alternative].

fibrous s. of tympanic membrane the middle layer of the membrane, consisting of radiating fibers externally *(stratum radiatum)* and circular fibers internally *(stratum circulare)*. Called also *fibrous layer of tympanic membrane.*

s. functiona′le functional layer of endometrium: the layer of endometrium facing the interior of the uterus, overlying the stratum basale; it is sometimes subdivided into the compact layer and the spongy layer. Its cells are cast off at menstruation and at parturition, and it is known as the *decidua* during pregnancy.

s. ganglio′nicum re′tinae [TA] official terminology for *ganglion cell layer of retina.*

s. germinati′vum 1. s. basale of epidermis. 2. sometimes, the stratum basale and stratum spinosum of the epidermis considered as a single layer. Called also *malpighian s.* or *layer.*

s. granula′re gy′ri denta′ti [TA] granular layer of dentate gyrus: the dense middle layer of the trilaminar dentate gyrus, composed mainly of granule cells.

s. granulo′sum cor′ticis cerebel′li [TA] granular layer of cerebellar cortex: the deep layer of the cortex of the cerebellum; it contains many small neurons (granule cells) and is separated from the molecular layer by the Purkinje cell layer.

s. granulosum of epidermis granular layer of epidermis: the layer of the epidermis between the stratum lucidum and stratum spinosum, containing keratohyalin granules. See figure at *epidermis.*

s. granulosum of ovary granular layer of ovary: the layer of follicle cells lining the theca of a vesicular ovarian follicle.

s. gri′seum interme′dium colli′culi superio′ris [TA] intermediate gray layer of superior colliculus: Layer IV, which together with the intermediate white layer constitutes the main afferent area of the colliculus. See also *layers of superior colliculus.*

s. gri′seum profun′dum colli′culi superio′ris [TA] deep gray layer of superior colliculus: Layer VI, which together with the deep white layer constitutes the main efferent area of the colliculus. See also *layers of superior colliculus.*

s. gri′seum superficia′le colli′culi superio′ris [TA] superficial gray layer of superior colliculus: a layer containing many small multipolar nerve cells which synapse with neurons from the overlying zonal layer and the underlying optic layer; it is Layer II of the colliculus. Called also *s. cinereum.*

stra′ta gy′ri denta′ti [TA] layers of dentate gyrus: the three layers of cell groups of the dentate gyrus of the hippocampus; from the outside inward they are the molecular layer (stratum moleculare), granular layer (stratum granulare), and multiform layer (stratum multiforme).

stra′ta hippocam′pi [TA] layers of hippocampus: the layers of cell groups of the hippocampus proprius, including the stratum moleculare et substratum lacunosum, stratum oriens, stratum pyramidale, and stratum radiatum. Called also *strata cornus ammonis* [TA alternative] and *layers of Ammon's horn.* See illustration at hippocampus.

s. interme′dium the layer of cells of the enamel organ of a tooth just peripheral to the ameloblastic layer.

s. inter′num longitudina′le mus′culi detruso′ris vesi′cae [TA] internal longitudinal layer of detrusor: the innermost layer of smooth muscle fibers of three ill-defined interlacing layers composing the detrusor muscle of the bladder, arranged in longitudinally oriented bundles.

stra′ta isocor′ticis [TA] official terminology for *layers of cerebral cortex.*

s. koniocellula′re nu′clei dorsa′lis cor′poris genicula′ti later-a′lis [TA] koniocellular layer of dorsal lateral geniculate nucleus: a sublayer of very small cell bodies located in the inner portion of each magnocellular and parvocellular layer of the dorsal lateral geniculate nucleus; believed to be involved in pathways for color vision.

s. lacuno′sum hippocam′pi the fibrous layer situated between the stratum radiatum and the stratum moleculare of the hippocampus, consisting chiefly of a dense fiber layer in association with Schaffer collaterals, axons ascending from the alveus, and axons and collaterals ascending from neurons of the stratum oriens. In official terminology, it is considered as a unit with the stratum moleculare and called *s. moleculare et substratum lacunosum hippocampi.*

s. lacuno′sum-molecula′re hippocam′pi s. moleculare et substratum lacunosum hippocampi.

s. lemnis′ci in the superior colliculus, the intermediate gray (stratum griseum intermedium), intermediate white (stratum medullare intermedium), deep gray (stratum griseum profundum), and deep white layers (stratum medullare profundum) considered as a unit.

s. li′mitans exter′num re′tinae [TA] official terminology for *external limiting membrane.*

s. li′mitans inter′num re′tinae [TA] official terminology for *internal limiting membrane.*

s. longitudina′le tu′nicae muscula′ris co′li [TA] longitudinal layer of muscular coat of colon: the outer layer of the muscular coat (tunica muscularis) of the colon, consisting of longitudinally coursing fibers; it is thick in the regions of the three teniae coli and very thin between them.

s. longitudina′le tu′nicae muscula′ris gas′tricae [TA] longitudinal layer of muscular coat of stomach: the layer of longitudinally coursing fibers in the muscular coat (tunica muscularis) of the stomach.

s. longitudina′le tu′nicae muscula′ris intesti′ni ten′uis [TA] longitudinal layer of muscular coat of small intestine: the outer layer of the muscular coat (tunica muscularis) of the small intestine, consisting of longitudinally coursing fibers.

s. longitudina′le tu′nicae muscula′ris par′tis interme′diae ure′thrae [TA] longitudinal layer of muscular coat of membranous urethra: the layer of longitudinally arranged bundles of smooth muscle fibers forming the majority of the muscular coat of the membranous urethra.

s. longitudina′le tu′nicae muscula′ris par′tis prosta′ticae ure′thrae [TA] longitudinal layer of muscular coat of prostatic urethra: the layer of longitudinally arranged bundles of smooth muscle fibers forming the majority of the muscular coat of the prostatic urethra.

s. longitudina′le tu′nicae muscula′ris par′tis spongio′sae ure′thrae [TA] longitudinal layer of muscular coat of spongy urethra: the layer of longitudinally arranged bundles of smooth muscle fibers forming the majority of the muscular coat of the spongy urethra.

s. longitudina′le tu′nicae muscula′ris rec′ti [TA] longitudinal layer of muscular coat of rectum: the outer layer of longitudinally coursing fibers of the muscular coat (tunica muscularis) of the rectum.

s. longitudina′le tu′nicae muscula′ris ure′thrae femini′nae [TA] longitudinal layer of muscular coat of female urethra: the layer of longitudinally arranged bundles of smooth muscle fibers forming the majority of the muscular coat of the female urethra.

s. lucidum of epidermis clear layer of epidermis: the clear translucent layer of the epidermis, just beneath the stratum corneum, particularly noticeable on the palms and soles. See figure at *epidermis.*

s. lucidum of hippocampus a clear layer between the stratum pyramidale and stratum radiatum of the hippocampus, containing mossy fibers that contact the proximal dendrites of the pyramidal cells in field CA3; it is not as prominent in humans as in other primates and is absent from official terminology.

stra′ta magnocellula′ria nu′clei dorsa′lis cor′poris genicula′ti latera′lis [TA] magnocellular layers of dorsal lateral geniculate nucleus: the two innermost ventral layers, laminae 1 and 2, of the lateral geniculate nucleus, composed of large neurons receiving retinal input from the contralateral (lamina 1) and ipsilateral sides (lamina 2), and projecting to the primary visual cortex.

malpighian s. s. germinativum (def. 2).

s. medulla′re interme′dium colli′culi superio′ris [TA] intermediate white layer of superior colliculus: Layer V of the superior colliculus, which together with the intermediate gray layer constitutes the main afferent area of the colliculus. See also *layers of superior colliculus.*

s. medulla′re profun′dum colli′culi superio′ris [TA] deep white layer of superior colliculus: Layer VII, which together with the deep gray layer constitutes the main efferent area of the colliculus. See also *layers of superior colliculus.*

s. membrano′sum te′lae subcuta′neae [TA] membranous layer of subcutaneous tissue: the deeper layer of subcutaneous tissue in certain areas of the body, underlying the panniculus adiposus.

s. membrano′sum te′lae subcuta′neae abdo′minis [TA] membranous layer of subcutaneous tissue of abdomen: the deeper layer of subcutaneous tissue of the skin of the abdomen. Called also *Scarpa fascia.*

Stratum *Continued*

s. membrano′sum te′lae subcuta′neae perine′i [TA] membranous layer of subcutaneous tissue of perineum: the deeper layer of subcutaneous tissue in the perineal area, where there is no panniculus adiposus.
s. molecula′re cor′ticis cerebel′li [TA] molecular layer of cerebellar cortex: the superficial layer of the cortex of the cerebellum, containing a relatively small number of stellate neurons, and separated from the granular layer by the Purkinje cell layer. Called also *plexiform layer of cerebellar cortex.*
s. molecula′re gy′ri denta′ti [TA] molecular layer of dentate gyrus: the outermost layer of the trilaminar dentate gyrus, which contains dendrites from the granule cells of the underlying granular layer (stratum granulare) and receives numerous afferent projections, primarily from the entorhinal cortex.
s. molecula′re hippocam′pi the most superficial layer of the hippocampus, in which the apical dendrites of the pyramidal cells terminate. In official terminology, it is considered as a unit with the stratum lacunosum and called *s. moleculare et substratum lacunosum hippocampi.*
s. molecula′re et sub′s. lacuno′sum hippocam′pi [TA] official terminology for the stratum moleculare hippocampi and stratum lacunosum hippocampi (qq.v.), considering them as a unit.
mucous s. of tympanic membrane mucous layer of tympanic membrane: the inner layer of the tympanic membrane, continuous with the mucosa lining the tympanic cavity.
s. multifor′me gy′ri denta′ti [TA] multiform layer of dentate gyrus: the innermost layer of the trilaminar dentate gyrus, a polymorphic layer containing cells that give rise primarily to ipsilateral association fibers.
s. musculo′sum panni′culi adipo′si te′lae subcuta′neae [TA] muscle layer of fatty layer of subcutaneous tissue: a layer of muscle fibers present within the fatty layer of the subcutaneous tissue in some parts of the body, which produces contraction or movement of the skin.
s. nervo′sum re′tinae [TA] neural layer of retina: the internal, transparent, light-sensitive portion of the optic nerve part of the retina (cf. *s. pigmentosum retinae*), comprising nine layers seen by light microscopy, named from within outward: internal limiting membrane, nerve fiber layer, ganglion cell layer, inner plexiform layer, inner nuclear layer, outer plexiform layer, outer nuclear layer, outer limiting membrane, and layer of rods and cones; the various layers are connected transversely by fibers of connective tissue *(Müller fibers).* See illustration at *retina.*
s. neurofibra′rum re′tinae [TA] official terminology for *nerve fiber layer of retina.*
s. nuclea′re exter′num re′tinae [TA] official terminology for *outer nuclear layer of retina.*
s. nuclea′re inter′num re′tinae [TA] official terminology for *inner nuclear layer of retina.*
s. op′ticum colli′culi superio′ris [TA] optic layer of superior colliculus: a layer of white fibers below the superficial gray layer and above the intermediate gray layer; many of its fibers are from the optic tract and it contains a few other large neurons.
s. o′riens hippocam′pi [TA] oriens layer of hippocampus: one of the layers of the hippocampus, lying between the alveus and the stratum pyramidalis; it is composed of neurons with ascending axons (basket cells), the ramifications of the basal dendrites of the pyramidal cells, and their axon collaterals.
s. papilla′re der′midis [TA] papillary layer: the outer layer of the dermis, characterized by ridges or papillae protruding into the epidermis. Called also *papillary dermis.*
stra′ta parvocellula′ria nu′clei dorsa′lis cor′poris genicula′ti latera′lis [TA] parvocellular layers of dorsal lateral geniculate nucleus: the outer dorsal layers (laminae 3, 4, 5, 6) of the lateral geniculate nucleus, which are composed of small neurons receiving input from the contralateral (4, 6) and ipsilateral (3, 5) sides and collectively projecting to the primary visual cortex.
s. pigmento′sum re′tinae [TA] pigmented layer of retina: a layer of pigmented epithelium that is the outer of the two parts of the optic part of the retina (cf. *stratum nervosum retinae*), extending from the entrance of the optic nerve to the pupillary margin of the iris. It is important in the turnover of rods and cones and functions as a blood-retina barrier to maintain the ionic environment of the retina. Called also *retinal pigment epithelium.* See illustration at *retina.*
s. plexifor′me exter′num re′tinae [TA] official terminology for *outer plexiform layer of retina.*
s. plexifor′me inter′num re′tinae [TA] official terminology for *inner plexiform layer of retina.*
s. purkinjen′se cor′ticis cerebel′li [TA] Purkinje cell layer: a layer of the cerebellar cortex containing the large neurons called Purkinje cells; it is bounded externally by the molecular layer and internally by the granular layer. Some consider it to be the deepest portion of the molecular layer.
s. pyramida′le hippocam′pi [TA] pyramidal layer of hippocampus: a well-defined double layer of pyramidal cells in the hippocampus; their dendrites extend from the stratum oriens to the stratum moleculare.
s. radia′tum hippocam′pi [TA] radiate layer of hippocampus: the superficial part of the pyramidal cell layer of the hippocampus, the bulk of which is formed by apical dendrites together with their axons and a few pyramidal cells.
s. radiatum of tympanic membrane radiate layer of tympanic membrane: the outer part of the fibrous stratum of the membrane, consisting of fibers radiating outward from the manubrium of the malleus to pass into the fibrocartilaginous ring.
s. reticula′re der′midis [TA] reticular layer: the inner layer of the dermis, consisting chiefly of dense fibrous tissue. Called also *reticular dermis.*
s. segmento′rum externo′rum et interno′rum re′tinae [TA] official terminology for *layer of rods and cones.*
s. spino′sum spinous layer: in the epidermis, the layer between the stratum granulosum and stratum basale; it contains the prickle cells. See figure at *epidermis.* Called also *prickle cell layer.*
s. submucosum of myometrium submucosal layer of myometrium: the inner layer of the myometrium, which is in contact with the endometrium.
s. subserosum of myometrium subserosal layer of myometrium: the outer layer of the myometrium, which is in contact with the serous coat of the uterus.
s. supravascula′re supravascular layer of myometrium: the layer of the myometrium that lies between the stratum vasculare and the stratum subserosum.
s. synovia′le cap′sulae articula′ris TA alternative for *membrana synovialis capsulae articularis.*
s. synovia′le vagi′nae ten′dinis [TA] synovial tendon sheath: the synovial layer of a tendon sheath. Called also *vagina synovialis* [TA alternative].
s. vascula′re vascular layer of myometrium: the middle layer of the myometrium, forming most of its bulk, and composed of circular and spiral fibers.
s. zona′le colli′culi superio′ris [TA] zonal layer of superior colliculus: the most external layer of the superior colliculus (Layer I), containing myelinated and unmyelinated fibers primarily from the occipital lobe.
s. zona′le tha′lami zonal layer of thalamus: a layer of myelinated fibers covering the superior aspect of the dorsal thalamus.

Straus reaction (phenomenon, test) (strous) [Isidore *Straus,* French physician, 1845–1896] see under *reaction.*

Strauss sign (shtrous) [Hermann *Strauss,* German physician, 1868–1944] see under *sign.*

streak (strēk) a line, stria, striation, or stripe.
angioid s's red to black irregular bands observed in the ocular fundus running outward from the region of the optic disk, which are seen in certain conditions, including pseudoxanthoma elasticum, osteitis deformans, and sickle-cell anemia. The lesions are thought to represent ruptures in the lamina basalis of the choroid.
fatty s. a small, flat, yellow-gray area, composed mainly of cholesterol-laden macrophages, within an artery; possibly an early stage of atherosclerosis.
germinal s. primitive s.
Knapp s's lines resembling blood vessels seen occasionally in the retina after hemorrhage.
medullary s. neural groove.
meningitic s. tache cérébrale.
Moore lightning s's a subjective sensation of vertical flashes of light resembling lightning, sometimes seen on the peripheral side of the field of vision when the eyes are moved; a benign condition.

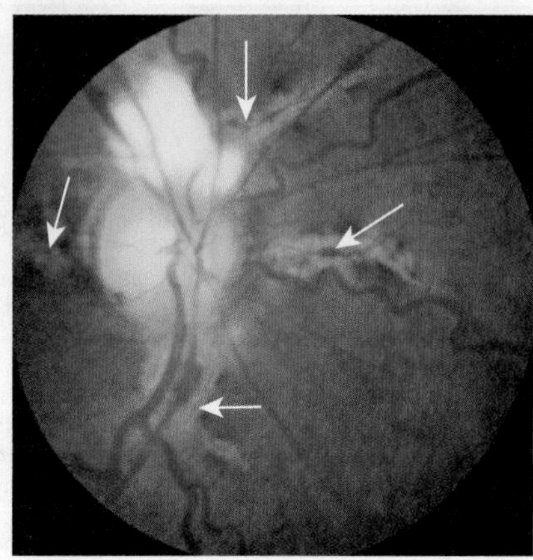

■ Angioid streaks *(arrows)* in Ehlers-Danlos syndrome.

primitive s. a faint white trace at the caudal end of the embryonic disc, formed by the movement of cells at the beginning of mesoderm formation; it provides the earliest evidence of the embryonic axis.

stream (strēm) a current or flow, usually of a fluid; called also *flumen.*
axial s. see under *current.*
blood s. bloodstream; see under *B.*
electron s. a stream of negatively charged particles (electrons) moving from cathode to anode across a potential difference in a low-pressure gas tube or a vacuum tube.
hair s's flumina pilorum.

stream·ing (strēm′ing) the movement of a current in a fluid.
cytoplasmic s., protoplasmic s. cyclosis.

Stree·ter horizons (stre′tər) [George Linius *Streeter*, American embryologist, 1873–1948] see *horizons.*

strength (strength) intensity or power.
electric field s. electric intensity.
fatigue s. the maximum stress at which a material will withstand cyclic loading for a given period.
ionic s. a quantity proportional to the amount of electrostatic interaction between ions in solution; equal to

$$\frac{1}{2}\sum m_i Z_i^2,$$

where m_i is the molar concentration of the medium i, and Z_i is the ionic charge. Symbol *I.*
magnetic field s. term used in magnetic resonance imaging to refer to the strength of induction of a given magnetic field.
muscle s. the greatest force that can be put forth by a muscle; it is measured with either isometric, isokinetic, or isotonic exercises.
yield s. an amount of deforming stress just above the elastic limit, when a substance begins to be permanently changed in shape.

streph(o)- [Gr. *strephein* to twist] a combining form meaning twisted.

strepho·po·dia (stref″o-po′de-ə) talipes equinus.

strepho·sym·bo·lia (stref″o-sim-bo′le-ə) [*strepho-* + *symbol* + *-ia*] 1. a disorder of perception in which objects seem reversed, as in a mirror. 2. a type of dyslexia in which letters are perceived as in a mirror; it begins with confusion between similar but oppositely oriented letters (b-d, q-p) and there may be a tendency to reverse direction in reading.

strep·i·tus (strep′ĭ-təs) [L.] a noise; a sound heard on auscultation.

strepo·gen·in (strep″o-jen′in) a factor present in casein and certain other proteins which is essential to optimal growth of animals.

Strep·tase (strep′tās) trademark for a preparation of streptokinase.

strep·tav·i·din (strep-tav′ĭ-din) a bacterial protein used as a probe in immunologic and biochemical assays because of its great affinity and specificity for biotin; it is frequently part of an indirect system in which specific substrates are biotinylated and then visualized by binding streptavidin to which is linked an easily detected compound, such as a fluorochrome.

strept(o)- [Gr. *streptos* twisted] a combining form meaning twisted.

strep·to·bac·il·lary (strep″to-bas′ĭ-lar″e) pertaining to or caused by streptobacilli.

Strep·to·ba·cil·lus (strep″to-bə-sil′əs) [*strepto-* + *bacillus*] a genus of gram-negative bacteria of the family Fusobacteriaceae, consisting of highly pleomorphic cells that vary from single rods with central swellings to chains or filaments resembling strings of beads; organisms are facultatively anaerobic, nonmotile, and non–spore-forming. The type species is *S. moniliformis.*
S. monilifor′mis a species, found in the throat and nasopharynx of wild and laboratory rats, that causes Haverhill fever and the bacillary form of rat-bite fever in humans.

strep·to·ba·cil·li (strep″to-bə-sil′i) plural of *streptobacillus.*

strep·to·ba·cil·lus (strep″to-bə-sil′əs) pl. *streptobacil′li.* A bacterium of the genus *Streptobacillus.*

strep·to·cer·ci·a·sis (strep″to-sər-ki′ə-sis) infection with *Mansonella streptocerca,* whose microfilariae produce a pruritic rash resembling that in onchocerciasis; transmitted by midges of the genus *Culicoides,* it occurs in Central Africa.

Strep·to·coc·ca·ceae (strep″to-kok-a′se-e) a family of gram-positive, facultatively anaerobic cocci of the order Lactobacillales; organisms are usually nonmotile and occur in pairs, chains, or tetrads. It includes the genera *Lactococcus* and *Streptococcus.*

strep·to·coc·ce·mia (strep″to-kok-se′me-ə) [*streptococcus* + *-emia*] the presence of streptococci in the blood.

strep·to·coc·ci (strep″to-kok′si) plural of *streptococcus.*

strep·to·coc·col·y·sin (strep″to-kŏ-kol′ĭ-sin) streptolysin.

strep·to·coc·co·sis (strep″to-kŏ-ko′sis) infection with streptococci.

Strep·to·coc·cus (strep″to-kok′əs) [*strepto-* + Gr. *kokkos* berry] a genus of gram-positive, homofermentative lactic acid bacteria of the family Streptococcaceae, consisting of nonmotile, non–spore-forming cocci occurring in pairs or chains; organisms are chemo-organotrophic, facultatively anaerobic, and cytochrome-, oxidase-, and catalase-negative. Many species are human or animal commensals or parasites, and some are pathogenic. Streptococci are most often classified according to patterns of hemolysis on blood agar (see *hemolytic streptococci,* under *streptococcus*), or by antigenic composition (see *Lancefield classification,* under *classification*). The type species is *S. pyo′genes.*
S. acidomi′nimus an α-hemolytic species with no Lancefield group antigen; it is found in the bovine vagina and in raw milk and occasionally causes human infection.
S. adja′cens former name for *Granulicatella adiacens.*
S. agalac′tiae a β-hemolytic species of Lancefield group B, found in raw milk; it causes mastitis in cattle and sometimes infection in human infants or less often older persons.
S. angino′sus a species that includes streptococci of Lancefield groups F and G. β-Hemolytic strains are found in several human sources including abscesses, while α-hemolytic and nonhemolytic strains are associated with primary atypical pneumonia.
S. bo′vis a species of α-hemolytic and nonhemolytic organisms, part of Lancefield group D; it is found in the bovine alimentary tract and sometimes in human feces, and has been associated with human infective endocarditis and urinary tract infections.
S. constella′tus a β-hemolytic species in Lancefield group F, microaerophilic or obligately anaerobic, found in purulent pleurisy and in the tonsils, appendix, nose, throat, gums, and infrequently the skin and vagina.
S. defecti′vus former name for *Abiotrophia defectiva.*
S. dysgalac′tiae a species containing both nonhemolytic and hemolytic organisms of Lancefield groups C, G, and L, divided into two subspecies on the basis of phenotypic and genotypic characterization.
S. dysgalac′tiae* subsp. *dysgalac′tiae a subspecies comprising nonhemolytic and α-hemolytic strains of Lancefield group C, commonly associated with bovine mastitis.
S. dysgalac′tiae* subsp. *equisi′milis a subspecies consisting of β-hemolytic strains belonging to Lancefield groups C, G, and L, occurring as part

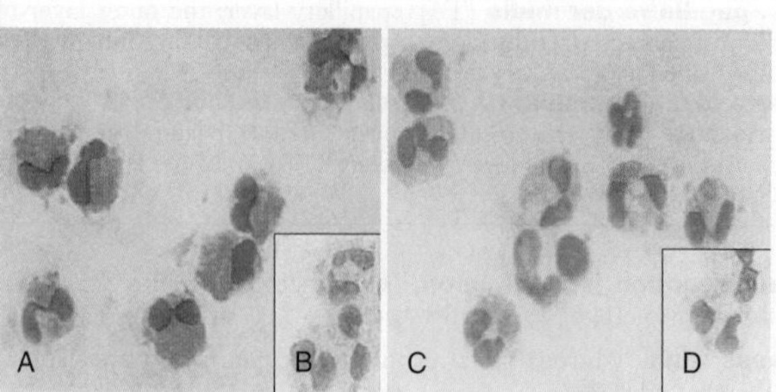

■ Streptavidin used to detect IL-9 protein, a cytokine expressed at high levels by eosinophils of individuals with asthma. Eosinophils from subjects with asthma *(A)* and nonasthmatic, nonatopic control subjects *(B)* were stained with goat polyclonal antibody to IL-9, followed by biotin-labeled rabbit anti-goat streptavidin alkaline phosphatase, then counterstained with hematoxylin. Goat IgG was used as a negative control *(B, D).* The intensity of red staining indicates the level of expression of IL-9 by the cells.

of the normal flora of the skin and mucous membranes and associated with infections in various animals. Formerly called *S. equisimilis.*

S. e'qui a β-hemolytic species of Lancefield group C, the specific etiologic agent of strangles in horses; it is usually not pathogenic for humans.

S. e'qui **subsp.** ***zooepide'micus*** a subspecies that can cause zoonotic infections in weak or immunocompromised humans.

S. equi'nus an α-hemolytic species of Lancefield group D, found in the alimentary tract of the horse and sometimes associated with human infection.

S. equisi'milis *S. dysgalactiae* subsp. *equisimilis.*

S. faeca'lis *Enterococcus faecalis.*

S. fae'cium *Enterococcus faecium.*

S. galloly'ticus a species in Lancefield group D, found most often in bovines and birds but occasionally in human endocarditis or other infections.

S. gordo'nii an α-hemolytic species that causes infective endocarditis.

S. infanta'rius a species in Lancefield group D, found normally in the intestines of various mammals and occasionally in cases of endocarditis.

S. interme'dius an α-hemolytic species in Lancefield group F, found in the human oral cavity and generally considered nonpathogenic.

S. lac'tis an α-hemolytic or nonhemolytic species of Lancefield group N, part of the lactic group and not considered pathogenic; it is found in dairy products and is commonly responsible for the souring of milk.

S. mi'tis an α-hemolytic species that has no specific Lancefield group antigen; it is found in the normal human upper respiratory tract and has been associated with subacute bacterial endocarditis.

S. mu'tans a species of variable hemolysis in Lancefield group K that is an important cause of dental caries and can also cause infective endocarditis. Organisms adhere to the tooth surface and, by fermentation of carbohydrates, produce acids that demineralize the enamel.

S. ora'lis an α-hemolytic species found normally in the human oral cavity, but sometimes causing opportunistic infections.

S. pneumo'niae the species known as *pneumococcus,* an α-hemolytic species with no specific Lancefield group antigen; it is the usual cause of lobar pneumonia and also causes other serious, acute, pyogenic disorders such as meningitis, septicemia, empyema, and peritonitis. There are many serovars, distinguished on the basis of specific capsular polysaccharides called *pneumococcal polysaccharides.*

S. pyo'genes a β-hemolytic species that comprises group A of the Lancefield classification and is toxigenic and pyogenic; it is separable into numbered serovars on the basis of the specificity and combination of the M, R, and T antigens. This species is the most frequent bacterial cause of acute pharyngitis and also causes a variety of cutaneous and systemic infections, including rheumatic fever, scarlet fever, puerperal sepsis, poststreptococcal acute glomerulonephritis, and necrotizing fasciitis.

S. saliva'rius a species of variable hemolysis with some strains in Lancefield group K; it is part of the normal flora of the upper respiratory tract and is occasionally associated with apical abscesses of the teeth and subacute bacterial endocarditis.

S. san'guinis, S. san'guis an α-hemolytic species in Lancefield group H; it is found in humans in dental plaque and the blood, and in subacute bacterial endocarditis.

S. su'is a β-hemolytic species of Lancefield group D, found in young pigs suffering from bacteremia and in asymptomatic older pigs; infection takes various forms, including streptococcal meningitis.

S. u'beris an α-hemolytic or nonhemolytic species with no specific Lancefield group antigen; it causes mastitis in cows, is found in milk, and occasionally causes human infections.

strep•to•coc•cus (strep″to-kok′əs) pl. *streptococ'ci.* An organism of the genus *Streptococcus.* **streptococ'cal, streptococ'cic** *adj*

α-hemolytic s., alpha-hemolytic s. see *hemolytic s.*

anhemolytic s. nonhemolytic s.

β-hemolytic s., beta-hemolytic s. see *hemolytic s.*

γ-hemolytic s., gamma-hemolytic s. nonhemolytic s.

group A, B, C (etc.) streptococci streptococci distinguished by the Lancefield classification into groups (Lancefield groups) on immunologic grounds according to the presence in the cell wall of specific antigenic carbohydrates called C carbohydrates. Those causing human infection are found primarily in groups A through G.

hemolytic s. any streptococcus capable of hemolyzing red blood cells or of producing a zone of hemolysis around the colonies on blood agar; the great majority of streptococci found in pathologic processes are of this type. They have been classified as the *α-hemolytic type,* which produces around the colony on blood agar a small greenish zone (see also *viridans s.*); and the *β-hemolytic type,* which produces around the colony on blood agar a clear zone of hemolysis that is larger than that of the α type.

indifferent s. nonhemolytic s.

nonhemolytic s. any streptococcus that does not cause a change in the medium when cultured on blood agar. Called also *γ-hemolytic* or *gamma-hemolytic s.*

nutritionally variant streptococci (NVS) a group of fastidious bacteria, formerly classified in the viridans group of the genus *Streptococcus,* that grow as satellite colonies around other bacteria. They are currently classified in the genera *Abiotrophia* and *Granulicatella.*

viridans streptococci in one classification, a group of streptococci other than *S. pneumoniae,* usually α-hemolytic but sometimes nonhemolytic; some are part of the normal flora of the respiratory tract, and some can cause dental caries, bacterial endocarditis, and various disorders in immunocompromised persons.

strep•to•dor•nase (strep″to-dor′nās) [*strepto*coccus + *deoxy*ribo*nucle*ase] a deoxyribonuclease produced by hemolytic streptococci; see also under *streptokinase.*

strep•to•gen•in (strep″to-jen′in) a growth-stimulating factor for certain microorganisms and laboratory animals, found in protein hydrolysates. Since a large number of peptides have streptogenin activity, they may serve simply as an accessible source of amino acids.

strep•to•gram•in (strep″to-gram′in) any in a group of antimicrobial agents derived from species of *Streptomyces.*

strep•to•he•mol•y•sin (strep″to-he-mol′ĭ-sin) streptolysin.

strep•to•ki•nase (SK) (strep″to-ki′nās) [*strepto*coccus + *kinase*] a protein produced by β-hemolytic streptococci; although it has no intrinsic enzymatic activity, it binds plasminogen and causes cleavage of that molecule to plasmin. It is used as a thrombolytic agent in the treatment of acute coronary arterial thrombosis, acute pulmonary embolism, deep vein thrombosis, and acute arterial thromboembolism or thrombosis, administered intravenously. It is also used to clear obstructed arteriovenous cannulae.

s.-streptodornase (SKSD) a mixture of the proteins streptokinase and streptodornase produced by hemolytic streptococci; used topically on surface lesions and by instillation in closed body cavities to remove clotted blood or fibrinous or purulent accumulations.

strep•tol•y•sin (strep-tol′ĭ-sin) [*strepto*coccus + hemo*lysin*] an exotoxin produced by certain strains of streptococci, particularly those of group A, that lyses red blood cells.

s. O an oxygen-labile and antigenic hemolysin produced by most group A streptococci and by some of groups C and G. It is inactive in the oxidized state but is readily activated by treatment with mild reducing agents, such as sulfite.

s. S an oxygen-stable and nonantigenic hemolysin and leukocidin produced by many strains of group A streptococci. It is sensitive to treatment with heat or acid, but is not inactivated by oxygen.

strep•to•mi•cro•dac•ty•ly (strep″to-mi″kro-dak′tə-le) [*strepto-* + *microdactyly*] camptodactyly in which the little fingers only are involved.

Strep•to•my•ces (strep″to-mi′sēz) [*strepto-* + Gr. *mykēs* fungus] a genus of bacteria of the family Streptomycetaceae, consisting of aerobic, gram-positive, non–acid-fast organisms that form a nonfragmented aerial mycelium. There are several hundred different species, usually soil forms but occasionally parasitic on plants or animals. Most species produce pigments. More than half of the antibiotics of practical value, including the aminoglycosides, tetracyclines, and macrolides, are produced from species of *Streptomyces.* The type species is *S. al'bus.*

S. al'bus a species that produces the antibiotic salinomycin.

S. ambofa'ciens a species that produces ambomycin, azotomycin, duazomycin, and spiramycin.

S. antibio'ticus a species that produces the antibiotic oleandomycin.

S. aureofa'ciens a species that produces the antibiotic partricin.

S. azu'reus a species that produces the antibiotic thiostrepton.

S. bambergien'sis a species that is a source of bambermycins.

S. cinnamonen'sis a species that produces the antibiotic monensin.

S. coeruleoru'bidus a species that produces the antineoplastic antibiotic daunorubicin.

S. ederen'sis a species that is a source of bambermycins.

S. eryth'reus *Saccharopolyspora erythraea.*

S. fra'diae a species that produces neomycin.

S. geysirien'sis a species that is a source of bambermycins.

S. ghanaen'sis a species that is a source of bambermycins.

S. grise'olus a species that produces the antibiotic sinefungin.

S. gri'seus a species that produces streptomycin.

S. hygrosco'picus a species that includes variants that produce the macrolide antibiotics pimecrolimus and sirolimus.

S. kanamyce'ticus a species that produces kanamycin.

S. kitasoen'sis a species that is the source of the antibiotic kitasamycin.

S. lasalien'sis a species that produces the antibiotic lasalocid.

S. lincolnen'sis a species that produces the antibiotic lincomycin.

S. ni'veus a species that produces the antibiotic novobiocin.

S. noboritoen'sis a species that produces the antibiotic hygromycin.

S. nodo'sus a species some strains of which produce amphotericin B.

S. noga'later a species including a variant that produces the antineoplastic substance nogalamycin.

S. nour'sei a species that produces the antibiotic nystatin.

S. orchida′ceus a species that is the source of cycloserine.

S. peuce′tius a species that produces the antineoplastic antibiotics daunorubicin and doxorubicin.

S. rimo′sus a species containing a variant, *S. rimo′sus* var. *paromomyci′nus*, that produces the antibiotic paromomycin.

S. roseospo′rus a species that produces the antibiotic daptomycin.

S. somalien′sis a species commonly found in Africa, North and South America, Israel, and India, causing actinomycotic mycetoma in which the granules in the discharged pus are white to yellow.

S. specta′bilis a species from which the antibiotic spectinomycin is derived.

S. tenebra′rius a species that produces nebramycin, the antibiotic complex from which tobramycin is derived.

S. tsukubaen′sis a species that produces the macrolide tacrolimus.

S. vina′ceus a species that produces vitamin B_{12}.

Strep•to•my•ce•ta•ceae (strep″to-mi″sə-ta′se-e) a family of aerobic, gram-positive bacteria of the suborder Streptomycineae; organisms of medical importance are contained in the genus *Streptomyces.*

strep•to•my•cin (strep″to-mi′sin) the first of the aminoglycoside antibiotics to be isolated, derived from *Streptomyces griseus;* it is effective against a wide variety of aerobic gram-negative bacilli and some gram-positive bacteria, including mycobacteria. Its use is now limited because of the emergence of resistant strains.

s. sulfate [USP] the sesquisulfate salt of streptomycin, used as a tuberculostatic in combination with other antituberculosis agents, and for the treatment of certain nontuberculous infections due to susceptible organisms, including plague, tularemia, and (in combination with other drugs) brucellosis, granuloma inguinale, chancroid, and bacterial endocarditis; administered intramuscularly.

Strep•to•my•ci•neae (strep″to-mi-sin′e-e) a suborder of bacteria of the order Actinomycetales, containing the single family Streptomycetaceae.

strep•to•my•co•sis (strep″to-mi-ko′sis) infection with bacteria of the genus *Streptomyces.*

Strep•to•neu•ra (strep″to-noor′ə) a subclass of gastropods, including snails found in salt water and occasionally fresh water habitats. A number of primary or intermediate hosts for trematodes and other pathogens are in this group in the order Mesogastropoda. A second order is the marine-dwelling Neogastropoda. Called also *Prosobranchiata.*

Strep•to•spo•ran•gi•neae (strep″to-spor″an-jin′e-e) [*strepto-* + Gr. *spora* seed + *angeion* vessel] a suborder of bacteria of the order Actinomycetales, consisting of gram-positive, aerobic, mesophilic or thermophilic organisms that produce an aerial mycelium. Medically important organisms are contained in the families Nocardiopsaceae and Thermomonosporaceae.

strep•to•zo•cin (strep″to-zo′sin) an antineoplastic antibiotic of the nitrosourea (q.v.) group, derived from *Streptomyces achromogenes* or produced by synthesis; used principally in the treatment of islet cell tumors as well as other endocrine tumors such as gastrinomas associated with Zollinger-Ellison syndrome and glucagonomas.

strep•to•zo•to•cin (strep″to-zo-to′sin) streptozocin.

stress (stres) 1. forcibly exerted influence; pressure. 2. force per unit area, which may cause strain (q.v.) on an object. 3. in dentistry, the pressure of the upper teeth against the lower in mastication. 4. a state of physiological or psychological strain caused by adverse stimuli, physical, mental, or emotional, internal or external, that tend to disturb the functioning of an organism and which the organism naturally desires to avoid; see also *stress reaction,* under *reaction.* 5. the stimuli that elicit such a state or stress reactions.

cold s. hypothermia.

heat s. the complications seen when persons undergo muscular exertion in conditions of excessive heat, such as when sweating does not cool off the body enough, or when heavy sweating depletes the body's supply of fluids and electrolytes. It may lead to heat exhaustion, heat cramps, and other conditions.

oxidative s. any of various pathological changes seen in living organisms in response to excessive levels of cytotoxic oxidants and free radicals in the environment.

stress-break•er (stres′brāk-ər) a device built into a removable partial denture that relieves the abutment teeth from excessive occlusal loads and stresses. Two basic types are recognized: one consisting of a movable joint between the direct retainer and the denture base *(hinge s.)* and the other consisting of a flexible connection between the direct retainer and the denture base or using a movable joint between two major connectors.

stretch•er (strech′ər) a portable couchlike or bedlike structure for carrying the sick or injured. Called also *litter.*

stretch•es (strech′əz) inherited periodic spasticity.

stria (stri′ə) pl. *stri′ae* [L. "a furrow, groove"] a band, line, streak, or stripe, especially one of various longitudinal collections of nerve fibers in the brain.

stri′ae al′bae, stri′ae albican′tes a later stage of striae distensae, particularly visible in light-skinned individuals, when the marks fade to a pale or white color. Called also *lineae albicantes.*

anterior acoustic s. s. cochlearis anterior.

atrophic striae, stri′ae atro′phicae striae distensae.

Baillarger external s. s. laminae granularis internae.

Baillarger inner s., Baillarger internal s. s. laminae pyramidalis internae.

Baillarger outer s. s. laminae granularis internae.

stri′ae cilia′res slight dark ridges running parallel with each other from the teeth of the ora serrata of the retina to the valleys between the ciliary processes.

s. cochlea′ris ante′rior [TA] anterior acoustic stria: axons from the ventral cochlear nucleus that course through the trapezoid body at the inferior aspect of the pontine tegmentum, cross the midline, and join the lateral lemniscus on the opposite side. En route they may project to the superior olive and trapezoid nuclei. Called also *ventral acoustic s.*

s. cochlea′ris interme′dia [TA] intermediate acoustic stria: axons from the posterior portion of the anterior cochlear nucleus that course through the dorsal cochlear nucleus, over the restiform body, and through the pontine tegmentum to the opposite lateral lemniscus. En route they terminate in the retro-olivary and periolivary nuclei of both sides.

s. cochlea′ris poste′rior [TA] posterior acoustic stria: axons from the dorsal cochlear nucleus that course over the surface of the restiform body, cross the midline below the medial longitudinal fasciculus, and enter the lateral lemniscus of the opposite side. En route these fibers may project to the superior olive and trapezoid nuclei. Called also *dorsal acoustic s.*

stri′ae cu′tis disten′sae striae distensae.

s. diagona′lis [TA], **s. diagona′lis (Bro′ca)** diagonal band: a band of nerve fibers that forms the caudal zone of the anterior perforated substance where it adjoins the optic tract, which is continuous caudolaterally with the periamygdaloid area and rostromedially passes above the optic chiasm to blend with the paraterminal gyrus; called also *band of Broca, bandaletta diagonalis (Broca), Broca's diagonal band,* and *diagonal band of Broca.*

stri′ae disten′sae linear, atrophic, pink to purple, scarlike lesions, which later become pale in light-skinned individuals *(striae albae* or *albicantes),* seen most often on the abdomen, breasts, buttocks, or thighs. They are due to weakening of the elastic tissues, and are associated with pregnancy *(striae gravidarum),* excessive obesity, rapid growth during puberty and adolescence, Cushing syndrome, or topical or prolonged treatment with corticosteroids. Called also *lineae atrophicae, linear atrophy, atrophic striae,* and *striae atrophicae.*

dorsal acoustic s. s. cochlearis posterior.

external s. of Baillarger s. laminae granularis internae.

s. of external granular layer s. laminae granularis externae.

s. exter′na zo′nae exter′nae medul′lae rena′lis [TA] outer stripe of outer zone of renal medulla: in the outer zone of the renal medulla, the part next to the cortex; it contains thick descending and thick ascending limbs of the loop of Henle.

s. of Gennari see under *line.*

stri′ae gravida′rum striae distensae seen during pregnancy.

inner s. of Baillarger s. laminae pyramidalis internae.

intermediate acoustic s. s. cochlearis intermedia.

internal s. of Baillarger s. laminae pyramidalis internae.

s. inter′na zo′nae exter′nae medul′lae rena′lis [TA] inner stripe of outer zone of renal medulla: in the outer zone of the renal medulla, the part next to the inner zone and away from the cortex; it contains thin descending and thick ascending limbs of the loop of Henle (ansa nephroni).

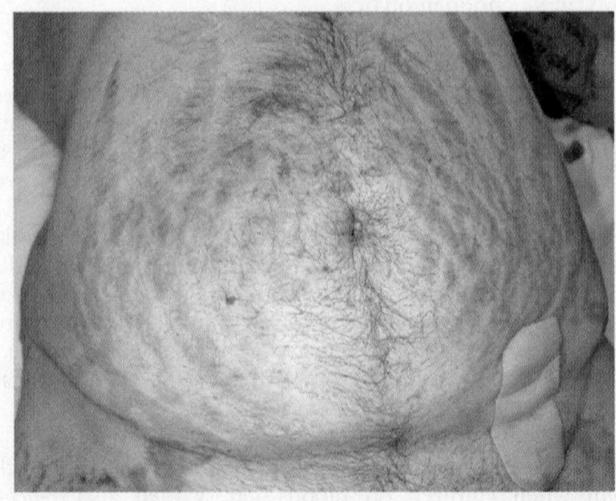

■ Striae distensae in a man with Cushing syndrome.

s. of internal granular layer s. laminae granularis internae.
s. of internal pyramidal layer s. laminae pyramidalis internae.
Kaes s., Kaes-Bekhterev s. Kaes-Bekhterev layer.
Knapp striae see under *streak.*
s. la′minae granula′ris exter′nae [TA] stria of external granular layer: a band of tangentially oriented nerve fibers in the external granular layer of the cerebral cortex.
s. la′minae granula′ris inter′nae [TA] stria of internal granular layer: a band of tangentially oriented white nerve fibers in the internal granular layer of the cerebral cortex. In the region of the calcarine sulcus, this stria is thick and highly visible and here is known as the *line of Gennari* (see also *striate cortex,* under *cortex*). Called also *external band, line, stria,* or *stripe of Baillarger.* See also *s. laminae pyramidalis internae.*
s. la′minae molecula′ris [TA], **s. la′minae plexifor′mis** stria of molecular layer: a band of tangentially oriented myelinated nerve fibers in the molecular layer of the cerebral cortex.
s. la′minae pyramida′lis inter′nae [TA] stria of internal pyramidal layer: a band of tangentially oriented white nerve fibers in the internal pyramidal layer of the cerebral cortex; called also *internal band, line, stria,* or *stripe of Baillarger.* See also *s. laminae granularis internae.*
s. of Lanci s. longitudinalis medialis corporis callosi.
Langhans s. cytotrophoblast.
Liesegang striae see under *phenomenon.*
longitudinal s. of corpus callosum, lateral s. longitudinalis lateralis corporis callosi.
longitudinal s. of corpus callosum, medial s. longitudinalis medialis corporis callosi.
s. longitudina′lis latera′lis cor′poris callo′si [TA] lateral longitudinal stria of corpus callosum: one of two slender bands of myelinated fibers which form longitudinal ridges in the indusium griseum on the superior aspect of each half of the corpus callosum.
s. longitudina′lis media′lis cor′poris callo′si [TA] medial longitudinal stria of corpus callosum: one of two slender bands of myelinated fibers which form longitudinal ridges in the indusium griseum on the superior aspect of each half of the corpus callosum. Called also *s. of Lanci.*
s. mallea′ris membra′nae tym′pani, s. mallea′ris membra′nae tympa′nicae [TA], **s. malleola′ris membra′nae tym′pani** malleolar stria of tympanic membrane: a nearly vertical radial band seen on the outer surface of the tympanic membrane; it extends from the umbo upward to the malleolar prominence and is produced by the manubrium mallei.
s. medulla′ris tha′lami [TA] medullary stria of thalamus: a fiber bundle that arises from the subcallosal and paraterminal gyri, the preoptic area, and amygdaloid area, and runs backward along the junction of the dorsal and medial surfaces of the thalamus to reach the habenular nucleus.
stri′ae medulla′res ventri′culi quar′ti [TA], **medullary striae of fourth ventricle** bundles of white fibers coursing transversely across the floor of the fourth ventricle; they arise from the arcuate nuclei, pass dorsally close to the midline, and after having reached the fourth ventricle finally enter the inferior cerebellar peduncle.
medullary s. of thalamus s. medullaris thalami.
meningitic s. tache cérébrale.
s. of molecular layer s. laminae molecularis.
Nitabuch s. see under *layer.*
stri′ae olfacto′riae [TA] olfactory striae: the radiating fibers of the olfactory tract, which diverge into a lateral and a medial band at the olfactory trigone and border the anterior perforated substance; the bands are covered by the lateral and medial olfactory gyri, respectively. See also *intermediate olfactory s.*
s. olfacto′ria latera′lis [TA] see *striae olfactoriae.*
s. olfacto′ria media′lis [TA] see *striae olfactoriae.*
olfactory striae see *striae olfactoriae* and *intermediate olfactory s.*
olfactory s., intermediate a small band of fibers that pass from the center of the olfactory trigone to penetrate the anterior perforated substance; its presence is variable. See also *striae olfactoriae.*
olfactory striae, lateral stria olfactoria lateralis.
olfactory s., medial stria olfactoria medialis.
outer s. of Baillarger s. laminae granularis internae.
posterior acoustic s. s. cochlearis posterior.
Retzius parallel striae incremental lines.
Rohr s. a layer of fibrin in the developing placenta, within the intervillous space at the fetal-maternal junction.
stri′ae ru′brae the earlier stage of striae distensae, particularly visible in light-skinned individuals, when the marks have a reddish color.
s. termina′lis [TA] terminal stria: a band of fibers along the lateral margin of the ventricular surface of the thalamus, covering the thalamostriate vein and, following the course of the vein, marking the line of separation between the thalamus and the caudate nucleus; it extends from the region of the interventricular foramen to the temporal horn of the lateral ventricle, carrying fibers from the amygdaloid nuclei to the septal, hypothalamic, and thalamic areas. Cf. *ventral amygdalofugal tract.*
transverse striae of corpus callosum transverse bands of fibers on the upper surface of the corpus callosum.
s. vascula′ris duc′tus cochlea′ris [TA] vascular stria of cochlear duct: a layer of vascular tissue consisting of epithelial cells, mesothelial cells, and probably some neuroectoderm; it covers the outer wall of the cochlear duct and is thought to secrete the endolymph.
ventral acoustic s. s. cochlearis anterior.
Vogt striae thin vertical lines seen on the posterior corneal surface in keratoconus.
Wickham striae pale grayish dots or lines forming a network on the surface of the papules in lichen planus.

striae (stri′e) [L.] plural of *stria.*

stri·a·tal (stri-a′təl) pertaining to the corpus striatum.

stri·ate (stri′āt) striated.

stri·at·ed (stri′āt-əd) [L. *striatus*] striped; marked by striae.

stri·a·tion (stri-a′shən) 1. the quality of being marked by stripes or striae. 2. a streak or scratch.
tabby cat s., tigroid s. a striation or marking on muscle tissue that has undergone marked fatty degeneration; seen especially in degenerated heart muscle.

stri·a·to·ni·gral (stri″ə-to-ni′grəl) projecting from the corpus striatum to the substantia nigra.

stri·a·tum (stri-a′təm) [L., neuter of *striatus* striped] 1. striped, or grooved. 2. corpus striatum. 3. neostriatum.

stric·ture (strik′chər) [L. *strictura*] stenosis.
annular s. a stricture which encircles the lumen of a tubular structure.
bridle s. a fold of membrane stretched across a canal, and partially closing it.
cicatricial s. see under *stenosis.*
contractile s. a stricture that can be mechanically dilated but soon returns to its previously contracted condition. Called also *recurrent s.*
false s., functional s. spasmodic s.
irritable s. a stricture through which the passage or attempted passage of an instrument produces pain.
organic s., permanent s. a stricture due to a structural change in or about a canal.
recurrent s. contractile s.
spasmodic s., spastic s. a stricture that is due to muscular spasm; called also *false s., functional s.,* and *temporary s.*
temporary s. spasmodic s.

stric·ture·plas·ty (strik′chər-plas″te) a type of enteroplasty in which the caliber of a constricted segment of intestine is enlarged by means of longitudinal incision and transverse suturing of the stricture. See illustration.

stric·tur·iza·tion (strik″chər-ĭ-za′shən) the process of decreasing in caliber or of becoming constricted.

stric·turo·plas·tic (strik′chər-o-plas″tik) pertaining to strictureplasty.

stric·turo·plas·ty (strik′chər-o-plas″te) strictureplasty.

stric·turo·tome (strik′chər-o-tōm″) a knife for cutting strictures.

stric·tur·ot·o·my (strik″chər-ot′ə-me) incision of a stricture.

stri·dor (stri′dər) [L.] a harsh, high-pitched breath sound such as the one often heard on inhalation with an acute laryngeal obstruction. Cf. *laryngismus stridulus.* **stri′dent, strid′ulous** *adj*
congenital laryngeal s. stridor and dyspnea of the newborn due to an indrawing or infolding of a congenitally flabby epiglottis and aryepiglottic folds (laryngomalacia) during inhalation; the condition is usually outgrown in two years.
laryngeal s. stridor due to laryngeal obstruction; see also *congenital laryngeal s.*
s. serra′ticus a sound like that made by filing a saw, caused by respiration through a tracheostomy tube.

strike (strīk) cutaneous myiasis (def. 1).
blowfly s. cutaneous blowfly myiasis.
body s. cutaneous myiasis on the back of an animal.

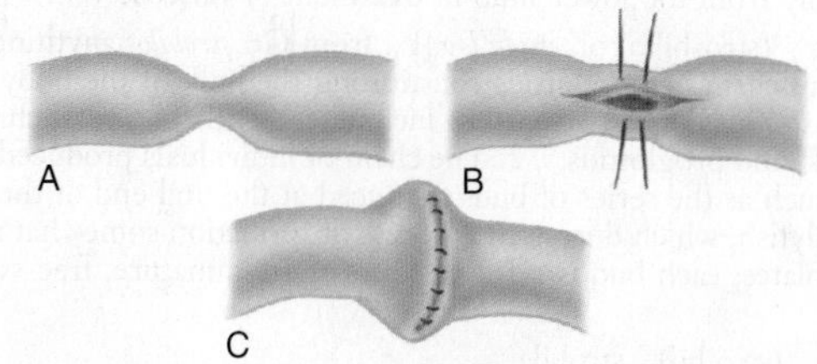

■ Strictureplasty. *(A),* Stricture; *(B),* longitudinal incision; *(C),* transverse closure.

breech s., crutch s., crutch s. cutaneous myiasis in the breech region of an animal. Called also *tail s.*
fly s. cutaneous blowfly myiasis.
pizzle s. cutaneous myiasis around the external genitals (particularly the prepuce) of a male animal.
poll s. cutaneous myiasis on the poll of an animal, either at a wound site (see *wound myiasis*) or in an area with folds of skin.
tail s. breech s.
wound s. traumatic myiasis in animals other than humans.

string·halt (string′hawlt) myoclonus of the hind leg of a horse, causing a gait in which the leg is suddenly raised and then stamped on the ground. Called also *spring hock.*

strio·cel·lu·lar (stri″o-sel′u-lər) [*stria* + *cellular*] composed of striated muscle fibers and cells.

strio·cer·e·bel·lar (stri″o-ser″ə-bel′ər) pertaining to or affecting both the corpus striatum and the cerebellum, as striocerebellar tremor.

strio·mo·tor (stri″o-mo′tər) pertaining to or affecting neurons supplying skeletal muscle.

strio·mus·cu·lar (stri″o-mus′ku-lər) pertaining to or composed of striated muscle.

strio·ni·gral (stri″o-ni′grəl) striatonigral.

strip (strip) 1. a thin, narrow, comparatively long piece of material. 2. to express the contents from a canal, such as a blood vessel, by running the finger along it. 3. to excise lengths of large veins and competent tributaries by subcutaneous dissection and a stripper. 4. to reduce the mesiodistal width of teeth, usually to make space to align crowded segments. 5. to remove metal from the inside of a crown electrochemically in order to increase the inside diameter.
abrasive s. a strip of linen or polymer film having abrasive material such as silica or garnet bonded to one side; used for polishing and contouring of the proximal surface of a tooth or denture.
linen s. an abrasive strip with a linen backing.
reagent s. a strip of paper impregnated with a reagent to a given substance, used in testing for that substance in a body fluid or other secretion.

stripe (strīp) a streak or stria.
Baillarger external s. stria laminae granularis internae.
Baillarger inner s., Baillarger internal s. stria laminae pyramidalis internae.
Baillarger outer s., external s. of Baillarger stria laminae granularis internae.
s. of Gennari see under *line.*
Hensen s. a band near the middle of the under surface of the membrana tectoria of the ear.
inner s. of Baillarger, internal s. of Baillarger stria laminae pyramidalis internae.
inner s. of outer zone of renal medulla stria interna zonae externae medullae renalis.
Mees s's diagonal white stripes on the fingernails in arsenic poisoning.
outer s. of Baillarger stria laminae granularis internae.
outer s. of outer zone of renal medulla stria externa zonae externae medullae renalis.
s's of Retzius incremental lines.
right paratracheal s. a thin stripe seen on an anterior radiograph of the chest, representing soft tissue between the right side of the trachea and the right upper lobe of the lung.
Vicq d'Azyr s. Kaes-Bekhterev layer.

strip·per (strip′ər) a surgical instrument for excision of veins, consisting of a flexible stainless steel cable with a stripping cup or disk at one end and a guide tip at the other; a rigid type of external stripper may also be used.

strip·ping (strip′ing) the pulling apart of two body parts that are normally adherent to each other.
Descemet s. removal of the posterior limiting lamina (Descemet membrane) along with the rest of the inner surface of the retina without removing other layers; see *Descemet stripping endothelial keratoplasty,* under *keratoplasty.*
vein s., venous s. the removal of a superficial vein or veins from a body part, usually from the lower limb in treatment of varicose veins.

stro·bi·la (stro-bi′lə) pl. *strobi′lae* [L., from Gr. *strobilos* anything twisted up] 1. the chain of proglottids constituting the bulk of the body of adult tapeworms; considered by some to include the entire body, including the head, neck, and proglottids. 2. The chain of individuals produced by strobilation, such as the series of buds produced at the oral end of the body of certain jellyfish, which during the process of formation somewhat resemble a pile of plates; each bud is released to form an immature, free-swimming jellyfish.

stro·bile (stro′bīl) strobila.

stro·bi·loid (stro′bĭ-loid) resembling a row of tapeworm segments.

stro·bi·lus (stro-bi′ləs) strobila.

stro·bo·scope (stro′bo-skōp) [Gr. *strobos* whirl + *-scope*] an instrument by which the successive phases of animal movements may be studied; motion may appear to come to rest. See also *laryngostroboscope.* **strobo·scop′ic** *adj*

stroke (strōk) 1. a sudden and severe attack; called also *ictus.* 2. stroke syndrome. 3. a pulsation.
back s. the recoil of the ventricles at the time the blood is forced into the aorta.
brainstem s. stroke syndrome affecting the brainstem, most often from ischemia in the distribution of the basilar or vertebral arteries; symptoms include partial or complete paralysis and breathing difficulties that can be fatal.
cardiogenic s. stroke syndrome resulting from heart disease when an embolus travels from the heart to the brain.
completed s. stroke syndrome reflecting the infarction of the vascular territory that is put at risk by a stenosis or occlusion of a feeding vessel.
developing s. s. in evolution.
effective s. the part of a ciliary beat in which the cilium stiffens and moves forward.
embolic s. stroke syndrome due to cerebral embolism; onset of symptoms is usually sudden, reflecting abrupt loss of blood flow to the region of the occluded artery.
s. in evolution a preliminary, unstable stage of stroke syndrome in which the blockage is present but the syndrome has not progressed to the stage of completed stroke.
heat s. a condition caused by exposure to excessive heat, natural or artificial, and marked by dry skin, vertigo, headache, thirst, nausea, and muscular cramps; body temperature may be dangerously elevated, contrasting with heat exhaustion in which the body temperature may be subnormal. Cf. *sunstroke.*
heat s., exertional heat stroke resulting from the production of heat by skeletal muscle during exercise faster than it can be dissipated by thermoregulatory mechanisms; it is usually accompanied by lactic acidosis.
ischemic s. stroke syndrome caused by ischemia of an area of the brain.
lacunar s. a lacunar infarct that causes symptoms; among the most common manifestations are pure motor hemiparesis, ataxic hemiparesis, pure sensory stroke, sensorimotor stroke, and clumsy-hand dysarthria. Called also *lacunar syndrome.*
light s. a fatal narcosis produced in sensitized mice by exposure to light.
lightning s. loss of consciousness and shock with burns, frequently fatal, caused by lightning.
middle cerebral artery s. the most common type of stroke syndrome, involving infarction or ischemia of part of the territory served by the middle cerebral artery.
paralytic s. stroke syndrome that produces paralysis.
pure sensory s. a lacunar stroke characterized by sensory loss over one side of the body without paralysis or other deficits, usually involving the face, upper limb, and lower limb.
recovery s. the part of a ciliary beat in which the cilium becomes flexible and bends, moving backward close to the cell surface.
sensorimotor s. a lacunar stroke characterized by sensory and motor deficits on one side of the body.
sun s. see *sunstroke.*
thrombotic s. stroke syndrome due to cerebral thrombosis, most often superimposed on a plaque of atherosclerosis; onset of symptoms ranges from minutes to days after the obstruction.

stro·ma (stro′mə) pl. *stro′mata* [Gr. *strōma* anything laid out for lying or sitting upon] the matrix or supporting tissue of an organ, as distinguished from its *parenchyma* or functional element. **stro′mal, stromat′ic** *adj*
s. of cornea substantia propria corneae.
s. gan′glii [TA], **s. ganglio′nicum** stroma of ganglion: the endoneurial stroma that permeates the capsule of a neural ganglion and surrounds and supports the neuronal and axonal components of the ganglion.
s. glan′dulae thyroi′deae [TA] stroma of thyroid gland: the tissue that forms the framework of the thyroid gland.
s. i′ridis [TA], **s. of iris** the soft mass of connective tissue fibers that make up the major portion of the iris.
ovarian s., s. ova′rii [TA], **s. of ovary** the fibrous tissue and smooth muscle composing the framework of the ovary.
Rollet s. the part of an erythrocyte left after removal of the hemoglobin.
s. of thyroid gland s. glandulae thyroideae.
vitreous s., s. vit′reum [TA] the framework of firmer material making up the vitreous body of the eye, and enclosing within its meshes the more fluid portion (humor vitreus).

stro·ma·tin (stro′mə-tin) a protein constituent of the stroma of erythrocytes.

stro·ma·tog·e·nous (stro″mə-toj′ə-nəs) [*stroma* + *-genous*] originating in the stroma or connective tissue of an organ.

stro·ma·tol·y·sis (stro″mə-tol′ĭ-sis) [*stroma* + *-lysis*] destruction of the stroma of a cell, especially that of a red blood cell.

stro·ma·to·sis (stro″mə-to′sis) adenomyosis in which the invading endometrial substance is stromal and not glandular; called also *stromal adenomyosis.*

Stro·mec·tol (stro-mek′tol) trademark for a preparation of ivermectin.

stro·me·lys·in (stro-mel′ĭ-sin) any of several matrix metalloproteinases that degrade proteoglycan, fibronectin, various types of collagen, and similar proteins. They are involved in breakdown of the extracellular matrix in normal physiologic processes (e.g., tissue remodeling) as well as in disease processes (e.g., metastasis). The group includes stromelysin 1 [EC 3.4.24.17], stromelysin 2 [EC 3.4.24.22], and stromelysin 3.

Stro·mey·er cephalhematocele (shtro′mi-ər) [Georg Friedrich Ludwig *Stromeyer*, German surgeon, 1804–1876] see under *cephalhematocele.*

stro·muhr (shtro′moor) [Ger. "stream clock"] an instrument for measuring the velocity of the blood flow; specifically one invented by Ludwig in 1867. It was superseded by the flowmeter. See also *thermostromuhr.*

stron·gy·li (stron′jə-li) plural of *strongylus.*

stron·gy·li·a·sis (stron″jə-li′ə-sis) strongylosis.

stron·gy·lid (stron′jə-lid) 1. of or pertaining to the superfamily Strongylidae. 2. strongylus.

Stron·gyl·i·dae (stron-jil′ĭ-de) a family of nematodes of the superfamily Strongyloidea; many are intestinal parasites in mammals. Genera of medical or veterinary interest include *Chabertia, Oesophagodontus, Oesophagostomum, Strongylus, Ternidens,* and *Triodontophorus.*

Stron·gy·loi·dea (stron″jə-loi′de-ə) a superfamily of phasmids, including the hookworms and related bursate nematodes. It comprises the families Ancylostomidae, Strongylidae, Trichostrongylidae, Metastrongylidae, and Syngamidae.

Stron·gy·loi·des (stron″jə-loi′dēz) a genus of phasmid nematodes of the family Rhabditidae, widely distributed as intestinal parasites of mammals.
S. intestina′lis *S. stercoralis.*
S. papillo′sus a species found in cows, pigs, sheep, goats, rabbits, and rats.
S. ranso′mi a species found in pigs.
S. rat′ti a species found in rats.
S. stercora′lis a species found in tropical and subtropical countries, the usual cause of strongyloidiasis. Called also *S. intestinalis.* Formerly called *Anguillula intestinalis* or *A. stercoralis.*

stron·gy·loi·di·a·sis (stron″jə-loi-di′ə-sis) infection with *Strongyloides stercoralis.* Adult female worms and larvae inhabit the mucosa and submucosa of the small intestine, and the larvae expelled in the feces develop in the soil and can penetrate skin on contact. They later are carried in the bloodstream to the lungs, and from there they travel to the intestine via the trachea and esophagus. Massive infection *(hyperinfection)* is occasionally seen in immunocompromised patients and those treated with corticosteroids or certain other agents. An endogenous cycle of development *(autoinfection)* may occur, allowing infections to persist for many years.
intestinal s. the stage of human strongyloidiasis in which the worms are in the intestines, causing ulceration and diarrhea; in some persons infection is subclinical for decades.
pulmonary s. the stage of human strongyloidiasis in which the worms are in the lungs, causing coughing, wheezing, and dyspnea; it occasionally progresses to sepsis or meningitis that can be fatal. Initial invasion from the bloodstream into the alveoli may be accompanied by hemorrhage and hemoptysis.

stron·gy·loi·do·sis (stron″jə-loi-do′sis) strongyloidiasis.

stron·gy·lo·sis (stron″jə-lo′sis) infection of a horse or other equid with worms of the genus *Strongylus.*

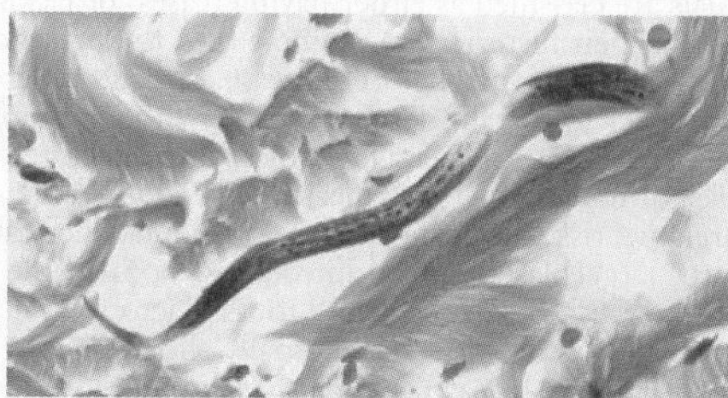

■ *Strongyloides stercoralis;* longitudinal section of larva in an intestinal biopsy section (H & E stain).

Stron·gy·lus (stron′jə-ləs) [Gr. *strongylos* round] a genus of parasitic nematodes of the family Strongylidae; several species infect horses and other equids.
S. edenta′tus a species found in horses.
S. equi′nus a species parasitic in the intestines of horses; called also *palisade worm.*
S. paradox′us *Metastrongylus elongatus.*
S. vulga′ris a species that causes verminous aneurysm in equines.

stron·gy·lus (stron′jə-ləs) pl. *stron′gyli.* An individual organism of the genus *Strongylus.*

stron·ti·um (Sr) (stron′she-əm) [*Strontian,* Scotland, where it was first found in lead mines] a dark yellowish metal; atomic number, 38; atomic weight, 87.62. See also *radiostrontium.*
s. 85 a radioactive isotope of strontium, atomic mass 85, having a half-life of 64.84 days and decaying by electron capture with emission of gamma rays (0.514 MeV); it is used in the form of the chloride or nitrate salt as a radioactive tracer in bone imaging.
s. 87m a metastable radioactive isotope of strontium, atomic mass 87, having a half-life of 2.80 hours and decaying with emission of gamma rays (0.388 MeV); it is used in the form of the chloride or nitrate salt as a radioactive tracer in bone imaging.
s. 89 a radioactive isotope of strontium, atomic mass 89, having a half-life of 50.55 days; it decays by beta emission (1.488 MeV) and is used as a radiation source in radiation therapy.
s. 90 a radioactive isotope of strontium, atomic mass 90, having a half-life of 28.5 years; it decays by emission of beta particles and forms yttrium 90 (q.v.) as a daughter product. It is used as a source of beta radiation in the treatment of a variety of benign ophthalmologic conditions.
s. chloride Sr 89 [USP] the chloride salt of strontium 89, a calcium analogue that concentrates in areas of increased osteogenesis; used as a local radiation source for palliative treatment of bone pain in patients with metastatic bone lesions; administered intravenously.
s. ranelate a salt of strontium that stimulates new bone formation and blocks breakdown of bone; used in treatment of osteoporosis in postmenopausal women. Administered orally.

stron·ti·ure·sis (stron″she-u-re′sis) the elimination of strontium from the body by way of the urine. **strontiuret′ic** *adj*

stro·phan·thin (stro-fan′thin) a glycoside or a mixture of steroidal glycosides obtained from *Strophanthus kombé;* a cardioactive poison.
G-s., s.-G ouabain.

Stro·phan·thus (stro-fan′thəs) [Gr. *strophos* a twisted band + *anthos* flower] a genus of shrubs, trees, and woody vines of the family Apocynaceae, found mostly in tropical Africa; several species are poisonous. *S. gra′tus* (Wall. & Hock.) Baill. yields ouabain; *S. his′pidus* DC. yields onaye and pseudostrophanthin; and *S. kom′bé* Oliv. yields strophanthidin and strophanthin.

Stro·pha·ri·a·ceae (strə-fa″re-a′se-e) a family of mushrooms (order Agaricales). Several genera are edible, and the genus *Psilocybe* is hallucinogenic.

stropho·so·mus (strof″o-so′məs) [Gr. *strophos* a twisted band + *sōma* body] a celosomus, especially in chicks, in which the extremities are reflexed onto the back with the distal ends resting on the head.

stroph·u·lus (strof′u-ləs) [L.] papular urticaria.

STRP short tandem repeat polymorphism; see *microsatellite polymorphism,* under *polymorphism.*

struck (struk) a usually fatal enterotoxemia of calves, lambs, and piglets, caused by *Clostridium perfringens* type C, occurring chiefly in the winter and spring and characterized by hemorrhagic enteritis and peritonitis. Called also *hemorrhagic enterotoxemia* and *Romney Marsh disease.*

struc·tu·ra (strək-too′rə) structure (def. 1).
structu′rae o′culi accesso′riae [TA] ocular adnexa.

struc·tur·al (struk′chər-əl) pertaining to or affecting the structure.

struc·ture (struk′chər) [L. *struere* to build] 1. something made up of arranged parts being held together in a given way, such as an *apparatus* or *organ.* 2. the manner of arrangement of the parts that constitute a whole.
accessory s's of eye, accessory visual s's ocular adnexa.
antigenic s. (of microorganisms), the mosaic of individual antigens present in cells of a microorganism.
β s. pleated sheet.
covalent s. primary s.
denture-supporting s's the tissues, either the teeth or residual ridges, or both, which serve as the foundation for removable partial or complete dentures.
fine s. ultrastructure.
primary s. the amino acid sequence of a polypeptide chain or the base sequence of a nucleic acid strand. Called also *covalent s.*
quaternary s. the geometric arrangement of the subunits of a macromolecule.

secondary s. aspects of the three-dimensional structure of macromolecules that have a regular geometric pattern, e.g., α helix or β sheet regions in proteins, double helix regions in nucleic acids, or the cloverleaf structure of transfer RNAs.

tertiary s. the three-dimensional structure of a monomeric macromolecule or of a subunit of a multimeric macromolecule.

stru·ma (stroo′mə) [L.] goiter.

s. aberra′ta aberrant goiter.

cast iron s. Riedel thyroiditis.

s. colloi′des colloid goiter.

s. endothora′cica intrathoracic goiter.

s. fibro′sa fibrous goiter.

s. follicula′ris parenchymatous goiter.

s. gelatino′sa colloid goiter.

Hashimoto s. see under *disease.*

ligneous s. Riedel thyroiditis.

s. lymphomato′sa Hashimoto disease.

s. nodo′sa multinodular goiter.

s. ova′rii a rare teratoid tumor of the ovary composed almost entirely of thyroid tissue, with large follicles containing abundant colloid; occasionally there are symptoms of hyperthyroidism.

s. parenchymato′sa parenchymatous goiter.

Riedel s. see under *thyroiditis.*

stru·mec·to·my (stroo-mek′tə-me) [*struma* + *-ectomy*] surgical removal of a goiter.

stru·mi·tis (stroo-mi′tis) thyroiditis.

Strüm·pell disease, sign (shtrēm′pəl) [Adolf von *Strümpell,* German physician, 1853–1925] see under *disease* and *sign.*

Strüm·pell-Leich·ten·stern encephalitis (disease) (shtrēm′pəl līk′tən-shtərn) [A. von *Strümpell;* Otto *Leichtenstern,* German physician, 1845–1900] hemorrhagic encephalitis.

Strüm·pell-Ma·rie disease (shtrēm′pəl mah-re′) [A. von *Strümpell;* Pierre *Marie,* French physician, 1853–1940] rheumatoid spondylitis.

Strüm·pell-West·phal pseudosclerosis (shtrēm′pəl vest′fahl) [A. von *Strümpell;* Carl Friedrich Otto *Westphal,* German neurologist, 1833–1890] Wilson disease; see under *disease.*

Strun·sky sign (strun′ske) [Max *Strunsky,* American orthopedic surgeon, 1873–1957] see under *sign.*

Struth·ers ligament (struth′ərz) [Sir John *Struthers,* Scottish anatomist, 1823–1899] see under *ligament.*

stru·vite (stroo′vīt) [Baron Heinrich Christian Gottfried von *Struve,* German-born Russian diplomat, 1772–1851] a hard crystalline mineral formed by interaction of magnesium salts with ammonium phosphate, closely allied to and often associated with triple phosphate. It is the main component of struvite calculi. Called also *magnesium ammonium phosphate.*

strych·nine (strik′nīn) a poisonous alkaloid obtained chiefly from *Strychnos nux-vomica* and other species of *Strychnos;* it is a central nervous stimulant that can cause fatal convulsions and respiratory arrest. See also *strychnine poisoning* and *strychninism.*

strych·nin·ism (strik′nin-iz-əm) chronic strychnine poisoning; symptoms include increased acuity of hearing, vision, touch, taste, and smell, followed by tonic convulsions and vomiting; in severe cases, it may culminate in respiratory paralysis and death.

strych·nino·ma·nia (strik″nin-o-ma′ne-ə) [*strychnine* + *-mania*] mental aberration due to strychnine poisoning.

strych·nism (strik′niz-əm) strychnine poisoning.

Strych·nos (strik′nos) [Gr. "nightshade"] a genus of tropical trees of the family Loganiaceae whose seeds contain strychnine and other toxic alkaloids. *S. nux-vo′mica* L. has seeds called *nux vomica. S. igna′tii* has seeds called *St. Ignatius beans.* See *strychnine poisoning,* under *poisoning.*

Stry·ker frame (stri′kər) [Homer H. *Stryker,* American orthopedic surgeon, 1894–1980] see under *frame.*

STS serologic test for syphilis; Society of Thoracic Surgeons.

Stu·dent *t*-test (stoo′dənt) ["*Student,*" pseudonym of William Sealy Gossett, British mathematician, 1876–1937] see *t-test,* under *test.*

Stu·der neobladder (shtoo′dər) [Urs E. *Studer,* Swiss urologist, late 20th century] see under *neobladder.*

study (stud′e) 1. an examination or procedure. 2. a research project; see also *examination, test,* and *trial.*

barium s. a radiographic examination of the gastrointestinal tract using barium as a contrast agent; cf. *barium enema, mucosal relief radiography,* and *upper gastrointestinal series.*

blind s. a clinical trial or other study in which participants are blinded; see *blind* (def. 2).

cardiac electrophysiologic s. see *cardiac electrophysiology* under *electrophysiology.*

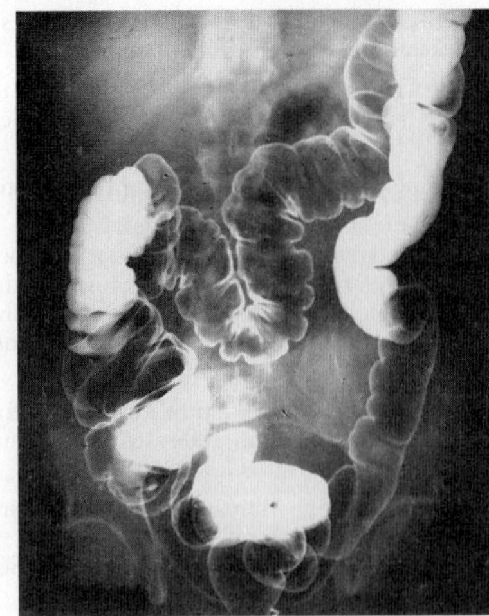

■ Barium study of the large intestine, using a double-contrast barium enema.

case s. a study that identifies and samples individuals with a particular disease or condition, noting characteristics of the disease or condition and persons afflicted. Case studies are often used to call attention to new diseases or to diseases entering new populations.

case-cohort s. an epidemiologic study in which samples of cases and surviving noncases of the condition being studied are drawn from the same cohort of a cohort study. The cases and noncases are matched for duration of survival and their histories are compared.

case-control s. retrospective s.

cohort s. prospective s.

cross-sectional s. a study that employs a single point of data collection for each participant or system being studied; used for examining phenomena expected to be static though the period of interest. Cf. *longitudinal s.*

ecological s. a statistical study exploring hypotheses by comparing groups, rather than individuals, e.g., comparing rates of breast cancer and levels of fat intake by country.

longitudinal s. a study in which participants, processes, or systems are studied over time, with data being collected at multiple intervals. The two main types are *prospective s.* and *retrospective s.* Cf. *cross-sectional s.*

nerve conduction s's electroneurography.

nested case-control s. a case-control study nested within a cohort study: a population is identified and baseline data obtained and stored; after following the cohort for some time, a case-control study is performed using the small percentage of people who develop the disease, with controls selected as a sample of those surviving members without disease who were at risk at the time of occurrence of each case. Baseline data can be analyzed solely for this small subset of the original population, and recall bias and other hazards of case-control studies are avoided.

prospective s. a longitudinal epidemiologic study in which the groups of individuals (cohorts) are selected on the basis of factors that are to be examined for their effects on outcomes, e.g., the effect of exposure to a specific risk factor on the eventual development of a particular disease, and are then followed over a period of time to determine the incidence rates of the outcomes in question in relation to the original factors. Called also *cohort s.* "Prospective" usually implies a cohort selected in the present and followed into the future, but the cohort method can also be applied to existing longitudinal historical data, such as insurance or medical records: a cohort is identified and classified as to exposure to some factor at some date in the past and followed up to the present to determine incidence rates of the outcome. This is called a historical prospective study, prospective study of past data, or retrospective cohort study. Cf. *retrospective s.*

repetitive stimulation s. repetitive nerve stimulation.

retrospective s. a longitudinal epidemiologic study in which participating individuals are classified as either having (cases) or lacking (controls) some outcome and their histories are examined for the presence of specific factors possibly associated with that outcome. Cases and controls are often matched with respect to certain demographic or other variables but need not be. As compared with prospective studies, retrospective studies suffer from drawbacks: although they can measure the odds ratio, which often approximates relative risk, they cannot reveal true incidence rates or attributable risk. Also, large biases can be introduced both in the selection of controls and in the recall of past exposure to risk factors. The advantage of the retrospective study is its small scale, usually short time for completion, and its applicability to rare diseases, which would require study of very large cohorts in prospective studies. See also *prospective s.*

stump (stump) the distal end of the limb left after amputation.

conical s. a cone-shaped amputation stump produced as a result of undue retraction of the muscles.

stun (stun) to knock senseless; to render unconscious by a blow or other force.

stun•ning (stun′ing) loss of function, analogous to unconsciousness.
myocardial s. temporarily impaired myocardial function, resulting from a brief episode of ischemia, that persists for some period after reperfusion. Cf. *myocardial hibernation.*

stunt (stunt) to retard the growth of.

stupe (sto͞op) [L. *stupa* oakum] a cloth, sponge, or the like, for external application, charged with hot water, wrung out nearly dry, and then made irritant or otherwise medicated.

stu•pe•fa•cient (stoo″pə-fa′shənt) [L. *stupefacere* to make senseless] 1. inducing stupor. 2. an agent that induces stupor.

stu•pe•fac•tive (stoo″pə-fak′tiv) stupefacient (def. 1).

stu•por (stoo′pər) [L.] 1. a lowered level of consciousness manifested by the subject's responding only to vigorous stimulation. See also *consciousness* 2. in psychiatry, a disorder marked by greatly reduced responsiveness, inattentiveness to the environment, and inaction. **stu′porous** *adj*
benign s. a condition of inattentiveness, inaction, and unresponsiveness from which recovery is likely; the term is often used to denote such symptoms occurring in the depressive phase of bipolar disorder, although it is now recognized that this condition has a poor prognosis and is more correctly termed a malignant stupor.
catatonic s. the extreme decrease in reactivity to the environment and in spontaneous activity characteristic of catatonic schizophrenia.
epileptic s. stupor following an epileptic convulsion; called also *postconvulsive s.*
malignant s. a condition of inattentiveness, inaction, and unresponsiveness from which recovery is unlikely; see also *benign s.*
postconvulsive s. epileptic s.

stupp (stup) a poisonous kind of soot which accumulates in the condensers of mercury smelters; it contains metallic mercury in a finely divided condition.

stur•dy (stur′de) gid.

Sturge syndrome (sturj) [William Allen *Sturge*, British physician, 1850–1919] Sturge-Weber syndrome.

Sturge-Kal•is•cher-Web•er syndrome (sturj′ kah′lish-ər va′bər) [W.A. *Sturge;* Siegfried *Kalischer*, German physician, late 19th century; Frederick Parkes *Weber*, British physician, 1863–1962] Sturge-Weber syndrome.

Sturge-Web•er syndrome (sturj′ va′bər) [W.A. *Sturge;* F.P. *Weber*] see under *syndrome.*

Sturm conoid, interval (shtoorm) [Johann Christoph *Sturm*, German mathematician and physician, 1635–1703] see under *conoid*, and see *focal interval*, under *interval.*

stut•ter•ing (stut′ər-ing) 1. a speech disorder involving three factors: (1) dysfluency with repetition of words and parts of words, prolongations of sounds, interjections of sounds or words, and long pauses; (2) listener reaction, considering the dysfluency to be abnormal or unacceptable; and (3) the speaker's reaction to the dysfluency and to the listener's reaction, with a self-conception as a stutterer. See also *stammering.* 2. something resembling this speech pattern.
urinary s. stuttering urination.

sty (sti) pl. *sties.* Hordeolum.

sty•co•sis (sti-ko′sis) the presence of calcium sulfate in the organs of the body, especially in the lymph nodes.

stye (sti) [L. *hordeolum*] hordeolum.
meibomian s. a stye involving a meibomian gland, usually draining through the conjunctival surface of the lid.
zeisian s. a stye involving a gland of Zeis, occurring on the surface of the skin at the edge of the lid.

style (stīl) 1. the way in which something is done or said. 2. stylet.
coping s. defense mechanism.

sty•let (sti′lət) [L. *stilus;* Gr. *stylos* pillar] 1. a wire run through a catheter or cannula to render it stiff or to remove debris from its lumen. 2. a slender probe.

sty•li•form (sti′lĭ-form) [*stilo-* + *form*] long and pointed; styloid.

sty•lis•cus (sti-lis′kəs) [L., from Gr. *styliskos* rod] a slender cylindrical tent.

styl(o)- [L. *stilus* a stake, pole] a combining form denoting resemblance to a stake or pole, used especially to denote relationship to the styloid process of the temporal bone.

sty•lo•hy•al (sti″lo-hi′əl) stylohyoid.

sty•lo•hy•oid (sti″lo-hi′oid) pertaining to the styloid process of the temporal bone and to the hyoid bone.

sty•loid (sti′loid) [*styl-* + *-oid*] resembling a pillar; long and pointed; styliform.

sty•loid•itis (sti″loi-di′tis) inflammation of tissues around the styloid process of the temporal bone.

sty•lo•man•dib•u•lar (sti″lo-man-dib′u-lər) pertaining to the styloid process of the temporal bone and the mandible.

sty•lo•mas•toid (sti″lo-mas′toid) pertaining to the styloid process of the temporal bone and the mastoid process.

sty•lo•max•il•lary (sti″lo-mak′sĭ-lar″e) pertaining to the styloid process of the temporal bone and to the maxilla.

Sty•lom•ma•to•pho•ra (sti-lom″ə-tof′ə-rə) a suborder of the order Pulmonata, including land snails and slugs. Families of medical importance include Helicellidae, Helicidae, and Pupillidae.

sty•lo•my•loid (sti″lo-mi′loid) [*stylo-* + Gr. *mylē* mill + *-oid*] pertaining to the styloid process of the temporal bone and to the region of the lower molar teeth.

sty•lo•po•di•um (sti″lo-po′de-əm) the second part of a fetal limb; see *limb.*

sty•lo•staph•y•line (sti″lo-staf′ə-līn) pertaining to the styloid process of the temporal bone and the velum palatinum.

sty•los•teo•phyte (sti-los′te-o-fīt) a pillar-shaped exostosis.

sty•lus (sti′ləs) [L. *stilus*] 1. a stylet. 2. a pencil-shaped medicinal preparation, as a stick of caustic.

styp•sis (stip′sis) [Gr. "contraction"] the action or application of a styptic.

styp•tic (stip′tik) [Gr. *styptikos*] 1. contracting the tissues or blood vessels; used particularly to denote that arresting hemorrhage or resulting in hemostasis. 2. an agent that contracts the tissues of blood vessels.
chemical s. a styptic that arrests hemorrhage by causing coagulation through chemical action.
mechanical s. a styptic that acts by causing coagulation mechanically, as a pledget of cotton.
vascular s. a styptic that acts by producing contraction of injured or divided blood vessels of small caliber.

Styp•ven (stip′vən) trademark for a preparation of Russell's viper venom; used as a hemostatic agent. See also under *test.*

Sty•rax (sti′raks) a genus of shrubs and trees of the family Styracaceae, most of which are native to Indonesia, Malaysia, or Thailand; *S. ben′zoin* and other species are sources of the resin benzoin.

sty•rax (sti′raks) storax.

sty•rene (sti′rēn) an unsaturated oily liquid hydrocarbon used in the manufacture of plastic, synthetic rubber, resins, as a dental filling component, and in drug manufacturing; it polymerizes spontaneously to form polystyrene. It is an irritant, toxic, possibly carcinogenic, and releases carbon monoxide on burning. Called also *cinnamene, cinnamol, styrol, styrolene,* and *vinyl benzene.*

sty•rol (sti′rol) styrene.

sty•ro•lene (sti′ro-lēn) styrene.

su. [L.] su′mat (let him take).

sub- [L. *sub* under] 1. a prefix meaning under, near, almost, partial, moderately, or subordinate. 2. in chemistry, a prefix denoting a basic compound or a compound containing less of an element or radical than another compound of the same elements.

sub•ab•dom•i•nal (sub″ab-dŏm′ĭ-nəl) inferior to the abdomen.

sub•ab•dom•i•no•peri•to•ne•al (sub″ab-dom″ĭ-no-per″ĭ-to-ne′əl) subperitoneal.

sub•ac•e•tab•u•lar (sub″as-ə-tab′u-lər) inferior to the acetabulum.

sub•ac•e•tate (səb-as′ə-tāt) any basic acetate.

sub•ac•id (səb-as′id) somewhat acid.

sub•a•cid•i•ty (sub″ə-sid′ĭ-te) deficient acidity.

sub•acro•mi•al (sub″ə-kro′me-əl) inferior to the acromion.

sub•acute (sub″ə-kūt′) somewhat acute; between acute and chronic.

sub•al•i•men•ta•tion (sub″al-ĭ-mən-ta′shən) hypoalimentation.

sub•anal (səb-a′nəl) inferior to the anus.

sub•aor•tic (sub″a-or′tik) below the aorta or the aortic valve.

sub•ap•i•cal (səb-ap′ĭ-kəl) inferior to an apex.

sub•apo•neu•rot•ic (sub″ap-o-no͞o-rot′ik) beneath an aponeurosis.

sub•arach•noid (sub″ə-rak′noid) between the arachnoid and the pia mater.

sub·ar·cu·ate (səb-ahr′ku-āt) [*sub-* + *arcuate*] somewhat arched or bent.

sub·are·o·lar (sub″ə-re′ə-lər) beneath an areola, particularly the areola of the breast.

sub·as·trag·a·lar (sub″əs-trag′ə-lər) subtalar.

sub·astrin·gent (sub″ə-strin′jənt) moderately astringent.

sub·at·loi·de·an (sub″at-loi′de-ən) inferior to the atlas.

sub·atom·ic (sub″ə-tom′ik) 1. smaller than an atom or occurring within an atom. 2. of or pertaining to the constituent parts of an atom as considered under the theory of the nuclear atom.

sub·au·ral (səb-aw′rəl) inferior to the ear.

sub·au·ra·le (sub″aw-ra′le) an anthropometric landmark, the lowest point on the inferior border of the ear lobule when the subject is looking straight ahead.

sub·au·ric·u·lar (sub″aw-rik′u-lər) inferior to the auricle of the ear.

sub·ax·i·al (səb-ak′se-əl) inferior to an axis.

sub·ax·il·lary (səb-ak′sĭ-lar″e) inferior to the axilla.

sub·ba·sal (səb-ba′səl) inferior to a base.

sub·bra·chi·al (səb-bra′ke-əl) pertaining to the brachium of the inferior (or caudal) colliculus.

sub·bra·chy·ce·phal·ic (sub″bra-ke-sə-fal′ik) somewhat brachycephalic; having a cephalic index of 78 to 79.

sub·cal·ca·re·ous (sub″kal-kar′e-əs) slightly calcareous.

sub·cal·car·ine (səb-kal′kər-īn) inferior to the calcarine fissure.

sub·cal·lo·sal (sub″kə-lo′səl) inferior to the corpus callosum.

sub·cap·su·lar (səb-kap′su-lər) beneath a capsule.

sub·cap·su·lo·peri·os·te·al (səb-kap″su-lo-per″e-os′te-əl) beneath the capsule and the periosteum of a joint.

sub·car·bo·nate (səb-kahr′bo-nāt) any basic carbonate.

sub·ca·ri·nal (sub″kə-ri′nəl) below the carina tracheae.

sub·car·ti·lag·i·nous (sub″kahr-tĭ-laj′ĭ-nəs) 1. beneath a cartilage. 2. partly cartilaginous.

sub·cep·tion (səb-sep′shən) perception below the level of awareness.

sub·chlo·ride (səb-klor′īd) that chloride of any series which contains the smallest proportion of chlorine.

sub·chon·dral (səb-kon′drəl) subcartilaginous (def. 1).

sub·chor·dal (səb-kor′dəl) 1. below the vocal folds (cords). 2. hypochordal.

sub·cho·ri·al (səb-kor′e-əl) beneath the chorion or some part of the chorion.

sub·cho·ri·on·ic (sub″kor-e-on′ik) beneath the chorion.

sub·cho·roi·dal (sub″ko-roi′dəl) beneath the choroid.

sub·chron·ic (səb-kron′ik) between chronic and subacute.

sub·class (sub′klas″) a taxonomic category sometimes established, subordinate to a class and superior to an order.

sub·cla·vi·an (səb-kla′ve-ən) inferior to the clavicle, such as the subclavian artery. Called also *infraclavicular* and *subclavicular*.

sub·cla·vic·u·lar (sub″klə-vik′u-lər) subclavian.

sub·clin·i·cal (səb-klin′ĭ-kəl) without clinical manifestations; said of the early stage(s) of an infection or other disease or abnormality before symptoms and signs become apparent or detectable by clinical examination or laboratory tests, or of a very mild form of an infection or other disease or abnormality. See also under *infection*.

sub·clone (sub′klōn) 1. the progeny of a mutant cell arising in a clone. 2. each new DNA population produced by cleaving DNA from a clonal population into fragments and cloning each fragment.

sub·com·mis·su·ral (səb-kə-mish′o͝o-rəl) beneath a commissure.

sub·con·junc·ti·val (sub″kən-junk′tĭ-vəl) beneath the conjunctiva.

sub·con·scious (səb-kon′shəs) 1. imperfectly or partially conscious. 2. a lay term used to include the preconscious and unconscious.

sub·con·scious·ness (səb-kon′shəs-nis) the state of being partially conscious.

sub·cor·a·coid (səb-kor′ə-koid) inferior to the coracoid process.

sub·cor·ne·al (səb-kor′ne-əl) 1. beneath the cornea. 2. beneath the stratum corneum of the skin.

sub·cor·tex (səb-kor′təks) the part of the brain substance underlying the cerebral cortex.

sub·cor·ti·cal (səb-kor′tĭ-kəl) beneath a cortex, such as the cerebral cortex.

sub·cos·tal (səb-kos′təl) inferior to or beneath a rib or all the ribs; called also *infracostal*.

sub·cos·ta·lis (sub″kos-ta′lis) pl. *subcosta′les* [L.] subcostal.

sub·cra·ni·al (səb-kra′ne-əl) beneath the cranium.

sub·crep·i·tant (səb-krep′ĭ-tənt) pertaining to a rale that is slightly more coarse than a crepitant rale; see under *rale*.

sub·crep·i·ta·tion (sub″krep-ĭ-ta′shən) the sound of a subcrepitant rale.

sub·cul·ture (sub′kul″chər) 1. a culture of bacteria derived from another culture. 2. the act of preparing a fresh culture from an existing one.

sub·cu·ta·ne·ous (SC, SQ) (sub″ku-ta′ne-əs) beneath the skin; called also *hypodermic*.

sub·cu·tic·u·lar (sub″ku-tik′u-lər) subepidermal.

sub·cu·tis (səb-ku′tis) tela subcutanea.

sub·de·lir·i·um (sub″də-lēr′e-əm) partial or mild delirium.

sub·del·toid (səb-del′toid) beneath the deltoid muscle.

sub·den·tal (səb-den′təl) [*sub-* + *dental*] beneath a tooth or teeth.

sub·di·a·phrag·mat·ic (sub″di-ə-frag-mat′ik) subphrenic.

sub·di·vi·sion (sub′dĭ-vĭ″zhən) in the classification of plants and fungi, a taxonomic category inferior to a division but superior to a class; equivalent to the subphylum of animal taxonomy.

sub·duct (səb-dukt′) [L. *subducere* to lead down] to depress or draw down; see *subduction*.

sub·duc·tion (səb-duk′shən) infraduction.

sub·du·ral (səb-doo′rəl) between the dura mater and the arachnoid.

sub·en·do·car·di·al (sub″en-do-kahr′de-əl) beneath the endocardium.

sub·en·do·car·di·um (sub″en-do-kahr′de-əm) subendocardial layer.

sub·en·do·the·li·al (sub″en-do-the′le-əl) beneath an endothelium.

sub·en·do·the·li·um (sub″en-do-the′le-əm) Debove membrane.

sub·ep·en·dy·mal (sub″ep-en′dĭ-məl) beneath the ependyma.

sub·ep·en·dy·mo·ma (sub″ep-en″dĭ-mo′mə) an ependymoma in which there is a diffuse proliferation of subependymal fibrillary astrocytes among the ependymal tumor cells. A few are malignant and others cause obstructive hydrocephalus, but many are clinically silent and are discovered only at autopsy.

sub·epi·car·di·al (sub″ep-ĭ-kahr′de-əl) below the epicardium.

sub·epi·car·di·um (sub″ep-ĭ-kahr′de-əm) subepicardial layer.

sub·epi·der·mal (sub″ep-ĭ-dur′məl) beneath the epidermis; called also *subcuticular*.

sub·epi·der·mic (sub″ep-ĭ-der′mik) subepidermal.

sub·epi·glot·tic (sub″ep-ĭ-glot′ik) inferior to the epiglottis.

sub·epi·the·li·al (sub″ep-ĭ-the′le-əl) beneath an epithelium.

su·ber·i·tin (soo-ber′ĭ-tin) [*Suberites*, a marine sponge (from L. *suber* cork) + chemical suffix *-in*] a toxic substance derived from the marine sponge, *Suberites domunculus*, which, when injected into dogs, produces intestinal hemorrhages and respiratory distress.

su·ber·o·sis (soo″bə-ro′sis) [L. *suber* cork + *-osis*] a type of hypersensitivity pneumonitis seen in those who work with cork, caused by inhalation

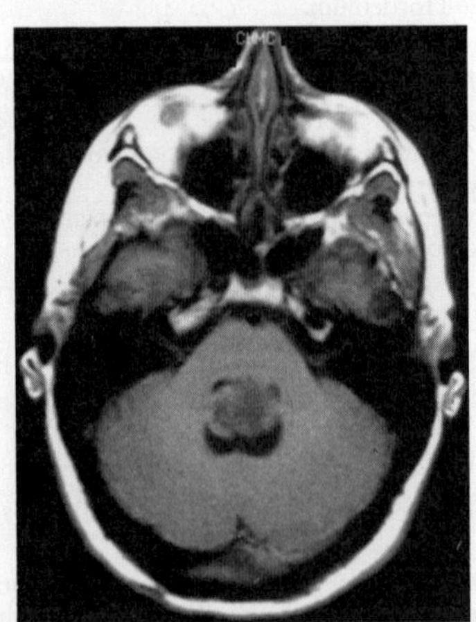

■ Subependymoma in fourth ventricle; appearing as a hypointense lesion in an axial T1-weighted MRI scan.

of moldy cork dust containing spores of various species of *Penicillium;* called also *cork handler's disease.*

sub·fam·i·ly (sub′fam″ĭ-le) a taxonomic category sometimes established, subordinate to a family and superior to a tribe or genus.

sub·fas·cial (səb-fash′əl) beneath a fascia.

sub·fer·tile (səb-fur′til) characterized by less than normal fertility; called also *hypofertile.*

sub·fer·til·i·ty (sub″fər-til′ĭ-te) the state of being less than normally fertile; relative sterility. Called also *hypofertility.*

Sub fin. coct. [L.] sub fi′nem coctio′nis (toward the end of boiling).

sub·fo·li·um (səb-fo′le-əm) [*sub-* + *folium*] any of the elementary divisions of the cerebellar folia.

sub·for·ni·cal (səb-for′nĭ-kəl) beneath a fornix.

sub·fron·tal (səb-frun′təl) inferior to or extending beneath the frontal lobe.

sub·ga·le·al (səb-ga′le-əl) beneath the galea aponeurotica.

sub·gem·mal (səb-jem′əl) [*sub-* + *gemma*] beneath a bud, such as a taste bud.

sub·ge·nus (sub′je″nəs) a taxonomic category between a genus and a species.

sub·ger·mi·nal (səb-jur′mĭ-nəl) below or under the germ or primordium.

sub·gin·gi·val (səb-jin′jĭ-vəl) beneath the gingiva.

sub·gle·noid (səb-gle′noid) inferior to the glenoid cavity of the scapula. Called also *infraglenoid.*

sub·glos·sal (səb-glos′əl) sublingual.

sub·glos·si·tis (sub″glos-i′tis) [*sub-* + *gloss-* + *-itis*] inflammation of the lower surface of the tongue.

sub·glot·tic (səb-glot′ik) inferior to the glottis; called also *infraglottic.*

sub·glot·tis (səb-glot′is) cavitas infraglottica.

sub·gran·u·lar (səb-gran′u-lər) somewhat granular.

sub·gron·da·tion (sub″gron-da′shən) [Fr.] a type of depressed skull fracture, with depression of one fragment of bone beneath another.

sub·gy·rus (səb-ji′rəs) any gyrus that is partly concealed or covered by another or by others.

sub·he·pat·ic (sub″hə-pat′ik) inferior to the liver.

sub·hu·mer·al (səb-hu′mər-əl) inferior to or beneath the humerus.

sub·hy·a·loid (səb-hi′ə-loid) beneath the hyaloid membrane.

sub·hy·oid (səb-hi′oid) inferior to the hyoid bone; called also *infrahyoid.*

sub·hy·oi·de·an (sub″hi-oi′de-ən) subhyoid.

sub·ic·ter·ic (sub″ik-ter′ik) somewhat jaundiced.

su·bic·u·lum (sə-bik′u-ləm) [L., from *subicere* to raise, lift] [TA] an underlying or supporting structure. **subic′ular** *adj*

s. cor′nu ammo′nis, s. hippocam′pi gyrus parahippocampalis.

s. promonto′rii tym′pani [TA] subiculum of promontory of tympanic cavity: a ridge of bone bounding the tympanic sinus inferiorly.

sub·il·i·ac (səb-il′e-ak) inferior to the ilium.

sub·il·i·um (səb-il′e-əm) the most inferior portion of the ilium.

sub·in·flam·ma·tion (sub″in-flə-ma′shən) a slight or mild inflammation.

sub·in·flam·ma·to·ry (sub″in-flam′ə-tor″e) pertaining to or causing only mild inflammation.

sub·in·ti·mal (səb-in′tĭ-məl) beneath the intima of a vessel.

sub·in·trance (səb-in′trans) recurrence of a paroxysm after a shorter period than usual.

sub·in·trant (səb-in′trənt) [L. *subintrans* entering by stealth] 1. beginning before the completion of a previous cycle or paroxysm; anticipating. 2. characterized by recurrence at lessening intervals.

sub·in·vo·lu·tion (sub″in-vo-loo′shən) incomplete involution; failure of a part to return to its normal size and condition after enlargement due to functional activity, such as with a uterus after delivery of the baby.

chronic s. of uterus a diffuse, symmetrical uterine enlargement commonly associated with painless menorrhagia and occurring soon after pregnancy.

sub·io·dide (səb-i′o-dīd) that iodide of any series which contains the smallest proportion of iodine.

sub·ja·cent (səb-ja′sənt) [*sub-* + L. *jacere* to lie] lying just beneath or underneath.

sub·ject[1] (səb-jekt′) [L. *subjectare* to throw under] to cause to undergo, or submit to; to render subservient.

sub·ject[2] (sub′jəkt) [L. *subjectus* cast under] a person or animal which has been the object of treatment, observation, or experiment.

sub·jec·tive (səb-jek′tiv) [L. *subjectivus*] pertaining to or perceived only by the affected individual; not perceptible to the senses of another person.

sub·jec·to·scope (səb-jek′to-skōp) [*subjective* + *-scope*] an instrument used in the study of subjective visual sensations.

sub·ju·gal (səb-joo′gəl) subzygomatic.

sub·la·tion (səb-la′shən) [L. *sublatio*] a lifting up, or elevation.

sub·le·sion·al (səb-le′zhən-əl) performed or occurring beneath a lesion.

sub·le·thal (səb-le′thəl) not quite fatal; insufficient to cause death.

sub·li·mate (sub′lĭ-māt) [L. *sublimare* to elevate] 1. a substance obtained or prepared by sublimation. 2. to divert consciously unacceptable instinctual drives into personally and socially acceptable channels through a mechanism operating outside of and beyond conscious awareness.

corrosive s. mercury bichloride.

sub·li·ma·tion (sub″lĭ-ma′shən) 1. the direct change of state from solid to vapor. 2. a type of defense mechanism in which consciously unacceptable instinctual drives are diverted into personally and socially acceptable channels.

Sub·li·maze (sub′lĭ-māz) trademark for a preparation of fentanyl citrate.

sub·lime (səb-līm′) [L. *sublimare* to elevate] to volatilize a solid body by heat and then to collect it in a purified form as a solid or powder.

sub·lim·i·nal (səb-lim′ĭ-nəl) [*sub-* + *liminal*] below the limen, or threshold, of sensation.

sub·li·mis (səb-li′mis) [L.] superficial.

sub·lin·gual (səb-ling′gwəl) beneath the tongue; called also *hypoglossal* and *subglossal.*

sub·lin·gui·tis (sub″ling-gwi′tis) inflammation of the sublingual gland.

sub·lobe (sub′lōb) a division of a lobe; see *lobule.*

sub·lob·u·lar (səb-lob′u-lər) beneath a lobule.

sub·lux·ate (səb-luk′sāt) to partially dislocate.

sub·lux·a·tion (sub″lək-sa′shən) [*sub-* + *luxation*] 1. an incomplete or partial dislocation. See illustration. 2. in chiropractic, any mechanical impediment to nerve function; originally, a vertebral displacement believed to impair nerve function. See also *vertebral subluxation complex*, under *complex.*

atlantoaxial s. a complication of rheumatoid arthritis of the cervical spine; degeneration of the atlas and axis causes malalignment and cervical myelopathy.

s. of lens partial dislocation of lens of the eye.

Volkmann s. a type of tuberculous arthritis marked by flexion contracture of the knee, external rotation of the leg, valgus position of the knee, and bending of the upper third of the tibia.

sub·lym·phe·mia (sub″lim-fe′me-ə) lymphocytopenia.

sub·mam·ma·ry (səb-mam′ə-re) located or occurring inferior to or deep to a mammary gland. Called also *inframammary.*

sub·man·dib·u·lar (sub″man-dib′u-lər) inferior to the mandible.

sub·mar·gi·nal (səb-mahr′jĭ-nəl) inferior to a margin or border.

sub·max·il·la (sub″mak-sil′ə) [*sub-* + *maxilla*] mandible.

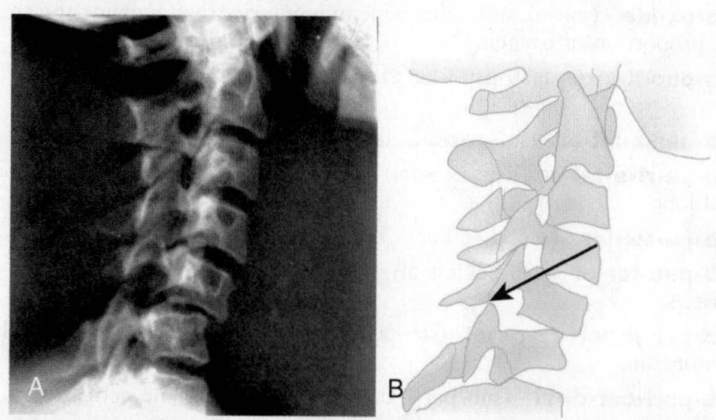

■ Severe subluxation of cervical vertebra C5 on C6, with bilateral "perched" facets, in a lateral radiograph *(A)*. The diagram *(B)* delineates the perching of the facets of C5 and C6 *(arrow)*.

sub·max·il·lar·itis (səb-mak″sĭ-lər-i′tis) inflammation of the submaxillary gland.

sub·max·il·lary (səb-mak′sĭ-lar″e) inferior to or beneath the maxilla; called also *inframaxillary.*

sub·me·di·al (səb-me′de-əl) submedian.

sub·me·di·an (səb-me′de-ən) beneath or near the middle; called also *submedial.*

sub·mem·bra·nous (səb-mem′brə-nəs) partly membranous.

sub·men·tal (səb-men′təl) [*sub-* + *mental*[2]] inferior to the chin.

sub·men·to·ver·tex (səb-ment″to-vur′teks) proceeding from underneath the chin toward the vertex of the head.

sub·mer·sion (səb-mur′zhən) [*sub-* + L. *mergere* to dip] the act of placing or the condition of being under the surface of a liquid.

sub·meta·cen·tric (sub″met-ə-sen′trik) having the centromere near, but not at, the center of the chromosome, so that one arm is shorter than the other. Cf. *acrocentric* and *metacentric.*

sub·mi·cro·scop·ic (sub″mi-kro-skop′ik) too small to be visible under the light microscope.

sub·mi·cro·scop·i·cal (sub″mi-kro-skop′ĭ-kəl) submicroscopic.

sub·mor·phous (səb-mor′fəs) neither amorphous nor perfectly crystalline.

sub·mu·co·sa (sub″mu-ko′sə) tela submucosa.
- **s. of bladder** tela submucosa vesicae urinariae.
- **s. of bronchus** tela submucosa bronchi.
- **s. of esophagus** tela submucosa oesophagi.
- **s. of large intestine** tela submucosa intestini crassi.
- **s. of pharynx** tela submucosa pharyngis.
- **s. of small intestine** tela submucosa intestini tenuis.
- **s. of stomach** tela submucosa gastrica.

sub·mu·co·sal (sub″mu-ko′səl) 1. pertaining to the submucosa. 2. beneath a mucous membrane.

sub·mu·cous (səb-mu′kəs) submucosal.

sub·nar·cot·ic (sub″nahr-kot′ik) moderately narcotic.

sub·na·sal (səb-na′zəl) inferior to the nose.

sub·na·sa·le (sub″na-sa′le) an anthropometric landmark situated at the point at which the nasal septum merges with the upper lip in the median plane. Called also *subnasion.*

sub·na·sion (səb-na′ze-on) subnasale.

sub·na·tant (səb-na′tənt) 1. situated below or at the bottom of something. 2. the liquid phase situated below another liquid or a solid phase, having a greater density than the upper layer.

sub·neu·ral (səb-noor′əl) beneath a nerve, such as the subneural clefts.

sub·ni·trate (səb-ni′trāt) a basic nitrate.

sub·nor·mal (səb-nor′məl) below or less than normal; characterized by qualities, such as intelligence, lower than the level usually observed.

sub·nor·mal·i·ty (sub″nor-mal′ĭ-te) the state of being subnormal.

sub·no·to·chor·dal (sub″no-to-kor′dəl) hypochordal.

sub·nu·cle·us (səb-noo′kle-əs) a partial or secondary nucleus into which a large nucleus of the central nervous system may be split up.

sub·nu·tri·tion (sub″noo-trĭ′shən) malnutrition.

sub·oc·cip·i·tal (sub″ok-sip′ĭ-təl) inferior to the occiput.

sub·or·bi·tal (səb-or′bĭ-təl) infraorbital.

sub·or·der (sub′or″dər) a taxonomic category sometimes established, subordinate to an order and superior to a family.

sub·ox·ide (səb-ok′sīd) the oxide in any series that contains the smallest proportion of oxygen.

sub·pap·il·lary (səb-pap′ĭ-lar-e) beneath the stratum papillare of the skin.

sub·par·a·lyt·ic (sub″par-ə-lit′ik) partially paralytic.

sub·pa·ri·e·tal (sub″pə-ri′ə-təl) inferior to the parietal bone or parietal lobe.

sub·pa·tel·lar (sub″pə-tel′ər) infrapatellar.

sub·pec·tor·al (səb-pek′tər-əl) inferior to the pectoral region or muscles.

sub·pel·vi·peri·to·ne·al (səb-pel″vĭ-per″ĭ-to-ne′əl) beneath the pelvic peritoneum.

sub·peri·car·di·al (sub″per-ĭ-kahr′de-əl) beneath the pericardium.

sub·peri·chon·dri·al (sub″per-ĭ-kon′dre-əl) beneath the perichondrium.

sub·peri·os·te·al (sub″per-e-os′te-əl) beneath the periosteum.

sub·peri·os·teo·cap·su·lar (sub″pər-e-os″te-o-kap′su-lər) subcapsuloperiosteal.

sub·peri·to·ne·al (sub″per-ĭ-to-ne′əl) beneath or deep to the peritoneum, such as a subperitoneal abscess.

sub·peri·to·neo·ab·dom·i·nal (sub″per-ĭ-to-ne″o-əb-dom′ĭ-nəl) subperitoneal.

sub·peri·to·neo·pel·vic (sub″pər-ĭ-to-ne″o-pel′vik) subpelviperitoneal.

sub·pha·ryn·ge·al (sub″fə-rin′je-əl) inferior to the pharynx.

sub·phren·ic (səb-fren′ik) inferior to the diaphragm; called also *hypophrenic, hypodiaphragmatic,* and *subdiaphragmatic.*

sub·phy·lum (səb-fi′ləm) pl. *subphy′la.* A taxonomic category sometimes established, subordinate to a phylum and superior to a class.

sub·pi·al (səb-pi′əl) beneath the pia mater.

sub·pla·cen·ta (sub″plə-sen′tə) decidua basalis.

sub·plas·ma·lem·mal (sub″plaz-mə-lem′əl) beneath the plasma membrane (plasmalemma).

sub·pleu·ral (səb-ploor′əl) beneath the pleura.

sub·pre·pu·tial (sub″pre-pu′shəl) beneath the prepuce.

sub·pu·bic (səb-pu′bik) inferior to the pubic arch.

sub·pul·mo·nary (səb-pool′mo-nar″e) inferior to a lung, usually meaning between the lung and the diaphragm.

sub·pul·pal (səb-pul′pəl) below the dental pulp.

sub·py·ram·i·dal (sub″pĭ-ram′ĭ-dəl) inferior to a pyramid.

sub·rec·tal (səb-rek′təl) inferior to the rectum.

sub·ret·i·nal (səb-ret′ĭ-nəl) below the retina.

sub·scapho·ceph·a·ly (sub″skaf-o-sef′ə-le) the condition of being moderately scaphocephalic.

sub·scap·u·lar (səb-skap′u-lər) inferior to the scapula.

sub·scle·ral (səb-skler′əl) beneath the sclera.

sub·scle·rot·ic (sub″sklə-rot′ik) 1. partly sclerosed. 2. subscleral.

sub·scrip·tion (səb-skrip′shən) the part of a prescription that gives the directions for compounding the ingredients.

sub·seg·men·tal (sub″seg-men′təl) involving less than a whole segment.

sub·seg·men·tec·to·my (sub″seg-men-tek′tə-me) resection of part of a segment of the liver.

sub·se·ro·sa (sub″sēr-o′sə) tela subserosa.
- **s. of bladder** tela subserosa vesicae urinariae.
- **s. of esophagus** tela subserosa oesophagi.
- **s. of gallbladder** tela subserosa vesicae biliaris.
- **s. of large intestine** tela subserosa intestini crassi.
- **s. of liver** tela subserosa hepatis.
- **s. of parietal pleura** tela subserosa pleurae parietalis.
- **s. of pericardium** tela subserosa pericardii.
- **s. of peritoneum** fascia extraperitonealis.
- **s. of small intestine** tela subserosa intestini tenuis.
- **s. of stomach** tela subserosa gastrica.
- **s. of testis** tela subserosa testis.
- **s. of urinary bladder** tela subserosa vesicae urinariae.
- **s. of uterine tube** tela subserosa tubae uterinae.
- **s. of uterus** tela subserosa uteri.
- **s. of visceral pleura** tela subserosa pleurae visceralis.

sub·se·ro·sal (sub″sēr-o′səl) 1. pertaining to the subserosa. 2. subserous.

sub·se·rous (səb-sēr′əs) beneath a serous membrane.

sub·sib·i·lant (səb-sib′ĭ-lənt) having a muffled, whistling sound.

sub·si·dence (sub′sĭ-dəns) settling of a component or components of the prosthesis after arthroplasty; a small amount is normal, but if it continues or is excessive the prosthesis has become loose.

sub·son·ic (səb-son′ik) infrasonic.

sub·spec·ial·ty (səb-spesh′əl-te) a branch of medicine subordinate to a specialty, as gastroenterology is a subspecialty of internal medicine.

sub·spe·cies (sub′spe″sēz) a taxonomic category subordinate to a species; its members differ morphologically from other members of the species but remain capable of interbreeding with them. See also *variety.*

sub·spi·na·le (sub″spi-na′le) the deepest midline point on the maxilla on the concavity between the anterior nasal spine and the prosthion. Called also *point A.*

sub·spi·nous (səb-spi′nəs) inferior to a spinous process.

sub·sple·ni·al (səb-sple′ne-əl) beneath the splenium of the corpus callosum.

sub·stage (sub′stāj) the part of the microscope located beneath the stage.

sub·stance (sub′stəns) [L. *substantia*] 1. matter with a particular set of characteristics; called also *material.* 2. the material constituting an organ or body; called also *substantia* [TA]. 3. psychoactive s.

black s. substantia nigra.

blood group s's see under *antigen.*

blood group specific s's A, B, and AB [USP] a sterile, isotonic solution of the polysaccharide–amino acid complexes that are capable of neutralizing the anti-A and the anti-B isoagglutinins of group O blood. Specific substance A is usually isolated from hog gastric mucin, and specific substance B usually from the glandular portion of horse gastric mucosa. Used for the immunization of plasma donors in the production of reagents for in vitro diagnosis.

cement s., cementing s. material which serves to hold together the different components of a tissue, as the intercellular substance in endothelium or the interprismatic substance in tooth enamel.

central gelatinous s. of spinal cord substantia gelatinosa centralis medullae spinalis.

chromophil s. Nissl bodies.

colloid s. a jelly-like material formed in colloid degeneration.

controlled s. any of the drugs regulated under the Controlled Substances Act (see under *C*).

depressor s. a substance that tends to decrease activity or blood pressure.

gelatinous s. of posterior horn of spinal cord substantia gelatinosa cornu posterioris medullae spinalis.

gray s. substantia grisea.

gray s., central substantia grisea centralis.

gray s. of spinal cord substantia grisea medullae spinalis.

ground s. the amorphous gel-like material in which connective tissue cells and fibers are embedded.

H s. H antigen (def. 2).

I s. an inhibitory substance which appears in the synapses of the vertebrate central nervous system, which seems generally to act as a hypopolarizer of the postsynaptic junction.

intermediate s. of spinal cord, central substantia intermedia centralis medullae spinalis.

intermediate s. of spinal cord, lateral substantia intermedia lateralis medullae spinalis.

interprismatic s. a cementing substance occupying the space between the round or polygonal enamel prisms; it is softer and more plastic than the enamel prism itself.

interstitial s. ground s.

s. of lens substantia lentis.

medullary s. 1. substantia alba. 2. the soft, marrowlike substance of the interior of an organ; see entries under *medulla.*

metachromatic s. fine particles seen in erythrocytes, especially after supravital staining.

müllerian inhibiting s. antimüllerian hormone.

Nissl s. Nissl bodies.

organ-forming s's specialized materials that become segregated in definite blastomeres, thus bringing about a mosaic type of development.

s. P a peptide composed of 11 amino acids, present in nerve cells throughout the body and in special endocrine cells in the intestine. It increases the contractions of gastrointestinal smooth muscle and causes vasodilatation, and is one of the most potent vasoactive substances known. It also serves as a sensory neurotransmitter, mediating pain, touch, and temperature.

perforated s., anterior substantia perforata anterior.

perforated s., interpeduncular, perforated s., posterior substantia perforata posterior.

perforated s., rostral substantia perforata anterior.

periaqueductal gray s., periventricular gray s. substantia grisea centralis.

prelipid s. degenerated nerve tissue which has not yet been converted into fat.

pressor s. any substance that tends to increase blood pressure.

psychoactive s., psychotropic s. any chemical compound that affects the mind or mental processes, usually referring to drugs used therapeutically in psychiatry; the major classes are the antipsychotics, antidepressants, anxiolytics-sedatives, and mood-stabilizing drugs, but also sometimes used to include other classes of mind-altering substances such as drugs of abuse and some toxins.

reticular s. 1. formatio reticularis. 2. the netlike mass seen in erythrocytes after vital staining.

sarcous s. the substance composing the sarcous element of muscle.

second visceral s. of spinal cord substantia visceralis secundaria medullae spinalis.

slow-reacting s. of anaphylaxis (SRS-A) an inflammatory agent released by mast cells in the anaphylactic reaction; it induces slow, prolonged contraction of certain smooth muscles and is a potent bronchoconstrictor and an important mediator of allergic bronchial asthma. It is composed of a mixture of leukotrienes C_4, D_4, and E_4.

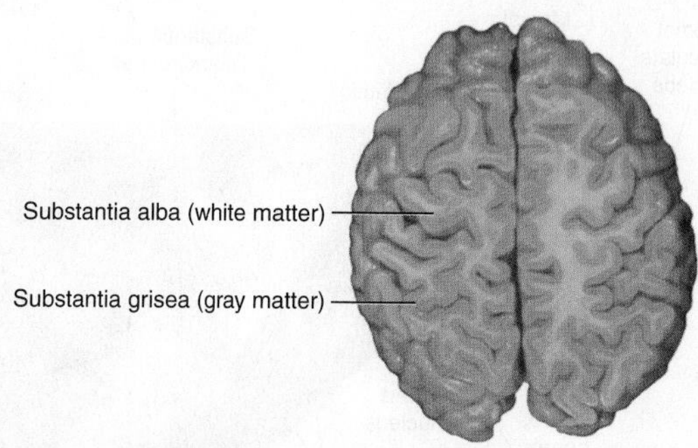

■ Substantia alba (white matter), consisting of axons, and substantia grisea (gray matter), consisting of the neuron dendrites and cell bodies, in an axial section of the brain.

specific soluble s. (SSS) the polysaccharide capsular material of pneumococci *(Streptococcus pneumoniae)*, which exhibits type-specific antigenic differences.

threshold s's those substances in the blood, such as glucose, that are excreted when they reach their renal threshold.

thromboplastic s. a general term for any material with procoagulant activity.

tigroid s. Nissl bodies.

white s. substantia alba.

white s. of cerebellum corpus medullare cerebelli.

white s. of spinal cord substantia alba medullae spinalis.

sub·stan·tia (səb-stan′she-ə) pl. *substan′tiae* [L.] substance: the material of which a tissue, organ, or body is composed. Called also *matter.*

s. adamanti′na den′tis dental enamel.

s. al′ba [TA] white substance: the white nervous tissue, constituting the conducting portion of the brain and spinal cord; it is composed mostly of myelinated nerve fibers arranged in anterior, posterior, and lateral funiculi in the spinal cord and in a number of named fasciculi in the brain. Called also *white matter.*

s. al′ba medul′lae spina′lis [TA] the white substance of the spinal cord, consisting of long myelinated nerve fibers arranged in parallel longitudinal bundles.

s. cine′rea s. grisea.

s. compac′ta os′sium [TA] compact bone: bone substance which is dense and hard.

s. cortica′lis len′tis cortex lentis.

s. cortica′lis os′sium [TA] cortical bone: the substance constituting the hard outer layer of a bone.

s. ebur′nea den′tis dentinum.

s. ferrugi′nea locus caeruleus.

s. gelatino′sa centra′lis medul′lae spina′lis [TA] central gelatinous substance of spinal cord: the zone of gelatinous-appearing substance consisting chiefly of neuroglia but also containing a few nerve fibers and cells, that encircles the central canal of the spinal cord and is surrounded by the central intermediate gray substance.

s. gelatino′sa cor′nu posterio′ris medul′lae spina′lis [TA] gelatinous substance of posterior horn of spinal cord: gelatinous-appearing material in Rexed laminae II of the posterior column of the spinal cord, consisting chiefly of Golgi type II neurons and some larger nerve cells.

s. glandula′ris pro′statae parenchyma prostatae.

s. gri′sea [TA] gray substance: the gray nervous tissue composed of nerve cell bodies, unmyelinated nerve fibers, and supportive tissue. See also *Rexed laminae*, under *lamina.* Called also *gray matter.*

s. gri′sea centra′lis [TA] periaqueductal gray substance: diffuse collections of small cells immediately surrounding the ependymal lining of the third ventricle of the brain, around the cerebral aqueduct, and in the floor of the fourth ventricle. Called also *central* or *periventricular gray substance* and *s. grisea periaqueductalis.*

s. gri′sea medul′lae spina′lis [TA] gray substance of spinal cord: it contains fewer myelinated fibers but more nerve cell bodies, unmyelinated nerve fibers, and blood vessels than the white substance.

s. gri′sea periaqueducta′lis s. grisea centralis.

s. innomina′ta [TA] nerve tissue immediately internal to the anterior perforated substance, and anterior to the globus pallidus and ansa lenticularis.

s. innominata of Reichert, s. innominata of Reil s. innominata.

s. interme′dia centra′lis medul′lae spina′lis [TA] central intermediate substance of spinal cord: the gray substance that makes up the gray commissure of the spinal cord.

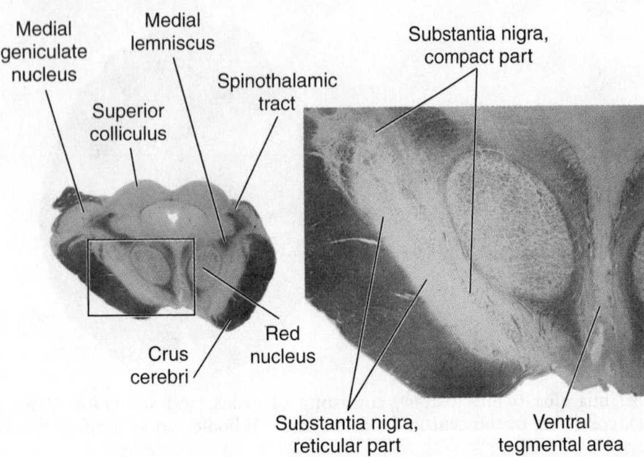

■ Substantia nigra in a section through the rostral midbrain.

s. interme′dia latera′lis medul′lae spina′lis [TA] lateral intermediate substance of spinal cord: the gray substance of the spinal cord that intervenes between the central intermediate substance, the intermediate column, and the anterior and posterior columns.

s. intertubula′ris den′tis dentinum.

s. len′tis [TA] substance of lens: the fibrous material making up the bulk of the lens of the eye.

s. muscula′ris pro′statae [TA] muscular tissue of prostate: the muscular stroma of the prostate, which is intimately blended with the fibrous capsule and permeates the glandular substance.

s. ni′gra [TA] black substance: the layer of melanin-containing neurons that separates the tegmentum of the midbrain from the crus cerebri; it includes a posterior compact part with many pigmented dopaminergic cells *(pars compacta)* and an anterior reticular part whose cells contain little pigment *(pars reticularis).*

s. os′sea den′tis cementum.

s. perfora′ta ante′rior [TA] anterior perforated substance: an area on the base of the brain anterior to each optic tract and lateral to the optic chiasm, containing numerous perforations through which small branches of the anterior and middle cerebral arteries are transmitted to deeper structures. Called also *olfactory area, s. perforata rostralis* [TA alternative], and *rostral perforated substance.*

s. perfora′ta poste′rior [TA] posterior perforated substance: the floor of the interpeduncular fossa, lying between the basis pedunculi of each side and pierced by central branches of the posterior cerebral artery; called also *interpeduncular perforated substance.*

s. perfora′ta rostra′lis TA alternative for *s. perforata anterior.*

s. pro′pria cor′neae [TA] proper substance of cornea: the fibrous, tough, and transparent main part of the cornea, between the anterior and the posterior limiting laminae; called also *stroma of cornea.*

s. pro′pria scle′rae [TA] proper substance of sclera: the chief part of the sclera, lying between the lamina fusca and the episcleral lamina, composed of dense bands of fibrous tissue, mostly parallel with the surface, and crossing each other in all directions. It is structurally continuous with the substantia propria corneae.

s. reticula′ris formatio reticularis.

s. reticulofilamento′sa reticular substance.

s. spongio′sa os′sium [TA] spongy bone: bone substance made up of thin intersecting lamellae, usually found internal to compact bone; called also *cancellated, cancellous,* or *trabecular bone,* and *s. trabecularis ossium* [TA alternative].

s. trabecula′ris os′sium TA alternative for *s. spongiosa ossium.*

s. viscera′lis secunda′ria medul′lae spina′lis [TA] second visceral substance of spinal cord: the gray substance lying ventral to the central intermediate substance.

sub•ster•nal (səb-stur′nəl) inferior to or deep to the sternum; called also *infrasternal.*

sub•ster•no•mas•toid (sub″stər-no-mas′toid) beneath or inferior to the sternocleidomastoid muscle.

sub•stit•u•ent (səb-stich′u-ənt) 1. of or pertaining to substitution. 2. substitute (def. 2). 3. the component substituted in a substitution reaction.

sub•sti•tute (sub′stĭ-to͞ot) [L. *substitutus,* past part. of *substituere* to substitute] 1. to put one thing in place of another. 2. a material used in place of another.

blood s., plasma s. a fluid which may be used instead of whole blood or plasma for replacement of circulating fluid in the body.

saliva s. a solution, such as methylcellulose and mouthwash in distilled water, used to lubricate the oral tissues in xerostomia.

skin s. a material used to cover wounds and burns where extensive areas of skin are missing, to promote healing; effective skin substitutes are bilaminar, with dermal analogue and epidermal analogue layers, and may be synthetic or manufactured from tissue elements.

sub•sti•tut•ed (sub′stĭ-to͞ot″əd) said of a chemical compound resulting from a substitution reaction.

sub•sti•tu•tion (sub″stĭ-too′shən) 1. the act of putting one thing in the place of another, such as in a substitution reaction. 2. a defense mechanism, operating unconsciously, in which an unattainable or unacceptable goal, emotion, or object is replaced by one that is attainable or acceptable.

creeping s. of bone the formation of new bone on the surfaces of necrotic trabeculae by osteoblasts, occurring after the revascularization of an area that has been disrupted by fracture, as at the head of the femur after fracture of the neck has disrupted the blood supply to the head of the bone.

sensory s. the substitution of one sense to compensate for deficits in a different one; this is popularly assumed in congenitally blind and deaf persons; it is sometimes used in rehabilitation techniques and apparatus for those who lose all or part of one of their senses.

sub•sti•tu•tive (sub″tĭ-too′tiv) bringing about a change or substitution.

sub•strate (sub′strāt) 1. a substance upon which an enzyme acts. Symbol S. 2. a neutral substance containing a nutrient solution. 3. a surface upon which a different material is deposited or adhered, usually in a coating or layer.

renin s. angiotensinogen.

sub•stra•tum (səb-stra′təm) [L.] 1. a substrate. 2. a lower layer or stratum.

sub•struc•ture (sub′struk″chər) 1. a structure that provides a foundation for another structure. 2. a basic underlying or supporting part of an organ or structure. Called also *infrastructure.* 3. implant s.

implant s. a metal framework implanted beneath the mucoperiosteum, in contact with bone, that retains, supports, and stabilizes the superstructural part of an implant denture. Called also *implant framework* and *implant infrastructure.*

sub•sul•cus (səb-sul′kəs) a sulcus concealed by another.

sub•sul•fate (səb-sul′fāt) a basic sulfate.

sub•syl•vi•an (səb-sil′ve-ən) beneath the sylvian fissure (sulcus lateralis cerebri).

sub•ta•lar (səb-ta′lər) [*sub-* + *talar*] inferior to the talus.

sub•tar•sal (səb-tahr′səl) inferior to the tarsus.

sub•telo•cen•tric (səb-tel″o-sen′trik) having the centromere almost, but not quite, at the telocentric position.

sub•tem•por•al (səb-tem′por-əl) infratemporal.

sub•te•ni•al (səb-te′ne-əl) beneath a taenia.

sub•ten•to•ri•al (sub″ten-tor′e-əl) beneath the tentorium of the cerebellum.

sub•ter•mi•nal (səb-tur′mĭn-əl) near an end or extremity.

sub•te•tan•ic (sub″tə-tan′ik) mildly tetanic.

sub•tha•lam•ic (sub″thə-lam′ik) 1. inferior to the thalamus. 2. pertaining to the subthalamus.

sub•thal•a•mot•o•my (səb-thal″ə-mot′ə-me) a stereotactic surgical technique that produces lesions in the subthalamic nucleus for treatment of symptoms of Parkinson disease.

sub•thal•a•mus (səb-thal′ə-məs) [TA] a large ovoid mass in the anterior part of the diencephalon interposed between the dorsal thalamus, hypothalamus, and tegmentum of the mesencephalon; it contains the nuclei of the lateral and medial geniculate bodies, the subthalamic and reticular nuclei, the zona incerta, and the Forel fields. Some authorities consider this to be part of the thalamus and refer to it as the *ventral thalamus.*

sub•tile (sut′əl) [L. *subtilis*] keen and acute.

sub•til•in (sub′til-in) an antibiotic substance isolated from strains of the soil bacteria *Bacillus subtilis;* it is chiefly effective against gram-positive bacteria and certain acid-fast bacilli.

sub•til•i•sin (səb-til′ĭ-sin) a proteolytic enzyme isolated from strains of the soil bacteria *Bacillus subtilis.* It catalyzes the hydrolysis of certain peptide bonds, and analysis has shown it to be composed of 274 amino acid residues.

sub•tle (sut′əl) [L. *subtilis*] 1. difficult to comprehend. 2. slight and almost imperceptible. 3. subtile.

sub•to•tal (səb-to′təl) less than complete, often something that is not much less than complete.

sub•trac•tion (səb-trak′shən) the removal of something from a group.

digital s. use of computerized digital methods to remove something unwanted, such as obscuring shadows in radiography after injection of contrast medium; see *digital subtraction radiography*, under *radiography*.

sub•tra•pe•zi•al (sub″trə-pe′ze-əl) beneath or inferior to the trapezius muscle.

sub•tribe (sub′trīb″) a taxonomic category sometimes established, subordinate to a tribe and superior to a genus.

sub•tro•chan•ter•ic (sub″tro-kan-ter′ik) inferior to a trochanter.

sub•troch•le•ar (səb-trok′le-ər) inferior to a trochlea.

sub•tu•ber•al (səb-too′bər-əl) beneath or inferior to a tuber.

sub•tym•pan•ic (sub″tim-pan′ik) 1. infratympanic. 2. having a somewhat tympanic quality.

sub•um•bil•i•cal (sub″əm-bil′ĭ-kəl) inferior to the umbilicus.

sub•un•gual (səb-ung′gwəl) [*sub-* + *ungual*] underneath a nail; called also *hyponychial.*

sub•ure•thral (sub″u-re′thrəl) inferior to the urethra.

sub•vag•i•nal (səb-vaj′ĭ-nəl) 1. inferior to the vagina. 2. inferior to a sheath.

sub•ver•te•bral (səb-vur′tə-brəl) beneath (deep to) the vertebral column.

sub•vit•ri•nal (səb-vit′rĭ-nəl) beneath the vitreous.

sub•vo•lu•tion (sub″vo-loo′shən) [*sub-* + L. *volvere* to turn] surgical reversal of a flap; especially, dissection and turning up of a pterygium so that its outer surface comes in contact with the raw surface of the dissection to prevent readhesion.

sub•wak•ing (səb-wāk′ing) intermediate between waking and sleeping.

sub•zo•nal (səb-zo′nəl) beneath or inferior to a zone, especially the zona pellucida.

sub•zy•go•mat•ic (sub″zi-go-mat′ik) inferior to the zygomatic arch.

suc•ca•gogue (suk′ə-gog) [L. *succus* juice or sap + *-agogue*] secretagogue.

suc•ce•da•ne•ous (suk″sə-da′ne-əs) 1. pertaining to a succedaneum. 2. coming after or replacing something else.

suc•ce•da•ne•um (suk″sə-da′ne-əm) [L. *succedaneus* taking another's place] a medicine or material that may be substituted for another of like properties.

suc•cen•tu•ri•ate (suk″sən-tu′re-āt) [L. *succenturiare* to substitute] accessory; serving as a substitute.

suc•ces•sion•al (sək-sesh′ən-əl) [L. *succcessus,* past part. of *succedere* to follow] pertaining to that which follows in order or sequence.

suc•ci•mer (DMSA) (suk′sĭ-mər) *meso*-2,3-dimercaptosuccinic acid; a chelating agent that is an analogue of dimercaprol, administered orally in the treatment of heavy metal poisoning; a complex with technetium 99m is used as a diagnostic aid in renal function testing. See table at *technetium.*

suc•ci•nate (suk′sĭ-nāt) any salt, ester, or anionic form of succinic acid.

s. semialdehyde γ-hydroxybutyric acid.

suc•ci•nate-CoA li•gase (GDP-form•ing) (suk′sĭ-nāt-ko-a′ li′gās form′ing) [EC 6.2.1.4] an enzyme of the ligase class that catalyzes the cleavage of succinate from succinyl CoA, using the energy so generated to form GTP from GDP. The reaction is part of the tricarboxylic acid cycle (see illustration under *cycle*). Called also *succinyl CoA synthetase.*

suc•ci•nate de•hy•dro•gen•ase (suk′sĭ-nāt de-hi′dro-jən-ās) [EC 1.3.99.1] an enzyme of the oxidoreductase class that catalyzes the oxidation of succinate to fumarate, using a variety of hydrogen acceptors. An iron-containing flavoprotein, it is a component of succinate dehydrogenase (ubiquinone), an enzyme complex of the tricarboxylic acid cycle.

suc•ci•nate de•hy•dro•gen•ase (ubiq•ui•none) (suk′sin-āt de-hi′dro-jən-ās u-bik′win-ōn″) [EC 1.3.5.1] an enzyme of the oxidoreductase class that catalyzes the oxidation of succinate to fumarate, using ubiquinone as an electron acceptor. It occurs in mitochondria as a membrane-bound complex, an iron-containing flavoprotein (FAD) with an associated iron-sulfur protein. The reaction is part of the tricarboxylic acid cycle (see illustration under *cycle*).

suc•ci•nate-semi•al•de•hyde de•hy•dro•gen•ase (suk′sĭ-nāt sem″e-al′də-hīd de-hi′dro-jən-ās) [EC 1.2.1.24] an enzyme of the oxidoreductase class that catalyzes the oxidation of γ-hydroxybutyric acid to succinate. The reaction is the final step in the inactivation of γ-aminobutyric acid (GABA); when enzyme activity is deficient, increased levels of GABA and γ-hydroxybutyric acid can be detected in urine, plasma, and cerebrospinal fluid.

suc•ci•nate-semi•al•de•hyde de•hy•dro•gen•ase de•fi•cien•cy (suk′sĭ-nāt sem″e-al′də-hīd de-hi′dro-jən-ās) an autosomal recessive aminoacidopathy caused by mutation in the succinate semialdehyde dehydrogenase gene (*ALDH5A1,* locus: 6p22), resulting in deficiency of the enzyme. The resulting increase in γ-aminobutyric acid and γ-hydroxybutyric acid causes mental retardation, hypotonia, and ataxia. Called also *γ-* or *4-hydroxybutyricaciduria.*

suc•cin•ic ac•id (sək-sin′ik) 1,4-butanedioic acid, an intermediate in the tricarboxylic acid cycle (q.v.).

suc•ci•ni•mide (sək-sin′ĭ-mīd) 1. an organic compound comprising a pyrrole ring with two carbonyl substitutions. 2. any of a class of anticonvulsants with such a basic structure, including ethosuximide, methsuximide, and phensuximide.

Suc•ci•ni•vib•ri•o•na•ceae (sək-sin″ĭ-vib″re-o-na′se-e) a family of bacteria tentatively assigned to the order Aeromonadales, consisting of anaerobic, gram-negative rods; it includes the genus *Anaerobiospirillum,* which can infect humans.

suc•ci•nyl (suk′sĭ-nəl) an acyl radical of succinic acid.

suc•ci•nyl•ac•e•to•ac•e•tate (suk″sin-əl-ə-se″to-as′ə-tāt) a compound formed by reduction of fumarylacetoacetate; it occurs at elevated levels in tyrosinemia type I, due to the deficiency of fumarylacetoacetase. It is readily decarboxylated to succinylacetone (q.v.); both compounds can cause hepatorenal damage.

suc•ci•nyl•ac•e•tone (suk″sin-əl-as′ə-tōn) the compound formed by decarboxylation of succinylacetoacetate, occurring at elevated levels in tyrosinemia type I, and believed to cause the characteristic hepatorenal damage. It competitively inhibits porphobilinogen synthase by being a structural analogue of δ-aminolevulinic acid, secondarily inhibits other enzymes of tyrosine metabolism, and is structurally similar to maleic acid, an inhibitor of renal tubular function.

suc•ci•nyl•cho•line chlo•ride (suk″sĭ-nəl-ko′lēn) [USP] a depolarizing neuromuscular blocking agent that produces skeletal muscle relaxation by blocking transmission at the myoneural junction; used for its muscle relaxant action during convulsive therapy and such procedures as endotracheal intubation and endoscopy, and as an adjunct to surgical anesthesia, administered intravenously and intramuscularly.

suc•ci•nyl CoA (suk′sĭ-nəl ko-a′) succinyl coenzyme A.

suc•ci•nyl CoA syn•the•tase (suk′sĭ-nəl ko-a′ sin′thə-tās) succinate-CoA ligase (GDP-forming).

suc•ci•nyl co•en•zyme A (suk″sĭ-nəl-ko-en′zīm) the succinate monothioester of coenzyme A, a high energy intermediate formed in the tricarboxylic acid cycle (q.v.). It is also a precursor in the synthesis of porphyrins.

suc•ci•nyl•di•hy•dro•lipo•am•ide (suk″sĭ-nəl-di-hi″dro-lip″o-am′īd) succinyl bound to lipoamide, an intermediate in the reaction catalyzed by the α-ketoglutarate dehydrogenase complex.

suc•cor•rhea (suk″o-re′ə) [L. *succus* juice or sap + *-rrhea*] an excessive flow of a juice or secretion, as in ptyalism.

suc•cus•sion (sə-kush′ən) [L. *succussio* a shaking from beneath, earthquake] 1. the shaking of the body during an examination; a splashing sound is indicative of the presence of fluid and air in a body cavity. 2. the vigorous shaking of a diluted homeopathic preparation in order to activate the medicinal substance.

hippocratic s. succussion to elicit a splashing sound in the chest; see *succussion sounds,* under *sound.*

suck (suk) [A.S. *sūcan*] 1. to draw liquid into a tube or the mouth by creating a partial vacuum, as in taking milk from the breast. 2. to use the lips or mouth parts in a manner resembling the motions of an infant at the breast.

suck•le (suk′əl) 1. to feed at the breast. 2. to breast-feed an infant; see *breast-feeding.*

Suc•quet-Hoy•er anastomosis (canal) (su-ka′ hoy′ər) [J.P. *Sucquet,* French anatomist, 1840–1870; Heinrich Friedrich *Hoyer,* Polish anatomist, 1834–1907] segmentum arteriale anastomosis arteriovenosae glomeriformis.

Su•craid (soo′krād) trademark for a preparation of sacrosidase.

su•cral•fate (soo-kral′fāt) [USP] a complex of aluminum and a sulfated polysaccharide, used as a gastrointestinal antiulcerative and gastric mucosa protectant; administered orally.

su•cra•lose (soo′krə-lōs) [NF] a chlorinated derivative of sucrose, used as a sweetening agent.

su•crase (soo′krās) an enzyme of the hydrolase class that catalyzes the cleavage of the glycosidic bond in the disaccharides sucrose and maltose to yield their component sugars. The enzyme occurs complexed with α-dextrinase in the brush border of the intestinal mucosa; deficiency of enzyme complex activity, an autosomal recessive trait called sucrase-isomaltase deficiency (see under *deficiency*), is a form of disaccharide intolerance. In EC nomenclature called *sucrose α-glucosidase.*

suc•rase-iso•mal•tase (soo′krās i″so-mawl′tās) see under *complex.*

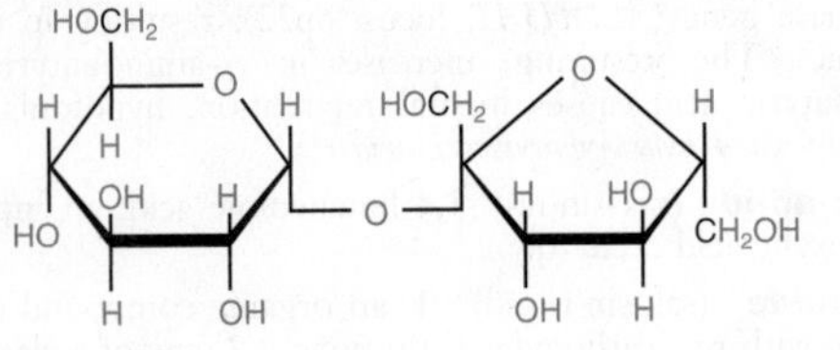

■ Sucrose.

su·crase-iso·mal·tase de·fi·cien·cy (soo′krās i″so-mawl′tās) see under *deficiency.*

su·crate (soo′krāt) a compound of a substance with sucrose.

su·cro·clas·tic (soo″kro-klas′tik) [*sucrose* + *-clastic*] splitting of sugar.

su·crose (soo′krōs) [Fr. *sucre* sugar] 1. a nonreducing disaccharide obtained from sugar cane *(Saccharum officinarum),* sugar beet *(Beta vulgaris),* and sorghum; it is composed of glucose and fructose linked via their anomeric carbons. It is used extensively as a food and a sweetener. 2. [NF] an official preparation used as a sweetening agent, tablet excipient, lozenge basis, and suspending and viscosity increasing agent.

s. octaacetate [NF] a white, almost odorless, hygroscopic powder, having an intensely bitter taste; used as an alcohol denaturant.

su·crose α-glu·co·si·dase (soo′krōs gloo-ko′sĭ-dās) [EC 3.2.1.48] EC nomenclature for *sucrase.*

su·cros·emia (soo″kro-se′me-ə) the presence of sucrose in the blood.

su·cros·uria (soo″kro-su′re-ə) presence of excessive sucrose in the urine, such as after ingestion of excessive sucrose or in congenital sucrose intolerance.

suc·tion (suk′shən) [L. *sugere* to suck] aspiration of gas or fluid by mechanical means.

post-tussive s. a sucking sound heard over a lung cavity just after a cough.

suc·to·ri·al (sək-tor′e-əl) fitted for performing suction.

Su·da·fed (soo′də-fed) trademark for preparations containing pseudoephedrine hydrochloride.

su·da·men (soo-da′mən) pl. *suda′mina* [L., from *sudare* to sweat] a whitish vesicle caused by the retention of sweat in the sweat ducts or the layers of the epidermis. **sudam′inal** *adj*

su·da·mi·na (soo-da′mĭ-nah) 1. miliaria crystallina. 2. plural of *sudamen.*

Su·dan (soo-dan′) a group of azo dyes used as stains for fats.

S. I a yellow fat-soluble azo dye that is an irritant and suspected carcinogen.

S. II an orange fat-soluble azo dye used in biological staining of fats; it is an irritant and suspected carcinogen.

S. III a red fat-soluble azo dye that is an important stain for demonstration of neutral fats.

S. IV scarlet red.

S. G S. III.

su·dano·phil (soo-dan′o-fil) an element that stains readily with Sudan.

su·dano·phil·ia (soo-dan″o-fil′e-ə) [*sudan* + *-philia*] affinity for Sudan stain.

su·dano·phil·ic (soo-dan″o-fil′ik) staining readily with Sudan.

su·dan·oph·i·lous (soo″dən-of′ĭ-ləs) sudanophilic.

su·da·tion (soo-da′shən) sweating.

Su·deck atrophy (disease) (soo′dek) [Paul Hermann Martin *Sudeck,* German surgeon, 1866–1938] posttraumatic osteoporosis; see under *osteoporosis.*

Su·deck-Le·riche syndrome (soo′dek lə-rēsh′) [P.H.M. *Sudeck;* René *Leriche,* French surgeon, 1879–1955] see under *syndrome.*

su·do·mo·tor (soo″do-mo′tər) [*sudor* + *motor*] stimulating the sweat glands.

su·do·re·sis (soo″do-re′sis) sweating.

su·do·rif·er·ous (soo″də-rif′ər-əs) [*sudor* + *-ferous*] 1. conveying sweat. 2. sudoriparous.

su·do·rif·ic (soo″də-rif′ik) diaphoretic.

su·do·rip·a·rous (soo″də-rip′ə-rəs) [*sudor* + *-parous*] secreting or producing sweat; called also *sudoriferous.*

SUDS sudden unexplained death syndrome.

su·et (soo′ət) [L. *sevum*] the fat from the abdominal cavity of a ruminant animal, especially the sheep or ox; used in the preparation of cerates and ointments and as an emollient. The preparation employed in pharmacy is the internal fat of the abdomen of the sheep.

prepared s. the internal fat of the abdomen of the sheep purified by melting and straining.

Su·fen·ta (soo-fen′tə) trademark for a preparation of sufentanil citrate.

su·fen·ta·nil cit·rate (soo-fen′tə-nil) [USP] an opioid analgesic derived from fentanyl, used as an analgesic adjunct in the maintenance of general anesthesia and as a primary agent for induction and maintenance of general anesthesia; administered intravenously. In combination with bupivacaine, it is administered epidurally for prevention and treatment of obstetric pain.

suf·fo·cant (suf′ə-kənt) an agent that causes suffocation.

suf·fo·ca·tion (suf″ə-ka′shən) [L. *suffocatio*] asphyxiation.

suf·fu·sion (sə-fu′zhən) [L. *suffusio*] 1. the process of overspreading, or diffusion. 2. the condition of being moistened or of being permeated through, as by blood.

sug·ar (shoog′ər) any of a class of sweet, water-soluble, crystallizable carbohydrates, which are the monosaccharides and smaller oligosaccharides; often used specifically for sucrose. In animals, they are the chief source of energy and their derivatives are universal constituents of structural materials (e.g., glycosaminoglycans, cellulose).

s. alcohol see under *alcohol.*

amino s. a sugar in which an amino group substituent has replaced a hydroxyl group; the amino sugars and their acyl derivatives are constituents of a variety of polysaccharides, glycoproteins, and glycolipids.

anhydrous s. anhydrosugar.

beet s. sucrose derived from the root of the beet.

blood s. 1. glucose occurring in the blood. 2. the amount of glucose in the blood.

burnt s. caramel.

cane s. sucrose obtained from sugar cane.

compressible s. [NF] a preparation which contains 95–98 per cent sucrose and which may contain starch, dextrin, and invert sugar; used as a sweetening agent and tablet excipient in pharmaceutical preparations.

confectioner's s. [NF] sucrose ground together with cornstarch to a fine powder, containing 95–97 per cent sucrose; used as a sweetening agent and tablet excipient in pharmaceutical preparations.

deoxy s. a sugar in which one or more carbon atoms have been reduced, thus losing their hydroxyl groups.

diabetic s. the glucose found in the urine in diabetes mellitus.

fasting blood s. fasting blood glucose; see under *glucose.*

fruit s. fructose.

invert s. a mixture of equal amounts of dextrose and fructose, obtained by hydrolyzing sucrose; used in solution as a parenteral nutrient.

reducing s. any sugar that can act as a reducing agent in an alkaline solution; included are all monosaccharides and di- or oligosaccharides in which at least one anomeric carbon is a free aldehyde or keto group.

simple s. monosaccharide.

threshold s. the lower limit of hyperglycemia at which glucose appears in the urine.

sug·ges·ti·bil·i·ty (səg-jes″tĭ-bil′ĭ-te) a condition of enhanced susceptibility to suggestion.

sug·ges·ti·ble (səg-jes′tĭ-bəl) highly susceptible to suggestion.

sug·ges·tion (səg-jes′chən) [L. *suggestio*] 1. the act of offering an idea for action or for consideration of action. 2. an idea so offered. 3. in psychiatry, the process of causing uncritical acceptance of an idea.

hypnotic s. a suggestion imparted to a person in the hypnotic state, by which the subject is induced to alter perceptions or memory or to perform actions.

posthypnotic s. implantation in the mind of a subject during hypnosis of a suggestion to be acted upon after recovery from the hypnotic state.

sug·gil·la·tion (sug″jĭ-la′shən) 1. ecchymosis. 2. contusion.

su·i·cide (soo′ĭ-sīd) [L. *sui* of himself + *-cide*] the taking of one's own life.

psychic s. the termination of one's own life without employment of physical agents.

su·i·ci·dol·o·gy (soo″ĭ-sīd-ol′ə-je) [*suicide* + *-logy*] the study of the causes and prevention of suicide.

su·id (soo′id) porcine.

suint (swint) a fat-like substance derivable from sheep's wool, from which anhydrous lanolin is prepared. Called also *s. de laine.*

Sui·pox·vi·rus (soo′ĭ-poks″vi′rəs) [L. *sus,* gen. *suis* pig + *poxvirus*] swinepox virus; a genus of viruses of the subfamily Chordopoxvirinae (family Poxviridae) that cause swinepox in piglets.

suit (so͞ot) an outer garment covering the entire body.

antiblackout s., anti-G s. G s.

antishock s. pneumatic antishock garment.

G s. a garment worn by pilots, designed to increase their ability to withstand ill effects of the acceleratory forces experienced in certain aerial maneuvers.

Su•ker sign (soo′kər) [George Franklin *Suker*, American ophthalmologist, 20th century] see under *sign.*

Sul•a•myd (sul′ə-mid) trademark for preparations of sulfacetamide.

Su•lar (soo′lahr) trademark for a preparation of nisoldipine.

sul•bac•tam (səl-bak′təm) a β-lactamase inhibitor.
s. sodium [USP] the sodium salt of sulbactam; a β-lactamase inhibitor used to increase the antibacterial activity of penicillins and cephalosporins against β-lactamase–producing organisms.

sul•ben•ox (səl-ben′ox) a veterinary growth stimulant.

sul•cate (sul′kāt) [L. *sulcatus*] furrowed or marked with sulci.

sul•ca•tion (səl-ka′shən) the formation of sulci; the state of being marked by sulci.

sul•ci (sul′si) [L.] genitive and plural of *sulcus.*

sul•ci•form (sul′sĭ-form) formed like a groove.

sul•con•a•zole ni•trate (səl-kon′ə-zōl) [USP] a broad-spectrum imidazole antifungal, applied topically in the treatment of tinea pedis, tinea corporis, tinea cruris, and tinea versicolor, and in the treatment of cutaneous *Candida albicans* infections.

sul•cu•lus (sul′ku-ləs) pl. *sul′culi* [L.] a small or minute sulcus.

sul•cus (sul′kəs) gen. and pl. *sul′ci* [L.] 1. [TA] anatomic terminology for a long groove or furrow, especially one of the cerebral sulci. 2. a linear depression or valley in the occlusal surface of a tooth, having sloping sides that meet at an angle.

Sulcus

Descriptions are given on TA terms, and include anglicized names of specific sulci.

alveololingual s. the depression between the dental arch and the tongue.
s. ampulla′ris [TA], **ampullary s.** ampullary groove: a transverse groove for the ampullary nerve on the membranous ampulla of each semicircular duct.
anterior interventricular s. s. interventricularis anterior.
anterior lateral s. of medulla oblongata s. anterolateralis medullae oblongatae.
anterior lateral s. of spinal cord s. anterolateralis medullae spinalis.
anterior parolfactory s. a sulcus on the medial surface of the cerebral hemisphere, between the area parolfactoria behind and the inferior frontal gyrus in front.
anterolateral s. of medulla oblongata s. anterolateralis medullae oblongatae.
anterolateral s. of spinal cord s. anterolateralis medullae spinalis.
s. anterolatera′lis medul′lae oblonga′tae [TA] anterolateral sulcus of medulla oblongata: a longitudinal sulcus on the anterior surface of the medulla oblongata, lateral to the pyramid, from which emerge the fibers of the hypoglossal nerve. Called also *ventrolateral s. of medulla oblongata.*
s. anterolatera′lis medul′lae spina′lis [TA] anterolateral sulcus of spinal cord: the longitudinal groove on the anterolateral surface of the spinal cord, from which the anterior nerve roots emerge; it separates the anterior and lateral funiculi. Called also *ventrolateral s. of spinal cord.*
s. anthe′licis transver′sus transverse sulcus of antihelix: the depression on the medial surface of the pinna corresponding to the lower crus of the antihelix.
s. arte′riae menin′geae me′diae [TA] groove for middle meningeal artery: either of two grooves in the parietal bone for branches of the meningeal artery; one, posterior to the coronal suture, lodges the frontal branch, and the other, anterior to the mastoid angle, lodges the parietal branch.
s. arte′riae occipita′lis [TA] occipital groove: the groove just medial to the mastoid notch on the temporal bone, lodging the occipital artery.
s. arte′riae subcla′viae [TA] groove for subclavian artery: a transverse groove on the cranial surface of the first rib, just posterior to the anterior scalene tubercle; it lodges the subclavian artery.
s. arte′riae tempora′lis me′diae [TA] groove for middle temporal artery: a nearly vertical groove running just superior to the external acoustic meatus on the external surface of the squamous part of the temporal bone; it lodges the middle temporal artery.
s. arte′riae vertebra′lis atlan′tis [TA] groove for vertebral artery: the groove on the cranial surface of the posterior arch of the atlas; it lodges the vertebral artery and the first spinal nerve.
arterial sulci sulci arteriosi.
sul′ci arterio′si [TA] arterial grooves: grooves on the internal surfaces of the cranial bones for the meningeal arteries.
atrioventricular s. s. coronarius cordis.
s. for auditory tube s. tubae auditivae.
basilar s. of pons, s. basila′ris pon′tis [TA] the anteromedian groove in the pons, lodging the basilar artery.
s. bicipita′lis latera′lis [TA] lateral bicipital groove: a longitudinal groove on the lateral side of the arm which marks the limit between the

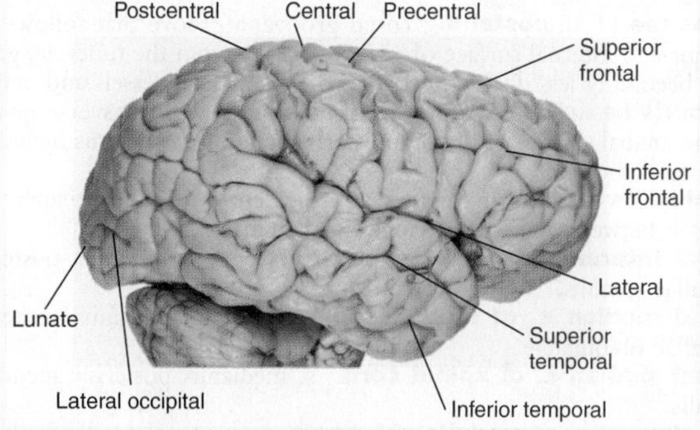

■ Sulci cerebri in a lateral view of the right hemisphere.

lateral border of the biceps muscle and the brachialis; called also *s. bicipitalis radialis* [TA alternative].
s. bicipita′lis media′lis [TA] medial bicipital groove: a longitudinal groove on the medial side of the arm that marks the limit between the medial border of the biceps muscle and the brachialis; called also *s. bicipitalis ulnaris* [TA alternative].
s. bicipita′lis radia′lis TA alternative for *s. bicipitalis lateralis.*
s. bicipita′lis ulna′ris TA alternative for *s. bicipitalis medialis.*
bulbopontine s., s. bulboponti′nus [TA] a transverse groove in front and on each side of the pons that demarcates it from the medulla oblongata, which is occupied by the abducent, facial, and vestibulocochlear nerves. Called also *medullopontine s.*
calcaneal s., s. calca′nei [TA] a rough, deep groove on the upper surface of the calcaneus, between the medial and the posterior articular surfaces and giving attachment to the interosseous talocalcaneal ligament.
calcarine s., s. calcari′nus [TA] a sulcus on the medial surface of the occipital lobe, separating the cuneus from the lingual gyrus; called also *calcarine fissure.*
callosal s. s. corporis callosi.
callosomarginal s. s. cinguli.
s. caro′ticus os′sis sphenoida′lis [TA], **carotid s.** the groove on the side of the body of the sphenoid bone that lodges the internal carotid artery and the cavernous sinus.
carpal s., s. car′pi [TA] carpal groove: a broad deep groove on the palmar surface of the carpal bones, which transmits the flexor tendons and the median nerve into the palm of the hand.
central s. of cerebrum s. centralis cerebri.
central s. of insula s. centralis insulae.
s. centra′lis ce′rebri [TA] central sulcus of cerebrum: a relatively deep, nearly vertical sulcus on the cerebral hemisphere, which separates the frontal from the parietal lobe.
s. centra′lis in′sulae [TA] central sulcus of insula: a deep, oblique furrow which divides the insula into a larger anterior and a smaller posterior part.
cerebral sulci, sul′ci ce′rebri [TA] the furrows on the surface of the brain between the cerebral gyri.
chiasmatic s., s. chias′matis s. prechiasmaticus.

cingulate s., s. cin′guli [TA] a long, irregularly shaped sulcus on the medial surface of a hemisphere, which separates the cingulate gyrus below from the medial surface of the superior frontal gyrus and the paracentral lobule above. At its posterior end it turns up to form a marginal part between the precuneus and the paracentral lobule.
circular s. of insula, s. circula′ris in′sulae [TA] a fissure that almost surrounds the insula (lobus insularis) and separates it from the opercula.
collateral s., s. collatera′lis [TA] a longitudinal sulcus on the inferior surface of the cerebral hemisphere between the fusiform gyrus and the hippocampal gyrus; called also *collateral fissure.*
s. corona′rius cor′dis [TA], **coronary s. of heart** a groove on the external surface of the heart, separating the atria from the ventricles; portions of it are occupied by the major arteries and veins of the heart; called also *atrioventricular groove.*
s. cor′poris callo′si [TA], **s. of corpus callosum** a sulcus in the convex aspect of a cerebral hemisphere, between the corpus callosum and the cingulate gyrus at the bottom of the longitudinal cerebral fissure.
s. cos′tae [TA], **costal s.** costal groove: a groove that follows the inferior and internal surface of a rib anteriorly from the tubercle, gradually becoming less distinct; it lodges the intercostal vessels and nerves.
s. cru′ris he′licis [TA] groove of crus of helix: a transverse groove on the medial surface of the pinna, corresponding to the crus helicis on the lateral surface.
sul′ci cu′tis [TA] skin furrows: the fine depressions on the surface of the skin between the dermal ridges. Called also *skin grooves.*
dorsal intermediate s. of spinal cord s. intermedius posterior medullae spinalis.
dorsal median s. of medulla oblongata s. medianus posterior medullae oblongatae.
dorsal median s. of spinal cord s. medianus posterior medullae spinalis.
dorsolateral s. of medulla oblongata s. posterolateralis medullae oblongatae.
dorsolateral s. of spinal cord s. posterolateralis medullae spinalis.
ethmoidal s. of nasal bone, s. ethmoida′lis os′sis nasa′lis [TA] ethmoidal groove: a groove that extends the entire length of the posteromedial surface of the nasal bone and lodges the external nasal branch of the anterior ethmoid nerve.
s. for eustachian tube s. tubae auditivae.
external spiral s. s. spiralis externus.
fimbriodentate s., s. fimbriodenta′tus [TA] a shallow groove between the medial parts of the dentate gyrus and fimbria hippocampi.
s. fronta′lis infe′rior [TA] inferior frontal sulcus: a short longitudinal sulcus that separates the inferior and middle frontal gyri.
s. fronta′lis supe′rior [TA] superior frontal sulcus: a longitudinal sulcus that separates the middle and superior frontal gyri.
gingival s., s. gingiva′lis [TA] a shallow V-shaped space around the tooth, bounded by the tooth surface on one side and the epithelium lining the free margin of the gingiva on the other; considered by some authorities to be the same as the gingival crevice. Called also *gingival groove.*
gluteal s., s. glutea′lis [TA] a curved transverse skin furrow on the posterior aspect of the upper thigh, separating the upper part of the thigh from the buttocks; called also *gluteal fold* or *furrow.*
habenular s., s. habenula′ris [TA] a groove separating the trigonum habenulae from the upper surface of the thalamus.
s. ha′muli pterygoi′dei [TA] groove of pterygoid hamulus: a smooth groove on the lateral surface of the medial pterygoid plate of the sphenoid bone, in the angle at the base of the pterygoid hamulus; it lodges the tendon of the tensor veli palatini muscle.
Harrison s. see under *groove.*
hippocampal s., s. hippocampa′lis [TA] the sulcus that extends from the splenium of the corpus callosum almost to the tip of the temporal lobe, and forms the medial boundary of the hippocampal gyrus; called also *hippocampal fissure.*
hypothalamic s., s. hypothala′micus [TA] a shallow curved sulcus on the wall of the third ventricle, extending from the interventricular foramen to the cerebral aqueduct.
inferior frontal s. s. frontalis inferior.
inferior interventricular s. s. interventricularis posterior.
inferior petrosal s., s. for inferior petrosal sinus s. sinus petrosi inferioris.
inferior temporal s. s. temporalis inferior.
infraorbital s., s. infraorbita′lis [TA] infraorbital groove: a groove in the orbital surface of the maxilla, commencing near the middle of the posterior edge of the surface and running anteriorly for a short distance to become continuous with the infraorbital canal.
infrapalpebral s., s. infrapalpebra′lis [TA] the skin furrow below the lower eyelid.
inner spiral s. s. spiralis internus.
interlobar sulci of cerebrum, sul′ci interloba′res ce′rebri [TA] the sulci that separate the lobes of the cerebrum from each other.
s. intermamma′rius [TA] intermammary cleft: the cleft between the left and right breasts.
s. interme′dius poste′rior medul′lae spina′lis [TA] posterior intermediate sulcus of spinal cord: a longitudinal sulcus in the cervical and upper thoracic parts of the spinal cord between the fasciculus gracilis and the fasciculus cuneatus. Called also *dorsal intermediate s. of spinal cord.*
internal spiral s. s. spiralis internus.
interparietal s. s. intraparietalis.
s. intersphincte′ricus ana′lis [TA] intersphincteric groove: an indistinct groove in the anal canal, forming the lower border of the pecten analis, marking the change between the subcutaneous part of the external anal sphincter and the border of the internal anal sphincter.
intertubercular s. of humerus, s. intertubercula′ris hu′meri [TA] a longitudinal groove on the anterior surface of the humerus, lying between the tubercles above and between the crests of the tubercles farther down, and lodging the tendon of the long head of the biceps muscle. Called also *bicipital* or *intertubercular groove.*
interventricular s. of heart the groove dividing the two ventricles, comprising the sulcus interventricularis anterior and the sulcus interventricularis posterior.
s. interventricula′ris ante′rior [TA] anterior interventricular sulcus: a groove on the sternocostal surface of the heart marking the position of the interventricular septum and the line of separation between the ventricles; called also *anterior interventricular groove.*
s. interventricula′ris poste′rior [TA] posterior interventricular sulcus: a groove on the diaphragmatic surface of the heart marking the position of the interventricular septum and the line of separation between the ventricles; called also *inferior interventricular groove.*
intraparietal s., s. intraparieta′lis [TA] an irregular sulcus on the convex surface of the parietal lobe of the cerebrum and between the inferior and superior parietal lobuli.
labiodental s. the arched groove in the embryo which separates off the anterior part of the mandibular prominence, thus helping to form the lower lip.
s. lacrima′lis [TA] lacrimal groove: a deep vertical groove in the medial wall of the orbit, formed by the lacrimal bone and the frontal process of the maxilla, bounded anteriorly by the anterior lacrimal crest and posteriorly by the posterior lacrimal crest, and lodging the lacrimal sac. It is continuous below with the nasolacrimal canal.
s. lacrima′lis maxil′lae [TA] lacrimal groove in maxilla: the part of the lacrimal groove (sulcus lacrimalis) contributed by the frontal process of the maxilla.
s. lacrima′lis os′sis lacrima′lis [TA] lacrimal groove in lacrimal bone: the part of the lacrimal groove (sulcus lacrimalis) contributed by the lacrimal bone.
lateral bicipital s. s. bicipitalis lateralis.
lateral s. of cerebrum s. lateralis cerebri.
lateral s. of mesencephalon s. lateralis mesencephali.
lateral occipital sulci a group of irregular sulci that divide the lateral occipital gyri into upper and lower portions.
s. latera′lis ce′rebri [TA] lateral sulcus of cerebrum: a deep cleft beginning at the anterior perforated substance, extending laterally between the temporal and frontal lobes, and turning posteriorly between the temporal and parietal lobes. It divides into posterior, ascending, and anterior branches. Called also *Sylvius s. or fissure* and *sylvian s.* or *fissure.*
s. latera′lis mesence′phali [TA] lateral groove of mesencephalon: a longitudinal groove on the side of the mesencephalon, separating the crus cerebri from the tegmentum.
s. li′mitans 1. [TA] a longitudinal groove on the lateral side of the medial eminence, extending the entire length of the floor of the fourth ventricle. 2. a groove midway on the inner surface of each lateral wall

of the neural tube, which separates it into a dorsal, alar plate and a ventral, basal plate.
lunate s., s. luna'tus [TA] a small semilunar furrow sometimes seen on the lateral surface of the occipital lobe of the cerebrum.
malleolar s. of fibula s. malleolaris fibulae.
malleolar s. of temporal bone a groove that runs obliquely downward and forward across the inner aspect of the anterior tympanic ring, which lodges the anterior process of the malleus, chorda tympani, and anterior tympanic artery at birth.
malleolar s. of tibia s. malleolaris tibiae.
s. malleola'ris fi'bulae [TA] malleolar groove of fibula: a groove on the posterior surface of the lateral malleolus of the fibula, which lodges the tendons of the peroneus muscles.
s. malleola'ris ti'biae [TA] malleolar groove of tibia: a short longitudinal groove on the posterior surface of the medial malleolus of the tibia, which lodges the tendons of the posterior tibial muscle and the long flexor muscles of the toes.
marginal s. ramus marginalis sulci cinguli.
s. margina'lis TA alternative for *ramus marginalis sulci cinguli.*
s. ma'tricis un'guis groove of nail matrix.
medial bicipital s. s. bicipitalis medialis.
medial s. of mesencephalon s. nervi oculomotorii.
median s. of fourth ventricle s. medianus ventriculi quarti.
median s. of tongue s. medianus linguae.
s. media'nus lin'guae [TA] median sulcus of tongue: a shallow groove on the dorsal surface of the tongue in the midline.
s. media'nus poste'rior medul'lae oblonga'tae [TA] posterior median sulcus of medulla oblongata: a narrow groove present only in the closed part of the medulla oblongata, separating the two fasciculi graciles; it is the continuation of the posterior median sulcus of the spinal cord. Called also *dorsal* or *posterior median fissure of medulla oblongata* and *dorsal median s. of medulla oblongata.*
s. media'nus poste'rior medul'lae spina'lis [TA] posterior median sulcus of spinal cord: a shallow vertical groove on the posterior median surface of the spinal cord, separating the two posterior funiculi; the posterior median septum extends out from it. Called also *dorsal* or *posterior median fissure of spinal cord* and *dorsal median s. of spinal cord.*
s. media'nus ventri'culi quar'ti [TA] median sulcus of fourth ventricle: a median groove in the floor of the fourth ventricle.
medullopontine s. s. bulbopontinus.
mentolabial s., s. mentolabia'lis [TA] the skin furrow between the lower lip and the chin. Called also *mentolabial furrow.*
s. of Monro s. hypothalamicus.
s. mus'culi subcla'vii [TA] groove for subclavius: a groove on the inferior surface of the clavicle into which the subclavian muscle is inserted by muscle fibers. Called also *subclavian groove.*
mylohyoid s. of mandible, s. mylohyoi'deus mandi'bulae [TA] mylohyoid groove: a groove on the medial surface of the ramus of the mandible, passing downward and forward from the foramen mandibulae and lodging the mylohyoid artery and nerve.
nasolabial s., s. nasolabia'lis [TA] the skin furrow between the nose and the upper lip.
s. ner'vi oculomoto'rii [TA] oculomotor sulcus: a longitudinal groove on the medial surface of the anterior part of the cerebral peduncle that lodges the oculomotor nerve.
s. ner'vi petro'si majo'ris [TA] groove for greater petrosal nerve: a small groove sometimes present on the anterior surface of the petrous part of the temporal bone (the floor of the middle cranial fossa), running anteromedially from the hiatus of the facial canal to the foramen lacerum, and lodging the greater petrosal nerve.
s. ner'vi petro'si mino'ris [TA] groove for lesser petrosal nerve: a small groove on the anterior surface of the petrous part of the temporal bone (the floor of the middle cranial fossa), running anteromedially just lateral to the groove for the greater petrosal nerve, and lodging the lesser petrosal nerve. Called also *innominate canaliculus.*
s. ner'vi radia'lis [TA] groove for radial nerve: a broad oblique groove on the posterior surface of the humerus for the radial nerve and the deep brachial artery; called also *radial groove* and *spiral s.*
s. ner'vi spina'lis [TA] groove for spinal nerve: the groove on the upper surface of each transverse process of a cervical vertebra, extending from the foramen transversarium lateralward and separating the anterior and posterior tubercles. It lodges the anterior ramus of a cervical nerve.
s. ner'vi ulna'ris [TA] groove for ulnar nerve: a shallow vertical groove on the posterior surface of the medial epicondyle of the humerus for the ulnar nerve; called also *ulnar groove.*
obturator s., s. obturato'rius [TA] obturator groove: a groove that obliquely crosses the inferior surface of the superior ramus of the pubis, giving passage to the obturator vessels and nerve.
s. occipita'lis transver'sus [TA] transverse occipital sulcus: a vertical sulcus in back of the angular gyrus, which may help to form the anterior boundary of the occipital lobe or may lie within it.
occipitotemporal s., s. occipitotempora'lis [TA] a longitudinal sulcus on the inferior surface of the temporal lobe that separates the inferior temporal gyrus.
oculomotor s., s. for oculomotor nerve s. nervi oculomotorii.
s. olfacto'rius lo'bi fronta'lis [TA] olfactory sulcus of frontal lobe: a straight parasagittal sulcus on the inferior surface of the frontal lobe, lodging the olfactory bulb and tract, and separating the gyrus rectus from the gyri orbitales.
s. olfacto'rius na'si [TA] olfactory groove: a shallow sulcus on the wall of the nasal cavity, passing upward from the level of the anterior end of the middle concha just above the agger nasi to the lamina cribrosa.
olfactory s. of frontal lobe s. olfactorius lobi frontalis.
olfactory s. of nose s. olfactorius nasi.
optic s. s. prechiasmaticus.
orbital sulci of frontal lobe, sul'ci orbita'les lo'bi fronta'lis [TA] irregular sulci between the orbital gyri of the frontal lobe.
outer spiral s. s. spiralis externus.
s. palati'nus ma'jor maxil'lae [TA] greater palatine groove of maxilla: the sulcus on the nasal surface of the maxilla which, along with the corresponding one on the perpendicular plate of the palatine bone, forms the canal for the greater palatine nerve.
s. palati'nus ma'jor os'sis palati'ni [TA] greater palatine groove of palatine bone: a vertical groove on the maxillary surface of the perpendicular plate of the palatine bone; it articulates with the maxilla to form the canal for the greater palatine nerve.
sul'ci palati'ni maxil'lae [TA] palatine grooves of maxilla: the laterally placed furrows, between the palatine spines on the inferior surface of the hard palate, that lodge the palatine vessels and nerves.
s. palatovagina'lis [TA] palatovaginal groove: the groove on the vaginal process of the sphenoid bone that participates in formation of the palatovaginal canal.
paracolic sulci, sul'ci paraco'lici [TA] paracolic gutters: small, shallow, and variable peritoneal pockets found lateral to the descending colon; called also *paracolic recesses.*
parieto-occipital s., s. parietooccipita'lis [TA] a sulcus in the medial surface of each cerebral hemisphere, running upward from the calcarine sulcus and marking the boundary between the cuneus and precuneus, and also between the parietal and occipital lobes. Called also *parieto-occipital fissure.*
s. for pharyngotympanic tube s. tubae auditivae.
s. popli'teus fe'moris [TA] groove for popliteus: a smooth, well-marked groove separated from the lateral femoral condyle by a prominent lip and extending superiorly and posteriorly to the posterior extremity of the lateral condyle; it lodges the tendon of the popliteus muscle.
postcentral s. of cerebrum, s. postcentra'lis ce'rebri [TA] a sulcus on the superolateral surface of the cerebrum, separating the postcentral gyrus from the remainder of the parietal lobe.
s. poste'rior auri'culae [TA], **posterior auricular s.** posterior auricular groove: the slight depression on the pinna that separates the antihelix from the antitragus.
posterior intermediate s. of spinal cord s. intermedius posterior medullae spinalis.
posterior interventricular s. s. interventricularis posterior.
posterior lateral s. of medulla oblongata s. posterolateralis medullae oblongatae.
posterior lateral s. of spinal cord s. posterolateralis medullae spinalis.
posterior median s. of medulla oblongata s. medianus posterior medullae oblongatae.
posterior median s. of spinal cord s. medianus posterior medullae spinalis.
posterior parolfactory s. a curved sulcus on the medial surface of the cerebral hemisphere, below the splenium of the corpus callosum and between the gyrus paraterminalis and the area parolfactoria.

posterolateral s. of medulla oblongata s. posterolateralis medullae oblongatae.
posterolateral s. of spinal cord s. posterolateralis medullae spinalis.
s. posterolatera′lis medul′lae oblonga′tae [TA] posterolateral sulcus of medulla oblongata: an upward extension of the posterolateral sulcus of the spinal cord; it gives attachment to the fibers of the glossopharyngeal and vagus nerves. Called also *posterolateral groove of medulla oblongata* and *dorsolateral s. of medulla oblongata.*
s. posterolatera′lis medul′lae spina′lis [TA] posterolateral sulcus of spinal cord: a longitudinal sulcus on the posterolateral surface of the spinal cord; it gives entrance to the posterior nerve roots and separates the lateral and posterior funiculi. Called also *posterolateral groove of spinal cord* and *dorsolateral s. of spinal cord.*
preauricular s. of ilium a slight, rough groove, anterior and inferior to the auricular surface of the ilium, that serves for attachment of the lower fibers of the anterior sacroiliac ligament; it is more apparent in females.
precentral s. of cerebrum, s. precentra′lis ce′rebri [TA] a vertical sulcus on the convex surface of a cerebral hemisphere, separating the precentral gyrus from the remainder of the frontal lobe.
prechiasmatic s., s. prechiasma′ticus [TA] a furrow on the superior surface of the sphenoid bone, located just anterior to the tuberculum sellae; it lodges the optic chiasm. Called also *chiasmatic s., s. chiasmatis, optic groove,* and *optic s.*
s. promonto′rii tym′pani [TA] groove of promontory of tympanic cavity: a groove in the surface of the promontory of tympanic cavity, lodging the tympanic nerve.
s. of pterygoid hamulus s. hamuli pterygoidei.
s. pulmona′lis [TA], **pulmonary s.** a large vertical groove in the posterior part of the thoracic cavity, one on either side of the bodies of the vertebrae posterior to the level of their ventral surface, lodging the posterior, bulky portion of the lung.
s. for radial nerve s. nervi radialis.
s. retrooliva′ris [TA] retro-olivary groove: a groove running longitudinally across the posterolateral surface of the upper medulla oblongata just behind the olive; it is the forward continuation of the sulcus posterolateralis medullae oblongatae.
rhinal s., s. rhina′lis [TA] a fissure on the inferior surface of the cerebral hemisphere, separating the anterior part of the parahippocampal gyrus from the rest of the temporal lobe.
sagittal s. s. sinus sagittalis superioris.
s. scle′rae [TA], **scleral s., sclerocorneal s.** the groove at the junction of the sclera and cornea.
sigmoid s., s. for sigmoid sinus s. sinus sigmoidei.
s. si′nus margina′lis [TA] groove for marginal sinus: a groove next to the foramen magnum on the inner surface of the occipital bone, lodging part of the marginal sinus.
s. si′nus occipita′lis [TA] groove for occipital sinus: a groove in the occipital bone that lodges the occipital sinus.
s. si′nus petro′si inferio′ris [TA] groove for inferior petrosal sinus: a groove continuous across the temporal and occipital bones, lodging the inferior petrosal sinus; it is located on the posteromedial edge of the internal surface of the petrous portion of the temporal bone and on the adjacent basilar part of the occipital bone.
s. si′nus petro′si superio′ris [TA] groove for superior petrosal sinus: a small posterolaterally directed sulcus that runs along the internal surface of the petrous part of the temporal bone on the angle separating the posterior and middle cranial fossae; it lodges the superior petrosal sinus.
s. si′nus sagitta′lis supe′rioris [TA] groove for superior sagittal sinus: a groove on the internal surface of the frontal, parietal, and occipital bones that lodges the superior sagittal sinus; called also *sagittal groove* and *sagittal s.*
s. si′nus sigmoi′dei [TA] groove for sigmoid sinus: an S-shaped sulcus beginning on the internal surface of the posteroinferior edge of the parietal bone and continuous with the lateral end of the groove for transverse sinus; it passes onto the internal surface of the mastoid part of the temporal bone, where it bends inferiorly and medially to continue onto the lateral portion of the occipital bone, ending at the jugular foramen. It lodges the sigmoid sinus.
s. si′nus transver′si [TA] groove for transverse sinus: a wide groove that passes horizontally, laterally, and anteriorly from the internal occipital protuberance to the parietal bone, where it becomes continuous with the sulcus of the sigmoid sinus; it lodges the transverse sinus.
skin sulci sulci cutis.
s. for spinal nerve s. nervi spinalis.
spiral s. 1. see *s. spiralis externus* and *s. spiralis internus.* 2. s. nervi radialis.
s. spira′lis exter′nus [TA] external spiral sulcus: a concavity within the cochlear duct immediately above the basilar crest. Called also *outer spiral s.*
s. spira′lis inter′nus [TA] internal spiral sulcus: the C-shaped concavity within the cochlear duct formed by the limbus laminae spiralis and its tympanic and vestibular labia along the edge of the osseous spiral lamina. Called also *inner spiral s.*
subclavian s. 1. s. arteriae subclaviae. 2. s. musculi subclavii. 3. s. venae subclaviae. 4. groove for subclavian artery (def. 2).
subparietal s., s. subparieta′lis [TA] a sulcus on the medial surface of a cerebral hemisphere, above the splenium of the corpus callosum, separating the precuneus from the cingulate gyrus.
superior frontal s. s. frontalis superior.
superior occipital sulci irregular sulci associated with the superior occipital gyri.
superior petrosal s., s. for superior petrosal sinus s. sinus petrosi superioris.
superior temporal s. s. temporalis superior.
s. supraacetabula′ris [TA] supra-acetabular groove: a sulcus located posterosuperior to the margin of the acetabulum, which is the site of attachment of the reflected head of the rectus femoris muscle.
supraorbital s. foramen supraorbitale.
suprapalpebral s., s. suprapalpebra′lis [TA] the skin furrow above the upper eyelid.
suprasplenial s. s. subparietalis.
sylvian s., Sylvius s. s. lateralis cerebri.
s. ta′li [TA], **s. of talus** a transverse groove on the inferior surface of the talus, between the medial and the posterior articular surface, which helps to form the sinus tarsi.
s. tempora′lis infe′rior [TA] inferior temporal sulcus: a longitudinal sulcus on the lateral surface of the temporal lobe, separating the middle and the inferior temporal gyri.
s. tempora′lis supe′rior [TA] superior temporal sulcus: a longitudinal sulcus on the lateral surface of a cerebral hemisphere, passing posteriorly from the temporal pole, separating the superior and the middle temporal gyri and ending in the gyrus angularis.
s. tempora′lis transver′sus [TA] transverse temporal sulcus: an irregularly vertical sulcus in the part of the temporal lobe that lies within the lateral sulcus; sometimes occurring as a pair.
s. ten′dinis mus′culi fibula′ris lon′gi [TA] groove for tendon of fibularis longus: a deep groove on the inferior surface of the cuboid bone, which in certain foot positions lodges the tendon of the peroneus longus muscle; called also *s. tendinis musculi peronei longi* [TA alternative] and *groove for tendon of peroneus longus.*
s. ten′dinis mus′culi flexo′ris hal′lucis lon′gi [TA] groove for tendon of flexor hallucis longus: a groove running successively across the posterior surface of the body of the talus and the inferior surface of the sustentaculum tali of the calcaneus, lodging the tendon of the flexoris hallucis longus muscle.
s. ten′dinis mus′culi perone′i lon′gi TA alternative for *s. tendinis musculi fibularis longi.*
terminal s. of heart s. terminalis cordis.
terminal s. of tongue s. terminalis linguae.
s. termina′lis cor′dis [TA] a shallow groove on the external surface of the right atrium of the heart between the superior and inferior venae cavae; it represents the junction of the sinus venosus with the primitive atrium in the embryo, and corresponds to a ridge on the internal surface, the crista terminalis.
s. termina′lis lin′guae [TA] terminal sulcus of tongue: a more or less distinct groove on the tongue, extending from the foramen cecum anteriorly and lateralward to the margin of the tongue on either side, and dividing the dorsum of the tongue from the root. It is marked by a row of vallate papillae.
transverse s. of antihelix s. anthelicis transversus.
transverse occipital s. sulcus occipitalis transversus.
s. for transverse sinus s. sinus transversi.
transverse temporal s. s. temporalis transversus.

Sulcus *Continued*

s. tu′bae auditi′vae [TA] sulcus for pharyngotympanic tube: a groove on the medial part of the base of the spine of the sphenoid bone; it lodges a portion of the cartilaginous part of the pharyngotympanic tube. Called also *s. tubae auditoriae* [TA alternative], and *groove* or *s. for auditory tube.*

s. tu′bae audito′riae TA alternative for *s. tubae auditivae.*

s. tympa′nicus os′sis tempora′lis [TA] tympanic sulcus of temporal bone: a narrow groove in the medial part of the external acoustic meatus of the temporal bone, into which the tympanic membrane fits; it is deficient above.

s. for ulnar nerve s. nervi ulnaris.

s. for vena cava, s. ve′nae ca′vae [TA] groove for vena cava: a groove on the posterior part of the diaphragmatic surface of the liver, separating the right lobe from the caudate lobe and lodging the inferior vena cava.

s. ve′nae subcla′viae [TA] groove for subclavian vein: a transverse groove on the cranial surface of the first rib, just anterior to the anterior scalene tubercle; it lodges the subclavian vein.

sul′ci veno′si [TA] venous grooves: grooves on the internal surfaces of the cranial bones for the meningeal veins.

ventrolateral s. of medulla oblongata s. anterolateralis medullae oblongatae.

ventrolateral s. of spinal cord s. anterolateralis medullae spinalis.

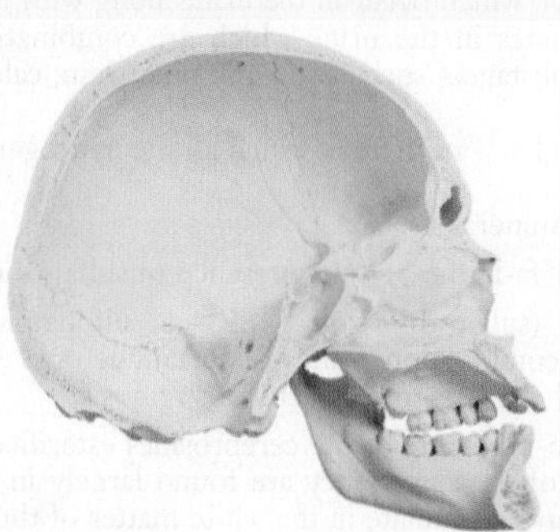

■ Sulci venosi (venous sulci) in an interior view of a sagittal section of the skull.

s. vo′meris [TA] vomerine groove: the cleft in the inferior half on the anterior border of the vomer that receives the inferior border of the septal cartilage of the nose.

s. vomerovagina′lis [TA] vomerovaginal groove: the groove on the vaginal process of the sphenoid bone that helps form the vomerovaginal canal.

sul•fa (sul′fə) of, related to, or containing sulfanilamide or other sulfonamide.

triple s. [USP] a combination of sulfathiazole, sulfacetamide, and sulfabenzamide, administered intravaginally in the treatment of bacterial vaginosis caused by *Gardnerella vaginalis.*

sul•fa•benz•a•mide (sul″fə-ben′zə-mīd) [USP] a sulfonamide antibacterial having properties similar to those of sulfamethoxazole; used topically in combination with sulfacetamide and sulfathiazole (as triple sulfa) in the treatment of bacterial vaginosis.

sul•fa•cet•a•mide (sul″fə-set′ə-mīd) [USP] a sulfonamide which has been used in the treatment of bacterial vaginosis.

s. sodium [USP] the sodium salt monohydrate of sulfacetamide, applied topically to the conjunctiva in the treatment of sulfonamide-responsive eye infections and to the skin in the treatment of acne vulgaris.

Sul•fa•cet-R (sul′fə-set) trademark for preparations of sulfacetamide sodium.

sul•fa•chlor•pyr•id•a•zine (sul″fə-klor″pir-id′ə-zēn) [USP] a sulfonamide used as an antibacterial in the treatment of veterinary enteric infections.

sulf•ac•id (səlf-as′id) thio acid.

sul•fa•cy•tine (sul″fə-si′tēn) a short-acting sulfonamide, used orally in the treatment of acute urinary tract infections.

sul•fa•di•a•zine (sul″fə-di′ə-zēn) [USP] a sulfonamide used, frequently in combination with other sulfonamides, in the treatment of infections due to susceptible organisms, including nocardiosis, toxoplasmosis, otitis media caused by susceptible strains of *Haemophilus influenzae*, streptococci, and pneumococci, and falciparum malaria caused by chloroquine-resistant plasmodia. It is administered orally. See also under *silver.*

silver s. see under *silver.*

s. sodium [USP] the monosodium salt of sulfadiazine, having the same actions and uses as the base; administered intravenously.

sul•fa•di•me•thox•ine (sul″fə-di″mə-thok′sēn) [USP] a long-acting sulfonamide, used as a veterinary antibacterial in a variety of infections; administered orally.

sul•fa•di•mi•dine (sul″fə-di′mĭ-dēn) INN and BAN for *sulfamethazine.*

sul•fa•dox•ine (sul″fə-dok′sēn) a long-acting sulfonamide used in combination with pyrimethamine in the prophylaxis and treatment of chloroquine-resistant falciparum malaria.

sul•fa•fu•ra•zole (sul″fə-fu′rə-zōl) INN and BAN for *sulfisoxazole.*

sul•fa•mer•a•zine (sul″fə-mer′ə-zēn) a readily absorbed sulfonamide antibacterial usually used in combination with other sulfonamides.

sul•fa•meth•a•zine (sul″fə-meth′ə-zēn) [USP] a sulfonamide used as an antibacterial in a variety of infections, usually in combination with other sulfonamides; administered orally. Called also *sulfadimidine.*

sul•fa•meth•i•zole (sul″fə-meth′ĭ-zōl) a sulfonamide used as an antibacterial, sometimes in combination with other antibacterials, in the treatment of urinary tract infections; administered orally.

sul•fa•meth•ox•a•zole (sul″fə-məth-ok′sə-zōl) [USP] a sulfonamide used as an antibacterial active against various gram-negative and gram-positive organisms, especially for the treatment of acute urinary tract infections, and as an antiprotozoal; administered orally, usually in combination with another agent such as trimethoprim.

sul•fam•i•do (səl-fam′ĭ-do) one of a group of compounds containing an aminosulfone group, $SO_2{\bullet}NH_2$.

sul•fam•ine (səl-fam′in) the univalent radical, $—SO_2NH_2$.

Sul•fa•my•lon (sul″fə-mi′lon) trademark for preparations of mafenide.

sul•fa•nil•a•mide (sul″fə-nil′ə-mīd) a potent antibacterial compound, the first of the sulfonamides discovered. Formerly used in the treatment of various infections, it has been replaced as a systemic agent by more effective and less toxic derivatives, and by antibiotics; it is still used vaginally in the treatment of vulvovaginal candidiasis.

sul•fan•i•late (səl-fan′ĭ-lāt) a salt of sulfanilic acid.

sul•fa•nil•ic ac•id (sul″fə-nil′ik) a white crystalline compound whose diazotized form (diazobenzenesulfonic acid) is used in Ehrlich diazo reaction.

sul•fa•ni•tran (sul″fə-ni′tran) an antibacterial sulfonamide and coccidiostat for poultry.

sul•fa•pyr•i•dine (sul″fə-pir′ĭ-dēn) [USP] a sulfonamide antibacterial used as an oral suppressant for dermatitis herpetiformis.

sul•fa•quin•ox•a•line (sul″fə-kwin-ok′sə-lēn) [USP] a sulfonamide used as a coccidiostat for poultry; administered orally or as a feed additive.

sul•fa•sal•a•zine (sul″fə-sal′ə-zēn) [USP] an antibacterial sulfonamide used orally or rectally in the prophylaxis and treatment of inflammatory bowel disease, and orally as a disease-modifying antirheumatic drug in the treatment of rheumatoid arthritis.

sul•fa•tase (sul′fə-tās) 1. a term used in the recommended and trivial names for the sulfuric ester hydrolases [EC 3.1.6], which catalyze the cleavage of inorganic sulfate from sulfate esters to form alcohols. 2. arylsulfatase.

multiple s. deficiency an autosomal recessive lysosomal storage disease caused by a mutation in the *SUMF1* gene (locus: 3p26), which encodes a factor necessary for catalytic activity of eukaryotic sulfatases, resulting in deficiency of at least nine lysosomal and microsomal sulfatases and leading to accumulation of sulfate-containing glycolipids, mucopolysaccharides, and steroids. The disorder generally manifests as metachromatic leukodystrophy and later also shows features of mucopolysaccharidoses, variably combining phenotypic features of the specific enzymatic defects. Neurologic deterioration is rapid. Called also *mucosulfatidosis.*

sul•fate (sul′fāt) [L. *sulphas*] any salt of sulfuric acid. For specific salts, see entries under the adjectival form, e.g., for *ferrous sulfate,* see under *ferrous.*

acid s. a sulfate in which only one half of the hydrogen of the sulfuric acid is replaced; a bisulfate.

basic s. a sulfate in which the normal sulfate of the base is combined with a hydroxide of the same base; a subsulfate.

conjugated s's, ethereal s's aromatic substances, such as phenol, skatoxyl, and indoxyl, which occur in the urine along with mineral sulfates.

mineral s's sulfates in the urine which are combinations of sulfuric acid with mineral substances such as sodium, potassium, calcium, and magnesium.

neutral s., normal s. a sulfate in which all the hydrogen of the sulfuric acid is replaced.

preformed s's mineral s's.

sul•fa•temia (sul″fə-te′me-ə) the presence of sulfates in the blood.

sul•fa•thi•a•zole (sul″fə-thi′ə-zōl) [USP] a sulfonamide antibacterial used topically in combination with sulfacetamide and sulfabenzamide (as triple sulfa) in the treatment of bacterial vaginosis.

sul•fa•tide (sul′fə-tīd) any of the cerebrosides esterified with a sulfate residue at the C-6 of the sugar; they are found largely in the medullated nerve fibers, and may accumulate in the white matter of the brain in metachromatic leukodystrophy.

sul•fa•tion (sul-fa′shən) addition of a sulfate group to a molecule.

Sul•fa•trim (sul′fə-trim″) trademark for combination preparations of trimethoprim and sulfamethoxazole.

sul•faz•a•met (səl-faz′ə-met) a veterinary sulfonamide antibacterial.

sulf•he•mo•glo•bin (sulf″he′mo-glo″bin) sulfmethemoglobin.

sulf•he•mo•glo•bin•emia (sulf″he″mo-glo″bin-e′me-ə) the presence of sulfmethemoglobin in the blood; the most significant symptom is cyanosis. It usually results from excessive exposure to sulfur-containing drugs or other chemicals.

sulf•hy•drate (səlf-hi′drāt) the HS^- anion or a salt containing this ion.

sulf•hy•dryl (səlf-hi′drəl) the univalent radical, —SH.

sul•fide (sul′fīd) any binary compound of sulfur; a compound of sulfur with another element or radical or base.

sul•fin•ic ac•id (səl-fin′ik) an organic compound containing an $—SO_2H$ group bonded to a carbon atom.

sul•fin•py•ra•zone (sul″fin-pi′rə-zōn) [USP] a sulfoxide analogue of phenylbutazone, used as a uricosuric agent in treatment of gout; administered orally. It also prolongs platelet survival and inhibits platelet adherence to subendothelial cells and prostaglandin synthesis and has been studied as an antithrombotic agent.

sul•fi•nyl (sul′fĭ-nəl) the bivalent radical, —SO—.

sul•fi•sox•a•zole (sul″fə-sok′sə-zōl) [USP] a short-acting sulfonamide used as an antibacterial in the treatment of a wide variety of infections, particularly of the urinary tract; administered orally. Called also *sulfafurazole.*

s. acetyl [USP] a tasteless derivative of sulfisoxazole having the same actions and uses as the base; usually used in infants and children; administered orally.

s. diolamine the diethanolamine salt of sulfisoxazole having the same actions as the base; administered topically in the treatment of susceptible eye infections.

sul•fite (sul′fīt) [L. *sulfis*] any salt of sulfurous acid.

sul•fite ox•i•dase (sul′fīt ok′sĭ-dās) [EC 1.8.3.1] an enzyme of the oxidoreductase class that catalyzes the final reaction in the degradation of sulfur-containing amino acids, oxidizing sulfite to sulfate; it also oxidizes and detoxifies sulfite and sulfur dioxide from exogenous sources. It is a mitochondrial molybdoenzyme that transfers electrons to cytochrome *c* via its b_5 heme. Deficiency of enzyme activity, due to defect in the enzyme protein or to molybdenum cofactor deficiency (q.v.), results in progressive neurologic abnormalities, lens dislocation, and mental retardation.

sulf•met•he•mo•glo•bin (sulf″mət-he′mo-glo″bin) hemoglobin with a sulfur atom on one of its porphyrin rings, so that it is ineffective for transporting oxygen and has a green color; see *sulfhemoglobinemia.* Called also *sulfhemoglobin.*

sulf(o)- [*sulfur*] a prefix used in naming chemical compounds, indicating the presence of divalent sulfur or of the group SO_2OH.

sul•fo•bro•mo•phthal•ein so•di•um (sul″fo-bro″mo-thal′ēn) a water-soluble triphenylmethane derivative bound by plasma proteins and excreted by the liver, used in liver function tests.

sul•fo•con•ju•ga•tion (sul″fo-kon″jə-ga′shən) the formation of conjugated sulfates; see under *sulfate.*

sul•fo•cy•a•nate (sul″fo-si′ə-nāt) thiocyanate.

sul•fo•cy•an•ic ac•id (sul″fo-si-an′ic) thiocyanic acid.

sul•fo•gel (sul′fo-jel) a gel in which sulfuric acid is the medium instead of water.

***N*-sul•fo•glu•cos•amine sul•fo•hy•dro•lase** (sul″fo-gloo-kōs′ə-mēn sul″fo-hi′dro-lās) [EC 3.10.1.1] an enzyme of the hydrolase class that catalyzes the cleavage of sulfate groups from the amino groups of sulfated glucosamine residues. The enzyme may be identical with *heparan N-sulfatase* (q.v.).

sul•fo•hy•drate (sul″fo-hi′drāt) sulfhydrate.

sul•fo•lip•id (sul″fo-lip′id) any lipid carrying a sulfate residue on its polar head group, usually a sphingolipid or steroid derivative.

sul•fo•litho•cho•lyl•gly•cine (sul″fo-lith″o-ko″ləl-gli′sēn) a bile salt, the sulfate ester at C-3 of lithocholylglycine.

sul•fo•litho•cho•lyl•tau•rine (sul″fo-lith″o-ko″ləl-taw′rēn) a bile salt, the sulfate ester at C-3 of lithocholyltaurine.

sul•fol•y•sis (səl-fol′ĭ-sis) [*sulfo-* + *-lysis*] a double decomposition, similar to hydrolysis, but in which sulfuric acid takes the place of water.

sul•fo•mu•cin (sul″fo-mu′sin) a mucin containing sulfated carbohydrate groups.

sul•fon•a•mide (səl-fon′ə-mīd) 1. an organic compound containing the $—SO_2NH_2$ group. 2. any of a class of drugs, the sulfa drugs, which are derivatives of sulfanilamide, competitively inhibiting folic acid synthesis in microorganisms and formerly bacteriostatic against gram-positive cocci (streptococci and pneumococci), gram-negative cocci (meningococci and gonococci), gram-negative bacilli (*Escherichia coli* and shigellae), a wide variety of other bacteria, and some protozoa. Because many strains of bacteria have developed resistance to sulfonamides, particularly to agents used singly, they have largely been supplanted by more effective and less toxic antibiotics, and when used are generally combined with another sulfonamide or other antimicrobial agent.

sul•fo•nate (sul′fo-nāt) a salt, ester, or anion of a sulfonic acid.

sul•fone (sul′fōn) 1. the radical SO_2. 2. any compound containing two hydrocarbon radicals attached to the radical SO_2, especially dapsone (4,4′-sulfonylbisbenzenamine) and its derivatives, which are potent antibacterials effective against many gram-positive and gram-negative organisms, and are widely used as leprostatics.

sul•fon•ic (səl-fon′ik) indicating chemical compounds containing the monovalent $—SO_2OH$ or $—SO_3H$ radical.

sul•fon•ic ac•id (səl-fon′ik) an organic compound having the formula RSO_2OH; used in synthesizing dyes and phenols.

sul•fo•nyl (sul′fo-nəl) the bivalent radical, $—SO_2—$.

sul•fo•nyl•urea (sul″fə-nəl-u-re′ə) any of a class of compounds that exert hypoglycemic activity by stimulating the islet tissue to secrete insulin; used to control hyperglycemia in patients with type 2 diabetes mellitus who cannot be treated solely by diet and exercise.

sul•fo•pro•tein (sul″fo-pro′tēn) any of a series of albumins containing loosely combined sulfur.

sul•fo•sa•lic•yl•ate (sul″fo-sə-lis′ĭ-lāt) a salt, anion, or ester of sulfosalicylic acid.

sul•fo•sal•i•cyl•ic ac•id (sul″fo-sal″ĭ-sil′ik) a protein precipitant used in qualitative tests for protein in urine and cerebrospinal fluid. See under *method.* Called also *salicylsulfonic acid.*

Sul•fose (sul′fōs) trademark for preparations of trisulfapyrimidines.

sul•fo•sol (sul′fo-sol) a sol in which sulfuric acid is the dispersion medium.

sul•fo•trans•fer•ase (sul″fo-trans′fər-ās) [EC 2.8.2] any member of a sub-subclass of enzymes of the transferase class that catalyze the transfer of a sulfate group.

sul•fox•i•da•tion (səl-fok″sĭ-da′shən) the addition of an oxygen atom to the sulfur atom of an organic compound of the form R—S—R or R—R—S to form a sulfoxide; in the liver, it is an important reaction, mediated by hepatic microsomal enzymes, in the metabolism of sulfur-containing compounds.

sul•fox•ide (səl-fok′sīd) 1. the bivalent radical ═SO. 2. any compound consisting of two organic radicals attached to the ═SO radical.

sul•fox•ism (səl-fok′siz-əm) sulfuric acid poisoning.

sul•fox•one so•di•um (səl-fok′sōn) an antibacterial derivative of dapsone having actions similar to those of the parent compound; used primarily as a leprostatic in the treatment of lepromatous and tuberculoid leprosy, administered orally.

Sul•fox•yl (sul-fok′sil) trademark for combination preparations of benzoyl peroxide and sulfur.

sul•fur (S) (sul′fər) [L.] a nonmetallic element existing in many allotropic forms; atomic number, 16; atomic weight, 32.064. It occurs in protein, being a constituent of the amino acids cysteine and methionine.

Sulfur is a laxative and diaphoretic and is used in diseases of the skin; it formerly was used for a variety of other medicinal purposes.

s. 35 a radioactive isotope of sulfur, atomic mass 35, having a half-life of 87.51 days and decaying by emission of beta particles (0.167 MeV); it has been used in the determination of extracellular fluid volume; administered intravenously.

colloidal s. sulfur in a state of extremely fine division.

s. dioxide [NF] a colorless, nonflammable, water soluble gas, SO_2, with a strong, irritating odor; used as an antioxidant in pharmaceutical preparations. It is also an important air pollutant, irritating to the eyes and respiratory tract, usually the product of incomplete combustion of coal, oil, and gasoline. Called also *sulfurous anhydride.*

flowers of s. sublimed s.

s. hydride H_2S, a poisonous gas having the smell of rotten eggs.

s. monochloride a lacrimating war gas, S_2Cl_2.

precipitated s. [USP] a form of sulfur obtained by adding acid to a solution containing a polysulfide and a thiosulfate; used topically as a scabicide, and also used in various dermatologic formulations for its antiparasitic, antibacterial, antifungal, and keratolytic effects.

sublimed s. [USP] a form of sulfur obtained by subliming elemental sulfur and condensing the vapor. It has been used topically as a scabicide and parasiticide. Called also *flowers of s.*

sul·fu·rat·ed (sul′fu-rāt″əd) combined or charged with sulfur.

sul·fu·ret·ted (sul′fu-ret″əd) sulfurated.

sul·fur·ic ac·id (səl-fūr′ik) a strong mineral acid, H_2SO_4, that is a strong oxidizing agent and is extremely corrosive to skin and mucous membranes; concentrated sulfuric acid can cause severe skin burns.

sul·fu·rize (sul′fu-rīz) to cause to combine with sulfur.

sul·fur·ous ac·id (səl-fūr′əs) the chemical species H_2SO_3, which is formed in aqueous solutions of sulfur dioxide, SO_2; its salts are sulfites.

sul·fur·trans·fer·ase (sul″fər-trans′fər-ās) [EC 2.8.1] any member of the sub-subclass of enzymes of the transferase class that catalyze the transfer of sulfur atoms.

sul·fu·ryl (sul′fu-rəl) the radical SO_2.

sul·fy·dryl (səl-fi′drəl) sulfhydryl.

sul·in·dac (səl-in′dak) [USP] a nonsteroidal antiinflammatory drug used in the treatment of osteoarthritis, rheumatoid arthritis, ankylosing spondylitis, bursitis or tendinitis of the shoulder, and acute attacks of gout or calcium pyrophosphate deposition disease.

su·lis·o·ben·zone (sə-lis″o-ben′zōn) a benzophenone compound used as a topical sunscreen; it absorbs UVB and some UVA rays.

sulph- for words beginning thus, see those beginning *sulf-*.

sul·pi·ride (sul′pĭ-rīd) a substituted benzamide that is a dopamine antagonist, used as an antidepressant and antipsychotic in the treatment of schizophrenia and other psychoses; administered orally and intramuscularly.

Sul·trin (sul′trin) trademark for a preparation of triple sulfa.

Sulz·ber·ger-Gar·be syndrome (sulz′bər-gər gahr′be) [Marion Baldur *Sulzberger*, American dermatologist, 1895–1983; William *Garbe*, Canadian dermatologist, 20th century] exudative discoid and lichenoid dermatitis.

sum. [L.] su′mat (let him take); sumen′dum (to be taken).

su·mac (soo′mak) any of various species of *Rhus*.

poison s., swamp s. *Rhus vernix*.

su·ma·trip·tan suc·ci·nate (soo″mə-trip′tan) a selective serotonin receptor agonist used in the acute treatment of migraine and cluster headaches; administered orally, subcutaneously, or intranasally.

sum·ma·tion (sə-ma′shən) [L. *summa* total] the cumulative effects of a number of stimuli applied to a muscle, nerve, or reflex arc.

central s. the condition in which successive subliminal stimuli accumulate in a reflex center until they finally produce a reflex discharge.

sum·mit (sum′it) [L. *summus*, superlative of *superus*] apex.

s. of bladder, s. of urinary bladder apex vesicae urinariae.

Sum·ner sign (sum′nər) [Franklin W. *Sumner*, British surgeon, 20th century] see under *sign*.

Su·my·cin (soo-mi′sin) trademark for preparations of tetracycline hydrochloride.

sun·block (sun′blok″) a topical protective agent, such as one containing zinc oxide or titanium dioxide, that prevents sunlight from reaching the skin; the term is often used interchangeably with *sunscreen*.

sun·burn (sun′burn″) a type of radiation burn to the skin, with erythema, tenderness, and sometimes blistering, following excessive exposure to sunlight; it is produced by ultraviolet rays that are not filtered out by clouds or water. Persons with lighter-colored skin are usually more susceptible.

SUNCT short-lasting unilateral neuralgiform headache attacks with conjunctival injection and tearing.

Sun·Dare (sun′dār) trademark for preparations of cinoxate.

sun·down·ing (sun′doun-ing) confusion, agitation, and other severely disruptive behavior coupled with inability to remain asleep, occurring solely or markedly worsening at night; sometimes seen in older patients with dementia or other mental disorders.

su·ni·ti·nib mal·ate (soo-nĭ′tĭ-nib) a tyrosine kinase inhibitor used in treatment for advanced renal cell carcinoma and gastrointestinal stromal tumor; administered orally.

sun·screen (sun′skrēn″) a topical agent that protects the skin from the effects of the sun's rays, either absorbing ultraviolet radiation or by reflecting the incident light, or both. Called also *solar screen* or *sun screen*. The term is often used interchangeably with *sunblock*.

sun·stroke (sun′strōk″) insolation, or thermic fever; a condition produced by exposure to the sun, and marked by convulsions, coma, and a high temperature of the skin. Cf. *heat exhaustion* and *heat stroke*.

super- [L. *super* above] a prefix meaning above, more than normal, excessive, or next above in rank. Cf. *hyper-*.

su·per·ab·duc·tion (soo″pər-əb-duk′shən) extreme or excessive abduction.

su·per·ac·id (soo″pər-as′id) excessively acid.

su·per·acid·i·ty (soo″pər-ə-sid′ĭ-te) excessive acidity.

su·per·acro·mi·al (soo″pər-ə-kro′me-əl) supra-acromial.

su·per·ac·tiv·i·ty (soo″pər-ak-tiv′ĭ-te) hyperactivity.

su·per·acute (soo″pər-ə-kūt′) extremely acute.

su·per·ag·o·nist (soo″pər-ag′ə-nist) a substance such as a drug or antibody that is an especially strong agonist and may elicit an immediate response when it enters the body.

su·per·al·i·men·ta·tion (soo″pər-al″ĭ-mən-ta′shən) therapeutic treatment by excessive feeding beyond the requirements of the appetite, done in treatment of wasting diseases. Called also *gavage*.

su·per·al·ka·lin·i·ty (soo″pər-al″kə-lin′ĭ-te) excessive alkalinity.

su·per·an·ti·gen (soo″pər-an′tĭ-jən) any of a group of powerful antigens occurring in various bacteria and viruses that binds outside of the normal T cell receptor site and is able to react with multiple T cell receptor molecules of a given β chain variable element, regardless of their α chain sequence, thus activating T cells nonspecifically. Included are staphylococcal enterotoxins and toxins causing toxic shock syndrome and exfoliative dermatitis.

su·per·au·ra·le (soo″pər-aw-ra′le) an anthropometric landmark, the highest point on the superior border of the helix of the ear.

su·per·car·bon·ate (soo″pər-kahr′bon-āt) bicarbonate.

su·per·cen·tral (soo″pər-sen′trəl) above or superior to a center.

su·per·cil·ia (soo″pər-sil′e-ə) [L., pl. of *supercilium*] 1. [TA] eyebrow (def. 2). 2. plural of *supercilium* (eyebrow, def. 1), i.e., the elevations upon which the hairs grow.

su·per·cil·i·ary (soo″pər-sil′e-ar-e) pertaining to the eyebrow.

su·per·cil·i·um (soo″pər-sil′e-əm) pl. *superci′lia* [L.] [TA] eyebrow (def. 1).

su·per·class (soo′pər-klas″) a taxonomic category that is sometimes used, subordinate to a phylum and superior to a class.

su·per·coil (soo′pər-koil) 1. a tertiary conformation characteristic of a DNA molecule with constrained ends, as a circular plasmid or closed loops of DNA in a chromosome; the molecule is over- or underwound, with the axis of the helix twisted upon itself. In negatively supercoiled DNA, the DNA axis twists in the direction opposite that of the normal helical turns, causing underwinding of the helix, while in positively supercoiled DNA, the DNA axis twists with the direction of the normal helical turns, causing overwinding. Supercoiling plays a role in a variety of processes, including replication, transcription, and recombination. Called also *superhelix*. 2. to form such a tertiary structure.

su·per·dis·ten·tion (soo″pər-dis-ten′shən) excessive distention.

su·per·duct (soo″pər-dukt′) [*super-* + *duct*] to carry up or elevate.

su·per·duc·tion (soo″pər-duk′shən) supraduction.

su·per·ego (soo″pər-e′go) [*super-* + *ego*] in psychoanalytic theory, the aspect of the personality acting as a monitor and evaluator of ego functioning, comparing it with an ideal standard (see *ego ideal*, under *ideal*) and including psychic functions expressed as social attitudes, self-criticism, and a concept of right and wrong (conscience or morality). Cf. *ego* and *id*.

su·per·ex·ten·sion (soo″pər-ək-sten′shən) hyperextension.

su·per·fam·i·ly (soo′pər-fam″ĭ-le) 1. a taxonomic category that is sometimes used, subordinate to an order and superior to a family.

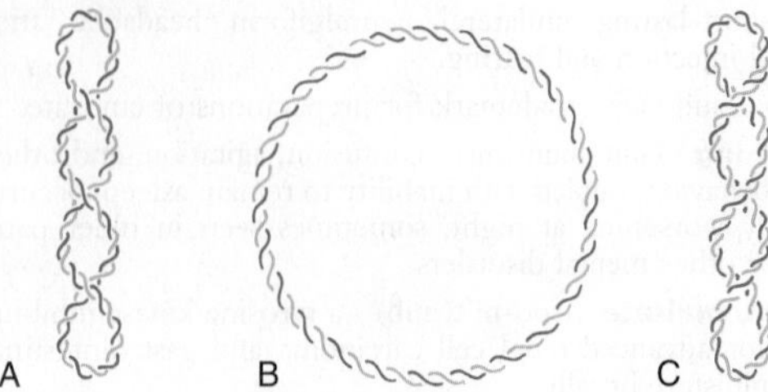

■ *(A)*, Positively supercoiled DNA; *(B)*, relaxed circle; *(C)*, negatively supercoiled DNA.

2. a group of proteins having similarities such as areas of structural homology and believed to descend from the same ancestral gene; e.g., integrins and immunoglobulins.

su·per·fe·cun·da·tion (soo″pər-fe″kən-da′shən) [*super-* + *fecundation*] fertilization of two or more oocytes during the same ovarian cycle by separate coital acts.

su·per·fe·ta·tion (soo″pər-fe-ta′shən) [*super-* + *fetation*] the fertilization and subsequent development of an oocyte when a fetus is already present in the uterus, a result of fertilization of oocytes during different ovarian cycles, yielding fetuses of different ages.

su·per·fi·cial (soo″pər-fish′əl) [L. *superficialis*] 1. pertaining to or situated near the surface. 2. external to the outermost layer of deep fascia.

su·per·fi·ci·a·lis (soo″pər-fish″e-a′lis) [TA] superficial; a term used to designate a structure situated closer than another to the surface of the body.

su·per·fi·ci·es (soo″pər-fish′e-ēz) [L.] an outer surface.

su·per·flex·ion (soo″pər-flek′shən) hyperflexion.

su·per·func·tion (soo″pər-funk′shən) hyperfunction.

su·per·fu·sate (soo″pər-fu′zāt) the fluid used for superfusion.

su·per·fuse (soo″pər-fūz′) [L. *superfundere* to pour over] to allow a fluid to drip or flow over the surface of an organ or tissue.

su·per·fu·sion (soo″pər-fu′zhən) the act or process of superfusing.

su·per·gen·u·al (soo″pər-jen′u-əl) superior to the knee.

su·per·group (soo′per-gro͞op) an unofficial designation for a group of viral serogroups that are related antigenically.

su·per·he·lix (soo″pər-he′liks) supercoil (def. 1).

su·per·im·preg·na·tion (soo″pər-im″preg-na′shən) [*super-* + *impregnation*] superfetation.

su·per·in·duce (soo″pər-in-do͞os′) to induce or bring on in addition to some already existing condition.

su·per·in·fec·tion (soo″pər-in-fek′shən) a new infection occurring in a patient having a preexisting one, such as bacterial superinfection in viral respiratory disease or infection of a chronic hepatitis B carrier with hepatitis D virus. Superinfection can complicate the course of antimicrobial therapy when the new infection is by organisms resistant to the drugs in use.

su·per·in·vo·lu·tion (soo″pər-in″vo-loo′shən) prolonged involution of the uterus after delivery, to a size much smaller than the normal, occurring in nursing mothers. Called also *hyperinvolution.*

su·pe·ri·or (soo-pēr′e-ər) [L. "upper"; neut. *superius*] 1. situated above, or directed upward. 2. [TA] a term used in reference to a structure occupying a position nearer the vertex.

su·per·ja·cent (soo″pər-ja′sənt) located immediately above; overlying.

su·per·lac·ta·tion (soo″pər-lak-ta′shən) hyperlactation.

su·per·lat·tice (soo′pər-lat″is) in a solid solution, an arrangement of atoms or molecules consisting of a lattice in which the different kinds of atoms or molecules have well-defined, regular locations with respect to each other.

su·per·le·thal (soo″pər-le′thəl) more than sufficient to cause death.

su·per·me·di·al (soo″pər-me′de-əl) superomedial.

su·per·mo·til·i·ty (soo″pər-mo-til′ĭ-te) hypermotility.

su·per·na·tant (soo″pər-na′tənt) [*super-* + L. *natare* to swim] 1. situated above or on top of something. 2. the overlying liquid after precipitation of a solid component of a system.

su·per·nate (soo′pər-nāt) supernatant (def. 2).

su·per·nor·mal (soo″pər-nor′məl) more than normal.

su·per·nu·mer·ary (soo″pər-noo′mər-ar″e) [L. *supernumerarius*] in excess of the regular or normal number.

su·per·nu·tri·tion (soo″pər-noo-trĭ′shən) excessive nutrition.

su·per·oc·cip·i·tal (soo″pər-ok-sip′ĭ-təl) supraoccipital.

su·pero·lat·er·al (soo″pər-o-lat′ər-əl) superior and at the side.

su·pero·me·di·al (soo″pər-o-me′de-əl) superior to the middle.

su·pero·tem·po·ral (so͞o″pər-o-tem′pərəl) supratemporal.

su·per·ov·u·la·tion (soo″pər-ov″u-la′shən) extraordinary acceleration of ovulation, producing a greater than normal number of oocytes, usually as a result of administration of exogenous gonadotropins.

su·per·ox·ide (soo″pər-ok′sīd) any compound containing the highly reactive superoxide radical, O_2^-, which is produced by reduction of molecular oxygen in many biological oxidations; this highly toxic free radical is continuously removed by the enzyme superoxide dismutase.

su·per·ox·ide dis·mu·tase (soo″pər-ok′sīd dis-mu′tās) [EC 1.15.1.1] an enzyme of the oxidoreductase class that catalyzes the reduction of superoxide anions to hydrogen peroxide, protecting cells against dangerous levels of superoxide.

su·per·par·a·site (soo″pər-par′ə-sīt) 1. a parasite involved in superparasitism. 2. hyperparasite.

su·per·par·a·sit·ism (soo″pər-par′ə-sit″iz-əm) 1. infestation with more parasites of one species than the host can support or bring to maturity. 2. hyperparasitic.

su·per·re·gen·e·ra·tion (soo″pər-re-jen″ə-ra′shən) the development of superfluous tissue, organs, or parts as a result of regeneration.

su·per·salt (soo′pər-sawlt) any salt obtained by reaction with an excess of acid; see *persalt* and *acid salt.*

su·per·sat·u·rate (soo″pər-sach′ər-āt) to add more of an ingredient than can be held in solution permanently.

su·per·scrip·tion (soo″pər-skrip′shən) [L. *superscriptio*] the heading of a prescription, i.e., the symbol ℞ or the word Recipe, meaning "take."

su·per·se·cre·tion (soo″pər-sə-kre′shən) excessive secretion.

su·per·sen·si·tiv·i·ty (soo″pər-sen″sĭ-tiv′ĭ-te) abnormally increased sensitivity; cf. *hypersensitivity.*

denervation s. increased sensitivity of a part to minor stimuli when its nerve supply is damaged or has its nutrient supply disrupted.

disuse s. increased activity of a neural pathway following chronic exposure to an antagonist drug caused by changes in postsynaptic receptors.

su·per·sen·si·ti·za·tion (soo″pər-sen″sĭ-tĭ-za′shən) hypersensitization.

su·per·soft (soo″pər-soft′) extremely soft; applied to x-rays of extremely long wavelengths, large absorption coefficients, and low penetrating power.

su·per·son·ic (soo″pər-son′ik) [*super-* + L. *sonus* sound] 1. having a speed greater than the velocity of sound, that is, faster than approximately one-fifth mile per second (or 720 miles an hour) in air. 2. ultrasonic.

su·per·son·ics (soo″pər-son′iks) the general science relating to phenomena associated with speed greater than the velocity of sound.

su·per·sphe·noid (soo″pər-sfe′noid) superior to the sphenoid bone.

su·per·struc·ture (soo′pər-struk″chər) 1. any structure built on something else. 2. the overlying or visible portion of a structure. 3. implant s.

implant s. a removable denture retained, supported, and stabilized by an abutment post protruding from the substructure of an implanted framework.

su·per·vas·cu·lar·iza·tion (soo″pər-vas″ku-lər-ĭ-za′shən) in radiotherapy, the relative increase in vascularity that occurs when tumor cells are destroyed so that the remaining tumor cells are better supplied by the (uninjured) capillary stroma.

su·per·ven·tion (soo″pər-ven′shən) the development of some condition in addition to an already existing one.

su·per·ver·sion (soo″pər-ver′zhən) sursumversion.

su·per·vis·or (soo′pər-vīz″ər) an individual who oversees the activities of others, such as a nurse who oversees the nursing activities in a specific ward or department of a hospital.

su·per·vi·ta·min·o·sis (soo″pər-vi″tə-min-o′sis) hypervitaminosis.

su·per·vol·tage (soo′pər-vōl″təj) in radiotherapy, voltage in the range of 500 kilovolts, as contrasted with orthovoltage (140 to 400 kilovolts) and megavoltage (greater than 1 megavolt).

su·pi·nate (soo′pĭ-nāt) to assume or place in a supine position.

su·pi·na·tion (soo″pĭ-na′shən) [L. *supinatio*] the act of assuming the supine position, or the state of being supine. Applied to the hand, the act of turning the palm forward (anteriorly) or upward, performed by lateral rotation of the forearm. Applied to the foot, it generally implies movements resulting in raising of the medial margin of the foot, hence of the longitudinal arch. Cf. *pronation.*

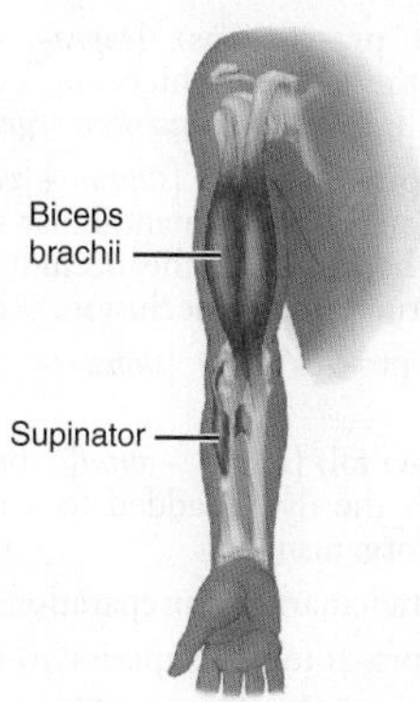

■ Supination: supinators contracted, the palm turned forward.

su•pi•na•tor (soo′pĭ-na-tər) 1. a muscle that serves to supinate. 2. musculus supinator.

su•pine (soo′pīn, soo-pīn′) [L. *supinus*] lying with the face upward.

sup•port (sə-port′) 1. to prevent weakening or failing. 2. a structure that bears the weight of something else. 3. a mechanism or arrangement that helps keep something else functioning. 4. the foundation upon which a denture rests.

extracorporeal life s. (ECLS) the provision of respiratory support by circulating the blood through an artificial lung consisting of two compartments separated by a gas-permeable membrane, with the blood on one side and the ventilating gas on the other; used in newborns and occasionally in adults with acute respiratory distress syndrome. Called also *extracorporeal membrane oxygenation.*

mechanical circulatory s. (MCS) the use of mechanical means, such as an intra-aortic balloon pump or a ventricular assist device, to help maintain the circulation in patients with heart failure.

sup•port•ive (sə-por′tiv) providing support or aid. See also *supportive treatment*, under *treatment*.

sup•pos•i•to•ry (sə-poz′ĭ-tor-e) [L. *suppositorium*] a medicated mass adapted for introduction into the rectal, vaginal, or urethral orifice of the body; suppository bases are solid at room temperature but melt or dissolve at body temperature. Commonly used bases are cocoa butter, glycerinated gelatin, hydrogenated vegetable oils, polyethylene glycols of various molecular weights, and fatty acid esters of polyethylene glycol.

Sup•prel•in (sə-prel′in) trademark for a preparation of histrelin acetate.

sup•pres•sant (sə-pres′ənt) 1. inducing suppression. 2. an agent that stops secretion, excretion, or normal discharge.

appetite s. anorectic (def. 2).

sup•pres•sion (sə-presh′ən) [L. *suppressus*, past part. of *supprimere* to hold back] 1. the act of holding back or checking. 2. sudden stoppage or inhibition, as of a secretion, excretion, normal discharge, or other function. 3. in psychiatry, conscious inhibition of an unacceptable impulse or idea as contrasted with repression, which is unconscious. 4. in genetics, masking of the phenotypic expression of a mutation by the occurrence of a second (suppressor) mutation at a different site from the first; the organism appears to be reverted but is in fact doubly mutant. Cf. *reversion* (def. 2). 5. cortical inhibition of perception of objects in all or part of the visual field of one eye during binocular vision.

bone marrow s. suppression of bone marrow activity, resulting in reduction in the number of platelets, red cells, and white cells, as in aplastic anemia or secondary to chemotherapy or radiation therapy. It may also be induced intentionally prior to bone marrow transplantation. See also *myeloablation*, and see *bone marrow failure*, under *failure*. Called also *myelosuppression*.

immune s. immunosuppression.

overdrive s. transient suppression of automaticity in a cardiac pacemaker following a period of stimulation by a more rapidly discharging pacemaker, proportional to the rate and duration of the dominating pacemaker. See also *overdrive pacing*, under *pacing*.

sup•pres•sor (sə-pres′ər) that which holds back or inhibits.

sup•pu•rant (sup′u-rənt) 1. suppurative (def. 1). 2. an agent that causes suppuration.

sup•pu•ra•tion (sup″u-ra′shən) [*sub-* + L. *puris* pus] 1. pyogenesis. 2. the act of becoming converted into and discharging pus.

alveodental s. periodontitis with the formation of pus.

sup•pu•ra•tive (sup′u-ra″tiv) characterized by suppuration; called also *purulent*.

supra- [L. "above"] a prefix signifying above or over.

su•pra•acro•mi•al (soo″prə-ə-kro′me-əl) above or over the acromion.

su•pra•anal (soo″prə-a′nəl) superior to the anus.

su•pra•au•ric•u•lar (soo″prə-aw-rik′u-lər) superior to the ear.

su•pra•ax•il•lary (soo″prə-ak′sĭ-lar″e) superior to the axilla.

su•pra•buc•cal (soo″prə-buk′əl) superior to the buccal region.

su•pra•bulge (soo′prə-bulj″) the surface or the crown of a tooth sloping toward the occlusal surface from the height of contour or survey line. Cf. *infrabulge*.

su•pra•ca•ri•nal (soo″prə-kə-ri′nəl) above the carina tracheae.

su•pra•ce•li•ac (soo″prə-se′le-ak) above the celiac trunk or plexus.

su•pra•cer•e•bel•lar (soo″prə-ser-ə-bel′ər) superior to or over the cerebellum.

su•pra•chi•as•mat•ic (soo″prə-ki-az-mat′ik) above the optic chiasm.

su•pra•cho•roid (soo″prə-kor′oid) superior to or over the choroid.

su•pra•cil•i•ary (soo″prə-sil′e-ar″e) superciliary.

su•pra•cla•vic•u•lar (soo″prə-klə-vik′u-lər) superior to the clavicle.

su•pra•cla•vic•u•la•ris (soo″prə-klə-vik″u-lar′is) [L.] supraclavicular.

su•pra•clu•sion (soo″prə-kloo′zhən) the condition in which the occluding surface of a tooth extends beyond the normal occlusal plane. Called also *overeruption* and *supraocclusion*.

su•pra•con•dy•lar (soo″prə-kon′də-lər) superior to a condyle or condyles.

su•pra•con•dy•loid (soo″prə-kon′də-loid) supracondylar.

su•pra•cos•tal (soo″prə-kos′təl) superior to or over a rib or ribs.

su•pra•cot•y•loid (soo″prə-kot′ə-loid) superior to the acetabulum.

su•pra•cra•ni•al (soo″prə-kra′ne-əl) on the superior surface of the cranium.

su•pra•di•a•phrag•mat•ic (soo″prə-di″ə-frag-mat′ik) superior to the diaphragm.

su•pra•duc•tion (soo″prə-duk′shən) [*supra-* + L. *duction*] 1. the upward rotation of an eye around its horizontal axis. 2. the upward rotation of one eye independent of the other by a basedown prism in testing for vertical divergence. See also *sursumversion*. Called also *superduction*, *sursumduction*, *supravergence*, and *sursumvergence*.

su•pra•epi•con•dy•lar (soo″prə-ep″ĭ-kon′də-lər) superior to an epicondyle.

su•pra•epi•troch•le•ar (soo″prə-ep″ĭ-trok′le-ər) superior to the medial epicondyle of the humerus.

su•pra•gin•gi•val (soo″prə-jin′jĭ-vəl) superior to the gingiva or to the gingival margin.

su•pra•gle•noid (soo″prə-gle′noid) superior to the glenoid cavity.

su•pra•glot•tic (soo″prə-glot′ik) 1. superior to the glottis. 2. pertaining to the supraglottis.

su•pra•glot•tis (soo″prə-glot′is) the area of the pharynx above the glottis as far as the epiglottis.

su•pra•glot•ti•tis (soo″prə-glŏ-ti′tis) inflammation of the supraglottis, most often as a result of infection with *Haemophilus influenzae* type B, but sometimes due to other bacterial, viral, or fungal infection or to thermal injury or other trauma; it is characterized by drooling, dysphagia, and swelling of the epiglottis that can progress to life-threatening upper airway obstruction. Called also *epiglottitis*.

su•pra•he•pat•ic (soo″prə-hə-pat′ik) superior to the liver.

su•pra•hy•oid (soo″prə-hi′oid) superior to the hyoid bone.

su•pra•in•gui•nal (soo″prə-ing′gwĭ-nəl) superior to the inguinal region, or groin.

su•pra•in•tes•ti•nal (soo″prə-in-tes′tĭ-nəl) superior to the intestine.

su•pra•lim•i•nal (soo″prə-lim′ĭ-nəl) above the limen of sensation; more than just perceptible.

su•pra•lum•bar (soo″prə-lum′bər, -bahr) superior to the loin or lumbar region.

su•pra•mal•le•o•lar (soo″prə-mə-le′o-lər) above a malleolus.

su•pra•mam•ma•ry (soo″prə-mam′ə-re) superior to a mammary gland.

su•pra•man•dib•u•lar (soo″prə-man-dib′u-lər) superior to the mandible.

su•pra•mar•gi•nal (soo″prə-mahr′jĭ-nəl) superior to a margin or border.

su•pra•mas•toid (soo″prə-mas′toid) superior to the mastoid process.

su•pra•max•il•lary (soo″prə-mak′sĭ-lar″e) superior to the maxilla.

su•pra•max•i•mal (soo″prə-mak′sĭ-məl) above the maximum.

su•pra•me•a•tal (soo″prə-me-a′təl) above a meatus.

su•pra•men•tal (soo″prə-men′təl) above the chin.

su•pra•men•ta•le (soo″prə-mən-ta′le) in radiographic cephalometry, the most posterior midline point in the concavity between the infradentale and pogonion, determined on the lateral head film.

su•pra•na•sal (soo″prə-na′səl) superior to the nose.

Sup•rane (soo′prān) trademark for a preparation of desflurane.

su•pra•nor•mal (soo″prə-nor′məl) greater than normal; present or occurring in excess of normal amounts or values.

su•pra•nu•cle•ar (soo″prə-noo′kle-ər) located or occurring superior to or on the cortical side of a nucleus in the nervous system.

su•pra•oc•cip•i•tal (soo″prə-ok-sip′ĭ-təl) above or in the superior portion of the occiput.

su•pra•oc•clu•sion (soo″prə-ŏ-kloo′zhən) supraclusion.

su•pra•oc•u•lar (soo″prə-ok′u-lər) superior to the eye.

su•pra•omo•hy•oid (soo″prə-o″mo-hi′oid) superior to the omohyoid muscle.

su•pra•op•tic (soo″prə-op′tik) superior to the optic chiasm.

su•pra•op•ti•mal (soo″prə-op′tĭ-məl) greater than optimal.

su•pra•op•ti•mum (soo″prə-op′tĭ-məm) a condition or quantity exceeding the optimum.

su•pra•or•bi•tal (soo″prə-or′bĭ-təl) superior to the orbit.

su•pra•pa•tel•lar (soo″prə-pə-tel′ər) superior to the patella.

su•pra•pel•vic (soo″prə-pel′vik) superior to the pelvis.

su•pra•phar•ma•co•log•ic (soo″prə-fahr″mə-ko-loj′ik) much greater than the usual therapeutic dose or pharmacologic concentration of a drug.

su•pra•phys•i•o•log•i•cal (soo″prə-fiz″e-o-loj′ĭ-kəl) [*supra-* + *physiological*] pertaining to an abnormal or artificially created state in which a naturally occurring substance is at a concentration greater than that occurring naturally.

su•pra•pon•tine (soo″prə-pon′tīn) above or in the upper part of the pons.

su•pra•pu•bic (soo″prə-pu′bik) superior to the pubic arch.

su•pra•re•nal (soo″prə-re′nəl) [*supra-* + *renal*] 1. superior to a kidney. 2. adrenal (def. 1).

su•pra•re•nal•ec•to•my (soo″prə-re″nəl-ek′tə-me) adrenalectomy.

su•pra•re•nal•ism (soo″prə-re′nəl-iz-əm) adrenalism.

su•pra•scap•u•lar (soo″prə-skap′u-lər) above or on the upper part of the scapula.

su•pra•scle•ral (soo″prə-sklēr′əl) on the outer surface of the sclera.

su•pra•scro•tal (soo″prə-skro′təl) superior to the scrotum.

su•pra•sel•lar (soo″prə-sel′ər) superior to the sella turcica.

su•pra•sep•tal (soo″prə-sep′təl) superior to a septum.

su•pra•spi•nal (soo″prə-spi′nəl) above or upon a spine.

su•pra•spi•nous (soo″prə-spi′nəs) 1. supraspinal. 2. superior to a spinous process.

su•pra•sta•pe•di•al (soo″prə-stə-pe′de-əl) superior to the stapes.

su•pra•ster•nal (soo″prə-stur′nəl) superior to the sternum.

su•pra•syl•vi•an (soo″prə-sil′ve-ən) superior to the sylvian fissure.

su•pra•tem•po•ral (soo″prə-tem′pə-rəl) superior to the temporal bone, fossa, or region; called also *superotemporal.*

su•pra•ten•to•ri•al (soo″prə-tən-tor′e-əl) superior to the tentorium of the cerebellum.

su•pra•tho•rac•ic (soo″prə-thə-ras′ik) superior to the thorax.

su•pra•thresh•old (soo″prə-thresh′ōld) above a threshold.

su•pra•ton•sil•lar (soo″prə-ton′sĭ-lər) superior to a tonsil.

su•pra•troch•le•ar (soo″prə-trok′le-ər) superior to a trochlea.

su•pra•tym•pan•ic (soo″prə-tim-pan′ik) superior to the tympanum.

su•pra•um•bil•i•cal (soo″prə-əm-bil′ĭ-kəl) superior to the umbilicus.

su•pra•vag•i•nal (soo″prə-vaj′ĭ-nəl) 1. superior to or outside a sheath. 2. superior to the vagina.

su•pra•val•var (soo″prə-val′vər) above a valve, particularly the aortic or pulmonary valve.

su•pra•ven•tric•u•lar (soo″prə-vən-trik′u-lər) situated or occurring superior to the ventricles, especially in an atrium or atrioventricular node.

su•pra•ver•gence (soo″prə-vur′jəns) [*supra-* + *vergence*] disjunctive reciprocal movement of the eyes in which one eye rotates upward while the other one remains still; called also *sursumvergence.*

su•pra•ver•sion (soo″prə-vur′zhən) [*supra-* + *version*] 1. malocclusion in which a tooth or other maxillary or mandibular structure extends farther away from the alveolus than normal, the occluding surfaces of the teeth extending beyond the normal line of occlusion. 2. sursumversion.

su•pra•ves•i•cal (soo″prə-ves′ĭ-kəl) [*supra-* + *vesical*] superior to the urinary bladder.

su•pra•vi•tal (soo″prə-vi′təl) [*supra-* + *vital*] beyond living; denoting a staining method in which the dye is added to a medium of cells already removed from the living organism.

Su•prax (soo′praks) trademark for preparations of cefixime.

su•pra•xi•phoid (soo″prə-zi′foid) superior to the xiphoid process.

su•pra•zy•go•mat•ic (soo″prə-zi″go-mat′ik) superior to the zygomatic bone.

su•preme (soo-prēm′) [L. *supremus* highest] ultimate, greatest, highest; used in anatomy to denote the one in a group having the most superior location.

su•pro•fen (soo-pro′fən) [USP] a nonsteroidal antiinflammatory drug applied topically to the conjunctiva to inhibit miosis during ophthalmic surgery.

su•ra (soo′rə) [TA] calf: the fleshy mass formed chiefly by the gastrocnemius muscle on the posterior aspect of the leg below the knee. See also *regio surae.* **su′ral** *adj*

Su•ra•gi•na (soo-rə-ji′nə) a genus of flies of the family Rhagionidae. *S. lon′gipes* of Mexico is a vicious biter.

sur•al•i•men•ta•tion (sur″al-ĭ-mən-ta′shən) superalimentation.

su•ra•min hexa•so•di•um (soo′rə-min) an antitrypanosomal and antifilarial agent, used in the prophylaxis and treatment of African trypanosomiasis and in the treatment of onchocerciasis (for which use it has largely been replaced by ivermectin). Called also *suramin sodium.*

surd (sərd) [L. *surdus*] voiceless.

sur•ex•ci•ta•tion (sur″ek-si-ta′shən) [L. *super* over + *excitation*] excessive excitation.

sur•face (sur′fəs) the outer part or external aspect of an object; for official names of anatomical surfaces, see entries under *facies.*

anterior s. the surface toward the front of the body; in humans this is toward the chest, and in quadrupeds it is toward the head. For official anatomical nomenclature, see terms beginning *facies anterior.*

anterior s. of adrenal gland facies anterior glandulae suprarenalis.

anterior s. of cornea facies anterior corneae.

anterior s. of eyelid facies anterior palpebrae.

anterior s. of heart facies sternocostalis cordis.

anterior s. of iris facies anterior iridis.

anterior s. of kidney facies anterior renis.

anterior s. of lens facies anterior lentis.

anterior s. of maxilla facies anterior corporis maxillae.

anterior s. of pancreas see *facies anteroinferior corporis pancreatis* and *facies anterosuperior corporis pancreatis.*

anterior s. of patella facies anterior patellae.

anterior s. of petrous part of temporal bone facies anterior partis petrosae ossis temporalis.

anterior s. of prostate facies anterior prostatae.

anterior s. of radius facies anterior radii.

anterior s. of sacrum facies pelvica ossis sacri.

anterior s. of scapula facies costalis scapulae.

anterior s. of suprarenal gland facies anterior glandulae suprarenalis.

anterior talar articular s. of calcaneus facies articularis talaris anterior calcanei.

anterior s. of tooth the proximal surface of a tooth that is closest to the midline of the dental arch.

anterior s. of ulna facies anterior ulnae.

anterior s. of uterus facies vesicalis uteri.

anteroinferior s. of body of pancreas facies anteroinferior corporis pancreatis.

anterolateral s. of arytenoid cartilage facies anterolateralis cartilaginis arytenoideae.

anterolateral s. of humerus facies anterolateralis humeri.

anteromedial s. of humerus facies anteromedialis humeri.

anterosuperior s. of body of pancreas facies anterosuperior corporis pancreatis.

approximal s. of tooth facies approximalis dentis.

articular s. facies articularis.

articular s. of arytenoid cartilage facies articularis cartilaginis arytenoidea.

articular s. for cuboid facies articularis cuboidea calcanei.

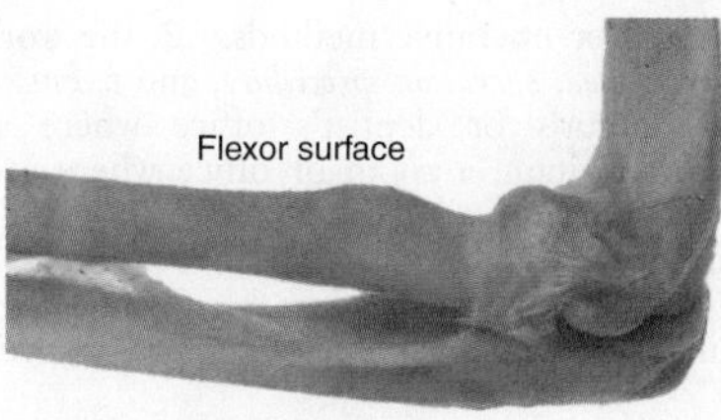

■ Flexor and extensor surfaces of the forearm.

articular s. of mandibular fossa facies articularis fossae mandibularis.
articular s. of patella facies articularis patellae.
arytenoid articular s. on cricoid cartilage facies articularis arytenoidea cartilaginis cricoideae.
auricular s. of ilium facies auricularis ossis ilii.
auricular s. of sacrum facies auricularis ossis sacri.
axial s. any surface parallel with an axis; in dentistry, any surface of a tooth that is parallel with its long axis, including the buccal, distal, labial, lingual, and mesial surfaces.
basal s. the surface of a denture that has detail determined by the impression and that rests upon the supporting tissues of the mouth. Called also *foundation s.* and *impression s.*
buccal s. of tooth facies buccalis dentis.
carpal articular s. of radius facies articularis carpalis radii.
cerebral s. of greater wing of sphenoid bone facies cerebralis alae majoris ossis sphenoidalis.
cerebral s. of temporal bone facies cerebralis ossis temporalis.
contact s. of tooth area contingens dentis.
costal s. of lung facies costalis pulmonis.
costal s. of scapula facies costalis scapulae.
diaphragmatic s. of heart facies diaphragmatica cordis.
diaphragmatic s. of liver facies diaphragmatica hepatis.
diaphragmatic s. of lung facies diaphragmatica pulmonis.
diaphragmatic s. of spleen facies diaphragmatica splenis.
distal s. the surface of a structure that is farther from a point of reference.
distal s. of tooth facies distalis dentis.
dorsal s. the surface toward the back of the body. In humans, synonymous with posterior surface. In quadrupeds, the superior surface.
dorsal s's of fingers facies dorsales digitorum manus.
dorsal s. of penis dorsum penis.
dorsal s. of sacrum facies dorsalis ossis sacri.
dorsal s. of scapula facies posterior scapulae.
dorsal s's of toes facies dorsales digitorum pedis.
extensor s. the aspect of a limb or joint on the side toward which extension is directed.
external s. of cranial base basis cranii externa.
external s. of frontal bone facies externa ossis frontalis.
external s. of parietal bone facies externa ossis parietalis.
facial s. of tooth facies vestibularis dentis.
flexor s. the aspect of a limb or joint on the side toward which flexion is directed.
foundation s. basal s.
gluteal s. of ilium facies glutea ossis ilii.
impression s. basal s.
incisal s. the cutting edges of the anterior teeth, the incisors and canines, which come into contact with those of the opposite teeth during the act of protrusive occlusion, in which they assume an edge-to-edge relationship. See also *facies occlusalis dentis.*
inferior s. that surface which is lower. In humans it is that directed away from the head; in quadrupeds, it is synonymous with *ventral surface.*
inferior articular s. of atlas facies articularis inferior atlantis.
inferior articular s. of tibia facies articularis inferior tibiae.
inferior s. of cerebral hemisphere facies inferior hemispherii cerebri.
inferior s. of heart facies diaphragmatis cordis.
inferior s. of liver facies visceralis hepatis.
inferior s. of petrous part of temporal bone facies inferior partis petrosae ossis temporalis.
inferior s. of tongue facies inferior linguae.
inferolateral s. of prostate facies inferolateralis prostatae.
infratemporal s. of greater wing of sphenoid bone facies infratemporalis alae majoris ossis sphenoidalis.
infratemporal s. of maxilla facies infratemporalis corporis maxillae.
interlobar s. of lung facies interlobaris pulmonis.
internal s. of cranial base basis cranii interna.
internal s. of frontal bone facies interna ossis frontalis.
internal s. of parietal bone facies interna ossis parietalis.
interproximal s. of tooth facies approximalis dentis.
intervertebral s. facies intervertebralis.
intestinal s. of uterus facies intestinalis uteri.
labial s. of tooth facies labialis dentis.
lateral s. a surface nearer to or directed toward the side of the body; for official anatomical nomenclature, see terms beginning *facies lateralis.*
lateral s. of fibula facies lateralis fibulae.
lateral s. of ovary facies lateralis ovarii.
lateral s. of radius facies lateralis radii.
lateral s. of testis facies lateralis testis.
lateral s. of tibia facies lateralis tibiae.
lateral s. of tooth the distal surface of an incisor or canine tooth. Cf. *posterior s. of tooth.*
lateral s. of zygomatic bone facies lateralis ossis zygomatici.
left s. of heart see *facies pulmonalis dextra/sinistra cordis.*
lingual s. of tooth facies lingualis dentis.
lunate s. of acetabulum facies lunata acetabuli.
masticatory s. of tooth 1. facies occlusalis dentis. 2. more specifically, the occlusal surfaces involved in mastication.
maxillary s. of greater wing of sphenoid bone facies maxillaris alae majoris ossis sphenoidalis.
maxillary s. of perpendicular plate of palatine bone facies maxillaris laminae perpendicularis ossis palatini.
medial s. a surface nearer to or directed toward the median plane of the body; for official anatomical nomenclature, see terms beginning *facies medialis.*
medial s. of arytenoid cartilage facies medialis cartilaginis arytenoideae.
medial s. of cerebral hemisphere facies medialis hemispherii cerebri.
medial s. of fibula facies medialis fibulae.
medial s. of ovary facies medialis ovarii.
medial s. of testis facies medialis testis.
medial s. of tibia facies medialis tibiae.
medial s. of ulna facies medialis ulnae.
mediastinal s. of lung facies mediastinalis pulmonis.
mesial s. of tooth facies mesialis dentis.
middle talar articular s. of calcaneus facies articularis talaris media calcanei.
morsal s. of tooth one of the occlusal surfaces of the mandibular and maxillary teeth which make contact in centric occlusion.
nasal s. of horizontal plate of palatine bone facies nasalis laminae horizontalis ossis palatini.
nasal s. of maxilla facies nasalis corporis maxillae.
nasal s. of perpendicular plate of palatine bone facies nasalis laminae perpendicularis ossis palatini.
navicular articular s. of talus facies articularis navicularis tali.
occlusal s. of tooth facies occlusalis dentis.
oral s. of tooth facies lingualis dentis.
orbital s. of frontal bone facies orbitalis ossis frontalis.
orbital s. of greater wing of sphenoid bone facies orbitalis alae majoris ossis sphenoidalis.
orbital s. of maxilla facies orbitalis corporis maxillae.
orbital s. of zygomatic bone facies orbitalis ossis zygomatici.
palatal s. of tooth facies palatinalis dentis.
palatine s. of horizontal plate of palatine bone facies palatina laminae horizontalis ossis palatini.
palmar s's of fingers facies palmares digitorum manus.
patellar s. of femur facies patellaris femoris.
pelvic s. of sacrum facies pelvica ossis sacri.
plantar s's of toes facies plantares digitorum pedis.
popliteal s. of femur facies poplitea femoris.
polished s. 1. a surface that has been smoothed to a fine finish. 2. in dentistry, the portion of the surface of a denture that is usually polished, including the palatal surface, and the buccal and lingual surfaces of the teeth.
posterior s. that surface which in humans is toward the back of the body, and in quadrupeds is toward the tail. For official anatomical nomenclature, see terms beginning *facies posterior.*
posterior s. of adrenal gland facies posterior glandulae suprarenalis.
posterior s. of arytenoid cartilage facies posterior cartilaginis arytenoideae.
posterior s. of body of pancreas facies posterior corporis pancreatis.
posterior s. of cornea facies posterior corneae.
posterior s. of eyelid facies posterior palpebrae.
posterior s. of fibula facies posterior fibulae.
posterior s. of humerus facies posterior humeri.
posterior s. of iris facies posterior iridis.
posterior s. of kidney facies posterior renis.
posterior s. of lens facies posterior lentis.
posterior s. of petrous part of temporal bone facies posterior partis petrosae ossis temporalis.
posterior s. of prostate facies posterior prostatae.

posterior s. of radius facies posterior radii.
posterior s. of sacrum facies dorsalis ossis sacri.
posterior s. of scapula facies posterior scapulae.
posterior s. of suprarenal gland facies posterior glandulae suprarenalis.
posterior talar articular s. of calcaneus facies articularis talaris posterior calcanei.
posterior s. of tibia facies posterior tibiae.
posterior s. of tooth the distal surface of a molar tooth. Cf. *lateral s. of tooth.*
posterior s. of ulna facies posterior ulnae.
posterior s. of uterus facies intestinalis uteri.
proximal s., proximate s. any surface nearer to a point of reference.
proximal s. of tooth, proximate s. of tooth facies approximalis dentis.
pulmonary s. of heart see *facies pulmonalis dextra/sinistra cordis.*
renal s. of adrenal gland, renal s. of suprarenal gland facies renalis glandulae suprarenalis.
right s. of heart see *facies pulmonalis dextra/sinistra cordis.*
sacropelvic s. of ilium facies sacropelvica ossis ilii.
sternocostal s. of heart facies sternocostalis cordis.
subocclusal s. of tooth a portion of the surface of a tooth that is directed toward but does not make contact with the occlusal surface of its opposite number in the other jaw.
superior s. that surface which is upper or higher. In humans, it is that directed toward the head; in quadrupeds, it is a synonym of *dorsal surface.*
superior articular s. of atlas facies articularis superior atlantis.
superior articular s. of tibia facies articularis superior tibiae.
superior s. of trochlea of talus facies superior trochleae tali.
superolateral s. of cerebral hemisphere facies superolateralis hemispherii cerebri.
symphysial s. of pubic bone facies symphysialis ossis pubis.
temporal s. of frontal bone facies temporalis ossis frontalis.
temporal s. of greater wing of sphenoid bone facies temporalis alae majoris ossis sphenoidalis.
temporal s. of squamous part of temporal bone facies temporalis partis squamosae ossis temporalis.
temporal s. of zygomatic bone facies temporalis ossis zygomatici.
tentorial s. the portion of the cerebral surface that is in contact with the tentorium cerebelli.
thyroid articular s. on cricoid cartilage facies articularis thyroidea cartilaginis cricoideae.
urethral s. of penis facies urethralis penis.
ventral s. the aspect of a structure that is toward the front of the body or on or nearer the abdomen. In humans, synonymous with anterior surface; in quadrupeds, the inferior surface.
ventral s. of penis facies urethralis penis.
ventral s. of scapula facies costalis scapulae.
vesical s. of uterus facies vesicalis uteri.
vestibular s. of tooth facies vestibularis dentis.
visceral s. of liver facies visceralis hepatis.
visceral s. of spleen facies visceralis splenis.

sur•fac•tant (sər-fak′tənt) 1. surface-active agent. 2. in pulmonary physiology, a mixture of phospholipids (chiefly lecithin and sphingomyelin) secreted by the alveolar type II cells into the alveoli and respiratory air passages, which reduces the surface tension of pulmonary fluids and thus contributes to the elastic properties of pulmonary tissue.

Sur•fak (sur′fak) trademark for a preparation of docusate calcium.

surge (surj) 1. to move like an advancing wave. 2. to increase suddenly. 3. a sudden sharp increase.
follicle-stimulating hormone s. a sharp increase in serum levels of follicle-stimulating hormone seen around the middle of the menstrual cycle about one to two days before ovulation.
luteinizing hormone s. a sharp increase in serum levels of luteinizing hormone seen around the middle of the menstrual cycle about one to two days before ovulation.
postnatal s. a temporary sharp rise in levels of circulating gonadotropins, sex hormones, and inhibin, seen in infants of both sexes in the first few weeks after birth.

sur•geon (sur′jən) [L. *chirurgio;* Fr. *chirurgien*] 1. a physician who specializes in surgery. 2. the senior medical officer of a military unit.
barber s. formerly a barber who was authorized to practice minor surgery, including bloodletting.
s. general 1. the chief of medical services in one of the armed forces. 2. the chief medical officer of the United States Public Health Service, or of a state public health agency.
house s. a surgeon who is an employee of a hospital and available there when on duty.
post s. the surgeon of an established army post.

sur•gery (sur′jər-e) [L. *chirurgia,* from Gr. *cheir* hand + *ergon* work] 1. the branch of medicine that treats diseases, injuries, and deformities by manual or operative methods. 2. the work performed by a surgeon; see also *method, operation, procedure,* and *technique.* 3. the place in a hospital or doctor's or dentist's office where surgery is performed. 4. in Great Britain, a room or office where a doctor sees and treats patients.
aesthetic s. cosmetic s.
ambulatory s. an operative procedure, performed either in a hospital or in a freestanding facility, that does not require an overnight stay in a hospital.
antiseptic s. surgery done using antiseptic principles; see also *aseptic s.*
aseptic s. surgery performed with aseptic techniques (q.v.).
bariatric s. surgery on part of the gastrointestinal tract as a treatment for morbid obesity.
bench s. surgery performed on an organ that has been removed from the body, after which it is reimplanted.
cineplastic s. creation of a skin-lined tunnel through a muscle adjacent to the stump of an amputated limb, to permit use of the muscle in operating a prosthesis.
clinical s. the study of surgical disease by symptomatic analysis, examination, and observation.
conservative s. surgery designed to preserve, or to remove with minimal risk, diseased or injured organs, tissues, or extremities. Cf. *radical s.*
cosmetic s. the branch of plastic surgery which deals with procedures designed to improve the patient's appearance by plastic restoration, correction, removal of blemishes, etc. Called also *aesthetic s.*
cytoreductive s. debulking.
dental s. oral and maxillofacial s.
dentofacial s. the branch of the healing arts which deals with the surgical and adjunctive treatment of diseases, injuries, and defects involving the face and structures of the mouth.
endoscopic s. surgery performed through an endoscope, such as various minimally invasive surgery techniques; called also *endosurgery.*
functional endoscopic sinus s. (FES) endoscopic surgery of the paranasal sinuses to correct problems causing sinus infection.
general s. the practice of surgery that deals with surgical problems of all kinds, rather than those in a restricted area, or in a surgical specialty such as neurosurgery.
keratorefractive s., lamellar refractive s. refractive keratoplasty.
lung volume reduction s. surgical removal of a nonfunctional area of the lung as a treatment of pulmonary emphysema.
major s. surgery that is particularly difficult or hazardous.
maxillofacial s. oral and maxillofacial s.
minimal access s., minimally invasive s. surgery performed through the smallest possible incision or no incision at all, as through a cannula with a laparoscope or endoscope.
minor s. surgery restricted to the management of minor problems and injuries.
Mohs s., Mohs micrographic s. a technique of microscopically controlled serial excision of high-risk, nonmelanoma skin cancers. Formerly the tissue was removed after being fixed in situ with zinc chloride paste *(Mohs chemosurgery);* later this was modified to a more tissue-sparing technique in which serial excisions of fresh tissue would be done with microscopic analysis. Called also *Mohs technique.*
open heart s. surgery that involves incision into one or more chambers of the heart, such as for repair or palliation of congenital heart defects, repair or replacement of defective heart valves, or coronary artery bypass.
operative s. the operative or mechanical aspect of surgery; that which deals with manual and manipulative methods or procedures.
oral s. oral and maxillofacial s.
oral and maxillofacial s. the branch of dental practice that deals with the diagnosis and the surgical and adjunctive treatment of diseases, injuries, and defects of the human mouth and dental structures. Called also *maxillofacial s.* and formerly *dental s.* and *oral s.*
orthognathic s. surgery to correct deformities of the jaw; see also *surgical orthodontics,* under *orthodontics.*
orthopedic s. orthopedics.
plastic s. surgery concerned with the restoration, reconstruction, correction, or improvement in the shape and appearance of body structures that are defective, damaged, or misshapen by injury, disease, or growth and development.
psychiatric s. psychosurgery.
radical s. surgery designed to extirpate all areas of locally extensive disease and adjacent zones of lymphatic drainage; cf. *conservative s.* Called also *radical operation.*
reconstructive s. plastic s.
sonic s. the use of focused ultrasonic waves to produce precisely circumscribed alterations within tissues at predetermined sites.
stereotactic s., stereotaxic s. any of several techniques for the production of sharply circumscribed lesions in specific areas of pathologic tissue in deep-seated structures. The site to be worked on is localized with three-dimensional coordinates; precise images are obtained with

computed tomography or magnetic resonance imaging. An arc guidance system may be used to direct an electrode or other lesion-producing instrument. Methods of producing lesions include heat, cold, x-rays, charged particles such as protons, and ultrasound. Called also *stereotaxy.*

structural s. surgery devoted to the correction of morphologic abnormalities.

veterinary s. the surgery of domestic animals.

video-assisted thoracic s., video-assisted thoracoscopic s. a minimally invasive surgical technique using a thoracoscope and other video assistive devices such as cameras and monitors, as well as specially designed instruments inserted through trocars for thoracic surgery. Abbreviated VATS.

sur·gi·cal (sur′jĭ-kəl) of, pertaining to, or correctable by surgery.

Sur·gi·cel (sur′jĭ-sel) trademark for an absorbable knitted fabric prepared by controlled oxidation of cellulose, used as a hemostatic agent to control intraoperative hemorrhage when other conventional methods are impractical or ineffective.

sur·ma (sur′mə) a lead sulfide traditionally applied to the eyelids in India for cosmetic and medical purposes; it can cause lead poisoning.

Sur·mon·til (sur′mon-til) trademark for a preparation of trimipramine maleate.

sur·ra (soor′ə) [Marathi *sūra* wheezing] a type of trypanosomiasis seen in domestic animals such as equines, camels, elephants, pigs, goats, and dogs, caused by *Trypanosoma evansi,* usually transmitted by tabanid flies. Common signs include fever, anemia, edema, progressive emaciation and weakness, and death. It occurs in East Asia, the Middle East, North Africa, and Central and South America; in the latter regions it is usually seen in horses, is spread by vampire bats as well as flies, and is called *murrina* or *derrengadera.*

sur·ro·gate (sur′o-gət) [L. *surrogatus* substituted] substitute; one put into the place of another.

sur·sum·duc·tion (sur″səm-duk′shən) supraduction.

sur·sum·ver·gence (sur″səm-vur′jəns) supravergence.

sur·sum·ver·sion (sur″səm-vur′zhən) [L. *sursum* upward + *version*] binocular conjugate upward rotation of both eyes; called also *supraversion* and *superversion.*

su·ru·çu·cu (soo″roo-soo′koo) bushmaster.

Sur·van·ta (sər-van′tə) trademark for a preparation of beractant.

sur·veil·lance (sər-vāl′əns) 1. watching or monitoring. 2. a procedure used instead of quarantine to control the spread of infectious disease, involving close supervision during the incubation period of possible contacts of individuals exposed to an infectious disease.

epidemiologic s. the ongoing and systematic collection, analysis, and interpretation of data about a disease or health condition; used in planning, implementing, and evaluating public health programs. It may be *passive,* requiring those parties responsible for reporting disease to do so on their own, or *active,* providing visits or other monitoring to those parties to ensure that information is obtained.

immune s., immunological s. a hypothesized monitoring function by which the immune system protects against cancer; according to the theory, tumor cells constantly arise throughout life by malignant transformation of normal cells but almost all are recognized and destroyed by the immune system, only a few somehow escaping or circumventing immune surveillance to grow and become clinically detectable cancers.

sur·vi·val (sər-vi′vəl) the act or process of remaining alive; the continuation of life.

sur·vi·vin (sər-vi′vin) a protein that neutralizes caspase activity and thus inhibits apoptosis, expressed during the G_2/M phase of the cell cycle in many tumors but not in most normal differentiated adult tissues.

sus·cep·ti·bil·i·ty (sə-sep″tĭ-bil′ĭ-te) 1. the state of being readily affected or acted upon. 2. diminished immunity to a disease, especially an infection.

antibiotic s., antimicrobial s. the vulnerability of a strain of a microorganism to being inhibited or killed by a given antibiotic or antimicrobial agent; see *antimicrobial susceptibility test,* under *test.* Called also *antibiotic* or *antimicrobial sensitivity.*

differential s. nonhomogeneity in response by the various regions of an embryo when subjected to a diffusely applied injurious agent.

sus·cep·ti·ble (sə-sep′tĭ-bəl) 1. capable of impression; readily acted on. 2. not having immunity to an infectious disease and thus at risk of infection.

Sush·rut Sam·hi·ta (shoosh′rooth-thə sung′hee-tah) the classic surgical text of ayurveda, written 1000 BCE by the surgeon Sushruta and adapted from the sacred Indian texts known as the Vedas (approximately 3000 BCE).

sus·lik (sōōs′lik) Russian ground squirrel.

sus·pen·si·om·e·ter (səs-pen″se-om′ə-tər) nephelometer.

sus·pen·sion (səs-pen′shən) [L. *suspensio*] 1. a condition of temporary cessation, as of animation, of pain, or of any vital process. 2. attachment of an organ or other body part to a supporting structure, as of the uterus or bladder in the correction of a hernia or prolapse. 3. a liquid preparation consisting of solid particles dispersed throughout a liquid phase in which they are not soluble.

bladder neck s. any of various methods of surgical fixation of the urethrovesical junction area and the bladder neck to restore the neck to a high retropubic position for relief of stress incontinence. The group includes the Marshall-Marchetti-Krantz operation and the Burch, Pereyra, and Stamey procedures. Called also *colposuspension, cystourethropexy, urethrocystopexy,* and *urethropexy.*

colloid s. a colloid system; see *colloid* (def. 2). Sometimes used specifically for a sol in which the dispersed phase is solid and the particles are large enough to settle out of solution.

corticotropin zinc hydroxide injectable s. [USP] a sterile suspension of corticotropin with prolonged action, adsorbed on zinc hydroxide; administered intramuscularly as an anticonvulsant in the treatment of infantile spasms.

urethrovesical s. bladder neck s.

sus·pen·soid (səs-pen′soid) lyophobic colloid.

sus·pen·so·ri·us (sus″pən-sor′e-əs) [L.] suspensory.

sus·pen·so·ry (səs-pen′sə-re) [L. *suspensorius*] 1. serving to hold up a part. 2. a ligament, bone, muscle, sling, or bandage which serves to hold up a part.

Sus-Phrine (sus′frin) trademark for a preparation of epinephrine.

sus·ten·tac·u·lar (sus″tən-tak′u-lər) [L. *sustentare* to support] 1. pertaining to a sustentaculum. 2. serving to support.

sus·ten·tac·u·lum (sus″tən-tak′u-ləm) pl. *sustentac′ula* [L.] a support.

s. lie′nis ligamentum splenorenale.

s. ta′li [TA], **s. of talus** a process of the calcaneus which supports the talus.

Sus·ti·va (sus-te′və) trademark for a preparation of efavirenz.

sus·to (soos′to) [Sp. "fright, shock"] a culture-specific syndrome seen in Latin America consisting of symptoms attributed to a severe fright that causes the soul to leave the body. It is characterized by anxiety, sadness, altered sleep and eating habits, and somatic symptoms such as headache, stomachache, muscle aches, and diarrhea.

Su·tent (soo′tent) trademark for a preparation of sunitinib malate.

su·ti·lains (soo′tĭ-lāns) a substance containing proteolytic enzymes derived from *Bacillus subtilis,* used as a proteolytic agent for débridement of wounds.

Sut·ton disease (sut′ən) [Richard Lightburn *Sutton,* Jr., American dermatologist, 1908–1990] granuloma fissuratum.

Sut·ton nevus (disease) (sut′ən) [Richard Lightburn *Sutton,* American dermatologist, 1878–1952] halo nevus; see under *nevus.*

Sut·to·nel·la (sut″ə-nel′ə) a genus of gram-negative, nonmotile, aerobic or facultatively anaerobic rod-shaped bacteria of the family Cardiobacteriaceae that are normal inhabitants of the human oropharynx. The type species is *S. indolo′genes.*

S. indolo′genes a species of uncertain pathogenicity, isolated from eye infections and endocarditis; formerly called *Kingella indologenes.*

su·tu·ra (soo-tu′rə) pl. *sutu′rae* [L. "a seam"] [TA] suture: a type of fibrous joint in which the apposed bony surfaces are so closely united by a thin layer of fibrous connective tissue that no movement can occur; found only in the skull. Called also *s. vera* and *true suture.*

s. corona′lis [TA] coronal suture: the line of junction of the frontal bone with the two parietal bones.

sutu′rae cra′nii [TA] cranial sutures: the sutures between the various bones of the skull, named generally for the specific components participating in their formation.

s. denta′ta s. serrata.

s. ethmoidolacrima′lis [TA] ethmoidolacrimal suture: the vertical line of junction, on the medial wall of the orbit, between the lacrimal bone and the orbital plate of the ethmoid bone; called also *lacrimoethmoidal suture.*

s. ethmoidomaxilla′ris [TA] ethmoidomaxillary suture: the line of junction between the orbital lamina of the ethmoid bone and the orbital surface of the maxilla.

s. fronta′lis frontal suture: the usually transient line of junction between the right and left halves of the frontal bone. The inferior part may persist in the adult, in which case it is called the *metopic suture* (sutura frontalis persistens [TA]).

s. fronta′lis meto′pica TA alternative for *s. frontalis persistens.*

s. fronta′lis persis′tens [TA] the name given to the inferior part of the frontal suture when it persists in the adult; called also *s. frontalis metopica* [TA alternative] and *metopic s.*

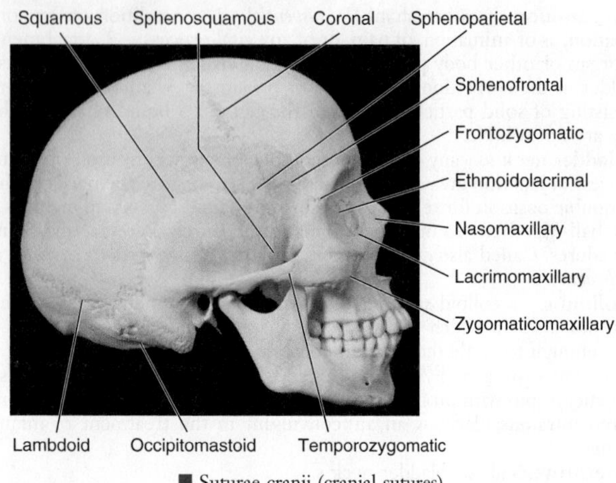

■ Suturae cranii (cranial sutures).

s. frontoethmoida'lis [TA] frontoethmoidal suture: the line of junction in the anterior cranial fossa between the frontal bone and the cribriform plate of the ethmoid bone.
s. frontolacrima'lis [TA] frontolacrimal suture: the line of junction between the upper edge of the lacrimal bone and the orbital part of the frontal bone.
s. frontomaxilla'ris [TA] frontomaxillary suture: the line of junction between the frontal bone and the frontal process of the maxilla.
s. frontonasa'lis [TA] frontonasal suture: the line of junction between the frontal and the two nasal bones; called also *nasofrontal suture*.
s. frontozygoma'tica [TA] frontozygomatic suture: the line of junction between the zygomatic bone and the zygomatic process of the frontal bone; called also *zygomaticofrontal suture*.
s. harmo'nia s. plana.
s. incisi'va [TA] incisive suture: an indistinct suture sometimes seen extending laterally from the incisive fossa to the space between the canine tooth and the lateral incisor, indicating the line of fusion between the premaxilla and the maxilla.
s. infraorbita'lis TA alternative for *s. zygomaticomaxillaris*.
s. intermaxilla'ris [TA] intermaxillary suture: the line of junction between the maxillary bones of either side, just inferior to the anterior nasal spine.
s. internasa'lis [TA] internasal suture: the line of junction between the two nasal bones.
s. lacrimoconcha'lis [TA] lacrimoconchal suture: the line of junction between the lacrimal bone and the inferior nasal concha.
s. lacrimomaxilla'ris [TA] lacrimomaxillary suture: a suture on the inner wall of the orbit, between the lacrimal bone and the maxilla.
s. lambdoi'dea [TA] lambdoid suture: the line of junction between the occipital and parietal bones, shaped like the Greek letter lambda.
s. limbo'sa [TA] limbous suture: a type of squamous suture in which there is interlocking of the beveled surfaces of the bones.
s. nasofronta'lis s. frontonasalis.
s. nasomaxilla'ris [TA] nasomaxillary suture: the line of junction between the lateral edge of the nasal bone and the frontal process of the maxilla.
s. occipitomastoi'dea [TA] occipitomastoid suture: an extension of the lambdoid suture between the occipital bone and the posterior edge of the mastoid portion of the temporal bone.
s. palati'na media'na [TA] median palatine suture: the line of junction between the horizontal part of the palatine bones of either side.
s. palati'na transver'sa [TA] transverse palatine suture: the line of junction between the palatine processes of the maxillae and the horizontal parts of the palatine bones.
s. palatoethmoida'lis [TA] palatoethmoidal suture: the line of junction between the orbital process of the palatine bone and the orbital lamina of the ethmoid bone.
s. palatomaxilla'ris [TA] palatomaxillary suture: the suture in the floor of the orbit, between the orbital processes of the palatine bone and the orbital portion of the maxilla.
s. parietomastoi'dea [TA] parietomastoid suture: the line of junction between the posterior inferior angle of the parietal bone and the mastoid process of the temporal bone.
s. pla'na [TA] flat suture: a type of suture in which there is simple apposition of the contiguous surfaces, with no interlocking of the edges of the participating bones. Called also *false suture*.
s. sagitta'lis [TA] sagittal suture: the line of junction between the two parietal bones.
s. serra'ta [TA] serrated suture: a type of suture in which the participating bones are united by interlocking processes resembling the teeth of a saw.
s. sphenoethmoida'lis [TA] sphenoethmoidal suture: the line of junction between the body of the sphenoid bone and the orbital lamina of the ethmoid bone.
s. sphenofronta'lis [TA] sphenofrontal suture: a long suture joining the orbital part of the frontal bone to the greater and lesser wings of the sphenoid bone on either side of the skull.
s. sphenomaxilla'ris [TA] sphenomaxillary suture: a suture occasionally seen between the pterygoid process of the sphenoid bone and the maxilla.
s. sphenoorbita'lis sphenoorbital suture: the line or junction between the orbital process of the palatine bone and the body of the sphenoid bone.
s. sphenoparieta'lis [TA] sphenoparietal suture: the line of junction between the greater wing of the sphenoid bone and the parietal bone.
s. sphenosquamo'sa [TA] sphenosquamous suture: the line of junction between the greater wing of the sphenoid bone and the squamous part of the temporal bone.
s. sphenovomera'lis [TA], **s. sphenovomeria'na** sphenovomerine suture: the line of junction between the vaginal processes of the medial pterygoid plates of the sphenoid and the ala of the vomer.
s. sphenozygoma'tica [TA] sphenozygomatic suture: the line of junction between the greater wing of the sphenoid bone and the zygomatic bone.
s. squamomastoi'dea [TA] squamomastoid suture: a suture existing early in life between the squamous and mastoid portions of the temporal bone. Called also *s. squamosomastoidea*.
s. squamo'sa [TA] squamous suture: a type of suture formed by overlapping of the broad beveled edges of the participating bones.
s. squamo'sa cra'nii [TA] squamous suture of cranium: the suture between the squamous part of the temporal bone and the parietal bone.
s. squamosomastoi'dea s. squamomastoidea.
s. temporozygoma'tica [TA] temporozygomatic suture: the line of junction between the zygomatic process of the temporal bone and the temporal process of the zygomatic bone.
s. ve'ra sutura.
s. zygomaticomaxilla'ris [TA] zygomaticomaxillary suture: the line of junction between the zygomatic bone and the zygomatic process of the maxilla.

su•tur•al (soo'chə-rəl) of or pertaining to a suture.

su•tur•a•tion (soo″chə-ra'shən) the act or process of suturing.

su•ture (soo'chər) [L. *sutura* a seam] 1. sutura. 2. one loop of thread or similar material used to secure apposition of the edges of a surgical or accidental wound; called also *stitch*. 3. the material used in thus closing a wound; see *absorbable s.* and *nonabsorbable s.* 4. to unite the edges of a wound using loops of thread or other material; called also *stitch*.

Suture

For descriptions of specific anatomic structures not listed here, see under *sutura*.

absorbable s. a surgical suture that closes a wound and later either is digested by proteolytic enzymes derived from inflammatory cells or is hydrolyzed by water.
absorbable surgical s. [USP] a sterile absorbable suture made of collagen derived from healthy mammals or from a synthetic polymer, available in various diameters and tensile strengths; it may be treated to modify its resistance to absorption, impregnated with a suitable antimicrobial agent, and colored.
Albert s. a form of Czerny suture in which the first row of stitches is passed through the entire thickness of the intestine.

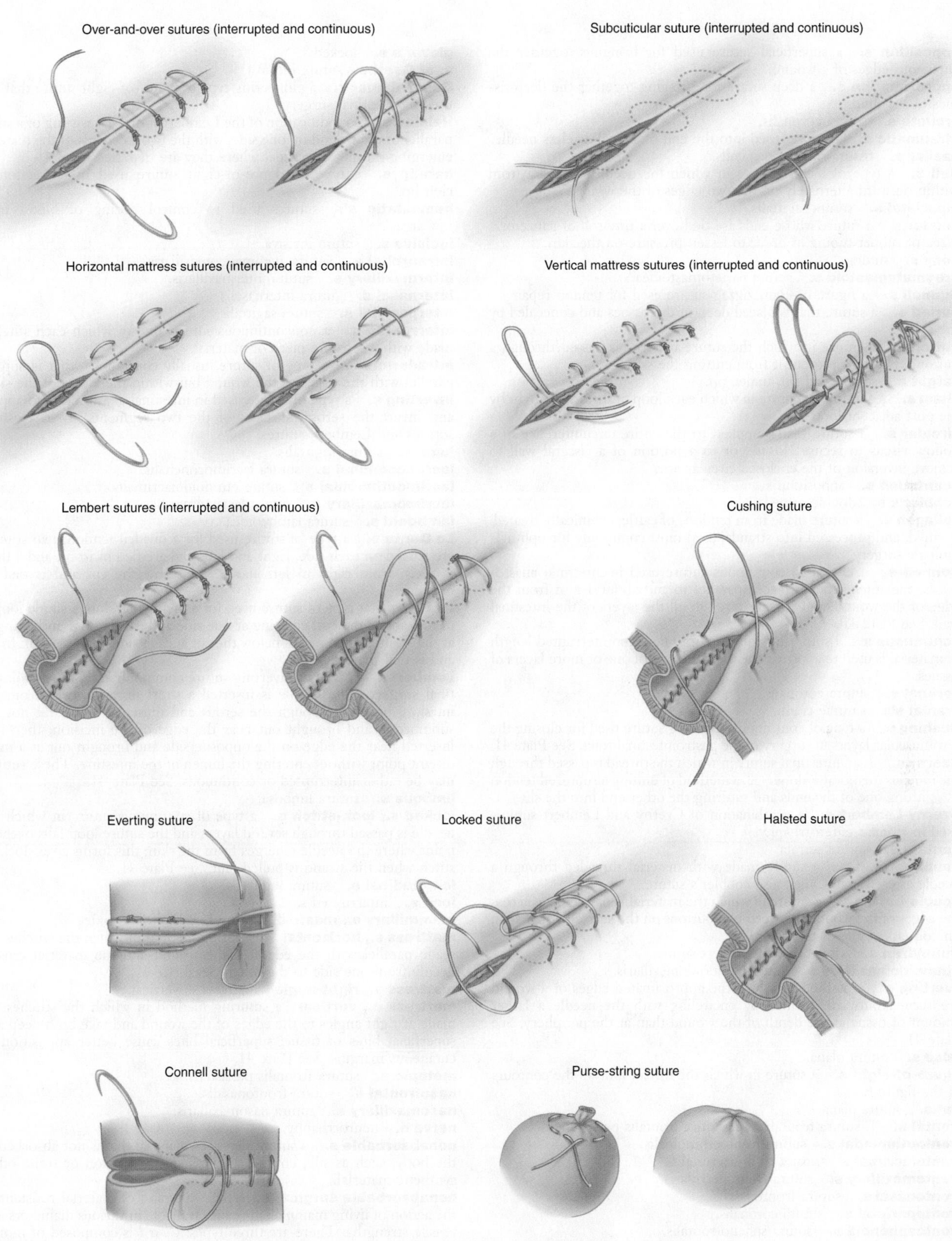

■ **PLATE 41—VARIOUS TYPES OF SUTURES**

Suture *Continued*

apposition s. a superficial suture used for bringing together the cutaneous edges of a wound.
approximation s. a deep suture for bringing together the deep tissues of a wound.
arcuate s. sutura coronalis.
atraumatic s. a suture fused into the end of a small eyeless needle.
basilar s. fissura sphenooccipitalis.
Bell s. a type of locked suture in which the needle is passed from within outward alternately on the two edges of the wound.
biparietal s. sutura sagittalis.
bolster s. a suture whose ends are tied over a tiny roll of gauze or a piece of rubber tubing in order to lessen pressure on the skin.
bony s. sutura.
bregmatomastoid s. sutura parietomastoidea.
Bunnell s. a figure-of-eight zigzag suture used for tendon repair.
buried s. a suture that is placed deep in the tissues and concealed by the skin.
button s. a suture in which the suture material is passed through a buttonlike disk to prevent it from cutting the skin.
catgut s. see *surgical gut,* under *gut.*
chain s. a continuous suture in which each loop of thread is caught by the next adjacent loop.
circular s. a suture that is applied to the entire circumference of a hollow viscus to secure closure, or to a portion of a visceral wall to achieve inversion of the enclosed circular area.
coaptation s. apposition s.
cobbler's s. double-armed s.
collagen s. a suture made from tendons of cattle, chemically treated, purified, and processed into strands; used most commonly for ophthalmologic surgery.
Connell s. a U-shaped continuous suture used in intestinal anastomosis, the stitches being placed parallel to and about 4 mm from the edge of the wound, and passing through all the layers of the intestinal wall. See Plate 41.
continuous s. a suture in which a continuous, uninterrupted length of material is used to approximate the cut edges of one or more layers of tissues.
coronal s. sutura coronalis.
cranial s's suturae cranii.
Cushing s. a type of continuous inverting suture used for closing the seromuscular layers in surgery of the gastrointestinal tract. See Plate 41.
Czerny s. 1. an intestinal suture in which the thread is passed through the mucous membrane alone. 2. a method of uniting a ruptured tendon by splitting one of the ends and suturing the other end into the slit.
Czerny-Lembert s. a combination of Czerny and Lembert sutures used in circular enterorrhaphy.
dentate s. sutura serrata.
double-armed s. a suture made with material threaded through a needle at each end. Called also cobbler's suture.
double-button s. a suture in which the material is passed deep across the edges of the wound, between two buttons on the surface of the skin, one on either side of the suture line.
Dupuytren s. a continuous Lembert suture.
ethmoidomaxillary s. sutura ethmoidomaxillaris.
everting s. a method by which the approximated edges of a wound are turned outward; formed by encircling with the needle a larger amount of tissue at the depth of the wound than at the periphery. See Plate 41.
false s. sutura plana.
figure-of-eight s. a suture in which the thread follows the contours of the figure 8.
flat s. sutura plana.
frontal s. 1. sutura frontalis. 2. sutura frontalis persistens.
frontoethmoidal s. sutura frontoethmoidalis.
frontolacrimal s. sutura frontolacrimalis.
frontomaxillary s. sutura frontomaxillaris.
frontonasal s. sutura frontonasalis.
frontoparietal s. sutura coronalis.
frontosphenoid s. sutura sphenofrontalis.
frontozygomatic s. sutura frontozygomatica.
Gaillard-Arlt s. a suture used in correction of entropion.
Gély s. a type of continuous suture used for repair of intestinal wounds, made by a thread with a needle at each end, and consisting of a series of cross-stitches closing the wound.
glover's s. locked s.
s. of Goethe sutura incisiva.
Gussenbauer s. a pioneering type of figure-of-eight suture that was used in intestinal surgery.
Halsted s. a modification of the Lembert suture, consisting of a stitch parallel to the wound on one side, with the two free ends of the material emerging on the other side, where they are tied. See Plate 41.
harelip s. a type of figure-of-eight suture used in correction of cleft lip.
hemostatic s's sutures used to control oozing of blood from raw areas.
incisive s. sutura incisiva.
infraorbital s. sutura zygomaticomaxillaris.
intermaxillary s. sutura intermaxillaris.
internasal s. sutura internasalis.
interparietal s. sutura sagittalis.
interrupted s. a noncontinuous suture; one in which each stitch is made with a separate piece of material.
intradermic s. a type of suture, usually continuous, that is applied parallel with the edges of the wound but within the layers of the skin.
inverting s. a type of suture used in intestinal anastomosis to appose and invert the serosal surfaces of the two segments, as in Cushing sutures and Lembert sutures.
jugal s. sutura sagittalis.
lacrimoconchal s. sutura lacrimoconchalis.
lacrimoethmoidal s. sutura ethmoidolacrimalis.
lacrimomaxillary s. sutura lacrimomaxillaris.
lambdoid s. sutura lambdoidea.
Le Dentu s. a type of suture used for a divided tendon; two stitches are passed on each side, right and left, and are tied in front, and a third is taken from right to left above and below the cut and is tied on one side.
Le Fort s. a type of suture used for a divided tendon; a single loop is passed above the cut, entering at one side and coming out and going in at the front; it then passes below the cut at each side, comes out in front, and is tied there.
Lembert s. a type of inverting suture commonly used in gastrointestinal surgery. The needle is inserted a short distance away from the incision, brought through the serous and muscular coats but not the submucosa, and brought out near the edge of the incision; then it is inserted near the edge on the opposite side and brought out at a more distant point without entering the lumen of the intestine. These sutures may be either interrupted or continuous. See Plate 41.
limbous s. sutura limbosa.
locked s., lock-stitch s. a type of continuous suture in which the needle is passed through several layers and the suture loop falls over the point where the needle emerges from the skin; this forms a self-locking stitch when the strand is pulled taut. See Plate 41.
longitudinal s. sutura sagittalis.
loop s. interrupted s.
mammillary s., mastoid s. sutura occipitomastoidea.
mattress s., horizontal a suturing method in which the stitches are made parallel with the edges of the wound and the material crosses deeply from one side to the other. See Plate 41.
mattress s., right-angle mattress s., vertical.
mattress s., vertical a suturing method in which the stitches are made at right angles to the edges of the wound and take both deep and superficial bites of tissue; superficial bites cause better apposition of cutaneous margins. See Plate 41.
metopic s. sutura frontalis persistens.
nasofrontal s. sutura frontonasalis.
nasomaxillary s. sutura nasomaxillaris.
nerve s. neurorrhaphy.
nonabsorbable s. a suture that uses material that is not absorbed in the body, such as silk, cotton, stainless steel, or nylon or some other synthetic material.
nonabsorbable surgical s. [USP] a strand of material resistant to the action of living mammalian tissue, available in various diameters and tensile strengths. There are three types: *Class I* is composed of monofilament, twisted, or braided silk or synthetic fibers; if there is a coating, it does not significantly affect the thickness. *Class II* is composed of cotton or linen fibers or of coated natural or synthetic fibers having a coating that significantly affects the thickness but not the strength. *Class III* is monofilament or multifilament wire.

Suture *Continued*

occipital s. sutura lambdoidea.
occipitomastoid s. sutura occipitomastoidea.
occipitoparietal s. sutura lambdoidea.
occipitosphenoidal s. fissura sphenooccipitalis.
over-and-over s. a suturing method in which equal bites of tissue are taken on each side of the wound; it may be either interrupted or continuous. See Plate 41.
palatine s., anterior sutura incisiva.
palatine s., median, palatine s., middle sutura palatina mediana.
palatine s., transverse sutura palatina transversa.
palatoethmoidal s. sutura palatoethmoidalis.
palatomaxillary s. sutura palatomaxillaris.
Paré s. a type of suture that uses strips of cloth applied along the edges of a wound and then stitched together to bring the wound margins into apposition.
parietal s. sutura sagittalis.
parietomastoid s. sutura parietomastoidea.
parietooccipital s. sutura lambdoidea.
petrobasilar s., petrosphenobasilar s. synchondrosis petrooccipitalis.
petrosphenooccipital s. of Gruber fissura petrooccipitalis.
petrosquamous s. fissura petrosquamosa.
plastic s. a suturing method in which a tongue is cut in one lip of the wound and a groove in the other, the tongue and groove are stitched together, and the ends of the thread are tied over a roll of adhesive plaster. Called also *tongue-and-groove s.*
premaxillary s. sutura incisiva.
presection s. a stitch or series of stitches placed in the tissues before an incision is made.
primary s. prompt surgical closure of a wound.
purse-string s. a continuous suture placed around a circular opening that is to be inverted; commonly used for the stump of the appendix or a hernia sac. See Plate 41.
quilt s., quilted s. a mattress suture that is continuous.
relaxation s. a suture that closes a wound but can be loosened in case tension becomes too great.
retention s. a suture in which a large amount of tissue is included in each stitch, using strong material such as braided silk or stainless steel; this type is especially for reinforcing of abdominal wounds, relieving pressure on the primary suture line, and preventing postoperative wound disruption and evisceration.
rhabdoid s. sutura sagittalis.
running s. an unbroken series of sutures used to close a long wound in which tension has been minimized and approximation of the edges is good.
sagittal s. sutura sagittalis.
secondary s. 1. delayed closure of an operative or accidental wound, usually because of the presence or expectation of infection. 2. resuture of an operative wound following disruption.
seroserous s. a suture that brings together two serous surfaces.
serrated s. sutura serrata.
shotted s., Sims s. a suture in which the two ends of the suture wire are passed through a split or perforated lead shot that is then compressed.
s's of skull suturae cranii.
sphenoethmoidal s. 1. sutura sphenoethmoidalis. 2. a craniometric landmark, being the most superior point of the sutura sphenoethmoidalis. Called also *point SE.* Abbreviated SE.
sphenofrontal s. sutura sphenofrontalis.
sphenomaxillary s. sutura sphenomaxillaris.
sphenooccipital s. fissura sphenooccipitalis.
sphenoorbital s. sutura sphenoorbitalis.
sphenoparietal s. sutura sphenoparietalis.
sphenopetrosal s. synchondrosis petrooccipitalis.
sphenosquamous s., sphenotemporal s. sutura sphenosquamosa.
sphenovomerine s. sutura sphenovomeralis.
sphenozygomatic s. sutura sphenozygomatica.
squamomastoid s., squamosomastoid s. sutura squamomastoidea.
squamosoparietal s. sutura squamosa cranii.
squamososphenoid s. sutura sphenosquamosa.
squamous s. sutura squamosa.
squamous s. of cranium sutura squamosa cranii.
subcuticular s. a method of skin closure with stitches in subcutaneous tissues parallel with the line of the wound; it may be either continuous or interrupted. See Plate 41.
superficial s. a suture placed through superficial fascia only.
temporal s. sutura squamosa cranii.
temporozygomatic s. sutura temporozygomatica.
tongue-and-groove s. plastic s.
transverse s. of Krause sutura zygomaticomaxillaris.
true s. sutura.
uninterrupted s. continuous s.
zygomaticofrontal s. sutura frontozygomatica.
zygomaticomaxillary s. sutura zygomaticomaxillaris.
zygomaticotemporal s. sutura temporozygomatica.

sux•a•me•tho•ni•um chlo•ride (suk″sə-mə-tho′ne-əm) INN and BAN for *succinylcholine chloride.*

Su•zanne gland (su-zahn′) [Jean Georges *Suzanne*, French physician, late 19th century] see under *gland.*

SUZI subzonal insemination.

SV stroke volume; sinus venosus; simian virus.

SV40 simian virus 40.

Sv sievert.

svas•tha (swus′thyə) [Sanskrit "established in oneself"] the term for health used in ayurveda.

SVC superior vena cava.

Sved•berg unit, flotation unit (sfed′bərg) [Theodor *Svedberg*, Swedish chemist, 1884–1971, inventor of the ultracentrifuge and winner of the Nobel prize for chemistry in 1926 for his work on disperse systems] see under *unit.*

sved•berg (sfed′bərg) Svedberg unit.

SVT supraventricular tachycardia.

swab (swahb) a wad of cotton or other absorbent material firmly attached to the end of a wire or stick, used for applying medication, removing material, collecting bacteriological material, etc.

swad•dler (swahd′lər) a wrapping for an infant's body.
silver s. a swaddler composed of polyester laminated on the inside surface with a thin layer of aluminum, used to prevent hypothermia in the newborn.

swage (swāj) 1. to shape metal by hammering or by adapting it to a die. 2. to fuse suture material to a needle, especially an eyeless needle. 3. a tool or form, often one of a pair, for shaping metal by pressure.

swag•er (swāj′ər) a device or apparatus for shaping metal to a desired form by using simultaneous pressures from various angles.

Swain•so•na (swān′sə-nə) the Darling peas, a genus of Australian legumes related to *Astragalus*; they contain a chemical that inhibits mannosidase activity and causes mannosidosis with potentially fatal neurological symptoms (similar to those of loco poisoning) in livestock grazing on them for extended periods.

swal•low•ing (swahl′o-ing) the taking in of a substance through the mouth and pharynx, past the cricopharyngeal sphincter through the esophagus and into the stomach. The oral phase is a voluntary act, whereas the remainder is a reflex act mediated by an integrating swallowing center in the medulla oblongata. Called also *deglutition.*

Swan-Ganz catheter (swahn′ ganz′) [Harold James C. (Jeremy) *Swan*, American cardiologist, 1922–2005; William *Ganz*, American cardiologist, born 1919] see under *catheter.*

swarm•ing (swawr′ming) spreading in a swarm; a term applied to bacteria, especially *Proteus* species, which spread over the surface of the colony.

sway•back (swa′bak) 1. lordosis (def. 2). 2. abnormal downward curvature of the vertebral column in the dorsal region in horses. 3. enzootic ataxia.

sweat (swet) 1. the liquid secreted by the sweat glands (glandulae sudoriferae), having a salty taste and a pH that varies from 4.5 to 7.5. That produced by the eccrine sweat glands is clear with a faint characteristic odor, and contains water, sodium chloride, and traces of albumin, urea, and other compounds; its composition varies according to factors such as fluid intake, external temperature and humidity, and some hormonal activity. Sweat produced by the larger, deeper, apocrine sweat glands of the axillae contains, in addition, organic material which on bacterial decomposition produces a strong odor. Called also *perspiration.* Cf. *diaphoresis.* 2. to secrete this fluid.

bloody s. hematidrosis.

blue s. chromhidrosis in which the sweat has a blue color, such as in copper workers.

green s. chromhidrosis in which the sweat has a green color, such as in copper workers.

night s's sweating during sleep, a symptom frequently occurring in tuberculosis and acquired immune deficiency syndrome.

sweat•ing (swet′ing) the secretion of sweat; see also *hyperhidrosis.* Called also *perspiration, diaphoresis,* and *sudoresis.*

gustatory s. 1. auriculotemporal syndrome. 2. see under *hyperhidrosis.*

thermal s., thermoregulatory s. the normal mechanism by which a warm external environment causes sweating, as opposed to conditions such as emotional hyperhidrosis and gustatory hyperhidrosis.

Swe•di•aur (Schwe•di•auer) disease (sva′dyour) [François Xavier *Swediaur* (or *Schwediauer*), Austrian physician, 1748–1824] see *Albert disease,* under *disease.*

swee•ney (swe′ne) suprascapular paralysis.

swee•ny (swe′ne) suprascapular paralysis.

Sweet syndrome (swēt) [Robert Douglas *Sweet,* English dermatologist, 20th century] acute febrile neutrophilic dermatosis.

swell•head (swel′hed) 1. lechuguilla fever. 2. bighead (def. 2).

swell•ing (swel′ing) 1. a transient abnormal enlargement or increase in volume of a body part or area not caused by proliferation of cells. See also *tumor* (def. 1). Called also *turgescence, tumescence,* and *tumefaction.* 2. an eminence or elevation.

arytenoid s. an eminence on each side of the embryonic laryngeal orifice that presages the future larynx.

Calabar s's edematous areas seen in loiasis, appearing suddenly on the surface of the body and lasting a few days, sometimes accompanied by fever, pruritus, and urticaria. Called also *Calabar edema* and *fugitive s's.*

capsular s. the development of a swollen appearance of capsulated pneumococci on exposure to type-specific antibody, due to the binding of antibody with capsular polysaccharide; called also *Neufeld reaction.*

cloudy s. hydropic degeneration.

fugitive s's Calabar s's.

genital s's labioscrotal s's.

hypo-osmotic s. swelling of sperm in a hypo-osmotic solution; see *hypo-osmotic swelling test,* under *test.*

labial s's the primordia of the labia majora.

labioscrotal s's a pair of elevations, one on each side of the embryonic phallus and urogenital orifice; they become either the labia majora or the scrotum. Called also *genital s's.*

lingual s., lateral either of a pair of oval elevations in the floor of the mouth in the embryo, at the level of the first pharyngeal arch; the two merge to form the anterior two-thirds of the tongue. Called also *distal tongue bud.*

lingual s., median tuberculum impar.

scrotal s's the primordia of the scrotum.

tympanic s. intumescentia tympanica.

Swen•son operation (swen′sən) [Orvar *Swenson,* American surgeon, born 1909] see under *operation.*

Swift disease (swift) [H. *Swift,* Australian physician, 1858–1937] acrodynia.

Swift-Feer disease (swift′ fār′) [H. *Swift;* Emil *Feer*-Sulzer, Swiss pediatrician, 1864–1955] acrodynia.

swim-up (swim′up) the migration of something into culture medium.

sperm s.-u. the migration of spermatozoa into culture medium; see *sperm swim-up technique,* under *technique.*

swine•pox (swīn-poks) an acute infectious, eruptive disease of piglets, marked by lesions of the skin of the abdomen, flanks, and head, caused by a poxvirus; it is usually mild but occasionally serious or fatal.

switch (swich) 1. a transfer, shift, or change. 2. a device that makes or breaks an electric circuit.

class s. the mechanism by which a B cell or plasma cell changes from production of IgM to production of IgG, IgA, or IgE. See *immunoglobulin genes,* under *gene.*

duodenal s. a surgical treatment for morbid obesity consisting of resection of the greater curvature of the stomach, leaving in place the pylorus and a little of the duodenum, which are anastomosed to the ileum; the rest of the duodenum and jejunum simply empty their secretions into the distal ileum through a new stoma.

isotype s. the mechanism by which a B cell changes from the production of one isotype to another in response to stimulation by various cytokines.

Swy•er syndrome (swi′ər) [Gerald Isaac MacDonald *Swyer,* British endocrinologist, 1917–1995] 46,XY gonadal dysgenesis.

Swy•er-James syndrome (swi′ər jāmz′) [Paul R. *Swyer,* English physician in Canada, born 1921; G.C.W. *James,* American physician, 20th century] see under *syndrome.*

sy•co•si•form (si-ko′sĭ-form) resembling sycosis.

sy•co•sis (si-ko′sis) [Gr. *sykōsis,* from *sykon* fig] a disease marked by inflammation of the hair follicles.

s. bar′bae inflammation of hair follicles, usually occurring on the neck of a male patient with tightly curled beard hair. This condition should not be confused with *pseudofolliculitis barbae* (the so-called "razor bumps"), which is usually seen in shaved areas. Called also *barber's itch.*

lupoid s. a chronic, scarring form of deep sycosis barbae, characterized by a slowly enlarging patch with follicular papulopustules in the active, advancing border, and healing in the central area leaving scars.

s. nu′chae acne keloidalis.

s. vulga′ris s. barbae.

Syd•en•ham chorea, cough (sid′ən-əm) [Thomas *Sydenham,* English physician, sometimes called "the English Hippocrates," 1624–1689] see under *chorea.*

syl•vat•ic (sil-vat′ik) sylvan; pertaining to, located in, or living in the woods. See under *plague.*

Syl•vest disease (səl-vest′) [Ejnar *Sylvest,* Norwegian physician, 1880–1931] epidemic pleurodynia.

syl•vi•an (sil′ve-ən) 1. described by or named for Franciscus *Sylvius.* 2. described by or named for Jacobus *Sylvius.*

Syl•vi•us (sil′ve-əs) Jacobus (Fr. *Jacques Dubois*), 1478–1555, French physician. Confusion exists as to whether some terms ascribed to Franciscus Sylvius should be ascribed instead to this man, particularly the aqueductus mesencephali and related terms.

Syl•vi•us angle, fissure, etc. (sil′ve-əs) [Franciscus *Sylvius* (François de la Böe), Dutch physician, anatomist, and physiologist, 1614–1672] see under *angle,* and see *aqueductus mesencephali, fossa lateralis cerebri, cavum septi pellucidi, sulcus lateralis cerebri,* and *valvula venae cavae inferioris.* Cf. Jacobus *Sylvius.*

Sym•bi•cort (sim′bĭ-kort) trademark for a combination preparation of budesonide and formoterol fumarate.

sym•bi•ol•o•gy (sim″bi-ol′ə-je) the scientific study of symbiosis and symbiotic organisms.

sym•bi•on (sim′bi-on) symbiont.

sym•bi•on•ic (sim-bi-on′ik) pertaining to or characterized by symbiosis.

sym•bi•ont (sim′bi-ont, sim′be-ont) [*syn-* + Gr. *bioun* to live] an organism which lives in a state of symbiosis.

sym•bi•o•sis (sim″bi-o′sis) pl. *symbio′ses* [Gr. *symbiōsis*] 1. in parasitology, the living together or close association of two dissimilar organisms, each of the organisms being known as a *symbiont.* The association may be beneficial to both (mutualism), beneficial to one without effect on the other (commensalism), beneficial to one and detrimental to the other (parasitism), detrimental to one without effect on the other (amensalism), or detrimental to both (synnecrosis). 2. in psychiatry, a mutually reinforcing relationship between two persons who are dependent on each other; a normal characteristic of the relationship between the mother and infant child.

antagonistic s., antipathetic s. an association between two organisms which is to the disadvantage of one of them; parasitism.

conjunctive s. association between two different organisms, with bodily union between them.

constructive s. an association between two organisms which is of benefit to the physiologic processes of one of them.

disjunctive s. symbiosis without actual union of the organisms.

sym•bi•ote (sim′bi-ōt) symbiont.

sym•bi•ot•ic (sim″bi-ot′ik) associated in symbiosis; living together.

sym•bleph•a•ron (sim-blef′ə-ron) [*syn* + Gr. *blepharon* eyelid] an adhesion between the tarsal conjunctiva and the bulbar conjunctiva.

anterior s. attachment of the lid to the eyeball by fibrous bands.

posterior s. adhesion between the lid and the eyeball extending into the fornix.

total s. adhesion of the entire conjunctival surface between the lid and the eyeball.

sym•bleph•a•rop•ter•yg•i•um (sim-blef″ə-ro-tər-ij′e-əm) a combination of symblepharon and pterygium; a form of symblepharon in which the lid is joined to the eyeball by a cicatricial band resembling a pterygium.

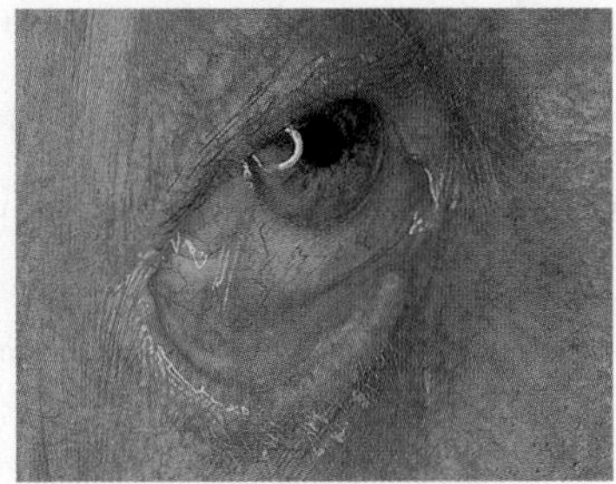

■ Symblepharon.

sym·bol (sim′bəl) [Gr. *symbolon*, from *symballein* to interpret] 1. something, particularly an object, representing something else. 2. in chemistry, a letter or combination of letters representing an atom or a group of atoms. 3. in psychoanalytic theory, a representation or perception that replaces unconscious mental content.

phallic s. in psychoanalysis, any pointed or upright object which may represent the phallus or penis.

sym·bo·lia (sim-bo′le-ə) ability to recognize the nature of objects by their distinctive forms.

sym·bol·ism (sim′bəl-iz-əm) 1. the act or process of representing something by a symbol. 2. in psychoanalytic theory, a mechanism of unconscious thinking characterized by substitution of a symbol for a repressed or threatening impulse or object, which is often of a sexual nature, so as to avoid censorship by the superego.

sym·bol·iza·tion (sim″bəl-ĭ-za′shən) a type of defense mechanism in which one idea or object comes to represent another because of similarity or association between them.

sym·brachy·dac·tyl·ia (sim-brak″e-dak-til′e-ə) symbrachydactyly.

sym·brachy·dac·tyl·ism (sim-brak″e-dak′təl-iz-əm) symbrachydactyly.

sym·brachy·dac·ty·ly (sim-brak″e-dak′tə-le) [Gr. *syn* together + *brachys* short + *daktylos* finger] a condition in which the fingers or toes are short and webbed.

***sym*·di·chlo·ro·meth·yl ether** (sim-di-klor″o-meth′əl e′thər) bis-(chloromethyl)ether.

Syme amputation (operation) (sīm) [James *Syme*, Scottish surgeon, 1799–1870] see under *amputation.*

sym·e·lus (sim′ə-ləs) symmelus.

Sy·ming·ton body (si′ming-tən) [Johnson *Symington*, Scottish anatomist, 1851–1924] the anococcygeal body; see under *body.*

Sym·lin (sim′lin) trademark for a preparation of pramlintide acetate.

sym·me·lia (sĭ-me′le-ə) [*syn-* + *-melia*] a developmental anomaly characterized by an apparent fusion of the lower limbs. There may be three feet *(tripodial s.)*, two feet *(dipodial s.)*, one foot *(monopodial s.)*, or no feet *(apodal s.* or *sirenomelia)*.

sym·me·lus (sim′ə-ləs) a fetus exhibiting symmelia.

Sym·mers disease (sim′ərz) [Douglas *Symmers*, American physician, 1879–1952] follicular lymphoma.

Sym·mers fibrosis (sim′ərz) [William St. Clair *Symmers*, Irish pathologist, 1863–1937] pipestem fibrosis.

Sym·me·trel (sim′ə-trəl) trademark for a preparation of amantadine hydrochloride.

sym·met·ri·cal (sĭ-met′rĭ-kəl) [Gr. *symmetrikos*] pertaining to or exhibiting symmetry; in chemistry, denoting compounds which contain atoms or groups at equal intervals in the molecule.

sym·me·try (sim′ə-tre) [Gr. *symmetria; syn* with + *metron* measure] the similar arrangement in form and relationships of parts around a common axis, or on each side of a plane of the body.

bilateral s. the configuration of an irregularly shaped body (as the human body or that of higher animals) that can be divided by a longitudinal plane into halves that are mirror images of each other.

helical s. an arrangement of capsomers seen in viruses with a rodlike or filamentous capsid, in which subunits form a coiled structure, with each subunit forming bonds with the subunit in each of the adjoining turns to provide stability.

icosahedral s. an arrangement of viral subunits in which the structure of the viral capsid is characterized by symmetry having the rotation axes of a regular polygon with 20 triangular surfaces (icosahedron); each face contains several subunits, the total number of subunits in the capsid being a multiple of 60.

inverse s. correspondence as between an object and its mirror image, in which one side of one object corresponds to the opposite side of another.

radial s. symmetry in which the body parts are arranged regularly around a central axis.

sym·pa·thec·to·mize (sim″pə-thek′tə-mīz) to subject to sympathectomy.

sym·pa·thec·to·my (sim″pə-thek′tə-me) [*sympathetic* + *-ectomy*] the transection or other interruption of any part of the sympathetic nervous pathways. Operations may be named according to the location of the nerve, ganglion, or plexus operated on, as *cervical, dorsal, lumbar,* or *thoracolumbar s.*, or in reference to the diaphragm, as *subdiaphragmatic, supradiaphragmatic,* or *transdiaphragmatic s.*

chemical s. suppression of the activity of the sympathetic nervous system by appropriate drugs.

sym·pa·the·tec·to·my (sim″pə-thə-tek′tə-me) sympathectomy.

sym·pa·thet·ic (sim″pə-thet′ik) [Gr. *sympathētikos*] 1. pertaining to, caused by, or exhibiting sympathy. 2. pertaining to the sympathetic nervous system or one of its nerves; see under *system.*

sym·pa·thet·i·co·mi·met·ic (sim″pə-thet″ĭ-ko-mi-met′ik) [*sympathetic* + *-mimetic*] sympathomimetic.

sym·pa·theto·blast (sim″pə-thet′o-blast) sympathoblast.

sym·path·ic (sim-path′ik) sympathetic.

sym·path·i·cec·to·my (sim-path″ĭ-sek′tə-me) sympathectomy.

sym·path·i·co·blast (sim-path′ĭ-ko-blast″) sympathoblast.

sym·path·i·co·blas·to·ma (sim-path″ĭ-ko-blas-to′mə) a neuroblastoma arising in one of the ganglia of the sympathetic nervous system; called also *sympathoblastoma.*

sym·path·i·co·go·ni·o·ma (sim-path″ĭ-ko-go″ne-o′mə) sympathicoblastoma.

sym·path·i·col·y·sis (sim-path″ĭ-kol′ĭ-sis) sympathectomy.

sym·path·i·co·lyt·ic (sim-path″ĭ-ko-lit′ik) sympatholytic.

sym·path·i·co·mi·met·ic (sim-path″ĭ-ko-mi-met′ik) sympathomimetic.

sym·path·i·cop·a·thy (sim-path″ĭ-kop′ə-the) any disease due to disorder of the sympathetic nervous system.

sym·path·i·co·trip·sy (sim-path″ĭ-ko-trip′se) [*sympathetic ganglion* + *-tripsy*] the surgical crushing of a nerve, ganglion, or plexus of the sympathetic nervous system.

sym·path·i·co·trope (sim-path′ĭ-ko-trōp) sympathicotropic (def. 2).

sym·path·i·co·tro·pic (sim-path″ĭ-ko-tro′pik) [*sympathetic* + *-tropic*] 1. having an affinity for the sympathetic nervous system. 2. an agent that has an affinity for or exerts its principal effect upon the sympathetic nervous system.

sym·pa·thism (sim′pə-thiz-əm) suggestibility.

sym·pa·tho·ad·re·nal (sim″pə-tho-ə-dre′nəl) 1. pertaining to the sympathetic nervous system and the adrenal medulla. 2. involving the sympathetic nervous system and the adrenal glands, such as the effects of the alarm reaction.

sym·patho·blast (sim-path′o-blast″) [*sympathetic* + *-blast*[1]] a pluripotential cell in the embryo that will develop into a sympathetic nerve cell or a chromaffin cell; called also *sympathetoblast, sympathicoblast,* and *sympathetic neuroblast.*

sym·pa·tho·blas·to·ma (sim″pə-tho-blas-to′mə) sympathicoblastoma.

sym·pa·tho·gone (sim′pə-tho-gōn″) sympathogonium.

sym·pa·tho·go·nia (sim″pə-tho-go′ne-ə) (sing. *sympathogo′nium*) [*sympathetic* + Gr. *gonē* seed] undifferentiated embryonic cells that develop into sympathetic neurons.

sym·pa·tho·go·ni·o·ma (sim″pə-tho-go″ne-o′mə) sympathicoblastoma.

sym·pa·tho·go·ni·um (sim″pə-tho-go′ne-əm) singular of *sympathogonia.*

sym·pa·tho·in·hib·i·to·ry (sim″pə-tho-in-hib′ĭ-to″re) causing inhibition of the activity of the sympathetic nervous system.

sym·pa·thol·y·sis (sim″pə-thol′ĭ-sis) sympathectomy.

sym·pa·tho·lyt·ic (sim″pə-tho-lit′ik) [*sympathetic* + *-lytic*] 1. opposing the effects of impulses conveyed by adrenergic postganglionic fibers of the

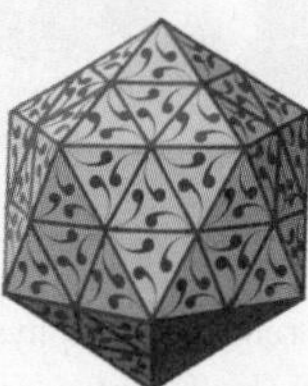

■ Icosahedral symmetry, the 20 faces of the figure each divided into 12 subunits (represented by apostrophes), for a total of 240 subunits.

sympathetic nervous system. 2. an agent that opposes the effects of impulses conveyed by adrenergic postganglionic fibers of the sympathetic nervous system; called also *antiadrenergic.*

sym·pa·tho·mi·met·ic (sim″pə-tho-mi-met′ik) [*sympathetic* + *-mimetic*] 1. mimicking the effects of impulses conveyed by adrenergic postganglionic fibers of the sympathetic nervous system. 2. an agent that produces effects similar to those of impulses conveyed by adrenergic postganglionic fibers of the sympathetic nervous system. See also *adrenergic.*

sym·pa·thy (sim′pə-the) [Gr. *sympatheia*] 1. compassion for another person's thoughts, feelings, and experiences; cf. *empathy.* 2. an influence produced in any organ by disease, disorder, or other change in another part. 3. a relation which exists between people or things such that change in the state of one is reflected in the other.

sym·pec·to·thi·ene (sim-pek″to-thi′ēn) ergothioneine.

sym·pec·to·thi·on (sim-pek″to-thi′on) ergothioneine.

sym·pha·lan·gia (sim″fə-lan′jə) [*syn-* + *phalang-* + *-ia*] congenital end-to-end fusion of contiguous phalanges of a digit, usually associated with other deformity of the hand or foot.

sym·phal·an·gism (sim-fal′ən-jiz-əm) symphalangia.

sym·phor·i·car·pus (sim″for-ĭ-kahr′pəs) [Gr. *symphorein* to bear together + *karpos* fruit] a homeopathic preparation of the fruit of *Symphoricarpos racemosus,* or snowberry, a shrub of North America.

Sym·pho·ro·my·ia (sim″for-o-mi′yə) a genus of snipe flies (family Rhagionidae), some of which are vicious biters.

sym·phys·e·or·rha·phy (sim-fiz″e-or′ə-fe) symphysiorrhaphy.

sym·phy·ses (sim′fĭ-sēz) [Gr.] plural of *symphysis.*

sym·phys·i·al (sim-fiz′e-əl) symphyseal.

sym·phys·ic (sim-fiz′ik) characterized by abnormal fusion of adjacent parts.

sym·phys·i·ol·y·sis (sim-fiz″e-ol′ĭ-sis) [*symphysis* + *-lysis*] separation or slipping of symphyses, especially the symphysis pubis.

sym·phys·i·or·rha·phy (sim-fiz″e-or′ə-fe) [*symphysis* + *-rrhaphy*] suture of a divided symphysis.

sym·phys·io·tome (sim-fiz′e-o-tōm) a knife used in performing symphysiotomy.

sym·phys·i·ot·o·my (sim-fiz″e-ot′ə-me) [*symphysis* + *-tomy*] the division of the fibrocartilage of the symphysis pubis, in order to facilitate delivery, by increasing the diameter of the pelvis.

sym·phy·sis (sim′fĭ-sis) pl. *sym′physes* [Gr. "a growing together, natural junction"] [TA] a type of cartilaginous joint in which the apposed bony surfaces are firmly united by a plate of fibrocartilage; called also *fibrocartilaginous joint.* **symphys′eal** *adj*

s. intervertebra′lis [TA] intervertebral symphysis: the union between the vertebral bodies, consisting of the anterior and posterior longitudinal ligaments, and the intervertebral disks.

s. mandi′bulae [TA] mandibular symphysis: the line of fusion in the median plane of the mandible that marks the union of the two halves of the mandible; called also *s. mentalis* and *s. menti.*

manubriosternal s., s. manubriosterna′lis [TA] manubriosternal joint: that uniting the manubrium with the body of the sternum, which begins as a synchondrosis *(synchondrosis manubriosternalis)* and later becomes a symphysis.

s. menta′lis, s. men′ti s. mandibulae.

pubic s., s. pu′bica [TA] the joint formed by union of the bodies of the pubic bones in the median plane by a thick mass of fibrocartilage.

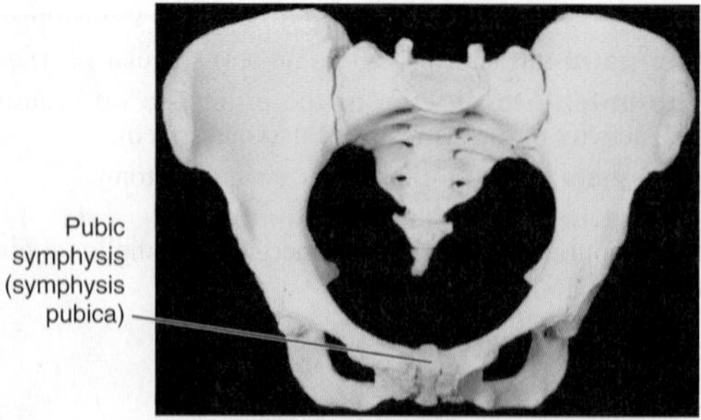

s. xiphosterna′lis [TA] xiphisternal joint: that uniting the xiphoid process with the body of the sternum. It is usually transformed to a synostosis by 40 years of age, but may remain a symphysis.

Sym·phy·tum (sim′fĭ-təm) [L., from Gr. *symphyton*] a genus of perennial Old World herbs of the family Boraginaceae, having coarse, hairy leaves and blue, yellow, or purple flowers. *S. officina′le* is comfrey, a species native to Europe and North America whose roots and leaves are demulcent and astringent.

sym·phy·tum (sim′fĭ-təm) a demulcent and astringent homeopathic preparation of *Symphytum officinale.*

sym·plasm (sim′plaz-əm) tissue in which there is no cellular structure.

sym·plast (sim′plast) symplasm.

sym·plex (sim′pleks) a chemical compound in which a high molecular substance is bound by residual valencies; included are activators, adsorbents, hemoglobin, and toxin-antitoxin.

sym·po·dia (sim-po′de-ə) symmelia.

sym·po·di·al (sim-po′de-əl) denoting a pattern of growth of conidiogenous cells in which after a spore breaks off at an apex the following apex and spore appear slightly farther back and to the side.

sym·pod·u·la (sim-pod′u-lə) a conidiogenous cell that grows in a sympodial pattern.

sym·port (sim′port) a cotransport mechanism that couples the movement of two substances across a membrane in the same direction. Cf. *antiport.*

sym·port·er (sim′port-ər) a membrane transport protein that mediates the cotransport of substances in the same direction.

symp·tom (simp′təm) [L. *symptoma;* Gr. *symptōma* anything that has befallen one] any subjective evidence of disease or of a patient's condition, i.e., such evidence as perceived by the patient; a noticeable change in a patient's condition indicative of some bodily or mental state. See also *sign.*

abstinence s's substance withdrawal.

accessory s. any symptom not necessarily characteristic of the patient's disease.

Bárány s. 1. in disturbances of equilibrium of the vestibular apparatus, the direction of the fall is influenced by changing the position of the patient's head. 2. caloric test; see under *test.*

Bonhoeffer s. loss of normal muscle tonus in chorea.

Buerger s. in thromboangiitis obliterans, with the patient lying down the pain in the affected lower limb is relieved only by lying with the limb hung over the side of the bed.

cardinal s. 1. a symptom of greatest significance to the physician, establishing the identity of the illness. 2. *(in the pl.)* the symptoms shown in the pulse, temperature, and respiration.

Castellani-Low s. a fine tremor of the tongue seen in sleeping sickness.

characteristic s. a symptom that is almost universally associated with a particular disease or condition.

concomitant s. a symptom not essential to a disease, but which may have an accessory value in its diagnosis.

constitutional s. a symptom indicative of or due to disorder of the whole body.

conversion s. symbolic representation of psychic conflict by alteration or absence of a voluntary motor or sensory function suggesting a neurological or general medical condition but not fully explained by either, and neither intentionally produced nor feigned.

crossbar s. of Fraenkel blocking of the peristaltic wave on the lesser curvature of the stomach at the site of an ulcer, on fluoroscopy of the stomach.

deficiency s. a symptom caused by a lack of something necessary for normal bodily functioning, such as an enzyme, vitamin, or hormone. See also *deficiency.*

delayed s. a symptom that does not appear for some time after the occurrence of the causes which produce it.

direct s. a symptom that is directly caused by the disease.

dissociation s. see under *anesthesia.*

Epstein s. in infants with certain neurologic conditions, failure of the upper eyelid to move downward, giving the child a frightened expression.

equivocal s. a symptom that may be produced by several different diseases.

factitious s. a symptom produced intentionally, usually by the patient; cf. *induced s.*

general s. constitutional s.

guiding s. characteristic s.

halo s. the seeing of colored rings around an individual light source; indicative of glaucoma.

indirect s. a symptom indicative of a condition that may or may not be due to a particular disease or lesion.

induced s. a symptom produced intentionally; cf. *factitious s.*

labyrinthine s's the symptoms of disease of the internal ear.

Liebreich s. a symptom of red-green color blindness in which light effects appear red and shadows green.

local s. a symptom caused by local disease or a particular lesion.

localizing s's symptoms that indicate the location of a lesion.

negative s. a symptom in which a characteristic of normal health is diminished or absent in disease, such as the flat affect or mutism sometimes occurring in schizophrenia.
objective s. a symptom that is obvious to the senses of the observer; see *sign.*
Oehler s. coldness and pallor of the feet in intermittent claudication.
pathognomonic s. a symptom that establishes with certainty the diagnosis of the disease.
precursory s., premonitory s. signal s.
presenting s. the symptom or group of symptoms of which the patient complains the most or from which they seek relief.
rainbow s. halo s.
rational s. subjective s.
reflex s. a symptom occurring in a part remote from that which is affected by the disease.
Roger s. a temperature below the normal in the third stage of tuberculous meningitis.
Séguin signal s. Sé sign.
signal s. a sensation, aura, or other subjective experience that gives warning of the approach of an epileptic or other seizure.
static s. a symptom that does not change.
subjective s. a symptom that is perceptible to the patient only.
sympathetic s. sympathetic pain or other disorder in a part separate from the part that is the seat of disease.
Trendelenburg s. see under *gait.*
withdrawal s's substance withdrawal.

symp·to·mat·ic (simp″tə-mat′ik) [Gr. *symptōmatikos*] 1. pertaining to or of the nature of a symptom. 2. indicative (of a particular disease or disorder). 3. exhibiting the symptoms of a particular disease but having a different cause. 4. directed at the allaying of symptoms, as symptomatic treatment.

symp·to·ma·tol·o·gy (simp″tə-mə-tol′ə-je) 1. the branch of medicine that deals with symptoms; the systematic discussion of symptoms. 2. the combined symptoms of a disease.

symp·to·ma·to·lyt·ic (simp″tə-mat″o-lit′ik) [*symptom* + *-lytic*] causing the disappearance of symptoms.

symp·to·mo·lyt·ic (simp″to-mo-lit′ik) symptomatolytic.

sym·pus (sim′pəs) symmelus.
s. a′pus sirenomelus.
s. di′pus a fetus with dipodial symmelia.
s. mo′nopus a fetus with monopodial symmelia.

Syms tractor (simz) [Parker *Syms,* American surgeon, 1860–1933] see under *tractor.*

syn- [Gr. *syn* with, together] a prefix signifying union or association.

Syn·a·cort (sin′ə-kort″) trademark for preparations of hydrocortisone.

syn·a·del·phus (sin″ə-del′fəs) [*syn-* + *-adelphus*] conjoined twins with a single body and eight limbs.

Syn·a·gis (sin′əjis) trademark for a preparation of palivizumab.

Syn·a·lar (sin′ə-lahr) trademark for preparations of fluocinolone acetonide.

syn·al·bu·min (sin″al-bu′min) a postulated competitive inhibitor of insulin, an insulin B chain bound to albumin; its significance in human diabetes mellitus is unknown.

syn·al·gia (sin-al′jə) referred pain. **synal′gic** *adj*

Syn·al·gos-DC (sin′əl-gos) trademark for a combination preparation of dihydrocodeine bitartrate, aspirin, and caffeine.

syn·ana·morph (sin-an′ə-morf″) [*syn-* + *anamorph*] any of two or more anamorphs having the same teleomorph.

syn·apse (sin′aps) [Gr. *synapsis* a conjunction, connection] the site of functional apposition between neurons, at which an impulse is transmitted from one neuron to another, usually by a chemical neurotransmitter (e.g., acetylcholine, norepinephrine, etc.) released by the axon terminal of the excited (presynaptic) cell. The neurotransmitter diffuses across the synaptic cleft to bind with receptors on the postsynaptic cell membrane, and thereby effects electrical changes in the postsynaptic cell which result in depolarization (excitation) or hyperpolarization (inhibition). Synapses also occur at sites of apposition between nerve endings and effector organs (e.g., the neuromuscular junction). A few synapses in the central nervous system are electrical synapses (q.v.). In official terminology called *synapsis.*
axoaxonic s. a synapse between the axon of one neuron and the axon of another neuron.
axodendritic s. a synapse between the axon of one neuron and dendrites of another.
axodendrosomatic s. a synapse between the axon of one neuron and the dendrites and body (soma) of another, as in motoneurons.
axosomatic s. a synapse between the axon of one neuron and the body (soma) of another.

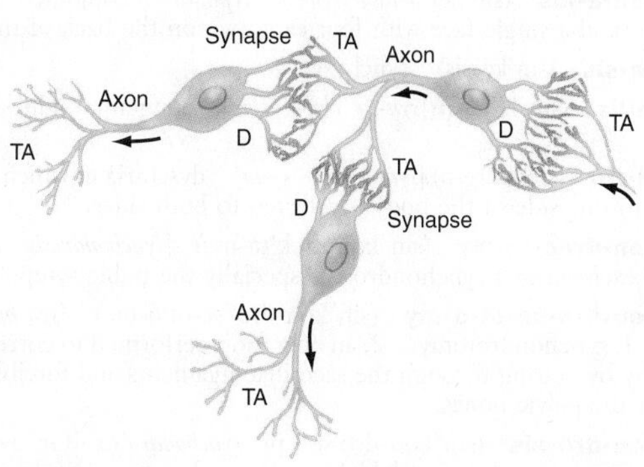

■ Diagram of three synapses. Nerve impulse is indicated by arrows, showing that the direction of passage is from the terminal arborization *(TA)* or nerve endings of the axon of one neuron to the dendrites *(D)* of another neuron.

chemical s. the usual type of synapse seen in vertebrates, in which the impulse is carried by a neurotransmitter. Cf. *electrical s.*
dendrodendritic s. a rare type of synapse involving transmission from a dendrite of one cell to a dendrite of another.
electrical s. a point of lateral contact (other than a synapse) between nerve fibers, across which impulses are conducted directly through the nerve membranes from one fiber to the other; it is common in invertebrates but in vertebrates it has been found at only a few central nervous system sites. Cf. *chemical s.* Called also *ephapse.*
electrotonic s. see *gap junction,* under *junction.*
en passant s. synaptic contact between nonterminal parts of axons; seen in coelenterates and among certain special cells in the central nervous system of vertebrates. Cf. *bouton en passant.*
loop s. a synapse having a relatively long area of contact of fiber membranes; seen in many invertebrates.

syn·ap·sis (sĭ-nap′sis) [Gr. "conjunction"] 1. the intimate association of homologous chromosomes, mediated by the synaptonemal complex, that occurs during the zygotene stage of meiosis I. 2. [TA] official terminology for *synapse.*

syn·ap·tic (sĭ-nap′tik) 1. pertaining to or affecting a synapse. 2. pertaining to synapsis.

syn·ap·to·brev·in (sə-nap″to-brev′in) a membrane protein associated with synaptic vesicles and playing a central role in exocytosis of neurons and docking and fusion of synaptic vesicles on plasma membranes.

syn·ap·tol·o·gy (sin″ap-tol′ə-je) a branch of neurology concerned with the synaptic correlations of the nervous system.

syn·ap·to·nem·al (sə-nap″to-ne′məl) [*synapsis* + Gr. *nēma* thread] see under *complex.*

syn·ap·to·phy·sin (sə-nap″to-fi′sin) an integral membrane glycoprotein found in the presynaptic vesicles of neurons.

syn·ap·to·some (sĭ-nap′to-sōm″) any of the membrane-bound sacs that break away from axon terminals at a synapse after brain tissue has been homogenized in sugar solution; it contains synaptic vessels and mitochondria.

syn·ap·to·tag·min (sə-nap″to-tag′min) an integral membrane protein of synaptic vesicles, thought to play a role in membrane interactions and the docking of the vesicles at postsynaptic sites.

Syn·a·rel (sin′ə-rel) trademark for a preparation of nafarelin acetate.

syn·ar·thro·dia (sin″ahr-thro′de-ə) synarthrosis.

syn·ar·thro·phy·sis (sin-ahr″thro-fi′sis) [*syn-* + *arthro-* + *physis* growth] any ankylosing process; progressive ankylosis of joints.

syn·ar·thro·ses (sin″ahr-thro′sēz) [Gr.] plural of *synarthrosis.*

syn·ar·thro·sis (sin″ahr-thro′sis) pl. *synarthro′ses* [*syn-* + *arthrosis*] [TA] a bony junction that is immovable and is connected by solid connective tissue; the two types are the fibrous joint *(juncture fibrosa)* and the cartilaginous joint *(junctura cartilaginea).* **synarthro′dial** *adj*

syn·can·thus (sin-kan′thəs) [*syn-* + *canthus*] adhesion of the eyeball to the orbital structures.

syn·cary·on (sin-kar′e-on) fertilization nucleus.

syn·ce·lom (sin-se′lom) the perivisceral cavities of the body considered as one structure, including the pleural, cardiac, and peritoneal cavities, as well as the tunica vaginalis testis.

Syn·ceph·a·las·trum (sin-sef″ə-las′trəm) a genus of fungi of the order Mucorales. *S. racemo′sum* has been found in cases of mucormycosis.

syn·ceph·a·lus (sin-sef′ə-ləs) [*syn-* + *-cephalus*] conjoined twins with one head and a single face with four ears, two on the back of the head.

syn·che·sis (sin′ke-sis) synchysis.

syn·chi·lia (sin-ki′le-ə) [*syn-* + *chil-* + *-ia*] congenital adhesion of the lips.

syn·chi·ria (sin-ki′re-ə) [*syn-* + *chir-* + *-ia*] dyschiria in which a stimulus applied to one side of the body is referred to both sides.

syn·chon·drec·to·my (sin″kon-drek′tə-me) [*synchondrosis* + *-ectomy*] surgical excision of a synchondrosis, especially the pubic symphysis.

syn·chon·dro·se·ot·o·my (sin″kon-dro″se-ot′ə-me) [*synchondrosis* + *-tomy*] 1. synchondrotomy. 2. an operation performed to correct bladder exstrophy by cutting through the sacroiliac ligaments and forcibly drawing together the pelvic bones.

syn·chon·dro·sis (sin″kon-dro′sis) pl. *synchondro′ses* [Gr. *synchondrōsis* a growing into one cartilage] [TA] a union between two bones formed by either hyaline cartilage or fibrocartilage; it is usually temporary, the intervening cartilage being converted into bone before adult life.

synchondro′ses colum′nae vertebra′lis [TA] synchondroses of vertebral column: the cartilaginous joints of the vertebral column, comprising the intervertebral disks (disci intervertabrales).

s. cos′tae pri′mae [TA] synchondrosis of first rib: the joint between the manubrium of the sternum and the first rib, in which the costal cartilage is united directly to the sternum.

cranial s's, synchondro′ses cra′nii [TA] the cartilaginous junctions between the bones of the cranium.

s. of first rib s. costae primae.

intraoccipital s., anterior s. intraoccipitalis anterior.

intraoccipital s., posterior s. intraoccipitalis posterior.

s. intraoccipita′lis ante′rior [TA] anterior intraoccipital synchondrosis: the cartilaginous union of the pars basilaris with the partes laterales of the occipital bone in the newborn.

s. intraoccipita′lis poste′rior [TA] posterior intraoccipital synchondrosis: the cartilaginous union of the squama with the partes laterales of the occipital bone in the newborn.

s. manubriosterna′lis [TA] manubriosternal synchondrosis: the joint uniting the manubrium with the body of the sternum, which begins as a synchondrosis and later becomes a symphysis *(symphysis manubriosternalis).*

neurocentral s. see under *joint.*

s. petrooccipita′lis [TA] petrooccipital synchondrosis: the plate of cartilage in the petrooccipital fissure which helps to unite the basilar portion of the occipital bone and the petrous portion of the temporal bone.

sphenobasilar s. s. sphenooccipitalis.

s. sphenoethmoida′lis [TA] sphenoethmoidal synchondrosis: the cartilaginous union between the body of the sphenoid and the labyrinth of the ethmoid bone.

sphenooccipital s. 1. s. sphenooccipitalis. 2. in cephalometric radiology, the uppermost point of the synchondrosis sphenooccipitalis. Called also *point SO.* Abbreviated SO.

s. sphenooccipita′lis [TA] sphenooccipital synchondrosis: the cartilaginous union of the anterior end of the basilar portion of the occipital bone with the posterior surface of the body of the sphenoid bone.

s. sphenopetro′sa [TA] sphenopetrosal synchondrosis: the cartilaginous union of the inferior border of the greater wing of the sphenoid bone with the petrous portion of the temporal bone in the sphenopetrosal fissure.

synchondro′ses sterna′les [TA] sternal synchondroses: the cartilaginous joints between different parts of the sternum, comprising the xiphisternal (symphysis xiphosternalis) and manubriosternal joints (symphysis manubriosternalis).

synchondro′ses tho′racis [TA] synchondroses of thorax: the cartilaginous joints uniting the various bones of the thorax, including those between the ribs and sternum and those between different parts of the sternum.

s's of vertebral column synchondroses columnae vertebralis.

syn·chon·drot·o·my (sin″kon-drot′ə-me) [*synchondrosis* + *-tomy*] 1. splitting of any synchondrosis. 2. symphysiotomy.

syn·cho·ri·al (sin-kor′e-əl) sharing a common placenta; said of multiple fetuses.

syn·chro·nia (sin-kro′ne-ə) 1. synchrony. 2. the formation of parts or tissues at the usual time. Cf. *heterochronia* (def. 1).

syn·chron·ic (sing-kron′ik) synchronous.

syn·chro·nism (sing′krə-niz-əm) synchrony.

syn·chro·ni·za·tion (sing″krə-nĭ-za′shən) 1. the achieving of a desired relationship among corresponding points of different signals (such as waves). 2. the achieving of synchronism.

syn·chro·nous (sing′krə-nəs) pertaining to or characterized by synchrony.

syn·chro·ny (sing′krə-ne) 1. the simultaneous occurrence of two events. 2. the linkage of two events (such as waves) by a fixed time interval. 3. a state in which corresponding points on two or more signals (such as waves) regularly occur simultaneously. Called also *synchronia* and *synchronism.*

atrioventricular s., AV s. in the heart, the physiological condition of atrial electrical activity followed by ventricular electrical activity, with the interval between being that necessary for impulse conduction from atria to ventricles.

bilateral s. the occurrence of a secondary synchronous discharge at a location in the brain exactly contralateral to a discharge caused by a lesion.

syn·chro·tron (sing′kro-tron) a machine for accelerating charged particles (electrons, protons) in circular orbits, by simultaneously manipulating the strength of the magnetic field and the frequency of the accelerating voltage. It combines features of the cyclotron and betatron and will produce 70 million volts.

syn·chy·sis (sin′kĭ-sis) [Gr. "a mixing together"] a softening or fluid condition of the vitreous body of the eye.

s. scintil′lans cholesterol crystals in the vitreous that develop as a degenerative change following inflammation or other ocular diseases.

syn·ci·ne·sis (sin″si-ne′sis) synkinesis.

syn·cli·nal (sin-kli′nəl) [Gr. *synklinein* to lean together] bent or inclined together.

syn·clit·ic (sin-klit′ik) pertaining to or marked by synclitism.

syn·clit·i·cism (sin-klit′ĭ-siz-əm) synclitism.

syn·clit·ism (sin′klit-iz-əm) [Gr. *synklinein* to lean together] 1. parallelism between the planes of the fetal head and those of the pelvis. 2. normal, synchronous maturation of the nucleus and cytoplasm of blood cells. Cf. *asynclitism.* Called also *syncliticism.*

syn·clo·nus (sin′klo-nəs) [*syn-* + *clonus*] 1. muscular tremor, or the successive clonic contraction of various muscles together. 2. any disease characterized by muscular tremors.

s. beribe′rica muscular tremors associated with beriberi.

syn·co·pe (sing′kə-pe) [Gr. *synkopē*] a temporary suspension of consciousness due to generalized cerebral ischemia; called also *faint.* **syn′copal, syncop′ic** *adj*

Adams-Stokes s. see under *syndrome.*

cardiac s. syncope due to cerebral anemia caused by obstructions to cardiac output or arrhythmias such as ventricular asystole, extreme bradycardia, or ventricular tachycardia; this type occurs suddenly, with no premonitory symptoms or only momentary ones.

carotid sinus s. see under *syndrome.*

convulsive s. syncope with convulsive movements that are milder than those seen in epilepsy.

cough s. tussive s.

deglutition s. swallow s.

digital s. a sudden, temporary loss of strength in the fingers.

laryngeal s. tussive s.

micturition s. brief syncope that occurs during or immediately after micturition, usually associated with rising from bed at night to urinate; it may be a form of orthostatic hypotension.

neurally mediated s., neurally mediated reflex s., neurocardiogenic s. a serious type of vasovagal syncope precipitated by a stimulus that causes either bradycardia, a decrease in vascular tone, or both at once.

postural s. syncope resulting from orthostatic hypotension.

Stokes-Adams s. Adams-Stokes syndrome.

stretching s. syncope associated with stretching upward of the upper limbs while the spine is extended.

swallow s. syncope associated with swallowing, a disorder of atrioventricular conduction mediated by the vagus nerve.

tussive s. syncope that is brief and associated with vigorous and explosive paroxysms of coughing; it is seen in men more often than women. Called also *cough s.*, *laryngeal s.*, and *laryngeal vertigo.*

vasodepressor s., vasovagal s. a transient vascular and neurogenic reaction marked by pallor, nausea, sweating, bradycardia, and rapid fall in arterial blood pressure which, when below a critical level, results in loss of consciousness and characteristic electroencephalographic changes. It is most often evoked by emotional stress associated with fear or pain. Called also *vagal* or *vasovagal attack, vasovagal reaction,* and *Gowers syndrome.*

syn·cre·tio (sin-kre′she-o) [L.] a growing together or adhesion, as between inflamed serous surfaces in contact.

syn·cyt·i·ol·y·sin (sin″sit-e-ol′ĭ-sin) a lysin destructive to the syncytium; formed in the blood of an animal into which matter from the placenta of another animal has been injected.

syn·cyt·i·o·ma (sin-sit″e-o′mə) syncytial endometritis.

s. malig′num choriocarcinoma.

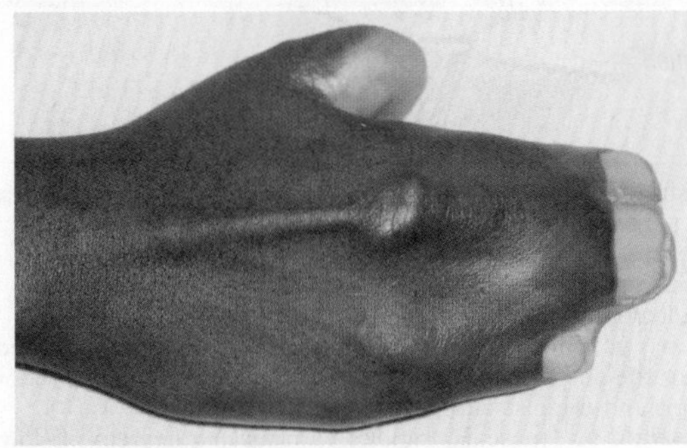

■ Syndactyly of the hand in Apert syndrome.

syn·cyt·io·tox·in (sin-sit′e-o-tok″sin) a toxin that has a specific action on the placenta.

syn·cyt·io·tro·pho·blast (sin-sit″e-o-tro′fo-blast) 1. the outer syncytial layer of the trophoblast; called also *syntrophoblast*. 2. syncytiotrophoblastic cell.

syn·cyt·io·tro·pho·blas·tic (sin-sit″e-o-tro″fo-blas′tik) pertaining to or of the nature of the syncytiotrophoblast.

syn·cy·ti·um (sin-sish′e-əm) a multinucleate mass of protoplasm produced by the merging of cells. **syncyt′ial** *adj*

syn·cy·toid (sin′sĭ-toid) resembling a syncytium.

syn·dac·tyl·ia (sin″dak-til′e-ə) syndactyly.

syn·dac·ty·lism (sin-dak′tə-liz-əm) syndactyly.

syn·dac·ty·ly (sin-dak′tə-le) [*syn-* + Gr. *daktylos* finger] the most common congenital anomaly of the hand or foot, marked by persistence of the webbing between distal phalanges of adjacent digits, so that they are more or less completely attached. Called also *webbed fingers* (in the hand) and *webbed toes* (in the foot). **syndac′tylous** *adj*

complete s. syndactyly in which the webbing extends from the base of the involved digits to the tip.

complex s. syndactyly in which the bones or nails of the involved digits are fused.

complicated s. the most severe form of syndactyly; in addition to the fusion of complex syndactyly, there are deformed and missing digits.

double s. syndactyly involving three digits (two webs).

incomplete s., partial s. syndactyly in which the connecting webbing does not extend all the way to the tips of the digits.

simple s. syndactyly in which the connecting webbing consists only of skin.

single s. syndactyly involving two digits (a single web).

triple s. syndactyly involving four digits (three webs).

syn·de·can (sin′də-kan) any of a group of integral membrane proteoglycans, consisting of a 33-kD core and a variable number of heparan sulfate and chondroitin sulfate chains; the extracellular domain binds a number of proteins of the extracellular matrix, and syndecans have roles in both cell signaling and cell adhesion.

syn·dec·to·my (sin-dek′tə-me) peritectomy.

syn·del·phus (sin-del′fəs) synadelphus.

syn·de·sis (sin′də-sis, sin-de′sis) 1. arthrodesis. 2. synapsis.

syn·des·mec·to·my (sin″dəz-mek′tə-me) [*syndesm-* + *-ectomy*] surgical removal of part or all of a ligament.

syn·des·mec·to·pia (sin″dəz-mək-to′pe-ə) [*syndesm-* + *ectopia*] unusual situation of a ligament.

syn·des·mi·tis (sin″dez-mi′tis) [*syndesm-* + *-itis*] 1. inflammation of a ligament or ligaments. 2. conjunctivitis.

s. metatar′sea inflammation of the metatarsal ligaments occurring during strenuous marches; called also *march tumor*.

syndesm(o)- [Gr. *syndesmos* band or ligament] a combining form denoting relationship to connective tissue, particularly the ligaments.

syn·des·mo·cho·ri·al (sin″dəz-mo-kor′e-əl) a type of placentation, occurring in ruminants, characterized by limited destruction of the endometrial epithelium.

syn·des·mog·ra·phy (sin″dəz-mog′rə-fe) [*syndesmo-* + *-graphy*] a description of the ligaments.

syn·des·mol·o·gy (sin″dəz-mol′ə-je) [*syndesmo-* + *-logy*] arthrology.

syn·des·mo·odon·toid (sin-dez″mo-o-don′toid) the posterior of the two atloaxoid articulations formed between the anterior surface of the transverse ligaments and the back of the odontoid process.

syn·des·mo·pexy (sin-dez′mo-pek″se) [*syndesmo-* + *-pexy*] the operative fixation of a dislocation by reattachment of the ligaments.

syn·des·mo·phyte (sin-dez′mo-fīt) [*syndesmo-* + *-phyte*] an osseous excrescence, or bony outgrowth, from a ligament.

syn·des·mo·plas·ty (sin-dez′mo-plas″te) [*syndesmo-* + *-plasty*] plastic operation on a ligament. **syndesmoplas′tic** *adj*

syn·des·mor·rha·phy (sin″dəz-mor′ə-fe) [*syndesmo-* + *-rrhaphy*] suture or repair of ligaments.

syn·des·mo·sis (sin″dəz-mo′sis) pl. *syndesmo′ses* [Gr. *syndesmos* band] [TA] a type of fibrous joint in which the intervening fibrous connective tissue forms an interosseous membrane or ligament.

syndesmo′ses colum′nae vertebra′lis [TA] syndesmoses of vertebral column: the fibrous joints holding the vertebral column in position, aided by ligaments including the interspinous, intertransverse, longitudinal, nuchal, supraspinous, and transverse ligaments, and the ligamenta flava.

s. dentoalveola′ris [TA] dentoalveolar syndesmosis: one of the fibrous joints by which a tooth is held in its socket. Called also gomphosis [TA alternative].

s. radioulna′ris [TA] radioulnar syndesmosis: the fibrous union of the radius and ulna, which consists of the interosseous membrane of the forearm and the oblique cord of the elbow; called also *middle radioulnar joint*.

syndesmo′ses tho′racis [TA] syndesmoses of thorax: the fibrous joints of the thorax, including the external and internal intercostal membranes.

s. tibiofibula′ris [TA] tibiofibular syndesmosis: a firm fibrous union formed at the distal ends of the tibia and fibula between the fibular notch of the tibia and a roughened triangular surface on the fibula, which frequently contains a synovial prolongation of the cavity of the talocrural articulation. Called also *distal* or *inferior tibiofibular joint*.

s. tympanostapedia′lis [TA] tympanostapedial syndesmosis: the connection of the base of the stapes with the secondary membrane in the fenestra vestibuli; see also *ligamentum anulare stapediale*.

s′s of vertebral column syndesmoses columnae vertebralis.

syn·des·mot·o·my (sin″dəz-mot′ə-me) [*syndesmo-* + *-tomy*] the dissection or cutting of a ligament.

syn·drome (sin′drōm) [Gr. *syndromē* concurrence] a set of symptoms that occur together; the sum of signs of any morbid state; a symptom complex. In genetics, a pattern of multiple malformations thought to be pathogenetically related. See also *disease*.

Syndrome

For terms not found here, see also under *disease*.

22q11 deletion s. hemizygous deletion of a 1.5 to 3.0 Mb region of chromosome 22q11.2 as a result of defective recombination in meiosis. It has a highly variable phenotype, partly as a function of the extent and precise location of the deletion, and includes various named syndromes with different presentations that have been shown to have the same genetic basis, including DiGeorge syndrome and velocardiofacial syndrome (qq.v.).

Aagenaes s. an autosomal recessive syndrome consisting of intrahepatic cholestasis and edema of the lower limbs.

Aarskog s., Aarskog-Scott s. an X-linked syndrome characterized by ocular hypertelorism, anteverted nostrils, broad upper lip, peculiar scrotal "shawl" above the penis, and small hands. Called also *faciogenital dysplasia* and *faciodigitogenital s.*

Aase s. a familial syndrome characterized by mild growth retardation, hypoplastic anemia, variable leukocytopenia, triphalangeal thumbs, narrow shoulders, and late closure of fontanels, and occasionally by cleft lip, cleft palate, retinopathy, and web neck. A recessive mode of inheritance has been suggested.

Syndrome *Continued*

abdominal muscle deficiency s. prune-belly s.
abstinence s. substance withdrawal.
achalasia-addisonian s. Allgrove s.
Achard s. arachnodactyly associated with receding mandible and joint laxity limited to the hands and feet.
Achard-Thiers s. masculinization with hirsutism and adult-onset diabetes mellitus in postmenopausal women resulting from overproduction of adrenocortical androgens.
acquired immune deficiency s., acquired immunodeficiency s. (AIDS) the most severe manifestation of disease due to infection with human immunodeficiency virus (HIV). The criteria established by the Centers for Disease Control and Prevention for the diagnosis of AIDS include (1) presence of certain opportunistic infections indicating an underlying defect in cell-mediated immunity in the absence of known causes of underlying immunodeficiency or other host defense defects; or (2) CD4$^+$ cell count of less than 200/mL; or (3) CD4$^+$ cell percentage of less than 14 per cent. See also *human immunodeficiency virus infection*, under *infection*.
actinic reticuloid s. chronic actinic dermatitis.
acute brain s. delirium.
acute chest s. a complex of symptoms seen in patients with sickle cell disease, often due to a bacterial infection or to infarction of lung tissue; characteristics include severe chest pain, dyspnea, tachypnea, fever, excessive leukocytosis, pulmonary edema, and sometimes petechiae on the chest or conjunctivae as well as fat emboli. Death may result from severe pulmonary complications.
acute coronary s. a classification encompassing clinical presentations ranging from unstable angina through non–Q wave infarction, sometimes also including Q wave infarction.
acute nephritic s. the sudden onset of hematuria, proteinuria, diminished urine production, azotemia, hypertension, and edema; the clinical manifestation of acute glomerulonephritis.
acute organic brain s. 1. delirium. 2. occasionally, a term used to denote the acute form of an organic mental syndrome.
acute radiation s. a syndrome caused by exposure to a whole-body dose of over 1 gray of ionizing radiation. Symptoms, whose severity and time of onset depend on the size of the dose, include erythema, nausea and vomiting, fatigue, diarrhea, fever, petechiae, bleeding from the mucous membranes, reduction in the number of lymphocytes, granulocytes, and platelets, gastrointestinal hemorrhage, epilation, hypotension, tachycardia, and dehydration; death may occur within hours or weeks of exposure.
acute respiratory distress s. (ARDS) fulminant pulmonary interstitial and alveolar edema, which usually develops within a few days after an initiating trauma; it is thought to result from alveolar injury that has led to increased capillary permeability. Called also *adult respiratory distress s.* and *shock lung*.
acute retinal necrosis s. acute retinal necrosis.
Adams-Stokes s. episodic cardiac arrest and syncope due to failure of normal and escape pacemakers, with or without ventricular fibrillation; it is the principal clinical manifestation of severe heart block. Called also *Adams-Stokes syncope*, *Morgagni-Adams-Stokes s.*, and *Stokes-Adams s.* or *syncope*.
addisonian s. the complex of symptoms resulting from adrenocortical insufficiency; see *Addison disease*, under *disease*.
addisonian-achalasia s. Allgrove s.
Adie s. a syndrome consisting of a pathological pupil reaction (tonic pupil) with a myotonic condition on accommodation; the pupil on the affected side contracts (for near vision) and dilates more slowly than the pupil on the opposite side. In direct or indirect light, the affected pupil either does not react at all or reacts in an abnormal fashion. Certain tendon reflexes are absent or diminished, usually the patellar reflexes, but there are no motor or sensory disturbances or other demonstrable changes indicating disease of the nervous system. Called also *Holmes-Adie s.*
adiposogenital s. see under *dystrophy*.
adrenogenital s. a general term for the group of syndromes in which inappropriate masculinization or feminization, sometimes with precocious puberty, results from disorders of adrenal function that also affect gonadal steroidogenesis; it includes congenital adrenal hyperplasia and tumors of the adrenal cortex.
adult respiratory distress s. (ARDS) acute respiratory distress s.
AEC s. Hay-Wells s.
afferent loop s. chronic partial obstruction of the proximal loop of duodenum and jejunum after partial gastrectomy and gastrojejunostomy, resulting in duodenal distention, pain, and nausea after the person ingests food.
aglossia-adactylia s. hypoglossia-hypodactyly s.
Ahumada-del Castillo s. galactorrhea-amenorrhea syndrome with low gonadotropin secretion.
Aicardi s. a syndrome affecting female infants, characterized by agenesis of the corpus callosum, large discrete areas of chorioretinopathy, spasms and tonic seizures, and mental retardation.
akinetic-rigid s. muscular rigidity with varying degrees of slowness of movement; seen in parkinsonism and disorders of the basal ganglia.
Alagille s. an autosomal dominant syndrome of neonatal jaundice, cholestasis with peripheral pulmonic stenosis, and occasionally septal defects or patent ductus arteriosus, due to paucity or absence of intrahepatic bile ducts; it is characterized by unusual facies and ocular, vertebral, and nervous system abnormalities.
Alajouanine s. symmetric lesions of the sixth and seventh cranial nerves with bilateral facial paralysis and bilateral lateral rectus palsy of the eyeball, associated with bilateral clubfoot. Cf. *Möbius s.*
albinism-deafness s. an X-linked syndrome consisting of deafness of varying degrees with piebaldism or albinism; some authorities consider it an allelic variant of Waardenburg syndrome type 2.
Albright s., Albright-McCune-Sternberg s. polyostotic fibrous dysplasia, patchy dermal pigmentation, and endocrine dysfunction. Called also *McCune-Albright s.*
Aldrich s. Wiskott-Aldrich s.
Alezzandrini s. a rare disorder of unknown pathogenesis, characterized by unilateral tapetoretinal degeneration followed by facial vitiligo and poliosis on the same side, sometimes associated with deafness.
"Alice in Wonderland" s. a delusional state manifested by depersonalization, alteration in the sense of the passage of time, distorted perception of objects, hallucinations, and other delusions or illusions. It may be associated with schizophrenia, epilepsy, migraine, diseases of the parietal lobe, hypnagogic states, or the use of hallucinogenic drugs.
alien hand s., alien limb s. involuntary but apparently purposeful movements of a hand or a limb, which is perceived by the patient to be controlled by an outside force; seen with lesions of the corpus callosum or frontal lobe and with corticobasal degeneration.
Allan-Herndon-Dudley s. an X-linked syndrome caused by mutations in the *SLC16A2* gene (locus: Xq13.2), which encodes a thyroid hormone transporter, characterized by severe mental retardation, dysarthria, athetoid movements, muscle hypoplasia, and spastic paraplegia.
Allemann s. the association of double kidney and clubbed fingers, sometimes associated with facial asymmetry and degeneration of various motor nerves.
Allgrove s. glucocorticoid deficiency with achalasia and alacrima; inherited as an autosomal recessive trait; called also *achalasia-addisonian s.*, *addisonian-achalasia s.*, and *triple-A s.*
Alport s. a hereditary disorder characterized by progressive sensorineural hearing loss, progressive pyelonephritis or glomerulonephritis, and occasionally ocular defects. There are various subtypes, some with autosomal dominant inheritance, some autosomal recessive, and others X-linked.
Alström s. an autosomal recessive syndrome of retinitis pigmentosa with nystagmus and early loss of central vision, deafness, obesity, and diabetes mellitus.
amnesic s., amnestic s., amnestic-confabulatory s. a mental disorder characterized by impaired memory with anterograde and sometimes retrograde amnesia in a normal state of consciousness; i.e., the syndrome does not include the impaired memory seen in dementia or delirium. There may be disorientation, confabulation, and lack of insight into the memory deficit. The most common cause is thiamine deficiency from chronic alcohol abuse *(Wernicke-Korsakoff syndrome)*, but it may also result from any pathological process causing bilateral damage to parts of the medial temporal lobe or diencephalon, such as the hippocampal formations, mammillary bodies, or dorsal medial nuclei of the thalamus. Other causes include head trauma, brain tumors, infarction, cerebral hypoxia, carbon monoxide poisoning, and herpes simplex encephalitis. Called also *dysmnesic s.*
amniotic band s. early rupture of the amnion with formation of fibrous strands of amnion that may adhere to or compress parts of the fetus, resulting in a wide variety of abnormalities, including craniofacial defects, limb distortions, amputation, and abdominal or thoracic evisceration. Called also *amniotic band sequence*, *amniotic band disruption complex*, and *constriction band s.*

amniotic infection s. of Blane a syndrome in which fetal sepsis follows swallowing and at times aspiration of contaminated amniotic fluid.
amyostatic s. Wilson disease.
Andersen s. 1. a syndrome consisting of bronchiectasis with cystic fibrosis and vitamin A deficiency. 2. Andersen-Tawil s.
Andersen-Tawil s. an autosomal dominant form of long QT syndrome characterized by periodic paralysis, ventricular arrhythmias, and dysmorphism of facial and skeletal bones. Called also *Andersen s.*
androgen insensitivity s. resistance of target organs in males to the action of androgens; the result is any of a spectrum from normal-appearing male phenotypes to female phenotype; see *complete androgen insensitivity s.*, *partial androgen insensitivity s.*, and *mild androgen insensitivity s.*
Angelman s. an autosomal recessive syndrome characterized by jerky puppetlike movements, frequent laughter, mental and motor retardation, peculiar open-mouthed facies, and seizures. It is caused by loss of expression of genes on maternally derived chromosome 15q11–13, usually as a result of a deletion; the same loss of gene function inherited from the father causes Prader-Willi syndrome.
Angelucci s. excitable temperament, palpitation, and vasomotor disturbance in patients with vernal conjunctivitis.
angry back s. excited skin s.
angular gyrus s. a syndrome resulting from an infarction or other lesion of the angular gyrus on the dominant side; symptoms may include alexia or agraphia or may feature the symptoms of Gerstmann syndrome.
ankyloblepharon–ectodermal dysplasia–clefting s. Hay-Wells s.
anorexia-cachexia s. a systemic response to conditions such as cancer or the acquired immunodeficiency syndrome, resulting from a poorly understood relationship between anorexia and cachexia, manifested by malnutrition, weight loss, muscular weakness, acidosis, and toxemia. The anorexia may be caused by a severe metabolic disturbance that contributes to development of cachectic wasting, which in turn reinforces anorexia by release from a tumor of a humoral product that stimulates the satiety center in the hypothalamus.
anterior chamber cleavage s. a term for several types of mesenchymal dysgenesis affecting neural crest derivatives in the iris, trabecula, and cornea. In ascending severity these disorders are: *Axenfeld anomaly*, *Axenfeld syndrome*, *Rieger anomaly*, and *Rieger syndrome*.
anterior cord s. anterior spinal artery s.
anterior cornual s. muscular atrophy due to lesions of the anterior horns of the spinal cord. Cf. *spinal muscular atrophy*.
anterior interosseous s., anterior interosseous nerve s. a complex of symptoms caused by a lesion of the anterior interosseous nerve, resulting usually from fracture or laceration but sometimes from an entrapment neuropathy; symptoms include pain in the proximal forearm and weakness of the muscles innervated by the nerve. Called also *Kiloh-Nevin s.*
anterior opercular s., anterior operculum s. intermittent or persistent loss of voluntary movements of the muscles of the lower face, throat, jaw, and tongue, characterized by dysarthria, sialorrhea, and dysphagia, and caused by bilateral lesions of the frontoparietal operculum. It most commonly results from sequential bilateral opercular strokes; other causes include congenital anomalies, epilepsy, and infection. Called also *Foix-Chavany-Marie s.*
anterior scalene s. scalenus anterior s.
anterior spinal artery s. injury to the ventral spinal cord caused by blockage of the anterior spinal artery and infarction of the areas it supplies. Below the level of the lesion complete paralysis, hypalgesia, and hypesthesia occur but there is relative preservation of the posterior sensations of touch, position, and vibration.
anterior tibial compartment s. rapid swelling, increased tension, pain, and ischemic necrosis of the muscles of the anterior tibial compartment of the leg; the skin becomes glossy, erythematous, and edematous as the necrosis occurs. The cause is unknown, but usually there is a history of excessive exertion.
anticholinergic s. the central and peripheral effects produced by overdosage or abnormal reaction to clinical dosage of anticholinergic drugs, e.g., atropine, phenothiazines, antihistamines, and tricyclic antidepressants; signs and symptoms include anxiety, delirium, disorientation, hallucinations, seizures, tachycardia, hyperpyrexia, mydriasis, vasodilation, gastric and urinary retention, and decreased salivary, sweat, bronchial, and nasopharyngeal secretions.

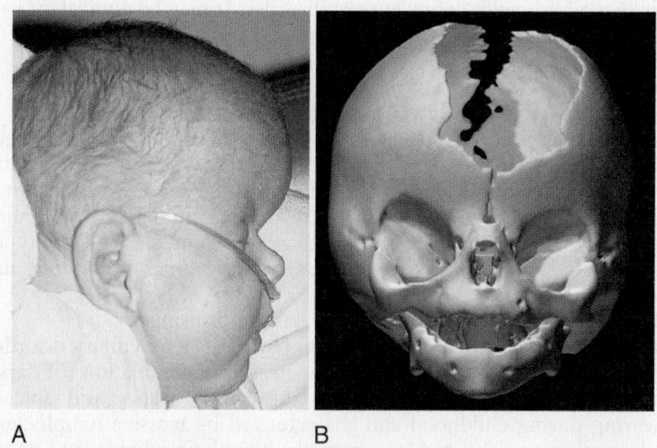

■ Apert syndrome in clinical view *(A)* and CT construction of the craniofacial skeleton *(B)*.

anticonvulsant hypersensitivity s. a life-threatening, multiorgan hypersensitivity reaction to anticonvulsant medications, especially phenytoin; manifestations include rash, arthralgia, eosinophilia, fever, lymphadenopathy, and liver dysfunction.
antiphospholipid s., antiphospholipid antibody s. (APS) a multisystem inflammatory disorder characterized by the presence of circulating antiphospholipid antibodies with thrombosis (including thrombotic microangiopathy), spontaneous abortion, thrombocytopenia, valvular heart disease, and other less frequent symptoms. A severe type called *catastrophic antiphospholipid syndrome* is characterized by infarctions of several different organs and is often fatal.
Anton s., Anton-Babinski s. a form of anosognosia in which the patient denies, and often is unaware of, the existence of clinically demonstrable blindness and may resort to confabulation to hide it; it may be the result of denial (q.v.) or of bilateral infarctions of the occipital lobes.
anxiety s. the physical symptoms accompanying anxiety, such as palpitation of the heart, rapid and shallow respiration, sweating, pallor, and a feeling of panic.
aortic arch s. any of a group of disorders leading to occlusion of the arteries arising from the aortic arch; causes include atherosclerosis, arterial embolism, syphilitic or tuberculous arteritis, and other conditions. See also *Takayasu arteritis*, under *arteritis*.
Apert s. an autosomal dominant disorder characterized by oxycephaly and syndactyly, often with other skeletal deformities and usually with mental retardation. Called also *acrocephalosyndactyly, type I* or, occasionally, *acrocephalosyndactyly*.
s. of apparent mineralocorticoid excess apparent mineralocorticoid excess.
ARN s. acute retinal necrosis.
Arnold-Chiari s. see under *malformation*.
Arnold nerve reflex cough s. a reflex cough due to irritation of the area supplied by Arnold nerve (the auricular branch of the vagus nerve); this area is the posterior and inferior portion of the external auditory canal and the posterior half of the tympanic membrane.
arthropathy-camptodactyly s. a rare autosomal recessive disorder characterized by arthropathy associated with congenital flexion contractures of the fingers and synovial and tendon abnormalities, and by constrictive pericarditis.
Ascher s. blepharochalasis occurring with goiter (adenoma of the thyroid) and redundancy of the mucous membrane and submucous tissue of the upper lip.
Asherman s. persistent amenorrhea and secondary sterility due to intrauterine adhesions and synechiae, usually as a result of uterine curettage.
Asherson s. a syndrome of dysphagia due to neuromuscular incoordination and achalasia of the cricopharyngeus muscle during the third stage of swallowing. It causes diversion of liquids into the air passages, precipitating paroxysms of coughing. Called also *cricopharyngeal achalasia s.*
Asperger s. [DSM-IV] a pervasive developmental disorder resembling autistic disorder, being characterized by severe impairment of social interactions and by restricted interests and behaviors, but lacking the delays in development of language, cognitive function, and self-help

skills that additionally define autistic disorder. It may be equivalent to a high-functioning form of autistic disorder.
asplenia s. Ivemark s.
ataxia-telangiectasia s. ataxia-telangiectasia; see under *ataxia.*
atypical mole s., atypical nevus s. dysplastic nevus s.
auriculotemporal s. redness and sweating on the cheek in connection with eating; many persons have mild cases, especially after eating spicy or sharp-tasting foods. Some individuals have more severe forms, such as after surgery or other damage to the parotid gland or auriculotemporal nerve, or in disease states such as syringomyelia or some types of encephalitis. Called also *Frey s., gustatory hyperhidrosis* or *sweating,* and *gustatory sweating s.*
autoerythrocyte sensitization s. painful bruising s.
autoimmune lymphoproliferative s. (ALPS) a hereditary disorder of lymphocyte apoptosis that results in the accumulation of large numbers of mature lymphocytes in the lymph nodes and spleen, appearing during childhood and characterized by massive lymphadenopathy, splenomegaly, and autoimmune hemolytic anemia and other cytopenias.
autoimmune polyendocrine s's, autoimmune polyglandular s's polyglandular autoimmune s's.
Avellis s. a syndrome in which a brainstem lesion limits vagal innervation unilaterally, resulting in ipsilateral paralysis of the vocal cord and soft palate and loss of sensitivity to pain and temperature in the contralateral leg, trunk, arm, and neck, and in the skin over the scalp; called also *Avellis paralysis.*
Axenfeld s. Axenfeld anomaly accompanied by glaucoma and defective development of the corneoscleral trabecular meshwork and other angle structures. See also *anterior chamber cleavage s.*
Ayerza s. pulmonary hypertension with dilatation of the pulmonary arteries, related to disease of the lungs; cf. *plexogenic pulmonary arteriopathy.*
Baastrup s. kissing spines.
Babinski s. the association of cardiac and arterial disorders with chronic syphilitic meningitis, tabes dorsalis, paralytic dementia, and other late syphilitic manifestations.
Babinski-Fröhlich s. adiposogenital dystrophy.
Babinski-Nageotte s. a syndrome due to multiple lesions affecting the medullary pyramid and sensory tracts, the cerebellar peduncle, and the reticular formation, and marked by contralateral hemiplegia and hemianesthesia (usually only of the pain and temperature senses), ipsilateral hemiasynergia, hemiataxia, and Horner syndrome.
Babinski-Vaquez s. Babinski s.
bacterial overgrowth s. stasis s.
BADS s. a rare congenital syndrome of unknown heritability characterized by *b*lack locks, oculocutaneous *a*lbinism, and *d*eafness of the *s*ensorineural type; see *oculocutaneous albinism.*
Balint s. gaze paralysis, ataxia of eye movements, and other disturbances of visual attention, with preservation of spontaneous and reflex eye movements, usually caused by bilateral lesions in the parietooccipital region.
Baller-Gerold s. an autosomal recessive syndrome characterized by craniosynostosis and radial aplasia. Called also *craniosynostosis–radial aplasia s.*
ballooning mitral valve s., ballooning posterior leaflet s. mitral valve prolapse s.
Bannayan-Zonana s. a rare autosomal dominant syndrome characterized by hemangiomas of the trunk, cutaneous lipomas, macrocephaly, and swelling of the abdomen with angiomas.
Bannwarth s. the European term for the meningopolyneuritis that may occur in Lyme disease.
Bardet-Biedl s. an autosomal recessive disorder characterized by mental retardation, pigmentary retinopathy, obesity, polydactyly, and hypogonadism; cf. *Laurence-Moon s.* and *Biemond s., II.*
Barlow s. mitral valve prolapse s.
Barraquer-Simons s. partial lipodystrophy.
Barrett s. peptic ulcer of the lower esophagus, often with stricture, due to the presence of columnar-lined epithelium in the esophagus (sometimes containing functional mucous cells, parietal cells, or chief cells) instead of the normal squamous cell epithelium. It is sometimes premalignant, followed by esophageal adenocarcinoma. Called also *Barrett esophagus.*
Bart s. a form of epidermolysis bullosa dystrophica inherited as an autosomal dominant trait, characterized by congenital localized absence of the skin, blister formation resulting from mechanical trauma, and nail dystrophy.
Barth s. an X-linked disorder caused by mutation in the *TAZ* gene (locus: q28), which encodes a protein of unknown function that is highly expressed in cardiac and skeletal muscle, characterized by dilated cardiomyopathy, hypotonia, neutropenia, and growth retardation, with moderately increased urinary excretion of 3-methylglutaconic and 3-methylglutaric acids. Called also *3-methylglutaconicaciduria type II.*
Bartter s. hypertrophy and hyperplasia of the juxtaglomerular cells, producing hypokalemic alkalosis and hyperaldosteronism, characterized by absence of hypertension in spite of markedly increased plasma renin concentrations, and by insensitivity to the pressor effects of angiotensin. It usually affects children, may be hereditary, and may be associated with other anomalies such as mental retardation and short stature. See also *Gitelman s.* Called also *juxtaglomerular cell hyperplasia.*
basal cell nevus s. nevoid basal cell carcinoma s.
basilar artery s. vertebrobasilar insufficiency.
BASM s. biliary atresia splenic malformation s.
Bassen-Kornzweig s. abetalipoproteinemia.
battered child s. unexplained or inappropriately explained physical trauma and other manifestations of severe, repeated physical abuse of children, usually by a parent or other caretaker.
Bazex s. eczematous and psoriasiform lesions on the ears, nose, cheeks, hands, feet, and knees in patients with carcinomas of the upper respiratory and digestive tracts. Called also *paraneoplastic acrokeratosis.*
Beals s. congenital contractural arachnodactyly.
Bean s. blue rubber bleb nevus s.
Bearn-Kunkel s., Bearn-Kunkel-Slater s. chronic active hepatitis.
Beckwith s., Beckwith-Wiedemann s. a congenital autosomal dominant syndrome with variable expressivity characterized by exomphalos, macroglossia, and gigantism, often associated with organomegaly, adrenocortical cytomegaly, and dysplasia of the renal medulla. Called also *EMG s.* and *exomphalos-macroglossia-gigantism s.*
Behçet s. a variant of neutrophilic dermatosis of unknown etiology, involving the small blood vessels, characterized by recurrent aphthous ulceration of oral and pharyngeal mucous membranes and genitalia, with skin lesions, severe uveitis, retinal vasculitis, optic atrophy, and often involvement of the joints, gastrointestinal system, and central nervous system.
Benedikt s. a syndrome consisting of ipsilateral oculomotor paralysis, contralateral hyperkinesia, contralateral tremor and paresis of the arm and leg, and ipsilateral ataxia; caused by lesions that damage the third nerve and involve the nucleus ruber and corticospinal tract. Called also *tegmental mesencephalic paralysis* and *tegmental s.*
benign hypermobility s., benign joint hypermobility s. Ehlers-Danlos syndrome, type III, inherited as an autosomal dominant trait and characterized by hypermobility of the joints with minimal abnormalities of the skin.
Berardinelli-Seip s. total lipodystrophy.
Berdon s. megacystis-microcolon–intestinal hypoperistalsis s.
Bernard s., Bernard-Horner s. Horner s.
Bernard-Sergent s. addisonian crisis.
Bernard-Soulier s. (BSS) an autosomal recessive disorder characterized by giant platelets with membranes lacking glycoprotein Ib, the probable receptor for plasma von Willebrand factor; this keeps the platelets from binding the factor, which is necessary for their adhesion to the subendothelial surfaces of blood vessels. Symptoms include mild to moderate mucocutaneous and visceral hemorrhaging, purpura, and prolonged bleeding time. Called also *giant platelet s.* See also *thrombasthenia* and *von Willebrand disease.*
Bernheim s. right ventricular heart failure due to left ventricular hypertrophy with bulging of the interventricular septum that causes obstruction to flow from the right atrium to ventricle, altering ventricular filling and capacity.
Bertolotti s. sacralization of the fifth lumbar vertebra together with sciatica and scoliosis.
bi s. in traditional Chinese medicine, a disease with pain caused by an obstruction in the body.
Biemond s., II an autosomal recessive disorder characterized by iris coloboma, obesity, mental retardation, hypogonadism, and postaxial polydactyly; cf. *Bardet-Biedl s.* and *Laurence-Moon s.*

biliary atresia splenic malformation s. a rare congenital condition of biliary atresia together with polysplenia or some other anomaly of the spleen. It may be associated with other anomalies, including defects of the portal vein, heart, lungs, and liver. Called also BASM s.

billowing mitral valve s., billowing posterior leaflet s. mitral valve prolapse s.

Bing-Neel s. the central nervous system manifestations of Waldenström macroglobulinemia; symptoms may include encephalopathy, hemorrhage, stroke, convulsions, delirium, and coma.

Birt-Hogg-Dube s. an autosomal dominant disorder of proliferation of ectodermal and mesodermal components, caused by a mutation on chromosome 17p and characterized by multiple acrochordons, trichodiscomas, and fibrofolliculomas on the head, chest, back, and arms; kidney tumors; spontaneous pneumothorax; and intestinal polyposis.

Björnstad s. an autosomal recessive disorder characterized by congenital sensorineural deafness and pili torti.

Blackfan-Diamond s. congenital hypoplastic anemia (def. 1).

Blau s. a rare, autosomal dominant type of autoinflammatory disease (q.v.) characterized by granulomatous arthritis, skin rash, and ocular symptoms that may include iritis or anterior uveitis.

blind loop s. stasis s.

Bloch-Sulzberger s. incontinentia pigmenti.

Bloom s. an autosomal recessive syndrome consisting of erythema and telangiectasia in a butterfly distribution on the face, photosensitivity, and well-proportioned dwarfism of prenatal onset. Immunoglobulins show abnormalities and there is a high incidence of malignancy, especially leukemia. Many patients are of Ashkenazi Jewish ancestry, due to a founder effect. The genome is unusually unstable in somatic cells, with an excess of sister chromatid exchange, and is characterized by chromosome abnormalities including breaks, gaps, rearrangements, and other mutations; it is caused by mutations in a gene *(BLM)* that encodes a specific DNA helicase.

blue diaper s. a defect of tryptophan absorption in which, because of intestinal bacterial action on the tryptophan, the urine contains abnormal indoles, giving it a blue color. It is similar to Hartnup disease and is thought to have autosomal recessive inheritance.

blue rubber bleb nevus s. a rare syndrome, sometimes autosomal dominant, of multiple blue rubber bleb nevi associated with hemangiomas of the gastrointestinal tract, which bleed readily and cause chronic iron deficiency anemia; most cases present in infancy or childhood, but some do not appear until later. Called also *Bean s.*

blue toe s. a blue color of the toes, sometimes bilateral, with skin necrosis and ischemic gangrene, resulting from arterial occlusion by emboli, thrombi, or injury.

body of Luys s. hemiballismus.

Boerhaave s. spontaneous rupture of the esophagus.

Bonnet-Dechaume-Blanc s. Wyburn-Mason s.

Böök s. PHC s.

BOR s. branchio-oto-renal s.

Börjeson s., Börjeson-Forssman-Lehmann s. an X-linked syndrome characterized by severe mental retardation, epilepsy, hypogonadism, hypometabolism, marked obesity, swelling of the subcutaneous tissues of the face, and large ears.

Bouillaud s. pericarditis and endocarditis accompanying rheumatic fever.

Bourneville-Pringle s. tuberous sclerosis complex.

Bouveret s. 1. paroxysmal supraventricular tachycardia. 2. obstruction of the gastric outlet by a gallstone passed into the duodenal bulb through a cholecystoduodenal or choledochoduodenal fistula.

bowel bypass s. a type of neutrophilic dermatosis with arthritis that may occur one to six years after jejunoileal bypass, characterized by rash, malaise, myalgia, joint pain, sterile skin pustules, and a flulike illness; it is probably caused by circulating immune complexes that include bacterial antigens resulting from overgrowth in the bypassed part of the intestine.

brachial s. see under *plexopathy.*

Brachmann-de Lange s. de Lange s.

Bradbury-Eggleston s. a syndrome of dysautonomia with orthostatic hypotension, visual disturbances, hypohidrosis, impotence, lowered basal metabolic rate, dizziness, syncope, presyncope, and a slow, unchanging pulse. It occurs predominantly in older males in the early morning hours during the summer and is due to impaired peripheral vasoconstriction; it usually has a progressive course. Called also *primary* or *pure autonomic failure.*

bradycardia-tachycardia s., brady-tachy s. a clinical manifestation of the sick sinus syndrome characterized by periods of atrial and ventricular bradycardia alternating with periods of rapid regular or irregular atrial or ventricular tachyarrhythmias.

branchio-oto-renal s. branchial arch anomalies (preauricular pits, branchial fistulas or pits) associated with Mondini deafness and renal dysplasia, inherited as an autosomal dominant trait with high penetrance and variable expression. Called also *BOR s.* and *Melnick-Fraser s.*

Brennemann s. mesenteric and retroperitoneal lymphadenitis as a sequel of throat infections.

Briquet s. somatization disorder.

Brissaud-Sicard s. spasmodic hemiplegia caused by lesions of the pons.

Bristowe s. a series of symptoms caused by a tumor of the corpus callosum, including hemiplegia and apraxia.

brittle cornea s. a rare autosomol recessive syndrome, characterized by brittle corneas, blue sclerae, skin hyperelasticity, and joint hypermobility.

Brock s. middle lobe s.

bronze baby s. brown discoloration of the skin in an infant undergoing phototherapy for neonatal hyperbilirubinemia, caused by failure to excrete bilirubin products properly.

Brooke-Spiegler s. an autosomal dominant syndrome (gene locus: 16q12-q13) characterized by multiple skin tumors such as cylindromas and trichoepitheliomas, usually in the head and neck region; some authorities consider this and multiple familial trichoepithelioma to be variants of the same condition. Called also *familial cylindromatosis.*

Brooks-Wisniewski-Brown s. an X-linked syndrome of characteristic facies, static encephalopathy, mental and growth retardation, ocular abnormalities, spastic diplegia, and behavioral problems; a mitochondrial defect has been suggested as the cause.

Brown vertical retraction s. adhesion of the muscles of the eye in the fetus.

Brown-Séquard s. a syndrome due to damage of one half of the spinal cord, resulting in ipsilateral paralysis and loss of discriminatory and joint sensation, and contralateral loss of pain and temperature sensation. Called also *Brown-Séquard paralysis* or *sign.*

Brown-Vialetto-van Laere s. an autosomal recessive syndrome consisting of progressive bulbar palsy with any of several cranial nerve disorders, including nerve deafness, facial weakness, dysarthria, and dysphagia.

Brueghel s. Meige s.

Brugada s. a type of ion channelopathy characterized by sudden, idiopathic ventricular fibrillation in an apparently healthy person, often resulting in death *(sudden adult* or *sudden arrhythmia death syndrome).* It is autosomal dominant and occurs most often in males of Southeast Asian origin.

Bruns s. intermittent headache, vertigo, vomiting, and visual disturbances on sudden movement of the head, characteristic of cysticercus infection of the fourth ventricle, lesion of the fourth ventricle, or tumors of the midline of the cerebellum and third or lateral ventricles. Called also *Bruns sign.*

Bruns-Garland s. diabetic amyotrophy.

Brunsting s., Brunsting-Perry s. a variant of cicatricial pemphigoid with lesions on the skin of the head and neck that heal and leave superficial scarring; if it is on the scalp, it causes cicatricial alopecia. Called also *Brunsting-Perry pemphigoid.*

Brushfield-Wyatt s. a congenital syndrome consisting of extensive unilateral nevus flammeus, homonymous hemianopia of both eyes, contralateral hemiplegia, cerebral angioma, and mental retardation; it may be related to the Sturge-Weber syndrome.

Buckley s. hyperimmunoglobulinemia E s.

Budd-Chiari s. symptomatic obstruction or occlusion of the hepatic veins, causing hepatomegaly, abdominal pain and tenderness, intractable ascites, mild jaundice, and, eventually, portal hypertension and liver failure. The obstruction is caused by thrombi or fibrous obliteration of the veins and has been associated with coagulation disorders; myeloproliferative disorders; invasion of hepatic veins by hepatic, renal, or adrenal carcinoma; and abdominal trauma. Onset may be acute with death in a few days in cases of complete occlusion, but more often there is a chronic course with survival for months or years. Called also *Chiari s.* and *endophlebitis hepatica obliterans.* Cf. *veno-occlusive disease of liver.*

Syndrome *Continued*

bulbar s. any syndrome caused by a lesion in the medulla and its nuclei, with paralysis of the cranial nerves originating there; cf. *progressive bulbar palsy.* Called also *Dejerine s.*
Bürger-Grütz s. familial hyperlipoproteinemia, type I.
Burnett s. milk-alkali s.
burning feet s. Gopalan s.
burning mouth s. any of various conditions of burning sensations and pain in the mouth (stomatalgia or glossalgia) having unknown etiologies; they occur most often in middle-aged, perimenopausal women or persons with candidiasis who have used antibiotics for prolonged periods.
Buschke-Ollendorff s. an autosomal dominant syndrome, present at birth or appearing before puberty, characterized by often symmetric connective tissue nevi of the elastic type on the limbs and lower trunk *(dermatofibrosis lenticularis disseminata)* in association with osteopoikilosis.
Butler-Albright s. a type of distal renal tubular acidosis occurring later than infancy and having autosomal dominant inheritance.
Bywaters s. crush s.
CADASIL s. [*c*erebral *a*utosomal *d*ominant *a*rteriopathy with *s*ubcortical *i*nfarcts and *l*eukoencephalopathy] a rare, autosomal dominant, adult-onset vascular condition affecting mainly the centrum semiovale of the cerebral hemispheres; characteristics include migraines and other neurologic symptoms, stroke and related conditions, and eventually subcortical dementia and death.
Caffey s., Caffey-Silverman s. infantile cortical hyperostosis.
camptomelic s. osteochondrodysplasia associated with flat facies, bowed tibiae with skin dimpling, hypoplastic scapulae, and short vertebrae.
Canada-Cronkhite s. Cronkhite-Canada s.
Canale-Smith s. autoimmune lymphoproliferative s.
cancer family s. type 2 hereditary nonpolyposis colorectal cancer.
Capgras s. a form of delusional misidentification in which the patient believes that other persons in the environment are not their real selves but doubles. Cf. *Frégoli phenomenon.*
capillary leak s. extravasation of plasma fluid and proteins into the extravascular space, resulting in sometimes fatal hypotension and reduced organ perfusion; an adverse effect of aldesleukin (interleukin-2) therapy.
Caplan s. pneumoconiosis associated with rheumatoid arthritis. Radiographically, multiple spherical nodular lesions with clearly demarcated borders are found throughout both lungs. Called also *rheumatoid pneumoconiosis.*
carcinoid s. a symptom complex associated with carcinoid tumors, characterized by attacks of severe cyanotic flushing of the skin and by watery diarrhea, bronchoconstrictive attacks, lesions of the heart valves, edema, ascites, and increased urinary excretion of 5-hydroxyindoleacetic acid. Symptoms are caused by secretion by the tumor of serotonin, prostaglandins, and other biologically active substances.
cardiac s. X a relatively benign syndrome of angina pectoris or anginalike chest pain associated with normal arteriographic appearance of the coronary arteries. Called also *s. X.*
Carney s. see under *complex.*
carotid sinus s. syncope sometimes associated with convulsive seizures due to overactivity of the carotid sinus reflex (q.v.) when pressure is applied to one or both carotid sinuses. Called also *carotid sinus syncope* and *Charcot-Weiss-Baker s.*
carpal tunnel s. an entrapment neuropathy characterized by pain and burning or tingling paresthesias in the fingers and hand, sometimes extending to the elbow. Symptoms result from compression of the median nerve in the carpal tunnel.

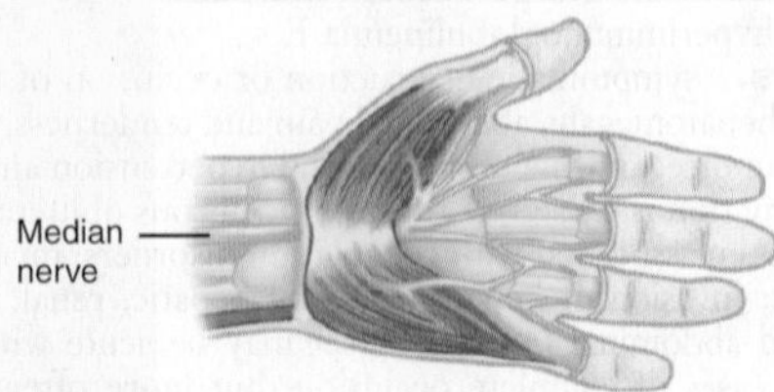

■ Median nerve entrapped in carpal tunnel in carpal tunnel syndrome.

Carpenter s. an autosomal recessive disorder characterized by acrocephaly with polysyndactyly, brachydactyly, mental retardation, mild obesity, hypogonadism, and other anomalies. It is believed to encompass disorders formerly distinguished as Goodman syndrome (q.v.). Called also *acrocephalopolysyndactyly, type II.*
cast s. superior mesenteric artery syndrome caused by enclosure in a body cast.
cat-eye s. an association of coloboma of the iris and anal atresia; there may also be many other anomalies, including preauricular skin tags or fistulas, hypertelorism, congenital heart disease, skeletal abnormalities, and renal malformations. It is associated with partial trisomy 22, i.e., the presence of a partial additional copy of chromosome 22.
cat's cry s. cri du chat s.
cat's eye s. cat-eye s.
cauda equina s. 1. a group of symptoms caused by compression of the spinal nerve roots, including dull, aching pain of the perineum, bladder, and sacrum that generally radiates in a sciatic fashion and is associated with paresthesias and areflexic paralysis. 2. see under *neuritis.*
caudal dysplasia s., caudal regression s. failure of formation of part or all of the coccygeal, sacral, and occasionally lumbar vertebral units and the corresponding segments of the caudal spinal cord, with resulting neurogenic dysfunction of bowel and bladder; called also *sacral agenesis.*
cavernous sinus s. edema of the conjunctiva, proptosis, edema of upper lid and root of the nose, together with paralysis of the third, fourth, and sixth cranial nerves and the ophthalmic branch of the fifth; it is usually due to thrombosis or tumor of the cavernous sinus. Cf. *Tolosa-Hunt s.* Called also *Foix s.*
celiac artery compression s., celiac axis compression s. compression of the celiac axis or trunk by crura of the diaphragm, which can interfere with the blood supply to the liver and spleen, resulting in intermittent postprandial pain in the upper abdomen.
central alveolar hypoventilation s. primary alveolar hypoventilation.
central cord s. a syndrome associated with injury to the cervical or upper thoracic portions of the spinal cord that results in damage to the central cord with sparing of the more external fibers that supply the lower extremity. It is characterized by disproportionately more weakness or paralysis in the upper extremity than in the lower, with varying sensory deficits below the level of the lesion, sometimes with bladder and bowel dysfunction.
central sleep apnea s. see under *apnea.*
centroposterior s. syringomyelia.
cerebellar s. see under *ataxia.*
cerebellopontine angle s. a syndrome caused by a tumor of the cerebellopontine angle or an acoustic tumor, characterized by hearing loss, subjective noises, ipsilateral cerebellar ataxia, and eventually ipsilateral impairment of function of the sixth and seventh cranial nerves accompanied by elevated intracranial pressure.
cerebral hyperperfusion s. hyperperfusion s.
cerebrocardiac s. Krishaber disease.
cerebrocostomandibular s. an autosomal recessive syndrome of severe micrognathia and costovertebral abnormalities, including small bell-shaped thorax, incompletely ossified aberrant rib structure, and abnormal rib attachment to vertebrae. Also present are palatal defects, glossoptosis, prenatal and postnatal growth deficiencies, and mental retardation, the last perhaps due to the neonatal respiratory distress which is frequently the presenting sign of the disorder.
cerebrohepatorenal s. an autosomal recessive disorder characterized by craniofacial abnormalities, hypotonia, hepatomegaly, polycystic kidneys, jaundice, and death in early infancy, and associated with absence of peroxisomes in the liver and kidneys; called also *Zellweger s.*
cervical s., cervical disk s. a condition caused by irritation or compression of the cervical nerve roots by a protruding disk; symptoms include neck pain radiating into the shoulder, arm, or forearm, paresthesias, and muscle weakness or spasm.
cervical rib s. a thoracic outlet syndrome caused by a cervical rib.
cervicobrachial s. brachial plexopathy.
Cestan s., Cestan-Chenais s. an association of contralateral hemiplegia and hemianesthesia, ipsilateral lateropulsion and hemiasynergia, Horner syndrome, and ipsilateral laryngoplegia, due to scattered lesions of the pyramid, sensory tract, inferior cerebellar peduncle, and nucleus ambiguus.

Cestan-Raymond s. Raymond-Cestan s.
Charcot s. 1. amyotrophic lateral sclerosis. 2. intermittent claudication.
Charcot-Marie s. Charcot-Marie-Tooth disease.
Charcot-Weiss-Baker s. carotid sinus s.
CHARGE s. a syndrome of associated defects caused by mutations in either of two genes that are important in embryonic development: *CHD7* (locus: 8q12.1) and *SEMA3E* (locus: 7q21.11). Defects include *c*oloboma of the eye, *h*eart anomaly, choanal *a*tresia, *r*etardation, and *g*enital and *e*ar anomalies. Facial palsy, cleft palate, and dysphagia are often present. Most cases are sporadic but some show a familial pattern.
Charlin s. pain, iritis, corneitis, rhinorrhea, and tenderness along the nose as a result of neuralgia of the nasociliary nerve. Called also *nasociliary neuralgia.*
Chédiak-Higashi s. a lethal autosomal recessive syndrome associated with oculocutaneous albinism, massive leukocyte inclusions (giant lysosomes), histiocytic infiltration of multiple body organs, development of pancytopenia, hepatosplenomegaly, recurrent or persistent bacterial infections, and a possible predisposition to development of malignant lymphoma. Called also *Béguez César disease* and *Chédiak-Higashi anomaly.*
Chiari s. Budd-Chiari s.
Chiari-Arnold s. Arnold-Chiari malformation.
Chiari-Frommel s. galactorrhea-amenorrhea syndrome occurring after pregnancy; called also *Frommel-Chiari s.*, *Chiari-Frommel disease*, and *Frommel disease.*
chiasma s., chiasmatic s. a syndrome indicative of lesions affecting the optic chiasma: impairment of vision, limitations of the field of vision, central scotoma, headache, vertigo, and syncope.
Chilaiditi s. interposition of the colon between the liver and diaphragm. Usually the condition is asymptomatic in adults, but symptoms are evident in children and include vomiting, abdominal pain, anorexia, constipation, and aerophagia. Signs include abdominal distention and absence of liver dullness.
CHILD s. [*c*ongenital *h*emidysplasia with *i*chthyosiform erythroderma and *l*imb *d*efects] a disorder of skin cornification characterized by unilateral erythema, scaling, and epidermal nevi; ipsilateral limb defects; and sometimes skeletal hypoplasia, brain defects, and visceral defects. It first appears in infancy and is believed to be an X-linked dominant trait.
Chinese restaurant s. a transient syndrome associated with arterial dilatation, due to ingestion of monosodium glutamate, which is sometimes used liberally in seasoning Chinese food; it is characterized by throbbing of the head, lightheadedness, tightness of the jaw, neck, and shoulders, and backache.
Chotzen s. an autosomal dominant disorder characterized by acrocephalosyndactyly in which the syndactyly is mild and by hypertelorism, ptosis, and sometimes mental retardation. Called also *acrocephalosyndactyly, type III* and *Saethre-Chotzen s.*
Christ-Siemens-Touraine s. anhidrotic ectodermal dysplasia.
Christian s. Hand-Schüller-Christian disease.
chronic fatigue s. persistent debilitating fatigue lasting longer than six months, with other known medical conditions having been ruled out by clinical diagnosis, accompanied by at least four of the following: significantly impaired short-term memory or concentration, muscle weakness, pain in multiple joints without swelling or redness, sore throat, tender lymph nodes, headaches, unrefreshing sleep, and malaise that lasts more than 24 hours following exertion. The cause is unknown and may be multifactorial; immune dysfunction has been suggested, and viral infection may be associated with it, although no causal relationship has been demonstrated. A number of names have been used for this syndrome, including *Iceland disease, myalgic* or *benign myalgic encephalomyelitis, chronic Epstein-Barr virus infection, chronic mononucleosis,* and *epidemic neuromyasthenia.*
chronic infantile neurologic cutaneous and articular s. neonatal-onset multisystem inflammatory disease.
chronic pelvic pain s. (CPPS) name given to nonspecific pain in pelvic organs or tissues, which has been continuous for at least six months and is not caused by malignancy, infection, or other obvious pathology.
Churg-Strauss s. a type of small vessel vasculitis that is also grouped with the systemic necrotizing vasculitides and has prominent lung involvement with severe asthma, eosinophilia, and granulomatous reactions. If present, cutaneous lesions consist of tender subcutaneous nodules, large ecchymotic plaques, and cutaneous infarcts. There are several different types; one is a type of ANCA-associated vasculitis. Called also *allergic granulomatosis, allergic granulomatous angiitis,* and *Churg-Strauss vasculitis.*
chylomicronemia s. familial hyperchylomicronemia.
CINCA s. neonatal-onset multisystem inflammatory disease.
Citelli s. mental dullness, loss of power of concentration, and drowsiness or insomnia, seen in persons with adenoids or sinus infection.
Clarke-Hadfield s. congenital pancreatic disease with infantilism; with enlarged liver, bulky fatty stools, and extensive atrophy of the pancreas in an undersized and underweight child.
Claude s. paralysis of the third (oculomotor) nerve on one side and asynergia on the other side, together with dysarthria; called also *inferior s. of red nucleus* and *rubrospinal cerebellar peduncle s.*
Claude Bernard–Horner s. Horner s.
click s., click-murmur s. mitral valve prolapse s.
closed head s. the complex of symptoms characteristic of cerebral injury without cranial penetration. See also *concussion* and *postconcussional s.*
Clouston s. hidrotic ectodermal dysplasia.
cloverleaf skull s. kleeblattschädel s.
Cockayne s. (CS) a rare, pleiotropic, autosomal recessive disorder characterized by a variety of cutaneous, neurologic, and somatic abnormalities that vary in severity, including growth failure; delayed psychomotor development, progressive hearing loss, and other neurologic manifestations; pigmentary retinal degeneration and other progressive ocular abnormalities; cutaneous photosensitivity, and calcification of basal ganglia. It is caused by mutations affecting the transcription-coupled repair subpathway of nucleotide excision repair.
Coffin-Lowry s. a condition with onset in the postnatal period characterized by incapability of speech, severe mental deficiency, and muscle, ligament, and skeletal abnormalities; it is transmitted with X-linked intermediate inheritance.
Coffin-Siris s. hypoplasia or absence of the nails of the fifth fingers and toes associated with growth and mental deficiencies, coarse facies, mild microcephaly, hypotonia, lax joints, mild hirsutism, and occasionally cardiac, vertebral, or gastrointestinal anomalies.
Cogan s. 1. nonsyphilitic interstitial keratitis with tinnitus and deafness; it usually occurs in children, often associated with polyarteritis nodosa. 2. Cogan oculomotor apraxia.
cold agglutinin s. the presence of circulating cold agglutinins, usually IgM, which are directed against three types of polysaccharide red cell antigens: *I antigens,* expressed primarily on adult red cells, *i antigens,* expressed primarily on cells of fetuses and infants, and *Pr antigens,* which, unlike I and i antigens, are protease sensitive. The primary clinical manifestations are intravascular hemolysis in exposed extremities and mild hemolytic anemia due to complement fixation, both occurring only upon exposure to cold. There are two major types: *chronic cold agglutinin disease,* a condition seen in the elderly with gradual onset and a chronic course; and *postinfectious cold agglutinin syndrome,* which usually follows *Mycoplasma pneumoniae* infection or infectious mononucleosis and lasts a few months. The syndrome can also develop secondary to malignancy.
Collet s., Collet-Sicard s. Vernet syndrome with ipsilateral paralysis of the tongue, due to complete lesion of the ninth, tenth, eleventh, and twelfth cranial nerves. Called also *Sicard s.*
combination s. a condition sometimes seen in patients with a mandibular distal extension partial denture opposing a complete maxillary denture; if there is not enough primary occlusal force, excessive load may be placed on the anterior part of the maxillary denture, causing loss of the anterior maxillary alveolus.
compartment s., compartmental s. a condition in which increased tissue pressure in a confined anatomical space causes decreased blood flow leading to ischemia and dysfunction of contained myoneural elements, marked by pain, muscle weakness, sensory loss, and palpable tenseness in the involved compartment. Ischemia can lead to necrosis resulting in permanent impairment of function.
complete androgen insensitivity s. (CAIS) an extreme type of androgen insensitivity syndrome with male pseudohermaphroditism, in which an individual is phenotypically female but has XY chromosomes; this results from mutations in the gene for the androgen receptor. There may be a rudimentary uterus and tubes, but the gonads are typically testes, which may be abdominal or inguinal in position.

Called also *complete androgen resistance, feminizing testes syndrome, Morris syndrome, testicular feminization,* and *testicular feminization syndrome.*
complex regional pain s. (CRPS) a chronic pain syndrome of uncertain pathogenesis, usually affecting an extremity, and characterized by intense burning pain, changes in skin color and texture, increased skin temperature and sensitivity, sweating, and edema. Type 1 (called also *reflex sympathetic dystrophy*) often follows tissue injury, but without demonstrable nerve injury, and may be accompanied by posttraumatic osteoporosis; when limited to the upper extremity it is called *shoulder-hand syndrome.* Type 2 (called also *causalgia*) is associated with injury to the peripheral nerves.
compression s. crush s.
concussion s. postconcussional s.
congenital central hypoventilation s. (CCHS) a congenital form of primary alveolar hypoventilation, generally resulting from a mutation in the short arm of chromosome 4 (4p12). Affected infants appear cyanotic, with symptoms of respiratory failure, within a few hours of birth, and hypoventilate during sleep but, unless the disease is severe, breathe normally when awake.
congenital high airway obstruction s. (CHAOS) a syndrome sometimes seen in utero, consisting of obstruction of the upper airway and dilation of the trachea and lungs; most fetuses with this condition die before birth.
congenital rubella s. developmental anomalies resulting from transplacental infection of the fetus with rubella, usually in the first trimester of pregnancy; maternal infection may be subclinical. The anomalies may include cardiac lesions, ocular lesions, deafness, microcephaly, mental retardation, and generalized growth retardation, sometimes associated with acute self-limited conditions such as thrombocytopenic purpura, anemia, hepatitis, encephalitis, and radiolucencies of long bones. Infected infants may shed virus to all contacts for an extended period. Called also *rubella s.*
congenital tremor s. any of several congenital neurological diseases of piglets characterized by noticeable trembling, often owing to defective myelination of nerves. Mild varieties may clear up within a month but in severe cases the animals cannot function normally and soon die. One variety is autosomal recessive; another is sex-linked; and others are caused by intrauterine viral infections such as with hog cholera virus. Affected pigs are called *dancing* or *shaker pigs.* Called also *congenital trembles* and *myoclonia congenita.*
congenital varicella s. developmental anomalies resulting from transplacental infection of the fetus with varicella during the first or second trimester of pregnancy; they may include eye abnormalities, brain damage, and moderate to severe limb abnormalities.
Conn s. primary aldosteronism.
Conradi s. chondrodysplasia punctata.
Conradi-Hünermann s. an autosomal dominant form of chondrodysplasia punctata, characterized by asymmetric shortening of the extremities and scoliosis; intelligence and life expectancy are normal. The syndrome is also associated with maternal use of warfarin sodium during pregnancy.
constriction band s. amniotic band s.
contiguous gene s. any syndrome known to be caused by the involvement of contiguous genes on a chromosome, e.g., aniridia–Wilms tumor association, which may also have genitourinary tract abnormalities, gonadoblastoma, and mental retardation; they are usually caused by chromosome deletions.
continuous muscle activity s., continuous muscle fiber activity s. Isaacs s.
conus medullaris s. a group of symptoms caused by compression of the conus medullaris, with diminished control of bowel and bladder functions, pain in the lower back, anesthesia in the pelvic region, and sometimes weakness in the lower limbs.
Cornelia de Lange s. de Lange s.
s. of corpus striatum Vogt s.
Costeff optic atrophy s. 3-methylglutaconicaciduria type III.
Costen s. temporomandibular disorder.
costoclavicular s. a thoracic outlet syndrome caused by compression or friction on nerves and blood vessels between a drooping clavicle and the first rib.
costosternal s. costochondritis.
Cotard s. paranoia with delusions of negation, a suicidal tendency, and sensory disturbances.
Courvoisier-Terrier s. dilatation of the gallbladder, retention jaundice, and discoloration of the feces, indicating obstruction due to a tumor of the ampulla of Vater.
cracked tooth s. a group of symptoms caused by presence of a cracked tooth, including pain on pressure or application of cold, with pulpitis if untreated.
cramp-fasciculation s. a relatively mild form of peripheral nerve hyperexcitability characterized by fasciculations, cramps, and intermittent myokymia, without neuromyotonia; it is usually idiopathic but in some cases is autoimmune in origin.
craniosynostosis–radial aplasia s. Baller-Gerold s.
crazy cow s. a type of neurotoxicity seen in cattle in the United States, Brazil, and South Africa after they have eaten any of various plants of the genus *Solanum;* characteristics include cerebellar damage with staggering and incoordination.
CREST s. a form of systemic scleroderma usually less severe than other forms, consisting of *c*alcinosis cutis, *R*aynaud phenomenon, *e*sophageal dysfunction, *s*clerodactyly, and *t*elangiectasia. When esophageal dysfunction is not prominent, it is known as *CRST s.*
cricopharyngeal achalasia s. Asherson s.
cri du chat s. a hereditary congenital syndrome characterized by hypertelorism, microcephaly, severe mental deficiency, and a plaintive catlike cry, due to deletion of part of the short arm of chromosome 5. Called also *cat's cry s.*
Crigler-Najjar s. an autosomal recessive form of nonhemolytic jaundice due to the absence of the hepatic enzyme glucuronosyltransferase. It is characterized by the presence in the blood of excessive amounts of unconjugated bilirubin, with kernicterus and severe disorders of the central nervous system. Called also *congenital hyperbilirubinemia* and *congenital nonhemolytic jaundice.*
s. of crocodile tears spontaneous lacrimation occurring parallel with the normal salivation of eating. It follows facial paralysis and seems to be due to inaccurate regrowth of the regenerating nerve fibers into the wrong nerve sheaths, with some of those destined for the salivary glands going to the lacrimal glands.
Cronkhite-Canada s. a rare syndrome of sporadic, widespread intestinal polyps and malabsorption accompanied by ectodermal defects such as alopecia and onychodystrophy; called also *Canada-Cronkhite s.*
Cross s., Cross-McKusick-Breen s. an autosomal recessive syndrome marked by cutaneous hypopigmentation, microphthalmos, small opaque corneas, gingival hypertrophy, and cerebral defect manifested by spasticity, mental and physical retardation, and athetoid movements. Called also *oculocerebral-hypopigmentation s.*
Crouzon s. an autosomal dominant disorder caused by mutations in the *FGFR2* gene (locus: 10q26), which encodes a fibroblast growth factor receptor, characterized by acrocephaly, exophthalmos, hypertelorism, strabismus, parrot-beaked nose, and hypoplastic maxilla with relative mandibular prognathism. Called also *craniofacial dysostosis.*
Crow-Fukase s. POEMS s.
crowned dens s. crystal-induced arthritis around the dens axis, often accompanied by fever and neck pain.
CRST s. see *CREST s.*
crush s. the edema, oliguria, and other symptoms of acute renal failure that follow the crushing of a part, especially a large muscle mass; see *acute tubular necrosis,* under *necrosis.*
Cruveilhier-Baumgarten s. cirrhosis with portal hypertension, associated with congenital patency of the umbilical or paraumbilical veins. It is characterized by hematemesis, ascites, splenomegaly, hypersplenism, esophageal varices, caput medusae, large tortuous veins in the abdominal wall, and a venous hum, often accompanied by a thrill, usually heard over the region of the xiphoid process. Called also *Cruveilhier-Baumgarten cirrhosis.*
cryopyrin-associated periodic s. any in a group of autoinflammatory diseases caused by mutations in the gene that codes for cryopyrin, resulting in fever, arthralgia, urticaria, and inflammation. Called also *cryopyrinopathy.*
cryptophthalmos s. an autosomal recessive abnormality, characterized by absence of the palpebral apertures, disorganization of one or both ocular globes, malformed ears, cleft palate, laryngeal stenosis, syndactyly, meningoencephalocele, imperforate anus, cardiac defects, and maldeveloped kidneys. Called also *Fraser s.*
cubital tunnel s. a type of entrapment neuropathy with a complex of symptoms resulting from injury or compression of the ulnar nerve at the

elbow, including pain and numbness along the ulnar aspect of the hand and forearm, and weakness of the hand.
culture-specific s. a form of disturbed behavior highly specific to certain cultural systems and that does not conform to Western nosologic entities; examples are amok, koro, piblokto, and windigo.
Currarino s. a complex of congenital anomalies in the anococcygeal region; it consists of partial sacral agenesis; presacral anterior meningocele, teratoma, or cyst; and rectal malformations such as stenosis, ectopia, or imperforation. Gynecologic and renal malformations are also common. In at least some cases it is caused by mutation of the *HLXB9* gene (locus: 7q36), a homeobox gene. Called also *Currarino triad.*
Currarino-Silverman s. premature obliteration of the sternal sutures with synostosis as well as a protruding manubrium, causing pectus carinatum; other abnormalities may also be present such as hyperostosis of ribs or hypotrophy of the anterior diaphragm. Called also *Silverman s.*
Curschmann-Batten-Steinert s. myotonic dystrophy.
Curtius s. hypertrophy of one side of the entire body or a portion of one side of the body, as of the face; called also *hemihypertrophy.*
Cushing s. 1. a complex of symptoms caused by hyperadrenocorticism due either to a neoplasm of the adrenal cortex or adenohypophysis, or to excessive intake of glucocorticoids. Symptoms may include adiposity of the face, neck, and trunk; kyphosis from osteoporosis of the spine; hypertension; diabetes mellitus; amenorrhea and hypertrichosis in females; impotence in males; dusky complexion with purple striae; polycythemia; and muscular wasting and weakness. When secondary to excessive pituitary secretion of corticotropin, it is known as *Cushing disease.* See also *ectopic ACTH s.* Called also *Cushing* or *pituitary basophilism.* 2. equine Cushing disease.
Cushing s., iatrogenic Cushing syndrome caused by prolonged excessive use of glucocorticoid medications; called also *Cushing s. medicamentosus.*
Cushing s. medicamentosus iatrogenic Cushing s.
cyclic vomiting s. cyclic vomiting.
Cyriax s. a syndrome due to slipped rib cartilages pressing on the nerves at the interchondral joint, resulting in pain in the region of the cartilage, radiation of pain to the shoulder and arm, or pain similar to that of angina pectoris.
Da Costa s. neurocirculatory asthenia.
Danbolt-Closs s. acrodermatitis enteropathica.
dancing eyes s. opsoclonus-myoclonus s.
Dandy-Walker s. see under *malformation.*
Debré-Sémélaigne s. autosomal recessive athyrotic cretinism associated with myotonia and muscular pseudohypertrophy. Called also *Kocher-Debré-Sémélaigne s.*
de Clérambault s. erotomania.
defibrination s. diffuse intravascular coagulation.
Dejean s. orbital floor s.
Dejerine s. 1. symptoms of radiculitis; namely, distribution of the pain, motor, and sensory defects in the region of the radicular or segmental disturbance of the nerve roots rather than along the course of the peripheral nerve. 2. bulbar s. 3. a polyneuropathy resembling tabes dorsalis, secondary to infection by *Corynebacterium diphtheriae* and the resultant lesions of peripheral nerves and of the posterior column of the spinal cord; deep sensibility is depressed but tactile sense is normal. Called also *diphtheritic polyneuropathy.*

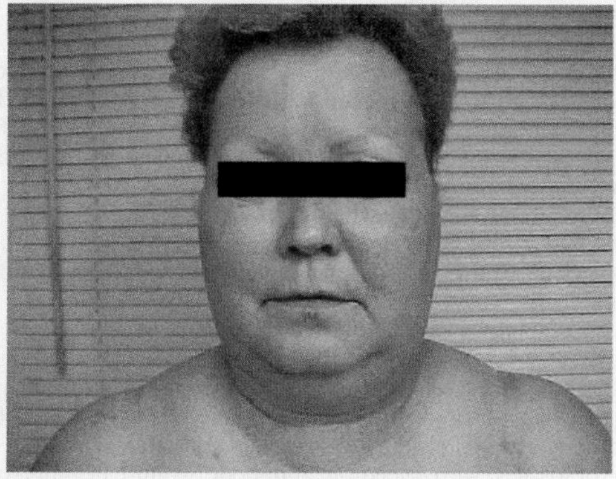
■ Moon facies, plethora, and supraclavicular fat associated with Cushing syndrome.

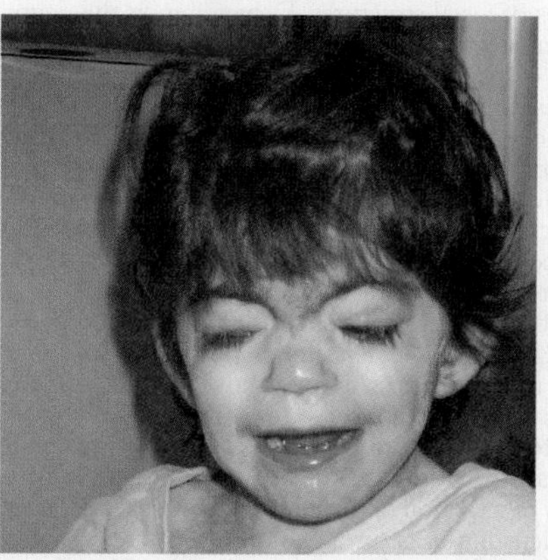
■ de Lange syndrome. Child showing typical facial features including finely arched heavy eyebrows, long eyelashes, small upturned nose, and long smooth philtrum.

Dejerine-Klumpke s. Klumpke paralysis.
Dejerine-Roussy s. thalamic s.
Dejerine-Thomas s. olivopontocerebellar atrophy.
de Lange s. a congenital syndrome in which severe mental retardation is associated with many abnormalities, including short stature (Amsterdam dwarf), brachycephaly, low-set ears, webbed neck, Cupid's-bow mouth, depressed bridge of the nose with the end tilted up and forward-directed nostrils, arched heavy eyebrows meeting at the midline, unruly coarse hair growing low on the forehead and neck, and flat spadelike hands with short tapering fingers. Called also *Brachmann-de Lange* or *Cornelia de Lange s.*
del Castillo s. Sertoli-cell–only s.
dementia s. of depression reversible dementia occurring in association with depression in the elderly, the cognitive deficits resolving with treatment of the depression.
de Morsier s. septo-optic dysplasia.
dengue shock s. see *hemorrhagic dengue,* under *dengue.*
Dennie-Marfan s. spastic paralysis and mental retardation in association with congenital syphilis.
Denys-Drash s. a rare syndrome that includes male pseudohermaphroditism, nephropathy leading to renal failure, and, in most cases, Wilms tumor. It is caused by a genetic abnormality in the p13 region of chromosome 11.
depressive s. depression (def. 3).
De Sanctis-Cacchione s. an autosomal recessive syndrome consisting of xeroderma pigmentosum associated with mental retardation, retarded growth, gonadal hypoplasia, and sometimes neurologic complications and photosensitivity.
descending perineum s. sagging of the perineum and levator plate, which causes constipation and other problems in the perineal region; it is seen most often after years of straining, vaginal deliveries, or surgical procedures in the area.
de Toni-Fanconi s. see *Fanconi s.* (def. 2).
dialysis dysequilibrium s. a group of symptoms seen during or after overly rapid hemodialysis or peritoneal dialysis, resulting from an osmotic shift of water into the brain; usually there is headache and less often nausea, muscle cramps, nervous irritability, drowsiness, and convulsions.
Diamond-Blackfan s. congenital hypoplastic anemia (def. 1).
diarrheogenic s. Verner-Morrison s.
DIDMOAD s. [*di*abetes *i*nsipidus, *d*iabetes *m*ellitus, *o*ptic *a*trophy, *d*eafness] Wolfram s.
diencephalic s. failure to thrive, emaciation, and sometimes nevus unius lateralis.
DiGeorge s. a congenital disorder in which defective development of the third and fourth pharyngeal pouches results in hypoplasia or aplasia of the thymus and parathyroid glands, often associated with congenital heart defects, anomalies of the great vessels, esophageal atresia, and

abnormalities of facial structures. Depending on the degree of parathyroid and thymic hypoplasia, there are hypocalcemic tetany or seizures due to lack of parathyroid hormone and deficiency of cell-mediated immunity resulting in increased susceptibility to low-grade or opportunistic pathogens. The syndrome is usually a phenotype of 22q11 deletion syndrome (q.v.) and is associated with loss of the T-box gene Tbx1, and even within the phenotype shows variability. A small number of cases have other causes, notably a defect in chromosome 10p13. Called also *thymic aplasia* or *hypoplasia* and *pharyngeal pouch s.*
Di Guglielmo s. erythroleukemia.
disconnection s. any neurologic disorder caused by an interruption in impulse transmission along cerebral fiber pathways; one result may be an inability to carry out a desired movement in response to a given sensory input, as in the apraxias.
disseminated intravascular coagulation s. see under *coagulation.*
distal intestinal obstruction s. a complication of cystic fibrosis consisting of obstruction of the intestine by thickened feces; it resembles meconium ileus but lasts throughout life.
Dobrin s. TINU s.
Donohue s. a rare, lethal, autosomal recessive condition caused by mutation in the *INSR* gene (locus: 19p13.2), which encodes the insulin receptor, characterized by slow physical and mental development, elfin facies, and endocrine abnormalities such as hyperinsulinemia and precocious puberty. Death usually occurs in utero or in the first year of life. Called also *leprechaunism.*
DOOR s. a rare syndrome of congenital *d*eafness, *o*nycho-*o*steodystrophy, and mental *r*etardation, existing in autosomal dominant and recessive forms.
dorsal midbrain s. Parinaud s.
double cortex s. band heterotopia.
double crush s. compression or other damage of the same nerve at two different points, such as carpal tunnel syndrome with cervical radiculopathy. Some authorities believe that damage at one point makes a nerve group more vulnerable to injury somewhere else.
Down s. a chromosome disorder characterized by a small, anteroposteriorly flattened skull, short, flat-bridge nose, epicanthal fold, short phalanges, widened spaces between the first and second digits of hands and feet, and moderate to severe mental retardation, with Alzheimer disease developing in the fourth or fifth decade. The chromosomal aberration is trisomy of chromosome 21 associated with late maternal age. Called also *trisomy 21* and *nondisjunction;* formerly called *mongolism.*
downer cow s. parturient paresis in a cow that is intractable to treatment and usually fatal.
Drash s. Denys-Drash s.
Dresbach s. hereditary elliptocytosis.
Dressler s. post–myocardial infarction s.
dropped head s. weakness of posterior neck muscles, especially late in the day, so that the head drops forward; seen most often in polymyositis and certain motor neuron diseases.
dry eye s. keratoconjunctivitis sicca.

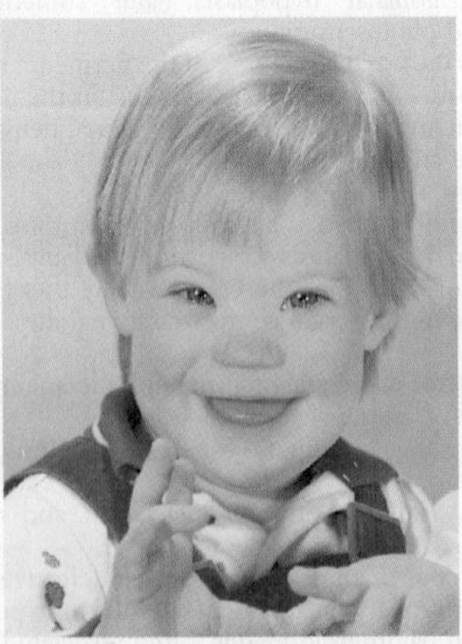

■ Boy with typical facial features and small hands of Down syndrome.

Duane s. a hereditary congenital syndrome in which the affected eye shows limitation or absence of abduction, restriction of adduction, retraction of the globe on adduction, narrowing of the palpebral fissure on adduction and widening on abduction, and deficient convergence. It is transmitted as an autosomal dominant trait. Called also *retraction, Stilling,* or *Stilling-Türk-Duane s.*
Dubin-Johnson s., Dubin-Sprinz s. a familial chronic form of nonhemolytic jaundice thought to be due to a defect in the excretion of conjugated bilirubin and certain other organic anions (such as sulfobromophthalein) by the liver. It is characterized by the presence of a brown, coarsely granular pigment in the hepatic cells, which is pathognomonic of the condition. Called also *Sprinz-Dubin s.* and *Sprinz-Nelson s.*
Dubreuil-Chambardel s. dental caries of the incisors, in most instances only the upper ones, usually appearing during adolescence; within a few years the teeth are irreparably damaged. Some authorities do not consider this syndrome a legitimate entity.
Duchenne s. progressive bulbar palsy.
Duchenne-Erb s. Erb-Duchenne paralysis.
dumping s. a complex reaction seen with rapid gastric emptying (see under *emptying*). Characteristics include nausea, weakness, sweating, palpitation, varying degrees of syncope, often a sensation of warmth, and sometimes diarrhea. It occurs most often in patients who have had partial gastrectomy with gastrojejunostomy. Called also *jejunal s.* and *postgastrectomy s.*
Duncan s. X-linked lymphoproliferative s.
Dyke-Davidoff-Masson s. a syndrome possibly due to injury to or severe disease affecting one side of the brain during the neonatal period, characterized by mental retardation, asymmetry of the face, and varying degrees of hemiplegia, neurological impairment, and atrophy of the side of the body contralateral to the lesion.
dysarthria–clumsy hand s. clumsy-hand dysarthria.
dyscontrol s. a pattern of episodic, abnormal, and often violent and uncontrollable social behavior with little or no provocation; it may result from diseases of the limbic system or the temporal lobe or may accompany abuse of alcohol or some other psychoactive substance. Called also *episodic dyscontrol.*
dyskinetic cilia s. primary ciliary dyskinesia.
dysmaturity s. postmaturity s.
dysmnesic s. amnestic s.
dysplastic nevus s. the occurrence of dysplastic nevi in persons having or at risk for having familial malignant melanoma. Called also *atypical mole s., atypical nevus s., familial atypical mole–malignant melanoma s.,* and *FAMMM s.*
Eagle-Barrett s. prune-belly s.
Eaton-Lambert s. Lambert-Eaton myasthenic s.
ectopic ACTH s. a condition caused by production of corticotropin by cells outside the pituitary, such as those of carcinoma of the lung; depending on its duration, it may be subtle, resembling true Cushing disease, but hypokalemic alkalosis and weakness are often prominent.
ectopic corticotropin-releasing hormone s. a disorder clinically indistinguishable from ectopic ACTH syndrome but caused by ectopic secretion of corticotropin-releasing hormone by a variety of tumors, generally bronchial carcinoid tumors.
ectrodactyly–ectodermal dysplasia–clefting s. EEC s.
Edwards s. trisomy 18 s.
EEC s. a congenital syndrome inherited as an autosomal dominant trait involving both ectodermal and mesodermal tissues, which consists of ectodermal dysplasia associated with hypopigmentation of the skin and hair, scanty hair and eyebrows, absence of lashes, nail dystrophy, hypo- and microdontia, ectrodactyly, and cleft lip and palate. Called also *ectrodactyly–ectodermal dysplasia–clefting s.*
effort s. neurocirculatory asthenia.
egg drop s. a viral disease of ducks and geese, caused by an adenovirus; apparently healthy birds begin laying eggs with thin or soft shells or without shells.
egg white s. biotin deficiency; see *biotin.*
Ehlers-Danlos s. a group of inherited disorders of the connective tissue; they were formerly classified into ten types, but more recently only six types are distinguished, varying widely in severity. The major manifestations include hyperextensible skin and joints, easy bruisability, friability of tissues with bleeding and poor wound healing, calcified subcutaneous spheroids, and pseudotumors. The *hypermobility type* (formerly type III) is autosomal dominant and the most common type;

mitral valve prolapse accompanies the skin and joint anomalies. The *classical type* (formerly types I and II) has both autosomal dominant and autosomal recessive subtypes; it includes mitral valve prolapse as well as fibrous growths on pressure areas such as the knees and elbows. The *vascular type* (formerly type IV) is autosomal dominant and is characterized by fragile blood vessels and organs that may rupture, as well as distinctive facial features such as protruding eyes and thin nose and lips. The *kyphoscoliosis type* (formerly type VI) is a rare, autosomal recessive type characterized by kyphoscoliosis and eye fragility accompanying the bone and joint anomalies. The *arthrochalasis type* (formerly types VIIA and VIIB) is a rare, autosomal dominant type in which joints are particularly loose and prone to dislocation; patients also suffer from arthritis and bone loss. The *dermatosparaxis type* (formerly type VIIC) is an autosomal recessive type characterized by particularly fragile and sagging skin. Most types are related to defects in procollagen, and the kyphoscoliosis type is caused by a deficiency in the enzyme lysyl hydroxylase. Called also *cutis hyperelastica*.

Eisenmenger s. ventricular septal defect with pulmonary hypertension and cyanosis due to right-to-left (reversed) shunt of blood. Sometimes defined as pulmonary hypertension (pulmonary vascular disease) and cyanosis with the shunt being at the atrial, ventricular, or great vessel area.

Ekbom s. restless legs s.

Ekman-Lobstein s. osteogenesis imperfecta, type I.

elfin facies s. Williams s.

Ellis-van Creveld s. an autosomal recessive disorder caused by mutation in either of two genes, *EVC* or *EVC2* (locus for both: 4p12), the functions of whose products are unknown. It is characterized by short limbs, polydactyly, defective development of skin, hair, and teeth, and cardiac defects, most commonly affecting the atrial septum. Called also *chondroectodermal dysplasia*.

embryonic testicular regression s. vanishing testes s.

EMG s. [exomphalos-*m*acroglossia-gigantism] Beckwith-Wiedemann s.

empty sella s. a syndrome diagnosed radiologically in which the diaphragma sellae is vestigial and the enlarged sella turcica forms an extension of the subarachnoid space and is filled with cerebrospinal fluid. The pituitary fossa appears empty, although the pituitary gland is present in a flattened form; pituitary hormone secretion may be normal, deficient, or excessive. Sometimes there is downward herniation of the optic chiasm, which leads to defects in the visual field.

encephalotrigeminal vascular s. Sturge-Weber s.

eosinophilia-myalgia s. a sometimes fatal combined syndrome of eosinophilia and severe generalized myalgia in patients ingesting L-tryptophan, occurring in the absence of infection, neoplasm, or other known causes of eosinophilia; other characteristics may include subjective weakness, fever, arthralgia, shortness of breath, rash, peripheral edema, and pneumonia.

epidermal nevus s. any of several syndromes that combine epidermal nevi with involvement of other body systems, such as CHILD syndrome, Proteus syndrome, and sebaceous nevus syndrome.

epiphyseal s. precocious development of external genitalia and sexual function, precocious abnormal growth of long bones, appearance of signs of internal hydrocephalus, in the absence of all other motor and sensory symptoms. It has been attributed to pineal body dysfunction and to mechanical effects on the brain caused by tumors of the pineal body. Called also *Pellizzi s.*, *pineal s.*, and *macrogenitosomia praecox*.

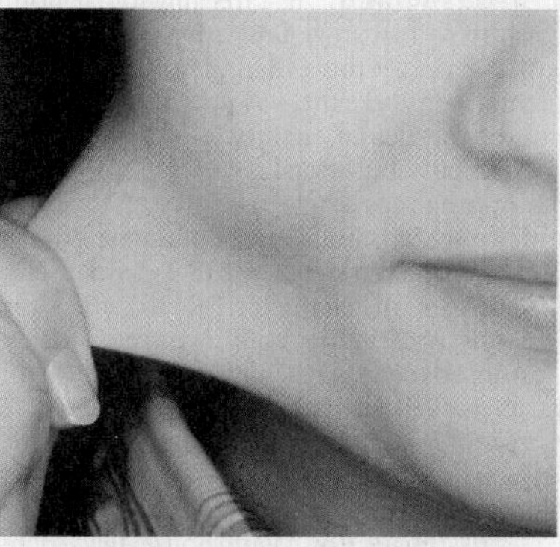

■ Hyperextensible skin of Ehlers-Danlos syndrome.

Epstein s. nephrotic s.

equine Cushing s. (ECS) see under *disease*.

erythrocyte autosensitization s. painful bruising s.

Escobar s. multiple pterygium s. (def. 1).

euthyroid sick s. subnormal levels of triiodothyronine in patients who have systemic illnesses but do not manifest symptoms of hypothyroidism. Called also *low* T_3 *s.* and *sick euthyroid s.*

Evans s. autoimmune hemolytic anemia accompanied by immune thrombocytopenia.

excited skin s. nonspecific cutaneous hyperirritability of the back, sometimes occurring when multiple positive reactions are elicited in patch tests screening a battery of substances. Called also *angry back*.

exfoliation s. degenerative alterations of anterior ocular tissues, first presenting as disturbances of pigmentary distribution in the iris, with partial atrophy of the iris pigmentary epithelium and deposition of liberated pigment granules on the lens capsule, papillary margin, ciliary body, and zonule. In later stages, gray, flakelike material increasingly covers the same areas, and glaucoma is a frequent sequela. The incidence of the syndrome increases markedly with age. Called also *pseudoexfoliation*.

exomphalos-macroglossia-gigantism s. Beckwith-Wiedemann s.

exploding head s. a rare, benign disturbance of the transition between waking and sleeping in which the person is aroused by the sensation of a loud explosion in the head, sometimes accompanied by flashing lights.

extrapyramidal s. any of a group of clinical disorders considered to be due to malfunction in the extrapyramidal system and characterized by abnormal involuntary movements; included are parkinsonism, athetosis, and chorea.

Faber s. hypochromic anemia.

facet s., facet joint s. pain in the facet joints of the vertebral column, usually owing to degeneration of intervertebral cartilages.

faciodigitogenital s. Aarskog s.

familial atypical mole s., familial atypical mole–melanoma s., familial atypical mole–malignant melanoma s., FAMMM s. dysplastic nevus s.

familial cold autoinflammatory s. an autosomal dominant autoinflammatory disease (q.v.) in the cryopyrin-associated periodic syndromes subgroup, characterized by fever, polyarthralgia, myalgia, urticarial rash, leukocytosis, headache, and conjunctivitis.

Fanconi s. 1. a rare recessive disorder with a poor prognosis, characterized by pancytopenia, bone marrow hypoplasia, and patchy brown skin discoloration due to deposition of melanin, as well as multiple congenital anomalies of the musculoskeletal and genitourinary systems. Called also *Fanconi anemia*, *pancytopenia*, or *panmyelopathy; congenital hypoplastic anemia; congenital pancytopenia;* and *pancytopenia-dysmelia s.* 2. a general term for a group of diseases marked by dysfunction of the proximal renal tubules (see *proximal renal tubular acidosis*, under *acidosis*) with generalized hyperaminoaciduria, renal glycosuria, hyperphosphaturia, and bicarbonate and water loss. The most common cause is cystinosis (q.v.), but it is also associated with other genetic diseases and occurs in idiopathic and acquired forms. When unassociated with cystinosis, the disorder is also called *de Toni-Fanconi syndrome*.

Farber s., Farber-Uzman s. see under *disease*.

fat cow s. a syndrome seen in overly fat cows just after they have given birth; loss of appetite postpartum leads to mobilization of body fat stores with deposition of fat in the liver and ketosis, sometimes ending in coma and death. Called also *fatty liver disease* and *pregnancy toxemia in cows*.

fat emboli s. (FES), fat embolism s. dyspnea, altered mental state, and petechiae caused by the entrance of fat into the vascular system, most often following trauma, especially that involving the fracture of long bones. It may also follow nontraumatic events, including lipid infusion and corticosteroid administration.

Favre-Racouchot s. a type of actinic elastosis usually seen in elderly men, in which giant comedones, pilosebaceous cysts, and large folds of furrowed and yellowish skin are seen in the periorbital region. Called also *nodular elastosis* or *elastoidosis*.

feline urological s. (FUS) dysfunction of the feline lower urinary tract. In male cats there is usually partial or complete obstruction from uroliths or other plugs, and in females there is more often cystitis or

urethritis. There may be various causes, including decreased physical activity and excessive dietary magnesium.
Felty s. a syndrome of splenomegaly with chronic rheumatoid arthritis and leukopenia; there are usually pigmented spots on the skin of the lower extremities, and sometimes there is other evidence of hypersplenism such as anemia or thrombocytopenia.
feminizing testes s. complete androgen insensitivity s.
fertile eunuch s. a syndrome of hypogonadotropic hypogonadism, with variable development of secondary sex characters, associated with normal spermatogenesis, normal levels of follicle-stimulating hormone, and variably low levels of luteinizing hormone.
fetal alcohol s. a syndrome of altered prenatal growth and morphogenesis seen in infants born to mothers who were chronically alcoholic during pregnancy; it includes facial anomalies such as maxillary hypoplasia, prominent forehead and mandible, short palpebral fissures, microphthalmia, and epicanthal folds, as well as growth retardation, microcephaly, and mental retardation.
fetal face s. Robinow s.
fetal hydantoin s. a symptom complex characterized by poor growth and development with craniofacial and skeletal abnormalities, produced by prenatal exposure to hydantoin analogues, including phenytoin.
Feuerstein-Mims s. sebaceous nevus s.
Fèvre-Languepin s. popliteal webbing associated with cleft lip and palate, fistula of the lower lip, syndactyly, onychodysplasia, and pes equinovarus. Called also *popliteal pterygium s.*
FG s. an X-linked recessive syndrome of mental retardation, megalencephaly, imperforate anus and other gastrointestinal defects, delayed motor development, congenital hypotonia, characteristic facies and personality, short stature, skeletal anomalies, and congenital cardiac defects.
Fiessinger-Leroy-Reiter s. Reiter s.
first arch s. anomalies, including macrostomia, hemignathia, and deformities of the external ear, resulting from an inhibitory process occurring toward the seventh week of embryonic life and affecting the facial bones derived from the first pharyngeal (branchial) arch.
first bite s. pain in the parotid region upon initiation of mastication, caused by denervation supersensitivity of salivary gland myoepithelial cells following loss of sympathetic innervation to the parotid gland.
Fisher s. 1. a variant of Guillain-Barré syndrome characterized by areflexia, ataxia, and ophthalmoplegia. Called also *Miller Fisher s.* 2. one-and-a-half s.
Fitz-Hugh–Curtis s. acute perihepatitis, occurring as a complication of gonorrhea or chlamydial infection; it is usually seen in women, secondary to extension of infection from the fallopian tube to the hepatic capsule and overlying peritoneum. It is marked by fever, hepatic tenderness, abdominal pain, and signs of right upper quadrant peritoneal inflammation.
floppy infant s. abnormal posture in an infant suspended in the prone position, the limbs and head hanging limply. It may be due to any of numerous conditions, including disorders of the brain, spinal cord, peripheral nerves, neuromuscular junction, muscles, or ligaments, and only sometimes is characterized by true limb weakness; the most common causes are perinatal injury to the brain or spinal cord, spinal muscular atrophy, and genetic disorders.
floppy valve s. mitral valve prolapse s.

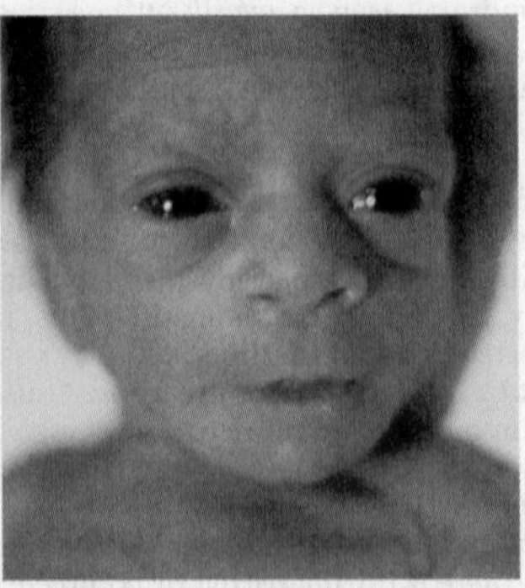

■ Typical facial features of an infant with fetal alcohol syndrome.

Flynn-Aird s. a rare autosomal dominant syndrome with abnormalities of the nervous system and ectodermal structures, including cataracts, retinitis pigmentosa, myopia, dental caries, skin atrophy and ulceration, peripheral neuropathy, ataxia, deafness, and cystic bone changes.
Foix s. cavernous sinus s.
Foix-Alajouanine s. a necrotizing myelopathy characterized by necrosis of the gray matter of the spinal cord, thickening of the walls of the spinal vessels, and abnormal spinal fluid; symptoms include subacute spastic paraplegia of the lower extremities that progresses to flaccid paralysis, often ascending, loss of sphincter control, and progressive sensory loss. Death occurs in one to two years. Called also *subacute necrotic myelitis.*
Foix-Chavany-Marie s. anterior opercular s.
folded lung s. round atelectasis.
follicular degeneration s. a type of cicatricial alopecia, usually beginning in the vertex of the scalp and extending outwards, caused by inflammation of hair follicles. It is sometimes called *hot comb alopecia* because it was originally seen in African-American women and thought to be related to hair relaxing procedures.
Forbes-Albright s. galactorrhea-amenorrhea syndrome not associated with pregnancy; usually a prolactin-secreting pituitary tumor is present.
Forsius-Eriksson s. X-linked tapetoretinal degeneration, formerly thought to be a form of ocular albinism, caused by a mutation in the *CACNA1F* gene (locus: Xp11.23), which encodes a voltage-gated calcium channel subunit. Symptomatic males exhibit foveal hypoplasia, axial myopia, and protanomaly; female carriers have slightly defective color discrimination and latent nystagmus, but no mosaic pigment pattern in the fundus. Called also *Aland eye disease.*
Förster s., Förster atonic-astatic s. atonic-astatic diplegia.
Foster Kennedy s. Kennedy s.
Foville s. a syndrome similar to the Millard-Gubler syndrome, except that, in addition to paralysis of the outward movement of the eye, there is paralysis of conjugate movement.
fragile X s. an X-linked syndrome associated with a fragile site on the X chromosome at q27.3, associated with mental retardation, enlarged testes, high forehead, and enlarged jaw and ears in most males and mild mental retardation in many heterozygous females. It is a triplet repeat disorder, associated with expansion of CGG triplet repeat sequences in the promoter region of a gene expressed in human brain cells, the *FMR1* (fragile X mental retardation 1) gene, with triplet repeats expanding from the normal 50 to as many as several thousand in the full syndrome. Between 50 and 200 copies, the sequence is unstable and prone to expansion; individuals appear normal, but are said to carry a (heritable) premutation, and when over 200 copies are present, abnormalities of methylation occur in the promoter region and prevent expression of the gene, and clinical symptoms are apparent. The expansion and methylation abnormalities also appear to interfere with chromosome replication, producing the characteristic fragile site.
Fraley s. nephralgia with dilation of the renal calices around the upper pole of the kidney due to compression of the adjacent infundibulum, usually caused by pressure from vessels serving that part of the kidney.
Franceschetti s. the complete form of mandibulofacial dysostosis.
Franceschetti-Jadassohn s. a rare autosomal dominant disorder characterized by gray to brown reticular hyperpigmentation beginning after infancy without preceding inflammatory changes; characteristics include palmoplantar keratoderma, vasomotor changes with hypohidrosis, and yellowing of the dental enamel.
François s. oculomandibulofacial s.
Fraser s. cryptophthalmos s.
Freeman-Sheldon s. an autosomal dominant syndrome caused by mutation in the *MYH3* gene (locus: 17p13.1), which encodes a myosin heavy chain. It consists of characteristic flattened, masklike facies; microstomia, the lips protruding as in whistling; deep-set eyes with hypertelorism; camptodactyly with ulnar deviation of the fingers; and talipes equinovarus. Called also *distal arthrogryposis type 2A, craniocarpotarsal dystrophy, whistling face syndrome,* and *whistling face–windmill vane hand syndrome.*
Frey s. auriculotemporal s.
Friderichsen-Waterhouse s. Waterhouse-Friderichsen s.
Fröhlich s. adiposogenital dystrophy.

Froin s. a condition of the lumbar spinal fluid consisting of a transparent clear yellow color (xanthochromia), with the finding of large amounts of protein, rapid coagulation, and the absence of an increased number of cells. It is seen in certain organic nervous diseases in which the lumbar fluid is cut off from communication with the fluid in the ventricles. Called also *loculation s.*
Frommel-Chiari s. Chiari-Frommel s.
Fuchs s. unilateral heterochromia, fine keratic precipitates, and secondary cataract.
Fukuhara s. MERRF s.
Fukuyama s. Fukuyama type congenital muscular dystrophy; see under *dystrophy.*
functional prepubertal castrate s. vanishing testes s.
G s. Opitz s.
Gailliard s. dextrocardia from retraction of lungs and pleura to the right.
galactorrhea-amenorrhea s. amenorrhea accompanied by galactorrhea, sometimes associated with increased levels of prolactin; several different types are known. See *Abumada-del Castillo s., Chiari-Frommel s.,* and *Forbes-Albright s.*
Ganser s. the giving of inappropriate, ridiculous, or approximate answers to questions, sometimes associated with amnesia, disorientation, perceptual disturbances, and conversion symptoms; it is most commonly seen in malingering prisoners feigning psychosis.
Garcin s. unilateral paralysis of all or most of the cranial nerves due to a tumor at the base of the skull or in the nasopharynx; called also *half base s.*
Gardner s. a phenotypic variant of familial adenomatous polyposis characterized by extracolonic lesions, including supernumerary teeth, fibrous dysplasia of the skull, retinal pigmentation, osteomas, fibromas, and epithelial cysts.
Gardner-Diamond s. painful bruising s.
gas bloat s. excessive gas in the gastrointestinal tract because of incompetence of the lower esophageal sphincter, such as after an operation to correct gastroesophageal reflux disease.
Gasser s. hemolytic uremic s.
gay bowel s. term coined in the 1970s for an assortment of sexually transmitted bowel and rectal diseases affecting homosexual males and others who engage in frequent anal intercourse; it is caused by a wide variety of infectious agents.
Gélineau s. narcolepsy.
gender dysphoria s. a group of psychological problems associated with discrepancy between the physical sex assignment and the psychological gender identity.
general adaptation s. a syndrome defined by Hans Selye to include all nonspecific systemic reactions of the body to prolonged exposure to systemic stress; he described three stages in the reacting: the alarm reaction, resistance, and exhaustion.
genital ulcer s. any of the diseases or conditions causing ulcerations of the genitalia, most commonly syphilis or herpes simplex, but also chancroid, lymphogranuloma venereum, granuloma inguinale, or trauma.
Gerstmann s. a combination of finger agnosia, right-left disorientation, agraphia, acalculia, and often constructional apraxia; it was formerly attributed to a lesion in the angular gyrus of the dominant hemisphere, but now that etiology is in doubt.
Gerstmann-Sträussler s., Gerstmann-Sträussler-Scheinker s. (GSS) a group of rare prion diseases, of autosomal dominant inheritance but linked to different mutations of the prion protein gene, having the common characteristics of cognitive and motor disturbances and the presence of multicentric amyloid plaques in the brain. In the *ataxic* form, there are progressive cerebellar ataxia and dementia; in the *telencephalic* form, there are dysarthria, dementia, rigidity, tremor, and hyperreflexia; in *GSS with neurofibrillary tangles,* there are progressive short-term memory loss and clumsiness. Death occurs in 1 to 5 years.
Gianotti-Crosti s. a viral disease of young children, generally benign and self-limited, characterized by skin-colored or reddish, flat-topped, firm papules forming a symmetrical eruption in an acral distribution, usually on the face, buttocks, or limbs, including the palms and soles. Symptoms are mild; the child may have malaise and a low grade fever. Several different viruses may cause it, but most commonly the hepatitis B virus. Called also *infantile acrodermatitis* and *papular acrodermatitis of childhood.*
giant platelet s. Bernard-Soulier s.

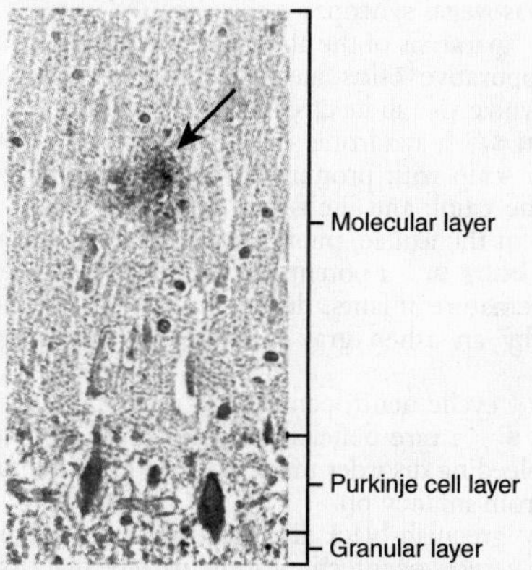

■ Gerstmann-Sträussler syndrome; immunostaining of a section through the cerebellum with antibodies to prion protein demonstrates an amyloid plaque *(arrow)* in the molecular layer.

Gilbert s. an inborn error of bilirubin metabolism, probably autosomal dominant, characterized by a benign elevation of unconjugated bilirubin without liver damage or hematologic abnormalities. Called also *familial* or *Gilbert cholemia, hyperbilirubinemia I, constitutional hyperbilirubinemia,* and *familial nonhemolytic jaundice.*
Gilles de la Tourette s. a syndrome comprising both multiple motor and one or more vocal tics, occurring over a period of at least one year, at least intermittently but sometimes as frequently as many times daily. Obsessions, compulsions, hyperactivity, distractibility, and impulsivity are often associated. Onset is in childhood and tics often lessen in severity and frequency and may even remit during adolescence and adulthood. Called also *Guinon disease, maladie des tics,* and *Tourette s.*
Gillespie s. a rare autosomal recessive syndrome consisting of aniridia, cerebellar ataxia, and mental retardation.
Gitelman s. a syndrome of hypertrophy of juxtaglomerular cells similar to Bartter syndrome but with hypocalciuria and hypomagnesemia; usually seen in adolescents or adults.
Gjessing s. recurrent episodes of stupor or excitement occurring in catatonic schizophrenia in association with variations in nitrogen metabolism and thyroid hormone level; it is related to nitrogen retention caused by inadequate metabolism of dietary protein.
glioma-polyposis s. Turcot s.
glucagonoma s. the spectrum of symptoms caused by a glucagonoma, associated with high blood levels of glucagon, mild diabetes mellitus, weight loss, anemia, glossitis, stomatitis, angular cheilitis, blepharitis, and necrolytic migratory erythema.
Goldberg s. galactosialidosis.
Goldenhar s. oculoauriculovertebral dysplasia.
Goltz s., Goltz-Gorlin s. focal dermal hypoplasia.
Good s. immunodeficiency with thymoma.
Goodman s. an autosomal recessive disorder resembling Carpenter syndrome but characterized also by congenital heart defects, clinodactyly, camptodactyly, and ulnar deviation; it is now generally believed to be a variant of Carpenter syndrome. Called also *acrocephalopolysyndactyly, type IV.*
Goodpasture s. a syndrome of glomerulonephritis, pulmonary hemorrhage, and circulating anti-GBM antibodies; it usually occurs in young men and is characterized by rapidly progressing renal failure as well as hemoptysis, pulmonary infiltrates, and dyspnea. Cf. *anti–GBM antibody nephritis* and *pulmonary renal s.*
Gopalan s. a symptom complex resulting from malnutrition, probably from deficiency of riboflavin or pantothenic acid; it consists of a burning sensation in the extremities, a feeling of "pins and needles" in the distal parts, and hyperhidrosis. Called also *burning feet* and *burning feet s.*
Gordon s. 1. pseudohypoaldosteronism type 2. 2. an autosomal dominant disorder characterized by camptodactyly, talipes, and cleft palate; called also *distal arthrogryposis type 3.*
Gorlin s., Gorlin-Goltz s. nevoid basal cell carcinoma s.
Gougerot-Blum s. pigmented purpuric lichenoid dermatitis.
Gougerot-Carteaud s. confluent and reticulate papillomatosis.
Gougerot-Nulock-Houwer s. Sjögren s.

Gowers s. vasovagal syncope.
Gradenigo s. paralysis of the abducens nerve and unilateral headache in chronic suppurative otitis media, caused by direct spread of the infection to involve the abducens and trigeminal nerves.
Graham Little s. a syndrome characterized by cicatricial patches of alopecia of the scalp with prominent follicular plugging and follicular keratoses on the trunk and limbs, sometimes associated with noncicatricial alopecia of the axillae, pubic region, trunk, and limbs.
gray s., gray baby s. a potentially fatal condition seen in neonates, particularly premature infants, due to a reaction to chloramphenicol, characterized by an ashen gray cyanosis, listlessness, weakness, and hypotension.
gray collie s. cyclic neutropenia.
gray platelet s. a rare deficiency of the alpha granules of platelets, resulting in a bleeding disorder that may include ecchymoses, petechiae, and epistaxis from infancy on.
green nail s. greenish-black discoloration of the nail plate secondary to *Pseudomonas aeruginosa* infection of the paronychial tissues, caused by the diffusion of pyocyanin produced by the bacteria into the nail bed.
Greig s. ocular hypertelorism.
Griscelli s. an albinoidism of autosomal recessive inheritance, marked by hypomelanosis, frequent pyogenic infection, hepatosplenomegaly, neutro- and thrombopenia, and possible immunodeficiency. Called also *hypopigmentation-immunodeficiency disease.*
Grisel s. subluxation of the atlantoaxial joint after an upper respiratory tract infection or an adenoidectomy, usually seen in children.
Grönblad-Strandberg s. angioid streaks in the retina together with pseudoxanthoma elasticum of the skin.
Gruber s. Meckel s.
Guillain-Barré s. (GBS) rapidly progressive ascending motor neuron paralysis of unknown etiology, frequently seen after an enteric or respiratory infection. An autoimmune mechanism following viral infection has been postulated. It begins with paresthesias of the feet, followed by flaccid paralysis of the entire lower limbs, ascending to the trunk, upper limbs, and face; other characteristics include slight fever, bulbar palsy, absent or lessened tendon reflexes, and increased protein in the cerebrospinal fluid without a corresponding increase in cells. Variant forms include acute autonomic neuropathy, Miller-Fisher syndrome, acute motor axonal neuropathy, and acute motor-sensory axonal neuropathy. Called also *Guillain-Barré polyneuritis* or *polyneuropathy; Landry paralysis* or *syndrome;* and *acute idiopathic, acute infectious,* or *acute postinfectious polyneuritis.*
Gulf War s. a group of symptoms of unknown cause, seen in military personnel of the United States and its allies in the Persian Gulf conflict of the early 1990s, consisting of widespread pain including fibromyalgia and headaches, sometimes gastrointestinal distress, and memory disorders.
Gunn s. unilateral ptosis of the eyelid, with the association of movements of the affected upper eyelid with those of the jaw; called also *Gunn phenomenon, Marcus Gunn s.* or *phenomenon,* and *jaw-winking s.* or *phenomenon.*
gustatory sweating s. auriculotemporal s.
Haddad s. a rare association of congenital central hypoventilation syndrome and Hirschsprung disease.
Hadfield-Clarke s. Clarke-Hadfield s.
Hakim s. normal-pressure hydrocephalus.
half base s. Garcin s.
Hallermann-Streiff s., Hallermann-Streiff-François s. oculomandibulofacial s.
Hallopeau-Siemens s. recessive epidermolysis bullosa dystrophica.
halzoun s. halzoun.
Hamman s. pneumomediastinum.
Hamman-Rich s. acute interstitial pneumonia.
hand-arm vibration s. a common occupational disease consisting of acrocyanosis in a person experiencing prolonged repetitive hand and arm vibrations. Called also *dead finger* and *vibration white finger.*
hand-foot s. a syndrome of erythema and dysesthesias of touch in the palms and soles, followed by desquamation; seen as a reaction to certain chemotherapeutic agents. Called also *acral, palmar-plantar,* or *palmoplantar erythrodysesthesia* and *palmar-plantar erythrodysesthesia syndrome.*
hand-foot-uterus s. a congenital syndrome consisting of small feet with unusually short great toes, abnormal thumbs, and, in females, duplication of the genital tract.
hand-shoulder s. shoulder-hand s.
Hanhart s. any of several syndromes of variable inheritance, characterized chiefly by severe micrognathia, high nose root, small eyelid fissures, low-set ears, and variable absence of digits or limbs, usually below the elbow or knee.
Hanot-Chauffard s. hypertrophic cirrhosis with pigmentation and diabetes mellitus.
hantavirus pulmonary s. a sometimes fatal febrile illness caused by viruses of the genus *Hantavirus,* spread to humans by various species of mice and rats; characteristics include variable respiratory symptoms followed by acute respiratory distress that may progress to respiratory failure.
happy puppet s. Angelman s.
Harada s. Vogt-Koyanagi-Harada s.
HARD s. Walker-Warburg s.
Hare s. Pancoast s. (def. 1).
Harris s. hyperinsulinism due to organic endogenous factors, such as insulinoma, manifested by hypoglycemia, weakness, perspiration, jitteriness, tachycardia, mental confusion, and disturbances of vision.
Hartnup s. see under *disease.*
haw s. protrusion of one or both of the nictitating membranes of a dog or cat. Called also *haw.*
Haw River s. an autosomal dominant neurodegenerative disorder characterized by ataxia, chorea, seizures, and dementia, with onset usually between ages 15 to 30 years, and death within 15 to 25 years. It is a triplet repeat disorder caused by expansion of the CAG triplet repeat in the *DPRLA* gene encoding the atrophin-1 protein, as occurs in dentatorubral-pallidoluysian atrophy (q.v.), although there are some differences in clinical expression and pathology, including lack of myoclonic seizures, and extensive demyelinization of the subcortical white matter, basal ganglia calcifications, and neuroaxonal dystrophy.
Hay-Wells s. an autosomal dominant syndrome of ectodermal dysplasia, cleft lip and palate, and ankyloblepharon filiforme adnatum; it is also characterized by hypodontia, palmar and plantar keratoderma, partial anhidrosis, sparse wiry hair, and sometimes otologic defects. Called also *AEC s.* and *ankyloblepharon–ectodermal dysplasia–clefting s.*
Hayem-Widal s. former name for *hemolytic anemia.*
heart-hand s. Holt-Oram s.
Hecht s., Hecht-Beals s., Hecht-Beals-Wilson s. trismus-pseudocamptodactyly s.
Heerfordt s. an occasional manifestation of sarcoidosis consisting of enlargement of the parotid and lacrimal glands, anterior uveitis, Bell palsy, and fever. Called also *uveoparotid fever.*
Heidenhain s. a rapidly progressive degenerative disease manifested by cortical blindness, presenile dementia, dysarthria, ataxia, athetoid movements, and generalized rigidity.
HELLP s. *h*emolysis, *el*evated *l*iver enzymes, and *l*ow *p*latelet count occurring in association with preeclampsia.
Helweg-Larsen s. an autosomal dominant syndrome consisting of anhidrosis present from birth and labyrinthitis later in life.
hemangioma-thrombocytopenia s. Kasabach-Merritt s.
hemolytic uremic s. a form of thrombotic microangiopathy usually seen in children, characterized by renal failure, hemolytic anemia, and severe thrombocytopenia and purpura. Some authorities consider it identical to thrombotic thrombocytopenic purpura. Called also *Gasser s.*
hemophagocytic s. see under *lymphohistiocytosis.*
hemopleuropneumonic s. a syndrome of dyspnea, hemoptysis, tachycardia, fever, pneumonia, and hydrothorax occurring after a puncture wound of the chest.
Hench-Rosenberg s. palindromic rheumatism.
Henoch-Schönlein s. see under *purpura.*
hepatopulmonary s. arterial hypoxemia caused by pulmonary vasodilation in conjunction with chronic liver disease, usually occurring as a result of portal hypertension in cirrhosis.
hepatorenal s. functional renal failure, oliguria, and low urinary sodium concentration, without pathological renal changes, associated with cirrhosis and ascites or with obstructive jaundice.
hereditary mixed polyposis s. an autosomal dominant syndrome characterized by the occurrence of atypical juvenile polyps of mixed histologic type, colonic adenomas, and colorectal carcinomas.
hereditary periodic fever s's autoinflammatory diseases.
Hermansky-Pudlak s. a rare, genetically heterogeneous, multisystem disorder characterized by oculocutaneous albinism, hemorrhagic diathesis secondary to a platelet defect, pulmonary fibrosis, colitis, and

accumulation of ceroid in the reticuloendothelial system and oral mucosa and its excretion in urine; cardiomyopathy and renal failure may also occur. Eight types have been identified, and its inheritance is autosomal recessive.

Herrmann s. an autosomal dominant syndrome characterized initially by photomyogenic seizures and progressive deafness, with later development of diabetes mellitus, nephropathy, and mental deterioration progressing to dementia.

heterotaxy s. a variable set of complex congenital anomalies of the gastrointestinal and cardiovascular systems that results from heterotaxia of the abdominal and thoracic viscera.

HHH s. hyperornithinemia-hyperammonemia-homocitrullinuria s.

high-pressure neurologic s. a group of neurologic and neuropsychiatric signs and symptoms seen in deep sea divers below 100 meters, especially in those breathing heliox mixtures; symptoms vary, depending on the depth and gas mixture, and include tremor, incoordination, myoclonus, opsoclonus, headache, vertigo, nausea, euphoria, and cognitive disturbances.

Hines-Bannick s. intermittent attacks of low temperature and disabling sweating.

Hinman s. a psychogenic disorder seen in children, imitating a neurogenic bladder, consisting of detrusor-sphincter dyssynergia without evidence of any neural lesions. Called also *nonneurogenic neurogenic bladder*.

HIV wasting s. wasting s.

Hoffmann-Werdnig s. Werdnig-Hoffmann disease.

holiday heart s. paroxysms of arrhythmias, most commonly atrial fibrillation, in patients without overt cardiomyopathy after a weekend bout of alcoholic consumption, especially during the year-end holiday season.

Holmes-Adie s. Adie s.

Holt-Oram s. autosomal dominant heart disease of varying severity, usually an atrial or ventricular septal defect, in association with upper limb malformation consisting of narrow shoulders, hypoplasia of the radius, and phocomelia, most commonly absence of the thumb and radius. Called also *heart-hand s.*

honker s. a disease of feedlot cattle, of unknown etiology, characterized by edema of the lower trachea with dyspnea and a honking sound during inspiration.

Horner s., Horner-Bernard s. sinking in of the eyeball, ptosis of the upper eyelid, slight elevation of the lower lid, constriction of the pupil, narrowing of the palpebral fissure, and anhidrosis and flushing of the affected side of the face; caused by a brainstem lesion on the ipsilateral side that interrupts sympathetic nerve fibers. See also *Horner ptosis.* Called also *Bernard* or *Bernard-Horner s.* and *oculosympathetic palsy.*

Horton s. giant cell arteritis.

hot foot s. *Pseudomonas* hot foot s.

Howel-Evans s. a rare type of diffuse palmoplantar keratoderma usually seen in children and associated with development of esophageal cancer later in life.

Hughes-Stovin s. thrombosis of the pulmonary arteries and peripheral veins, characterized by headache, fever, cough, papilledema, and hemoptysis.

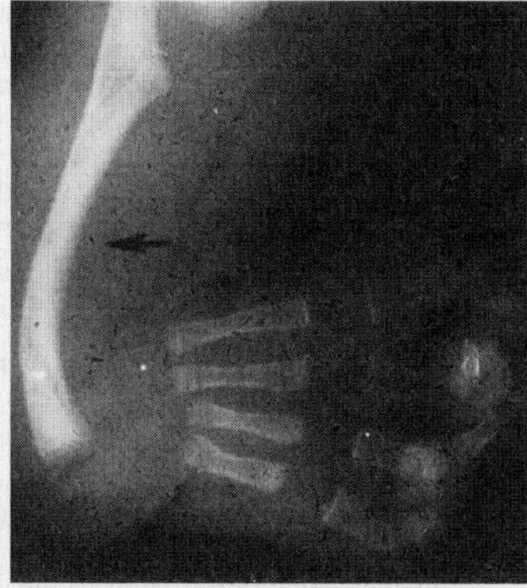

■ Holt-Oram syndrome. Radiograph shows the absence of a radius shadow *(arrow)* and missing thumb.

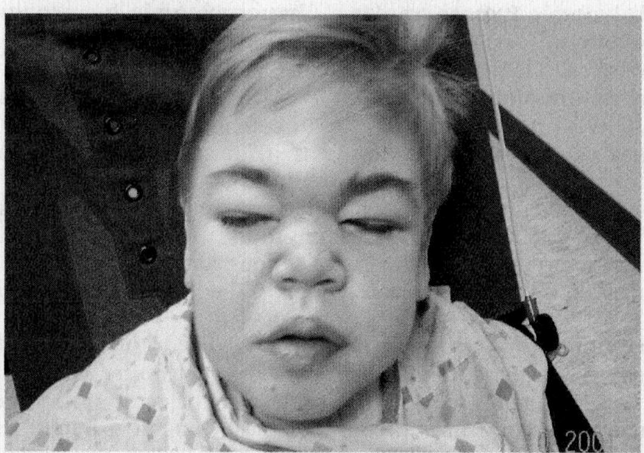

■ Hurler syndrome. Child showing typical coarsening of facial features including prominent forehead, flattened nasal bridge, short broad nose, and widening of the lips.

hungry bone s. a condition seen after parathyroidectomy in patients who had had hyperparathyroidism; rapid deposition of calcium in bones leads to hypocalcemia.

Hunt s. Ramsay Hunt s.

Hunter s. a mucopolysaccharidosis caused by deficiency of iduronate-2-sulfatase, characterized by excretion of dermatan sulfate and heparan sulfate in the urine; it differs clinically from Hurler syndrome by (1) X-linked inheritance; (2) slower progression, less severity, and longer survival (thus resembling the Hurler-Scheie syndrome); and (3) absence of corneal clouding. Two clinical forms exist: the severe form has Hurler-Scheie–like symptoms with death before 15, usually from heart disease; the mild form has onset in the first decade, reduced somatic involvement, and near-normal intelligence and lifespan. Called also *mucopolysaccharidosis II.*

Hurler s. the prototype of the mucopolysaccharidoses, and the gravest of the three allelic disorders of mucopolysaccharidosis I. It is caused by deficiency of L-iduronidase, and onset is after the first year with progressive physical and mental deterioration; there is corneal clouding, with death usually by age 10 caused by respiratory infection and heart failure. Further symptoms include gargoyle-like facies with hypertelorism, depressed nasal bridge, large tongue, and widely spaced teeth; dwarfism; severe somatic and skeletal changes, including short neck and trunk, scaphocephaly, and kyphosis with gibbus; short broad hands with short fingers; progressive opacities of the cornea; deafness; cardiovascular defects; hepatosplenomegaly; and joint contractures. Called also *mucopolysaccharidosis IH.*

Hurler-Scheie s. one of the three allelic disorders of mucopolysaccharidosis I, with clinical features intermediate between the Hurler and the Scheie syndromes, caused by deficiency of L-iduronidase, and specifically characterized by receding chin (micrognathism). Symptoms include mental retardation, dwarfism, dysostosis multiplex, corneal clouding, deafness, hernia, stiff joints (claw hand), and valvular heart disease. Patients survive until their late teens or twenties. Called also *mucopolysaccharidosis IH/S.*

Hutchinson s. see under *triad.*

Hutchinson-Gilford s. progeria.

Hutchison s. neuroblastoma with metastases to the skull.

17-hydroxylase deficiency s. 17α-hydroxylase deficiency; see under *H.*

hyperabduction s. a thoracic outlet syndrome due to compression of the brachial plexus trunk roots and axillary vessels by the pectoralis minor muscle and the coracoid process when the arms are stretched above the head, as during sleep. Called also *Wright s.*

hyperactive child s. former name for *attention-deficit/hyperactivity disorder.*

hypercalcemia s. milk-alkali s.

hypereosinophilic s. any of several diseases characterized by a massive increase in the number of eosinophils in the blood and bone marrow, with eosinophilic infiltration of other organs. Symptoms vary, depending on the organ involved, and may include pruritic skin ulcers or erythroderma, endomyocarditis, lymph node or spleen enlargement, and ophthalmologic or gastrointestinal complications. Eosinophilic leukemia is a potentially fatal member of the group.

hyperglycemic hyperosmolar s., hyperglycemic hyperosmolar nonketotic s. see under *state.*
hyper-IgE s. hyperimmunoglobulinemia E s.
hyperimmunoglobulinemia D s. (HIDS), hyperimmunoglobulinemia D with periodic fever s. an autoinflammatory disease (q.v.) inherited as an autosomal recessive trait, caused by mutations in the gene for mevalonate kinase, with onset usually before one year of age. It is characterized by attacks of high fever preceded by chills, occurring about every 4 to 8 weeks and lasting 4 to 6 days, often with headache, arthritis and arthralgia, erythematous lesions, and hepatosplenomegaly; serum IgD levels are continuously high. Called also *Dutch type periodic fever.*
hyperimmunoglobulinemia E s. (HIES) hyper-IgE syndrome: 1. a primary immunodeficiency disorder caused by mutations of the STAT3 gene (see *STAT*). It is usually of autosomal dominant inheritance but sometimes occurs sporadically and is characterized by recurrent staphylococcal abscesses of skin, lungs, joints, and other sites; pruritic dermatitis; distinctive coarse facies; retained primary dentition; skeletal abnormalities; eosinophilia; and very high serum immunoglobulin E (IgE) levels. Called also *Buckley s.* and *Job s.* 2. an autosomal recessive syndrome that is clinically similar to the autosomal dominant form but lacks the skeletal abnormalities.
hyperinfection s. a highly fatal form of strongyloidiasis, most often occurring in immunocompromised persons and characterized by massive infection and widespread hematogenous dissemination of parasites to organs not normally affected. Manifestations are highly variable; pulmonary signs and symptoms resemble those of acute respiratory distress syndrome.
hyperkinetic s. former name for *attention-deficit/hyperactivity disorder.*
hyperkinetic heart s. increased cardiac output of unknown cause associated with slightly elevated systolic and pulse pressures, normal mean arterial pressure, and low systemic vascular resistance.
hyperlucent lung s. a syndrome simulating localized emphysema, but due to congenital absence or hypoplasia of pulmonary arteries; there may be lobar or segmental agenesis, as well as accessory lungs, lobes, or segments.
hypermobility s. benign joint hypermobility s.
hyperornithinemia-hyperammonemia-homocitrullinuria s. an autosomal recessive syndrome characterized by elevated plasma levels of ornithine, postprandial hyperammonemia and homocitrullinuria, and aversion to protein ingestion. It is believed to result from a defect in the transport of ornithine into mitochondria, which disturbs the cycle of ureagenesis. Called also *HHH s.*
hyperosmolar hyperglycemic s. hyperglycemic hyperosmolar state.
hyperperfusion s. a complex of symptoms that sometimes follows carotid endarterectomy procedures, consisting of headache, seizures, focal deficits, brain edema, and sometimes cerebral hemorrhage; the cause is believed to be loss of arterial regulatory ability on the side where an occlusion has been removed.
hyperreactive malarial spleen s. tropical splenomegaly s.
hypersomnia-bulimia s. Kleine-Levin s.
hypertelorism-hypospadias s. Opitz s.
hyperventilation s. a complex of symptoms that accompany hypocapnia caused by hyperventilation, including palpitations, shortness of breath, lightheadedness, profuse perspiration, and tingling sensations in the fingertips, face, or toes; prolonged overbreathing may result in vasomotor collapse and loss of consciousness. Hyperventilation unrecognized by the patient is a common cause of the subjective somatic symptoms associated with chronic anxiety or panic attacks (see *panic disorder*, under *disorder*).
hyperviscosity s. any of various syndromes associated with increased viscosity of the blood. One type is due to serum hyperviscosity and is characterized by spontaneous bleeding with neurologic and ocular disorders. Another type is characterized by polycythemia with retarded blood flow, organ congestion, reduced capillary perfusion, and increased cardiac effort. A third group includes conditions in which the deformability of erythrocytes is impaired, such as sickle cell anemia.
hypocomplementemic urticarial vasculitis s. (HUVS) a potentially severe vasculitis characterized by recurrent urticaria with hypocomplementemia and the presence of autoantibodies to complement component C1q. Extracutaneous involvement may occur and can be life-threatening.
hypoglossia-hypodactyly s. a rare syndrome consisting of partial to complete absence of the tongue and of the digits or one or more limbs. Called also *aglossia-adactylia s.*
hypoplastic left heart s. (HLHS) any of a group of congenital anomalies consisting of hypoplasia or atresia of the left ventricle and of the aortic or mitral valve or both and hypoplasia of the ascending aorta; it is characterized by respiratory distress and extreme cyanosis, with cardiac failure and death in early infancy.
hypothenar hammer s. traumatic aneurysm of the ulnar artery at the hypothenar in persons who repeatedly use the hypothenar to push or pound.
hypotonic s's a group of syndromes involving inadequate water excretion in comparison to the amount ingested, so that body fluids become hypotonic and hyponatremic; some are due to excessive water intake as in water intoxication, while others are caused by derangements of the excretory process such as the vasopressin excess in the syndrome of inappropriate diuretic hormone or complications of the nephrotic syndrome, congestive heart failure, or kidney failure.
hypotrichosis-lymphedema-telangiectasia s. a rare, autosomal recessive condition consisting of progressive hair loss, lymphedema of the lower limbs, and telangiectasias on various parts of the body.
IBIDS s. [*i*cthyosis, *b*rittle hair, *i*nfertility, *d*evelopmental delay, *s*hort stature] Tay s.
idiopathic postprandial s. the repeated occurrence of the clinical manifestations of hypoglycemia after meals; a controversial disease entity.
iliotibial band s. a type of overuse injury in athletes caused by repetitive rubbing of the iliotibial tract (or band) against the lateral femoral epicondyle as the hip is repetitively extended and flexed; the primary symptom is severe pain in the thigh and knee.
Imerslund s., Imerslund-Graesbeck s. a rare familial form of megaloblastic anemia, usually transmitted as an autosomal recessive trait, characterized by selective intestinal malabsorption of vitamin B_{12} uninfluenced by intrinsic factor, and associated with proteinuria and structural genitourinary tract anomalies.
immotile cilia s. primary ciliary dyskinesia.
impingement s. a type of overuse injury with progressive pathologic changes resulting from mechanical impingement by the acromion, coracoacromial ligament, coracoid process, or acromioclavicular joint against the rotator cuff; changes may include reversible edema and hemorrhage, fibrosis, tendinitis, pain, bone spur formation, and tendon rupture.
s. of inappropriate antidiuresis (SIAD) a disorder of sodium and water balance characterized by hyponatremia with hypovolemia and elevated urine osmolality in the absence of kidney disease; it may be caused by inappropriate secretion of vasopressin *(s. of inappropriate antidiuretic hormone)* or mutations affecting the ability of the renal collecting tubules to absorb water *(nephrogenic s. of inappropriate antidiuresis).*
s. of inappropriate antidiuretic hormone (SIADH) hyponatremia with decreased extracellular fluid osmolality, inability to produce dilute urine, normovolemia, and elevated urinary sodium excretion, in the absence of kidney disease or other cause of normovolemic hypo-osmolality. Causes include vasopressin-secreting tumor cells, neoplasms (especially oat cell carcinoma of the lung or pancreatic carcinoma), pulmonary disorders, central nervous system disease, and adverse drug reactions.
inferior s. of red nucleus Claude s.
inhibitory s. the manifestations produced by a somatostatinoma, including diabetes mellitus, cholecystolithiasis, steatorrhea, indigestion, hypochlorhydria, and occasionally anemia.
inspissated bile s. biliary obstruction caused by plugging of the outflow tract.
insulin autoimmune s. a rare condition in which hypoglycemia is produced by extremely high concentrations of autoantibodies to insulin, seen primarily in persons of Asian descent and in most cases associated with treatment with sulfhydryl-containing medications.
intersection s. a type of overuse injury with tenosynovitis about 4 cm proximal to the wrist, at the point where the tendons of the abductor pollicis longus and extensor pollicis brevis muscles cross over those of the extensor carpi radialis longus and brevis muscles; it is caused by

frequent, repetitive wrist movements such as in athletes. Symptoms are similar to those of de Quervain disease.
intrauterine parabiotic s. placental transfusion; see under *transfusion.*
irritable bowel s. (IBS), irritable colon s. a common, chronic, noninflammatory condition characterized by abdominal pain and altered bowel habits (diarrhea or constipation or both), but no detectable pathologic change; there may be spasms of the intestinal muscles. A variant form is characterized by painless diarrhea. It is usually due to a combination of psychologic and physiologic factors. Called also *irritable* or *spastic colon.*
Irukandji s. a clinical syndrome observed in Queensland, Australia, due to stinging by the jellyfish *Carukia barnesi;* symptoms include initial neuromuscular paralysis that can be fatal, and in survivors systemic symptoms with pulmonary edema and skin ulcers at the site of infection.
Isaacs s., Isaacs-Mertens s. a rare autoimmune form of peripheral nerve hyperexcitability that affects the potassium channels of motor nerve axons, resulting in abnormal nerve firing and consequent spontaneous muscle activity, characterized by progressive muscle stiffness, delayed muscle relaxation after contraction, cramping, myokymia, and hyperhidrosis. It may accompany a variety of other autoimmune disorders; it sometimes occurs as a paraneoplastic condition or secondary to infection. Called also *acquired neuromyotonia.*
Ivemark s. congenital splenic agenesis, cardiac defects, and partial situs inversus viscerum; called also *asplenia s.* and *Polhemus-Schafer-Ivemark s.*
IVIC s. a rare autosomal dominant syndrome of internal ophthalmoplegia, hearing impairment, and radial ray defects varying from a long slender thumb to deformity of an entire upper limb, first observed in Venezuela and later in Italy. Called also *oculo-oto-radial s.*
Jaccoud s. see under *arthropathy.*
Jackson s. paralysis of structures innervated by the tenth, eleventh, and twelfth cranial nerves, including the soft palate, larynx, half of the tongue, and the sternomastoid and trapezius muscles. Called also *Mackenzie s.* and *vagoaccessory-hypoglossal s.*
Jacod s. unilateral blindness and ophthalmoplegia with facial hemiplegia or trigeminal neuralgia as a result of damage to the second, third, fourth, fifth, and sixth cranial nerves, often from a tumor or other lesion just behind the sphenoid bone. Called also *Jacod triad, Negri-Jacod s.,* and *petrosphenoid s.*
Jadassohn-Lewandowsky s. pachyonychia congenita.
Jahnke s. a variant of Sturge-Weber syndrome in which glaucoma is absent.
Janz s. juvenile myoclonic epilepsy.
Jarcho-Levin s. an autosomal recessive disorder consisting of multiple vertebral defects, short thorax, rib abnormalities, camptodactyly, and syndactyly; urogenital abnormalities are sometimes present. Death, from respiratory insufficiency, usually occurs in infancy. Called also *spondylothoracic dysplasia.*
jaw-winking s. Gunn s.
Jefferson s. cavernous sinus s.
jejunal s. dumping s.
Jervell and Lange-Nielsen s. a rare, autosomal recessive form of the long QT syndrome, characterized by neural hearing loss and syncope, sometimes with ventricular fibrillation and sudden death.
Jeune s. asphyxiating thoracic dystrophy.
Job s. hyperimmunoglobulinemia E s.
Johanson-Blizzard s. a rare autosomal recessive syndrome characterized by a small, pointed nose with underdeveloped nostrils; malformed or absent teeth; sparse, coarse hair; and sometimes growth retardation or failure to thrive.
Joubert s. an autosomal recessive syndrome consisting of partial or complete agenesis of the cerebellar vermis, with hypotonia, episodic hyperpnea, mental retardation, and abnormal eye movements; most patients die in infancy.
jugular foramen s. Vernet s.
jumping Frenchmen of Maine s. a form of jumping disease observed in a group of lumbermen of French-Canadian descent working in a remote area of Maine; affected individuals had exaggerated startle responses, automatic obedience, and often echolalia. It is believed to have represented a form of operant conditioning rather than a true disease.
juvenile polyposis s. juvenile polyposis.
Kabuki make-up s. a congenital, possibly inherited, syndrome of mental retardation, dwarfism, scoliosis, peculiar facies resembling the makeup of Japanese actors of Kabuki, and frequently cardiovascular abnormalities.
Kallmann s. a type of hypogonadotropic hypogonadism caused by failure of fetal gonadotropin-releasing hormone neurons to migrate to the thalamus, usually associated with anosmia or hyposmia. It is usually passed by autosomal recessive inheritance, and some cases are X-linked.
Kanner s. autistic disorder.
Kartagener s. a hereditary disorder involving a combination of dextrocardia (situs inversus), bronchiectasis, and sinusitis, transmitted as an autosomal recessive trait.
Kasabach-Merritt s. a blood disorder usually occurring in the first few months of life in which severe thrombocytopenia and other evidence of intravascular coagulation are accompanied by rapidly expanding hemangiomas of the trunk, extremities, and abdominal viscera, sometimes associated with bleeding and anemia. Bleeding is thought to be due to trapping and destruction of platelets within the tumor and depletion of circulating clotting factors. Called also *hemangioma-thrombocytopenia s.*
Kast s. Maffucci s.
Kaufman-McKusick s. a rare autosomal recessive disorder of hydrometrocolpos accompanied by postaxial polydactyly, congenital cardiac defects, and sometimes subsequent bilateral hydronephrosis. Manifestations in males include hypospadias and prominent scrotal raphe. Called also *McKusick-Kaufman s.*
Kearns-Sayre s. progressive ophthalmoplegia, pigmentary degeneration of the retina, myopathy, ataxia, and cardiac conduction defect; onset is before age 20. Almost all patients have large mitochondrial DNA deletions, and ragged red fibers are seen on muscle biopsy. Called also *ophthalmoplegia plus.*
Kennedy s. retrobulbar optic neuritis, central scotoma, optic atrophy on the side of the lesion and papilledema on the opposite side, occurring in tumors of the frontal lobe of the brain which press downward. Called also *Foster Kennedy s.*
Kenny-Caffey s. a hereditary syndrome characterized by hypoparathyroidism with intermittent hypocalcemia, short stature, and medullary stenosis of tubular bones. It is usually autosomal dominant, but autosomal recessive cases have also been observed.
keratitis-ichthyosis-deafness s. a rare syndrome, often inherited in autosomal recessive fashion, consisting of erythroderma, lamellar ichthyosis, sensorineural hearing loss, and sometimes keratitis, inflammatory corneal vascularization, postnatal growth deficiency, alopecia, nail dystrophy, tooth malformations, and decreased sweating. Called also *KID s.* and *Senter s.*
Key-Gaskell s. feline dysautonomia.
KID s. keratitis-ichthyosis-deafness s.
Kiloh-Nevin s. 1. ocular myopathy in patients with ptosis and progressive external ophthalmoplegia. 2. anterior interosseous s.
Kimmelstiel-Wilson s. the nodular type of intercapillary glomerulosclerosis.
Kindler s. a rare type of genodermatosis of variable inheritance, characterized by acrokeratosis with blistering, photosensitivity, and poikiloderma. Called also *bullous* or *hereditary acrokeratotic poikiloderma.*
King s. a form of malignant hyperthermia (q.v.) in which patients also exhibit characteristic physical abnormalities including short stature, characteristic facies, kyphoscoliosis, pectus carinatum, cryptorchidism, delayed motor development, progressive myopathy, and cardiovascular structural defects.
kinky hair s. Menkes disease
Kinsbourne s. myoclonic encephalopathy of childhood; see under *encephalopathy.*
kleeblattschädel s. a congenital disorder, characterized by synostosis of multiple or all cranial sutures, hydrocephalus, and in some cases facial dysostosis and long bone anomalies.
Klein-Waardenburg s. Waardenburg s. type 3.
Kleine-Levin s. episodic periods of excessive sleep and overeating lasting for several weeks, with amnesia for the attacks; it usually occurs in adolescent boys.
Klinefelter s. a syndrome in males characterized by small testes, hyalinization of seminiferous tubules, azoospermia, variable degrees of masculinization, and increased urinary excretion of gonadotropin. Patients tend to be tall, with long legs, and about half have gynecomastia. It is associated typically with an XXY chromosome complement,

although variants include XXYY, XXXY, XXXXY, and several mosaic patterns. Called also *seminiferous tubule dysgenesis* and *XXY s.*

Klippel-Feil s. a condition characterized by shortness of the neck resulting from reduction in the number of cervical vertebrae or the fusion of multiple hemivertebrae into one osseous mass; the hairline is low and motion of the neck is limited.

Klippel-Trénaunay s., Klippel-Trénaunay-Weber s. a rare condition usually affecting one extremity, characterized by hypertrophy of the bone and related soft tissues, large cutaneous hemangiomas, persistent nevus flammeus (see *port-wine stain,* under *stain*), and skin varices.

Klumpke-Dejerine s. Klumpke paralysis.

Klüver-Bucy s. bizarre behavior disturbances seen in monkeys following experimental bilateral temporal lobectomy which destroys important limbic structures; reported in humans after large injuries, usually from trauma, affecting the undersurface of the anterior temporal lobes. It is characterized by a tendency to examine objects orally, depression of drive and emotional reactions, hypermetamorphosis, and lack of sexual inhibitions.

Kocher-Debré-Sémélaigne s. Debré-Sémélaigne s.

Koerber-Salus-Elschnig s. sylvian s.

König s. constipation alternating with diarrhea and attended with abdominal pain, tympanites, and gurgling sounds in the right iliac fossa.

Korsakoff s. a syndrome of anterograde and retrograde amnesia with confabulation associated with alcoholic or nonalcoholic polyneuritis described as "cerebropathia psychica toxemica" by Korsakoff; currently used synonymously with the term amnestic syndrome or, more narrowly, to refer to the amnestic component of the Wernicke-Korsakoff syndrome, i.e., an amnestic syndrome resulting from thiamine deficiency. Spelled also *Korsakov s.* Called also *Korsakoff psychosis.*

Kostmann s. an autosomal recessive form of severe congenital neutropenia (gene locus: 1q21.3), characterized by early onset of recurrent pyogenic infections of the skin and lung, absence of neutrophils in the blood, absolute monocytosis and eosinophilia, and early death. Called also *infantile genetic agranulocytosis* and *Kostmann neutropenia.*

Krause s. a retinal and cerebral dysplasia found in premature infants several months after birth, characterized by malformations of the choroid, retina, and optic nerve, and possible blindness, cataract, coloboma, glaucoma, and microphthalmos. Cerebral symptoms include aplasia, hyperplasia, and hypertrophy of the brain, hydrocephaly, microcephaly, and mental retardation. Called also *encephalo-ophthalmic dysplasia.*

Kugelberg-Welander s. type III spinal muscular atrophy (see under *atrophy*), an autosomal recessive condition caused by lesions of the anterior horns of the spinal cord. Onset is in the first or second decade, principally between two and seventeen years, with atrophy and weakness of the proximal muscles of the lower limbs and pelvic girdle, followed by involvement of the distal muscles and muscular twitching. Called also *juvenile* or *proximal spinal muscular atrophy* and *Wohlfart-Kugelberg-Welander s.*

Kunkel s. chronic active hepatitis.

lacrimo-auriculo-dento-digital s., LADD s. a syndrome of autosomal dominant inheritance, characterized by abnormalities of the nasolacrimal ducts, ears, limbs, and teeth, often with mixed hearing loss. Abnormalities of the salivary glands and urogenital system may also occur. Spelled also *lacrimoauriculodentodigital s.* Called also *Levy-Hollister s.*

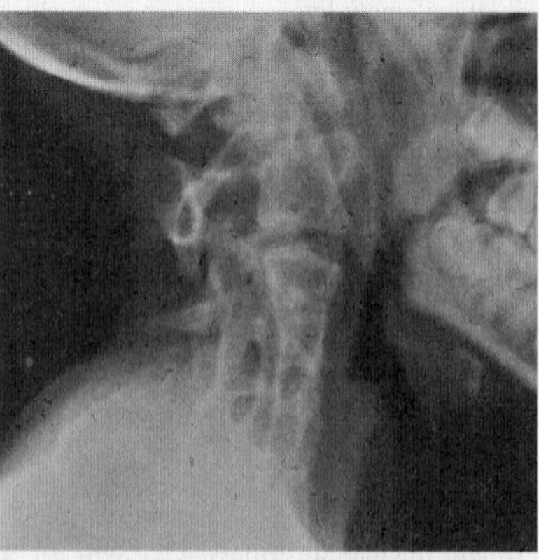

■ Klippel-Feil syndrome. Radiograph shows severe osseous involvement with fusion and hypoplasia of spinal segments C3–C7.

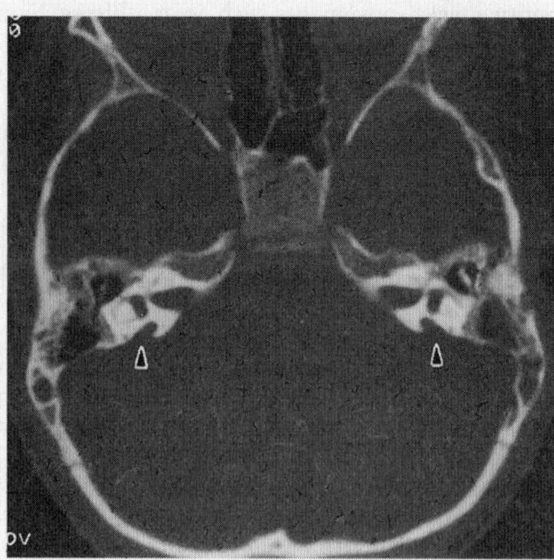

■ Large vestibular aqueduct syndrome showing bilateral enlargement of the vestibular aqueducts *(arrows)* on an axial CT scan.

lacunar s. see under *stroke.*

Ladd s. congenital obstruction of the duodenum due to peritoneal bands (Ladd bands) and cecal volvulus.

LAMB s. a syndrome of familial myxomas with cutaneous, cardiac, and endocrine involvement, manifested as *l*entigines, *a*trial *m*yxoma, and *b*lue nevi. Cf. *NAME s.*

Lambert-Eaton s., Lambert-Eaton myasthenic s. (LEMS) an autoimmune, myasthenialike syndrome caused by autoantibodies to the voltage-gated calcium channel (anna 1 antibodies) that interfere with the release of acetylcholine at the motor nerve terminal. Weakness usually affects the limbs, but ocular and bulbar muscles are spared; there is reduced muscle action potential on stimulation of its nerve but with repetitive stimulation it becomes augmented. It is often associated with oat-cell carcinoma of the lung. Called also *Eaton-Lambert s.* and *myasthenic s.*

Lance-Adams s. the chronic form of posthypoxic myoclonus.

Landau-Kleffner s. an epileptic syndrome of childhood characterized by partial or generalized seizures, psychomotor abnormalities, and aphasia progressing to mutism. The electroencephalogram from bilateral temporal regions is abnormal, with spikes like those of benign rolandic epilepsy. Called also *acquired epileptic aphasia.*

Landry s. Guillain-Barré s.

Langer-Giedion s. an inherited disorder characterized by mental retardation, microcephaly, multiple exostosis, characteristic facies with bulbous nose, sparse hair, cone-shaped epiphyses, loose redundant skin, joint laxity, and other anomalies.

Lannois-Gradenigo s. Gradenigo s.

large vestibular aqueduct s. symptoms resulting from enlargement of the vestibular aqueduct of the inner ear, with sensorineural hearing loss that may be progressive and become severe, and frequently vertigo.

Laron s. an autosomal recessive syndrome of skeletal growth retardation due to impaired inability to synthesize insulin-like growth factor I, usually because of growth hormone receptor defects. Called also *Laron dwarfism.*

Larsen s. a rare syndrome of variable inheritance, characterized by cleft palate, flattened facies, multiple congenital bone dislocations, and foot deformities.

lateral medullary s. Wallenberg s.

Launois s. pituitary gigantism.

Launois-Bensaude s. multiple symmetric lipomatosis.

Laurence-Moon s. an autosomal recessive disorder characterized by mental retardation, pigmentary retinopathy, hypogonadism, and spastic paraplegia; cf. *Bardet-Biedl s.* and *Biemond s., II.*

Lawrence-Seip s. total lipodystrophy.

lazy leukocyte s. a syndrome of unknown etiology, usually seen in children, marked by recurrent low-grade infections, associated with a defect in neutrophil chemotaxis and deficient random mobility of neutrophils.

Syndrome *Continued*

Legg-Calvé-Perthes s. osteochondrosis of the capital epiphysis.
Lemierre s. thrombophlebitis of the internal jugular vein with secondary spread of infection, resulting from an acute oropharyngeal infection. Called also *postanginal sepsis.*
Lemieux-Neemeh s. an autosomal dominant syndrome consisting of Charcot-Marie-Tooth disease with progressive deafness.
Lennox s., Lennox-Gastaut s. an atypical form of absence epilepsy characterized by diffuse slow spike waves, often with atonic, tonic, or clonic seizures and mental retardation; there may also be other neurological abnormalities or multiple seizure types. Unlike typical absence epilepsy, it may persist into adulthood. Called also *petit mal variant.*
lentiginosis profusa s. LEOPARD syndrome.
Lenz s. a hereditary syndrome, transmitted as an X-linked trait, consisting of microphthalmia or anophthalmos, unilateral or bilateral, and digital anomalies; narrow shoulders, double thumbs, and other skeletal abnormalities; dental, urogenital, and cardiovascular defects may also occur.
LEOPARD s. an autosomal dominant syndrome consisting of multiple *l*entigines, asymptomatic *e*lectrocardiographic abnormalities, and often *o*cular hypertelorism, *p*ulmonary stenosis, *a*bnormal genitalia, growth *r*etardation, and sensorineural *d*eafness. Patients have characteristic coarse facies. Called also *lentiginosis profusa, lentiginosis profusa s.,* and *multiple lentigines s.*
Leredde s. severe dyspnea on exertion, combined with advanced emphysema and recurrent attacks of acute febrile bronchitis; seen in children with congenital syphilis.
Léri-Weill s. see under *dyschondrosteosis.*
Leriche s. a syndrome caused by obstruction of the terminal aorta, usually occurring in males and characterized by fatigue in the hips, thighs, or calves on exercising, absence of pulsation in the femoral arteries, and impotence, and often pallor and coldness of the lower extremities.
Lermoyez s. tinnitus and hearing loss preceding an attack of vertigo and then subsiding after the vertigo has become established. Cf. *Meniere disease.*
Lesch-Nyhan s. a rare X-linked disorder of purine metabolism due to deficient hypoxanthine phosphoribosyltransferase, characterized by physical and mental retardation, compulsive self-mutilation of the fingers and lips by biting, choreoathetosis, spastic cerebral palsy, impaired renal function; and by excessive purine synthesis and consequent hyperuricemia and uricaciduria.
lethal multiple pterygium s. a lethal autosomal recessive disorder caused by mutations in any of several genes that encode acetylcholine receptor components, characterized by multiple pterygia, lung hypoplasia, flexion contractures of the limbs, characteristic facies, and other abnormalities.
levator s., levator ani s. a functional pain syndrome occurring chiefly in women under 45 years of age and consisting of chronic or recurrent episodes of vague, dull aching or pressure high in the rectum that last at least 20 minutes; the pain is often worse when sitting. It is attributed to spasm of the levator muscles. The term is often used interchangeably with *proctalgia fugax* (q.v.). Called also *pelvic tension myalgia, levator spasm,* and *piriformis* or *puborectalis s.*
Levy-Hollister s. lacrimo-auriculo-dento-digital s.
Lévy-Roussy s. Roussy-Lévy s.
Lewis-Sumner s. an immune-mediated multifocal neuropathy characterized by conduction blocks of sensory and motor nerves in asymmetric locations in the body, usually one upper limb, with sensory deficits, weakness, and wasting.
Leyden-Möbius s. limb-girdle muscular dystrophy; see under *dystrophy.*
Li-Fraumeni s. an autosomal dominant cancer syndrome with early onset of tumors, multiple tumors in individuals, and multiple affected family members; the most common tumors include soft tissue sarcomas and osteosarcomas, breast cancer, brain tumors, leukemia, and adrenocortical carcinoma. Most cases are caused by mutation in the p53 tumor suppressor gene.
Lichtheim s. subacute combined degeneration of spinal cord; see under *degeneration.*
licking s. a form of pica in cattle in which they lick their own or each other's hair and skin, or other surfaces; it is often due to dietary deficiency of copper or sodium.
Liddle s. a rare autosomal dominant syndrome resulting from epithelial sodium channel mutations that lead to abnormally increased channel function, characterized by hypertension with excessive renal reabsorption of sodium, depletion of potassium, and low activity of renin and aldosterone. Cf. *pseudoprimary aldosteronism.*
Lightwood s. a transient, nonhereditary type of distal renal tubular acidosis seen in infant boys.
Lignac s., Lignac-Fanconi s. 1. Fanconi s. (def. 2). 2. cystinosis.
linear nevus sebaceus s., linear sebaceous nevus s. sebaceous nevus s.
lissencephaly s. Miller-Dieker s.
Lobstein s. osteogenesis imperfecta, type I.
locked-in s. quadriplegia and mutism with intact consciousness and the preservation of voluntary vertical eye movements and blinking; usually due to a vascular lesion of the pars ventralis pontis. Called also *coma vigil, de-efferented state,* and *pseudocoma.* Cf. *akinetic mutism.*
loculation s. Froin s.
Löffler s. transient infiltrations and eosinophilia of the lungs, accompanied by cough, fever, and dyspnea; it may be idiopathic or due to infestation by parasites (particularly *Ascaris lumbricoides*), infection, or drug therapy. See also *Ascaris pneumonitis,* under *pneumonitis.* Called also *Löffler eosinophilia* or *pneumonia* and *simple pulmonary eosinophilia.*
Löfgren s. erythema nodosum in conjunction with bilateral adenopathy of hilar lymph nodes, seen as a manifestation of sarcoidosis.
loin pain–hematuria s. a syndrome of intense loin pain, either unilateral or bilateral, lasting from a few days to weeks, followed by hematuria, usually seen in young women; the etiology is unknown, but some cases have been linked to treatment with estrogen compounds.
long QT s. prolongation of the Q–T interval combined with torsades de pointes, one of the most common types of ion channelopathy. Acquired forms are usually due to a metabolic or cardiac abnormality or to drug administration. Congenital forms result from a variety of mutations in genes coding for channel subunits and are usually noted early in life. The condition may lead to serious arrhythmia and sudden cardiac death (sudden arrhythmia death syndrome).
loose anagen hair s. a syndrome of unknown etiology, usually seen in children, in which scalp hair can be plucked easily and painlessly during the anagen part of the hair cycle, owing to defective anchorage of the hair shaft to the follicle; there is also slowing of hair growth.
Looser-Milkman s. Milkman s.
Lorain-Lévi s. pituitary dwarfism.
Louis-Bar s. ataxia-telangiectasia.
low cardiac output s. the clinical manifestations of low-output heart failure (see under *failure*). Called also *low output s.*
Lowe s., Lowe-Terrey-MacLachlan s. oculocerebrorenal s.
lower radicular s. Klumpke paralysis.
Lown-Ganong-Levine s. a preexcitation syndrome of electrocardiographic abnormality characterized by a short P–R interval with a normal QRS complex, accompanied by atrial tachycardia.
low output s. low cardiac output s.
low T_3 s. euthyroid sick s.
Lucey-Driscoll s. a syndrome of retention jaundice due to defective bilirubin conjugation, occurring in infants; apparently the result of an unidentified factor, presumably a steroid in maternal blood, transmitted to the infant.
lupus-like s. see *systemic lupus erythematosus,* under *lupus.*
Lutembacher s. atrial septal defect associated with mitral stenosis. Called also *Lutembacher complex.*
Lyell s. toxic epidermal necrolysis.
lymphadenopathy s. a condition seen in immunocompromised persons, characterized by unexplained lymphadenopathy of extrainguinal sites that lasts for three or more months and on biopsy reveals nonspecific lymphoid hyperplasia; in some patients it may be a prodrome of acquired immunodeficiency syndrome.

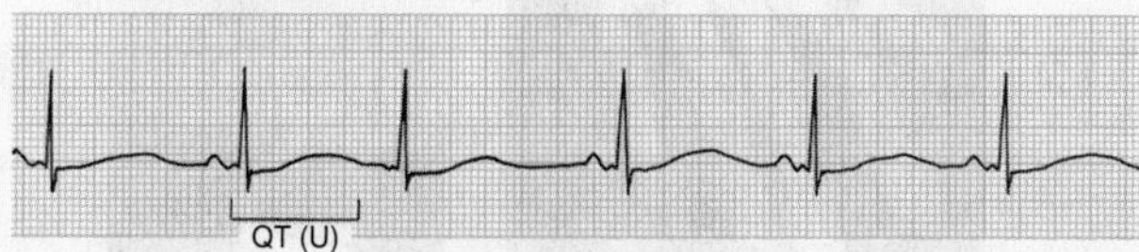

■ Quinidine-induced long QT syndrome. Patient on quinidine (monitor lead) developed marked prolongation of repolarization with low amplitude T–U waves. Cardiac arrest with torsades de pointes ventricular tachycardia later developed.

Syndrome *Continued*

lymphoproliferative s's see under *disorder.*
lymphoreticular s's see under *disorder.*
Lynch s. hereditary nonpolyposis colorectal cancer.
McCune-Albright s. Albright s.
Mackenzie s. Jackson s.
McKusick-Kaufman s. Kaufman-McKusick s.
McLeod s. a syndrome seen in some individuals having the McLeod phenotype of blood, characterized by mild hemolytic anemia with acanthocytes, elevated serum creatinine phosphokinase, and sometimes muscle wasting and neurological defects. A few cases have manifested as X-linked types of chronic granulomatous disease.
Macleod s. Swyer-James s.
macrophage activation s. hemophagocytic lymphohistiocytosis.
Maffucci s. enchondromatosis associated with multiple cutaneous or visceral hemangiomas. Called also *Kast s.*
magenblase s. excessive gas in the stomach, owing to habitual taking in of air with the food.
MAGIC s. an inflammatory syndrome of mouth and genital ulcers with inflamed cartilage; a term encompassing overlapping features of Behçet syndrome and relapsing polychondritis.
malabsorption s. any of a group of disorders characterized by subnormal absorption of dietary constituents, and thus excessive loss of nonabsorbed substances in the feces; the malabsorption may be due to an intraluminal (digestive) defect (e.g., pancreatic insufficiency), a mucosal abnormality (celiac disease or disaccharidase deficiency), or a lymphatic obstruction (intestinal lymphangiectasia). Unless there is a specific enzyme or transport defect, steatorrhea is usually present. Deficiency syndromes may result from excessive loss of vitamins, electrolytes, iron, calcium, or other substances.
malarial hyperreactive spleen s. tropical splenomegaly s.
Mallory-Weiss s. hematemesis or melena that follows typically upon many hours or days of severe vomiting and retching, traceable to one or several slitlike lacerations of the gastric mucosa, longitudinally placed at or slightly below the esophagogastric junction.
manic s. mania.
man-in-the-barrel s. brachial diplegia of proximal areas of the upper limbs, usually owing to an infarction in the blood supply to the area, giving the appearance of having the arms and trunk constrained by a barrel; it often begins with weakness and numbness and can progress to become life threatening.
Marchesani s. Weill-Marchesani s.
Marchiafava-Micheli s. paroxysmal nocturnal hemoglobinuria.
Marcus Gunn s. Gunn s.
Marfan s. one of the manifestations of abnormal fibrillin metabolism, a congenital disorder of connective tissue characterized by abnormal length of extremities, especially fingers and toes, subluxation of the lens, cardiovascular abnormalities (commonly dilatation of the ascending aorta), and other deformities. It is an autosomal dominant disorder with variable degrees of expression, caused by mutations in the *FBN1* gene, which encodes fibrillin-1.
Marie-Bamberger s. hypertrophic pulmonary osteoarthropathy.
Marinesco-Sjögren s. a hereditary syndrome transmitted as an autosomal recessive trait, consisting of cerebellar ataxia, mental and somatic growth retardation, congenital cataracts, inability to chew, thin brittle fingernails, and sparse, incompletely keratinized hair.

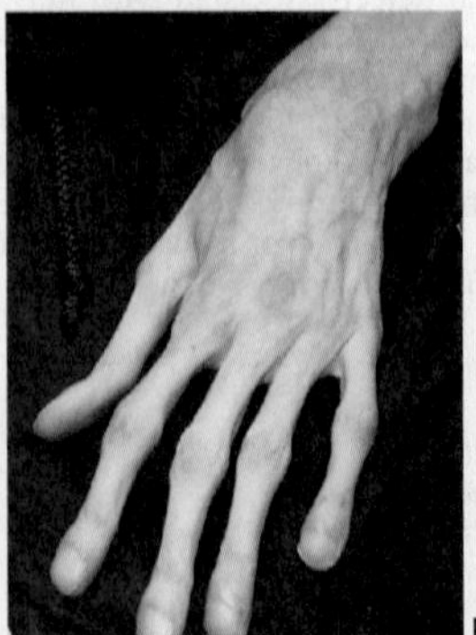

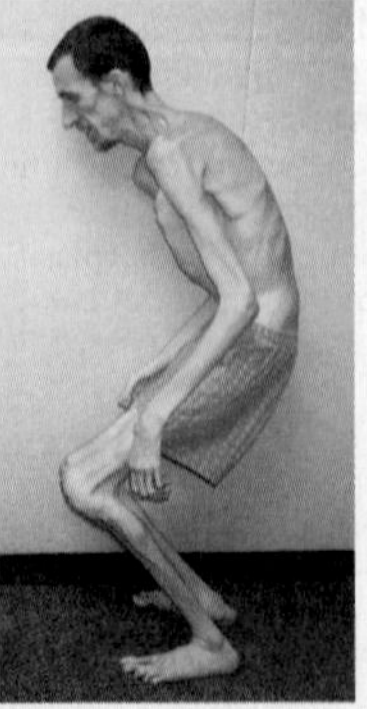

■ Marfan syndrome in a young man. *(A)*, Long, thin fingers, with clubbing due to associated cardiopulmonary problems; *(B)*, pectus carinatum, kyphosis, and joint contractures.

Maroteaux-Lamy s. a mucopolysaccharidosis caused by deficiency of *N*-acetylgalactosamine-4-sulfatase (arylsulfatase B), and characterized biochemically by the predominance of dermatan sulfate in the urine and the presence of coarse metachromatic granules in the leukocytes, and clinically by Hurler-like signs with normal intelligence. There are three clinical forms: the severe or classic form shows Hurler-like symptoms; the intermediate form has the same phenotype as mucolipidosis III (pseudo-Hurler polydystrophy); the mild form is difficult to distinguish from the Scheie syndrome. Called also *mucopolysaccharidosis VI* and *arylsulfatase B (ARSB) deficiency.*
marrara s. halzoun.
Marshall s. a rare, autosomal dominant syndrome characterized by ectodermal dysplasia, hypertelorism, myopia progressing to retinal detachment and blindness, and degenerative changes in the joints; sensorineural deafness may also occur. It resembles hereditary progressive arthro-ophthalmopathy, but has been found to be caused by a different genetic defect.
Martin-Bell s. fragile X s.
Martorell s. Takayasu arteritis.
mastocytosis s. an episodic syndrome occurring in certain patients with systemic mastocytosis, usually those with skin lesions, bone lesions, and hepatosplenomegaly, presumably associated with histamine release from degranulation of mast cells, and characterized mainly by intense pruritus, flushing, headache, tachycardia, hypotension, and syncope.
maternal deprivation s. failure to thrive with severe growth retardation (deprivation dwarfism), unresponsiveness to the environment, depression, retarded mental and emotional development, and behavioral problems resulting from loss of, absence of, or neglect by the mother or other primary caregiver.
Mauriac s. dwarfism, hepatomegaly, obesity, and retarded sexual maturation, in association with diabetes mellitus.
May-Thurner s. deep vein thrombosis of the left lower limb resulting from compression of the left common iliac vein between the right common iliac artery and the fifth lumbar vertebra, characterized by severe pain and swelling of the limb and venous claudication.
May-White s. a rare autosomal dominant syndrome of myoclonus, cerebellar ataxia, and deafness.
Mayer-Rokitansky-Küster-Hauser s. lack of müllerian development, congenital absence of the vagina, and a rudimentary uterus (typically bicornuate remnants), with normal uterine tubes, ovaries, and secondary female sex characteristics and normal growth. Called also *Rokitansky-Küster-Hauser s.*
Mazabraud s. a syndrome of fibrous dysplasia associated with soft tissue myxomas.
Meckel s., Meckel-Gruber s. a hereditary syndrome, transmitted as an autosomal recessive trait, usually characterized by sloping forehead, posterior meningoencephalocele, polydactyly, and polycystic kidneys, with death occurring in the perinatal period. Called also *Gruber s.* and *dysencephalia splanchnocystica.*
meconium aspiration s. the respiratory complications resulting from the passage and aspiration of meconium prior to or during delivery. Postterm infants and those who had hypoxia or acidosis in utero are at higher risk.
meconium plug s. intestinal obstruction in an infant due to unusually thick or hard meconium in which neither enzymatic nor ganglion cell deficiency can be demonstrated, most often seen in premature infants.
median arcuate ligament s. celiac artery compression syndrome.
median cleft facial s. a hereditary form of defective midline development of the head and face, including ocular hypertelorism, occult cleft nose and maxilla, and sometimes mental retardation or other defects. Called also *frontonasal dysplasia.*
megacystis-megaureter s. chronic ureteral dilatation (megaureter) associated with hypotonia and dilatation of the bladder (megacystis) and gaping of ureteral orifices, permitting vesicoureteral reflux of urine, and resulting in chronic pyelonephritis. Called also *megaureter-megacystis s.*
megacystis-microcolon–intestinal hypoperistalsis s. (MMIHS) a congenital syndrome with a female preponderance, usually autosomal recessive and fatal in the first year of life, consisting of an enlarged bladder (megacystis) and small colon with decreased or absent peristalsis (microcolon and intestinal hypoperistalsis); patients also have the

abdominal muscle defect seen in the prune-belly syndrome. Called also *Berdon s.* and *MMIH s.*

megaureter-megacystis s. megacystis-megaureter s.

Meige s. focal dystonia of facial and oromandibular muscles with blepharospasm, grimacing mouth movements, and protrusion of the tongue, usually occurring in older women. Called also *Brueghel s.*

Meigs s., Meigs-Salmon s. ascites and hydrothorax associated with ovarian fibroma or other pelvic tumor.

MELAS s. *m*itochondrial *e*ncephalopathy, *l*actic *a*cidosis, and *s*troke-like episodes; a familial syndrome, of maternal (mitochondrial) inheritance.

Melkersson s., Melkersson-Rosenthal s. an autosomal dominant condition usually beginning in childhood or adolescence, characterized chiefly by chronic noninflammatory facial swelling, usually confined to the lips in the form of *granulomatous cheilitis*, with recurrent facial palsy and sometimes fissured tongue. Associated ophthalmic symptoms may include lagophthalmos, blepharochalasis, swollen eyelids, burning sensation of the eyes, corneal opacities, retrobulbar neuritis, and exophthalmos.

Melnick-Fraser s. branchio-oto-renal s.

Melnick-Needles s. a rare X-linked disorder (gene locus: Xq28), caused by mutations in the gene encoding filamin A. It is characterized by severe congenital bone abnormalities manifested by distinctive facies (exophthalmos, full cheeks, micrognathia, and malalignment of the teeth), flaring of the metaphyses of long bones, S-like curvature of the bones of the lower limbs, irregular constrictions in the ribs, and sclerosis of the base of the skull. It is lethal in males, resulting in death in utero or during the first few months of life, but not in females. Called also *Melnick-Needles osteodysplasty.*

Mendelson s. pulmonary acid aspiration s.

Mendes da Costa s. erythrokeratodermia variabilis.

MERRF s. [*m*yoclonic *e*pilepsy with *r*agged *r*ed *f*ibers] a familial type of mitochondrial encephalopathy of maternal (mitochondrial) inheritance, characterized by myoclonic epilepsy and mitochondrial myopathy with ragged red fibers, and also by abnormal brainstem evoked responses, sensorineural hearing loss, ataxia, renal dysfunction, diabetes, cardiomyopathy, and dementia. It is usually caused by mutation within the mitochondrial gene encoding the tRNA specific for lysine. Called also *Fukuhara s.*

metabolic s., metabolic s. X a combination including at least three of the following: abdominal obesity, hypertriglyceridemia, low level of high-density lipoproteins, hypertension, and high fasting plasma glucose level. It is associated with an increased risk for development of diabetes mellitus and cardiovascular disease. Called also *s. X.*

metameric s. segmentary s.

methionine malabsorption s. an autosomal recessive disorder of methionine absorption in which the urine has a characteristic odor resembling that of the interior of an oasthouse (room where tobacco, hops, and malt are dried). It is due to alpha-hydroxybutyric acid formed by bacterial action on the unabsorbed methionine. Characteristics include white hair, mental retardation, convulsions, and attacks of hyperpnea. Called also *oasthouse urine disease* and *Smith-Strang disease.*

Meyer-Schwickerath and Weyers s. oculodentodigital dysplasia.

Michelin tire s., Michelin tire baby s. a rare, autosomal dominant syndrome characterized by deep creases in the skin, particularly around the limbs, resembling those between the treads on a tire; it is usually most pronounced in infants.

MIDAS s. MLS s.

middle lobe s. lobar atelectasis in the right middle lobe of the lung, with chronic pneumonitis; called also *Brock s.*

midsystolic click–late systolic murmur s. mitral valve prolapse s.

Mikulicz s. a chronic bilateral hypertrophy of the lacrimal, parotid, and salivary glands, associated with decreased or absent lacrimation and xerostomia, and often accompanied by chronic lymphocytic infiltration. It may be associated with other diseases, such as Sjögren syndrome, sarcoidosis, lupus erythematosus, leukemia, lymphoma, and tuberculosis. See also *benign lymphoepithelial lesion*, under *lesion.*

mild androgen insensitivity s. (MAIS) the least severe form of androgen insensitivity syndrome; affected males have normal male genitalia but may be infertile. Some develop gynecomastia and are at risk for breast cancer. Called also *minimal androgen insensitivity s.*

milk-alkali s. a syndrome characterized by hypercalcemia without hypercalciuria or hypophosphatemia, with only mild alkalosis, normal serum phosphatase, severe renal insufficiency with hyperazotemia, and calcinosis, attributed to ingestion of milk and absorbable alkali for long periods of time. Called also *Burnett* or *hypercalcemia s.*

Milkman s. a generalized bone disease marked by multiple transparent stripes of absorption in the long and flat bones; called also *Looser-Milkman s.*

Millard-Gubler s. crossed paralysis, affecting the limbs on one side of the body and the face on the opposite side, together with paralysis of outward movement of the eye; it is due to infarction of the pons, involving the sixth and seventh cranial nerves and the fibers of the corticospinal tract. Called also *Gubler hemiplegia* or *paralysis* and *Millard-Gubler paralysis.* Cf. *Foville s.*

Miller s. a syndrome of extensive facial and limb defects, characterized by malar hypoplasia, downslanting palpebral fissures, micrognathia, cleft lip and palate, cup-shaped ears, lower lid ectropion, postaxial limb deficiencies, and syndactyly. Less frequently present are heart defects and hearing loss. The syndrome is probably an autosomal recessive trait. Called also *postaxial acrofacial dysostosis.*

Miller-Dieker s. an autosomal recessive syndrome characterized by lissencephaly, microcephaly, mental retardation, dysmorphic facial appearance, and sometimes polydactyly, cryptorchidism, heart lesions, kidney defects, and defects of the gastrointestinal system. It is caused by hemizygous deletion of chromosome locus 17p13.3. Called also *lissencephaly s.*

Miller Fisher s. 1. Fisher s. (def. 1). 2. one-and-a-half s.

Milwaukee shoulder s. a type of crystal-induced arthropathy seen most often in older women, characterized by calcium phosphate crystals around the shoulder joint, often bilaterally, with pain that may be worse at night. Called also *apatite-associated destructive arthritis.*

minimal androgen insensitivity s. (MAIS) mild androgen insensitivity s.

minimal change nephrotic s. minimal change disease.

Minkowski-Chauffard s. hereditary spherocytosis.

Minot-von Willebrand s. von Willebrand disease.

Mirizzi s. a rare syndrome of extrahepatic obstruction of the common bile duct owing to impaction of a gallstone in the cystic duct; symptoms include recurring pain, fever, and jaundice.

mitral valve prolapse s. prolapse of the mitral valve, often with regurgitation, associated with myxomatous proliferation of the leaflets of the mitral valve, a common, usually benign, often asymptomatic condition characterized by midsystolic clicks and late systolic murmurs on auscultation. Palpitations and chest discomfort may occur, and in some cases progressive mitral regurgitation necessitates valve replacement. Called also *Barlow s., click-murmur s., floppy valve s., MVP s.,* and *systolic click–murmur s.*

MLS s. [*m*icrophthalmia, *l*inear *s*kin defects] a rare X-linked syndrome of linear defects on the face and neck with microphthalmia and sometimes brain defects such as agenesis of the corpus callosum and mental retardation. Most patients are female because it is lethal for male fetuses. Called also *MIDAS s.*

MMIH s. megacystis-microcolon–intestinal hypoperistalsis s.

Möbius s. agenesis or aplasia of the motor nuclei of the cranial nerves characterized by congenital bilateral facial palsy in various combinations, with unilateral or bilateral paralysis of the abductors of the eye, sometimes associated with involvement of the cranial nerves, particularly the oculomotor, trigeminal, and hypoglossal, and anomalies of the extremities. Called also *nuclear agenesis* or *aplasia, congenital facial diplegia, congenital abducens-facial paralysis,* and *congenital oculofacial paralysis.*

Mohr s. an autosomal recessive disorder characterized by brachydactyly, clinodactyly, polydactyly, syndactyly, and bilateral hallucal polysyndactyly; by cranial, facial, lingual, palatal, and mandibular anomalies; and by episodic neuromuscular disturbances. Called also *orodigitofacial dysostosis, oral-facial-digital s., type II,* and *orofaciodigital s., type II.* See also *oral-facial-digital s., type I.*

Monakow s. hemiplegia on the side opposite the lesion in occlusion of the anterior choroidal artery, sometimes with hemianesthesia and hemianopia.

monosomy 9p⁻ s. a rare chromosomal disorder in which a piece of the short arm of the ninth chromosome is broken and often lost. Symptoms include mental retardation, a triangular head with forward angulation of the frontal bone, and various other physical deformities.

Moore s. abdominal epilepsy.

Morel s. hyperostosis frontalis interna.

Morgagni-Adams-Stokes s. Adams-Stokes s.
morning glory s. a coloboma in which there is a funnel-shaped optic nerve head with a dot of whitish, fluffy material in the center, an elevated ring of pigment around the disk, and vessels radiating from the ring like spokes. Vision is severely affected.
Morquio s. either of two biochemically distinct, but clinically nearly indistinguishable, forms of mucopolysaccharidosis characterized by excretion of keratan sulfate in the urine. Clinical features, affecting primarily the skeletal and secondarily the nervous system, include genu valgum, pectus carinatum, progressive platyspondyly, short neck and trunk, normal but broad-mouthed facies with spacing between the teeth, progressive deafness, and very mild corneal clouding. Intelligence is normal. The two enzymatic types are *type A,* caused by N-acetylgalactosamine-6-sulfatase deficiency; and *type B,* caused by β-galactosidase deficiency. Called also *mucopolysaccharidosis IV.*
Morris s. complete androgen insensitivity s.
Morton s. a congenital insufficiency of the first metatarsal segment of the foot, characterized by metatarsalgia due to shortening or relaxation of the part.
Morvan s. 1. syringomyelia. 2. a manifestation of syringomyelia in which the subcutaneous tissues of the hands become thickened, edematous, soft, swollen, cyanotic, and cold (see *Marinesco succulent hand,* under *hand*), associated with analgesic ulceration of the fingertips and paresthesia and atrophy of the hands and forearms.
Mosse s. polycythemia vera with cirrhosis of the liver.
Mounier-Kuhn s. tracheobronchomegaly.
Mount s., Mount-Reback s. a rare autosomal dominant disorder characterized by paroxysmal attacks of choreoathetosis and dystonic movements with Kayser-Fleischer rings on the corneas. It appears in childhood or young adulthood and does not involve a change in consciousness. Called also *paroxysmal* or *familial paroxysmal choreoathetosis.* See also *paroxysmal kinesigenic choreoathetosis.*
Mowat-Wilson s. an autosomal dominant complex developmental disorder caused by a microdeletion or mutation in the long arm of chromosome 2 (2q22). It is characterized by a typical facies; mental retardation; delayed motor development; epilepsy; and multiple congenital anomalies, including agenesis of the corpus callosum and genital, cardiac, and eye defects. Hirschsprung disease is often present.
Moynahan s. 1. multiple symmetric lentigines, congenital mitral valve stenosis, dwarfism, genital hypoplasia, and mental retardation. Called also *progressive cardiomyopathic lentiginosis.* 2. a familial congenital syndrome consisting of delayed hair growth on the scalp, epilepsy, mental retardation, and unusual electroencephalogram.
Muckle-Wells s. an autosomal dominant autoinflammatory disease in the cryopyrin-associated periodic syndromes subgroup, characterized by amyloidosis involving the kidneys and causing nephritis, recurrent urticaria, deafness, and pain in the extremities.
mucocutaneous lymph node s. (MLNS) Kawasaki disease.
mucosal neuroma s. multiple endocrine neoplasia, type 2B.
Muir-Torre s. Torre s.
multiple endocrine deficiency s., multiple glandular deficiency s. primary failure of any combination of endocrine glands, including adrenals, thyroid, gonads, parathyroids, and endocrine pancreas, often accompanied by nonendocrine autoimmune abnormalities.
multiple hamartoma s. Cowden disease.
multiple lentigines s. LEOPARD s.
multiple pterygium s. 1. an autosomal recessive syndrome caused by mutations in the *CHRNG* gene (locus: 2q33-q34), which encodes an acetylcholine receptor subunit. It is characterized by pterygia of the neck, axillae, and popliteal, antecubital, and intercrural areas, accompanied by hypertelorism, cleft palate, micrognathia, ptosis of eyelids, and short stature. Skeletal abnormalities include camptodactyly, syndactyly, equinovarus, and rocker-bottom feet, as well as vertebral fusion and rib anomalies. Cryptorchidism is present in males and labia majora are absent in females. Called also *Escobar s.* and *pterygium s.* Cf. *lethal multiple pterygium s.* 2. an autosomal dominant syndrome that in its most severe forms resembles the recessive disorder; milder cases may present with contractures of the extremities and ptosis. Called also *distal arthrogryposis type 8.*
Munchausen s. a condition characterized by habitual presentation for hospital treatment of an apparent acute physical illness, the patient giving a plausible and dramatic history, all of which is false; it is a subtype of factitious disorder (q.v.).
Munchausen s. by proxy see *factitious disorder by proxy,* under *disorder.*
MVP s. mitral valve prolapse s.
myasthenic s. Lambert-Eaton myasthenic s.
myelodysplastic s. any of a group of related bone marrow disorders of varying duration preceding the development of overt acute myelogenous leukemia; they are characterized by abnormal hematopoietic stem cells, anemia, neutropenia, and thrombocytopenia. Splenomegaly, hepatomegaly, and lymphadenopathy may not occur until the onset of leukemia, which is sometimes sudden and fulminating. Called also *preleukemia.*
myelofibrosis-osteosclerosis s. agnogenic myeloid metaplasia.
myeloproliferative s's see under *disorder.*
myonephropathic s. myoglobinuria, hemodynamic instability, lactic acidosis, and hyperkalemia that occur during reperfusion of the lower limb, caused by release of the products of muscle breakdown.
Naegeli s. former name for *Franceschetti-Jadassohn s.*
Naffziger s. scalenus s.
Nager s., Nager-de Reynier s. Nager acrofacial dysostosis.
nail-patella s. a hereditary, autosomal dominant syndrome consisting of dystrophy of the nails, absence or hypoplasia of the patella, hypoplasia of the lateral side of the elbow joint, bilateral iliac horns, and often thickening of the lamina densa of the renal glomeruli. Called also *hereditary osteo-onychodysplasia.*
NAME s. a syndrome of familial myxomas with cutaneous, cardiac, and endocrine involvement, manifested as *n*evi, *a*trial *m*yxoma, and neurofibroma *e*phelides. Cf. *LAMB s.*
narcotic bowel s. a group of intestinal symptoms seen in persons who use narcotic analgesics over a long period, including intestinal pseudoobstruction, abdominal pain, vomiting, and weight loss.
neck-tongue s. pain in the neck, sometimes followed by numbness of the neck and tongue, on sudden turning of the head; it is thought to be due to compression of C2 nerve roots in the area of the atlantoaxial articulations because the C2 roots contain proprioceptive fibers from the tongue.
Negri-Jacod s. Jacod s.
Nelson s. the development of an ACTH-producing pituitary tumor after bilateral adrenalectomy for Cushing syndrome; it is characterized by aggressive growth of the tumor and hyperpigmentation of the skin.
neonatal abstinence s. signs of substance withdrawal, including tremor, sweating, yawning, poor feeding, sleep disturbance, and high-pitched cry, occurring in newborns exposed in utero to drugs taken by the mother.
neonatal maladjustment s. a disease of newborn foals, caused by perinatal hypoxia and characterized by behavioral disturbances such as inability to nurse, aimless wandering, apparent blindness, and uttering of a barklike sound; it may progress to convulsions, coma, and death. Affected foals are called *barkers, dummies,* or *wanderers.*
neonatal respiratory distress s. dyspnea with cyanosis in the newborn, a condition caused by deficiency of surfactant. Prodromal signs include dilatation of the alae nasi, expiratory grunt, and retraction of the suprasternal notch or costal margins. It is usually seen in infants who are premature, have diabetic mothers, or were delivered by cesarean section; sometimes there is no known cause. Some infants die of respiratory failure in the first few days of life and at autopsy have eosinophilic hyaline material lining the alveoli, alveolar ducts, and bronchioles. Called also *respiratory distress s. of newborn* and *idiopathic respiratory distress of newborn.*
nephrogenic s. of inappropriate antidiuresis (NSIAD) a hyponatremic syndrome, clinically resembling the syndrome of inappropriate diuretic hormone, caused by inability of the renal collecting tubules to absorb water in response to antidiuretic hormone. *Type I,* which accounts for 90 percent of cases, is an X-linked syndrome caused by loss of vasopressin receptor function as a result of mutations in the gene encoding the receptors (locus: Xq28). *Type II* is caused by a mutation in the gene encoding aquaporin-2 (locus: 12q13); inheritance may be autosomal dominant or recessive.
nephrotic s. general name for any of a large group of diseases involving defective renal glomeruli, characterized by massive proteinuria and lipiduria with varying degrees of edema, hypoalbuminemia, and hyperlipidemia. See also *glomerulonephropathy.*
nerve compression s. entrapment neuropathy.
Netherton s. a rare syndrome, believed to be autosomal recessive, consisting of lamellar ichthyosis or ichthyosis linearis circumflexa,

trichorrhexis invaginata, atopy, and sometimes mental retardation and aminoaciduria.

Nettleship-Falls s. see under *albinism.*

neurocutaneous s. phakomatosis.

neuroleptic malignant s. a rare, sometimes fatal reaction to antipsychotic (neuroleptic) agents, characterized by hyperthermia, rigidity, and coma.

nevoid basal cell carcinoma s., nevoid basalioma s. an autosomal dominant syndrome characterized by the development in early life of numerous basal cell carcinomas, associated with abnormalities of the skin (especially an unusual erythematous pitting edema of the hands and feet), bones, nervous system, eyes, and reproductive tract. Called also *basal cell nevus s., Gorlin s.,* and *Gorlin-Goltz s.*

nevus sebaceus s. sebaceous nevus s.

Nezelof s. any of a heterogeneous group of immunodeficiency disorders characterized by profoundly deficient cellular immunity and varying degrees of humoral immunodeficiency. Immunoglobulin levels may be normal or increased, but antibody response to immunization may be absent. Patients are highly susceptible to life-threatening infections with low-grade or opportunistic pathogens, such as *Candida albicans, Pneumocystis jiroveci,* and cytomegalovirus. Both autosomal recessive and X-linked inheritance have been described. Called also *cellular immunodeficiency with immunoglobulins.*

Nicolau s. a severe cutaneous reaction after intramuscular administration of medications, often in the gluteal region, because of ischemia from accidental arterial obliteration or vasculitis. Manifestations include severe local pain, swelling, livedoid changes, and increased skin temperature; there may also be fever, tachycardia, dyspnea, albuminuria, and eventually gangrene. Called also *livedoid dermatitis* and *embolia cutis medicamentosa.*

Noack s. Pfeiffer s.

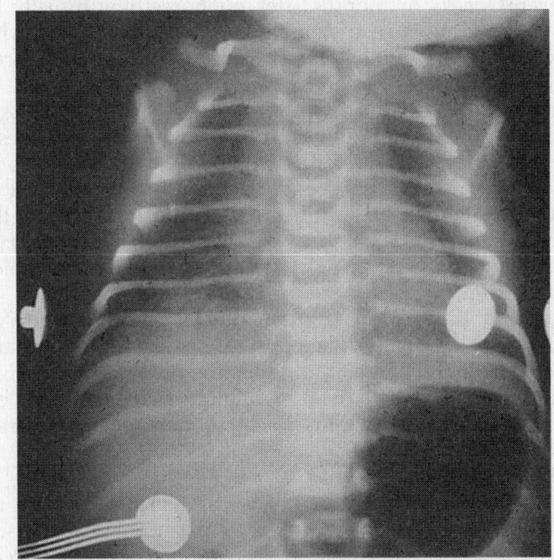

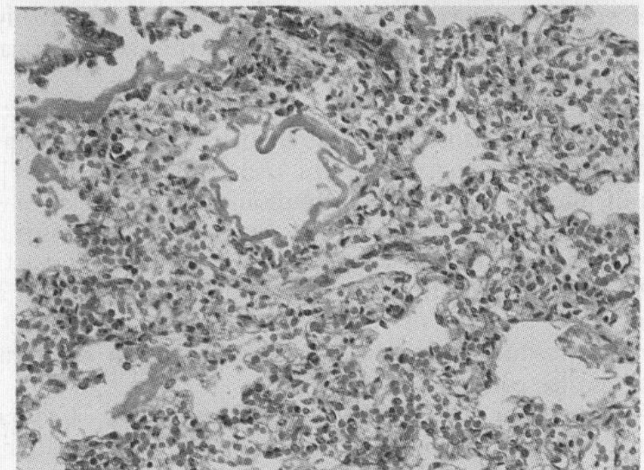

■ Neonatal respiratory distress syndrome. *(A),* Ground-glass appearance and air bronchograms. *(B),* Alveoli are collapsed and the alveolar ducts and respiratory bronchioles are dilated and lined by hyaline membrane.

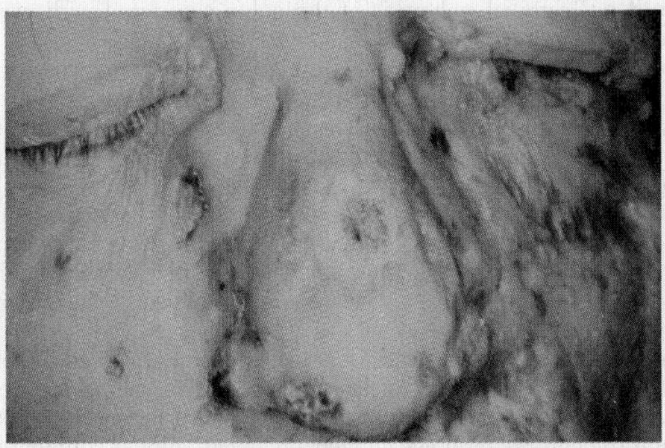

■ Nevoid basal cell carcinoma syndrome.

noninsulinoma pancreatogenous hypoglycemia s. (NIPHS) a rare syndrome of endogenous hyperinsulinemia and hypoglycemia in the postprandial period, resembling symptoms of an insulinoma; some patients develop this following a Roux-en-Y bypass.

Nonne-Milroy-Meige s. a name formerly given to hereditary lymphedema, now considered to be two disorders, Milroy disease and lymphedema praecox.

nonsense s. Ganser s.

nonstaphylococcal scalded skin s. toxic epidermal necrolysis.

Noonan s. the phenotype of Turner syndrome (webbed neck, ptosis, hypogonadism, congenital heart disease, and short stature) without gonadal dysgenesis; formerly called *male Turner syndrome* until the female counterpart was identified. Called also *Ullrich-Turner s.*

Nothnagel s. unilateral oculomotor paralysis combined with cerebellar ataxia, in lesions of the cerebral peduncles.

numb chin s. paresthesias or loss of sensation in the lower face and chin, owing to compression of the mental nerve, usually by a tumor.

nutcracker s. see under *phenomenon.*

Nyssen-van Bogaert s. the adult form of metachromatic leukodystrophy.

obesity-hypoventilation s. a complex of obesity, somnolence, hypoventilation, and erythrocytosis; called also *pickwickian s.*

obstructive sleep apnea s. (OSAS) see under *apnea.*

obstructive sleep apnea–hypopnea s. (OSAHS) obstructive sleep apnea and related hypopneas considered as one syndrome.

occipital horn s. a mild allelic variant of Menkes disease, characterized by hyperelastic and bruisable skin, hernias, bladder diverticula and dysfunction, hyperextensible joints, varicosities, multiple skeletal abnormalities, and relatively normal intelligence. Characteristic exostoses, resulting from calcification, occur at the sites of muscular attachment to the occipital skull. Called also *X-linked cutis laxa.*

Ochoa s. urofacial s.

oculocerebral-hypopigmentation s. Cross s.

oculocerebrorenal s. an X-linked disorder characterized by vitamin D–refractory rickets, hydrophthalmia, congenital glaucoma and cataracts, mental retardation, and tubule reabsorption dysfunction as evidenced by hypophosphatemia, acidosis, and aminoaciduria. Called also *Lowe disease* and *Lowe-Terrey-MacLachlan s.*

oculodentodigital s., oculodento-osseous s. see under *dysplasia.*

oculoglandular s. Parinaud oculoglandular s.

oculomandibulodyscephaly-hypotrichosis s. oculomandibulofacial s.

oculomandibulofacial s. a syndrome principally characterized by dyscephaly (usually brachycephaly), parrot nose, mandibular hypoplasia, proportionate nanism, hypotrichosis, bilateral congenital cataracts, and microphthalmia. Called also *mandibulo-oculofacial dyscephaly* and *Hallermann-Streiff, Hallermann-Streiff-François,* or *François s.*

oculo-oto-radial s. IVIC s.

oculopharyngeal s. see under *dystrophy.*

ODD s. oculodentodigital dysplasia.

OFD s. oral-facial-digital s.

Ogilvie s. distention of the colon resembling that caused by obstruction, but without evidence of mechanical obstruction; it is usually due to a defect in the sympathetic nerve supply. Called also *false colonic obstruction.*

Oldfield s. familial polyposis of the colon associated with extensive sebaceous cysts.
Olmsted s. a rare syndrome of unknown etiology in which infants develop keratoderma on the palms and soles as they begin to use their hands and feet; this increases in severity to cause contractures and sometimes fissuring of the skin. Many also have plaques of keratoderma around body orifices.
Omenn s. an autosomal recessive but genetically heterogeneous disorder combining immunodeficiency with inflammation; it is characterized by failure to thrive, pneumonitis, and chronic diarrhea beginning early in infancy as well as a variety of autoimmune and allergic inflammatory responses.
one-and-a-half s. a disorder of ocular movement caused by a brainstem lesion of one abducens nucleus and the nearby medial longitudinal fasciculus; the ipsilateral eye cannot move beyond the midline horizontally and the contralateral eye abducts on any attempt at conjugate gaze. Called also *Fisher s.* and *Miller Fisher s.*
Opitz s., Opitz-Frias s. an autosomal dominant syndrome consisting of hypertelorism and hernias, and in males hypospadias, cryptorchidism, and bifid scrotum. Cardiac anomalies, laryngotracheal malformations, imperforate anus, renal defects, lung hypoplasia, and downslanted palpebral fissures may also be present. Called also *G s.* and *hypertelorism-hypospadias s.*
opsoclonus-myoclonus s. a syndrome of movements of the eyes (opsoclonus) and trunk (myoclonus), occurring in conjunction with a number of conditions, including viral infections, trauma, drug toxicity, tumors, and hyperosmolar nonketotic coma. It also occurs as a paraneoplastic syndrome; in some cases of small cell lung carcinoma or breast or fallopian tube cancer, it is associated with an autoantibody (anti-Ri).
oral-facial-digital s., type I a male-lethal X-linked dominant disorder characterized by camptodactyly, polydactyly, and syndactyly; by cranial, facial, lingual, and dental anomalies; and by mental retardation, familial trembling, alopecia, and seborrhea of the face and milia. Called also *orodigitofacial dysostosis* and *orofaciodigital s., type I.* See also *Mohr s.*
oral-facial-digital s., type II Mohr s.
oral-facial-digital s., type III an autosomal recessive disorder characterized by postaxial hexadactyly of the hands and feet, by ocular, lingual, and dental anomalies, and by profound mental retardation. Called also *orodigitofacial dysostosis* and *orofaciodigital s., type III.*
orbital apex s. ophthalmoplegia with impairment of vision that may lead to blindness, swelling of the eyelids, ptosis, hyper- or hypoesthesia of the upper eyelid, one half of the forehead, and cornea, and vasomotor disturbances; it is caused by traumatic, inflammatory, or neoplastic processes involving the sphenoidal fissure and optic canal or the structures they contain.
orbital floor s. exophthalmos, diplopia, and anesthesia in the areas innervated by the trigeminal nerve, occurring with a lesion in the floor of the orbit. Called also *Dejean s.*
organic anxiety s. a term used in a former system of classification, denoting an organic mental syndrome characterized by prominent, recurrent panic attacks or generalized anxiety caused by a specific organic factor and not associated with delirium. Such disorders are now mainly classified as *substance-induced anxiety disorders* and *anxiety disorders due to a general medical condition.*
organic brain s. organic mental s.
organic delusional s. a term used in a former system of classification, denoting an organic mental syndrome characterized by the presence of delusions caused by a specific organic factor and not associated with delirium. Such disorders are now mainly classified as *substance-induced psychotic disorders* and *psychotic disorders due to a general medical condition.*
organic dust toxic s. pneumonitis, usually hypersensitivity pneumonitis, resulting from an allergic reaction to inhaled organic dust, as in bagassosis and various other conditions.
organic mental s. former term for a constellation of psychological or behavioral signs and symptoms associated with brain dysfunction of unknown or unspecified etiology and grouped according to symptoms (cf. *organic mental disorder*). Designating certain conditions as having an organic basis, possibly implying that others do not, is currently discouraged.
organic mood s. a term used in a former system of classification, denoting an organic mental syndrome characterized by the presence of manic or depressive mood disturbance caused by a specific organic factor and not associated with delirium. Such disorders are now mainly classified as *substance-induced mood disorders* and *mood disorders due to a general medical condition.*
organic personality s. a term used in a former system of classification, denoting an organic mental syndrome characterized by a marked change in behavior or personality, caused by a specific organic factor and not associated with delirium or dementia. The most common causes are space-occupying lesions of the brain, head trauma, and cerebrovascular disease.
orofaciodigital s., type I oral-facial-digital s., type I.
orofaciodigital s., type II Mohr s.
orofaciodigital s., type III oral-facial-digital s., type III.
Ortner s. laryngeal paralysis associated with heart disease, due to compression of the recurrent laryngeal nerve between the aorta and a dilated pulmonary artery.
osmotic demyelination s. a form of central pontine myelinolysis that occurs when a patient with chronic hypernatremia has the condition corrected too quickly, so that cells of the central nervous system experience the cerebrospinal fluid as being hypertonic.
Ostrum-Furst s. congenital synostosis of the neck, platybasia, and Sprengel deformity.
Othello s. delusional belief in the infidelity of the sexual partner, often of sudden onset and usually affecting middle-aged men; it is characterized by repeated accusations, intense searches for evidence, and prolonged interrogation of the partner.
outlet s. thoracic outlet s.
ovarian hyperstimulation s. an iatrogenic condition seen in women undergoing ovulation induction, characterized by mild to severe ovarian enlargement with exudation of fluid and protein, leading to ascites, pleural or pericardial effusion, azotemia, oliguria, and thromboembolism.
ovarian remnant s. pelvic pain, sometimes cyclic, typically occurring several weeks or months after oophorectomy, usually associated with a pelvic mass, most frequently a corpus luteum cyst, which occasionally leads to unilateral ureteral obstruction. It is due to survival of an ovarian fragment after the operation.
ovarian vein s. obstruction of the ureter due to compression by an enlarged or varicose ovarian vein; typically the vein becomes enlarged during pregnancy, the symptoms being those of obstruction or infection of the upper urinary tract. The right side is usually affected.
overlap s. any of a group of connective tissue disorders that either combine scleroderma with polymyositis or systemic lupus erythematosus or combine systemic lupus erythematosus with rheumatoid arthritis or polymyositis. Cf. *mixed connective tissue disease.*
overtraining s. a group of symptoms seen in athletes who train beyond the body's ability to adapt; there is inability to sustain intense exercise, generalized fatigue, and sometimes mood or sleep disturbances that may last for weeks after the training has stopped or decreased. In some persons a contributing factor is hormonal imbalance caused by the physical stress.
overuse s. see under *injury.*
overwear s. extreme photophobia, pain, and lacrimation associated with contact lenses, particularly non–gas permeable hard lenses, usually caused by wearing them excessively. Prolonged lens-induced corneal hypoxia results in corneal epithelial edema and eventually erosion; it can be a chronic condition or an acute episode that usually occurs several hours after lenses are removed.
pacemaker s. vertigo, syncope, and hypotension, often accompanied by dyspnea, cough, nausea, peripheral edema, and palpitations, induced or exacerbated by abnormalities of the cardiac pacemaker so that it stimulates the ventricle. The symptoms occur because ventricular pacing does not maintain normal atrioventricular synchrony; retrograde ventriculoatrial conduction causes low cardiac output and activates cardiac reflexes that result in increased peripheral vasodilation and hypotension.
pacemaker twiddler s. twiddler's syndrome in a patient with an artificial cardiac pacemaker.
Paget-Schroetter s., Paget-von Schroetter s. a thoracic outlet syndrome in which a thrombus forms in the axillary vein after strenuous exercise; symptoms include pain, edema, and skin discoloration in the shoulder and upper arm. Called also *effort thrombosis.*
painful arc s. shoulder pain occurring at a particular portion of the arc described when the arm is abducted from the side to the fully raised position, as in inflammation of the tendons of the supraspinatus muscle.

painful bruising s. a purpuric reaction usually seen in young to middle-aged women, characterized by spontaneous, chronic, recurring painful ecchymoses, occurring singly or multiply, without significant prior trauma; it may be precipitated by emotional stress. Because some patients exhibit autoerythrocyte sensitization (q.v.), some authorities believe the etiology to be autosensitization to a component of the erythrocyte membrane; others believe it is a purely psychosomatic or factitious condition. Called also *autoerythrocyte sensitization s.*, *erythrocyte autosensitization s.*, and *Gardner-Diamond s.*
painful legs and moving toes s. a syndrome of neuropathic pain in the lower limbs with involuntary movements of the toes or feet; some cases accompany peripheral or central nervous system disorders, and others are idiopathic.
paleostriatal s., pallidal s. juvenile paralysis agitans (of Hunt).
Pallister-Killian s. a rare syndrome of mosaicism in which only the fibroblasts are aneuploid, having 47 chromosomes. This results in mental retardation, seizures, streaks of discoloration on the skin, various facial anomalies, and less often defects of limbs, heart, or other structures. Called also *tetrasomy 12p.*
palmar fasciitis and polyarthritis s. a syndrome of palmar fasciitis, which may be crippling, and polyarthritis in various parts of the body, seen most often as a paraneoplastic condition.
palmar-plantar erythrodysesthesia s. hand-foot s.
Pancoast s. 1. neuritic pain in the arm, atrophy of the muscles of the arm and hand, and Horner syndrome, observed with a pulmonary sulcus tumor, due to involvement of the brachial plexus and cervical sympathetic nerves. 2. osteolysis in the posterior part of one or more ribs, sometimes also involving the corresponding vertebra.
pancreatic cholera s. Verner-Morrison s.
pancreaticohepatic s. Zieve s.
pancytopenia-dysmelia s. Fanconi s. (def. 1).
PAPA s. a rare, autosomal dominant type of autoinflammatory disease (q.v.), characterized by pyogenic arthritis, pyoderma gangrenosum, and acne.
Papillon-Lefèvre s. an autosomal recessive disorder occurring between the first and fifth years of life, characterized by psoriasiform palmoplantar keratoderma, which may also involve the elbows, knees, tibias, external malleoli, and other areas; ectopic calcifications of the skull; and periodontitis and premature shedding of both the deciduous and permanent teeth.
papular-purpuric gloves-and-socks s. a syndrome resulting from parvovirus B19 infection, characterized by pruritus, edema, and erythema of the hands and feet, often with shallow ulcerations in and around the mouth, accompanied by fever and leukopenia.
paraganglioma s. (PGL) an autosomal dominant disorder characterized by tumors of the paraganglia, most frequently of the carotid body, classified into four forms (PGL1–PGL4) on the basis of the site of the mutation; three result from mutations in genes coding for subunits of succinate dehydrogenase, while the site of mutation in the fourth (PGL2) is unknown.
paraneoplastic s. a symptom-complex arising in a cancer-bearing patient that cannot be explained by local or distant spread of the tumor.
paratrigeminal s. Raeder paratrigeminal s.
Parinaud s. paralysis of conjugate upward movement of the eyes without paralysis of convergence, associated with lesions of the midbrain, such as a lesion in the superior colliculi or a tumor of the pineal gland.
Parinaud oculoglandular s. conjunctivitis, most often unilateral and of the follicular type, followed by tenderness and enlargement of the preauricular lymph nodes; it is often associated with other infections, such as cat-scratch fever, lymphogranuloma venereum, or tularemia.
Parkes Weber s. Sturge-Weber s.
parkinsonian s. any disorder manifesting the symptoms of Parkinson disease.
Parry-Romberg s. facial hemiatrophy.
Parsonage-Turner s. neuralgic amyotrophy.
partial androgen insensitivity s. a type of androgen insensitivity syndrome of less severity than the complete androgen insensitivity syndrome, with genetic males having decreased sensitivity of target tissues to androgen. Affected boys are often born with ambiguous genitalia, such as hypospadias and a small vaginal pouch, a hooded phallus, or a bifid scrotum that may or may not contain gonads. Called also *incomplete testicular feminization* and *partial androgen resistance.*
Patau s. trisomy 13 s.
Paterson s., Paterson-Brown Kelly s., Paterson-Kelly s. Plummer-Vinson s.
Pearson s. a rare, often fatal, congenital syndrome characterized by transfusion-dependent sideroblastic anemia with vacuolation of bone marrow precursors and pancreatic dysfunction; it is caused by a large deletion in the mitochondrial genome.
peeling skin s. keratolysis exfoliativa.
Pellizzi s. epiphyseal s.
Pendred s. an autosomal recessive syndrome of congenital bilateral nerve deafness with development in middle childhood of goiter without hypothyroidism; the main biochemical feature is dyshormonogenesis of thyroxine.
PEP s. [*p*lasma cell dyscrasia, *e*ndocrinopathy, *p*olyneuropathy] POEMS s.
Pepper s. neuroblastoma with metastases to the liver.
pericolic membrane s. symptoms resembling those of chronic appendicitis, owing to the pressure of pericolic membranes.
Perlman s. a rare, lethal syndrome consisting of renal dysplasia, nephroblastoma, fetal gigantism, and hypertrophy of the islets of Langerhans with hyperinsulinism. It may be transmitted by autosomal recessive inheritance.
persistent müllerian duct s. (PMDS) a hereditary syndrome in males, either X-linked or autosomal recessive, consisting of persistence of müllerian structures in addition to male genital ducts, with undescended testes and bilateral uterine tubes, a uterus, and an upper vagina. There may be cryptorchidism on just one side with a contralateral inguinal hernia that contains a testis, uterus, and uterine tube *(hernia uteri inguinalis).*
pertussis s. pertussis.
pertussis-like s. a syndrome clinically indistinguishable from pertussis, but without evidence of infection with *Bordetella pertussis* or *B. parapertussis;* the most common infectious agents are adenoviruses. Cf. *parapertussis.*
petrosphenoid s. Jacod s.
Peutz-Jeghers s. an autosomal dominant polyposis syndrome characterized by hamartomas of the small intestine and excessive melanin pigmentation of the skin and mucous membranes; gastrointestinal bleeding and intussusception are common complications.
Pfeiffer s. an autosomal dominant disorder characterized by acrocephalosyndactyly associated with broad short thumbs and great toes. Called also *acrocephalopolysyndactyly, type I, acrocephalosyndactyly, type V,* and *Noack s.*
PHACES s. a congenital syndrome of *p*osterior fossa malformations, *h*emangioma, *a*rterial anomalies, *c*ardiac defects, *e*ye anomalies, and *s*ternal defects.
pharyngeal pouch s. DiGeorge s.
PHC s. an autosomal dominant syndrome consisting of premolar aplasia, hyperhidrosis, and premature canities. Called also *Böök s.*
pickwickian s. obesity-hypoventilation s.
PIE s. [*p*ulmonary *i*nfiltration with *e*osinophilia] 1. any syndrome characterized by pulmonary infiltrates with eosinophilia, such as Löffler syndrome or chronic eosinophilic pneumonia. 2. a syndrome of diffuse pulmonary infiltration and peripheral eosinophilia, seen in dogs and sometimes cats; the cause varies but sometimes it may be an allergic reaction. Affected animals are dyspneic with decreased exercise tolerance. Called also *eosinophilic pneumonia.*
Pierre Robin s. see under *sequence.*
pineal s. epiphyseal s.
piriformis s. levator ani s.
placental dysfunction s. postmaturity s.
plica s. pain, tenderness, crepitus, and swelling of the knee joint, sometimes accompanied by weakness or locking of the joint, caused by fibrosis and calcification of the synovial plicae, usually the mediopatellar plica.
Plummer-Vinson s. a syndrome usually seen in middle-aged women with hypochromic anemia, characterized by cracks or fissures at the corners of the mouth, painful tongue with atrophy of filiform and later fungiform papillae, and dysphagia due to esophageal webs or stenosis. Called also *Paterson, Paterson-Kelly,* or *Vinson s.* and *sideropenic dysphagia.*
POEMS s. a multisystem syndrome combining *p*olyneuropathy, *o*rganomegaly, *e*ndocrinopathy, *M* component, and *s*kin changes. It may be linked to a dysproteinemia such as the presence of unusual monoclonal proteins and light chains. Called also *Crow-Fukase s.* and *PEP s.*

Poland s. unilateral absence of the sternocostal head of the pectoralis major muscle and ipsilateral syndactyly; called also *Poland anomaly.*
Polhemus-Schafer-Ivemark s. Ivemark s.
polyangiitis overlap s. a systemic form of necrotizing vasculitis with clinicopathologic signs overlapping those of polyarteritis nodosa and allergic granulomatous angiitis, but also showing features of hypersensitivity vasculitis. Immunoglobulins are often deposited in involved organs. Called also *overlap vasculitis.*
polycystic ovary s. (PCOS) a clinical symptom complex associated with polycystic ovaries, characterized by oligomenorrhea or amenorrhea, anovulation (hence infertility), and hirsutism. Both hyperestrogenism (from peripheral conversion of androgen) and hyperandrogenism are present. Called also *polycystic ovary disease* and *Stein-Leventhal s.*
polyendocrine autoimmune s's, polyglandular autoimmune s's syndromes comprising combinations of endocrine and nonendocrine autoimmune diseases. *Type I* is caused by mutations in the autoimmune regulator gene (*AIRE*, locus: 21q22.3) and occurs in infants and children. It is characterized by the presence of two of three major clinical symptoms: candidiasis, hypoparathyroidism, and adrenal insufficiency. Pernicious anemia, vitiligo, gonadal failure, alopecia, insulin-dependent diabetes, or thyroid autoimmune disease may also occur. *Type II* is *Schmidt s.* Called also *autoimmune polyendocrine* or *autoimmune polyglandular s's.*
polyglandular deficiency s. multiple endocrine deficiency s.
polysplenia s. a congenital syndrome characterized by multiple splenic masses, left-sidedness, abnormal position and development of visceral organs, complex cardiovascular defects, and abnormal, usually bilobate, lungs; it may be related to Ivemark syndrome.
pontine s. Raymond-Cestan s.
popliteal pterygium s. 1. popliteal web s. 2. Fèvre-Languepin s.
popliteal web s. a congenital syndrome consisting chiefly of popliteal webs, cleft palate, lower lip pits, and dysplasia of the toenails; a wide variety of other abnormalities may be associated. Called also *popliteal pterygium s.*
porcine epidemic abortion and respiratory s. (PEARS) a disease caused by a virus of the genus *Arterivirus*, affecting pregnant pigs and characterized by fever, anorexia, and respiratory distress followed by unusually high numbers of stillbirths and other piglets born with respiratory distress, weakness, and neurological conditions such as splayleg. Called also *mystery pig disease.*
porcine stress s. sudden death of a pig in response to a stressor such as fighting, transport, or malignant hyperthermia, or as part of a drug reaction. Susceptibility in most cases is inherited as an autosomal recessive gene. Called also *herztod.*
post–cardiac injury s. fever, chest pain, pleuritis, and pericarditis occurring several weeks to months after injury to the heart, including that inflicted by surgery (often called *postpericardiotomy s.*) or myocardial infarction (often called *post–myocardial infarction s.*).
postcardiotomy s. postpericardiotomy s.
postcardiotomy psychosis s. anxiety, confusion, and perceptual disturbances occurring three or more days after open heart surgery.
postcholecystectomy s. a type of sphincter of Oddi dysfunction (see under *dysfunction*) seen after cholecystectomy.
postcommissurotomy s. postpericardiotomy s.
postconcussion s., postconcussional s. physical and personality changes that sometimes occur after concussion of the brain (q.v.); they include amnesia, headache, dizziness, tinnitus, irritability, fatigability, sweating, palpitations of the heart, disordered sleep, and difficulty in concentrating. Called also *traumatic encephalopathy* and *concussion, posttraumatic,* or *posttraumatic brain s.* Cf. *boxer's dementia* and *chronic traumatic encephalopathy.*
posterior column s., posterior cord s. sensory deficits and ataxic phenomena derived from a lesion of the posterior columns of the spinal cord.
posterior inferior cerebellar artery s. Wallenberg s.
posterior leukoencephalopathy s., posterior reversible encephalopathy s., posterior reversible leukoencephalopathy s. reversible posterior leukoencephalopathy s.
postgastrectomy s. dumping s.
postirradiation s. a symptom complex caused by massive irradiation, with hemorrhage, anemia, and malnutrition. See also *acute radiation s.*
post–lumbar puncture s. the lumbar puncture headache and other symptoms, which may include pain at the back of the neck, nausea, vomiting, sweating, and malaise, felt in the erect position and relieved when the person lies down, lasting from several hours after lumbar puncture for sometimes a few days; it is due to lowering of intracranial pressure by leakage of cerebrospinal fluid through the needle tract.
postmastectomy pain s. chronic pain in the breast, axilla, or proximal part of the upper limb after a mastectomy, aggravated by movement of the shoulder and sometimes by stretching or other exertion of the arm muscles; it is usually neuropathic, caused by trauma to a nerve in the area, particularly the intercostobrachial nerve or superior lateral cutaneous nerve.
postmaturity s. a syndrome due to placental insufficiency that causes chronic stress and hypoxia, seen in fetuses and newborn infants in postterm pregnancies and characterized by decreased subcutaneous fat, skin desquamation, and long fingernails, often with yellow meconium staining of the nails, skin, and vernix. Called also *dysmaturity, dysmaturity s.*, and *placental dysfunction s.*
post–myocardial infarction s. pericarditis with fever, leukocytosis, pleurisy, and pneumonia occurring after myocardial infarction; called also *Dressler s.*
postperfusion s. a type of cytomegalovirus mononucleosis sometimes seen about 3 to 6 weeks after extracorporeal circulation or multiple blood transfusions.
postpericardiotomy s. pericardial or pleural reaction occurring more than one week after opening of the pericardium, characterized by fever, chest pain, and signs of pleural and/or pericardial inflammation.
postphlebitic s. the various complications associated with deep vein thrombosis which are caused by greatly increased pressure in the deep and communicating veins, resulting in chronic venous insufficiency, and principally characterized by persistent edema, pain, purpura and increased cutaneous pigmentation, eczematoid dermatitis, pruritus, ulceration, and indurated cellulitis. Called also *postthrombotic s.*
postpolio s., postpoliomyelitis s. a group of symptoms of unknown etiology seen in patients several years to many years after they have recovered from the major illness of poliomyelitis; it includes new weakness, fatigue, and pain, either generalized or limited to the parts that were affected by the poliomyelitis. Called also *postpoliomyelitis sequela.*
postpump s. a series of complications occasionally seen in patients after heart surgery that involved cardiopulmonary bypass, with pulmonary edema and other signs of acute respiratory distress syndrome and damage to kidneys, brain, and other organs that can be fatal.
postthrombotic s. postphlebitic s.
posttransfusion s. former name for *postperfusion s.*
posttraumatic s., posttraumatic brain s. postconcussional s.
postural orthostatic tachycardia s. (POTS) a group of symptoms (not including hypotension) that sometimes occur when a person assumes an upright position, including tachycardia, tremulousness, lightheadedness, sweating, and hyperventilation; this is seen more often in women than in men, and the etiology is uncertain.
Potter s. oligohydramnios sequence.
Prader-Willi s. a congenital disorder characterized by obesity, short stature, lack of muscle tone, hypogonadism, and central nervous system dysfunction; there is often a characteristic rounded face with almond-shaped eyes and a low forehead. Mental retardation is common. It is caused by loss of expression of genes on paternally derived chromosome 15q11–13, usually as a result of a deletion; the same loss of gene function inherited from the mother causes Angelman syndrome.
preexcitation s. any syndrome characterized by electrocardiographic evidence of preexcitation, such as Wolff-Parkinson-White syndrome or Lown-Ganong-Levine syndrome; sometimes used as a synonym of the former.
premenstrual s. (PMS) a syndrome of unknown cause, typically occurring in the period between ovulation and the onset of menstruation, marked by some or all of the following symptoms: feelings of depression, hopelessness, anxiety, or anger, emotional lability, bloating, edema, headache, increased fatigue or lethargy, changes in appetite or cravings for selected foods, breast swelling and tenderness, constipation, and decreased ability to concentrate.
premotor s. the association of spastic hemiplegia with increased reflexes, disturbances of skilled movements, forced grasping, and transient vasomotor disturbance; occurring in very large lesions of the premotor cortex.
progeroid s. Werner s.

prolonged QT interval s. long QT s.
pronator s., pronator teres s. an entrapment neuropathy in which the median nerve or its anterior interosseous branch is compressed by the structures of the cubital fossa or by its passage between the heads of the pronator teres muscle, causing pain in the forearm and weakness or sensory deficits in the radial aspect of the hand.
Proteus s. a rare congenital disorder with highly variable manifestations, including partial gigantism of the hands and feet with hypertrophy of the palms and soles, epidermal nevi, hemihypertrophy, subcutaneous tumors, macrocephaly and other skull abnormalities, and abdominal or pelvic lipomatosis. The etiology is unknown, although a genetic origin, possibly of autosomal dominant transmission, has been conjectured.
prune-belly s. a syndrome in which the lower part of the rectus abdominis muscle and the lower and medial parts of the oblique muscles are absent, the bladder and ureters are usually greatly dilated, the kidneys are small and dysplastic, with hydronephrosis, and the testes are undescended. The abdomen is protruding and thin-walled, with wrinkled skin, giving the syndrome its name. Called also *abdominal muscle deficiency s.* and *Eagle-Barrett s.*
pseudo–Cushing s. the presence of clinical or biochemical features of Cushing syndrome in patients with certain nonendocrine disorders, such as alcoholism or depression.
***Pseudomonas* hot foot s.** a skin eruption characterized by painful, erythematous nodules on the soles of the feet, seen in persons exposed to *Pseudomonas aeruginosa*, such as children using a wading pool with abrasive strips of tape on the bottom. Called also *hot foot s.*
pterygium s. multiple pterygium s.
puborectalis s. levator ani s.
pulmonary acid aspiration s. the disorder produced, as a complication of anesthesia, by inhalation of gastric content with a pH of less than 2.5, including bronchoconstriction and destruction of tracheal mucosa, progressing to a syndrome resembling acute respiratory distress syndrome. Called also *Mendelson s.*
pulmonary dysmaturity s. Wilson-Mikity s.
pulmonary renal s. any of several conditions in which diffuse alveolar hemorrhage occurs in patients with glomerulonephritis , such as with anti-GBM nephritis, lupus nephritis, or immune complex glomerulonephritis.
pulmonary sling s. a constellation of unilateral aeration disturbances caused by a pulmonary artery sling with tracheal stenosis. See also *sling ring complex*, under *complex.*
punch drunk s. chronic traumatic encephalopathy.
Purtilo s. X-linked lymphoproliferative s.
Putnam-Dana s. subacute combined degeneration of spinal cord (see under *degeneration*).
quadrilateral space s. a rare type of entrapment neuropathy caused by compression of the axillary nerve as it passes through the quadrilateral space; symptoms are paresthesias and shoulder pain upon abduction of the arm.
rabbit s. a side effect of certain antipsychotic drugs, especially neuroleptics, characterized by involuntary facial movements resembling those of a rabbit chewing.
Rabson-Mendenhall s. a rare syndrome seen in children, characterized by a mutation or other defect in an insulin receptor gene, with severe insulin resistance and acanthosis nigricans as well as thick hair, abnormalities of teeth and nails, and hyperplasia of the pineal gland.
radial tunnel s. a type of radial neuropathy in which the posterior interosseous nerve is compressed in the radial tunnel, causing paresthesias and paralysis in the wrist and hand.

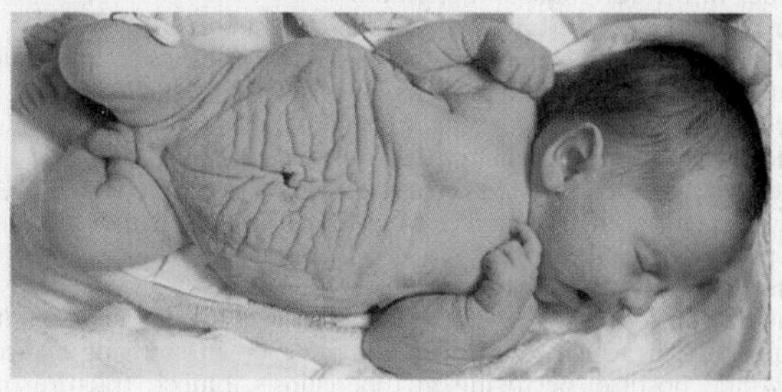
■ Prune-belly syndrome.

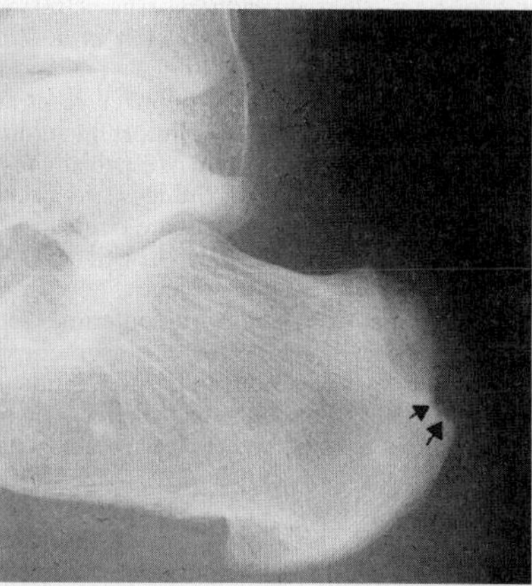
■ Reiter syndrome, with bony erosion at the insertion of the Achilles tendon on the posterosuperior margin of the calcaneus *(arrows)*.

radicular s. a syndrome due to lesion of the roots of the spinal nerves, consisting of restricted mobility of the spine and root pain.
Raeder s., Raeder paratrigeminal s. paroxysmal neuralgic pain on one side of the face associated with blockage of sympathetic nerve impulses; see also *Horner s.* Called also *paratrigeminal s.*
Ramsay Hunt s. 1. herpes zoster involving the facial and vestibulocochlear nerves, often associated with transitory ipsilateral facial paralysis and herpetic vesicles of the external ear or tympanic membrane; there may or may not be tinnitus, vertigo, and hearing disorders. Called also *geniculate* or *Hunt neuralgia* and *herpes zoster oticus.* 2. juvenile paralysis agitans (of Hunt). 3. dyssynergia cerebellaris progressiva.
Rapp-Hodgkin s. an autosomal dominant syndrome caused by mutations in the *TP63* gene (locus: 3q27), which encodes a regulatory protein important in stem cell maintenance in stratified epithelial tissues, characterized by anhidrotic ectodermal dysplasia, cleft lip and palate, and mid face hypoplasia.
Rasmussen s. see under *encephalitis.*
Raymond-Cestan s. a syndrome due to obstruction of twigs of the basilar artery causing lesions of the pontine region; it is characterized by quadriplegia, anesthesia, and nystagmus. Called also *Cestan-Raymond s.* and *pontine s.*
reactive airways dysfunction s. a rare asthmalike disorder consisting of persistent coughing, wheezing, and dyspnea upon only slight irritation, lasting for months after a person has inhaled a high concentration of irritating fumes.
red man s. sudden flushing of the skin, usually of the head and upper body, often with pruritus, following administration of medication; it is most common with vancomycin and has been observed with certain other drugs. It is thought to be related to release of histamine and mast cells.
redundant supraglottic mucosa s. redundancy of the aryepiglottic folds, the mucosa overlying the arytenoid cartilages, and the interarytenoid region of the larynx, associated with obstructive sleep apnea, with or without stridor.
Reed s. leiomyomatosis cutis et uteri.
refeeding s. moderate to severe electrolyte and fluid shifts occurring during a period of refeeding (q.v.); hypophosphatemia is common, and heart failure sometimes occurs.
Reichel s. Henderson-Jones disease.
Reifenstein s. a syndrome of male hypergonadotropic hypogonadism, due to partial androgen insensitivity syndrome, with hypospadias, gynecomastia, primary hypogonadism, and postpubertal testicular atrophy and azoospermia.
Reiter s. the triad of acute aseptic arthritis, nongonococcal urethritis, and conjunctivitis; there may also be mucocutaneous manifestations such as keratoderma blennorrhagicum, circinate balanitis, and stomatitis. It usually affects young men and runs a self-limited but relapsing course. Some authorities now consider this symptom complex to be more appropriately classified as reactive arthritis and not distinguished or named separately. Called also *Fiessinger-Leroy-Reiter s.*
renal-retinal s. Senior-Loken s.

Rendu-Osler-Weber s. hereditary hemorrhagic telangiectasia.
respiratory distress s. see *acute respiratory distress s.* and *neonatal respiratory distress s.*
respiratory distress s. of newborn neonatal respiratory distress s.
restless legs s. unpleasant deep discomfort including paresthesias inside the calves when sitting or lying down, especially just before sleep, producing an irresistible urge to move the legs; the cause is unknown, but in some cases it may be due to inadequate circulation, a reaction to medication, or a complication of uremia. Called also *restless legs* and *Ekbom s.*
retained gastric antrum s. a syndrome sometimes seen after partial gastrectomy in the Billroth II operation, if a segment of antrum was retained. Lack of the usual acid-secreting gastric glands means that the antral segment is continually exposed to the alkaline environment of the duodenum, which causes it to secrete excessive acid and be prone to form ulcers.
retraction s. Duane s.
Rett s. [DSM-IV] a pervasive developmental disorder affecting the gray matter of the brain, occurring exclusively in females and present from birth; it is progressive and is characterized by autistic behavior, ataxia, dementia, seizures, and loss of purposeful use of the hands, with cerebral atrophy, mild hyperammonemia, and decreased levels of biogenic amines. It is an X-linked dominant disorder caused by a loss-of-function mutation in the *MEP2* gene, which encodes a methyl-CpG-binding protein that regulates transcription of other genes. Called also *cerebroatrophic hyperammonemia.*
reversible posterior leukoencephalopathy s. a syndrome resulting from leukoencephalopathy with edema in posterior parts of the occipital and parietal lobes, characterized by headaches, confusion, seizures, and visual disturbances; the brain lesions are most often related to hypertension, and sometimes to use of certain immunosuppressive drugs or to some other cause. Called also *posterior leukoencephalopathy s., posterior reversible encephalopathy s.,* and *posterior reversible leukoencephalopathy s.*
Reye s., Reye-Johnson s. a rare, acute, sometimes fatal disease of childhood, characterized by recurrent vomiting and elevated serum transaminase levels, with distinctive changes in the liver and other viscera; an encephalopathic phase may follow with acute brain swelling, disturbances of consciousness, and seizures. It most often occurs as a sequela of chickenpox or a viral upper respiratory infection.
Rh-null s. chronic hemolytic anemia in persons who lack all Rh factors (Rh_{null}); it is marked by spherocytosis, stomatocytosis, and increased osmotic fragility.
Richards-Rundle s. a congenital syndrome consisting of ketoaciduria, mental retardation, low development of secondary sex characters, deafness, lack of muscle coordination, and peripheral muscular wasting that progresses during childhood but eventually becomes static.
Richner-Hanhart s. type II tyrosinemia.
Richter s. chronic lymphocytic leukemia with diffuse histiocytic lymphoma.
Rieger s. Rieger anomaly accompanied by hypodontia, anal stenosis, hypertelorism, mental deficiency, and agenesis of the facial bones. See also *anterior chamber cleavage s.*
rigid spine s. a rare type of muscular dystrophy characterized by weak neck muscles, fibrous contractures of the vertebral column with scoliosis, and respiratory insufficiency.
Riley-Day s. familial dysautonomia.
Riley-Smith s. macrocephaly without hydrocephalus, multiple hemangiomas, and pseudopapilledema; presumed to be transmitted as an autosomal dominant trait.
Roberts s. a hereditary syndrome, transmitted as an autosomal recessive trait, consisting of imperfect development of the long bones of the limbs associated with cleft palate and lip and other anomalies.
Robinow s. dwarfism associated with increased interorbital distance, malaligned teeth, bulging forehead, depressed nasal bridge, and short limbs. Called also *Robinow dwarfism* and *fetal face s.*
Rochon-Duvigneaud s. superior orbital fissure s.
Rokitansky-Küster-Hauser s. Mayer-Rokitansky-Küster-Hauser s.
rolandic vein s. hemiplegia resulting from interference with the cerebral venous circulation.
Rollet s. orbital apex s.
Romano-Ward s. the more common, autosomal dominant form of the long QT syndrome, characterized by syncope and sometimes ventricular fibrillation and sudden death.
Rosenberg-Bergstrom s. an autosomal recessive syndrome characterized by hyperuricemia, renal insufficiency, ataxia, and deafness, probably due to deficiency of ribose-phosphate pyrophosphokinase.
Rosenberg-Chutorian s. a rare X-linked hereditary syndrome characterized by optic atrophy, progressive neural deafness, and polyneuropathy.
Rosenthal s. factor XI deficiency.
Rosenthal-Kloepfer s. a rare hereditary, autosomal dominant syndrome consisting of corneal opacities, features resembling those of acromegaly, and cutis verticis gyrata of the scalp.
Rosewater s. a mild form of hereditary X-linked hypergonadotropic hypogonadism in males, characterized by sterility and gynecomastia.
Ross s. a rare syndrome, sometimes considered a variant of Adie syndrome, characterized by tonic pupils, loss of deep tendon reflexes, and hypohidrosis on one side of the body; in some cases there is compensatory hyperhidrosis on the other side.
Roth (Rot) s., Roth-Bernhardt (Rot-Bernhardt) s. meralgia paresthetica.
Rothmann-Makai s. a rare syndrome of idiopathic circumscribed panniculitis with fat cell necrosis, lipophagic granuloma, and cyst formation; it usually subsides spontaneously.
Rothmund-Thomson s. an autosomal recessive syndrome characterized by reticulated, atrophic, hyperpigmented, telangiectatic cutaneous plaques, often with juvenile cataracts, saddle nose, congenital bone defects, disturbances in growth of hair, nails, and teeth, and hypogonadism. At least some cases appear to be caused by mutations affecting a particular DNA helicase. Called also *poikiloderma congenitale.* Cf. *Thomson disease.*
Rotor s. a type of chronic familial nonhemolytic jaundice that differs from Dubin-Johnson syndrome in the lack of liver pigmentation.
Roussy-Dejerine s. thalamic s.
Roussy-Lévy s. a slowly progressive autosomal dominant disorder in which sensory ataxia is associated with areflexia, atrophy of muscles of distal extremities, especially the peroneal muscles, static tremor of the hands, pes cavus or clawfoot, and sometimes kyphoscoliosis. Called also *hereditary areflexic dystasia, Lévy-Roussy s.,* and *Roussy-Lévy hereditary areflexic dystasia.*
Roux stasis s. a complication sometimes seen in persons who have had a Roux-en-Y procedure, consisting of intractable nausea and abdominal pain because of gastric paresis or failure of food to move through the anastomosis.
Rovsing s. horseshoe kidney with nausea, abdominal discomfort, and pain on hyperextension.
Rowell s. name given to a rare combination of systemic lupus erythematosus and erythema multiforme.
Rozycki s. a rare autosomal recessive syndrome characterized by deafness, vitiligo, short stature, and muscle wasting.
RS3PE s. [*r*emitting *s*eronegative *s*ymmetrical *s*ynovitis with *p*itting *e*dema] a rare syndrome of acute onset but self-limited course, primarily affecting the elderly, consisting of polyarthritis with seronegativity for rheumatoid factor, accompanied by pitting edema of the hands and sometimes the feet.
rubella s. congenital rubella s.
Rubinstein s., Rubinstein-Taybi s. a congenital condition characterized by mental and motor retardation, broad thumbs and great toes, short stature, characteristic facies including high-arched palate and straight or beaked nose, various eye abnormalities, pulmonary stenosis, keloid formation in surgical scars, large foramen magnum, and abnormalities of the vertebrae and sternum.
rubrospinal cerebellar peduncle s. Claude s.
Rud s. congenital syndrome consisting of ichthyosis simplex, mental deficiency, epilepsy, and infantilism.
rudimentary testis s. vanishing testes s.
Rundles-Falls s. hereditary sideroblastic anemia.
runting s. a type of graft-versus-host reaction characterized by diarrhea, dermatitis, enlargement of the liver and spleen, hemolytic anemia, and pancytopenia.
Russell s., Russell-Silver s. Silver-Russell s.
Rust s. stiff neck, stiff carriage of the head, with the necessity of grasping the head with both hands in lying down or rising up from a horizontal posture, occurring in tuberculosis, cancer, fracture of the spine, rheumatic or arthritic processes, or syphilitic periostitis.

Ruvalcaba s. a syndrome of unknown etiology but present from birth in males; it is characterized by microcephaly, skeletal abnormalities, hypoplastic genitalia, and mental and physical retardation.
Sabin-Feldman s. chorioretinitis and cerebral calcifications, similar to the manifestations of toxoplasmosis, but having all tests for toxoplasmosis negative.
Saethre-Chotzen s. Chotzen s.
Sakati-Nyhan s. an autosomal dominant disorder characterized by acrocephaly and polysyndactyly with hypoplastic tibias and deformed, displaced fibulas. Called also *acrocephalopolysyndactyly, type III.*
salt depletion s., salt-losing s. vomiting, dehydration, hypotension, and sudden death due to very large sodium losses from the body (salt wasting). It may be seen in abnormal losses of sodium into the urine (as in congenital adrenal hyperplasia, adrenocortical insufficiency, or one of the forms of salt-losing nephropathy) or in large extrarenal sodium losses, usually from the gastrointestinal tract. Called also *salt-depletion* or *salt-losing crisis* and *salt-losing defect.*
Sandifer s. intermittent torticollis occurring in children as a symptom of reflux esophagitis or hiatal hernia.
Sanfilippo s. four heterogeneous, biochemically distinct but clinically indistinguishable forms of mucopolysaccharidosis characterized biochemically by excretion of heparan sulfate in the urine and clinically by severe, rapid mental deterioration and relatively mild somatic symptoms. Onset is from 2 to 6 years of age; the head is large, height normal; Hurler-like features (dysostosis multiplex, hepatomegaly) are mild; hirsutism is generalized; death usually occurs before 20 years of age. The four enzymatic types are *type A*, the most severe, due to deficiency of heparan *N*-sulfatase; *type B*, due to deficiency of α-*N*-acetylglucosaminidase; *type C*, due to deficiency of heparan-α-glucosaminide *N*-acetyltransferase; and *type D*, due to deficiency of *N*-acetylglucosamine-6-sulfatase. Called also *mucopolysaccharidosis III.*
Santavuori s., Santavuori-Haltia s. Haltia-Santovuori disease.
SAPHO s. a syndrome of unknown etiology, consisting of *s*ynovitis, *a*cne, *p*ustulosis, *h*yperostosis, and *o*steitis; the osteitis is often painful and usually involves the sternum, ribs, or vertebral column, and less often the mandible or limbs.
scalenus s., scalenus anterior s., scalenus anticus s. a thoracic outlet syndrome caused by compression of nerves and vessels between a cervical rib and the scalenus anterior muscle; symptoms include pain over the shoulder, often extending down the arm *(brachial plexopathy)* or radiating up the back of the neck. Called also *Naffziger s.*
scapulocostal s. pain in the superior or posterior aspect of the shoulder girdle, radiating to contiguous regions, as a result of long-standing alteration of the relationship of the scapula and the posterior thoracic wall.
Schäfer s. pachyonychia congenita associated with retardation of physical and mental development.
Schanz s. a series of symptoms indicating spinal weakness, consisting of a sense of fatigue, pain on pressure over the spinous processes, pain on lying prone, and indications of spinal curvature.
Schaumann s. sarcoidosis.
Scheie s. a relatively mild allelic variant of Hurler syndrome and the mildest of the three allelic disorders of mucopolysaccharidosis I, characterized by corneal clouding, claw hand, involvement of the aortic valve, somewhat coarse facies with a broad mouth, genu valgum, and pes cavus. Stature, intelligence, and life span are normal; it is caused by a deficiency of L-iduronidase. Called also *mucopolysaccharidosis IS;* formerly called *mucopolysaccharidosis V.*
Schiff-Sherrington s. paraplegia in dogs with rigid extension of the hind limbs, usually associated with acute severe compression of the thoracolumbar spinal cord.
Schimmelpenning s. sebaceous nevus s.
Schinzel-Giedion s. a rare syndrome, probably of autosomal recessive inheritance, of hydronephrosis, skeletal abnormalities, flattened midface, hypertrichosis, seizures, and profound growth and developmental retardation.
Schirmer s. a variant of the Sturge-Weber syndrome in which glaucoma occurs early in the course of the disease.
Schmidt s. 1. [A. Schmidt] paralysis on one side, affecting the vocal cord, the velum palati, the trapezius muscle, and the sternocleidomastoid muscle, due to a brain lesion affecting the vagus nerve and the spinal accessory nerve. Called also *vagoaccessory s.* 2. [M. B. Schmidt] hypofunction of more than one endocrine gland, such as the thyroid, adrenals, gonads, parathyroids, and endocrine pancreas (in any combination), along with nonendocrine abnormalities of presumed autoimmune origin, such as vitiligo, alopecia, and pernicious anemia; it occurs primarily in adult females. The term was originally applied to primary failure of the adrenal and thyroid glands. Called also *polyglandular autoimmune syndrome, type II.*
Schnitzler s. a rare, usually benign syndrome consisting of elevated levels of immunoglobulin M and chronic, nonpruritic urticaria, fever, and pain in the bones and joints.
Schönlein-Henoch s. Henoch-Schönlein purpura.
Schüller s., Schüller-Christian s. Hand-Schüller-Christian disease.
Schultz s. agranulocytosis.
Schwartz-Jampel s., Schwartz-Jampel-Aberfeld s. an autosomal recessive disorder characterized by muscle abnormalities, dwarfism, blepharophimosis, joint contractures, and flat facies. Called also *chondrodystrophic myotonia.*
scimitar s. complete or partial venous drainage of the right lung into the inferior vena cava, usually with hypoplasia of the right lung; the anomalous vein has a scimitar shape on a radiograph; see *scimitar sign,* under *sign.*
sea-blue histiocyte s. a rare disorder characterized by the presence of abnormal histiocytes that stain blue with Wright and Giemsa stains *(sea-blue histiocytes)*, accompanied by splenomegaly. Clinically it may range from a benign course with mild purpura secondary to thrombocytopenia, to progressive cirrhosis, hepatic failure, and death. The etiology is unknown, but sometimes it is inherited as an autosomal recessive condition. Called also *sea-blue histiocytosis.*
Seabright bantam s. pseudohypoparathyroidism.
sebaceous nevus s. a syndrome characterized by a sebaceous nevus or nevi in a linear formation, present at birth and changing progressively throughout life. Some patients have neurologic symptoms (retardation or seizures) or ophthalmologic abnormalities. After puberty the nevi become thickened and verrucous, often with projections and numerous other skin changes; eventually some lesions become nodular and may develop benign or malignant adnexal tumors or basal cell carcinoma. Called also *Feuerstein-Mims, Schimmelpenning,* or *Solomon s., linear nevus sebaceus s.,* and *linear sebaceous nevus syndrome.*
Seckel s. a syndrome of unknown etiology, characterized by intrauterine growth retardation and postnatal dwarfism with a small head, narrow birdlike face with a beaklike nose, large eyes with palpebral fissures higher medially than temporally, receding mandible, and mild mental retardation. Called also *bird-headed dwarfism, Seckel dwarfism,* and *Virchow-Seckel s.*
second impact s. acute, usually fatal, brain swelling and increased cranial pressure, caused by repeated head trauma in a short space of time, so that a second concussion occurs before recovery from a previous concussion is complete.
Segawa s. dopa-responsive dystonia, particularly that due either to an autosomal dominant defect in GTP cyclohydrolase I or an autosomal recessive defect in tyrosine hydroxylase.
segmental aneusomy s. contiguous gene s.
segmentary s. a syndrome produced by a lesion of the gray matter of the spinal cord, and marked by weakness and wasting in the affected segment; called also *metameric s.*
Seip-Berardinelli s. total lipodystrophy.
Selye s. general adaptation s.
Senear-Usher s. pemphigus erythematosus.
Senior-Loken s. a rare autosomal recessive syndrome of tapetoretinal degeneration and familial juvenile nephronophthisis; it is considered by some authorities to be a part of the juvenile nephronophthisis–medullary cystic disease complex. Called also *renal-retinal s.*
s. of sensory dissociation with brachial amyotrophy see *syringomyelia.*
Senter s. keratitis-ichthyosis-deafness s.
serotonin s. a symptom complex caused by hyperserotonemia, usually owing to a person's taking selective serotonin reuptake inhibitors along with some other drug that increases serotonin levels. Symptoms are variable but may include mental status changes, autonomic hyperactivity, and irregular muscular movements; severe cases can be fatal.
Sertoli-cell-only s. congenital absence of the germinal epithelium of the testes, so that the seminiferous tubules contain only Sertoli cells and the testes are smaller than normal; there is azoospermia with elevated

titers of follicle-stimulating hormone and sometimes of luteinizing hormone. Called also *del Castillo s.* and *germinal* or *germinal cell aplasia.*

serum sickness–like s. see *serum sickness,* under *sickness.*

Setleis s. a rare, autosomal recessive type of ectodermal dysplasia characterized by scarlike depressions on the temples, sometimes missing or supernumerary eyelashes, and redundant skin around the nasal and chin areas.

severe acute respiratory s. (SARS) an infectious respiratory illness caused by a coronavirus and characterized by fever, dry cough, and breathing difficulties, often accompanied by headache and body aches.

Sézary s. a form of cutaneous T-cell lymphoma manifested by generalized exfoliative erythroderma, intense pruritus, peripheral lymphadenopathy, and *Sézary cells* (abnormal T lymphocytes) in the skin, lymph nodes, and peripheral blood. Called also *Sézary erythroderma.*

Shah-Waardenburg s. Waardenburg s. type 4.

shaker foal s. a type of botulism in young horses, accompanied by flaccid tetraparesis and inability to swallow, so that there is risk of aspiration pneumonia.

Shapiro s. a rare syndrome of periodic hyperhidrosis and hypothermia owing to agenesis or dysplasia of the corpus callosum, sometimes accompanied by hydrocephalus and mental retardation.

Sheehan s. postpartum pituitary necrosis.

Sheldon-Hall s. an autosomal domininant syndrome caused by mutations in any of several genes that encode for troponin or a mysoin heavy chain, with characteristics similar to those of Freeman-Sheldon syndrome but without the severe deformity of the mouth and chin. Called also *distal arthrogryposis 2B.*

short bowel s., short gut s. any of the malabsorption conditions resulting from massive resection of the small intestine, the degree and kind of malabsorption depending on the site and extent of the resection; it is characterized by diarrhea, steatorrhea, and malnutrition.

short PR s. Lown-Ganong-Levine syndrome.

shoulder-hand s. reflex sympathetic dystrophy limited to the upper extremity; see under *dystrophy.*

Shprintzen s., Shprintzen-Goldberg s. velocardiofacial s.

shrinking lung s. a rare complication of systemic lupus erythematosus, usually because of weakened chest muscles or diaphragm; the diaphragm may be elevated, but radiography of the chest appears normal, although lung volumes are decreased and the patient has dyspnea.

Shulman s. eosinophilic fasciitis.

Shwachman s., Shwachman-Diamond s. a syndrome, believed to be hereditary and autosomal recessive, characterized by primary pancreatic insufficiency and bone marrow failure, with normal sweat chloride values and neutropenia. It may be associated with dwarfism and metaphyseal dysostosis of the hips.

Shy-Drager s. a form of multiple system atrophy that begins with symptoms of autonomic insufficiency (orthostatic hypotension, impotence in males, constipation, urinary urgency or retention, and anhidrosis); these are followed by signs of generalized neurologic dysfunction, (parkinsonism, cerebellar incoordination, muscle wasting and fasciculations, and coarse tremors of the legs). Called also *chronic, chronic idiopathic,* or *idiopathic orthostatic hypotension.*

Shy-Magee s. central core disease.

Sicard s. Collet s.

sicca s. keratoconjunctivitis and xerostomia without connective tissue disease; cf. *Sjögren s.*

sick euthyroid s. euthyroid sick s.

sick sinus s. (SSS) a syndrome of bradycardia, generally intermittent and sometimes mixed with episodes of atrial tachyarrhythmias (see *bradycardia-tachycardia s.*) or periods of sinus arrest, due to malfunction originating in the supraventricular portion of the cardiac conduction system.

Silfverskiöld s. a form of eccentro-osteochondrodysplasia in which the skeletal changes are chiefly in the extremities and which is inherited as a dominant character.

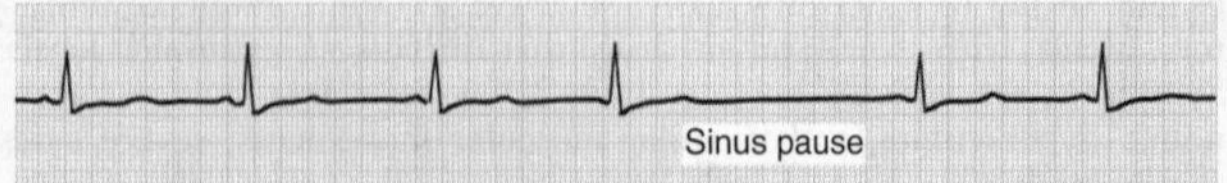

■ Sick sinus syndrome; the monitor lead shows sinus bradycardia with a long sinus pause.

Silver s., Silver-Russell s. a syndrome consisting of low birth weight despite normal length of gestation, short stature, lateral asymmetry, and slight to moderate increase in excretion of gonadotropins, which may be associated with incurved fifth fingers, café-au-lait spots, syndactyly, triangular face, downturned corners of the mouth, and precocious puberty. Called also *Russell s.* or *dwarfism, Russell-Silver s.* or *dwarfism,* and *Silver-Russell dwarfism.*

Silverman s. Currarino-Silverman s.

Silvestrini-Corda s. a rare syndrome seen in certain persons with cirrhosis, consisting of eunuchoid body type, loss of body hair, decreased libido, and sterility; affected males have atrophy of the testes and gynecomastia, and affected females have menstrual disorders such as menorrhagia or amenorrhea. It results from abnormally high estrogenic activity due to failure of the liver to inactivate the circulating estrogens.

Simmonds s. panhypopituitarism.

Sipple s. multiple endocrine neoplasia, type 2A.

Sjögren s. a symptom complex of unknown etiology, usually occurring in middle-aged or older women, marked by the triad of keratoconjunctivitis sicca with or without lacrimal gland enlargement, xerostomia with or without salivary gland enlargement, and the presence of a connective tissue disease, usually rheumatoid arthritis but sometimes systemic lupus erythematosus, scleroderma, or polymyositis. An abnormal immune response has been implicated. See also *sicca s.*

Sjögren-Larsson s. a congenital syndrome of mental retardation, ichthyosis, and spastic pyramidal symptoms.

sleep apnea s. sleep apnea.

sleeper s. thromboembolic meningoencephalitis.

SLE-like s. see *systemic lupus erythematosus,* under *lupus.*

slipping rib s. weakness or rupture of the medial fibrous attachments of the eighth, ninth, or tenth ribs, so that their cartilage tip slips upward and impinges on the intercostal nerve, causing chest pain.

Sluder s. see under *neuralgia.*

Sly s. a mucopolysaccharidosis caused by deficiency of β-glucuronidase and characterized biochemically by excretion of dermatan sulfate, heparan sulfate, and chondroitin sulfates A and C in the urine and by granular inclusions in granulocytes. Onset is between 1 and 2 years with mild to moderate Hurler-like features including dysostosis multiplex, pectus carinatum, visceromegaly, cardiac murmurs, short stature, and moderate mental retardation. Milder forms exist. Called also *mucopolysaccharidosis VII.*

Smith-Lemli-Opitz s. a hereditary syndrome, transmitted as an autosomal recessive trait, characterized by multiple congenital anomalies, including microcephaly, mental retardation, hypotonia, incomplete development of male genitalia, short nose with anteverted nostrils, and syndactyly of second and third toes.

Sneddon s. a rare condition in which cerebral arteriopathy and ischemia are accompanied by diffuse noninflammatory livedo reticularis.

SO s. orbital apex s.

social breakdown s. deterioration of social and interpersonal skills, work habits, and behavior in persons confined in institutions for extended periods with little productive activity, such as long-term psychiatric patients or prisoners; it is caused by the effects of long-term institutionalization rather than any diagnosed mental disorder. Symptoms include excessive passivity, assumption of the chronic sick role, withdrawal, and apathy.

Sohval-Soffer s. a congenital syndrome in males, consisting of hypogonadism with abnormalities of the cervical spine and ribs, as well as mental retardation.

solitary rectal ulcer s. prolapse or internal intussusception of the rectal mucosa with a single ulcer on the anterior aspect 4 to 12 cm from the anal verge, accompanied by constipation and hematochezia; the condition may sometimes be confused with malignancy, infection, or Crohn disease. It is most common in persons 20 to 40 years old who have a history of straining at evacuation.

Solomon s. sebaceous nevus s.

somnolence s. a transient condition of drowsiness, lethargy, anorexia, and irritability with electroencephalographic changes, occurring in children after irradiation of the head in the treatment of brain tumors, acute leukemia, or non-Hodgkin lymphoma.

Sorsby s. an autosomal dominant condition consisting of bilateral macular colobomas associated with dystrophic changes of the hands and feet, usually brachydactyly of the distal two phalanges of certain fingers or toes.

Sotos s., Sotos s. of cerebral gigantism cerebral gigantism.
space adaptation s. a form of motion sickness occurring in a weightless environment during space flight, with nausea, vomiting, anorexia, headache, malaise, drowsiness, and lethargy. It is probably caused by conflicting signals concerning motion from the otolith (whose proper function depends on the presence of gravity) and the visual system (which affects the autonomic nervous system). Called also *space sickness.*
Spanish toxic oil s. name given to an epidemic of acute pneumonia with pulmonary edema, fever, and pseudoscleroderma (rash, myalgia, and eosinophilia), sometimes with neuromuscular damage or fatal respiratory failure. It occurred in Spain in 1981 after contaminated cooking oil was sold by traveling salesmen. The toxin has not been identified. Called also *toxic oil s.*
Spens s. Adams-Stokes s.
sphenoidal fissure–optic canal s. orbital apex s.
spherophakia-brachymorphia s. Weill-Marchesani s.
splenic flexure s. constipation with left upper quadrant pain attributed to kinking of an adhesion between the transverse and descending colon with obstruction; probably a manifestation of the irritable colon syndrome rather than an organic lesion. Called also *Payr disease.*
split brain s. an association of symptoms produced by disruption of or interference with the connection between the hemispheres of the brain. See also *split brain,* under *brain.*
Sprinz-Dubin s., Sprinz-Nelson s. Dubin-Johnson s.
spun glass hair s. uncombable hair s.
stagnant loop s. stasis s.
staphylococcal scalded skin s. an infectious disease of infants, young children, and occasionally older children and adults, seen after infection with certain strains of *Staphylococcus aureus* (phage group II), which elaborate exfoliatin (q.v.). Clinical signs are localized or widespread fine vesicles and bullae that rupture easily to cause exfoliation of large sheets of skin, leaving raw, denuded areas that make the skin surface look scalded. Called also *dermatitis exfoliativa neonatorum* and *Ritter disease.* Cf. *toxic epidermal necrolysis.*
stasis s. overgrowth of bacteria within the small intestine resulting from a variety of conditions causing stasis. The most common causes are disturbances to intestinal motility or decreased acid secretion; it may also be caused by structural abnormalities such as diverticula, fistulae between the colon and small intestine, or chronic obstruction. Characteristics include malabsorption of vitamin B_{12}, steatorrhea, and anemia. Called also *bacterial overgrowth s., blind loop s.,* and *stagnant loop s.*
Stauffer s. a paraneoplastic syndrome seen in patients with renal cell carcinoma, marked by biochemical hepatic abnormalities without hepatic metastasis of the tumor.
Steele-Richardson-Olszewski s. progressive supranuclear palsy.
steely hair s. Menkes disease.
Stein-Leventhal s. polycystic ovary s.
Steinbrocker s. shoulder-hand s.
Steiner s. Curtius s.
Stevens-Johnson s. a syndrome traditionally considered to be a severe form of erythema multiforme. A respiratory prodrome precedes characteristic mucocutaneous lesions and other symptoms. Large areas of the skin and oronasal, genital, and colonic mucous membranes develop macules and become necrotic; hemorrhagic crusts appear on the lips. Ocular lesions may include conjunctivitis, iritis, keratitis, and corneal perforations and opacities leading to blindness. The lungs, heart, kidneys, and gastrointestinal system may also become involved, sometimes with a fatal outcome. Called also *erythema multiforme majus.*

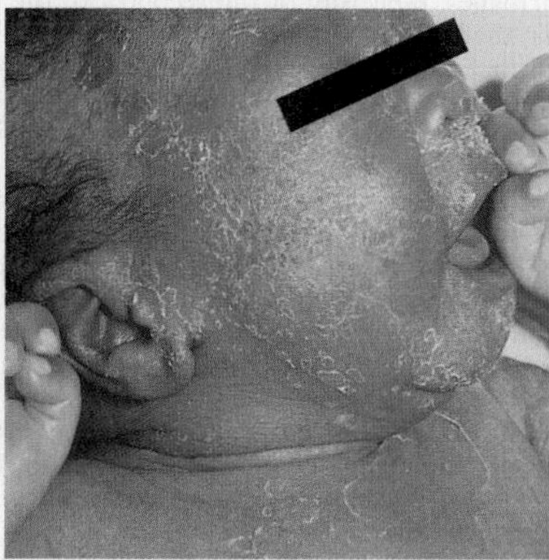
■ Staphylococcal scalded skin syndrome.

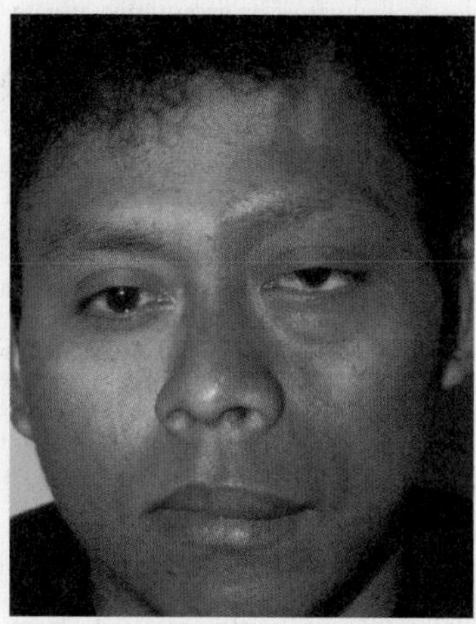
■ Sturge-Weber syndrome.

Stewart-Treves s. lymphangiosarcoma which occurs as a late complication of severe lymphedema of the arm following excision of lymph nodes, usually associated with radical mastectomy.
Stickler s. hereditary progressive arthro-ophthalmopathy.
stiff heart s. any cardiac disease characterized by restrictive hemodynamics; it may result from any pathologic process that renders the myocardial fibers abnormally rigid or that externally applies a constricting pressure and as a consequence impedes flow of blood into the ventricular cavities.
stiff man s., stiff person s. a condition of unknown etiology characterized by progressive fluctuating rigidity of axial and limb muscles in the absence of signs of cerebral and spinal cord disease but with continuous electromyographic activity; some cases have been linked to autoimmune conditions.
Stilling s., Stilling-Türk-Duane s. Duane s.
Stokes s., Stokes-Adams s. Adams-Stokes s.
Stokvis-Talma s. enterogenous cyanosis.
stomatitis-pneumoenteritis s. peste des petits ruminants.
Strachan s., Strachan-Scott s. a nutritional polyneuropathy of unknown etiology found in impoverished areas of Jamaica and other countries, possibly due to a deficiency in dietary thiamine or riboflavin; characterized by amblyopia, paresthesias, dizziness, glossitis, stomatitis, lesions of the sensory pathways, and various other symptoms.
straight back s. a skeletal deformity characterized by loss of the anterior concavity of the vertebral column in the upper thoracic region, with consequent reduction in the anteroposterior diameter of the thorax and compression of the heart between the dorsal spine and the sternum.
stroke s. a condition with sudden onset caused by acute vascular lesions of the brain, such as infarction from hemorrhage, embolism, or thrombosis, or rupturing aneurysm. It may be marked by any of a variety of symptoms reflecting the focus of infarction or hemorrhage, including hemiparesis, vertigo, numbness, aphasia, and dysarthria; it is often followed by permanent neurologic damage. Called also *cerebrovascular accident* and *stroke.*
Sturge s., Sturge-Kalischer-Weber s. Sturge-Weber s.
Sturge-Weber s. a congenital syndrome of unknown etiology consisting of a port-wine stain distributed over the trigeminal nerve, usually unilaterally, with a similar vascular disorder of underlying meninges and cerebral cortex. Called also *encephalofacial* or *encephalotrigeminal angiomatosis, Sturge* or *Sturge-Kalischer-Weber s.,* and *Weber disease.*
subclavian steal s. cerebral or brainstem ischemia resulting from vertebrobasilar insufficiency in cases of subclavian steal.
sudden adult death s., sudden arrhythmia death s., sudden arrhythmic death s. (SADS) any of various conditions in which

sudden cardiac death results from an arrhythmia, usually tachycardia but occasionally severe bradycardia.
sudden infant death s. (SIDS) the sudden and unexpected death of an apparently healthy infant, typically occurring between the ages of three weeks and five months, and not explained by careful postmortem studies; called also *cot death* and *crib death.*
sudden unexplained death s. (SUDS) 1. death for which no underlying cause can be found of a person two years old or older. 2. Brugada s.
Sudeck-Leriche s. post-traumatic osteoporosis associated with vasospasm.
Sulzberger-Garbe s. exudative discoid and lichenoid dermatitis.
sump s. an occasional complication of choledochoduodenostomy when the anastomosis becomes stenosed and the common bile duct acts as a diverticulum; food and other debris collects in the duct, causing infection.
sundown s. sundowning.
superior mesenteric artery s. compression of the third, or transverse, portion of the duodenum against the aorta by the superior mesenteric artery, resulting in complete or partial obstruction that may be chronic, intermittent, or acute; symptoms range from mild to severe, including nausea and vomiting, pain, and extreme distention of the stomach and duodenum.
superior orbital fissure s. deep orbital and unilateral frontal headache with progressive sixth, third, and fourth cranial nerve palsies, with oculomotor paralysis, diminution of the field of vision, and other ocular changes; it occurs either as a result of a meningioma of the sphenoid bone that compresses nearby nerves or as an extension of infection from sphenoid sinusitis into the superior orbital fissure. Cf. *Tolosa-Hunt s.*
superior sulcus tumor s. Pancoast s. (def. 1).
superior thoracic aperture s. thoracic outlet s.
superior vena cava s. a complex of symptoms caused by compression of the superior vena cava, such as by a bronchial tumor or by metastatic mediastinal lymph nodes in lung cancer; characteristics include suffusion and brawny edema of the face, neck, or upper arms; central nervous system disturbances; cyanosis; conjunctival edema; and edema of the trachea and esophagus leading to dyspnea and dysphagia.
supine hypotension s., supine hypotensive s. partial occlusion of the inferior vena cava and the descending aorta by the uterus, especially when a woman is pregnant, resulting in hypotension when in a supine position; it is corrected by assuming a side-lying position. Called also *vena caval s.*
supraspinatus s. tenderness over the supraspinatus tendon, a painful arc on movement of the arm, and a reversal of scapulohumeral rhythm.
supravalvular aortic stenosis s. Williams s.
sweat retention s. 1. the dermatologic symptoms caused by occlusion of sweat ducts; dependent on factors such as extent of blockage, environmental temperature, and duration of the sweating stimulus. See also *miliaria.* 2. tropical anhidrotic asthenia.
Sweet s. acute febrile neutrophilic dermatosis.
Swyer s. 46,XY gonadal dysgenesis.
Swyer-James s. acquired unilateral emphysema, with severe airway obstruction during exhalation, oligemia, and a small hilum; called also *Macleod s.*
sylvian s., sylvian aqueduct s. impairment of vertical gaze, retraction nystagmus, convergence nystagmus, convergence spasms, and poor or absent reaction of the pupils (which are usually of normal size) to light or near vision. It is caused by a neoplasm, inflammation, or vascular lesion adjacent to the periductal gray matter of the aqueduct of Sylvius. Called also *Koerber-Salus-Elschnig s.* and *retraction nystagmus.*
syringomyelic s. syringomyelia.
systolic click–murmur s. mitral valve prolapse s.
Takayasu s. see under *arteritis.*
Tapia s. unilateral paralysis of the tongue and larynx, the soft palate being unaffected. It follows injury to the vagus and hypoglossal nerves, most often from trauma or a tumor.
TAR s. thrombocytopenia–absent radius s.
tarsal tunnel s. a syndrome of overuse injury with a complex of symptoms resulting from compression of the posterior tibial nerve or of the plantar nerves in the tarsal tunnel, with pain, numbness, and tingling paresthesia of the sole of the foot.
Taussig-Bing s. a rare congenital malformation of the heart characterized by transposition of the great vessels and a ventricular septal defect straddled by a large pulmonary artery; hemodynamically it is characterized by pulmonary hypertension, pulmonary plethora, cyanosis, and greater O_2 saturation of blood in the pulmonary artery than in the aorta.
Tay s. a rare autosomal recessive syndrome characterized by trichothiodystrophy, ichthyosis, infertility, developmental delay, and short stature; called also *IBIDS s.*
tegmental s. Benedikt s.
temporomandibular joint s. temporomandibular disorder.
Terry s. retinopathy of prematurity.
Terson s. vitreous hemorrhage caused by spreading of an intracranial, subarachnoid, or subdural hemorrhage.
testicular feminization s. complete androgen insensitivity s.
tethered cord s. a congenital anomaly resulting from defective closure of the neural tube; the conus medullaris is abnormally low and is tethered by one or more forms of intradural abnormality such as a short, thickened filum terminale, fibrous bands or adhesions, or an intraspinal lipoma.
thalamic s., thalamic pain s. a syndrome caused by a lesion in the thalamus and characterized by contralateral hemianesthesia; some later develop persistent severe pain and choreoathetoid movements on the affected side, mild hemiataxia, and astereognosis. Called also *Dejerine-Roussy s.* and *thalamic hyperesthetic anesthesia.*
Thibierge-Weissenbach s. calcinosis.
Thiele s. tenderness and pain in the region of the lower portion of the sacrum and coccyx, or in contiguous soft tissues and muscles.
Thiemann s. see under *disease.*
thin ewe s. chronic caseous lymphadenitis in a ewe, with weight loss and reproductive failure.
thoracic insufficiency s. inability of the thorax to support normal respiration and lung growth, resulting from a variety of conditions that cause thoracic deformities, such as progressive scoliosis or asphyxiating thoracic dystrophy.
thoracic outlet s. any of a variety of neurovascular syndromes resulting from compression of the subclavian artery, the brachial plexus nerve trunks, or less often the axillary vein or subclavian vein, by thoracic outlet abnormalities such as a drooping shoulder girdle, a cervical rib or fibrous band, an abnormal first rib, or occasionally compression of the edge of the scalenus anterior muscle. Continual hyperabduction of the arm may cause another variety *(hyperabduction s.).* Arterial compression leads to ischemia, paresthesias, numbness, and weakness of the affected arm, sometimes with Raynaud phenomenon of the arm. Nerve compression causes atrophy and weakness of the muscles of the hand and, in advanced cases, of the forearm, with pain and sensory disturbances in the arm. Venous obstruction usually takes the form of the Paget-Schroetter syndrome. Other types include *cervical rib s., costoclavicular s.,* and *scalenus anticus s.*
Thorn s. salt-losing nephropathy.
thrombocytopenia–absent radius s. an autosomal recessive syndrome consisting of thrombocytopenia associated with absence or hypoplasia of the radius and sometimes congenital heart disease and renal anomalies. Called also *TAR s.*
thromboembolic s. the association between the formation of thrombi in the deep veins of the leg and pulmonary embolism.
Tietze s. 1. idiopathic painful nonsuppurative swellings of one or more costal cartilages, especially of the second rib; the anterior chest pain may mimic that of coronary artery disease. Called also *costal chondritis.* 2. albinism, except for normal eye pigment, deafness, and hypoplasia of the eyebrows.
TINU s. a rare syndrome of tubulointerstitial nephritis and uveitis, often with immunologic alterations; called also *Dobrin s.*
TMJ s. [*t*emporo*m*andibular *j*oint] temporomandibular disorder.
TNF-receptor–associated periodic s. (TRAPS) an autoinflammatory disease (q.v.) of autosomal dominant inheritance, caused by mutations in the gene for tumor necrosis factor and characterized by febrile attacks lasting one or two days to two weeks. It may be accompanied by myalgia, abdominal pain and gastrointestinal disturbances, headache, testicular pain, conjunctivitis, periorbital edema, pleuritis, erythematous skin lesions, and arthralgia. There is neutrophilia, and serum C-reactive protein is elevated while the soluble type 1 receptor for TNF-α is decreased. Called also *tumor necrosis factor receptor–associated periodic s.* and *familial Hibernian fever.*
Tolosa-Hunt s. unilateral ophthalmoplegia associated with pain behind the orbit and in the area supplied by the first division of the

trigeminal nerve; it is thought to be due to nonspecific inflammation and granulation tissue in the superior orbital fissure or cavernous sinus. Cf. *cavernous sinus s.* and *superior orbital fissure s.*

Tommaselli s. see under *disease.*

TORCH s. [*t*oxoplasmosis, *o*ther agents, *r*ubella, *c*ytomegalovirus, *h*erpes simplex] any of a group of infections seen in neonates that occurs when organisms causing one of the infections cross the placental barrier; they all have similar symptoms in babies and may be clinically silent in the mothers. Called also *TORCH infection.*

Torre s. multiple carcinomas, primarily of the gastrointestinal tract, in association with large numbers of sebaceous neoplasms ranging from sebaceous hyperplasia to sebaceous carcinoma. Called also *Muir-Torre s.*

Touraine-Solente-Golé s. pachydermoperiostosis.

Tourette s. Gilles de la Tourette s.

Townes s. an autosomal dominant syndrome of auricular anomalies, anal defects, limb and digit—particularly thumb—anomalies, and renal deficiencies; it occasionally includes cardiac disease, deafness, or cystic ovary.

toxic fat s. toxicity in 3- to 10-week old chickens that have been fed diets supplemented with fat containing any of several toxins; symptoms are edema of the pericardium and abdomen, waddling gait, and sudden death.

toxic hypoglycemic s. Jamaican vomiting sickness.

toxic oil s. Spanish toxic oil s.

toxic shock s. a severe illness caused by a bacterial infection, characterized by high fever of sudden onset, vomiting, diarrhea, and myalgia, followed by hypotension and, in severe cases, shock. A sunburnlike rash with peeling of the skin, especially of the palms and soles, occurs during the acute phase. It was originally observed almost exclusively in menstruating women using tampons, with the infective agent being *Staphylococcus aureus,* but a nearly identical syndrome has subsequently been seen in males and females of different ages infected with group A streptococcus.

translocation Down s. Down syndrome in which the excess chromosomal material (the long arm of chromosome 21) is translocated to another acrocentric chromosome (in standard trisomy 21 there is an additional chromosome 21). A carrier of the translocation chromosome has 45 chromosomes including the translocation chromosome and may be at increased risk of having a child with Down syndrome.

transurethral resection s. severe hyponatremia caused by absorption of fluids used to irrigate the bladder during transurethral resection of the prostate. Called also *TUR s.*

Treacher Collins s. the incomplete form of mandibulofacial dysostosis.

Treacher Collins–Franceschetti s. mandibulofacial dysostosis.

trichorhinophalangeal s. an autosomal recessive syndrome consisting of sparse, slowly growing hair, pear-shaped nose with high philtrum, and brachyphalangia with deformity of the fingers and wedge-shaped epiphyses.

triparanol s. alopecia, poliosis, ichthyosis, irreversible cataracts, and impotence, due to the use of triparanol, a drug formerly used to depress the synthesis of cholesterol.

triple-A s. [*a*lacrima-*a*chalasia-*a*ddisonian] Allgrove s.

trismus-pseudocamptodactyly s. a rare autosomal dominant disorder caused by mutation in the *MYH8* gene (locus: 17p13.1), which encodes a myosin heavy chain, characterized by inability to open the mouth fully, facultative camptodactyly resulting from shortened finger-flexor tendons, and short stature. Called also *distal arthrogryposis type* 7 and *Hecht, Hecht-Beals,* or *Hecht-Beals-Wilson s.*

trisomy 8 s. a syndrome associated with an extra chromosome 8, usually mosaic (trisomy 8/normal), characterized by mild to severe mental retardation, prominent forehead, deep-set eyes, thick lips, prominent ears, and camptodactyly.

trisomy 11q s. a rare syndrome resulting from the presence of an extra long arm of chromosome 11; because different segments may be involved, the associated anomalies are highly variable and include preauricular fistulas, hypoplasia of the gallbladder, micropenis, bicornuate uterus, microphthalmos, malformations of the heart, lung, and brain, seizures, and recurrent infection.

trisomy 13 s. a chromosome aberration in which an extra chromosome 13 causes severe central nervous system defects, such as arhinencephalia and holoprosencephaly, and mental retardation, together with cleft palate and lip, polydactyly, dermal pattern anomalies, and abnormalities of the heart, viscera, and genitalia. Called also *Patau s.*

trisomy 18 s. a condition characterized by mental retardation, scaphocephaly or other skull abnormality, micrognathia, blepharoptosis, low-set ears, corneal opacities, deafness, webbed neck, short digits, ventricular septal defects, Meckel diverticulum, and other deformities. It is due to the presence of an extra chromosome 18. Called also *Edwards* or *trisomy E s.*

trisomy 21 s. Down s.

trisomy 22 s. a rare syndrome due to an extra chromosome 22, characterized typically by mental and growth retardation, microcephaly, low-set or malformed ears, micrognathia, long philtrum, preauricular skin tag or sinus, and congenital heart disease. In males, there is often a small penis or undescended testes.

trisomy C s. trisomy 8 s.

trisomy D s. trisomy 13 s.

trisomy E s. trisomy 18 s.

Troisier s. bronzed cachexia occurring in diabetes associated with hemochromatosis.

tropical splenomegaly s. a syndrome of massive splenomegaly, hepatomegaly, anemia, and elevated serum IgM levels that occurs in some areas where malaria is endemic, such as parts of sub-Saharan Africa and New Guinea. Lymphocytic infiltrates are present in hepatic sinusoids, and the association with chronic malarial infection is suggested by a polyclonal increase in IgM, a very high titer of IgM antibodies to *Plasmodium falciparum,* and often by a therapeutic response to malarial chemoprophylaxis. Called also *tropical splenomegaly.*

Trousseau s. thrombophlebitis migrans occurring primarily as a paraneoplastic syndrome in association with carcinoma of the abdominal viscera, but also with some types of metastatic neoplasms and chemotherapy.

tumor lysis s. severe hyperphosphatemia, hyperkalemia, hyperuricemia, and hypocalcemia occurring after effective induction chemotherapy of rapidly growing malignant neoplasms; thought to be due to release of intracellular products after cell lysis.

tumor necrosis factor receptor–associated periodic s. TNF-receptor–associated periodic syndrome.

TUR s. transurethral resection s.

Turcot s. familial adenomatous polyposis of the colon associated with malignant tumors (gliomas) of the central nervous system.

Turner s. a disorder of gonadal differentiation in patients phenotypically female, marked by short stature, undifferentiated (streak) gonads, and variable abnormalities that may include webbing of the neck, low posterior hairline, cubitus valgus, and cardiac defects; it is typically associated with absence of the second sex chromosome (XO or 45,X), although structural abnormality of one X chromosome or mosaicism (e.g., XX/XX or X/XXX) may also be responsible. Called also *gonadal dysgenesis.*

Turner s., male Noonan s.

twiddler's s. dislodgement, breakdown, or other malfunction of an artificial cardiac pacemaker, chemotherapy port, drip infusion valve, or similar implanted diagnostic or therapeutic device as a result of unconscious or habitual manipulation by the patient.

twin transfusion s., twin-twin transfusion s. a syndrome caused by twin-to-twin transfusion (q.v.); the donor twin develops hypovolemia, hypotension, anemia, microcardia, and growth retardation, while the recipient develops hypervolemia, hypertension, polycythemia,

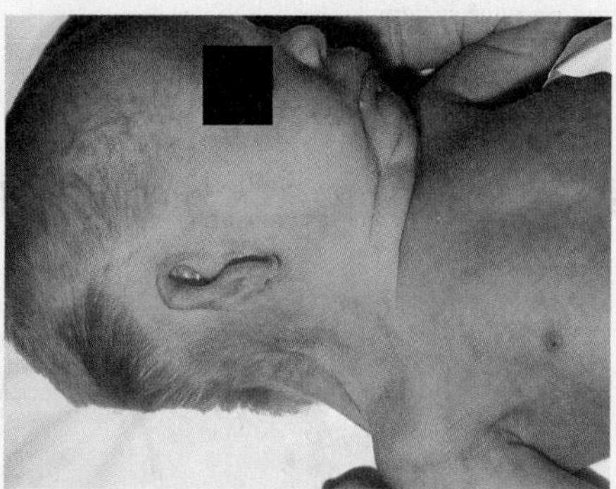

■ Turner syndrome; newborn showing webbed neck with low hairline, shield-shaped chest with widespread nipples, abnormal ears, and micrognathia.

cardiomegaly, and congestive heart failure; polyhydramnios frequently occurs.
tying-up s. azoturia (def. 2).
Uberreiter s. chronic superficial keratitis.
Ullrich-Feichtiger s. a condition of micrognathia, hexadactyly, and genital abnormalities, with depressed nose, small eyes, hypertelorism, and protuberant ears, along with other defects.
Ullrich-Turner s. Noonan s.
uncombable hair s. an abnormality of the hair inherited as an autosomal dominant trait, in which the individual hairs are triangular in cross section, with a longitudinal groove; the hair has a spun-glass appearance and is arranged in bundles that stand out in different directions. Called also *pili canaliculi, pili trianguli et canaliculi,* and *spun glass hair s.*
unilateral nevoid telangiectasia s. unilateral nevoid telangiectasia.
Unna-Thost s. nonepidermolytic palmoplantar keratoderma.
upper airway resistance s. an incomplete form of obstructive sleep apnea in which the upper airway resists air flow and becomes partially obstructed during sleep.
uremic s. the spectrum of symptoms accompanying uremia; see *uremia* (def. 2).
urethral s. a nonspecific group of symptoms considered to arise from a urethral problem other than urinary tract infection; it may include suprapubic aching and cramping, urinary frequency, and such bladder complaints as dysuria, straining on urination, and low back pain.
urofacial s. a rare hereditary syndrome, usually autosomal recessive, consisting of hydronephrosis, hydroureter, and an inverted facial expression, so that affected children appear to be crying when they try to smile. Called also *Ochoa s.*
Usher s. an autosomal recessive syndrome in which congenital deafness is accompanied by retinitis pigmentosa, often ending in blindness; sometimes mental retardation and disturbances of gait also occur.
vagoaccessory s. Schmidt s. (def. 1).
vagoaccessory-hypoglossal s. Jackson s.
Vail s. vidian neuralgia.
van Bogaert-Nyssen s., van Bogaert-Nyssen-Peiffer s. the adult form of metachromatic leukodystrophy.
van Buchem s. hyperostosis corticalis generalisata.
Van der Woude s. an autosomal dominant syndrome consisting of cleft lip with or without cleft palate, with cysts of the lower lip.
vanishing bile duct s. progressive destruction of intrahepatic bile ducts with cholestasis; some cases are a reaction to medications, and others are idiopathic.
vanishing testes s. a disorder in males characterized by absence of testes and gonadal tissue (usually unilateral but sometimes bilateral) and a small penis; when it is bilateral the individual will not undergo puberty or adolescent masculinization without testosterone supplements. The testes are thought to have been present in the embryo but to have "vanished" before completion of male sexual differentiation. Called also *embryonic testicular regression s.*
vanishing twin s. the disappearance of one fetus following the sonographic diagnosis of a twin pregnancy, with only one twin eventually being delivered; the vanished twin may be resorbed or incorporated into the placental membrane.
Van Lohuizen s. cutis marmorata telangiectatica congenita.
vascular s. any syndrome due to occlusion or stenosis of vessels supplying the nervous system.
vascular leak s. a disorder caused by extravasation of plasma through vessel walls, causing edema in surrounding tissues; the most common cause is a reaction to therapy with interleukin-2.

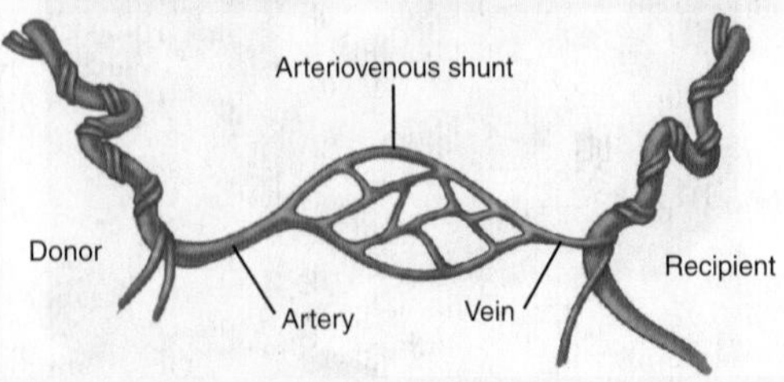

■ Twin transfusion syndrome characterized by arteriovenous shunt at a shared placental cotyledon in diamniotic monochorionic twins.

VCF s., velocardiofacial s. a rare autosomal dominant syndrome of cardiac defects and characteristic craniofacial abnormalities including cleft palate, jaw abnormalities, and prominent nose. Learning disabilities occur often; short stature, slender hyperextensible hands and digits, scoliosis, mental retardation, inguinal hernia, auricular abnormalities, and microcephaly occur less frequently. It is a phenotype of 22q11 deletion syndrome (q.v.). Called also *Shprintzen* or *Shprintzen-Goldberg s.*
vena caval s. supine hypotension s.
Verner-Morrison s. a rare syndrome of profuse watery diarrhea, hypokalemia, and achlorhydria, usually associated with excess levels of vasoactive intestinal polypeptide resulting from a VIPoma in the pancreas; called also *diarrheogenic s., pancreatic cholera, pancreatic cholera s.,* and *WDHA s.*
Vernet s. paralysis of the ninth, tenth, and eleventh cranial nerves due to a lesion in the region of the jugular foramen, and marked by paralysis of the superior constriction of the pharynx and difficulty in swallowing solids; paralysis of the soft palate and fauces with anesthesia of these parts and of the pharynx, and loss of taste in the posterior third of the tongue; paralysis of the vocal cords and anesthesia of the larynx; and paralysis of the sternocleidomastoid and trapezius muscles. Called also *jugular foramen s.*
vertebrobasilar s. see under *insufficiency.*
Villaret s. unilateral paralysis of the ninth, tenth, eleventh, and twelfth cranial nerves and sometimes the seventh, due to a lesion behind the parotid glands. This causes paralysis of the superior constriction of the pharynx and difficulty swallowing solids; paralysis of soft palate and fauces with anesthesia there and in the pharynx; loss of taste in the posterior third of the tongue; paralysis of the vocal cords with anesthesia of the larynx; paralysis of the sternocleidomastoid and trapezius; and paralysis of the cervical sympathetic nerves *(Horner syndrome).*
Vinson s. Plummer-Vinson s.
Virchow-Seckel s. Seckel s.
vitamin E–selenium deficiency s. a deficiency disease of pigs whose diet is low in vitamin E and selenium, most commonly rapidly growing, recently weaned piglets. It usually manifests as either hepatosis dietetica or mulberry heart disease, and affected animals may die suddenly during exercise.
Vogt s. a syndrome associated with birth trauma, characterized by bilateral athetosis, walking difficulties, spasmodic outbursts of laughing or crying, speech disorders, excessive myelination of the nerve fibers of the corpus striatum, giving it a marbled appearance *(status marmoratus),* and sometimes mental deficiency. Called also *s. of corpus striatum.*
Vogt-Koyanagi s. uveomeningitis characterized by exudative iridocyclitis and choroiditis associated with patchy depigmentation of the skin and hair; the lashes and eyebrows also become whitened, and there may also be retinal detachment and associated deafness and tinnitus. Cf. *Vogt-Koyanagi-Harada s.*
Vogt-Koyanagi-Harada s. bilateral uveitis with exudative iridocyclitis, choroiditis, meningism, and temporary or permanent retinal detachment, occurring in association with alopecia, vitiligo, poliosis, loss of visual acuity, headache, vomiting, deafness, and sometimes vertigo or glaucoma. The syndrome may be an inflammatory autoimmune disorder. Called also *Harada s.*
Vohwinkel s. an autosomal dominant, progressive form of palmoplantar keratoderma that begins in childhood, characterized by a stellate pattern of hyperkeratosis on the backs of the hands and feet, linear keratoses on elbows and knees, and annular constrictions of digits like those of ainhum. In some patients it is associated with scarring alopecia and deafness. Called also *keratoderma* or *keratoma hereditarium mutilans.*
Volkmann s. see under *contracture.*
vulvar vestibulitis s. (VVS) severe pain and tenderness of the vulvar vestibule upon touch or attempted vaginal entry; a major cause of dyspareunia.
Waardenburg s. any of several hereditary conditions characterized principally by a combination of auditory and pigmentary abnormalities, including hypopigmented or heterochromatic irides and sometimes hypopigmented fundi; pigmentation defects of the skin and hair, particularly white forelock, white eyelashes, and leukoderma; and cochlear hearing loss. The underlying cause is disruption of various genes associated with the development, migration, or differentiation of melanocytes and neural crest cells; four types have been distinguished on clinical and genetic bases.

Syndrome *Continued*

type 1 an autosomal dominant form caused by mutation in the transcription factor gene *PAX3*, and additionally characterized by wide bridge of the nose due to dystopia canthorum.

type 2 an autosomal dominant form similar to type 1, but lacking dystopia canthorum. It is subdivided into types 2A and 2B; mutation in the transcription factor gene *MITF* causes type 2A, but the mutation associated with type 2B has not been identified.

type 3 a form clinically similar to type 1 but characterized also by upper limb defects. It is caused by mutation of the transcription factor gene *PAX3*, and autosomal dominant and recessive inheritance have both been observed. Called also *Klein-Waardenburg s.*

type 4 a form clinically similar to type 2, but characterized also by Hirschsprung disease. It may be either autosomal dominant, caused by mutation in the transcription factor gene *SOX10*, or autosomal recessive, caused by mutation in the gene encoding either endothelin-3 or a specific receptor for it.

Waardenburg-Shah s. Waardenburg s. type 4.

WAGR s. a syndrome of *W*ilms' tumor, *a*niridia, *g*enitourinary abnormalities or *g*onadoblastoma, and mental *r*etardation, due to a small interstitial deletion of the p13 region of chromosome 11.

Walker-Warburg s. a congenital syndrome, usually fatal before the age of one year, consisting of hydrocephalus, agyria, various ocular anomalies such as retinal dysplasia, corneal opacity, and microphthalmia, and sometimes an encephalocele. Called also *Walker lissencephaly, HARD s.*, and *Warburg s.*

Wallenberg s. a syndrome due usually to occlusion of the vertebral artery, and less often to occlusion of its branch, the posterior inferior cerebellar artery; marked by ipsilateral loss of temperature and pain sensations of the face and contralateral loss of these sensations of the extremities and trunk, ipsilateral ataxia, dysphagia, dysarthria, nystagmus, and Horner syndrome. Called also *lateral medullary s.* and *posterior inferior cerebellar artery s.*

Warburg s. Walker-Warburg s.

Ward-Romano s. Romano-Ward s.

wasting s. the wasting condition seen in persons infected with the human immunodeficiency virus (HIV), consisting of weight loss, muscle wasting, and often fever, due to a variety of causes including nutritional deficiencies and chronic diarrhea. Called also *HIV wasting s.*

Waterhouse-Friderichsen s. a fulminating complication of meningococcemia, with bilateral adrenal hemorrhages, characterized by sudden onset and short course, cyanosis with petechial hemorrhages of the skin and mucous membranes, fever, and hypotension that can lead to shock and coma.

Watson s. a rare, autosomal dominant condition characterized by pulmonary stenosis, café au lait spots, subnormal intelligence, and sometimes neurofibromas; some authorities consider it a variant of neurofibromatosis 1.

WDHA s. [*w*atery *d*iarrhea, *h*ypokalemia, *a*chlorhydria] Verner-Morrison s.

WDHH s. [*w*atery *d*iarrhea, *h*ypokalemia, *h*ypochlorhydria] Verner-Morrison s.

Weber s. a syndrome caused by a lesion in a cerebral peduncle, with paralysis of the oculomotor nerve on the same side as the lesion, producing ptosis, strabismus, and loss of light reflex and of accommodation, as well as spastic hemiplegia on the side opposite the lesion with increased reflexes and loss of superficial reflexes. Called also *alternating oculomotor hemiplegia* and *Weber paralysis.*

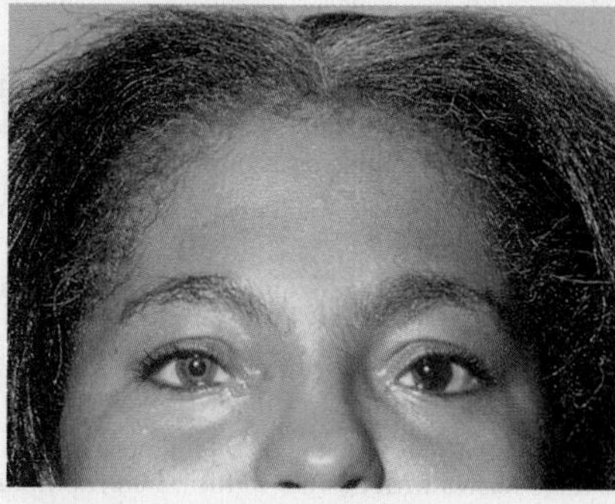

■ Waardenburg syndrome type 1.

Weber-Cockayne s. the localized form of epidermolysis bullosa simplex.

Weber-Gubler s., Weber-Leyden s. Weber s.

Wegener s. see under *granulomatosis.*

Weil s. a severe form of leptospirosis characterized by jaundice usually with azotemia, hemorrhages, anemia, disturbances of consciousness, and fever. It is usually caused by *Leptospira interrogans* serovar *icterohaemorrhagiae* but may be caused by other serovars. Called also *Fiedler disease, icterohemorrhagic leptospirosis*, and *infectious* or *leptospiral jaundice.*

Weill-Marchesani s. a congenital disorder of connective tissue transmitted as an autosomal dominant or recessive trait, characterized by brachycephaly, brachydactyly, short stature with a broad chest and heavy musculature, reduced joint mobility, spherophakia, ectopia lentis, myopia, and glaucoma; called also *dystrophia mesodermalis congenita hyperplastica, Marchesani s.*, and *spherophakia-brachymorphia s.*

Weingarten s. tropical eosinophilia.

Wellens s. electrocardiographic signs indicating critical left anterior descending artery stenosis in patients with unstable angina: biphasic or symmetric, often deeply inverted, T waves in the anterior precordial leads, no pathologic precordial Q waves, little or no ST segment elevation, no loss of precordial R waves, and little or no cardiac enzyme elevation.

Wells s. cellulitis with erythema, edema, and often blistering of the skin accompanied by eosinophilia, flame figures, and a mild fever; a single episode lasts 2 to 6 weeks and recurrences or exacerbations are common. Called also *eosinophilic cellulitis.*

Wermer s. multiple endocrine neoplasia, type 1.

Werner s. an autosomal recessive syndrome of premature aging in the adult, caused by mutations in the *RECQL2* gene (locus: 8p12-p11.2), which encodes a helicase important in maintaining genome stability. Characteristics include short stature with slender limbs and a stocky trunk, scleroderma-like skin changes (especially on the limbs), cataracts, subcutaneous calcification, muscular atrophy, a tendency to diabetes mellitus, prematurely aged face, canities, baldness, and a high incidence of malignancy.

Wernicke-Korsakoff s. the behavioral disorder caused by thiamine deficiency, most commonly due to chronic alcohol abuse and associated with other nutritional polyneuropathies. *Wernicke encephalopathy* (confusion, ataxia of gait, nystagmus, and ophthalmoplegia) occurs as an acute attack and is reversible, except for some residual ataxia or nystagmus, by administration of thiamine; *Korsakoff syndrome* (severe anterograde and retrograde amnesia) may occur in conjunction with Wernicke encephalopathy or may become apparent later; only about 20 per cent of patients recover completely from the amnesia.

West s. infantile spasms.

Weyers oligodactyly s. a congenital syndrome consisting of deficiency of the ulna and ulnar rays, antecubital pterygia, reduced sternal segments, malformations of the kidney and spleen, and cleft lip and palate.

whiplash shake s. a constellation of injuries to the brain and eye that may occur when a very young child is shaken vigorously while being held by the trunk or limbs with the head unsupported. This causes stretching and tearing of the cerebral blood vessels and brain substance, often with subdural hematomas and retinal hemorrhages, and sometimes with cerebral contusion. It may result in blindness and other visual disturbances, as well as paralysis, convulsions, and even death.

whistling face s., whistling face–windmill vane hand s. Freeman-Sheldon s.

white clot s. heparin-induced thrombocytopenia.

Widal s. former name for *hemolytic anemia.*

Wilkie s. superior mesenteric artery s.

Willebrand s. von Willebrand disease.

Williams s., Williams-Beuren s. a neurodevelopmental disorder caused by a deletion on chromosome 7, characterized by supravalvular aortic stenosis, mental retardation, elfin facies, transient idiopathic hypercalcemia, musculoskeletal defects, growth deficiency, hypersensitivity to sound, visual impairment, and a hoarse voice; sometimes inherited in an autosomal recessive pattern. Called also *elfin facies s.*

Williams-Campbell s. congenital bronchomalacia and bronchiectasis, resulting from absence of annular cartilage distal to the first division of the peripheral bronchi.

Wilson-Mikity s. a rare form of pulmonary insufficiency in low-birth-weight infants, marked by hyperpnea and cyanosis of

Syndrome *Continued*

insidious onset during the first month of life and often resulting in death. Radiographically, there are multiple cystlike foci of hyperaeration throughout the lung with coarse thickening of the interstitial supporting structures. The disorder has been attributed to disparity of maturation of parenchymal elements, especially of alveoli proliferation, and hence has been called *pulmonary dysmaturity*.

Winchester s. an autosomal recessive syndrome consisting of short stature, joint contractures, osteoporosis, corneal opacities, and changes in the joints resembling rheumatoid arthritis.

Winter s. a congenital syndrome consisting of renal hypoplasia or aplasia, anomalies of the internal genitalia, especially vaginal atresia, and anomaly of the ossicles of the middle ear.

Wiskott-Aldrich s. an X-linked immunodeficiency syndrome characterized by eczema, thrombocytopenia, and recurrent pyogenic infection. Patients cannot produce antibodies to polysaccharide antigens and have increased susceptibility to infection with encapsulated bacteria (*Haemophilus influenzae*, meningococcus, pneumococcus). Typically IgM is low, IgA and IgE are elevated, and there is anergy of the skin. Many affected persons also have lymphoreticular disorders. Called also *Aldrich s.*

withdrawal s. substance withdrawal.

wobbler s. 1. in large to giant dogs, malformation of the lower cervical vertebrae with compression of the spinal cord so that the animal has ataxia of the hind limbs and a swaying gait; it may progress to paralysis. Called also *wobbles.* 2. in young horses, incoordination of the hind legs with a swaying gait progressing to stumbling, inability to walk, and sometimes paralysis; causes are varied and include stenosis of the spinal canal, malformation of the cervical vertebrae with demyelination, and inflammation of the cord. Called also *equine sensory ataxia* and *wobbles.*

Wohlfart-Kugelberg-Welander s. Kugelberg-Welander s.

Wolf-Hirschhorn s. a syndrome associated with partial deletion of the short arm of chromosome 4, characterized by microcephaly, ocular hypertelorism, epicanthus, cleft palate, micrognathia, low-set ears simplified in form, cryptorchidism, and hypospadias.

Wolff-Parkinson-White s. the association of paroxysmal tachycardia or atrial fibrillation with preexcitation; the electrocardiogram displays a short P–R interval and a wide QRS complex, usually with an early QRS vector (delta wave). The term is sometimes used synonymously with *preexcitation s.* Called also *WPW s.*

Wolfram s. an autosomal recessive syndrome, first evident in childhood, consisting of diabetes mellitus, diabetes insipidus, optic atrophy, and neural deafness. Called also *DIDMOAD s.*

WPW s. Wolff-Parkinson-White s.

Wright s. 1. hyperabduction s. 2. a condition marked by multifocal areas of osteitis fibrosa, patchy cutaneous pigmentation, and precocious puberty.

Wyburn-Mason s. arteriovenous aneurysms on one or both sides of the brain, with ocular anomalies, especially in the retina, facial nevi, and sometimes mental retardation.

s. X 1. cardiac s. X. 2. metabolic s.

X-linked lymphoproliferative s. an X-linked immunodeficiency disorder caused by mutation in either the *SHD2D1A* or *XIAP* gene (both at locus Xq25), which are involved in T-cell development and apoptosis; the disorder is characterized by defective cellular or humoral immune response to infection with Epstein-Barr virus.

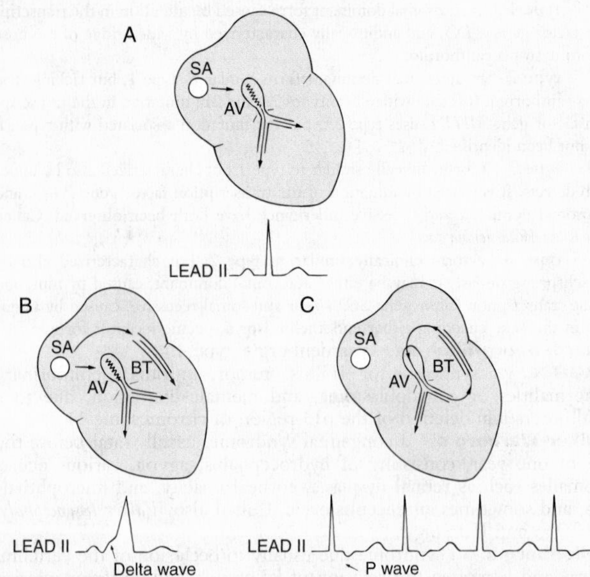

■ Wolff-Parkinson-White (WPW) syndrome. *(A)*, Normal sinus rhythm, traveling from the sinoatrial (SA) node to the atrioventricular (AV) node and then down the bundle branches, with physiologic slowing in the AV node *(jagged line)*. *(B)*, In sinus rhythm in WPW syndrome, conduction down the bypass tract *(BT)* preexcites the ventricles ahead of impulse arrival at the AV node; the PR interval is short and the QRS complex is wide, with slurring at its onset (delta wave). *(C)*, Atrioventricular reentrant tachycardia (AVRT) in WPW syndrome, caused by spread of the premature atrial beat back up the bypass tract to create a repeating reentrant loop; characterized by a normal QRS complex and a negative P wave in lead II.

Fulminant infectious mononucleosis, fatal B cell malignancies, or hypogammaglobulinemia can result from viral infection. Called also *Duncan s.* and *Purtilo s.*

XXY s. Klinefelter s.

yellow nail s. a syndrome consisting of a yellow to greenish discoloration of the nails, which may be smooth, thickened, excessively curved on the long axis, and slow growing, and may become loose and be shed. It is often associated with lymphedema, especially of the lower limbs.

Young s. obstructive azoospermia associated with chronic respiratory infections of sinuses and lungs.

Zellweger s. cerebrohepatorenal s.

Zieve s. a syndrome of hypercholesterolemia, hepatosplenomegaly, fatty liver, hemolytic anemia, and hypertriglyceridemia seen in alcoholics.

Zinsser-Cole-Engman s. dyskeratosis congenita.

Zollinger-Ellison s. (ZES) a triad comprising extreme gastric hyperacidity; peptic ulcers that are intractable and sometimes fulminating; and gastrinomas (gastrin-secreting islet cell tumors) that may appear outside the pancreas, such as in the duodenum. See also *multiple endocrine neoplasia, type 1.*

syn·drom·ic (sin-drom′ik) occurring as a syndrome or as part of a syndrome.

syn·drom·ol·o·gy (sin″drə-mol′ə-je) the field concerned with the taxonomy, etiology, and patterns of congenital malformations.

syn·ech·ia (sĭ-nek′e-ə) pl. *syne′chiae* [Gr. *synecheia* continuity] adhesion of parts, especially adhesion of the iris to the cornea or to the lens.
 annular s. adhesion of the whole rim of the iris to the lens.
 anterior s. adhesion of the base of the iris to the cornea, producing occlusion of the chamber angle; it may be caused by glaucoma, cataract, or intraocular tumors, or occur after perforation resulting from keratitis, iridocyclitis, trauma, or surgery.
 circular s. annular s.
 s. pericar′dii concretio cordis.
 posterior s. adhesion of the iris to the capsule of the lens or to the surface of the vitreous body, producing an irregularly shaped pupil.
 total anterior s. adhesion of the entire surface of the iris to the cornea.
 total posterior s. adhesion of the entire surface of the iris to the lens.
 s. vul′vae fused vulva: a congenital condition in which the labia minora are sealed in the midline, with only a small opening below the clitoris through which urination and menstruation may occur.

syn·echo·tome (sin-ek′o-tōm) a cutting instrument for use in synechotomy.

syn·echot·o·my (sin″ə-kot′ə-me) [*synechia* + *-tomy*] the operation of cutting a synechia.

syn·ecol·o·gy (sin″ə-kol′ə-je) the study of the environment of organisms in the mass, as distinguished from *autecology*.

syn·e·min (sin′ə-min) an intermediate filament protein expressed in muscle, where it associates with desmin to form heteropolymeric intermediate filaments.

Syn·e·mol (sin′ə-mol) trademark for a preparation of fluocinolone acetonide.

syn·en·ceph·a·lo·cele (sin″ən-sef′ə-lo-sēl″) [*syn-* + *encephalocele*] an encephalocele with adhesions to the adjoining parts.

syn·en·ceph·a·lus (sin″ən-sef′ə-ləs) a fetus with synencephaly.

syn·en·ceph·a·ly (sin″ən-sef′ə-le) [*syn-* + Gr. *enkephalos* brain] a developmental anomaly in which there are two bodies and one head.

Syn·er·cid (sin′ər-sid) trademark for a combination preparation of quinupristin and dalfopristin.

syn·er·e·sis (sĭ-ner′ə-sis) [Gr. *synairesis* a taking or drawing together] a drawing together of the particles of the dispersed phase of a gel, with separation of some of the disperse medium and shrinkage of the gel, such as occurs in the clotting of blood.

syn·er·get·ic (sin″ər-jet′ik) synergic.

syn·er·gia (sin-er′je-ə) synergy.

syn·er·gic (sin-ur′jik) acting together or in harmony.

syn·er·gism (sin′ər-jizm) synergy.

syn·er·gist (sin′ər-jist) 1. a medicine that aids or cooperates with another; an adjuvant. 2. an organ that acts in concert with another. 3. a synergistic muscle.

syn·er·gis·tic (sin″ər-jis′tik) 1. acting together. 2. enhancing the effect of another force or agent.

syn·er·gy (sin′ər-je) [L. *synergia;* Gr. *syn* together + *ergon* work] 1. correlated action or cooperation on the part of two or more structures or drugs. 2. in neurology, the faculty by which movements are properly grouped for the performance of acts requiring special adjustments.

syn·es·the·sia (sin″es-the′zhə) [*syn-* + *esthesia*] 1. a secondary sensation accompanying an actual perception. 2. a dysesthesia in which a stimulus of one sense is perceived as a sensation of a different sense, as when a sound produces a sensation of color. 3. a dysesthesia in which a stimulus to one part of the body is experienced as being at a different location.
 s. al′gica synesthesialgia.

syn·es·the·si·al·gia (sin″es-the″ze-al′jə) a painful synesthesia.

Syn·gam·i·dae (sin-gam′ĭ-de) a family of nematodes that includes the genera *Cyathostoma*, *Mammomonogamus*, and *Syngamus*. Many parasitize the respiratory tracts of mammals and birds.

syn·ga·mous (sing′gə-məs) [*syn-* + *gam-* + *-ous*] 1. pertaining to or characterized by syngamy. 2. syngonic.

Syn·ga·mus (sin′gə-məs) a genus of nematode worms of the family Syngamidae that are usually parasitic in birds.
 S. laryn′geus a species that infects the upper respiratory tract, usually of ruminants but occasionally of humans.
 S. tra′chea the gapeworm, a species of parasitic worm found in the trachea of birds, sometimes interfering with respiration and causing gapes (q.v.).

syn·ga·my (sing′gə-me) [*syn-* + Gr. *gamos* marriage] 1. sexual reproduction. 2. the union of two gametes in fertilization to form a zygote.

syn·ge·ne·ic (sin″jə-ne′ik) [*syn-* + *geno-* + *-ic*] denoting individuals or tissues that have identical genotypes and thus could participate in a syngraft. Cf. *allogeneic* and *xenogeneic.* Called also *isogeneic* and *isogenic.*

syn·ge·ne·sio·plas·tic (sin″jə-ne″ze-o-plas′tik) [*syn-* + *genesis* + *plastic*] pertaining to a living related donor; see under *transplantation.*

syn·ge·ne·sio·trans·plan·ta·tion (sin″jə-ne″ze-o-trans″plan-ta′shən) living related donor transplantation.

syn·gen·e·sis (sin-jen′ə-sis) 1. the origin of an individual from a germ cell derived from both parents, as occurs in nearly all higher animals, and not from just one alone. 2. the state of having descended from a common ancestor.

syn·gna·thia (sĭ-na′the-ə) [*syn-* + *gnath-* + *-ia*] a congenital condition characterized by the presence of fibrous bands extending from the maxilla to the mandible.

syn·gon·ic (sin-gon′ik) [*syn-* + *gon-*[1] + *-ic*] having the sex of the individual determined at the time the oocyte is fertilized; called also *syngamous.*

syn·graft (sin′graft) a graft between genetically identical individuals. Typically, syngrafts are grafts between identical twins, between animals of a single highly inbred strain, or between F_1 hybrids produced by crossing inbred strains. Called also *isograft* and *isogeneic, isologous,* or *syngeneic graft.*

syn·i·ze·sis (sin″ĭ-ze′sis) [Gr. *synizēsis*] occlusion.
 s. pupil′lae occlusion of the pupil.

syn·kary·on (sin-kar′e-on) [*syn-* + *karyon*] fertilization nucleus.

syn·ki·ne·sia (sin″ki-ne′zhə) synkinesis.

syn·ki·ne·sis (sin″kĭ-ne′sis) [*syn-* + *-kinesis*] an unintentional movement accompanying a volitional movement, such as the facial contortions accompanying severe exertion. Called also *associated* or *synkinetic movement.* **synkinet′ic** *adj*
 imitative s. an involuntary movement on the healthy side accompanying an attempt at movement on the paralyzed side.
 mouth-and-hand s. Saunders sign; see under *sign.*
 spasmodic s. contralateral associated movement.

syn·ne·cro·sis (sin″ə-kro′sis) [*syn-* + *necro-* + *-sis*] a relationship between populations (or individuals) resulting in mutual depression or death.

syn·ne·ma (sin-e′mə) a group of erect, sometimes fused conidiophores that produce conidia at or near the apex. Called also *coremium.*

syn·neu·ro·sis (sin″u-ro′sis) syndesmosis.

syn·onych·ia (sin″o-nik′e-ə) [*syn-* + *onych-* + *-ia*] fusion of the nails of two or more digits in complicated syndactyly.

syn·oph·rys (sin-of′ris) [Gr. “with meeting eyebrows”] the growing together of the eyebrows.

syn·oph·thal·mia (sin″of-thal′me-ə) [*syn-* + *ophthalm-* + *-ia*] the usual form of cyclopia, in which the two eyes are more or less completely fused into one.

syn·oph·thal·mus (sin″of-thal′məs) cyclops.

syn·op·to·phore (sin-op′to-for) [*syn-* + *opto-* + Gr. *phora* movement, range] an instrument for diagnosing strabismus and for treating it by orthoptic methods.

syn·or·chi·dism (sin-or′kĭ-diz-əm) fusion of the two testes into one mass, which may be located in the scrotum or in the abdomen.

syn·or·chism (sin′or-kiz-əm) synorchidism.

syn·os·che·os (sin-os′ke-os) [*syn-* + Gr. *oscheon* scrotum] penoscrotal fusion.

syn·os·te·ol·o·gy (sin″os-te-ol′ə-je) [*syn-* + *osteo-* + *-logy*] the sum of knowledge regarding the joints and articulations.

syn·os·te·o·sis (sin″os-te-o′sis) synostosis. **synosteot′ic** *adj*

syn·os·te·ot·o·my (sin″os-te-ot′ə-me) [*syn-* + *osteo-* + *-tomy*] the dissection of the joints.

syn·os·to·sis (sin″os-to′sis) pl. *synosto′ses* [*syn-* + *oste-* + *-osis*] the osseous union of bones that are normally distinct. **synostot′ic** *adj*
 radioulnar s. bony fusion of the proximal ends of the radius and ulna.
 sagittal s. premature fusion of the sagittal suture, usually a sporadic disorder but sometimes inherited with autosomal dominance; it results in anteroposterior elongation and reduction in width of the skull (scaphocephaly), often with bossing and a ridge along the suture. Fusion may be confined predominantly to one end of the suture or may be complete. Brain development is usually normal.
 tarsal s. fusion of various tarsal bones.
 tribasilar s. fusion in infancy of the three bones at the base of the skull, producing mental retardation.

sy·no·tia (sĭ-no′she-ə) [*syn-* + *-ot-* + *-ia*] a developmental anomaly characterized by persistence of the ears in their initial fetal position (horizontal, beneath the mandible).

sy·no·tus (sĭ-no′təs) a fetus with synotia.

syn·o·vec·to·my (sin″o-vek′tə-me) [*synovi-* + *-ectomy*] excision of a synovial membrane, as of that lining the capsule of the knee joint, performed in treatment of rheumatoid arthritis of the knee, or of the synovial sheath of a tendon.
 radiation s., radioisotope s. synoviorthesis.

sy·no·via (sĭ-no′ve-ə) [L., from Gr. *syn* with + *ōon* egg] [TA] a transparent alkaline viscid fluid, resembling the white of an egg, secreted by the synovial membrane, and contained in joint cavities, bursae, and tendon sheaths; called also *synovial fluid.*

sy·no·vi·al (sĭ-no′ve-əl) [L. *synovialis*] 1. pertaining to a synovium. 2. pertaining to or secreting synovia.

sy·no·vi·a·lis (sĭ-no″ve-a′lis) [L.] synovial.

sy·no·vi·a·lo·ma (sĭ-no″ve-ə-lo′mə) synovioma.

sy·no·vi·anal·y·sis (sĭ-no″ve-ə-nal′ĭ-sis) the laboratory examination of joint fluid (synovia).

syn·o·vin (sin′o-vin) the mucin found in synovia.

synovi(o)- [L. *synovia,* q.v.] a combining form denoting relationship to the synovia, or to a synovial membrane.

sy·no·vio·blast (sĭ-no′ve-o-blast) a fibroblast of synovial membrane.

sy·no·vio·cyte (sĭ-no′ve-o-sīt) a cell of the synovial membrane.

sy·no·vi·o·ma (sĭ-no″ve-o′mə) [*synovi-* + *-oma*] a tumor of synovial membrane origin.
 benign s. giant cell tumor of tendon sheath.
 malignant s. synoviosarcoma.

sy·no·vi·or·the·sis (sĭ-no″ve-or-the′sis) [*synovi-* + *ortho-* + *-esis*] irradiation of the synovium by intra-articular injection of radiocolloids to destroy inflamed synovial tissue.

sy·no·vio·sar·co·ma (sĭ-no″ve-o-sahr-ko′mə) [*synovio-* + *sarcoma*] a malignant neoplasm arising in the synovial membrane of the joints and also in synovial cells of tendons and bursae; called also *malignant synovioma* and *synovial sarcoma.*

syn·o·vip·a·rous (sin″o-vip′ə-rəs) [*synovi-* + *-parous*] producing synovia.

syno·vi·tis (sin″o-vi′tis) inflammation of a synovium; it is usually painful, particularly on motion, and is characterized by a fluctuating swelling due to effusion within a synovial sac. Some types are named for accompanying tissue changes, such as *fibrinous, hyperplastic,* or *lipomatous synovitis;* others are named for accompanying disease processes or complications, such as *gonorrheal, metritic, puerperal, rheumatic, scarlatinal, syphilitic,* or *tuberculous synovitis.*

dendritic s. synovitis characterized by villous growths within the synovial sac.

detritic s. synovitis with fibrosis, metaplasia of cartilage and bone, and solid fragments of bone as a result of osteolysis.

dry s. synovitis with but little effusion.

foreign body s. synovitis due to presence of a foreign body, usually from outside the body; cf. *silicone s.*

fungous s. mycotic arthritis.

hemophilic s. proliferation of microvasculature in a joint cavity in hemophilia with bleeding into the cavity, causing inflammation and sometimes leading to hemophilic arthropathy (q.v.).

infectious s., infectious avian s. a disease of young chickens and turkeys caused by infection with *Mycoplasma synoviae*; it ranges from a subclinical respiratory infection to swollen leg joints with lameness and anorexia.

localized nodular s. lesions of the tendon sheaths that give histological evidence of evolution from a number of smaller nodules, or from villous structures.

pigmented villonodular s. synovial proliferation forming brown nodular masses, probably caused by hemangiomas of synovial membrane that become traumatized, resulting in synovial hyperplasia and inflammation; it is characterized by episodic monoarticular pain and swelling, with joint locking and hemorrhagic effusions.

purulent s. synovitis in which there is an effusion of pus in a synovial sac.

remitting seronegative symmetrical s. a symmetric type of polyarthritis and synovitis in which patients are seronegative for rheumatoid factor; onset is typically acute, but it has a self-limited course. It usually affects the elderly, and is almost always accompanied by pitting edema; see *RS3PE syndrome*, under *syndrome.*

serous s. synovitis with copious nonpurulent effusion.

s. sic′ca dry s.

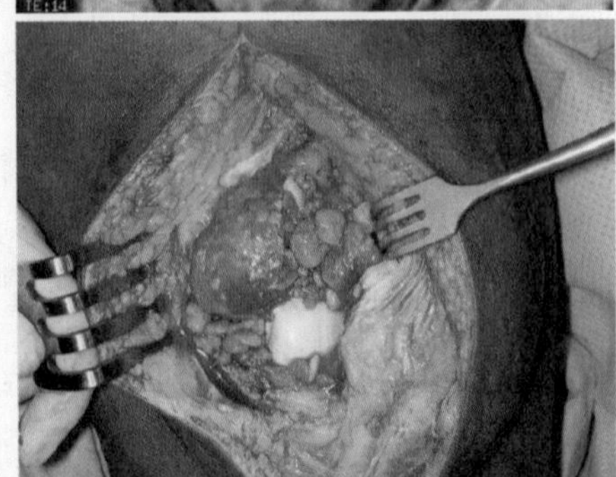

■ Pigmented villonodular synovitis in a 31-year old woman with lytic lesion in the distal femur and degenerative changes in the knee. *(A)*, MRI showing effusion with intra-articular and intraosseous masses *(dark)*; *(B)*, intraoperative view.

silicone s. a type of foreign body synovitis occurring as an inflammatory reaction to particulate debris that has been dislodged by wear from a silicone prosthesis.

simple s. synovitis in which the effusion is clear or only slightly turbid.

tendinous s. tenosynovitis.

transient s. a common cause of hip pain, usually seen in children, often accompanying a viral infection, and lasting for only a few days. It is characterized by sudden onset of pain, occasionally with mild fever, that disappears with rest.

vaginal s. tenosynovitis.

vibration s. synovitis produced by the passage of a missile through the tissues near a joint, but without actually wounding the joint.

villonodular s. proliferation of synovial tissue, especially of the knee joint, composed of synovial villi and fibrous nodules infiltrated by giant cells and by macrophages containing lipids and hemosiderin.

sy·no·vi·um (sĭ-no′ve-əm) membrana synovialis capsulae articularis.

syn·phal·an·gism (sin-fal′ən-jiz-əm) symphalangia.

syn·pneu·mon·ic (sin″noo-mon′ik) occurring in association with pneumonia.

syn·poly·dac·ty·ly (sin-pol″e-dak′tə-le) association of polydactyly and syndactyly of varying degrees of the hand and foot.

syn·re·flex·ia (sin″re-flek′se-ə) the association existing between various reflexes.

syn·tac·tic (sin-tak′tik) pertaining to or affecting syntax, or the proper arrangement of words in speech.

syn·tax·is (sin-tak′sis) [Gr. "a putting together in order"] articulation (def. 1).

syn·ten·ic (sin-ten′ik) pertaining or relating to synteny.

syn·te·no·sis (sin″tə-no′sis) [*syn-* + *teno-* + *-osis*] a hinge joint surrounded by tendons.

syn·te·ny (sin′tə-ne) [*syn-* + Gr. *tainia* ribbon] 1. the presence together on the same chromosome of two or more gene loci whether or not in such proximity that they may be subject to linkage (q.v.). 2. conservation of gene order between the chromosome of different species.

syn·tex·is (sin-tek′sis) [Gr. *syntēxis* colliquation] wasting or emaciation. **syntec′tic** *adj*

syn·thase (sin′thās) a term used in the trivial or recommended names of some enzymes, particularly those of the lyase class [EC 4], when the synthetic aspect of the reaction is dominant or emphasized. Cf. *synthetase.*

syn·the·sis (sin′thə-sis) [Gr. "a putting together, composition"] 1. the creation of an integrated whole by the combining of simpler parts or entities. 2. the formation of a chemical compound by the union of its elements or from other suitable components. 3. in psychiatry, the integration of the various elements of the personality.

s. of continuity union of the edges of a wound or the ends of a fractured bone.

morphologic s. histogenesis.

syn·the·size (sin′thə-sīz) to produce by means of synthesis.

syn·the·tase (sin′thə-tās) a term used in the trivial names of most enzymes of the ligase class [EC 6]; formerly part of the recommended name, it is no longer favored because of confusion with the term synthase and because it emphasizes reaction products rather than substrates. Cf. *synthase.*

syn·thet·ic (sin-thet′ik) [L. *syntheticus;* Gr. *synthetikos*] 1. pertaining to, of the nature of, or participating in synthesis. 2. produced by synthesis; artificial.

syn·tho·rax (sin-thor′aks) thoracopagus.

Syn·throid (sin′throid) trademark for a preparation of levothyroxine sodium.

syn·to·nin (sin′to-nin) an acid metaprotein which precipitates from a gastric digestion mixture at or near the neutral point.

syn·to·py (sin′tə-pe) [*syn-* + Gr. *topos* place] the position of an organ in relation to neighboring organs.

syn·trip·sis (sin-trip′sis) [*syn-* + *tripsis*] 1. the comminution or crushing of a bone. 2. comminuted fracture.

syn·tro·phin (sin′trə-fin) any of a heterogeneous group comprising five different phosphorylated proteins; one α (α-1, acidic), two β (β-1 and β-2, basic), and two γ (γ-1 and γ-2) components. The proteins bind to and are believed to organize the subcellular localization of a variety of membrane proteins; in muscle they mediate the interaction of signaling proteins with the dystrophin and utrophin complexes at the neuromuscular junction.

syn·troph·ism (sin′trōf-iz-əm) [*syn-* + *troph-* + *-ism*] crossfeeding; the stimulation of growth of a cell or organ by a factor released by another cell or organ; especially, growth stimulation of a bacterium resulting from admixture with or nearness of another strain or species, e.g., the growth of *Haemophilus influenzae* as satellite colonies of *Staphylococcus.*

syn·tropho·blast (sin-trof′o-blast) syncytiotrophoblast (def. 1).

syn·tro·pic (sin-tro′pik) [*syn-* + *-tropic*] 1. turning or pointing in the same direction, as the ribs or the vertebral spinous processes. 2. denoting the correlation of several factors, as the relation of one disease to the development or incidence of another disease.

syn·tro·py (sin′trə-pe) the state of being syntropic.

sy·nuc·le·in (sĭ-noo′kle-in) a family of abundant, structurally related brain proteins of uncertain function, comprising three types designated α, β, and γ. Abnormal aggregations of α-synuclein are characteristic of certain neurodegenerative diseases (see *α-synucleinopathy).*

α-sy·nuc·le·in·op·a·thy (sĭ-noo″kle-in-op′ə-the) any of a group of neurodegenerative disorders, including multiple system atrophy, Lewy body dementia, and Parkinson disease, that are characterized by the aggregation of α-synuclein to form inclusion bodies. Called also *synucleopathy.*

Syn·u·ra (sin-u′rə) [*syn-* + G. *oura* tail] a genus of free-swimming, colonial, plantlike biflagellate freshwater organisms, formerly considered to be protozoa but now classified as algae in the class Synurophyceae, phylum Phaeophyta; they may impart an unpleasant taste to drinking water.

Syn·u·ro·phy·ce·ae (sin-u″ro-fi′se-e) a class of free-swimming, flagellate, ameboid, plantlike organisms, formerly considered part of the class Chrysophyceae. All of these organisms were formerly considered protozoa but are now assigned to the algae phylum Phaeophyta. The genus *Synura* in this group can be a water contaminant.

Syn·visc (syn′visk) trademark for a preparation of hylan G-F 20.

syn·xen·ic (sin-zen′ik) [*syn-* + *xen-* + *-ic*] associated with a known number of microbic species; applied to laboratory animals whose microfauna and microflora are known (gnotobiotes).

Sy·pha·cia (si-fa′se-ə) a genus of nematodes of the family Oxyuridae. *S. obveola′ta* is a common intestinal parasite of laboratory rats that has occasionally been reported in human infants.

syph·i·lid (sif′ĭ-lid) one of the skin lesions of secondary syphilis, appearing six weeks to two years after infection in a series of crops lasting a few days to months. Mucous membrane lesions in this stage are clinically the most contagious lesions of the disease.

syph·i·lis (sif′ĭ-lis) [*Syphilus,* a shepherd infected with the disease in a poem by Fracastorius (Girolamo Fracastorio, Italian physician and poet, 1483–1553); the poet may have derived the name from Gr. *syn* together + *philein* to love, or from Gr. *siphlos* crippled, maimed] a subacute to chronic infectious disease caused by the spirochete *Treponema pallidum,* usually transmitted by sexual contact or acquired in utero, although it can be contracted by direct contact with infected tissues or blood or with contaminated fomites. Untreated syphilis usually progresses through three clinical stages (*primary, secondary,* and *tertiary s.),* with a latent period *(latent syphilis)* intervening between the first two and the last. The time of duration of each stage varies, and they are often noticeably shortened in immunocompromised patients. There is also an endemic variety of syphilis (see *endemic s.*). **syphilit′ic** *adj*

cardiovascular s. a form of tertiary syphilis in which aortic insufficiency and aortic aneurysm, usually of the ascending aorta, occur as a result of obliterative endarteritis of the vasa vasorum, causing damage to the intima and media of the great vessels, and may result in congestive heart failure. Cf. *syphilitic aortitis.*

cerebrospinal s. Erb spastic paraplegia.

congenital s. syphilis acquired in utero, manifested by any of several characteristic malformations of the teeth or bones known as stigmata, with active mucocutaneous symptoms at the time of birth or shortly afterward, ocular changes such as interstitial keratitis, or neurologic changes such as deafness.

early s. the stage comprising primary, secondary, and early latent syphilis.

endemic s. a chronic, inflammatory, non–sexually transmitted treponemal infection caused by a subspecies of *Treponema pallidum;* it mainly affects children in dry regions around the Mediterranean and nearby desert areas in Africa and the Middle East. Characteristics include early mucous patches of the secondary type localized to the oral and faucial mucosa, followed by the appearance of moist papules in the axillae and skin folds, a latent period, and late complications that may include osseous and cutaneous gummata. Called also *bejel* and *nonvenereal s.*

equine s. dourine.

gummatous s. late benign s.

horse s. dourine.

late s. tertiary s.

late benign s. a form of tertiary syphilis whose typical lesion is the gumma (q.v.); it responds rapidly to treatment and is therefore relatively benign. Called also *gummatous s.*

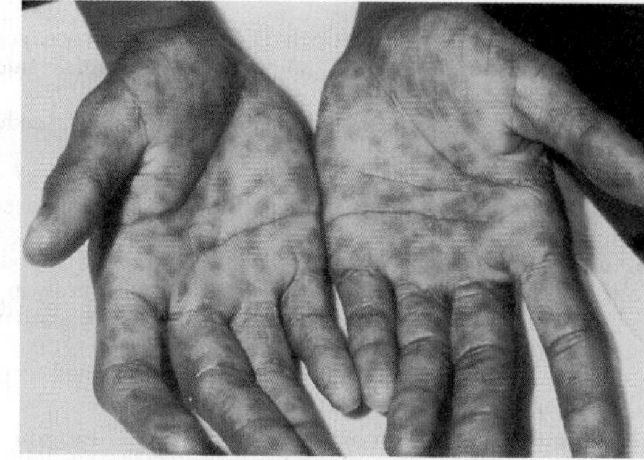

■ Palmar rash of secondary syphilis.

latent s. a stage after secondary syphilis when an infected patient is free of overt symptoms but has a positive serologic test for syphilis; it may last a short time or many years and may be subdivided into *early latent* and *late latent syphilis,* distinguished by the time since initial infection, degree of infectiousness of the disease, and certain other characteristics.

latent s., early the first period of latent syphilis, when relapses of secondary syphilis are most likely to occur and the patient is considered to be more infectious than at later stages; this usually lasts until one to two years after the initial infection.

latent s., late the later period of latent syphilis, beginning one to two years after the initial infection; relapses of secondary syphilis are rare and patients are resistant to infection. The disease is now usually not infectious, although fetuses in utero may contract congenital syphilis from their mothers.

meningovascular s. see under *neurosyphilis.*

nonvenereal s. endemic s.

parenchymatous s. see under *neurosyphilis.*

primary s. the first stage of syphilis, in which a painless primary lesion called a chancre appears at the site of inoculation and is associated with regional adenopathy and bubo formation. Chancres usually appear two to four weeks after infection and heal spontaneously within two weeks. Untreated patients soon develop secondary syphilis.

rabbit s. a venereal disease of rabbits consisting of lesions with scabs around the external genitalia, and sometimes elsewhere on the body, caused by infection with *Treponema paraluiscuniculi;* called also *vent disease.*

secondary s. the second stage of syphilis, usually occurring two to eight weeks after appearance of the primary chancre; characterized chiefly by widespread mucocutaneous lesions (see *syphilid)* and generalized regional lymphadenopathy. It is usually followed by latent syphilis (q.v.).

spinal s. syphilis primarily affecting the spinal cord; see *tabes dorsalis, meningovascular neurosyphilis,* and *Erb spastic paraplegia.* Called also *myelosyphilis.*

tertiary s. the third and last stage of syphilis, which may develop soon or many years after the lesions of secondary syphilis have resolved; it is marked by destructive lesions involving many tissues and organs and occurs in three principal forms: *cardiovascular s., late benign syphilis,* and *neurosyphilis.* Called also *late s.*

syph·i·lo·ma (sif″ĭ-lo′mə) gumma.

syph·i·lo·pho·bia (sif″ĭ-lo-fo′be-ə) [*syphilis* + *-phobia*] 1. irrational fear of syphilis. 2. the delusion of being infected with syphilis.

Syp·rine (sip′rēn) trademark for a preparation of trientine hydrochloride.

Syr. [L.] sy′rupus (syrup).

sy·rig·mus (sĭ-rig′məs) [Gr. *syrigmos* a shrill piping sound] tinnitus.

sy·rin·gad·e·no·ma (sə-ring″gad-ə-no′mə) syringocystadenoma.

papillary s., s. papilli′ferum see under *syringocystadenoma.*

sy·rin·gad·e·no·car·ci·no·ma (sə-ring″gad-ə-no-kahr″sĭ-no′mə) hidradenocarcinoma.

sy·ringe (sĭ-rinj′, sir′inj) [L. *syrinxe;* Gr. *syrinx*] an instrument for injecting liquids into or withdrawing them from any vessel or cavity.

air s. a small fine-nozzled syringe connected by a hose to the compressed air tank in the dental unit; used to direct a current of air into a tooth cavity during excavation, to remove the small chips detached from the teeth, or to dry the cavity. Called also *chip s.*

Anel s. a delicate syringe for the treatment of the lacrimal passages.

bulb s. a syringe with a bulb on one end; compression of the bulb creates a vacuum for gentle suction of small amounts of bodily drainage.

chip s. air s.

dental s. a small syringe into which is fitted a hermetically sealed cartridge containing an anesthetic solution for intraoral injection anesthesia.

fountain s. an apparatus which injects a liquid by the action of gravity.

hypodermic s. a syringe, usually of small caliber, by means of which drugs in solution or other liquids are injected through a hollow needle of small bore into the subcutaneous tissues.

Luer s., Luer-Lok s. a glass syringe for intravenous and hypodermic use, with a metallic tip and locking device to hold the needle firmly in place.

probe s. a syringe whose point may be used also as a probe; used mostly in treating the lacrimal passages.

water s. a syringe that is part of the dental unit, designed to permit controlled spraying of water in a desired area.

syr•in•gec•to•my (sir″in-jek′tə-me) [*syring-* + *-ectomy*] excision of the walls of a fistula.

syr•in•gi•tis (sir″in-ji′tis) inflammation of the auditory tube.

syring(o)- [Gr. *syrinx*, gen. *syringos* pipe, tube, fistula] a combining form denoting relationship to a tube or a fistula.

sy•rin•go•acan•tho•ma (sə-ring″go-ak″an-tho′mə) [*syringo-* + *acanthoma*] a rare epithelial neoplasm resembling seborrheic keratosis, characterized by multiple nests of small basaloid cells within the acanthotic epidermis.

sy•rin•go•ad•e•no•ma (sĭ-ring′go-ad″ə-no′mə) syringocystadenoma.

sy•rin•go•bul•bia (sĭ-ring′go-bul′be-ə) [*syringo-* + *bulb-* + *-ia*] syringomyelia in which the cavity extends to involve the medulla oblongata. Cf. *hydromyelia.*

sy•rin•go•car•ci•no•ma (sĭ-ring″go-kahr″sĭ-no′mə) hidradenocarcinoma.

sy•rin•go•cele (sĭ-ring′go-sēl) 1. a cystlike swelling in a tubular structure of the body. 2. myelocele.

Cowper s. a cystlike swelling of a bulbourethral gland (Cowper gland) or one of its ducts, seen in infant boys or occasionally in older males; those in the duct are caused by obstruction of its orifice. Called also *Cowper cyst.*

sy•rin•go•coele (sĭ-ring′go-sēl) [*syringo-* + *-coele*] canalis centralis medullae spinalis.

sy•rin•go•cys•tad•e•no•car•ci•no•ma (sə-ring″go-sis-tad″ə-no-kahr-sĭ-no′mə) hidradenocarcinoma.

sy•rin•go•cys•tad•e•no•ma (sĭ-ring″go-sis-tad″ə-no′mə) [*syringo-* + *cyst-* + *adenoma*] an adnexal adenoma of the sweat glands. Called also *syringadenoma, syringoadenoma,* and *syringocystoma.*

papillary s., s. papilli′ferum an adenoma arising from an apocrine sweat gland, occurring as a grouping of firm, rose red papules, usually on the scalp but sometimes on the face, trunk, or skin of the genital or inguinal region, and characterized by papillary projections extending into the lumina of dilated cystic sweat glands and ducts.

sy•rin•go•cys•to•ma (sə-ring″go-sis-to′mə) syringocystadenoma.

sy•rin•go•en•ce•pha•lia (sĭ-ring″go-en″sə-fa′le-ə) [*syringo-* + *enkephal* + *-ia*] the formation of abnormal cavities in the brain substance.

sy•rin•go•en•ceph•a•lo•my•elia (sĭ-ring″go-ən-sef″ə-lo-mi-e′le-ə) [*syringo-* + *encephal-* + *myel-* + *-ia*] the existence of cavities in the substance of the brain and spinal cord.

sy•rin•go•fi•bro•ad•e•no•ma (sə-ring″go-fi″bro-ad″ə-no′mə) a type of eccrine adenoma that resembles a syringoma but also has fibroadenomatous tissue.

sy•rin•go•hy•dro•my•elia (sə-ring″go-hi″dro-mi-e′le-ə) hydrosyringomyelia.

sy•rin•goid (sĭ-ring′goid) [L. *syringoides,* from Gr. *syrinx* pipe + *eidos* form] resembling a pipe or tube; fistulous.

sy•rin•go•ma (sir″ing-go′mə) [*syring-* + *-oma*] 1. a benign adnexal adenoma originating from an eccrine duct and consisting of dilated cystic duct segments in a fibrous stroma. Syringomas occur as multiple, small, flesh-colored papules on the face, neck, and upper chest, most often in postpubertal females. 2. syringocystadenoma.

chondroid s. a usually benign tumor originating in the sweat glands, occurring as a solitary, firm, deep-seated intradermal or subcutaneous nodule on the head or neck, and characterized by ductal and glandular proliferation.

eruptive s. a condition in which syringomas arise in large numbers in successive crops, usually on the anterior trunk or abdomen. Called also *eruptive hidradenoma.*

sy•rin•go•my•elia (sĭ-ring″go-mi-e′le-ə) [*syringo-* + *myel-* + *-ia*] a slowly progressive syndrome of cavitation in the central segments of the spinal cord, generally in the cervical region, but sometimes extending up into the medulla oblongata *(syringobulbia)* or down into the thoracic region; it may be of developmental origin, arise secondary to tumor, trauma, infarction, or hemorrhage, or be of unknown cause. It results in neurologic deficits, usually segmental muscular weakness and atrophy with a dissociated sensory loss (loss of pain and temperature sensation, with preservation of the sense of touch), and thoracic scoliosis is often present. Sometimes the use of the term *syringomyelia* is restricted to this condition, with the terms *segmental sensory dissociation with brachial muscular atrophy* and *syndrome of sensory dissociation with brachial amyotrophy* being used for a similar condition that may be associated with other pathological lesions or states. Called also *cavitary myelitis, hydrosyringomyelia, Morvan syndrome, syringomyelic syndrome,* and *syringomyelus.* See also *Morvan syndrome* (def. 2).

posttraumatic s., traumatic s. syringomyelia resulting from trauma.

sy•rin•go•my•elus (sĭ-ring″go-mi′ə-ləs) syringomyelia.

sy•rin•go•tome (sĭ-ring′go-tōm) fistulatome.

sy•rin•got•o•my (sir″in-got′ə-me) [*syringo-* + *-tomy*] incision of a fistula, particularly an anal fistula.

syr•inx (sir′inks) [Gr. "a pipe"] 1. a tube or pipe. 2. fistula. 3. the lower or posterior part of the trachea of birds in which vocal sounds are produced. 4. an abnormal cavity in the spinal cord in syringomyelia.

Syr•phi•dae (sir′phĭ-de) a family of flies, the hover flies, of the order Diptera, including the genera *Eristalis* and *Helophilus.*

syr•up (sir′əp) [L. *syrupus,* from Arabic *sharāb*] 1. a concentrated solution of a sugar, such as sucrose, in water or other aqueous liquid, sometimes with a medicinal agent added. 2. more generally, any liquid dosage form in a sweet and viscid vehicle, including oral suspensions. 3. [NF] a solution of sucrose in purified water, used as a flavored vehicle in pharmaceutical preparations.

acacia s. [NF] a preparation of powdered acacia, sodium benzoate, vanilla tincture, sucrose, and purified water, used as a flavored vehicle and demulcent for drugs.

aromatic eriodictyon s., aromatic yerba santa s. a solution of eriodictyon fluidextract, potassium hydroxide, compound cardamom tincture, sassafras oil, lemon oil, clove oil, alcohol, sucrose, and magnesium carbonate, in purified water; used as a vehicle for drugs.

cacao s. chocolate s.

cherry s. [NF] a mixture of cherry juice, sucrose, alcohol, and purified water, used as a flavored vehicle for drugs.

chocolate s. [NF] a preparation of chocolate, sucrose, liquid glucose, glycerin, sodium chloride, vanillin, sodium benzoate, and purified water; used as a flavored vehicle for drugs.

citric acid s. a preparation of lemon tincture, citric acid, and purified water, in syrup, used as a flavored vehicle for drugs.

cocoa s. chocolate s.

ipecac s. [USP] a preparation of powdered ipecac, glycerin, and syrup, used as an emetic.

lactulose s. see under *solution.*

medicated s. a syrup to which a medicinal substance has been added.

orange s. [NF] a syrup prepared from sweet orange peel tincture, citric acid, talc, and sucrose, in purified water, used as a flavored vehicle for drugs.

raspberry s. a syrup consisting of raspberry juice, sucrose, and alcohol, in purified water, used as a flavored vehicle for drugs.

senna s. [USP] a syrup prepared from senna fluidextract, sucrose, suitable essential oils, and purified water; used as a cathartic.

simple s. syrup (def. 3).

s. of tolu, tolu balsam s. a mixture of tolu balsam tincture, magnesium carbonate, sucrose, and purified water; used as a flavored vehicle for drugs.

wild cherry s. a mixture of a percolate of wild cherry, glycerin, sucrose, alcohol, and water; used as a flavored vehicle, chiefly for cough syrups.

sys•sar•co•sis (sis″ahr-ko′sis) [*syn-* + *sarc-* + *-osis*] the union or connection of bones by means of muscle, as the connection between the hyoid bone and the mandible, the scapula, and the breast bone. **sysarco′sic, syssarcot′ic** *adj*

sys•so•mus (sĭ-so′məs) [Gr. *syn* with + *sōma* body] conjoined twins with two heads and with the bodies united. Cf. *dicephalus.*

sys•tal•tic (sis-tawl′tik) [Gr. *systaltikos* drawing together] alternately contracting and expanding; pulsating.

sys•tat•ic (sis-tat′ik) affecting several of the sensory faculties at the same time.

sys•tem (sis′təm) [Gr. *systēma* a complex or organized whole] a set or series of interconnected or interdependent parts or entities (objects, organs, or organisms) that function together in a common purpose or produce results impossible to achieve by one of them acting or operating alone.

System

AJCC s. a method of staging malignant tumors proposed by the American Joint Committee on Cancer, based on TNM staging; it divides cancers into five stages.
alimentary s. systema digestorium.
anterolateral s. lemniscus spinalis.
APUD s. neuroendocrine s.
arc guidance s. an apparatus used in stereotactic surgery consisting of a metal arc-shaped band or bar with degree markings and an attachment for an electrode that is positioned by moving through the arc to aim at a precise location in the brain. Cf. *arc-quadrant.*
articular s. juncturae; see *junctura* (def. 2).
association s. the cortex and related tracts of fibers in the brain by means of which perceptions are associated and thought rendered possible.
auditory s. the series of structures by which sounds are received from the environment and conveyed as signals to the central nervous system; it consists of the external, middle, and internal ear as well as the tracts in the auditory pathways.
autonomic nervous s. the portion of the nervous system concerned with regulation of the activity of cardiac muscle, smooth muscle, and glandular epithelium; usually restricted to the two visceral efferent peripheral components, the sympathetic nervous system and the parasympathetic nervous system. Called also *divisio autonomica systematis nervosi peripherici* [TA], *pars autonomica systematis nervosi peripherici* [TA alternative], *visceral nervous system, autonomic division of peripheral nervous system,* and *autonomic part of peripheral nervous system.* See Plate 42.
Bethesda S. a classification of cervical and vaginal cytology that provides a standardized nomenclature for cytopathologic diagnosis of diseases of the cervix and vagina. it encompasses three elements: comment on the adequacy of the specimen, a general categorization of the specimen, and a descriptive diagnosis.
biological s. a system composed of living material; such systems range from a collection of separate molecules to an assemblage of separate organisms.
blood group s. blood group.
blood-vascular s. the blood vessels of the body; see *circulatory s.*
brain cooling s. thermoregulated equipment for sensing and controlling brain temperature in neurophysiological and neuropsychological applications.
buffer s. see *buffer.*
cardiovascular s. the heart and blood vessels, by which blood is pumped and circulated through the body. Called also *systema cardiovasculare* [TA].
case s. a method of teaching based on the logical analysis of, and deductions formed from, reported cases of disease.
CD s. [*c*luster *d*esignation] a system for classifying cell-surface markers expressed by lymphocytes based on a computer analysis of monoclonal antibodies against human leukocyte antigens, with antibodies having similar specificity characteristics being grouped together and assigned a number (CD1, CD2, CD3, etc.); these CD numbers are also applied to the specific antigens recognized by the various groups of monoclonal antibodies. See also *CD antigen,* under *antigen.*
cell-free s. a subcellular fraction that retains biologic function, created in vitro in order to study cellular processes in isolation. Called also *cell-free extract.*
centimeter-gram-second s. (CGS, cgs) a system of measurements in which the units are based on the centimeter as the unit of length, the gram as the unit of mass, and the second as the unit of time.
central nervous s. (CNS) the part of the nervous system consisting of the brain and spinal cord. In TA terminology, called *pars centralis systematis nervosi.* See Plates 9 and 10.
centrencephalic s. the system of neurons located in the central core of the upper brainstem from the thalamus down to the medulla oblongata, and connecting the two hemispheres of the brain.
chemoreceptor s. the system of body structures, principally the carotid, para-aortic, and tympanic bodies, that respond to variations in oxygen tension and carbon dioxide tension of the blood and may play a role in the regulation of respiration.
chromaffin s. the chromaffin cells of the body considered collectively; see under *cell.*
circulatory s. the cardiovascular and lymphatic systems considered together. However, the term is occasionally used to denote one of the systems only, particularly the former.
collecting s. a group of renal calices and its pelvis considered as a unit.
colloid s., colloidal s. see *colloid* (def. 2).
complement s. see *complement.*
conducting s. of heart, conduction s. of heart, conductive s. of heart complexus stimulans cordis.
coordinate s. a method by which a point, a line, a plane, or a geometric solid can be located in space by a set of numbers.
dentinal s. all the tubules radiating from a single pulp cavity.
dermal s. integumentum commune.
digestive s. systema digestorium.
dioptric s. a system of lenses or of different media for refracting light.
disperse s., dispersion s. a colloid system; see *colloid* (def. 2).
dosimetric s. a regular and determinate system of administration of a therapeutic agent.
double collecting s., duplex collecting s. a collecting system involving a double ureter; there may be either a duplex kidney or an ectopic kidney.
ecological s. see *ecosystem.*
endocrine s. the system of glands and other structures that elaborate internal secretions (hormones) that are released directly into the circulatory system, and also elaborate paracrine, autocrine, and possibly intracrine regulators that are not released to the blood stream, all of which influence metabolism and other body processes. It includes organs such as the hypothalamus, pituitary, thyroid, parathyroids, adrenal glands, gonads, pancreas, paraganglia, and pineal body; the intestines and the lung also secrete substances that have hormonal functions. See Plate 17.
endothelial s. see *reticuloendothelial s.*
enteric nervous s. the plexus entericus, sometimes considered separately from the autonomic nervous system because it has independent local reflex activity.
exteroceptive nervous s. the part of the afferent elements of the somatic nervous system that is sensitive to stimuli originating outside the body.
extracorticospinal s. extrapyramidal s.
extralemniscal s. a group of multisynaptic pathways in the spinothalamic tracts, projecting to the intralaminar nuclei of the thalamus.
extrapyramidal s. an imprecise term referring to a functional rather than an anatomical part of the central nervous system that controls motor activities and is not part of the pyramidal tract; it includes the corpus striatum, subthalamic nucleus, substantia nigra, and red nucleus along with their interconnections with the reticular formation, cerebrum, and cerebellum; they control and coordinate especially the postural, static, supporting, and locomotor mechanisms. Since the term is imprecise and applies literally to all structures outside the corticospinal system, it has largely fallen into disuse. Called also *extracorticospinal s.* or *tract* and *extrapyramidal tract.*
FDI tooth numbering s. *[Fédération Dentaire Internationale]* a tooth numbering system that uses two digits to identify each tooth. The first digit denotes the quadrant, with the numerals 1 through 4 used for the permanent teeth and 5 through 8 used for the primary teeth; the second denotes tooth position within the quadrant, numbering from the midline posteriorly. See illustration at *tooth number,* under *number,* and see also *International Standards Organization S. for Teeth.*
Frank lead s. in spatial vectorcardiography, the most commonly used corrected system of orthogonal leads, consisting of seven electrodes placed and connected to form leads X, Y, and Z, which describe the transverse, vertical, and sagittal planes, respectively. See also *spatial vectorcardiography,* under *vectorcardiography.*
genital s., female systema genitale femininum.
genital s., male systema genitale masculinum.
genitourinary s. urogenital s.
glandular s. the glandular tissue of the body considered collectively.
glycine cleavage s. a group of four mitochondrial enzymes, designated P, H, T, and L, that together catalyze the conversion of glycine to CO_2 and a one-carbon unit that can be transferred to tetrahydrofolate. Deficiency of one or more of the proteins, an autosomal recessive trait, results in nonketotic hyperglycinemia.
haversian s. a haversian canal and its concentrically arranged lamellae, constituting the basic unit of structure of compact bone; see *osteon.*

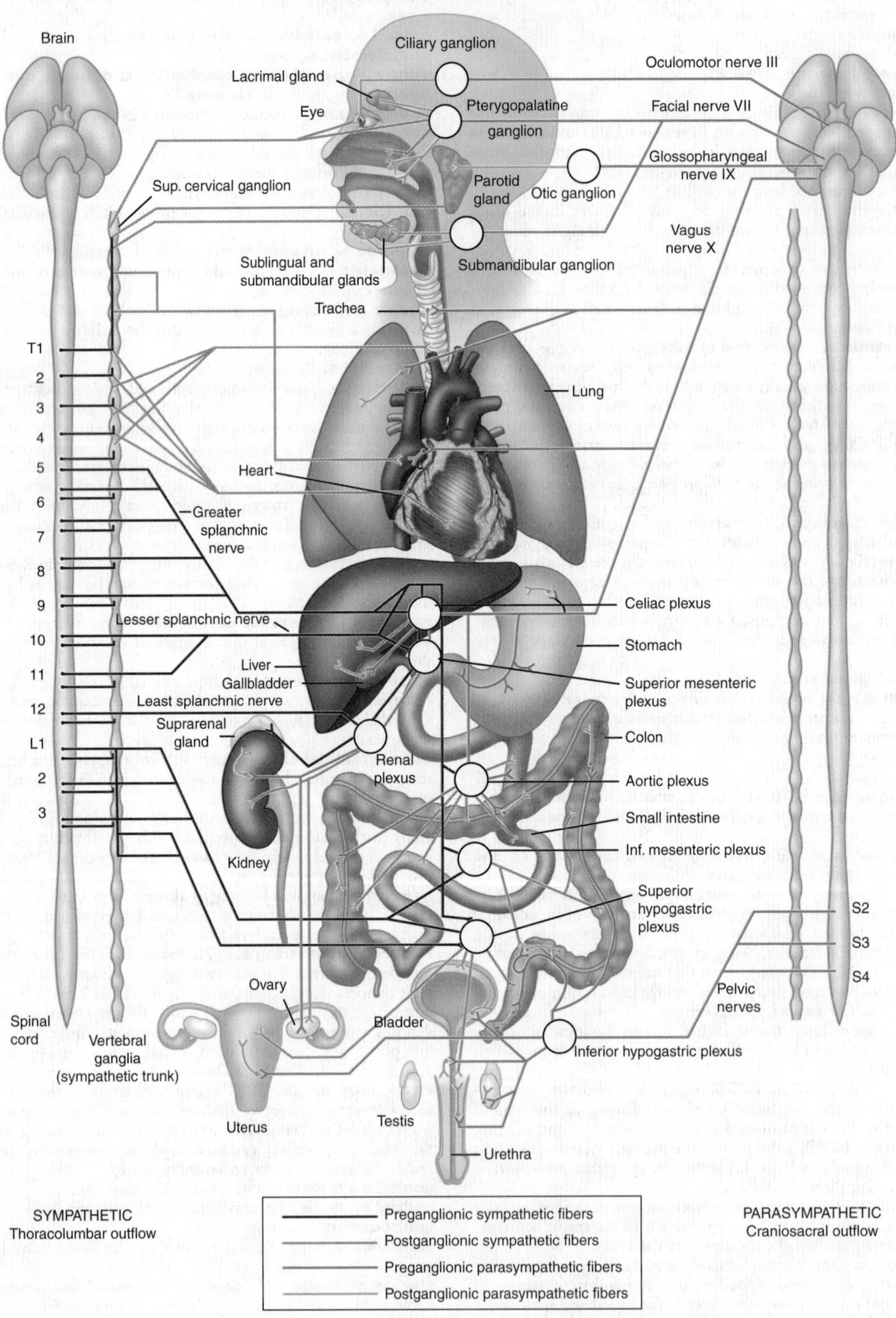

■ **PLATE 42—AUTONOMIC NERVOUS SYSTEM**

hematopoietic s. the tissues concerned in production of the blood, including the bone marrow, liver, lymph nodes, spleen, and thymus. See also *hematopoiesis.*
heterogeneous s. a system or structure made up of mechanically separable parts, as an emulsion.
hexaxial reference s. a series of lines used in electrocardiography to describe the potentials of the heart in the frontal plane by diagramming vectors that represent the standard bipolar limb leads and the augmented unipolar limb leads. See illustration.
His-Purkinje s. a portion of the conducting system of the heart (systema conducens cordis), usually referring specifically to the segment beginning with the bundle of His and ending at the terminus of the Purkinje fiber network within the ventricles.
homogeneous s. a system or structure made up of parts that cannot be mechanically separated, as a solution.
humoral amplification s's a collective term for the four enzyme cascades that serve as amplification and control mechanisms in hemostasis, inflammation, and tissue repair, including the complement, coagulation, fibrinolytic, and kinin systems.
hypophyseoportal s., hypophysioportal s. hypothalamo-hypophysial portal s.
hypothalamic hypophysial portal s., hypothalamic-pituitary s., hypothalamic-pituitary portal s. hypothalamo-hypophysial portal s.
hypothalamo-hypophysial portal s. the venules connecting the capillaries (gomitoli) in the median eminence of the hypothalamus with the sinusoidal capillaries of the adenohypophysis. See *venae portales hypophysiales.* Called also *hypophysial portal* or *hypophysioportal circulation, hypothalamic hypophysial portal s., hypothalamic-pituitary s.,* and *pituitary portal s.*
immune s. a complex system of cellular and molecular components having the primary function of distinguishing self from nonself and defense against foreign organisms or substances. The primary cellular components are lymphocytes and macrophages, and the primary molecular components are antibodies and lymphokines; granulocytes and the complement system are also involved in immune responses but are not always considered part of the immune system per se.
integumentary s. integumentum commune.
International Standards Organization S. for Teeth a tooth numbering system based on the Fédération Dentaire Internationale system (q.v.) and adding also two-digit numbering denoting areas of the oral cavity and letters designating surfaces of the teeth. Called also *ISO s.*
International S. of Units see *SI unit,* under *unit.*
interoceptive nervous s. the system that transmits afferent impulses from viscera by fibers that run centrally in either autonomic or somatic nerves.
interstitial s. see under *lamella.*
involuntary nervous s. autonomic nervous s.
ISO s. International Standards Organization S. for Teeth.

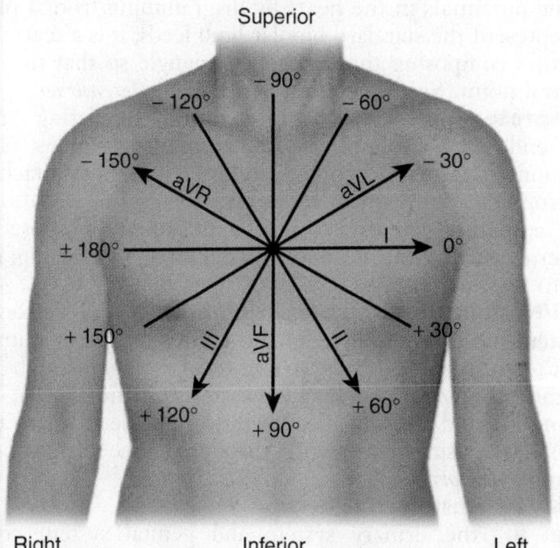

■ Hexaxial reference system and axes of deviation. The triaxial reference system comprises the vectors I, II, and III (standard dipolar limb leads) only.

kallikrein s. kinin s.
keratinizing s. the cells composing the bulk of the epithelium of the epidermis; they are of ectodermal origin and undergo death and keratinization to form the stratum corneum.
kinin s. the system of proteins involved in the production and destruction of kinins such as bradykinin and kallidin. Kinins are cleaved from precursor substances called kininogens by kallikreins and are rapidly destroyed by kininases. Plasma kallikrein circulates as a proenzyme called prekallikrein and is converted to active form by factor XIIa, which cleaves HMW kininogen, an α_2-globulin, to produce bradykinin. Called also *kallikrein s.*
labyrinthine s. the parts of the vestibulocochlear organ concerned with hearing and the maintenance of equilibrium.
lemniscal s. an oligosynaptic pathway in the ventral spinothalamic tract, projecting to the ventral posterolateral and ventral mediolateral nuclei of the thalamus.
limbic s. a term loosely applied to a group of brain structures common to all mammals (including the hippocampus and dentate gyrus with their archaeocortex, the cingulate gyrus and septal areas, and the amygdala), associated with olfaction but of greater importance in other activities, such as autonomic functions and certain aspects of emotion and behavior; see also *rhinencephalon.*
locomotor s. the structures in a living organism responsible for locomotion; in humans these consist of the muscles, joints, and ligaments of the lower limbs as well as the arteries and nerves that supply them.
lymphatic s., lymphoid s. the lymphatic vessels and lymphoid tissue considered collectively. Called also *systema lymphoideum* [TA].
lymphoreticular s. the tissues of the lymphatic (lymphoid) and reticuloendothelial systems considered together as one system; see also lymphoreticular disorders, under *disorder.*
macrophage s. mononuclear phagocyte s.
masticatory s. see under *apparatus.*
mastigont s. an ultrastructural complex characteristic of mastigophorans, comprising all of the organelles associated with the flagella, including basal bodies, axostyle, and Golgi body; it may or may not be associated with a nucleus (see also *karyomastigont* and *akaryomastigont*).
melanocyte s. pigmentary s.
mesocortical s. dopaminergic nerve fibers originating in the ventral tegmental area and projecting to the prefrontal cortex; important in cognition and stimulus processing.
mesolimbic s. dopaminergic nerve fibers originating in the ventral tegmental area and projecting to various structures of the limbic system; important in memory, stimulus processing, and motivation.
meter-kilogram-second s. (MKS) a system of measurements in which the units are based on the meter as the unit of length, the kilogram as the unit of mass, and the second as the unit of time.
metric s. a decimal system of weights and measures based on the meter. See also *SI unit,* under *unit,* and see Appendix 7.
mononuclear phagocyte s. (MPS) the collection of cells consisting of macrophages and their precursors (blood monocytes and their precursor cells in bone marrow). The term has been proposed as a replacement for reticuloendothelial system, which does not include all macrophages and does include other unrelated cell types. Called also *macrophage s.* See also *macrophage.*
muscular s. musculi; see *musculus* (def. 2).
musculoskeletal s. the muscles (muscular system) and bones (skeletal system) of the body considered as one unit.
nervous s. the organ system which, along with the endocrine system, correlates the adjustments and reactions of an organism to internal and environmental conditions. It comprises the central and peripheral nervous systems: the former is composed of the brain and spinal cord, and the latter includes all the other neural elements. Called also *systema nervosum* [TA]. See also *central nervous s., peripheral nervous s.,* and *autonomic nervous s.*
neuroendocrine s. the APUD cells considered as a system, having endocrine effects on the structures of the central and peripheral nervous systems. Called also *APUD s.*
orthogonal lead s. a system for placing the electrocardiographic leads in spatial vectorcardiography so that ideally the three leads used are mutually perpendicular, each is parallel to one of the rectilinear coordinates of the body, and each is of equal amplitude vectorially. In corrected systems, the lead vectors also retain the same magnitude

and direction for all points of cardiac electromotive force generation. See also *Frank lead s.*
Palmer tooth notation s. a tooth numbering system in which each quadrant is designated 1 through 8 (permanent teeth) or A through E (primary teeth), working from the midline laterally, with the quadrant specified by a bracket made up of a combination of a vertical and a horizontal line that is specific to each quadrant. See illustration at *tooth number*, under *number*.
parasympathetic nervous s. the craniosacral division of the autonomic nervous system, its preganglionic fibers traveling with cranial nerves III, VII, IX, and X, and with the second to fourth sacral ventral roots; it innervates the heart, the smooth muscle and glands of the head and neck, and the thoracic, abdominal, and pelvic viscera. The ganglion cells with which these fibers synapse are in or near the organs innervated. In TA terminology, called *pars parasympathica divisionis autonomici systematis nervosi.* Called also *craniosacral division* and *craniosacral part of autonomic nervous system.* See Plate 42.
pelvicalyceal s. collecting s.
peripheral nervous s. (PNS) the part of the nervous system consisting of nerves and ganglia outside the brain and spinal cord. In TA terminology, called *pars peripherica systematis nervosi.* See Plates 33 to 38.
periventricular s. collective name for the efferent pathways of the hypothalamus that arise mainly in the supraoptic, posterior, and tuberal nuclei and descend in the periventricular gray matter.
pigmentary s. the melanocytes, collectively.
pituitary portal s. hypothalamo-hypophysial portal s.
plenum s. a system of ventilation based on the mechanical propulsion of air into the room.
portal s. an arrangement of vessels whereby blood collected from one set of capillaries passes through a large vessel or vessels and then through a second set of capillaries before it returns to the systemic circulation, such as in the hepatic portal circulation and the hypothalamo-hypophysial portal system.
properdin s. former name for the *alternative complement pathway.*
proprioceptive nervous s. the portion of the afferent elements of the somatic nervous system that is sensitive to stimuli originating inside the body (from muscles, bones, joints, and ligaments).
Purkinje s. a portion of the conducting system of the heart (systema conducens cordis), usually referring specifically to the Purkinje network (rami subendocardiales).
pyelocalyceal s. collecting s.
pyramidal s. tractus pyramidalis (def. 1).
renin-angiotensin s. (RAS), renin-angiotensin-aldosterone s. (RAAS) the regulation of sodium balance, fluid volume, and blood pressure by renal secretions: in response to reduced perfusion, renin is secreted, which hydrolyzes a plasma globulin to release angiotensin I, which is rapidly hydrolyzed to angiotensin II; this in turn stimulates aldosterone secretion, which brings about sodium retention, increase in blood pressure, and restoration of renal perfusion, which shuts off the signal for renin release.
respiratory s. the tubular and cavernous organs and structures by means of which pulmonary ventilation and gas exchange between ambient air and the blood are brought about; the chief organs involved are the nose, larynx, trachea, bronchi, bronchioles, and lungs. Called also *systema respiratorium* [TA] and *respiratory apparatus* or *tract.* See Plate 43.
reticular activating s. (RAS) the system of cells of the reticular formation of the medulla oblongata that receive collaterals from the ascending sensory pathways and project to higher centers; they control the overall degree of central nervous system activity, including wakefulness, attentiveness, and sleep.
reticuloendothelial s. (RES) a group of cells having the ability to take up and sequester inert particles and vital dyes; it includes macrophages and macrophage precursors; specialized endothelial cells lining the sinusoids of the liver, spleen, and bone marrow; and reticular cells of lymphatic tissue (macrophages) and of bone marrow (fibroblasts). See also *mononuclear phagocyte s.*
sensory storage s. the shortest type of memory, maintaining for less than a second briefly perceived stimuli; see *echoic memory* and *iconic memory*, under *memory*.
SI s. see under *unit.*
skeletal s. ossa; see *os*[2] (def. 2).
somatic nervous s. the parts of the peripheral nervous system that are concerned with the transmission of impulses to and from the nonvisceral components of the body, such as the skeletal muscles, bones, joints, ligaments, skin, and eye and ear. Called also *voluntary nervous s.*
stomatognathic s. the structures of the mouth and jaws, considered collectively, as they subserve the functions of mastication, deglutition, respiration, and speech. See also *masticatory apparatus*, under *apparatus.*
stress s. the parts of the neuroendocrine system that mediate the physiologic changes that occur in response to stress; they include the corticotropin-releasing hormone–secreting neurons in the hypothalamus and noradrenergic neurons in the brainstem, the hypothalamic-pituitary-adrenal axis, and the peripheral and autonomic nervous systems.
superficial musculoaponeurotic s. superficial fascia of the head and neck, tissue important in the making of facial expressions and commonly manipulated in plastic surgery.
sympathetic nervous s. (SNS) the portion of the autonomic nervous system that receives its fibers of connection with the central nervous system through the thoracolumbar outflow of visceral efferent fibers. These fibers (preganglionic fibers) arise from cells in the thoracic and upper lumbar levels of the spinal cord, leave by way of ventral roots, and, by way of rami communicantes, enter sympathetic trunks, where some synapse with ganglion cells. Distal to these ganglia, there are postganglionic fibers that either return to spinal nerves by way of rami communicantes to supply blood vessels, smooth muscles, and glands of the trunk and limbs, or go as visceral branches to blood vessels, smooth muscles, glands of the head and neck, and viscera of the thorax, abdomen, and pelvis. Some preganglionic fibers pass through the sympathetic trunks and synapse in the prevertebral ganglia; postganglionic fibers from those ganglia supply adjacent viscera. In TA terminology, called *pars sympathica divisionis autonomici systematis nervosi.* Called also *thoracolumbar division* and *thoracolumbar part of autonomic nervous system.* See Plate 42.
T s. a system of transverse tubular invaginations *(T,* or *transverse, tubules)* of the sarcolemma, each of which penetrates deep into the muscle fiber. In mammalian skeletal muscle, they are located at the junction of the A band with the I band, and in mammalian cardiac muscle at the level of the Z band; the system plays a role in the excitation and relaxation of muscle and provides an important additional surface for the exchange of metabolites between muscle and the extracellular space. Called also *triad s.* See also *triad of skeletal muscle; terminal cisterns,* under *cistern;* and *T tubule,* under *tubule.*
tooth numbering s. any of several systems used to uniquely identify individual teeth by position in the jaw; see *Fédération Dentaire Internationale tooth numbering s., International Standards Organization S. for Teeth, Palmer tooth notation s.,* and *Universal Numbering S.*
transdermal delivery s. any means by which a drug is applied to the surface of the skin for transdermal absorption, such as a transdermal patch.
triad s. T s.
triaxial reference s. a series of lines used in electrocardiography to describe the potentials in the heart by diagramming frontal plane vectors that represent the standard bipolar limb leads; it is a rearrangement of the vectors composing the Einthoven triangle so that they bisect a single central point. See illustration at *hexaxial reference s.*
ubiquitin-proteasome s. a mechanism regulating receptor-mediated endocytosis of selected membrane proteins, involving ubiquitination of targeted proteins followed by their attachment to the proteasome and subsequent internalization and degradation.
UICC s. a method of staging malignant tumors proposed by the Union Internationale Contre Cancer, based on TNM staging; it divides cancers into five stages.
Universal/National S., Universal Numbering S. the tooth numbering system most widely used in the United States; it numbers the permanent teeth from 1 (maxillary right third molar) through 32 (mandibular right third molar), working leftward across the maxilla, dropping to the mandible and working back rightward. The primary teeth are denoted similarly, using the letters A through T. See illustration at *tooth number*, under *number*.
urinary s. systema urinarium.
urogenital s. the urinary system and genital system considered together; see *systema urinaria, systema genitale femininum,* and *systema genitale masculinum.* See Plate 44.

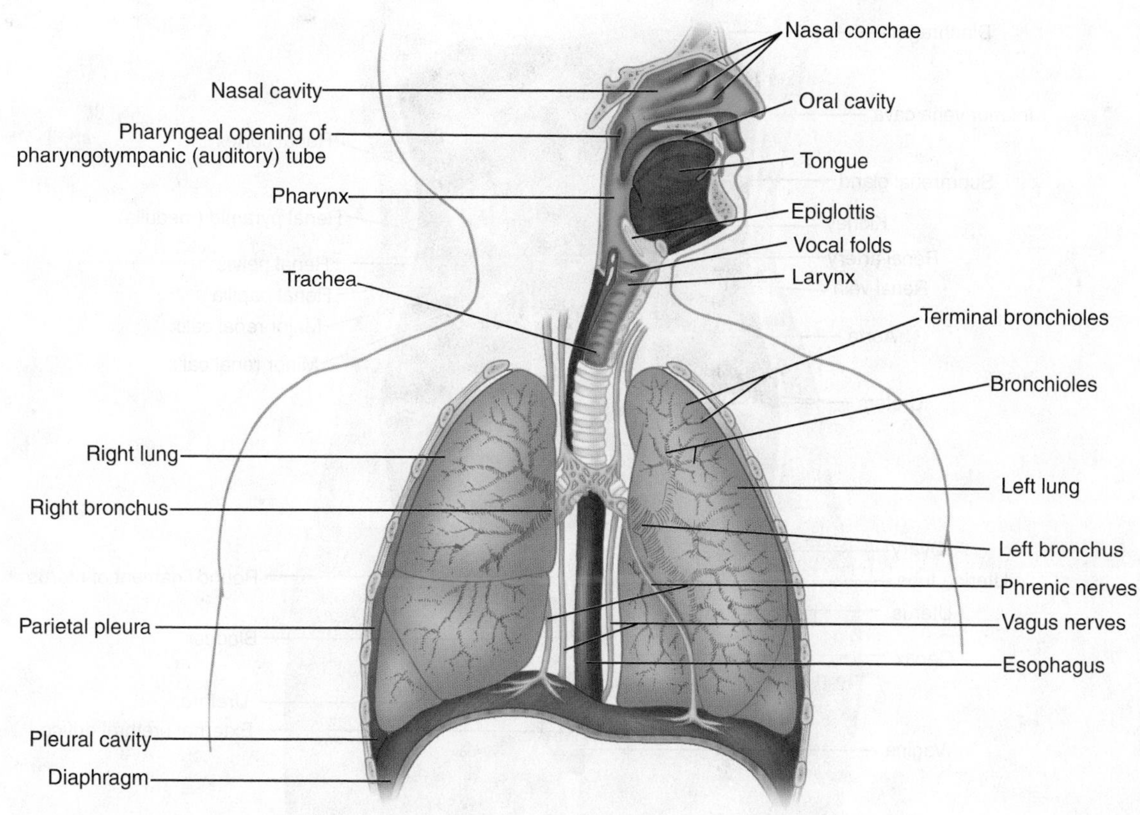

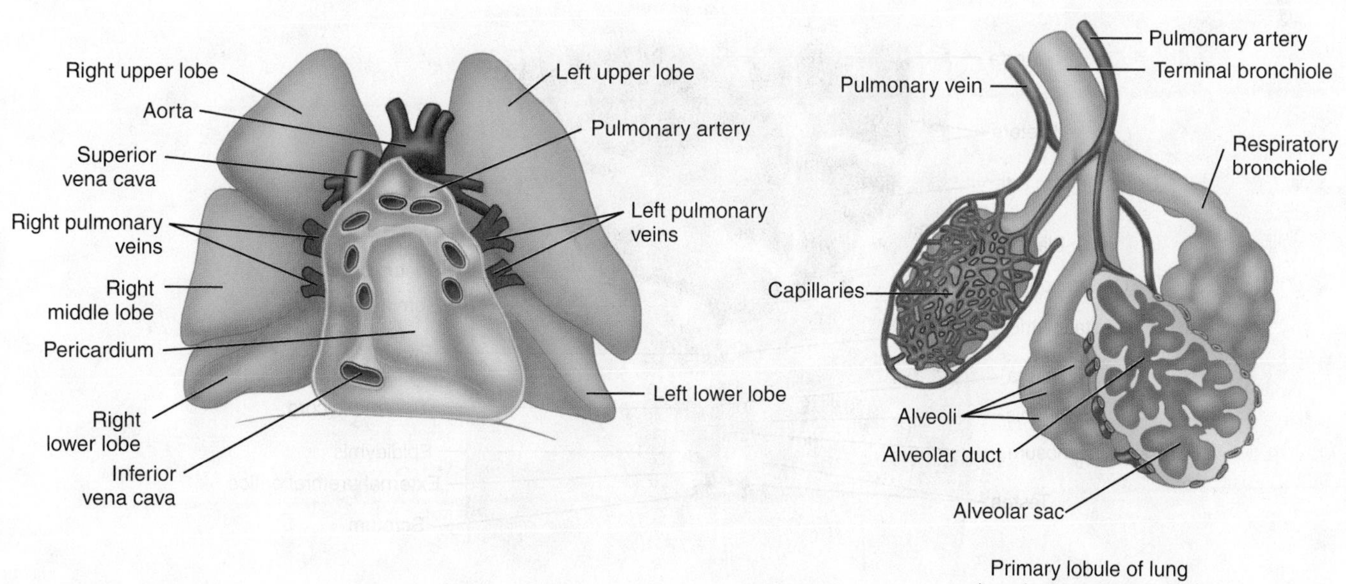

■ **PLATE 43**—ORGANS OF THE RESPIRATORY SYSTEM

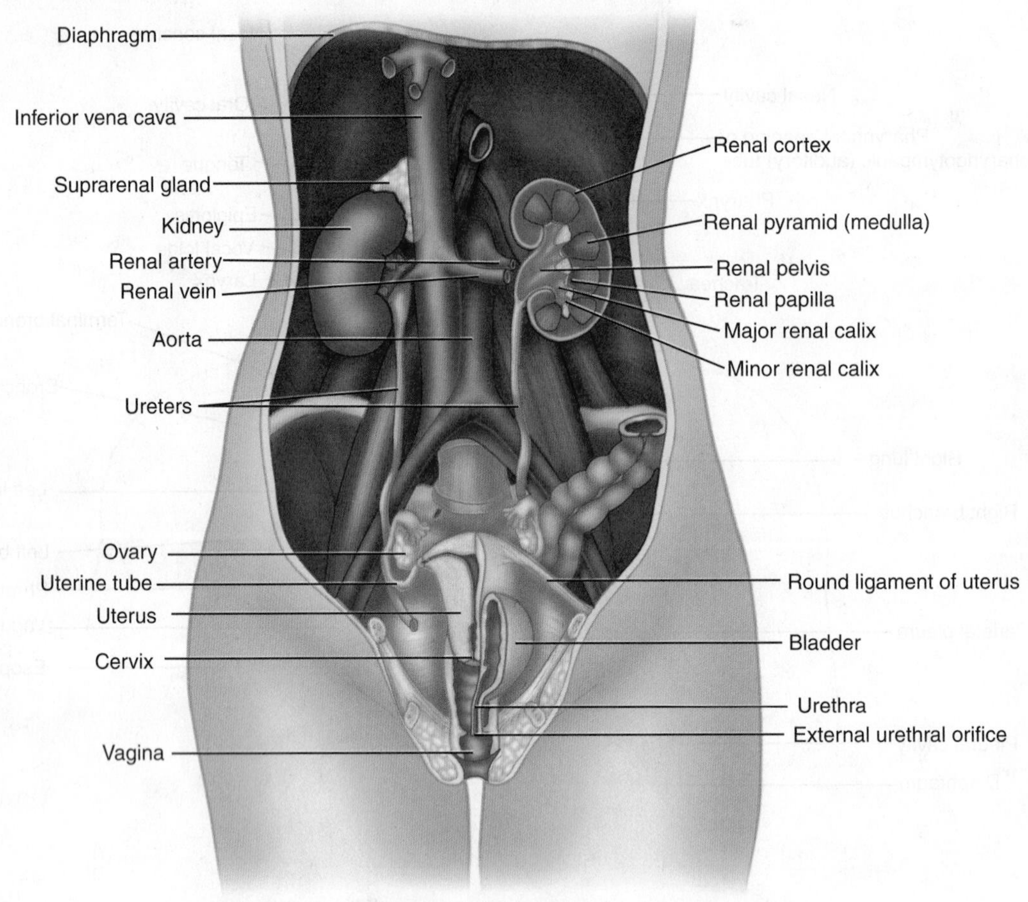

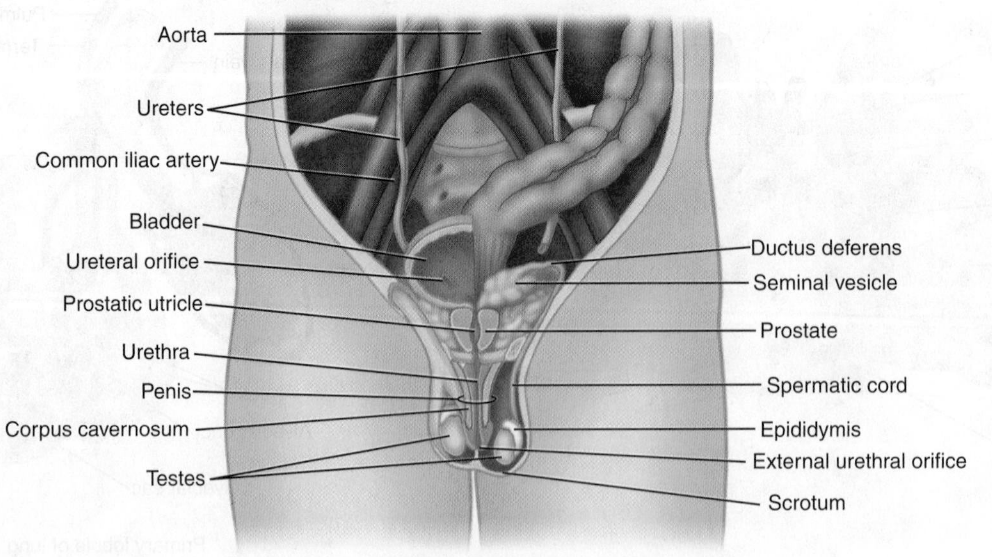

■ **PLATE 44**—ORGANS OF THE UROGENITAL SYSTEM

System *Continued*

vascular s. the blood and lymphatic vessels of the body and all their ramifications, considered collectively. The term is sometimes used specifically to denote either the blood or lymphatic vessels and their respective ramifications, particularly the former.
vestibular s. the bodily structures connected with receiving and processing sensations of the sense of equilibrium; they include the vestibular labyrinths, the sensory pathways of the vestibular nerves, and the vestibular nuclei.
visceral nervous s. autonomic nervous s.
visual s. the series of structures by which visual sensations are received from the environment and conveyed as signals to the central nervous system; it consists of the photoreceptors in the retina and the afferent fibers in the optic nerve, chiasm, and tract.
voluntary nervous s. somatic nervous s.

sys•te•ma (sis-te′mə) [Gr. *systēma* a complex or organized whole] system: a series of interconnected or interdependent organs which together accomplish a specific function.
s. articula′re TA alternative for *juncturae;* see *junctura* (def. 2).
s. cardiovascula′re [TA] official terminology for *cardiovascular system;* see under *system.*
s. condu′cens cor′dis TA alternative for *complexus stimulans cordis.*
s. digesto′rium [TA] digestive system: the organs associated with the ingestion and digestion of food, including the mouth and associated structures, pharynx, and components of the digestive tube, as well as the associated organs and glands. See also *digestive tract,* under *tract.* Called also *alimentary system.*
syste′mata genita′lia [TA] the male and female genital systems considered together; see *s. genitale masculinum* and *s. genitale femininum.*
s. genita′le femini′num [TA] female genital system: the internal and external reproductive organs in the female; see *organa genitalia feminina interna* and *organa genitalia feminina externa,* under *organum.*
s. genita′le masculi′num [TA] male genital system: the internal and external reproductive organs in the male; see *organa genitalia masculina interna* and *organa genitalia masculina externa.*
s. lymphoi′deum [TA] official terminology for *lymphatic system;* see under *system.*
s. muscula′re TA alternative for *musculi;* see *musculus* (def. 2).
s. nervo′sum [TA] the nervous system: the chief organ system that correlates the adjustments and reactions of the organism to internal and environmental conditions; see under *system.*
s. nervo′sum centra′le TA alternative for *pars centralis systematis nervosi.*
s. nervo′sum periphe′ricum TA alternative for *pars peripherica systematis nervosi.*
s. respirato′rium [TA] official terminology for *respiratory system;* see under *system.*
s. skeleta′le TA alternative for *ossa;* see *os*[2] (def. 2).
s. urina′rium [TA] urinary system: the organs and passageways concerned with the production and excretion of urine, including the kidneys, ureters, urinary bladder, and urethra.

sys•te•mat•ic (sis″tə-mat′ik) [Gr. *systēmatikos*] pertaining or according to a system.

sys•tem•a•ti•za•tion (sis-tem″ə-tĭ-za′shən) arrangement according to a system. In psychiatry, the arrangement of ideas into a logical sequence, or of delusions into a superficially coherent system.

sys•te•ma•tol•o•gy (sis″tə-mə-tol′ə-je) [*system* + *-logy*] the science of classification.

sys•tème sé•cant (sis-tem′ sa-kahn′) [Fr. "cutting system"] one of the suture lines seen in ciliate protozoa where fields of kineties from different body areas converge.

sys•tem•ic (sis-tem′ik) pertaining to or affecting the body as a whole.

sys•te•moid (sis′tə-moid) [*system* + *-oid*] 1. resembling a system. 2. denoting tumors made up of various kinds of tissue.

sys•to•le (sis′to-le) [Gr. *systolē* a drawing together, contraction] the contraction, or period of contraction, of the heart, especially that of the ventricles; sometimes divided into components, as preejection and ejection periods, or isovolumic and ejection.
aborted s. a weak systole, usually premature, not associated with pulsation of a peripheral artery.
atrial s. the contraction of the atria by which blood is propelled from them into the ventricles.
electromechanical s. the interval from the onset of the QRS complex on the electrocardiogram to the aortic component of the second heart sound; it is one of the systolic time intervals (q.v.), encompassing the left ventricular ejection time and the preejection period, and is used to assess left ventricular performance. Symbol QS_2.
extra s. extrasystole.
premature s. extrasystole.
total electromechanical s. electromechanical s.
ventricular s. the contraction of the ventricles of the heart by which the blood is forced into the aorta and the pulmonary trunk.

sys•tol•ic (sis-tol′ik) 1. pertaining to or produced by systole. 2. occurring during systole.

sys•trem•ma (sis-trem′ə) [Gr. "anything twisted up together"] a cramp in the muscles of the calf.

Sy•to•bex (si′to-beks) trademark for preparations of cyanocobalamin.

Sy•zy•gi•um (sĭ-zĭ′je-əm) [Gr. *syzygos* yoked together] a genus of tropical trees of the family Myrtaceae. *S. aroma′ticum* (called also *Eugenia caryophyllus*) is the clove, a species with aromatic flowers that yields the spice clove as well as clove oil.

sy•zy•gi•um (sĭ-zĭ′je-əm) syzygy.

syz•y•gy (siz′ĭ-je) [Gr. *syzygos* yoked together] the conjunction and fusion of organs without loss of identity. **syzyg′ial** *adj*

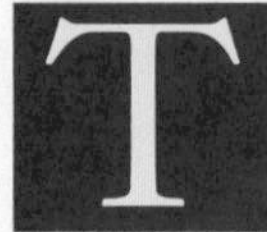

T tera-; tesla; tetanus toxoid; thoracic vertebrae (T1–T12); threonine; thymine or thymidine; triangulation number; intraocular tension (see under *pressure*). Normal intraocular tension is indicated by the symbol Tn.

T absolute temperature; transmittance; twisting number.

$T_{1/2}$ half-life; half-time.

T_1 tricuspid valve closure; see *first heart sound*, under *sound*.

T_3 triiodothyronine.

T_4 thyroxine.

T_m melting temperature; transport (or tubular) maximum.

2,4,5-T a toxic herbicide (2,4,5-trichlorophenoxyacetic acid) that acts as a growth-regulating hormone killing broadleaf plants by overstimulation.

T-1824 Evans blue.

t translocation.

t time; temperature (measured on a customary scale). See *t-test* under *test*.

$t_{1/2}$ half-life; half-time.

θ theta, the eighth letter of the Greek alphabet. Symbol for *angle* (def. 2).

τ tau, the nineteenth letter of the Greek alphabet. Symbol for *mean life* and *torque*.

TA *Terminologia Anatomica*; toxin-antitoxin.

Ta tantalum.

TAA tumor-associated antigen.

tab•a•co•sis (tab″ə-ko′sis) a form of pneumoconiosis seen in workers who cut up dried tobacco by hand and inhale tobacco dust.

tab•a•cum (tab′ə-kəm) [L., from Amerindian] tobacco.

tab•a•gism (tab′ə-jiz-əm) tobacco poisoning.

tab•a•nid (tab′ə-nid) any member of the family Tabanidae; called also *gadfly* or *gad fly* and *horsefly*.

Ta•ba•ni•dae (tə-ban′ĭ-de) the tabanids or horseflies, a family of insects that bite mammals to get blood. It includes the genera *Chrysops*, *Diachlorus*, *Goniops*, *Haematopota*, *Hybomitra*, *Silvius*, and *Tabanus*. Many species are vectors of disease.

Ta•ba•nus (tə-ba′nəs) [L. "gadfly"] a genus of biting, bloodsucking flies of the family Tabanidae, which transmit trypanosomes and anthrax.

T. atra′tus the common black horsefly of North America.

T. bovi′nus a species that attacks cattle in Asia, Africa, and South America.

T. ditaenia′tus, *T. fascia′tus*, *T. gra′tus* the Seroot fly of the Sudan, which bites mammals.

tab•ar•di•llo (tab″ər-de′yo) [Sp.] murine typhus.

ta•ba•tière ana•to•mique (tah-bah″te-ār′ ah-nah-to-mēk′) [Fr. "anatomical snuff box"] anatomical snuff box; see under *box*.

ta•bel•la (tə-bel′ə) pl. *tabel′lae* [L.] a medicated tablet or troche.

ta•bes (ta′bēz) [L. "wasting away, decay, melting"] 1. wasting of the body or a part of it. 2. t. dorsalis.

diabetic t. see under *pseudotabes*.

t. dorsa′lis parenchymatous neurosyphilis in which there is slowly progressive degeneration of the posterior columns and posterior roots and ganglia of the spinal cord, occurring 15 to 20 years after the initial infection of syphilis, characterized by lancinating lightning pains, urinary incontinence, ataxia, impaired position and vibratory sense, optic atrophy, hypotonia, hyperreflexia, and trophic joint degeneration (Charcot joints). Called also *Duchenne disease*, *locomotor ataxia*, and *tabetic neurosyphilis*.

t. ergo′tica a condition resembling tabes dorsalis, due to ergotism.

t. infan′tum tabes as seen in infants with congenital syphilis.

t. mesente′rica, t. mesara′ica tuberculosis of the mesenteric glands in children, resulting in digestive derangement and wasting of the body.

t. spina′lis t. dorsalis.

ta•bes•cent (tə-bes′ənt) [L. *tabescere* to waste away] wasting away; see *wasting*.

ta•bet•ic (tə-bet′ik) pertaining to or affected with tabes.

ta•bet•i•form (tə-bet′ĭ-form) resembling tabes.

tab•la•ture (tab′lə-chər) the separation of the chief cranial bones into inner and outer tables, which are separated by a diploë.

ta•ble (ta′bəl) [L. *tabula*] 1. a flat surface or layer. 2. an arrangement of data in rows and columns.

2 × 2 contingency t. a contingency table having two rows and two columns.

Aub-Dubois t. a table of normal basal metabolic rates for persons of various ages.

cohort life t. a table giving the survival data of a cohort of individuals in a clinical study or trial, i.e., the number alive and under observation (not lost to follow-up) at the beginning of each year, the number dying in each year, the number lost to follow-up each year, the conditional probability of survival for each year, and the cumulative probabilities of survival from the beginning of the study to the end of each year.

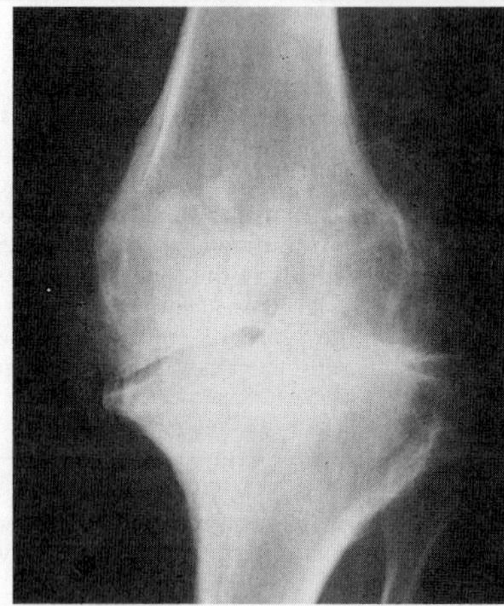

■ Advanced tabes dorsalis.

contingency t. a table used to display statistical data according to two characteristics, each having a number of mutually inclusive categories; categories of one characteristic are listed in rows and categories of the other characteristic are listed in columns. Statistical analysis (often using chi-squared or exact tests) can be readily applied to the rows and columns of the table. The most common is the *2 × 2 contingency t.*, having two rows and two columns. See also *r × c contingency t.*

external t. of calvaria lamina externa calvariae.

inner t. of calvaria lamina interna calvariae.

inner t. of frontal bone facies interna ossis frontalis.

internal t. of calvaria lamina interna calvariae.

life t. any of various tables describing mortality and survival data for groups of individuals at specific times or over defined intervals; tables may summarize combined mortality experience by age over a brief period or may follow a cohort over time *(cohort life t.)*. See also *survival curve*, under *curve*.

Mendeleev (Mendeléef, Mendeléeff) t. periodic t.

outer t. of calvaria lamina externa calvariae.

outer t. of frontal bone facies externa ossis frontalis.

periodic t. an ordering of all the known chemical elements in the form of a chart according to the periodic law, in which corresponding elements from the several periods form groups with similar properties; called also *Mendeleev t.*

***r* × *c* contingency t.** a contingency table having more than two categories for at least one of the variables of interest, *r* standing for the number of rows and *c* standing for the number of columns.

tilt t. a plinth, equipped with a footboard for support, to which a patient can be strapped for rotation to a nearly upright position; used in cases of spinal cord injury and other neurological disorders to enhance blood circulation to the lower limbs, improve posture, and aid in muscle training and sense of balance.

vitreous t. lamina interna calvariae.

water t. the upper surface of the impervious strata on which the ground water lies below the surface of the earth.

ta•ble•spoon (ta′bəl-spo͞on) a household unit of capacity, approximately equivalent to 4 fluid drams, or 15 milliliters.

tab•let (tab′lət) a solid dosage form of a medicinal substance, of varying weight, size, and shape, which may be molded or compressed. In addition to the active drug, it contains a diluent (or filler) and an excipient to give the mass adhesiveness, firmness, and plasticity, so that the tablet can be worked by hand or machine to the desired form. Called also *pill*.

buccal t. a small, flat, oval tablet to be held between the cheek and gum, permitting direct absorption through the oral mucosa of the medicinal substance contained therein.

dispensing t. a compressed or molded tablet containing a large quantity of a drug, used by dispensing pharmacists in compounding prescriptions.

enteric-coated t. a tablet coated with material that delays release of the medication until after it leaves the stomach.

hypodermic t. a tablet containing a medicinal substance to be dissolved in water for hypodermic injection.

sublingual t. a small, flat, oval tablet to be held beneath the tongue, permitting direct absorption of the medicinal substance contained therein.

t. triturate a small, usually cylindrical, molded disk containing a medicinal substance diluted with a mixture of lactose and powdered sucrose, in varying proportions, with a moistening agent.

Tab·loid (tab′loid) trademark for a preparation of thioguanine.

ta·boo (tă-boo′) [Tongan *tabu* forbidden, set apart] 1. any of the negative traditions, objects, or behaviors that are generally regarded as harmful to social welfare and are therefore prohibited. Cf. *mores.* 2. excluded from use; prohibited.

ta·bo·pa·ral·y·sis (ta″bo-pə-ral′ĭ-sis) taboparesis.

ta·bo·pa·re·sis (ta″bo-pə-re′sis) general paresis occurring concomitantly with tabes dorsalis; called also *taboparalysis.*

tab·u·lar (tab′u-lər) [L. *tabula* a board or table] resembling or shaped like a table.

ta·bun (ta′bən) an organophosphorus compound that is a potent cholinesterase inhibitor and is used as a nerve gas; symptoms of poisoning include bronchial constriction, convulsions, and often death. See *organophosphorus compound poisoning,* under *poisoning.*

TAC tetracaine, epinephrine (adrenaline), and cocaine (see under *solution*); trigeminal autonomic cephalalgia.

tache (tahsh) [Fr.] spot.

t. cérébrale (sa-ra-brahl′) ["cerebral spot"] a congested streak produced by drawing the nail across the skin, seen in various neurological diseases. Called also *Trousseau sign* and *meningitic streak* or *stria.*

t. noire (nwahr) ["black spot"] an ulcer covered with a black adherent crust, a characteristic local reaction occurring at the presumed site of the infective bite in certain tick-borne rickettsioses, such as scrub typhus or boutonneuse fever.

ta·chis·to·scope (tə-kis′kə-skōp) [Gr. *tachistos* swiftest + *-scope*] a device used in physiological psychology to demonstrate iconic memory; it displays images for controlled times, usually less than one-tenth of a second.

tach(o)- [Gr. *tachos* speed] a combining form denoting relationship to speed.

tacho·gram (tak′o-gram) [*tacho-* + *-gram*] a graphic record of the movement and velocity of the blood current.

tach·og·ra·phy (tə-kog′rə-fe) [*tacho-* + *-graphy*] the recording of the speed of the blood current.

tachy- [Gr. *tachys* swift] a combining form meaning swift or rapid.

tachy·al·i·men·ta·tion (tak″e-al″ĭ-mən-ta′shən) [*tachy-* + *alimentation*] a complication of the dumping syndrome consisting of hypoglycemia after the person eats; the cause is accelerated passage of glucose into the small intestine, from which it enters the bloodstream more rapidly than normal, stimulating production of insulin by the pancreas.

tachy·ar·rhyth·mia (tak″e-ə-rith′me-ə) [*tachy-* + *arrhythmia*] any disturbance of the heart rhythm in which the heart rate is abnormally increased, usually to greater than 100 beats per minute in an adult.

tachy·aux·e·sis (tak″e-awk-ze′sis) [*tachy-* + *auxesis*] heterauxesis in which the part grows more rapidly than the whole.

tachy·car·dia (tak″ĭ-kahr′de-ə) [*tachy-* + *cardia*] excessive rapidity in the action of the heart; the term is usually applied to a heart rate above 100 beats per minute in an adult and is often qualified by the locus of origin as well as by whether it is paroxysmal or nonparoxysmal.

antidromic atrioventricular reciprocating t., antidromic circus movement t. a reentrant tachycardia in which the reentrant circuit involves anterograde conduction over the accessory pathway and retrograde conduction over the normal pathway through the AV node and the His bundle. Cf. *orthodromic atrioventricular (AV) reciprocating t.*

atrial t. tachycardia originating from an atrial locus, usually having between 160 and 190 beats per minute; it may result from enhanced automaticity or impulse reentry.

atrioventricular junctional t., atrioventricular nodal t. junctional t.

atrioventricular nodal reentrant t. tachycardia resulting from reentry in or around the atrioventricular node, characterized by a QRS complex of supraventricular origin, sudden onset and termination, and a regular rhythm at a rate of 150 to 250 beats per minute. See also *antidromic atrioventricular (AV) reciprocating t.* and *orthodromic atrioventricular (AV) reciprocating t.*

atrioventricular reciprocating t. (AVRT) a reentrant tachycardia in which the reentrant circuit contains both the normal pathway through the AV node and the His bundle and an accessory pathway as integral parts. See *antidromic atrioventricular reciprocating t.* and *orthodromic atrioventricular reciprocating t.*

benign ventricular t. ventricular tachycardia that is not associated with structural heart disease or significant hemodynamic symptoms.

bidirectional ventricular t., bifascicular ventricular t. ventricular tachycardia with heart rates of 90 to 160 beats per minute, alternating right and left axis deviation, ectopic focus that alternates between the anterior superior and posterior inferior fascicles, and a right bundle branch block pattern in lead V_1; seen in digitalis toxicity and other conditions.

chaotic atrial t. tachycardia characterized by atrial rates of 100 to 130 beats per minute, markedly variable P wave morphology, and irregular P–P intervals; it occurs predominantly in patients with chronic obstructive pulmonary disease, diabetics, and the elderly, and may lead to atrial fibrillation. Called also *multifocal atrial t.*

circus movement t. reentrant t.

double t. the occurrence of two types of ectopic tachycardia at the same time, such as nodal and ventricular tachycardia.

ectopic t. abnormally rapid heart action in response to impulses arising outside the sinoatrial node.

endless loop t. see *pacemaker-mediated t.*

junctional t. tachycardia arising in response to impulses originating in the atrioventricular junction, with a heart rate greater than 75 beats per minute. It may be nonparoxysmal *(nonparoxysmal junctional t.)* or paroxysmal; if the latter, it may be due to reentry (e.g., *atrioventricular nodal reentrant t.*) or to enhanced automaticity.

monomorphic ventricular t. ventricular tachycardia that has a uniform beat-to-beat QRS morphology.

multifocal atrial t. (MAT) chaotic atrial t.

nodal t. junctional t.

nonparoxysmal junctional t. a junctional tachycardia of slow onset, with a heart rate of 70 to 130 beats per minute. It is due to enhanced automaticity of the atrioventricular junctional tissue and is often associated with digitalis toxicity, acute myocardial infarction, acute carditis, or surgical trauma.

nonsustained ventricular t. ventricular tachycardia that terminates spontaneously within 30 seconds and does not lead to hemodynamic collapse.

orthodromic atrioventricular reciprocating t., orthodromic circus movement t. a nodal reentrant tachycardia in which the reentrant circuit involves anterograde conduction over the usual pathway through the AV node and His bundle, and retrograde conduction over an accessory pathway. Cf. *antidromic atrioventricular (AV) reciprocating t.*

orthostatic t. tachycardia that occurs when a person rises from a reclining to a standing position.

pacemaker-mediated t. in patients with dual chamber pacemakers, tachycardia caused by retrograde conduction of ventricular impulses, either premature ventricular complexes or impulses triggered by ventricular pacing which are sensed by the atria and trigger a subsequent ventricular impulse. An endless loop may develop, in which case it is called *endless loop tachycardia.*

paroxysmal t. attacks of tachycardia having sudden onset and cessation; it is usually qualified by the locus of impulse origin as either ventricular or supraventricular. Some classifications subdivide the latter into atrial and junctional tachycardias.

paroxysmal atrial t., paroxysmal supraventricular t. (PSVT) supraventricular tachycardia occurring in attacks of rapid onset and cessation; it usually is due to a reentrant circuit.

permanent junctional reciprocating t. (PJRT) a chronic orthodromic atrioventricular nodal reciprocating tachycardia in which retrograde conduction on a posteroseptal accessory pathway is much slower than anterograde conduction along the normal conduction pathway.

polymorphic ventricular t. ventricular tachycardia whose beat-to-beat QRS configuration is constantly changing, sometimes subtly.

reciprocating t. a tachycardia due to a reentrant mechanism and characterized by a reciprocating rhythm (q.v.).

reentrant t. any tachycardia characterized by a reentrant circuit; called also *circus movement t.*

reflex t. tachycardia initiated through a reflex neural arc by an event occurring elsewhere in the body.

sinus t. (ST) tachycardia originating in the sinus node; it is normal during exercise or anxiety and occurs abnormally associated with shock, hypotension, hypoxia, congestive heart failure, fever, and various high output states.

sinus node reentrant t., sinus node reentry t., sinus reentrant t. tachycardia arising from a reentrant circuit that encompasses the sinus node.

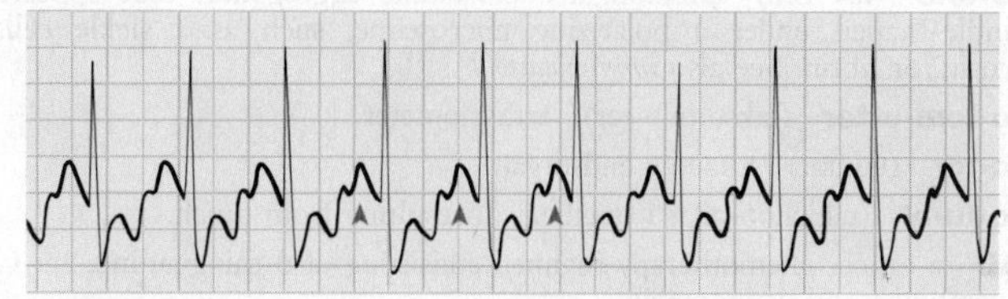

■ Sinus tachycardia (150 beats per minute) during acute myocardial ischemia. P waves are indicated by arrowheads.

supraventricular t. (SVT) any regular tachycardia in which the point of stimulation is located above the bundle branches, either in the sinus node, atria, or atrioventricular junction; it may also include those arising from large reentrant circuits encompassing both atrial and ventricular sites.

sustained ventricular t. ventricular tachycardia lasting more than 30 seconds leading to shock that can be fatal.

ventricular t. (VT) an abnormally rapid ventricular rhythm with aberrant ventricular excitation (wide QRS complexes), usually in excess of 150 per minute, which is generated within the ventricle and is most commonly associated with atrioventricular dissociation. Minor irregularities of rate may also occur. Evidence implicates a reentrant pathway as the usual cause.

tachy•car•di•ac (tach″ĭ-kahr′de-ak) 1. pertaining to, characterized by, or causing tachycardia. 2. an agent that acts to accelerate the pulse.

tachy•car•dic (tak″ĭ-kahr′dik) having a rapid heart rate.

tachy•dys•rhyth•mia (tak″e-dis-rith′me-ə) [*tachy-* + *dysrhythmia*] an abnormal heart rhythm with rate greater than 100 beats per minute in an adult; the term *tachyarrhythmia* is usually used instead.

tachy•gas•tria (tak″ĭ-gas′tre-ə) a dysrhythmia of the electric potentials in the stomach wall, with abnormally increased frequency.

tachy•gen•e•sis (tak″ĭ-jen′ə-sis) [*tachy-* + *-genesis*] the acceleration and compression of ancestral stages in embryonic development.

tachy•ki•nin (tak″e-ki′nin) any member of the tachykinin family of hormones; see under *family*.

tachy•lal•ia (tak″e-la′le-ə) logorrhea.

tachy•lo•gia (tak″e-lo′jə) logorrhea.

ta•chym•e•ter (tə-kim′ə-tər) [*tachy-* + *-meter*] any instrument for measuring rapidity of motion of any body.

tachy•pha•gia (tak″ĭ-fa′je-ə) [*tachy-* + *-phagia*] rapid or hasty eating; seen in some forms of regressed schizophrenia.

tachy•pha•sia (tak″e-fa′zhə) logorrhea.

tachy•phe•mia (tak″e-fe′me-ə) logorrhea.

tachy•phra•sia (tak″e-fra′zhə) logorrhea.

tachy•phy•lax•is (tak″e-fə-lak′sis) [*tachy* + *phylaxis*] 1. rapid immunization against the effect of toxic doses of an extract or serum by previous injection of small doses. 2. rapidly decreasing response to a drug or physiologically active agent after administration of a few doses.

tach•yp•nea (tak″ip-ne′ə, tak″e-ne′ə) [*tachy-* + *-pnea*] excessive rapidity of breathing. See also *hyperpnea* and *hyperventilation*.

tachy•rhyth•mia (tak″ĭ-rith′me-ə) [*tachy-* + *rhythm* + *-ia*] tachycardia, especially when the mechanism is obscure.

tach•ys•te•rol (tak-is′tə-rol) an isomer of ergosterol produced by irradiation.

tachy•tro•phism (tak″ĭ-tro′fiz-əm) [*tachy-* + *trophism*] rapid metabolism.

tachy•zo•ite (tak″ĭ-zo′īt) [*tachy-* + *zo-* + *-ite*] the crescent or oval, quickly multiplying trophozoite of *Toxoplasma gondii*, found in all tissues except non-nucleated erythrocytes during the acute stage of toxoplasmosis. Called also *endozoite*. Cf. *bradyzoite* and *pseudocyst* (def. 2).

tac•rine hy•dro•chlo•ride (tak′rēn) a cholinesterase inhibitor used to improve cognitive performance in patients with mild to moderate dementia of the Alzheimer type, administered orally.

tac•ro•li•mus (tak″ro-li′məs) a macrolide immunosuppressant of the calcineurin inhibitor group, derived from *Streptomyces tsukubaensis* and having actions similar to those of cyclosporine. Administered orally or intravenously to prevent rejection of organ transplants, especially liver; applied topically to treat moderate to severe atopic dermatitis.

tac•tic (tak′tik) 1. exhibiting tacticity. 2. pertaining to or characterized by taxis.

tac•tic•i•ty (tak-tis′ĭ-te) the condition of having a regular chemical arrangement of the units making up the main chain of a polymer.

tac•tile (tak′til) [L. *tactilis*, from *tangere* to touch] pertaining to touch.

tac•tion (tak′shən) [L. *tactio*] touch.

tac•toid (tak′toid) an elongated crystallike aggregation that appears spindle-shaped under a polarizing microscope, such as a sickle cell, myosin, or fibrin. See also *immunotactoid*.

tac•tom•e•ter (tak-tom′ə-tər) esthesiometer.

tac•tor (tak′tər) a tactile end-organ.

tac•tu•al (tak′choo-əl) 1. tactile. 2. resulting from touch.

TAD a cancer chemotherapy regimen consisting of 6-thioguanine, ara-C (cytarabine), and daunomycin.

ta•dal•a•fil (tə-dal′ə-fil) a phosphodiesterase inhibitor that relaxes the smooth muscle of the penis, thereby facilitating blood flow to the corpus cavernosum; used to treat erectile dysfunction in impotence therapy. Administered orally.

Tae•nia (te′ne-ə) [L. "a flat band," "bandage," "tape"] a genus of large tapeworms of the family Taeniidae.

T. africa′na *T. saginata.*

T. antarc′tica a species found in dogs in Antarctic regions.

T. bala′niceps a species found in dogs and bobcats in the southwestern United States.

T. brachyso′ma a species found in dogs in Italy.

T. brem′neri *T. confusa.*

T. cer′vi a species found in dogs in Denmark.

T. confu′sa a species found in the Mississippi Valley and in East Africa, believed by some to be a variant of *T. saginata*. Called also *T. bremneri*.

T. cras′siceps a species infecting foxes in Alaska and Canada, found in rodents as an intermediate host.

T. crassicol′lis *T. taeniaeformis.*

T. cucurbiti′na *T. saginata.*

T. demararien′sis *Raillietina demarariensis.*

T. echinococ′cus *Echinococcus granulosus.*

T. ellip′tica *Dipylidium caninum.*

T. hydati′gena a species found in dogs and other carnivores; the larval stage (cysticercus) is found in the liver and abdominal cavity of ruminants, rodents, and occasionally other animals. Called also *T. marginata*.

T. krab′bei a species that infects the bobcat, dog, and wolf in the northern United States, Canada, Alaska, and Iceland.

T. madagascarien′sis *Raillietina madagascariensis.*

T. margina′ta *T. hydatigena.*

T. mediocanella′ta *T. saginata.*

T. mul′ticeps a species whose adult stage is parasitic in the dog; its larval stage *(Coenurus cerebralis)* infests goats, sheep, and occasionally humans, usually in the central nervous system but sometimes elsewhere, producing coenurosis or gid.

T. na′na *Hymenolepis nana.*

T. o′vis a species parasitic in dogs; found in the musculature of sheep and goats as intermediate hosts.

T. philippi′na *T. saginata.*

T. pisifor′mis a tapeworm found most often in carnivores, but occasionally in other animals; the cysticercus (larval stage) is found in the liver and peritoneal cavity of rabbits.

T. sagina′ta the most common of the large tapeworms infecting humans, a species 4 to 8 meters long, found in the adult form in the intestine. The cysticerci (larval stage) develop in the muscles and other tissues of ruminants, and humans become infected by eating raw or rare meat. Called also *beef* or *unarmed tapeworm* and *T. africana*.

T. sagina′ta asia′tica a genetically distinct subspecies of *T. sagina′ta*, found only in Southeast and East Asia and nearby islands, with intermediate hosts being various wild and domestic mammals.

T. seria′lis a species whose adult stage is parasitic in dogs; its larval stage develops in the connective tissues of rodents and occasionally humans.

T. so′lium the pork tapeworm, a species 1 to 2 meters long found in the adult form in the human intestine; the cysticerci (larval stage) occur most often in muscle and other tissues of pigs, but are also found in other mammals. Humans may become infested if they eat inadequately cooked or measly pork; see also *cysticercosis*. Called also *armed* or *measly tapeworm*.

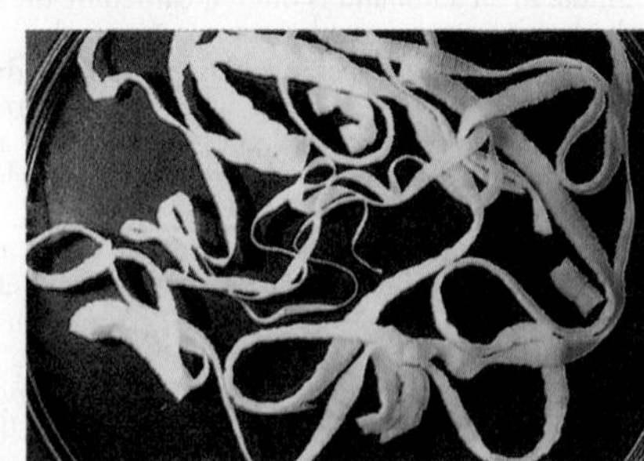

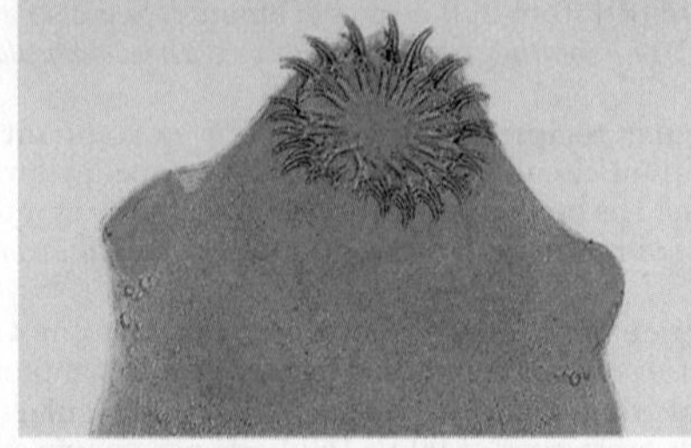

■ *Taenia solium:* *(A)*, adult; *(B)*, scolex, showing suckers and hooks.

T. taeniaefor′mis a species found most often in cats and sometimes in other animals; rats, mice, and other rodents are intermediate hosts. Called also *T. crassicollis.*

tae•nia (te′ne-ə) gen. and pl. *tae′niae* [L. "band, tape"] 1. in anatomy, a flat band or strip of soft tissue. 2. an individual organism of the genus *Taenia.* Spelled also *tenia.*

t. choroi′dea [TA] choroid line: the line of attachment of the lateral choroid plexus to the medial wall of the cerebral hemisphere; specifically, the line of attachment of the ependyma of the ventricle to the ependyma of the choroid plexus.

t. cine′rea [TA] the line of attachment of the ependymal cells of the choroid plexus to the ependyma along the edge of the caudal part of the fourth ventricle. Called also *t. of fourth ventricle.*

tae′niae co′li [TA], **taeniae of colon** three thickened bands, about 0.6 cm wide and one-sixth shorter than the colon, formed by the longitudinal fibers in the tunica muscularis of the large intestine; they extend from the root of the vermiform appendix to the rectum, where the fibers spread out and form a continuous layer encircling the tube. The three taeniae are the *t. libera, t. mesocolica,* and *t. omentalis.*

t. for′nicis [TA] taenia of fornix: the line of attachment of the choroid plexus of the lateral ventricle to the fornix, including the line of its attachment to the fimbria of the hippocampus.

t. of fourth ventricle t. cinerea.

t. li′bera [TA] the thickened band formed by anterior longitudinal muscle fibers of the large intestine, almost equidistant from the taenia mesocolica and the taenia omentalis.

medullary t. of thalamus t. thalami.

t. mesoco′lica [TA] the thickened band of longitudinal muscle fibers of the large intestine along the site of attachment of the mesocolon.

t. omenta′lis [TA] the band of longitudinal muscle fibers of the large intestine along the site of attachment of the greater omentum.

t. tha′lami [TA] the line of attachment of the ependymal cells of the roof of the third ventricle to the dorsal margin of the thalamus; called also *medullary t. of thalamus,* and *t. of third ventricle.*

t. of third ventricle t. thalami.

t. tu′bae a thickened band of peritoneum along the upper border of the uterine tube.

taenia- [L. *taenia* tape] a combining form denoting relationship to tapeworms or to bands or strips of soft tissue. For words beginning thus, see also those beginning *tenia-.*

tae•ni•a•cide (te′ne-ə-sīd″) [*taenia-* + *-cide*] 1. destruction of tapeworms. 2. an agent lethal to tapeworms. Called also *teniacide* and *tenicide.*

tae•niae (te′ne-e) genitive and plural of *taenia.*

tae•ni•a•fu•gal (te″ne-ə-fu′gəl) expelling tapeworms.

tae•ni•a•fuge (te′ne-ə-fūj″) [*taenia* + *-fuge*] an agent that expels tapeworms. Called also *teniafuge* and *tenifuge.*

tae•ni•al (te′ne-əl) 1. of or pertaining to tapeworms of the genus *Taenia.* 2. tenial (def. 1).

tae•ni•a•sis (te-ni′ə-sis) infection with any of the tapeworms of the genus *Taenia.*

tae•ni•form (te′nĭ-form) [*taenia* + *form*] resembling the organism *Taenia,* or a tapeworm.

Tae•ni•i•dae (te-ni′ĭ-de) a family of medium-sized or large tapeworms of the order Cyclophyllidea, subclass Cestoda, which are parasitic in mammals. Genera found in humans include *Taenia* and *Echinococcus.*

tag (tag) 1. a small appendage, flap, or polyp. 2. label.

auricular t. preauricular t.

cutaneous t. acrochordon.

expressed sequence t. (EST) a short (several hundred base pairs) DNA sequence obtained by randomly sequencing a clone from a cDNA library; the sequence thus represents a portion of an expressed gene and is sufficient to identify the gene to which it corresponds uniquely. It is equivalent to a sequence tagged site, but specifically obtained from cDNA.

preauricular t. a rudimentary appendage of auricular tissue sometimes found on the face along the line of union of the first pharyngeal arch; it may or may not be accompanied by microtia. Called also *accessory tragus.*

radioactive t. see under *label.*

skin t. acrochordon.

Tag•a•met (tag′ə-met) trademark for preparations of cimetidine.

tag•a•tose (tag′ə-tōs) [NF] chemical name: D-tagatose; a low-calorie ketohexose epimeric with fructose, used as a bulk sweetener.

ta•gli•a•co•tian (tal-yə-ko′shən) named for Gasparo *Tagliacozzi,* Italian surgeon, 1546–1599.

tai chi (ti′ che′) [Chinese] a system of postures linked by elegant and graceful movements, originating in China and existing in a number of styles, whose purpose is to balance yin and yang, creating inner and outer harmony. Physiologically, tai chi improves cardiovascular, musculoskeletal, and respiratory function; because it demands intense concentration, it increases central nervous system function and is useful for the treatment of stress-related conditions, obesity, and chronic pain.

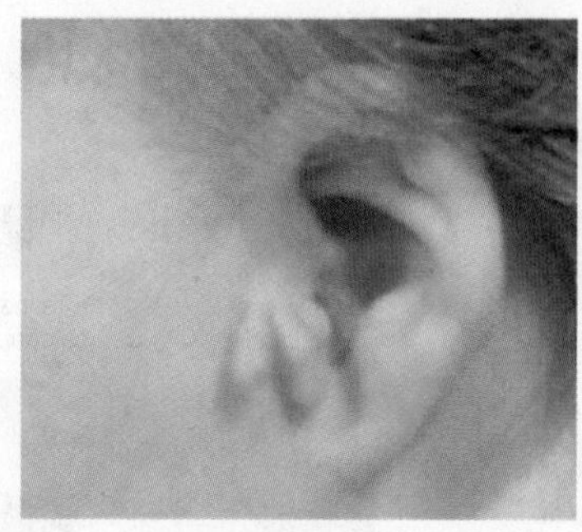

■ Preauricular tags.

tail (tāl) [L. *cauda;* Gr. *oura*] 1. any slender appendage; called also *cauda* [TA]. 2. the appendage that extends from the posterior trunk of animals.

axillary t. processus axillaris glandulae mammariae.

t. of caudate nucleus cauda nuclei caudati.

t. of dentate gyrus Giacomini band.

t. of epididymis cauda epididymidis.

t. of helix cauda helicis.

occult t. supernumerary segments of the coccyx, present in the buttock.

t. of pancreas cauda pancreatis.

poly A t., polyadenylate t. a sequence of about 200 adenylate residues that is added to the 3′ end of many primary mRNA transcripts during post-transcriptional processing in eukaryotes. Its function seems to be protection of the RNA from enzymatic degradation.

t. of Spence the projection of mammary glandular tissue extending into the axillary region, sometimes forming a visible mass which may enlarge premenstrually or during lactation.

t. of spermatozoon the flagellum of a spermatozoon, which contains the axoneme; it has four regions: the *neck, middle piece, principal piece,* and *end piece.*

t. of spleen extremitas anterior splenis.

tail•bud (tāl′bud″) caudal eminence.

tail•gut (tāl′gut″) a prolongation of the hindgut into the caudal eminence (tailbud) of the early embryo; it usually undergoes complete obliteration.

Tail•le•fer valve (ti″yə-fa′) [Louis Auguste Horace Sydney Timeléon *Taillefer,* French physician, 1802–1868] see under *valve.*

tai•pan (ti-pan′) *Oxyuranus scutellatus,* a venomous snake found in northern Australia and New Guinea.

Ta•ka-di•as•tase (tah′kah-di″əs-tās) [Jokichi *Takamine,* Japanese-born chemist in United States, 1854–1922] trademark for an amylolytic enzyme formed by the action of the spores of the fungus *Aspergillus oryzae* on the bran of wheat; used as a digestant.

Ta•ka•ha•ra disease (tah″kah-hah′rah) [Shigeo *Takahara,* Japanese otolaryngologist, 20th century] acatalasia.

Ta•ka•ya•su arteritis (disease, syndrome) (tah-kah-yah′soo) [Mikito *Takayasu,* Japanese surgeon, 1860–1938] see under *arteritis.*

Ta•la•cen (tal′ə-sen) trademark for a preparation of pentazocine hydrochloride and acetaminophen.

tal•al•gia (tal-al′jə) pain in the heel or ankle.

tal•amp•i•cil•lin hy•dro•chlo•ride (tal-amp″ĭ-sil′in) the monohydrochloride salt of the phthalidyl ester of ampicillin, having the actions and uses of ampicillin (q.v.).

talc (talk) 1. a powdered hydrous form of magnesium silicate, sometimes containing a small proportion of aluminum silicate; solid lumps found in nature are called *soapstone* or *steatite.* Inhalation of the powder can cause talc pneumoconiosis. 2. [USP] a purified form of talc used as a dusting powder and pharmaceutic aid. Called also *purified t.*

tal•co•sis (tal-ko′sis) talc pneumoconiosis.

pulmonary t. talc pneumoconiosis.

tal•cum (tal′kəm) [L.] talc.

ta•li (ta′li) genitive and plural of *talus.*

tal•i•a•co•tian (tal″e-ə-ko′shən) tagliacotian.

ta•lin (ta′lin) an actin-binding protein that also binds to β-integrins and vinculin; it is associated with adhesion plaques and with vinculin mediates cell-cell and cell–extracellular matrix adhesion by linking actin filaments of the cytoskeleton to the cytoplasmic domains of β-integrins.

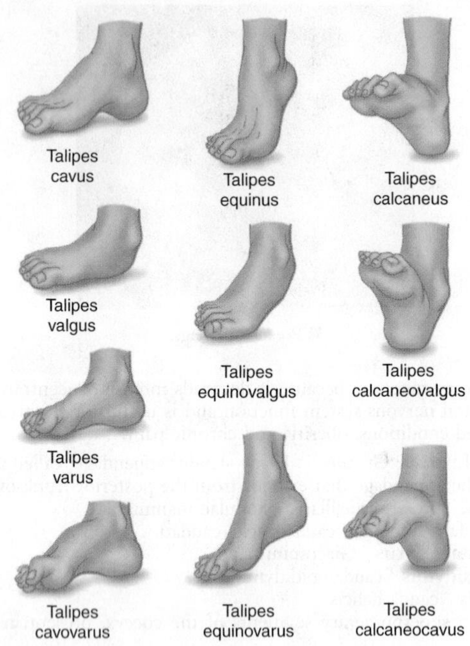

■ Various forms of talipes.

tal•i•ped (tal′ĭ-ped) 1. talipedic. 2. a person with talipes (clubfoot).

tal•i•pes (tal′ĭ-pēz) [L.] a congenital deformity of the foot, which is twisted out of shape or position; called also *clubfoot* and *reel foot.* See also under *pes.* **talipe′dic** *adj*

t. calcaneoca′vus a deformity in which the anterior part of the foot is elevated and the longitudinal arch of the foot is abnormally high.

t. calcaneoval′gus a deformity of the foot in which the heel is turned outward from the midline of the body and the anterior part of the foot is elevated.

t. calcaneova′rus a deformity of the foot in which the heel is turned toward the midline of the body and the anterior part is elevated.

t. calca′neus a deformity in which the foot is dorsiflexed.

t. cavoval′gus a deformity in which the longitudinal arch of the foot is abnormally high, and the heel is turned outward from the midline of the body.

t. cavova′rus a deformity of the foot in which the longitudinal arch is abnormally high and the heel is turned inward from the midline of the leg.

t. ca′vus exaggerated height of the longitudinal arch of the foot; it may be congenital or secondary to contractures or disturbed balance of the muscles.

t. equinoval′gus a deformity of the foot in which the heel is elevated and turned outward from the midline of the body.

t. equinova′rus a deformity of the foot in which the heel is turned inward from the midline of the leg and the foot is plantar flexed. This is associated with the raising of the inner border of the foot (supination) and displacement of the anterior part of the foot so that it lies medially to the vertical axis of the leg (adduction). With this type of foot the arch is higher (cavus) and the foot is in equinus (plantar flexion). This is a typical clubfoot.

t. equi′nus a deformity in which the foot is plantar flexed, causing the person to walk on the toes without touching the heel.

t. planoval′gus a deformity of the foot in which the heel is turned outward from the midline of the leg and the outer border of the anterior part of the foot is higher than the inner border. This results in a lowering of the longitudinal arch. The condition may be congenital and permanent, or it may be spasmodic as a result of reflex spasm of the muscles controlling the foot.

t. val′gus a deformity of the foot in which the heel is turned outward from the midline of the leg. See also *flatfoot.*

t. va′rus a deformity of the foot in which the heel is turned inward from the midline of the leg.

tal•i•pom•a•nus (tal″ĭ-pom′ə-nəs) [*talipes + manus*] clubhand.

ta•lo•cal•ca•ne•al (ta″lo-kal-ka′ne-əl) pertaining to the talus and calcaneus; called also *astragalocalcanean.*

ta•lo•cal•ca•ne•an (ta″lo-kal-ka′ne-ən) talocalcaneal.

ta•lo•cru•ral (ta″lo-kroo′rəl) [*talus + crural*] pertaining to the talus and the bones of the leg.

ta•lo•fib•u•lar (ta″lo-fib′u-lər) pertaining to the talus and the fibula.

tal•on (tal′on) [Fr. "bird's claw," from L. *talus* ankle] 1. the claw of a bird of prey or other predatory animal. 2. a structure or part resembling such a claw.

t. noir (tah-law′ nwahr′) [Fr. "black claw"] black heel.

ta•lo•na•vic•u•lar (ta″lo-nə-vik′u-lər) pertaining to the talus and the navicular bone.

ta•lo•scaph•oid (ta″lo-skaf′oid) talonavicular.

ta•lo•tib•i•al (ta″lo-tib′e-əl) pertaining to the talus and tibia; called also *astragalotibial.*

ta•lus (ta′ləs) pl. *ta′li* [L. "ankle"] [TA] the highest of the tarsal bones and the one that articulates with the tibia and fibula to form the ankle joint; called also *ankle bone, astragalus, astragaloid bone,* and *os tarsi tibiale.* **ta′lar** *adj*

Tal•win (tal′win) trademark for preparations containing pentazocine.

ta•mas (tah-mus′) [Sanskrit] according to ayurveda, one of the three gunas, characterized by inertia and responsible for stability, lethargy, and retentiveness in the mind and body, in contrast to activity (rajas) and equilibrium (sattva).

Tam•bo•cor (tam′bo-kor) trademark for a preparation of flecainide acetate.

tam•bour (tam-bo͝or′) [Fr. "drum"] a drum-shaped appliance used in transmitting movements in a recording instrument. It consists of a cylinder having an elastic membrane stretched over it, from which passes a tube that transmits the changes in air pressure to a recording device.

Tam•i•flu (tam′ĭ-floo) trademark for a preparation of oseltamivir phosphate.

Tamm-Hors•fall mucoprotein (protein) (tam′ hors′fal) [Igor *Tamm,* American virologist, born 1922; Frank Lappin *Horsfall,* Jr., American virologist, 1906–1971] see under *mucoprotein.*

ta•mox•i•fen cit•rate (tə-mok′sĭ-fən) [USP] a nonsteroidal oral antiestrogen also having weak estrogenic effects; used as an antineoplastic in the prophylaxis and treatment of breast cancer.

tam•pan (tam′pan) 1. *Argas persicus.* 2. *Ornithodoros moubata.*

tam•pon (tam′pon) [Fr. "stopper, plug"] a pack; a pad or plug made of cotton, sponge, or other material; variously used in surgery to plug the nose, vagina, etc., for the control of hemorrhage or the absorption of secretions.

tam•pon•ade (tam″pon-ād′) [Fr. *tamponner* to stop up] 1. surgical use of a tampon. 2. pathologic compression of a part.

balloon t. esophagogastric tamponade by means of a device with a triple-lumen tube and two inflatable balloons, the third lumen providing for aspiration of blood clots.

cardiac t. acute compression of the heart caused by increased intrapericardial pressure due to the collection of blood or fluid in the pericardium from rupture of the heart, penetrating trauma, or progressive effusion.

chronic t. chronic compression of the heart caused by chronic pericardial effusion and pericardial thickening.

esophagogastric t. the exertion of direct pressure against bleeding esophageal varices by insertion of a tube with a sausage-shaped balloon in the esophagus and a globular one in the stomach and inflating the balloons.

heart t. cardiac t.

pericardial t. cardiac t.

tam•po•nage (tahm-po-nahzh′) tamponade.

tam•pon•ing (tam′pon-ing) tamponade.

tam•pon•ment (tam-pon′mənt) the act of plugging with a tampon.

tam•su•lo•sin hy•dro•chlo•ride (tam-soo′lo-sin) an α_1-adrenergic blocking agent specific for the receptors in the prostate; used to improve urine flow rate and reduce symptoms of benign prostatic hyperplasia, administered orally.

Ta•mus (ta′məs) [L.] a genus of plants of the family Dioscoreaceae, having tuberous roots. *T. commu′nis* L. is black bryony, a species native to Europe and Asia whose root is used in homeopathy as a rubefacient and diuretic.

tan (tan) 1. a light brown color. In persons with light-colored skin, this color is acquired by sun or ultraviolet exposure. The change results from darkening of preformed melanin (the Meirowsky phenomenon), accelerated formation of new melanin, and retention of melanin in the epidermis as a result of retardation of keratinization. 2. to become such a light brown color from exposure to sun or to ultraviolet radiation; said of the skin of persons having naturally white to light brown skin.

Tan•a•ce•tum (tan″ə-se′təm) a genus of strongly aromatic, chiefly Old World herbs of the family Compositae.

T. parthe′nium [NF] feverfew (q.v.); a species native to southeastern Europe and now widely distributed throughout Europe, North America, and Australia; the dried leaves are used medicinally.

tan•a•pox (tan′ə-poks″) [*Tana* River, Kenya] a viral disease seen in Central and East Africa, caused by a poxvirus and characterized by fever and isolated papulovesicular lesions on the limbs.

tan•dem (tan′dəm) consisting of two similar components arranged one in front of the other.

tan•gen•ti•al•i•ty (tan-jen″she-al′ĭ-te) a pattern of speech characterized by oblique, digressive, or irrelevant replies to questions; the responses never approach the point of the questions. It differs from *circumstantiality*, in which the responder eventually reaches the point.

tan•ghin (tan′gēn) 1. *Tanghinia venenifera.* 2. the poisonous seed of *T. venenifera.*

Tan•ghin•ia (tang-gin′e-ə) a genus of trees of the family Apocyanaceae. *T. veneni′fera* and other species found in southern Africa and Madagascar have seeds called tanghin that are highly toxic.

Tan•gier disease (tan-jēr′) [*Tangier* Island, in Chesapeake Bay, USA, where the disease was first described in 1961] see under *disease.*

tan•gle (tang′gəl) a knot or snarl.

neurofibrillary t's intracellular knots or clumps of neurofibrils seen in the cerebral cortex in Alzheimer disease.

tank (tank) an artificial receptacle for liquids.

Hubbard t. a tank in which a patient may be immersed in order to take underwater exercise.

tan•nase (tan′ās) an esterase found in various tannin-bearing plants and produced in cultures by various fungi and some strains of bacteria; it catalyzes the hydrolysis of various ester linkages in gallic acid components of tannins.

tan•nate (tan′āt) [L. *tannas*] any salt of tannic acid; all the tannates are astringent.

Tan•ner stages (tan′ər) [James Mourilyan *Tanner*, British pediatrician, born 1920] see under *stage.*

tan•nic ac•id (tan′ik) [USP] a substance obtained from nutgalls, used as an ingredient of dermatological preparations. It was formerly used as an astringent for oral and pharyngeal mucous membranes, as suppositories for treatment of hemorrhoids, and in treatment of burns, but it has fallen into disuse because of the possibility of severe liver damage. Called also *gallotannic acid, tannin,* and, erroneously, *digallic acid.*

tan•nin (tan′in) tannic acid.

tan•ta•lum (Ta) (tan′tə-ləm) a rare metallic element; atomic number, 73; atomic weight, 180.948. It is a noncorrosive and malleable metal which has been used for plates or disks to replace cranial defects, for wire sutures, and for making prosthetic appliances.

tan•trum (tan′trəm) a violent display of bad temper.

tan•y•cyte (tan′ĭ-sīt) [Gr. *tanyein* to stretch + *-cyte*] a modified ependymal cell of the median eminence, having a body that lies near the third ventricle and sending out processes that extend to the capillary plexus of the portal circulation. Its function is unknown, but it may transport hormones from the cerebrospinal fluid into the portal circulation or from hypothalamic neurons to the cerebrospinal fluid.

TAO (ta′o) trademark for preparations of troleandomycin.

tap (tap) 1. a quick, light blow. 2. to drain off fluid by paracentesis.

bloody t. a lumbar puncture in which the fluid obtained is bloody or pinkish.

front t. a tap on the muscles of the front of the lower limb; in cases of spinal irritability this produces contraction of the gastrocnemius muscle.

spinal t. lumbar puncture.

Tap•a•zole (tap′ə-zōl) trademark for a preparation of methimazole.

tape (tāp) a long, narrow strip of fabric or other flexible material.

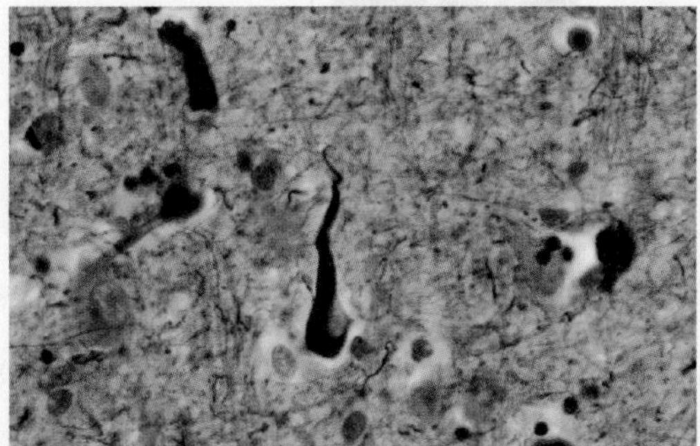

■ Neurofibrillary tangle within neuronal cytoplasm (silver stain).

adhesive t. [USP] a strip of fabric and/or film evenly coated on one side with a pressure-sensitive, adhesive mixture, the whole having high tensile strength, used for the application of dressings and sometimes to produce immobilization.

flurandrenolide t. [USP] flexible polyethylene tape having an adhesive layer impregnated with flurandrenolide; the tape acts as both a vehicle and an occlusive dressing.

Montgomery t's see under *strap.*

sterile adhesive t. adhesive tape, the adhesive surface of which is covered by strips of a protective material of equal width, and which is sterilized after packaging.

tap•ei•no•ceph•a•ly (tap″ĭ-no-sef′ə-le) [Gr. *tapeinos* low-lying + *-cephaly*] a low form of the skull, which is also flattened at front, having a vertical index below 72. **tapeinocephal′ic** *adj*

ta•pe•tal (tə-pe′təl) pertaining to a tapetum, especially to the tapetum lucidum.

ta•pe•to•ret•i•nal (tə-pe″to-ret′ĭ-nəl) [*tapetum oculi,* former name for the stratum pigmentosum retinae + *retinal*] pertaining to the stratum pigmentosum retinae.

ta•pe•tum (tə-pe′təm) pl. *tape′ta* [L., from Gr. *tapētion,* dim. of *tapēs* a carpet, rug] 1. a covering structure, or layer of cells. 2. t. corporis callosi.

t. cellulo′sum a type of tapetum lucidum, being the more complex, more cellular type found in all but two species of carnivores and in seals.

t. choroi′deae t. lucidum.

t. cor′poris callo′si [TA] a stratum of commissural fibers of the corpus callosum on the superolateral aspect of the occipital horn of the lateral ventricle.

t. fibro′sum a type of tapetum lucidum, being the simpler, fibrous type found in hoofed animals, marsupials, elephants, whales, and a few fish.

t. lu′cidum the iridescent pigment epithelium of the choroid of animals, which gives their eyes the property of shining in the dark; the two primary types are the tapetum cellulosum and the tapetum fibrosum. Called also *t. choroideae.*

tape•worm (tāp′wərm) any flatworm of the class Cestoidea; many are intestinal parasites. Those infecting humans are principally of the genera *Taenia, Diphyllobothrium, Dipylidium, Echinococcus,* and *Hymenolepis.* The eggs are ingested by the intermediate host and make their way into the tissues, where their larval stages are produced (see *hydatid cyst, plerocercoid,* and *cysticercus*). When a person or animal eats the flesh of one of these intermediate hosts, the larvae develop within the alimentary canal of this second (definitive) host and become adult tapeworms, which consist of an attachment organ, or scolex, an undifferentiated neck, and a strobila made up of a variable number of separate segments, or proglottids, each of which is hermaphroditic and produces eggs. Called also *cestode.*

African t. *Taenia saginata.*

armed t. *Taenia solium.*

beef t. *Taenia saginata.*

broad t. *Diphyllobothrium latum.*

dog t. 1. *Echinococcus granulosus.* 2. *Dipylidium caninum.*

double-pored dog t. *Dipylidium caninum.*

dwarf t. *Hymenolepis nana.*

fish t. *Diphyllobothrium latum.*

fringed t. *Thysanosoma actinioides.*

heart-headed t. *Diphyllobothrium cordatum.*

hydatid t. *Echinococcus granulosus.*

Madagascar t. *Raillietina madagascariensis.*

Manson larval t. *Diphyllobothrium mansonoides.*

measly t. *Taenia solium.*

pork t. *Taenia solium.*

rat t. *Hymenolepis diminuta.*

Swiss t. *Diphyllobothrium latum.*

unarmed t. *Taenia saginata.*

taph•e•pho•bia (taf″ə-fo′be-ə) [Gr. *taphos* grave + *-phobia*] irrational fear of being buried alive.

tapho•phil•ia (taf″o-fil′e-ə) morbid attraction to graves or cemeteries.

Ta•pia syndrome (tah′pyah) [Antonio García *Tapia*, Spanish otolaryngologist, 1875–1950] see under *syndrome.*

tap•i•no•ce•phal•ic (tap″ĭ-no-sə-fal′ik) tapeinocephalic.

tap•i•no•ceph•a•ly (tap″ĭ-no-sef′ə-le) tapeinocephaly.

ta•pi•roid (ta′pĭ-roid) resembling the snout of a tapir.

ta•pote•ment (tah-pōt-maw′) [Fr.] a tapping or percussing movement in massage.

Taq po•lym•er•ase (tak′ pə-lim′ər-ās) a DNA-directed DNA polymerase [EC 2.7.7.7] from the bacillus *Thermus aquaticus,* which lives in hot springs; it is thermostable and thus can be used in the polymerase chain reaction.

tar (tahr) a dark brown or black viscid liquid, obtained by roasting the wood of various species of pine, or as a by-product of the destructive distillation of bituminous coal (see *coal t.*). It is a mixture of complex composition, and is the source of organic substances such as cresol, creosol, guaiacol, naphthalene, paraffin, phenol, toluene, and xylene. Once used in chronic bronchitis, diarrhea, and diseases of the urinary organs, it now has only limited use in certain skin diseases, notably psoriasis and chronic eczematous disorders. If it is ingested or its fumes are inhaled, it is toxic and carcinogenic. See also *pitch* and *pitch poisoning*.

coal t. 1. tar obtained as a by-product of the destructive distillation of bituminous coal, used as a raw material for plastics, solvents, waterproofing compounds, sealants, and various other organic chemicals. If it is ingested or its fumes are inhaled it is toxic and carcinogenic; see also *pitch* and *pitch poisoning*. 2. [USP] a preparation of coal tar used as a topical antieczematic and antipsoriatic.

juniper t. [USP] a volatile thick brown oil with a bitter taste, obtained from the woody portions of *Juniperus oxycedrus*, used as a pharmaceutic necessity and for the topical therapy of dermatoses. Called also *cade oil*.

pine t. a viscid, blackish brown liquid obtained by destructive distillation of the wood of various pine trees, used as a local antieczematic and rubefacient; applied topically.

ta•ran•tu•la (tə-ran′tu-lə) 1. any of numerous large venomous spiders whose bite causes local inflammation and pain. 2. European t.

American t. *Eurypelma hentzii*, a large, dark, ferocious-looking spider with a poisonous bite.

black t. *Sericopelma communis*, a black venomous species found in Panama.

European t. *Lycosa tarentula*, a large hairy spider whose bite causes pain and was formerly believed to be deadly. Called also *European wolf spider*.

Ta•rax•a•cum (tə-rak′sə-kəm) [L., from Ar. *tarakhshaqūn* wild chicory] a widespread genus of perennial weedy herbs of the family Compositae, having long taproots, toothed leaves, and usually yellow flowers. *T. officina′le*, the dandelion, is used medicinally.

tar•ba•gan (tahr′bə-gən) *Marmota bobak*, a reddish-brown marmot found on the steppes of Central Asia; it is a natural reservoir of the plague.

Tar•ce•va (tahr′sə-və) trademark for a preparation of erlotinib hydrochloride.

Tar•dieu spots (tahr-dyoo͝′) [Auguste Ambroise *Tardieu*, French physician, 1818–1879] see under *spot*.

tar•dive (tahr′div) [Fr. "tardy, late"] marked by lateness, late; said of a disease in which the characteristic lesion is late in appearing.

tare (tār) 1. the weight of the vessel in which a substance is weighed. 2. to take the weight of a vessel which is to contain a substance, in order to allow for it when the vessel and the substance are weighed together.

tar•get (tahr′gət) 1. an object or area toward which something is directed, such as the metal or plate of an x-ray tube on which the electrons impinge and from which the x-rays are sent out. 2. denoting a cell or organ that is selectively affected by a particular agent, e.g., a hormone or drug.

tar•get•ing (tahr′gət-ing) the process of aiming at a specified object or area.

gene t. a process for making precise alterations in a genome, by inducing homologous recombination between newly introduced DNA sequences and the same sequences residing in the chromosome.

Tar•gret•in (tar-gret′in) trademark for preparations of bexarotene.

Ta•ri•cha (tə-re′kə) a genus of amphibious newts. *T. toro′sa* contains the poison tarichatoxin (tetrodotoxin) in its body.

tar•ich•a•tox•in (tar′ik-ə-tok″sin) a neurotoxin from the newt *Taricha torosa*, identical with tetrodotoxin (q.v.).

Ta•rin recess (space) (tah-ră′) [Pierre *Tarin (Tarini, Tarinus)*, French anatomist, 1725–1761] see *anterior recess of interpeduncular fossa*, under *recess*.

Tar•ka (tahr′kə) trademark for a combination preparation of trandolapril and verapamil hydrochloride.

Tar•lov cyst (tahr′lov) [Isadore Max *Tarlov*, American surgeon, 1905–1977] perineurial cyst.

Tar•nier forceps (tahr-nya′) [Etienne Stéphane *Tarnier*, French obstetrician, 1828–1897] see under *forceps*.

tar•ry (tahr′e) 1. filled with or covered by tar. 2. thick, dark; resembling tar.

tar•sad•e•ni•tis (tahr″sad-ə-ni′tis) inflammation of the meibomian glands and tarsus; cf. *blepharadenitis*.

tar•sal (tahr′səl) [L. *tarsalis*] 1. pertaining to the tarsus of the foot. 2. pertaining to the tarsus of an eyelid. 3. any of the bones of the tarsus.

tar•sal•gia (tahr-sal′jə) pain in the ankle or foot.

tar•sa•lia (tahr-sa′le-ə) the bones of the tarsus.

tar•sa•lis (tahr-sa′lis) [L.] tarsal.

tar•sec•to•my (tahr-sek′tə-me) [*tarso-* + *-ectomy*] 1. excision of the tarsus of the foot. 2. excision of all or part of the tarsus of an eyelid.

tar•sec•to•pia (tahr″sek-to′pe-ə) [*tarso-* + *ectopia*] dislocation of the tarsus of the foot.

tar•si•tis (tahr-si′tis) blepharitis.

tars(o)- [Gr. *tarsos* a broad flat surface] a combining form denoting relationship to the edge of the eyelid, or to the instep of the foot.

tar•so•chei•lo•plas•ty (tahr″so-ki′lo-plas″te) [*tarso-* + *cheilo-* + *-plasty*] plastic surgery on the edge of the eyelid, such as for treatment of trichiasis.

tar•soc•la•sis (tahr-sok′lə-sis) [*tarso-* + Gr. *klasis* breaking] the operation of fracturing the tarsus of the foot.

tar•so•con•junc•ti•val (tahr″so-kən-junk′tĭ-vəl) pertaining to the tarsus of an eyelid and the conjunctiva.

tar•so•ma•la•cia (tahr″so-mə-la′shə) [*tarso-* + *malacia*] softening of the tarsus of an eyelid.

tar•so•meg•a•ly (tahr″so-meg′ə-le) enlargement of the os calcis.

tar•so•meta•tar•sal (tahr″so-met″ə-tahr′səl) pertaining to the tarsus and the metatarsus.

tar•so•or•bi•tal (tahr″so-or′bĭ-təl) pertaining to the tarsus of the eyelid and to the orbit.

tar•so•pha•lan•ge•al (tahr″so-fə-lan′je-əl) pertaining to the tarsus and the phalanges of the toes.

tar•so•pla•sia (tahr″so-pla′zhə) blepharoplasty.

tar•so•plas•ty (tahr′so-plas″te) blepharoplasty.

tar•sop•to•sis (tahr″sop-to′sis, tahr″so-to′sis) flatfoot.

tar•sor•rha•phy (tahr-sor′ə-fe) [*tarso-* + *-rrhaphy*] suturing together of the upper and lower eyelids in order to shorten or close the palpebral fissure. See also *partial t.* and *total t.* Called also *blepharorrhaphy*.

external t. partial tarsorrhaphy involving the external part of the fissure.

internal t. partial tarsorrhaphy involving the internal part of the fissure.

median t. partial tarsorrhaphy involving the middle part of the fissure.

partial t. tarsorrhaphy that closes only part of a palpebral fissure. See also *external t.*, *median t.*, and *internal t.*

total t. tarsorrhaphy that entirely closes a palpebral fissure.

tar•so•tar•sal (tahr″so-tahr′səl) pertaining to the articulation between the two rows of tarsal bones.

tar•so•tib•i•al (tahr″so-tib′e-əl) tibiotarsal.

tar•sot•o•my (tahr-sot′ə-me) [*tarso-* + *-tomy*] blepharotomy.

tar•sus (tahr′səs) [L., from Gr. *tarsos* a frame of wickerwork; any broad flat surface] 1. [TA] the region of the foot adjacent to the articulation between the foot and the leg, composed of seven tarsal bones *(ossa tarsi)*. Called also *ankle*. 2. one of the plates of connective tissue forming the framework of an eyelid; see *t. inferior palpebrae* and *t. superior palpebrae*.

t. infe′rior pal′pebrae [TA] the firm framework of connective tissue that gives shape to the lower eyelids.

t. supe′rior pal′pebrae [TA] the firm framework of connective tissue that gives shape to the upper eyelids.

tar•tar (tahr′tər) [L. *tartarum*; Gr. *tartaron*] 1. dental calculus. 2. crude potassium bitartrate.

tar•tar•at•ed (tahr′tər-āt″əd) charged with tartaric acid.

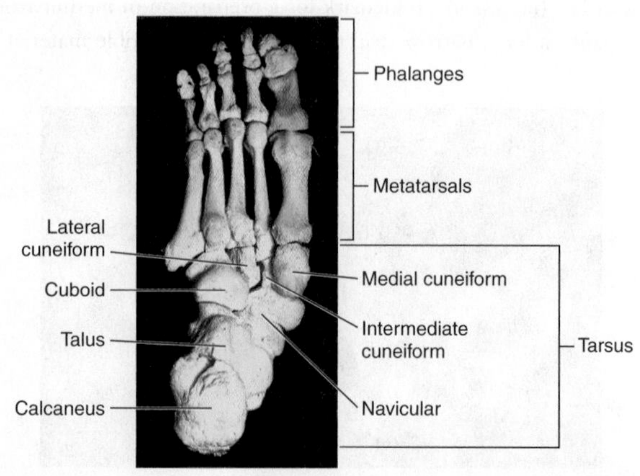

■ Tarsus, comprising the seven tarsal bones.

tar•tar•ic ac•id (tahr-tar′ik) 2,3-dihydroxybutanedioic acid, a dicarboxylic acid; its salts (tartrates) are used in food preparation (cream of tartar) and have been used as cathartics. Tartaric acid has two asymmetric carbon atoms and has three structural isomers: two enantiomers, *d*- and *l*-tartaric acid, and one meso compound, *meso*-tartaric acid, which is a diastereomer of the other two.

tar•tar•ized (tahr′tər-īzd) tartarated.

tar•trate (tahr′trāt) [L. *tartras*] any salt of tartaric acid.

acid t. a bitartrate; any salt of tartaric acid in which one atom only of hydrogen is replaced by a base.

ferric ammonium t. see under *ammonium*.

normal t. a salt of tartaric acid in which two hydrogen atoms are replaced; various tartrates are employed as remedial agents.

tar•trat•ed (tahr′trāt-əd) [L. *tartratus*] containing tartar or tartaric acid.

Ta•rui disease (tah′roo-e) [Seiichiro *Tarui*, Japanese physician, born 1927] glycogen storage disease, type VII.

Tas•mar (tas′mahr) trademark for a preparation of tolcapone.

tas•tant (tās′tənt) any substance, e.g., salt, capable of eliciting gustatory excitation, i.e., stimulating the sense of taste.

taste (tāst) [L. *gustus*] 1. the sense effected by the gustatory receptors in the tongue. Four qualities are distinguished by taste: sweet, sour, salty, and bitter. 2. the act of perceiving by this sense.

color t. a pseudogeusia in which tastes are associated with colors; called also *colored gustation*.

franklinic t. a sour taste produced by stimulating the tongue with static electricity.

tast•er (tās′tər) an individual capable of tasting a particular test substance, such as phenylthiourea, used in certain genetic studies.

TAT Thematic Apperception Test; toxin-antitoxin (see under *reaction*).

Tat•lock•ia mic•da•dei (tat-lok′e-ə mik-da′de-i) *Legionella micdadei*.

tat•too•ing (tă-too′ing) [from Polynesian] the insertion of permanent colors in the skin by introducing them through punctures.

t. of the cornea the permanent coloring of the cornea chiefly to conceal spots of leukoma.

Ta•tu•mel•la (ta″tə-mel′ə) [Harvey W. *Tatum*, American bacteriologist, 1919–2001] a genus of gram-negative bacteria of the family Enterobacteriaceae, consisting of facultatively anaerobic, nonpigmented, catalase-positive, oxidase-negative rods; it is isolated from human clinical specimens, primarily from the respiratory tract and is probably an infrequent opportunistic pathogen. The sole species is *T. pty′seos*.

tau (tou, taw) [Τ, τ] the nineteenth letter of the Greek alphabet.

Kendall t. Kendall rank correlation coefficient.

tau•op•a•thy (tou-, taw-op′ə-the) a neurodegenerative disease in which there are neurofibrillary tangles containing abnormal tau proteins.

tau-pro•tein ki•nase (tou, taw pro′tēn ki′nās) [EC 2.7.11.26] a protein-serine/threonine kinase that phosphorylates serine and threonine residues in tau proteins; it is activated by tubulin. Altered enzyme activity, leading to hyperphosphorylation of tau proteins, is involved in the formation of the paired helical filaments found in the neurofibrillary tangles characteristic of Alzheimer disease.

tau•rine (taw′rēn) an oxidized sulfur-containing amine, found conjugated in the bile, such as with cholic acid as cholyltaurine; it is also thought to be a central nervous system neurotransmitter or neuromodulator. It is excreted excessively in the urine in hyper-β-alaninemia.

taur(o)- [L. *taurus* bull] a combining form denoting relationship to a bull, or to taurine.

tau•ro•che•no•de•oxy•cho•late (taw″ro-ke″no-de-ok″se-ko′lāt) chenodeoxycholyltaurine.

tau•ro•che•no•de•oxy•cho•lic ac•id (taw″ro-ke″no-de-ok″se-ko′lik) chenodeoxycholyltaurine.

tau•ro•cho•late (taw″ro-ko′lāt) cholyltaurine.

tau•ro•cho•le•mia (taw″ro-ko-le′me-ə) [*taurocholic* acid + *-emia*] the presence of cholyltaurine (taurocholic acid) in the blood.

tau•ro•cho•lic ac•id (taw″ro-ko′lik) cholyltaurine.

tau•ro•don•tism (taw″ro-don′tiz-əm) [*taur-* + *odont-* + *-ism*] a variation in tooth form characterized by prism-shaped molars with large pulp spaces, resulting from branching of the root only in the middle (*mesotaurodontism*), or in the apical third or not at all (*hypertaurodontism*).

Taus•sig-Bing syndrome (tou′sig bing′) [Helen Brooke *Taussig*, American pediatrician, 1898–1986; Richard John *Bing*, German-born American cardiac physiologist, born 1909] see under *syndrome*.

taut(o)- [Gr. *tautos*, from *to auto* the same] a combining form meaning the same.

tau•to•me•ni•al (taw″to-me′ne-əl) [*tauto-* + Gr. *mēniaia* menses] pertaining to the same menstrual period.

tau•to•mer (taw′to-mər) a chemical compound exhibiting, or capable of exhibiting, tautomerism.

tau•tom•er•al (taw-tom′ər-əl) [*tauto-* + *mer-*[1] + *-al*[1]] pertaining to the same part, especially sending processes to help in the formation of the white matter in the same side of the spinal cord; said of certain neurons and neuroblasts. See *tautomeral cells*, under *cell*.

tau•tom•er•ase (taw-tom′ər-ās) [EC 5.3.2] any member of a sub-subclass of enzymes of the isomerase class that catalyze the interconversion of the keto and enol forms of a substrate. See also *enol*.

tau•to•mer•ic (taw″to-mer′ik) exhibiting, or capable of exhibiting, tautomerism.

tau•tom•er•ism (taw-tom′ər-iz-əm) [*tauto-* + *mer-*[1] + *-ism*] the relationship that exists between two structural isomers that are in chemical equilibrium and freely change from one form to the other.

keto-enol t. tautomerism between two compounds, one an enol and the other a ketone, that equilibrate by transfer of a proton. The keto form usually predominates except where the enol form is stabilized by conjugation with other double bonds.

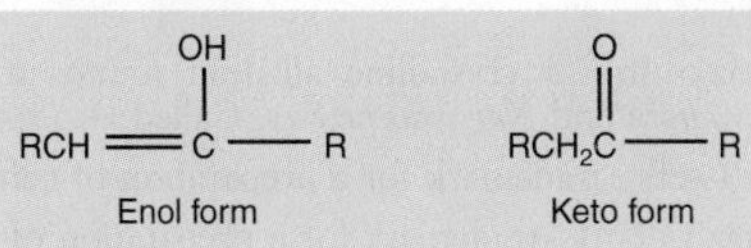

proton t. tautomerism in which an acidic proton is transferred from one position to another in the same molecule, e.g., keto-enol tautomerism. Called also *prototropy*.

ring-chain t. tautomerism involving open-chain and ring forms, as occurs with sugars. See *mutarotation*.

Tav•ist (tav′ist) trademark for a preparation of clemastine fumarate.

Ta•wa•ra node (tah-wah′rah) [K. Sunao *Tawara*, Japanese pathologist, 1873–1938] nodus atrioventricularis.

taxa (tak′sə) plural of *taxon*.

tax•ane (tak′sān) any of a group of chemical substances with antitumor activity of varying degrees, acting by promoting and stabilizing the polymerization of microtubules; it includes paclitaxel, docetaxel, and related compounds.

tax•ine (tak′sēn) a mixture of alkaloids (*taxine-1* and *taxine-2*) from members of the genus *Taxus*, responsible for their toxicity.

tax•is (tak′sis) [Gr. "a drawing up in rank and file"] 1. an orientation movement of a motile organism in response to an external stimulus. Such a response may be either positive (toward) or negative (away from the stimulus). Cf. *tropism*. 2. exertion of force in the manual replacement of a displaced or injured organ or structure, as in the reduction of a fracture or dislocation, or the replacement of a protruded intestine in hernia.

-taxis a word termination used to describe an orientation movement of a motile organism in response to a stimulus, affixed to a stem denoting the nature of the stimulus (e.g., chemotaxis, phototaxis).

tax•oid (tak′soid) any of a group of chemical substances with antitumor activity of varying degrees, acting by promoting and stabilizing the polymerization of microtubules; it includes paclitaxel, docetaxel, and related compounds.

Tax•ol (tak′sol) trademark for a preparation of paclitaxel.

tax•ol•o•gy (taks-ol′ə-je) taxonomy.

tax•on (tak′son) pl. *tax′a* [*taxis* + *-on* Gr. neuter ending] a particular group (category) into which related organisms are classified; the main categories are (in ascending order): species, genus, family, order, class, phylum, and kingdom.

tax•on•o•mist (taks-on′ə-mist) a specialist in taxonomy.

tax•on•o•my (tak-son′ə-me) [L. *taxinomia; taxis* + Gr. *nomos* law] the orderly classification of organisms into appropriate categories (taxa) on the basis of relationships among them, with the application of suitable and correct names. **taxonom′ic** *adj*

numerical t. an arithmetic method of classifying large numbers of bacterial strains on the basis of their overall similarity to one another, according to the number of phenotypic characters they share, each character being given equal weight. Called also *adansonian*, or *numerical classification*.

polyphasic t. a multidisciplinary method of classifying bacteria that uses a wide range of data, including genotypic, phenotypic, and ecologic, to create a consensus classification.

Tax•o•tere (tak′so-tēr) trademark for a preparation of docetaxel.

Tax•us (tak′səs) [L.] the yews, a genus of evergreen trees or shrubs of the family Taxaceae, having brown scaly bark, green needles, and red berries. All plant parts are toxic, sometimes deadly; symptoms of poisoning include nausea, vomiting, abdominal pain, dyspnea, and circulatory failure, with death from cardiac or respiratory failure.

T. brevifo'lia the Pacific yew, a species that grows along the Pacific coast of Canada and the United States and is the source of the antitumor agent paclitaxel.

Tay spot (sign) (ta) [Warren *Tay*, English physician, 1843–1927] cherry-red spot; see under *spot*.

Tay-Sachs disease (ta' saks') [W. *Tay;* Bernard Parney *Sachs*, New York neurologist, 1858–1944] see under *disease*.

Tay·lor brace (apparatus, splint) (ta'lər) [Charles Fayette *Taylor*, American orthopedic surgeon, 1827–1899] see under *brace*.

Tay·lo·rel·la (ta″lər-el'ə) [C.E.D. *Taylor*, English bacteriologist, 20th century] a genus of gram-negative bacteria of the family Alcaligenaceae, consisting of nonmotile, micro-aerophilic, oxidase-positive, short rods. The type species is *T. equigenita'lis*.

T. equigenita'lis a species that causes contagious equine metritis. Formerly called *Haemophilus equigenitalis*.

ta·zar·o·tene (tə-zar'o-tēn) a prodrug that undergoes hydrolysis to a retinoid in the skin; used topically in the treatment of acne vulgaris and psoriasis.

taz·et·tine (tāz'ə-tin) a crystalline alkaloid found in the poisonous bulbs of *Lycoris radiata* and *Narcissus tazetta*. Called also *sekisanine*.

Taz·i·cef (taz'ĭ-sef) trademark for a preparation of ceftazidime.

Taz·i·dime (taz'ĭ-dēm) trademark for a preparation of ceftazidime.

taz·o·bac·tam (taz″o-bak'tam) a penicillanic acid sulfone derivative similar to sulbactam that acts as a beta-lactamase inhibitor.

t. sodium the sodium salt of tazobactam, used in combination with piperacillin sodium to broaden its spectrum of activity against beta-lactamase–producing organisms.

Taz·o·rac (taz'o-rak) trademark for preparations of tazarotene.

TB popular abbreviation for *tuberculosis*.

Tb terbium.

TBG thyroxine-binding globulin.

TBI traumatic brain injury; total body irradiation.

TBII TSH-binding inhibitory immunoglobulins.

TBW total body water.

TC transcobalamin.

Tc technetium.

TCA tricyclic antidepressant.

TCDD 2,3,7,8-tetrachlorodibenzo-*p*-dioxin.

$TCID_{50}$ median tissue culture infective dose.

TCM traditional Chinese medicine.

TCMI T cell–mediated immunity.

TCR T cell antigen receptor; transcription-coupled repair.

TCV total cell volume.

TD_{50} median toxic dose.

Td tetanus and diphtheria toxoids.

TDA TSH-displacing antibody.

Tdap tetanus toxoid, reduced diphtheria toxoid, and acellular pertussis vaccine.

TDE tetrachlorodiphenylethane, a moderately toxic chlorinated hydrocarbon pesticide; called also *DDD* (dichlorodiphenyldichloroethane).

TDI toluene diisocyanate.

T1DM type 1 diabetes mellitus.

T2DM type 2 diabetes mellitus.

t.d.s. [L.] ter di'e sumen'dum (to be taken three times a day).

TdT terminal deoxynucleotidyl transferase; see *DNA nucleotidylexotransferase*.

Te tellurium.

tea (te) [L. *thea*] 1. *Camellia sinensis.* 2. the dried leaves of *C. sinensis*, which contain caffeine, theophylline, tannic acid, and a volatile oil. Tea is either *green* or *black* depending on the curing method. 3. a decoction of these leaves, used as a stimulating beverage or soothing drink for various abdominal discomforts. Green tea has been used for prevention of dental caries and is also used in traditional Chinese medicine, ayurveda, and homeopathy. Excessive consumption can cause theaism. 4. any decoction or infusion.

Teale amputation (operation) (tēl) [Thomas Pridgin *Teale*, Sr., English surgeon, 1801–1868] see under *amputation*.

tear (tār) 1. to pull apart or in pieces by force. 2. to wound or injure, especially by ripping apart or rending; lacerate. 3. laceration.

cemental t., cementum t. complete or partial detachment of a fragment of cementum from the root surface of a tooth, especially when associated with occlusal trauma. Called also *cemental* or *cementum fracture*.

Mallory-Weiss t. a small, slitlike laceration in the gastric mucosa, longitudinally placed at or slightly below the esophagogastric junction, seen in Mallory-Weiss syndrome

tears (tērz) [L. *lacrimae;* Gr. *dakrya*] 1. the watery secretion of the lacrimal glands which serves to moisten the conjunctiva; the secretion is slightly alkaline and saline. 2. small, naturally formed, droplike masses of a gum or resin.

crocodile t. lacrimation on chewing and eating; see *syndrome of crocodile tears*.

teart (tert) 1. soil or plants that contain unusually high amounts of molybdenum. 2. molybdenosis in ruminants that graze on teart plants; see also *teart disease of cattle*.

tease (tēz) to pull a tissue apart with needles for microscopical examination.

tea·spoon (te'spo͞on) a household unit of capacity, containing about 5 milliliters.

teat (tēt) papilla mammae.

TeBG testosterone-estradiol–binding globulin.

te·bor·ox·ime (teb″ə-rok'sēm) a compound which, complexed with technetium 99m, constitutes a BATO that is used as a marker of local perfusion in cardiovascular imaging. See table at *technetium*.

teb·u·tate (teb'u-tāt) USAN contraction for tertiary butyl acetate.

Tech·ne·plex (tek'nə-pleks″) trademark for a kit for the preparation of technetium Tc 99m pentetate.

Techne·Scan (tek'nə-skan″) trademark for a series of kits used in the preparation of radiolabeled technetium-containing compounds.

T. Gluceptate trademark for a kit for the preparation of technetium Tc 99m gluceptate.

T. HDP trademark for a kit for the preparation of technetium Tc 99m oxidronate.

T. HIDA trademark for a kit for the preparation of technetium Tc 99m lidofenin.

T. MAA trademark for a kit for the preparation of technetium Tc 99m albumin aggregated.

T. MAG3 trademark for a kit for the preparation of technetium Tc 99m mertiatide.

T. MDP trademark for a kit for the preparation of technetium Tc 99m medronate.

T. PYP trademark for a kit for the preparation of technetium Tc 99m pyrophosphate.

T. Sulfur Colloid trademark for a kit for the preparation of technetium Tc 99m sulfur colloid.

tech·ne·ti·um (Tc) (tek-ne'she-əm) a metallic element, atomic number 99, having no stable isotopes or naturally occurring radioactive isotopes.

t. 99m a metastable isotope of technetium, atomic mass 99, having a half-life of 6.01 hours; it decays by isomeric transition emitting gamma rays (0.141 MeV), and is the most commonly used radionuclide in nuclear medicine.

t. Tc 99m HSA trademark for a preparation of technetium Tc 99m albumin.

t. 99m pertechnetate the ionic form of technetium 99m, TcO_4^-, having a variety of uses as an imaging agent (see table) and in the preparation of other ^{99m}Tc radiopharmaceuticals.

tech·nic (tek'nik) technique.

tech·ni·cal (tek'nĭ-kəl) 1. pertaining to technique. 2. having particular training or knowledge.

tech·ni·cian (tek-nish'ən) a person skilled in the performance of the technical or procedural aspects of a health care profession; the minimum requirement is usually an associate degree. The technician carries out routine work under the supervision of a physician, therapist, technologist, or other health care professional.

tech·nique (tek-nēk') [Fr.] the method of procedure and the details of any mechanical process or surgical operation. See also under *maneuver, method, operation, procedure, treatment, stain, test*, etc.

Alexander t. a bodywork technique that uses psychophysical reeducation to correct dysfunctional habits of posture and movement, based on the principle that human movement is most fluid when the head leads and the spine follows, in order to improve postural balance, coordination, and breathing function; relieve stress and chronic pain; and improve general well-being.

Selected Technetium Tc 99m Radiopharmaceuticals

Radiopharmaceutical		Other Names	Selected Uses	Administration Mode
Tc 99m albumin	USP	Tc 99m-labeled human serum albumin Tc 99m-labeled HSA	Cardiac blood pool imaging; assessment of pericardial effusion and ventricular aneurysm (adjunct)	IV
Tc 99m albumin aggregated	USP	Tc 99m-labeled MAA	Lung imaging; radionuclide venography; assessment of peritoneovenous shunt patency	IV; intraperitoneal
Tc 99m albumin colloid	USP		Liver imaging; spleen imaging; bone marrow imaging	IV
Tc 99m albumin microaggregated			Liver imaging; assessment of regional blood flow	IV
Tc 99m apcitide	USP		Diagnosis of lower extremity acute venous thrombosis	IV
Tc 99m arcitumomab	USP		Detection of recurrent or metastatic colorectal carcinoma	IV
Tc 99m bectumomab			Diagnosis of non-Hodgkin lymphoma	IV
Tc 99m biciromab			Diagnosis of deep vein thrombosis	IV
Tc 99m bicisate		Tc 99m ethyl cysteinate dimer Tc 99m ECD	Brain imaging	IV
Tc 99m depreotide	USP		Diagnosis of non-small cell lung carcinoma	IV
Tc 99m disofenin	USP	Tc 99m diisopropyl-IDA Tc 99m DISIDA	Hepatobiliary imaging; hepatic function studies	IV
Tc 99m etidronate	USP	Tc 99m hydroxyethylidene diphosphonate Tc 99m EHDP	Skeletal imaging	IV
Tc 99m exametazime	USP	Tc 99m hexamethylpropyleneamine oxime Tc 99m HMPAO	Imaging of cerebral regional blood flow; leukocyte labeling for diagnosis of inflammatory lesions and bowel disease	IV
Tc 99m ferpentetate			Renal imaging	IV
Tc 99m furifosmin			Myocardial perfusion imaging	IV
Tc 99m gluceptate	USP	Tc 99m glucoheptonate Tc 99m GHP; Tc 99m GHA; Tc 99m GH	Brain and renal imaging or perfusion studies	IV
Tc 99m lidofenin	USP	Tc 99m HIDA	Hepatobiliary imaging; hepatic function studies	IV
Tc 99m mebrofenin	USP	Tc 99m trimethylbromo-IDA Tc 99m BrIDA	Hepatobiliary imaging; hepatic function studies	IV
Tc 99m medronate	USP	Tc 99m methylene diphosphonate Tc 99m MDP	Skeletal imaging	IV
Tc 99m mertiatide	USP	Tc 99m mercaptoacetyltriglycine Tc 99m MAG3	Renal imaging; renal function studies	IV
Tc 99m nofetumomab merpentan	USP		Evaluation of small cell lung cancer	IV
Tc 99m oxidronate	USP	Tc 99m hydroxymethylene diphosphonate Tc 99m HMDP; Tc 99m HDP	Skeletal imaging	IV
Tc 99m pamidronate		Tc 99m aminohydroxypropane diphosphonate Tc 99m ADP	Skeletal imaging	IV
Tc 99m pentetate	USP	Tc 99m diethylenetriamine pentaacetic acid Tc 99m DTPA	Renal imaging and perfusion studies; determination of glomerular filtration rate; brain imaging; lung imaging; radionuclide cisternography	IV
Tc 99m pertechnetate			Brain, parathyroid, salivary glands, thyroid stomach, heart, joints, and Meckel diverticulum imaging; assessment of shunt patency	IV; oral
Tc 99m pyrophosphate	USP	Tc 99m, PPi; Tc 99m PYP	Cardiac imaging; skeletal imaging	IV
Tc 99m (pyro- and trimeta-) phosphates	USP		Cardiac imaging; skeletal imaging	IV
Tc 99m red blood cells	USP	Tc 99m RBC	Cardiac blood pool imaging; detection of gastrointestinal bleeding	IV
Tc 99m sestamibi	USP	Tc 99m (hexakis) methoxyisobutyl isonitrile Tc 99m MIBI; Tc 99m hexamibi	Myocardial perfusion and cardiac function studies; parathyroid imaging; thyroid imaging	IV
Tc 99m siboroxime			Brain imaging	IV
Tc 99m succimer	USP	Tc 99m dimercaptosuccinic acid Tc 99m DMSA	Renal imaging	IV
Tc 99m sulesomab			Detection of osteomyelitis and soft tissue infections	IV
Tc 99m sulfur colloid	USP	Tc 99m SC	Spleen, liver, bone marrow, and esophageal imaging; assessment of gastrointestinal bleeding; gastric emptying studies; assessment of peritoneovenous shunt patency	IV; oral; intraperitoneal; intra-arterial; percutaneous transtubal
Tc 99m teboroxime			Myocardial perfusion imaging	IV
Tc 99m tetrofosmin	USP		Myocardial perfusion imaging	IV

Amplatz t. a femoral approach for coronary arteriography similar to the Judkins technique but using preformed Amplatz right or left coronary catheters.

aseptic t. any procedure designed to keep a surgical field as nearly aseptic as possible, e.g., gloving of the surgeon and aides, draping of the patient, autoclaving of instruments, and proper disposal of waste. Called also *sterile t.*

Begg t. an orthodontic technique employing a fixed multibanded appliance that incorporates a concept of differential light forces and uses a modified ribbon arch attachment and elastics (Begg appliance). Tipping the crowns of teeth to be moved, rather than moving them laterally, is used in the technique, thereby minimizing the use of orthodontic force.

Bowen t. a bodywork technique in which soft tissue mobilization is performed by gentle pressure from the thumb and fingers; used primarily for musculoskeletal conditions and stress-related disorders and for symptomatic relief in chronic conditions.

Bricker t. see under *procedure.*

Brown-Roberts-Wells t. a technique for stereotactic neurosurgery that uses a ring to hold the head in position, a ring for localization of a computed tomography image, and an arc guidance system.

clamp t. see *clamping.*

Cohen t., cross-trigonal t. a type of ureteroneocystostomy in which the ureter is excised from its attachment to the bladder and reimplanted in a new submucosal tunnel slightly above the bladder trigone.

dilution-filtration t. a blood culture technique in which any culture inhibitors present in the blood are diluted out and red blood cells are removed before the sample is filtered and cultured, thereby permitting the identification of organisms in about 24 hours.

DNA amplification t. see *nucleic acid amplification t.*

dye dilution t. see under *method.*

enzyme-multiplied immunoassay t. see *EMIT.*

fluorescent antibody t. an immunofluorescence technique in which antigen in tissue sections is located by homologous antibody labeled with fluorochrome (the single-layer technique) or by treating the antigen with unlabeled antibody followed by a second layer of labeled antiglobulin which is reactive with the unlabeled antibody (double-layer technique). Variations include direct, indirect, inhibition, and complement staining techniques.

gene amplification t. a term sometimes used to denote a nucleic acid amplification technique, although the segment of DNA or RNA undergoing amplification does not necessarily correspond to a single, entire gene.

Gil-Vernet t. a type of ureteroneocystostomy in which both ureters are excised from their normal attachments to the bladder and reattached medially near each other within the trigone.

Glenn-Anderson t. a type of ureteroneocystostomy in which a damaged ureteral attachment site is repaired in the original location.

hanging drop t. a method of microscopic examination of organisms suspended in a drop on a special concave microscope slide.

immunoperoxidase t. a method of histologic staining in which a peroxidase-labeled antibody that binds to antigen is added to tissue, and the sites of its localization are revealed by addition of a chromogenic substrate system that produces a colored reaction product visible by light microscopy. Cf. *peroxidase-antiperoxidase (PAP) t.*

indicator dilution t. see under *method.*

Irving t. a method of tubal ligation in which the uterine tubes are ligated and severed and the proximal ends are sewn into the myometrium. Called also *Irving operation.*

isolation-perfusion t. a technique for administering high doses of a chemotherapy agent to a region while protecting the patient from toxicity: the blood flow of the region is isolated, as by application of a tourniquet to an extremity, and the region is perfused by means of a pump-oxygenator; the drug is added to the perfusate, which may be heated by a heat exchanger to provide hyperthermia.

Jerne plaque t. a hemolytic technique for detecting antibody-producing cells: a suspension of presensitized lymphocytes is mixed in an agar gel with erythrocytes; after a period of incubation, complement is added and a clear area of lysis of red cells can be seen around each of the antibody-producing cells.

Judkins t. a femoral approach for coronary arteriography, in which a preformed Judkins right or left coronary catheter is inserted into the right or left coronary artery, respectively, via percutaneous cannulation of the femoral artery.

Kleinschmidt t. rupture of the virion by osmotic shock so that viral DNA is exposed.

Laurell t. 1. crossed immunoelectrophoresis (Laurell first technique). 2. rocket immunoelectrophoresis (Laurell second technique).

Leboyer t. see under *method.*

LeDuc t. a type of ureterointestinal anastomosis in which the ureter is brought through the bowel wall and the end is spatulated and sutured to a T-shaped incision in the bowel mucosa. Called also *LeDuc implantation.*

Leksell t. a technique for stereotactic neurosurgery that uses an arc guidance system and a cube-shaped frame that holds the head in position and is marked with X, Y, and Z coordinates for three-dimensional orientation.

Lich t., Lich-Gregoir t. a type of ureteroneocystostomy in which the ureter is excised from its attachment to the bladder and reattached to a submucosal tunnel created within the bladder.

membrane filter t. a technique for detecting bacteria in a sample of water: the sample is passed through a membrane filter, leaving bacteria on the filter surface; that surface is then placed on culture medium, incubated, and analyzed for bacterial colonies.

Mohs t. see under *surgery.*

needle-through-needle t. a technique of anesthetic administration in which a narrow spinal needle is advanced through the lumen of a larger-gauge needle such as a Tuohy needle and past its tip to puncture the dura so that spinal and epidural anesthesia can be administered at the same time.

nucleic acid amplification t. any of various in vitro methods by which a DNA or RNA sequence is amplified, making it more readily detectable for various procedures or tests. The original, and still most commonly used, is the polymerase chain reaction. See also under *test.*

Oakley-Fulthorpe t. double diffusion in one dimension; see under *diffusion.*

Ouchterlony t. double diffusion in two dimensions; see under *diffusion.*

Oudin t. a single diffusion (see under *diffusion*) technique in which agar containing antiserum is placed in a test tube and antigen is layered over it; precipitin lines form where the concentrations of each antigen and antibody are equivalent.

PAP t. peroxidase-antiperoxidase t.

Paquin t. a type of ureteroneocystostomy in which the ureter is excised from its attachment to the bladder and reattached in a more posteromedial position.

peroxidase-antiperoxidase t. a technique for detecting antigen or antibody in tissue sections. The tissue section is incubated with rabbit antibody specific for the antigen to be detected, followed by an excess of anti-rabbit IgG. A complex of horseradish peroxidase and rabbit antiperoxidase is added; these are linked to the antigen-bound antibody by the antirabbit IgG. The PAP complexes are then stained by incubation with a chromogenic substrate to produce a colored reaction product. Called also *PAP t.*

Politano-Leadbetter t. a type of ureteroneocystostomy in which the ureter is excised from its attachment to the bladder and reattached in a more medial and superior position.

Pomeroy t. a method of tubal ligation in which a loop of fallopian tube is picked up and ligated at its base with an absorbable suture, about 5 cm from the uterine cornua, and the tied loop is then resected. Called also *Pomeroy operation.*

push-back t. a surgical procedure designed to reposition the soft palate posteriorly and reestablish velopharyngeal competence. Called also *push-back procedure.*

Ravitch t. a surgical technique for the repair of pectus excavatum, in which the deformed costal cartilages are resected with preservation of the perichondrium, from which new cartilage regenerates, and correction of the sternal deformity.

Rebuck skin window t. a technique used to study the inflammatory process; an area of skin is abraded until capillary bleeding occurs and a coverslip or chamber containing balanced salt solution is applied. This permits direct observation of inflammatory cells migrating into the site; polymorphonuclear leukocytes predominate at about 10 hours; macrophages predominate at about 4 days.

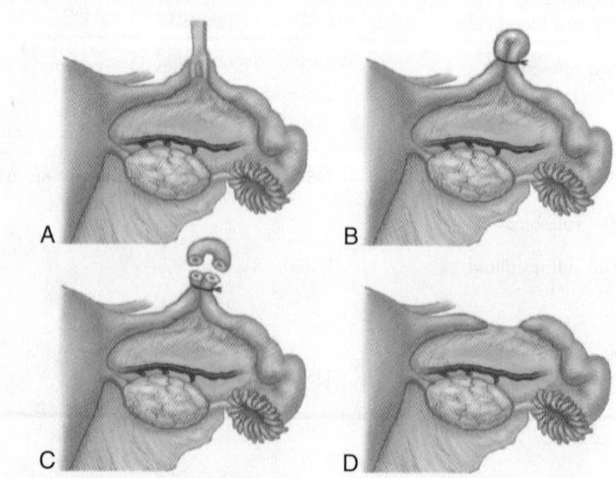

■ Pomeroy technique. *(A)*, Tube is grasped with forceps; *(B)*, a loop is ligated; *(C)*, the loop is excised; *(D)*, several months later, the fibrosed ends of the tube separate.

Riechert-Mundinger t. a technique for stereotactic neurosurgery that uses a semicircular arc guidance system and a ring to hold the head in position.

RNA amplification t. see *nucleic acid amplification t.*

sandwich t. 1. detection of a specific molecule, as a protein or nucleic acid, by sandwiching it between two layers of a different molecule or material, the second of which is radiolabeled or otherwise tagged for detection. The term is sometimes used specifically to denote detection of an antigen using two layers of antibody. 2. any technique that places something of interest between two layers of something else more easily detected or performed, or otherwise useful.

Schuster t. a method for repair of an omphalocele consisting of covering the sac with prosthetic sheeting followed by progressive reduction of the contents into the abdominal cavity.

scintillation counting t. a method of determining the amount of radioactivity by use of a scintillation counter (q.v.).

Seldinger t. a method for introducing a catheter into a hollow lumen structure or body cavity; a narrow needle is used to enter the structure, a guidewire is passed through the needle, the needle is removed, and the catheter is advanced over the wire. Used in angiography, cardiac catheterization, and cannulation of the central venous system.

shoelace t. a technique for delayed primary closure of fasciotomy: skin staples placed 2 cm apart serve as eyes for a loop of suture material that serves as the lace; daily tightening produces gradual reapproximation of the skin edges.

Sones t. a brachial approach for coronary arteriography, in which the catheter is inserted via a brachial arteriotomy; usually a single Sones catheter can be used in either coronary artery or for entry into the left ventricle.

sperm swim-up t. any of several methods of checking sperm for motility; a semen sample is centrifuged to form pellets, which are then covered with culture medium. The spermatozoa with greatest motility will swim up into the culture medium and be more suitable for use in in vitro fertilization.

squash t. any of a variety of techniques for preparation of a tissue or other histologic sample for microscopic examination, including treatment and staining of the sample, placement on a slide, and finally "squashing" down of the coverslip to flatten and spread the material.

squeeze t. a technique used for treatment of premature ejaculation; the patient is repeatedly aroused almost to the point of ejaculatory inevitability and then the thumb and first two fingers are used to forcibly squeeze the head of the penis, preventing ejaculation.

sterile t. aseptic t.

thermal dilution t., thermodilution t. thermodilution.

Todd-Wells t. a technique for stereotactic neurosurgery that uses an arc-quadrant, a ring around the head to steady the head and provide one set of reference angles, and a ring around the neck to provide a second set of reference angles.

transfixion t. a percutaneous approach for arterial or venous access; using a needle within a catheter, the posterior wall of the artery is punctured, the needle removed, and the catheter slowly withdrawn until blood flows freely.

Uchida t. a method of tubal ligation with injection of saline solution beneath the tubal mucosa to separate it from the underlying tube; a portion of mucosa is removed and the mucosa-free tube then retracts to form a stump that is closed with sutures.

ultrasound dilution t. a technique for measuring blood flow and access recirculation in hemodialysis patients: ultrasound sensors are attached to the venous and arterial catheters in their normal positions and blood flow is checked; then they are reversed, the ultrafiltration is turned off, and at a known pumped blood flow rate a bolus of saline is released into the venous catheter to dilute the blood; the velocity of the dilution as it passes through the access apparatus is measured by ultrasonography.

Western blot t. see *Western blot,* under *blot.*

tech•no•cau•sis (tek″no-kaw′sis) [Gr. *technē* art + *kausis* burning] use of the actual cautery.

tech•nol•o•gist (tek-nol′ə-jist) a person skilled in the theory and practice of a technical profession, usually with at least a baccalaureate degree; in several allied health fields, technologist is the highest professional rank.

tech•nol•o•gy (tek-nol′ə-je) [Gr. *technē* art + *-logy*] scientific knowledge; the sum of the study of a technique.

assisted reproductive t. (ART) any procedure involving manipulation of eggs or sperm to establish pregnancy in treatment of infertility.

gene t. genetic engineering.

recombinant DNA t. a body of techniques that isolate specific DNA sequences, create recombinant molecules by splicing together segments of DNA from different sources, introduce the recombinant sequences into cells and amplify them, and employ the products in a variety of analytic, therapeutic, and industrial applications.

tec•to•ce•phal•ic (tek″to-sə-fal′ik) scaphocephalic.

tec•to•ceph•a•ly (tek″to-sef′ə-le) scaphocephaly.

tec•tol•o•gy (tek-tol′ə-je) [Gr. *tektōn* builder + *-logy*] a branch of biology concerned with the building up of organisms from structured elements; the doctrine of structure, a division of morphology.

tec•ton•ic (tek-ton′ik) [Gr. *tektonikos* skilled in building] pertaining to construction; used in denoting the mechanics underlying tectonic keratoplasty.

tec•to•ri•al (tek-tor′e-əl) pertaining to a roof or covering.

tec•to•ri•um (tek-tor′e-əm) pl. *tecto′ria* [L. "roof"] membrana tectoria ductus cochlearis.

tec•to•spi•nal (tek″to-spi′nəl) extending from the tectum mesencephali to the spinal cord; see also under *tract.*

tec•tum (tek′təm) [L. "roof"] any rooflike structure.

t. mesence′phali [TA] mesencephalic tectum: that part of the mesencephalic tegmentum comprising the tectal lamina and the inferior and superior colliculi.

t. of midbrain t. mesencephali.

TED threshold erythema dose.

TEE transesophageal echocardiography.

teeth (tēth) see *tooth.*

teeth•ing (tēth′ing) the entire process which results in the eruption of the teeth.

Tef•lon (tef′lon) trademark for preparations of polytef (polytetrafluoroethylene).

teg•a•fur (teg′ə-fər) an investigational cancer chemotherapeutic agent, which is 5-fluorouracil (5-FU) attached to a tetrahydrofuran moiety analogous to the ribose and deoxyribose moieties in the active metabolites of 5-FU. It acts like a depot form of 5-FU and potential uses are the same as those of 5-FU.

teg•a•ser•od maleate (teg″ə-ser′od) a selective serotonin antagonist, used in the treatment of irritable bowel syndrome and other gastrointestinal motility disorders. It has been withdrawn from the market in the United States.

Te•ge•na•ria (te″jə-nar′e-ə) a genus of spiders of the family Agelenidae that build funnel-shaped webs.

T. agres′tis the hobo spider, a species of the Pacific Northwest whose bite can cause slow-healing ulcers at the site of the bite, headache, nausea, fever, and altered mentation; potentially fatal hematologic changes, including aplastic anemia, pancytopenia, and thrombocytopenia, may rarely result.

teg•men (teg′mən) pl. *teg′mina* [L. "cover"] a covering structure or roof.

t. mastoid′eum the part of the tegmen tympani that forms a bony roof of the mastoid cells.

t. tym′pani [TA] roof of tympanum: the thin layer of translucent bone, on the petrous part of the temporal bone in the floor of the middle cranial fossa, separating the epitympanum from the cranial cavity; see also *paries tegmentalis cavitatis tympani.*

t. ventri′culi quar′ti [TA] roof of fourth ventricle: the superior part of the ventricle, formed by the superior and inferior medullary vela.

teg•men•tal (təg-men′təl) pertaining to or of the nature of a tegmen or tegmentum.

teg•men•tum (təg-men′təm) pl. *tegmen′ta* [L.] 1. a covering. 2. t. mesencephali. 3. the dorsal part of each cerebral peduncle; see also *t. mesencephali* and *pedunculus cerebri.*

hypothalamic t. subthalamic t.

t. mesence′phali [TA] tegmentum of midbrain: the posterior part of the mesencephalon, formed by continuation of the posterior parts of the cerebral peduncles across the median plane, and extending on each side from the substantia nigra to the level of the mesencephalic aqueduct. Called also *tegmentum* and *t. of mesencephalon.*

t. of mesencephalon, t. of midbrain t. mesencephali.

pontine t., t. pon′tis [TA] tegmentum of pons: the posterior part of the pons, which resembles the medulla oblongata in structure and is continuous with the tegmentum of the mesencephalon.

subthalamic t. the portion of the tegmentum of the cerebral peduncle extending beneath the thalamus.

Teg•re•tol (teg′rə-tol) trademark for preparations of carbamazepine.

teg•u•ment (teg′u-ment) [L. *tegumentum* or *tegmentum* covering] 1. integument. 2. a structure lying between the capsid and envelope of herpesvirus, varying in thickness and often distributed asymmetrically.

Teich•mann crystals, test (tīk′mahn) [Ludwig Carl *Teichmann*-Stawiarski, German histologist, 1823–1895] see under *crystal* and *test.*

tei•cho•ic ac•id (ti-ko′ik) any of a diverse group of polymers found in the cell wall and cell membrane of gram-positive bacteria. They consist of phosphate-linked backbones of sugar alcohol residues, to which are attached various sugars and D-alanine residues. The sugar alcohol may be glycerol *(glycerol teichoic acids)* or ribitol *(ribitol teichoic acids);* the first type occurs in both the cell wall and cell membrane, the second only in the cell wall. They can also be classified as *lipoteichoic acids* or *wall teichoic acids* on the basis of their site of attachment in the cell. In certain bacteria, at least some of the teichoic acids serve as major antigenic determinants.

wall t. a. any of various teichoic acids that are attached to *N*-acetylmuramic acid residues of the peptidoglycan of gram-positive bacteria; they may serve as antigenic determinants for certain bacteria. Cf. *lipoteichoic acid.*

tei•chop•sia (ti-kop′se-ə) [Gr. *teichos* wall + *-opsia*] the sensation of a luminous appearance before the eyes, with a zigzag, wall-like outline; it may be a migraine aura. Called also *fortification spectrum, flittering scotoma,* and *scintillating scotoma.*

tei•co•pla•nin (ti-ko-pla′nin) a glycopeptide antibiotic produced by the bacterium *Actinoplanes teichomyceticus,* used as a less toxic alternative to vancomycin in the treatment of moderate to severe infections caused by gram-positive bacteria where other antibiotics cannot be used.

Tek•tur•na (tek-ter′nə) trademark for a preparation of aliskiren.

te•la (te′lə) pl. *te′lae* [L. "something woven," "web"] tissue: a thin weblike layer or membrane.

t. choroidea of fourth ventricle t. choroidea ventriculi quarti.

t. choroidea of lateral ventricle t. choroidea ventriculi lateralis.

t. choroidea of third ventricle t. choroidea ventriculi tertii.

t. choroi′dea ventri′culi latera′lis tela choroidea of lateral ventricle: the lateral extension of the tela choroidea of the third ventricle into the choroid fissure of the lateral ventricle of the brain; from it, vascular folds invaginate the ventricular ependyma to form the choroid plexus of the lateral ventricle.

t. choroi′dea ventri′culi quar′ti [TA] tela choroidea of fourth ventricle: a double layer or fold of pia mater between the cerebellum and the lower part of the roof of the fourth ventricle; the anterior layer of the fold, together with the ventricular ependyma, contains vascular fringes which constitute the choroid plexus.

t. choroi′dea ventri′culi ter′tii [TA] tela choroidea of third ventricle: a double layer or fold of pia mater which, together with the ventricular ependyma, forms the roof of the third ventricle; from the lower fold two vascular fringes invaginate the roof to form the choroid plexuses.

t. subcuta′nea [TA] subcutaneous tissue: the layer of loose connective tissue situated just beneath the skin; called also *hypodermis* [TA alternative] and *superficial fascia.*

t. subcuta′nea abdo′minis [TA] subcutaneous tissue of abdomen: the loose connective tissue just below the skin of the abdomen, consisting of an adipose layer (Camper fascia) overlying a membranous layer (Scarpa fascia).

t. subcuta′nea pe′nis [TA] subcutaneous tissue of penis: the loose external layer of fascial tissue of the penis, continuous with the tunica dartos and the tela subcutanea perinei. Called also *superficial penile fascia.*

t. subcuta′nea perine′i [TA] subcutaneous tissue of perineum: the subcutaneous tissue of the urogenital region, consisting almost entirely of the stratum membranosum with little overlying fat. Called also *superficial perineal fascia* and *superficial fascia of perineum.*

t. submuco′sa submucosa: the layer of loose connective tissue between the lamina muscularis mucosae and the tunica muscularis in most parts of the digestive, respiratory, urinary, and genital tracts.

t. submuco′sa bron′chi [TA] that underlying the mucosa of a bronchus.

t. submuco′sa gas′trica [TA] that underlying the mucosa of the stomach.

t. submuco′sa intesti′ni cras′si [TA] that underlying the mucosa of the large intestine.

t. submuco′sa intesti′ni te′nuis [TA] that underlying the mucosa of the small intestine.

t. submuco′sa oeso′phagi [TA] that underlying the mucosa of the esophagus.

t. submuco′sa pharyn′gis [TA] that underlying the mucosa of the pharynx.

t. submuco′sa vesi′cae urina′riae [TA] that underlying the mucosa of the wall of the urinary bladder.

t. subsero′sa subserosa or subserous layer: a layer of loose areolar tissue underlying the tunica serosa of various organs.

t. subsero′sa gas′trica [TA] that underlying the serosa of the stomach.

t. subsero′sa he′patis [TA] that underlying the serosa of the liver.

t. subsero′sa intesti′ni cras′si [TA] that underlying the serosa of the large intestine.

t. subsero′sa intesti′ni te′nuis [TA] that underlying the serosa of the small intestine.

t. subsero′sa oeso′phagi [TA] that underlying the serosa of the esophagus.

t. subsero′sa pericar′dii [TA] that underlying the serosa of the serous pericardium.

t. subsero′sa peritone′i [TA] fascia extraperitonealis.

t. subsero′sa pleu′rae parieta′lis [TA] that underlying the serosa of the parietal pleura.

t. subsero′sa pleu′rae viscera′lis [TA] that underlying the serosa of the visceral pleura.

t. subero′sa tes′tis [TA] that underlying the serosa of the testis.

t. subsero′sa tu′bae uteri′nae [TA] that underlying the serosa of the uterine (fallopian) tube.

t. subsero′sa u′teri [TA] that underlying the serosa of the uterus.

t. subsero′sa vesi′cae bilia′ris [TA] that underlying the serosa of the gallbladder.

t. subsero′sa vesi′cae urina′riae [TA] that underlying the serosa of the urinary bladder.

Te•la•dor•sa•gia (te″lə-dor-sa′jə) a genus of nematode stomach worms of the family Trichostrongylidae, closely resembling *Ostertagia* but found primarily in the abomasum of sheep and goats.

te•lae (te′le) [L.] genitive and plural of *tela.*

tel•al•gia (tə-lal′jə) referred pain.

tel•an•gi•ec•ta•sia (tə-lan″je-ək-ta′zhə) [*tele-* + *angi-* + *ectasia*] permanent dilation of preexisting small blood vessels (capillaries, arterioles, venules) to form focal, discolored lesions, usually in the skin or mucous membranes. See also *capillary fragility,* under *fragility.* Called also *telangiectasis.*

generalized essential t. that involving the entire body or localized to a large area; lesions may be discrete or confluent and macular, plaquelike, or retiform.

hereditary hemorrhagic t. an autosomal dominant vascular anomaly characterized by multiple small telangiectases of the skin, mucous membranes, gastrointestinal tract, and other organs, associated with recurrent episodes of bleeding from affected sites and gross or occult melena. Called also *Osler disease, Osler-Weber-Rendu disease,* and *Rendu-Osler-Weber syndrome.*

t. macula′ris erupti′va per′stans a rare form of mastocytosis, usually affecting adults, characterized by multiple hyperpigmented telangiectatic macules on the skin of the trunk or limbs.

periungual t. telangiectasia near the nails, seen in persons with dermatomyositis.

spider t. see under *angioma.*

unilateral nevoid t. patches of essential telangiectasia in a unilateral, linear distribution; it may be either congenital or acquired. The acquired form is more common in women and represents a latent vascular nevus that becomes manifest; causes are thought to be increased estrogen in the body (such as in pregnancy or at menarche) or increased venous pressure (such as in liver disease). Called also *unilateral nevoid telangiectasia syndrome.*

tel•an•gi•ec•ta•sis (tə-lan″je-ek′tə-sis) pl. *telangiec′tases* [*tele-* + *angi-* + *ectasis*] 1. the lesion produced by telangiectasia, which may present as a coarse or fine red line or as a punctum with radiating limbs (spider). 2. telangiectasia.

tel•an•gi•ec•tat•ic (tə-lan″je-ək-tat′ik) pertaining to or characterized by telangiectasia.

tel•an•gi•ec•to•des (tə-lan″je-ek-to′dēz) marked by telangiectasia.

tel•an•gi•itis (tə-lan″je-i′tis) [*tele-* + *angi-* + *-itis*] capillaritis.

tel•an•gi•on (tə-lan′je-on) [*tele-* + Gr. *angeion* vessel] a terminal artery.

tel•an•gi•o•sis (tə-lan″je-o′sis) [*tele-* + *angi-* + *-osis*] capillaropathy.

te•lar (te′lər) pertaining to, affecting, or resembling tela.

tel•biv•u•dine (tel-biv′u-dēn) a synthetic thymidine analogue with antiviral activity against hepatitis B virus; administered orally.

Tel•drin HBP (tel′drin) trademark for a preparation of chlorpheniramine maleate.

tele- [Gr. *tēle* far off, at a distance] a combining form meaning operating at a distance, or far away.

tele•bi•noc•u•lar (tel″ə-bi-nok′u-lər) a prism-refracting instrument for use in orthoptic training.

tele•can•thus (tel″ə-kan′thəs) [*tele-* + *canthus*] abnormally increased distance between the medial canthi of the eyelids.

tele•car•dio•gram (tel″ə-kahr′de-o-gram) [*tele-* + *cardio-* + *-gram*] the tracing obtained by telecardiography.

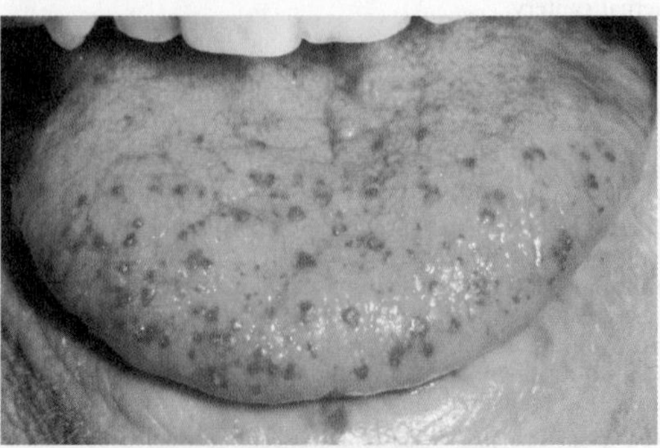

■ Hereditary hemorrhagic telangiectasia.

tele·car·di·og·ra·phy (tel″ə-kahr″de-og′rə-fe) [*tele-* + *cardio-* + *-graphy*] electrocardiography done by telemetry.

tele·car·dio·phone (tel″ə-kahr′de-o-fōn) [*tele-* + *cardio-* + Gr. *phōnē* sound] an apparatus for rendering heart sounds audible to listeners at a distance from the patient.

tele·cep·tor (tel′ə-sep″tər) [*tele-* + *receptor*] a sensory nerve terminal which is sensitive to stimuli originating at a distance; such nerve endings exist in the eyes, ears, and nose. **telecep′tive** *adj*

tele·cord (tel′ə-kord) an apparatus for attachment to an x-ray machine; by means of it each cardiac phase can be photographed in series.

tele·cu·rie·ther·a·py (tel″ə-ku″re-ther′ə-pe) external beam radiotherapy.

tele·der·ma·tol·o·gy (tel″ədur″mə-tol′ə-je) the use of telemedicine techniques in dermatology.

tele·di·ag·no·sis (tel″ə-di″əg-no′sis) [*tele-* + *diagnosis*] determination of the nature of a disease at a site remote from the patient on the basis of telehealth methods of transmitted data.

tele·echo·car·di·og·ra·phy (tel″e-ek″o-kahr″de-og′rə-fe) echocardiography performed under the direction of a remotely located consultant by means of a transmitted signal.

tele·flu·o·ros·co·py (tel″ə-floo-ros′kə-pe) [*tele-* + *fluoroscopy*] a telehealth technique consisting of electronic transmission of fluoroscopic images.

tele·health (tel′ə-helth) the use of electronic information and telecommunications technologies to support long-distance clinical health care, professional health-related education, public health, and health administration.

tele·ki·ne·sis (tel″ə-kĭ-ne′sis) [*tele-* + *-kinesis*] the power claimed by certain persons of moving objects without contact with the object moved; also motion produced without contact with a moving body. **telekinet′ic** *adj*

tel·elec·tro·car·dio·gram (tel″ə-lek″tro-kahr′de-o-gram) telecardiogram.

tel·elec·tro·car·dio·graph (tel″ə-lek″tro-kahr′de-o-graf) [*tele-* + *electrocardiograph*] a device for transmission and remote reception of electrocardiographic signals.

tele·med·i·cine (tel″ə-med′ĭ-sin) [*tele-* + *medicine*] a branch of telehealth consisting of provision of consultant services by off-site health care professionals to those on the scene; diagnosis and treatment can be done at a great distance through methods such as the videoconference or rapid transmission of digital files.

te·lem·e·try (tə-lem′ə-tre) [*tele-* + *-metry*] the making of measurements at a distance from the subject, with measurable evidence of the phenomena under investigation being transmitted by radio signals, wires, or other means. See *radiotelemetry*, *telefluoroscopy*, and *telecardiography*.

tele·mne·mon·i·ke (tel″ə-ne-mon′ĭ-ke) [*tele-* + Gr. *mnēmonikos* pertaining to memory] the gaining of consciousness of things in the memory of another person.

tel·en·ce·phal·ic (tel″en-sə-fal′ik) pertaining to the telencephalon.

tel·en·ceph·al·iza·tion (tel″en-sef″əl-ĭ-za′shən) the transfer to the telencephalon, during the process of evolution, of the direction of the more complex nerve reactions.

tel·en·ceph·a·lon (tel″en-sef′ə-lon) [*tele-* + *encephalon*] 1. [TA] one of the two divisions of the prosencephalon, composing the cerebrum (q.v.). 2. in the developing embryo, the anterior of the two brain vesicles formed by specialization of the prosencephalon, consisting of the anterolateral evaginations of the prosencephalon, together with the median, unpaired portion, the lamina terminalis; from it the cerebral hemispheres are derived. Called also *endbrain*. See Plates 9 and 10.

tele·neu·rite (tel″ə-noor′īt) the end expansion of an axon.

tele·neu·ron (tel″ə-noor′on) [*tele(o)-* + *neuron*] a nerve ending.

tele(o)- [Gr. *telos* end] a combining form denoting relationship to the end.

te·leo·log·i·cal (te″le-ə-log′ĭ-kəl) 1. pertaining to teleology. 2. serving an ultimate purpose in development.

te·le·ol·o·gy (te″le-ol′ə-je) [*teleo-* + *-logy*] the doctrine of final causes, or of adaptation to a definite purpose.

te·leo·morph (te′le-o-morf″) [*teleo-* + *-morph*] the stage of a fungus where reproduction results from plasmogamy followed by karyogamy, with sexual spores, as opposed to an anamorph. See also *perfect fungus*, under *fungus*. Called also *perfect stage* or *state* and *sexual stage* or *state*.

te·leo·nom·ic (te″le-o-nom′ik) pertaining to or having evolutionary survival value.

te·le·on·o·my (te″le-on′ə-me) [*teleo-* + Gr. *nomos* law] the doctrine that the existence of a structure or a function in an organism implies that it has had evolutionary survival value.

tele·op·sia (tel″e-op′se-ə) [*tele-* + *-opsia*] a visual disturbance in which objects appear to be farther away than they actually are.

te·le·or·gan·ic (te″le-or-gan′ik) necessary to life.

tele·ost (tel′e-ost) a member of the Teleostei, comprising the higher bony fishes.

Tele·paque (tel′ə-pāk) trademark for a preparation of iopanoic acid.

tele·pa·thol·o·gy (tel″ə-pə-thol′ə-je) [*tele-* + *pathology*] the practice of pathology at a remote location using telecommunications technology to transmit digital images for display on a high-resolution video monitor; images may be static or may be real-time images obtained by a video-equipped remote-control microscope.

te·lep·a·thy (tə-lep′ə-the) [*tele-* + *-pathy*] extrasensory perception of the mental activity of another person. Cf. *clairvoyance*.

tele·ra·dio·gram (tel″ə-ra′de-o-gram) the picture or film obtained by teleradiography.

tele·ra·di·og·ra·phy (tel″ə-ra″de-og′rə-fe) 1. a telehealth technique consisting of electronic transmission of radiographic images. 2. radiography with the radiation source about 2 meters from the subject, more nearly securing parallelism of the rays and minimizing distortion.

tele·ra·dio·ther·a·py (tel″ə-ra″de-o-ther′ə-pe) external beam radiotherapy.

tele·ra·di·um (tel″ə-ra′de-əm) [*tele-* + *radium*] a radium source located at a distance from the body, as for use in external beam radiotherapy.

tele·re·cep·tor (tel″ə-rə-sep′tər) teleceptor.

tele·roent·gen·ther·a·py (tel″ə-rent″gən-ther′ə-pe) external beam radiotherapy.

tel·e·steth·o·scope (tel″ə-steth′ə-skōp) [*tele-* + *stethoscope*] a combination of stethoscope and electrical amplification by which persons at a distance from the patient can hear the heart and lung sounds, as in demonstrating to a class or to a medical audience.

tel·es·the·sia (tel″es-the′zhə) [*tele-* + *esthesia*] extrasensory perception of objects or conditions.

tele·tac·tor (tel′ə-tak″tər) [*tele-* + L. *tangere* to touch] an instrument for communicating with the deaf by means of touch on a vibrating plate.

tele·ther·a·py (tel″ə-ther′ə-pe) [*tele-* + *therapy*] treatment in which the source of the therapeutic agent is at a distance from the body, as in external beam radiotherapy; cf. *brachytherapy*.

tele·ther·mom·e·ter (tel″ə-thər-mom′ə-tər) an apparatus for determining temperature on which the reading is made at a distance from the object or subject being studied.

tele·thon·in (tel″ə-thon′in) a 19 kDa sarcomeric protein of the Z band of striated and cardiac muscle. It is a substrate of and binds to titin, and acts as a muscle assembly regulating factor. Mutations in the gene encoding telethonin have been associated with types of limb-girdle muscular dystrophy and dilated cardiomyopathy.

Te·lio·my·ce·tes (te″le-o-mi-se′tēz) a class of perfect fungi of the subphylum Basidiomycotina, including those that have teliospores. It includes the orders Uredinales and Ustilaginales.

te·lio·spore (te′le-o-spor) a type of resting spore seen in fungi of the orders Uredinales and Ustilaginales, which afterwards produces a basidium.

te·lith·ro·my·cin (tə-lith′ro-mi″sin) a ketolide antibiotic used in the treatment of mild to moderate community-acquired respiratory tract infections, including those caused by multi-drug resistant *Streptococcus pneumoniae;* administered orally.

tel·lu·ric (tə-lu′rik) 1. pertaining to or originating from the earth. 2. pertaining to the element tellurium.

tel·lu·ri·um (Te) (tə-lu′re-əm) [L. *tellus* earth] a nonmetallic or metalloid element; specific gravity, 6.24; atomic weight, 127.60; atomic number, 52.

tel·mi·sar·tan (tel″mĭ-sahr′tan) an angiotensin II receptor antagonist, used as an antihypertensive; administered orally.

tel(o)- [Gr. *telos* end] a combining form denoting relationship to an end.

telo·bran·chi·al (tel″o-brang′ke-əl) ultimobranchial.

telo·cen·tric (tel″o-sen′trik) having the centromere at the extreme end of the chromosome, which thus consists of only one arm.

telo·coele (tel′o-sēl) [*telo-* + *-coele*] the cavity of the telencephalon.

telo·den·dron (tel″o-den′dron) pl. *teloden′dra* [*telo-* + Gr. *dendron* tree] one of the many fine twiglike terminal branches of an axon; called also *end-brush*.

tel·o·gen (tel′o-jən) the quiescent or resting third phase of the hair cycle following catagen; the hair has become a club hair and does not grow further.

tel·og·lia (təl-og′le-ə) terminal Schwann cells associated with the motor nerve endings.

tel•og•no•sis (tel″og-no′sis) [from *tele*phonic dia*gnosis*] diagnosis based on interpretation of radiograms transmitted by telephonic or radio communication. See also *teleradiography* (def. 1).

telo•lec•i•thal (tel″o-les′ĭ-thəl) [*telo-* + *-lecithal*] having a medium to large amount of yolk, with the yolk concentrated toward one pole (thus designated the vegetal pole); characteristic of the eggs of fish, amphibians, birds, and reptiles.

telo•mer•ase (tə-lo′mər-ās) a specialized RNA-directed DNA polymerase [EC 2.7.7.49] involved in the formation of telomeres, using RNA of the enzyme as a template to synthesize the tandem repeating DNA sequences that are added to the 3′ protruding ends of the telomeres, and also in maintaining telomere sequences during replication.

telo•mere (tel′o-mēr) [*telo-* + *-mere*] either of the ends of a eukaryotic chromosome, consisting of many repeats of a short DNA sequence in specific orientation (5′-TTAGGG-3′ in humans); their functions include protection of the ends of the chromosome and preservation of their linear integrity, facilitation of replication of the extreme ends of the chromosome (by telomerase), and maintenance of the three-dimensional positioning of the chromosomes within the nucleus. The number of repeats of telomeric DNA at the end of a chromosome decreases with age.

telo•phase (tel′o-fāz) [*telo-* + *phase*] the stage of cell division following metaphase, beginning when the daughter chromatids reach the poles; it is the final stage of mitosis and meiosis and immediately precedes cytokinesis. The chromatids separate from the kinetochore microtubules and the nuclear membrane reforms. In plant cells the new cell wall that separates the daughter cells begins to form during this stage.

telo•phrag•ma (tel″o-frag′mə) [*telo-* + Gr. *phragmos* a fencing in] name proposed for the Z band; cf. *inophragma*.

telo•re•cep•tor (tel′o-re-sep″tər) teleceptor.

telo•tax•is (tel″o-tak′sis) the tendency of an organism to maintain a constant angle to the source of a stimulus while it moves; observed in the behavior of social insects, such as bees and ants.

telo•tism (tel′o-tiz-əm) the complete performance of a function.

tel•son (tel′sən) an appendage on the terminal segment of some arthropods, especially the stinging organ of a scorpion.

TEM transanal endoscopic microsurgery.

Tem•a•ril (tem′ə-ril) trademark for preparations of trimeprazine tartrate.

te•maz•e•pam (tə-maz′ə-pam) [USP] a benzodiazepine used as a sedative and hypnotic in the treatment of insomnia; administered orally.

tem•e•fos (tem′ə-fos) USAN for *temephos*.

tem•e•phos (tem′ə-fos″) an organophosphorus insecticide used as a larvicide for control of mosquitoes and blackflies and as a veterinary ectoparasiticide; it can also cause organophosphorus compound poisoning (q.v.).

Tem•o•dar (tem′o-dahr) trademark for a preparation of temozolomide.

tem•o•dox (tem′o-doks) a veterinary growth stimulant.

Tem•o•vate (tem′ə-vāt″) trademark for preparations of clobetasol propionate.

tem•o•zo•lo•mide (tem″ə-zo′lə-mīd) a cytotoxic alkylating agent used as an antineoplastic in the treatment of refractory anaplastic astrocytoma; administered orally.

tem•per•a•ment (tem′pər-ə-mənt) [L. *temperamentum* mixture] an inherent, constitutional predisposition to react to stimuli in a certain way. The term is often used synonymously with *personality* (q.v.); cf. *character*.

tem•per•ate (tem′pər-ət) [L. *temperatus*, past part. of *temperare* to temper] restrained; characterized by moderation; as a temperate bacteriophage, which infects but does not lyse its host.

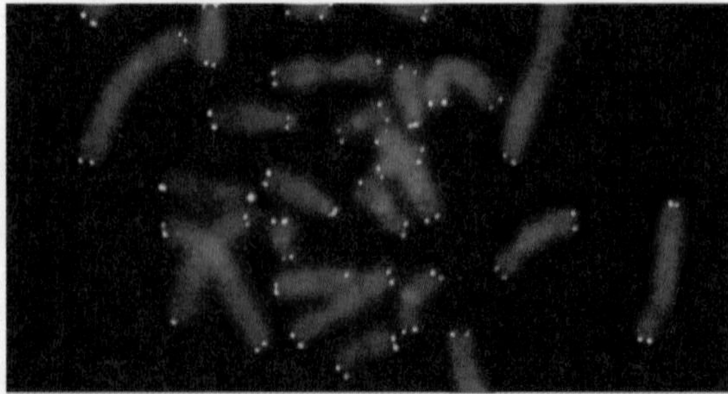

■ Detection of telomeres at the ends of each chromosome by fluorescence in situ hybridization (FISH) using a repeated TTAGGG probe. The two sister chromatids are evident by the double yellow hybridization signal at the end of most chromosome arms.

tem•per•a•ture (tem′pər-ə-chər) [L. *temperatura*, from *temperare*, to regulate] 1. the degree of sensible heat or cold; the property of a system that determines whether or not the system is in thermal equilibrium with other systems; a measure of the average kinetic energy due to thermal agitation of the particles in a system. Symbol *t*. 2. the level of heat natural to a living being. 3. colloquial term for *fever*.

absolute t. (*T*) temperature reckoned from absolute zero (−273.15°C or −459.67°F), expressed on an absolute scale (Kelvin or Rankine).

basal body t. (BBT) the temperature of the body under conditions of absolute rest; it has a slight sustained rise during the luteal phase of the menstrual cycle and can be used as an indirect indicator of when ovulation has occurred.

body t. the temperature of the body: in cold-blooded animals it varies with environmental temperature; in warm-blooded animals it is usually constant within a narrow range. See *normal t.*

core t. the temperature of structures deep within the body, as opposed to peripheral temperature such as that of the skin.

critical t. a temperature below which a gas may be liquefied by increased pressure.

fusion t. the temperature at which a metal or alloy changes from a solid to a liquid (melts or undergoes fusion). Cf. *melting point*.

maximum t. in bacteriology, the temperature above which growth does not take place.

melting t. (T_m) in molecular biology, the temperature at which half the length of a double-stranded nucleic acid becomes single-stranded; it is a function of the degree of match or mismatch between the two strands, the percentage of guanine-cytosine pairs in the molecule, and other variables. Cf. *melting point*.

minimum t. in bacteriology, temperature below which growth does not take place.

normal t. the temperature of the human body in health, about 37°C (98.6°F) when measured orally. This is maintained by the thermotaxic nerve mechanism, which maintains a balance between the thermogenetic, or heat-producing, and the thermolytic, or heat-dispelling, processes.

optimum t. the temperature promoting the most rapid growth of a given species of microorganism, or the temperature at which a reaction proceeds at maximum velocity.

room t. the temperature considered most comfortable for a room, defined as being between 18° and 27°C (65° and 80°F).

subnormal t. temperature below the normal.

tem•plate (tem′plət) [Old Fr. *templet* a weaver's bar] 1. a pattern or mold. 2. in genetics, a strand of DNA or RNA that specifies the base sequence of the strand of DNA or RNA to be synthesized in replication or transcription, the newly synthesized strand being complementary to the template. 3. in dentistry, a curved or flat plate used as an aid in setting teeth in a denture.

surgical t. a thin transparent resin base shaped to duplicate the form of the impression surface of an immediate denture and used as a guide for surgically shaping the alveolar process and its soft tissue covering to fit an immediate denture.

tem•ple (tem′pəl) [L. *tempula*, dim. of *tempora*, pl. of *tempus*] the lateral region on either side of the superior part of the head superior to the zygomatic arch; see *tempora*.

tem•po•la•bile (tem″po-la′bəl, -la′bīl) [L. *tempus* time + *labile*] subject to change with the passage of time.

tem•po•ra (tem′pə-rə) [L., pl. of *tempus*] [TA] the temples: the regions on each side of the head superior to the zygomatic arches.

tem•po•ral (tem′pə-rəl) [L. *temporalis*] 1. pertaining to the lateral region of the head, superior to the zygomatic arch. 2. pertaining to time; limited as to time; temporary.

tem•po•ra•lis (tem-pə-ra′lis) [L.] pertaining to the lateral region of the head, superior to the zygomatic arch.

tempor(o)- [L. *tempus*, gen. *temporis* time, temple] a combining form denoting relationship to time or to the temporal region.

tem•po•ro•au•ric•u•lar (tem″pə-ro-aw-rik′u-lər) pertaining to the temporal and auricular regions of the head.

tem•po•ro•fa•cial (tem″pə-ro-fa′shəl) pertaining to a temple and the face.

tem•po•ro•fron•tal (tem″pə-ro-fron′təl) pertaining to the temporal and frontal bones or regions.

tem•po•ro•hy•oid (tem″pə-ro-hi′oid) pertaining to the temporal and hyoid bones.

tem•po•ro•ma•lar (tem″pə-ro-ma′lər) temporozygomatic.

tem•po•ro•man•dib•u•lar (tem″pə-ro-mən-dib′u-lər) pertaining to the temporal bone and the mandible.

tem•po•ro•max•il•lary (tem″pə-ro-mak′sĭ-lar″e) pertaining to the temporal bone, or region, and the maxilla.

tem•po•ro•oc•cip•i•tal (tem″pə-ro-ok-sip′ĭ-təl) pertaining to the temporal and occipital bones or regions.

tem•po•ro•pa•ri•e•tal (tem″pə-ro-pə-ri′ə-təl) pertaining to the temporal and parietal bones or regions.

tem•po•ro•pa•ri•e•ta•lis (tem″pə-ro-pə-ri″ə-ta′lis) [L.] temporoparietal; see under *musculus.*

tem•po•ro•pon•tile (tem″pə-ro-pon′tīl) pertaining to or connecting the temporal lobe and the pons.

tem•po•ro•spa•tial (tem″pə-ro-spa′shəl) [L. *tempus* time + *spatial*] pertaining to both time and space.

tem•po•ro•sphe•noid (tem″pə-ro-sfe′noid) pertaining to the temporal and sphenoid bones.

tem•po•ro•zy•go•mat•ic (tem″pə-ro-zi″go-mat′ik) pertaining to the temporal and zygomatic bones, or to the region of the zygomatic arch.

tem•po•sta•bile (tem″po-sta′bəl, -sta′bīl) [L. *tempus* time + *stabile*] not subject to change with the passage of time.

tem•sir•ol•i•mus (tem″sir-ol′ĭməs) a kinase inhibitor used in treatment of advanced renal cell carcinoma; administered by intravenous infusion.

te•na•cious (tə-na′shəs) [L. *tenax*] holding fast; adhesive.

te•nac•u•lum (tə-nak′u-ləm) [L.] 1. a hooklike instrument for seizing and holding tissues. 2. a fibrous band that holds structures in place; see also *retinaculum.*

te•nal•gia (te-nal′jə) [*ten-* + *-algia*] pain in a tendon; called also *tenodynia.*

ten•as•cin (ten-as′in) any of a family of at least three glycoproteins of the extracellular matrix, designated C, R, and X, originally found in rat fetal tissues and mammary tumors. In humans they have been isolated from a variety of embryo and adult tissues including some epithelial sites and smooth muscles, as well as being found in new granulation tissue and some tumors such as carcinoma of the breast.

Tenck•hoff catheter (tengk′of) [H. *Tenckhoff,* American nephrologist, 20th century] see under *catheter.*

ten•der•ness (ten′dər-nis) abnormal sensitiveness to touch or pressure.
 pencil t. local tenderness on pressure with the rubber tip of a pencil, signifying the location of underlying pathology.
 rebound t. a sensation of pain felt on the release of pressure.

ten•di•nes (ten′dĭ-nēz) plural of *tendo.*

ten•di•ni•tis (ten″dĭ-ni′tis) inflammation of tendons and of tendon-muscle attachments; called also *tendonitis* and *tenonitis.*
 Achilles t. see under *tendinopathy.*
 adductor t. tendinitis affecting a tendon of one of the adductor muscles of the inner thigh, with pain when the limb is adducted; it is usually sports-related.
 biceps t., bicipital t. an overuse injury consisting of inflammation of the tendon of the long head of the biceps brachii muscle, often associated with rotator cuff tendinitis or glenohumeral instability.
 calcific t. inflammation and calcification of the subacromial or subdeltoid bursa, resulting in pain, tenderness, and limitation of motion in the shoulder. Called also *calcific bursitis* and *scapulohumeral bursitis.*
 t. ossi′ficans trauma′tica a condition in which areas of ossification develop in tendons as a result of trauma.
 patellar t. see under *tendinopathy.*
 rotator cuff t. an overuse injury consisting of inflammation of tendons of one or more of the muscles forming the rotator cuff, usually owing to repetitive elevation and abduction of the upper limb; it can lead to tendon degeneration and bony changes of the acromial head. Called also *rotator cuff tendinopathy.*
 t. steno′sans, stenosing t. stenosing tenosynovitis of the flexor tendons of the finger.

tendin(o)- [L. *tendo,* pl. *tendines* tendon] a combining form denoting relationship to a tendon; see also terms beginning *tend(o)-*, *ten(o)-*, and *tenont(o)-*.

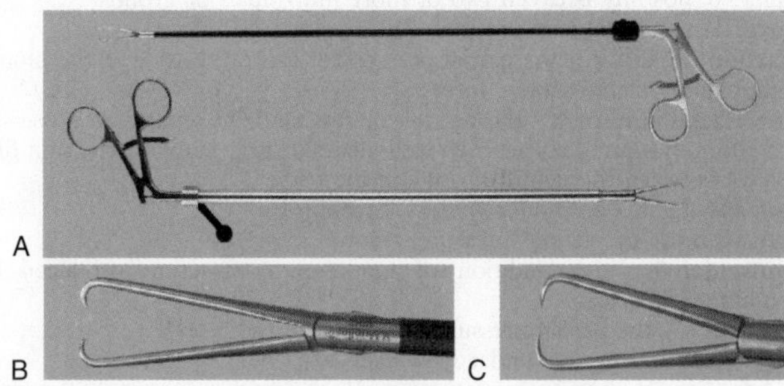

■ *(A),* Tenaculums; *(B, C),* tips.

ten•di•nop•a•thy (ten″dĭ-nop′ə-the) any pathologic condition of a tendon; see also *tendinitis.*
 Achilles t. injury to the Achilles (calcaneal) tendon, most often an overuse injury, such as in athletes, persons who strain their legs excessively, or sometimes those who wear high heels. Called also *Achilles tendinitis.*
 patellar t. an overuse injury of the patellar tendon, seen in activities that involve vigorous jumping, such as soccer, basketball, volleyball, and ballet; the predominant symptom is pain at the lower end of the patella, made worse by bending of the knee. Called also *jumper's knee* and *patellar tendinitis.*
 rotator cuff t. see under *tendinitis.*

ten•di•no•plas•ty (ten′dĭ-no-plas″te) [*tendino-* + *-plasty*] tenoplasty.

ten•di•no•sis (ten-dĭ-no′sis) tendinopathy.

ten•di•no•su•ture (ten″dĭ-no-soo′chər) [*tendino-* + *-suture*] the suturing of a tendon.

ten•di•nous (ten′dĭ-nəs) [L. *tendinosus*] pertaining to, resembling, or of the nature of a tendon.

ten•do (ten′do) pl. *ten′dines* [L.] [TA] tendon: a fibrous cord of connective tissue in which the fibers of a muscle end and by which the muscle is attached to a bone or other structure.
 t. calca′neus [TA] calcaneal tendon: a powerful tendon at the back of the heel which attaches the triceps surae muscle to the tuberosity of the calcaneus; called also *Achilles tendon.*
 t. conjuncti′vus TA alternative for *falx inguinalis.*
 t. cricooesopha′geus [TA] cricoesophageal tendon: the tendon giving origin to the longitudinal fibers of the esophagus that come from the upper part of the lamina of the cricoid cartilage.
 t. infundi′buli [TA] tendon of infundibulum: a collagenous band connecting the posterior surface of the pulmonary valve and the muscular infundibulum to the root of the aorta; called also *conus ligament.*

tend(o)- [L. *tendo* tendon] a combining form denoting relationship to a tendon; see also terms beginning *tendin(o)-*, *ten(o)-*, and *tenont(o)-*.

ten•dol•y•sis (ten-dol′ə-sis) [*tendo-* + *-lysis*] tenolysis.

ten•do•mu•cin (ten″do-mu′sin) a mucin derivable from tendons.

ten•don (ten′dən) [L. *tendo;* Gr. *tenōn*] a fibrous cord of connective tissue by which a muscle is attached; see *tendo.* Tendons are usually named after the muscle to which they attach.
 Achilles t. tendo calcaneus.
 bowed t. tendinitis of the flexor tendons in a horse, usually in the foreleg and due to strain from overwork; the tendons become enlarged and palpable.
 calcaneal t. tendo calcaneus.
 central t. of diaphragm centrum tendineum diaphragmatis.
 central t. of perineum corpus perineale.
 common t. a tendon that serves more than one muscle.
 common annular t. anulus tendineus communis.
 conjoined t., conjoint t. falx inguinalis.
 t. of conus tendo infundibuli.
 cordiform t. of diaphragm centrum tendineum diaphragmatis.
 coronary t's the anuli fibrosi cordis (fibrous rings) surrounding the aortic and pulmonary trunk orifices.
 cricoesophageal t. tendo cricooesophageus.
 hamstring t. see *hamstring.*
 t. of Hector, heel t. tendo calcaneus.
 t. of infundibulum tendo infundibuli.
 intermediate t. of diaphragm centrum tendineum diaphragmatis.
 membranaceous t. aponeurosis.
 patellar t., anterior, patellar t., inferior ligamentum patellae.
 pulled t. disruption of the fibers attaching a muscle to its point of origin, occurring as the result of unusual muscular effort.
 riders' t. injury to the adductor tendons of the thigh incurred in horseback riding.
 slipped t. perosis.
 t. of Todaro a palpable subendocardial collagen bundle in the wall of the right atrium, extending from the central fibrous body across the torus aorticus toward the medial extremity of the valve of the inferior vena cava.
 trefoil t. centrum tendineum [diaphragmatis].
 t. of Zinn zonula ciliaris.

ten•do•ni•tis (ten″də-ni′tis) tendinitis.

ten•do•plas•ty (ten′do-plas″te) [*tendo-* + *-plasty*] tenoplasty.

ten•do•syn•o•vi•tis (ten″do-sin″o-vi′tis) tenosynovitis.

ten•do•tome (ten′do-tōm) tenotome.

ten•dot•o•my (ten-dot′ə-me) tenotomy.

ten•do•vag•i•nal (ten″do-vaj′ĭ-nəl) [*tendo-* + *vaginal*] pertaining to a tendon and its sheath.

ten•do•vag•i•ni•tis (ten″do-vaj″ĭ-ni′tis) 1. inflammation of a tendon and its sheath. 2. tenosynovitis.

Te•neb•rio (tə-nēb′re-o) a genus of vegetable-eating beetles, the grain beetles; their larvae are called *mealworms.*

te•nec•te•plase (tə-nek′tə-plās) a modified form of human tissue plasminogen activator (see under *activator*) produced by recombinant DNA technology; used as a thrombolytic agent in the treatment of myocardial infarction, administered intravenously.

te•nec•to•my (tə-nek′tə-me) [*ten-* + *-ectomy*] excision of a lesion of a tendon or of a tendon sheath.

te•nes•mus (tə-nez′məs) [L., from Gr. *teinesmos*] straining, especially ineffectual and painful straining at stool or in urination. **tenes′mic** *adj*
rectal t. painful, ineffective, and long-continuing straining to defecate.
vesical t. straining to urinate.

Ten•ex (ten′eks) trademark for a preparation of guanfacine hydrochloride.

te•nia (te′ne-ə) gen. and pl. *te′niae* [L. *taenia*] taenia.

te•ni•a•cide (te′ne-ə-sīd″) taeniacide.

te•niae (te′ne-e) genitive and plural of *tenia.*

te•ni•a•fu•gal (te″ne-ə-fu′gəl) taeniafugal.

te•ni•a•fuge (te′ne-ə-fūj″) taeniafuge.

te•ni•al (te′ne-əl) 1. pertaining to taenia of anatomical nomenclature. 2. taenial (def. 1).

te•ni•a•sis (te-ni′ə-sis) taeniasis.

ten•i•cide (ten′ĭ-sīd) taeniacide.

ten•i•form (ten′ĭ-form) taeniform.

te•nif•u•gal (te-nif′u-gəl) taeniafugal.

ten•i•fuge (ten′ĭ-fūj) taeniafuge.

te•ni•oid (te′ne-oid) taeniform.

te•nio•tox•in (te″ne-o-tok′sin) a poisonous principle occurring in tapeworms.

ten•i•po•side (VM-26) (ten-ĭ-po′sīd) a semisynthetic derivative of podophyllotoxin, closely related to etoposide, that causes DNA strand breakage and crosslinking, resulting in inhibition of mitosis in the late S and G_2 phases of the cell cycle; used as an antineoplastic in the treatment of neuroblastoma, non-Hodgkin lymphoma, and acute lymphoblastic leukemia, administered intravenously.

Ten•i•vac (ten′ĭ-vak) trademark for a preparation of tetanus and diphtheria toxoids.

ten(o)- [Gr. *tenōn* tendon] a combining form denoting relationship to a tendon. See also terms beginning *tend(o)-*, *tendin(o)-*, and *tenont(o)-*.

te•nod•e•sis (tə-nod′ə-sis) [*teno-* + *-desis*] the stabilization of a joint by anchoring a tendon to a bone, done either surgically or through use of an orthosis (see *tenodesis orthosis,* under *orthosis*).

ten•odyn•ia (ten″o-din′e-ə) [*ten-* + *-odynia*] tenalgia.

te•no•fo•vir (tə-no′fo-vir″) a nucleotide analogue that acts as an antiretroviral agent by inhibiting reverse transcriptase.
t. disoproxil fumarate a prodrug of tenofovir, used in the treatment of HIV-1 (human immunodeficiency virus-1) infection.

te•nol•y•sis (tə-nol′ĭ-sis) [*teno-* + *-lysis*] the operation of freeing a tendon from adhesions; called also *tendolysis.*

teno•myo•plas•ty (ten″o-mi′o-plas″te) [*teno-* + *myo-* + *-plasty*] a plastic operation involving tendon and muscle. **tenomyoplas′tic** *adj*

teno•my•ot•o•my (ten″o-mi-ot′ə-me) [*teno-* + *myo-* + *-tomy*] excision of a portion of tendon and muscle.

Te•non capsule (fascia, membrane), space (tə-naw′) [Jacques René *Tenon,* French surgeon, 1724–1816] see *vagina bulbi* and *spatium intervaginale.*

teno•nec•to•my (ten″ə-nek′tə-me) [*teno-* + *-ectomy*] excision of a part of a tendon for the purpose of shortening it.

teno•ni•tis (ten″ə-ni′tis) 1. tendinitis. 2. inflammation of the Tenon capsule.

teno•nom•e•ter (ten″ə-nom′ə-tər) tonometer.

ten•on•os•to•sis (ten″on-os-to′sis) tenostosis.

tenont(o)- [Gr. *tenōn,* gen. *tenontos* tendon] a combining form denoting relationship to a tendon; see also terms beginning *tend(o)-*, *tendin(o)-*, and *ten(o)-*.

te•non•to•lem•mi•tis (tə-non″to-lem-i′tis) tenosynovitis.

ten•on•tol•o•gy (ten″on-tol′ə-je) the sum of what is known regarding the tendons.

teno•phyte (ten′o-fīt) [*teno-* + *-phyte*] a growth or concretion in a tendon.

teno•plas•ty (ten′o-plas″te) [*teno-* + *-plasty*] plastic surgery of the tendons; operative repair of a defect in a tendon. Called also *tendinoplasty, tendoplasty.* **tenoplas′tic** *adj*

teno•re•cep•tor (ten′o-re-sep″tər) [*teno-* + *receptor*] a proprioceptor situated in tendon; such receptors are stimulated by contraction.

Teno•ret•ic (ten″o-ret′ik) trademark for a combination preparation of atenolol and chlorthalidone.

Ten•or•min (ten′or-min) trademark for preparations of atenolol.

te•nor•rha•phy (tə-nor′ə-fe) [*teno-* + *-rrhaphy*] the union of a divided tendon by a suture.

teno•si•tis (ten″o-si′tis) tendinitis.

ten•os•to•sis (ten″os-to′sis) [*teno-* + *oste-* + *-osis*] ossification of a tendon.

teno•su•ture (ten″o-soo′chər) [*teno-* + *suture*] tenorrhaphy.

teno•syn•o•vec•to•my (ten″o-sin″o-vek′tə-me) surgical removal of a tendon sheath.

teno•syn•o•vi•tis (ten″o-sin″o-vi′tis) inflammation of a tendon sheath. Called also *tendinous synovitis, tendosynovitis, tendovaginitis,* and *tenovaginitis.*
t. acu′ta purulen′ta tenosynovitis with pus formation.
adhesive t. tenosynovitis in which the tendons become bound in an inflammatory mass.
t. cre′pitans tenosynovitis accompanied by a crackling sound in the soft tissues on movement.
gonococcic t., gonorrheal t. inflammation of a tendon sheath due to metastatic gonococcal infection.
t. granulo′sa tuberculosis of tendon sheaths, which become filled with granulation tissue.
t. hypertro′phica an inflammatory condition marked by swellings of the tendons and their sheaths.
infectious t. a disease of chickens and turkeys caused by a reovirus; the tendons of the legs become infected and inflamed and often rupture.
nodular t. giant cell tumor of tendon sheath; see under *tumor.*
t. sero′sa chro′nica tenosynovitis with serous effusion.
t. steno′sans a painful condition of the wrist, marked by thickening and narrowing of the tendon sheath of the extensor brevis and abductor longus pollicis.
tuberculous t. chronic tuberculous infection of tendon sheaths and bursae.
villonodular t. a condition characterized by proliferation of synovial membrane cells, producing a solid tumorlike mass, usually in periarticular soft tissues and less often in joints.
villous t. chronic infection of tendon sheaths and bursae, with proliferation of villous projections from the surface of the membranes.

teno•tome (ten′o-tōm) a cutting instrument used in tenotomy.

te•not•o•my (tə-not′ə-me) [*teno-* + *-tomy*] 1. the surgical cutting of any tendon. 2. the cutting of an extraocular tendon for strabismus. Called also *tendotomy* and *tendon release.*
curb t. the operation of cutting an eye muscle in strabismus and inserting it farther back on the globe of the eye.

teno•vag•i•ni•tis (ten″o-vaj″ĭ-ni′tis) inflammation of a tendon sheath; tenosynovitis.

ten•ox•i•cam (ten-ok′sĭ-kam) a nonsteroidal antiinflammatory drug used in the treatment of various rheumatic and nonrheumatic inflammatory conditions; administered orally.

TENS transcutaneous electrical nerve stimulation.

tense (tens) drawn tight; rigid.

Ten•si•lon (ten′sĭ-lon) trademark for a solution of edrophonium chloride.

ten•sio-ac•tive (ten″se-o-ak′tiv) having an effect on surface tension.

ten•si•om•e•ter (ten″se-om′ə-tər) [*tension* + *-meter*] an apparatus for measuring the surface tension of liquids.

ten•sion (ten′shən) [L. *tensio;* Gr. *tonos*] 1. the act of stretching. 2. the condition of being stretched or strained; the degree to which anything is stretched or strained. 3. the partial pressure of a gas in a fluid, e.g., of oxygen in blood. 4. voltage. 5. mental, emotional, or nervous strain. 6. hostility between two or more individuals or groups.
arterial t. blood pressure (def. 2).
carbon dioxide t. the partial pressure of carbon dioxide in the blood.
electric t. electromotive force.
interfacial surface t. the tension or resistance to separation possessed by the film of liquid between two well-adapted surfaces, as by the thin film of saliva between the denture base and the tissues.
intraocular t. see under *pressure.* Symbol T.
intravenous t. venous pressure.
muscular t. the condition of moderate contraction produced by stretching a muscle.
oxygen t. the partial pressure of oxygen in the blood.
premenstrual t. see under *syndrome.*
surface t. the tension or resistance which acts to preserve the integrity of a surface, such as the tension or resistance to rupture possessed by the

surface film of a liquid, or the tension or strain upon the surface of a liquid in contact with another substance with which it does not mix.

tissue t. a state of equilibrium between tissues and cells that prevents overaction of any part.

wall t. the circumferential stretching force in a vessel wall, usually expressed as a function of intraluminal pressure and the radius according to the Laplace equation.

ten•sor (ten′sor) [L., "stretcher," "puller"] any muscle that stretches or makes tense.

tent (tent) [L. *tenta*, from *tendere* to stretch] 1. a covering of fabric designed to enclose an open space, especially such an arrangement over a patient's bed for the purpose of administering oxygen or vaporized medication by inhalation. 2. a conical and expansible plug of soft material, as lint, gauze, etc., for dilating an orifice or for keeping a wound open, so as to prevent its healing except at the bottom.

oxygen t. a tent erected over a bed into which a constant flow of oxygen can be maintained.

steam t. a tent erected over a bed into which steam is passed; used in certain respiratory conditions.

ten•ta•cle (ten′tə-kəl) a slender whiplike appendage in animals that may function in prehension and feeding or as a sense organ.

ten•to•ria (ten-tor′e-ə) plural of *tentorium.*

ten•to•ri•al (ten-tor′e-əl) pertaining to the tentorium of the cerebellum.

ten•to•ri•um (ten-tor′e-əm) pl. *tento′ria* [L. "tent"] an anatomical part resembling a tent or a covering.

t. cerebel′li [TA], **t. of cerebellum** the process of dura mater that supports the occipital lobes and covers the cerebellum. Its internal border is free and bounds the tentorial notch; its external border is attached to the skull and encloses the transverse sinus behind.

t. of hypophysis diaphragma sellae.

Ten•u•ate (ten′u-āt) trademark for preparations of diethylpropion hydrochloride.

TEOAE transient evoked otoacoustic emissions.

Tep•a•nil (tep′ə-nil) trademark for preparations of diethylpropion hydrochloride.

TEPP tetraethyl pyrophosphate.

Te•quin (te′kwin) trademark for preparations of gatifloxacin.

ter- [L. *ter* thrice] a prefix meaning three, three-fold.

tera- [Gr. *teras* monster] a prefix used in naming units of measurement to indicate a quantity one trillion (10^{12}) times the unit specified by the root with which it is combined. Symbol T.

ter•a•tism (ter′ə-tiz-əm) [Gr. *teratisma*] an anomaly of formation or development; see *developmental anomaly*, under *anomaly*. **terat′ic** *adj*

terat(o)- [Gr. *teras*, gen. *teratos* monster] a combining form denoting relationship to a monster.

ter•a•to•blas•to•ma (ter″ə-to-blas-to′mə) teratoma.

ter•a•to•car•ci•no•gen•e•sis (ter″ə-to-kahr″sĭ-no-jen′ə-sis) the production of teratocarcinomas.

ter•a•to•car•ci•no•ma (ter″ə-to-kahr″sĭ-no′mə) a malignant neoplasm consisting of elements of teratoma with those of embryonal carcinoma or choriocarcinoma, or both; occurring most often in the testis.

ter•a•to•gen (ter′ə-to-jən) any agent or factor that induces or increases the incidence of abnormal prenatal development.

ter•a•to•gen•e•sis (ter″ə-to-jen′ə-sis) [*terato-* + *-genesis*] the production of birth defects in embryos and fetuses. **teratogenet′ic** *adj*

ter•a•to•gen•ic (ter″ə-to-jen′ik) tending to produce congenital anomalies.

ter•a•tog•e•nous (ter″ə-toj′ə-nəs) developed from fetal remains.

ter•a•tog•e•ny (ter″ə-toj′ə-ne) teratogenesis.

ter•a•toid (ter′ə-toid) teratomatous.

ter•a•tol•o•gy (ter″ə-tol′ə-je) the branch of embryology and pathology which deals with abnormal development and the production of congenital anomalies. **teratolog′ic, teratolog′ical** *adj*

ter•a•to•ma (ter″ə-to′mə) pl. *teratomas, terato′mata* [*terat-* + *-oma*] a type of germ cell tumor derived from pluripotent cells and made up of elements of different types of tissue from one or more of the three germ cell layers; most often found in the ovary or testis in adults and in the sacrococcygeal region in children. Teratomas range from benign (mature, dermoid, and cystic) to malignant (immature and solid). Called also *dysembryoma, teratoblastoma, organoid tumor*, and *teratoid tumor.* **teratom′atous** *adj*

benign cystic t., cystic t. dermoid cyst (def. 2).

immature t. malignant t.

malignant t. 1. a solid, malignant ovarian tumor resembling a dermoid cyst but composed of immature embryonal or extraembryonal elements derived from all three germ layers. Called also *immature t.* and *solid t.* 2. teratocarcinoma.

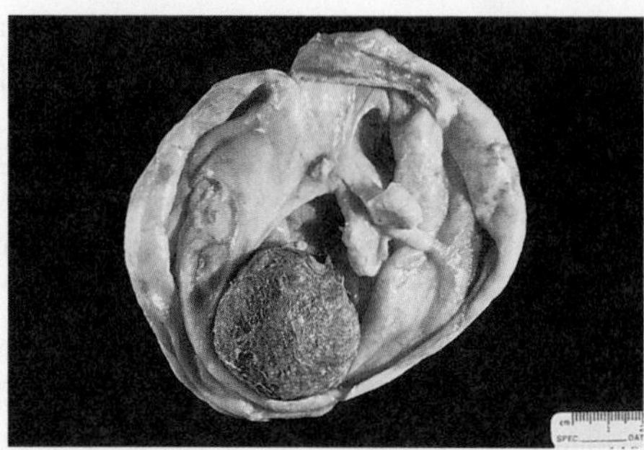

■ Opened mature cystic teratoma (dermoid cyst) of the ovary, containing a mixture of tissues, including hair *(bottom).*

mature t. dermoid cyst (def. 2).

sacrococcygeal t. a solid tumor containing derivatives of one or more of the embryonic germ layers, arising from the pluripotent cells of the primitive node and usually presenting as a protruding mass between the coccyx and rectum; the most common teratoma in the newborn.

solid t. malignant t.

ter•a•to•ma•ta (ter″ə-to′mə-tə) plural of *teratoma.*

ter•a•to•sis (ter″ə-to′sis) teratism.

ter•a•to•sper•mia (ter″ə-to-spur′me-ə) teratozoospermia.

ter•a•to•zo•o•sper•mia (ter″ə-to-zo″o-spur′me-ə) the presence of malformed spermatozoa in the semen; called also *teratospermia.*

Ter•a•zol (ter′ə-zol) trademark for preparations of terconazole.

ter•a•zo•sin hy•dro•chlo•ride (tər-a′zo-sin) [USP] an alpha$_1$-adrenergic blocking agent used in the treatment of hypertension and benign prostatic hyperplasia, administered orally.

ter•bi•na•fine hy•dro•chlo•ride (tur′bĭ-nə-fēn″) a synthetic antifungal compound that interferes with biosynthesis of ergosterol and so disrupts fungal cell membrane function; used topically and orally in the treatment of various forms of tinea and onychomycosis.

ter•bi•um (Tb) (tur′be-əm) a rare metallic element; atomic number, 65; atomic weight, 158.924.

ter•bu•ta•line sul•fate (tər-bu′tə-lēn) [USP] a β_2-adrenergic receptor agonist, used as a bronchodilator for the treatment of asthma-associated bronchospasm and the treatment and prophylaxis of bronchospasm associated with chronic bronchitis, pulmonary emphysema, or other chronic obstructive airway disease; administered by oral inhalation, subcutaneously, or orally. It is also used as a tocolytic in the prevention of premature labor; administered intravenously.

ter•chlo•ride (tər-klor′īd) trichloride.

ter•co•na•zole (tər-kon′ə-zōl) an imidazole derivative used as a topical antifungal, applied intravaginally in the treatment of vulvovaginal candidiasis.

ter•e•ben•thene (ter″ə-ben′thēn) turpentine oil.

ter•e•bin•thi•nate (ter″ə-bin′thĭ-nāt) resembling or containing turpentine.

ter•e•bin•thi•nism (ter″ə-bin′thĭ-niz-əm) [L. *terebinthina* turpentine] poisoning with oil of turpentine; symptoms include hemoglobinemia, pulmonary edema, convulsions, and damage to nervous system and kidneys.

ter•e•brant (ter′ə-brənt) [L. *terebrans* boring] of a boring or piercing quality.

ter•e•brat•ing (ter′ə-brāt″ing) terebrant.

ter•e•bra•tion (ter″ə-bra′shən) [L. *terebratio*] a boring pain.

te•res (te′rēz) [L.] long and round, as a muscle or ligament.

ter•fen•a•dine (tər-fen′ə-dēn) a nonsedating antihistamine (H_1 receptor antagonist) formerly used in the treatment of allergic conditions but withdrawn in the United States because of possible cardiotoxic effects.

Ter•gi•tol 4 (tur′jĭ-tol) trademark for a preparation of sodium tetradecyl sulfate.

ter in die (ter in de′a) [L.] three times a day.

ter•i•par•a•tide (ter″ĭ-par′ə-tīd) a recombinant form of parathyroid hormone, administered by subcutaneous injection in treatment of osteoporosis.

ter•li•pres•sin ac•e•tate (ter-lĭ-pres′in) a prodrug of lypressin, used primarily to control bleeding of esophageal varices.

ter·m (turm) [L. *terminus*, from Gr. *terma*] 1. a word or combination of words commonly used to designate a specific entity. 2. a limit or boundary. 3. a definite period or specified time of duration, such as the culmination of pregnancy at the end of 40 weeks from the last menstrual period or 38 weeks from conception.

ter·mi·nad (tur′mĭ-nəd) [*terminus* + *-ad*[1]] toward the end or terminus.

ter·mi·nal (tur′mĭ-nəl) [L. *terminalis*] 1. forming or pertaining to an end; placed at the end. 2. a termination, end, or extremity; see *ending*.

C t. C-terminal.

central t. of Wilson in electrocardiography, a terminal created by connecting the standard limb leads through 5000-ohm resistors in series, forming a common reference electrode.

N t. N-terminal.

nerve t's terminationes nervorum.

ter·mi·nal ad·di·tion en·zyme (tur′mĭ-nəl ə-dĭ′shən en′zīm) DNA nucleotidylexotransferase.

ter·mi·nal de·oxy·nu·cleo·ti·dyl trans·fer·ase (TdT) (tur′mĭ-nəl de-ok″se-noo″kle-o-ti′dəl trans′fər-ās) DNA nucleotidylexotransferase.

ter·mi·na·tio (tur″mĭ-na′she-o) pl. *terminatio′nes* [L. "a limiting, bounding"] ending: the site of discontinuation of a structure.

terminatio′nes nervo′rum [TA] nerve terminals: sensory (or afferent) nerve endings and their receptors in the periphery; the term may also be used more broadly to denote the ending of any nerve fiber, including motor nerves, and synapses.

ter·mi·na·tion (tur″mĭ-na′shən) [L. *terminatio*] 1. a distal end. 2. the ending or cessation of an activity or process.

ter·mi·na·ti·o·nes (tur″mĭ-na″she-o′nēz) [L.] plural of *terminatio*.

ter·mi·ni (tur′mĭ-ni) [L.] plural of *terminus*.

Ter·mi·no·lo·gia Ana·to·mi·ca (TA) (tur″mĭ-no-lo′je-ə an″ə-tom′ĭ-kə) [L. "anatomical terminology"] *International Anatomical Terminology:* the official body of anatomical nomenclature created jointly by the Federative Committee on Anatomical Terminology and the 56 Member Associations of the International Associations of Anatomists and published in 1998. It supersedes the *Nomina Anatomica* [NA].

ter·mi·nol·o·gy (tur″mĭ-nol′ə-je) [*terminus* + *-logy*] 1. the vocabulary of an art or science. 2. the science that deals with the investigation, arrangement, and construction of terms.

International Anatomical T. *Terminologia Anatomica.*

ter·mi·nus (tur′mĭ-nəs) pl. *ter′mini* [L. "boundary"] a terminal or ending.

ter·mo·lec·u·lar (tur″mo-lek′u-lər) involving three molecules.

ter·na·ry (tur′nə-re) [L. *ternarius*] 1. third in order. 2. made up of three distinct chemical elements.

Ter·ni·dens (ter′nĭ-dənz) a genus of nematodes of the family Strongylidae. *T. diminu′tus* is found in the large intestines of monkeys and occasionally humans.

ter·ni·trate (tər-ni′trāt) a trinitrate.

ter·ox·ide (tər-ok′sīd) [*ter-* + *oxide*] trioxide.

ter·pene (tur′pēn) any hydrocarbon of the formula $C_{10}H_{16}$, derivable chiefly from essential oils, resins, and other vegetable aromatic products. They may be acyclic, bicyclic, or monocyclic, and differ somewhat in physical properties.

ter·pen·ism (tur′pən-iz-əm) poisoning with a terpene, resulting in vomiting, convulsions, unconsciousness, pulmonary edema, and tachycardia.

ter·pin (tur′pin) a product obtained by the action of nitric acid on turpentine oil and alcohol.

t. hydrate [USP] the monohydrate of terpin, used as an expectorant; administered orally.

ter·ra (ter′ə) [L.] earth.

t. sili′cea purifica′ta purified infusorial earth that has been boiled, washed, and calcined and is used in certain pharmaceutical operations.

Ter·ra-Cor·tril (ter″ə-kor′tril) trademark for a combination preparation of oxytetracycline hydrochloride and hydrocortisone acetate.

Ter·ra·my·cin (ter″ə-mi′sin) trademark for preparations of oxytetracycline.

ter·ri·to·ri·al·i·ty (ter″ĭ-tor″ĭ-al′ĭ-te) a pattern of behavior in which an individual organism or a group of organisms delineates a territory and vigorously defends it against intrusion by other members of the same or competing species.

ter·ri·to·ry (ter′ĭ-tor″e) [L. *terra* earth] an area or region.

chromosome t's discrete, compact regions within the cell nucleus that are occupied by individual chromosomes during interphase and separated by the interchromosomal domain.

ter·ror (ter′ər) intense fright.

day t's pavor diurnus.

night t's, sleep t's pavor nocturnus.

Ter·ry syndrome (ter′e) [Theodore Lasater *Terry*, American ophthalmologist, 1899–1946] retinopathy of prematurity.

Ter·son syndrome (ter-saw′) [Albert *Terson*, French ophthalmologist, 1867–1935] see under *syndrome*.

ter·sul·fide (tər-sul′fīd) trisulfide.

ter·tian (tur′shən) [L. *tertianus*] recurring every third day, counting the day of occurrence as the first day; applied to the type of fever caused by *Plasmodium vivax*.

ter·ti·ary (tur′she-ar-e) [L. *tertiarius*] third in order.

ter·ti·grav·i·da (tər-tĭ-grav′ĭ-də) [L. *tertius* third + *gravida*] a woman pregnant for the third time; also written *gravida III*.

ter·tip·a·ra (tər-tip′ə-rə) [L. *tertius* third + *para*] a woman who has had three pregnancies which resulted in viable offspring; also written *para III*.

Tesch·en disease (tesh′ən) [*Teschen* district in Czechoslovakia, where it was described in 1929] infectious porcine encephalomyelitis.

TESE testicular sperm extraction.

tes·la (T) (tes′lə) [Nikola *Tesla*, Serbian-born American physicist, 1856–1943] the SI unit of magnetic flux density, calculated as webers per square meter.

Tes·lac (tes′lak) trademark for preparations of testolactone.

Tes·la·scan (tes′lə-skan) trademark for a preparation of mangafodipir trisodium.

TESPA thiotepa.

Tes·sa·lon (tes′ə-lon) trademark for a preparation of benzonatate.

tes·sel·lat·ed (tes′ə-lāt″əd) [L. *tessellatus; tessella* a square] divided into squares, like a checker board.

test[1] (test) [L. *testa* shell] a loose or rigid, secreted or agglutinated, protective shell or shell-like covering or exoskeleton, seen in various invertebrates, including certain protozoa and echinoderms.

test[2] (test) [L. *testum* crucible] 1. an examination or trial. 2. a significant chemical reaction. 3. a reagent.

Test

See also under *method*, *phenomenon*, *reaction*, *reagent*, *sign*, and *symptom*.

abduction–external rotation t. Roos t.

ABLB t. alternate binaural loudness balance t.

abortus Bang ring t., ABR t. *(screening for brucellosis in cattle)* since *Brucella* agglutinins, as well as the organisms, are shed in the milk of infected cattle, a drop of hematoxylin-stained brucellae is mixed in a sample of pooled milk from the herd. After incubation, agglutinated bacteria are adsorbed by the globules of fat that rise to the surface to form a colored ring. Called also *milk ring t.*

acetate breath t. a breath test for gastric emptying: the patient is administered a test meal containing acetate labeled with carbon 13, and the breath is assessed at intervals for levels of labeled carbon dioxide; excessive carbon dioxide is seen when gastric emptying is inadequate.

acid elution t. *(for fetal hemoglobin)* air-dried blood smears on a glass slide are fixed in 80 per cent methanol and immersed in a buffer at pH 3.3 (citric acid and sodium phosphate); all hemoglobins are eluted except fetal hemoglobin, which remains fixed in the red cells and can be detected after staining. Called also *Kleihauer* or *Kleihauer-Betke t.*

acidified serum t. *(for paroxysmal nocturnal hemoglobinuria)* the patient's washed red cells are incubated at 37°C in acidified normal serum or the patient's acidified serum; after centrifugation the supernatant is examined colorimetrically for hemolysis. In paroxysmal nocturnal hemoglobinuria the red cells are abnormally susceptible to lysis by complement, which is activated by the alternate pathway in acidified serum. Called also *Ham t.*

acid-lability t. a test to distinguish rhinoviruses from enteroviruses on the basis of their activity at various pH levels, rhinoviruses being inactivated by incubation at pH 3 to 5 for one to three hours.

acid perfusion t. Bernstein t.

acoustic reflex t. *(for hearing)* measurement of the acoustic reflex threshold by testing for contraction of the stapedial muscle in response to sound; used to differentiate between conductive and sensorineural deafness and to diagnose acoustic neuroma.

ACTH stimulation t. *(for adrenal insufficiency)* in a fasting patient, blood levels of corticotropin are determined and cosyntropin is administered by intravenous or intramuscular injection. This should cause a significant rise in plasma cortisol levels by 4 hours after the injection; persons with little or no rise have adrenal insufficiency. Called also *corticotropin stimulation t.*

Addis t. after the patient is given a dry diet for 24 hours, the specific gravity of the urine is determined.

Adson t. *(for thoracic outlet syndrome)* the sitting patient breathes in deeply and holds the breath, then hyperextends the neck and turns the head toward the affected side. If the radial pulse on that side is significantly diminished, the result is considered positive. The test has been found to be nonspecific. Called also *Adson maneuver*.

agglutination t. *(for presence of antibody)* cells containing antigens to a given antibody are mixed into the solution being tested; agglutination indicates presence of the antibody. See also *agglutination reaction* and *latex agglutination t.*

AL t. a type of patch test in which the materials being tested are applied to cellulose disks arrayed on polyethylene-coated aluminum paper, which is affixed to the skin for several days.

alkali denaturation t. *(for fetal hemoglobin)* a spectrophotometric method for determining the concentration of hemoglobin F, which depends on the resistance of the hemoglobin molecule to denaturation of its globin moiety when exposed to alkali.

Allen t. *(for occlusion of ulnar or radial arteries)* the patient makes a tight fist so as to express the blood from the skin of the palm and fingers; the examiner digitally compresses either the radial or the ulnar artery. When the patient unclenches the fist, if blood fails to return to the palm and fingers, there is indicated obstruction to blood flow in the artery that has not been compressed.

Allen-Doisy t. *(for estrogens)* a formerly common test in which the material being tested was injected into spayed laboratory mice and a change from leukocytes to cornified cells in their vaginal secretions was a positive result.

alternate binaural loudness balance t. *(for hearing)* comparison of the intensity levels at which a given pure tone sounds equally loud to the normal ear and the ear with hearing loss; done to determine recruitment with unilateral sensorineural loss. Called also *ABLB t.*

alternate cover t. a test for determining the type of tropia and/or phoria done by alternately covering each eye and noting the movement of the uncovered eye.

alternate loudness balance t. *(for hearing)* a test done with pure tones that compares the loudness perceived in one ear with that perceived in the other, with the frequency kept constant.

Ames t. a test for mutagenicity of chemical compounds, using special strains of the bacteria serovar *Salmonella enterica* subsp. *enterica* serovar Typhimurium. The bacteria are incubated on a histidine-deficient medium in the presence of the suspected mutagen and rat liver microsomal cell fraction, which contains mixed-function oxidases known to activate many procarcinogens. Growth of bacterial colonies indicates mutagenicity (reverse mutations restoring the ability to synthesize histidine have occurred). About 90–95 per cent of demonstrated mutagens are also carcinogenic.

aminopyrine breath t. *(for liver function)* a breath test in which the patient is given a dose of ^{14}C-labeled aminopyrine and at 15-minute intervals for two hours the amount of ^{14}C-labeled carbon dioxide in the patient's breath is measured. Excessively low levels of carbon dioxide indicate impaired liver function, such as cirrhosis.

anterior drawer t. see *drawer t's.*

antibiotic sensitivity t., antibiotic susceptibility t. antimicrobial susceptibility t.

anti-DNA t., anti–double-stranded DNA t. an enzyme immunoassay that uses native double-stranded DNA as an antigen to detect and monitor increased serum levels of anti-DNA antibodies, a sign of systemic lupus erythematosus; used in both detection and management of disease.

antiglobulin t. (AGT) a test for the presence of nonagglutinating antibodies against red blood cells, using antihuman globulin antibody to agglutinate cells coated with the nonagglutinating antibody. The *direct antiglobulin test* detects antibodies bound to circulating red cells in vivo. It is used in the evaluation of autoimmune and drug-induced immune hemolytic anemia and erythroblastosis fetalis. The *indirect antiglobulin test* detects serum antibodies that bind to red cells in an in vitro incubation step. It is used in typing of erythrocyte antigens and in compatibility testing (cross-match). Called also *Coombs t.*

antiglobulin consumption t. a test for serum antibodies against cellular antigens. Cells are incubated with the serum sample and then with antiglobulin; any serum antibody that binds to the cells will take up antiglobulin. The amount of antiglobulin consumed is determined by testing the supernatant with antibody-coated red cells; the amount of agglutination is inversely proportional to the antiglobulin consumption.

antihuman globulin (AHG) t. direct antiglobulin test; see *antiglobulin test.*

antimicrobial sensitivity t., antimicrobial susceptibility t. any of numerous tests of how susceptible bacteria are to antimicrobial agents; the bacteria are classified as either *sensitive* or *susceptible, indeterminate* or *intermediate*, or *resistant.* Called also *antibiotic sensitivity* or *antibiotic susceptibility t.*

Apley t. *(for torn meniscus)* the patient lies prone and flexes the knee of the leg being examined to 90 degrees, with the thigh stabilized by the examiner. For the *Apley compression test,* the examiner places one or both hands firmly on the heel of the flexed leg and opposes the tibia to the femur, then rotates the tibia externally and internally. An increase in pain, clicking, or locking on compression indicates a torn meniscus. For the *Apley distraction test,* the ankle is grasped with one or both hands, and the tibia is pulled upward, away from the femur, and then rotated externally and internally. Lessening of pain on distraction indicates a torn meniscus, while increase in pain indicates ligament injury.

apprehension t. any of various provocative tests of joints, either active or passive, in which the patient is observed for signs of apprehension or resistance as the joint is moved; such signs or the production of pain constitutes a positive test.

Apt t. *(for differentiating fetal from adult hemoglobin)* a specimen from an infant's vomitus or stool is mixed with 5 volumes of water and centrifuged so that a clear pink supernatant separates. Sodium hydroxide solution is added to the supernatant; if hemoglobin F (fetal blood) is present, the pink color persists for more than 2 minutes, whereas if hemoglobin A (from swallowed maternal blood) is present, the supernatant turns from pink to yellow within 2 minutes.

aptitude t's tests given to determine aptitude or ability to undertake study or training in a particular field.

arginine stimulation t. *(for pituitary function and growth hormone production)* in a fasting patient, baseline levels are measured for growth hormone. Arginine is injected intravenously for 30 minutes and growth hormone levels are measured at 30, 60, 90, and 120 minutes. A normal response is at least 5 ng/mL of growth hormone.

arm ergometry exercise t. a variant of the bicycle ergometer exercise test in which the patient uses the arms to pedal the bicycle.

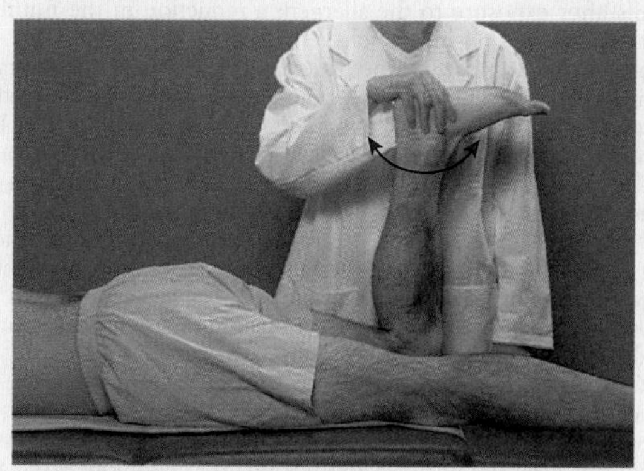

■ Apley test for detection of a meniscal tear of the knee.

arylsulfatase t. *(for differentiating species of rapid-growing mycobacteria)* a sample from a Tween-albumin broth culture of the suspected organism is incubated with tripotassium phenolphthalein disulfate for three days and then alkalinized. Those species producing arylsulfatase *(Mycobacterium fortuitum* and *M. chelonae)* show a pink to red positive reaction; a colorless reaction is negative.
aspirin tolerance t. any of various bleeding time tests in which aspirin is administered and its effect on bleeding time is assessed; aspirin prolongs bleeding time in patients with von Willebrand disease and certain other platelet disorders.
association t. a test based on associative reaction. It is usually performed by mentioning words to a subject and noting what other words they will give as the ones called to mind. Their reaction time is also noted.
atrial pacing stress t. a stress test in which temporary immediately reversible atrial pacing is used to stress coronary reserve; used for patients incapable of exercise or in whom an exercise stress test is contraindicated.
augmented histamine t. *(for gastric function)* a newer type of histamine test; after a 12-hour fast, residual gastric contents are aspirated. Basal gastric secretion is then collected every 15 minutes for 1 hour; at the 30-minute point, antihistamine is given intramuscularly. At the end of the hour, histamine acid phosphate (0.04 mg per kg of body weight) is given subcutaneously, and gastric contents are collected every 15 minutes for another hour. Volume, pH, and titratable acidity are measured on each sample.
autohemolysis t. *(for hereditary spherocytosis)* a sample of blood is defibrinated and incubated at 37°C for 24 and 48 hours; if hereditary spherocytosis is present, spontaneous hemolysis is increased.
automated reagin t. (ART) a modification of the rapid plasma reagin test for syphilis, used with automated analyzers in clinical chemistry.
Ayer-Tobey t. Tobey-Ayer t.
Babinski t. see under *sign.*
Babinski-Weil t. *(for labyrinthine disease)* the patient, with eyes shut, walks forward and backward ten times; with labyrinthine disease there will be deviation from the straight path, bending to one side when walking forward and to the other when walking backward.
bacteriolytic t. Pfeiffer phenomenon.
Baermann t. *(for nematodes and larvae in soil or feces)* a specimen of soil or feces is suspended over gauze or wire mesh in a water-filled funnel to which a piece of rubber tubing is attached; larval nematodes such as *Strongyloides stercoralis* will migrate from the specimen to the water, and collect in the rubber tubing.
balloon expulsion t. *(for constipation)* a small balloon with a weight on the distal end is inserted into the rectum and the patient is asked to sit on the toilet and try to evacuate it.
Bang t. abortus Bang ring t.
Bárány t. caloric t.
Bárány pointing t. the patient points at a fixed object alternately with the eyes open and closed; a constant error with the eyes closed indicates a brain lesion. Called also *pointing t.*
bar-reading t. *(for binocular and stereoscopic vision)* a ruler is held midway between the patient's eyes and the printed page; this may also be used as an exercise to develop stereoscopic vision. Called also *Welland t.*
basophil degranulation t. an in vitro procedure testing allergic sensitivity to a specific allergen at the cellular level by measuring staining of basophils after exposure to the allergen; a reduction in the number of granulated cells is a positive result.
Becker t. *(for astigmatism)* the patient looks at a test card containing lines radiating in sets of three and points out which seem blurred.
Bekhterev (Bechterew) t. *(for sciatica)* the patient seated in bed is directed to stretch out both legs; in sciatica they cannot do this, but can stretch out each leg in turn.
Bender Gestalt t., Bender Visual-Motor Gestalt t. a psychological test used for evaluating perceptual-motor coordination, for assessing personality dynamics, as a test of organic brain impairment, and for measuring neurological maturation. The subject is asked to make free-hand copies of nine simple geometric designs presented separately on cards or sometimes to reproduce the design from memory.
Benedict t. *(for glucose in urine)* a test for glucose in the urine using Benedict reagent.
bentiromide t. *(for pancreatic function)* bentiromide is administered orally and its cleavage into benzoyl-tyrosyl and *p*-aminobenzoic acid is monitored as a measure of pancreatic production of chymotrypsin.
bentonite flocculation t. any agglutination test using antigen adsorbed on particles of bentonite; when the antigen is added to serum containing specific antibodies, flocculation occurs.
benzidine t. *(for occult blood in urine or feces)* benzidine, acetic acid, and hydrogen peroxide are added to the specimen; hemoglobin catalyzes the oxidation of benzidine by hydrogen peroxide, giving a blue color. This is the most sensitive screening test for occult blood, but it is seldom used because benzidine is a carcinogen, and its use is restricted.
Bernstein t. *(for diagnosis of gastroesophageal reflux)* 0.1 N hydrochloric acid infused at a rate of 120 drops per minute produces pain and other symptoms. Called also *acid perfusion t.* and *esophageal acid perfusion t.*
Bial t. *(for pentoses in urine)* the specimen is heated with a solution of orcinol, hydrochloric acid, and ferric chloride; pentoses are converted to furfural, which reacts with orcinol to form a green product.
bicycle ergometer exercise t. an exercise test in which the patient pedals a stationary bicycle ergometer; the test is usually graded, with incremental or continuous increases in power produced by increases in pedal resistance at a given pedal speed. Cf. *treadmill exercise t.*
Bielschowsky head-tilting t. *(for types of paresis)* tilting the head to the right and the left shoulder with the patient looking at a distance fixation device permits distinction between superior rectus paresis and contralateral superior oblique paresis.
bile acid breath t. *(for overgrowth of bacteria in the intestine)* a breath test in which the patient is given a dose of a conjugated bile acid labeled with carbon 14 and the amount of radioactively labeled carbon dioxide in the breath is measured at hourly intervals. Excessive labeled carbon dioxide in the breath indicates excessive bacteria in the intestine breaking down the bile acids.
bile solubility t. *(for differentiation of pneumococci from other streptococci)* a sample of a broth culture is incubated at pH 7.4 to 7.6 with sodium deoxycholate. A decrease in turbidity (positive test) indicates lysing of the cells. Pneumococci give a positive result, whereas other viridans streptococci give a negative one.
biliary drainage t. examination of the contents of the duodenum at the site where the common bile duct empties into it; this is done when other, more conventional diagnostic tests for gallbladder disease reveal no pathology but the patient's symptoms persist. Specimens are collected with a special tube and examined for leukocytes, cholesterol crystals, and parasites.
bilirubin t. see specific tests, including *Fouchet t.* and *Harrison spot t.*
binaural distorted speech t's tests of the capacity of the central nervous system to coordinate two incoming speech patterns, each of which is incomplete.
Binet t., Binet-Simon t. a method of testing the mental capacity of children and youth by asking a series of questions adapted to, and standardized on, the capacity of normal children at various ages. According to the answers given, the mental age of the subject is ascertained.
Bing t. *(for hearing)* a vibrating tuning fork is held to the mastoid process and the auditory meatus is alternately occluded and left open: changes in loudness (positive Bing) are perceived by the normal ear and in sensorineural hearing loss, but in conduction hearing loss no difference is perceived (negative Bing).
biuret t. a colorimetric test for protein that makes use of the biuret reaction (q.v.).
bleeding time t. a test of bleeding time, assessing capillary function and platelet function, such as *Duke t., Ivy t.,* or the *template method.*
bone conduction t's tests of bone conduction; see *tuning fork t's.*
Bozicevich t. a serologic test for the detection of trichinosis.
breath t. any of various tests in which a person's breath is analyzed for presence of something abnormal. Subgroups called the *13C breath tests* and *14C breath tests* involve administration of organic compounds labeled with carbon 13 (heavy carbon) or carbon 14 (radioactive carbon) and measuring the subsequent levels of labeled carbon dioxide in the patient's breath; the labeled compound may be found to be metabolized normally, too fast, or too slow in the gastrointestinal tract.
breath hydrogen t. hydrogen breath t.
Broadbent t. *(for cerebral dominance of language function)* different numbers (or words) are presented simultaneously to the two ears; right-handed persons tend to report first the words going into the right ear.
bronchial challenge t. see under *challenge.*
buccal smear t. sex chromatin t.
Burchard-Liebermann t. Liebermann-Burchard t.
χ^2 t. chi-square t.

caffeine breath t. *(for liver function)* a breath test in which the patient is given a dose of caffeine labeled with carbon 13; excessively low levels of labeled carbon dioxide in the patient's breath indicate inadequate metabolism of it by the liver, as in patients who have cirrhosis or who smoke.
caffeine halothane contracture t. measurement of the force of contraction of a muscle tissue sample when exposed to caffeine and to halothane; response to halothane or to low concentrations of caffeine indicates increased susceptibility to malignant hyperthermia.
calcium infusion t. *(for hyperglycinemia)* calcium gluconate is administered to the fasting patient for 180 minutes. Serum samples are obtained 30 minutes before infusion, at its initiation, and every 30 minutes for two hours afterwards. The patient with a gastrinoma will show a sharp rise in production of gastrin.
calcium stimulation t. *(for localization of an insulinoma)* the patient is administered calcium gluconate, a secretagogue for insulin; veins around the suspected tumor are monitored for increased levels of insulin.
California mastitis t. (CMT) *(for subclinical mastitis in cows)* equal amounts of milk, bromcresol purple, and an anionic surface-active substance are mixed in four separate cups within a plastic paddle by rapidly rotating the paddle horizontally; a positive reaction is indicated by various degrees of gel formation, according to the degree of abnormality of the milk.
caloric t. *(for ocular and vestibular functioning)* irrigation of the normal ear with warm water produces rotatory nystagmus (*caloric nystagmus*) toward the irrigated side; irrigation with cold water produces similar nystagmus away from that side. Called also *Bárány t., sign,* or *symptom* and *nystagmus t.*
CAMP t. [*C*hristie, *A*tkins, and *M*unch-*P*etersen, discoverers of the phenomenon] *(for the presumptive identification of Group B beta-hemolytic streptococci)* a culture of streptococcus is streaked on a blood agar plate near a streak of beta-lysin–producing *Staphylococcus aureus.* Group B streptococci produce a substance (CAMP factor) that enlarges the zone of lysis formed by the staphylococcal beta-hemolysin.
capillary fragility t., capillary resistance t. tourniquet t. (def. 1).
captopril t. *(for renovascular hypertension)* the angiotensin-converting enzyme inhibitor captopril is administered to a patient with hypertension. If the patient's plasma renin level increases sharply within one hour, this indicates that the hypertension has a renovascular cause such as renal artery stenosis (see under *stenosis*).
carbohydrate utilization t. any of several tests for identification of yeasts and certain other organisms according to a profile of carbohydrate assimilation.
card t. a type of laboratory test that uses nonmicroscopic techniques; tissue or fluid to be examined is placed on a plastic-coated card with a reagent and visible reactions such as color changes or agglutination are noted.
Casoni intradermal t. *(for hydatid disease)* after injection into the skin of hydatid fluid, if there is immediate or delayed production of a wheal and flare reaction, this denotes hydatid infection. The test is now little used because of low specificity.
catalase t. *(for the production of heat-stable catalase by bacteria)* a culture is treated with hydrogen peroxide and heated. The presence of gas bubbles indicates a positive reaction. Micrococci, staphylococci, most species of *Bacillus,* and anaerobic diphtheroids are catalase-positive; streptococci, pneumococci, and most *Actinomyces* are catalase-negative. Catalase quantity and heat stability are species-dependent; inclusion of the detergent Tween-80 makes the test semiquantitative.

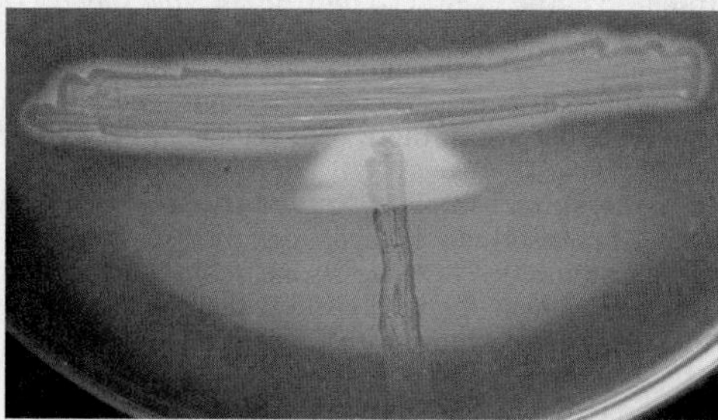

■ CAMP test, positive result. *Streptococcus agalactiae* shows an arrowhead-shaped area of enhanced hemolysis where it approaches the staphylococcal streak.

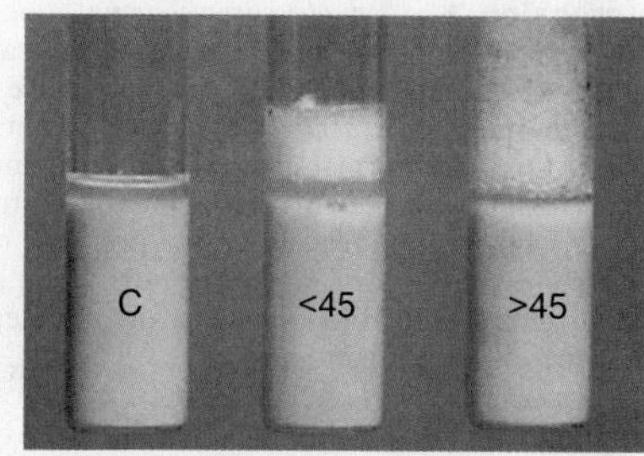

■ Semiquantitative catalase test, the column height recorded as greater than or less than 45 mm.

catoptric t. *(for cataract)* observations are done of the reflections from the cornea and the surfaces of the crystalline lens.
CCK t. cholecystokinin t.
cellobiose/mannitol t. *(for celiac disease)* cellobiose and mannitol are administered and their relative degrees of absorption are compared. Because of the relative permeability of the intestine to large molecules like cellobiose and small ones like mannitol, in celiac disease there is greater absorption of cellobiose and less absorption of mannitol.
challenge t. challenge (def. 3).
chemiluminescence t. *(for neutrophil microbicidal function)* a sensitive test that involves detection of the chemiluminescent energy emitted by unstable and highly reactive oxygen metabolites, e.g., singlet oxygen, produced during the respiratory burst following phagocytosis. It is able to detect heterozygous carriers of chronic granulomatous disease as well as homozygotes and also patients with myeloperoxidase deficiency.
Chick-Martin t. a method for determining the phenol coefficient of disinfectants in water contaminated by organic matter; serial dilutions of disinfectant are incubated with a specified quantity of yeast and bacteria for a period of 30 minutes to see how many of the microorganisms have been killed.
Chimani-Moos t. a test for detecting simulated deafness.
chi-square t. any statistical hypothesis test that employs the chi-square (χ^2) distribution (q.v.), especially two tests applied to categorical data: the χ^2-test of goodness of fit, which tests whether an observed frequency distribution fits a specified theoretical model, and the χ^2-test of independence or homogeneity, which tests whether two or more series of frequencies (the rows and columns of a contingency table) are independent. In both cases the test statistic is the sum over all categories of the squared difference between the observed and expected frequencies divided by the expected frequency, under the null hypothesis. The sampling distribution of this χ^2-statistic approaches the χ^2-distribution as the sample size increases, under the null hypothesis.
cholecystokinin t. *(for pancreatic function)* CCK test; after intravenous administration of cholecystokinin, the resultant pancreatic secretion of amylase, trypsin, and lipase is measured by collection through a tube in the duodenum. This test is often combined with the secretin test and called the secretin-cholecystokinin test.
cholesterol t. see specifc tests, including *Liebermann-Burchard t.* and *Salkowski t.* (def. 1).
***cis-trans* t.** in microbial genetics, a test to determine whether two (recessive) mutations are alleles (located in the same gene) or pseudoalleles (located in different genes). A heterozygote carrying the mutations on the same chromosome (*cis* configuration) will show a wild-type phenotype in either case, but one carrying the mutations on different chromosomes (*trans* configuration) will show a wild-type phenotype if they are pseudoalleles and a mutant phenotype if they are alleles.
citrate t. *(for differentiation of organisms of the Enterobacter group of bacteria)* the test organism is grown on a medium containing citrate as its sole carbon source (Simmons citrate agar). The metabolism of citrate (positive reaction) turns the medium from green to blue. The Enterobacteriaceae are mostly positive; *Edwardsiella, Escherichia, Morganella, Shigella,* and *Yersinia* are negative.
clomiphene citrate challenge t. *(for female factor infertility)* the patient's blood levels of follicle-stimulating hormone are measured on the third day of her menstrual cycle and she takes clomiphene citrate on days 5 through 9. If her levels of follicle-stimulating hormone are elevated on day 10, she probably has a diminished ovarian reserve.

clonidine suppression t. *(for pheochromocytoma)* one hour after injection of glucagon, base levels of norepinephrine are calculated and the patient is given clonidine; norepinephrine levels are determined over three hours to monitor for expected decreases. Patients with pheochromocytomas will not have normal decreases in norepinephrine.
coagulase t. *(for coagulase activity)* bacteria are added to citrated or oxalated (human or rabbit) blood plasma; in the presence of coagulase, the plasma gels within three hours. Coagulase activity is also demonstrable by mixing bacteria with blood plasma on a slide; if positive, clumping occurs, with fibrin formation.
cocaine t. *(for Horner syndrome)* after instillation of a cocaine solution in each eye, the pupil of a person who has Horner syndrome remains smaller than that of the normal eye.
coccidioidin t. *(for coccidioidomycosis)* an intracutaneous test that makes use of the antigen coccidioidin. Because most individuals in endemic areas are skin test positive, this test is not useful in diagnosis. A negative skin test (cutaneous anergy) occurs in many patients with disseminated disease and indicates a poor prognosis.
cold pressor t. immersion of one hand in ice water for several minutes, causing vasoconstriction, tachycardia, and transient hypertension; it is used as an alternative stress test for detection of coronary artery disease in patients incapable of undergoing an exercise stress test and as a test of vasomotor function.
collateral circulation t. see specific tests, including *Korotkoff t.*, *Pachon t.*, and *tourniquet t.* (defs. 2, 3).
color perception t. see specific tests, including the Ishihara test and the lantern test.
combined anterior pituitary t. *(for functioning of the anterior pituitary)* four exogenous hypothalamic hormones are administered intravenously (corticotropin-releasing hormone, growth hormone–releasing hormone, luteinizing hormone–releasing hormone, and thyrotropin-releasing hormone) and levels of the corresponding pituitary hormones in the blood are assessed at intervals for about two hours.
complement fixation t. see under *fixation.*
concentration t. 1. *(for renal function)* the patient is placed under conditions that cause the normal person to elaborate urine containing one or more constituents in high concentration, and the results are observed to see whether the patient is able to attain this concentration. 2. *(for renal tubular function)* water restriction to measure urine concentration as reflected in specific gravity or osmolality.
conglutinating complement absorption t. (CCAT) a test resembling the complement fixation test (see under *fixation*), using as the indicator of antigen-antibody reaction the disappearance of conglutinin (q.v.) activity.

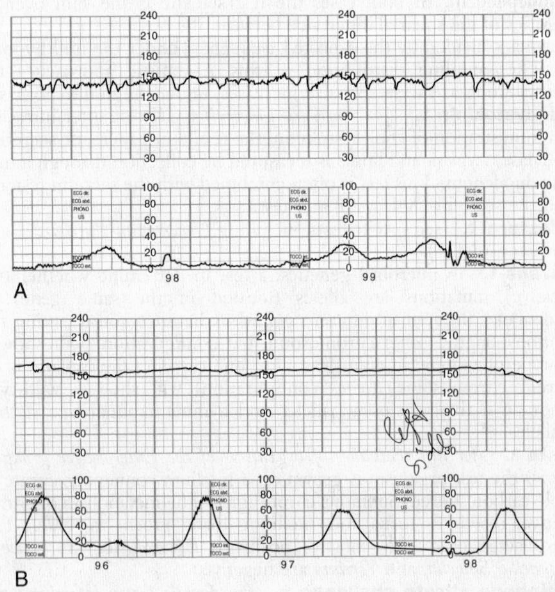

■ Contraction stress test. The top tracing of each pair shows the fetal heart rate; the bottom shows uterine contractions. *(A)*, A negative (normal) result, with uterine contractions followed by an unchanged fetal heart rate. *(B)*, A positive result, showing late deceleration with uterine contractions.

Congo red t. *(for amyloidosis)* Congo red is injected intravenously; if more than 60 per cent of the dye disappears after 1 hour, amyloidosis is indicated.
conservative t. a test having a type I error probability that is at most a stated nominal level.
contact t's patch t's.
contraction stress t. (CST) the monitoring of the response of the fetal heart rate to uterine contractions by cardiotocography; uterine contractions may be spontaneous or induced by maternal nipple stimulation or by intravenous infusion of oxytocin (oxytocin challenge test). A negative (normal) test consists of three contractions within a 10-minute period with no deceleration of the fetal heart rate; a late deceleration pattern may reflect fetal hypoxia.
Coombs t. antiglobulin t.
copper reduction t. any of various tests that use copper compounds as reagents for detecting sugars in urine, such as the Benedict test or Clinitest.
corticotropin stimulation t. ACTH stimulation t.
cover t. see *alternate cover t.* and *cover-uncover t.*
cover-uncover t. *(for determining type of phoria)* one eye is covered and its movement is assessed as it is uncovered.
Crampton t. a test for physical resistance and condition based on the difference between the pulse and blood pressure in the recumbent position and in the standing position. A difference of 75 or more indicates good condition; one of 65 or less shows a poor condition.
creatinine t. see *Jaffe t.* and see also *creatinine, methods for*, under *method.*
crossed straight-leg raising t. *(for disk herniation)* with the patient supine, the unaffected leg is lifted with the knee straight; pain in the affected leg indicates presence of herniation.
Cuignet t. *(for simulated unilateral blindness)* the bar-reading test used to detect simulated unilateral blindness or malingering.
cycle ergometer t. bicycle ergometer exercise t.
cysteine t. see *nitroprusside t.*
dark-adaptation t. *(for vitamin A deficiency)* a test based on the fact that with a deficient intake of vitamin A the ability to see a dimly illuminated object in a dark room is diminished.
darkroom t. *(for tendency to develop acute angle-closure glaucoma)* ocular pressure is measured by the applanation tonometer, the subject is placed in a darkroom for one hour, and applanation tonometry is then repeated.
Davidsohn differential absorption t. Paul-Bunnell-Davidsohn t.
D-dimer t. see under *assay.*
dehydrocholate t. *(for speed of blood circulation)* sodium dehydrocholate solution is injected intravenously; the usual time elapsing until a bitter taste in the mouth occurs is between 10 and 14 seconds.
Denver Developmental Screening t. a test for identification of infants and preschool children with developmental delay.
deoxyribonuclease t. *(for deoxyribonuclease in bacteria)* a nutrient agar plate containing deoxyribonucleic acid and toluidine blue is inoculated from a young agar slant; after incubation a red zone around the inoculum indicates the presence of deoxyribonuclease. Called also *DNase t.*
deoxyuridine suppression t. *(for folate or cobalamin deficiency)* lack of 5,10-methylene tetrahydrofolate inhibits incorporation of deoxyuridine into DNA, so that deoxyuridine fails to inhibit incorporation of ^{3}H-thymidine.
dexamethasone suppression t., high-dose *(for Cushing syndrome)* urinary levels of cortisol and 17-hydroxycorticosteroid are measured following administration of dexamethasone at 16 times the level used in replacement therapy; cortisol secretion is suppressed in patients with Cushing syndrome but not in those with ectopic ACTH syndrome or adrenal tumors.
dexamethasone suppression t., low-dose *(for Cushing syndrome)* urinary levels of cortisol and 17-hydroxycorticosteroid are measured following administration of dexamethasone at three to four times the level used in replacement therapy; cortisol secretion is suppressed in normal patients but not in those with Cushing syndrome.
dextrose t. glucose t.
DFA-TP t. direct fluorescent antibody–*Treponema pallidum* t.
diabetes t. any of various tests for diabetes mellitus; see *glucose t.* and *glucose tolerance t.*

diacetyl t. *(for urea)* the solution to be tested is mixed with concentrated hydrochloric acid and diacetyl monoxime, a more stable precursor of diacetyl; condensation of diacetyl and urea forms the yellow chromogen diazine, particularly at an elevated temperature (usually 45 °C).
dial t. *(for instability of posterolateral structures of the knee)* with the patient lying either prone or supine, each knee is flexed at 30° and rotated externally, and rotation of the tibial tubercles between the injured and normal contralateral limb are compared; a difference of more than 10° indicates abnormal laxity. The test is often repeated with the knees flexed at 90°. Called also *tibial external rotation t.*
Dick t. *(for susceptibility to scarlet fever)* purified erythrogenic toxin from group A streptococci is injected intradermally; appearance within 24 to 48 hours of a small area of reddening of the skin indicates susceptibility of the subject.
differential t. for infectious mononucleosis Paul-Bunnell-Davidsohn t.
dilution t. see under *method.*
dimethylglyoxime t. *(for nickel)* the object or substance being tested is placed in a solution of dimethylglyoxime; if nickel is present, the solution will turn brown.
diphtheria t. see *Schick t.*
direct antiglobulin t., direct Coombs t. see *antiglobulin t.*
direct fluorescent antibody–*Treponema pallidum* t. DFA-TP test; a serologic test for syphilis that uses direct immunofluorescence.
disk diffusion t., disk sensitivity t. a type of antimicrobial susceptibility test in which agar plates are inoculated with a standardized suspension of a microorganism and then antibiotic-containing disks are applied to the agar surface. Following overnight incubation, the diameters of the zones of inhibition or clearing surrounding the disks are measured to calculate how susceptible or resistant the microorganism is.
Dix-Hallpike t. see under *maneuver.*
DNase t. deoxyribonuclease t.
Donath-Landsteiner t. *(for paroxysmal cold hemoglobinuria)* a test based on the fact that the blood of patients with this disease contains complement-dependent iso- and autohemolysin (Donath-Landsteiner antibody) which unites with red cells only at low temperatures (2° to 10°C), hemolysis occurring only after warming to 37°C.
double glucagon t. *(for deficiency of amylo-1-6-glucosidase)* glucagon is administered after a 12-hour fast and again shortly after a meal; if the blood sugar fails to rise after the first administration but has a normal rise after the second, the test is positive.
Draw-a-Person t. a commonly used projective test for assessing personality style and psychopathology by interpretation of a drawing of a person done by the subject, based on the assumption that their personality characteristics will be introjected onto the drawing.
drawer t's *(for integrity of cruciate ligaments of knee)* the knee is flexed to a 90° angle; at the femoral-tibial junction, if the tibia can be drawn too far forward there is rupture of the anterior ligaments *(anterior drawer t.)* and if it can be drawn too far back there is rupture of the posterior ligaments *(posterior drawer t.)*. Called also *drawer signs.*
drinking t. *(for glaucoma)* one liter of water is ingested as rapidly as possible into an empty stomach. The intraocular pressure is measured every 15 minutes; a rise of 8 to 15 mm Hg in less than 30 minutes indicates glaucoma. Called also *water provocative t.*

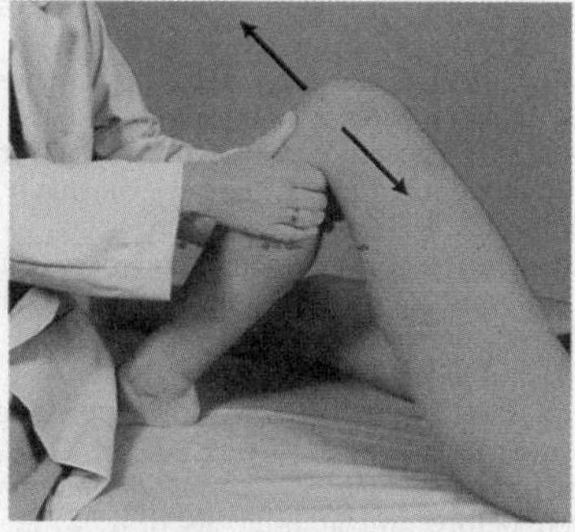

■ Anterior and posterior drawer tests.

Dugas t. *(for dislocation of the shoulder)* the patient's hand on the affected side is placed on the opposite shoulder and the elbow is brought to the side of the chest; if this cannot be accomplished (Dugas sign), dislocation of the shoulder exists.
Duke t. a type of bleeding time test in which the incision is made in the earlobe.
dye exclusion t. *(for cell viability in vitro)* following exposure of a cell preparation to trypan blue or eosin, dead cells take up the dye from the medium whereas living cells remain unstained.
dynamic t. a test of some physiologic process in the body, such as a challenge, a stimulation test, or a suppression test.
E t. a variation of the dilution method for testing antimicrobial susceptibility. A plastic strip is used that has a defined concentration of drug on one side and an interpretive scale of minimal inhibitory concentrations on the other side; it is put on the surface of an agar medium inoculated with the microorganism to be tested. This method is most useful for fastidious bacteria such as *Streptococcus pneumoniae*, *Haemophilus influenzae*, and certain anaerobic bacteria.
early pregnancy t. a do-it-yourself immunologic test for pregnancy performed in the home as early as one day after menstruation was expected (missed period); a variety of tests exist, all based on an increase in urinary levels of human chorionic gonadotropin after fertilization.
ECG stress t's stress t's.
Ehrlich t. Ehrlich diazo reaction; see under *reaction.*
Elek t. toxigenicity t.
Elsberg t. *(for sense of smell)* variations in function of the sense of smell, or in rate of fatigue, may be used to distinguish between intracerebral and extracerebral tumors or other lesions.
Ely t. *(for contracture)* with the patient prone, if flexion of the leg on the thigh causes the buttocks to arch away from the table and the leg to abduct at the hip joint, there is contracture of the lateral fascia of the thigh.
EP t. erythrocyte protoporphyrin t.
Erichsen t. see under *sign.*
erythrocyte protoporphyrin t. *(for lead poisoning)* EP test; a screening test in which erythrocyte protoporphyrin levels are determined by direct fluorometry of whole blood or fluorescence analysis of whole blood extracts; levels are increased in lead poisoning and iron deficiency.
esophageal acid perfusion t. Bernstein t.
euglobulin lysis t. *(for hemorrhagic tendencies)* the time of fibrinolysis is measured by determining the time required to dissolve an incubated clot composed of precipitated plasma euglobulin and exogenous thrombin. Lysis in less than 90 minutes indicates abnormally enhanced fibrinolytic activity.
exact t. a statistical test based on the actual probability distribution of the data in the study, rather than on an approximation of it.
exercise t's, exercise stress t's any of various stress tests in which exercise is used in the electrocardiographic assessment of cardiovascular health and function, particularly in the diagnosis of myocardial ischemia. The most widely used forms are the treadmill and bicycle ergometer exercise tests; they are usually graded, consisting of a series of incrementally increasing work loads sustained for defined intervals.
***F*-t.** a statistical test comparing the means of more than two groups simultaneously by comparing two different measures of variance of the observations. One statistic measures the variations between the means of the groups (the between-groups variation), the other the variations within the groups (the within-group variation). If the two measures of variance yield similar results and their ratio, the *F*-ratio, approximates 1.0, the null hypothesis that all observations came from the same population cannot be rejected, whereas under the alternative hypothesis, the *F*-ratio is expected to be larger than 1.0. The test is the first step in the analysis of variance (ANOVA).
FAB t. fluorescent antibody t.
Farber t. *(for infantile intestinal blockage)* presence of swallowed vernix cells in the meconium of a newborn baby indicates partial intestinal stenosis; their absence indicates intestinal atresia.
Farr t. *(a radioimmunoassay for measuring absolute amounts of antibody)* antibody is reacted with radiolabeled antigen and precipitated with ammonium sulfate; bound antigen or hapten is precipitated while free antigen remains in solution. This test is based on the capacity of antibody to combine with antigen rather than on such secondary properties as precipitation and therefore measures all immunoglobulin classes and subclasses.
FENa t. see *fractional excretion of sodium,* under *excretion.*

femoral nerve stretch t., femoral stretch t. *(for lesions of third or fourth lumbar disk)* the patient lies prone and the knee is passively flexed; the location of pain in the back or thighs indicates which disk is herniated.
fermentation t. *(for glucose and other sugars in urine)* boil a specimen to destroy bacteria, then add baker's yeast and incubate; perform Benedict test for reducing sugars on this specimen and an unfermented specimen. Glucose, fructose, and maltose are fermented and give a reaction in the unfermented specimen but not in the fermented specimen.
fern t. see *ferning.*
ferric chloride t. ferric chloride in acidic solution is added to a urine specimen; many substances are oxidized giving colored products. Positive reactions are given by melanin, acetoacetic acid, bilirubin, phenothiazines, salicylates, and the keto acids present in phenylketonuria, alkaptonuria, maple syrup urine disease, and oasthouse urine disease.
fetal acoustic stimulation t. *(for assessing fetal health)* a vibroacoustic stimulus such as an electronic artificial larynx is applied either externally or directly to the fetus and resultant fetal movements, cardioacceleration, and alterations in respiration are evaluated.
FIGLU excretion t. histidine loading t.
finger-to-finger t. similar to finger-nose test, for testing coordinated movements of the extremities.
finger-nose t., finger-to-nose t. *(for coordinated movements of the upper limbs)* with arm extended to one side the patient is asked to slowly try to touch an index finger to the end of the nose.
Finn chamber t. a type of patch test in which the materials being tested are held in shallow aluminum cups (Finn chambers) that are taped against the skin, usually for several days.
Fishberg concentration t. *(for kidney function)* the patient's evening meal includes not more than 200 mL of fluid, and nothing else is consumed before morning. Urine voided during the night is discarded. The morning urine is saved, the patient kept in bed, and the urine of 1 hour later and 2 hours later is saved. If the specific gravity of any of these 3 specimens is less than 1.024 there is impairment of renal concentration.
Fisher exact t. a statistical hypothesis test of independence of rows and columns in a 2×2 contingency table based on the exact sampling distribution of the observed frequencies, useful when any expected value in the table is small.
fistula t. *(for perilymph fistula in the ear)* the air in the external auditory canal is compressed or rarefied: if there is erosion of the inner osseous wall of the tympanum exposing the membranous labyrinth, nystagmus will be produced, provided the labyrinth still functions.
Flack t. *(for physical efficiency of lungs)* after a full inhalation the subject blows as long as possible into a mercury manometer with a force of 40 mm mercury.
flocculation t. any serologic test in which a flocculent agglomerate is formed; usually referring to a variant form of the precipitin reaction, and sometimes to types of agglutination tests.
fluorescein dilaurate t. pancreolauryl t.
fluorescent antibody t. FAB test; a test for the distribution of cells expressing a specific protein by binding antibody specific for the protein and detecting complexes by fluorescent labeling of the antibody; if it is combined with cell sorting, determinations can be quantitative.

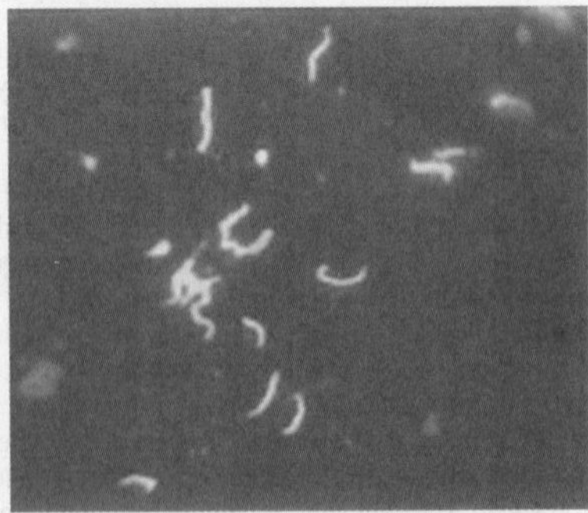

■ Fluorescent treponemal antibody absorption test (FTA-ABS) showing a positive result for syphilis.

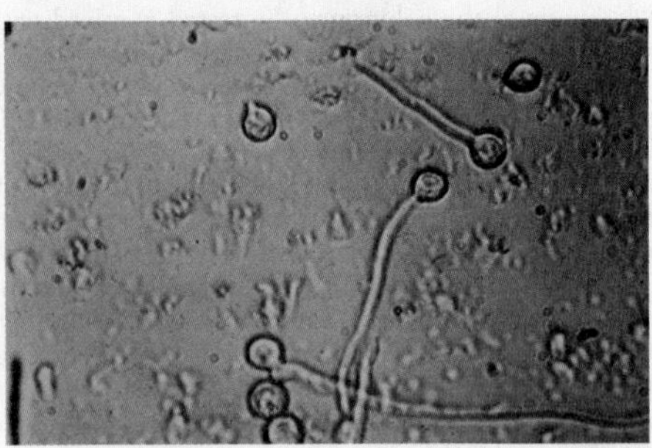

■ Positive germ tube test; a true germ tube, as here, lacks a constriction at its base.

fluorescent treponemal antibody absorption t. FTA-ABS test; a highly specific treponemal antigen serologic test for syphilis; patient serum is absorbed with other treponemes to remove nonspecific antibodies, then reacted with a strain of *Treponema pallidum* fixed to a glass slide; specific antibodies adhering to the treponemes are demonstrated with fluorescein-labeled antihuman globulin.
food challenge t. food challenge.
Fouchet t. *(for bilirubin in urine)* a few drops of Fouchet reagent are added to the specimen; a green color is produced if bilirubin is present.
Fournier t. *(for ataxic gait)* from a sitting position, the patient is asked to rise, walk, and stop quickly at a given signal, and then to walk and turn around quickly when a signal is given.
Friberg t. tray agglutination t.
Friderichsen t. *(for vitamin A deficiency)* determination of the weakest light stimulus which will give rise to an oculomotor reflex. A variation from normal indicates vitamin A deficiency.
fructosamine t. determination of the serum fructosamine level by measurement of the reduction of nitroblue tetrazolium to purple under alkaline conditions; it is used as an index of the average glycemic state over the preceding two to three weeks and is used to monitor glycemic control in diabetes.
fructose t. see *Selivanoff t.*
fructose tolerance t. *(for liver function)* a large quantity of fructose is administered and the power of the liver to absorb it is monitored.
FTA-ABS t. fluorescent treponemal antibody absorption t.
Gaenslen t. see under *sign.*
galactose breath t. *(for liver function)* a breath test in which the fasting subject is given a dose of galactose labeled with carbon 13 and levels of labeled carbon dioxide in the breath are measured at specific time intervals. Low levels of carbon dioxide indicate that the galactose is not being metabolized properly, indicating either an enzyme deficiency or liver dysfunction such as the fibrosis accompanying hepatitis.
galactose tolerance t. *(for liver function)* a test of the liver's ability to convert galactose into glycogen. Two methods may be used; the *oral method,* which requires about 5 hours to complete, and the *intravenous method,* which requires about 2 hours and is more accurate. With the oral method, elimination of more than 3 g of galactose in the urine during a 5-hour period indicates liver damage. With the intravenous method, all galactose should have been eliminated from the blood 45 minutes after its injection.
gastric function t. see specific tests, such as *augmented histamine t.* and *pentagastrin t.* Abnormal results on the Schilling test may indicate defective gastric secretion of intrinsic factor.
gaze t. *(for ocular and vestibular functioning)* movements of the eye are recorded with the patient gazing straight at an object and at positions off to different sides of it; then with eyes closed for 20 seconds, the patient must perform a small mental exercise. The eyes normally should assume a center gaze while they are closed.
gelatin agglutination t. a sperm agglutination test in which the sperm and serum are put in a gelatin solution. Called also *Kibrick t.*
gel diffusion t. see *immunodiffusion.*
germ tube t. *(for Candida albicans)* an inoculum of *Candida* is incubated in serum for 2 to 3 hours at 37°C; formation of germ tubes is a positive result.
glucagon stimulation t. *(for epinephrine and norepinephrine)* blood samples are taken before and at intervals of 1, 2, 2.5, and 3 hours after subcutaneous or intramuscular injection of glucagon, and blood

levels of epinephrine and norepinephrine are determined. Excessive levels of those hormones indicate a possible pheochromocytoma.
glucose t. any of various laboratory tests for glucose in the urine; many formerly common ones are no longer used. See *Benedict t.* and *saccharimeter t.*
glucose tolerance t. (GTT) a metabolic test of carbohydrate tolerance, measuring active insulin, a hepatic function based on the power of the normal liver to absorb and store large quantities of glucose, and the effectiveness of intestinal absorption of glucose. The most common method is the *oral glucose tolerance test* (q.v.).
glucose tolerance t., oral (OGTT) the most common kind of glucose tolerance test. Glucose is ingested into a fasting stomach and measurements of plasma glucose are taken over time; if glucose levels do not return to normal within 2 to 2.5 hours the patient may have impaired glucose tolerance or diabetes mellitus.
glycosylated hemoglobin t. *(for diabetes mellitus)* the percentage is determined of hemoglobin A molecules that have formed a stable keto–amine linkage between the terminal amino acid position of the β-chains and a glucose group; in normal persons this amounts to about 7 per cent of the total, in diabetics about 14.5 per cent.
Goodenough draw-a-man t., Goodenough draw-a-person t. *(for intelligence)* the general intelligence of the child is assessed by asking him or her to draw a picture of a person as well as possible.
Goodenough-Harris drawing t. a revision of the Goodenough draw-a-man test, in which scoring emphasizes the presence or absence of body and clothing detail rather than artistic skill.
graded exercise t's (GXT) see *exercise t's.*
Graefe t. *(for heterophoria)* when a prism is held at 10 degrees before one eye, base up or down, two images are formed; if the patient has heterophoria, one of these images will be displaced laterally.
Graham t. the intravenous or oral administration of iodophthalein sodium prior to radiographic examination of the gallbladder.
Griess t. 1. *(for nitrate-reducing bacteria in a fluid)* a formerly common test in which sulfuric acid and an indicator were added to a dilute solution and color change was assessed. 2. the same name is now applied to nitrite tests for bacteriuria in which a urine specimen collected when the patient wakes in the morning is tested for nitrites using a special tape or dipstick.
group t. a test of intelligence or aptitude given to a number of persons at one time.
guaiac t. *(for occult blood)* glacial acetic acid and a solution of gum guaiac are mixed with the specimen; on addition of hydrogen peroxide, the presence of blood is indicated by a blue tint.
Guerreiro-Machado t. Machado-Guerreiro t.
Guthrie t. *(for phenylketonuria)* blood from an infant suspected of having abnormally high levels of phenylalanine is placed on filter paper, which is then put on an agar plate with a strain of *Bacillus subtilis* that requires phenylalanine for growth. In the presence of blood containing phenylalanine, a halo will form around the filter paper.
HAI t. hemagglutination inhibition t.
hair perforation t. *(for identification of dermatophytes)* sterile pieces of hair are floated on the surface of a mixture of water and yeast extract, and the fungal sample in question is inoculated onto this. After a week the hairs are removed; different dermatophytes cause specific types of erosions.
halothane caffeine contracture t. caffeine halothane contracture test.
Ham t. acidified serum t.
hapten inhibition t. serologic characterization of an antigenic determinant by employing known haptens to mask the antigen binding site of antibody specific for it.
harmonic acceleration t. *(for vestibuloocular reflex)* rotation of a patient seated in a chair in complete darkness, with monitoring of eye movements; with normal vestibuloocular reflexes the eyes will undergo rotatory nystagmus to the same degree in both eyes in the direction opposite to that of the rotation.
Harrison spot t. *(for bilirubin in urine)* add to 10 mL of urine 5 mL of a 10 per cent solution of barium chloride, mix, and filter. Spread filter paper on dry filter paper. Add one to two drops of Fouchet reagent (trichloroacetic acid 25 g, water 100 mL, and 10 per cent solution of ferric chloride 10 mL); a positive reaction gives a blue to green color.
hatching t. *(for schistosomiasis)* live schistosome eggs in urine or feces can be detected when they hatch to produce miracidia when placed in water; the miracidia are attracted to light and can readily be identified.
Heaf t. a type of intracutaneous tuberculin test; needle points of a multiple-puncture apparatus are dipped into 1 to 2 drops of tuberculin PPD, then placed on the forearm and made to penetrate the skin to a depth of 1 mm, depositing tuberculin in the outer layer of the skin. In three to seven days, a positive reaction is palpable, coalescing induration (edema) extending more than 5 mm around the puncture wounds.
heel-knee t., heel-shin t. *(for coordinated movements of lower limbs)* the patient, lying supine, is asked to touch the knee on one side with the opposite heel and then to pass the heel slowly down the front of the shin to the ankle. Called also *heel-to-knee* or *heel-to-shin t.*
heel-tap t. see under *reflex.*
heel-to-knee t., heel-to-shin t. heel-knee t.
hemadsorption t. *(for hemagglutinating viruses)* an in vitro test based on the adherence of red blood cells to cells of the infected tissue in the presence of hemagglutinin.
hemagglutination inhibition t. 1. a highly sensitive procedure for the measurement of soluble antigens in biologic specimens; the specimen is first incubated with homologous antibody and then incubated with antigen-coated red blood cells; the amount of hemagglutination reflects the amount of free antibody present after reaction with the specimen and thus varies inversely with the amount of antigen in the specimen. 2. a procedure for the measurement of serum antibodies directed against a hemagglutinating virus; the highest dilution of serum that completely inhibits hemagglutination by a standardized viral preparation is reported as the hemagglutination titer. Called also *HAI* or *HI t.*
Henshaw t. a test to aid in the selection of the appropriate homeopathic remedy in a given case of disease. A visible zone of flocculation develops in the patient's blood serum when it is brought into contact with a potentized remedy homeopathically indicated in the case.
hepatic function t. liver function t.
Hering t. *(for binocular versus monocular vision)* the subject looks with both eyes through a tube blackened within and having a thread running vertically across the farther end. A small round body is placed either before or behind the thread. If vision is binocular, the subject can immediately tell whether the ball is nearer than the thread or farther away; if vision is monocular, this distinction cannot be made.
Hess capillary t. tourniquet t. (def. 1).
heterophil antibody t., heterophile antibody t. any of several tests for heterophile antibodies associated with infectious mononucleosis; the most common ones are the monospot test and the Paul-Bunnell-Davidsohn test.
HI t. hemagglutination inhibition t.
Hickey-Hare t. *(for diabetes insipidus)* after the patient has been given enough water to establish diuresis, a hypertonic saline solution is administered. Under normal conditions, this should suppress the diuresis, but if the patient has diabetes insipidus, that will not happen.
high-sensitivity C-reactive protein (hs-CRP) t. an extremely sensitive test to determine the level of C-reactive protein in the blood; as the hs-CRP rises, the risk of cardiovascular disease increases.
Hines and Brown t. cold pressor t.
histamine t. 1. histamine flare t. 2. any of several formerly common gastric function tests in which histamine was injected to stimulate gastric secretion and measure output of gastric acid; see also *augmented histamine test.* 3. a formerly used test for presence of a pheochromocytoma; persons with such a tumor would show first a fall and then a marked rise in blood pressure.
histamine flare t. *(for leprosy and postherpetic neuralgia)* a drop of 1:1000 histamine acid phosphate solution is placed on the skin and a needle puncture is made through it; the test is positive if there is no erythema flare when the puncture is made within the suspected lesion area, or if the flare stops at the border of the lesion when it is made slightly outside it.
histidine loading t. *(for folic acid deficiency)* a loading dose of histidine is given, and the resultant urinary excretion of excess formiminoglutamic acid (FIGLU) is measured, because that is dependent on the amount of tetrahydrofolic acid that is present. Called also *FIGLU excretion t.*
hock t. spavin t.
Hoppe-Seyler t. 1. *(for carbon monoxide in the blood)* add to blood twice its volume of a solution of sodium hydroxide of 1.3 specific gravity: normal blood will form a dingy brown mass with a green shade if spread thin on a white surface; but if carbon monoxide is present, the mass is red, and so is the thin layer. 2. *(for xanthine)* add the substance to be tested to a mixture of chlorinated lime in a porcelain dish; a dark-green ring is formed at first.

horse cell t. monospot t.
Hotis t. *(for mastitis in cows)* fresh milk containing bromcresol purple is incubated for 24 hours; a positive reaction is the formation of yellow flakes on the sides of the test tube.
Huddleson t. an agglutination test for human brucellosis.
Huhner t. postcoital t.
hydrogen breath t. *(for deficiency of lactase or other hydrolases, or colonic overgrowth of bacteria)* a breath test in which a known quantity of carbohydrate is administered and the subject's exhalations measured at timed intervals; in patients who are unable to digest or absorb carbohydrates in the small intestine, bacterial fermentation of excess carbohydrate in the colon causes an increase in blood hydrogen and thus in hydrogen exhaled by the lungs.
hydrogen peroxide t. *(for blood)* a 20 per cent solution of hydrogen peroxide is added to the suspected fluid; if blood is present even in minute proportion, bubbles will rise, forming foam on the surface of the fluid.
hydrostatic t. floating of the lungs of a dead infant when placed in water indicates that the child was born alive.
hyperabduction t. *(for thoracic outlet syndrome)* the patient elevates and hyperabducts the arms; reproduction of symptoms is a positive indication for thoracic outlet syndrome, but the results must be confirmed by other tests.
hyperventilation t. *(for Prinzmetal angina)* the patient hyperventilates (breathes rapidly and deeply) for five minutes and an electrocardiogram is recorded before, during, and for ten minutes after this. Abnormal coronary vasoconstriction, demonstrated by ST segment changes, indicates Prinzmetal angina.
hypo-osmotic swelling t. *(for viability of sperm)* a sperm sample is put into a hypo-osmotic solution; spermatozoa with normal plasma membranes should undergo swelling and curling of their tails. If less than 50 per cent of the spermatozoa show this change, the sample is abnormal.
hypothesis t. an abstract procedure for determining whether a set of observations is consistent with a hypothesis under consideration; it is the theoretical basis of most statistical tests. A hypothesis test decides between two hypotheses, one stating that the effect under investigation does not exist (the *null hypothesis*, H_0), and the other that some specified effect does exist (the *alternative hypothesis*, H_a or H_1), based on the observed value of a test statistic whose sampling distribution is completely determined by H_0. When the test statistic falls in a set of values known as the critical region, H_0 is rejected. The level of probability of incorrectly rejecting H_0 may be set before the data are collected, usually at 0.05 or 0.01; this is called the *significance level* or *α level*. It is now more common to report the smallest α at which the null hypothesis can be rejected; this is called the *significance probability* or P *value*.
ICG t. indocyanine green t.
IFA t. indirect fluorescent antibody test; see *immunofluorescence*.
immobilization t. detection of antibody based on its ability to inhibit the motility of a bacterial cell or protozoon.
IMViC t. [modified acronym from *i*ndole, *m*ethyl red, *V*oges-Proskauer, *c*itrate] a series of metabolic tests used as standard procedure to differentiate genera of the family Enterobacteriaceae. See also *methyl red t.* and *Voges-Proskauer t.*
indirect antiglobulin t., indirect Coombs' t. see *antiglobulin t.*
indirect fluorescent antibody t. see *immunofluorescence*.
indocyanine green t. *(for liver function)* indocyanine green is administered intravenously and the blood concentration is monitored to track hepatic clearance. Called also *ICG t.*
indole t. see *Salkowski t.* (def. 2).
inhalational challenge t. see under *challenge*.
inkblot t. Rorschach t.
insulin sensitivity t. *(for differentiation of diabetes mellitus from pituitary and adrenal diabetes)* a test dose of exogenous insulin will produce a rapid and marked decrease in blood glucose levels if the pancreas is not secreting enough insulin. A much less dramatic response is produced if hyperglycemia is due to excessive secretion of either anterior pituitary or adrenocortical hormones.
insulin tolerance t. (ITT) *(for growth hormone deficiency)* insulin is administered to a fasting, nondiabetic individual and levels of growth hormone are measured. Blood levels of growth hormone should increase in the presence of insulin; if their rise is less than 3 mmol/L, the person has significant growth hormone deficiency.
intelligence t. a set of problems or tasks posed to assess an individual's innate ability to judge, comprehend, and reason.

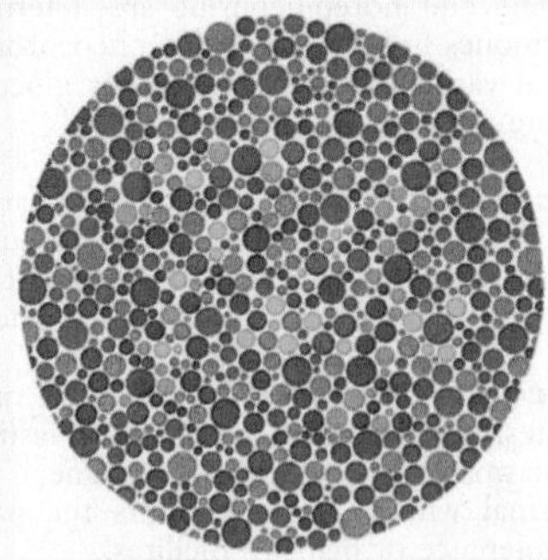

■ A pseudoisochromatic plate used in the Ishihara test. Persons with normal vision can see the *74*, whereas persons with red-green color blindness cannot.

intracutaneous t. intradermal t.
intradermal t. a skin test in which the antigen is injected below the skin. Called also *intracutaneous t.*
intradermal tuberculin t. a tuberculin test in which tuberculin is injected below the skin; see specific tests, including *Heaf t.*, *Mantoux t.*, and *tine t.*
intravenous secretin t. secretin t.
inulin clearance t. see under *clearance*.
iodine t. *(for starch)* when a compound solution of iodine is added to starch, and especially to an acid or neutral solution of cooked starch paste, a deep blue color is produced that disappears on heating and reappears on cooling.
Iowa pressure articulation t. a test of the ability to produce the consonant sounds in isolated words, particularly the pressure sounds.
irresistible impulse t. see under *impulse*.
ischemic forearm t. *(for metabolic myopathies)* blood flow in the forearm is impeded using a blood pressure cuff, blocking oxidative phosphorylation and causing dependence on anaerobic processes; normal subjects will show rises in ammonia, lactate, and pyruvate, whereas those with metabolic myopathies will not.
Ishihara t. a color perception test that makes use of a series of pseudoisochromatic plates.
Isojima t. sperm immobilization t.
isopropanol precipitation t. *(for unstable hemoglobins)* a drop of blood is mixed with the nonpolar solvent isopropanol; most unstable hemoglobins precipitate more readily than other hemoglobins. Addition of potassium cyanide reduces false-positive results.
Ivy t. a bleeding time test in which incisions are made on the forearm, a sphygmomanometer is inflated around the upper arm, and the time until cessation of bleeding is recorded. Called also *Ivy method*.
Jaffe t. *(for creatinine)* to the liquid add trinitrophenol and then make alkaline with sodium hydroxide. A red color indicates presence of creatinine.
Kato t. *(for estimation of worm burden)* a standard 50-mg sample of fresh feces is collected, cleared with glycerine, and examined for worms.
Kibrick t. gelatin agglutination t.
kidney function t. a test of kidney function, such as of renal clearance or of the glomerular filtration rate; see also specific tests, including *Fishberg concentration t.*, *radioisotope renal excretion t.*, *Rehberg t.*, and D-*xylose absorption t.* Called also *renal function t.*
King-Devick t. *(for evaluation of saccade)* the patient looks at a series of charts of numbers that become progressively harder to read, arranged in a flowing manner with increasing space between the numbers. Both errors in reading and speed of reading are included in deriving a score.
Kirby-Bauer t. disk diffusion t.
Kjeldahl t. *(for nitrogen)* see under *method*.
Kleihauer t., Kleihauer-Betke t. acid elution t.
Knott t. *(for microfilariae or worm larvae in blood)* a blood sample is subjected to lysis in a dilute (2 per cent) formalin solution, followed by centrifugation and examination of the stained sediment for microfilariae or larvae.
Kolmogorov-Smirnov t. a statistical test of goodness of fit of a sample to a specified theoretical distribution function, based on the size of the maximum difference between the cumulative distribution functions of the sample and theoretical distributions and using the

exact sampling distribution of this difference to determine the significance level. The test can also be used to determine whether two samples are drawn from the same population by examining the maximum difference between the cumulative distribution functions of the two samples.

Korotkoff t. *(for collateral circulation)* in aneurysm, if the blood pressure in the peripheral circulation remains fairly high while the artery above the aneurysm is compressed, the collateral circulation is good.

Kremer t. SCMC t.

Kruskal-Wallis t. a nonparametric test for ordinal data, comparing three or more groups simultaneously: all data are ranked numerically and then the rank values are summed and averaged for each group. If the null hypothesis that all groups are drawn from the same population is true, then the mean ranks should be similar across all groups.

Kuhlmann t. a modification of the Binet test of intelligence for use in infants.

Kveim t. *(for sarcoidosis)* a skin test using antigen from human sarcoid tissue injected intradermally; any palpable nodule developing at the inoculation site within 6 weeks is biopsied, and histopathologic evidence of epithelioid cell granulomas constitutes a positive reaction. The test is positive in about 60 to 80 per cent of patients.

Lachman t. an anterior drawer test for cases of severe knee injury, performed at 20 degrees of flexion.

lactulose-mannitol t. *(for intestinal permeability)* a solution containing lactulose, mannitol, and physiologic saline is administered orally to a fasting patient; urine is then collected for six hours and the urinary ratio between lactulose and mannitol is measured.

Lancefield precipitation t. a ring precipitation test for identification and classification of streptococci. Group-specific antibody reacts in vitro with group-specific polysaccharide to produce a ring of precipitation where the two reagents react at the interface.

lantern t. a color perception test that uses a set of specially devised lanterns to test the patient's color vision.

Lasègue t. straight leg–raising test.

lateral pivot shift t. *(for integrity of the anterior cruciate ligament)* the patient lies prone with the hip flexed and the knee extended; the examiner gradually flexes the knee while pushing the outside of the knee medially and internally rotating the tibia. A thud or jerk at 30°–40° of flexion indicates deficiency of the anterior cruciate ligament.

latex agglutination t., latex fixation t. *(for presence of antibody)* a type of agglutination test in which antigen to a given antibody is adsorbed to latex particles and mixed with a solution to observe for agglutination of the latex.

leishmanin t. *(for leishmaniasis)* leishmanin is injected intradermally; a positive reaction consists of a palpable nodule developing in 48 to 72 hours and indicates delayed hypersensitivity, but not necessarily immunity, to *Leishmania* organisms. The positive result appears early in some forms of cutaneous and mucocutaneous leishmaniasis, but only after recovery in the case of visceral leishmaniasis. Called also *Montenegro t.*

lepromin t. *(for certain types of leprosy)* after intradermal injection of lepromin (q.v.), a positive reaction consists of either a tuberculin-type reaction at 48 to 72 hours *(Fernandez reaction)* or a nodular, occasionally ulcerated, lesion at 3 to 4 weeks *(Mitsuda reaction).* The test is not diagnostic; a large fraction of the normal population exhibits positive reactivity owing to sensitivity to cross-reacting antigens. In individuals known to have leprosy, a positive result on this test is indicative of tuberculoid or borderline tuberculoid leprosy, and lack of reactivity is indicative of lepromatous or borderline lepromatous leprosy.

Lewis and Pickering t. *(for peripheral circulation)* vasodilation of a part is produced by warming it and applying a sphygmomanometer cuff; return of blood to the part is assessed when the cuff is released.

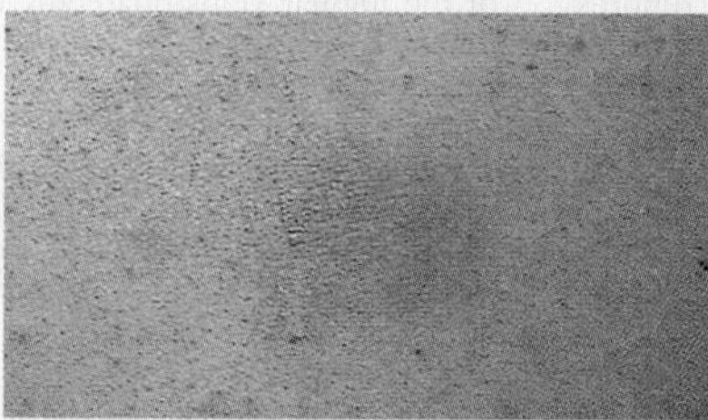

■ Lepromin test; positive reaction at four weeks.

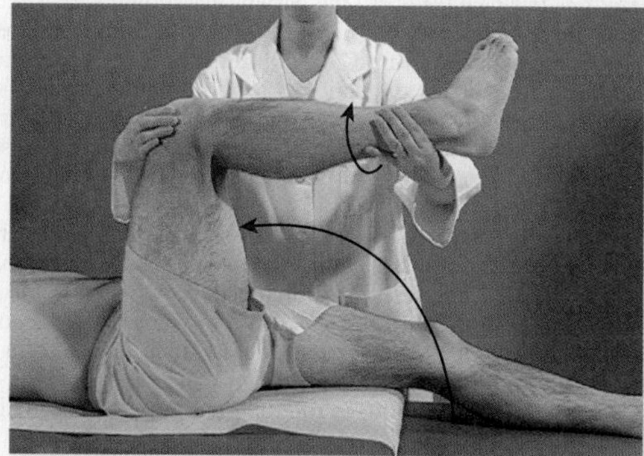

■ McMurray test being used to detect a torn lateral meniscus.

Lichtheim t. *(for aphasia)* if a patient is able to indicate the number of syllables in a word they cannot utter, it indicates that the cortex is less involved than the association fibers.

Liebermann-Burchard t. *(for cholesterol)* dissolve the sample in chloroform and add acetic anhydride plus concentrated sulfuric acid; cholesterol can be quantitated by the intensity of the resulting blue-green color.

likelihood ratio t. in statistics, a test using the ratio of the maximum value of the likelihood function from one statistical model to that from another model, a smaller ratio indicating a stronger relationship between the variables.

limulus t. *(for gram-negative endotoxin)* a blood sample from a patient is exposed to an extract of blood cells from the horseshoe crab *(Limulus polyphemus);* if the sample contains gram-negative endotoxin, gel formation will occur.

lipase t. *(for liver function and pancreatitis)* lipase levels in the blood are measured; elevated levels are seen in impaired liver function and pancreatitis.

liver function t. see specific tests, such as *aminopyrine breath t., fructose tolerance t., galactose breath t., lipase t., methacetin breath t., monoethylglycinexylidide t., rose bengal t.,* and *sulfobromophthalein excretion t.* Increased levels of alanine aminotransferase, aspartate aminotransferase, alkaline phosphatase, γ-glutamyl transpeptidase, and 5′-nucleotidase, and decreased levels of bilirubin, are often seen with impaired liver function.

log-rank t. a statistical test used to test the null hypothesis that two groups have the same distribution of survival by analyzing and comparing the number of observed and expected deaths for each group each time a death occurs in either group.

Lundh t. *(for pancreatic function)* a liquid test meal is administered, containing protein, fat, and sugar; the trypsin concentration in duodenal aspirates is then measured for several hours. A decrease in trypsin concentration indicates abnormally low pancreatic secretion. Called also *Lundh test meal.*

lupus band t. *(for diagnosis of systemic lupus erythematosus)* an immunofluorescence test to determine the presence and extent of immunoglobulin and complement deposits at the dermal-epidermal junction of skin specimens from patients suspected of having systemic lupus erythematosus.

lymphocyte proliferation t. a functional test of the ability of lymphocytes to respond to mitogens, specific antigens, or allogenic cells. Lymphocytes are cultured both with and without the stimulant for several days and then are cultured for several hours with ^{3}H-labeled thymidine. The ratio of the thymidine uptake in the stimulated and control cultures is reported as the "stimulation index" (SI) or "stimulation ratio" (SR). The test with allogenic cells, called a mixed lymphocyte culture (MLC), is commonly performed for transplantation tissue typing; all three types of stimulants are used in investigation of immunodeficiency. Commonly used mitogens are phytohemagglutinin (PHA), concanavalin A (ConA), and pokeweed mitogen (PWM); commonly used antigens are PPD (tuberculin), *Candida* antigen, and streptokinase-streptodornase. Called also *blastogenesis assay* and *lymphocyte proliferation assay.*

Machado-Guerreiro t. *(for Chagas disease)* a complement fixation test, using as antigen an extract of the spleen of puppies infected with *Trypanosoma cruzi.*

McMurray t. *(for torn meniscus)* the patient lies supine with knee fully flexed and foot flat on the table near the buttocks. The examiner stabilizes the flexion with the thumb and index finger, then holds the heel with the other hand, rotates the patient's foot fully outward, and slowly extends the knee to a 90° angle; a palpable or audible "click," grinding, pain, or limitation of extension indicates a tear of the medial meniscus of the knee joint. The lateral meniscus is tested by repeating the maneuver but rotating the foot inward.
McNemar t. a modified chi-squared test performed on data with one degree of freedom to compare findings in a matched analysis or in a before and after study on the same individual.
maintenance of wakefulness t. (MWT) measurement of the length of time for which an individual can remain awake in a dark, quiet room; used as a measure of physiological sleepiness.
mallein t. a skin test analogous to the tuberculin test, using mallein to test whether an animal has been exposed to glanders.
Mann-Whitney t., Mann-Whitney *U* t., Mann-Whitney-Wilcoxon t. rank sum t.
Mantoux t. a type of intradermal tuberculin test; 0.1 mL of PPD containing 5 TU is administered, usually into the forearm; the size of the area of any induration on the second or third day, combined with risk factors, is used to determine whether the patient has had exposure to or infection with *Mycobacterium tuberculosis* or a related organism.
manual muscle t. *(for muscle function)* the therapist manually puts the patient's body part through a range of motion and records the extent of function and limitations.
Marlow t. *(for heterophoria)* one eye is occluded by a bandage for some time; after the bandage is removed, measurements for heterophoria are made.
Master "2-step" exercise t. *(for coronary insufficiency)* an early exercise test in which a patient stepped on and off a set of two stairs for a number of trips standardized for age, weight, and sex, with electrocardiograms recorded immediately after test cessation. It has been supplanted by graded exercise tests that can induce higher levels of stress.
Matas t. *(for collateral circulation)* after hyperemia of the limb has been induced with a tourniquet, the tourniquet is removed and the extent of collateral circulation is determined by compressing the main artery. Called also *tourniquet t.*
maximal exercise t. an exercise test that continues until the maximal capability of the subject to exercise has been reached; the endpoint is usually subjective fatigue, shortness of breath, or chest pain.
Mayer t. a method for determining the presence of certain plant alkaloids.
Mazzotti t. *(for onchocerciasis)* a small dose of diethylcarbamazine is administered orally; the death of microfilariae in the skin causes an intensely pruritic rash within 20 minutes to 24 hours.
MEGX t. monoethylglycinexylidide t.
melanin t. see *Thormählen t.*
methacetin breath t. *(for liver function)* a breath test in which the fasting patient is administered a dose of methacetin labeled with carbon 13 and breath levels of carbon dioxide are measured at regular intervals; low levels of carbon dioxide indicate liver dysfunction such as cirrhosis.
methyl red t. *(for differentiation of Enterobacteriaceae)* the organism is inoculated into a buffered glucose-peptone broth containing methyl red. In a positive reaction, the medium remains red after incubation owing to acid metabolic products. Most Enterobacteriaceae are positive, and *Klebsiella* and related genera are negative.
metyrapone t. *(for Cushing syndrome)* plasma 11-deoxycortisol or urinary 17-hydroxycorticosteroids are measured after the administration of metyrapone; levels are increased in patients with Cushing disease but not in patients with ectopic ACTH syndrome.
microprecipitation t. a precipitin test in which a minute quantity of the serum is employed.
MIF t., migration inhibitory factor t. an in vitro test for the production of migration inhibitory factor (MIF) by lymphocytes in response to specific antigens; used for evaluation of cell-mediated immunity. MIF production is absent in certain immunodeficiency disorders, such as DiGeorge syndrome, Wiskott-Aldrich syndrome, and Hodgkin disease.
milk ring t. abortus Bang ring t.
Millon t. *(for proteins and nitrogenous compounds)* a solution of 10 g of mercury and 20 g of nitric acid is diluted with water and decanted after standing 24 hours. This reagent gives a red color with proteins and other substances, such as tyrosine, phenol, and thymol, which contain the hydroxyphenyl group.
Mills t. *(for tennis elbow)* with the wrist and fingers fully flexed and the forearm pronated, complete extension of the elbow is painful.
Mitsuda t. lepromin t.
mixed lymphocyte culture t. see under *culture*, and see *lymphocyte proliferation t.*
mixed meal t. *(for carbohydrate tolerance)* the fasting patient is given a liquid meal of 55 percent carbohydrate, 25 percent protein, and 20 percent fat; blood samples are drawn at 0, 15, 30, 60, 90, 120, and 180 minutes and tested for levels of glucose, insulin, and C peptide.
mixed triglyceride breath t. *(for pancreatic function)* a breath test in which a mixture of synthetic triglycerides labeled with carbon 13 is administered to the fasting patient and levels of labeled carbon dioxide in the breath are subsequently measured at regular time intervals; excessively low carbon dioxide indicates inadequate pancreatic lipase in the intestine.
MLB t. monaural loudness balance t.
Molisch t. 1. *(for glucose in urine)* add 2 mL of urine, 2 drops of a 15 per cent solution of thymol, and an equal volume of strong sulfuric acid; a deep red color results. Called also *Molisch reaction.* 2. *(for glucose in urine)* to 1 mL of urine add 2 or 3 drops of a 5 per cent solution of α-naphthol in alcohol, then add 2 mL of strong sulfuric acid; a deep violet color is produced, and a violet precipitate follows if water is added. 3. *(for proteins)* the substance is treated with a 15 per cent alcoholic solution of α-naphthol and then with concentrated sulfuric acid; a violet color is formed if proteins are present. Called also *Molisch reaction;* defs. 2 and 3 called also *alpha-naphthol reaction.*
Moloney t. *(for delayed sensitivity to diphtheria toxoid)* 0.1 mL of 1:10 dilution of fluid toxoid is injected intradermally on the flexor surface of the forearm; the appearance in 12 to 24 hours of an area of redness with induration of more than 12 mm in diameter is a positive reaction.
monaural loudness balance t. *(for hearing)* MLB test; a test that measures recruitment in bilateral sensorineural hearing loss; the loudness sensation at impaired frequencies is compared with that at normal frequencies.
monoethylglycinexylidide t. *(for liver function)* MEGX test; the plasma concentration of monoethylglycinexylidide (MEGX) is measured 15 or 30 minutes after the intravenous injection of lidocaine; MEGX levels are reduced in impaired liver function.
mononucleosis spot t., monospot t. a type of heterophile antibody test for infectious mononucleosis, a modification of the Paul-Bunnell-Davidsohn test, using horse erythrocytes instead of sheep erythrocytes; no centrifugation step is needed and the whole test is performed in minutes.
Montenegro t. leishmanin t.
Morton t. *(for metatarsalgia)* transverse pressure is exerted across the heads of the metatarsals; in metatarsalgia this will cause a sharp pain, especially between the second and third metatarsals.
multiple-puncture t. a skin test in which the material used (e.g., tuberculin) is introduced into the skin by pressure of several needles or pointed tines or prongs. See also *tine t.* and *Heaf t.*
multiple sleep latency t. (MSLT) measurement of the speed at which an individual falls asleep when given multiple opportunities to sleep throughout the day and instructed not to resist doing so; used as a measure of physiological sleepiness.
mumps skin t. *(for immunity to mumps)* an intradermal test formerly widely used to determine previous exposure to mumps virus; killed virus (mumps skin test antigen) is injected intradermally; a positive response is development of tuberculin-type delayed hypersensitivity.
Naffziger t. *(for nerve root compression)* increase or aggravation of pain or sensory disturbance over the distribution of the involved nerve root upon manual compression of the jugular veins bilaterally confirms the presence of an extruded intervertebral disk or other mass.
Nagler t. see under *reaction.*
NBT t. nitroblue tetrazolium t.
neostigmine t. *(for myasthenia gravis)* used in children, and in adults suspected of having myasthenia gravis but with a negative Tensilon test; neostigmine methylsulfate mixed with atropine sulfate is injected intramuscularly. This will relieve symptoms of myasthenia gravis if that is what is causing the patient's symptoms. Called also *Prostigmin t.*
Neufeld t. see under *reaction.*
neutralization t. a test for the power of an antiserum, antibiotic, antitoxin, antiviral, or other substance to antagonize the pathogenic

properties of a microorganism, virus, bacteriophage, or toxic substance. Called also *protection t.* and *serum neutralization t.*
niacin t. (*for* Mycobacterium tuberculosis) either of two tests to distinguish strains of *M. tuberculosis* by adding aniline, ethanol, and cyanogen bromide to a culture; this will turn human *M. tuberculosis* yellow because of its niacin content.
Nickerson-Kveim t. Kveim t.
Ninhydrin t. (*for free carboxyl or alpha-amino groups*) to a solution of aminoacetic acid and water, a solution of sodium acid is added, followed by a solution of triketohydrindene hydrate. The suspected matter is then added and the mixture is boiled. A violet color indicates a free carboxyl and alpha-amino group from a protein, peptone, peptide, or amino acid. Called also *triketohydrindene hydrate t.*
nitrate reduction t. (*for bacteriuria or presence of bacteria in other fluids*) a type of nitrite test that identifies the reduction of nitrate to nitrite by a bacterial culture. The fluid under investigation is cultured in a broth containing nitrate and the medium is tested for nitrite by mixing with solutions containing sulfanilic acid and alpha-naphthylamine in 5 N acetic acid; a red color indicates the presence of nitrite. The test is useful in identifying doubtful strains of Enterobacteriaceae, mycobacteria, and certain aerobic bacteria.
nitrite t. 1. (*for nitrites in saliva*) to the saliva add 1 or 2 drops of sulfuric acid, a few drops of potassium iodide solution, and some starch paste; a blue color indicates nitrites. 2. a test for nitrites in any fluid; see specific tests, including *Griess t.* and *nitrate reduction t.*
nitroblue tetrazolium t. (*for neutrophil microbicidal function*) neutrophils are incubated with latex particles and nitroblue tetrazolium (NBT). Normally phagocytosis of the particles is accompanied by reduction of NBT to a blue formazan pigment; absence of NBT reduction indicates a defect in some of the metabolic pathways involved in intracellular microbial killing, as seen in chronic granulomatous disease. Called also *NBT t.*
nitrogen washout t. (*for functional residual capacity of lungs*) with the patient inhaling pure oxygen, the concentration of exhaled nitrogen is obtained for each breath until it falls below 1 per cent of the gas being exhaled (usually about seven minutes' time); the total volume of nitrogen that has been exhaled at this point is assumed to be 0.8 of the functional residual capacity.
nitrogen washout t., single breath the patient inhales a vital capacity's volume of pure oxygen and then slowly exhales. The nitrogen concentration of the exhaled gas is measured over the entire breath and a curve is generated; different parts of the curve represent nitrogen concentrations of gas in different components of the vital capacity, and can be analyzed for uniformity of ventilation and determination of anatomic dead space and closing volume. Called also *single breath t.* and *single breath oxygen t.*
nitroprusside t. (*for cysteine*) if a protein containing cysteine is dissolved in water and 2 to 4 drops of a 4 or 5 per cent solution of sodium nitroprusside and then a few drops of ammonia are added, a deep purple-red color appears.
nocturnal penile tumescence t. monitoring of erections occurring during sleep; in the differential diagnosis of psychogenic and organic impotence, the former is generally associated with the presence of normal patterns of nocturnal erection while the latter is not. Called also *NPT t.*
nonparametric t. a statistical test using nonparametric statistics, such as the rank sum test or signed rank test; nonparametric tests are often less powerful than parametric tests but are valid in cases where parametric tests are not.
nonstress t. (NST) the monitoring of the response of the fetal heart rate to fetal movements by cardiotocography; a reactive (normal) test consists of two or more fetal movements occurring within 20 minutes accompanied by acceleration of the fetal heart rate by at least 15 beats per minute for at least 15 seconds with a long-term variability of at least 10 beats per minute.
nontreponemal antigen t. see *serologic t. for syphilis.*
NPT t. nocturnal penile tumescence t.
nucleic acid t. any of various tests that use molecular biology techniques to detect and identify microorganisms, including viruses, on the basis of their nucleic acids. It includes culture confirmation tests, which identify organisms grown in culture, and direct tests, which can identify the organisms directly in a specimen. Direct tests can be further subdivided on the basis of whether their target nucleic acids are nonamplified or amplified for the test; the former are based on identification of a unique target sequence using a labeled probe; the latter are classified as nucleic acid amplification tests (q.v.).
nucleic acid amplification t. (NAAT) any nucleic acid test (q.v.) that uses nucleic acid amplification techniques in a direct test for the presence of a specific pathogen in a sample; such tests do not depend on the production of antibody by the pathogen, and can be rapid, highly sensitive, and very specific.
nystagmus t. caloric t.
Oakley-Fulthorpe t. see under *technique.*
Ober t. (*for hip contracture*) the patient lies on the side opposite that to be tested, with the underneath hip and knee flexed; with the upper knee flexed to a right angle, the upper hip is flexed to 90 degrees, fully abducted, brought into full hyperextension, and allowed to adduct; the angle that the thigh makes above the horizontal is the degree of abduction contracture.
occult blood t. see specific tests, including *guaiac t.*, and *Hemoccult.*
octanoate breath t., octanoic acid breath t. (*for gastric emptying*) a breath test in which the patient is given a test meal containing octanoic acid labeled with carbon 13, and the breath is assessed at intervals for levels of labeled carbon dioxide; excessive carbon dioxide is seen when gastric emptying is inadequate.
one-stage prothrombin t., one-stage prothrombin time t. prothrombin time.
one-tailed t. a hypothesis test (q.v.) in which the critical region is one tail of the distribution of the test statistic and the null hypothesis is tested against a one-sided alternative that includes deviations from the null hypothesis only in one direction, deviations in the other direction being of no consequence.
ONPG t. (*for β-galactosidase in bacteria*) a pure culture of a bacterial isolate is grown on a lactose-rich medium, then transferred to a substrate containing the test substance *o*-nitrophenyl-β-D-galactopyranoside (ONPG). ONPG does not require permease to enter the cell, so the test is independent of the presence of permease in the bacteria being tested, and is useful for identification of late lactose fermenters. If the bacterial strain possesses β-galactosidase, the ONPG will be split to form *o*-nitrophenol, yielding a yellow color. The test is used in diagnostic microbiology, particularly in identification of Enterobacteriaceae, such as in distinguishing certain *Citrobacter* species and *Salmonella enterica* subsp. *arizonae* from other species of *Salmonella.*
opticokinetic drum t., optokinetic t., optokinetic drum t. (*for vision*) a rotating drum or other figure is used, painted with vertical black and white stripes; because the eye involuntarily follows such a figure, this can be used in the differential diagnosis of psychogenic blindness, to detect the presence of vision in infants, and to check for normality of opticokinetic nystagmus.
optochin susceptibility t. (*for differentiation of pneumococci from other streptococci*) an SBA plate is inoculated with a sample of α-hemolytic streptococci, and a filter paper disk containing optochin is added to the surface of the plate, which is then incubated overnight. The size of the observed zone of inhibition determines whether *Streptococcus pneumoniae* is present.
orcinol t. Bial t.
orientation t. testing whether the patient can correctly give the time of day, the day of the week, month, and year, and the place.
osmotic fragility t. (*for spherocytosis*) heparinized or defibrinated blood is placed in tubes of sodium chloride solution (pH 7.4) varying in concentration from 0.85 to 0.00 per cent (w/v); the amount of hemolysis in each tube is determined colorimetrically. Increased fragility indicates spherocytosis.
Ouchterlony t. double diffusion in two dimensions; see under *diffusion.*
Oudin t. see under *technique.*
oxytocin challenge t. (OCT) a contraction stress test in which uterine contractions are stimulated by intravenous infusion of oxytocin.
Pachon t. (*for collateral circulation*) measuring of the blood pressure in cases of aneurysm to determine the state of the collateral circulation.
Paget t. a solid tumor is hardest in its center, whereas with a cyst the softest part is the center.
pancreatic function t. see specific tests, such as *bentiromide t.*, *cholecystokinin t.*, *Lundh t.*, *mixed triglyceride breath t.*, *pancreolauryl t.*, *secretin t.*, and *triolein breath t.*
pancreolauryl t. (*for pancreatic function*) fluorescein dilaurate is administered orally and its cleavage to yield lauric acid is monitored as a measure of pancreatic esterase activity.

Pap t., Papanicolaou t. an exfoliative cytological staining procedure for detection and diagnosis of various conditions, particularly malignant and premalignant conditions of the female genital tract (cancer of the vagina, cervix, or endometrium). Cells that have been desquamated from the genital epithelium are obtained by smears, fixed and stained, and examined under the microscope for evidence of pathologic changes. The test is also used in detection of human papillomavirus infection, evaluation of endocrine function, and diagnosis of malignancies of other organs, such as the breast or organs of the respiratory tract and lungs, gastrointestinal tract, or urinary tract. Called also *Pap* or *Papanicolaou smear*. See also *Papanicolaou stain*, at *Stains and Staining Methods* under *stain*.
parametric t. a statistical test using parametric statistics, i.e., one that depends upon assumptions about the distribution of the data.
partial thromboplastin time t. see under *time*.
passive cutaneous anaphylaxis t. see *passive cutaneous anaphylaxis*, under *anaphylaxis*.
passive protection t. a test in which antiserum is tested for protective antibody by parenteral inoculation of groups of animals with graded doses in constant volume.
passive transfer t. see *Prausnitz-Küstner reaction*, under *reaction*.
patch t's skin tests, used primarily in the diagnosis of allergies, in which small pieces of gauze or filter paper impregnated with suspected allergens are applied to the skin for fixed time periods; swelling or redness constitutes a positive reaction.
Patrick t. *(for arthritis of the hip)* with the patient supine, the thigh and knee are flexed and the external malleolus is placed over the patella of the opposite leg; the knee is depressed, and if pain is produced, arthritis of the hip is indicated. Patrick called this test *fabere sign*, from the initial letters of movements that are necessary to elicit it, namely, flexion, abduction, external rotation, extension.
Paul-Bunnell t. the original heterophile antibody test, which determined the highest dilution of the patient's serum that was capable of agglutinating sheep red blood cells.
Paul-Bunnell-Davidsohn t. a type of heterophile antibody test for infectious mononucleosis, a modification of the Paul-Bunnell test that differentiates among three types of heterophile sheep erythrocyte agglutinins: those associated with infectious mononucleosis, those associated with serum sickness, and natural antibodies against Forssman antigen. The patient's serum is absorbed with guinea pig kidney cells or with beef erythrocytes and centrifuged. Unabsorbed serum has an abnormally high heterophile antibody titer in infectious mononucleosis and serum sickness. Absorption with guinea pig kidney removes Forssman antibodies and serum sickness heterophile antibodies. Absorption with beef erythrocytes removes heterophile antibodies associated with infectious mononucleosis and serum sickness. Called also *Davidsohn differential absorption t.*
PCA t. see *passive cutaneous anaphylaxis*.
pentagastrin t., pentagastrin stimulation t. *(for gastric function)* after the patient fasts overnight, a basal acid output and its pH are obtained for secretion of stomach acid. Then pentagastrin is administered into the stomach through a nasogastric tube and maximal acid output and peak acid output values are obtained. See *basal*, *maximal*, and *peak acid outputs*, under *output*.

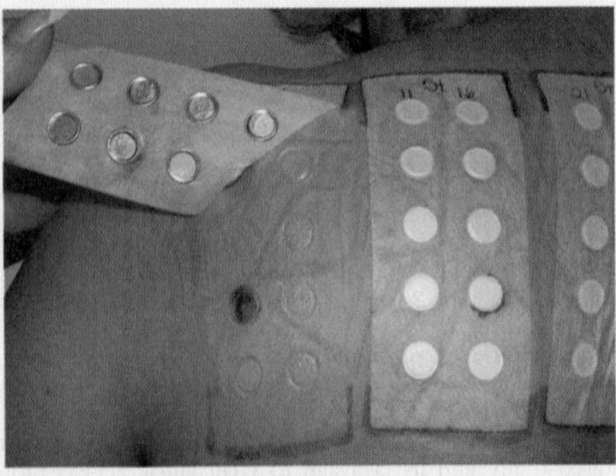

■ Patch tests with one positive result.

peptide t. see *Ninhydrin t.*
peptone t. see *Ninhydrin t.*
perchlorate discharge t. *(for thyroid function)* one to two hours after administration of radioiodine, perchlorate is administered to block further iodine uptake and flush from the thyroid gland any that has not bound to thyroid proteins. In euthyroid patients only trace amounts will be flushed out; the discharge of significant amounts indicates a defect in thyroid iodine binding.
performance t. an intelligence test in which the subject is required to do a series of tasks rather than to answer questions.
peritoneal equilibration t. *(for adequacy of peritoneal dialysis)* after a certain specific dwell time of the dialysis solution, ratios are calculated of the difference in plasma and dialysis solution concentrations of solutes such as creatinine, glucose, other small solutes, and proteins at different times during the remainder of the procedure.
Perthes t. *(for collateral circulation in patients with varicose veins)* a bandage is applied just below the knee and the patient walks around with it on; varicose veins of the leg will become evacuated from continuous compression if there is sufficient collateral circulation in the deep veins. Called also *tourniquet t.*
Phalen t. *(for carpal tunnel syndrome)* the size of the carpal tunnel is reduced by holding the affected hand with the wrist fully flexed or extended for 30 to 60 seconds, or by placing a sphygmomanometer cuff on the involved arm and inflating to a point between diastolic and systolic pressure; appearance of numbness or paresthesias indicates carpal tunnel syndrome. Called also *Phalen maneuver* and *wrist flexion t.*
phenacetin t. *(for phenacetin in urine)* to the urine add a little concentrated hydrochloric acid, a small amount of 1 per cent solution of sodium nitrate, and a small amount of alkaline α-naphthol solution; make alkaline and a red color indicates phenacetin.
phenolphthalein t. *(for blood)* boil a thin fecal suspension, cool, and add it to half as much reagent (made by dissolving 1 to 2 g of phenolphthalein and 25 g of potassium hydroxide in water). Add 10 g of metallic zinc and heat until decolorized. A pink color indicates the presence of blood.
photopatch t. a type of patch test for assessing the photosensitization potential of medications and other chemicals. On the patient's back, each substance is applied in two different locations; then one spot of each substance is irradiated. A positive reaction at only the irradiated site of a substance indicates photoallergy; reaction at both the irradiated and the nonirradiated sites indicates a different type of allergic reaction.
pinch t. *(for hand dexterity)* a test measuring any of the various pinches of the hand.
Pirquet t. a formerly much used tuberculin test in which the tuberculin is applied by scarification.
pivot shift t. see under *phenomenon*.
P-K t. see *Prausnitz-Küstner reaction*, under *reaction*.
pointing t. Bárány pointing t.
Politzer t. see under *method*.
porphobilinogen t. a test for the presence of porphobilinogen; see *Watson-Schwartz t.*
Porteus maze t. a performance test in which the subject is required to trace with a pencil through printed mazes of increasing difficulty.
postcoital t. *(for infertility)* examination of secretions aspirated from the vaginal fornix and endocervical canal after coitus, to determine the number and condition of spermatozoa present and the extent to which they have penetrated the cervical mucus. Called also *Huhner t.* and *Sims t.*
posterior drawer t. see *drawer t's*.
Prausnitz-Küstner t. see under *reaction*.
precipitin t. any serologic test based on a precipitin reaction (q.v.).
pregnancy t. a test for detection or confirmation of pregnancy; currently it is usually an immunologic test measuring the level of human chorionic gonadotropin in the urine, which rises to detectable levels soon after fertilization; see also *early pregnancy t.*
Proetz t. *(for acuity of sense of smell)* use of a series of substances each in 10 different concentrations in a liter of petroleum of specific gravity 0.880, to determine the least concentration at which the substance can be recognized, termed *olfactory coefficient* or *minimal identifiable odor*.
projective t. any of various psychological tests in which an individual interprets ambiguous stimulus situations according to subjective, unconscious dispositions, which yields information about the person's personality structure, its underlying dynamics, and possible psychopathology. See *Rorschach t.* and *Thematic Apperception T.*
Prostigmin t. neostigmine t.

protection t. neutralization t.
protein t. see specific tests, including *biuret reaction, Ninhydrin t.*, and *sulfur t.*
protein-bound iodine t. *(for thyroid function)* a formerly common test in which the amount of iodine firmly bound to protein in the serum was determined by precipitating the proteins, yielding an estimate of serum thyroid hormone concentration. Errors were introduced if iodine compounds from nonthyroid sources were present.
protein truncation t. a method for detection of one or more translation termination mutations in a gene that cause a truncated, usually inactive, protein to be synthesized; the appropriate genomic DNA or mRNA is isolated, amplified by polymerase chain reaction, and used as a template for in vitro transcription and translation. The size of the resulting protein is compared to that of a wild type protein by means of SDS–polyacrylamide gel electrophoresis.
prothrombin t. 1. prothrombin time. 2. two-stage prothrombin time t.
prothrombin consumption t. a test formerly much used to measure the formation of intrinsic thromboplastin by determining the residual serum prothrombin after the completion of blood coagulation.
prothrombin-proconvertin t. a test formerly used in the control of coumarin-type anticoagulants, employing a saline extract of brain as a thromboplastin and requiring presence of excess blood coagulation factor V.
provocative t. challenge (def. 3).
psychological t. any test to measure a subject's development, achievement, personality, intelligence, thought processes, etc.
psychomotor t. a test that assesses the subject's ability to perceive instructions and perform motor responses, often including measurement of the speed of the reaction.
pull t. *(for postural stability)* with a patient who has a movement disorder such as Parkinson disease, the examiner stands behind and asks the patient to maintain balance when briskly pulled backwards.
pulmonary function t. any of numerous tests that measure aspects of the respiratory system in order to assess functional state and presence or nature of any disease process. Factors evaluated include lung mechanics (capacities, flow rates, and volumes), gas exchange, pulmonary blood flow, blood gases, and pH of blood.
pulp t. a diagnostic test to determine tooth pulp vitality or abnormality, usually by means of electric pulp testers or by application of a hot or cold stimulus.
Queckenstedt t. see under *sign.*
quellung t. Neufeld reaction; see under *reaction.*
Quick t. prothrombin time.
radioactive iodine uptake t. *(for thyroid function)* a known quantity of radioiodine is administered and 24 hours later the per cent is calculated that has been absorbed by the thyroid gland. Patients who have recently been exposed to iodine compounds, such as in dietary supplements, contrast media, medications, or antiseptics, may not be good candidates for this test.
radioallergosorbent t. (RAST) *(for measurement of IgE antibodies in serum)* allergen extract is coupled to a solid matrix (paper, cellulose particles); this immunosorbent is reacted with serum and washed and then reacted with radiolabeled anti–human IgE antibody and washed. Uptake of the labeled antibody is proportional to the level of specific serum IgE antibodies to the allergen. This test may be used as an alternative to skin tests to determine sensitivity to suspected allergens.
radioimmunosorbent t. (RIST) a highly sensitive radioimmunoassay for measuring the total IgE antibody concentration in serum; the serum sample is reacted with radiolabeled IgE and anti–human IgE antibody coupled to an insoluble support. The amount of labeled IgE remaining bound to the immunosorbent varies inversely with the amount of (unlabeled) IgE present in the sample.
radioiodine uptake t. radioactive iodine uptake t.
radioisotope renal excretion t. *(for kidney function)* radioisotopic material diluted with saline is rapidly injected into a well-hydrated patient; urine collected through a catheter is examined at known intervals and the radioactivity of each specimen is determined and recorded.
Ramon flocculation t. a test formerly widely used to assess the quality of toxoid-based vaccines; to a series of tubes containing a constant amount of toxin, such as diphtheria toxin, antitoxin is added in increasing amounts; when flocculation occurs, it indicates a neutralized mixture of toxin and antitoxin.
rank sum t. a nonparametric statistical test for ordinal data, testing the null hypothesis that two samples are drawn from the same population versus the alternative hypothesis that the two samples are drawn from two populations having probability distributions of the same shape but different locations. It is based on the value of the rank sum statistic, which is calculated as the sum of the ranks of each sample after the observations in both samples are jointly ranked in ascending order; if and only if the null hypothesis is true, the average ranks of the two samples will be similar. Called also *Mann-Whitney U t.*, *Mann-Whitney-Wilcoxon t.*, and *Wilcoxon rank sum t.*
rapid plasma reagin t. RPR test; a type of card test that is a flocculation test widely used in screening for syphilis. Unheated serum and a modified VDRL antigen containing choline chloride and charcoal particles are placed on a plastic-coated white card, followed by macroscopic identification of the flocculation.
Rebuck t. Rebuck skin window technique.
red glass t. *(for ocular deviation)* a red glass is placed over the right eye while the patient looks at a light; the position at which the patient sees the red image reveals any affected muscle.
Rehberg t. a formerly used test of creatinine clearance.
Reinsch t. *(for heavy metals, including arsenic, mercury, bismuth, antimony, and large amounts of selenium, tellurium, and sulfide)* insert a strip of clean copper into the suspected acidified liquid or finely ground tissue, and boil; if one or more heavy metals are present, a coating will form on the copper strip.
renal function t. kidney function t.
resorcinol–hydrochloric acid t. Selivanoff t.
rheumatoid arthritis t. see specific tests, such as the *latex agglutination t.*, *Rose-Waaler t.*, and *sheep cell agglutination t.*
Rideal-Walker t. see under *method.*
RIF t. Rubin t. (def. 2).
ring t., ring precipitation t., ring precipitin t. a type of precipitin test in which a solution containing antigen is carefully layered over a solution of antibody in a test tube; if the antigen and antibody are specific for one another, a precipitin reaction will happen and a ring of precipitate will form on the surface where the two solutions meet.
Rinne t. *(for hearing)* with the opposite ear masked, vibrating tuning forks of 256, 512, and 1024 Hz alternately have their stems placed on the mastoid process and just outside the external auditory meatus until nothing is heard at one of these positions. When air conduction is

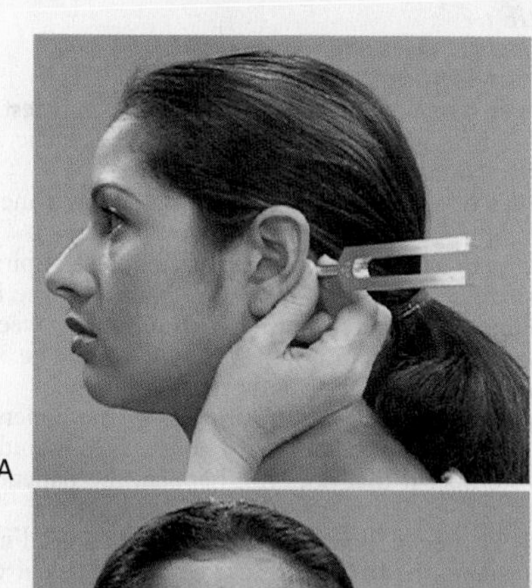

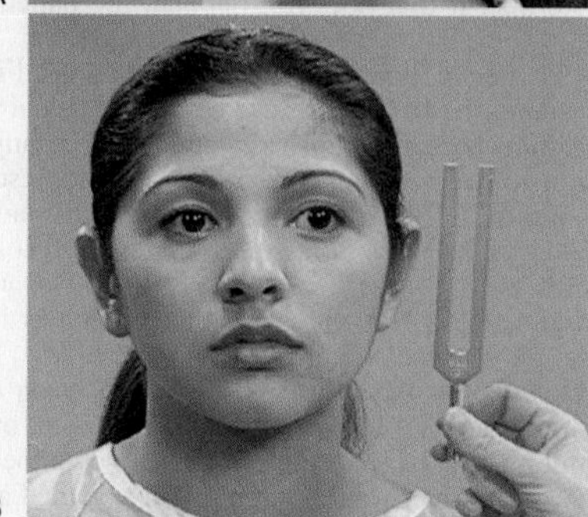

■ Rinne test. Tuning fork placed on mastoid bone for bone conduction *(A)* and held in front of ear for air conduction *(B)*.

greater than bone conduction *(positive Rinne test)*, it indicates normal hearing or sensorineural hearing loss. When bone conduction is greater than air conduction *(negative Rinne test)*, it indicates conductive hearing loss.

Rivalta t. see under *reaction.*

rollover t. *(for risk of preeclampsia in pregnant women)* a comparison of blood pressure is made with the woman lying on her left side and on her back; an excessive increase in blood pressure when she rolls to the supine position indicates increased risk of preeclampsia.

Romberg t. see under *sign.*

Roos t. *(for thoracic outlet syndrome)* the patient raises the arms to 180° above the shoulders, abducts them, bends the elbows, and opens and closes the fists for 3 minutes; reproduction of symptoms is a positive outcome. This test has been found to be nonspecific. Called also *abduction–external rotation t.*

Rorschach t. a projective test in which the subject is asked to relate his associations to a series of inkblot designs.

rose bengal t. *(for liver function)* a solution of radiolabeled rose bengal sodium I 131 is injected into the bloodstream. It should disappear from the blood rapidly; delayed clearance time points to diminished activity of the liver.

Rose-Waaler t. an agglutination test for rheumatoid factor (RF) using tanned sheep red blood cells (SRBC) coated with subagglutinating amounts of rabbit anti-SRBC IgG antibody. These cells agglutinate when exposed to RF (anti-IgG autoantibodies) owing to cross-reaction between human and rabbit IgG.

Rothera t. *(for acetone)* to 5 mL of urine add a little solid ammonium sulfate and add 2 to 3 drops of a fresh 5 per cent solution of sodium nitroprusside and 1 to 2 mL of ammonium hydroxide; a purple color forms if acetone is present.

RPR t. rapid plasma reagin t.

Rubin t. 1. *(for patency of uterine tubes)* transuterine insufflation is done with carbon dioxide. If the tubes are patent the gas enters the peritoneal cavity and may be demonstrated by the fluoroscope or radiograph. This subphrenic pneumoperitoneum may cause pain in one or both shoulders of the patient. If the manometer registers not over 100 mm Hg the tubes are patent; if between 120 and 130, there may be stenosis or stricture, but not complete occlusion; if it rises to 200, the tubes are completely occluded. 2. *(for avian leukosis viruses in egg-culture vaccines)* if the viruses are present, they induce a cellular resistance to Rous sarcoma viruses subsequently inoculated (resistance-inducing factor). Called also *RIF t.*

Rumpel-Leede t. see under *phenomenon.*

Russell's viper venom t. Stypven time t.

Sabin-Feldman dye t. *(for toxoplasmosis)* a serologic test based on the failure of living toxoplasmas, in the presence of specific antibody and accessory factor, to take up methylene blue dye.

saccharimeter t. glucose in solution rotates the plane of polarized light to the right, while fructose turns it to the left.

saccharin t. *(for mucociliary clearance)* the upper respiratory tract is cleaned and small crystals of saccharin are placed on the inferior nasal mucosa. The time is measured until the patient has a sweet taste in the mouth. With normal ciliary transport the time should be 30 minutes or less; a time of more than 1 hour indicates pathology.

saline infusion t. *(for primary aldosteronism)* the patient is administered 2 liters of 0.9 percent saline over 4 hours. This should cause a drop in serum aldosterone; if that does not happen, the patient has primary aldosteronism.

Salkowski t. 1. *(for cholesterol)* the sample is dissolved in chloroform and an equal volume of strong sulfuric acid is added; if cholesterol is present, the solution becomes bluish red and slowly changes to a violet red, and the sulfuric acid becomes red with a green fluorescence. 2. *(for indole)* to the solution to be tested, a little nitric acid is added and then slowly a solution of 2 per cent potassium nitrite; a red color shows that indole is present.

scarification t. a skin test in which the antigen is introduced by scarification.

Schamroth t., Schamroth window t. *(for clubbing of fingers)* the patient holds the fingers back to back against each other; there is normally a diamond-shaped space between the two nailbeds and fingernails. If the space is missing, clubbing is present. Called also *Schamroth sign.*

Schick t. *(for reactivity or immunity to diphtheria toxin)* an intradermal test in which diphtheria toxin equal to one-fiftieth of the minimum lethal dose for a guinea pig is injected into one of the subject's arms (the test site) and an equal quantity of heat-inactivated diphtheria toxin is injected into the other arm (the control site). A positive reaction consists of redness at the test site only, appearing in 24 to 36 hours and persisting for 4 to 5 days, leaving a brown spot on the skin; this indicates lack of immunity to diphtheria. Immunity is indicated by either a *pseudoreaction* (redness at both sites, usually disappearing in 48 hours without residual pigmentation) or a *negative reaction.*

Schiller t. *(for cancer of cervix)* a test for early squamous cell cancer by treating the tissue with a solution of 1 g of iodine and 2 g of potassium iodide in 300 mL of water: if the cervix is healthy, the surface turns brown; if there is cancer, the treated area turns white or yellow, because cancer cells do not contain glycogen and therefore do not stain with iodine.

Schilling t. *(for gastrointestinal absorption of vitamin B_{12})* a measured amount of radioactively labeled cyanocobalamin is given orally, followed by a parenteral flushing dose of the nonradioactive vitamin, and the percentage of radioactivity is determined in the urine excreted over a 24-hour period. The test is usually done three times: first with added intrinsic factor, then without it, and then after antibiotic therapy. The results are used in the diagnosis of pernicious anemia and other disorders of vitamin B_{12} metabolism.

Schirmer t. *(for keratoconjunctivitis sicca)* a test of tear production in which a piece of filter paper is inserted over the conjunctival sac of the lower lid, with the end of the paper hanging down on the outside. The range of normal wetting, determined by measuring the area of moisture on the projecting paper, depends on age, sex, and disease processes.

Schlichter t. serum bactericidal activity t.

Schober t. *(for range of motion of lumbar spine)* with the patient standing erect, marks are drawn 5 cm above and 10 cm below the posterior superior iliac spine; when the patient bends at the waist to the most flexion possible, the distance between the two marks should increase to at least 20 cm; if the distance is less, there is decreased range of motion, such as with ankylosing spondylitis.

Schumm t. *(for heme in plasma)* a given volume of plasma is covered with a layer of ether; one-tenth the volume of concentrated ammonium sulfide (analar) is then run in with a pipette and subsequently mixed by shaking. A positive reaction is indicated by the appearance of a hemochromogen with a sharply defined α band at 558 nm in a depth up to 4 cm of plasma.

Schwabach t. *(for hearing)* with the patient's opposite ear masked, vibrating tuning forks of 256, 512, 1024, and 2048 Hz have their stems placed first on the patient's mastoid process and then on that of the examiner (whose hearing should be normal), until sound is no longer heard by one of them. The result is expressed as "Schwabach prolonged" if heard longer by the patient (indicative of conductive hearing loss), as "Schwabach shortened or diminished" if heard longer by the examiner (indicative of sensorineural hearing loss), and as "Schwabach normal" if heard for the same time by both.

sciatic nerve stretch t. a variant of the straight leg–raising test in which after the leg is raised, the ankle is dorsiflexed; if this increases pain, it indicates abnormal tension of the sciatic nerve root.

SCMC t. [sperm–cervical *m*ucus contact] *(for cervical factor infertility)* fresh sperm is put both on a slide with cervical mucus and on a slide without mucus, and motility of the two sperm samples is assessed over time. If the sperm shows irregularities of motility through the mucus, there is cervical factor infertility. Called also *Kremer t.*

scratch t. a skin test in which the antigen is applied on a superficial scratch.

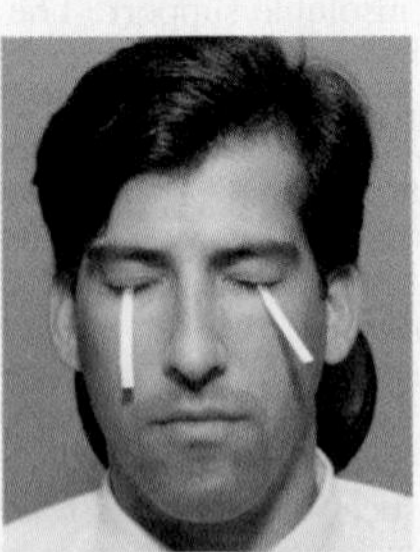

■ Schirmer test.

screen t. 1. alternate cover t. 2. cover-uncover t.
screening t. any test used to eliminate those who are definitely not affected by the disease in question, the remainder (those with positive reactions) being subjected to more refined diagnostic tests.
secretin t. 1. *(for pancreatic function)* after intravenous injection of secretin, pancreatic secretions are measured by collection through a tube in the duodenum. 2. *(for hypergastrinemia)* basal values of gastrin are obtained and secretin is administered intravenously; levels of gastrin are then measured at short intervals to assess whether its secretion is normal or abnormal. Defs. 1 and 2 called also *intravenous secretin t.* and *secretin injection* or *secretin stimulation t.*
secretin-cholecystokinin t. *(for pancreatic function)* a combination of the secretin test and the cholecystokinin test, measuring pancreatic secretion volume and secretion of bicarbonate, amylase, lipase, and trypsin. Called also *secretin-pancreozymin t.*
secretin injection t. secretin t.
secretin-pancreozymin t. secretin-cholecystokinin t.
secretin stimulation t. secretin t.
SeHCAT t. *(for absorption of bile salts)* the bile acid analogue SeHCAT (75 selenium homocholic acid, labeled with radioactive selenium-75) is administered; seven days later, the amount left in the body is measured.
Selivanoff t. *(for fructose in urine)* to the urine is added an equal volume of hydrochloric acid containing resorcinol; formation of a dark red color after boiling for 10 seconds indicates fructose. Called also *resorcinol–hydrochloric acid t.* and *Selivanoff reaction.*
sentence completion t. a projective test for assessing personality and possible psychopathology, in which the individual is asked to provide endings for unfinished sentences.
Sereny t. *(for invasiveness of bacteria)* the organism is inoculated into the eye of a guinea pig; invasiveness is determined by the organism's ability to produce conjunctivitis. The test is used particularly for determining the invasiveness of strains of *Escherichia coli* and *Listeria monocytogenes.*
serologic t. a laboratory test involving seroreactions (precipitin reaction, agglutination, complement fixation, etc.), especially one measuring serum antibody titer.
serologic t. for syphilis (STS) any test for serum antibodies indicative of *Treponema pallidum* infection. There are two types: *nontreponemal antigen tests* detect antibodies to substance (reagin) derived from host tissues, now known to consist of the phospholipids cardiolipin and lecithin; they originated with the Wassermann test and are now represented by the VDRL and RPR (rapid plasma reagin) tests. *Treponemal antigen tests* detect specific antitreponemal antibodies; they originated with the TPI (*T. pallidum* immobilization) test and are now represented by the DFA-TP (direct fluorescent antibody–*T. pallidum*) test, the FTA-ABS (fluorescent treponemal antibody absorption) test, the MHA-TP (microhemagglutination assay–*T. pallidum*), and assays using ELISA (enzyme-linked immunosorbent assay) methods. The term "serologic tests for syphilis" is occasionally used with reference only to nontreponemal antigen tests.
serum bactericidal t., serum bactericidal activity t. a type of antimicrobial susceptibility test for determining, by serial dilution, the titer of serum (and antimicrobial in serum) that has effective serum bactericidal activity (see under *activity*). Called also *Schlichter t.*
serum gastrin t. any test that measures blood levels of gastrin; see *fasting serum gastrin,* under *gastrin.*
serum neutralization t. neutralization t.
set t. a screening tool for the presence of dementia.
sex chromatin t. *(for determination of chromosomal sex)* examination of somatic cells for presence of a Barr body at the periphery of the nucleus; an index of the presence of two X chromosomes, as in a normal XX female, but also giving a positive result with certain chromosomal anomalies. Called also *buccal smear t.*
sham feeding t. *(for assessment of completeness of a vagotomy)* an appetizing meal is served and chewed but not swallowed, stimulating gastric acid secretion solely by vagal pathways; if vagotomy has been successful, there will be no acid secretion.
sheep cell agglutination t. (SCAT) any agglutination test using sheep red blood cells, such as the Rose-Waaler test.
short increment sensitivity index t. see under *index.*
shuttle walk t., shuttle walking t. an exercise test for cardiac function in which the person walks laps (shuttles) at least 10 meters long on a flat, nonslippery surface, keeping pace with audio signals; there are different levels of difficulty in which the patient walks faster until the point of becoming breathless.
Sia t. *(for macroglobulinemia)* a simple screening test performed by adding a drop of serum to 10 to 100 mL of cold distilled water; a positive reaction is indicated by the formation of a heaving cloud of precipitate at the bottom of the container. It is not diagnostic, because it may be positive in other conditions, as in rheumatoid arthritis.
sickling t. *(for hemoglobin S and sickling in erythrocytes)* a test particularly useful for heterozygotes, done by reducing the environmental oxygen around the erythrocytes, which may be done by simply sealing a drop of blood under a coverslip or may be speeded up by adding 2 per cent sodium metabisulfite or sodium dithionite to the preparation.
sign t. a nonparametric statistical test based on a null hypothesis that by chance the experimental group should outperform the control group for half the outcome variables and vice versa. Results are scored as a series of pluses and minuses awarded to the experimental group depending on its performance relative to that of the control group, a binomial distribution of scores with $p = 0.5$ being expected under the null hypothesis.
signed rank t. a nonparametric statistical test for ordinal data, comparing two populations of data by examining the differences between matched pairs in the two populations. It is based on the signed rank statistic, calculated by arranging all samples in order without regard to which population they are drawn from, identifying pairs, assessing the difference in rankings for the members of each pair, and summing these differences for all pairs. If the null hypothesis is true and there is no difference between the two populations, the median difference in rankings between matched pairs in the population approximates 0. Called also *Wilcoxon signed rank t.*
Sims t., Sims-Huhner t. postcoital t.
single breath t., single breath oxygen t. nitrogen washout t., single breath.
SISI t. see *short increment sensitivity index,* under *index.*
skin t. any test in which an antigen is applied to the skin in order to observe the response of the patient, described according to method of application, such as patch tests, scratch tests, and intradermal tests. Skin tests are used to determine prior exposure or immunity to an infectious disease (e.g., tuberculin test), to identify allergens producing allergic reactions, and to assess ability to mount a cellular immune response (using a battery of antigens that give positive test results in most normal individuals).
skin window t. Rebuck skin window technique.
smear t. Papanicolaou t.
Snellen t. determination of visual acuity by means of Snellen test types.
sniff t. *(for paralysis of one side of the diaphragm)* the patient sniffs under radiographic examination; with paralysis of part of the diaphragm, the paralyzed half is seen to rise and the intact half to descend.
sodium-loading t. *(for primary aldosteronism)* the patient is given a high-sodium diet supplemented by sodium tablets for 4 days. This should suppress serum levels of aldosterone; if that does not happen, the patient has primary aldosteronism.
solubility t. see *bile solubility t.*
sorting t. *(for assessing abstract thinking)* the patient must arrange objects or cards into groups based on some abstract relationship. Schizophrenics and patients with cortical lesions show impaired performance.
soybean t. urease t. (def. 1).
spavin t. *(for spavin in horses)* the limb with the hock is held up and bent sharply; the horse is then started suddenly, and in cases of spavin the first steps are very lame. Called also *hock t.*
specific gravity t. see specific tests, including *Fishberg concentration t.* and *urine concentration t.*
sperm agglutination t. *(for male factor infertility)* any of various tests for presence of antisperm antibodies as a cause of infertility, based on the fact that large multivalent isotypes such as IgM or secretory IgA may be able to cross-link and agglutinate spermatozoa that have such antibodies. Serum or seminal plasma is mixed with a known concentration of sperm; immunoglobulins in the mixture then begin agglutinating the sperm. After a given period of time at 37°C, the amount of agglutination is assessed.
sperm–cervical mucus contact t. SCMC t.

sperm immobilization t. *(for male factor infertility)* a test for antisperm antibodies as a cause of infertility, based on the fact that spermatozoa with such surface antibodies lose their ability to move if complement is present (as it normally is in the female reproductive tract). Serum from the patient is incubated with motile sperm and complement is added. After one hour the mixture is checked to calculate the percentage of formerly motile sperm that can no longer move; a 50 per cent reduction in motility is a positive result for presence of antisperm antibodies. Called also *Isojima t.*
Spurling t. *(for cervical radiculopathy)* the examiner presses down on the top of the head while the patient rotates the head laterally and into hyperextension; pain radiating into the upper limb ipsilateral to a rotation position of the head indicates radiculopathy.
STA t., standard tube agglutination t. *(for brucellosis)* a serologic test using *Brucella abortus* antigens to detect infections with *B. abortus, B. melitensis,* and *B. suis.*
Stanford-Binet t. a modification of the Binet test, translated, adapted, and standardized on children in the United States.
starch t. see *iodine t.*
Staub-Traugott t. see under *effect.*
Stenger t. *(for simulated unilateral hearing loss)* a signal is presented at an intensity less than the admitted threshold to the affected ear, and a less intense signal of the same frequency is presented simultaneously to the unaffected ear. If the subject is feigning a loss of hearing, the signal in the unaffected ear will not be heard.
stimulation t. a type of challenge or provocative test used when hypofunction of an endocrine gland is suspected that cannot be detected by other means; either an exogenous releasing hormone or some other substance is administered to stimulate release of the hormone under investigation and levels of it are subsequently measured to assess whether the patient had a normal response.
Stoll t. *(for estimation of worm burden)* a 24-hour stool specimen is collected and the number of eggs present in an aliquot is calculated.
straight leg-raising t. *(for lumbar radiculopathy)* with the patient lying supine, the symptomatic leg is lifted with the knee fully extended; pain in the lower extremity between 30 and 90 degrees of elevation indicates lumbar radiculopathy, with the distribution of the pain indicating the nerve root involved. Called also *Lasègue t.* See also *Lasègue sign,* under *sign.*
Straus biological t. Straus reaction; see under *reaction.*
stress t's any of various tests that assess cardiovascular health and function after application of a stress to the heart, usually exercise but sometimes others such as atrial pacing, the cold pressor test, or specific drugs. Subjects are monitored electrocardiographically, symptomatically, by blood pressure and heart rate, and often by recordings of ventilation and tidal volume recordings as well as other applicable noninvasive or invasive methods. See also *exercise t's.*
Student *t*-t. *t*-t.
Stypven time t. a prothrombin test similar to the (one-stage) prothrombin time, but performed with Russell's viper venom (Stypven) as the thromboplastic agent; useful in defining deficiencies of blood coagulation factor X. Called also *Russell's viper venom t.* or *time* and *Stypven time.*
submaximal exercise t. an exercise test that is stopped at a predetermined point less than the maximal exercise capability of the subject, usually at a particular percentage of the maximal heart rate or after a set time interval.
sucrose hemolysis t. *(for paroxysmal nocturnal hemoglobinuria)* the patient's whole blood is mixed with isotonic sucrose solution, which promotes binding of complement to red cells, then incubated and examined for hemolysis; greater than 10 per cent hemolysis is indicative of paroxysmal nocturnal hemoglobinuria.
sulfobromophthalein excretion t. *(for liver function)* sulfobromophthalein, a dye that in normal individuals is almost completely cleared from the blood by the liver, is administered intravenously and its rate of disappearance from the blood is determined colorimetrically; of historic interest.
sulfur t. *(for protein)* the suspected liquid is heated with an excess of sodium hydroxide and a small quantity of acetate of lead; if proteins are present, a black precipitate of lead sulfide is formed.
suppression t. a type of dynamic test used when hyperfunction of an endocrine gland or presence of a hormone-secreting tumor is suspected; a substance is administered that is normally antagonistic to glandular secretion of a given hormone and hormonal levels are measured to assess whether they drop in the normal fashion.
susceptibility t. antimicrobial susceptibility t.
sweat t. 1. *(for cystic fibrosis)* sweating is induced in a small area on an upper or lower limb and sweat is collected and analyzed for chlorine content; a chlorine concentration at or greater than 60 mmol/L indicates that the person has cystic fibrosis. 2. any test for sudomotor function in which heat is applied to the skin and the amount of sweating is measured.
swinging flashlight t. *(for damage to the optic nerve or retina)* with the patient's eyes fixed at a distance and a strong light shining before the intact eye, a crisp bilateral contraction of the pupil is noted. If when the light is moved to the affected eye, both pupils dilate for a short period, but when it is returned to the intact eye, both pupils contract promptly and remain contracted, this indicates damage to the optic nerve or retina. See also *Marcus Gunn pupillary phenomenon,* under *phenomenon.*
syphilis t. see *serologic t. for syphilis.*
t-t. a statistical hypothesis test based on the *t*-distribution (q.v.) used to test for a difference between the means of two groups. Called also *Student t-t.* Written also *t test.*
Teichmann t. *(for blood)* the suspected liquid is put under a coverglass with a crystal of sodium chloride and a little glacial acetic acid; heat carefully without boiling and then cool. If blood is present, rhombic crystals of hemin will appear.
Tensilon t. *(for myasthenia gravis)* after administration of Tensilon (edrophonium chloride), the patient's eye signs (ptosis and extraocular muscle abnormalities) markedly decrease within two minutes in cases of myasthenia gravis.
thallium stress t. *(for coronary artery disease)* stress is placed on the cardiovascular system by exercising the patient on a treadmill or bicycle ergometer. Thallous chloride Tl-201 is injected intravenously when stress is maximal, just prior to exercise cessation. Immediate (stress) and delayed (redistribution) images are obtained with a gamma camera (see *thallium-201 myocardial perfusion scintigraphy*); then abnormalities of radionuclide distribution and redistribution are assessed, compared with electrocardiograms obtained during exercise, and used to diagnose areas of ischemia and coronary artery disease. In patients incapable of exercise, stress is induced by injection of dipyridamole or adenosine.
Thematic Apperception T. (TAT) a projective test in which the subject tells a story based on each of a series of standard ambiguous pictures; his or her responses reflect a projection of some aspect of the personality and current psychological preoccupations and conflicts.
thin layer rapid use epicutaneous t. TRUE t.
Thomas t. *(for flexion contracture of the hip)* the patient lies supine and flexes one leg to bring the knee as close to the chest as possible, with the lumbar spine kept flattened. With normal hip function, the opposite leg

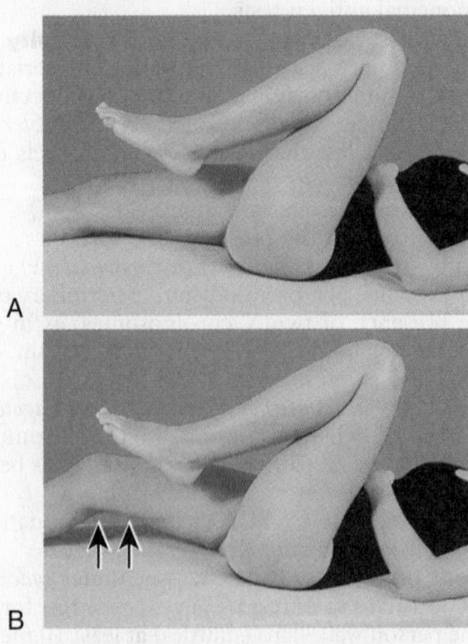

■ Thomas test. *(A),* Normal hip function. *(B),* Flexion contracture of hip, the extent indicated by the degree of flexion of the opposite leg *(arrows).*

will remain flat on the table; with flexion contracture, the opposite hip and leg will flex also, with the angle taken approximating the degree of flexion deformity.
Thormählen t. *(for melanin in urine)* treat urine with a solution of sodium nitroprusside, potassium hydroxide, and acetic acid; if melanin is present, a deep blue color will form.
thromboplastin generation t. a test formerly used in the detection of defects in formation of prothrombinase and hence deficiencies of the factors involved.
thyroid function t. any of various diagnostic procedures measuring the functioning of the thyroid gland, such as the *perchlorate discharge test, protein-bound iodine test, radioactive iodine uptake test, thyroid-stimulating hormone test, thyroid suppression test, thyrotropin-releasing hormone test, triiodothyronine resin uptake test,* and measurement of *pertechnetate uptake.*
thyroid-stimulating hormone t., thyroid-stimulating hormone stimulation t. *(for thyroid function)* TSH test; thyrotropin (thyroid-stimulating hormone) is administered intramuscularly and the thyroid gland is monitored over time with scintiscanning or radioimmunoassays for a response or areas of decreased responsiveness. The test was formerly also much used for determining whether hypothyroidism was caused by thyroid gland failure or by deficiency in thyrotropin. Called also *TSH stimulation t.*
thyroid suppression t. *(for thyroid function)* after administration of liothyronine for several days, radioactive iodine uptake is decreased in normal persons but not in those with hyperthyroidism.
thyrotropin-releasing hormone t., thyrotropin-releasing hormone stimulation t. *(for thyroid function)* pituitary release of thyrotropin is assessed by administration of a bolus of thyrotropin-releasing hormone and measurement of serum concentrations of thyrotropin at intervals. If serum levels do not increase within 30 to 40 minutes, the pituitary thyrotrophs are dysfunctional. Called also *TRH stimulation t.*
tibial external rotation t. dial t.
tilt t., tilt table t. measurement of various bodily responses while the patient is tilted to different angles on a tilt table, usually head up, such as monitoring of circulatory, cardiac, and neurologic responses.
tine t., tine tuberculin t. a type of intradermal tuberculin test; four small tines on a plastic handle, coated with dip-dried tuberculin, are pressed into the outer layer of skin on the forearm. The skin is checked 48 to 72 hours later for induration; if the induration around one or more of the puncture wounds is 2 mm or more in diameter or if there is vesiculation, the test is considered positive. If positive, it is usually confirmed with the more specific Mantoux test (q.v.).
Tobey-Ayer t. *(for sinus thrombosis)* the jugular vein on the side of the suspected thrombosis is compressed. A rise in spinal fluid pressure should occur; its absence indicates presence of thrombosis. Called also *Ayer-Tobey t.*
tolbutamide t. *(for insulinoma)* one gram of tolbutamide is administered intravenously and plasma levels of glucose and insulin are monitored for 3 hours; prolonged hypoglycemia with hyperinsulinemia indicates presence of an insulinoma.
tolerance t. 1. an exercise test to determine the efficiency of the circulation. 2. a test to determine the body's ability to metabolize a substance or to endure administration of a drug.
tone decay t. *(for hearing)* with an audiometer, the patient is asked to raise one hand as long as they hear a continuous tone at threshold level and to lower it when the tone becomes inaudible; whenever the patient lowers their hand before 60 seconds, the intensity is raised by 5 decibels and the amount of tone decay from the initial threshold level in decibels is determined.
tourniquet t. 1. *(for capillary fragility)* pressure is applied midway between diastole and systole for 5 minutes by a manometer cuff; the cuff is released and petechiae are counted in an area 2.5 cm in diameter, on the inner aspect of the forearm. A number between 10 and 20 is marginal; above 20 is abnormal. Called also *capillary fragility t.* and *Hess capillary t.* 2. Matas t. 3. Perthes t.

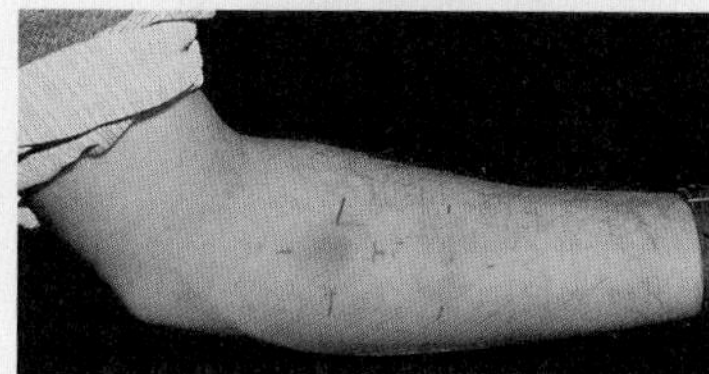

■ Positive tine test for tuberculosis.

toxigenicity t. *(for toxigenic strains of* Corynebacterium diphtheriae*)* a primary culture is streaked onto a plate of tellurite agar containing a strip of filter paper perfused with diphtheria antitoxin. The exotoxin produced by the bacteria forms a band of precipitation with antitoxin diffusing from the filter paper. Called also *Elek t.*
Toynbee t. *(for patency of the auditory tube)* the Toynbee maneuver is done, and pressure changes in the middle ear are monitored. Middle ear negative pressure or negative pressure followed by ambient pressure usually indicates normal function of the auditory tube.
TPI t. *Treponema pallidum* immobilization t.
Trail Making T. a test of cognitive performance in two parts: part A consists of circles containing the numbers 1 to 25 in random order with instructions to connect them in ascending order, and part B has circles with either a number or a letter and the task of drawing a trail that ascends alternating numbers and letters, as 1-A-2-B, etc.
tray agglutination t. a type of sperm agglutination test in which a small amount of sperm and serum is mixed on a microscopic tray for examination. Called also *Friberg t.*
treadmill exercise t. (TET), treadmill stress t. (TMST) any of various graded exercise tests in which the patient walks on an inclined treadmill, which is generally increased in speed and incline through the test; see also specific test protocols, e.g., *Bruce protocol.* Cf. *bicycle ergometer exercise t.*
Trendelenburg t. 1. *(for varicosity and condition of heart valves)* the leg is raised above the level of the heart until the veins are empty, and then quickly lowered. If the veins become distended at once, varicosity and valve incompetence are indicated. 2. *(for gluteus medius function)* the patient, standing erect with back to the examiner, lifts first one leg and then the other. If when weight is supported by an affected limb, the pelvis on the sound side falls instead of rising, this indicates disturbance of the gluteus medius mechanism, such as deformity of the femoral neck, dislocation of the hip joint, or weakness or paralysis of the gluteus medius muscle. Called also *Trendelenburg sign.*
treponemal antigen t. see *serologic t. for syphilis.*
***Treponema pallidum* complement fixation t's** nontreponemal antigen serologic tests for syphilis using complement fixation rather than flocculation as the indicator reaction. Once widely used to confirm positive results of flocculation procedures, they have now been replaced by treponemal antigen tests.
***Treponema pallidum* immobilization t.** TPI test; the first (1949) treponemal antigen serologic test for syphilis; live *Treponema pallidum* was mixed with patient serum and complement and examined to see what proportion of treponemes were immobilized by antibodies in the serum.
T_3 resin uptake t. triiodothyronine resin uptake t.
TRH t., TRH stimulation t. thyrotropin-releasing hormone t.
trichophytin t. *(for Trichophyton infection)* a type of intradermal test in which trichophytin (a broth filtrate of the fungus) is injected into an infected person; if a reaction similar to the tuberculin reaction is produced, the patient is having a cell-mediated hypersensitivity reaction.
triiodothyronine resin uptake t. *(for thyroid function)* determination of the number of sites on thyroxine-binding globulin (TBG) that are occupied by endogenous triiodothyronine (T_3) and how many sites remain available. An excess of radioactive exogenous triiodothyronine is added to the sample, followed by the addition of a resin that also binds T_3. A portion of the radioactive T_3 binds to sites on TBG not already occupied by endogenous thyroid hormones, and the remainder binds to the resin. The amount of labeled hormones bound to the resin (the triiodothyronine resin uptake) can be subtracted from the total that was added and the remainder is the amount that bound to the unoccupied binding sites on the thyroxine-binding globulin. Called also T_3 resin uptake t.
triketohydrindene hydrate t. Ninhydrin t.
triolein breath t. *(for pancreatic function)* a breath test in which the fasting patient is given triolein labeled with either carbon 13 or carbon 14 and levels of labeled carbon dioxide in the exhaled breath are subsequently measured at regular time intervals; low levels of carbon dioxide indicate inadequate pancreatic lipase, such as with a pancreatic disease or cystic fibrosis.
triple t. *(for evaluation of breast masses)* the use of physical examination, mammography, and fine needle aspiration to evaluate palpable breast masses. Results of each method are given point values of 1 (benign), 2

(suspicious), or 3 (malignant) and the points are totaled; a total score of 4 or less indicates a probably benign lesion, and 6 or more indicates one that is probably malignant.

TRUE t. [thin layer rapid use epicutaneous test] a ready-to-use method for patch testing, consisting of a desiccated mixture of allergen and hydrophilic gel printed on a mylar backing; after application the gel absorbs water from the skin and releases allergen.

tryptophan load t. *(for vitamin B_6 deficiency)* a single large dose of tryptophan is administered orally and a 24-hour urine sample is analyzed for xanthurenic acid, and sometimes also kynurenine, hydroxykynurenine, and kynurenic acid. If vitamin B_6 deficiency exists, kynureninase activity will be decreased and these metabolites will accumulate in the urine.

TSH t., TSH stimulation t. thyroid-stimulating hormone t.

tuberculin t. a skin test for tuberculosis using any of various different types of tuberculin and methods of application. See also *Heaf t.*, *intradermal tuberculin t.*, *Mantoux t.*, and *tine t.*

tuberculosis t. a test for the presence of *Mycobacterium tuberculosis;* see *tuberculin t.* and *niacin t.*

tube-slide agglutination t. a type of sperm agglutination test in which sperm and serum are mixed in a tube and then transferred to a slide for examination.

Tuffier t. in aneurysm, when the main artery and vein of a limb are compressed, swelling of the veins of the hand or foot will occur only if the collateral circulation is free.

tuning fork t's hearing tests using a vibrating tuning fork of known frequency as a source of sound. See *Bing t.*, *Rinne t.*, *Schwabach t.*, and *Weber t.* (def. 1).

two-stage prothrombin t., two-stage prothrombin time t. *(for prothrombin)* the quantity of prothrombin can be measured after tissue thromboplastin and excess factor V have converted it to thrombin, by determining the clotting time of a standard fibrinogen solution to which the previously generated thrombin has been added.

two step exercise t. Master "2-step" exercise t.

two-tailed t. a hypothesis test (q.v.) in which the critical region comprises both tails of the distribution of the test statistic and the null hypothesis is tested against a two-sided alternative that includes deviation from the null hypothesis in both directions.

Tzanck t. examination of tissue from the floor of a vesicular or bullous lesion; the presence of multinucleated giant cells (Tzanck cells) is pathognomonic of chickenpox, herpes simplex, herpes zoster, and pemphigus.

unheated serum reagin t. *(for syphilis)* a modification of the VDRL test done with unheated serum, used primarily for screening. Called also USR test.

urea t. see specific tests, including *diacetyl t.* and *urease t.* (def. 1). See also *urea, methods for*, under *method.*

urea breath t. *(for* Helicobacter pylori *in the stomach)* a breath test in which the patient is given an oral dose of urea labeled with carbon 13 or carbon 14 and at fixed time intervals the breath is analyzed for presence of labeled carbon dioxide. Excessive levels of carbon dioxide indicate presence of *H. pylori*, since it is accompanied by bacterial urease that converts the urea to ammonia and carbon dioxide.

urease t. 1. a test for urea based on the conversion of urea into ammonium carbonate by the urease of soybean. 2. *(for the production of urease by bacteria)* urease test broth (see under *culture medium*) is prepared in slants. After inoculation of the surface and incubation, urease-positive cultures produce an alkaline reaction (red color) in the medium. *Proteus* cultures show an early urease-positive reaction; other bacteria (such as *Salmonella* and *Shigella*) usually have a delayed response.

Urecholine supersensitivity t. *(for neurogenic bladder)* 2.5 mg of Urecholine (bethanechol) is administered subcutaneously; the bladder is neurogenic if it exhibits a rise in intravesical pressure more than 15 cm greater than that of a control.

urine concentration t. *(for kidney function)* the patient is deprived of fluids for a given period and the concentration of the urine is checked. Cf. *water deprivation t.*

USR t. unheated serum reagin t.

Valsalva t. Valsalva maneuver (def. 2).

Van Slyke t. *(for amide nitrogen)* nitrous acid acting on amide nitrogen sets free nitrogen gas, which is collected and its volume determined.

VDRL t. [*V*enereal *D*isease *R*esearch *L*aboratory] the standard nontreponemal antigen serologic test for syphilis, a flocculation test on a slide using heat-inactivated serum and VDRL antigen. Positive tests are seen in about 70 per cent of cases in primary syphilis, 100 per cent in secondary syphilis, and 70 per cent in tertiary syphilis. There is a 20 to 40 per cent false positive rate.

ventilation t. a pulmonary function test that measures the quantity of air exhaled by a person during a period of exercise.

vitamin t. see specific tests, including *dark-adaptation t.*, *deoxyuridine suppression t.*, *Friderichsen t.*, *histidine loading t.*, and *Schilling t.*

Voges-Proskauer t. *(for differentiation of Enterobacteriaceae)* a test for the production of acetylmethylcarbinol from glucose in bacterial cultures. An appropriate culture is treated with a solution of potassium hydroxide and creatine. Development of a red color indicates a positive reaction. *Enterobacter*, *Klebsiella*, *Pantoea*, and *Serratia* are V-P positive; *Erwinia*, *Pectobacterium*, and *Yersinia* are variable; *Escherichia* and other genera of Enterobacteriaceae are V-P negative.

Waaler-Rose t. Rose-Waaler t.

Wada t. *(for cerebral dominance of language function)* amobarbital is injected into an internal carotid artery to produce transient hemiparesis of the contralateral limbs. Injection into the artery of the hemisphere dominant for language produces a transient aphasia, into that of the nondominant hemisphere does not interfere with language function.

walking t. an exercise test used to assess exercise tolerance in very disabled patients by measuring the distance walked in a set time interval.

Wassermann t. the original (1906) nontreponemal antigen test for syphilis; see *serologic t. for syphilis.*

water deprivation t. *(for ability to concentrate urine when plasma osmolality is increased)* without fasting, the patient is deprived of water for at least eight hours. Patient weight and measurements of plasma and urine osmolalities are obtained before the test and each hour after the four-hour point. In a normal individual, the osmolality of the urine should increase to two to four times that of the plasma with eight hours of water deprivation. After eight hours, vasopressin is administered and the patient is allowed to drink as usual; in normal persons this should increase the urine osmolality no more than 9 per cent in the first hour; in those with diabetes insipidus and other abnormalities the osmolality may increase between 10 and 50 per cent.

water-loading t. *(for syndrome of inappropriate antidiuretic hormone)* the patient is given a large quantity of water to drink over a 30-minute period; under normal conditions, within 4 hours 80 to 90 percent of the water should be excreted.

water provocative t. drinking t.

Watson-Schwartz t. a simple qualitative procedure for differentiating porphobilinogen from urobilinogen and other Ehrlich reactors, based on the insolubility of porphobilinogen aldehyde in chloroform and butanol; it is useful in diagnosis of acute porphyria.

Weber t. 1. *(for hearing)* the stem of a vibrating tuning fork is placed on the vertex or midline of the forehead; if the sound is heard best in the affected ear, conductive hearing loss is probable; if sound is heard best in the normal ear, there is probably sensorineural hearing loss. (F. E. Weber.) 2. *(for blood)* mix the sample with 30 per cent acetic acid and extract with ether; to the ether extract add an alcoholic solution of guaiac and hydrogen peroxide. A blue color indicates blood. (E. H. Weber.)

Weil-Felix t. *(for typhus and certain other rickettsial diseases)* the blood serum of a patient with suspected rickettsial disease is tested

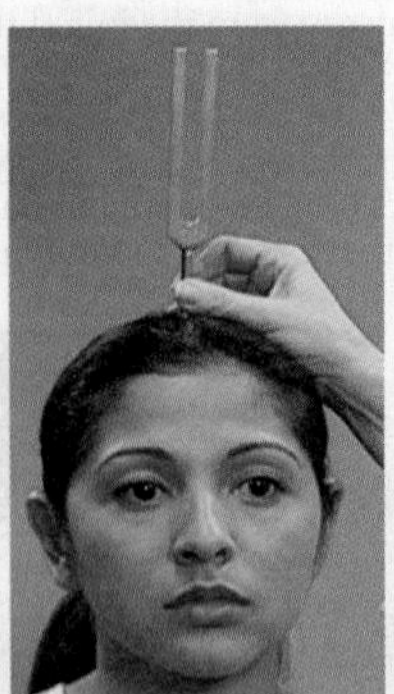

■ Weber test for hearing loss.

Test *Continued*

against certain strains of *Proteus vulgaris* (OX-2, OX-19, OX-K). The agglutination reactions, based on antigens common to both organisms, determine the presence and type of rickettsial infection.
Welland t. bar-reading t.
Wernicke t. see *hemiopic pupillary reaction,* under *reaction.*
Western blot t. Western blot.
Whitaker t. *(for resistance of ureters)* a pressure-flow study measuring resistance of the ureters to a given flow rate of urine by antegrade pyelography of the renal pelvis and a catheter in the bladder.
Widal t., Widal serum t. *(for typhoid and paratyphoid fevers)* a test of serum of patients with suspected *Salmonella* infection, for the presence of agglutinins to O antigens and H antigens of the *Salmonella enterica* serovars causing typhoid and paratyphoid fevers.
Wilcoxon rank sum t. rank sum t.
Wilcoxon signed rank t. signed rank t.
Wormley t. *(for alkaloids)* the suspected solution is treated with an alcoholic solution of picric acid; if a yellow precipitate forms, the result is positive.
wrist flexion t. Phalen t.
xanthine t. see *Hoppe-Seyler t.* (def. 2).
D-xylose absorption t. *(for malabsorption syndromes)* D-xylose dissolved in water is given orally to a fasting adult, followed immediately by additional water, and the amount excreted in the urine during a 5-hour period is determined. Since poor renal function may also result in low xylose absorption, blood levels are also determined at two hours. Less than normal excretion of xylose suggests intestinal malabsorption. Called also *D-xylose tolerance t.*
D-xylose breath t. *(for bacterial overgrowth in the intestine)* a breath test in which the fasting patient is administered D-xylose labeled with carbon 14 and the amount of radiolabeled carbon dioxide in the breath is measured at regular time intervals. Excessive levels of carbon dioxide mean that there are high levels of anaerobic bacteria in the intestines breaking down the xylose.
D-xylose tolerance t. D-xylose absorption t.
Young t. *(for cataract)* on a disk with a varied number of pinholes in different portions, the patient's ability to recognize the number of holes is a test of the integrity of macular function.
***z* t.** a statistical test using normalized data (*z* values) to compare differences in proportions between sets of data or between individual members of different sets of data.

tes·ta (tes′tə) [L. "shell"] test[1].

Tes·ta·cea (tes-ta′she-ə) [L. *testa* shell] Arcellinida.

Tes·ta·ce·a·lo·bo·sia (tes-ta″she-ə-lo-bo′shə) [Gr. *testa* shell + L. *lobus* lobe] the testate amebae when they are considered as a subclass; see under *ameba.*

tes·ta·ce·an (tes-ta′she-ən) 1. any protozoan of the subclass Testacealobosia. 2. pertaining to protozoa of the subclass Testacealobosia.

tes·ta·ceous (tes-ta′shəs) [L. *testa* shell] of the nature of shell; having a shell.

tes·tal·gia (tes-tal′jə) [*testis* + *-algia*] orchialgia.

Test·aq·ua (test-ah′kwə) trademark for a preparation of testosterone.

test card (test kahrd) a card printed with various letters or symbols, used in testing vision.
  stigmometric t. c. a card with dots and squares arranged in groups, for testing vision (Fridenberg).

test·cross (test′kros) test cross; see under *cross.*

tes·tec·to·my (təs-tek′tə-me) orchiectomy.

tes·tes (tes′tēz) [L.] plural of *testis.*

tes·ti·cle (tes′tĭ-kəl) [L. *testiculus*] testis. **testic′ular** *adj*

tes·ti·cond (tes′tĭ-kond) [*testis* + L. *condere* to hide] having the testes retained within the abdominal cavity, as occurs normally in many mammals, such as the elephant and armadillo.

tes·tic·u·lo·ma (tes-tik″u-lo′mə) testicular tumor; see under *tumor.*
  t. ova′rii arrhenoblastoma.

tes·tic·u·lus (tes-tik′u-ləs) gen. and pl. *testi′culi* [L., dim. of *testis*] testis.

test·ing (test′ing) administration of a test or tests.
  autonomic t. testing for effective functioning of the autonomic nervous system and autonomic reflexes.
  compatibility t. determination of the compatibility of the recipient's serum and the donor's red blood cells by pretransfusion testing to ensure that the product will survive in and improve the clinical condition of the recipient.
  quantitative sensory t. various tactile stimuli are applied to the skin, such as light touch, heat, cold, and vibrations, and the patient's responses are monitored and compared either with stimuli to the opposite side of the body or with the responses of a control subject known not to have impairment.
  reality t. objective evaluation of the external world and differentiation between it and the ego or self. Impaired reality testing is seen in psychological defense mechanisms that falsify reality, such as projection and denial, and it is a major criterion for psychosis.

tes·tis (tes′tis) pl. *tes′tes* [L.] [TA] testicle: the male gonad; either of the paired egg-shaped glands normally situated in the scrotum. Each testis is surrounded by an outer mesothelial layer *(tunica vaginalis)* and an inner white capsule *(tunica albuginea),* and is composed of compartments *(lobuli testis)* containing the seminiferous tubules, in which the spermatozoa are produced. Specialized interstitial cells *(Leydig cells)* secrete testosterone. Called also *orchis* [TA alternative] and *testiculus.*
  abdominal t. an undescended testis located in the abdominal cavity.
  ascending t. a testis that is in the scrotum in the infant boy but later ascends to a suprascrotal position; called also *acquired cryptorchidism.*
  canalicular t. an undescended testis located between the internal and external inguinal rings.
  cryptorchid t. undescended t.
  ectopic t. a testis lodged in a location outside of the normal pathway of descent.
  gliding t. an undescended testis that can reach the top of the scrotum but then glides back up.
  intra-abdominal t. abdominal t.
  obstructed t. an ectopic testis whose descent was prevented by a fascial sheet at the entrance to the scrotum.
  peeping t. an undescended testis in the peritoneal cavity that moves slightly across the internal inguinal ring.
  t. re′dux retractile t.
  retained t. undescended t.
  retractile t. a testis that can descend fully into the scrotum but moves freely up into the inguinal canal, usually because of an exaggerated cremasteric reflex.
  undescended t. 1. a testis in the normal pathway of descent but failing to descend into the scrotum; see also *cryptorchidism.* Called also *cryptorchid* or *retained t.* 2. cryptorchidism.
  vanishing t. a testis that was originally present in the fetus but atrophied in utero because of torsion.

tes·ti·tis (tes-ti′tis) orchitis.

test let·ter (test let′ər) see *test type.*

Tes·to·derm (tes′to-derm) trademark for preparations of testosterone.

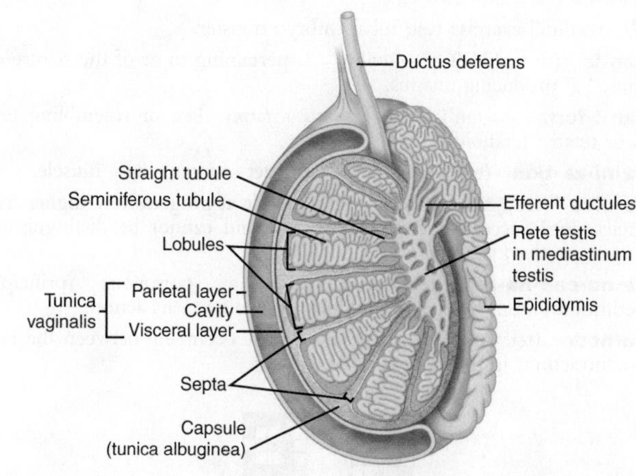

■ Testis and surrounding structures.

tes·toid (tes′toid) an older term applied to testicular hormones and other natural or synthetic androgens.

tes·to·lac·tone (tes″to-lak′tōn) [USP] a synthetic anabolic-androgenic steroid derived from testosterone, having antineoplastic properties, used as an adjunct in palliative treatment of advanced or disseminated breast cancer in postmenopausal women; administered orally.

tes·top·a·thy (təs-top′ə-the) [*testes* + *-pathy*] orchiopathy.

Tes·to·pel (tes′to-pel) trademark for a preparation of testosterone.

tes·tos·te·rone (tes-tos′tə-rōn) 1. the major androgenic hormone produced by the interstitial cells (Leydig cells) of the testes in response to stimulation by the luteinizing hormone of the adenohypophysis; it regulates gonadotropic secretion and wolffian duct differentiation (formation of the epididymis, vas deferens, and seminal vesicle), and stimulates skeletal muscle. It is also responsible for other male characteristics and spermatogenesis after its conversion to dihydrotestosterone (q.v.) by 5α-reductase in peripheral tissue. In addition, testosterone possesses protein anabolic properties, manifested by retention of nitrogen, calcium, phosphorus, and potassium, and is important in maintaining muscle mass and bone tissue in the adult male. It is also converted by aromatization to estradiol in peripheral tissue. See also *anabolic-androgenic steroids*, under *steroid.* 2. [USP] the same principle prepared synthetically from cholesterol or isolated from bull testes, used as the base or various esters in treating primary and secondary male hypogonadism and delayed male puberty, and in palliation of metastatic breast carcinoma in postmenopausal women; its derivatives may be used for their anabolic properties. Administered by subcutaneous implantation, transdermal delivery, or intramuscular injection.

t. cypionate [USP] an ester of testosterone, having the same actions and uses as the base but a prolonged duration of effect; administered by intramuscular injection.

t. enanthate [USP] an ester of testosterone, having the same actions and uses as the base but a prolonged duration of effect; administered by intramuscular injection.

t. heptanoate t. enanthate.

methyl t. see *methyltestosterone.*

t. propionate an ester of testosterone, having the same actions and uses as the base, and with a shorter duration of effect than those of the cypionate and enanthate esters; administered intramuscularly.

tes·tos·te·rone 17β-de·hy·dro·gen·ase (NADP⁺) (tes-tos′tər-ōn de-hi′dro-jən-ās) [EC 1.1.1.64] a microsomal enzyme of the oxidoreductase class that catalyzes the reduction of Δ^4-androstenedione to testosterone using NADPH as an electron donor; it also catalyzes the conversion of estrone to estradiol. Deficiency of the enzyme, an autosomal recessive trait, is called 17β-hydroxysteroid dehydrogenase deficiency. Called also *17β-hydroxysteroid dehydrogenase* and *17-ketosteroid reductase.*

tes·to·tox·i·co·sis (tes″to-tok″sĭ-ko′sis) a type of isosexual precocious puberty in males occurring at about age three, caused by excessive amounts of circulating testosterone; it has autosomal dominant inheritance, and patients usually have normal fertility as adults.

Tes·tred (tes′tred) trademark for a preparation of methyltestosterone.

test type (test tīp) printed letters of varying size, used in the testing of visual acuity; see also under *chart.*

Jaeger t. t. ordinary printer's type of seven different sizes imprinted on a card; used in testing near vision.

Landolt t. t. see under *ring.*

Snellen t. t. block letters used in testing visual acuity, so designed that the whole letter subtends, at the appropriate distance, a visual angle usually of 5 minutes, and each component part subtends an angle of 1 minute. See also *Snellen chart,* under *chart.*

TET treadmill exercise test; tubal embryo transfer.

te·tan·ic (tə-tan′ik) [Gr. *tetanikos*] 1. pertaining to or of the nature of tetanus. 2. producing tetanus.

te·tan·i·form (tə-tan′ĭ-form) [*tetanus* + *form*] like or resembling tetanus or tetany; tetanoid.

tet·a·ni·za·tion (tet″ə-nĭ-za′shən) the act of tetanizing a muscle.

tet·a·nize (tet′ə-nīz) to stimulate a muscle at progressively higher frequencies until successive contractions fuse and cannot be distinguished from one another; see *tetanus* (def. 2).

tet·a·no·can·na·bin (tet″ə-no-kan′ə-bin) a poisonous principle sometimes found in hemp; it resembles strychnine in its action.

tet·a·node (tet′ə-nōd) the unexcited stage occurring between the tetanic contractions in tetanus.

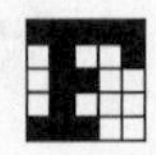
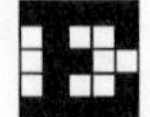

■ Two Snellen test types.

tet·a·noid (tet′ə-noid) [*tetanus* + *-oid*] like or resembling tetanus or tetany; tetaniform.

tet·a·nol·y·sin (tet″ə-nol′ĭ-sin) [*tetanus* + *lysin*] the hemolytic exotoxin produced by *Clostridium tetani;* its importance in the pathogenesis of tetanus is uncertain. Cf. *tetanospasmin.*

tet·a·nom·e·ter (tet″ə-nom′ə-tər) [*tetanus* + *-meter*] an apparatus for measurement and analysis of physiological tetanus.

tet·a·no·spas·min (tet″ə-no-spaz′min) [*tetanus* + *spasm-* + *-in* chemical suffix] the neurotoxic exotoxin produced by *Clostridium tetani,* a highly potent protein that binds to gangliosides and blocks the synaptic terminals of the central nervous system, causing the typical muscle spasms of tetanus. It is one of the most powerful poisons known. Called also *tetanus toxin.* See also *tetanolysin.*

tet·a·nus (tet′ə-nəs) [Gr. *tetanos,* from *teinein* to stretch] 1. an acute, often fatal infectious disease caused by the bacillus *Clostridium tetani,* which produces the exotoxins tetanospasmin and tetanolysin; it usually enters the body through a contaminated puncture wound such as from a metal nail, wood splinter, or insect bite, although other portals of entry include burns, surgical wounds, ulcers, and the umbilical stump of neonates. 2. a state of sustained muscular contraction without periods of relaxation caused by repetitive stimulation of the motor nerve trunk at frequencies so high that individual muscle twitches are fused and cannot be distinguished from one another; called also *physiological t., tetanic* or *tonic contraction* and *tetanic* or *tonic spasm.*

cephalic t., cerebral t. a rare, sometimes fatal form of tetanus sometimes seen after injury to the head or face or a bout of otitis media where *Clostridium tetani* has invaded the middle ear; it is characterized by isolated or combined dysfunction of the cranial nerves, especially the seventh cranial, and may remain localized or progress to generalized tetanus.

cryptogenic t. tetanus in which the source of infection can not be ascertained.

generalized t. the most common type of *Clostridium tetani* infection, characterized by tetanic muscular contractions and hyperreflexia, resulting in trismus (lockjaw), laryngospasm, generalized muscle spasm, opisthotonos, respiratory spasm, seizures, and paralysis that can be fatal.

localized t. *Clostridium tetani* infection characterized by localized muscular twitching and spasms near the site of injury; it may be mild and self-limited or may progress to the generalized form.

neonatal t., t. neonato′rum a severe form of *Clostridium tetani* infection seen during the first few days of life, owing to contamination of the umbilical stump because of factors such as unhygienic delivery practices and lack of maternal immunization; in some parts of the world this is a common cause of infant mortality.

physiological t. tetanus (def. 2).

tet·a·ny (tet′ə-ne) hyperexcitability of nerves and muscles due to decrease in concentration of extracellular ionized calcium, which may be associated with such conditions as parathyroid hypofunction, vitamin D deficiency, and alkalosis or result from ingestion of alkaline salts; it is characterized by carpopedal spasm, muscular twitching and cramps, laryngospasm with inspiratory stridor, hyperreflexia, and choreiform movements.

duration t. a continuous tetanic contraction in response to a very strong continuous current; it occurs especially in degenerated muscles; abbreviated Dt.

gastric t. a severe form due to disease of the stomach, attended by difficult respiration and painful tonic spasms of the extremities.

grass t. lactation t.

hyperventilation t. tetany produced by forced inhalation and exhalation continued for a considerable time.

hypomagnesemic t. 1. lactation t. 2. hypomagnesemia in calves fed only milk (which lacks magnesium); it is often fatal, with symptoms like those of lactation tetany in cows.

lactation t. 1. an often fatal condition seen in cows and sheep in the first few weeks after lactation has begun, when they are turned out into lush pastures, due to deficiency of magnesium in the diet. Symptoms include muscular spasms and convulsions. Called also *grass staggers* and *grass* or *hypomagnesemic t.* 2. puerperal t.

latent t. tetany elicited by the application of electrical and mechanical stimulation.

neonatal t., t. of newborn hypocalcemic tetany occurring in the first few days of life, often marked by irritability, muscular twitchings, jitteriness, tremors, and convulsions, and less frequently by laryngospasm and carpopedal spasm.

parathyroid t., parathyroprival t. tetany due to removal of the parathyroids.

puerperal t. tetany in a nursing mother dog or cat as a result of hypocalcemia; small dogs with large litters are particularly susceptible. Called also *lactation t.* and *eclampsia.*

transit t., transport t. a condition sometimes seen in livestock shipped for long distances, especially well-fed cows and ewes in advanced pregnancy or lactating mares; it may result in paralysis, unconsciousness, and death unless treatment is begun early. The etiology is unknown, but it may be due to acute hypocalcemia associated with improper care and feeding. Called also *railroad disease* or *sickness.*

tet·ar·ta·no·pia (tet″ər-tə-no′pe-ə) [Gr. *tetartos* fourth + *an-*[1] + *-opia*] 1. a very rare type of dichromatic vision characterized by retention of the sensory mechanism for two hues only (red and green), lacking that for blue and yellow, which are replaced in the spectrum by an achromatic (gray) band. Some authorities doubt its existence. 2. quadrantanopia.

tet·ar·ta·nop·sia (tet″ər-tə-nop′se-ə) tetartanopia.

te·tio·thal·ein so·di·um (te″she-o-thal′ēn) iodophthalein sodium.

tetr(a)- [Gr.] a combining form meaning *four.*

tet·ra·ba·sic (tet″rə-ba′sik) [*tetra-* + *basic*] containing four atoms of replaceable hydrogen.

tet·ra·ben·a·zine (tet″rə-ben′ə-zēn) an antispasmodic drug used to treat Huntington disease; administered orally.

tet·ra·blas·tic (tet″rə-blas′tik) having four germ layers.

tet·ra·bo·ric ac·id (tet″rə-bor′ik) pyroboric acid.

tet·ra·bra·chi·us (tet″rə-bra′ke-əs) [*tetra-* + Gr. *brachiōn* arm] conjoined twins having four upper limbs.

tet·ra·bro·mo·flu·o·res·ce·in (tet″rə-bro″mo-flo͞o-res′ēn) eosin.

tet·ra·bro·mo·phe·nol·phthal·ein (tet″rə-bro″mo-fe″nol-thal′ēn) an indicator which is colorless with acids and violet with alkalis.

tet·ra·bro·mo·phthal·ein so·di·um (tet″rə-bro″mo-thal′ēn) the sodium salt of tetrabromophenolphthalein, used for radiologic examination of the gallbladder, in which organ it appears after intravenous injection.

tet·ra·caine (tet′rə-kān) [USP] a local anesthetic applied topically to the skin, mucous membranes, and conjunctiva. Called also *amethocaine.*

t. hydrochloride [USP] the hydrochloride salt of tetracaine, applied topically to the conjunctiva, to the mucous membranes of the nose, throat, and respiratory tract, and to the skin to produce surface anesthesia and also used parenterally for spinal, and occasionally infiltration, anesthesia.

tet·ra·chi·rus (tet″rə-ki′rəs) [*tetra-* + Gr. *cheir* hand] a fetus having four hands.

tet·ra·chlor·eth·ane (tet″rə-klor-eth′ān) tetrachloroethane.

tet·ra·chlo·ride (tet″rə-klor′īd) a compound of a radical with four atoms of chlorine.

tet·ra·chlor·meth·ane (tet″rə-klor-meth′ān) carbon tetrachloride, CCl_4.

2,3,7,8-tet·ra·chlo·ro·di·ben·zo-*p*-di·ox·in (TCDD) (tet″rə-klor″o-di-ben″zo-di-ok′sin) a teratogenic and carcinogenic dioxin that contaminates the herbicide 2,4,5-T.

tet·ra·chlo·ro·eth·ane (tet″rə-klor″o-eth′ān) acetylene tetrachloride, formed by the reaction of acetylene and chlorine; an industrial solvent and intermediate in the synthesis of chlorinated hydrocarbons. If ingested it causes a hepatotoxic condition called *tetrachloroethane poisoning* (see under *poisoning*).

tet·ra·chlo·ro·eth·y·lene (tet″rə-klor″o-eth′ə-lēn) a moderately toxic chlorinated hydrocarbon, formerly used as an anthelmintic but now used only as a dry cleaning solvent and for other industrial uses. Called also *perchloroethylene.*

tet·ra·chlor·phen·ox·ide (tet″rə-klor″fən-ok′sīd) a fungicide used for the preservation of lumber; it may cause a dermatitis in workmen.

tet·ra·chro·mic (tet″rə-kro′mik) [*tetra-* + *chrom-* + *-ic*] 1. pertaining to or exhibiting four colors. 2. able to distinguish only four of the seven colors of the spectrum according to the Eldridge-Green classification of color blindness.

tet·rac·id (tet′ras-id) capable of replacing four atoms of hydrogen in an acid, or having four atoms of hydrogen replaceable by acid radicals.

tet·ra·co·sac·tide (tet″rə-ko-sak′tīd) cosyntropin.

tet·ra·co·sa·no·ic ac·id (tet″rə-ko″sə-no′ik) systematic name for *lignoceric acid*; see also table at *fatty acid.*

tet·ra·crot·ic (tet″rə-krot′ik) [*tetra-* + Gr. *krotos* beat] showing four elevations in the sphygmographic tracing of the pulse.

tet·ra·cyc·lic (tet″rə-sik′lik, -si′klik) containing four fused rings or closed chains in the molecular structure.

tet·ra·cy·cline (tet″rə-si′klēn) 1. [USP] a semisynthetic broad-spectrum antibiotic produced from chlortetracycline; administered orally. 2. any of a group of related broad-spectrum antibiotics; some are isolated from certain species of *Streptomyces* and others are produced semisynthetically. The group includes chlortetracycline, demeclocycline, doxycycline, methacycline, minocycline, oxytetracycline, and rolitetracycline. Tetracyclines are effective against a wide range of aerobic and anaerobic gram-positive and gram-negative bacteria, and are used particularly for rickettsiae, mycoplasmas, and chlamydiae; they are also effective against certain protozoa.

t. hydrochloride [USP] a salt of tetracycline, having the same actions and uses as the base; administered orally, intramuscularly, or intravenously, or applied topically to the skin or conjunctiva.

t. phosphate complex a salt of tetracycline, used as an antibacterial, administered orally, intramuscularly, or intravenously.

Tet·ra·cyn (tet′rə-sin) trademark for preparations of tetracycline.

tet·rad (tet′rad) [Gr. *tetra-* four] a group of four similar or related entities, as (1) any element or radical having a valence, or combining power, of four; (2) a group of four homologous chromatids formed in the pachytene state of the first meiotic prophase; (3) a square of cells produced by the division into two planes of certain cocci *(Sarcina).*

Fallot t. tetralogy of Fallot.

narcoleptic t. the combination of daytime sleepiness, cataplexy, sleep paralysis, and hypnagogic hallucinations.

tet·ra·dac·ty·ly (tet″rə-dak′tə-le) [*tetra-* + Gr. *daktylos* finger] the condition of having four digits on the hand or foot. **tetradac′tylous** *adj*

tet·ra·dec·a·no·yl phor·bol ac·e·tate (tet″rə-dek′ə-no-əl for′bol as′ə-tāt) a phorbol ester that is a cancer promoter and is used to produce skin cancer in laboratory animals.

-tetraene a suffix denoting a chemical compound in which there are four conjugated double bonds.

tet·ra·eth·yl py·ro·phos·phate (TEPP) (tet″rə-eth′il pi″ro-fos′fāt) a highly toxic organophosphorus agricultural insecticide; see *organophosphorus compound poisoning*, under *poisoning.*

tet·ra·eth·yl·thi·uram di·sul·fide (tet″rə-eth″əl-thi′u-ram″) disulfiram.

tet·ra·fil·con A (tet″rə-fil′kon) a hydrophilic contact lens material.

tet·ra·go·num (tet″rə-go′nəm) [L., from Gr. *tetragōnon*] quadrilateral.

t. lumba′le the four-sided space bounded by the four lumbar muscles: the serratus posterior inferior superiorly, the internal oblique inferiorly, the erector spinae internally, and the external oblique externally.

tet·ra·hy·dric (tet″rə-hi′drik) containing four atoms of ionizable hydrogen: said of an acid or alcohol.

tet·ra·hy·dro·bi·op·ter·in (BH4, BH_4) (tet″rə-hi″dro-bi-op′tər-in) a reduced form of dihydrobiopterin that functions as a coenzyme in the reactions hydroxylating phenylalanine, tryptophan, and tyrosine by carrying electrons to oxygen. Defects in the biosynthesis or regeneration of the coenzyme affect all three hydroxylation reactions, interfere with production of the corresponding neurotransmitter precursors, and result in hyperphenylalaninemia unresponsive to a low-phenylalanine diet unless the missing neurotransmitters can also be supplied; see also *tetrahydrobiopterin deficiency*, under *deficiency.*

tet·ra·hy·dro·can·nab·i·nol (THC) (tet″rə-hi″dro-kə-nab′ĭ-nol) the active principle of cannabis, occurring in two isomeric forms, both considered psychotomimetically active.

tet·ra·hy·dro·fo·late (THF) (tet″rə-hi″dro-fo′lāt) an ester or dissociated form of tetrahydrofolic acid.

tet·ra·hy·dro·fo·lic ac·id (THF) (tet″rə-hi″dro-fo′lik) a form of folic acid in which the pteridine ring is fully reduced; it is the parent compound of a variety of coenzymes that serve as carriers of one-carbon groups in metabolic reactions. Tetrahydrofolic acid and its derivatives are required for the metabolism of several amino acids, the formation of creatine and choline, the methylation of RNA molecules, the synthesis of purines, and the synthesis of deoxythymidine monophosphate. Called also *tetrahydropteroylglutamic acid.*

tet·ra·hy·dro·pter·o·yl·glu·ta·mate meth·yl·trans·fer·ase (tet″rə-hi″dro-ter″o-əl-gloo′tə-māt meth″əl-trans′fər-ās) methionine synthase.

tet·ra·hy·dro·pter·o·yl·glu·tam·ic ac·id (tet″rə-hi″dro-ter″o-əl-gloo-tam′ik) tetrahydrofolic acid.

tet·ra·hy·droz·o·line hy·dro·chlo·ride (tet″rə-hi-droz′ə-lēn) [USP] an adrenergic, applied topically to the nasal mucosa and to the conjunctiva to produce vasoconstriction.

Tet·ra·hy·me·na (tet″rə-hi′mə-nə) [*tetra-* + Gr. *hymēn* membrane] a genus of ciliate protozoa (suborder Tetrahymenina, order Hymenostomatida) used extensively in physiologic and genetic studies; they have been shown to be capable of parasitic existence when experimentally injected into various hosts. *T. lima′cis* and *T. pyrifor′mis* are representative species.

Tet·ra·hy·me·ni·na (tet″rə-hi″mə-ni′nə) a suborder of ciliate protozoa (order Hymenostomatida, subclass Hymenostomatia), characterized by the presence of uniform ciliation, three oral membranelles on the left and an undulating or paroral membrane on the right, and mucocysts. Most are free-living in fresh water, but a few species are symbiotic, mainly in invertebrates. *Tetrahymena* is a representative genus.

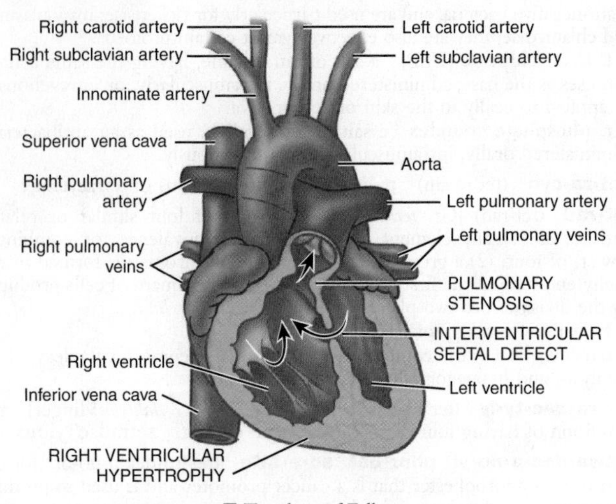

■ Tetralogy of Fallot.

tet·ra·iodo·phe·nol·phthal·ein (tet″rə-i″o-do-fe″nol-thal′ēn) a dye which after intravenous injection is excreted in the bile in sufficient amount to make possible radiography of the gallbladder.

tet·ra·iodo·phthal·ein so·di·um (tet″rə-i″o-do-thal′ēn) iodophthalein sodium.

L-3,5,3′,5′-tet·ra·iodo·thy·ro·nine (tet″rə-i″o-do-thi′ro-nēn) thyroxine.

te·tral·o·gy (tě-tral′ə-je) a combination of four elements or factors, such as four concurrent symptoms or defects.

t. of Eisenmenger Eisenmenger complex.

t. of Fallot a combination of congenital cardiac defects consisting of pulmonary stenosis, interventricular septal defect, dextroposition of the aorta so that it overrides the interventricular septum and receives venous as well as arterial blood, and right ventricular hypertrophy. See illustration.

tet·ra·mer (tet′rə-mur″) a compound composed of four identical simpler molecules.

Te·tram·er·es (tě-tram′ər-ēz) a genus of nematodes parasitic in the alimentary tract of chickens and other fowl. *T. america′na* is found in the proventriculus of chickens and other birds; heavy infestations may be fatal to young birds.

tet·ra·mer·ic (tet″rə-mer′ik) having four parts.

tet·ra·meth·yl (tet″rə-meth′əl) a chemical compound each molecule of which contains four methyl groups.

tet·ra·meth·yl·am·mo·ni·um hy·drox·ide (tet″rə-meth″əl-ə-mo′ne-əm hi-drok′sīd) a toxic fraction isolated from the sea anemone, *Actinia equina*, and from the salivary glands of whelks.

tet·ra·meth·yl·ben·zi·dine (tet″rə-meth″əl-ben′zĭ-dēn) an analog of benzidine; it acts as a chromogen to detect horseradish peroxidase activity in biochemical assays.

tet·ra·meth·yl·ene·di·amine (tet″rə-meth″əl-ēn-di′a-mēn) putrescine.

tet·ra·meth·yl·pu·tres·cine (tet″rə-meth″əl-pu-tres′in) an extremely poisonous crystalline base derivable from putrescine; it produces symptoms like those of muscarine poisoning.

tet·ra·mine (tet′rə-mēn) tetramethylammonium hydroxide.

te·tram·i·sole hy·dro·chlo·ride (tě-tram′ĭ-sōl) a veterinary anthelmintic effective against roundworms, hookworms, and strongyloids.

tet·ran·oph·thal·mos (tet″ran-of-thal′mos) [*tetra-* + Gr. *ophthalmos* eye] a fetus having four eyes.

tet·ra·nop·sia (tet″rə-nop′se-ə) quadrantanopia.

Tet·ra·nych·i·dae (tet″rə-nik′ĭ-de) a family of mites. Genera that infest humans include *Bryobia* and *Tetranychus*.

Tet·ran·y·chus (tet-ran′ĭ-kəs) [*tetra-* + Gr. *onyx* nail] a genus of mites of the family Tetranychidae.

T. urti′cae the two-spotted spider mite, a species that infests and damages many different types of food plants and occasionally causes allergic reactions in susceptible persons.

Tet·ra·odon (tet″rə-o′don) a genus of poisonous puffer fish of the family Tetraodontidae. Their bodies contain tetrodotoxin, and ingestion without special preparation can cause fatal tetrodotoxism.

Tet·ra·odon·ti·dae (tet″rə-o-don′tĭ-de) a family of bony tropical marine fish, including puffers and sunfish; it includes the genera *Fugu*, *Sphaeroides*, and *Tetraodon*. See also *tetrodotoxin* and *tetrodotoxism*.

tet·ra·odon·tox·in (tet′rə-o-don-tok″sin) tetrodotoxin.

tet·ra·odon·tox·ism (tet″rə-o-don-tok′siz-əm) tetrodotoxism.

tet·ra·otus (tet″rə-o′təs) [Gr. *tetraōtos* four-eared] a fetus with two nearly separate heads, two faces, four eyes, and four ears.

tet·ra·pa·re·sis (tet″rə-pə-re′sis) [*tetra-* + *paresis*] muscular weakness affecting all four limbs; called also *quadriparesis*.

tet·ra·pep·tide (tet″rə-pep′tīd) a peptide which on hydrolysis yields four amino acids.

tet·ra·ple·gia (tet″rə-ple′jə) [*tetra-* + *-plegia*] quadriplegia.

tet·ra·ploid (tet′rə-ploid″) 1. pertaining to or characterized by tetraploidy. 2. an individual or cell having four sets of chromosomes.

tet·ra·ploi·dy (tet′rə-ploi″de) the state of having four sets of chromosomes (4*n*).

tet·ra·pus (tet′rə-pəs) [*tetra-* + Gr. *pous* foot] a human fetus having four feet.

tet·ra·pyr·role (tet″rə-pə-rōl′) a compound containing four pyrrole rings, e.g., heme or chlorophyll.

tet·ra·sac·cha·ride (tet″rə-sak′ə-rīd) any of a class of carbohydrates composed of four glycosidically linked monosaccharide groups.

te·tras·ce·lus (tě-tras′ə-ləs) [*tetra-* + Gr. *skelos* leg] a human fetus with four lower limbs.

tet·ra·so·my (tet′rə-so″me) [*tetra-* + Gr. *sōma* body] the presence of two additional chromosomes of one type in an otherwise diploid cell (2*n* + 2). **tetraso′mic** *adj*

t. 12p Pallister-Killian syndrome.

tet·ra·spore (tet′rə-spor) in fungi, one of the spores of a four-spored basidium. Cf. *dispore*.

tet·ra·sti·chi·a·sis (tet″rə-stĭ-ki′ə-sis) [*tetra-* + Gr. *stichos* row + *-iasis*] an extremely rare condition in which there are four rows of eyelashes.

tet·ra·tom·ic (tet″rə-tom′ik) 1. consisting of four atoms. 2. having four replaceable atoms.

Tet·ra·tricho·mo·nas (tet″rə-trik″o-mo′nəs) a genus of protozoa of the order Trichomonadida, phylum Parabasalia, including certain species with four anterior flagella that were formerly included in *Trichomonas*.

T. gallina′rum a species found in the lower digestive tract of chickens, turkeys, and other domestic birds in which it sometimes causes a fatal form of avian trichomoniasis.

tet·ra·va·lent (tet″rə-va′lənt) having a valence of four.

tet·ro·don·ic ac·id (tet″ro-don′ik) a poisonous acid from various puffer fish (family Tetraodontidae).

tet·ro·do·tox·in (tet′ro-do-tok″sin) a pure, crystalline, highly lethal neurotoxin present in puffer fish of the order Tetraodontidae and in newts of the genus *Taricha* (in which it is called *tarichatoxin*). Ingestion of improperly cooked flesh may result in tetrodotoxism within minutes. Called also *tetraodontoxin*.

tet·ro·do·tox·ism (tet″ro-do-tok′siz-əm) [*Tetraodon* + *toxin*] 1. the most severe form of ichthyosarcotoxism, produced by ingestion of puffer fish or other animals containing tetrodotoxin; symptoms include malaise, dizziness, and tingling around the mouth, which may be followed within a short time by ataxia, convulsions, respiratory paralysis, and death. Called also *fugu poisoning* and *puffer* or *puffer fish poisoning*. 2. poisoning from tetrodotoxin after being bitten or stung by an animal such as the blue-ringed octopus. Defs. 1 and 2 called also *tetraodontoxism*.

tet·ro·fos·min (tet″ro-foz′min) a phosphine which when labeled with technetium 99m is used in myocardial perfusion imaging; see table at *technetium*.

tet·roph·thal·mos (tet″rof-thal′mos) [*tetra-* + Gr. *ophthalmos* eye] tetranophthalmos.

tet·rose (tet′rōs) a monosaccharide containing four carbon atoms in a molecule.

tet·ro·tus (tet-ro′təs) tetraotus.

te·trox·ide (tě-trok′sīd) a compound of an element or a radical with four oxygen atoms, as osmium tetroxide.

tet·ru·lose (tet′roo-lōs) ketotetrose.

tet·ryl (tet′rəl) an organic explosive and expellant which may cause an industrial dermatitis.

tet·ter (tet′ər) a formerly popular name for various eczematous skin diseases.

milky t. crusta lactea.

Teut·le·ben ligament (toit′la-bən) [Friedrich Ernst Karl von *Teutleben*, German anatomist, 19th century] see under *ligament*.

Tev·e·ten (tev′ə-ten) trademark for a preparation of eprosartan mesylate.

tex•ti•form (teks′tĭ-form) [L. *textum* any material put together + *form*] formed like a tissue, network, or web.

tex•to•blas•tic (teks″to-blas′tik) [L. *textum* any material put together + *blast*[1] + *-ic*] forming adult tissue; regenerative; said of cells.

tex•ture (teks′chər) [L. *textura*] the structure or organization of a tissue or organ. **tex′tural** *adj*

tex•tus (teks′təs) gen. and pl. *tex′tus* [L., from *texere* to weave] tissue.
 t. connec′tivus lax′us [TA] loose connective tissue: a type of connective tissue made up largely of interlacing collagen and elastin fibers; it provides connections between adjacent organs or structures but allows them to move independently. Cf. *dense connective tissue.* Called also *areolar, areolar connective*, or *cribriform tissue.*

TF transfer factor.

TFF trefoil factor.

6-TG 6-thioguanine.

Tg thyroglobulin.

TGE transmissible gastroenteritis.

TGF transforming growth factor.

TGN trans-Golgi network.

T-group training group; see *sensitivity group*, under *group*.

TGT thromboplastin generation test.

TH tyrosine hydroxylase.

Th thorium.

THA total hip arthroplasty.

Thal fundoplication (procedure) (thal) [Alan P. *Thal*, American surgeon, born 1925] see under *fundoplication*.

thal•a•mec•to•my (thal″ə-mek′tə-me) [*thalamus* + *-tomy*] thalamotomy.

thal•a•mi (thal′ə-mi) [L.] genitive and plural of *thalamus*.

thal•a•mo•cor•ti•cal (thal″ə-mo-kor′tĭ-kəl) pertaining to the thalamus and cerebral cortex.

thal•a•mo•len•tic•u•lar (thal″ə-mo-lən-tik′u-lər) pertaining to the thalamus and the lenticular nucleus.

thal•a•mo•mam•mil•lary (thal″ə-mo-mam′ĭ-lar-e) pertaining to the thalamus and mammillary bodies.

thal•a•mo•teg•men•tal (thal″ə-mo-təg-men′təl) pertaining to the thalamus and tegmentum.

thal•a•mot•o•my (thal″ə-mot′ə-me) [*thalamus* + Gr. *-otomy*] a stereotactic surgical technique for the discrete destruction of specific groups of cells within the thalamus; done to relieve pain, to alleviate the tremor and rigidity of Parkinson disease, and as psychosurgery to relieve certain anxiety states, psychoses, and obsessive-compulsive states.
 anterior t. production of lesions in the anterior nucleus of the thalamus.
 dorsomedial t. production of lesions in the dorsomedial nucleus of the thalamus, a psychosurgical technique for the relief of certain anxiety states, psychoses, and obsessive-compulsive states.

thal•a•mus (thal′ə-məs) pl. *thal′ami* [L., from Gr. *thalamos* inner chamber] [TA] a large ovoid mass in the posterior part of the diencephalon forming most of each lateral wall of the third ventricle, composed chiefly of gray substance and associated laminae of white substance. It is divided into anterior, medial, and lateral parts, each part containing groups of nuclei that function as relay centers for sensory impulses and cerebellar and basal ganglia projections to the cerebral cortex. The main groups of thalamic nuclei are the reticular, anterior, median, medial, medullary, intralaminar, ventrolateral, and posterior nuclei. Some authorities consider the subthalamus part of the thalamus and refer to it as the *ventral thalamus*, calling the posterior part the *dorsal thalamus*. **thalam′ic** *adj*
 dorsal t., t. dorsa′lis see *thalamus*.
 optic t. corpus geniculatum laterale.
 ventral t., t. ventra′lis name given to the subthalamus when it is considered part of the thalamus.

tha•las•sa•ne•mia (thə-las″ə-ne′me-ə) thalassemia.

thal•as•se•mia (thal″ə-se′me-ə) [Gr. *thalassa* sea (because it was observed originally in persons of Mediterranean stock) + *-emia*] a heterogeneous group of hereditary hemolytic anemias that have in common a decreased rate of synthesis of one or more hemoglobin polypeptide chains and are classified according to the chain involved (α, β, δ); the two major categories are α- and β-thalassemia. Homozygous forms are manifested by profound anemia or death in utero, and heterozygous forms by erythrocyte anomalies ranging from mild to severe.
 α-t. a group of thalassemias caused by decreased rate of synthesis of the alpha chains of hemoglobin relative to that of the beta chains. The homozygous form is incompatible with life, the stillborn infant displaying severe hydrops fetalis; the heterozygous form may be asymptomatic or marked by mild anemia.

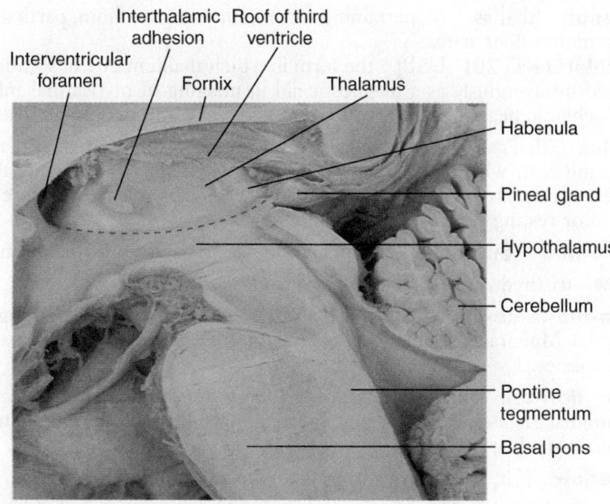

■ Thalamus and adjacent structures in a median sagittal section of the diencephalon and part of the brainstem.

 β-t. a group of thalassemias caused by decreased synthesis of beta chains of hemoglobin relative to that of alpha chains. The homozygous form is known as *t. major* and the heterozygous form is known as *t. minor*.
 δ-t. thalassemia involving suppression of the delta chains of hemoglobin; it is usually symptom-free.
 δβ-t. a form of heterozygous thalassemia in which synthesis of both delta and beta chains of hemoglobin is decreased; clinically it resembles thalassemia minor.
 hemoglobin C–t. see under *disease*.
 hemoglobin E–t. see under *disease*.
 hemoglobin S–t. sickle cell–thalassemia disease.
 t. interme′dia β-thalassemia whose clinical appearance is intermediate between thalassemia major and thalassemia minor.
 t. ma′jor the homozygous form of β-thalassemia, a severe condition evident from the neonatal period with complete absence of hemoglobin A; characteristics include hemolytic, hypochromic, microcytic anemia, pronounced hepatosplenomegaly, skeletal deformation, mongoloid facies, and cardiac enlargement. Called also *Cooley anemia* or *disease*.
 t. mi′nor the heterozygous form of β-thalassemia; it is usually asymptomatic, although hemoglobin A synthesis may be retarded and there is sometimes moderate anemia and splenomegaly.
 sickle cell–t. see under *disease*.

tha•las•sin (thə-las′in) a toxic substance derived from tentacles of the sea anemone, *Anemonia sulcata*, which, when injected into dogs, produces allergic symptoms.

tha•lid•o•mide (thə-lid′o-mīd) [USP] a sedative and hypnotic commonly used in Europe in the late 1950′s and 1960′s. Its use was discontinued because it was discovered to cause serious congenital anomalies in the fetus, notably amelia and phocomelia, when taken by a woman during early pregnancy. It is currently used in the treatment of erythema nodosum leprosum.

Thal•i•tone (thal′ĭ-tōn) trademark for a preparation of chlorthalidone.

thal•lic (thal′ik) 1. pertaining to a thallus. 2. pertaining to conidiogenesis in which formation of conidia begins with formation of a septum and progresses to separation of a whole section of the parent cell.

thal•li•tox•i•co•sis (thal″ĭ-tok″sĭ-ko′sis) thallium poisoning.

thal•li•um (Tl) (thal′e-əm) [Gr. *thallos* green shoot] a heavy, soft, bluish white metal; atomic number, 81; atomic weight, 204.37; specific gravity, 11.85; used in some manufacturing processes and formerly used as a rodenticide. Its salts are active poisons, causing thallium poisoning; see under *poisoning*.
 t. 201 a radioactive isotope of thallium, atomic mass 201, having a half-life of 3.05 days; it decays by electron capture with emission of gamma rays (0.135, 0.167 MeV) and is used as a diagnostic aid in the form of thallous chloride (q.v.).

thall(o)- [Gr. *thallos* green shoot] a combining form denoting a relationship to a branch or shoot, or to thallium.

thal•lo•phyte (thal′o-fīt) [*thallo-* + *-phyte*] an individual of the Thallophyta.

thal•lo•spore (thal′o-spor) [*thallo-* + *spore*] a thallus modified to serve as an organ of reproduction.

thal•lo•tox•i•co•sis (thal″o-tok″sĭ-ko′sis) thallium poisoning.

thal•lous (thal′əs) of, pertaining to, or containing thallium, particularly in the monovalent state.

t. chloride Tl 201 [USP] the form in which thallium 201 in solution is injected intravenously as a diagnostic aid in imaging of myocardial infarction, ischemic heart disease, parathyroid disorders, and neoplastic disease.

thal•lus (thal′əs) 1. a simple plant body not differentiated into root, stem, and leaf, which is characteristic of mycelial fungi and some algae. 2. the actively growing vegetative organism as distinguished from reproductive or resting portions, as in fungi.

Thal•o•mid (thal′o-mid″) trademark for a preparation of thalidomide.

THAM tris(hydroxymethyl)aminomethane; see *tromethamine.*

Tham•nid•ia•ce•ae (tham-nid″e-a′se-e) a family of perfect fungi of the order Mucorales. Genera *Cokeromyces* and *Thamnidium* contain pathogenic species.

Tham•nid•i•um (tham-nid′e-əm) a genus of fungi of the family Thamnidiaceae. Some species contain trichothecenes and can cause alimentary toxic aleukia.

thanat(o)- [Gr. *thanatos* death] a combining form denoting death.

than•a•to•bi•o•log•ic (than″ə-to-bi″ə-loj′ik) [*thanato-* + *biologic*] pertaining to death and life.

than•a•to•gno•mon•ic (than″ə-to-no-mon′ik) [*thanato-* + Gr. *gnōmonikos* decisive] indicating the approach of death.

than•a•toid (than′ə-toid) [*thanato-* + *-oid*] resembling death.

than•a•tol•o•gy (than″ə-tol′ə-je) the medicolegal study of death and conditions affecting dead bodies.

than•a•tom•e•ter (than″ə-tom′ə-tər) [*thanato-* + *-meter*] a thermometer used to prove the occurrence of death by registering the reduction of the bodily temperature.

than•a•to•phid•ia (than″ə-to-fid′e-ə) [*thanato-* + Gr. *ophis* snake] venomous snakes. **thanatophid′ial** *adj*

than•a•to•pho•bia (than″ə-to-fo′be-ə) [*thanato-* + *-phobia*] irrational fear of death.

than•a•to•pho•ric (than″ə-to-for′ik) [*thanato-* + Gr. *pherein* to bear] deadly; lethal.

than•a•to•sis (than″ə-to′sis) 1. necrosis. 2. gangrene.

thau•mat•ro•py (thaw-mat′rə-pe) [Gr. *thauma* wonder + *-tropy*] the transformation of an organ or structure into another organ or structure.

Thay•sen disease (ti′sen) [Thornwald Einar Hess *Thaysen*, Danish physician, 1883–1936] nontropical sprue.

THC tetrahydrocannabinol.

thea•ism (the′ə-iz-əm) [L. *thea* tea] caffeinism resulting from ingestion of excessive quantities of tea.

the•ba•ic (the-ba′ik) [L. *Thebaicus* Theban, named for Thebes, where opium was once prepared] pertaining to or derived from opium.

the•baine (the-ba′in) a crystalline, poisonous, and anodyne alkaloid from opium, having properties similar to those of strychnine; called also *dimethyl morphine.*

the•be•sian (thə-be′zhən) named for Adam Christian *Thebesius*, German physician, 1686–1732.

the•ca (the′kə) pl. *the′cae* [L., from Gr. *thēkē* case] an enclosing case or sheath, as of an ovarian follicle or tendon. **the′cal** *adj*

t. exter′na the outer, fibrous layer of the theca folliculi. Called also *tunica externa thecae folliculi.*

t. folli′culi an envelope of condensed connective tissue surrounding a vesicular ovarian follicle, comprising an internal vascular layer (t. interna) and an external fibrous layer (t. externa).

t. inter′na the inner, vascular layer of secretory cells of the theca folliculi. Called also *tunica interna thecae folliculi.*

t. medulla′re spina′lis dura mater of the spinal cord.

t. vertebra′lis dura mater of the spinal cord.

the•cae (the′se) [L.] genitive and plural of *theca.*

the•ci•tis (the-si′tis) tenosynovitis.

the•co•dont (the′ko-dont) [*theca* + Gr. *odous* tooth] having the teeth inserted in sockets or alveoli.

the•co•ma (the-ko′mə) theca cell tumor.

the•co•ma•to•sis (the″ko-mə-to′sis) diffuse hyperplasia of the ovarian stroma; called also *ovarian stromal hyperplasia.*

the•co•steg•no•sis (the″ko-stəg-no′sis) [*theca* + *stegnosis*] contraction of a tendon sheath.

Thei•le canal, muscle (ti′lə) [Friedrich Wilhelm *Theile*, German anatomist, 1801–1879] see *musculus transversus perinei superficialis*, and see *sinus transversus pericardii.*

Thei•ler disease, virus (ti′lər) [Max *Theiler*, South African–born American physician, microbiologist, and Nobel prize winner, 1899–1972] see *Theilovirus* and see under *disease.*

Thei•lo•vi•rus (ti′lo-vi″rəs) a species of the genus *Cardiovirus* that is normally found in the intestines of mice but sometimes invades the central nervous system to cause Theiler disease. Called also *murine poliovirus* and *Theiler virus.*

Thei•le•ria (thi-lēr-e-ə) [Sir Arnold *Theiler*, Swiss microbiologist, 1867–1936] a genus of minute tick-borne protozoa (order Piroplasmida, subclass Piroplasmia) parasitic in the erythrocytes, lymphocytes, and endothelial cells of mammals; some species cause economically important diseases in cattle, sheep, and goats. See *theileriasis.*

T. annula′ta a species causing tropical theileriasis in cattle, transmitted by ticks of the genus *Hyalomma*. Called also *T. dispar.*

T. dis′par *T. annulata.*

T. hir′ci a species found in North Africa and from Eastern Europe across Central Asia to India, causing a highly fatal disease in adult sheep and goats; the vector is unknown.

T. lawren′cei the etiologic agent of corridor disease in African cattle; it is antigenically related to and may be a variant of *T. parva.*

T. mu′tans a species parasitic in African cattle and African and Indian water buffaloes; it is usually nonpathogenic or only mildly so but has been known to cause a severe form of theileriasis known as Tzaneen disease.

T. o′vis a species parasitic in sheep and goats in Africa, Europe, and Asia from the Middle East to Sri Lanka; it sometimes causes a mild disease manifested by fever, slight anemia, and lymphadenopathy at the site of the tick bite.

T. par′va the etiologic agent of East Coast fever, a highly fatal disease of African cattle, transmitted by ticks of the genera *Rhipicephalus* and *Hyalomma.*

thei•le•ri•a•sis (thi″lə-ri′ə-sis) a group of febrile infections, including both acute and chronic conditions, caused by protozoa of the genus *Theileria*. Called also *theileriosis.*

bovine t. 1. East Coast fever. 2. any of various febrile diseases of cattle caused by species of *Theileria.*

tropical t. an infection in cattle similar to but milder than East Coast fever, caused by *Theileria annulata*, transmitted by *Hyalomma* spp.; it occurs in North Africa, Mediterranean coastal regions, and many parts of Asia, including Turkey, Central Asia, the Middle East, and the Indian subcontinent. Called also *Mediterranean Coast fever*, and *tropical piroplasmosis.*

thei•le•ri•o•sis (thi-le″re-o′sis) theileriasis.

Thei•mich lip sign (ti′mik) [Martin *Theimich*, German pediatrician, late 19th century] see under *sign.*

the•in•ism (the′in-iz-əm) theaism.

the•lal•gia (the-lal′jə) [*thel-* + *-algia*] pain in the nipple.

the•lar•che (the-lahr′ke) [*thel-* + Gr. *archē* beginning] the beginning of development of the breasts at puberty.

premature t. breast development occurring in girls under the age of 8 years without other signs of sexual maturation.

The•la•zia (the-la′zhə) a genus of nematodes of the family Thelaziidae. Several species, such as *T. callipae′da* and *T. californien′sis*, are eye worms parasitic in domestic animals.

the•la•zi•a•sis (the″lə-zi′ə-sis) infection of the eye of a domestic animal with a species of *Thelazia.*

The•la•zi•i•dae (the″lə-zi′ĭ-de) a family of nematodes of the superfamily Spiruroidea; some parasitize the eyes of domestic animals. It includes the genus *Thelazia.*

thele- [Gr. *thēlē* nipple] a combining form denoting a relationship to the nipple or to a nipplelike structure.

the•le•plas•ty (the′le-plas″te) [*thele-* + *-plasty*] a plastic operation upon the nipple.

the•ler•e•thism (thə-ler′ə-thiz″əm) [*thele-* + *erethisma* a stirring up] erection or protrusion of the nipple.

the•lio•lym•pho•cyte (the″le-o-lim′fo-sīt) intraepithelial lymphocyte; a small lymphocyte found within the epithelium, especially intestinal epithelium.

the•li•tis (the-li′tis) [*thel-* + *-itis*] mammillitis.

the•li•um (the′le-əm) pl. *the′lia* [L.] 1. a papilla. 2. a nipple.

thel(o)- see *thele-.*

The•lo•ha•nia (the″lo-ha′ne-ə) a genus of protozoa (suborder Pansporoblastina, order Microsporida) parasitic in the larvae of certain culicine and anopheline mosquitoes and crane flies and in the brains of rodents.

the•lor•rha•gia (the″lo-ra′jə) [*thelo-* + *-rrhagia*] hemorrhage from the nipple.

the•lo•thism (the′lo-thiz-əm) thelerethism.

the•lo•tism (the′lo-tiz-əm) thelerethism.

thel•y•blast (thel′ə-blast) [Gr. *thēlys* female + *-blast*] female pronucleus. thelyblas′tic *adj*

thel•y•gen•ic (thel″ə-jen′ik) [Gr. *thēlys* female + *-genic*] producing only female offspring.

thel•y•to•cia (thel″ə-to′shə) [Gr. *thēlys* female + *toc-* + *-ia*] normal parthenogenesis producing females only. Called also *thelytoky*. **thelyt′ocous** *adj*

the•lyt•o•ky (the-lit′ə-ke) thelytocia.

Them•i•son of Lao•di•cea (them′ĭ-son) a first century B.C. Greek physician who founded the Methodist school of medicine.

the•nad (the′nad) toward the thenar eminence or toward the palm.

the•nal (the′nəl) pertaining to the palm or thenar.

the•nar (the′nər) [Gr.] 1. [TA] the mound on the palm at the base of the thumb; called also *eminentia thenaris* [TA alternative] and *thenar eminence*.

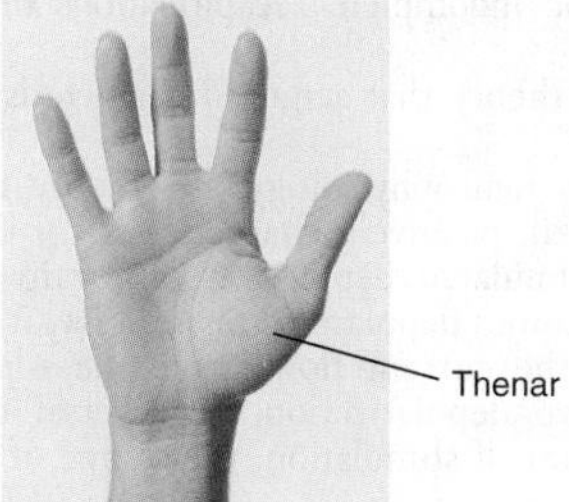

2. pertaining to the palm.

then•i•um clo•sy•late (then′e-əm klo′sə-lāt) an anthelmintic formerly widely used to treat hookworm infestations in dogs.

Theo-24 (the′o) trademark for preparations of theophylline.

The•o•bal•dia (the″o-bawl′de-ə) [Frederic Vincent *Theobald*, British zoologist, 1868–1930] *Culiseta*.

The•o•bro•ma (the″o-bro′mə) [Gr. *theos* god + *brōma* food] a genus of trees of the family Sterculiaceae, native to tropical parts of the Americas. *T. caca′o* L. is the cacao plant, whose seeds (cacao) contain the alkaloid theobromine, and yield cocoa, chocolate, and cocoa butter.

the•o•bro•mine (the″o-bro′min) one of the methylxanthines, a white crystalline alkaloid found in cocoa or made synthetically from xanthine. It has physiologic properties similar to those of caffeine, and is used as a diuretic, smooth muscle relaxant, myocardial stimulant, and vasodilator. Derivatives such as t. calcium salicylate, t. sodium acetate, t. sodium salicylate, t. sodium formate, and t. salicylate are available for use. Dogs consuming excessive amounts of cocoa sometimes suffer toxic effects from the theobromine, such as vomiting, diarrhea, muscle spasms, and coma.

Theo-Dur (the′o-dur) trademark for a preparation of theophylline.

Theo•lair (the′o-lār) trademark for a preparation of theophylline.

the•oph•yl•line (the-of′ə-lin) [USP] a methylxanthine compound occurring in tea leaves and prepared synthetically; theophylline, its salts, and its derivatives act as smooth muscle relaxants, central nervous system and cardiac muscle stimulants, and bronchodilators. Used as a bronchodilator in the prevention and treatment of symptoms of asthma and of reversible airway obstruction associated with chronic bronchitis, emphysema, or other chronic obstructive pulmonary disease; administered orally and intravenously.

t. cholinate oxtriphylline.

t. sodium the sodium salt of theophylline, used in the preparation of theophylline sodium glycinate.

t. sodium glycinate [USP] an equimolar mixture of theophylline sodium and glycine buffered with an additional mole of glycine, having the same actions and uses as the base; administered orally.

the•o•rem (the′ə-rəm, thēr′əm) [Gr. *theorēma* a principle arrived at by speculation] a proposition capable of demonstration or proof.

Bayes t. a theorem used to interconvert conditional probabilities:

$$P(B|A) = \frac{P(A|B)P(B)}{P(A|B)P(B) + P(A|notB)P(notB)}$$

where *P(A)* and *P(B)* are the probabilities of two events, *A* and *B*, and *P(A|B)* and *P(B|A)* are the conditional probabilities of *A* given *B* and of *B* given *A*. For example, if *A* denotes a positive laboratory test result and *B* denotes the actual presence of disease in a tested patient, then *P (A|B)* is the "diagnostic sensitivity" of the test (true positive rate) and *P(B)* is the prevalence of the disease (*P(A)* is the frequency of positive test results). *P(B|A)* is the "predictive value of a positive test," the probability that a patient testing positive will actually have the disease. The denominator of the equation, representing the sum of the true positives and false positives, is sometimes simplified to the equivalent function *P(A)*, representing all those with positive results, both true and false.

Bernoulli t. in an experiment involving probability, the larger the number of trials, the closer the observed probability of an event approaches its theoretical probability.

central limit t. if random samples of size *n* are taken from a population having a normally distributed variable with mean μ and standard deviation σ, the distribution of the sample means is normal, with mean μ and standard deviation

$$\sigma/\sqrt{n};$$

if the variable in the population is not normally distributed, the sampling distribution of means approximates the normal distribution and the approximation gets better as the sample size increases.

Gibbs t. substances which lower the surface tension of the pure dispersion medium tend to collect on its surface.

the•o•ry (the′ə-re, thēr′e) [Gr. *theōria* speculation as opposed to practice] 1. the doctrine or the principles underlying an art as distinguished from the practice of that particular art. 2. a formulated hypothesis, or, loosely speaking, any hypothesis or opinion not based upon actual knowledge.

Theory

acidogenic t. a theory of the etiology of dental caries, according to which acids produced by bacteria cause decalcification and softening of the residue.

aging t. of atherosclerosis a theory that atherosclerosis is an inevitable consequence of aging and therefore an irreversible process.

apposition t. the theory that tissues grow by the deposit of cells from without.

Arrhenius' t. the theory of electrolytic dissociation, proposed in 1887, which explained the properties of electrolytes based on the presence of free ions in solution and also defined acids and bases as compounds that dissociate to release hydrogen and hydroxide ions, respectively, in solution.

atomic t. the theory that the molecules of a substance are made up of one or more atoms, each representing a definite amount of the element, which amount does not vary in the molecule, whatever combinations the molecule may enter.

avalanche t. the theory that nervous influence increases in force as it descends along an efferent nerve.

Buergi's t. two different substances causing identical therapeutic manifestations when combined are increased in their effects if they possess identical pharmacologic points of attack.

Cannon's t., Cannon-Bard t. emergency t.

cell t. the doctrine that all living matter is composed of cells and that cell activity is the essential process of life.

cellular immunity t. Metchnikoff's cellular immunity t.

clonal deletion t. a theory of immunologic tolerance to self antigens according to which "forbidden clones" of immunocytes, those reactive with self antigens, are eliminated on contact with antigen during fetal life. The terms "clonal abortion," "clonal anergy," "clonal silencing," and "clonal purging" have also been used for this phenomenon. See also *clonal selection t.*

clonal selection t. a modification of the natural selection theory (q.v.): there are in each adult several million clones of antibody-producing cells, each programmed to make antibody of a single specificity and bearing cell-surface receptors capable of reacting with specific antigens; exposure to antigen induces cells of antigen-reactive clones to proliferate and differentiate to produce large quantities of specific antibody. This theory has been found to be essentially correct. See *clonal deletion t.* and *recombinational germline t.*

closed circulation t. one of the theories explaining how the blood in the spleen gets from the arteries to the venous sinuses; it holds that

Theory *Continued*

the capillaries empty directly into the venous sinuses. Cf. *open circulation t.* and *closed-open circulation t.* Called also *fast circulation t.*
closed-open circulation t. the theory that both an open and a closed circulation are present in the spleen; e.g., a closed circulation in a contracted spleen may become an open circulation when the organ is distended. Cf. *closed circulation t.* and *open circulation t.*
Cohnheim's t. the theory that tumors develop from embryonic rests that do not participate in formation of normal surrounding tissue.
convergence-projection t. a theory advanced as an explanation for reference of pain, according to which some visceral afferent nerve fibers converge with cutaneous pain afferents to end upon the same neuron at some point in the sensory pathway.
core conductor t. a theory regarding the development of electrotonic potentials and their associated currents along nerve fibers, according to which the nerve fibers are considered to be core conductors, i.e., cylinders of conducting fluid material with a sheath of high electrical resistance, surrounded by a layer of conducting medium.
darwinian t. darwinism.
dimer t. the theory that the tooth organ of primates is composed of two halves, each of which is a representative of an independent tooth in the lower orders of animals.
dualistic t. a variant of the polyphyletic theory that holds that blood cells arise from two distinct types of stem cells, the myeloblasts and lymphoblasts. Cf. *monophyletic t.* and *trialistic t.* Called also *dualism.*
Ehrlich's t., Ehrlich's side-chain t. the first (1896) comprehensive theory of antibody production, which proposed that antibody-producing cells have surface molecules (side chains) that can bind to antigens and that binding to a specific side chain causes the cell to produce more of the same side chain and to release these side chains into the serum as antibodies. Two of Ehrlich's postulates, that antibodies are identical to the antigen receptors and that antigen binding triggers the synthesis of antibody with the same specificity as the receptor, are now known to be essentially correct. Cf. *clonal selection t.*
electron t. all bodies are complex structures composed of small particles called atoms together with still smaller particles called electrons.
emergency t. the theory that the adrenal medulla is stimulated during emotional excitement, pain, and bodily emergencies; see also *alarm reaction,* under *reaction.* Called also *Cannon's t.* and *Cannon-Bard t.*
equilibrium t. a theory that the number of breeding species in a biome is a result of the rate of immigration of new species and the rate of extinction.
fast circulation t. closed circulation t.
frequency t. an early theory of hearing that postulated that the pattern of excitation of auditory nerve fibers was more important in perception of pitch than was the excitation of fibers in any particular area of the cochlear basilar membrane. Called also *Rutherford's t.* Cf. *place t.*
gate t., gate-control t. neural impulses generated by noxious painful stimuli and transmitted to the spinal cord by small-diameter C-fibers and A-delta fibers are blocked at their synapses in the dorsal horn by the simultaneous stimulation of large-diameter myelinated A-fibers, thus inhibiting pain by preventing pain impulses from reaching higher levels of the central nervous system. Called also *gate hypothesis.*
germ t. the doctrine that infectious diseases are caused by microorganisms.
germ layer t. the theory that the embryo develops three primary germ layers, each of which gives rise to definite organ derivatives.
gestalt t. see *gestaltism.*
Helmholtz t. an early theory of sound perception, now disproved; it held that each basilar fiber responded sympathetically to a definite tone and stimulated the hair cells of Corti organ, causing nerve impulses that were then carried to the brain. Called also *place t.* and *resonance t.*
Hering's t. the doctrine that color sensation depends on decomposition and restitution of the visual substance: disassimilation producing red, yellow, and white, and restitution producing blue, green, and black. Called also *opponent colors t.*
hit t. target t.
information t. a system for analyzing, chiefly by statistical methods, the characteristics of communicated messages and the systems that encode, transmit, distort, receive, and decode them.
instructive t. template t.
ionic t. a theory that, on going into solution, the molecules of an electrolyte either completely or partially break up or dissociate into two or more portions, these portions being positively and negatively charged electrically, the positively charged portions being different chemically from those negatively charged. When an electric current is passed through the solution of an electrolyte, the positively charged portions are attracted by the negative pole or electrode, and move toward it; the negatively charged portions are attracted by and migrate toward the positive electrode. From this property of moving toward one of the electrodes, these charged molecular fractions of electrolytes are called ions, from the Greek verb meaning "to move."
Ladd-Franklin's t. a theory of the evolution of color vision: first, light stimulates a substance in the visual cells, producing a sensation of white light; next, molecular changes from the first reaction produce two reactive products, one for each end of the spectrum, for blue and yellow; finally, the reactive product from the yellow becomes two products for red and green. Dichromasies and anomalous trichromasies are considered to be incomplete recapitulations of the evolutionary development.
Lamarck's t. the theory that acquired characteristics may be transmitted.
local circuit t. in neurophysiology, the theory that current flows from the unstimulated, positively charged areas of the cell membrane of a neuron to the stimulated, depolarized or negative portion, and that as each new area becomes depolarized or negative, it in turn acts as the sink toward which the current flows from the adjacent area, which results in progressive depolarization, or reversal charge, along the neuron from the point of stimulation; the source of the current is the flow of Na^+ into the cell.
mendelian t. see *Mendel's laws,* under *law.*
metabolic t. of atherosclerosis a theory that atherosclerosis is caused by a disturbance in lipid metabolism, specifically cholesterol metabolism.
Metchnikoff's (Mechnikov's) cellular immunity t. the theory, proposed in the 1880s, that phagocytosis by macrophages and polymorphonuclear leukocytes is the main mechanism of host defense against bacterial infection and that inflammation is the result of the enzymatic digestion process occurring with phagocytosis.
monophyletic t. the theory that all forms of blood cells have their origin in a single type of cell, the blast cell (which develops into a pluripotential stem cell), with the different types of cells arising from there by a process of differentiation. Cf. *dualistic t., polyphyletic t.,* and *trialistic t.* Called also *monophyletism* and *unitarian t.*
myogenic t. the theory that the muscle fibers of the heart possess in themselves the power of originating and maintaining the contraction of the heart.
natural selection t. the first selective theory of antibody formation, according to which about a million different antibody molecules are constantly being produced at low levels; when an antibody combines with a complementary antigen the complex is taken up by antibody-producing cells and the antibody is replicated. This theory explained many features of the immune response but incorrectly located immunologic memory in serum rather than cells. See *clonal selection t.*
neuron t. (Waldeyer, 1891) the theory that the nervous system consists of innumerable neurons in contiguity, but not in continuity. See *neuron.*
open circulation t. one of the theories explaining how the blood in the spleen gets from the arteries to the venous sinuses; it holds that the capillaries open directly into the pulp reticulum, and that the blood gradually filters back into the venous sinuses. Called also *slow circulation t.* Cf. *closed circulation t.* and *closed-open circulation t.*
open-closed circulation t. see *closed-open circulation t.*
opponent colors t. Hering's t.
overflow t. a theory of ascites formation similar to the *underfilling theory* but proposing that the primary event is sodium and water retention resulting in portal hypertension; plasma volume expansion to the point of overflow from the hepatic sinusoids then causes ascites formation.
overproduction t. see *Weigert's law,* under *law.*
pithecoid t. the theory that humans are descended from apelike ancestors.
place t. an early theory of pitch perception which postulated that excitation of specific areas of the basilar membrane of the cochlea determined the pitch perceived. Cf. *frequency t.*
Planck's t. quantum t.
polyphyletic t. the theory that the various blood cells have their origin from two or more types of stem cells. Cf. *dualistic t., monophyletic t.,* and *trialistic t.* Called also *polyphyletism.*

Theory *Continued*

proteolysis-chelation t. a theory of the etiology of dental caries, according to which keratolytic microorganisms cause formation of chelates, which in turn cause decalcification.
proteolytic t. a theory of the etiology of dental caries, according to which microorganisms destroy enamel protein.
quantum t. the theory that the radiation and absorption of energy take place in definite quantities called quanta (E) which vary in size and are defined by the equation $E = h\nu$, in which h is Planck constant and ν is the frequency of the radiation.
recapitulation t. ontogeny recapitulates phylogeny; that is, an organism in the course of its development goes through the same successive stages as did the species in developing from the lower to the higher forms of animal life. Called also *Haeckel's law.*
recombinational germline t. a theory of the origin of antibody diversity, according to which the DNA coding for a single immunoglobulin chain is assembled by a somatic recombinational event from two genes, one a unique constant region gene and the other one of several million variable region genes. The first theory to propose that two genes might code for a single polypeptide chain, it is now known to be essentially correct, although more than two types of genes are actually involved. Called also *Dreyer and Bennett hypothesis.*
resonance t. 1. Helmholtz t. 2. the theory of specificity which assumes that the surface forces of reacting substances must harmonize.
Ribbert's t. a tumor is formed from the development of cell rests owing to reduced tension in the surrounding tissues.
Rutherford's t. frequency t.
Schön's t. the theory (of ocular accommodation) that the ciliary muscle exerts on the lens the same effect as is produced on a rubber ball held in both hands and compressed by the fingers.
side-chain t. Ehrlich's side-chain t.
single hit t. the theory that hemolysis results from a single complement-induced lesion of the erythrocyte surface, rather than that lesions at several sites are necessary.
sliding filament t. see under *mechanism.*
slow circulation t. open circulation t.
Spitzer's t. the formation of the septa in the heart are teleologically conditioned, phylogenetically brought about, and mechanically achieved by the appearance and development of the lungs through phylogeny.
target t. the theory advanced to explain some biological effects of radiation on the basis of ionization occurring in a very small sensitive region within the cell, which postulates that one or more ionizing events, or "hits," within the sensitive volume are necessary to bring about the biological end-effect; called also *hit t.*
template t. a theory of the mechanism of antibody specificity, current during the 1930s and 40s, which proposed that the shape of an antibody molecule is determined as it is synthesized by being molded on an antigen molecule. The antigen thus "instructs" a cell to make specific antibody. Called also *instructive t.*
thermostat t. a theory which suggests that the feeding and satiety centers of the brain, like the thermoregulatory centers, are sensitive to body temperature; a decrease in body temperature activates the feeding center and depresses the satiety center, whereas increased temperature acts on the centers in the opposite way.
Traube's resonance t. resonance t. (def. 2).
trialistic t. a variant of the polyphyletic theory that holds that blood cells arise from three distinct types of stem cells, the myeloblasts, lymphoblasts, and monocytes. Cf. *dualistic t.* and *monophyletic t.* Called also *trialism.*
underfilling t. the theory that ascites associated with portal hypertension causes hypovolemia and so both a lowering of portal pressure and retention of sodium and water. The higher sodium concentration causes increases in the plasma volume and portal pressure, and the subsequent formation of ascites renews the cycle. See also *overflow t.*
undulatory t. wave t.
unitarian t. monophyletic t.
wave t. the theory that light, heat, and electricity are transmitted through space in the form of waves.
Weismann's t. see *weismannism.*
Woods-Fildes t. the theory that the antibacterial activity of at least some drugs (especially the sulfonamides) is a consequence of a competitive inhibition of essential metabolic reactions of the microorganism.
Young-Helmholtz t. the doctrine that color vision depends on three sets of retinal fibers, corresponding to the colors red, green, and violet.

theo·ther·a·py (the″o-ther′ə-pe) [Gr. *theos* god + *therapy*] the treatment of disease by prayer and religious exercises.

theque (tek) [Fr. a "box or small chest"] junctional nest.

Thera·Cys (ther′ə-sis) trademark for a preparation of live BCG (bacille Calmette-Guérin) for intravesical use.

ther·a·peu·sis (ther″ə-pu′sis) therapeutics.

ther·a·peu·tic (ther″ə-pu′tik) [Gr. *therapeutikos* inclined to serve] 1. pertaining to therapeutics or to therapy. 2. curative.

ther·a·peu·tics (ther″ə-pu′tiks) 1. the branch of medical science concerned with the treatment of disease. 2. therapy.

Ther·a·pho·si·dae (ther″ə-fo′sĭ-de) a family of large, hairy spiders of the suborder Orthognatha, found in temperate and tropical areas. Some species have painful bites, but *Sericopelma communis*, the black tarantula, is the only one whose bite is toxic. Various other members of this family have been erroneously called tarantulas (q.v.). See also *bird spider.*

ther·a·pist (ther′ə-pist) [Gr. *therapeutēs* one who attends to the sick] a person skilled in the treatment of disease; often combined with a term indicating the specific type of disorder treated (as *speech t.*) or a particular type of treatment rendered (as *physical t.*).

physical t. a person skilled in the techniques of physical therapy and qualified to administer treatments prescribed by a physician and under his supervision; called also *physiotherapist.*

respiratory t. a person who has graduated from an approved respiratory therapist program or is registered by the National Board for Respiratory Care and is qualified to provide respiratory care under the supervision of a physician.

speech t. a person specially trained to assist patients in overcoming speech and language disorders. Cf. *speech pathologist.*

ther·a·py (ther′ə-pe) [Gr. *therapeia* service done to the sick] the treatment of disease; called also *therapeutics.*

Therapy

See also under *treatment.*

ablation t. the destruction of small areas of myocardial tissue, usually by application of electrical or chemical energy, in the treatment of some tachyarrhythmias. See also *electrical* and *chemical ablation,* under *ablation.*
add-back t. endocrine therapy to restore a hormone that is depleted by some other prescribed therapy.
adjuvant t. the use of chemotherapy or radiotherapy in addition to surgical resection in the treatment of cancer.
aerosol t. inhalation therapy using an aerosol.
androgen ablation t., androgen deprivation t. androgen deprivation.
anticoagulant t. the use of anticoagulants such as heparin, warfarin, or dicumarol to discourage thrombosis.
antiplatelet t. the use of platelet inhibitors such as aspirin, dipyridamole, sulfinpyrazone, or ticlopidine hydrochloride to inhibit platelet

Therapy *Continued*

adhesion or aggregation and so prevent thrombosis, alter the course of atherosclerosis, or prolong vascular graft patency.
art t. the use of art media and images, the creative process, and patient response to the products created for the treatment of psychiatric and psychologic conditions, often as an adjunct to psychotherapy, and for rehabilitation.
autolymphocyte t. autopheresis.
autoserum t. treatment of disease by the injection of the patient's own blood serum.
aversion t., aversive t. a form of behavior therapy using aversive conditioning, pairing undesirable behavior or symptoms with unpleasant stimulation in order to reduce or eliminate the behavior or symptoms. The term is sometimes used synonymously with *aversive conditioning.*
B-cell–targeted t. a type of immunotherapy that decreases the immune response caused by B lymphocytes, using monoclonal antibodies for treatment of autoimmune conditions.
beam t. external beam radiotherapy.
behavior t. a therapeutic approach in which the focus is on the patient's observable behavior, rather than on conflicts and unconscious processes presumed to underlie his maladaptive behavior. This is accomplished through systematic manipulation of the environmental and behavioral variables related to the specific behavior to be modified; operant conditioning, systematic desensitization, token economy, aversive control, flooding, and implosion are examples of techniques that may be used in behavior therapy. Called also *behavior modification* and *conditioning t.*
behavioral marital t. (BMT) a form of marital therapy using principles and techniques from behavior therapy; it attempts to alleviate marital distress by increasing positive, pleasant interactions between the members of a couple.
bile acid t., bile acid replacement t. administration of bile acids for treatment of hyperliposis.
biological t. treatment of disease by injection of substances that produce a biological reaction in the organism, such as sera, antitoxins, vaccines, and nonspecific proteins.
buffer t. intravenous injection of buffer substances, such as sodium bicarbonate, with the object of lowering the hydrogen ion concentration.
cardiac resynchronization t. cardiac pacing in which a lead is used to deliver current directly to the left ventricle, in addition to those used to deliver current to the right atrium and ventricle, so that the ventricles can be induced to pump in synchrony. Called also *bilateral pacing.*
Chaoul t. x-ray therapy with a short source-to-tissue distance and low voltage; see also *Chaoul tube,* under *tube.*
chelation t. the use of a chelating agent to remove toxic metals from the body, used in the treatment of heavy metal poisoning. In complementary medicine, also used for the treatment of atherosclerosis and other disorders.
client-centered t. a form of psychotherapy in which the emphasis is on the patient's self-discovery, interpretation, conflict resolution, and reorganization of values and life approach, which are enabled by the warm, nondirective, unconditionally accepting support of the therapist, who reflects and clarifies the patient's discoveries.
cognitive t., cognitive behavior t. a directive form of psychotherapy based on the theory that emotional problems result from distorted attitudes and ways of thinking that can be corrected. Using techniques drawn in part from behavior therapy, the therapist actively seeks to guide the patient in altering or revising negative or erroneous perceptions and attitudes.
cold t. cryotherapy.
collapse t. a treatment for pulmonary tuberculosis, formerly widely used, in which the diseased lung was collapsed in order to immobilize it and allow it to rest. Common methods were oleothorax, plombage, pneumonolysis, artificial pneumothorax, and thoracoplasty. Pneumonolysis and thoracoplasty are still sometimes done to collapse a lung and allow access during thoracic surgery.
color t. the therapeutic use of light of specific colors. It encompasses a number of methods used in complementary medicine, including the direction of light of specific colors at the chakras associated with the colors, the stimulation of acupoints, and the use of light of specific wavelengths to facilitate healing. Called also *chromotherapy.*
combined t. 1. psychotherapy in which the patient sees the same therapist for both individual and group therapies concurrently. Cf. *conjoint t.* 2. psychotherapy and medication used together.
combined modality t. treatment of cancer using two or more types of therapy, such as radiation therapy, chemotherapy, or surgery in an effort to achieve additive or synergistic effects; see also *chemoradiotherapy.* Called also *multimodality t.*
compression t. treatment of venous insufficiency, varicose veins, or venous ulceration of the lower limbs by having the patient wear compressing garments such as elastic support stockings.
conditioning t. behavior t.
conjoint t. psychotherapy in which a patient is involved in both group and individual therapy concurrently, seeing separate therapists for each. Cf. *combined t.*
continuous renal replacement t. (CRRT) hemodialysis or hemofiltration done 24 hours a day for an extended period, usually in a critically ill patient.
continuous sleep t. treatment of certain mental disorders by inducing prolonged sleep (18 to 20 hours a day for about two weeks) with drugs, usually barbiturates; it is no longer used in the United States.
convulsive t. treatment of mental disorders, primarily depression, by induction of convulsions. The type now almost universally used is electroconvulsive therapy (ECT), in which the convulsions are induced by electric current. In earlier forms, convulsions were induced pharmacologically, at first by pentylenetetrazol and later by flurothyl.
corrective t. the planning and administration of progressive physical exercise and activities most effective in improving or maintaining general physical and emotional health, through individual or group participation.
couples t. a form of therapy that parallels marital therapy, but used to include the treatment of two adults in a committed relationship, not restricted to those who are married.
craniosacral t. a system of manipulation by light touch whose purpose is to facilitate the body's self-healing capacity by finding and correcting cerebrospinal fluid blockages and imbalances within the craniosacral system (the dura mater of the central nervous system and the cerebrospinal fluid within it) that are supposed to cause sensory, motor, or intellectual dysfunction.
dance t., dance/movement t. the therapeutic use of movement to further the emotional, social, cognitive, and physical integration of the individual; used in the treatment of a variety of social, emotional, cognitive, and physical disorders.
deep roentgen-ray t. orthovoltage radiotherapy.
deleading t. the use of chelating agents in the mobilization and excretion from the body of a heavy metal such as lead or radium.
diathermic t. diathermy.
diet t. treatment of disease by regulation of the diet; called also *dietotherapy, nutritional t.,* and *trophotherapy.*
drug t. pharmacotherapy.
electric convulsive t., electric shock t. electroconvulsive t.
electroconvulsive t. (ECT) a treatment for mental disorders, primarily depression, in which a seizure in the brain is induced by application of a brief pulse of low-voltage alternating current to the brain via scalp electrodes. A general anesthetic and a muscle relaxant, generally succinylcholine, are used to prevent injury during the seizure. Awakening usually occurs within 5 to 10 minutes and may be followed by a temporary confusional state; transient memory impairment may be present for weeks to as much as a year after treatment. ECT produces a therapeutic response in a majority of cases of major depression.
electrodermal activity t. a type of biofeedback therapy in which sensors attached to the palm or the palmar aspect of the fingers are used to monitor sweat output in response to stress; used in the treatment of stress, anxiety disorders, chronic pain, and hyperhidrosis.
electroshock t. (EST) electroconvulsive t.
emotionally focused t. a form of couples therapy in which the couple increases intimacy and improves their relationship by each assessing, acknowledging, and expressing their underlying emotions and unmet feelings and needs.
empiric t. administration of therapy when there are signs and symptoms of infection but the specific disease-causing agent has not yet been proven by a test.
endocrine t. treatment of disease by the use of hormones; called also *hormonal* or *hormone t., endocrinotherapy,* and *hormonotherapy.*
enzyme t. in complementary medicine, the oral administration of proteolytic enzymes for the purpose of improving immune system function; used for a wide variety of disorders, including trauma,

Therapy *Continued*

inflammation, autoimmune diseases, and viral infection, and as adjunctive therapy in cancer treatment.
estrogen replacement t. administration of an estrogen to treat estrogen deficiency, such as that following menopause; indications include the prevention of postmenopausal osteoporosis and coronary artery disease. In women with a uterus, a progestational agent is usually included to prevent endometrial hyperplasia. Called also *hormone replacement t.*
external beam t. see under *radiotherapy.*
family t. *group therapy* of the members of a family, exploring and improving family relationships and processes, understanding and modifying home influences that contribute to mental disorder in one or more family members, and improving communication and collective, constructive methods of problem solving.
fever t. pyretotherapy.
fibrinolytic t. the use of fibrinolytic agents (prourokinase, streptokinase, t-plasminogen activator, u-plasminogen activator) to lyse thrombi in patients with acute peripheral arterial occlusion, deep venous thrombosis, pulmonary embolism, and acute myocardial infarction. Called also *thrombolytic t.*
first line t. induction t.
fluidized t. application of a dry whirlpool of solid particles suspended in warm air for treatment of traumatic or nontraumatic musculoskeletal disorders, especially of the limbs.
gene t. manipulation of the genome of an individual to prevent, mask, or lessen the effects of a genetic disorder. The defective function may be replaced by introduction of genetic material into targeted cells, or the defective gene itself may be corrected by targeting a recombinational event to replace all or part of the defective gene with a normal DNA sequence.
Goeckerman t. see under *treatment.*
gold t. chrysotherapy.
grid t. therapeutic application of ionizing radiations through a metal grid having a pattern of small, evenly spaced perforations.
group t. a form of psychotherapy in which a group of people meet regularly with a group leader, usually a therapist. The group uses therapeutic forces within the group, interactions between members, and the interventions of the trained leader to achieve insight into the cause of problems, provide emotional support, or effect changes in maladaptive behavior, thoughts, or feelings of the individual members. Called also *group psychotherapy.*
highly active antiretroviral t. (HAART) the aggressive use of extremely potent antiretroviral agents in the treatment of human immunodeficiency virus infection; it generally includes three such agents, two of which are nucleoside reverse transcriptase inhibitors and the other either an HIV protease inhibitor or a nonnucleoside reverse transcriptase inhibitor.
high-voltage roentgen t. high-voltage radiotherapy.
hormonal t., hormone t. endocrine t.
hormone replacement t. (HRT) the administration of hormones to correct a deficiency; usually used to denote *estrogen replacement therapy* after menopause.
humidification t. inhalation therapy using air supersaturated with moisture in treatment of congestive conditions of the upper and lower respiratory tract.
immunization t. treatment with antiserum and with actively antigenic substances, e.g., vaccines.
immunosuppressive t. treatment with agents, such as x-rays, corticosteroids, and cytotoxic chemicals, which suppress the immune response to antigen(s); it is used in various conditions, including autoimmune disease, allergy, multiple myeloma, and chronic nephritis, and in organ transplantation.
induction t. the first therapeutic measure used to treat a disease, especially when combined modality therapy is planned. Called also *first line t.*
inhalation t. respiratory care (def. 3).
intradiscal electrothermal t. (IDET) a minimally invasive procedure for treatment of discogenic low back pain: heat is administered to the disc wall, contracting and thickening its collagen fibers and destroying afferent nociceptors.
intraosseous t. the infusion of blood or other solutions into the circulation by injection through the bone marrow.
intravenous t. the introduction of therapeutic liquid agents directly into the venous circulation.
light t. 1. phototherapy (def. 1). 2. photodynamic t.
locoregional t. therapy that affects only a localized area rather than being systemic; said particularly of chemotherapy.
magnetic field t. the application of permanent or pulsed magnetic fields to specific areas of the body or to acupoints for therapeutic purposes; in addition to the FDA-approved use of pulsed magnetic fields for the treatment of nonunion fractures, it has been tried for a large number of other conditions, usually self-administered by patients.
maintenance t. therapy of chronically ill patients that is aimed at keeping the pathology at its present level and preventing exacerbation.
manual t. physical therapy or chiropractic techniques done by hand.
marital t., marriage t. a type of family therapy aimed at understanding and treating one or both members of a couple in the context of a distressed relationship. The term may be used more generally to include unmarried couples in a committed relationship, more properly called *couples t.*
massage t. the manipulation of the soft tissues of the body for the purpose of normalizing them, thereby enhancing health and healing. Massage therapy includes a number of methods, such as acupressure, classical Western massage, and shiatsu.
metatrophic t. administration of a diet that acts as an adjunct to the drug taken.
milieu t. treatment, usually in a psychiatric hospital, that emphasizes the provision of an environment and activities appropriate to the patient's emotional and interpersonal needs.
molecularly targeted t. chemotherapy with molecularly targeted agents.
Morita t. a school of psychotherapy originating in Japan, based on the essential elements of conduct in Zen Buddhism. It emphasizes the combating of egocentricity and the correction of alienation from nature.
movement t. see *dance/movement t.*
multimodality t. combined modality t.
music t. the use of music to effect positive changes in the psychological, physical, cognitive, or social functioning of individuals with health or educational problems; used for a wide variety of indications, including mental disorders, developmental and learning disabilities, neurologic disabilities, and the management of pain or stress.
myofunctional t. training of the orofacial musculature, including modification of habits, in edentulous conditions, malocclusion, or temporomandibular joint disorders.
neoadjuvant t. in combined modality therapy for cancer, initial use of one modality, such as chemotherapy or radiotherapy, to decrease the tumor burden prior to treatment by another modality, usually surgery. Called also *preoperative t.* and *presurgical t.*
nutritional t. diet t.
occupational t. the therapeutic use of self-care, work, and play activities to increase function, enhance development, and prevent disability; it may include modification of tasks or the environment to enable the patient to achieve maximum independence and to enhance the quality of the patient's life.
oral rehydration t. (ORT) oral administration of a solution of electrolytes and carbohydrates in the treatment of dehydration.
orthomolecular t. treatment of disease based on the theory that restoration of optimal concentrations of substances normally present in the body, such as vitamins, trace elements, and amino acids, will effect a cure. See also under *medicine,* and *psychiatry.*
oxygen t. respiratory care involving inhalation of oxygen.
pancreatic enzyme t., pancreatic enzyme replacement t. replacement therapy for conditions of pancreatic insufficiency with malabsorption, such as cystic fibrosis.
photodynamic t. (PDT) intravenous administration of a photosensitizing agent such as hematoporphyrin derivative, which concentrates selectively in metabolically active tumor tissue, followed by exposure of the tumor tissue to red laser light of a specific wavelength, to bring about production of cytotoxic free radicals that selectively destroy the photosensitized tissue. Called also *photochemotherapy, photoradiation, phototherapy,* and *light therapy.*
physical t. 1. treatment by physical means. 2. the health profession concerned with the promotion of health, with the prevention of physical disability, with the evaluation and rehabilitation of patients disabled by pain, disease, or injury, and with treatment using physical therapeutic measures as opposed to medical, surgical, or radiologic measures.
plasma t. the therapeutic use of blood plasma.

Therapy *Continued*

play t. a method of psychotherapy used in treating children, in which play is used to a considerable extent as the means of communication between the child and therapist, enabling self-expression and the revealing of unconscious material.
poetry t. a form of bibliotherapy in which a selected poem is used to evoke feelings and responses for discussion in a therapeutic setting. The poem may be a published work or one created by the patient, and poetic devices such as rhythm, image, and metaphor contribute to the therapeutic effect.
polarity t. a bodywork technique that combines tissue manipulation with theories of vital energy derived from ayurveda and acupuncture. It is believed that energy blockages within the body result in imbalances, which in turn manifest as pain. Manipulation, using light touch and medium and deep pressure, is used to release these energy blockages and restore balance. Exercise and nutritional and lifestyle counseling may also be included in the therapy.
preoperative t., presurgical t. neoadjuvant t.
primal t. psychotherapy in which the patient is encouraged to relive his early traumatic experiences and so relieve the painful emotions with which they are associated.
protective t. prophylaxis.
proton beam t. radiotherapy using a beam of protons, which penetrates tissues with minimal energy deposition before the beam reaches a certain depth (Bragg peak), thus localizing the dose to the target area and minimizing irradiation of surrounding tissues.
pulp canal t. root canal t.
pulse t. administration of medication in short intensive courses at regular intervals.
PUVA t. [*p*soralen + *u*ltra*v*iolet *A*] a form of photochemotherapy for skin disorders such as psoriasis and vitiligo; oral psoralen administration is followed two hours later by exposure to ultraviolet A.
radiation t. radiotherapy.
radiofrequency t. the use of radiofrequency ablation for therapeutic purposes, such as the treatment of pain syndromes and arrhythmias.
radium t. the treatment of disease by means of radium.
recreational t. programs designed to help persons with illnesses or other disabling conditions increase their functioning and sense of well-being through recreation, games, and group activities.
reflex t. treatment by producing a reflex action; called also *reflexotherapy.*
relaxation t. any of a number of techniques for inducing the relaxation response (q.v.), used for the reduction of stress; such techniques are helpful in the management of a wide variety of chronic illnesses that are caused or exacerbated by stress.
renal replacement t. therapy such as hemodialysis or transplantation that takes the place of nonfunctioning kidneys. See also *continuous renal replacement t.*
replacement t. 1. treatment to replace deficiencies in body products by administration of natural or synthetic substitutes. Called also *substitution t.* 2. treatment such as hemodialysis or transplantation that replaces or compensates for a nonfunctioning organ.
respiratory t. see under *care.*
root canal t. the aspect of endodontics concerned with the treatment of diseases of the dental pulp, consisting of partial *(pulpotomy)* or complete *(pulpectomy)* extirpation of the diseased pulp, cleaning and sterilization of the empty root canal, enlarging and shaping of the canal to receive sealing material, and obturation of the canal with a nonirritating hermetic sealing agent. Called also *pulp canal t.*
rotation t. in radiotherapy, circular movement of the patient or of the radiation source and beam around a fixed anatomical axis during a treatment exposure; it may entail complete, partial, or skip-field exposure.
salvage t. the use of experimental or strong therapeutic measures in patients whose prognosis is poor after they have failed other therapies.
serum t. see *serotherapy.*
short wave t. short wave diathermy.
solar t. heliotherapy.
sparing t. treatment directed to the protecting and sparing of an organ by allowing it to rest as much as possible.
specific t. see under *treatment.*
speech t. the use of special techniques for correction of speech and language disorders. Cf. *speech pathology.*
strategic t. a directive form of psychotherapy in which the therapist helps couples or families to change their interactions and behavior by noticing where maladaptive patterns are occurring, then eliminating them by demanding deliberate attempts to behave in ways that, paradoxically, would normally be expected to cause them instead.
substitution t. replacement t. (def. 1).
substitutive t. substitutive medication.
suggestion t. a form of psychotherapy characterized by suggestion, reassurance, and sometimes also hypnosis.
thrombolytic t. fibrinolytic t.
thyroid replacement t., thyroxine replacement t. treatment of hypothyroidism by administration of thyroxine, usually in the form of levothyroxine sodium. Called also *thyroidotherapy* and *thyrotherapy.*
Trager t. see under *approach.*
virus-directed enzyme/prodrug t. a method of treating tumors by the introduction of a suicide gene (q.v.) into tumor cells by a viral vector, followed by the administration of a nontoxic prodrug that is converted to a toxic agent, resulting in tumor cell death.

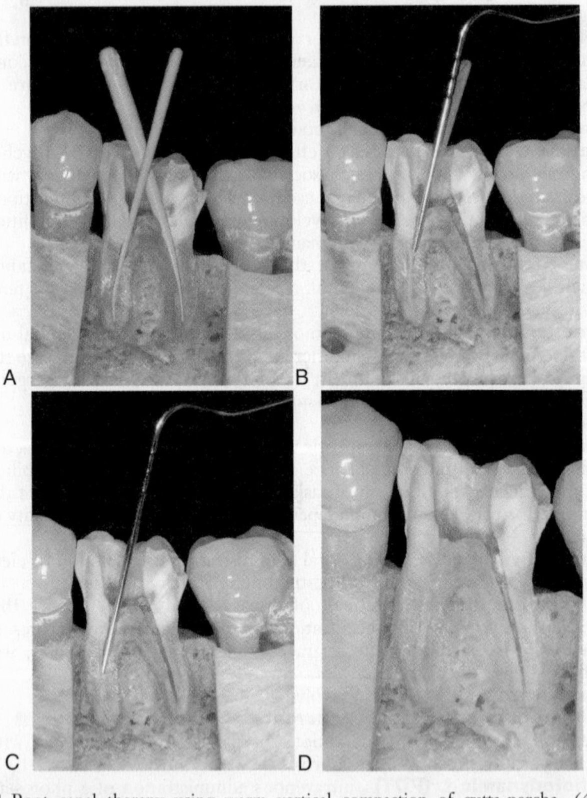

A B C D

■ Root canal therapy using warm vertical compaction of gutta-percha. *(A),* Conventional cones are selected and fitted short of the prepared canal length. *(B),* Heated pluggers or spreaders are used to apply heat to the master cone and remove excess coronal material; *(C),* Room temperature plugger is used to compact the heated gutta-percha (the process is then repeated for the coronal portion of the canal; *not shown*). *(D),* Completed obturation.

The•ria (the′re-ə) [Gr. *thērion* beast, animal] in some systems of classification, a subclass of the Mammalia, including the infraclasses Eutheria and Metatheria, the members of which are viviparous.

Ther•i•di•i•dae (ther″ĭ-di′ĭ-de) the comb-footed spiders, a family of small dark spiders of the suborder Labidognatha, whose venomous bite may be fatal to humans. It includes the genus *Latrodectus.*

the•rio•gen•ol•o•gist (the″re-o-jən-ol′ə-jist) a specialist in theriogenology.

the•rio•gen•ol•o•gy (the″re-o-jən-ol′ə-je) [Gr. *thērion* beast + *geno-* + *-logy*] the branch of veterinary medicine concerned with reproduction, including the physiology and pathology of male and female reproductive systems and the clinical practice of veterinary obstetrics, gynecology, and semenology. **theriogenolog′ic, theriogenolog′ical** *adj*

therm (thurm) [Gr. *thermē* heat] a unit of heat. The word has been used as equivalent to *(a)* large calorie; *(b)* small calorie; *(c)* 1000 large calories; *(d)* 100,000 British thermal units.

ther·ma·co·gen·e·sis (thur″mə-ko-jen′ə-sis) [*therm-* + *-genesis*] the production of elevated body temperature by a drug.

ther·mal (thur′məl) pertaining to or characterized by heat.

ther·mal·ge·sia (thur″məl-je′ze-ə) [*therm-* + *algesia*] a dysesthesia in which the application of heat produces pain; called also *thermoalgesia.* Cf. *thermohyperalgesia.*

ther·mal·gia (thər-mal′jə) causalgia.

therm·an·al·ge·sia (thurm″an-əl-je′ze-ə) thermoanesthesia.

therm·an·es·the·sia (thurm″an-es-the′zhə) thermoanesthesia.

ther·ma·tol·o·gy (thur″mə-tol′ə-je) the scientific study of heat as a therapeutic agent.

Ther·ma·zene (thur′mə-zēn) trademark for a preparation of silver sulfadiazine.

ther·mel·om·e·ter (thur′məl-om′ə-tər) an electric thermometer, used particularly for recording very small temperature variations.

therm·es·the·sia (thurm″es-the′zhə) temperature sense.

therm·es·the·si·om·e·ter (thurm″əs-the″ze-om′ə-tər) [*thermesthesia* + *-meter*] an instrument for measuring sensibility to heat.

therm·hy·per·es·the·sia (thurm″hi-pər-es-the′zhə) thermohyperesthesia.

therm·hy·pes·the·sia (thurm″hi-pes-the′zhə) thermohypesthesia.

ther·mic (thur′mik) of or pertaining to heat.

ther·mi·on (thur′me-on) a particle containing an electric charge emitted by an incandescent substance, such as the electrons emitted from the cathode in a Coolidge tube.

ther·mi·on·ics (thur″me-on′iks) the science of the phenomena exhibited by thermions.

ther·mis·tor (thər-mis′tər) a temperature-sensitive semiconductor whose resistance decreases as the ambient temperature increases; it is used to measure extremely small changes in temperature.

therm(o)- [Gr. *thermē* heat] a combining form denoting relationship to heat.

Ther·mo·ac·ti·no·my·ces (thur″mo-ak″tĭ-no-mi′sēz) [*thermo-* + Gr. *aktis, aktinos* a ray + *mykēs* fungus] a genus of gram-positive, aerobic, chemo-organotrophic bacteria of the family Thermoactinomycetaceae, consisting of thermophilic (45° to 60° C) organisms having single spores on the aerial and substrate mycelia. They occur as soil and water saprophytes. The type species is *T. vulga′ris.*

T. vulga′ris a species isolated from soils, manure, and hay; one of the causative organisms of farmer's lung.

Ther·mo·ac·ti·no·my·ce·ta·ceae (thur″mo-ak″tĭ-no-mi″sə-ta′se-e) a family of gram-positive, endospore-forming bacteria of the order Bacillales; medically important organisms are contained in the genus *Thermoactinomyces.*

ther·mo·al·ge·sia (thur″mo-al-je′ze-ə) thermalgesia.

ther·mo·an·al·ge·sia (thur″mo-an″əl-je′ze-ə) thermoanesthesia.

ther·mo·an·es·the·sia (thur″mo-an″es-the′zhə) [*thermo-* + *anesthesia*] inability to recognize sensations of heat and cold; loss or lack of temperature sense. Called also *thermanalgesia, thermoanalgesia, thermanesthesia,* and *thermal anesthesia.*

ther·mo·cau·ter·ec·to·my (thur″mo-kaw″tər-ek′tə-me) [*thermocautery* + *-ectomy*] excision of an organ by thermocautery.

ther·mo·cau·tery (thur″mo-kaw′tər-e) cauterization by means of a hot wire or point. See also *electrocautery.*

ther·mo·chem·is·try (thur″mo-kem′is-tre) the aspect of physical chemistry dealing with heat changes that accompany chemical reactions.

ther·mo·chro·ic (thur″mo-kro′ik) [*thermo-* + Gr. *chroa* color] reflecting some of the heat rays and absorbing or transmitting others.

ther·mo·chro·ism (thur″mo-kro′iz-əm) the state or condition of being thermochroic.

ther·mo·chro·sis (thur″mo-kro′sis) thermochroism.

ther·mo·co·ag·u·la·tion (thur″mo-ko-ag″u-la′shən) coagulation of tissue by the action of electromagnetic energy; used in removal of growths and in stereotactic surgery.

radiofrequency t. the use of low-frequency electromagnetic waves for precisely controlled coagulation of tissue in stereotactic surgery and rhizotomy.

ther·mo·cou·ple (thur′mo-kup″əl) a device used for measuring temperature differences, consisting of a pair of dissimilar electrical conductors (such as platinum and platinum-rhodium) joined in such a way that an electromotive force is developed by the thermoelectric effects when the junctions are at different temperatures. See also *thermocouple thermometer,* under *thermometer.*

ther·mo·cur·rent (thur″mo-kur′ent) a thermoelectric current.

ther·mo·cyc·ler (ther″mo-si′klər) an apparatus that delivers heat varying in intensity over time in a predetermined cycle for processes that require annealing, such as polymerase chain reactions.

ther·mo·dif·fu·sion (thur″mo-dĭ-fu′zhən) diffusion under the influence of a temperature gradient.

ther·mo·di·lu·tion (thur″mo-dĭ-loo′shən) a method of measuring blood flow by injection of a known quantity of a cool or cold indicator, such as a saline solution or distilled water, into the cardiovascular system and measuring with a thermistor the temperature over time at a specific point in the system.

ther·mo·du·ric (thur″mo-du′rik) [*thermo-* + L. *durus* enduring] capable of withstanding high temperature.

ther·mo·dy·nam·ics (thur″mo-di-nam′iks) [*thermo-* + *dynamics*] the branch of science which deals with heat, energy, work, and the interconversion of these, and with related problems. See also under *law.*

equilibrium t. the classic form of thermodynamics, that dealing with the application of the laws of thermodynamics to macroscopic systems in equilibrium states, or undergoing transformations between two equilibrium states.

laws of t. see under *law.*

nonequilibrium t. the branch of thermodynamics that deals with irreversible processes of macroscopic systems and their rates.

statistical t. that correlating the properties of individual atoms and molecules with macroscopic systems.

ther·mo·elec·tric (thur″mo-e-lek′trik) pertaining to electricity generated by heat.

ther·mo·elec·tric·i·ty (thur″mo-e″lek-tris′ĭ-te) electricity generated by heat.

ther·mo·es·the·sia (thur″mo-es-the′zhə) temperature sense.

ther·mo·es·the·si·om·e·ter (thur″mo-əs-the″ze-om′ə-tər) thermesthesiometer.

ther·mo·ex·ci·to·ry (thur″mo-ek-si′tə-re) exciting or stimulating the production of heat in the body.

ther·mo·gen·e·sis (thur″mo-jen′ə-sis) [*thermo-* + *-genesis*] the production of heat, especially within the animal body.

nonshivering t. the production of heat in the animal body without shivering, primarily through the uncoupling of oxidative phosphorylation in brown adipose tissue; it is most important in small mammals with a large surface to mass ratio and in neonates.

obligatory t. the energy required to digest, absorb, and metabolize nutrients; called also *calorigenic effect* and *thermic effect.*

shivering t. the production of heat in the animal body by shivering (q.v.).

ther·mo·ge·net·ic (thur″mo-jə-net′ik) 1. pertaining to thermogenesis. 2. thermogenic.

ther·mo·gen·ic (thur″mo-jen′ik) producing heat.

ther·mo·gen·ics (thur″mo-jen′iks) the science relating to heat production.

ther·mog·e·nin (thər-moj′ə-nin) uncoupling protein.

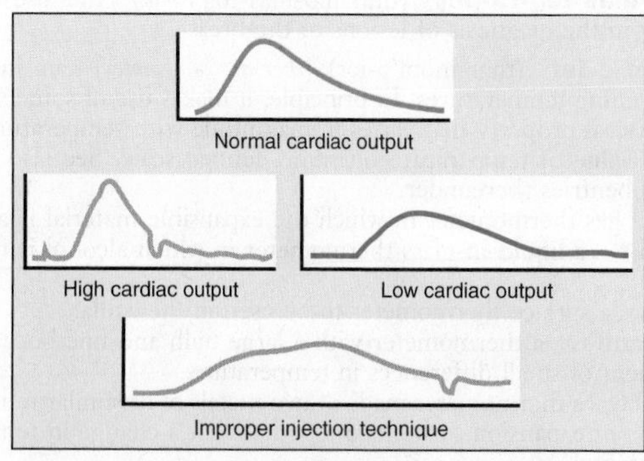

■ Thermodilution cardiac output curves. The area under the curve is inversely related to output. In the normal state, saline injection is followed by a sharp upstroke and a smooth curve with a mildly prolonged downslope to baseline. In a high cardiac output state, the saline injectate moves faster through the right side of the heart and temperature returns to baseline more quickly, reducing the area under the curve. In a low cardiac output state, the return to baseline is prolonged, increasing the area under the curve.

ther•mog•e•nous (thər-moj′ə-nəs) pertaining to or caused by heat or elevation of temperature.

ther•mo•gram (thur′mo-gram) 1. a graphic record of variations in temperature (heat). 2. the visual record obtained by thermography.

ther•mo•graph (thur′mo-graf) 1. an instrument for recording variations in temperature (heat). 2. a thermogram (def. 2). 3. the apparatus or device employed in thermography.

continuous scan t. a thermograph that presents a continuous scan image of the thermal pattern (thermogram) of a patient or object on cathode ray tube.

ther•mo•graph•ic (thur″mo-graf′ik) pertaining to a thermogram or to thermography.

ther•mog•ra•phy (thər-mog′rə-fe) [*thermo-* + *-graphy*] a technique wherein an infrared camera is used to photographically portray the surface temperatures of the body, based on the self-emanating infrared radiation; sometimes employed as a means of diagnosing underlying pathologic processes, such as breast tumors.

infrared tympanic t. determination of body temperature by measuring the infrared radiation emanating from the tympanic membrane, using a probe introduced into the external acoustic meatus.

ther•mo•gra•vim•e•ter (thur″mo-grə-vim′ə-tər) an analytical instrument for measuring change in mass of a substance at changing temperature.

ther•mo•hy•per•al•ge•sia (thur″mo-hi″pər-al-je′ze-ə) a condition in which the application of moderate heat causes extreme pain.

ther•mo•hy•per•es•the•sia (thur″mo-hi″pər-es-the′zhə) a dysesthesia marked by increased sensibility to heat and cold; called also *thermhyperesthesia.*

ther•mo•hy•pes•the•sia (thur″mo-hi″pes-the′zhə) [*thermo-* + *hyp-* + *esthesia*] a dysesthesia marked by decreased sensibility to heat and cold; see also *thermoanesthesia.* Called also *thermhypesthesia* and *thermohypoesthesia.*

ther•mo•hy•po•es•the•sia (thur″mo-hi″po-es-the′zhə) thermohypesthesia.

ther•mo•in•ac•ti•va•tion (thur″mo-in-ak″tĭ-va′shən) destruction of the power to act by exposure to heat.

ther•mo•in•hib•i•to•ry (thur″mo-in-hib′ĭ-tor-e) inhibiting or retarding the production of bodily heat.

ther•mo•in•te•gra•tor (thur″mo-in′tə-gra″tər) an apparatus for recording environmental warmth.

ther•mo•ker•a•to•plasty (thur″mo-ker′ə-to-plas″te) reshaping of the cornea by the application of heat, either by means of a heated probe or a laser, which shrinks the collagen of the corneal stroma, resulting in flattening of the cornea in the area of heating. **thermokeratoplas′tic** *adj*

ther•mo•la•bile (thur″mo-la′bəl, -la′bīl) easily altered or decomposed by heat; called also *heat labile.*

ther•mol•o•gy (thər-mol′ə-je) [*thermo-* + *-logy*] the science of heat.

ther•mo•lu•mi•nes•cence (thur″mo-loo″mĭ-nes′əns) the production of light by a substance when its temperature is increased.

ther•mol•y•sis (thər-mol′ĭ-sis) [*thermo-* + *-lysis*] 1. chemical dissociation by means of heat. 2. the dissipation of bodily heat by radiation, evaporation, or some other means.

ther•mo•lyt•ic (thur″mo-lit′ik) [*thermo-* + *-lytic*] 1. pertaining to, characterized by, or promoting thermolysis. 2. an agent that promotes thermolysis.

ther•mo•mas•sage (thur″mo-mə-sahzh′) massage with heat.

ther•mo•mas•tog•ra•phy (thur″mo-mas-tog′rə-fe) the use of thermography in the diagnosis of lesions of the breast.

ther•mom•e•ter (thər-mom′ə-tər) [*thermo-* + *-meter*] an instrument for determining temperatures. In principle, it makes use of some substance with a physical property that varies in magnitude with temperature, to determine a value of temperature on some defined scale. See also *scale* and selected subentries thereunder.

air t. a gas thermometer in which the expansible material is air.

alcohol t. a liquid-in-glass thermometer in which alcohol is the liquid used.

axilla t. a surface thermometer to be used in the axilla.

Beckmann t. a thermometer with a large bulb and fine bore stem for measurement of small differences in temperature.

bimetal t. a thermometer made of two metals of dissimilar temperature coefficients of expansion so bonded together that a change in temperature causes it to curl.

Celsius t. a thermometer employing the Celsius scale (q.v.).

centigrade t. a thermometer in which the interval between two established reference points is divided into 100 units; usually specifically denoting a *Celsius t.*

clinical t. a thermometer for use in determining temperature of the human body.

depth t. a thermometer whose sensitive element may be introduced into the tissues, for registering the actual temperature of a tissue.

differential t. a thermometer for measuring small differences in temperature.

Fahrenheit t. a thermometer employing the Fahrenheit scale (q.v.).

fever t. clinical t.

gas t. a thermometer in which the expansible material is a gas, such as air, carbon dioxide, helium, neon, nitrogen, or oxygen.

half-minute t. a clinical thermometer with a short time lag.

infrared tympanic t. a clinical thermometer inserted into the external acoustic meatus to measure body temperature by infrared tympanic thermography.

kata t. see *katathermometer.*

Kelvin t. a thermometer employing the Kelvin scale (q.v.).

liquid-in-glass t. the common type of thermometer, containing a liquid which expands with increase in temperature; most of the liquid is in a bulb, but its free surface is in a capillary tube graduated to indicate the degree of temperature causing expansion to each particular point.

maximum t. a thermometer which registers the highest temperature to which it has been exposed.

mercury t. a liquid-in-glass thermometer in which mercury is the liquid used.

metallic t. a thermometer in which some solid metal is used as the expansible element.

metastatic t. differential t.

minimum t. a thermometer that registers the lowest temperature to which it has been exposed.

oral t. a clinical thermometer which is placed under the tongue, to record the temperature in the mouth; characteristically the bulb containing the mercury is elongated.

Rankine t. a thermometer employing the Rankine scale (q.v.).

Réaumur t. a thermometer employing the Réaumur scale (q.v.).

recording t. a temperature-sensitive instrument by which the temperature to which it has been exposed is continuously recorded on a specially designed chart.

rectal t. a clinical thermometer which is inserted in the rectum, for determining body temperature; characteristically the bulb containing the mercury is pear shaped.

resistance t. a thermometer which uses the electric resistance of metals for determining temperature; it consists of a resistance bulb of platinum or other metal wire, and uses a Wheatstone bridge.

self-registering t. 1. recording t. 2. a thermometer that registers the maximum or minimum temperature attained with a single measurement.

surface t. a clinical thermometer for determining the temperature on the surface of the body.

thermocouple t. a combination of a thermocouple with some device for measuring its electromotive force, such as a potentiometer; in use the thermocouple's reference junction is kept at a reference temperature (such as the ice point) and its measuring junction at the temperature being measured.

tympanic t. infrared tympanic t.

wet-and-dry-bulb t. psychrometer.

ther•mo•met•ric (thur″mo-met′rik) pertaining to a thermometer or to the measurement of degrees of temperature.

ther•mom•e•try (thər-mom′ə-tre) the measurement of temperatures.

Ther•mo•mo•no•spo•ra•ceae (thur″mo-mo-nos″pə-ra′se-e) [*thermo-* + Gr. *monos* single + *sporos* seed] a family of aerobic, gram-positive, non–acid-fast, chemo-organotrophic bacteria of the suborder Streptosporangineae, order Actinomycetales, that produce a branched substrate mycelium bearing aerial hyphae. Medically important organisms are contained in the genus *Actinomadura.*

ther•mo•pal•pa•tion (thur″mo-pal-pa′shən) palpation for the purpose of determining differences of temperature at different portions of the body.

ther•mo•pen•e•tra•tion (thur″mo-pen″ə-tra′shən) medical diathermy.

ther•mo•phile (thur′mo-fīl) 1. an organism that grows best at elevated temperatures. 2. a bacterium with an optimal growth temperature of 50° to 70° C.

ther•mo•phil•ic (thur″mo-fil′ik) [*thermo-* + *-philic*] growing best at or having a fondness for high temperatures. Cf. *mesophilic* and *psychrophilic.*

ther•mo•phore (thur′mo-for) [*thermo-* + *-phore*] a device or apparatus for retaining heat; used in therapeutic local application.

ther•mo•pile (thur′mo-pīl) [*thermo-* + *pile* (def. 1)] a number of thermocouples in series; used to increase the sensitivity of a temperature-measuring device, or for the direct conversion of heat into electric energy.

ther•mo•plac•en•tog•ra•phy (thur″mo-plas″ən-tog′rə-fe) the use of thermography for determining the site of placental attachment.

ther·mo·plas·tic (thur′mo-plas′tik) softening under heat and capable of being molded into shape with pressure, then hardening on cooling without undergoing chemical change.

ther·mo·pre·cip·i·ta·tion (thur″mo-pre-sip″ĭ-ta′shən) precipitation by heat.

ther·mo·ra·dio·ther·a·py (thur″mo-ra″de-o-ther′ə-pe) application of ionizing radiation to an anatomical site whose tissue temperature has been elevated by artificial means on the theory of increasing its radiosensitivity.

ther·mo·re·cep·tor (thur″mo-re-sep′tər) a nerve ending, usually in the skin, that is sensitive to a change in temperature; see *cold receptor* and *warmth receptor*, under *receptor*.

ther·mo·reg·u·la·tion (thur″mo-reg″u-la′shən) the regulation of heat, such as the body heat of a warm-blooded animal; see also *thermostasis*.

ther·mo·reg·u·la·tor (thur″mo-reg′u-la″tər) thermostat.

ther·mo·re·sis·tance (thur″mo-re-zis′təns) the quality of being little affected by heat. **thermoresis′tant** *adj*

ther·mo·scope (thur′mo-skōp) [*thermo-* + *-scope*] differential thermometer.

ther·mo·set (ther′mo-set″) having undergone thermosetting.

ther·mo·set·ting (ther′mo-set″ing) becoming hard or solid when heat is applied and remaining that way upon being recooled; the change is not reversible. Said of resins.

ther·mo·sta·bile (thur″mo-sta′bəl, -sta′bīl) unaffected by heat; able to withstand the effects of heat without undergoing change; in immunology, the term usually refers to substances that are not inactivated by heating to 56°C for 30 minutes, which inactivates complement. Called also *heat stabile*.

ther·mo·sta·bil·i·ty (thur″mo-stə-bil′ĭ-te) the quality of withstanding the effects of heat without undergoing change.

ther·mo·sta·sis (thur″mo-sta′sis) [*thermo-* + *stasis*] the maintenance of body temperature in warm-blooded animals.

ther·mo·stat (thur′mo-stat) [*thermo-* + *-stat*] a device interposed in a heating system by which the temperature can be automatically maintained between certain levels.

hypothalamic t. the mechanism for control of body temperature, which involves two thermoregulatory centers of the hypothalamus: the preoptic area of the anterior hypothalamus, which senses core temperature and compares it to the set-point, and an area in the posterior hypothalamus that integrates signals from the preoptic area and from cold and warmth receptors in the skin and controls mechanisms of heat dissipation (skin vasodilation, sweating) and production and conservation (skin vasoconstriction, release of epinephrine and thyroid hormones, sympathetic stimulation).

ther·mo·ste·re·sis (thur″mo-stə-re′sis) [*thermo-* + Gr. *sterēsis* deprivation] the deprivation of heat.

ther·mo·stro·muhr (thur″mo-stro′moor) an instrument for measuring the amount of blood flowing in a blood vessel by noting temperature changes.

ther·mo·sys·tal·tic (thur″mo-sis-tawl′tik) [*thermo-* + *systaltic*] contracting under the influence or stimulus of heat; pertaining to thermosystaltism.

ther·mo·sys·tal·tism (thur″mo-sis′təl-tiz-əm) [*thermo-* + Gr. *systellein* to contract] muscular contraction in response to temperature changes.

ther·mo·tac·tic (thur″mo-tak′tik) pertaining to thermotaxis.

ther·mo·tax·ic (thur″mo-tak′sik) thermotactic.

ther·mo·tax·is (thur″mo-tak′sis) [*thermo-* + *-taxis*] 1. the normal adjustment of body temperature; see also *thermoregulation*. 2. taxis in response to increased temperature.

ther·mo·ther·a·py (thur″mo-ther′ə-pe) [*thermo-* + *therapy*] treatment of disease by the application of heat; usually defined as that which raises body temperature to above 45° C. Cf. *hyperthermia* (def. 2).

transurethral microwave t. (TUMT) delivery of microwave energy to the prostatic fossa using an antenna attached to a Foley-type catheter, which is inserted through the urethra; used to destroy hyperplastic tissue in the treatment of benign prostatic hyperplasia.

ther·mot·ics (thər-mot′iks) the science of heat.

ther·mo·tol·er·ant (thur″mo-tol′ər-ənt) enduring heat; said of bacteria whose activity is not checked by high temperature.

ther·mo·to·nom·e·ter (thur″mo-to-nom′ə-tər) [*thermo-* + *tono-* + *-meter*] an instrument for measuring the amount of muscular contraction caused by heat.

ther·mot·ro·pism (thər-mot′ro-piz-əm) [*thermo-* + *tropism*] tropism of an organism in response to an increase in temperature. **thermotrop′ic** *adj*

the·ro·morph (the′ro-morf) [Gr. *thēr* wild beast + *morph*] a morphologic part of an organism or individual with supernumerary, teratic, or absent parts, giving it a resemblance to a different animal.

the·ro·mor·phism (the″ro-mor′fiz-əm) the abnormal resemblance of some part of the organism to the normal structure of the corresponding part of an animal of lower type.

Ther·o·my·zon (ther-o′mĭ-zon) a genus of leeches of the family Gnathobdellidae; they parasitize the nasal passages and sometimes the conjunctivae of geese.

the·ront (the′ront) [Gr. *thēr* wild beast + *on*, *ontos* being] the free-swimming stage or form in the life cycle of certain ciliate protozoa that arises from a tomite and searches ("hunts") for a new host or food source necessary for the development into the trophont.

the·sau·ro·cyte (thə-saw′ro-sīt) an abnormal plasma cell that is distended with homogeneous cytoplasm that stains gray or red, possibly owing to a disturbance in synthesis of immunoglobulin A.

the·ta (tha′tə) [Θ, θ] the eighth letter of the Greek alphabet.

THF tetrahydrofolic acid or tetrahydrofolate.

thi·a·ben·da·zole (thi″ə-ben′də-zōl) [USP] a broad-spectrum benzimidazole anthelmintic with activity against roundworms, pinworms, threadworms, whipworms, and hookworms; used in the treatment of strongyloidiasis, cutaneous larva migrans, visceral larva migrans, and trichinosis, administered orally.

thi·ac·et·ar·se·mide so·di·um (thi-as″ət-ahr′sə-mīd) [USP] a trivalent arsenical used in veterinary practice for the treatment of dirofilariasis.

thi·a·di·a·zine (thi″ə-di′ə-zēn) thiazide.

thi·am·a·zole (thi-am′ə-zōl) INN and BAN for *methimazole*.

thi·a·min (thi′ə-min) thiamine.

thi·am·i·nase (thi-am′ĭ-nās) [EC 3.5.99.2] an enzyme of the hydrolase class that catalyzes the cleavage of thiamine into its component pyrimidine and thiazole moieties, inactivating it. The enzyme is present in intestinal microorganisms. Called also *t. II*.

t. I thiamine pyridinylase.

t. II thiaminase.

thi·a·mine (thi′ə-min) vitamin B_1, a heat-labile, water-soluble bicyclic compound comprising a substituted pyrimidine linked to a thiazole moiety. It is found particularly in pork, organ meats, legumes, nuts, and whole grain or enriched cereals and breads. The active form is thiamine pyrophosphate (q.v.). Deficiency of the vitamin can result in beriberi and is a factor in alcoholic neuritis and Wernicke-Korsakoff syndrome. Written also *thiamin*.

t. hydrochloride [USP] the monohydrochloride salt of thiamine, administered orally and intramuscularly for the prophylaxis and treatment of thiamine deficiency states.

t. mononitrate [USP] the mononitrate salt of thiamine, used in the preparation of various multivitamin dosage forms.

t. pyrophosphate (TPP) the active form of thiamine, which serves as a coenzyme in a variety of reactions, particularly those involving oxidative decarboxylation of certain important intermediates in carbohydrate metabolism.

thi·a·mine pyr·i·din·yl·ase (thi′ə-min pir-ĭ-din′ə-lās) [EC 2.5.1.2] an enzyme of the transferase class that catalyzes the transfer of the pyrimidine moiety of thiamine from the thiazole ring component to pyridine or another base or thiol compound. The reaction inactivates thiamine. The enzyme occurs in the gastrointestinal tract of many freshwater animals. Called also *thiaminase I*.

thi·am·phen·i·col (thi-əm-fen′ĭ-kōl) a broad-spectrum antibacterial, effective against a wide range of gram-positive and gram-negative organisms.

thi·am·y·lal (thi-am′ə-lal) a very short-acting barbiturate used as an anesthetic.

t. sodium the sodium salt of thiamylal, administered intravenously to produce general anesthesia of brief duration, for induction of anesthesia, to supplement other anesthetics, or to induce hypnosis.

Thi·a·ra (thi-ah′rə) a genus of fresh water snails of the family Thiaridae, found mostly in tropical regions of Africa and Asia; formerly called *Melania*. Some species, such as *T. grani′fera* and *T. tubercula′ta*, act as the main snail hosts of various trematode parasites, including *Paragonimus*, *Metagonimus*, and *Haplorchis*.

Thi·ar·i·dae (thi-ar′ĭ-de) a family of fresh water snails of the subclass Streptoneura, order Mesogastropoda, found in warm regions of Africa, Asia, and various Pacific islands. It includes the genera *Hua* and *Thiara*.

thi·a·sine (thi′ə-sin) ergothioneine.

thi·a·zide (thi′ə-zīd) any of a group of benzothiadiazene sulfonamide derivatives, typified by chlorothiazide, that act as diuretics by inhibiting the reabsorption of sodium in the proximal renal tubule and stimulating chloride excretion, with resultant increase in excretion of water. They also increase the excretion of potassium, which can cause hypokalemia requiring potassium supplementation, and some increase in bicarbonate excretion. Thiazides are used for the treatment of edema due to congestive heart failure or chronic hepatic or renal disease and, alone or in combination with other drugs, in the treatment of hypertension. Called also *benzothiadiazide, benzothiadiazine,* and *thiadiazine.*

-thiazide a suffix indicating a thiazide diuretic.

thi·a·zine (thi′ə-zēn) any of a class of organic heterocyclic chemical compounds containing a six-membered ring having one sulfur and one nitrogen in the ring; used as dyes.

thi·a·zole (thi′ə-zōl) the chemical ring:

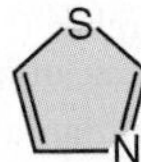

or any substituted derivative containing such a ring.

thi·a·zol·i·dine·di·one (TZD) (thi″ə-zōl″ə-dēn-di′ōn) any of a group of structurally related oral antihyperglycemic agents that increase insulin-stimulated glucose uptake by skeletal muscle cells, reducing insulin resistance in peripheral tissues, and decrease lipolysis in adipocytes.

Thi·bi·erge-Weis·sen·bach syndrome (te-be-erzh′ vīs′ən-bahk) [Georges *Thibierge,* French physician, 1856–1926; Raymond Joseph Emil *Weissenbach,* French physician, 1885–1963] calcinosis.

thick·ness (thik′nis) a measurement across the smallest dimension of an object.

half-value t. see under *layer.*

Breslow t. a method of estimating the prognosis of a melanoma of the skin by determining how far into the skin the lesion extends; thicker tumors have a poorer prognosis.

triceps skinfold (TSF) t. a measurement of subcutaneous fat taken by measuring a fold of skin running parallel to the length of the upper limb over the triceps muscle midway between the acromion and olecranon; used as a means of estimating percentage of body fat.

Thiele syndrome (thēl) [George Henry *Thiele,* American proctologist, 20th century] see under *syndrome.*

Thie·mann disease (te′mahn) [H. *Thiemann,* German physician, early 20th century] see under *disease.*

thi·emia (thi-e′me-ə) [*thi-* + *-emia*] an excess of sulfur in the blood.

thi·en·a·my·cin (thi-en″ə-mi′sin) an antibacterial produced by *Streptomyces cattleya;* it is a precursor of the carbapenems.

Thiersch graft, operation (tērsh) [Karl *Thiersch,* German surgeon, 1822–1895] see *Ollier-Thiersch graft,* under *graft,* and see under *operation.*

thi·eth·yl·per·a·zine (thi-eth″əl-par′ə-zēn) a phenothiazine derivative with sedating antihistaminic effects; used as an antiemetic in the treatment and prophylaxis of nausea and vomiting, particularly that associated with surgery, chemotherapy, radiation therapy, or toxins.

t. malate the malate salt of thiethylperazine, having the same actions and uses as the base; administered intramuscularly.

t. maleate [USP] the maleate salt of thiethylperazine, having the same actions and uses as the base; administered orally or rectally.

thigh (thi) the portion of the lower extremity extending from the hip above to the knee below; in official terminology called *femur.*

cricket t. rupture of some of the fibers of the rectus femoris, which may occur in playing cricket or football; sometimes the tendon of the quadriceps or that of the patella is also ruptured.

drivers' t. sciatic neuralgia caused by pressure from the use of the accelerator in driving an automobile.

Heilbronner t. broadening and flattening of the thigh, seen in cases of organic paralysis but not in hysterical paralysis when the patient lies on his back on a hard mattress.

thig·mes·the·sia (thig″mes-the′zhə) [*thigm-* + *esthesia*] touch (def. 1).

thigm(o)- [Gr. *thigma* touch] a combining form denoting relationship to touch or physical contact.

thig·mo·tax·is (thig″mo-tak′sis) [*thigmo-* + *taxis*] taxis of an organism in response to the stimulus of contact or touch; called also *stereotaxis.* **thigmotac′tic** *adj*

thig·mot·ro·pism (thig-mot′ro-piz-əm) [*thigmo-* + *tropism*] tropism of an organism elicited by touch or direct contact with a solid or rigid surface; called also *stereotropism.* **thigmotrop′ic** *adj*

thim·ble (thim′bəl) 1. coping. 2. see *thimbling.*

thim·bling (thim′bling) horizontal cracks or fissures in the hoof of an animal, such as those resulting from laminitis.

thi·mero·sal (thi-mer′o-səl) [USP] an organomercurial antiseptic, which is actively antifungal and bacteriostatic for many nonsporulating bacteria; used as a topical antiinfective and as a preservative in pharmaceutical preparations. Called also *thiomersalate.*

think·ing (thingk′ing) ideational mental activity (in contrast to emotional activity); the flow of ideas, symbols, and associations that brings forth concepts and reasons.

abstract t. thinking characterized by the ability to appreciate and use metaphors, concepts, and generalizations, to think symbolically, to reason and predict, and to formulate hypotheses and draw conclusions. Cf. *concrete t.*

autistic t. self-absorption; preoccupation with inner thoughts, drives, and idiosyncratic logic; egocentric, subjective thinking lacking objectivity and preferring a narcissistic, inner, private reality to that which is externally validated. Used interchangeably with *dereistic t.,* although differing in emphasis. Called also *autism.*

concrete t. thinking grounded in the literal, limited in the use or understanding of metaphor or nuance, and representing objects or ideas as specific items rather than as abstractions, generalizations, or totalities. Cf. *abstract t.*

dereistic t. thinking not in accordance with the facts of reality and experience and following illogical, idiosyncratic reasoning. Used interchangeably with *autistic thinking,* although not an exact synonym: dereistic emphasizes disconnection from reality and autistic emphasizes preoccupation with inner experience. Called also *dereism.*

magical t. thinking characterized by the belief that thinking or wishing something can cause it to occur; it is normal in childhood and dreams but also occurs in schizophrenia and other mental disorders.

preoperational t. a type of thinking usually characteristic of children between the ages of approximately 2 and 7; it is characterized by a capability for symbolic representation but also by egocentricity and by lack of true understanding of relational terms, the principles of conservation, or the ability to arrange series of objects in order.

primary process t. in psychoanalytic theory, the primitive thought processes deriving from the id and marked by illogical form, preverbal content, an emphasis on immediate wish fulfillment, and an equating of thought and action; characteristic of childhood and of dreams.

secondary process t. in psychoanalytic theory, the more sophisticated thought processes, based on logic, obeying the rules of causality, and consistent with external reality; characteristic of mature conscious thought.

thi(o)- [Gr. *theion* sulfur] a prefix denoting the presence of sulfur. In systematic chemical nomenclature, it indicates the replacement of oxygen by sulfur as in thiophosphoric acid (H_3PSO_3) or ethanethio (CH_3CH_2SH).

thio ac·id (thi″o) an organic compound produced by replacement of one of the oxygens of the carboxyl group by divalent sulfur.

thio·al·co·hol (thi″o-al′kə-hol) mercaptan.

thio·ar·se·nite (thi″o-ahr′sə-nīt) any compound of sulfur and arsenic of the type K_3AsS_3.

thio·bar·bit·u·rate (thi″o-bahr-bit′u-rāt) a salt or derivative of thiobarbituric acid.

thio·bar·bi·tu·ric ac·id (thi″o-bahr″bĭ-tu′rik) a condensation of malonic acid and thiourea, differing from barbituric acid only by the presence of a sulfur atom instead of an oxygen atom at the number 2 carbon; it is the parent compound of a class of drugs, the thiobarbiturates. Thiobarbiturates and barbiturates are analogous in their effects.

thio·car·ba·mide (thi″o-kahr′bə-mīd) thiourea.

thio·cy·a·nate (thi″o-si′ə-nāt) the $S{=}C{=}N^-$ anion or a salt or ester containing this ion. Thiocyanate is produced in the metabolism of cysteine and detoxification of cyanide and is excreted in the urine.

thio·cy·an·ic ac·id (thi″o-si-an′ik) the molecular species $H{-}S{=}C{=}N$; aqueous solutions are an equilibrium mixture of thiocyanic and isothiocyanic acid and are very strong acids. Called also *sulfocyanic acid.*

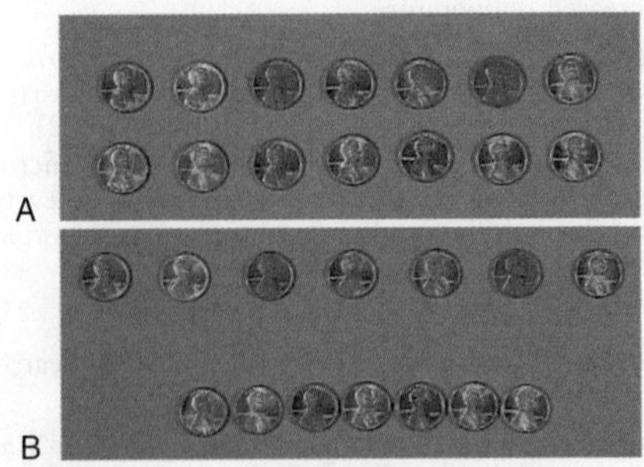

■ Demonstration of preoperational thinking. *(A),* A three- or four-year-old child agrees the two rows have the same number of pennies. *(B),* After seeing the pennies rearranged to this configuration, the child will say the top row has more pennies because it is longer.

thio·cy·a·nide (thi″o-si′ə-nīd) thiocyanate.

thio·di·phen·yl·amine (thi″o-di-fen″əl-am′ēn) phenothiazine (def. 1).

thio·es·ter (thi″o-es′tər) a carboxylic acid and a thiol group in ester linkage, e.g., acetyl coenzyme A.

thio·ether (thi″o-e′thər) a sulfur ether; an ether in which sulfur replaces oxygen.

thio·eth·yl·amine (thi″o-eth″əl-am′in) an amine, $SH(CH_2)_2NH_2$, formed from cysteine by the loss of CO_2.

thio·fla·vine (thi″o-fla′vin) any of several related yellow basic dyes of the thiazole class that fluoresce yellow to yellowish-green when excited by ultraviolet energy; thioflavines S and T are used as histologic stains to detect amyloid.

thio·glu·cose (thi″o-gloo′kōs) a synthetic derivative of glucose in which a sulfhydryl group has replaced the oxygen of the aldehyde group.

thio·gua·nine (6-TG) (thi″o-gwah′nēn) [USP] a thiopurine drug, closely related to mercaptopurine, having multiple metabolic effects that lead to blockade of purine nucleotide synthesis and utilization. 6-TG is cell cycle–specific for the S phase and is used for the treatment of acute myelogenous leukemia, administered orally. Called also *6-thioguanine.*

thio·ki·nase (thi″o-ki′nās) a term used in the trivial names of some enzymes of the ligase class that catalyze the formation of a thioester by joining a carboxylic acid and coenzyme A, coupled to cleavage of a high-energy phosphate bond.

thi·ol (thi′ol) 1. sulfhydryl. 2. any organic compound containing the —SH group; the analogue of an alcohol, which contains the —OH group.

Thi·o·la (thi-ol′ə) trademark for a preparation of tiopronin.

thi·o·lase (thi′o-lās) an enzyme that cleaves a carbon-carbon bond of a thiol compound to form a thioester. See *acetyl-CoA C-acetyltransferase,* and *acetyl-CoA C-acyltransferase.*

thi·ol en·do·pep·ti·dase (thi′ol en″do-pep′tĭ-dās) cysteine endopeptidase.

thi·ol·his·ti·dine (thi″ol-his′tĭ-din) the sulfur derivative of histidine occurring in the betaine form as ergothioneine.

thio·mer·sa·late (thi″o-mur′sə-lāt) thimerosal.

thio·ne·ine (thi″o-ne′in) ergothioneine.

thi·o·nine (thi′o-nēn) a dark green powder, giving a purple color in solution, and used as a metachromatic stain in microscopy. Called also *Lauth violet.*

thi·o·nyl (thi′o-nəl) the radical SO.

thio·pan·ic ac·id (thi″o-pan′ik) pantoyltaurine.

thio·pen·tal so·di·um (thi″o-pen′təl) [USP] an ultra–short-acting barbiturate, administered intravenously or rectally to produce general anesthesia of brief duration, for induction of anesthesia prior to administration of other anesthetics, or to supplement regional anesthesia, and intravenously as an anticonvulsive and for narcoanalysis in psychiatric disorders.

thio·pen·tone (thi″o-pen′tōn) thiopental; see thiopental sodium.

Thio·plex (thi′o-pleks″) trademark for a preparation of thiotepa.

thi·o·pu·rine (thi″o-pu′rēn) 1. a purine base in which a thiol group is found in place of one of the hydroxyl groups. 2. any of a group of drugs that include such a compound as part of their structure.

thi·o·re·dox·in (thi″o-rə-dok′sin) any of a group of small disulfide-containing proteins that serve as oxidoreductases for protein disulfides. Thioredoxin-1 occurs in the cytosol and is important in DNA synthesis and the regulation of transcription factors that control cell growth.

thi·o·rid·a·zine (thi″o-rid′ə-zēn) [USP] a phenothiazine compound having antipsychotic and sedative effects, used in the treatment of schizophrenia and acute psychotic episodes, for the relief of anxiety, agitation, and depression in mood disorders, and for the treatment of disruptive behavior disorders in children; administered orally.

t. hydrochloride [USP] the monohydrochloride salt of thioridazine, having the same actions and uses as the base; administered orally.

thio·strep·ton (thi″o-strep′ton) [USP] an antibacterial compound produced by *Streptomyces azureus,* used in topical antibacterial preparations for veterinary use.

thio·sul·fate (thi″o-sul′fāt) the $S_2O_3^{2-}$ anion or a salt containing this ion. Thiosulfate is produced in the metabolism of cysteine and excreted in the urine. It has also been used as a tracer for measuring extracellular fluid volume and is a commonly used reducing agent in laboratory chemistry and photography. Called also *hyposulfite.* See also *sodium thiosulfate.*

thio·sul·fate sul·fur·trans·fer·ase (thi-o-sul′fāt sul″fər-trans′fər-ās) [EC 2.8.1.1] a mitochondrial enzyme of the transferase class that catalyzes the conversion of cyanide to thiocyanate, using thiosulfate as a sulfur donor. The reaction is the major physiologic mechanism for detoxifying cyanide.

thio·sul·fur·ic ac·id (thi″o-səl-fūr′ik) the molecular species $H_2S_2O_3$.

thio·tepa (thi″o-tep′ə) [USP] an alkylating agent used as an antineoplastic in the treatment of adenocarcinoma of the breast or ovary, papillary carcinoma of the bladder, pericardial or pleural effusions secondary to malignancy, and Hodgkin disease; used by intracavitary, intratumor, intravesical, or intravenous administration. Called also *triethylenethiophosphoramide.*

thio·thix·ene (thi″o-thik′sēn) [USP] a thioxanthene derivative used for the treatment of symptoms of psychotic disorders; administered orally.

t. hydrochloride [USP] the dihydrate dihydrochloride salt of thiothixene, having the same actions and uses as the base; administered orally or intramuscularly.

Thio·tri·cha·les (thi″o-trĭ-ka′lēz) [*thio-* + Gr. *thrix,* gen. *trichos,* hair] a diverse order of bacteria of the class Gammaproteobacteria, phylum Proteobacteria, grouped on the basis of 16S rRNA sequence analysis; some members are obligate parasites of animals. Genera of medical interest are contained in the family Francisellaceae.

thio·ura·cil (thi″o-u′rə-sil) 1. a thiourea derivative that affects adversely the synthesis of the thyroid hormones. It was used as an antithyroid agent in hyperthyroidism. 2. any of several drugs structurally related to thiouracil, e.g., propylthiouracil, which are used in the treatment of hyperthyroidism.

thio·urea (thi″o-u-re′ə) urea in which the oxygen is replaced by sulfur; used as a photographic fixing agent, as an accelerator in vulcanization, and for other purposes. It was formerly used to treat hyperthyroidism but was withdrawn because it is carcinogenic and is a contact allergen. Called also *thiocarbamide.*

alphanaphthyl t., α-naphthyl t. ANTU.

thio·xan·thene (thi″o-zan′thēn) 1. a three-ring compound structurally related to phenothiazine but having the nitrogen atom at position 10 replaced by a carbon atom with a double bond. 2. any of a class of structurally related antipsychotic agents derived from thioxanthene, including flupenthixol and thiothixene.

thi·ram (thi′ram) an antifungal, applied topically and sometimes used to treat seed corn; if animals consume excessive amounts of the corn they may suffer weight loss, dyspnea, lethargy, and convulsions.

thirst (thurst) [L. *sitis,* Gr. *dipsa*] a sensation, often referred to the mouth and throat, associated with a craving for drink; ordinarily interpreted as a desire for water. Called also *dipsia.*

insensible t. subliminal t.

real t. true t.

subliminal t. a sensation of need for water that is not strong enough to prompt the ingestion of water but may be enough to maintain drinking once it is initiated.

true t. thirst which is associated with a bodily need for water and is satisfied by the ingestion of water.

twilight t. subliminal t.

Thi·ry fistula (te′re) [Ludwig *Thiry,* Austrian physiologist, 1817–1897] see under *fistula.*

this·tle (this′əl) any of a number of weedy plants of the family Compositae, having spiny leaves and flower heads surrounded by spiny bracts.

blessed t. 1. a tall, branched, thistlelike herb with pale yellow composite flowers, *Cnicus benedictus,* native to southern Europe. 2. the dried flowers, leaves, and upper stems of *C. benedictus,* used for dyspepsia and loss of appetite; used also in folk medicine for fever and colds and as a diuretic.

milk t. 1. a tall thistle, *Silybum marianum,* native to southern Europe and naturalized in North America. 2. [NF] the dried ripe fruit of *S. marianum,* used for loss of appetite and for supportive treatment in gallbladder and liver disorders.

thix·o·la·bile (thik″so-la′bəl, -la′bīl) easily affected by shaking or stirring.

thix·ot·ro·pism (thik-sot′ro-piz-əm) thixotropy.

thix·ot·ro·py (thik-sot′rə-pe) [Gr. *thixis* a touch + *-tropy*] the property, exhibited by certain gels, of becoming fluid when shaken or otherwise agitated and then becoming semisolid again at rest. **thixotrop′ic** *adj*

Tho·go·to virus (tho-go′to) [*Thogoto* Forest, Kenya, where it was first isolated] see under *virus.*

Tho·ma ampulla, fluid (to′mah) [Richard *Thoma,* German histologist, 1847–1923] see under *ampulla* and *fluid.*

Tho·ma-Zeiss counting chamber (counting cell) (to′mah tsīs′) [R. *Thoma;* Carl *Zeiss,* German optician, 1816–1888] see under *chamber.*

Thom·as shunt (tom′əs) [G.I. *Thomas,* American nephrologist, 20th century] see under *shunt.*

Thom·as sign, splint, test (tom′əs) [Hugh Owen *Thomas,* English orthopedic surgeon, 1834–1891] see under *sign, splint,* and *test.*

Thomp·son arthroplasty, prosthesis (tomp′sən) [Frederick Roeck *Thompson*, American orthopedic surgeon, 1907–1983] see under *arthroplasty* and *prosthesis.*

Thom·sen disease (tom′sen) [Asmus Julius Thomas *Thomsen*, Danish physician, 1815–1896] the autosomal dominant form of myotonia congenita (q.v.).

Thom·son disease (tom′sən) [Mathew Sidney *Thomson*, English dermatologist, 1894–1969] see under *disease.*

Thom·son scattering (tom′sən) [Sir Joseph John *Thomson*, English physicist, 1856–1940] see under *scattering.*

thon·zo·ni·um bro·mide (thon-zo′ne-əm) a cationic detergent used as an additive to ear drops to enhance tissue contact by dispersion and penetration of cellular debris.

tho·ra·cal (thor′ə-kəl) thoracic.

tho·ra·cal·gia (thor″ə-kal′jə) [*thorac-* + *-algia*] 1. pain in the chest; see also *pleurodynia* and *costalgia.* Called also *pectoralgia, stethalgia,* and *thoracodynia.* 2. pectoralgia (def. 1).

tho·ra·cec·to·my (thor″ə-sek′tə-me) [*thorac-* + *-ectomy*] thoracotomy with resection of a portion of a rib.

tho·ra·cen·te·sis (thor″ə-sen-te′sis) [*thorac-* + *-centesis*] paracentesis of the thoracic cavity for aspiration of fluids; called also *pleuracentesis, pleurocentesis,* and *thoracocentesis.*

tho·ra·ces (tho′rə-sēz) plural of *thorax.*

tho·rac·ic (thə-ras′ik) [L. *thoracicus;* Gr. *thōrakikos*] pertaining to or affecting the thorax (chest). Called also *pectoral.*

tho·rac·i·co·ab·dom·i·nal (thə-ras″ĭ-ko-ab-dom′ĭ-nəl) thoracoabdominal.

tho·rac·i·co·hu·mer·al (thə-ras″ĭ-ko-hu′mər-əl) pertaining to the thorax and the humerus.

tho·raci·spi·nal (thə-ras″ĭ-spi′nəl) pertaining to the thoracic portion of the vertebral column (thoracic spine).

thorac(o)- [Gr. *thōrax*, gen. *thōrakos* chest] a combining form denoting relationship to the chest.

tho·ra·co·ab·dom·i·nal (thor″ə-ko-ab-dom′ĭ-nəl) pertaining to the thorax and the abdomen. Called also *abdominothoracic* and *thoracicoabdominal.*

tho·ra·co·acro·mi·al (thor″ə-ko-ə-kro′me-əl) pertaining to the thorax and the acromion.

tho·ra·co·cen·te·sis (thor″ə-ko-sen-te′sis) thoracentesis.

tho·ra·co·cyl·lo·sis (thor″ə-ko-sĭ-lo′sis) [*thoraco-* + Gr. *kyllōsis* crippling] deformity of the chest.

tho·ra·co·cyr·to·sis (thor″ə-ko-sir-to′sis) [*thoraco-* + *cyrtosis*] abnormal curvature of the thorax, or unusual prominence of the chest.

tho·ra·co·del·phus (thor″ə-ko-del′fəs) [*thoraco-* + *-adelphus*] conjoined twins with one head, two upper limbs, and four lower limbs, the bodies being joined superior to the umbilicus.

tho·ra·co·did·y·mus (thor″ə-ko-did′ĭ-məs) thoracopagus.

tho·ra·co·dyn·ia (thor″ə-ko-din′e-ə) 1. thoracalgia (def. 1). 2. pectoralgia (def. 1).

tho·ra·co·gas·tros·chi·sis (thor″ə-ko-gas-tros′kĭ-sis) [*thoraco-* + *gastro-* + *-schisis*] congenital fissure of the thorax and abdomen; cf. *celosomia.*

tho·ra·co·lap·a·rot·o·my (thor″ə-ko-lap″ə-rot′ə-me) [*thoraco-* + *laparo-* + *-tomy*] incision through both the thorax and abdomen to gain access to the subphrenic space and adjoining regions.

tho·ra·co·lum·bar (thor″ə-ko-lum′bər, -bahr) pertaining to the thoracic and lumbar parts of the spine.

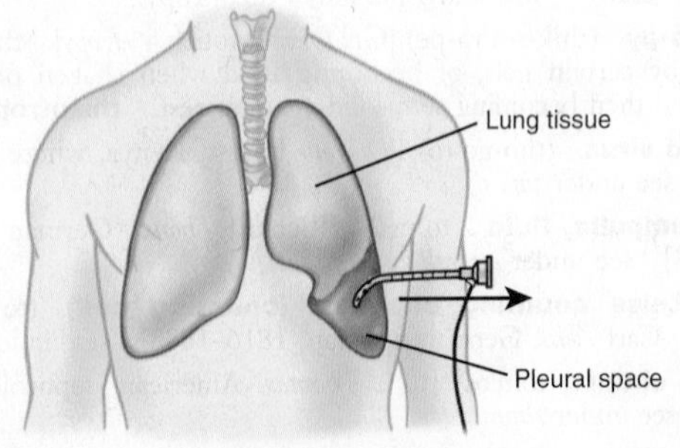

■ Thoracentesis.

tho·ra·col·y·sis (thor″ə-kol′ĭ-sis) [*thoraco-* + *-lysis*] the freeing of adhesions of the chest wall.

tho·ra·com·e·lus (thor″ə-kom′ə-ləs) [*thoraco-* + Gr. *melos* limb] a fetus with a supernumerary limb attached to the thorax.

tho·ra·com·e·ter (tho″rə-kom′ə-tər) [*thoraco-* + *-meter*] stethometer.

tho·ra·com·e·try (thor″ə-kom′ə-tre) measurement of the thorax.

tho·ra·co·om·pha·lop·a·gus (thor″ə-ko-om″fə-lop′ə-gəs) conjoined twins united at the sternum and umbilicus.

tho·ra·cop·a·gus (thor″ə-kop′ə-gəs) [*thoraco-* + *-pagus*] conjoined twins united in or near the sternal region, so that the two components are face to face. Called also *thoracodidymus.*

t. epigas′tricus asymmetrical conjoined twins in which the parasitic twin is attached to the epigastric region of the larger twin.

t. parasi′ticus asymmetrical conjoined twins in which the parasitic twin is attached to the thorax of the larger twin.

tho·ra·co·para·ceph·a·lus (thor″ə-ko-par″ə-sef′ə-ləs) [*thoraco-* + *para-* + *-cephalus*] asymmetrical conjoined twins, a parasitic twin with rudimentary head being attached to the thorax of the larger twin.

tho·ra·cop·a·thy (thor″ə-kop′ə-the) [*thoraco-* + *-pathy*] any disorder of the thorax or of the thoracic organs.

tho·ra·co·plas·ty (thor′ə-ko-plas″te) [*thoraco-* + *-plasty*] surgical removal of several ribs in order for the chest wall to move inward and collapse the lung; it was formerly a common method of collapse therapy (q.v.) and is still sometimes done to allow access during thoracic surgery. **thoracoplas′tic** *adj*

costoversion t. thoracoplasty in which several ribs are removed and replaced inside out in order to prevent outward movement of the chest wall.

tho·ra·cos·chi·sis (thor″ə-kos′kĭ-sis) [*thoraco-* + *-schisis*] congenital fissure of the thorax, which may result in herniation of lung tissue. Called also *schizothorax.*

tho·raco·scope (thə-rak′o-skōp) an endoscope for examining the pleural cavity; it is inserted into the cavity through a skin incision in an intercostal space.

tho·ra·cos·co·py (thor″ə-kəs′kə-pe) [*thoraco-* + *-scopy*] the diagnostic examination of the pleural cavity through an endoscope. Called also *pleuroscopy.*

tho·ra·co·ste·no·sis (thor″ə-ko-stə-no′sis) [*thoraco-* + *stenosis*] abnormal contraction of the chest wall.

tho·ra·cos·to·my (thor″ə-kos′tə-me) [*thoraco-* + *-stomy*] 1. surgical creation of an opening in the wall of the chest for the purpose of drainage. 2. the opening so created.

tube t. thoracostomy with insertion of a chest tube for drainage of air or fluid from the pleural space.

tho·ra·cot·o·my (thor″ə-kot′ə-me) [*thoraco-* + *-tomy*] surgical incision into the pleural space through the wall of the chest. Called also *pleuracotomy* and *pleurotomy.*

tho·ra·del·phus (thor″ə-del′fəs) thoracodelphus.

tho·rax (thor′aks) gen. *tho′racis* pl. *tho′races* [Gr. *thōrax*] 1. [TA] chest: the part of the body between the neck and the thoracic diaphragm, encased by the ribs. 2. cavitas thoracis.

amazon t. a chest with only one breast.

barrel-shaped t. barrel chest.

cholesterol t. see under *pleurisy.*

Peyrot t. a chest that is obliquely oval; seen in large pleural effusions.

pyriform t. a pear-shaped thorax, large above, small below.

Thor·a·zine (thor′ə-zēn) trademark for preparations of chlorpromazine.

Tho·rel bundle (to′rəl) [Christen *Thorel*, German physician, 1868–1935] see under *bundle.*

tho·ri·um (Th) (thor′e-əm) [*Thor*, a Norse deity] a rare, heavy, gray metal, atomic number, 90; atomic weight, 232.038. The naturally occurring radioactive isotope ^{232}Th has a half-life of 1.4×10^{10} years and is the parent element of a radioactive disintegration series.

t. dioxide a contrast medium formerly used in radiography of the alimentary tract; its use was discontinued after it was linked to hepatic angiosarcoma.

sodium t. tartrate a contrast medium used especially in radiography of the gastrointestinal tract.

Thor·mäh·len test (tor′ma-lən) [Johann *Thormählen*, German physician, late 19th century] see under *test.*

Thorn syndrome (thorn) [George Widmer *Thorn*, American physician, 1906–2004] salt-losing nephropathy.

Thorn·waldt see *Tornwaldt.*

thor·ough·pin (thur′o-pin) a distention of the synovial sheath of the flexor perforans tendon of the horse at the hock joint. Called also *knee-gall.*

thought broad•cast•ing (thawt brawd′kast-ing) the delusion that one's thoughts are being broadcast to the environment.

thought in•ser•tion (thawt in-sur′shən) the delusion that thoughts that are not one's own are being inserted into one's mind.

thought with•draw•al (thawt with-draw′əl) the delusion that someone or something is removing thoughts from one's mind.

Thr threonine.

thread (thred) a long slender structure, such as a continuous filament of some substance used as suture material.

Simonart t. a band formed by the stretching of adhesions between the amnion and fetus when the amniotic cavity is distended with its fluid; called also *Simonart band.*

thread•worm (thred′wərm) any long slender nematode, such as members of the genera *Capillaria* and *Strongyloides.* Called also *hairworm.*

thready (thred′e) weak, thin; shallow.

thre•o•nine (Thr, T) (thre′o-nēn) 1. α-amino-β-hydroxybutyric acid, a natural essential amino acid necessary for optimal growth in infants and for nitrogen equilibrium in adults. See also table at *amino acid.* 2. [USP] a preparation of threonine used as a dietary supplement.

thre•o•nine de•hy•dra•tase (thre′o-nēn de-hi′drə-tās) an enzyme of the lyase class that catalyzes the dehydration and deamination of threonine, an irreversible step in the degradation of this amino acid.

thre•o•nyl (thre′o-nəl) the acyl radical of threonine.

thre•ose (thre′ōs) an aldotetrose epimeric with erythrose at the 2 carbon.

thresh•old (thresh′ōld) 1. the minimum level of input required to cause some event to occur. 2. limen; that value at which a stimulus just produces a sensation, is just appreciable, or comes just within the limits of perception; see also *absolute t.* and *differential t.* 3. renal t. 4. in anatomy, limen (def. 2).

absolute t. the lowest possible limit of stimulation that is capable of producing sensation; called also *stimulus t.*

achromatic t. the least intensity of the spectrum that produces a sensation of color; reduction of intensity below this point produces a sensation of brightness only, without any color distinction.

anaerobic t. the point during exercise at which the ratio of ventilation to oxygen consumption begins to increase as a result of lactic acidosis.

arousal t. the minimal stimulation necessary to awaken a sleeper.

auditory t. the slightest perceptible sound; called also *minimum audible.*

t. of consciousness the lowest limit of sensibility; the point of consciousness at which a stimulus is barely perceived. Called also *minimum sensibile.*

convulsant t. the minimum amount of electric current or drug required to produce a convulsion in convulsive therapy.

defibrillation t. (DFT) the minimum amount of energy in joules that will consistently terminate ventricular fibrillation.

differential t. the lowest limit of discriminative sensibility; the ratio which the difference of two stimuli must bear to half their sum in order that their difference may be just perceptible.

displacement t. the threshold of perception of a break in the continuity of a contour or of a border; called also *Vernier acuity.*

double point t. the smallest distance apart at which two stimuli of touch are felt as distinct.

erythema t. the size of the radiation dose that is required to cause erythema of the skin.

fibrillation t. the least intensity of an electrical impulse that will cause cardiac tissue to begin fibrillation.

flicker fusion t. critical fusion frequency.

insular t. limen insulae.

neuron t. the degree of stimulation of a neuron that just suffices to call forth a response.

t. of nose limen nasi.

pacing t. the minimal level of electrical stimulation necessary to induce cardiac depolarization consistently.

relational t. the ratio that two stimuli must have to each other in order for the difference between them to be just perceptible.

renal t. the concentration of any of certain substances *(threshold substances)* in the blood plasma above which the substance is excreted by the kidneys and below which it is not excreted.

renal t. for glucose the point of glucose concentration in the blood (180 mg per dL is normal) at which the kidney will excrete glucose (see *glycosuria*). Called also *transport maximum for glucose.*

resolution t. the least distance that two objects may be apart and still be distinguished as two; called also *minimum separabile.*

sensing t. the minimal level of electrical activity necessary for recognition by the cardiac pacemaker as a signal of depolarization.

sensitivity t. absolute t.

speech reception t., speech recognition t. (SRT) the minimum intensity in decibels at which a patient can understand 50 per cent of spoken words; used in tests of speech audiometry.

stimulus t. absolute t.

swallowing t. the minimal stimulation necessary to elicit the reflex action that leads to swallowing.

t. of visual sensation the least possible amount of stimulus that gives rise to the sensation of sight.

thrill (thril) a sensation of vibration felt by the examiner on palpation of the body, such as over the heart during loud, harsh cardiac murmurs; cf. *fremitus.*

aneurysmal t. a thrill felt on palpation of an aneurysm.

aortic t. a thrill felt over the aortic orifice in disease of its valves.

diastolic t. a thrill felt over the precordium during ventricular diastole, as in advanced aortic insufficiency.

fat t. a peculiar thrill sometimes felt in abdominal examinations due to excessive fatness of the parietes.

hydatid t. a tremulous impulse sometimes felt on palpation of the body surface over a hydatid cyst.

presystolic t. a thrill felt just before the systole by the hand placed over the apex of the heart.

purring t. a thrill that resembles the purring of a cat.

systolic t. a thrill felt over the precordium on systole, as in aortic stenosis, pulmonary stenosis, and ventricular septal defect.

thrix (thriks) [Gr.] hair.

-thrix a word termination denoting relationship to hair.

throat (thrōt) 1. pharynx. 2. fauces. 3. the anterior part of the neck.

sore t. see *sore throat,* under *S.*

throb (throb) a pulsating movement or sensation.

throb•bing (throb′ing) beating; attended with a rhythmic beating sensation.

Throck•mor•ton reflex (sign) (throk′mor-tən) [Thomas Bentley *Throckmorton,* American neurologist, 1885–1961] see under *reflex.*

throe (thro) a severe pain or paroxysm.

throm•ba•phe•re•sis (throm″bə-fə-re′sis) thrombocytapheresis.

throm•base (throm′bās) thrombin.

throm•bas•the•nia (throm″bəs-the′ne-ə) [*thrombocyte* + *astheneia*] 1. decreased platelet function; called also *thromboasthenia.* 2. Glanzmann t.

Glanzmann t. a hereditary platelet abnormality characterized by defective clot retraction, prolonged bleeding time, and related symptoms such as epistaxis and inappropriate bleeding. Clinically there is abnormal glass adhesion and impaired aggregation to ADP, collagen, and thrombin. Most cases are autosomal recessive, but a few are autosomal dominant. Called also *thrombasthenia* and *Glanzmann disease.*

Throm•bate III (throm′bāt) trademark for a preparation of antithrombin III.

throm•bec•to•my (throm-bek′tə-me) [*thromb-* + *-ectomy*] excision of a thrombus from a blood vessel.

throm•bi (throm′bi) plural of *thrombus.*

throm•bin (throm′bin) 1. the activated form of coagulation factor II (prothrombin); it converts fibrinogen to fibrin. Called also *fibrinogenase* and *thrombase.* 2. [USP] a sterile protein substance *(topical t.)* prepared from prothrombin of bovine origin through interaction with added thromboplastin in the presence of calcium; used therapeutically as a local hemostatic.

Throm•bin-JMI (throm′bin) trademark for preparations of thrombin of bovine origin.

throm•bin•o•gen (throm-bin′o-jən) factor II; see under *coagulation factors,* at *factor.*

thromb(o)- [Gr. *thrombos* clot] a combining form denoting relationship to a clot, or thrombus.

throm•bo•ag•glu•ti•nin (throm″bo-ə-gloo′tĭ-nin) platelet agglutinin.

throm•bo•an•gi•itis (throm″bo-an″je-i′tis) [*thrombo-* + *angiitis*] inflammation of a blood vessel (vasculitis) with thrombosis.

t. obli′terans an inflammatory and obliterative disease of the blood vessels of the extremities, primarily the lower extremities, occurring chiefly in young men and leading to ischemia of the tissues and gangrene; called also *Buerger* or *Winiwarter-Buerger disease.*

throm•bo•ar•ter•i•tis (throm″bo-ahr″tər-i′tis) thrombosis occurring in association with inflammation of an artery.

t. purulen′ta purulent softening of an arterial thrombosis, with infiltration of the artery walls.

throm•bo•as•the•nia (throm″bo-əs-the′ne-ə) thrombasthenia.

throm•boc•la•sis (throm-bok′lə-sis) thrombolysis.

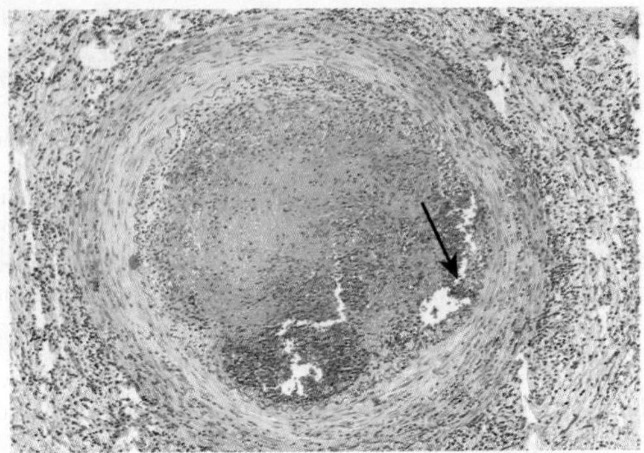

■ Thromboangiitis obliterans. The lumen of the vessel is occluded by a thrombus containing two abscesses *(arrow)*, and the vessel wall is infiltrated with leukocytes.

throm•bo•clas•tic (throm″bo-klas′tik) thrombolytic.

throm•bo•cyst (throm′bo-sist) [*thrombo-* + *cyst*] the chronic sac which may form around a thrombus in a hematoma.

throm•bo•cys•tis (throm″bo-sis′tis) thrombocyst.

throm•bo•cy•ta•phe•re•sis (throm″bo-si″tə-fə-re′sis) [*thrombocyte* + *apheresis*] the selective separation and removal of platelets (thrombocytes) from withdrawn blood, the remainder of the blood then being retransfused into the donor. Called also *plateletpheresis* and *thrombapheresis.*

throm•bo•cyte (throm′bo-sīt) [*thrombo-* + *-cyte*] platelet.

throm•bo•cy•the•mia (throm″bo-si-the′me-ə) [*thrombocyte* + *-emia*] 1. an increase in the number of circulating platelets; called also *thrombocytosis.* 2. essential t.

essential t., hemorrhagic t. a myeloproliferative disorder characterized by a sharp increase in the number of circulating platelets, with repeated spontaneous hemorrhages either externally or into the tissues. Called also *idiopathic* or *primary t.* and *megakaryocytic leukemia.*

idiopathic t., primary t. hemorrhagic t.

throm•bo•cyt•ic (throm″bo-sit′ik) 1. pertaining to, characterized by, or of the nature of a platelet (thrombocyte). 2. pertaining to the thrombocytic series.

throm•bo•cy•tol•y•sis (throm″bo-si-tol′ĭ-sis) destruction of platelets (thrombocytes).

throm•bo•cy•to•path•ia (throm″bo-si″to-path′e-ə) thrombocytopathy.

throm•bo•cy•top•a•thy (throm″bo-si-top′ə-the) any qualitative disorder of the platelets, due most often to deficiency of platelet factor 3. **thrombocytopath′ic** *adj*

constitutional t. thrombasthenia.

throm•bo•cy•to•pe•nia (throm″bo-si″to-pe′ne-ə) [*thrombocyte* + *-penia*] decrease in the number of platelets, such as in thrombocytopenic purpura. See also *pancytopenia.*

essential t. idiopathic thrombocytopenic purpura.

heparin-induced t. a complication of heparin therapy characterized by intravascular clots composed of platelet aggregates. In some sensitive individuals heparin stimulates formation of antibody to the person's own platelets; the antigen-antibody reaction causes clumping of the affected cells and formation of a clot. Called also *white clot syndrome.*

immune t. thrombocytopenia associated with the presence of anti-platelet antibodies (IgG).

infectious cyclic t. thrombocytopenia in dogs recurring every one to two weeks, caused by infection with *Anaplasma platys*; it usually resolves spontaneously in time.

neonatal t., neonatal alloimmune t. immune thrombocytopenia that results when platelets of the fetus express an antigen that is lacking on maternal platelets; fetal platelets enter the maternal circulation and stimulate the production of antibodies, which in turn cross the placenta and destroy fetal platelets.

throm•bo•cy•to•poi•e•sis (throm″bo-si″to-poi-e′sis) [*thrombocyte* + *-poiesis*] the production of platelets. **thrombocytopoiet′ic** *adj*

throm•bo•cy•to•sis (throm″bo-si-to′sis) an increase in the number of circulating platelets; called also *thrombocythemia.*

primary t. essential thrombocythemia.

reactive t., secondary t. thrombocytosis occurring in reaction to some other disease process such as an infection, neoplasm, inflammatory process, or rheumatoid process.

throm•bo•elas•to•gram (throm″bo-e-las′to-gram) the graphic record of the values determined by thromboelastography.

throm•bo•elas•to•graph (throm″bo-e-las′to-graf) an apparatus used in study of the rigidity of blood or plasma during coagulation.

throm•bo•elas•tog•ra•phy (throm″bo-e″las-tog′rə-fe) determination of the rigidity of the blood or plasma during coagulation, by use of the thromboelastograph.

throm•bo•em•bo•lia (throm″bo-əm-bo′le-ə) thromboembolism.

throm•bo•em•bo•lism (throm″bo-em′bo-liz-əm) obstruction of a blood vessel with thrombotic material carried by the blood stream from the site of origin to plug another vessel. **thromboembol′ic** *adj*

throm•bo•end•ar•ter•ec•to•my (throm″bo-end″ahr-tər-ek′tə-me) [*thrombo-* + *endarterectomy*] removal of thrombus and atherosclerotic inner lining from an obstructed artery.

throm•bo•end•ar•ter•i•tis (throm″bo-end-ahr″tər-i′tis) inflammation of the innermost coat of an artery, with thrombus formation.

throm•bo•en•do•car•di•tis (throm″bo-en″do-kahr-di′tis) [*thrombo-* + *endocarditis*] a term formerly used for nonbacterial thrombotic endocarditis or sometimes incorrectly for nonbacterial verrucous endocarditis.

throm•bo•gen•e•sis (throm″bo-jen′ə-sis) the formation of thrombi or blood clots.

throm•bo•gen•ic (throm″bo-jen′ik) [*thrombo-* + *-genic*] producing a thrombus or blood clot.

β-throm•bo•glob•u•lin (throm″bo-glob′u-lin) a platelet-specific protein released with platelet factor 4 on platelet activation; it mediates several reactions of the inflammation process, binds and inactivates heparin, and blocks the endothelial cell release of prostacyclin.

throm•boid (throm′boid) [Gr. *thromboeidēs*] resembling a thrombus.

throm•bo•ki•nase (throm″bo-ki′nās) activated factor X; see under *coagulation factors,* at *factor.*

throm•bo•ki•ne•sis (throm″bo-ki-ne′sis) [*thrombo-* + *kinesis*] blood coagulation.

throm•bo•ki•net•ics (throm″bo-kĭ-net′iks) the dynamics of blood coagulation.

throm•bo•lym•phan•gi•tis (throm″bo-lim″fan-ji′tis) inflammation of a lymph vessel due to a thrombus.

throm•bol•y•sis (throm-bol′ĭ-sis) [*thrombo-* + *-lysis*] lysis of a thrombus or thrombi; it involves a complex series of events, of which the most important involves local action of plasmin within the substance of the thrombus.

intracoronary t. lysis of clots by thrombolytic agents introduced into the coronary arteries; used in thrombolytic therapy after myocardial infarction.

throm•bol•y•so•an•gi•o•plas•ty (throm-bol″ĭ-so-an′je-o-plas″te) the dissolution of arterial thrombi by intra-arterial infusion of a thrombolytic agent followed by balloon angioplasty.

throm•bo•lyt•ic (throm″bo-lit′ik) 1. dissolving or splitting up thrombi. 2. an agent that dissolves or splits up thrombi. Cf. *antithrombotic.*

throm•bo•mod•u•lin (throm″bo-mod′u-lin) an endothelial cell protein that binds protein C and thrombin, allowing the creation of activated protein C.

throm•bon (throm′bon) [*thrombo-* + Gr. *on* neuter ending] the platelets and their precursors; it is the counterpart of *erythron* and *leukon.*

throm•bop•a•thy (throm-bop′ə-the) thrombocytopathy.

throm•bo•pe•nia (throm″bo-pe′ne-ə) thrombocytopenia.

throm•bo•phil•ia (throm″bo-fil′e-ə) [*thrombo-* + *-philia*] a tendency to the occurrence of thrombosis. It can be familial, occurring as a multifactorial trait and resulting from mutation in any of numerous

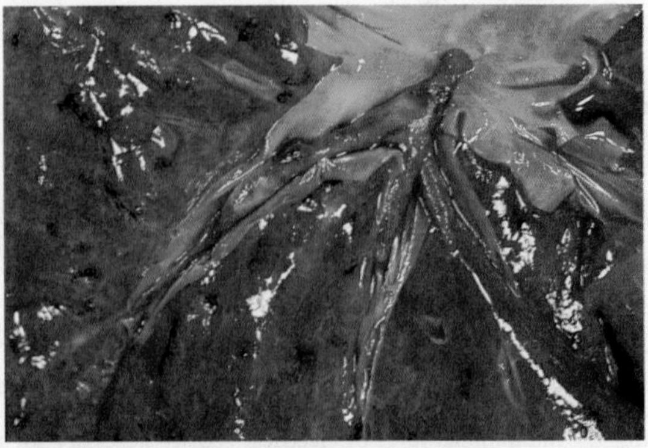

■ Thromboembolism; the main branches of the pulmonary artery are occluded with multiple emboli.

clotting, anticoagulant, or thrombolytic factors, either alone or in combination with each other or with various environmental factors.

throm·bo·phle·bi·tis (throm″bo-flə-bi′tis) [*thrombo-* + *phlebitis*] inflammation of a vein (phlebitis) associated with thrombus formation (thrombosis).

intracranial t. thrombophlebitis in one of the sinuses of the dura mater; see also *sinus thrombosis*.

t. mi′grans, migratory t. a recurring phlebitis usually affecting segments of superficial peripheral veins, and sometimes involving major and visceral veins; it may occur in multiple sites simultaneously or at intervals. Called also *phlebitis migrans*.

postpartum iliofemoral t. thrombophlebitis of the iliofemoral vein following childbirth; see also *phlegmasia alba dolens*.

throm·bo·plas·tic (throm″bo-plas′tik) [*thrombo-* + *-plastic*] causing or accelerating clot formation in the blood.

throm·bo·plas·tid (throm″bo-plas′tid) platelet.

throm·bo·plas·tin (throm″bo-plas′tin) factor III; see under *coagulation factors*, at *factor*.

tissue t. factor III; see under *coagulation factors*, at *factor*. So called because it is released by or derived from extravascular tissues.

throm·bo·poi·e·sis (throm″bo-poi-e′sis) 1. thrombogenesis. 2. thrombocytopoiesis.

throm·bo·poi·et·ic (throm″bo-poi-et′ik) 1. pertaining to or characterized by thrombopoiesis. 2. thrombogenic.

throm·bo·poi·e·tin (throm″bo-poi′ə-tin) a colony-stimulating factor that is the humoral regulator of the production of platelets.

throm·bo·pro·phy·lax·is (throm″bo-pro″fə-lak′sis) the prevention of formation of thrombi. **thromboprophylac′tic** *adj*

throm·bo·re·sis·tance (throm″bo-re-zis′təns) resistance by a blood vessel to thrombus formation; see also *anticoagulation*.

throm·bosed (throm′bōzd) affected with thrombosis.

throm·bo·si·nus·itis (throm″bo-si″nəs-i′tis) sinus thrombosis.

throm·bo·sis (throm-bo′sis) [Gr. *thrombōsis*] the formation, development, or presence of a thrombus. **thrombot′ic** *adj*

atrophic t. marasmic t.

cardiac t. thrombosis in the heart.

caudal vena caval t. thrombosis of the caudal vena cava in cattle, usually because of emboli from a hepatic abscess; it often progresses to embolic pneumonia, which can be fatal.

cavernous sinus t. thrombosis affecting the cavernous sinus.

cerebral t. thrombosis of a cerebral vessel, which may result in a cerebral infarction or thrombotic stroke.

coronary t. development of an obstructive thrombus in a coronary artery, usually associated with atherosclerosis and often causing sudden death or a myocardial infarction.

creeping t. thrombosis gradually involving one portion of a vein after another. See also *propagating t.*

deep vein t., deep venous t. (DVT) thrombosis of one or more deep veins, usually of the lower limb, characterized by swelling, warmth, and erythema; it is frequently a precursor of pulmonary embolism.

dilatation t., dilation t. thrombosis due to the slowing of circulation on account of dilation of a vein.

dural sinus t. sinus t.

effort t. Paget-Schroetter syndrome.

infective t. thrombosis associated with an infection such as septic phlebitis.

intracranial t., intracranial sinus t. sinus t.

marantic t., marasmic t. thrombosis, usually of one of the sagittal sinuses, occurring in the wasting diseases of infancy and of old age; called also *atrophic t.*

mesenteric arterial t. formation of a clot in an artery or arteriole of the mesentery.

mesenteric venous t. formation of a clot in one of the mesenteric veins, leading to ischemia and infarction of the small bowel or colon.

placental t. 1. a normal formation of thrombi in the placenta. 2. an abnormal extension of the placental thrombus formation to the veins of the uterus.

plate t., platelet t. the presence or development of a platelet thrombus.

propagating t. progressive clot formation upon an occlusive thrombus, producing an elongated mass sometimes extending into other blood vessels. See also *creeping t.*

puerperal t. coagulation of blood in the veins after childbirth; see also *postpartum iliofemoral thrombophlebitis*.

sagittal sinus t. sinus thrombosis in a superior sagittal sinus, which can cause stroke syndrome.

sinus t. thrombosis of a sinus of the dura mater, usually secondary to head injury or to infection of a nearby structure; called also *intracranial t.* and *intracranial sinus t.*

traumatic t. thrombosis following injury to a part.

venous t. phlebothrombosis.

throm·bo·spon·din (throm″bo-spon′din) a 450-kilodalton multifunctional glycoprotein secreted by endothelial cells and by the alpha granules of platelets following activation by thrombin; it interacts with a wide variety of molecules, including heparin, fibrin, fibrinogen, platelet cell membrane receptors, collagen, and fibronectin, and plays a role in platelet aggregation, tumor metastasis, adhesion of *Plasmodium falciparum*, vascular smooth muscle growth, and tissue repair in skeletal muscle following crush injury.

throm·bos·ta·sis (throm-bos′tə-sis) stasis of blood in a part, with formation of a thrombus.

throm·bo·sthe·nin (throm″bo-sthe′nin) [*thrombo-* + *stheno-* + *-in* chemical suffix] a contractile protein of platelets, active in clot retraction.

throm·box·ane (throm-bok′sān) [*thrombocyte* + *oxane* ring] either of two compounds related to prostaglandins and derived from arachidonic acid. *Thromboxane* A_2 *(*TXA_2*)* is an extremely potent inducer of platelet aggregation and platelet release reactions and is also a vasoconstrictor; it is thus a physiologic antagonist of prostacyclin. It is synthesized by platelets and is very unstable, with a half-life of 30 seconds, undergoing nonenzymatic hydrolysis to *thromboxane* B_2 *(*TXB_2*)*, which is inactive.

throm·box·ane-A syn·thase (throm-bok′sān sin′thās) [EC 5.3.99.5] an enzyme of the isomerase class that catalyzes the conversion in platelets of prostaglandin G_2 to thromboxane A_2, a potent vasoconstrictor and platelet agonist. Deficient enzyme activity, an autosomal dominant trait, causes defects in the release of platelets. See illustration at *prostaglandin*.

throm·bus (throm′bəs) pl. *throm′bi* [Gr. *thrombos* clot] a stationary blood clot along the wall of a blood vessel, frequently causing vascular obstruction. Some authorities differentiate thrombus formation from simple coagulation or clot formation. Cf. *embolus*.

agonal t. see under *clot*.

annular t. a thrombus which has an opening through its center, while the circumference is attached to the wall of the vessel.

antemortem t. see under *clot*.

ball t. a roughly spherical, organized thrombus which may obstruct an orifice (usually the mitral valve) intermittently like a ball valve.

bile t. a plug in one of the intrahepatic bile ducts, causing cholestasis.

blood plate t., blood platelet t. platelet t.

calcified t. phlebolith.

coral t. a coral-colored thrombus formed by coagulated fibrin and erythrocytes.

currant jelly t. see under *clot*.

fibrin t. a parietal thrombus composed mainly of fibrin.

hyaline t. a thrombus composed of erythrocytes which have lost their hemoglobin, forming a colorless translucent mass.

infective t. the thrombus seen with infective thrombosis.

laminated t. a thrombus whose substance is in layers, suggesting different periods of formation. Called also *mixed t.* and *stratified t.*

lateral t. parietal t.

marantic t., marasmic t. a thrombus associated with severe wasting diseases, often a terminal event; see also under *thrombosis*.

mixed t. laminated t.

mural t. a thrombus attached to the wall of the heart adjacent to an area of diseased endocardium, or to the aortic wall overlying an intimal lesion. Cf. *parietal t.*

obstructive t. occlusive t.

occluding t., occlusive t. a thrombus that occupies the entire lumen of a vessel and obstructs blood flow. Called also *obstructive t.*

organized t. a thrombus that has been invaded by fibroblasts and thereby changed to loose fibrous tissue with varying degrees of vascularity.

pale t. white t.

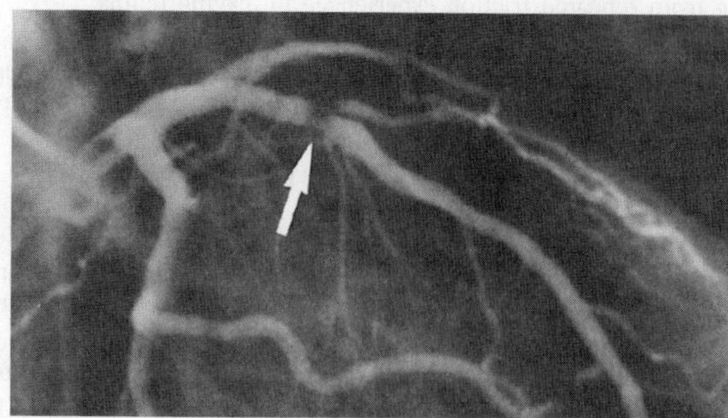

■ Coronary artery thrombus in a patient with unstable angina; coronary angiography shows a globular thrombus *(arrow)* in the anterior interventricular branch of the left coronary artery at the level of, and extending into, the second diagonal branch.

parasitic t. an accumulation of the pigmented bodies of free malarial parasites and their spores in the capillaries of the brain, causing cerebral malaria (q.v.).

parietal t. a thrombus attached to the wall of a vessel. Cf. *mural t.* Called also *lateral t.*

plate t., platelet t. a thrombus formed by an abnormal accumulation of platelets; see also *white t.* (def. 3).

postmortem t. see under *clot.*

primary t. a thrombus that remains at its place of origin.

propagated t. a thrombus that has grown beyond its original limits.

red t. a dark red thrombus formed by the coagulation of blood and composed mainly of erythrocytes.

stratified t. laminated t.

traumatic t. the thrombus seen in traumatic thrombosis.

white t. 1. a thrombus containing few or no red cells. 2. a thrombus composed chiefly of leukocytes. 3. a thrombus composed chiefly of platelets and fibrin, usually seen in arterial thrombosis. Called also *pale t.*

thrush (thrush) 1. candidiasis of the oral mucosa, usually the buccal mucosa and tongue, and sometimes the palate, gingivae, and floor of the mouth. It is characterized by white plaques of soft curdlike material that may be stripped off, leaving a raw bleeding surface. It usually affects sick or weak infants, individuals in poor health, and immunocompromised patients, and less often those who have had treatment with antibiotics. Called also *mycotic stomatitis, acute pseudomembranous candidiasis,* and *oral candidiasis.* 2. an infection of the foot of a horse, with degeneration of the horn and production of a fetid discharge.

thrust (thrust) a sudden forceful movement forward.

paraspinal t. a variant of the spinal thrust in which the therapist's hands are placed on either side of the spinous processes with fingers pointing toward the head.

spinal t. a treatment for lumbosacral strain: with the patient in the prone position on the examining table, the health care provider stands on the right, facing the patient, and places the right palm over the patient's lumbosacral joint perpendicular to the spinal axis. Using the left hand as reinforcement, the worker makes a series of short rapid thrusts downward and toward the head, progressing along each interspace to the midthoracic spine.

tongue t. the infantile pattern of the suckle-swallow in which the tongue is placed between the incisor teeth or alveolar ridges during the initial stages of deglutition, resulting sometimes in anterior open bite, deformation of the jaws, and abnormal function.

thryp·sis (thrip′sis) [Gr. "a breaking in small pieces"] a comminuted fracture.

Thu·ja (thu′jə) [L., from Gr. *thyia*] a genus of coniferous trees of the family Cupressaceae. *T. occidenta′lis* is the white cedar (also called *arbor vitae*), a species native to eastern North America; its leafy twigs contain the medicinal substance thuja but can be poisonous. Oil from its leaves has been used as an expectorant, antirheumatic, and emmenagogue, and externally as a counterirritant and for dermatological diseases. *T. plica′ta* is the western red cedar, which can cause western red cedar asthma in wood products workers.

thu·ja (thu′jə) the fresh tops of *Thuja occidentalis;* used in some topical dermatologic preparations and also in homeopathy.

thu·jone (thu′jōn) an aromatic terpene ketone present in many essential oils and in plants such as species of *Thuja;* it can cause symptoms of neurotoxicity if ingested.

thu·li·um (Tm) (thoo′le-əm) [*Thule*, ancient name of Shetland] a very rare metallic element; atomic number, 69; atomic weight, 168.934.

thumb (thum) pollex.

bifid t. a deformed thumb in which the distal phalanx is divided or bifurcated.

tennis t. tendinitis with calcification in the flexor pollicis longus, resulting from repeated friction experienced in playing tennis.

thumb·print·ing (thum′print″ing) a radiographic sign appearing as smooth indentations on the barium-filled colon, as though made by depression with the thumb; seen in ischemic colitis and various other disorders of the colon.

thump (thump) 1. to strike or beat with a blunt instrument. 2. the blow so incurred.

precordial t. thumpversion.

thumps (thumps) 1. a disease of swine caused by *Ascaris* larvae in the lungs. 2. a kind of singultus, or hiccup, of horses, due to spasm of the diaphragm.

thump·ver·sion (thump-vur′zhən) delivery of one or two blows to the chest in initiating cardiopulmonary resuscitation, in order to initiate a pulse or to convert ventricular fibrillation to a normal rhythm.

thyme (tīm) [L. *thymus*, from Gr. *thymon*] 1. a plant of the genus *Thymus.* Garden thyme is *Thymus vulgaris.* 2. a preparation of the leaves and flowers of *T. vulgaris,* used for cough and bronchitis, often in combination with other herbal preparations.

thy·mec·to·mize (thi-mek′tə-mīz) to remove the thymus gland.

thy·mec·to·my (thi-mek′tə-me) [*thym-*[1] + *ectomy*] surgical removal of the thymus gland.

-thymia [Gr. *thymos* mind + *-ia*] a word termination denoting a condition of mind.

thy·mic (thi′mik) [L. *thymicus*] 1. pertaining to the thymus. 2. contained in or derived from thyme.

thy·mi·co·lym·phat·ic (thi″mĭ-ko-lim-fat′ik) pertaining to the thymus and the lymphatic glands.

thy·mi·dine (thi′mĭ-dēn) a pyrimidine nucleoside, thymine linked by its N1 nitrogen to the C1 carbon of ribose; symbol T. The term is commonly used as a synonym for deoxythymidine (dT), for it was thought that thymidine-containing ribonucleosides do not exist, which would make the prefix deoxy- unnecessary. However, it is now known that thymine, produced by post-transcriptional methylation of uracil, occurs as a rare base in rRNAs and tRNAs; therefore the term should be restricted to the ribonucleoside and ribonucleotide forms.

t. monophosphate a nucleotide, the 5′-phosphate of thymidine, occurring as a rare base in rRNAs and tRNAs.

thy·mi·dine ki·nase (TK) (thi′mĭ-dēn ki′nās) [EC 2.7.1.21] an enzyme of the transferase class that catalyzes the ATP-dependent phosphorylation of thymine deoxyribonucleoside, a reaction of pyrimidine salvage. Because the reaction produces an easily selectable phenotype, the gene and promoter are used extensively in genetic research.

thy·mi·dyl·ate (thi″mĭ-dil′āt) 1. deoxythymidylate; see *thymidine.* 2. a dissociated form of thymidylic acid.

thy·mi·dyl·ate syn·thase (thi″mĭ-dil′āt sin′thās) [EC 2.1.1.45] an enzyme of the transferase class that catalyzes the transfer of a methyl group from 5,10-methylenetetrahydrofolate to deoxyuridine monophosphate, forming deoxythymidine monophosphate and dihydrofolate in the synthesis of deoxythymidine triphosphate. Improperly called *thymidylate synthetase* in older literature.

thy·mi·dyl·ic ac·id (thi″mĭ-dil′ik) 1. deoxythymidylic acid. 2. thymidine monophosphate.

thy·mi·dyl·yl (thi″mĭ-dil′əl) 1. deoxythymidylyl. 2. the radical formed by removal of OH from the phosphate group of thymidine monophosphate.

thy·mine (thi′mēn) a pyrimidine base, in animal cells usually occurring condensed with deoxyribose to form the nucleoside deoxythymidine, a component of deoxyribonucleic acid. The corresponding ribonucleoside, thymidine, is a rare constituent of ribonucleic acids. See also illustration of *purine and pyrimidine bases,* under *base.* Called also *5-methyluracil.*

thy·mine-ura·cil·uria (thi″mēn-ūr″ə-sil-u′re-ə) excess of the pyrimidines thymine and uracil in the urine, as occurs in dihydropyrimidine dehydrogenase deficiency.

thy·min·ic ac·id (thi-min′ik) an acid formed by the splitting up of deoxyribonucleic acid.

thy·mi·tis (thi-mi′tis) inflammation of the thymus.

thym(o)-[1] [Gr. *thymos* thymus] a combining form denoting relationship to the thymus gland.

thym(o)-[2] [Gr. *thymos* mind, spirit] a combining form denoting relationship to the emotions.

thy·mo·cyte (thi′mo-sīt) [*thymo-*[1] + *-cyte*] a lymphocyte found in the thymus; about 10 per cent are mature T cells, and the rest are immature precursors in various stages of maturation.

Thy·mo·glob·u·lin (thi″mo-glob′u-lin) trademark for a preparation of antithymocyte globulin (rabbit).

thy·mo·hy·dro·quin·one (thi″mo-hi″dro-kwin-ōn′) a compound occurring in the urine after the administration of thymol, and also found in various essential oils.

thy·mo·ke·sis (thi″mo-ke′sis) enlargement of the remnant of the thymus that is found in the adult.

thy·mo·ki·net·ic (thi″mo-ki-net′ik) tending to stimulate the thymus.

thy·mol (thi′mol) [NF] a phenol obtained from thyme oil or other volatile oils; used as a stabilizer in pharmaceutical preparations. It has been used for its antiseptic, antibacterial, and antifungal actions.

t. phthalein see *thymolphthalein.*

thy·mo·lep·tic (thi″mo-lep′tik) [*thymo-*[2] + Gr. *lēpsis* a taking hold] any drug that favorably modifies mood in serious affective disorders such as depression or mania; the main categories of thymoleptics include the tricyclic antidepressants, monoamine oxidase inhibitors, and lithium compounds.

thy•mol•phthal•ein (thi″mo-thal′ēn) an indicator with a pH range of 9.3 to 10.5, being colorless at 9.3 and blue at 10.5.

thy•mol•y•sis (thi-mol′ĭ-sis) [*thymo-*[1] + *lysis*] involution or dissolution of the thymus. **thymolyt′ic** *adj*

thy•mo•ma (thi-mo′mə) [*thymo-*[1] + *-oma*] a tumor derived from the epithelial or lymphoid elements of the thymus.

thy•mop•a•thy (thi-mop′ə-the) any disease of the thymus. thymopath′ic *adj*

thy•mo•pen•tin (thi″mo-pen′tin) a pentapeptide immunostimulant, corresponding to amino acids 32–36 of thymopoietin.

thy•mo•poi•e•tin (thi″mo-poi′ĕ-tin) a 5500-dalton polypeptide hormone secreted by thymic epithelial cells that promotes differentiation of precursor lymphocytes into thymocytes.

thy•mo•priv•ic (thi″mo-priv′ik) thymoprivous.

thy•mop•ri•vous (thi-mop′rĭ-vəs) [*thymo-*[1] + L. *privus* without] pertaining to or caused by removal or atrophy of the thymus.

thy•mo•sin (thi′mo-sin) any of several thymic humoral factors, the most active being thymosin α_1, a 3100-dalton polypeptide; it is secreted by thymic epithelial cells, maintains immune system functions, and can restore T cell function in thymectomized animals.

t. β_4 a small (5 kD) actin-binding protein that forms a complex with G-actin and prevents it from polymerizing to form F-actin. See also *profilin.*

thy•mo•tox•ic (thi′mo-tok″sik) toxic for thymus tissue.

thy•mo•tox•in (thi′mo-tok″sin) an element that exerts a deleterious effect on the thymus.

thy•mo•tro•phic (thi″mo-tro′fik) having an influence on the thymus.

Thy•mus (thi′məs) thyme; a genus of herbs of the family Labiatae, native to south central Europe and grown extensively elsewhere. *T. vulga′ris* L. is garden thyme, a source of thyme oil and thymol.

thy•mus (thi′məs) [L., from Gr. *thymos*] [TA] a bilaterally symmetric lymphoid organ consisting of two pyramidal lobes situated in the anterior superior mediastinum. It develops as an outgrowth of the epithelium of the third branchial pouch, which is invaded by lymphoid stem cells that migrate via the blood from the yolk sac and later from the bone marrow. Each lobe is surrounded by a fibrous capsule from which septa penetrate to divide the parenchyma into lobules; each lobule consists of an outer zone, the cortex, relatively rich in lymphocytes (thymocytes), and an inner zone, the medulla, relatively rich in epithelial cells. The thymus is the site of production of T lymphocytes. Precursor cells migrate into the outer cortex, where they actively proliferate. As they mature and acquire T cell surface markers they move through the inner cortex, where approximately 90 per cent die (possibly as part of the acquisition of self-tolerance). The remainder move on to the medulla, become mature T cells, and enter the circulation. T cell maturation is regulated by hormones, including thymopoietin and thymosin, produced by thymic epithelial cells. Congenital athymia or neonatal thymectomy results in complete lack of functional T cells. The thymus reaches its maximal development at about puberty and then undergoes a gradual process of involution (replacement of parenchyma by fat and fibrous tissue), resulting in a slow decline of immune function throughout adulthood.

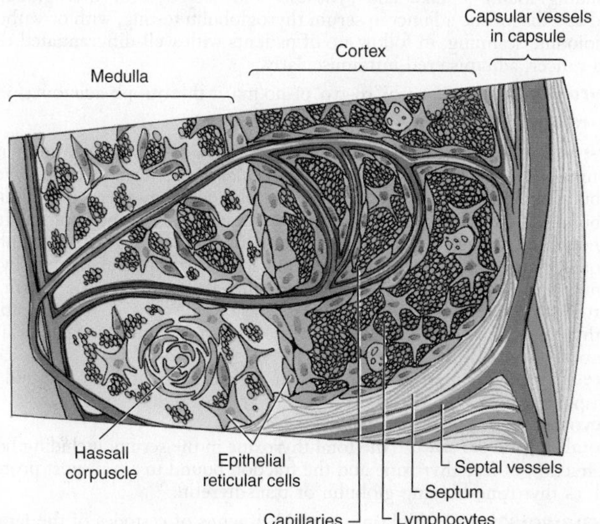

■ Diagram of the thymus demonstrating its blood supply and its histological arrangement.

accessory t. ectopic thymic tissue, separated from the thymus during its descent into the mediastinum during fetal development, occasionally found in the neck.

persistent t., t. persis′tens hyperplas′tica a thymus which persists into adult life, sometimes even becoming hypertrophied.

thy•mus-de•pen•dent (thi″məs-de-pen′dənt) pertaining to T lymphocytes (see under *lymphocyte*). See also under *area.*

thy•mus•ec•to•my (thi″məs-ek′tə-me) thymectomy.

thy•mus-in•de•pen•dent (thi″məs-in-de-pen′dənt) pertaining to B lymphocytes (see under *lymphocyte*). See also under *area.*

thy•ra•tron (thi′rə-tron) a form of discharge tube containing mercury vapor and a multiplicity of electrodes, used as an electric valve to rectify alternating current.

Thy•rel (thi′rel) trademark for a preparation of protirelin.

thyre(o)- for words beginning thus, see those beginning *thyr(o)-*.

thyr(o)- [*thyroid*, q.v.] a combining form denoting relationship to the thyroid gland.

thy•ro•ac•tive (thi″ro-ak′tiv) 1. thyromimetic. 2. thyrotropic.

thy•ro•ad•e•ni•tis (thi″ro-ad″ə-ni′tis) thyroiditis.

thy•ro•apla•sia (thi″ro-ə-pla′zhə) [*thyro-* + *aplasia*] defective development of the thyroid gland with hypothyroidism.

thy•ro•ar•y•te•noid (thi″ro-ar″ĭ-te′noid) pertaining to the thyroid and arytenoid cartilages.

thy•ro•cal•ci•to•nin (thi″ro-kal″sĭ-to′nin) calcitonin.

thy•ro•car•di•ac (thi″ro-kahr′de-ak) pertaining to actions of the thyroid hormones on the heart.

thy•ro•chon•drot•o•my (thi″ro-kon-drot′ə-me) [*thyro-* + *chondrotomy*] median laryngotomy.

thy•ro•col•loid (thi″ro-kol′oid) thyroid colloid.

thy•ro•cri•cot•o•my (thi″ro-kri-kot′ə-me) incision of the cricothyroid membrane.

thy•ro•cyte (thi′ro-sīt) thyroid follicular cell.

thy•ro•epi•glot•tic (thi″ro-ep″ĭ-glot′ik) pertaining to the thyroid and to the epiglottis.

thy•ro•fis•sure (thi″ro-fish′ər) median laryngotomy.

Thy•ro•gen (thi′ro-jən) trademark for a preparation of thyrotropin alfa.

thy•ro•gen•ic (thi″ro-jen′ik) thyrogenous.

thy•rog•e•nous (thi-roj′ə-nəs) [*thyro-* + *-genous*] originating in the thyroid gland.

thy•ro•glob•u•lin (Tg) (thi-ro-glob′u-lin) an iodine-containing glycoprotein of high molecular weight found in the colloid of thyroid gland follicles; it is made by thyroid follicular cells and secreted into the follicular lumen where it is iodinated, after which its iodinated tyrosyl moieties form the iodothyronines thyroxine and triiodothyronine. Thyroglobulins are then taken up by endocytosis into the follicular cells, where the iodothyronines are liberated by proteolysis, followed by release into the extracellular fluid and thence to the bloodstream.

thy•ro•glos•sal (thi″ro-glos′əl) pertaining to the thyroid gland and the tongue.

thy•ro•hy•al (thi″ro-hi′əl) 1. pertaining to the thyroid cartilage and the hyoid bone. 2. cornu majus ossis hyoidei.

thy•ro•hy•oid (thi″ro-hi′oid) pertaining to the thyroid gland or cartilage and the hyoid bone.

thy•roid (thi′roid) [Gr. *thyreoeidēs*, from *thyreos* oblong shield + *eidos* form] 1. glandula thyroidea. 2. pertaining to the thyroid gland *(glandula thyroidea)*. 3. scutiform. 4. [USP] a preparation of cleaned, dried, powdered thyroid gland obtained from domesticated food animals and free of connective tissue and fat; it contains levothyroxine and liothyronine and is used as replacement therapy in the diagnosis and treatment of hypothyroidism, to prevent and treat goiter, and to prevent and treat thyroid carcinoma, administered orally.

aberrant t′s, accessory t′s, ectopic t′s glandulae thyroideae accessoriae.

intrathoracic t. an accessory thyroid gland or thyroid tissue located within the thoracic cavity.

lingual t. an accessory thyroid gland or thyroid tissue located at the base of the tongue, between the foramen cecum and the hyoid bone. It may project into the pharynx, be entirely within the tongue, or be just beneath it; sometimes the normally located thyroid is lacking and this is the only thyroid tissue present.

retrosternal t., substernal t. an accessory thyroid gland or thyroid tissue situated in the thorax behind the sternum.

suprahyoid t. an accessory thyroid gland or thyroid tissue found above the hyoid bone.

thy•roid•ec•to•mize (thi″roid-ek′tə-mīz) to remove the thyroid gland or otherwise suppress its function.

thy•roid•ec•to•my (thi″roid-ek′tə-me) [*thyroid* + *-ectomy*] 1. surgical removal of the thyroid gland. 2. ablation of thyroid function.

chemical t., medical t. pharmacologic suppression of thyroid function.

thy•roid•itis (thi″roid-i′tis) inflammation of the thyroid gland; called also *thyroadenitis.*

acute pyogenic t., acute suppurative t. see *suppurative t.*

atrophic t., atrophic autoimmune t. a type of autoimmune thyroiditis with atrophy of the follicles and without goiter; called also *nongoitrous autoimmune t.* and *primary myxedema.*

autoimmune t. 1. any of various types of thyroiditis characterized by the presence of Askanazy cells and autoantibodies that destroy the gland and cause hypothyroidism; they may occur in any age or sex but particularly affect middle-aged to elderly women. A distinction is made between types with goiter *(Hashimoto disease)* and those without goiter *(atrophic* or *atrophic autoimmune thyroiditis). Riedel thyroiditis* is a less common type, and *Graves disease* is a closely related condition. 2. Hashimoto disease. 3. any of various experimental animal models of thyroiditis.

chronic t., chronic fibrous t. Riedel t.

chronic lymphadenoid t., chronic lymphocytic t. Hashimoto disease.

chronic sclerosing t. Riedel t.

de Quervain t. subacute granulomatous t.

giant cell t., giant follicular t. subacute granulomatous t.

goitrous t. Hashimoto disease.

granulomatous t. subacute granulomatous t.

Hashimoto t. see under *disease.*

invasive t., invasive fibrous t., ligneous t. Riedel t.

lymphocytic t., lymphoid t. Hashimoto disease.

nongoitrous autoimmune t. atrophic t.

painless t. painless, self-limited hyperthyroidism with lymphocytic infiltration of the thyroid gland but without the nonthyroidal features of Graves disease. Called also *silent t.* and *subacute lymphocytic t.*

postpartum t. a type of autoimmune thyroiditis occurring in women after childbirth.

pseudotuberculous t. subacute granulomatous t.

pyogenic t. suppurative t.

radiation t. thyroiditis during or soon after radioiodine therapy, with painful epithelial swelling and narcosis, edema, and disruption of follicular architecture.

Riedel t., sclerosing t. a rare chronic type of autoimmune thyroiditis characterized by a proliferating, fibrosing, inflammatory process that involves usually one but sometimes both lobes, with adhesions to the trachea and other adjacent structures. Called also *chronic fibrous, invasive fibrous, invasive,* or *ligneous t.* and *Riedel disease.*

silent t. painless t.

subacute granulomatous t. a condition characterized by fever and painful enlargement of the thyroid gland, often following a viral infection, especially of the respiratory tract, with granulomas in the gland consisting of masses of colloid surrounded by giant cells and mononuclear cells, and a moderate amount of fibrosis. Called also *de Quervain, giant cell, granulomatous,* or *pseudotuberculous t.*

subacute lymphocytic t. painless t.

suppurative t. a rare, painful inflammation of the thyroid gland caused by an infectious process such as with *Staphylococcus, Streptococcus,* other bacteria, or fungi. Pathogens may invade through a puncture wound or a channel open during fetal life that has remained patent. It is characterized by suppuration and abscess formation and may progress to a subacute or acute stage. In immunocompromised patients it can be caused by opportunistic pathogens.

woody t. Riedel t.

thy•roid•iza•tion (thi″roid-ĭ-za′shən) 1. thyroid replacement therapy. 2. in histopathology, the thyroidlike appearance of a tissue.

thy•roido•ther•a•py (thi″roid-o-ther′ə-pe) thyroid replacement therapy.

thy•roid•ot•o•my (thi″roid-ot′ə-me) 1. median laryngotomy. 2. thyrotomy.

thy•roido•tox•in (thi′roid-o-tok″sin) a toxin specific for thyroid tissue.

thy•roid per•ox•i•dase (thi′roid pər-ok′sĭ-dās) iodide peroxidase.

thy•ro•in•tox•i•ca•tion (thi″ro-in-tok″sĭ-ka′shən) thyrotoxicosis.

Thy•ro•lar (thi′ro-lahr) trademark for a preparation of liotrix.

thy•ro•lib•er•in (thi″ro-lib′ər-in) [*thyro*tropin + *-liberin*] thyrotropin-releasing hormone.

thy•ro•lin•gual (thi″ro-ling′gwəl) thyroglossal.

thy•ro•lyt•ic (thi″ro-lit′ik) [*thyro-* + *-lytic*] destructive to thyroid tissue.

thy•ro•meg•a•ly (thi″ro-meg′ə-le) [*thyro-* + *-megaly*] goiter.

thy•ro•mi•met•ic (thi″ro-mi-met′ik) producing effects similar to those of thyroid hormones or the thyroid gland.

thy•ro•nine (thi′ro-nēn) the *p*-hydroxyphenol ether of tyrosine found in nature as its iodinated derivatives, the iodothyronines.

thy•ro•para•thy•roid•ec•to•my (thi″ro-par″ə-thi″roi-dek′tə-me) excision of the thyroid and parathyroids.

thy•ro•para•thy•ro•priv•ic (thi″ro-par″ə-thi″ro-priv′ik) lacking thyroid and parathyroid glands or secretions.

thy•rop•a•thy (thi-rop′ə-the) [*thyro-* + *-pathy*] any disease of the thyroid gland.

thy•ro•per•ox•i•dase (thi″ro-pər-ok′sĭ-dās) iodide peroxidase.

thy•ro•pri•val (thi″ro-pri′vəl) hypothyroid.

thy•ro•priv•ia (thi″ro-priv′e-ə) hypothyroidism.

thy•ro•priv•ic (thi″ro-priv′ik) hypothyroid.

thy•ro•priv•ous (thi″ro-priv′us) hypothyroid.

thy•rop•to•sis (thi″rop-to′sis, thi″ro-to′sis) [*thyro-* + *-ptosis*] downward displacement of the thyroid gland into the thorax.

thy•ro•ther•a•py (thi″ro-ther′ə-pe) thyroid replacement therapy.

thy•ro•tome (thi′ro-tōm) an instrument for cutting the thyroid cartilage.

thy•rot•o•my (thi-rot′ə-me) [*thyro-* + *-tomy*] 1. median laryngotomy. 2. the operation of cutting the thyroid gland. 3. biopsy of the thyroid gland. Called also *thyroidotomy.*

thy•ro•tox•ic (thi′ro-tok″sik) 1. pertaining to the effects of thyroid hormone excess. 2. affected by thyrotoxicosis.

thy•ro•tox•i•co•sis (thi″ro-tok″sĭ-ko′sis) the condition caused by excessive quantities of thyroid hormones (see *hyperthyroidism*); it may be due to overproduction by the thyroid gland as in Graves disease, overproduction originating outside the thyroid, or loss of storage function and leakage from the gland.

factitious t. thyrotoxicosis caused by accidental or deliberate ingestion of thyroid hormones.

gestational t. thyrotoxicosis during pregnancy, owing to an excess of the normal increase in thyroid gland stimulation. It is usually transient, but if it persists, such as in a woman with Graves disease, she is at higher risk for complications such as preterm delivery or preeclampsia.

thy•ro•trope (thi′ro-trōp) thyrotroph.

thy•ro•troph (thi′ro-trōf) a basophil of the adenohypophysis that secretes thyrotropin; called also *beta basophil* and *thyrotrope* or *thyrotropic cell.*

thy•ro•tro•phic (thi″ro-tro′fik) thyrotropic.

thy•rot•ro•phin (thi-rot′rə-fin) thyrotropin.

thy•ro•tro•pic (thi″ro-tro′pik) having an influence on the thyroid gland.

thy•rot•ro•pin (thi-rot′rə-pin) a glycoprotein anterior pituitary hormone (28,000 daltons) that promotes the growth of, sustains, and stimulates hormonal secretion of the thyroid gland. Called also *thyroid-stimulating hormone.*

t. alfa a recombinant form of human thyrotropin; it binds to thyrotropin receptors and stimulates the steps in thyroid hormone synthesis, including iodine uptake and synthesis and secretion of thyroglobulin; used as a diagnostic adjunct in serum thyroglobulin testing, with or without radioiodine scanning, in follow-up of patients with well-differentiated thyroid cancer, administered intramuscularly.

thy•ro•tro•pi•no•ma (thi″ro-tro″pĭ-no′mə) thyrotroph adenoma.

thy•rox•in (thi-rok′sin) thyroxine.

thy•rox•ine (T_4) (thi-rok′sin) L-3,5,3′,5′-tetraiodothyronine, the major hormone elaborated by the thyroid follicular cells, formed from thyroglobulin and transported mainly in the blood serum thyroxine-binding globulin. Its chief function is to increase the rate of cell metabolism. It is also essential for central nervous system maturation and regulates a number of other functions. Thyroxine is deiodinated in peripheral tissues (liver, kidney, and heart) to form triiodothyronine, the active "tissue" form of thyroid hormone, which is much more biologically active. A preparation of thyroxine, levothyroxine (q.v.), is used pharmaceutically. Spelled also *thyroxin.* **thyroxin′ic** *adj*

free t. the fraction of thyroxine in the serum that is not bound to transport protein.

levo t. see *levothyroxine sodium.*

total t., total serum t. the total thyroxine in the serum, including both the fraction of free thyroxine and the fraction bound to a transport protein such as thyroxine-binding globulin or transthyretin.

Thys•a•no•so•ma (this″ə-no-so′mə) a genus of cestodes of the family Anoplocephalidae. *T. actinoi′des,* the fringed tapeworm, is found in the bile ducts and small intestines of ungulates in the western United States and in Africa.

Thy•tro•par (thi′tro-pahr) trademark for a preparation of thyrotropin.

Ti titanium.

TIA transient ischemic attack.

ti·ag·a·bine hy·dro·chlo·ride (ti-ag′ə-bēn) an anticonvulsant agent used as an adjunct to other anticonvulsants in the treatment of partial seizures, administered orally.

ti·a·pro·fen·ic ac·id (ti″ə-pro-fen′ik) a nonsteroidal antiinflammatory drug used for treatment of rheumatoid arthritis and osteoarthritis; administered orally.

Ti·a·zac (ti′ə-zak) trademark for a preparation of diltiazem hydrochloride.

ti·az·ur·il (ti-az′ur-il) a coccidiostat for poultry.

TIBC total iron-binding capacity.

tib·ia (tib′e-ə) [L. "a pipe, flute"] [TA] the shin bone: the inner and larger bone of the leg below the knee; it articulates with the femur and head of the fibula above and with the talus below. **tib′ial** *adj*

saber t., saber-shaped t. a tibia curved outward as a result of gummatous periostitis.

t. val′ga a bowing of the leg in which the angulation is away from the midline of the body.

t. va′ra medial angulation of the tibia in the metaphyseal region, due to a growth disturbance of the medial aspect of the proximal tibial epiphysis; there are both infantile and adolescent types. Called also *Blount disease* and *osteochondrosis deformans tibiae*.

tib·i·ad (tib′e-ad) toward the tibial aspect.

tib·i·a·le (tib″e-a′le) a bone on the tibial side of the tarsus of the embryo, partly represented in the adult by the astragalus.

t. exter′num, t. posti′cum a sesamoid bone found in the tendon of the tibialis posterior muscle.

tib·i·al·gia (tib″e-al′jə) pain in the tibia (shin).

tib·i·a·lis (tib″e-a′lis) [TA] tibial.

tib·io·cal·ca·ne·an (tib″e-o-kal-ka′ne-ən) calcaneotibial.

tib·io·fem·or·al (tib″e-o-fem′ə-rəl) pertaining to the tibia and the femur.

tib·io·fib·u·lar (tib″e-o-fib′u-lər) pertaining to the tibia and the fibula; called also *tibioperoneal*.

tib·io·na·vic·u·lar (tib″e-o-nə-vik′u-lər) pertaining to the tibia and the navicular bone.

tib·io·per·o·ne·al (tib″e-o-per″o-ne′əl) tibiofibular.

tib·io·scaph·oid (tib″e-o-skaf′oid) tibionavicular.

tib·io·tar·sal (tib″e-o-tahr′səl) pertaining to the tibia and the tarsus.

ti·bo·lone (ti′bo-lōn) an anabolic steroid with weak estrogenic, androgenic, and progestogenic properties, used in the treatment of menopausal and postmenopausal symptoms; administered orally.

tic (tik, Fr. tēk) [Fr.] an involuntary, compulsive, rapid, repetitive, stereotyped movement or vocalization, experienced as irresistible although it can be suppressed for some length of time; occurrence is exacerbated by stress and diminished during sleep or engrossing activities. Tics may be psychogenic or neurogenic in origin and are subclassified as either simple, such as eye blinking, shoulder shrugging, coughing, grunting, snorting, or barking, or complex, such as facial gestures, grooming motions, coprolalia, echolalia, or echokinesis.

convulsive t. facial spasm.

diaphragmatic t. spasmodic twitching movements of the diaphragm.

t. douloureux (doo-loo-roo′) [Fr. "painful tic"] trigeminal neuralgia.

facial t. see under *spasm*.

t. de Guinon (də ge-naw′) [Fr.] Gilles de la Tourette syndrome.

habit t. any tic that is psychogenic in origin; called also *habit spasm*.

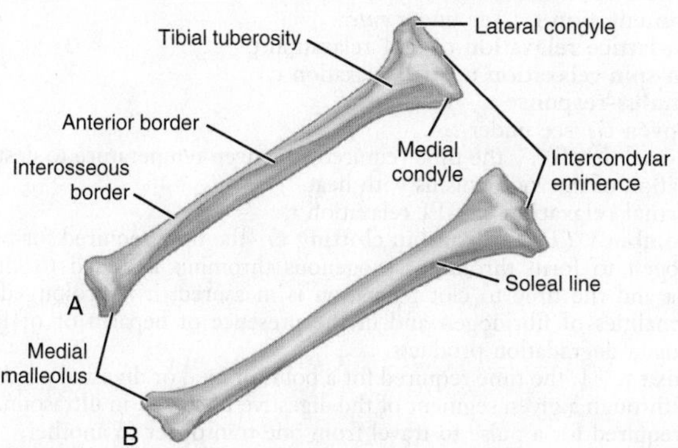

■ Tibia. Anterior *(A)* and posterior *(B)* views of the right tibia.

local t. a tic affecting only a limited locality, as the eye.

mimic t. facial spasm.

rotatory t. see under *spasm*.

saltatory t. see under *spasm*.

t. de sommeil (də so-ma′) [Fr. "tic of sleep"] an involuntary movement of the head during sleep.

Ti·car (ti′kahr) trademark for a preparation of ticarcillin disodium.

ti·car·cil·lin (ti″kahr-sil′in) a semisynthetic broad-spectrum penicillin effective against both gram-negative and gram-positive organisms.

t. disodium [USP] the disodium salt of ticarcillin, used primarily in the treatment of severe systemic infections, septicemia, and infections of the genitourinary tract, the respiratory tract, or the soft tissues due to susceptible strains of bacteria; administered intramuscularly or intravenously.

t. monosodium [USP] the monosodium salt of ticarcillin, having the same actions and uses as the disodium salt.

t. sodium t. disodium.

Tice (tīs) trademark for a preparation of live BCG (bacille Calmette-Guérin) for intravesical use.

tick (tik) a blood-sucking, parasitic arachnid arthropod of the suborder Ixodides, superfamily Ixodoidea. The ticks are larger than their relatives, the mites. There are two families: Argasidae (soft ticks) and Ixodidae (hard ticks).

adobe t. *Argas persicus*.

American dog t. *Dermacentor variabilis*.

argasid t. argasid (def. 2).

bandicoot t. *Haemaphysalis humerosa*.

black-legged t. either of two species of *Ixodes; I. scapularis* is the eastern black-legged tick and *I. pacificus* is the western black-legged tick.

black pitted t. *Rhipicephalus simus*.

bont t. *Amblyomma hebraeum*.

brown dog t. *Rhipicephalus sanguineus*.

brown ear t. *Rhipicephalus appendiculatus*.

castor bean t. *Ixodes ricinus*.

cattle t. any tick that parasitizes cattle, such as species of *Boophilus* or *Rhipicephalus*.

Cayenne t. *Amblyomma cajennense*.

deer t. any of the ticks that infest deer, especially species of *Ixodes* in North America that are vectors for Lyme disease and babesiosis.

dog t. any of the ticks that parasitize dogs, such as *Dermacentor variabilis, Haemaphysalis leachi*, or *Rhipicephalus sanguineus*.

ear t. *Otobius megnini*.

Gulf Coast t. *Amblyomma maculatum*.

hard t., hard-bodied t., ixodid t. ixodid (def. 2).

Kenya t. *Rhipicephalus appendiculatus*.

Lone Star t. *Amblyomma americanum*.

miana t. *Argas persicus*.

Pacific Coast t. *Dermacentor occidentalis*.

pajaroello t. *Ornithodoros coriaceus*.

pigeon t. *Argas reflexus*.

rabbit t. *Haemaphysalis leporispalustris*.

Rocky Mountain wood t. *Dermacentor andersoni*.

scrub t. *Ixodes holocyclus*.

seed t. the young six-legged larva of a tick: after molting it emerges as an eight-legged nymph.

soft t., soft-bodied t. argasid (def. 2).

spinose ear t., spinous ear t. *Otobius megnini*.

taiga t. *Ixodes persulcatus*.

tampan t. 1. *Ornithodoros moubata*. 2. *Argas persicus*.

winter t. *Dermacentor albipictus*.

wood t. *Dermacentor andersoni*.

tick·ling (tik′ling) 1. light stimulation of a body surface, such as stroking the skin, causing a tingling sensation. 2. the sensation of being so stimulated, which may cause reflex responses such as involuntary laughter and withdrawal of the body part; called also *gargalesthesia*. Defs. 1 and 2 called also *titillation*.

tick·over (tik′o-vər) a continuous, low-level activity needing an additional factor to produce any measurable effect, analogous to the idle of an engine; used in describing regulation of the alternative pathway of complement.

Ti·clid (ti′klid) trademark for a preparation of ticlopidine hydrochloride.

ti·clo·pi·dine hy·dro·chlo·ride (ti-klo′pĭ-dēn) a platelet inhibitor used in the prophylaxis of stroke syndrome; administered orally.

tic·po·lon·ga (tik″po-long′ə) [Sinhalese] Russell's viper.

t.i.d. [L.] ter in di′e (three times a day).

ti·dal (ti′dəl) ebbing and flowing like the waters of the oceans.

tide (tīd) 1. the periodic fluctuation in the surface level of the ocean and related bodies of water, caused by the gravitational pull of the moon and sun, or a specific occurrence of such fluctuation. 2. anything that fluctuates in a similar manner, as a physiological variation or increase of a certain constituent in body fluids.

acid t. temporary increase in the acidity of the urine, which sometimes follows fasting.

alkaline t. temporary increase in the alkalinity of the urine during gastric digestion.

red t. a tremendous overabundance of protozoa of the phylum Dinoflagellata in ocean waters, giving them a red tint; some species simply deplete oxygen in the water, but many species contain neurotoxins that can kill fish and other marine life and cause shellfish poisoning (q.v.) in humans who eat contaminated seafood.

Tie•de•mann nerve (te′də-mahn) [Friedrich *Tiedemann*, German anatomist, 1781–1861] see under *nerve*.

Tiet•ze syndrome (tēt′sə) [Alexander *Tietze*, German surgeon, 1864–1927] see under *syndrome*.

Ti•gan (ti′gan) trademark for preparations of trimethobenzamide hydrochloride.

ti•ge•cy•cline (ti″gə-si′klēn) an antibiotic of the glycylcycline group that inhibits bacterial protein synthesis and is effective against a variety of gram-positive and gram-negative organisms; administered intravenously for treatment of complicated skin and intra-abdominal infections.

tig•lic ac•id (tig′lik) an unsaturated fatty acid, *trans*-2-methyl-2-butanoic acid, occurring in triglycerides in croton oil.

tig•li•um (tig′le-əm) gen. *tig′lii* [L.] *Croton tiglium.*

ti•groid (ti′groid) [Gr. *tigroeidēs* tiger-spotted] striped like a tiger, as Nissl bodies or a tigroid fundus oculi.

ti•grol•y•sis (ti-grol′ĭ-sis) chromatolysis.

Tik•o•syn (tik′o-sin) trademark for a preparation of dofetilide.

ti•let•amine hy•dro•chlo•ride (ti-let′ə-mēn) [USP] an anesthetic used in veterinary practice in combination with zolazepam hydrochloride.

Til•ia (til′e-ə) the lindens, a genus of deciduous trees of the family Tiliaceae, native to Europe and eastern North America, which have heart-shaped leaves and fragrant flowers. The wood, leaves, and flowers of *T. corda′ta* (small-leaved linden) and *T. platyphyl′los* (large-leaved linden) are used as folk remedies, particularly as diaphoretics.

Til•laux disease, fracture (te-yo′) [Paul Jules *Tillaux*, French physician, 1834–1904] see under *disease* and *fracture*.

Til•le•tia (tĭ-le′she-ə) a genus of fungi of the family Tilletiaceae, causing smut on cereals. *T. tri′tici* (called also *T. ca′ries*) causes wheat smut.

Til•le•ti•a•ceae (tĭ-le″she-a′se-e) a family of fungi of the order Ustilaginales, including the genera *Tilletia* and *Urocystis.*

til•mi•co•sin (til-mi′kə-sin) [USP] a macrolide antibiotic used as a veterinary antibacterial.

til•mus (til′məs) [Gr. *tilmos* a plucking] floccillation.

til•tom•e•ter (til-tom′ə-tər) an instrument for measuring the degree of tilting of the operating table in spinal anesthesia and other procedures.

ti•lu•dro•nate di•so•di•um (ti-loo′drə-nāt) an inhibitor of bone resorption, used in the treatment of osteitis deformans; administered orally.

tim•bre (tam′bər) [Fr.] a musical quality in a tone or sound.

t. métallique a high-pitched tympanic second sound heard in dilatation of the aorta. When heard in persons under 55 years old, it has been considered suggestive of syphilitic aortitis. Called also *Potain sign* and *bruit de tabourka.*

time (*t*) (tīm) [A.S. tīma] a measure of duration.

Achilles tendon reflex t. assessment of the duration of the triceps surae reflex (Achilles tendon reflex); the phase from the initial tap to half relaxation is prolonged in hypothyroidism, diabetes mellitus, hypothermia, propranolol therapy, local edema, and a few other conditions.

activated partial thromboplastin t. (APTT; aPTT) the period required for clot formation in recalcified blood plasma after contact activation and the addition of platelet substitutes (e.g., brain cephalin or similar phospholipids); used to assess the intrinsic and common pathways of coagulation. A prolonged aPTT can indicate a deficiency of a number of factors, including prekallikrein, high-molecular-weight kininogen, factors XII, XI, IX, VIII, X, V, and II, and fibrinogen.

apex t. the interval at which the apex of the summated twitches of a muscle succeeds the second stimulus applied to the same muscle.

bleeding t. the duration of bleeding that follows puncture of the skin; see *bleeding time test*, under *test*.

central motor conduction t. the conduction time of a motor stimulus through pathways in the central nervous system; abnormal increases or decreases indicate pathology.

circulation t. the time required for blood to flow between two designated points, as arm-to-tongue time.

clot retraction t. the time required for 50 per cent of a blood clot to retract from the wall of the vessel containing it; it is prolonged in thrombasthenia and certain other conditions.

clotting t., coagulation t. the time required for blood to clot in a glass tube.

cold ischemia t. the time between the placement of a traumatically amputated body part in ice and the time of surgical replantation.

conduction t. latency (def. 2).

dead t. the amount of time that a system remains unresponsive after the occurrence of some event.

decimal reduction t. the time of heat sterilization required for a 10-fold reduction of viable microorganisms. Symbol D. Called also *D value.*

dextrinizing t. the time required for saliva to convert starch into sugar.

doubling t. generation t. (def. 3).

dwell t. the time that something therapeutic or diagnostic remains inside a patient's body; in peritoneal dialysis, the time needed for the dialysis solution to remain in the body in order for equilibration to be reached on the two sides of the membrane.

generation t. 1. the period of time between the receipt of an infection by a host and the maximal infectivity of that host. 2. the time elapsing from one generation to the next. 3. the time required for all components of a cell culture to multiply by two. Called also *doubling t.*

inertia t. the time required to overcome the inertia of a muscle after the reception of a stimulus from a nerve.

isovolumic relaxation t. (IVRT) the duration of the period of isovolumic relaxation (see under *period*), normally 50 to 70 msec.

lead t. the interval in the natural history of a disease which can be gained by diagnosing it earlier; the interval between the early and usual times of diagnosis.

left ventricular ejection t. (LVET) the interval from systole to closure of the aortic valve, measured on the carotid pulse tracing from the beginning upstroke to the dicrotic notch; it is one of the systolic time intervals (q.v.) measured to assess left ventricular performance.

longitudinal relaxation t. T1 relaxation t.

median survival t. the length of time at which 50 per cent of the patients have died and 50 per cent still survive.

one-stage prothrombin t. prothrombin t.

partial thromboplastin t. (PTT) a measure of the coagulation factors of the intrinsic pathway of coagulation in plasma; now largely superseded by the test of *activated partial thromboplastin t.*

prothrombin t. (PT) the rate at which prothrombin is converted to thrombin in citrated blood with added calcium; used to assess the extrinsic pathway of coagulation. Results indicate the integrity of the prothrombin complex, i.e., of factors II, V, VII, and X, and the test is often used to monitor administration of coumarin-type anticoagulants. Called also *one-stage prothrombin t., one-stage prothrombin time test*, and *Quick test.*

reaction t. the time elapsing between the application of a stimulus and the resulting reaction.

recalcification t. an insensitive measure of hemostasis, calculating the interval required for clot formation when calcium ion is replaced in anticoagulated platelet-rich plasma.

relaxation t. any of several measures of loss of energy by magnetized materials (particularly hydrogen ions) after a magnetizing current is cut off; in magnetic resonance imaging two particularly useful measures are *T1 relaxation t.* and *T2 relaxation t.* (q.v.).

reptilase t. a test of coagulation time similar to the thrombin time, measuring coagulation time of blood to which reptilase has been added; since reptilase is not affected by the presence of heparin, the test can be used in patients receiving heparin therapy.

rise t. 1. the length of time a waveform takes to rise from 10 per cent to 90 per cent of its peak amplitude. 2. in neurophysiology, the time between the start of a change in potential and when it reaches its positive peak.

R peak t. intrinsicoid deflection.

Russell viper venom t. Stypven time test.

sedimentation t. see under *rate.*

spin-lattice relaxation t. T1 relaxation t.

spin-spin relaxation t. T2 relaxation t.

stimulus-response t. reaction t.

Stypven t. see under *test.*

thermal death t. the time required at a given temperature to destroy a population of microorganisms with heat.

thermal relaxation t. T1 relaxation t.

thrombin t. (TT), thrombin clotting t. the time required for plasma fibrinogen to form thrombin: exogenous thrombin is added to citrated plasma and the time to clot formation is measured; it is prolonged with abnormalities of fibrinogen and in the presence of heparin or of fibrin/fibrinogen degradation products.

transit t. 1. the time required for a bolus of food or digested product to travel through a given segment of the digestive tract. 2. in ultrasound, the time required for a pulse to travel from one transducer to another.

transverse relaxation t. T2 relaxation t.

T1 relaxation t. a component of relaxation time representing the time required for longitudinal magnetization of a substance to return to equilibrium with its surroundings after administration of a pulse of radiofrequency energy; different substances have different times that are measured in magnetic resonance imaging. Called also *longitudinal relaxation t., spin-lattice relaxation t.,* and *thermal relaxation t.*

T2 relaxation t. a component of relaxation time representing the time required for decay or loss of transverse magnetization after administration of a pulse of radiofrequency energy; different substances have different times that are measured in magnetic resonance imaging. Called also *spin-spin relaxation t.* and *transverse relaxation t.*

utilization t. latency of activation.

Ti•men•tin (ti-men′tin) trademark for combination preparations of ticarcillin disodium and clavulanate potassium.

tim•er (tīm′ər) a clock mechanism that can be set to automatically signal the end of a given interval of time or to activate or cut off some apparatus at a desired time.

Ti•mo•feew corpuscles (te-mo-fa′ef) [Dmitri Aleksandrovich *Timofeew*, Russian anatomist, late 19th century] see under *corpuscle*.

Ti•mo•lide (ti′mo-līd) trademark for a preparation of timolol maleate and hydrochlorothiazide.

ti•mo•lol (ti′mo-lol) a nonselective beta-adrenergic blocking agent, used topically as the hemihydrate to lower intraocular pressure in treatment of glaucoma.

t. maleate the maleate salt of timolol; used topically to lower intraocular pressure in the treatment of glaucoma and ocular hypertension; also used orally in the treatment of hypertension, the treatment and prophylaxis of recurrent myocardial infarction, and the prophylaxis of migraine.

Ti•mop•tic (ti-mop′tik) trademark for a preparation of timolol maleate.

tim•o•thy (tim′ə-the) *Phleum pratense.*

tin (Sn) (tin) a white metallic element; atomic number, 50; atomic weight, 118.69; valence 2 or 4. Some of its salts are reagents, others are stains, while some of its compounds, particularly the oxide, have been tried in medicine. Its organic compounds exhibit moderate but variable toxicity.

t. chloride stannous chloride.

t. oxide stannic oxide.

Tin•ac•tin (tin-ak′tin) trademark for preparations of tolnaftate.

tinct. [L.] tinctura (tincture).

tinc•ta•ble (tink′tə-bəl) stainable or tingible.

tinc•tion (tink′shən) [L. *tingere* to dye] 1. the act of staining. 2. the addition of coloring or flavoring agents to a prescription.

tinc•to•ri•al (tink-tor′e-əl) pertaining to dyeing or staining.

tinc•tu•ra (tink-tu′rə) gen. and pl. *tinctu′rae* [L.] tincture.

tinc•tur•a•tion (tink″chər-a′shən) the preparation of a tincture; the treatment of a drug with a menstruum, such as alcohol or ether, for the purpose of preparing a tincture.

tinc•ture (tink′chər) [L. *tingere* to wet, to moisten] an alcoholic or hydroalcoholic solution prepared from vegetable materials or from chemical substances.

belladonna t. [USP] an alcoholic preparation containing, in each 100 mL, between 27 and 33 mg of alkaloids of belladonna leaf and having anticholinergic and antimuscarinic effects; it has been used as an antispasmodic for disorders of the gastrointestinal tract. Cf. *belladonna extract.*

camphorated opium t. paregoric.

compound benzoin t. [USP] a preparation of benzoin, aloe, storax, and tolu balsam in alcohol, used as a topical skin protectant.

compound cardamom t. [NF] a preparation of powdered cardamom seed, cinnamon, and caraway in glycerin and diluted alcohol; used as a flavoring agent.

deodorized opium t. opium t.

green soap t. [USP] a preparation of green soap, lavender or other essential oil, and alcohol; used as a skin detergent.

iodine t. [USP] a preparation of iodine and sodium iodide in diluted alcohol, used as a topical antiinfective.

lemon t. a preparation produced by the maceration in alcohol of the outer, yellow rind of the fresh ripe fruit of *Citrus limon*; used as a flavoring agent.

opium t. [USP] a preparation containing between 0.90 g and 1.10 g of anhydrous morphine per 100 mL, obtained by percolation of granulated or sliced opium.

strong iodine t. an alcoholic solution containing 6.8–7.5 g of iodine and 4.7–5.5 g of potassium iodide in each 100 mL; used as an irritant, antibacterial, and antifungal agent.

sweet orange peel t. [NF] a preparation produced by the maceration in alcohol of the outer rind of the nonartificially colored fresh ripe fruit of *Citrus sinensis;* used as a flavoring agent.

tolu balsam t. a preparation of tolu balsam in alcohol; used in expectorant mixtures and in the preparation of tolu balsam syrup.

vanilla t. [NF] a preparation of vanilla and sucrose in equal parts of diluted alcohol and purified water; used as a flavor.

tine (tīn) [A.S. *tind* a prong] a prong or pointed projection on an implement, as on a fork.

tin•ea (tin′e-ə) [L. "grub," "moth larva," "worm"] any of various dermatophytoses of humans, usually designated by a modifying term depending on appearance of lesions, etiologic agent, or site. Popularly called *ringworm.*

t. amianta′cea misnomer for an inflammatory condition of the scalp, not caused by a fungus, characterized by a dense concentration of white to gray scales that extend upwards to form an asbestoslike encasement on the hair shafts.

t. axilla′ris misnomer for trichomycosis axillaris, which is not a form of tinea.

t. bar′bae tinea of the bearded area of the face and neck. There are three types: in the *inflammatory type*, usually caused by *Trichophyton mentagrophytes* or *T. verrucosum*, lesions are usually kerions or nodules and may produce crusting; in the *ringworm type*, the annular lesions resemble those of tinea corporis; and in the *sycosiform type (t. sycosis)*, caused by *T. violaceum* or less often *T. rubrum*, lesions are follicular pustules containing hairs that may break off and leave a stub or may become epilated. Called also *barber's itch* and *ringworm of the beard.*

t. ca′pitis tinea of the scalp, or sometimes the eyebrows and eyelashes, caused by species of *Microsporum* and *Trichophyton;* it sometimes occurs in epidemics. Depending upon the etiologic agent, it may vary from a subclinical or benign, scaly infection to an inflammatory disease. The latter is marked by scaly, erythematous, papular eruptions with loose and broken-off hairs causing areas of alopecia that can become severely inflamed and form deep, ulcerative kerions resulting in keloid formation, scarring, and permanent alopecia. It has two common types, known as *black dot ringworm* and *gray patch ringworm* (see under *ringworm*). Called also *t. tonsurans* and *ringworm of the scalp.*

t. cilio′rum tinea capitis involving the eyelashes.

t. circina′ta t. corporis.

t. cor′poris tinea involving glabrous skin areas other than hands and feet, usually caused by *Microsporum canis, Trichophyton rubrum*, or *T. mentagrophytes.* The typical lesion is a well demarcated, erythematous, scaly macule with a raised border and central healing that leaves an annular outline. There may also be vesicular, eczematous, psoriasiform, verrucous, plaquelike, and deep lesions. Called also *ringworm of the body* and *t. circinata.*

t. cru′ris tinea in the groin or perineal area, sometimes spreading to nearby regions, seen most often in males who have tinea pedis and have the same etiologic agent for both infections. Characteristics include circumscribed pruritic lesions with raised erythematous margins and thin, dry scaling. Popularly called *jock itch.* Called also *eczema marginatum, ringworm of the groin,* and *t. inguinalis.*

t. fa′ciei tinea of the nonhairy areas of the face, often with a similar presentation to that of t. corporis. Called also *ringworm of the face.*

t. favo′sa favus.

t. fla′va t. versicolor.

t. glabro′sa t. corporis.

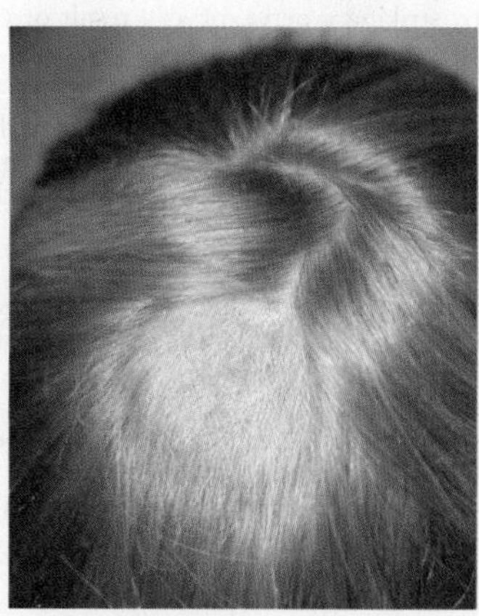

■ Tinea capitis.

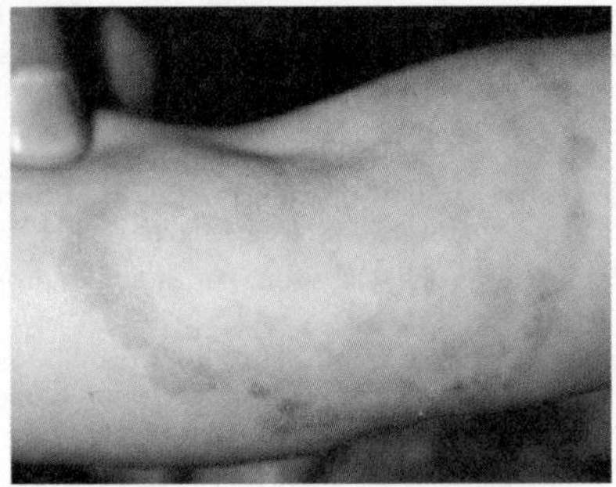

■ Tinea corporis in the cubital fossa.

t. imbrica'ta a chronic tropical type of tinea corporis due to *Trichophyton concentricum*, found on certain South Pacific islands and in Southeast Asia, Central America, and South America. It is seen almost exclusively in persons of Indonesian or Polynesian descent and is characterized by confluent, polycyclic, concentric rings of scaly patches, sometimes over large areas of the body. Called also *Oriental* or *Tokelau ringworm.*

t. inguina'lis tinea cruris.

t. ma'nus, t. ma'nuum tinea of the hands, usually between the fingers or on the palms; it almost always accompanies tinea pedis and has the same etiologic agent. It usually presents as hyperkeratosis of affected skin and may be unilateral, but it may also present as skin exfoliation, circumscribed vesicular patches, discrete, red, papulofollicular patches, or red, scaly sheets on the dorsum. Called also *ringworm of the hand.*

t. ni'gra a minor fungal infection, caused by *Hortaea werneckii*, having dark lesions that look like spattered silver nitrate on the skin of the hands or occasionally other areas. Called also *pityriasis nigra.*

t. pe'dis tinea on the feet, usually between the toes or on the soles, most often caused by *Trichophyton rubrum*, *T. mentagrophytes*, or *Epidermophyton floccosum*. It is characterized by intensely pruritic lesions varying from mild, chronic, and scaling to acute, exfoliative, pustular, and bullous. It may be spread to other parts of the body by autoinoculation; see *t. cruris* and *t. manuum.* Called also *athlete's foot* and *ringworm of the foot.*

t. profun'da trichophytic granuloma.

t. syco'sis the sycosiform type of tinea barbae.

t. tonsu'rans t. capitis.

t. un'guium onychomycosis.

t. versi'color a common, chronic, usually symptomless disorder, characterized by macular patches of various sizes and shapes, with colors from white in pigmented skin to tan or brown in pale skin. It is caused by *Malassezia furfur* and is usually seen in hot, humid tropical regions. Called also *dermatomycosis furfuracea, liver spots, pityriasis versicolor*, and *t. flava.*

Ti•nel sign (te-nel') [Jules *Tinel*, French neurologist, 1879–1952] see under *sign.*

tin•foil (tin'foil) tin foil.

tin•gi•bil•i•ty (tin″jĭ-bil'ĭ-te) the quality of being tingible.

tin•gi•ble (tin'jĭ-bəl) [L. *tingere* to stain] susceptible of being tinged or stained.

ting•ling (ting'gling) a sensation as of repetitive moving pin pricks, caused by cold or by striking a nerve, or as a result of various diseases of the central or peripheral nervous system.

distal t. on percussion Tinel sign; see under *sign.*

ti•nid•a•zole (ti-nid'ə-zōl) [USP] an antimicrobial having properties and uses similar to those of metronidazole, effective against *Trichomonas vaginalis, Entamoeba histolytica*, and *Giardia intestinalis;* administered orally and intravenously.

tin•ni•tus (tin'ĭ-təs, tĭ-ni'təs) [L. "a ringing"] a noise in the ears, such as ringing, buzzing, roaring, or clicking. It is usually subjective in type (see *subjective t.*). Most classifications stress distinctions between *vibratory* and *nonvibratory* types. Called also *t. aurium.*

t. au'rium tinnitus.

central t., t. ce'rebri subjective tinnitus that is experienced as being inside the head rather than in an ear.

clicking t. a type of objective tinnitus in which the patient hears a clicking sound, usually a sign of serous otitis media.

cochlear t. vibratory tinnitus in which the cochlea has been damaged.

Leudet t. a type of objective tinnitus in which the patient hears a crackling sound, produced by involuntary contraction of an internal muscle, coinciding with a tic of fibers of the mandibular division of the trigeminal nerve.

nonvibratory t. a type of subjective tinnitus produced by biochemical changes in the nerve mechanism of hearing. Cf. *vibratory t.*

objective t. a rare type of tinnitus that is audible to others, such as to an examiner with a stethoscope. Cf. *subjective t.*

pulsatile t. vibratory tinnitus in which the sound is rhythmic and synchronous with the heartbeat.

sensorineural t. subjective t.

subjective t. the usual type of tinnitus, in which the sound cannot be heard by an examiner or measured by objective instruments. Subtypes include *vibratory* and *nonvibratory t.* Cf. *objective t.*

tonal t. nonvibratory t.

vibratory t. tinnitus caused by transmission to the cochlea of vibrations from adjacent tissues or organs, most often from blood in vascular malformations. It is usually a type of subjective tinnitus, but occasionally the vibrations are loud enough to be heard by an examiner. Cf. *nonvibratory t.*

tin•tom•e•ter (tin-tom'ə-tər) [*tint* + *-meter*] an instrument used in determining the relative proportion of coloring matter in a liquid.

tin•tom•e•try (tin-tom'ə-tre) the use of the tintometer. **tintomet'ric** *adj*

tin•zap•a•rin so•di•um (tin-zap'ə-rin) a low molecular weight heparin obtained by depolymerization of heparin from porcine intestinal mucosa using an enzyme from *Flavobacterium heparinum;* it acts as an anticoagulant and antithrombotic and is used as an adjunct to warfarin sodium in the treatment of deep vein thrombosis with or without pulmonary embolism, administered subcutaneously.

ti•o•con•a•zole (ti″o-kon'ə-zōl) an imidazole derivative used as a topical antifungal in the treatment of cutaneous candidiasis, tinea corporis, tinea cruris, tinea pedis, and tinea versicolor; also used intravaginally in the treatment of vulvovaginal candidiasis.

ti•o•pro•nin (ti-o'pro-nin) a thiol compound that reacts with cystine to form a soluble mixed disulfide, which can be readily excreted; used in the treatment of cystinuria and the prophylaxis of renal cystine calculi, administered orally.

ti•o•tro•pi•um bro•mide (ti″o-tro'pe-əm) an anticholinergic compound used for the treatment of chronic obstructive pulmonary disease; administered by inhalation.

tip (tip) a pointed extremity of a body part; called also *apex.*

t. of nose apex nasi.

t. of sacral bone apex ossis sacri.

t. of tongue apex linguae.

Woolner t. tuberculum auriculare.

tip•ping (tip'ing) 1. a tooth movement in which its vertical position is altered, either spontaneously or as a result of orthodontic therapy. See also *uprighting.* 2. cusp restoration.

ti•pran•a•vir (ti-pran'ə-vir) an HIV protease inhibitor used in treatment of human immunodeficiency virus infection and the acquired immunodeficiency syndrome; administered orally.

TIPS transjugular intrahepatic portosystemic shunt.

ti•queur (te-kur') [Fr.] a person subject to a tic.

tir•ing (tīr'ing) the operation of passing a wire around a fractured patella, like a tire around a wheel; cerclage.

ti•ro•fi•ban hy•dro•chlo•ride (ti″ro-fi'ban) a platelet inhibitor used in the prophylaxis of thrombosis in patients with acute coronary syndrome (unstable angina or non–Q wave myocardial infarction); administered intravenously.

Ti•se•li•us apparatus (te-sa'le-əs) [Arne Wilhelm Kaurin *Tiselius*, Swedish biochemist, 1902–1971, winner of the Nobel prize for chemistry in 1948] see under *apparatus.*

Tis•seel (tis'ēl) trademark for a fibrin-based sealant.

Tis•si•er•el•la (tis″e-ə-rel'ə) a genus of gram-negative bacteria of the family Peptostreptococcaceae, anaerobic, non–spore-forming, motile rods with peritrichous flagella. The type species is *T. praeacu'ta.*

T. praeacu'ta a bile-sensitive, nonpigmented, nonfermentative or weakly fermentative species isolated from the blood, from gangrenous lesions, and from the intestinal tract of infants and adults; formerly called *Bacteroides praeacutus.*

tis•sue (tish'oo) [Fr. *tissu*] an aggregation of similarly specialized cells united in the performance of a particular function. **tis'sular** *adj*

Tissue

accidental t. a tissue growing in or upon a part to which it is foreign; it may be either *analogous* or *heterologous.*
adenoid t. lymphoid t.
adipose t. connective tissue made up of fat cells in a meshwork of areolar tissue; see *brown adipose t.* and *white adipose t.* Called also *fatty t.*
adrenogenic t. fetal zone of adrenal cortex.
analogous t. accidental tissue that is similar to one found normally in other parts of the body.
areolar t., areolar connective t. textus connectivus laxus.
basement t. the substance of a basement membrane.
bony t. osseous t.
bronchial-associated lymphoid t., bronchus-associated lymphoid t. (BALT) lymphoid tissue associated with the lungs.
brown adipose t. a thermogenic type of adipose tissue containing a dark pigment. It arises during embryonic life in certain specific areas in many mammals, and is prominent in newborn babies. It remains distinct and conspicuous in adults in only certain species, especially those that hibernate. Cf. *white adipose t.* Called also *brown fat.*
bursa-equivalent t., bursal equivalent t. a hypothesized lymphoid tissue in nonavian vertebrates including human beings, equivalent to the bursa of Fabricius in birds: the site of B lymphocyte maturation. It now appears that B lymphocyte maturation occurs primarily in the bone marrow.
cancellous t. the loose spongy tissue of the interior and articular ends of bone.
cartilaginous t. the substance of the cartilages.
cavernous t. erectile t.
cellular t. loose connective tissue with large interspaces.
chondroid t. an embryonic form of cartilage composed of vesicular cells provided with elastic capsules and having collagenous fibers in its interstitial substance. Called also *fibrohyaline t.* and *pseudocartilage.*
chordal t. the tissue of the notochord.
chromaffin t. tissue composed largely of chromaffin cells, well supplied with nerves and vessels; it occurs in the adrenal medulla and also forms the paraganglia of the body.
cicatricial t. the dense fibrous tissue forming a scar or cicatrix and derived directly from granulation tissue; called also *scar t.*
compact t. the hard external portion of a bone.
connective t. the tissue that binds together and is the support of the various structures of the body. It is made up of fibroblasts, fibroglia, collagen fibrils, and elastic fibers, is derived from the mesoderm, and in a broad sense includes the collagenous, elastic, mucous, reticular, osseous, and cartilaginous tissue. Some authorities also include the blood. Two primary types are distinguished according to concentration of fibers: loose (TA, *textus connectivus laxus*) and dense.
cribriform t. textus connectivus laxus.
dartoic t., dartoid t. tissue that resembles the tunica dartos, such as in a tumor with muscular elements; see *leiomyoma cutis.*
dense connective t. connective tissue that has closely packed fibers and does not allow extensive movement of adjacent organs and other structures, in contrast to loose connective tissue.
elastic t. connective tissue made up of elastic fibers, frequently massed into sheets. Called also *yellow elastic t.*
endothelial t. endothelium.
episcleral t. the loose connective tissue over the sclera, between it and the conjunctiva.
epithelial t. epithelium.
epivaginal connective t. connective tissue surrounding the sheath of the optic nerve.
erectile t. tissue containing large venous spaces with which arteries communicate directly, as in the penis and clitoris. Another type formed of dilated venules occurs in the nasal mucosa. The smooth muscle of the nipples constitutes another erectile organ.
extracellular t. the total of tissues and body fluids outside the cells, including the plasma volume and all plasma components, the extracellular fluid volume and its components, plus the intercellular and extracellular tissue solids, most notably the collagen, cartilage, bone, elastin, and other connective tissues of the body framework and viscera.
extraperitoneal t. fascia extraperitonealis.
fatty t. adipose t.
fibrohyaline t. chondroid t.
fibrous t. the ordinary connective tissue of the body, made up largely of yellow or white fibers.
Gamgee T. trademark for a surgical dressing consisting of a thick layer of absorbent cotton between two layers of absorbent gauze.

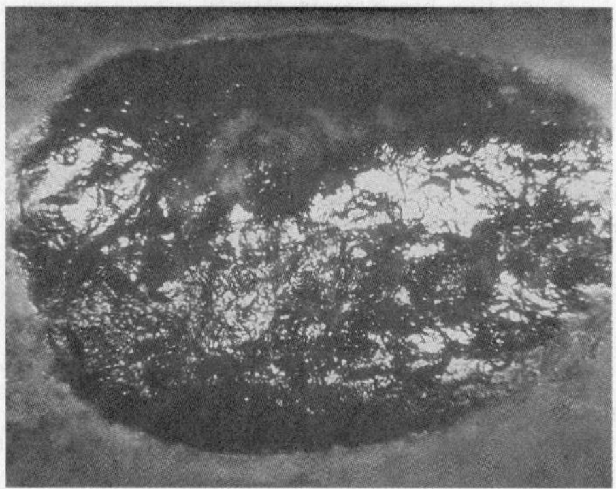

■ Granulation tissue.

gelatiginous t. tissue which yields gelatin on boiling with water.
gelatinous t. mucous t.
glandular t. an aggregation of epithelial cells that elaborate secretions.
granulation t. the newly formed vascular tissue normally produced in the healing of wounds of soft tissue and ultimately forming the cicatrix; it consists of small, translucent, red, nodular masses or granulations that have a velvety appearance.
gut-associated lymphoid t. (GALT) lymphoid tissue associated with the gut (primordial digestive tube), including the tonsils, Peyer patches, lamina propria of the gastrointestinal tract, and appendix.
hematopoietic t. see under *system.*
heterologous t. tissue unlike any other that is normal to the organism.
heterotopic t. choristoma.
homologous t. tissue identical with another tissue in structural type.
hyperplastic t. 1. tissue affected by hyperplasia. 2. in dentistry, an overgrowth of tissue about the maxilla or mandible that is excessively movable, or more readily displaced than is normal.
indifferent t. undifferentiated embryonic tissue.
interstitial t. stroma.
junctional t. the portion of the conducting system of the heart forming a bridge between the atrium and ventricle of the heart, comprising the atrioventricular node and the bundle of His.
Kuhnt intermediary t. glial tissue surrounding the optic nerve and separating it from the retina.
lardaceous t. tissue having the appearance of lard as a result of a degenerative process.
loose connective t. textus connectivus laxus.
lymphadenoid t. tissue resembling that of the lymph nodes, found in the spleen, bone marrow, tonsils, and other organs.
lymphatic t., lymphoid t. a latticework of reticular tissue the interspaces of which contain lymphocytes; lymphoid tissue may be diffuse, or densely aggregated as in lymph nodules and nodes. See also under *system.*
mesenchymal t. mesenchyme.
metanephrogenic t. the nephrogenic tissue of the metanephros; it gives rise to the nephrons of the permanent kidney.
mucosa-associated lymphoid t. (MALT) a type of specialized lymphoid tissue found in association with certain types of epithelia; it usually has prominent B-cell follicles and sometimes has zones of T cells.
mucous t. a jellylike mucoid connective tissue, such as occurs in the umbilical cord.
muscle t., muscular t. tissue specialized for contraction, which produces movement of the body and its parts; it consists of muscle fibers, muscle cells, connective tissue, and extracellular material. Called also *flesh.* See also *muscle.*
myeloid t. medulla ossium rubra.
nephrogenic t. see under *cord.*
nerve t., nervous t. the specialized tissue making up the central and peripheral nervous systems; it consists of neurons with their processes, other specialized or supporting cells such as the neuroglia, and extracellular material.
nodal t. tissue made up of nerve and muscle fibers, such as that composing the sinoatrial node of the heart.

Tissue *Continued*

osseous t. bone that has become ossified, whether normal or of a pathologic change to soft tissue. Called also *bony t.*
osteogenic t. 1. that part of the periosteum adjacent to bone and concerned in the formation of osseous tissue. 2. any tissue capable of generating bone.
osteoid t. uncalcified bone tissue.
parenchymatous t. parenchyma.
protochondral t. centers of chondrification.
reticular t., reticulated t. connective tissue consisting of reticular cells and fibers.
rubber t. rubber in sheets for use in surgery.
scar t. cicatricial t.
sclerous t's a category that includes cartilaginous, fibrous, and osseous tissues.
shock t. the tissue in the animal body that bears the brunt of the antigen-antibody reaction in anaphylaxis.
skeletal t. the bony, ligamentous, fibrous, and cartilaginous tissue forming the skeleton and its attachments.
splenic t. pulpa splenica.
subcutaneous t. tela subcutanea.
subcutaneous t. of abdomen tela subcutanea abdominis.
subcutaneous fatty t. panniculus adiposus.
subcutaneous t. of penis tela subcutanea penis.
subcutaneous t. of perineum tela subcutanea perinei.
sustentacular t. a non-nervous structure of the retina composed of its Müller fibers.
symplastic t. symplasm.
target t. 1. tissue, either in vivo or in vitro, against which humoral or cell-mediated immunity is directed. 2. the tissue that responds specifically to a given hormone.
tuberculous granulation t. the tissue that forms the characteristic tubercle in tuberculosis, composed of epithelioid cells in concentric masses, lymphocytes, and often Langhans giant cells.
vesicular supporting t. chondroid t.
white adipose t. the adipose tissue comprising the bulk of the body fat; called also *yellow adipose t.* Cf. *brown adipose t.*
white fibrous t. fibrous tissue that is composed almost wholly of collagenous fibers.
yellow adipose t. white adipose t.
yellow elastic t. elastic t.

ti•ta•ni•um (Ti) (ti-ta′ne-əm) [L., from Gr. *Titan* a child of Uranus and Gaia] a dark gray metallic element of widespread distribution but occurring in small amounts; atomic number, 22; atomic weight, 47.90; specific gravity, 4.5; used for fixation of fractures. Titanium and its alloys are the most common metals used in dental implants because of their excellent biocompatibility when in contact with hard or soft tissues and their low corrosion rate due to formation of a stable oxide surface film through passivation.

t. dioxide 1. TiO_2, an oxide of titanium used as a white pigment, primarily in paints; workers inhaling excessive amounts of its dust may suffer from titanium dioxide pneumoconiosis. 2. [USP] a purified form of this substance, used as a topical skin protectant and in sunscreens; it is also an ingredient of dusting powders and of pigments for artificial teeth.

ti•ter (ti′tər) [Fr. *titre* standard] the quantity of a substance required to produce a reaction with a given volume of another substance, or the amount of one substance required to correspond with a given amount of another substance.

agglutination t. the highest dilution of a serum that causes agglutination (clumping) of microorganisms or other particulate antigens.

bacteriophage t. the concentration of viable bacteriophage in a given solution.

whole complement t. see *CH50 assay*, under *assay.*

tit•il•la•tion (tit″ĭ-la′shən) [L. *titillatio*] tickling (defs. 1, 2).

ti•tin (ti′tin) an extremely large (about 3000 kDa), flexible polypeptide that occurs in striated muscle, spanning half the length of a sarcomere, and serves as a scaffold to which myofibrils and other muscle-related proteins are attached, also providing elasticity by connecting the ends of the thick filaments to the Z band. It is activated by phosphorylation and by calmodulin binding, facilitates assembly of the sarcomere by providing defined binding sites for other sarcomeric proteins, and has kinase activity. Called also *connectin.*

ti•trant (ti′trənt) the solution of known strength that is added in titration.

ti•trate (ti′trāt) to determine by titration.

ti•tra•tion (ti-tra′shən) [Fr. *titre* standard] determination of a given component in solution by addition of a liquid reagent of known strength until a given endpoint (e.g., change in color) is reached.

colorimetric t. a method of determining hydrogen ion concentration by adding an indicator to the unknown and then comparing the color with a set of tubes containing this same indicator in solutions of known hydrogen ion concentration.

complexometric t. titration of a substance (e.g., the calcium in clear serum) with a complexing agent (e.g., EDTA); the endpoint of the titration is generally observed as a change in color of the solution.

coulometric t. titration by determining the amount of electricity required to electrochemically generate a titrant which reacts with the substance in question. If the current is kept constant, the amount of electricity (coulombs) used is proportional to the elapsed time.

Dean and Webb t. a test for measuring antibody in which varying dilutions of antigen are mixed with a constant quantity of antiserum; antibody activity is determined by the dilution in which flocculation occurs most rapidly, i.e., the endpoint. In this dilution, antigen and antibody are together at a ratio of optimal proportions.

potentiometric t. a method of determining hydrogen ion concentration by placing a hydrogen electrode in unknown solution and measuring the potential developed as compared with some standard electrode by means of a potentiometer.

ti•tre (ti′tər) [Fr.] titer.

ti•trim•e•try (ti-trim′ə-tre) [*titration* + *-metry*] analysis by titration. **titrimet′ric** *adj*

tit•u•bant (tit′u-bant) pertaining to or characterized by titubation.

tit•u•ba•tion (tit″u-ba′shən) [L. *titubatio*] 1. the act of staggering or reeling. 2. a tremor of the head and sometimes trunk, commonly seen in cerebellar disease.

lingual t. 1. stuttering (def. 1). 2. stammering.

Tit•y•us (tit′e-əs) a genus of scorpions of the family Buthidae, found in Central and South America. *T. serrula′tus* is a yellow Brazilian species with a severe sting that can kill children.

ti•ux•e•tan (ti-uks′ə-tan) a linker-chelator that is conjugated with the monoclonal antibody ibritumomab to provide a chelation site for indium 111 or yttrium 90; see *ibritumomab tiuxetan*, under *ibritumomab.*

TIV trivalent inactivated influenza vaccine; see *influenza virus vaccine* (def. 1), under *vaccine.*

tix•o•cor•tol piv•a•late (tik-so′kor-tol) a glucocorticoid with antiinflammatory action, administered rectally in the treatment of ulcerative colitis.

ti•zan•i•dine hy•dro•chlo•ride (ti-zan′ĭ-dēn″) an α_2-adrenergic agonist used as a short-acting agent to manage the increased muscle tone associated with spasticity, as that related to multiple sclerosis or spinal cord injury; administered orally.

TJA total joint arthroplasty.

TK thymidine kinase.

TKA total knee arthroplasty.

TKD tocodynamometer.

TKG tocodynagraph.

Tl thallium.

TLC total lung capacity; thin-layer chromatography.

TLI total lymphoid irradiation.

TLSO thoracolumbosacral orthosis.

TLV threshold limit value.

Tm thulium.

TMA trimellitic anhydride.

TMD temporomandibular disorder.

TME total mesorectal excision.

TMI transmandibular implant.

TMJ temporomandibular joint.

TMJD temporomandibular joint disorder.

TMST treadmill stress test.

Tn normal intraocular tension; see *intraocular pressure*, under *pressure*.

TND transmissible neurodegenerative disease; see *prion disease*, under *disease*.

TNF tumor necrosis factor.

TNKase (te″en-kās′) trademark for a preparation of tenecteplase.

TNM tumor-nodes-metastasis; see under *staging*.

TNS transcutaneous nerve stimulation.

TNT trinitrotoluene.

toad (tōd) any of various tailless leaping amphibians of the order Anura, having rough skin and webbed feet and often used in laboratory experiments. Cf. *frog*. The most common genus is *Bufo*.

clawed t. *Xenopus laevis*.

fire t. *Bombinator igneus*.

fire-bellied t. *Bombina bombina*.

toad•skin (tōd′skin) follicular hyperkeratosis.

toad•stool (tōd′sto͞ol) popular name for a poisonous mushroom.

to•bac•co (tə-bak′o) [L. *tabacum*] 1. any of various plants of the genus *Nicotiana*, especially *N. tabacum*. 2. the dried and prepared leaves of *N. tabacum*; it contains various alkaloids, the principal one being *nicotine*, has qualities of both a sedative narcotic and an emetic and diuretic, and is also a heart depressant and antispasmodic. See also *tobacco poisoning* and *nicotine poisoning*, under *poisoning*.

mountain t. 1. Arnica. 2. arnica.

to•bac•co•ism (tə-bak′o-iz-əm) tobacco poisoning.

To•bey-Ayer test (to′be a′ər) [George L. *Tobey*, Jr., American otolaryngologist, 1881–1947; James Bourne *Ayer*, American neurologist, 1882–1963] see under *test*.

To•bi (to′be) trademark for a preparation of tobramycin.

To•bra•Dex (to′brə-deks) trademark for combination preparations of tobramycin and dexamethasone.

to•bra•my•cin (to″brə-mi′sin) [USP] an aminoglycoside antibiotic, part of the nebramycin complex, effective against a wide range of aerobic gram-negative bacilli and some gram-positive bacteria, having a range of antibacterial activity similar to that of gentamicin; used topically in the treatment of external infections of the eye and its adnexa. It is also inhaled orally in the treatment of *Pseudomonas aeruginosa* infection in patients with cystic fibrosis.

t. sulfate [USP] the sulfate salt of tobramycin, used for the treatment of a wide variety of infections caused by susceptible gram-negative organisms; administered intravenously and intramuscularly.

Tob•rex (to′breks) trademark for preparations of tobramycin.

to•cai•nide hy•dro•chlo•ride (to-ka′nīd) [USP] an oral antiarrhythmic agent, similar to lidocaine in structure and action, used in the treatment of ventricular arrhythmias.

to•cam•phyl (to-kam′fəl) a choleretic obtained from turmeric, $C_{19}H_{26}O_4{\cdot}C_4H_{11}NO_2$.

to•cer•a•nib phos•phate (to-ser′ə-nib) a tyrosine kinase inhibitor with antitumor and antiangiogenic activity, used to treat mast cell tumors in dogs.

toc(o)- [Gr. *tokos* childbirth] a combining form denoting relationship to childbirth, or labor; see also words beginning *tok(o)-*.

to•co•dy•na•graph (to″ko-di′nə-graf) the record obtained with a tocodynamometer.

to•co•dy•na•mom•e•ter (to″ko-di″nə-mom′ə-tər) an instrument for measuring uterine contractions.

to•co•graph (to′ko-graf) a recording tocodynamometer.

to•cog•ra•phy (to-kog′rə-fe) [*toco-* + *-graphy*] the graphic recording of uterine contractions.

to•col (to′kol) the basic unit of the tocopherols and tocotrienols, hydroquinone with a saturated polyisoprenoid side chain at the 6 position; it is an antioxidant.

to•col•y•sis (to-kol′ĭ-sis) [*toco-* + *lysis*] inhibition of uterine contractions.

to•co•lyt•ic (to″ko-lit′ik) 1. pertaining to or causing tocolysis. 2. an agent having such an action.

to•com•e•ter (to-kom′ə-tər) [*toco-* + *-meter*] tocodynamometer.

to•coph•er•ol (to-kof′ər-ol) [*toco-* + Gr. *pherein* to carry + *-ol*] any of a series of structurally similar compounds, methyl-substituted tocols, some of which have biological vitamin E activity.

α-t., alpha t. a doubly methylated tocopherol isomer; it is the most prevalent form of vitamin E occurring in the body and the form administered as a supplement. In nature, it usually occurs with β- and γ-tocopherols. The term is often used synonymously with vitamin E.

to•coph•er•yl (to-kof′ər-əl) the acyl radical of tocopherol.

α-t. acetate a substituted form of α-tocopherol having the same actions and uses; see also *vitamin E*.

α-t. acid succinate a substituted form of α-tocopherol having the same actions and uses; see also *vitamin E*.

to•co•pho•bia (to″ko-fo′be-ə) [*toco-* + *-phobia*] irrational fear of childbirth.

to•co•tri•en•ol (to″ko-tri′ə-nol) any of a series of structurally similar compounds derived from tocol, at least some of which have biological vitamin E activity; they are similar to tocopherols but their isoprenoid side chains are unsaturated.

To•da•ro tendon (to-dah′ro) [Francesco *Todaro*, Italian physician, 1839–1918] see under *tendon*.

Todd bodies (tod) [John Launcelot *Todd*, Canadian physician, 1876–1949] see under *body*.

Todd paralysis (palsy) (tod) [Robert Bentley *Todd*, Irish physician, 1809–1860] see under *paralysis*.

Todd-Wells apparatus, technique (tod′ welz′) [Edwin M. *Todd*, American neurosurgeon, 20th century; T.H. *Wells*, Jr., American neurosurgeon, 20th century] see under *apparatus* and *technique*.

Tod•dal•ia (to-dal′e-ə) a genus of shrubs of the family Rutaceae. *T. aculea′ta* Pers. is an East Indian species whose root is a stomachic and whose root bark is antimalarial and antipyretic.

toe (to) 1. any of the five digits of the foot. See *hallux*, *digitus secundus pedis*, *digitus tertius pedis*, *digitus quartus pedis*, and *digitus minimus pedis*. 2. the anterior part of a horse's hoof.

claw t. a toe deformity in which the metatarsophalangeal joint is held in extension while the proximal interphalangeal joint is fixed in flexion and the distal joint is held in the neutral or slightly flexed position. When a cause is known, it is often an underlying neurologic disorder, such as tethered cord syndrome or Charcot-Marie-Tooth disease; sometimes it may be a complication of rheumatoid arthritis. The metatarsal heads bear weight and become painful during walking so that the patient has a shuffling gait. Called also *cock-up deformity*.

curly t′s a condition affecting chicks, in which the toes curl underneath the feet, due to a deficiency of riboflavin.

fifth t. digitus minimus pedis.

first t. hallux.

fourth t. digitus quartus pedis.

great t. hallux.

hammer t. a condition in which the proximal phalanx of a toe, usually the second, is extended and the more distal phalanges are flexed, causing a clawlike appearance.

little t. digitus minimus pedis.

mallet t. flexion contracture of the distal interphalangeal joint of any of the lesser toes.

Morton t. see under *neuralgia*.

pigeon t. a permanent toeing-in position of the feet.

second t. digitus secundus pedis.

seedy t. a disease of horses' hoofs marked by a horny, honeycombed texture between the coffin bone and the wall. Called also *hollow wall* and *dystrophia ungulae*.

tennis t. pain in the great toe or second toe from a subungual hematoma resulting from trauma to the toe such as in tennis players who repeatedly have sudden stops that force their feet forward in tennis shoes.

third t. digitus tertius pedis.

webbed t′s syndactyly of the toes.

toe•nail (to′nāl) the nail on a toe; see *unguis* [TA].

ingrowing t., ingrown t. aberrant growth of a toenail, with one, or occasionally both, of the lateral margins pushing deeply into adjacent soft tissues. Called also *ingrown nail*, *onychocryptosis*, and *unguis incarnatus*.

To•fra•nil (to-fra′nil) trademark for preparations of imipramine hydrochloride.

To•fra•nil-PM (to-fra′nil) trademark for a preparation of imipramine pamoate.

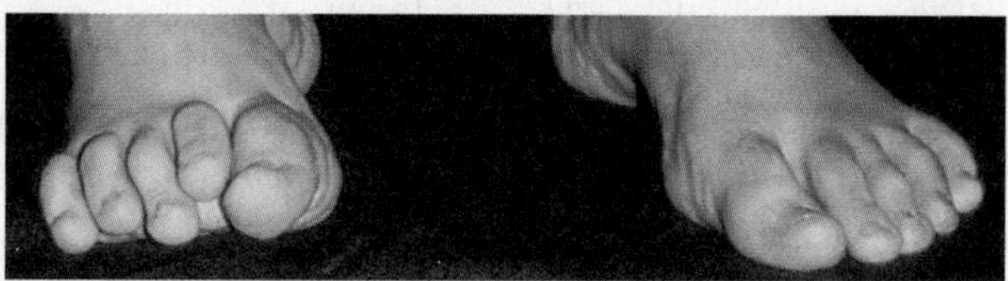

■ Unilateral claw toes in a child with a tethered spinal cord.

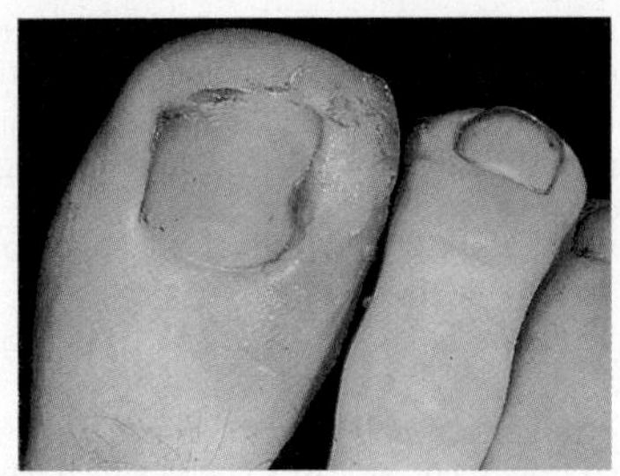

■ Ingrown toenail.

To•ga•vi•ri•dae (to″gə-vir′ĭ-de) the togaviruses, a family of RNA viruses having a spherical virion 60–70 nm in diameter consisting of a lipid-containing envelope, with five peplomers, surrounding an icosahedral nucleocapsid. The genome consists of a single molecule of polyadenylated positive-sense single-stranded RNA (MW 4×10^6, size 9.7–11.8 kb). Viruses contain three or four major structural proteins and are sensitive to lipid solvents, detergents, and ultraviolet radiation. Replication occurs in the cytoplasm and assembly occurs by budding through the plasma membrane. There are two genera: *Alphavirus* and *Rubivirus*.

to•ga•vi•rus (to′gə-vi″rəs) [L. *toga* robe + *virus*] any virus of the family Togaviridae.

toi•let (toi′lət) [Fr. *toilette*] cleansing, as of an accidental wound and the surrounding skin, or of an obstetrical patient after childbirth.

Toi•son solution (fluid) (twah-zaw′) [J. *Toison*, French histologist, 1858–1900] see under *solution*.

To•ke•lau ringworm (to-kĕ-lou′) [*Tokelau*, Islands in the South Pacific, part of New Zealand, where it is commonly observed] tinea imbricata.

tok(o)- [Gr. *tokos* childbirth] for words beginning thus, see also those beginning *toc(o)-*.

to•ko•dy•na•graph (TKG) (to″ko-di′nə-graf) tocodynagraph.

to•ko•dy•na•mom•e•ter (TKD) (to″ko-di″nə-mom′ə-tər) [*toko-* + *dynamometer*] tocodynamometer.

to•la•mo•lol (to-lă′mə-lol) a beta-adrenergic blocking agent which has been used as a coronary vasodilator in the treatment of angina of effort and as a cardiac depressant in the treatment of arrhythmias.

tol•az•a•mide (tol-az′ə-mīd) [USP] a sulfonylurea compound used as a hypoglycemic in the treatment of type 2 diabetes mellitus; administered orally.

tol•az•o•line hy•dro•chlo•ride (tol-az′o-lēn) [USP] an adrenergic blocking agent and peripheral vasodilator used in the treatment of peripheral vascular disorders due to vasospasm, administered orally, and as a vasodilator in pharmacoangiography, administered by intra-arterial infusion.

tol•bu•ta•mide (tol-bu′tə-mīd) [USP] a sulfonylurea compound used as a hypoglycemic in the treatment of type 2 diabetes mellitus; administered orally.

t. sodium the monosodium salt of tolbutamide, having the same actions as the base; used as a diagnostic test for insulinoma (tolbutamide test, q.v.) and for diabetes mellitus and other pancreatic disorders, administered intravenously.

tol•ca•pone (tōl′kə-pōn″) [USP] a reversible inhibitor of catechol *O*-methyltransferase; when administered with levodopa and carbidopa or some other aromatic amino acid decarboxylase inhibitor, it produces more sustained plasma levels of levodopa; used as a treatment adjunct in Parkinson disease; administered orally.

Toldt membrane (tōlt) [Karl *Toldt*, Austrian anatomist, 1840–1920] see under *membrane*.

Tol•ec•tin (tol′ek-tin) trademark for a preparation of tolmetin sodium.

tol•er•ance (tol′ər-əns) [L. *tolerare* to endure] 1. diminution of response to a stimulus after prolonged exposure. 2. the ability to endure unusually large doses of a poison or toxin. 3. drug t. 4. immunologic t.

acquired drug t. drug t.

adoptive t. immunologic tolerance induced by the passive transfer to an irradiated recipient animal of lymphoid cells from a donor rendered tolerant to an antigen.

alkali t. ability of the body to endure the administration of alkalis, measured by the amount of alkali that must be given to cause an alkaline urine; this forms a rough measure of the degree of acidosis.

crossed t. the lessened susceptibility which persons who have acquired a tolerance for one drug or poison may thereafter exhibit toward another drug.

drug t. a decreasing response to repeated constant doses of a drug or the need for increasing doses to maintain a constant response.

glucose t. ability of the body to properly metabolize an administered glucose load; see also *impaired glucose t.*, and see *glucose tolerance test*, under *test*.

high-dose t., high-zone t. see *immunologic t.*

immunologic t. an immune response consisting of the development of specific nonreactivity of the lymphoid tissues to a given antigen that in other circumstances can induce cell-mediated or humoral immunity; it results from previous contact with the antigen and has no effect on the response to non–cross-reacting antigens. Tolerance is readily induced by administration of antigen to immunologically immature animals (fetuses, neonates). In adults tolerance may be induced by repeated administration of very large doses of antigen (*high-dose* or *high-zone t.*), or of small doses that are below the threshold required for stimulation of an immune response (*low-dose* or *low-zone t.*). Tolerance is most readily induced by soluble antigens administered intravenously; immunosuppression also facilitates the induction of tolerance.

impaired glucose t. (IGT) a term denoting values of fasting plasma glucose or results of an oral glucose tolerance test that are abnormal but not high enough to be diagnostic of diabetes mellitus. Formerly called *chemical, latent, preclinical,* or *subclinical diabetes.*

ischemic t. the development of a degree of resistance to the effects of a second transient ischemic attack in certain patients after the first attack.

low-dose t., low-zone t. see *immunologic t.*

self t. immunologic unresponsiveness to autoantigens (self antigens), acquired during fetal life by a process of "self recognition." Theories of tolerance induction include deletion of antigen-responsive clones of B cells, antigen-induced inactivation of B or T cells, and induction of antigen-specific T suppressor cells.

split t. 1. following induction of immunologic tolerance to allogeneic cells, tolerance to an antigen or group of antigens on the cell surface occurs, while there is an immune response to other antigens on the cell surface. 2. immunologic tolerance that affects either the humoral immune system or the cell-mediated immune system, but not both simultaneously. Called also *immunodeviation.*

transplantation t. immunologic tolerance of transplanted tissue.

tol•er•ant (tol′ər-ənt) able to endure, without effect, the action of any particular drug or other agent; exhibiting tolerance.

tol•er•a•tion (tol″ər-a′shən) tolerance.

tol•ero•gen (tol′ər-o-jən) an antigen used to introduce tolerance, particularly a form of an antigen (usually a soluble form) that induces tolerance, as distinguished from an immunogen, another form (usually an insoluble form) that induces immunity.

tol•ero•gen•e•sis (tol″ər-o-jen′ə-sis) induction of immunologic tolerance.

tol•ero•gen•ic (tol″ər-o-jen′ik) capable of inducing immunologic tolerance.

o-to•li•dine (tol′ĭ-dēn) a compound related to benzidine and formerly used in testing for occult blood; its use is now restricted because it is a carcinogen.

Tol•in•ase (tōl′in-ās) trademark for a preparation of tolazamide.

tol•le cau•sam (tol′ə kaw′zam) [L. "remove the cause"] a principle of naturopathic medicine, stating that the goal of treatment is to identify and remove the cause of the disease, often involving the removal of multiple causes in the proper order.

tol•met•in so•di•um (tol′met-in) [USP] a nonsteroidal antiinflammatory drug used in the treatment of osteoarthritis, rheumatoid arthritis, ankylosing spondylitis, and other rheumatic inflammatory disorders; administered orally.

tol•naf•tate (tol-naf′tāt) [USP] a synthetic antifungal used topically in the treatment of various forms of tinea of the skin.

to•lo•ni•um chlo•ride (to-lo′ne-əm) an antiheparin compound that has been used in the treatment of menstrual disorders, in the detection of oral and gastric carcinomas, and to stain the parathyroid glands. It is a thiazine dye chemically related to methylene blue; when used nonpharmaceutically, it is usually called *toluidine blue O* (q.v.).

To•lo•sa-Hunt syndrome (to-lo′sah hunt′) [Eduardo S. *Tolosa*, Spanish neurosurgeon, 1900–1981; William Edward *Hunt*, American neurosurgeon, born 1921] see under *syndrome.*

tol•ter•o•dine tar•trate (tol-ter′ə-dēn) a muscarinic receptor antagonist used in the treatment of overactive bladder with symptoms of urinary frequency, urgency, or urge incontinence; administered orally.

tol•u•ene (tol′u-ēn) the hydrocarbon methylbenzene, $C_6H_5{\bullet}CH_3$; a colorless liquid derived by the catalytic reforming of petroleum on the fractional distillation of cal-tar light oil. It is an organic solvent used in rubber and plastic cements, paint removers, etc. Poisoning may result from ingesting the solvent or inhaling its concentrated vapors. Called also *methyl benzene.*

t. diisocyanate (TDI) a pale yellow liquid with a sharp, pungent odor used in the manufacture of polyurethane foams and elastomers; it is highly toxic and a strong irritant of the skin, eyes, and respiratory system.

tol•u•i•dine (tol-u′ĭ-din) a compound homologous with aniline, made by reducing nitrotoluene; used in dyemaking and chemical manufacturing. It has several different isomers, all of which are toxic if inhaled, ingested, or absorbed through the skin. Called also *aminotoluene.*

t. blue O see under *blue.*

***o*-t.** the *ortho-* isomer of toluidine, a yellow liquid used in dyemaking and chemical manufacture; it is more carcinogenic than the other isomers. Called also *o-aminotoluene.*

tol•vap•tan (tol-vap′tan) a selective vasopressin receptor antagonist used in treatment of euvolemic or hypervolemic hyponatremia; administered orally.

tol•yl (tol′əl) the univalent radical, $CH_3 \cdot C_6H_4$, derived from toluene and occurring in three isomeric forms.

t. hydroxide cresol.

to•mac•u•lous (to-mak′u-ləs) [L. *tomaculum* sausage] resembling a sausage, usually because of swelling.

to•ma•tine (to-ma′tin) an antibiotic substance with antifungal properties, isolated from tomato plants affected with wilt.

-tome [Gr. *tomē* a cutting] a word termination signifying *(a)* an instrument for cutting or *(b)* a segment.

to•men•tum (to-men′təm) a little-used term for a network of minute blood vessels of the pia mater and the cortex cerebri.

Tomes layer, process (fiber, fibril) (tōmz) [Sir John *Tomes,* English anatomist and dentist, 1815–1895] see *odontoblastic process,* under *process,* and see *granular layer of Tomes,* under *layer.*

Tomes process (tōmz) [Charles Sissmore *Tomes,* English anatomist and dentist, 1846–1928] see under *process* (def. 1).

to•mite (to′mīt) [*tom-* + Gr. *mitos* thread] the free-swimming nonfeeding stage or form in the life cycle of certain ciliate protozoa, produced by a tomont and, depending on the species, developing into a phoront, theront, or trophont.

Tom•ma•sel•li disease (syndrome) (tom″ə-sel′e) [Salvatore *Tommaselli,* Italian physician, 1834–1906] see under *disease.*

tom(o)- [Gr. *tomē* a cutting] a combining form denoting relationship to a cutting, or to a designated layer, as might be achieved by cutting or slicing.

to•mo•gram (to′mo-gram) a radiograph of a selected layer of the body made by tomography.

to•mo•graph (to′mo-graf) an apparatus for moving an x-ray source in one direction as the film is moved in the opposite direction, thus showing in detail a predetermined plane of tissue while blurring or eliminating detail in other planes.

to•mog•ra•phy (to-mog′rə-fe) [*tomo-* + *-graphy*] the recording of internal body images at a predetermined plane by means of the tomograph; called also *body section radiography.*

computed t. (CT), computerized axial t. (CAT) tomography in which the emergent x-ray beam is measured by a scintillation counter; the electronic impulses are recorded digitally and then are processed by a computer for reconstruction display. Called also *CAT* or *CT scan.*

electron beam computed t. (EBCT) ultrafast computed tomography done with a scanner in which the patient is surrounded by a large circular anode that emits x-rays as the electron beam is guided around it.

helical computed t. spiral computed t.

high-resolution computed t. (HRCT) computed tomography that produces images with a high degree of spatial resolution and anatomic detail using a high-speed scanner, thin slices, and a special algorithm for reconstructing the image.

hypocycloidal t. tomography in which the path of the x-ray source is a hypocycloid, i.e., the path traced by a point on one circle rolling along inside the circumference of another circle.

linear t. tomography in which the tube and film move in the same direction.

narrow angle t. zonography.

optical coherence t. (OCT) the creation of high-resolution (close to that of light microscopy) cross-sectional images of body structures by recording the reflection of infrared waves from the tissues, using an energy source and a detector in a method similar to that used in B-mode ultrasonography.

optical Doppler t. optical coherence tomography in which shifts in frequency caused by interaction between the infrared waves and moving particles in tissue are used to measure the particle velocities (e.g., in the imaging of blood flow), based on the principle of the Doppler effect.

positron emission t. (PET) tomography accomplished by detection of gamma rays emitted from tissues after administration of a natural biochemical substance (e.g., glucose, fatty acids) into which positron-emitting isotopes have been incorporated. The paths of the gamma rays, which result from collisions of positrons and electrons, are interpreted by a computer, and the resultant tomogram represents local concentrations of the isotope-containing substance.

single-photon emission computed t. (SPECT) a type of tomography in which gamma photon–emitting radionuclides are administered to patients and then detected by one or more gamma cameras rotated around the patient. From the series of two-dimensional images produced, a three-dimensional image can be created by computer reconstruction. The technique improves resolution of, and decreases interference by, overlapping organs.

spiral computed t. computed tomography in which the patient is moved through the scanner continuously rather than in increments, so that the path of the beam through the patient is a continuous spiral. Called also *helical computed t.*

ultrasonic t. the ultrasonographic visualization of a cross-section of a predetermined plane of the body by linear scanning with an ultrasonic probe across the desired site and displaying on a B-scan.

to•mont (to′mont) [*tom-* + Gr. *ontos* beings] the nonfeeding, dividing stage or form in the life cycle of certain protozoa that typically encysts and produces tomites by fission.

-tomy [Gr. *tomē* a cutting] a word termination signifying the operation of cutting, or incision.

ton•a•pha•sia (ton″ə-fa′zhə) [*tono-* + *aphasia*] amusia.

tone (tōn) [Gr. *tonos;* L. *tonus*] 1. the normal degree of vigor and tension. 2. tonus. 3. a particular quality of sound or of voice. 4. to make permanent, or to change, the color of silver stain by chemical treatment, usually with a heavy metal.

feeling t. the condition or state of mind and feeling which accompanies every thought or act.

jecoral t. the sound produced by percussion over the liver.

parasympathetic t. continual background discharge of parasympathetic nerve fibers, which normally decreases as the sympathetic tone increases; when the sympathetic tone is chronically elevated, it may rise to compensate for the increased sympathetic activity.

sympathetic t. continual background discharge of sympathetic nerve fibers, leading to resting contractions of cardiac and vascular smooth muscles. It normally increases and decreases in inverse proportion to parasympathetic tone.

tongs (tongs) an instrument for grasping and holding, consisting of two arms joined by a hinge or pivot.

skull t. tongs used to exert traction on the skull, as in surgery for fractures of cervical vertebrae; many forms are available, including Crutchfield t., Gardner-Wells t., Barton t., and Vinke t.

tongue (tung) [L. *lingua;* Gr. *glōssa*] 1. lingua. 2. lingula. 3. any structure or organ having a shape similar to the oral organ of the same name.

adherent t. ankyloglossia.

amyloid t. enlargement of the tongue due to amyloidosis.

antibiotic t. glossitis caused by sensitivity to an antibiotic.

baked t. the dry, brown tongue of typhoid fever.

bald t. Moeller glossitis.

beefy t. erythematous and/or atrophic glossitis, characterized by red, irregular ulcerations on the dorsal surface of the tongue.

bifid t. a tongue that is divided in its anterior part by a longitudinal fissure; called also *cleft t.*

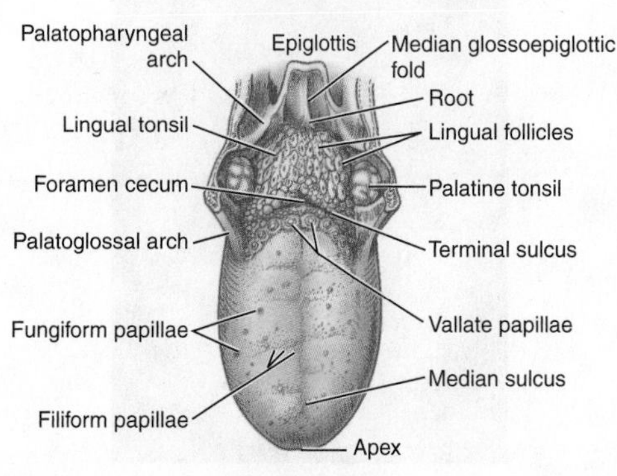

■ The tongue, showing principal structures.

black t. 1. black hairy t. 2. niacin deficiency in dogs, which is accompanied by severe stomatitis and a dark-colored tongue.
black hairy t. hairy tongue (q.v.) in which the hypertrophied filiform papillae are brown or black. Called also *black t.*, *lingua nigra*, *melanoglossia*, *melanotrichia linguae*, and *nigrities linguae*.
blue t. bluetongue.
burning t. glossopyrosis.
cardinal t. a tongue whose surface is denuded of epithelium, giving it a bright red appearance.
cerebriform t. fissured t.
cleft t. bifid t.
coated t. a tongue covered with a whitish or yellowish layer consisting of desquamated epithelium, debris, bacteria, fungi, or other material, which is readily removed by scraping.
cobble-stone t. a condition marked by interstitial glossitis with hypertrophy of the papillae and a verrucous white coating on the tongue, such as seen in riboflavin deficiency.
dotted t. stippled t.
double t. bifid t.
earthy t. a tongue that is coated with a deposit of rough, calcareous matter.
encrusted t. a heavily coated tongue.
fern leaf t. a tongue with a central furrow having lateral branches.
filmy t. a tongue marked with symmetrical whitish patches.
fissured t. a sometimes familial condition characterized by the presence on the dorsal surface of the tongue of numerous furrows, which may radiate outwardly from the median raphe. Called also *cerebriform t.*, *furrowed t.*, *grooved t.*, *plicated t.*, *scrotal t.*, *sulcated t.*, *wrinkled t.*, and *lingua plicata*.
flat t. a condition in which the borders of the tongue cannot be rolled; it is due to paralysis of the transverse lingual muscles occurring as a result of congenital syphilis.
furred t. a tongue with papillae so changed as to give the mucous membrane the appearance of whitish fur.
furrowed t. fissured t.
geographic t. benign migratory glossitis.
grooved t. fissured t.
hairy t. a benign condition characterized by hypertrophy of the filiform papillae, giving the dorsum of the tongue a furry appearance. The color of the elongated papillae varies from yellowish white to brown or black *(black hairy t.)*, depending upon staining by substances such as tobacco, foods, or drugs. Called also *glossotrichia* and *trichoglossia*.
lobulated t. a congenital condition marked by a secondary lobe arising from the surface of the tongue.
magenta t. the magenta-colored tongue seen in cases of riboflavin deficiency.
plicated t. fissured t.
raspberry t., red strawberry t. the dark red tongue with a glistening smooth surface and prominent filiform papillae seen after desquamation of the white coating characteristic of the early stage of scarlet fever. See also *white strawberry t.*
Sandwith bald t. an extremely clean tongue sometimes seen in the late stages of pellagra.
scrotal t. fissured t.
smokers' t. oral leukoplakia of the tongue.
smooth t. congenital absence of papillae on the dorsum of the tongue in cattle, with hypersalivation and velvety body hair; called also *epitheliogenesis imperfecta linguae bovis*.

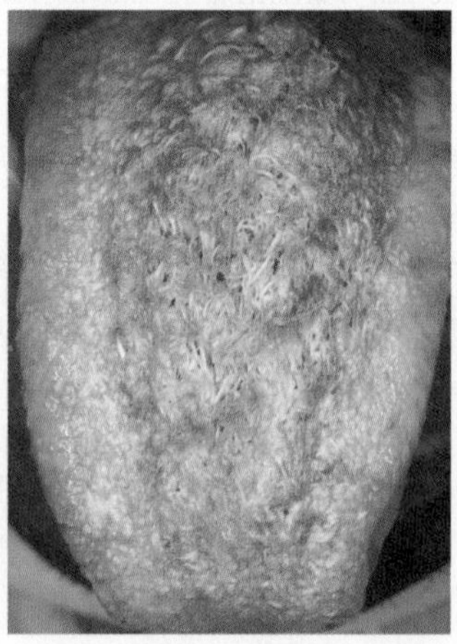
■ Hairy tongue.

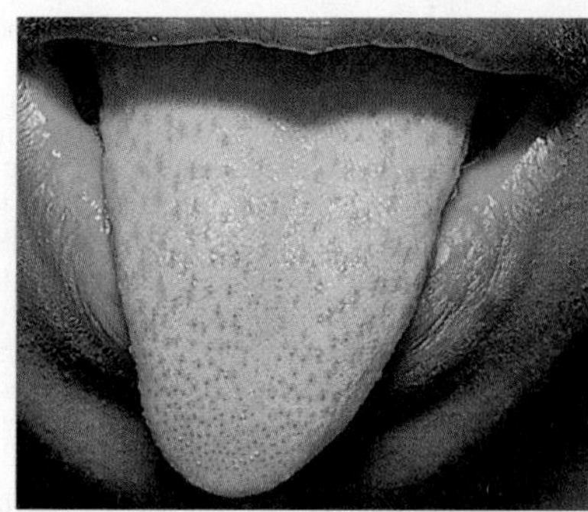
■ White strawberry tongue of early scarlet fever.

t. of sphenoid bone lingula sphenoidalis.
split t. bifid t.
stippled t. a tongue on which each papilla is covered with a separate white patch of epithelium; called also *dotted t.*
strawberry t. 1. a tongue that is dark red colored and whose surface resembles the surface of a strawberry; seen in conditions such as *Staphylococcus aureus* infection, mucocutaneous lymph node syndrome, and streptococcal pharyngitis. 2. raspberry t.
sulcated t. fissured t.
timber t. wooden t.
white t. a condition in which all or part of the papillae and epithelium of the tongue have a dull white color.
white strawberry t. the white-coated tongue with prominent red papillae characteristic of the early stage of scarlet fever; the coating desquamates, leaving a beefy red tongue *(raspberry t.)*.
wooden t. actinobacillosis of cattle in which hard tumor-like nodules form inside the tongue; called also *timber t.*
wrinkled t. fissured t.

tongue-tie (tung'ti") ankyloglossia.

ton•ic (ton'ik) [Gr. *tonikos*] 1. producing and restoring the normal tone. 2. characterized by continuous tension. 3. a term formerly used for a class of medicinal preparations believed to have the power of restoring normal tone to tissue; named for the organ or system on which they acted, e.g., cardiac tonic, digestive tonic.
bitter t. a tonic of bitter taste, used for stimulating the appetite and improving digestion, such as quinine, quassia, and gentian.

ton•ic-clon•ic (ton'ik klon'ik) tonicoclonic.

to•nic•i•ty (to-nis'ĭ-te) 1. the state of tissue tone or tension. 2. in body fluid physiology, the effective osmotic pressure equivalent.

ton•i•co•clon•ic (ton"ĭ-ko-klon'ik) both tonic and clonic; said of a spasm or seizure consisting of a convulsive twitching of the muscles. Called also *tonic-clonic* and *tonoclonic*.

ton(o)- [Gr. *tonos* tension] a combining form denoting relationship to tone or tension.

Tono•card (to'no-kahrd) trademark for a preparation of tocainide hydrochloride.

tono•clon•ic (ton"o-klon'ik) tonicoclonic.

tono•fi•bril (ton'o-fi"bril) a bundle of tonofilaments occurring in epithelial cells, the individual strands of which traverse the cytoplasm in all directions and extend into the cell processes to converge and insert on the desmosomes.

tono•fil•a•ment (ton"o-fil'ə-mənt) an intermediate filament composed of cytokeratin and occurring in epithelial cells, particularly those of the epidermis; tonofilaments participate in the formation of desmosomes and hemidesmosomes. The term is often used synonymously with *keratin filament*. See also *tonofibril*.

to•no•gram (to'no-gram) the record produced by tonography.

to•no•graph (to'no-graf) [*tono-* + *-graph*] a recording tonometer.

to•nog•ra•phy (to-nog'rə-fe) [*tono-* + *-graphy*] the recording of changes in intraocular pressure produced by the constant application of a known weight on the globe of the eye, reflecting the facility of outflow of the aqueous humor from the anterior chamber.
carotid compression t. a test for occlusion of the carotid artery by measuring the intraocular pressure and pulse before, while, and after the proximal portion of the carotid artery is compressed by the fingers.

to·nom·e·ter (to-nom′ə-tər) [*tono-* + *-meter*] 1. an instrument for measuring tension or pressure. 2. specifically, an instrument by which intraocular pressure is measured.

air-puff t. an instrument for measuring intraocular pressure; it does not touch the eye, but rather senses deflections of the cornea in reaction to a puff of pressurized air.

applanation t. an instrument that measures intraocular pressure by determination of the force necessary to flatten a corneal surface of constant size.

electronic t. a tonometer having an electronic readout.

Gärtner t. an instrument for measuring blood pressure by means of a compressing ring applied to the finger.

gastric t. a tonometer, drainage tube, and vent that are incorporated into one device with three separate lumens.

Goldmann applanation t. an instrument for measuring intraocular pressure which eliminates the effects of scleral resistance.

impression t., indentation t. an instrument that measures intraocular pressure by direct pressure on the eyeball, such as the Schiøtz, McLean, or MacKay-Marg electronic tonometer.

MacKay-Marg electronic t. an electronic applanation tonometer equipped with a flat plunger which measures intraocular pressure by direct application to the cornea.

McLean t. impression t.

Recklinghausen t. an instrument for observing oscillatory blood pressure.

Schiøtz t. an instrument that registers intraocular pressure by direct application to the cornea, the reading on the scale being translated into millimeters of mercury by means of a conversion table.

to·nom·e·try (to-nom′ə-tre) [*tono-* + *-metry*] the measurement of tension or pressure, particularly intraocular pressure.

digital t. estimation of the degree of intraocular pressure by pressure exerted on the eyeball by the finger of the examiner.

gastric t. monitoring of the gastric intramucosal pH to obtain early indications of inadequate tissue oxygenation; the sensitive nature of the mucosa allows for monitoring of metabolic changes produced by hypoxia well in advance of other, more common indices of hypoxia.

tono·top·ic (ton″o-top′ik) having a spatial arrangement such that certain tone frequencies are transmitted along a particular portion of the structure, as in the cochlear nuclei.

tono·top·ic·i·ty (ton″o-top-is′ĭ-te) the property of being tonotopic.

ton·sil (ton′sil) 1. a small rounded mass of tissue, especially lymphoid tissue. Called also *tonsilla.* 2. tonsilla palatina.

adenoid t. tonsilla pharyngealis.

buried t. submerged t.

t. of cerebellum tonsilla cerebelli.

eustachian t. tonsilla tubaria.

faucial t. tonsilla palatina.

Gerlach t. tonsilla tubaria.

lingual t. tonsilla lingualis.

Luschka t. tonsilla pharyngealis.

palatine t. tonsilla palatina.

pharyngeal t. tonsilla pharyngealis.

submerged t. a palatine tonsil that is shrunken and atrophied and is partly or entirely hidden by the palatoglossal arch.

third t. tonsilla pharyngealis.

t. of torus tubarius, tubal t. tonsilla tubaria.

ton·sil·la (ton-sil′ə) pl. *tonsil′lae* [L.] tonsil: a small rounded mass of tissue, especially lymphoid tissue.

t. cerebel′li [TA] tonsil of cerebellum (HIX): a rounded mass forming part of the hemisphere of the cerebellum, continuous with the uvula vermis in the posterior lobe; called also *ventral paraflocculus* and *paraflocculus ventralis* [TA alternative].

t. lingua′lis [TA] lingual tonsil: an aggregation of lymph follicles on the floor of the oropharyngeal passageway, at the root of the tongue.

t. palati′na [TA] palatine tonsil: either of two small, almond-shaped masses located between the palatoglossal and palatopharyngeal arches, one on either side of the oropharynx, composed mainly of lymphoid tissue, covered with mucous membrane, and containing various crypts and many lymph follicles. Called also *tonsil* and *faucial tonsil.*

t. pharyngea′lis [TA] pharyngeal tonsil: the diffuse lymphoid tissue and follicles in the roof and posterior wall of the nasopharynx; called also *adenoid tonsil.* See also *adenoid* (def. 2).

t. tuba′ria [TA] tubal tonsil: a collection of lymphoid tissue associated with the pharyngeal opening of the auditory tube; called also *eustachian tonsil, Gerlach tonsil,* and *tonsil of torus tubarius.*

ton·sil·lar (ton′sĭ-lər) [L. *tonsillaris*] of or pertaining to a tonsil; called also *amygdaline.*

ton·sil·lec·to·my (ton″sĭ-lek′tə-me) [*tonsill-* + *-ectomy*] surgical removal of a tonsil or tonsils.

ton·sil·lith (ton′sĭ-lith) tonsillolith.

ton·sil·li·tis (ton″sĭ-li′tis) [*tonsill-* + *-itis*] inflammation of the tonsils, especially the palatine tonsils. **tonsillit′ic** *adj*

acute t. tonsillitis of abrupt onset, usually due to infection with a bacteria (commonly a beta-hemolytic streptococcus) or a virus. Characteristics include swelling, chills and fever, headache, and pain in the throat with dysphagia. See also *lacunar t.* and *streptococcal pharyngitis.*

caseous t. lacunar tonsillitis in which the crypts contain caseous material.

chronic t. persistent inflammation of the tonsils resulting from recurrent infections.

follicular t. lacunar t.

herpetic t. a local manifestation of herpes on the tonsil.

lacunar t. acute tonsillitis affecting the crypts of the tonsils; see also *caseous t.* Called also *follicular t.*

lingual t. inflammation of the lingual tonsils.

mycotic t. tonsillomycosis.

streptococcal t. acute tonsillitis resulting from streptococcal pharyngitis that infects the tonsils.

tonsill(o)- [L. *tonsilla* tonsil] a combining form denoting relationship to a tonsil or to the tonsils.

ton·sil·lo·ad·e·noid·ec·to·my (ton″sĭ-lo-ad″ə-noid-ek′tə-me) adenotonsillectomy.

ton·sil·lo·lith (ton-sil′o-lith) [*tonsillo-* + *-lith*] a concretion or calculus in a tonsil. Called also *tonsillar calculus.*

ton·sil·lo·my·co·sis (ton-sil″o-mi-ko′sis) a fungal infection of the tonsils. Called also *mycotic tonsillitis.*

ton·sil·lop·a·thy (ton″sĭ-lop′ə-the) [*tonsillo-* + *-pathy*] any disease of the tonsil.

ton·sil·lo·phar·yn·gi·tis (ton″sil-o-far″in-ji′tis) pharyngotonsillitis.

ton·sil·lo·tome (ton-sil′o-tōm) guillotine.

ton·sil·lot·o·my (ton″sĭ-lot′ə-me) [*tonsillo-* + *-tomy*] incision of a tonsil; the surgical removal of a part of a tonsil.

to·nus (to′nəs) [L., from Gr. *tonos*] the slight, continuous contraction of muscle, which in skeletal muscles aid in the maintenance of posture and in the return of blood to the heart. Called also *tone.* See also *hypertonia* and *hypotonia.*

Tooth disease (atrophy) (tōōth) [Howard Henry *Tooth*, English physician, 1856–1925] Charcot-Marie-Tooth disease.

tooth (tōōth) pl. *teeth* [L. *dens;* Gr. *odous*] 1. any of the hard calcified structures set in the alveolar processes of the mandible and maxilla for mastication of food. In humans, there are two sets of teeth (*dentes* [TA]), *deciduous* and *permanent.* Each tooth consists of three parts: the *crown* (see *corona dentis*), the *neck* (see *cervix dentis*), and the *root* (see *radix dentis*). The solid part includes *dentin,* forming most of the tooth and resembling true bone; *enamel,* a very hard inorganic substance, covering the crown; and *cementum,* covering the root. In the center is the soft pulp (see *pulpa dentis*). See also *dentition.* 2. a structure resembling the tooth of an animal.

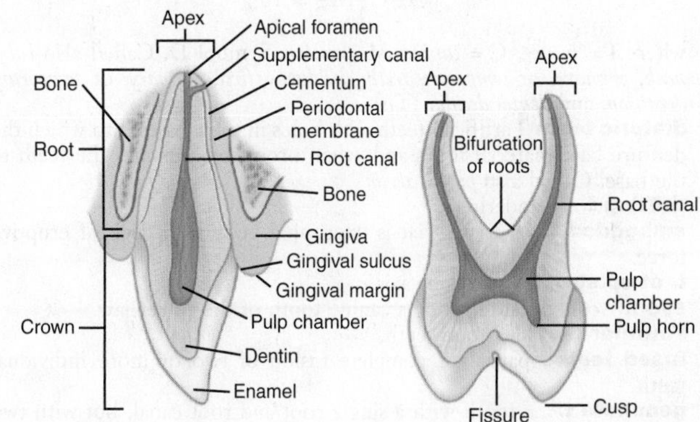

■ Schematic cross section of an anterior *(left)* and a posterior *(right)* tooth in the maxilla.

Tooth

abutment t. a tooth selected to support a bridge on the basis of the total surface area of a healthy attachment apparatus. See also *abutment* (def. 2).
accessional teeth the molar teeth of the permanent dentition, so called because they do not supplant any deciduous predecessors in the dental arch. Cf. *succedaneous teeth.*
anatomic teeth 1. artificial teeth that duplicate the anatomic forms of natural teeth. 2. teeth that have prominent pointed or rounded cusps on the masticating surfaces and are designed to occlude with the teeth of the opposing denture or natural dentition.
ankylosed t. submerged t.
anterior teeth the incisor and canine teeth, which are in the anterior parts of the dental arches. Called also *labial* or *morsal teeth.*
artificial t. a tooth fabricated for use as a substitute for a natural tooth in a prosthesis, usually made of porcelain or resin. See also *denture.*
auditory teeth, auditory teeth of Huschke dentes acustici.
t. of axis dens axis.
baby teeth deciduous teeth.
bicuspid teeth premolar teeth.
buccal teeth posterior teeth.
canine t. the tooth immediately lateral to the lateral, or second, incisor; it has a long conical crown and the longest, most powerful root of all the teeth. Called also *canine, cuspid, cuspid t.,* and *dens caninus* [TA].
carnassial t. a large molar or premolar of a carnivore, specialized for shearing and tearing.
cheek teeth posterior teeth.
cog t. of malleus spur of malleus.
conical t. peg t.
connate t. geminate t.
corner t. the third incisor on either side of each jaw in the horse. Called also *corner.*
cross-bite teeth artificial posterior teeth designed to permit positioning of the modified buccal cusps of the upper teeth in the fossae of the lower teeth.
cross-pin teeth artificial teeth in which the pins are inserted horizontally.
cuspid t. canine t.
cuspless t. any tooth deprived of a cusp; particularly an artificial tooth designed without cuspal prominences on the occlusal surface.
deciduous teeth the 20 teeth of the first dentition, which are shed and replaced by the permanent teeth. They begin to calcify at about the fourth month of fetal life, and near the end of the sixth month they all have begun to develop. The first incisors appear at about the age of $6\frac{1}{2}$ months; they are followed by the second incisors $\frac{1}{2}$ month later; and, within $1\frac{1}{2}$ months, by the maxillary incisors. The deciduous molars begin eruption at about 1 year, and the deciduous canines approximately 4 months later. All the deciduous teeth are expected to erupt by the time the child is $2\frac{1}{2}$ years of age. The deciduous dentition formula (one side) is as follows:

$$I\frac{2}{2}C\frac{1}{1}M\frac{2}{2} = 10$$

where I = *incisor;* C = *canine;* M = *molar.* Symbol D. Called also *baby, milk, primary,* or *temporary teeth; deciduous, first, primary,* or *temporary dentition;* and *dentes decidui* [TA].
diatoric teeth artificial teeth with holes in their bases into which the denture base material flows and, when processed, attaches the teeth to the base. Called also *pinless teeth.*
drifting t. wandering t.
embedded t. a tooth that is unerupted because of lack of eruptive force.
t. of epistropheus dens axis.
eye t. colloquial term for a canine tooth of the upper jaw.
Fournier teeth Moon teeth.
fused teeth partial or complete fusion of two or more individual teeth.
geminate t. a tooth with a single root and root canal, but with two completely or incompletely separated crowns, resulting from invagination of a single tooth germ, causing incomplete formation of two teeth. Called also *connate t.*
Goslee t. an interchangeable artificial tooth attached to a metal base.
hag teeth upper medial incisors that are widely separated.

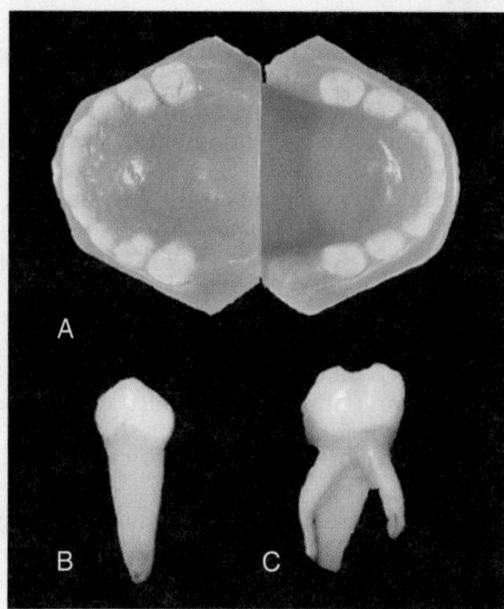

■ Models of deciduous teeth *(A);* deciduous canine *(B);* and deciduous second molar *(C).*

Horner teeth incisor teeth that are horizontally grooved owing to a deficiency of enamel.
Hutchinson teeth a tooth abnormality seen in congenital syphilis, in which the permanent incisors have a screwdriverlike shape, sometimes with notching of the incisal edges or depressions in the labial surfaces above the cutting edge. Called also *Hutchinson incisors* and *screwdriver teeth.*
impacted t. a tooth that is prevented from erupting by a physical barrier. See also *unerupted t.*
incisor t. either of the four most frontal teeth in each jaw, two on either side of the midline; this tooth has a long root and is adapted for cutting. Symbol I. Called also *incisor* and *dens incisivus* [TA].
labial teeth anterior teeth.
malacotic teeth teeth that are soft in structure and are abnormally susceptible to caries.
malposed t. a tooth out of its normal position.
mandibular teeth the teeth of the mandible, or lower jaw.
maxillary teeth the teeth of the maxilla, or upper jaw.
metal insert t. an artificial tooth, usually of acrylic resin, containing an inserted ribbon of metal or a cutting blade in the occlusal surface, with one edge exposed; sometimes used in removable dentures.
milk t. 1. predeciduous t. 2. neonatal t. 3. deciduous t.
molar teeth the most posterior teeth on either side in each jaw, totaling 8 in the deciduous dentition (2 on each side, upper and lower), and usually 12 in the permanent dentition (3 on each side, upper and lower). They are the grinding teeth, having large crowns with broad chewing surfaces. The upper molars characteristically have 4 major cusps and three roots. The lower first molars characteristically have 5 cusps, and the remaining lower molars 4 cusps. Normally all lower molars have two roots. The third molars ("wisdom teeth") are often malformed, but when developed normally their crown and root form corresponds in general with neighboring molars in the same jaw. Symbol M. Called also *molars* and *dentes molares* [TA].
molar t., third the tooth most distal to the medial line on either side in each jaw, so called because it is the last of the permanent dentition to erupt, usually at the age of 17 to 21 years. Called also *wisdom t., third molar, dens molaris tertius* [TA], and *dens serotinus* [TA alternative].
Moon teeth small, domed first molars observed in patients with congenital syphilis.
morsal teeth [L. *morsus* a seizing] anterior teeth.
mottled teeth see under *enamel.*
mulberry t. mulberry molar.
natal t. predeciduous t.
neonatal t. a tooth that erupts within the first month of life. Called also *milk t.*
nonanatomic teeth a term applied to artificial teeth whose occlusal surfaces are especially designed on the basis of engineering concepts, without regard to the features of natural teeth.

Tooth *Continued*

peg t., peg-shaped t. a tooth having a conical form, with sides that converge or taper together incisally instead of being parallel or diverging mesially and distally; a condition frequently observed in the maxillary lateral incisor. Called also *conical t.*

permanent teeth the 32 teeth of the second dentition, which begin to appear in humans at about 6 years of age. The first molars appear first, followed by the mandibular central and lateral incisors, maxillary central incisors, maxillary lateral incisors, mandibular canines, first premolars, second premolars, maxillary canines, second molars, and third molars. They take their position posterior to the deciduous teeth and erupt in succession, whenever the jaws grow sufficiently to accommodate them. Exfoliation of the deciduous teeth is brought about by resorption of their roots, and the succedaneous permanent teeth take their place. The permanent dentition formula (one side) is as follows:

$$I\frac{2}{2}C\frac{1}{1}P\frac{2}{2}M\frac{3}{3} = 16$$

where I = *incisor;* C = *canine;* P = *premolar;* M = *molar.* Called also *dentes permanentes* [TA] and *permanent* or *secondary dentition.*

pink t. of Mummery internal tooth resorption (def. 1).

pinless teeth diatoric teeth.

posterior teeth the premolar and molar teeth, which are in the posterior parts of the dental arches. Called also *buccal* or *cheek teeth.*

predeciduous t. any tooth present at birth, which may be normal in all respects or may represent a hornified epithelial rootless structure, found on the gingivae over the crest of the ridge before eruption of the deciduous teeth. Called also *dentia praecox, milk* or *natal t.,* and *predeciduous dentition.*

premature teeth deciduous teeth that erupt prior to the end of the third month of life, or permanent teeth that erupt prior to the end of the fourth year of life. Called also *dentia praecox* and *precocious* or *premature dentition.* See also *predeciduous teeth.*

premolar teeth 1. the permanent teeth between the canines and the molars; there are two on either side in each jaw. The upper premolars are bicuspid and the lower have from one to three cusps. Premolars are succedaneous to the deciduous molar teeth. Symbol P. Called also *dentes premolares* [TA], *premolars, bicuspids,* and *bicuspid teeth.* 2. in animals other than humans, the teeth that succeed the deciduous molars regardless of the number to be succeeded.

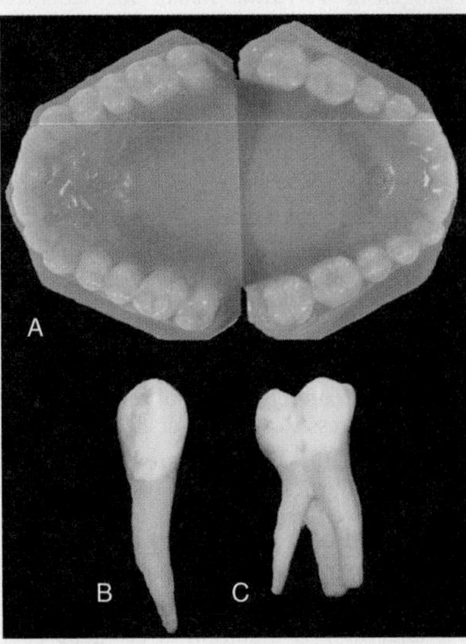

■ Models of permanent teeth *(A);* permanent canine *(B);* and permanent first molar *(C).*

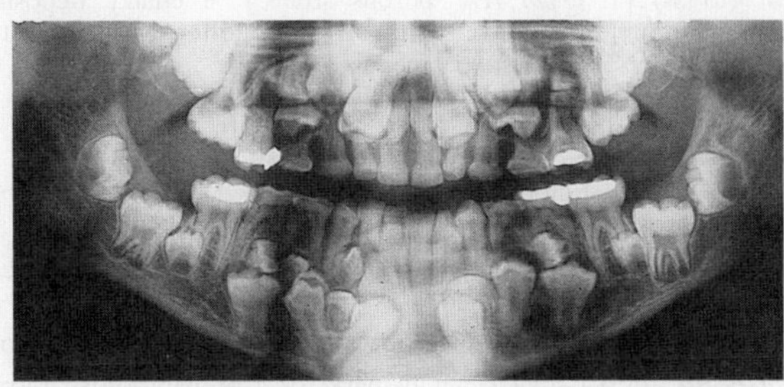

■ Supernumerary teeth in cleidocranial dysplasia.

primary teeth deciduous teeth.

pulpless t. a tooth from which the pulp has been extirpated.

rake teeth teeth that are widely separated.

rootless teeth dentinal dysplasia.

sclerotic teeth teeth that are hard in structure and resistant to caries.

screwdriver teeth Hutchinson teeth.

shell t. a condition characterized by dysplasia of the dentin, associated with essentially normal enamel, thus resulting in an extremely large pulp chamber and root canal that give the affected tooth the appearance of a shell.

snaggle t. a tooth out of proper line with the others.

stomach t. a canine tooth of the mandible.

straight-pin teeth artificial teeth in which the pins are inserted vertically.

submerged t. a deciduous tooth, usually a second mandibular molar, that has undergone resorption and has become ankylosed to the bone, thus preventing its exfoliation and replacement by a permanent tooth; it appears to be submerged below the level of occlusion in relation to the adjacent permanent teeth. Called also *ankylosed t.*

succedaneous teeth, successional teeth the permanent teeth that have deciduous predecessors in the dental arch. Cf. *accessional teeth.*

superior teeth maxillary teeth.

supernumerary teeth, supplemental teeth natural teeth in excess of the number normally present in the jaw.

temporary teeth deciduous teeth.

tube teeth artificial teeth having a vertical, cylindrical aperture from the center of the base up into the body of the tooth, into which a pin may be placed or cast for attachment of the tooth to the denture base.

Turner t. enamel hypoplasia of a single tooth, most commonly one of the permanent maxillary incisors or a maxillary or mandibular premolar, resulting from local infection or trauma. Called also *Turner hypoplasia.*

unerupted t. a tooth that has failed to break out of its crypt and emerge through the gingiva; the presence of multiple unerupted permanent teeth is sometimes referred to as *pseudoanodontia.* See also *embedded t.* and *impacted t.*

vital teeth teeth that have vital pulp, i.e. to which the nerve and vascular supply is intact.

wandering t. a tooth that drifts from its normal position in the dental arch. Called also *drifting t.*

wisdom t. third molar t.

wolf t. a vestigial first premolar tooth sometimes present in the jaw of a horse.

zero degree teeth artificial teeth which have no cusp angles in relation to the horizontal on their occlusal surfaces.

tooth•ache (to͞oth′āk″) pain in a tooth. Called also *dentagra, dentalgia,* and *odontalgia.*

tooth-borne (to͞oth′born) supported entirely by the teeth; said of a prosthesis or part of a prosthesis entirely supported by the abutment teeth.

top•ag•no•sia (top″ag-no′zhə) [*topo-* + *agnosia*] atopognosia.

top•ag•no•sis (top″ag-no′sis) atopognosia.

to•pal•gia (to-pal′jə) [*top-* + *-algia*] pain fixed in one spot, a common feature of pain without organic basis, as seen in conversion disorder.

To•pa•max (to′pə-maks) trademark for a preparation of topiramate.

-tope [Gr. *topos* place, position] a word termination denoting place or position.

to•pec•to•my (to-pek′tə-me) [*top-* + *-ectomy*] ablation of a small and specific area of the frontal cortex, for the treatment of certain forms of epilepsy and psychiatric disorders; called also *corticectomy* and *frontal gyrectomy.*

top•es•the•sia (top″es-the′zhə) [*topo-* + *esthesia*] the power of localizing a tactile sensation.

to·pha·ceous (to-fa′shəs) [L. *tophaceus: tophus* porous stone] hard or gritty; of the nature of or characterized by tophi.

to·phi (to′fi) [L.] plural of *tophus.*

topho·li·po·ma (tof″o-lĭ-po′mə) a lipoma containing tophi.

to·phus (to′fəs) pl. *to′phi* [L. "porous stone"] a chalky deposit of sodium urate occurring in gout; tophi form most often around joints in cartilage, bone, bursae, and subcutaneous tissue and in the external ear, producing a chronic, foreign-body inflammatory response.
 auricular t. a tophus on the ear.
 dental t. dental calculus.
 t. syphili′ticus syphilitic node.

top·i·cal (top′ĭ-kəl) [Gr. *topikos*] pertaining to a particular surface area, as a topical antiinfective applied to a certain area of the skin and affecting only the area to which it is applied.

Top·i·cort (top′ĭ-kort) trademark for preparations of desoximetasone.

Top·i·cy·cline (top″ĭ-si′klēn) trademark for a preparation of tetracycline hydrochloride.

To·pi·nard angle, line (to″pe-nahr′) [Paul *Topinard*, French physician and anthropologist, 1830–1911] see *ophryospinal angle*, under *angle*, and see under *line.*

to·pi·ra·mate (to-pi′rə-māt) a substituted monosaccharide used as an anticonvulsant in the treatment of partial seizures; administered orally.

top(o)- [Gr. *topos* place] a combining form meaning place.

topo·an·es·the·sia (top″o-an″es-the′zhə) atopognosia.

topo·chem·is·try (top″o-kem′is-tre) the chemical composition at specific sites of a structure, as at the surface membrane of a cell.

top·og·no·sis (top″og-no′sis) [*topo-* + Gr. *gnōsis* recognition] topesthesia.

topo·graph·ag·no·sia (top″o-graf″ag-no′zhə) inability to orient to an abstract representation of a familiar place, usually owing to a lesion in the parietal lobe of the brain. Cf. *environmental agnosia.*

to·pog·ra·phy (to-pog′rə-fe) [*topo-* + *-graphy*] the description of an anatomical region or of a special part. **topograph′ic, topograph′ical** *adj*

topo·iso·mer (to″po-i′so-mər) a DNA molecule that differs from another only in linking number, the number of times one strand of the helix wraps around the other in a right-hand direction.

topo·isom·er·ase (to″po-i-som′ə-rās) an enzyme that interconverts topoisomers of DNA by breaking and rejoining one or more phosphodiester bonds and altering the degree of supercoiling of the DNA.
 type I t. DNA topoisomerase.
 type II t. DNA topoisomerase (ATP-hydrolyzing).

topo·log·i·cal (top-o-loj′ĭ-kəl) pertaining to topology.

to·pol·o·gy (tə-pol′ə-je) [*topo-* + *-logy*] 1. the relation between the presenting part of the fetus and the birth canal. 2. regional anatomy. 3. in molecular biology, mathematical description of the tertiary structure of a DNA helix whose ends are not capable of free rotation; it is defined as $L = I \times W$ where L is the linking number, the total number of times one strand winds around the other in a right-hand direction, I is the twisting number, the number of helical turns, and W is the writhing number, the number of superhelical turns.

topo·nym (top′o-nim) the name of a region as distinguished from an organ.

to·pon·y·my (to-pon′ĭ-me) [*topo-* + Gr. *onoma* name] terminology pertaining to the regions of the body.

To·po·sar (to′po-sahr) trademark for a preparation of etoposide.

topo·scop·ic (to″po-skop′ik) pertaining to endoscopic delivery to a specific site.

to·po·te·can hy·dro·chlo·ride (to″po-te′kan) a cytotoxic topoisomerase inhibitor derived from camptothecin, acting by preventing the rejoining of DNA strands following breakage by DNA topoisomerase; this leads to double-strand DNA breakage and cell death. Used as a secondary agent in treatment of metastatic ovarian carcinoma and refractory small cell lung carcinoma; administered by intravenous infusion.

topo·therm·es·the·si·om·e·ter (top″o-thərm″əs-the-ze-om′ə-tər) [*topo-* + *thermesthesiometer*] an apparatus for measuring the local temperature sense.

Top·rol-XL (top′rol) trademark for a preparation of metoprolol succinate.

To·ra·dol (tor′ə-dol) trademark for preparations of ketorolac tromethamine.

TORCH toxoplasmosis, other agents, rubella, cytomegalovirus, herpes simplex; see under *syndrome.*

tor·cu·lar (tor′ku-lər) [L. "wine-press"] a hollow, or expanded area.
 t. Hero′phili confluens sinuum.

To·rek operation (to′rek) [Franz J. A. *Torek*, American surgeon, 1861–1938] see under *operation.*

to·re·mi·fene cit·rate (tor′ə-mĭ-fēn″) an analogue of tamoxifen that acts as an estrogen antagonist, used in the palliative treatment of metastatic carcinoma of the breast; administered orally.

to·ri (to′ri) [L.] plural of *torus.*

to·ric (tor′ik) pertaining to or resembling a torus.

Tori·sel (tor′ĭ-sel) trademark for a preparation of temsirolimus.

Tor·kild·sen shunt (operation) (tor′kild-sen) [Arne *Torkildsen*, Norwegian neurosurgeon, 1899–1968] ventriculocisternal shunt.

Torn·waldt (Thorn·waldt) abscess, bursa (cyst), etc. (torn′vahlt) [Gustav Ludwig *Tornwaldt* (or *Thornwaldt*), German physician, 1843–1910] see under *abscess* and *bursitis*, and see *bursa pharyngealis.*

to·rose (to′rōs) [L. *torosus* muscular, brawny] bulging or knobby; called also *torous.*

to·rous (to′rəs) torose.

Tor·o·vi·rus (tor″o-vi′rəs) [*torus* + *virus*] the toroviruses; a genus of viruses of the family Coronaviridae having a tubular nucleocapsid that may bend into an open torus; organisms cause gastrointestinal disease. It includes Berne and Breda viruses, as well as human and porcine toroviruses.

tor·o·vi·rus (tor′o-vi″rəs) any virus belonging to the genus *Torovirus.* torovi′ral *adj*

tor·pent (tor′pənt) [L. *torpere* to be sluggish] 1. torpid. 2. an agent that reduces irritation.

tor·pid (tor′pid) [L. *torpidus* numb, sluggish] not acting with normal vigor and facility.

tor·pid·i·ty (tor-pid′ĭ-te) torpor.

tor·por (tor′pər) [L.] lack of response to normal or ordinary stimuli.
 t. re′tinae a condition in which the retina is excited to action only by stimuli of considerable luminous power.

torque (tork) [L. *torquēre* to twist] 1. a rotatory force causing part of a structure to twist about an axis. Symbol τ. 2. the rotation of a tooth on its long axis, especially moving the root apex in a buccal or lingual direction through the application of force produced by torsion within the arch wire. See also *torsion.*

torqu·ing (tork′ing) the twisting of a tooth into position, as in the correction of malposition.

torr (tor) [Evangelista *Torricelli*, Italian mathematician and physicist, 1608–1647] a unit of pressure equal to one millimeter of mercury (mm Hg), or 133.3 pascals.

Tor·re syndrome (tor′a) [Douglas Paul *Torre*, American dermatologist, 1919–1996] see under *syndrome.*

tor·re·fac·tion (tor″ə-fak′shən) [L. *torrefactio*] the act of roasting or parching.

tor·re·fy (tor′e-fi) [L. *torrefacere*] to parch, roast, or dry by the aid of heat.

tor·ri·cel·li·an (tor″e-chel′e-ən) named for Evangelista *Torricelli*, Italian mathematician, 1608–1647, as *torricellian vacuum.*

tor·sades de pointes (tor-sahd′ də pwant) [Fr. "fringe of pointed tips"] an atypical rapid ventricular tachycardia with periodic waxing and waning of amplitude of the QRS complexes on the electrocardiogram as well as rotation of the complexes about the isoelectric line; it may be self-limited or may progress to ventricular fibrillation.

tor·se·mide (tor′sə-mīd) [USP] a diuretic and antihypertensive related to sulfonylurea; used in the treatment of hypertension and of edema associated with congestive heart failure, hepatic disease, or kidney disease; administered orally or intravenously.

tor·sin (tor′sin) any of a family of molecular chaperones of the AAA protein family residing in the endoplasmic reticulum and nuclear envelope; their function is uncertain. A mutation in the gene coding for torsinA is responsible for early-onset torsion dystonia.

tor·sion (tor′shən) [L. *torsio*, from *torquēre* to twist] 1. the act or process of twisting; turning or rotating about an axis. 2. a type of mechanical

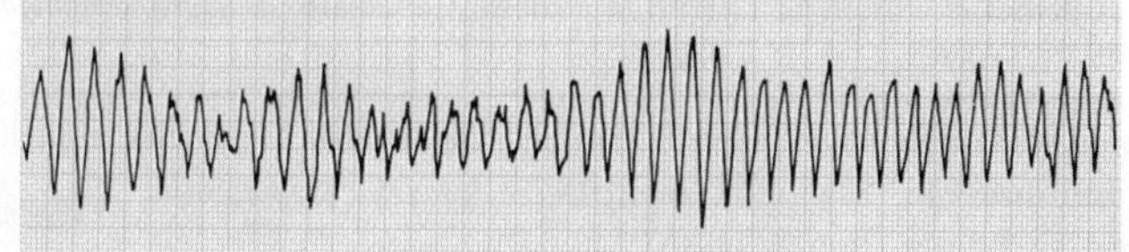

■ Sustained torsades de pointes; the QRS axis appears to rotate cyclically, pointing downward for several beats then twisting and pointing upward in the same lead.

stress, whereby the external forces (load) twist an object about its axis. See also *torque.* 3. in ophthalmology, any rotation of the vertical corneal meridians; such movements are severely limited under normal conditions. See also *extorsion* and *intorsion.* Called also *cyclorotation* and *wheel rotation.*

abomasal t., t. of the abomasum twisting of the abomasum of a cow, often three to six weeks after birth of a calf and after subclinical right displacement of the abomasum (see under *displacement*); symptoms include distention of the abdomen, acute abdominal pain, shock, and (if untreated) circulatory failure and death within 48 hours. Called also *abomasal volvulus.*

negative t. rotation in a counterclockwise direction.

positive t. rotation in a clockwise direction.

tibial t. inward twisting of the tibia so that the foot turns inward.

tor•sion•om•e•ter (tor″shən-om′ə-tər) [*torsion* + *-meter*] an apparatus for estimating the degree of rotation of the vertebral column.

tor•sive (tor′siv) twisted.

tor•si•ver•sion (tor″sĭ-vur′zhən) [L. *torquēre* to twist + *version*] the turning or rotation of a tooth on its long axis.

tor•so (tor′so) truncus (def. 1).

tor•ti•col•lis (tor″tĭ-kol′is) [L. *tortus* twisted + *collum* neck] abnormal contraction of the muscles of the neck, producing twisting of the neck and an unnatural position of the head. Called also *wryneck.* **torticol′lar** *adj*

congenital t. torticollis due to injury to the sternocleidomastoid muscle on one side at the time of birth and its transformation into a fibrous cord which cannot lengthen with the growing neck.

fixed t. torticollis due to persistent shortening of muscles.

intermittent t. spasmodic t.

mental t. torticollis with spasmodic contraction of neck muscles and deviation of the head that may cease when the patient lies down or applies slight pressure.

myogenic t. a transient condition due to muscular contraction in rheumatism, and to cold.

neurogenic t. spasmodic t.

ocular t. torticollis due to a high degree of astigmatism or to paralysis of ocular muscles.

psychogenic t. torticollis that is psychogenic in origin.

reflex t. torticollis caused by inflammation or suppuration in the neck, enlarged cervical lymph nodes, or tumor in the tonsil, neck, or pharynx.

spasmodic t., symptomatic t. a type of focal dystonia with spasms of neck muscles, particularly the sternocleidomastoid and trapezius muscles. The cause is unknown, although irritation of the accessory nerve has been implicated in some cases. Cf. *retrocollis* and *rotatory spasm.* Called also *intermittent* or *neurogenic t.* and *cervical* or *idiopathic cervical dystonia.*

tor•ti•pel•vis (tor″tĭ-pel′vis) dystonia musculorum deformans.

tor•tu•ous (tor′choo-əs) twisted; full of turns and twists.

To•ru•la (tə-roo′lə) a genus of Fungi Imperfecti of the form-class Hyphomycetes, form-family Dematiaceae. *T. jeansel′mei* is a former name for *Exophiala jeanselmei.*

tor•u•li (tor′u-li) [L.] plural of *torulus.*

Tor•u•lop•sis (tor″u-lop′sis) a genus of Fungi Imperfecti of the family Cryptococcaceae; it is closely related to *Candida* and some authorities have considered it the same genus. Some species are normal inhabitants of the skin, respiratory tract, gastrointestinal tract, and urogenital region but may also cause opportunistic infections.

T. glabra′ta a species that is part of the normal flora of the human mouth, intestine, and urinary tract but that in weak or immunocompromised patients may cause opportunistic infections such as torulopsosis, meningitis, pneumonia, cystitis, and fungemia. Called also *Candida glabrata.*

tor•u•lop•so•sis (tor″u-lop′so-sis) infection by *Torulopsis glabrata*; symptoms resemble those of histoplasmosis.

tor•u•lo•sis (tor″u-lo′sis) [*Torula* + *-osis*] former name for *cryptococcosis.*

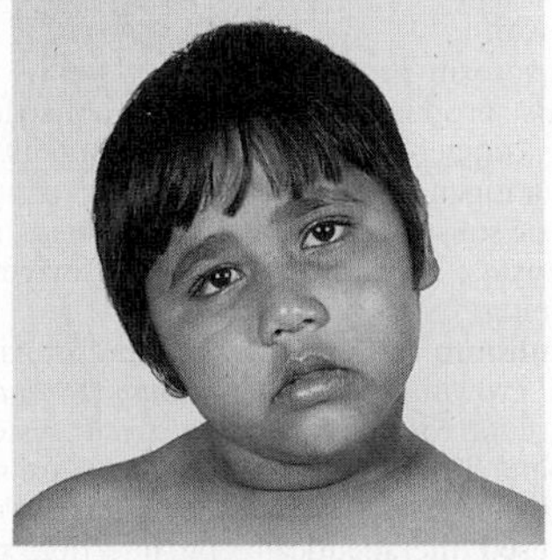

■ Torticollis.

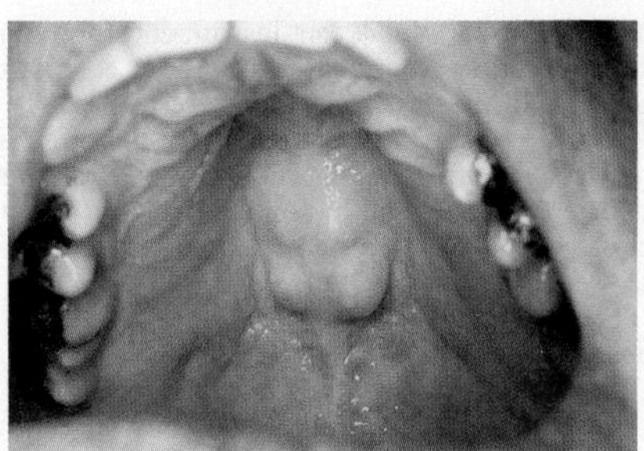

■ Torus palatinus.

tor•u•lus (tor′u-ləs) pl. *to′ruli* [L., dim. of *torus*] a small elevation or papilla.

to′ruli tac′tiles [TA] tactile elevations: the small elevations on the skin of the palm and the sole, richly supplied with sensory nerve endings.

to•rus (tor′əs) pl. *to′ri* [L. "a round swelling," "protuberance"] 1. a bulging projection or swelling. 2. the doughnut-shaped geometric figure produced by rotating a circle about an axis that lies in the same plane as the circle but does not cut the circle.

t. aor′ticus a bulge in the anterosuperior part of the right coronary wall, caused by the proximity of the right aortic cusp and sinus.

t. fronta′lis a protuberance in the middle line of the root of the nose, on the external surface of the skull.

t. levato′rius [TA] the mucosal fold covering the levator veli palatini muscle in the lateral wall of the nasal part of the pharynx.

t. mandibula′ris [TA] mandibular torus: a prominence sometimes seen on the lingual aspect of the mandible at the base of its alveolar part, adjacent to the postcanine teeth.

t. occipita′lis a rounded edge occasionally seen on the occipital bone in the region of the superior nuchal line.

t. palati′nus [TA] palatine torus: a bony protuberance sometimes found on the hard palate at the junction of the intermaxillary suture and the transverse palatine suture.

t. tuba′rius [TA] tubal prominence: the projecting posterior lip of the pharyngeal opening of the auditory tube. Called also *eustachian cushion* and *tubal protuberance.*

tos•i•tu•mo•mab (tos″ĭ-too′mo-mab) a murine monoclonal antibody with actions similar to those of rituximab, binding the CD20 antigen; it is used as an antineoplastic in the treatment of CD20-positive, B-cell non-Hodgkin lymphoma; administered intravenously.

to•sy•late (to′sə-lāt) USAN contraction for *p*-toluenesulfonate.

To•ta•cil•lin (to″tə-sil′in) trademark for preparations of ampicillin.

to•ti•po•ten•cy (to″tĭ-po′tən-se) [L. *totus* all + *potency*] the ability to differentiate along any line or into any type of cell. **totip′otent, totipoten′tial** *adj*

to•ti•po•ten•ti•al•i•ty (to″tĭ-po-ten″she-al′ĭ-te) totipotency.

touch (tuch) [L. *tactus;* Old Fr. *touchier*] 1. the sense (actually a group of senses) by which contact with objects gives evidence as to certain of their qualities, as registered by mechanoreceptors in the skin and mucous membranes. Types of touch include light touch, coarse touch, tickling, pressure sense, vibration sense, tissue distortion sense, and pain sense. Called also *tactile sense* and *taction.* 2. palpation or exploration with the finger.

therapeutic t. (TT) a healing method based on the premise that the body possesses an energy field that can be affected by the focused intention of the healer, using a consciously directed exchange of energy between practitioner and patient. The practitioner uses the hands as a focus in order to assess the patient's energy field, to release areas where the free flow of energy is blocked, and to balance the patient's energy, by transferring energy from a universal life energy force to the patient.

touch•er•ism (tuch′ər-iz-əm) a paraphilia in which sexual arousal or orgasm is achieved by touching or fondling or by such fantasies. See also *frotteurism.*

Tou•pet fundoplication (operation) (too-pa′) [André *Toupet*, French surgeon, born 1915] see under *fundoplication.*

Tou•raine-So•lente-Go•lé syndrome (too-ren′ so-lahnt′ go-la′) [Albert *Touraine*, French dermatologist, 1883–1961; G. *Solente*, French physician, 20th century; L. *Golé*, French physician, 20th century] pachydermoperiostosis.

Tou•rette see *Gilles de la Tourette.*

Tour•nay sign (tōōr-na′) [Auguste *Tournay*, French ophthalmologist, 1878–1969] see under *sign.*

tour•ni•quet (toor′nĭ-kət) [Fr.] an instrument for compression of a blood vessel by application around an extremity to control the circulation and prevent the flow of blood to or from the distal area.

automatic rotating t. a system consisting of a motor, air compressor, and four blood pressure cuffs for application to the extremities; the cuffs are inflated and deflated in series and in sequence for treatment of acute pulmonary edema.

Esmarch t. see under *bandage.*

garrote t. Spanish windlass.

pneumatic t. a narrow rubber bag to be wound around a limb, pressure being applied by pumping air into the inflatable cuff.

scalp t. a tourniquet placed around the scalp with enough pressure to occlude the superficial blood vessels and thereby to lessen the risk of drug-induced alopecia.

Spanish t., torcular t. Spanish windlass.

Tou•ro (too′ro) trademark for a preparation of guaifenesin.

Tou•ton giant cell (too′ton) [Karl *Touton*, German dermatologist, 1858–1934] see under *cell.*

Towne projection (toun) [Edward Bancroft *Towne*, American physician, 1883–1957] see under *projection.*

Townes syndrome (tounz) [Philip Leonard *Townes*, American pediatrician, born 1927] see under *syndrome.*

Town•send ionization (toun′zənd) [John *Townsend*, Irish physicist, 1868–1957] see *avalanche ionization*, under *ionization.*

tox•ane•mia (tok″sə-ne′me-ə) toxic hemolytic anemia.

tox•a•phene (toks′ə-fēn) a chlorinated hydrocarbon used as an agricultural insecticide; if ingested or absorbed through the skin by a human or other animal, it may cause neurotoxicity such as tremors and potentially fatal convulsions. Called also *camphechlor.*

Tox•as•ca•ris (tok-sas′kə-ris) a genus of parasitic nematodes of the family Ascarididae.

T. leoni′na a species found commonly in large felines such as lions and tigers, and in domestic dogs and cats, especially older ones. Its larvae differ from those of *Toxocara canis* and *T. cati* by not passing through the lungs of the infected animal.

tox•emia (tok-se′me-ə) [*tox-* + *-emia*] any condition resulting from the spread of toxins or toxic bacterial products by the bloodstream. **toxe′mic** *adj*

pregnancy t. in cows fat cow syndrome.

pregnancy t. in ewes an acute disorder in ewes caused by ketosis during the last few weeks of pregnancy, especially when they are carrying twins, triplets, or a large single lamb; the usual cause is undernutrition associated with stress. It can lead to impaired nervous function, coma, and death. Called also *twin-lamb disease* and *lambing paralysis.*

tox•en•zyme (toks-en′zīm) any poisonous enzyme.

toxi- see *tox(o)-.*

tox•i•cant (tok′sĭ-kənt) [L. *toxicans* poisoning] 1. poisonous. 2. a poisonous agent.

tox•i•ca•tion (tok″sĭ-ka′shən) poisoning.

tox•i•ce•mia (tok″sĭ-se′me-ə) toxemia.

tox•ic•i•ty (tok-sis′ĭ-te) 1. the quality of being poisonous. 2. the degree of virulence of a toxic microbe or of a poison.

developmental t. the extent to which a toxin crosses the placental barrier and produces adverse effects on a developing embryo or fetus; see also *teratogenesis.*

fetal t. developmental toxicity in a fetus.

glucose t. glucotoxicity.

O_2 t., oxygen t. the effects of hyperoxia due to the breathing of high partial pressures of oxygen for prolonged periods; they include serious, sometimes irreversible, damage to the pulmonary capillary endothelium, followed by cerebral edema and convulsions that can be fatal. Called also *oxygen poisoning.*

radiation t. the degree of virulence of a given exposure or dose of ionizing radiation; see also *radiation sickness*, under *sickness.* Called also *radiotoxicity.*

toxic(o)- [Gr. *toxikon (pharmakon)* poison for arrows, from *toxon* bow] a combining form meaning poisonous or denoting relationship to poison. See also *tox(o)-.*

tox•i•co•den•drol (tok″sĭ-ko-den′drol) a poisonous, nonvolatile oil found in certain plants of the genus *Rhus (Toxicodendron).*

Tox•i•co•den•dron (tok″sĭ-ko-den′dron) [*toxico-* + Gr. *dendron* tree] name often used for only the poisonous species of *Rhus.*

T. diversilo′bum *Rhus diversiloba.*

T. pubes′cens Atlantic poison oak, a variant of *Rhus toxicodendron.*

T. quercifo′lium *Rhus quercifolia.*

T. ra′dicans *Rhus radicans.*

T. rydber′gii *Rhus rydbergii.*

T. toxica′rium, T. toxicoden′dron *Rhus toxicodendron.*

T. ver′nix *Rhus vernix.*

tox•i•co•gen•ic (tok″sĭ-ko-jen′ik) toxigenic.

tox•i•coid (tok′sĭ-koid) resembling a poison.

tox•i•col•o•gist (tok″sĭ-kol′ə-jist) a specialist in toxicology.

tox•i•col•o•gy (tok″sĭ-kol′ə-je) the sum of what is known regarding poisons; the scientific study of poisons, their actions, their detection, and the treatment of the conditions produced by them. **toxicolog′ic** *adj*

developmental t. the study of the effects of toxins on embryos in utero. Cf. *teratology.*

tox•i•cop•a•thy (tok″sĭ-kop′ə-the) [*toxico-* + *-pathy*] toxicosis.

tox•i•co•pex•is (tok″sĭ-ko-pek′sis) [*toxico-* + *pexis*] the fixing or neutralizing of a poison in the body. **toxicopec′tic, toxicopex′ic** *adj*

tox•i•co•pexy (tok′sĭ-ko-pek″se) toxicopexis.

tox•i•co•phid•ia (tok″sĭ-ko-fid′e-ə) [*toxico-* + Gr. *ophis* snake] venomous snakes.

tox•i•co•pho•bia (tok″sĭ-ko-fo′be-ə) [*toxico-* + *-phobia*] irrational fear of being poisoned.

tox•i•co•sis (tok″sĭ-ko′sis) [*toxic-* + *-osis*] any disease condition due to poisoning. See also entries under *poisoning.*

exogenic t. poisoning by the ingestion of toxic material, as in the food. See *food poisoning*, under *poisoning.*

fescue t. fescue foot.

gestational t. preeclampsia.

hemorrhagic capillary t. Henoch-Schönlein purpura.

proteinogenous t. an acute and fatal intoxication seen in laboratory mice fed a diet consisting exclusively of protein.

retention t. toxicosis that is due to failure to excrete noxious waste products.

T_3 t. thyrotoxicosis in which the production of triiodothyronine (T_3) is increased disproportionately to that of thyroxine (T_4).

T_4 t. thyrotoxicosis in which the serum levels of thyroxine (T_4) are increased, while serum levels of triiodothyronine (T_3) are normal or decreased; it may be caused by ingestion of iodine-containing compounds or may accompany severe illness.

tick t. sweating sickness.

toxi•cyst (tok′sĭ-sist) [*toxi-* + *cyst*] one of the numerous toxic subpellicular organelles occurring as slender extrusible tubular structures located apically in certain ciliate protozoa, especially certain of the Kinetofragminophorea, with which the organism penetrates the body of and cytolyzes its prey. Cf. *trichocyst.*

tox•i•drome (tok′sĭ-drōm) a specific syndromelike group of symptoms associated with exposure to a given poison.

tox•if•er•ous (tok-sif′ər-əs) [*toxi-* + *-ferous*] 1. carrying or conveying a poison. 2. toxicogenic.

tox•i•gen•e•sis (tok″sĭ-jen′ə-sis) the elaboration of a poison.

tox•i•gen•ic (tok″sĭ-jen′ik) 1. producing or elaborating toxins. 2. derived from or containing toxins.

tox•i•ge•nic•i•ty (tok″sĭ-jə-nis′ĭ-te) the property of producing toxins.

tox•ig•nom•ic (tok″sig-nom′ik) [*toxin* + Gr. *gnōmē* a means of knowing] characteristic of the toxic action of a poison.

tox•in (tok′sin) [Gr. *toxikon (pharmakon)* poison for arrows, from *toxon* bow] a poison; frequently used to refer specifically to a protein that is produced by some higher plants, certain animals, or pathogenic bacteria and is highly toxic for other living organisms. Such substances are differentiated from the simple chemical poisons and the vegetable alkaloids by their high molecular weight and antigenicity. **tox′ic** *adj*

A-B t's a class of exotoxins consisting of an active (A) component that crosses the cell membrane and a binding (B) component that binds to cell surface receptors.

***Amanita* t.** amatoxin.

animal t. zootoxin.

anthrax t. an exotoxin produced by most strains of *Bacillus anthracis* that is immunogenic, produces edema, and is lethal for mice. It consists of three heat-labile, antigenically distinct components: edema factor (EF, factor I), protective antigen (PA, factor II), and lethal factor (LF, factor III).

bacterial t's toxic substances produced by bacteria, including exotoxins, endotoxins, enterotoxins, neurotoxins, and toxic enzymes, such as seen in cases of food poisoning.

botulinal t., botulinum t., botulinus t. an exotoxin produced by germinating spores and growing cells of *Clostridium botulinum.* The toxin binds to presynaptic terminals of the central nervous system and blocks the release of acetylcholine, leading to paralysis. There are seven immunologically distinct types (A–G). Type A is one of the most powerful poisons known; it is also used therapeutically by injection to inhibit muscular spasm in the treatment of dystonic disorders such as blepharospasm and strabismus, to treat wrinkles of the upper face, and to reduce anal sphincter pressure to promote healing of chronic anal fissure. Type B is used therapeutically by injection in the treatment of cervical dystonia. See also *botulism.*

cholera t. an exotoxin produced by *Vibrio cholerae;* a protein enterotoxin that binds to the membrane of enteric cells and stimulates the adenylate cyclase system, causing the hypersecretion of chloride and bicarbonate ions seen in cholera. Called also *choleragen* and *cholera enterotoxin.*

clostridial t. a toxin elaborated by species of *Clostridium,* such as botulinus toxin, gas gangrene toxin, or tetanus toxin. *C. difficile* also produces an exotoxin that causes intestinal necrosis, and *C. perfringens* produces exotoxins that cause gas gangrene, intestinal necrosis, and hemolysis, others that have cardiotoxic, deoxyribonuclease, and hyaluronidase activity, and an enterotoxin that causes acute food poisoning.

Dick t. a type of streptococcal toxin used in the Dick test.

diphtheria t. a protein exotoxin produced by virulent (lysogenic) strains of *Corynebacterium diphtheriae* that is primarily responsible for the pathogenesis of diphtheritic infection. It is an enzyme that inhibits protein synthesis by inactivating a factor (EF-2) required for the transfer of polypeptidyl-tRNA from acceptor to donor sites on ribosomes.

diphtheria t., diagnostic diphtheria t. for Schick test.

diphtheria t., inactivated diagnostic Schick test control.

diphtheria t. for Schick test [USP] a standardized preparation of diphtheria toxin used in the Schick test (q.v.). Formerly called *diagnostic diphtheria t.*

dysentery t. any of various exotoxins produced by species of *Shigella.* The one formed by *S. dysenteriae* serovar 1 (Shiga toxin) is a potent neurotoxin with hemorrhagic and paralytic properties.

erythrogenic t. streptococcal pyrogenic exotoxin.

extracellular t. exotoxin.

fatigue t. kenotoxin.

fugu t. tetrodotoxin.

fusarial t. any mycotoxin produced by molds of the genus *Fusarium.* See also *fusariotoxicosis.*

gas gangrene t. any of the exotoxins produced by *Clostridium perfringens* and associated with gas gangrene. At least 10 types have been identified. The α toxin is a lethal, necrotizing lecithinase (phospholipase-C) that splits lecithin in cell membranes, is hemolytic, and causes capillary damage. *C. novyi* and *C. septicum* produce similar toxins that cause gas gangrene.

intracellular t. endotoxin.

plague t. a necrotizing exotoxin produced by *Yersinia pestis;* its significance in the pathology of plague is unclear.

plant t. phytotoxin.

pseudomonal t. an exotoxin produced by *Pseudomonas aeruginosa.* It is a protein, lethal for mice and rats and toxic for fibroblast cultures, which inhibits protein synthesis by inactivating elongation factor EF_2.

Shiga t. the exotoxin formed by *Shigella dysenteriae* 1; it is also produced by some strains of *Escherichia coli.*

Shiga-like t. verocytotoxin.

soluble t. exotoxin.

staphylococcal t. a mixture of exotoxins produced by *Staphylococcus aureus.* There are four chemically and serologically distinct hemolysins, called α, β, γ, and δ, variously having dermonecrotic activity (α-hemolysin), sphingomyelinase activity (β-hemolysin), necrotizing activity (γ-hemolysin), and leukocidin activity (δ-hemolysin). Other toxins produced are leukocytal and exfoliative (causing scalded skin syndrome). Strains of *S. aureus* also produce five serologically distinct enterotoxins: types A and D are major factors in staphylococcal food poisoning.

streptococcal t. a mixture of exotoxins formed by *Streptococcus pyogenes,* including two distinct hemolysins *(streptolysin O* and *streptolysin S),* an erythrogenic toxin (causing scarlet fever rash), and a DPNase that is cardiotoxic.

T-2 t. a trichothecene mycotoxin produced by *Fusarium poae, F. sporotrichioides,* and *F. tricinctum,* which contaminates grain and other foodstuffs, causing fusariotoxicosis with hemorrhaging in livestock and alimentary toxic aleukia in humans.

tetanus t. tetanospasmin.

tox•in-an•ti•tox•in (TA) (tok″sin-an′tĭ-tok″sin) a nearly neutral mixture of diphtheria toxin with its antitoxin; formerly used for immunization against diphtheria.

tox•in•emia (tok″sĭ-ne′me-ə) toxemia.

tox•in•ol•o•gy (tok″sin-ol′ə-je) the science dealing with the toxins produced by certain higher plants and animals and by pathogenic bacteria.

tox•in•o•sis (tok″sĭ-no′sis) toxicosis.

toxi•pho•bia (tok″sĭ-fo′be-ə) toxicophobia.

tox•is•ter•ol (tok-sis′tər-ol) [*toxi-* + *sterol*] a poisonous isomer of ergosterol, produced by ultraviolet irradiation of ergosterol.

tox(o)- [Gr. *toxikon (pharmakon)* poison for arrows, from *toxon* bow] a combining form denoting relationship to a toxin, or poison. Also *toxi-, toxic(o)-.*

Tox•o•ca•ra (tok″so-kar′ə) a genus of nematodes of the family Ascarididae.

T. ca′nis a species usually parasitic in the intestine of dogs; migrating larvae may cause lesions of the lung, liver, kidney, brain, and eye. In human infections, the larvae do not complete their cycle but cause visceral larva migrans (see under *larva*).

T. ca′ti a species closely related to *T. canis* but usually found in cats; it has also been reported in humans as an accidental intestinal parasite that may cause visceral larva migrans (see under *larva*). Called also *T. mystax.*

T. mys′tax *T. cati.*

tox•o•car•al (tok″so-kar′əl) pertaining to or caused by *Toxocara.*

tox•o•car•i•a•sis (tok″so-kə-ri′ə-sis) infection by roundworms of the genus *Toxocara,* such as in ocular or visceral larva migrans.

tox•o•gen (tok′so-jən) something that produces a poison.

toxo•glob•u•lin (tok″so-glob′u-lin) a poisonous globulin.

tox•oid (tok′soid) [*toxo-* + *-oid*] a modified or inactivated bacterial exotoxin that has lost toxicity but retains the properties of combining with, or stimulating the formation of, antitoxin.

***Clostridium perfringens* t.** see under *bacterin-toxoid.*

diphtheria t. the formaldehyde-inactivated toxin of *Corynebacterium diphtheriae,* used for immunization against diphtheria. It is generally used in mixtures with tetanus toxoid and acellular pertussis vaccine (DTaP or Tdap vaccines) or with tetanus toxoid alone (DT or Td) when pertussis vaccine is contraindicated.

diphtheria and tetanus t's adsorbed (DT) [USP] a combination of full-strength doses of diphtheria toxoid and tetanus toxoid which are adsorbed either before or after being combined; used for immunization of pediatric patients under seven years of age when pertussis vaccine is contraindicated.

tetanus t. (T) the formaldehyde-inactivated toxins of *Clostridium tetani,* used for immunization against tetanus; both fluid (tetanus toxoid [USP]) and adsorbed (on alum, aluminum hydroxide, or aluminum phosphate) (tetanus toxoid adsorbed [USP]) forms are available. It is used in mixtures with diphtheria toxoid and acellular pertussis vaccine (DTaP and Tdap), with diphtheria toxoid (DT and Td), or by itself (T); routine childhood immunization is generally with the first (diphtheria and tetanus toxoids and acellular pertussis vaccine).

tetanus and diphtheria t's (Td) a combination of tetanus toxoid and (reduced) diphtheria toxoid used for immunization of patients at least seven years of age when pertussis vaccine is contraindicated; it contains 5- to 10-fold less diphtheria toxoid than does the diphtheria and tetanus toxoid combination (DT) used for younger patients. It is available as *tetanus and diphtheria toxoids adsorbed for adult use* [USP].

tox•oid-an•ti•tox•oid (tok″soid-an′tĭ-tok″soid) a toxoid mixed with an equivalent amount of antitoxic serum, the precipitate being suspended in saline.

toxo•lec•i•thid (tok″so-les′ĭ-thid) toxolecithin.

toxo•lec•i•thin (tok″so-les′ĭ-thin) a lecithin compounded with a toxin, as cobra venom.

toxo•neme (tok′so-nēm) rhoptry.

toxo•phil (tok′so-fil) [*toxo-* + *-phil*] having an affinity for toxins.

toxo•phil•ic (tok″so-fil′ik) [*toxo-* + *-philic*] easily susceptible to a poison; having an affinity for toxins (like certain haptophore groups).

tox•oph•i•lous (tok-sof′ĭ-ləs) toxophilic.

toxo•phore (tok′so-for) [*toxo-* + *-phore*] the group of atoms in the molecule of a toxin that is responsible for the toxic effect. **toxoph′orous** *adj*

Toxo•plas•ma (tok″so-plaz′mə) [*toxo-* + *plasma*] a genus of coccidian protozoa (suborder Eimeriina, order Eucoccidiida) comprising intracellular parasites of many organs and tissues of birds and mammals. The only known complete hosts are cats and other felines, in which both asexual and sexual developmental cycles occur in the intestinal epithelium, culminating in the passage of oocysts in the feces. The intestinal stages do not occur in other hosts.

T. cuni′culi *T. gondii.*

T. gon′dii an obligate intracellular species found in a wide range of mammals and birds. The sexual cycle of the organism takes place in the intestinal epithelium of the cat, which is the definitive host. It exists in three forms: tachyzoite, tissue cysts (pseudocysts), and oocysts. Infection (see *toxoplasmosis*) occurs chiefly by ingestion of oocytes shed in cat feces or by ingestion of cysts in raw or uncooked meat.

toxo•plas•mic (tok″so-plaz′mik) pertaining to *Toxoplasma* or to toxoplasmosis.

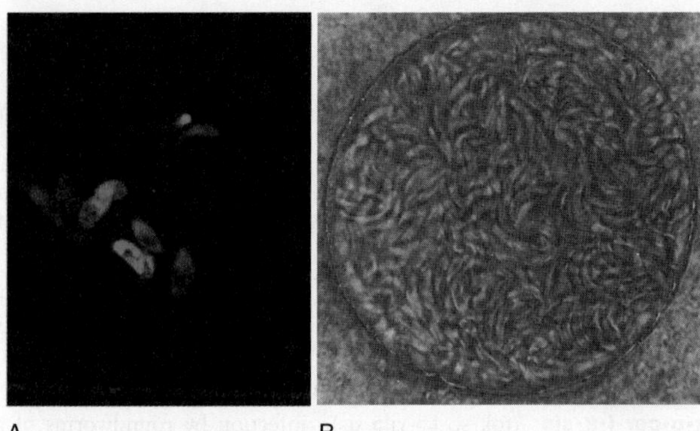

■ *Toxoplasma gondii. (A),* Tachyzoites; *(B),* tissue cyst containing bradyzoites.

tox•o•plas•mo•sis (tok″so-plaz-mo′sis) [*toxo-* + *plasma* + *-osis*] infection by the protozoon *Toxoplasma gondii,* transmitted in oocysts in the feces of cats (the definitive host), usually by contaminated soil, exposure to feces, tissue cysts in infected meat, or tachyzoites in blood. Most human infections are asymptomatic; when symptoms do occur, they are often a mild disease resembling mononucleosis. Occasionally toxoplasmosis becomes a fulminating, disseminated disease, usually in an immunocompromised patient or a fetus infected transplacentally; this may cause extensive damage to the brain, eyes, skeletal muscles, heart, liver, or lungs. See also *toxoplasmic meningoencephalitis* and *toxoplasmic chorioretinitis.* Chorioretinitis may occur with any form but is most often a late sequel of the congenital type. In domestic animals toxoplasmosis may be any of several nonfatal conditions such as a type of infectious abortion in ewes.

ocular t. toxoplasmic chorioretinitis.

pulmonary t. infection of the lungs by *Toxoplasma gondii,* usually seen in immunocompromised patients; symptoms resemble those of pneumocystis pneumonia, with fever, coughing, and dyspnea.

toxo•pro•tein (tok″so-pro′tēn) 1. a toxic protein; see *toxin.* 2. a mixture of a toxin and a protein.

Toyn•bee corpuscles, law, etc. (toin′be) [Joseph *Toynbee,* English otologist, 1815–1866] see under *maneuver* and *test;* see *corneal corpuscles,* under *corpuscle;* and see *Gull-Toynbee law,* under *law.*

TPA, t-PA tissue plasminogen activator.

TPHA *Treponema pallidum* hemagglutination assay.

t-plas•min•o•gen ac•ti•va•tor (plaz-min′o-jən″ ak′tĭ-va-tər) [EC 3.4.21.68] see under *activator.*

TPN total parenteral nutrition.

TPP thiamine pyrophosphate.

TR tricuspid regurgitation.

TRA tumor-specific transplantation antigen (tumor rejection antigen).

tra•be•cu•la (trə-bek′u-lə) pl. *trabe′culae* [L., dim. of *trabs* beam, timber] a supporting or anchoring strand of connective tissue, such as one extending from a capsule into the substance of the enclosed organ. **trabec′ular** *adj*

arachnoid trabeculae, trabe′culae arachnoi′deae [TA] delicate fibrous threads connecting the inner surface of the arachnoid to the pia mater.

trabeculae of bone anastomosing bony spicules in cancellous bone which form a meshwork of intercommunicating spaces that are filled with bone marrow.

trabe′culae car′neae cor′dis [TA] irregular bundles and bands of muscle projecting from a great part of the interior of the walls of the ventricles of the heart. They occur as three types: as simple muscular ridges, as bundles attached at both ends but free in the middle, or as papillary muscles (q.v.), projecting from the heart wall and attaching to the chordae tendineae cordis.

trabe′culae car′neae ventri′culi dex′tri [TA] the trabeculae carneae cordis in the right cardiac ventricle.

trabe′culae car′neae ventri′culi sinis′tri [TA] the trabeculae carneae cordis in the left cardiac ventricle.

trabe′culae cor′porum cavernoso′rum pe′nis [TA] trabeculae of corpora cavernosa of penis: numerous bands and cords of fibromuscular tissue traversing the interior of the corpora cavernosa of the penis, attached to the tunica albuginea and septum and creating the cavernous spaces that become filled with blood during erection.

trabe′culae cor′poris spongio′si pe′nis [TA] trabeculae of corpus spongiosum of penis: numerous bands and cords of fibromuscular tissue traversing the interior of the corpus spongiosum of the penis, creating the cavernous spaces that give the structure its spongy character.

trabe′culae cra′nii a pair of longitudinal cranial bars of cartilage in the embryo, bounding the pituitary space that becomes the sella turcica.

trabe′culae no′di lymphoi′dei trabeculae of lymph node: strands of dense connective tissue radiating out from the capsule through the interior of the node.

Rathke trabeculae trabeculae cranii.

t. septomargina′lis [TA] septomarginal trabecula: a bundle of muscle at the apical end of the right ventricle of the heart, connecting the base of the anterior papillary muscle to the interventricular septum; it usually contains a branch of the atrioventricular bundle. It has been thought to prevent ventricular overdistention and thus is called also *moderator band.*

trabe′culae sple′nicae [TA] trabeculae of spleen: fibrous bands that pass into the spleen from the tunica fibrosa and form the supporting framework of the organ.

tra•be•cu•lae (trə-bek′u-le) [L.] plural of *trabecula.*

tra•bec•u•lar•ism (trə-bek′u-lar-iz-əm) trabeculation (def. 2).

tra•bec•u•late (trə-bek′u-lāt) [L. *trabecula* a small beam or bar] marked with transverse or radiating bars or trabeculae.

tra•bec•u•la•tion (trə-bek″u-la′shən) 1. the formation of trabeculae in a part. 2. the condition of being trabeculated.

tra•bec•u•lec•to•my (trə-bek″u-lek′tə-me) [*trabecula* + *-ectomy*] creation of a fistula between the anterior chamber of the eye and the subconjunctival space by surgical removal of a portion of the trabecular meshwork, performed to facilitate drainage of the aqueous humor in glaucoma.

tra•bec•u•lo•plas•ty (trə-bek′u-lo-plas″te) plastic surgery of a trabecula.

laser t. an operation for open-angle glaucoma, in which surface burns are placed in the trabecular meshwork of the eye to lower intraocular pressure.

trace (trās) 1. a very small amount. 2. a sign of the former presence of something.

memory t. engram (def. 3).

trac•er (trās′ər) 1. a means or agent by which certain substances or structures can be identified or followed, as a radioactive tracer. 2. a mechanical device by which the outline of an object or the direction and extent of movement of a part may be graphically recorded; see also *tracing.* 3. a dissecting instrument for isolating vessels and nerves.

arrow point t., gothic arch t., needle point t. a mechanical device used in recording jaw movements, in which the tracing is made on a horizontal plate by a weighted or a spring-loaded needle attached to the jaw. See also under *tracing.*

radioactive t. a radioactive isotope replacing a stable chemical element in a compound (said to be *radiolabeled*) and so able to be followed or tracked through one or more reactions or systems by means of a radiation detector; used especially for such a compound that is introduced into the body for study of the compound's metabolism, distribution, and passage through the body.

stylus t. gothic arch t.

tra•chea (tra′ke-ə) pl. *tra′cheae* [L., from Gr. *tracheia artēria*] 1. [TA] the cartilaginous and membranous tube descending from the larynx and branching into the right and left main bronchi. It is kept patent by a series of about twenty transverse horseshoe-shaped cartilages. Called also *windpipe.* 2. one of a system of minute tubes ramifying throughout the body of a terrestrial arthropod and delivering air to the tissues; called also *tracheal tubule.* See also *tracheole.*

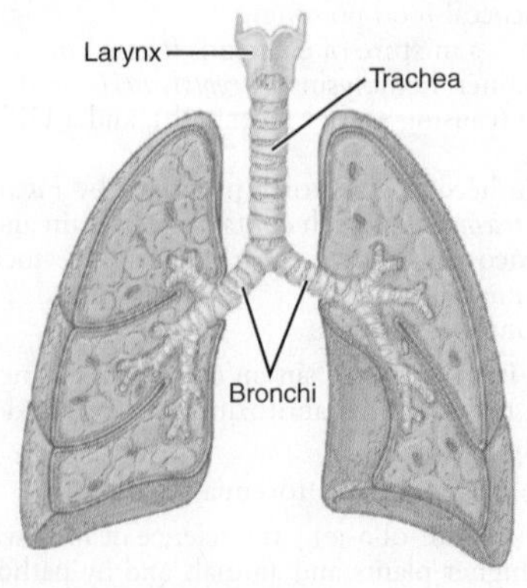

scabbard t. a trachea which is flattened by approximation of its lateral walls.

tra•cheae (tra′ke-e) [L.] plural of *trachea.*

tra•chea•ec•ta•sy (tra″ke-ə-ek′tə-se) dilatation of the trachea.

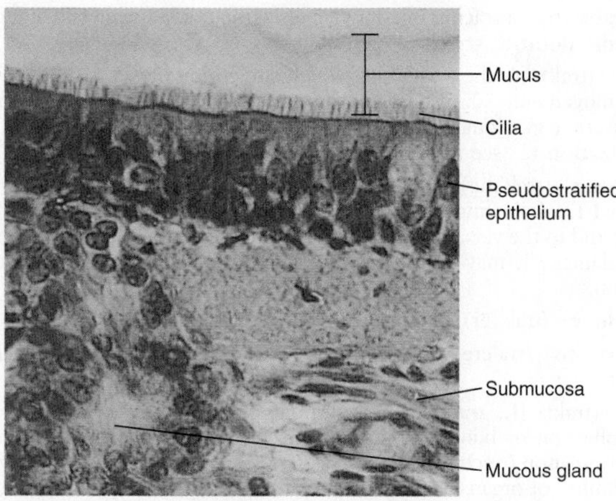

■ Trachea, transverse section.

tra·che·al (tra′ke-əl) [L. *trachealis*] pertaining to the trachea.

tra·che·al·gia (tra″ke-al′jə) [*trache-* + *-algia*] pain in the trachea.

tra·che·itis (tra″ke-i′tis) inflammation of the trachea.

bacterial t. an acute crouplike bacterial infection of the upper airway in children, characterized by coughing and high fever; common causative organisms are *Haemophilus influenzae* type B, *Moraxella catarrhalis, Staphylococcus aureus,* and species of *Streptococcus.* Called also *bacterial, membranous,* and *pseudomembranous croup.*

tra·che·lec·to·my (tra″kə-lek′tə-me) cervicectomy.

tra·che·lism (tra′kə-liz-əm) [Gr. *trachēlismos*] spasm of the neck muscles; spasmodic retraction of the head in epilepsy.

tra·che·lis·mus (tra″kə-liz′məs) trachelism.

tra·che·li·tis (tra″kə-li′tis) cervicitis.

trachel(o)- [Gr. *trachēlos* neck] a combining form denoting relationship to the neck or to a necklike structure.

tra·che·lo·cys·ti·tis (tra″kə-lo-sis-ti′tis) cystitis colli.

tra·che·lo·dyn·ia (tra″kə-lo-din′e-ə) cervicodynia.

tra·che·lo·pexy (tra′kə-lo-pek″se) cervicopexy.

tra·che·lo·plas·ty (tra′kə-lo-plas″te) cervicoplasty (def. 2).

tra·che·lor·rha·phy (tra″kə-lor′ə-fe) suture of the lacerated cervix uteri; called also *Emmet operation.*

tra·che·los·chi·sis (tra″kə-los′kĭ-sis) congenital fissure of the neck.

tra·che·lot·o·my (tra″kə-lot′ə-me) cervicotomy.

trache(o)- [L. *trachea,* q.v.] a combining form denoting relationship to the trachea.

tra·cheo·bron·chi·al (tra″ke-o-brong′ke-əl) pertaining to the trachea and bronchi. Called also *bronchotracheal.*

tra·cheo·bron·chi·tis (tra″ke-o-brong-ki′tis) inflammation of the trachea and bronchi.

canine infectious t. a contagious disease of the respiratory tract, seen in dogs that are confined together in close quarters and spread by aerosol droplets; characteristics include mild cough, laryngitis, and swelling of the air passages. In puppies and weakened animals it may progress to pneumonia. Etiologic agents include *Bordetella bronchiseptica,* adenoviruses, canine parainfluenza virus, and occasionally other bacteria or viruses.

tra·cheo·bron·cho·meg·a·ly (tra″ke-o-brong″ko-meg′ə-le) great enlargement of the lumen of the trachea and the larger bronchi, a rare, usually congenital condition. Called also *Mounier-Kuhn syndrome.*

tra·cheo·bron·chos·co·py (tra″ke-o-brong-kos′kə-pe) inspection of the interior of the trachea and bronchi.

tra·cheo·cele (tra′ke-o-sēl″) [*tracheo-* + *-cele*[1]] hernial protrusion of the tracheal mucous membrane.

tra·cheo·cu·ta·ne·ous (tra″ke-o-ku-ta′ne-əs) connecting the trachea and the skin surface, as a fistula.

tra·cheo·esoph·a·ge·al (tra″ke-o-ə-sof″ə-je′əl) pertaining to or communicating with both the trachea and esophagus. Called also *esophagotracheal.*

tra·cheo·fis·tu·li·za·tion (tra″ke-o-fis″tu-lĭ-za′shən) surgical creation of an opening in the trachea communicating with the cervical skin. See also *tracheostomy* and *tracheotomy.*

tra·che·o·gen·ic (tra″ke-o-jen′ik) originating in the trachea.

tra·cheo·la·ryn·ge·al (tra″ke-o-lə-rin′je-əl) laryngotracheal.

tra·che·ole (tra′ke-ōl) one of the minute, fluid-filled tubules in which the tracheae of a terrestrial arthropod terminate, which contain air cells and permeate all the body tissues.

tra·cheo·ma·la·cia (tra″ke-o-mə-la′shə) softening of the tracheal cartilages, often as a congenital condition in infants or in patients of any age after prolonged intubation, and usually accompanied by a barking cough and expiratory stridor or wheezing; nearby organs such as the esophagus or aorta may compress the trachea and cause apnea.

tra·cheo·path·ia (tra″ke-o-path′e-ə) tracheopathy.

t. osteoplas′tica a condition marked by the formation of a bony and cartilaginous deposit in the tracheal mucosa.

tra·che·op·a·thy (tra″ke-op′ə-the) [*tracheo-* + *-pathy*] disease of the trachea; called also *tracheopathia.*

tra·cheo·pha·ryn·ge·al (tra″ke-o-fə-rin′je-əl) pertaining to the trachea and pharynx.

Tra·che·o·phi·lus (tra″ke-ŏ′fĭ-ləs) a genus of trematodes. *T. cym′bius* is parasitic in the trachea of ducks in Europe and Asia. *T. cucumeri′nus* is parasitic in the trachea, esophagus, and thoracic cavity of chickens and ducks in Brazil and Madagascar.

tra·che·oph·o·ny (tra″ke-of′ə-ne) [*tracheo-* + Gr. *phōnē* voice] a voice sound heard over the trachea.

tra·cheo·plas·ty (tra′ke-o-plas″te) [*tracheo-* + *-plasty*] plastic repair of the trachea. **tracheoplas′tic** *adj*

slide t. surgical treatment of tracheal stenosis by dividing the stenosis at the midpoint, incising the segments vertically on opposite anterior and posterior surfaces, and sliding the segments together to create an anastomosis with a widened lumen.

tra·che·or·rha·gia (tra″ke-o-ra′jə) [*tracheo-* + *-rrhagia*] hemorrhage from the trachea.

tra·che·or·rha·phy (tra″ke-or′ə-fe) [*tracheo-* + *-rrhaphy*] repair of an incised or wounded trachea.

tra·che·os·chi·sis (tra″ke-os′kĭ-sis) [*tracheo-* + *-schisis*] fissure of the trachea.

tra·che·os·co·py (tra″ke-os′kə-pe) [*tracheo-* + *-scopy*] the inspection of the interior of the trachea. **tracheoscop′ic** *adj*

tra·cheo·ste·no·sis (tra″ke-o-stə-no′sis) [*tracheo-* + *stenosis*] contraction or narrowing of the trachea.

tra·che·os·to·ma (tra″ke-os′to-mə) [*tracheo-* + *stoma*] an opening into the trachea through the neck. Cf. *tracheostomy* (def. 3).

tra·che·os·to·mize (tra″ke-os′tə-mīz) to perform tracheostomy upon.

tra·che·os·to·my (tra″ke-os′tə-me) [*tracheo-* + *-stomy*] 1. tracheotomy. 2. creation of an opening in the anterior trachea for insertion of a tube to relieve upper airway obstruction and facilitate ventilation. 3. the opening created by either of these processes.

tra·cheo·tome (tra′ke-o-tōm) an instrument for use in incising the trachea.

tra·che·ot·o·mize (tra″ke-ot′ə-mīz) to perform tracheotomy upon.

tra·che·ot·o·my (tra″ke-ot′ə-me) [*tracheo-* + *-tomy*] surgical creation of an opening into the trachea through the neck, with the tracheal mucosa being brought into continuity with the skin. Called also *tracheostomy.*

inferior t. a tracheotomy below the isthmus of the thyroid.

superior t. a tracheotomy above the isthmus of the thyroid.

Tra·chin·i·dae (trə-kin′ĭ-de) the weever fishes (q.v.), a family of small stinging bony fishes.

Tra·chi·pleis·toph·o·ra (tra-kĭ-plīs-tof′ə-rə) a genus of parasitic protozoa (suborder Pansporoblastina, order Microsporida), usually found in the muscles of tropical freshwater fish; they have been found in immunocompromised persons, causing microsporidiosis with myositis.

T. ho′minis the most common species in the genus, found in cases of opportunistic myositis and other infections.

tra·chi·tis (trə-ki′tis) tracheitis.

tra·cho·ma (trə-ko′mə) pl. *tracho′mata* [Gr. *trachōma* roughness] a chronic infectious disease of the conjunctiva and cornea, producing photophobia, pain, and lacrimation, caused by a strain of *Chlamydia trachomatis.* Tiny follicles and later papillae form on the eyelid and conjunctiva, leading to contraction and scarring with symblepharon, entropion, trichiasis, and corneal scarring that can result in blindness. Called also *Arlt t.* and *granular* or *trachomatous conjunctivitis.* **tracho′matous** *adj*

Arlt t. trachoma.

tra·cho·ma·ta (trə-ko′mə-tə) [Gr.] plural of *trachoma.*

tra·chy·chro·mat·ic (tra″ke-kro-mat′ik) [Gr. *trachys* rough + *chromat-* + *-ic*] strongly or deeply staining.

tra·chy·onych·ia (tra″ke-o-nik′e-ə) [Gr. *trachys* rough + *onych-* + *-ia*] roughness of the nails with brittleness and splitting, usually associated with psoriasis, alopecia areata, or lichen planus. Called also *twenty-nail dystrophy.*

tra•chy•pho•nia (tra″kĭ-fo′ne-ə) hoarseness.

trac•ing (trās′ing) 1. a record of movements of the mandible produced by a tracer; the shape of the tracing depends on the relative location of the marking point and the tracing plate, and the apex of a properly made tracing is considered to indicate the most retruded unstrained position of the mandible in relation to the maxilla (centric jaw relation). 2. cephalometric t.

arrow point t. gothic arch t.

cephalometric t. a line drawing of structural outlines of craniofacial landmarks and facial bones made directly from a cephalometric radiogram.

extraoral t. a tracing of mandibular movements made outside the oral cavity.

gothic arch t. a tracing of the movements of the mandible, resembling an arrowhead or a Gothic arch, made by means of a device attached to the opposing arches, the exact shape depending on the location of the marking point relative to the tracing table; the apex of the tracing is considered as an indication of the centric relation. Called also *arrow point* or *needle point t.* See also *gothic arch tracer,* under *tracer.*

intraoral t. a tracing of condylar direction made within the oral cavity.

needle point t., stylus t. gothic arch t.

track (trak) 1. the path along which something moves, or the mark left by its movement. 2. of pus, to follow the path of least resistance through the tissues, e.g., along an intermuscular septum.

ionization t. see under *path.*

track•ing (trak′ing) pursuing or following.

visual t. following an object with one's gaze; it is fundamental to focusing and to the visual aspects of maintaining equilibrium. In patients with brain damage it may be assessed as a test for neurologic status and eye function.

Trac•leer (trak′lēr) trademark for a preparation of bosentan.

Tra•cri•um (tra′cre-əm) trademark for a preparation of atracurium besylate.

tract (trakt) [L. *tractus*] 1. a region, principally one of some length. 2. a collection or bundle of nerve fibers having the same origin, function, and termination (tractus [TA]); see also under *bundle, fasciculus,* and *lemniscus.* 3. a number of organs, arranged in series, subserving a common function.

Tract

For descriptions of specific anatomic structures not listed here, see under *tractus,* and see under the entries listed above.

aerodigestive t., upper the respiratory cavities of the head and neck considered together, including the nasal cavity, oral cavity, pharynx, and larynx.

alimentary t. digestive t.

anterolateral t's lemniscus spinalis.

ascending t. any bundle of nerve fibers conveying impulses toward the brain.

atriohisian t's myocardial fibers that bypass the physiologic delay of the atrioventricular node and connect the atrium directly to the bundle of His, allowing preexcitation of the ventricle.

Bekhterev (Bechterew) t. tractus tegmentalis centralis.

biliary t. the organs, ducts, and other structures that participate in the secretion, storage, and delivery of bile into the duodenum.

Bruce t., t. of Bruce and Muir fasciculus septomarginalis.

bulbar t. any of the bundles of nerve fibers of the medulla oblongata.

bulboreticulospinal t. tractus bulboreticulospinalis.

Burdach t. fasciculus cuneatus medullae spinalis.

central t. of auditory nerve a group of fibers passing from the cochlear nuclei to the superior olive, to the lateral lemniscus on the same and the opposite side and then up through the brachium of the inferior colliculus into the medial geniculate body and from there to the cortex of the transverse temporal gyri.

cerebellorubral t. a group of fibers arising chiefly in the dentate nucleus of the cerebellum and projecting to the opposite red nucleus via the superior cerebellar peduncle; impulses are then relayed to the reticular formation and spinal cord.

cerebellorubrospinal t. a group of fibers passing from one dentate nucleus of the cerebellum to the contralateral red nucleus, and thence to the spinal cord.

cerebellospinal t. uncinate fasciculus of the cerebellum, from the fastigial nucleus to the cervical cord.

cerebellotegmental t's of bulb fastigiobulbar t's.

cerebellothalamic t. dentatothalamic t.

ceruleospinal t. tractus caeruleospinalis.

comma t. of Schultze fasciculus interfascicularis.

conariohypophyseal t., conariohypophysial t. a portion of the cavity of the embryonic brain connecting the pineal gland (body) and the pituitary gland.

corticobulbar t. corticonuclear t.

corticohypothalamic t. a diffuse collection of fibers arising from various parts of the frontal lobe and are distributed directly to the hypothalamus.

corticonuclear t. the nerve fiber tract formed by fibers (corticonuclear fibers) associated with the pyramidal tract that arise in the cerebral cortex, descend in the internal capsule, and synapse in the various motor nuclei of the mesencephalon, pons, and medulla oblongata. Called also *corticobulbar t.*

corticopontine t. tractus corticopontinus.

corticorubral t. a group of fibers passing from the cerebral cortex to the red nucleus.

corticospinal t., anterior tractus corticospinalis anterior.

corticospinal t., crossed tractus corticospinalis lateralis.

corticospinal t., direct tractus corticospinalis anterior.

corticospinal t., lateral tractus corticospinalis lateralis.

corticospinal t., ventral tractus corticospinalis anterior.

corticospinal t. of medulla oblongata tractus pyramidalis (def. 1).

corticospinal t's of spinal cord the two spinal cord tracts that are continuations of the pyramidal tract of the medulla oblongata; see *tractus corticospinalis lateralis* and *tractus corticospinalis anterior.* Called also *pyramidal t's of spinal cord.*

corticotectal t., external a tract of efferent fibers from visual association areas of the cortex, running transversely into the zonal layer of the superior colliculus.

corticotectal t., internal a tract of efferent fibers from visual association areas of the cortex, running through the intermediate gray and white layers of the superior colliculus and carrying impulses to muscles controlling eye coordination.

cuneocerebellar t. the dorsal external arcuate fibers considered as a unit.

Deiters t. tractus vestibulospinalis.

dentatothalamic t. a group of fibers arising chiefly in the dentate nucleus of the cerebellum and projecting to the ventral lateral nucleus of the opposite thalamus via the cranial cerebellar peduncle; impulses are then relayed to the frontal lobe. Called also *cerebellothalamic tract.*

descending t. any bundle of nerve fibers conveying impulses from the brain toward target nuclei at lower levels of the nervous system.

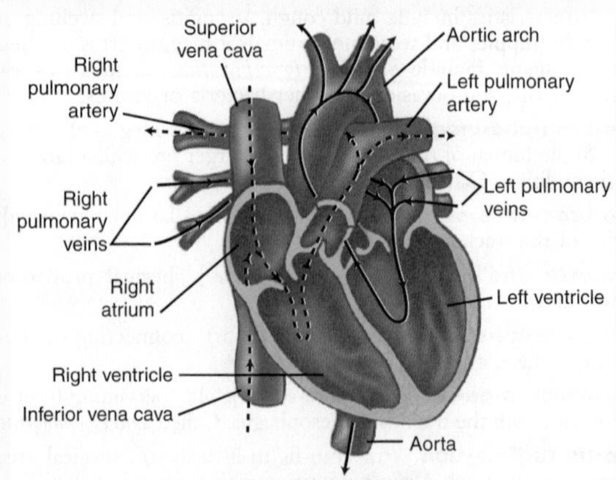

■ Flow tracts of the heart, left *(solid line)* and right *(dotted line).*

Tract *Continued*

digestive t. the part of the digestive system (TA, *systema digestorium*) consisting of the esophagus, stomach, and small and large intestines. Called also *alimentary t.* or *canal* and *digestive canal.*
dorsolateral t. tractus posterolateralis.
extracorticospinal t., extrapyramidal t. extrapyramidal system.
fastigiobulbar t's bundles of efferent fibers running from the nucleus fastigii to the medulla oblongata.
fastigiospinal t. tractus fastigiospinalis.
fiber t's of spinal cord distinct bundles in the white substance of the spinal cord, made up of fibers which have similar origin, termination, and function.
Flechsig t. tractus spinocerebellaris posterior.
flow t's of the heart the paths of the blood within the chambers of the heart. In the *left flow tract,* oxygenated blood from the pulmonary circulation enters the left atrium through the pulmonary veins, flows through the mitral valve into the left ventricle, and passes out through the aortic valve into the aorta and systemic circulation. In the *right flow tract,* deoxygenated blood from the systemic circulation enters the right atrium through the venae cavae, flows through the tricuspid valve into the right ventricle, and passes through the pulmonary valve and on into the pulmonary artery and the pulmonary circulation.
frontopontine t. tractus frontopontinus.
gastrointestinal t. the stomach and intestines in continuity.
geniculocalcarine t., geniculostriate t. radiatio optica.
genitourinary t. urogenital system.
Goll t. fasciculus gracilis medullae spinalis.
Gowers t. tractus spinocerebellaris anterior.
habenulointerpeduncular t., habenulopeduncular t. tractus habenulointerpeduncularis.
Helweg t. olivospinal t.
hypothalamicohypophysial t., hypothalamohypophysial t. tractus hypothalamohypophysialis.
iliotibial t. tractus iliotibialis.
intermediolateral t. columna intermediolateralis medullae spinalis.
internodal t's specialized conduction pathways, designated anterior, middle, and posterior, that preferentially transmit the cardiac impulse through the atria; their existence and details remain controversial.
internuncial t. a fiber tract connecting two nuclei or centers.
intersegmental t. of spinal cord, anterior fasciculus proprius anterior medullae spinalis.
intersegmental t. of spinal cord, dorsal fasciculus proprius posterior medullae spinalis.
intersegmental t. of spinal cord, lateral fasciculus proprius lateralis medullae spinalis.
intersegmental t. of spinal cord, posterior fasciculus proprius posterior medullae spinalis.
intersegmental t. of spinal cord, ventral fasciculus proprius anterior medullae spinalis.
interstitiospinal t. tractus interstitiospinalis.
intestinal t. the small and large intestines in continuity.
Lissauer t. tractus posterolateralis.
Löwenthal t. tractus tectospinalis.
Maissiat t. tractus iliotibialis.
mammillopeduncular t. a fiber tract from the mammillary body to nuclei in the interpeduncular fossa.
mammillotegmental t. fasciculus mammillotegmentalis.
mammillothalamic t. fasciculus mammillothalamicus.
Marchi t. tractus tectospinalis.
mesencephalic t. of trigeminal nerve tractus mesencephalicus nervi trigemini.
Meynert t. tractus habenulointerpeduncularis.
Monakow t. tractus rubrospinalis.
motor t. any bundle of nerve fibers within the central nervous system conveying impulses to neurons that innervate muscle.
nigrostriatal t. a bundle of nerve fibers extending from the substantia nigra to the globus pallidus and putamen in the corpus striatum; injury to it may be a cause of parkinsonism. Its interlacing pattern with fibers of the internal capsule gives it a comblike appearance. Called also *comb bundle.*
occipitopontile t., occipitopontine t. see *occipitopontine fibers,* under *fiber.*
olfactory t. tractus olfactorius.
olivocerebellar t. tractus olivocerebellaris.
olivocochlear t. tractus olivocochlearis.
olivospinal t. a group of nerve fibers in the lateral funiculus, seen as a triangular area in transverse section of the spinal cord; it descends from the olivary nucleus through the medulla oblongata to the upper cervical segments. Recent studies have drawn its existence into question. Called also *Helweg* or *triangular t.*
optic t. tractus opticus.
outflow t. ventricular outflow t.
paraventriculohypophysial t. tractus paraventriculohypophysialis.
parietopontine t. see *fibrae parietotemporopontinae,* under *fibra.*
peduncular t., transverse a small band of fibers passing from the brachium of the inferior colliculus to the sulcus medialis cruris cerebri.
Philippe-Gombault t. Gombault-Philippe triangle.
pontoreticulospinal t. tractus pontoreticulospinalis.
portal t. a channel through an acinus of the liver, containing terminal branches of three vessels: a hepatic artery proper, a hepatic portal vein, and a bile duct.
posterolateral t. tractus posterolateralis.
pyramidal t. tractus pyramidalis.
pyramidal t., anterior tractus corticospinalis anterior.
pyramidal t., crossed tractus corticospinalis lateralis.
pyramidal t., direct tractus corticospinalis anterior.
pyramidal t., lateral tractus corticospinalis lateralis.
pyramidal t., ventral tractus corticospinalis anterior.
pyramidal t. of medulla oblongata tractus pyramidalis (def. 1).
pyramidal t's of spinal cord corticospinal t's of spinal cord; see *tractus corticospinalis lateralis* and *tractus corticospinalis anterior.*
respiratory t. see under *system.*
reticulospinal t., reticulospinal t., anterior tractus reticulospinalis anterior.
reticulospinal t., lateral, reticulospinal t., medullary tractus bulboreticulospinalis.
reticulospinal t., medial tractus pontoreticulospinalis.
reticulospinal t., ventral tractus reticulospinalis anterior.
rubrobulbar t. tractus rubrobulbaris.
rubroreticular t. a group of fibers extending from the red nucleus to the reticular formation of the pons and medulla oblongata.
rubrospinal t. tractus rubrospinalis.
Schultze t., semilunar t. fasciculus interfascicularis.
Schütz t. fasciculus longitudinalis posterior.
sensory t. any bundle of nerve fibers within the central nervous system that conveys sensory information originating from peripheral receptors.
septomarginal t. fasciculus septomarginalis.
sinus t. a pathological passage in the body resembling a fistula but open at only one end; it may later develop infection that drains through the tract.
solitary t. of medulla oblongata tractus solitarius medullae oblongatae.
spinal t. of trigeminal nerve tractus spinalis nervi trigemini.
spinocerebellar t., anterior tractus spinocerebellaris anterior.
spinocerebellar t., direct, spinocerebellar t., dorsal, spinocerebellar t., posterior tractus spinocerebellaris posterior.
spinocerebellar t., ventral tractus spinocerebellaris anterior.
spinocervical t. tractus spinocervicalis.
spinocervicothalamic t. a tract ascending uncrossed in the posterior part of the lateral funiculus to the lateral cervical nucleus, which relays to the thalamus by way of the opposite medial lemniscus.
spinoolivary t. tractus spinoolivaris.
spinoreticular t. tractus spinoreticularis.
spinotectal t. tractus spinotectalis.
spinothalamic t. tractus spinothalamicus lateralis.
spinothalamic t., anterior tractus spinothalamicus anterior.
spinothalamic t., lateral tractus spinothalamicus lateralis.
spinothalamic t., ventral tractus spinothalamicus anterior.
Spitzka t., Spitzka-Lissauer t. tractus posterolateralis.
strionigral t. a bundle of fibers from the corpus striatum to the substantia nigra.
sulcomarginal t. fasciculus sulcomarginalis.
supraopticohypophysial t. tractus supraopticohypophysialis.
tectobulbar t. tractus tectobulbaris.
tectocerebellar t. a bundle of fibers from the tectum of the mesencephalon to the cerebellum.
tectospinal t. tractus tectospinalis.
tegmental t. a tract of fibers in the tegmentum, back of the nucleus posterior corporis trapezoidei, believed to connect the latter with the midbrain.
tegmental t., central tractus tegmentalis centralis.
tegmentospinal t. tractus reticulospinalis anterior.

Tract *Continued*

temporopontine t. see *fibrae parietotemporopontinae* and *fibrae temporopontinae*, under *fibra.*
thalamo-olivary t. a bundle of fibers descending from the thalamus to the olivary nucleus.
triangular t. olivospinal t.
triangular t. of Philippe and Gombault Gombault-Philippe triangle.
trigeminothalamic t. lemniscus trigeminalis.
tuberohypophysial t., tuberoinfundibular t. a group of nerve fibers arising in the cells of the infundibular nucleus and related nuclei of the intermediate hypothalamic region, believed to provide a neurosecretory pathway associated with the control of secretory activity by the adenohypophysis.
urinary t. 1. systema urinarium. 2. sometimes more specifically the conduits leading from the pelvis of the kidneys to the urinary meatus.
urogenital t. see under *system.*
uveal t. tunica vasculosa bulbi.
ventral amygdalofugal t. a diffuse fiber tract connecting the basolateral part of the amygdaloid body with the lateral preoptic and hypothalamic regions. Cf. *stria terminalis.*
ventricular outflow t. the portion of the flow tract of the heart in which blood flows out of a ventricle; called also *outflow t.*
vestibulocerebellar t. a group of fibers of the pars vestibularis nervi octavi that extends to the cortex of the cerebellum.
vestibulospinal t., lateral tractus vestibulospinalis lateralis.
vestibulospinal t., medial tractus vestibulospinalis medialis.
Vicq d'Azyr t. fasciculus mammillothalamicus.
vocal t. the passages from the glottis through the nose and throat that influence the quality of the voice.

trac·tel·lum (trak-tel'əm) pl. *tractel'la* [L.] an anterior locomotive flagellum.

trac·tion (trak'shən) [L. *tractio*] the act of drawing or exerting a pulling force, as along the long axis of a structure.
  Bryant t. overhead vertical traction for fracture of the femoral shaft.
  cervical t. traction applied to the neck, usually by means of a sling that fits under the chin and behind the occiput; used in the treatment of osteoarthritis, rheumatoid arthritis, and other disorders of the cervical spine.
  controlled cord t. Brandt-Andrews method.
  elastic t. traction by an elastic force or by means of an elastic appliance.
  external t. traction applied by means of a fixed anchorage (as by a headgear) outside the oral cavity; used principally in the management of midfacial fractures.
  halo-pelvic t. traction applied to the spine by means of two metal hoops, one (the halo) applied to the skull and the other to the pelvis, connected by four extension rods which can be lengthened by turn screws.
  intermaxillary t. maxillomandibular t.
  internal t. traction applied by using one of the cranial bones above the point of fracture for anchorage; used in the management of facial fractures.
  lumbar t. traction applied to the lumbar spine.
  maxillomandibular t. traction applied by means of elastic or wire ligatures and interdental wiring and/or splints; called also *intermaxillary t.*
  Russell t. traction incorporating a sling beneath the knee that is connected to an overhead pulley.
  skeletal t. traction applied directly upon the long bones by means of pins, Kirschner wire, or some other mechanism.
  skin t. traction on a body part maintained by an apparatus affixed by dressings to the body surface.
  tongue t. the pulling forward of the tongue to improve the airway.

trac·tor (trak'tər) [L. "drawer"] an instrument for applying traction.
  prostatic t. a straight instrument with a traction apparatus on the end, formerly used to draw the prostate down in perineal prostatectomy.
  Syms t. a type of prostatic tractor having an inflatable rubber bag at the end to bring down the prostate.

trac·tot·o·my (trak-tot'ə-me) surgical severing or incising of a nerve tract.
  medullary t. interruption of one or more tracts in the medulla oblongata for the relief of pain.
  mesencephalic t. mesencephalotomy.
  stereotactic t. production of lesions in the fibers of the caudate nucleus; used as a psychosurgical technique to relieve intractable depression, anxiety, or obsessional states.

trac·tus (trak'təs) pl. *trac'tus* [L. "track, trail"] 1. a tract; a region, principally one of some length. 2. [TA] a collection or bundle, especially of nerve fibers, having the same origin and termination, and serving the same function. See also under *bundle, fasciculus,* and *lemniscus.*

Tractus

Descriptions are given on the TA terms, and include anglicized names of specific tracts.

trac'tus anterolatera'les TA alternative for *lemniscus spinalis.*
t. bulboreticulospina'lis [TA] bulboreticulospinal tract: a group of reticulospinal nerve fibers in the lateral funiculus of the spinal cord, whose axons are derived from nerve cells of the medulla oblongata. Called also *lateral reticulospinal tract* and *medullary reticulospinal tract.*
t. caeruleospina'lis [TA] ceruleospinal tract: a tract arising from the nucleus caeruleus and nucleus subcaeruleus and projecting to spinal laminae, predominately laminae VII to IX, at all levels; it includes projections to the intermediolateral cell column and sacral parasympathetic cell groups. The tract is bilateral with most fibers remaining ipsilateral.
t. corticoponti'nus [TA] corticopontine tract: the collection of corticopontine fibers (fibrae corticopontinae), arising in various areas of the cerebral cortex, particularly from areas involved in movement, and projecting to the pons.
t. corticospina'lis ante'rior [TA] anterior corticospinal tract: a group of nerve fibers in the anterior funiculus of the spinal cord, originating in the cerebral cortex; called also *t. pyramidalis anterior; direct* or *ventral corticospinal tract;* and *anterior, direct,* or *ventral pyramidal tract.*
t. corticospina'lis latera'lis [TA] lateral corticospinal tract: a group of nerve fibers in the lateral funiculus of the spinal cord, originating in the cerebral cortex; called also *crossed corticospinal tract, crossed* or *lateral pyramidal tract,* and *t. pyramidalis lateralis.*
t. fastigiospina'lis [TA] fastigiospinal tract: a tract arising in the fastigial nucleus, projecting to the contralateral side, and descending to terminate predominately in the intermediate zone and medial regions of the anterior horn of the spinal cord.
t. frontoponti'nus [TA] frontopontine tract: a collection of nerve fibers arising in the frontal lobe of the cerebrum, traversing the internal capsule and peduncle, and ending in the pontine nuclei.
t. habenulointerpeduncula'ris [TA] habenulointerpeduncular tract: a bundle of nerve fibers arising in the habenular nuclei and extending rostroventrally to the interpeduncular nucleus to relay fibers to the reticular formation of the mesencephalon; called also *fasciculus retroflexus* [TA alternative], *habenulopeduncular tract,* and *Meynert bundle, fasciculus,* or *tract.*
t. hypothalamohypophysia'lis [TA] hypothalamicohypophysial tract: the group of nerve fibers making up the efferent pathways of the hypothalamus, arising in the hypothalamic nuclei and ending at various levels in the median eminence, infundibulum, and neurohypophysis (posterior pituitary). It contains subgroups of fibers; see *t. paraventriculohypophysialis* and *t. supraopticohypophysialis.* See also *tuberohypophysial tract.*
t. iliopu'bicus [TA] iliopubic tract: a thickened band of tissue that strengthens the lower part of the deep inguinal ring and forms the base of the internal spermatic fascia.

Tractus *Continued*

t. iliotibia′lis [TA] iliotibial tract: a thickened longitudinal band of fascia lata extending from the tensor muscle downward along the lateral side of the thigh to the lateral condyle of the tibia.
t. interstitiospina′lis [TA] interstitiospinal tract: a tract of nerve fibers descending from the interstitial nucleus into the spinal cord as part of the medial longitudinal fasciculus.
t. mesencepha′licus ner′vi trigemina′lis, t. mesencepha′licus ner′vi trige′mini [TA] mesencephalic tract of trigeminal nerve: a group of sensory fibers of the entering trigeminal nerve; they continue rostrally along the medial aspect of the superior cerebellar peduncle and their cell bodies are located in the nucleus of the mesencephalic tract.
t. olfacto′rius [TA] olfactory tract: a narrow triangular band in the olfactory sulcus of the frontal lobe, which arises from the olfactory bulb and extends posteriorly, to end by dividing into medial and lateral olfactory striae, the latter ending in the primary olfactory cortex.
t. olivocerebella′ris [TA] olivocerebellar tract: a fiber tract that arises from the olive, crosses to the opposite side to pierce the other olive, and enters the cerebellum through its inferior peduncle.
t. olivocochlea′ris [TA] olivocochlear tract: a group of fibers derived from the nucleus of the superior olive that terminates in relation to the hair cells in the spiral organ of the cochlea; called also *olivocochlear fasciculus.*
t. op′ticus [TA] optic tract: the tract arising from the optic chiasma, proceeding backward, around the cerebral peduncle, and dividing into a lateral and a medial root; the roots end in the superior colliculus and lateral geniculate body, respectively.
t. paraventriculohypophysia′lis [TA] paraventriculohypophysial tract: the part of the hypothalamicohypophysial tract that arises in the paraventricular nucleus of the hypothalamus; some of the fibers end in the infundibulum and others reach the neurohypophysis (posterior pituitary), where their neurosecretory material is stored as oxytocin before being released into the systemic circulation. See also *t. supraopticohypophysialis.*
t. pontoreticulospina′lis [TA] pontoreticulospinal tract: a group of reticulospinal nerve fibers in the lateral funiculus of the spinal cord, arising in the pontobulbar region. Called also *medial reticulospinal tract.*
t. posterolatera′lis [TA] posterolateral tract: a group of nerve fibers in the lateral funiculus of the spinal cord immediately external to the posterior horn, composed in part of primary pain and temperature fibers which enter the spinal cord, travel the distance of a few segments in the dorsolateral tract, and then synapse in the posterior horn. Called also *dorsolateral fasciculus* or *tract* and *Lissauer marginal zone.*
t. pyramida′lis 1. [TA] pyramidal tract: a term generally applied to several groups of fibers (corticonuclear, corticospinal, and corticoreticular) arising chiefly in the sensorimotor regions of the cerebral cortex and descending in the internal capsule, cerebral peduncle, and pons to the medulla oblongata, the corticoreticular fibers descending with the corticospinal fibers and synapsing with cells of the reticular formation and the corticonuclear fibers synapsing with motor nuclei throughout the brainstem. Most of the corticospinal fibers cross in the decussation of the pyramids and descend in the spinal cord as the lateral corticospinal tract; most of the uncrossed fibers form the anterior corticospinal tract; both end by synapsing with internuncial and motor neurons. The pyramidal tract is a phylogenetically new tract, most prominent in humans, and provides for direct cortical control and initiation of skilled movements, especially those related to speech and involving the hand and fingers. Called also *corticospinal tract of medulla oblongata, fasciculus pyramidalis medullae oblongatae,* and *pyramidal system.* 2. either of the corticospinal tracts of the spinal cord; see *t. corticospinalis anterior* and *t. corticospinalis lateralis.*
t. pyramida′lis ante′rior t. corticospinalis anterior.
t. pyramida′lis latera′lis t. corticospinalis lateralis.
t. pyramida′lis ventra′lis t. corticospinalis anterior.
t. reticulospina′lis ante′rior [TA], **t. reticulospina′lis ventra′lis** anterior reticulospinal tract: a group of fibers arising mostly from the reticular formation of the pons and medulla oblongata; chiefly homolateral, the fibers descend in the ventral and lateral funiculi to most levels of the spinal cord; called also *ventral reticulospinal tract* and *tegmentospinal tract.*
t. rubrobulba′ris [TA] rubrobulbar tract: a group of nerve fibers arising in the red nucleus and terminating at several different parts of the brainstem including the nucleus of the facial nerve, the motor nucleus of the trigeminal nerve, and the inferior olivary nucleus.
t. rubrospina′lis [TA] rubrospinal tract: a group of nerve fibers in the lateral funiculus of the spinal cord, arising in the large cells of the red nucleus of the mesencephalon and terminating predominantly in the cervical region of the spinal cord. Called also *Monakow bundle, fasciculus,* or *tract.*
t. solita′rius medul′lae oblonga′tae [TA] solitary tract of medulla oblongata: a descending tract in the medulla oblongata, ventrolateral to the caudal part of the fourth ventricle, near the dorsal nucleus of the vagus and glossopharyngeal nerves, and comprising primary visceral afferent fibers from the facial, glossopharyngeal, and vagus nerves.
t. spina′lis ner′vi trigemina′lis, t. spina′lis ner′vi trige′mini [TA] spinal tract of trigeminal nerve: a descending tract of the trigeminal nerve extending from the level of entrance of the sensory root of the trigeminal nerves into the pons to the upper cervical segments of the spinal cord. It lies lateral to the nucleus of the spinal tract of the trigeminal nerve, in which its fibers synapse, and carries mainly pain and temperature impulses from the face.
t. spinocerebella′ris ante′rior [TA] anterior spinocerebellar tract: a group of nerve fibers in the lateral funiculus of the spinal cord, arising mostly in the opposite gray matter and ascending to the cerebellum by way of the anterior part of the lateral funiculus and then the superior cerebellar peduncle; they carry sensory impulses activated by nerve endings in skin, muscles, tendons, and joints. Called also *Gowers column, fasciculus,* or *tract, ventral spinocerebellar tract,* and *t. spinocerebellaris ventralis.*
t. spinocerebella′ris dorsa′lis t. spinocerebellaris posterior.
t. spinocerebella′ris poste′rior [TA] posterior spinocerebellar tract: a group of nerve fibers in the lateral funiculus of the spinal cord, arising chiefly from the columna thoracica and ascending to the cerebellum by way of the posterior part of the lateral funiculus and then the inferior cerebellar peduncle; they carry sensory impulses activated by nerve endings in skin, muscles, tendons, and joints. Called also *direct* or *dorsal spinocerebellar tract* and *t. spinocerebellaris dorsalis.*
t. spinocerebella′ris ventra′lis t. spinocerebellaris anterior.
t. spinocervica′lis [TA] spinocervical tract: a somatosensory pathway consisting of fibers that pass out of the posterior spinocerebellar tract, pass through the lateral cervical nucleus, and ascend with the medial lemniscus to the nucleus ventralis posterolateralis of the thalamus.
t. spinooliva′ris [TA] spinoolivary tract: an ascending tract of nerve fibers in the lateral funiculus of the spinal cord, arising from the posterior gray columns of the spinal cord and running to the olivary nucleus.
t. spinoreticula′ris [TA] spinoreticular tract: an ascending tract of nerve fibers in the lateral funiculus of the spinal cord, passing to the reticular formation of the brainstem.
t. spinotecta′lis [TA] spinotectal tract: a group of nerve fibers in the lateral funiculus of the spinal cord, mostly crossed from their origin; they ascend as part of the anterolateral system to the superior and inferior colliculi and carry somatic sensory impulses.
t. spinothala′micus t. spinothalamicus lateralis.
t. spinothala′micus ante′rior [TA] anterior spinothalamic tract: a group of nerve fibers in the anterior funiculus of the spinal cord, continuous with the spinothalamic tract. They arise in the contralateral gray substance and ascend to the thalamus; in the rostral pons and midbrain they are located adjacent to the medial lemniscus. The fibers are part of the anterolateral system and carry sensory impulses activated by light touch. Called also *ventral spinothalamic tract.*
t. spinothala′micus latera′lis [TA] lateral spinothalamic tract: a group of nerve fibers in the lateral funiculus of the spinal cord; they arise in the opposite gray matter and ascend to the thalamus, running with the lateral lemniscus in the rostral brainstem. The fibers are part of the anterolateral system and carry sensory impulses activated by pain and temperature.
t. spira′lis foramino′sus [TA] foraminous spiral tract: a spiral area on the fundus of the internal acoustic meatus, below the crista transversa and in front of the area vestibularis inferior; it corresponds to the base of the cochlea and is perforated with numerous holes for the passage of branches of the vestibulocochlear nerve.
t. supraopticohypophysia′lis [TA] supraopticohypophysial tract: the group of fibers of the hypothalamicohypophysial tract arising in the supraoptic nucleus; some of the fibers descend to end in the infundibulum and others reach the neurohypophysis (posterior pituitary), where their neurosecretory material is stored as vasopressin before

Tractus *Continued*

being released into the systemic circulation. The term has also been used to denote either the entire set of fibers of the hypothalamicohypophysial tract entering the infundibulum without regard to point of termination, or only the parts of that tract that arise in the supraoptic nucleus and the paraventricular nucleus (see *t. paraventriculohypophysialis*).

t. tectobulba′ris [TA] tectobulbar tract: a bundle of fibers arising mostly in the superior colliculus; it descends to the lower border of the pons where it ends in the nuclei of the brainstem and in the reticular formation.

t. tectospina′lis [TA] tectospinal tract: a group of nerve fibers, chiefly crossed, arising mostly in the superior colliculus and descending to the cervical cord, where they lie in the ventral funiculus.

t. tegmenta′lis centra′lis [TA] central tegmental tract: a composite nerve tract arising from the midbrain tegmentum, periaqueductal gray matter, and red nucleus; it descends in the tegmentum and reticular formation to end in the inferior olivary complex. The tract includes an ascending component from the reticular formation. Called also *Bekhterev tract.*

t. trigeminothala′micus TA alternative for *lemniscus trigeminalis.*

t. vestibulospina′lis latera′lis [TA] lateral vestibulospinal tract: a group of nerve fibers arising from the lateral vestibular nucleus and descending first ipsilaterally in the periphery of the anterolateral funiculus and then through the medial part of the anterior funiculus at lower levels of the spinal cord, ending ipsilaterally in the medial part of the anterior gray column.

t. vestibulospina′lis media′lis [TA] medial vestibulospinal tract: a group of nerve fibers arising mainly from the medial vestibular nucleus and descending via the medial longitudinal fasciculus into the anterior funiculus of the spinal cord, close to the midline; it contains both crossed and uncrossed fibers and projects mainly to the cervical cord segments, ending at the midthoracic cord level.

---

traf•fick•ing (traf′ik-ing) [Old It. *trafficare* to trade] the carrying on of trade or communication.

vesicular t. the intracellular transport of proteins and lipids between organelles by means of vesicles; see *vesicular transport,* under *transport.*

trag•a•canth (trag′ə-kanth) [NF] the dried gummy exudation from *Astragalus gummifer* or other Asian species of *Astragalus;* used as a suspending agent for drugs. Called also *gum tragacanth.*

tra•gal (tra′gəl) pertaining to the tragus.

Tra•ger Approach (tra′gər) [Milton *Trager,* American physician, 1908–1997] see under *approach.*

Tra•gia (tra′je-ə) a genus of poisonous plants of the family Euphorbiaceae. *T. u′rens* and other species are weeds of the southern United States.

trag•i•on (traj′e-on) a cephalometric landmark located at the superior margin of the tragus of the ear.

trag•o•pho•nia (trag″o-fo′ne-ə) egophony.

tra•goph•o•ny (trə-gof′ə-ne) [Gr. *tragos* goat + *phōne* voice] egophony.

trag•o•po•dia (trag″o-po′de-ə) genu valgum.

tra•gus (tra′gəs) pl. *tra′gi* [L., from Gr. *tragos* goat] 1. [TA] the cartilaginous projection anterior to the external opening of the ear. 2. [TA] *(in the pl.)* hairs growing on the pinna of the external ear, especially on the cartilaginous projection anterior to the external opening.

accessory t. preauricular tag.

train•ing (trān′ing) a system of instruction or teaching; preparation by instruction and practice.

assertiveness t. a form of behavior therapy in which individuals are taught appropriate interpersonal responses involving direct, forthright expression of their feelings, needs and wishes, both negative and positive.

bladder t. the training of a child or an incontinent adult in habits of urinary continence.

bowel t. the training of a child or an incontinent adult in habits of fecal continence.

cognitive t. rehabilitation techniques aimed at restoring or preserving cognitive functions, such as in the elderly or persons with brain damage or schizophrenia.

tilt t. standing upright against a wall, with the ankles close together and 15 cm from the wall, for increasing periods each day, used for therapy for recurrent syncope.

train-of-four (trān′ əv fŏr′) a test for measuring the level of neuromuscular blockade: four consecutive stimuli are delivered along the path of a nerve and the response of the muscle is measured in order to evaluate stimuli that are blocked versus those that are delivered. Four equal muscle contractions will result if there is no neuromuscular blockade, but if nondepolarizing blockade is present, there will be a loss of twitch height and number, which will indicate the degree of blockade.

trait (trāt) 1. any genetically determined characteristic; see also entries under *character, gene,* and *inheritance.* 2. sometimes, more specifically, the condition prevailing in the heterozygous state of a recessive disorder, as in sickle cell anemia. 3. a distinctive behavior pattern.

dominant t. an inherited trait that is phenotypically expressed even when the mutant allele is present in the heterozygous state. Cf. *recessive t.*

hemoglobin C t. the heterozygous state for hemoglobin C; it is asymptomatic although individuals have increased numbers of target cells in the blood. See also *hemoglobin C–thalassemia disease,* under *disease.*

personality t. a consistent pattern of acting, feeling, and thinking that occurs across a variety of situations and endures, and so characterizes a person.

qualitative t. an inherited trait for which the phenotype falls into different categories, which are not necessarily ordered, e.g., blood type. It is usually caused by a single gene and expression is minimally influenced by the environment. Cf. *quantitative t.*

quantitative t. an inherited trait for which the phenotype falls anywhere along a continuum of values, e.g., height or weight. It is usually caused by the interaction of multiple genes. Cf. *qualitative t.*

recessive t. an inherited trait that is phenotypically expressed only when the mutant allele is present in the homozygous state. Cf. *dominant t.*

sex-influenced t. an inherited trait carried on an autosome but expressed more often or to a greater extent in one sex; e.g., androgenetic alopecia.

sex-limited t. an inherited trait carried on an autosome but expressed in one sex only, e.g., lactation.

sex-linked t. an inherited trait determined by a gene on a sex chromosome, and therefore having a different pattern of expression in males and females; the term is usually used to denote an X-linked trait.

sickle cell t. the condition, usually asymptomatic, caused by heterozygosity for hemoglobin S.

threshold t. a quantitative trait in which although expression can be said to fall along a continuum, the trait is usually evaluated as a function of whether the value crosses a defined threshold of observation, e.g., canine hip dysplasia.

X-linked t. an inherited trait determined by a gene on the X chromosome (X-linked gene); see also under *inheritance.*

Y-linked t. an inherited trait determined by a gene on the Y chromosome (Y-linked gene); see also under *inheritance.*

tra•jec•tor (trə-jek′tər) an instrument for locating a bullet in a wound.

TRALI transfusion-related acute lung injury.

tra•ma•dol hy•dro•chlo•ride (tram′ə-dol″) an opioid analgesic used for the treatment of moderate to moderately severe pain following surgical procedures and oral surgery; administered orally.

tra•maz•o•line hy•dro•chlo•ride (trə-maz′o-lēn) an adrenergic compound used intranasally as a decongestant.

trance (trans) a state of altered consciousness characterized by heightened focal awareness and reduced peripheral awareness; a sleeplike state of reduced consciousness and activity.

hypnotic t. the state induced by hypnosis.

Tran•date (tran′dāt) trademark for a preparation of labetalol hydrochloride.

tran•do•la•pril (tran-do′lə-pril″) an angiotensin-converting enzyme inhibitor used in the treatment of hypertension and post–myocardial infarction congestive heart failure or left ventricular dysfunction; administered orally.

tran•ex•am•ic ac•id (tran″ək-sam′ik) an antifibrinolytic that acts by competitively inhibiting activation of plasminogen; it is used as a hemostatic in the prophylaxis and treatment of severe hemorrhage associated with excessive fibrinolysis, such as that following oral surgery in patients with hemophilia; administered orally or intravenously.

tran·qui·liz·er (trang″kwĭ-līz′ər) [L. *tranquillus* quiet, calm + *-ize* + *-er* agent] a drug with a calming, soothing effect; currently it is usually used to denote a *minor t.*

major t. former name for antipsychotic agent; see *antipsychotic*.

minor t. antianxiety agent.

trans (tranz) [L., through] 1. in organic chemistry, having certain atoms or radicals on opposite sides. 2. in genetics, denoting two or more loci, particularly pseudoalleles, occurring on opposite chromosomes of a homologous pair. Cf. *cis*. See also *cis-trans test*, under *test*.

trans- a prefix meaning through, across, or beyond.

trans·ab·dom·i·nal (trans″ab-dom′ĭ-nəl) through the abdominal wall.

trans·ac·e·tyl·ase (trans-ə-set′ə-lās) acetyltransferase.

trans·ac·e·tyl·a·tion (trans″ə-set″ə-la′shən) a chemical reaction involving the transfer of an acetyl group. It occurs in many metabolic reactions.

trans·ac·ti·va·tion (trans-ak″tĭ-va′shən) stimulation of gene transcription by a specific protein.

trans·ac·y·lase (trans-a′sə-lās) acyltransferase.

trans·ac·y·la·tion (trans-a″sə-la′shən) a chemical reaction involving the transfer of the acyl radical between acetic and higher carboxylic acids.

trans·al·do·lase (trans-al′do-lās) [EC 2.2.1.2] an enzyme of the transferase class that catalyzes the transfer of a dihydroxyacetone group from a ketose phosphate to an aldose phosphate in a reaction of the pentose phosphate pathway.

trans·am·i·din·ase (trans″ə-mid′in-ās) amidinotransferase.

trans·am·i·nase (trans-am′ĭ-nās) [EC 2.6.1] a sub-subclass of enzymes of the transferase class that catalyze the transfer of an amino group from a donor (generally an amino acid) to an acceptor (generally a 2-keto acid). Most are pyridoxal phosphate proteins. Called also *aminotransferase*.

trans·am·i·na·tion (trans″am-ĭ-na′shən) the reversible transfer of an amino group from an amino acid to what was originally an α-keto acid, forming a new keto acid and a new amino acid, without the appearance of ammonia in the free state.

trans·anal (trans-a′nəl) performed through the anus.

trans·an·tral (trans-an′trəl) performed across or through an antrum, such as brain surgery done through the ethmoid antrum.

trans·aor·tic (trans″a-or′tik) performed through the aorta; used especially in reference to surgical procedures on the aortic valve, performed through an incision in the wall of the aorta.

trans·atri·al (trans-a′tre-əl) performed through the atrium; used especially in reference to surgical procedures on a cardiac valve, performed through an incision in the wall of the atrium.

trans·au·di·ent (trans-aw′de-ənt) permitting passage of the mechanical vibrations perceived as sound.

trans·ax·i·al (trans-ak′se-əl) directed at right angles to the long axis of the body or a part.

trans·ba·sal (trans-ba′səl) through the base, as a surgical approach through the base of the skull.

trans·bron·chi·al (trans-brong′ke-əl) performed through a bronchus.

trans·ca·lent (trans-ka′lənt) [*trans-* + L. *calere* to be hot] permitting the passage of radiant heat.

trans·cal·lo·sal (trans-kə-lo′səl) performed across or through the corpus callosum.

trans·cal·var·i·al (trans″kal-var′e-əl) through or across the calvaria.

trans·can·al (trans-kə-nal′) done through a canal, such as surgery done through the auditory canals.

trans·car·bam·o·yl·ase (trans″kahr-bam′o-ə-lās) carbamoyltransferase.

trans·car·boxy·lase (trans″kahr-bok′sə-lās) carboxyltransferase.

trans·cath·e·ter (trans-kath′ə-tər) performed through the lumen of a catheter.

trans·cel·lu·lar (trans-sel′u-lər) through a cell.

trans·cer·vi·cal (trans-sur′vĭ-kəl) performed through the cervical opening of the uterus.

trans·clo·mi·phene (trans-clo′mĭ-fēn) zuclomiphene.

trans·co·bal·a·min (TC) (trans″ko-bal′ə-min) any of three plasma glycoproteins, transcobalamin I, II, and III, that bind and transport cobalamin (vitamin B_{12}).

t. I (TCI) a plasma glycoprotein synthesized by granulocytes; it binds most of the endogenous cobalamin but its function is uncertain. Deficiency of the glycoprotein results in low levels of serum cobalamin but does not cause abnormalities of metabolism. Its concentration is increased in myeloproliferative disorders.

t. II (TCII) the plasma glycoprotein that binds vitamin B_{12} absorbed into the blood from the ileum then transports it to the tissues, predominantly the liver, where the complex is absorbed by the cells via receptor-mediated endocytosis. Deficiency of TCII results in failure of immunoglobulin production, megaloblastic anemia, granulocytopenia, thrombocytopenia, and intestinal villous atrophy, all correctable with vitamin B_{12} therapy.

t. III (TCIII) a plasma glycoprotein synthesized by granulocytes, differing from TCI only in its carbohydrate content. The serum concentration of TCIII is increased in myeloproliferative disorders, but its function is unknown.

trans·coch·le·ar (trnas-kok′le-ər) done through the cochlea, such as removal of a tumor. Cf. *translabyrinthine*.

trans·coe·lom·ic (trans-se-lom′ik) spreading by extension through a visceral cavity; said of tumor metastasis.

trans·con·dy·loid (trans-kon′də-loid) through the condyles.

trans·cor·ti·cal (trans-kor′tĭ-kəl) connecting two different parts of the cerebral cortex; also, dependent on disease of the tracts connecting different parts of the cerebral cortex.

trans·cor·tin (trans-kor′tin) an α-globulin that specifically and avidly binds and transports in plasma the unconjugated and presumably biologically active cortisol. Called also *corticosteroid-* or *cortisol-binding globulin*.

trans·cra·ni·al (trans-kra′ne-əl) performed through the cranium.

trans·cri·co·thy·roid (trans-kri″ko-thi′roid) through or across the cricothyroid membrane.

trans·cript (trans′kript) a strand of nucleic acid that has been synthesized using another nucleic acid strand as a template.

primary t. the initial RNA transcript of a eukaryotic gene, before post-transcriptional modifications and processing take place.

trans·crip·tase (trans-krip′tās) a general term denoting a DNA-directed RNA polymerase.

reverse t. RNA-directed DNA polymerase.

trans·crip·tion (trans-krip′shən) [L. *transcriptio* transfer, copy] the process by which a single-stranded RNA with a base sequence complementary to one strand of a double-stranded DNA is synthesized. The enzymes involved are called DNA-dependent RNA polymerases (see under *polymerase*).

reverse t. the synthesis of a DNA molecule complementary to RNA molecule, the RNA acting as a template; catalyzed by reverse transcriptase.

trans·crip·tome (trans-krip′tōm) [*transcript*ion + *-ome*] the complete population of mRNA transcripts produced by the genome at a particular time and under particular conditions, weighted by their expression levels.

trans·crip·to·mics (trans″krip-to′miks) the qualitative and quantitative study of the transcriptome.

trans·crur·al (trans-krōōr′əl) done through a crus.

trans·cu·ta·ne·ous (trans″ku-ta′ne-əs) transdermal.

trans·cy·to·sis (trans″si-to′sis) a means of transporting a substance across a cell, occurring mainly in sheets of polarized epithelial cells: the substance is taken up by endocytosis, sorted in the endosomal compartment, and delivered to the opposite side of the cell where it is released by exocytosis.

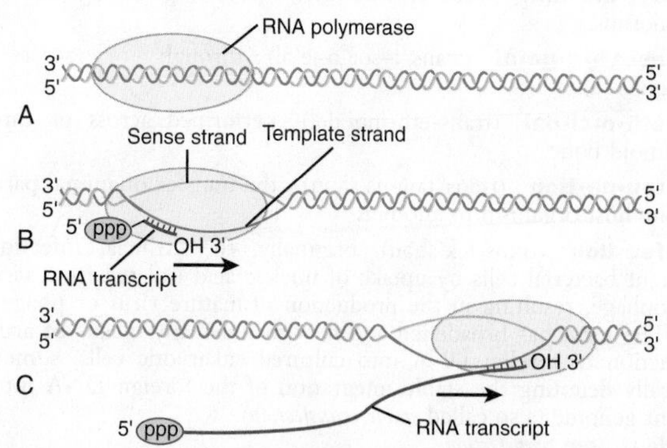

■ Transcription. Binding of the RNA polymerase at a specific site on DNA to be transcribed *(A)* is followed by unwinding of a region of the DNA helix and initiation of transcription in a 5′ to 3′ direction *(B)*, producing an RNA transcript complementary to, and hydrogen-bonded with, the template strand of the DNA. The transcript elongates as the polymerase proceeds down the DNA *(C)*, with the helix unwinding before and rewinding after it.

trans·der·mal (trans-dur′məl) entering through the dermis, or skin, as in administration of a drug applied to the skin in ointment or in a transdermal patch. Cf. *percutaneous.* Called also *transcutaneous.*

Trans·derm-Ni·tro (trans′dərm-ni′tro) trademark for a preparation of nitroglycerin.

Trans·derm-Scōp (trans′dərm-skōp′) trademark for a preparation of scopolamine.

trans·dif·fer·en·ti·a·tion (trans-dif″ər-en″she-a′shən) the irreversible conversion of differentiated cells of one type to normal cells of another type.

trans·du·cer (trans-doo′sər) a receptor or artificial device that translates one form of energy to another, such as pressure, temperature, or pulse to an electrical signal.

neuroendocrine t. a neuron having the properties of both nerve and gland, such as a neurohypophysial neuron, that on stimulation secretes a hormone, thereby translating neural information into endocrine information, with consequent inhibition or stimulation of hormonal secretion.

pressure t. an electronic device that converts pressure (such as blood pressure) into electrical signals that can be recorded graphically and monitored.

ultrasound t. a transducer used in ultrasonography, containing a piezoelectric crystal that can translate mechanical energy into electrical signals or electrical signals into mechanical energy.

trans·du·cin (trans-doo′sin) a G protein of the disk membrane of the retinal rods that interacts with activated rhodopsin and participates in the triggering of a nerve impulse in vision; it stimulates hydrolysis of cyclic guanosine monophosphate, beginning the cascade that closes specific ion channels and generates an action potential.

trans·duc·tion (trans-duk′shən) [L. *transducere* to lead across] 1. the transfer of genetic information from one bacterium to another via a bacteriophage vector. 2. the transforming of one form of energy into another, such as by the sensory mechanisms of the body; see also *sensory t.* and *transducer.*

generalized t. a form of bacterial transduction in which the phage head forms around a random piece of bacterial DNA and transports it to the recipient bacterial cell, where it integrates into the genome via recombination. Cf. *specialized t.*

mechanoelectrical t. transduction of a mechanical stimulus into an electrical impulse, as in the excitation of hair cells in the internal ear.

sensory t. the process by which a sensory receptor converts a stimulus from the environment into an action potential for transmission to the brain. See also *organa sensuum* under *organum.*

signal t. the process by which a cell receives and acts on some external chemical or physical signal, such as a hormone, including receiving the information at specific receptors in the plasma membrane, conveying the signal across the plasma membrane into the cell, and subsequently inducing an intracellular chain of other signaling molecules, thereby stimulating a specific cellular response.

specialized t. a form of bacterial transduction in which a temperate bacteriophage packages and carries some DNA from the region surrounding its integration site in the donor cell, transferring it to the recipient. Cf. *generalized t.*

visual t. the transducing of light energy to afferent nerve impulses, such as takes place in the retinal rods and cones.

trans·du·ral (trans-doo′rəl) through or across the dura mater.

tran·sec·tion (tran-sek′shən) [*trans-* + *section*] a section made across a long axis; a cross section; division by cutting transversely.

trans·epi·der·mal (trans″ep-ĭ-dur′məl) occurring through or across the epidermis.

trans·esoph·a·ge·al (trans″ə-sof″ə-je′əl) through or across the esophagus.

trans·eth·moi·dal (trans-eth-moi′dəl) performed across or through the ethmoid bone.

trans·fau·na·tion (trans″faw-na′shən) the transfer of animal parasites from one host organism to another.

trans·fec·tion (trans-fek′shən) originally, the artificial infection of competent bacterial cells by uptake of nucleic acid isolated from virus or bacteriophage, resulting in the production of mature virus or phage particles. The term has broadened and now includes any means of artificial introduction of foreign DNA into cultured eukaryotic cells; sometimes specifically denoting the stable integration of the foreign DNA into the recipient genome (also called *stable transfection*).

stable t. see *transfection.*

trans·fec·to·ma (trans″fek-to′mə) lymphoid cells transfected with immunoglobulin genes; they are capable of producing antibody molecules separate from the specificity encoded by their own genes.

trans·fem·o·ral (trans-fem′ə-rəl) 1. across or through the femur. 2. through the femoral artery.

trans·fer (trans′fər) [*trans-* + L. *ferre* to carry] the taking or moving of something from one place to another.

adoptive t. see under *immunization.*

fluorescence resonance energy t. (FRET) a process used to study protein-protein interactions in living cells when two proteins are in extremely close proximity. Light energy emitted by a fluorochrome is absorbed by an adjacent acceptor fluorochrome, which then emits light at a wavelength different from that of the light it received. The difference between the wavelengths can be analyzed to measure the spacing between the two proteins in ângstroms.

gamete intrafallopian t. (GIFT) a method of assisted reproductive technology consisting of retrieval of oocytes from the ovary, followed by laparoscopic placement of the oocytes and sperm in the fallopian tubes.

linear energy t. (LET) the energy dissipation of ionizing radiation over a given linear distance. Highly penetrating radiations, such as gamma rays, cause very low ion concentration and thus have a relatively low LET, beta particles and x-rays have an intermediate LET, and alpha particles have a relatively high LET.

passive t. the conferring of immunity to a nonimmune host by injection of antibody or lymphocytes from an immune or sensitized donor.

tendon t. surgical relocation of the insertion of a tendon of a normal muscle to a different site to take over the function of a muscle inactivated by trauma or disease.

tubal embryo t. (TET) 1. a method of assisted reproductive technology consisting of retrieval of oocytes from the ovary, followed by their fertilization and culture in the laboratory with placement of the resulting embryos in the fallopian tubes by laparoscopy more than 24 hours after the original retrieval. 2. laparoscopic transfer of cryopreserved embryos to the fallopian tubes.

viral gene t. in gene therapy, the use of a virus to deliver a new DNA sequence to a defective cell; called also *viral gene delivery.*

zygote intrafallopian t. (ZIFT) a method of assisted reproductive technology consisting of retrieval of oocytes from the ovary, followed by their fertilization and culture in the laboratory with placement of the resulting zygotes in the fallopian tubes by laparoscopy 24 hours after the original retrieval.

trans·fer·ase (trans′fər-ās) [EC 2] a class of enzymes that transfer a chemical group from one compound (the donor) to another compound (the acceptor).

trans·fer·ence (trans-fer′əns) in psychotherapy, the unconscious tendency to assign to others in one's present environment feelings and attitudes associated with significant persons in one's early life, especially the patient's transfer to the therapist of feelings and attitudes associated with a parent. The feelings may be affectionate *(positive t.)* or hostile *(negative t.).*

counter t. see *countertransference.*

trans·fer·rin (trans-fer′in) [*trans-* + *ferrum* + *-in* chemical suffix] a nonheme serum glycoprotein of molecular weight 79,500, which binds and transports iron; most is produced in the liver. A similar substance called apoferritin is produced in the small intestine. Called also *siderophilin.*

trans·fer·rin·uria (trans-fer″in-u′re-ə) excessive increase in transferrin in the urine, seen in the nephrotic syndrome.

trans·fix (trans′fiks) [*trans-* + L. *figere* to fix] to pierce through and through.

trans·fix·ion (trans-fik′shən) a cutting through from within outward, as in amputation.

trans·fo·ram·i·nal (trans″fo-ram′ĭ-nəl) through or across a foramen.

trans·for·ma·tion (trans″for-ma′shən) [*trans-* + *formation*] 1. change of form or structure; conversion from one form to another. 2. in oncology, the change that a normal cell undergoes as it becomes malignant. 3. in eukaryotes, the conversion of normal cells to malignant cells in cell culture. 4. bacterial t.

asbestos t. the deposition of extraneous fibers in hyaline cartilage, which gives it a silky, glossy appearance.

bacterial t. the exchange of genetic material between strains of bacteria by the transfer of a fragment of naked DNA from a donor cell to a recipient cell, followed by recombination in the recipient chromosome.

blast t., lymphocyte t. the morphologic changes accompanying lymphocyte activation, in which small, resting lymphocytes are transformed into large, active lymphocytes (lymphoblasts).

nodular t. of the liver nodular regenerative hyperplasia.

trans·fron·tal (trans-frun′təl) through the frontal bone.

trans·fu·sion (trans-fu′zhən) [L. *transfusio*] the introduction of whole blood or blood components directly into the bloodstream. Cf. *infusion.*

autologous t. autotransfusion.

direct t. immediate t.

exchange t., exsanguination t. repetitive withdrawal of small amounts of blood and replacement with donor blood, until a large proportion of the blood volume has been exchanged; used primarily in newborn infants with erythroblastosis fetalis and sometimes in patients with various other blood conditions. Called also *replacement t.* and *substitution t.*

fetomaternal t. transplacental passage of fetal blood into the circulation of the mother; in small amounts it may go unnoticed, but in larger amounts it can cause anemia or edema in the fetus.

immediate t. the transfer of blood from one person to another without use of an intermediate container or anticoagulant. Called also *direct t.*

indirect t. transfer of blood from a donor to a flask or other container, and then to the recipient. Called also *mediate t.*

intraperitoneal t. infusion of blood into the peritoneal cavity; see *intrauterine t.*

intrauterine t. transfusion performed on an unborn infant in utero, often referring to transfusion of Rh-negative blood into the infant's peritoneal cavity in the treatment of erythroblastosis fetalis in utero.

mediate t. indirect t.

placental t. return to the newborn, through the umbilical vessels, of some of the blood contained in the fetal placenta.

replacement t., substitution t. exchange t.

twin-to-twin t. an abnormality of fetal circulation occurring between two monozygotic twins, in which blood is shunted directly from one twin to the other.

trans·gene (trans′jēn) a segment of recombinant DNA that has been transferred from one genome to another; the term is sometimes used specifically to denote one that has been integrated into the germline of the recipient and is transmissible to future generations.

trans·gen·ic (trans-jen′ik) [*trans-* + *genic*] pertaining to the experimental incorporation of a segment of DNA from one genome into a different genome; often used specifically to denote transfer across species.

trans·glu·co·syl·ase (trans″gloo-ko′sə-lās) glucosyltransferase.

trans·glu·tam·in·ase (trans″gloo-tam′in-ās) protein-glutamine γ-glutamyltransferase.

trans·gly·co·si·da·tion (trans″gli-kōs″ĭ-da′shən) the transfer of a sugar residue from a glycoside to a suitable free hydroxyl group to form a new glycosidic bond, such as is catalyzed by glycosyltransferases.

trans·gly·co·syl·ase (trans″gli-ko′sə-lās) glycosyltransferase.

trans·gre·di·ent (trans-gre′de-ənt) [L. *transgrediens*, transgressing or stepping across a line] spreading outside the usual area; said of skin lesions that begin on the palms or soles and spread to the back of the hand or foot.

trans·hi·a·tal (trans″hi-a′təl) across or through a hiatus.

trans·hu·mer·al (trans-hu′mər-əl) across or through the humerus.

tran·sient (tran′shent, tran′se-ənt) [L. *transiens* present participle of *transire* to go across] an isolated wave or complex seen on an electroencephalogram.

trans·il·i·ac (trans-il′e-ak) across or between the two ilia.

tran·sil·i·ent (tran-sil′e-ənt) [*trans-* + L. *salire* to leap] leaping or passing across.

trans·il·lu·mi·na·tion (trans″ĭ-loo″mĭ-na′shən) the passage of light through body tissues for the purpose of examination, the object or part under examination being interposed between the observer and the light source; called also *diaphanoscopy.*

trans·in·su·lar (trans-in′su-lər) across the insula; crossing the insula.

trans·is·chi·ac (trans-is′ke-ak) between the two ischia.

trans·isth·mi·an (trans-is′me-ən) across an isthmus, especially the isthmus of the gyrus fornicatus.

trans·is·tor (tran-zis′tər) a small wafer of semiconducting material having three electrodes, called the emitter, base, and collector, which perform functions similar to those of the cathode, grid, and plate of a vacuum tube.

tran·sit (tran′sit) passage across or through.

colonic t. passage of feces through the colon.

gastrointestinal t. passage of food through the gastrointestinal tract.

intestinal t. passage of feces through the intestines.

tran·si·tion (tran-zĭ′shən) [L. *transitio* crossing over] 1. a passage or change from one state or condition to another. 2. in molecular genetics, a point mutation in which one purine base replaces another purine or one pyrimidine base replaces another pyrimidine. Cf. *transversion.*

glass t. the change in a crystalline polymer or ceramic material from a rubbery or viscous state to a hard, brittle state, usually as a result of a decrease in temperature.

isobaric t. a radioactive decay process in which the daughter and parent are isobars, possessing the same mass number but differing in atomic number. Included are beta decay, positron emission, and electron capture.

trans·jug·u·lar (trans-jug′u-lər) through a jugular vein, such as a diagnostic procedure.

trans·ke·to·lase (trans-ke′to-lās) [EC 2.2.1.1] an enzyme of the transferase class that catalyzes the transfer to aldose phosphates of glycolaldehyde groups from specific ketose phosphates, reactions that occur in the pentose phosphate pathway. The enzyme contains thiamine pyrophosphate and Mg^{2+} and has displayed reduced thiamine-binding capacity in patients with Wernicke-Korsakoff syndrome.

trans·lab·y·rin·thine (trans-lab″ə-rin′thēn) done through the labyrinth, such as otologic surgery. Cf. *transcochlear.*

trans·lat·er·al (trans-lat′ər-əl) from side to side; in radiography, referring to the view obtained with the patient supine and the radiation directed horizontally.

trans·la·tion (trans-la′shən) [L. *translatio* transfer] 1. conversion or transformation. 2. in genetics, the process by which the series of codons (triplet bases) in a messenger RNA (mRNA) is converted to the ordered sequence of amino acids that constitutes a specific polypeptide chain; it involves also ribosomes, transfer RNA (tRNA), and numerous soluble proteins.

nick t. a process by which radiolabeled nucleotides are incorporated into duplex DNA at single-strand nicks or cleavage points created enzymatically along its two strands.

trans·lo·case (trans-lo′kās) 1. transport protein. 2. the prokaryotic elongation factor, involved in protein synthesis.

trans·lo·ca·tion (trans″lo-ka′shən) [*trans-* + L. *locus* place] 1. movement of a substance from one place to another; used particularly for movement within a biological fluid or across a biological membrane. 2. movement of the ribosome from one codon to the next along the messenger RNA (mRNA) in protein synthesis. 3. a structural chromosome aberration in which one segment of a chromosome is transferred to a nonhomologous chromosome, the result of breakage of both chromosomes with repair in abnormal arrangement. Called also *interchange.* Abbreviated t. See *insertion* (def. 3), and see illustration at *aberration.*

balanced t. translocation that results in no more or no less than the normal chromosomal complement. The phenotype is usually normal, but there will be partial aneuploidy in a percentage of the gametes, with a risk of an unbalanced chromosomal complement in offspring.

reciprocal t. (rcp) the complete mutual exchange of fragments between two broken nonhomologous chromosomes, one part of one uniting with part of the other, with no fragments left over. See illustration at *aberration.*

robertsonian t. (rob) translocation involving two acrocentric chromosomes (13, 14, 15, 21, and 22), which fuse at the centromere region and lose their heterochromatic short arms; since these short arms contain no essential genetic material, the rearrangement is considered to be a functionally balanced one. A carrier of a robertsonian translocation involving chromosomes 14 and 21 has a virtually complete chromosomal complement but only 45 chromosomes (including the translocation chromosome), is phenotypically normal, but risks producing offspring with trisomy 21 (translocation Down syndrome). See illustration at *aberration.*

unbalanced t. translocation that results in a net gain or loss of chromosomal material, usually with serious clinical effects and often incompatible with life.

trans·lo·con (tranz-lo′kon) [*translo*cation + *-on*] a complex of transmembrane proteins of the endoplasmic reticulum, through which nascent polypeptides pass into the lumen during protein synthesis and which regulates ribosome–endoplasmic reticulum interaction.

trans·lu·cent (trans-loo′sənt) [*trans-* + L. *lucens* shining] transmitting light, but diffusing it so that objects beyond are not clearly distinguished.

trans·lu·mi·nal (trans-loo′mĭ-nəl) through or across a lumen, particularly the lumen of a blood vessel.

trans·man·dib·u·lar (trans″man-dib′u-lər) through or across the mandible.

trans·me·a·tal (trans″me-at′əl) through a meatus.

trans·mem·brane (trans-mem′brān) crossing a membrane, such as the plasma membrane.

trans·meta·tar·sal (trans-met″ə-tahr′səl) across the metatarsal bones.

trans·meth·y·lase (trans-meth′ə-lās) methyltransferase.

trans·meth·y·la·tion (trans″məth-ə-la′shən) the transfer of a methyl group from one compound to another.

trans·mi·gra·tion (trans″mi-gra′shən) 1. a wandering, especially a change of place from one side of the body to the other. 2. diapedesis.

external t. see under *migration.*

internal t. see under *migration.*

trans·mis·si·ble (trans-mis′ĭ-bəl) capable of being transmitted from one individual, part, or species to another.

trans·mis·sion (trans-mish′ən) [*trans-* + L. *missio* a sending] 1. a passage or transfer, as of a disease from one individual to another, or of neural impulses from one neuron to another. 2. the communication of genetic traits from parent to offspring.

airborne t. transmission of an airborne infection (see under *infection*).

duplex t. the transmission of neural impulses in two directions along a nerve.

ephaptic t. the conduction of a nerve impulse across an ephapse, as opposed to synaptic transmission.

horizontal t. the spread of infection from one individual to another, usually through contact with bodily excretions or fluids containing the agent. Cf. *vertical t.*

iatrogenic t. transmission through treatment by a health care professional.

neurochemical t., neurohumoral t. transmission of an impulse across a synaptic junction through the medium of a chemical substance (neurotransmitter).

neuromuscular t. the chemically mediated transmission of an action potential from nerve to muscle across the myoneural junction.

nosocomial t. transmission of an infection within a hospital; see *nosocomial infection*, under *infection*.

synaptic t. the communication of a neural impulse from one neuron to another neuron, a muscle fiber, or a gland across a synapse.

vector-borne t. transmission of a vector-borne infection.

vertical t. transmission from one generation to another. The term is restricted by some to genetic transmission and extended by others to include also transmission of infection from one generation to the next, as by maternal milk or through the placenta. Cf. *horizontal t.*

waterborne t. transmission of a waterborne infection.

trans•mi•tral (trans-mi′trəl) through the mitral valve.

trans•mit•tance (*T*) (trans-mit′əns) 1. in analytical chemistry, the ratio I/I_0 of the light intensity transmitted by the solution under analysis (I) to that transmitted by the pure solvent or other reference solution (I_0). 2. in physics, the ratio I/I_0 of the radiant energy transmitted by an object divided by the incident radiant energy.

trans•mit•ter (trans-mit′ər) something that transmits; see also *neurotransmitter*.

trans•mu•co•sal (trans″mu-ko′səl) entering through, or across, a mucous membrane, as the administration of a drug via the buccal cavity.

trans•mu•ral (trans-mu′rəl) [*trans-* + *mural*] through the wall of an organ; extending through or affecting the entire thickness of the wall of an organ or cavity.

trans•mu•ta•tion (trans″mu-ta′shən) 1. evolutionary change of one species into another. 2. the change of one chemical element into another; nucleonics, the changing of an atomic nucleus to one of a different atomic number by nuclear bombardment, causing rearrangement of the protons and neutrons.

trans•neu•ro•nal (trans-noor′ə-nəl) between or across neurons.

trans•oc•u•lar (trans-ok′u-lər) across the eye.

tran•so•nance (tran′so-nəns) [*trans-* + L. *sonans* sounding] transmission of a sound originating in one organ through the substance of another organ.

trans•ovar•i•al (trans″o-var′e-əl) through the ovary; referring to transmission of pathogens from the maternal organism, by invasion of the ovary and infection of eggs, to individuals of the next generation, as may occur in infections of arthropods, especially mites and ticks.

trans•ovar•i•an (trans″o-var′e-ən) transovarial.

trans•pal•a•tal (trans-pal′ə-təl) performed through the roof of the mouth, or palate.

trans•par•ent (trans-par′ənt) [*trans-* + L. *parere* to appear] permitting the passage of rays of light, so that objects may be seen through the substance.

trans•pa•ri•e•tal (trans″pə-ri′ə-təl) [*trans-* + *parietal*] through or across a wall, as through the intact body wall.

trans•peri•to•ne•al (trans″per-ĭ-to-ne′əl) through or across the peritoneum.

trans•phos•phor•y•la•tion (trans-fos″for-ə-la′shən) the exchange of phosphate groups between organic phosphates, without their going through the stage of inorganic phosphate.

tran•spi•ra•tion (tran″spĭ-ra′shən) [*trans-* + L. *spiratio* exhalation] the discharge of air, sweat, or vapor through the skin.

pulmonary t. the exhalation of water vapor from the blood circulating through the lungs.

trans•pla•cen•tal (trans″plə-sen′təl) through the placenta.

trans•plant[1] (trans′plant) 1. an organ or tissue taken from the body for grafting into another area of the same body or into another individual. 2. the process of removing and grafting such an organ or tissue. See also *transplantation*. Called also *graft*.

Gallie t. strips of fascia lata employed as sutures in the repair of hernias.

trans•plant[2] (trans-plant′) to transfer tissue from one part to another.

trans•plan•tar (trans-plan′tər) [*trans-* + *plantar*] across the sole.

trans•plan•ta•tion (trans″plan-ta′shən) [*trans-* + *plantation*] the grafting of tissues taken from the patient's own body or from another; called also *graft*, *grafting*, and *transplant*.

allogeneic t. transplantation of an allograft; the three types are *cadaveric donor t.*, *living related donor t.*, and *living unrelated donor t.* Called also *allotransplantation*.

autologous t. autotransplantation.

autologous bone marrow t. see *bone marrow t.*

autologous stem cell t. (ASCT) a treatment for advanced or refractory solid tumors such as neuroblastomas, lymphomas, and Ewing sarcoma. Stem cells from the bone marrow or blood are withdrawn prior to high-dose irradiation or chemotherapy that destroys many of the remaining cells; afterwards the removed cells are reinfused to form a new population of blood cells.

bone marrow t. (BMT) intravenous infusion of autologous, syngeneic, or allogeneic bone marrow or stem cells (see *peripheral blood progenitor cells*, under *cell*); done to treat malignancies such as leukemia, lymphoma, myeloma, and selected solid tumors, as well as nonmalignant conditions such as aplastic anemia, immunologic deficiencies, inborn errors of metabolism, and the myeloablation resulting from chemotherapy or radiotherapy.

cadaveric donor t. allogeneic transplantation using a cadaveric donor (see under *donor*).

corneal t. keratoplasty.

domino t. a combination of two transplantation operations, with a patient receiving a donor organ and having the removed organ transplanted into another patient; this is possible when the organ removed from the first person is not functional for reasons that do not exist in the recipient.

double autologous stem cell t. tandem autologous stem cell t.

heterotopic t. transplantation of tissue typical of one area to a different recipient site.

homotopic t. orthotopic t.

living nonrelated donor t. living unrelated donor t.

living related donor t. allogeneic transplantation using a living related donor (see under *donor*).

living unrelated donor t. allogeneic transplantation using a living unrelated donor (see under *donor*).

orthotopic t. transplantation of tissue from a donor into its normal position in the body of the recipient.

skin t. see under *grafting*.

syngeneic t. transplantation of a syngraft; called also *isotransplantation*.

syngenesioplastic t. living related donor t.

tandem autologous stem cell t. two autologous stem cell transplantations performed on the same patient within a short period of time, such as when the response is not adequate to the first one. Called also *double autologous stem cell t.*

tendon t. 1. surgical replacement of a damaged segment of tendon by a free tendon graft. 2. tendon transfer.

tooth t. the insertion into a prepared dental alveolus of an autogenous or homologous tooth; it may be a developing tooth germ from the same mouth, a homologous transplant, or a tooth with or without vital pulp, or one having had endodontic treatment, transplanted from one site to another in the same individual or from one individual to another.

xenogeneic t. transplantation of a xenograft; called also *heterotransplantation*.

trans•pleu•ral (trans-ploor′əl) through the pleura; by way of the pleural sac.

trans•port (trans′port) [L. *transportare* to carry across] the movement of substances in biological systems, particularly into and out of cells and across epithelial layers.

active t. the movement of substances across the cell membrane, usually up a concentration gradient, produced by the expenditure of metabolic energy. See *primary active t.* and *secondary active t.* and cf. *passive t.*

anterograde t. fast axonal transport from the nerve cell body to the axon terminal, occurring at a rate of about 400 mm/day; besides providing molecular transport, it also furnishes large amounts of membrane for renewal of the terminal and axolemma and for vesicles for retrograde transport.

cotranslational t. transport of a protein across the membrane of the endoplasmic reticulum as it is being synthesized, before translation is complete.

exchange t. transport in which one substance is moved into the cell while another is moved out, as by Na^+,K^+-ATPase or by antiport.

fast axonal t. the rapid bidirectional movement of vesicles containing glycoproteins and neurotransmitters along microtubules between the nerve cell body and the axon terminal.

oxygen t. the carrying of oxygen through the bloodstream bound to hemoglobin (see *oxyhemoglobin*).

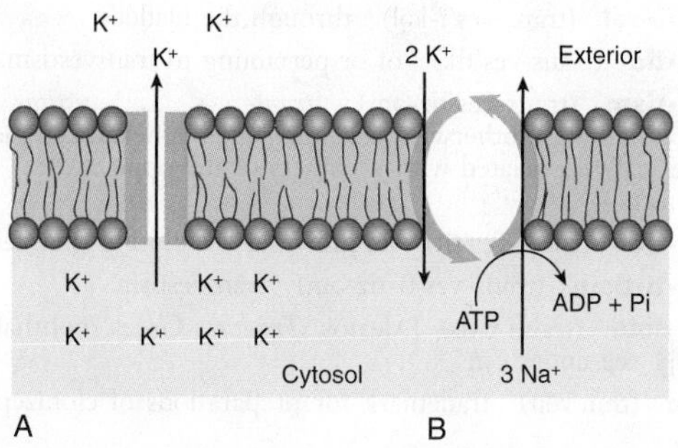

■ *(A)* Passive transport exemplified by diffusion of potassium ions across the plasma membrane, through specific ion channels, down a concentration gradient; *(B)* active transport exemplified by the cellular sodium pump, which uses ATP hydrolysis to create gradients of sodium and potassium across the plasma membrane.

paracellular t. transport of molecules around cells and through tight junctions in an epithelial cell layer. Cf. *transcellular t.*

passive t. the movement of substances, usually across cell membranes, by processes not requiring expenditure of metabolic energy. Cf. *active t.*

primary active t. active transport in which the energy that drives the process is derived from the breakdown of ATP or another high-energy phosphate compound, e.g., the movement of sodium and potassium by Na^+,K^+-ATPase.

retrograde t. fast axonal transport from the axon terminal to the nerve cell body, occurring at a rate of about 250 mm/day; it provides for the movement of endogenous and extracellular elements from the synaptic cleft to the cell body for sampling.

reverse cholesterol t. the process by which high-density lipoproteins (HDL) facilitate the movement of cholesterol from peripheral cells back to the liver for excretion in the bile. Cholesterol released into plasma during cell turnover is adsorbed to HDL where it is esterified by lecithin–cholesterol acyltransferase; most of the cholesteryl esters then are transferred to intermediate-density or very-low-density lipoproteins by a specific transfer protein and these lipoproteins are ultimately taken up by the liver.

secondary active t. active transport in which the movement of a second substance is coupled to the movement of a substance undergoing primary active transport, as in cotransport and countertransport

slow axonal t. the movement of cytoskeletal elements *(component a)* and glycolytic enzymes and actin *(component b)* along an axon away from the nerve cell body, occurring at a rate of 0.2 to 2 mm/day, depending on the species and age of the animal and on the particular nerve. Its function is to renew the cytoskeleton, regulate the axonal caliber, and transport energy-related enzymes.

transcellular t. transport of molecules through the cells of an epithelial cell layer. Cf. *paracellular t.*

vesicular t. intracellular transport of substances by means of membrane-bound vesicles that bud from the donor compartment and are delivered to a specific target compartment, where they fuse with the compartment membrane and release their cargo.

trans•port•er (trans-por′tər) transport protein; often specifically a transport protein that after binding one to several molecules of substrate, undergoes a conformational change that moves only the substrate across the membrane. Different types facilitate movement with (symport) and against (antiport) concentration gradients.

ABC t's [*A*TP-*b*inding *c*assette] a large family of transport proteins, consisting of two transmembrane and two cytoplasmic domains, that use energy released by ATP hydrolysis to transport a variety of substances across cell membranes.

trans•pos•a•ble (trans-poz′ə-bəl) capable of being interchanged or put in a different place or order.

trans•po•sase (trans-poz′ās) an enzyme that mediates the movement of a transposable element to a new location.

trans•po•si•tion (trans″po-zĭ′shən) [*trans-* + *position*] 1. any of various congenital anomalies in which organs are displaced to the opposite side from normal. 2. the operation of carrying a tissue flap from one situation to another without severing its connection entirely until it is united at its new location. 3. the exchange of position of two atoms within a molecule. 4. movement of genetic information from one locus to another, such as via a transposable element.

conservative t. transposition in which the transposable element excises from the genome and integrates elsewhere; cf. *replicative t.*

corrected t. of great vessels a developmental anomaly of the heart characterized by transposition of the great vessels with inversion of the ventricles and atrioventricular valves; termed "corrected" because the inverted ventricles compensate for the transposition, producing a mirror-image blood flow in the heart. Called also *mixed levocardia.*

gastric t. surgical relocation of the stomach into the mediastinum, with creation of a pharyngogastric or gastroesophageal anastomosis, performed to restore continuity of the gastrointestinal tract after esophagectomy or to correct esophageal atresia.

t. of great arteries, t. of great vessels a congenital anomaly of the cardiovascular system in which the aorta arises entirely from the right ventricle and the pulmonary artery from the left ventricle, so that the venous return from the peripheral circulation is recirculated by the right ventricle via the aorta to the systemic circulation without being oxygenated in the lungs. Life then depends on a crossflow of blood between blood in the right heart and that in the left heart, as through a ventricular septal defect or a patent ductus arteriosus. Cyanosis is the chief symptom.

partial t. of great vessels Taussig-Bing syndrome.

penoscrotal t. a developmental anomaly in which the two halves of the scrotum are found lateral to the shaft of the penis or sometimes higher, often accompanied by hypospadias.

replicative t. transposition in which the transposable element replicates itself into the target location while leaving a copy at the original site; cf. *conservative t.*

trans•po•son (tranz-po′zon) a transposable element that carries additional genes, such as for drug resistance, besides merely those for transposition, particularly a complex one occurring in prokaryotes. The term, however, is sometimes used interchangeably with *transposable element.*

trans•pu•bic (trans-pu′bik) performed through the pubic bone after removal of a segment of the bone.

trans•ra•di•al (trans-ra′de-əl) 1. through the radial artery. 2. across the radius.

trans•re•pres•sion (trans″re-presh′ən) inhibition of gene transcription by a specific protein.

trans•sa•cral (tran-sa′krəl) through or across the sacrum.

trans•sec•tion (tran-sek′shən) transection.

trans•seg•men•tal (tran″səg-men′təl) extending across a segment.

trans•sep•tal (tran-sep′təl) through or across a septum.

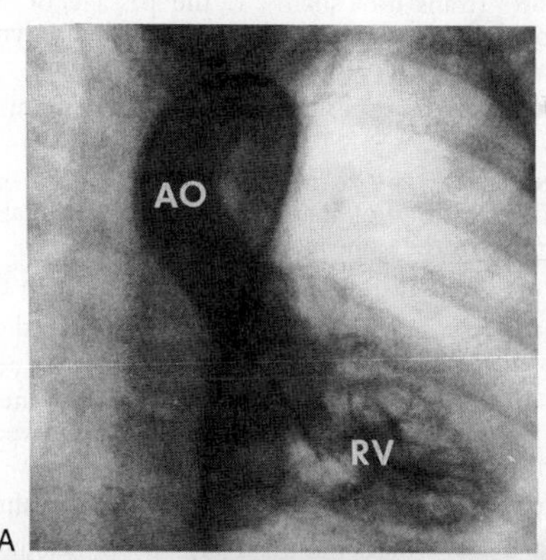

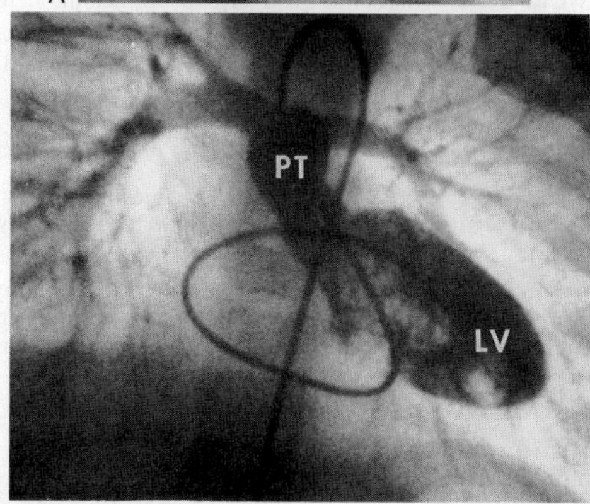

■ Complete transposition of great arteries, patent foramen ovale, intact ventricular septum, and closed ductus arteriosus in an 8-month-old boy. A balloon atrial septostomy was performed at 6 days of age. *(A)*, The right ventricle *(RV)* gives rise to the ascending aorta *(AO)*, which is convex to the right. *(B)*, The left ventricle *(LV)* gives rise to a centrally placed pulmonary trunk *(PT)* with a rightward inclination. The great arteries parallel each other and do not cross.

trans·sex·u·al (tran-sek′shoo-əl) 1. a person affected by transsexualism. 2. a person whose external anatomy has been changed to that of the opposite sex.

trans·sex·u·al·ism (tran-sek′shoo-əl-iz-əm) 1. the most severe manifestation of gender identity disorder in adults, being a prolonged, persistent desire to relinquish their primary and secondary sex characters and acquire those of the opposite sex; particularly describing those persons who go so far as to live as members of the opposite sex through dress, hormonal treatments, or surgical reassignment. 2. the state of being a transsexual.

trans·sphe·noi·dal (trans″sfe-noi′dəl) performed through the sphenoid bone.

trans·sphinc·ter·ic (trans-sfingk-ter′ik) crossing a sphincter, as a fistula.

trans·ster·nal (trans-stur′nəl) through the sternum.

trans·suc·ci·ny·lase (trans″sək-sĭ′nə-lās) dihydrolipoyllysine-residue succinyltransferase.

trans·tem·po·ral (trans-tem′por-əl) 1. crossing the temporal lobe. 2. through the temporal bone, such as otologic surgery.

trans·tha·lam·ic (trans″thə-lam′ik) crossing the thalamus.

trans·tho·rac·ic (trans″thə-ras′ik) performed through the wall of the thorax, or through the thoracic cavity.

trans·thy·re·tin (trans″thi-ret′in) an α-globulin secreted by the liver that transports retinol-binding protein and thyroxine in the blood. Numerous mutations in the gene encoding transthyretin have been associated with ATTR amyloidosis, the most common form of hereditary amyloidosis.

trans·tib·i·al (trans-tib′e-əl) across or through the tibia.

trans·tra·che·al (trans-tra′ke-əl) through the wall of the trachea.

trans·tro·chan·ter·ic (trans″tro-kan-ter′ik) through a trochanter; said of surgical procedures.

trans·tym·pan·ic (trans″tim-pan′ik) across the tympanic membrane or the cavity of the middle ear.

tran·su·date (trans′u-dāt) [*trans-* + L. *sudare* to sweat] a fluid substance which has passed through a membrane or been extruded from the blood as a result of hydrodynamic forces. A transudate, in contrast to an exudate, is characterized by high fluidity and a low content of protein, cells, or of solid materials derived from cells.

tran·su·da·tion (trans″u-da′shən) 1. the passage of serum or other body fluid through a blood vessel as a result of hydrodynamic forces; it may be the result of inflammation. 2. transudate.

trans·ura·ni·um (trans″u-ra′ne-əm) beyond uranium; see *transuranic elements*, under *element.*

trans·ure·tero·ure·ter·os·to·my (trans″u-re″tər-o-u-re″tər-os′tə-me) urinary diversion consisting of anastomosis of the proximal portion of one ureter to the ureter of the opposite side.

trans·ure·thral (trans″u-re′thrəl) performed through the urethra.

trans·vag·i·nal (trans-vaj′ĭ-nəl) performed through the vagina.

trans·vec·tor (trans-vek′tər) an organism that conveys or transmits a poison which is not generated in its own body but is obtained from another source, such as the mussel, *Mytilus,* which serves as a transvector of paralytic shellfish poison derived from the dinoflagellate *Gonyaulax.*

trans·ve·nous (trans-ve′nəs) performed or inserted through a vein.

trans·ven·tric·u·lar (trans″vən-trik′u-lər) performed through a ventricle.

trans·ver·sa·lis (trans″vər-sa′lis) [*trans-* + L. *vertere, versum* to turn] 1. transverse. 2. [TA] a term designating a structure situated at a right angle to the long axis of the body or of an organ.

trans·verse (trans-vurs′) [L. *transversus*] placed crosswise; situated at right angles to the long axis of a part.
 t. abdominal see *musculus transversus abdominis*, under *musculus.*

trans·ver·sec·to·my (trans″vər-sek′tə-me) [*transverse* + *-ectomy*] surgical removal of the transverse process of a vertebra.

trans·ver·sion (trans-vur′zhən) [L. *transvertere* to turn away] 1. displacement of a tooth from its proper numerical position in the jaw. 2. in molecular genetics, a point mutation in which a purine base replaces a pyrimidine base or vice versa. Cf. *transition.*

trans·ver·so·cos·tal (trans-vur″so-kos′təl) costotransverse.

trans·ver·sot·o·my (trans″vər-sot′ə-me) [*transverse* + *-tomy*] the operation of cutting the transverse process of a vertebra.

trans·ver·so·ure·thral·is (trans-vur″so-u″re-thral′is) the transverse fibers of the sphincter urethrae muscle.

trans·ver·sus (trans-vur′səs) [L.] [TA] transverse; a general term designating a position at right angles to a long axis.
 t. abdo′minis see under *musculus.*
 t. nu′chae see under *musculus.*

trans·ves·i·cal (trans-ves′ĭ-kəl) through the bladder.

trans·ves·tic (trans-ves′tik) of or pertaining to transvestism.

trans·ves·tism (trans-ves′tiz-əm) [*trans-* + L. *vestitus* clothed] 1. cross-dressing and otherwise assuming the appearance, manner, or roles traditionally associated with members of the opposite sex. 2. transvestic fetishism.

trans·ves·tite (trans-ves′tīt) an individual exhibiting transvestism.

trans·ves·ti·tism (trans-ves′tĭ-tiz-əm) transvestism.

Tran·tas dots (trahn′tahs) [Alexios *Trantas,* Greek ophthalmologist, 1867–1960] see under *dot.*

Tran·xene (tran′zēn) trademark for preparations of clorazepate dipotassium.

tran·yl·cy·pro·mine sul·fate (tran″əl-si′pro-mēn) a monoamine oxidase inhibitor with rapid onset of action; administered orally as an antidepressant in patients who have not responded to other antidepressant agents. It is also used in the prophylaxis of migraine.

tra·pe·zi·al (trə-pe′ze-əl) pertaining to a trapezium.

tra·pez·i·form (trə-pez′ĭ-form) trapezoid (def. 1).

tra·pe·zio·meta·car·pal (trə-pe′ze-o-met″ə-kahr′pəl) pertaining to or connecting the trapezium and the metacarpus.

tra·pe·zi·um (trə-pe′ze-əm) [L., from Gr. *trapezion*] 1. an irregular four-sided figure. 2. os trapezium.

trap·e·zoid (trap′ə-zoid) [L. *trapezoides;* Gr. *trapezoeidēs* table shaped] 1. having the shape of a four-sided plane, with two sides parallel and two diverging. 2. the trapezoid bone (os trapezoideum [TA]).

TRAPS TNF-receptor–associated periodic syndrome.

tras·tuz·u·mab (tras-tuz′u-mab) a recombinant DNA-derived humanized monoclonal antibody that binds to human growth factor receptor 2 (HER2), a protein overexpressed in some breast cancers; used as an antineoplastic in the treatment of metastatic breast cancer with overexpression of HER2, administered intravenously.

Tras·y·lol (tras′ə-lol) trademark for a preparation of aprotinin.

Trau·be sign, space (trou′bə) [Ludwig *Traube,* German physician, 1818–1876] see under *sign* and *space.*

Trau·be-Her·ing waves (trou′bə her′ing) [L. *Traube;* Edwald *Hering,* German physiologist, 1834–1918] see under *wave.*

trau·ma (traw′mə, trou′mə) pl. *traumas, trau′mata* [Gr.] 1. injury. 2. psychological or emotional damage.
 birth t. 1. an injury to the infant received in or due to the process of being born; called also *birth injury.* 2. in some psychiatric theories, the psychic shock produced in an infant by the experience of being born.
 occlusal t. injury to any part of the masticatory system as a result of occlusal dysfunction. See also *traumatic occlusion,* under *occlusion.*
 potential t. in dentistry, an alteration in tissue that may occur at any time as a result of an existing dental disharmony.
 psychic t. a psychologically upsetting experience that produces an emotional or mental disorder or otherwise has lasting negative effects on a person's thoughts, feelings, or behavior.

trau·ma·ther·a·py (traw′mə-ther′ə-pe) [*trauma* + *therapy*] treatment of wounds and injuries.

trau·mat·ic (trə-mat′ik) pertaining to, occurring as the result of, or causing trauma.

trau·ma·tism (traw′mə-tiz-əm) 1. the physical or psychic state resulting from an injury or wound. Called also *traumatosis.* 2. a wound or injury.

trau·ma·tize (traw′mə-, trou′mə-tīz) to subject to trauma.

traumat(o)- [Gr. *trauma,* gen. *traumatos* wound] a combining form denoting relationship to trauma, or to a wound or injury.

trau·ma·to·gen·ic (traw″mə-to-jen′ik) [*traumato-* + *-genic*] 1. caused by or due to a wound or wounds. 2. capable of causing trauma.

trau·ma·tol·o·gist (traw″mə-tol′ə-jist) a surgeon experienced in treating accidental injuries.

trau·ma·tol·o·gy (traw″mə-tol′ə-je) [*traumato-* + *-logy*] the branch of surgery which deals with wounds and disability from injuries.

trau·ma·top·a·thy (traw″mə-top′ə-the) [*traumato-* + *-pathy*] any pathological condition due to wound or injury.

trau·ma·top·nea (traw″mə-top′ne-ə) [*traumato-* + *-pnea*] open pneumothorax.

trau·ma·to·ther·a·py (traw″mə-to-ther′ə-pe) traumatherapy.

trau·mat·ro·pism (trə-mat′ro-piz-əm) [*trauma* + *tropism*] the growth or movement of organisms in relation to injury.

Traut·mann triangle (trout′mahn) [Moritz Ferdinand *Trautmann,* German surgeon, 1832–1902] see under *triangle.*

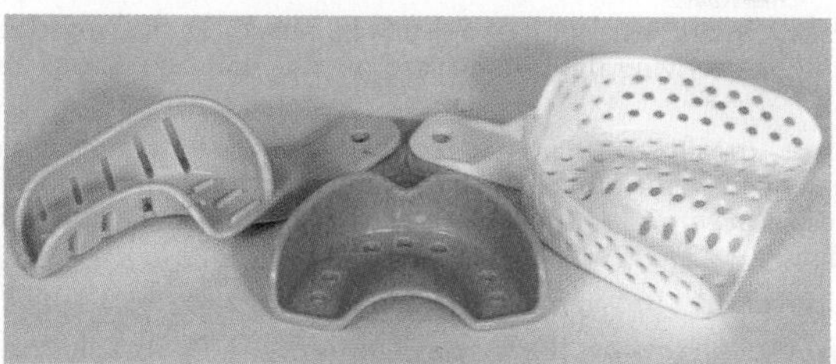

■ Impression trays.

Trav·a·sol (trav′ə-sol) trademark for a crystalline amino acid solution for intravenous administration, containing a mixture of essential and nonessential amino acids but no peptides.

Trav·a·tan (trav′ə-tan″) trademark for a preparation of travoprost.

trav·o·prost (trav′o-prost) a synthetic prostaglandin analogue used in the treatment of elevated intraocular pressure in patients with open-angle glaucoma or ocular hypertension; administered topically to the conjunctiva.

tray (tra) a flat-surfaced utensil for the conveyance of various objects or material.
acrylic resin t. an impression tray made of acrylic resin.
impression t. a horseshoe-shaped receptacle made of metal or other suitable material used to carry the impression material to the mouth, to confine the material in apposition to the surfaces to be recorded, and to control the impression material while it sets to form the impression.

tra·zo·done hy·dro·chlo·ride (tra′zo-dōn) [USP] an antidepressant used to treat major depressive episodes with or without prominent anxiety; administered orally.

Trea·cher Col·lins syndrome (tre′chər kol′inz) [Edward *Treacher Collins*, British surgeon, 1862–1932] see under *syndrome.*

Trea·cher Col·lins–Fran·ce·schet·ti syndrome (tre′chər kol′inz frahn″cha-sket′e) [E. *Treacher Collins;* Adolphe *Franceschetti*, Swiss ophthalmologist, 1896–1968] mandibulofacial dysostosis; see under *dysostosis.*

tread (tred) injury of the coronet of a horse's hoof, such as from being repeatedly struck with the shoe of the opposite side.

treat·ment (trēt′mənt) the management and care of a patient for the purpose of combating disease or disorder. See also under *care, maneuver, method, technique, test,* and *therapy.*
active t. curative t.
causal t. treatment directed against the cause of a disease.
conservative t. treatment designed to avoid radical medical therapeutic measures or operative procedures; often reserved for elderly or debilitated patients.
curative t. treatment designed to cure an existing disease, as opposed to *palliative t.* Called also *active t.*
drug t. pharmacotherapy.
electroconvulsive t., electroshock t. see under *therapy.*
empiric t. treatment by means which experience has proved to be beneficial.
expectant t. treatment designed only to relieve untoward symptoms, leaving the cure mainly to nature.
fever t. pyretotherapy.
Goeckerman t. treatment of psoriasis by applying ointments of tar followed by irradiation with ultraviolet B.
Hartel t. alcoholic injection for trigeminal neuralgia in which the needle is passed through the mouth into the region of the foramen ovale of the sphenoid bone.
medicinal t. pharmacotherapy.
neurodevelopmental t. Bobath method.
palliative t. treatment designed to relieve pain and distress, but not attempting a cure. See also *curative t.* Called also *supportive t.* and *palliative care.*
preventive t., prophylactic t. prophylaxis.
root canal t. see under *therapy.*
slush t. the treatment of acne by the application of a mixture of carbon dioxide snow, acetone, and sulfur.
specific t. treatment particularly adapted to a given disease.
supporting t., supportive t. palliative t.
surgical t. therapy using chiefly surgical methods. Cf. *pharmacotherapy* and *physical therapy.*
symptomatic t. expectant t.

Trec·a·tor (trek′ə-tor) trademark for a preparation of ethionamide.

tree (tre) 1. a perennial of the plant kingdom characterized by having a main stem or trunk and numerous branches. 2. something resembling such a plant, such as an anatomical structure that has branches. Called also *arbor.*
bronchial t. arbor bronchialis.
chaste t. 1. *Vitex agnus-castus,* a shrub native to the Mediterranean region, having blue or pink flowers and reddish black berries. 2. [USP] an extract prepared from the berries and root bark of *V. agnus-castus,* used for the symptomatic treatment of premenstrual syndrome and menopause; it is also used in homeopathy.
decision t. a graph resembling a tree in having an increasingly more complex branching structure flowing off an initial stem or point; used in decision analysis (q.v.) to represent choices and outcomes as the results of series of sequential decisions.
dendritic t. the branching arrangement of a dendrite.
tea t. *Melaleuca alternifolia,* a tree native to eastern Australia; its leaves and branches yield tea tree oil.
tracheobronchial t. the trachea and the bronchial tree considered as a unit.

tree-in-bud (tree-in-bud′) exhibiting a pattern of centrilobular nodular and branching linear opacities, resembling a tree in bud; a nonspecific radiographic finding seen in a number of pulmonary conditions.

tre·foil (tre′foyl) 1. clover; see *Trifolium.* 2. any of various cloverlike plants, such as certain species of *Medicago* and *Lotus.*
bird's foot t. 1. *Lotus americanus.* 2. *Lotus corniculatus.*
burr t. *Medicago polymorpha.*

Treg T-regulatory; see *regulatory T cells,* under *cell.*

α,α-tre·hal·ase (tre-ha′lās) [EC 3.2.1.28] an enzyme of the hydrolase class that catalyzes cleavage of the glycosidic bond in trehalose to yield two molecules of glucose. Deficiency of the enzyme, an autosomal recessive disorder, causes trehalose malabsorption, which may be manifested as vomiting and diarrhea after ingestion of large amounts of edible mushrooms.

tre·ha·lose (tre-ha′lōs) a disaccharide occurring mainly in insects, algae, and some mushrooms; when hydrolyzed by acids or enzymes it yields glucose.

Treitz arch, hernia, etc. (trīts) [Wenzel *Treitz,* Czech physician, 1819–1872] see under *arch* and *hernia* and see *musculus suspensorius duodeni* and *recessus duodenalis superior.*

Trel·star (trel′stahr) trademark for a preparation of triptorelin pamoate.

Trem·a·to·da (trem″ə-to′də) [Gr. *trēmatōdēs* pierced] the flukes, a class of the phylum Platyhelminthes. Most are parasitic, with animals becoming infected by eating uncooked or undercooked fish, crustaceans, or vegetation. All flukes require a mollusk as their first intermediate host, in which a complex developmental cycle takes place. The larval stage, which escapes from the mollusk, may either enter a second intermediate host (fish, crustacean, or another mollusk), encyst on vegetation, or penetrate directly into the skin of the definitive host. Important trematodes infecting humans belong to the genera *Clonorchis, Dicrocoelium, Echinostoma, Fasciola, Fasciolopsis, Gastrodiscoides, Heterophyes, Metagonimus, Opisthorchis, Paragonimus,* and *Schistosoma.*

trem·a·tode (trem′ə-tōd) any member of the class Trematoda; called also *fluke.*

trem·a·to·di·a·sis (trem″ə-to-di′ə-sis) infection with trematodes.

trem·ble (trem′bəl) [L. *tremulus* trembling] to shake or quiver involuntarily, as with anger or fear.

trem·bles (trem′bəlz) 1. any of various neurological diseases of domestic animals in which tremors are a prominent symptom. 2. poisoning in cattle and sheep that feed on the plants *Eupatorium rugosum* and *Haplopappus heterophyllus,* which contain the toxin tremetol; the animal has muscular tremors, becomes weak, and may suddenly stumble and fall. Humans who consume milk, milk products, or flesh from an animal so affected may develop the acute condition called *milk sickness.*
congenital t. congenital tremor syndrome.

trem·el·loid (trem′ə-loid) like jelly; gelatinous.

tre·mel·lose (trem′ə-lōs) tremelloid.

trem·e·tol (trem′ə-tol) a toxin found in the white snakeroot, *Eupatorium rugosum,* and the rayless goldenrod, *Haplopappus heterophyllus,* which causes trembles in cattle and sheep and milk sickness in humans. Called also *tremetone.*

trem·e·tone (trem′ə-tōn) tremetol.

tre·mo·gram (tre′mo-gram) [*tremor* + *-gram*] the tracing or record made by a tremograph; a graphic tracing of a tremor. See *ataxiameter.*

tre·mo·graph (tre′mo-graf) [*tremor* + *-graph*] an instrument for recording tremors.

trem·or (trem′ər) [L., from *tremere* to shake] an involuntary trembling or quivering. **trem′ulous** *adj*
action t. rhythmic, oscillatory, involuntary motion of a part during voluntary movements, as of the outstretched upper limb when writing or lifting a cup. Called also *intention t., kinetic t., postural t.,* and *volitional t.*

cerebellar t. a type of action tremor in a limb or limbs owing to a lesion or other damage to the cerebellum, such as from a stroke, a tumor, or a disease such as multiple sclerosis.
coarse t. a tremor in which the vibrations are slow.
continuous t. persistent t.
darkness t. involuntary movements of the eyes, resembling nystagmus, which occur in young animals kept in the dark.
enhanced physiologic t. a tremor that may appear in normal individuals under conditions of stress, such as cold, excitement, hunger, or exercise; it represents an intensification of physiologic tremor to detectable levels.
epidemic t. avian encephalomyelitis.
essential t. a hereditary tremor with onset at varying ages, usually at about 50 years of age, beginning with a fine rapid tremor (as distinct from that of parkinsonism) of the hands, followed by tremor of the head, tongue, limbs, and trunk; it is aggravated by emotional factors, is accentuated by volitional movement, and in some cases is temporarily improved by alcohol. Called also *familial t.*, *heredofamilial t.*, and *hereditary essential t.*
familial t. essential t.
fine t. a tremor in which the vibrations are rapid.
flapping t. asterixis.
hereditary essential t. essential t.
heredofamilial t. essential t.
Holmes t. an irregular tremor of low frequency caused by a lesion in the midbrain, usually in the vicinity of the red nucleus; it persists during both activity and rest. Called also *midbrain* or *rubral t.*
intention t. action t.
kinetic t. action t.
t. lin′guae trembling of the tongue, as seen in alcoholism, typhoid fever, and general paresis.
metallic t. a tremor seen in various metallic poisonings.
midbrain t. Holmes t.
orthostatic t. a rare tremor of the lower limbs noted when standing but not when walking or sitting.
palatal t. see under *myoclonus*.
parkinsonian t. the resting tremor commonly seen with parkinsonism, consisting of slow, regular movements of the hands and sometimes the lower limbs, neck, face, or jaw; it typically stops upon voluntary movement of the part and is intensified by stimuli such as cold, fatigue, and strong emotions.
passive t. resting t.
persistent t. a tremor occurring whether the patient is at rest or in motion.
physiologic t. a rapid tremor of extremely low amplitude found in the limbs and sometimes the neck or face of normal individuals, only subtly detectable on an electromyogram and seldom visible to the naked eye; it may become accentuated and visible under certain conditions. Cf. *enhanced physiologic t.*
pill-rolling t. a parkinsonian tremor of the hand consisting of flexion and extension of the fingers in conjunction with adduction and abduction of the thumb. Called also *pill-rolling*.
postural t. action t.
purring t. a thrill, like the purring of a cat, felt by the hand placed over the heart.
rest t., resting t. a tremor occurring when a limb or other body part is at rest; it may be normal, as in some physiologic tremors, or abnormal, as in parkinsonian tremors. Called also *passive t.*
rubral t. Holmes t.
senile t. a tremor resulting from the infirmities of age.
static t. a tremor occurring on effort to hold one of the limbs in a definite position.
striocerebellar t. a combined form of tremor with both striatal and cerebellar components, usually due to diffuse degeneration of the central nervous system.
toxic t. a tremor seen in states of chronic poisoning.
trombone t. of tongue Magnan movement.
volitional t. action t.
wing-beating t. a symptom seen in Wilson disease, in which the patient flexes the arm at the elbow and flaps the hands similarly to how a bird beats its wings.

trem•or•gram (trem′ər-gram) tremogram.

Tren•de•len•burg operation, etc. (tren′de-lən-bərg) [Friedrich *Trendelenburg*, German surgeon, 1844–1924] see under *operation, position, symptom*, and *test*.

Tren•tal (tren′tal) trademark for a preparation of pentoxifylline.

trep•a•na•tion (trep″ə-na′shən) [L. *trepanatio*] trephination.

treph•i•na•tion (tref″ĭ-na′shən) surgery with a trephine.
corneoscleral t. a method of trephining the sclerocornea for the relief of increased tension in glaucoma.
dental t. surgical creation of a fistula by puncturing the soft tissue and cortical bone overlying the root apex to provide drainage. Called also *apicostomy*.

tre•phine (trə-fīn′, trə-fēn′) [L. *trephina*] 1. a saw for removing a disk of bone, chiefly from the skull. 2. an instrument for removing a circular area of cornea, as in corneal transplant operations. 3. to operate upon with this instrument.

tre•phine•ment (trĕ-fīn′mənt) trephination.

trepho•cyte (tref′o-sīt) [Gr. *trephein* to feed + *-cyte*] trophocyte.

trep•i•dant (trep′ĭ-dənt) tremulous.

trep•i•da•tion (trep″ĭ-da′shən) [L. *trepidatio*] 1. tremor. 2. nervous anxiety and fear.

trepo- [Gr. *trepein* to turn] a combining form denoting a relationship to a turning movement.

Trep•o•mo•nas (trep″o-mo′nəs) [*trepo-* + Gr. *monas* unit, from *monos* single] a genus of flagellate protozoa (suborder Diplomonadina, order Diplomonadida) free-living in fresh water, coprophilic, or parasitic in amphibians, fish, and turtles, and characterized by the presence of one long and three short flagella on each side of the body.

Trep•o•ne•ma (trep″o-ne′mə) [*trepo-* + Gr. *nēma* thread] a genus of gram-negative bacteria of the family Spirochaetaceae, consisting of microaerophilic, spiral microorganisms that exhibit motility with a flexing, bending, snapping motion and divide by transverse fission. The outer surfaces have polar flagella that wind around the organism. They are found in the oral, intestinal, and genital mucosa. Pathogenic species, which cause syphilis, yaws, and pinta, have not been cultured in vitro.
T. cara′teum the species that causes pinta.
T. cuni′culi *T. paraluiscuniculi.*
T. denti′cola a nonpathogenic species found in the oral cavity of humans and chimpanzees, usually in calculus occurring at the gingival margin.
T. hyodysente′riae *Brachyspira hyodysenteriae*.
T. microden′tium *T. denticola*.
T. muco′sum a species of uncertain status found in the oral cavity of a person with periodontitis.
T. pal′lidum the species that causes syphilis in humans.
T. paraluiscuni′culi a species causing syphilis in guinea pigs and rabbits; not pathogenic for humans. Called also *T. cuniculi*.
T. perte′nue the species that causes yaws.
T. vincen′tii a species isolated from the human oral cavity, especially in necrotizing ulcerative gingivitis in association with *Fusobacterium nucleatum*.

trep•o•ne•ma (trep″o-ne′mə) an organism of the genus *Treponema*. Called also *treponeme*.

trep•o•ne•mal (trep″o-ne′məl) of, pertaining to, or caused by treponemas.

trep•o•ne•ma•to•sis (trep″o-ne-mə-to′sis) any infection with a species of *Treponema*, such as syphilis.

trep•o•neme (trep′o-nēm) treponema.

trep•o•ne•mi•a•sis (trep″o-ne-mi′ə-sis) treponematosis.

trep•o•ne•mi•ci•dal (trep″o-ne″mĭ-si′dəl) killing *Treponema* species; see *antisyphilitic*.

tre•pop•nea (tre″pop-ne′ə) [*trepo-* + *-pnea*] dyspnea that is relieved when a person is in a lateral recumbent position.

trep•pe (trep′ə) [Ger. "staircase"] the phenomenon of gradual increase in the extent of muscular contraction following rapid repeated stimulation; called also *staircase phenomenon*.

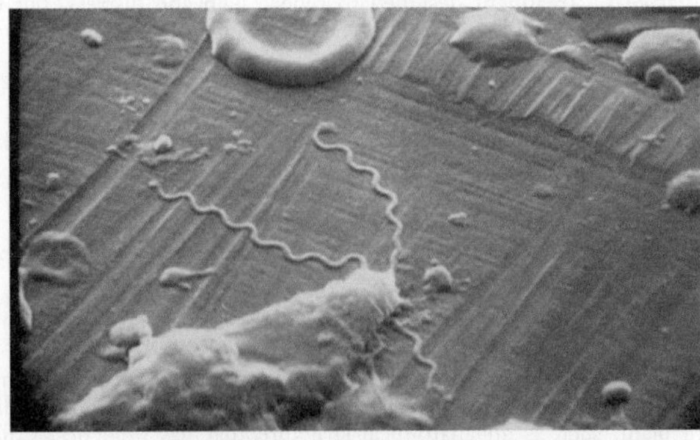

■ *Treponema pallidum*. Scanning electron micrograph of two treponemes.

tre•pros•ti•nil so•di•um (trə-pros′tĭ-nil) a prostacyclin analog that acts as a vasodilator and is used in treatment of pulmonary arterial hypertension; administered by continuous subcutaneous or intravenous infusion.

Tre•sil•i•an sign (trə-sil′e-ən) [Frederick James *Tresilian*, English physician, 1862–1926] see under *sign*.

tret•i•noin (tret′ĭ-noin″) all-*trans*-retinoic acid, applied topically in the treatment of acne vulgaris and as a keratolytic in the treatment of disorders of keratinization, and administered orally as an antineoplastic in the treatment of acute promyelocytic leukemia. Called also *retinoic acid* and *vitamin A acid*.

Treves fold (trēvz) [Sir Frederick *Treves*, English surgeon, 1853–1923] see *plica ileocaecalis*.

Trev•or disease (trev′ər) [David *Trevor*, British orthopedic surgeon, 1906–1988] dysplasia epiphysealis hemimelica; see under *dysplasia*.

TRH thyrotropin-releasing hormone.

tri- [Gr. *treis;* L. *tres* three] a prefix meaning *three* or *thrice*.

tri•ac•e•tate (tri-as′ə-tāt) an acetate containing three molecules of the acetic acid radical.

tri•ac•e•tin (tri-as′ə-tin) [USP] an antifungal agent used topically in the treatment of superficial fungal infections of the skin. Called also *glyceryl triacetate*.

tri•ace•tyl•ole•an•do•my•cin (tri-as″ə-təl-o″le-an″do-mi′sin) troleandomycin.

tri•ac•id (tri-as′id) a base capable of neutralizing three equivalents of monobasic acid.

tri•acyl•glyc•er•ol (tri-a″səl-glis′ər-ol) triglyceride.

tri•acyl•glyc•er•ol li•pase (tri-a″səl-glis′ə-rol li′pās) [EC 3.1.1.3] an enzyme of the hydrolase class that catalyzes the cleavage of the two outer fatty acyl groups from triglycerides in the digestion of dietary fats. Individual enzymes are frequently named for the tissues with which they are associated; see entries under *lipase*. The term is sometimes used specifically to denote pancreatic lipase.

tri•ad (tri′ad) [L. *trias:* Gr. *trias* group of three] 1. any trivalent element. 2. a group of three entities or objects, as an association of three symptoms.

acute compression t. Beck t.

adrenomedullary t. the symptoms caused by excessive amounts of adrenomedullary catecholamines: tachycardia, vasoconstriction, and sweating.

Beck t. three symptoms characteristic of cardiac tamponade: a high venous pressure, a low arterial pressure, and a small, quiet heart.

Bezold t. prolonged bone conduction (negative Rinne test) and lessened perception of low tones, indicating otosclerosis.

Borchardt t. three symptoms that indicate gastric volvulus: upper abdominal pain, retching, and blockage against placement of a nasogastric tube.

Carney t. a rare syndrome of gastrointestinal stromal tumor, pulmonary chondromas, and functional extra-adrenal paragangliomas, seen chiefly in young females.

Charcot t. 1. the combination of nystagmus, intention tremor, and staccato speech, three cerebellar symptoms that sometimes accompany multiple sclerosis. 2. the symptom complex of biliary colic, jaundice, and fever and chills characteristic of intermittent cholangitis.

Currarino t. see under *syndrome*.

Cushing t. decreased pulse, increased blood pressure, and a widening pulse pressure associated with increased intracranial pressure; it is a late clinical sign and may indicate brainstem herniation.

Dieulafoy t. hypersensitivity of the skin, reflex muscular contraction, and tenderness at the McBurney point in appendicitis.

female athlete t. low energy availability, menstrual disorders, and low bone mineral density in females engaged in sports or fitness training. The low energy availability may be due to inadequate caloric consumption or other disordered eating, such as fasting or purging, or to excessive energy output, or to a combination of these behaviors.

hepatic t's the grouping of the tributaries of the hepatic artery, vein, and bile duct at the angles of the lobules of the liver.

Hutchinson t. the combination of diffuse interstitial keratitis, disease of the labyrinth, and Hutchinson teeth, seen in congenital syphilis.

Jacod t. see under *syndrome*.

Kartagener t. see under *syndrome*.

Osler t. the telangiectasis, capillary fragility, and hereditary hemorrhagic diathesis seen in hereditary hemorrhagic telangiectasia.

portal t's hepatic t's.

t. of retinal cone the tip of two horizontal cell dendrites and one midget cell dendrite, enclosed in a synaptic invagination of a retinal cone pedicle.

Saint t. hiatus hernia, colonic diverticula, and cholelithiasis, occurring concomitantly.

t. of skeletal muscle a pair of terminal cisterns in close apposition to the T tubule, running transversely across a myofibril of skeletal muscle; in mammalian muscle there are two triads to each sarcomere, situated at the A band–I band junction. See also *T system*, under *system* and *T tubule*, under *tubule*.

Virchow t. three factors predisposing to vascular thrombosis: changes in the vascular wall, changes in the local pattern of blood flow, and changes in the blood constituents.

Whipple t. three essential clinical features of insulin-producing tumors: (1) spontaneous hypoglycemia with blood sugar levels below 50 mg per 100 mL; (2) central nervous system or vasomotor symptoms; and (3) relief of symptoms by oral or intravenous administration of glucose.

tri•ad•i•tis (tri″ad-i′tis) inflammation of a group of three.

portal t. inflammation of the hepatic triads and adjacent connective tissue.

tri•age (tre-ahzh′, tre′ahzh) [Fr. "sorting"] 1. the sorting out and classification of casualties of war or other disaster, to determine priority of need and proper place of treatment. 2. by extension, the sorting and prioritizing of patients for treatment in nonemergency health care settings.

tri•al (tri′əl, trīl) a test, study, or experiment.

Bernoulli t's in statistics, a series of independent trials, each having only two mutually exclusive outcomes, commonly called "success" and "failure," so that if the probability of success is p and that of failure is q, then $p + q = 1$ and the probability of success remains the same throughout the trials. Cf. *Bernoulli distribution*.

blind t. a clinical trial with blinding, as opposed to an open trial. See *single blind*, *double blind*, and *triple blind*. Called also *masked t.*

clinical t. an experiment performed on human beings in order to evaluate the comparative efficacy of two or more therapies. The most reliable results are usually considered to be those from randomized controlled trials (q.v.). Well-designed trials are usually done with blinding or masking; see *single blind*, *double blind*, and *triple blind*.

crossover t. a multipart clinical trial in which each subject is tested with each (or most) of the treatments being compared in turn, in random order.

masked t. blind t.

open t. a clinical trial that is not blind; i.e., the administrators and subjects know which testing group the subjects are in.

phase I t. a clinical trial on normal volunteers, designed to determine the biological activities and range of toxicity or other safety factors of a given therapy.

phase II t. a clinical trial on a small group of patients, designed to determine the effectiveness of the given regimen in treating the disorder in question.

phase III t. a clinical trial that uses a large sample of patients and is designed to compare the overall course of their disorder under the new treatment with its course untreated and treated with standard therapies previously used; studies are also done on the relative morbidities of the different treatments.

phase IV t. additional studies done after a drug has been approved for distribution or marketing, which could include examination of long-term effects, adverse effects, or specific aspects of a drug's action.

randomized controlled t. (RCT) a test in which subjects are assigned to groups in a random manner. In a clinical trial, an appropriate control group is used, such as to receive placebo or sham treatment or the standard well-established therapy, and this is compared with a group receiving experimental therapy; patients are assigned in a random manner to one of the groups, usually with blinding (see *blind t.*). This method is generally considered to yield the strongest scientific evidence of any well-designed trial.

tri•al•ism (tri′əl-iz-əm) trialistic theory; see under *theory*.

tri•al•lyl•am•ine (tri″ə-ləl-am′in) a volatile, oily, liquid amine, used as an intermediate; it is an irritant and a fire risk.

tri•am•cin•o•lone (tri″am-sin′ə-lōn) [USP] a synthetic glucocorticoid used in replacement therapy for adrenocortical insufficiency and as an antiinflammatory and immunosuppressant in a wide variety of disorders; administered orally.

t. acetonide [USP] an ester of triamcinolone; applied topically to the skin or oral mucosa as an antiinflammatory, and administered by inhalation for the chronic treatment of asthma, intranasally in the treatment of allergic rhinitis and other inflammatory nasal conditions, and by intra-articular, intradermal, intralesional, intramuscular, intrabursal, or tendon sheath injection as an antiinflammatory and immunosuppressant in a wide variety of disorders.

t. diacetate [USP] the diacetate ester of triamcinolone, having actions similar to those of the base and used as an antiinflammatory and immunosuppressant in a wide variety of disorders; administered orally and by intra-articular, intrasynovial, intralesional, sublesional, soft tissue, or intramuscular injection.

t. hexacetonide [USP] an ester of triamcinolone having actions similar to those of the base and used as an antiinflammatory and immunosuppressant in a wide variety of disorders; administered by intra-articular, intralesional, or sublesional injection.

tri•am•ine (tri-am′in) a compound containing three amino (—NH_2) groups.

tri•am•ter•ene (tri-am′tər-ēn) [USP] a potassium-sparing diuretic that blocks the reabsorption of sodium in the distal convoluted tubules; used for the treatment of edema and hypertension, either alone or in conjunction with a loop or thiazide diuretic; administered orally.

tri•an•gle (tri′ang-gəl) [L. *triangulum; tres* three + *angulus* angle] a three-cornered area or figure; called also *trigone* and *trigonum.* **triang′ular** *adj*

Triangle

Alsberg t. an equilateral triangle with its apex upward, formed by a line passing through the long axis of the femur, a second line passing through the long axis of the neck of the femur, and a third line on a plane passing through the base of the head of the femur. The angle at the apex is known as the *Alsberg* or *elevation angle.*
anal t. regio analis.
Assézat t. facial t.
auricular t. a triangle bounded by lines drawn from the tip of the auricle and the two ends of its base of insertion.
t. of auscultation, auscultatory t. trigonum auscultationis.
axillary t. the triangular area formed by the inner aspect of the arm, the axilla, and the pectoral region.
Béclard t. the area lying between the posterior edge of the hyoglossal muscle, the posterior belly of the digastric muscle, and the greater cornu of the hyoid bone.
Bolton t. the triangle formed by drawing a line from the nasion to the sella turcica to the Bolton point.
Bonwill t. a triangle formed by a line connecting the centers of the mandibular condyles and lines connecting either center with the mesial contact area of the mandibular medial incisors, each side being approximately 10 cm long.
brachial t. axillary t.
Bryant t. iliofemoral t.
Burger scalene t. a triangle providing a reference frame to represent the quantitative relationships between the electromotive forces of the heart and the extremity leads of the electrocardiograph. The lines representing leads I and II are considerably shorter on this than those of the Einthoven triangle.
Calot t. trigonum cystohepaticum.
cardiohepatic t. the triangular region in the fifth intercostal space of the right side, separating the heart from the superior edge of the liver.
carotid t. trigonum caroticum.
carotid t., inferior trigonum musculare.
carotid t., superior trigonum caroticum.
cephalic t. a triangle formed on the anteroposterior plane of the skull by two lines extending from the occiput, one to the forehead and one to the chin, and a third line extending from the chin to the forehead.
cervical t., anterior regio cervicalis anterior.
cervical t., posterior regio cervicalis lateralis.
clavipectoral t. trigonum clavipectorale.
Codman t. a triangular area visible radiographically where the periosteum, elevated by a bone tumor, rejoins the cortex of normal bone.
color t. a plane figure with red, green, and blue located at the three apices, and gray at the center, with lines drawn from side to side, as a guide to the color mixing equation needed to produce any intermediate hue.
crural t. the triangular area formed by the inner aspect of the thigh and the lower abdominal, inguinal, and genital regions.
cystohepatic t. trigonum cystohepaticum.
deltopectoral t. trigonum clavipectorale.
digastric t. trigonum submandibulare.
t. of doom a triangular area in the inguinal region, encountered in hernia repair, bounded medially by the ductus deferens and laterally by testicular vessels; the external iliac artery and vein pass through the area, and must be avoided during surgery.
Einthoven t. an equilateral triangle used as a mathematical model of the standard electrocardiographic limb leads, in which the instantaneous heart vector in the frontal plane may be projected on the sides of the triangle thereby demonstrating that the algebraic sum of the potential differences as recorded in electrocardiographic leads I and III will equal that potential difference recorded in lead II.
Elaut t. a triangular area whose base is the promontory of the sacrum and whose sides are the left and right common iliac arteries.
t. of elbow a triangular area on the front of the elbow, having the brachioradialis muscle on the lateral side and the pronator teres on the medial side, the base being toward the humerus.
facial t. a triangular area whose points are the basion, the alveolar point, and the nasion; called also *Assézat t.*
Farabeuf t. a triangular area on the superior part of the neck whose sides are formed by the internal jugular vein and facial vein and whose base is formed by the hypoglossal nerve.
femoral t. trigonum femorale.
fetal t. a triangular space made by the side of the fetal trunk, the thigh above, and the arm below.
frontal t. a triangle bounded by the maximum frontal diameter and lines from either end of this diameter to the glabella.
Garland t. a triangular area of relative resonance in the lower back, close to the spine on the diseased side; seen in pleurisy with effusion.
Gerhardt t. a triangular area of dullness to percussion above the third left rib, an inconstant sign in patent ductus arteriosus.
Gombault-Philippe t. a triangular field formed in the conus medullaris by the fibers of the septomarginal tract.
Grocco t. a triangular area of dullness on the back, on the side opposite to that of a pleural effusion. Called also *Grocco sign* and *paravertebral t.*
Grynfeltt t., Grynfeltt-Lesshaft t. Lesshaft t.
Guillain-Mollaret t. a triangular neuronal pathway in the brain, connecting the dentate nucleus on one side with the red nucleus and the olive on the other side. Called also *dentato-rubro-olivary pathway.*
Henke t. a triangular area between the descending portion of the inguinal fold, the lateral portion of the inguinal fold, and the lateral border of the rectus muscle.
Hesselbach t. trigonum inguinale.
hypoglossohyoid t. the triangular space in the subhyoid region, bounded superiorly by the hypoglossal nerve, anteriorly by the posterior border of the mylohyoid muscle, and posteriorly and inferiorly by the tendon of the digastric muscle. Called also *Pinaud* or *Pirogoff t.*
iliofemoral t. a triangular area bounded by the Nélaton line, a line through the anterior superior iliac spine, and one extending from this spine to the greater trochanter of the femur. Called also *Bryant t.*
infraclavicular t. fossa infraclavicularis.
inguinal t. 1. trigonum inguinale. 2. trigonum femorale.
Jackson safety t. a triangular space bounded above by the lower end of the thyroid cartilage, its apex in the suprasternal notch, and its sides the inner edges of the sternocleidomastoid muscle; so called because it marks the limits of the area through which the trachea may safely be incised in tracheostomy.
Kanavel t. a triangular area in the middle of the palm beneath which lies the common tendon sheath of the digital flexor tendons.
Killian t. Killian dehiscence.
t. of Koch a roughly triangular area on the septal wall of the right atrium, bounded by the base of the septal leaflet of the tricuspid valve, the anteromedial margin of the orifice of the coronary sinus, and the tendon of Todaro; it marks the site of the atrioventricular node.
Labbé t. a triangle bounded by a horizontal line along the inferior border of the cartilage of the ninth rib, the line of the false ribs, and the

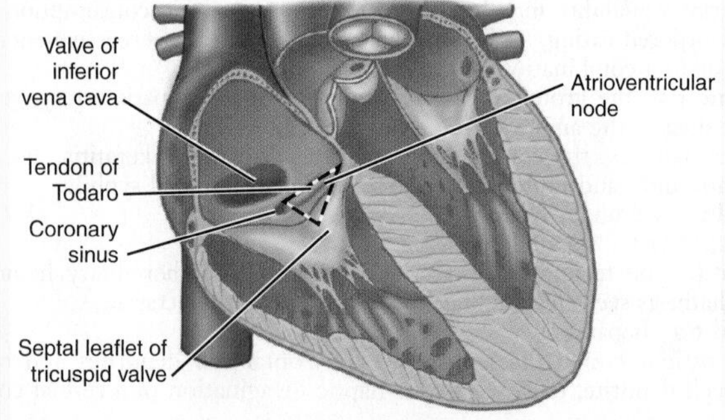

■ Triangle of Koch, at the apex of which lies the atrioventricular node.

Triangle *Continued*

line of the liver; it marks the area where the stomach lies in contact with the anterior abdominal wall.
Langenbeck t. a triangle having its apex at the anterior superior spine of the ilium, its base along the anatomical neck of the femur, and its external side by the external face of the greater trochanter of the femur.
Lesser t. a triangle bounded by the hypoglossal nerve superiorly and the two bellies of the digastricus muscle on the other two sides.
Lesshaft t. a triangular space (sometimes quadrangular) between the external oblique muscle in front, the latissimus dorsi behind, the serratus posticus above, and the internal oblique below, frequently the site of a hernia or of pointing of an abscess. Called also *Lesshaft space* and *Grynfeltt t.*
Lieutaud t. trigonum vesicae urinariae.
lumbar t., lumbar t., inferior trigonum lumbale inferius.
lumbar t., superior trigonum lumbale superius.
lumbocostoabdominal t. a space between the obliquus externus abdominis muscle, the serratus posterior inferior, the erector spinae, and the obliquus internus abdominis.
Macewen t. foveola suprameatica.
Malgaigne t. trigonum caroticum.
Minor t. an angular defect posterior to the anus, produced by attachment of the superficial portion of the external sphincter to the coccyx.
Mohrenheim t. fossa infraclavicularis.
muscular t. trigonum musculare.
occipital t. the area bounded by the sternocleidomastoid muscle anteriorly, the trapezius muscle posteriorly, and the omohyoid muscle inferiorly.
occipital t., inferior a triangular area having a line between the two mastoid processes as its base and the inion as its apex.
omoclavicular t. trigonum omoclaviculare.
omotracheal t. trigonum musculare.
t. of pain a triangular area in the inguinal region, encountered during surgery for inguinal hernias, bounded inferomedially by gonadal vessels and superolaterally by the iliopubic tract; the lateral femoral cutaneous nerve and the femoral branch of the genitofemoral nerve pass through this area and could be entrapped by staples during surgical procedures.
palatal t. a triangle bounded by the greatest transverse diameter of the palate and lines from either end of this diameter to the alveolar point.
paravertebral t. Grocco t.
Petit t. trigonum lumbale inferius.
Pinaud t., Pirogoff t. hypoglossohyoid t.
pubourethral t. a triangle in the perineum bounded externally by the ischiocavernosus muscle, internally by the bulbocavernosus, and posteriorly by the transversus perinei superficialis.
Reil t. trigonum lemnisci.
retromandibular t., retromolar t. trigonum retromolare.
sacral t. a shallow triangular depression overlying the sacrum.
t. of safety the fifth or sixth left intercostal space, considered a safe site for pericardial aspiration.
Scarpa t. trigonum femorale.
sternocostal t. trigonum sternocostale.
subclavian t. trigonum omoclaviculare.
subinguinal t. trigonum femorale.
submandibular t., submaxillary t. trigonum submandibulare.
submental t. trigonum submentale.
suboccipital t. a triangular area lying between the rectus capitis posterior major and the obliquus capitis superior and obliquus capitis inferior muscles.
supraclavicular t. trigonum omoclaviculare.
suprameatal t. foveola suprameatica.
surgical t. any triangular area or region in which certain nerves, vessels, or organs are located; established for reference in surgical operations.
Trautmann t. a space with its anterior angle at the prominence containing the labyrinth, bounded posteriorly by the transverse sinus and superiorly by the inferior temporal line. When the bone is surgically removed, the superior petrosal sinus will be encountered at the superior posterior angle of this triangle.
Tweed t. a triangle defined by facial and dental landmarks on a lateral cephalometric film, using the Frankfort horizontal plane as a base.
umbilicomammillary t. a triangle having its base formed by the line joining the nipples and its apex at the umbilicus.
urogenital t. 1. urogenital diaphragm. 2. regio urogenitalis.
vesical t. trigonum vesicae urinariae.
von Weber t. a region on the sole of the foot formed by lines connecting the head of the first metatarsal, the head of the fifth metatarsal, and the center of the undersurface of the heel.
Ward t. the space formed by the angle of the trabeculae in the neck of the femur; a vulnerable point for fracture.
Wernicke t. the area within the posterior limb on the internal capsule in which the optic radiation, having just left the lateral geniculate body, comes into close proximity to the auditory and somesthetic radiations.

tri•an•gu•la•ris (tri-ang″gu-lar′is) [L.] triangular.

tri•an•te•bra•chia (tri″an-te-bra′ke-ə) [*tri-* + *antebrachium* + *-ia*] a developmental anomaly characterized by tripling of the forearm.

Tri•at•o•ma (tri-at′o-mə) the cone-nose bugs, a genus of insects of the family Reduviidae; many species are important vectors of *Trypanosoma cruzi*, the etiologic agent of Chagas disease. These include *T. dimidia′ta*, *T. genicula′ta*, and *T. mexica′na* in Mexico and Central America; *T. gerstacek′eri*, *T. protrac′ta*, and *T. sanguisu′ga* in the southern United States; *T. recu′va* and *T. rubi′da* in Arizona; and *T. infes′tans* (the unchuca or great black bug), *T. nigrova′rius*, *T. sor′dida*, and *T. vit′ticeps* in South America. Several of the species in the United States and Mexico are called *Mexican bedbugs* and inflict painful bites that cause swelling and nausea. Species *T. megista* has been renamed *Panstrongylus megistus*.

tri•a•tome (tri′ə-tōm) cone-nose bug (def. 1).

tri•atom•ic (tri″ə-tom′ik) made up of three atoms.

tri•at•o•mid (tri-at′o-mid) 1. cone-nose bug (def. 1). 2. triatomine.

tri•at•o•mine (tri-at′o-mēn) pertaining to bugs of the genus *Triatoma;* called also *triatome* and *triatomid.*

Tri•a•vil (tri′ah-vil) trademark for a combination preparation of perphenazine and amitriptyline hydrochloride.

Tri•az (tri′az) trademark for preparations of benzoyl peroxide.

tri•a•zene (tri′ə-zēn) 1. the chemical species HN═N—NH_2. 2. a group of cytotoxic alkylating agents containing this moiety, typified by dacarbazine.

tri•a•zo•lam (tri-a′zə-lam) [USP] a benzodiazepine used as a sedative and hypnotic in the treatment of insomnia; administered orally.

tri•a•zole (tri′ə-zōl, tri-a′zōl) 1. a five-membered heterocyclic ring containing two carbon and three nitrogen atoms:

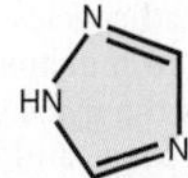

It is a type of azole. 2. any of a class of fungistatic compounds containing such a ring, a subset of the class of azole antifungals, effective against a wide range of fungi; they alter cell membrane functions and permeability by inhibiting the biosynthesis of ergosterol.

trib•a•dism (trib′ə-diz-əm) [Gr. *tribein* to rub] 1. lesbianism; usually used to denote that in which heterosexual intercourse is simulated; sometimes used to refer to the use of an artificial penis. 2. mutual friction of the genitals between women.

tri•ba•sic (tri-ba′sik) [*tri-* + *basic*] having three replaceable hydrogen atoms.

tribe (trīb) a taxonomic category subordinate to a family (or subfamily) and superior to a genus (or subtribe).

tri•ben•o•side (tri-ben′o-sīd) a sclerosing agent which has been used in inflammatory and varicose disorders of the veins.

Tri•bo•li•um (tri-bo′le-əm) a genus of small beetles that live in and are destructive to flour and other cereal products. The most common species, *T. confu′sum* and *T. casta′neum*, are reddish brown and 3.5 mm long.

tri•bol•o•gy (trĭ-bol′ə-je) [Gr. *tribē* a rubbing + *-logy*] the study of the lubrication, friction, and wear of the joints.

tri•bo•lu•mi•nes•cence (tri″bo-loo″mĭ-nes′əns) [Gr. *tribein* to rub + *luminescence*] luminescence produced by mechanical energy, as by the grinding, rubbing, or breaking of certain crystals.

tri•bra•chia (tri-bra′ke-ə) [*tri-* + *brachia*] a developmental anomaly characterized by tripling of the upper limb.

tri•bra•chi•us (tri-bra′ke-əs) 1. a fetus exhibiting tribrachia. 2. conjoined twins having only three upper limbs.

trib•u•lo•sis (trib″u-lo′sis) poisoning in sheep in Australia and South Africa caused by eating wilted plants of the species *Tribulus terrestris;* symptoms include hepatic injury, photosensitization, and encephalopathy.

Trib•u•lus (trib′u-ləs) a genus of tropical and subtropical herbs. *T. terres′tris* is the puncture vine, which causes tribulosis in sheep.

tri•bu•tyl cit•rate (tri-bu′təl) [NF] the ester of *n*-butyl alcohol and citric acid, used as a plasticizer in pharmaceutical preparations.

tri•bu•tyr•in (tri-bu′tər-in) the triglyceride formed from butyric acid and occurring in butter; it is a liquid fat with an acrid taste. Called also *butyrin.*

tri•cal•cic (tri-kal′sik) containing three atoms of calcium.

tri•ceph•a•lus (tri-sef′ə-ləs) [*tri-* + *-cephalus*] a fetus having three heads.

tri•ceps (tri′seps) [L., from *tri-* + *caput* head] having three heads, as a triceps muscle.

t. su′rae see under *musculus.*

tri•chei•ria (tri-ki′re-ə) [*tri-* + *cheir-* + *-ia*] a developmental anomaly characterized by tripling of a hand.

trich•es•the•sia (trik″es-the′zhə) trichoesthesia.

trichi- see *trich(o)-*.

tri•chi•a•sis (trĭ-ki′ə-sis) [*trich-* + *-iasis*] 1. a condition of ingrowing hairs about an orifice, such as of ingrowing eyelashes in cases of entropion. 2. the appearance of hairlike filaments in the urine.

trich•i•lem•ma (trik′ĭ-lem′ə) the outer root sheath. **trichilem′mal** *adj*

trich•i•lem•mo•ma (trik″ĭ-ləm-o′mə) [*trichi-* + Gr. *lemma* rind, husk + *-oma*] a benign adnexal tumor of the lower outer root sheath of the hair; called also *tricholemmoma.*

Tri•chi•na (trĭ-ki′nə) *Trichinella.*

tri•chi•na (trĭ-ki′nə) pl. *trichi′nae.* An individual organism of the genus *Trichinella.*

Trich•i•nel•la (trik″ĭ-nel′ə) [Gr. *trichinos* of hair] a genus of nematode parasites of the family Trichinellidae.

T. brito′vi a species found in temperate regions; it infests the human intestine but has low pathogenicity.

T. murrel′li a species found most often in forest carnivores in southern Arctic regions of North America, and sometimes in human intestines; it has moderate to severe pathogenicity and is not resistant to freezing.

T. nati′va a species that infects the human intestine in Arctic and Subarctic regions; its pathogenicity is high and it has high resistance to freezing.

T. nelso′ni a species that infects the human intestine in hot regions, especially in Africa, and is moderately pathogenic.

T. pseudospira′lis a widespread species usually found in birds; it does not encyst, and its pathogenicity in humans has not been established.

T. spira′lis the species that is the usual etiologic agent of trichinosis; it is small, usually around 1.5 mm long, and is found coiled in cysts in the muscles of bears, rats, pigs, and humans. When infected meat is eaten without proper cooking, the cyst dissolves and the parasite matures and deposits its larvae in the deep mucosa; larvae then enter the lymphatics, are carried to all parts of the body, and again encyst. Called also *pork worm.*

trich•i•nel•li•a•sis (trik″ĭ-nə-li′ə-sis) trichinosis.

Trich•i•nel•li•dae (trik″ĭ-nel′ĭ-de) a family of nematodes of the superfamily Trichuroidea; it contains the genus *Trichinella.*

trich•i•nel•lo•sis (trik″ĭ-nə-lo′sis) trichinosis.

trich•i•ni•a•sis (trik″ĭ-ni′ə-sis) trichinosis.

trich•i•nif•er•ous (trik″ĭ-nif′ər-əs) [*trichina* + *-ferous*] containing trichinae.

trich•i•ni•za•tion (trik″ĭ-nĭ-za′shən) trichinosis.

trich•i•no•sis (trik″ĭ-no′sis) a disease due to infection with *Trichinella spiralis,* seen following the eating of undercooked contaminated meat; early symptoms are diarrhea, nausea, colic, and fever, followed later by stiffness, pain, muscle swelling, fever, eosinophilia, edema around the eyes, splinter hemorrhages, sweating, and insomnia. Called also *trichinellosis.*

trich•i•nous (trik′ĭ-nəs) affected with or containing trichinae.

trich•i•on (trik′e-on) pl. *trich′ia* [Gr.] a cephalometric landmark, the point at which the midsagittal plane of the head intersects the hairline.

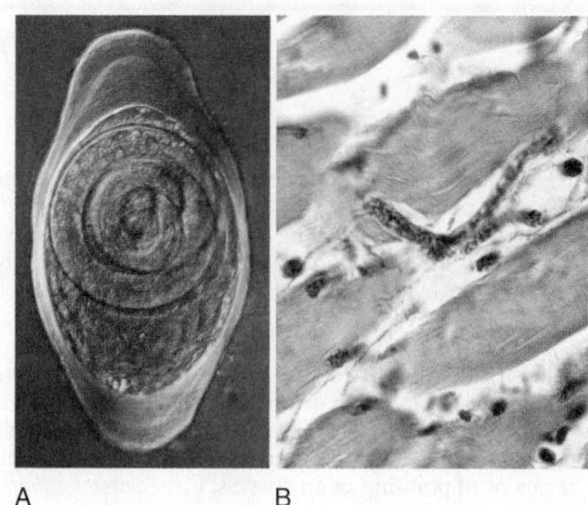

■ *Trichinella spiralis* nurse cell–larva complex *(A)* and larva migrating outward in muscle from a capillary *(B).*

tri•chite (tri′kīt) [Gr. *thrix* hair] 1. trichocyst. 2. nematodesma. 3. a hollow, rodlike, subpellicular component of the skeleton of oligotrich ciliates.

tri•chlor•fon (tri-klor′fon) metrifonate.

tri•chlo•ride (tri-klor′īd) any combination of three atoms of chlorine with one of another element.

tri•chlor•me•thi•a•zide (tri-klor″mə-thi′ə-zīd) [USP] a thiazide diuretic used in the treatment of hypertension and edema; administered orally.

tri•chlo•ro•ac•et•al•de•hyde (tri-klor″o-as″ət-al′də-hīd) chloral (def. 1).

tri•chlo•ro•ace•tic ac•id (tri-klor″o-ə-se′tik) 1. acetic acid with all three of its hydrogen ions exchanged for chlorine atoms; it is a strong organic acid and is used as a protein precipitant in clinical chemistry. 2. a preparation of this acid, used as a caustic in the removal of warts and in chemabrasion; administered topically.

tri•chlo•ro•eth•y•lene (tri-klor″o-eth′ə-lēn) a toxic liquid widely used as an industrial solvent; formerly used as an inhalation anesthetic.

tri•chlo•ro•meth•yl•chlo•ro•for•mate (tri-klor″o-meth″əl-klor″o-for′māt) a chlorine-containing gas which is irritating to lung tissue.

tri•chlo•ro•mono•flu•o•ro•meth•ane (tri-klor″o-mon″o-floor′o-meth′ān) [NF] chemical name: trichlorofluoromethane. A clear, colorless gas having a faint, ethereal odor, CCl_3F, used as an aerosol propellant.

2,4,5-tri•chlo•ro•phen•oxy•ace•tic ac•id (tri-klor″o-fən-ok″se-ə-se′tik) 2,4,5-T.

tri•chlo•ro•tri•vi•nyl•ar•sine (tri-klor″o-tri-vi″nəl-ahr′sin) a sternutatory war gas.

tri•chlor•phon (tri-klor′fon) metrifonate.

trich(o)- [Gr. *thrix,* gen. *trichos,* hair] a prefix denoting relationship to hair.

tricho•ad•e•no•ma (trik″o-ad″ə-no′mə) [*tricho-* + *adenoma*] a type of adnexal adenoma on the face or trunk, with histologic features midway between those of trichofolliculoma and trichoepithelioma, having large cystic spaces lined by squamous epithelium and squamous cells.

tricho•bac•te•ria (trik″o-bak-tēr′e-ə) [*tricho-* + *bacteria*] 1. a group of bacteria including the forms that have flagella. 2. the filamentous or threadlike bacteria.

tricho•be•zoar (trik″o-be′zor) [*tricho-* + *bezoar*] a concretion within the stomach or intestines formed of hairs; called also *hairball* or *hair ball.*

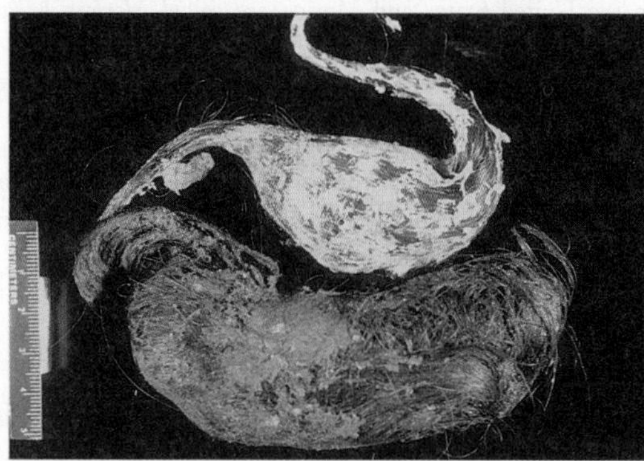

■ Trichobezoar, consisting of an agglomeration of hair, food, and mucus within the gastric lumen.

Tricho·bil·har·zia (trik″o-bil-hahr′ze-ə) a genus of flukes of the family Schistosomatidae. *T. ocella′ta* is found in the portal veins of ducks in Europe and North America and can cause cercarial dermatitis in humans.

tricho·blas·to·ma (trik″o-blas-to′mə) any of a large group of benign adnexal tumors that differentiate toward hair germ epithelium. Cf. *trichoepithelioma.*

tricho·car·dia (trik″o-kahr′de-ə) [*tricho-* + Gr. *kardia* heart] shaggy pericardium.

tricho·ceph·a·li·a·sis (trik″o-sef″ə-li′ə-sis) trichuriasis.

tricho·ceph·a·lo·sis (trik″o-sef″ə-lo′sis) trichuriasis.

Tricho·ceph·a·lus (trik″o-sef′ə-ləs) *Trichuris.*

tricho·cla·sia (trik″o-kla′zhə) trichorrhexis nodosa.

trich·oc·la·sis (trik-ok′lə-sis) trichorrhexis nodosa.

Tricho·co·ma·ceae (trik″o-ko-ma′se-e) [Gr. *trichokomos* hairdresser] a family of fungi of the order Eurotiales, containing the perfect (sexual) stage of certain species of *Aspergillus, Paecilomyces,* and *Penicillium.* Medically important genera include *Emericella* and *Eurotium.*

tricho·cyst (trik′o-sist) [*tricho-* + *-cyst*] one of the extrusible and explosive, nontoxic, spindle-shaped subpellicular organelles occurring in many protozoa, which can discharge long, striated, fibrous shafts. Its true function is unknown, but it may serve to anchor the organism during feeding, serve an offensive or defensive function, or serve in prey capture. Called also *trichite.*

Tricho·dec·tes (trik″o-dek′tēz) [*tricho-* + Gr. *dēktēs* biter] a genus of parasitic biting lice of the order Mallophaga.

T. ca′nis a species that infests dogs and is an intermediate host for the tapeworm *Dipylidium caninum.*

T. e′qui *Damalinia equi.*

T. herm′si *Damalinia hermsi.*

T. la′tus a species that infests dogs.

T. sphaeroce′phalus a species that infests the wool of sheep in Europe and North America.

Tricho·der·ma (trik″o-dur′mə) [*tricho* + *derma* skin] a genus of soil-inhabiting Fungi Imperfecti of the form-class Hyphomycetes, form-family Moniliaceae; some species contain trichothecenes and cause alimentary toxic aleukia. Its perfect (sexual) stage when found is in the genera *Hypocrea* and *Pododerma.*

tricho·dis·co·ma (trik″o-dis-ko′mə) [*tricho-* + *disc-* + *-oma*] a benign adnexal tumor arising from the mesodermal portion of the hair disk, now thought to be a variety of fibrofolliculoma.

tricho·dys·pla·sia (trik″o-dis-pla′zhə) [*tricho-* + *dysplasia*] 1. abnormal hair growth. 2. t. spinulosa.

hereditary t. Marie Unna hypotrichosis.

t. spinulo′sa eruption of spiny papules on the skin of the face with abnormalities of the hair follicles; it is a cutaneous viral infection associated with immunosuppression.

tricho·dys·tro·phy (trik″o-dis′trə-fe) any disorder of the hair marked by defects in the structure of the hair shaft, frequently manifested by alopecia with lusterless, fractured hair.

tricho·epi·the·li·o·ma (trik″o-ep″ĭ-the-le-o′mə) [*tricho-* + *epithelioma*] a benign adnexal tumor originating in the hair matrix, usually on the face; histologically there are strands of basal cells surrounded by fibrocellular stroma. There are two types, the multiple type and the solitary type. Some authorities consider this to be a subgroup of the trichoblastomas.

desmoplastic t. a benign, solitary, pale, hard nodule with a central nonulcerated depression, usually on the face of a young to middle-aged woman; it contains strands of basaloid cells and epidermal cysts infiltrating fibrotic stroma. Called also *sclerosing epithelial hamartoma.*

multiple t., multiple familial t. an autosomal dominant condition (gene locus: 6q12-q13), usually seen in young women, characterized by the occurrence of multiple smooth, flesh-colored, cystic and solid nodules or papules, primarily on the face. Some authorities consider this and Brooke-Spiegler syndrome to be variants of the same condition. Called also *Brooke epithelioma* or *tumor.*

solitary t. an uncommon type of trichoepithelioma that occurs as a solitary lesion; it does not seem to be hereditary and is usually seen in young adult women.

tricho·es·the·sia (trik″o-es-the′zhə) [*tricho-* + *esthesia*] the perception that one of the hairs of the skin has been touched, caused by stimulation of a hair follicle receptor.

tricho·es·the·si·om·e·ter (trik″o-əs-the″ze-om′ə-tər) [*tricho-* + *esthesio-* + *-meter*] an electric apparatus for measuring the hair sensibility, or the sensitiveness of the scalp by means of the hairs.

tricho·fol·lic·u·lo·ma (trik″o-fə-lik″u-lo′mə) [*tricho-* + *folliculus* + *-oma*] a type of benign adnexal tumor, a hamartoma of the hair follicle, usually solitary, dome-shaped, and nodular with a central pore containing a woolly, hairlike tuft. It usually occurs on the head or neck and is characterized histologically by a central keratinous cystic cavity into which numerous abortive hair follicles radiate. Called also *hair follicle nevus.*

tricho·glos·sia (trik″o-glos′e-ə) [*tricho-* + *gloss-* + *-ia*] hairy tongue.

tricho·hy·a·lin (trik″o-hi′ə-lin) [*tricho-* + *hyalin*] a protein found in granules in the cytoplasm of the cells of the Huxley layer of a hair follicle.

trich·oid (trik′oid) [*tricho-* + *-oid*] like or resembling a hair, or the hair.

tricho·lem·mo·ma (trik″o-lem-o′mə) trichilemmoma.

tricho·leu·ko·cyte (trik″o-loo′ko-sīt) hairy cell.

tricho·lith (trik′o-lith) [*tricho-* + *-lith*] a hairy concretion.

trich·ol·o·gy (trĭ-kol′ə-je) the study of hair, or the sum of what is known about the hair.

tricho·meg·a·ly (trik″o-meg′ə-le) [*tricho-* + *-megaly*] elongation of the eyelashes, which can be acquired, usually during treatment with certain drugs; it is also seen as part of an inherited syndrome associated with dwarfism, mental retardation, and pigmentary degeneration of the retina.

tricho·mo·na·ci·dal (trik″o-mo″nə-si′dəl) destructive to trichomonads.

tricho·mo·na·cide (trik″o-mo′nə-sīd) something that kills *Trichomonas;* cf. *antitrichomonal.*

tricho·mo·nad (trik″o-mo′nad, trik″o-mon′ad) [*tricho-* + *monad*] any protozoan of the order Trichomonadida.

Tricho·mo·nad·i·da (trik″o-mo-nad′e-də) an order of chiefly parasitic protozoa of the phylum Parabasalia, typically having karyomastigonts with three to six flagella, one of which is recurrent or free or has a proximal segment or the entire length adherent to the body surface. An undulating membrane (if present) is associated with adherent segments of recurrent flagellum, and there are a pelta and noncontractile axostyle in each mastigont. Representative genera include *Dientamoeba, Histomonas, Pentatrichomonas, Tetratrichomonas, Trichomonas,* and *Tritrichomonas.*

tricho·mo·nal (trik″o-mo′nəl) pertaining to or caused by trichomonads.

Tricho·mo·nas (trik″o-mo′nəs) [*tricho-* + Gr. *monas* unit, from *monas* single] a genus of parasitic flagellated protozoa of the order Trichomonadida, phylum Parabasalia, found in the intestinal and genitourinary tracts of various invertebrates and vertebrates, and characterized by the presence of a pelta, an axostyle, an undulating membrane, and three to five anterior flagella. In newer systems of classification, those with three flagella have been assigned to genus *Tritrichomonas,* and those with five to genus *Pentatrichomonas.*

T. bucca′lis *T. tenax.*

T. foe′tus *Tritrichomonas foetus.*

T. galli′nae a species found in birds, having four anterior flagella and usually inhabiting the upper digestive tract and related structures or other organs such as the liver; it causes a form of avian trichomoniasis. Infection varies from mild to a rapidly fatal disease manifested by caseous accumulations and necrosis in involved tissues and severe weight loss.

T. gallina′rum *Tetratrichomonas gallinarum.*

T. ho′minis *Pentatrichomonas hominis.*

T. te′nax a commensal species found in the mouths of primates, having four anterior flagella; it is most often seen in the tartar around teeth, cavities of carious teeth, pockets associated with periodontal disease, and tonsillar crypts. Called also *T. buccalis.*

T. vagina′lis a species with four flagella found in the vagina and male genital tract, the cause of trichomoniasis vaginalis.

tricho·mo·ni·a·sis (trik″o-mo-ni′ə-sis) infection with protozoa of the genus *Trichomonas.*

avian t. trichomoniasis in birds and poultry, especially pigeons, caused by either *Trichomonas gallinae* or *Tetratrichomonas gallinarum;* characteristics include necrotic lesions of the upper digestive tract and liver, with diarrhea, anorexia, and weight loss, often ending fatally.

bovine t. venereal trichomoniasis in cattle, caused by *Tritrichomonas foetus* and marked by abortion and pyometra.

vaginal t., t. vagina′lis *Trichomonas* vaginitis.

Tricho·my·ce·tes (trik″o-mi-se′tēs) [*tricho-* + Gr. *mykēs* fungus] a class of perfect fungi of the phylum Zygomycota, most of whose members

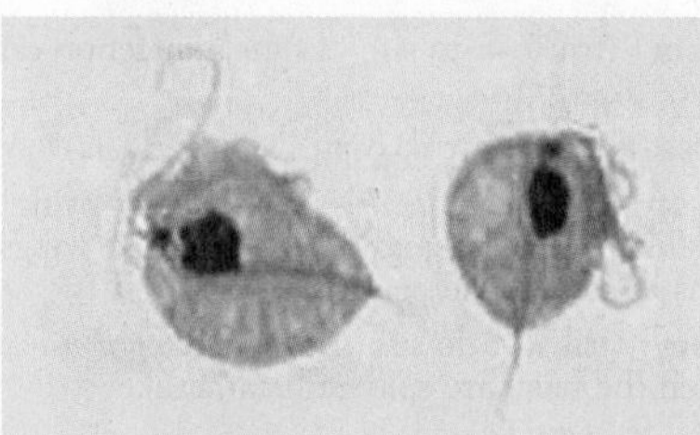

■ *Trichomonas vaginalis.* Flagellated trophozoites (Giemsa stain).

are found as parasites in the digestive tract or on the external cuticle of living arthropods.

tricho·my·co·sis (trik″o-mi-ko′sis) [*tricho-* + *mycosis*] 1. any disease of the hair due to infection by a fungus. 2. t. axillaris.

t. axilla′ris a common, superficial infection of the axillary or pubic hair in which yellow, black, or red nodular concretions form around the hair shaft; it is caused by any of several species of *Corynebacterium.*

t. nodo′sa, t. nodula′ris piedra.

tricho·no·do·sis (trik″o-no-do′sis) [*tricho-* + L. *nodus* knot + *-osis*] a rare condition characterized by apparent or actual knotting of the hair, thought to be the result of inability of new hairs to grow freely from their follicles, because of toughness of the surrounding tissues.

trich·op·a·thy (trĭ-kop′ə-the) trichosis.

tricho·pha·gia (trik″o-fa′jə) [*tricho-* + *-phagia*] the habit of eating hair, a form of pica.

trich·oph·a·gy (trĭ-kof′ə-je) trichophagia.

tricho·phyt·ic (trik″o-fit′ik) pertaining to trichophytosis.

tri·choph·y·tid (trĭ-kof′ĭ-tid) [*Trichophyton* + *-id*] a dermatophytid associated with trichophytosis; applied especially to allergic manifestations of any ringworm infection.

tri·choph·y·tin (trĭ-kof′ĭ-tin) the soluble broth culture products of various species of *Trichophyton;* used in the trichophytin test.

tricho·phy·to·be·zoar (trik″o-fi″to-be′zor) [*tricho-* + *phyto-* + *bezoar*] a bezoar composed of animal hair and vegetable fibers; called also *phytotrichobezoar.*

Tri·choph·y·ton (tri-kof′ĭ-ton) [*tricho-* + Gr. *phyton* plant] a genus of Fungi Imperfecti of the form-class Hyphomycetes, form-family Moniliaceae, consisting of flat, branched filaments. Many species are dermatophytes and attack the skin, nails, and hair, and most are either of the large-spored ectothrix or endothrix type. As the perfect (sexual) stages are identified they are classified in the genus *Arthroderma.*

T. concen′tricum a species that is the usual cause of tinea imbricata in humans.

T. equi′num a species that causes dermatophytosis in horses.

T. erina′cei a species closely related to *T. mentagrophytes* and usually found in hedgehogs but sometimes causing ringworm (tinea) in humans.

T. ferrugi′neum *Microsporum ferrugineum.*

T. galli′nae a species that is a large-spored ectothrix and causes favus in fowls. Called also *Microsporum gallinae.*

T. gourvi′lii a species closely related to *T. rubrum,* found in cases of ringworm (tinea).

T. interdigita′le a species closely related to *T. mentagrophytes* and sometimes causing ringworm (tinea) in humans.

T. mentagrophy′tes a small-spored ectothrix species that causes ringworm (tinea) of various types in humans and dermatophytosis in farm animals. It has perfect (sexual) stages in genus *Arthroderma.*

T. quinckea′num a species closely related to *T. mentagrophytes* and usually found in mice with favus, but sometimes causing tinea (ringworm) in humans.

T. ru′brum a species that commonly causes various types of ringworm (tinea).

T. schoenlei′nii a species that causes favus in humans.

T. si′mii a geophilic species found in India that causes ringworm in monkeys and chickens and tinea corporis in humans. Its perfect (sexual) stage is *Arthroderma simii.*

T. soudanen′se a species closely related to *T. rubrum,* found in cases of ringworm (tinea).

T. tonsu′rans a species that is an endothrix and causes human tinea capitis and tinea corporis; it occurs throughout the world but is particularly prevalent in the Americas.

T. verruco′sum a species that causes ringworm (tinea) in farm animals and humans.

T. viola′ceum a species that is an endothrix and usually causes tinea capitis but sometimes also causes tinea corporis and onychomycosis.

T. yaoun′dei a species closely related to *T. rubrum,* found in cases of ringworm (tinea).

tricho·phy·to·sis (trik″o-fi-to′sis) a fungal infection caused by species of *Trichophyton*; see also *favus.*

tricho·po·lio·dys·tro·phy (trik″o-po″le-o-dis′trə-fe) Menkes disease.

Tri·chop·tera (tri-kop′tər-ə) [*tricho-* + Gr. *pteron* wing] an order of flies, the caddis flies. The hair and scales from the wings may produce allergic symptoms in susceptible persons.

trich·op·ti·lo·sis (trik″o-tĭ-lo′sis) [*tricho-* + Gr. *ptilon* feather + *-osis*] a condition in which the hairs are split and featherlike.

trich·or·rhex·is (trik″o-rek′sis) [*tricho-* + *-rrhexis*] breaking of the hairs; cf. *trichoschisis.*

t. invagina′ta a rare condition in which there is invagination of the end of one segment into the adjacent segment in ball-and-socket fashion to resemble a light-colored nodule, seen especially in Netherton syndrome. Called also *bamboo hair.*

t. nodo′sa a hair condition in which the shafts appear to have nodes but actually have splitting of the cortex into strands; it usually affects the proximal part of the shaft, so that hairs grow a few centimeters and break off. It may be either congenital or acquired; the acquired form is usually in persons with curly hair who repeatedly straighten their hair.

trich·os·chi·sis (trik-os′kĭ-sis) [*tricho-* + *-schisis*] splitting of the hairs; cf. *trichorrhexis.*

tricho·sid·er·in (trik″o-sid′ər-in) [*tricho-* + Gr. *sidēros* iron] an iron-containing brown pigment found in normal human red hair.

tri·cho·sis (trĭ-ko′sis) [Gr. *trichōsis* growth of hair] any disease of the hair; called also *trichopathy.*

t. carun′culae abnormal development of the hair on the lacrimal caruncle.

Tricho·so·ma (trik″o-so′mə) former name for *Capillaria.*

Tricho·so·moi·des (trik″o-so-moi′dēz) a genus of nematodes of the family Trichuridae. *T. crassicau′da* is parasitic in rats; the male is much smaller than the female and lives inside the uterus.

Tri·chos·po·ron (tri-kos′pə-ron) [*tricho-* + Gr. *sporos* seed] a genus of Fungi Imperfecti of the form-family Cryptococcaceae, closely related to *Geotrichum.* Called also *Trichosporum.*

T. asa′hii a species that can cause serious or fatal mycosis in immunocompromised persons.

T. asteroi′des a species that causes superficial skin infections.

T. bei′gelii a former species now considered to be several different species; these organisms are normal inhabitants of the skin, respiratory tract, and digestive tract, but can also cause white piedra and potentially fatal opportunistic infections.

T. capita′tum *Blastoschizomyces capitatus.*

T. cuta′neum a species formerly considered part of *T. beigelii,* found most often in superficial infections but sometimes in serious opportunistic infections.

T. in′kin a species usually seen in cases of white piedra but occasionally in more serious opportunistic infections.

T. mucoi′des a species usually seen in persons with white piedra but sometimes causing a severe or even fatal opportunistic infection.

T. ovoi′des a species usually seen in cases of white piedra but occasionally in more serious opportunistic infections.

tri·chos·po·ro·no·sis (tri-kos″pə-rə-no′sis) infection by species of *Trichosporon,* usually referring to opportunistic infections and not including white piedra. Called also *trichosporosis.*

tricho·spo·ro·sis (trik″o-spə-ro′sis) 1. trichosporonosis. 2. white piedra.

Tri·chos·po·rum (tri-kos′pə-rəm) *Trichosporon.*

tri·chos·ta·sis spin·u·lo·sa (trĭ-kos′tə-sis spin″u-lo′sə) [*tricho-* + *stasis* + L. *spinulosus* thorny] a condition in which the hair follicles contain a dark, horny, comedolike keratin plug that contains a bundle of vellus hair.

Tricho·sto·mat·i·da (trik″o-sto-mat′ĭ-də) [*tricho-* + Gr. *stoma* mouth] an order of ciliate protozoa (subclass Vestibuliferia, class Kinetofragminophorea), many of which are endocommensals in vertebrates; most have uniform somatic ciliature, sometimes asymmetrical, and no buccal ciliature in the oral region is present. It comprises two suborders: Trichostomatina and Blepharocorynthina.

Tricho·sto·ma·ti·na (trik″o-sto″mə-ti′nə) a suborder of ciliate protozoa (order Trichostomatida, subclass Vestibuliferia) in which the somatic ciliature is not reduced. *Balantidium* and *Isotricha* are representative genera.

tricho·stron·gy·li·a·sis (trik″o-stron″jə-li′ə-sis) infection by nematodes of the genus *Trichostrongylus;* it is usually asymptomatic, but diarrhea may occur. Called also *trichostrongylosis.*

Tricho·stron·gyl·i·dae (trik″o-stron-jil′ĭ-de) a family of nematodes that includes many parasites of animals. Genera of medical or veterinary interest include *Cooperia, Dictyocaulus, Hyostrongylus, Mecistocirrus, Nematodirus, Nippostrongylus, Ostertagia, Teladorsagia,* and *Trichostrongylus.*

tricho·stron·gy·lo·sis (trik″o-stron″jə-lo′sis) trichostrongyliasis.

Tricho·stron·gy·lus (trik″o-stron′jə-ləs) a genus of nematodes of the family Trichostrongylidae, comprising some species formerly included in the genus *Strongylus.* Adult worms are small and embed their heads in the mucosa of the small intestines of mammals; their eggs are often mistaken for those of the hookworm. See *trichostrongyliasis.*

T. caprico′la a species commonly found in ruminants.

T. colubrifor′mis a species frequently present in sheep and goats and occasionally in humans; called also *T. instabilis.*

T. insta′bilis *T. colubriformis.*

T. orienta′lis a species found in humans and sheep in Asia.

T. probolu′rus a species found in ruminants and occasionally humans in Europe, Africa, and North America.

T. vitri′nus a species found in ruminants and occasionally humans.

tri•choth•e•cene (tri-koth′ə-sēn) any of a group of mycotoxins found contaminating grain and other foods; those from species of *Fusarium* cause fusariotoxicosis and those from species of *Stachybotrys* cause stachybotryotoxicosis. The group includes deoxynivalenol, diacetoxyscirpenol, roridins, satratoxins, T-2 toxin, and verrucarins.

Tricho•the•ci•um (trik″o-the′se-əm) [*tricho-* + Gr. *thēkē* case] a genus of Fungi Imperfecti of the form-class Hyphomycetes, form-family Moniliaceae. Certain species contain trichothecenes and can cause alimentary toxic aleukia. *T. ro′seum* causes pinkrot on apples and lumber and is occasionally recovered from human otitis externa and mycotic keratitis.

tricho•thio•dys•tro•phy (trik″o-thi″o-dis′trə-fe) any of several autosomal recessive disorders in which hair is sparse and brittle, has an unusually low sulfur content, and has a banded appearance under polarized light; ichthyotic skin and physical and mental retardation are also present. The disorders are categorized on the basis of whether photosensitivity is also present; the photosensitive form is caused by mutations affecting either subunit of a DNA helicase involved in transcription and nucleotide excision repair; there are multiple nonphotosensitive forms caused by varying mutations.

tricho•til•lo•ma•nia (trik″o-til″o-ma′ne-ə) [*tricho-* + Gr. *tillein* to pull + *-mania*] [DSM-IV] compulsive pulling out of one's hair, associated with tension or an irresistible urge before pulling and followed by pleasure or relief.

tri•chot•o•mous (tri-kot′ə-məs) [Gr. *tricha* three-fold + *tom-* + *-ous*] divided into three parts.

tri•cho•tox•in (tri′ko-tok″sin) an antibody that has a toxic action on epithelial cells.

tri•chro•ism (tri′kro-iz-əm) [*tri-* + Gr. *chroa* color] the exhibition of three different colors in three different aspects. **trichro′ic** *adj*

tri•chro•ma•cy (tri-kro′mə-se) trichromatic vision.
  anomalous t. anomalous trichromatic vision.

tri•chro•ma•sy (tri-kro′mə-se) trichromatic vision.

tri•chro•mat (tri′kro-mat) a person with trichromatic vision.

tri•chro•mat•ic (tri″kro-mat′ik) [*tri-* + Gr. *chrōma* color] 1. pertaining to or exhibiting three colors. 2. able to distinguish the three primary colors of light (red, blue, and green); see *trichromatic vision.* Called also *trichromic.*

tri•chro•ma•tism (tri-kro′mə-tiz-əm) trichromatic vision.
  anomalous t. anomalous trichromatic vision.

tri•chro•ma•top•sia (tri″kro-mə-top′se-ə) trichromatic vision.

tri•chro•mic (tri-kro′mik) trichromatic.

trich•ter•brust (trich′ter-broost) [Ger.] pectus excavatum.

trich•u•ri•a•sis (trik″u-ri′ə-sis) infection with nematodes of the genus *Trichuris,* seen most often in humans and dogs. The worm inhabits the large intestine, often without symptoms, although heavy infestations may cause diarrhea, vomiting, rectal bleeding, and prolapse.

Tri•chu•ri•dae (trĭ-ku′rĭ-de) a family of nematodes of the superfamily Trichuroidea. It includes the genera *Capillaria, Trichosomoides,* and *Trichuris.*

Tri•chu•ris (trĭ-ku′ris) [*tricho-* + Gr. *oura* a tail] the whipworms, a genus of nematodes of the family Trichuridae; several species parasitize the intestines of mammals.

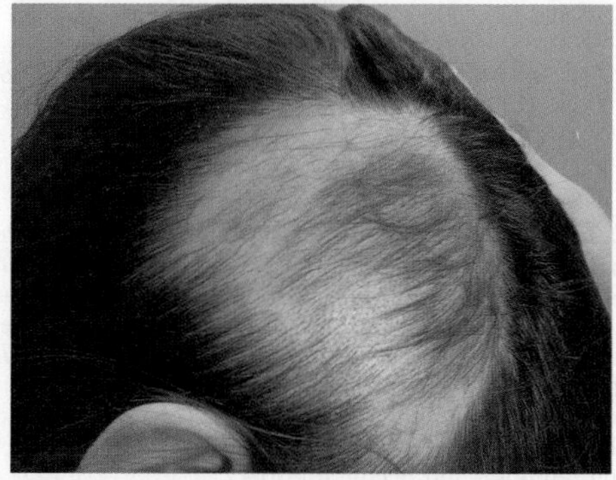

■ Trichotillomania.

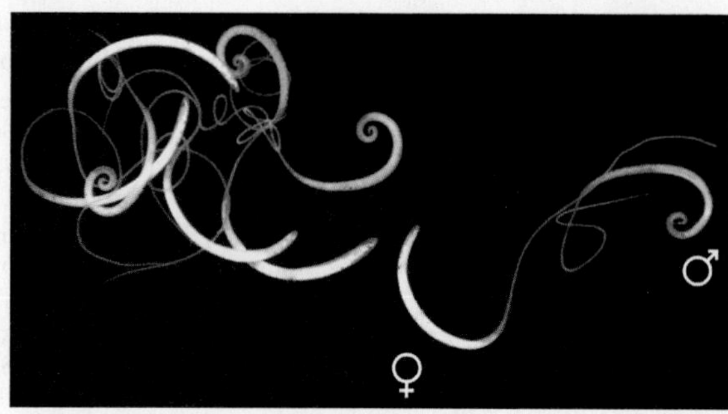

■ *Trichuris trichiura* adults. Their anterior region is tapered; the posterior end of the male is coiled and that of the female is straight.

T. trichiu′ra the species that principally infects humans; it is about 5 cm long, with the front part of its body (the esophageal zone) thin like a hair.

T. vul′pis the species that most often causes trichuriasis in dogs.

Trich•u•roi•dea (trik″u-roi′de-ə) a superfamily of aphasmid nematodes including the families *Trichinellidae* and *Trichuridae.*

tri•cip•i•tal (tri-sip′ĭ-təl) [L. *tricipitis*] 1. pertaining to a triceps muscle. 2. having three heads.

tri•cit•rates (tri-sit′rāts) [USP] a solution of sodium citrate, potassium citrate, and citric acid; used as a systemic or urinary alkalizer, antiurolithic, and neutralizing buffer.

tri•cla•ben•da•zole (tri″klə-ben′də-zōl) a benzimidazole used as an anthelmintic in the treatment of fascioliasis and paragonimiasis; administered orally.

tri•clo•car•ban (tri″klo-kahr′ban) a disinfectant, effective against gram-positive bacteria and to a lesser extent against gram-negative bacteria and against fungi; used in the preparation of soaps and other cleansing products and dermatological compositions to control skin infections.

tri•clo•san (tri-klo′san) [USP] an antibacterial effective against gram-positive and most gram-negative organisms and exhibiting slight activity against yeasts and fungi; used as a detergent in surgical scrubs, soaps, and deodorants.

Tri•co•fu•ron (tri″ko-fu′ron) trademark for preparations of furazolidone.

Tri•cor (tri′kor) trademark for a preparation of fenofibrate.

tri•cor•nute (tri-kor′nūt) [*tri-* + L. *cornutus* horned] having three horns, cornua, or processes.

tri•cre•sol (tri-kre′sol) cresol.

tri•cres•yl phos•phate (tri-kres′əl) tritolyl phosphate.

tri-o-cres•yl phos•phate (tri-kres′əl) tri-*o*-tolyl phosphate.

tri•crot•ic (tri-krot′ik) [Gr. *trikrotos* rowed with a triple stroke; triple beating] pertaining to or characterized by tricrotism. See also *anatricrotic* and *catatricrotic.*

tri•cro•tism (tri′kro-tiz-əm) presence of a tricrotic pulse.

tri•cus•pid (tri-kus′pid) [*tri-* + *cuspid*] 1. having three points or cusps. 2. pertaining to the tricuspid valve of the heart.

tri•cy•cla•mol chlo•ride (tri-si′klə-mol) a quaternary ammonium anticholinergic derived from procyclidine which inhibits gastrointestinal hypermotility and reduces secretion of gastric juices; it has been used in the treatment of peptic ulcer and as a gastrointestinal antispasmodic.

tri•cyc•lic (tri-sik′lik, -si′klik) containing three fused rings or closed chains in the molecular structure; see also under *antidepressant.*

Trid. [L.] trid′uum (three days).

tri•dac•ty•lism (tri-dak′tə-liz-əm) [*tri-* + *dactyl-* + *-ism*] the condition of having three digits on the hands or feet. **tridac′tylous** *adj*

tri•dent (tri′dent) tridentate.

tri•den•tate (tri-den′tāt) three-pronged.

tri•der•mal (tri-der′məl) pertaining to or possessing all three germ layers.

tri•der•mic (tri-dur′mik) [*tri-* + *dermic*] derived from all three germ layers (ectoderm, endoderm, and mesoderm).

tri•der•mo•gen•e•sis (tri″dər-mo-jen′ə-sis) [*tri-* + *dermo-* + *-genesis*] the formation of the three germ layers (gastrulation) and, by extension, the stage in embryonic development during which it occurs.

tri•der•mo•ma (tri″dər-mo′mə) [*tri-* + *derm-* + *-oma*] a teratoma containing representatives of all three germ layers.

Tri•des•i•lon (tri-des'ĭ-lon) trademark for preparations of desonide.

-triene a chemical suffix indicating the presence of three double bonds.

tri•en•tene hy•dro•chlo•ride (tri'en-tēn) a chelating agent used to chelate and facilitate the excretion of excess copper in Wilson disease; administered orally.

tri•es•ter (tri'es-tər) a compound containing three ester groups.

tri•eth•a•nol•amine (tri″eth-ə-nol'ə-mēn) an ethanolamine carrying three ethanol substituents, produced by ammonolysis of ethylene oxide. A pharmaceutical preparation is called *trolamine* (q.v.).

tri•eth•yl•amine (tri″eth-əl-am'in) a liquid ptomaine with a fishy, ammoniacal smell, occurring during putrefaction, especially in fish; it is also synthesized for use in a variety of industrial processes. It is an irritant to tissue and is toxic by inhalation and ingestion.

tri•eth•yl cit•rate (tri-eth'əl) [NF] the ethyl ester of citric acid, used as a plasticizer in pharmaceutical preparations.

tri•eth•yl•ene•thio•phos•pho•ra•mide (tri-eth″ə-lēn-thi″o-fos-for'ə-mīd) thiotepa.

tri•fa•cial (tri-fa'shəl) [L. *trifacialis*] designating the fifth cranial nerve (nervus trigeminus [TA]).

tri•fas•cic•u•lar (tri″fə-sik'u-lər) pertaining to three bundles, or fasciculi.

tri•fid (tri'fid) [L. *trifidus*, from *tres* three + *findere* to split] split into three parts.

tri•flu•o•per•a•zine hy•dro•chlo•ride (tri-floo″o-per'ə-zēn) [USP] a phenothiazine derivative, used in the treatment of symptoms of psychotic disorders; administered orally or intramuscularly.

tri•flu•o•ro•thy•mi•dine (tri-floor″o-thi'mĭ-dēn) trifluridine.

tri•flu•per•i•dol (tri-floo-per'ĭ-dol) a butyrophenone used in the treatment of mania and schizophrenia; administered orally.

tri•flu•pro•ma•zine (tri″floo-pro'mə-zēn) [USP] a phenothiazine derivative with antipsychotic and antiemetic actions.
  t. hydrochloride [USP] the monohydrochloride salt of triflupromazine, having the same actions and uses as the base; administered intramuscularly or intravenously.

tri•flur•i•dine (tri-floor'ĭ-dēn) [USP] an antiviral compound that interferes with viral DNA synthesis, used in the treatment of keratitis and keratoconjunctivitis caused by human herpesviruses 1 and 2; applied topically to the conjunctiva.

tri•flu•tate (tri'floo-tāt″) USAN contraction for trifluoroacetate.

tri•fo•cal (tri-fo'-, tri'fo-kəl) 1. having three foci. 2. containing one part for near vision, one for intermediate, and a third for distant vision; see under *lens.*

tri•fo•cals (tri'fo-kəlz) trifocal glasses.

tri•fo•li•o•sis (tri″fo-le-o'sis) a disease usually seen in horses, marked by photosensitization and irritation of the oral mucous membranes, sometimes with liver damage; attributed to the eating of *Trifolium hybridum* (hybrid clover) and related plants.

Tri•fo•li•um (tri-fo'le-əm) the clovers, a genus of herbs commonly fed to livestock. *T. hy'bridum*, the hybrid clover, can cause trifoliosis. *T. re'pens*, the white clover, contains cyanogenetic compounds and can cause cyanide poisoning. The flower heads of *T. praten'se*, the red clover, are used medicinally.

tri•fur•ca•tion (tri″fər-ka'shən) [*tri-* + *furcation*] 1. division into three branches or parts, such as with blood vessels, or teeth that have three roots. 2. the site of such division.

tri•gas•tric (tri-gas'trik) [*tri-* + Gr. *gastēr* belly] having three bellies; said of a muscle.

tri•gem•i•nal (tri-jem'ĭ-nəl) [*tri-* + L. *geminus* twin] 1. triple. 2. pertaining to the fifth cranial nerve (nervus trigeminus [TA]). 3. pertaining to trigeminy.

tri•gem•i•nus (tri-jem'ĭ-nəs) [L.] triple; see *nervus trigeminus.*

tri•gem•i•ny (tri-jem'ĭ-ne) [*tri-* + L. *geminus* twin] 1. occurrence in threes. 2. the occurrence of a trigeminal pulse.
  ventricular t. an arrhythmia consisting of the repetitive sequence of one ventricular premature complex followed by two normal beats.

trig•gered (trig'ərd) having an output that is set in motion by a smaller input.

Tri•glo•chin (tri-glo'kin) arrow grass, a genus of grasses (family Gramineae), some species of which have pollen that can cause hay fever.

tri•glyc•er•ide (tri-glis'ər-īd) a compound consisting of three molecules of fatty acid esterified to glycerol; it is a neutral fat synthesized from carbohydrates for storage in animal adipose cells. On enzymatic hydrolysis, it releases free fatty acids in the blood.

tri•glyc•er•ide lip•ase (tri-glis'ə-rīd li'pās) triacylglycerol lipase.

tri•go•na (tri-go'nə) [L.] plural of *trigonum.*

tri•go•nal (tri'go-nəl) 1. triangular. 2. pertaining to a trigone.

tri•gone (tri'gōn) 1. triangle. 2. the first three cusps of an upper molar tooth; see *hypocone*, *paracone*, and *protocone.*
  bladder t., t. of bladder trigonum vesicae urinariae.
  carotid t. trigonum caroticum.
  cerebral t. fornix (def. 2).
  collateral t. of fourth ventricle trigonum nervi vagi.
  collateral t. of lateral ventricle trigonum collaterale ventriculi lateralis.
  fibrous t. of heart, left trigonum fibrosum sinistrum cordis.
  fibrous t. of heart, right trigonum fibrosum dextrum cordis.
  habenular t. trigonum habenulare.
  Henke t. see under *triangle.*
  hypoglossal t., t. of hypoglossal nerve trigonum nervi hypoglossi.
  iliopectineal t. fossa iliopectinea.
  interpeduncular t. fossa interpeduncularis.
  t. of lateral lemniscus trigonum lemnisci lateralis.
  olfactory t. trigonum olfactorium.
  omoclavicular t. trigonum omoclaviculare.
  pontocerebellar t. trigonum pontocerebellare.
  t. of Reil trigonum lemnisci.
  retromolar t. see under *triangle.*
  t. of urinary bladder trigonum vesicae urinariae.
  urogenital t. urogenital diaphragm.
  vagal t., t. of vagus nerve trigonum nervi vagi.
  vesical t. trigonum vesicae urinariae.

Tri•go•nel•la (tri-gə-nel'ə) a genus of leguminous plants. *T. foe'num-grae'cum* L. is fenugreek, a species found in Southern Europe, North Africa, and India whose seeds are the medicinal substance fenugreek; if eaten in large quantities it is toxic to livestock.

trig•o•nel•line (trig″o-nel'in) an alkaloid found in fenugreek, cannabis, strophanthus, and various other plants, in sea urchins and jellyfish, and also in the urine after administration of nicotinic acid. It is a betaine of methyl nicotinic acid.

tri•gon•id (tri-gon'id) the first three cusps of a lower molar tooth. See *hypoconid*, *paraconid*, and *protoconid.*

trig•o•ni•tis (trig″o-ni'tis) [*trigone* + *-itis*] inflammation or localized hyperemia of the trigone of the bladder.

trig•o•no•ce•pha•lia (trig″o-no-sə-fa'le-ə) trigonocephaly.

trig•o•no•ceph•a•lus (trig″o-no-sef'ə-ləs) an individual exhibiting trigonocephaly.

trig•o•no•ceph•a•ly (trig″o-no-sef'ə-le) [Gr. *trigonos* triangular + *-cephaly*] a deformity of the head characterized by sharp angulation ventrad of the squamous portion of the frontal bones at the site of the suture between them. **trigonocephal'ic** *adj*

tri•go•num (tri-go'nəm) pl. *trigo'na* [L., from Gr. *trigōnon* triangle] triangle.
  t. auscultatio'nis [TA] triangle of auscultation: the area limited by the lower edge of the trapezius muscle, the latissimus dorsi, and the medial margin of the scapula.
  t. caro'ticum [TA] carotid triangle: the triangular region bounded by the posterior belly of the digastric muscle and the stylohyoid, the sternocleidomastoid muscle, and the superior belly of the omohyoid; called also *superior carotid triangle.*

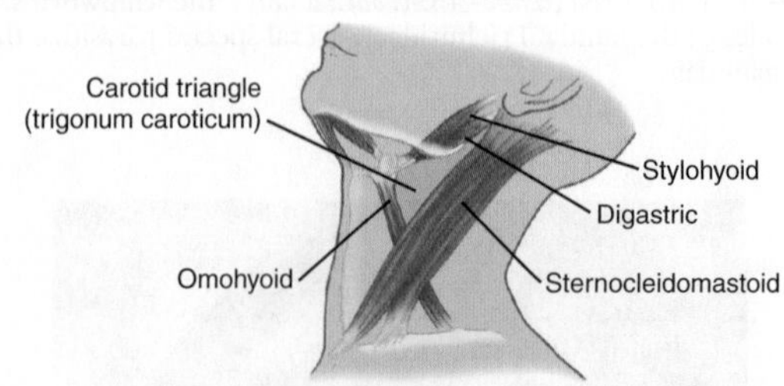

  t. cervica'le ante'rius TA alternative for *regio cervicalis anterior.*
  t. cervica'le poste'rius TA alternative for *regio cervicalis lateralis.*
  t. clavipectora'le [TA] clavipectoral triangle: the triangular region separating the upper border of the pectoralis minor muscle from the clavicle, which contains the clavipectoral fascia. Called also *t. deltopectorale* [TA alternative] and *deltopectoral triangle.*
  t. collatera'le ventri'culi latera'lis [TA] collateral trigone of lateral ventricle: the triangular area in the floor of the lateral ventricle between the diverging temporal and occipital horns.
  t. col'li ante'rius TA alternative for *regio cervicalis anterior.*

t. col'li latera'le TA alternative for *regio cervicalis lateralis.*

t. coracoacromia'le a triangle bounded by the coracoid process, the apex of the acromion, and the concave border of the clavicle.

t. cystohepa'ticum [TA] cystohepatic triangle: the triangle formed by the cystic artery superiorly, the cystic duct inferiorly, and the hepatic duct medially. Called also *Calot triangle.*

t. deltopectora'le TA alternative for *t. clavipectorale.*

t. femora'le [TA] femoral triangle: a triangular area just distal to the inguinal fold, bounded superiorly by the inguinal ligament, laterally by the medial border of the sartorius muscle, and medially by the medial border of the adductor longus muscle; called also *Scarpa triangle.*

t. fibro'sum dex'trum cor'dis [TA] right fibrous trigone of heart: a thickened, irregularly triangular portion of the fibrous skeleton of the base of the heart, located between the right and left atrioventricular fibrous rings, posterior to the aortic orifice. Called also *central fibrous body of heart.*

t. fibro'sum sinis'trum cor'dis [TA] left fibrous trigone of heart: a thickened and irregularly triangular portion of the fibrous skeleton of the base of the heart, located between the left atrioventricular fibrous ring and the left posterior margin of the aortic fibrous ring.

t. habenula're [TA] habenular trigone: the small, depressed triangular area on the dorsomedial aspect of the posterior part of the thalamus which contains the habenular nuclei and marks the habenular commissure.

t. hypoglossa'le TA alternative for *t. nervi hypoglossi.*

t. inguina'le [TA] inguinal triangle: the triangular area on the anteroinferior abdominal wall bounded by the rectus abdominis muscle, the inguinal ligament, and the inferior epigastric vessels: the site in which a direct inguinal hernia begins.

t. lemnis'ci latera'lis [TA] trigone of lateral lemniscus: a small, more or less distinct triangular area lateral to the isthmus and the inferior colliculus, bounded inferiorly by the superior cerebellar peduncle and the lateral lemniscus, posteromedially by the brachium of the inferior colliculus, and anterolaterally by the lateral sulcus of the mesencephalon.

t. lumba'le infe'rius [TA] inferior lumbar triangle: a small triangular interval between the inferolateral margin of the latissimus dorsi muscle and the external oblique muscle of the abdomen, just superior to the ilium; called also *trigonum lumbare, lumbar triangle,* and *Petit triangle.*

t. lumba'le supe'rius [TA] superior lumbar triangle: an inconstant triangle or rhombus bounded by the twelfth rib and the serratus posterior inferior, erector spinae, and internal oblique muscles, and overlapped by the latissimus dorsi and the external oblique, with the thoracolumbar fascia as its floor. When present it is sometimes a site through which abscesses point or hernias occur.

t. lumba're trigonum lumbale inferius.

t. lumbocosta'le [TA] a triangular opening of variable size between the lateral arcuate ligament and the pars costalis diaphragmatis.

t. muscula're [TA] muscular triangle: the part of the trigonum caroticum medial to the omohyoid muscle; called also *t. omotracheale* [TA alternative], *inferior carotid triangle,* and *omotracheal triangle.*

t. ner'vi hypoglos'si [TA] trigone of hypoglossal nerve: the tapering lower end of the medial eminence of the rhomboid fossa just superficial to the position of the hypoglossal nucleus. Called also *hypoglossal trigone.*

t. ner'vi va'gi [TA] trigone of vagus nerve: an area in the floor of the fourth ventricle immediately lateral to the trigonum nervi hypoglossi; beneath it lies the dorsal nucleus of the vagus nerve. Called also *t. vagale* [TA alternative] and *vagal trigone.*

t. olfacto'rium [TA] olfactory trigone: the area of the anterior perforated substance between the diverging lateral and medial olfactory striae, and bounded posteriorly by the diagonal band.

t. omoclavicula're [TA] omoclavicular triangle: a deep region of the neck, corresponding to the fossa supraclavicularis major on the surface, in which the brachial plexus may be palpated, and by downward pressure the subclavian artery can be compressed against the first rib; called also *subclavian triangle.*

t. omotrachea'le TA alternative for *t. musculare.*

t. pontocerebella're pontocerebellar triangle: the angular depression between the inferior border of the pons, the interior cerebellar peduncle, and the flocculus of the cerebellum.

t. retromola're [TA] retromolar triangle: a triangular shallow area on the mandible posterior to the third molar, forming the anterior, horizontal portion of the retromolar fossa.

t. sternocosta'le [TA] sternocostal triangle: a triangular opening between the pars costalis and the pars sternalis diaphragmatis; beyond this point the internal thoracic vessels become the superior epigastric vessels. Called also *Larrey cleft.*

t. submandibula're [TA] submandibular triangle: the triangular region of the neck bounded by the mandible, the stylohyoid muscle and posterior belly of the digastric muscle, and the anterior belly of the digastric muscle.

t. submenta'le [TA] submental triangle: a triangle bounded on either side by the anterior belly of the digastric muscle and below by the hyoid bone.

t. urogenita'le urogenital diaphragm.

t. vaga'le TA alternative for *t. nervi vagi.*

t. vesi'cae urina'riae [TA] trigone of urinary bladder: a smooth triangular portion of the mucous membrane in the fundus of the bladder; two of its corners are the ureteral orifices, with the interureteric fold between them, and its third corner is the internal urethral orifice. Called also *bladder trigone, trigone of bladder,* and *Lieutaud* or *vesical triangle.*

tri•hex•o•syl•cer•a•mide (tri-hek″so-səl-ser′ə-mīd) ceramide trihexoside.

tri•hex•y•phen•i•dyl hy•dro•chlo•ride (tri-hek″sĭ-fen′ĭ-dəl) [USP] an antidyskinetic with a direct antispasmodic effect on smooth muscle; believed to act by partially blocking central cholinergic receptors, so that cholinergic and dopaminergic activity in the basal ganglia is more balanced. It is used in the treatment of parkinsonism and for the control of drug-induced extrapyramidal reactions (except tardive dyskinesia), administered orally.

Tri•HIB•it (tri-hib′it) trademark for a preparation that combines diphtheria and tetanus toxoids and acellular pertussis (DTaP) vaccine and *Haemophilus* b conjugate vaccine.

tri•hy•drate (tri-hi′drāt) trihydroxide; a compound containing three hydroxyl groups.

tri•hy•dric (tri-hi′drik) containing three hydrogen atoms that are replaceable by bases.

tri•hy•drol (tri-hi′drol) the associated water or ice molecule, $(H_2O)_3$.

tri•hy•drox•ide (tri″hi-drok′sīd) trihydrate.

tri•hy•droxy (tri″hi-drok′se) a term denoting a compound containing three molecules of the hydroxy (OH) radical; used also as a prefix (trihydroxy-) to denote such a compound.

tri•hy•droxy•es•trin (tri″hi-drok″se-es′trin) estriol.

tri•in•i•od•y•mus (tri″in-e-od′ĭ-məs) [*tri-* + *inio-* + *-didymus*] a fetus with a single body and three heads united posteriorly.

tri•io•dide (tri-i′o-dīd) a compound containing three atoms of iodine to one of another element.

tri•io•do•eth•i•on•ic ac•id (tri-i″o-do-eth″e-on′ik) iophenoxic acid.

tri•io•do•meth•ane (tri-i″o-do-meth′ān) iodoform.

tri•io•do•thy•ro•nine (T_3) (tri-i″o-do-thi′ro-nēn) 3,5,3′-triiodothyronine, an iodine-containing thyroid hormone secreted in smaller amounts than thyroxine; most circulating triiodothyronine is produced by the deiodination of thyroxine in the peripheral tissues, chiefly the liver. It has several times the biological activity of thyroxine and is the "tissue-active" form of thyroid hormone.

free t. the fraction of triiodothyronine in the serum that is not bound to a transport protein.

reverse t. (rT_3) 3,3′,5′-triiodothyronine, a thyroxine derivative that has little if any biologic activity; it is produced in increased amounts in hypothyroidism, hyperthyroidism, and the euthyroid sick syndrome, as well as during febrile illness or carbohydrate deprivation.

total t., total serum t. the total triiodothyronine in the serum, including both the fraction of free triiodothyronine and the fraction bound to a transport protein such as thyroxine-binding globulin or transthyretin.

tri•kates (tri′kāts) [USP] a solution of potassium acetate, potassium bicarbonate, and potassium citrate in purified water; used as a potassium supplement in the treatment and prophylaxis of hypokalemia, administered orally.

tri•ke•to•hy•drin•dene hy•drate (tri-ke″to-hi-drin′dēn) chemical name: 1,2,3-indantrione monohydrate. A compound, $C_9H_4O_3{\cdot}H_2O$, occurring as white to brownish white crystals or crystalline powder, used as a reagent. See under *tests.*

tri•ke•to•pu•rine (tri″ke-to-pu′rēn) uric acid.

tri•labe (tri′lāb) [*tri-* + Gr. *labē* a handle] a three-pronged instrument for taking calculi from the bladder.

Tri•la•fon (tri′lə-fon) trademark for preparations of perphenazine.

tri•lam•i•nar (tri-lam′ĭ-nər) consisting of three layers.

tri•lat•er•al (tri-lat′ər-əl) [*tri-* + *lateral*] having three sides; see *triangle.*

tri•lau•rin (tri-law′rin) the triglyceride formed from lauric acid residues, forming the principal constituent of coconut oil, and found in bayberry oil and palm nut oil.

Tri•lep•tal (tri-lep′təl) trademark for a preparation of oxcarbazepine.

Tri-Lev•len (tri″lev′lən) trademark for therapeutic regimens containing levonorgestrel and ethinyl estradiol.

tri•lin•o•le•in (tri″lin-o′le-in) an unsaturated triglyceride formed from linoleic acid, found in drying oils such as linseed or sunflower oil.

Tri•lip•ix (tri-lip′iks) trademark for a preparation of fenofibric acid.

Tril•i•sate (tril′ĭ-sāt) trademark for a preparation of choline magnesium trisalicylate.

tri•lo•bate (tri-lo′bāt) [*tri-* + *lobate*] having three lobes.

tri•lobed (tri′lōbd) trilobate.

tri•loc•u•lar (tri-lok′u-lər) [*tri-* + *locular*] having three compartments or cells.

tril•o•gy (tril′ə-je) a combination of three elements, such as three concurrent defects or symptoms.

t. of Fallot a term sometimes applied to the combination of pulmonic stenosis, atrial septal defect, and right ventricular hypertrophy.

tri•lo•stane (tri′lo-stān) an adrenocortical suppressant that has been used as an aldosterone antagonist to raise potassium levels in patients with hyperadrenalism or Cushing syndrome.

tri•mag•ne•si•um phos•phate (tri″mag-ne′ze-əm) tribasic magnesium phosphate; see *magnesium phosphate.*

tri•men•su•al (tri-men′su-əl) occurring every three months.

tri•mep•ra•zine tar•trate (tri-mep′rə-zēn) [USP] a phenothiazine derivative having mild central nervous system depressant, moderate antiemetic and anticonvulsant properties, and powerful antihistaminic actions; used as an antipruritic, administered orally.

tri•mer (tri′mər) 1. a compound formed by combination of three identical simpler molecules. 2. a capsomer having three structural units.

tri•mer•cu•ric (tri″mər-ku′rik) containing three atoms of bivalent mercury.

Trim•e•re•su•rus (trim″ə-re-su′rəs) a genus of venomous pit vipers of the family Crotalidae, found in East and Southeast Asia and nearby islands; they are usually green with a prehensile tail. *T. flavovi′ridis* and *T. mucrosqua′matus* are both known as *habu.* See table at *snake.*

tri•mer•ic (tri′mər-ik) exhibiting the characteristics of a trimer.

tri•mes•ter (tri-mes′tər) a period of three months.

tri•meth•a•di•one (tri″meth-ə-di′ōn) an anticonvulsant with analgesic properties, used for the control of petit mal seizures, administered orally. In veterinary medicine, used as an anticonvulsant and analgesic for cats. Called also *troxidone.*

tri•meth•a•phan cam•sy•late (tri-meth′ə-fən) a short-acting ganglionic blocking agent with direct vasodilator action, used as an antihypertensive to produce controlled hypotension during surgery and for the emergency treatment of hypertensive crises and pulmonary edema due to hypertension, administered intravenously.

tri•meth•o•ben•za•mide hy•dro•chlo•ride (tri-meth″o-ben′zə-mīd) [USP] a sedating antihistamine used as an antiemetic, administered orally, intramuscularly, or rectally.

tri•meth•o•prim (tri-meth′o-prim) [USP] an antibacterial closely related to the antimalarial pyrimethamine, acting by inhibiting a step in bacterial folate biosynthesis and effective against various gram-negative and gram-positive bacteria; administered orally in the prophylaxis and treatment of urinary tract infections and the treatment of pneumocystis pneumonia. It is usually administered in combination with a sulfonamide because the two drugs markedly potentiate each other, and in such combination (e.g., co-trimoxazole) has additional uses including treatment of bronchitis, *Shigella* enterocolitis, acute otitis media, and traveler's diarrhea. In certain countries, it is used alone as an antimalarial.

t. sulfate [USP] the sulfate salt of trimethoprim, having the same actions as the base; administered topically to the conjunctiva, in combination with polymyxin B sulfate, in the treatment of ocular bacterial infections caused by susceptible organisms.

tri•meth•y•lene (tri-meth′ə-lēn) cyclopropane.

tri•meth•yl•xan•thine (tri-meth″əl-zan′thin) caffeine.

tri•me•trex•ate (tri″mə-trek′sāt) a folic acid antagonist structurally related to methotrexate; it competitively inhibits dihydrofolate reductase. Used investigationally as an antineoplastic; also used in combination with leucovorin to treat pneumocystis pneumonia in acquired immunodeficiency syndrome, administered intravenously as the glucuronate salt.

tri•mip•ra•mine (tri-mip′rə-mēn) a tricyclic antidepressant of the dibenzazepine class.

t. maleate the maleate salt of trimipramine, used particularly in the treatment of endogenous depression; used also in the treatment of peptic ulcer and of chronic severe pain. Administered orally.

tri•mor•phous (tri-mor′fəs) [*tri-* + *morph-* + *-ous*] existing in three different forms.

Tri•mox (tri′moks) trademark for a preparation of amoxicillin.

Tri-Na•sal (tri-na′zəl) trademark for a preparation of triamcinolone acetonide.

tri•neg•a•tive (tri-neg′ə-tiv) having three negative valences or charges.

tri•ni•trate (tri-ni′trāt) a nitrate containing three radicals of nitric acid.

tri•ni•trin (tri-ni′trin) nitroglycerin.

tri•ni•tro•glyc•er•in (tri-ni″tro-glis′ər-in) nitroglycerin.

tri•ni•tro•glyc•er•ol (tri-ni″tro-glis′ər-ol) nitroglycerin.

tri•ni•tro•phe•nol (tri″ni-tro-fe′nol) a yellow crystalline substance used as a dye and a tissue fixative; its toxic effects are similar to those of dinitrophenol. It can be detonated by percussion or heating above 300°C. Called also *picric acid.*

tri•ni•tro•tol•u•ene (tri″ni-tro-tol′u-ēn) a high explosive obtained by nitrating toluene; called also TNT.

tri•no•mi•al (tri-no′me-əl) [*tri-* + L. *nomen* name] composed of three names or terms.

Tri-Nor•i•nyl (tri-nor′ĭ-nəl) trademark for a therapeutic regimen of norethindrone and ethinyl estradiol.

tri•nu•cle•ate (tri-noo′kle-āt) having three nuclei.

tri•nu•cleo•tide (tri-noo′kle-o-tīd) a polymer made up of three mononucleotides.

trio•ceph•a•lus (tri″o-sef′ə-ləs) [*tri-* + *-cephalus*] a fetus in which the structures of the mouth, nose, and eyes are absent and the head is a shapeless mass.

Trio•don•toph•o•rus (tri″o-don-tof′ə-rəs) a genus of nematodes of the family Strongylidae. *T. tenuicol′lis* is found in ulcers in the colons of horses.

tri•o•ki•nase (tri″o-ki′nās) [EC 2.7.1.28] an enzyme of the transferase class that catalyzes the phosphorylation of glyceraldehyde to form glyceraldehyde 3-phosphate. The reaction occurs in the liver and is part of the series funneling fructose into the Embden-Meyerhof pathway. Called also *triose kinase.*

tri•o•le•in (tri-o′le-in) olein.

tri•op•a•thy (tri-op′əthe) three morbid conditions appearing together, especially as part of a disease process.

diabetic t. the combination of diabetic nephropathy, diabetic neuropathy, and diabetic retinopathy, three conditions commonly found as part of diabetes mellitus.

tri•oph•thal•mos (tri″of-thal′mos) [*tri-* + Gr. *ophthalmos* eye] a double-faced fetus with three eyes.

tri•o•pod•y•mus (tri″o-pod′ĭ-məs) triprosopus.

tri•or•chid (tri-or′kid) [*tri-* + Gr. *orchis* testis] 1. having three testes; see *triorchidism.* 2. an individual with three testes.

tri•or•chi•dism (tri-or′ki-diz-əm) the condition of having three testes; called also *triorchism.*

tri•or•chism (tri-or′kiz-əm) triorchidism.

tri•or•tho•cres•yl phos•phate (tri-or″tho-kres′əl) tri-*o*-tolyl phosphate.

tri•or•tho•tol•yl phos•phate (tri-or″tho-tol′əl) tri-*o*-tolyl phosphate.

tri•ose (tri′ōs) a monosaccharide containing three atoms of carbon in the molecule.

t. phosphate a phosphorylated triose, particularly glyceraldehyde 3-phosphate and dihydroxyacetone phosphate, two important intermediates in glycolysis, alcoholic fermentation, and gluconeogenesis. Called also *phosphotriose.*

tri•ose ki•nase (tri′ōs ki′nās) triokinase.

tri•ose•phos•phate de•hy•dro•gen•ase (tri′ōs fos′fāt de-hi′dro-jən-ās) glyceraldehyde-3-phosphate dehydrogenase.

tri•ose-phos•phate isom•er•ase (tri′ōs fos′fāt i-som′ər-ās) [EC 5.3.1.1] an enzyme of the isomerase class that catalyzes the reversible interconversion of glyceraldehyde 3-phosphate and dihydroxyacetone phosphate in the Embden-Meyerhof pathway (see illustration under *pathway*). Deficiency of the enzyme, an autosomal recessive trait, causes hemolytic anemia, neuromuscular dysfunction, and susceptibility to infection.

Tri•o•stat (tri′o-stat) trademark for a preparation of liothyronine sodium.

tri•otus (tri-o′təs) [*tri-* + Gr. *ous* ear] an individual with a supernumerary external ear.

tri•ox•ide (tri-ok′sīd) a compound containing three atoms of oxygen to one of another element.

tri•ox•sa•len (tri-ok′sə-lən) [USP] a synthetic psoralen used orally in conjunction with exposure to ultraviolet radiation to facilitate repigmentation and increase tolerance to sunlight in vitiligo.

tri•oxy•pu•rine (tri″ok-se-pu′rēn) uric acid.

tri•pal•mi•tin (tri-pal′mĭ-tin) palmitin.

trip•a•ra (trip′ə-rə) [*tri-* + *para*] tertipara.

tri•par•tite (tri-pahr′tīt) having three parts.

Tri•pe•dia (tri-pe′de-ə) trademark for a preparation of diphtheria and tetanus toxoids and acellular pertussis vaccine.

tri·pe·len·na·mine (tri″pə-len′ə-min) an ethylenediamine derivative with antihistaminic (H_1 receptor antagonist), anticholinergic, and sedative effects.

t. citrate the citrate salt of tripelennamine, used as an antihistamine in the symptomatic treatment of allergic disorders, administered orally.

t. hydrochloride [USP] the monohydrochloride salt of tripelennamine, having the same actions and uses as the citrate salt; administered orally.

tri·pep·tide (tri-pep′tid) a peptide which on hydrolysis yields three amino acids.

tri·pep·ti·dyl-pep·ti·dase (tri-pep″tĭ-dəl-pep′tĭ-dās) [EC 3.4.14] any member of a sub-subclass of enzymes of the hydrolase class that catalyze the cleavage of a tripeptide residue from a free N-terminal end of a peptide or polypeptide.

tri·pha·lan·gia (tri″fə-lan′jə) triphalangism.

tri·phal·an·gism (tri-fal′ən-jiz-əm) the presence of three phalanges in the longitudinal axis of a digit normally composed of only two. **triphalan′geal** *adj*

tri·pha·sic (tri-fa′zik) [*tri-* + Gr. *phasis* phase] triply varied or triply phasic; used in describing the electromotive actions of muscles. Cf. *diphasic* and *monophasic.*

Tri·pha·sil (tri-fa′zil) trademark for therapeutic regimens containing levonorgestrel and ethinyl estradiol.

tri·phen·yl·meth·ane (tri-fen″əl-meth′ān) a substance obtained from coal tar, the basis of various dyes and stains, including aurin, rosaniline, basic fuchsin, and gentian violet.

tri·phos·phate (tri-fos′fāt) a salt containing three phosphate radicals.

tri·phos·pho·pyr·i·dine nu·cle·o·tide (tri-fos″fo-pir′ĭ-dēn noo′kle-o-tid″) former name for *nicotinamide adenine dinucleotide phosphate (NADP).* Abbreviated TPN.

Tri·pier amputation (tre″pya′) [Léon *Tripier,* French surgeon, 1842–1891] see under *amputation.*

trip·le-an·gle (trip′əl-ang″gəl) having three angles; a dental instrument having three angulations in the shank connecting the handle, or shaft, with the working portion of the instrument, known as the blade, or nib. Cf. *binangle, monangle,* and *quadrangle* (def. 2).

trip·le blind (trip′əl blīnd) pertaining to a clinical trial or other experiment in which neither the subject nor the person administering treatment nor the person evaluating the response to treatment knows which treatment any particular subject is receiving.The term *triple masked* is sometimes preferred to avoid confusion associated with the use of the term "blind."

tri·ple·gia (tri-ple′jə) [*tri-* + *-plegia*] paralysis of three limbs.

trip·le masked (trip′əl maskt) triple blind.

trip·let (trip′lət) 1. one of three individuals having coextensive gestation periods and produced at the same birth. 2. a combination of three objects or entities occurring or acting together, as three lenses constituting a microscope eyepiece or objective. 3. codon. 4. triple discharge.

tri·plex (tri′pleks, trip′leks) [Gr. *triploos* triple] triple or three-fold.

trip·lo·blas·tic (trip″lo-blas′tik) [Gr. *triploos* triple + *blast-* + *-ic*] having three germ layers or blastodermic membranes; said of an embryo.

trip·loid (trip′loid) 1. pertaining to or characterized by triploidy. 2. an individual or cell having three sets of chromosomes.

trip·loi·dy (trip′loi-de) the presence in humans of 69 chromosomes, or three full sets.

trip·lo·ko·ria (trip″lo-kor′e-ə) [Gr. *triploos* triple + *cor-* + *-ia*] the presence of three pupils in one eye.

trip·lo·pia (trip-lo′pe-ə) [Gr. *triploos* triple + *-opia*] the perception of three images of a single object; triple vision.

tri·pod (tri′pod) [*tri-* + Gr. *pous* foot] anything having three feet or supports.

Haller t. truncus coeliacus.

tri·po·dia (tri-po′de-ə) [*tri-* + *pod-* + *-ia*] tripodial symmelia.

tri·po·di·al (tri-po′de-əl) having three feet; see *symmelia.*

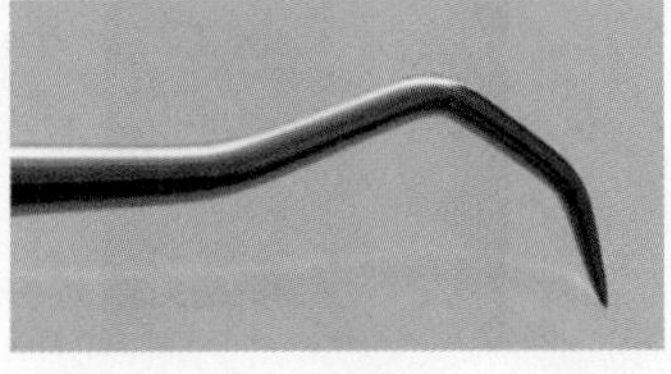

■ Triple-angle.

tri·pod·ing (tri′pod-ing) the use of three points of support, as adopted by paralyzed patients when changing from a sitting or standing position. See also *tripod position,* under *position.*

trip·o·li (trip′o-le) [*Tripoli,* Libya] a granulated porous siliceous rock originally mined in North Africa and presently produced from silica; used as a dental polishing agent.

tri·pos·i·tive (tri-pos′ĭ-tiv) having three positive valences or charges.

tri·pro·li·dine hy·dro·chlo·ride (tri-pro′lĭ-dēn) [USP] an antihistamine (H_1 receptor antagonist) with sedative and anticholinergic effects; used in the treatment of allergic rhinitis, allergic conjunctivitis, and cutaneous manifestations of allergic reactions, and particularly used as an ingredient in cough and cold preparations, administered orally.

tri·pro·so·pus (tri″pro-so′pəs) [*tri-* + Gr. *prosōpon* face] a fetus having a triple face.

trip·tans (trip′təns) a group of serotonin receptor agonists used in treatment of migraines.

-tripsy [Gr. *tripsis* a rubbing, friction] a word termination designating a surgical procedure in which a structure is intentionally crushed.

trip·to·ko·ria (trip″to-kor′e-ə) triplokoria.

trip·to·rel·in pam·o·ate (trip″tə-rel′in) a synthetic analogue of gonadorelin that on prolonged administration suppresses gonadotropin release, used as an antineoplastic in the palliative treatment of prostatic carcinoma and also used in the treatment of precocious puberty and endometriosis; administered intramuscularly.

tri·pus (tri′pəs) [*tri-* + *pous* foot] 1. tripod. 2. conjoined twins with tripodial symmelia.

tri·que·trous (tri-kwe′trəs) [L. *triquetrus*] triangular; three cornered.

tri·que·trum (tri-kwe′trəm) [L.] three cornered; see *os triquetrum.*

tri·ra·di·al (tri-ra′de-əl) triradiate.

tri·ra·di·ate (tri-ra′de-āt) [*tri-* + L. *radiatus* rayed] having three rays; radiating in three directions; called also *triradial.*

tri·ra·di·a·tion (tri″ra-de-a′shən) radiation in three directions.

TRIS tris(hydroxymethyl)aminomethane; see *tromethamine.*

tris (tris) 1. tris(hydroxymethyl)aminomethane; see *tromethamine.* 2. tris(2,3-dibromopropyl) phosphate.

tri·sac·cha·ride (tri-sak′ə-rīd) any of a class of carbohydrates composed of three glycosidically linked monosaccharide groups.

tri·sal·i·cyl·ate (tri″sal-ĭ-sil′āt, tri″sə-lis′ə-lāt) a compound containing three salicylate ions.

choline magnesium t. a combination of choline salicylate and magnesium salicylate, used as an analgesic, antipyretic, antiinflammatory, and antirheumatic; administered orally.

tris·(2,3-di·bro·mo·pro·pyl) phos·phate (tris″di-bro″mo-pro′pəl fos′fāt) a yellow liquid flame retardant, formerly used in children's clothing but now restricted in use because it is carcinogenic. Called also *tris.*

tri·seg·men·tec·to·my (tri″seg-men-tek′tə-me) resection of the liver in which three segments are removed.

left t. trisegmentectomy in which the left lobe and anterior segment of the right lobe are removed.

right t. trisegmentectomy in which the right lobe and medial segment of the left lobe are removed.

Tri·se·nox (tri′sə-noks) trademark for a preparation of arsenic trioxide.

Tri·se·tum (tri-se′tum) a genus of grasses found in pastures. *T. flaves′cens* is yellow or golden oat grass, a European variety that causes enzootic calcinosis in ruminants.

tris·(hy·droxy·meth·yl)·am·i·no·meth·ane (TRIS, THAM) (tris″hi-drok″se-meth″əl-ə-me″no-meth′ān) tromethamine.

tris·mic (triz′mik) of the nature of or pertaining to trismus.

tris·mus (triz′məs) [Gr. *trismos* grating, grinding] motor disturbance of the trigeminal nerve, especially spasm of the masticatory muscles, with difficulty in opening the mouth; a characteristic early symptom of tetanus. Called also *lockjaw.*

tri·so·di·um phos·pho·no·for·mate (tri-so′de-əm fos″fon-o-for′māt) foscarnet sodium.

tri·so·mia (tri-so′me-ə) trisomy.

tri·so·my (tri′so-me) [*tri* + Gr. *sōma* body] the presence of an extra chromosome of one type in an otherwise diploid cell (2n +1). See specific trisomy syndromes under *syndrome.* **triso′mic** *adj*

Tri·sor·a·len (tri-sor′ə-lən) trademark for a preparation of trioxsalen.

tri·splanch·nic (tri-splangk′nik) [*tri-* + *splanchnic*] pertaining to or supplying the three great body cavities and their viscera.

tri•ste•a•rin (tri-ste′ə-rin) the saturated triglyceride formed from stearic acid; it occurs mainly in harder fats such as tallow and cacao butter and can be prepared by hydrogenation of oils. Called also *stearin.*

tri•stich•ia (tri-stik′e-ə) [Gr. *treis* three + *stichos* row] the existence of three rows of eyelashes.

tri•sub•sti•tut•ed (tri-sub′stĭ-to͞ot″əd) having three molecules or atoms replaced by three other molecules or atoms.

tri•sul•cate (tri-sul′kāt) having three furrows.

tri•sul•fa•py•rim•i•dines (tri-sul″fə-pĭ-rim′ĭ-dēnz) [USP] preparations containing a mixture of the sulfonamides sulfadiazine, sulfamerazine, and sulfamethazine.

tri•sul•fate (tri-sul′fāt) a binary compound containing three sulfate (SO_4) groups in the molecule.

tri•sul•fide (tri-sul′fīd) a sulfur compound containing three atoms of sulfur to one of the base.

Trit. [L.] tri′tura (triturate).

tri•tan (tri′tən) 1. pertaining to tritanomaly or tritanopia. 2. a person with tritanomaly or tritanopia.

tri•ta•nom•al (tri″tə-nom′əl) a person with tritanomaly.

tri•ta•nom•a•ly (tri″tə-nom′ə-le) [Gr. *tritos* third + *anomaly*] a very rare anomalous trichromasy in which the third, blue-sensitive, cones have decreased sensitivity; therefore a greater than normal proportion of blue light to green light is required to match a blue-green stimulus. Tritanomaly is an X-linked trait and occurs in about 0.0001 per cent of white males; it is therefore of little clinical importance. **tritanom′alous** *adj*

tri•ta•nope (tri′tə-nōp″) an individual exhibiting tritanopia.

tri•ta•no•pia (tri″tə-no′pe-ə) [Gr. *tritos* third + *an-*[1] + *-opia*] a rare type of dichromatic vision characterized by retention of the sensory mechanism for two hues only (red and green) of the normal 4-primary quota, and lacking blue and yellow, with loss of luminance and shift of brightness and hue curves toward the long-wave end of the spectrum. Often associated with drug administration, retinal detachment, or diseases of the nervous system. **tritanop′ic** *adj*

tri•ta•nop•sia (tri″tə-nop′se-ə) tritanopia.

tri•ter•pene (tri-tur′pēn) any of a class of compounds biosynthesized from or comprising six isoprene, and thus three terpene, units; most are tetra- or pentacyclic steroids.

tri•ti•ceous (tri-tish′əs) [L. *triticeus*] resembling a grain of wheat.

tri•tic•e•um (tri-tis′e-əm) [L.] cartilago triticea.

Trit•i•ra•chi•um (trit″ĭ-ra′ke-əm) a genus of Fungi Imperfecti of the form-class Hyphomycetes. *T. ory′zae* has been isolated from human infections such as corneal ulcers.

trit•i•um (^{3}H) (trit′e-əm) [Gr. *tritos* third] the mass three isotope of hydrogen, a radioactive gas with a half-life of 12.33 years and emitting beta particles (0.0186 MeV); it has been used as a tracer in metabolic studies. Cf. *deuterium* and *protium.*

tri•tol•yl phos•phate (tri-tol′əl) a mixture of isomers prepared from creosote and other organic compounds; used as a flame retardant, in the manufacture of vinyl plastics, and for other industrial purposes. One of the isomers, tri-*o*-tolyl phosphate, is highly toxic. Called also *tricresyl phosphate.*

tri-o-tol•yl phos•phate (tri-tol′əl) the highly toxic ortho isomer of tritolyl phosphate; when ingested, it can cause paralysis. See *Jamaica ginger paralysis,* under *paralysis.* Called also *triorthotolyl phosphate, tri-o-cresyl phosphate* and *triorthocresyl phosphate.*

Tri•tricho•mo•nas (tri″trik-o-mo′nas) [*tri-* + *tricho-* + Gr. *monas* unit, from *monos* single] a genus of protozoa of the order Trichomonadida, phylum Parabasalia, including species formerly in *Trichomonas* that have three anterior flagella.

T. foe′tus a species found in the genital tract of cattle, the cause of the venereal disease bovine trichomoniasis, transmitted from bulls to cows by coitus or by artificial insemination. Formerly called *Trichomonas foetus.*

trit•ur•ate (trich′ər-āt) 1. to rub to a powder. 2. to create a homogeneous whole by mixing; see trituration (def. 3). 3. a triturated substance.

trit•ur•a•tion (trich″ər-a′shən) [L. *tritura* the treading out of corn] 1. the reduction of solid bodies to a powder by continuous rubbing. 2. a triturated drug, especially one rubbed up with lactose. 3. the creation of a homogeneous whole by mixing, as the combining of particles of an alloy with mercury to form dental amalgam; called also *amalgamation.*

trit•ur•a•tor (trich′ūr-a″tər) an apparatus in which substances can be continuously rubbed, as in the process of amalgamating an alloy with mercury. Called also *amalgamator.*

tri•va•lence (tri-va′ləns) the condition or quality of being trivalent.

tri•va•lent (tri-va′lənt) 1. having a valence of three. 2. effective against three different entities, as diseases or strains of a pathogen.

tri•valve (tri′valv) having three valves or three blades, as a speculum.

Tri•vo•ra (tri-vor′ə) trademark for a therapeutic regimen containing levonorgestrel and ethinyl estradiol.

Tri•zi•vir (tri′zĭ-vir) trademark for a combination preparation of abacavir sulfate, zidovudine, and lamivudine.

tri•zo•nal (tri-zo′nəl) arranged in three zones.

tRNA transfer RNA.

Tro•bi•cin (tro-bi′sin) trademark for a preparation of spectinomycin hydrochloride.

tro•car (tro′kahr) [Fr. *trois quarts* three quarters] a sharp-pointed instrument equipped with a cannula, used to puncture the wall of a body cavity and withdraw fluid.

troch. [L.] trochiscus (troche).

tro•chan•ter (tro-kan′tər) [L., from Gr. *trochantēr*] either of the two processes below the neck of the femur. **trochanter′ian, trochanter′ic** *adj*

greater t. t. major.

lesser t. t. minor.

t. ma′jor [TA] greater trochanter: a broad, flat process at the upper end of the lateral surface of the femur, to which several muscles are attached.

t. mi′nor [TA] lesser trochanter: a short conical process projecting medially from the lower part of the posterior border of the base of the neck of the femur.

rudimentary t. t. tertius.

small t. t. minor.

t. ter′tius [TA] third trochanter: a term applied to the gluteal tuberosity of the femur when it is unusually prominent.

tro•chan•ter•plas•ty (tro-kan′tər-plas″te) surgical excision of a ridge of bone to form a new femoral neck.

tro•chan•tin (tro-kan′tin) trochanter minor.

tro•chan•tin•i•an (tro″kən-tin′e-ən) pertaining to the lesser trochanter.

tro•che (tro′ke) [Gr. *trochos* a round cake or pill] lozenge (def. 1).

troch•lea (trok′le-ə) pl. *troch′leae* [L., from Gr. *trochilia* pulley] a pulley-shaped part or structure.

t. fibula′ris calca′nei [TA] fibular trochlea of calcaneus: a small eminence on the lateral surface of the calcaneus, separating the tendons of the peroneus brevis and longus muscles; called also *t. peronealis calcanei* [TA alternative].

t. hu′meri [TA], **t. of humerus** the pulleylike medial portion of the distal end of the humerus for articulation with the semilunar notch of the ulna.

t. muscula′ris [TA] muscular trochlea: an anatomical part that serves to change the direction of pull of a tendon; it may be fibrous or bony.

t. mus′culi obli′qui superio′ris bul′bi [TA], **t. mus′culi obli′qui superio′ris o′culi** trochlea of superior oblique muscle: the fibrocartilaginous pulley near the internal angular process of the frontal bone, through which the tendon of the superior oblique muscle of the eyeball passes.

peroneal t. of calcaneus t. fibularis calcanei.

t. peronea′lis calca′nei TA alternative for *t. fibularis calcanei.*

t. phalan′gis ma′nus [TA] trochlea of phalanx of hand: the pulleylike concavity of the head of a proximal or middle phalanx, to which the base of the articulating phalanx is adapted.

t. phalan′gis pe′dis [TA] trochlea of phalanx of foot: the pulleylike concavity of the head of a proximal or middle phalanx (except in the big toe, which has only two phalanges), to which the base of the articulating phalanx is adapted.

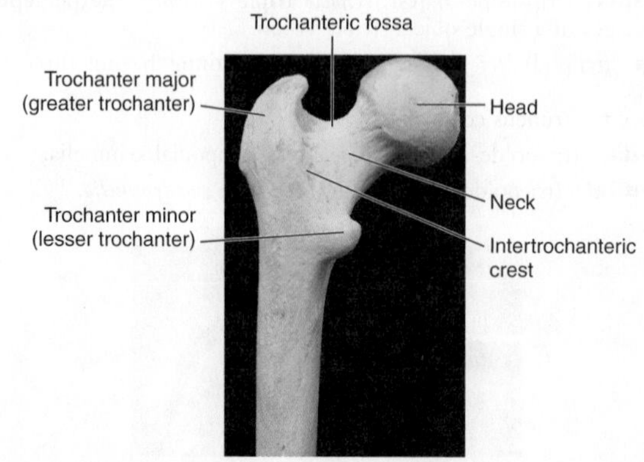

■ Posterior aspect of left femur, showing the greater and lesser trochanters.

t. of superior oblique muscle t. musculi obliqui superioris bulbi.

t. ta'li [TA] trochlea of talus: the rounded part of the talus that articulates with the tibia and fibula.

troch·le·ar (trok'le-ər) [L. *trochlearis*] 1. of the nature of or resembling a pulley. 2. pertaining to a trochlea.

troch·le·ar·i·form (trok″le-ar'ĭ-form) pulley-shaped.

troch·le·a·ris (trok″le-ar'is) [L.] trochlear.

troch·le·i·tis (trok″le-i'tis) inflammation of the trochlear nerve.

tro·cho·ce·pha·lia (tro″ko-sə-fa'le-ə) trochocephaly.

tro·cho·ceph·a·ly (tro″ko-sef'ə-le) [Gr. *trochos* wheel + *-cephaly*] a rounded appearance of the head caused by synostosis of the frontal and parietal bones.

tro·choid (tro'koid) [Gr. *trochos* wheel + *-oid*] resembling a pivot or a pulley.

tro·choi·des (tro-koi'dēz) articulatio trochoidea.

tro·gli·ta·zone (tro″glĭ-ta'zōn) an antihyperglycemic that lowers insulin resistance, formerly used in the treatment of type 2 diabetes mellitus; withdrawn because of hepatotoxicity.

Trog·lo·stron·gy·lus (trog″lo-stron'jə-ləs) a genus of nematodes of the family Crenosomatidae. Some species infect the respiratory tract or lungs of cats.

Trog·lo·tre·ma (trog″lo-tre'mə) *Nanophyetus.*

Trog·lo·tre·ma·ti·dae (trog″lo-tre-mat'ĭ-de) a family of trematodes that includes the genera *Nanophyetus* and *Paragonimus.*

Troi·sier node (ganglion, sign), syndrome (trwah-sya') [Charles Emile *Troisier*, French physician, 1844–1919] see under *syndrome* and see *signal node*, under *node.*

tro·la·mine (tro'lə-mēn) 1. [NF] a pharmaceutical preparation of triethanolamine with small amounts of other ethanolamines; used as an alkalizer in pharmaceutical preparations. 2. USAN contraction for triethanolamine.

t. salicylate [USP] a mixture of trolamine and salicylic acid in propylene glycol having analgesic and anesthetic properties and also absorbing ultraviolet A; used topically as an analgesic and as a sunscreen.

tro·land (tro'lənd) [for Leonard Thompson *Troland*, American psychologist and physicist, 1889–1932] the retinal illuminance produced by the image of an object the luminance of which is 1 lumen per square meter for an area of the entrance pupil of 1 square millimeter.

Tro·lard plexus, vein (tro-lahr') [Paulin *Trolard*, French anatomist, 1842–1910] see *plexus venosus canalis nervi hypoglossi* and *vena anastomotica inferior.*

tro·le·an·do·my·cin (tro″le-an-do-mi'sin) [USP] a macrolide antibiotic, the synthetically prepared triacetyl ester of oleandomycin, to which it is converted in the body, used in the treatment of pneumococcal pneumonia and Group A β-hemolytic streptococcal infections resistant to other systemic antibiotics; administered orally.

trol·ni·trate phos·phate (trol-ni'trāt) an organic nitrate having vasodilating actions, which has been used to reduce the frequency and severity of anginal attacks.

Tröltsch corpuscles, recesses (spaces) (trurlch) [Anton Friedrich von *Tröltsch*, German otologist, 1829–1890] see under *corpuscle*, and see *recessus membranae tympani anterior* and *recessus membranae tympani posterior.*

Trom·bic·u·la (trom-bik'u-lə) a genus of mites of the family Trombiculidae; it is further divided into the subgenera *Eutrombicula* and *Leptotrombidium.* Their larvae, called *chiggers*, cause an irritating dermatitis in many vertebrates; some species spread scrub typhus.

T. akamu'shi the kedani mite, whose larvae (chiggers) transmit *Orientia tsutsugamushi* and are the chief vector for scrub typhus in Japan. Called also *Microtrombidium akamushi.*

T. alfreddugè'si *Eutrombicula alfreddugèsi.*

T. autumna'lis *Neotrombicula autumnalis.*

T. delien'sis a species whose larvae (chiggers) transmit *Orientia tsutsugamushi* and are the chief vector for scrub typhus outside of Japan.

T. flet'cheri a species whose larvae (chiggers) transmit *Orientia tsutsugamushi*, and are vectors for scrub typhus.

T. holoseri'ceum *Neotrombicula autumnalis.*

T. interme'dia a species whose larvae (chiggers) transmit *Orientia tsutsugamushi*, and are vectors for scrub typhus.

T. ir'ritans *Eutrombicula alfreddugèsi.*

T. mus'cae domes'ticae a red acarid parasite on the housefly.

T. musca'rum *T. muscae domesticae.*

T. pal'lida a species whose larvae (chiggers) transmit *Orientia tsutsugamushi*, and are vectors for scrub typhus.

T. scutella'ris a species whose larvae (chiggers) transmit *Orientia tsutsugamushi*, and are vectors for scrub typhus.

T. splen'dens *Eutrombicula splendens.*

T. tsalsahua'tl *Eutrombicula alfreddugèsi.*

trom·bic·u·li·a·sis (trom-bik″u-li'ə-sis) infestation with mites of the family Trombiculidae, usually in the form of dermatitis when the larval forms attach to the skin of a mammal or bird. Called also *trombidiosis.*

trom·bic·u·lid (trom-bik'u-lid) a mite of the family Trombiculidae; called also *chigger mite.*

Trom·bic·u·li·dae (trom-bik'u-lĭ″de) a family of mites found in many parts of the world; their larvae are parasitic on vertebrates. Genera of medical significance include *Trombicula* and *Neotrombicula.*

trom·bic·u·li·di·a·sis (trom-bik″u-lĭ-di'ə-sis) trombiculiasis.

trom·bid·i·o·sis (trom-bid″e-o'sis) trombiculiasis.

Trom·bid·i·um (trom-bid'e-əm) a name formerly given a genus of mites, now included in the genus *Trombicula.*

tro·meth·amine (tro-meth'ə-mēn) 1. an organic amine proton acceptor, used to make buffer solutions (see *TRIS buffer*, under *buffer*). 2. [USP] an aqueous preparation of tromethamine used intravenously as an alkalizer for the correction of metabolic acidosis. Called also *tris(hydroxymethyl)aminomethane* (*TRIS* or *THAM*).

tromo·pho·nia (trom″o-fo'ne-ə) a type of dysphonia characterized by a tremulous voice.

Tron·o·thane (tron'o-thān) trademark for preparations of pramoxine hydrochloride.

tro·pate (tro'pāt) a salt of tropic acid.

troph·ec·to·derm (trof-ek'to-dərm) [*tropho-* + *ectoderm*] the outer layer of cells of the early blastocyst; the earliest trophoblast.

troph·ede·ma (trof″ə-de'mə) [*tropho-* + *edema*] permanent edema of the lower limbs or feet.

Tro·phe·ry·ma (tro-fer'ĭ-mə) [*troph-* + Gr. *eryma* barrier] a genus of gram-positive, soil-dwelling bacteria of the family Cellulomonadaceae, consisting of aerobic, nonmotile, short, filamentous rods. *T. whip'plei*, the type species, is the cause of Whipple disease.

tro·phic (tro'fik) [Gr. *trophikos*] nutritional.

-trophic [Gr. *trophikos* nourishing] a word termination denoting relationship to nutrition.

tro·phic·i·ty (tro-fis'ĭ-te) a trophic function or relation.

-trophin see *-tropin.*

troph·ism (trof'iz-əm) direct trophic influence.

troph(o)- [Gr. *trophē* nutrition] a combining form denoting relationship to food or nourishment.

tro·pho·blast (tro'fo-blast) [*tropho-* + *-blast*] a layer of extraembryonic ectodermal tissue on the outside of the blastocyst. It attaches the blastocyst to the endometrium of the uterine wall and supplies nutrition to the embryo. From it are derived the chorion and amnion. The inner cellular layer of the trophoblast covering a chorionic villus is called *cytotrophoblast* and its outer syncytial layer *syncytiotrophoblast.* The mesoblast, once thought to be trophoblastic, is now traced in primates to the caudal end of the primitive streak. **trophoblas'tic** *adj*

tro·pho·cyte (tro'fo-sīt) a cell that furnishes nutrition to other cells, as a Sertoli cell; called also *trephocyte.*

tro·pho·derm (tro'fo-dərm) [*tropho-* + *-derm*] trophoblast.

tro·pho·der·ma·to·neu·ro·sis (tro″fo-der″mə-to-noŏ-ro'sis) acrodynia.

tro·pho·dy·nam·ics (tro″fo-di-nam'iks) the study of the forces engaged in nutrition.

tro·pho·ede·ma (tro″fo-ə-de'mə) trophedema.

tro·phol·o·gy (tro-fol'ə-je) nutriology.

tro·pho·neu·ro·sis (tro″fo-noŏ-ro'sis) any functional disease due to the failure of nutrition in part because of defective nerve supply. **trophoneurot'ic** *adj*

facial t. facial hemiatrophy.

lingual t. progressive lingual hemiatrophy.

t. of Romberg facial hemiatrophy.

tro·pho·no·sis (tro″fo-no'sis) [*tropho-* + *nos-* + *-sis*] any disease or disorder due to nutritional causes.

tro·phont (tro'font) [*troph-* + Gr. *on, ontos* being] the active, motile, feeding stage or form in the life cycle of certain ciliate protozoa, especially that produced by a tomite and developing into a theront. Cf. *trophozoite.*

tro·pho·nu·cle·us (tro″fo-noo'kle-əs) macronucleus.

tro·pho·path·ia (tro″fo-path'e-ə) trophopathy.

tro·phop·a·thy (tro-fop'ə-the) [*tropho-* + *-pathy*] any derangement of nutrition.

tro·pho·tax·is (tro″fo-tak'sis) [*tropho-* + *taxis*] chemotaxis of an organism in response to nutritive material.

tro·pho·ther·a·py (tro″fo-ther′ə-pe) diet therapy.

tro·pho·tro·pism (tro″fo-tro′piz-əm) [*tropho-* + *tropism*] chemotropism of an organism in response to nutritive material.

tro·pho·zo·ite (tro″fo-zo′īt) [*tropho-* + Gr. *zōon* animal] the active, motile, feeding stage of protozoa, as contrasted with the nonmotile encysted stage. In the malarial parasite, this is the stage between the merozoite and the mature schizont. Trophozoites of *Toxoplasma gondii* (tachyzoites) are found in the tissues during the acute stage of toxoplasmosis. Cf. *trophont.*

-trophy [Gr. *trophē* nutrition] a word termination denoting food or nutrition.

tro·pia (tro′pe-ə) [Gr. *tropē* a turning] a manifest deviation of an eye from the normal position when both eyes are open and uncovered; strabismus, or squint. See *cyclotropia, esotropia, exotropia, hypertropia,* and *hypotropia.*

-tropic [Gr. *tropikos* turning] a word termination denoting turning toward, changing, or tending to turn or change; see *tropism.*

tro·pic ac·id (tro′pik) 2-phenyl-3-hydroxypropanoic acid, a degradation product of atropine and scopolamine.

tro·pic·a·mide (tro-pik′ə-mīd) [USP] an anticholinergic applied topically to the conjunctiva to produce mydriasis and cycloplegia.

-tropin [Gr. *tropos* a turning] a word termination denoting an affinity for the structure or thing indicated by the stem to which it is affixed, as gonadotropin. Also, *-trophin.*

tro·pism (tro′piz-əm) [Gr. *tropē* a turn, turning] the turning, bending, movement, or growth of an organism or part of an organism in response to an external stimulus. Such response may be either positive (toward) or negative (away from) the stimulus. Cf. *taxis* (def. 1).

-tropism a word termination affixed to a stem denoting the nature of the stimulus (phototropism) or the material or entity for which an organism or substance shows a special affinity (neurotropism), usually applied to nonmotile organisms.

trop(o)- [Gr. *tropos* a turn, turning] a combining form denoting a turn, reaction, or change.

tro·po·chrome (tro′po-krōm″) [*tropo-* + *-chrome*] refusing to stain with mucin stains after formol-bichromate fixation, as applied to certain serous cells of the salivary glands. Cf. *homeochrome.*

tro·po·col·la·gen (tro″po-kol′ə-jən) [*tropo-* + *collagen*] the basic structural unit of collagen; a helical structure consisting of three polypeptide chains, each chain composed of about a thousand amino acids, coiled around each other to form a spiral and stabilized by inter- and intrachain covalent bonds. It is rich in glycine, which occurs nearly one residue out of three, as well as in proline, hydroxyproline, and hydroxylysine; the last two rarely occur in other proteins.

tro·po·elas·tin (tro″po-e-las′tin) the precursor of elastin.

tro·pom·e·ter (tro-pom′ə-tər) [*tropo-* + *-meter*] an instrument for measuring the twist or torsion of a long bone.

tropo·mod·u·lin (tro″po-mod′u-lin) an actin-binding protein that caps the minus ends of actin filaments, protecting them from depolymerizing.

tro·po·my·o·sin (tro″po-mi′o-sin) muscle protein of the I band, occurring in several tissue-specific isoforms, that inhibits contraction unless its position is modified by troponin so that the myosin molecules can make contact with the actin molecules. See Plate 32.

tro·po·nin (tro′po-nin) a complex of globular muscle proteins of the I band that inhibits contraction by blocking the interaction of actin and myosin; when combined with Ca^{2+}, it so modifies the position of the tropomyosin molecules that contraction takes place. See Plate 32.

-tropy [Gr. *tropos* a turn, turning] a word termination denoting a turn, turning, or change in response to a stimulus.

trough (trof) a shallow longitudinal depression or channel.

synaptic t. an invagination of the membrane of a striated muscle fiber, surrounding a motor end plate at a neuromuscular junction. Called also *synaptic cleft* and *primary synaptic cleft.*

Trous·seau phenomenon, sign, syndrome, twitching (troo-so′) [Armand *Trousseau*, French physician, 1801–1867] see under *phenomenon, sign, syndrome,* and *twitching.*

tro·va·flox·a·cin mes·y·late (tro″və-flok′sə-sin) a fluoronaphthyridone antibacterial, effective against a broad spectrum of gram-positive and gram-negative organisms, used in the treatment of serious infections caused by susceptible organisms; administered orally.

Tro·van (tro′van) trademark for preparations of trovafloxacin mesylate or its prodrug alatrofloxacin mesylate.

trox·i·done (trok′sĭ-dōn) trimethadione.

troy (troi) a system of weights commonly used in England and the United States for expressing quantities of gold and silver; for equivalents see Appendix 7.

Trp tryptophan.

TRU turbidity reducing unit.

trun·cal (trung′kəl) pertaining to the trunk.

trun·cate (trung′kāt) [L. *truncatus*] having the end cut squarely off.

trun·cus (trung′kəs) pl. *trun′ci* [L. "trunk"] trunk: 1. [TA] the main part of the body, to which the head and limbs are attached; called also *torso.* 2. anatomical nomenclature for a major, undivided, usually short portion of a nerve, blood vessel, lymphatic vessel, or duct.

t. arterio′sus an arterial trunk, especially the artery connected with the embryonic heart, which gives off the arteries of the pharyngeal arches and develops into the aortic and pulmonary arteries.

t. brachiocepha′licus [TA] brachiocephalic trunk: the first branch of the arch of the aorta, which behind the right sternoclavicular joint divides into the right common carotid and right subclavian arteries, with distribution to the right side of the head and neck and to the right upper limb; the lowest thyroid artery may arise from this trunk. Called also *brachiocephalic artery* and *innominate artery.*

t. bronchomediastina′lis [TA] bronchomediastinal trunk: either of the two lymphatic trunks (right and left) that drain the pulmonary, bronchopulmonary, tracheobronchial, tracheal, and parasternal lymph nodes: that on the right side into the right lymphatic duct or subclavian vein, and that on the left into the thoracic duct or the subclavian vein.

t. coeli′acus [TA] celiac trunk: the arterial trunk that arises from the abdominal aorta, gives off the left gastric, common hepatic, and splenic arteries, and supplies the esophagus, stomach, duodenum, spleen, pancreas, liver, and gallbladder.

t. cor′poris callo′si [TA] trunk of corpus callosum: the main central portion of the corpus callosum as distinguished from the rostrum and the splenium.

t. costocervica′lis [TA] costocervical trunk: an artery that arises from the back of the subclavian artery, arches backward, and at the neck of the first rib divides into the deep cervical and highest intercostal arteries, thus supplying blood to the structures of the first two intercostal spaces, the vertebral column, the muscles of the back, and the deep neck muscles.

t. ence′phali [TA], **t. encepha′licus** encephalic trunk: the stemlike portion of the brain connecting the cerebral hemispheres with the spinal cord and comprising the pons, medulla oblongata, and mesencephalon; the diencephalon is considered part of the truncus encephalicus by some. Called also *brainstem.*

t. fasci′culi atrioventricula′ris trunk of atrioventricular bundle: the undivided portion of the atrioventricular bundle, from its origin at the atrioventricular node to the point of division into the right and left bundle branches at the superior end of the muscular part of the interventricular septum. It contains the penetrating portion of the bundle, a short segment of multiple small fascicles that penetrate the fibrous tissue of the atrioventricular septum.

t. infe′rior plex′us brachia′lis [TA] inferior trunk of brachial plexus: the trunk of the brachial plexus that is formed by the anterior branches of the eighth cervical and first thoracic nerves; medial pectoral nerves may arise from it. Its anterior division becomes the medial cord of the plexus, and its posterior division helps form the posterior cord; *modality,* general sensory and motor. Called also *lower trunk of brachial plexus.*

trun′ci intestina′les [TA] intestinal trunks: short lymphatic trunks that leave the gastrointestinal tract and participate in formation of the thoracic duct.

t. jugula′ris [TA] jugular trunk: either of the two lymphatic trunks (right and left) that drain the deep cervical lymph nodes; on the right side they drain into the right lymphatic duct or subclavian vein, and on the left side into the thoracic duct or subclavian vein.

t. linguofacia′lis [TA] linguofacial trunk: the common trunk by which the facial and lingual arteries often arise from the external carotid artery.

t. lumba′lis [TA], **t. lumba′ris** lumbar trunk: either of the two lymphatic trunks (right and left) that drain lymph upward from the lumbar lymph nodes and help form the thoracic duct.

t. lumbosacra′lis [TA] lumbosacral trunk: a trunk formed by union of the lower division of the anterior branch of the fourth lumbar nerve with the anterior branch of the fifth lumbar nerve; it descends to the sacral plexus.

trun′ci lympha′tici lymphatic trunks: the lymphatic vessels that drain lymph from various regions of the body into the right lymphatic duct or the thoracic duct; they include the intestinal trunks and the right and left bronchomediastinal, jugular, lumbar, and subclavian trunks. See *t. bronchomediastinalis, trunci intestinales, t. jugularis, t. lumbalis,* and *t. subclavius.*

t. me′dius plex′us brachia′lis [TA] middle trunk of brachial plexus: the trunk of the brachial plexus that is formed by the anterior branch of the seventh cervical nerve. Its anterior division, from which lateral pectoral nerves may arise, helps form the lateral cord of the plexus, and its posterior division helps form the posterior cord; *modality,* general sensory and motor.

t. ner′vi accesso′rii [TA] trunk of accessory nerve: the nerve trunk formed by joining of the cranial and spinal roots of the accessory nerve;

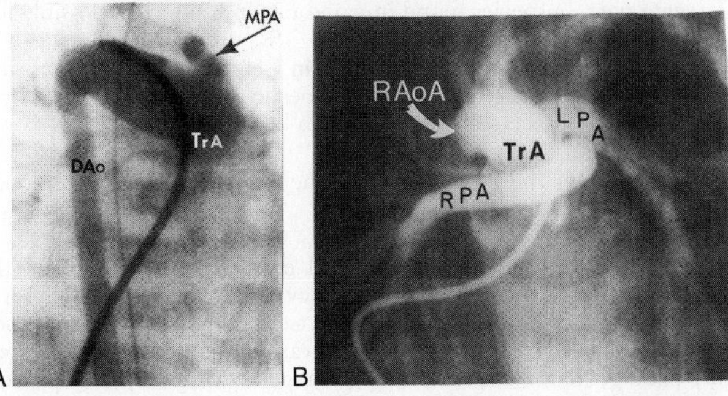

■ Persistent truncus arteriosus. *(A)*, Angiogram from a 1-week-old girl with truncus arteriosus type 1 *(TrA)*. A main pulmonary artery *(MPA)* arises from the truncus. *DAo*, Descending aorta. *(B)*, Angiogram from a 4-month-old girl with truncus arteriosus type 2. Separate right and left pulmonary arteries *(RPA, LPA)* arise by separate ostia from the truncus. *RAoA*, Right aortic arch.

after traversing the jugular foramen, the cranial root splits from the spinal root, becoming in official terminology the internal (ramus internus nervi accessorii) and external branches (ramus externus nervi accessorii), respectively. See also *nervus accessorius.*

t. ner′vi spina′lis [TA] trunk of spinal nerve: the usually very short nerve trunk formed by the ventral and dorsal roots of a spinal nerve.

persistent t. arteriosus a congenital anomaly in which a single arterial trunk with a single semilunar valve arises from the heart, receives blood from both ventricles, and supplies blood to the coronary, pulmonary, and systemic circulations. It is often subclassified anatomically; in the most common type, type 1, incomplete formation of the aorticopulmonary septum results in a partially separate main pulmonary artery of variable length, which gives rise to separate left and right pulmonary arteries. In types 2 and 3, the aorticopulmonary septum is absent, there is no separate main pulmonary artery, and the left and right pulmonary branches arise separately, directly from the truncus; in type 2, they arise close to each other from the posterior aspect of the truncus, and in type 3, each arises from a lateral aspect. Type 3 is sometimes considered as part of type 2.

trun′ci plex′us brachia′lis [TA] trunks of brachial plexus: the three trunks (superior, middle, and inferior) of the brachial plexus, arising from the anterior branches of the lower four cervical nerves and the first thoracic nerve near the lateral border of the scalenus anterior muscle; they continue laterally and downward, above and behind the subclavian artery, and near the clavicle each splits into an anterior and a posterior division. The anterior divisions of the superior and medial trunks unite to form the lateral fasciculus and that of the inferior trunk forms the medial fasciculus of the plexus; and the posterior divisions of the three trunks form the posterior fasciculus of the plexus.

t. pulmona′lis [TA] pulmonary trunk: the vessel arising from the conus arteriosus of the right ventricle, extending upward obliquely to divide into the right and left pulmonary arteries beneath the arch of the aorta, and conveying unaerated blood toward the lungs. Called also *pulmonary artery.*

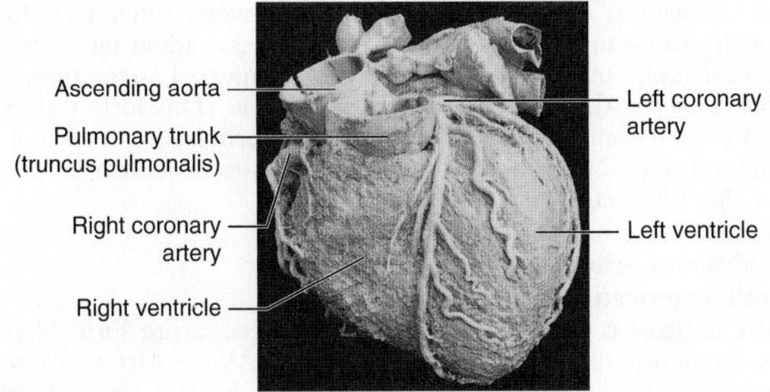

t. subcla′vius [TA] subclavian trunk: either of two lymphatic trunks (right and left) that drain the axillary lymph nodes; the one on the right drains into the right lymphatic duct or subclavian vein, and the one on the left drains into the thoracic duct or the subclavian vein.

t. supe′rior plex′us brachia′lis [TA] superior trunk of brachial plexus: the trunk of the brachial plexus that is formed by the anterior branches of the fifth and sixth cervical nerves. Its anterior division helps form the lateral cord of the plexus, its posterior division helps form the posterior cord, and it gives rise directly to the suprascapular and subclavian nerves; *modality,* general sensory and motor. Called also *upper trunk of brachial plexus.*

t. sympathe′ticus, t. sympa′thicus [TA] sympathetic trunk: two long nerve strands, one on each side of the vertebral column, extending from the base of the skull to the coccyx. Interconnected by nerve strands, each has cervical, thoracic, lumbar, and sacral sympathetic ganglia. These receive preganglionic fibers from thoracic and upper lumbar anterior roots by way of rami communicantes, send postganglionic fibers to anterior roots by rami communicantes, and give branches to prevertebral plexuses and adjacent viscera and blood vessels.

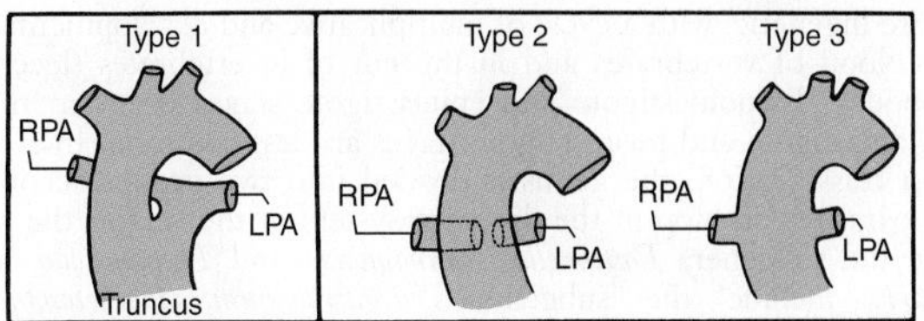

■ Three types of persistent truncus arteriosus. *LPA*, Left pulmonary artery; *RPA*, right pulmonary artery.

t. thyrocervica′lis [TA] thyrocervical trunk: a short artery that arises from the convex side of the subclavian artery just medial to the anterior scalene muscle and at once divides into the inferior thyroid, transverse cervical, and suprascapular arteries, supplying thyroid, neck, and scapular regions.

t. vaga′lis ante′rior [TA] anterior vagal trunk: a nerve trunk (or trunks) formed by fibers from both left and right vagus nerves, collected from the anterior part of the esophageal plexus; it descends through the esophageal opening of the diaphragm to supply branches to the anterior surface of the stomach.

t. vaga′lis poste′rior [TA] posterior vagal trunk: a nerve trunk or trunks formed by fibers from both left and right vagus nerves, collected from the posterior part of the esophageal plexus; it descends through the esophageal opening of the diaphragm to supply branches to the posterior surface of the stomach.

trunk (trungk) [L. *truncus* the stem or trunk of a tree] truncus.
t. of accessory nerve truncus nervi accessorii.
t. of atrioventricular bundle truncus fasciculi atrioventricularis.
t's of brachial plexus trunci plexus brachialis.
brachiocephalic t. truncus brachiocephalicus.
bronchomediastinal t. truncus bronchomediastinalis.
t. of bundle of His truncus fasciculi atrioventricularis.
celiac t. truncus coeliacus.
t. of corpus callosum truncus corporis callosi.
costocervical t. truncus costocervicalis.
encephalic t. truncus encephali.
inferior t. of brachial plexus truncus inferior plexus brachialis.
intestinal t's trunci intestinales.
jugular t. truncus jugularis.
lower t. of brachial plexus truncus inferior plexus brachialis.
lumbar t. truncus lumbalis.
lumbosacral t. truncus lumbosacralis.
lymphatic t's trunci lymphatici.
middle t. of brachial plexus truncus medius plexus brachialis.
pulmonary t. truncus pulmonalis.
t. of spinal nerve truncus nervi spinalis.
subclavian t. truncus subclavius.
superior t. of brachial plexus truncus superior plexus brachialis.
sympathetic t. truncus sympathicus.
thyrocervical t. truncus thyrocervicalis.
upper t. of brachial plexus truncus superior plexus brachialis.
vagal t., anterior truncus vagalis anterior.
vagal t., posterior truncus vagalis posterior.

TRUS transrectal ultrasonography.

Tru•sopt (troo′sopt) trademark for a preparation of dorzolamide hydrochloride.

truss (trus) an elastic, canvas, or metallic device for retaining a hernia reduced within the abdominal cavity.

try-in (tri′in) a preliminary insertion of a dental prosthesis or orthodontic appliance to determine its fit and suitability.

try•pan•id (tri′pan-id) trypanosomid (def. 1).

try•pano•ci•dal (tri-pan″o-si′dəl) lethal to trypanosomes; cf. *antitrypanosomal.*

try•pano•cide (tri-pan′o-sīd) an antitrypanosomal agent that kills the parasites; called also *trypanosomicide.*

try•pan•ol•y•sis (tri″pan-ol′ĭ-sis) destruction of trypanosomes by lysis. **trypanolyt′ic** *adj*

Try•pano•so•ma (tri-pan″o-so′mə) [Gr. *trypanon* borer + *sōma* body] a genus of hemoflagellate protozoa of the order Kinetoplastida, phylum Euglenozoa, parasitic in invertebrates and vertebrates (see *trypanosomiasis*).

Most are digenetic, with a cycle of multiplicative and developmental stages in the blood of vertebrates and in the gut of invertebrates (leeches and arthropods). Trypomastigote and epimastigote stages occur in most life cycles; amastigote and promastigote stages are less common. In some systems of classification, the genus is divided into two groups according to where parasites develop in the digestive system of the vector: the *salivaria* include the subgenera *Duttonella*, *Nannomonas*, and *Trypanozoon;* and the *stercoraria* include the subgenera *Megatrypanum*, *Herpetosoma*, and *Schizotrypanum*. Another system classifies the genus into four groups based on biological similarities: (1) the *lewisi group* includes *T. cruzi*, *T. lewisi*, and various nonpathogenic species; (2) the *vivax group* includes *T. vivax* and *T. uniforme;* (3) the *congolense group* includes *T. congolense*, *T. dimorphon*, and *T. simiae;* and (4) the *brucei group* includes *T. brucei*, *T. gambiense*, *T. rhodesiense*, *T. evansi*, *T. equinum*, and *T. equiperdum*.

T. bru′cei a salivarian species widely distributed in Africa where it is transmitted by the bites of tsetse flies from a reservoir in wild animals to domestic animals, especially cattle, in which it causes nagana. Some systems of classification divide this species into three subspecies, although they are morphologically indistinguishable: *T. brucei brucei*, which causes nagana; *T. brucei gambiense*, which causes West African trypanosomiasis; and *T. brucei rhodesiense*, which causes East African trypanosomiasis. Other authorities prefer to grant species status to *T. gambiense* and *T. rhodesiense* because of their biologic and epidemiologic differences.

T. bru′cei bru′cei a subspecies of *T. brucei* that is transmitted from a reservoir in wild animals to domestic animals, especially cattle, in which it causes nagana. Called also *T. brucei*.

T. bru′cei gambien′se a polymorphic subspecies of *T. brucei* that causes West African trypanosomiasis and is transmitted by the bite of infected tsetse flies, chiefly *Glossina palpalis*, *G. tachinoides*, and *G. fuscipes*. Humans are the only important reservoir. Called also *T. gambiense*, *T. hominis*, and *T. ugandense*.

T. bru′cei rhodesien′se a polymorphic subspecies of *T. brucei* that causes East African trypanosomiasis and is transmitted by the bite of infected tsetse flies, chiefly *Glossina morsitans*, *G. pallidipes*, and *G. swynnertoni*. The most important reservoirs are types of antelopes; domestic animals, particularly cattle, may also serve as reservoirs. Transmission to humans is usually via these animals, although infection between humans is also possible. Called also *T. rhodesiense*.

T. congolen′se a tsetse fly–transmitted salivarian species found in Central Africa that is a cause of nagana in domestic animals, particularly cattle. Called also *T. nanum*.

T. cru′zi a species found in feces of many wild and domestic animals throughout the Americas; it is usually transmitted by reduviid bugs of the genera *Panstrongylus*, *Triatoma*, and *Rhodnius*. It is the etiologic agent of Chagas disease in humans. Called also *T. triatomae* and *Schizotrypanum cruzi*.

T. dimor′phon a tsetse fly–transmitted salivarian species widely distributed in Central Africa that causes nagana.

T. equi′num a salivarian species transmitted mechanically primarily by tabanid flies and causing mal de caderas in horses in Central and South America. Except for the absence of a kinetoplast, it is identical with *T. evansi*.

T. equiper′dum a salivarian species structurally indistinguishable from *T. evansi* that causes dourine in horses and other equines. Called also *T. rougeti*.

T. evan′si a salivarian species transmitted mechanically, usually by tabanid flies in East Asia, the Middle East, North Africa, and certain parts of Central and South America (where the vampire bat is also a vector). It causes surra in domestic animals. Called also *T. hippicum*.

T. gambien′se *T. brucei gambiense*.

T. hip′picum *T. evansi*.

T. ho′minis *T. brucei gambiense*.

T. lew′isi a stercorarian species found in the blood of rats, usually nonpathogenic in adults but sometimes causing lethal infection in nursing babies. It is transmitted by the rat flea, *Nosopsyllus fasciatus*. This species is much used in laboratory research.

T. na′num *T. congolense*.

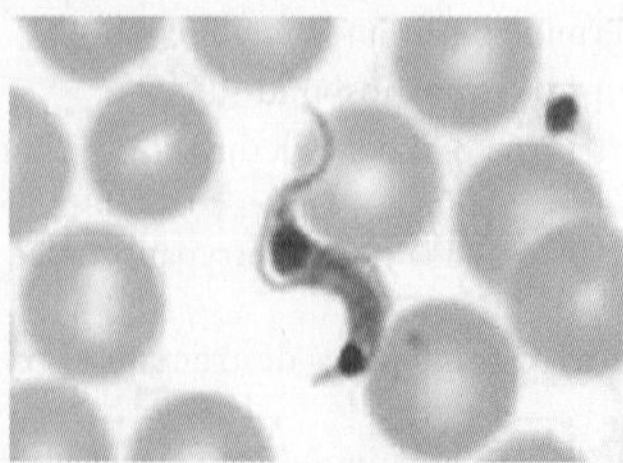

■ *Trypanosoma cruzi* in a thin blood smear. The flagellum leaves the body at the anterior end and runs along the undulating membrane (Giemsa stain).

T. neoto′mae a species found in wood rats in California, possibly identical with *T. cruzi*.

T. range′li a salivarian species found in Central America and northern South America, infecting humans and domestic animals, transmitted by the bites of reduviid insects, but not known to be pathogenic.

T. rhodesien′se *T. brucei rhodesiense*.

T. rotato′rium the type species of the genus, found in the blood of several species of frogs.

T. rouge′ti *T. equiperdum*.

T. si′miae a salivarian species found especially in Central and East Africa. It was first reported in the monkey although its natural reservoir is the warthog; it is usually transmitted by tsetse flies but sometimes also by bloodsucking flies. It causes nagana in various domestic animals, being highly pathogenic for camels, mildly pathogenic for goats, and apparently nonpathogenic for cattle, horses, and dogs.

T. su′is a species that causes nagana in pigs.

T. tria′tomae *T. cruzi*.

T. uganden′se *T. brucei gambiense*.

T. unifor′me a tsetse fly–transmitted salivarian species similar to but smaller than *T. vivax;* it causes nagana in ruminants in Central Africa.

T. vi′vax a tsetse fly–transmitted salivarian species found in many mammals in tropical and subtropical Africa and the Americas; it is a cause of nagana that may be fatal in cattle and is less serious in other species.

try•pano•so•mal (tri-pan″o-so′məl) pertaining to or caused by trypanosomes.

try•pano•so•ma•tid (tri-pan″o-so′mə-tid) 1. any protozoan of the suborder Trypanosomatina. 2. trypanosomal.

Try•pano•so•ma•ti•na (tri-pan″o-so″mə-ti′nə) a suborder of parasitic protozoa of the order Kinetoplastida, phylum Euglenozoa, comprising hemoflagellates that are found in the hosts' blood, lymph, and tissues. They have a leaflike or rounded body with one nucleus, one flagellum that is free or attached to the body by an undulating membrane, and a relatively small, compact kinetoplast, and pass through at least two morphologically distinct stages in their life cycles (see *amastigote*, *choanomastigote*, *epimastigote*, *opisthomastigote*, *promastigote*, and *trypomastigote*). Genera causing disease in humans include *Leishmania* and *Trypanosoma*.

try•pano•some (tri-pan′o-sōm) an individual of the genus *Trypanosoma* or of the suborder Trypanosomatina.

try•pano•so•mi•a•sis (tri-pan″o-so-mi′ə-sis) infection with protozoa of the genus *Trypanosoma*. In humans this can cause East African trypanosomiasis, West African trypanosomiasis, and Chagas disease. In domestic animals, trypanosomal diseases include nagana, dourine, mal de caderas, and surra.

African t. human trypanosomiasis endemic in tsetse fly–infested areas of tropical Africa. The early stage is manifested by hemolymphatic involvement with intermittent fever, anemia, rash, and transitory, localized edema. Later, invasion of the central nervous system occurs, with resultant meningoencephalitis, leading to extreme mental and physical lethargy, tremors, convulsions, and eventually coma and death. The disease occurs in two forms: *East African* and *West African*. Called also *sleeping sickness* or *African sleeping sickness*.

American t. Chagas disease.

East African t. the usually acute, more severe, often fatal form of African trypanosomiasis, occurring in East Africa, caused by *Trypanosoma brucei rhodesiense*, transmitted by the bites of infected tsetse flies, chiefly *Glossina pallidipes*, *G. morsitans*, and *G. swynnertoni*. This form differs from West African trypanosomiasis in that the acute form has a duration of 3 to 9 months and central nervous system involvement occurs earlier in its course. Called also *Rhodesian t.* and *rhodesiense t.*

Gambian t., gambiense t. West African t.

Rhodesian t., rhodesiense t. East African t.

South American t. Chagas disease.

West African t. the usually chronic and less severe form of African trypanosomiasis, occurring in Central and West Africa, caused by *Trypanosoma brucei gambiense*, and transmitted by the bites of infected tsetse flies, chiefly *Glossina palpalis*, *G. tachinoides*, and *G. fuscipes*. This form differs from East African trypanosomiasis in that the duration of the chronic disease is several months to years and central nervous system involvement usually occurs later in its course. Called also *Gambian* or *gambiense t.*

try•pano•so•mi•ci•dal (tri-pan″o-so″mĭ-si′dəl) trypanocidal.

try•pano•so•mi•cide (tri-pan″o-so′mĭ-sīd) trypanocide.

try•pano•so•mid (tri-pan′o-so-mid) 1. a skin eruption occurring in trypanosomiasis; called also *trypanid*. 2. trypanosomal.

Try•pano•zo•on (tri-pan″o-zo′ən) [Gr. *trypanon* borer + *zoon* animal] in some systems of classification, a salivarian subgenus of the genus

Trypanosoma, including *T. brucei*, *T. equinum*, *T. equiperdum*, *T. evansi*, *T. gambiense*, and *T. rhodesiense*.

try·pe·sis (tri-pe′sis) [Gr. *trypēsis*] trephination.

try·po·mas·ti·gote (tri″po-mas′tĭ-gōt) [Gr. *trypanon* borer + *mastix* whip] a morphologic stage in the life cycle of certain trypanosomatid protozoa; the slender elongate cell has a kinetoplast and basal body at the posterior end and a flagellum running anteriorly along an undulating membrane to become a free-flowing structure. Cf. *amastigote*, *choanomastigote*, *epimastigote*, *opisthomastigote*, and *promastigote*.

tryp·sin (trip′sin) [EC 3.4.21.4] a serine endopeptidase that catalyzes cleavage of peptide bonds on the carboxyl side of either arginine or lysine. It is secreted by the pancreas as the proenzyme trypsinogen and converted to the active form in the small intestine by enteropeptidase; the active enzyme catalyzes the cleavage and activation of additional trypsinogen and other pancreatic proenzymes important to protein digestion.

crystallized t. [USP] a purified, crystallized preparation from an extract of the pancreas of the ox, *Bos taurus;* used topically for its proteolytic effect in the débridement of necrotic wounds and ulcers, abscesses, fistulas, and sinuses, and in the treatment of empyema.

tryp·sin·o·gen (trip-sin′o-jən) the inactive proenzyme of trypsin secreted by the pancreas, activated in the duodenum via cleavage by enteropeptidase.

tryp·ta·mine (trip′tə-mēn) a product of the decarboxylation of tryptophan, occurring in plants and certain foods such as cheese; it raises blood pressure via vasoconstriction by causing the release of norepinephrine at postganglionic nerve endings. It is also a precursor of many natural and synthetic compounds, including psychoactive ones such as diethyltryptamine and dimethyltryptamine.

Tryp·tar (trip′tahr) trademark for a preparation of crystallized trypsin.

tryp·tic (trip″tik) relating to or produced as a result of digestion by trypsin.

tryp·tone (trip′tōn) a peptone produced by proteolytic digestion with trypsin.

tryp·to·phan (Trp, W) (trip′to-fan) 1. an essential amino acid, α-amino-3-indolepropionic acid, existing in proteins, from which it is set free by tryptic digestion; necessary for optimal growth in infants and for nitrogen equilibrium in human adults. It is a precursor of serotonin. Adequate levels of tryptophan in the diet may compensate for deficiencies of niacin and thus mitigate pellagra. See also table at *amino acid*. 2. [USP] a preparation of tryptophan used as a dietary supplement.

tryp·to·phan 2,3-di·oxy·gen·ase (trip′to-fan di-ok′sə-jən-ās) [EC 1.13.11.11] an enzyme of the oxidoreductase class that catalyzes the first step in tryptophan catabolism, the oxidation of tryptophan to formylkynurenine. The enzyme is a heme protein.

tryp·to·phan 5-mono·oxy·ge·nase (trip′to-fan mon″o-ok′sə-jən-ās) [EC 1.14.16.4] a monooxygenase that activates molecular oxygen to catalyze the hydroxylation of tryptophan to hydroxytryptophan, a precursor of serotonin; it requires the cofactor tetrahydrobiopterin. The enzyme occurs in the central nervous system and is inactivated in malignant hyperphenylalaninemia.

tryp·to·phan hy·droxy·lase (trip′to-fan hi-drok′sə-lās) tryptophan 5-monooxygenase.

tryp·to·phan pyr·ro·lase (trip′to-fan pə-rōl′ās) tryptophan 2,3-dioxygenase.

tryp·to·phan·uria (trip″to-fə-nu′re-ə) an aminoaciduria consisting of excessive tryptophan in the urine, such as in persons taking tryptophan-containing drugs. The symptoms resemble those of pellagra.

tryp·to·phyl (trip′to-fəl) the acyl radical of tryptophan.

TS test solution; tricuspid stenosis.

TSA tumor-specific antigen.

TSC tuberous sclerosis complex.

TSD Tay-Sachs disease.

TSE transmissible spongiform encephalopathy; see *prion disease*, under *disease*.

tset·se (tset′se) any member of the genus *Glossina*.

TSF triceps skinfold; see under *thickness*.

TSH thyroid-stimulating hormone; see *thyrotropin*.

T-spine thoracic spine.

TSTA tumor-specific transplantation antigen.

T-Stat (te′stat) trademark for a preparation of erythromycin.

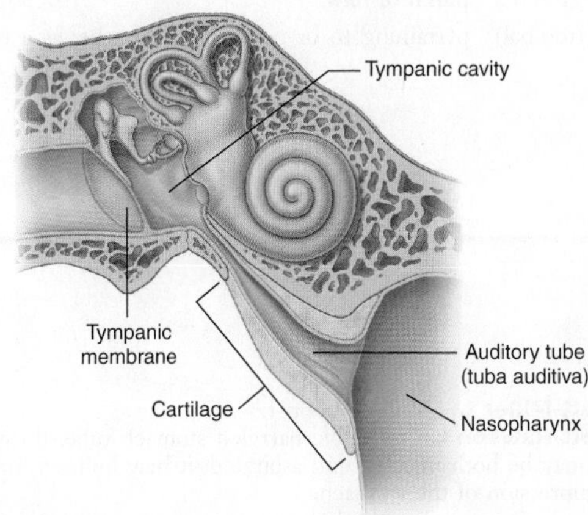

■ Tuba auditiva (auditory tube), connecting the middle ear with the nasopharynx.

Tsu·ga (tsoo′gə) the hemlocks, a genus of coniferous trees of the family Pinaceae. *T. canaden′sis* L. Carr. is the eastern hemlock, a source of Canada pitch, of the volatile oil of hemlock, and of an astringent extract.

Tsu·ka·mu·rel·la (tsoo-kə-mu-rel′ə) a genus of gram-positive, aerobic, rod-shaped bacteria of the family Tsukamurellaceae.

T. paurometa′bola a species that has been isolated from skin infections, lung infections, bacteremia, and peritonitis.

Tsu·ka·mu·rel·la·ceae (tsoo-kə-mu-rel-a′se-e) a family of gram-positive, rod-shaped bacteria of the order Actinomycetales, suborder Corynebacterineae.

TT therapeutic touch; thrombin time.

TTV thrombotic threshold velocity.

TU tuberculin unit.

Tu·a·mine (too′ə-min) trademark for preparations of tuaminoheptane.

tu·am·i·no·hep·tane (too″ə-me″no-hep′tān) an adrenergic administered by inhalation to produce vasoconstriction of the nasal mucosa for relief of congestion.

t. sulfate the sulfate of tuaminoheptane, having the same actions and uses as the base; applied topically to the nasal mucosa.

tu·ba (too′bə) pl. *tu′bae* [L. "trumpet"] tube: an elongated hollow cylindrical organ.

t. auditi′va [TA] pharyngotympanic tube: a channel about 3.6 cm long, lined with mucous membrane, that establishes communication between the tympanic cavity and the nasopharynx and serves to adjust the pressure of gas in the cavity to the external pressure, as well as for mucociliary clearance of the middle ear. It comprises a bony part (pars ossea), located in the temporal bone, and a cartilaginous part (pars cartilaginea), ending in the nasopharynx. Called also *t. auditoria* [TA alternative], *eustachian canal* or *tube*, *otopharyngeal tube*, and *auditory tube*.

t. audito′ria TA alternative for *t. auditiva*.

t. uteri′na [TA] uterine tube: a long slender tube that extends from the upper lateral cornu of the uterus to the region of the ovary of the same side; it is attached to the broad ligament by the mesosalpinx, and consists of an ampulla, an infundibulum, an isthmus, two ostia, and a pars uterina. Called also *fallopian tube*, *oviduct*, and *salpinx* [TA alternative].

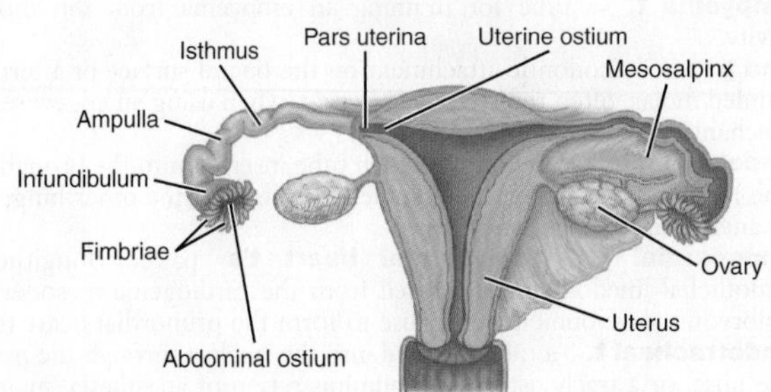

■ Tuba uterina (uterine, or fallopian, tube), divisible into the infundibulum and fimbriae, ampulla, isthmus, and pars uterina.

tu•bae (too′be) plural of *tuba*.

tu•bal (too′bəl) pertaining to or occurring in a tube, as a tubal pregnancy.

tu•ba•tor•sion (too″bə-tor′shən) torsion or twisting of the uterine tube.

tube (tōōb) [L. *tubus*] an elongated hollow cylindrical organ or instrument.

Tube

Abbott-Miller t. Miller-Abbott t.
Abbott-Rawson t. a double-barreled stomach tube, through which fluid may be both injected and aspirated; it may be used for lavage or decompression of the stomach.
air t. 1. airway. 2. any tubular passage of the respiratory system; see *trachea, bronchus,* and *bronchiolus.*
auditory t. tuba auditiva.
balloon t. see under *catheter.*
Bouchut t's a set of tubes for use in the intubation of the larynx.
Bowman t's tubes formed artificially between the lamellae of the cornea in the process of injection; called also *corneal t's.*
buccal t. see *end t.*
Cantor t. a mercury-weighted intestinal tube for decompression of the small intestine or removal of an obstruction.
Carlens t. an early type of endobronchial tube equipped with a small hook to hold it in position at the tracheal bifurcation; used for ventilation of the left lung.
cathode-ray t. a vacuum tube in which the cathode rays are accelerated as a beam to form luminous spots on a fluorescent screen.
Celestin t. a plastic tube used to keep the esophagus open in inoperable esophageal carcinoma.
cerebromedullary t. neural t.
Chaoul t. a low voltage x-ray tube designed with the anode at 2 cm from the body, allowing intense but superficial tissue penetration of the ionizing radiation beam.
chest t. a tube inserted into the thoracic cavity for the purpose of removing air or fluid, or both; it is attached to a closed drainage system so that normal pressures within the alveoli and the pleural cavity can be restored. These pressures are essential to adequate expansion and reinflation of the lung.
Coolidge t. a vacuum tube for the generation of x-rays in which the cathode consists of a spiral filament of incandescent tungsten and the anode (the target) of massive tungsten.
corneal t's Bowman t's.
Craigie t. a tube apparatus used for separating motile from nonmotile bacteria; it consists of a length of glass tubing with slanted bottom inserted into a larger tube of semisolid culture medium with the top of the smaller tube protruding above the medium. The medium is inoculated by stab inside the smaller tube. Organisms isolated from the medium outside the tubing are motile; nonmotile types remain inside.
digestive t. see under *tract.*
discharge t. a vessel of insulating material (usually glass) provided with metal electrodes which is exhausted to a low gas pressure and permits the passage of electricity through the residual gas when a moderately high voltage is applied to the electrodes.
drainage t. a tube used in surgery to facilitate the escape of fluids.
Durham t. 1. [Arthur Edward *Durham*] a jointed tracheostomy tube. 2. [Herbert Edward *Durham*] a small inverted test tube used in determining bacterial gas production.
empyema t. a tube for draining an empyema from the thoracic cavity.
end t. an orthodontic attachment on the buccal surface of a terminal banded molar; often referred to as *buccal t.* when using an edgewise arch mechanism.
endobronchial t. a double-lumen tube inserted into the bronchus of one lung and permitting the complete deflation of the other lung; used in anesthesia and thoracic surgery.
endocardial t's, endocardial heart t's paired, longitudinal, endothelial-lined channels formed from the cardiogenic mesoderm in embryonic development; they fuse to form the primordial heart tube.
endotracheal t. a tube inserted into the trachea through the mouth, the nose, or a tracheostomy for administration of anesthesia, maintenance of an airway, aspiration of secretions, ventilation of the lungs, or prevention of entrance of foreign material into the tracheobronchial tree. Called also *tracheal t.*
esophageal t. 1. a tube going into or through the esophagus. 2. stomach t.
eustachian t. tuba auditiva.
Ewald t. a stomach tube of large bore, used to evacuate the stomach.
fallopian t. tuba uterina.
feeding t. a stomach tube used to introduce fluids of high caloric value.
fermentation t. a U-shaped tube with one arm closed for determining gas production by bacteria.
fusion t's heteroscope.
gastrostomy t. a tube inserted through a stoma on the body surface into the stomach in a gastrostomy.
germ t. the short tube formed by a germinating hypha, conidium, or yeast cell; see also *germ tube test,* under *test.*
Harris t. a single-lumen intestinal tube with a mercury weight, similar to the Miller-Abbott tube, used as a diagnostic aid in study of the small intestine.
heart t. primordial heart t.
horizontal t. a metal tube attachment placed in a horizontal position on the buccal surface of each anchor molar.
hot-cathode t. a vacuum tube in which the cathode is electrically heated to incandescence and in which the stream of electrons depends on the temperature of the cathode.
intestinal t. a tube into the intestines, inserted for therapeutic measures.
laryngotracheal t. the embryonic endodermal tube that is split off from the primordium of the oropharynx and esophagus when the tracheoesophageal septum divides the cranial part of the foregut; it constitutes the primordium of the larynx, trachea, bronchi, and lungs.
Levin t. a type of nasogastric tube used for decompression of the stomach.
medullary t. neural t.
Miller-Abbott t. a double-channel intestinal tube with an inflatable balloon at its distal end, for use in the treatment of obstruction of the small intestine; occasionally used also as a diagnostic aid.
nasogastric t. a flexible tube inserted through a nostril and into the stomach for instilling liquid foods or other substances, or for withdrawing gastric contents.
nasotracheal t. an endotracheal tube that passes through the nose.
nephrostomy t. a tube inserted into the renal pelvis for direct drainage of the urine through a percutaneous nephrostomy opening.

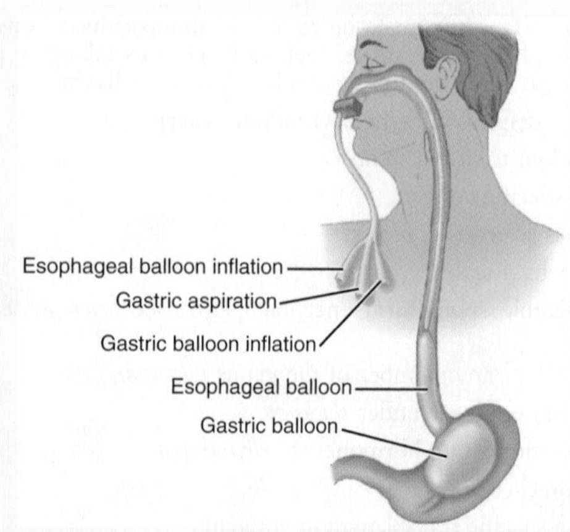

■ Sengstaken-Blakemore tube for esophagogastric tamponade.

Tube *Continued*

neural t. the neuroepithelial tube developed from the neural plate and forming the central nervous system of the embryo; called also *medullary t.* and *cerebromedullary t.*
orogastric t. a flexible tube inserted through the mouth and into the stomach for instilling liquid foods or other substances, or for withdrawing gastric contents.
orotracheal t. an endotracheal tube that passes through the mouth.
otopharyngeal t. tuba auditiva.
ovarian t's groups of cells that grow down and are cut off from the thickened surface layer of the ovary; they surround the primordial sex cells, which develop into primary oocytes, each with a follicular layer.
pharyngotympanic t. tuba auditiva.
photomultiplier t. a vacuum tube that converts electromagnetic radiation signals into electrical pulses, consisting of a light-sensitive surface that emits electrons when light is incident on it, the electrons then passing through successive stages with electron multiplication at each stage.
polar t. a hollow, extensible, filamentous tubular organelle found coiled in the spore of microsporidan protozoa, through which the sporoplasm is injected into the host's tissues. Called also *polar injecting filament.*
primitive heart t., primordial heart t. the primordium of the heart, formed by fusion of the two lateral endocardial tubes.
Robertshaw t. an endobronchial tube that has various improvements over the Carlens tube such as lack of the positioning hook and availability for ventilation of either lung.
Roida t. a tube designed for the separation of motile from nonmotile bacteria; the motile organisms make their way through sand, glass-wool, and other obstructions.
roll t. see *roll-tube culture*, under *culture*.
Ruysch t. a very small tubular opening on the nasal septum, just anterior and inferior to the nasopalatine foramen: it is a relic of the fetal Jacobson organ.
Ryle t. a thin, flexible stomach tube with an olive-shaped end, used in giving a test meal.
Sengstaken-Blakemore t. a multilumen esophageal tube used for the tamponade of bleeding esophageal varices. One lumen leads to a balloon that is inflated in the stomach, to retain the instrument in place, and to compress the vessels around the cardia; another leads to a long narrow balloon by which pressure is exerted against the varices in the wall of the esophagus; and a third provides for aspirating contents of the stomach.
sputum t. a graduated capillary tube for containing sputum to be rotated in the centrifuge.
stomach t. a *nasogastric* or *orogastric tube.*
T t. a self-retaining drainage tube in the shape of a T.
test t. a tube of thin glass closed at one end, used for various procedures in chemistry and for the growth of bacterial or viral cultures.
thoracostomy t. a tube inserted through an opening in the chest wall, for application of suction to the pleural cavity; used to drain fluid or blood or to reexpand the lung in pneumothorax.
tracheal t. endotracheal t.
tracheostomy t. a curved endotracheal tube inserted into the trachea through the opening made in tracheostomy.
tympanostomy t. ventilation t.
uterine t. tuba uterina.
vacuum t. a glass tube from which the air has been exhausted to a high degree of vacuum.
valve t. a vacuum tube used to rectify an alternating current.
Veillon t. a piece of glass tubing with a rubber cork at one end and a plug of cotton at the other, used in bacterial culture work.
ventilation t. a tube inserted after myringotomy in chronic cases of middle ear effusion, such as in secretory or mucoid otitis media; it provides ventilation and drainage for the middle ear during healing. Called also *tympanostomy t.*
vertical t. an orthodontic attachment usually placed on the lingual surface of the anchor band to allow for the insertion of the lingual arch wire.
Westergren t. a straight glass pipette 30 cm long and 2.5 mm in internal diameter, marked in millimeters from 0 to 200 and used in the Westergren method of determining the erythrocyte sedimentation rate.
Wintrobe hematocrit t. a thick-walled glass tube with a uniform internal bore, a flat bottom, and millimeter calibrations from 0 to 105; used in the Wintrobe method of calculating hematocrit.
x-ray t. a glass vacuum bulb containing two electrodes. Electrons are obtained either from gas in the tube or from a heated cathode. When suitable potential is applied, electrons travel at high velocity from cathode to anode, where they are suddenly arrested, giving rise to x-rays.

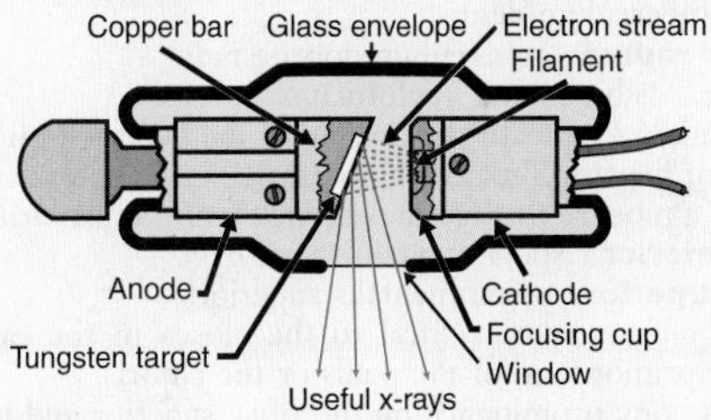

■ Standard stationary anode x-ray tube; diagram in longitudinal section.

tu•bec•to•my (too-bek′tə-me) salpingectomy.

tu•ber (too′bər) pl. *tubers* or *tu′bera* [L.] 1. [TA] a swelling or protuberance. Called also *tuberosity.* 2. the essential lesion of tuberous sclerosis, presenting as a pale, firm, nodular phakomalike glial hamartomatous brain lesion that sometimes becomes calcified, which develops predominantly in the cerebral hemispheres, cerebellum, medulla oblongata, and spinal cord.

t. calca′nei [TA] calcaneal tuberosity: the posteroinferior projection of the calcaneus that forms the heel.

t. cine′reum [TA] a layer of gray matter that is part of the hypothalamus; forming a part of the floor of the third ventricle, it lies in front of and between the corpora mammillaria and merges anteriorly into the infundibulum.

frontal t., t. fronta′le [TA] one of the slight rounded prominences on the frontal bone on either side superior to the eyes, forming the most prominent portions of the forehead; called also *eminentia frontalis* [TA alternative] and *frontal eminence.*

t. ischia′dicum [TA] ischial tuberosity: a large elongated mass on the inferior part of the posterior margin of the body of the ischium, to which several muscles are attached.

t. maxil′lae [TA] maxillary tuberosity: a rounded eminence at the posteroinferior angle of the infratemporal surface of the maxilla; called also *maxillary eminence* and *eminentia maxillae* [TA alternative].

t. omenta′le he′patis [TA] omental tuberosity of liver: the rounded prominence on the posteroinferior surface of the left liver, just cranial to the lesser curvature of the stomach.

t. omenta′le pancre′atis [TA] omental eminence of pancreas: a rounded prominence chiefly on the anterior surface of the neck of the pancreas.

t. parieta′le [TA] parietal tuber: the somewhat laterally bulging prominence just superior to the superior temporal line on the external surface of the parietal bone. Called also *eminentia parietalis* [TA alternative] and *parietal eminence.*

sciatic t. t. ischiadicum.

t. ver′mis [TA], **t. of vermis** (VII B); the part of the vermis of the cerebellum between the folium vermis and the pyramis vermis, continuous with the inferior semilunar lobule on each side.

tu•be•ra (too′bə-rə) [L.] plural of *tuber.*

tu•ber•cle (too′bər-kəl) 1. a nodule or small eminence; in official nomenclature called *tuberculum* [TA]. Similar structures may be called tubers or tuberosities. 2. the characteristic lesion of tuberculosis, a small round gray translucent granulomatous lesion, usually with central caseation; it is made up of modified macrophages called epithelioid cells, surrounded by a rim of mononuclear cells, principally lymphocytes, and sometimes a center of giant cells called Langhans giant cells.

Tubercle

For descriptions of specific anatomic structures not found here, see under *tuberculum*.

acoustic t. auditory t.
adductor t. of femur tuberculum adductorium femoris.
anatomical t. see *tuberculosis verrucosa cutis*.
anomalous t. of tooth 1. Carabelli cusp. 2. tuberculum dentis.
anterior t. of atlas tuberculum anterius atlantis.
anterior t. of cervical vertebrae tuberculum anterius vertebrarum cervicalium.
areolar t's Montgomery t's.
articular t. of temporal bone tuberculum articulare ossis temporalis.
auditory t. an eminence in the lateral recess of the fourth ventricle, formed by an extension of the vestibular area and the underlying dorsal nucleus and the cochlear part of the vestibulocochlear nerve; called also *acoustic t.*
auricular t. tuberculum auriculare.
Babès t's see under *nodule*.
calcaneal t. tuberculum calcanei.
Carabelli t. see under *cusp*.
carotid t. tuberculum caroticum.
caseous t. a tubercle with central caseation, such as in tuberculosis.
cervical t's two small eminences on the femur, a *superior* one on the upper and anterior part of the neck at its junction with the greater trochanter, and an *inferior* one at the junction with the lesser trochanter.
Chassaignac t. tuberculum caroticum.
conglomerate t. a mass made up of an aggregation of many smaller tubercles or nodules.
conoid t. tuberculum conoideum.
corniculate t. tuberculum corniculatum.
cuneate t. tuberculum cuneatum.
cuneiform t. tuberculum cuneiforme.
Darwin t., darwinian t. tuberculum auriculare.
deltoid t. 1. tuberculum deltoideum. 2. a prominence on the clavicle for attachment of the deltoid muscle. 3. tuberositas deltoidea.
dental t. tuberculum dentis.
dorsal t. of radius tuberculum dorsale radii.
epiglottic t. tuberculum epiglotticum.
Farre t's masses beneath the capsule of the liver, felt on palpation in some cases of hepatocellular carcinoma.
fibrous t. a tubercle that has undergone chronic inflammatory scarring.
genial t., inferior spina mentalis inferior.
genial t., superior spina mentalis superior.
genital t. an eminence ventral to the cloaca in the early embryo, which is the primordium of the penis or the clitoris.
Gerdy t. a bony prominence on the tibia, superior and lateral to the tibial tuberosity, to which the proximal end of the tibialis anterior muscle is attached; it is a reference point in some knee surgery.
Ghon t. see under *focus*.
gracile t. tuberculum gracile.
gray t. 1. tuberculum trigeminale. 2. tuber cinereum.
greater t. of humerus tuberculum majus humeri.
hard t. a noncaseating tubercle, the characteristic lesion of sarcoidosis, composed of discrete aggregations of large, pale-staining, epithelioid cells intermingled with histiocytes, lymphocytes, and Langhans giant cells, sometimes surrounded by a narrow band of lymphocytes; when necrosis is present, it is minimal. Similar lesions may be seen in association with foreign bodies in the tissues and in such conditions as tuberculoid leprosy, tuberculosis, cutaneous leishmaniasis, and deep fungal infections.
iliac t., t. of iliac crest tuberculum iliacum.
iliopectineal t. eminentia iliopubica.
infraglenoid t. tuberculum infraglenoidale.
intercolumnar t. organum subfornicale.
intercondylar t., lateral tuberculum intercondylare laterale.
intercondylar t., medial tuberculum intercondylare mediale.
intervenous t. tuberculum intervenosum.
jugular t. tuberculum jugulare.
labial t. tuberculum labii superioris.
lacrimal t. papilla lacrimalis.
lateral orbital t. tuberculum orbitale.
lateral t. of posterior process of talus tuberculum laterale processus posterioris tali.
lesser t. of humerus tuberculum minus humeri.

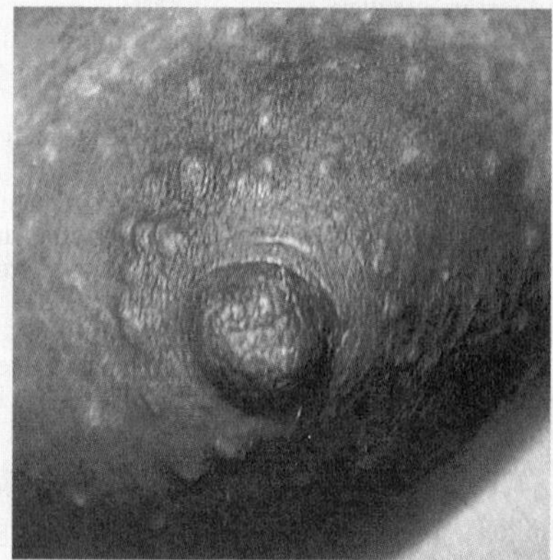

■ Montgomery tubercles.

Lisfranc t. tuberculum musculi scaleni anterioris.
Lister t. tuberculum dorsale radii.
Lower t. tuberculum intervenosum.
mammillary t. of hypothalamus corpus mammillare.
marginal t. of zygomatic bone tuberculum marginale ossis zygomatici.
medial t. of posterior process of talus tuberculum mediale processus posterioris tali.
mental t. tuberculum mentale.
miliary t. one of the minute tubercles formed in organs in miliary tuberculosis.
molar t. tuberculum molare.
Montgomery t's swellings at the openings of the areolar glands on the surface of the areola of the breast, which hypertrophy and become prominent during pregnancy. In official terminology, called *tubercula areolae* [TA].
Müller t., müllerian t. sinus t.
nuchal t. the prominence formed by the tip of the spinous process of the seventh cervical vertebra.
obturator t., anterior tuberculum obturatorium anterius.
obturator t., posterior tuberculum obturatorium posterius.
olfactory t. tuberculum olfactorium.
orbital t. tuberculum orbitale.
paramolar t. cuspis paramolaris.
pharyngeal t. tuberculum pharyngeum.
posterior t. of atlas tuberculum posterius atlantis.
posterior t. of cervical vertebrae tuberculum posterius vertebrarum cervicalium.
postglenoid t. a small conical tubercle projecting inferiorly from the zygomatic process of the temporal bone between the mandibular fossa and the external auditory meatus.
pterygoid t. tuberositas pterygoidea.
pubic t. tuberculum pubicum.
quadrate t. tuberculum quadratum.
t. of rib tuberculum costae.
t. of Rolando tuberculum trigeminale.
t. of Santorini tuberculum corniculatum.
scalene t. tuberculum musculi scaleni anterioris.
t. of scaphoid bone tuberculum ossis scaphoidei.
t. of sella turcica tuberculum sellae turcicae.
sinus t. a protrusion into the urogenital sinus caused by the caudal growing of the paramesonephric ducts; it is the primordium of the uterus. Called also *Müller* or *müllerian t.*
supraglenoid t. tuberculum supraglenoidale.
supratragic t. tuberculum supratragicum.
thalamic t., anterior tuberculum anterius thalami.
thalamic t., posterior pulvinar.
thyroid t., inferior tuberculum thyroideum inferius.
thyroid t., superior tuberculum thyroideum superius.
t. of trapezium tuberculum ossis trapezii.

Tubercle *Continued*

trigeminal t. tuberculum trigeminale.
t. of upper lip tuberculum labii superioris.
Whitnall t. tuberculum orbitale.
Wrisberg t. tuberculum cuneiforme.
zygomatic t., t. of zygomatic root tuberculum articulare ossis temporalis.

tu•ber•cu•la (too-bur′ku-lə) [L.] plural of *tuberculum.*

tu•ber•cu•lar (too-bur′ku-lər) 1. pertaining to or resembling tubercles. 2. tuberculous.

Tu•ber•cu•lar•i•a•ceae (too-ber″ku-lar″ĭ-a′se-e) in some systems of classification, a form-family of Fungi Imperfecti of the form-order Moniliales; it includes the genus *Fusarium.*

tu•ber•cu•late (too-bur′ku-lāt″) having tubercles; called also *tuberculated.*

tu•ber•cu•lat•ed (too-bur′ku-lāt″əd) tuberculate.

tu•ber•cu•la•tion (too-bur″ku-la′shən) development of tubercles.

tu•ber•cu•lid (too-bur′ku-lid) any of a group of recurrent skin eruptions, usually followed by spontaneous involution. Some authorities consider them local hyperergic reactions to mycobacteria or their antigens that are spread hematogenously to the skin from foci of active tuberculosis; others believe they are unrelated to tuberculosis. The group includes erythema induratum, lichen scrofulosorum, and papulonecrotic tuberculid; some also include lupus miliaris disseminatus faciei.

papulonecrotic t. a grouped symmetric eruption of papules appearing in successive crops and healing spontaneously with depressed scars. They are found chiefly on the extensor surfaces of the limbs, cause few symptoms, and occur mainly in children and young adults.

rosacealike t. granulomatous rosacea.

tu•ber•cu•lin (too-bur′ku-lin) [USP] a sterile solution containing growth products of *Mycobacterium tuberculosis* or *M. bovis,* used in skin tests for tuberculosis (see *tuberculin test,* under *test*) and also a commonly used antigen in laboratory immunology. It is provided as either Old tuberculin or purified protein derivative (PPD) tuberculin.

Koch t. Old t.

Old t. (OT) [USP] a form of tuberculin prepared as a culture filtrate adjusted to a standard potency by addition of glycerin and isotonic sodium chloride solution; used for tuberculin tests. Called also *Koch t.*

PPD t., purified protein derivative t. [USP] a form of tuberculin prepared by precipitation of a purified protein fraction from a culture filtrate; used for tuberculin tests.

tu•ber•cu•li•tis (too-bur″ku-li′tis) [*tubercle* + *-itis*] inflammation of or near a tubercle.

tu•ber•cu•li•za•tion (too-bur″ku-lĭ-za′shən) 1. conversion into tubercles. 2. tuberculation.

tu•ber•cu•lo•ci•dal (too-bur″ku-lo-si′dəl) lethal to *Mycobacterium tuberculosis;* cf. *antitubercular.*

tu•ber•cu•lo•der•ma (too-bur″ku-lo-der′mə) [*tuberculo-* + *derma*] 1. any tuberculous condition or disease of the skin. 2. cutaneous tuberculosis.

tu•ber•cu•loid (too-bur′ku-loid) 1. resembling a tubercle. 2. resembling tuberculosis.

tu•ber•cu•lo•ma (too-bur″ku-lo′mə) a tumorlike mass resulting from aggregation or enlargement of caseous tubercles.

t. en plaque a flat plaque on the surface of the frontoparietal cortex in tuberculous meningitis, producing the symptoms of brain tumor.

tu•ber•cu•lo•sil•i•co•sis (too-bur″ku-lo-sil″ĭ-ko′sis) silicotuberculosis.

tu•ber•cu•lo•sis (too-bur″ku-lo′sis) 1. any of the infectious diseases caused by species of *Mycobacterium* and characterized by tubercle formation with caseous necrosis in the tissues. The usual causative species are *M. tuberculosis* and *M. bovis.* Tuberculosis occurs in various different animal species and can vary widely in its manifestations, with a tendency to long chronicity. Any organ may be affected, but in humans the lung is the major seat of the disease (see *pulmonary t.*) and is the usual portal of entry into the body. See also *nontuberculous mycobacteria,* under *mycobacterium.* 2. pulmonary t.

anthracotic t. tuberculosis associated with anthracosis.

atypical t. any of various types of mycobacteriosis not caused by *Mycobacterium tuberculosis;* the incidence is sharply increased in immunocompromised persons.

avian t. a variety of tuberculosis affecting birds, caused by *Mycobacterium avium,* and characterized by tubercles consisting principally of epithelioid cells. It can be communicated to other animals and humans.

basal t. pulmonary tuberculosis in the lower part of a lung.

t. of bones and joints skeletal t.

bovine t. tuberculosis in cattle caused by infection with *Mycobacterium bovis,* which is transmissible to other animals. Characteristics include tubercles or nodular lesions in lymph nodes and various organs, such as the udder, kidneys, uterus, and meninges.

cerebral t. tuberculous meningitis.

t. colliquati′va, t. colliquati′va cu′tis scrofuloderma.

cutaneous t., t. cu′tis tuberculosis affecting the skin; it may be from exogenous infection such as autoinoculation, or endogenous infection such as by extension of an existing infection or hematogenous spread of pulmonary tuberculosis. It can present with any of numerous clinical expressions, including lupus vulgaris, tuberculosis verrucosa cutis, scrofuloderma, tuberculous chancre, or papulonecrotic tuberculid. Called also *t. of skin.*

cutaneous miliary t. a severe, acute form of miliary tuberculosis involving the skin, seen in children and immunocompromised or otherwise debilitated adults. It occurs as a generalized cutaneous eruption of brown, cone-shaped papules that become necrotic and may form minute circular ulcers with red borders and pale granulating bases covered by a seropurulent exudate. Called also *t. cutis miliaris disseminata.*

t. cu′tis milia′ris dissemina′ta cutaneous miliary t.

t. cu′tis verruco′sa t. verrucosa cutis.

disseminated t. 1. tuberculosis that has spread to other organs from a primary focus (usually pulmonary tuberculosis) through hematogenous or lymphohematogenous channels; its incidence is increased among immunocompromised patients. 2. miliary t.

disseminated miliary t. cutaneous miliary t.

exudative t. the simplest form of pulmonary tuberculosis, often the earliest type seen, in which alveolar spaces and smaller bronchi become filled with a cellular exudate consisting mainly of large mononuclear cells. See also *tuberculous pneumonia.*

genital t. tuberculosis of the genital tract; see tuberculous endometritis, under *endometritis,* and *tuberculous epididymitis,* under *epididymitis.*

genitourinary t. tuberculosis involving the genitourinary tract, often the result of hematogenous dissemination of pulmonary tuberculosis. It usually begins as renal tuberculosis (q.v.) and spreads downward to cause tuberculous endometritis, tuberculous epididymitis, or other less common conditions.

hematogenous t. disseminated tuberculosis that is carried through the bloodstream.

hilar t. pulmonary tuberculosis involving the hilum of the lung.

intestinal t., t. of intestines tuberculosis involving the intestines, usually from hematogenous spread of pulmonary tuberculosis; characteristics

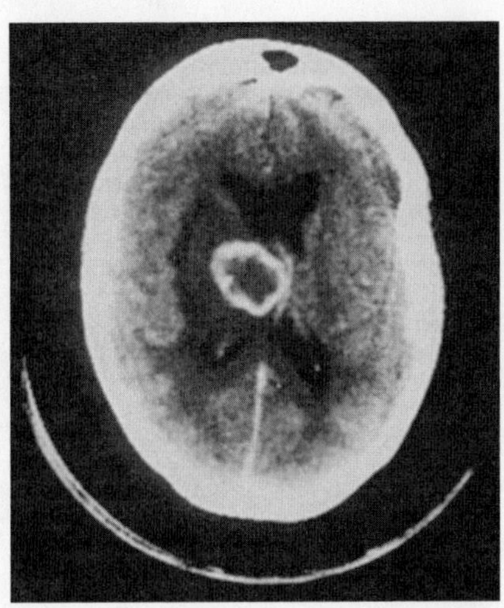

■ Tuberculoma, appearing as a ring-enhancing mass lesion with surrounding edema in a CT scan.

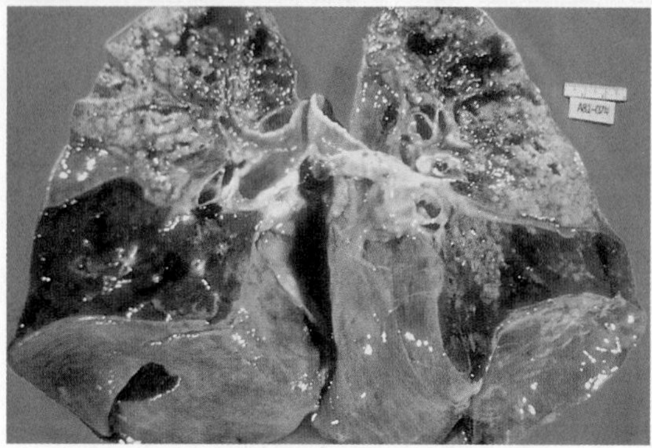

■ Postprimary tuberculosis. The upper parts of both lungs are riddled with gray-white areas of caseation and multiple areas of softening and cavitation.

include diarrhea, spreading ulcers (especially of lymphoid tissue), and sometimes scarring with stricture formation.

laryngeal t., t. of larynx tuberculosis involving the larynx, from either direct spread or hematogenous dissemination of pulmonary tuberculosis; symptoms include ulceration of the vocal cords and mucosa, hoarseness, cough, pain on swallowing, and hemoptysis.

t. of lungs pulmonary t.

t. milia′ris dissemina′ta cutaneous miliary t.

miliary t. a type of tuberculosis that varies from a chronic, slowly progressive, debilitating infection to an acute fulminating disease; it is caused by hematogenous or lymphohematogenous dissemination of infected material into the bloodstream with seeding of many organs with miliary tubercles. See also *t. miliaris disseminata.* Called also *disseminated t.*

open t. 1. tuberculosis with lesions that are discharging tubercle bacilli from the body. 2. pulmonary tuberculosis with cavitation.

oral t. a rare type of tuberculosis in the mouth, most often resulting from hematogenous spread of pulmonary tuberculosis; it usually involves the gingivae and tongue, with small, crateriform, painless ulcers that bleed readily and are surrounded by edema or reddish nodules. See also *tuberculous gingivitis*, under *gingivitis.*

orificial t. a rare form of cutaneous tuberculosis on mucous membranes and adjacent skin around orifices, occurring either by direct hematogenous or lymphatic extension from an internal organ or by inoculation; it forms nodules that break down to form painful, shallow ulcers with undermined bluish edges. It is usually a manifestation of advanced systemic disease in the middle-aged and elderly.

peritoneal t. tuberculous peritonitis.

postprimary t. pulmonary tuberculosis that is typical of a fresh infection but in which the person has actually had an earlier, probably subclinical, attack; it is distinguished by caseation and cavitation with healing that results in fibrosis. Called also *reactivation* or *secondary t.*

primary t. pulmonary tuberculosis when a person is first infected, usually seen in children or immunocompromised adults. It is often asymptomatic, with simply a positive result on a tuberculin test. In children there may be exudation (see *exudative t.*), with the primary complex consisting of a parenchymal pulmonary lesion and a corresponding lymph node focus.

primary inoculation t. cutaneous tuberculosis at the site of inoculation of tubercle bacilli in a person with no previous exposure to *Mycobacterium tuberculosis*, usually with prominent involvement of regional lymph nodes and a tuberculous chancre. Called also *primary inoculation complex* and *primary tuberculous complex.*

productive t. pulmonary tuberculosis in which a new type of tissue appears at the site of infection, consisting of epithelioid cells in concentric masses, lymphocytes, and often Langhans giant cells.

pulmonary t. infection of the lungs by *Mycobacterium tuberculosis.* The usual course of untreated disease is tuberculous pneumonia, formation of granulation tissue, caseation, calcification, and cavity formation. It may spread to other lung segments via the bronchi, or to other organs via the blood or lymph vessels. Symptoms may include weight loss, lassitude and fatigue, night sweats, and wasting, with purulent sputum, hemoptysis, and chest pain. See also *primary t.* and *postprimary t.* Called also *t. of lungs.*

reactivation t. postprimary t.

reinfection t. a new infection with tuberculosis in a patient who was previously infected and cured.

renal t. disseminated tuberculosis that has spread to the kidney, often the first manifestation of genitourinary tuberculosis. Pathological changes include granulomatous inflammation and caseous necrosis of kidney tissue. Called also *nephrotuberculosis.*

secondary t. postprimary t.

skeletal t. disseminated tuberculosis that has spread to bones and joints, leading to conditions such as spinal tuberculosis and tuberculous arthritis. Called also *t. of bones and joints.*

t. of skin cutaneous t.

spinal t., t. of spine skeletal tuberculosis of the vertebral column, with osteitis or caries of the vertebrae; characteristics include back stiffness, pain on motion, tenderness on pressure, prominence of certain vertebral spines, and occasionally abdominal pain, abscess formation, and paralysis. Called also *David disease, Pott disease, spondylitis tuberculosa,* and *tuberculous spondylitis.*

surgical t. tuberculosis that can be treated by surgical means.

tracheobronchial t. tuberculosis involving the bronchi, characterized by wheezing, mucosal redness and edema, granulation tissue, and sometimes ulceration and bronchial stricture due to cicatrization.

t. ulcero′sa orificial t.

t. verruco′sa cu′tis, warty t. a type of cutaneous tuberculosis consisting of a wartlike lesion, acquired accidentally by inoculation from an infected source; usually seen in those having a degree of immunity or tuberculin sensitivity because of previous infection or contact with *Mycobacterium* spp. Called also *t. cutis verrucosa.* It has been called by many names referring to the mode of transmission, such as *anatomical, necrogenic, postmortem, prosector's,* and *tuberculous wart.*

tu•ber•cu•lo•stat•ic (too-bur″ku-lo-stat′ik) inhibiting growth of *Mycobacterium tuberculosis.* Cf. *antitubercular.*

tu•ber•cu•lot•ic (too-bur″ku-lot′ik) tuberculous.

tu•ber•cu•lous (too-bur′ku-ləs) pertaining to or affected with tuberculosis: caused by *Mycobacterium tuberculosis.* Called also *tubercular* and *tuberculotic.*

tu•ber•cu•lum (too-bur′ku-ləm) pl. *tuber′cula* [L., dim. of *tuber*] [TA] tubercle; anatomical nomenclature for a nodule, or small eminence, such as a rough, rounded eminence on a bone; similar structures may be called tubers or tuberosities.

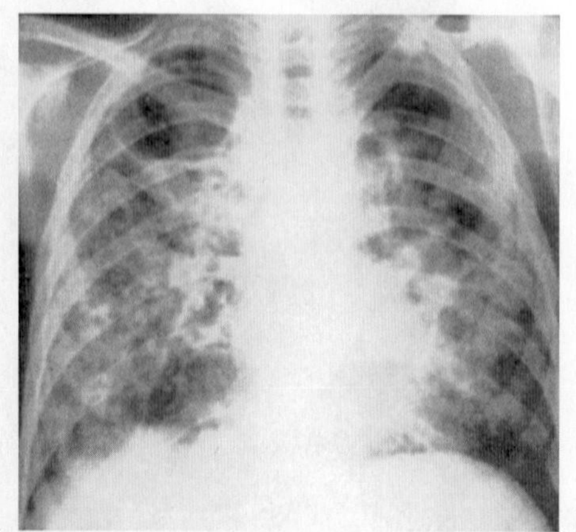

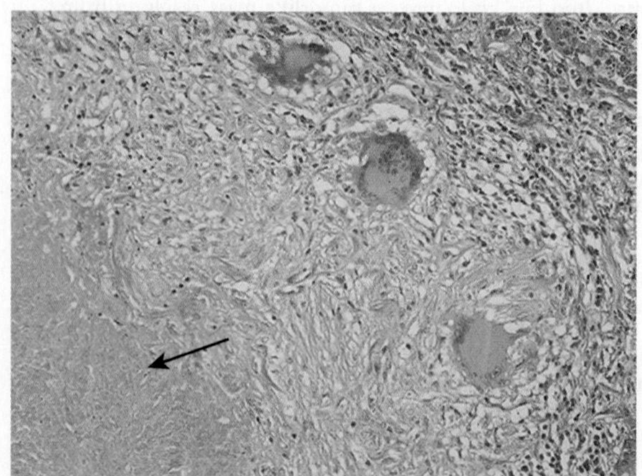

■ Pulmonary tuberculosis. *(A),* Frontal view chest radiograph showing extensive tuberculosis that resulted in respiratory failure. *(B),* Detail view of tubercle, characterized by caseation *(arrow)* surrounded by epithelioid and multinucleated giant cells.

Tuberculum

Descriptions of tubercles are given on TA terms, and include anglicized names of specific tubercles.

t. adducto′rium fe′moris [TA] adductor tubercle of femur: a small projection from the upper part of the medial epicondyle of the femur, to which the tendon of the adductor magnus muscle is attached.
t. ano′male den′tis [TA] official terminology for *Carabelli cusp.*
t. ante′rius atlan′tis [TA] anterior tubercle of atlas: the conical eminence on the front of the anterior arch of the atlas.
t. ante′rius tha′lami [TA] anterior thalamic tubercle: a distinct enlargement on the dorsal surface of the most rostral part of the thalamus; it contains the anterior nuclear group.
t. ante′rius ver′tebrae cervica′lis [TA] anterior tubercle of cervical vertebra: a tubercle on the anterior part of the extremity of each transverse process, lying lateral to the posterior tubercle and at a slightly higher level in all except the sixth vertebra, to which are attached the scalenus anterior, longus capitis, and longus colli muscles.
tuber′cula areo′lae [TA] official terminology for *Montgomery tubercles.*
t. arthri′ticum a gouty concretion in a joint.
t. articula′re os′sis tempora′lis [TA] articular tubercle of temporal bone: an enlargement of the inferior border of the zygomatic process of the temporal bone, forming the anterior boundary of the mandibular fossa and marking the termination of the anterior root of the zygomatic arch; it gives attachment to the lateral ligament of the temporomandibular articulation. Called also *tubercle of zygomatic root.*
t. auricula′re [TA] auricular tubercle: a small projection sometimes found on the edge of the helix, and conjectured by some to be a relic of a simian ancestry. Called also *darwinian* or *Darwin tubercle.* Cf. *apex auriculae.*
t. calca′nei [TA] calcaneal tubercle: the eminence, often double, on the inferior surface of the calcaneus at the anterior extremity of the rough area for the attachment of the long plantar ligament.
t. caro′ticum [TA] carotid tubercle: the large anterior tubercle of the transverse process of the sixth cervical vertebra, which lies lateral to and at a slightly higher level than the posterior tubercle. Called also *Chassaignac tubercle.*
t. cine′reum t. trigeminale.
t. conoi′deum [TA] conoid tubercle: a prominent elevation on the inferior aspect of the lateral part of the clavicle, to which the conoid part of the coracoclavicular ligament is attached.
t. cornicula′tum [TA] corniculate tubercle: a rounded eminence near the posterior end of the aryepiglottic fold, posterior to the cuneiform tubercle, corresponding to the corniculate cartilage. Called also *tubercle of Santorini.*
t. cos′tae [TA] tubercle of rib: a small eminence on the posterior surface of a rib where the neck and body join; it protrudes inferiorly and posteriorly, and bears on its medial part a surface that articulates with the transverse process of the corresponding vertebra.
t. cunea′tum [TA] cuneate tubercle: an enlargement of the fasciculus cuneatus in the medulla oblongata, just lateral to the tuberculum gracile, produced by the underlying nucleus cuneatus.
t. cuneifor′me [TA] cuneiform tubercle: a rounded eminence in the posterior portion of the aryepiglottic fold, anterior to the corniculate tubercle, corresponding to the cuneiform cartilage; called also *Wrisberg tubercle.*

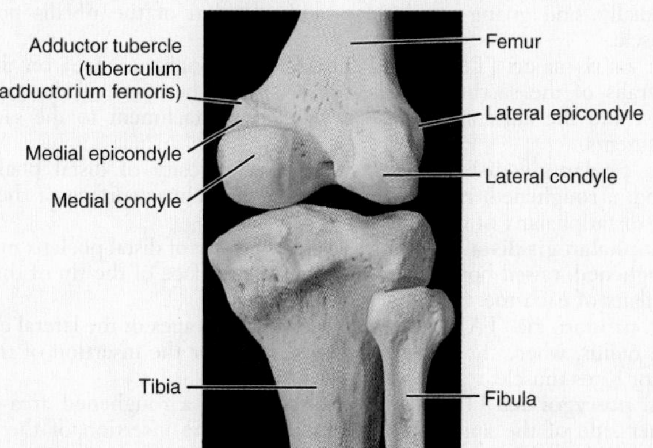

■ Tuberculum adductorium femoris (adductor tubercle).

t. deltoi′deum [TA] deltoid tubercle: a rough prominence on the dorsal or subcutaneous aspect of the spine of the scapula, into which the lowest fibers of the trapezius muscle insert.
t. den′tis [TA] dental tubercle: a small elevation of indiscriminate size on some portion of the crown of a tooth, produced by extra formation of enamel.
t. doloro′sum a painful nodule or tubercle, such as one situated in the subcutaneous tissue near a joint, produced by enlargement of the end of a sensory nerve.
t. dorsa′le ra′dii [TA] dorsal tubercle of radius: an easily palpable prominence on the distal dorsal aspect of the radius; it is grooved by the tendon of the extensor pollicis longus muscle. Called also *Lister tubercle.*
t. epiglot′ticum [TA] epiglottic tubercle: a posterior projection on the inferior part of the posterior surface of the epiglottic cartilage.
t. gra′cile [TA] gracile tubercle: an enlargement of the nucleus gracilis in the medulla oblongata, forming the lower lateral border of the posterior part of the fourth ventricle, produced by the underlying nucleus gracilis.
t. ilia′cum [TA] iliac tubercle: a prominence on the iliac crest about 5 cm behind the anterior superior iliac spine. Called also *tubercle of iliac crest.*
t. im′par a small elevation in the midline on the floor of the pharynx of the embryo, between the ends of the first and second pharyngeal arches (mandibular and hyoid arches); it is overgrown by the lateral lingual swellings and forms a small unrecognizable part of the adult tongue. Called also *median tongue bud.*
t. infraglenoida′le [TA] infraglenoid tubercle: a roughened area, just below the glenoid cavity of the scapula, that gives origin to the long head of the triceps muscle; called also *infraglenoid tuberosity.*
t. intercondyla′re latera′le [TA] lateral intercondylar tubercle: a lateral spur projecting upward from the intercondylar eminence at the proximal end of the tibia.
t. intercondyla′re media′le [TA] medial intercondylar tubercle: a medial spur projecting upward from the intercondylar eminence at the proximal end of the tibia.
t. interveno′sum [TA] intervenous tubercle: a more or less distinct ridge across the inner surface of the right atrium between the openings of the venae cavae. Called also *Lower tubercle.*
t. jugula′re [TA] jugular tubercle: a smooth eminence overlying the hypoglossal canal on the superior surface of the lateral part of the occipital bone.
t. la′bii superio′ris [TA] tubercle of upper lip: the central prominence of the superior border between the skin and the mucous membrane of the upper lip, marking the distal termination of the philtrum. Called also *procheilon* and *labial tubercle.*
t. latera′le proces′sus posterio′ris ta′li [TA] the lateral tubercle of the posterior process of the talus.
t. ma′jus hu′meri [TA] greater tubercle of humerus: a large flattened prominence at the upper end of the lateral surface of the humerus, just lateral to the highest part of the anatomical neck, giving attachment to the infraspinatus, the supraspinatus, and the teres minor muscles.
t. margina′le os′sis zygoma′tici [TA] marginal tubercle of zygomatic bone: a process on the superior part of the temporal border of the zygomatic bone to which a strong slip of the temporal fascia is attached.
t. media′le proces′sus posterio′ris ta′li [TA] the medial tubercle of the posterior process of the talus.
t. menta′le [TA] mental tubercle: a more or less distinct prominence on the inferior border of either side of the mental protuberance of the mandible.
t. mi′nus hu′meri [TA] lesser tubercle of humerus: a distinct prominence at the proximal end of the anterior surface of the humerus, just lateral to the anatomical neck; it gives insertion to the subscapular muscle.
t. mola′re [TA] molar tubercle: the prominent bulge occurring at the mesiobuccal corner of the crown of a deciduous molar, particularly a maxillary first molar.
t. mus′culi scale′ni anterio′ris [TA] scalene tubercle: the tubercle on the cranial surface of the first rib for the insertion of the anterior scalene muscle.

Tuberculum *Continued*

t. obturato′rium ante′rius [TA] anterior obturator tubercle: a small spur sometimes present on the margin of the obturator foramen, projecting from the superior ramus of the pubis.
t. obturato′rium poste′rius [TA] posterior obturator tubercle: a small protuberance often present on the margin of the obturator foramen, projecting from the free edge of the acetabular fossa near the junction of the pubis and ischium.
t. olfacto′rium [TA] olfactory tubercle: a small oval area on the base of the cerebral hemisphere between the medial and lateral olfactory striae; it incorporates the intermediate stria when present, portions of the anterior perforated substance, and structures located immediately internal to this area.
t. orbita′le [TA] orbital tubercle: a small eminence on the internal aspect of the orbital surface of the zygomatic bone, inferior to the frontozygomatic suture; it provides attachment for the lateral palpebral ligament, suspensory ligament of the eye, and levator palpebrae superioris muscle; called also *lateral orbital tubercle*.
t. os′sis scaphoi′dei [TA] tubercle of scaphoid bone: a projection on the palmar surface of the scaphoid bone of the wrist, giving attachment to the flexor retinaculum and abductor pollicis brevis.
t. os′sis trape′zii [TA] tubercle of trapezium: a prominent ridge on the palmar surface of the trapezium bone, forming the lateral margin of the groove that transmits the tendon of the flexor carpi radialis muscle.
t. paramola′re TA alternative for *cuspis paramolaris*.
t. pharyn′geum [TA] pharyngeal tubercle: a midline eminence on the inferior surface of the basilar part of the occipital bone, for attachment of the pharynx (superior constrictor and pharyngeal raphe).
t. poste′rius atlan′tis [TA] posterior tubercle of atlas: a variable prominence on the posterior surface of the posterior arch of the atlas, which represents a spinous process and gives attachment to the rectus capitis posterior minor muscle.
t. poste′rius ver′tebrae cervica′lis [TA] posterior tubercle of cervical vertebra: a tubercle on the posterior part of the extremity of each transverse process of a cervical vertebra, lying lateral to the anterior tubercle and at a slightly lower level in all except the sixth vertebra, to which are attached the splenius, longissimus and iliocostalis cervicis, levator scapulae, and scalenus posterior and medius muscles.
t. pu′bicum [TA] pubic tubercle: a prominent tubercle at the lateral end of the pubic crest and the medial end of the superior border of the superior ramus of the pubic bone; it is the anterior medial terminal of the obturator crest and of the pecten of the pubic bone.

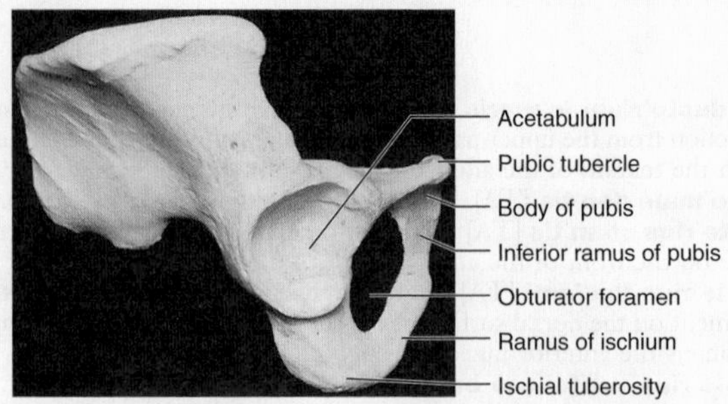

■ Tuberculum pubicum (pubic tubercle).

t. quadra′tum [TA] quadrate tubercle: an elevation on the femur just above the intertrochanteric crest that gives attachment to the quadratus femoris muscle.
t. sel′lae tur′cicae [TA] tubercle of sella turcica: a transverse ridge on the superior surface of the body of the sphenoid bone; it is anterior to the sella turcica, posterior to the prechiasmatic sulcus, and between the anterior clinoid processes.
t. sep′ti a tubercle or prominence on the superior anterior part of the nasal septum.
t. supraglenoida′le [TA] supraglenoid tubercle: a raised roughened area, just superior to the glenoid cavity of the scapula, that gives attachment to the long head of the biceps muscle of the arm.
t. supratra′gicum [TA] supratragic tubercle: a small tubercle sometimes seen on the pinna just superior to the tragus.
t. thyroi′deum infe′rius [TA] inferior thyroid tubercle: a more or less distinct tubercle at the inferior end of the oblique line of the thyroid cartilage.
t. thyroi′deum supe′rius [TA] superior thyroid tubercle: a more or less distinct tubercle at the superior extremity of the oblique line of the thyroid cartilage.
t. trigemina′le [TA] trigeminal tubercle: an elevation in the caudal part of the posterior surface of the medulla oblongata located between the fasciculus cuneatus and the roots of the accessory nerve, overlying the descending spinal tract of the trigeminal nerve and a small portion of the restiform body. Called also *t. cinereum* and *tubercle of Rolando*.

tu•be•ro•hy•po•phys•i•al (too″bə-ro-hi″po-fiz′e-əl) pertaining to or connecting the tuber cinereum with the hypophysis.

tu•be•ro•in•fun•dib•u•lar (too″-bə-ro-in″fən-dib′u-lər) pertaining to or connecting the tuber cinereum with the infundibulum.

tu•ber•o•sis (too″bər-o′sis) a condition characterized by the development of nodules.

tu•be•ros•i•tas (too″bə-ros′ĭ-təs) pl. *tuberosita′tes* [L.] [TA] tuberosity: a general term in anatomical nomenclature for an elevation or protuberance. See also *tuber*, *tubercle*, and *tuberculum*.
t. deltoi′dea [TA] deltoid tuberosity: a rough, triangular elevation, about the middle of the anterolateral border of the shaft of the humerus, for attachment of the deltoid muscle.
t. glu′tea [TA] gluteal tuberosity: an elevation on the upper part of the shaft of the femur for attachment of the gluteus maximus muscle.
t. ili′aca [TA] iliac tuberosity: a roughened area on the sacropelvic surface of the ilium, between the iliac crest and the auricular surface, for the attachment of muscles and ligaments.
t. ligamen′ti coracoclavicula′ris [TA] tuberosity for coracoclavicular ligament: a protuberance on the inferior surface of the acromial extremity of the clavicle, giving attachment to the coracoclavicular ligament and including the surface for the acromial joint.
t. massete′rica [TA] masseteric tuberosity: an elongated, raised and roughened area on the lateral side of the angle of the mandible, for the insertion of tendinous bundles of the masseter muscles.
t. mus′culi serra′ti anterio′ris [TA] tuberosity for serratus anterior: a roughened, raised area on the second rib that gives attachment to a slip of the serratus anterior muscle.
t. os′sis cuboi′dei [TA] tuberosity of cuboid: a transverse ridge on the lower surface of the cuboid bone over which the tendon of the peroneus longus muscle plays.
t. os′sis metatar′si pri′mi [TA] tuberosity of first metatarsal: a blunt process projecting downward and laterally from the lower surface of the base of the first metatarsal bone, to which the tendon of the peroneus longus muscle is attached.
t. os′sis metatar′si quin′ti [TA] tuberosity of fifth metatarsal: a large conical protuberance projecting backward and laterally from the base of the fifth metatarsal bone, to which the tendon of the peroneus brevis muscle is attached.
t. os′sis navicula′ris [TA] tuberosity of navicular: a rough protuberance on the navicular bone of the foot, projecting downward and medially, and giving attachment to the tendon of the tibialis posterior muscle.
t. os′sis sa′cri [TA] sacral tuberosity: a roughened area on the pars lateralis of the sacrum, on the dorsal surface between the lateral sacral crest and the auricular surface, which gives attachment to the sacroiliac ligaments.
t. phalan′gis dista′lis ma′nus [TA] tuberosity of distal phalanx of hand: a roughened, raised bony mass on the palmar surface of the tip of the distal phalanx of each finger.
t. phalan′gis dista′lis pe′dis [TA] tuberosity of distal phalanx of foot: a roughened, raised bony mass on the plantar surface of the tip of the distal phalanx of each toe.
t. pronato′ria [TA] pronator tuberosity: the apex of the lateral curve of the radius, where there is a roughened ridge for the insertion of the pronator teres muscle.
t. pterygoi′dea [TA] pterygoid tuberosity: a roughened area on the inner side of the angle of the mandible for the insertion of the medial pterygoid muscle.
t. ra′dii [TA] radial tuberosity: the tuberosity on the anterior inner surface of the neck of the radius, for the insertion of the tendon of the biceps muscle.

t. ti′biae [TA] tibial tuberosity: a longitudinally elongated, raised and roughened area on the anterior crest of the tibia, located just distal to the intercondylar eminence, and giving attachment to the patellar ligament.

t. ul′nae [TA] tuberosity of ulna: a large roughened area on the volar surface of the ulna, located just distal to the coronoid process, and giving attachment to the brachialis muscle.

tu·be·ros·i·ta·tes (too″bər-os′ĭ-tah′tēs) [L.] plural of *tuberositas.*

tu·be·ros·i·ty (too″bə-ros′ĭ-te) an elevation or protuberance; called also *tuber* and *tuberositas.*

bicipital t. tuberositas radii.

calcaneal t. tuber calcanei.

t. for coracoclavicular ligament tuberositas ligamenti coracoclavicularis.

coracoid t. tuberculum conoideum.

costal t. of clavicle impressio ligamenti costoclavicularis.

t. of cuboid tuberositas ossis cuboidei.

deltoid t. tuberositas deltoidea.

t. of distal phalanx of foot tuberositas phalangis distalis pedis.

t. of distal phalanx of hand tuberositas phalangis distalis manus.

t. of fifth metatarsal tuberositas ossis metatarsi quinti.

t. of first metatarsal tuberositas ossis metatarsi primi.

gluteal t. tuberositas glutea.

greater t. of humerus tuberculum majus humeri.

iliac t. tuberositas iliaca.

infraglenoid t. tuberculum infraglenoidale.

ischial t. tuber ischiadicum.

lesser t. of humerus tuberculum minus humeri.

masseteric t. tuberositas masseterica.

maxillary t. tuber maxillae.

t. of navicular tuberositas ossis navicularis.

omental t. of liver tuber omentale hepatis.

pronator t. tuberositas pronatoria.

pterygoid t. tuberositas pterygoidea.

pubic t. tuberculum pubicum.

radial t. tuberositas radii.

sacral t. tuberositas ossis sacri.

scaphoid t. tuberculum ossis scaphoidei.

t. for serratus anterior tuberositas musculi serrati anterioris.

tibial t. tuberositas tibiae.

t. of ulna tuberositas ulnae.

ungual t. see *tuberositas phalangis distalis manus* and *tuberositas phalangis distalis pedis.*

tu·ber·ous (too′bər-əs) covered with tubers; called also *tubiferous.*

Tu·ber·sol (too′ber-sol) trademark for a preparation of purified protein derivative tuberculin.

tu·bi (too′bi) [L.] genitive and plural of *tubus.*

Tu·bif·era (too-bif′ər-ə) *Eristalis.*

tu·bif·er·ous (too-bif′ər-əs) tuberous.

tub(o)- [L. *tubus* pipe, tube] a combining form denoting relationship to a tube.

tu·bo·ab·dom·i·nal (too″bo-ab-dom′ĭ-nəl) pertaining to the uterine tube and the abdomen.

tu·bo·ad·nexo·pexy (too″bo-ad-nek′so-pek″se) the operation of suturing the uterine adnexa in a fixed position.

tu·bo·cu·ra·rine (too″bo-ku-rah′rēn) an alkaloid isolated from the bark and stems of *Chondodendron tomentosum* R. & P. (Menispermaceae), and an active principle of curare from this source; it is a nondepolarizing neuromuscular blocking agent. Cf. *curare.*

t. chloride [USP] a nondepolarizing neuromuscular blocking agent used for relaxation of skeletal muscles in surgery and convulsive therapy and in the diagnosis of myasthenia gravis. Administered intravenously or intramuscularly.

tu·bo·lig·a·men·tous (too″bo-lig″ə-men′təs) pertaining to a uterine tube and a broad ligament.

tu·bo-ovar·i·an (too″bo-o-var′e-ən) of or pertaining to a uterine tube and ovary. Called also *ovariotubal.*

tu·bo-ovar·i·ot·o·my (too″bo-o-var″e-ot′ə-me) salpingo-oophorectomy.

tu·bo-ova·ri·tis (too″bo-o″və-ri′tis) salpingo-oophoritis.

tu·bo·peri·to·ne·al (too″bo-per″ĭ-to-ne′əl) pertaining to a uterine tube and the peritoneum.

tu·bo·plas·ty (too′bo-plas″te) 1. plastic repair of a tube, such as the uterine tube (salpingoplasty) or auditory tube (eustachian tuboplasty). 2. salpingoplasty. **tuboplas′tic** *adj*

eustachian t. plastic repair of the eustachian tube.

transcervical balloon t. recanalization of an obstructed uterine tube by inflation of a balloon catheter introduced through the cervix under fluoroscopic guidance.

tu·bor·rhea (too″bo-re′ə) [*tubo-* + *-rrhea*] a fluid discharge from the auditory tube.

tu·bos·co·py (too-bos′kə-pe) endoscopic visualization of the uterine tubes; often used specifically to denote salpingoscopy.

tu·bo·tor·sion (too″bo-tor′shən) a twisting of a tube, especially of the auditory tube.

tu·bo·tym·pa·nal (too″bo-tim′pə-nəl) tubotympanic.

tu·bo·tym·pan·ic (too″bo-tim-pan′ik) pertaining to the auditory tube and tympanic cavity.

tu·bo·tym·pa·num (too″bo-tim′pə-nəm) the auditory tube and tympanic cavity considered together.

tu·bo·uter·ine (too″bo-u′tər-in) pertaining to a uterine tube and the uterus.

tu·bo·vag·i·nal (too″bo-vaj′ĭ-nəl) pertaining to a uterine tube and the vagina.

tu·bu·lar (too′bu-lər) [L. *tubularis*] 1. shaped like a tube. 2. of or pertaining to a tubule.

tu·bule (too′būl) a small tube; called also *tubulus.*

arcuate renal t. tubulus renalis arcuatus.

attenuated t. thin t.

biliferous t's ductuli biliferi.

caroticotympanic t's canaliculi caroticotympanici.

collecting t. a channel through which fluids pass from the secreting cells; see *tubulus renalis colligens.*

connecting t. tubulus renalis arcuatus.

convoluted t. a channel that follows a tortuous course; see *tubulus contortus distalis, tubulus contortus proximalis,* and *tubuli seminiferi contorti.*

convoluted seminiferous t's tubuli seminiferi contorti.

cortical collecting t. the more proximal parts of the renal tubule, lying within the cortex.

dental t's, dentinal t's dental canaliculi; see under *canaliculus.*

discharging t's channels by which a fluid is discharged from the substance of the gland or organ in which it is secreted, such as tubuli renales recti.

distal convoluted t. tubulus contortus distalis.

distal straight t. tubulus rectus distalis.

Ferrein t's the portions of the renal tubules making up the radii medullares.

first convoluted t. tubulus contortus proximalis.

Henle t. ansa nephroni.

junctional t. tubulus renalis arcuatus.

Kobelt t's the outer series of tubules in the epoöphoron.

lactiferous t's ductus lactiferi.

malpighian t. one of the tubular or hairlike excretory organs arising from the midgut-hindgut junction of many arthropods; two to several hundred such tubules may be present.

medullary collecting t. the distal part of the renal tubule, including the loop of Henle, lying within the medulla.

mesonephric t's the tubules constituting the mesonephros of the embryo of an amniote.

metanephric t's the tubules constituting the metanephros of an amniote.

pronephric t's the rudimentary tubules constituting the pronephros of an amniote.

proximal convoluted t. tubulus contortus proximalis.

proximal straight t. tubulus rectus proximalis.

renal t. tubulus renalis.

renal collecting t. tubulus renalis colligens.

second convoluted t. tubulus contortus distalis.

segmental t's mesonephric t's.

seminiferous t's channels in the testis in which the spermatozoa develop and through which they leave the gland; see *tubuli seminiferi contorti* and *tubuli seminiferi recti.*

spiral t. convoluted t.

straight t. a channel that follows a comparatively straight course; see *tubulus rectus distalis, tubulus rectus proximalis,* and *tubuli seminiferi recti,* under *tubulus.*

straight collecting t. tubulus colligens rectus.

straight seminiferous t's tubuli seminiferi recti.

T t's the transverse intracellular tubules invaginating from the cell membrane and surrounding the myofibrils of the T system of skeletal and cardiac muscle, serving as a pathway for the spread of electrical excitation within a muscle cell, enabling the nearly simultaneous activation of all myofibrils; in skeletal muscle, a T tubule is the intermediate element of a triad of tubular structures, the other elements being a pair of terminal cisterns. See also *T system*, under *system*, *terminal cistern*, under *cistern*, and *triad of skeletal muscle*.

thin t. part of the renal tubule where the walls are especially thin, extending from the proximal straight tubule to the distal straight tubule; this concept is now considered outdated. Called also *tubulus attenuatus*.

tracheal t. trachea (def. 2).

transverse t. T t.

uriniferous t., uriniparous t. tubulus renalis.

vertical t's the inner set of tubules in the epoophoron.

tu•bu•li (too′bu-li) [L.] plural of *tubulus*.

tu•bu•lin (too′bu-lin) a globular 55-kD protein found in all eukaryotes, existing in several isoforms; a heterodimer of α- and β-tubulin is the subunit from which microtubules are assembled.

Tu•bu•li•na (too″bu-li′nə) [L. *tubulus*, dim. of *tubus* tube] in older classifications, a suborder of ramicristate amebae, protozoa of the order Amoebida, having a branched or unbranched cylindrical body.

tu•bu•li•tis (too″bu-li′tis) inflammation of a renal tubule.

tu•bu•li•za•tion (too″bu-lĭ-za′shən) a method of treating injured nerves by isolating the nerve stump in an absorbable cylinder, which serves as a guide for new growth.

tu•bu•lo•ac•i•nar (too″bu-lo-as′ĭ-nər) composed of tubular acini; said of glands.

tu•bu•lo•cyst (too′bu-lo-sist) any cystic dilatation of a vestigial canal or functionless duct.

tu•bu•lo•glo•mer•u•lar (too″bu-lo-glo-mer′u-lər) 1. glomerulotubular. 2. going from a renal tubule to a glomerulus.

tu•bu•lo•in•ter•sti•tial (too″bu-lo-in″tər-stĭ′shəl) pertaining to the renal tubules and interstitial tissues.

tu•bu•lo•ne•phri•tis (too″bu-lo-nə-fri′tis) tubulointerstitial nephritis.

tu•bu•lop•a•thy (too″bu-lop′ə-the) any disease of the renal tubules.

tu•bu•lo•rac•e•mose (too″bu-lo-ras′ə-mōs) both tubular and racemose.

tu•bu•lo•re•tic•u•lar (too″bu-lo-rə-tik′u-lər) both tubular and reticular.

tu•bu•lor•rhex•is (too″bu-lo-rek′sis) [*tubule* + *-rrhexis*] disruption of continuity of renal tubules, with the basement membrane being suddenly interrupted or disintegrated into fibrils.

tu•bu•lo•sac•cu•lar (too″bu-lo-sak′u-lər) both tubular and saccular.

tu•bu•lous (too′bu-ləs) containing tubules.

tu•bu•lo•ves•icle (too″bu-lo-ves′ĭ-kəl) a saclike membranous inclusion of nonsecreting parietal cell cytoplasm that contains the hydrogen pump mechanism. Upon stimulation of acid secretion, the tubulovesicles coalesce to form canaliculi with elongated microvilli, which have the greater surface area conducive to rapid secretion.

tu•bu•lo•ve•sic•u•lar (too″bu-lo-və-sik′u-lər) 1. composed of small tubes and sacs. 2. pertaining to tubulovesicles.

tu•bu•lus (too′bu-ləs) pl. *tu′buli* [L., dim. of *tubus*] a tubule or small tube.

t. attenua′tus thin tubule.

t. col′ligens rec′tus straight collecting tubule: the lower straight part of the renal collecting tubule, extending from the arcuate renal tubule to the papillary duct.

t. contor′tus dista′lis distal convoluted tubule: a distal, convoluted part of the ascending limb of the renal tubule, extending from the distal straight tubule to the connecting tubule.

t. contor′tus proxima′lis proximal convoluted tubule: the most proximal part of the renal tubule, extending from the glomerular capsule to the proximal straight tubule.

t. rec′tus dista′lis distal straight tubule: part of the renal tubule that is primarily on ascending limb and extends from the thin tubule to the distal convoluted tubule. Called also *thick ascending limb*.

t. rec′tus proxima′lis proximal straight tubule: part of the descending limb of the renal tubule that extends from the proximal convoluted tubule to the thin tubule. Called also *pars recta tubuli renalis*.

t. rena′lis renal tubule: one of the minute, reabsorptive, secretory, and collecting canals, made up of basement membrane lined with epithelium, that form the substance of a kidney. See also *nephron*. See Plate 20.

t. rena′lis arcua′tus arcuate renal tubule: a short, curved part of the distal end of the renal tubule, extending from the distal convoluted tubule to the straight collecting tubule. Called also *connecting tubule* or *junctional tubule*.

t. rena′lis col′ligens renal collecting tubule: the arcuate renal tubule, straight collecting tubule, and papillary duct considered together. Called also *collecting duct*.

tu′buli semini′feri contor′ti [TA] convoluted seminiferous tubules: the numerous delicate, contorted canals within each lobule of the testis; their epithelial linings contain Sertoli cells and germ cells.

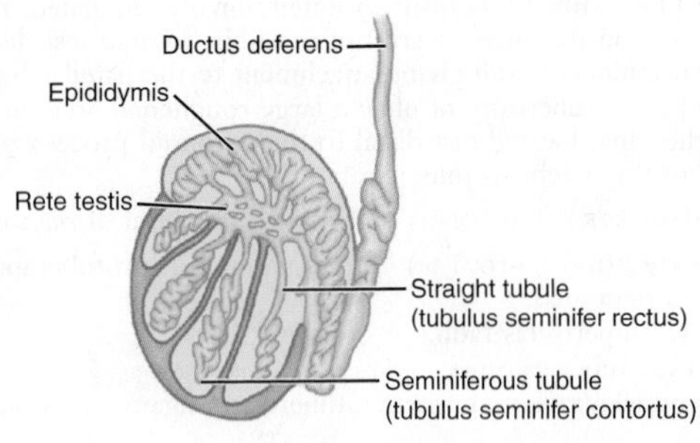

■ Tubuli seminiferi (seminiferous tubules) and associated structures.

tu′buli semini′feri rec′ti [TA] straight seminiferous tubules: the straight terminal portion of the seminiferous tubules; they join to form the rete testis.

tu•bus (too′bəs) gen. and pl. *tu′bi* [L.] tube; used as a general term in anatomical nomenclature.

Tuerck see *Türck*.

tuft (tuft) a small clump or cluster.

enamel t's bunches of tuftlike structures extending from the dentinoenamel junction through about one third of the thickness of the enamel, representing defects in mineralization; confined to the innermost 20–30 per cent of the enamel.

hair t's groups of several hairs from one follicle, consisting of one main hair and some secondary hairs.

synovial t's villi synoviales.

tuft•sin (tuft′sin) [*Tufts* University + *-in*] a tetrapeptide (Thr-Lys-Pro-Arg) cleaved from IgG that stimulates phagocytosis by neutrophils. It is produced primarily in the spleen; hereditary tuftsin deficiency and tuftsin deficiency following splenectomy result in increased susceptibility to certain infections.

tug•ging (tug′ing) a pulling sensation.

tracheal t. a pulling sensation in the trachea, due to aneurysm of the arch of the aorta; it is most apparent when the head is extended and a finger is placed on the thyroid cartilage. Called also *Oliver* or *Porter sign*.

tui na (too′e nah′) [Chinese "pushing and pulling"] a Chinese system of massage, acupoint stimulation, and manipulation using forceful maneuvers, including pushing, rolling, kneading, rubbing, and grasping, sometimes in conjunction with acupuncture.

Tui•nal (too′ĭ-nəl) trademark for a combination preparation of secobarbital sodium and amobarbital sodium.

TUIP transurethral incision of prostate.

tu•la•re•mia (too″lə-re′me-ə) [*Tulare* County, California, where it was first described in 1911] a plaguelike, zoonotic disease caused by infection with the bacillus *Francisella tularensis*, whose hosts include sheep and various species of lagomorphs and rodents such as rabbits, squirrels, and muskrats. It is transmitted by the bites of deerflies, fleas, and ticks; by contact with contaminated animals or their products; by inhalation of aerosolized *F. tularensis;* and by ingestion of contaminated food or water. In addition to a marked reaction at the portal of entry of the pathogen, which has led to classification of the various forms of tularemia, most cases are characterized by abrupt onset of fever, chills, weakness, headache, backache, and malaise. Called also *deer fly*, *Pahvant Valley*, or *rabbit fever* and *Francis disease*. **tulare′mic** *adj*

gastrointestinal t. a rare form of tularemia that follows ingestion of large numbers of *Francisella tularensis*, characterized by cramping abdominal pain, acute watery diarrhea, fever, and, infrequently, superficial ulcerations of the colon resulting in bloody diarrhea or acute hemorrhage with minimal diarrhea.

glandular t. a type of tularemia similar to ulceroglandular tularemia, with lymphadenopathy but no visible primary skin lesion.

oculoglandular t. a type of tularemia whose primary site of entry is the conjunctival sac, characterized by conjunctivitis, itching, lacrimation, pain, enlargement of preauricular lymph nodes, and granulomatous corneal lesions that if untreated may result in perforation of the cornea and optic atrophy.

oropharyngeal t., pharyngeal t. a type of ulceroglandular tularemia, usually seen in children and resulting from direct inoculation from eating contaminated food such as inadequately cooked meat; characteristics include ulcerative pharyngitis with pustular lesions on the tonsils, with or without membrane formation, cervical lymph node involvement resembling the bull neck of diphtheria, and dysphagia.

pneumonic t., pulmonary t., pulmonic t. tularemia with lung involvement, caused by either lymphohematogenous spread of a primary infection or by inhalation of aerosolized bacteria; characteristics include nonproductive cough, headache, fever, substernal pain, and bloody, mucoid sputum. Called also *tularemic pneumonia.*

septicemic t., typhoidal t. the most serious form of tularemia, which may be caused by swallowing an inoculum of the pathogen or by inhaling the organisms while chewing contaminated food; symptoms include abdominal pain, high fever, and other symptoms similar to those of typhoid fever. Oropharyngeal involvement and pneumonia and pleural effusion are also sometimes seen.

ulceroglandular t. the most common form of tularemia in humans, beginning as a painful, swollen, erythematous papule at the point of inoculation with *Francisella tularensis* that becomes pustular and then ruptures to form a shallow ulcer; mild, generalized lymphadenopathy, hepatosplenomegaly, and pneumonia may be associated.

TULIP transurethral laser-induced prostatectomy.

tulle gras (tūl grah′) [Fr. "fatty tulle"] a close-meshed net cut into squares and impregnated with soft paraffin, Peruvian balsam, and vegetable oil; used in treating raw surfaces.

Tul•lio phenomenon (too′le-o) [Pietro *Tullio*, Italian physician, 20th century] see under *phenomenon.*

Tul•pi•us valve (tul′pe-əs) [Nicolas *Tulpius* (Nikolaas *Tulp*), Dutch physician, 1593–1674] ileocecal valve.

tul•si (tool′se) a type of basil, *Ocimum sanctum*, considered sacred in India and having immunostimulant, antibacterial, antifungal, and antiviral properties, used for a wide variety of indications in ayurvedic medicine.

tu•me•fa•cient (too″mə-fa′shənt) [L. *tumefaciens*] tending to cause or causing a swelling.

tu•me•fac•tion (too″mə-fak′shən) [L. *tumefactio*] swelling (def. 1).

tu•men•tia (too-men′shə) [L.] swelling (def. 1).

tu•mes•cence (too-mes′əns) swelling (def. 1). **tumes′cent** *adj*

nocturnal penile t. tumescence or erection of the penis when sleeping at night; see under *test.*

tu•mid (too′mid) [L. *tumidus*] swollen or edematous.

tu•mor (too′mər) [L., from *tumere* to swell] 1. swelling, one of the cardinal signs of inflammation; morbid enlargement. 2. a new growth of tissue in which the multiplication of cells is uncontrolled and progressive; called also *neoplasm.*

Tumor

See also under specific types of tumors, e.g., *angioma, sarcoma.*

Abrikosov (Abrikossoff) t. granular cell t.

acinar cell t., acinic cell t. acinar carcinoma; see under *carcinoma.*

acoustic nerve t. acoustic neuroma.

acute splenic t. a swelling resulting from acute splenitis.

adenoid t. adenoma.

adenomatoid t. a small, circumscribed, benign tumor of the genital tract (the epididymis, testicular tunicae, uterine corpus, or uterine tube), composed of small glandlike spaces lined by flattened or cuboidal mesothelium-like cells.

adenomatoid odontogenic t. a benign odontogenic tumor characterized by ductlike or glandlike arrangements of columnar epithelial cells; it usually occurs in the anterior jaw region in children and young adults. Formerly called *adenoameloblastoma.*

adipose t. lipoma.

adnexal t's neoplasms of the skin adnexa, a large group that includes both benign lesions such as hamartomas and adnexal adenomas, and malignant lesions such as adnexal carcinomas.

adrenal rest t. 1. a rare neoplasm of the testis of young boys, consisting of adrenal tissue; it may be secondary to hyperplasia of an adrenal gland. 2. lipoid cell t. of ovary.

aldosterone-producing t., aldosterone-secreting t. aldosteronoma.

alveolar cell t. bronchioloalveolar carcinoma.

ameloblastic adenomatoid t. adenomatoid odontogenic t.

appendage t's adnexal t's.

Askin t. a malignant small-cell tumor of soft tissue in the thoracopulmonary region in children, one of the peripheral neuroectodermal tumors.

Bednar t. a pigmented variant of dermatofibrosarcoma protuberans.

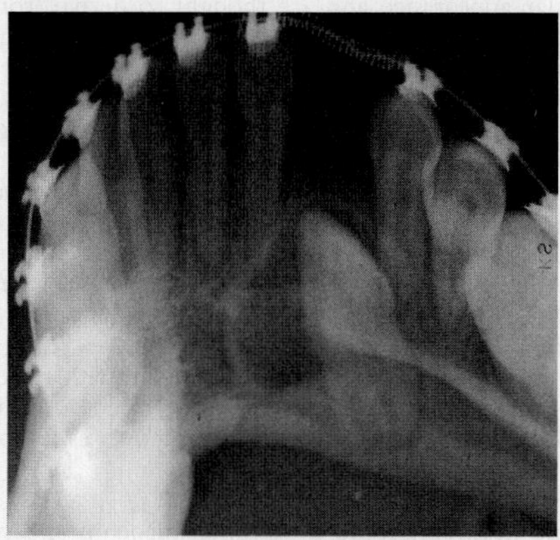

■ Adenomatoid odontogenic tumor surrounding the crown of an impacted tooth.

benign t. a tumor that lacks the properties of invasiveness and metastasis and is usually surrounded by a fibrous capsule; its cells also show a lesser degree of anaplasia than those of malignant tumors. Called also *innocent t.*

benign epithelial odontogenic t. squamous odontogenic t.

benign mixed t. pleomorphic adenoma.

borderline ovarian t's a group of ovarian tumors whose appearance and behavior are between those of adenomas and carcinomas; it includes some Brenner tumors, as well as endometrioid, mucinous borderline, and serous borderline tumors.

Brenner t. a rare type of ovarian tumor whose structure consists of groups of epithelial cells lying in a fibrous connecting tissue stroma; it may be either an adenoma or a borderline ovarian tumor. When small, it may be solid and resemble a fibroma; when large it may resemble a cystadenoma with nodular masses called Brenner nodules in the cyst wall.

Brooke t. multiple trichoepithelioma.

brown t. a giant-cell granuloma produced in and replacing bone, occurring in osteitis fibrosa cystica and due to hyperparathyroidism.

Burkitt t. see under *lymphoma.*

Buschke-Löwenstein t. a destructive tumor resembling squamous cell carcinoma but actually a form of condyloma acuminatum, usually on the penis but sometimes elsewhere in the anogenital area in either men or women. It presents as a large verrucous to fungating, cauliflowerlike mass that erodes the involved skin and progresses to penetrate and destroy deeper tissues. Called also *giant condyloma* and *verrucous carcinoma.*

calcifying epithelial odontogenic t. a rare, benign type of odontogenic tumor, usually of the mandible, believed to arise from epithelial elements of the enamel organ. It is slow growing but potentially invasive and is characterized histologically by sheets of polyhedral epithelial cells with occasional Liesegang rings. Called also *Pindborg t.*

canine transmissible venereal t. a venereal tumor found on the external genitalia of male or female dogs, usually wartlike or pedunculated and varying in size from less than 1 cm to 10 cm. Ulceration and hemorrhaging sometimes occur. Called also *canine venereal granuloma.*

carcinoid t. a small, slow-growing neuroendocrine tumor arising from enterochromaffin cells and occurring most often in the gastrointestinal tract and lung; it consists of nests of cells of uniform size containing finely stippled chromatin and electron-dense secretory granules. Such tumors produce a variety of humoral mediators that are normally metabolized by the liver; if they escape into the blood stream, the carcinoid syndrome results.

carcinoma ex mixed t. carcinoma ex pleomorphic adenoma.

carotid body t. a chemodectoma of the carotid body; a benign, encapsulated, firm round mass at the bifurcation of the common carotid artery, with nests of large polyhedral cells in alveolar or organoid arrangement; usually asymptomatic, but sometimes causing dizziness and nausea or vomiting. Called also *potato t.*

Tumor *Continued*

cartilaginous t. a chondroma or an enchondroma.
cavernous t. see under *hemangioma.*
cellular t. a tumor made up chiefly of cells in a homogeneous stroma.
chromaffin cell t. pheochromocytoma.
clear cell odontogenic t. a rare type of odontogenic tumor found in the jaw, usually in older women, consisting of a locally aggressive, poorly circumscribed lesion with sheets of clear cells.
Codman t. chondroblastoma.
collision t. an area of mixing of malignant cells from two distinct tumors (such as a carcinoma and a sarcoma) that have developed separately but near each other.
colloid t. myxoma.
connective tissue t. any tumor developed from some structure of the connective tissue, such as a lipoma, fibroma, glioma, chondroma, or sarcoma.
corticotrope t., corticotroph t. see under *adenoma.*
craniopharyngeal duct t. craniopharyngioma.
cutaneous adnexal t's, cutaneous appendage t's adnexal t's.
cutaneous mixed t. chondroid syringoma.
cystic t. a tumor that contains cysts; it may be either benign or malignant. Called also *cystoma.*
Dabska t. endovascular papillary angioendothelioma.
dermal analogue t. membranous adenoma.
dermal duct t. a small, intradermal, papular, eccrine lesion occurring on the head and neck in older adults.
dermoid t. dermoid cyst (def. 2).
desmoid t. a fibromatous tumor arising in the musculoaponeurotic tissue, usually of the abdominal wall, and often closely resembling fibrosarcoma; desmoid tumors are not encapsulated, are locally invasive, and rarely metastasize. Extraabdominal desmoid tumors occur most frequently in the shoulder girdle, arm, thigh, neck, pelvis, forearm, and popliteal fossa.
diarrheogenic t. VIPoma.
dumbbell t. hourglass t.
embryonal t., embryoplastic t. embryoma.
endodermal sinus t. yolk sac t.
endometrioid t. a type of borderline ovarian tumor that contains elements resembling endometrium.
endolymphatic sac t. a tumor arising in the endolymphatic sac; these are histologically benign, but if they extend into the adjacent temporal bone they may cause symptoms such as hearing loss, tinnitus, and vertigo. Some are associated with von Hippel-Lindau disease and others are primary or idiopathic.
epidermoid t. epidermoid cyst (def. 2).
erectile t. cavernous hemangioma.
Ewing t. see under *sarcoma.*
false t. pseudotumor.
familial bilateral giant cell t. cherubism.
fatty t. lipoma.
fecal t. fecaloma.
feminizing t. a functional tumor that produces feminization in boys and men or precocious sexual development in girls; common types are germinomas, tumors of the anterior pituitary, and tumors of the adrenal cortex. Cf. *virilizing t.*

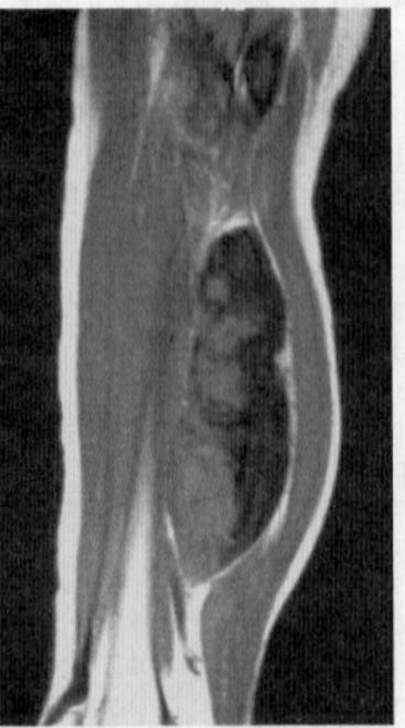

■ Desmoid tumor of the posterior thigh; sagittal MRI shows a lobular mass along the sciatic nerve.

fibrocellular t. fibroma.
fibrohistiocytic t. 1. a tumor containing cells resembling fibroblasts and cells resembling histiocytes in varying proportions. 2. malignant fibrous histiocytoma.
fibroid t. 1. fibroma. 2. leiomyoma.
fibroplastic t. 1. fibroma. 2. fibrosarcoma.
follicular infundibulum t., t. of follicular infundibulum a rare type of smooth papular lesion arising from the follicular infundibulum, usually seen on the face and neck of older patients, characterized by platelike proliferation of squamous cells that are connected at many points to the lower surface of the epidermis.
Frantz t. solid pseudopapillary t. of pancreas.
functional t., functioning t. a hormone-secreting tumor in an endocrine gland; cf. *endocrine-active adenoma.*
gastrointestinal stromal t. (GIST) any of a group of leiomyosarcomas that arise in the lamina muscularis of the stomach or intestine; some have epithelioid cells and others have spindle cells.
gelatinous t. myxoma.
germ cell t. any of a group of tumors arising from primitive germ cells, usually of the testis or ovary; they range from benign to highly malignant. Types include embryonal carcinoma, germinoma, gonadoblastoma, polyembryoma, teratoma, and yolk sac or endodermal sinus tumor, as well as some types of choriocarcinoma. Many tumors are mixtures of types.
giant cell t. a benign or malignant tumor containing giant cells; see under *carcinoma, granuloma,* and *sarcoma.*
giant cell t. of bone a bone tumor composed of cellular spindle cell stroma containing scattered multinucleated giant cells resembling osteoclasts; symptoms may include local pain and tenderness, functional disability, and, occasionally, pathologic fractures. The tumors remain benign or progress to frankly malignant lesions. See also *giant cell sarcoma,* under *sarcoma.* Called also *osteoclastoma.*
giant cell t. of tendon sheath a benign tumorlike lesion of tendon sheath origin forming a small, yellow, discrete nodule, usually on the wrist and fingers or the ankle and toes. The tissue is laden with lipophages and contains multinucleated giant cells. This is sometimes considered a variant or subtype of benign fibrous histiocytoma (q.v). Called also *benign synovioma* and *nodular tenosynovitis.*
glomus t. 1. a benign but painful tumor involving the arterial portion of a glomus body, usually found on the skin of the distal part of a finger or toe, especially beneath the nail, and sometimes in the stomach or nasal cavity. Called also *glomangioma.* 2. chemodectoma.
glomus jugulare t. a chemodectoma involving the tympanic body (glomus jugulare). It may cause symptoms in the ear (see *glomus tympanicum t.*) or in the mouth (hoarseness, dysphagia, aspiration, or tongue atrophy).
glomus tympanicum t. a type of glomus jugulare tumor involving the glomus tympanicum adjacent to the promontory of the tympanic cavity. When large, the tumor may fill the tympanic cavity, causing tinnitus and conductive hearing loss.
glomus vagale t. a chemodectoma of a glomus vagale. Those along the auricular branch of the nerve often cause vocal cord paralysis with subsequent tinnitus and deafness.
gonadal stromal t. androblastoma (def. 1).
granular cell t. a common, usually benign neoplasm whose cells have a granular appearance and are thought to derive from Schwann cells. It may be found anywhere in the body, but most often in the oral cavity, especially the tongue; sometimes there are multiple tumors. It was formerly called *granular cell myoblastoma* because it was thought to be derived from muscle cells. Called also *Abrikosov t.* and *granular cell schwannoma.* See also *congenital epulis,* under *epulis.*
granulosa t., granulosa cell t. an ovarian tumor originating in the cells of the primordial membrana granulosa; it may be associated with excessive production of estrin, inducing endometrial hyperplasia with menorrhagia. See also *granulosa-theca cell t.* and *granulosa cell carcinoma.*
granulosa-theca cell t. an ovarian tumor predominantly composed of either granulosa cells (follicular cells) or theca cells, and often associated with excessive production of estrogen, with hyperplasia and carcinoma of the endometrium. When luteinized, i.e., having cells resembling those of the corpus luteum, it is known as luteoma.
Grawitz t. renal cell carcinoma.
gummy t. gumma.
heterologous t., heterotypic t. a tumor made up of tissue different from the tissue it is growing in.

hilar cell t., hilum cell t., hilus cell t. a rare benign neoplasm of the hilum of the ovary, histologically resembling Leydig cell tumor of the testis; it may cause virilization. Sometimes this tumor is called *Leydig cell t.*
histioid t. a tumor formed of a single tissue resembling that of the surrounding parts.
homoiotypic t., homologous t. a tumor that resembles the surrounding parts in its structure.
hourglass t. a spinal tumor made up of intradural and extradural masses joined by a narrow pedicle passing through an enlarged intervertebral foramen.
Hürthle cell t. a new growth of the thyroid gland composed wholly or predominantly of large cells *(Hürthle,* or *Askanazy, cells)* that have abundant granular, eosinophilic cytoplasm. Such tumors are usually benign (Hürthle cell adenoma) but on occasion may be locally invasive or may metastasize (Hürthle cell carcinoma or malignant Hürthle cell tumor). Called also *oxyphil cell t.*
hyalinizing trabecular t. a type of thyroid tumor having nests and trabeculae of elongated cells within a fibrovascular, hyaline stroma. Some are well-encapsulated adenomas, and others are invasive and may be a type of papillary thyroid carcinoma.
innocent t. benign t.
interstitial cell t. Leydig cell t. (def. 1).
intraductal papillary mucinous t. see under *neoplasm.*
islet cell t. any of various types of tumor of the islets of Langerhans; many cause excessive hormone secretion by islet cells. Types include *gastrinoma, glucagonoma, insulinoma, somatostatinoma,* and *VIPoma.* Called also *nesidioblastoma.*
ivorylike t. osteoma durum.
Jensen t. see under *sarcoma.*
juxtaglomerular t., juxtaglomerular cell t. a rare benign tumor of renal juxtaglomerular cells in young men, causing hyperreninemia. Called also *hemangiopericytoma of kidney* and *reninoma.*
Klatskin t. hilar cholangiocarcinoma.
Koenen t. periungual fibroma.
Krukenberg t. a special type of carcinoma of the ovary, usually metastatic from cancer of the gastrointestinal tract, especially of the stomach. It is characterized by areas of mucoid degeneration and signet ring cells. Called also *carcinoma mucocellulare.*
Leydig cell t. 1. the most common nongerminal tumor of the testis, derived from the Leydig cells of the testis; such tumors are rarely malignant. Called also *interstitial cell t.* 2. hilar cell t.
Lindau t. hemangioblastoma.
lipoid cell t. of ovary a rare, usually benign, ovarian tumor composed of eosinophilic cells or cells with lipoid vacuoles, arising from ovarian cells or embryonic rest cells of the adrenals; it causes masculinization. Called also *adrenal rest t.*
luteinized granulosa-theca cell t. luteoma.
malignant t. a tumor that has the properties of invasiveness and metastasis and that shows a greater degree of anaplasia than do benign tumors.
malignant mixed t. a type of malignant pleomorphic adenoma usually occurring in the salivary glands of older adults in one of two forms: in the first both epithelial and mesenchymal components are malignant and may metastasize *(carcinosarcoma)* and in the second a histologically benign appearance persists in both the primary tumor and metastatic foci. The term is sometimes used synonymously with *carcinoma ex pleomorphic adenoma* or with the more general term *malignant pleomorphic adenoma.*
malignant peripheral nerve sheath t. a malignant type of schwannoma whose appearance is superficially similar to that of a fibrosarcoma; it may occur in association with neurofibromatosis that is undergoing malignant transformation. Called also *malignant schwannoma, neurofibrosarcoma,* and *neurogenic sarcoma.*

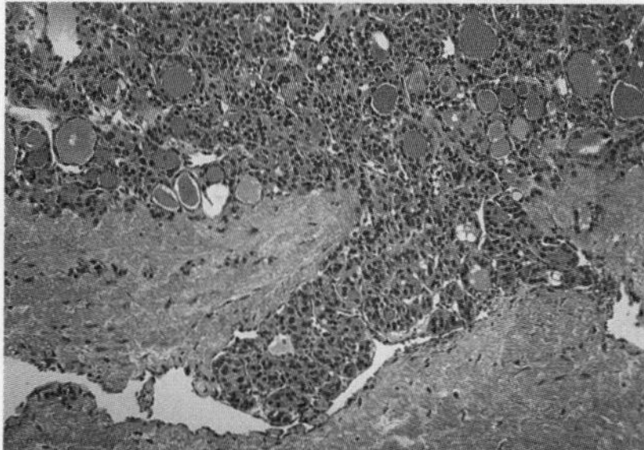

■ Hürthle cell tumor, tumor cells invading capsular vessels.

march t. syndesmitis metatarsea.
margaroid t. a cholesteatoma.
Masson t. intravascular papillary endothelial hyperplasia.
mast cell t. mastocytoma.
melanotic neuroectodermal t. a benign, rapidly growing, deeply pigmented tumor of the jaw or occasionally other sites, consisting of an infiltrating mass of cells arranged in an alveolar pattern, and occurring almost exclusively in infants. Its source of origin is in dispute, the various theories giving rise to its different names. Called also *melanoameloblastoma, melanotic ameloblastoma, pigmented ameloblastoma, melanotic progonoma,* and *retinal anlage t.*
Merkel cell t. see under *carcinoma.*
mesodermal mixed t. müllerian mixed t.
mixed t., mixed-cell t. a tumor composed of more than one type of neoplastic tissue, such as a mixed-cell adenoma, pleomorphic adenoma, or chondroid syringoma.
mixed t. of skin chondroid syringoma.
mucinous borderline t. a type of borderline ovarian tumor consisting of large multilocular cysts and producing mucin.
mucoepidermoid t. see under *carcinoma.*
mucous t. myxoma.
müllerian mixed t. a malignant mixed tumor of the uterus containing both endometrial adenocarcinoma and sarcomatous cells that may be of either uterine or extrauterine origin.
multilocular cystic renal t. multilocular cyst of kidney.
muscular t. myoma.
Nélaton t. a dermoid tumor of the wall of the abdomen.
nerve sheath t. a tumor of the myelin sheath, such as an acoustic neuroma or a schwannoma; called also *sheath t.*
neuroectodermal t. of infancy melanotic neuroectodermal t.
neuroendocrine t., neuroendocrine cell t. any of a diverse group of tumors containing neurosecretory cells that cause endocrine dysfunction; most are carcinoids or carcinomas. They occur most often in the gastrointestinal tract, in bronchial and tracheal mucous membranes, and in teratoid ovarian tumors.
neuroepithelial t. any of several closely related types of highly malignant tumors that develop from elements derived from the neural crest and are seen mainly in children. They may be found outside the central nervous system but resemble central nervous system tumors. Included are ependymoblastoma, medulloblastoma, medulloepithelioma, neuroblastoma, pinealoblastoma, and spongioblastoma. They compose the majority of the proposed new category, the *primitive neuroectodermal tumors.*
nonfunctional t., nonfunctioning t. a tumor located in an endocrine gland but not secreting hormones; cf. *endocrine-inactive adenoma.*
odontogenic t. any of various tumors derived from epithelial or mesenchymal elements normally associated with development of the teeth; they are usually found in the mandible or maxilla, and occasionally in the gingiva.
organoid t. teratoma.
oxyphil cell t. 1. oncocytoma. 2. Hürthle cell t.
Pancoast t. pulmonary sulcus t.
papillary t. papilloma.
papillary cystic t. of pancreas solid pseudopapillary t. of pancreas.
pearl t., pearly t. cholesteatoma.
Pepper t. see under *syndrome.*
peripheral neuroectodermal t. (PNET) a primitive neuroectodermal tumor occurring outside of the central nervous system, such as on a limb, the pelvis, or the chest wall; seen most often in adolescents and young adults, frequently with widespread metastases.
phyllodes t. 1. a large fibroadenoma in the breast, with an unusually cellular, sarcomalike stroma; it is locally aggressive and sometimes metastasizes. Called also *cystosarcoma phyllodes* and *giant fibroadenoma of the breast.* 2. a rare benign tumor of the prostate having a leaflike appearance similar to that of the phyllodes tumor of the breast; in some cases it may be premalignant.
Pindborg t. calcifying epithelial odontogenic t.
Pinkus t. premalignant fibroepithelioma.
plasma cell t. 1. plasma cell dyscrasias. 2. solitary myeloma.
pleomorphic t. mixed t.
potato t. carotid body t.

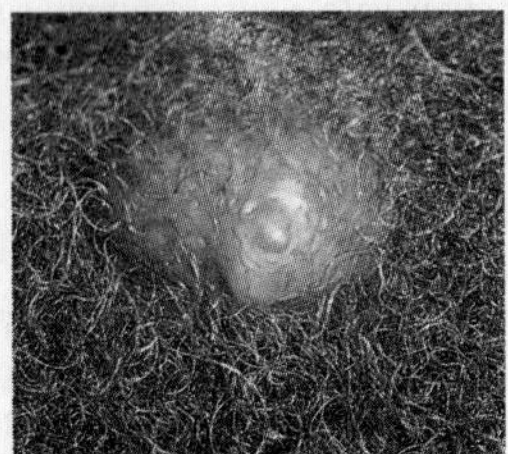

■ Proliferating trichilemmal tumor on the scalp of an elderly woman.

Pott puffy t. a circumscribed area of edema surrounding lesions of osteomyelitis of the skull.
pregnancy t. a tumorous type of gingivitis, histologically and clinically identical to angiogranuloma or pyogenic granuloma. It is most common in pregnant women, especially in the third trimester, resulting from minor trauma or irritation that is probably intensified by the endocrine alteration of pregnancy; it may or may not regress after delivery. Identical lesions are sometimes seen in men and in nonpregnant women. Called also *granuloma gravidarum.*
premalignant fibroepithelial t. premalignant fibroepithelioma.
primitive neuroectodermal t. (PNET) a heterogeneous group of neoplasms thought to derive from undifferentiated neuroglial cells of the neural crest. Some occur in the brain and some (the *peripheral neuroectodermal tumors*) elsewhere, such as on a limb, the pelvis, or the chest wall. The classification also includes the neuroepithelial tumors of childhood.
primitive neuroepithelial t. neuroepithelial t.
prolactin-secreting t. prolactinoma.
proliferating pilar t., proliferating trichilemmal t. a type of adnexal tumor, usually benign, consisting of a solitary, multilobulated lesion of the hair follicle, arising from the root sheath; it is often confused with squamous cell carcinoma. It usually occurs on the scalp of middle-aged or older women. Called also *proliferating pilar* or *proliferating trichilemmal cyst.*
pulmonary sulcus t. a tumor at the apex of the lung, extending outward to destroy the ribs and vertebrae and invading the brachial plexus; see also *Pancoast syndrome* (def. 1), under *syndrome.* Called also *Pancoast t.* and *superior sulcus t.*
Rathke t., Rathke pouch t. craniopharyngioma.
Recklinghausen t. an adenomatoid tumor of the posterior uterine wall or of the wall of a uterine tube.
Regaud t. lymphoepithelioma.
renomedullary interstitial cell t. small, round, grayish white, benign nodules consisting of medullary interstitial cells and spindle cells, found occasionally in the renal medulla at autopsy.
retinal anlage t. melanotic neuroectodermal t.
rhabdoid t. of the kidney a malignant kidney tumor similar to Wilms tumor but with a poorer prognosis; it has large cells with large nuclei and eosinophilic fibrils in the cytoplasm. It often metastasizes to the brain.
sand t. psammoma.
Schmincke t. lymphoepithelioma.
Schwann cell t. schwannoma.
serous borderline t. the most common type of borderline ovarian tumor, having a serous histology and thought to originate from germinal epithelium.
Sertoli cell t. androblastoma (def. 1).
Sertoli-Leydig cell t. androblastoma (def. 2).
sex cord–stromal t's stromal t's.
sheath t. nerve sheath t.
solid-cystic t. of pancreas, solid pseudopapillary t. of pancreas a rare, low-grade tumor of endothelial origin, predominantly affecting young women beginning in adolescence, consisting of a well-circumscribed mass containing both solid and cystic elements; tumor cells are small, polygonal, and eosinophilic and form solid sheets or papillary projections. Called also *Frantz t.* and *papillary cystic t. of pancreas.*
solitary fibrous t. a usually benign, localized tumor of mesenchymal origin with a wide range of histologic growth patterns, arising most often in the pleura but also occurring in the mediastinum, upper respiratory tract, head and neck, and abdomen. Called also *localized fibrous mesothelioma.*
spinal axis t. any of various tumors of the spinal axis, which may be metastatic or primary. Primary types include chordomas, which may be either intradural or extradural; schwannomas and meningiomas, which are intradural but extramedullary; and astrocytomas and ependymomas, which are intramedullary.
squamous odontogenic t. a benign epithelial odontogenic tumor in the mandible or maxilla, believed to derive from transformation of Malassez rests; it is characterized by islands of mature squamous epithelium surrounded by flattened or cuboidal cells.
stercoral t. fecaloma.
stromal t's a diverse group of tumors derived from the ovarian stroma; many of them secrete sex hormones. Included are granulosa-theca cell tumor, hilar cell tumor, lipoid cell tumor, arrhenoblastoma, and gynandroblastoma. Called also *sex cord–stromal t's.*
superior sulcus t. pulmonary sulcus t.
teratoid t. teratoma.
testicular t. general term for any tumor of the testis; in adults these are nearly always malignant germinomas, whereas in children many are yolk sac tumors or benign varieties such as teratomas, Leydig cell tumors, or androblastomas. Called also *testiculoma.*
theca cell t. a fibroidlike tumor of the ovary containing yellow areas of lipoid material derived from theca cells. It may be associated with excessive production of estrogen and have a tendency to cystic degeneration. These tumors are rarely composed entirely of theca cells; commonly both theca and granulosa cells are found. Called also *thecoma* and *fibroma thecocellulare xanthomatodes.* See also *granulosa-theca cell t.*
thyrotrope t., thyrotroph t. see under *adenoma.*
tomato t. a cylindroma or trichoepithelioma, particularly a large one.
tridermic t. tridermoma.
Triton t. a variant of the malignant peripheral nerve sheath tumor, associated with neurofibromatosis 1, having rhabdomyoblastic differentiation.
turban t. multiple cylindromas of the scalp.
vascular t. 1. angioma. 2. any tumor with a copious blood supply.
villous t. papilloma.
virilizing t. a functional tumor that produces virilization in girls and women or precocious sexual development in boys; common types are germinomas, tumors of the anterior pituitary, and tumors of the adrenal cortex. Cf. *feminizing t.*
Warthin t. adenolymphoma.
white t. chronic tuberculous arthritis.
Wilms t. a rapidly developing malignant mixed tumor of the kidneys, made up of embryonal elements; it usually affects children before the fifth year, but may occur in the fetus and rarely in later life. Called also *embryonal adenomyosarcoma* or *adenosarcoma, embryonal carcinosarcoma* or *nephroma,* and *nephroblastoma.*
yolk sac t. a malignant germ cell tumor of children that represents a proliferation of both yolk sac endoderm and extraembryonic mesenchyme. It is characterized by a labyrinthine glandular pattern with a papillary projection into a sinuslike space; frequently there are hyaline bodies and Schiller-Duval bodies. It produces α-fetoprotein and most often occurs in the testes, but is also seen in the ovaries and some extragonadal sites. Called also *infantile embryonal carcinoma, juvenile embryonal carcinoma, yolk sac carcinoma, orchioblastoma,* and *endodermal sinus t.*

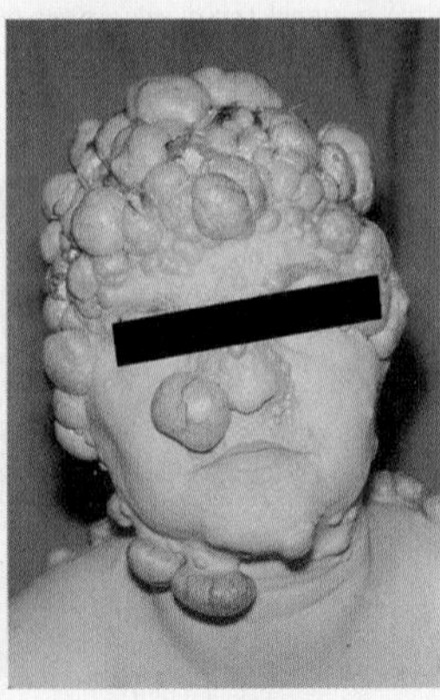

■ Turban tumor.

tu•mor•af•fin (too″mər-af′in) oncotropic.

tu•mor•ec•to•my (too-mər-ek′tə-me) [*tumor* + *-ectomy*] an imprecise term usually used to denote either debulking or removal of most or all of a primary tumor, particularly of the breast, with only minimal removal of surrounding tissue.

tu•mor•i•ci•dal (too″mər-ĭ-si′dal) oncolytic.

tu•mor•i•gen•e•sis (too″mər-ĭ-jen′ə-sis) the production of tumors. Called also *oncogenesis.*

tu•mor•i•gen•ic (too″mər-ĭ-jen′ik) giving rise to either benign or malignant tumors; said especially of a cell or group of cells capable of producing a tumor. Cf. *oncogenic.*

tu•mor•let (too′mər-lət) a type of tiny, often microscopic, benign neoplasm occurring singly or multiply in bronchial and bronchiolar mucosa of middle-aged to elderly people; it often occurs in areas of scarring or chronic irritation and is asymptomatic.

tu•mor•ous (too′mər-əs) neoplastic (def. 1).

TUMT transurethral microwave thermotherapy.

tu•mul•tus (too-mul′təs) [L.] excessive organic action or motility.

TUNA transurethral needle ablation.

Tun•ga (tung′gə) a genus of fleas of the family Hectopsyllidae, found in hot parts of the world. *T. pe′netrans* is the chigoe (q.v.).

tun•gi•a•sis (təng-gi′ə-sis) infestation of the skin with chigoes *(Tunga penetrans).*

tung•sten (W) (tung′stən) [Swed. "heavy stone"] the chemical element of atomic number 74, and atomic weight 183.85; used in electric light filaments and in steel alloys to secure hardness.

t. carbide WC, an extremely hard material used for dental drills and burs. Inhalation of its fine dust during manufacturing can cause hard metal disease (see under *disease*).

tu•ni•ca (too′nĭ-kə) pl. *tu′nicae* [L.] a membrane or other structure covering or lining a body part or organ. Called also *coat* and *layer.*

Tunica

Descriptions of coats are given on TA terms, and include anglicized names of specific coats.

t. abdomina′lis the aponeurosis of the abdominal muscles in certain quadrupeds, as the horse.

t. adventi′tia adventitia: the outermost covering of an organ, vessel, or other structure, which is made up of connective tissue and elastic fibers and may be in contact with surrounding structures.

t. adventi′tia duc′tus deferen′tis [TA] that of the ductus deferens.

t. adventi′tia glan′dulae vesiculo′sae [TA] that of a seminal vesicle.

t. adventi′tia oeso′phagi [TA] that of the esophagus.

t. adventi′tia pel′vis rena′lis [TA] that of the renal pelvis.

t. adventi′tia ure′teris [TA] that of the ureter.

t. albugi′nea corpo′rum cavernoso′rum pe′nis [TA], **t. albuginea of corpora cavernosa of penis** the dense, white, fibroelastic sheath that encloses the corpora cavernosa penis. Its superficial, longitudinal fibers form a tunic surrounding both corpora, and the deep circularly coursing fibers surround them separately, uniting medially to form the septum of the penis.

t. albugi′nea cor′poris spongio′si pe′nis [TA], **t. albuginea of corpus spongiosum of penis** the dense, white, fibroelastic sheath that encloses the corpus spongiosum of the penis.

t. albugi′nea ova′rii [TA], **t. albuginea of ovary** the layer of dense, white, connective tissue beneath the surface epithelium of the ovary.

t. albugi′nea tes′tis [TA], **t. albuginea of testis** the dense, white, inelastic tissue immediately covering the testis, beneath the visceral layer of the tunica vaginalis.

t. conjuncti′va [TA] official terminology for *conjunctiva.*

t. conjuncti′va bul′bi [TA] official terminology for *bulbar conjunctiva.*

t. conjuncti′va palpebra′rum [TA] official terminology for *palpebral conjunctiva.*

t. dar′tos dartos fascia: the thin layer of subcutaneous tissue underlying the skin of the scrotum, consisting mainly of nonstriated muscle fibers *(musculus dartos).* Called also *dartos, superficial fascia of scrotum,* and *dartos muscle.*

t. exter′na the′cae folli′culi theca externa.

t. exter′na vaso′rum [TA] external coat of vessels: the outer, fibroelastic coat of the blood vessels, sometimes in contact with surrounding tissues.

t. fibro′sa fibrous tunic or coat: an enveloping fibrous membrane or capsule.

t. fibro′sa bul′bi [TA] fibrous layer of eyeball: the outer of the three layers of the eye, comprising the cornea and the sclera.

t. fibro′sa he′patis [TA] fibrous capsule of liver: the fibroelastic layer that surrounds the liver beneath the peritoneum; at the hepatic portal it is continuous with the perivascular fibrous capsule.

t. fibro′sa sple′nica TA alternative for *capsula splenica.*

t. inter′na bul′bi [TA] inner layer of eyeball: the innermost of the three layers of the eye; it is nervous and sensory and consists primarily of the retina and its blood vessels. See also *retina.*

t. inter′na the′cae folli′culi theca interna.

t. in′tima vaso′rum [TA] the inner coat of the blood vessels, made up of endothelial cells surrounded by longitudinal elastic fibers and connective tissue. Called also *intima.*

t. me′dia vaso′rum [TA] the middle coat of the blood vessels, made up of transverse elastic and muscle fibers.

t. muco′sa mucous membrane: the mucous lining of various tubular structures, facing the lumen, comprising the epithelium, basement membrane, lamina propria mucosae, and lamina muscularis mucosae. Called also *mucous coat* and *mucosa.*

t. muco′sa bronchio′rum [TA] that lining the bronchi.

t. muco′sa cavita′tis tympa′nicae [TA] that covering the walls and most of the internal structures of the tympanic cavity.

t. muco′sa duc′tus deferen′tis [TA] that lining the ductus deferens.

t. muco′sa gas′trica [TA] that lining the stomach.

t. muco′sa glan′dulae vesiculo′sae [TA] that lining the seminal vesicle.

t. muco′sa intesti′ni cras′si [TA] that lining the large intestine.

t. muco′sa intesti′ni te′nuis [TA] that lining the small intestine.

t. muco′sa laryn′gis [TA] that lining the larynx.

t. muco′sa lin′guae [TA] that covering the tongue.

t. muco′sa na′si [TA] that lining the nasal cavity; called also *schneiderian membrane.*

t. muco′sa oeso′phagi [TA] that lining the esophagus.

t. muco′sa o′ris [TA] that lining the oral cavity.

t. muco′sa par′tis interme′diae ure′thrae [TA] that lining the membranous urethra.

t. muco′sa par′tis prosta′ticae ure′thrae [TA] that lining the prostatic urethra.

t. muco′sa par′tis spongio′sae ure′thrae [TA] that lining the spongy urethra.

t. muco′sa pel′vis rena′lis [TA] that lining the renal pelvis.

t. muco′sa pharyn′gis [TA] that lining the pharynx.

t. muco′sa tra′cheae [TA] that lining the trachea.

t. muco′sa tu′bae auditi′vae [TA] that lining the auditory tube.

t. muco′sa tu′bae uteri′nae [TA] that lining the uterine tube, arranged in longitudinal rugae or folds, and continuous with the mucosa of the uterus. Called also *endosalpinx.*

t. muco′sa ure′teris [TA] that lining the ureter.

t. muco′sa ure′thrae femini′nae [TA] that lining the female urethra.

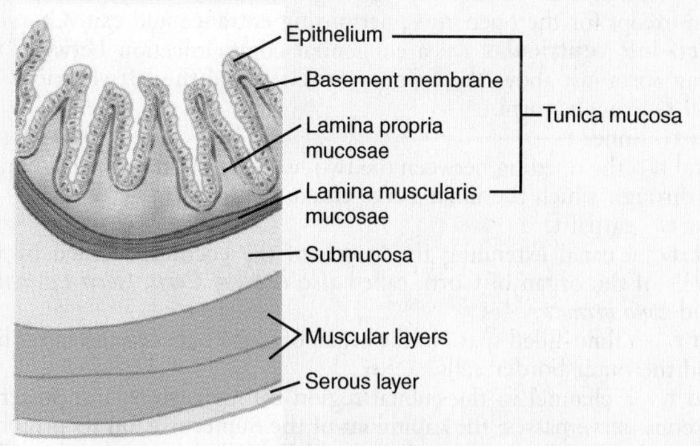

■ Tunica mucosa lining the walls of the small intestine.

Tunica *Continued*

t. **muco′sa u′teri** [TA] that lining the uterus, whose thickness and structure vary with the phase of the menstrual cycle. It is divided into two layers, the stratum basale and stratum functionale. Called also *endometrium* [TA alternative].

t. **muco′sa vagi′nae** [TA] that lining the vagina.

t. **muco′sa vesi′cae bilia′ris** [TA] that lining the gallbladder.

t. **muco′sa vesi′cae urina′riae** [TA] that lining the urinary bladder, representing the innermost layer of the bladder wall.

t. muscula′ris muscular layer or coat: the layer of smooth muscle lying between the mucosa and the serosa or the adventitia in many portions of the digestive, respiratory, urinary, and genital tracts.

t. **muscula′ris co′li** [TA] that of the colon, with sublayers of longitudinal and circular fibers.

t. **muscula′ris duc′tus deferen′tis** [TA] that of the ductus deferens.

t. **muscula′ris gas′trica** [TA] that of the stomach, with sublayers of longitudinal, circular, and oblique fibers.

t. **muscula′ris glan′dulae vesiculo′sae** [TA] that of the seminal vesicle.

t. **muscula′ris intesti′ni cras′si** [TA] that of the large intestine.

t. **muscula′ris intesti′ni te′nuis** [TA] that of the small intestine, with sublayers of longitudinal and circular fibers.

t. **muscula′ris oeso′phagi** [TA] that of the esophagus.

t. **muscula′ris par′tis interme′diae ure′thrae** [TA] that of the membranous urethra.

t. **muscula′ris par′tis prosta′ticae ure′thrae** [TA] that of the prostatic urethra.

t. **muscula′ris par′tis spongio′sae ure′thrae** [TA] that of the spongy urethra.

t. **muscula′ris pel′vis rena′lis** [TA] that of the renal pelvis.

t. **muscula′ris pharyn′gis** TA alternative for *musculi pharyngis.*

t. **muscula′ris rec′ti** [TA] that of the rectum, having two sublayers or strata, an outer longitudinal and an inner circular one.

t. **muscula′ris tu′bae uteri′nae** [TA] that of the uterine tube.

t. **muscula′ris ure′teris** [TA] that of the ureter.

t. **muscula′ris ure′thrae femini′nae** [TA] that of the female urethra, with an inner sublayer of circular fibers and an outer sublayer of longitudinal fibers.

t. **muscula′ris u′teri** [TA] that of the uterus, which forms the mass of the organ; called also *myometrium* [TA alternative] and *mesometrium.*

t. **muscula′ris vagi′nae** [TA] that of the vagina.

t. **muscula′ris vesi′cae bilia′ris** [TA] that of the gallbladder.

t. **muscula′ris vesi′cae urina′riae** [TA] that of the bladder wall.

t. pro′pria tunic proper: anatomical nomenclature for the actual coat or layer of a part, as distinguished from an investing membrane.

t. sero′sa serosa: the membrane lining the exterior of the walls of various body cavities, reflected over the surfaces of protruding organs; it consists of mesothelium lying upon a connective tissue layer, and it secretes a watery exudate. Called also *serous coat* or *membrane.*

t. **sero′sa gas′trica** [TA] that of the stomach.

t. **sero′sa he′patis** [TA] that of the liver.

t. **sero′sa intesti′ni cras′si** [TA] that of the large intestine.

t. **sero′sa intesti′ni te′nuis** [TA] that of the small intestine.

t. **sero′sa oeso′phagi** [TA] that of the esophagus.

t. **sero′sa pericar′dii** [TA] that of the serous pericardium.

t. **sero′sa peritone′i** [TA] that of the peritoneum.

t. **sero′sa pleu′rae parieta′lis** [TA] that of the parietal pleura.

t. **sero′sa pleu′rae viscera′lis** [TA] that of the visceral pleura.

t. **sero′sa sple′nica** [TA] that of the spleen.

t. **sero′sa tes′tis** [TA] that of the testis.

t. **sero′sa tu′bae uteri′nae** [TA] that of the uterine (fallopian) tube.

t. **sero′sa u′teri** [TA] that of the uterus; called also *perimetrium* [TA alternative].

t. **sero′sa vesi′cae bilia′ris** [TA] that of the gallbladder.

t. **sero′sa vesi′cae urina′riae** [TA] that of the bladder wall.

t. spongio′sa ure′thrae femini′nae [TA] spongy layer of female urethra: a thin layer of spongiose erectile tissue, located just beneath the mucosa and containing a plexus of large veins.

t. spongio′sa vagi′nae [TA] spongy layer of vagina: a thin layer of spongiose erectile tissue, located between the muscular layer and the mucosa of the vagina and containing a large plexus of blood vessels.

testicular tunicae the coverings of the testis; see *tunica albuginea testis, tunica vaginalis testis,* and *tunica vasculosa testis.*

t. vagina′lis tes′tis [TA] the serous membrane covering the front and sides of the testis and epididymis, composed of a visceral layer *(lamina visceralis)* and a parietal layer *(lamina parietalis).*

t. vasculo′sa a vascular coat, or a layer well supplied with blood vessels.

t. vasculo′sa bul′bi [TA] vascular layer of eyeball: the middle, pigmented, vascular coat of the eye, comprising the choroid, the ciliary body, and the iris; called also *uvea* and *uveal tract.*

t. vasculo′sa len′tis the vascular envelope that encloses and nourishes the developing lens of the fetus; it consists of the *pupillary membrane* in the region of the pupil, the *capsulopupillary membrane* around the edge of the lens, and the *capsular membrane* at the back of the lens. It normally degenerates during the late fetal period when the hyaloid artery degenerates.

t. vasculo′sa tes′tis [TA] vascular layer of testis: the layer of blood vessels and loose connective tissue immediately surrounding the testis, underlying the tunica albuginea.

---

tu•ni•cary (too″nĭ-kar′e) tunicate (def. 1).

Tu•ni•ca•ta (too″nĭ-ka′tə) [L. "clothed with a tunic"] Urochordata.

tu•ni•cate (too′nĭ-kāt) 1. having a tunic. 2. urochordate.

tu•ni•cin (too′nĭ-sin) a substance resembling cellulose occurring in the body covering of some of the lowest vertebrates, such as the tunicates or ascidians; animal cellulose.

tun•nel (tun′əl) a passageway through a solid body, completely enclosed except for the open ends, permitting entrance and exit. Cf. *canal.*

aortico–left ventricular t. a congenital communication between the ascending aorta just above the coronary arteries, and the left ventricle.

carpal t. canalis carpi.

Corti t. inner t.

cubital t. the opening between the two heads of the flexor carpi ulnaris muscle through which the ulnar nerve enters the forearm.

flexor t. carpal t.

inner t. a canal extending the length of the cochlea, formed by the pillar cells of the organ of Corti; called also *canal of Corti, Corti t., arcuate zone,* and *zona arcuata.*

outer t. a fluid-filled space in the organ of Corti between the outer hair cells and the outer border cells.

radial t. a channel in the cubital region through which the posterior interosseous nerve passes; the capitulum of the humerus is on its posterior surface proximally, the brachioradialis and brachialis muscles border it laterally, and the supinator muscle borders it distally.

tarsal t. the osseofibrous passage for the posterior tibial vessels, tibial nerve, and flexor tendons, formed by the flexor retinaculum and tarsal bones.

Tuo•hy needle (too′e) [Edward B. *Tuohy,* American anesthesiologist, 1908–1959, who popularized but did not invent it] see under *needle.*

TUR transurethral resection.

tu•ra•nose (tōōr′ə-nōs) a reducing disaccharide composed of fructose and glucose; it is isomeric with sucrose and is part of the trisaccharide melezitose.

tur•ban (tur′bən) [Turkish *tülbend* gauze] a headdress made of a long strip of material wound around the head.

ice t. a soft head wrapping filled with ice, used to promote scalp hypothermia and prevent alopecia during chemotherapy.

Tur•ba•trix (tər-ba′triks) a genus of nematodes. *T. ace′ti* (formerly called *Anguillula aceti*) is the vinegar eel, a species found in vinegar and

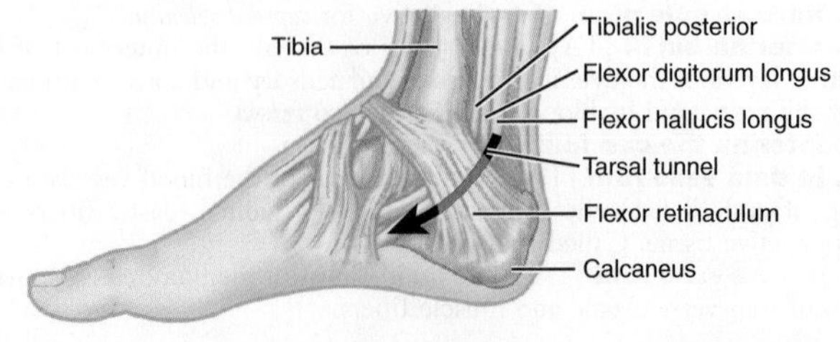

■ Tarsal tunnel.

fermenting vegetable substances, and sometimes in the urine of patients who have used vinegar douches.

tur•bid (tur′bid) [L. *turba* a tumult] cloudy; showing turbidity.

tur•bi•dim•e•ter (tur″bĭ-dim′ə-tər) an instrument that measures the turbidity of a solution by measuring the loss of intensity of a beam of light as it passes through the solution. Cf. *nephelometer*.

tur•bid•i•met•ric (tur″bid-ĭ-met′rik) performed by the turbidimeter.

tur•bi•dim•e•try (tur″bĭ-dim′ə-tre) measurement of the turbidity of a fluid.

tur•bid•i•ty (tər-bid′ĭ-te) cloudiness of a solution caused by the scattering of light by colloidal particles or by suspended precipitate or sediment.

tur•bi•nal (tur′bĭ-nəl) [L. *turbinalis*, from *turbo* a child's top] turbinate.

tur•bi•nate (tur′bĭ-nāt) [L. *turbineus*] 1. shaped like a top. 2. any of the nasal conchae; see terms beginning *concha nasalis*. Called also *turbinal*.
 inferior t. concha nasalis inferior.
 middle t. concha nasalis media.
 sphenoid t. concha sphenoidalis.
 superior t. concha nasalis superior.
 supreme t. concha nasalis suprema.

tur•bi•nat•ed (tur′bĭ-nāt″əd) shaped like a top.

tur•bi•nec•to•my (tur″bĭ-nek′tə-me) [*turbinate* + *-ectomy*] the surgical removal of a nasal concha (turbinate bone).

tur•bino•tome (tər-bin′ə-tōm) an instrument used for removal or cutting of a nasal concha (turbinate bone). Called also *conchotome*.

tur•bi•not•o•my (tur″bĭ-not′ə-me) [*turbinate* + *-tomy*] the surgical cutting of a nasal concha (turbinate bone). Called also *conchotomy*.

Tur•bo•hal•er (tur′bo-hāl″ər) trademark for a type of dry powder inhaler that can deliver multiple doses of medication.

TURBT transurethral resection of bladder tumor.

Türck bundle, column (tērk) [Ludwig *Türck*, Austrian neurologist and laryngologist, 1810–1868] see *tractus corticospinalis anterior* and *fibrae temporopontinae*.

Tur•cot syndrome (tēr-ko′) [Jacques *Turcot*, Canadian physician, 20th century] see under *syndrome*.

tur•ges•cence (tər-jes′əns) [L. *turgescens* swelling] swelling (def. 1).

tur•ges•cent (tər-jes′ənt) [L. *turgescens*] 1. swollen. 2. beginning to swell.

tur•gid (tur′jid) [L. *turgidus*] swollen and congested.

tur•gid•iza•tion (tur″jid-ĭ-za′shən) the creation of turgor in a tissue by the injection of fluid.

tur•gom•e•ter (tər-gom′ə-tər) [*turgor* + *-meter*] an instrument for measuring the amount of turgescence.

tur•gor (tur′gər) [L.] the condition of being turgid; normal or other fullness. See also *swelling* (def. 1).
 skin t. a reflection of the skin's elasticity, measured by monitoring the time it takes for the skin of the forearm to return to position after it is lightly pinched between the examiner's thumb and forefinger. Normal turgor is a return to normal contour within three seconds; if the skin remains elevated (tented) more than three seconds, turgor is decreased.
 t. vita′lis the normal consistency of living tissue.

Turi•cel•la (to͝or″ĭ-sel′ə) a genus of gram-positive, club-shaped bacteria of the order Bifidobacteriales that has not been assigned to a family.
 T. oti′tidis a species that is a normal colonizer of the human auditory canal and occasionally causes opportunistic infections.

tu•ris•ta (too-rēs′tah) [Sp.] Mexican name for *traveler's diarrhea*.

Türk cell (tērk) [Wilhelm *Türk*, Austrian physician, 1871–1916] see under *cell*.

tur•mer•ic (tur′mər-ik) 1. *Curcuma longa*. 2. the rhizome of *C. longa*, which contains curcumin, an orange-yellow coloring principle, and several aromatic principles that give it a pepperlike and bitter taste; used as a coloring agent, chemical indicator, and condiment (as curry powder). Medicinally it is used for the treatment of dyspepsia and anorexia, and it has a wide variety of uses in traditional Chinese medicine, ayurveda, and folk medicine

turm•schä•del (toorm′sha-dəl) [Ger.] a developmental anomaly in which the skull is high and rounded, due to early synostosis of the three major sutures of the skull.

Tur•ner sign (tur′nər) [George Grey *Turner*, British surgeon, 1877–1951] see under *sign*.

Tur•ner syndrome (tur′nər) [Henry Hubert *Turner*, American endocrinologist, 1892–1970] see under *syndrome*.

Tur•ner tooth (hypoplasia) (tur′nər) [Joseph George *Turner*, British dentist, died 1955] see under *tooth*.

tur•nera (tur′nər-ə) damiana.

turn•over (turn′o-vər) 1. the movement of something into, through, and out of a place. 2. the rate at which something is depleted and replaced.
 bone t. see under *remodeling*.
 erythrocyte iron t. (EIT) the rate at which iron moves from the bone marrow into circulating red cells, calculated as: plasma iron turnover (PIT) × red cell utilization (RCU). Called also *red blood cell iron t.*
 plasma iron t. (PIT) the rate at which iron leaves the blood plasma for bone marrow or other tissues, expressed in mg/day; calculated as: (plasma iron concentration) × (plasma volume) × 0.693 ÷ (plasma iron clearance half-time).
 red blood cell iron t. (RBC IT) erythrocyte iron t.

turn•sick (tərn′sik) gid.

turn•sick•ness (tərn′sik-nis) gid.

TURP transurethral resection of the prostate.

tur•pen•tine (tur′pən-tīn) [L. *terebinthina*] the concrete oleoresin obtained from *Pinus palustris* and other species of *Pinus*. It contains a volatile oil, turpentine oil (q.v.) to which its properties are due, and in which form it is generally used.

tur•ri•ceph•a•ly (tur″ĭ-sef′ə-le) oxycephaly.

tu•run•da (tu-run′də) [L. "a roll of lint"] 1. tent (def. 2). 2. a suppository.

Tu•ryn sign (too′rin) [Felix *Turyn*, Polish physician, 20th century] see under *sign*.

tus. [L.] tus′sis (a cough).

tus•sal (tus′əl) [L. *tussis* cough] tussive.

tus•sic•u•la (tə-sik′u-lə) [L., dim. of *tussis* cough] a slight cough.

tus•sic•u•lar (tə-sik′u-lər) [L. *tussicula*] tussive.

tus•sic•u•la•tion (tə-sik″u-la′shən) hacking cough.

tus•si•gen•ic (tus″ĭ-jen′ik) [*tussis* + *-genic*] causing cough.

Tus•si•o•nex Penn•ki•net•ic (tus′e-ə-neks″ pen″kĭ-net′ik) trademark for a combination preparation of hydrocodone polistirex and chlorpheniramine polistirex.

tus•sis (tus′is) [L.] cough.

tus•sive (tus′iv) pertaining to or due to a cough; called also *tussal*, and *tussicular*.

tu•ta•men (tu-ta′mən) pl. *tuta′mina* [L.] a protective covering or structure.
 tuta′mina o′culi ocular adnexa.

TUVP transurethral vaporization of the prostate.

Tween (twēn) trademark for preparations of polysorbates, used with a numerical suffix; e.g., *Tween 80* is a trademark for polysorbate 80.

twig (twig) in anatomy, a final ramification, as of branches of nerves or blood vessels.

twin (twin) one of two offspring produced in the same pregnancy; see *monozygotic t's* and *dizygotic t's*.
 acardiac t. acardius.
 allantoidoangiopagous t's twins joined by the vessels of the umbilical cord only; called also *omphaloangiopagous t's*.
 asymmetrical conjoined t's see *conjoined t's*.
 binovular t's dizygotic t's.
 conjoined t's monozygotic twins whose bodies are joined, ranging from two well-developed individuals joined by a superficial connection of varying extent, usually in the frontal, transverse, or sagittal body plane (*symmetrical* or *equal conjoined t's*), to those in which only a small part of the body is duplicated or one small and incompletely developed parasitic twin is attached to a much larger and more fully developed twin (*asymmetrical* or *unequal conjoined t's*). Called also *Siamese t's*.
 diamnionic t's, diamniotic t's twins developing within separate amniotic cavities; such twins may be monochorionic or dichorionic.
 dichorial t's, dichorionic t's twins having distinct chorions; this includes monozygotic twins separated within 72 hours of fertilization and all dizygotic twins.
 dissimilar t's, dizygotic t's, dizygous t's twins developed from two separate oocytes that were fertilized at the same time, resulting in two zygotes; they may be of the same or different sex, and they have different genomes. Called also *binovular*, *false*, *fraternal*, *heterologous*, *hetero-ovular*, *two-egg*, and *unlike t's*.
 enzygotic t's monozygotic t's.
 equal conjoined t's see *conjoined t's*.
 false t's, fraternal t's dizygotic t's.
 heterologous t's, hetero-ovular t's dizygotic t's.
 identical t's monozygotic t's.

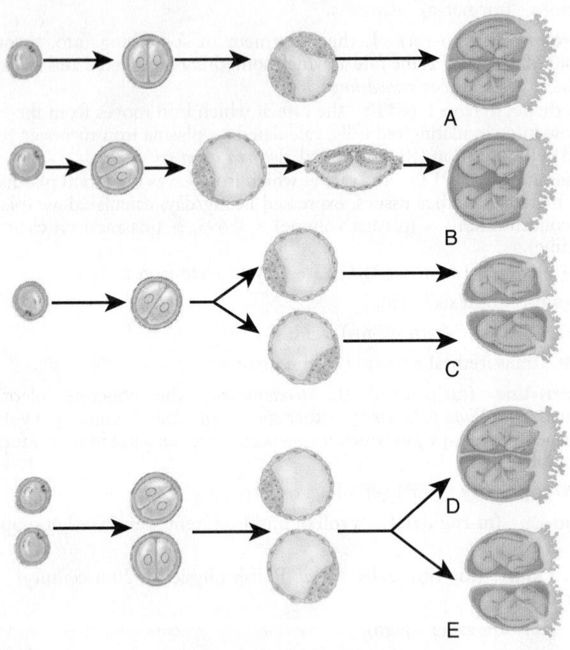

■ Twins. *(A)*, The most common type of monozygotic twinning, with division of the inner cell mass of the blastocyst resulting in separate amnions but a single chorion and placenta; *(B)*, a rare form of monozygotic twinning, with complete division of the embryonic disc resulting in two embryos in a single amniotic sac with a single placenta and chorionic sac; *(C)*, monozygotic twinning with division occurring between the two-cell and morula stages to produce identical blastocysts, resulting in separate amniotic and chorionic sacs and either separate *(shown)* or fused placentas; *(D,E)*, dizygotic twinning, with *(D)* or without *(E)* fusion of the placenta and chorion.

impacted t's, locked t's twins so situated during delivery that the pressure of one against the other prevents simultaneous engagement of both.

membranous t. fetus papyraceus.

monoamnionic t's, monoamniotic t's twins developing within a single amniotic cavity; they are always monozygotic and monochorionic.

monochorial t's, monochorionic t's twins developing with a single chorion; such twins are almost always monozygotic and may be monoamniotic or diamniotic.

mono-ovular t's, monovular t's monozygotic t's.

monozygotic t's, monozygous t's two individuals developed from one zygote that divided into two embryos at an early stage (usually during the first eight days); the twins therefore have identical genomes. Called also *enzygotic, identical, mono-ovular, monovular, similar, true,* and *uniovular t's.*

omphaloangiopagous t's allantoidoangiopagous t's.

one-egg t's monozygotic t's.

Siamese t's conjoined t's.

similar t's, true t's monozygotic t's.

symmetrical conjoined t's see *conjoined t's.*

two-egg t's dizygotic t's.

unequal conjoined t's see *conjoined t's.*

uniovular t's monozygotic t's.

unlike t's dizygotic t's.

twinge (twinj) a short, sharp pain.

twin•ning (twin′ing) 1. the simultaneous production of two (or more) offspring. 2. the production of symmetrical structures or parts by division.

experimental t. embryonic duplication produced by purposeful external intervention.

spontaneous t. embryonic duplication without external intervention, as occurs in nature.

Twin•rix (twin′riks) trademark for a combination preparation of hepatitis A vaccine inactivated and hepatitis B vaccine (recombinant).

twin•ship (twin′ship) the state of being a twin.

Twis•ton (twis′ton) trademark for preparations of rotoxamine tartrate.

twitch (twich) 1. a brief contractile response of a skeletal muscle elicited by a single maximal volley of impulses in the motor neurons supplying it. 2. a noose passed around the lip or ear and through a perforation in a board, used for restraining a horse during minor surgery.

fast t. see *muscle fibers,* under *fiber.*

slow t. see *muscle fibers,* under *fiber.*

twitch•ing (twich′ing) the occurrence of a single contraction or a series of contractions of a muscle; see *twitch.*

fascicular t. repetitive brief contraction of large groups of bundles of muscle fibers.

fibrillar t. repetitive brief contraction of single bundles of muscle fibers.

Trousseau t. repetitive brief contraction involving muscles of the face.

Twort-d'He•relle phenomenon (twort′ dĕ-rel′) [Frederick William *Twort,* English bacteriologist, 1877–1950; Félix Hubert *d'Herelle,* Canadian bacteriologist in France, 1873–1949] see under *phenomenon.*

TWZ triangular working zone; see *Kambin triangular working zone,* under *zone.*

TXA_2, TXB_2 thromboxanes A_2 and B_2; see *thromboxane.*

Ty•ga•cil (ti′gə-sil) trademark for a preparation of tigecycline.

ty•ing up (ti′ing up) azoturia (def. 2).

ty•lec•to•my (ti-lek′tə-me) [Gr. *tylos* knot + *-ectomy*] lumpectomy.

Ty•le•nol (ti′lə-nol) trademark for preparations of acetaminophen.

tyl•i•on (til′e-on) [Gr. *tyleion* cushion] the point on the anterior edge of the optic groove in the median line.

ty•lo•ma (ti-lo′mə) callus (def. 1).

ty•lo•sin (ti′lo-sin) [USP] a macrolide antibiotic, similar to erythromycin, used in veterinary practice.

ty•lo•sis (ti-lo′sis) [Gr. *tylōs* a knob or callus] formation of a callus. **tylot′ic** *adj*

t. cilia′ris thickening of the eyelids due to long-term ulcerative blepharitis.

t. palma′ris et planta′ris palmoplantar keratoderma.

Ty•los•ter•one (ti-los′tə-rōn) trademark for a combination preparation of diethylstilbestrol and methyltestosterone.

Ty•lox (ti′loks) trademark for a combination preparation of oxycodone hydrochloride and acetaminophen.

ty•lox•a•pol (ti-lok′sə-pol) [USP] a nonionic liquid polymer of the alkyl aryl polyether alcohol type; used as a surfactant to aid liquefaction and removal of mucopurulent bronchopulmonary secretions, administered by inhalation through a nebulizer or with a stream of oxygen.

Tym•pa•ge•sic (tim″pə-je′zik) trademark for a preparation of antipyrine, benzocaine, and phenylephrine hydrochloride otic solution.

tym•pa•nal (tim′pə-nəl) 1. tympanic (def. 1). 2. tympanitic (def. 1).

tym•pa•nec•to•my (tim″pə-nek′tə-me) [*tympan-* + *-ectomy*] excision of the tympanic membrane. Called also *myringectomy.*

tym•pan•ia (tim-pan′e-ə) tympanites.

tym•pan•ic (tim-pan′ik) [L. *tympanicus,* from Gr. *tympanon* drum] 1. of or pertaining to the tympanic cavity or the tympanic membrane. 2. bell-like or resonant; called also *tympanitic.* 3. tympanitic (def. 1).

tym•pa•nic•i•ty (tim″pə-nis′ĭ-te) a tympanic (hollow or resonant) quality.

tym•pa•nism (tim′pə-niz-əm) tympanites.

tym•pa•ni•tes (tim″pə-ni′tēz) [Gr. *tympanitēs,* from *tympanon* drum] distention of the abdomen from gas or air in the intestine or peritoneal cavity, as in peritonitis and typhoid fever. Called also *meteorism.*

uterine t. physometra.

tym•pa•nit•ic (tim″pə-nit′ik) 1. pertaining to or affected with tympanites. 2. tympanic (def. 2).

tympan(o)- [Gr. *tympanon* drum] a combining form denoting relationship to the tympanic cavity or to the tympanic membrane.

tym•pa•no•cen•te•sis (tim″pə-no-sen-te′sis) surgical puncture of the tympanic membrane for removal of fluid from the middle ear. Cf. *myringotomy.*

tym•pa•no•eu•sta•chi•an (tim″pə-no-u-sta′ke-ən) pertaining to the tympanic cavity and auditory tube.

tym•pa•no•gen•ic (tim″pə-no-jen′ik) [*tympano-* + *-genic*] arising from the tympanic cavity.

tym•pa•no•gram (tim-pan′o-gram″) [*tympano-* + *-gram*] a graphic representation of the relative compliance and impedance of the tympanic membrane and ossicles of the middle ear obtained by tympanometry.

tym•pa•no•hy•al (tim″pə-no-hi′əl) 1. pertaining to the tympanic cavity and the second pharyngeal (hyoid) arch. 2. a small bone or cartilage at the base of the styloid process of the temporal bone; in early life it becomes a part of the temporal bone.

tym•pa•no•mal•le•al (tim″pə-no-mal′e-əl) pertaining to the tympanic membrane and the malleus.

tym•pa•no•man•dib•u•lar (tim″pə-no″man-dib′u-lər) pertaining to the tympanic cavity and the mandible.

tym•pa•no•mas•toid•ec•to•my (tim″pə-no-mas″toid-ek′tə-me) mastoidectomy with tympanectomy.

canal wall down t. open-cavity t.

canal wall up t. closed-cavity t.

closed-cavity t. tympanomastoidectomy with tympanoplasty and maintenance of an intact posterior wall of the ear canal. Called also *closed-cavity mastoidectomy*, *canal wall up t.* or *mastoidectomy*, and *intact canal wall t.* or *mastoidectomy*. Cf. *open-cavity t.*

intact canal wall t. closed-cavity t.

open-cavity t. tympanomastoidectomy with removal of the posterior wall of the ear canal, such as radical mastoidectomy and modified radical mastoidectomy. Called also *open-cavity mastoidectomy*, and *canal wall down t.* or *mastoidectomy*. Cf. *closed-cavity t.*

tym•pa•no•mas•toid•itis (tim″pə-no-mas″toi-di′tis) inflammation of the tympanic cavity and the mastoid air cells.

tym•pa•no•me•a•tal (tim″pə-no-me-a′təl) pertaining to the tympanum and the external acoustic meatus.

tym•pa•nom•e•try (tim″pə-nom′ə-tre) indirect measurement of the compliance (mobility) and impedance of the tympanic membrane and ossicles of the middle ear; it is done by subjecting the external acoustic meatus to positive, normal, and negative air pressure and monitoring the resultant sound energy flow. **tympanomet′ric** *adj*

tym•pa•no•plas•ty (tim′pə-no-plas″te) [*tympano-* + *-plasty*] surgical reconstruction of the hearing mechanism of the middle ear, with restoration of the drum membrane to protect the round window from sound pressure, and establishment of ossicular continuity between the tympanic membrane and the oval window. See also *myringoplasty*. **tympanoplas′tic** *adj*

tym•pa•no•scle•ro•sis (tim″pə-no-sklə-ro′sis) the presence of masses of hard, dense connective tissue around the auditory ossicles. **tympanosclerot′ic** *adj*

tym•pa•no•squa•mo•sal (tim″pə-no-skwah-mo′səl) pertaining to the pars tympanica and pars squamosa of the temporal bone.

tym•pa•no•sta•pe•di•al (tim″pə-no-stə-pe′de-əl) pertaining to the tympanic cavity and the stapes.

tym•pa•nos•to•my (tim″pə-nos′tə-me) myringotomy.

tym•pa•no•tem•po•ral (tim″pə-no-tem′pə-rəl) pertaining to the tympanic cavity and the region over the temporal bone or region.

tym•pa•not•o•my (tim″pə-not′ə-me) [*tympano-* + *-tomy*] 1. tympanocentesis. 2. myringotomy.

facial recess t. posterior t.

posterior t. tympanotomy with exenteration of the air cells posterior to the facial recess. Called also *facial recess t.*

tym•pa•nous (tim′pə-nəs) tympanitic (def. 1).

tym•pa•num (tim′pə-nəm) [L., from Gr. *tympanon* drum] 1. membrana tympanica. 2. cavitas tympani.

tym•pa•ny (tim′pə-ne) [Gr. *tympanias*] 1. tympanites. 2. a tympanic, or bell-like, percussion note.

bell t. a modified tympanitic note heard on percussion of the chest in some cases of pneumothorax.

ruminal t. a kind of indigestion in cattle and sheep, marked by an abnormal collection of gas in the rumen; the usual cause is a diet too high in carbohydrates. As gas volume increases, the rumen presses against adjacent organs; it may occlude the vena cava and cause circulatory problems or press against the diaphragm and lungs and cause death from asphyxia. Called also *bloat*.

ruminal t., primary ruminal tympany caused by eating too much wet or frothy legume, particularly alfalfa or clover, which forms a stable foam in the rumen. Called also *frothy bloat*.

ruminal t., secondary ruminal tympany caused by an esophageal obstruction that prevents eructation; called also *free gas bloat*.

Skoda t., skodaic t. skodaic resonance.

t. of the stomach bloat (def. 1).

Tyn•dall cone, effect (phenomenon), light (tin′dəl) [John *Tyndall*, British physicist, 1820–1893] see under *cone*, *effect*, and *light*.

tyn•dal•li•za•tion (tin″dəl-ĭ-za′shən) [John *Tyndall*] fractional sterilization.

type (tīp) [Gr. *typos* type] something with particular characteristics, such as a person, substance, or case of a disease.

ampullary t. of renal pelvis a type of renal pelvis in which the calices open into a saclike central chamber.

blood t. blood group; see under *B*.

body t. somatotype.

branching t. of renal pelvis a type of renal pelvis without a central chamber, but simply formed by the merger of several calices at the opening into the ureter.

Fitzpatrick skin t. one of the six skin types according to the Fitzpatrick scale.

mating t. in ciliate protozoa, certain bacteria, and certain fungi, the equivalent of a sex; as many as eight sexes are present in some species of protozoa.

personality t. any of various categories of both normal and abnormal personality variants; usually they derive from a theory-based topology, such as introvert/extrovert or oral/anal/phallic.

phage t. an intraspecies type of bacterium demonstrated by phage typing (see under *typing*); called also *phagotype*.

test t. see *test type*.

wild t. the typical form occurring in a natural population or in the standard laboratory stock, as a strain, phenotype, or gene, and therefore designated as representative of the group.

Ty•phim Vi (ti′fim) trademark for a preparation of typhoid Vi polysaccharide vaccine.

typh•lec•to•my (tif-lek′tə-me) cecectomy.

typh•li•tis (tif-li′tis) cecitis.

neutropenic t. former name for *necrotizing enterocolitis*.

typhl(o)-[1] [Gr. *typhlos* blind] a combining form denoting relationship to blindness.

typhl(o)-[2] [Gr. *typhlon* cecum, from *typhlos* blind] a combining form denoting relationship to the cecum; see also terms beginning with *cec(o)-*.

Typh•lo•coe•lum (tif″lo-se′ləm) former name for a genus of trematodes, now classified as part of *Tracheophilus*.

typh•lol•o•gy (tif-lol′ə-je) [*typhlo-*[1] + *-logy*] the study of blindness.

typh•lot•o•my (tif-lot′ə-me) [*typhlo*[2] + *-tomy*] cecotomy.

ty•phoid (ti′foid) [Gr. *typhōdes* like smoke; delirious] 1. resembling typhus. 2. see under *fever*. 3. typhoidal.

fowl t. an acute infectious disease of fowl caused by *Salmonella enterica* subspecies *enterica* serovar Gallinarum, marked by drowsiness, anorexia, extreme weakness, usually diarrhea, and death.

provocation t. the systemic reaction to the endotoxin of killed typhoid bacilli in typhoid vaccine.

ty•phoid•al (ti-foid′əl) pertaining to or resembling typhoid fever; called also *typhoid*.

ty•phous (ti′fəs) pertaining to or resembling typhus.

ty•phus (ti′fəs) [Gr. *typhos* stupor arising from fever] any of a group of acute, arthropod-borne infections caused by rickettsiae, closely related clinically and pathologically but differing in signs and symptoms and severity; all are characterized by severe headache, chills, high fever, stupor, and a macular, maculopapular, petechial, or papulovesicular eruption. The most common conditions in the group are epidemic typhus, its recrudescent form known as Brill-Zinsser disease, murine typhus, and scrub typhus. Called also *typhus fever*. In English-speaking countries, often used alone to refer to epidemic typhus, whereas in several European languages it refers to typhoid fever.

Australian tick t. Queensland tick t.

canine t. Stuttgart disease.

cat flea t. a flea-borne form of typhus clinically similar to murine typhus, caused by *Rickettsia felis* and transmitted by the cat flea (*Ctenocephalides felis*).

classic t. epidemic t.

endemic t. murine t.

epidemic t. the classic, louse-borne form of typhus, caused by *Rickettsia prowazekii*, which is transmitted from person to person by the human body louse, *Pediculus humanus humanus*, although the organism can also grow in the head louse, *P. humanus capitis*. Characteristics include abrupt onset; chills, fever, and malaise; headache that progresses in severity; backache and myalgia; a skin eruption that spreads from the trunk to cover much of the body; and central nervous system symptoms from dullness to stupor and sometimes coma and death. Recrudescences occur (see *Brill-Zinsser disease*, under *disease*). Outbreaks usually occur in crowded or unsanitary environments, so that it has been called by names such as *camp fever*, *prison fever*, and *war fever*.

European t., exanthematous t. epidemic t.

flea-borne t. murine t.

flying squirrel t., flying squirrel–associated t. an acute infectious disease occurring in the southeastern United States, particularly during the winter months, caused by *Rickettsia prowazekii*, which is transmitted to humans by the fleas and lice of the flying squirrel; it is clinically similar to epidemic typhus but has a lower mortality rate.

Indian tick t., Israeli tick t. boutonneuse fever.

Kenya t., Kenyan tick t., Kenya tick t. boutonneuse fever.

louse-borne t. epidemic t.

mite-borne t. scrub t.

murine t. an acute, flea-borne endemic infectious disease clinically similar to but milder than epidemic typhus; caused by *Rickettsia typhi*,

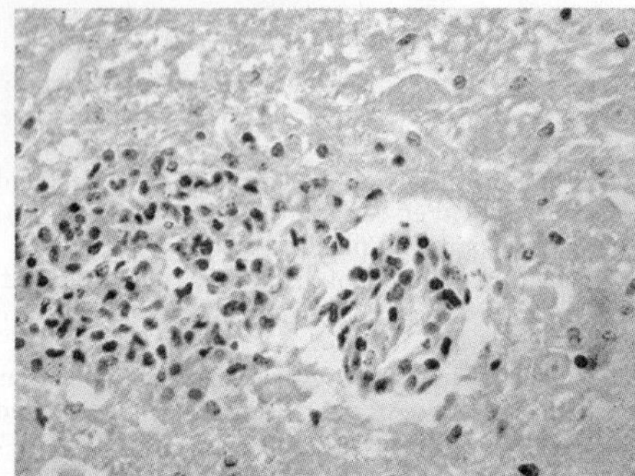

■ Epidemic typhus. Nodule in the brain.

which is transmitted from rats to humans chiefly by the rat flea, *Xenopsylla cheopis*. The condition has been seen in many parts of the world and given a variety of local names. Called also *endemic*, *flea-borne*, or *rat t.*

North Asian tick t. a mild type of spotted fever, characterized by high fever, headache, malaise, conjunctival injection, a maculopapular rash, and a primary ulcerative lesion at the site of the tick bite. Besides Siberia, it has also been observed in Central and East Asia and a few other parts of the world. It is caused by *Rickettsia sibirica*, which is transmitted by ticks of the genera *Dermacentor* and *Haemaphysalis*. Called also *Siberian tick t.*

North Queensland tick t. Queensland tick t.

Queensland tick t. an acute type of spotted fever marked by a primary lesion (tache noire), caused by *Rickettsia australis*, and transmitted by the Australian ticks *Ixodes holocyclus* and *I. tasmani*. Called also *Australian* or *North Queensland tick t.*

rat t., rat flea t. murine t.

recrudescent t. Brill-Zinsser disease.

São Paulo t. Rocky Mountain spotted fever.

scrub t. an acute infectious disease resembling epidemic typhus, caused by *Orientia tsutsugamushi* and transmitted by the bite of infected mite larvae (chiggers) of the species *Trombicula*. It occurs chiefly in Asia and the southern and western Pacific, and is characterized by a pathognomonic primary cutaneous lesion or eschar (tache noire) at the site of inoculation, with regional lymphadenopathy, fever, and a maculopapular rash. Called also *island*, *Japanese flood*, *Japanese river*, or *tsutsugamushi fever*; and *mite-borne* or *tropical t.*, as well as by many local names.

shop t. urban t.

Siberian tick t. North Asian tick t.

tick t., tick-borne t. 1. see under *fever*. 2. spotted fever.

tropical t. scrub t.

urban t. a mild form of murine typhus observed in indoor workers in Malaysia and the Mediterranean region; called also *shop t.*

typ·i·cal (tip′ĭ-kəl) [Gr. *typikos*] presenting the distinctive features of any type.

typ·ing (tīp′ing) determination of the type category to which an individual, object, or other entity belongs; e.g., bacteria, blood cells, cell cultures, or tissues.

t. of blood classification of the blood with reference to various erythrocytic membrane antigens. See *blood group*.

HLA t. determination of the human leukocyte antigens (HLA) possessed by an individual. Class I antigens (HLA-A, -B, and -C) are detected by lymphocyte microcytotoxicity assay using standard typing sera. Class II antigens are detected by one-way mixed lymphocyte cultures using panels of homozygous typing cells; they may also be identified by primed lymphocyte typing (q.v.). DR Class II antigens are also detected by lymphocyte microtoxicity assay using B lymphocytes and anti-DR antibody types. HLA typing is used to identify compatible donors and recipients for transplantation or platelet or granulocyte transfusion, to establish associations of human leukocyte antigens with diseases, and in paternity testing.

phage t. characterization of bacteria, extending to strain differences, by demonstration of susceptibility to a race or races (a spectrum) of bacteriophage; this is widely applied to staphylococci, typhoid bacilli, and other bacteria for epidemiological purposes.

primed lymphocyte t. (PLT) a technique used for typing of Class II HLA antigens: unknown cells are exposed to a panel of lymphocytes primed against specific HLA antigens by prior coculture with stimulator cells that matched the primed cells at all but one HLA locus; when restimulated by the same HLA antigen the primed cells give a secondary proliferative response, which shows that the unknown cells bear the same antigen as the stimulator cells.

tissue t. HLA t.

ty·po·dont (ti′po-dont) an artificial model that contains artificial teeth or natural teeth that are used for teaching exercises.

ty·pol·o·gy (ti-pol′ə-je) the study of types; the science of classifying, as bacteria according to type.

ty·po·scope (ti′po-skōp) [Gr. *typos* type + *-scope*] an instrument to aid amblyopia and help cataract patients in reading.

ty·pus (ti′pəs) [L.] type.

t. ampulla′ris pel′vis rena′lis [TA] ampullary type of renal pelvis; see under *type*.

t. dendri′ticus pel′vis rena′lis [TA] branching type of renal pelvis; see under *type*.

Tyr tyrosine.

ty·ra·mine (ti′rə-mēn) a decarboxylation product of tyrosine, which may be converted to cresol and phenol; closely related structurally to epinephrine and norepinephrine, it has a similar but weaker action. It is found in decayed animal tissue, ripe cheese, and ergot.

ty·re·sin (ti-re′sin) a principle derivable from the venom of serpents and from the juice of mushrooms; it was thought to be an antidote for snake poisoning.

tyr(o)- [Gr. *tyros* cheese] a combining form denoting relationship to cheese.

ty·ro·ci·dine (ti″ro-si′din) a polypeptide antibiotic that is the major component of tyrothricin, the lesser component being gramicidin. It can be separated into three components, tyrocidines A, B, and C.

Ty·rode solution (ti′rōd) [Maurice Vejux *Tyrode*, American pharmacologist, 1878–1930] see under *solution*.

ty·rog·e·nous (ti-roj′ə-nəs) [*tyro-* + *-genous*] originating in cheese.

Ty·rog·ly·phus (ti-rog′lĭ-fəs) [*tyro-* + Gr. *glyphein* to carve] *Tyrophagus*.

T. si′ro *Acarus siro*.

ty·roid (ti′roid) caseous.

ty·ro·ma·to·sis (ti″ro-mə-to′sis) a condition characterized by caseous degeneration.

ty·ro·pa·no·ate so·di·um (ti″ro-pə-no′āt) a diagnostic radiopaque medium for use in cholecystography.

Ty·roph·a·gus (ti-rof′ə-gəs) the meal mites, a genus of pale, soft-bodied mites of the family Acaridae; called also *Tyroglyphus*.

T. castella′ni the copra mite, the species that causes copra itch.

T. fari′nae the flour mite, found in flour mills and granaries.

T. lon′gior the cheese mite, which has been reported from the human urinary and digestive tracts and feces.

T. si′ro *Acarus siro*.

ty·ros·amine (ti-rōs′ə-mēn) tyramine.

ty·ro·sin·ase (ti-ro′sin-ās) a monophenol monooxygenase that can also act as a catechol oxidase; absence of enzyme activity, an autosomal recessive trait, leads to oculocutaneous albinism type 1a.

ty·ro·sine (Tyr, Y) (ti′ro-sēn) 1. a nonessential amino acid, β-*p*-hydroxyphenylalanine, found in most proteins and synthesized metabolically from phenylalanine; it is a precursor of thyroid hormones, catecholamines, and melanin. See also table at *amino acid*. 2. [USP] a preparation of tyrosine used as a dietary supplement.

ty·ro·sine ami·no·trans·fer·ase (ti′ro-sēn ə-me″no-trans′fər-ās) tyrosine transaminase.

ty·ro·sine hy·droxy·lase (TH) (ti′ro-sēn hi-drok′sə-lās) a monooxygenase that activates molecular oxygen to catalyze the hydroxylation of tyrosine to dopa; it is found in adrenal medulla and catecholaminergic neurons and requires the cofactor tetrahydrobiopterin. Deficiency of the enzyme, an autosomal recessive trait caused by mutation of the *TH* gene, which encodes the enzyme, results in dopa-responsive dystonia. In official nomenclature, called *tyrosine 3-monooxygenase* [EC 1.14.16.2].

ty·ro·sine ki·nase (ti′ro-sēn ki′nās) protein-tyrosine kinase.

ty·ro·sin·e·mia (ti″ro-sĭ-ne′me-ə) any of several aminoacidopathies of tyrosine metabolism characterized by hypertyrosinemia, tyrosyluria, and urinary excretion of related metabolites such as *p*-hydroxyphenylpyruvic acid. See also *hawkinsinuria* and *hyperphenylalaninemia*.

hepatorenal t., hereditary t. t. type I.

neonatal t. a transitory, usually asymptomatic, neonatal disorder caused by a combination of immaturity of the enzyme 4-hydroxyphenylpyruvate dioxygenase, elevated dietary intake of tyrosine and phenylalanine, and a relative ascorbate deficiency. It occurs most often in premature infants and usually has no sequelae; a causal relationship with mild mental retardation is possible.

t. type I an autosomal recessive disorder due to mutation in the *FAH* gene (locus: 15q23-q25), which encodes fumarylacetoacetase, an enzyme important in tyrosine catabolism. It is characterized by accumulation of succinylacetoacetate and succinylacetone, leading to secondary deficiencies in porphobilinogen synthase and other enzymes and subsequent hepatorenal damage. The *acute* form shows onset soon after birth, with cabbagelike odor and death from liver failure in infancy; the *chronic* form is characterized by chronic liver disease, renal tubular dysfunction, hypophosphatemic rickets, and death in childhood.

t. type II a rare autosomal recessive disorder due to mutation in the *TAT* gene (locus: 16q22.1-q22.3), which encodes tyrosine transaminase, an enzyme important in tyrosine catabolism. Clinical characteristics include crystallization of the accumulated tyrosine in the epidermis as palmoplantar hyperkeratosis and in the corneas as herpetiform ulcers; frequently patients have mental retardation. Called also *Richner-Hanhart syndrome.*

t. type III an extremely rare autosomal recessive disorder caused by homozygous mutation in the *HPD* gene (locus: 12q24-qter), which encodes 4-hydroxyphenylpyruvate dioxygenase, an enzyme important in tyrosine catabolism. It is characterized by hypertyrosinemia and massive urinary excretion of its derivatives, mild mental retardation, seizures, but absence of liver damage. Cf. *hawkinsinuria.*

ty·ro·sine 3-mono·oxy·ge·nase (ti′ro-sēn mon″o-ok′sə-jən-ās) [EC 1.14.16.2] official nomenclature for *tyrosine hydroxylase.*

ty·ro·sine trans·am·i·nase (ti′ro-sēn trans-am′ĭ-nās) [EC 2.6.1.5] an enzyme of the transferase class that catalyzes the transamination of tyrosine to form the keto acid *p*-hydroxyphenylpyruvate as the first step in the catabolism of tyrosine. Deficiency of the enzyme, an autosomal recessive trait, causes tyrosinemia, type II.

ty·ro·sin·o·sis (ti″ro-sĭ-no′sis) abnormal accumulation of tyrosine; the term is usually used to denote type I tyrosinemia. However, it is sometimes used to describe a single case of abnormal tyrosine metabolism characterized by myasthenia gravis but neither hepatorenal nor oculocutaneous signs and elevated urinary 4-hydroxyphenylpyruvic acid; the presentation was atypical but it was never biochemically classified.

ty·ro·sis (ti-ro′sis) caseation (def. 2).

ty·ro·syl (ti′ro-səl) the acyl radical of tyrosine.

ty·ro·syl·uria (ti″ro-səl-u′re-ə) the increased urinary excretion of *p*-hydroxyphenyl compounds derived from tyrosine, as in tyrosinemia.

ty·ro·thri·cin (ti″ro-thri′sin) an antibiotic substance isolated from the soil bacillus *Bacillus brevis,* consisting principally of two polypeptides, the major one being tyrocidine and the other gramicidin. It is effective against many gram-positive bacteria, and is applied topically in pyodermic, ocular, and other localized infections due to susceptible organisms.

Tyr·rell fascia, hook (tir′əl) [Frederick *Tyrrell,* English anatomist, 1793–1843] see *fascia rectoprostatica* and see under *hook.*

Ty·sab·ri (ti-sab′re) trademark for a preparation of natalizumab.

Ty·son glands (crypts) (ti′sən) [Edward *Tyson,* English physician and anatomist, 1650–1708] glandulae preputiales.

ty·so·ni·an (ti-so′ne-ən) named for Edward *Tyson.*

ty·so·ni·tis (ti″sə-ni′tis) inflammation of the preputial (Tyson) glands.

ty·vel·ose (ti′vəl-ōs) an unusual sugar found in the lipopolysaccharides of certain serovars of *Salmonella.* It is the determinant of somatic (O) antigen factor 9 of group D salmonellae.

Ty·ze·ka (ti-ze′kə) trademark for a preparation of telbivudine.

Ty·zine (ti′zēn) trademark for preparations of tetrahydrozoline hydrochloride.

Tyz·ze·ria (ti-zēr′e-ə) a genus of coccidian protozoa (suborder Eimeriina, order Eucoccidiida), characterized by the presence of oocysts containing eight naked sporozoites. *T. pernicio′sa* is highly pathogenic for domestic ducklings, being parasitic in the small intestine, especially in the upper half.

Tzanck cell, test (tsahngk) [Arnault *Tzanck,* Russian dermatologist in France, 1886–1954] see under *cell* and *test.*

Tza·neen disease (tsah-nēn′) [*Tzaneen,* South Africa, where the disease was first reported] see under *disease.*

TZD thiazolidinedione.

tzet·ze (tset′se) tsetse.

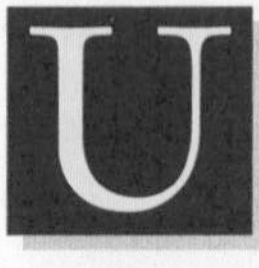

U uranium; uracil; uridine; international unit of enzyme activity; unit *(on the JCAHO "Do Not Use" List).*

u atomic mass unit.

uar·thri·tis (u″ahr-thri′tis) gouty arthritis.

ubi·deca·re·none (u″bĭ-dek″ə-re′nōn) [NF] ubiquinone.

ubi·qui·nol (u″bĭ-kwĭ-nol′) the reduced form of a ubiquinone.

ubi·qui·nol–cy·to·chrome-c re·duc·tase (u″bĭ-kwĭ-nol′ si′to-krōm rē-duk′tās) [EC 1.10.2.2] an enzyme complex of the inner mitochondrial membrane that catalyzes the transfer of electrons from ubiquinol to cytochrome *c*, oxidizing the former and reducing the latter in a reaction of the electron transport chain (q.v.). The enzyme contains cytochromes *b* and c_1 and iron-sulfur prosthetic groups and is associated with proton translocation and the resultant synthesis of ATP. Called also *ubiquinol dehydrogenase.*

ubi·qui·nol de·hy·dro·gen·ase (u″bĭ-kwĭ-nol′ de-hi′dro-jən-ās) ubiquinol–cytochrome-*c* reductase.

ubi·qui·none (u″bĭ-kwĭ-nōn′) a quinone derivative with a variable length side chain of isoprene units; in mammals it usually contains ten such units. It occurs in the lipid core of inner mitochondrial membranes and functions in the electron transport chain (q.v.), acting as a point of entry for electrons from FAD and transferring them to ubiquinol–cytochrome-*c* reductase. In naturopathic practice it is administered for a wide variety of indications, and it is used as a dietary supplement for its antioxidant properties. Abbreviated Q or Q_{10}. Called also *coenzyme Q, coenzyme* Q_{10}, and *ubidecarenone.*

ubiq·ui·tin (u-bik′wĭ-tin) a 76–amino acid polypeptide that is present in the cells of all higher animals and plants; it attaches to proteins during intracellular proteolysis, marking them for degradation by proteasomes.

ubiq·ui·ti·na·tion (u-bik″wĭ-tĭ-na′shən) attachment of ubiquitin to proteins during intracellular proteolysis. **ubiquitinat′ed** *adj*

ubiq·ui·tin·yl·a·tion (u-bik″wĭ-tin″ə-la′shən) ubiquitination.

Uchi·da technique (oo-che′də) [Hajime *Uchida*, Japanese obstetrician and gynecologist, 20th century] see under *technique.*

ud·der (ud′ər) the mammary organ of cattle and certain other mammals; within the large baglike envelope are two or more glands, each having a teat.

UDP uridine diphosphate.

UDP-*N*-ac·e·tyl·ga·lac·to·sa·mine (as″ə-tēl-gal″ak-tōs′ə-mēn) a nucleotide derivative of *N*-acetylgalactosamine; it donates acetylgalactosamine groups in the synthesis of glycosaminoglycans.

UDP-*N*-ac·e·tyl·glu·co·sa·mine (as″ə-tēl″gloo-kōs′ə-mēn) a nucleotide derivative of *N*-acetylglucosamine; it donates acetylglucosamine groups in the synthesis of glycosaminoglycans and is the parent compound for other hexosamines.

UDP-*N*-ac·e·tyl·glu·co·sa·mine 4-epim·er·ase (as″ə-tēl″gloo-kōs′ə-mēn ə-pim′ə-rās) [EC 5.1.3.7] an enzyme of the isomerase class that catalyzes the interconversion of the epimers UDP-*N*-acetylglucosamine and UDP-*N*-acetylgalactosamine.

UDP-*N*-ac·e·tyl·glu·co·sa·mine–ly·so·so·mal-en·zyme *N*-ac·e·tyl·glu·co·sa·mine·phos·pho·trans·fer·ase (as″ə-tēl″gloo-kōs′ə-mēn li″so-so′məl en′zīm as″ə-tēl″gloo-kōs″ə-mēn-fos″fo-trans′fər-ās) [EC 2.7.8.17] an enzyme of the transferase class that catalyzes a step in the synthesis of the mannose 6-phosphate recognition markers necessary on most lysosomal enzymes for internalization of the enzymes into lysosomes. It is a hexameric protein comprising two alpha, two beta, and two gamma subunits; the subunits are encoded by two separate genes. Deficiency of the enzyme results in mucolipidosis type II or III, with the specific type related to the subunit or subunits affected as well as to the level of enzyme activity remaining. Called also *N-acetylglucosaminylphosphotransferase.*

UDP-*N*-ac·e·tyl·glu·co·sa·mine py·ro·phos·phor·y·lase (as″ə-tēl-gloo-kōs′ə-mēn pi″ro-fos-for′ə-lās) [EC 2.7.7.23] an enzyme of the transferase class that catalyzes the attachment of a UMP group from UTP to *N*-acetylglucosamine 1-phosphate, forming UDP-*N*-acetylglucosamine (UDP-GlcNAc), the final step in the biosynthetic pathway of UDP-GlcNAc from fructose-6-phosphate. It is a sperm-associated antigen that has been implicated in antibody-mediated infertility in men. Called also *antigen X.* In official nomenclature, the preferred name is now *UDP-N-acetylglucosamine diphosphorylase.*

UDP-ga·lac·tose (gə-lak′tōs) a nucleotide derivative of galactose; it donates galactosyl groups in the synthesis of lactose, polysaccharides, and glycosaminoglycans and is an intermediate in the metabolism of galactose.

UDP-ga·lac·tose 4-epim·er·ase (gə-lak′tōs ə-pim′ər-ās) UDP-glucose 4-epimerase.

UDP-glu·cose (gloo′kōs) a nucleotide derivative of glucose; it donates glucosyl groups in the synthesis of glycogen and other polysaccharides. It is the parent compound from which the other UDP-hexoses are synthesized.

UDP-glu·cose 6-de·hy·dro·gen·ase (gloo′kōs de-hi′dro-jən-ās) [EC 1.1.1.22] an enzyme of the oxidoreductase class that catalyzes the oxidation of UDP-glucose to UDP-glucuronate, using NAD^+ as an electron acceptor.

UDP-glu·cose 4-epim·er·ase (gloo′kōs ə-pim′ər-ās) [EC 5.1.3.2] an enzyme of the isomerase class that catalyzes the interconversion of UDP-galactose and UDP-glucose in the metabolism of galactose, requiring NAD^+ as a cofactor. Deficiency of the enzyme in erythrocytes, an autosomal recessive trait, causes accumulation in red cells of galactose 1-phosphate. Called also *UDP-galactose 4-epimerase.*

UDP-glu·cose 4-epim·er·ase de·fi·cien·cy (gloo′kōs ə-pim′ər-ās) a form of galactosemia caused by mutations in the *GALE* gene (locus: 1p36-p35), which encodes UDP-glucose 4-epimerase. There are two forms: one is benign and characterized by the accumulation of galactose 1-phosphate in erythrocytes and leukocytes, while the other is severe and clinically resembles classic galactosemia, with the addition of hypotonia and sensorineural hearing loss.

UDP-glu·cose–hex·ose-1-phos·phate uri·dyl·yl·trans·fer·ase (gloo′kōs hek′sōs fos′fāt u″rĭ-dil″əl-trans′fər-ās) [EC 2.7.7.12] an enzyme of the transferase class that catalyzes the exchange of galactose 1-phosphate for the glucose 1-phosphate moiety of UDP-glucose, forming UDP-galactose and glucose 1-phosphate. The reaction is the second step in the utilization of galactose as a fuel. Lack of enzyme activity, an autosomal recessive trait, causes galactosemia. Called also *galactose 1-phosphate uridyltransferase, hexose 1-phosphate uridylyltransferase,* and *uridyl transferase.*

UDP-glu·cose py·ro·phos·pho·ry·lase (gloo′kōs pi″ro-fos-for′ə-lās) UTP–glucose-1-phosphate uridylyltransferase.

UDP-glu·cu·ro·nate (gloo-ku′ro-nāt) a nucleotide derivative of glucuronate; it donates glucuronate groups for the synthesis of glucuronides, polysaccharides, and glycosaminoglycans, as well as for the reduction and solubilization of bilirubin and the detoxification of foreign phenols and amines in the liver.

UDP-glu·cu·ro·nate de·car·boxy·lase (gloo-ku′ro-nāt de-kahr-bok′sə-lās) [EC 4.1.1.35] an enzyme of the lyase class that catalyzes the decarboxylation of UDP-glucuronate to form UDP-xylose.

UDP-hex·ose (hek′sōs) a nucleotide consisting of hexose linked to the terminal phosphoryl group of uridine diphosphate (q.v.). The UDP-hexoses act as activated intermediates in the syntheses of polysaccharides, glycosaminoglycans, and glycolipids.

UDP-id·uron·ate (īd″u-ron′āt) a nucleotide derivative of iduronate, synthesized from UDP-glucuronate; it donates iduronate groups in proteoglycan synthesis.

UDP-xy·lose (zi′lōs) a nucleotide derivative of xylose, synthesized from UDP-glucuronate; it donates xylose groups in the synthesis of proteoglycans.

Uhl anomaly (yo͞ol) [Henry Stephen Magraw *Uhl*, American physician, born 1921] see under *anomaly.*

UK urokinase.

ulag·an·ac·te·sis (u-lag″an-ak-te′sis) [*ul-*[2] + Gr. *aganaktēsis* irritation] irritation or itching of the gingiva.

ulal·gia (u-lal′jə) [*ul-*[2] + *-algia*] gingivalgia.

ulat·ro·phy (u-lat′ro-fe) [*ul-*[2] + *atrophy*] atrophy of the gingiva associated with its recession and exposure of the root portion of the tooth.

afunctional u. ulatrophy occurring in congenital malocclusion.

atrophic u. ischemic u.

calcic u. ulatrophy that is caused by the presence of salivary concretions.

ischemic u. ulatrophy due to deficient blood supply. Called also *atrophic u.*

traumatic u. ulatrophy due to gingival trauma.

ul·cer (ul′sər) [L. *ulcus*, gen. *ulceris*] a local defect, or excavation, of the surface of an organ or tissue, which is produced by the sloughing of inflammatory necrotic tissue.

Ulcer

acute vulvar u. a nonvenereal, usually shallow lesion of the vulva, often associated with a febrile illness; its etiology is uncertain. Called also *Lipschütz disease* or *ulcer*.
Aden u. Old World cutaneous leishmaniasis.
amebic u. the ulcerous lesion of amebiasis cutis.
anastomotic u. a peptic ulcer near the site of a gastrectomy or gastroenterostomy; see also *stomal u.*
aphthous u. the ulcerative lesion on the oral mucosa seen in recurrent aphthous stomatitis.
atheromatous u. loss of intima over an atheroma, often causing thrombus formation.
Bairnsdale u. Buruli u.
Barrett u. chronic peptic ulcer of the esophagus, usually with heterotopic gastric mucosa; see *Barrett syndrome*, under *syndrome*.
burrowing phagedenic u. 1. progressive synergistic gangrene. 2. Meleney u. (def. 1).
Buruli u. cutaneous infection by *Mycobacterium ulcerans*, manifested by a small, firm, painless, movable subcutaneous nodule that enlarges, becomes fluctuant, and ulcerates, leaving an undermined edge. It was first seen in Uganda and Zaire but has now been seen across Western and Central Africa, in Australia, and in many other tropical and subtropical regions.
Cameron u. a peptic ulcer within a sliding hiatal hernia; it may be accompanied by chronic bleeding or be clinically silent.
catarrhal corneal u. a corneal ulcer found near the limbus in catarrhal conjunctivitis.
chancroid u. chancroid.
chicle u., chiclero u. an endemic, zoonotic form of New World cutaneous leishmaniasis, found mainly in forest workers in southeastern Mexico, Belize, and Guatemala. It is caused by *Leishmania mexicana*, transmitted by *Lutzomyia olmeca*. There are usually just a few lesions, self-limited and healing within six months; sometimes the pinna of the ear is involved, and lesions are chronic, lasting many years and slowly destroying the cartilage of the ear.
chrome u. an ulcer on the skin or a mucous membrane produced by chromium or its salts; seen in persons who work with chromium or its compounds. Called also *tanner's u.*
contact u. see under *granuloma*.
corneal u. ulcerative keratitis.
corneal marginal u. Mooren u.
Curling u. a duodenal ulcer associated with a lesion on the surface of the body, such as a burn.
Cushing u., Cushing-Rokitansky u. a small peptic ulcer, usually occurring in groups, associated with manifest or occult lesions of the central nervous system. Called also *Rokitansky-Cushing u.*
decubital u., decubitus u. an ulcer caused by arterial occlusion or prolonged pressure, such as when a patient lies still in bed for a long period or is confined to a wheelchair; called also *decubitus*, *bed sore*, and *pressure u.* or *sore*.
dendriform u., dendritic u. a corneal ulcer that branches in various directions, usually caused by herpes simplex infection.
diabetic u. an ulcer associated with diabetes mellitus, usually on the lower limb, as in diabetic gangrene.

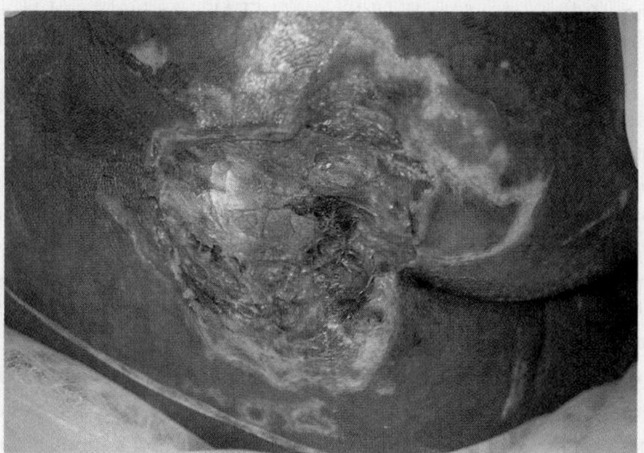

■ Decubitus ulcer of the sacral area in an 85-year-old man, with exposure of the sacrum and necrosis of surrounding muscles.

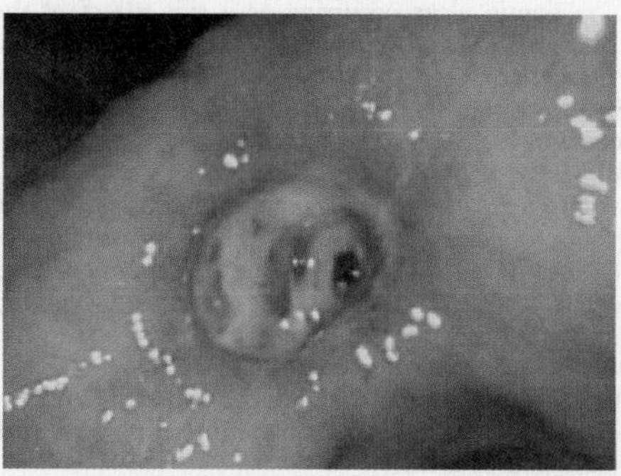

■ Endocsopic appearance of gastric ulcer at the angular notch.

Dieulafoy u. see under *lesion*.
diphtheritic u. an ulcer whose surface is partly or entirely covered by a gray membrane, as in cutaneous diphtheria.
duodenal u. a peptic ulcer in the duodenum.
elusive u. Hunner u.
eosinophilic u. a type of rodent ulcer in cats, usually on the upper lip near a canine tooth and seldom pruritic or painful; it is part of the eosinophilic granuloma complex and may progress to a more serious lesion.
Fenwick-Hunner u. Hunner u.
fistulous u. the ulcerated superficial end of a fistula.
flask u. an ulcer of the intestine in amebic dysentery.
follicular u. a small ulcer on the mucous membrane having its origin in a lymph follicle.
gastric u. a peptic ulcer of the gastric mucosa.
giant peptic u. a rare type of peptic ulcer that is particularly large.
girdle u. a rare type of ulcer seen in tuberculosis, spreading along the wall of the intestine in an encircling manner.
gouty u. a superficial ulcer of the skin over a gouty joint.
gummatous u. a broken-down superficial gumma.
Hunner u. an ulcer in the bladder, occurring in interstitial cystitis, and involving all the layers of the bladder wall; it appears as a small brown to red patch on the mucosa. It tends to heal superficially and is therefore often difficult to detect.
hypertensive ischemic u. a manifestation of infarction of the skin due to arteriolar occlusion as part of a longstanding vascular disease, seen especially in women in late middle age, and presenting as a red painful plaque on the lower limb or ankle that later breaks down into a superficial ulcer surrounded by a zone of purpuric erythema.
hypopyon u. a type of corneal ulcer with creeping central suppurative ulceration and hypopyon, often due to a pneumococcal infection. Called also *Saemisch ulcer*, *serpiginous corneal ulcer*, *ulcus corneae serpens*, and *ulcus serpens corneae*.
Jacob u. rodent ulcer, especially one on an eyelid.
jejunal u. a rare type of peptic ulcer caused by gastric acid in the jejunum, such as when there is ectopic stomach mucosa secreting acid there; sometimes one develops secondary to a gastroenterostomy that has bypassed the duodenum.
kissing u's gastric ulcers on directly opposing surfaces of the stomach, as on opposite sides of the lesser curvature.
Lipschütz u. acute vulvar u.
Mann-Williamson u. a progressive peptic ulcer produced in experimental animals by means of a gastric resection or gastroenterostomy.
marginal u. stomal u.
marginal corneal u. Mooren u.
Marjolin u. an ulcer located over an old scar; it may degenerate into squamous cell carcinoma with a propensity for metastasis.
Meleney u. 1. a variety of progressive synergistic gangrene associated with formation of burrowing cutaneous fissures and sinus tracts that open at distant sites. Called also *burrowing phagedenic u.* and *undermining burrowing u.* 2. progressive synergistic gangrene.
Mooren u. a chronic type of corneal ulcer of the marginal part, having a serpiginous, usually bilateral formation. These are usually seen in elderly individuals and have unknown etiology.
neurogenic u., neurotrophic u. an ulcer resulting from separation of tissue from its nerve supply, such as in sensory neuropathy.

Ulcer *Continued*

NSAID u. a peptic ulcer occurring as a side effect of therapy with nonsteroidal antiinflammatory drugs (NSAIDs), usually either a gastric ulcer or a duodenal ulcer.
penetrating u. an ulcer that extends to involve the wall or substance of an adjacent organ.
penetrating u. of foot plantar u.
peptic u. an ulcer of the mucous membrane of the alimentary tract, caused by action of acidic gastric juice. The most common locations are the stomach (see *gastric u.*) and duodenum (see *duodenal u.*); less often they may occur in the esophagus or in a part of the small intestine that has ectopic gastric mucosa and hence secretion of acid.
perambulating u. phagedenic u. (def. 1).
perforating u. an ulcer that involves the entire thickness of an organ, such as the foot, the stomach wall, or the intestinal wall, with openings both internally and externally.
phagedenic u. 1. any of a group of conditions due to bacterial invasion of a cutaneous lesion or of the intact skin of a person with impaired resistance; it is characterized by necrotic ulceration and prominent tissue destruction. The group includes desert sore, Meleney ulcer, and tropical phagedenic ulcer. Called also *perambulating* or *sloughing u.* 2. tropical phagedenic u.
plantar u. a deep neurotrophic ulcer of the sole of the foot, resulting from repeated injury because of lack of sensation in the part; seen with diseases such as diabetes mellitus and leprosy. Called also *penetrating u. of foot* and *mal perforant du pied.*
postbulbar u. a duodenal ulcer distal to the ampulla duodeni (duodenal bulb).
pressure u. decubitus u.
pudendal u. granuloma inguinale.
ring u. in a corneal ulcer, fusion of foci of ulceration to form a peripheral ring.
rodent u. an ulcerating basal cell carcinoma.
Rokitansky-Cushing u. Cushing u.
Saemisch u. hypopyon u.
serpiginous corneal u. hypopyon u.
sloughing u. phagedenic u. (def. 1).
soft u. chancroid.
stasis u. venous u.
stercoraceous u., stercoral u. 1. an ulcer caused by the pressure of impacted feces. 2. a fistulous ulcer through which fecal matter escapes.
stoma u., stomal u. a jejunal ulcer located near the margin of a gastroenterostomy stoma; called also *marginal u.*
stress u. a peptic ulcer, usually gastric, resulting from stress; possible predisposing factors include changes in the microcirculation of the gastric mucosa, increased permeability of the gastric mucosal barrier to hydrogen ions, and impaired cell proliferation.
sublingual u. an ulcer on the frenum of the tongue.
submucous u. Hunner u.; so called because of the tendency of the lesion to heal superficially.
symptomatic u. an ulcer that indicates some general disease.
tanner's u. chrome u.
trophic u. an ulcer due to imperfect nutrition of the part.
trophoneurotic u. neurotrophic u.
tropical u. 1. a lesion of cutaneous leishmaniasis. 2. tropical phagedenic u.
tropical phagedenic u. a chronic, painful phagedenic ulcer usually seen on the lower limbs of persons in the tropics. The etiology is unknown but spirochetes, fusiform bacilli, and other bacteria are often present in the developing lesion. Protein and vitamin deficiency with lowered resistance to infection may play a role; many patients are malnourished children. Called also *phagedenic u.* and *tropical u.*, as well as local names and names with only geographic significance.
undermining burrowing u. 1. progressive synergistic gangrene. 2. Meleney u. (def. 1).
varicose u. an ulcer on the leg due to varicose veins, such as a stasis ulcer.
venereal u. a nonspecific term referring to ulcers resembling chancre or chancroid around the external genitalia; some may be from a cause other than sexual transmission.
venous u., venous stasis u. ulceration on the skin of the ankle due to venous insufficiency and venous stasis.

---

ul•cera (ul′sər-ə) [L.] plural of *ulcus.*

ul•cer•ate (ul′sər-āt) [L. *ulcerare, ulceratus*] to become affected with ulceration.

ul•cer•a•tion (ul″sər-a′shən) [L. *ulceratio*] 1. the formation or development of an ulcer. 2. an ulcer.

ul•cer•a•tive (ul′sə-ra″tiv, ul′sər-ə-tiv) pertaining to or characterized by ulceration.

ul•cero•cav•er•nous (ul″sər-o-kav′ər-nəs) ulcerated and cavernous.

ul•cero•gan•gre•nous (ul″sər-o-gang′rə-nəs) characterized by both ulceration and gangrene; pertaining to a gangrenous ulcer.

ul•cero•gen•ic (ul″sər-o-jen′ik) causing ulceration; leading to the production of ulcers.

ul•cero•mem•bra•nous (ul″sər-o-mem′brə-nəs) characterized by ulceration and by a membranous exudation.

ul•cer•ous (ul′sər-əs) ulcerative.

ul•cus (ul′kəs) pl. *ul′cera* [L.] ulcer.
u. am′bulans phagedenic ulcer.
u. cor′neae ser′pens hypopyon ulcer.
u. interdigita′le keratolysis of the stratum corneum of the skin between the toes, a disease similar to pitted keratolysis.
u. ser′pens cor′neae hypopyon ulcer.
u. vul′vae acu′tum acute vulvar u.

ule- see *ul(o)-*[1].

ulec•to•my[1] (u-lek′tə-me) [*ul-*[1] + *-ectomy*] excision of scar tissue.

ulec•to•my[2] (u-lek′tə-me) [*ul-*[2] + *-ectomy*] gingivectomy.

ule•gy•ria (u″le-ji′re-ə) [*ule-* + *gyr-* + *-ia*] a condition in which the cerebral gyri are narrow and distorted by scars, resulting from lesions existing in fetal life or early infancy.

uler•y•the•ma (u-ler″ə-the′mə) [*ul-*[1] + *erythēma* redness] an erythematous disease of the skin characterized by scarring and atrophy.
u. ophryo′genes a type of keratosis pilaris that affects the follicles of the eyebrow hairs of young persons, associated with erythema and often resulting in scarring and atrophy; it is transmitted as an autosomal dominant trait.

ulig•i•nous (u-lij′ĭ-nəs) [L. *uliginosus* moist] muddy or slimy.

Ull•mann line (ool′mahn) [Emerich *Ullmann*, Hungarian surgeon, 1861–1937] see under *line.*

Ull•rich-Feich•ti•ger syndrome (ool′rik fik′tĭ-gər) [Otto *Ullrich*, German pediatrician, 1894–1957; H. *Feichtiger*, German physician, 20th century] see under *syndrome.*

Ull•rich-Tur•ner syndrome (ool′rik tur′nər) [O. *Ullrich;* Henry Hubert *Turner*, American endocrinologist, 1892–1970] Noonan syndrome.

Ul•mus (ul′məs) [L. "elm"] the elms, a genus of trees of the family Ulmaceae. *U. ru′bra* Muhlenberg (*U. ful′va* Micheaux) is the slippery elm, source of slippery elm bark (see under *bark* and see *elm*, def. 2).

ul•na (ul′nə) pl. *ul′nae* [L. "the arm"] [TA] the inner and larger bone of the forearm, on the side opposite that of the thumb; it articulates with the humerus and with the head of the radius at its proximal end and with the radius and bones of the carpus at the distal end. See illustration and Plate 40.

ul•nad (ul′nad) toward the ulna.

ul•nar (ul′nər) [L. *ulnaris*] pertaining to the ulna or to the medial (ulnar) aspect of the forearm as compared with the lateral (radial) aspect.

ul•na•re (əl-na′re) [L.] os triquetrum.

ul•na•ris (əl-na′ris) [L., from *ulna*, q.v.] [TA] ulnar; a general term denoting relationship to the ulna or to the ulnar aspect of the forearm.

ul•nen (ul′nən) pertaining to the ulna alone.

ul•no•car•pal (ul″no-kahr′pəl) pertaining to the ulna and carpus.

ul•no•ra•di•al (ul″no-ra′de-əl) pertaining to the ulna and radius.

ul(o)-[1] [Gr. *oulē* scar] a combining form denoting relationship to a scar, or cicatrix. Also, *ule-*.

ul(o)-[2] [Gr. *oulon* gum] for terms beginning thus, see also those beginning *gingiv(o)-*.

-ulose a suffix indicating that the substance is a ketose.

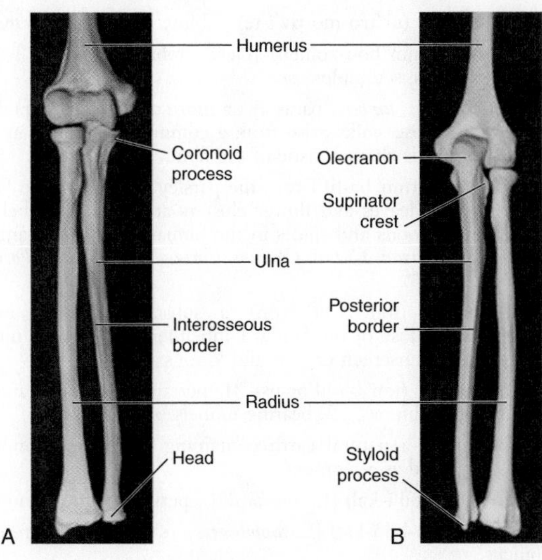

■ Ulna and radius. *(A)*, Anterior view; *(B)*, posterior view.

Ulo•cla•di•um (u″lo-kla′de-um) a genus of fungi of the form-family Dematiaceae, usually found growing on plants, but implicated as the cause of human skin infections after traumatic inoculation.

ulot•o•my[1] (u-lot′ə-me) [*ulo-*[1] + *-tomy*] the cutting or division of scar tissue.

ulot•o•my[2] (u-lot′ə-me) [*ulo-*[2] + *-tomy*] incision of the gingivae.

ulo•trip•sis (u″lo-trip′sis) [*ulo-*[2] + *tripsis*] revitalization of the gingivae by massage.

Ul•tane (ul′tān) trademark for a preparation of sevoflurane.

ul•ti•mate (ul′tĭ-mət) [L. *ultimus* last] the last or farthest; final or most remote.

ul•ti•mo•bran•chi•al (ul″tĭ-mo-brang′ke-əl) [L. *ultimus* last + *branchial*] pertaining to or derived from the fourth pharyngeal pouch. Called also *ultimopharyngeal.*

ul•ti•mo•pha•ryn•ge•al (ul″tĭ-mo-fə-rin′je-əl) ultimobranchial.

ul•ti•mum mo•ri•ens (ul′tĭ-məm mo′re-ənz) [L. "last to die"] the right atrium; said to be the last part of the body to cease moving in death.

Ul•ti•va (ul-te′vah) trademark for a preparation of remifentanil hydrochloride.

ult. praes. [L.] ul′timum prae′scriptus (last prescribed).

ultra- [L. "beyond"] a prefix denoting excess, or beyond.

ul•tra•brachy•ce•phal•ic (ul″trə-brak″e-sə-fal′ik) pertaining to or characterized by an extremely broad, short skull, with a cephalic index of more than 90.0.

ul•tra•cen•trif•u•ga•tion (ul″trə-sən-trif″u-ga′shən) subjection to the action of an ultracentrifuge.

ul•tra•cen•tri•fuge (ul″trə-sen′trĭ-fūj) a centrifuge with an exceedingly high rate of rotation, which will separate and sediment the molecules of a substance.

Ul•tra•cet (ul′trə-set) trademark for a preparation of tramadol hydrochloride and acetaminophen.

ul•tra•di•an (ul″trə-de′ən) [*ultra-* + L. *dies* day] pertaining to the rhythmic repetition of certain phenomena in living organisms occurring in cycles of greater frequency than circadian, that is, more frequently than once a day. Cf. *circadian* and *infradian.*

ul•tra•dol•i•cho•ce•phal•ic (ul″trə-dol″ĭ-ko-sə-fal′ik) [*ultra-* + *dolichocephalic*] pertaining to or characterized by an extremely long, narrow head, with a cephalic index of not more than 64.9.

ul•tra•fil•ter (ul″trə-fil′tər) an apparatus for performing ultrafiltration through a semipermeable membrane.

ul•tra•fil•trate (ul″trə-fil′trāt) the liquid that has passed through an ultrafilter.

ul•tra•fil•tra•tion (ul″trə-fil-tra′shən) filtration through filters with minute pores, which allows separation of extremely minute particles. It occurs naturally, as in the filtration of plasma at the capillary membrane, and is also performed clinically and in the laboratory, such as in hemodialysis. In hemodialysis it involves bulk movement of solute and solvent across a membrane down pressure gradients and is usually performed under pressure to accelerate the process.

Ul•tram (ul′tram) trademark for a preparation of tramadol hydrochloride.

ul•tra•mi•cro•chem•is•try (ul″trə-mi″kro-kem′is-tre) the chemical study of materials in extremely minute quantities.

ul•tra•mi•cro•pi•pet (ul″trə-mi″kro-pi-pet′) a pipet designed to handle extremely small quantities of liquid (less than 0.005 mL).

ul•tra•mi•cro•scope (ul″trə-mi′kro-skōp) a special darkfield microscope for the examination of particles of colloidal size. See *darkfield illumination*, under *illumination*, and *darkfield microscope*, under *microscope.*

ul•tra•mi•cro•scop•ic (ul″trə-mi″kro-skop′ik) 1. pertaining to the ultramicroscope. 2. too small to be seen with an ordinary microscope.

ul•tra•mi•cros•co•py (ul″trə-mi-kros′kə-pe) use of the ultramicroscope.

ul•tra•mi•cro•tome (ul″trə-mi′kro-tōm) an instrument for making very thin tissue sections for electron microscopy.

ul•tra•pas•teur•iza•tion (ul″trə-pas″chər-ĭ-za′shən) a modified form of pasteurization, generally of milk or milk products, that uses much higher heat for a very brief period; used to extend shelf life.

Ul•trase (ul′trās) trademark for preparations of pancrelipase.

ul•tra•son•ic (ul″trə-son′ik) [*ultra-* + L. *sonus* sound] pertaining to sound waves having a frequency beyond the upper limit of perception by the human ear, that is, beyond about 20,000 Hz (20 kHz); called also *supersonic.* See also *ultrasonics.*

ul•tra•son•ics (ul″trə-son′iks) the study and use of ultrasonic waves; these could include any frequencies above 20 kHz, but the term is usually restricted to those above 500 kHz. Such waves are injurious to living tissue because of their thermal effects, but controlled doses may be used therapeutically to break down pathologic tissue or diagnostically in ultrasonography.

ul•tra•sono•gram (ul″trə-son′o-gram) the record obtained by ultrasonography.

ul•tra•so•nog•ra•phy (ul″trə-sə-nog′rə-fe) the visualization of deep structures of the body by recording the reflections of (echoes of) pulses of ultrasonic waves directed into the tissues. Diagnostic ultrasonography, as in echocardiography, uses a frequency range of 1 million to 10 million hertz (cycles per second), or 1 to 10 MHz. Such sound waves are transmissible only in liquids and solids. See also *scan* (def. 2). Called also *echography* and *sonography.* **ultrasonograph′ic** *adj*

A-mode u. ultrasonography in which one axis of the display represents the time required for the return of the echo and the other corresponds to the strength of the echo.

B-mode u. ultrasonography in which the position of a spot on the display corresponds to the time elapsed (and thus to the position of the echogenic surface), and the brightness of the spot corresponds to the strength of the echo; movement of the transducer produces a sweep of the ultrasound beam and a tomographic scan of a cross section of the body.

continuous wave Doppler u. Doppler ultrasonography using two transducers, with one continually transmitting and the other continually recording the ultrasonic waves. It is used to record signals with very high velocities, such as occur in severely stenotic valves, but cannot provide spatial resolution of the signals. Cf. *pulsed wave Doppler u.*

Doppler u. ultrasonography in which the shifts in frequency between emitted ultrasonic waves and their echoes are used to measure the velocities of moving objects, based on the principle of the Doppler effect. The waves may be continuous or pulsed; the technique is frequently used to examine cardiovascular blood flow (Doppler echocardiography). See also *color flow Doppler imaging*, under *imaging*, *pulsed wave Doppler u.*, and *continuous wave Doppler u.*

duplex u. the combination of real-time and Doppler ultrasonography.

endorectal u. 1. endosonography of the rectum with a transducer on a rigid rectal probe, used particularly in the staging of rectal cancer. 2. transrectal u.

endoscopic u. endosonography of the esophagus, stomach, or duodenum to provide views of the mediastinum or abdominal organs.

gray-scale u. a B-scan technique in which a television video-scan converter amplifies and processes echoes according to their strength into a visual display ranging from white for the strongest echoes to varying shades of gray.

intravascular u. visualization of the interior of blood vessels by ultrasound; the transducer is mounted on the end of a catheter that is introduced percutaneously.

pulsed wave Doppler u. Doppler ultrasonography in which a single transducer alternately transmits and records ultrasonic waves. It can be used to determine the site of signal origin precisely but cannot record signals with high velocities. Cf. *continuous wave Doppler u.*

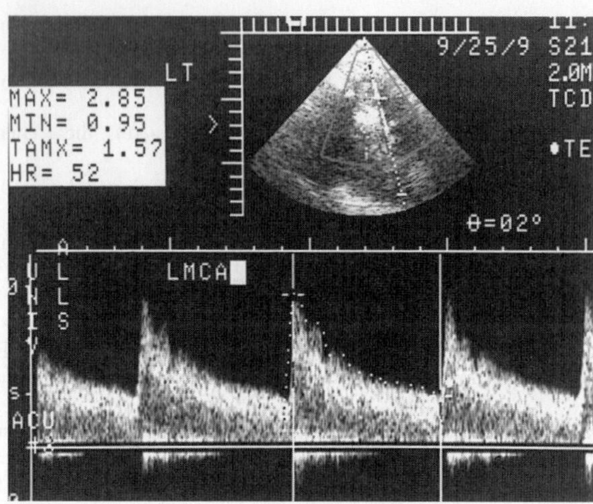

■ Transcranial Doppler ultrasonographic image of left middle cerebral artery after subarachnoid hemorrhage, showing elevated flow velocities consistent with vasospasm.

real-time u. a series of ultrasound images produced in rapid succession so that the video display shows motion of an organ or part.

transcranial Doppler u. a form of Doppler ultrasonography in which pulses of ultrasound are directed at vascular formations in the base of the skull, allowing measurements of blood flow velocity in the major basal intracranial arteries on a real time basis.

transrectal u. (TRUS) the sonographic visualization of structures adjacent to the rectum using an endorectal probe; used particularly in the diagnosis and evaluation of disorders of the prostate.

ul•tra•so•nom•e•try (ul″trə-sə-nom′ə-tre) the measurement of certain physical properties of biologic fluids by means of ultrasound.

ul•tra•sound (ul′trə-sound) 1. sound waves with a frequency above the range of human hearing (greater than 20,000 Hz); see *ultrasonics.* 2. ultrasonography.

ul•tra•struc•ture (ul′trə-struk″chər) the arrangement of the smallest elements making up a body; the structure beyond the resolution power of the light microscope, i.e., the structure visible only under the ultramicroscope and electron microscope. Called also *fine structure.*

Ultra•Tag RBC (ul′trə-tag″) trademark for a kit for the preparation of technetium Tc 99m red blood cells.

Ul•tra•vate (ul′trə-vāt) trademark for preparations of halobetasol propionate.

ul•tra•vi•o•let (ul″trə-vi′ə-lət) beyond the violet end of the spectrum; said of electromagnetic rays or radiation between the violet rays and the x-rays, that is, with wavelengths between 200 and 400 nm. These rays have powerful actinic and chemical properties, inducing sunburn and tanning of the skin and producing ergocalciferol (vitamin D_2) by their action on ergosterol in the skin.

u. A (UVA) ultraviolet radiation with wavelengths between 320 and 400 nm; this constitutes over 99 per cent of the ultraviolet radiation reaching the surface of the earth. UVA enhances the harmful effects of ultraviolet B radiation and is also responsible for some photosensitivity reactions; it is used therapeutically in the treatment of a variety of skin disorders (see *PUVA therapy*, under *therapy*).

u. B (UVB) ultraviolet radiation with wavelengths between 290 and 320 nm; this constitutes less than 1 per cent of the ultraviolet radiation reaching the earth's surface. UVB causes sunburn and a number of damaging photochemical changes within cells, including damage to DNA, leading to premature aging of the skin, premalignant and malignant changes, and a variety of photosensitivity reactions; it is also used therapeutically in the treatment of skin disorders.

u. C (UVC) ultraviolet radiation with wavelengths between 200 and 290 nm; all UVC radiation is filtered out by the ozone layer so that none reaches the earth's surface. UVC is germicidal and is also used in ultraviolet phototherapy.

far u. the ultraviolet radiation that has the shortest wavelengths and is farthest from the visible spectrum; its wavelengths are between 200 and 300 nm.

near u. the ultraviolet radiation that has the longest wavelengths and is nearest to the visible spectrum; its wavelengths are between 300 and 400 nm.

ul•tra•vis•i•ble (ul″trə-viz′ĭ-bəl) ultramicroscopic.

Ul•tra•vist (ul′trə-vist″) trademark for a preparation of iopromide.

ul•tro•mo•tiv•i•ty (ul″tro-mo-tiv′ĭ-te) ability to move spontaneously.

um•bau•zo•nen (um″bou-zo′nen) [Ger., "rebuilding zones"] Looser transformation zones; see under *zone.*

um•bel (um′bəl) [L. *umbella* parasol] a more or less flat-topped cluster of small flowers whose stalks arise from a common small area at the top of the main stem; it is characteristic of the family Umbelliferae.

Um•bel•li•fe•rae (um″bə-lif′ĭ-re) the parsley family, a large family of plants with fragrant leaves and flower clusters arranged in umbels; many species are used as foods and spices in the human diet. Important genera include *Anethum, Carum, Cicuta, Conium, Coriandrum, Daucus, Foeniculum,* and *Pimpinella.*

um•bel•lif•er•one (um″bə-lif′ər-ōn) a substance present in many plants, particularly those of the family Umbelliferae; it absorbs ultraviolet rays and is used in sunscreen creams and lotions.

um•bel•lif•er•ous (um″bə-lif′ər-us) 1. pertaining to or characteristic of the family Umbelliferae. 2. bearing umbels.

um•ber (um′bər) a natural earth containing chiefly manganese, iron oxide, and silica; used as a pigment.

um•bil•i•cal (əm-bil′ĭ-kəl) [L. *umbilicalis*] pertaining to the umbilicus.

um•bil•i•cate (əm-bil′ĭ-kāt) [L. *umbilicatus*] shaped like or resembling the umbilicus.

um•bil•i•cat•ed (əm-bil′ĭ-kāt″əd) marked by depressed areas resembling the umbilicus.

um•bil•i•ca•tion (əm-bil″ĭ-ka′shən) a pit or depression resembling the umbilicus.

um•bil•i•co•plas•ty (əm-bil′ĭ-ko-plas′te) [*umbilicus* + *-plasty*] a plastic surgical operation on the umbilicus.

um•bil•i•cus (əm-bil′ĭ-kəs) [L.] 1. the navel: the cicatrix marking the site of attachment of the umbilical cord in the fetus. Called also *omphalus.* 2. [TA] the region of the abdomen surrounding the umbilicus; called also *regio umbilicalis* [TA alternative] and *umbilical region.*

amniotic u. the oval aperture formed by converging amniotic folds.

um•bo (um′bo) gen. *umbo′nis*, pl. *umbo′nes* [L. "a boss"] a round projection; the projecting center of any rounded surface.

u. membra′nae tympa′nicae umbo of tympanic membrane: the slight projection at the center of the outer surface of the tympanic membrane, corresponding to the point of attachment of the tip of the manubrium of the malleus. Called also *spatula mallei.*

um•bo•nate (um′bo-nāt) [L. *umbo* a knob] knoblike; buttonlike; having a buttonlike, raised center.

um•bo•nes (əm-bo′nēz) [L.] plural of *umbo.*

um•bra (um′brə) [L. "shadow"] 1. the area of a shadow where there is no illumination; cf. *penumbra.* 2. in radiography, the area of sharp contrast.

UMP uridine monophosphate.

UMP syn•thase (sin′thās) the combined activities of the enzymes orotate phosphoribosyltransferase and orotidine-5′-phosphate decarboxylase, which together catalyze the last steps in pyrimidine nucleotide biosynthesis.

UMP syn•thase de•fi•cien•cy (sin′thās) oroticaciduria, type I.

uña de ga•to (oo′nyah da gah′to) [Sp. "cat's claw"] cat's claw.

Un•a•syn (u′nə-sin) trademark for a combination preparation of ampicillin sodium and sulbactam sodium.

un•azo•tized (ən-a′zo-tīzd) containing no nitrogen.

un•bal•ance (ən-bal′əns) lack or loss of normal balance.

un•cal (ung′kəl) of or pertaining to the uncus.

Un•ca•ria (ən-kar′e-ə) [L.] a genus of shrubs of the family Rubiaceae, native to Asia.

***U. gam′bier*, U. gam′bir** gambir, a species whose twigs and bark are used medicinally and called gambir.

U. tomento′sa a woody vine of the South American rain forest, whose root bark is used medicinally as uña de gato or cat's claw.

un•car•thro•sis (ung″kahr-thro′sis) bone disease involving the uncinate processes of vertebrae.

un•ci (un′si) [L.] genitive and plural of *uncus.*

un•ci•form (un′sĭ-form) [*uncus* (def. 1) + *form*] uncinate.

un•ci•for•me (un″sĭ-for′me) [L.] uncinate.

un•ci•nal (un′sĭ-nəl) uncinate.

Un•ci•na•ria (un″sĭ-nar′e-ə) [L. *uncus* hook] a genus of hookworms of the family Ancylostomatidae.

U. america′na *Necator americanus.*

U. duodena′lis *Ancylostoma duodenale.*

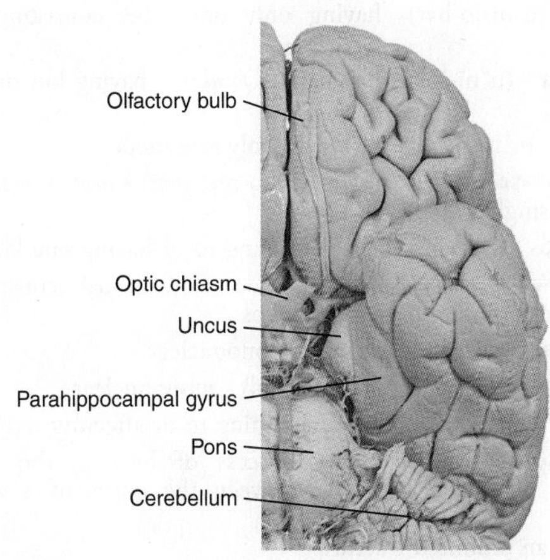

■ Uncus, in an inferior view of a cerebral hemisphere.

U. stenoce'phala a species that commonly causes hookworm disease in dogs; also parasitic in foxes, cats, and other carnivores.

un•ci•na•ri•al (un″sĭ-nar′e-əl) of, pertaining to, or caused by a hookworm.

un•cin•a•ri•a•sis (un″sin-ə-ri′ə-sis) a type of hookworm disease in carnivores caused by infection with worms of the genus *Uncinaria.* uncinariat′ic *adj*

un•ci•nate (un′sĭ-nāt) 1. shaped like a hook (uncus). Cf. *hamate.* Called also *unciform* and *uncinal.* 2. pertaining to or affecting the uncinate gyrus.

un•ci•na•tum (un″sĭ-na′təm) [L.] uncinate.

un•ci•pres•sure (un′sĭ-presh″ər) [*uncus* (def. 1) + *pressure*] pressure with a hook to control hemorrhage.

un•com•ple•ment•ed (ən-kom′plə-ment″əd) not joined with complement, and therefore not active.

un•con•di•tioned (un″kən-dish′ənd) not a result of conditioning; unlearned; occurring naturally or spontaneously.

un•con•scious (ən-kon′shəs) 1. insensible; incapable of responding to sensory stimuli and of having subjective experiences; see also *coma* and *consciousness.* 2. the part of the mind that is not readily accessible to conscious awareness by ordinary means but whose existence may be manifested in symptom formation, in dreams, or under the influence of drugs; it is one of the systems of Freud's topographic model of the mind. Cf. *conscious* and *preconscious.*

collective u. in jungian psychology, the elements of the unconscious that are theoretically common to all human beings.

un•co-os•si•fied (un″ko-os′ĭ-fīd) not united into one bone.

un•cot•o•my (əng-kot′ə-me) [*uncus* (def. 2) + *-tomy*] the production of a circumscribed lesion in the uncus in the treatment of psychotic states.

un•co•ver•te•bral (ung″ko-vur′tə-brəl) pertaining to or affecting the uncinate processes of a vertebra.

unc•tion (ungk′shən) [L. *unctio*] 1. ointment. 2. inunction.

unc•tu•ous (ungk′choo-əs) greasy or oily; oleaginous.

un•cus (ung′kəs) [L. "hook"] 1. hook; an anatomical structure that is long, thin, and curved like a hook. 2. [TA] the medially curved anterior end of the parahippocampal gyrus; called also *u. gyri parahippocampalis.*

u. of body of cervical vertebra u. corporis vertebrae cervicalis.

u. of body of first thoracic vertebra u. corporis vertebrae thoracicae primae.

u. cor′poris ver′tebrae cervica′lis [TA] uncus of body of cervical vertebra: a hooklike projection found on each side of the superior surface of the third to seventh cervical vertebral bodies. It is a frequent site of formation of spurs (osteophytes), leading to spondylosis uncovertebralis. Called also *processus uncinatus vertebrae cervicalis* [TA alternative] and *uncinate process of cervical vertebra.*

u. cor′poris ver′tebrae thora′cicae pri′mae [TA] uncus of body of first thoracic vertebrae: a raised lateral margin on each side of the body of the first thoracic vertebra. Called also *processus uncinatus vertebrae thoracicae primae* [TA alternative] and *uncinate process of first thoracic vertebrae.*

u. gy′ri parahippocampa′lis uncus (def. 2).

un•dec•e•no•ic ac•id (ən-des″ə-no′ik) systematic name for *undecylenic acid.*

un•dec•yl•en•ic ac•id (un″des-əl-en′ik) [USP] an unsaturated fatty acid used as a topical fungicide, effective against *Epidermophyton, Trichophyton,* and *Microsporum* spp.

un•der•bite (un′dər-bīt) popular name for *retrognathism.*

un•der•cut (un′dər-kət) 1. the portion of a tooth that lies between the survey line (height of contour) and the gingivae. 2. the contour of a cross-section of a residual ridge or dental arch which would prevent the insertion of a denture. 3. the contour of flasking stone which interlocks in such a way as to prevent the separation of the parts. 4. a depressed or intaglio irregularity in the wall of a prepared tooth that prevents the ready withdrawal and seating of a wax pattern and the metal alloy casting.

un•der•drive (un′dər-drīv″) pertaining to a rate less than normal; see under *pacing.*

un•der•horn (un′dər-horn) cornu temporale ventriculi lateralis.

un•der•nu•tri•tion (un″dər-noo-trish′ən) malnutrition due to inadequate food supply or to inability to metabolize or use necessary food elements.

un•der•sens•ing (un′dər-sens″ing) missed sensing of cardiac electrical signals by an artificial cardiac pacemaker, resulting in too frequent or irregular delivery of stimuli; causes include head dislodgment, malfunctioning of the pulse generator, fibrosis, infarct, and drugs.

un•der•stain (un′dər-stān) to stain less deeply than usual.

un•der•toe (un′dər-to) hallux valgus in which the great toe is displaced under the others.

Un•der•wood disease (un′dər-wood) [Michael *Underwood,* English obstetrician and pediatrician, 1737–1820] sclerema.

un•dif•fer•en•ti•at•ed (ən-dif″ər-en′she-āt-əd) anaplastic.

un•dif•fer•en•ti•a•tion (un″dif-ər-en″she-a′shən) anaplasia.

un•dine (ən-dēn′, un′din) [L. *unda* wave, water] a small glass flask for irrigating the eye.

un•din•ism (un′din-iz-əm) [from *Undine* a water nymph, from L. *unda* wave] the association of sexual ideas with water, including urine and urination.

un•do•ing (ən-doo′ing) a defense mechanism aimed at negating or atoning for some disapproved act or impulse by performing an action that is somehow opposite to that feared; most commonly seen in the rituals accompanying obsessive-compulsive disorder.

Un•dritz anomaly (oon′drits) [E. *Undritz,* Swiss physician, 20th century] hereditary hypersegmentation of neutrophils; see under *hypersegmentation.*

un•du•lant (un′jə-, un′dyə-lənt) [L. *unda* wave] characterized by wavelike fluctuations; see also under *fever.*

un•du•late[1] (un′jə-, un′dyə-lāt) [L. *undulatus,* from *unda* wave] 1. to move in waves or in a wavelike motion. 2. to have a wavelike appearance, outline, or form.

un•du•late[2] (un′jə-, un′dyə-lət) having a wavy, curved border, as a colony of microorganisms.

un•du•la•tion (un′jə-, un″dyə-la′shən) [L. *undulatio*] 1. a wavelike motion; see also *pulsation.* 2. a wavelike appearance, outline, or form.

respiratory u. the variation of the blood pressure curve due to respiration.

ung. [L.] unguen′tum (ointment).

un•gual (ung′gwəl) [L. *unguis* nail] pertaining to the unguis (nail).

un•guent (ung′gwənt) [L. *unguentum*] ointment.

un•guen•tum (əng-gwen′təm) gen. *unguen′ti* pl. *unguen′ta* [L.] ointment.

un•gues (ung′gwēz) [L.] plural of *unguis.*

un•guic•u•late (əng-gwik′u-lāt) 1. provided with claws or nails. 2. resembling a claw.

un•guic•u•lus (əng-gwik′u-ləs) [L., dim. of *unguis*] claw.

un•guis (ung′gwis) pl. *un′gues* [L.] 1. [TA] nail: the horny cutaneous plate on the dorsal surface of the distal end of the terminal phalanx of a finger or toe, made up of flattened epithelial scales developed from the stratum lucidum of the skin. 2. a naillike part or structure.

u. incarna′tus ingrown toenail; see under *toenail.*

un•gu•la (ung′gu-lə) [L. "hoof," "claw," "talon"] hoof.

un•gu•late (ung′gu-lāt) [L. *ungula* hoof] a hoofed mammal. Formerly all classified into one order, they are now divided into the orders Artiodactyla and Perissodactyla.

un•gu•li•grade (ung′gu-lĭ-grād″) [*ungula* + L. *gradi* to walk] characterized by standing or walking on hooves (the tips of the toes); applied to certain quadrupeds known as *ungulates*, including horses, cattle, pigs, sheep, and deer. Cf. *digitigrade* and *plantigrade*.

uni- [L. *unus* one] a prefix meaning one.

uni·ar·tic·u·lar (u″ne-ahr-tik′u-lər) [*uni-* + *articular*] pertaining to a single joint.

uni·au·ral (u″ne-aw′rəl) monaural.

uni·ax·i·al (u″ne-ak′se-əl) [*uni-* + *axial*] 1. having but one axis; said of a joint. 2. developing in an axial direction only, as a uniaxial organism.

uni·ba·sal (u″nĭ-ba′səl) [*uni-* + *basal*] having only one base.

uni·ca·lyc·e·al (u″nĭ-kə-lis′e-əl) having just one calyx; said of an anomalous type of kidney. Spelled also *unicaliceal*.

uni·cam·er·al (u″nĭ-kam′ər-əl) [*uni-* + *camera* + *-al*[1]] having only one cavity or compartment.

uni·cel·lu·lar (u″nĭ-sel′u-lər) [*uni-* + *cellular*] made up of but a single cell, as the bacteria.

uni·cen·tral (u″nĭ-sen′trəl) [*uni-* + *central*] pertaining to or having a single center.

uni·cen·tric (u″nĭ-sen′trik) unicentral.

uni·ceps (u″nĭ-seps) [*uni-* + L. *caput* head] having one head or origin; said of a muscle.

uni·col·lis (u″nĭ-kol′is) [*uni-* + L. *collum* neck] having a single cervix; see *uterus bicornis unicollis*, under *uterus*.

uni·cor·nous (u″nĭ-kor′nəs) unicornuate.

uni·cor·nu·ate (u″nĭ-kor′nu-āt) [*uni-* + L. *cornu* horn] having only one horn or cornu.

uni·cus·pid (u″nĭ-kus′pid) a tooth with only one cusp.

uni·cus·pi·date (u″nĭ-kus′pĭ-dāt) having only one cusp.

uni·di·rec·tion·al (u″nĭ-di-rek′shən-əl) flowing in only one direction.

Uni·Dur (u′nĭ-dur) trademark for a preparation of theophylline.

uni·fas·cic·u·lar (u″nĭ-fə-sik′u-lər) pertaining to a single bundle, or fasciculus.

uni·flag·el·late (u″nĭ-flaj′ə-lāt) having one flagellum.

uni·fo·cal (u″nĭ-fo′kəl) arising from or pertaining to a single focus.

uni·fo·rate (u″nĭ-for′āt) [*uni-* + L. *foratus* pierced] having only one opening.

uni·gem·i·nal (u″nĭ-jem′ĭ-nəl) [*uni-* + *geminus*] pertaining to or affecting one twin of a pair.

uni·ger·mi·nal (u″nĭ-jur′mĭ-nəl) 1. pertaining to a single germ or ovum. 2. monozygotic.

uni·glan·du·lar (u″nĭ-glan′du-lər) pertaining to or affecting only one gland.

uni·grav·i·da (u″nĭ-grav′ĭ-də) primigravida.

uni·lam·i·nar (u″nĭ-lam′ĭ-nər) having only one layer or lamina.

uni·lat·er·al (u″nĭ-lat′ər-əl) [*uni-* + *lateral*] affecting but one side.

uni·lo·bar (u″nĭ-lo′bər) having only one lobe; consisting of a single lobe.

uni·loc·u·lar (u″nĭ-lok′u-lər) [*uni-* + *locular*] having but one cavity or compartment.

uni·mo·dal (u″nĭ-mo′dəl) having only one mode.

uni·ne·phrec·to·my (u″nĭ-nə-frek′tə-me) [*uni-* + *nephrectomy*] surgical removal of a single kidney.

uni·neph·ric (u-ne-nef′rik) pertaining to or having one kidney only.

un·in·hib·it·ed (un″in-hib′ĭ-təd) free from usual constraints; not subject to normal inhibitory mechanisms.

uni·nu·cle·ar (u″nĭ-noo′kle-ər) mononuclear.

uni·nu·cle·at·ed (u″nĭ-noo′kle-āt″əd) mononuclear.

uni·oc·u·lar (u″ne-ok′u-lər) pertaining to or affecting only one eye.

un·ion (ūn′yən) [L. *unio*] the process of healing; the renewal of continuity in a broken bone or between the edges of a wound. See *healing*.

faulty u. an ununited fracture.

primary u. healing by first intention.

radioulnar u., middle syndesmosis radioulnaris.

vicious u. union of the ends of a fractured bone so as to produce deformity.

uni·ov·u·lar (u″ne-ov′u-lər) 1. monozygotic. 2. monovular.

uni·pap·il·lary (u″nĭ-pap′ĭ-lar-e) having just one papilla; said of an anomalous type of kidney.

unip·a·ra (u-nip′ə-rə) primipara.

uni·pa·ren·tal (u″nĭ-pə-ren′təl) pertaining to one of the parents only.

unip·a·rous (u-nip′ə-rəs) [*uni-* + *-parous*] 1. producing only one offspring or egg at one time. 2. primiparous.

Uni·phyl (u′nĭ-fəl) trademark for a preparation of theophylline.

uni·po·lar (u″nĭ-po′lər) [*uni-* + *polar*] 1. having a single pole or process, as a nerve cell. 2. pertaining to mood disorders in which only depressive episodes occur.

uni·port (u′nĭ-port) facilitated diffusion.

uni·port·er (u′nĭ-port-ər) a cell membrane transport protein that facilitates the passage of small hydrophilic ions and molecules through a cell membrane down a concentration gradient. See also *facilitated diffusion*, under *diffusion*.

uni·po·ten·cy (u″nĭ-po′tən-se) [*uni-* + *potency*] the ability of a part to develop in one manner only, or of a cell to develop into only one type of cell. **unip′otent, unipoten′tial** *adj*

Uni·ret·ic (u-nĭ-ret′ik) trademark for a combination preparation of moexipril hydrochloride and hydrochlorothiazide.

un·ir·ri·ta·ble (un-ir′ĭ-tə-bəl) not irritable; not capable of being stimulated.

uni·sep·tate (u″nĭ-sep′tāt) having only one septum.

uni·sex·u·al (u″nĭ-sek′shoo-əl) [*uni-* + *sexual* (def. 1)] 1. pertaining to only one sex. 2. having the sexual organs of one sex only.

unit (u′nit) [L. *unus* one] 1. a single thing. 2. a quantity assumed as a standard of measurement. Symbol U.

Unit

Allen-Doisy u. in the Allen-Doisy test, the least amount of estrogen that causes cornification of vaginal epithelium in a spayed laboratory mouse. Called also *mouse u.*

amboceptor u. in complement fixation tests, the smallest amount of anti-RBC antibody (amboceptor) that produces complete red cell lysis in the presence of an excess of complement.

Angström u. angstrom.

Ansbacher u. a unit of vitamin K dosage.

antigen u. in complement fixation tests, the smallest amount of antigen that will fix one unit of complement.

antitoxic u. a unit for expressing the strength of an antitoxin. The unit of diphtheria antitoxin is approximately the amount that will preserve the life of a guinea pig weighing 250 g for at least four days after it is injected subcutaneously with a mixture of 100 times the minimum lethal dose of diphtheria toxin. The unit of tetanus antitoxin is approximately ten times the amount that will preserve the life of a guinea pig weighing 350 g for at least 96 hours after injection of a mixture with 100 times minimum lethal dose of tetanus toxin.

atomic mass u. (u, amu) the unit mass equal to $\frac{1}{12}$ the mass of the nuclide of carbon-12, equivalent to 1.657×10^{-24} gm. Called also *atomic weight u.* and *dalton.*

atomic weight u. atomic mass u.

Bethesda u. a measure of the level of inhibitor to coagulation factor VIII; equal to the amount of inhibitor in patient plasma that will inactivate 50 percent of factor VIII in an equal volume of normal plasma following a 2-hour incubation period.

Bodansky u. the quantity of alkaline phosphatase that liberates 1 mg of phosphate ion from glycerol 2-phosphate in 1 hour at 37°C and under other standardized conditions.

British thermal u. (BTU) the amount of heat necessary to raise the temperature of one pound of water one degree Fahrenheit, usually from 39°F to 40°F.

Unit *Continued*

burst-forming u.–erythroid (BFU-E) the earliest erythrocyte precursor in the erythrocytic series, detectable mainly in vitro and having a high requirement for erythropoietin; it gets its name from the fact that its growth is composed of subcolonies resembling bursts. It is followed by the colony-forming unit–erythroid.
CGS u. any unit in the centimeter-gram-second system.
CH50 u. the amount of complement that will lyse 50 percent of a standard preparation of sheep red blood cells coated with antisheep erythrocyte antibody.
colony-forming u. 1. any of several hematopoietic stem cells identified by their ability to give rise to monoclonal colonies in the spleen when transplanted into isogeneic, lethally irradiated mice. 2. in microbiology, estimation of the number of bacteria or yeasts by counting the colonies on a solid medium, with one bacterium being considered equal to one colony; some colonies develop from two or more organisms attached to or lying close to each other when inoculated. Abbreviated *CFU*.
colony-forming u.–culture (CFU-C) colony-forming u.–granulocyte-macrophage.
colony-forming u.–erythroid (CFU-E) an erythrocyte precursor in the erythrocyte series that follows the burst-forming unit–erythroid and precedes the proerythroblast; detectable mainly in vitro.
colony-forming u.–granulocyte-macrophage (CFU-GM) a precursor cell in the granulocytic series that can grow into a myeloblast in the presence of appropriate stimulators in vitro. Called also *colony forming u.–culture.*
colony-forming u.–spleen (CFU-S) a name for the hematopoietic stem cell, based on the fact that in mice whose marrow has been ablated by irradiation this cell gives rise to colonies of marrow cells in the spleen.
complement u. in complement fixation tests, the smallest amount of complement or serum that will produce complete hemolysis of sensitized red cells. Called also *hemolytic u.*
coronary care u. (CCU) a specially designed and equipped hospital area containing a small number of private rooms, with all facilities necessary for constant observation and possible emergency treatment of patients with severe heart disease.
critical care u. (CCU) intensive care u.
dental u. 1. a single tooth and its adnexa, considered as a unit in the physiology of mastication. 2. a mobile or fixed article of dental equipment, which may be combined with a chair, consisting of items and attachments needed for dental examination and operations, and housing the electrical, mechanical, and plumbing facilities needed to operate the equipment and fixtures of the unit.
elbow u. in an upper limb prosthesis for an amputation above the elbow, a component, often with a hinge, that goes at the level of the elbow.
electromagnetic u's a system of units based on the fundamental definition of a unit magnetic pole as one which will repel an exactly similar pole with a force of one dyne when the poles are 1 cm apart.
electrostatic u's (esu) a system of units based on the fundamental definition of a unit charge as one which will repel an equal and like charge with a force of one dyne when the two charges are 1 cm apart in a vacuum.
enzyme u. see *international u. of enzyme activity*.
French u. a linear unit for diameter size in the French scale, equivalent to 0.33 mm.
Hampson u. a unit of radiation exposure, equal to one fourth of the erythema dose.
hemolytic u. complement u.
hemorrhagin u. the amount of snake venom necessary to produce hemorrhages in the vascular network of a three-day-old chick embryo.
Hounsfield u. a unit of x-ray attenuation used for CT scans, each pixel being assigned a value on a scale on which air is −1000, water is 0, and compact bone is +1000. Symbol H.
intensive care u. (ICU) a hospital unit in which are concentrated special equipment and skilled personnel for the care of seriously ill patients requiring immediate and continuous attention. Many such units are specialized, such as burn, cardiac or coronary, neonatal, neurologic, and pediatric intensive care units. Called also *critical care u.*
International u. (IU) a unit of biological material, as of enzymes, hormones, vitamins, etc., established by the International Conference for the Unification of Formulas.
international u. of enzyme activity the amount of an enzyme that will catalyze the transformation of 1 micromole of substrate per minute under standard conditions of temperature, optimal pH, and optimal substrate concentration. Symbol U.
international insulin u. one twenty-second of a milligram (.045 mg) of the pure crystalline product of insulin, now adopted as the standard.
international u. of penicillin the specific penicillin activity contained in 0.6 microgram of the international standard sodium salt of penicillin II or G.
international u. of vitamin A an older unit of vitamin A activity, equal to the activity of 0.3 microgram retinol or 0.6 microgram β-carotene; because the provitamin A carotenoids are absorbed less efficiently than is retinol, the source must be specified. Although largely supplanted by retinol equivalent (q.v.), the unit is still used in labeling. When the source is retinol, the unit is officially *vitamin A u.*
international u. of vitamin D the specific biological activity of 0.025 microgram of cholecalciferol.
international u. of vitamin E the specific biological activity of 0.671 milligram of *d*-alpha-tocopherol or 1.0 milligram of *dl*-alpha-tocopherol acetate. See also *alpha-tocopherol equivalent.*
Karmen u. the amount of transaminase that under specified conditions will cause a change of 0.001 in the absorbance of NADH when measured at 340 nm in a 1 cm light path.
Kienböck u. a unit of x-ray exposure equal to 0.1 erythema dose; symbol X.
King u., King-Armstrong u. the amount of phosphatase that liberates 1 mg of phenol from an excess of disodium phenylphosphate under defined conditions; alkaline phosphatase can be measured under alkaline conditions and acid phosphatase under acidic conditions.
Lf u. see under *dose.*
map u. centimorgan.
motor u. the unit of motor activity formed by a motor nerve cell and its many innervated muscle fibers.
mouse u. Allen-Doisy u.
neurocritical care u., neurointensive care u., neuroscience intensive care u. a neurologic intensive care unit; one specializing in patients with serious or life-threatening neurologic conditions.
Noon pollen u. the activity present in the saline extract from one millionth of a grain of pollen.
u. of oxytocin a USP unit expressing the uterus-stimulating activity of preparations of synthetic oxytocin; one unit is approximately equivalent to the strength of 2 μg of pure hormone.
pepsin u. a unit for measuring the proportion of pepsin in the gastric juice.
peripheral resistance u. (PRU) a conventional unit of vascular resistance equal to the resistance that produces a pressure difference of 1 mm Hg, corresponding to a blood flow of 1 mL/sec.
pilosebaceous u. the complex consisting of a hair follicle, its sebaceous (pilosebaceous) gland, and the arrector pili muscle. Called also *pilosebaceous apparatus.*
plaque-forming u. an estimate of the titer of a bacteriophage solution, determined by mixing the bacteriophage with a solution of susceptible bacteria, plating, incubating, and counting the number of plaques present on the bacterial lawn, with each plaque representing a viable bacteriophage.
postanesthesia care u. (PACU) a specialized unit adjoining an operating room, equipped and staffed for giving postoperative care to patients recovering from anesthesia and intravenous sedation; called also *recovery room.*
quantum u. see *Planck constant*, under *constant.*
SI u. any of the units of the Système International d'Unités, or International System of Units, adopted in 1960 at the Eleventh General Conference of Weights and Measures. SI units are based on the metric system and many are derived from natural constants. For units and for multiples and submultiples of these units formed by the use of prefixes, see table and Appendix 7.
Somogyi u. the amount of amylase that will liberate reducing equivalents equal to 1 mg of glucose per 30 minutes under defined conditions.
sudanophobic u. the smallest amount of corticotropin that will cause the disappearance of the sudanophobic zone of the adrenal

Unit *Continued*

SI UNITS

Quantity	Unit	Symbol	Derivation
Base Units			
length	meter	m	
mass	kilogram	kg	
time	second	s	
electric current	ampere	A	
temperature	kelvin	K	
luminous intensity	candela	cd	
amount of substance	mole	mol	
Supplementary Units			
plane angle	radian	rad	
solid angle	steradian	sr	
Derived Units			
force	newton	N	$kg{\cdot}m/s^2$
pressure	pascal	Pa	N/m^2
energy, work	joule	J	N·m
power	watt	W	J/s
electric charge	coulomb	C	A·s
electric potential	volt	V	J/C
electric capacitance	farad	F	C/V
electric resistance	ohm	Ω	V/A
electric conductance	siemens	S	Ω^{-1}
magnetic flux	weber	Wb	V·s
magnetic flux density	tesla	T	Wb/m^2
inductance	henry	H	Wb/A
frequency	hertz	Hz	s^{-1}
luminous flux	lumen	lm	cd·sr
illumination	lux	lx	lm/m^2
temperature	degree celsius	°C	K − 273.15
radioactivity	becquerel	Bq	s^{-1}
absorbed dose	gray	Gy	J/kg
absorbed dose equivalent	sievert	Sv	J/kg

cortex in at least two of three hypophysectomized rats when they are injected morning and evening on eight consecutive days.

Svedberg u. (S) a unit equal to 10^{-13} second used for expressing sedimentation coefficients (q.v.) of macromolecules.

Svedberg flotation u. (S_f) a unit equal to 10^{-13} second used for expressing negative sedimentation coefficients of macromolecules that float rather than sink in a centrifuge, e.g., lipoproteins.

terminal respiratory u. the part of the lung distal to a single terminal bronchiole; it is the anatomical and functional unit of the lung and consists of a respiratory bronchiole, two or more alveolar ducts, and alveoli. Called also *primary lobule of lung, pulmonary acinus,* and *transitional and respiratory zone.* See Plate 43.

toxic u., toxin u. the smallest dose of toxin which will kill a guinea pig weighing about 250 g in three to four days.

tuberculin u. (TU) an arbitrary unit of tuberculin dosage defined by comparison of clinical response with a standard preparation of PPD tuberculin.

turbidity reducing u. (TRU) the amount of hyaluronidase which is just sufficient to reduce the turbidity produced by 0.2 mg of hyaluronan to that produced by 0.1 mg after addition of acidified horse serum.

USP u. a unit used in the United States Pharmacopeia in expressing the potency of antibiotic, pharmacodynamic, and endocrine preparations, as well as most of the sera, toxins, vaccines, and related products, corresponding to units established internationally, by the Food and Drug Administration, or by the National Institutes of Health.

vitamin A u. [USP] the specific biological activity of 0.3 mg of the all-*trans* isomer of retinol. See also *international u. of vitamin A* and *retinol equivalent.*

vitamin D u. see *international u. of vitamin D.*

Wood u. peripheral resistance u.

wrist u. the part of a prosthetic upper limb that the terminal device attaches to.

x-ray u. Kienböck u.

unit·age (u′nit-əj) a statement of the unit quantity in any system of measurement.

uni·tary (u′nĭ-tar″e) [L. *unitas* oneness] composed of or pertaining to a single unit.

Unit·ed States Phar·ma·co·peia (USP) a legally recognized compendium of standards for drugs, published by The United States Pharmacopeial Convention, Inc., and revised periodically. It includes also assays and tests for the determination of strength, quality, and purity.

uni·ter·mi·nal (u″nĭ-tur′mĭ-nəl) 1. monopolar. 2. a monopolar apparatus.

Uni·throid (u′nĭ-throid″) trademark for a preparation of levothyroxine sodium.

unit·less (u′nit-ləs) lacking units.

Uni·tu·ni·ca·tae (u″ne-too″nĭ-ka′te) in fungal taxonomy, a series of the subphylum Ascomycotina, consisting of those having a unitunicate ascus. It is usually subdivided into operculate and inoperculate groups according to whether or not the ascus has an operculum (small cap that pops open for ejection of spores).

uni·va·lence (u″nĭ-va′ləns) the state or condition of being univalent.

uni·va·lent (u″nĭ-va′lənt) monovalent.

uni·var·i·ate (u″nĭ-vār′e-ət) pertaining to only one variable.

Uni·vasc (u′nĭ-vask″) trademark for a preparation of moexipril hydrochloride.

uni·vi·tel·line (u″nĭ-vi-tel′in) pertaining to or derived from a single oocyte or ovum.

un·med·ul·lat·ed (ən-med′u-lāt″əd) unmyelinated.

un·my·eli·nat·ed (ən-mi′ə-lĭ-nāt″əd) not possessing a myelin sheath; said of a nerve fiber. Called also *nonmedullated, nonmyelinated,* and *unmedullated.*

Un·na paste boot, alkaline methylene blue (oon′ah) [Paul Gerson *Unna,* German dermatologist, 1850–1929] see under *boot,* and *blue.*

Un·na-Pap·pen·heim stain (oon′ah pah′pən-hīm) [P.G. *Unna;* Artur *Pappenheim,* German physician, 1870–1916] see *Stains and Staining Methods,* under *stain.*

Un·na-Thost syndrome (oon′ah tost′) [P.G. *Unna;* Arthur *Thost,* German physician, late 19th century] nonepidermolytic palmoplantar keratoderma.

uno·pros·tone iso·pro·pyl (u″no-pros′tōn) an antiglaucoma agent that decreases elevated intraocular pressure by increasing the outflow of aqueous humor; used in the treatment of open-angle glaucoma and ocular hypertension, applied topically to the conjunctiva.

un·or·ga·nized (ən-or′gən-īzd) not developed into an organic structure; not having organs.

un·phys·i·o·log·ic (un″fiz-e-o-loj′ik) not physiologic in character.

un·sat·u·rat·ed (ən-sach′ə-rāt″əd) not saturated; applied to a chemical compound in which two or more atoms are united by double or triple bonds, which contain multiple pairs of shared electrons. Such compounds may still add atoms or groups to the unsaturated bonding atoms up to a limit of bonding power, or saturation. Most commonly refers to carbon-carbon bonds, as in unsaturated fatty acids. Also applied to a solution in which more solute may still be dissolved under stated conditions.

Un·schuld sign (oon′shoolt) [Paul *Unschuld,* German internist, 1835–c. 1905] see under *sign.*

un·sharp·ness (ən-shahrp′nis) in radiology, the measure or degree to which sharp boundaries of an object or person being imaged are blurred in that image.

un·spe·cif·ic mono·oxy·ge·nase (un″spə-sif′ik mon″o-ok′sə-jən-ās) [EC 1.14.14.1] a broadly specific monooxygenase for which the hydrogen donor is a reduced flavoprotein; it contains cytochrome P-450 as its oxygen

A Ethylene B Ethane

■ Unsaturated *(A)* and saturated *(B)* two-carbon hydrocarbons.

activator. It acts on a wide range of substrates, including xenobiotics, steroids, fatty acids, vitamins, and prostaglandins.

un·stri·at·ed (ən-striʹāt-əd) having no striations or striae; see under *muscle.*

un·thrif·ti·ness (ən-thrifʹte-nis) failure of a young animal to grow or gain weight at a normal rate in spite of an adequate diet and lack of overt illness. Called also *ill thrift.*

Un·ver·richt disease (oonʹfer-ikt) [Heinrich *Unverricht,* German physician, 1853–1912] myoclonic epilepsy.

Un·ver·richt-Lund·borg disease (oonʹfer-ikt loondʹborg) [H. *Unverricht;* Herman Bernhard *Lundborg,* Swedish physician, 1868–1943] see under *disease.*

un·voiced (un-voistʹ) voiceless.

upa·dha·tu (ooʺpə-thŭʹtoo) [Sanskrit *upa* above + *dhatu* to support] according to ayurveda, secondary, temporary tissue that arises from the metabolism and waste of primary tissues (dhatus); for example, feces provide temporary strength and structure to the colon and sweat lubricates the skin.

u-plas·min·o·gen ac·ti·va·tor (plaz-minʹə-jənʺ akʹtĭ-vaʺtər) [EC 3.4.21.73] see under *activator.*

UPP urethral pressure profile.

UPPP uvulopalatopharyngoplasty.

up·reg·u·la·tion (upʺreg-u-laʹshən) increase in expression of a gene; in the narrowest sense, that in which transcription of a specific mRNA is increased, but also used more broadly to refer to increase in mRNA levels for a particular gene from any cause, such as increased stability of the specific mRNA.

up·right·ing (upʹrīt-ing) tipping inclined teeth to a more vertical axial inclination. See also *tipping* (def. 1).

up·si·loid (upʹsĭ-loid) [Gr. *upsilon* + *-oid*] shaped like the Greek upsilon (υ or Y); see *hyoid* (def. 1) and *hypsiloid.*

up·si·lon (upʹsi-lon) [Y, υ] the twentieth letter of the Greek alphabet.

up·stream (upʹstrēm) in molecular biology, a term used to denote a region of nucleic acid to the 5′ side of a gene or region of interest.

up·take (upʹtāk) absorption and incorporation of a substance by living tissue.

pertechnetate u. a thyroid function test in which, along with radioiodine, radioactive technetium is administered in the form of the pertechnetate ion (technetium 99m pertechnetate) to measure early uptake and trapping of the ion by the thyroid gland.

radioactive iodine u. (RAIU), radioiodine u. uptake of radioiodine from the blood by the thyroid gland; see under *test.*

triiodothyronine resin u. the uptake of radioactive triiodothyronine at binding sites on resin, contrasted to uptake at sites on thyroxine-binding globulin in the triiodothyronine resin uptake test (see under *test*).

ura·cho·ves·i·cal (uʺrə-ko-vesʹĭ-kəl) pertaining to the urachus and the urinary bladder.

ura·chus (uʹrə-kəs) [Gr. *ourachos*] the derivative of the allantoic stalk in the fetus that connects the urinary bladder with the umbilicus; it persists throughout life as a fibrous cord, the *median umbilical ligament,* into which a patent canal may extend for part of the distance to the umbilicus. **uʹrachal** *adj*

patent u. a congenital anomaly in which the urachus remains patent from the bladder to the umbilicus, with a channel that may be small or large and leakage of urine at the umbilicus.

ura·cil (ūrʹə-sil) a pyrimidine base, in animal cells usually occurring condensed with ribose to form the ribonucleoside uridine, a component of ribonucleic acid and of free nucleotides with functions in metabolism. The corresponding deoxyribonucleoside, deoxyuridine, is a component of free nucleotides involved in pyrimidine biosynthesis. See illustration of *purine and pyrimidine bases,* under *base.* Symbol U.

ura·cra·sia (uʺrə-kraʹzhə) [*ur-* + *a-*^{1} + *-crasia*] a disordered state of the urine.

uranisc(o)- [Gr. *ouraniskos,* the roof of the mouth] for words beginning thus, see *palat(o)-.*

ura·nis·cus (uʺrə-nisʹkəs) [Gr. *ouraniskos*] palate.

ura·ni·um (U) (u-raʹne-əm) [L. *Uranus* a planet] a hard and heavy radioactive metallic element; atomic number, 92; atomic weight, 238.03; specific gravity, 18.68. Naturally occurring uranium is composed of three isotopes of mass numbers 234, 235, and 238. Uranium 235 separated from U 238 undergoes fission with slow neutrons, giving up neutrons which can join the nucleus of U 238 to form neptunium, which in turn decays by beta particle emission to form plutonium. Cf. *neptunium* and *plutonium.*

uran(o)- [Gr. *ouranos* the vault of heaven, or the roof of the mouth] a combining form denoting relationship to the palate; see also *palat(o)-.*

ura·no·plas·ty (uʹrə-no-plasʺte) palatoplasty. **uranoplasʹtic** *adj*

ura·no·ple·gia (uʺrə-no-pleʹjə) palatoplegia.

ura·nor·rha·phy (uʺrə-norʹə-fe) palatorrhaphy.

ura·nos·chi·sis (uʺrə-nosʹkĭ-sis) cleft palate.

ura·no·staph·y·lo·plas·ty (uʺrə-no-stafʹə-lo-plasʺte) an operation for repairing a defect of both the soft and hard palate. See also *palatoplasty.*

ura·no·staph·y·lor·rha·phy (uʺrə-no-stafʺə-lorʹə-fe) [*urano-* + *staphylo-* + *-rrhaphy*] suture of both the soft and hard palate. See also *palatorrhaphy.*

ura·no·staph·y·los·chi·sis (uʺrə-no-stafʺə-losʹkĭ-sis) cleft palate involving both the soft palate and the hard palate.

Ura·no·tae·nia (uʺrə-no-teʹne-ə) a genus of culicine mosquitoes. *U. sappariʹnus* is found in the eastern United States.

ura·nyl (uʹrə-nəl) the UO_2^{2+} ion.

urar·thri·tis (uʺrahr-thriʹtis) gouty arthritis.

urate (ūrʹāt) any salt or anion of uric acid; the salts are insoluble in water and can form crystals, stones, and calculi.

calcium u. the calcium salt of uric acid; it is a less common type of renal calculus.

monosodium u. monohydrate, sodium u. the monosodium salt of uric acid, deposited as needle-shaped crystals (tophi, q.v.) in the joints and other sites in gout.

ura·te·mia (uʺrə-teʹme-ə) the presence of urates in the blood.

urate ox·i·dase (ūrʹāt okʹsĭ-dās) [EC 1.7.3.3] an enzyme of the oxidoreductase class that catalyzes the oxidation of uric acid to allantoin with liberation of CO_2 and H_2O_2. It is a copper enzyme, found in most mammals but not in primates; it is frequently used in clinical assays of uric acid concentrations. Called also *uricase.*

urat·ic (u-ratʹik) 1. pertaining to urates. 2. pertaining to gout.

ura·to·his·tech·ia (uʺrə-to-his-tekʹe-ə) [*urate* + *hist-* + Gr. *echein* to hold] the presence of an excessive amount of urate, urea, or uric acid in a tissue.

ura·to·ma (uʺrə-toʹmə) a tophus or concretion made up of urates.

ura·to·sis (uʺrə-toʹsis) the deposition of crystalline urates in the tissues.

ura·tu·ria (uʺrə-tuʹre-ə) hyperuricosuria.

Ur·bach-Wiethe disease (urʹbak veʹtə) [Erich *Urbach,* American dermatologist, 1893–1946; Camillo *Wiethe,* Austrian otologist, 1888–1949] lipoid proteinosis, see under *proteinosis.*

ur·ce·i·form (ər-seʹĭ-form) [L. *urceus* pitcher + *form*] pitcher-shaped.

ur·ce·o·late (ər-seʹə-lāt) urceiform.

urea (u-reʹə) 1. a compound, $CO(NH_2)_2$, formed in the liver via the urea cycle (q.v.) from ammonia produced by the deamination of amino acids and later excreted by the kidney; it is the principal end product of protein catabolism and constitutes about one half of the total urinary solids. Elevation of the blood levels of urea and other nitrogenous compounds (azotemia) occurs with decreased glomerular filtration rate due to inadequate renal perfusion, acute or chronic renal disease, or urinary tract obstruction (see *uremia*). Called also *carbamide.* 2. [USP] a preparation of urea administered intravenously as an osmotic diuretic to reduce intracranial or intraocular pressure; injected transabdominally into the amniotic sac as a hypertonic solution to induce abortion of a second trimester pregnancy, and used in topical preparations to moisten and soften rough dry skin. 3. a preparation of urea used as a feed additive for ruminants, enhancing protein synthesis from dietary roughage and stimulating multiplication of microorganisms that digest cellulose.

u. nitrogen the urea concentration of blood or serum stated in terms of nitrogen content; converted to urea concentration by multiplying by 60/28 or 2.14. The serum or plasma urea nitrogen is traditionally referred to as *blood urea nitrogen (BUN).*

urea·gen·e·sis (u-reʺə-jenʹə-sis) the formation or production of urea; called also *ureapoiesis.*

urea·ge·net·ic (u-reʺə-jə-netʹik) [*urea* + Gr. *gennan* to produce] pertaining to ureagenesis.

ure·al (uʹre-əl) pertaining to urea.

Urea·phil (u-reʹə-fil) trademark for preparations of urea.

Urea·plas·ma (u-reʺə-plazʹmə) [*urea* + Gr. *plasma* anything formed or molded] a genus of gram-negative bacteria of the family Mycoplasmataceae, consisting of pleomorphic, nonmotile, microaerophilic, coccoid or coccobacillary organisms that lack a cell wall, form extremely small colonies, and hydrolyze urea; they occur most commonly in the oropharynx and respiratory and urogenital tracts. The type species is *U. urealyʹticum.* Called also *T-strain mycoplasma* (T for *tiny*).

U. par′vum a species having the same habitat and pathogenicity as *U. urealyticum*, of which it was formerly considered a biovar.

U. urealy′ticum a species that is a normal commensal of the genitourinary tract, but can also be an opportunistic pathogen and cause genitourinary and respiratory infections; it is sometimes transmitted perinatally from mother to infant, resulting in prematurity and neonatal disease.

urea•plas•ma (u-re″ə-plaz′mə) an individual organism of the genus *Ureaplasma*.

urea•poi•e•sis (u-re″ə-poi-e′sis) [*urea* + *-poiesis*] ureagenesis.

ure•ase (u′re-ās) [EC 3.5.1.5] an enzyme of the hydrolase class that catalyzes the hydrolysis of urea to CO_2 and ammonia; it is a nickel protein found in microorganisms and plants that is frequently used in clinical assays of plasma urea concentrations.

Urech•i•tes (u-rek′ĭ-tēz) a genus of plants of the family Apocyanaceae, native to tropical parts of the Americas. *U. lu′tea* is a Cuban plant that causes fatal heart failure in cattle. *U. suberec′ta* is the Savannah flower, whose leaves are poisonous and antipyretic.

urech•i•tin (u-rek′ĭ-tin) a poisonous glycoside from *Urechites suberecta.*

urech•i•tox•in (u-rek′ĭ-tok″sin) a poisonous glycoside from *Urechites suberecta.*

Ure•cho•line (u″re-ko′lēn) trademark for preparations of bethanechol chloride.

Ure•di•na•les (u″rə-dĭ-na′lēz) the rusts, an order of perfect fungi of the class Teliomycetes; they cause damage to numerous different economically important food plants.

ure•ic (u-re′ik) ureal.

ure•ide (u-re′īd) a compound of urea and an acid or aldehyde. Those from one molecule of urea, as alloxan, are monoureides; those derived from two, as uric acid, are diureides.

ure•id•o•pen•i•cil•lin (u-re″ĭ-do-pen″ĭ-sil′in) [*ureide* + *penicillin*] any in a group of penicillin derivatives in which a urea has replaced an amino side chain.

ure•mia (u-re′me-ə) [*ur-* + *-emia*] 1. azotemia. 2. in current usage, the entire constellation of signs and symptoms of chronic renal failure, including nausea, vomiting, anorexia, a metallic taste in the mouth, a characteristic odor of the breath, pruritus, urea frost on the skin, neuromuscular disorders, pain and twitching in the muscles, hypertension, edema, mental confusion, and acid-base and electrolyte imbalances. Some authorities prefer to call this the *uremic syndrome.*

ure•mic (u-re′mik) pertaining to or characterized by uremia.

ure•mi•gen•ic (u-re″mĭ-jen′ik) 1. caused by or due to uremia. 2. causing uremia.

ure(o)- [*urea,* q.v.] for words beginning thus, see also those beginning *urea-*.

ure•ol•y•sis (u″re-ol′ĭ-sis) [*ureo-* + *-lysis*] the decomposition of urea to carbon dioxide and ammonia. **ureolyt′ic** *adj*

ureo•tel•ic (u″re-o-tel′ik) [*ureo-* + *tel-* + *-ic*] having urea as the chief excretory product of nitrogen metabolism.

ure•sis (u-re′sis) [Gr. *ourēsis*] urination.

-uresis a word termination denoting excretion in the urine of the substance indicated by the stem to which it is affixed, as chloruresis, cupruresis, or saluresis.

ure•ter (u-re′tər, u′rə-tər) [Gr. *ourētēr*] [TA] the fibromuscular tube that conveys the urine from the kidney to the bladder. It begins with the renal pelvis, a funnel-like dilatation, and empties into the base of the bladder. It is 40 to 46 cm long and is divided into an abdominal part *(pars abdominalis)* and a pelvic part *(pars pelvica).* See Plate 44. **ure′teral, ureter′ic** *adj*

bifid u. a ureter in which proximal segments come from two different collecting systems but join before reaching the bladder.

circumcaval u. postcaval u.

double u., duplex u. existence of a second ureter on one side; it may be a complete connection from the kidney to the bladder or a partial tube forming a blind pouch. Most are asymptomatic, but some are accompanied by ectopic ureterocele. Called also *ureteral duplication.*

ectopic u. a ureter that opens elsewhere than in the bladder wall, usually arising from the upper segment of a double kidney. In women it may open in the vestibule, terminal urethra, vagina, cervix, or uterine cavity; in men it invariably enters the genital or urinary tract above the level of the external sphincter.

lower pole u. the ureter draining the lower pole of a duplex kidney.

pipestem u. stenosis and calcification of a ureter, seen as a complication of renal tuberculosis that has spread into the ureter.

postcaval u., retrocaval u. a congenital anomaly in which the right ureter passes posterior to the inferior vena cava and curves around it back to the usual anterior position for descent to the bladder. Called also *circumcaval u.*

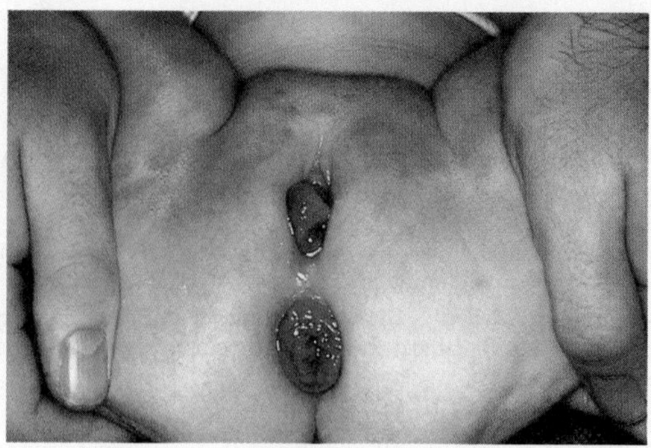

■ Ureterocele.

retroiliac u. a congenital anomaly in which a ureter passes behind the iliac artery.

upper pole u. the ureter draining the upper pole of a duplex kidney.

ure•ter•al•gia (u-re″tər-al′jə) pain in the ureter; neuralgia of the ureter.

ure•ter•ec•ta•sia (u-re″tər-ək-ta′zhə) ureterectasis.

ure•ter•ec•ta•sis (u-re″tər-ek′tə-sis) [*ureter* + *ectasis*] distention of the ureter, such as in megaureter or hydroureter. Called also *ureterectasia.*

ure•ter•ec•to•my (u-re″tər-ek′tə-me) [*ureter* + *-ectomy*] surgical removal of all or part of a ureter.

ure•ter•itis (u-re″tər-i′tis) inflammation of a ureter.

u. cys′tica ureteritis with formation of multiple submucosal cysts; see also *pyeloureteritis cystica.*

u. glandula′ris ureteritis characterized by conversion of transitional mucosal into cylindrical epithelium, with formation of glandular acini.

ureter(o)- [*ureter,* q.v.] a combining form denoting relationship to the ureter.

ure•tero•ar•te•ri•al (u-re″tər-o-ahr-te′re-əl) pertaining to or connecting a ureter and an artery, such as a fistula.

ure•tero•cele (u-re′tər-o-sēl″) [*uretero-* + *-cele*[1]] sacculation of the terminal portion of the ureter into the bladder, as a result of stenosis of the ureteral meatus. See illustration.

double system u., duplex system u. a ureterocele involving a double collecting system; seen most often in girls in an ectopic ureter.

ectopic u. an intravesical ureterocele located distal to the trigone of the bladder, so that it may extend into the urethra.

intravesical u. a ureterocele located entirely inside the bladder; it may be either orthotopic or ectopic.

orthotopic u. an intravesical ureterocele in which the ureter is in the proper position in the trigone of the bladder; it may be small and asymptomatic or large and extending deeply into the bladder.

prolapsed u., prolapsing u. an intravesical ureterocele that extends beyond the bladder neck down into the urethra; usually seen in females.

single system u. a ureterocele involving the ureter of a collecting system that is not double; it is usually orthotopic, intravesical, and seen in adults

ure•tero•ce•lec•to•my (u-re″tər-o-se-lek′tə-me) excision of a ureterocele.

ure•tero•cer•vi•cal (u-re″tər-o-ser′vĭ-kəl) pertaining to a ureter and to the cervix uteri.

ure•ter•o•col•ic (u-re″tər-o-kol′ik) pertaining to or communicating between a ureter and the colon; called also *ureterocolonic.*

ure•tero•co•lon•ic (u-re″tər-o-ko-lon′ik) ureterocolic.

ure•tero•co•los•to•my (u-re″tər-o-kə-los′tə-me) ureterocolonic anastomosis.

ure•tero•cu•ta•ne•os•to•my (u-re″tər-o-ku-ta″ne-os′tə-me) an ileal conduit or other means of urinary diversion by which the ureter is surgically connected with the body surface instead of to the bladder.

ure•tero•cys•to•ne•os•to•my (u-re″tər-o-sis″to-ne-os′tə-me) ureteroneocystostomy.

ure•tero•cys•tos•to•my (u-re″tər-o-sis-tos′tə-me) ureteroneocystostomy.

ure•tero•du•o•de•nal (u-re″tər-o-doo″o-de′nəl) pertaining to or communicating between a ureter and the duodenum.

ure•tero•en•ter•ic (u-re″tər-o-ən-ter′ik) ureterointestinal.

ure·tero·en·tero·anas·to·mo·sis (u-re″tər-o-en″tər-o-ə-nas″tə-mo′sis) ureterointestinal anastomosis.

ure·tero·en·ter·os·to·my (u-re″tər-o-en″tər-os′tə-me) ureterointestinal anastomosis.

ure·tero·gram (u-re′tər-o-gram) a radiograph of the ureter.

ure·ter·og·ra·phy (u-re″tər-og′rə-fe) [*uretero-* + *-graphy*] radiography of the ureter after injection of an opaque medium.

ure·tero·hy·dro·ne·phro·sis (u-re″tər-o-hi″dro-nə-fro′sis) hydroureteronephrosis.

ure·tero·il·e·al (u-re″tər-o-il′e-əl) pertaining to or communicating between the ileum and a ureter. Called also *ileoureteral.*

ure·tero·il·e·os·to·my (u-re″tər-o-il″e-os′tə-me) urinary diversion consisting of anastomosis of the ureters to an isolated loop of ileum, drained through a stoma on the abdominal wall. See also *ileal conduit*, under *conduit.*

ure·tero·in·tes·ti·nal (u-re″tər-o-in-tes′tĭ-nəl) pertaining to or connecting a ureter and the intestine; called also *ureteroenteric.*

ure·tero·lith (u-re′tər-o-lith) [*uretero-* + *-lith*] a calculus lodged or formed in a ureter.

ure·tero·li·thi·a·sis (u-re″tər-o-lĭ-thi′ə-sis) the formation or presence of calculi in the ureter.

ure·tero·li·thot·o·my (u-re″tər-o-lĭ-thot′ə-me) [*uretero-* + *litho-* + *-tomy*] the removal of a calculus from the ureter by incision.

ure·ter·ol·y·sis (u-re″tər-ol′ĭ-sis) [*uretero-* + *-lysis*] 1. the operation of freeing the ureter from adhesions. 2. rupture of the ureter.

ure·tero·me·a·tot·o·my (u-re″tər-o-me″ə-tot′ə-me) incision of the opening of the ureter in the bladder wall.

ure·tero·neo·cys·tos·to·my (u-re″tər-o-ne″o-sis-tos′tə-me) [*uretero-* + *neo-* + *cystostomy*] surgical transplantation of the ureter to a different site of attachment to the bladder. Called also *ureteral reimplantation, ureterocystostomy, ureterocystoneostomy,* and *ureterovesicostomy.*

ure·tero·neo·py·elos·to·my (u-re″tər-o-ne″o-pi″ə-los′tə-me) ureteropyelostomy.

ure·tero·ne·phrec·to·my (u-re″tər-o-nə-frek′tə-me) nephroureterectomy.

ure·tero·ne·phros·co·py (u-re″tər-o-nə-fros′kə-pe) ureterorenoscopy.

ure·ter·op·a·thy (u-re″tər-op′ə-the) [*uretero-* + *-pathy*] any disease of the ureter.

ure·tero·pel·vic (u-re″tər-o-pel′vik) pertaining to or affecting the ureter and the renal pelvis.

ure·tero·pel·vio·ne·os·to·my (u-re″tər-o-pel″ve-o-ne-os′tə-me) ureteropyelostomy.

ure·tero·plas·ty (u-re′tər-o-plas″te) [*uretero-* + *-plasty*] plastic surgery of a ureter. ureteroplas′tic *adj*

reduction u. surgical tapering or plication of the ureter for treatment of megaureter.

ure·tero·proc·tos·to·my (u-re″tər-o-prok-tos′tə-me) ureterorectostomy.

ure·tero·py·eli·tis (u-re″tər-o-pi-ə-li′tis) pyeloureteritis.

ure·tero·py·elog·ra·phy (u-re″tər-o-pi-ə-log′rə-fe) radiography of the ureter and renal pelvis.

ure·tero·py·elo·ne·os·to·my (u-re″tər-o-pi″ə-lo-ne-os′tə-me) ureteropyelostomy.

ure·tero·py·elo·ne·phros·to·my (u-re″tər-o-pi″ə-lo-nə-fros′tə-me) ureteropyelostomy.

ure·tero·py·elo·plas·ty (u-re″tər-o-pi′ə-lo-plas″te) ureteropyelostomy. ureteropyeloplas′tic *adj*

ure·tero·py·elos·to·my (u-re″tər-o-pi″ə-los′tə-me) surgical formation of a new passage from a renal pelvis to a ureter to replace a damaged ureteropelvic junction. Called also *pyeloureteroplasty* and *ureteropyeloplasty.*

ure·tero·py·o·sis (u-re″tər-o-pi-o′sis) pyoureter.

ure·tero·rec·tal (u-re″tər-o-rek′təl) pertaining to or communicating between a ureter and the rectum.

ure·tero·rec·to·ne·os·to·my (u-re″tər-o-rek″to-ne-os′tə-me) ureterorectostomy.

ure·tero·rec·tos·to·my (u-re″tər-o-rek-tos′tə-me) urinary diversion consisting of surgical creation of an anastomosis between a ureter and the lower rectum.

ure·tero·re·no·scope (u-re″tər-o-re′no-skōp) a fiberoptic endoscope used in ureterorenoscopy.

ure·tero·re·nos·co·py (u-re″tər-o-re-nos′kə-pe) visual inspection of the interior of the ureter and kidney by means of a fiberoptic endoscope for such purposes as a biopsy or removal or crushing of stones.

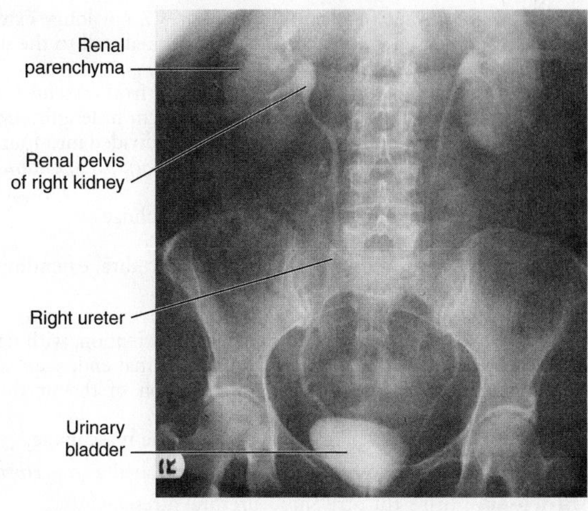

■ Ureteropyelography showing kidneys, ureters, and bladder.

ure·ter·or·rha·gia (u-re″tər-o-ra′jə) [*uretero-* + *-rrhagia*] a discharge of blood from the ureter.

ure·ter·or·rha·phy (u-re″tər-or′ə-fe) [*uretero-* + *-rrhaphy*] suture of a ureter.

ure·tero·scope (u-re′tər-o-skōp″) a fiberoptic endoscope used in ureteroscopy.

ure·ter·os·copy (u-re″tər-os′kə-pe) examination of the ureter by means of a ureteroscope.

ure·tero·sig·moi·dos·to·my (u-re″tər-o-sig″moi-dos′tə-me) ureterosigmoid anastomosis.

ure·tero·ste·no·sis (u-re″tər-o-stə-no′sis) stricture of the ureter.

ure·ter·os·to·ma (u-re″tər-os′to-mə) [*uretero-* + *stoma*] the opening of a ureterostomy on the body surface.

ure·ter·os·to·my (u-re″tər-os′tə-me) [*uretero-* + *-stomy*] any of various channels artificially created for urinary diversion with part or all of the ureter left intact.

cutaneous u. ureterocutaneostomy.

ure·ter·ot·o·my (u-re″tər-ot′ə-me) [*uretero-* + *-tomy*] surgical incision of a ureter.

Davis u. an open procedure combining a ureteral incision with intubation, usually for long or multiple strictures below the ureteropelvic junction.

ure·tero·ure·ter·al (u-re″tər-o-u-re′tər-əl) connecting two parts of the ureter.

ure·tero·ure·ter·os·to·my (u-re″tər-o-u-re″tər-os′tə-me) end-to-end anastomosis of the two portions of a transected ureter; called also *ureteroureteral anastomosis* and *van Hook operation.*

ure·tero·uter·ine (u-re″tər-o-u′tər-in) pertaining to or communicating with a ureter and the uterus.

ure·tero·vag·i·nal (u-re″tər-o-vaj′ĭ-nəl) pertaining to or communicating with a ureter and the vagina.

ure·tero·vas·cu·lar (u-re″tər-o-vas′ku-lər) pertaining to a ureter and a blood vessel.

ure·tero·ves·i·cal (u-re″tər-o-ves′ĭ-kəl) pertaining to a ureter and the bladder; called also *vesicoureteral.*

ure·tero·ves·i·co·plas·ty (u-re″tər-o-ves′ĭ-ko-plas″te) plastic repair of the ureterovesical junction for correction of an obstruction or vesicoureteral reflux.

ure·tero·ves·i·cos·to·my (u-re″tər-o-ves″ĭ-kos′tə-me) ureteroneocystostomy.

ure·thra (u-re′thrə) [Gr. *ourēthra*] the membranous canal conveying urine from the bladder to the exterior of the body. See *u. feminina* and *u. masculina* and see Plate 44. ure′thral *adj*

anterior u. the distal portion of the male urethra, extending from the bulb to the meatus.

bulbar u., bulbous u. the part of the male urethra where it passes through the bulb of the penis.

double u. congenital complete or partial duplication of the urethra, seen almost exclusively in males. In complete duplication, the urethral openings may be side by side or one above the other; in partial duplication, there may be a blind tube ending in the periurethral tissue or there may be an accessory opening on the shaft of the penis. Called also *urethral duplication.*

female u., u. femini′na [TA] a canal about 3.7 cm long, extending from the neck of the bladder above the anterior vaginal wall to the urinary meatus.

male u., u. masculi′na [TA] a canal extending from the neck of the bladder to the urinary meatus, measuring about 20 cm in length, and presenting a double curve when the penis is flaccid; it is divided into four parts: the *pars spongiosa*, *pars intermedia* (or *pars membranacea*), *pars prostatica*, and *pars intramuralis* (or *pars preprostatica*).

membranous u. pars intermedia urethrae masculinae.

penile u. pars spongiosa urethrae masculinae.

posterior u. the proximal portion of the male urethra, extending from the bladder to the bulb.

prostatic u. pars prostatica urethrae masculinae.

spinning top u. deformity of the urethra upon urination, with narrowing at the urinary meatus and dilatation at the proximal end; seen sporadically in conditions such as prolonged inflammation of the urethra and detrusor instability. Called also *spinning top deformity*.

spongiose u., spongy u. pars spongiosa urethrae masculinae.

ure·thral·gia (u″re-thral′jə) pain in the urethra; called also *urethrodynia*.

ure·thra·tre·sia (u-re″thrə-tre′zhə) urethral atresia.

ure·threc·to·my (u″rə-threk′tə-me) [*urethr-* + *-ectomy*] surgical removal of all or part of the urethra.

ure·threm·phrax·is (u″rə-thrəm-frak′sis) [*urethr-* + *emphraxis*] obstruction of the urethra.

ure·thrism (u′rə-thriz-əm) urethrospasm.

ure·thri·tis (u″rə-thri′tis) inflammation of the urethra.

u. cys′tica urethritis with formation of multiple submucosal cysts.

u. glandula′ris urethritis with conversion of transitional mucosal into cylindrical epithelium and formation of glandular acini.

gonococcal u., gonorrheal u. gonorrhea in the male urethra.

nongonococcal u., nonspecific u. urethritis without evidence of gonococcal infection, such as that caused by *Chlamydia trachomatis* or *Trichomonas vaginalis*. Called also *simple u.*

simple u. nongonococcal u.

urethr(o)- [*urethra*, q.v.] a combining form denoting relationship to the urethra.

ure·thro·anal (u-re″thro-a′nəl) anourethral.

ure·thro·bul·bar (u-re″thro-bul′bər) bulbourethral.

ure·thro·cele (u-re′thro-sēl) [*urethro-* + *-cele*[1]] 1. prolapse of the urethral mucosa. 2. a diverticulum of the urethral walls encroaching upon the vaginal canal.

ure·thro·cys·ti·tis (u-re″thro-sis-ti′tis) inflammation of the urethra and bladder; called also *cystourethritis*.

ure·thro·cys·to·gram (u-re″thro-sis′to-gram) a radiograph of the urethra and bladder.

ure·thro·cys·tog·ra·phy (u-re″thro-sis-tog′rə-fe) [*urethro-* + *cysto-* + *-graphy*] radiography of the urethra and bladder after the injection of a contrast medium.

ure·thro·cys·tom·e·try (u-re″thro-sis-tom′ĕ-tre) simultaneous measurement of pressures in the urinary bladder and urethra.

ure·thro·cys·to·pexy (u-re″thro-sis′to-pek″se) bladder neck suspension.

ure·thro·cys·tos·co·py (u-re″thro-sis-tos′kə-pe) cystourethroscopy.

ure·thro·dyn·ia (u-re″thro-din′e-ə) urethralgia.

ure·throg·ra·phy (u″rə-throg′rə-fe) radiography of the urethra after the injection of an opaque medium.

retrograde u. radiographic examination of the urethra after obstruction of its external orifice and injection of contrast material that travels in a retrograde direction towards the bladder; used for evaluation of strictures, diverticula, and trauma.

ure·thro·il·e·al (u-re″thro-il′e-əl) ileourethral.

ure·throm·e·ter (u″rə-throm′ə-tər) [*urethro-* + *-meter*] an instrument for measuring the urethra.

ure·throm·e·try (u″rə-throm′ə-tre) 1. determination of the resistance of various segments of the urethra to retrograde flow of fluid. 2. measurement of the urethra.

ure·thro·pe·nile (u-re″thro-pe′nīl) pertaining to the urethra and the penis.

ure·thro·peri·ne·al (u-re″thro-per″ĭ-ne′əl) pertaining to or communicating with the urethra and the perineum.

ure·thro·peri·neo·scro·tal (u-re″thro-per″ĭ-ne″o-skro′təl) pertaining to or communicating with the urethra, perineum, and scrotum.

ure·thro·pexy (u-re′thro-pek″se) [*urethro-* + *-pexy*] bladder neck suspension.

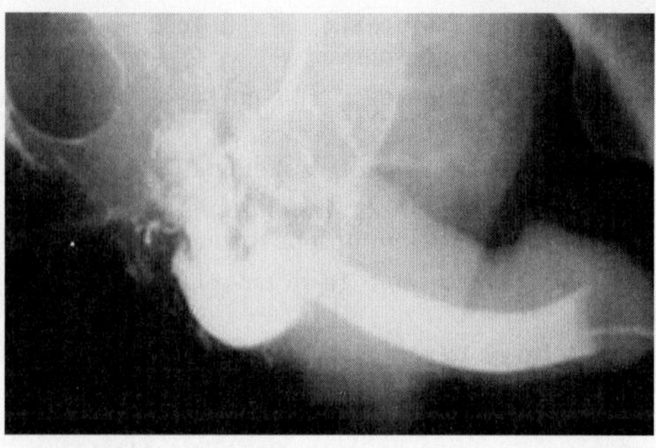

■ Retrograde urethrography showing complete disruption of posterior urethra secondary to pelvic fracture.

ure·thro·plas·ty (u-re′thro-plas″te) [*urethro-* + *-plasty*] plastic surgery of the urethra. **urethroplas′tic** *adj*

Cecil u. see under *operation*.

ure·thro·pros·tat·ic (u-re″thro-pros-tat′ik) pertaining to the urethra and the prostate.

ure·thro·rec·tal (u-re″thro-rek′təl) rectourethral.

ure·thror·rha·gia (u-re″thro-ra′jə) [*urethro-* + *-rrhagia*] a flow of blood from the urethra.

ure·thror·rha·phy (u″rə-thror′ə-fe) [*urethro-* + *-rrhaphy*] suture of the urethra.

ure·thror·rhea (u-re″thro-re′ə) [*urethro-* + *-rrhea*] an abnormal discharge from the urethra.

ure·thro·scope (u-re′thro-skōp) [*urethro-* + *-scope*] an endoscope for viewing the interior of the urethra.

ure·thro·scop·ic (u-re″thro-skop′ik) 1. pertaining to a urethroscope. 2. pertaining to urethroscopy.

ure·thros·co·py (u″rə-thros′kə-pe) inspection of the interior of the urethra with a urethroscope.

ure·thro·scro·tal (u-re″thro-skro′təl) pertaining to or communicating with the urethra and scrotum.

ure·thro·spasm (u-re′thro-spaz″əm) [*urethro-* + *spasm*] spasm of the urethra; called also *urethrism*.

ure·thro·stax·is (u-re″thro-stak′sis) [*urethro-* + *staxis*] oozing of blood from the urethra.

ure·thro·ste·no·sis (u-re″thro-stə-no′sis) [*urethro-* + *stenosis*] stricture or stenosis of the urethra.

ure·thros·to·my (u″rə-thros′tə-me) [*urethro-* + *-stomy*] surgical formation of a permanent opening of the urethra at the perineal surface.

ure·thro·tome (u-re′thro-tōm) an instrument for cutting a urethral stricture.

Maisonneuve u. a urethrotome in which the knife is concealed until it reaches the stricture.

ure·throt·o·my (u″rə-throt′ə-me) [*urethro-* + *-tomy*] incision of the urethra, usually for relief of a stricture.

external u. urethrotomy performed through the perineum; called also *perineal u.*

internal u. urethrotomy performed from within, either blindly or with an instrument that permits direct visualization.

perineal u. external u.

ure·thro·tri·go·ni·tis (u-re″thro-tri″go-ni′tis) inflammation of the urethra and trigone of the bladder.

ure·thro·vag·i·nal (u-re″thro-vaj′ĭ-nəl) pertaining to or communicating with the urethra and the vagina.

ure·thro·ves·i·cal (u-re″thro-ves′ĭ-kəl) vesicourethral.

uret·ic (u-ret′ik) 1. ureteric. 2. urinary.

Urex (u′reks) trademark for a preparation of methenamine hippurate.

ur·gen·cy (ur′jən-se) a sudden compelling need to do something.

bowel u. the sudden, almost uncontrollable, need to defecate.

urinary u. the sudden, almost uncontrollable, need to urinate.

Ur·gin·ea (ər-jin′e-ə) [L.] a genus of plants of the family Liliaceae. *U. mari′tima* (L.) Baker, a white Mediterranean species, and *U. in′dica* Kunth., an Indian species, are varieties of squill.

urhi·dro·sis (u″rĭ-dro′sis) [*ur-* + *hidro-* + *-sis*] the presence in the sweat of urinous materials, such as uric acid, urea, etc. Called also *uridrosis*.

u. crystal′lina uremic frost.

-uria [Gr. *ouron* urine + *-ia*] a word termination denoting a characteristic or constituent of the urine, indicated by the stem to which it is affixed, as oliguria, proteinuria.

uri·an (u′re-an) urochrome.

uric (u′rik) [Gr. *ourikos*] urinary. See also *uric acid.*

uric ac·id (u′rik) the end product of purine catabolism in primates; elevated blood levels are associated with gout and nephrolithiasis. Its salts, urates, are insoluble in water and can form crystals, stones, or calculi. Called also *lithic acid.*

uric·ac·i·de·mia (u″rik-as″ĭ-de′me-ə) hyperuricemia.

uric·ac·i·du·ria (u″rik-as″ĭ-du′re-ə) hyperuricosuria.

uri·case (u′rĭ-kās) urate oxidase.

uri·ce·mia (u″rĭ-se′me-ə) hyperuricemia.

uric(o)- [Gr. *ouron* urine] of or pertaining to the urine or to uric acid.

uri·co·cho·lia (u″rĭ-ko-ko′le-ə) [*urico-* + *chol-* + *-ia*] the presence of uric acid in the bile.

uri·col·y·sis (u″rĭ-kol′ĭ-sis) [*urico-* + *-lysis*] the cleavage of uric acid or of urates. **uricolyt′ic** *adj*

uri·co·poi·e·sis (u″rĭ-ko-poi-e′sis) the formation of uric acid.

uri·co·su·ria (u″rĭ-ko-su′re-ə) excretion of uric acid in the urine.

uri·co·su·ric (u″rĭ-ko-su′rik) 1. pertaining to, characterized by, or promoting uricosuria. 2. an agent that promotes uricosuria.

uri·co·tel·ic (u″rĭ-ko-tel′ik) [*urico-* + *tel-* + *-ic*] having uric acid as the chief excretory product of nitrogen metabolism, as in reptiles and birds.

uri·co·tel·ism (u″rĭ-ko-tel′iz-əm) the excretion of uric acid as the end product of nitrogen metabolism, as in reptiles and birds.

Uri·cult (u′rĭ-kəlt) trademark for a bacterial culture device, consisting of a glass slide in a sterile plastic container. On one face of the slide a 13 cm^2 area is coated with MacConkey medium; on the other a similar area is coated with nutrient agar. The slide is dipped into freshly voided urine, removed, and replaced in the container, where growth takes place.

uri·dine (ūr′ĭ-dēn) a pyrimidine nucleoside, uracil linked by its N1 nitrogen to the C1 carbon of ribose. It is a component of ribonucleic acid, and its nucleotides participate in the biosynthesis of polysaccharides and some polysaccharide-containing compounds. Symbol U.

u. diphosphate (UDP) a nucleotide, the 5′-pyrophosphate of uridine, which serves as a carrier for hexoses, hexosamines, and hexuronic acids in the synthesis of glycogen, glycoproteins, and glycosaminoglycans. UDPglucose and UDP-*N*-acetylglucosamine are the parent compounds from which are synthesized the other UDP-linked hexoses, hexosamines, and hexuronic acids. See also specific UDP-linked compounds (e.g., UDPgalactose).

u. monophosphate (UMP) a nucleotide, the 5′-phosphate of uridine; it is a component of ribonucleic acid. Called also *uridylic acid.*

u. triphosphate (UTP) a nucleotide, the 5′-triphosphate of uridine; it is an activated precursor in the synthesis of ribonucleic acid and of UDP-linked hexoses involved in glycogen and glycoprotein metabolism.

uri·dro·sis (u″rĭ-dro′sis) urhidrosis.

uri·dyl·ate (u″rĭ-dil′āt) a dissociated form of uridylic acid.

uri·dyl·ic ac·id (u″rĭ-dil′ik) phosphorylated uridine; uridine monophosphate unless otherwise specified.

uri·dyl trans·fer·ase (u′ri-dəl trans′fər-ās) UDP-glucose–hexose-1-phosphate uridylyltransferase.

uri·dyl·yl (u′rĭ-dil′əl) the radical formed by removal of OH from the phosphate group of uridine monophosphate.

Uri·max (u′rĭ-maks) trademark for a combination preparation of methenamine, sodium biphosphate, phenyl salicylate, methylene blue, and hyoscyamine sulfate.

urin·ac·i·dom·e·ter (u″rin-as″ĭ-dom′ə-tər) an instrument for estimating the pH of urine.

uri·nal (u′rĭ-nəl) [L. *urinalis* urinary] a vessel or other receptacle for urine.

uri·nal·y·sis (u″rĭ-nal′ĭ-sis) physical, chemical, or microscopic analysis or examination of urine.

uri·nary (u′rĭ-nar″e) 1. pertaining to urine. 2. containing or secreting urine.

uri·nate (u′rĭ-nāt) to discharge urine.

uri·na·tion (u″rĭ-na′shən) the discharge or passage of urine. Called also *micturition* and *uresis.*

precipitant u. urinary urgency.

stuttering u. an intermittent flow of urine, due to vesical spasm. Called also *urinary stuttering.*

urine (u′rin) [L. *urina;* Gr. *ouron*] the fluid excreted by the kidneys, passed through the ureters, stored in the bladder, and discharged through the urethra; its constituents and volume vary widely from day to day in order to maintain normal fluid and electrolyte homeostasis.

black u. urine colored black by melanin (melanuria), or by derivatives of homogentisic acid (ochronosis).

chylous u. chyluria.

cloudy u. urine having a cloudy appearance, usually due to phosphaturia or uraturia, but sometimes caused by pyuria; called also *nebulous u.*

crude u. light-colored, watery urine, which deposits little sediment.

diabetic u. urine that contains an excess of glucose.

dyspeptic u. the urine in dyspepsia, frequently containing calcium oxalate crystals.

febrile u. strong, odorous, high-colored, concentrated urine, such as is secreted in fever.

gouty u. scanty, high-colored urine containing large quantities of urates.

milky u. urine having a milky appearance, which may be due to chyluria or pyuria.

nebulous u. cloudy u.

residual u. the urine that remains in the bladder after urination in disease of the bladder and hypertrophy of the prostate.

uri·ni·dro·sis (u″rĭ-nĭ-dro′sis) urhidrosis.

uri·nif·er·ous (u″rĭ-nif′ər-əs) [*urine* + *-ferous*] transporting or conveying the urine.

uri·nip·a·rous (u″rĭ-nip′ə-rəs) urogenous (def. 1).

urin(o)- [L. *urina,* q.v.] a combining form denoting relationship to urine; see also *ur(o)-.*

uri·no·cry·os·co·py (u-ri″no-kri-os′kə-pe) cryoscopy of the urine.

uri·no·gen·i·tal (u″rĭ-no-jen′ĭ-təl) genitourinary.

uri·nog·e·nous (u″rĭ-noj′ə-nəs) urogenous.

uri·no·glu·co·som·e·ter (u″rĭ-no-gloo″ko-som′ə-tər) an instrument for measuring the glucose in the urine.

uri·nol·o·gy (u″rĭ-nol′ə-je) urology.

uri·no·ma (u″rĭ-no′mə) [*urine* + *-oma*] a collection of urine encapsulated by fibrous tissue, resulting from leakage of urine from a tear in the ureter, renal pelvis, or renal calices because of obstruction of the ureter; it may be a result of external trauma or a postoperative complication. Called also *paranephric, pararenal,* or *uriniferous pseudocyst.*

uri·nom·e·ter (u″rĭ-nom′ə-tər) [*urino-* + *-meter*] an instrument for determining the specific gravity of the urine.

uri·nom·e·try (u″rĭ-nom′ə-tre) the ascertainment of the specific gravity of the urine.

uri·noph·i·lous (u″rĭ-nof′ĭ-ləs) [*urino-* + Gr. *philein* to love] having an affinity for urine, as a microorganism that grows best in urine.

uri·nos·co·py (u″rĭ-nos′kə-pe) uroscopy.

uri·no·sex·u·al (u″rĭ-no-sek′shoo-əl) genitourinary.

uri·no·tho·rax (u″rĭ-no-tho′raks) hydrothorax in which the fluid is urine, secondary to an obstruction in the renal pelvis or urinary tract.

uri·nous (u′rĭ-nəs) urinary.

uri·po·sia (u″rĭ-po′ze-ə) [*ur*ine + *-posia*] the drinking of urine.

Uri·sed (u′rĭ-sed) trademark for a combination preparation of methenamine, phenyl salicylate, methylene blue, benzoic acid, atropine sulfate, and hyoscyamine sulfate.

urish·i·ol (u-rish′e-ol) urushiol.

Uri·spas (u′rĭ-spaz) trademark for a preparation of flavoxate hydrochloride.

ur(o)- [Gr. *ouron* urine] a combining form denoting relationship to urine, the urinary tract, or urination. See also *urin(o)-.*

uro·ac·i·dim·e·ter (u″ro-as″ĭ-dim′ə-tər) an instrument for measuring the acidity of the urine.

uro·am·mo·ni·ac (u″ro-ə-mo′ne-ak) containing uric acid and ammonia.

uro·az·o·tom·e·ter (u″ro-az″o-tom′ə-tər) an apparatus for measuring the nitrogenous matter of the urine.

uro·ben·zo·ic ac·id (u″ro-ben-zo′ik) hippuric acid.

uro·bi·lin (u″ro-bi′lin) [*uro-* + *bilin*] a brown pigment, an oxidized form of urobilinogen, found in the feces and sometimes in urine left standing in the air.

uro·bil·in·emia (u″ro-bil″ĭ-ne′me-ə) [*urobilin* + *-emia*] the presence of urobilin in the blood.

uro·bi·lino·gen (u″ro-bĭ-lin′o-jən) [*urobilin* + *-gen*] a colorless compound formed in the intestines by the reduction of bilirubin. Some is excreted in the feces, where by oxidation it becomes urobilin, and some is reabsorbed and re-excreted either in the bile as bilirubin or in the urine, where it is later oxidized to urobilin.

uro•bi•lino•gen•emia (u″ro-bĭ-lin″o-jə-ne′me-ə) the presence of urobilinogen in the blood.

uro•bi•lino•gen•uria (u″ro-bĭ-lin″o-jə-nu′re-ə) excessive urobilinogen in the urine, as in liver dysfunction or the jaundice from hemolytic anemia.

uro•bil•i•noid (u″ro-bil′ĭ-noid) resembling urobilin.

uro•bil•in•uria (u″ro-bil″ĭ-nu′re-ə) [*urobilin* + *-uria*] excessive urobilin in the urine, as in cirrhosis or certain other liver conditions.

Uro•bi•ot•ic (u′ro-bi-ot″ik) trademark for a combination preparation of oxytetracycline hydrochloride, sulfamethizole, and phenazopyridine hydrochloride.

uro•can•ase (u″ro-kan′ās) urocanate hydratase.

uro•can•ase de•fi•cien•cy (u″ro-kan′ās) an inherited disorder of histidine catabolism caused by mutation in the *UROC1* gene (locus 3q21.3), which encodes urocanate hydratase. It is characterized by excess urinary excretion of urocanic acid and growth retardation and may also be associated with mental retardation.

uro•can•ate (u″ro-kan′at) the anionic form of urocanic acid.

uro•can•ate hy•dra•tase (u″ro-kan′āt hy′drə-tās) [EC 4.2.1.49] an enzyme of the lyase class that catalyzes the reduction of urocanate to forminiminoglutamate, a step in the catabolism of histidine. Deficiency of the enzyme, presumed to be an autosomal recessive trait, causes urocanase deficiency. Called also *urocanase.*

uro•can•ic ac•id (u″ro-kan′ik) a product of the direct deamination of histidine, one of the pathways of histidine catabolism; it is accumulated and excreted in the urine in urocanase deficiency.

uro•cele (u′ro-sēl) [*uro-* + *-cele*[1]] distention of the scrotum with extravasated urine.

uro•che•zia (u″ro-ke′zhə) [*uro-* + Gr. *chezein* to defecate + *-ia*] presence of urine in the feces.

Uro•chor•da•ta (u″ro-kor-da′tə) [Gr. *oura* tail + L. *chorda* string] a subphylum of chordates intermediate between the invertebrates and true vertebrates, including the sea squirts and their allies, the members of which have a saclike body and a leathery tunic; the notochord is present only during the larval stage. Called also *Tunicata.*

uro•chor•date (u-ro-kor′dāt) any member of the Urochordata; called also *tunicate.*

uro•chrome (u′ro-krōm) [*uro-* + *-chrome*] the end product of hemoglobin breakdown, found in the urine and responsible for its yellow color.

uro•chro•mo•gen (u″ro-kro′mo-jən) an intermediate formed in the breakdown of hemoglobin to urochrome.

Uro•cit-K (ūr′o-sit-ka) trademark for a preparation of potassium citrate.

Uro•cys•tis (u″ro-sis′tis) a genus of fungi of the family Tilletiaceae. *U. tri′tici* causes flag smut on wheat in Australia and southern and eastern Asia.

uro•cys•ti•tis (u″ro-sis-ti′tis) cystitis.

uro•di•al•y•sis (u″ro-di-al′ĭ-sis) [*uro-* + *dialysis*] partial or complete suppression of the urine.

uro•dil•a•tin (u″ro-dil′ə-tin) a 32–amino acid peptide isolated from human urine, chemically related to atrial natriuretic peptide and having similar chemical activities.

uro•dy•nam•ic (u″ro-di-nam′ik) pertaining to the flow and motion of liquids in the urinary tract.

uro•dy•nam•ics (u″ro-di-nam′iks) the dynamics of the propulsion and flow of urine in the urinary tract.

uro•dyn•ia (u″ro-din′e-ə) [*ur-* + *-odynia*] pain accompanying urination.

uro•ede•ma (u″ro-ə-de′mə) [*uro-* + *edema*] edema caused by infiltration of extravasated urine.

uro•er•y•thrin (u″ro-er′ĭ-thrin) [*uro-* + Gr. *erythros* red] a dark reddish coloring matter found in the urine, giving it the red color seen in deposits of urates. Called also *purpurin.*

uro•flo•me•ter (u″ro-flo′me-tər) uroflowmeter.

uro•flow (u′ro-flo) flow of urine.

uro•flow•me•ter (u″ro-flo′me-tər) a device for the continuous recording of urine flow in milliliters per second, consisting of a cylinder placed on a transducer that weighs the urine entering the cylinder and records it on a time scale. Spelled also *uroflometer.*

uro•fol•li•tro•pin (u″ro-fol′ĭ-tro″pin) a preparation of gonadotropins from the urine of postmenopausal women; it contains follicle-stimulating hormone and is used in conjunction with human chorionic gonadotropin to induce ovulation in the treatment of female infertility and to stimulate multiple oocyte development in ovulatory patients utilizing assisted reproductive technologies. Administered by subcutaneous injection.

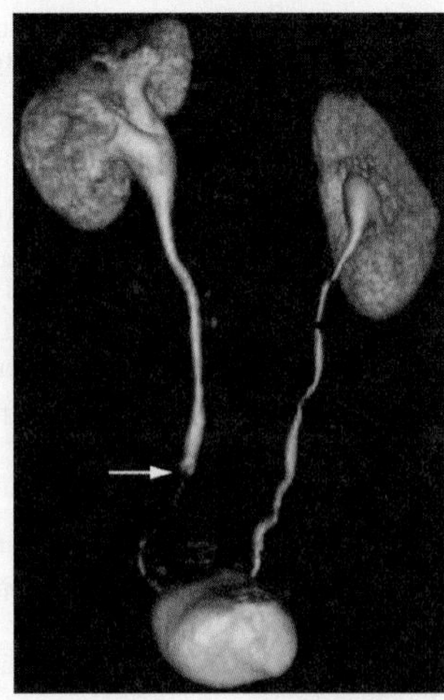

■ Magnetic resonance urography; 3D post-processing techniques used to mimic intravenous urography show a non-occluding distal ureteral stone *(arrow).*

uro•gas•ter (u″ro-gas′tər) [*uro-* + Gr. *gastēr* stomach] part of the allantoic cavity of the embryo.

uro•gas•trone (u″ro-gas′trōn) human epidermal growth factor.

uro•gen•e•sis (u″ro-jen′ə-sis) uropoiesis.

uro•gen•i•tal (u″ro-jen′ĭ-təl) genitourinary.

urog•e•nous (u-roj′ə-nəs) [*uro-* + *-genous*] 1. producing urine. 2. produced from or in the urine. Called also *urinogenous.*

Uro•ge•sic (u″ro-je′zik) trademark for a preparation of phenazopyridine hydrochloride.

Uro•gra•fin (ūr-o-graf′in) trademark for a contrast medium containing diatrizoate meglumine and diatrizoate sodium.

uro•gram (u′ro-gram) a radiograph of part of the urinary tract.

urog•ra•phy (u-rog′rə-fe) radiography of a part of the urinary tract that has been made opaque by an opaque medium.

ascending u., cystoscopic u. retrograde u.

descending u., excretion u., excretory u., intravenous u. radiographic examination of the urinary tract after the intravenous injection of an opaque medium that is rapidly excreted in the urine.

magnetic resonance u. imaging of the urinary tract using magnetic resonance imaging, such as to detect obstructions and dilations during pregnancy when other methods are ineffective or undesirable.

oral u. urography in which the opaque medium is given by mouth.

retrograde u. urography in which the contrast medium is injected into the bladder through the urethra. Called also *ascending* or *cystoscopic u.*

uro•gra•vim•e•ter (u″ro-grə-vim′ə-tər) [*uro-* + *gravimeter*] urinometer.

uro•gy•ne•col•o•gy (u″ro-gi″nə-kol′ə-je) a subspecialty of gynecology that deals with pelvic floor disorders, originally applied only to the lower female urinary tract but now including a wide range of disorders, such as fecal or urinary incontinence or prolapse of the bladder or uterus.

uro•hem•a•tin (u″ro-he′mə-tin) the coloring matter or pigments of the urine; regarded as identical with heme.

uro•hem•a•to•por•phy•rin (u″ro-he″mə-to-por′fĭ-rin) hematoporphyrin derived from the urine.

uro•ki•nase (UK) (u″ro-ki′nās) u-plasminogen activator; the term is used particularly to denote a pharmaceutical preparation of the enzyme, administered intravenously as a thrombolytic agent in the treatment of acute coronary arterial thrombosis and acute pulmonary embolism; also used to restore patency to intravenous catheters.

Uro-KP-Neu•tral (ūr′o ka-pe noo′trəl) trademark for preparations of potassium and sodium phosphates.

uro•lag•nia (u″ro-lag′ne-ə) [*uro-* + Gr. *lagneia* lust] sexual excitement associated with the sight or thought of urine or urination. Cf. *urophilia.*

Uro•lene Blue (u′ro-lēn bloo′) trademark for a preparation of methylene blue.

uro•lith (u′ro-lith) [*uro-* + *-lith*] urinary calculus. **urolith′ic** *adj*

uro·li·thi·a·sis (u″ro-lĭ-thi′ə-sis) 1. the formation of urinary calculi (see under *calculus*). 2. the diseased condition associated with the presence of urinary calculi. Called also *urinary lithiasis.*

feline u. urolithiasis in cats, usually males; it is one type of feline urological syndrome.

uro·li·thol·o·gy (u″ro-lĭ-thol′ə-je) the sum of knowledge regarding urinary calculi.

urol·o·gist (u-rol′ə-jist) a physician who specializes in urology.

urol·o·gy (u-rol′ə-je) the medical specialty concerned with the urinary tract in both male and female, and with the genital organs in the male. **urolog′ic, urolog′ical** *adj*

uro·man·cy (u′ro-man″se) [*uro-* + Gr. *manteia* a divination] prognosis based on examination of urine.

uro·mel·a·nin (u″ro-mel′ə-nin) [*uro-* + *melanin*] a black pigment sometimes found in urine; it results from the decomposition of urochrome.

urom·e·ter (u-rom′ə-tər) [*uro-* + *-meter*] urinometer.

uro·met·ric (u″ro-met′rik) pertaining to urometry.

urom·e·try (u-rom′ə-tre) 1. the measurement and recording of pressure changes caused by contraction of the ureter during ureteral peristalsis. 2. urinometry.

uro·mod·u·lin (u″ro-mod′u-lin) Tamm-Horsfall protein.

uro·nate (u′ro-nāt) a salt, anion, or ester of a uronic acid.

ur·on·ic ac·id (ūr-on′ik) a carboxylic acid produced by oxidation of the terminal —CH_2OH group in a sugar farthest from the carbonyl group to a carboxyl (=COOH) group, e.g., glucuronic acid.

uron(o)- for words beginning thus, see *ur(o)-*.

uro·patho·gen (u″ro-path′o-jən) a microorganism which causes diseases of the urinary tract.

urop·a·thy (u-rop′ə-the) [*uro-* + *-pathy*] any disease or other pathologic change in the urinary tract.

obstructive u. uropathy resulting from an obstruction in the tract; see also *obstructive nephropathy*, under *nephropathy*.

uro·pep·sin·o·gen (u″ro-pep-sin′o-jən) pepsinogen occurring in the urine.

uro·phe·in (u″ro-fe′in) [*uro-* + Gr. *phaios* gray] an odoriferous gray pigment of the urine.

uro·phil·ia (u″ro-fil′e-ə) [*uro-* + *-philia*] a paraphilia in which sexual arousal or activity is linked to urine. Cf. *urolagnia.*

uro·phos·phom·e·ter (u″ro-fos-fom′ə-tər) an instrument for measuring the quantity of phosphorus in the urine.

uro·pod (u′ro-pod) [Gr. *oura* tail + *pous*, gen. *podos* foot] the cytoplasmic footlike process that trails behind locomoting leukocytes; the term is used particularly of lymphocytes, in which the trailing process and large nucleus produce a characteristic "hand mirror" shape. The uropod serves as a point of attachment to the substrate and may also be involved in cell-cell interactions.

uro·poi·e·sis (u″ro-poi-e′sis) [*uro-* + *-poiesis*] the production of the urine; called also *urogenesis.*

uro·poi·et·ic (u″ro-poi-et′ik) 1. pertaining to uropoiesis. 2. urogenous (def. 1).

uro·por·phyr·ia (u″ro-por-fir′e-ə) porphyria in which there is excessive excretion of uroporphyrin.

erythropoietic u. congenital erythropoietic porphyria.

uro·por·phy·rin (u″ro-por′fə-rin) the porphyrin (q.v.) produced by oxidation of the methylene bridges in uroporphyrinogen. Excessive amounts of uroporphyrin I are excreted in congenital erythropoietic porphyria, and both types I and III are excreted in porphyria cutanea tarda. See *uroporphyrinogen.*

uro·por·phy·rin·o·gen (u″ro-por″fə-rin′ə-jən) a porphyrinogen (q.v.) in which each pyrrole ring has one acetate side chain and one propionate side chain; it is formed by condensation of four molecules of porphobilinogen. Four isomers are possible but only two exist naturally, types I and III; the latter is a functional intermediate in heme biosynthesis while the former is produced in an abortive side reaction.

uro·por·phy·rin·o·gen III co·syn·thase (u″ro-por″fə-rin′ə-jən ko-sin′thās) uroporphyrinogen-III synthase.

uro·por·phy·rin·o·gen de·car·boxy·lase (u″ro-por″fə-rin′ə-jən de-kahr-bok′sə-lās) [EC 4.1.1.37] an enzyme of the lyase class that catalyzes the decarboxylation of uroporphyrinogen III to coproporphyrinogen III in the biosynthesis of heme. Decreased enzyme activity is associated with porphyria cutanea tarda and the variant hepatoerythropoietic porphyria.

uro·por·phy·rin·o·gen I syn·thase (u″ro-por″fə-rin′ə-jən sin′thās) hydroxymethylbilane synthase.

uro·por·phy·rin·o·gen-III syn·thase (u″ro-por″fə-rin′ə-jən sin′thās) [EC 4.2.1.75] an enzyme of the lyase class that acts concertedly with hydroxymethylbilane synthase to convert porphobilinogen to uroporphyrinogen III in the biosynthesis of porphyrins and heme. Deficiency of the enzyme, an autosomal recessive trait, causes congenital erythropoietic porphyria. Called also *uroporphyrinogen III cosynthase.*

uro·pro·tec·tion (u″ro-pro-tek′shən) protection of the urinary tract, especially against urotoxic substances. **uroprotec′tive** *adj*

uro·psam·mus (u″ro-sam′əs) [*uro-* + *psammous*] sediment or gravel in the urine.

urop·ter·in (u-rop′tər-in) a pigment, identical with xanthopterin, isolated from human urine; see *pterin.*

Uro·qid-Ac·id (u′ro-kid as′id) trademark for a combination preparation of methenamine mandelate and sodium acid phosphate, monohydrate.

uro·ra·di·ol·o·gy (u″ro-ra″de-ol′ə-je) radiology of the urinary tract.

uro·sac·cha·rom·e·try (u″ro-sak″ə-rom′ə-tre) the measurement or estimation of sugar in the urine.

uros·che·sis (u-ros′kə-sis) [*uro-* + *-schesis*] urinary retention.

uros·co·py (u-ros′kə-pe) [*uro-* + *-scopy*] diagnostic examination of the urine. **uroscop′ic** *adj*

uro·se·mi·ol·o·gy (u″ro-se″me-ol′ə-je) diagnostic study of the urine.

uro·sep·sis (u″ro-sep′sis) [*uro-* + *sepsis*] a term used imprecisely to denote infection ranging from urinary tract infection to generalized sepsis which may result from such infection.

uro·sep·tic (u″ro-sep′tik) pertaining to or marked by urosepsis.

uro·stal·ag·mom·e·try (u″ro-stal″əg-mom′ə-tre) the use of the stalagmometer in the study of the urine.

uro·the·li·um (u″ro-the′le-əm) [*uro-* + *thelium*] a layer of transitional epithelium in the wall of the bladder, ureter, and renal pelvis, external to the lamina propria. **urothe′lial** *adj*

uro·tox·ic (u′ro-tok″sik) harmful to the bladder. **urotoxic′ity** *n*

uro·tox·in (u′ro-tok″sin) a urotoxic substance.

Urox·a·tral (u-rok′sə-tral) trademark for a preparation of alfuzosin hydrochloride.

urox·in (u-rok′sin) alloxantin.

URR urea reduction ratio.

Ur·so (ur′so) trademark for a preparation of ursodiol.

ur·so·de·oxy·cho·late (ur″so-de-ok″se-ko′lāt) a salt, ester, or anionic form of ursodeoxycholic acid.

ur·so·de·oxy·cho·lic ac·id (ur″so-de-ok″se-ko′lik) a secondary bile acid formed in the intestine from chenodeoxycholic acid; it is a choleretic and decreases the concentration of cholesterol in the bile. The pharmaceutical preparation is called *ursodiol.*

ur·so·de·oxy·cho·lyl·gly·cine (ur″so-de-ok″se-ko″ləl-gli′sēn) a bile salt, the glycine conjugate of ursodeoxycholic acid.

ur·so·de·oxy·cho·lyl·tau·rine (ur″so-de-ok″se-ko″ləl-taw′rēn) a bile salt, the taurine conjugate of ursodeoxycholic acid.

ur·so·di·ol (ur″so-di′ol) [USP] ursodeoxycholic acid used as an anticholelithic to dissolve radiolucent, noncalcified gallstones; administered orally.

Ur·ti·ca (ər-ti′kə) [L.] the nettles, a genus of plants of the family Urticaceae that are covered with stinging hairs and secrete a poisonous fluid. *U. dio′ica* is a type of stinging nettle that grows in temperate regions and is stimulating, diuretic, and hemostatic.

ur·ti·cant (ur′tĭ-kənt) 1. causing an itching or stinging sensation. 2. causing a wheal.

ur·ti·ca·ria (ur″tĭ-kar′e-ə) [*Urtica* + *-ia*] a vascular reaction in the upper dermis, usually transient, consisting of localized edema caused by dilatation and increased capillary permeability with wheals. Most types are named for the causative stimulus or mechanism, such as *physical urticaria* and *contact urticaria. Angioedema* is the same physiological response in the deep dermis or subcutaneous or submucosal tissues. Called also *hives.* **urticar′ial, urticar′ious** *adj*

acute u. urticaria taking place within hours to a few days of the stimulus; some cases evolve into chronic urticaria.

allergic contact u. a type of contact urticaria seen as part of allergic contact dermatitis, particularly in children.

aquagenic u. contact urticaria caused by contact with water or sweat. In some persons this is from an urticariogenic substance dissolved in the sweat; it was formerly thought to be in the sebum, but now it appears to be an antigen from the stratum corneum.

u. bullo′sa, bullous u. any urticaria in which bullae are superimposed over the characteristic wheals.

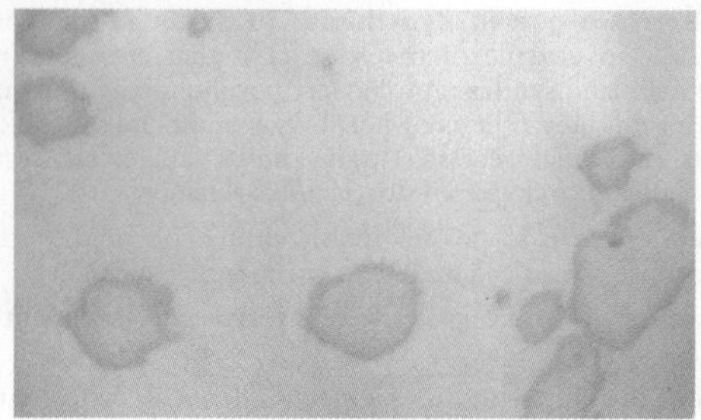

■ Urticaria.

cholinergic u. a type of physical urticaria, usually evoked by exertion, stress, or increased environmental heat. It is thought to be a nonimmunologic hypersensitivity reaction in which acetylcholine released from parasympathetic or motor nerve terminals induces release of mediators from mast cells. On the skin there are punctate wheals surrounded by areas of erythema.

chronic u. urticaria that either is continuous or develops over a period of six weeks or more; most cases are idiopathic.

cold u. a type of physical urticaria precipitated by cold air, water, or objects, with wheals appearing on cold-exposed areas when they have been rewarmed; lesions are erythematous, burning papules and macules. There are two types: The more common *acquired form* is usually self-limited, occurs most often in young adults, and has an unknown etiology. The *familial form* is much rarer and better known as *familial cold autoinflammatory syndrome* (see under *syndrome*).

colonic u. a pattern of the mucosal surface of the colon resembling urticaria of the skin, seen radiographically; the mucosa is lifted up owing to edema and has a characteristic mosaic pattern.

complement-mediated u. urticaria caused by the excessive circulating complement found in conditions such as angioedema, serum sickness, and necrotizing vasculitis.

contact u. a type of immune-mediated urticaria that is a form of allergic reaction, consisting of a localized or generalized, transient wheal and flare reaction after exposure to the causative substance. See also *contact dermatitis.*

delayed pressure u. pressure u.

dermatographic u., dermographic u. dermographism.

drug-induced u. a type of immune-mediated urticaria in reaction to a medication; see also *drug eruption,* under *eruption.* Called also *u. medicamentosa.*

exercise u. cholinergic urticaria caused by strenuous physical exercise.

factitious u. dermographism.

giant u. angioedema.

heat u. cholinergic urticaria produced by application of heat to the skin or by exposure to high environmental temperature; it may be associated with cramps, weakness, flushing, salivation, and collapse.

idiopathic u. urticaria whose cause is unknown; most of these cases are chronic (see *chronic u.*).

immune-mediated u. acute urticaria that is an immune response to antigenic stimulation.

light u. solar u.

u. medicamento'sa drug-induced u.

u. multifor'mis endem'ica harara.

papular u. acute urticaria consisting of a persistent cutaneous eruption that is a hypersensitivity reaction to bites of insects such as mites, fleas, bedbugs, gnats, mosquitoes, or lice, seen primarily in atopic children. Characteristics include small papules, wheals, and combinations of the two, which may become infected or lichenified by rubbing or excoriation. Cf. *prurigo mitis.* Called also *lichen urticatus* and *strophulus.*

physical u. acute urticaria caused by a physical stimulus such as heat, cold, sunlight, or rubbing or light scratching of the skin.

u. pigmento'sa the most common form of mastocytosis, seen primarily in children, characterized by multiple persistent small, hyperpigmented, pruritic macules and papules. The usual site is on the trunk, although some cases are on the limbs, head, or neck. Lesions tend to produce urticaria upon mild mechanical trauma or chemical irritation (Darier sign). See also *mastocytoma.*

pressure u. a type of physical urticaria with pain, occurring hours after local pressure on the skin, usually on the feet after walking or on the buttocks after sitting; the exact mechanism behind the reaction and why it is delayed is not clear. Called also *delayed pressure u.*

solar u., u. sola'ris a type of idiopathic photodermatosis characterized by rapidly developing physical urticaria in reaction to ultraviolet radiation, sometimes after only brief exposure to sunlight. Called also *light u.*

stress u. cholinergic urticaria caused by emotional stress.

vibratory u. see under *angioedema.*

ur•ti•car•i•o•gen•ic (ur″tĭ-kar″e-o-jen′ik) causing urticaria.

ur•ti•cate (ur′tĭ-kāt) 1. characterized by wheals. 2. to produce urtication.

ur•ti•ca•tion (ur″tĭ-ka′shən) [L. *urtica* a stinging nettle] 1. development or formation of urticaria. 2. a burning sensation as of stinging with nettles.

uru•shi•ol (u-roo′she-ol) a mixture of oleoresins found in the leaves and stems of various plants; it is one of the most common causes of allergic contact dermatitis (see *urushiol dermatitis,* under *dermatitis*). The most common urushiol-containing plants are in the family Anacardiaceae, such as in the genera *Rhus (Toxicodendron), Anacardium, Mangifera, Schinus,* and *Semecarpus.*

US ultrasound.

USAN (u′san) United States Adopted Name.

USDA United States Department of Agriculture.

Ush•er syndrome (ush′ər) [Charles Howard *Usher,* British ophthalmologist, 1865–1942] see under *syndrome.*

Us•nea (us′ne-ə) a genus of lichens of the family Usneaceae. *U. barba′ta* (L.) Wigg. is a species that grows on forest trees and contains usnic acid; it is used as a homeopathic preparation.

us•ne•in (us′ne-in) usnic acid.

us•nic ac•id (us′nik) an antibacterial compound occurring in the lichen *Usnea barbata.*

USP *United States Pharmacopeia.*

USPHS United States Public Health Service.

USRDS United States Renal Data System.

Us•ti•lag•i•na•ceae (us″tĭ-laj″ĭ-na′se-e) a family of smuts, fungi of the order Ustilaginales. It includes the genus *Ustilago.*

Us•ti•lag•i•na•les (us″tĭ-laj″ĭ-na′lēz) the smuts, an order of perfect fungi of the class Teliomycetes, characterized by lack of a basidiocarp; it includes the families Ustilaginaceae and Tilletiaceae.

us•ti•lag•i•nism (us″tĭ-laj′ĭ-niz-əm) a condition resembling ergotism, seen in animals that have eaten corn contaminated with *Ustilago maydis* or *U. zeae.*

Us•ti•la•go (us″tĭ-la′go) [L.] a genus of smuts, fungi of the family Ustilaginaceae that are parasitic on plants. *U. may′dis* and *U. ze′ae* cause corn smut, and the ingestion of contaminated seeds causes ustilaginism.

us•tion (us′chən) [L. *ustio*] burning with the actual cautery.

us•tu•la•tion (us″tu-la′shən) [L. *ustulare* to scorch] the drying of a moist drug by heat.

uta (oo′tah) [from Peruvian Indian name for the disease] a form of New World cutaneous leishmaniasis occurring in the Peruvian Andes, caused by *Leishmania peruviana,* probably transmitted by *Lutzomyia verrucarum* and *L. peruensis,* and characterized by the presence of just a few ulcerlike, self-limited lesions.

Ut dict. [L.] ut dic′tum (as directed).

Utend. [L.] uten′dus (to be used).

uter•al•gia (u″tər-al′jə) hysteralgia.

uteri (u′tər-i) [L.] genitive and plural of *uterus.*

uter(o)- [L. *uterus,* q.v.] a combining form denoting relationship to the uterus. See also words beginning with *hyster(o)-* and *metr(o)-.*

utero•ab•dom•i•nal (u″tər-o-ab-dom′ĭ-nəl) pertaining to the uterus and the abdomen.

utero•cer•vi•cal (u″tər-o-ser′vĭ-kəl) pertaining to the uterus and the cervix uteri.

utero•fix•a•tion (u″tər-o-fik-sa′shən) hysteropexy.

utero•gen•ic (u″tər-o-jen′ik) formed in the uterus.

utero•ges•ta•tion (u″tər-o-jəs-ta′shən) [*utero-* + *gestation*] 1. uterine pregnancy; any pregnancy which is not extrauterine. 2. the full period of time of normal pregnancy.

utero•glo•bin (u′tər-o-glo″bin) a globulin found in the uterine lumen of some mammals and in the blood and urine of humans; in mice it stimulates and regulates blastocyst implantation. Other biological activities, including antiinflammatory actions and an ability to act as a binding protein, are under investigation. Called also *blastokinin.*

utero•glob•u•lin (u″tər-o-glob′u-lin) uteroglobin.

uter•og•ra•phy (u″tər-og′rə-fe) hysterography.

utero•lith (u′tər-o-lith″) [*utero-* + *-lith*] uterine calculus.

uter•om•e•ter (u″tər-om′ə-tər) an instrument for measuring the uterus.

uter•om•e•try (u″tər-om′ə-tre) measurement of the uterus.

utero·ovar·i·an (u″tər-o-o-var′e-ən) pertaining to the uterus and ovary.

utero·pel·vic (u″tər-o-pel′vik) pertaining to or connecting the uterus and the pelvis.

utero·pexy (u′tər-o-pek″se) hysteropexy.

utero·pla·cen·tal (u″tər-o-plə-sen′təl) pertaining to the uterus and the placenta.

utero·plas·ty (u′tər-o-plas″te) metroplasty. **uteroplas′tic** *adj*

utero·rec·tal (u″tər-o-rek′təl) rectouterine.

utero·sa·cral (u″tər-o-sa′krəl) pertaining to the uterus and the sacrum.

utero·sal·pin·gog·ra·phy (u″tər-o-sal″ping-gog′rə-fe) hysterosalpingography.

utero·scle·ro·sis (u″tər-o-sklə-ro′sis) sclerosis of the uterus.

utero·scope (u′tər-o-skōp″) hysteroscope.

utero·ther·mom·e·try (u″tər-o-thər-mom′ə-tre) the measurement of the temperature in the uterus.

uter·ot·o·my (u″tər-ot′ə-me) hysterotomy.

utero·ton·ic (u″tər-o-ton′ik) 1. giving muscular tone to the uterus. 2. an agent that increases the tonus of the uterine muscle.

utero·tro·pic (u″tər-o-tro′pik) having a special affinity for or exerting its principal influence upon the uterus.

utero·tu·bal (u″tər-o-too′bəl) tubouterine.

utero·vag·i·nal (u″tər-o-vaj′ĭ-nəl) pertaining to the uterus and the vagina.

utero·ven·tral (u″tər-o-ven′trəl) pertaining to the uterus and the abdominal cavity.

uter·o·ves·i·cal (u″tər-o-ves′ĭ-kəl) vesicouterine.

uter·us (u′tər-əs) pl. *u′teri* [L., from Gr. *hystera*] [TA] the hollow muscular organ in female mammals in which the blastocyst normally becomes embedded and in which the developing embryo and fetus is nourished. In the nongravid human, it is a pear-shaped structure, about 8 cm in length, consisting of a fundus, body, isthmus, and cervix. Its cavity opens into the vagina below, and into the uterine tube on either side at the cornu. It is supported by direct attachment to the vagina and by indirect attachment to various other nearby pelvic structures. Called also *metra*. **u′terine** *adj*

u. arcua′tus a uterus with a depressed fundus.

u. bicor′nis a uterus with two horns or cornua.

u. bicor′nis bicol′lis a uterus with two horns and two cervices.

u. bicor′nis unicol′lis a uterus with two horns and a single cervix.

bicornuate u. u. bicornis.

u. bi′foris a uterus in which the external os is divided by a septum.

u. bilocula′ris a uterus whose cavity is divided into two parts by a septum; called also *bipartite* or *septate u.*

bipartite u., u. biparti′tus u. bilocularis.

cochleate u. a small adult uterus with a conical cervix and a body that is small, globular, and acutely flexed.

u. cordifor′mis a heart-shaped uterus.

u. didel′phys the existence of two distinct uteri in the same individual; called also *didelphia* and *u. duplex*.

duplex u., u. du′plex 1. u. didelphys. 2. a double uterus, as occurs normally in marsupial mammals.

fetal u. a uterus in which the cervical canal is longer than the cavity of the corpus.

gravid u. the pregnant uterus.

u. incudifor′mis a uterus bicornis that is broad between the two horns.

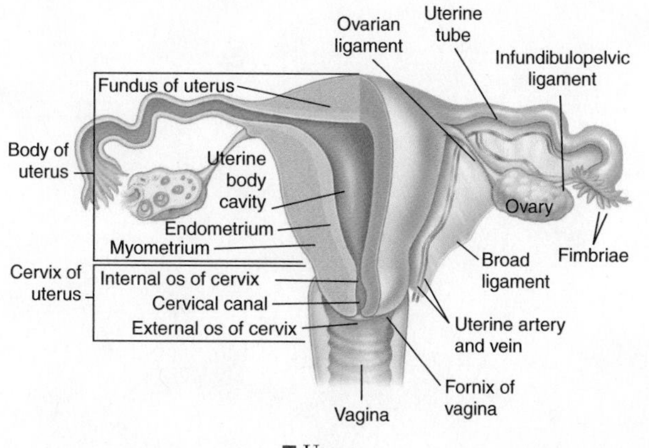

■ Uterus.

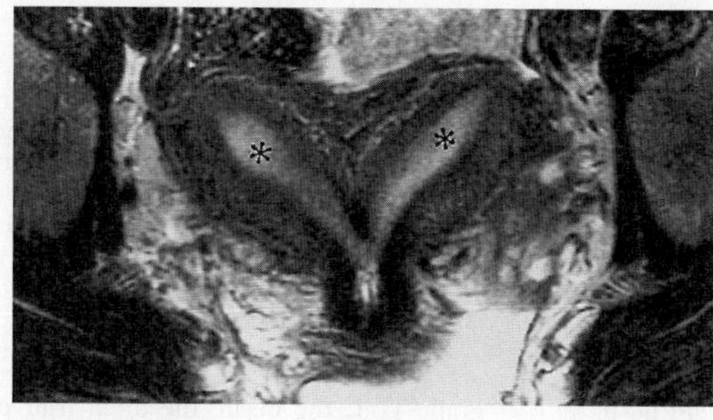

■ Uterus bicornis (bicornuate uterus). MRI demonstrates the presence of two endometrial canals *(asterisks)*.

infantile u. pubescent u.

masculine u., u. masculi′nus utriculus prostaticus.

u. parvicol′lis a uterus in which the cervical portion is very small, but the corpus is of normal size.

u. planifunda′lis u. incudiformis.

pubescent u. a uterus that is adult in type but is undeveloped; called also *infantile u.*

ribbon u. an aplastic uterus found as a transverse ribbon of fibromuscular tissue between the blind ends of the uterine tubes and the bladder.

u. rudimenta′rius a hypoplastic uterus measuring 1 to 3 cm in length; affected women are amenorrheic and sterile.

saddle-shaped u. u. arcuatus.

septate u., u. sep′tus u. bilocularis.

u. simplex a uterus that is single throughout its length, as in humans.

u. subsep′tus u. bicornis.

u. triangula′ris u. incudiformis.

u. unicor′nis, unicornuate u. a uterus with only one cornu, one lateral half being undeveloped or imperfectly developed.

UTI urinary tract infection.

Uti·bid (u′tĭ-bid) trademark for a preparation of oxolinic acid.

Uti·cort (u′tĭ-kort″) trademark for preparations of betamethasone benzoate.

util·iza·tion (u″til-ĭ-za′shən) the use of something.

red cell u. (RCU) the fraction of iron leaving the blood plasma that is incorporated in circulating red blood cells; iron-59 bound to the patient's own transferrin is administered, and the red cell utilization is calculated as: (radioactive iron/mL blood at 10–14 days) ÷ (extrapolated radioactive iron/mL blood at time zero) × 100 per cent.

UTP uridine triphosphate.

UTP–glu·cose-1-phos·phate uri·dyl·yl·trans·fer·ase (gloo′kōs fos′fāt u″rĭ-dil′əl-trans′fər-ās) [EC 2.7.7.9] an enzyme of the transferase class that catalyzes the reaction UTP + glucose 1-phosphate = pyrophosphate + UDP-glucose, a reaction in the glycogen storage mechanism. Called also *UDP-glucose pyrophosphorylase*.

UTP–hex·ose-1-phos·phate uri·dyl·yl·trans·fer·ase (hek′sōs fos′fāt u″rĭ-dil″əl-trans′fər-ās) [EC 2.7.7.10] an enzyme of the transferase class that catalyzes the transfer of galactose 1-phosphate to UTP to form UDP-galactose. The reaction is an alternative minor pathway for producing UDP-galactose for galactose utilization (cf. *UDP-glucose–hexose-1-phosphate uridylyltransferase*). The enzyme is present in the liver of adults, but is lacking in infants. Called also *galactose 1-phosphate uridylyltransferase*.

utri·cle (u′trĭ-kəl) [L. *utriculus*] 1. any small sac. 2. utriculus (def. 2).

prostatic u., urethral u. utriculus prostaticus.

utric·u·lar (u-trik′u-lər) 1. pertaining to a utricle. 2. resembling a bladder.

utric·u·li (u-trik′u-li) [L.] genitive and plural of *utriculus*.

utric·u·li·tis (u-trik″u-li′tis) 1. inflammation of the prostatic utricle. 2. inflammation of the utricle of the labyrinth.

utric·u·lo·sac·cu·lar (u-trik″u-lo-sak′u-lər) pertaining to the utricle and saccule of the labyrinth.

utric·u·lus (u-trik′u-ləs) pl. *utric′uli* [L., dim. of *uter*] 1. a small sac. 2. [TA] utricle: the larger of the two vestibular sacs, located in the posterosuperior region of the vestibule. It is the major organ of the vestibular system, which gives information about position and movements of the head. Called also *u. vestibularis*.

u. masculi′nus, u. prosta′ticus [TA] prostatic utricle: the remains in the male of the lower part of the müllerian (paramesonephric) duct; it is a small blind pouch arising in the parenchyma of the prostate and opening onto the seminal colliculus. Called also *masculine uterus, uterus masculinus, sinus pocularis*, and *Weber corpuscle* or *organ*.

u. vestibula′ris utriculus (def. 2).

utri•form (u′trĭ-form) having the shape of a bottle.

u•tro•phin (u′trə-fin) a homologue of dystrophin with similar structure and function; it contains an actin-binding N-terminus and a C-terminus that interacts with dystroglycan protein components, links the actin cytoskeleton to the extracellular matrix, and is ubiquitously expressed. In muscle tissue, it is located at the neuromuscular synapse and myotendinous junctions, and participates in postsynaptic membrane maintenance and acetylcholine receptor clustering.

UV ultraviolet.

UVA ultraviolet A.

uva (u′və) pl. *u′vae* [L. "grape"] 1. the raisin; the dried fruit of *Vitis vinifera.* 2. any of various other fruits resembling that of *V. vinifera.*

u. ur′si [L. "bear's grapes"] 1. *Arctostaphylos uva-ursi.* 2. the leaves of *A. uva-ursi*, used medicinally as a tea for urinary tract inflammation and as a homeopathic preparation for the same indication.

Uva•dex (u′və-deks) trademark for a preparation of methoxsalen.

UVB ultraviolet B.

UVC ultraviolet C.

uvea (u′ve-ə) tunica vasculosa bulbi. **u′veal** *adj*

uve•itis (u″ve-i′tis) [*uvea* + *-itis*] an inflammation of part or all of the uvea, commonly involving the other tunics of the eye (sclera, cornea, and retina). **uveit′ic** *adj*

anterior u. uveitis involving the structures of the iris and/or ciliary body, including iritis, cyclitis, and iridocyclitis.

equine recurrent u. periodic ophthalmia.

Förster u. syphilitic involvement of the entire uvea.

granulomatous u. uveitis of any part of the uveal tract but particularly the posterior portion, characterized by nodular collections of epithelioid cells and giant cells surrounded by lymphocytes.

heterochromic u. see under *iridocyclitis.*

lens-induced u. a type of granulomatous uveitis that has a zonular pattern and is induced by lens protein after the lens capsule has ruptured. Called also *phacoantigenic u.*

nongranulomatous u. inflammation of the anterior portion of the uveal tract (iris and ciliary body).

phacoantigenic u. lens-induced u.

phacotoxic u. a rare type of lens-induced uveitis that is a low-grade reaction to lens protein.

posterior u. uveitis involving the posterior segment of the eyeball, such as choroiditis and chorioretinitis.

sympathetic u. see under *ophthalmia.*

toxoplasmic u. chorioretinitis as a complication of toxoplasmosis.

tuberculous u. granulomatous uveitis due to infection with the tubercle bacillus, usually a severe, caseating type of chorioretinitis.

uveo•me•nin•gi•tis (u′ve-o-men″in-ji′tis) a disorder characterized by lesions of the uvea accompanied by meningeal inflammation.

uveo•pa•rot•id (u″ve-o-pə-rot′id) affecting the uvea and the parotid gland; see under *fever.*

uveo•scle•ri•tis (u″ve-o-sklə-ri′tis) scleritis resulting from an extension of the inflammation from the uvea to the sclera.

uvi•form (u′vĭ-form) [*uva* + *form*] having the form of a grape.

uvu•la (u′vu-lə) pl. *u′vulae* [L. "little grape"] 1. a pendent, fleshy mass. 2. u. palatina.

bifid u. bifurcation of the uvula, considered an incomplete form of cleft palate. Called also *cleft, forked,* or *split u.* and *staphyloschisis.*

u. of bladder u. vesicae urinariae.

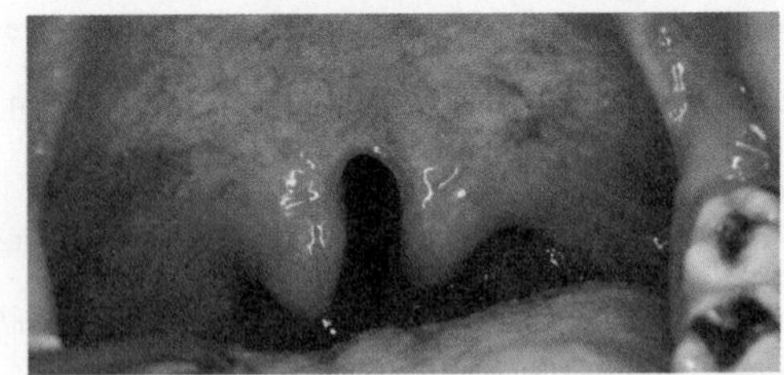

■ Bifid uvula.

u. of cerebellum u. vermis.

cleft u., forked u. bifid u.

u. palati′na [TA], **palatine u.** palatine uvula: the small, fleshy mass hanging from the soft palate above the root of the tongue, composed of the levator and tensor palatini muscles and the muscle of the uvula, connective tissue, and mucous membrane.

split u. bifid u.

u. of urinary bladder u. vesicae urinariae.

u. ver′mis [TA] uvula of vermis (IX): the lobule of the vermis of the cerebellum between the pyramis and the nodulus; it is part of the posterior lobe.

u. vesi′cae urina′riae [TA] uvula of urinary bladder: a rounded elevation at the bladder neck, seen mainly in adult males, formed by convergence of many fibers of the trigonal muscle as they pass through the encircling internal sphincter muscle to terminate in the urethra.

uvu•lar (u′vu-lər) pertaining to the uvula; called also *staphyline.*

uvu•la•ris (u″vu-lar′is) [L., from *uvula*] uvular.

uvu•lec•to•my (u″vu-lek′tə-me) [*uvula* + *-ectomy*] excision of the uvula.

uvu•li•tis (u″vu-li′tis) [*uvula* + *-itis*] inflammation of the uvula; staphylitis.

uvu•lo•pal•a•to•phar•yn•go•plas•ty (UPPP) (u″vu-lo-pal″ə-to″fə-ring′go-plas″te) palatopharyngoplasty.

uvu•lo•pal•a•to•plas•ty (u″vu-lo-pal′ə-to-plas″te) palatopharyngoplasty. **uvulopalatoplas′tic** *adj*

uvu•lop•to•sis (u″vu-lop-to′sis, u″vu-lo-to′sis) [*uvula* + *-ptosis*] elongation or relaxation of the palate.

uvu•lo•tome (u′vu-lo-tōm) an instrument for cutting the uvula.

uvu•lot•o•my (u″vu-lot′ə-me) [*uvula* + *-tomy*] surgical removal of all or part of the uvula; cf. *uvulectomy.*

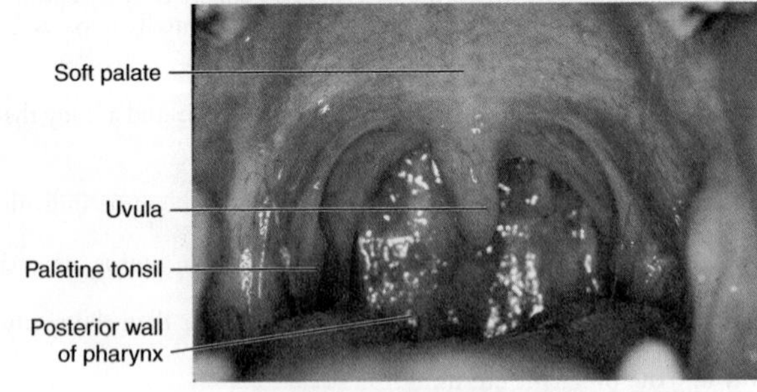

■ Uvula and pharynx.

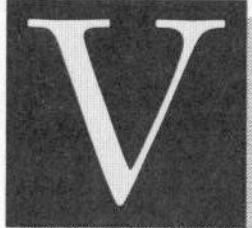

V valine; vanadium; visual acuity; volt; volume.

V voltage; volume.

V_H see *variable region,* under *region.*

V_L see *variable region,* under *region.*

V_{max} the maximum velocity of an enzyme-catalyzed reaction; see *Michaelis-Menten equation* under *equation.*

V_T tidal volume (in pulmonary ventilation).

v. [L.] ve′na (vein).

v velocity; voltage.

VA visual acuity; Veterans Administration (now the Department of Veterans Affairs [DVA]).

VAC a cancer chemotherapy regimen consisting of vincristine, dactinomycin, and cyclophosphamide.

vac•cen•ic ac•id (vak-sen′ik) a monounsaturated fatty acid isomeric with oleic and elaidic acids; it occurs naturally in both *cis* and *trans* configurations, the former in bacteria and the latter in beef fat and butterfat. See table accompanying *fatty acid.*

vac•ci•na (vak-si′nə) vaccinia.

vac•ci•nal (vak′sĭ-nəl) [L. *vaccinus*] 1. pertaining to vaccinia, to vaccine, or to vaccination. 2. having protective qualities when used by way of inoculation.

vac•ci•nate (vak′sĭ-nāt) to inoculate with vaccine for the purpose of producing immunity.

vac•ci•na•tion (vak″sĭ-na′shən) [L. *vacca* cow] the introduction of vaccine into the body for the purpose of inducing immunity. Coined originally to apply to the injection of smallpox vaccine, the term has come to mean any immunizing procedure in which vaccine is injected.

vac•ci•na•tor (vak′sĭ-na″tər) 1. one who vaccinates. 2. an instrument for use in vaccination.

vac•cine (vak-sēn′) [L. *vaccinus* pertaining to cows, from *vacca* cow (from the use of cowpox virus inoculation for immunization against smallpox)] a suspension of attenuated or killed microorganisms (bacteria, viruses, or rickettsiae), or of antigenic proteins derived from them, administered for the prevention, amelioration, or treatment of infectious diseases.

Vaccine

acellular v. a cell-free vaccine prepared from purified antigenic components of pathogenic microorganisms, thus carrying less risk of adverse reactions than whole-cell preparations.

acellular pertussis v. a preparation of purified antigenic components of *Bordetella pertussis;* used for routine immunization against pertussis (whooping cough). It is administered in combination preparations with diphtheria and tetanus toxoids; see *diphtheria and tetanus toxoids and acellular pertussis v.* and *tetanus toxoid, reduced diphtheria toxoid, and acellular pertussis v.*

anthrax v. adsorbed (AVA) [USP] a cell-free filtrate of cultures of an avirulent nonencapsulated strain of *Bacillus anthracis,* adsorbed on aluminum hydroxide, concentrated, and resuspended; used for immunization of persons with potential occupational exposure to anthrax, e.g., those working with imported animal hides or hair; administered subcutaneously.

anthrax spore v. a live vaccine consisting of *Bacillus anthracis* spores in saponified diluent, used for vaccination of domestic farm animals against anthrax.

attenuated v., attenuated live v. a vaccine prepared from live microorganisms or viruses cultured under adverse conditions leading to loss of their virulence but retention of their ability to induce protective immunity.

autogenous v. a vaccine prepared from a culture of microorganisms taken from the person to be treated with it.

avian encephalomyelitis v. a live virus vaccine of chick embryo origin, used for immunization of layer or breeder replacement pullets against avian encephalomyelitis.

bacterial v. a preparation of killed or attenuated bacteria used as an active immunizing agent. Called also *bacterin.*

BCG v. [*bacille Calmette-Guérin*] [USP] a vaccine made from the Calmette-Guérin strain of *Mycobacterium bovis,* which was made avirulent by culture by Calmette and Guérin for many years on a medium enriched in beef bile; it is administered by scarification or intradermal or intracutaneous injection to tuberculin-negative individuals for prevention of tuberculosis. It is used for routine vaccination of children only in regions where there is a high incidence of tuberculosis. In the United States it is recommended only for immunization of high-risk individuals. BCG vaccine is also administered intravesically in the treatment of carcinoma of the bladder.

bluetongue v. a modified live virus vaccine of bovine tissue culture origin, used for prevention of bluetongue in sheep.

bovine rhinotracheitis v. a modified live virus vaccine of tissue culture origin used for immunization of healthy cattle against infectious bovine rhinotracheitis.

bovine virus diarrhea v. a modified live virus vaccine of tissue culture origin, used for immunization of cattle against bovine virus diarrhea.

bronchitis v. a modified live virus vaccine of chick embryo origin prepared from the Massachusetts or Connecticut variant strains of bronchitis virus, used for prevention of infectious bronchitis in chickens and other birds.

***Brucella abortus* v.** a modified live virus vaccine of *Brucella abortus* strain 19, used for immunization of healthy calves against brucellosis.

bursal disease v. a modified live virus vaccine of chick embryo origin, used for immunization of chicks against infectious bursal disease.

Calmette v. BCG v.

canine distemper v. a modified live virus vaccine consisting of an attenuated strain of canine distemper virus propagated in tissue culture, used for immunization of dogs against canine distemper.

coccidiosis v. live sporulated oocysts of chicken origin, used to introduce subclinical coccidial infection in chickens in order to establish immunity against clinical infections.

conjugate v. a vaccine composed of an immunogenic polysaccharide conjugated with a protein carrier.

diphtheria and tetanus toxoids v. diphtheria and tetanus toxoids.

diphtheria and tetanus toxoids and acellular pertussis v. DTaP vaccine; a combination of diphtheria toxoid, tetanus toxoid, and acellular pertussis vaccine; adsorbed on an aluminum-adsorbing agent. It is administered intramuscularly to children younger than seven years of age, for simultaneous immunization against diphtheria, tetanus, and pertussis. Cf. *tetanus toxoid, reduced diphtheria toxoid, and acellular pertussis v.*

diphtheria and tetanus toxoids and pertussis v. DTP vaccine; a combination of diphtheria toxoid, tetanus toxoid, and whole-cell pertussis vaccine; administered intramuscularly for simultaneous immunization against diphtheria, tetanus, and pertussis. It is no longer used in the United States. See *diphtheria and tetanus toxoids and acellular pertussis v.* and *tetanus toxoid, reduced diphtheria toxoid, and acellular pertussis v.*

distemper v.–mink a modified live virus vaccine of chick embryo of tissue culture origin, used for prevention of canine distemper in mink.

DNA v. a vaccine consisting of a modified form of the DNA of an infectious organism that codes for an antigenic protein to stimulate immunity in the host.

DTaP v. diphtheria and tetanus toxoids and acellular pertussis v.

DTP v. diphtheria and tetanus toxoids and pertussis v.

duck virus enteritis v. a modified live virus vaccine of chick embryo origin, used for prevention of duck virus enteritis.

duck virus hepatitis v. a modified live virus vaccine of chick embryo origin, used for prevention of duck virus hepatitis.

encephalomyelitis v. a bivalent killed virus vaccine of chicken tissue culture origin, used for immunization of horses against eastern and western equine encephalomyelitis.

equine influenza v. a bivalent killed virus vaccine of chick embryo origin, used for immunization of horses against equine influenza due to influenza virus A equine strains 1 and 2.

equine rhinopneumonitis v. a modified live virus vaccine of tissue culture origin or a killed virus vaccine, used for immunization of horses against equine viral rhinopneumonitis due to equine herpesvirus type 1.

***Erysipelothrix rhusiopathiae* v.** an avirulent live culture of *Erysipelothrix rhusiopathiae,* used for prevention of erysipelas in pigs.

feline panleukopenia v. a modified live virus vaccine or killed virus vaccine of tissue culture origin, used for immunization of cats against feline panleukopenia.

feline pneumonitis v. an attenuated vaccine of chick embryo origin, used for immunization of cats against *Chlamydophila psittaci.*

Vaccine *Continued*

feline rhinotracheitis v. a modified live virus vaccine of tissue culture origin, used for immunization of cats against feline rhinotracheitis.

fowl laryngotracheitis v. a modified live virus vaccine of chick embryo origin, used for prevention of laryngotracheitis in chickens.

fowlpox v. a modified live virus vaccine of chicken embryo or tissue culture origin, used to immunize chickens and turkeys against fowlpox.

***Haemophilus* b conjugate v. (HbCV)** a preparation of *Haemophilus influenzae* type b capsular polysaccharide covalently bound to a specific diphtheria protein or meningococcal protein, or to tetanus toxoid. Administered intramuscularly as a routine immunizing agent in children between the ages of 2 months and 5 years.

hepatitis A v. inactivated an inactivated whole-virus vaccine derived from an attenuated strain of hepatitis A virus grown in cell culture; administered intramuscularly as an immunizing agent for preexposure prophylaxis in susceptible persons at least two years of age.

hepatitis B v. (recombinant) an inactivated virus vaccine derived by recombination from hepatitis B surface antigen and cloned in yeast cells; administered intramuscularly for immunization of children and adolescents and of persons at increased risk for infection.

heptavalent pneumococcal conjugate v. pneumococcal 7-valent conjugate v.

heterologous v., heterotypic v. a vaccine that confers protective immunity against a pathogen not present in the vaccine, because it contains microorganisms that possess cross-reacting antigens which they share in common with that pathogen. For example, vaccinia virus protects against smallpox.

human diploid cell v. (HDCV) an inactivated viral vaccine prepared from rabies virus grown in cultures of human diploid embryo lung cells and inactivated with propiolactone; administered intramuscularly or intradermally for pre- and postexposure prophylaxis against rabies. In official terminology, called *rabies v.* [USP].

human papillomavirus quadrivalent v., recombinant a quadrivalent vaccine prepared from the viruslike particles of the major capsid protein of human papillomavirus types 6, 11, 16, and 18, which are responsible for the great majority of cases of condyloma acuminatum and cervical cancer; administered intramuscularly to girls and young women between the ages of 9 and 26 for the prevention of condyloma acuminatum and neoplastic diseases caused by susceptible types.

inactivated poliovirus v. poliovirus v. inactivated.

influenza virus v. 1. TIV; an inactivated trivalent virus vaccine, containing two influenza A virus strains and one influenza B virus strain, usually prepared from virus subunits; administered intramuscularly. The composition of the vaccine is changed each year in response to antigenic shifts and changes in prevalence of influenza virus strains. Annual immunization before November is recommended for children more than 6 months of age, adults over 50 years of age, persons who work in the healthcare industry, and persons at increased risk of developing complications from influenza. 2. LAIV; a live, attenuated, cold-adapted trivalent vaccine containing temperature-sensitive type A and B strains of influenza virus that can replicate in the nasal passages but not in the lower respiratory tract; administered intranasally for immunzation against influenza in persons ages 2 through 49 years.

Japanese encephalitis virus v. a formaldehyde-inactivated vaccine prepared from infected mouse brains, used for immunization against Japanese encephalitis; recommended for persons staying a month or more in endemic or epidemic regions of Asia during transmission season and for laboratory workers who may be exposed to Japanese encephalitis virus.

live v. attenuated v.

live, attenuated influenza v. (LAIV) influenza virus v. (def. 2).

Marek disease v. a modified live virus vaccine of tissue culture origin, used for immunization of 1-day-old chicks against Marek disease, prepared from one or more of the three serovars of Marek disease virus.

measles v. 1. measles virus v. live. 2. a modified live virus vaccine of canine tissue culture origin, used to induce resistance to canine distemper in 3- to 6-week-old puppies in which response to canine distemper vaccine would be neutralized because of interference by maternal antibody.

measles, mumps, rubella, and varicella virus v. live (MMRV) a combination of live attenuated measles, mumps, rubella, and human herpesvirus 3 (varicella-zoster virus), administered subcutaneously for simultaneous immunization against measles, mumps, rubella, and varicella in children between the ages of 12 months and 12 years.

measles, mumps, and rubella virus v. live (MMR) [USP] a combination of live attenuated measles, mumps, and rubella viruses, administered subcutaneously for simultaneous immunization against measles, mumps, and rubella in persons 12 months of age or older.

measles and rubella virus v. live [USP] a combination of live attenuated measles and rubella viruses, which has been used for simultaneous immunization against measles and rubella. See *measles, mumps, and rubella virus v.*

measles virus v. live [USP] a live virus vaccine prepared from an attenuated line of measles virus; used for immunization against measles, usually as the combination measles, mumps, and rubella virus vaccine (MMR).

meningococcal conjugate v. (MCV, MCV4) a preparation of capsular polysaccharide antigens of *Neisseria meningitidis* serovars A, C, Y, and W-135, covalently bound to diphtheria toxoid; administered intramuscularly for the prevention of meningococcal disease. It is recommended for routine immunization of adolescents ages 11 through 18 years and for persons ages 2 to 55 years in certain high risk groups.

meningococcal polysaccharide v. (MPSV) a preparation of capsular polysaccharide antigens of *Neisseria meningitidis* serovars A, C, Y, and W-135; used for the prevention of meningococcal disease. The vaccine is administered subcutaneously to persons over 2 years of age in certain high-risk groups, including all military recruits, persons deficient in any of the late complement components, and those with asplenia.

mink enteritis v. a killed virus vaccine of feline tissue culture origin, used for immunization of mink against mink viral enteritis.

mixed v. polyvalent v.

modified live viral v., modified live virus v. a vaccine containing live virus that is still capable of reproducing in the recipient's body but has had its disease-causing ability restricted or removed.

mumps virus v. live [USP] a live virus vaccine prepared from an attenuated strain of mumps virus; used for immunization against mumps, usually as the combination measles, mumps, and rubella virus vaccine (MMR).

Newcastle disease v. modified live virus vaccine or chemically inactivated, adsorbed killed virus vaccine, both of chick embryo origin, used for immunization of chickens against Newcastle disease, the live vaccine for mass immunization in drinking water, aerosol spray, or eye drops, the killed vaccine for immunization by injection.

ovine ecthyma v. a modified live virus vaccine of ovine origin, used for immunization of sheep and goats against contagious ecthyma (orf).

***Pasteurella multocida* v.** a live bacterial vaccine, used for prevention of pasteurellosis in turkeys due to *Pasteurella multocida,* types 3 and 4.

pertussis v. a suspension of killed *Bordetella pertussis* organisms (whole-cell vaccine) or a fraction thereof (acellular pertussis vaccine, q.v.). In the United States, it is available as the latter.

pigeonpox v. a modified live virus vaccine of chick embryo origin, used for prevention of fowlpox in chickens and turkeys.

plague v. a suspension of killed *Yersinia pestis* bacilli, used for immunization of persons having occupational or avocational exposure to wild rodents in plague enzootic areas, administered intramuscularly.

pneumococcal conjugate v. (PCV), pneumococcal 7-valent conjugate v. (PCV7) a heptavalent vaccine containing purified polysaccharides of the capsular antigens of *Streptococcus pneumoniae* serovars 4, 6B, 9V, 14, 18C, 19F, 23F individually coupled to a nonpathogenic variant of diphtheria toxin, diphtheria CRM_{197} protein; used for routine immunization of children aged less than 23 months as well as children aged 24 to 59 months who are at high risk for pneumococcal infection. Administered intramuscularly.

pneumococcal v. polyvalent (PPSV) a 23-valent vaccine containing capsular polysaccharide from the 23 most prevalent or invasive serovars of *Streptococcus pneumoniae,* which are responsible for about 90 per cent of pneumococcal disease in the United States. Administered intramuscularly or subcutaneously for immunization of persons over 2 years of age at increased risk for the disease or its complications.

poliovirus v. inactivated (IPV) [USP] a suspension of formalin-inactivated poliovirus, types I, II, and III, grown in monkey kidney cell tissue culture, administered intramuscularly or subcutaneously for immunization against poliomyelitis in infants, children, and adolescents, as well as adults at increased risk of exposure. Called also *Salk v.*

Vaccine *Continued*

poliovirus v. live oral (OPV) a live virus vaccine containing attenuated poliovirus, types I, II, and III, grown in monkey kidney cell tissue culture and used for immunization against poliomyelitis; administered orally. OPV induces both humoral and intestinal immunity and is excreted in the feces for at least several weeks after immunization. Because it can cause vaccine-associated paralytic poliomyelitis in those vaccinated and also their contacts, it is used only under special circumstances or in countries in which wild polioviruses have not been eradicated. OPV should not be administered to immunocompromised individuals or their household contacts. Called also *Sabin v.*

polyvalent v. a vaccine prepared from cultures or antigens of more than one strain or species.

pseudorabies v. any of several vaccines used for immunization of swine against pseudorabies. Four types are used: one using an attenuated virus, one with an inactivated virus, one with a thymidine kinase–deficient virus, and a subunit vaccine.

purified chick embryo cell v. (PCECV) an inactivated viral vaccine prepared from rabies virus grown in primary cultures of chicken fibroblasts and inactivated with propiolactone; used for pre- and post-exposure rabies prophylaxis, administered intramuscularly.

rabies v. any of several inactivated viral vaccines against rabies; used for preexposure immunization to persons at high risk of exposure, such as veterinarians, and for postexposure prophylaxis in conjunction with rabies immune globulin. The currently available preparations are *human diploid cell vaccine* and *purified chick embryo cell vaccine.* In official terminology, the term is used specifically to denote the human diploid cell vaccine.

reo-corona viral calf diarrhea v. a modified live virus vaccine of bovine tissue culture origin, used for immunization of newborn calves against enteric disease caused by reoviruses and coronaviruses.

replicative v. any vaccine containing organisms that are able to reproduce, including live and attenuated viruses and bacteria.

rotavirus v. (RV) a live attenuated vaccine administered orally to immunize infants against rotaviral gastroenteritis.

rotavirus v., live, oral an oral solution containing a live, attenuated human rotavirus strain; active against serotypes G1, G3, G4, and G9.

rotavirus v., live, oral, pentavalent an oral solution containing five live human–bovine reassortant rotavirus strains; active against serotypes G1, G2, G3, and G4.

rubella virus v. live [USP] a live virus vaccine prepared from an attenuated strain of rubella virus; used for immunization against rubella, usually as the combination measles, mumps, and rubella virus vaccine (MMR).

Sabin v. poliovirus v. live oral.

Salk v. poliovirus v. inactivated.

shingles v. zoster v. live.

smallpox v. [USP] a live viral vaccine prepared from vaccinia virus grown in the skin of a vaccinated bovine calf; used for immunization against smallpox, administered by scarification. Now recommended only for laboratory workers exposed to smallpox virus; certain countries continue to vaccinate those in the military forces. Complications that result from smallpox vaccination include vaccinia, secondary bacterial infections, and encephalomyelitis.

split-virus v. subunit v.

streptococcus group E v. an oral modified live virus vaccine of Lancefield group E streptococcus, used for prevention of streptococcal lymphadenitis (jowl or cervical abscesses) in pigs.

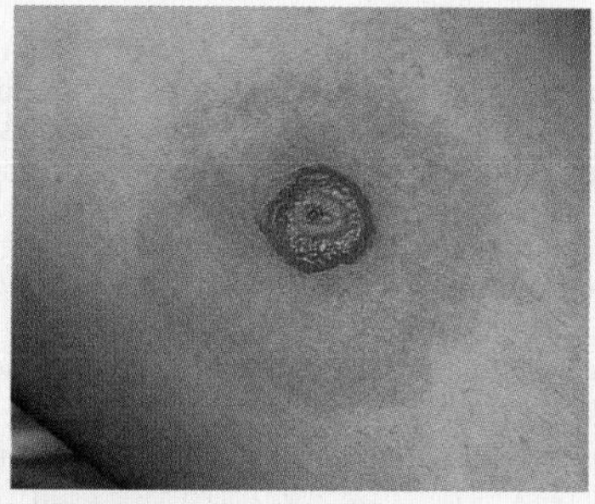

■ Smallpox vaccination, primary reaction.

subunit v., subvirion v. a vaccine produced from specific protein subunits of a virus and thus having less risk of adverse reactions than live or killed whole virus vaccines, e.g., hepatitis B vaccine and some influenza vaccines. Called also *split-virus v.*

Tdap v. tetanus toxoid, reduced diphtheria toxoid, and acellular pertussis v.

tetanus and diphtheria toxoids v. tetanus and diptheria toxoids.

tetanus toxoid, reduced diphtheria toxoid, and acellular pertussis v. Tdap vaccine; a combination of tetanus toxoid, a reduced dose of diphtheria toxoid, and acellular pertussis vaccine; adsorbed on an aluminum-adsorbing agent. It is administered intramuscularly to adolescents and adults, for simultaneous immunization against diphtheria, tetanus, and pertussis. Cf. *diphtheria and tetanus toxoids and acellular pertussis v.*

tenosynovitis v. a modified live virus vaccine of chick embryo origin, administered to broiler-breeder replacement chickens for prevention of infectious tenosynovitis.

transmissible gastroenteritis v. a modified live virus vacine of porcine tissue culture origin, used for prevention of transmissible gastroenteritis in pigs.

trivalent inactivated influenza v. (TIV) influenza virus v. (def. 1).

tuberculosis v. BCG v.

typhoid v. live oral a preparation of the attenuated strain *Salmonella enterica* subsp. *enterica* serovar Typhi Ty21a; administered orally for immunization against typhoid fever.

typhoid Vi polysaccharide v. a preparation of the cell surface Vi polysaccharide extracted from the strain *Salmonella enterica* subsp. *enterica* serovar Typhi Ty2, administered intramuscularly for immunization against typhoid fever.

varicella virus v. live a live attenutated virus vaccine prepared from human herpesvirus 3 (varicella-zoster virus); administered subcutaneously for production of immunity to varicella.

yellow fever v. [USP] a live virus vaccine prepared from an attenuated strain of yellow fever virus cultured in chick embryos; administered subcutaneously for prevention of yellow fever. It is recommended for persons over the age of 9 months residing or traveling in endemic areas of Africa, Central America, and South America.

zoster v. live a live attenuated virus vaccine prepared from human herpesvirus 3 (varicella-zoster virus); used to renew immunity in older adults for prevention of herpes zoster, administered subcutaneously.

---

vac•cin•ia (vak-sin′e-ə) [L., from *vacca* cow] the cutaneous and sometimes systemic reactions associated with vaccination with smallpox vaccine. Cf. *cowpox* and *paravaccinia.* **vaccin′ial** *adj*

fetal v. vaccinia of the fetus due to bloodborne dissemination of vaccinia virus in the pregnant woman after primary smallpox vaccination; it is frequently lethal to the fetus.

v. gangreno′sa progressive v.

generalized v. a usually self-limited generalized skin eruption resembling smallpox, sometimes occurring after primary smallpox vaccination, caused by transient viremia with localization of the virus in the skin.

progressive v. a rare but often fatal complication of smallpox vaccination, seen most often in immunodeficient persons, characterized by tissue necrosis that spreads from the inoculation site and may result in metastatic vaccinial lesions in the skin, bones, and viscera. Called also *v. gangrenosa.*

vac•cin•i•form (vak-sin′ĭ-form) resembling vaccinia.

Vac•ci•ni•um (vak-sin′e-əm) [L.] a genus of low, dedicuous shrubs with white to reddish flowers and edible red or blue to blue-black berries, common in central and northern Europe, Asia, and North America, including the bilberry (blueberry), and cranberry; the leaves and fruit of *V. myrtil′lus* and the fruit of *V. uligino′um* are used medicinally.

vac•cino•gen (vak-sin′o-jən) a source from which vaccine is derived.

vac•ci•nog•e•nous (vak″sĭ-noj′ə-nəs) producing vaccine.

vac•ci•no•ther•a•py (vak″sĭ-no-ther′ə-pe) therapeutic use of vaccines.

VACOP-B a cancer chemotherapy regimen consisting of VePesid (etoposide), Adriamycin (doxorubicin), cyclophosphamide, Oncovin (vincristine), prednisone, and bleomycin.

VACTERL [*v*ertebral, *a*nal, *c*ardiac, *t*racheal, *e*sophageal, *r*enal, and *l*imb] see under *association.*

vac•u•o•late (vak′u-o-lāt″) to form vacuoles.

vac·u·o·lat·ed (vak′u-o-lāt″əd) containing vacuoles.

vac·u·o·la·tion (vak″u-o-la′shən) 1. the process of forming vacuoles; called also *vacuolization.* 2. the condition of being vacuolated.

vac·u·ole (vak′u-ōl) [L. *vacuus* empty + *-ole* diminutive ending] any membrane-bound space or cavity within a cell. **vacuo′lar** *adj*

autophagic v. autophagosome.

condensing v's membrane-bound spherical vacuoles in the trans-Golgi network of secretory cells, which contain secretory products in varying degrees of condensation and mature into secretory granules.

contractile v. an osmoregulatory organelle of protozoa and sponges that alternately fills with water extracted from the adjacent cytoplasm and then ejects the water to the outside; thus it acts as a pumping mechanism to remove excess water from the cell. Called also *water expulsion vesicle.*

digestive v. secondary lysosome.

food v. a fluid-containing intracytoplasmic space in which food material is suspended; it occurs in holozoic protozoa.

vac·u·o·li·za·tion (vak″u-o-lĭ-za′shən) vacuolation (def. 1).

vac·u·ome (vak′u-ōm) the system of vacuoles in a cell which stain with neutral red.

vac·u·um (vak′ūm) [L.] a space devoid of air or of other gas; a space from which the air has been exhausted.

high v. a vacuum in which the attenuation is extreme.

torricellian v. the vacuum in a barometric tube.

VAD ventricular assist device.

va·dum (va′dəm) [L. "a shallow"] an occasional elevation from the bottom of a cerebral sulcus, rendering the sulcus more or less shallow.

va·gal (va′gəl) pertaining to the vagus nerve.

va·gec·to·my (va-jek′tə-me) surgical vagotomy.

va·gi (va′ji) [L.] genitive and plural of *vagus.*

Vag·i·fem (vaj′ə-fem) trademark for a preparation of estradiol.

va·gi·na (və-ji′nə) pl. *vagi′nae* [L.] 1. sheath; a tubular enveloping structure. 2. [TA] the genital canal in the female, extending from the vulva to the cervix uteri, which receives the penis in copulation.

v. bul′bi [TA] sheath of eyeball: connective tissue that forms the capsule enclosing the posterior part of the eyeball, extending anteriorly to the conjunctival fornix, and continuous with the muscular fascia of the eye; called also *bulbar fascia, bulbar sheath,* and *Bonnet, ocular,* or *Tenon capsule.*

v. caro′tica fas′ciae cervica′lis [TA] carotid sheath of cervical fascia: the portion of the cervical fascia that encloses the carotid vessels and vagus nerve.

v. commu′nis ten′dinum musculo′rum fibula′rium [TA] common tendon sheath of peronei: the tendon sheath for the peroneus longus and brevis muscles; it is single proximally and double distally, and extends about 4 cm proximally and distally from the tip of the lateral malleolus. Called also *v. communis musculorum peroneorum* [TA alternative].

v. commu′nis ten′dinum musculo′rum flexo′rum ma′nus [TA] the common sheath for the flexor tendons as they pass through osteofibrous canals of the fingers.

v. commu′nis ten′dinum musculo′rum peroneo′rum TA alternative for *v. communis musculorum fibularium.*

v. exter′na ner′vi op′tici [TA] external sheath of optic nerve: the thick outer sheath of the optic nerve, continuous with the dura mater and connecting it with the sclera; called also *fibrous* or *outer sheath of optic nerve* and *dural sheath.*

v. fibro′sa TA alternative for *stratum fibrosum vaginae tendinis.*

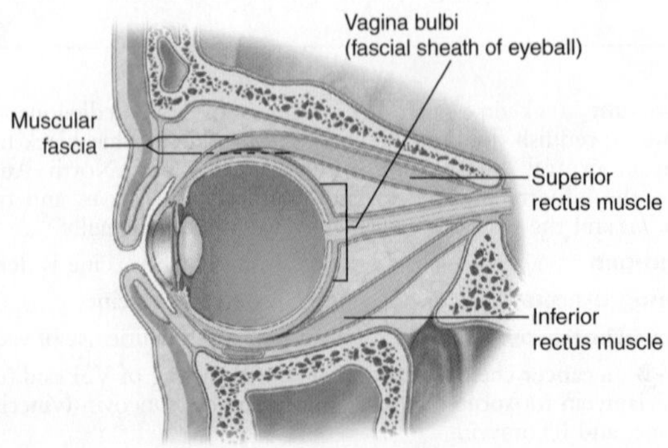

■ Section through the eyeball, showing the vagina bulbi continuous with the muscular fascia.

vagi′nae fibro′sae digito′rum ma′nus [TA] fibrous sheaths of fingers: strong fibrous, semicylindrical sheaths investing the grooved palmar surface of the proximal and middle phalanges of the fingers.

vagi′nae fibro′sae digito′rum pe′dis [TA] fibrous sheaths of toes: more or less complete fascial sheaths surrounding the phalanges of the toes, for attachment of the tendons and their synovial membranes.

v. inter′na ner′vi op′tici [TA] internal sheath of optic nerve: the inner sheath of the optic nerve, continuous with the pia mater and arachnoidea mater; called also *inner sheath of optic nerve.* See also *arachnoid sheath* and *pial sheath,* under *sheath.*

v. mus′culi rec′ti abdo′minis [TA] sheath of rectus abdominis muscle: a sheath formed by the aponeuroses of other abdominal muscles, within which the rectus abdominis can move. Called also *rectus sheath.*

v. planta′ris ten′dinis mus′culi fibula′ris lon′gi [TA] plantar tendon sheath of peroneus longus: a tendon sheath beginning in the fibular groove of the cuboid bone. Called also *v. plantaris tendinis musculi peronei longi* [TA alternative].

v. planta′ris ten′dinis mus′culi pero′nei lon′gi TA alternative for *v. plantaris tendinis musculi fibularis longi.*

v. proces′sus styloi′dei [TA] sheath of styloid process: a ridge on the inferior surface of the temporal bone, partly enclosing the base of the styloid process.

v. synovia′lis 1. synovial sheath: a double-layered, fibrous sheath with synovial fluid present between the layers. 2. TA alternative for stratum synoviale vaginae tendinis.

vagi′nae synovia′les digito′rum ma′nus [TA] the synovial sheaths surrounding the tendons of the fingers.

vagi′nae synovia′les digito′rum pe′dis [TA] the synovial sheaths surrounding the tendons of the toes.

v. ten′dinis [TA] tendon sheath: a sheath of tissue that covers a tendon; it has both fibrous and synovial layers (*stratum fibrosum vaginae tendinis* and *stratum synoviale vaginae tendinis*).

vagi′nae ten′dinum carpa′les dorsa′les [TA] tendon sheaths enclosing the tendons of extensor muscles of the wrist, thumb, and fingers as they pass into the hand along the medial, lateral, and posterior sides of the wrist.

vagi′nae ten′dinum carpa′les palma′res [TA] tendon sheaths enclosing the tendons of flexor muscles on the palmar aspect of the wrist and allowing free motion of the tendons; they occur deep to or within the flexor retinaculum.

vagi′nae ten′dinum digito′rum pe′dis [TA] tendon sheaths enclosing the tendons of the flexor muscles of the toes.

v. ten′dinis intertubercula′ris [TA] intertubercular tendon sheath: the tendon sheath that surrounds the long head of the biceps brachii muscle as it passes through the intertubercular sulcus.

v. ten′dinum musculo′rum abducto′ris lon′gi et extenso′ris pol′licis bre′vis [TA] the tendon sheath enclosing the tendons of the abductor pollicis longus and extensor pollicis brevis muscles, passing into the hand on the lateral side of the wrist.

v. ten′dinum musculo′rum extenso′rum car′pi radia′lium [TA] the tendon sheath enclosing the tendons of the extensor carpi radialis brevis and extensor carpi radialis longus muscles as they pass into the hand along the lateral side of the wrist.

v. ten′dinis mus′culi extenso′ris car′pi ulna′ris [TA] the tendon sheath enclosing the tendon of the extensor carpi ulnaris muscle, passing into the hand along the medial side of the wrist.

v. ten′dinum musculo′rum extenso′ris digito′rum et extenso′ris in′dicis [TA] the tendon sheath enclosing the tendons of the extensor digitorum and extensor indicis muscles, passing into the hand along the posterior side of the wrist.

v. ten′dinis mus′culi extenso′ris di′giti mi′nimi [TA] the tendon sheath enclosing the tendon of the extensor digiti minimi muscle, passing into the hand along the medial side of the wrist.

v. ten′dinum mus′culi extenso′ris digito′rum lon′gi [TA] the tendon sheath enclosing the tendons of the extensor digitorum longus muscle, extending from just above the malleoli to the base of the fifth metatarsal.

v. ten′dinis mus′culi extenso′ris hal′lucis lon′gi [TA] the tendon sheath of the extensor hallucis longus muscle, extending from the level of the malleoli and reaching the base of the first metatarsal.

v. ten′dinis mus′culi extenso′ris pol′licis lon′gi [TA] the tendon sheath enclosing the tendon of the extensor pollicis longus muscle, passing into the hand on the lateral side of the wrist.

v. ten′dinis mus′culi flexo′ris car′pi radia′lis [TA] the tendon sheath enclosing the tendon of the flexor carpi radialis muscle, which passes through a tubular compartment formed by attachment of the lateral aspect of the flexor retinaculum to the margins of a groove on the medial side of the tubercle of trapezium, on the palmar aspect of the wrist.

v. ten′dinum mus′culi flexo′ris digito′rum lon′gi [TA] the tendon sheath enclosing the tendons of the flexor digitorum longus muscle, extending from the medial malleolus to below the navicular bone.

v. ten′dinis mus′culi flexo′ris hal′lucis lon′gi [TA] the tendon sheath of the flexor hallucis longus muscle, extending from the medial malleolus to the base of the first metatarsal.

v. ten′dinis mus′culi flexo′ris pol′licis lon′gi [TA] the tendon sheath enclosing the tendon of the flexor pollicis longus muscle, passing into the hand on the lateral side of the wrist.

v. ten′dinis mus′culi obli′qui superio′ris bul′bi [TA] the tendon sheath of the superior oblique muscle of the eye, particularly where its tendon passes through the trochlea.

v. ten′dinis mus′culi tibia′lis anterio′ris [TA] the tendon sheath of the tibialis anterior muscle, extending from the proximal margin of the superior extensor retinaculum to the region between the diverging limbs of the inferior extensor retinaculum, passing deep to the retinacula.

v. ten′dinis mus′culi tibia′lis posterio′ris [TA] the tendon sheath of the tibialis posterior muscle, beginning at the medial malleolus and extending into the foot.

vagi′nae ten′dinum tarsa′les anterio′res [TA] the group of tendon sheaths enclosing tendons passing into the foot along the anterior region of the ankle.

vagi′nae ten′dinum tarsa′les fibula′res [TA] the group of tendon sheaths enclosing tendons passing into the foot along the lateral side of the ankle.

vagi′nae ten′dinum tarsa′les tibia′les [TA] the group of tendon sheaths enclosing tendons passing into the foot along the medial side of the ankle.

v. vaso′rum a fibrous sheath that encloses any of various arteries, sometimes along with their veins and nerves.

va•gi•nae (və-ji′ne) genitive and plural of *vagina.*

vag•i•nal (vaj′ĭ-nəl) 1. of the nature of a sheath; ensheathing. 2. pertaining to the vagina. 3. pertaining to the tunica vaginalis testis.

vag•i•na•li•tis (vaj″ĭ-nə-li′tis) periorchitis.

vag•i•na•pexy (vaj″ĭ-nə-pek′se) colpopexy.

vag•i•nate (vaj′ĭ-nāt) enclosed in a sheath.

vag•i•nec•to•my (vaj″ĭ-nek′tə-me) excision of the vagina.

vag•i•ni•peri•ne•ot•o•my (vaj″ĭ-nĭ-per″ĭ-ne-ot′ə-me) paravaginal incision.

vag•i•nis•mus (vaj″ĭ-niz′məs) [L.] painful spasm of the vagina due to involuntary contraction of the vaginal musculature, usually severe enough to prevent intercourse; the cause may be organic or psychogenic.

vag•i•ni•tis (vaj″ĭ-ni′tis) 1. inflammation of the vagina; it is marked by pain and by a purulent discharge. Called also *colpitis.* 2. inflammation of a sheath.

v. adhaesi′va, adhesive v. atrophic vaginitis with ulceration and exfoliation of the mucosa resulting in adhesions of the membranes; opposite surfaces may adhere to each other, causing obliteration of the vaginal canal. Called also *senile v.*

atrophic v. vaginitis occurring in postmenopausal women, associated with estrogen deficiency. The two most common types are *senile vulvovaginitis* and *adhesive vaginitis.*

***Candida* v., candidal v.** vulvovaginal candidiasis.

desquamative inflammatory v. vaginitis of unknown etiology, resembling atrophic vaginitis clinically and microscopically, but occurring in the absence of estrogen deficiency, and characterized chiefly by recrudescent reddened superficial ulcerations.

v. emphysemato′sa, emphysematous v. inflammation of the vagina and adjacent cervix, characterized by numerous, asymptomatic, gas-filled cystlike lesions; the gas filling the lesions has been shown to have a carbon dioxide content.

granular v. vaginitis in cows with small nodules on the vulvar mucosa, apparently a nonspecific response of lymphatic tissue to irritation.

senile v. see *atrophic v.*

v. tes′tis periorchitis.

***Trichomonas* v.** vaginitis produced by *Trichomonas vaginalis;* it is usually transmitted by coitus and is often asymptomatic. The symptomatic condition may take the form of severe vaginal irritation associated with discharge, burning, pruritus, and chafing. Male partners of infected women may have signs of nonspecific urethritis, enlarged prostate, and epididymitis. Called also *vaginal trichomoniasis.*

vagin(o)- [L. *vagina,* q.v.] a combining form denoting relationship to the vagina (def. 2).

vag•i•no•ab•dom•i•nal (vaj″ĭ-no-ab-dom′ĭ-nəl) pertaining to the vagina and the abdomen.

vag•i•no•cele (vaj′ĭ-no-sēl″) [*vagina* + *-cele*[1]] prolapse or falling of the vagina; called also *colpoptosis, vaginal hernia,* and *vaginal prolapse.*

vag•i•no•cer•vi•cal (vaj″ĭ-no-sər′vĭ-kəl) cervicovaginal.

vag•i•no•cu•ta•ne•ous (vaj″ĭ-no-ku-ta′ne-əs) pertaining to or communicating between the vagina and skin.

vag•in•odyn•ia (vaj″ĭ-no-din′e-ə) [*vagina* + *-odynia*] pain in the vagina; called also *colpodynia.*

vag•i•no•fix•a•tion (vaj″ĭ-no-fik-sa′shən) colpopexy.

vag•i•no•gram (vaj′ĭ-no-gram) a radiograph of the vagina.

vag•i•nog•ra•phy (vaj″ĭ-nog′rə-fe) radiography of the vagina.

vag•i•no•la•bi•al (vaj″ĭ-no-la′be-əl) pertaining to the vagina and the labia.

vag•i•nom•e•ter (vaj″ĭ-nom′ə-tər) [*vagina* + *-meter*] an instrument for measuring the length and diameter of the vagina.

vag•i•no•my•co•sis (vaj″ĭ-no-mi-ko′sis) [*vagina* + *mycosis*] fungal disease of the vagina; see also *vulvovaginal candidiasis,* under *candidiasis.*

vag•i•nop•a•thy (vaj″ĭ-nop′ə-the) any disease of the vagina.

vag•i•no•per•i•ne•al (vaj″ĭ-no-per″ĭ-ne′əl) pertaining to the vagina and perineum.

vag•i•no•peri•neo•plas•ty (vaj″ĭ-no-per″ĭ-ne′o-plas″te) [*vagino-* + *perineoplasty*] plastic surgery of the vagina and perineum.

vag•i•no•peri•ne•or•rha•phy (vaj″ĭ-no-per″ĭ-ne-or′ə-fe) suture repair of the vagina and perineum.

vag•i•no•peri•ne•ot•o•my (vaj′ĭ-no-per″ĭ-ne-ot′ə-me) paravaginal incision.

vag•i•no•peri•to•ne•al (vaj″ĭ-no-per″ĭ-to-ne′əl) pertaining to the vagina and peritoneum.

vag•i•no•pexy (vaj′ĭ-no-pek″se) colpopexy.

vag•i•no•plas•ty (vaj′ĭ-no-plas″te) [*vagina* + *-plasty*] plastic surgery of the vagina; called also *colpoplasty.* **vaginoplas′tic** *adj*

vag•i•no•rec•tal (vaj″ĭ-no-rek′təl) rectovaginal.

vag•i•no•scope (vaj′ĭ-no-skōp) [*vagina* + *-scope*] a vaginal speculum; called also *colposcope.*

vag•i•nos•co•py (vaj″ĭ-nos′kə-pe) colposcopy.

vag•i•no•sis (vaj″ĭ-no′sis) vaginopathy.

bacterial v. a type of vaginitis characterized by high concentrations of anaerobic bacteria in the vaginal flora, with greatly lowered concentrations of lactobacilli and by increased malodorous (fishy) thin gray vaginal discharge that cannot be attributed to other cause; it is frequently associated with positive cultures for *Gardnerella vaginalis* or *mobiluncus.*

vag•i•not•o•my (vaj″ĭ-not′ə-me) colpotomy.

vag•i•no•ves•i•cal (vaj″ĭ-no-ves′ĭ-kəl) vesicovaginal.

vag•i•no•vul•var (vaj″ĭ-no-vul′vər) vulvovaginal.

Va•gi•stat (vaj′ĭ-stat″) trademark for a preparation of tioconazole.

va•gi•tus (və-ji′təs) [L.] the cry of an infant.

v. uteri′nus the crying of a child in the uterus.

v. vagina′lis the crying of a child while its head is still within the vagina.

va•go•glos•so•pha•ryn•ge•al (va″go-glos″o-fə-rin′je-əl) pertaining to the vagus and glossopharyngeal nerves.

va•go•gram (va′go-gram) [*vagus* + *-gram*] a tracing showing the electrical variations of the vagus nerve; called also *electrovagogram.*

va•gol•y•sis (va-gol′ĭ-sis) [*vagus* + *-lysis*] surgical destruction of the vagus nerve.

va•go•lyt•ic (va″go-lit′ik) 1. pertaining to or caused by vagolysis. 2. having an effect resembling that produced by interruption of impulses transmitted by the vagus nerve; cf. *parasympatholytic.*

va•go•mi•met•ic (va″go-mĭ-met′ik) having an effect which resembles that produced by vagal stimulation.

va•go•splanch•nic (va″go-splank′nik) vagosympathetic.

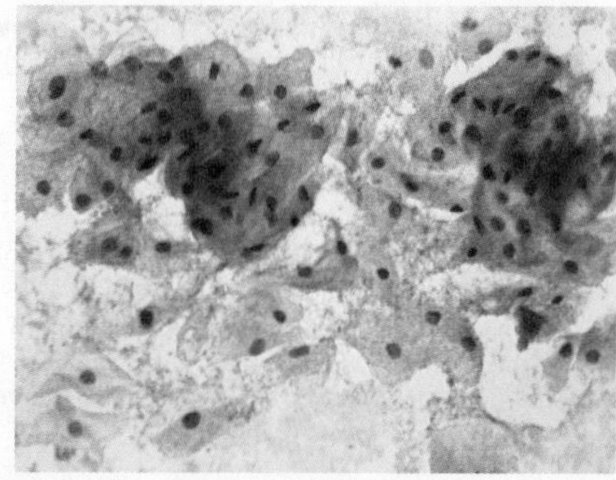

■ Minute basophilic coccobacilli cover the epithelial cells and are present throughout the proteinaceous background in bacterial vaginosis.

va·go·sym·pa·thet·ic (va″go-sim″pə-thet′ik) pertaining to both the vagus and sympathetic innervation.

va·got·o·my (va-got′ə-me) [*vagus* + *-tomy*] interruption of the impulses carried by the vagus nerve or nerves.

bilateral v. truncal v.

highly selective v. a treatment for peptic ulcers less extensive than the selective vagotomy, consisting of division of only those vagal fibers supplying the acid-secreting glands of the stomach, with preservation of those supplying the antrum as well as the hepatic and celiac branches.

medical v. vagal block.

parietal cell v. a type of highly selective vagotomy consisting of severing of the vagus nerve fibers supplying the proximal two-thirds (parietal area) of the stomach. Called also *proximal gastric v.*

posterior truncal v. a variation of the highly selective vagotomy in which the posterior vagal trunk is surgically cut for treatment of severe intractable gastric ulcers.

proximal gastric v. parietal cell v.

selective v. a treatment for peptic ulcers less extensive than the truncal vagotomy, consisting of division of the vagal fibers to the stomach only with preservation of hepatic and celiac branches.

truncal v. surgical division of the two main trunks of the abdominal vagus nerve just below the esophageal hiatus, done to treat peptic ulcers; because of the resultant atony of the stomach, this is usually combined with a drainage procedure.

va·go·to·nia (va″go-to′ne-ə) [*vagus* + *ton-* + *-ia*] hyperexcitation of the vagus nerve, resulting in increased parasympathetic tone. **vagoton′ic** *adj*

malignant v. severe bradycardia, hypotension, and syncope resulting from increased parasympathetic tone.

va·go·tro·pic (va″go-tro′pik) having an effect on the vagus nerve.

va·go·va·gal (va″go-va′gəl) arising as a result of afferent and efferent impulses which are both mediated through the vagus nerve.

va·gus (va′gəs) pl. *va′gi* [L. "wandering"] designating the tenth cranial nerve; see *nervus vagus.*

Vahl·kamp·fia (vahl-kamp′fe-ah) a genus of freshwater or parasitic ameboid protozoa of the class Lobosa, phylum Sarcomastigophora, having one broad pseudopodium; some species may cause keratitis.

vai·dya (vi′dyah) [Sanskrit "one who knows"] in ayurveda, a physician.

Vail neuralgia (syndrome) (vāl) [Harris Holmes *Vail,* American otorhinolaryngologist, 1892–1939] vidian neuralgia.

Val valine.

val·a·cy·clo·vir hy·dro·chlo·ride (val″a-si′klo-vir) the hydrochloride salt of the L-valyl ester of acyclovir, used as an antiviral agent in the treatment of genital herpes and herpes zoster in immunocompetent adults; administered orally. Following absorption, valacyclovir is converted by intestinal and hepatic metabolism to the active drug acyclovir.

Val·cyte (val′sīt) trademark for a preparation of valganciclovir hydrochloride.

val·de·cox·ib (val″də-kok′sib) a nonsteroidal antiinflammatory drug of the COX-2 inhibitors group, used for symptomatic treatment of osteoarthritis, rheumatoid arthritis, and primary dysmenorrhea; administered orally.

va·lence (va′lens) [L. *valēre* to be strong] 1. a positive number that represents the combining power of an element in a chemical compound, i.e., the number of bonds each atom of that element makes with other atoms. In this most general sense "valence" has been superseded by the concept "oxidation number." However, "valence" is still used to indicate *(a)* the number of covalent bonds formed by an atom in a covalent compound or *(b)* the charge on a monatomic or polyatomic molecule. 2. in immunology, *(a)* the number of antigen-binding sites possessed by an antibody molecule, two per immunoglobulin monomer, or *(b)* the number of antigenic determinants possessed by an antigen, usually a large number.

va·len·cy (va′lən-se) 1. strength; ability. 2. valence.

Val·en·tin corpuscles, ganglion (pseudoganglion), nerve (val′ən-tin) [Gabriel Gustav *Valentin,* German physiologist, 1810–1883] see under *corpuscle* and *nerve,* and see *intumescentia tympanica.*

Val·en·tine position (val′ən-tīn) [Ferdinand C. *Valentine,* American surgeon, 1851–1909] see under *position.*

val·er·ate (val′ər-āt) a salt or ester of valeric acid.

Val·er·gen (val′ər-gen) trademark for preparations of estradiol valerate.

va·le·ri·an (və-lēr′e-ən) [L. *valeriana*] 1. any plant of the genus *Valeriana.* 2. [NF] the dried roots, rhizome, and stolons of *V. officinalis,* which are antispasmodic and sedative and are used for nervousness and insomnia.

Greek v. Jacob's ladder.

Va·le·ri·a·na (və-leēr′e-a-nə) [L. *Valeria,* a Roman province (present day Hungary)] valerian; a widespread genus of perennial herbs having white or pink flowers, including *V. officinalis,* whose dried roots are used medicinally.

va·le·ric ac·id (və-lēr′ik) a monobasic organic acid derived from valerian, used as an intermediate in pharmaceutical manufacture.

val·gan·ci·clo·vir hy·dro·chlo·ride (val″gan-si′klo-vir) a prodrug of ganciclovir (q.v.); used in the treatment of cytomegalovirus retinitis in patients with acquired immunodeficiency syndrome, administered orally.

val·gus (val′gəs) [L.] bent or twisted outward; denoting a deformity in which the angulation of the part is away from the midline of the body; the term is an adjective and should be used only in connection with the noun it describes, such as talipes valgus, genu valgum, and coxa valga. The meanings of *valgus* and *varus* are often reversed, so that genu valgum is knock-knee, not bowleg. Cf. *varus.*

val·i·da·tion (val″ĭ-da′shən) confirmation or corroboration; the declaration of validity.

consensual v. the confirmation of reality by comparison of one's own perceptions and concerns with those of others, including the recognition and modification of distortions.

va·lid·i·ty (və-lid′ĭ-te) the extent to which a measurement, test, or study measures what it purports to measure.

construct v. the degree to which an instrument measures the characteristic being investigated; the extent to which the conceptual definition matches the operational definition.

content v. verification that the method of measurement actually measures what it is expected to measure, covering all areas under investigation reasonably and thoroughly.

criterion v. verification that the instrument correlates with external criteria of the phenomenon under study, either concurrently or predictively.

external v. the extent to which study results can be generalized beyond the sample used in the study.

face v. a type of content validity, determining the suitability of a given instrument as a source of data on the subject under investigation, using common-sense criteria.

internal v. the extent to which the effects detected in a study are truly caused by the treatment or exposure in the study sample, rather than being due to other biasing effects of extraneous variables.

predictive v. the effectiveness of one set of test or research results as a predictor of the outcome of future experiments or tests.

val·ine (Val, V) (va′lēn, val′ēn) 1. an essential amino acid, α-aminoisovaleric acid, produced by the digestion or hydrolytic decomposition of proteins; it is essential for optimal growth in infants and for nitrogen equilibrium in human adults. See also table at *amino acid.* 2. [USP] a preparation of valine used as a dietary supplement.

val·in·emia (val″in-e′me-ə) hypervalinemia.

val·ine trans·am·i·nase (va′lēn trans-am′ĭ-nās) a branched-chain-amino-acid transaminase acting on valine.

Val·i·sone (val′ĭ-sōn) trademark for preparations of betamethasone valerate.

Val·i·um (val′e-əm) trademark for preparations of diazepam.

val·late (val′āt) [L. *vallatus* walled] having a wall or rim; cup-shaped.

val·lec·u·la (və-lek′u-lə) pl. *vallec′ulae* [dim. of L. *valles* a hollow] 1. a depression or furrow. 2. v. epiglottica.

v. cerebel′li [TA], **v. of cerebellum** the longitudinal hollow on the inferior surface of the cerebellum, between the hemispheres, in which the medulla oblongata rests.

epiglottic v., v. epiglot′tica [TA] a depression between the lateral and median glossoepiglottic folds on each side.

val·lec·u·lar (və-lek′u-lər) pertaining to or affecting a vallecula.

val·lic·e·po·bu·fa·gin (və-lis″ə-po-bu′fə-jin) a cardiac poison from the skin glands of the toad, *Bufo valliceps.*

val·lum (val′əm) [L. "rampart"] a wall.

v. un′guis [TA] nail wall: the fold of skin overlapping the lateral and proximal edges of the nail; called also *nail fold* and *paronychium.*

Val·nac (val′nak) trademark for preparations of betamethasone valerate.

val·one (val′ōn) an indanedione anticoagulant used as an insecticide and rodenticide; it can cause fatal anticoagulant rodenticide poisoning (q.v.) in many mammalian species.

Val·pin (val′pin) trademark for preparations of anisotropine methylbromide.

val·pro·ate so·di·um (val-pro′āt) the sodium salt of valproic acid, having the same uses as the parent compound.

val·pro·ic ac·id (val-pro′ik) [USP] a simple eight-carbon branched-chain fatty acid used as an anticonvulsant in the treatment of epileptic seizures, particularly absence seizures; administered orally.

val·ru·bi·cin (val-roo′bĭ-sin″) an antineoplastic that interferes with various interrelated biological functions, most involving nucleic acid metabolism; it inhibits incorporation of nucleosides into nucleic acids, causes chromosomal damage, and arrests the cell cycle in the G_2 phase. Administered intravesically for treatment of bladder carcinoma.

Val·sal·va maneuver (experiment, method, test), etc. (vahl-sahl′və) [Antonio Maria *Valsalva*, Italian anatomist, 1666–1723] see under *maneuver*, and see *sinus aortae.*

val·sar·tan (val-sahr′tan) an angiotensin II receptor antagonist, used as an antihypertensive; administered orally.

Val·star (val′stahr) trademark for a preparation of valrubicin.

Val·trex (val′treks) trademark for a preparation of valacyclovir hydrochloride.

val·ue (val′u) 1. a measure of worth or efficiency. 2. a quantitative measurement of the activity, concentration, or some other quality of a substance; see *normal v's.*

acetyl v. see under *number.*

acid v. see under *number.*

buffer v. a numerical expression of the degree of change in pH of a solution in response to the addition of acid or alkali.

D v. decimal reduction time.

expected v. in statistics, the value of an estimate that is the mean of its sampling distribution.

fuel v. the potential heat energy of a food.

Hehner v. see under *number.*

liminal v. that intensity of a stimulus which produces a just noticeable impression.

negative predictive v. see *predictive v.*

normal v's see *reference v's.*

***P* v., *p* v.** the probability of obtaining by chance a result at least as extreme as that observed, even when the null hypothesis is true and no real difference exists; when $P \leq 0.05$ the sample results are usually deemed significant at a statistically important level and the null hypothesis rejected. See also *Type I error;* under *error.*

positive predictive v. see *predictive v.*

predictive v. the conditional probability that a clinical test result correctly identifies a patient as having or not having a disease, i.e., the predictive value of a positive test *(positive predictive v.)* is the probability that a person with a positive test is a true positive (i.e., does have the disease) and the predictive value of a negative test *(negative predictive v.)* is the probability that a person with a negative test does not have the disease. Cf. *sensitivity* and *specificity.* The predictive value of a screening test is determined by the sensitivity and specificity of the test, and by the prevalence of the condition for which the test is used.

reference v's a set of values of a quantity measured in the clinical laboratory that characterize a specified population in a defined state of health. The values obtained from a statistical sample are used to establish a *reference interval* that covers 95 per cent of the values of the healthy general population or of specific subpopulations differing in age and sex. These concepts were originally and are still widely referred to as "normal values" and the "normal range," but the use of these terms is now discouraged because of their implication that values falling outside of the reference interval are "abnormal" or "unhealthy," which has led to much confusion. It must be remembered that, by definition, 5 per cent of healthy individuals fall outside of the reference interval.

saponification v. see under *number.*

threshold v. liminal v.

threshold limit v. (TLV) a value assigned to an industrial chemical by the American Conference of Governmental Hygienists, representing the maximum concentration to which most workers can be repeatedly exposed without adverse health effects.

valence v. the number obtained by multiplying the lowering of the freezing point in degrees by the amount of urine in milliliters.

***z* v.** a normalized value created from a member of a set of data by expressing it in terms of standard deviations from the mean, using the equation

$$z = \frac{x - \bar{x}}{\sigma}$$

where x is an item of data, $\bar{x}$ is the mean of the data, and σ is the standard deviation. The mean and standard deviation of the set of such z values are 0 and 1, respectively.

val·va (val′və) pl. *val′vae* [sing. of L. *valvae* folding doors] [TA] valve: a membranous fold in a canal or passage that prevents reflux of the contents passing through it.

v. aor′tae [TA] aortic valve: the valve that guards the aortic orifice in the left ventricle of the heart and prevents backflow into the left ventricle; it is composed of three semilunar cusps or segments called the semilunar cusps of the aortic valve.

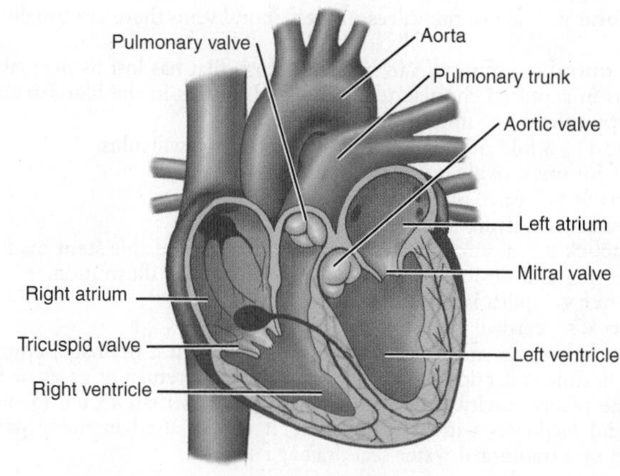

■ Valves of the heart.

v. atrioventricula′ris dex′tra [TA] tricuspid valve: the valve between the right atrium and right ventricle of the heart; it usually has three cusps (anterior, posterior, and septal), but additional small cusps may be present. Called also *v. tricuspidalis* [TA alternative] and *right atrioventricular valve.*

v. atrioventricula′ris sinis′tra [TA] mitral valve: the valve between the left atrium and left ventricle of the heart; it usually has two cusps (anterior and posterior), but additional small cusps may be present. Called also *v. mitralis* [TA alternative] and *left atrioventricular valve.*

v. mitra′lis TA alternative for *v. atrioventricularis sinistra.*

v. tricuspida′lis TA alternative for *v. atrioventricularis dextra.*

v. trun′ci pulmona′lis [TA] valve of pulmonary trunk: the valve that guards the pulmonary orifice of the right ventricle of the heart and prevents backflow of blood into the ventricle; it is composed of three semilunar cusps or segments (semilunar cusps of pulmonary valve). Called also *pulmonary* or *pulmonic valve.*

val·vate (val′vāt) pertaining to or having valves.

valve (valv) a membranous fold in a canal or passage that prevents reflux of the contents passing through it; see also *valva* and *valvula.* **val′val, val′var, val′vular** *adj*

anal v's valvulae anales.

anterior urethral v. a rare type of obstructing fold in the distal part of the male urethra, usually a type of diverticulum in the corpus spongiosum.

v. of aorta, aortic v. valva aortae.

artificial cardiac v., artificial heart v. prosthetic heart v.

ball v. caged-ball v.

Bauhin v. papilla ilealis.

Béraud v. a fold of mucous membrane sometimes found at the junction of the lacrimal sac and the nasolacrimal duct; called also *Krause v.*

bicuspid aortic v. a congenital anomaly of the aortic valve, caused by incomplete separation of two of the three cusps; it is generally asymptomatic early in life but is predisposed to calcification and stenosis later on.

bileaflet v. a type of prosthetic heart valve consisting of a sewing ring surrounding a circular valve seat, to which are attached two semicircular occluding disks that swing open and closed to regulate blood flow.

bioprosthetic v. a prosthetic heart valve composed of biological tissue, sterilized and mounted on a plastic or metallic supporting structure; it is inaudible and does not require anticoagulation; a common type is the porcine valve. Called also *tissue v.*

Björk-Shiley v. a tilting-disk valve consisting of a cobalt alloy cage, a Teflon fabric–covered sewing ring, and a disk made of pyrolytic carbon that opens to an angle of 60 degrees.

Bochdalek v. a fold within the lacrimal duct near the punctum lacrimale.

caged-ball v. a type of prosthetic heart valve consisting of a sewing ring to which is attached a cage made of curved struts; a ball within the cage floats freely, allowing passage of blood or occluding the orifice to prevent reflux.

cardiac v's valves that control the flow of blood through and from the heart; they are the atrioventricular, aortic, and pulmonary trunk valves.

Carpentier-Edwards v. a porcine valve mounted on an Elgiloy alloy stent with a Teflon cloth–covered sewing ring. See illustration.

caval v. valvula venae cavae inferioris.

Cooley-Cutter v. a caged-ball valve consisting of an open cage with four metal struts forming foot-like projections into the orifice, a cloth-covered sewing ring, and a disk-shaped or biconical poppet.

coronary v., v. of coronary sinus valvula sinus coronarii.

eustachian v. valvula venae cavae inferioris.

femoral v. one of the valves of the femoral vein; there are usually four or five.

flail mitral v. a mitral valve having a cusp that has lost its normal support (as in ruptured chordae tendineae) and flutters in the bloodstream.

floppy mitral v. mitral valve prolapse.

Foltz v. a fold of membrane at the lacrimal canaliculus.

v. of foramen ovale valvula foraminis ovalis.

Gerlach v. valve of vermiform appendix.

Guérin v. valvula fossae navicularis.

Hancock v. a porcine valve mounted on a semiflexible stent made of a Stellite ring and flexible struts of polypropylene. See illustration.

Hasner v. plica lacrimalis.

heart v's cardiac v's.

Heimlich v. a small one-way valve used for chest drainage, emptying into a flexible collection device; the valve prevents return of gases or fluids into the pleural cavity. The Heimlich valve is less than 13 cm (5 inches) long and facilitates patient ambulation; it can be used in many patients instead of a traditional water seal drainage system.

Heister v. plica spiralis.

Hoboken v's foldlike thickenings of the vessels of the umbilical cord, especially the arteries, which protrude into the lumen of the vessels.

homograft v. a transplanted cardiac valve obtained from a human donor and antibiotic-sterilized or cryopreserved, then sewn into the native anulus.

Houston v's plicae transversae recti.

Huschke v. plica lacrimalis.

ileal v. 1. ileocecal v. 2. papilla ilealis.

ileocecal v., ileocolic v. a valvelike structure formed by the flaps or lips, one above and one below, of the ileal (ileocecal) orifice. In the cadaver the flaps project into the lumen of the large intestine as thickened folds, but in the living individual there is only a conical or papillary projection called the *papilla ilealis.*

v. of inferior vena cava valvula venae cavae inferioris.

Ionescu-Shiley v. a type of prosthetic heart valve consisting of glutaraldehyde-fixed bovine pericardium constructed as a three-cusp valve mounted on a Dacron-covered titanium frame.

Kerckring v's, Kerkring v's plicae circulares.

Krause v. Béraud v.

left atrioventricular v. valva atrioventricularis sinistra.

Lillehei-Kaster v. a tilting-disk valve consisting of a titanium valve housing, Teflon sewing ring, and flat, free-floating, pivoting pyrolytic carbon disk that opens to 80 degrees.

lymphatic v. valvula lymphatica.

Medtronic-Hall v. a type of tilting-disk valve consisting of a titanium valve housing an S-shaped disk guide strut, a Teflon cloth sewing ring, and a centrally perforated pyrolytic carbon–coated graphite disk that opens to an angle of 75 degrees. See illustration.

mitral v. valva atrioventricularis sinistra.

Morgagni v's valvulae anales.

nasal v. limen nasi.

v. of navicular fossa valvula fossae navicularis.

O'Beirne v. rectosigmoid sphincter.

Omnicarbon v. a type of tilting-disk valve similar to the Omniscience valve but entirely coated with pyrolytic carbon, including the sewing ring.

Omniscience v. a type of tilting-disk valve that is a modification of the Lillehei-Kaster valve, with a curvilinear pyrolytic carbon disk suspended in a one-piece titanium frame with finlike projections and a Teflon sewing ring.

porcine v. a type of prosthetic heart valve made from a pig aortic valve cured in glutaraldehyde and mounted on a supporting structure.

posterior urethral v. an abnormal congenital obstructing membrane present in the proximal part of the male urethra; it is the most common cause of bladder outlet obstruction in male infants.

prosthetic cardiac v., prosthetic heart v. a substitute for a cardiac valve, composed of either artificial material or tissue. See illustration. Called also *artificial heart v.* and *heart valve prosthesis.*

pulmonary v., v. of pulmonary trunk, pulmonic v. valva trunci pulmonalis.

pyloric v. a prominent circular fold of mucous membrane in the stomach near the pyloric orifice.

right atrioventricular v. valva atrioventricularis dextra.

Rosenmüller v. plica lacrimalis.

St. Jude Medical v. a type of bileaflet valve consisting of a Dacron sewing ring and pyrolytic carbon leaflets and housing, with the leaflets opening to 85 degrees. See illustration.

semilunar v. 1. a valve having semilunar cusps, such as the aortic valve or pulmonary valve. 2. by extension, one of the semilunar cusps composing such a valve; see entries beginning *valvula semilunaris.*

sinoatrial v., sinuatrial v. the valve at the opening of the sinus venosus into the primordial right atrium.

spiral v. of cystic duct, spiral v. of Heister plica spiralis.

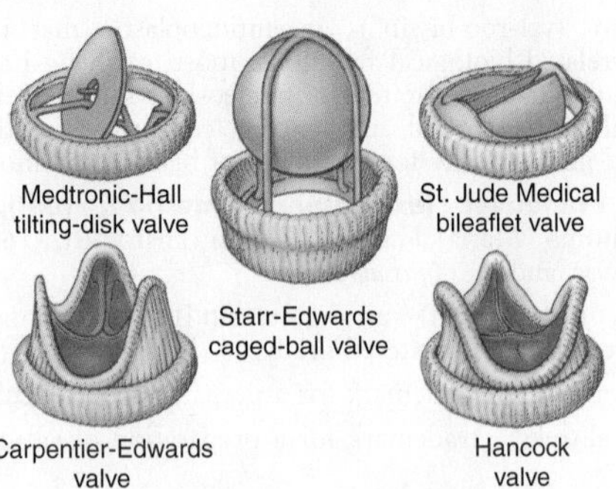

■ Prosthetic cardiac valves.

Starr-Edwards v. a type of caged-ball valve consisting of a Stellite retaining cage containing a Silastic ball and a Teflon and polypropylene cloth–covered sewing ring. See illustration.

v. of Sylvius valvula venae cavae inferioris.

Taillefer v. a fold of the mucous membrane of the nasolacrimal duct near the middle of its course.

Tarinus v. velum medullare inferius.

thebesian v. valvula sinus coronarii.

tilting-disk v. a type of prosthetic heart valve consisting of a sewing ring and a valve housing containing a suspended disk that swings between closed and open positions.

tissue v. bioprosthetic v.

tricuspid v. valva atrioventricularis dextra.

v. of Tulpius ileocecal v.

ureteral v. a congenital transverse fold across the lumen of the ureter, composed of redundant mucosa prominent by circular muscle fibers; it usually disappears in time but may rarely cause urinary obstruction. Pathological valves or kinks also occur.

v. of Varolius ileocecal v.

v. of veins, venous v. valvula venosa.

v. of vermiform appendix an inconstant fold of mucous membrane at the orifice of the vermiform appendix.

v. of Vieussens velum medullare superius.

valved (valvd) having valves; opening by valves.

val·vi·form (val′vĭ-form) shaped like a valve.

val·vo·tome (val′vo-tōm) a surgical instrument for incising a valve.

val·vot·o·my (val-vot′ə-me) [*valve* + *-tomy*] incision of a valve. Called also *valvulotomy.*

mitral v. dilation of the left atrioventricular (mitral) valve, the commissures being split with or without the aid of a knife or a mechanical dilator.

pulmonary v. incision of the pulmonary valve to correct valvular stenosis.

transventricular closed v. correction of pulmonary valvular stenosis by passage of a valvotome through the wall of the right ventricle into the pulmonary artery to open the valve; called also *Brock operation.*

val·vu·la (val′vu-lə) pl. *val′vulae* [L., dim of *valva*] [TA] valvule: a small valve; formerly used in official nomenclature to designate any valve, but now restricted to certain small valves in the body and cusps of heart valves.

val′vulae ana′les [TA] anal valves: archlike folds of mucous membrane connecting the caudal ends of the anal columns.

val′vulae conniven′tes plicae circulares.

v. corona′ria dex′tra val′vae aor′tae TA alternative for *v. semilunaris dextra valvae aortae.*

v. corona′ria sinis′tra val′vae aor′tae TA alternative for *valvula semilunaris sinistra valvae aortae.*

v. fora′minis ova′lis 1. [TA], valve of foramen ovale: in the adult, a crescentic ridge on the left side of the interatrial septum, representing the edge of what was the septum primum before fusion of the septum; called also *falx septi.* 2. a fold in the left atrium of the fetal heart, derived from the embryonic septum primum.

v. fos′sae navicula′ris [TA] valve of navicular fossa: a fold of mucous membrane occasionally found in the roof of the navicular fossa of the male urethra; called also *Guérin fold* or *valve.*

v. lympha′tica [TA] lymphatic valve: any of the usually doubled cusps in the collecting lymphatic vessels, serving to ensure flow in only one direction.

v. non corona′ria val′vae aor′tae TA alternative for *v. semilunaris posterior valvae aortae.*

v. semiluna′ris ante′rior val′vae trun′ci pulmona′lis [TA] anterior semilunar cusp of pulmonary valve: the left anterior cusp of the valve of the pulmonary trunk; named for its position in fetal anatomy. See illustration at *cusp.*

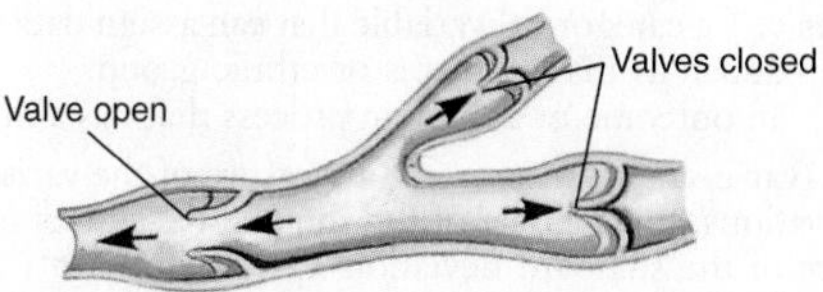

■ Valvulae venosae (venous valves). Pooled blood is moved toward the heart as valves are forced open by the pressure from the volume of blood below; closure of the valves prevents backflow.

v. semiluna´ris dex´tra val´vae aor´tae [TA] right semilunar cusp of aortic valve: the anterior cusp of the aortic valve; named for its position in fetal anatomy. Called also *v. coronaria dextra valvae aortae* [TA alternative] and *right coronary cusp of aortic valve*. See illustration at *cusp*.

v. semiluna´ris dex´tra val´vae trun´ci pulmona´lis [TA] right semilunar cusp of pulmonary valve: the right anterior cusp of the valve of the pulmonary trunk; named for its position in fetal anatomy. See illustration at *cusp*.

v. semiluna´ris poste´rior val´vae aor´tae [TA] posterior semilunar cusp of aortic valve: the right posterior cusp of the aortic valve; named for its position in fetal anatomy. Called also *v. non coronaria valvae aortae* [TA alternative] and *noncoronary cusp of aortic valve*. See illustration at *cusp*.

v. semiluna´ris sinis´tra val´vae aor´tae [TA] left semilunar cusp of aortic valve: the left posterior cusp of the aortic valve; named for its position in fetal anatomy. Called also *v. coronaria sinistra valvae aortae* [TA alternative] and *left coronary cusp of aortic valve*. See illustration at *cusp*.

v. semiluna´ris sinis´tra val´vae trun´ci pulmona´lis [TA] left semilunar cusp of pulmonary valve: the posterior cusp of the valve of the pulmonary trunk; named for its position in fetal anatomy. See illustration at *cusp*.

v. si´nus corona´rii [TA] valve of coronary sinus: a fold of endocardium along the right and inferior margins of the opening of the coronary sinus into the right atrium of the heart; it covers the lower part of the sinus and prevents regurgitation into the sinus during atrial contractions.

v. ve´nae ca´vae inferio´ris [TA] valve of inferior vena cava: the variably sized crescentic fold of endocardial tissue, enclosing a few muscle fibers, that is attached to the anterior margin of the opening of the inferior vena cava into the right atrium of the heart. Rudimentary in the adult, in the fetus it directs blood flow from the inferior vena cava into the left atrium via the foramen ovale. Called also *caval* or *eustachian valve* and *valve of Sylvius*.

v. veno´sa [TA] venous valve: any of the small cusps or folds found in the tunica intima of many veins, serving to prevent backflow of blood.

val•vu•lae (val´vu-le) [L.] genitive and plural of *valvula*.

val•vule (val´vūl) [L. *valvula*, q.v.] a small valve; see *valvula*.

val•vu•li•tis (val″vu-li´tis) inflammation of a valve or valvula, especially a cardiac valve.

rheumatic v. valvulitis due to rheumatic fever, characterized by numerous small, translucent vegetations, composed of fibrin and platelets, located on the edges of the valve cusps along the lines of closure. The mitral valve is most frequently involved. It is sometimes incorrectly called *rheumatic endocarditis* (q.v.).

val•vu•lop•a•thy (val″vu-lop´ə-the) abnormality of a valve or valvula, especially a cardiac valve.

val•vu•lo•plas•ty (val´vu-lo-plas″te) plastic repair of a cardiac or venous valve. **valvuloplas´tic** *adj*

balloon v. dilation of a stenotic cardiac valve by means of a balloon-tip catheter that is introduced into the valve and inflated.

internal v. repair of a venous valve through a venotomy incision, using sutures to shorten the floppy cusps.

val•vu•lo•tome (val´vu-lo-tōm″) valvotome.

val•vu•lot•o•my (val″vu-lot´ə-me) valvotomy.

val•yl (val´əl, va´ləl) the acyl radical of valine.

VAMP a cancer chemotherapy regimen consisting of vincristine, methotrexate, 6-mercaptopurine, and prednisone.

vam•pire (vam´pīr) vampire bat.

van•a•date (van´ə-dāt) any salt of vanadic acid; the salts have various industrial applications and many are toxic.

va•nad•ic ac•id (və-nad´ik) an inorganic acid produced by dissolving vanadium pentoxide in water; there are various degrees of hydration, HVO_3, H_3VO_4, $H_4V_2O_7$, etc., seen in salts (vanadates).

va•na•di•um (V) (və-na´de-əm) [*Vanadis*, a Norse deity] a rare, gray, metallic element; atomic number, 23; atomic weight, 50.942. Its salts have been used in treating various diseases. See also *vanadiumism*.

v. pentoxide a yellow to brown oxide of vanadium, used to add color and ultraviolet blocking to glass and as a component of photographic developers; its fumes can cause vanadiumism and vanadium bronchitis.

va•na•di•um•ism (və-na´de-əm-iz-əm) a chronic intoxication caused by absorption of vanadium compounds, usually via the lungs; symptoms include irritation of the respiratory tract *(vanadium bronchitis)*, pneumonitis, conjunctivitis, and anemia.

van Bo•gaert encephalitis, sclerosing leukoencephalitis (vahn bo´gärt) [Ludo *van Bogaert*, Belgian neuropathologist, 1897–1989] subacute sclerosing panencephalitis.

van Bo•gaert-Nys•sen syndrome (vahn bo´gärt ni´sen) [L. *van Bogaert;* René *Nyssen*, Belgian neurologist, 20th century] metachromatic leukodystrophy (adult form); see under *leukodystrophy*.

van Bo•gaert-Nys•sen-Peif•fer syndrome (vahn bo´gärt ni´sen pi´fer) [L. *van Bogaert;* R. *Nyssen;* Jürgen *Peiffer*, German physician, born 1922] metachromatic leukodystrophy (adult form); see under *leukodystrophy*.

van Bu•chem syndrome (vahn boo´kem) [Francis Steven Peter *van Buchem*, Dutch physician, 20th century] hyperostosis corticalis generalisata; see under *hyperostosis*.

van Bu•ren disease (van bu´rən) [William Holme *van Buren*, American surgeon, 1819–1883] Peyronie disease; see under *disease*.

Van•ce•nase (van´sə-nāz″) trademark for preparations of beclomethasone dipropionate.

Van•cer•il (van´sər-il″) trademark for a preparation of beclomethasone dipropionate.

Van•co•cin (van´ko-sin) trademark for preparations of vancomycin hydrochloride.

van•co•my•cin hy•dro•chlo•ride (van″ko-mi´sin) [USP] an antibiotic produced by the soil bacillus *Amycolatopsis orientalis*, which is highly effective against cocci, especially staphylococci, and other gram-positive bacteria; administered intravenously in the treatment of severe staphylococcal infections resistant to other antibiotics. It is administered orally in the treatment of staphylococcal enterocolitis and antibiotic-associated pseudomembranous enterocolitis caused by *Clostridium difficile*.

van den Bergh disease (vahn dən burg´) [A.A. Hymans *van den Bergh*, Dutch physician, 1869–1943] see under *disease*.

van der Kolk's law (vahn där kolks) [Jacob Ludwig Conrad Schroeder *van der Kolk*, Dutch physiologist, 1797–1862] Schroeder van der Kolk's law; see under *law*.

van der Waals forces (vahn dər vahlz´) [Johannes Diderik *van der Waals*, Dutch physicist, 1837–1923] see under *force*.

Van der Woude syndrome (van der wo´də) [Anne *Van der Woude*, American physician, 20th century] see under *syndrome*.

van Ge•huch•ten method (vahn ga-hook´ten) [Arthur *van Gehuchten*, Belgian anatomist, 1861–1914] see under *method*.

van Gie•son stain (van ge´sən) [Ira *van Gieson*, American neuropathologist, 1865–1913] see *Stains and Staining Methods*, under *stain*.

Van•gue•ria (van-ger´e-ə) a genus of shrubs of the family Rubiaceae. *V. pygmo´ra* is a shrub of southern Africa that is poisonous to sheep and cattle, causing gousiekte.

van Hook operation (van hook´) [Weller *van Hook*, American surgeon, 1862–1933] ureteroureterostomy.

van Hoorne canal (vahn horn´) [Jan *van Hoorne*, Dutch anatomist, 1621–1670] see *ductus thoracicus*.

Va•nil•la (və-nil´ə) [L.] a genus of climbing plants of the family Orchidaceae, native to hot climates. *V. planifo´lia* Andr. is Mexican or Bourbon vanilla and *V. tahiten´sis* Moor. is Tahitian vanilla; both have fruits called vanilla beans, which are sources of the flavoring vanilla.

va•nil•la (və-nil´ə) [Sp. *vainilla* little sheath] 1. any plant of the genus *Vanilla*. 2. the fruit of *Vanilla planifolia* or *V. tahitensis*, an elongated pod that is the source of the flavoring called vanilla. Called also *vanilla bean*. 3. [NF] a preparation of the cured unripe fruit of *V. planifolia* or *V. tahitensis*, used in medicine as a flavoring agent, usually in the form of vanilla tincture (see under *tincture*).

Bourbon v., Mexican v. *Vanilla planifolia*.

Tahitian v. *Vanilla tahitensis*.

va•nil•lal (və-nil´əl) ethyl vanillin.

va•nil•lic ac•id (və-nil´ik) 4-hydroxy-3-methoxybenzoic acid, an oxidation product of vanillin.

va•nil•lin (və-nil´in, van´ĭ-lin) [NF] a constituent of vanilla and other plants, which also may be prepared synthetically; used as a flavor in pharmaceutical preparations.

ethyl v. [NF] a synthetic compound closely related to vanillin, having a more intense vanilla odor and taste but a slightly different taste; used as a flavor in pharmaceutical preparations.

va·nil·lism (və-nil′iz-əm) a type of acarodermatitis with rhinitis and malaise, seen in persons working with raw vanilla, caused by the mite *Acarus siro.*

va·nil·lyl·man·del·ic ac·id (və-nil′əl-mən-del′ik) the primary end-product of catecholamine metabolism excreted in the urine; urinary levels are used in screening patients for pheochromocytoma. Abbreviated VMA.

va·nil·man·del·ic ac·id (van″əl-man-del′ik) vanillylmandelic acid.

Van·i·qa (van′ĭ-kə) trademark for a preparation of eflornithine hydrochloride.

Van Lo·hui·zen syndrome (vahn lo′hou-zen) [Cato *Van Lohuizen*, Dutch pediatrician, early 20th century] cutis marmorata telangiectatica congenita.

Van·sil (van′sil) trademark for a preparation of oxamniquine.

Van Slyke formula, test (method) (van slīk′) [Donald Dexter *Van Slyke*, American biochemist, 1883–1971] see under *formula* and *test.*

van't Hoff's law, rule (vahnt hofs′) [Jacobus Hendricus *van't Hoff*, Dutch chemist, 1852–1911; winner of the Nobel prize for chemistry in 1901] see under *law* and *rule.*

Van·tin (van′tin) trademark for preparations of cefpodoxime proxetil.

Van·zet·ti sign (vahn-tset′e) [Tito *Vanzetti*, Italian surgeon, 1809–1888] see under *sign.*

va·por (va′pər) pl. *vapo′res, vapors* [L.] 1. an atmospheric dispersion of a substance that in its normal state is a liquid or solid. 2. steam, gas, or an exhalation.

va·por·iza·tion (va″pər-ĭ-za′shən) 1. the conversion of a solid or liquid into a vapor without chemical change. See also *nebulization.* 2. distillation.

transurethral v. of prostate (TUVP) destruction of hyperplastic prostatic tissue using an electrode introduced through the urethra. The leading edge of the electrode uses high heat to cause vaporization of tissue, and the trailing edge uses lower heat to cause coagulation-induced desiccation of tissue.

va·por·ize (va′pər-īz) to convert into vapor or to be transformed into vapor.

va·por·iz·er (va″por-īz′ər) a device for producing an aerosol or mist, as from a solution containing a medication to ease breathing. Cf. *nebulizer.*

Vap·ri·sol (vap′rĭ-sol) trademark for a preparation of conivaptan hydrochloride.

Vaqta (vak′tə) trademark for a preparation of hepatitis A vaccine inactivated.

Va·quez disease (vah-ka′) [Louis Henri *Vaquez*, French physician, 1860–1936] polycythemia vera.

var. variety.

var·den·a·fil hy·dro·chlo·ride (vahr-den′ə-fil) a phosphodiesterase inhibitor that relaxes the smooth muscle of the penis, thereby facilitating blood flow to the corpus cavernosum; used to treat erectile dysfunction in impotence therapy. Administered orally.

va·ren·i·cline tar·trate (və-ren′ĭ-klēn) a partial agonist of one type of nicotinic receptor, used as an aid in smoking cessation; administered orally.

var·i·a·bil·i·ty (var″e-ə-bil′ĭ-te) the state of being variable.

var·i·a·ble (var′e-ə-bəl) [L. *variare* to change] 1. changing from time to time. 2. in mathematics, a symbol that represents an arbitrary number or an arbitrary element of a set.

categorical v. one of the variables that are not continuous but instead put data into categories.

confounding v. confounder.

continuous v. a variable that can assume the complete continuum of values (a theoretically infinite variety) through its distribution; cf. *discrete v.*

dependent v. in a mathematical equation or relationship between two or more variables, a variable whose value depends on those of others; e.g., in the formula $x = 3y + z^2$, x is the dependent variable.

dichotomous v. a categorical variable that can assign data to one of only two groups, such as male versus female.

discrete v. an experimental variable that can assume only certain specific values in its distribution; the possible list of values is finite and often countable; cf. *continuous v.*

extraneous v. a factor that is not itself under study but affects the measurement of the study variables or the examination of their relationships.

independent v. in a mathematical equation or relationship between two or more variables, any variable whose value determines that of others; e.g., in the formula $x = 3y + z^2$, y and z are the independent variables.

nested v. a variable located entirely within another variable, such as the rate of a given disease in one specific city.

outcome v. a variable that measures consequences or results; it may be primary, ancillary, or incidental to a particular study.

polytomous v. a categorical variable that can assign data to any of three or more groups, such as marital status or ethnic group.

random v. an outcome of a random process that has a numerical value.

var·i·ance (var′e-əns) in statistics, a measure of the variation shown by a set of observations: the average of the squared deviations from the mean; it is the square of the standard deviation (q.v.). Symbol σ^2.

genetic v. the observable (phenotypic) variance that is due to the presence of different genotypes in the population.

phenotypic v. the total observable variance of a measured quantity in a population; it is the sum of that contributed by the genotype and the environment.

var·i·ant (var′e-ənt) 1. something that differs in some characteristic from the class to which it belongs, as a variant of a disease, trait, species, etc. 2. exhibiting such variation.

L-phase v. a variant phase of certain bacteria, induced by osmotic shock, temperature shock, or the presence of antibiotics, and consisting of a spherical or ellipsoidal body without a rigid cell wall. The cells are capable of growth and multiplication; they may be stable or may revert to a normal bacterial cell. Called also *L-form.*

migraine v. migraine associated with non-neurologic symptoms, such as occurs in ophthalmic migraine, basilar migraine, or abdominal migraine.

petit mal v. Lennox-Gastaut syndrome.

var·i·ate (var′e-āt) a variable or random variable.

var·i·a·tion (var″e-a′shən) 1. the act or process of changing. 2. the state or fact of differing. 3. in genetics, deviation in phenotype of an individual from that typical of the group to which it belongs; also, deviation in phenotype of the offspring from that of its parents.

allotypic v. the antigenic differences that characterize immunoglobulin allotypes.

antigenic v. 1. a mechanism whereby microorganisms or parasites, such as trypanosomes, plasmodia, and *Borrelia*, are enabled to escape immune surveillance of a host by modifying or completely altering their surface antigens. 2. a phenomenon occurring in the influenza virus, in which the virus spontaneously exhibits both slow antigenic drift and sharp antigenic changes at intervals.

contingent negative v. (CNV) a small negative potential recorded on an electroencephalogram over the front central scalp of some subjects who perform tasks requiring close attention or who have just received a warning stimulus. Called also *E wave* and *expectancy wave.*

continuous v. variation in which the differences form a continuous spectrum, and none predominates.

discontinuous v. variation in which the differences are marked, do not grade into one another, and form two or more separate, discontinuous classes.

idiotypic v. the antigenic differences that characterize the different amino acid sequences and structures of immunoglobulin variable regions (idiotypes) and corresponding differences in antigen specificity.

isotypic v. the antigenic differences that characterize the immunoglobulin classes and subclasses (isotypes).

meristic v. change in the number or the geometrical relation of parts or segments of an organism.

microbial v. the range of characteristics within a species used in identification and differentiation.

smooth-rough v., S-R v. a genetic mutation or an adaptation seen in bacteria, most often evidenced by a change in the surface of colonies from smooth (S, glossy) to rough (R, dull). The change correlates with pathogenicity, S strains being generally more virulent and R strains less so. The cells in S colonies have polysaccharide capsules and are more antigenically complete; R cells contain little or no capsule. The term may also refer to changes in other cell structures such as flagella and somatic antigens, as well as susceptibility to bacteriophage. Variations are often reversible and tend to result in mixed types on repeated subculture. See also *bacterial dissociation*, under *dissociation.*

var·i·ca·tion (var″ĭ-ka′shən) 1. the formation of a varix. 2. varicosity (def. 1).

var·i·ce·al (var″ĭ-se′əl) varicose.

var·i·cel·la (var″ĭ-sel′ə) [L.] chickenpox.

v. gangreno′sa a rare form of chickenpox in which the eruption leads to a gangrenous ulceration, occurring mainly in children with leukemia, immunodeficiency, or some other severe underlying disease.

var·i·cel·li·form (var″ĭ-sel′ĭ-form) resembling chickenpox (varicella); called also *varicelloid.*

var·i·cel·loid (var″ĭ-sel′oid) varicelliform.

Var·i·cel·lo·vi·rus (var″ĭ-sel′o-vi″rəs) [*varicella* + *virus*] varicella and pseudorabies-like viruses; a genus of viruses of the subfamily Alphaherpesvirinae (family Herpesviridae) that infect mammals, including human herpesvirus 3 and, tentatively, pseudorabies virus, bovine herpesvirus 1, and equid herpesviruses 1 and 4. **varicellovi′ral** *adj*

var·i·ces (var′ĭ-sēz) [L.] plural of *varix.*

var·ic·i·form (var-is′ĭ-form) 1. varicoid. 2. varicose.

varic(o)- [L. *varix* a varicose vein] a combining form denoting relationship to a varix, or meaning twisted and swollen.

var·i·co·bleph·a·ron (var″ĭ-ko-blef′ə-ron) [*varico-* + Gr. *blepharon* eyelid] a varicose swelling of the eyelid.

var·i·co·cele (var′ĭ-ko-sēl″) [*varico-* + *-cele*[1]] 1. a condition in males characterized by varicosity of the veins of the pampiniform plexus, forming a swelling that feels like a "bag of worms;" it appears bluish through the skin of the scrotum and is accompanied by a constant pulling, dragging, or dull pain in the scrotum. Since the presence of excess blood in the scrotum increases temperature, the condition is thought to be linked to male factor infertility. 2. a similar condition in females, with varicosity of the veins of the broad ligament of the uterus.

ovarian v., pelvic v., utero-ovarian v. varicocele (def. 2).

var·i·co·ce·lec·to·my (var″ĭ-ko-sə-lek′tə-me) [*varicocele* + *-ectomy*] ligation and excision of the enlarged veins of a varicocele.

var·i·cog·ra·phy (var″ĭ-kog′rə-fe) [*varico-* + *-graphy*] radiographic visualization of varicose veins.

var·i·coid (var′ĭ-koid) [*varico-* + *-oid*] resembling a varix; called also *variciform.*

var·i·com·pha·lus (var″ĭ-kom′fə-ləs) [*varico-* + *omphalus*] a varicose tumor at the umbilicus.

var·i·co·phle·bi·tis (var″ĭ-ko-flə-bi′tis) varicose veins with inflammation.

var·i·cose (var′ĭ-kōs) [L. *varicosus*] pertaining to a varix; unnaturally and permanently distended. Called also *variceal* and *variciform.*

var·i·co·sis (var″ĭ-ko′sis) [L.] varicosity (def. 1).

var·i·cos·i·ty (var″ĭ-kos′ĭ-te) 1. a varicose condition; the state of being varicose. Called also *varication, varicosis,* and *phlebectasia.* 2. varix. 3. varicose vein.

var·i·cot·o·my (var″ĭ-kot′ə-me) [*varico-* + *-tomy*] incision into a varix or a varicose vein.

va·ric·u·la (və-rik′u-lə) [L.] a varix of the conjunctiva.

var·i·e·gate (var′e-ĭ-gāt″) [L. *varius* diverse] 1. marked by variety; diversified. 2. having patchy spots or streaks of different colors.

va·ri·e·ty (və-ri′ə-te) in taxonomy, a subcategory of a species; see *subspecies.*

va·ri·o·la (və-ri′o-lə) [L.] smallpox. **vari′olar, vari′olous** *adj*

v. capri′na goatpox.

v. haemorha′gica hemorrhagic smallpox.

v. ma′jor the classic severe form of smallpox.

v. mi′nor a mild form of smallpox that was found only in certain parts of South America and Africa.

v. ovi′na sheep-pox.

v. si′ne eruptio′ne modified smallpox in which no rash is present.

Va·ri·o·la·ria ama·ra (va″re-o-lar′e-ə ə-ma′rə) a febrifugal and anthelmintic lichen of the Old World; it is a source of litmus.

va·ri·o·late (var′e-o-lāt) 1. having the nature or appearance of smallpox. 2. to inoculate with variola virus; see *variolation.*

va·ri·o·la·tion (var″e-o-la′shən) deliberate inoculation with the virus of unmodified smallpox to produce immunity to the naturally occurring disease; this was done in China and elsewhere in the region from ancient times to the 20th century. Dried crusts of smallpox lesions were applied to the skin or nasal mucous membranes, or were ingested. A modified method used in Europe in the eighteenth century consisted of subcutaneous injection of material from the lesions. Variolation is now used only experimentally in animals.

va·ri·ol·i·form (var″e-o′lĭ-form) varioloid.

va·ri·o·li·za·tion (var″e-o-lĭ-za′shən) variolation.

va·ri·o·loid (və-ri′o-loid″) resembling smallpox; called also *varioliform.*

va·ris·tor (və-ris′tər) a voltage-variable resistor; a resistor, usually a semiconductor, designed to change its resistance with the voltage applied across it.

Vari·vax (var′ĭ-vaks) trademark for a preparation of varicella virus vaccine live.

va·rix (var′iks) pl. *va′rices* [L.] an enlarged and tortuous vein, artery, or lymphatic vessel.

anastomotic v. aneurysmal v. (def. 2).

aneurysmal v., aneurysmoid v. 1. a markedly dilated tortuous vessel. 2. a form of arteriovenous aneurysm in which the blood flows directly into a neighboring vein without the intervention of a connecting sac; called also *anastomotic v.* and *Pott aneurysm.*

arterial v. a racemose aneurysm or varicose artery.

cirsoid v. racemose aneurysm.

esophageal varices varicosities of the branches of the azygos vein which anastomose with tributaries of the portal vein in the lower esophagus, occurring in patients with portal hypertension.

esophagogastric varices gastroesophageal varices.

gastric varices varices in the stomach, classified as either *gastroesophageal varices* or *isolated gastric varices.*

gastroesophageal varices gastric varices that are associated with esophageal varices, cross the esophagogastric junction, and extend along the lesser or greater curvatures.

isolated gastric varices gastric varices that are not near the esophagogastric junction or associated with esophageal varices; the usual location is in the gastric fundus.

lymph v., v. lympha′ticus a soft, lobulated swelling of a lymph node, resulting from obstruction and dilatation of the lymphatic vessels.

var·nish (vahr′nish) 1. a solution of resin or of natural gum, such as copal or rosin, in a suitable solvent, such as acetone, ether, or chloroform, which is capable of hardening into a thin film. 2. cavity v.

cavity v. a cavity lining agent consisting of a solution of one or more natural or synthetic resins, gums, and rosin in an organic solvent such as chloroform, ethanol, acetone, or benzene; applied to the floor and walls of the prepared cavity.

va·ro·li·an (və-ro′le-ən) 1. described by or named for Costanzo *Varolius.* 2. pertaining to the pons.

Va·ro·li·us valve (və-ro′le-əs) [Costanzo *Varolius (Varoli, Varolio),* Italian anatomist, 1543–1575] ileocecal valve; see under *valve.*

va·rus (var′əs) [L. "knock-kneed"] bent or twisted inward; denoting a deformity in which the angulation of the part is toward the midline of the body. The term varus is an adjective and should be used only in connection with the noun it describes, such as talipes varus, genu varum, and coxa vara. The meanings of *varus* and *valgus* are often reversed, so that genu varum is bowleg, not knock-knee. Cf. *valgus.*

vas (vas) pl. *va′sa* [L.] vessel; a canal for carrying fluid, especially one carrying blood, lymph, or spermatozoa.

v. aber′rans 1. ductulus aberrans superior 2. any anomalous or unusual vessel.

va′sa aberran′tia he′patis numerous vessels found in the fibrous capsule of the liver and the inconstant fibrous appendix.

v. anastomo′ticum [TA] anastomotic vessel: a vessel that serves to interconnect other vessels; such communications are present in the palm of the hand, sole of the foot, base of the brain, and other regions.

va′sa bre′via arteriae gastricae breves.

v. capilla′re [TA] capillary.

v. collatera′le [TA] collateral vessel: a vessel that parallels another vessel, nerve, or other structure.

v. de′ferens ductus deferens.

v. lympha′ticum [TA] lymphatic vessel: one that collects lymph from the tissues and through which the lymph passes to reach the bloodstream.

v. lympha′ticum profun′dum [TA] deep lymphatic vessel: any lymphatic vessel that drains lymph from deep body structures; deep lymphatic vessels accompany the deeply placed blood vessels.

v. lympha′ticum superficia′le [TA] superficial lymphatic vessel: any lymphatic vessel located under the skin and superficial fascia, in the submucous areolar tissue of the digestive, respiratory, and genitourinary tracts, and in the subserous tissue of the walls of the abdomen and thorax.

v. lymphocapilla′re [TA] lymphocapillary vessel: one of the minute vessels of the lymphatic system, having a caliber greater than a blood capillary; they form closed networks (sing. *rete lymphocapillare*) by which they communicate freely with one another.

va′sa nervo′rum [TA] blood vessels supplying the nerves.

va′sa prae′via presentation, in front of the fetal head during labor, of the blood vessels of the umbilical cord where they enter the placenta.

v. pro′minens duc′tus cochlea′ris [TA] a small vessel often seen deep to the spiral prominence in the cochlear duct.

va′sa rec′ta re′nis TA alternative for *arteriolae rectae renis.*

v. sangui′neum [TA] blood vessel.

va′sa sangui′nea au′ris inter′nae [TA] the blood vessels of the internal ear.

va′sa sangui′nea choroi′deae [TA] the blood vessels of the choroid.

va′sa sangui′nea intrapulmona′lia [TA] the blood vessels within the parenchyma of the lungs.

va′sa sangui′nea re′tinae [TA] the blood vessels of the retina, including all the arterioles, derived from the central artery of the retina, and the venules, which return blood to the central vein.

v. sinusoi′deum [TA] sinusoid: a form of terminal blood channel consisting of a large, irregular anastomosing vessel, having a lining of reticuloendothelium but little or no adventitia; sinusoids are found in the liver, adrenals, heart, parathyroid, carotid gland, spleen, and pancreas. Those in the anterior pituitary gland, adrenal cortex, and islets of Langerhans have a continuous basal lamina and a thin endothelium penetrated by pores closed

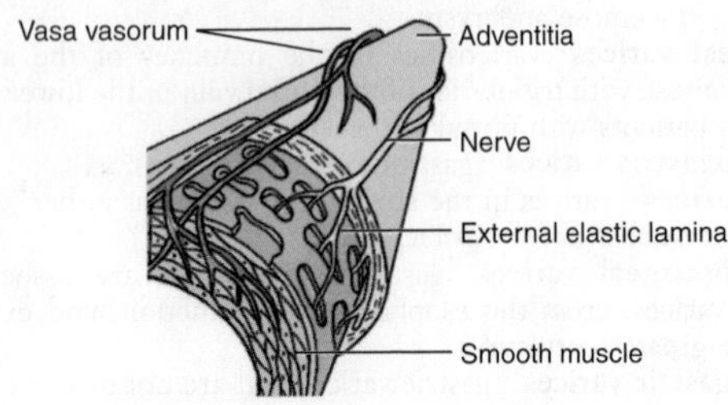

■ Vasa vasorum entering an artery.

by thin diaphragms *(fenestrated sinusoids);* in many mammals the endothelial cells lining sinusoids of the liver meet and overlap in some areas, but have gaps between the cells in other areas *(discontinuous sinusoids)*. Called also *sinusoidal capillary*.

v. spira′le [TA] a prominent vessel in the basilar membrane near the osseous spiral lamina.

va′sa vaso′rum [TA] the small nutrient arteries and the veins in the walls of the larger blood vessels.

va•sa (va′sə) [L.] plural of *vas*.

va•sal (va′səl) 1. pertaining to a vas. 2. vascular.

Vas•cor (vas′kor) trademark for a preparation of bepridil hydrochloride.

Vas•co•ray (vas′ko-ra) trademark for a combination preparation of iothalamate meglumine and iothalamate sodium.

vas•cu•lar (vas′ku-lər) 1. pertaining to vessels, particularly blood vessels; called also *vasal*. 2. having a copious blood supply.

vas•cu•lar•i•ty (vas″ku-lar′ĭ-te) the condition of being vascular.

vas•cu•lar•iza•tion (vas″ku-lər-ĭ-za′shən) 1. the process of becoming vascular. 2. angiogenesis. 3. the surgically induced development of vessels in a tissue.

vas•cu•lar•ize (vas′ku-lər-īz) to supply with vessels.

vas•cu•la•ture (vas′ku-lə-chər) the vascular system (q.v.) of the body, or any specific part of it.

vas•cu•li•tis (vas″ku-li′tis) pl. *vasculi′tides* [*vasculum* + *-itis*] inflammation of a blood or lymph vessel; see *arteritis*, *lymphangitis*, and *phlebitis*. Called also *angiitis*. **vasculit′ic** *adj*

allergic v. hypersensitivity v.

ANCA-associated v., ANCA-associated systemic v. a subgroup of small vessel vasculitis in which there are circulating antineutrophil cytoplasmic autoantibodies (ANCA), including microscopic polyangiitis, Wegener granulomatosis, and some types of Churg-Strauss syndrome.

Churg-Strauss v. see under *syndrome*.

consecutive v. vasculitis caused by extension of inflammation from neighboring tissues.

cryoglobulinemic v. vasculitis in small vessels with cryoglobulin immune deposits. Some types accompany chronic bacterial or viral infections; one type occurs with Sjögren syndrome; and an idiopathic group is referred to as *essential mixed cryoglobulinemia*.

cutaneous leukocytoclastic v. vasculitis affecting the small vessels of the skin, with infiltration by polymorphonuclear leukocytes, red blood cell extravasation, and dermal necrosis, manifesting first as a rash on the lower extremity or buttocks, usually accompanied by a tingling or burning sensation; a wide variety of skin lesions may develop later. It usually resolves in 1 to 4 weeks, often with residual hyperpigmentation, though some individuals may develop recurrent disease. Because there is frequently a known or presumed precipitating antigen, it is often called hypersensitivity vasculitis. Called also *cutaneous leukocytoclastic angiitis*.

granulomatous central nervous system v. primary central nervous system angiitis.

hypersensitivity v. 1. a group of systemic necrotizing vasculitides thought to represent hypersensitivity to an antigenic stimulus, such as a drug, infectious agent, or exogenous or endogenous protein; all disorders in this group involve the small vessels. Types include varieties of Henoch-Schönlein purpura and serum sickness, as well as urticarial v. Called also *allergic* or *leukocytoclastic v.* and *hypersensitivity* or *leukocytoclastic angiitis*. 2. cutaneous lymphcytoclastic vasculitis, so called because of the hypersensitivity reaction sometimes, but not always, seen.

hypocomplementemic v. vasculitis accompanied by hypocomplementemia.

isolated central nervous system v. primary central nervous system angiitis.

leukocytoclastic v. hypersensitivity v.

livedo v., livedoid v. a chronic, relapsing vasculitis of the lower legs, usually affecting middle-aged persons, characterized by nodular or purpuric skin lesions at the onset that later become ulcerated and leave scars (atrophie blanche); histologically, there are endothelial proliferations, hyaline degeneration, and thrombosis in the middle and lower dermis. Called also *livedoid vasculopathy* and *segmental hyalinizing v.*

mesenteric v. a complication sometimes seen in systemic lupus erythematosus, characterized by inflammation of mesenteric arteries with pain in the lower abdomen, bleeding from the rectum, and sometimes later intestinal perforation.

necrotizing v. systemic necrotizing v.

nodular v. vasculitis of subcutaneous tissues of the lower legs, a condition of unknown etiology, almost identical to erythema induratum but without evidence of tuberculosis; it is usually seen in young or middle-aged women. There are painful, red to blue, nodular lesions that may ulcerate and leave scars or resorb and leave atrophic depressions. In late stages, the subcutaneous fat is replaced by fibrosis and atrophy.

overlap v. polyangiitis overlap syndrome.

primary central nervous system v. see under *angiitis*.

pulmonary v. any of numerous inflammatory conditions of the walls of the pulmonary vessels; the most common ones are allergic granulomatous angiitis and Wegener granulomatosis.

rheumatoid v. systemic vasculitis associated with rheumatoid arthritis, affecting small and medium-sized vessels, and generally occurring in patients with long-standing disease, rheumatoid nodules, and a high titer of rheumatoid factor.

segmental hyalinizing v. livedoid v.

small vessel v. any of a group of vascular diseases of the small vessels, including microscopic polyangiitis, Wegener granulomatosis, Churg-Strauss syndrome, and pauci-immune crescentic glomerulonephritis.

systemic v., systemic necrotizing v. any of a group of disorders characterized by inflammation and necrosis of blood vessels, occurring in a broad spectrum of cutaneous and systemic disorders. It includes Churg-Strauss syndrome, polyarteritis nodosa, polyangiitis overlap syndrome, the various kinds of hypersensitivity vasculitis, and other conditions. Called also *necrotizing v.* or *angiitis*.

urticarial v. a group of cutaneous vasculitides characterized by urticaria lasting longer than 24 hours. There are three types: a normocomplementemic, generally idiopathic and benign manifestation of cutaneous leukocytoclastic angiitis; a hypocomplementemic type that is often associated with systemic inflammatory disease; and the potentially life-threatening hypocomplementemic urticarial vasculitis syndrome (q.v.).

vas•cu•lo•gen•e•sis (vas″ku-lo-jen′ə-sis) angiogenesis.

vas•cu•lo•gen•ic (vas″ku-lo-jen′ik) angiogenic (def. 1).

vas•cu•lo•lym•phat•ic (vas″ku-lo-lim-fat′ik) pertaining to blood or lymphatic vessels.

vas•cu•lo•mo•tor (vas″ku-lo-mo′tər) vasomotor.

vas•cu•lop•a•thy (vas″ku-lop′ə-the) any disorder of the blood vessels; cf. *angiopathy*.

livedoid v. see under *vasculitis*.

vas•cu•lo•pro•lif•er•a•tive (vas-ku-lo-pro-lif′ər-ə-tiv) characterized by the proliferation of blood vessels or their constituents.

vas•cu•lo•tox•ic (vas′ku-lo-tok″sik) pertaining to or characterized by a deleterious or toxic effect on the vessels of the body.

vas•cu•lum (vas′ku-ləm) [L., dim. of *vas*] a small vessel.

va•sec•to•mized (və-sek′tə-mīzd) having undergone removal of the ductus deferentes (vasa deferentia) by surgical means.

va•sec•to•my (və-sek′tə-me) [*vas* + *-ectomy*] surgical removal of all or part of the ductus deferens (vas deferens), done to induce infertility or in association with prostatectomy. Called also *vasoresection*.

Va•se•ret•ic (vas-ə-ret′ik) trademark for a combination preparation of enalapril maleate and hydrochlorothiazide.

vas•i•form (vas′ĭ-form) [*vas* + *form*] having the appearance of a vessel.

va•si•tis (və-si′tis) deferentitis.

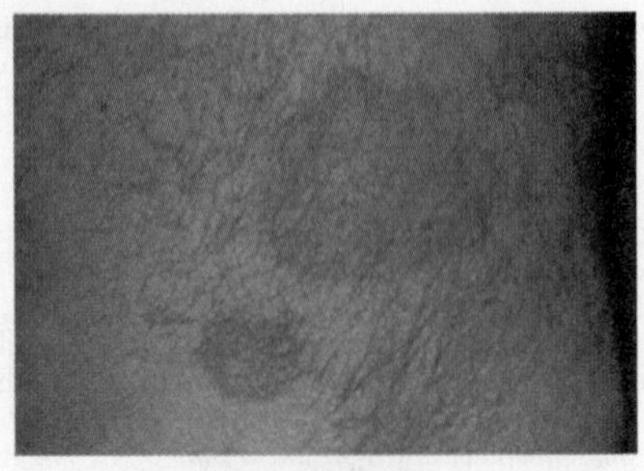

■ Urticarial vasculitis.

vas(o)- [L. *vas,* q.v.] a combining form denoting relationship to a vessel or to a duct.

vaso·ac·tive (va″zo-, vas″o-ak′tiv) exerting an effect upon the caliber of blood vessels.

vaso·con·stric·tion (va″zo-, vas″o-kən-strik′shən) the diminution of the caliber of vessels, especially constriction of arterioles leading to decreased blood flow to a part. **vasoconstric′tive** *adj*

vaso·con·stric·tor (va″zo-, vas″o-kən-strik′tər) 1. causing constriction of the blood vessels. 2. a motor nerve or chemical compound that causes constriction of the blood vessels.

vaso·co·ro·na [*vaso-* + *corona*] an arrangement of vessels resembling a crown or circle.

arterial v. a vascular ring encircling the spinal cord, formed by anastomosis between branches of the anterior and posterior arteries.

vaso·de·pres·sion (va″zo-, vas″o-de-presh′ən) decrease in vascular resistance with hypotension.

vaso·de·pres·sor (va″zo-, vas″o-de-pres′ər) 1. having the effect of lowering the blood pressure through reduction in peripheral resistance. 2. an agent that causes vasodepression.

Va·so·di·lan (va″zo-di′lan) trademark for preparations of isoxsuprine hydrochloride.

vaso·di·la·ta·tion (va″zo-, vas″o-dĭ-lə-ta′shən) vasodilation.

vaso·di·la·tion (va″zo-, vas″o-di-la′shən) dilation of a vessel, especially dilation of arterioles leading to increased blood flow to a part; extreme, abnormal vasodilation is called *angiectasis.* Called also *vasodilatation.* **vaso-di′lative** *adj*

reflex v. vasodilation occurring as a reflex response to stimuli applied elsewhere, or subsequent to an initial vasoconstrictive response.

vaso·di·la·tor (va″zo-, vas″o-di′la-tər) 1. causing dilation of the blood vessels. 2. a motor nerve or chemical compound that causes dilation of the blood vessels.

vaso·epi·did·y·mog·ra·phy (va″zo-, vas″o-ep″ĭ-did″ĭ-mog′rə-fe) radiography of the vas deferens and epididymis after injection of a contrast medium.

vaso·epi·did·y·mos·to·my (va″zo-, vas″o-ep″ĭ-did-ĭ-mos′tə-me) operative formation of a communication between the ductus deferens (vas deferens) and the epididymis to correct an obstruction or as a means of vasectomy reversal. Called also *epididymovasostomy.*

vaso·for·ma·tive (va″zo-, vas″o-for′mə-tiv) angiogenic (def. 1).

vaso·gan·gli·on (va″zo-, vas″o-gang′gle-on) any vascular ganglion or rete.

vaso·gen·ic (va″zo-jen′ik) originating in the blood vessels.

va·sog·ra·phy (va-zog′rə-fe) [*vaso-* + *-graphy*] angiography.

vaso·hy·per·ton·ic (va″zo-, vas″o-hi″pər-ton′ik) vasoconstrictor (def. 1).

vaso·hy·po·ton·ic (va″zo-, vas″o-hi″po-ton′ik) vasodilator (def. 1).

vaso·in·ert (va″zo-, vas″o-in-ərt′) exerting no effect on the caliber of blood vessels.

vaso·in·hib·i·tor (va″zo-, vas″o-in-hib′ĭ-tər) an agent that inhibits the action of the vasomotor nerves.

vaso·in·hib·i·to·ry (va″zo-, vas″o-in-hib′ĭ-tor-e) hindering the action of the vasomotor nerves.

vaso·li·ga·tion (va″zo-, vas″o-li-ga′shən) ligation of the ductus (vas) deferens.

vaso·mo·tion (va″zo-, vas″o-mo′shən) [*vaso-* + *motion*] change in the caliber of a vessel, especially of a blood vessel.

vaso·mo·tor (va″zo-, vas″o-mo′tər) [*vaso-* + *motor*] affecting the caliber of a vessel, especially of a blood vessel. Cf. *vasoactive.*

vaso·mo·tor·ic·i·ty (va″zo-, vas″o-mo-tər-is′ĭ-te) the power of producing change in the caliber of blood vessels.

vaso·neu·rop·a·thy (va″zo-, vas″o-nōō-rop′ə-the) angioneuropathy.

vaso·neu·ro·sis (va″zo-, vas″o-nōō-ro′sis) angioneuropathy.

vaso·oc·clu·sion (va″zo-, vas″o-ə-kloo′zhən) occlusion of a blood vessel or vessels. Cf. *ischemia.* **vasoocclu′sive** *adj*

vaso·pa·re·sis (va″zo-, vas″o-pə-re′sis) [*vaso-* + *paresis*] partial vasomotor paralysis (q.v.); called also *angioparesis.*

vaso·per·me·a·bil·i·ty (va″zo-, vas″o-pur″me-ə-bil′ĭ-te) the permeability of a blood vessel; the extent to which a blood vessel is permeable.

vaso·pres·sin (va″zo-, vas″o-pres′in) 1. one of two nonapeptide hormones (the other being oxytocin) that are formed by neuronal cells of hypothalamic nuclei and stored as posterior pituitary hormones. It stimulates contraction of muscles of capillaries and arterioles, raising blood pressure; promotes contraction of the intestinal musculature, increasing peristalsis; exerts contractile influence on the uterus; and has a specific effect on the epithelial cells of renal collecting tubules, augmenting resorption of water independently of solutes to cause concentration of urine and dilution of blood serum. Its rate of secretion is regulated chiefly by the osmolarity of the plasma. 2. [USP] a synthetic pharmaceutical preparation of the same principle, used as an antidiuretic in treatment of central diabetes insipidus, administered intranasally or by injection. It is also used to induce vasoconstriction to treat hemorrhage or administered intramuscularly as a test of hypothalamo-neurohypophysial-renal function in distinguishing central from nephrogenic diabetes insipidus. Called also *antidiuretic hormone.*

arginine v. (AVP) vasopressin containing arginine, the type found in most mammals; for medicinal uses, see *vasopressin* (def. 2). Called also *argipressin.*

lysine v. the antidiuretic hormone of the pig family, differing from arginine vasopressin in having lysine instead of arginine at position 8; used pharmaceutically as the synthetic preparation lypressin (q.v.).

vaso·pres·sin·ase (va″zo-, vas″o-pres′in-ās) cystinyl aminopeptidase.

vaso·pres·sor (va″zo-, vas″o-pres′ər) 1. stimulating contraction of the muscular tissue of the capillaries and arteries. 2. an agent that stimulates contraction of the muscular tissue of the capillaries and arteries.

vaso·punc·ture (va″zo-, vas″o-punk′chər) vasotomy.

vaso·re·flex (va″zo-, vas″o-re′fleks) a reflex involving a blood vessel.

vaso·re·lax·a·tion (va″zo-, vas″o-re-lak-sa′shən) decrease of vascular pressure.

vaso·re·sec·tion (va″zo-, vas″o-re-sek′shən) vasectomy.

vaso·sec·tion (va″zo-, vas″o-sek′shən) [*vaso-* + *section*] the severing of a vessel or vessels.

vaso·sen·so·ry (va″zo-, vas″o-sen′sər-e) supplying sensory filaments to the vessels.

vaso·spasm (va′zo-, vas′o-spaz″əm) spasm of the blood vessels, resulting in vasoconstriction. Called also *angiospasm.*

cerebral v. spasm of cerebral arteries, occurring sometimes as a complication of a subarachnoid hemorrhage; symptoms include decrease in level of consciousness and often hemiparesis.

vaso·spas·mo·lyt·ic (va″zo-, vas″o-spaz″mo-lit′ik) arresting spasm of the vessels.

vaso·spas·tic (va″zo-, vas″o-spas′tik) producing or affected by vasospasm.

vaso·stim·u·lant (va″zo-, vas″o-stim′u-lənt) vasotonic.

va·sos·to·my (vas-os′tə-me) [*vas* deferens + *-stomy*] 1. surgical formation of an opening into the ductus deferens (vas deferens). 2. vasotomy.

Vaso·tec (vaz′o-tek) trademark for preparations of enalapril maleate and enalaprilat.

vaso·to·cin (va″zo-, vas″o-to′sin) a nonapeptide hormone having some properties similar to those of vasopressin and oxytocin, produced in the supraoptico-neurohypophysial unit of birds, reptiles, amphibians, and fishes. It is found in the pituitary gland and hypothalamus of the human fetus but amounts in humans after birth are minute to indetectable.

va·sot·o·my (va-zot′ə-me) [*vaso-* + *-tomy*] incision into or cutting of the ductus deferens (vas deferens); called also *vasopuncture* and *vasostomy.*

vaso·to·nia (va″zo-, vas″o-to′ne-ə) [*vaso-* + *ton-* + *-ia*] tone or tension of the vessels; called also *angiotonia.*

vaso·ton·ic (va″zo-, vas″o-ton′ik) pertaining to, characterized by, or promoting vasotonia. Called also *angiotonic* and *vasostimulant.*

vaso·tro·phic (va″zo-, vas″o-tro′fik) [*vaso-* + *-trophic*] pertaining to the nutrition of blood vessels.

vaso·tro·pic (va″zo-, vas″o-tro′pik) tending to act on blood vessels.

vaso·va·gal (va″zo-, vas″o-va′gəl) vascular and vagal; see *vasovagal syncope,* under *syncope.*

vaso·va·sos·to·my (va″zo-, vas″o-va-zos′tə-me) reanastomosis of the ends of the severed ductus deferens (vas deferens), done to correct an obstruction or as a form of vasectomy reversal.

vaso·ve·sic·u·lec·to·my (va″zo-, vas″o-və-sik″u-lek′tə-me) excision of the ductus deferens (vas deferens) and seminal vesicles.

vaso·ve·sic·u·li·tis (va″zo-, vas″o-və-sik″u-li′tis) inflammation of ductus deferentes (vasa deferentia) and seminal vesicles.

Vas·ox·yl (va-zok′səl) trademark for preparations of methoxamine hydrochloride.

vas·tu (vahs′too) [Sanskrit] a traditional Hindu system of space design whose purpose is to promote well-being by constructing buildings in harmony with natural forces.

vas·tus (vas′təs) [L.] great or vast; description of muscles, as musculus vastus lateralis.

va·ta (vah′tah) [Sanskrit "wind"] according to ayurveda, one of the three doshas, or principles of constitution of the body, condensed from the elements air and ether. Vata is the principle of kinetic energy in the body and is concerned with the nervous system and with circulation, movement, and pathology at all levels—cell, organ, and body. It is eliminated from the body through defecation.

VATER *v*ertebral defects, imperforate *a*nus, *t*racheo*e*sophageal fistula, *r*adial and *r*enal dysplasia; see under *association*.

Va·ter ampulla, fold, etc. (fah′ter) [Abraham *Vater*, German anatomist, 1684–1751] see under *fold* and see *ampulla hepatopancreatica* and *papilla duodeni major*.

Va·ter-Pa·ci·ni corpuscle (fah′ter pah-che′ne) [A. *Vater;* Filippo *Pacini*, Italian anatomist, 1812–1883] pacinian corpuscle; see under *corpuscle*.

VATS video-assisted thoracic (or thoracoscopic) surgery.

vault (vawlt) 1. any arched or domelike structure. See also *fornix*. 2. the longest palatal border obtainable through a coronal section of the maxilla. 3. a cavity or a prepared area within a bone for an implant.
 cranial v. calvaria.
 vaginal v. fornix vaginae, used to denote the entire recess without reference to its parts.

VBG vertical banded gastroplasty.

VC vital capacity.

VCG vectorcardiogram.

V-Cil·lin K (ve-sil′in) trademark for preparations of penicillin V potassium.

VCU voiding cystourethrography.

VCUG voiding cystourethrogram; voiding cystourethrography.

VD venereal disease.

VDH valvular disease of the heart.

VDRL Venereal Disease Research Laboratories; see also under *antigen* and *test*.

Vec·ti·bix (vek′tĭ-biks) trademark for a preparation of panitimumab.

vec·tion (vek′shən) [L. *vectio* a carrying] the carrying of disease germs from an infected individual to a well one by a vector.

vec·tor (vek′tər) [L. "one who carries," from *vehere* to carry] 1. a carrier, especially the animal (usually an arthropod) that transfers an infective agent from one host to another. 2. cloning v. 3. a quantity possessing magnitude and direction and commonly represented by a straight line resembling an arrow: the length of the line denotes magnitude and the arrowhead and the position of the line with respect to an axis of reference denote direction. 4. in mathematics, an ordered set of values. For example, the vector x denotes the ordered set $(x_1, x_2, \ldots x_n)$.
 biological v. an animal vector in whose body the pathogenic organism develops and multiplies before being transmitted to the next host.
 cloning v. a DNA molecule, as a plasmid, bacteriophage, or cosmid, that can carry a fragment of foreign DNA into a host cell and create many copies of itself and the foreign DNA; it must include a cloning site into which the DNA fragment can be inserted, sequences for autonomous replication, and one or more selectable markers. See also *expression v*.
 expression v. a cloning vector designed such that the inserted DNA is efficiently transcribed and translated in the host cell.
 mechanical v. an animal vector not essential to the life cycle of the parasite.
 recombinant v. a cloning vector into which a foreign DNA fragment has been inserted; i.e., that contains both the vector and foreign insert sequences.
 retroviral v. a cloning vector that contains retroviral material.
 shuttle v. a vector capable of replicating in at least two different types of host cells; used for transfer of specific segments of DNA among various hosts.
 spatial v. a vector representing a three-dimensional force; see *vectorcardiography*.
 viral v. a cloning vector that contains viral material.

vec·tor-borne (vek′tər-born″) spread or transmitted from one host to another by a vector, as an infectious disease.

vec·tor·car·dio·gram (VCG) (vek″tər-kahr′de-o-gram″) the record, usually a photograph, of the loop formed on the oscilloscope in vectorcardiography, the inscribed loop representing the ends of the instantaneous vectors.

vec·tor·car·dio·graph (vek″tər-kahr′de-o-graf) the instrument used in vectorcardiography.

vec·tor·car·di·og·ra·phy (vek″tər-kahr″de-og′rə-fe) the registration, usually by formation of a loop display on an oscilloscope, of the direction and magnitude (vector) of the moment-to-moment electromotive forces of the heart during one complete cycle, as transmitted by electrocardiographic leads.
 spatial v. vector cardiography in which the potential vectors of cardiac excitation are projected upon three mutually perpendicular coordinates, usually designated X, Y, and Z, where X is the transverse (right or left), Y the vertical (up or down), and Z the sagittal (anterior or posterior). See also *orthogonal lead system*, under *system*.

vec·to·ri·al (vek-tor′e-əl) pertaining to a vector.

Vec·trin (vek′trin) trademark for preparations of minocycline hydrochloride.

vec·u·ro·ni·um bro·mide (vek″u-ro′ne-əm) a nondepolarizing neuromuscular blocking agent, used as an adjunct to general anesthesia to induce relaxation of skeletal muscle and to facilitate endotracheal intubation and mechanical ventilation; administered intravenously.

VEE Venezuelan equine encephalomyelitis.

Vee·tids (ve′tidz) trademark for a preparation of penicillin V potassium.

ve·gan (ve′gən, vej′ən) an extreme vegetarian who excludes all food of animal origin from the diet.

ve·gan·ism (ve′gən-iz-əm) strict limitation to a vegetable diet, with exclusion of all food of animal origin.

veg·e·ta·ble (vej′ə-tə-bəl) [L. *vegetabilis* quickening] 1. pertaining to or derived from plants. 2. any plant or species of plant, especially one cultivated as a source of food.

veg·e·tal (vej′ə-təl) vegetative (defs. 1, 2, and 3).

veg·e·tal·i·ty (vej″ə-tal′ĭ-te) the aggregate of phenomena that are common to plants.

veg·e·tar·i·an (vej″ə-tar′e-ən) 1. one who practices vegetarianism. 2. pertaining to vegetarianism.

veg·e·tar·i·an·ism (vej″ə-tar′e-ən-iz″əm) restriction of the diet to disallow some or all foods of animal origin, consuming mainly or wholly foods of plant origin. See also *lactovegetarianism*, *ovolactovegetarianism*, *ovovegetarianism*, and *veganism*.

veg·e·ta·tion (vej″ə-ta′shən) [L. *vegetatio*] any plantlike fungoid neoplasm or growth; a luxuriant fungus-like growth of pathologic tissue.
 bacterial v's irregular excrescences formed on the cardiac valves or endocardium by bacteria, frequently associated with valve destruction.
 dendritic v. 1. the shaggy appearance of a villous cancer. 2. the arachnoidal tufts and villous neoplasms on the pleura and other serous membranes.
 Libman-Sacks v's the vegetations seen on cardiac valves in Libman-Sacks endocarditis.
 marantic v's small, sterile, verrucous, fibrinous excrescences occurring in the left-side heart valves in nonbacterial thrombotic (marantic) endocarditis.
 verrucous v's small irregular fibrinous excrescences usually occurring along the line of closure of the cardiac valve cusps, sometimes extending into the mural endocardium or chordae tendineae, and rarely also present on the left ventricular papillary muscles.

veg·e·ta·tive (vej′ə-ta″tiv) 1. of, pertaining to, or characteristic of plants. 2. concerned with growth and with nutrition, as opposed to reproduction. 3. of or pertaining to asexual reproduction, as by budding or fission. 4. functioning involuntarily or unconsciously.

veg·e·to·an·i·mal (vej″ə-to-an′ĭ-məl) common to plants and animals.

VEGF vascular endothelial growth factor.

ve·hi·cle (ve′ĭ-kəl) [L. *vehiculum*] 1. excipient. 2. a structure for conveyance.

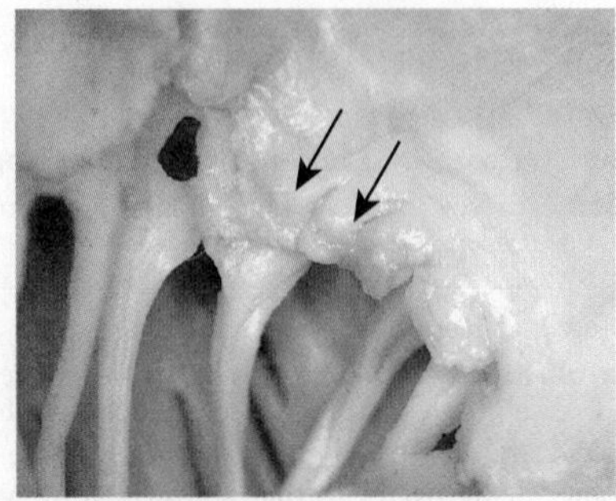

■ Verrucous vegetations *(arrows)* along the line of closure of the mitral valve leaflet in acute rheumatic mitral valvulitis superimposed on chronic rheumatic heart disease.

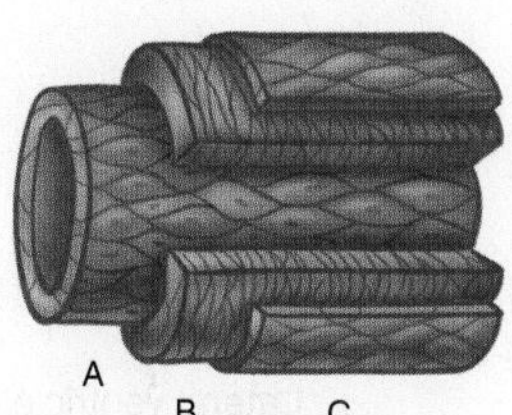

■ The three coats of a vein: *(A)*, tunica intima (endothelium); *(B)*, tunica media; *(C)*, tunica externa.

cloning v. see under *vector.*

structured v. an aqueous solution of a polymer used to increase the viscosity of a pharmaceutical supension and thereby decrease the sedimentation rate of the dispersed particles.

sugar-free suspension structured v. [NF] a structured vehicle prepared from potassium sorbate, xanthan gum, citric acid, saccharin sodium, sorbitol, mannitol, glycerin, and purified water.

suspension structured v. [NF] a structured vehicle prepared from potassium sorbate, xanthan gum, anhydrous citric acid, sucrose, and purified water.

veil (vāl) 1. a covering structure; see *velum.* 2. caul.

Fick v. see under *phenomenon.*

Jackson v. see under *membrane.*

Sattler v. Fick phenomenon.

Veil•lon tube (va-yaw′) [Adrien *Veillon,* Paris bacteriologist, 1864–1931] see under *tube.*

Veil•lon•el•la (va″on-el′ə) [Adrien *Veillon*] a genus of gram-negative bacteria of the family Acidaminococcaceae consisting of small, non-spore-forming cocci occurring in pairs or short chains; organisms are anaerobic, chemo-organotrophic, and oxidase- and catalase-negative, and do not ferment carbohydrates. They are found as normal inhabitants of the mouth and gastrointestinal tract, and vagina and have been implicated in a variety of infections, especially in immunocompromised persons. The type species is *V. par′vula.*

V. par′vula the species most commonly isolated from human specimens, usually as part of a polymicrobial process.

vein (vān) [L. *vena*] a vessel through which blood passes from various organs or parts back to the heart; all veins except the pulmonary veins carry blood low in oxygen. Like arteries, veins have three coats, an *inner, middle,* and *outer,* but the coats are not so thick, and they collapse when the vessel is cut. Many veins have *valves* formed of reduplications of their lining membrane, which prevent the backward flow of blood away from the heart. Called also *vena* [TA].

Vein

For descriptions of specific veins, see under *vena.*

accompanying v. vena comitans.

accompanying v. of hypoglossal nerve vena comitans nervi hypoglossi.

afferent v's veins that carry blood to an organ.

allantoic v's paired vessels arising from the dorsal aorta that accompany the allantois; they enter the connecting stalk of the early embryo with the allantois and later form the umbilical veins.

anastomotic v., inferior vena anastomotica inferior.

anastomotic v., superior vena anastomotica superior.

angular v. vena angularis.

antebrachial v., median vena mediana antebrachii.

anterior v's of heart, anterior v's of right ventricle venae ventriculi dextri anteriores.

anterior v. of septum pellucidum vena anterior septi pellucidi.

apical v. vena apicalis.

apicoposterior v. vena apicoposterior.

appendicular v. vena appendicularis.

aqueous v's microscopic, blood vessel–like pathways on the surface of the eye, containing aqueous humor or diluted blood and connecting the sinus venosus sclerae (Schlemm canal) with conjunctival or subconjunctival veins.

arciform v's of kidney, arcuate v's of kidney venae arcuatae renis.

articular v's venae articulares.

atrial v's of heart, left venae atriales sinistrae.

atrial v's of heart, right venae atriales dextrae.

auditory v's, internal venae labyrinthi.

auricular v's, anterior venae auriculares anteriores.

auricular v., posterior vena auricularis posterior.

axillary v. vena axillaris.

azygos v. vena azygos.

basal v. 1. vena basalis. 2. see *vena basalis communis, vena basalis inferior,* and *vena basalis superior.*

basal v., anterior vena basalis anterior.

basal v., common vena basalis communis.

basal v., inferior vena basalis inferior.

basal v., superior vena basalis superior.

basilic v. vena basilica.

basilic v., intermediate, basilic v., median vena basilica antebrachii.

basivertebral v's venae basivertebrales.

brachial v's venae brachiales.

brachiocephalic v. vena brachiocephalica.

Breschet v's venae diploicae.

bronchial v's venae bronchiales.

Browning v. vena anastomotica inferior.

v. of bulb of penis vena bulbi penis.

v. of bulb of vestibule vena bulbi vestibuli.

Burow v. an inconstant vessel formed by the two inferior epigastric veins and a branch from the bladder; it joins the portal vein.

v. of canaliculus of cochlea vena aqueductus cochleae.

capsular v's venae capsulares.

cardiac v's venae cordis.

cardiac v's, anterior venae ventriculi dextri anteriores.

cardiac v., great vena cardiaca magna.

cardiac v., middle vena cardiaca media.

cardiac v., small vena cardiaca parva.

cardiac v's, smallest venae cardiacae minimae.

cardinal v's embryonic vessels that include the precardinal, postcardinal, and common cardinal veins.

cardinal v's, anterior precardinal v's.

cardinal v's, common two short venous trunks in the embryo that open into the primordial atrium of the heart; the right one combines with the anterior cardinal vein to become the superior vena cava.

cardinal v's, posterior postcardinal v's.

v's of caudate nucleus venae nuclei caudati.

cavernous v's of penis venae cavernosae penis.

central v's of hepatic lobules, central v's of liver venae centrales hepatis.

central v. of retina vena centralis retinae.

central v. of suprarenal gland vena centralis glandulae suprarenalis.

cephalic v. vena cephalica.

cephalic v., accessory vena cephalica accessoria.

cephalic v., intermediate, cephalic v., median vena cephalica antebrachii.

cerebellar v's venae cerebelli.

cerebellar v's, inferior see *venae cerebelli.*

cerebellar v., precentral vena precentralis cerebelli.

cerebellar v's, superior see *venae cerebelli.*

cerebral v's venae encephali.

cerebral v's, anterior venae anteriores cerebri.

cerebral v's, deep venae profundae cerebri.

cerebral v., deep middle vena media profunda cerebri.

cerebral v., great vena magna cerebri.

cerebral v's, inferior venae inferiores cerebri.

cerebral v's, internal venae internae cerebri.

cerebral v's, superficial venae superficiales cerebri.

cerebral v's, superficial middle vena media superficialis cerebri.

cerebral v's, superior venae superiores cerebri.

cervical v., deep vena cervicalis profunda.

cervical v's, transverse venae transversae cervicis.

choroid v., inferior vena choroidea inferior.

choroid v., superior vena choroidea superior.

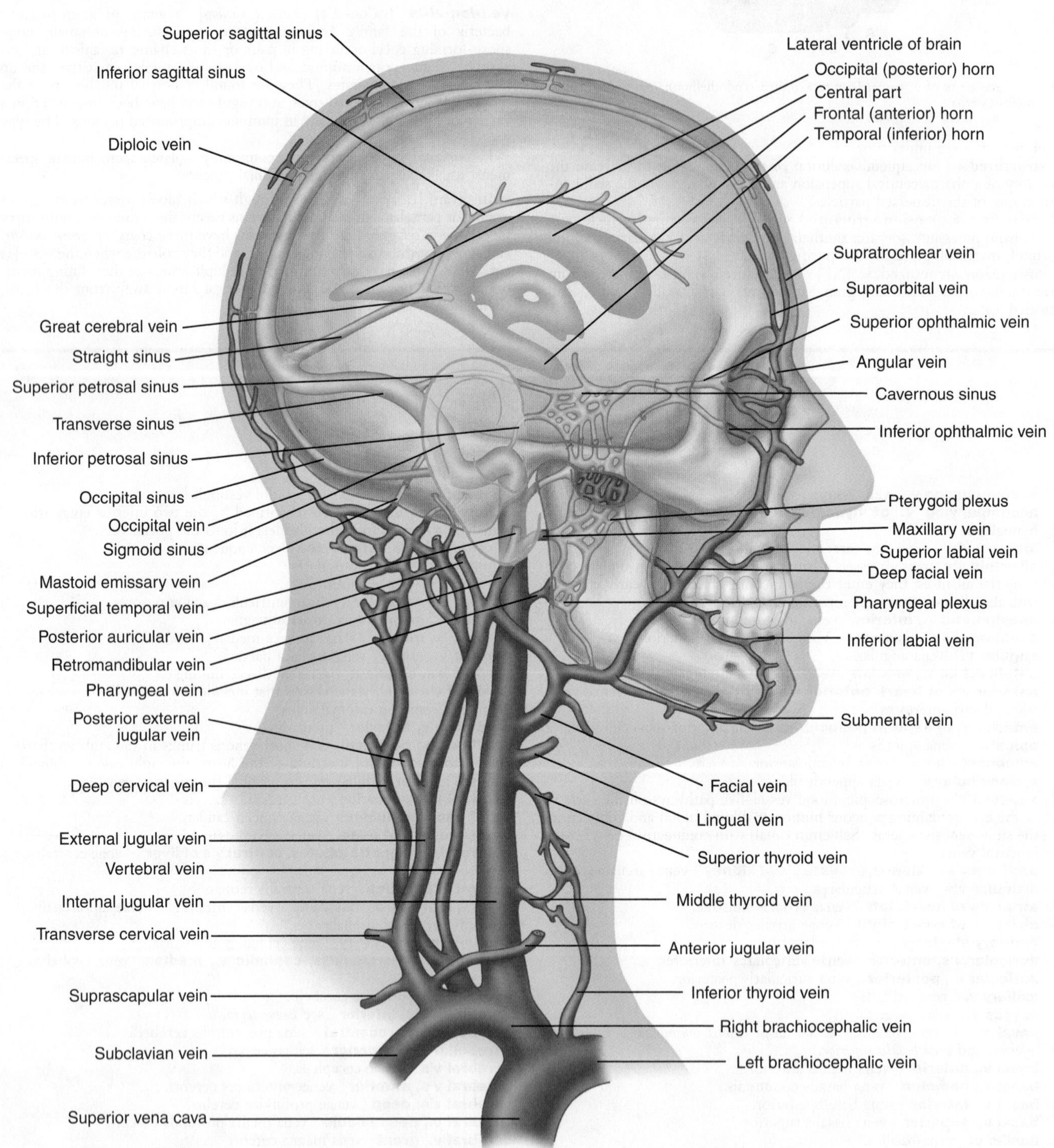

■ **PLATE 45**—VEINS OF THE HEAD AND NECK

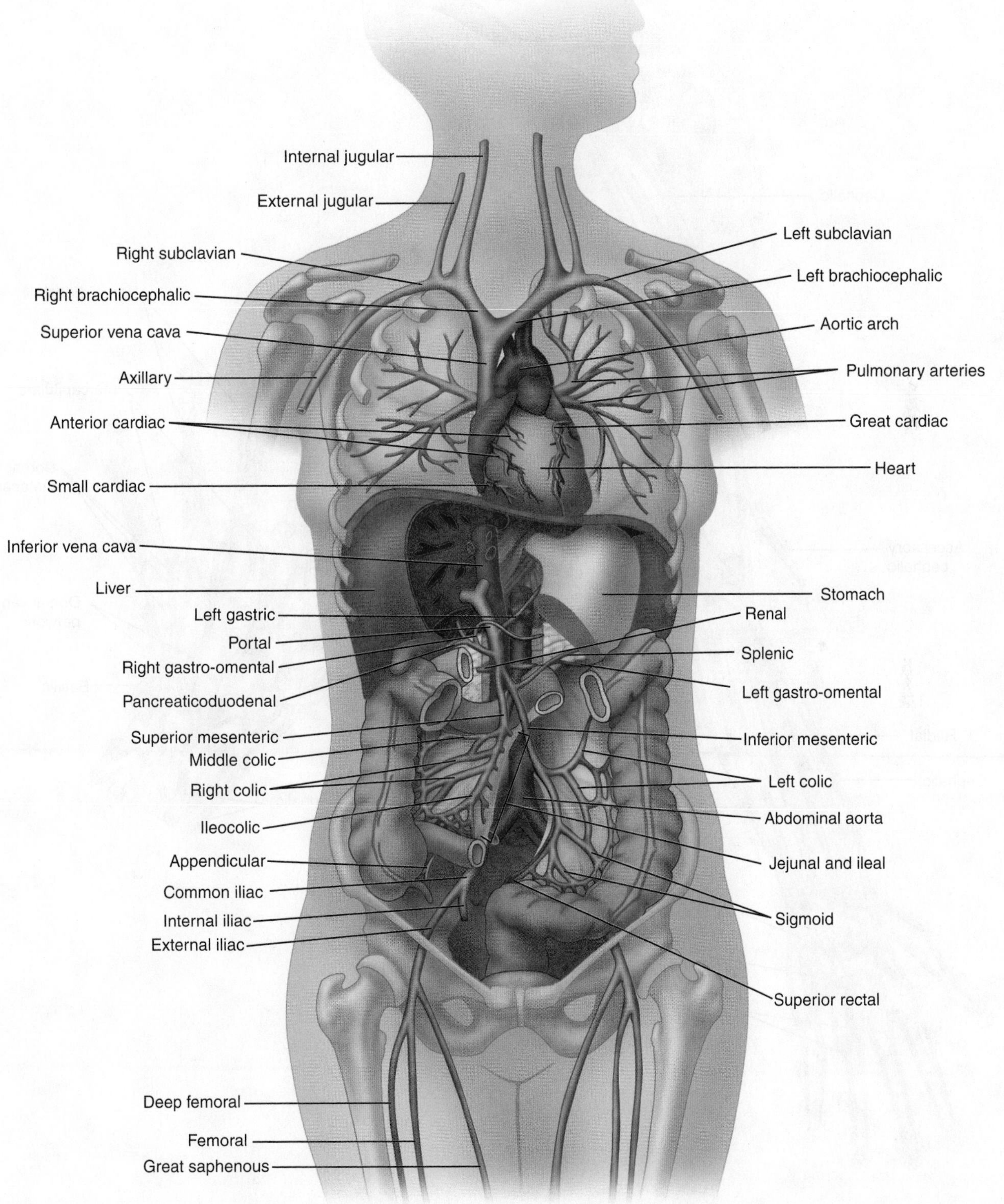

■ **PLATE 46**—PRINCIPAL VEINS OF THE BODY

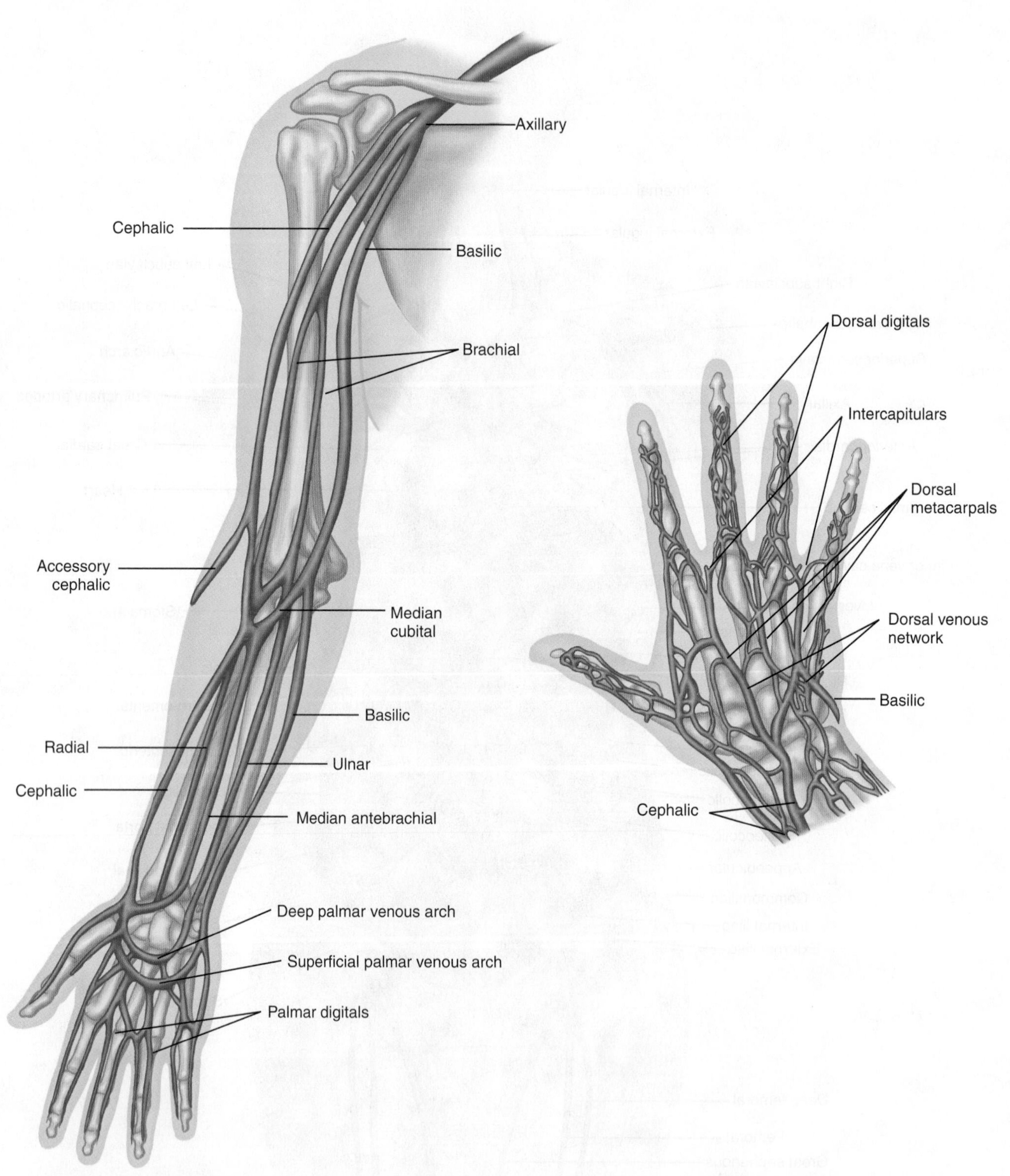

■ **PLATE 47**—SUPERFICIAL VEINS OF THE UPPER LIMB

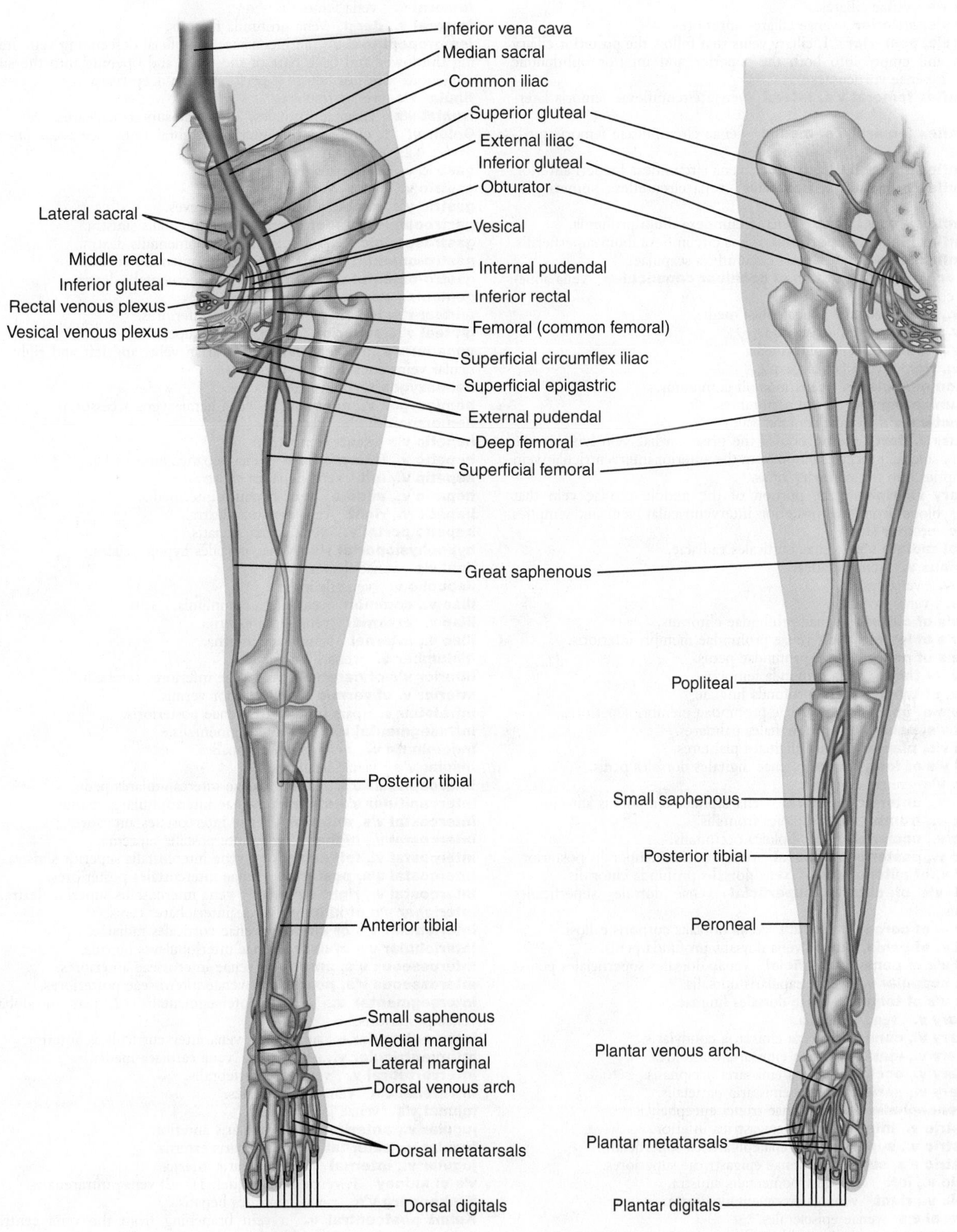

■ **PLATE 48**—SUPERFICIAL VEINS OF THE LOWER LIMB

Vein *Continued*

ciliary v's venae ciliares.
ciliary v's, anterior venae ciliares anteriores.
ciliary v's, posterior 1. ciliary veins that follow the posterior ciliary arteries and empty into both the superior and inferior ophthalmic veins. 2. venae vorticosae.
circumflex femoral v's, lateral venae circumflexae femoris laterales.
circumflex femoral v's, medial venae circumflexae femoris mediales.
circumflex humeral v., anterior vena circumflexa humeri anterior.
circumflex humeral v., posterior vena circumflexa humeri posterior.
circumflex iliac v., deep vena circumflexa ilium profunda.
circumflex iliac v., superficial vena circumflexa ilium superficialis.
circumflex scapular v. vena circumflexa scapulae.
v. of cochlear aqueduct, v. of cochlear canaliculus vena aqueductus cochleae.
colic v., intermediate vena colica media.
colic v., left vena colica sinistra.
colic v., middle vena colica media.
colic v., right vena colica dextra.
common modiolar v. vena modioli communis.
communicating v's venae perforantes.
conjunctival v's venae conjunctivales.
coronary v., left the portion of the great cardiac vein lying in the coronary sulcus; it receives blood from the anterior interventricular vein and empties into the coronary sinus.
coronary v., right the portion of the middle cardiac vein that receives blood from the posterior interventricular vein and empties into the coronary sinus.
cortical radiate v's venae corticales radiatae.
cutaneous v. vena cutanea.
cystic v. vena cystica.
deep v. vena profunda.
deep v's of clitoris venae profundae clitoridis.
deep v's of lower limb venae profundae membri inferioris.
deep v's of penis venae profundae penis.
deep v. of thigh vena profunda femoris.
deep v. of tongue vena profunda linguae.
deep v's of upper limb venae profundae membri superioris.
digital v's, palmar venae digitales palmares.
digital v's, plantar venae digitales plantares.
digital v's of foot, dorsal venae digitales dorsales pedis.
diploic v's venae diploicae.
diploic v., anterior temporal vena diploica temporalis anterior.
diploic v., frontal vena diploica frontalis.
diploic v., occipital vena diploica occipitalis.
diploic v., posterior temporal vena diploica temporalis posterior.
dorsal v. of clitoris, deep vena dorsalis profunda clitoridis.
dorsal v's of clitoris, superficial venae dorsales superficiales clitoridis.
dorsal v. of corpus callosum vena dorsalis corporis callosi.
dorsal v. of penis, deep vena dorsalis profunda penis.
dorsal v's of penis, superficial venae dorsales superficiales penis.
dorsal scapular v. vena scapularis dorsalis.
dorsal v's of tongue venae dorsales linguae.
emissary v. vena emissaria.
emissary v., condylar vena emissaria condylaris.
emissary v., mastoid vena emissaria mastoidea.
emissary v., occipital vena emissaria occipitalis.
emissary v., parietal vena emissaria parietalis.
v's of encephalic trunk venae trunci encephalici.
epigastric v., inferior vena epigastrica inferior.
epigastric v., superficial vena epigastrica superficialis.
epigastric v's, superior venae epigastricae superiores.
epiploic v., left vena gastroomentalis sinistra.
epiploic v., right vena gastroomentalis dextra.
episcleral v's venae episclerales.
esophageal v's venae oesophageales.
ethmoidal v's venae ethmoidales.
facial v. vena facialis.
facial v., deep vena profunda faciei.
facial v., posterior vena retromandibularis.
facial v., transverse vena transversa faciei.
femoral v. vena femoralis.
femoral v., deep vena profunda femoris.
femoropopliteal v. an inconstant superficial descending vein draining the lower and back part of the thigh and opening into the small saphenous vein just before it perforates the deep fascia.
fibular v's venae fibulares.
frontal v's 1. venae frontales. 2. venae supratrochleares.
Galen v. 1. either of the internal cerebral veins; see *venae internae cerebri.* 2. vena magna cerebri.
gastric v., left vena gastrica sinistra.
gastric v., right vena gastrica dextra.
gastric v's, short venae gastricae breves.
gastroepiploic v., left vena gastroomentalis sinistra.
gastroepiploic v., right vena gastroomentalis dextra.
gastro-omental v., left vena gastroomentalis sinistra.
gastro-omental v., right vena gastroomentalis dextra.
genicular v's venae geniculares.
gluteal v's, inferior venae gluteae inferiores.
gluteal v's, superior venae gluteae superiores.
gonadal v's the left and right ovarian veins and left and right testicular veins considered as a group.
hemiazygos v. vena hemiazygos.
hemiazygos v., accessory vena hemiazygos accessoria.
hemorrhoidal v's rectal v's.
hepatic v's venae hepaticae.
hepatic v., intermediate vena hepatica intermedia.
hepatic v., left vena hepatica sinistra.
hepatic v., middle vena hepatica intermedia.
hepatic v., right vena hepatica dextra.
hepatic portal v. vena portae hepatis.
hypophysioportal v's venae portales hypophysiales.
ileal v's venae ileales.
ileocolic v. vena ileocolica.
iliac v., common vena iliaca communis.
iliac v., external vena iliaca externa.
iliac v., internal vena iliaca interna.
iliolumbar v. vena iliolumbalis.
inferior v's of cerebellum venae inferiores cerebelli.
inferior v. of vermis vena inferior vermis.
infralobar v. pars infralobaris venae posterioris.
infrasegmental v. pars intersegmentalis.
innominate v. vena brachiocephalica.
insular v's venae insulares.
intercapitular v's of foot venae intercapitulares pedis.
intercapitular v's of hand venae intercapitulares manus.
intercostal v's, anterior venae intercostales anteriores.
intercostal v., highest vena intercostalis suprema.
intercostal v., left superior vena intercostalis superior sinistra.
intercostal v's, posterior venae intercostales posteriores.
intercostal v., right superior vena intercostalis superior dextra.
interlobar v's of kidney venae interlobares renis.
interlobular v's of kidney venae corticales radiatae.
interlobular v's of liver venae interlobulares hepatis.
interosseous v's, anterior venae interosseae anteriores.
interosseous v's, posterior venae interosseae posteriores.
intersegmental v. 1. pars intersegmentalis. 2. pars intralobaris venae posterioris.
interventricular v., anterior vena interventricularis anterior.
interventricular v., posterior vena cardiaca media.
intervertebral v. vena intervertebralis.
intrarenal v's venae intrarenales.
jejunal v's venae jejunales.
jugular v., anterior vena jugularis anterior.
jugular v., external vena jugularis externa.
jugular v., internal vena jugularis interna.
v's of kidney 1. venae renales (def. 1). 2. venae intrarenales.
Krukenberg v's venae centrales hepatis.
Kuhnt postcentral v. a vein branching from the vena centralis retina, extending posteriorly from the center of the optic nerve, and draining into the canalis opticus.
Labbé v. vena anastomotica inferior.
labial v's, anterior venae labiales anteriores.
labial v's, inferior venae labiales inferiores.
labial v's, posterior venae labiales posteriores.

Vein *Continued*

labial v., superior vena labialis superior.
v's of labyrinth, labyrinthine v's venae labyrinthi.
lacrimal v. vena lacrimalis.
laryngeal v., inferior vena laryngea inferior.
laryngeal v., superior vena laryngea superior.
lateral direct v's venae directae laterales.
v. of lateral recess of fourth ventricle vena recessus lateralis ventriculi quarti.
v. of lateral ventricle, lateral vena lateralis ventriculi lateralis.
v. of lateral ventricle, medial vena medialis ventriculi lateralis.
lingual v. vena lingualis.
lingual v., deep vena profunda linguae.
lingual v's, dorsal venae dorsales linguae.
lingular v. vena lingularis.
v's of lower limb venae membri inferioris.
lumbar v's venae lumbales.
lumbar v., ascending vena lumbalis ascendens.
mammary v's, internal venae thoracicae internae.
marginal v., lateral vena marginalis lateralis.
marginal v., left vena marginalis sinistra.
marginal v., medial vena marginalis medialis.
marginal v., right vena marginalis dextra.
v. of Marshall, Marshall oblique v. vena obliqua atrii sinistri.
masseteric v's veins from the masseter muscle that empty into the facial vein.
maxillary v's venae maxillares.
Mayo v. vena prepylorica.
median cubital v., median v. of elbow vena mediana cubiti.
median v. of forearm vena mediana antebrachii.
median v. of neck a vein sometimes formed when the anterior jugular veins unite as they pass down the neck.
mediastinal v's venae mediastinales.
v's of medulla oblongata venae medullae oblongatae.
meningeal v's venae meningeae.
meningeal v's, middle venae meningeae mediae.
mesencephalic v's venae trunci encephalici.
mesenteric v., inferior vena mesenterica inferior.
mesenteric v., superior vena mesenterica superior.
metacarpal v's, dorsal venae metacarpales dorsales.
metacarpal v's, palmar venae metacarpales palmares.
metatarsal v's, dorsal venae metatarsales dorsales.
metatarsal v's, plantar venae metatarsales plantares.
middle lobe v., middle lobe v., right vena lobi medii.
musculophrenic v's venae musculophrenicae.
nasal v's, external venae nasales externae.
nasofrontal v. vena nasofrontalis.
nutrient v. vena nutricia.
oblique v. of left atrium vena obliqua atrii sinistri.
obturator v's venae obturatoriae.
occipital v. 1. vena occipitalis. 2. *(in the pl.)* venae occipitales.
v. of olfactory gyrus vena gyri olfactorii.
omphalomesenteric v's vitelline v's.
ophthalmic v., inferior vena ophthalmica inferior.
ophthalmic v., superior vena ophthalmica superior.
ophthalmomeningeal v. a small inferior meningeal vein that opens usually into the superior ophthalmic vein, or occasionally into the superior petrosal sinus.
v's of orbit venae orbitae.
ovarian v., left vena ovarica sinistra.
ovarian v., right vena ovarica dextra.
palatine v., palatine v., external vena palatina externa.
palpebral v's venae palpebrales.
palpebral v's, inferior venae palpebrales inferiores.
palpebral v's, superior venae palpebrales superiores.
pancreatic v's venae pancreaticae.
pancreaticoduodenal v's venae pancreaticoduodenales.
paraumbilical v's venae paraumbilicales.
parietal v's venae parietales.
parietal v. of Santorini vena emissaria parietalis.
parotid v's venae parotideae.
pectoral v's venae pectorales.
peduncular v's venae pedunculares.
perforating v's venae perforantes.
pericardiac v's venae pericardiacae.
pericardiacophrenic v's venae pericardiacophrenicae.
pericardial v's venae pericardiacae.
peroneal v's venae fibulares.
petrosal v. vena petrosa.
pharyngeal v's venae pharyngeae.
phrenic v's, inferior venae phrenicae inferiores.
phrenic v's, superior venae phrenicae superiores.
v's of pons, pontine v's venae pontis.
pontomesencephalic v. vena pontomesencephalica.
popliteal v. vena poplitea.
portal v. vena portae hepatis.
portal v's of hypophysis venae portales hypophysiales.
postcardinal v's paired vessels in the embryo caudal to the heart; called also *posterior cardinal v's.*
posterior v. of corpus callosum vena posterior corporis callosi.
posterior v. of left ventricle vena ventriculi sinistri posterior.
posterior v. of septum pellucidum vena posterior septi pellucidi.
precardinal v's paired venous trunks in the embryo cranial to the heart; called also *anterior cardinal v's.*
precentral v. of cerebellum vena precentralis cerebelli.
prefrontal v's venae prefrontales.
prepyloric v. vena prepylorica.
primary head v's vessels alongside the embryonic brain that continue into the precardinal veins.
v. of pterygoid canal vena canalis pterygoidei.
pubic v. vena pubica.
pudendal v's, external venae pudendae externae.
pudendal v., internal vena pudenda interna.
pulmonary v's venae pulmonales.
pulmonary v., left inferior vena pulmonalis sinistra inferior.
pulmonary v., left superior vena pulmonalis sinistra superior.
pulmonary v., right inferior vena pulmonalis dextra inferior.
pulmonary v., right superior vena pulmonalis dextra superior.
pulp v's vessels draining the splenic sinuses.
pyloric v. vena gastrica dextra.
radial v's venae radiales.
ranine v. vena sublingualis.
rectal v's, inferior venae rectales inferiores.
rectal v's, middle venae rectales mediae.
rectal v., superior vena rectalis superior.
renal v's 1. venae renales (def. 1). 2. venae intrarenales.
retinal v., central vena centralis retinae.
retromandibular v. vena retromandibularis.
Retzius v's inconstant venous anastomoses that connect veins from the walls of the intestine to the tributaries of the inferior vena cava rather than to the superior mesenteric vein.
revehent v's venae revehentes.
Rosenthal v. vena basalis.
v. of round window vena fenestrae cochleae.
sacral v's, lateral venae sacrales laterales.
sacral v., median vena sacralis mediana.
saphenous v., accessory vena saphena accessoria.
saphenous v., great vena saphena magna.
saphenous v., small vena saphena parva.
v's of Sappey venae para-umbilicales.
v. of scala tympani vena scalae tympani.
v. of scala vestibuli vena scalae vestibuli.
scleral v's venae sclerales.
scrotal v's, anterior venae scrotales anteriores.
scrotal v's, posterior venae scrotales posteriores.
segmental v., anterior see *vena anterior lobi superioris pulmonis dextri* and *vena anterior lobi superioris pulmonis sinistri.*
segmental v., apical vena apicalis.
segmental v., apicoposterior vena apicoposterior.
segmental v., inferior lingular pars inferior venae lingularis.
segmental v., lateral pars lateralis venae lobi medii.
segmental v., medial pars medialis venae lobi medii.
segmental v., posterior vena posterior lobi superioris pulmonis dextri.
segmental v., superior see *vena superior lobi inferioris pulmonis dextri* and *vena superior lobi inferioris pulmonis sinistri.*
segmental v., superior lingular pars superior venae lingularis.
v's of semicircular ducts venae ductuum semicircularium.
sigmoid v's venae sigmoideae.

Vein *Continued*

small v. of heart vena cardiaca parva.
spermatic v. either of the testicular veins; see *vena testicularis dextra* and *vena testicularis sinistra.*
spinal v's, anterior venae spinales anteriores.
spinal v's, posterior venae spinales posteriores.
v's of spinal cord venae medullae spinalis.
splenic v. vena splenica.
stellate v's of kidney venae stellatae renis.
Stensen v's venae vorticosae.
sternocleidomastoid v. vena sternocleidomastoidea.
striate v's venae thalamostriatae inferiores.
stylomastoid v. vena stylomastoidea.
subcardinal v's paired vessels in the embryo, replacing the postcardinal veins and persisting to some degree as definitive vessels.
subclavian v. vena subclavia.
subcostal v. vena subcostalis.
subcutaneous v's of abdomen venae subcutaneae abdominis.
sublingual v. vena sublingualis.
sublobular v's tributaries of the hepatic veins that receive the central veins of hepatic lobules.
submental v. vena submentalis.
subscapular v. vena subscapularis.
superficial v. vena superficialis.
superficial v's of lower limb venae superficiales membri inferioris.
superficial v's of upper limb venae superficiales membri superioris.
superior v's of cerebellum venae superiores cerebelli.
superior v. of inferior lobe of left lung vena superior lobi inferioris pulmonis sinistri.
superior v. of inferior lobe of right lung vena superior lobi inferioris pulmonis dextri.
superior v. of vermis vena superior vermis.
supracardinal v's paired vessels in the embryo, developing later than the subcardinal veins and persisting chiefly as the inferior segment of the inferior vena cava.
supraorbital v. vena supraorbitalis.
suprarenal v., left vena suprarenalis sinistra.
suprarenal v., right vena suprarenalis dextra.
suprascapular v. vena suprascapularis.
supratrochlear v's venae supratrochleares.
sural v's venae surales.
sylvian v's, v's of sylvian fossa see *vena media superficialis cerebri.*
temporal v's, deep venae temporales profundae.
temporal v., middle vena temporalis media.
temporal v's, superficial venae temporales superficiales.
temporomandibular articular v's venae articulares.
terminal v. vena thalamostriata superior.
testicular v., left vena testicularis sinistra.
testicular v., right vena testicularis dextra.
thalamostriate v's, inferior venae thalamostriatae inferiores.
thalamostriate v., superior vena thalamostriata superior.
thebesian v's, v's of Thebesius venae cardiacae minimae.
thoracic v's, internal venae thoracicae internae.
thoracic v., lateral vena thoracica lateralis.
thoracoacromial v. vena thoracoacromialis.
thoracodorsal v. vena thoracodorsalis.
thoracoepigastric v's venae thoracoepigastricae.
thymic v's venae thymicae.
thyroid v., inferior vena thyroidea inferioris.
thyroid v's, middle venae thyroideae mediae.
thyroid v., superior vena thyroidea superior.
thyroid ima v. vena thyroidea ima.
tibial v's, anterior venae tibiales anteriores.
tibial v's, posterior venae tibiales posteriores.

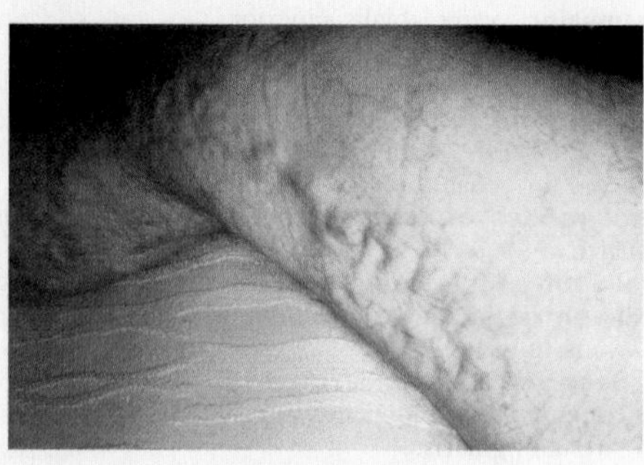
■ Varicose veins.

trabecular v's vessels coursing in splenic trabeculae, formed by tributary pulp veins.
tracheal v's venae tracheales.
transverse v. of face vena transversa faciei.
transverse v's of neck venae transversae cervicis.
transverse v. of scapula vena suprascapularis.
Trolard v. vena anastomotica superior.
tympanic v's venae tympanicae.
ulnar v's venae ulnares.
umbilical v. 1. vena umbilicalis. 2. *(in the pl.)* the pair of left and right umbilical veins (qq.v.) in the early embryo, before the right umbilical vein degenerates.
umbilical v., left the left of the two veins in the umbilical cord that carry blood from the placenta to the sinus venosus of the heart in the early embryo; after the right umbilical vein degenerates, the left is referred to as the umbilical vein (see *vena umbilicalis*).
umbilical v., right the right of the two veins in the umbilical cord that carry blood from the placenta to the sinus venosus of the heart in the early embryo; it degenerates during the seventh week.
v. of uncus vena uncalis.
v's of upper limb venae membri superioris.
uterine v's venae uterinae.
varicose v. a dilated tortuous vein, usually in the subcutaneous tissues of the leg, often associated with incompetency of the venous valves.
ventricular v's of heart, left venae ventriculares sinistrae.
ventricular v's of heart, right venae ventriculares dextrae.
ventricular v., inferior vena ventricularis inferior.
vertebral v. vena vertebralis.
vertebral v., accessory vena vertebralis accessoria.
vertebral v., anterior vena vertebralis anterior.
vertebral v's, superficial the veins of the external vertebral plexuses; see *plexus venosus vertebralis externus anterior* and *posterior.* Called also *external v's of vertebral column.*
v's of vertebral column venae columnae vertebralis.
v's of vertebral column, external superficial vertebral v's.
vesalian v. an emissary vein connecting the cavernous sinus with the pterygoid venous plexus, sometimes passing through an opening in the great wing of the sphenoid bone.
vesical v's venae vesicales.
vestibular v., anterior vena vestibularis anterior.
vestibular v., posterior vena vestibularis posterior.
v. of vestibular aqueduct vena aqueductus vestibuli.
vestibulocochlear v. vena vestibulocochlearis.
vidian v. vena canalis pterygoidei.
v's of Vieussens venae ventriculi dextri anteriores.
vitelline v's veins that return the blood from the yolk sac to the primordial heart of the early embryo. Called also *omphalomesenteric v's.*
vorticose v's venae vorticosae.

VeIP a cancer chemotherapy regimen consisting of vinblastine, ifosfamide, and Platinol (cisplatin).

Vel blood group (vel) [from part of the name of the propositus first described in 1952] see under *blood group.*

ve•la (ve′lə) [L.] plural of *velum.*

ve•la•men (ve-la′mən) pl. *vela′mina* [L. "a covering"] a membrane, velum, meninx, or tegument.

vel•a•men•ta (vel″ə-men′tə) [L.] plural of *velamentum.*

vel•a•men•tous (vel″ə-men′təs) [L. *velamen* veil] membranous and pendant; like a veil.

vel•a•men•tum (vel″ə-men′təm) pl. *velamen′ta* [L.] any covering, velum, or envelope.

velamen′ta ce′rebri the meninges.

ve•lar (ve′lər) 1. pertaining to a velum, especially to the velum palatinum (palatum molle). 2. of consonantal speech sounds, produced with the tongue near the soft palate, such as *g* and *k.*

Vel•ban (vel′ban) trademark for a preparation of vinblastine sulfate.

Vel•cade (vel′kād) trademark for a preparation of bortezomib.

vel•i•form (vel′ĭ-form) velamentous.

Vel•la fistula (va′lah) [Luigi *Vella*, Italian physiologist, 1825–1886] see under *fistula.*

vel•lo•sine (və-lo′sin) a poisonous alkaloid from the bark of *Geissospermum laeve* and *G. vellosii.*

vel•lus (vel′əs) [L. "fleece"] 1. the fine hair that succeeds the lanugo over most of the body. 2. a structure resembling this fine hair.

ve•lo•cim•e•try (ve″lo-sim′ə-tre) measurement of speed, such as speed of flow. See also *flowmeter.*

laser-Doppler v. measurement of the flow of red cells in a microcirculatory bed by means of laser light delivered to and detected from the region of interest by fiberoptic probes.

ve•loc•i•ty (*v*) (və-los′ĭ-te) [L. *velox* swift] the rate of movement of a body in a given direction.

nerve conduction v. (NCV) the speed, in meters per second, at which an impulse moves along the largest fibers of a peripheral nerve.

PSA v. the annual rate of increase of prostate-specific antigen (PSA) in a man's blood.

thrombotic threshold v. (TTV) the minimum velocity of blood flow through a vascular graft or prosthesis, below which thrombogenicity would begin along the intimal surface; variables affecting it include lumen diameter and type of material the graft or prosthesis is made of.

ve•lo•pha•ryn•ge•al (ve″lo-fə-rin′je-əl) pertaining to the soft palate (velum palatinum) and pharynx.

Vel•o•sef (vel′o-sef) trademark for preparations of cephradine.

Ve•lo•su•lin (ve-lo′soo-lin) trademark for preparations of buffered insulin human.

Vel•peau bandage, canal, deformity, hernia (vel-po′) [Alfred Armand Louis Marie *Velpeau*, French surgeon, 1795–1867] see under *bandage;* see *canalis inguinalis;* see *silver fork fracture*, under *fracture;* and see *prevascular femoral hernia*, under *hernia.*

ve•lum (ve′ləm) pl. *ve′la* [L.] a veil or veillike structure.

artificial v. an artificial palate (q.v.) for the soft palate.

v. interpo′situm ce′rebri tela choroidea ventriculi tertii.

v. medulla′re infe′rius [TA] inferior medullary velum: either of two thin layers of white substance symmetrically located on the sides of the nodule of the vermis; their internal surface forms the lower wall of the lateroposterior recess of the fourth ventricle. On the sides the velum is continuous with the pedunculus flocculi and the taenia, and anteriorly it is fused with the choroid plexus. Called also *posterior medullary v.*

v. medulla′re supe′rius superior medullary velum: a thin layer of white substance forming the roof of the superior part of the fourth ventricle, and extending from the tectal lamina in front to the fastigium behind, and between the superior cerebellar peduncles; called also *anterior medullary v.*

medullary v., anterior v. medullare superius.

medullary v., inferior, medullary v., posterior v. medullare inferius.

medullary v., superior v. medullare superius.

v. palati′num TA alternative for *palatum molle.*

v. transver′sum a transverse fold of the tela choroidea marking the boundary between the diencephalon and the telencephalon in the embryonic brain.

ve•na (ve′nə) pl. *ve′nae* [L.] [TA] vein.

Vena

Descriptions of veins are given on TA terms, and include anglicized names of specific veins.

ve′nae advehen′tes channels in the early embryo that convey blood to the sinusoids of the liver and later join to form the portal vein.

v. anastomo′tica infe′rior [TA] inferior anastomotic vein: a vein that interconnects the superficial middle cerebral vein and the transverse sinus. Called also *Browning vein.*

v. anastomo′tica supe′rior [TA] superior anastomotic vein: a vein that interconnects the superficial middle cerebral vein and the superior sagittal sinus. Called also *Trolard vein.*

v. angula′ris [TA] angular vein: a short vein between the eye and the root of the nose; it is formed by union of the supratrochlear and supraorbital veins and continues inferiorly as the facial vein.

ve′nae anterio′res ce′rebri [TA] anterior cerebral veins: veins that accompany the anterior cerebral artery and join the basal vein.

v. ante′rior lo′bi supe′rioris pulmo′nis dex′tri [TA] anterior vein of superior lobe of right lung: a vein draining the anterior segment of the superior lobe of the right lung and emptying into the right superior pulmonary vein; called also *ramus anterior venae pulmonalis dextrae superioris* [TA alternative] and *anterior segmental vein.*

v. ante′rior lo′bi supe′rioris pulmo′nis sinis′tri [TA] anterior vein of superior lobe of left lung: a vein draining the anterior segment of the superior lobe of the left lung and emptying into the left superior pulmonary vein; called also *ramus anterior venae pulmonalis sinistrae superioris* [TA alternative] and *anterior segmental vein.*

v. ante′rior sep′ti pellu′cidi [TA] anterior vein of septum pellucidum: a vein that drains the anterior septum pellucidum into the superior thalamostriate vein.

v. apica′lis [TA] apical vein: a vein draining the apical segment of the superior lobe of the right lung and emptying into the right superior pulmonary vein; called also *ramus apicalis venae pulmonalis dextrae superioris* [TA alternative] and *apical segmental vein.*

v. apicoposte′rior [TA] apicoposterior vein: a vein draining the apicoposterior segment of the superior lobe of the left lung and emptying into the left superior pulmonary vein. Called also *ramus apicoposterior venae pulmonalis dextrae superioris* [TA alternative] and *apicoposterior segmental vein.*

v. appendicula′ris [TA] appendicular vein: the vena comitans of the appendicular artery; it drains into the ileocolic vein.

v. aqueduc′tus coch′leae [TA] vein of cochlear aqueduct: a vein along the aqueduct of the cochlea that empties into the superior bulb of the internal jugular vein; called also *vein of cochlear canaliculus.*

v. aqueduc′tus vesti′buli [TA] vein of vestibular aqueduct: a small vein from the internal ear that passes through the aqueduct of the vestibule and empties into the superior petrosal sinus.

ve′nae arcua′tae re′nis [TA] arcuate veins of kidney: a series of complete arches across the bases of the renal pyramids; they are formed by union of the interlobular veins and the venulae rectae and drain into the interlobar veins.

ve′nae articula′res [TA] articular veins: small vessels that drain the plexus around the temporomandibular joint into the retromandibular vein; called also *temporomandibular articular veins.*

ve′nae atria′les dex′trae [TA] right atrial veins: the smallest cardiac veins (venae cardiacae minimae) emptying into the right atrium of the heart.

ve′nae atria′les sinis′trae [TA] left atrial veins: inconstant smallest cardiac veins (venae cardiacae minimae) emptying into the left atrium of the heart.

ve′nae auricula′res anterio′res [TA] anterior auricular veins: branches from the anterior part of the pinna that enter the superficial temporal vein.

v. auricula′ris poste′rior [TA] posterior auricular vein: a vein that begins in a plexus on the side of the head, passes down behind the pinna, and joins with the retromandibular vein to form the external jugular vein.

v. axilla′ris [TA] axillary vein; the venous trunk of the upper limb; it begins at the lower border of the teres major muscle by junction of the basilic and brachial veins, and at the lateral border of the first rib is continuous with the subclavian vein.

v. a′zygos [TA] azygos vein: an intercepting trunk for the right intercostal veins as well as a connecting branch between the superior and inferior venae cavae: it arises from the ascending lumbar vein, passes up in the posterior mediastinum to the level of the fourth thoracic vertebra, where it arches over the root of the right lung *(arcus venae azygou)*, and empties into the superior vena cava.

v. basa′lis [TA] basal vein: a vein that arises at the anterior perforated substance, passes backward and around the cerebral peduncle, and empties into the internal cerebral vein; called also *Rosenthal vein.*

v. basa′lis ante′rior [TA] anterior basal vein: either of two veins, each draining the anterior basal segment of the inferior lobe of a lung and emptying into the corresponding superior basal vein. Called also *ramus basalis anterior venae basalis communis* [TA alternative].

Vena *Continued*

v. basa′lis commu′nis [TA] common basal vein: either of two veins, each draining the inferior lobe of a lung, via the superior and inferior basal veins, and emptying into the corresponding inferior pulmonary vein.

v. basa′lis infe′rior [TA] inferior basal vein: either of two veins, each draining the medial and posterior basal segments of the inferior lobe of a lung and emptying into the corresponding common basal vein.

v. basa′lis supe′rior [TA] superior basal vein: either of two veins, each draining the lateral and anterior basal segments of the inferior lobe of a lung and emptying into the corresponding common basal vein.

v. basi′lica [TA] basilic vein: the superficial vein that arises from the ulnar side of the dorsal rete of the hand, passes up the forearm, and joins with the brachial veins to form the axillary vein.

v. basi′lica antebra′chii [TA] median basilic vein: a vein sometimes present as the medial branch, ending in the basilic vein, of a bifurcation of the median antebrachial vein.

ve′nae basivertebra′les [TA] basivertebral veins: venous sinuses in the cancellous tissue of the bodies of the vertebrae, which communicate with the plexus of veins on the anterior surface of the vertebrae and with the anterior internal and anterior external vertebral plexuses.

ve′nae brachia′les [TA] brachial veins: the venae comitantes of the brachial artery, which join with the basilic vein to form the axillary vein.

v. brachiocepha′lica [TA] brachiocephalic vein: either of the two veins that drain blood from the head, neck, and upper limbs, and unite to form the superior vena cava. Each is formed at the root of the neck by union of the ipsilateral internal jugular and subclavian veins. The right vein *(v. brachiocephalica dextra)* passes almost vertically downward in front of the brachiocephalic artery, and the left vein *(v. brachiocephalica sinistra)* passes from left to right behind the upper part of the sternum. Each vein receives the vertebral, deep cervical, deep thyroid, and internal thoracic veins. The left vein also receives intercostal, thymic, tracheal, esophageal, phrenic, mediastinal, and pericardiac branches, as well as the thoracic duct; and the right vein receives the right lymphatic duct. Called also *innominate vein.*

ve′nae bronchia′les [TA] bronchial veins: vessels that drain blood from the larger subdivisions of the bronchi; on the left they drain into the azygos vein and on the right they drain into the hemiazygos vein or superior intercostal vein.

v. bul′bi pe′nis [TA] vein of bulb of penis: a vein draining blood from the bulb of the penis into the internal pudendal vein.

v. bul′bi vesti′buli [TA] vein of bulb of vestibule: a vein draining blood from the bulb of the vestibule of the vagina into the internal pudendal vein.

v. cana′lis pterygoi′dei [TA] vein of pterygoid canal: one of the veins that pass through the pterygoid canal and empty into the pterygoid plexus; called also *vidian vein.*

ve′nae capsula′res [TA] capsular veins: veins draining the renal capsules and emptying into the renal veins.

ve′nae cardi′acae anterio′res TA alternative for *venae ventriculi dextri anteriores.*

v. cardi′aca mag′na [TA] great cardiac vein: a vein that collects blood from the anterior surface of the ventricles, follows the anterior longitudinal sulcus, and empties into the coronary sinus; called also *v. cordis magna* [TA alternative]. See also *v. interventricularis anterior* and see *left coronary vein,* under *vein.*

v. cardi′aca me′dia [TA] middle cardiac vein: a vein that collects blood from the diaphragmatic surface of the ventricles, follows the posterior longitudinal sulcus, and empties into the coronary sinus; called also *v. cordis media* [TA alternative]. See also *v. interventricularis posterior* and see *right coronary vein,* under *vein.*

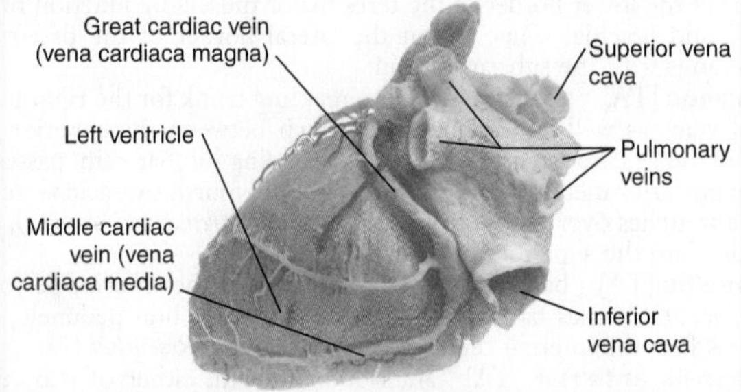

■ Vena cardiaca magna and vena cardiaca media (great and middle cardiac veins) in a posterior view of the heart.

ve′nae cardi′acae mi′nimae [TA] smallest cardiac veins: numerous small veins arising in the muscular walls and draining independently into the cavities of the heart, particularly the right atrium and ventricle; called also *thebesian veins* and *venae cordis minimae* [TA alternative].

v. cardi′aca par′va [TA] small cardiac vein: a vein that collects blood from both parts of the right heart, follows the coronary sulcus to the left, and opens into the coronary sinus; called also *v. cordis parva* [TA alternative].

v. ca′va see *v. cava inferior* and *v. cava superior.*

v. ca′va infe′rior [TA] inferior vena cava: the venous trunk for the lower extremities and for the pelvic and abdominal viscera; it begins at the level of the fifth lumbar vertebra by union of the common iliac veins, passes upward on the right of the aorta, and empties into the right atrium of the heart.

v. ca′va supe′rior [TA] superior vena cava: the venous trunk draining blood from the head, neck, upper extremities, and chest; it begins by union of the two brachiocephalic veins, passes directly downward, and empties into the right atrium of the heart.

ve′nae caverno′sae pe′nis [TA] cavernous veins of penis: veins that return the blood from the corpora cavernosa to the deep veins and the dorsal vein of the penis.

v. centra′lis glan′dulae suprarena′lis [TA] central vein of suprarenal gland: the large single vein into which the various veins within the substance of the gland empty, and which continues at the hilum as the suprarenal vein.

ve′nae centra′les he′patis [TA] central veins of liver: veins in the middle of the hepatic lobules, draining into the hepatic vein. Called also *central veins of hepatic lobules* and *Krukenberg veins.*

v. centra′lis re′tinae [TA] central retinal vein: the vein that is formed by union of the retinal veins; it passes out of the eyeball in the optic nerve to empty into the superior ophthalmic vein. Called also *central vein of retina.*

v. cepha′lica [TA] cephalic vein: the superficial vein that arises from the radial side of the dorsal rete of the hand, and winds anteriorly to pass along the anterior border of the brachioradialis muscle; above the elbow it ascends along the lateral border of the biceps muscle and the pectoral border of the deltoid muscle, and opens into the axillary vein.

v. cepha′lica accesso′ria [TA] accessory cephalic vein: a vein arising from the dorsal rete of the hand, passing up the forearm to join the cephalic vein just above the elbow.

v. cepha′lica antebra′chii [TA] median cephalic vein: a vein sometimes present as the lateral branch, ending in the cephalic vein, of a bifurcation of the median antebrachial vein. Called also *intermediate cephalic vein.*

ve′nae cerebel′li [TA] cerebellar veins: the veins on the surface of the cerebellum; see *venae inferiores cerebelli* and *venae superiores cerebelli.*

ve′nae ce′rebri venae encephali.

v. cervica′lis profun′da [TA] deep cervical vein: a vein that arises from a plexus in the suboccipital triangle, follows the deep cervical artery down the neck, and empties into the vertebral or the brachiocephalic vein.

v. choroi′dea infe′rior [TA] inferior choroid vein: a vein that drains the inferior choroid plexus into the basal vein.

v. choroi′dea supe′rior [TA] superior choroid vein: the vein that runs along the whole length of the choroid plexus, draining it and the hippocampus, fornix, and corpus callosum; it unites with the superior thalamostriate vein to form the internal cerebral vein.

ve′nae cilia′res [TA] ciliary veins: veins that arise inside the eyeball by branches from the ciliary muscle and drain into the superior ophthalmic vein; they are subdivided into anterior and posterior ciliary veins.

ve′nae cilia′res anterio′res [TA] anterior ciliary veins: ciliary veins that follow the anterior ciliary arteries, receiving branches from the sinus venosus, sclerae, the episcleral veins, and the tunica conjunctiva bulbi, and draining into the superior ophthalmic vein.

ve′nae circumflex′ae fe′moris latera′les [TA] lateral circumflex femoral veins: venae comitantes of the lateral circumflex femoral artery, emptying into the femoral or the deep femoral vein.

ve′nae circumflex′ae fe′moris media′les [TA] medial circumflex femoral veins: venae comitantes of the medial circumflex femoral artery, emptying into the femoral or the deep femoral vein.

v. circumflex′a hu′meri ante′rior [TA] anterior circumflex humeral vein: a vena comitans of the homonymous artery, passing anteriorly around the neck of the humerus and draining into the axillary vein.

v. circumflex′a hu′meri poste′rior [TA] posterior circumflex humeral vein: a vena comitans of the homonymous artery, passing posteriorly around the neck of the humerus and draining into the axillary vein.

v. circumflex′a i′lium profun′da [TA] deep circumflex iliac vein: a common trunk formed from the venae comitantes of the homonymous artery and emptying into the external iliac vein.

v. circumflex′a i′lium superficia′lis [TA] superficial circumflex iliac vein: a vein that follows the homonymous artery and empties into the great saphenous vein.

v. circumflex′a sca′pulae [TA] circumflex scapular vein: a vena comitans of the homonymous artery, draining the lateral region of the scapula and joining with the thoracodorsal vein to form the subscapular vein.

v. co′lica dex′tra [TA] right colic vein: a vein that follows the distribution of the right colic artery and empties into the superior mesenteric vein.

v. co′lica me′dia [TA] middle colic vein: a vein that follows the distribution of the middle colic artery and empties into the superior mesenteric vein; called also *intermediate colic vein.*

v. co′lica sinis′tra [TA] left colic vein: a vein that follows the left colic artery and opens into the inferior mesenteric vein.

ve′nae colum′nae vertebra′lis [TA] veins of the vertebral column: a plexiform venous network extending the entire length of the vertebral column, outside or inside the vertebral canal; the anterior and posterior external and anterior and posterior internal groups freely anastomose and end in the intervertebral veins. See terms beginning *plexus venosus vertebralis.*

v. co′mitans [TA] accompanying vein: a vein, usually occurring in a pair (venae comitantes), that closely accompanies its homonymous artery and is found especially in the extremities.

v. co′mitans ner′vi hypoglos′si [TA] accompanying vein of hypoglossal nerve: a vessel, formed by union of the deep lingual vein and the sublingual vein, that accompanies the hypoglossal nerve; it empties into the facial, lingual, or internal jugular vein.

ve′nae conjunctiva′les [TA] conjunctival veins: small veins that drain blood from the conjunctiva to the superior ophthalmic vein.

ve′nae cor′dis [TA] cardiac veins: the veins of the heart, which drain blood from the various tissues making up the organ.

ve′nae cor′dis anterio′res TA alternative for *venae ventriculi dextri anteriores.*

v. cor′dis mag′na TA alternative for *v. cardiaca magna.*

v. cor′dis me′dia TA alternative for *v. cardiaca media.*

ve′nae cor′dis mi′nimae TA alternative for *venae cardiacae minimae.*

v. cor′dis par′va TA alternative for *v. cardiaca parva.*

ve′nae cortica′les radia′tae [TA] cortical radiate veins: veins that collect blood from the capillary network of the renal cortex and empty into the arcuate veins. Called also *venae interlobulares renis* [TA alternative] and *interlobular veins of kidney.*

v. cuta′nea [TA] cutaneous vein: one of the small veins that begin in the papillae of the skin, form subpapillary plexuses, and open into the subcutaneous veins.

v. cys′tica [TA] cystic vein: a small vein that returns the blood from the gallbladder to the right branch of the portal vein, within the substance of the liver.

ve′nae digita′les dorsa′les pe′dis [TA] dorsal digital veins of foot: the veins on the dorsal surfaces of the toes that unite in pairs around each cleft to form the dorsal metatarsal veins.

ve′nae digita′les palma′res [TA] palmar digital veins: the venae comitantes of the proper and common palmar digital arteries, which join the superficial palmar venous arch.

ve′nae digita′les planta′res [TA] plantar digital veins: veins from the plantar surfaces of the toes which unite at the clefts to form the plantar metatarsal veins of the foot.

ve′nae diplo′icae [TA] diploic veins: veins of the skull, including the frontal, occipital, anterior temporal, and posterior temporal diploic veins, which form sinuses in the cancellous tissue between the laminae of the cranial bones. They send branches to the external and the internal lamina, the periosteum, and the dura mater, and empty in part inside and in part outside the skull, communicating with meningeal veins, dural sinuses, pericranial veins, and each other.

v. diplo′ica fronta′lis [TA] frontal diploic vein: a vein that drains the frontal bone, emptying externally into the supraorbital vein and internally into the superior sagittal sinus.

v. diplo′ica occipita′lis [TA] occipital diploic vein: the largest of the diploic veins, which drains blood from the occipital bone and empties into the occipital vein or the transverse sinus.

v. diplo′ica tempora′lis ante′rior [TA] anterior temporal diploic vein: a vein that drains the lateral portion of the frontal and the anterior part of the parietal bone, opening internally into the sphenoparietal sinus and externally into a deep temporal vein.

v. diplo′ica tempora′lis poste′rior [TA] posterior temporal diploic vein: a vein that drains the parietal bone and empties into the transverse sinus.

ve′nae direc′tae latera′les [TA] lateral direct veins: veins of the lateral ventricle, draining into the great cerebral vein.

v. dorsa′lis cor′poris callo′si [TA] dorsal vein of corpus callosum: a vein that drains the superior surface of the corpus callosum into the great cerebral vein.

ve′nae dorsa′les lin′guae [TA] dorsal lingual veins: veins that unite with a small vena comitans of the lingual artery and join the main lingual trunk.

v. dorsa′lis profun′da clito′ridis [TA] deep dorsal vein of clitoris: a vein that follows the course of the dorsal artery of clitoris and opens into the vesical plexus.

v. dorsa′lis profun′da pe′nis [TA] deep dorsal vein of penis: a vein lying subfascially in the midline of the penis between the dorsal arteries; it begins in small veins around the corona glandis, is joined by the deep veins of the penis as it passes proximally, and passes between the arcuate pubic and transverse perineal ligaments where it divides into a left and right vein to join the prostatic plexus.

ve′nae dorsa′les superficia′les clito′ridis [TA] superficial dorsal veins of clitoris: veins that collect blood subcutaneously from the clitoris and drain into the external pudendal vein.

ve′nae dorsa′les superficia′les pe′nis [TA] superficial dorsal veins of penis: veins that collect blood subcutaneously from the penis and drain into the external pudendal vein.

v. dorsa′lis ve′nae intercosta′lis posterio′ris [TA] dorsal branch of posterior intercostal vein: the vena comitans of the dorsal branch of the posterior intercostal artery, receiving blood from the muscles and skin of the back. Called also *ramus dorsalis venae intercostalis posterioris* [TA alternative].

ve′nae duc′tuum semicircula′rium [TA] veins of semicircular ducts: small veins that collect blood from the semicircular ducts and empty into the vein of vestibular aqueduct.

v. emissa′ria [TA] emissary vein: one of the small, valveless veins that pass through foramina of the skull, connecting the dural venous sinuses with scalp veins or with deep veins below the base of the skull. Called also *emissary.*

v. emissa′ria condyla′ris [TA] condylar emissary vein: a small vein running through the condylar canal of the skull, connecting the sigmoid sinus with the vertebral or the internal jugular vein.

v. emissa′ria mastoi′dea [TA] mastoid emissary vein: a small vein passing through the mastoid foramen of the skull and connecting the sigmoid sinus with the occipital or the posterior auricular vein.

v. emissa′ria occipita′lis [TA] occipital emissary vein: an occasional small vein running through a minute foramen in the occipital protuberance of the skull and connecting the confluence of the sinuses with the occipital vein.

v. emissa′ria parieta′lis [TA] parietal emissary vein: a small vein passing through the parietal foramen of the skull and connecting the superior sagittal sinus with the superficial temporal veins.

ve′nae ence′phali [TA] cerebral veins: veins that drain the surfaces or inner regions of the cerebral hemispheres; they are divided into superficial and deep groups (see *venae superficiales cerebri* and *venae profundae cerebri*).

v. epigas′trica infe′rior [TA] inferior epigastric vein: a vein that accompanies the inferior epigastric artery and opens into the external iliac vein.

v. epigas′trica superficia′lis [TA] superficial epigastric vein: a vein that follows its homonymous artery and opens into the great saphenous or the femoral vein.

ve′nae epigas′tricae superio′res [TA] superior epigastric veins: the venae comitantes of the superior epigastric artery, which open into the internal thoracic vein.

ve′nae episclera′les [TA] episcleral veins: the veins that ring the cornea and drain into the vorticose and ciliary veins.
ve′nae esophagea′les venae oesophageales.
ve′nae ethmoida′les [TA] ethmoidal veins: veins that follow the anterior and posterior ethmoidal arteries, emerge from the ethmoidal foramina, and empty into the superior ophthalmic vein.
v. facia′lis [TA] facial vein: the vein that begins at the medial angle of the eye as the angular vein, descends behind the facial artery, and usually ends in the internal jugular vein; this vessel sometimes joins the retromandibular vein to form a common trunk.
v. femora′lis [TA] femoral vein: a vein that lies in the proximal two-thirds of the thigh; it is a direct continuation of the popliteal vein, follows the course of the femoral artery, and at the inguinal ligament becomes the external iliac vein. NOTE: Vascular surgeons refer to the portion of the femoral vein proximal to the branching of the deep femoral vein as the *common femoral vein,* and to its continuation distal to the branching as the *superficial femoral vein.*
v. fenes′trae coch′leae [TA] vein of round window: a small vein of the internal ear, draining the round window and emptying into the vestibulocochlear vein.
ve′nae fibula′res [TA] peroneal veins: the venae comitantes of the peroneal artery, emptying into the posterior tibial vein; called also *venae peroneae* [TA alternative].
ve′nae fronta′les [TA] frontal veins: a group of superior cerebral veins, superficial cerebral veins that drain the cortex of the frontal lobe.
ve′nae gas′tricae bre′ves [TA] short gastric veins: small vessels draining the left portion of the greater curvature of the stomach and emptying into the splenic vein.
v. gas′trica dex′tra [TA] right gastric vein: the vena comitans of the right gastric artery, emptying into the portal vein.
v. gas′trica sinis′tra [TA] left gastric vein: the vena comitans of the left gastric artery, emptying into the portal vein.
v. gastroepiplo′ica dex′tra TA alternative for *v. gastroomentalis dextra.*
v. gastroepiplo′ica sinis′tra TA alternative for *v. gastroomentalis sinistra.*
v. gastroomenta′lis dex′tra [TA] right gastro-omental vein: a vein that follows the distribution of its homonymous artery and empties into the superior mesenteric vein; called also *right epiploic vein, right gastroepiploic vein,* and *v. gastroepiploica dextra* [TA alternative].
v. gastroomenta′lis sinis′tra [TA] left gastro-omental vein: a vein that follows the distribution of its homonymous artery and empties into the splenic vein; called also *left epiploic vein, left gastroepiploic vein,* and *v. gastroepiploica sinistra* [TA alternative].
ve′nae genicula′res [TA] genicular veins: veins accompanying the genicular arteries and draining into the popliteal vein.
ve′nae glu′teae inferio′res [TA] inferior gluteal veins: venae comitantes of the inferior gluteal artery; they drain the subcutaneous tissue of the back of the thigh and the muscles of the buttock, unite into a single vein after passing through the greater sciatic foramen, and empty into the internal iliac vein.
ve′nae glu′teae superio′res [TA] superior gluteal veins: venae comitantes of the superior gluteal artery; they drain the muscles of the buttock, pass through the greater sciatic foramen, and empty into the internal iliac vein.
v. gy′ri olfacto′rii [TA] vein of olfactory gyrus: a vein that drains the olfactory gyrus into the basal vein.
v. hemia′zygos [TA] hemiazygos vein: an intercepting trunk for the lower left posterior intercostal veins; it arises from the ascending lumbar vein, passes up on the left side of the vertebrae to the eighth thoracic vertebra, where it may receive the accessory branch, and crosses over the vertebral column to open into the azygos vein.
v. hemia′zygos accesso′ria [TA] accessory hemiazygos vein: the descending intercepting trunk for the upper, often the fourth through the eighth, left posterior intercostal veins. It lies on the left side and at the eighth thoracic vertebra joins the hemiazygos vein or crosses to the right side to join the azygos vein directly; above, it may communicate with the left superior intercostal vein.
ve′nae hepa′ticae [TA] hepatic veins: veins that receive blood from the central veins of the liver. The upper group usually consists of three large veins (left, middle, and right hepatic veins), and the lower group consists of six to twenty small veins, which come from the right and caudate lobes; all are contiguous with the hepatic tissue and valveless, and open into the inferior vena cava on the posterior aspect of the liver.
v. hepa′tica dex′tra [TA] right hepatic vein: the large hepatic vein that drains the central veins in the right side of the liver and empties into the inferior vena cava.
v. hepa′tica interme′dia [TA] intermediate hepatic vein: the large hepatic vein that drains the central veins in the middle part of the liver and empties into the inferior vena cava. Called also *middle hepatic vein.*
v. hepa′tica sinis′tra [TA] left hepatic vein: the large hepatic vein that drains the central veins in the left side of the liver and empties into the inferior vena cava.
ve′nae ilea′les [TA] ileal veins: veins draining blood from the ileum into the superior mesenteric vein.
v. ileoco′lica [TA] ileocolic vein: a vein that follows the distribution of its homonymous artery and empties into the superior mesenteric vein.
v. ili′aca commu′nis [TA] common iliac vein: a vein that arises at the sacroiliac joint by union of the external iliac and the internal iliac veins, and passes upward to the right side of the fifth lumbar vertebra where it unites with its fellow of the opposite side to form the inferior vena cava.
v. ili′aca exter′na [TA] external iliac vein: the continuation of the femoral vein from the inguinal ligament to the sacroiliac joint, where it joins with the internal iliac vein to form the common iliac vein.
v. ili′aca inter′na [TA] internal iliac vein: a short trunk formed by union of parietal branches; it extends from the greater sciatic notch to the brim of the pelvis, where it joins the external iliac vein to form the common iliac vein.
v. iliolumba′lis [TA] iliolumbar vein: a vein that follows the distribution of the iliolumbar artery and opens into the internal iliac or the common iliac vein, or it may divide to end in both.
ve′nae inferio′res cerebel′li [TA] inferior veins of cerebellum: veins that drain the inferior surface of the cerebellum and empty into the straight or sigmoid sinus, or into the inferior petrosal and occipital sinuses.
ve′nae inferio′res ce′rebri [TA] inferior cerebral veins: rather large superficial cerebral veins that ramify on the base and the inferolateral surface of the brain: those on the inferior surface of the frontal lobe drain into the inferior sagittal sinus and the cavernous sinus; those on the temporal lobe, into the superior petrosal sinus and the transverse sinus; those on the occipital lobe into the straight sinus.
v. infe′rior ver′mis [TA] inferior vein of vermis: a vein that drains the inferior surface of the cerebellum; it runs backward on the inferior vermis to empty into the straight sinus or one of the sigmoid sinuses.
ve′nae insula′res [TA] insular veins: veins that drain the insula and join the deep middle cerebral vein.
ve′nae intercapitula′res ma′nus [TA] intercapitular veins of hand: veins at the clefts of the finger that pass between the heads of the metacarpal bones and establish communication between the dorsal and palmar venous systems of the hand.
ve′nae intercapitula′res pe′dis [TA] intercapitular veins of foot: veins at the clefts of the toes that pass between the heads of the metatarsal bones and establish communication between the dorsal and plantar venous systems of the foot.
ve′nae intercosta′les anterio′res [TA] anterior intercostal veins: the twelve paired venae comitantes of the anterior thoracic arteries, which drain into the internal thoracic veins.
ve′nae intercosta′les posterio′res [TA] posterior intercostal veins: the veins that accompany the corresponding intercostal arteries and drain the intercostal spaces posteriorly; the first ends in the brachiocephalic or the vertebral vein, the second and third join the superior intercostal vein, and the fourth to eleventh join the azygos vein on the right and the hemiazygos or accessory hemiazygos vein on the left.
v. intercosta′lis supe′rior dex′tra [TA] right superior intercostal vein: a common trunk formed by union of the second, third, and sometimes fourth posterior intercostal veins, which drains into the azygos vein.
v. intercosta′lis supe′rior sinis′tra [TA] left superior intercostal vein: the common trunk formed by union of the second, third, and sometimes fourth posterior intercostal veins, which crosses the arch of the aorta and joins the left brachiocephalic vein.
v. intercosta′lis supre′ma [TA] highest intercostal vein: the first posterior intercostal vein of either side, which passes over the apex of the lung and ends in the brachiocephalic, vertebral, or superior intercostal vein.

ve′nae interloba′res re′nis [TA] interlobar veins of kidney: veins that drain the arcuate veins, pass down between the renal pyramids, and unite to form the renal vein.
ve′nae interlobula′res he′patis [TA] interlobular veins of liver: the veins that arise as tributaries of the hepatic veins between the hepatic lobules.
ve′nae interlobula′res re′nis TA alternative for *venae corticales radiatae.*
ve′nae inter′nae ce′rebri [TA] internal cerebral veins: two veins that arise at the interventricular foramen by the union of the thalamostriate and the choroid veins; they pass backward through the tela choroidea, collecting blood from the basal nuclei, and unite at the splenium of the corpus callosum to form the great cerebral vein.
ve′nae interos′seae anterio′res [TA] anterior interosseous veins: the veins accompanying the anterior interosseous artery, which join the ulnar veins near the elbow.
ve′nae interos′seae posterio′res [TA] posterior interosseous veins: the veins accompanying the posterior interosseous artery, which join the ulnar veins near the elbow.
v. interventricula′ris ante′rior [TA] anterior interventricular vein: the portion of the great cardiac vein ascending in the anterior interventricular sulcus and emptying into the left coronary vein.
v. interventricula′ris poste′rior TA alternative for *v. cardiaca media.*
v. intervertebra′lis [TA] intervertebral vein: any one of the veins that drain the vertebral plexuses, passing out through the intervertebral foramina and emptying into the regional veins: in the neck, into the vertebral; in the thorax, the intercostal; in the abdomen, the lumbar; and in the pelvis, the lateral sacral veins.
ve′nae intrarena′les [TA] intrarenal veins: the veins within the kidney, including the interlobar, arcuate, interlobular, and stellate veins, and the straight venules. Called also *renal veins.*
ve′nae jejuna′les [TA] jejunal veins: veins draining blood from the jejunum into the superior mesenteric vein.
v. jugula′ris ante′rior [TA] anterior jugular vein: a vein that arises under the chin, passes down the neck, and opens into the external jugular or the subclavian vein or into the jugular venous arch.
v. jugula′ris exter′na [TA] external jugular vein: the vein that begins in the parotid gland behind the angle of the jaw by union of the retromandibular and the posterior auricular vein, passes down the neck, and opens into the subclavian, the internal jugular, or the brachiocephalic vein.
v. jugula′ris inter′na [TA] internal jugular vein: the vein that begins as the superior bulb in the jugular fossa, draining much of the head and neck; it descends with first the internal carotid and then the common carotid artery in the neck, and joins with the subclavian vein to form the brachiocephalic vein.
ve′nae labia′les anterio′res [TA] anterior labial veins: veins that collect blood from the anterior aspect of the labia and drain into the external pudendal vein; they are homologues of the anterior scrotal veins in the male.
ve′nae labia′les inferio′res [TA] inferior labial veins: veins that drain the region of the lower lip into the facial vein.
ve′nae labia′les posterio′res [TA] posterior labial veins: small branches from the labia which open into the vesical venous plexus; they are homologues of the posterior scrotal veins in the male.
v. labia′lis supe′rior [TA] superior labial vein: the vein that drains blood from the region of the upper lip into the facial vein.
ve′nae labyrin′thi [TA] veins of labyrinth: several small veins that pass through the internal acoustic meatus from the cochlea into the inferior petrosal or the transverse sinus; called also *internal auditory veins* and *labyrinthine veins.*
v. lacrima′lis [TA] lacrimal vein: the vein that drains blood from the lacrimal gland into the superior ophthalmic vein.
v. laryn′gea infe′rior [TA] inferior laryngeal vein: a vein draining blood from the larynx into the inferior thyroid vein.
v. laryn′gea supe′rior [TA] superior laryngeal vein: a vein that drains blood from the larynx into the superior thyroid vein.
v. latera′lis ventri′culi latera′lis [TA] lateral vein of lateral ventricle: a vein passing through the lateral wall of the lateral ventricle to drain the temporal and parietal lobes into the superior thalamostriate vein.
v. liena′lis TA alternative for *v. splenica.*
v. lingua′lis [TA] lingual vein: the deep vein that follows the distribution of the lingual artery and empties into the internal jugular vein.
v. lingula′ris [TA] lingular vein: a vein draining the lingular segments of the superior lobe of the left lung, emptying into the left superior pulmonary vein and formed by the union of superior and inferior parts. Called also *ramus lingularis venae pulmonalis sinistrae superioris* [TA alternative].
v. lo′bi me′dii [TA] middle lobe vein: a vein draining the middle lobe of the right lung, emptying into the right superior pulmonary vein and formed by the union of lateral and medial parts. Called also *ramus lobi medii venae pulmonalis dextrae superior* [TA alternative] and *right middle lobe vein.*
ve′nae lumba′les [TA] lumbar veins: the veins, four or five on each side, that accompany the corresponding lumbar arteries and drain the posterior wall of the abdomen, vertebral canal, spinal cord, and meninges; the first four usually end in the inferior vena cava, although the first may end in the ascending lumbar vein; the fifth is a tributary of the iliolumbar or of the common iliac vein; and all are generally united by the ascending iliac vein.
v. lumba′lis ascen′dens [TA] ascending lumbar vein: an ascending intercepting vein for the lumbar veins of either side; it begins in the lateral sacral veins and passes up the spine to the first lumbar vertebra, where by union with the subcostal vein it becomes on the right side the azygos vein, and on the left side, the hemiazygos vein.
v. mag′na ce′rebri [TA] great cerebral vein: a short median trunk formed by union of the two internal cerebral veins, which curves around the splenium of the corpus callosum and empties into, or is continued as, the straight sinus.
v. margina′lis dex′tra [TA] right marginal vein: a vein ascending along the right margin of the heart, draining adjacent parts of the right ventricle and opening into the right atrium or anterior cardiac veins.
v. margina′lis latera′lis [TA] lateral marginal vein: a vein running along the lateral side of the dorsum of the foot, returning blood from the dorsal venous arch, dorsal venous network, and superficial veins of the sole and draining into the small saphenous vein.
v. margina′lis media′lis [TA] medial marginal vein: a vein running along the medial side of the dorsum of the foot, returning blood from the dorsal venous arch, the dorsal venous network, and superficial veins of the sole and draining into the great saphenous vein.
v. margina′lis sinis′tra [TA] left marginal vein: a vein ascending along the left margin of the heart, draining the left ventricle and emptying into the great cardiac vein.
ve′nae maxilla′res [TA] maxillary veins: veins from the pterygoid plexus, usually forming a single short trunk, passing back and uniting with the superficial temporal vein in the parotid gland to form the retromandibular vein.
v. me′dia profun′da ce′rebri [TA] deep middle cerebral vein: the vein that accompanies the middle cerebral artery in the floor of the lateral sulcus, and joins the basal vein.
v. me′dia superficia′lis ce′rebri [TA] superficial middle cerebral vein: either of the two veins, one in each hemisphere, that drain the lateral surface of the cerebrum, follow the lateral cerebral fissure, and empty into the cavernous sinus; they are fed by the inferior and superior anastomotic veins. Called also *sylvian vein and vein of sylvian fossa.*
v. media′lis ventri′culi latera′lis [TA] medial vein of lateral ventricle: a vein passing through the medial wall of the lateral ventricle to drain the parietal and occipital lobes into the internal cerebral or great cerebral vein.
v. media′na antebra′chii [TA] median antebrachial vein: a vein that arises from a palmar venous plexus and passes up the forearm between the cephalic and the basilic veins to the elbow, where it either joins one of these, bifurcates to join both, or joins the median cubital vein; called also *median vein of forearm.*
v. media′na cu′biti [TA] median cubital vein: the large connecting branch that arises from the cephalic vein below the elbow and passes obliquely upward over the cubital fossa to join the basilic vein; called also *median vein of elbow.*
ve′nae mediastina′les [TA] mediastinal veins: numerous small branches that drain blood from the anterior mediastinum into the brachiocephalic vein, azygos vein, or the superior vena cava.
ve′nae medul′lae oblonga′tae [TA] veins of medulla oblongata: the veins that drain the medulla oblongata, which empty into the veins of the spinal cord, the adjacent dural venous sinuses, or along the last four cranial nerves to the inferior petrosal sinus or superior bulb of the jugular vein.

Vena *Continued*

ve′nae medul′lae spina′lis [TA] veins of spinal cord: longitudinal veins that drain the spinal cord and empty into the anterior internal vertebral venous plexus.
ve′nae mem′bri inferio′ris [TA] veins of lower limb: veins that drain the thigh, leg, and foot, divided into *superficial veins* (those in the superficial fascia) and *deep veins* (those that accompany arteries). See also *venae profundae membri inferioris* and *venae superficiales membri inferioris.*
ve′nae mem′bri superio′ris [TA] veins of upper limb: veins that drain the arm, forearm, and hand, divided into *superficial veins* (those in the superficial fascia) and *deep veins* (those that accompany arteries); there are frequent anastomoses between the two groups. See also *venae profundae membri superioris* and *venae superficiales membri superioris.*
ve′nae menin′geae [TA] meningeal veins: the venae comitantes of the meningeal arteries, which drain the dura mater, communicate with the lateral lacunae, and empty into the regional sinuses and veins.
ve′nae menin′geae me′diae [TA] middle meningeal veins: the venae comitantes of the middle meningeal artery, which end in the pterygoid venous plexus.
v. mesente′rica infe′rior [TA] inferior mesenteric vein: a vein that follows the distribution of its homonymous artery and empties into the splenic vein.
v. mesente′rica supe′rior [TA] superior mesenteric vein: a vein that follows the distribution of its homonymous artery and joins with the splenic vein to form the hepatic portal vein.
ve′nae metacarpa′les dorsa′les [TA] dorsal metacarpal veins: veins that arise from the union of dorsal veins of adjacent fingers and pass proximally to join in forming the dorsal venous rete of the hand.
ve′nae metacarpa′les palma′res [TA] palmar metacarpal veins: the venae comitantes of the palmar metacarpal arteries, which open into the deep palmar venous arch.
ve′nae metatarsa′les dorsa′les [TA] dorsal metatarsal veins: veins that are formed by the dorsal digital veins of the toes at the clefts of the toes, joining the dorsal venous arch.
ve′nae metatarsa′les planta′res [TA] plantar metatarsal veins: deep veins of the foot that arise from the plantar digital veins at the clefts of the toes and pass back to open into the plantar venous arch.
v. modio′li commu′nis [TA] common modiolar vein: a vein receiving blood from the vein of scala tympani and vein of scala vestibuli, running a spiral course in the modiolus of the cochlea, and draining into the vein of cochlear aqueduct.
ve′nae musculophre′nicae [TA] musculophrenic veins: the venae comitantes of the musculophrenic artery, draining blood from parts of the diaphragm and from the wall of the thorax and abdomen and emptying into the internal thoracic veins.
ve′nae nasa′les exter′nae [TA] external nasal veins: small ascending branches from the nose that open into the angular and facial veins.
v. nasofronta′lis [TA] nasofrontal vein: a vein that begins at the supraorbital vein, enters the orbit, and joins the superior ophthalmic vein.
ve′nae nu′clei cauda′ti [TA] the veins of the caudate nucleus, located within the corpus striatum; they drain into the superior thalamostriate vein.
v. nutri′cia [TA] nutrient vein: a vein that drains blood from a bone, accompanying the nutrient artery and emerging through the nutrient foramen. Called also *v. nutriens* [TA alternative].
v. nu′triens TA alternative for *v. nutricia.*
v. obli′qua a′trii sinis′tri [TA] oblique vein of left atrium: a small vein from the left atrium that opens into the coronary sinus. Called also *vein of Marshall* and *Marshall oblique vein.*
ve′nae obturato′riae [TA] obturator veins: veins that drain the hip joint and the regional muscles, enter the pelvis through the obturator canal, and empty into the internal iliac or the inferior epigastric vein, or both.
ve′nae occipita′les [TA] occipital veins: a group of superior cerebral veins, superficial cerebral veins that drain the cortex of the occipital lobe.
v. occipita′lis [TA] occipital vein: a vein in the scalp that follows the distribution of the occipital artery and opens under the trapezius muscle into the suboccipital venous plexus; it may continue with the occipital artery and end in the internal jugular vein.
ve′nae oesophagea′les [TA] esophageal veins: small veins that drain blood from the esophagus into the hemiazygos and azygos veins, or into the left brachiocephalic vein; spelled also *venae esophageales.*
v. ophthal′mica infe′rior [TA] inferior ophthalmic vein: a vein formed by confluence of muscular and ciliary branches, and running backward either to join the superior ophthalmic vein or to open directly into the cavernous sinus; it sends a communicating branch through the inferior orbital fissure to join the pterygoid venous plexus.
v. ophthal′mica supe′rior [TA] superior ophthalmic vein: a vein that begins at the medial angle of the eye, where it communicates with the frontal, supraorbital, and angular veins; it follows the distribution of the ophthalmic artery, and may be joined by the inferior ophthalmic vein at the superior orbital fissure before opening into the cavernous sinus.
ve′nae or′bitae [TA] veins of orbit: the veins that drain the orbit and its structures, including the superior ophthalmic vein and its tributaries and the inferior ophthalmic vein.
v. ova′rica dex′tra [TA] right ovarian vein: a vein that drains the right pampiniform plexus of the broad ligament and empties into the inferior vena cava.
v. ova′rica sinis′tra [TA] left ovarian vein: a vein that drains the left pampiniform plexus of the broad ligament and empties into the left renal vein.
v. palati′na exter′na [TA] external palatine vein: the vein that drains blood from the tonsils and the soft palate into the facial vein.
ve′nae palpebra′les [TA] palpebral veins: small branches from the eyelids that open into the superior ophthalmic vein.
ve′nae palpebra′les inferio′res [TA] inferior palpebral veins: branches that drain the blood from the lower eyelid into the facial vein.
ve′nae palpebra′les superio′res [TA] superior palpebral veins: branches that drain the blood from the upper eyelid to the angular vein.
ve′nae pancrea′ticae [TA] pancreatic veins: numerous branches from the pancreas which open into the splenic and the superior mesenteric veins.
ve′nae pancreaticoduodena′les [TA] pancreaticoduodenal veins: four veins that drain blood from the pancreas and duodenum, closely following the homonymous arteries. A superior and an inferior vein originate from both an anterior and a posterior venous arcade. The anterior superior vein joins the right gastro-omental vein; the posterior superior vein joins the hepatic portal vein. The anterior and posterior inferior veins join, sometimes as one trunk and other times singly, the uppermost jejunal vein or the superior mesenteric vein.
ve′nae paraumbilica′les [TA] paraumbilical veins: veins that communicate with the portal vein and anastomose with the superior and inferior epigastric and the superior vesical veins in the region of the umbilicus. They form a part of the collateral circulation of the portal vein in the event of hepatic obstruction. Called also *veins of Sappey.*
ve′nae parieta′les [TA] parietal veins: a group of superior cerebral veins, superficial cerebral veins that drain the cortex of the parietal lobe.
ve′nae paroti′deae [TA] parotid veins: small veins from the parotid gland that open into the facial vein or into the retromandibular vein. Those opening into the facial vein are called also *rami parotidei venae facialis* [TA alternative].
ve′nae pectora′les [TA] pectoral veins: collective term for branches of the subclavian vein that drain the pectoral region.
ve′nae peduncula′res [TA] peduncular veins: veins that drain the cerebral peduncle into the basal vein.
ve′nae perforan′tes [TA] perforating veins: valved veins that drain blood from the superficial to the deep veins in the leg and foot. Called also *communicating veins.*
ve′nae pericardi′acae [TA] pericardial veins: numerous small branches that drain blood from the pericardium into the brachiocephalic, inferior thyroid, and azygos veins, and the superior vena cava; called also *pericardiac veins.*
ve′nae pericardiacophre′nicae [TA] pericardiacophrenic veins: small veins that drain blood from the pericardium and diaphragm into the left brachiocephalic vein.
ve′nae perone′ae TA alternative for *venae fibulares.*
v. petro′sa [TA] petrosal vein: a short trunk arising from the union of four or five cerebellar and pontine veins opposite the middle cerebellar peduncle and terminating in the superior petrosal sinus.
ve′nae pharyn′geae [TA] pharyngeal veins: veins that drain the pharyngeal plexus and empty into the internal jugular vein.
ve′nae phre′nicae inferio′res [TA] inferior phrenic veins: veins that follow the homonymous arteries, the one on the right entering

the inferior vena cava, and the one on the left entering the left suprarenal or renal vein or the inferior vena cava.
ve′nae phre′nicae superio′res [TA] superior phrenic veins: small veins on the superior surface of the diaphragm that drain into the azygos and hemiazygos veins.
ve′nae pon′tis [TA] pontine veins: the veins that drain the pons, which empty into the basal vein, cerebellar veins, petrosal or venous sinuses, or venous plexus of the foramen ovale.
v. pontomesencepha′lica [TA] pontomesencephalic vein: a vein lying on the superior and anterior aspects of the pons in the midline of the interpeduncular fossa, communicating superiorly with the basal vein and inferiorly with the petrosal vein.
v. popli′tea [TA] popliteal vein: a vein following the popliteal artery, and formed by union of the venae comitantes of the anterior and posterior tibial arteries; at the adductor hiatus it becomes continuous with the femoral vein.
v. por′tae he′patis [TA] hepatic portal vein: a short thick trunk formed by union of the superior mesenteric and the splenic veins behind the neck of the pancreas; it passes upward to the right end of the porta hepatis, where it divides into successively smaller branches, following the branches of the hepatic artery, until it forms a capillary-like system of sinusoids that permeates the entire substance of the liver. Called also *portal vein.*
ve′nae porta′les hypophysia′les [TA] hypophysioportal veins: a system of venules connecting capillaries in the hypothalamus with sinusoidal capillaries in the anterior lobe of the hypophysis. Called also *portal veins of hypophysis.*
v. poste′rior cor′poris callo′si [TA] posterior vein of corpus callosum: a vein that drains the posterior surface of the corpus callosum into the great cerebral vein.
v. poste′rior lo′bi superio′ris pulmo′nis dex′tri [TA] posterior vein of superior lobe of right lung: a vein draining the posterior segment of the superior lobe of the right lung and emptying into the right superior pulmonary vein; called also *ramus posterior venae pulmonalis dextrae superioris* [TA alternative] and *posterior segmental vein.*
v. poste′rior sep′ti pellu′cidi [TA] posterior vein of septum pellucidum: a vein that drains the posterior septum pellucidum into the superior thalamostriate vein.
v. precentra′lis cerebel′li [TA] precentral vein of cerebellum: a vein arising in the precentral cerebellar fissure and passing anterior and superior to the culmen, terminating in the great cerebral vein.
ve′nae prefronta′les [TA] prefrontal veins: a group of superior cerebral veins, superficial cerebral veins that drain the prefrontal area of the cerebral cortex.
v. prepylo′rica [TA] prepyloric vein: a vein that passes upward over the anterior surface of the junction between the pylorus and the duodenum and empties into the right gastric vein. Called also *Mayo vein.*
v. profun′da [TA] deep vein: any deeply situated vein.
ve′nae profun′dae ce′rebri [TA] deep cerebral veins: the veins that drain the inner regions of the cerebral hemispheres, consisting of the basal veins, the great cerebral veins, the veins of the encephalic trunk, and their tributaries.
ve′nae profun′dae clito′ridis [TA] deep veins of clitoris: small veins of the clitoris that drain into the vesical venous plexus.
v. profun′da facie′i [TA] deep facial vein: a vein draining from the pterygoid plexus to the facial vein.
v. profun′da fe′moris [TA] deep femoral vein: a vein that follows the distribution of the deep femoral artery and opens into the femoral vein.
v. profun′da lin′guae [TA] deep lingual vein: a vein that drains blood from the deep aspect of the tongue and joins the sublingual vein to form the vena comitans of the hypoglossal nerve.
ve′nae profun′dae mem′bri inferio′ris [TA] deep veins of lower limb: veins that drain the lower limb, found accompanying homonymous arteries, and anastomosing freely with the superficial veins; the principal deep veins are the femoral and popliteal veins.
ve′nae profun′dae mem′bri superio′ris [TA] deep veins of upper limb: veins that drain the upper limb, found accompanying homonymous arteries, and anastomosing freely with the superficial veins; they include the brachial, ulnar, and radial veins, and their tributaries, all of which ultimately drain into the axillary vein.
ve′nae profun′dae pe′nis [TA] deep veins of penis: veins that follow the distribution of the homonymous artery and empty into the dorsal vein of the penis.
v. pu′bica [TA] pubic vein: a vein connecting the external iliac and obturator veins, ascending on the pelvic surface of the pubis and accompanying the pubic branch of the inferior epigastric artery. Called also *ramus pubicus venae epigastricae inferioris* [TA alternative] and *pubic branch of inferior epigastric vein.*
ve′nae puden′dae exter′nae [TA] external pudendal veins: veins that follow the distribution of the external pudendal arteries, drain anterior parts of the labia or scrotum, and open into the great saphenous vein and femoral vein.
v. puden′da inter′na [TA] internal pudendal vein: a vein that follows the course of the internal pudendal artery, and drains into the internal iliac vein.
ve′nae pulmona′les [TA] pulmonary veins: the four veins, right and left superior and right and left inferior, that return aerated blood from the lungs to the left atrium of the heart. See also *segmenta bronchopulmonalia.*
v. pulmona′lis dex′tra infe′rior [TA] right inferior pulmonary vein: the vein that returns blood from the lower lobe of the right lung (from the superior segmental and common basal veins) to the left atrium of the heart.
v. pulmona′lis dex′tra supe′rior [TA] right superior pulmonary vein: the vein that returns blood from the upper and middle lobes of the right lung (from the middle lobe, apical, anterior segmental, and posterior segmental veins) to the left atrium of the heart.
v. pulmona′lis sinis′tra infe′rior [TA] left inferior pulmonary vein: the vein that returns blood from the lower lobe of the left lung (from the superior segmental and common basal veins) to the left atrium of the heart.
v. pulmona′lis sinis′tra supe′rior [TA] left superior pulmonary vein: the vein that returns blood from the upper lobe of the left lung (from the apicoposterior, anterior segmental, and lingular veins) to the left atrium of the heart.
ve′nae radia′les [TA] radial veins: the venae comitantes of the radial artery, which open into the brachial veins.
v. reces′sus latera′lis ventri′culi quar′ti [TA] vein of lateral recess of fourth ventricle: a small vein arising in the tonsil of the cerebellum, passing the lateral recess of the fourth ventricle, and terminating in the petrosal vein.
ve′nae recta′les inferio′res [TA] inferior rectal veins: veins that drain the rectal plexus into the internal pudendal vein.
ve′nae recta′les me′diae [TA] middle rectal veins: veins that drain the rectal plexus and empty into the internal iliac and superior rectal veins.
v. recta′lis supe′rior [TA] superior rectal vein: the vein that drains the upper part of the rectal plexus into the inferior mesenteric vein and thus establishes connection between the portal system and the systemic circulation.
ve′nae rena′les 1. renal veins: two veins, one from each kidney, that receive blood from the interlobar veins, with the left also receiving blood from the left testicular (or ovarian), left suprarenal, and (sometimes) inferior phrenic veins; they empty into the inferior vena cava at the level of the second lumbar vertebra. 2. former name for *venae intrarenales.*
v. retromandibula′ris [TA] retromandibular vein: the vein that is formed in the upper part of the parotid gland behind the neck of the mandible by union of the maxillary and superficial temporal veins; it passes downward through the gland, communicates with the facial vein, and emerging from the gland joins with the posterior auricular vein to form the external jugular vein.
ve′nae revehen′tes revehent veins: channels in the early embryo that convey blood from the sinusoids of the liver to the sinus venosus and later become the hepatic veins.
ve′nae sacra′les latera′les [TA] lateral sacral veins: veins that follow the homonymous arteries, help to form the lateral sacral plexus, and empty into the internal iliac vein or the superior gluteal veins.
v. sacra′lis media′na [TA] median sacral vein: a vein that follows the median sacral artery and opens into the common iliac vein.
v. saphe′na accesso′ria [TA] accessory saphenous vein: a vein that, when present, drains the medial and posterior superficial parts of the thigh and opens into the great saphenous vein.
v. saphe′na mag′na [TA] great saphenous vein: the longest vein in the body, extending from the dorsum of the foot to just below the inguinal ligament, where it opens into the femoral vein. It drains

the foot and leg through many tributaries, including the medial marginal, accessory saphenous, superficial external pudendal, superficial circumflex iliac, superficial epigastric, and numerous cutaneous veins.
v. saphe′na par′va [TA] small saphenous vein: the vein that continues the lateral marginal vein from behind the malleolus and passes up the back of the leg to the knee joint, where it opens into the popliteal vein.
v. sca′lae tym′pani vein of scala tympani: a tributary of the common modiolar vein draining the scala tympani of the cochlea.
v. sca′lae vesti′buli vein of scala vestibuli: a tributary of the common modiolar vein draining the scala vestibuli of the cochlea.
v. scapula′ris dorsa′lis [TA] dorsal scapular vein: an occasional branch that contributes to the subclavian vein.
ve′nae sclera′les [TA] scleral veins: tributaries of the anterior ciliary veins that drain the sclera.
ve′nae scrota′les anterio′res [TA] anterior scrotal veins: veins that collect blood from the anterior aspect of the scrotum and drain into the external pudendal vein.
ve′nae scrota′les posterio′res [TA] posterior scrotal veins: small branches from the posterior aspect of the scrotum that open into the vesical venous plexus.
ve′nae sigmoi′deae [TA] sigmoid veins: veins from the sigmoid colon that empty into the inferior mesenteric vein.
ve′nae spina′les anterio′res [TA] anterior spinal veins: a group of longitudinal veins forming a plexus on the anterior surface of the spinal cord, comprising a median vein lying anterior to the anterior median fissure and two anterolateral veins lying slightly posterior to the anterior nerve roots; they drain the anterior spinal cord. See also *plexus venosus vertebralis externus anterior* and *plexus venosus vertebralis internus anterior.*
ve′nae spina′les posterio′res [TA] posterior spinal veins: a group of longitudinal, usually discontinuous, veins forming a plexus on the posterior surface of the spinal cord, comprising a median vein lying behind the posterior median septum and two posterolateral veins lying posterior to the posterior nerve roots; they drain the posterior spinal cord. See also *plexus venosus vertebralis externus posterior* and *plexus venosus vertebralis internus posterior.*
v. spina′lis ve′ae intercosta′lis posterio′ris [TA] spinal branch of posterior intercostal vein: a vessel, the vena comitans of the arterial spinal branch, that emerges from the vertebral canal and contributes to the dorsal branch of each posterior intercostal vein. Called also *ramus spinalis venae intercostalis posterioris* [TA alternative].
v. sple′nica [TA] splenic vein: the vein formed by union of several branches at the hilum of the spleen, passing from left to right to the neck of the pancreas, where it joins the superior mesenteric vein to form the portal vein; called also *v. lienalis* [TA alternative].
ve′nae stella′tae re′nis [TA] stellate veins of kidney: veins on the surface of the kidney that collect blood from the superficial parts of the renal cortex and empty into the interlobular veins. Called also *Verheyen stars* or *stellulae.*
v. sternocleidomastoi′dea [TA] sternocleidomastoid vein: a vein that follows the course of the homonymous artery and opens into the internal jugular vein.
v. stylomastoi′dea [TA] stylomastoid vein: a vein following the stylomastoid artery and emptying into the retromandibular vein.
v. subcla′via [TA] subclavian vein: the vein that continues the axillary as the main venous stem of the upper limb, follows the subclavian artery, and joins with the internal jugular vein to form the brachiocephalic vein.
v. subcosta′lis [TA] subcostal vein: the vena comitans of the subcostal artery on the left or right side; it joins the ascending lumbar vein to form the azygos vein on the right or the hemiazygos vein on the left.
ve′nae subcuta′neae abdo′minis [TA] subcutaneous veins of abdomen: the superficial veins of the abdominal wall.
v. sublingua′lis [TA] sublingual vein: a vein that follows the sublingual artery and opens into the lingual vein.
v. submenta′lis [TA] submental vein: a vein that follows the submental artery and opens into the facial vein.
v. subscapula′ris [TA] subscapular vein: a vena comitans of the homonymous artery, formed by the union of the circumflex scapular and thoracodorsal veins and draining into the axillary vein.
v. superficia′lis [TA] superficial vein: any superficially situated vein.
ve′nae superficia′les ce′rebri [TA] superficial cerebral veins: the veins that drain the surfaces of the cerebral hemispheres, comprising the superior, inferior, and middle superficial cerebral veins and their tributaries.
ve′nae superficia′les mem′bri inferio′ris [TA] superficial veins of lower limb: veins that drain the lower limb, found immediately beneath the skin, and anastomosing freely with the deep veins; the principal superficial veins are the great and small saphenous veins.
ve′nae superficia′les mem′bri superio′ris [TA] superficial veins of upper limb: veins that drain the upper limb, found immediately beneath the skin, and anastomosing freely with the deep veins; they include the cephalic, basilic, and median cubital and antebrachial veins, and their tributaries, all of which ultimately drain into the axillary vein.
superior v. cava, persistent left a developmental anomaly in which the left superior vena cava persists into postnatal life, usually draining into the left atrium; it is due to failure of the upper part of the left anterior cardinal vein to become obliterated. It may be an isolated anomaly or accompany other cardiovascular defects, such as tetralogy of Fallot.
ve′nae superio′res cerebel′li [TA] superior veins of cerebellum: veins that drain the superior surfaces of the cerebellar hemisphere and empty into the straight sinus or great cerebral vein, or into the transverse and superior petrosal sinuses.
ve′nae superio′res ce′rebri [TA] superior cerebral veins: the 8 to 12 superficial cerebral veins (prefrontal, frontal, parietal, and occipital) that drain the superior, lateral, and medial surfaces of the cerebrum toward the longitudinal cerebral fissure, where they open into the superior sagittal sinus.
v. supe′rior lo′bi inferio′ris pulmo′nis dex′tri [TA] superior vein of inferior lobe of right lung: a vein draining the superior segment of the inferior lobe of the right lung and emptying into the right inferior pulmonary vein. Called also *ramus superior venae pulmonalis dextrae inferioris* [TA alternative] and *superior segmental vein.*
v. supe′rior lo′bi inferio′ris pulmo′nis sinis′tri [TA] superior vein of inferior lobe of left lung: a vein draining the superior segment of the inferior lobe of the left lung and emptying into the left inferior pulmonary vein. Called also *ramus superior venae pulmonalis sinistrae inferioris* [TA alternative] and *superior segmental vein.*
v. supe′rior ver′mis [TA] superior vein of vermis: a vein that drains the superior surface of the cerebellum; it runs forward and medially across the superior vermis to empty into the straight sinus or the great cerebral vein.
v. supraorbita′lis [TA] supraorbital vein: the vein that passes down the forehead lateral to the supratrochlear vein, joining it at the root of the nose to form the angular vein.
v. suprarena′lis dex′tra [TA] right suprarenal vein: a vein that drains the right suprarenal gland into the inferior vena cava.
v. suprarena′lis sinis′tra [TA] left suprarenal vein: the vein that returns blood from the left suprarenal gland to the left renal vein.
v. suprascapula′ris [TA] suprascapular vein: the vein that accompanies the homonymous artery (sometimes as two veins that unite), opening usually into the external jugular, or occasionally into the subclavian vein; called also *transverse vein of scapula.*
ve′nae supratrochlea′res [TA] supratrochlear veins: two veins, each beginning in a venous plexus high up on the forehead and descending to the root of the nose, where it joins with the supraorbital vein to form the angular vein. Called also *frontal veins.*
ve′nae sura′les [TA] sural veins: veins that ascend with the sural arteries and drain blood from the calf into the popliteal vein.
v. tempora′lis me′dia [TA] middle temporal vein: the vein that arises in the substance of the temporal muscle and passes down under the fascia to the zygoma, where it breaks through to join the superficial temporal vein.
ve′nae tempora′les profun′dae [TA] deep temporal veins: veins that drain the deep portions of the temporal muscle and empty into the pterygoid plexus.
ve′nae tempora′les superficia′les [TA] superficial temporal veins: veins that drain the lateral part of the scalp in the frontal and parietal regions, the tributaries forming a single superficial temporal vein in front of the ear, just above the zygoma. This descending vein receives the middle temporal and transverse facial veins and, entering the parotid gland, unites with the maxillary vein deep to the neck of the mandible to form the retromandibular vein.

Vena *Continued*

v. termina′lis TA alternative for *v. thalamostriata superior*.

v. testicula′ris dex′tra [TA] right testicular vein: a vein that drains the right pampiniform plexus and empties into the inferior vena cava.

v. testicula′ris sinis′tra [TA] left testicular vein: a vein that drains the left pampiniform plexus and empties into the left renal vein.

ve′nae thalamostria′tae inferio′res [TA] inferior thalamostriate veins: veins that pass through the anterior perforated substance and join the deep middle cerebral and anterior cerebral veins to form the basal vein; called also *striate veins*.

v. thalamostria′ta supe′rior [TA] superior thalamostriate vein: a vein that collects blood from the corpus striatum and thalamus, and joins with the choroid vein to form the internal cerebral vein; called also *terminal vein* and *v. terminalis* [TA alternative].

ve′nae thora′cicae inter′nae [TA] internal thoracic veins: two veins formed by junction of the venae comitantes of the internal thoracic artery of either side; each continues along the artery to open into the brachiocephalic vein. Called also *internal mammary veins*.

v. thora′cica latera′lis [TA] lateral thoracic vein: a large vein accompanying the lateral thoracic artery and draining into the axillary vein.

v. thoracoacromia′lis [TA] thoracoacromial vein: the vein that follows the homonymous artery and opens into the subclavian vein.

v. thoracodorsa′lis [TA] thoracodorsal vein: a vena comitans of the homonymous artery, draining the latissimus dorsi and joining with the circumflex scapular vein to form the subscapular vein.

ve′nae thoracoepigas′tricae [TA] thoracoepigastric veins: long, longitudinal, superficial veins in the anterolateral subcutaneous tissue of the trunk, which empty superiorly into the lateral thoracic and inferiorly into the femoral vein.

ve′nae thy′micae [TA] thymic veins: small branches from the thymus gland that open into the left brachiocephalic vein.

v. thyroi′dea i′ma thyroid ima vein: an occasional vein formed by high junction of the right and left inferior thyroid veins, and usually emptying into the left brachiocephalic vein.

v. thyroi′dea inferio′ris [TA] inferior thyroid vein: either of two veins, left and right, that drain the thyroid plexus into the left and right brachiocephalic veins; occasionally they may unite into a common trunk to empty, usually, into the left brachiocephalic vein.

ve′nae thyroi′deae me′diae [TA] middle thyroid veins: veins that drain blood from the thyroid gland into the internal jugular vein.

v. thyroi′dea supe′rior [TA] superior thyroid vein: a vein arising from the upper part of the thyroid gland on either side, opening into the internal jugular vein, occasionally in common with the facial vein.

ve′nae tibia′les anterio′res [TA] anterior tibial veins: venae comitantes of the anterior tibial artery, which unite with the posterior tibial veins to form the popliteal vein.

ve′nae tibia′les posterio′res [TA] posterior tibial veins: accompanying veins of the posterior tibial artery, which unite with the anterior tibial veins to form the popliteal vein.

ve′nae trachea′les [TA] tracheal veins: small branches that drain blood from the trachea into the brachiocephalic vein.

ve′nae transver′sae cer′vicis [TA] transverse cervical veins: veins that follow the transverse cervical artery and open into the subclavian vein. Called also *venae transversae colli* [TA alternative].

ve′nae transver′sae col′li TA alternative for *venae transversae cervicis*.

v. transver′sa facie′i [TA] transverse facial vein: a vein that passes backward with the transverse facial artery just below the zygomatic arch to join the retromandibular vein.

ve′nae trun′ci encepha′lici [TA] veins of encephalic trunk: the veins that drain the brainstem and empty into the basal or great cerebral vein; see *v. pontomesencephalica anterior*, *venae pontis*, *venae medullae oblongatae*, and *v. recessus lateralis ventriculi quarti*.

ve′nae tympa′nicae [TA] tympanic veins: small veins from the tympanic cavity that pass through the petrotympanic fissure, open into the plexus around the temporomandibular joint, and finally drain into the retromandibular vein.

ve′nae ulna′res [TA] ulnar veins: the venae comitantes of the ulnar artery, which unite with the radial veins at the elbow to form the brachial veins.

v. umbilica′lis [TA] umbilical vein: the vein formed from the left umbilical vein after degeneration of the right umbilical vein; it carries the blood from the placenta to the ductus venosus.

v. unca′lis [TA] vein of uncus: a vein that drains the uncus into the ipsilateral inferior cerebral vein.

ve′nae uteri′nae [TA] uterine veins: veins that drain the uterine plexus into the internal iliac veins.

ve′nae vaso′rum small veins that return blood from the tissues making up the walls of the blood vessels themselves.

ve′nae ventricula′res dex′trae [TA] right ventricular veins: the smallest cardiac veins (venae cardiacae minimae) emptying into the right ventricle of the heart.

v. ventricula′ris infe′rior [TA] inferior ventricular vein: a vein that drains the temporal lobe into the basal vein.

ve′nae ventricula′res sinis′trae [TA] left ventricular veins: rarely occurring smallest cardiac veins (venae cardiacae minimae) emptying into the left ventricle of the heart.

ve′nae ventri′culi dex′tri anterio′res [TA] anterior veins of right ventricle: small veins that drain blood from the anterior aspect of the right ventricle, ascend in subepicardial tissue to cross the right part of the atrioventricular sulcus, and empty into the right atrium. Called also *venae cardiacae anteriores* [TA alternative], *venae cordis anteriores* [TA alternative], *anterior cardiac veins*, and *anterior veins of heart*.

v. ventri′culi sinis′tri poste′rior [TA] posterior vein of left ventricle: the vein that drains blood from the posterior surface of the left ventricle into the coronary sinus. It may occur as several veins *(venae ventriculi sinistri posteriores)*.

v. vertebra′lis [TA] vertebral vein: a vein that arises from the suboccipital venous plexus, passes with the vertebral artery through the foramina of the transverse processes of the upper six cervical vertebrae, and opens into the brachiocephalic vein.

v. vertebra′lis accesso′ria [TA] accessory vertebral vein: a vein that sometimes arises from a plexus formed around the vertebral artery by the vertebral vein, descends with the vertebral vein, and emerges through the transverse foramen of the seventh cervical vertebra to empty into the brachiocephalic vein.

v. vertebra′lis ante′rior [TA] anterior vertebral vein: a small vein accompanying the ascending cervical artery; it arises in a venous plexus adjacent to the more cranial cervical transverse processes, and descends to end in the vertebral vein.

ve′nae vesica′les [TA] vesical veins: veins passing from the vesical plexus to the internal iliac vein.

v. vestibula′ris ante′rior [TA] anterior vestibular vein: the anterior of a pair of veins draining blood from the vestibule into the labyrinthine veins.

v. vestibula′ris poste′rior [TA] posterior vestibular vein: the posterior of a pair of veins draining blood from the vestibule into the labyrinthine veins.

v. vestibulocochlea′ris [TA] vestibulocochlear vein: a vena comitans of the vestibulocochlear artery, emptying into the vein of cochlear aqueduct.

ve′nae vortico′sae [TA] vorticose veins: four veins that pierce the sclera and carry blood from the choroid to the superior ophthalmic vein; called also *posterior ciliary veins*.

---

ve•na•ca•val (ve″nə-ka′vəl) caval.

ve•na ca•val (ve′nə ka′vəl) caval.

ve•na•ca•vo•gram (ve″nə-ka′vo-gram) the film obtained byn venacavography.

ve•na•ca•vog•ra•phy (ve″nə-ka-vog′rə-fe) radiography of a vena cava, usually of the inferior vena cava.

ve•nae (ve′ne) [L.] genitive and plural of *vena*.

ve•na•tion (ve-na′shən) [L. *vena*, q.v.] the manner of distribution of the veins of a part.

ve•nec•ta•sia (ve″nək-ta′zhə) a varicosity of a vein.

ve•nec•to•my (ve-nek′tə-me) phlebectomy.

ve•neer (və-nēr′) a thin layer of tooth-colored material, usually porcelain, some other ceramic, or acrylic resin, attached to the surface by direct fusion, cementation, or mechanical retention in the construction of crowns or pontics, or cemented directly to the prepared surface of a tooth to modify its shape or color.

full v. full crown.

ven•e•na•tion (ven″ə-na′shən) poisoning.

ven•e•nif•er•ous (ven″ə-nif′ər-əs) toxiferous.

ven•e•no•sal•i•vary (ven′ə-no-sal′ĭ-var-e) venomosalivary.

ven•e•nos•i•ty (ven″ə-nos′ĭ-te) toxicity.

ven•e•nous (ven′ə-nəs) [L. *venenosus*] venomous.

vene•punc•ture (ven′ə-punk″chər) phlebotomy (def. 2).

ve•ne•re•al (və-nēr′e-əl) [L. *venereus*] pertaining or related to or transmitted by sexual contact; see *sexually transmitted disease*, under *disease*.

ve•ne•re•ol•o•gist (və-nēr″e-ol′ə-jist) a specialist in venereology.

ve•ne•re•ol•o•gy (və-nēr″e-ol′ə-je) the branch of medicine that deals with sexually transmitted diseases.

vene•sec•tion (ven″ə-sek′shən) [*vena* + *section*] phlebotomy.

vene•su•ture (ven″ə-soo′chər) phleborrhaphy.

veni•punc•ture (ven′ĭ-punk″chər) phlebotomy (def. 2).

veni•sec•tion (ven″ĭ-sek′shən) phlebotomy.

veni•su•ture (ven″ĭ-soo′chər) phleborrhaphy.

ven•la•fax•ine hy•dro•chlo•ride (ven″lə-fak′sēn) a serotonin-norepinephrine reuptake inhibitor; used as an antidepressant and antianxiety agent, administered orally.

ven(o)- [L. *vena*, q.v.] a combining form denoting relationship to a vein. See also words beginning *phleb(o)-*.

ve•no•at•ri•al (ve″no-a′tre-əl) pertaining to the vena cava and the right atrium.

ve•noc•ly•sis (ve-nok′lĭ-sis) [*veno-* + *clysis*] phleboclysis.

Ve•no•fer (ve′no-fer) trademark for a preparation of iron sucrose.

ve•no•fi•bro•sis (ve″no-fi-bro′sis) phlebosclerosis.

Ve•no•glob•u•lin (ve″no-glob′u-lin) trademark for preparations of immune globulin intravenous (human).

ve•no•gram (ve′no-gram) 1. phlebogram. 2. a venous-pulse tracing.

ve•nog•ra•phy (ve-nog′rə-fe) phlebography (def. 1).

intraosseous v. radiography of the veins after injection of the contrast medium into bone marrow at an appropriate site, such as the iliac crest, ischium, pubic bones, greater trochanter, spinous processes of the vertebrae, or sternum.

portal v. portography.

splenic v. splenic portography.

ven•om (ven′əm) [L. *venenum* poison] a poison, especially one secreted by an animal such as a snake or arthropod.

Russell's viper v. the venom of Russell's viper, *Vipera russelli*, which acts in vitro as an intrinsic thromboplastin and is useful in defining deficiencies of coagulation factor X.

snake v. the poisonous secretion of snakes, containing hemotoxins, hemagglutinins, neurotoxins, leukotoxins, or endotheliotoxins. The venoms of various species have been used as hemostatics.

spider v. the venom of a spider such as *Atrax*, *Ctenus*, *Latrodectus*, or *Lycosa*.

ven•o•mo•sal•i•vary (ven″ə-mo-sal′ĭ-var″e) secreting a poisonous saliva.

ve•no•mo•tor (ve″no-mo′tər) pertaining to or producing constriction or dilatation of the veins.

ven•o•mous (ven′ə-məs) secreting venom; cf. *toxic*.

ve•no•oc•clu•sion (ve″no-ə-kloo′zhən) venous occlusion. **venoocclu′sive** *adj*

ve•no•peri•to•ne•os•to•my (ve″no-per″ĭ-to″ne-os′tə-me) [*veno-* + *peritoneostomy*] anastomosis of the saphenous vein with the peritoneum for permanent drainage of the peritoneal cavity in ascites.

ve•no•pres•sor (ve″no-pres′ər) 1. pertaining to venous blood pressure. 2. an agent that causes venous constriction.

ve•nor•rha•phy (ve-nor′ə-fe) [*veno-* + *-rrhaphy*] phleborrhaphy.

lateral v. suture of the lateral aspect of a vein after traumatic injury.

ve•no•scle•ro•sis (ve″no-sklə-ro′sis) phlebosclerosis.

ve•nose (ve′nōs) provided with veins.

ve•no•si•nal (ve″no-si′nəl) pertaining to the venae cavae and the right atrium of the heart.

ve•nos•i•ty (ve-nos′ĭ-te) 1. the condition of being venous. 2. excess of venous blood in a part. 3. a plentiful supply of veins.

ve•no•sta•sis (ve″no-sta′sis) [*veno-* + *-stasis*] venous stasis.

ve•not•o•my (ve-not′ə-me) phlebotomy.

ve•nous (ve′nəs) [L. *venosus*] of or pertaining to the veins.

ve•no•ve•nos•to•my (ve″no-ve-nos′tə-me) phlebophlebostomy.

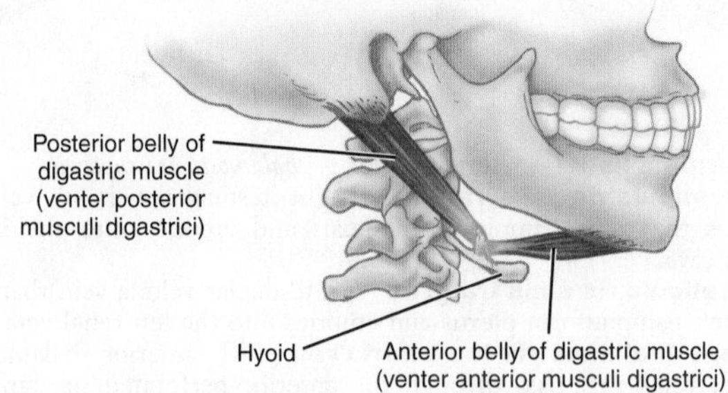

■ Venter anterior and ventor posterior (anterior and posterior bellies) of digastric muscle.

ve•no•ve•nous (ve″no-ve′nəs) beginning at a vein and ending at a vein, such as a tube for access in hemodialysis or hemofiltration.

vent (vent) [Fr. *fente* slit] 1. any opening or outlet; especially the anus. 2. an opening that discharges pus. 3. cloacal aperture.

Ven•ta•vis (ven′tə-vis) trademark for a preparation of iloprost.

ven•ter (ven′tər) pl. *ven′tres* [L. "belly"] 1. [TA] belly: anatomic terminology for a fleshy contractile part of a muscle. 2. abdomen. 3. any hollowed part or cavity.

v. ante′rior mus′culi digas′trici [TA] anterior belly of digastric muscle: the shorter belly of the digastric muscle, arising from the digastric fossa on the mandible and extending posteriorly to join the posterior belly through an intermediate tendon attached to the hyoid bone.

v. fronta′lis mus′culi occipitofronta′lis [TA] frontal belly of occipitofrontal muscle: a part that originates from the galea aponeurotica and inserts into the skin of the eyebrows and the root of the nose. Called also *musculus frontalis*.

v. infe′rior mus′culi omohyoi′dei [TA] inferior belly of omohyoid muscle: a narrow band that attaches to the superior margin of the scapula.

v. occipita′lis mus′culi occipitofronta′lis [TA] occipital belly of occipitofrontal muscle: a part that originates from the highest nuchal line of the occipital bone and inserts into the galea aponeurotica; called also *musculus occipitalis*.

v. poste′rior mus′culi digas′trici [TA] posterior belly of digastric muscle: the longer belly of the digastric muscle, arising from the mastoid notch of the temporal bone and extending anteriorly to join the anterior belly through an intermediate tendon attached to the hyoid bone.

v. supe′rior mus′culi omohyoi′dei [TA] superior belly of omohyoid muscle: a part that ascends and attaches to the hyoid bone.

ven•ti•la•tion (ven″tĭ-la′shən) [L. *ventilare* to fan, from *ventus* wind] 1. circulation, replacement, or purification of air or other gas in a defined or enclosed space. 2. in respiratory physiology, the process of exchange of air between the lungs and the environment, including *inhalation* and *exhalation*. See also *alveolar v.* and *pulmonary v.* Called also *breathing*, *pneusis*, and *respiration*. 3. in psychiatry, verbalization of one's problems, emotions, or feelings.

alveolar v. a fraction of the pulmonary ventilation, being the amount of air that reaches the alveoli and is available for gas exchange with the blood.

artificial v. see under *respiration*.

assist/control mode v. positive pressure ventilation in the assist-control mode (see under *mode*); if the spontaneous ventilation rate falls below a preset level, the ventilator enters the control mode.

assisted v. artificial respiration.

assist mode v. positive pressure ventilation in which the ventilator is in assist mode (see under *mode*); cf. *control mode v.* and *assist/control mode v.*

collateral v. the entrance of air into alveoli through pulmonary alveolar pores and other pathways so that a lobule may remain aerated even though its bronchiole is obstructed. Called also *collateral respiration*.

continuous positive pressure v. control mode ventilation using continuous positive airway pressure.

controlled v., controlled mechanical v. control mode v.

control mode v. positive pressure ventilation in which the ventilator is in control mode, with its cycle entirely controlled by the apparatus and not influenced by the patient's efforts at spontaneous ventilation. Called also *controlled* or *controlled mechanical v.*

downward v. ventilation of a building or room in which the outlets have places lower than those of the inlets.

exhausting v. ventilation of a building or room by means of an exhaust fan or some other process that withdraws the foul air.

expired air v. see under *resuscitation*.

high-frequency v. mechanical ventilation in which small tidal volumes are delivered at a high respiration rate; it may either be positive pressure ventilation or be delivered in the form of frequent jets of air.

intermittent mandatory v. (IMV) a type of control mode ventilation in which the patient breathes spontaneously while the ventilator delivers a positive-pressure breath at preset intervals. Cf. *intermittent positive-pressure breathing.*

intermittent mandatory v., synchronized (SIMV) positive pressure ventilation in which the patient breathes spontaneously while the ventilator delivers a positive-pressure breath at intervals that are predetermined but synchronized with the patient's breathing.

intermittent positive pressure v. see under *breathing.*

inverse ratio v. a type of assisted ventilation in which the length of inhalations is artificially increased until it is longer than the length of exhalations; it is believed to improve distribution of ventilation at lower airway-inflating pressures and to decrease intrapulmonary shunting. Used for patients with acute lung injury or acute respiratory distress syndrome that is refractory to other methods.

mandatory minute v. a type of intermittent positive pressure breathing designed to maintain a constant minute ventilation.

maximal voluntary v., maximum voluntary v. (MVV) the greatest volume of gas that can be breathed per minute by voluntary effort. Called also *maximal breathing capacity.*

mechanical v. ventilation accomplished by extrinsic means, usually distinguished as either *negative pressure v.* or *positive pressure v.* Cf. *spontaneous v.*

minute v. the total volume of gas in liters exhaled from the lungs per minute. See also *minute volume,* under *volume.* Called also *total v.*

natural v. ventilation of a building or room done without the aid of any special appliance.

negative pressure v. a type of mechanical ventilation in which negative pressure is generated on the outside of the patient's chest and transmitted to the interior of the thorax in order to expand the lungs and allow air to flow in; used primarily with patients having extreme weakness or paralysis of the chest muscles. See also *negative pressure ventilator,* under *ventilator.*

partial liquid v. ventilatory support in which the lungs are filled to the level of the functional residual capacity with a liquid perfluorocarbon; mechanical ventilation is then superimposed and oxygen and carbon dioxide are transferred through the liquid.

plenum v. ventilation of an entire building by fan blowers.

positive pressure v. any of numerous types of mechanical ventilation in which gas is delivered into the airways and lungs under positive pressure, producing positive airway pressure during inhalation; it may be done via either an endotracheal tube or a nasal mask.

pressure control v. positive pressure ventilation in which breaths are augmented by air at a fixed rate and amount of pressure, with tidal volume not being fixed; used particularly for patients with acute respiratory distress syndrome.

pressure support v. positive pressure ventilation in which the patient breathes spontaneously and breathing is augmented with air at a preset amount of pressure, with tidal volume not being fixed.

proportional assist v. positive pressure ventilation in which the ventilator can sense the patient's level of inspiratory flow and deliver pressure support to achieve a given tidal volume.

pulmonary v. a measure of the rate of ventilation, referring to the total exchange of air between the lungs and the ambient air, usually in liters per minute.

spontaneous v. breathing accomplished naturally, without artificial aids, as opposed to mechanical ventilation and other forms of artificial respiration.

total v. minute v.

upward v. ventilation of a building or room in which air is introduced below the place of its withdrawal.

vacuum v. ventilation of a room or building by the forced extraction of air.

ven·ti·la·tor (ven′tĭ-la″tər) 1. an apparatus designed to qualify the air that passes through it. 2. an apparatus used in artificial respiration, usually in mechanical ventilation (see under *ventilation*). Called also *inhaler* and *respirator.*

cuirass v. a type of negative pressure ventilator in which a cuirasslike apparatus either completely surrounds the trunk or is applied only to the front of the chest and abdomen, and allows intermittent negative pressure by evacuation of air to force the chest to expand. Called also *cuirass respirator.*

negative pressure v. a type of ventilator that uses negative pressure ventilation (q.v.) for patients having extreme weakness or paralysis of the chest muscles; the most common types are the Drinker respirator and the cuirass ventilator.

tank v. Drinker respirator.

ven·ti·la·to·ry (ven′tĭ-lə-tor″e) pertaining to ventilation.

Ven·to·lin (ven′tə-lin) trademark for preparations of albuterol.

ven·trad (ven′trad) [*ventr-* + *-ad*[1]] toward the abdomen, a venter, or a ventral aspect.

ven·tral (ven′trəl) [L. *ventralis*] 1. pertaining to the abdomen or to any venter. 2. denoting a position more toward the belly surface than some other object of reference; a synonym of *anterior* in human anatomy and of *inferior* in quadruped anatomy.

ven·tra·lis (vən-tra′lis) [TA] ventral.

ven·tral·ward (ven′trəl-wərd) ventrad.

ventri- see *ventr(o)-.*

ven·tri·cle (ven′trĭ-kəl) ventriculus (def. 1).

v. of Arantius the fossa rhomboidea, especially its lower end.

auxiliary v. an implanted pumping mechanism designed to assist the left ventricle of the heart in maintaining normal output, rate, and blood pressure; called also *booster heart.*

v's of brain, cerebral v's cavities within the brain that are filled with cerebrospinal fluid, including two lateral ventricles (see *ventriculus lateralis cerebri*), the third ventricle (see *ventriculus tertius cerebri*), and the fourth ventricle (see *ventriculus quartus cerebri*).

common v. a congenital anomaly caused by failure of formation of the interventricular septum, the heart having two atria and a single ventricle; called also *cor triloculare biatriatum* and *single v.*

double-inlet v. a congenital anomaly in which both atrioventricular valves or a single common atrioventricular valve open into a single heart ventricle, which usually resembles the left ventricle morphologically *(double-inlet left v.)* but may resemble the right *(double-inlet right v.)* or neither or both ventricles.

double-outlet left v. a rare congenital anomaly in which both great arteries arise from the left ventricle of the heart; it is often associated with a hypoplastic right ventricle, ventricular septal defect, valvular or subvalvular pulmonic stenosis, and a variety of associated malformations.

double-outlet right v. incomplete transposition of the great vessels in which both the aorta and the pulmonary artery arise from the right ventricle of the heart, associated with a ventricular septal defect. The defect may be remote from or close to either or both semilunar valves; it may be related to the aorta *(subaortic),* to the pulmonary trunk *(subpulmonic),* to both vessels *(doubly committed),* or to neither *(uncommitted);* and it may be associated with pulmonary stenosis.

Duncan v., fifth v. cavum septi pellucidi.

first v. of brain, first cerebral v. ventriculus lateralis cerebri.

fourth v. of brain, fourth cerebral v. ventriculus quartus cerebri.

Galen v. ventriculus laryngis.

v's of heart ventriculus cordis dexter and ventriculus cordis sinister (qq.v.).

laryngeal v. ventriculus laryngis.

lateral v. of brain, lateral cerebral v. ventriculus lateralis cerebri.

left v. of heart ventriculus cordis sinister.

Morgagni v. ventriculus laryngis.

pineal v. recessus pinealis.

right v. of heart ventriculus cordis dexter.

second v. of brain, second cerebral v. ventriculus lateralis cerebri.

single v. common ventricle.

sixth v. Verga v.

v. of Sylvius cavum septi pellucidi.

terminal v. of spinal cord ventriculus terminalis medullae spinalis.

third v. of brain, third cerebral v. ventriculus tertius cerebri.

Verga v. an occasional space (not a true ventricle) between the corpus callosum and the fornix; called also *sixth v.*

Vieussens v. cavum septi pellucidi.

ven·tri·cose (ven′trĭ-kōs) having an expansion or belly on one side.

ven·tric·u·lar (ven-trik′u-lər) pertaining to a ventricle.

ven·tric·u·li (ven-trik′u-li) [L.] genitive and plural of *ventriculus.*

ven·tric·u·li·tis (ven-trik″u-li′tis) inflammation of a ventricle, especially of a ventricle of the brain.

ventricul(o)- [L. *ventriculus,* dim. of *venter* belly] a combining form denoting relationship to a ventricle, of the heart or brain.

ven·tric·u·lo·atri·al (ven-trik″u-lo-a′tre-əl) connecting a cerebral ventricle with a cardiac atrium, as a shunt in the treatment of hydrocephalus.

ven·tric·u·lo·atri·os·to·my (ven-trik″u-lo-a″tre-os′tə-me) ventriculoatrial shunt.

ven·tric·u·lo·cis·ter·nos·to·my (ven-trik″u-lo-sis″tər-nos′tə-me) ventriculocisternal shunt.

ven·tric·u·lo·en·ceph·a·li·tis (ven-trik″u-lo-en-sef″ə-li′tis) [*ventriculo-* + *encephalitis*] ventriculitis accompanied by encephalitis.

cytomegalovirus v. a late-appearing type of cytomegalovirus encephalitis seen in immunocompromised patients, characterized by high protein levels and pleocytosis of the cerebrospinal fluid, encephalitis, cranial nerve deficits, ventriculomegaly with necrotizing ventriculitis, and sometimes ascending muscle weakness with nystagmus.

ven•tric•u•lo•gram (ven-trik′u-lo-gram) a radiograph of the cerebral ventricles or of the ventricles of the heart.

ven•tric•u•log•ra•phy (ven-trik″u-log′rə-fe) [*ventriculo-* + *-graphy*] 1. radiography of the head following removal of cerebrospinal fluid from the cerebral ventricles and its replacement by air or other contrast medium. 2. radiography of a ventricle of the heart after injection of a contrast medium.

first pass v. see under *angiocardiography*.

gated blood pool v. equilibrium radionuclide angiocardiography.

left v. cineangiography of the heart after insertion of a catheter into the left ventricle, usually retrograde across the aortic valve, and injection of iodinated contrast material; used to assess various ventricular function parameters and to detect regurgitation through the atrioventricular valves.

radionuclide v. see under *angiocardiography*.

ven•tric•u•lo•meg•a•ly (ven-trik″u-lo-meg′ə-le) [*ventriculo-* + *-megaly*] gross enlargement of a ventricle of the brain, as by hydrocephalus.

ven•tric•u•lom•e•try (ven-trik″u-lom′ə-tre) [*ventriculo-* + *-metry*] the measurement of the intraventricular (intracranial) pressure.

ven•tric•u•lo•my•ot•o•my (ven-trik″u-lo-mi-ot′ə-me) incision of the muscular wall of the heart.

ven•tric•u•lo•peri•to•ne•al (ven-trik″u-lo-per″ĭ-to-ne′əl) connecting a cerebral ventricle with the peritoneum, as a shunt in the treatment of hydrocephalus.

ven•tric•u•lo•punc•ture (ven-trik′u-lo-pungk″chər) ventricular puncture.

ven•tric•u•lo•scope (ven-trik′u-lo-skōp) an endoscope for examining the cerebral ventricles and for cauterizing the choroid plexus.

ven•tric•u•los•co•py (ven-trik″u-los′kə-pe) [*ventriculo-* + *-scopy*] direct examination of the cerebral ventricles by means of an endoscope or cystoscope.

ven•tric•u•los•ti•um (ven-trik″u-los′te-əm) [*ventriculo-* + *ostium*] an artificial opening created between one of the cerebral ventricles and the external surface of the brain; see also *shunt*.

ven•tric•u•los•to•my (ven-trik″u-los′tə-me) [*ventriculo-* + *-stomy*] the operation of establishing a free communication or shunt between the floor of the third ventricle and the underlying cisterna interpeduncularis; for the treatment of hydrocephalus.

ven•tric•u•lo•sub•arach•noid (ven-trik″u-lo-sub″ə-rak′noid) pertaining to the cerebral ventricles and the subarachnoid spaces.

ven•tric•u•lot•o•my (ven-trik″u-lot′ə-me) [*ventriculo-* + *-tomy*] incision of a ventricle of the brain or heart.

partial encircling endocardial v. the encompassing and isolation of visible areas of endocardial fibrosis in the left ventricle by an incision extending partway through the endocardium; done to relieve ventricular tachycardia in patients with ischemic heart disease.

ven•tric•u•lo•ve•nos•to•my (ven-trik″u-lo-ve-nos′tə-me) ventriculovenous shunt.

ven•tric•u•lus (ven-trik′u-ləs) pl. *ventri′culi* [L., dim. of *venter* belly] 1. ventricle: a small, normal cavity in an organ such as the heart or brain. 2. gaster. 3. the midgut of an invertebrate.

v. cor′dis dex′ter [TA] right ventricle of heart: the lower chamber of the right side of the heart, which pumps venous blood through the pulmonary trunk and arteries to the capillaries of the lungs. See illustration and Plate 18.

v. cor′dis sinis′ter [TA] left ventricle of heart: the lower chamber of the left side of the heart, which pumps oxygenated blood out through the aorta into the systemic arteries. See illustration and Plate 18.

v. laryn′gis [TA] laryngeal ventricle: a lateral evagination of mucous membrane between the vocal and vestibular folds, reaching nearly to the angle of the thyroid cartilage.

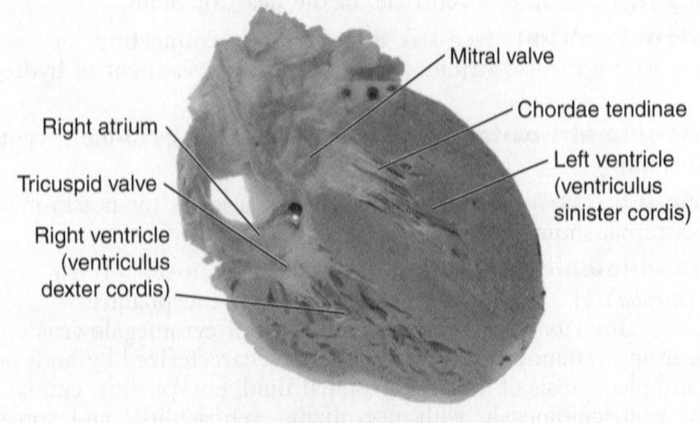

■ Ventricles of the heart.

v. latera′lis ce′rebri [TA] lateral ventricle of brain: the cavity in each cerebral hemisphere, derived (developed) from the cavity of the embryonic neural tube; it consists of a central part or body (pars centralis) and three horns: the frontal horn (cornu frontale), temporal horn (cornu temporale), and occipital horn (cornu occipitale) in the frontal, temporal, and occipital lobes, respectively. The body and occipital and temporal horns meet at the atrium of the lateral ventricle. The two lateral ventricles are separated from each other by the septum pellucidum, and each communicates with the third ventricle by an interventricular foramen, through which the choroid plexuses of the lateral ventricles become continuous with that of the third ventricle; these foramina also allow cerebrospinal fluid formed in the lateral ventricle to flow into the third ventricle. Called also *lateral cerebral ventricle*.

v. quar′tus ce′rebri [TA] fourth ventricle of brain: an irregularly shaped cavity in the rhombencephalon, between the medulla oblongata, the pons, and the isthmus in front, and the cerebellum behind; it is continuous with the central canal of the cord below and with the cerebral aqueduct above, and through its lateral and median apertures it communicates with the subarachnoid space. Called also *fourth cerebral ventricle*.

v. termina′lis medul′lae spina′lis [TA] terminal ventricle of spinal cord: a saclike expansion of the central canal of the spinal cord within the conus medullaris.

v. ter′tius ce′rebri [TA] third ventricle of brain: a narrow cleft below the corpus callosum, within the diencephalon between the two thalami. Its floor is formed by the optic chiasm and infundibular area, its anterior wall by the lamina terminalis, and its roof by ependyma. It communicates with the lateral ventricles by the interventricular foramina, and with the fourth ventricle by the cerebral aqueduct. Called also *third cerebral ventricle*.

ven•tri•cum•bent (ven″trĭ-kum′bənt) [*ventri-* + L. *cumbere* to lie] lying upon the belly; prone.

ven•tri•duct (ven′trĭ-dukt) [*ventri-* + *duct*] to bring or carry ventrad.

ven•tri•duc•tion (ven″trĭ-duk′shən) the act of drawing a part ventrad.

ven•tri•flex•ion (ven″trĭ-flek′shən) [*ventri-* + *flexion*] flexion toward the belly or ventral surface.

ven•tri•me•sal (ven″trĭ-me′səl) pertaining to the ventrimeson.

ven•trim•e•son (vən-trim′ə-son) [*ventri-* + *meson*] the middle line on the ventral surface.

ventr(o)- [L. *venter* belly or abdomen] a combining form denoting relationship to the belly, or to the front (anterior) aspect of the body. Also, *ventri-*.

ven•tro•cys•tor•rha•phy (ven″tro-sis-tor′ə-fe) the stitching of a cyst, or of the bladder, to the abdominal wall.

ven•tro•dor•sad (ven″tro-dor′sad) from the ventral toward the dorsal aspect.

ven•tro•dor•sal (ven″tro-dor′səl) pertaining to the ventral and dorsal surfaces.

ven•tro•fix•a•tion (ven″tro-fik-sa′shən) [*ventro-* + *fixation*] the operation of suspending the retroplaced uterus to the abdominal wall. Cf. *hysteropexy*.

ven•tro•hys•tero•pexy (ven″tro-his′tər-o-pek″se) ventrofixation.

ven•tro•in•gui•nal (ven″tro-ing′gwĭ-nəl) inguinoabdominal.

ven•tro•lat•er•al (ven″tro-lat′ər-əl) both ventral and lateral.

ven•tro•me•di•an (ven″tro-me′de-ən) both ventral and median.

ven•tro•pos•te•ri•or (ven″tro-pos-tēr′e-ər) both ventral and posterior.

ven•trop•to•sis (ven″trop-to′sis, ven″tro-to′sis) gastroptosis.

ven•tros•co•py (ven-tros′kə-pe) peritoneoscopy.

ven•trose (ven′trōs) having a bellylike expansion.

ven•tro•sus•pen•sion (ven″tro-səs-pen′shən) ventrofixation.

ven•trot•o•my (ven-trot′ə-me) laparotomy.

Ven•tu•ri mask (ven-too′re) [Giovanni Battista *Venturi*, Italian physicist, 1746–1822] see under *mask*.

ven•tu•rim•e•ter (ven″tu-rim′ə-tər) [G.B. *Venturi* + *-meter*] an instrument for measuring the flow of liquids, as of the blood in vessels, by relating difference of pressures between a constricted and a nonconstricted portion of a tube through which fluid is flowing.

ven•u•la (ven′u-lə) pl. *ven′ulae* [L., dim. of *vena*] [TA] venule.

v. macula′ris infe′rior [TA] inferior macular venule: the inferior venule draining blood from the macula lutea.

v. macula′ris me′dia [TA] medial macular venule: a small branch draining blood from the central region of the retina to the central retinal vein.

v. macula′ris supe′rior [TA] superior macular venule: the superior venule draining blood from the macula lutea.

v. nasa′lis re′tinae infe′rior [TA] inferior nasal venule of retina: a small vein returning blood from the inferior nasal region of the retina to the central vein.

v. nasa′lis re′tinae supe′rior [TA] superior nasal venule of retina: a small vein returning blood from the superior nasal region of the retina to the central vein.

ve′nulae rec′tae re′nis [TA] straight venules of kidney: venules that drain the papillary part of the kidney and empty into the arcuate veins.

v. tempora′lis re′tinae infe′rior [TA] inferior temporal venule of retina: a small vein returning blood from the inferior temporal region of the retina to the central vein.

v. tempora′lis re′tinae supe′rior [TA] superior temporal venule of retina: a small vein returning blood from the superior temporal region of the retina to the central vein.

ven•u•lae (ven′u-le) [L.] genitive and plural of *venula.*

ven•ule (ven′ūl) venula; any of the small vessels that collect blood from the capillary plexuses and join to form veins. ven′ular *adj*

high endothelial v's specialized postcapillary venules with tall cuboidal endothelial cells, found in lymph nodes and gut-associated lymphoid tissue; they are the sites where lymphocytes recirculate from blood to lymph, binding specifically to the endothelial cells and then passing between them. Called also *postcapillary v's.*

macular v. see *venula macularis inferior* and *venula macularis superior.*

nasal v. of retina see *venula nasalis retinae inferior* and *venula nasalis retinae superior.*

postcapillary v. venous capillary.

stellate v's of kidney venae stellatae renis.

straight v's of kidney venulae rectae renis.

temporal v. of retina see *venula temporalis retinae inferior* and *venula temporalis retinae superior.*

ven•u•lec•ta•sia (ven″u-lek-ta′zhə) a type of telangiectasia formed by a venule that has become distended and protrudes as a blue lesion on the skin.

ven•u•li•tis (ven″u-li′tis) inflammation of a venule or venules.

cutaneous necrotizing v. necrotizing vasculitis of venules of the skin, usually of the limbs, caused by deposition of circulating immune complexes; it may be associated with infection, chronic disease, or drug administration, or be idiopathic. Manifestations are variable, the most common being palpable purpura, angioedema, urticaria, and deposition of fibrinoid material and cellular infiltrates.

VEP visual evoked potential.

Ve•Pe•sid (ve″pe′sid) trademark for a preparation of etoposide.

Ver•al•ba (vər-al′bə) trademark for a mixture of protoveratrines A and B.

ve•rap•a•mil hy•dro•chlo•ride (və-rap′ə-mil) a calcium channel blocking agent that dilates coronary arteries and decreases myocardial oxygen demand, administered orally in the treatment and prophylaxis of angina pectoris, in the treatment of hypertension, and in the prophylaxis of supraventricular tachyarrhythmias, and used intravenously in the treatment of supraventricular tachyarrhythmias.

Ve•ra•trum (ve-ra′trəm) [L.] a genus of plants of the genus Liliaceae. Some species contain antihypertensive alkaloids that are used medicinally; most are poisonous when eaten.

V. al′bum the European or white hellebore, a poisonous variety that is a source of the protoveratrines; it is also used in folk medicine and homeopathy.

V. califor′nicum skunk cabbage, a variety found in the western United States that contains teratogenic alkaloids, causing cyclopia and other conditions in fetal sheep when their mothers eat the plant.

V. viri′de the American or green hellebore, a poisonous variety formerly important in folk medicine and homeopathy but no longer used because of its high toxicity.

ver•bal (vur′bəl) consisting of words; pertaining to words or speech.

Ver•be•na (vər-be′nə) a genus of herbs of the family Verbenaceae, mostly native to the Americas. *V. triphyl′la* L. is the source of verbenone.

ver•be•none (vər-be′nōn) a terpene ketone from *Verbena triphylla,* an American herb.

ver•big•er•a•tion (vər-bij″ər-a′shən) [L. *verbigerare* to chatter] stereotyped and meaningless repetition of words and phrases; seen in some cases of schizophrenia. See also *logorrhea* and *perseveration.* Called also *cataphasia.*

ver•bo•ma•nia (vur″bo-ma′ne-ə) logorrhea.

Ver•cyte (vur′sīt) trademark for a preparation of pipobroman.

ver•do•he•mo•glo•bin (ver″do-he″mo-glo″bin) choleglobin.

ver•do•per•ox•i•dase (ver″do-pər-ok′sĭ-dās) peroxidase (def. 2).

Ver•e•lan (ver′ə-lan) trademark for a preparation of verapamil hydrochloride.

Ve•ress needle (və-res′) [J. *Veress,* German surgeon, 20th century] see under *needle.*

Ver•ga lacrimal groove, ventricle (ver′gah) [Andrea *Verga,* Italian neurologist, 1811–1895] see under *groove* and *ventricle.*

verge (vurj) a circumference, or ring.

anal v. linea anocutanea.

ver•gence (vur′jəns) [L. *vergere* to bend] 1. the amount of convergence or divergence of a pencil of rays entering or leaving a lens or mirror, expressed as the reciprocal of the distance from the lens or mirror to the focus of the rays. For rays through a principal focus, the vergence is equal to the focal power of the lens or mirror. See *convergence* (def. 2) and *divergence* (def. 1). 2. a disjunctive reciprocal rotation of both eyes around their horizontal, vertical, or anteroposterior axes such that the axes of fixation are not parallel. The kind of vergence is indicated by a prefix. See *convergence* (def. 3), *divergence* (def. 2), *infravergence, supravergence,* and see *duction* and *version* (def. 5).

ver•gen•cy (vur′jən-se) vergence.

Ver•hey•en stars (ver-hi′en) [Philippe *Verheyen,* Flemish anatomist, 1648–1710] venae stellatae renis.

Ver•hoeff stain (vur′hef) [Frederick Herman *Verhoeff,* American ophthalmologist, 1874–1968] see *Stains and Staining Methods,* under *stain.*

Ver•hoeff-van Gie•son stain (vur′hef van ge′sən) [F.H. *Verhoeff;* Ira *van Gieson,* American neuropathologist, 1865–1913] see *Stains and Staining Methods,* under *stain.*

ver•mes (vur′mēz) [L.] plural of *vermis.*

ver•mi•an (vur′me-ən) pertaining to the vermis cerebelli.

Ver•mi•cel•la (vur″mĭ-sel′ə) [L.] a genus of mildly venomous Australian snakes.

ver•mi•ci•dal (vur″mĭ-si′dəl) anthelmintic (def. 1).

ver•mi•cide (vur′mĭ-sīd) anthelmintic (def. 2).

ver•mic•u•lar (vər-mik′u-lər) [L. *vermicularis*] wormlike in shape or appearance; called also *helminthoid* and *vermiculous.*

ver•mic•u•la•tion (vər-mik″u-la′shən) [L. *vermiculatio,* from *vermis* worm] 1. wormlike movement. 2. peristalsis.

ver•mi•cule (vur′mĭ-kūl) a wormlike structure; see also *ookinete.*

ver•mic•u•lous (vər-mik′u-ləs) 1. vermicular. 2. verminous.

ver•mi•form (vur′mĭ-form) [L. *vermiformis,* from *vermis* worm + *forma* shape] shaped like a worm.

ver•mif•u•gal (vər-mif′u-gəl) anthelmintic (def. 1).

ver•mi•fuge (vur′mĭ-fūj) anthelmintic (def. 2).

ver•mil•ion•ec•to•my (vər-mil″yon-ek′tə-me) excision of the vermilion border of the lip, the surgically created defect being resurfaced by advancement of the undermined labial mucosa.

ver•min (vur′min) [L. *vermis* worm] 1. any small animal, insect, or worm that is a nuisance to humans; sometimes limited to parasitic animals. 2. nuisance animals or ectoparasites collectively.

ver•mi•nal (vur′mĭ-nəl) verminous.

ver•mi•na•tion (vur″mĭ-na′shən) 1. infestation with vermin; called also *verminosis.* 2. helminthiasis.

ver•mi•no•sis (vur″mĭ-no′sis) 1. vermination (def. 1). 2. helminthiasis.

ver•mi•nous (vur′mĭ-nəs) [L. *verminosus*] 1. pertaining to, due to, or abounding in worms. 2. pertaining to, due to, or abounding in vermin. Called also *verminal.*

ver•mis (vur′mis) [L. "worm"] a wormlike structure, particularly the vermis cerebelli.

cerebellar v., v. cerebel′li [TA] the narrow median part of the cerebellum, between the two lateral hemispheres; the *cranial* or *superior* portion extends from the lingula to the folium vermis, and the *inferior* or *caudal* portion from the tuber vermis to the nodulus. It is subdivided into lobules, designated I–X; see also *cerebellum.*

ver•mix (vur′miks) appendix vermiformis.

Ver•mox (vur′moks) trademark for preparations of mebendazole.

ver•nal (vur′nəl) [L. *vernalis* of the spring] pertaining to or occurring in the spring.

Ver•ner-Mor•ri•son syndrome (vur′nər mor′ĭ-sən) [John Victor *Verner,* American physician, born 1927; Ashton Byrom *Morrison,* American physician, born 1922] see under *syndrome.*

Ver•net syndrome (vār-na′) [Maurice *Vernet,* French neurologist, 1887–1974] see under *syndrome.*

Ver•neuil canals, disease, neuroma (vār-nwe′) [Aristide August Stanislaus *Verneuil,* French surgeon, 1823–1895] see under *canal;* see *hidradenitis suppurativa;* and see *plexiform neurofibroma,* under *neurofibroma.*

Ver•nier acuity (vār-nya′) [Pierre *Vernier,* French physicist, 1580–1637] see *displacement threshold,* under *threshold.*

ver•ni•er (vur′ne-ər) [Pierre *Vernier*] a finely graduated scale accessory to a more coarsely graduated one for measuring fractions of the divisions of the latter.

ver•nix (vur′niks) [L. "sandarac" (resin), from Gr. *Berenikē* (now *Benghazi*) where first made] varnish.
v. **caseo′sa** ["cheesy varnish"] an unctuous substance composed of sebum and desquamated epithelial cells, which covers the skin of the fetus.

Ver•no•nia (vər-no′ne-ə) a genus of mostly tropical herbs and shrubs of the family Compositae. *V. anthelmin′tica* Willd. is an Indian species used as an anthelmintic, abortifacient, and treatment for skin diseases.

Ver•o•cay bodies (ver′o-ka) [José *Verocay,* Czechoslovakian pathologist, 1876–1927] see under *body.*

ver•o•cy•to•tox•in (ver″o-si′to-tok″sin) either of two toxins closely related to the Shiga toxin, found in *Shigella dysenteriae* type I and some strains of *Escherichia coli;* they cause one type of hemolytic uremic syndrome. Humans are infected by ingesting undercooked meat, unpasteurized milk, and foods contaminated with cattle feces. Called also *Shiga-like toxin.*

Ve•ron•i•cel•la (və-ron″ĭ-sel′ə) a genus of slugs of the family Veronicellidae, order Pulmonata. *V. leydi′gi* and other species are intermediate hosts of *Angiostrongylus cantonensis* on various islands in the Pacific.

ver•o•tox•in (ver′o-tok″sin) [*Vero* cells, q.v.] either of two enterotoxins, designated I and II, elaborated by certain enterohemorrhagic serovars of *Escherichia coli;* both are cytotoxic to intestinal villi and colonic epithelial cells and v. I is also cytotoxic to vascular endothelial cells. They are similar to toxins of *Shigella dysenteriae* and have been implicated in at least some cases of hemorrhagic colitis and enterocolitis.

ver•ru•ca (və-roo′kə) gen. and pl. *verru′cae* [L.] wart.
v. **acumina′ta** condyloma acuminatum.
v. **filifor′mis** filiform wart.
v. **necroge′nica** see *tuberculosis verrucosa cutis.*
v. **perua′na, v. peruvia′na** verruga peruana.
v. **pla′na, v. pla′na juveni′lis** a type of small, smooth, flat, usually skin colored wart seen on the hands, arms, or face in children and less often in adults, caused by a human papillomavirus; they sometimes occur in large numbers and in linear distributions. Called also *flat* or *plane wart.* See also *epidermodysplasia verruciformis.*
v. **planta′ris** plantar wart.
v. **seborrhe′ica** seborrheic keratosis.
v. **vulga′ris** common wart.

ver•ru•cae (və-roo′se) [L.] genitive and plural of *verruca.*

ver•ru•ca•rin (və-roo′kə-rin) any of several trichothecene mycotoxins found in species of *Stachybotrys,* especially *S. alternans,* causing stachybotryotoxicosis.

ver•ru•ci•form (və-roo′sĭ-form) [*verruca* + *form*] resembling a wart.

ver•ru•cose (və-roo′kōs) warty.

ver•ru•co•sis (ver″oo-ko′sis) the presence of multiple warts.

ver•ru•cous (və-roo′kəs) warty.

ver•ru•ga (və-roo′gə) [Sp.] wart.
v. **perua′na** the second or chronic stage of bartonellosis; called also *verruca peruana* or *peruviana, hemorrhagic pian,* and *Peruvian wart.*

Ver•sa•pen (vur′sə-pen) trademark for preparations of hetacillin.

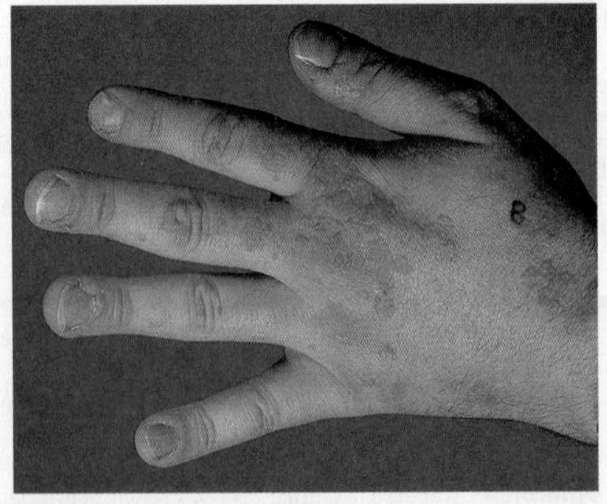

■ Verrucae planae.

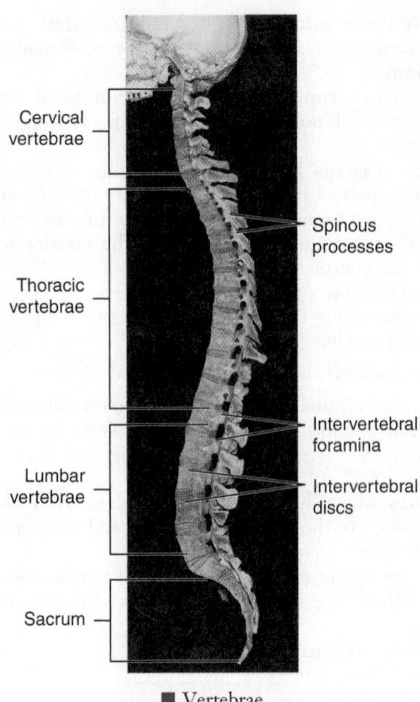

■ Vertebrae.

Ver•sed (ver-sed′) trademark for a preparation of midazolam.

ver•si•can (vur′sĭ-kan) a small proteoglycan of the extracellular matrix, consisting of a 260-kD core with associated chondroitin sulfate and oligosaccharide chains; it plays a role in cell signaling.

ver•si•co•lor (vur″si-kul′ər) [L. *vertere* to turn + *color*] 1. variegated; having a variety of colors. 2. changing in color.

ver•sion (vur′zhən) [L. *versio,* turning] 1. the act or process of turning something or of changing direction. 2. the situation of an organ or part in relation to an established normal position. 3. in gynecology, the tilting of the uterus; cf. *flexion* (def. 2). 4. in obstetrics, the manual conversion of or changing of the polarity of the fetus with reference to the mother; cf. *presentation.* 5. in ophthalmology, the conjugate rotation of both eyes in the same direction. See *infraversion* and *sursumversion,* and see *duction* and *vergence* (def. 2).
abdominal v. external v.
bimanual v. version done by combined external and internal manipulation, the cervix being open enough to admit the hand; called also *combined v.*
bipolar v. version done by purely external manipulation or by combined internal and external manipulation.
Braxton Hicks v. internal podalic version performed through a partially but not completely dilated cervix; done only on a nonviable fetus.
cephalic v. version in which the fetal head is brought down into the maternal pelvis.
combined v. bimanual v.
external v. manipulation of the fetal body applied through the abdominal wall of the mother.
Hicks v. Braxton Hicks v.
internal v. turning of the fetus with the obstetrician's hand or fingers inserted through the dilated cervix.
pelvic v. version done by manipulating the buttocks of the fetus.
podalic v. version in which one or both lower limbs of the fetus are brought down into the maternal pelvis.
Potter v. podalic version in head presentation when the cervix is fully effaced and dilated.
spontaneous v. conversion of an abnormal position of the fetus into a relatively normal one without use of manipulation.
Wigand v. external conversion of a transverse lie into a cephalic presentation, accomplished by pushing the fetal head down with one hand and buttocks up with the other; called also *Wigand maneuver.*

ver•te•bra (vur′tə-brə) gen. and pl. *ver′tebrae* [L.] [TA] any of the thirty-three bones of the vertebral column (columna vertebralis), comprising the seven *cervical,* twelve *thoracic,* five *lumbar,* five *sacral,* and four *coccygeal* vertebrae. **ver′tebral** *adj*
abdominal vertebrae vertebrae lumbales.
basilar v. the lowest or last of the lumbar vertebrae.
caudal vertebrae, caudate vertebrae 1. coccygeal vertebrae. 2. the vertebrae in the tail of an animal.

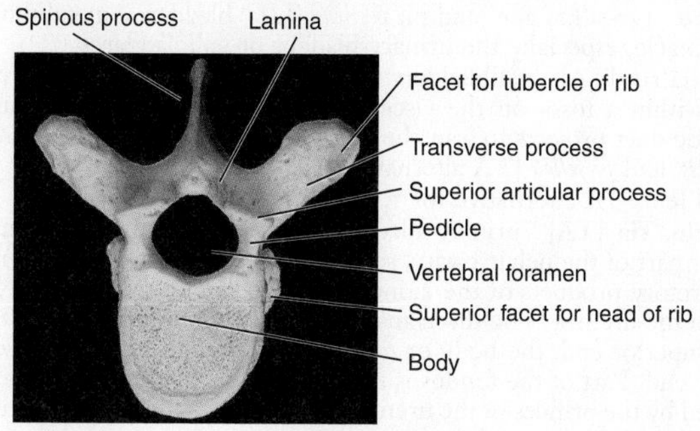

■ Typical (seventh) thoracic vertebra viewed from above.

cervical vertebrae, ver′tebrae cervica′les [TA] the upper seven vertebrae, constituting the skeleton of the neck. Symbols C1 through C7.

ver′tebrae coccy′geae, coccygeal vertebrae the lowest segments of the vertebral column, comprising three to five fused rudimentary vertebrae that constitute the coccyx.

v. denta′ta the second cervical vertebra (*axis* [TA]).

dorsal vertebrae vertebrae thoracicae.

false vertebrae the vertebrae that become fused, i.e., the sacral and coccygeal vertebrae.

ver′tebrae lumba′les [TA], **lumbar vertebrae** [TA] the five vertebrae between the thoracic vertebrae and the sacrum. Symbols L1 through L5.

v. mag′na os sacrum.

odontoid v. the second cervical vertebra (*axis* [TA]).

v. pla′na a condition of spondylitis in which the body of the vertebra is reduced to a sclerotic disk; often due to eosinophilic granuloma.

v. pro′minens [TA] prominent vertebra: the seventh cervical vertebra, so called because of the length of its spinous process, although it is only the spine that is prominent. NOTE: The spinous process of the first thoracic vertebra is often more prominent.

sacral vertebrae, ver′tebrae sacra′les the segments (usually five) below the lumbar vertebrae, which are normally fused, forming the sacrum. Symbols S1–S5.

sternal v. sternebra.

thoracic vertebrae, ver′tebrae thora′cicae [TA] the vertebrae, usually twelve in number, situated between the cervical and the lumbar vertebrae, giving attachment to the ribs and forming part of the posterior wall of the thorax. Symbols T1 through T12.

true vertebrae the vertebrae that normally remain unfused throughout life, i.e., the cervical, thoracic, and lumbar vertebrae.

ver•te•brae (vur′tə-bre) [L.] genitive and plural of *vertebra.*

ver•te•brar•te•ri•al (vur″tə-brahr-tēr′e-əl) vertebroarterial.

Ver•te•bra•ta (vur″tə-bra′tə) a subphylum of the Chordata comprising all animals that have a vertebral column, including mammals, birds, reptiles, amphibians, and fishes.

ver•te•brate (vur′tə-brāt) [L. *vertebratus*] 1. having a vertebral column. 2. any member of the subphylum Vertebrata.

ver•te•brate col•la•gen•ase (vur′tə-brāt kol′ə-jen-ās) see under *collagenase.*

ver•te•brat•ed (vur′tə-brāt′əd) made up of joints resembling the vertebrae.

ver•te•brec•to•my (vur″tə-brek′tə-me) [*vertebr-* + *-ectomy*] excision of a vertebra.

vertebr(o)- [L. *vertebra,* q.v.] a combining form denoting relationship to a vertebra, or to the vertebral column.

ver•te•bro•ar•te•ri•al (vur″tə-bro-ahr-tēr′e-əl) 1. pertaining to vertebrae and arteries. 2. pertaining to the vertebral artery. Called also *vertebrarterial.*

ver•te•bro•bas•i•lar (vur″tə-bro-bas′ĭ-lər) pertaining to or involving the vertebral and basilar arteries.

ver•te•bro•ca•rot•id (vur″tə-bro-kə-rot′id) caroticovertebral.

ver•te•bro•chon•dral (vur″tə-bro-kon′drəl) pertaining to a vertebra and a costal cartilage.

ver•te•bro•cos•tal (vur″tə-bro-kos′təl) [*vertebro-* + *costal*] pertaining to a vertebra and a rib.

ver•te•bro•did•y•mus (vur″tə-bro-did′ĭ-məs) [*vertebro-* + *-didymus*] conjoined twins united in the region of the vertebral column.

ver•te•bro•fem•or•al (vur″tə-bro-fem′ə-rəl) relating to the vertebrae and the femur.

ver•te•bro•gen•ic (vur″tə-bro-jen′ik) arising in a vertebra or in the vertebral column.

ver•te•bro•il•i•ac (vur″tə-bro-il′e-ak) pertaining to the vertebrae and the ilium.

ver•te•bro•mam•ma•ry (vur″tə-bro-mam′ə-re) pertaining to or extending between the vertebral column and the pectoral region.

ver•te•bro•plas•ty (vur′tə-bro-plas″te) [*vertebro-* + *-plasty*] plastic repair of a vertebra. **vertebroplas′tic** *adj*

percutaneous v. injection of polymethacrylate cement into a vertebra for spinal stabilization and relief of pain in the treatment of osteoporotic compression fractures.

ver•te•bro•sa•cral (vur″tə-bro-sa′krəl) pertaining to the vertebrae and the sacrum.

ver•te•bro•ster•nal (vur″tə-bro-stur′nəl) pertaining to the vertebrae and the sternum.

ver•te•por•fin (vur″tə-por′fin) [USP] a photosensitizer that accumulates preferentially in blood vessels formed through neovascularization, such as those in the choroid; it is activated by nonthermal light (689 nm) in the presence of oxygen, and causes local damage to the neovascular endothelium followed by vessel occlusion; administered intravenously prior to irradiation of the lesion with 689 nm wavelength light from a compatible laser in the treatment of neovascularization due to disciform macular degeneration, presumed ocular histoplasmosis, or pathologic myopia.

ver•tex (vur′teks) pl. *ver′tices* [L.] 1. a summit or top. 2. [TA] the top or crown of the head.

v. cor′neae [TA] vertex of cornea: the central, thinner portion of the cornea.

ver•ti•cal (vur′tĭ-kəl) 1. perpendicular to the plane of the horizon; see also *verticalis.* 2. relating to the vertex. 3. relating to or occupying different levels in a hierarchy, as the spread from one generation to another in vertical transmission.

ver•ti•ca•lis (vur″tĭ-ka′lis) [L.] [TA] vertical: a term denoting relationship to this orientation when the body is in the anatomical, i.e., the upright, position.

ver•tic•il•late (vər-tis′ĭ-lāt) [L. *vertex* a whorl] arranged in the form of a whorl.

Ver•ti•cil•li•um (vur″tĭ-sil′e-əm) a genus of Fungi Imperfecti of the form-class Hyphomycetes, form-family Moniliaceae. Some species cause apple wilt, and some contain trichothecenes and can cause alimentary toxic aleukia. A species called *V. gra′phii,* isolated from otitis externa and mycotic keratitis, may actually be a species of *Trichosporon.*

ver•ti•co•men•tal (vur″tĭ-ko-men′təl) pertaining to the vertex and the chin.

ver•ti•go (vur′tĭ-go) [L. *vertigo*] an illusory sense that either the environment or one's own body is revolving; it may result from diseases of the internal ear or may be due to disturbances of the vestibular centers or pathways in the central nervous system. The term is sometimes erroneously used to mean any form of dizziness. Cf. *dysequilibrium.* **vertig′inous** *adj*

alternobaric v. a transient vertigo sometimes affecting those such as caisson workers and members of airplane crews who are subjected to large, rapid variations in barometric pressure; see also *barotrauma.* Called also *pressure v.*

angiopathic v. vertigo due to arteriosclerosis of cerebral vessels, particularly the vertebral or basilar arteries; called also *arteriosclerotic v.*

apoplectic v. scotodinia.

arteriosclerotic v. angiopathic v.

benign paroxysmal v. of childhood a form of paroxysmal vertigo occurring in young children otherwise in good health; sudden attacks are accompanied by pallor, sweating, and immobility and less often by vomiting and nystagmus.

benign paroxysmal positional v., benign paroxysmal postural v. recurrent brief periods of positional vertigo and nystagmus occurring when the head is placed in certain positions such as with one ear down. It is due to otolithiasis that causes exaggerated movement of the endolymph.

benign positional v., benign postural v. benign paroxysmal positional v.

central v. vertigo due to disease of the central nervous system. See also *cerebral v.*

cerebral v. vertigo resulting from a brain lesion, such as a cerebellar infarct. Called also *organic v.*

cervical v. vertigo after injury to the neck such as whiplash.

disabling positional v. constant positional vertigo or dysequilibrium and nausea in the upright position, without hearing disturbance or loss of vestibular function.

encephalic v. a sensation of movement of tissues within the skull, as of the brain turning over and over.

endemic paralytic v. vestibular neuronitis.

epidemic v. vestibular neuronitis.
epileptic v. vertigo that accompanies epilepsy, usually as part of an aura. See also *vertiginous epilepsy.*
essential v. vertigo whose cause is unknown.
gastric v. vertigo associated with stomach disease.
height v. dizziness (not a true vertigo) felt on looking down from a high location.
horizontal v. positional vertigo experienced when a person lies down.
labyrinthine v. Meniere disease.
laryngeal v. tussive syncope.
lateral v. vertigo caused by rapidly passing a row of similar objects, such as a fence or a series of pillars.
mechanical v. vertigo due to long-continued turning or vibration of the body, as in motion sickness.
nocturnal v. a sensation of falling occurring as the subject is going to sleep.
objective v. vertigo experienced as objects moving around the observer, in contrast to subjective vertigo.
ocular v. vertigo due to eye disease, especially paralysis of or lack of balance in the eye muscles.
organic v. cerebral v.
paralytic v. vestibular neuronitis.
paralyzing v. vertigo so severe that the patient is afraid to move.
paroxysmal v. vertigo occurring in sudden, brief attacks; see *benign paroxysmal positional v.* and *benign paroxysmal v. of childhood.*
peripheral v. vestibular v.
pilot's v. spatial disorientation.
positional v. vertigo associated with a specific position of the head in space or changes in the position of the head in space. See also *benign paroxysmal positional v., disabling positional v., horizontal v.,* and *vertical v.* Called also *postural v.*
posttraumatic v. vertigo following some injury, such as fracture of the temporal bone, whiplash (see *cervical v.*), or lesions of the cerebral cortex or cerebellum.
postural v. positional v.
pressure v. alternobaric v.
primary v. vestibular v.
recurrent aural v. Meniere disease.
residual v. 1. vertigo in the aftermath of some disease process. 2. vertigo associated with motion, resulting from hypofunction or absence of vestibular sensory or neural elements; see also *positional v.*
riders' v. motion sickness.
rotary v., rotatory v. subjective v.
subjective v. vertigo in which the patient has a sensation of turning round and round, in contrast to objective vertigo. Called also *rotatory v.* and *systematic v.*
systematic v. subjective v.
tenebric v. scotodinia.
toxic v. vertigo as a result of ototoxicity; see also *acute serous labyrinthitis.*
vertical v. 1. height v. 2. positional vertigo experienced when a person is in an upright position.
vestibular v. vertigo due to disturbances of the vestibular system, such as in Meniere disease. Called also *peripheral* or *primary v.*

ver•tig•ra•phy (vər-tig′rə-fe) [*vertigo* + *-graphy*] tomography.

ve•ru•mon•ta•num (ver″u-mon-ta′nəm) [L. "mountain ridge"] colliculus seminalis.

ve•sa•li•an (və-sa′le-ən) named for Andreas *Vesalius,* as the *vesalian bone* or *vein.*

ve•sa•li•a•num (və-sa″le-a′nəm) [Andreas *Vesalius*] a name applied to several sesamoid bones: one on the outer border of the foot between the cuboid and fifth metatarsal bone, and one (sometimes more) in the tendon of origin of the gastrocnemius muscle.

Ve•sa•li•us (və-sa′le-əs) Andreas, 1514–1564. Flemish physician and professor of anatomy in Padua, Italy; in 1543 he produced his *De humani corporis fabrica libri septem* (Seven Books on the Structure of the Human Body), which founded the modern science of anatomy. Following Galen's exhortations to dissect and observe, Vesalius dissected and observed and overthrew Galen's anatomy, which was founded on nonhuman dissection. Vesalius standardized anatomical nomenclature and made important contributions in osteology and myology; in cardiology he rejected Galen's doctrine of the pervious septum. The flood of criticism for the old orthodoxy and against Vesalius drove him from Padua to Spain, where he became physician to Emperor Charles V.

Ve•sa•li•us foramen, ligament (və-sa′le-əs) [A. *Vesalius*] see *foramen venosum* and *ligamentum inguinale.*

Ves•a•noid (ves′ə-noid) trademark for a preparation of tretinoin.

Vesic. [L.] vesi′cula (a blister).

ve•si•ca (və-si′kə) gen. and pl. *vesi′cae* [L.] bladder: a membranous sac or receptacle, especially the urinary bladder or gallbladder.
v. bilia′ris [TA] gallbladder: the pear-shaped reservoir for the bile, found within a fossa on the visceral surface of the liver. From its neck, the cystic duct projects to join the common bile duct. Called also *cholecyst, cholecystis,* and *v. fellea* [TA alternative].
v. fel′lea TA alternative for *v. biliaris.*
v. urina′ria [TA] urinary bladder: a musculomembranous sac in the anterior part of the pelvic cavity, serving as a reservoir for urine; it receives the excretory products of the kidneys through the ureters and expels them through the urethra. The three anatomical areas of the bladder are the *apex* at the superior end, the body or *corpus* in the center, and the *fundus* at the inferior end. Part of the fundus is the *trigone of the bladder,* a triangular area bounded by the orifices of the ureters and the internal orifice of the urethra. Called also *bladder.*

ve•si•cae (və-si′se) [L.] genitive and plural of *vesica.*

ves•i•cal (ves′ĭ-kəl) pertaining to the urinary bladder. Cf. *cystic.*

ves•i•cant (ves′ĭ-kənt) [L. *vesica* blister] 1. causing blisters (vesicles). 2. a chemical that causes blistering.

VESI•care (ves′ĭ-kār) trademark for a preparation of solifenacin succinate.

ves•i•ca•tion (ves″ĭ-ka′shən) vesiculation.

ves•i•ca•to•ry (ves″ĭ-kə-tor′e) vesicant.

ves•i•cle (ves′ĭ-kəl) [L. *vesicula*] 1. a small bladder or sac containing liquid; called also *vesicula.* 2. a small circumscribed epidermal elevation, usually containing a clear fluid; called also *blister.* Cf. *bulla.* 3. a small membrane-bound sac, derived mainly from the plasma membrane, Golgi complex, or endoplasmic reticulum, occurring in eukaryotic cells. 4. the swollen end of a conidiophore from which sterigmata are produced.
acoustic v. otic v.
acrosomal v. a membrane-bounded vacuolelike structure containing the enlarging acrosomal granule, which undergoes collapse and spreads over the upper two-thirds of the head of a spermatozoon to form the head cap.
allantoic v. see under *diverticulum.*
amniocardiac v's fissures in the mesoderm of the early embryo representing the paired primordia of the pericardial sac and the heart.
auditory v. otic v.
blastodermic v. blastocyst.
brain v's the five divisions of the closed neural tube in the head of the developing embryo, including, in craniocaudal sequence, the telencephalon, diencephalon, mesencephalon, metencephalon, and myelencephalon.
brain v's, primary the three earliest subdivisions of the embryonic neural tube, including the prosencephalon, mesencephalon, and rhombencephalon.
brain v's, secondary the five brain vesicles formed by specialization of the prosencephalon (telencephalon and diencephalon), mesencephalon, and rhombencephalon (metencephalon and myelencephalon) in later embryonic development.
cephalic v's, cerebral v's brain v's.
cervical v. a sac in the cervical region of the embryo formed by the closing off of the cervical sinus; it usually disappears, but may persist as a cervical cyst.
chorionic v. see under *sac.*
clathrin-coated v. a transport vesicle having a clathrin coat, involved in the transport of products from the Golgi complex to lysosomes, the transport of molecules taken up by endocytosis, and the retrieval of synaptic vesicle membrane following neurotransmitter release.
COP-coated v. a transport vesicle having a COP (coat protein) coat; COPI-coated vesicles transport cargo within the Golgi complex and from the Golgi complex to the endoplasmic reticulum, while COPII-coated vesicles transport cargo from the endoplasmic reticulum to the Golgi complex.
encephalic v's brain v's.
germinal v. the fluid-filled nucleus of an oocyte toward the end of prophase of its first meiotic division.
lens v. a vesicle formed by fusion of the edges of the lens pit of the embryo; it later develops into the crystalline lens.
matrix v's small membrane-limited structures at sites of calcification of the cartilage matrix.
metanephric v's comma- and S-shaped vesicles that arise from the mesenchyme of the metanephros and develop into metanephric nephrons.
ocular v. optic v.
olfactory v. 1. the vesicle in the embryo that later develops into the olfactory bulb and tract. 2. a bulbous expansion at the distal end of an olfactory cell, from which the olfactory hairs project.
ophthalmic v., optic v. an evagination developing on either side of the forebrain of the early embryo, from which the percipient parts of the eye are formed.

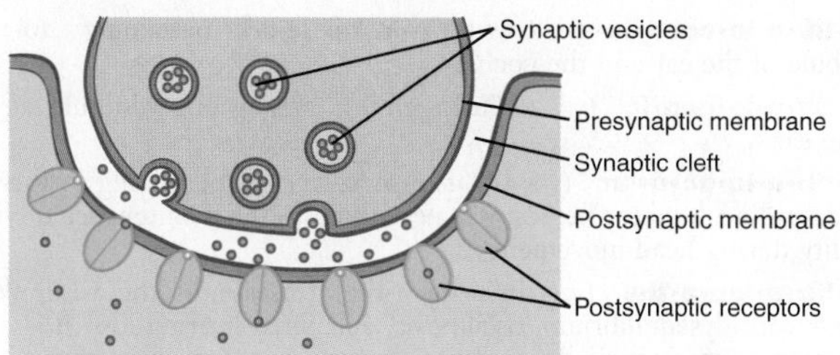

■ Diagram of synaptic vesicles in a synapse.

otic v. a detached ovoid sac formed by closure of the otic pit in embryonic development of the external ear; called also *acoustic* or *auditory v.*
phagocytotic v. phagosome.
pinocytotic v. pinosome.
pituitary v. Rathke pouch.
plasmalemmal v. caveola.
Purkinje v. germinal v.
secretory v's secretory granules.
seminal v. glandula vesiculosa.
sense v. the vesicular primordium of a sense organ in the embryo.
synaptic v's small membrane-bound structures behind a presynaptic membrane, containing neurotransmitters; when depolarization occurs they fuse with the presynaptic membrane and release the neurotransmitter into the synaptic cleft.
transport v. a vesicle, coated with clathrin or coat protein (COP), that carries substances between intracellular compartments.
umbilical v. the yolk sac in a human embryo.
water expulsion v. contractile vacuole.

vesic(o)- [L. *vesica* bladder] a combining form denoting relationship to the bladder, or to a blister.

ves•i•co•ab•dom•i•nal (ves″ĭ-ko-ab-dom′ĭ-nəl) abdominovesical.

ves•i•co•cav•er•nous (ves″ĭ-ko-kav′ər-nəs) both vesicular and cavernous.

ves•i•co•cele (ves′ĭ-ko-sēl″) [*vesico-* + *-cele*[1]] cystocele.

ves•i•co•cer•vi•cal (ves″ĭ-ko-sur′vĭ-kəl) [*vesico-* + *cervical*] pertaining to or communicating between the urinary bladder and the cervix uteri or cervical canal. Called also *cervicovesical.*

ves•i•coc•ly•sis (ves″ĭ-kok′lĭ-sis) [*vesico-* + *clysis*] irrigation of the urinary bladder.

ves•i•co•col•ic (ves″ĭ-ko-kol′ik) vesicocolonic.

ves•i•co•co•lon•ic (ves″ĭ-ko-ko-lon′ik) pertaining to or communicating with the urinary bladder and colon. Called also *colovesical* and *vesicocolic.*

ves•i•co•en•ter•ic (ves″ĭ-ko-en-ter′ik) enterovesical.

ves•i•co•il•e•al (ves″ĭ-ko-il′e-əl) ileovesical.

ves•i•co•in•tes•ti•nal (ves″ĭ-ko-in-tes′tĭ-nəl) enterovesical.

ves•i•co•li•thot•o•my (ves″ĭ-ko-lĭ-thot′ə-me) cystolithotomy.

ves•i•co•per•i•ne•al (ves″ĭ-ko-per″ĭ-ne′əl) pertaining to or communicating with the urinary bladder and perineum.

ves•i•co•pexy (ves′ĭ-ko-pek″se) cystopexy.

ves•i•co•pros•tat•ic (ves″ĭ-ko-pros-tat′ik) pertaining to the urinary bladder and the prostate; called also *prostatovesical.*

ves•i•co•pu•bic (ves″ĭ-ko-pu′bik) pertaining to the urinary bladder and the pubic region. Called also *pubovesical.*

ves•i•co•pus•tu•lar (ves″ĭ-ko-pus′choo-lər) 1. both vesicular and pustular. 2. pertaining to a vesicopustule.

ves•i•co•pus•tule (ves″ĭ-ko-pus′tūl) a vesicle that is developing into a pustule by entry of leukocytes into its contents.

ves•i•co•rec•tal (ves″ĭ-ko-rek′təl) rectovesical.

ves•i•co•re•nal (ves″ĭ-ko-re′nəl) pertaining to the urinary bladder and the kidney.

ves•i•co•sig•moid (ves″ĭ-ko-sig′moid) sigmoidovesical.

ves•i•co•sig•moid•os•to•my (ves″ĭ-ko-sig″moi-dos′tə-me) [*vesico-* + *sigmoidostomy*] surgical creation of an opening between the urinary bladder and the sigmoid colon.

ves•i•co•spi•nal (ves″ĭ-ko-spi′nəl) pertaining to the urinary bladder and the spinal cord.

ves•i•cos•to•my (ves″ĭ-kos′tə-me) cystostomy.
cutaneous v. urinary diversion consisting of anastomosis of the bladder mucosa to an opening in the skin below the umbilicus, creating a stoma for bladder drainage; done in infants as a temporary alternative to suprapubic cystotomy.

ves•i•cot•o•my (ves″ĭ-kot′ə-me) cystotomy.

ves•i•co•um•bil•i•cal (ves″ĭ-ko-əm-bil′ĭ-kəl) pertaining to the urinary bladder and the umbilicus.

ves•i•co•ura•chal (ves″ĭ-ko-u′rə-kəl) pertaining to the urinary bladder and the urachus.

ves•i•co•ure•ter•al (ves″ĭ-ko-u-re′tər-əl) ureterovesical.

ves•i•co•ure•ter•ic (ves″ĭ-ko-u″rə-ter′ik) ureterovesical.

ves•i•co•ure•thral (ves″ĭ-ko-u-re′thrəl) pertaining to or communicating with the urinary bladder and the urethra.

ves•i•co•uter•ine (ves″ĭ-ko-u′tər-in) pertaining to or communicating between the urinary bladder and the uterus; called also *uterovesical.*

ves•i•co•utero•vag•i•nal (ves″ĭ-ko-u″tər-o-vaj′ĭ-nəl) pertaining to or communicating with the urinary bladder, uterus, and vagina.

ves•i•co•vag•i•nal (ves″ĭ-ko-vaj′ĭ-nəl) pertaining to or communicating with the urinary bladder and vagina.

ves•i•co•vag•i•no•rec•tal (ves″ĭ-ko-vaj″ĭ-no-rek′təl) pertaining to or communicating between the urinary bladder, vagina, and rectum.

ve•sic•u•la (və-sik′u-lə) pl. *vesic′ulae* [L., dim. of *vesica*] vesicle (def. 1).
v. germinati′va germinal vesicle.
v. ophthal′mica optic vesicle.
v. semina′lis TA alternative for glandula vesiculosa.
v. sero′sa chorion.

ve•sic•u•lae (və-sik′u-le) [L.] genitive and plural of *vesicula.*

ve•sic•u•lar (və-sik′u-lər) 1. pertaining to or composed of vesicles. 2. having a low pitch; said of a breath sound.

ve•sic•u•lat•ed (və-sik′u-lāt″əd) having vesicles.

ve•sic•u•la•tion (və-sik″u-la′shən) 1. the process of blistering. 2. a blistered spot or surface. Called also *vesication.*

ve•sic•u•lec•to•my (və-sik″u-lek′tə-me) [*vesicle* + *-ectomy*] removal of a vesicle, especially the seminal vesicle.

ve•sic•u•li•tis (və-sik″u-li′tis) 1. inflammation of a seminal vesicle; called also *seminal v.* 2. inflammation of any vesicle.
seminal v. vesiculitis (def. 1).

ve•sic•u•lo•bron•chi•al (və-sik″u-lo-brong′ke-əl) characterized by both vesicular and bronchial sounds, said of breath sounds.

ve•sic•u•lo•bul•lous (və-sik″u-lo-bul′əs) containing both vesicles and bullae.

ve•sic•u•lo•cav•er•nous (və-sik″u-lo-kav′ər-nəs) having both vesicular and cavernous qualities, such as abnormal respiration.

ve•sic•u•lo•gram (və-sik′u-lo-gram″) a radiograph of the seminal vesicles.

ve•sic•u•log•ra•phy (və-sik″u-log′rə-fe) radiography of the seminal vesicles.

ve•sic•u•lo•pap•u•lar (və-sik″u-lo-pap′u-lər) papulovesicular.

ve•sic•u•lo•pus•tu•lar (və-sik″u-lo-pus′tu-lər) consisting of or pertaining to vesicles and pustules.

ve•sic•u•lot•o•my (və-sik″u-lot′ə-me) [*vesicle* + *-tomy*] incision of a vesicle, especially the seminal vesicle.

ve•sic•u•lo•tu•bu•lar (və-sik″u-lo-too′bu-lər) having both a vesicular and a tubular quality; said of auscultatory sounds.

ve•sic•u•lo•tym•pan•ic (və-sik″u-lo-tim-pan′ik) vesiculotympanitic.

ve•sic•u•lo•tym•pa•nit•ic (və-sik″u-lo-tim-pə-nit′ik) having both a vesicular and tympanitic quality; said of auscultatory sounds or resonance. Called also *vesiculotympanic.*

Ves•ic•u•lo•vi•rus (və-sik′u-lo-vi″rəs) [L. *vesicula* vesicle + *virus*] vesicular stomatitis-like viruses: a genus of viruses of the family Rhabdoviridae that includes viruses that cause vesicular stomatitis in swine, cattle, and horses and related viruses that infect other animals. Mosquitoes, sandflies, and ticks are vectors, and some viral species have been isolated only from arthropods. **vesiculovi′ral** *adj*

Ves•i•vi•rus (ves′ĭ-vi″rəs) a genus of viruses of the family Caliciviridae comprising a wide range of animal pathogens, including vesicular exanthema of swine virus, the type species, and feline calicivirus. **vesivi′ral** *adj*

Ves•pa (ves′ə) a genus of wasps and hornets of the family Vespidae; several species live in Europe or North America and have painful stings.

ves•per•al (ves′pər-əl) [L. *vespera* evening] pertaining to or occurring in the evening.

Ves•pi•dae (ves′pĭ-de) the social wasps, a family of flying insects of the order Hymenoptera that have a long thin body and delicate wings; many species can sting. Members of this family live in complicated social units with castes. Genera include *Polistes, Vespa,* and *Vespula.*

Ves·pu·la (ves′pu-lə) a genus of wasps and hornets of the family Vespidae; several species are common in North America and have painful stings.

ves·sel (ves′əl) any channel for carrying a fluid, such as the blood or lymph; see also *vas.*

absorbent v. see vas lymphaticum.
afferent v. of glomerulus arteriola glomerularis afferens.
afferent v's of lymph node lymphatic vessels that carry lymph to a lymph node, entering through the capsule.
anastomotic v. vas anastomoticum.
arterioluminal v's small branches of coronary arterioles that lie near the endocardium, and after a short course open directly into the lumen of the heart.
arteriosinusoidal v's small branches of coronary arterioles that soon break up into sinusoids that lie between bundles or individual muscle fibers of the heart.
bile v's ductuli biliferi.
blood v. any of the vessels conveying the blood; an artery, arteriole, capillary, venule, or vein. Called also *vas sanguineum* [TA].
chyliferous v. lacteal (def. 3).
collateral v. 1. vas collaterale. 2. a vessel important in establishing and maintaining collateral circulation (q.v.).
efferent v. of glomerulus arteriola glomerularis efferens.
efferent v's of lymph node lymphatic vessels that carry lymph away from a lymph node, emerging at the hilus.
ghost v. a blood vessel that persists as a remnant after neovascularization of the cornea has ended or has regressed.
great v's the large vessels entering the heart, including the aorta, the pulmonary arteries and veins, and the venae cavae.
hemorrhoidal v's veins of the rectum that have become dilated and swollen; see *hemorrhoid.*
lacteal v. lacteal (def. 3).
lymphatic v. vas lymphaticum.
lymphatic v., deep vas lymphaticum profundum.
lymphatic v., superficial vas lymphaticum superficiale.
lymphocapillary v. vas lymphocapillare.
nutrient v's vessels that supply nutritive elements to special tissues, such as arteries entering the substance of bone, or supplying walls of the blood vessels themselves. See also *arteria nutricia.*
sinusoidal v. vas sinusoideum.

ves·tib·u·la (ves-tib′u-lə) [L.] plural of *vestibulum.*

ves·tib·u·lar (ves-tib′u-lər) [L. *vestibularis*] 1. pertaining to or toward a vestibule. 2. in dental anatomy, pertaining to the tooth surface directed toward the vestibule of the mouth; see *facies vestibularis dentis.*

ves·ti·bule (ves′tĭ-būl) a space or cavity at the entrance to a canal; called also *vestibulum* [TA].

v. of aorta, aortic v. vestibulum aortae.
v. of bony labyrinth vestibulum labyrinthi ossei.
buccal v. the portion of the vestibule of the mouth that lies between the cheeks and the teeth and gingivae or residual alveolar ridges.
v. of ear vestibulum labyrinthi ossei.
labial v. the portion of the vestibule of the mouth that lies between the lips and the teeth and gingivae, or residual alveolar ridges.
v. of larynx vestibulum laryngis.
v. of mouth vestibulum oris.
nasal v., v. of nose vestibulum nasi.
v. of omental bursa vestibulum bursae omentalis.
oral v. vestibulum oris.
Sibson v. v. of aorta.
v. of vagina, v. of vulva vestibulum vaginae.

Ves·ti·bu·li·fer·ia (vəs-tib″u-lĭ-fer′e-ə) [*vestibule* + Gr. *phōros* bearing] a subclass of free-living or parasitic (especially in the digestive tract of vertebrates and invertebrates) ciliate protozoa (class Kinetofragminophorea, phylum Ciliophora), characterized by the presence of a cytosome within a groove (vestibulum) bearing distinct ciliature at or near the apical end of the body and a cytopharynx. It comprises three orders: Trichostomatida, Entodiniomorphida, and Colpodida.

ves·tib·u·li·tis (ves-tib″u-li′tis) inflammation of the vulvar vestibule and the periglandular and subepithelial stroma; it results in a burning sensation and dyspareunia.

ves·tib·u·lo·cer·e·bel·lum (vəs-tib″u-lo-ser″ə-bel′əm) [*vestibular system* + *cerebellum*] [TA] the portion of the cerebellum serving as the primary site of termination of the vestibular afferents, roughly corresponding to the flocculonodular lobe; therefore, the term is sometimes equated with archicerebellum, which is the anatomical division of the cerebellum comprising the flocculonodular lobe. Cf. *spinocerebellum* and *pontocerebellum.*

ves·tib·u·lo·coch·le·ar (ves-tib″u-lo-kok′le-ər) pertaining to the vestibule of the ear and the cochlea.

ves·tib·u·lo·gen·ic (vəs-tib″u-lo-jen′ik) arising in a vestibule, as that of the ear.

ves·tib·u·lo·oc·u·lar (vəs-tib″u-lo-ok′u-lər) 1. pertaining to the vestibular and oculomotor nerves. 2. pertaining to the maintenance of visual stability during head movements.

ves·tib·u·lop·a·thy (vəs-tib″u-lop′ə-the) disease of the vestibule of the ear with dysequilibrium, oscillopsia, and often hearing loss; it is often a reaction to an ototoxic drug, although many cases are idiopathic.

ves·tib·u·lo·plas·ty (vəs-tib′u-lo-plas″te) the surgical modification of the gingival–mucous membrane relationships in the vestibule of the mouth, including deepening of the vestibular trough, repositioning of the frenum or muscle attachments, and broadening of the zone of attached gingiva, after periodontal treatment. **vestibuloplas′tic** *adj*

ves·tib·u·lot·o·my (vəs-tib″u-lot′ə-me) [*vestibule* + *-tomy*] surgical opening of the vestibule of the internal ear.

ves·tib·u·lo·ure·thral (vəs-tib″u-lo-u-re′thrəl) pertaining to the vestibulum vaginae and to the urethra.

ves·tib·u·lo·vag·i·nal (vəs-tib″u-lo-vaj′ĭ-nəl) pertaining to the vestibule of the vagina (vestibulum vaginae [TA]).

ves·ti·bu·lum (vəs-tib′u-ləm) pl. *vesti′bula* [L.] 1. vestibule: anatomic nomenclature for a space or cavity at the entrance to a canal. 2. a depression, invagination, chamber, or cavity in the body of an organism that gives access to another such space, e.g., as the preoral chamber of certain ciliate protozoa.

v. aor′tae [TA] vestibule of aorta: a space within the left ventricle of the heart at the root of the aorta. Called also *aortic vestibule.*
v. bur′sae omenta′lis [TA] vestibule of omental bursa: that part of the omental bursa posterior to the lesser omentum and adjacent to the epiploic foramen.
v. labyrin′thi os′sei [TA] vestibule of bony labyrinth: an oval cavity in the middle of the bony labyrinth, communicating anteriorly with the cochlea and posteriorly with the semicircular canals, and containing perilymph surrounding the sacculus and utriculus. Called also *vestibule of ear.*
v. laryn′gis [TA] vestibule of larynx: the portion of the laryngeal cavity above the vestibular folds.
v. na′si [TA] vestibule of nose: the anterior part of the nasal cavity, just inferior to the nares and limited posteriorly by the limen nasi. It is lined with stratified squamous epithelium and contains hairs (vibrissae) and sebaceous glands. Called also *nasal vestibule.*
v. o′ris [TA] oral vestibule: the portion of the oral cavity bounded on one side by the teeth and gingivae, or the residual alveolar ridges, and on the other side by the lips *(labial vestibule)* and cheeks *(buccal vestibule);* called also *external oral cavity.*
v. vagi′nae [TA] vestibule of vagina: the space between the labia minora into which the urethra and vagina open.

ves·tige (ves′tij) the remnant of a structure that functioned in a previous stage of species or individual development; called also *vestigium.*

coccygeal v. the remnant of the caudal end of the neural tube.
v. of ductus deferens ductus deferens vestigialis.
v. of vaginal process vestigium processus vaginalis.

ves·tig·ia (vəs-tij′e-ə) [L.] plural of *vestigium.*

ves·tig·i·al (vəs-tij′e-əl) of the nature of a vestige, trace, or relic; rudimentary.

ves·ti·gi·um (vəs-tĭ′je-əm) pl. *vesti′gia* [L. "a trace"] vestige.

v. proces′sus vagina′lis [TA] vestige of vaginal process: a band of connective tissue in the spermatic cord that is a vestige of the processus vaginalis.

ve·su·vine (ve-su′vēn) Bismark brown R.

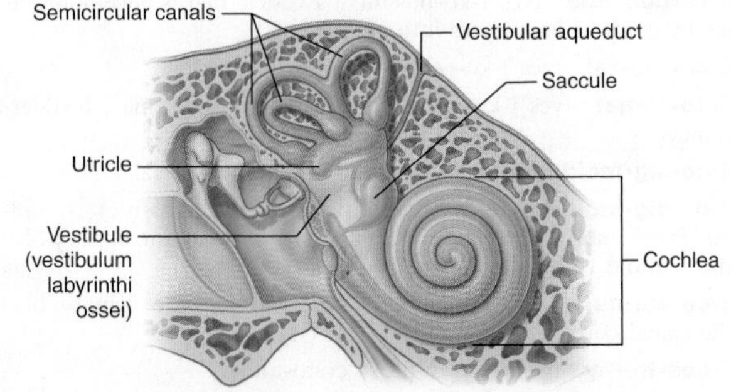

■ Vestibulum labyrinthi ossei (vestibule of bony labyrinth).

vetch (vech) 1. any plant of the genus *Vicia.* 2. any of several plants of the genus *Lathyrus.*

vet•er•i•nar•i•an (vet″ər-ĭ-nar′e-ən) a doctor of veterinary medicine, trained and authorized to practice veterinary medicine and surgery.

vet•er•i•nary (vet′ər-ĭ-nar″e) [L. *veterinarius*] pertaining to the diseases and other disorders of domestic animals.

Vex•ol (vek′sol) trademark for a preparation of rimexolone.

VF vocal fremitus.

vf visual field.

Vfend (vee′fend) trademark for a preparation of voriconazole.

VFib (ve′fib) ventricular fibrillation.

VFl ventricular flutter.

VHDL very-high-density lipoprotein.

vi•a•bil•i•ty (vi″ə-bil′ĭ-te) ability to live after birth.

vi•a•ble (vi′ə-bəl) capable of living; especially said of a fetus that has reached such a stage of development that it can live outside of the uterus. This usually connotes a fetus that weighs at least 500 gm and has reached a gestational age of 20 weeks (22 weeks after fertilization).

Via•dur (vi′ə-dur) trademark for preparations of leuprolide acetate.

Vi•ag•ra (vi-ag′rə) trademark for a preparation of sildenafil citrate.

vi•al (vi′əl) [Gr. *phialē*] a small bottle.

Vi•an•nia (ve-an′e-ə) a subgenus of the genus *Leishmania* (q.v.), comprising the species that develop initially in the hindgut of the sandfly, migrating forward to the midgut and foregut before transmission by bite.

vi•bex (vi′beks) [L. *vibix* mark of a blow] singular of *vibices.*

vi•bi•ces (vĭ-bi′sēz) (sing. *vibex*) [L.] streaks on the skin from subcutaneous effusions of blood.

Vi•bra•my•cin (vi-brə-mi′sin) trademark for preparations of doxycycline.

Vi•bra-Tabs (vi′brə-tabz) trademark for preparations of doxycycline hyclate.

vi•bra•tile (vi′brə-til) [L. *vibratilis*] having an oscillatory motion; swaying or moving to and fro.

vi•bra•tion (vi-bra′shən) [L. *vibratio,* from *vibrare* to shake] 1. a rapid movement to and fro; cf. *oscillation.* 2. massage in which a light, rhythmic, quivering effect is achieved; often performed with a mechanical device (electrovibratory or vibratory massage).

vi•bra•tor (vi′bra-tər) an instrument for producing vibrations.

vi•bra•to•ry (vi′brə-tor″e) [L. *vibratorius*] vibrating or causing vibration.

Vib•rio (vib′re-o) [L. *vibrare* to move rapidly, vibrate] a genus of mainly aquatic, gram-negative, facultatively anaerobic bacteria of the family Vibrionaceae, consisting of straight, curved, or comma-shaped rods that are motile by means of one or more polar flagella. Some species (the *cholera vibrios*) cause cholera; others (the *noncholera vibrios*) cause milder forms of diarrhea in humans; and others infect only animals other than humans. The type species is *V. cho′lerae.*

V. alginoly′ticus a halophilic species found in seawater and seafood that is sometimes associated with diarrhea, septicemia, and wound infections.

V. cho′lerae the etiologic agent of human cholera, found in the intestinal tract of normal and diseased humans and animals and in water. The species is divided into serogroups on the basis of somatic (O) antigens; serogroups are further divided into serovars and biogroups. Only serogroups O1 and O139 cause clinical disease, producing an enterotoxin that promotes secretion of fluid and electrolytes by the small intestine.

V. cho′lerae* biovar *El Tor a pathogenic strain belonging to serogroup O1, first isolated in Egypt in 1960; it is the cause of the present cholera pandemic. Called also *El Tor vibrio.*

V. cincinnatien′sis a halophilic species that is associated with bacteremia and meningitis.

V. co′li *Campylobacter coli.*

V. dam′sela *Photobacterium damselae.*

V. fluvia′lis a halophilic species that frequently occurs in estuaries and causes diarrhea.

V. furnis′sii a halophilic species that occurs in estuaries and has been associated with sporadic cases of diarrhea.

V. hol′lisae a halophilic species that is a cause of sporadic diarrhea and of cellulitis.

V. jeju′ni *Campylobacter jejuni.*

V. metschniko′vii a halophilic species that is widespread in marine and freshwater environments and found in the intestinal tract or feces of mammals and birds; it causes gastroenteritis and bacteremia in humans and guinea pigs.

V. mi′micus a nonhalophilic species that causes diarrhea in animals that eat raw seafood and occasionally causes otitis in saltwater swimmers.

V. parahaemoly′ticus a halophilic species that is a major cause of gastroenteritis when raw or improperly cooked fish or seafood is eaten, especially in Japan.

V. vulni′ficus a halophilic species whose strains are similar to *V. parahaemolyticus* and *V. alginolyticus* but differ in that they can ferment lactose. Infection by eating raw seafood causes septicemia and cellulitis, and may be especially severe or even fatal in those with preexisting hepatic disease. Wound infection may occur following exposure to sea water or from injury when handling crabs.

vib•rio (vib′re-o) pl. *vibrios, vibrio′nes.* An organism of the genus *Vibrio.*

Celebes v. *Vibrio cholerae,* biovar *El Tor.*

cholera v. *Vibrio cholerae.*

El Tor v. *Vibrio cholerae* biovar *El Tor.*

v. group EF-6, v. group F a group of vibrios isolated from individuals with diarrheal disease.

NAG v's, nonagglutinating v's nonpathogenic paracholera vibrios, unrelated to the cholera vibrio O antigenic group.

noncholera v's (NCVs) a group of microorganisms similar to *Vibrio cholerae,* but differing from it immunologically; they have variable pathogenic properties. Many have been isolated from water or from the feces of persons with mild diarrhea and have been named for the place of their discovery.

paracholera v's noncholera v's.

vib•rio•ci•dal (vib″re-o-si′dəl) destructive to organisms of the genus *Vibrio,* especially *V. cholerae.*

vib•ri•oid (vib′re-oid) resembling a vibrio; having a curved, rod-shaped morphology.

Vib•rio•na•ceae (vib″re-o-na′se-e) a family of primarily aquatic, gram-negative, facultatively anaerobic, motile, straight or curved, rod-shaped bacteria of the order Vibrionales. Medically important organisms are contained in the genera *Photobacterium* and *Vibrio.*

Vib•ri•o•na•les (vib″re-o-na′lēz) an order of gram-negative, rod-shaped bacteria of the class Gammaproteobacteria, phylum Proteobacteria; it contains the single family Vibrionaceae.

vib•ri•o•nes (vib″re-o′nēz) plural of *vibrio.*

vib•ri•o•sis (vib″re-o′sis) infection with bacteria of the genus *Vibrio.*

bovine genital v. see under *campylobacteriosis.*

ovine genital v. see under *campylobacteriosis.*

vi•bris•sa (vi-bris′ə) [L.] singular of *vibrissae.*

vi•bris•sae (vi-bris′e) (sing. *vibris′sa*) [L. pl. of *vibrissa*] 1. [TA] the hairs growing in the vestibular region of the nasal cavity. 2. long coarse hairs growing around the nose (muzzle) of an animal, as of the dog or cat.

vi•bro•acous•tic (vi″bro-ə-kōōs′tik) 1. containing both vibratory and acoustic elements. 2. referring to sound associated with tactile vibration as well as, or instead of, auditory stimuli.

Vi•bur•num (vi-bur′nəm) [L.] a genus of trees and shrubs of the family Caprifoliaceae.

V. o′pulus the cranberry bush or tree, whose dried bark is medicinal; see *cramp bark,* under *bark.*

V. prunifo′lium the black haw, whose root and stem have bark that has been used as a uterine sedative.

vi•car•i•ous (vi-kar′e-əs) [L. *vicarius*] 1. acting in the place of another or of something else. 2. occurring at an abnormal site.

Vic•ia (vish′e-ə) the vetches, a genus of climbing plants of the family Leguminosae.

***V. fa′ba,* V. fa′va** a species whose beans or pollen contain a component that causes favism (q.v.) in susceptible individuals; called also *fava, fava bean,* and *broad bean.*

V. sati′va a common species of vetch that contains cyanogenetic compounds and also causes photosensitization and liver damage in livestock.

vi•cine (vi′sin) a pyrimidine-based glycoside occurring in species of *Vicia*; in fava beans it is cleaved by an endogenous β-glucosidase to form the toxic compound divicine.

Vi•co•din (vi′ko-din″) trademark for combination preparations of hydrocodone bitartrate and acetaminophen.

Vi•co•din Tuss (vi′ko-din″ tus) trademark for a combination preparation of hydrocodone bitartrate and guaifenesin.

Vi•co•pro•fen (vi-ko-pro′fen) trademark for a combination preparation of hydrocodone bitartrate and ibuprofen.

Vicq d'Azyr band (stripe), fasciculus, foramen (vĕk dah-zēr′) [Félix *Vicq d'Azyr,* French anatomist, 1748–1794] see *fasciculus mammillothalamicus* and *foramen caecum medullae oblongatae,* and see *Kaes-Bekhterev layer,* under *layer.*

Vi•cryl (vi′krəl) trademark for polyglactin 910.

vi•dar•a•bine (vi-dar′ə-bēn) [USP] a purine analogue that inhibits DNA synthesis; used as a topical antiviral agent in the treatment of herpes simplex keratitis or keratoconjunctivitis and intravenously in the treatment of herpes simplex encephalitis. Called also *adenine arabinoside* or *ara-A.*

Vi•da•za (vĭ-da′zə) trademark for a preparation of 5-azacytidine.

video- [L. *videre* to see] a combining form denoting relationship to an electrical signal carrying timing, intensity, and often color, information such that when displayed on an appropriate device it gives a visual image representing the original information.

vid•eo•den•si•tom•e•try (vĭ″de-o-den″sĭ-tom′ə-tre) densitometry using a video camera to record the images to be analyzed.

vid•eo•en•do•scope (vid″e-o-en′do-skōp) a flexible endoscope whose tip is equipped with a video camera that transmits a signal that is converted to an image on a color monitor; written also *video endoscope.*

vid•eo•en•dos•co•py (vid″e-o-en-dos′kə-pe) endoscopy performed under the guidance of a video camera in the tip of the endoscope.

vid•eo•flu•o•rog•ra•phy (vid″e-o-flo͞o-rog′rə-fe) a radiographic technique in which an image displayed on an intensifying screen is scanned by a television camera and displayed on a television monitor.

vid•eo•flu•o•ros•co•py (vid″e-o-flo͞o-ros′kə-pe) the recording on videotape of the images appearing on a fluoroscopic screen.

vid•e•og•no•sis (vid″e-og-no′sis) [*video-* + dia*gnosis*] diagnosis based on the interpretation of radiographs transmitted by television techniques to a radiologic center.

vid•eo•ky•mog•ra•phy (vid″e-o-ki-mog′rə-fe) recording of vibrations (see *kymography*) using a high-speed video camera.

vid•eo•lap•a•ro•scope (vid″e-o-lap′ə-ro-skōp″) a laparoscope whose tip is equipped with a video camera that transmits a signal that is converted to an image on a color monitor; written also *video laparoscope.*

vid•eo•lap•a•ros•co•py (vid″e-o-lap″ə-ros′kə-pe) laparoscopic surgery performed under the guidance of a video camera in the tip of the laparoscope.

vid•eo•la•ser•os•co•py (vid″e-o-la-zər-os′kə-pe) [*video-* + *laser* + *-scopy*] a modification of laser laparoscopy in which the inside of the cavity is visualized through a video camera that projects an enlarged image onto a video monitor.

vid•eo•mi•cros•co•py (vid″e-o-mi-kros′kə-pe) television microscopy.

Vi•dex (vi′deks) trademark for a preparation of didanosine.

vid•i•an (vid′e-ən) named for Vidus *Vidius* (It. Guido *Guidi*), Italian physician and anatomist, 1500–1567, as *vidian artery.*

Vieus•sens ansa, etc. (vyo͞o-sah′) [Raymond de *Vieussens,* French anatomist, 1641–1715] see *ansa subclavia, cavum septi pellucidi, foramina venarum minimarum, limbus fossae ovalis,* and *venae ventriculi dextri anteriores.*

view (vu) projection (def. 5).

VIG vaccinia immune globulin.

vi•ga•ba•trin (vi-ga′bə-trin) an anticonvulsant used as an adjunct in the treatment of epilepsy refractory to conventional treatment and to control infantile spasms; administered orally.

vig•il•am•bu•lism (vij″il-am′bu-liz-əm) an ambulatory automatism resembling somnambulism but occurring in the waking state.

vig•i•lance (vij′ĭ-ləns) [L. *vigilantia*] alert watchfulness, particularly with regard to danger or other changes in the environment; attentiveness; readiness to respond to stimuli.

Vig•nal cells (ve-nyahl′) [Guillaume *Vignal,* French physiologist, 1852–1893] see under *cell.*

vig•or (vig′ər) [L. *vigere* to flourish] a combination of attributes of living organisms which expresses itself in rapid growth, high fertility and fecundity, and long life.

hybrid v. heterosis.

vi•kri•ti (vik′rĭ-te) in ayurveda, a disordered physical constitution, resulting from an imbalance of the doshas; cf. *prakriti.*

Vi•la•no•va disease (ve″lah-no′vah) [Xavier *Vilanova* i Montiu, Spanish dermatologist and venereologist, 1902–1965] subacute nodular migratory panniculitis.

Vil•la•ret syndrome (ve-yah-ra′) [Maurice *Villaret,* French neurologist, 1877–1946] see under *syndrome.*

vil•li (vil′i) [L.] genitive and plural of *villus.*

vil•lif•er•ous (vĭ-lif′ər-əs) having or bearing villi.

vil•li•ki•nin (vil″ĭ-ki′nin) [*villi* + Gr. *kinein* to move] a hormone hypothesized to exist in the duodenum, stimulating villus movement and being released by action of hydrochloric acid on the mucous membrane.

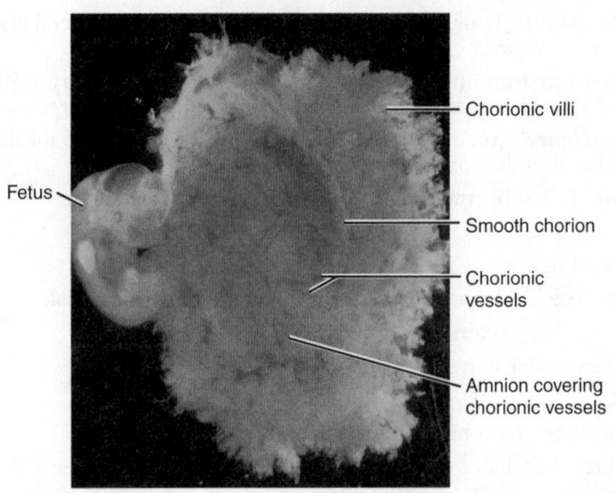

■ Chorionic villi covering the entire chorionic sac in an embryo at Carnegie stage 15, about 36 days.

vil•lin (vil′in) an actin-binding protein, found in the intestinal epithelium and elsewhere, that severs actin filaments at high calcium concentrations and caps them at low calcium concentrations; in microvilli it crosslinks F-actin to form the microvillus core.

vil•li•tis (vĭ-li′tis) [*villi* + *-itis*] 1. villositis. 2. inflammation of the villous tissue of the coronet and of the plantar substance of a horse's foot.

vil•lo•nod•u•lar (vil″o-nod′u-lər) characterized by villous and nodular thickening; said of a proliferative disorder of the synovial tissue.

vil•lose (vil′ōs) [L. *villosus*] shaggy with soft hairs; covered with villi.

vil•lo•si•tis (vil″o-si′tis) a bacterial disease characterized by alterations in the villi of the placenta. Called also *villitis.*

vil•los•i•ty (vĭ-los′ĭ-te) 1. the condition of being covered with villi. 2. a villus.

vil•lous (vil′əs) villose.

vil•lus (vil′əs) pl. *vil′li* [L. "tuft of hair"] 1. a small protrusion resembling a tuft of hair. 2. a small vascular process or protrusion, especially one on the free surface of a membrane.

amniotic v. one of the irregular, flat, opaque areas of imperfect skin on the amnion near the distal end of the umbilical cord.

anchoring v. a chorionic villus that attaches to the decidua basalis.

arachnoid villi 1. granulationes arachnoideae. 2. numerous microscopic projections of the arachnoid into some of the venous sinuses, which are thought by some to enlarge in persons with advancing age to become the granulationes arachnoideae (q.v.).

branch v. a branch of a tertiary (stem) villus through which the main transport of substances between the mother and fetus occurs.

chorionic v. one of the threadlike projections growing in tufts on the external surface of the chorion; see *primary, secondary,* and *tertiary v.*

villi of choroid plexus tiny hairlike processes of varying sizes along the edges of the choroid plexus, containing blood vessels; their exact function is unknown.

free v. a chorionic villus that projects into the intervillous space; it is not attached to the decidua basalis.

intestinal villi, vil′li intestina′les [TA] the multitudinous threadlike projections that cover the surface of the mucosa of the small intestine and serve as the sites of absorption (by active transport and diffusion) of fluids and nutrients.

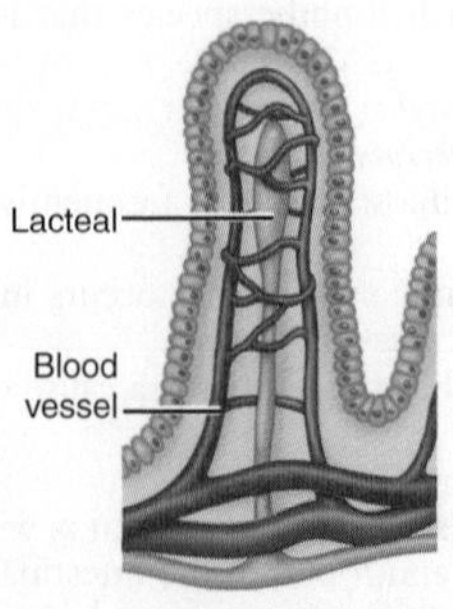

■ Intestinal villus.

lingual villi papillae filiformes.
primary v. the first stage of development of chorionic villi; it is composed of trophoblast only.
secondary v. an intermediate stage of development of chorionic villi, having a core of connective tissue (mesoblast) covered with trophoblast.
villi of small intestine villi intestinales.
stem v. tertiary v.
vil'li synovia'les [TA] synovial villi: slender projections of the synovial membrane from its free inner surface into the joint cavity.
tertiary v. the definitive stage of development of chorionic villi, having a trophoblastic cover, connective tissue (mesoblastic) core, and blood vessels. Called also *stem v.*

vil•lus•ec•to•my (vil″əs-ek′tə-me) synovectomy.

vi•men•tin (vĭ-men′tin) a protein that forms the vimentin filaments (q.v.); it is used as an immunohistochemical marker for cells derived from the embryonic mesenchyme.

vin•blas•tine sul•fate (vin-blas′tēn) [USP] the sulfate salt of a vinca alkaloid, used as an antineoplastic in treatment of lymphomas, including generalized Hodgkin disease, Kaposi sarcoma, advanced mycosis fungoides, Letterer-Siwe disease, choriocarcinoma resistant to other agents, breast carcinoma unresponsive to other therapy, and embryonal carcinoma of the testis. Administered intravenously.

Vin•ca (vin′kə) [L. pervinca *periwinkle*] a genus of woody herbs of the family Apocynaceae, including periwinkles. *V. mi′nor* L. is the common, or lesser, periwinkle. *V. ro′sea* L. is the Madagascar periwinkle, source of the vinca alkaloids (see under *alkaloid*).

vin•ca (ving′kə) any plant of the genus *Vinca.*

vin•ca•mine (vin′kə-mēn) a major alkaloid obtained from *Vinca minor*, used to help improve intellectual capacity in patients with cerebrovascular disorders.

Vin•ca•sar (vin′kə-sahr) trademark for a preparation of vincristine sulfate.

Vin•cent angina, gingivitis (vă-sah′) [Henri *Vincent*, French physician, 1862–1950] see under *angina*, and see *necrotizing ulcerative gingivitis*, under *gingivitis.*

vin•cris•tine sul•fate (vin-kris′tēn) [USP] the sulfate salt of a vinca alkaloid, used as an antineoplastic agent, primarily as a component of combination chemotherapy regimens for Hodgkin disease, acute lymphoblastic leukemia, and non-Hodgkin lymphomas, as well as in the treatment of other neoplastic disorders including Wilms tumor, neuroblastoma, AIDS-associated Kaposi sarcoma, and rhabdomyosarcoma. Administered intravenously.

vin•cu•lin (vin′ku-lin) a 130-kD protein, found in muscle, fibroblasts, and epithelial cells, that binds to α-actinin and talin; it is associated with attachment plaques and with talin mediates cell-cell and cell–extracellular matrix adhesion by linking actin filaments of the cytoskeleton to the cytoplasmic domains of β-integrins.

vin•cu•lum (ving′ku-ləm) pl. *vin′cula* [L.] a term used in anatomy to denote a band or bandlike structure.
v. bre′ve digito′rum ma′nus [TA] either of two fan-shaped expansions near the ends of the flexor tendons of a finger, one connecting the superficial tendon to the proximal interphalangeal joint and the other connecting the deep tendon to the intermediate interphalangeal joint.
v. lon′gum digito′rum ma′nus [TA] either of two independent pairs of slender bands in each finger, one connecting the deep flexor tendon to the superficial tendon after the latter becomes subjacent, and the other connecting the superficial tendon to the proximal phalanx.
vin′cula ten′dinum digito′rum ma′nus [TA] vincula of tendons of fingers: small vascular bands that connect the tendons of the flexor digitorum profundus and flexor digitorum superficialis muscles to the phalanges and interphalangeal articulations of the hand. The tendon blood supply is also carried in them. See *v. breve digitorum manus* and *v. longum digitorum manus.*
vin′cula ten′dinum digito′rum pe′dis [TA] vincula of tendons of toes: bands connecting the tendons of the flexor digitorum longus and flexor digitorum brevis muscles to the phalanges and interphalangeal articulations of the foot. They are similar to the vincula found in the hand.
vincula of tendons of fingers vincula tendinum digitorum manus.
vincula of tendons of toes vincula tendinum digitorum pedis.

vin•de•sine sul•fate (vin′də-sēn) a synthetic vinca alkaloid derived from vinblastine sulfate, used as an antineoplastic in the treatment of acute lymphoblastic leukemia and non–small cell carcinoma; administered intravenously.

Vine•berg operation (vīn′bərg) [Arthur M. *Vineberg*, Canadian surgeon, 1903–1988] see under *operation.*

vin•e•gar (vin′ə-gər) [Fr. *vinaigre* sour wine] 1. a weak and impure dilution of acetic acid; especially a sour liquid consisting chiefly of acetic acid, formed by the fermentation of cider, wine, etc., or by the distillation of wood. 2. a medicinal solution of a drug in dilute acetic acid.

vin•e•ga•roon (vin″ə-gə-ro͞on′) *Mastigoproctus giganteus*, a species of whip scorpion so called because it produces an irritating excretion with an odor resembling that of vinegar.

vi•no•rel•bine tar•trate (vĭ-nor′el-bēn) [USP] a semisynthetic vinca alkaloid derived from vinblastine, used as an antineoplastic in the treatment of non–small cell lung carcinoma; administered intravenously.

Vin•son syndrome (vin′sən) [Porter Paisley *Vinson*, American surgeon, 1890–1959] Plummer-Vinson syndrome; see under *syndrome.*

vi•nyl (vi′nəl) the univalent group CH_2═CH—.
v. acetate a vinyl group to which the monovalent radical CH_3COO— is attached, the monomer which polymerizes to polyvinyl acetate.
v. benzene styrene.
v. chloride a vinyl group to which an atom of chlorine is attached, the monomer which polymerizes to polyvinyl chloride, used in organic synthesis and in the plastics industry; it is toxic and carcinogenic. Called also *chloroethylene.* See also *vinyl chloride disease*, under *disease.*
v. cyanide acrylonitrile.

Vi•o•kase (vi′o-kās) trademark for preparations of pancrelipase.

vi•o•la•ce•in (vi″o-la′se-in) a violet pigment with antibiotic properties produced by species of *Chromobacter.* It is soluble in ethanol but not in water or chloroform.

vi•o•la•ceous (vi″o-la′shəs) having a violet color, usually describing a discoloration of the skin.

vi•o•les•cent (vi″o-les′ənt) somewhat violet in color.

vi•o•let (vi′o-lət) 1. the color produced by the shortest waves of the visible spectrum, beyond indigo, approximately 380 to 420 nm. 2. a dye or stain with this color.
cresyl v. acetate a basic violet dye used as a stain for the central nervous system.
cresyl v., cresylecht v. a dye used in pathologic staining.
crystal v., gentian v., hexamethyl v. gentian violet; see under *gentian.*
Hofmann v., iodine v. dahlia.
Lauth v. thionine.
methyl v. gentian violet; see under *gentian.*
methylene v. Bernthsen an uncharged thiazine dye produced when methylene blue is converted to polychrome methylene blue.. It is unrelated to various other dyes which are also called methylene violets.

vi•os•ter•ol (vi-os′tər-ol) ergocalciferol.

Vi•oxx (vi′oks) trademark for a preparation of rofecoxib.

VIP vasoactive intestinal polypeptide.

vi•per (vi′pər) 1. any member of the families Viperidae and Crotalidae. 2. any venomous snake. See table at *snake.*
carpet v. saw-scaled v.
European v. *Vipera berus*, a venomous snake native to Europe, North Africa, and the Middle East; it may be either red, brown, or gray with dark markings, or completely black. Called also *adder.*
Gaboon v. *Bitis gabonica*, a deadly, brightly marked, viperine snake found in tropical West Africa.
horned v. *Cerastes cerastes*, a venomous species found in the Sahara Desert and from Lebanon south to the Arabian peninsula.
nose-horned v. sand v.
Old World v. true v.
palm v. any of various small, greenish, arboreal pit vipers of the genera *Bothrops* and *Trimeresurus*, which have prehensile tails that enable them to move from tree to tree.
pit v. crotalid (def. 1).
pit v., Malayan *Calloselasma rhodostoma.*
rhinoceros v. *Bitis nasicornis*, a venomous, brightly colored, viperine snake found in tropical Africa, characterized by the presence of a pair of hornlike growths on its snout.
Russell's v. *Vipera russelli*, an extremely venomous, brightly colored, viperine snake of southeastern Asia and Indonesia. Called also *daboia* and *ticpolonga.*
sand v. *Vipera ammodytes*, a venomous snake found in southern Europe and Turkey that has a hornlike protuberance on its snout for burrowing; called also *nose-horned v.*
saw-scaled v. either of two venomous snakes, *Echis carinatus* and *E. coloratus*; called also *carpet v.*
true v. any of the snakes of the family Viperidae.

Vi•pera (vi′pər-ə) a genus of venomous snakes of the family Viperidae. *V. ammody′tes* is the sand viper; *V. be′rus* is the European viper; and *V. rus′selli* is Russell's viper.

vi·per·id (vi′pər-id) viperine.

Vi·per·i·dae (vi-per′ĭ-de) a family of venomous snakes, the true or Old World vipers, characterized by front, movable, hollow fangs. It includes the genera *Bitis, Cerastes, Echis,* and *Vipera.* Cf. *Crotalidae.* See table at *snake.*

vi·per·ine (vi′pər-in, vi′pər-īn) 1. of or pertaining to the family Viperidae. 2. true viper.

VIP·oma (vĭ-po′mə) [*v*asoactive *i*ntestinal *p*olypeptide + *-oma*] an endocrine tumor, usually a type of islet cell tumor, that produces excessive vasoactive intestinal polypeptide, causing severe diarrhea and other symptoms of the Verner-Morrison syndrome. Called also *diarrheogenic tumor.* Written also *vipoma.*

Vira-A (vi′rə-a) trademark for a preparation of vidarabine.

Vi·ra·cept (vi′rə-sept) trademark for a preparation of nelfinavir mesylate.

vi·ra·gin·i·ty (vi″rə-jin′ĭ-te) [L. *virago* a manlike woman] the adoption by a woman of qualities and behaviors usually considered masculine.

vi·ral (vi′rəl) pertaining to, caused by, or of the nature of virus.

Vi·ra·mune (vi′rə-mūn) trademark for a preparation of nevirapine.

Vi·ra·zole (vi′rə-zōl) trademark for a preparation of ribavirin.

Vir·chow (fĕr′ko) Rudolf Ludwig Karl, 1821–1902. German writer and editor, politician and statesman, anthropologist, ethnologist, archaeologist, and pathologist; his *Cellularpathologie* (1858) finally overthrew humoralism and marked the beginning of modern pathology. He made valuable contributions to anatomy, parasitology, the history of medicine, public health, histology, and anatomic pathology. He regarded the body as a cell-state in which every cell is a citizen, with disease being a civil war brought about by external forces among the cells; he thought all cells arose from other cells (implicitly rejecting spontaneous generation), and that cell theory applied to diseased tissue. He opposed Pasteur's theory of germs, Darwin's theory of natural selection and evolution, and Semmelweiss's washing of hands to prevent puerperal fever.

Vir·chow angle, etc. (fĕr′ko) [R.L.K. *Virchow*] see under *angle, crystal, granulation, line* and *triad;* see *lepra cell,* under *cell;* see *corneal corpuscles,* under *corpuscle;* and see *signal node,* under *node.*

Vir·chow-Rob·in spaces (fĕr′ko ro-bă′) [R.L.K. *Virchow;* Charles Philippe *Robin,* French anatomist, 1821–1885] see under *space.*

Vir·chow-Seck·el syndrome (fĕr′ko sek′əl) [R.L.K. *Virchow;* Helmut Paul George *Seckel,* American physician, 1900–1960] Seckel syndrome; see under *syndrome.*

Vir·e·ad (vir′e-ad) trademark for a preparation of tenofovir disoproxil fumarate.

vi·re·mia (vi-re′me-ə) the presence of viruses in the blood. vire′mic *adj*

vir·gin (vur′jin) [L. *virgo*] 1. a person who has not had sexual intercourse. 2. a laboratory animal that has been kept free from sexual intercourse.

vir·gin·al (vir′jĭ-nəl) pertaining to a virgin or to virginity.

vir·gin·ia·my·cin (vir-jin′yə-mi′sin) a streptogramin antibiotic produced by *Streptomyces virginiae* or by other means, consisting chiefly of two components, virginiamycin M_1 (factor M_1) and virginiamycin S_1 (factor S); administered as a feed additive to pigs as a growth stimulant and to combat infections, especially those with gram-positive cocci.

vir·gin·i·ty (vir-jin′ĭ-te) [L. *virginitas*] the condition of being a virgin.

vi·ri·ci·dal (vi″rĭ-si′dəl) virucidal.

vi·ri·cide (vi′rĭ-sīd) virucide.

vir·i·do·bu·fa·gin (vir″ĭ-do-bu′fə-jin) a cardiac poison from the skin glands of the toad *Bufo viridis.*

vir·ile (vir′il) [L. *virilis*] 1. masculine. 2. specifically, having male copulative power.

vir·i·les·cence (vir″ĭ-les′əns) the development of masculine characteristics in a female. Cf. *masculinization.*

vir·i·lism (vir′ĭ-liz-əm) the development or possession of male secondary sex characters in a female or prepubertal male. Cf. *masculinization.*

adrenal v. virilism due to inappropriate adrenal cortical androgen production.

vi·ril·i·ty (vĭ-ril′ĭ-te) [L. *virilitas,* from *vir* man] masculinity.

vir·il·iza·tion (vir″il-ĭ-za′shən) masculinization; usually used for that occurring inappropriately in a female or prepubertal male.

vir·i·liz·ing (vir′ĭ-līz″ing) producing virilization.

Vir·i·lon (vir′ĭ-lon) trademark for a preparation of methyltestosterone.

vi·ri·on (vi′re-on) the complete viral particle, found extracellularly and capable of surviving in crystalline form and infecting a living cell; it comprises the nucleoid (genetic material) and the capsid. Called also *viral particle.*

vi·ro·gene (vi′ro-jēn) [*virus* + *gene*] in theoretical genetics, an RNA tumor virus assembled by the normal genetic complement of a cell.

vi·ro·ge·net·ic (vi″ro-jə-net′ik) having a viral origin; caused by a virus.

vi·roid (vi′roid) any of a class of infectious agents consisting of a small strand of RNA not associated with any protein. The RNA does not code for proteins and is not translated; it is replicated by host cell enzymes. Viroids are known to cause several plant diseases.

vi·ro·lac·tia (vi″ro-lak′shə) secretion of viruses in the milk.

vi·ro·log·ic (vi″ro-loj′ik) 1. pertaining to virology. 2. pertaining to therapy for viral infections; sometimes this is a synonym for *antiviral.*

vi·rol·o·gist (vi-rol′ə-jist) a microbiologist specializing in virology.

vi·rol·o·gy (vi-rol′ə-je) the branch of microbiology that is concerned with viruses and viral diseases.

vi·ro·mi·cro·some (vi″ro-mi′kro-sōm) a name sometimes applied to an incomplete virus particle released by premature disruption of the host cell.

vi·ro·pex·is (vi″ro-pek′sis) [*virus* + *pexis*] the fixation of virus to the membrane of an animal cell and its subsequent engulfment by the cell.

vi·ro·plasm (vi′ro-plaz″əm) plaques of very fine granular substance that appear in cells before virions are observed and which correspond to the DNA material, as in poxvirus infections.

Vi·rop·tic (vi-rop′tik) trademark for a preparation of trifluridine.

vi·ro·sis (vi-ro′sis) pl. *viro′ses.* A disease caused by a virus.

vi·ro·some (vi′ro-sōm) a liposome into which viral proteins have been incorporated; virosomes containing viral surface proteins can be used as antigens for vaccine manufacture.

vi·ro·stat·ic (vi″ro-stat′ik) 1. said of an antiviral agent that inhibits the replication of viruses. 2. an agent that inhibits the replication of viruses; called also *virustatic.*

vir·tu·al (vir′choo-əl) 1. having the essence or effect, although not the actual fact or form. 2. created by, carried on, or performed by means of computers.

vi·ru·cide (vi′rə-sīd) an agent that neutralizes or destroys a virus. viruci′dal *adj*

vir·u·lence (vir′u-ləns) [L. *virulentia,* from *virus* poison] 1. the degree of pathogenicity of a microorganism as indicated by the severity of the disease produced and its ability to invade the tissues of a host. It is measured experimentally by the median lethal dose (LD_{50}) or median infective dose (ID_{50}). 2. by extension, the competence of any infectious agent to produce pathologic effects.

vir·u·lent (vir′u-lənt) [L. *virulentus,* from *virus* poison] pertaining to or characterized by virulence; exceedingly pathogenic or deleterious.

vir·u·lif·er·ous (vir″u-lif′ər-əs) [*virus* + *-ferous*] conveying or producing a virus.

vir·uria (vi-roo′re-ə) the presence of viruses in the urine.

vi·rus (vi′rəs) [L.] one of a group of minute infectious agents, usually not resolvable under a light microscope, although there are certain exceptions such as poxviruses. Viruses are characterized by lack of independent metabolism and by the ability to replicate only within living host cells. Like living organisms, they can reproduce with genetic continuity and the possibility of mutation. They range from 200–300 nm to 15 nm in size and are morphologically heterogeneous, occurring as rod-shaped, spherical, or polyhedral, and tadpole-shaped forms; masses of the spherical or polyhedral forms may be made up of orderly arrays to give a crystalline structure. The individual particle, or virion, consists of nucleic acid (the nucleoid), DNA or RNA (but not both) and a protein shell, or capsid, which contains and protects the nucleic acid and may be multilayered. Viruses are customarily separated into three subgroups on the basis of host specificity, namely bacterial viruses, animal viruses, and plant viruses. They are also classified as to their origin (e.g., reoviruses), mode of transmission (arboviruses, tick-borne viruses), or the manifestations they produce (polioviruses, polyomaviruses, poxviruses). They are sometimes named for the geographical location in which they were first isolated (e.g., coxsackievirus).

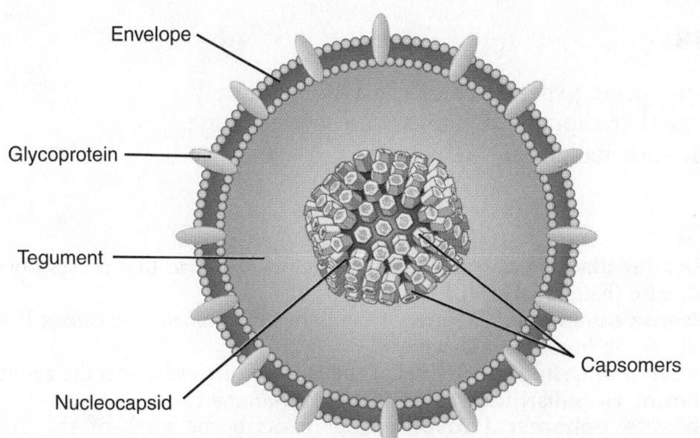

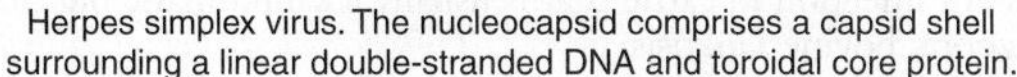
Herpes simplex virus. The nucleocapsid comprises a capsid shell surrounding a linear double-stranded DNA and toroidal core protein.

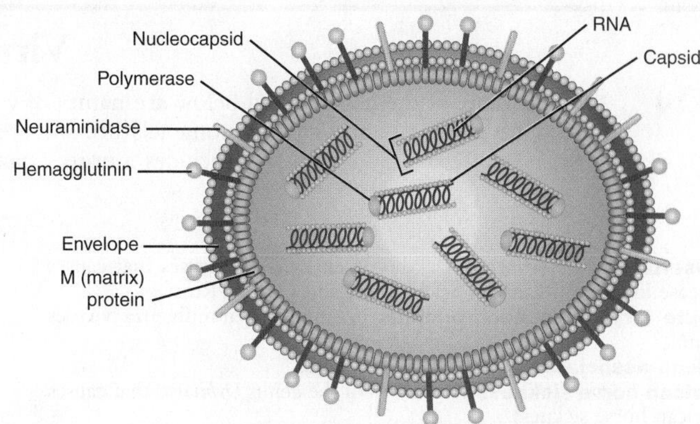

Influenza virus. The nucleocapsids, helical assemblies of single-stranded RNA and nucleoprotein capsids, are twisted on themselves to form tightly coiled helical superstructures (not shown).

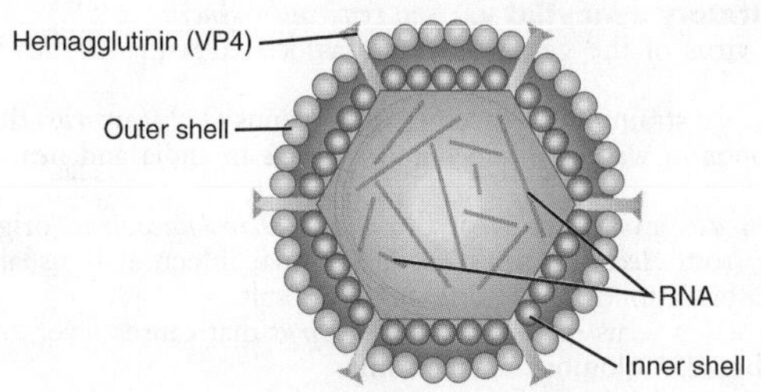

Rotavirus. The double-stranded RNA genome occurs in 11 segments.

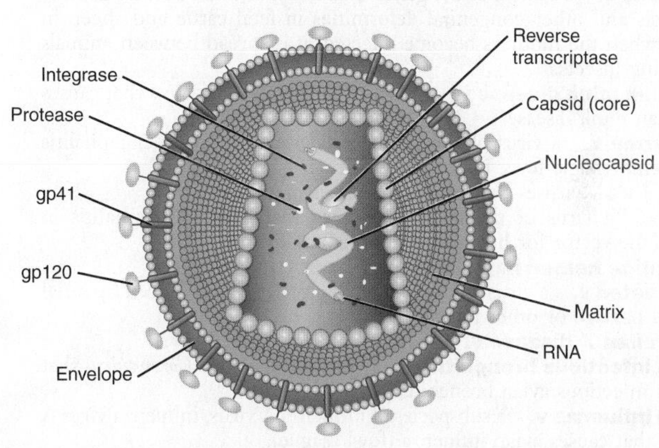

Human immunodeficiency virus (HIV). Within the core capsid, the diploid, single-stranded, positive-sense RNA is complexed to nucleoprotein.

Life cycle of the human immunodeficiency virus. The extracellular envelope protein gp120 binds to CD4 on the surface of T lymphocytes or mononuclear phagocytes, while the transmembrane protein gp41 mediates the fusion of the viral envelope with the cell membrane (gp = glycoprotein).

■ PLATE 49—STRUCTURE OF VARIOUS VIRUSES AND LIFE CYCLE OF HUMAN IMMUNODEFICIENCY VIRUS

Virus

Many of the names listed below are names of virus species; species names in viral taxonomy do not use Latin binomial nomenclature and are neither capitalized (unless the species name includes a proper name) nor italicized.

Absettarov v. a strain of tick-borne encephalitis viruses that causes disease in Central Europe, Scandinavia, and western Russia.
acute laryngotracheobronchitis v. human parainfluenza viruses 1 and 2.
adeno-associated v. (AAV) *Dependovirus.*
African horse sickness v. a virus of the genus *Orbivirus* that causes African horse sickness.
African swine fever v. a double-stranded DNA virus that is the etiological agent of African swine fever; it was formerly classified as a member of the Iridoviridae but is now assigned to the genus African swine fever–like viruses, which belongs to no family and of which it is the only member.
Akabane v. a species of the genus *Orthobunyavirus* that causes arthrogryposis and other congenital deformities in fetal cattle and sheep in utero when the mothers become infected; it is spread between animals by biting insects.
Aleutian mink disease v. a virus of the genus *Parvovirus* that causes Aleutian mink disease.
Alkhurma v. a virus of the genus *Flavivirus* that causes encephalitis and hemorrhagic fever in Saudi Arabia.
animal v's viruses that produce diseases in animals.
Apoi v. a virus of the genus *Flavivirus* that causes encephalitis in Japan; the vector for human infection is unknown.
Argentine hemorrhagic fever v. Junin v.
attenuated v. a virus whose pathogenicity has been reduced by serial animal passage or other means.
Australian X disease v. Murray Valley encephalitis v.
avian infectious bronchitis v. a virus of the genus *Coronavirus* that causes infectious avian bronchitis.
avian influenza v. a subspecies of influenza A virus, influenza virus A avian, that causes avian influenza (fowl plague).
avian leukosis v. a species of the genus *Alpharetrovirus* that causes avian leukosis in chickens.
B v. herpesvirus B.
B19 v. a species belonging to the genus *Erythrovirus* that binds to the erythrocyte P blood group antigen and is the cause of erythema infectiosum. In patients with hemolytic anemia or sickle cell disease it causes aplastic crisis; it can also cause acute arthritis. Fetal infection can cause hydrops fetalis and spontaneous abortion or death in utero. Persistent infection in immunocompromised patients can lead to chronic bone marrow failure. Called also *human parvovirus B19.*
bacterial v. a virus capable of producing transmissible lysis of bacteria; the virus particle attaches to the bacterial cell wall and viral nucleoprotein enters the cell, resulting in the synthesis of virus and its liberation on physical disruption of the cell. Bacterial viruses are usually specific for bacterial species, but they may be strain-specific or may infect more than one species of bacteria. Called also *bacteriophage* or *phage.* See *Twort-d'Herelle phenomenon,* under *phenomenon.*
Banna v. a tick-associated virus of the genus *Seadornavirus* that has been linked to cases of encephalitis in China.
Banzi v. a virus of the genus *Flavivirus,* antigenically related to yellow fever virus; it causes febrile illness in southern and eastern Africa.
Barmah Forest v. a species of togavirus of the genus *Alphavirus* that causes rash, fever, and arthritis in Queensland, Australia; it is transmitted to humans by mosquitoes of the genus *Aedes.*
Bayou v. a virus of the genus *Hantavirus* that causes hantavirus pulmonary syndrome on the Gulf Coast of Texas; the natural host is the rice rat, *Oryzomys palustris.*
Belgrade v. see *Dobrava-Belgrade v.*
Berne v. a virus of the genus *Torovirus* associated with diarrhea in horses.
Bittner v. mouse mammary tumor v.
BK v. see under *polyomavirus.*
Black Creek Canal v. a virus of the genus *Hantavirus* that causes hantavirus pulmonary syndrome, found in warm regions of the Americas; the vectors are rodents, especially cotton rats of genus *Sigmodon.*
bluetongue v. a virus of the genus *Orbivirus,* separable into at least 24 serotypes, that causes bluetongue.
Bolivian hemorrhagic fever v. Machupo v.
border disease v. a virus of the genus *Pestivirus* that causes border disease (hairy shaker disease).
Borna disease v. a virus of the genus *Bornavirus* that causes Borna disease in horses and sheep.
bovine diarrhea v. a virus of the genus *Pestivirus* that is the agent of bovine virus diarrhea; called also *mucosal disease v.*
bovine ephemeral fever v. an insect-borne virus of the genus *Ephemerovirus* that causes bovine ephemeral fever.
bovine leukemia v. a virus of the genus *Deltaretrovirus* that causes a persistent infection in cattle that is usually asymptomatic but may result in enzootic bovine leukosis.
bovine papillomatosis v. bovine papillomavirus.
bovine papular stomatitis v. a virus of the genus *Parapoxvirus* that causes bovine papular stomatitis.
bovine respiratory syncytial v. see *respiratory syncytial v's.*
Breda v. a virus of the genus *Torovirus* associated with diarrhea in calves.
buffalopox v. a strain of the vaccinia virus (genus *Orthopoxvirus*) that causes buffalopox in water buffaloes and humans in India and nearby countries.
Bunyamwera v. an arbovirus of the genus *Orthobunyavirus,* originally isolated from *Aedes* mosquitoes in Uganda; infection is usually asymptomatic, but a mild febrile disease may result.
Bussuquara v. a virus of the genus *Flavivirus* that causes fever and arthralgia in Brazil, Colombia, and Panama.
Bwamba v. an arbovirus of the genus *Orthobunyavirus,* which was originally isolated in Uganda but is prevalent in much of Africa and causes a mild febrile disease.
C v. coxsackievirus.
CA v. croup-associated v.; see *human parainfluenza v. 1* and *human parainfluenza v. 2.*
California encephalitis v. a mosquito-borne virus of the genus *Orthobunyavirus* occurring in the western United States and Canada; it is the cause of California encephalitis.
camelpox v. a virus of the genus *Orthopoxvirus* that causes camelpox.
cancer-inducing v. oncovirus.
canine distemper v. a virus of the genus *Morbillivirus* that causes canine distemper.
Cantagalo v. a strain of the vaccinia virus (genus *Orthopoxvirus*) that causes pustular lesions in cattle and humans in parts of Brazil.
caprine arthritis-encephalitis v. a species of the genus *Lentivirus* that in young goats causes acute encephalitis and in older goats causes chronic arthritis, sometimes with mastitis, pneumonia, or glomerulonephritis.
Catu v. a species of viruses of the genus *Orthobunyavirus* closely related to *Guama virus,* isolated from a Brazilian patient with a febrile illness.
CELO v. [*c*hicken-*e*mbryo-*l*ethal *o*rphan] fowl adenovirus.
Central European encephalitis v's old classification for those tick-borne encephalitis viruses (genus *Flavivirus*) occurring in Central Europe and nearby areas.
Chagres v. an arbovirus of the genus *Phlebovirus,* causing fever associated with malaise, headache, and pains of localized and generalized distribution, in Panama.
Chandipura v. a virus of the genus *Vesiculovirus* that causes encephalitis in parts of India; infections can be fatal in children.
chikungunya v. a species of togavirus of the genus *Alphavirus* transmitted chiefly by mosquitoes of the genus *Aedes* that causes chikungunya in Africa and Asia.
Coe v. former name for *coxsackievirus A21.*
Colorado tick fever v. a virus of the family Reoviridae that causes a febrile disease occurring in regions of the Rocky Mountains where the tick vector, *Dermacentor andersoni,* is prevalent.
Columbia SK v. a strain of encephalomyocarditis virus that was originally isolated from a monkey previously inoculated with the Yale SK strain of poliovirus.
common cold v's viruses such as rhinoviruses considered to cause the common cold.
conditionally replicative v's mutant viruses that can replicate only inside certain types of tumor cells and may disrupt those cells; the most common kind are adenoviruses.

coryza v. rhinovirus.
cowpox v. a virus of the genus *Orthopoxvirus* that causes cowpox; it is closely related to vaccinia virus.
Coxsackie v. coxsackievirus.
Crimean-Congo hemorrhagic fever v. a virus of the genus *Nairovirus* that causes Crimean-Congo hemorrhagic fever.
croup-associated v. human parainfluenza viruses 1 and 2.
defective v. a virus that cannot be completely replicated or cannot form a protein coat; in some cases replication can proceed if missing gene functions are supplied by other (helper) viruses; see *helper v.*
dengue v. a species of the genus *Flavivirus* existing as four antigenically related but distinct types (designated 1, 2, 3, and 4) that causes classic dengue and hemorrhagic dengue.
Desert Shield v. a calicivirus of the genus *Norovirus* that can cause gastroenteritis.
DNA v. a virus whose genome consists of DNA; called also *deoxyribovirus.*
Dobrava v. see *Dobrava-Belgrade v.*
Dobrava-Belgrade v. a virus of the genus *Hantavirus*, originally isolated as Dobrava virus in Slovenia and Belgrade virus in Serbia; it causes severe epidemic hemorrhagic fever in various Balkan countries. The reservoir is the yellow-necked field mouse, *Apodemus flavicollis.*
duck hepatitis B v. a virus of the genus *Avihepadnavirus* that causes duck virus hepatitis.
Duvenhage v. a virus of the genus *Lyssavirus* that is widely distributed in bats in Europe and Africa and causes a rabies-like disease; fatal human infection has occurred.
eastern equine encephalitis v., eastern equine encephalomyelitis v. a species of togavirus of the genus *Alphavirus*, which causes eastern equine encephalomyelitis. Called also *EEE v.*
EB v. Epstein-Barr v.
Ebola v. a virus of the genus *Filovirus* that causes Ebola virus disease, first isolated near the Ebola River in Zaire; there are four subtypes: Zaire, Sudan, Reston, and Côte d'Ivoire. The natural reservoir and mode of transmission of primary infection are unknown, but secondary infection is by direct contact with infected blood and other body secretions and by airborne particles.
ectromelia v. a virus of the genus *Orthopoxvirus* that causes infectious ectromelia in mice.
Edge Hill v. a virus of the genus *Flavivirus*, antigenically related to yellow fever virus; it causes fever and polyarthritis and is spread from marsupials to humans by mosquitoes of the genus *Aedes.*
EEE v. eastern equine encephalitis v..
egg drop syndrome 1976 v. an adenovirus (duck adenovirus 1), first recognized in 1976, that causes apparently healthy ducks and geese to lay eggs with thin or soft shells or without shells.
EMC v., encephalomyocarditis v. a virus of the genus *Cardiovirus* found in Africa, South America, and elsewhere, which causes mild aseptic meningitis in humans and encephalomyocarditis in pigs and certain nonhuman primates. There are several different strains that are substantially identical in immunologic and other respects, including the Columbia SK virus and the Mengo virus.
enteric v's an epidemiologic class of viruses that are normally acquired by ingestion and replicate in the intestinal tract, causing local rather than generalized infection. Enteric viruses are included in the families Adenoviridae, Astroviridae, Caliciviridae, Coronaviridae, and Reoviridae.
enteric orphan v's viruses isolated from the intestinal tracts of animals, called orphan viruses because they are often not specifically associated with illness; they include such viruses isolated from cattle (ecboviruses), dogs (ecdoviruses), humans (echoviruses), monkeys (ecmoviruses), and swine (ecsoviruses).
enveloped v. a virus having an outer lipoprotein bilayer acquired by budding through the host cell membrane.
epidemic keratoconjunctivitis v. human adenovirus type 8; see *Mastadenovirus.*
Epstein-Barr v. (EBV) a virus of the genus *Lymphocryptovirus* that causes infectious mononucleosis and is associated with Burkitt lymphoma and nasopharyngeal carcinoma. Called also *human herpesvirus 4.*
equine arteritis v. a virus of the genus *Arterivirus* that causes equine viral arteritis.
equine encephalitis v's, equine encephalomyelitis v's a group of togavirus species of the genus *Alphavirus*, each named for the type of encephalomyelitis it causes in horses, other equines, and humans; birds serve as a reservoir and transmission is by mosquitoes. The most common types are *eastern, western,* and *Venezuelan equine encephalitis* or *encephalomyelitis viruses.*
equine infectious anemia v. a virus of the genus *Lentivirus* that causes equine infectious anemia.
Everglades v. a species of togavirus of the genus *Alphavirus*, transmitted by mosquitoes of the genus *Culex;* it has been isolated from rodents in the Everglades National Park and causes febrile illness in humans.
exanthematous disease v. any of a group of dermotropic viruses, including poxviruses, that cause exanthematous disease.
Eyach v. a tickborne virus of the genus *Coltivirus* that has caused neurologic illness in France, Germany, and the former Czechoslovakia.
FA v. a strain of Theiler v.
feline immunodeficiency v. a virus of the genus *Lentivirus* that causes a wasting syndrome with lymphadenopathy and lymphopenia in cats.
feline infectious peritonitis v. a species of the genus *Coronavirus* that causes feline infectious peritonitis.
feline leukemia v. a retrovirus of the genus *Gammaretrovirus* that is found in domestic cats and can cause any of various types of contagious leukemias and lymphomas and other conditions such as anemia, glomerulonephritis, spontaneous abortion, and immunosuppression. See also *feline leukemia*, under *leukemia.*
feline panleukopenia v. a virus of the genus *Parvovirus* that causes panleukopenia in cats and infections in other animals; it is antigenically closely related to canine parvovirus and mink enteritis virus. See also *feline parvovirus.*
feline rhinotracheitis v. felid herpesvirus 1.
v. fixé, fixed v. 1. rabies virus whose virulence and incubation period have been stabilized by serial passage and remain fixed during further transmission; used for inoculating animals from which rabies vaccine is prepared. Cf. *street v.* 2. a virus whose virulence and incubation period have been stabilized by serial passage and remained fixed during further transmission; used for research, testing, and vaccine production.
foamy v's *Spumavirus.*
foot-and-mouth disease v. a species of the genus *Aphthovirus* that causes foot-and-mouth disease.
fowlpox v. a virus of the genus *Avipoxvirus* that causes fowlpox.
Friend v., Friend murine leukemia v. a strain of murine leukemia virus that causes erythroleukemia in mice.
Germiston v. a virus in the serogroup Bwamba virus, genus *Orthobunyavirus*, the cause of mild febrile disease in South Africa.
goatpox v. a virus of the genus *Capripoxvirus* that causes goatpox.
Gross v. a strain of murine leukemia virus that induces lymphomas in mice.
Guama v. a virus of the genus *Orthobunyavirus* isolated in the region of Belem, Brazil, from foresters suffering from hyperthermia, headache, muscular and articular pains, and occasionally nausea and vertigo.
Guanarito v. an arenavirus of the Tacaribe complex, first isolated from patients in Guanare, Venezuela, that causes Venezuelan hemorrhagic fever.
Guaroa v. an arbovirus of the genus *Orthobunyavirus* isolated in Colombia from the blood of patients with a febrile disease.
Hantaan v. a virus of the genus *Hantavirus* that causes severe epidemic hemorrhagic fever in Asia. The reservoir is mice of the genus *Apodemus.*
Hanzalova v. a strain of tick-borne encephalitis viruses that causes disease in the Czech Republic.
Hawaii v. a species of the genus *Norovirus* that causes gastroenteritis, which can be severe in children.
helper v. a virus (e.g., the Rous-associated virus) that aids the development of a defective virus by supplying or restoring the activity of a viral gene or enabling a defective virus (e.g., the Rous sarcoma virus) to form a protein coat.
hemadsorption v., type 1 (HA1) former name for human parainfluenza virus 3.
hemadsorption v., type 2 (HA2) former name for human parainfluenza virus 1.
hemagglutinating encephalomyelitis v. of pigs porcine hemagglutinating encephalomyelitis v.
Hendra v. a paramyxovirus of the genus *Henipavirus* that causes encephalitis and pneumonia in horses and humans having contact with infected animals.

Virus *Continued*

hepatitis A v. (HAV) the sole species of the genus *Hepatovirus*, the etiologic agent of hepatitis A.
hepatitis B v. (HBV) a virus of the genus *Orthohepadnavirus*, that causes hepatitis B.
hepatitis C v. a species of the genus *Hepacivirus* that causes hepatitis C.
hepatitis C–like v's *Hepacivirus*.
hepatitis D v. (HDV) a satellite virus of the genus *Deltavirus* that causes hepatitis D. The presence of hepatitis B virus is required to provide helper functions, and the viral envelope is composed of hepatitis B surface antigen. Called also *hepatitis delta v.*
hepatitis delta v. hepatitis D v.
hepatitis E v. a species of the genus *Hepevirus*, family Caliciviridae, the enterically transmitted etiologic agent of hepatitis E. It consists of a spherical virion 27–34 nm in diameter with a positive-sense single-stranded RNA genome.
hepatitis G v. (HGV) a parenterally transmitted flavivirus originally isolated from a patient with chronic hepatitis and considered to be identical to hepatitis GB virus-C; most infections are benign, and the role of HGV in the etiology of liver disease is uncertain.
hepatitis GB v. (HGBV) a group of viruses isolated from a patient with hepatitis and classified as HGBV-A, HGBV-B, and HGBV-C; HGBV-C belongs to the same species as hepatitis G virus. The name is derived from the patient's initials (G.B.).
hepatotropic v. a virus that primarily affects the liver, such as the hepatitis viruses.
herpangina v. any of several viruses that cause herpangina, primarily in children; these are most often coxsackieviruses and less often echoviruses.
herpes v. see *herpesvirus*.
herpes simplex v. (HSV) see human herpesvirus 1 and human herpesvirus 2, under *herpesvirus*.
Highlands J v. a mosquito-born species of togavirus of the genus *Alphavirus;* it causes encephalitis in birds and horses in Florida, but has not been known to cause disease in humans.
H1N1 v. an antigenic variant of *Influenzavirus A*, arising from recombination of genetic material from human, avian, and swine influenza viruses, that causes disease in humans.
hog cholera v. a virus of the genus *Pestivirus* that causes hog cholera.
human immunodeficiency v. (HIV) either of two species of the genus *Lentivirus* (HIV-1 and HIV-2), which cause the acquired immunodeficiency syndrome (AIDS). HIV-1, which comprises at least three subgroups (M, N, and O), is of worldwide distribution, while HIV-2 is largely confined to West Africa. Transmission and manifestations are similar for both. HIV-1 was formerly called *human T-cell lymphotropic v. type III* and *lymphadenopathy-associated v.* See Plate 49.
human parainfluenza v. 1 a paramyxovirus of the genus *Respirovirus* that causes croup in young children and mild upper respiratory infections in older children and adults. Called also *acute laryngotracheobronchitis v., CA v.*, and *croup-associated v.*
human parainfluenza v. 2 a virus of the genus *Rubulavirus* that causes croup in young children. Called also *acute laryngotracheobronchitis v., CA v.*, and *croup-associated v.*
human parainfluenza v. 3 a paramyxovirus of the genus *Respirovirus* that causes croup and lower respiratory tract infections in young children.
human parainfluenza v. 4 a virus of the genus *Rubulavirus* that causes upper respiratory infections, chiefly in young children.
human respiratory syncytial v. see *respiratory syncytial v's.*
human T-cell leukemia v. synonym for *human T-lymphotropic v.*; see there for entries for specific strains.
human T-cell lymphotropic v. type I (HTLV-I) human T-lymphotropic virus 1.
human T-cell lymphotropic v. type II (HTLV-II) human T-lymphotropic virus 2.
human T-cell lymphotropic v. type III (HTLV-III) former name for *human immunodeficiency v. 1.*
human T-lymphotropic v. 1 (HTLV-1) a virus of the genus *Deltaretrovirus* with a worldwide distribution, having an affinity for the helper cell type of T lymphocytes; it causes chronic infection and is associated with adult T-cell leukemia/lymphoma and chronic progressive myelopathy. Called also *human T-cell leukemia v. type I* and *human T-cell lymphotrophic virus type I.*
human T-lymphotropic v. 2 (HTLV-2) a virus of the genus *Deltaretrovirus*, having extensive serologic cross-reactivity with HTLV-1, isolated from an atypical T cell variant of hairy cell leukemia and from patients with other hematologic disorders; no clear association with disease has been established. Called also *human T-cell leukemia v. type II* and *human T-cell lymphotropic v. type II.*
human T-lymphotropic v. 3 (HTLV-3) a virus of the genus *Deltaretrovirus*, found among persons in southern Cameroon living in close contact with monkeys or apes; its pathogenic significance is unknown.
human T-lymphotropic v. 4 (HTLV-4) a virus of the genus *Deltaretrovirus*, found among persons in southern Cameroon living in close contact with monkeys or apes; its pathogenic significance is unknown.
Hypr v. a strain of tick-borne encephalitis virus seen in Central Europe and Scandinavia, possibly identical to Hanzalova virus.
igbo-ora v. an arbovirus of the genus *Alphavirus*, closely related to chikungunya virus and o'nyong-nyong virus, that has been associated with a denguelike disease in Nigeria and other West African countries.
Ilheus v. an arbovirus of the genus *Flavivirus*, first isolated from species of *Aedes* and *Psorophora* in Brazil; also found in Panama, where birds may be hosts. It is related to St. Louis encephalitis virus, Japanese encephalitis virus, and West Nile virus.
infectious bovine rhinotracheitis v. bovine herpesvirus 1.
infectious bursal disease v. a virus of the genus *Avibirnavirus* that causes infectious bursal disease in chickens.
infectious ectromelia v. a virus of the genus *Orthopoxvirus* that causes infectious ectromelia in mice.
infectious laryngotracheitis v. gallid herpesvirus 1.
infectious pancreatic necrosis v. a virus of the genus *Aquabirnavirus* that causes infectious pancreatic necrosis in fish.
infectious porcine encephalomyelitis v. porcine enterovirus.
influenza v. any of a group of orthomyxoviruses that cause influenza, including at least three genera: *Influenzavirus A, Influenzavirus B*, and *Influenzavirus C*. Antigenic variants are classified on the basis of their surface antigens (hemagglutinin and neuraminidase) as H1N1, H2N2, etc. Serotype A viruses are subject to major antigenic changes (antigenic shifts) as well as minor gradual antigenic changes (antigenic drift) and cause the major pandemics. Serotype B viruses appear to undergo only antigenic drift and cause more localized epidemics. Serotype C viruses appear to be antigenically stable and cause only sporadic disease. See Plate 49.
influenza A v., influenza B v., influenza C v. species in the genera *Influenzavirus A, Influenzavirus B*, and *Influenzavirus C;* see *influenza v.*
Jamestown Canyon v. a strain of California encephalitis virus that can cause encephalitis.
Japanese encephalitis v. a mosquito-borne virus of the genus *Flavivirus*, antigenically related to Murray Valley and St. Louis encephalitis virus; it causes Japanese encephalitis.
JC v. see under *polyomavirus.*
Junin v. an arenavirus of the Tacaribe complex that causes Argentine hemorrhagic fever, transmitted by contact with infected rodents, especially of the genus *Calomys*. Called also *Argentine hemorrhagic fever v.*
K v. a virus of the genus *Polyomavirus* that infects mice, particularly newborns, and causes pneumonia.
Karshi v. a tick-borne virus of the genus *Flavivirus* that causes fever in Uzbekistan; various species of ticks spread it from rodents to humans.
Kemerovo v. a tick-borne virus of the genus *Orbivirus* that causes a benign febrile disease in western Siberia and Egypt.
Kokobera v. a virus of the genus *Flavivirus* that causes fever and arthralgia in Australia and Papua New Guinea; mosquitoes of the genus *Culex* spread it from rodents to humans.
Korean hemorrhagic fever v. Hantaan v.
Koutango v. a mosquito-borne virus of the genus *Flavivirus* that causes fever, rash, and arthralgia in West and Central Africa; various species of ticks spread it from rodents to humans. It is antigenically related to the Japanese, Murray Valley, and St. Louis encephalitis viruses.
Kumba v. a strain of Semliki Forest virus isolated from mosquitoes in the Kumba region of Cameroon.
Kumlinge v. a strain of tick-borne encephalitis virus that causes fever and encephalitis in Finland.
Kunjin v. a mosquito-borne virus of the genus *Flavivirus*, antigenically related to Japanese encephalitis virus, that causes febrile disease and encephalitis in Australia and Malaysia.

Virus *Continued*

Kyasanur Forest disease v. a tick-borne virus of the genus *Flavivirus*, antigenically related to Omsk hemorrhagic fever virus, transmitted by ticks of the genus *Haemaphysalis;* it causes Kyasanur Forest disease in forest workers in India.
La Crosse v. a strain of California encephalitis virus that causes La Crosse encephalitis.
Langat v. a tick-borne virus of the genus *Flavivirus* that causes fever and encephalitis in Malaysia, Thailand, and Russia; the vector spreading it from rodents to humans is ticks of the genus *Ixodes.*
Lansing v. the prototype strain of poliovirus type 2.
Lassa v. an arenavirus of the LCMV-LASV complex, existing in several serologically distinct strains and distributed throughout West and Central Africa. The natural reservoir is the multimammate mouse, in which it causes an inapparent infection; human infection (Lassa fever) results from contact with mouse urine.
latent v. masked v.
LCM v. lymphocytic choriomeningitis v.
Leon v. the prototype strain of poliovirus type 3.
Lordsdale v. a calicivirus of the genus *Norovirus* that can cause gastroenteritis.
louping ill v. a tick-borne virus of the genus *Flavivirus*, transmitted by the tick *Ixodes ricinus;* it causes louping ill of sheep, and is transmissible to humans, in whom it may cause meningitis and encephalitis.
lumpy skin disease v. a virus of the genus *Capripoxvirus* that causes lumpy skin disease in African cattle.
lymphadenopathy-associated v. (LAV) former name for *human immunodeficiency v. 1.*
lymphocystis v's *Lymphocystivirus.*
lymphocyte-associated v. any virus of the subfamily Gammaherpesvirinae, members of which are specific for either B or T lymphocytes; infection is often arrested at a prelytic or lytic stage without production of infectious virions. Latent virus may frequently be demonstrated in lymphoid tissue. Host range is very narrow.
lymphocytic choriomeningitis v. an arenavirus of the LCMV-LASV complex that causes lymphocytic choriomeningitis. Called also *LCM v.*
lytic v. a virus that is replicated in the host cell and causes death and lysis of the cell.
Machupo v. an arenavirus of the Tacaribe complex that causes Bolivian hemorrhagic fever, transmitted by contact with infected rodents of the species *Calomys callosus.* Called also *Bolivian hemorrhagic fever v.*
maedi/visna v. visna/maedi v.
Makonde v. Uganda S v.
mammary tumor v. mouse mammary tumor v.
Marburg v. a virus of the genus *Filovirus* that causes Marburg virus disease, transmitted by direct physical contact with African green monkeys or their organs or with an infected person.
Marek disease v. either of two herpesviruses that cause Marek disease in chickens; see *gallid herpesvirus 2* and *gallid herpesvirus 3*, under *herpesvirus.*
masked v. a virus that ordinarily occurs in a noninfective state and is demonstrable by indirect methods that activate it, such as by blind passage in experimental animals.
Mayaro v. a species of togavirus of the genus *Alphavirus*, originally isolated in Mayaro County, Trinidad; it causes a denguelike illness in Central and South America and is transmitted by mosquitoes of the genus *Haemagogus.*
measles v. a virus of the genus *Morbillivirus* that causes measles.
measles-like v's *Morbillivirus.*
Menangle v. a paramyxovirus of the genus *Rubulavirus*, the cause of spontaneous abortion and other diseases in pigs and fruit bats; it may be zoonotic to humans having contact with infected animals, causing influenzalike symptoms.
Mengo v. a strain of encephalomyocarditis virus that was first isolated in Uganda from a monkey with encephalomyelitis, and later from mosquitoes and a mongoose in the same area; it was later found to be the cause of an epizootic disease of pigs in Panama.
milker's node v. pseudocowpox v.
mink enteritis v. a virus of the genus *Parvovirus* that causes mink viral enteritis; it is sometimes considered to be a species-specific variant of feline parvovirus.
MM v. a strain of encephalomyocarditis virus that was first isolated from the brain of a hamster previously inoculated with material from a human case of paralytic disease.
Modoc v. a virus of the genus *Flavivirus* that causes aseptic meningitis in the western United States and Canada.
Mokola v. a virus of the genus *Lyssavirus* that is found in South Africa and can cause a rabieslike illness, sometimes fatal, in domestic animals and humans.
molluscum contagiosum v. the single species of the genus *Molluscipoxvirus*, the etiologic agent of molluscum contagiosum.
Moloney v. a strain of murine leukemia virus that causes lymphoid leukemia in mice.
monkeypox v. a virus of the genus *Orthopoxvirus* that produces a mild, epidemic, exanthematous disease in monkeys and a smallpox-like disease in humans.
mouse mammary tumor v. the sole member of the mammalian type B retroviruses, which induces mammary adenocarcinoma in certain strains of mice, usually transmitted from mother to offspring through the milk; viral expression and carcinogenesis are influenced by estrogen stimulation. Called also *Bittner v.*
mucosal disease v. bovine diarrhea v.
mumps v. a virus of the genus *Rubulavirus* that causes mumps and, in some cases, tenderness and swelling of the testes, pancreas, ovaries, or other organs.
murine leukemia v. a species of the genus *Gammaretrovirus* that infects mice; it includes a number of strains that can be grouped by their envelope antigens or by the antigens induced on the surface of the infected cell; some strains cause leukemia or solid tumors.
Murray Valley encephalitis v. a mosquito-borne virus of the genus *Flavivirus*, antigenically related to Japanese encephalitis virus, that causes Murray Valley encephalitis.
myxoma v. a virus of the genus *Leporipoxvirus* that causes infectious myxomatosis in rabbits.
Nairobi sheep disease v. a tick-borne virus of the genus *Nairovirus* that causes Nairobi sheep disease.
naked v. a virus lacking an outer lipoprotein bilayer.
Nakiwogo v. Semunya v.
Negishi v. a tick-borne virus of the genus *Flavivirus* that was isolated from fatal cases of encephalitis in Japan.
Neudoerfl v. a strain of tick-borne encephalitis virus that causes disease in Europe.
neurotropic v. a virus that has a predilection for and causes infection in nerve tissue, such as the rabies virus.
newborn pneumonitis v. human parainfluenza v. 1.
Newcastle disease v. a virus of the genus *Avulavirus* that causes Newcastle disease in birds; human infection is mild and characterized by conjunctivitis and brief generalized symptoms. Called also *avian paramyxovirus 1.*
Nipah v. a paramyxovirus of the genus *Henipavirus* that causes Nipah encephalitis.
non-A, non-B hepatitis v. a hepatitis virus other than hepatitis A virus or hepatitis B virus, usually referring to hepatitis C virus.
nonenveloped v. naked v.
non-oncogenic v. a virus that does not induce cell transformation or malignancy.
Norwalk v. the type species of the genus *Norovirus;* it is a common cause of epidemics of acute gastroenteritis, with diarrhea and vomiting lasting 24 to 48 hours.
Norwalk-like v. *Norovirus.*
Omsk hemorrhagic fever v. a tick-borne virus of the genus *Flavivirus* that has been isolated from patients with Omsk hemorrhagic fever and is transmitted by ticks of the genera *Dermacentor* and *Ixodes.*
oncogenic v's an epidemiologic class of viruses that are acquired by close contact (including sexual contact) or injection and cause usually persistent infection; they may induce cell transformation and malignancy. Oncogenic viruses are included in the families Adenoviridae, Hepadnaviridae, Herpesviridae, Papovaviridae, and Retroviridae.
o'nyong-nyong v. a species of togavirus of the genus *Alphavirus*, closely related to chikungunya virus; it causes o'nyong-nyong in East Africa and Senegal and is transmitted by anopheline mosquitoes.
orf v. a virus of the genus *Parapoxvirus* that causes contagious ecthyma (orf).
Oropouche v. a member of the Simbu serogroup of the genus *Orthobunyavirus* that causes illness in Brazil; infection may be severe and is characterized by fever, chills, malaise, headache, myalgia, and arthralgia, sometimes with nausea and vomiting, and occasionally with central nervous system involvement.

Virus *Continued*

orphan v's viruses which when isolated originally in tissue culture showed no specific association with disease, such as the enteric orphan viruses; some have since been found to occur in association with human disease.
Orungo v. a mosquito-borne virus of the genus *Orbivirus* that causes a febrile illness in Nigeria and Uganda.
pantropic v. a virus that affects or has an affinity for many different kinds of tissue or organs.
papilloma v. papillomavirus.
pappataci fever v. see *Phlebovirus.*
parainfluenza v. any of various species of viruses of the family Paramyxoviridae that cause upper respiratory tract disease in humans and other animals. Those infecting humans have been classified in two genera: *Paramyxovirus* (human parainfluenza viruses 1 and 3) and *Rubulavirus* (human parainfluenza viruses 2 and 4). Also included here are simian parainfluenza viruses and Sendai virus.
paravaccinia v. pseudocowpox v.
peste-des-petits-ruminants v. a virus of the genus *Morbillivirus* that causes peste des petits ruminants.
pharyngoconjunctival fever v. human adenovirus type 3; see *Mastadenovirus.*
Pichinde v. a virus of the Tacaribe complex infecting rodents in Colombia, and isolated from human subclinical infections.
Piry v. a virus of the genus *Vesiculovirus,* related to vesicular stomatitis virus, isolated from an opossum in Brazil; laboratory infections have occurred, marked by fever, myalgia, and abdominal tenderness.
plant v's viruses that replicate and sometimes produce disease in plants.
poliomyelitis v. see *poliovirus.*
polyoma v. polyomavirus.
Pongola v. a virus in the serogroup Bwamba virus, genus *Orthobunyavirus,* occurring in central and southern Africa. Natural hosts are donkeys, horses, and monkeys; human infection is asymptomatic.
porcine hemagglutinating encephalomyelitis v. a virus of the genus *Coronavirus* that causes vomiting and wasting disease (q.v.) in piglets.
porcine transmissible gastroenteritis v. a virus of the genus *Coronavirus* that causes transmissible gastroenteritis of swine.
Powassan v. a tick-borne virus of the genus *Flavivirus* that causes Powassan encephalitis in eastern Canada and the northeastern United States.
pox v. see *poxvirus.*
pseudocowpox v. a virus of the genus *Parapoxvirus* that produces paravaccinia (pseudocowpox) on the udders and teats of milk cows and the oral mucosa of suckling calves and milker's nodules in humans. Called also *milker's node v.* and *paravaccinia v.*
pseudorabies v. a virus of the genus *Varicellovirus* that causes pseudorabies. Called also *suid herpesvirus 1.*
Puumala v. a virus of the genus *Hantavirus* that causes nephropathia epidemica in Scandinavia, Russia, and several other European countries; the natural host is the bank vole, *Clethrionomys glareolus.*
Quaranfil v. an arbovirus found in Egypt, where it was isolated from the blood of children with febrile disease, from the blood of young egrets, and from ticks (*Argas arboreus* and *A. hermanni*). It is ether-sensitive and presumed to contain RNA.
rabbit fibroma v. a virus of the genus *Leporipoxvirus* that causes rabbit fibroma.
rabbit hemorrhagic disease v. a calicivirus of the genus *Lagovirus* that causes rabbit hemorrhagic disease.
rabies v. a virus of the genus *Lyssavirus* that causes rabies.
rabies-like v's *Lyssavirus.*
Rauscher v. a strain of murine leukemia virus that causes lymphoid leukemia in mice.
respiratory v's an epidemiologic class of viruses that are acquired by inhalation of fomites and replicate in the respiratory tract, causing local rather than generalized infection. Respiratory viruses are included in the families Adenoviridae, Coronaviridae, Orthomyxoviridae, Paramyxoviridae, and Picornaviridae.
respiratory syncytial v. (RSV) any of a group of viruses belonging to the genus *Pneumovirus,* isolated originally from chimpanzees with coryza. In humans, they cause respiratory disease that is particularly severe in infants, in whom it causes bronchiolitis (q.v.) and sometimes pneumonia. Other viruses (bovine respiratory syncytial virus) cause respiratory disease in cattle. In tissue RSV causes syncytium formation. RSV is separable into two groups (A and B) on the basis of the antigenic structure of the G protein and into subgroups within the two groups.
Rift Valley fever v. a virus of the genus *Phlebovirus,* which causes Rift Valley fever in domestic animals and humans, first seen in the Rift Valley of Kenya, but now widespread in southern and eastern Africa to Egypt; transmitted by mosquitoes of the genera *Aedes, Culex,* and *Erethmapodites* or by contact with tissues and secretions of infected animals.
rinderpest v. a virus of the genus *Morbillivirus* that causes cattle plague (rinderpest).
Rio Bravo v. a virus of the genus *Flavivirus,* first isolated from bats in Mexico and the southwestern United States, which causes fever and sometimes meningitis in humans; no arthropod vector is known.
RNA v. a virus whose genome consists of RNA; called also *ribovirus.*
Rocio v. a mosquito-borne virus of the genus *Flavivirus,* found in Brazil, the cause of sometimes fatal encephalitis.
Ross River v. a species of togavirus of the genus *Alphavirus* that causes epidemic polyarthritis.
Rous-associated v. (RAV) a helper virus in whose presence a defective Rous sarcoma virus is able to form a protein coat.
Rous sarcoma v. (RSV) a usually defective virus of the genus *Alpharetrovirus* that produces Rous sarcoma in birds and sometimes tumors in other animals.
RS v. respiratory syncytial v.
rubella v. a species of togavirus, the sole species of the genus *Rubivirus;* it causes rubella.
Russian spring-summer encephalitis v. the strain of *Flavivirus* that causes Russian spring-summer encephalitis.
SA v. a parainfluenza virus isolated from the hamster brain following inoculation with a chick embryo allantoic culture of nasal washings from a person with acute upper respiratory infection; identical to simian virus SV5.
Sabia v. a species of arenavirus of the Tacaribe complex, isolated from a fatal case of hemorrhagic fever in São Paulo, Brazil; the reservoir is unknown but assumed to be a rodent.
St. Louis encephalitis v. a virus of the genus *Flavivirus,* antigenically related to Japanese encephalitis virus, that causes St. Louis encephalitis; transmitted by mosquitoes.
salivary gland v. cytomegalovirus.
sandfly fever v's see *Phlebovirus.*
sandfly fever-Naples v. a virus of the Naples serogroup of the genus *Phlebovirus,* an etiologic agent of phlebotomus fever.
sandfly fever-Sicilian v. a virus of the Sicilian serogroup of the genus *Phlebovirus,* an etiologic agent of phlebotomus fever.
Sapporo-like v. *Sapovirus.*
satellite v. a strain of virus that cannot replicate except in the presence of helper virus; considered to be deficient in coding for capsid formation.
Schwartz leukemia v. a virus that causes lymphoid leukemia in mice in Switzerland.
Semliki Forest v. a species of togavirus of the genus *Alphavirus,* originally isolated from *Aedes* mosquitoes in Uganda and later found in many parts of Africa; infection is usually mild or asymptomatic.
Semunya v. an arbovirus isolated from East African patients with an acute febrile syndrome; called also *Nakiwogo v.*
Sendai v. a paramyxovirus of the genus *Respirovirus* that causes latent infection in laboratory mice and asymptomatic infection in other animals, used experimentally as a model for paramyxoviruses in molecular studies and to induce syncytium formation in tissue culture.
Seoul v. a virus of the genus *Hantavirus* that causes mild to moderately severe epidemic hemorrhagic fever. *Rattus rattus* and *Rattus norvegicus* are the natural hosts.
Sepik v. a mosquito-borne virus of the genus *Flavivirus,* antigenically related to yellow fever virus; it causes febrile disease in Papua New Guinea.
sheeppox v. a virus of the genus *Capripoxvirus* that causes sheeppox.
sigma v. a congenitally transmitted genus of rhabdoviruses that induces carbon dioxide sensitivity in *Drosophila melanogaster* and other fruit flies.
Simbu v. a species of the genus *Orthobunyavirus* isolated from the mosquito *Aedes circumluteolis* in Africa; serologically related species infect mammals.
simian v's viruses that have been recovered from monkeys; these belong to many different groups, including adenoviruses, enteroviruses, herpesviruses, and reoviruses.

Virus *Continued*

simian v. 40 (SV40) a species of the genus *Polyomavirus* that was isolated from *Rhesus* monkey kidney tissue and produces transformation in human and newborn hamster kidney cell cultures and has caused progressive multifocal leukoencephalopathy in humans.
simian immunodeficiency v. (SIV) a species of the genus *Lentivirus*, closely related to human immunodeficiency virus, that causes inapparent infection in African green monkeys and a disease resembling acquired immunodeficiency syndrome in macaques.
Sindbis v. a species of togavirus of the genus *Alphavirus;* it is transmitted by *Culex* mosquitoes and causes Sindbis fever from East Africa to the Philippines and in Scandinavia.
Sin Nombre v. a virus of the genus *Hantavirus* that causes hantavirus pulmonary syndrome in the western United States; the natural host is the deer mouse, *Peromyscus maniculatus*.
slow v. any virus causing a disease characterized by a long preclinical course and gradual progression once the symptoms appear.
smallpox v. variola v.
Snow Mountain v. a species of the genus *Norovirus* that causes gastroenteritis, which can be severe in children.
Spondweni v. a mosquito-borne virus of the genus *Flavivirus*, antigenically related to Zika virus; it has caused febrile illness and hepatitis in several different parts of Africa.
street v. virus from a naturally infected animal, as opposed to a laboratory-adapted strain of the virus. Cf. *fixed v.*
swine infertility and respiratory syndrome v. a virus of the genus *Arterivirus* that causes porcine epidemic abortion and respiratory syndrome.
swine influenza v. a type A influenza virus that causes swine influenza; direct transmission to humans has occasionally caused infection that can be fatal.
swinepox v. the sole species of the genus *Suipoxvirus*, which causes swinepox.
Tacaribe v. an arenavirus of the Tacaribe complex, isolated from bats in Trinidad.
Tahyna v. a virus belonging to the California serogroup of the genus *Orthobunyavirus* that causes a febrile illness in Russia and Central Europe.
Tamiami v. an arenavirus of the Tacaribe complex, first found in bats in Trinidad and later found to be serologically linked to human infection.
tanapox v. a virus of the genus *Yatapoxvirus* that causes tanapox.
temperate v. see under *bacteriophage*.
Teschen v. porcine enterovirus.
Theiler v., Theiler murine encephalomyelitis v. Theilovirus.
Thogoto v. a species of tick-borne orthomyxoviruses that infect humans, cattle, and sheep in Africa. Human infection results in sometimes severe encephalitis and optic neuritis.
Thogoto-like v's a genus of tick-borne viruses of the family Orthomyxoviridae that cause infection in vertebrates in Africa, Europe, and Asia.
tick-borne v's viruses that are transmitted by ticks.
tick-borne encephalitis v's a serogroup of the genus *Flavivirus*, consisting of viruses that are transmitted by ticks and cause encephalitis in humans and animals that ranges in severity from subclinical to fatal. It was formerly divided into Central European and Far Eastern subtypes.
torque teno v. a virus of the genus *Anellovirus* that can cause liver damage or hepatitis; it was originally observed in Japan but was later found in other parts of the world. Called also *TT v.*
Toscana v. a virus of the Naples serogroup of the genus *Phlebovirus*, an etiologic agent of phlebotomus fever.
Tribec v. a tickborne virus of the genus *Orbivirus* that is found in Slovakia and sometimes causes encephalitis.
TT v. Torque teno v.
tumor v. oncovirus.
turkey rhinotracheitis v. a species of the genus *Pneumovirus* that causes upper respiratory tract disease in turkeys; called also *avian pneumovirus*.
U v. echovirus 11; isolated from children with subglottic laryngitis, it causes respiratory and gastrointestinal disease and rashes. Called also *Uppsala v.*
Uganda S v. a mosquito-borne virus of the genus *Flavivirus*, antigenically related to yellow fever virus; it causes mild febrile disease in various parts of Africa, especially Nigeria.
Uppsala v. U v.
Usutu v. a mosquito-borne virus of the genus *Flavivirus* that causes rash and fever in Central and southern Africa. It is spread from birds to humans by mosquitoes of the genus *Culex*.
Uukuniemi v. the type species of the Uukuniemi group of the genus *Phlebovirus* (q.v.).
vaccinia v. a virus of the genus *Orthopoxvirus* that does not occur in nature, being propagated only in the laboratory. It is used to prepare vaccine against smallpox and is also used as in research as a vector for antigens of other microorganisms. The present virus is derived from the original one used by Jenner, obtained from the lesions of cowpox, but the origin of the original virus remains unclear. Some believe that vaccinia virus is a derivative of the immunologically similar but antigenically different viruses of cowpox and variola (smallpox), while others think that it may be a recombinant of these viruses.
varicella-zoster v. human herpesvirus 3.
variola v. the virtually extinct virus, belonging to the genus *Orthopoxvirus*, that causes smallpox. No natural infection has occurred since 1977, and no reservoir of the virus now exists.
VEE v. Venezuelan equine encephalitis v.
Venezuelan equine encephalitis v., Venezuelan equine encephalomyelitis v. a species of togavirus of the genus *Alphavirus*, which causes Venezuelan equine encephalomyelitis.
vesicular exanthema of swine v. a calicivirus of the genus *Vesivirus* having at least 13 serotypes, designated A–M, which causes vesicular exanthema in swine.
vesicular stomatitis v. any of several antigenically distinct species of the genus *Vesiculovirus* (vesicular stomatitis Alagoas, vesicular stomatitis Indiana, and vesicular stomatitis New Jersey viruses) that cause vesicular stomatitis in swine, cattle, and horses.
vesicular stomatitis–like v's *Vesiculovirus*.
visna/maedi v. a species of the genus *Lentivirus* that causes ovine progressive pneumonia (maedi or visna). Called also *maedi/visna v.*
WEE v. western equine encephalitis v.
Wesselsbron v. a mosquito-borne virus of the genus *Flavivirus*, antigenically related to yellow fever virus; it causes Wesselsbron disease in sheep and cattle and a mild febrile illness in humans.
western equine encephalitis v., western equine encephalomyelitis v. a species of togavirus of the genus *Alphavirus*, which causes western equine encephalomyelitis.
West Nile v. a virus of the genus *Flavivirus* antigenically closely related to the Japanese, Murray Valley, and St. Louis encephalitis viruses; it causes West Nile encephalitis and is transmitted by *Culex* mosquitoes, with wild birds serving as the reservoir. It occurs widely in Africa, Europe, the Middle East, and Asia, and sometimes in the eastern, southern, and midwestern United States.
Wyeomyia v. a virus belonging to the Bunyamwera serogroup of the genus *Orthobunyavirus*, originally isolated from the mosquito *Wyeomyia melanocephala* and occurring in Central and South America and Trinidad, that causes a febrile illness.
Yaba monkey tumor v. a virus of the genus *Yatapoxvirus* that causes yabapox.
Yale SK v. a strain of poliovirus.
yellow fever v. a mosquito-borne virus of the genus *Flavivirus* that causes yellow fever in Central and South America and Africa.
Zika v. a mosquito-borne virus of the genus *Flavivirus*, antigenically related to Spondweni virus; it occurs in Central Africa, where it causes a febrile illness with rash.

Selected Tick-Borne Encephalitis Viruses

European Subtypes	Far Eastern Subtypes
Hanzalova virus	Absettarov virus
Hypr virus	Kyasanur forest disease virus
Kumlinge virus	Louping ill virus
Neudoerfl virus	Negishi virus
	Omsk hemorrhagic fever virus
	Powassan virus
	Russian spring-summer encephalitis virus

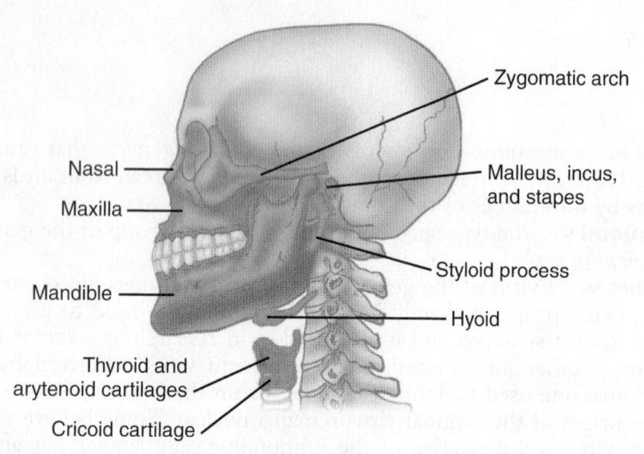

■ Viscerocranium, comprising the membranous viscerocranium *(gray)* and cartilaginous viscerocranium *(red).*

viru•stat•ic (vir″u-stat′ik) virostatic.

VISA vancomycin-intermediate *Staphylococcus aureus,* denoting strains that have an intermediate level of vancomycin resistance on the basis of the minimal inhibitory concentration.

vis•ce•ra (vis′ər-ə) [L.] plural of *viscus.*

vis•cer•ad (vis′ər-ad) toward the viscera.

vis•cer•al•gia (vis″ər-al′jə) [*viscer-* + *-algia*] pain in the viscera or in any bodily organ.

vis•ceri•mo•tor (vis″ər-ĭ-mo′tər) visceromotor.

viscer(o)- [L. *viscus,* gen. *visceris*] a combining form denoting relationship to the organs (viscera) of the body.

vis•cero•cra•ni•um (vis″ər-o-kra′ne-əm) [*viscero-* + *cranium*] [TA] the parts of the cranium that are derived from the branchial (or pharyngeal) arches and comprise the bones of the face; cf. *neurocranium.* Called also *splanchnocranium* and *visceral cranium.*

cartilaginous v. the part of the viscerocranium formed by endochondral ossification of the pharyngeal (branchial) arch cartilages. It includes the malleus, incus, stapes, styloid process of temporal bone, hyoid bone, and laryngeal cartilages other than the epiglottis.

membranous v. the part of the viscerocranium formed by intramembranous ossification in the first pharyngeal (branchial) arch. It includes the maxilla, mandible, nasal bone, and zygomatic arch.

vis•cer•og•ra•phy (vis″ər-og′rə-fe) radiography of the viscera.

vis•cero•in•hib•i•to•ry (vis″ər-o-in-hib′ĭ-tor-e) inhibiting the essential movements of any viscus or organ.

vis•cero•meg•a•ly (vis″ər-o-meg′ə-le) organomegaly.

vis•cero•mo•tor (vis″ər-o-mo′tər) [*viscero-* + *motor*] conveying or concerned with motor impulses to the viscera.

vis•cero•pa•ri•e•tal (vis″ər-o-pə-ri′ə-təl) pertaining to the viscera and the abdominal wall.

vis•cero•peri•to•ne•al (vis″ər-o-per″ĭ-to-ne′əl) pertaining to the viscera and the peritoneum.

vis•cero•pleu•ral (vis″ər-o-ploor′əl) pertaining to both the viscera and the pleura.

vis•cero•sen•so•ry (vis″ər-o-sen′sə-re) pertaining to sensation in the viscera.

vis•cero•skel•e•tal (vis″ər-o-skel′ə-təl) pertaining to the visceral skeleton.

vis•cero•so•mat•ic (vis″ər-o-so-mat′ik) pertaining to the viscera and body.

vis•cero•tome (vis′ər-o-tōm) 1. an instrument designed for obtaining specimens of liver tissue from cadavers by simple puncture. 2. an area on an abdominal viscus which is supplied with afferent nerve fibers by a single posterior root.

vis•cer•ot•o•my (vis″ər-ot′ə-me) [*viscero-* + *-tomy*] incision of an organ, especially postmortem excision of a portion of the liver.

vis•cero•to•nia (vis″ər-o-to′ne-ə) [*viscero-*+ *ton-* + *-ia*] a temperament type characterized by love of physical comfort, sociability, tolerance for others, and extroversion; the behavioral counterpart of endomorphy.

vis•cero•tro•phic (vis″ər-o-tro′fik) trophic and dependent upon the viscera.

vis•cer•o•tro•pic (vis″ər-o-tro′pik) [*viscero-* + *-tropic*] primarily acting on the viscera; having a predilection for the abdominal or thoracic viscera.

vis•cid (vis′id) [L. *viscidus*] glutinous or sticky.

vis•cid•i•ty (vĭ-sid′ĭ-te) the quality of being viscid.

vis•co•elas•tic (vis″ko-e-las′tik) both viscous and elastic; said of viscous substances used to restore or maintain the shape of the eye, especially the anterior chamber, during cataract surgery or other procedures performed on the anterior chamber.

vis•co•gel (vis′ko-jel) a gel which on melting gives a sol of high viscosity.

vis•com•e•ter (vis-kom′ə-tər) viscosimeter.

vis•com•e•try (vis-kom′ə-tre) viscosimetry.

vis•cose (vis′kōs) 1. viscous. 2. a form of cellulose acetate, used in dialysis membranes and other products.

vis•co•sim•e•ter (vis″ko-sim′ə-tər) an instrument used to determine the viscosity of a substance. Called also *viscometer.*

Ostwald v. an instrument that measures relative viscosity by comparing the time required for the meniscus of the solution under study to fall a fixed distance in a capillary tube with the time required for the same movement by a meniscus of a liquid of known viscosity.

Stormer v. an apparatus for determining viscosity by measurement of the time required, under controlled conditions, for a definite number of revolutions of a rotating cylinder immersed in the substance to be tested.

vis•co•sim•e•try (vis″ko-sim′ə-tre) the measurement of the viscosity of a substance. Called also *viscometry.*

vis•cos•i•ty (vis-kos′ĭ-te) resistance to flow; a physical property of a substance that depends on the friction of its component molecules as they slide past one another.

absolute v. the frictional resistance generated in a fluid when two parallel planes are flowing at different velocities, defined as the frictional force per unit area times the separation of the planes divided by the relative velocity of the planes; measured in poises. Called also *dynamic v.* Symbol η.

dynamic v. absolute v.

kinematic v. absolute viscosity divided by the density of the fluid; measured in stokes as the time for an exact quantity of liquid to flow by gravity through a capillary tube. Symbol ν.

vis•co•sup•ple•men•ta•tion (vis″ko-sup″lə-mən-ta′shən) injection of hyaluronan into a joint as treatment for the pain of osteoarthritis.

vis•cous (vis′kəs) [L. *viscosus*] sticky or gummy; characterized by a high degree of viscosity.

Vis•cum (vis′kəm) a genus of parasitic plants of the family Loranthaceae, native to Europe and Asia. *V. al′bum* is European mistletoe, preparations of which are used medicinally.

vis•cus (vis′kəs) pl. *vis′cera* [L. "internal organs"] any large interior organ in one of the three great cavities of the body, especially in the abdomen; see Plate 50. **vis′ceral** *adj*

Visi•col (viz′ĭ-kol) trademark for a combination preparation of monobasic sodium phosphate and dibasic sodium phosphate.

vis•ile (viz′īl) 1. pertaining to vision. 2. understanding or recalling most readily what has been seen. Cf. *audile.*

Vi•sine (vi-zēn′) trademark for a preparation of tetrahydrozoline hydrochloride.

vi•sion (vizh′ən) [L. *visio,* from *vidēre* to see] 1. the special sense by which objects in the external environment are perceived by means of light they give off or reflect, which stimulates the photoreceptors in the retina; called also *sight.* 2. the act of seeing. 3. an apparition; a subjective sensation of vision not elicited by actual visual stimuli. 4. visual acuity.

achromatic v. monochromatic vision.

anomalous trichromatic v. defective color vision in which a person has all three cone pigments, but one is deficient or anomalous (but not absent). There are three types: protanomaly, deuteranomaly, and tritanomaly; they may be either *acquired* (resulting from a retinal, cerebral, systemic, or toxic disorder) or *congenital* (inherited as an X-linked recessive trait). Called also *anomalous trichromacy.*

binocular v. the use of both eyes together without diplopia.

central v. vision that is elicited by stimuli impinging directly on the macula lutea.

chromatic v. color v.

color v. 1. perception of the different colors making up the spectrum of visible light; it is mediated by the retinal cones. 2. chromatopsia.

day v. visual perception in the daylight, or under conditions of bright illumination; see also *light adaptation.*

dichromatic v. a color vision deficiency (q.v.) in which one of the three cone pigments is missing altogether. The most common forms are protanopia and deuteranopia, each of which is transmitted by X-linked inheritance and affects about 1 per cent of white males. The third form, tritanopia, is very rare; and a fourth, tetartanopia, is of doubtful existence.

direct v. central v.

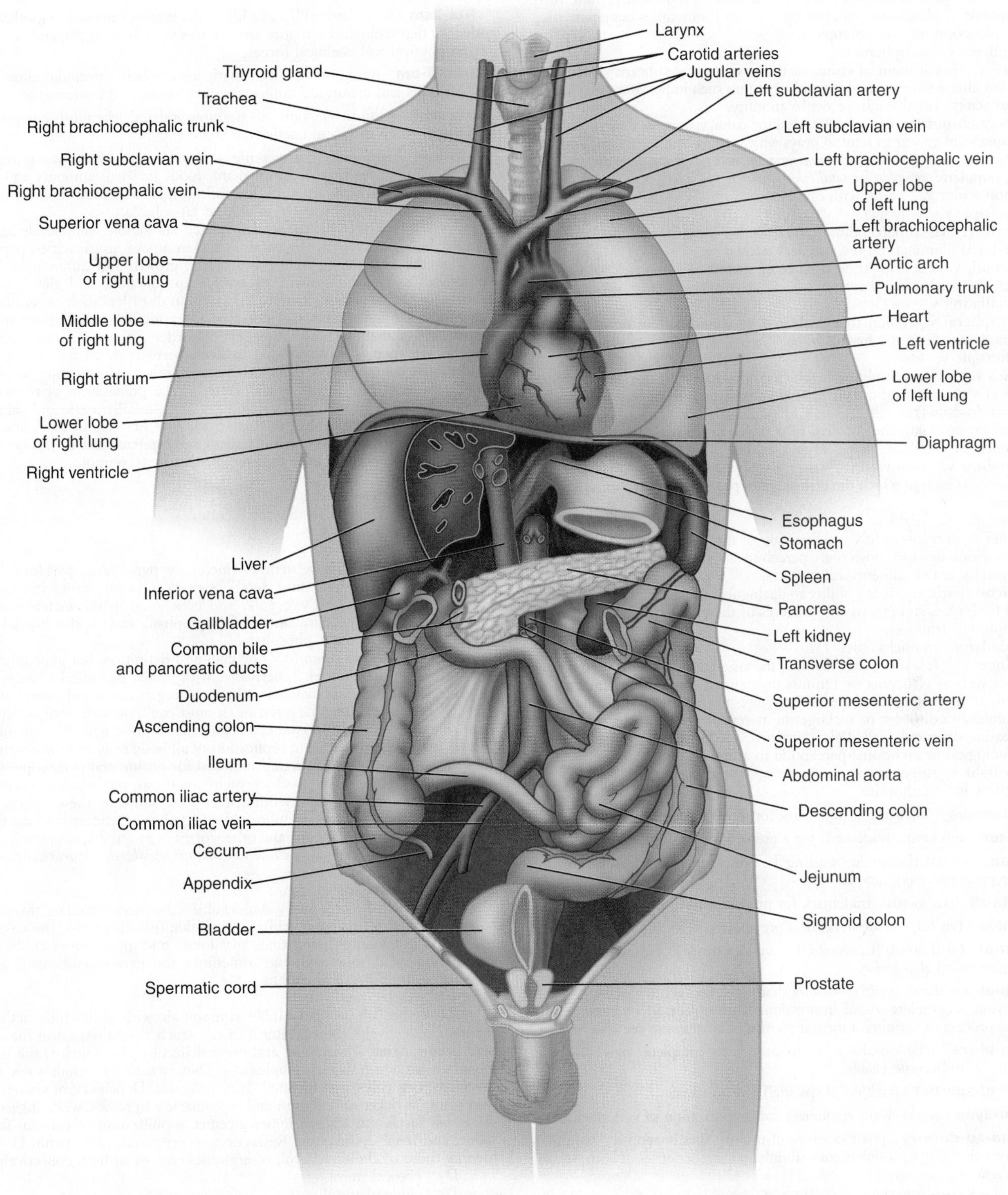

■ **PLATE 50**—THORACIC AND ABDOMINAL VISCERA

double v. diplopia.
facial v. the ability, formerly thought to be possessed by some blind people, to judge distance, direction, etc., of objects in one's environment by sensation felt in the skin of the face.
foveal v. central v.
gun-barrel v. tunnel v.
halo v. perception of a colored halo about a light source, one of the symptoms of glaucoma, punctate cataract, and sometimes conjunctivitis.
haploscopic v. stereoscopic v.
indirect v. peripheral v.
low v. impairment of vision such that there is significant visual handicap but also significant usable residual vision; such impairment may involve visual acuity, visual fields, or ocular motility.
monochromatic v. complete lack of color vision, so that all colors of the spectrum appear as neutral grays with varying shades of light and dark. Called also *achromatism, achromatopsia, monochromatism, monochromatopsia,* and, popularly, *complete* or *total color blindness.*
monocular v. vision with one eye.
multiple v. polyopia.
night v. visual perception in the darkness of night, or under conditions of reduced illumination; see also *dark adaptation.*
v. null, v. obscure the existence of scotomas in the field of vision of which the patient is not aware.
oscillating v. oscillopsia.
peripheral v. vision that is elicited by stimuli falling on areas of the retina distant from the macula lutea.
photopic v. day v.
Pick v. a visual condition in which objects lose their normal horizontal-vertical alignment and converge toward or diverge from one another.
pseudoscopic v. the reverse of stereoscopic vision, an illusion produced by reversing the pictures in a stereoscope, with apparent reversal of concavity and convexity, near and far, etc.
rainbow v. halo v.
rod v. vision in which the retinal cones play little or no part, as in night vision.
scotopic v. night v.
solid v., stereoscopic v. perception of the relief of objects or of their depth; vision in which objects are perceived as having three dimensions, and not merely as two-dimensional pictures.
trichromatic v. 1. any ability to distinguish the three primary colors of light (red, blue, and green) and mixtures of them. 2. normal color vision.
triple v. triplopia.
tubular v. tunnel v. (def. 1).
tunnel v. 1. severe constriction of the visual field. When due to organic causes such as glaucoma or retinitis pigmentosa the field expands as it is tested at increasing distances; when due to functional disorders such as conversion disorder or malingering it remains constant or contracts at increasing distances. Called also *tubular v.* 2. in psychiatry, restriction of psychological or emotional perception to a limited range.
twilight v. night v.
yellow v. xanthopsia.

Vis·i·paque (viz′ĭ-pāk) trademark for a preparation of iodixanol.

Vis·ken (vis′ken) trademark for a preparation of pindolol.

vis·na (vis′nə) [Icelandic "wasting"] the meningoencephalitic form of ovine progressive pneumonia.

Vis·ta·ril (vis′tə-ril) trademark for preparations of hydroxyzine.

Vis·tide (vis′tīd) trademark for a preparation of cidofovir.

vis·u·al (vizh′oo-əl) [L. *visualis,* from *videre* to see] pertaining to vision or sight; called also *optical.*

vis·u·al·iza·tion (vizh″oo-əl-ĭ-za′shən) 1. the act of viewing, or of achieving a complete visual impression of an object, as by radiography. 2. the process of forming a mental picture of something; see also *imagery.*

vis·u·al·ize (vizh′oo-əl-īz) 1. to achieve a complete view of something. 2. to become visible.

vis·u·al-spa·tial (vizh′oo-əl spa′shəl) visuospatial.

Vis·u·dyne (viz′u-dīn) trademark for a preparation of verteporfin.

vis·uo·au·di·to·ry (vizh″oo-o-aw′dĭ-tor″e) simultaneously stimulating, or pertaining to simultaneous stimulation of, the senses of both hearing and sight.

visu·og·no·sis (vizh″oo-og-no′sis) [L. *visus* sight + Gr. *gnōsis* knowledge] the recognition and interpretation of visual impressions.

vis·uo·mo·tor (vizh″oo-o-mo′tər) pertaining to connections between visual and motor processes, such as the use of visual cues to maintain coordinated movements.

vis·uo·psy·chic (vizh″oo-o-si′kik) visual and psychic; a term applied to that area of the cerebral cortex concerned in the judgment of visual sensations.

vis·uo·sen·so·ry (vizh″oo-o-sen′sə-re) pertaining to the perception of stimuli giving rise to visual impressions.

vis·uo·spa·tial (vizh″oo-o-spa′shəl) pertaining to the ability to understand visual representations and their spatial relationships; called also *visual-spatial.* Cf. *visual-spatial agnosia.*

vi·tal (vi′təl) [L. *vitalis,* from *vita* life] necessary to or pertaining to life.

vi·ta·lism (vi′tə-liz-əm) [L. *vita* life] the theory, opposed to mechanism (def. 3), that biological activities are due to a vital force or principle distinct from physical and chemical forces.

Vi·tal·li·um (vi-tal′e-əm) trademark for a cobalt-chromium alloy used in dentures and in surgical appliances, prostheses, and instruments.

vi·ta·mer (vi′tə-mər) one of multiple related chemical compounds possessing a given vitamin activity.

vi·ta·min (vi′tə-min) [L. *vita* life + *amine*] any of various unrelated organic substances that occur in many foods in small amounts and that are necessary in trace amounts for the normal metabolic functioning of the body. They may be water-soluble or fat-soluble.
v. A 1. retinol or any of several related fat-soluble compounds having similar biological activity; the vitamin acts in numerous capacities, particularly in the functioning of the retina, the growth and differentiation of epithelial tissue, the growth of bone, reproduction, and the immune response. Deficiency of vitamin A causes skin disorders such as xeroderma and follicular hyperkeratosis, increased susceptibility to infection, nyctalopia, xerophthalmia, and other eye disorders, anorexia, and sterility. As vitamin A, it is mostly found in liver, particularly of fish, egg yolks, and the fat component of dairy products; its other major dietary source is the provitamin A carotenoids of plants. 2. a preparation of retinol or esters of retinol formed from edible fatty acids, usually acetic and palmitic acids, used in the prophylaxis and treatment of vitamin A deficiency. Vitamin A is toxic when taken in excess; see *hypervitaminosis A.* The term vitamin A is sometimes used to refer specifically to retinol.
v. A_1 retinol.
v. A_2 dehydroretinol.
v. B a member of the vitamin B complex.
v. B_1 thiamine.
v. B_2 riboflavin.
v. B_6 water-soluble substances (including pyridoxine, pyridoxal, and pyridoxamine) found in most foods, especially meats, liver, vegetables, whole grain cereals, and egg yolk, and concerned in the metabolism of amino acids, in the degradation of tryptophan, and in the breakdown of glycogen to glucose-1-phosphate.
v. B_{12} cyanocobalamin (q.v.) by chemical definition, but generally any substituted cobalamin (def. 2) derivative with similar biological activity; it is a water-soluble hematopoietic vitamin occurring in meats and animal products. To be absorbed by the intestine, it must combine with intrinsic factor, and its metabolism is interconnected with that of folic acid. The vitamin is necessary for the growth and replication of all body cells and the functioning of the nervous system, being required for purine and pyrimidine (and hence DNA, protein, and nucleoprotein) synthesis, methylation reactions, hematopoiesis, and myelin synthesis; at least some of these effects are mediated through its role in folic acid metabolism. Deficiency of the vitamin causes pernicious anemia and other forms of megaloblastic anemia, and neurologic lesions. See also *adenosylcobalamin, cobalamin, hydroxocobalamin,* and *methylcobalamin.*
v. B_{12a} hydroxocobalamin.
v. B complex a group of water-soluble substances including thiamine, riboflavin, niacin (nicotinic acid), niacinamide (nicotinamide), the vitamin B_6 group (including pyridoxine, pyridoxal, and pyridoxamine), biotin, pantothenic acid, folic acid, and sometimes also para-aminobenzoic acid, inositol, vitamin B_{12}, and choline.
v. C ascorbic acid.
v. D either of two fat-soluble compounds with antirachitic activity, or both collectively: cholecalciferol (q.v.), which is synthesized in the skin and is considered a hormone, and ergocalciferol (q.v.), which is the form generally used as a dietary supplement. Dietary sources include some fish liver oils, egg yolks, and fortified dairy products. Deficiency of vitamin D can result in rickets in children and osteomalacia in adults, while ingestion of excess levels can lead to hypercalcemia, mobilization of calcium from bone, and renal dysfunction. References to metabolites of vitamin D may denote those of cholecalciferol, of ergocalciferol, or of both collectively.
v. D_2 ergocalciferol.
v. D_3 cholecalciferol.
v. E 1. any of a group of at least eight related compounds with similar biological antioxidant activity, particularly α-tocopherol but also including other isomers of tocopherol and the related compound tocotrienol. It occurs naturally in wheat germ oil, cereal germs, egg yolk, liver, green plants, milk fat, and vegetable oils and is also prepared synthetically. In various species, it is important for normal reproduction, muscle development, and resistance of erythrocytes to hemolysis, but deficiency in human children and adults is rare except in severe cases of malabsorption.

Deficiency is rare and is seen more often in children than in adults, with symptoms such as hemolytic anemia and neurologic disorders including gait ataxia, weakness, incoordination, loss of tendon reflexes, ophthalmoplegia, and dysarthria. The term is sometimes used synonymously with α-tocopherol. 2. an official preparation comprising some combination of the *d*- or *dl*-isomers of α-tocopherol, α-tocopheryl acid succinate, and α-tocopheryl acetate; used as dietary supplement, administered orally.

fat-soluble v's vitamins (A, D, E, and K) that are soluble in fat solvents and are absorbed along with dietary fats; they are not normally excreted in the urine and tend to be stored in the body in moderate amounts.

v. K any of a group of structurally similar fat-soluble compounds that promote blood clotting by increasing hepatic biosynthesis of prothrombin and other coagulation factors, activating these factors by γ-carboxylation of glutamic acid moieties in inactive precursor proteins. Two forms exist naturally, phytonadione (vitamin K_1) and menaquinone (vitamin K_2), as well as one synthetic provitamin form, menadione (vitamin K_3). The best sources are green leafy vegetables, liver, cheese, butter, and egg yolk, and as menaquinone it is synthesized by the intestinal flora. Deficiency, usually seen only in neonates, in disorders of absorption, or during antibiotic therapy, is characterized by hemorrhage.

v. K_1 phytonadione.

v. K_2 menaquinone.

v. K_3 menadione.

water-soluble v's all the vitamins soluble in water (i.e., all but vitamins A, D, E, and K); they are excreted in the urine and are not stored in the body in appreciable quantities.

vi•ta•min A ac•id (vi′tə-min) tretinoin.

vi•tan•i•tion (vi″tə-nĭ′shən) hypovitaminosis.

vi•tel•la•ri•um (vi″tə-lar′e-əm) an accessory genital gland found in flukes and tapeworms which secretes the yolk and shell for the fertilized egg; called also *vitelline gland.*

vit•el•lary (vit′ə-lar″e) vitelline.

vi•tel•lin (vĭ-tel′in) [L. *vitellus* yolk] a phosphoprotein found in the yolk of eggs.

vi•tel•line (vĭ-tel′ēn) [L. *vitellus* yolk] pertaining to or resembling a yolk.

vi•tel•lo•gen•e•sis (vi″təl-o-jen′ə-sis) production of yolk.

vi•tel•lo•lu•te•in (vi″təl-o-loo′tēn) [*vitellus* + *lutein*] a yellow pigment obtainable from lutein.

vi•tel•lose (vi-tel′ōs) a form of proteose derived from vitellin.

vi•tel•lus (vĭ-tel′əs) [L.] yolk (def. 1).

Vi•tex [L. "chaste tree"] a widespread genus of mainly tropical trees and shrubs, including *V. agnus castus,* the chaste tree, whose dried fruit and leaves are used medicinally

vi•ti•a•tin (vi-ti′ə-tin) a compound sometimes occurring in the urine along with creatine and creatinine; it is a homologue of choline.

vi•ti•a•tion (vish″e-a′shən) [L. *vitiatio*] impairment of efficiency; the perversion of any process so as to render it faulty or ineffective.

vit•i•lig•i•nes (vit″ĭ-lij′ĭ-nēz) [pl. of *vitiligo*] depigmented areas of the skin.

vit•i•lig•i•nous (vit″ĭ-lij′ĭ-nəs) pertaining to or characterized by vitiligo.

vit•i•li•go (vit″ĭ-li′go) [L.] 1. a chronic, usually progressive, type of hypomelanosis in which melanocytes are destroyed, resulting in white patches on the skin that may be surrounded by a hyperpigmented border; there is an autosomal dominant predisposition to the condition, and the etiology is thought to be an autoimmune mechanism. 2. depigmentation.

acrofacial v. a common type of generalized vitiligo, with depigmentation on the face and hands.

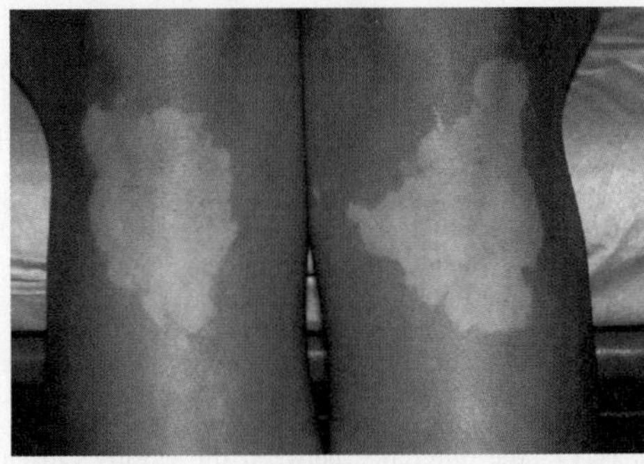

■ Vitiligo.

generalized v. vitiligo over wide areas of the body surface, often distributed symmetrically, but less extensive than universal vitiligo. See also *acrofacial v.* and *v. vulgaris.*

v. i′ridis depigmentation of the iris.

localized v. vitiligo in just one area of the skin.

occupational v. loss of pigment in the skin owing to contact with, ingestion of, or inhalation of certain chemicals, usually in the workplace, such as monobenzyl ether of hydroquinone or phenol-containing compounds.

segmental v. localized vitiligo on a band of skin, often on the face.

universal v. vitiligo over all or nearly all of the body surface.

v. vulga′ris the most common type of vitiligo, in which depigmentation is in a generalized pattern on only certain parts of the body, usually the face and hands.

Vi•tis (vi′tis) [L.] a genus of plants of the family Vitaceae, including grapes. *V. vini′fera* L. is the species most widely cultivated as fruit and wine grapes for human consumption.

Vit•rase (vit′rās) trademark for a preparation of hyaluronidase.

Vit•ra•sert (vit′rə-sərt) trademark for a preparation of ganciclovir.

Vit•ra•vene (vit′rə-vēn) trademark for a preparation of fomivirsen sodium.

vi•trec•to•my (vĭ-trek′tə-me) [*vitreum* + *-ectomy*] surgical extraction of the contents of the vitreous chamber of the eye, usually via the pars plana.

vit•re•i•tis (vit″re-i′tis) hyalitis.

vit•reo•cap•su•li•tis (vit″re-o-kap″su-li′tis) hyalitis.

vit•reo•ret•i•nal (vit″re-o-ret′ĭ-nəl) of or pertaining to the vitreous body and retina.

vit•re•ous (vit′re-əs) 1. glasslike or hyaline. 2. vitreous body (corpus vitreum [TA]).

detached v. a vitreous body separated from its usual attachments; see *vitreous detachment,* under *detachment.*

persistent hyperplastic primary v. a congenital anomaly, usually unilateral, due to persistence of embryonic remnants of the primary vitreous and part of the adjacent vascular structures. Clinically, there is a white pupil, elongated ciliary processes, and often microphthalmia; the lens, although clear initially, may become completely opaque.

primary v. the earliest vitreous in the embryo, formed from a mass of ectodermal and mesodermal fibrils between the optic cup and the lens vesicle and vascularized by the proliferating hyaloid system. It ceases to be formed when the lens capsule is formed, and is then enveloped by secondary vitreous.

secondary v. embryonic vitreous composed of densely packed fine fibrils formed around the primary vitreous by the inner layer of the optic cup.

tertiary v. embryonic zonular fibers derived from the primary vitreous and the basement membrane of the nonpigmented epithelium of the ciliary body; the fibers eventually attach to the lens capsule, giving rise to the zonule of Zinn.

vit•re•um (vit′re-əm) corpus vitreum.

vit•ri•fi•ca•tion (vit″rĭ-fĭ-ka′shən) [L. *vitrum* glass] the forming of a supercooled liquid such as glass.

vit•ri•tis (vĭ-tri′tis) hyalitis.

Vit•ta•for•ma (vi″tə-for′mə) a genus of parasitic protozoa (suborder Apansporoblastina, order Microsporida); some species cause microsporidiosis.

V. cor′neae a species that causes corneal infections in immunocompromised persons.

vit•ro•nec•tin (vit″ro-nek′tin) a multifunctional adhesive glycoprotein occurring in serum and various tissues and having binding sites for integrins, collagen, heparin, complement components and perforin. Its functions include regulation of the coagulation, fibrinolytic, and complement cascades, and it plays a role in hemostasis, wound healing, tissue remodeling, and cancer. It binds plasminogen activator inhibitor (PAI-1); mediates the inflammatory and repair reactions occurring at sites of tissue injury; and promotes adhesion, spreading, and migration of cells. It has been shown to be identical to *S protein,* which was identified as an inhibitor of complement activation, binding the membrane attack complex and preventing its insertion into the membrane.

Vi•vac•til (vi-vak′til) trademark for preparations of protriptyline hydrochloride.

Vi•velle (vi-vel′) trademark for a preparation of estradiol.

vivi- [L. *vivus* alive] a combining form meaning alive or denoting relationship to life.

vivi•par•i•ty (viv″ĭ-par′ĭ-te) the quality of being viviparous.

vi•vip•a•rous (vi-vip′ə-rəs) [*vivi-* + *-parous*] bearing living young which derive nutrition directly from the maternal organism.

Vi·vip·a·rus (vi-vip′ə-rəs) a genus of freshwater snails of the family Viviparidae, order Mesogastropoda. *V. java′nicus* is a second intermediate host of the fluke *Echinostoma ilocanum* in Indonesia.

vivi·pa·tion (viv″ĭ-pa′shən) the form of reproduction in which the embryo develops within and derives nutrition directly from the maternal organism.

vivi·sec·tion (viv″ĭ-sek′shən) the performance of surgical procedures upon living animals for purposes of research.

vivi·sec·tion·ist (viv″ĭ-sek′shən-ist) an individual who practices or defends vivisection.

Vivo·tif (viv′o-tif ber′nə) trademark for a preparation of typhoid vaccine live oral.

VLA very late activation (antigen); see *β_1 integrin*, under *integrin*.

Vla·di·mir·off-Mi·ku·licz amputation (vlah″dĭ-mir′of me′koo-lich) [Alexander A. *Vladimiroff*, Russian surgeon, 1837–1903; Johann von *Mikulicz*-Radecki, Polish surgeon in Germany, 1850–1905] see under *amputation*.

VLBW very low birth weight; see under *infant*.

VLCD very low calorie diet.

VLDL very-low-density lipoprotein.

β-VLDL, beta VLDL a mixture of lipoproteins with diffuse electrophoretic mobility approximately that of β-lipoproteins but having lower density; they are remnants derived from mutant chylomicrons and very-low-density lipoproteins that cannot be metabolized completely and therefore accumulate in plasma. Called also *floating beta lipoproteins*. See also *familial dysbetalipoproteinemia*.

pre-β-VLDL very-low-density lipoprotein; the term is used to emphasize its normal electrophoretic mobility.

VM-26 teniposide.

VMA vanillylmandelic acid.

VMD [L.] Veterina′riae Medici′nae Doc′tor (Doctor of Veterinary Medicine).

VNS vagal nerve stimulation.

VNTR variable number tandem repeats or variable number of tandem repeats.

vo·cal (vo′kəl) [L. *vocalis*, from *vox* voice] pertaining to the voice.

Vo·ges-Pros·kau·er test (reaction) (fo′ges pros′kou-er) [Daniel Wilhelm Otto *Voges*, German physician, early 20th century; Bernhard *Proskauer*, German hygienist, 1851–1915] see under *test*.

Vogt angle (fōkt) [Karl *Vogt*, German naturalist and physiologist, 1817–1895] see under *angle*.

Vogt point (fōkt) [Paul Frederick Emmanuel *Vogt*, German surgeon, 1844–1885] see under *point*.

Vogt striae (fōkt) [Alfred *Vogt*, Swiss ophthalmologist, 1879–1943] see under *stria*.

Vogt syndrome (fōkt) [Cécile *Vogt*, French physician in Germany, 1875–1962, and Oskar *Vogt*, German neurologist, 1870–1959] see under *syndrome*.

Vogt-Hue·ter point (fōkt′ he′ter) [P.F.E. *Vogt;* Karl *Hueter*, German surgeon, 1838–1882] Vogt point; see under *point*.

Vogt-Ko·ya·na·gi syndrome (fōkt′ ko-yah-nah′ge) [A. *Vogt;* Yoshizo *Koyanagi*, Japanese ophthalmologist, 1880–1954] see under *syndrome*.

Vogt-Ko·ya·na·gi-Ha·ra·da syndrome (fōkt′ ko-yah-nah′ge hah-rah′dah) [A. *Vogt;* Y. *Koyanagi;* Einosuke *Harada*, Japanese surgeon, 1892–1947] see under *syndrome*.

Vogt-Spiel·mey·er disease (fōkt′ shpēl′mi-ər) [Heinrich *Vogt*, German physician, early 20th century; Walter *Spielmeyer*, German physician, 1879–1935] see under *disease*.

Voh·win·kel syndrome (fo-ving′kəl) [Karl Hermann *Vohwinkel*, German dermatologist, 20th century] see under *syndrome*.

voice (vois) [L. *vox* voice] a sound produced by the larynx and modified by the vocal cords and other structures in the pharynx and oral cavity.

amphoric v. cavernous v.

cavernous v. a type of pectoriloquy consisting of hollow voice sounds heard over a lung cavity when the patient speaks. Called also *amphoric v.*, *amphoriloquy*, and *amphorophony*.

double v. diphonia.

eunuchoid v. a high falsetto voice in a man, resembling that of a eunuch or a woman.

whispered v. see under *pectoriloquy*.

voiced (voist) produced with vibration of the vocal cords, said of speech sounds such as *b, d,* or *z*. Called also *sonant* and *sonorant*.

voice·less (vois′ləs) produced without vibration of the vocal cords, said of speech sounds such as *p, t,* or *s*. Called also *surd* and *unvoiced*.

void (void) excrete.

Voigt line (foit) [Christian August *Voigt*, Austrian anatomist, 1809–1890] see under *line*.

Voit nucleus (foit) [Karl von *Voit*, German physiologist, 1831–1908] see under *nucleus*.

voix (vwah) [Fr.] voice.

v. de Polichinelle (də po-le-she-nel′) ["Punch's voice"] egophony.

vo·la (vo′lə) gen. and pl. *vo′lae* [L.] 1. a concave or hollow surface. 2. TA alternative for *palma*.

vo·lar (vo′lər) [L. *volaris*] pertaining to the palm or sole; see *palmar* and *plantar*.

vo·lar·dor·sal (vo″lər-dor′səl) from the volar to the dorsal surface.

vo·la·ris (vo-lar′is) [L., from *vola* (q.v.)] volar; TA alternative for *palmaris*.

vol·a·tile (vol′ə-til) [L. *volatilis*, from *volare* to fly] tending to evaporate rapidly; readily vaporizable at low temperature.

vol·a·til·iza·tion (vol″ə-til″ĭ-za′shən) the conversion into vapor or gas without chemical change.

vol·a·til·ize (vol′ə-til-īz) to convert into vapor.

vol·a·til·iz·er (vol′ə-til-īz″ər) an apparatus for producing volatilization.

vole (vōl) any of various small rodents of the family Muridae found in northern Europe, Asia, and North America, including the genera *Clethrionomys* and *Microtus;* some serve as reservoirs for disease.

bank v. *Clethrionomys glareolus*.

field v. either of two species of *Microtus*, vectors of leptospirosis.

vo·li·tion (vo-lish′ən) [L. *velle* to will] a conscious choice or decision, or the act or power of performing such. **voli′tional** *adj*

Volk·mann canal (fōk′mahn) [Alfred Wilhelm *Volkmann*, German physiologist, 1800–1877] see under *canal*.

Volk·mann contracture (ischemic paralysis, syndrome), etc. (fōk′-mahn) [Richard von *Volkmann*, German surgeon, 1830–1889] see under *contracture*, *disease*, *paralysis*, and *spoon*.

vol·ley (vol′e) [Fr. *volée* flight] a number of simultaneous muscle twitches or nerve impulses all caused by the same stimulus.

antidromic v. a volley of nerve impulses that travel in a direction opposite to normal, usually under experimental stimulation.

Vol·max (vol′maks) trademark for a preparation of albuterol sulfate.

vol·sel·la (vol-sel′ə) [L.] vulsella.

volt (V) (vōlt) [Alessandro *Volta*, Italian physiologist and physicist, 1745–1827] the SI unit of electric potential or electromotive force (EMF), equivalent to the EMF that will move a current of one ampere through a resistance of one ohm; i.e., one watt per ampere (or one joule per coulomb).

electron v. (eV) the energy acquired by an electron accelerated through a potential difference of one volt, equal to 1.6022×10^{-19} joule. Larger units, used for specifying rest masses and kinetic energies of particles, are obtained by attaching SI prefixes, giving *kiloelectron volt* (keV = 10^3 eV), *megaelectron volt* (MeV = 10^6 eV), and *gigaelectron volt* (GeV = 10^9 eV).

vol·tage (vōl′təj) electromotive force measured in volts. Symbol *V* or *v*.

vol·ta·ic (vol-ta′ik) galvanic (def. 2).

vol·tam·me·ter (vōl-tam′ə-tər) an instrument for measuring both volts and amperes.

volt·am·pere (vōlt-am′pēr) the product of multiplying a volt by an ampere; equivalent to a watt.

Vol·ta·ren (vōl′tə-ren) trademark for preparations of diclofenac sodium.

volt·me·ter (vōlt′me-tər) an instrument for measuring electromotive force in volts.

Vol·to·li·ni disease (vol″to-le′ne) [Friedrich Edward Rudolf *Voltolini*, German otorhinolaryngologist, 1819–1889] see under *disease*.

vol·ume (vol′ūm) the measure of the quantity or capacity of a substance. Symbol V or *V*.

atomic v. the value obtained by dividing the atomic weight of an element by its specific gravity in the solid condition.

blood v. the plasma volume added to the red cell volume.

circulation v., v. of circulation the amount of blood pumped through the lungs and out to all the organs of the body by the heart, expressed in liters of blood flow per minute.

closing v. (CV) the difference between the closing capacity and the residual volume; the volume of gas still in the lungs in excess of the residual volume when dependent small airways are assumed to have closed. Seen in the test results (such as with the single breath nitrogen washout test) near the end of the vital capacity period as a sharp rise in nitrogen concentration, indicating that most gas at this point is coming from the upper lung areas. It has sometimes been analyzed for indications of early lung disease.

v. of distribution a dilution method for determining the volume of fluids, e.g., plasma, in a body fluid compartment. A solute (e.g., inulin) is injected into the compartment and, after it is equally distributed, a sample is taken. The quantity of solute removed (as by metabolism, excretion, etc.) is then subtracted from the quantity administered, and the result is divided by the concentration per milliliter in the sample.

end-diastolic v. (EDV) the volume of blood in each ventricle at the end of diastole, usually about 120–130 mL but sometimes reaching 200–250 mL in the normal heart; it is a measure of preload (q.v.) and is the sum of the stroke volume and the end-systolic volume.

end-systolic v. (ESV) the volume of blood remaining in each ventricle at the end of systole, usually about 50–60 mL but sometimes as little as 10–30 mL in the normal heart; it is the difference between the end-diastolic volume and the stroke volume and is determined by the contractility of the ventricles and the state of the venous system.

expiratory reserve v. (ERV) the maximal amount of gas that can be exhaled from the resting end-expiratory level. See illustration at *capacity*.

forced expiratory v. the fraction of the forced vital capacity that is exhaled in a specific number of seconds; abbreviated FEV, with a subscript telling how many seconds the measurement lasted. See also *forced expiratory flow*, under *flow*.

functional venous v. the increase in volume of blood in veins of the legs, measured in milliliters, when a patient who has been supine with legs elevated changes to a standing position.

inspiratory reserve v. (IRV) the maximal amount of gas that can be inhaled from the end-inspiratory position.

mean corpuscular v. (MCV) the average volume of erythrocytes, conventionally expressed in cubic micrometers or femtoliters per red cell, obtained by multiplying the hematocrit (in L/L) by 1000 and dividing by the red cell count (in millions per μL): MCV = Hct/RBC. Automated electronic blood cell counters generally obtain the MCV directly from the average pulse height of the voltage pulses produced during the red cell count. These instruments obtain the hematocrit indirectly from the equation Hct = MCV × RBC.

minute v. (MV) the quantity of gas exhaled from the lungs per minute; tidal volume multiplied by respiratory rate.

packed-cell v. (PCV), v. of packed red cells (VPRC) hematocrit.

plasma v. the total volume of blood plasma, i.e., the extracellular fluid volume of the vascular space, measured by tracer dilution using ^{125}I- or ^{131}I-labeled albumin or T-1824 Evans blue dye as the tracer.

red cell v. the total volume of red cells in the body measured by isotopic dilution methods, usually with ^{51}Cr-labeled autologous red cells.

residual v. (RV) the amount of gas remaining in the lung at the end of a maximal exhalation. See illustration at *capacity*.

stroke v. the amount of blood ejected from a ventricle at each beat of the heart, equal to the difference between the end-diastolic volume and the end-systolic volume.

tidal v. (V_T) the amount of gas that is either inhaled or exhaled during one respiratory cycle. See *ventilation* (def. 2) and see illustration at *capacity*. Called also *tidal air*.

total cell v. (TCV) a measure of the adequacy of urea clearance of a hemodialyzer, calculated as the volume of saline necessary to fill its blood compartment; it declines slightly with each reuse of the dialyzer.

vol·u·men·om·e·ter (vol″u-mən-om′ə-tər) volumometer.

vol·u·met·ric (vol″u-met′rik) [*volume* + *metric*] pertaining to or accomplished by measurement in volumes.

vol·u·mette (vol″u-met′) an instrument for delivering repeatedly quantities of fluid in accurate predetermined amounts.

vol·u·mom·e·ter (vol″u-mom′ə-tər) [*volume* + *-meter*] an instrument for measuring volume or changes in volume.

vol·un·tary (vol′ən-tar″e) [L. *voluntas* will] accomplished in accordance with the will.

vol·un·to·mo·to·ry (vo″lən-to-mo′tə-re) [L. *voluntas* will + *motor*] subject to voluntary motor influence.

vo·lute (vo-lūt′) rolled up.

vo·lu·tin (vo-lu′tin) a complex molecule containing large amounts of orthophosphate polymers, nucleoprotein, and lipid, occurring as cytoplasmic granular inclusions (granules) in certain bacteria, yeasts, yeastlike fungi, and protozoa, and serving as an intracellular phosphate reserve. Because volutin granules stain red with blue basic dyes they are sometimes called *metachromatic granules*.

vol·u·trau·ma (vol′u-traw″mə) damage to the lung caused by overdistension by a mechanical ventilator set for an excessively high tidal volume.

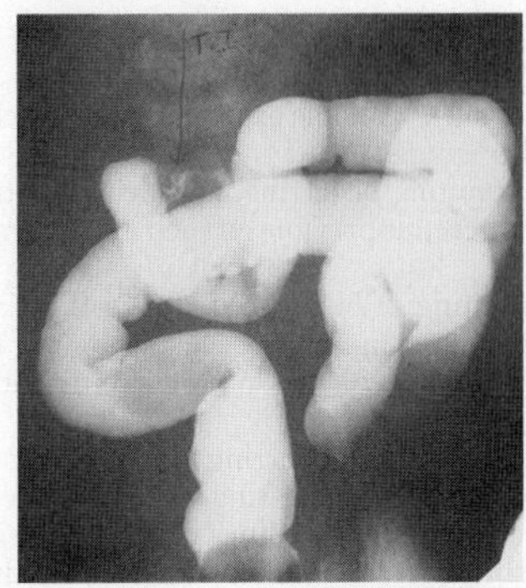

■ Volvulus of the colon, visualized by means of a barium enema.

vol·vu·late (vol′vu-lāt) [L. *volvere* to twist round] to twist or form a knot; see also *volvulus*.

vol·vu·lo·sis (vol″vu-lo′sis) onchocerciasis.

vol·vu·lus (vol′vu-ləs) [L. *volvere* to twist round] obstruction due to a knotting and twisting of part of the gastrointestinal tract.

abomasal v. see under *torsion*.

cecal v. a type of colonic volvulus consisting of twisting and anomalous rotation of the cecum, such as in volvulus neonatorum or Ladd syndrome.

colonic v. volvulus involving any portion of the colon; the most common types are cecal volvulus, sigmoid volvulus, and transverse colon volvulus.

gastric v. twisting of the stomach, usually due to laxity of one of its ligaments; this may or may not result in obstruction. The two most common types are mesenteroaxial volvulus and organoaxial volvulus.

gastric dilatation-v. a condition in dogs, consisting of excessive dilatation of the stomach; it is usually seen in large deep-chested breeds, the result of swallowing of air. If untreated, the dilatation can progress to fatal volvulus.

mesenteroaxial v. the less common of the two types of gastric volvulus, in which the stomach twists transversely around its mesenteric axis; this type is more common in children.

midgut v. volvulus neonatorum involving the entire part of the intestines derived from the midgut.

neonatal v., v. neonato′rum volvulus in the newborn, usually cecal volvulus or midgut volvulus.

organoaxial v. the more common of the two types of gastric volvulus, in which the stomach twists around its longitudinal axis; this type is more common in the elderly.

sigmoid v. a type of colonic volvulus consisting of twisting of an elongated section of sigmoid colon on its mesenteric axis; usually seen in the elderly.

transverse colon v., transverse colonic v. a rare type of colonic volvulus involving the transverse colon.

vo·mer (vo′mər) [L. "plowshare"] [TA] the unpaired flat bone that forms the inferior and posterior part of the nasal septum, articulating with the ethmoid and sphenoid bones and both maxillae and palatine bones. **vo′merine** *adj*

vo·mero·bas·i·lar (vo″mər-o-bas′ĭ-lər) pertaining to the vomer and to the basilar portion of the cranium.

vo·mero·na·sal (vo″mər-o-na′səl) pertaining to the vomer and the nasal bone.

vom·it (vom′it) [L. *vomitare*] 1. to cast up from the stomach by the mouth. 2. matter cast up from the stomach; vomited matter.

bilious v. vomited matter stained with bile.

black v. vomit discolored black, seen in conditions in which blood collects in the stomach, such as ulcers or yellow fever.

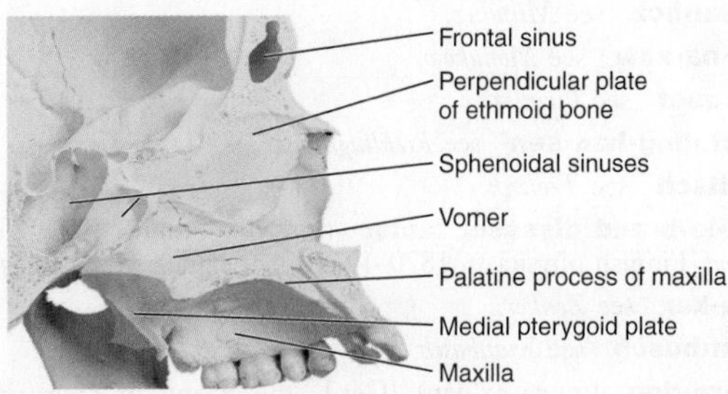

■ Vomer, in a median section of the anterior portion of the interior of the skull.

coffee-ground v. a type of black vomit in which the consistency is granular owing to mixture with stomach contents.

vom•it•ing (vom′it-ing) forcible expulsion of stomach contents through the mouth; called also *emesis.*

anticipatory v. vomiting occurring in anticipation of a second episode of something that triggered it previously, such as a migraine or chemotherapy.

bilious v. the vomiting of bile; called also *cholemesis.*

central v., cerebral v. vomiting due to a disorder of the central nervous system, especially stimulation of the vomiting center; it is usually without preceding nausea.

cyclic v. severe vomiting recurring at irregular intervals, usually occurring in childhood and disappearing in adolescence; it may result in dehydration and electrolyte abnormalities and may persist for several days. The etiology is variable and often unknown; some children seem to have a hereditary tendency, others have psychogenic conditions, and others have various underlying gastrointestinal or neurological conditions. Called also *cyclic vomiting syndrome, periodic v.,* and *recurrent v.*

delayed v. vomiting occurring much later than its stimulus, such as several hours after a meal or several days after a course of chemotherapy.

dry v. retching.

epidemic v. former name for viral gastroenteritis.

fecal v., feculent v. the vomiting of fecal matter, such as in appendicitis or intestinal obstruction or when bacterial overgrowth in the upper intestine has modified intestinal contents. Called also *stercoraceous v.*

functional v. vomiting whose physiologic cause is unknown.

obstructive v. vomiting caused by an obstruction in the gastrointestinal tract; if there is an intestinal obstruction, the vomit will contain bile (see *bilious v.*).

periodic v. cyclic v.

pernicious v. severe morning sickness, sometimes so severe as to threaten the life of the mother.

v. of pregnancy morning sickness.

projectile v. vomiting in which the vomitus is ejected with force.

psychogenic v. vomiting due to emotional anxiety or other psychological factors.

recurrent v. cyclic v.

stercoraceous v. fecal v.

vom•i•tive (vom′ĭ-tiv) emetic.

vom•i•to•ry (vom′ĭ-tor″e) emetic.

vom•i•tox•in (vom′ĭ-tok″sin) deoxynivalenol.

vom•it•u•ri•tion (vom″it-u-rish′ən) retching.

vom•i•tus (vom′ĭ-təs) [L.] 1. vomiting. 2. matter vomited.

v. cruen′tus bloody vomit.

von Arlt see *Arlt.*

von Behr•ing see *Behring.*

von Be•zold see *Bezold.*

v-*onc* (ve′onk″) [*v*iral *onc*ogene] a nucleic acid sequence in a virus responsible for the oncogenicity of the virus; it is derived from the cellular proto-oncogene and acquired from the host by recombination. Cf. *c-onc.*

von Econ•o•mo see *Economo.*

von Gier•ke see *Gierke.*

von Grae•fe see *Graefe.*

von Hal•ler see *Haller.*

von Han•se•mann cells (fōn hahn′sə-mahn) [David Paul von *Hansemann,* German pathologist, 1858–1920] see under *cell.*

von Hip•pel disease (von hip′əl) [Eugen *von Hippel,* German ophthalmologist, 1867–1939] see under *disease.*

von Hip•pel-Lin•dau disease (von hip′əl lin′dou) [E. *von Hippel;* Arvid *Lindau,* Swedish pathologist, 1892–1958] see under *disease.*

von Lan•gen•beck see *Langenbeck.*

von Mi•ku•licz see *Mikulicz.*

von Mo•na•kow see *Monakow.*

von Pir•quet see *Pirquet.*

von Reck•ling•hau•sen see *Recklinghausen.*

von Tröltsch see *Tröltsch.*

von Wil•le•brand disease, factor (fōn vil′ə-brahnt) [Erik Adolf *von Willebrand,* Finnish physician, 1870–1949] see under *disease* and *factor.*

von Zen•ker see *Zenker.*

von Zum•busch see *Zumbusch.*

vor•bei•re•den (for′bi-ra″dən) [Ger.] the giving of approximate or otherwise ridiculous answers or talking past the point, as occurs in Ganser syndrome and other mental disorders but which also may occur in tired or stressed but otherwise mentally healthy individuals.

vo•ri•co•na•zole (vor″ĭ-ko′nə-zōl) a triazole antifungal compound used for the treatment of invasive aspergillosis, administered orally.

Vör•ner disease (vur′nər) [Hans *Vörner,* German dermatologist, early 20th century] epidermolytic palmoplantar keratoderma; see under *keratoderma.*

vor•tex (vor′teks) pl. *vor′tices* [L. "whirl"] 1. a spiral or whorl. 2. an anatomical structure arranged in a spiral or whorl.

v. cor′dis [TA] vortex of heart: the whorled arrangement of muscle fibers at the apex in the left ventricle of the heart, through which the more superficial fibers pass to the interior of the left ventricle toward the base.

Fleischer v. a rare congenital opacity characterized by ochre-colored whorls which radiate from the center of the cornea at the level of Bowman membrane; called also *cornea verticillata.*

v. len′tis a spiral figure on the surface of the lens of the eye produced by the concentric arrangement of the fibers composing it; called also *nuclear arc* or *zone.*

vor′tices pilo′rum [TA] hair whorls: coiled patterns of hair growth on the body, such as on the crown of the head.

vor•ti•ces (vor′tĭ-sēz) [L.] plural of *vortex.*

Vō•Sol (vo′sol) trademark for a preparation of acetic acid.

Vō•Sol HC (vo′sol) trademark for a combination preparation of hydrocortisone and acetic acid.

Vos•si•us ring (fos′e-əs) [Adolf *Vossius,* German ophthalmologist, 1855–1925] see under *ring.*

vox•el (vok′sel) [*vo*lume *el*ement, by analogy with *pixel*] each defined volume unit of an element being scanned in computerized axial tomography. Cf. *pixel.*

vo•yeur (voi-yoor′) a person who practices voyeurism.

vo•yeur•ism (voi′yər-iz-əm) [DSM-IV] a paraphilia characterized by recurrent, intense sexual urges or arousal involving real or fantasized observation of unsuspecting people who are naked, disrobing, or engaging in sexual activity.

VP variegate porphyria.

VP-16 etoposide.

VPB ventricular premature beat; see *ventricular premature complex,* under *complex.*

VPC ventricular premature complex.

VPD ventricular premature depolarization; see *ventricular premature complex,* under *complex.*

VPF vascular permeability factor; see *vascular endothelial growth factor,* under *factor.*

VPRC volume of packed red cells.

VR vocal resonance.

VRE vancomycin-resistant enterococci.

Vro•lik disease (vro′lik) [Willem *Vrolik,* Dutch anatomist, 1801–1863] osteogenesis imperfecta (type II); see under *osteogenesis.*

VRSA vancomycin-resistant *Staphylococcus aureus,* denoting strains that have a high level of vancomycin resistance on the basis of the minimal inhibitory concentration.

VS volumetric solution.

VSG variable surface glycoprotein.

VT ventricular tachycardia.

vu•er•om•e•ter (vu″ər-om′ə-tər) [Fr. *vue* sight + *-meter*] an instrument for measuring the interpupillary distance.

vul•ca•nize (vul′kə-nīz) to subject raw rubber, in the presence of sulfur, to heat and high steam pressure, producing a flexible or hard rubber.

vul•ga•ris (vəl-ga′ris) [L.] ordinary or common; used especially in species names and names of pathologic conditions.

vul•ner•a•bil•i•ty (vul″nər-ə-bil′ĭ-te) susceptibility to injury or to contagion.

vul•ner•ant (vul′nər-ənt) 1. inflicting injury or causing a wound. 2. an agent that causes injury.

vul•ner•ary (vul′nər-ar″e) [L. *vulnerarius,* from *vulnus* wound] 1. pertaining to wounds or the healing of wounds. 2. an agent that promotes the healing of wounds.

vul•ner•ate (vul′nər-āt) [L. *vulnerare*] to wound.

vul•nus (vul′nəs) pl. *vul′nera* [L.] wound.

vul•sel•la (vəl-sel′ə) [L.] a forceps with clawlike hooks at the extremity of each blade.

vul·sel·lum (vəl-sel′əm) [L.] vulsella.

vul·va (vul′və) [L.] TA alternative for pudendum femininum. vul′val, vul′var *adj*

fused v. synechia vulvae.

vul·vec·to·my (vəl-vek′tə-me) excision of the vulva.

vul·vis·mus (vəl-viz′məs) vaginismus.

vul·vi·tis (vəl-vi′tis) [*vulva* + *-itis*] inflammation of the vulva.

atrophic v. *lichen sclerosus* (q.v.) of the vulvar region.

diabetic v. vulvitis occurring in diabetes.

eczematiform v. vulvitis marked by the formation of vesicular pustules.

erosive v. inflammation of the vulva due to mixed microbial infection with development of gangrenous ulcerations similar to those of noma of the oral tissues; it usually affects one labium majus and then the other. Called also *noma vulvae* and *phlegmonous v.*

leukoplakic v. *lichen sclerosus* (q.v.) of the vulvar region.

phlegmonous v. erosive v.

plasma cell v., v. plasmocellula′ris the counterpart in women of Zoon balanitis in men; the vulva has a lacquerlike appearance with erosions, punctate hemorrhage, synechiae, and sometimes grayish or tan discoloration.

ulcerative v. inflammation of the vulva marked by ulceration, pain, and lymphangitis.

vul·vo·cru·ral (vul″vo-kroo′rəl) pertaining to the vulva and the thigh.

vul·vo·dyn·ia (vul″vo-din′e-ə) pain affecting the vulva.

vul·vop·a·thy (vəl-vop′ə-the) [*vulva* + *-pathy*] any disease of the vulva.

vul·vo·rec·tal (vul″vo-rek′təl) rectovulvar.

vul·vo·uter·ine (vul″vo-u′tər-in) pertaining to the vulva and uterus.

vul·vo·vag·i·nal (vul″vo-vaj′ĭ-nəl) pertaining to the vulva and vagina.

vul·vo·vag·i·ni·tis (vul″vo-vaj″ĭ-ni′tis) inflammation of the vulva and vagina, or of the vulvovaginal glands.

Candida **v., candidal v.** vulvovaginal candidiasis.

infectious pustular v. a venereal infection of cows, caused by bovine herpesvirus I and characterized by inflammation, necrosis, and pustule formation of varying degree in the vulva and vagina. It is the female counterpart of infectious pustular balanoposthitis.

senile v. atrophic vaginitis in which there is intense itching around the vagina, almost complete lack of vaginal secretions, and tissue atrophy.

Vu·mon (voo′mon) trademark for a preparation of teniposide.

vv. [L.] ve′nae (veins).

v/v volume (of solute) per volume (of solvent).

VVS vulvar vestibulitis syndrome.

VW vessel wall.

VX an organophosphorus compound that is a potent cholinesterase inhibitor and is used as a nerve gas; symptoms of poisoning include bronchial constriction, convulsions, and often death. See *organophosphorus compound poisoning*, under *poisoning*.

vWF von Willebrand factor.

V-Y plas·ty (ve′wi′plas-te) V-Y procedure.

Vy·tone (vi′tōn) trademark for a combination preparation of hydrocortisone and iodoquinol.

Vy·to·rin (vi-tor′in) trademark for a preparation of ezetimibe and simvastatin.

VZIG varicella-zoster immune globulin.

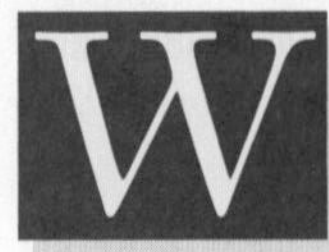

W tryptophan; tungsten (Ger. *Wolfram*); watt.

W writhing number; work.

Waar·den·burg syndrome (vahr′den-boorg) [Petrus Johannes *Waardenburg*, Dutch ophthalmologist, 1886–1979] see under *syndrome.*

Waar·den·burg-Shah syndrome (vahr′den-boorg shah′) [P.J. *Waardenburg*; Krishnakumar N. *Shah*, Indian physician, late 20th century] Waardenburg syndrome type 4; see under *syndrome.*

Wach·en·dorf membrane (vahk′en-dorf) [Eberhard Jacob *Wachendorf*, Dutch physician, 1703–1758] see under *membrane.*

Wa·da test (wah′də) [Juhn Atsushi *Wada*, Japanese-born Canadian neurosurgeon, born 1924] see under *test.*

Wag·staffe fracture (wag′staf) [William Warwick *Wagstaffe*, English surgeon, 1843–1910] see under *fracture.*

WAIS Wechsler Adult Intelligence Scale.

waist (wāst) the portion of the body between the thorax and the hips.

wake·ful·ness (wāk′fəl-nis) 1. a condition of alertness or watchfulness. 2. a state marked by indisposition to sleep; sleeplessness; see also *consciousness.*

Wal·den·ström disease (vahl′den-strəm) [Johan Henning *Waldenström*, Swedish orthopedic surgeon, 1877–1972] Legg-Calvé-Perthes disease; see under *disease.*

Wal·den·ström macroglobulinemia, purpura (vahl′den-strəm) [Jan Gosta *Waldenström*, Swedish physician, 1906–1996] see under *macroglobulinemia* and *purpura.*

Wal·dey·er fossa, etc. (vahl′di-er) [Heinrich Wilhelm Gottfried von *Waldeyer*, German anatomist, 1836–1921] see under *fossa, gland, layer,* and *ring.*

walk (wawk) 1. to move on foot. 2. gait.

Walk·er lissencephaly (wawk′ər) [Arthur Earl *Walker*, American surgeon, 1907–1995] Walker-Warburg syndrome.

Walk·er-War·burg syndrome (wawk′ər vahr′boorg) [A.E. *Walker;* Mette *Warburg*, Danish ophthalmologist, 20th century] see under *syndrome.*

Wa·ters position, projection (waw′tərz) [Charles Alexander *Waters*, American radiologist, 1888–1961] see under *position* and *projection.*

walk·er (wawk′ər) an enclosing framework made of lightweight metal tubing, sometimes with wheels (rollator), for patients who need more support for walking than that given by a cane or a crutch.

walk·ing (wawk′ing) 1. progressing on foot; called also *ambulation.* 2. gait.

chromosome w. in molecular genetics, the sequential isolation of clones carrying overlapping DNA sequences so that the isolation "walks" along part of a chromosome; it is important for isolation of a specific locus for which there is no probe but which is linked to a gene that has been identified and cloned.

heel w. a gait marked by walking on the heels to avoid the pain of pressure upon the hyperalgesic soles of the feet in cases of peripheral neuritis.

sleep w. somnambulism.

wall (wawl) 1. the limiting structure of a space, hollow organ, or definitive mass of material. See also *paries.* 2. the rigid external surface of a horse's hoof.

anterior w. of stomach paries anterior gastrica.

anterior w. of tympanic cavity paries caroticus cavitatis tympani.

anterior w. of vagina paries anterior vaginae.

axial w. a cavity wall approximating the pulp tissue, parallel with the long axis of the tooth.

bladder w. the surrounding structure of the urinary bladder, consisting of the serosa, subserosa, muscular layer, submucosa, and mucosa.

carotid w. of tympanic cavity paries caroticus cavitatis tympani.

cavity w. the walls of a prepared cavity, named according to the surface of a tooth toward which they are placed, extracoronal walls being named after surfaces that have been reduced, and intracoronal ones after surfaces from which they derive.

cell w. a rigid structure that lies just outside of and is joined to the plasma membrane of plant cells and most prokaryotic cells; it protects the cell and maintains its shape.

chest w. the bony and muscular structures that form the outer framework of the thorax and move during breathing.

external w. of cochlear duct paries externus ductus cochlearis.

gastric w. stomach w.

gastric w., anterior paries anterior gastrica.

gastric w., posterior paries posterior gastrica.

germ w. a ringlike thickening around the blastoderm of the bird, consisting of the advancing boundary zone at its margin.

gingival w. a peripheral cavity wall near the apical end of the crown of the tooth.

hollow w. seedy toe.

inferior w. of orbit paries inferior orbitae.

inner w. of glomerular capsule visceral layer of glomerular capsule.

jugular w. of tympanic cavity paries jugularis cavitatis tympani.

labyrinthic w. of tympanic cavity paries labyrinthicus cavitatis tympani.

lateral w. of nasal cavity the lateral surface of the cavity, containing the nasal conchae and meatus.

lateral w. of orbit paries lateralis orbitae.

lateral w. of tympanic cavity paries membranaceus cavitatis tympani.

mastoid w. of tympanic cavity paries mastoideus cavitatis tympani.

medial w. of nasal cavity septum nasi.

medial w. of orbit paries medialis orbitae.

medial w. of tympanic cavity paries labyrinthicus cavitatis tympani.

membranous w. of trachea paries membranaceus tracheae.

membranous w. of tympanic cavity paries membranaceus cavitatis tympani.

nail w. vallum unguis.

outer w. of glomerular capsule parietal layer of glomerular capsule.

parietal w. somatopleure.

parietal w. of glomerular capsule see under *layer.*

party w. a bony septum in the nose.

periotic w. the wall of the otic vesicle.

posterior w. of stomach paries posterior gastrica.

posterior w. of tympanic cavity paries mastoideus cavitatis tympani.

posterior w. of vagina paries posterior vaginae.

pulpal w. the cavity wall on the occlusal surface that covers the pulp in a plane at right angles to the long axis of the tooth.

splanchnic w. splanchnopleure.

stomach w. the layered structure that makes up the stomach, consisting of a serous coat, a muscular coat, a mucous membrane, and other tissue layers in between. See *gaster* and see also *paries anterior gastrica* and *paries posterior gastrica.* Called also *gastric wall.*

stomach w., anterior paries anterior gastrica.

stomach w., posterior paries posterior gastrica.

subpulpal w. the floor of a prepared cavity formed when the pulp is removed and the cavity is extended to include the pulp chamber.

superior w. of orbit paries superior orbitae.

tegmental w. of tympanic cavity paries tegmentalis cavitatis tympani.

tympanic w. of cochlear duct paries tympanicus ductus cochlearis.

vestibular w. of cochlear duct paries vestibularis ductus cochlearis.

visceral w. of glomerular capsule see under *layer.*

Wal·len·berg syndrome (vahl′ən-bərg) [Adolf *Wallenberg*, German physician, 1862–1949] see under *syndrome.*

wal·le·ri·an (wah-le′re-ən) named for Augustus Volney *Waller*, English physiologist, 1816–1870, as *wallerian degeneration.*

wall·eye (wawl′i) 1. leukoma of the cornea. 2. exotropia.

Wal·thard islets (cell nests, cell rests, inclusions) (vahl′tahrd) [Max *Walthard*, Swiss gynecologist, 1867–1933] see under *islet.*

Wal·ther oblique ligament (vahl′ter) [August Friedrich *Walther*, German anatomist, 1688–1746] see *ligamentum talofibulare posterius.*

wan·der·er (wahn′dər-ər) a foal with neonatal maladjustment syndrome.

wan·der·ing (wahn′dər-ing) 1. moving about freely, as a wandering (ameboid) cell. 2. abnormally movable; too loosely attached.

pathologic tooth w. see under *migration.*

Wang·i·el·la (wang″e-el′ə) former name for *Exophiala.*

war·bles (wor′bəlz) 1. larvae of the flies *Hypoderma bovis* and *H. lineatum.* 2. cysts containing these larvae, especially on the backs of cattle near the spinal canal. 3. infection of cattle by these larvae, a type of larva migrans seen around the world in the Northern Hemisphere. Symptoms include damage to the hide, periesophagitis, sometimes anaphylaxis, and, if the larvae invade the nervous system, partial paralysis; serious cases may prove fatal. Called also *ox w.*

ox w. warbles.

War·burg syndrome (vahr′boorg) [Mette *Warburg*, Danish ophthalmologist, born 1926] Walker-Warburg syndrome.

Ward-Ro·ma·no syndrome (word′ ro-mah′no) [Owen Conor *Ward*, Irish pediatrician, born 1923; Cesarino *Romano*, Italian pediatrician, born 1924] Romano-Ward syndrome.

ward (word) 1. a large room in a hospital for the accommodation of several patients. 2. a division within a hospital for the care of numerous patients having the same condition, e.g., a maternity ward.

war·fa·rin (wor′fər-in) [*Wisconsin Alumni Research Foundation*] a synthetic coumarin anticoagulant that acts by inhibiting the hepatic synthesis of vitamin K–dependent coagulation factors (prothrombin and factors VII,

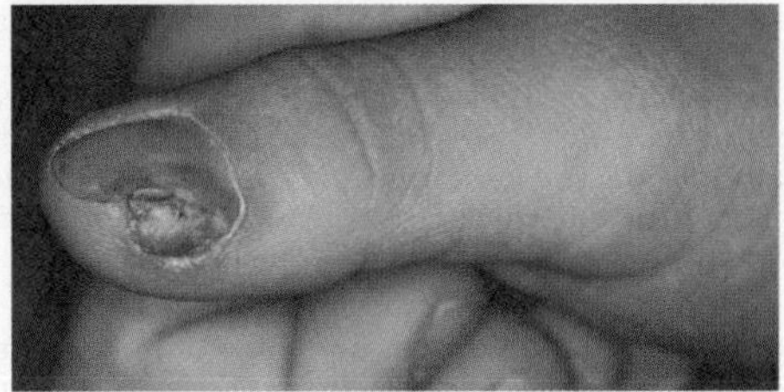

■ Periungual wart with disruption of nail growth.

IX, and X) and proteins C and S. It also acts as a rodenticide, causing fatal hemorrhaging in any mammal that consumes a sufficient dose.

w. potassium the potassium salt of warfarin, which has been used as an oral anticoagulant.

w. sodium [USP] the sodium salt of warfarin, having the same actions as the base; administered orally, intravenously, or intramuscularly in the treatment and prophylaxis of thromboembolic disorders.

War•ren incision (wor′ən) [John Collins *Warren*, American surgeon, 1778–1856] see under *incision.*

War•ren shunt (wor′ən) [W. Dean *Warren*, American surgeon, 1924–1989] see under *shunt.*

wart (wort) [L. *verruca*] 1. a hyperplastic lesion of the skin or a mucous membrane caused by a human papillomavirus; called also *verruca.* 2. any of various nonviral epidermal proliferations resembling this lesion. **war′ty** *adj*

acuminate w. condyloma acuminatum.

anatomical w. see *tuberculosis verrucosa cutis.*

butcher's w. a type of wart seen on the hands of persons working with raw meat, caused by human papillomavirus type 7.

cadaver w. see *tuberculosis verrucosa cutis.*

cattle w. one of the lesions of bovine papillomatosis.

common w. a lobulated, hyperplastic skin lesion with a horny surface, usually found on the back of a hand or finger. Called also *verruca vulgaris.*

filiform w. a wart with soft, thin, threadlike projections on its surface, seen most often on the face. Called also *verruca filiformis.*

flat w. verruca plana.

genital w. condyloma acuminatum.

Hassall-Henle w's hyaline excrescences in the periphery of the Descemet membrane, which occur with advancing age.

juvenile w. verruca plana.

moist w. condyloma latum.

mosaic w. an irregularly shaped wart with a granular surface, found most often on the palm or sole, formed by an aggregation of several contiguous warts.

necrogenic w. see *tuberculosis verrucosa cutis.*

Peruvian w. verruga peruana.

pitch w. a type of precancerous, keratotic, epidermal tumor seen in individuals who work in gas, tar, pitch, or various oils derived from coal.

plane w. verruca plana.

plantar w. a painful wart on the sole, usually transmitted by a human papillomavirus. Called also *verruca plantaris.*

pointed w. condyloma acuminatum.

postmortem w., prosector's w. see *tuberculosis verrucosa cutis.*

seborrheic w. seborrheic keratosis.

seed w. common w.

soot w. a precancerous lesion on the skin caused by long-term exposure to soot; see *chimney-sweeps' cancer*, under *cancer.*

telangiectatic w. misnomer for the wartlike papule of angiokeratoma.

tuberculous w. see *tuberculosis verrucosa cutis.*

venereal w. condyloma acuminatum.

War•ten•berg disease, sign (wor′tən-bərg) [Robert *Wartenberg*, American neurologist, 1887–1956] see *cheiralgia paresthetica* and see under *sign.*

War•thin tumor (wor′thin) [Aldred Scott *Warthin*, American pathologist, 1866–1931] see *papillary adenocystoma lymphadenomatosum*, under *adenocystoma.*

War•thin-Fin•kel•dey cell (wor′thin fing′kəl-da) [A.S. *Warthin*; Wilhelm *Finkeldey*, German pathologist, 20th century] see under *cell.*

wash (wahsh) 1. to clean or bathe. 2. a solution used for cleaning or bathing a part; see also *bath, irrigation*, and *lavage.*

eye w. collyrium.

mouth w. see *mouthwash.*

wash•ing (wahsh′ing) 1. cleaning or bathing. 2. the process of doing this; see *irrigation* and *bath.*

sperm w. the bathing of fresh sperm with a special solution to remove antibodies and other contaminants so that it can be used for in vitro fertilization or some other technique of artificial insemination.

wash•out (wahsh′out) a thorough washing.

nitrogen w. see under *test.*

wasp (wahsp) [L. *vespa*] 1. a general term for almost any member of the families Vespidae and Sphecidae, flying hymenopteran insects with long thin bodies, many of which have painful stings. Some live in complicated social colonies and others live in solitary social settings. Cf. *hornet* and *yellowjacket.* 2. any of various other animals thought to resemble these insects.

sea w. any of various venomous stinging cubomedusan jellyfish; species dangerous to humans include *Chironex fleckeri* and *Chiropsalmus quadrigatus.*

was•ser•hel•le (vahs′ər-hel″ĕ) [Ger. "water-clear"] see *water-clear cell*, under *cell.*

Was•ser•mann test (reaction) (vahs′er-mahn) [August Paul von *Wassermann*, German bacteriologist, 1866–1925] see under *test.*

Was•ser•mann-fast (vahs′er-mahn-fast) showing a persistent positive reaction to the Wassermann test despite antisyphilitic treatment.

waste (wāst) 1. gradual loss, decay, or diminution of bulk. 2. useless material, unfit for further use within the organism. 3. to pine away or dwindle.

wast•ing (wāst′ing) 1. gradual loss or decay; emaciation. See also *wasting disease*, under *disease*, and *wasting syndrome*, under *syndrome.* 2. excessive depletion.

salt w. inappropriate sodium excretion in the urine (natriuresis) with hyponatremia and hyperkalemia; see also *salt-losing syndrome*, under *syndrome.*

wa•ter (waw′tər, wah′tər) 1. a tasteless, odorless, colorless liquid, $(H_2O)_n$, used as the standard of specific gravity and of specific heat. It freezes at 0°C (32°F) and boils at 100°C (212°F). It is present in all organic tissues and in many other substances and is the most universal of the solvents. 2. aromatic w. 3. purified w.

ammonia w. dilute ammonia solution.

aromatic w. an aqueous solution, usually saturated, of a volatile oil or other aromatic or volatile substance; it may be prepared by distillation or solution.

bacteriostatic w. for injection [USP] water for injection, sterilized and containing one or more suitable antimicrobial agents.

bound w. water in the tissues of the body bound to macromolecules or organelles.

capillary w. the water contained in the soil above the water table of the ground water.

w. of combustion metabolic w.

w. of crystallization water that is chemically combined in many salts; it forms a structural part of the crystal but can be removed by heating.

distilled w. water that has been purified by distillation.

egg w. 1. water that has bathed eggs of various invertebrates and acquired one or another substance detectable by a physiological reaction; e.g., oyster egg water may stimulate spawning of male oysters. 2. water containing fertilizin exuded from the ripe eggs of sea urchins and other aquatic animals, by which the spermatozoa are agglutinated.

free w. that portion of the water in body tissues which is not bound by macromolecules or organelles.

ground w. the water which lies in the depth of soils, being carried along underground over impervious strata.

hamamelis w. witch hazel (def. 2).

heavy w. a compound analogous to water but containing deuterium, the mass two isotope of hydrogen, the formula being D_2O or ^2H_2O. It differs from ordinary water in having a higher freezing point (3.8°C) and boiling point (101.4°C), and in the fact that it is incapable of supporting life. It is the stable isotope used as a moderator in nuclear reactors. Called also *deuterium oxide.*

w. for hemodialysis [USP] water for use in hemodialysis, produced by subjecting water meeting the requirements of drinking water regulations to further treatment to reduce chemical and microbiological components; it contains no added antimicrobials and is not intended for injection.

w. for injection [USP] water for parenteral use, prepared by distillation or reverse osmosis, containing no added substance, and meeting certain standards as to sterility and clarity.

lime w. calcium hydroxide topical solution.

metabolic w. water in the body derived from metabolism of a food element such as starch, glucose, or fat; called also *w. of combustion.*

w. O 15 [USP] water in which a portion of the molecules are labeled with ^{15}O; used for positron emission tomography in the diagnosis of vascular disorders.

potable w. water that is suitable for drinking purposes.

purified w. [USP] water obtained by distillation or deionization, used for pharmaceutical or other purposes requiring mineral-free water. Not for parenteral administration.

rose w. a solution prepared by diluting stronger rose water with an equal volume of purified water; used as a perfuming agent in pharmaceutical preparations.

sterile w. for inhalation [USP] water for injection, sterilized and containing no antimicrobial agents, except where used in devices in which it is liable to contamination over a period of time (e.g., humidifiers), or other added substances. It is for inhalation therapy only, not for parenteral administration.

sterile w. for injection [USP] water for injection, sterilized and containing no antimicrobial agents or other added substances.

sterile w. for irrigation [USP] water for injection, sterilized and containing no antimicrobial agents or other added substances; used for irrigation but not for parenteral administration.

sterile purified w. [USP] purified water, sterilized and containing no antimicrobial agents. It is not for parenteral administration.

stronger ammonia w. strong ammonia solution.

stronger rose w. [NF] a saturated solution of the odoriferous principles of the flowers of *Rosa centifolia* Linné, used as a perfuming agent in pharmaceutical preparations.

total body w. (TBW) any of various estimates of the water content of the human body, taking into consideration the person's height, weight, and age; used in urea kinetic modeling calculations.

wa•ter-borne (waw′tər-born″) conveyed or spread by water, as an infectious disease; see under *infection*.

Wa•ter•house-Fri•der•ich•sen syndrome (waw′tər-hous frid′rik-sən) [Rupert *Waterhouse*, British physician, 1873–1958; Carl *Friderichsen*, Danish pediatrician, 20th century] see under *syndrome*.

wa•ter-jet (waw′tər-jet″) see under *dissector*.

wa•ters (waw′tərz) popular name for amniotic fluid.

wa•ter•shed (waw′tər-shed) 1. a ridge that directs drainage toward either side. 2. an area where the peripheries of two vascular beds meet, particularly in the brain; small anastomoses link the adjoining beds. See also *watershed area*, under *area*.

abdominal w's the ridges formed in the supine position by the forward projection of the lumbar vertebrae and the projecting brim of the pelvis, causing free effusions to gravitate into the lumbar fossae and pelvis.

Wa•ter•ston operation (anastomosis, shunt) (waw′tər-stən) [David J. *Waterston*, British thoracic and pediatric surgeon, 20th century] see under *operation*.

Wat•son-Schwartz test (waht′sən shworts′) [Cecil James *Watson*, American physician, 1901–1983; Samuel *Schwartz*, American physician, 1916–1983] see under *test*.

Wat•so•ni•us (waht-so′ne-əs) [Malcolm *Watson*, British physician, 1873–1955] a genus of pear-shaped trematodes of the family Paramphistomatidae. *W. watso′ni* (formerly called *Amphistoma watsoni*) is a cause of paramphistomiasis in humans and monkeys in Africa.

watt (W) (waht) [James *Watt*, British engineer and inventor, 1736–1819] the SI unit of power, being the work done at the rate of 1 joule per second. In electric power, it is equivalent to a current of 1 ampere under a pressure of 1 volt.

watt•age (waht′əj) the power output or consumption of an electrical device; expressed in watts.

watt-hour (waht′our) a unit of electrical work or energy, equal to the wattage multiplied by the time in hours.

watt•me•ter (waht′me-tər) an instrument for measuring electric activity in watts.

wave (wāv) 1. a uniformly advancing disturbance in which the parts move while undergoing a double oscillation. 2. anything having this pattern.

Wave

A w. 1. a compound muscle action potential evoked by a submaximal stimulus to the motor nerve of a muscle, occurring because of an axon reflex and due to axonal branching; it has an amplitude similar to that of the F wave but a shorter, more constant latency. Called also *axon w.* 2. in an intracardiac electrogram, the complex waveform due to depolarization of the atria, usually specifically the lower atrial septum in the His bundle electrogram. See illustration at *electrogram*.

a w. 1. in a tracing of the venous pulse, a positive deflection representing contraction of the right atrium, occurring just prior to the carotid arterial pulse and first heart sound. See also illustration at *pulse*. 2. in the electroretinogram, the small negative deflection occurring after stimulus presentation, related to the photoreceptor processes of the rods and cones. 3. in the apexcardiogram, a small positive deflection in late diastole, coinciding with the third heart sound; it represents the passage of blood into the left ventricle as a result of atrial systole.

alpha w's brain waves in the electroencephalogram which have a frequency of 8 to 13 per second; they are typical of the normal person awake and in a quiet resting state and occur principally in the occipital region.

anacrotic w. the wave on a tracing of an anacrotic pulse.

anadicrotic w. the wave on a tracing of an anadicrotic pulse.

atrial pressure w's the three elevations commonly seen on the graphic representation of the cardiac cycle, known as the *a wave*, *c wave*, and *v wave*. See illustration at *cardiac cycle*, under *cycle*.

axon w. A w. (def. 1).

b w. in the electroretinogram, a high-amplitude, positive deflection occurring immediately after the a wave and representing complex activity of the retinal bipolar layer.

beta w's brain waves in the electroencephalogram, which have a frequency of 18 to 30 per second; they are typical during periods of intense activity of the nervous system and occur principally in the parietal and frontal regions.

brain w's the fluctuations of electrical potential in the brain, as recorded by electroencephalography. See *alpha*, *beta*, *delta*, and *theta w's*.

c w. 1. in a tracing of the venous pulse, a small positive deflection representing the bulging back toward the atria of the tricuspid valve at the onset of ventricular contraction. See also illustration at *pulse*. 2. in the electroretinogram, the positive deflection representing

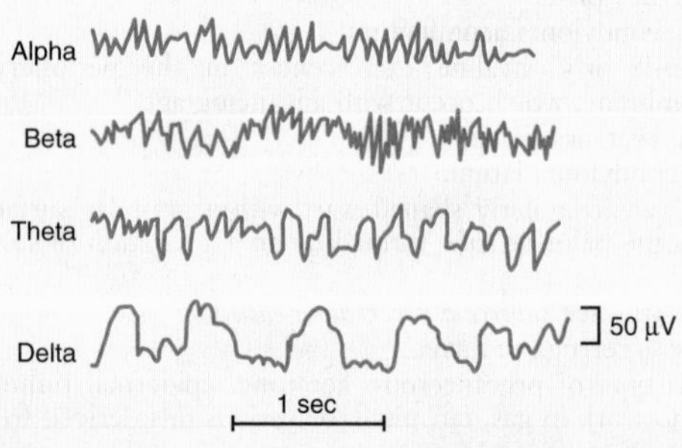

■ Brain waves characteristic of a normal electroencephalogram.

the response of the pigmented epithelium of the retina to photoreceptor-induced changes in extracellular potassium.

cannon a w's in tracings of the jugular venous pulse, abnormal tall a waves seen in rhythm disturbances in which the atrium contracts against a closed tricuspid valve. See also *giant a w's*.

catacrotic w. the wave of a tracing of a catacrotic pulse.

catadicrotic w. the wave of a tracing of a catadicrotic pulse.

contraction w. the wave of progression of the contraction in a muscle from the point of stimulation; also the graphic representation of a contracting muscle.

d w. in the electroretinogram, a small positive deflection produced by cone receptors in the latent period after stimulus termination.

delta w. 1. a small hump occurring on the upstroke of the QRS complex in electrocardiography; it is characteristic of preexcitation. 2. *(in the pl.)* waves in the electroencephalogram that have a frequency below 4 per second; they are typical in deep sleep, in infancy, and in serious brain disorders.

dicrotic w. the second portion of the arterial pulse or arterial pressure recording after the dicrotic notch, attributed to the reflected impulse of closure of the aortic valves. Called also *recoil w.*

E w. contingent negative variation.

electroencephalographic w's see *brain w's*.

electromagnetic w's the spectrum of waves propagated through space or matter by the oscillation of an electric field and a magnetic

Wave *Continued*

field at right angles to one another; they travel perpendicularly to both the electric and magnetic fields and have a velocity in a vacuum of 3×10^8 m/s. They include, in order of decreasing wavelength, radio waves, microwaves, infrared rays, visible light, ultraviolet rays, x-rays, gamma rays, and cosmic rays.
excitation w. an electric wave flowing from a muscle just previous to its contraction.
expectancy w. contingent negative variation.
F w's 1. rapid sawtooth-edged atrial waves without isoelectric intervals between them, seen in the electrocardiogram in atrial flutter. Written also *f w's.* Called also *flutter w's.* 2. compound muscle action potentials with a smaller amplitude and a longer latency than the corresponding M waves; caused by antidromic activation of the motor neuron. 3. f w's (def. 1).
f w's 1. small, irregular, rapid deflections in the electrocardiogram in atrial fibrillation. Written also *F w's.* Called also *fibrillary w's.* 2. F w's (def. 1).
fibrillary w's f w's (def. 1).
flutter w's F w's (def. 1).
giant a w's abnormally tall a waves in tracings of the jugular venous pulse; they occur when either inflow resistance to or outflow resistance from the right ventricle is increased or when atrial contractions occur out of phase, during the period the tricuspid valve is closed (cannon a waves).
H w. 1. a compound muscle action potential of consistently longer latency and smaller amplitude than the corresponding M wave; evoked primarily from extensor muscles, usually in the calf, and thought to be due to a spinal reflex (the H-reflex). It is evoked only by submaximal stimulation and disappears when the stimulation increases to the supramaximal level. 2. His bundle deflection.
J w. a deflection occurring in the electrocardiogram between the QRS complex and the onset of the ST segment; it occurs prominently in hypothermia and in hypercalcemia.
lambda w's electropositive sharp waves of medium amplitude sometimes seen on an electroencephalogram of the occipital region during concentration on a visual stimulus or during saccadic eye movements.
Liesegang w's see under *phenomenon.*
light w's the electromagnetic waves that produce sensations in the retina; see *light.*
longitudinal w. a wave whose oscillatory motion is parallel to the direction of its propagation.
M w. a compound muscle action potential evoked from a muscle by a single electric stimulus to its motor nerve; the waveform is usually biphasic and relatively similar on repeated stimulations.
Mayer w's regular variations in blood pressure over intervals longer than those of Traube-Hering waves, associated with pathologic mechanisms such as abnormal oscillations in the baroreceptor system or activation of vasopressor reflexes.
Osborn w's prominent electrocardiographic J waves; usually associated with hypothermia, hypercalcemia, or other pathology.
P w. in the electrocardiogram, the initial deflection of the cardiac cycle, representing excitation of the atria. See illustration at *electrocardiogram.*
papillary w., percussion w. the chief ascending portion of a sphygmographic tracing.
plateau w. a wave seen during intracranial pressure monitoring in advanced stages of increased pressure with hypoxia of brain cells; a rapid increase in pressure is followed by a plateau of high pressure lasting for 5 to 30 minutes before the decline in pressure begins.

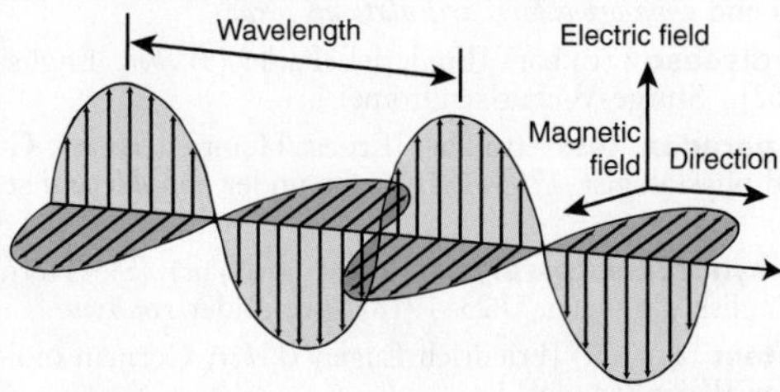

■ Diagrammatic representation of electromagnetic waves.

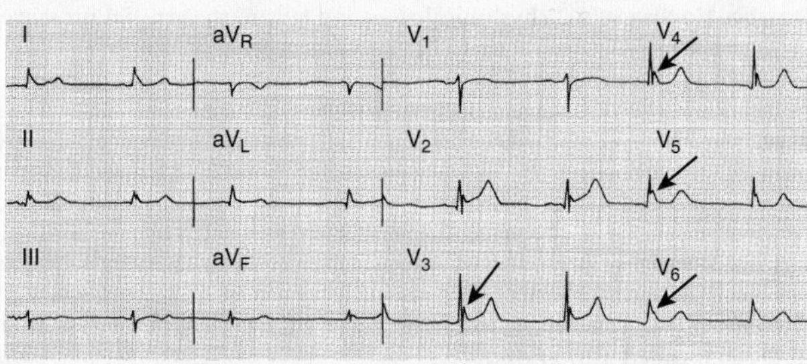

■ Osborn waves *(arrows)* associated with hypothermia.

positive sharp w. a short burst of biphasic electrical activity recorded from a muscle fiber, usually evoked by stimulation or injury by electrode insertion or other electrode movement; spontaneous occurrence of such waves at other times may be a sign of a myopathic disorder or a denervated muscle.
pulse w. the elevation of the pulse felt by the finger or shown graphically in a recording of pulse or pressure.
Q w. in the QRS complex, the initial downward (negative) deflection, related to the initial phase of depolarization (excitation) of the ventricular myocardium and the depolarization of the interventricular septum. See illustration at *electrocardiogram.*
R w. the initial upward deflection of the QRS complex, following the Q wave in the normal electrocardiogram and representing early depolarization of the ventricles. See illustration at *electrocardiogram.*
R_1 w. the earlier of the two blink responses.
R_2 w. the later of the two blink responses.
radio w's electromagnetic radiation of wavelength between 10^{-1} and 10^6 cm and frequency of about 10^{11} to 10^4 hertz.
random w's brain waves showing irregular changes in potential and no fixed frequency.
rapid filling w. in the apexcardiogram, the steep positive deflection following the O point, or mitral valve opening, representing the period of rapid blood flow into the left ventricle. Its transition to the slow filling wave is marked by the third heart sound.
recoil w. dicrotic w.
S w. a downward deflection of the QRS complex following the R wave in the normal electrocardiogram and representing late depolarization of the ventricles. See illustration at *electrocardiogram.*
sharp w. a wave on an electroencephalogram that has a sharp peak but is longer in duration than a spike.
short w. a wave having a wavelength of 60 meters or less.
sine w. the waveform of an alternating current characterized by a rise from zero to maximum positive potential, descending back through zero to its maximum negative value, and then rising back to zero. Called also *sinusoidal w.* and *sinusoidal waveform.*
sinusoidal w. sine w.
slow filling w. in the apexcardiogram, the shallow-sloped positive deflection following the rapid filling wave; it represents continued, but slowed, blood flow into the left ventricle.
sonic w's audible sound waves.
sound w's longitudinal waves of mechanical energy that transmit the vibrations interpreted as sound (def. 2).
stimulus w. excitation w.
T w. the deflection of the normal electrocardiogram following the QRS complex; it represents repolarization, or recovery, of the ventricles. See illustration at *electrocardiogram.*
Ta w. a small asymmetric wave, of opposite polarity to the P wave, representing atrial repolarization; together with the P wave it defines atrial electrical systole. In most electrocardiograms, it is obscured by the QRS complex.
theta w's brain waves in the electroencephalogram which have a frequency of 4 to 7 per second; they occur mainly in children but also in adults during periods of emotional stress.
tidal w. the sphygmographic wave after the percussion wave; the second elevation of the sphygmographic tracing between the percussion and dicrotic waves.
transverse w. a wave in which the oscillatory motion is perpendicular to the direction of propagation.

Wave *Continued*

Traube-Hering w's rhythmical rises and falls in the arterial pressure, attributed to rhythmical activity of the vasoconstrictor center.
tricrotic w. a third wave in the sphygmographic curve in addition to the tidal and dicrotic waves, occurring during systole.
U w. in the electrocardiogram, a small positive deflection usually immediately following the T wave but often poorly separated from it and so concealed; it is postulated to represent repolarization of the Purkinje fibers or a mechanical event such as ventricular relaxation. It is not invariably present and is most often seen in tachyarrhythmias and electrolyte disturbances. See also illustration at *electrocardiogram.*
ultrashort w. an electromagnetic wave of wavelength of less than 10 meters; called also *microwave.*
ultrasonic w's waves similar to sound waves but of such high frequency (20,000 hertz or higher) that the human ear does not perceive them as sound; see *ultrasonics.*
v w. in a tracing of the venous pulse, a positive deflection representing the filling of the right atrium against the closed tricuspid valve during ventricular contraction. See also illustration at *pulse.*
x w. in a tracing of the venous pulse, a negative deflection representing relaxation of the atria. See also illustration at *pulse.*
y w. in a tracing of the venous pulse, a negative deflection representing emptying of the right atrium upon right ventricular relaxation and opening of the tricuspid valve. See also illustration at *pulse.*

wave•form (wāv′form) the shape of a wave on a graph; sometimes used as a synonym for *wave.*
sinusoidal w. sine wave.

wave•length (λ) (wāv′length) the distance between the top of one wave and the identical phase of the succeeding one.
effective w., equivalent w. in radiology, the wavelength of monochromatic x-rays which would undergo the same percentage attenuation in a specified absorber as the heterogeneous beam under consideration.
minimum w. the shortest wavelength in an x-ray spectrum.

wax (waks) [L. *cera*] a low-melting, high-molecular-weight, organic mixture or compound, similar to fats and oils but lacking glycerides; it may be deposited by insects, obtained from plants, or prepared synthetically. Most are esters of fatty acids and alcohols, with some hydrocarbons. The wax of pharmacy is principally *yellow w.* and its bleached form *white w.*
baseplate w. a dental wax containing about 75 per cent paraffin or ceresin with additions of beeswax and other waxes and resins; used chiefly to establish the initial arch form in making trial plates for the construction of complete dentures. Called also *try-in w.*
blockout w. a dental wax used as a blockout (q.v.) material to eliminate undercuts on master casts prior to duplication.
bone w. a waxy substance used for packing small bone cavities, as in bones of the skull, and for controlling bleeding from them.
boxing w. a dental wax used for boxing (q.v.) impressions in the fabrication of restorations and appliances.
carding w. dental wax used as a base for mounting artificial teeth, organized by standard sizes, shades, and so forth.
carnauba w. [NF] a wax obtained from the leaves of the palm *Copernicia cerifera*, used as a tablet coating agent.
casting w. a mixture of several dental waxes; used for making patterns to determine the shape of the metallic framework and other parts of removable partial dentures.
cetyl esters w. [NF] a mixture consisting primarily of esters of saturated fatty alcohols and saturated fatty acids; used as a stiffening agent in pharmaceutical preparations. Called also *synthetic spermaceti.*
dental w. a mixture of two or more natural and synthetic waxes, resins, coloring agents, and other additives; used for pattern making for casting purposes and in the construction of nonmetallic denture bases, for registering jaw relations, and as aids in laboratory work.
dental inlay casting w. a mixture of waxes used to make a pattern for an inlay (wax pattern), containing various waxes, usually including paraffin, carnauba wax, and beeswax; synthetic waxes are sometimes used to replace the carnauba wax. Called also *inlay casting w.* and *inlay pattern w.*
ear w. cerumen.
emulsifying w. [NF] a waxy solid prepared from cetostearyl alcohol, containing a polyoxyethylene derivative of a fatty acid ester of sorbitan; used as an emulsifying and stiffening agent in pharmaceutical preparations.
inlay casting w., inlay pattern w. dental inlay casting w.
microcrystalline w. [NF] a mixture of straight chain, branched chain, and cyclic hydrocarbons obtained from the still bottom fraction of petroleum; used as a pharmaceutical stiffening agent and tablet and capsule coating agent.
paraffin w. paraffin (def. 1).
set-up w. a dental wax used in laboratories to align artificial teeth in dentures.
try-in w. baseplate w.
tubercle bacillus w. a high-molecular-weight phosphatidic glycolipid extracted from the cell walls of *Mycobacterium tuberculosis*, made up of arabinoglycans and mycolic and muramic acids. It is used as an adjuvant to enhance the immunogenicity of tuberculin preparations.
utility w. a soft, pliable, adhesive dental wax used for various purposes in the laboratory, such as to give the desired contour to a perforated tray to be used with hydrocolloids.
vegetable w. a waxy substance, resembling beeswax, derived from various vegetable sources.
white w. [NF] the bleached, purified wax from the honeycomb of the bee, *Apis mellifera*, used as a stiffening agent in pharmaceutical preparations.
yellow w. [NF] the purified wax from the honeycomb of the bee *Apis mellifera;* used as a stiffening agent in pharmaceutical preparations. Called also *beeswax.*

wax•ing (wak′sing) the contouring of a wax pattern or the wax base of a trial denture into the desired shape. Called also *waxing up.*

wax•ing up (wak′sing up) waxing.

waxy (wak′se) 1. composed of or covered by wax. 2. resembling wax, especially denoting some combination of pliability, paleness, and smoothness and luster.

Wb weber.

WBC white blood cell (see *leukocyte*); white blood cell count.

wean (wēn) to discontinue the breast feeding of an infant, with substitution of other feeding habits.

wean•ling (wēn′ling) 1. recently weaned. 2. a recently weaned human infant or other animal.

web (web) a tissue or membrane.
antral w. see under *membrane.*
esophageal w. a fibrous circumferential fold of the mucous membrane of the esophagus, seen in esophageal atresia, Plummer-Vinson syndrome, and other conditions.
interdigital w. the free border of the web connecting the bases of adjoining digits; called also *interdigital fold.*
laryngeal w. a common congenital malformation of the larynx that may be thin and translucent or thicker and more fibrotic; it is spread between the vocal folds near the anterior commissure and may cause hoarseness, aphonia, and other symptoms. See also *laryngeal atresia*, under *atresia.*
pyloric w. see under *membrane.*
subsynaptic w. a system of filaments or fine canaliculi, seen to penetrate at a varying distance into the postsynaptic cell.
terminal w. a cytoplasmic network of actin, spectrin, and intermediate filaments at the base of the microvilli of certain epithelial cells such as the absorptive cells of the intestine; it provides anchorage and support for the microvilli.

webbed (webd) connected by a membrane.

We•ber corpuscle (organ), glands, zone (va′bər) [Moritz Ignatz *Weber*, German anatomist, 1795–1875] see under *gland*, and see *utriculus prostaticus* and *zona orbicularis articulationis coxae.*

Web•er disease (va′bər) [Frederick Parkes *Weber*, English physician, 1863–1962] Sturge-Weber syndrome.

We•ber paradox, test (va′bər) [Ernest Heinrich *Weber*, German anatomist and physiologist, 1795–1878] see under *paradox* and see *Weber test* (def. 2).

Web•er syndrome (paralysis, sign) (web′ər) [Sir Hermann David *Weber*, English physician, 1823–1918] see under *syndrome.*

We•ber test (va′bər) [Friedrich Eugen *Weber*, German otologist, 1832–1891] see *Weber test* (def. 1).

web•er (Wb) (web′ər) the SI unit of magnetic flux which, linking a circuit of one turn, produces in it an electromotive force of one volt as it is reduced to zero at a uniform rate in one second.

Web•er-Chris•tian panniculitis (disease) (va′bər kris′chən) [F.P. *Weber;* Henry Asbury *Christian,* American physician, 1876–1951] relapsing febrile nodular nonsuppurative panniculitis.

Web•er-Cock•ayne syndrome (va′bər kok-ān′) [F.P. *Weber;* Edward Alfred *Cockayne,* English physician, 1880–1956] the localized form of epidermolysis bullosa simplex.

Web•er-Gub•ler syndrome (web′ər g o͞ ob′lər) [Sir H.D. *Weber;* Adolphe Marie *Gubler,* French physician, 1821–1879] Weber syndrome.

We•ber-Ley•den syndrome (web′ər li′dən) [Sir H.D. *Weber;* Ernst Victor von *Leyden,* German physician, 1832–1910] Weber syndrome.

Web•ster operation (web′stər) [John Clarence *Webster,* American gynecologist, 1863–1950] see under *operation.*

Wechs•ler Adult Intelligence Scale, Intelligence Scale for Children (weks′lər) [David *Wechsler,* Romanian-born American psychologist, 1896–1981] see under *scale.*

wed•dell•ite (wed′ə-līt) [*Weddell* Sea in the Antarctic, where minute quantities were first found] a dihydrate of calcium oxalate, seen in urinary calculi.

We•den•sky facilitation, inhibition, phenomenon (və-den′ske) [Nikolai Yevgenyevich *Wedensky,* Russian neurologist, 1852–1922] see under *facilitation, inhibition,* and *phenomenon.*

wedge (wej) [A.S. *wecg*] 1. a piece of material thick at one end and tapering to a thin edge at the other end. 2. to force something into a space of limited size; see under *pressure.*

step w. penetrometer; a block of an absorber, usually aluminum, machined in steps of increasing thickness, used to measure the penetrability of x-rays.

WEE western equine encephalomyelitis.

Weeks bacillus (wēks) [John Elmer *Weeks,* New York ophthalmologist, 1853–1949] *Haemophilus aegyptius.*

Week•sel•la (wēk-sel′ə) a genus of bacteria of the family Flavobacteriaceae, consisting of gram-negative rods; species are found most often in mammals other than humans.

W. viro′sa a species usually found in the genital tracts of women and not causing symptoms; if it contaminates the peritoneal cavity, it can cause peritonitis.

weep (wēp) 1. to shed tears. Called also *cry.* 2. to ooze serum.

wee•vil (we′vəl) any of various beetles, some of which are highly destructive to plants and food.

wheat w. *Sitophilus granarius.*

We•ge•ner granulomatosis (syndrome) (veg′ĕ-ner) [Friedrich *Wegener,* German pathologist, 1907–1990] see under *granulomatosis.*

Wei•bel-Pa•lade bodies (vi′bəl pah-lād′) [Ewald Rudolf *Weibel,* Swiss physician, born 1929; George Emil *Palade,* Romanian-born American cytologist, winner of 1974 Nobel prize in physiology or medicine, 1912–2008] see under *body.*

Wei•gert law, stain (method) (vi′gert) [Carl *Weigert,* German pathologist, 1845–1904] see under *law,* and see *Stains and Staining Methods,* under *stain.*

Wei•gert-Mey•er rule (law) (vi′gert mi′er) [C. *Weigert;* R. *Meyer,* American physician, mid-20th century] see under *rule.*

weight (wāt) 1. heaviness; the degree to which a body is drawn toward the earth by gravity. See also Appendix 7. Abbreviated wt. 2. in statistics, the process of assigning greater importance to some observations than to others, or a mathematical factor used to apply such a process.

apothecaries' w. a system of weights used in compounding prescriptions, based on the grain (64.8 mg). Its units are the scruple (20 grains), dram (3 scruples), ounce (8 drams), and pound (12 ounces). See Appendix 7.

atomic w. the sum of the masses of the constituents of an atom, either that of a single isotope or that obtained using weighted averages of the masses of the natural isotopes. It can be expressed in atomic mass units (or daltons), in SI units (i.e., kilograms), or as a dimensionless ratio derived by comparing the mass to the mass of the ^{12}C isotope of carbon, which is defined as exactly 12.000. Abbreviated at wt. Called also *atomic mass.*

avoirdupois w. the system of weight commonly used for ordinary commodities in English-speaking countries; its units are the grain (64.8 mg), dram (27.344 grains), ounce (16 drams), and pound (16 ounces). See Appendix 7.

combining w. equivalent w.

equivalent w. the amount of a substance that combines with or displaces 8.0 g of oxygen (or 1.008 g of hydrogen), usually expressed in grams; for acid-base reactions, one equivalent donates or receives a mole of protons, and the equivalent weight is the ratio of the molecular weight to the number of protons involved in the reaction. For redox reactions, one equivalent donates or receives a mole of electrons, and the equivalent weight is the ratio of the molecular weight to the number of electrons involved in the reaction.

gram molecular w. the molecular weight of a substance expressed in grams; one gram molecular weight of any molecular substance contains one mole of the molecules. Cf. *mole*[1].

molecular w. the weight of a molecule of a substance as compared with that of an atom of carbon 12; it is equal to the sum of the atomic weights of its constituent atoms and is dimensionless (cf. *molecular mass* and *molar mass*). Abbreviated Mol wt or MW. Although widely used, the term is not technically correct; relative molecular mass (M_r) is preferable.

Weil basal layer (zone) (vīl) [Ludwig A. *Weil,* German dentist, 1849–1895] see under *layer.*

Weil stain (wīl) [Arthur *Weil,* American neuropathologist, 1887–1969] see *Stains and Staining Methods,* under *stain.*

Weil syndrome (vīl) [Adolf *Weil,* German physician, 1848–1916] see under *syndrome.*

Weil-Fe•lix test (reaction) (vīl′ fa′liks) [Edmund *Weil,* Austrian physician in Czechoslovakia, 1880–1922; Arthur *Felix,* Polish-born bacteriologist in England, 1887–1956] see under *test.*

Weill sign (vīl) [Edmond *Weill,* French pediatrician, 1858–1924] see under *sign.*

Weill-Mar•che•sa•ni syndrome (vīl′ mahr-kə-sah′ne) [Georges *Weill,* French ophthalmologist, 1866–1952; Oswald *Marchesani,* German ophthalmologist, 1900–1952] see under *syndrome.*

Wein•gar•ten syndrome (wīn′gahr-tən) [R.J. *Weingarten,* American physician, 20th century] tropical eosinophilia; see under *eosinophilia.*

Weir Mitch•ell (wēr′ mich′əl) see *Mitchell.*

Weis•bach angle (vīs′bahk) [Albin *Weisbach,* Austrian anthropologist, 1837–1914] see under *angle.*

Weis•mann's theory (vīs′mahnz) [August Friedrich Leopold *Weismann,* German biologist, 1834–1914] weismannism.

weis•mann•ism (wīs′man-iz-əm) [August *Weismann*] the doctrine of the noninheritance of acquired characters, with only changes in the germ plasm being passed from generation to generation.

Weiss reflex (vīs) [Leopold *Weiss,* German oculist, 1848–1901] see under *reflex.*

Weit•brecht cartilage, cord (ligament), etc. (vīt′brekt) [Josias *Weitbrecht,* German anatomist in Russia, 1702–1747] see *chorda obliqua membranae interosseae antebrachii* and *discus articularis articulationis acromioclavicularis,* and see under *foramen* and *retinaculum.*

We•lan•der distal myopathy (myopathy) (va′lahn-dər) [Lisa *Welander,* Swedish neurologist, 1909–2001] see under *myopathy.*

Welch bacillus (welch) [William Henry *Welch,* American pathologist, 1850–1934] *Clostridium perfringens.*

Wel•Chol (wel′kol) trademark for a preparation of colesevelam hydrochloride.

Wel•cker angle (vel′kər) [Hermann *Welcker,* Austrian physician, 1822–1897] see *angulus sphenoidalis ossis parietalis.*

Well•bu•trin (wel′bu-trin) trademark for a preparation of bupropion hydrochloride.

Well•co•vo•rin (wel″ko-vo′rin) trademark for preparations of leucovorin calcium.

Wel•lens syndrome (wel′enz) [Hein J. J. *Wellens,* Dutch cardiologist, born 1935] see under *syndrome.*

Wells syndrome (welz) [G.C. *Wells,* British dermatologist, 20th century] see under *syndrome.*

welt (welt) wheal.

wen (wen) pilar cyst.

Wen•cke•bach block, period, phenomenon (veng′kə-bahk) [Karel Frederik *Wenckebach,* Dutch internist in Austria, 1864–1940] see under *block, period,* and *phenomenon.*

Werd•nig Hoff•mann disease (verd′nig hof′mahn) [Guido *Werdnig,* Austrian neurologist, 1844–1919; Johann *Hoffmann,* German neurologist, 1857–1919] see under *disease.*

Werl•hof disease (verl′hof) [Paul Gottlieb *Werlhof,* German physician, 1699–1767] idiopathic thrombocytopenic purpura.

Wer•mer syndrome (wur′mər) [Paul *Wermer,* American internist, 1898–1975] multiple endocrine neoplasia, type 1; see under *neoplasia.*

Wer•ner syndrome (ver′ner) [C.W. Otto *Werner,* German physician, 1879–1936] see under *syndrome.*

Wer•ner Schultz disease (ver′ner shooltz′) [*Werner Schultz,* German internist, 1878–1947] agranulocytosis.

Wer•ni•cke area (field, zone), encephalopathy, etc. (ver′nĭ-kə) [Karl *Wernicke*, German neurologist, 1848–1905] see under *area*, *encephalopathy*, and *triangle*, and see *receptive aphasia*, under *aphasia*.

Wer•ni•cke-Kor•sa•koff syndrome (ver′nĭ-kə kor′sə-kof) [K. *Wernicke;* Sergei Sergeivich *Korsakoff*, Russian neurologist, 1854–1900] see under *syndrome*.

Wer•ni•cke-Mann hemiplegia (ver′nĭ-kə mahn) [K. *Wernicke;* Ludwig *Mann*, German neurologist, 1866–1936] see under *hemiplegia*.

Wert•heim operation (vert′hīm) [Ernst *Wertheim*, German gynecologist, 1864–1920] see under *operation*.

West syndrome (west) [Charles *West*, British physician, 1816–1898] infantile spasms.

West•berg space (vest′bərg) [Friedrich *Westberg*, German physician, late 19th century] see under *space*.

West•cort (west′kort) trademark for a preparation of hydrocortisone valerate.

Wes•ter•gren method, tube (ves′ter-gren) [Alf Vilhelm Albertsson *Westergren*, Swedish physician, 1891–1968] see under *method* and *tube*.

Wes•ter•mark sign (ves′ter-mahrk) [Nils Johan Hugo *Westermark*, Swedish radiologist, 1892–1980] see under *sign*.

Wes•tern blot (blot analysis, blot hybridization, blot technique, blot test) (wes′tərn) [facetious coinage by analogy with *Southern blot*] see under *blot*.

West Nile encephalitis (fever), virus (west′ nīl′) [*West Nile* River valley and region in northern Uganda, where the disease was first observed in 1937] see under *encephalitis* and *virus*.

West•phal nucleus, sign (phenomenon) (vest′fahl) [Carl Friedrich Otto *Westphal*, German neurologist, 1833–1890] see under *sign*, and see *nucleus nervi accessorii*.

West•phal phenomenon, pupillary reflex (vest′fahl) [Alexander Karl Otto *Westphal*, German neurologist, 1863–1941] orbicularis pupillary reflex.

West•phal-Piltz phenomenon, reflex (vest′fahl pilts′) [A.K.O. *Westphal;* Jan *Piltz*, Austrian neurologist, 1870–1930] orbicularis pupillary reflex.

West•phal-Strüm•pell disease, pseudosclerosis (vest′fahl strēm′pel) [C.F.O. *Westphal;* Ernst Adolf Gustav Gottfried von *Strümpell*, German physician, 1853–1925] Wilson disease; see under *disease*.

wet-nurse (wet′nərs) see under *nurse*.

wet•pox (wet′poks) a form of fowlpox, with lesions occurring in the mouth and surrounding region, frequently causing death by suffocation.

Wet•zel grid (wet′səl) [Norman Carl *Wetzel*, American pediatrician, 1897–1984] see under *grid*.

We•ver-Bray phenomenon (we′vər bra′) [Ernest Glen *Wever*, American psychologist, 1902–1991; Charles William *Bray*, American otologist, 1904–1982] cochlear microphonic.

Wey•ers oligodactyly syndrome (vi′ərz) [Helmut *Weyers*, German pediatrician, 20th century] see under *syndrome*.

Whar•ton duct, jelly (gelatin) (hwor′tən) [Thomas *Wharton*, English physician and anatomist, 1614–1673] see *ductus submandibularis*, and see under *jelly*.

wheal (hwēl, wēl) the typical lesion of urticaria, the dermal evidence of allergy; it is a smooth, slightly elevated, discolored area on the body surface, often accompanied by severe itching. In sensitive persons it may also be provoked by mechanical irritation of the skin. Called also *hive* and *welt*.

wheel (hwēl) [A.S. *hwēol*] 1. a circular frame or disk designed to revolve around a central axis. 2. any of various round, engine-driven cutting or polishing dental instruments that may be of uniform thickness or knife-edge.

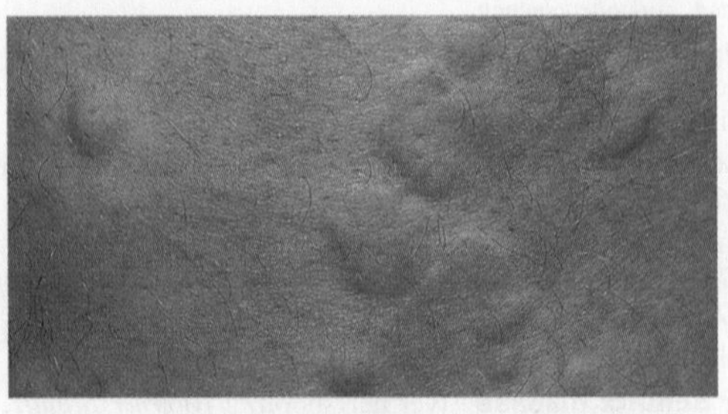

■ Wheals.

rag w. a dental disk made up of several layers of cloth stitched together and wetted down with pumice; used to polish dentures. Called also *cloth disk*.

wheeze (hwēz) 1. a continuous sound (q.v.) consisting of a whistling noise with a high pitch, thought to be generated by gas flowing through narrowed airways. Called also *sibilant* or *whistling rhonchus*. 2. to breathe making such a high-pitched sound.

asthmatoid w. a sound similar to the wheezing of an asthmatic, heard in cases of foreign body in the trachea or bronchus.

whelk (hwelk) any of various large ocean-dwelling snails with pointed spiral shells. Some are edible, but others are poisonous; see under *poison* and *poisoning*.

whelp (hwelp) 1. to give birth to; said of the female dog. 2. an unweaned puppy.

whe•well•ite (hu′wə-līt) [William *Whewell*, English philosopher, 1794–1866] a monohydrate of calcium oxalate, found in urinary calculi.

whey (hwa) the thin serum of milk remaining after the casein and fat have been removed; it contains proteins and the bulk of the lactose and water-soluble vitamins and minerals. The whey proteins, chiefly lactalbumins and lactoglobulins, constitute the majority of the protein content of human milk.

WHHL Watanabe heritable hyperlipidemic; see under *rabbit*.

whip (hwip) 1. to move suddenly and quickly. 2. a sudden, quick, thrashing movement.

catheter w. excessive mobility of the tip of an intracardiac catheter due to cardiac contraction, causing pressure measurements to be alternately artificially elevated and reduced.

whip•lash (hwip′lash) see under *injury*.

Whip•ple disease (hwip′əl) [George Hoyt *Whipple*, American pathologist and Nobel prize winner, 1878–1976] see *intestinal lipodystrophy*, under *lipodystrophy*.

Whip•ple procedure (operation), triad (hwip′əl) [Allen Oldfather *Whipple*, American surgeon, 1881–1963] see under *procedure* and *triad*.

whip•worm (hwip′wurm″) any member of the genus *Trichuris*.

whis•per (hwis′pər) a soft, low, sibilant breathing sound produced by the unvoiced passage of the breath through the glottis. Cf. *hypophonia*.

Whit•a•ker test (hwit′ə-kər) [Robert H. *Whitaker*, British urologist, born 1939] see under *test*.

white (hwīt) [A.S. *hwīt*] 1. the color, as of new snow, that results from reflection of all the rays of the spectrum; it is the opposite of black. 2. something having this color. 3. being of the color white.

visual w. exhausted or decolorized rhodopsin; called also *leukopsin*.

White•head operation (hwīt′hed) [Walter *Whitehead*, English surgeon, 1840–1913] see under *operation*.

white•head (hwīt′hed) 1. milium. 2. closed comedo.

white•leg (hwīt′leg) phlegmasia alba dolens.

Whit•field ointment (hwit′fēld) [Arthur *Whitfield*, British dermatologist, 1868–1947] benzoic and salicylic acids ointment.

whit•lock•ite (hwit′lə-kīt) [Herbert P. *Whitlock*, American mineralogist, 1868–1948] a type of tribasic calcium phosphate found in urinary calculi.

whit•low (hwit′lo) a painful abscess on the palmar aspect of a fingertip, occurring as the result of infection in the closed space of the terminal phalanx; it often follows inoculation into the skin of a pathogenic microorganism. Called also *pulp abscess* and *felon*.

herpetic w. cutaneous herpes simplex on the terminal segment of a finger, resulting in formation of deep coalescing vesicles with tissue destruction. Called also *herpetic paronychia*.

melanotic w. subungual melanoma.

thecal w. suppurative tenosynovitis of the terminal phalanx of a finger.

Whit•more disease (hwit′mor) [Major Alfred *Whitmore*, English surgeon in India, 1876–1946] melioidosis.

Whit•nall tubercle (hwit′nawl) [Samuel Ernest *Whitnall*, English anatomist, 1876–1950] tuberculum orbitale.

WHO World Health Organization; wrist-hand orthosis.

whoop (hoop) the sonorous and convulsive inhalation heard in pertussis (whooping cough).

whorl (hwurl) a spiral turn or twist, such as in a fingerprint or the hair.

bone w. an enostosis.

hair w′s vortices pilorum.

Whytt disease (hwit) [Robert *Whytt*, Scottish physician, 1714–1766] see under *disease*.

Wick•ers•hei•mer fluid (medium) (vik′ərz-hi″mər) [J. *Wickersheimer*, German anatomist, 1832–1896] see under *fluid*.

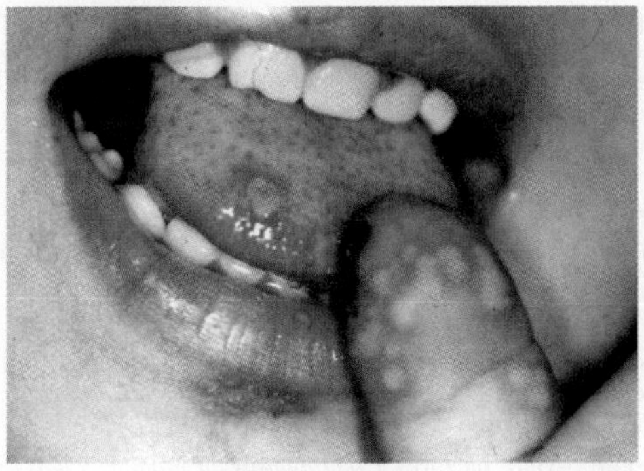

■ Herpetic whitlow.

Wick•ham striae (vik′ahm) [Louis-Frédéric *Wickham*, French dermatologist, 1861–1913] see under *stria*.

Wi•dal syndrome, test (reaction, serum test) (ve-dahl′) [Georges Fernand Isidore *Widal*, French physician, 1862–1929] see *hemolytic anemia*, under *anemia*, and see under *test*.

width (width) the extent of something from side to side.
biasteric w. the shortest distance between the two asteria.
bistephanic w. the shortest distance between the two stephanions.
window w. the energy range of gamma radiation that, once detected, will be accepted by the detection system; determined by the upper and lower window settings of the pulse height analyzer.

Wi•gand version (maneuver) (ve′gahnt) [Justus Heinrich *Wigand*, German gynecologist, 1766–1817] see under *version*.

Wig•gers di•a•gram (wig′ərz) [Carl John *Wiggers*, American surgeon, 1883–1963] see under *diagram*.

Wi•graine (wi′grān) trademark for combination preparations of ergotamine tartrate and caffeine.

Wil•cox•on rank sum test, signed rank test (wil-kok′sən) [Frank *Wilcoxon*, American chemist and statistician, 1892–1962] see *rank sum test* and *signed rank test*, under *test*.

wild (wīld) raised in a natural environment and not in captivity or a laboratory.

Wil•der sign (wīl′dər) [William Hamlin *Wilder*, American ophthalmologist, 1860–1935] see under *sign*.

Wil•der•muth ear (vil′der-moot) [Hermann A. *Wildermuth*, German neurologist, 1852–1907] see under *ear*.

wild-type (wīld′tīp″) typical of a natural population or standard laboratory stock; see under *type*.

Wil•liams syndrome (wil′yəmz) [J.C.P. *Williams*, New Zealand cardiologist, 20th century] see under *syndrome*.

Wil•liams-Beu•ren syndrome (wil′yəmz boi′rən) [J.C.P. *Williams*; Alois J. *Beuren*, German cardiologist, 1919–1984] see under *syndrome*.

Wil•liams-Camp•bell syndrome (wil′yəmz kam′bəl) [Howard *Williams*, Australian physician, 20th century; Peter E. *Campbell*, Australian physician, 20th century] see under *syndrome*.

Wil•liam•son sign (wil′yəm-sən) [Oliver K. *Williamson*, English physician, 1866–1941] see under *sign*.

Wil•lis circle, cord, etc. (wil′is) [Thomas *Willis*, English anatomist and physician, 1621–1675] see *circulus arteriosus cerebri* and *nervus accessorius*, and see under *cord* and *paracusis*.

wil•low (wil′o) [A.S. *welig*] any plant of the genus *Salix*. White willow bark (see under *bark*) contains salicin, the precursor of salicylic acid, and is used as an herbal remedy.

Wilms tumor (vilmz) [Max *Wilms*, German surgeon, 1867–1918] see under *tumor*.

Wil•son disease (degeneration, syndrome) (wil′sən) [Samuel Alexander Kinnier *Wilson*, English neurologist, 1877–1937] see under *disease*.

Wil•son muscle (wil′sən) [James *Wilson*, English surgeon, 1765–1821] see *musculus sphincter urethrae externus urethrae femininae* and *musculus sphincter urethrae externus urethrae masculinae*.

Wil•son-Mik•i•ty syndrome (wil′sən mik′ĭ-te) [Miriam Geisendorfer *Wilson*, American pediatrician, born 1922; Victor G. *Mikity*, American radiologist, born 1919] see under *syndrome*.

Wim•ber•ger sign (vim′ber-ger) [Heinrich *Wimberger*, German radiologist, 20th century] see under *sign*.

Win•ches•ter syndrome (win′ches-tər) [Patricia *Winchester*, American physician, 20th century] see under *syndrome*.

Win•ckel disease (ving′kəl) [Franz Karl Ludwig Wilhelm von *Winckel*, German gynecologist, 1837–1911] see under *disease*.

wind•burn (wind′bərn) chapping of the skin caused by excessive exposure to wind.

wind•chill (wind′chil) loss of heat from bodies subjected to wind.

wind•gall (wind′gawl) distention of the joint capsule or of a tendon sheath in the region of the fetlock of a horse, caused by a collection of synovial fluid; it is unsightly but usually does not interfere with functioning. Also written *wind gall*. Called also *windpuff*.

win•di•go (win′dĭ-go) [Ojibwa name for a cannibalistic monster of the mythology of Eskimos and certain Native Americans] a culture-specific syndrome characterized by delusions of being possessed by the windigo, with fears of becoming cannibalistic, and agitated depression. Called also *witigo*.

wind•lass (wind′ləs) an apparatus for lifting or hauling, consisting of a bar that can be turned to reel in a cable attached to a load.
Spanish w. an improvised tourniquet consisting of a handkerchief tied around a body part and twisted by a stick passed under it.

win•dow (win′do) [L. *fenestra*] 1. a circumscribed opening in a surface; called also *fenestra*. 2. the upper and lower voltage limits that determine which pulses a pulse height analyzer will accept and pass on. 3. the range of Hounsfield units over which the gray scale is spread in a particular CT scan; there are different windows for different types of tissues, such as bone and soft tissue.
aortic w. a radiolucent region below the aortic arch and above the pulmonary artery that contains mediastinal lymph nodes, visible on a radiograph.
aorticopulmonary w. aortic septal defect.
w. of cochlea, cochlear w. fenestra cochleae.
nasoantral w. a surgically created opening between the maxillary sinus and the nasal cavity; see *nasoantrostomy*.
oval w. fenestra vestibuli.
round w. fenestra cochleae.
skin w. see *Rebuck skin window technique*, under *technique*.
therapeutic w. the range between the minimum and maximum doses of an agent. See also *therapeutic index*, under *index*.
vestibular w., w. of vestibule fenestra vestibuli.

wind•pipe (wind′pīp) the trachea.

wind•puff (wind′pəf) windgall.

wind•suck•ing (wind′sək-ing) cribbing.

wing (wing) [L. *ala*] 1. either of the paired anterior appendages of birds, which are modified for flight. 2. a structure or part resembling the wing of a bird; called also *ala*.
w. of central lobule ala lobuli centralis.
great w. of sphenoid bone, greater w. of sphenoid bone ala major ossis sphenoidalis.
w. of ilium ala ossis ilii.
w. of Ingrassia ala minor ossis sphenoidalis.
lateral w. of sacrum pars lateralis ossis sacri.
lesser w. of sphenoid bone ala minor ossis sphenoidalis.
major w. of sphenoid bone ala major ossis sphenoidalis.
minor w. of sphenoid bone ala minor ossis sphenoidalis.
w. of nose ala nasi.
orbital w. of sphenoid bone, small w. of sphenoid bone ala minor ossis sphenoidalis.
w's of sphenoid bone the laterally projecting processes of the sphenoid bone; see *ala major ossis sphenoidalis* and *ala minor ossis sphenoidalis*.
temporal w. of sphenoid bone ala major ossis sphenoidalis.
w. of vomer ala vomeris.

Win•i•war•ter-Buer•ger disease (vin′ĭ-vahr″ter bēr′gər) [Felix von *Winiwarter*, German physician, 1848–1917; Leo *Buerger*, American physician, 1879–1943] thromboangiitis obliterans.

wink•ing (wingk′ing) [A.S. *wincian*] quick closing and opening of the eyelids, particularly of only one eye.
jaw w. Gunn syndrome.

Wink•ler disease (vingk′ler) [Max *Winkler*, Swiss physician, 1875–1952] chondrodermatitis nodularis chronica helicis.

Win•Rho (win′ro) trademark for preparations of $Rh_0(D)$ immune globulin.

Wins•low foramen, ligament, stars (winz′lo) [Jacob Benignus *Winslow*, Danish anatomist in Paris, 1669–1760] see under *star* and see *foramen epiploicum* and *ligamentum popliteum obliquum*.

Win•strol (win′strol) trademark for a preparation of stanozolol.

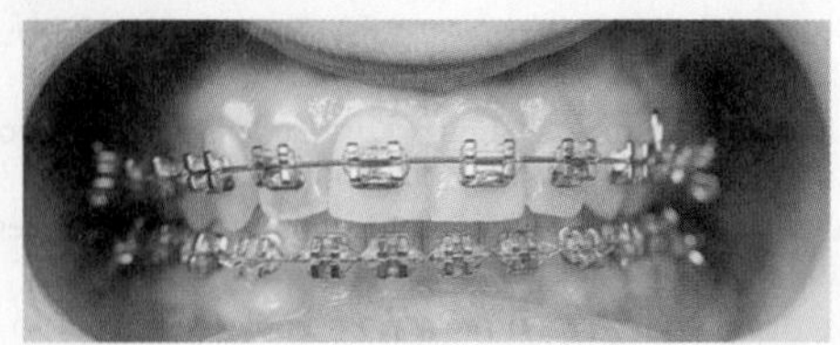

■ Arch wire connecting attachments on each dental arch.

Win•ter syndrome (win′tər) [Jeremy Stephen Drummond *Winter*, Canadian physician, born 1937] see under *syndrome.*

win•ter•ber•ry (win′tər-ber″e) *Ilex verticillata.*

Win•ter•bot•tom sign (win′tər-bot″əm) [Thomas Masterman *Winterbottom*, English physician, 1765–1859] see under *sign.*

win•ter•green (win′tər-grēn) *Gaultheria procumbens.*

Win•ter•nitz sound (vin′ter-nits″) [Wilhelm *Winternitz*, German physician in Austria, 1835–1917] see under *sound.*

Win•trobe hematocrit tube, method (win′trōb) [Maxwell Myer *Wintrobe*, American hematologist, 1901–1986] see under *tube* and *method.*

wire (wīr) 1. a long, slender, flexible structure of metal, used in surgery and dentistry. 2. to insert such strands into a body structure, as into a broken bone to immobilize fragments, or into an aneurysm to promote clot formation.

arch w. a wire attached to molar bands or an orthodontic appliance and applied around the dental arch to control and force tooth movement in orthodontic therapy. Called also *orthodontic w.*

arch w., ideal the configuration of an arch wire that conforms as closely as possible to the desired ultimate shape of the arch for a particular individual.

Kirschner w. a steel wire for skeletal fixation of fractured bones and for obtaining skeletal traction in fractures; it is inserted through the soft tissues and the bone.

ligature w. a soft, thin wire used to tie an arch wire to band attachments or brackets in an orthodontic appliance.

orthodontic w. arch w.

separating w. a brass wire threaded between two teeth having tight contact in an effort to wedge them slightly apart before fitting a band in the application of an orthodontic appliance.

twin w. see under *appliance.*

wire•worm (wīr′werm) *Haemonchus contortus.*

wir•ing (wīr′ing) the fixing into position by means of wire, as of segments of fractured bone.

circumferential w. a technique for fixation of mandibular fractures in which wires are passed around a section of bone with the ends exiting into the oral cavity and then around a fixed intraoral splint.

continuous loop w. wiring of the teeth for the reduction and fixation of fractures, by using a single length of wire to form wire loops on both the maxillary and mandibular teeth, over which intermaxillary elastics can be placed; called also *Stout w.*

craniofacial suspension w. wiring of noncontiguous areas of bone (piriform aperture, zygomatic arch, zygomatic process of the frontal bone) for the support of fractured jaw segments.

Gilmer w. a method of intermaxillary fixation in which single opposing teeth are wired circumferentially and the wires twisted together.

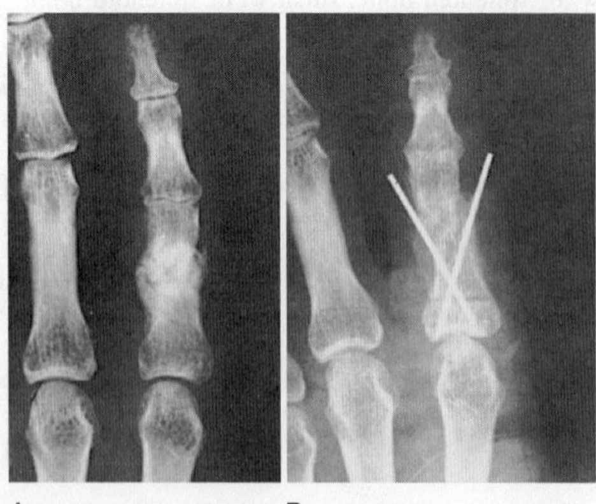

■ Kirschner wire. Malunited phalangeal fracture with rotational deformity *(A)* after osteotomy through the proximal end of the bone and fixation with two Kirschner wires *(B).*

Ivy loop w. wiring of adjacent teeth in groups of two to provide an attachment for intermaxillary elastics.

perialveolar w. the fixing of a splint to the maxillary arch by passing a wire through the alveolar process from the buccal plate to the palate.

piriform aperture w. wiring through the nasal bones at the piriform aperture for the stabilization of fractures of the jaws.

Stout w. continuous loop w.

Wir•sung duct (vēr′soong) [Johann Georg *Wirsung*, German physician in Italy, 1600–1643] see *ductus pancreaticus.*

WISC Wechsler Intelligence Scale for Children.

Wis•kott-Al•drich syndrome (vis′kot awl′drich) [Alfred *Wiskott*, German pediatrician, 1898–1978; Robert Anderson *Aldrich*, American pediatrician, 1917–1999] see under *syndrome.*

witch ha•zel (wich′ ha′zəl) 1. *Hamamelis virginiana.* 2. [USP] a clear, colorless distillate prepared from recently cut, partially dried twigs of *H. virginiana* macerated in water, used topically as a mild astringent. Called also *hamamelis water.*

Wi•tha•nia (wĭ-tha′ne-ə) a genus of Old World shrubs of the family Solanaceae, having woolly leaves and clustered bell-shaped flowers; *W. somni′fera* (ashwagandha) is used medicinally in ayurveda.

with•draw•al (with-draw′əl) 1. a pathological retreat from interpersonal contact and social involvement, as may occur in schizophrenia, depression, or schizoid, avoidant, or schizotypal personality disorders. 2. substance w.

substance w. [DSM-IV] a substance-specific mental disorder that follows the cessation of use or reduction in intake of a psychoactive substance that had been regularly used to induce a state of intoxication. DSM-IV includes specific withdrawal syndromes for alcohol; amphetamines or similarly acting sympathomimetics; cocaine; nicotine; opioids; and sedatives, hypnotics, or anxiolytics. Called also *withdrawal, withdrawal symptoms* or *syndrome,* and *abstinence symptoms* or *syndrome.*

with•ers (with′ərz) the top of the shoulders of the horse.

fistulous w. distention and rupture of the bursa in the withers region of horses, with suppuration; it is caused by a dual infection with *Brucella* species and *Actinomyces* species and is virtually identical to poll evil.

wi•ti•go (wĭ-ti′go) windigo.

Wit•kop disease (wit′kop) [Carl J. *Witkop*, American oral pathologist and geneticist, 1920–1993] see under *disease.*

Wit•kop-von Sall•mann disease (wit′kop von sahl′mən) [C. J. *Witkop*; Ludwig J. K. *von Sallmann*, Austrian-born American ophthalmologist, 1892–1975] see under *disease.*

wit•kop (wit′kop) [Afrikaans "whitehead"] a South African term for *favus.*

Wit•zel gastrostomy (operation) (vit′səl) [Friedrich Oskar *Witzel*, German surgeon, 1856–1925] see under *gastrostomy.*

wit•zel•sucht (vit′sel-zo͞okt) [Ger.] a mental condition characteristic of frontal lobe lesions and marked by the making of poor jokes and puns and the telling of pointless stories, which the patient finds intensely amusing.

WMA World Medical Association.

WNV West Nile virus.

wob•ble (wob′əl) to move unsteadily or unsurely back and forth or from side to side. See under *hypothesis.*

wob•bles (wob′əlz) wobbler syndrome, defs. 1 and 2.

Wohl•fart-Ku•gel•berg-We•lan•der syndrome (vōl′fahrt koo′gəl-bārg va′lahn-dər) [Karl Gunnar Vilhelm *Wohlfart*, Swedish neurologist, 1910–1961; Eric Klas Henrik *Kugelberg*, Swedish neurologist, 1913–1983; Lisa *Welander*, Swedish neurologist, 1909–2001] Kugelberg-Welander syndrome.

Wohl•fahr•tia (vōl-fahr′te-ə) [Peter *Wohlfahrt*, German medical writer, 1675–1726] a genus of flesh flies of the family Sarcophagidae.

W. magni′fica a species found in Russia and the Middle East that causes wound myiasis.

W. opa′ca a North American species that causes cutaneous myiasis.

W. vi′gil a North American species that causes cutaneous myiasis.

Wol•bach•ia (wol-bak′e-ə) [S. Burt *Wolbach*, American pathologist, 20th century] a genus of bacteria of the family Anaplasmataceae, consisting of small rods and cocci that grow in vacuoles of the host cells. Organisms are symbionts in a wide variety of invertebrates, including insects, spiders, crustaceans, and nematodes such *Onchocerca*, and play a major role in the clinical manifestations of filariasis. The type species is *W. pipien′tis.*

Wolf-Hirsch•horn syndrome (voolf′ hursh′horn) [Ulrich *Wolf*, German physician, born 1933; Kurt *Hirschhorn*, American physician, born 1926] see under *syndrome.*

Wolfe graft (woolf) [John Reissberg *Wolfe*, Scottish ophthalmologist, 1824–1904] Krause-Wolfe graft.

Wolfe-Krause graft (woolf′ krou′zə) [J.R. *Wolfe;* Fedor *Krause*, German surgeon, 1857–1937] Krause-Wolfe graft.

Wolff duct (voolf) [Kaspar Friedrich *Wolff*, German anatomist and physiologist, 1733–1794] see *mesonephric duct*, under *duct*.

Wolff's law (voolfs) [Julius *Wolff*, German anatomist, 1836–1902] see under *law*.

Wolff-Chai•koff effect (woolf′ cha′kof) [J. *Wolff*, American physiologist, 20th century; Israel Lyon *Chaikoff*, British-born American physiologist, 1902–1966] see under *effect*.

Wolff-Par•kin•son-White syndrome (woolf′ pahr′kin-sən hwīt′) [Louis *Wolff*, American cardiologist, 1898–1972; Sir John *Parkinson*, English physician, 1885–1976; Paul Dudley *White*, American cardiologist, 1886–1973] see under *syndrome*.

wolf•fi•an (wool′fe-ən) described by Kaspar Friedrich *Wolff*, as wolffian body (mesonephros), cyst, duct (mesonephric duct), and ridge (mesonephric ridge).

Wöl•fler glands (vurl′flər) [Anton *Wölfler*, Austrian surgeon, 1850–1917] glandulae thyroideae accessoriae.

Wol•fram syndrome (wool′frəm) [D.J. *Wolfram*, American physician, 20th century] see under *syndrome*.

Wolf•ring glands (volf′ring) [Emilij Franzevic von *Wolfring*, Polish ophthalmologist, 1832–1906] see under *gland*.

wolfs•bane (woolfs′bān) 1. *Arnica*. 2. arnica. 3. *Aconitum napellus*. 4. aconite.

Wol•hy•nia fever (vōl-hi′ne-ə) [*Wolhynia* (or Volhynia), region divided between Russia and Ukraine, where it was found to be endemic] trench fever; see under *fever*.

Woll•as•ton doublet (wool′əs-tən) [William Hyde *Wollaston*, English physician, 1766–1828] see under *doublet*.

Wol•man disease (wol′mən) [Moshe *Wolman*, Polish-born neuropathologist in Israel, 20th century] see under *disease*.

Wo•mack procedure (wo′mak) see under *procedure*.

womb (wo͞om) the uterus.

Wood filter (glass), lamp, light (wood) [Robert Williams *Wood*, American physicist, 1868–1955] see under *filter*, *lamp*, and *light*.

Wood sign (wood) [Horatio Charles *Wood*, American physician and pharmacologist, 1874–1958] see under *sign*.

wood•chuck (wood′chuk) *Marmota monax*, a large, fat, brown rodent of northeastern North America, sometimes a natural reservoir of the plague. Called also *groundhog*.

wool (wool) [L. *lana*] 1. the hair of sheep. Called also *lana*. 2. by extension, any material existing as fine threads.

lumpy w. dermatophilosis in sheep.

Wool•ner tip (wool′nər) [Thomas *Woolner*, English sculptor and poet, 1825–1892] tuberculum auriculare.

word sal•ad (wurd′ sal′əd) a meaningless mixture of words and phrases characteristic of advanced schizophrenia; called also *schizophasia*.

Wo•rin•ger-Ko•lopp disease (vo″rin-zhār′ ko-lop′) [Frédéric *Woringer*, French dermatologist, 1903–1964; P. *Kolopp*, French dermatologist, 20th century] pagetoid reticulosis; see under *reticulosis*.

work (*W*) (wurk) in physics, the force applied to an object times the distance traveled in the direction of the force. The SI unit of work is the joule.

stroke w. a measure of the performance of the heart, usually referring to the left ventricle and cardiac output; it is increased in hypovolemia and hypertension and decreased in aortic stenosis, shock, and heart failure.

work-up (wurk′əp) the procedures done to arrive at a diagnosis, including history taking, laboratory tests, x-rays, and so on.

World Health Or•ga•ni•za•tion (WHO) an agency of the United Nations, devoted to attainment of the highest level of health by all peoples of the world; the permanent secretariat is located in Geneva, Switzerland.

worm (wurm) [L. *vermis*] any of the soft-bodied, naked, elongated invertebrates of the phyla Platyhelminthes, Annelida, Acanthocephala, and Aschelminthes. See also *helminth*.

barber's pole w. *Haemonchus contortus.*
bilharzia w. *Schistosoma.*
bladder w. 1. cysticercus. 2. coenurus.
case w. *Echinococcus.*
cayor w. the larva of *Cordylobia anthropophaga.*
dragon w. *Dracunculus medinensis.*
eel w. nematode.
eye w. any of various parasitic nematodes that infest the conjunctivae and conjunctival glands or sacs of animals, such as *Loa loa* and species of *Onchocerca* and *Thelazia.*
flat w. platyhelminth.
fleece w. wool maggot.
giant kidney w. *Dioctophyma renale.*
guinea w. *Dracunculus medinensis.*
heart w. *Dirofilaria immitis.*
horsehair w. *Gordius.*
kidney w. *Dioctophyma renale.*
lung w. see *lungworm.*
maw w. *Ascaris.*
meal w. mealworm.
Medina w. *Dracunculus medinensis.*
nodular w. any nematode of the genus *Oesophagostomum.*
palisade w. *Strongylus equinus.*
pork w. *Trichinella spiralis.*
round w. nematode.
scour w. a parasitic worm that causes diarrhea (scours) in ruminants, such as a nematode of one of the genera *Cooperia, Nematodirus, Ostertagia,* or *Trichostrongylus.*
screw w. see *screwworm.*
serpent w. *Dracunculus medinensis.*
spinyheaded w. acanthocephalan.
stomach w. any parasitic worm that lives in the stomach of an animal, such as species of *Haemonchus, Ostertagia,* and *Teladorsagia.*
thorny-headed w. acanthocephalan.
tongue w. pentastome.
trichina w. *Trichinella.*
wire w. *Haemonchus contortus.*

wor•mi•an (wur′me-ən) named for Ole *Worm* (Olaus Wormius), Danish physician and humanist, 1588–1654, as *wormian bones.*

Worm•ley test (worm′le) [Theodore George *Wormley*, American chemist, 1826–1897] see under *test.*

worm•wood (wurm′wood″) a plant of the genus *Artemisia*, especially *A. absinthium* (common wormwood), which yields the extract used to make absinthe.

sweet w. *Artemisia annua.*

Woulfe bottle (woolf) [Peter *Woulfe*, English chemist, 1727–1803] see under *bottle.*

wound (wo͞ond) [L. *vulnus*] an injury or damage, usually restricted to those caused by physical means with disruption of normal continuity of structures. Called also *injury* and *trauma.*

aseptic w. a wound that is not infected with pathogens.
blowing w. open pneumothorax.
contused w. nonpenetrating w.
incised w. a wound made by a cutting instrument.
lacerated w. laceration.
nonpenetrating w. a wound in which there is no disruption of the skin but there is injury to underlying structures. See also *contusion.*
open w. a wound that communicates with the atmosphere by direct exposure.
penetrating w. a wound caused by a sharp, usually slender object, such as a nail or ice pick, which passes through the skin into the underlying tissues. Called also *puncture w.*
perforating w. a penetrating wound which extends into a viscus or bodily cavity.
puncture w. penetrating w.
septic w. a wound that is infected with pathogens.
seton w. a wound that enters and exits on the same side of the injured part.
subcutaneous w. a wound that involves only the skin and subcutaneous tissue.
sucking w. a penetrating wound of the chest through which air is drawn in and out. See also *open pneumothorax.*
tangential w. an oblique glancing wound which results in one edge being undercut.

W-plas•ty (dub′əl-u-plas″te) a technique in plastic surgery used mainly in the repair of straight scars that require the redistribution of tension. It consists of excising a series of consecutive small triangular areas of tissue on each side of the wound or scar and imbricating the resultant triangular flaps.

wrap•ping (rap′ing) the act or process of putting a cover around a thing.

fundic w. fundoplication.
vein w. the wrapping of an injured nerve with an autologous vein (usually saphenous vein) graft to provide insulation and cushioning following decompression in treatment of entrapment neuropathy.

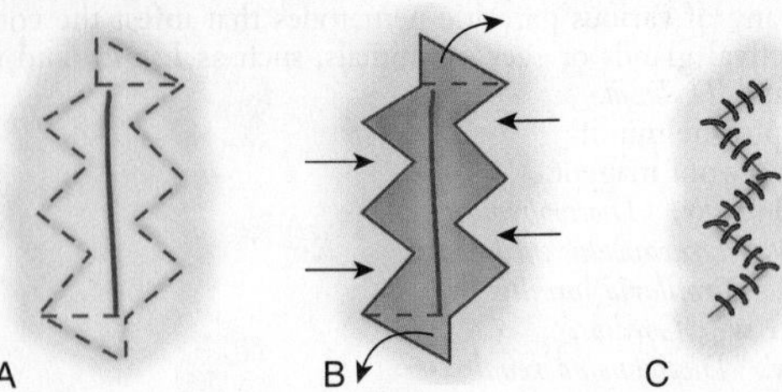

■ W-plasty. *(A)*, lines of excision; *(B)*, removal of triangular end flaps and apposition of segments; *(C)*, after suturing.

Wright blood group (rīt) [*Wright*, surname of the English propositus first reported on in 1953] see under *blood group.*

Wright inbreeding coefficient (rīt) [Sewall Green *Wright*, American geneticist, 1889–1988] coefficient of inbreeding.

Wright stain (rīt) [James Homer *Wright*, American pathologist, 1869–1928] see *Stains and Staining Methods*, under *stain.*

Wright syndrome (rīt) [Irving Sherwood *Wright*, American physician, 1901–1997] see under *syndrome.*

wrin•kle (ring′kəl) a furrow or fold in the skin or a mucous membrane; see also *rhytid.*

  dynamic w's see under *line.*
  glabellar w's see under *line.*

Wris•berg cartilage, etc. (ris′bərg) [Heinrich August *Wrisberg*, German anatomist, 1739–1808] see *cartilago cuneiformis, ganglia cardiaca, ligamentum meniscofemorale posterius, nervus intermedius, nervus cutaneus brachii medialis,* and *tuberculum cuneiforme.*

wrist (rist) 1. carpus, defs. 1 and 3. 2. articulatio radiocarpalis.

  SLAC w. a wrist affected by scapholunate advanced collapse (SLAC).
  tennis w. tenovaginitis of the tendons of the wrist in tennis players.

wrist•drop (rist′drop) a condition resulting from paralysis of the extensor muscles of the hand and fingers. Called also *carpoptosis* and *drop hand.*

writ•ing (rīt′ing) the inscription of letters or other symbols, and of words, phrases, and sentences, so that they may be perceived by the eyes or, by the blind, through the fingertips.

  mirror w. writing in which the right and left relationships of letters and words are reversed, as if seen in a mirror.

wry (ri) abnormally twisted; bent to one side; crooked or contorted.

wry•neck (ri′neck) torticollis.

wt weight.

Wu•cher•e•ria (voo″kər-er′e-ə) [Otto *Wucherer*, German physician in Brazil, 1820–1873] a genus of nematodes of the superfamily Filarioidea that affect mainly humans in warm regions of the world.

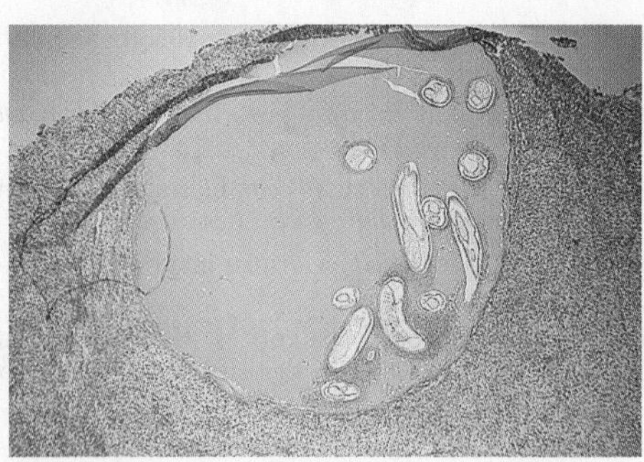

■ Cross-section of adult *Wuchereria bancrofti* in human lymph node, showing extensive inflammatory reaction (H & E stain).

  W. bancrof′ti a white threadlike worm that causes elephantiasis, lymphangitis, and chyluria by interfering with the lymphatic circulation. The immature forms, or microfilariae, are found in the circulating blood, especially at night, and are carried by *Culex* and other mosquitoes. In the Pacific strain of *W. bancrofti*, sometimes called *W. bancrofti* var. *pacifica*, the microfilariae do not show the nocturnal periodicity seen elsewhere.
  W. ma′layi *Brugia malayi.*

wu•cher•e•ri•a•sis (voo-ker″e-ri′ə-sis) any infection with nematodes of the genus *Wuchereria;* see *bancroftian filariasis.*

Wun•der•lich curve (voon′der-lik) [Carl Reinhold August *Wunderlich*, German physician, 1815–1877] see under *curve.*

w/v weight (of solute) per volume (of solvent).

Wy•a•mine (wi′ə-min) trademark for preparations of mephentermine sulfate.

Wy•burn-Ma•son syndrome (wi′bərn-ma′sən) [Roger *Wyburn-Mason*, British physician, 1911–1983] see under *syndrome.*

Wy•cil•lin (wi-sil′lin) trademark for preparations of penicillin G procaine.

Wy•dase (wi′dās) trademark for preparations of hyaluronidase for injection.

Wye•o•my•ia (we″o-mi′yə) a genus of mosquitoes of the subfamily Culicinae, native to Central and South America, the vector of the Wyeomyia virus.

Wy•mox (wi′moks) trademark for a preparation of amoxicillin.

Wynn method (win) [Sidney Keith *Wynn*, American plastic surgeon, born 1917] see under *method.*

Wy•ten•sin (wi-ten′sin) trademark for a preparation of guanabenz acetate.

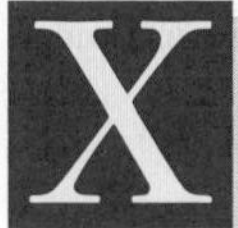

X Kienböck unit; xanthine; xanthosine.

X reactance.

X̄ sample mean.

x abscissa.

ξ xi, the fourteenth letter of the Greek alphabet.

Xal·a·tan (zal′ə-tan) trademark for a preparation of latanoprost.

Xan·ax (zan′aks) trademark for a preparation of alprazolam.

xan·chro·mat·ic (zan″kro-mat′ik) xanthochromic.

xan·thel·as·ma (zan″thəl-az′mə) [*xanth-* + Gr. *elasma* plate] a common type of planar xanthoma found on the eyelid. Called also *xanthoma palpebrarum*.

xan·thel·as·ma·to·sis (xan″thəl-az″mə-to′sis) xanthomatosis.

xan·them·a·tin (zan-them′ə-tin) a yellow substance derivable from hematin by the action of nitric acid.

xan·thene (zan′thēn) the compound, $(C_6H_4)_2(O)CH_2$, or dibenzpyran, from which the xanthene dyes and indicators are derived.

xan·thic (zan′thik) 1. yellow. 2. pertaining to xanthine.

xan·thin (zan′thin) any of the yellow pigments obtained from yellow flowers and other plants, probably consisting of oxygen-containing carotenoids.

xan·thine (X) (zan′thēn) [Gr. *xanthos* yellow, from the yellow color of its nitrate] a purine base found in most body tissues and fluids, certain plants, and some urinary calculi. It is an intermediate in the degradation of adenosine monophosphate to uric acid, being formed by oxidation of hypoxanthine. Methylated xanthines (see *methylxanthine*) are used medicinally. Xanthine also occurs complexed with ribose as xanthose.

xan·thine de·hy·dro·gen·ase (zan′thēn de-hi′dro-jən-ās) [EC 1.17.1.4] an enzyme of the oxidoreductase class that catalyzes the hydroxylation of xanthine to urate, using NAD^+ as an electron acceptor; it also acts on a variety of other purines and aldehydes, including hypoxanthine. The enzyme is a molybdoflavoprotein with a bound FAD and two iron-sulfur centers. Under certain conditions the enzyme from animal tissues interconverts with the form, xanthine oxidase (q.v.). Deficiency of enzyme activity, due to isolated defect in the enzyme or to molybdenum cofactor deficiency, results in xanthinuria and deposition of xanthine calculi.

xan·thine ox·i·dase (zan′thēn ok′sĭ-dās) [EC 1.17.3.2] an enzyme of the oxidoreductase class that catalyzes the oxidation of xanthine to urate, with oxygen as an acceptor, and generating peroxide; it also oxidizes hypoxanthine, some other purines and pterins, and aldehydes. Under some conditions the product is mainly superoxide rather than peroxide. It is a molybdoflavoprotein with a bound FAD and two iron-sulfur centers. Under certain conditions, the enzyme from animal tissues interconverts with xanthine dehydrogenase (q.v.).

xan·thin·uria (zan″thin-u′re-ə) any of several disorders of purine metabolism in which deficiency of xanthine dehydrogenase (XDH) activity results in urinary secretion of excessive xanthine and a tendency to formation of xanthine calculi in the urinary tract. Xanthinuria type I is an autosomal recessive disorder caused by mutation in the *XDH* gene (locus 2p23-p22), which encodes xanthine dehydrogenase; xanthinuria type II is a combined deficiency of both xanthine dehydrogenase and aldehyde oxidase activity. Xanthinuria is also a feature of molybdenum cofactor deficiency (q.v.).

xan·thin·uric (zan″thin-u′rik) pertaining to or resulting from xanthinuria.

xan·thism (zan′thiz-əm) [Gr. *xanthos* auburn] oculocutaneous albinism type 3.

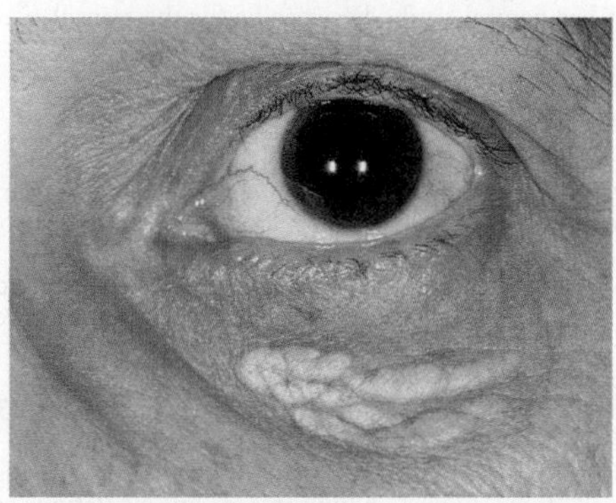

■ Xanthelasma.

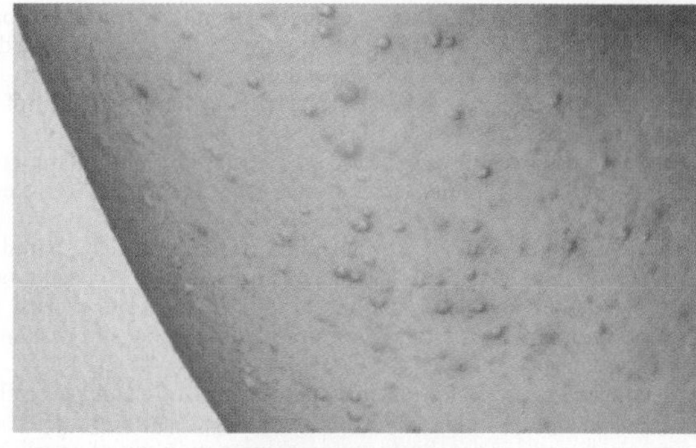

■ Eruptive xanthomas.

Xan·thi·um (zan′the-um) the cockleburrs, a genus of composite plants. In several species, the small new shoots that appear after rainstorms are poisonous, causing hepatic necrosis and fatal encephalopathy in livestock.

xan·thi·uria (zan″the-u′re-ə) xanthinuria.

xanth(o)- [Gr. *xanthos* yellow] a combining form meaning yellow.

xan·tho·chro·mia (zan″tho-kro′me-ə) [*xantho-* + *chrom-* + *-ia*] any yellowish discoloration, as of the cerebrospinal fluid or skin. **xanthochromat′ic, xanthochromic** *adj*

x. stria′ta palma′ris a type of planar xanthoma involving the volar creases of the palms and finger joints, with yellowish brown discoloration in light-skinned persons. Some authorities think that it gradually progresses to xanthoma striatum palmare.

xan·tho·cy·a·nop·sia (zan″tho-si″ə-nop′se-ə) [*xantho-* + *cyano-* + *-opsia*] ability to discern yellow and blue tints, but not red or green.

xan·tho·cyte (zan′tho-sīt) a cell that contains yellow pigment.

xan·tho·der·ma (zan″tho-der′mə) [*xantho-* + *derma*] any yellowish discoloration of the skin, such as in carotenemia or jaundice.

xan·tho·eryth·ro·der·mia (zan″tho-ə-rith″ro-der′me-ə) yellow to red discoloration of the skin.

x. per′stans small plaque parapsoriasis.

xan·tho·gran·u·lo·ma (zan″tho-gran″u-lo′mə) [*xanthoma* + *granuloma*] a tumor having the histologic characteristics of both granuloma and xanthoma.

juvenile x. a rare, benign, self-limited skin tumor, usually present at birth on the head, trunk, or proximal part of a limb, consisting of discolored papules or nodules caused by lipid-laden macrophages, inflammatory cells, and Touton giant cells in the dermis. Some authorities consider this a variant of benign fibrous histiocytoma.

necrobiotic x. a xanthogranuloma characterized by nodules or plaques overlying necrobiosis in the dermis, usually occurring on the face but occasionally on the trunk or a limb. It is typically accompanied by plasma cell dyscrasias and other systemic manifestations.

xan·tho·ky·an·o·py (zan″tho-ki-an′ə-pe) xanthocyanopsia.

xan·tho·ma (zan-tho′mə) [*xanth-* + *-oma*] a benign tumor composed of lipid-laden foam cells (macrophages containing lipid material). The most common types are in the skin, but xanthomas also appear elsewhere in the body. Called also *lipoid granuloma*. See also *xanthomatosis*. **xantho′matous** *adj*

craniohypophyseal x., craniohypophysial x. deposits of cholesterol esters in bones around the hypophysis in Hand-Schüller-Christian disease.

diabetic x., x. diabetico′rum eruptive x.

disseminated x., x. dissemina′tum a rare type of xanthomatosis that is normolipidemic and is characterized by yellow to brown papules and nodules that may coalesce to form furrowed plaques. The most common locations are in flexural creases; on mucous membranes of the mouth and respiratory tract; on the cornea or sclera; and in the central nervous system, such as the pituitary gland (in which case it may produce diabetes insipidus). Called also *x. multiplex*.

eruptive x., x. erupti′vum a benign skin tumor consisting of a group of small yellow to orange papules surrounded by a reddish halo, usually on the buttocks, posterior thighs, knees, or elbows. Onset is sudden; lesions may be intensely pruritic and may ulcerate. It is caused by high concentrations of plasma triglycerides, such as with a deficiency of lipoprotein lipase, uncontrolled diabetes mellitus, pancreatitis, or certain other conditions, and it usually disappears when the underlying condition is corrected. See also *tuberoeruptive x.* Called also *diabetic x.*

fibrous x. benign fibrous histiocytoma.

x. mul′tiplex disseminated x.

x. palpebra′rum xanthelasma.

planar x., plane x., x. pla′num a benign skin tumor consisting of soft macules or plaques of a variety of colors; there are both localized and generalized types. Sometimes the condition is associated with other types of xanthomas, certain types of hyperlipoproteinemia, lymphoma, or multiple myeloma.

x. stria′tum palma′re a type of planar xanthoma found in the creases of the palms and finger joints, characterized by linear, slightly elevated papules.

x. tendino′sum, tendinous x. xanthoma characterized by papules or nodules in the tendons, ligaments, fascia, and periosteum, especially on the hands, elbows, knees, or heels. It often occurs in association with types of hyperlipoproteinemia, tuberous xanthoma, xanthelasma, and cerebrotendinous xanthomatosis.

tuberoeruptive x. a condition in which lesions of eruptive xanthoma develop in association with already existing tuberous xanthoma and have a tendency to coalesce; this usually occurs in combination with hyperlipoproteinemia type III.

x. tubero′sum, x. tubero′sum mul′tiplex, tuberous x. a skin tumor consisting of groups of large, yellow to orange, indurated nodules on extensor surfaces and areas subjected to trauma, particularly on the elbows and knees; lesions tend to coalesce. It is often associated with conditions such as hyperlipoproteinemia, biliary cirrhosis, and myxedema. See also *tuberoeruptive x.*

verruciform x. an uncommon, solitary type of xanthoma of the oral mucosa; it is covered with a rough parakeratinized layer and usually occurs on the lower alveolar ridge.

xan•tho•ma•to•sis (zan″tho-mə-to′sis) any of various conditions characterized by the presence of xanthomas.

x. bul′bi fatty degeneration of the cornea.

cerebrotendinous x. an autosomal recessive lipid storage disease caused by mutation in the *CYP27A1* gene (locus: 2q33-qter), which encodes sterol 27-hydroxylase, an enzyme important in the bile synthesis pathway. It is characterized by xanthomas of the tendons, the white matter of the brain, and the lungs, as well as by spasticity, ataxia, pyramidal paresis, mental retardation, dementia, early cataracts, and atherosclerosis. It is associated with elevated plasma and tissue levels of cholestanol and defective bile synthesis, with deposition of cholestanol and cholesterol in virtually all tissues.

chronic idiopathic x. Hand-Schüller-Christian disease.

x. cor′neae dystrophia adiposa corneae.

x. generalisa′ta os′sium Hand-Schüller-Christian disease

hypercholesterolemic x. any of the types caused by excessive cholesterol levels in the blood.

x. i′ridis the formation of yellow patches in the discolored iris of an eye blinded as the result of protracted iritis or glaucoma.

primary familial x., Wolman x. Wolman disease.

Xan•tho•mo•na•da•ceae (zan″tho-mo″nə-da′se-e) the sole family of the order Xanthomonadales; organisms of medical interest are included in the genera *Stenotrophomonas* and *Xanthomonas.*

Xan•tho•mo•na•da•les (zan″tho-mo″nə-da′lēz) an order of gram-negative, catalase-positive bacteria of the class Gammaproteobacteria, phylum Proteobacteria, consisting of motile or nonmotile, non-spore-forming, straight rods lacking prosthecae; organisms are obligately anaerobic with a strictly respiratory metabolism. It contains the single family Xanthomonadaceae.

Xan•tho•mo•nas (zan″tho-mo′nəs) [Gr. *xanthos* yellow + Gr. *monas* unit, from *monos* single] a genus of gram-negative, aerobic, rod-shaped bacteria of the family Xanthomonadaceae. The organisms produce a yellow pigment; most species are plant pathogens. The type species is *X. campes′tris.*

X. campes′tris a species that is used in the production of xanthan gum.

X. maltophi′lia *Stenotrophomonas maltophilia.*

xan•tho•phore (zan′tho-for) [*xantho-* + *-phore*] a type of chromatophore containing granules of yellow or red pigment, found in cold-blooded animals.

xan•tho•phyll (zan′tho-fəl) [*xantho-* + Gr. *phyllon* leaf] a yellow coloring matter of plants, one of a group of oxygenated carotenoids occurring along with carotene in green leaves, grass, egg yolks, human plasma, and other organic matter.

xan•tho•pia (zan-tho′pe-ə) xanthopsia.

xan•tho•pro•te•ic ac•id (zan″tho-pro-te′ik) the product of treating protein with nitric acid.

xan•tho•pro•tein (zan″tho-pro′tēn) an orange pigment produced by heating proteins with nitric acid.

xan•thop•sia (zan-thop′se-ə) [*xantho-* + *-opsia*] a form of chromatopsia in which objects appear yellow.

xan•thop•ter•in (zan-thop′tər-in) [*xantho-* + *pterin*] a yellow pigment from the integument of wasps and hornets and from butterfly wings, which has some hematopoietic activity in anemic animals. It is an inhibitor of xanthine oxidase. See *pterin.*

xan•tho•sar•co•ma (zan″tho-sahr-ko′mə) a tumor in the inflammatory subtype of malignant fibrous histiocytoma.

xan•tho•sine (zan′tho-sēn) a pyrimidine nucleoside; xanthine linked by its N1 nitrogen to the C1 carbon of ribose. Symbol X.

x. monophosphate (XMP) a nucleotide, the 5′-phosphate of xanthosine, that is an intermediate in the synthesis of guanosine monophosphate (GMP).

xan•tho•sis (zan-tho′sis) a yellowish discoloration; degeneration with yellowish pigmentation.

xan•thous (zan′thəs) yellow or yellowish.

xanth•u•ren•ic ac•id (zanth″u-ren′ik) a bicyclic aromatic compound formed as a minor catabolite of tryptophan and present in increased amounts in the urine in vitamin B_6 deficiency and some disorders of tryptophan catabolism.

xan•thu•ria (zan-thu′re-ə) xanthinuria.

xan•thyl (zan′thəl) the monovalent radical of xanthene.

xan•thyl•ic ac•id (zan-thil′ik) phosphorylated xanthine, usually xanthosine monophosphate.

X-bite (kros′bīt″) crossbite.

Xe xenon.

Xe•lo•da (zel′ə-də) trademark for a preparation of capecitabine.

Xen•a•zine (zen′ə-zēn) trademark for a preparation of tetrabenazine.

Xen•i•cal (zen′ĭ-cal) trademark for a preparation of orlistat.

xen(o)- [Gr. *xenos* strange, foreign] a combining form meaning strange, or denoting relationship to foreign material.

xeno•an•ti•gen (zen″o-an′tĭ-jən) an antigen occurring in organisms of more than one species, e.g., the A and B antigens of the ABO blood group.

xeno•bi•ot•ic (zen″o-bi-ot′ik) a chemical foreign to a given biologic system.

xeno•cy•to•phil•ic (zen″o-si″to-fil′ik) [*xeno-* + *cyto-* + *-philic*] having an affinity for cells derived from a different species.

xeno•di•ag•no•sis (zen″o-di″əg-no′sis) [*xeno-* + *diagnosis*] a method of animal inoculation using laboratory-bred reduviids and larger animals for diagnosis of parasitic infections when it is not possible to demonstrate the infecting organism in blood films. Originally used for diagnosis of *Trypanosoma cruzi* infection (Chagas disease), the method is also used in *Trichinella spiralis* infections. In the original method, bugs are fed or offered the patient's blood through a membrane, and their feces or intestinal contents are examined later for trypanosomes. For the diagnosis of trichinosis, a muscle tissue sample from the patient is fed to laboratory rats to detect larvae of the parasite. **xenodiagnos′tic** *adj*

xeno•es•tro•gen (zen″o-es′trə-jen) a chemical from outside the body, such as an industrial contaminant or pollutant, that has estrogenlike qualities when ingested.

xeno•ge•ne•ic (zen″o-jə-ne′ik) [*xeno-* + *gennan* to produce] in transplantation biology, denoting individuals from different species or tissues transplanted between species; called also *heterogenic, heterogenous,* and *heterologous.* See *xenograft* and see *xenogeneic transplantation,* under *transplantation.*

xen•og•e•nous (zen-oj′ə-nəs) [*xeno-* + *-genous*] caused by a foreign body, or originating outside the organism.

xeno•graft (zen′o-graft″) a graft of tissue transplanted between animals of different species. Called also *heterograft, heterologous graft,* and *heteroplastic graft.*

Carpentier-Edwards porcine x. see under *valve.*

concordant x. a graft between members of closely related species, in which the recipient lacks natural antibodies specific for the transplanted tissue.

discordant x. a graft between members of divergent species, in which the recipient has natural antibodies specific for the transplanted tissue.

Hancock porcine x. see under *valve.*

Ionescu-Shiley pericardial x. see under *valve.*

xen•ol•o•gy (ze-nol′ə-je) the science of the relations of parasites to their hosts.

xe•non (Xe) (ze′non) [Gr. *xenos* stranger] a chemically unreactive gaseous element found in the atmosphere; atomic number, 54; atomic weight, 131.30.

x. Xe 127 [USP] a radioactive isotope of xenon, atomic mass 127, having a half-life of 36.41 days and decaying by electron capture with emission of gamma rays (0.172, 0.203 MeV); administered by inhalation as a gas for assessment of respiratory perfusion and in lung imaging.

x. Xe 133 [USP] a radioisotope of xenon, atomic mass 133, having a half-life of 5.25 days and emitting beta particles (0.346 MeV) and gamma rays (0.081 MeV); used for assessment of respiratory perfusion and in cerebral blood flow studies, administered by inhalation as a gas or intra-arterially or intramuscularly as a gas in solution.

xeno·para·site (zen″o-par′ə-sīt) an organism not usually parasitic on the host but that becomes so because of a weakened condition of the host.

xeno·pho·bia (zen″o-fo′be-ə) [*xeno-* + *-phobia*] irrational fear of strangers.

xeno·pho·nia (zen″o-fo′ne-ə) [*xeno-* + *phon-* + *-ia*] an abnormal alteration of the accent and intonation of a person's speech.

xen·oph·thal·mia (zen″of-thal′me-ə) [*xen-* + *ophthalmia*] ophthalmia caused by a foreign body in the eye.

Xen·op·syl·la (zen″op-sil′ə) [*xeno-* + Gr. *psylla* flea] a genus of fleas that infest primarily rats; many species transmit disease-producing microorganisms.

X. as′tia a rat flea of parts of Sri Lanka and India that has been implicated in the transmission of plague.

X. brasilien′sis a rat flea of Africa, Brazil, and India, a transmitter of plague.

X. cheo′pis a rat flea of worldwide distribution that transmits plague and murine typhus; called also *Pulex cheopis.*

X. hawaiien′sis *X. vexabilis.*

X. vexa′bilis a species infesting field rats in Hawaii; called also *X. hawaiiensis.*

Xeno·pus (zen′o-pəs) a genus of frogs and toads that have large clawed hindlimbs and weak forelimbs. *X. lae′vis* is the clawed frog or clawed toad, an African species used extensively in research.

xeno·tro·pic (zen″o-tro′pik) [*xeno-* + *-tropic*] pertaining to a virus that is found benignly in cells of one animal species but will replicate into complete virus particles only when it infects cells of a different species. Cf. *ecotropic.*

xen·yl (zen′əl) the univalent chemical group $C_6H_5•C_6H_4$—.

xen·yl·amine (zə-nil′ə-mēn) *p*-aminobiphenyl.

Xe·rac (ze′rak) trademark for a preparation of aluminum chloride.

xer(o)- [Gr. *xēros* dry] a combining form meaning dry, or denoting relationship to dryness.

xe·ro·col·lyr·i·um (zēr″o-ko-lir′e-əm) [*xero-* + *collyrium*] a dry collyrium; an eye salve.

xe·ro·cyte (ze′ro-sīt) an erythrocyte that is dehydrated and has decreased cations due to abnormal permeability of the membrane that allows leakage of potassium ions and water out of the cell. See also *xerocytosis.* **xerocyt′ic** *adj*

xe·ro·cy·to·sis (ze″ro-si-to′sis) presence of xerocytes in the blood.

hereditary x. dehydrated hereditary stomatocytosis.

xe·ro·der·ma (zēr″o-der′mə) [*xero-* + *derma*] a mild form of ichthyosis, marked by a dry, rough, discolored state of the skin, with the formation of a scaly desquamation.

x. pigmento′sum a rare, autosomal recessive, pigmentary and atrophic condition characterized by extreme cutaneous photosensitivity to ultraviolet radiation, as a result of defects in mechanisms of repair of ultraviolet-damaged DNA. It begins in childhood with senile changes in sun-exposed skin, including excessive freckling, telangiectases, keratoses, papillomas, and increased risk of all major types of skin cancer; there are also ocular disorders, including photophobia, lacrimation, keratitis, opacities, and tumors of the lid and cornea. Some patients have mental retardation, areflexia, or other neurological disorders. Multiple complementation groups exist, representing various mutations interfering with different proteins in the global genome repair subpathway of nucleotide excision repair; a variant form *(xeroderma pigmentosum variant)* is instead defective in a DNA polymerase important in postreplication repair of damaged DNA.

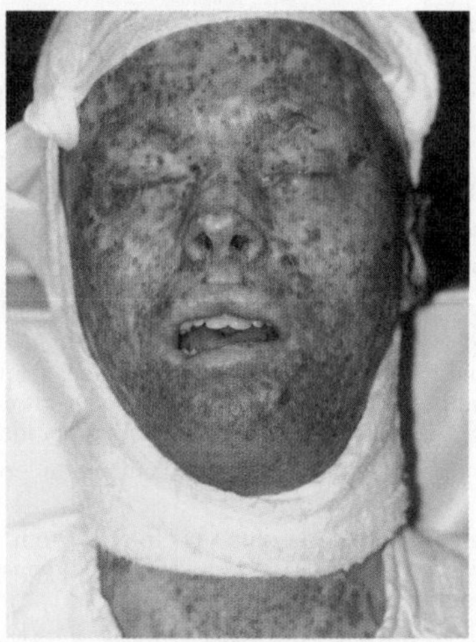

■ Xeroderma pigmentosum, showing atrophic changes and pigment disturbances.

xe·ro·der·mia (zēr″o-der′me-ə) xeroderma.

xe·ro·der·moid (zēr″o-der′moid) [*xeroderma* + *-oid*] resembling xeroderma.

xe·ro·gel (zēr′o-jəl) a gel containing little liquid. Cf. *lyogel.*

xe·rog·ra·phy (ze-rog′rə-fe) xeroradiography.

xe·ro·ma (zēr-o′mə) xerophthalmia.

xe·ro·mam·mog·ra·phy (zēr″o-mə-mog′rə-fe) xeroradiography of the breast.

xe·ro·me·nia (zēr″o-me′ne-ə) [*xero-* + *men-* + *-ia*] a condition in which the bodily symptoms of menstruation occur without any bloody flow.

xe·ro·myc·te·ria (zēr″o-mik-tēr′e-ə) [*xero-* + Gr. *myktēr* nose] dryness of the nasal mucous membrane.

xe·roph·thal·mia (zēr″of-thal′me-ə) [*xero-* + *ophthalmia*] dryness of the conjunctiva and cornea due to vitamin A deficiency. The condition begins with night blindness and conjunctival xerosis and progresses to corneal xerosis and, in the late stages, to keratomalacia.

xe·roph·thal·mus (zēr″of-thal′məs) xerophthalmia.

xe·ro·ra·di·og·ra·phy (zēr″o-ra″de-og′rə-fe) a dry, totally photoelectric process for recording x-ray images, using metal plates coated with a semiconductor such as selenium.

xe·ro·si·a·log·ra·phy (zēr″o-si″ə-log′rə-fe) sialography in which the images are recorded by xeroradiography.

xe·ro·sis (zēr-o′sis) [Gr. *xērosis*] abnormal dryness, as of the eye, skin, or mouth. Cf. *dehydration.* **xerot′ic** *adj*

x. conjuncti′vae, conjunctival x. dryness of the conjunctiva. When associated with Bitot spots, it is due to vitamin A deficiency and may progress to xerophthalmia and keratomalacia.

x. cor′neae, corneal x. dryness of the cornea, giving it a hazy or milky appearance; see *xerophthalmia.*

x. cu′tis asteatotic eczema.

generalized x. dryness of the skin, with pruritus and branny scaling, seen in patients with acquired immunodeficiency syndrome.

x. parenchymato′sa xerophthalmia due to trachoma.

x. superficia′lis xerophthalmia due to abnormal exposure of the eyeball to the air.

xe·ro·sto·mia (zēr″o-sto′me-ə) [*xero-* + *stom-* + *-ia*] dryness of the mouth from salivary gland dysfunction, as in Sjögren syndrome.

xe·ro·to·mog·ra·phy (zēr″o-tə-mog′rə-fe) tomography in which the images are recorded by xeroradiography.

xe·ro·trip·sis (zēr″o-trip′sis) [*xero-* + *tripsis*] dry friction.

X-His di·pep·ti·dase (di-pep′tĭ-dās) [EC 3.4.13.3] an enzyme of the hydrolase class that catalyzes the cleavage of the dipeptide carnosine into component amino acids β-alanine and histidine; it also acts on some other aminoacyl-L-histidine dipeptides. The tissue isozyme requires zinc ions and does not hydrolyze anserine or homocarnosine; the serum isozyme requires cadmium and does hydrolyze anserine and homocarnosine. Deficiency of the serum isozyme causes serum carnosinase deficiency. Called also *carnosinase* and *aminoacyl-histidine dipeptidase.* See also *carnosinemia* and *homocarnosinase.*

xi (zi, kse) [Ξ, ξ] the fourteenth letter of the Greek alphabet.

Xi·fax·an (zĭ-fak′ən) trademark for a preparation of rifaximin.

Xi·gris (zi′gris) trademark for a preparation of drotrecogin alfa.

xip·a·mide (zip′ə-mīd) a diuretic and antihypertensive with actions and uses similar to those of the thiazide diuretics; administered orally.

xiphi- see *xiph(o)-.*

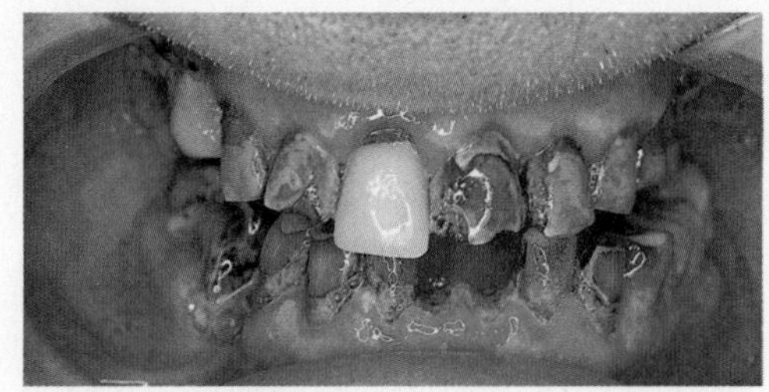

■ Caries associated with radiation-induced xerostomia.

xiphi•ster•num (zif″ĭ-stur′nəm) [*xiphi-* + *sternum*] processus xiphoideus. **xiphister′nal** *adj*

xiph(o)- [Gr. *xiphos* sword] a combining form denoting relationship to the xiphoid process. Also, *xiphi-*.

xipho•cos•tal (zi″fo-, zif″o-kos′təl) [*xipho-* + *costal*] pertaining to the xiphoid process and the ribs.

xipho•did•y•mus (zi″fo-, zif″o-did′ĭ-məs) xiphopagus.

xi•phod•y•mus (zi-fod′, zĭ-fod′ĭ-məs) xiphopagus.

xiph•odyn•ia (zi″fo-, zif″o-din′e-ə) [*xiph-* + *-odynia*] pain in the xiphoid process.

xiph•oid (zif′oid, zi′foid) [Gr. *xiphoeidēdes* sword-shaped, from *xiphos* sword + *eidos* form] 1. shaped like a sword; called also *ensiform.* 2. processus xiphoideus. 3. pertaining to the processus xiphoideus.

xiph•oi•di•tis (zi″foi-, zif″oi-di′tis) inflammation of the xiphoid process.

xi•pho•om•pha•lo•is•chi•op•a•gus (zi″fo-, zif″o-om″fə-lo-is″ke-op′ə-gəs) [*xipho-* + *omphalo-* + *ischio-* + *-pagus*] conjoined twins united from the level of the xiphoid process to the ischia.

xi•phop•a•gus (zi-fop′-, zĭ-fop′ə-gəs) [*xipho-* + *-pagus*] symmetrical conjoined twins fused in the region of the xiphoid process.

XIST [*X-i*nactivation–*s*pecific *t*ranscript] see under *gene.*

X-linked (eks′linkt) carried on the X chromosome, as an X-linked gene; by extension, determined by such a gene, as an X-linked trait or X-linked inheritance.

XMP xanthosine monophosphate.

XO symbol used to indicate the presence of only one X chromosome, the other X or the Y chromosome being absent.

Xo•lair (zo′lār) trademark for a preparation of omalizumab.

Xo•pe•nex (zo′pə-neks) trademark for a preparation of levalbuterol hydrochloride.

X-Pro di•pep•ti•dase (di-pep′tĭ-dās″) [EC 3.4.13.9] a dipeptidase that catalyzes the cleavage of a C-terminal proline or another imino acid from imidodipeptides, an important step in intestinal absorption of the imino acid portion of dipeptides. Reduced enzyme activity, an autosomal recessive trait, causes prolidase deficiency. Called also *prolidase* and *proline dipeptidase.*

x-ray (eks′ra) see under *ray.*

XU excretory urography.

xy•lan (zi′lan) any of a group of pentosans composed of xylose residues; they are major structural constituents of wood, straw, and bran.

xy•la•zine hy•dro•chlo•ride (zi′lə-zēn) [USP] a veterinary analgesic, sedative, and muscle relaxant, used in most domestic animals except pigs.

xy•lene (zi′lēn) [Gr. *xylon* wood] 1. any of three isomeric hydrocarbons, $C_6H_4(CH_3)_2$, from methyl alcohol or coal tar; usually qualified by the substituent positions. Called also *dimethylbenzene.* 2. a mixture of all three isomers, with uses including solvent and clarifier for microscopy, protective coating, and in various syntheses.

xy•li•dine (zi′lĭ-din) a compound, dimethylaniline $(CH_3)_2C_6H_3{\cdot}NH_2$, used as a dyestuff intermediate and for blending gasoline.

xy•li•tol (zi′lĭ-tol) [NF] a five-carbon sugar alcohol derived from xylose by reduction of the carbonyl group; it is as sweet as sucrose and is used as a noncariogenic sweetener and also as a sugar substitute in diabetic diets.

xy•li•tol de•hy•dro•gen•ase (zi′lĭ-tol de-hi′dro-jən-ās) L-xylulose reductase.

xyl(o)- [Gr. *xylon* wood] a combining form denoting relationship to wood.

Xy•lo•caine (zi′lo-kān) trademark for preparations of lidocaine.

Xy•lo•hy•pha (zi″lo-hi′fə) a genus of Fungi Imperfecti of the form-class Hyphomycetes, form-family Dematiaceae.

X. bantia′na former name for *Cladophialophora bantiana.*

xy•lol (zi′lol) xylene.

xy•lo•met•a•zo•line hy•dro•chlo•ride (zi″lo-met″ə-zo′lēn) [USP] an adrenergic used topically as a vasoconstrictor to reduce swelling and congestion of the nasal mucosa.

xy•lo•py•ra•nose (zi″lo-pi′rə-nōs) xylose in the cyclic pyranose form.

Xy•lor•rhi•za (zi″lə-ri′zə) a genus of plants of the family Compositae; all species preferentially seek seleniferous soil and may be high in selenium, causing selenium poisoning in livestock.

xy•lose (zi′lōs) 1. an aldopentose epimeric with ribose at the 3 carbon and occurring in pyranose form; it is found in plants in the form of xylans. 2. [USP] an official preparation of xylose, used as a diagnostic aid in testing for intestinal function and malabsorption syndromes, such as the D-xylose absorption test.

xy•lo•side (zi-lo-sīd) a glycoside of xylose.

xy•lu•lose (zi′lu-lōs) a ketopentose epimeric with ribulose at the 3 carbon, occurring naturally as both the D- and L- isomers. The latter is excreted in the urine in essential pentosuria; the former, phosphorylated at the 5 carbon *(D-xylulose 5-phosphate)*, is an intermediate in the pentose phosphate pathway.

L-xy•lu•lose re•duc•tase (zi′lu-lōs re-duk′tās) [EC 1.1.1.10] an enzyme of the oxidoreductase class that catalyzes the reduction of xylulose to xylitol, using NADPH as an electron donor. Deficiency of the enzyme, an autosomal recessive trait, leads to essential pentosuria.

xy•lyl (zi′ləl) the hydrocarbon radical $CH_3C_6H_4CH_2$—.

xyph•oid (zif′oid, zi′foid) xiphoid (def. 1).

xys•ma (zis′mə) [Gr. "that which is scraped or shaved off"] bits of membrane found in the feces in diarrhea.

xys•ter (zis′tər) [Gr. *xystēr* scraper] rasp (def. 1).

Xy•zal (zi′zal) trademark for a preparation of levocetirizine dihydrochloride.

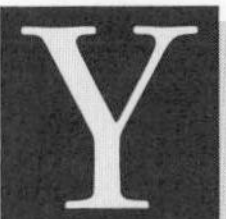

Y tyrosine; yttrium.

y ordinate.

Υ the Greek capital letter upsilon.

υ upsilon, the twentieth letter of the Greek alphabet.

yab·a·pox (yab′ə-poks″) [*Yaba*, Nigeria, where the disease was first recognized in a rhesus monkey colony] a viral disease caused by the Yaba monkey tumor virus that causes subcutaneous tumorlike growths in rhesus and cynomolgus monkeys; accidental human infection has occurred, characterized by localized skin nodules that resolve spontaneously.

YAC yeast artificial chromosome.

yang (yang) [Mandarin Chinese] in Chinese philosophy, the active, positive, masculine principle that is complementary to yin; see *yin/yang principle*, under *principle*.

yar·row (yar′o) 1. any of several plants of the genus *Achillea*, especially *A. millefolium*. 2. a preparation of the above-ground parts of *A. millefolium*, used for loss of appetite and dyspepsia and for liver and gallbladder complaints; it is also used in homeopathy.

Yas·min (yaz′min) trademark for a combination preparation of drospirenone and ethinyl estradiol.

Yat·a·pox·vi·rus (yat′ə-poks-vi″rəs) [*ya*bapox + *ta*napox + *virus*] a genus of viruses of the subfamily Chordopoxvirinae (family Poxviridae) comprising tanapox virus and Yaba monkey tumor virus.

yaw (yaw) a lesion of yaws (q.v.).

guinea corn y. a lesion of yaws that resembles a grain of corn (maize).

mother y. the initial cutaneous lesion of yaws; called also *frambesioma* and *framboesioma*.

ringworm y. a circular or ring-shaped lesion of yaws.

yawn·ing (yawn′ing) a deep, involuntary inhalation with the mouth open, often accompanied by the act of stretching. Cf. *pandiculation*. Called also *hiation* and *oscitation*.

yaws (yawz) [from Caribbean Indian name for the disease] an endemic, infectious, tropical disease caused by *Treponema pertenue*, usually affecting persons under age 15, and spread by direct contact with skin lesions or contaminated fomites. The spirochete initially appears at the site of inoculation and then enters the body through abraded or otherwise compromised skin; then a painless papule appears and grows into a papilloma (mother yaw); when that heals, it leaves a scar, followed by crops of generalized secondary granulomatous papules that may relapse repeatedly. Late manifestations include destructive and deforming lesions of the skin, bones, and joints. Called also *frambesia* or *framboesia* and *frambesia tropica*.

crab y. yaws characterized by hyperkeratosis with fissuring and ulceration of the soles of the feet, and less commonly involving the palms of the hands.

forest y. pian bois.

Yb ytterbium.

yeast (yēst) an imprecise term used to refer to a member of one of the two largest groupings of fungi (the other being *molds*); yeasts are single-celled, usually rounded fungi that produce by budding (blastospore formation). Some transform to a mycelial (mold) stage under certain environmental conditions, while others always remain single-celled. Many of the perfect yeasts are classified in the order Endomycetales, and many imperfect ones are classified in the form-family Moniliaceae. A few yeasts are pathogenic for humans.

dried y. the dry cells of any suitable strain of *Saccharomyces cerevisiae*, usually a by-product of the brewing industry; used as a natural source of protein and B-complex vitamins.

imperfect y. any yeast whose perfect (sexual) stage is unknown; these are classified in the subphylum Deuteromycotina.

perfect y. any yeast whose perfect (sexual) stage is known; these are classified in the subphyla Ascomycotina and Basidiomycotina, or the phylum Zygomycota.

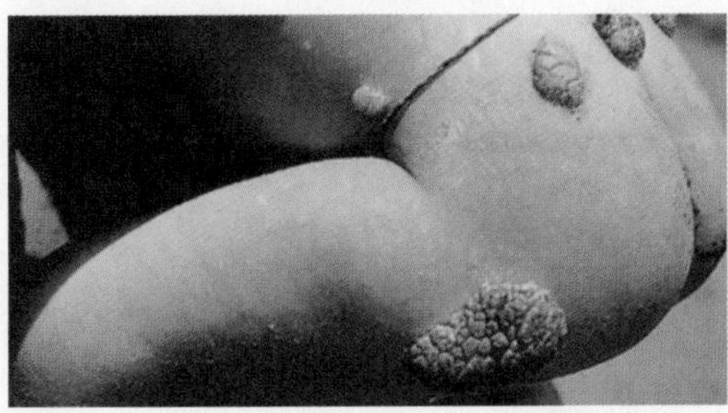

■ Secondary lesions of yaws in a child.

yel·low (yel′o) 1. a color between orange and green, produced by energy of wavelengths between 570 and 590 nm. 2. a dye or stain with this color.

acid y. fast y.

alizarin y. an indicator used in the determination of hydrogen ion concentration with a pH range of 10.1–12.1.

brilliant y. an indicator used in determining hydrogen ion concentration, with a pH range of 6–8.

butter y. *p*-dimethylaminoazobenzene.

corallin y. yellow corallin.

fast y. a yellow, acid azo dye used in staining bone.

imperial y. aurantia.

Manchester y., Martius y. a poisonous yellow azo dye used as a stain and in preparation of light filters.

metanil y., metaniline y. (extra) an indicator used in the determination of hydrogen ion concentration, with a pH range of 1.2–2.3.

methyl y. *p*-dimethylaminoazobenzene.

naphthol y. Manchester y.

Philadelphia y. phosphine (def. 3).

Sudan y. G a brown powder used as a stain for fats.

yel·low·jack·et (yel′o-jak″ət) any of various wasps that have dark bodies with yellow or brown markings.

yel·lows (yel′ōz) 1. a form of canine leptospirosis resembling the human condition Weil syndrome, caused by *Leptospira interrogans*; formerly believed to be caused specifically by the serovar *L. icterohaemorrhagiae*. 2. hepatogenous photosensitization seen in sheep and goats in Scotland in the summertime, usually after ingestion of *Narthecium ossifragum* (the bog asphodel).

yer·ba san·ta (yer′bə sahn′tə) [Sp. "sacred herb"] *Eriodictyon californicum*.

Yer·kes discrimination box (yur′kēz) [Robert Mearns *Yerkes*, American psychobiologist, 1876–1956] see under *box*.

Yer·kes-Dod·son law (yur′kēz dod′sən) [R.M. *Yerkes*; John D. *Dodson*, American psychologist, early 20th century] see under *law*.

Yer·sin·ia (yər-sin′e-ə) [Alexandre J.E. *Yersin*, Swiss bacteriologist in France, 1863–1943] a genus of gram-negative bacteria of the family Enterobacteriaceae, consisting of facultatively anaerobic, non–spore-forming, nonencapsulated straight rods to coccobacilli; organisms are nonmotile at 37°C, but most species are motile by means of peritrichous flagella below 30°C. It contains the organism responsible for bubonic plague (see *Y. pestis*) and other species that cause gastroenteritis and mesenteric lymphadenitis. Numerous serovars based on the presence of an O antigen have been described. The type species is *Y. pes′tis*.

Y. enterocoli′tica a ubiquitous species isolated from mammals, birds, and frogs, and material contaminated by feces; it is transmitted by infected food and water and by person-to-person contact and can cause yersiniosis in humans.

Y. frederikse′nii an opportunistic pathogen, a species that resembles *Y. enterocolitica* except that it ferments L-rhamnose.

Y. interme′dia an opportunistic pathogen, a species that resembles *Y. enterocolitica* except that it ferments L-rhamnose, raffinose, and melibiose.

Y. kristense′nii an opportunistic pathogen, a species that resembles *Y. enterocolitica* except that it does not ferment sucrose.

Y. pes′tis the etiologic agent of plague in humans and various rodents, transmitted from rat to rat and from rat to humans by the rat flea, and from human to human by the human body louse.

Y. pseudotuberculo′sis a species found in the intestinal tract of birds, rodents, and other animals; it can cause mesenteric lymphadenitis in humans and pseudotuberculosis in various rodent species and other animals. Human infection occurs from contact with infected food or animals.

Y. ruc′keri a species that resembles *Y. enterocolitica* except that it does not ferment cellobiose. It is found in fresh waters and causes disease in fish.

yer·sin·ia (yər-sin′e-ə) a bacterium of the genus *Yersinia*.

yer·sin·i·o·sis (yər-sin″e-o′sis) 1. infection with bacteria of the genus *Yersinia*. 2. specifically, infection with *Yersinia enterocolitica*; symptoms include acute gastroenteritis and mesenteric lymphadenitis in children and arthritis, septicemia, and erythema nodosum in adults. 3. pseudotuberculosis caused by *Yersinia pseudotuberculosis*, seen in guinea pigs, white rats, rabbits, and birds.

enteric y., intestinal y. *Yersinia* enteritis.

yew (yu) any of the evergreens of the genus *Taxus*.

Pacific y. *Taxus brevifolia*.

YF-Vax (wi-ef-vaks′) trademark for a preparation of yellow fever vaccine.

yin (yin) [Mandarin Chinese] in Chinese philosophy, the passive, negative, feminine principle that is complementary to yang; see *yin/yang principle*, under *principle*.

-yl [Gr. *hylē* matter, substance] a chemical suffix signifying a radical, particularly a univalent hydrocarbon radical.

-ylene a suffix used in chemistry to denote a bivalent hydrocarbon radical.

Y-linked (wi′linkt) carried on the Y chromosome, as a Y-linked gene; by extension, determined by such a gene, as a Y-linked trait or Y-linked inheritance.

Yo·dox·in (yo-dok′sin) trademark for a preparation of iodoquinol.

yo·ga (yo′gə) [Sanskrit "union"] an ancient system of Indian philosophy incorporated into the ayurvedic system of medicine and well-being, whose goal is the attainment of ultimate balance of mind and body, or self-realization. A number of different systems of yoga have developed, all sharing certain basic principles: control of the body through correct posture and breathing, control of the emotions and mind, and meditation. There are four main paths: *raja yoga* (or *classical yoga*), a systematic classification of yoga practices into eight "limbs" set forth in the Yoga Sutras of Patanjali about 300 BCE; *bhakti yoga*, which is the surrender of the self to the divine spirit; *karma yoga*, which aims at union with the divine spirit through selfless actions; and *jnana yoga*, which seeks union through knowledge and truth. In the West, yoga is often reduced to the practice of postures, breath control, and meditation for healing and well-being, without attention to the larger philosophy.

ashtanga y. a physically demanding style of yoga in which breathing is synchronized with movement between asanas (postures); it encourages profuse sweating for the purpose of purification and detoxification and it produces strength, flexibility, and stamina.

hatha y. the limb of raja yoga best known in the West, based on physical purification and strengthening as a means of self-transformation. It encompasses a system of over 1000 asanas (postures), designed to promote mental and physical well-being and to allow the mind to focus and become free from distraction for long periods of meditation, along with pranayama (breath control). A number of styles of yoga founded on hatha yoga have been developed.

Iyengar y. a style of yoga that emphasizes correct body alignment in the asanas (postures) and holding the asanas for extended periods of time; it also uses props such as wooden blocks and belts to help achieve and support the asanas.

kundalini y. a style of yoga whose purpose is controlled release of latent kundalini (q.v.) energy.

yo·him·bine hy·dro·chlo·ride (yo-him′bēn) [USP] an alkaloid chemically similar to reserpine, from *Pausinystalia yohimbe* (=*Corynanthe yohimbi*) and from *Rauwolfia serpentina.* It possesses alpha-adrenergic blocking properties and is used as a sympathicolytic and mydriatic, and for the treatment of impotence; administered orally.

yoke (yōk) 1. a connecting structure. 2. jugum.

alveolar y's of mandible juga alveolaria mandibulae.

alveolar y's of maxilla juga alveolaria maxillae.

sphenoidal y. jugum sphenoidale.

yoked (yōkt) joined together, and so acting in concert.

yolk (yōk) [L. *vitellus*] 1. the stored nutrient of an oocyte or ovum. 2. crude wool fat or suint.

accessory y. the part of the yolk that serves for the nutrition of the formative portion.

egg y. the yellow portion of the egg of a bird.

formative y. the part of the ovum from which the embryo is developed, as in birds.

nutritive y. accessory y.

Yo·me·san (yo′mə-san) trademark for preparations of niclosamide.

Young operation (yung) [Hugh Hampton *Young*, American urologist, 1870–1945] see under *operation.*

Young-Helm·holtz theory (yung′ helm′hōlts) [Thomas *Young*, English physician, physicist, and philologist, 1773–1829; Herman Ludwig Ferdinand von *Helmholtz*, German physiologist, 1821–1894] see under *theory.*

yper·ite (i′pər-īt) dichlorodiethyl sulfide.

yp·sil·i·form (ip-sil′ĭ-form) upsiloid.

yp·si·loid (ip′sĭ-loid) upsiloid.

yt·ter·bi·um (Yb) (ĭ-tur′be-əm) [from *Ytterby*, Sweden] a very rare metal; atomic number, 70; atomic weight, 173.04.

yt·tri·um (Y) (ĭ′tre-əm) [from *Ytterby*, Sweden] a very rare metal, allied to cerium; atomic number, 39; atomic weight, 88.905.

y. 90 a radioactive isotope of yttrium, atomic mass 90, having a half-life of 64.1 hours and emitting beta particles (2.288 MeV); it localizes predominantly to bone, and also liver, and has been used in radiation synovectomy and, linked to antibody, in radioimmunotherapy.

y. Y 90 ibritumomab tiuxetan [USP] a chelate of ^{90}Y and the immunoconjugate ibritumomab tiuxetan, used in the treatment of non-Hodgkin lymphoma; administered intravenously.

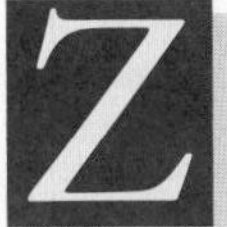

Z atomic number; impedance.

Z- [Ger. *zusammen* together] a stereodescriptor used to specify the absolute configuration of compounds having double bonds. See *E-*.

ζ zeta, the sixth letter of the Greek alphabet.

Zad•i•tor (zad′ĭ-tor) trademark for a preparation of ketotifen fumarate.

za•fir•lu•kast (zə-fir′loo-kast) a leukotriene receptor antagonist used as an antiasthmatic agent; administered orally.

Za•gam (za′gam) trademark for a preparation of sparfloxacin.

Zahn infarct, lines (tsahn) [Friedrich Wilhelm *Zahn*, German-born pathologist in Switzerland, 1845–1904] see under *infarct* and *line.*

Za•hor•sky disease (zə-hor′ske) [John *Zahorsky*, Hungarian-born American physician, 1871–1963] exanthema subitum.

zal•ci•ta•bine (zal-si′tə-bēn) [USP] 2′3′-dideoxycytidine, a nucleoside analogue of 2′-deoxycytidine; an antiretroviral agent that is converted intracellularly into the active metabolite dideoxycytidine 5′-triphosphate, which inhibits the action of reverse transcriptase and so inhibits viral replication; used in the treatment of human immunodeficiency virus (HIV) infection, administered orally. Formerly called *dideoxycytidine (ddC).*

zal•e•plon (zal′ə-plon) a nonbenzodiazepine sedative and hypnotic used in the short-term treatment of insomnia; administered orally.

Za•mia (za′me-ə) a genus of zamia palms whose leaves and seeds contain macrozamin and other toxic glycosides and cause hepatotoxicity, spinal cord degeneration, and cancer. See also *zamia staggers,* under *staggers.*

za•mia (za′me-ə) 1. a poisonous cycad palm of genus *Zamia, Macrozamia*, or related genera; these trees contain toxic glycosides such as macrozamin. 2. misnomer for any cycad. See also *zamia staggers,* under *staggers.*

Zan•a•flex (zan′ə-fleks) trademark for a preparation of tizanidine hydrochloride.

za•nam•i•vir (zə-nam′ĭ-vir) an inhibitor of viral neuraminidase used for the prophylaxis and treatment of influenza A and influenza B, administered by inhalation.

Zan•o•sar (zan′o-sahr) trademark for preparations of streptozocin.

Zan•tac (zan′tak) trademark for preparations of ranitidine hydrochloride.

Zap•pert chamber (tsah′pert) [Julius *Zappert*, Czechoslovakian physician in Austria, 1867–1942] see under *chamber.*

Za•ron•tin (zə-ron′tin) trademark for preparations of ethosuximide.

Za•rox•o•lyn (zə-rok′so-lin) trademark for a preparation of metolazone.

Z-DNA see under *DNA.*

Zea (ze′ə) [Gr. *zeia* single-grained wheat] a genus of large grasses (family Gramineae), originally native to the Americas. *Z. mays* is maize or corn, a tall cereal plant that produces seeds or kernels on large ears. See also *corn oil,* under *oil.*

zea•ral•e•nol (zə-ral′ə-nol) zeranol.

zea•ral•e•none (zə-ral′ə-nōn) an estrogenic mycotoxin produced by the fungus *Fusarium roseum*; animals eating contaminated grain or flour products may develop fertility problems or vulvovaginitis. See also *zeranol.*

Ze•be•ta (ze-ba′tə) trademark for a preparation of bisoprolol fumarate.

Ze•bu•tal (zə-bu′tal) trademark for a combination preparation of butalbital, acetaminophen, and caffeine.

zed•o•ary (zed′o-ar″e) [L. *zedoaria*] the rhizome of *Curcuma zedoaria*, a plant of India, which resembles ginger; used medicinally as an aromatic stimulant and carminative.

Zee•man effect (tsa′mahn) [Pieter *Zeeman*, Dutch physicist, 1865–1943] see under *effect.*

Zeg•er•id (zeg′ər-id) trademark for a preparation of omeprazole.

zein (ze′in) a protein of the prolamin group, molecular weight about 40,000, found in corn; it does not contain tryptophan or lysine.

zei•o•sis (zi-o′sis) [Gr. *zein* to boil, seethe + *-osis*] bubbling or blebbing activity, giving the appearance of boiling in slow motion, observed in apoptosis and at the periphery of cells cultured in artificial media.

Zeis gland (tsīs) [Eduard *Zeis*, German ophthalmologist, 1807–1868] see under *gland.*

zei•si•an (zi′se-ən) named for Eduard *Zeis*, as *zeisian stye.*

ze•ism (ze′iz-əm) [L. *zea* maize, corn] any condition attributed to excessive use of maize in the diet, most commonly pellagra.

ze•is•mus (ze-is′məs) zeism.

zeit•ge•ber (zīt′ga-ber) [Ger. "time giver"] any of a number of periodic natural fluctuations, such as the cycle of light and darkness, that act as signals to control circadian rhythms.

Zell•weg•er syndrome (zel′weg-ər) [Hans Ulrich *Zellweger*, American pediatrician, 1909–1990] cerebrohepatorenal syndrome; see under *syndrome.*

Zel•norm (zel′norm) trademark for a preparation of tegaserod maleate.

Zem•plar (zem′plahr) trademark for a preparation of paricalcitol.

Zem•u•ron (zem′u-ron) trademark for a preparation of rocuronium bromide.

Zen•a•pax (zen′ə-paks) trademark for a preparation of daclizumab.

Zen•ker degeneration (necrosis), diverticulum (tseng′ker) [Friedrich Albert von *Zenker*, German pathologist, 1825–1898] see under *degeneration* and *diverticulum.*

Zen•ker fixative (fluid, solution) (tseng′ker) [Konrad *Zenker*, German histologist, died 1894] see under *fixative.*

zen•ker•ism (zeng′kər-iz-əm) [F.A. von *Zenker*] Zenker degeneration; see under *degeneration.*

zen•ker•ize (zeng′kər-īz) [K. *Zenker*] to treat with Zenker fixative.

ze•o•lite (ze′o-lit) any of a group of hydrated aluminum silicate minerals; some have ion-exchange properties and others are used as absorbents or filters. See also *erionite.*

zeo•scope (ze′o-skōp) [Gr. *zein* to boil, seethe + *-scope*] an apparatus for determining the alcoholic strength of a liquid by means of its boiling point.

Zeph•i•ran (zef′ĭ-rən) trademark for preparations of benzalkonium chloride.

ze•ra•nol (zer′ə-nol) a reduction product of zearalenone; an anabolic-estrogenic agent that has been used for estrogen replacement in humans but is used primarily in veterinary medicine as a growth stimulant. Called also *zearalenol.*

Zer•it (zer′it) trademark for preparations of stavudine.

ze•ro (ze′ro) [Ital. "naught"] 1. the absence of all quantity or magnitude; naught. 2. the point on a thermometer scale at which the graduation begins; the ice point on the Celsius and Réaumur scales and 32° below the ice point on the Fahrenheit.

absolute z. the lowest possible temperature, designated as 0 on the Kelvin or Rankine scale; by definition this is equivalent to −273.15°C or −459.67°F.

limes z. limes nul dose.

physiologic z. the temperature at which a thermal stimulus ceases to cause a sensation.

Ze•ro Bal•anc•ing (ze′ro bal′əns-ing) a bodywork system, based on a combination of Western anatomical principles and Eastern concepts of body energy, that uses gentle manipulation at key areas of the skeleton to align the energy of the body with the body's physical structure; used for stress reduction and to promote general well-being.

ZES Zollinger-Ellison syndrome.

Zes•to•ret•ic (zes″tə-ret′ik) trademark for a combination preparation of lisinopril and hydrochlorothiazide.

Zes•tril (zes′tril) trademark for a preparation of lisinopril.

ze•ta (za′tə) [Z, ζ] the sixth letter of the Greek alphabet.

ze•ta•crit (za′tə-krit) the packed-cell volume produced by the zeta sedimentation ratio procedure (see under *ratio*).

Ze•ta•fuge (za′tə-fūj) trademark for a specially designed centrifuge used in determination of the zeta sedimentation ratio.

Ze•tar (ze′tahr) trademark for a preparation of coal tar.

Zet•ia (zet′e-ə) trademark for a preparation of ezetimibe.

zeu•go•po•di•um (zoo″go-po′de-əm) zygopodium (see *limb*).

Zev•a•lin (zev′ə-lin) trademark for a preparation of ibritumomab tiuxetan.

Zi•ac (zi′ak) trademark for a combination preparation of bisoprolol fumarate and hydrochlorothiazide.

Zi•a•gen (zi′ə-jen) trademark for a preparation of abacavir sulfate.

zi•do•vu•dine (zi-do′vu-dēn) [USP] a synthetic nucleoside analogue, of thymidine, that inhibits replication of some retroviruses, including the human immunodeficiency virus (HIV); used in the management of HIV infection and acquired immunodeficiency syndrome (AIDS), administered orally or intravenously.

Zieg•ler operation (zēg′lər) [Samuel Louis *Ziegler*, American ophthalmologist, 1861–1926] see under *operation.*

Ziehl-Neel•sen carbolfuchsin, staining method (tsēl′ nāl′sen) [Franz *Ziehl*, German bacteriologist, 1857–1926; Friedrich Karl Adolf *Neelsen*, German pathologist, 1854–1894] see under *carbolfuchsin*, and at *Stains and Staining Methods*, under *stain*.

Ziel•ke instrumentation (tsēl′kə) [K. *Zielke*, German orthopedic surgeon, 20th century] see under *instrumentation*.

Ziems•sen motor point (tsēm′sen) [Hugo Wilhelm von *Ziemssen*, German physician, 1829–1902] see under *point*.

Zieve syndrome (zēv) [Leslie *Zieve*, American physician, 1915–2000] see under *syndrome*.

ZIFT zygote intrafallopian transfer.

zi•leu•ton (zi-loo′tən) an antiasthmatic agent of the leukotriene pathway modifier type that inhibits the enzymatic action of arachidonate 5-lipoxygenase; used in prophylaxis and treatment of symptoms of chronic asthma, administered orally.

zimb (zim) a fly of the genus *Pangonia*.

Zim•mer•lin atrophy (tsĭ′mer-lin) [Franz *Zimmerlin*, Swiss physician, 1858–1932] see under *atrophy*.

Zim•mer•mann arch (tsĭ′mer-mahn) [Karl Wilhelm *Zimmermann*, German histologist, 1861–1935] see under *arch*.

Zin•a•cef (zin′ə-sef) trademark for a preparation of cefuroxime sodium.

zinc (Zn) (zingk) [L. *zincum*] a blue-white metal, many of whose salts are used in medicine; atomic number, 30; atomic weight, 65.37. Zinc is necessary in trace amounts in the body, and hence in the diet; it forms an essential part of many enzymes (e.g., carbonic anhydrase, important in carbon dioxide metabolism) and plays an important role in protein synthesis and in cell division. Deficiency in zinc is associated with anemia, short stature, hypogonadism, impaired wound healing, and geophagia. Excessive exposure to zinc is toxic, and can interfere with the use of copper by the body; ingestion causes gastrointestinal irritation and vomiting, and inhalation of zinc dust, generally associated with welding or other industrial exposure, causes metal fume fever.

z. acetate [USP] a salt produced by the reaction of zinc oxide with acetic acid, used as a pharmaceutic necessity for zinc oxide–eugenol cement and as an astringent and styptic.

z. carbonate [USP] a zinc salt used as a topical antiseptic and astringent. It may be used in the preparation of calamine (calamine [USP] contains zinc oxide).

z. chloride [USP] a salt, $ZnCl_2$, used as a nutritional supplement in total parenteral nutrition; also used topically as an astringent and desensitizer for dentin.

z. gluconate [USP] a zinc salt used as a dietary supplement; administered orally.

z. oxide [USP] a salt, ZnO, used topically as an astringent, skin protectant, and sunscreen, and as an ingredient in calamine. It is also found in several dental cements. Called also *white z.*

z. phosphide the phosphide salt of zinc, a rodenticide that is toxic to most mammals and causes vomiting, convulsions, and pulmonary edema with dyspnea.

z. stearate [USP] a compound of zinc with a mixture of solid organic acids obtained from fats, consisting predominantly of variable proportions of palmitate and stearate salts of zinc; used as a topical skin protectant, antiseptic, and astringent, and in the manufacture of tablets.

z. sulfate [USP] the heptahydrate or the monohydrate zinc salt of sulfuric acid, used as a topical astringent for the mucous membranes, especially for those of the eye. It is also used as a nutritional supplement, administered orally or parenterally.

z. undecylenate [USP] the zinc salt of undecylenic acid, used as a topical antifungal in the treatment and prevention of dermatophytoses.

white z. z. oxide.

zinc•al•ism (zingk′əl-iz-əm) zinc poisoning; see under *poisoning*.

zin•cif•er•ous (zing-kif′ər-əs) containing zinc.

zin•coid (zing′koid) [*zinc* + *-oid*] pertaining to or resembling zinc.

Zin•e•card (zin′ə-kahrd) trademark for a preparation of dexrazoxane.

Zin•gi•ber (zin′jĭ-bər) a genus of leafy herbs of the family Zingiberaceae, native to southern Asia and southern Pacific islands. *Z. officina′le* is ginger, whose rhizome is ground into the spice also called ginger.

Zinn artery, etc. (tsin) [Johann Gottfried *Zinn*, German anatomist, 1727–1759] see *anulus tendineus communis, arteria centralis retinae, circulus vasculosus nervi optici, fibrae zonulares*, and *zonula ciliaris;* and see under *cap*.

Zins•ser-Cole-Eng•man syndrome (tsin′ser kōl′ eng′mən) [Ferdinand *Zinsser*, German dermatologist, 1865–1952; Harold Newton *Cole*, American dermatologist, 1884–1966; Martin Feeney *Engman*, American dermatologist, 1869–1953] dyskeratosis congenita.

zip•per (zip′ər) a fastener made of two rows of protruding teeth that may be made to interdigitate, linking the rows, or something resembling such a fastener.

leucine z. a stretch of amino acids consisting of four to seven leucine residues, each separated by six amino acids, occurring adjacent to a highly basic stretch of amino acids in some DNA-binding proteins. The configuration of the region is a helix, arranged such that leucine residues from two separate helices can interdigitate or interact to form dimers; the basic regions are arranged so as to recognize and bind specific DNA sequences.

zi•pra•si•done hy•dro•chlo•ride (zĭ-pra′sĭ-dōn) an antipsychotic used in the treatment of schizophrenia; administered orally.

zir•co•ni•um (Zr) (zir-ko′ne-əm) a rather rare metallic element; atomic number, 40; atomic weight, 91.22; chiefly obtained from a mineral called zircon.

Zith•ro•max (zith′ro-maks) trademark for preparations of azithromycin.

Zmax (ze′maks) trademark for a preparation of azithromycin.

Zn zinc.

zo•an•thro•py (zo-an′thro-pe) [*zo-* + Gr. *anthrōpos* man] the delusion that one has become an animal. **zoanthrop′ic** *adj*

Zo•cor (zo′kor) trademark for preparations of simvastatin.

Zo•fran (zo′fran) trademark for preparations of ondansetron hydrochloride.

zo•ic (zo′ik) [Gr. *zōikos* of or proper to animals] pertaining to or characterized by animal life.

Zo•la•dex (zo′lə-deks) trademark for preparations of goserelin acetate.

zo•la•ze•pam hy•dro•chlo•ride (zo′la-zə-pam) [USP] a sedative-hypnotic compound used in veterinary practice in combination with tiletamine hydrochloride.

zo•le•dro•nate (zo′lə-dro″nāt) any salt of zoledronic acid (q.v.).

zo•le•dron•ic ac•id (zo′lə-dron″ik) a bisphosphonate inhibitor of osteoclastic bone resorption, used for the treatment of hypercalcemia of malignancy, multiple myeloma, bone metastases from solid tumors, and osteitis deformans; administered intravenously.

Zol•lin•ger-El•li•son syndrome (zol′in-jər el′ĭ-sən) [Robert Milton *Zollinger*, American surgeon, 1903–1992; Edwin H. *Ellison*, American surgeon, 1918–1970] see under *syndrome*.

Zöll•ner lines (figures) (tsurl′nər) [Johann Karl Friedrich *Zöllner*, German physicist, 1834–1882] see under *line*.

zol•mi•trip•tan (zōl″mĭ-trip′tan) a selective serotonin receptor agonist used to relieve acute migraine, with or without aura; administered orally.

Zo•loft (zo′loft) trademark for preparations of sertraline hydrochloride.

zol•pi•dem tar•trate (zōl-pi′dem) a non-benzodiazepine sedative-hypnotic administered orally in the short-term treatment of insomnia.

Zo•meta (zo′met-ə) trademark for a preparation of zoledronic acid.

Zo•mig (zo′mig) trademark for preparations of zolmitriptan.

zo•na (zo′nə) gen. and pl. *zo′nae* [L. "a girdle"] 1. zone: an anatomical area with a specific boundary or characteristics. 2. herpes zoster.

z. arcua′ta inner tunnel.

z. cilia′ris ciliary zone.

z. derma′tica an elevation of thick skin around the protruding mass in spina bifida.

z. epitheliosero′sa an area of membranous tissue inside the zona dermatica.

z. exter′na medul′lae rena′lis [TA] outer zone of renal medulla: the part of the renal medulla nearest to the cortex, containing part of the distal straight tubule and the medullary collecting tubule. It is subdivided into the *inner stripe* and the *outer stripe*.

z. fascicula′ta fascicular zone: the thick middle layer of the adrenal cortex; it is the major source of glucocorticoids.

z. glandula′rum periurethra′lium a narrow area of the prostate consisting of the short ducts adjacent to the prostatic urethra; it is also a site of benign prostatic hyperplasia, but not as commonly as the transitional zone.

z. glomerulo′sa glomerular zone: the thin outer layer of the adrenal cortex, contiguous with the capsule; it is the source of aldosterone.

z. granulo′sa the peripheral stratified cuboidal epithelium of the ovarian follicle.

zo′nae hypothala′micae [TA] zones of hypothalamus; the zones into which the hypothalamus can be divided mediolaterally, being the zona periventricularis, zona medialis, and zona lateralis.

z. incer′ta [TA] a narrow layer of gray matter extending throughout most of the diencephalon, ventral to and separated from the thalamus by the thalamic fasciculus and laterally continuous with the reticular nucleus of the thalamus. See also *fields of Forel*, under *field*.

z. inter'na medul'lae rena'lis [TA] inner zone of renal medulla: the part of the renal medulla farthest in from the cortex, containing the innermost part of the loop of Henle and of the medullary collecting tubule.

z. latera'lis hypothala'micae [TA] lateral zone of hypothalamus; a longitudinal division of the hypothalamus, containing part of the preoptic nuclei as well as the supraoptic and tuberal nuclei and the nuclei of the mammillary body.

z. media'lis hypothala'micae [TA] medial zone of hypothalamus; a longitudinal division of the hypothalamus, containing part of the preoptic nuclei as well as the anterior, dorsomedial, and ventromedial hypothalamic nuclei.

z. ophthal'mica herpes zoster ophthalmicus.

z. orbicula'ris articulatio'nis cox'ae [TA] orbicular zone of hip joint: circular fibers of the articular capsule of the hip joint which form a ring around the neck of the femur; they are especially prominent at the inferior and posterior part of the capsule.

z. pectina'ta pectinate zone: the outer part of the lamina basilaris ductus cochlearis, running from the rods of Corti to the spiral ligament.

z. pellu'cida 1. pellucid zone: a thick, transparent, noncellular layer or envelope of uniform thickness surrounding an oocyte; called also *oolemma.* Under the light microscope it appears as a radially striated layer; under the electron microscope this can be seen to be microvillous, so that it is called the *z. radiata, z. striata,* or *striated membrane.* 2. area pellucida.

z. perfora'ta the inner portion of the lamina basilaris ductus cochlearis.

z. periventricula'ris hypothala'micae [TA] periventricular zone of hypothalamus; a longitudinal division of the hypothalamus, containing part of the preoptic nuclei as well as the periventricular, infundibular, and posterior nuclei.

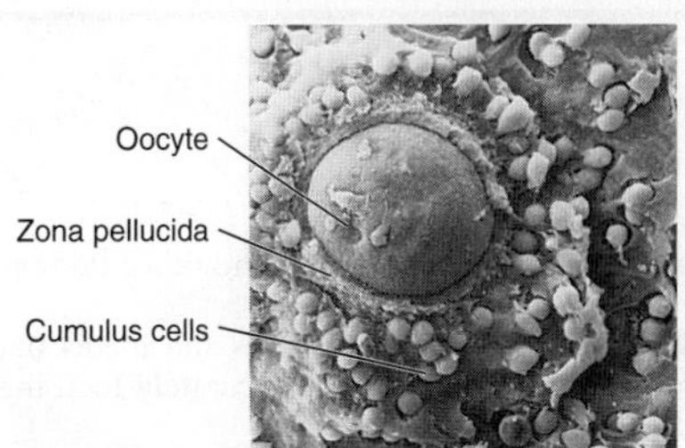

z. radia'ta see *z. pellucida* (def. 1).

z. reticula'ris reticular zone: the inner layer of the adrenal cortex, consisting of cells arranged as clearly anastomosing cords, and abutting the medulla.

z. stria'ta see *z. pellucida* (def. 1).

z. transitiona'lis ana'lis [TA] anal transitional zone: the transitional zone around the anocutaneous line, where the simple columnar epithelium of the anus changes to the stratified squamous epithelium typical of external skin.

zo•nae (zo'ne) [L.] genitive and plural of *zona.*

Zon•a•lon (zon'ə-lon) trademark for a preparation of doxepin hydrochloride.

zo•na•ry (zo'nə-re) zonal.

zone (zōn) [Gr. *zōnē* a belt, girdle] a region or area, especially one with specific characteristics or boundary; called also *zona.* **zo'nal** *adj*

Zone

active z. a site in a presynaptic membrane that is especially adapted for the release of synaptic vesicles.
adoral z. of membranelles an area of serially arranged membranelles (three or more) along the left side of the oral area, typically in a buccal cavity or peristome, in ciliate protozoa.
anal transitional z. zona transitionalis analis.
androgenic z. fetal z. of adrenal cortex.
anelectrotonic z. polar z.
z. of antibody excess prozone.
z. of antigen excess in a precipitin reaction, the region of relatively high antigen concentration, in which soluble complexes are formed and the reaction is inhibited. Called also *postzone.*
apical z. a narrow area along the mucous membrane over the apexes of the roots of the teeth.
arcuate z. inner tunnel.
border z. a zone at the boundary of two contiguous structures, as that where the trophoblast and the endometrium meet.
cell-free z., cell-poor z. Weil basal layer.
cell-rich z. the layer of the dental pulp lying inside the Weil basal layer, containing reticular fibers and abundant cellular elements, such as fibroblasts, macrophages, and mesenchymal cells, as well as blood vessels and nerves.
central z. a cone-shaped area of the prostate composed mainly of stromal cells, found deep to the peripheral zone and extending from there to the base of the prostate.
cervical z. that third of the coronal zone which is nearest the cervix of the tooth, marked by the cementoenamel junction of crown and root.
chemoreceptor trigger z. a trigger zone in the area postrema in the fourth ventricle. It mediates physiological reactions to various chemicals and drugs, plays an indirect role in stimulation of vomiting, and mediates some impulses that in turn stimulate the vomiting center in the medulla.
ciliary z. the outer of two regions of the anterior surface of the iris, separated from the pupillary zone by the collarette.
cloacogenic z. zona transitionalis analis.
comfort z. an environmental temperature between 13° and 21°C (55° to 70°F) with a humidity of 30 to 55 per cent.
contact area z. the zone which includes the contact area of adjoining teeth; usually it is in the middle third of the coronal zone between the occlusal and the cervical zones.
cornuradicular z. the outer part of the fasciculus cuneatus medullae spinalis.
coronal z. the entire enamel area of the tooth crown above the cementoenamel junction, the demarcation between crown and root. The coronal zone is subdivided horizontally into three areas: the occlusal zone, the contact area zone, and the cervical zone. These divisions are also spoken of as the occlusal third, the middle third, and the cervical third.
Cozzolino z. fissula ante fenestram.
definitive z. of adrenal cortex the smaller outer zone of the primordial adrenal cortex and that of the fetus and newborn; this part develops into the zona fasciculata and zona glomerulosa. See also *fetal z. of adrenal cortex.*
dentofacial z. the entire lower part of the face; the region of the face overlying the teeth and the alveolar processes of the jaws.
z's of discontinuity zones of varying optic density, seen with the slit lamp, in the lens of the eye; these zones are formed at particular periods in the prenatal development of the lens.
dolorogenic z. a trigger zone that when stimulated causes pain or an attack of neuralgia.
dorsal z. of His the smaller upper thickening of the dorsal portion of the embryonic spinal cord projecting into the central canal.
entry z. the area where the dorsal roots enter the spinal cord on the brainstem.
ependymal z. see under *layer.*
epigastric z. epigastrium.
epileptogenic z. see under *focus.*
z. of equivalence z. of optimal proportions.
erogenous z., erotogenic z. in psychoanalytic theory, an area of the body through which the libido expresses itself and which is therefore susceptible to erotic excitation upon stimulation; the primary sites are

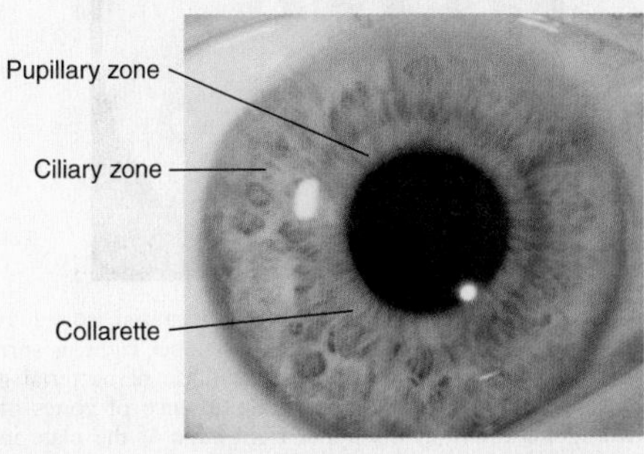

■ Iris showing the pupillary and ciliary zones separated by the collarette.

the oral, anal, and genital regions, but the other body orifices, breasts, and skin are also included.
extravisual z's those dioptric surfaces and media outside the visual zone that are practically incapable of accurately focusing light.
fascicular z. zona fasciculata.
fetal z. of adrenal cortex the inner zone of the primordial adrenal cortex and that of the fetus and newborn; it begins involuting shortly after birth. See also *definitive z. of adrenal cortex*. Called also *fetal adrenal cortex* and *provisional cortex*.
Flechsig primordial z's the cortex of the ascending frontal gyrus and the ascending parietal gyrus of the brain.
glomerular z. zona glomerulosa.
Golgi z. the part of the cytoplasm containing the Golgi complex; in most secretory cells, it is located between the nucleus and the apical surface.
grenz z. a narrow layer in the upper dermis just below the epidermis, made up of densely packed collagen fibrils, which is not infiltrated in the same way other layers of the dermis are. It is seen in granuloma faciale, lepromatous leprosy, and a few other conditions.
Head z's areas of cutaneous sensitiveness associated with diseases of the viscera; called also *z's of hyperalgesia*.
hemorrhoidal z. the part of the anal canal that extends from the anal valves to the anus and contains the rectal venous plexus.
His z's four thickenings running the entire length of the embryonic spinal cord.
z's of hyperalgesia Head z's.
hyperesthetic z. a region of the body surface marked by abnormal sensibility.
hypogastric z. hypogastrium.
z's of hypothalamus zonae hypothalamicae.
z. of inhibition in the disk diffusion test, the area in which an antimicrobial agent inhibits growth of the isolate being tested; beyond that area, the concentration of the agent in the medium is insufficient for inhibition of bacterial growth. See illustration.
inner z. of renal medulla zona interna medullae renalis.
intermediate z. of spinal cord columna intermedia medullae spinalis.
interpalpebral z. the part of the cornea not covered by the eyelids when the eye is open.
Kambin triangular working z. a triangular space free of significant vascular and neural structures that allows safe access to a lumbar disk in microdiskectomy; it is bounded anteriorly by the spinal nerve, inferiorly by the upper rim of the next lower vertebral plate, and posteriorly by the lateral edge of the superior articular process.
keratogenous z. an area where keratin is formed, such as in the nail matrix or just above the papilla pili in the hair bulb.
language z. see under *area*.
lateral z. of hypothalamus zona lateralis hypothalamicae.
Lissauer marginal z. tractus posterolateralis.
Looser transformation z's dark lines seen on radiographs of bones, thought to represent pathological healing phases of fatigue fractures occurring in certain bone diseases.

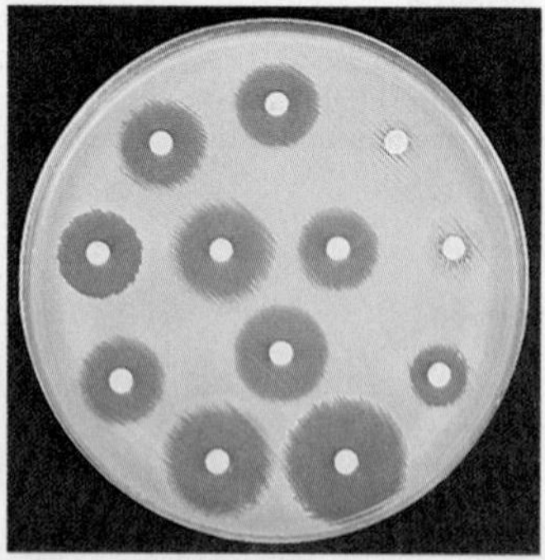

■ Zones of inhibition in disk diffusion test of a bacterial isolate. Each of the antimicrobial agents tested, except the two at the upper right, is surrounded by a zone of some diameter in which there is inhibition of bacterial growth; the isolate is thus susceptible to these agents. The absence of zones of inhibition around the two agents tested at the upper right edge of the plate indicates the isolate is resistant to them.

mantle z. 1. see under *layer*. 2. a dense area of lymphocytes encircling a germinal center.
marginal z. 1. border z. 2. see under *layer*. 3. a loosely packed region of T and B lymphocytes and macrophages encircling periarterial lymphatic sheaths in the mammalian spleen.
medial z. of hypothalamus zona medialis hypothalamicae.
motor z. see under *area*.
neutral z. the potential space between the lips and cheeks on one side and the tongue on the other, natural or artificial teeth in this zone being subject to equal and opposite forces from the surrounding musculature.
neutral z. of His a thickening of the dorsal portion of the embryonic spinal cord projecting into the central canal.
Nitabuch z. see under *layer*.
nuclear z. vortex lentis.
occlusal z. that third of the coronal zone of the teeth which is nearest the occlusal plane.
z. of optimal proportions in a precipitin reaction, the region of maximal precipitation, the antigen and antibody combining to form a cross-linked lattice. Called also *z. of equivalence*.
orbicular z. of hip joint zona orbicularis articulationis coxae.
outer z. of renal medulla zona externa medullae renalis.
z. of oval nuclei a narrow band of sustentacular cells with oval nuclei in the olfactory mucosa.
z. of partial preservation in spinal cord injury, a region where there may be only partial damage to nerves, including one to three spinal segments below the level of the injury.
pectinate z. zona pectinata.
pellucid z. zona pellucida.
peripheral z. a large area of the prostate just beneath the capsule, covering the posterior and lateral aspects and composed mainly of acinar glandular tissue; its ducts drain into the prostatic urethra along most of its length.
peripolar z. the region surrounding a polar zone.
periurethral z., periurethral gland z. zona glandularum periurethralium.
periventricular z. of hypothalamus zona periventricularis hypothalamicae.
placental z. the area of the uterus to which the placenta is attached.
polar z. the region immediately around an electrode applied to the body.
pupillary z. the inner of two regions of the anterior surface of the iris, separated from the ciliary zone by the collarette.
reticular z. zona reticularis.
retinal z's three zones on the retina used for determining the location of retinopathy. *Zone I* is a circular area around the optic disc; *zone II* is a doughnut-shaped area around zone I; and *zone III* is a crescent-shaped area that partially encircles zone II.
Rolando z. primary somatomotor area.
root z. entry z.
z. of round nuclei a broad band of olfactory cells with round nuclei in the olfactory mucosa.
rugae z. see under *area*.
segmental z. a zone of undifferentiated mesoderm between somites already formed and the primitive node, from which additional somites will be produced.
sudanophobic z. a broad zone of cells that appears in the adrenal cortex of rats following hypophysectomy and does not stain with Sudan; see also *sudanophobic unit*, under *unit*.
tendinous z's of heart see anulus fibrosus dexter/sinister cordis.
thymus-dependent z. see under *area*.
thymus-independent z. see under *area*.
transformation z. the area of the uterine cervix between the original squamocolumnar junction and the active one as it moves in response to puberty, pregnancy, menopause, and hormonal changes.
transition z., transitional z. 1. any anatomical region that marks the point at which the constituents of a structure change from one type to another. 2. either of two bilobed areas of the prostate found deep to the central zone and surrounding the prostatic urethra near its angle with the preprostatic part of the urethra; this zone enlarges through the male life cycle and is the site of benign prostatic hyperplasia.
transitional and respiratory z. terminal respiratory unit.
triangular working z. (TWZ) Kambin triangular working zone.
trigger z. an area to which stimulation may cause physiological or pathological changes. See also *dolorogenic z.* and *trigger point*.
umbau z's Looser transformation z's.

Zone *Continued*

visual z. those dioptric surfaces and media around an optic axis in which there is practically no aberration of light rays.
Weber z. zona orbicularis articulationis coxae.
Weil basal z. see under *layer*.
Wernicke z. see under *area*.
Westphal z. a zone of the posterior gray column of the spinal cord in the lumbar region; it is said to contain the exodic fibers concerned in the patellar reflex.
X z. fetal z. of adrenal cortex.
z. of Zinn zonula ciliaris.

Zo•neg•ran (zo′nə-gran) trademark for a preparation of zonisamide.

zo•nes•the•sia (zo″nes-the′zhə) [*zone* + *-esthesia*] a dysesthesia consisting of a sensation of constriction, as by a girdle. Called also *cincture sensation*, *girdle sensation*, and *strangalesthesia*.

zo•nif•u•gal (zo-nif′ə-gəl) [*zona* + *-fugal*[2]] passing outward from any area or region.

zon•ing (zōn′ing) the occurrence of a stronger fixation of complement in a lesser amount of suspected serum.

zo•nip•e•tal (zo-nip′ə-təl) [*zona* + *-petal*] passing from outside into any area or region.

zo•nis•a•mide (zo-nis′ə-mīd″) a sulfonamide that acts as an anticonvulsant, used as an adjunct in the treatment of partial seizures in adults; administered orally.

zo•nog•ra•phy (zo-nog′rə-fe) a type of tomography that has a particularly thick area of focus, resulting in thicker sections for examination. Called also narrow angle tomography.

zo•no•skel•e•ton (zo″no-skel′ə-ton) the most proximal part of a fetal limb; see *limb*.

zo•nu•la (zo′nu-lə) gen. and pl. *zo′nulae* [L., dim. of *zona*] a small zone, or zonule.

z. adhe′rens an adherens junction occurring between columnar epithelial cells near their apical surface, where it forms a complete band around the cell surface and maintains the physical integrity of the epithelium. Cells are bound together by E-cadherins and the plasma membranes are separated by 15–30 nm and linked by and to actin filaments of the terminal web.

z. cilia′ris [TA] ciliary zonule: a system of fibers extending between the ciliary body and the equator of the lens, holding the lens in place; called also *Zinn membrane* and *tendon* or *zonule of Zinn*.

z. occlu′dens tight junction.

zo•nu•lae (zo′nu-le) [L.] genitive and plural of *zonula*.

zo•nule (zo′nūl) a small zone; called also *zonula*. **zon′ular** *adj*

ciliary z., lens z., z. of Zinn zonula ciliaris.

zo•nu•li•tis (zo″nu-li′tis) inflammation of the zonula ciliaris.

zo•nu•lol•y•sis (zo″nu-lol′ĭ-sis) [*zonule* + *lysis*] dissolution of the zonula ciliaris in surgery by means of enzymes such as chymotrypsin.

zon•u•lot•o•my (zon″u-lot′o-me) [*zonule* + *-tomy*] incision of the zonula ciliaris.

zo•nu•ly•sis (zo″nu-li′sis) zonulolysis.

zo(o)- [Gr. *zōon* animal] a combining form denoting relationship to an animal other than a human.

zoo•bi•ol•o•gy (zo″o-bi-ol′ə-je) [*zoo-* + *bio-* + *-logy*] zoology.

zoo•chem•is•try (zo″o-kem′is-tre) the study of the chemical reactions occurring in animal tissues. **zoochem′ical** *adj*

zoo•der•mic (zo″o-dur′mik) [*zoo-* + *derm-* + *-ic*] performed with the skin of an animal; said of skin grafting in which the grafts are from the skin of an animal.

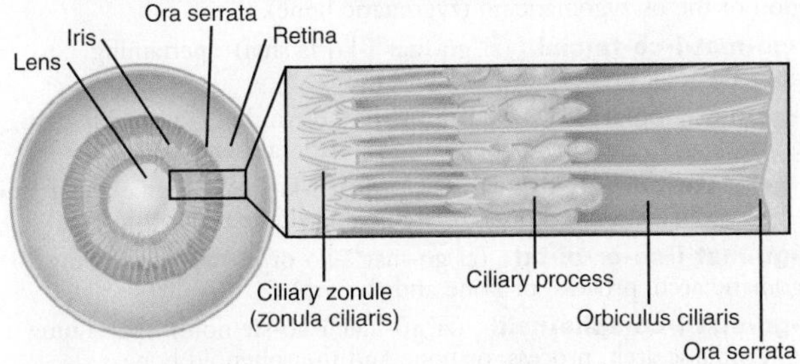

■ Zonula ciliaris (ciliary zonule), the system of suspensory ligaments holding the lens in position.

zoo•de•tri•tus (zo″o-de-tri′təs) biodetritus produced by the disintegration and decomposition of animal organisms. Cf. *phytodetritus*.

zoo•eras•tia (zo″o-e-ras′te-ə) [*zoo-* + Gr. *erastēs* lover] bestiality.

zoo•flag•el•late (zo″o-flaj′ə-lāt) [*zoo-* + *-flagellate*] any protozoan of a large group exhibiting animallike behavior, formerly classified in the class Zoomastigophorea.

zoo•gen•e•sis (zo″o-jen′ə-sis) zoogeny.

zo•og•e•nous (zo-oj′ə-nəs) 1. acquired from animals. 2. viviparous.

zo•og•e•ny (zo-oj′ə-ne) [*zoo-* + *-geny*] the development and evolution of animals.

zoo•ge•og•ra•phy (zo″o-je-og′rə-fe) the study of the distribution of animal life on the earth.

zo•og•o•ny (zo-og′ə-ne) [*zoo-* + Gr. *gonē* offspring] viviparity.

zoo•graft•ing (zo′o-graft″ing) xenografting of tissue from a different species into a human.

zoo•hor•mone (zo″o-hor′mōn) an animal hormone.

zo•oid (zo′oid) [*zoo-* + *-oid*] 1. resembling an animal. 2. an object or form which resembles an animal. 3. one of the individuals in a united colony of animals. See *blastozooid* and *oozooid*.

zoo•lag•nia (zo″o-lag′ne-ə) [*zoo-* + Gr. *lagneia* lust] sexual attraction toward animals. Cf. *bestiality* and *zoophilia*.

zo•ol•o•gy (zo-ol′ə-je) [*zoo-* + *-logy*] the biology of animals; the sum of what is known regarding animals other than humans. Called also *zoobiology*.

experimental z. the study of animals by means of experiments performed upon them.

Zoo•mas•ti•goph•o•ra (zo″o-mas″tĭ-gof′ə-rə) Zoomastigophorea.

Zoo•mas•ti•go•pho•rea (zo″o-mas″tĭ-gə-for′e-ə) [*zoo-* + Gr. *mastix* whip + *phōros* bearing] in older systems of classification, a class of protozoa of the phylum Sarcomastigophora comprising all of the animallike (as opposed to plantlike) members of the phylum; collectively called zooflagellates. Members of this group lack chromatophores and are heterotrophic, and most are either commensal or parasitic. They have one to many flagella and some are capable of ameboid movement with or without flagella. Cf. *Phytomastigophorea*.

zoo•mas•ti•go•pho•re•an (zo″o-mas″tĭ-gə-for′e-ən) zooflagellate.

Zoon balanitis (erythroplasia) (zōn) [Johannes Jacobus *Zoon*, Dutch dermatologist, 1902–1958] see under *balanitis*.

zoo•no•sis (zo″o-no′sis, zo-on′ə-sis) pl. *zoono′ses* [*zoo-* + *nos-* + *-is*] a disease of nonhuman animals that may be transmitted to humans under natural conditions. **zoonot′ic** *adj*

Zoo•pa•ga•les (zo″ə-pə-ga′lēz) an order of perfect fungi of the phylum Zygomycota, class Zygomycetes, many of which are saprobes; it includes the genus *Piptocephalis*, which can infect humans.

zoo•para•site (zo″o-par′ə-sīt) animal parasite. **zooparasit′ic** *adj*

zoo•pa•thol•o•gy (zo″o-pə-thol′ə-je) animal pathology; the study of the diseases of animals. Cf. *veterinary medicine*.

zo•oph•a•gous (zo-of′ə-gəs) carnivorous.

zoo•phile (zo′o-fīl) 1. zoophilic. 2. an antivivisectionist.

zoo•phil•ia (zo″o-fil′e-ə) 1. fondness or preference for animals other than humans. 2. a paraphilia in which intercourse or other sexual activity with animals is the preferred method of achieving sexual excitement.

zoo•phil•ic (zo″o-fil′ik) 1. pertaining to or characterized by zoophilia. 2. preferring other animals to human beings, such as certain mosquitoes and dermatophytes. Cf. *anthropophilic* and *anthropozoophilic*.

zoo•phil•ism (zo-of′ĭ-liz-əm) 1. fondness for animals; antivivisection. 2. the state of being zoophilic.

erotic z. sexual pleasure experienced in the fondling of animals.

zo•oph•i•lous (zo-of′ĭ-ləs) zoophilic.

zoo•pho•bia (zo″o-fo′be-ə) [*zoo-* + *-phobia*] irrational fear of animals.

zoo•phys•i•ol•o•gy (zo″o-fiz″e-ol′ə-je) animal physiology.

zoo•phyte (zo′o-fīt) [*zoo-* + *-phyte*] any plantlike animal, such as a sponge or hydroid.

zoo•plank•ton (zo″o-plangk′ton) [*zoo-* + *plankton*] the minute animal organisms which, with those of the vegetable kingdom (phytoplankton), make up the plankton of natural waters.

zoo•plas•ty (zo′o-plast″te) [*zoo-* + *-plasty*] zoografting. **zooplas′tic** *adj*

zoo•pre•cip•i•tin (zo″o-pre-sip′ĭ-tin) a precipitin obtained by injections of protein substances of animal origin.

zoo•pro•phy•lax•is (zo″o-pro″fi-lak′sis) 1. prophylaxis applied to animals; veterinary prophylaxis. Cf. *veterinary medicine.* 2. the prevention or amelioration of disease (e.g., smallpox) in humans as a result of previous exposure to heterologous infection of animal origin (e.g., cowpox). 3. protection of humans from bites of mosquitoes by providing cattle or other animals for the mosquitoes to feed on.

zo•op•sia (zo-op′se-ə) [*zoo-* + *-opsia*] a hallucination in which patients think they see animals.

zoo•psy•chol•o•gy (zo″o-si-kol′ə-je) animal psychology.

zoo•sa•dism (zo″o-sa′diz-əm) cruelty to animals; sadism directed toward animals.

zoo•sper•mia (zo″o-spur′me-ə) the presence of live spermatozoa in the ejaculated semen.

zoo•spo•ran•gi•um (zo″o-spə-ran′je-əm) pl. *zoosporan′gia* [*zoo-* + *sporangium*] the case within which zoospores are developed.

zoo•spore (zo′o-spor) [*zoo-* + *spore*] a motile spore, such as an asexual flagellate of certain algae and lower fungi, or a minute sexual or asexual flagellate or ameboid spore produced by certain protozoa; it forms within a case called a zoosporangium. Called also *flagellospore.*

zoo•ste•rol (zo″o-ste′rol) any sterol of animal origin.

zoo•tech•nics (zo″o-tek′niks) the raising, breeding, and handling of animals in domestication or captivity. Called also *zootechny.*

zoo•tech•ny (zo″o-tek′ne) zootechnics.

zo•ot•ic (zo-ot′ik) pertaining to animals other than humans.

zoo•tox•in (zo′o-tok″sin) [*zoo-* + *toxin*] a toxic substance of animal origin, such as the venoms of snakes, spiders, and scorpions.

zo•pic•lone (zo′pĭ-klōn″) a sedative-hypnotic used in the short-term treatment of insomnia; administered orally.

ZOR•prin (zor′prin) trademark for a preparation of aspirin.

Zos•ta•vax (zos′tə-vaks) trademark for a preparation of zoster vaccine live.

zos•ter (zos′tər) [Gr. *zōstēr* a girdle] herpes zoster.
z. si′ne eruptio′ne, z. si′ne her′pete pain typical of herpes zoster in an appropriate sensory area but not followed by the development of characteristic lesions.
ophthalmic z. herpes zoster ophthalmicus.

zos•ter•i•form (zos-ter′ĭ-form) resembling herpes zoster.

zos•ter•oid (zos′tər-oid) zosteriform.

Zos•trix (zos′triks) trademark for a preparation of capsaicin.

Zo•syn (zo′sin) trademark for combination preparations of piperacillin sodium and tazobactam sodium.

Zo•to-HC (zo′to) trademark for a combination preparation of chloroxylenol, pramoxine hydrochloride, and hydrocortisone.

Zo•via (zo′ve-ə) trademark for combination preparations of ethynodiol diacetate and ethinyl estradiol.

Zo•vir•ax (zo-vi′raks) trademark for preparations of acyclovir.

Z-plas•ty (ze′plas″te) a type of skin flap procedure used for relaxation of contracted scar tissue; a Z-shaped incision is made with its middle bar over the contracted scar, and the triangular flaps are rotated so that their apices cross the line of contraction. Called also Z-*flap.*

Zr zirconium.

ZSR zeta sedimentation ratio.

Zuck•er•kan•dl bodies (organs), convolution, fascia (tsook′er-kahn″dəl) [Emil *Zuckerkandl,* Hungarian-born anatomist in Germany and Austria, 1849–1910] see *corpora paraaortica,* under *corpus,* see *gyrus paraterminalis,* and see under *fascia.*

zu•clo•mi•phene (zoo-klo′mĭ-fēn) the *trans*-isomer of the gonad-stimulating principle clomiphene citrate (q.v.); called also *transclomiphene.* Cf. *enclomiphene.*

Zum•busch psoriasis (tsoom′boosh) [Leo von *Zumbusch,* German dermatologist, 1874–1940] generalized pustular psoriasis.

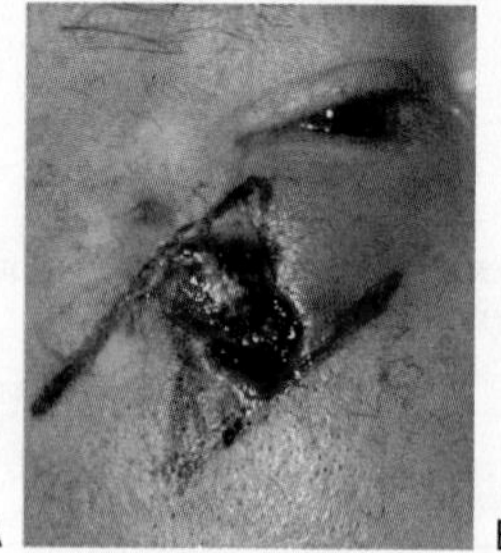
A

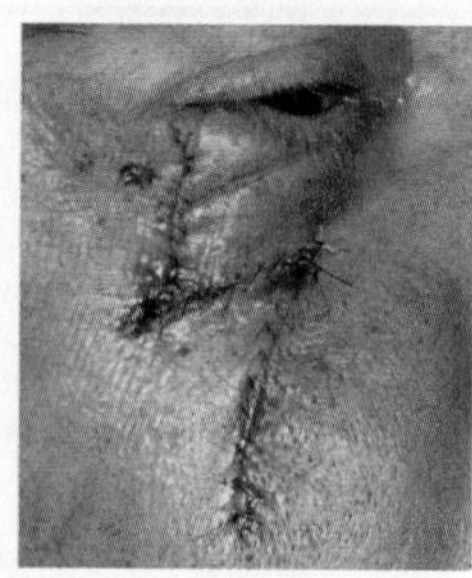
B

■ Z-plasty.

zwit•ter•ion (tsvit′er-i″on) a dipolar ion, i.e., an ion that has both positive and negative regions of charge; amino acids, for example, occur as zwitterions in neutral solution, and the pH value at which the zwitterion state is at a maximum is the isoelectric point.

Zy•ban (zi′ban) trademark for a preparation of bupropion hydrochloride.

Zy•done (zi′dōn) trademark for a combination preparation of hydrocodone bitartrate and acetaminophen.

Zy•flo (zi′flo) trademark for a preparation of zileuton.

zy•gal (zi′gəl) [*zyg-* + *-al*[1]] shaped like a yoke.

zy•ga•poph•y•sis (zi″gə-pof′ĭ-sis) pl. *zygapoph′yses* [*zyg-* + *apophysis*] an articular process of a vertebra. **zygapophyse′al** *adj*
z. inferior TA alternative for *processus articularis inferior vertebrae.*
z. superior TA alternative for *processus articularis superior vertebrae.*

zyg•ia (zij′e-ə) plural of *zygion.*

zyg•i•on (zij′e-on) pl. *zyg′ia* [Gr.] a craniometric and cephalometric landmark, being the most laterally situated point on either zygomatic arch.

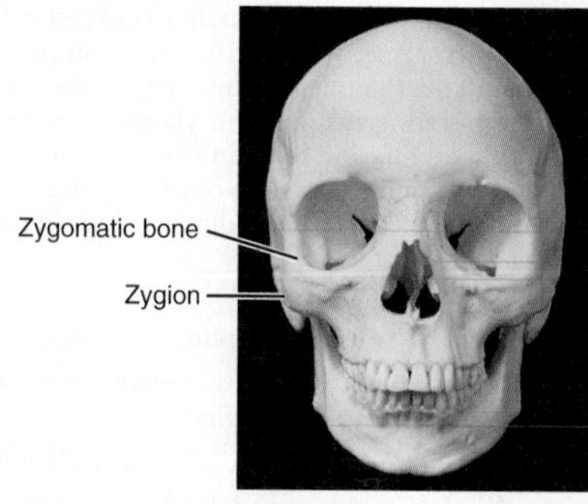

zyg(o)- [Gr. *zygon* yoke] a combining form meaning yoked or joined, or denoting relationship to a junction.

Zy•go•co•ty•le lu•na•tum (zi″go-ko′tə-le loo-na′təm) a trematode parasitic in the intestine of a variety of hosts, including rats, cattle, and ducks in North America.

zy•go•dac•ty•ly (zi″go-dak′tə-le) [*zygo-* + Gr. *daktylos* finger] a term sometimes used to designate simple syndactyly, as distinguished from syndactyly in which there is bony fusion between the phalanges of the digits involved; usually occurring in the hand between the third and fourth digits and in the foot between the fourth and fifth.

zy•go•ma (zi-go′mə) [Gr. *zygōma* bolt or bar] 1. processus zygomaticus ossis temporalis. 2. arcus zygomaticus. 3. a term sometimes applied to the os zygomaticum.

zy•go•mat•ic (zi″go-mat′ik) pertaining to, connecting with, or in the region of the os zygomaticum (zygomatic bone).

zy•go•mat•i•co•fa•cial (zi″go-mat″ĭ-ko-fa′shəl) pertaining to the zygomatic arch, process, or bone and the face.

zy•go•mat•i•co•fron•tal (zi″go-mat″ĭ-ko-frun′təl) pertaining to the zygomatic arch, process, or bone and the frontal bone.

zy•go•mat•i•co•max•il•lary (zi″go-mat″ĭ-ko-mak′sĭ-lar″e) pertaining to the zygomatic arch, process, or bone and the maxilla.

zy•go•mat•i•co•or•bi•tal (zi″go-mat″ĭ-ko-or′bĭ-təl) pertaining to the zygomatic arch, process, or bone and the orbit.

zy•go•mat•i•co•sphe•noid (zi″go-mat″ĭ-ko-sfe′noid) pertaining to the zygomatic arch, process, or bone and the sphenoid bone.

zy•go•mat•i•co•tem•po•ral (zi″go-mat″ĭ-ko-tem′pər-əl) pertaining to the zygomatic arch, process, or bone and the temporal bone.

zy•go•max•il•la•re (zi″go-mak′sĭ-lar″e) [L.] a craniometric point at the inferior end of the zygomatic suture.

zy•go•max•il•lary (zi″go-mak′sĭ-lar″e) zygomaticomaxillary.

Zy•go•my•ce•tes (zi″go-mi-se′tēz) [*zygo-* + Gr. *mykēs* fungus] a class of saprobic and parasitic fungi of the phylum Zygomycota, having a mycelial thallus, coenocytic hyphae, and chitinous cell walls; sexual reproduction is by means of zygospores. Pathogenic organisms are included in the orders Entomophthorales, Mucorales, and Zoopagales.

zy•go•my•co•sis (zi″go-mi-ko′sis) 1. mucormycosis. 2. any fungal infection with members of the class Zygomycetes, including entomophthoromycosis and mucormycosis.

rhinocerebral z. zygomycosis that has spread from the paranasal sinuses to the brain; see *rhinocerebral mucormycosis* and *conidiobolomycosis.*

rhinofacial z. rhinoentomophthoromycosis.

subcutaneous z. basidiobolomycosis.

Zy•go•my•co•ta (zi″go-mi-ko′tə) a phylum of perfect fungi consisting of soil saprobes and invertebrate parasites; it includes the classes Zygomycetes and Trichomycetes. Organisms may cause human or animal infection in debilitated or highly stressed individuals. In some systems of classification, it is considered a subphylum, Zygomycotina, and placed under the phylum Eumycota.

Zy•go•my•co•ti•na (zi″go-mi″ko-ti′nə) name given to Zygomycota when it is seen as a subphylum under Eumycota.

zy•gon (zi′gon) [Gr. "bar" or "yoke"] the bar or stem connecting the two branches of a zygal fissure.

zy•go•phore (zi′go-for) a specialized branch of a hypha containing isogametes (zygospheres) that unite to form a zygospore.

zy•go•po•di•um (zi″go-po′de-əm) the third part of a fetal limb; see *limb.*

zy•go•sis (zi-go′sis) [Gr. *zygōsis* a balancing] conjugation; the sexual union of two unicellular organisms.

zy•gos•i•ty (zi-gos′ĭ-te) [*zygon* + *-ity* state or condition] the genetic condition or characteristics of a zygote.

-zy•gos•i•ty a word termination denoting relationship to the zygote.

zy•go•sperm (zi′go-spərm) zygospore.

zy•go•sphere (zi′go-sfēr) a gamete arising from a zygophore which unites with another to form a zygospore.

zy•go•spore (zi′go-spor) a sexual spore formed by the conjugation of two isogametes (zygospheres) that are morphologically identical, or in the Zygomycetes, from the fusion of like gametangia.

zy•go•style (zi′go-stīl) the last coccygeal vertebra.

zy•gote (zi′gōt) [Gr. *zygōtos* yoked together] the diploid cell resulting from union of a male and a female gamete (spermatozoon and oocyte). More precisely, the cell after synapsis at the completion of fertilization until first cleavage. Also, used loosely to refer to the fertilized oocyte and early derivatives for an indefinite period. Cf. *conceptus.* **zygot′ic** *adj*

zy•go•tene (zi′go-tēn) [Gr. *zygōtos* yoked together] the second stage of prophase in meiosis I, during which homologous chromosomes begin to pair off by the process of synapsis.

Zy•lo•prim (zi′lo-prim) trademark for a preparation of allopurinol.

zym(o)- [Gr. *zymē* leaven] a combining form denoting relationship to an enzyme, or to fermentation.

zy•mo•chem•is•try (zi″mo-kem′is-tre) the chemistry of fermentation.

zy•mo•gen (zi′mo-jən) a proenzyme, particularly of a proteolytic enzyme.

zy•mo•gen•ic (zi″mo-jen′ik) pertaining to a zymogen (proenzyme) or to its transformation into an active enzyme form.

zy•mog•e•nous (zi-moj′ə-nəs) zymogenic.

zy•mo•san (zi′mo-sən) a mixture of polysaccharides, proteins, and ash, of variable concentration, derived from the cell walls or the entire cell of yeast, commonly *Saccharomyces cerevisiae.* It is anticomplementary, absorbing the C3 component of complement, and is used in assaying properdin.

zy•mos•ter•ol (zi-mos′tər-ol) a mycosterol occurring in yeast as an intermediate in the synthesis of cholesterol.

Zy•prex•a (zi-prek′sə) trademark for preparations of olanzapine.

Zyr•tec (zur′tek) trademark for preparations of cetirizine hydrochloride.

Zy•vox (zi′voks) trademark for preparations of linezolid.

Zz. [L.] zin′giber (ginger).

APPENDICES

APPENDIX 1

FREQUENTLY USED STEMS

The following list includes those Greek and Latin words occurring most frequently in this Dictionary, arranged alphabetically under their English combining forms as rubrics. The dash appended to a combining form indicates that it is not a complete word and, if the dash precedes the combining form, that it commonly appears as the terminal element of a compound. Infrequently a combining form is both preceded and followed by a dash, showing that it usually appears between two other elements. Closely related forms are shown in one entry by the use of parentheses: thus carbo(n)-, showing it may be either carbo-, as in *carbo*hydrate, or carbon-, as in *carbon*uria.

Following each combining form the first item of information is the Greek or Latin word, identified by [Gr.] or [L.], from which it is derived. Occasionally both a Greek and a Latin word are given. Presence of a dash before or after such an element indicates that it does not occur as an independent word in the original language. Information necessary to the understanding of the form appears next in parentheses. Then the meaning or meanings of the word are given, followed where appropriate by reference to a synonymous combining form. Finally, an example is given to illustrate use of the combining form in a compound English derivative.

If this list is used in close conjunction with the etymological information given in the body of the Dictionary, no confusion should be caused by the similarity of elements in such words as *mel*algia, *mel*ancholia, and *mel*icera, where the similarity is only apparent and the derivation of each word is different.

a-[1] *a-* [Gr.] (*n* is added before words beginning with a vowel) negative prefix. Cf. in-[3]. *a*metria

a-[2] *a-* [L.] separation, away from. *a*vulsion

ab- *ab* [L.] away from. Cf. apo-. *ab*ducent

abdomin- *abdomen, abdominis* [L.] abdomen. *abdomino*scopy

abs- *abs* [L.] variant of ab. *abs*cess

ac- See ad-. *ac*cretion

acanth- *akantha* [Gr.] thorny, spiny. *acantho*cyte

acar- *akari* [Gr.] mite. *acaro*dermatitis

acet- *acetum* [L.] vinegar. *acet*ic acid

acid- *acidus* [L.] sour. *acid*uric

acou- *akouō* [Gr.] hear. *acou*stic. (Also spelled acu-)

acr- *akron* [Gr.] extremity, peak. *acro*megaly

act- *ago, actus* [L.] do, drive, act. re*act*ion

actin- *aktis, aktinos* [Gr.] ray, radius. Cf. radi-. *Actino*bacillus

acu- See acou-. dys*acu*sis

ad- *ad* [L.] (*d* changes to *c, f, g, p, s,* or *t* before words beginning with those consonants) to. *ad*renal

-ad[1] *-ad* [L.] toward. cephal*ad*

-ad[2] *-as, ados* [Gr.] group, derivation from, connection with. pseudomon*ad*

-adelphus *adelphos* [Gr.] brother. der*adelphus*

aden- *adēn* [Gr.] gland. Cf. gland-. *aden*oma

adip- *adeps, adipis* [L.] fat. Cf. lip- and stear-. *adipo*cellular

aer- *aēr* [Gr.] air. an*aero*biosis

af- See ad-. *af*ferent

ag- See ad-. *ag*glutinant

agam- *agamos* [Gr.] unmarried. *agam*ous

-agogue *agōgos* [Gr.] leading, inducing. galact*agogue*

-agra *agra* [Gr.] catching, seizure. pod*agra*

-al[1] *-alis* [L.] pertaining to, characterized by. arteri*al*, diarrhe*al*

-al[2] *-alia* [L.] act, process. deni*al*

alb- *albus* [L.] white. Cf. leuk-. *alb*iduria

alg- *algos* [Gr.] pain. neur*alg*ia

algesi- *algēsis* [Gr.] sense of pain. an*alges*ia, *algesi*meter

all- *allos* [Gr.] other, different. *all*ergy

allant- *allas, allantos* [Gr.] sausage, *allant*iasis. *allant*oid

allel- *allēlōn* [Gr.] of one another. *allel*ic

allotri- *allotrios* [Gr.] strange. *allotrio*geustia

alve- *alveus* [L.] trough, channel, cavity. *alveo*bronchiolitis

alveol- *alveolus*, dim. of *alveus* [L.] alveolus. *alveol*itis

ambi- *ambi-* [L.] (*i* may be dropped before words beginning with a vowel) on all sides. *ambi*dexterity

ambly- *amblys* [Gr.] dull. *ambly*opia

ambo- *ambo* [L.] both. *ambo*sexual

ameb- *amoibē* [Gr.] change. *ameb*oid

amni- *amnion* [Gr.] bowl, membrane enveloping the fetus. *amnio*centesis

amphi- *amphi* [Gr.] (*i* is dropped before words beginning with a vowel) on both sides. *amphi*centric

ampho- *amphō* [Gr.] both. *ampho*genic

amygdal- *amygdalē* [Gr.] almond. *amygdal*in, *amygdal*oid

amyl- *amylon* [Gr.] starch. *amyl*uria

an-[1] See a-[1]. *an*iridia

an-[2] See ana-. *an*ode

ana- *ana* [Gr.] (final *a* is dropped before words beginning with a vowel) up, positive. *ana*bolism

ancyl- See ankyl-. *ancylo*stomiasis

andr- *anēr, andros* [Gr.] man. *andr*ogen

angi- *angeion* [Gr.] vessel. Cf. vas-. *angi*oma

anis- *anisos* [Gr.] unequal, uneven. *aniso*coria

ankyl- *ankylos* [Gr.] crooked, looped. *ankyl*osis. (Also spelled ancyl-)

anomal- *anōmalos* [Gr.] irregular. *anomal*ous

ant- See anti-. *ant*acid

ante- *ante* [L.] before. *ante*flexion

anthrac- *anthrax* [Gr.] coal, charcoal. *anthraco*silicosis

anthrop- *anthrōpos* [Gr.] man, human being. *anthropo*morphism

anti- *anti* [Gr.] (*i* may be dropped before words beginning with a vowel) against, counter. Cf. contra. *anti*pruritic

antr- *antron* [Gr.] cavern. *antro*cele

ap-[1] See apo-. *ap*eidosis

ap-[2] See ad-. *ap*pendage

aph- *haptō, haph-* [Gr.] touch. dys*aph*ia. (See also hapt-)

apic- *apex* [L.] top, summit. *apic*oectomy

apo- *apo* [Gr.] (*o* may be dropped before words beginning with a vowel) away from, detached. Cf. ab-. *apo*lipoprotein

appendic- *appendix, appendicis* [L.] appendix. *appendic*itis

arachn- *arachnē* [Gr.] spider. *arachno*dactyly

arch- *archē* [Gr.] beginning, origin. *arch*enteron

arteri- *arteria* [Gr.] (*i* is sometimes dropped) windpipe, artery. *arterio*sclerosis, peri*arter*itis

arteriol- *arteriola*, dim. of *arteria* [L.] arteriole. *arteriolo*pathy

arthr- *arthron* [Gr.] joint. Cf. articul-. syn*arthr*osis

articul- *articulus* [L.] joint. Cf. arthr-. dis*articul*ation

as- See ad-. *as*similation

asthen- *asthenēs* [Gr.] weak. *astheno*coria

astr- *astron* [Gr.] star. *astro*cyte

at- See ad-. *at*tenuate

atel- *atelēs* [Gr.] incomplete. *atelo*cardia

ather- *athērē* [Gr.] gruel. *athero*sclerosis

atlant- *atlas, atlantos* [Gr.] atlas. *atlanto*axial

atm- *atmos* [Gr.] steam, vapor. *atmo*sphere

atret- *atrētos* [Gr.] not perforated. *atreto*stomia

atri- *atrium* [L.] atrium. *atrio*ventricular

atroph- *atrophia* [Gr.] ill-fed. *atropho*derma

Appendix 1

audi- *audire* [L.] to hear. *audi*ometry

aur- *auris* [L.] ear. Cf. ot-. *aur*inasal

aut- *autos* [Gr.] self. *aut*oimmunity

aux- *auxō* [Gr.] increase. *aux*otrophic

ax- *axōn* [Gr.] or *axis* [L.] axis. *ax*olemma

axon- *axōn* [Gr.] axis. *axon*opathy

ba- *bainō, ba-* [Gr.] go, walk, stand. *aba*sia

bacill- *bacillus* [L.] small staff, rod. Cf. bacter-. actino*bacill*osis

bacter- *bactērion* [Gr.] small staff, rod. Cf. bacill-. *bacter*iophage

balan- *balanos* [Gr.] acorn. *balan*itis

ball- *ballō, bol-* [Gr.] throw. *ball*ismus. (See also bol-)

bar- *baros* [Gr.] weight. *bar*osinusitis

bas- See basi-. *bas*ophil

basi- *basis* [Gr.] base. *basi*oglossus, *basi*hyoid

bath(y)- *bathys* [Gr.] deep. *bath*orhodopsin, *bathy*pnea

bi-[1] *bios* [Gr.] life Cf. vit-. aero*bic*

bi-[2] *bi-* [L.] (an *n* may be added before words beginning with a vowel) two. *bi*cornuate. (See also di-[1])

bil- *bilis* [L.] bile. Cf. chol-. *bil*iary

bin- See bi-[2]. *bin*ocular

bis- *bis* [L.] twice. *bis*ferious

blast- *blastos* [Gr.] bud, child, a growing thing in its early stages. Cf. germ-. *blast*oma, mono*blast*

blenn- *blenna* [Gr.] mucus. *blenn*orrhea

blep- *blepō* [Gr.] look, see. mono*blep*sia

blephar- *blepharon* [Gr.] (from *blepō*; see blep-) eyelid. Cf. cili-. *blephar*itis

bol- See ball-. em*bol*ism

brachi- *brachiōn* [Gr.] arm. *brachi*ocephalic

brachy- *brachys* [Gr.] short. *brachy*dactyly

brady- *bradys* [Gr.] slow. *brady*cardia

breph- *brephos* [Gr.] embryo, newborn infant. *breph*oplastic

brevi- *brevis* [L.] short. *brevi*collis

brom- *brōmos* [Gr.] stench. *brom*hidrosis

bronch- *bronchos* [Gr.] windpipe. *bronch*oscopy

bronchiol- *bronchiolus*, dim. of *bronchus* [Gr.] bronchiole. *bronchiol*ectasis

bry- *bryō* [Gr.] be full of life. em*bry*onic

bucc- *bucca* [L.] cheek. *bucc*oclusion

bulb- *bulbus* [L.] bulb. *bulb*ospiral

butyr- *boutyron* [Gr.] butter. *butyr*oid

cac- *kakos* [Gr.] bad, abnormal. Cf. mal-. *cac*ogeusia. (See also dys-)

calc-[1] *calx, calcis* [L.] stone (cf. lith-), limestone, lime. *calc*ipexy

calc-[2] *calx, calcis* [L.] heel. *calc*aneodynia

calor- *calor* [L.] heat. Cf. therm-. *calor*imeter

campt- *camptos* [Gr.] bent. *campt*odactyly

cancr- *cancer, cancri* [L.] crab, cancer. Cf. carcin-. *cancr*oid. (Also spelled chancr-)

canth- *kanthos* [Gr.] foreign. *canth*oplasty

capit- *caput, capitis* [L.] head. Cf. cephal-. de*capit*ation

capn- *kapnos* [Gr.] smoke. *capn*ography

caps- *capsa* [L.] (from *capio*; see cept-) container. *caps*ule

carbo(n)- *carbo, carbonis* [L.] coal, charcoal. *carbo*hydrate, *carbon*ic acid

carcin- *karkinos* [Gr.] crab, cancer. Cf. cancr-. *carcin*oma

cardi- *kardia* [Gr.] heart. lipo*cardi*ac

cari- *caries* [L.] rottenness. *cari*ogenesis

cary- See kary-. Eu*cary*otae

cata- *kata* [Gr.] (final *a* is dropped before words beginning with a vowel) down, negative. *cata*crotism, *cat*ion

caud- *cauda* [L.] tail. *caud*ad

cav- *cavus* [L.] hollow. Cf. coel-. con*cav*e

cec- *caecus* [L.] blind. Cf. typhl-. *cec*otomy

cel-[1] See -cele. varico*cel*ectomy

cel-[2] See coel-. a*cel*omate

cel-[3] See celi-. *cel*itis

-cele[1] *kēlē* [Gr.] tumor, hernia. gastro*cele*

-cele[2] *koilos* [Gr.] hollow. rhino*cele*

celi- *koilia* [Gr.] belly. *celi*otomy

cell- *cella* [L.] room, cell. Cf. cyt-. *cell*ular

cement- *caementum* [L.] rough stone. *cement*oblast

cen- *koinos* [Gr.] common. *cen*esthesia

cente- *kenteō* [Gr.] to puncture. Cf. punct-. entero*cente*sis

centi- *centum* [L.] hundred. Cf. hect-. Indicates fraction in metric system. [This exemplifies the custom in the metric system of identifying fractions of units by stems from the Latin, as centimeter, decimeter, millimeter, and multiples of units by the similar stems from the Greek, as hectometer, decameter, and kilometer.] *centi*meter, *centi*pede

centr- *kentron* [Gr.] or *centrum* [L.] point, center. *centr*ifugal, *centr*omere

cephal- *kephalē* [Gr.] head. Cf. capit-. en*cephal*itis, *cephal*ocentesis

cept- *capio, -cipientis, -ceptus* [L.] take, receive. re*cept*or

cer- *kēros* [Gr.] or *cera* [L.] wax. *cer*oplasty, *cer*umen

cerat- See kerat-. *cerat*ocricoid

cerc- *kerkos* [Gr.] tail. Oncho*cerc*a

cerebell- *cerebellum* [L.] dim. of *cerebrum* little brain. *cerebell*ifugal

cerebr- *cerebrum* [L.] brain. *cerebr*ospinal

cervic- *cervix, cervicis* [L.] neck. Cf. trachel-. *cervic*itis

chancr- See cancr-. *chancr*oid

cheil- *cheilos* [Gr.] lip. Cf. labi-. *cheil*oschisis

cheir- *cheir* [Gr.] hand. Cf. man-. macro*cheir*ia. (Also spelled chir-)

chem- *chēmeia* [Gr.] alchemy. *chem*istry, *chem*otherapy

chir- See cheir-. *chir*opractic

chlor- *chlōros* [Gr.] green. *chlor*ophyll

choan- *choanē* [Gr.] funnel. *choan*omastigote

chol- *cholē* [Gr.] bile. Cf. bil-. *chol*angitis

chondr- *chondros* [Gr.] cartilage. *chondr*omalacia

chondri- *chondrion* [Gr.] granule. mito*chondri*a

chord- *chordē* [Gr.] string, cord. peri*chord*al

chore- *choreia* [Gr.] dance. *chore*oathetosis

chori- *chorion* [Gr.] membrane. *chori*ocarcinoma

chro- *chrōs* [Gr.] color. poly*chro*matic

chron- *chronos* [Gr.] time. syn*chron*ous

chrys- *chrysos* [Gr.] gold. *chrys*otherapy

chy- *cheō, chy-* [Gr.] pour. ec*chy*mosis

chyl- *chylos* [Gr.] juice. *chyl*iform, *chyl*opericardium

-cid(e) *caedo, -cisus* [L.] cut, kill. fungi*cide*, germi*cid*al

cili- *cilium* [L.] eyelid. Cf. blephar-. super*cili*ary

cine- See kine-. acro*cine*sis

-cipient See cept-. ex*cipient*

circum- *circum* [L.] around. Cf. peri-. *circum*ferential

cirs- *kirsos* [Gr.] varix. *cirs*ophthalmia

cis- *cis* [L.] on this side. *cis*platin

-cis- *caedo, -cisus* [L.] cut, kill. ex*cis*ion

-clast *klaō* [Gr.] break. osteo*clast*

cleid- *kleis, kleidos* [Gr.] key, clavicle. *cleid*ocranial

-cleisis *kleiein* [Gr.] to enclose. colpo*cleisis*

clin- *klinō* [Gr.] bend, incline, make lie down. *clin*ocephaly

clus- *claudo, -clusus* [L.] shut. maloc*clus*ion

cnid- *knidē* [Gr.] nettle. *cnid*oblast

co- See con-[1]. *co*hesion

cocc- *kokkos* [Gr.] berry. gono*cocc*us

coel- *koilos* [Gr.] hollow. Cf. cav-. *coel*ozoic. (Also spelled cel-)

-coele See coel-. blasto*coele*

coen- See cen-. *coen*ocyte

coin- See cen-. *coin*osite

col-[1] See colon-. *col*ic

col-[2] See con-[1]. *col*lapse

colon- *kalon* [Gr.] lower intestine. *colon*ic

colp- *kolpos* [Gr.] hollow, vagina. Cf. sin- and vagin-. *colp*itis

com- See con-[1]. *com*mensal

con-[1] *con-* [L.] (becomes co- before vowels or *h*; col- before *l*; com- before *b*, *m*, or *p*; cor- before *r*) with, together. Cf. syn-. *con*traction

con-[2] *kōnos* [Gr.] cone. *con*otruncal

coni- *konis* [Gr.] dust. *coni*ofibrosis

contra- *contra* [L.] against, counter. Cf. anti-. *contra*indication

copr- *kopros* [Gr.] dung, feces. Cf. sterco-. *copr*ophilia

cor-[1] *korē* [Gr.] doll, little image, pupil. iso*cor*ia

cor-[2] See con-[1]. *cor*relation

cord- See chord-. *cord*otomy

corpor- *corpus, corporis* [L.] body. Cf. somat-. intra*corpor*eal

cortic- *cortex, corticis* [L.] bark, rind. *cortic*osterone

cost- *costa* [L.] rib. Cf. pleur-. inter*cost*al

counter- See contra-. *counter*traction

crani- *kranion* [Gr.] or *cranium* [L.] skull, peri*crani*um

-crasia *krasis* [Gr.] mixture. dys*crasia*

creat- *kreas, kreato-* [Gr.] meat, flesh. *creat*ine

-crescence *cresco, crescentis, cretus* [L.] grow. ex*crescence*

cret-[1] *cerno, cretus* [L.] distinguish, separate off. Cf. crin-. dis*cret*e

cret-[2] See -crescence. ac*cret*ion

crin- *krinō* [Gr.] distinguish, separate off. Cf. cret-[1]. endo*crin*ology

crur- *crus, cruris* [L.] shin, leg. talo*crur*al

cry- *kryos* [Gr.] cold. *cry*esthesia. (See also crym-)

Appendix 1

crym- *krymos* [Gr.] frost. *crym*odynia. (See also cry-)
crypt- *kryptō* [Gr.] hide, conceal. *crypt*orchidism
cult- *colo, cultus* [L.] tend, cultivate. *cult*ure
cune- *cuneus* [L.] wedge. Cf. sphen-. *cune*iform
cut- *cutis* [L.] skin. Cf. derm(at)-. sub*cut*aneous
cyan- *kyanos* [Gr.] blue. *cyan*ophil
cycl- *kyklos* [Gr.] circle, cycle. *cycl*ophoria
-cyesis *kyēsis* [Gr.] pregnancy. pseudo*cyesis*
cymb- *kymbē* [Gr.] boat. *cymb*ocephaly
cyn- *kyōn, kynos* [Gr.] dog. *cyn*ophobia
cyst- *kystis* [Gr.] bladder. Cf. vesic-. *cyst*algia
cyt- *kytos* [Gr.] cell. Cf. cell-. *cyt*otaxis
dacry- *dakry* [Gr.] tear. *dacry*ocyst
dactyl- *daktylos* [Gr.] finger, toe. Cf. digit-. hexa*dactyly*
de- *de* [L.] down from. *de*composition
deca- *deka* [Gr.] ten. Indicates multiple in metric system. Cf. deci-. *deca*gram
deci- *decem* [L.] ten. Indicates fraction in metric system (one-tenth). Cf. deca-. *deci*bel, *deci*liter
demi- *demi* [Fr.], from *dimidius* [L.] half. *demi*gauntlet
dendr- *dendron* [Gr.] tree. *dendr*ite
dent- *dens, dentis* [L.] tooth. Cf. odont-. inter*dent*al
derm(at)- *derma, dermatos* [Gr.] skin. Cf. cut-. endo*derm*, *dermat*itis
-desis *desis* [Gr.] a binding together. arthro*desis*
desm- *desmos* [Gr.] band, ligament. syn*desm*oplasty
deut(er)- *deuteros* [Gr.] second. *deuter*anopia, *deut*an
dextr- *dexter, dextr-* [L.] right-hand. ambi*dextr*ous
di-[1] *di* [Gr.] two. *di*morphism. (See also bi-[2])
di-[2] See dia-. *di*uresis
di-[3] See dis-[1]. *di*vergent
dia- *dia* [Gr.] (*a* is dropped before words beginning with a vowel) through, apart. Cf. per-. *dia*gnosis
dicty- *diktyon* [Gr.] nest. *dicty*otene
didym- *didymos* [Gr.] twin. Cf. gemin-. epi*didym*al
digit- *digitus* [L.] finger, toe. Cf. dactyl-. *digit*igrade
diplo- *diploos* [Gr.] double. *diplo*myelia
dips- *dipsa* [Gr.] thirst. poly*dips*ia, *dips*ogen
dis-[1] *dis-* [L.] (*s* may be dropped before a word beginning with a consonant) apart, away from. *dis*location
dis-[2] *dis* [Gr.] twice. *dis*diaclast
disc- *diskos* [Gr.] or *discus* [L.] disk. *disc*oplacenta. (Also spelled disk-)
dolich- *dolichos* [Gr.] long. *dolich*ocephalic
dors- *dorsum* [L.] back. *dors*oventral
drom- *dromos* [Gr.] course. *drom*ograph
-ducent See duct-. ad*ducent*
-duct *duco, ducentis, ductus* [L.] lead, conduct. ovi*duct*
dur- *durus* [L.] hard. Cf. scler-. in*dur*ation
dynam- *dynamis* [Gr.] power. *dynam*ometer, thermo*dynam*ics
dys- *dys-* [Gr.] bad, improper. Cf. mal-. *dys*trophic. (See also cac-)
e- *e* [L.] out from. Cf. ec-[1] and ex-. *e*mission
ec-[1] *ek* [Gr.] out of. Cf. e- and ex-. *ec*centric
ec-[2] *oikos* [Gr.] house. *ec*ogenetics
-ech- *echō* [Gr.] have, hold, be. syn*ech*otomy
echin- *echinos* [Gr.] hedgehog. *echin*ophthalmia
ect- *ektos* [Gr.] outside. Cf. extra-. *ect*oderm. (See also exo-)
ectr- *ektrōsis* [Gr.] miscarriage. *ectr*odactyly
ede- *oideō* [Gr.] swell. *ede*matous
ef- See ex-. *ef*florescent
elast- *elasticus* [L.] elastic. *elast*ofibroma
elc- See helc-. cyst*elc*osis
electro- *ēlektron* [Gr.] amber. *electro*therapy
em- See en-. *em*bolism, *em*pathy
-em- *haima* [Gr.] blood, an*em*ia. (See also hem(at)-)
-emesis *emein* [Gr.] to vomit. hyper*emesis*
en- *en* [Gr.] (*n* changes to *m* before *b*, *m*, *p*, or *ph*) in, on. Cf. in-[1]. *en*arthosis
encephal- *enkephalos* [Gr.] brain. *encephal*opathy
end- *endon* [Gr.] inside. Cf. intra-. *end*angitis. (See also eso-)
ent- *entos* [Gr.] inside. *ent*optic
enter- *enteron* [Gr.] intestine. dys*enter*y
entom- *entomon* [Gr.] insect. *entom*ology
epi- *epi* [Gr.] (*i* is dropped before words beginning with a vowel) upon, after, in addition. *epi*glottis, *ep*axial
epipl- *epiploon* [Gr.] omentum. gastro*epipl*oic
episi- *epision* [Gr.] pubic region. *episi*otomy
erg- *ergon* [Gr.] work, deed. en*erg*y
erot- *erōs, erōtos* [Gr.] sexual desire. *erot*omania
erythr- *erythros* [Gr.] red. Cf. rub(r)-. *erythr*ocyte
eso- *esō* [Gr.] inside. Cf. intra-. *eso*gastritis. (See also end-)
esthe- *aisthanomai, aisthē-* [Gr.] perceive, feel. Cf. sens-. an*esthe*sia
etio- *aitia* [Gr.] cause. *etio*logy
eu- *eu* [Gr.] good, normal. *eu*pepsia
eury- *eurys* [Gr.] wide. *eury*gnathism
ex- *ex* [Gr.] or *ex* [L.] out of. Cf. e- and ec-[1]. *ex*cretion
exo- *exō* [Gr.] outside. Cf. extra-. *exo*skeleton. (See also ect-)
extra- *extra* [L.] outside of, beyond. Cf. ect- and exo-. *extra*cellular. (Also written extro-)
extro- See extra-. *extro*vert
faci- *facies* [L.] face. Cf. prosop-. *faci*olingual
-facient *facio, facientis, factus, -fectus* [L.] make. Cf. poie-. cale*facient*
-fact- See -facient. arti*fact*
fasci- *fascia* [L.] band. *fasci*otomy
febr- *febris* [L.] fever. Cf. pyr-. *febr*icity
-fect- See -facient. de*fect*ive
femor- *femur* [L.] femur. *femor*otibial
-ferent *fero, ferentis, latus* [L.] bear, carry. Cf. phor-. ef*ferent*
-ferous *ferre* [L.] to bear. lacti*ferous*
ferr- *ferrum* [L.] iron. *ferr*oprotein
fet- *fetus* [L.] fetus. *fet*oscope
fibr- *fibra* [L.] fiber. Cf. in-[3]. chondro*fibr*oma
fil- *filum* [L.] thread. *fil*iform
fiss- *findo, fissus* [L.] split. Cf. schis-. *fiss*ion
flagell- *flagellum* [L.] whip. *flagell*ation
flav- *flavus* [L.] yellow. Cf. xanth-. ribo*flav*in. (See also lute-)
-flect- *flecto, flexus* [L.] bend, divert. de*flect*ion
-flex- See -flect-. re*flex*ometer
flu- *fluo, fluxus* [L.] flow. Cf. rhe-. *flu*id
flux- See flu-. de*flux*ion
for- *foro* [L.] bore. imper*for*ate
-form *forma* [L.] shape. Cf. -oid. cruci*form*
fract- *frango, fractus* [L.] break. re*fract*ion
front- *frons, frontis* [L.] forehead, front. naso*front*al
-fug(e) *fugio* [L.] flee, avoid. vermi*fuge*, centri*fug*al
funct- *fungor, functus* [L.] perform, serve. mal*funct*ion
fund- *fundo, fusus* [L.] pour. in*fund*ibulum
fus-[1] See fund-. dif*fus*ion
fus-[2] *fusus* [L.] spindle. *fus*ocellular
galact- *gala, galactos* [Gr.] milk. Cf. lact-. *galact*orrhea
gam- *gamos* [Gr.] marriage, reproductive union. *gam*ete
gangli- *ganglion* [Gr.] swelling, plexus. *gangli*itis
gastr- *gastēr, gastros* [Gr.] stomach. cholangio*gastr*ostomy
ge- *gē* [Gr.] earth. *ge*ophagia
gelat- *gelo, gelatus* [L.] freeze, congeal. *gelat*in
gemin- *geminus* [L.] twin, double. Cf. didym-. quadri*gemin*al
gen-[1] *gignomai, gen-, gon-* [Gr.] become, be produced, originate. endo*gen*ous
gen-[2] *gennaō* [Gr.] produce, originate. cyto*gen*ic
geni- *geneion* [Gr.] chin. *geni*oplasty
genit- *genitalis* [L.] pertaining to birth. *genit*ourinary
ger- *gēras* [Gr.] old age. *ger*oderma
germ- *germen, germinis* [L.] bud, a growing thing in its early stages. Cf. blast-. *germ*inal
geront- *gerōn, gerontos* [Gr.] old man. *geront*ology
gest- *gero, gerentis, gestus* [L.] bear, carry. con*gest*ion
gingiv- *gingiva* [L.] gum. *gingiv*itis
gland- *glans, glandis* [L.] acorn. Cf. aden-. uni*gland*ular
gli- *glia* [Gr.] glue. neuro*gli*a, *gli*oma
glomerul- *glomerulus*, dim. of *glomus* [L.] little ball. *glomerul*onephritis
gloss- *glōssa* [Gr.] tongue. Cf. lingu-. tricho*gloss*ia
glott- *glōtta* [Gr.] tongue, language. *glott*ic
gluc- See glyc(y)-. *gluc*ophore
glutin- *gluten, glutinis* [L.] glue. ag*glutin*ation
glyc(y)- *glykys* [Gr.] sweet. *glyc*emia, *glycy*rrhiza. (Also spelled gluc-)
gnath- *gnathos* [Gr.] jaw. ortho*gnath*ous
gno- *gignōsō, gnō-* [Gr.] know, discern. dia*gno*sis
gon-[1] *gonē* [Gr.] offspring, seed, genitalia. *gon*ocyte, *gon*orrhea
gon-[2] *gony* [Gr.] knee. *gon*arthrosis, *gon*ocampsis
gonad- *gonas, gonadis* [L.] gonad. *gonad*oblastoma
goni- *gōnia* [Gr.] angle. *goni*ometer, *goni*otomy
grad- *gradior* [L.] walk, take steps. retro*grad*e
-gram *gramma* [Gr.] letter, drawing. cardio*gram*
gran- *granum* [L.] grain, particle. lipo*gran*uloma
graph- *graphō* [Gr.] scratch, write, record. angio*graph*y
grav- *gravis* [L.] heavy. multi*grav*ida
gymn- *gymnos* [Gr.] naked. *gymn*ospore

gyn(ec)- *gynē, gynaikos* [Gr.] woman, wife. andro*gyny*, *gynec*ologic

gyr- *gyros* [Gr.] ring, circle. *gyro*spasm

haem(at)- See hem(at)-. *Haem*aphysalis, *Haemat*oxylon

hamart- *hamartia* [Gr.] fault. *hamart*oma

hapl- *haploos* [Gr.] simple, single. *haplo*type

hapt- *haptō* [Gr.] touch, *haptics*

hect- *hekaton* [Gr.] hundred. Cf. centi-. Indicates multiple in metric system. *hecto*gram

hel- *hēlos* [Gr.] nail, corn, callus. *hel*oma

helc- *helkos* [Gr.] sore, ulcer. kerato*helc*osis

heli- *hēlios* [Gr.] sun. *helio*taxis

helic- *helix, helikos* [Gr.] coil. *helico*trema

hem(at)- *haima, haimatos* [Gr.] blood. Cf. sanguin-. *hem*angioma, *hemato*cele. (See also -em-) [Also written haem(at)-]

hemi- *hēmi* [Gr.] half. Cf. semi-. *hemi*ageusia

hen- *heis, henos* [Gr.] one. Cf. un-. *heno*genesis

hepat(ic)- *hēpar, hēpatos* [Gr.] liver. *hepato*cele, *hepatic*olithotomy

hept(a)- *hepta* [Gr.] seven. Cf. sept-[2]. *hepta*valent, *hept*ose

hered- *heres, heredis* [L.] heir. *heredo*familial

herpet- *herpo, herpet-* [Gr.] creep, crawl. *herpeto*phobia, *herpeti*form

heter- *heteros* [Gr.] other, different. *hetero*chromia

hex- *echō, hech-* [Gr.] (*hech-* added to *s* becomes *hex-*) have, hold, be. cac*hexia*

hex(a)- *hex* [Gr.] six. Cf. sex-[1]. *hex*ose, *hexa*dactyly

hidr- *hidros* [Gr.] sweat. hyper*hidr*osis

hipp- *hippos* [Gr.] horse. *hippo*campus

hist- *histos* [Gr.] web, tissue. *histo*compatibility

hod- *hodos* [Gr.] road, path. *hodo*neuromere. (See also od- and -ode[1])

hol- *holos* [Gr.] entire. *holo*systolic

hom- *homos* [Gr.] common, same. *homo*graft

home- *homoios* [Gr.] like, resembling. *homeo*stasis

horm- *hormē* [Gr.] impetus, impulse. *horm*one

hyal- *hyalos* [Gr.] glass. *hyalo*plasm

hydat- *hydōr, hydatos* [Gr.] water. *hydat*oid

hydr- *hydōr, hydr-* [Gr.] water. achlor*hydr*ia. (See also lymph-)

hygr- *hygros* [Gr.] moist. *hygro*metry

hyl- *hylē* [Gr.] matter. *hylo*tropy

hymen- *hymēn* [Gr.] membrane. *hymen*opteran, *hymen*ectomy

hyp- See hypo-. *hyp*axial

hyper- *hyper* [Gr.] above, beyond, extreme. Cf. super-. *hyper*trophy

hypn- *hypnos* [Gr.] sleep. *hypn*otic

hypo- *hypo* [Gr.] (*o* is dropped before words beginning with a vowel) under, below. Cf. sub-. *hypo*calcemia

hyps- *hypsos* [Gr.] height. *hyps*arrhythmia

hyster- *hystera* [Gr.] womb. Cf. uter-. *hystero*pexy. (See also metr-[2])

iatr- *iatros* [Gr.] physician. ped*iatr*ics

ichthy- *ichthys* [Gr.] fish. *ichthy*osis

icter- *ikteros* [Gr.] jaundice. *ictero*hepatitis

id- *eidos* [Gr.] form, shape. homin*id*, dermatophyt*id*

idi- *idios* [Gr.] peculiar, separate, distinct. *idio*syncrasy

il-[1] See in-[1]. *il*lumination

il-[2] See in-[2]. *il*legible

ile- See ili- [ile- is commonly used to refer to the portion of the intestines known as the ileum]. *ile*ostomy

ili- *ilium (ileum)* [L.] lower abdomen, intestines [ili- is commonly used to refer to the flaring part of the hip bone known as the ilium]. *ilio*femoral

im-[1] See in-[1]. *im*mersion

im-[2] See in-[2]. *im*perforate

in-[1] *in* [L.] (*n* changes to *l* before *l*, *m* before *b*, *m*, or *p*, and *r* before *r*) in, on. Cf. en-. *in*sertion

in-[2] *in-* [L.] (*n* changes to *l* before *l*, *m* before *b*, *m*, or *p*, and *r* before *r*) negative prefix. Cf. a-. *in*compatible

in-[3] *is, inos* [Gr.] fiber. Cf. fibr-. *ino*tropic

infra- *infra* [L.] beneath. *infra*orbital

ini- *inion* [Gr.] occiput. *ini*encephaly

insul- *insula* [L.] island. *insul*in

inter- *inter* [L.] among, between. *inter*costal

intra- *intra* [L.] inside. Cf. end- and eso-. *intra*venous

intro- *intro* [L.] within. *intro*spection

ipsi- *ipse* [L.] self. *ipsi*lateral

ir-[1] See in-[1]. *ir*radiation

ir-[2] See in-[2]. *ir*reducible

irid- *iris, iridos* [Gr.] rainbow, colored circle. *irido*cyclitis

is- *isos* [Gr.] equal. *iso*tope

isch- *ischein* [Gr.] to suppress. *isch*emia

ischi- *ischion* [Gr.] hip, haunch. *ischio*pubic

-ism *-ismos* [Gr.] noun-forming suffix. vegetarian*ism*, thigmotrop*ism*, alcohol*ism*

-itis *-itis* [Gr.] inflammation. dermat*itis*, phleb*itis*

-ize *-izein* [Gr.] verb-forming suffix. cauter*ize*, oxid*ize*

jact- *iacio, iactus* [L.] throw. *jact*itation

-ject *iacio, -iectus* [L.] throw. in*ject*ion

jejun- *ieiunus* [L.] empty. gastro*jejuno*stomy

jug- *iugum* [L.] yoke. con*jug*ation

junct- *iungo, junctus* [L.] yoke, join. con*junct*iva

juxta- *juxta* [L.] near, close by. *juxta*glomerular

kary- *karyon* [Gr.] nut, kernel, nucleus. Cf. nucle-. mega*kary*ocyte. (Also spelled cary-)

kerat- *keras, keratos* [Gr.] horn. *kerato*lysis. (Also spelled cerat-)

kilo- *chilioi* [Gr.] one thousand. Cf. milli-. Indicates multiple in metric system. *kilo*gram

kine- *kineō* [Gr.] move. *kine*scope. (Also spelled cine-)

klept- *kleptein* [Gr.] to steal. *klepto*mania

koil- *koilos* [Gr.] hollow. *koil*onychia

labi- *labium* [L.] lip. Cf. cheil-. *labio*mental

lact- *lac, lactis* [L.] milk. Cf. galact-. *lact*iferous

lal- *laleō* [Gr.] talk, babble. glosso*lal*ia

lapar- *lapara* [Gr.] flank. *laparo*tomy

laryng- *larynx, laryngos* [Gr.] windpipe. *laryng*ectomy

lat- *fero, latus* [L.] bear, carry. See -ferent. trans*lat*ion

later- *latus, lateris* [L.] side. ventro*later*al

lecith- *lekithos* [Gr.] yolk. iso*lecith*al

leio- *leios* [Gr.] smooth. *leio*myoma

-lemma *lemma* [Gr.] rind, husk. axo*lemma*

lent- *lens, lentis* [L.] lentil. Cf. phac-. *lent*iconus

lep- *lambanō, lēp* [Gr.] take, seize. cata*lep*sy

lept- *leptos* [Gr.] slender. *lepto*meninges

leuc- See leuk-. *leuc*ine

leuk- *leukos* [Gr.] white. Cf. alb-. *leuk*orrhea. (Also spelled leuc-)

lev- *laevus* [L.] left. *levo*cardia, *levo*rotatory

lien- *lien* [L.] spleen. Cf. splen-. *lieno*cele

lig- *ligo* [L.] tie, bind. *lig*ature

lingu- *lingua* [L.] tongue. Cf. gloss-. sub*lingu*al

lip- *lipos* [Gr.] fat. Cf. adip-. glyco*lip*id

lith- *lithos* [Gr.] stone. Cf. calc-[1]. nephro*litho*tomy

loc- *locus* [L.] place. Cf. top-. *loco*motion

log- *legō, log-* [Gr.] speak, give an account. *log*orrhea, embryo*logy*

loph- *lophos* [Gr.] ridge, tuft. *lopho*trichous

lumb- *lumbus* [L.] loin. *lumb*ago

lute- *luteus* [L.] yellow. Cf. xanth-. *lute*oma. (See also flav-)

lymph- *lympha* [Gr.] water. *lymph*adenopathy. (See also hydr-)

lyo- *lyō* [Gr.] loose, dissolve. Cf. solut-. *lyo*philization

lys- *lysis* [Gr.] dissolution. kerato*lys*is, *lys*ogen

macr- *makros* [Gr.] long, large. *macro*myeloblast

mal- *malus* [L.] bad, abnormal. Cf. cac- and dys-. *mal*formation

malac- *malakos* [Gr.] soft. osteo*malac*ia

mamm- *mamma* [L.] breast. Cf. mast-. sub*mamm*ary

man- *manus* [L.] hand. Cf. cheir-. *man*ipulation

mani- *mania* [Gr.] mental aberration. klepto*mania*

mast- *mastos* [Gr.] breast. Cf. mamm-. hyper*mast*ia

mechan- *mēchanē* [Gr.] machine. *mechano*receptor

medi- *medius* [L.] middle. Cf. mes-. *medio*lateral

mega- *megas* [Gr.] great, large. Also indicates multiple (one million) in metric system. *mega*colon, *mega*volt. (See also megal-)

megal- *megas, megalou* [Gr.] great, large. acro*megaly*

mel-[1] *melos* [Gr.] limb, member. sym*mel*ia

mel-[2] *mēlon* [Gr.] cheek. *melo*plasty

melan- *melas, melanos* [Gr.] black. *melano*cyte

meli(t)- *meli, melitos* [Gr.] honey. *meli*biose, *melit*uria

men- *mēn* [Gr.] month. dys*men*orrhea

mening- *mēninx, mēningos* [Gr.] membrane. *mening*itis

ment- *mens, mentis* [L.] mind. Cf. phren-, psych-, and thym-[2]. de*ment*ia

mer-[1] *meros* [Gr.] part. poly*mer*ic

mer-[2] *mēros* [Gr.] thigh. *mer*algia

mes- *mesos* [Gr.] middle. Cf. medi-. *meso*derm

mesi- *mesos* [Gr.] in the middle. *mesio*dens

meta- *meta* [Gr.] (*a* is dropped before words beginning with a vowel) after, beyond, accompanying. *meta*carpal, *met*encephalon

metr-[1] *metron* [Gr.] measure. audio*metry*

metr-[2] *metra* [Gr.] womb. Cf. uter-. endo*metr*itis. (See also hyster-)

mi- *meiōn* [Gr.] smaller. *mi*osis
micr- *mikros* [Gr.] small. Also indicates fraction in metric system (one-millionth). photo*micro*graph, *micro*gram
milli- *mille* [L.] one thousand. Also indicates fraction in metric system (one-thousandth). Cf. kilo-. *milli*gram, *milli*pede
-mimetic *mimētikos* [Gr.] mimetic. sympatho*mimetic*
mis- *misos* [Gr.] hatred. *mis*ogamy
miss- See -mittent. intro*miss*ion
mit- *mitos* [Gr.] thread. *mit*ochondria
-mittent *mitto, mittentis, missus* [L.] send. inter*mittent*
mne- *mimnēskō, mnē-* [Gr.] remember. a*mne*sia
mogi- *mogis* [Gr.] with difficulty. *mogi*arthria
mon- *monos* [Gr.] only, sole. *mono*plegia
morph- *morphē* [Gr.] from, shape. poly*morph*onuclear
mot- *moveo, motus* [L.] move. vaso*mot*or
muc- *mucus* [L.] mucus. *muc*ilage, *muc*ogingival, *muc*oprotein
multi- *multus* [L.] many, much. *multi*para
my- *mys, myos* [Gr.] muscle. leio*my*oma
-myces *mykēs, mykētos* [Gr.] fungus. Strepto*myces*
myc(et)- See -myces. strepto*myc*in, *mycet*oma
myel- *myelos* [Gr.] marrow. polio*myel*itis
myring- *myringa* [L.] membrane. *myring*otomy
myx- *myxa* [Gr.] mucus. *myx*edema
nan- *nanos* [Gr.] dwarf. Also indicates fraction (one-billionth) in metric system. *nan*ophthalmos, *nan*ometer
narc- *narkē* [Gr.] numbness. *narc*olepsy
nas- *nasus* [L.] nose. Cf. rhin-. *nas*opalatine
ne- *neos* [Gr.] new, young. *ne*onate
necr- *nekros* [Gr.] corpse. *necr*ophilia
nemat- *nēma, nēmatos* [Gr.] thread. *nemat*ocyst
nephel- *nephelē* [Gr.] cloud, mist. *nephel*ometer
nephr- *nephros* [Gr.] kidney. Cf. ren-. para*nephr*ic
neur- *neuron* [Gr.] nerve. *neur*algia
neutr- *neuter* [Gr.] neither. *neutr*ophil
nev- *naevus* [L.] mole. *nev*olipoma
noci- *noceo* [L.] to injure. *noci*ceptor
nod- *nodus* [L.] knot. *nod*osity
nom- *nomos* [Gr.] (from *nemō* deal out, distribute) law, custom. taxo*nom*y
non-^{1} *non* [L.] not. *non*disjunction
non-^{2} *nona* [L.] nine. *non*apeptide
norm- *norma* [L.] rule. *norm*otensive
nos- *nosos* [Gr.] disease. *nos*ology
not- *nōton* [Gr.] back. *not*ochord
nucle- *nucleus* [L.] (from *nux, nucis* nut) kernel. Cf. kary-. *nucle*ocapsid
nutri- *nutrio* [L.] nourish. mal*nutri*tion
nyct- *nyx, nyctos* [Gr.] night. *nyct*ophobia
nymph- *nymphē* [Gr.] bride. *nymph*omania, *nymph*otomy
ob- *ob* [L.] (*b* changes to *c* before words beginning with that consonant) against, toward. *ob*tusion
oc- See ob-. *oc*clude
oct- *oktō* [Gr.] or *octo* [L.] eight. *oct*igravida
ocul- *oculus* [L.] eye. Cf. ophthalm-. *ocul*omotor
-od- See –ode^{1}. esthes*od*ic
-ode^{1} *hodos* [Gr.] road, path. cath*ode*. (See also hod-)
-ode^{2} See -oid. nemat*ode*
odont- *odous, odontos* [Gr.] tooth. Cf. dent-. orth*odont*ia
odyn- *odynē* [Gr.] pain, distress. gastr*odyn*ia, *odyn*ophagia
-oid *eidos* [Gr.] form. Cf. -form. hy*oid*
-ol See ole-. choleste*rol*
ole- *oleum* [L.] oil. *ole*oresin
olig- *oligos* [Gr.] few, small. Cf. pauci-. *olig*ospermia
om- *ōmos* [Gr.] shoulder. *om*algia
-oma *ōma* [Gr.] noun-forming suffix. Used to denote a neoplasm. hepat*oma*, carcin*oma*
omphal- *omphalos* [Gr.] navel. *omphal*ectomy
-on *iōn* [Gr.] something that goes. neutr*on*
onc-^{1} *onkos* [Gr.] bulk, mass. *onc*ogenesis
onc-^{2} *onkos* [Gr.] barb, hook. *onc*osphere
onch- See onc-^{2}. *Onch*ocerca
oneir- *oneiros* [Gr.] dream. *oneir*ogenic
onych- *onyx, onychos* [Gr.] claw, nail. an*onych*ia
oo- *ōon* [Gr.] egg. Cf. ov-. *oo*genesis
oophor- *ōophoros* [Gr.] bearing eggs. Cf. ovari-. *oophor*ectomy
op- *hōraō, op-* [Gr.] see. hetero*op*sia
ophthalm- *ophthalmos* [Gr.] eye. Cf. ocul-. ex*ophthalm*os
opisth- *opisthen* [Gr.] behind, at the back. *opisth*otonos
or- *os, oris* [L.] mouth. Cf. stom(at)-. intra*or*al
orb- *orbis* [L.] circle. sub*orb*ital
orchi- *orchis* [Gr.] testicle. Cf. test-. *orchi*opathy
organ- *organon* [Gr.] implement, instrument. *organ*omegaly
orth- *orthos* [Gr.] straight, right, normal. *orth*opedics
oscill- *oscillare* [L.] to swing. *oscill*opsia
-osis *-osis* [Gr.] noun-forming suffix. Used to denote a process, particularly a disease. dermat*osis*, bacteri*osis*
osm-^{1} *osmē* [Gr.] odor. *osm*ophore
osm-^{2} *ōsmos* [Gr.] impulse. *osm*oregulation
oss- *os, ossis* [L.] bone. Cf. ost(e)-. *oss*iferous
ost(e)- *osteon* [Gr.] bone. Cf. oss-. en*ost*osis, *oste*oarthritis
-ostomy *stoma* [Gr.] mouth. col*ostomy*
ot- *ous, ōtos* [Gr.] ear. Cf. aur-. par*ot*id, *ot*otoxic
ov- *ovum* [L.] egg. Cf. oo-. syn*ov*ia, *ov*ovegetarian
ovari- *ovarium* [L.] ovary. Cf. oophor-. *ovari*opexy
oxy- *oxys* [Gr.] (y is sometimes dropped, often denoting relationship to oxygen). sharp. *oxy*cephalic, *ox*idation
pachy- *pachys* [Gr.] thick. *pachy*derma
pag- *pēgnymi, pag-* [Gr.] fix, make fast. thoraco*pag*us
palat- *palatum* [L.] palate. Cf. uran-. *palat*orrhaphy
pale- *palaios* [Gr.] old. *pale*ocortex
pali(n)- *palin* [Gr.] backward, again. *pali*kinesia, *palin*genesis
pan- *pan* [Gr.] all. *pan*demic
par-^{1} *pario* [L.] bear, give birth to. primi*par*a
par-^{2} See para-. *par*occipital
para- *para* [Gr.] (final *a* is sometimes dropped before words beginning with a vowel) beside, beyond. *para*cervical, *para*oral, *par*amnesia
pariet- *paries, parietis* [L.] wall. *pariet*ofrontal
part- *pario, partus* [L.] bear, give birth to. *part*urition
path- *pathos* [Gr.] that which one undergoes, sickness. psycho*path*ic, cardio*path*y
pauci- *paucus* [L.] few. Cf. olig-. *pauci*articular
pec- *pēgnymi, pēg-* [Gr.] (*pēk-* before *t*) fix, make fast. amylo*pec*tin. (See also pex-)
ped-^{1} *pais, paidos* [Gr.] child. *ped*iatrics
ped-^{2} *pes, pedis* [L.] foot. *ped*icure, *ped*ometer
pell- *pellis* [L.] skin, hide. *pell*agra
-pellent *pello, pellentis, pulsus* [L.] drive. chemore*pellent*
pen- *penomai* [Gr.] need, lack. neutro*pen*ia
pend- *pendeo* [L.] hang down. ap*pend*ix
pent(a)- *pente* [Gr.] five. Cf. quint-. *pent*ose, *penta*logy
peps- *peptō, peps-* [Gr.] digest. eu*peps*ia
pept- *peptō* [Gr.] digest. dys*pept*ic
per- *per* [L.] through. Cf. dia-. *per*oral
peri- *peri* [Gr.] around. Cf. circum-. *peri*phery
pero- *pēros* [Gr.] maimed. *pero*splanchnia
pet- *peto* [L.] seek, tend toward. centri*pet*al
pex- *pēgnymi, pēg-* [Gr.] (*pēg-* added to *s* becomes *pēx-*) fix, make fast. hepato*pex*y
pha- *phēmi, pha-* [Gr.] say, speak. dys*pha*sia
phac- *phakos* [Gr.] lentil, lens. Cf. lent-. *phac*osclerosis. (Also spelled phak-)
phag- *phagein* [Gr.] eat. dys*phag*ia
phak- See phac-. *phak*itis
phalang- *phalanx, phalangos* [Gr.] a line or array of soldiers. *phalang*ectomy
phall- *phallos* [Gr.] penis. *phall*oplasty
phan- See phen-. *phan*erosis
pharmac- *pharmakon* [Gr.] drug. *pharmac*ognosy
pharyng- *pharynx, pharyng-* [Gr.] throat. *pharyng*ocele
-phas- *phasis* [Gr.] speech. a*phas*ia.
phe- *phaios* [Gr.] dun, dusky. *phe*omelanin
phen- *phainō, phan-* [Gr.] show, be seen. phos*phen*e, *phen*ocopy
pher- *pherō, phor-* [Gr.] bear, support. peri*pher*y
phil- *phileō* [Gr.] like, have affinity for. eosino*phil*ia
phleb- *phleps, phlebos* [Gr.] vein. Cf. ven-. peri*phleb*itis
phleg- *phlegō, phlog-* [Gr.] burn, inflame. *phleg*mon
phlog- See phleg-. *phlog*ogenic
phob- *phobos* [Gr.] fear, dread. claustro*phob*ia
phon- *phōne* [Gr.] sound. *phon*ocardiography
phor- See pher-. Cf. -ferent. exo*phor*ia
phos- See phot-. *phos*phorus
phot- *phōs, phōtos* [Gr.] light. *phot*ophobia
phrag- *phrassō, phrag-* [Gr.] fence, wall off, stop up. Cf. sept-^{1}. dia*phrag*m
phrax- *phrassō, phrag-* [Gr.] (*phrag-* added to *s* becomes *phrax-*) fence, wall off, stop up. urethro*phrax*is
phren- *phrēn* [Gr.] mind, midriff. Cf. ment-. *phren*oplegia, *phren*otropic. (See also psych- and thym-^{2})
phthi- *phthinō* [Gr.] decay, waste away. *phthi*sis

phy- *phyō* [Gr.] beget, bring forth, produce, be by nature. osteo*phyte*
phyc- *phykos* [Gr.] seaweed. *phyc*ochrome
phyl- *phylon* [Gr.] tribe, kind. *phyl*ogeny
phylac- *phylax* [Gr.] guard. pro*phylac*tic
phyll- *phyllon* [Gr.] leaf. chloro*phyll*, *phyll*oerythrin
phys- *physaō* [Gr.] blow, inflate. *phys*ometra
physe- *physaō*, *physē* [Gr.] blow, inflate. em*physe*ma
physi- *physis* [Gr.] nature. *physi*ology
phyt- *phyton* [Gr.] plant. *phyt*obezoar, dermato*phyte*
picr- *pikros* [Gr.] bitter. *picr*ogeusia
-piesis *piesis* [Gr.] a pressing or squeezing. aniso*piesis*
piez- *piezo* [Gr.] press. *piez*oelectricity
pil- *pilus* [L.] hair. e*pil*ation
pituit- *pituita* [L.] phlegm, rheum. *pituit*ary
placent- *placenta* [L.] (from *plakous* [Gr.]) cake. extra*placent*al
plas- *plassō* [Gr.] mold, shape. rhino*plas*ty
platy- *platy-* [Gr.] broad, flat. *platy*podia
pleg- *plēssō*, *pleg-* [Gr.] strike. di*pleg*ia
pleo- *pleiōn* [Gr.] more. *pleo*morphism, *pleio*tropy. (Also spelled pleio-)
plet- *pleo*, *-pletus* [L.] fill. *plet*hora
pleur- *pleura* [Gr.] rib, side. Cf. cost-. *pleur*algia
plex- *plēssō*, *plēg-* [Gr.] (*plēg-* added to *s* becomes *plēx-*) strike. apo*plex*y
plic- *plico* [L.] fold. com*plic*ation, *plic*ate
pluri- *plus*, *pluris* [L.] more. *pluri*glandular
pne- *pneuma*, *pneumatos* [Gr.] breathing. ortho*pne*a
pneum(at)- *pneuma*, *pneumatos* [Gr.] breath, air. *pneum*arthrosis, *pneumat*ocele
pneumo(n)- *pneumōn* [Gr.] lung. Cf. pulmo(n)-. *pneumo*enteritis, *pneumon*otomy
pod- *pous*, *podos* [Gr.] foot. *pod*iatry
poie- *poieō* [Gr.] make, produce. Cf. -facient. sarco*poie*tic
poikil- *poikilos* [Gr.] spotted, mottled, varied. *poikil*oderma
pol- *polos* [Gr.] axis of a sphere. uni*pol*ar
poli- *polios* [Gr.] gray. *poli*omyelopathy
poly- *polys* [Gr.] much, many. *poly*spermy
pont- *pons*, *pontis* [L.] bridge. *pont*ocerebellar
por-[1] *poros* [Gr.] passage. *por*adenitis
por-[2] *pōros* [Gr.] callus. *por*okeratosis
-pos- *posis* [Gr.] a drink. hyper*pos*ia
posit- *pono*, *positus* [L.] put, place. re*posit*or
post- *post* [L.] after, behind in time or place. *post*natal, *post*renal
pre- *prae* [L.] before in time or place. *pre*natal, *pre*vesical
presby- *presbys* [Gr.] old man. *presby*opia
press- *premo*, *pressus* [L.] press. *press*oreceptive
pro- *pro* [Gr.] or *pro* [L.] before in time or place. *pro*hormone, *pro*labium, *pro*lapse
proct- *prōktos* [Gr.] anus. Cf. rect-. *proct*ology
pros- *prosō* [Gr.] forward. *pros*odemic
prosop- *prosōpon* [Gr.] face. Cf. faci- *prosop*agnosia
prot- *prōtos* [Gr.] first. *prot*oplasm, *prot*otype
psamm- *psammos* [Gr.] sand. *psamm*oma
pseud- *pseudēs* [Gr.] false. *pseud*oparaplegia
psych- *psychē* [Gr.] soul, mind. Cf. ment-. *psych*osomatic. (See also phren- and thym-[2])
psychr- *psychros* [Gr.] cold. *psychr*oalgia
pto- *piptō*, *ptō* [Gr.] fall. nephro*pto*sis
ptyal- *ptyalon* [Gr.] saliva. *ptyal*ism
pub- *pubes* [L.] adult. ischio*pub*ic. (See also puber-)
puber- *puber* [L.] adult. *puber*ty
pulmo(n)- *pulmo*, *pulmonis* [L.] lung. Cf. pneumo(n)-. *pulmo*gram, cardio*pulmon*ary
puls- *pello*, *pellentis*, *pulus* [L] drive. pro*puls*ion
punct- *pungo*, *punctus* [L.] prick, pierce. Cf. cente-. *punct*iform
pupill- *pupilla* [L.] girl or pupil. *pupill*ometry
pur- *pus*, *puris* [L.] pus. Cf. py-. sup*pur*ation
py- *pyon* [Gr.] pus. Cf. pur-. spondylo*py*osis
pyel- *pyelos* [Gr.] trough, basin, pelvis. nephro*pyel*itis
pyg- *pygē* [Gr.] rump. *pyg*algia
pykn- *pyknos* [Gr.] thick, frequent. *pykn*omorphous, *pykn*ophrasia
pyl- *pylē* [Gr.] door, orifice. *pyl*ephlebitis
pyr- *pyr* [Gr.] fire. Cf. febr-. *pyr*ogen
quadr- *quadr-* [L.] four. Cf. tetr(a)-. *quadr*igeminal
quasi- *quasi* [L.] as if, as though. *quasi*dominance
quint- *quintus* [L.] fifth. Cf. pent(a)-. *quint*uplet
rachi- *rachis* [Gr.] spine. Cf. spin-. *rachi*odynia
radi- *radius* [L.] ray. Cf. actin-. ir*radi*ation, *radi*ocarpal
re- *re-* [L.] back, again. *re*traction
rect- *rectum* [L.] rectum. Cf. proct-. *rect*ocele
ren- *renes* [L.] kidney. Cf. nephr-. ad*ren*al, *ren*ography
ret- *rete* [L.] net. *ret*iform
retr- *retro* [L.] backwards. *retr*odeviation
rhabd- *rhabdos* [Gr.] rod. *rhabd*omyolysis
rhag- *rhēgnymi*, *rhag-* [Gr.] break, burst. hemor*rhag*ic
rhaph- *rhaphē* [Gr.] suture. arterior*rhaph*y
rhe- *rheos* [Gr.] flow. Cf. flu-. diar*rhe*al
rhex- *rhēgnymi*, *rhēg-* [Gr.] (*rhēg-* added to *s* becomes *rhēx-*) break, burst. metror*rhex*is
rhin- *rhis*, *rhinos* [Gr.] nose. Cf. nas-. *rhin*oplasty
rhiz- *rhiza* [Gr.] root. *rhiz*otomy
rhod- *rhodon* [Gr.] rose. *rhod*opsin
rhytid- *rhytis*, *rhytidos* [Gr.] wrinkle. *rhytid*ectomy
rot- *rota* [L.] wheel. *rot*ation
rub(r)- *ruber*, *rubri* [L.] red. Cf. erythr-. bili*rub*in, *rubr*ospinal
sacchar- *sakcharon* [Gr.] sugar. *sacchar*imeter
sacr- *sacrum* [L.] sacred, sacrum. *sacr*algia
salping- *salpinx*, *salpingos* [Gr.] tube, trumpet. *salping*itis
sangui(n)- *sanguis*, *sanguinis* [L.] blood. Cf. hem(at)-. *sangui*facient, *sanguin*eous
sapr- *sapros* [Gr.] rotten. *sapr*ophyte
sarc- *sarx*, *sarkos* [Gr.] flesh. *sarc*oma
scaph- *skaphē* [Gr.] skiff, light boat. *scaph*ocephaly
scat- *skōr*, *skatos* [Gr.] dung. *scat*ology
schis- *schizō*, *schid-* [Gr.] (*schid-* before *t* or added to *s* becomes *schis-*) split. Cf. fiss-. *schis*tocyte, thoraco*schis*is. (Also spelled *schiz-*)
schiz- See schis-. *schiz*onychia
scirrh- *skirrhos* [Gr.] hard. *scirrh*ous
scler- *sklēros* [Gr.] hard. Cf. dur-. *scler*osis
scoli- *skolios* [Gr.] twisted. *scoli*okyphosis
scop- *skopeō* [Gr.] look at, observe. endo*scop*e
scot- *skotos* [Gr.] darkness. *scot*ophobia
sect- *seco*, *sectus* [L.] cut. Cf. tom-. *sect*ion
semi- *semi* [L.] half. Cf. hemi-. *semi*flexion
sens- *sentio*, *sensus* [L.] perceive, feel. Cf. esthe-. *sens*ory
sep- *sepō* [Gr.] rot, decay. *sep*sis
sept-[1] *saepio*, *saeptus* [L.] fence, wall off, stop up. Cf. phrag-. *sept*onasal
sept-[2] *septum* [L.] seven. Cf. hept(a)-. *sept*uplet
ser- *serum* [L.] whey, watery substance. *ser*osynovitis
sex-[1] *sex* [L.] six. Cf. hex(a)-. *sex*tuplet
sex-[2] *sexus* [L.] sex. *sex*opathy
sial- *sialon* [Gr.] saliva. *sial*adenitis
sider- *sidēros* [Gr.] iron. *sider*oblast
sin- *sinus* [L.] hollow, fold. Cf. colp-. *sin*obronchitis
sinistr- *sinister* [L.] left. *sinistr*ocerebral
-sis *-sis* [Gr.] suffix of action. amebia*sis*, psycho*sis*, diagno*sis*
sit- *sitos* [Gr.] food. para*sit*ic
solen- *sōlēn* [Gr.] channel, gutter, pipe. *solen*onychia
solut- *solvo*, *solventis*, *solutus* [L.] loosen, dissolve, set free. Cf. ly-. dis*solut*ion
-solvent See solut-. re*solvent*
som(at)- *sōma*, *somatos* [Gr.] body. Cf. corpor-. psycho*somat*ic, chromo*some*
somn- *somnus* [L.] sleep. *somn*ambulism
spas- *spaō*, *spas-* [Gr.] draw, pull. *spas*m, *spas*tic
spectr- *spectrum* [L.] appearance, what is seen. micro*spectr*oscope
sperm(at)- *sperma*, *spermatos* [Gr.] seed. *sperm*icide, *spermat*ozoon
spers- *spargo*, *-spersus* [L.] scatter. di*spers*ion
sphen- *sphēn* [Gr.] wedge. Cf. cune-. *sphen*oid
spher- *sphaira* [Gr.] ball. hemi*sphere*
sphygm- *sphygmos* [Gr.] pulsation. *sphygm*omanometer
spin- *spina* [L.] spine. Cf. rachi-. *spin*ocerebellar
spir- *speira* [Gr.] coil. *spir*ochete
spir(at)- *spiro*, *spiratus* [L.] breathe. *spir*ometry, in*spirat*ory
splanchn- *splanchna* [Gr.] entrails, viscera. neuro*splanchn*ic
splen- *splēn* [Gr.] spleen. Cf. lien-. *splen*omegaly
spondyl- *spondylos* [Gr.] vertebra. *spondyl*olisthesis
spongi- *spongia* [L.] sponge. *spongi*oblastoma
spor- *sporos* [Gr.] seed. *spor*ocyst, zoo*spor*e
squam- *squama* [L.] scale. de*squam*ation
sta- *histēmi*, *sta-* [Gr.] make stand, stop. hemo*sta*sis
stal- *stellō*, *stal-* [Gr.] send. peri*stal*sis. (See also -stol-)
staphyl- *staphylē* [Gr.] bunch of grapes, uvula. *staphyl*ococcus, *staphyl*edema
stear- *stear*, *steatos* [Gr.] fat. Cf. adip-. *stear*ate. (See also lip-)
steat- See stear-. *steat*orrhea
sten- *stenos* [Gr.] narrow, compressed. *sten*othorax
ster- *stereos* [Gr.] solid. chole*ster*ol

sterc- *stercus* [L.] dung, feces. Cf. copr-. *stercoroma*
stern- *sternon* [Gr.] sternum. *sternalgia*, *sternoschisis*
steth- *stēthos* [Gr.] chest. *stethoscope*
sthen- *sthenos* [Gr.] strength. a*sthenia*
-stol- *stellō*, *stol-* [Gr.] send. dia*stole*
stom(at)- *stoma*, *stomatos* [Gr.] mouth, orifice. Cf. or-. ana*stomosis*, *stomatalgia*
strep(h)- *strephō*, *strep-* (before *t*) [Gr.] twist. Cf. tors-. *strephosymbolia*, *streptomycin*. (See also stroph-)
strict- *stringo*, *stringentis*, *strictus* [L.] draw tight, compress, cause pain. con*striction*
-stringent See strict-. a*stringent*
stroph- *strephō*, *stroph-* [Gr.] twist. Cf. tors-. angio*strophe*. (See also strep(h)-)
struct- *struo*, *structus* [L.] pile up (against). ob*struction*
styl- *stilus* [L.] stake, pole. *stylohyoid*, *stylosteophyte*
sub- *sub* [L.] (*b* changes to *f* and *p* before words beginning with those consonants) under, below. Cf. hypo-. *sublingual*
suf- See sub-. *suffusion*
sup- See sub-. *suppository*
super- *super* [L.] above, beyond, extreme. Cf. hyper-. *supermotility*
supra- *supra* [L.] above. *supraduction*
sy- See syn-. *systole*
sym- See syn-. *symbiosis*, *symmetry*, *sympathetic*, *symphysis*
syn- *syn* [Gr.] (*n* disappears before *s*, changes to *l* before *l*, and changes to *m* before *b*, *m*, *p*, and *ph*) with, together. Cf. con-. *synarthrosis*
syring- *syrinx*, *syringos* [Gr.] pipe, tube, fistula. *syringocystadenoma*
ta- See ton-. ec*tasia*
tac- *tassō*, *tag-* [Gr.] (*tag-* changes to *tak-*, which becomes *tac-*, before *t*) order, arrange. a*tactiform*
tach(y)- *tachys* [Gr.] swift. *tachography*, *tachycardia*
tact- *tango*, *tactus* [L.] touch. con*tact*
taenia- *taenia* [L.] tape. *taeniafuge*. (Also spelled tenia-)
tars- *tarsos* [Gr.] a broad, flat surface. *tarsorrhaphy*, *tarsoclasis*
taur- *taurus* [L.] bull. *taurodontism*
taut- *tautos* [Gr.] same. *tautomerism*
tax- *tassō*, *tag-* [Gr.] (*tag-* added to *s* becomes *tax-*) order, arrange. a*taxia*
tect- See teg-. pro*tective*
teg- *tego*, *tectus* [L.] cover. in*tegument*
tel- *telos* [Gr.] end. *telomere*
tele- *tēle* [Gr.] at a distance. *teleceptor*
tempor- *tempus*, *temporis* [L.] time, temple. *temporomandibular*
tend(in)- *tendo*, *tendines* [L.] tendon. *tendovaginal*, *tendinitis*
ten(ont)- *tenōn*, *tenontos* [Gr.] (from *teinō* stretch) tightly stretched band. *tenodynia*, *tenontology*
tens- *tendo*, *tensus* [L.] stretch. Cf. ton-. ex*tensor*
terat- *teras*, *teratos* [Gr.] monster. *teratoma*
ter(ti)- *ter* [L.] thrice. Cf. tri-. *termolecular*, *tertigravida*
test- *testis* [L.] testicle. Cf. orchi-. *testitis*
tetr(a)- *tetra-* [Gr.] four. Cf. quadr-. *tetradactyly*, *tetroxide*
thanat- *thanatos* [Gr.] death, *thanatophobia*
the- *tithēmi*, *thē-* [Gr.] put, place. syn*thesis*
thec- *thēkē* [Gr.] repository, case. *thecostegnosis*
thel(e)- *thēlē* [Gr.] teat, nipple. *thelerethism*, *theleplasty*
therap- *therapeia* [Gr.] treatment. chemo*therapy*
therm- *thermē* [Gr.] heat. Cf. calor-. dia*thermy*
thi- *theion* [Gr.] sulfur. *thiazole*, *thiocyanate*
thigm- *thigma* [Gr.] touch. *thigmotaxis*
thorac- *thōrax*, *thōrakos* [Gr.] chest. *thoracoplasty*
-thrix See trich-. monile*thrix*
thromb- *thrombos* [Gr.] lump, clot. *thrombocytopenia*
thym-[1] *thymos* [Gr.] thymus. *thymoma*
thym-[2] *thymos* [Gr.] spirit. Cf. ment-. dys*thymia*, *thymoleptic*. (See also phren- and psych-)
thyr- *thyreos* [Gr.] shield (shaped like a door [*thyra*]). *thyroid*
-tme- *temnō*, *tmē-* [Gr.] cut. axono*tmesis*
toc- *tokos* [Gr.] childbirth. dys*tocia*
tom- *temnō*, *tom-* [Gr.] cut. Cf. sect-. appendec*tomy*, *tomography*
ton- *teino*, *ton-*, *ta-* [Gr.] stretch, put under tension. Cf. tens-. peri*toneum*
top- *topos* [Gr.] place. Cf. loc-. *topesthesia*, iso*tope*
tors- *torqueo*, *torsus* [L.] twist. Cf. strep(h)- and stroph-. *torsion*
tox(ic)- *toxikon* [Gr.] (from *toxon* bow) arrow poison, poison. *toxemia*, *toxicology*
trache- *tracheia* [Gr.] windpipe. *tracheotomy*
trachel- *trachēlos* [Gr.] neck. Cf. cervic-. *trachelopexy*
tract- *traho*, *tractus* [L.] draw, drag. pro*traction*
trans- *trans* [L.] through, *transaortic*, *transfection*
traumat- *trauma*, *traumatos* [Gr.] wound. *traumatic*
trepo- *trepō* [Gr.] turn. *trepopnea*, *treponema*
tri- *treis*, *tria* [Gr.] or *tri-* [L.] three. Cf. ter(ti)-. *trilaminar*
trich- *thrix*, *trichos* [Gr.] hair. *trichobezoar*
trip- *tribō* [Gr.] rub. litho*tripsy*
trop- *trepō*, *trop-* [Gr.] turn, react. sito*tropism*
troph- *trepō*, *troph-* [Gr.] nurture. a*trophy*
tub- *tubus* [L.] pipe. *tuboplasty*
tuber- *tuber* [L.] swelling, node. *tubercle*
tympan- *tympanon* [Gr.] drum. *tympanocentesis*
typ- *typos* [Gr.] (from *typto* strike) type. a*typical*
typh- *typhos* [Gr.] fog, stupor. *typhus*
typhl- *typhlos* [Gr.] blind. Cf. cec-. *typhlectomy*
tyr- *tyros* [Gr.] cheese. *tyrogenous*
ul-[1] *oulē* [Gr.] scar. *ulerythema*
ul-[2] *oulon* [Gr.] gum. *ulatrophy*
ultra- *ultra* [L.] beyond. *ultrastructure*
uni- *unus* [L.] one. Cf. hen-. *unilateral*
ur- *ouron* [Gr.] urine. poly*uria*
uran- *ouranos* [Gr.] the vault of heaven, or the roof of the mouth. Cf. palat-. *uranostaphyloplasty*
ureter- *ourētēr* [Gr.] ureter. *ureterography*
urethr- *ourēthra* [Gr.] urethra. *urethropexy*
uter- *uterus* [L.] womb. Cf. hyster- and metr-[2]. *uterorectal*
vacc- *vacca* [L.] cow. *vaccine*
vagin- *vagina* [L.] sheath. in*vagination*, *vaginitis*
varic- *varix*, *varicis* [L.] varicose vein. *varicocele*
vas- *vas* [L.] vessel. Cf. angi-. *vascular*
ven- *vena* [L.] vein. Cf. phleb-. *venopressor*
ventr- *venter* [L.] belly. *ventrocystorrhaphy*, *ventriculotomy*
vers- See vert-. in*version*
vert- *verto*, *versus* [L.] turn. di*verticulum*
vesic- *vesica* [L.] bladder. Cf. cyst-. *vesicovaginal*
video- *video* [L.] see. *videolaparoscopy*
viscer- *viscus*, *visceris* [L.] internal organs. *visceromotor*
vit- *vita* [L.] life. Cf. bi-[1]. de*vitalize*
vivi- *vivus* [L.] alive. *viviparous*
vuls- *vello*, *vulsus* [L.] pull, twitch. con*vulsion*
xanth- *xanthos* [Gr.] yellow, blond. Cf. flav- and lute-. *xanthochromia*
xen- *xenos* [Gr.] strange, foreign. *xenograft*
xer- *xēros* [Gr.] dry. *xeroderma*
xiph- *xiphos* [Gr.] sword, xiphoid process. *xiphodynia*
-yl- *hyle* [Gr.] substance. carbox*yl*
zo- *zoē* [Gr.] life or *zōon* [Gr.] animal. micro*zoon*
zyg- *zygon* [Gr.] yoke, union. *zygodactyly*
zym- *zymē* [Gr.] ferment. en*zyme*

APPENDIX 2

SELECTED ABBREVIATIONS USED IN MEDICINE

A accommodation; adenine; adenosine; alanine; alveolar gas (as subscript); ampere; anode; anterior
A. L. annum (year)
A absorbance; activity; admittance; area; mass number
AI secondary auditory cortex
AII second auditory area
A_2 aortic second sound
Å angstrom
a accommodation; arterial blood (as subscript); atto-
a. L. annum (year); L. aqua (water); L. arteria (artery)
a acceleration; activity; specific absorptivity
ā L. ante (before)
α alpha chain of hemoglobin; Bunsen coefficient; heavy chain of IgA; the probability of Type I error
AA achievement age; amino acid
aa. L. arteriae (arteries)
AAO amino acid oxidase
AAS anabolic-androgenic steroid
AAV adeno-associated virus
AB L. Artium Baccalaureus (Bachelor of Arts)
Ab antibody
ABC argon beam coagulator; aspiration biopsy cytology; avidin-biotin complex
ABCD Adriamycin (doxorubicin), bleomycin, CCNU (lomustine), and dacarbazine
ABE acute bacterial endocarditis
ABG arterial blood gases
ABI ankle-brachial index
ABLE alternate binatural loudness balance
ABMT autologous bone marrow transplantation
ABP arterial blood pressure
ABR auditory brainstem response
abs. feb. L. absente febre (while fever is absent)
abst, abstr abstract
ABVD Adriamycin (doxorubicin), bleomycin, vinblastine, and dacarbazine
AC acromioclavicular; air conduction; alternating current; axiocervical; Adriamycin (doxorubicin) and cyclophosphamide
Ac actinium
a.c. L. ante cibum (before meals)
ACAT acyl CoA:cholesterol acyltransferase
Acc accommodation
ACD acid citrate dextrose
ACE angiotensin-converting enzyme
ACG angiocardiography; apexcardiogram
AcG accelerator globulin (factor V)
ACh acetylcholine
AchE acetylcholinesterase
ACP acid phosphatase
ACPS acrocephalopolysyndactyly
ACTH adrenocorticotropic hormone
AD alcohol dehydrogenase; L. auris dextra (right ear)
ADA adenosine deaminase
ADCC antibody-dependent cell-mediated cytotoxicity
add. L. adde (add); L. addatur (let there be added)
ADH alcohol dehydrogenase; antidiuretic hormone
Adhib. L. adhibendus (to be administered)
ADL activities of daily living
ad lib. L. ad libitum (at pleasure)
admov. L. admove (add); L. admoveatur (let there be added)
AdoCbl adenosylcobalamin
ADP adenosine diphosphate
ADPKD autosomal dominant polycystic kidney disease
Ad pond. om. L. ad pondus omnium (to the weight of the whole)
adst. feb. L. adstante febre (while fever is present)
Adv. L. adversum (against)
Ad 2 vic. L. ad duas vices (at two times, for two doses)
A-E, AE above-elbow
AED automatic external defibrillator
Aeg. L. aeger, aegra (the patient)
AEP auditory evoked potential
aet. L. aetas (age)
AF atrial fibrillation
AFib atrial fibrillation
AFl atrial flutter
AFO ankle-foot orthosis
AFP alpha fetoprotein
AFX atypical fibroxanthoma
AG atrial gallop
Ag antigen; silver (L. argentum)
AGE advanced glycation end product
AGEP acute generalized exanthematous pustulosis
AGEPC acetyl glyceryl ether phosphoryl choline
aggred. fed. L. aggrediente febre (while the fever is coming on)
Agit. vas. L. agitato vase (the vial being shaken)
AGT antiglobulin test
ah hyperopic astigmatism
AHA acetohydroxamic acid
AHF antihemophilic factor (factor VIII)
AHG antihemophilic globulin (factor VIII)
AHP Assistant House Physician
AHS Assistant House Surgeon
AI anaphylatoxin inactivator; aortic incompetence; aortic insufficiency; apical impulse; aromatase inhibitor; artificial insemination
AICC anti-inhibitor coagulant complex
AICD activation-induced cell death; automatic implantable cardioverter-defibrillator
AID artificial insemination by donor
AIDS acquired immunodeficiency syndrome
AIH artificial insemination by husband
AIHA autoimmune hemolytic anemia
AILD angioimmunoblastic lymphadenopathy with dysproteinemia
AIP acute intermittent porphyria
AIS androgen insensitivity syndrome
A-K, AK above-knee
Al aluminum
ALA aminolevulinic acid
Ala alanine
ALARA as low as reasonably achievable (exposure dose of radiation)
ALAS 5-aminolevulinate synthase
ALAT alanine aminotransferase
ALG antilymphocyte globulin
ALL acute lymphoblastic leukemia
ALM acral-lentiginous melanoma
ALP alkaline phosphatase
ALS amyotrophic lateral sclerosis; antilymphocyte serum
ALT alanine transaminase
Alt. dieb. L. alternis diebus (every other day)
Alt. hor. L. alternis horis (every other hour)
AM L. Artium Magister (Master of Arts)
Am americium
am ametropia; meter angle; myopic astigmatism
AMAN acute motor axonal neuropathy
AME apparent mineralocorticoid excess
Amh mixed astigmatism with myopia predominating over hyperopia
AMI acute myocardial infarction
AML acute myelogenous leukemia
AMP adenosine monophosphate
3′,5′-AMP cyclic AMP; cyclic adenosine monophosphate
ams amount of a substance
amu atomic mass unit
An anodal; anode
ANA antinuclear antibodies
anat. anatomical; anatomy
ANCA antineutrophil cytoplasmic autoantibody (or antibody)
ANCOVA analysis of covariance

Appendix 2

ANF antinuclear factor
ANNA-1 type 1 antineuronal antibody
ANNA-2 type 2 antineuronal antibody
ANOVA analysis of variance
ANP atrial natriuretic peptide
ANS anterior nasal spine; autonomic nervous system
ant. anterior
ANTU alphanaphthyl thiourea
ANUG acute necrotizing ulcerative gingivitis
AO ankle orthosis; opening of the atrioventricular valves
AP action potential; angina pectoris; anterior pituitary; anteroposterior; arterial pressure
Apaf-1 apoptotic protease activating factor 1
APB atrial premature beat
APC atrial premature complex; activated protein C
APCA anti–Purkinje cell antibody
APCC anti-inhibitor coagulant complex
APD atrial premature depolarization; pamidronate (aminohydroxypropylidene diphosphonate)
APECED autoimmune polyendocrinopathy-candidiasis-ectodermal dysplasia; autoimmune polyendocrinopathy-candidiasis-ectodermal dystrophy
APF acidulated phosphate fluoride
APN advanced practice nurse
APP amyloid precursor protein
APRI AST to platelet ratio index
APRN advanced practice registered nurse
APS antiphospholipid (antibody) syndrome
APTT, aPTT activated partial thromboplastin time
APUD amine precursor uptake (and) decarboxylation
AQ achievement quotient
Aq. L. aqua (water)
Aq. dest. L. aqua destillata (distilled water)
Aq. pur. L. aqua pura (pure water)
Aq. tep. L. aqua tepida (tepid water)
AR alarm reaction; aortic regurgitation; artificial respiration
Ar argon
ara-A adenine arabinoside
ara-C arabinosylcytosine
ARC AIDS-related complex; anomalous retinal correspondence
ARD acute respiratory disease (of any undefined form); acute respiratory distress
ARDS acute respiratory distress syndrome; adult respiratory distress syndrome
ARF acute renal failure
Arg arginine
ARN acute retinal necrosis
AROA autosomal recessive ocular albinism
ARPKD autosomal recessive polycystic kidney disease
ART Accredited Record Technician; assisted reproductive technology; automated reagin test
AS aortic stenosis; arteriosclerosis; L. auris sinistra (left ear)
As arsenic; astigmatism
ASA acetylsalicylic acid; argininosuccinic acid; antisperm antibody
5-ASA 5-aminosalicylic acid
ASAT aspartate aminotransferase
ASCT autologous stem cell transplantation
ASCVD arteriosclerotic cardiovascular disease
ASF aniline, formaldehyde, and sulfur
ASH asymmetrical septal hypertrophy
ASHD arteriosclerotic heart disease
ASI Addiction Severity Index
ASL antistreptolysin
Asn asparagine
ASO arteriosclerosis obliterans
Asp aspartic acid
asRNA antisense RNA
ASS anterior superior spine (of ilium)
AST aspartate transaminase
Ast. astigmatism
Asth. asthenopia
AT atrial tachycardia
At astatine
ATA alimentary toxic aleukia
ATCC American Type Culture Collection
ATG antithymocyte globulin
ATL adult T-cell leukemia/lymphoma
atm atmosphere
ATN tyrosinase-negative (ty-neg) oculocutaneous albinism
at no atomic number
ATP adenosine triphosphate
ATPase adenosinetriphosphatase
ATS antitetanic serum
at vol atomic volume
at wt atomic weight
AU L. aures unitas (both ears together); L. auris uterque (each ear)
Au Australia antigen; gold (L. aurum)
AUC area under the curve
AUL acute undifferentiated leukemia
AV, A-V atrioventricular; arteriovenous
av avoirdupois
AVA anthrax vaccine adsorbed
AVN atrioventricular node
AVP arginine vasopressin
AVRT atrioventricular reciprocating tachycardia
awu atomic weight unit
ax. axis
Az azote
AZOOR acute zonal occult outer retinopathy
AZQ diaziquone
AZT zidovudine
B bel; boron
B magnetic flux density
b barn; base (nucleic acids); born
β beta chain of hemoglobin
BA Bachelor of Arts
Ba barium
BAC bacterial artificial chromosome
BACOP bleomycin, Adriamycin (doxorubicin), cyclophosphamide, Oncovin (vincristine), and prednisone
BAEP brain stem auditory evoked potential
BAL British antilewisite; biphenotypic acute leukemia
BAN British Approved Name
BAO basal acid output
BATO boronic acid adduct of technetium oxime
BBB blood-brain barrier; bundle branch block
BBBB bilateral bundle branch block
BBT basal body temperature
BC bone conduction
BCAA branched-chain amino acids
B-CAVe bleomycin, CCNU (lomustine), Adriamycin (doxorubicin), and vinblastine
BCDF B cell differentiation factors
BCF basophil chemotactic factor
BCG bacille Calmette-Guérin; bicolor guaiac test; ballistocardiogram
BCGF B cell growth factors
BDNF brain-derived neurotrophic factor
BCNU carmustine
b.d. L. bis die (twice a day)
BDS Bachelor of Dental Surgery
BDSc Bachelor of Dental Science
B-E, BE below-elbow
Be beryllium
BF blastogenic factor
BFP biologic false-positive
BFU-E burst-forming unit-erythroid
BH4 tetrahydrobiopterin
BHA butylated hydroxyanisole
BHC benzene hexachloride
BHT butylated hydroxytoluene
Bi bismuth
Bib. L. bibe (drink)
b.i.d. L. bis in die (twice a day)
B-K, BK below-knee
Bk berkelium
BKV BK virus
BMI body mass index
BMP bone morphogenetic protein
BMR basal metabolic rate
BMS Bachelor of Medical Science
BMT behavioral marital therapy; bone marrow transplantation
BNA *Basle Nomina Anatomica*
BNP brain natriuretic peptide
Bol. L. bolus (pill)
BOOP bronchiolitis obliterans with organizing pneumonia
BP blood pressure; British Pharmacopoeia
bp base pair; boiling point
BPD bronchopulmonary dysplasia
BPH benign prostatic hyperplasia
B Ph British Pharmacopoeia

BPI	bactericidal permeability increasing protein
BPIG	bacterial polysaccharide immune globulin
BPRS	Brief Psychiatric Rating Scale
Bq	becquerel
Br	bromine
BrdU	5-bromodeoxyuridine
BrIDA	mebrofenin
BRM	biologic response modifier
BS	Bachelor of Surgery; Bachelor of Science; blood sugar; breath sounds
BSA	body surface area
BSF	B lymphocyte stimulatory factor
BSS	Bernard-Soulier syndrome
BTK	Bruton tyrosine kinase
BTU	British thermal unit
BUDR	5-bromodeoxyuridine
Bull.	L. bulliat (let it boil)
BUN	blood urea nitrogen
But.	L. butyrum (butter)
BVAD	biventricular assist device
C	canine (tooth); carbon; cathode; Celsius (scale); cervical vertebrae (C1–C7); clonus; closure; color sense; complement (C1–C9); compliance (subscripts denote the structure, e.g., C_L lung compliance); contraction; coulomb; cylinder; cylindrical lens; cytidine; cytosine; large calorie
C	capacitance; clearance (subscripts denote the substance, e.g., C_I or C_{In} inulin clearance); heat capacity
°C	degree Celsius
c	centi-; small calorie
c.	L. cibus (food); L. cum (with)
c	molar concentration; specific heat capacity; velocity of light in a vacuum
$\bar{c}$	L. cum (with)
χ^2	chi-square
CA	cardiac arrest; chronologic age; cold agglutinin; coronary artery; croup-associated (virus)
CA 125	cancer antigen 125
Ca	calcium
ca	L. circa (about)
CABG	coronary artery bypass graft
CAD	coronary artery disease; chronic actinic dermatitis
CAH	congenital adrenal hyperplasia
CAIS	complete androgen insensitivity syndrome
Cal	large calorie (kilocalorie)
cal	calorie
Calef.	L. calefac (make warm); L. calefactus (warmed)
CALLA	common acute lymphoblastic leukemia antigen
CAM	cell adhesion molecules; complementary and alternative medicine
cAMP	cyclic adenosine monophosphate
CAP	catabolite (gene) activator protein
Cap.	L. capiat (let him take)
CAPD	continuous ambulatory peritoneal dialysis
Capsul.	L. capsula (capsule)
CAR	cancer-associated retinopathy
CASA	computer-aided (or assisted) semen analysis
CAT	computerized axial tomography
Cath.	L. catharticus (cathartic)
CAVB	complete atrioventricular block
CB	L. Chirurgiae Baccalaureus (Bachelor of Surgery)
cbc	complete blood count
CBF	cerebral blood flow
CBG	corticosteroid-binding globulin
Cbl	cobalamin
CC	chief complaint
cc	cubic centimeter *(on the JCAHO "Do Not Use" List)*
CCA	congenital contractural arachnodactyly
CCAT	conglutinating complement absorption test
CCF	crystal-induced chemotactic factor
CCHS	congenital central hypoventilation syndrome
CCK	cholecystokinin
CCP	complement control protein; cyclic citrullinated peptide
CCPD	continuous cycling peritoneal dialysis
CCU	coronary care unit; critical care unit
CD	cadaveric donor; cluster designation; conjugata diagonalis; curative dose
CD$_{50}$	median curative dose
Cd	cadmium; caudal; coccygeal
cd	candela
2-CdA	cladribine
CDC	Centers for Disease Control and Prevention
CDDP	cisplatin (*cis*-diamminedichloroplatinum)
cdf	cumulative distribution function
CDG	congenital disorder of glycosylation
CDH	congenital dislocation of the hip
cDNA	complementary DNA; copy DNA
CDP	cytidine diphosphate
Ce	cerium
CEA	carcinoembryonic antigen
Cel	Celsius
CEM	contagious equine metritis
CEP	congenital erythropoietic porphyria
ces	central excitatory state
CESD	cholesteryl ester storage disease
CETP	cholesteryl ester transfer protein
CF	carbolfuchsin; cardiac failure; Christmas factor; citrovorum factor
Cf	californium
CFAP	chronic functional abdominal pain
CFC	chlorofluorocarbon
cff	critical fusion frequency
CFT	complement fixation test
CFTR	cystic fibrosis transmembrane regulator
CFU	colony-forming unit
CFU-C	colony-forming unit-culture
CFU-E	colony-forming unit-erythroid
CFU-GM	colony-forming unit-granulocyte-macrophage
CFU-S	colony-forming unit-spleen
CGD	chronic granulomatous disease
CGH	comparative genomic hybridization
cGMP	cyclic guanosine monophosphate
CGS, cgs	centimeter-gram-second system
cGy	centigray
CH	crown-heel (length of fetus)
CH50, CH$_{50}$	total hemolytic complement
CHAOS	congenital high airway obstruction syndrome
CJD	Creutzfeldt-Jakob disease
Chart.	L. charta (paper)
ChB	L. Chirurgiae Baccalaureus (Bachelor of Surgery)
CHD	congenital heart disease; coronary heart disease
ChD	L. Chirurgiae Doctor (Doctor of Surgery)
ChE	cholinesterase
CHF	congestive heart failure
CHL	crown-heel length (of fetus)
ChM	L. Chirurgiae Magister (Master of Surgery)
CHO	Chinese hamster ovary (cell)
CHOP	cyclophosphamide, hydroxydaunomycin (doxorubicin), Oncovin (vincristine), and prednisone
CHOP-BLEO	cyclophosphamide, hydroxydaunomycin (doxorubicin), Oncovin (vincristine), prednisone, and bleomycin
Chr	chromosome
CHS	cholinesterase
CI	cardiac index; Colour Index
Ci	curie
cib.	L. cibus (food)
CIDP	chronic inflammatory demyelinating polyneuropathy
CIE	counterimmunoelectrophoresis
CIH	Certificate in Industrial Health
Ci-hr	curie-hour
CIN	cervical intraepithelial neoplasia
C1 INH	C1 inhibitor
CK	creatine kinase
Cl	chlorine
ClC	chloride channel
CLIP	corticotropin-like intermediate lobe peptide
CM	L. Chirurgiae Magister (Master of Surgery)
Cm	curium
cM	centimorgan
cm	centimeter
cm^2	square centimeter
cm^3	cubic centimeter
CMA	Certified Medical Assistant
CMAP	compound muscle action potential
CMD	cerebromacular degeneration
CMF	cyclophosphamide, methotrexate, and 5-fluorouracil
CMHC	community mental health center
cm H_2O	centimeter(s) of water
CMI	cell-mediated immunity
CML	cell-mediated lympholysis
c mm	cubic millimeter
C-MOPP	cyclophosphamide, Oncovin (vincristine), procarbazine, and prednisone
CMP	cytidine monophosphate

Appendix 2

c.m.s. L. cras mane sumendus (to be taken tomorrow morning)
CMT California mastitis test; Certified Medical Transcriptionist; Charcot-Marie-Tooth disease
CMV cytomegalovirus
CN chloroacetophenone
c.n. L. cras nocte (tomorrow night)
CN-Cbl cyanocobalamin
C3 NeF C3 nephritic factor
CNM Certified Nurse-Midwife
CNS central nervous system
c.n.s. L. cras nocte sumendus (to be taken tomorrow night)
CNV contingent negative variation
CO cardiac output
Co cobalt; coccygeal (in vertebral formulas)
CoA coenzyme A
CoA-SH coenzyme A
COBS cesarean-obtained barrier–sustained
COC calcifying odontogenic cyst
cochl. L. cochleare (a spoonful)
cochl. amp. L. cochleare amplum (a heaping spoonful)
cochl. mag. L. cochleare magnum (a tablespoonful)
cochl. med. L. cochleare medium (a dessertspoonful)
cochl. parv. L. cochleare parvum (a teaspoonful)
Coct. L. coctio (boiling)
Col. L. cola (strain)
Colat. L. colatus (strained)
COLD chronic obstructive lung disease
Colet. L. coletur (let it be strained)
Collut. L. collutorium (mouth wash)
Collyr. L. collyrium (an eye wash)
Color. L. coloretur (let it be colored)
COMP cartilage oligomeric matrix protein
Comp. L. compositus (compound)
ConA concanavalin A
Concis. L. concisus (cut)
Cons. L. conserva (keep)
Cont. L. contusus (bruised)
Contin. L. continuetur (let it be continued)
Cont. rem. L. continuetur remedium (let the medicine be continued)
COP cyclophosphamide, Oncovin (vincristine), and prednisone
COP-BLAM cyclophosphamide, Oncovin (vincristine), prednisone, bleomycin, Adriamycin (doxorubicin), and Matulane (procarbazine)
COPD chronic obstructive pulmonary disease
COPP cyclophosphamide, Oncovin (vincristine), procarbazine, and prednisone
Coq. L. coque (boil)
Coq. in s. a. L. coque in sufficiente aqua (boil in sufficient water)
Coq. s. a. L. coque secundum artem (boil properly)
Cort. L. cortex (bark)
CP candle power; chemically pure
cp centipoise
C3PA C3 proactivator (former name for factor B)
CPAP continuous positive airway pressure
CPC clinicopathological conference
CPD citrate phosphate dextrose
CPDA-1 citrate phosphate dextrose adenine
CPDD calcium pyrophosphate deposition disease
C Ped Certified Pedorthist
CPH Certificate in Public Health
CPI California Personality Inventory; congenital palatopharyngeal incompetence
CPK creatine phosphokinase
CPM central pontine myelinolysis; cyclophosphamide
cpm counts per minute
CPP cerebral perfusion pressure
CPPD calcium pyrophosphate dihydrate
CPPS chronic pelvic pain syndrome
CPR cardiopulmonary resuscitation
CPS carbamoyl phosphate synthetase
CPSI carbamoyl phosphate synthetase I
CPSII carbamoyl phosphate synthetase II
cps cycles per second
CR complement receptor; conditioned response; crown-rump (length of fetus)
CR3 complement receptor type 3
Cr chromium
Crast. L. crastinus (for tomorrow)
CREG cross-reactive group (of HLA antigens)
CRF chronic renal failure
CRH corticotropin-releasing hormone
CRL crown-rump length (of fetus)
CRM cross-reacting material
CRNA Certified Registered Nurse Anesthetist
cRNA complementary RNA
CRP C-reactive protein
CRPS complex regional pain syndrome
CRRT continuous renal replacement therapy
Crys. crystal
CS cesarean section; conditioned stimulus; coronary sinus; *o*-chlorobenzylidenemalononitrile
Cs cesium
CSC Fr. coup sur coup (blow on blow)
CSF cerebrospinal fluid; colony-stimulating factor
CSF-1 macrophage colony-stimulating factor
CSII continuous subcutaneous insulin infusion
CSM cerebrospinal meningitis
C-spine cervical spine
CST contraction stress test
CT computed tomography
CTBA cetrimonium bromide
CTL cytotoxic T lymphocytes
CTP cytidine triphosphate
Cu copper (L. cuprum)
Cuj. L. cujus (of which)
CV cardiovascular; closing volume; coefficient of variation
C.V. L. cras vespere (tomorrow evening); L. conjugata vera (true conjugate diameter of the pelvic inlet)
CVA cerebrovascular accident; costovertebral angle
CVID common variable immunodeficiency
CVP central venous pressure; cyclophosphamide, vincristine, and prednisone
CVS cardiovascular system; chorionic villus sampling
CX circumflex artery
Cx cervix; convex
Cy cyanogen
Cyath. L. cyathus (a glassful)
CYC cyclophosphamide
cyclic AMP cyclic adenosine monophosphate
cyclic GMP cyclic guanosine monophosphate
cyl cylinder; cylindrical lens
Cys cysteine
Cys-Cys cystine
D dalton; deciduous (teeth); decimal reduction time; density; deuterium; died; diffusing capacity; diopter; distal; dorsal vertebrae (D1–D12); dose; duration; dwarf (colony)
D. L. da (give); L. detur (let it be given); L. dexter (right); L. dosis (dose)
D_L diffusing capacity of the lung
d day; deci-; deoxyribose
d. L. da (give); L. detur (let it be given); L. dexter (right); L. dosis (dose)
d density; diameter
Δ change (as in temperature); increment
δ delta chain of hemoglobin; heavy chain of IgD
DA developmental age; diphenylchlorarsine
Da dalton
DAC decitabine
DACT dactinomycin
DAD delayed afterdepolarization
dADP deoxyadenosine diphosphate
DAEC diffusely adherent *Escherichia coli*
DAF decay accelerating factor
DAG diacylglycerol
dAMP deoxyadenosine monophosphate
D and C dilatation and curettage
dATP deoxyadenosine triphosphate
DAy Doctor of Ayurvedic Medicine
dB, db decibel
DBA dibenzanthracene
DBS deep brain stimulation
DC direct current; Doctor of Chiropractic
D & C dilatation and curettage
dC deoxycytidine
DCA desoxycorticosterone acetate
DCc double concave
dCDP deoxycytidine diphosphate
DCF direct centrifugal flotation
DCH Diploma in Child Health
DCIS ductal carcinoma in situ
dCMP deoxycytidine monophosphate

DCOG Diploma of the College of Obstetricians and Gynaecologists (British)
dCTP deoxycytidine triphosphate
DCx double convex
d.d. L. detur ad (let it be given to)
ddC dideoxycytidine
DDH developmental dysplasia of the hip
ddI dideoxyinosine
DDP, *cis*-DDP cisplatin (*cis*-diamminedichloroplatinum)
DDS diaminodiphenylsulfone (dapsone); Doctor of Dental Surgery
DDSc Doctor of Dental Science
Deb. spis. L. debita spissitudine (of the proper consistency)
Dec. L. decanta (pour off)
Decoct. L. decoctum (a decoction)
Decub. L. decubitus (lying down)
de d. in d. L. de die in diem (from day to day)
DEF decayed, extracted, filled
Deg degeneration; degree
Deglut. L. deglutiatur (let it be swallowed)
del deletion
Dep. L. depuratus (purified)
DES diethylstilbestrol
dest. L. destilla (distill); L. destillatus (distilled)
destil. L. destilla (distill)
DET diethyltryptamine
Det. L. detur (let it be given)
Det. in dup., Det. in 2 plo L. detur in duplo (let twice as much be given)
D. et s. L. detur et signetur (let it be given and labeled)
DFDT difluoro-diphenyl-trichloroethane
DFP diisopropyl fluorophosphate
DFT defibrillation threshold
dG deoxyguanosine
DGC dystrophin-glycoprotein complex
dGDP deoxyguanosine diphosphate
dGMP deoxyguanosine monophosphate
dGTP deoxyguanosine triphosphate
DH delayed hypersensitivity
DHA 2,8-dihydroxyadenine; docosahexaenoic acid
DHAD mitoxantrone hydrochloride (dihydroanthracenedione dihydrochloride)
DHEA dehydroepiandrosterone
DHF dihydrofolate; dihydrofolic acid
DHFR dihydrofolate reductase
DHg Doctor of Hygiene
DHom Doctor of Homeopathic Medicine
DHPG 3,4-dihydroxyphenylglycol; ganciclovir (9-[(1,3-dihydroxy-2-propoxy)methyl] guanine)
DHPR 6,7-dihydropteridine reductase
DHS dehydrated hereditary stomatocytosis
DHT dihydrotestosterone
DHy Doctor of Hygiene
DIC diffuse intravascular coagulation; disseminated intravascular coagulation
Dieb. alt. L. diebus alternis (on alternate days)
Dieb. tert. L. diebus tertiis (every third day)
Dig. L. digeratur (let it be digested)
dil. L. dilue (dilute, dissolve)
Diluc. L. diluculo (at daybreak)
dilut. L. dilutus (diluted)
dim. L. dimidius (one half)
D. in p. aeq. L. divide in partes aequales (divide into equal parts)
DIP distal interphalangeal
Dir. prop. L. directione propria (with proper direction)
DIS Diagnostic Interview Schedule
DISH diffuse idiopathic skeletal hyperostosis
DISIDA disofenin (diisopropyl iminodiacetic acid)
Dist. L. distilla (distill)
Div. L. divide (divide)
DJD degenerative joint disease
dk deca-
DKA diabetic ketoacidosis
DL diffusing capacity of the lung
dL deciliter
DLE discoid lupus erythematosus
DM diabetes mellitus; diphenylamine chlorarsine
DMAPN dimethylaminopropionitrile
DMARD disease-modifying antirheumatic drug
DMBA 7,12-dimethylbenz[a]anthracene
DMD Doctor of Dental Medicine
DMF decayed, missing, filled; dimethylformamide
DMPE 3,4-dimethoxyphenylethylamine
DMRD Diploma in Medical Radio-Diagnosis (British)
DMRT Diploma in Medical Radio-Therapy (British)
DMSA succimer (*meso*-2,3-dimercaptosuccinic acid)
DMSO dimethyl sulfoxide
DMT dimethyltryptamine
DN dibucaine number
DNA deoxyribonucleic acid
DNase deoxyribonuclease
DNB dinitrobenzene; Diplomate of the National Board (of Medical Examiners)
DNCB dinitrochlorobenzene
DNFB dinitrofluorobenzene
DNOC dinitro-*o*-cresol
DNR do not resuscitate
DO Doctor of Osteopathy
DOA dead on arrival
DOC 11-deoxycorticosterone
DOM 2,5-dimethoxy-4-methylamphetamine
Donec alv. sol. fuerit L. donec alvus soluta fuerit (until the bowels are opened, i.e., until a bowel movement occurs)
DP Doctor of Pharmacy; Doctor of Podiatry; L. directione propria (with proper direction)
DPH Diploma in Public Health
DPM Diploma in Psychological Medicine; Doctor of Podiatric Medicine
DPT diphtheria and tetanus toxoids and pertussis vaccine
DR reaction of degeneration
dr dram
DRE digital rectal examination
DRG Diagnosis-Related Group
DrPH Doctor of Public Health
DRPLA dentatorubral-pallidoluysian atrophy
DSC Doctor of Surgical Chiropody
DSD disorder of sexual development
dsDNA double-stranded DNA
DSM Diagnostic and Statistical Manual of Mental Disorders
dsRNA double-stranded RNA
DT diphtheria and tetanus toxoids
Dt duration tetany
dT deoxythymidine
DTaP diphtheria and tetanus toxoids and acellular pertussis vaccine
D.T.D. L. datur talis dosis (give of such a dose)
dTDP deoxythymidine diphosphate
DTH delayed-type hypersensitivity
DTIC, Dtic dacarbazine
dTMP deoxythymidine monophosphate
DTP diphtheria and tetanus toxoids and pertussis vaccine
DTPA diethylenetriamine pentaacetic acid
dTTP deoxythymidine triphosphate
dU deoxyuridine
DUB dysfunctional uterine bleeding
DUH dyschromatosis universalis hereditaria
dUMP deoxyuridine monophosphate
Dur. dolor. L. durante dolore (while the pain lasts)
dUTP deoxyuridine triphosphate
dv double vibrations
DVM Doctor of Veterinary Medicine
DVT deep vein thrombosis; deep venous thrombosis
Dy dysprosium
dyn dyne
E enzyme
E elastance; energy; expectancy; electromotive force; illumination; electric intensity; redox potential
E_1 estrone
E_2 estradiol
E_3 estriol
E_4 estetrol
E_h redox potential
E° standard reduction potential
e electron
e elementary unit of electric charge; the base of natural logarithms
e^+ positron
e^- electron
ε epsilon chain of hemoglobin; heavy chain of IgE; molar absorptivity
η absolute viscosity
EAC erythrocyte, antibody, and complement
EACA epsilon-aminocaproic acid
EAD early afterdepolarization

Appendix 2

ead. L. eadem (the same)
EAE experimental allergic encephalomyelitis
EAEC enteroadherent *Escherichia coli*
EAggEC enteroaggregative *Escherichia coli*
EAHF eczema, asthma, hay fever
EAP epiallopregnanolone
EAR expired air resuscitation
Ea. R. Ger. Entartungs-Reaktion (reaction of degeneration)
EAV electroacupuncture after Voll
EB elementary body
EBCT electron beam computed tomography
EBL enzootic bovine leukosis
EBV Epstein-Barr virus
EC Enzyme Commission
ECD ethyl cysteinate dimer
ECF extracellular fluid; eosinophil chemotactic factor; extended care facility
ECF-A eosinophil chemotactic factor of anaphylaxis
ECG electrocardiogram
ECI electrocerebral inactivity
ECLS extracorporeal life support
ECM extracellular matrix
ECMO extracorporeal membrane oxygenation
ECS electrocerebral silence
ECT electroconvulsive therapy
ED effective dose; emergency department; erectile dysfunction; erythema dose
ED$_{50}$ median effective dose
EDR effective direct radiation; electrodermal response
EDRF endothelium-derived relaxing factor
EDTA ethylenediaminetetraacetic acid
EDV end-diastolic volume
EEE eastern equine encephalomyelitis
EEG electroencephalogram
EEJ electroejaculation
EENT eyes, ears, nose, and throat
EERP extended endocardial resection procedure
EFA essential fatty acid
EGD esophagogastroduodenoscopy
EGF epidermal growth factor
EGTA egtazic acid
EHBF estimated hepatic blood flow
EHDP etidronate (ethane-1-hydroxy-1,1-diphosphonate)
EHEC enterohemorrhagic *Escherichia coli*
EI erythema infectiosum
EIA enzyme immunoassay
EIEC enteroinvasive *Escherichia coli*
EIT erythrocyte iron turnover
Ejusd. L. ejusdem (of the same)
EKG electrocardiogram
EKY electrokymogram
ELBW extremely low birth weight
ELISA enzyme-linked immunosorbent assay
Em emmetropia
EMB eosin–methylene blue
EMC encephalomyocarditis
EMF electromotive force
EMG electromyogram
Emp. L. emplastrum (a plaster)
EMS Emergency Medical Service
emul. L. emulsum (emulsion)
ENA extractable nuclear antigens
ENaC epithelial sodium channel
ENG electronystagmography
ENT ears, nose, and throat
EOG electro-olfactogram
EP evoked potential
EPA eicosapentaenoic acid
EPEC enteropathogenic *Escherichia coli*
EPM progressive myoclonic epilepsy
EPP erythropoietic protoporphyria
EPR electron paramagnetic resonance; electrophrenic respiration
EPSP excitatory postsynaptic potential
ER emergency room; endoplasmic reticulum; estrogen receptor
Er erbium
ERBF effective renal blood flow
ERCP endoscopic retrograde cholangiopancreatography
ERG electroretinogram
ERGIC endoplasmic reticulum–Golgi intermediate compartment
ERM egrin, radixin, and moiesin
ERP endocardial resection procedure
ERPF effective renal plasma flow
ERV expiratory reserve volume
Es einsteinium
ESE Ger. elektrostatische Einheit (electrostatic unit)
ESF erythropoietic stimulating factor
ESP extrasensory perception
ESR electron spin resonance; erythrocyte sedimentation rate
ESRD end-stage renal disease
EST electric shock therapy; electroshock therapy; expressed sequence tag
esu electrostatic unit
ESV end-systolic volume
Et ethyl
ETEC enterotoxigenic *Escherichia coli*
ETF electron transfer flavoprotein
ET-NANB enterically transmitted non-A, non-B hepatitis
Eu europium
eV electron volt
EWHO elbow-wrist-hand orthosis
Exhib. L. exhibeatur (let it be given)
ext. extract
F Fahrenheit (scale); farad; fertility (plasmid); fluorine; formula; French (scale); phenylalanine; visual field
F. L. fiat (let there be made)
F coefficient of inbreeding; faraday; force
F$_1$ first filial generation
F$_2$ second filial generation
°F degree Fahrenheit
f femto-; focal length
f frequency
FA fatty acid; fluorescent antibody
FAB French-American-British (classification)
Fab fragment, antigen-binding
Facb fragment, antigen-and-complement-binding
FACD Fellow of the American College of Dentists
FACOG Fellow of the American College of Obstetricians and Gynecologists
FACP Fellow of the American College of Physicians
FACR Fellow of the American College of Radiology
FACS Fellow of the American College of Surgeons; fluorescence-activated cell sorter
FACSM Fellow of the American College of Sports Medicine
FAD flavin adenine dinucleotide
FADH$_2$ the reduced form of flavin adenine dinucleotide
F and R force and rhythm (of pulse)
FAP familial adenomatous polyposis
FAPHA Fellow of the American Public Health Association
fasc. L. fasciculus (bundle)
FBG fasting blood glucose
FC fragment, crystallizable
5-FC flucytosine
fCi femtocurie
FDA Food and Drug Administration; L. fronto-dextra anterior (right frontoanterior [position of the fetus])
FDH familial dysalbuminemic hyperthyroxinemia
FDP fibrin degradation products; fibrinogen degradation products; L. fronto-dextra posterior (right frontoposterior [position of the fetus])
FDT L. fronto-dextra transversa (right frontotransverse [position of the fetus])
F-dUMP 5-fluorodeoxyuridine monophosphate
FE$_{Na}$ fractional excretion of sodium
Fe$_{Na}$ excreted fraction of filtered sodium
Fe iron (L. ferrum)
Feb. dur. L. febre durante (while the fever lasts)
FEF forced expiratory flow
Fem. intern. L. femoribus internus (at the inner side of the thighs)
FEP free erythrocyte protoporphyrin
Ferv. L. fervens (boiling)
FES fat embolism syndrome; functional electrical stimulation; functional endoscopic sinus surgery
FEV forced expiratory volume
FFA free fatty acids
FFT flicker fusion threshold
F.h. L. fiat haustus (let a draft be made)
FIA fluorescence immunoassay; fluorescent immunoassay; fluoroimmunoassay
FIAC Fellow of the International Academy of Cytology
FICD Fellow of the International College of Dentists
FICS Fellow of the International College of Surgeons

FIGLU formiminoglutamic acid
FIGO Fédération Internationale de Gynécologie et d'Obstétrique (International Federation of Gynecology and Obstetrics) (classification)
FISH fluorescence in situ hybridization
FITC fluorescein isothiocyanate
Fl. fluid
FLA L. fronto-laeva anterior (left frontoanterior [position of the fetus])
F.l.a. L. fiat lege artis (let it be done according to rule)
fld fluid
fl dr fluid dram
Flor. L. flores (flowers)
fl oz fluid ounce
FLP L. fronto-laeva posterior (left frontoposterior [position of the fetus])
FLT L. fronto-laeva transversa (left frontotransverse [position of the fetus])
F.M. L. fiat mistura (make a mixture)
Fm fermium
FMN flavin mononucleotide
$FMNH_2$ the reduced form of flavin mononucleotide
FNH focal nodular hyperplasia
FNS functional neuromuscular stimulation
FNTC fine needle transhepatic cholangiography
F.p. L. fiat potio (let a potion be made)
fp freezing point
FPG fasting plasma glucose
F.pil. L. fiant pilulae (let pills be made)
Fr francium
Fract. dos. L. fracta dosi (in divided doses)
FRC functional residual capacity
FRCP Fellow of the Royal College of Physicians
FRCP(C) Fellow of the Royal College of Physicians of Canada
FRCPE Fellow of the Royal College of Physicians of Edinburgh
FRCP(Glasg) Fellow of the Royal College of Physicians and Surgeons of Glasgow *qua* Physician
FRCPI Fellow of the Royal College of Physicians in Ireland
FRCS Fellow of the Royal College of Surgeons
FRCS(C) Fellow of the Royal College of Surgeons of Canada
FRCSEd Fellow of the Royal College of Surgeons of Edinburgh
FRCS(Glasg) Fellow of the Royal College of Physicians and Surgeons of Glasgow *qua* Surgeon
FRCSI Fellow of the Royal College of Surgeons in Ireland
FRCVS Fellow of the Royal College of Veterinary Surgeons
FRET fluorescence resonance energy transfer
FRFPSG Fellow of the Royal Faculty of Physicians and Surgeons of Glasgow
FRS Fellow of the Royal Society
Frust. L. frustillatim (in small pieces)
F.s.a. L. fiat secundum artem (let it be made skillfully)
FSF fibrin-stabilizing factor (factor XIII)
FSG focal segmental glomerulosclerosis
FSGS focal segmental glomerulosclerosis
FSH follicle-stimulating hormone
FSH/LH-RH follicle-stimulating hormone and luteinizing hormone–releasing hormone
FSH-RH follicle-stimulating hormone–releasing hormone
Ft. L. fiat, fiant (let there be made)
ft foot
Ft. mas. div. in pil. L. fiat massa dividenda in pilulae (let a mass be made and divided into pills)
Ft. pulv. L. fiat pulvis (let a powder be made)
5-FU 5-fluorouracil
FUDR, FUdR floxuridine (5-fluorouracil deoxyribonucleoside)
FUO fever of unknown origin
FUS feline urological syndrome
FVC forced vital capacity
G gauss; giga-; glycine; gravida; guanine; guanosine
G conductance; G force; Gibbs free energy; gravitational constant
g gram
g standard gravity
γ gamma chain of fetal hemoglobin; heavy chain of IgG
Ga gallium
GABA γ-aminobutyric acid
GAD generalized anxiety disorder; glutamic acid decarboxylase
GAG glycosaminoglycan
GalNAc *N*-acetylgalactosamine
GALT gut-associated lymphoid tissue
Galv. galvanic
GAPD glyceraldehyde-3-phosphate dehydrogenase
Garg L. gargarisma (gargle)
GAVE gastric antral vascular ectasia
GBM glomerular basement membrane
GBS Guillain-Barré syndrome
GC gas chromatography
g-cal. gram calorie
GCS Glasgow Coma Scale
G-CSF granulocyte colony–stimulating factor
Gd gadolinium
GDM gestational diabetes mellitus
GDP guanosine diphosphate
Ge germanium
Gel. quav. L. gelatina quavis (in any kind of jelly)
GERD gastroesophageal reflux disease
GES gastric electrical stimulation
GeV gigaelectron volt (one billion electron volts)
GFAP glial fibrillary acidic protein
GFR glomerular filtration rate
GGR global genome repair
GGT γ-glutamyltransferase
GH growth hormone
GHA glucoheptonate (gluceptate)
GH-RH growth hormone–releasing hormone
GI gastrointestinal
GIFT gamete intrafallopian transfer
GIP gastric inhibitory polypeptide
GIST gastrointestinal stromal tumor
GL greatest length
gl. L. glandula (gland)
GLC gas-liquid chromatography
GlcNAc *N*-acetylglucosamine
GLI glucagon-like immunoreactivity
Gln glutamine
GLP glucagon-like peptide
Glu glutamic acid
Gly glycine
gm gram
GMC General Medical Council (British)
GM-CSF granulocyte-macrophage colony–stimulating factor
GMK green monkey kidney (cells)
GMO genetically modified organism
GMP guanosine monophosphate
3′,5′-GMP, cyclic GMP cyclic guanosine monophosphate
GMS Gomori methenamine silver
Gn-RH gonadotropin-releasing hormone
GOT glutamic-oxaloacetic transaminase
GP general paresis; general practitioner
GPCR G protein–coupled receptor
G6PD glucose-6-phosphate dehydrogenase
GPT glutamic-pyruvic transaminase
gr grain
Grad. L. gradatim (by degrees)
GRH growth hormone–releasing hormone
GSC gas-solid chromatography
GSH reduced glutathione
GSS Gerstmann-Sträussler-Scheinker syndrome
GSSG oxidized glutathione
gt. L. gutta (drop)
GTH gonadotropic hormone
GTN gestational trophoblastic neoplasia
GTP guanosine triphosphate
GTT glucose tolerance test
gtt. L. guttae (drops)
GU genitourinary
Guttat. L. guttatim (drop by drop)
Gutt. quibusd. L. guttis quibusdam (with a few drops)
GVH graft-versus-host (disease)
GVHD graft-versus-host disease
GXT graded exercise test
Gy gray
H Ger. Hauch (breath, used to describe bacterial colonies henry; histidine; Hounsfield unit; hydrogen; hyperopi
H enthalpy
H_0 null hypothesis
H_1 alternative hypothesis
H_a alternative hypothesis
h hecto-; hour
h. L. hora (hour)
h Planck's constant; height
HA hemadsorbent; hemagglutinin; hepatitis A

Appendix 2

HAA	hepatitis-associated antigen
HAART	highly active antiretroviral therapy
HAI	bemagglutination inhibition (test)
H and E	hematoxylin-eosin (stain)
HANE	hereditary angioneurotic edema
HAPE	high-altitude pulmonary edema
HAT	hypoxanthine-aminopterin-thymidine (medium)
Haust.	L. haustus (a draft)
HAV	hepatitis A virus
HB	hepatitis B
Hb	hemoglobin
HBc	hepatitis B core (antigen)
HBcAg	hepatitis B core antigen
HbCV	*Haemophilus* b conjugate vaccine
HBE	His bundle electrogram
HBe	hepatitis B e (antigen)
HBeAg	hepatitis B e antigen
HbO_2	oxyhemoglobin
HbPV	*Haemophilus* b polysaccharide vaccine
HBs	hepatitis B surface (antigen)
HBsAg	hepatitis B surface antigen
HBV	hepatitis B virus
HC	Hospital Corps
HCG, hCG	human chorionic gonadotropin
HCM	hypertrophic cardiomyopathy
HCP	hereditary coproporphyria
Hct	hematocrit
HCV	hepatitis C virus
HD	hemodialysis; Huntington disease
H.d.	L. hora decubitus (at bedtime)
HDCV	human diploid cell (rabies) vaccine
HDL	high-density lipoprotein
HDL-C	high-density-lipoprotein cholesterol
HDN	hemolytic disease of the newborn
HDP	oxidronate (hydroxymethylene diphosphonate)
HDV	hepatitis D virus
H & E	hematoxylin-eosin (stain)
He	helium
HED	Ger. Haut-Einheits-Dosis (unit skin dose)
HeGF	human epidermal growth factor
HEK	human embryo kidney (cell culture)
HEL	human embryo lung (cell culture)
HEMPAS	hereditary erythroblastic multinuclearity with positive acidified serum
HEP	hepatoerythropoietic porphyria
Herb. recent.	L. herbarium recentium (of fresh herbs)
HERV	human endogenous retroviruses
HETE	hydroxyeicosatetraenoic acid
HEV	hepatitis E virus
HF	Hageman factor (factor XII); high frequency
Hf	hafnium
Hfr	high frequency of recombination
Hg	mercury (L. hydrargyrum)
HGA	human granulocytic anaplasmosis
Hgb	hemoglobin
HGBV	hepatitis GB virus
HGE	human granulocytic ehrlichiosis
HGF	hepatocyte growth factor
HGG	human gamma globulin
HGH, hGH	human growth hormone
hGHr	human growth hormone recombinant
HGPRT	hypoxanthine-guanine phosphoribosyltransferase
HGV	hepatitis G virus
HHT	hydroxyheptadecatrienoic acid
HI	hemagglutination inhibition (test)
5-HIAA	5-hydroxyindoleacetic acid
HIDA	hepatobiliary iminodiacetic acid
HIDS	hyperimmunoglobulinemia D syndrome
HIES	hyper-immunoglobulin E syndrome
His	histidine
HIV	human immunodeficiency virus
HKAFO	hip-knee-ankle-foot orthosis
Hl	latent hyperopia
HLA	human leukocyte antigens
HLHS	hyoplastic left heart syndrome
Hm	manifest hyperopia
HMDP	oxidronate (hydroxymethylene diphosphonate)
HMG	3-hydroxy-3-methylglutaryl
hMG	human menopausal gonadotropin
HMM	hexamethylmelamine
HMO	health maintenance organization
HMPA	hexamethylphosphoramide
HMPAO	hexamethylpropyleneamine oxime
HMSN	hereditary motor and sensory neuropathy
HMWK	high-molecular-weight kininogen
HMW-NCF	high-molecular-weight neutrophil chemotactic factor
HNPCC	hereditary nonpolyposis colorectal cancer
hnRNA	heterogeneous nuclear RNA
hnRNP	heterogeneous nuclear ribonucleoprotein
HO	hand orthosis; hip orthosis
Ho	holmium
HOCM	hypertrophic obstructive cardiomyopathy
HOP	hydroxydaunomycin (doxorubicin), Oncovin (vincristine), and prednisone
Hor. decub.	L. hora decubitus (at bedtime)
Hor. interm.	L. horis intermediis (at the intermediate hours)
Hor. un. spatio	L. horae unius spatio (at the end of one hour)
HP	house physician
Hp	haptoglobin
HPA	hyperphenylalaninemia
HPETE	hydroperoxyeicosatetraenoic acid
HPF	high-power field
HPL, hPL	human placental lactogen
HPLC	high-performance liquid chromatography
HPRT	hypoxanthine phosphoribosyltransferase
HPTA	hepatopoietin A
HPV	human papillomavirus
HRA	high right atrial (electrogram)
HRCT	high-resolution computed tomography
HRF	histamine-releasing factor; homologous restriction factor
HRP	horseradish peroxidase
HRT	hormone replacement therapy
HS	house surgeon
h.s.	L. hora somni (at bedtime)
HSA	human serum albumin
HSAN	hereditary sensory and autonomic neuropathy
hs-CRP	high-sensitivity C-reactive protein
HSR	homogeneously staining regions
HSV	herpes simplex virus
5-HT	5-hydroxytryptamine (serotonin)
Ht	total hyperopia
HTACS	human thyroid adenylate cyclase stimulators
HTC	homozygous typing cells
^{3}H-TdR	tritium-labeled thymidine
HTLV-1	human T-lymphotropic virus 1
HTLV-2	human T-lymphotropic virus 2
HTLV-III	human T-cell lymphotropic virus type III (human immunodeficiency virus)
HuIFN	human interferon
HUVS	hypocomplementemic urticarial vasculitis syndrome
HVA	homovanillic acid
HVL	half-value layer
Hz	hertz
I	incisor; inosine; iodine; isoleucine
I	electric current; intensity (of radiant energy); ionic strength
IAB	infra-aortic balloon (counterpulsation)
IABP	infra-aortic balloon pump
IADL	instrumental activities of daily living
IAEA	International Atomic Energy Agency
IAHA	immune adherence hemagglutination assay
IAP	inhibitor of apoptosis protein
IAPP	islet amyloid polypeptide
IB	inclusion body
IBC	iron-binding capacity
IBD	inflammatory bowel disease
IBF	immunoglobulin-binding factor
IBS	irritable bowel syndrome
IC	inspiratory capacity; irritable colon
ICAM-1	intercellular adhesion molecule 1
ICAM-2	intercellular adhesion molecule 2
ICCs	interstitial cells of Cajal
ICD	implantable cardioverter-defibrillator; International Classification of Diseases (of the World Health Organization); intrauterine contraceptive device
ICF	intracellular fluid
ICP	intracranial pressure
ICSH	interstitial cell–stimulating hormone (luteinizing hormone)
ICSI	intracytoplasmic sperm injection
ICT	insulin coma therapy
ICU	intensive care unit
ID	intradermal; inside diameter; infective dose

Appendix 2

ID_{50}	median infective dose
Id.	L. idem (the same)
IDA	iminodiacetic acid
IDD, IDDM	insulin-dependent diabetes mellitus (type 1 diabetes mellitus)
IDL	intermediate-density lipoprotein
IDU	idoxuridine
IEP	immunoelectrophoresis
IF	intrinsic factor
IFA	immunofluorescence assay
IFN	interferon
Ig	immunoglobulin
IgA	immunoglobulin A
IgD	immunoglobulin D
IgE	immunoglobulin E
IGF	insulin-like growth factor
IgG	immunoglobulin G
IGIV	immune globulin intravenous (human)
IgM	immunoglobulin M
IGT	impaired glucose tolerance
IHD	ischemic heart disease
IHSS	idiopathic hypertrophic subaortic stenosis
IL	interleukin
Ile	isoleucine
ILT	infectious laryngotracheitis
ILVEN	inflammatory linear verrucous epidermal nevus
IM	intramuscular
ImD_{50}	median immunizing dose
IMF	inframammary fold
IMPA	incisal mandibular plane angle
IMV	intermittent mandatory ventilation
IMViC, imvic	indole, methyl red, Voges-Proskauer, and citrate
In	indium
in	inch
in d.	L. in dies (daily)
Inf.	L. infunde (pour in)
INH	isonicotine hydrazine (isoniazid)
INN	International Nonproprietary Name
$InsP_3$	inositol 1,4,5-triphosphate
IOL	intraocular lens
IOP	intraocular pressure
IORT	intraoperative radiotherapy
IP	intraperitoneal; isoelectric point
IP_3	inositol 1,4,5-triphosphate
IPD	intermittent peritoneal dialysis
IPPB	intermittent positive pressure breathing
IPSID	immunoproliferative small intestine disease
IPSP	inhibitory postsynaptic potential
IPSS	inferior petrosal sinus sampling
IPV	poliovirus vaccine inactivated
IQ	intelligence quotient
Ir	iridium
IRMA	immunoradiometric assay
IRV	inspiratory reserve volume
IS	insertion sequence; intercostal space
ISA	intrinsic sympathomimetic activity
ISO	International Standards Organization
ITP	idiopathic thrombocytopenic purpura; inosine triphosphate
IU	International unit *(on the JCAHO "Do Not Use" List)*
IUD	intrauterine device
IUGR	intrauterine growth restriction; intrauterine growth retardation
IUI	intrauterine insemination
IV	intravenous
IVC	inferior vena cava
IVF	in vitro fertilization
IVP	intravenous pyelogram; intravenous pyelography
IVRT	isovolumic relaxation time
IVS	interventricular septum (of heart)
J	joule
JAK	Janus kinase
JCV	JC virus
JIA	juvenile idiopathic arthritis
JRA	juvenile rheumatoid arthritis
juscul.	L. jusculum (soup or broth)
K	kelvin; lysine; potassium (L. kalium)
K	equilibrium constant
K_a	acid dissociation constant
K_b	base dissociation constant
K_d	dissociation constant
K_{eq}	equilibrium constant
K_M, K_m	Michaelis constant
K_{sp}	solubility product constant
K_W	ion product of water
k	kilo-
k	Boltzmann constant; rate constant
κ	dielectric constant; one of the two types of immunoglobulin light chains
KAFO	knee-ankle-foot orthosis
kat	katal
kb	kilobase
kbp	kilobase pairs (1000 base pairs)
kcal	kilocalorie
kCi	kilocurie
kD, kDa	kilodalton
keV	kiloelectron volt (1000 electron volts)
kg	kilogram
kg-cal	large calorie
kHz	kilohertz
kj	knee jerk
km	kilometer
KP	keratic precipitates
Kr	krypton
KS	Kaposi sarcoma
17-KS	17-ketosteroid
KUB	kidney, ureter, and bladder
kV	kilovolt
kVp	kilovolts peak
L	lambert; left; leucine; light chain; liter; lung; lumbar vertebra (L1-L5)
L.	L. libra (pound)
L	luminance; self-inductance
L_0	limes nul (dose)
L+, L_+	limes tod (dose)
L0	limes nul (dose)
l	former symbol for liter (now replaced by L)
l.	L. ligamentum (ligament)
l	length; levo-
λ	decay constant; one of the two types of immunoglobulin light chains; wavelength
L0	limes nul (dose)
L & A	light and accommodation (reaction of pupils)
La	lanthanum
LAC	laparoscopic-assisted colectomy
LAD	left axis deviation; leukocyte adhesion deficiency
LAE	left atrial enlargement
Lag.	L. lagena (flask)
LAH	left anterior hemiblock
LAIV	live, attenuated influenza vaccine
LAM	lymphangiomyomatosis
LAO	left anterior oblique (position of the fetus)
LAP	leukocyte adhesion protein; leukocyte alkaline phosphatase
LAS	lymphangioscintigraphy
LASIK	laser-assisted in-situ keratomileusis
Lat. dol.	L. lateri dolenti (to the painful side)
LATS	long-acting thyroid stimulator
LATS-p	long-acting thyroid stimulator protector
LAV	lymphadenopathy-associated virus (human immunodeficiency virus)
LAVH	laparoscopically assisted vaginal hysterectomy
lb	pound (L. libra)
LBBB	left bundle branch block
LBP	low back pain
LBW	low birth weight (infant)
LCA	left coronary artery; leukocyte common antigens
LCAT	lecithin-cholesterol acyltransferase
LCIS	lobular carcinoma in situ
LCM	lymphocytic choriomeningitis
LCR	locus control region
LD	lethal dose; light difference
LD_{50}	median lethal dose
LDA	left displacement of the abomasum; left dorsoanterior (position of the fetus)
LDH	L-lactate dehydrogenase
LDL	low-density lipoprotein
LE	left eye; lupus erythematosus
LEMS	Lambert-Eaton myasthenic syndrome
les	local excitatory state
LET	linear energy transfer
Leu	leucine
Lf	limes flocculating (dose)
LFA	left frontoanterior (position of the fetus)

LFA-1	leukocyte function–associated antigen 1
LFA-2	leukocyte function–associated antigen 2
LFA-3	leukocyte function–associated antigen 3
LFP	left frontoposterior (position of the fetus)
LFT	left frontotransverse (position of the fetus)
LGA	large for gestational age
LGB	laparoscopic gastric banding
LH	luteinizing hormone
LH-RH	luteinizing hormone–releasing hormone
Li	lithium
LIA	leukemia-associated inhibitory activity
LIF	left iliac fossa; leukocyte inhibitory factor
lig.	ligament; ligamentum
ligg.	L. ligamenta (ligaments)
Liq.	L. liquor (liquid)
LLL	left lower lobe (of lung)
LM	light minimum; linguomesial
lm	lumen
LMA	left mentoanterior (position of the fetus)
LMF	lymphocyte mitogenic factor
LMO	living modified organism
LMP	left mentoposterior (position of the fetus); last menstrual period; latent membrane protein
LMT	left mentotransverse (position of the fetus)
LMWK	low-molecular-weight kininogen
ln	natural logarithm
LNG	levonorgestrel
LNMP	last normal menstrual period
LNPF	lymph node permeability factor
LOA	left occipitoanterior (position of the fetus)
LOAEL	lowest observed adverse effect level
Loc. dol.	L. loco dolenti (to the painful spot)
LOEL	lowest observed effect level
LOH	loss of heterozygosity
LOP	left occipitoposterior (position of the fetus)
LOS	lipooligosaccharide
LOT	left occipitotransverse (position of the fetus)
Lot.	L. lotio (lotion)
LP	lumbar puncture
LPF	low-power field
LPH	left posterior hemiblock; lipotropic hormone
LPN	licensed practical nurse
LPR	laryngopharyngeal reflux
LPS	lipopolysaccharide
LPV	lymphotropic papovavirus
Lr	limes reacting (dose)
LRD	living related donor
LRR	leucine-rich repeat
LSA	left sacroanterior (position of the fetus)
LScA	left scapuloanterior (position of the fetus)
LScP	left scapuloposterior (position of the fetus)
LSD	lysergic acid diethylamide
LSO	lumbosacral orthosis
LSP	left sacroposterior (position of the fetus)
L-spine	lumbar spine
LST	left sacrotransverse (position of the fetus)
LT	lymphotoxin
LTF	lymphocyte-transforming factor
LTR	long terminal repeats
Lu	lutetium
LUL	left upper lobe (of lung)
LVAD	left ventricular assist device
LVEDP	left ventricular end-diastolic pressure
LVEDV	left ventricular end-diastolic volume
LVET	left ventricular ejection time
LVH	left ventricular hypertrophy
LVN	licensed vocational nurse
Lw	lawrencium
lx	lux
Lys	lysine
M	low frequency component of the first heart sound; methionine; molar; morgan; mucoid (colony); myopia
M.	L. misce (mix); L. mistura (a mixture)
M	mutual inductance; molar mass; molar
M_1	mitral valve closure
M_r	relative molecular mass
m	median; meter; milli-
m.	L. musculus (muscle); minim
m	mass; molal
m-	meta-
μ	electrophoretic mobility; heavy chain of IgM; linear attenuation coefficient; micro-; micron; population mean
MA	Master of Arts; mental age; meter angle
mA	milliampere
μA	microampere
MAA	macroaggregated albumin
MAC	membrane attack complex; minimal alveolar concentration; *Mycobacterium avium* complex
Mac.	L. macerare (macerate)
MADD	multiple acyl CoA dehydrogenation deficiency
MAF	macrophage-activating factor
Mag.	L. magnus (large)
MAIS	mild androgen insensitivity syndrome; minimal androgen insensitivity syndrome
MALT	mucosa-associated lymphoid tissue
Man., Manip.	L. manipulus (a handful)
Man. pr.	L. mane primo (early in the morning)
MAO	maximal acid output; monoamine oxidase
MAOI	monoamine oxidase inhibitor
MAP	mean arterial pressure; microtubule-associated protein
MAPK	mitogen-activated protein kinase
masc	mass concentration
Mas. pil.	L. massa pilularum (pill mass)
MAST	military (or medical) anti-shock trousers
MAT	multifocal atrial tachycardia
Matut.	L. matutinus (in the morning)
MB	Medicinae Baccalaureus (Bachelor of Medicine)
Mb	megabase
m.b.	L. misce bene (mix well)
MBC	minimal bactericidal concentration
MBL	mannose-binding lectin
MBP	major basic protein; myelin basic protein
MBq	megabecquerel
MC	L. Magister Chirurgiae (Master of Surgery); Medical Corps
mC	millicoulomb
μC	microcoulomb
MCA	3-methylcholanthrene
MCD	mean of consecutive differences
MCE	myocardial contrast echocardiography
MCF	macrophage chemotactic factor
MCFA	medium-chain fatty acid
mcg	microgram
MCH	mean corpuscular hemoglobin
MCHC	mean corpuscular hemoglobin concentration
MCi	megacurie
mCi	millicurie
μCi	microcurie
MCI/MI	methylchloroisothiazolinone and methylisothiazolinone
MCMI	Millon Clinical Multiaxial Inventory
MCP	membrane cofactor protein
Mcps	megacycles per second (million cycles per second)
MCS	mechanical circulatory support
M-CSF	macrophage colony–stimulating factor
MCT	mean circulation time
MCV	meningococcal conjugate vaccine; mean corpuscular volume
MD	L. Medicinae Doctor (Doctor of Medicine)
Md	mendelevium
MDA	methylenedioxyamphetamine; L. mento-dextra anterior (right mentoanterior [position of the fetus])
MDF	myocardial depressant factor
MDMA	3,4-methylenedioxymethamphetamine
MDP	methylene diphosphonate; L. mento-dextra posterior (right mentoposterior [position of the fetus])
MDR	multidrug resistance; multiple drug resistance
MDS	myelodysplasia
MDT	L. mento-dextra transversa (right mentotransverse [position of the fetus])
2-ME	2-mercaptoethanol
Me	methyl
MeCbl	methylcobalamin
MED	minimal effective dose; minimal erythema dose
MEDLARS	Medical Literature Analysis and Retrieval System
MEDLINE	MEDLARS on line
MEG	magnetoencephalograph
MEGX	monoethylglycinexylidide
MEN	multiple endocrine neoplasia
MEP	maximum expiratory pressure
mEq, meq	milliequivalent

Appendix 2

MESA microsurgical epididymal sperm aspiration
MeSH Medical Subject Headings
Met methionine
M. et sig. L. misce et signa (mix and write a label)
MeV megaelectron volt (one million electron volts)
μF microfarad
M. flac. L. membrana flaccida (pars flaccida membranae tympanicae)
MFR monthly fecundity rate
M. ft. L. mistura fiat (let a mixture be made)
Mg magnesium
mg milligram
μg microgram
MGUS monoclonal gammopathy of undetermined significance
3MH 3-methylhistidine
MHA-TP microhemagglutination assay–*Treponema pallidum*
MHC major histocompatibility complex
MHz megahertz
MI myocardial infarction
MIBG, mIBG iobenguane (*m*-iodobenzylguanidine)
MIBI sestamibi
MIC minimal inhibitory concentration
MID minimum infective dose
MIF migration inhibition factor; migration inhibitory factor
min. L. minimum (a minim)
MIO minimal identifiable odor
MIP maximum inspiratory pressure
MIRL membrane inhibitor of reactive lysis (protectin)
miRNA microRNA
mist. L. mistura (a mixture)
MIT monoiodotyrosine
Mit. L. mitte (send)
MJD Machado-Joseph disease
MK monkey lung (cell culture)
MKS meter-kilogram-second system
mL milliliter
μL microliter
MLA L. mento-laeva anterior (left mentoanterior [position of the fetus])
MLBW moderately low birth weight (infant)
MLC mixed lymphocyte culture; minimal lethal concentration
MLD median lethal dose; minimum lethal dose
MLNS mucocutaneous lymph node syndrome
MLP L. mento-laeva posterior (left mentoposterior [position of the fetus])
MLR mixed lymphocyte reaction
MLT L. mento-laeva transversa (left mentotransverse [position of the fetus])
MM mucous membrane
mM millimolar
mm millimeter
μM micromolar
μm micrometer
MMF mycophenolate mofetil
mm Hg millimeter of mercury
MMIHS megacystis-microcolon–intestinal hypoperistalsis syndrome
mmol millimole
MMP matrix metalloproteinase
MMPI Minnesota Multiphasic Personality Inventory
MMR measles-mumps-rubella (vaccine)
MMRV measles, mumps, rubella, and varicella vaccine live
Mn manganese
MNGIE mitochondrial neurogastrointestinal encephalomyopathy
MO Medical Officer
Mo molybdenum
Mod. praesc. L. modo praescripto (in the way directed)
MODY maturity-onset diabetes of youth
Mol wt, mol wt molecular weight
MOPP mechlorethamine, Oncovin (vincristine), procarbazine, and prednisone
MORC Medical Officers Reserve Corps
Mor. dict. L. more dicto (in the manner directed)
Mor. sol. L. more solito (in the usual way)
mOsm milliosmole
MOTT mycobacteria other than tubercle bacilli
6-MP 6-mercaptopurine
mp melting point
MPD maximum permissible dose
MPH Master of Public Health
MPO myeloperoxidase
MPS mononuclear phagocyte system; mucopolysaccharidosis
MPSV meningococcal polysaccharide vaccine
MR mitral regurgitation
mR milliroentgen
μR microroentgen
MRA Medical Record Administrator; magnetic resonance angiography
MRACP Member of Royal Australasian College of Physicians
mrad millirad
MRCP Member of the Royal College of Physicians
MRCPE Member of the Royal College of Physicians of Edinburgh
MRCP(Glasg) Member of Royal College of Physicians and Surgeons of Glasgow *qua* Physician
MRCPI Member of the Royal College of Physicians of Ireland
MRCS Member of the Royal College of Surgeons
MRCSEd Member of the Royal College of Surgeons of Edinburgh
MRCSI Member of the Royal College of Surgeons of Ireland
MRCVS Member of the Royal College of Veterinary Surgeons
MRD minimum reacting dose
MRDM malnutrition-related diabetes mellitus
mrem millirem
MRI magnetic resonance imaging
mRNA messenger RNA
MRSA methicillin-resistant *Staphylococcus aureus*
MS Master of Science; Master of Surgery; mitral stenosis; multiple sclerosis
ms millisecond
μs microsecond
MSA multiple system atrophy
MSE Mental Status Examination
msec millisecond
MSG monosodium glutamate
MSH melanocyte-stimulating hormone
MSI microsatellite instability
MSL midsternal line
MSLT multiple sleep latency test
MS/MS tandem mass spectrometry
MSUD maple syrup urine disease
MT Medical Technologist
MTC medullary thyroid carcinoma
MTD maximum tolerated dose
mtDNA mitochondrial DNA
MTHFR methylenetetrahydrofolate reductase
MTOC microtubule organizing center
MTP microsomal triglyceride transfer protein
MTX methotrexate
mU milliunit
m.u. mouse unit
μU microunit
MUAP motor unit action potential
MUC maximum urinary concentration
Muc. L. mucilago (mucilage)
MUGA multiple gated acquisition (scanning)
MUP motor unit potential
MV megavolt (million electron volts); minute volume; L. Medicus Veterinarius (veterinary physician)
mV millivolt
μV microvolt
M-VAC methotrexate, vinblastine, Adriamycin (doxorubicin), and cisplatin
MVP mitral valve prolapse
MVV maximal (or maximum) voluntary ventilation
MW molecular weight
μW microwatt
Mx Medex
My myopia
N newton; nitrogen; normal (solution)
N Avogadro's number; neutron number; normal (solution number; population size
N_A Avogadro's number
n nano; neutron; refractive index
n. L. nervus (nerve)
n (haploid) chromosome number; refractive index; samp size
***n*-** normal
n_D refractive index
ν degrees of freedom; frequency; kinematic viscosity; neutrino
NA *Nomina Anatomica*; numerical aperture
Na sodium (L. natrium)
NAAT nucleic acid amplification test

Appendix 2

NAD nicotinamide adenine dinucleotide; no appreciable disease
NAD$^+$ the oxidized form of nicotinamide adenine dinucleotide
NADH the reduced form of nicotinamide adenine dinucleotide
NADP nicotinamide adenine dinucleotide phosphate
NADP$^+$ the oxidized form of nicotinamide adenine dinucleotide phosphate
NADPH the reduced form of nicotinamide adenine dinucleotide phosphate
NAN N-acetylneuraminic acid
NANBH non-A, non-B hepatitis
NAP nasion, point A, pogonion
NASH nonalcoholic steatohepatitis
NAT nucleic acid test
Nb niobium
NBS National Bureau of Standards (National Institute of Standards and Technology)
NBT nitroblue tetrazolium
NBTE nonbacterial thrombotic endocarditis
NCF neutrophil chemotactic factor
NCHS National Center for Health Statistics
NCI National Cancer Institute
nCi nanocurie
NCV nerve conduction velocity
ND Doctor of Naturopathy
Nd neodymium
nDNA nuclear DNA
NDV Newcastle disease virus
Nd:YAG neodymium:yttrium-aluminum-garnet (laser)
Ne neon
NED no evidence of disease
NEFA nonesterified fatty acids
NER nucleotide excision repair
NF *National Formulary*
ng nanogram
NGF nerve growth factor
Ni nickel
NIDD, NIDDM non–insulin-dependent diabetes mellitus (type 2 diabetes mellitus)
NIPHS noninsulinoma pancreatogenous hypoglycemia syndrome
nL nanoliter
nm nanometer
NMDA *N*-methyl-D-aspartate
NMN nicotinamide mononucleotide
NMR nuclear magnetic resonance
NMS neuroleptic malignant syndrome
nn. L. nervi (nerves)
NNRTI non-nucleoside reverse transcriptase inhibitor
No nobelium
No. numero (to the number of)
NOAEL no observed adverse effect level
Noct. L. nocte (at night)
Noct. maneq. L. nocte maneque (at night and in the morning)
NOEL no observed effect level
NOMID neonatal-onset multisystem inflammatory disease
non repetat. L. non repetatur (do not repeat)
NOR nucleolar organizing region
Np neptunium
NPN nonprotein nitrogen
NPO L. nil per os (nothing by mouth)
NRC normal retinal correspondence
NREM non-rapid eye movement
NRI selective norepinephrine reuptake inhibitor
NS normal saline
ns nanosecond
NSAIA nonsteroidal antiinflammatory analgesic (or agent)
NSAID nonsteroidal antiinflammatory drug
NSCLC non-small cell lung carcinoma
nsec nanosecond
NSIAD nephrogenic syndrome of inappropriate antidiuresis
NSILA nonsuppressible insulin-like activity
NSR normal sinus rhythm
NST nonstress test
NTP normal temperature and pressure; National Toxicology Program
nU nanounit
NUG necrotizing ulcerative gingivitis
nvCJD new variant Creutzfeldt-Jakob disease
NVS nutritionally variant streptococci
NYD not yet diagnosed

O Ger. ohne Hauch (without breath, used to describe bacterial colonies); oxygen
O. L. oculus (eye)
***o*-** ortho-
Ω ohm
OA ocular albinism
OAE otoacoustic emissions
OAF osteoclast activating factor
OAP Oncovin (vincristine), ara-C (cytarabine), and prednisone
ODDD oculodentodigital dysplasia
OAT ornithine aminotransferase
OB obstetrics
OCA oculocutaneous albinism
OCD obsessive-compulsive disorder
OCT optical coherence tomography; ornithine carbamoyltransferase; oxytocin challenge test
OD L. oculus dexter (right eye); Doctor of Optometry; optical density; outside diameter; overdose
ODA L. occipito-dextra anterior (right occipitoanterior [position of the fetus])
ODC orotidine 5-phosphate decarboxylase
ODP L. occipito-dextra posterior (right occipitoposterior [position of the fetus])
ODT L. occipito-dextra transversa (right occipitotransverse [position of the fetus])
OFD oral-facial-digital (syndrome)
OGTT oral glucose tolerance test
OH-Cbl hydroxocobalamin
17-OHCS 17-hydroxycorticosteroid
OI osteogenesis imperfecta; oxygenation index
OIC osteogenesis imperfecta congenita
OIH orthoiodohippurate
OIT osteogenesis imperfecta tarda
OL L. oculus laevus (left eye)
Ol. L. oleum (oil)
OLA L. occipito-laeva anterior (left occipitoanterior [position of the fetus])
OLP L. occipito-laeva posterior (left occipitoposterior [position of the fetus])
OLT L. occipito-laeva transversa (left occipitotransverse [position of the fetus])
o.m. L. omni mane (every morning)
OMD Doctor of Oriental Medicine
Omn. bih. L. omni bihora (every two hours)
Omn. hor. L. omni hora (every hour)
Omn. noct. L. omni nocte (every night)
OMPA octamethyl pyrophosphoramide
Om. quar. hor. L. omni quadrante hora (every quarter of an hour)
o.n. L. omni nocte (every night)
OPG osteoprotegerin
OPRT orotate phosphoribosyltransferase
OPV poliovirus vaccine live oral
OR operating room
ORF open reading frame
Orn ornithine
ORS oral rehydration salts
ORT oral rehydration therapy
OS L. oculus sinister (left eye)
Os osmium
OSA obstructive sleep apnea
OSAS obstructive sleep apnea syndrome
OSHA Occupational Safety and Health Administration
OT old term (anatomy); Old tuberculin
OTC over the counter; ornithine transcarbamoylase
OTD organ tolerance dose
OU L. oculus uterque (each eye)
OVD occlusal vertical dimension
oz ounce (It. onza)
P para; peta-; phosphate group; phosphorus; poise; posterior; premolar; proline; pupil
P power; pressure; probability
P_1 parental generation
P_2 pulmonic second sound
P_{CO_2} carbon dioxide partial pressure (carbon dioxide tension)
P_i orthophosphate
P_{O_2} oxygen partial pressure (oxygen tension)
p pico-; proton; short arm of a chromosome
p150,95 glycoprotein p150,95
p momentum; (in statistics) the probability that a specific event will occur

Appendix 2

p- para-
Π product (in mathematics)
π the ratio of the circumference to the diameter of a circle, approximately 3.1415926536; osmotic pressure
Φ magnetic flux
ϕ pseudouridine
PA physician assistant; posteroanterior; pulmonary artery
Pa pascal; protactinium
PAB, PABA *p*-aminobenzoic acid
PAC premature atrial complex
PACU postanesthesia care unit
PAF platelet activating factor
PAGE polyacrylamide gel electrophoresis
PAH *p*-aminohippuric acid; phenylalanine hydroxylase
PAHA *p*-aminohippuric acid
PAI plasminogen activator inhibitor
PAIS partial androgen insensitivity syndrome
PALS periarterial lymphoid sheath
PAM primary amebic meningoencephalitis
L-PAM L-phenylalanine mustard
PAN polyarteritis nodosa
PAO peak acid output
PAP peroxidase-antiperoxidase (technique)
PAR pseudoautosomal region
Par. aff. L. pars affecta (the part affected)
Part. aeq. L. partes aequales (equal parts)
Part. vic. L. partitis vicibus (in divided doses)
PAS *p*-aminosalicylic acid; periodic acid–Schiff (reaction)
PASA *p*-aminosalicylic acid
PASG pneumatic antishock garment
PAT paroxysmal atrial tachycardia
PAWP pulmonary artery wedge pressure
PB *Pharmacopoeia Britannica*
Pb lead (L. plumbum)
PBB polybrominated biphenyl
PBG porphobilinogen
PBI protein-bound iodine
PBPC peripheral blood progenitor cells
PC phosphocreatine; phosphatidylcholine
p.c. L. post cibum (after meals)
PCA passive cutaneous anaphylaxis
PCB polychlorinated biphenyl
PcB near point of convergence
PCC prothrombin complex concentrate
PCD pterin-4α-carbinolamine dehydratase
PCE pseudocholinesterase
PCEC purified chick embryo cell (vaccine)
PCG phonocardiogram
PCI percutaneous coronary intervention
pCi picocurie
P_{CO_2} carbon dioxide partial pressure (carbon dioxide tension)
PCOS polycystic ovary syndrome
PCP phencyclidine hydrochloride; *Pneumocystis carinii* pneumonia
PCR polymerase chain reaction; protein catabolic rate
PCT porphyria cutanea tarda
PCV packed-cell volume
PCV7 pneumococcal 7-valent conjugate vaccine
PCWP pulmonary capillary wedge pressure
PD prism diopter; interpupillary distance; peritoneal dialysis
Pd palladium
PDA patent ductus arteriosus; posterior descending (coronary) artery
PDT photodynamic therapy
PE phosphatidylethanolamine; phycoerythrin; pulmonary embolism
PEA pulseless electrical activity
PEARS porcine epidemic abortion and respiratory syndrome
PEEP positive end-expiratory pressure
PEF peak expiratory flow
PEFR peak expiratory flow rate
PEG percutaneous endoscopic gastrostomy; pneumoencephalography; polyethylene glycol
PEG-ADA PEG-adenosine deaminase
PEM protein-energy malnutrition
PEN pharmacy equivalent name
PEP phospho*enol*pyruvate; preejection period
PET positron emission tomography
PETN pentaerythritol tetranitrate
PFES pelvic floor electrical stimulation
PFO patent foramen ovale
PG prostaglandin; *Pharmacopoeia Germanica*
pg picogram
PGAD persistent genital arousal disorder
PGD preimplantation genetic diagnosis
PGD_2, PGE_2, $PGF_{2\alpha}$, PGI_2 symbols for various prostaglandins
PGL paraganglioma syndrome
Ph Pharmacopeia; phenyl
PHA phytohemagglutinin
PHA1 pseudohypoaldosteronism type 1
phar pharmaceutical; pharmacopeia; pharmacy
Phar B L. Pharmaciae Baccalaureus (Bachelor of Pharmacy)
Phar C Pharmaceutical Chemist
Phar D L. Pharmaciae Doctor (Doctor of Pharmacy)
Phar G Graduate in Pharmacy
Phar M L. Pharmaciae Magister (Master of Pharmacy)
pharm pharmaceutical; pharmacopeia; pharmacy
Pharm D L. Pharmaciae Doctor (Doctor of Pharmacy)
PhB British Pharmacopoeia
PhD L. Philosophiae Doctor (Doctor of Philosophy)
Phe phenylalanine
PhG Graduate in Pharmacy; *Pharmacopoeia Germanica*
PHN postherpetic neuralgia; public health nurse
PHP pseudohypoparathyroidism
PMDS persistent müllerian duct syndrome
PHPPA *p*-hydroxyphenylpyruvic acid
PI phosphatidylinositol; protease inhibitor
PID pelvic inflammatory disease
PIE pulmonary interstitial emphysema; pulmonary infiltration with eosinophilia
PIF prolactin-inhibiting factor; peak inspiratory flow
Pil. L. pilula (pill); L. pilulae (pills)
PIP proximal interphalangeal
PIP_2 phosphatidylinositol 4,5-bisphosphate
PIT plasma iron turnover
PJRT permanent junctional reciprocating tachycardia
PJT paroxysmal junctional tachycardia
PK pyruvate kinase
PKU, PKU1 phenylketonuria
PLED periodic lateralized epileptiform discharge
PLEVA pityriasis lichenoides et varioliformis acuta
PLP proteolipid protein
PLT primed lymphocyte typing
PLTP phospholipid transfer protein
Pm promethium
PMI point of maximal impulse
PMMA polymethyl methacrylate
PMN polymorphonuclear; polymorphonuclear neutrophil
PMR proportionate mortality ratio
PMS premenstrual syndrome
PNS peripheral nervous system
PNET peripheral neuroectodermal tumor; primitive neuro-ectodermal tumor
PNH paroxysmal nocturnal hemoglobinuria
PO L. per os (by mouth, orally)
Po_2, P_{O_2} oxygen partial pressure (oxygen tension)
Po polonium
pO_2, pO_2 oxygen partial pressure (oxygen tension)
POA pancreatic oncofetal antigen
Pocill. L. pocillum (a small cup)
Pocul. L. poculum (cup)
poly A polyadenylate; polyadenylic acid
POMC pro-opiomelanocortin
POMP prednisone, Oncovin (vincristine), methotrexate, and Purinethol (6-mercaptopurine)
Pond. L. pondere (by weight)
POR problem-oriented record
Post sing. sed. liq. L. post singulas sedes liquidas (after every watery bowel movement)
pot AGT potential abnormality of glucose tolerance
POTS postural orthostatic tachycardia syndrome
PP L. punctum proximum (near point of accommodation)
PP_i pyrophosphate
PPD purified protein derivative (tuberculin)
PPI proton pump inhibitor
PPLO pleuropneumonia-like organisms
ppm parts per million
PPR peste des petits ruminants
PPSV pneumococcal vaccine polyvalent
Ppt precipitate; prepared
PR prosthion; pulmonic regurgitation; L. punctum remotum (far point of accommodation)

Appendix 2

Pr praseodymium; presbyopia; prism

PRA panel-reactive antibody

P. rat. aetat. L. pro ratione aetatis (in proportion to age)

prev AGT previous abnormality of glucose tolerance

PRF prolactin-releasing factor

PRK photorefractive keratectomy

PRL, Prl prolactin

p.r.n. L. pro re nata (according to circumstances)

PRO Peer Review Organization; Professional Review Organization

Pro proline

PROM premature rupture of membranes

pro-UK prourokinase

PrP prion protein

PRPP phosphoribosylpyrophosphate

PRU peripheral resistance unit

PS phosphatidylserine; pulmonary stenosis

ps per second

PSA prostate-specific antigen

P_{450}SCC cholesterol monooxygenase (side-chain-cleaving)

PSE portal-systemic encephalopathy; portosystemic encephalopathy

psi pounds per square inch

PSM presystolic murmur

PSMA prostate-specific membrane antigen

PSP phenolsulfonphthalein

PSRO Professional Standards Review Organization

PSTI pancreatic secretory trypsin inhibitor

PSVT paroxysmal supraventricular tachycardia

PT prothrombin time

Pt platinum

pt pint

PTA plasma thromboplastin antecedent (factor XI)

PTC phenylthiocarbamide; plasma thromboplastin component (factor IX)

PTCA percutaneous transluminal coronary angioplasty

PteGlu pteroylglutamate; pteroylglutamic acid

pter the end of the short arm of a chromosome

PTFE polytetrafluoroethylene (polytef)

PTH parathyroid hormone

PTPS 6-pyruvoyltetrahydropterin synthase

PTRA percutaneous transluminal renal angioplasty

PTS 6-pyruvoyltetrahydropterin synthase

PTSD posttraumatic stress disorder

PTT partial thromboplastin time

Pu plutonium

PUBS percutaneous umbilical blood sampling

PUFA polyunsaturated fatty acid

pulv. L. pulvis (powder)

PUO pyrexia of unknown origin

PUPPP pruritic urticarial papules and plaques of pregnancy

PUVA psoralen plus ultraviolet A (therapy)

PVC polyvinyl chloride

PVL periventricular leukomalacia

PVP polyvinylpyrrolidone (povidone)

PVP-I povidone-iodine

PVS persistent vegetative state; persistent vegetative state

PWA person with AIDS

PWM pokeweed mitogen

PZA pyrazinamide

PZD partial zona dissection

PZI protamine zinc insulin

Q ubiquinone

Q electric charge; heat; reaction quotient

Q_{10} temperature coefficient; ubiquinone

Q rate of blood flow

q the long arm of a chromosome

q. L. quaque (each, every)

q electric charge, ubiquinone; (in statistics) the probability of an alternative event occurring

q.d. L. quaque die (every day) *(on the JCAHO "Do Not Use" List)*

q.h. L. quaque hora (every hour)

q.i.d. L. quater in die (four times a day)

q.l. L. quantum libet (as much as desired)

QNS Queen's Nursing Sister (of Queen's Institute of District Nursing)

qns quantity not sufficient

q.p. L. quantum placeat (as much as desired)

q.q.h. L. quaque quarta hora (every four hours)

Qq.hor. L. quaque hora (every hour)

QS_2 electromechanical systole

q.s. L. quantum satis (sufficient quantity)

q.suff. L. quantum sufficit (as much as suffices)

qt quart

qter the end of the long arm of a chromosome

quadrupl. L. quadruplicato (four times as much)

Quat., quat. L. quattuor (four)

Quinq. L. quinque (five)

Quint. L. quintus (fifth)

Quotid. L. quotidie (daily)

q.v. L. quantum vis (as much as you please); L. quod vide (which see)

R arginine; organic radical; Rankine (scale); rate; expiratory exchange ratio; Réaumur scale; resistance; respiration; rhythm; right; roentgen; rough (colony)

R. L. remotum (far)

R resistance; gas constant

R_A, R_{AW} airway resistance

R_e Reynolds number

R_x L. recipe (take)

r drug resistance; ring chromosome

r correlation coefficient; distance; radius; drug resistance

r_s Spearman rank correlation coefficient

ρ correlation coefficient

RA rheumatoid arthritis

Ra radium

RAAS renin-angiotensin-aldosterone system

RAD right axis deviation

rad radian; radiation absorbed dose

rad. L. radix (root)

RAE right atrial enlargement

RAIU radioactive iodine uptake

RAO right anterior oblique (position of the fetus)

RAS renal artery stenosis; renin-angiotensin system

RAST radioallergosorbent test

RAV Rous-associated virus

Rb rubidium

RBBB right bundle branch block

RBC red blood cell; red blood (cell) count

RBC IT red blood cell iron turnover

RBD REM sleep behavior disorder

RBE relative biological effectiveness

RBP retinol binding protein

RCA regulator of complement activation; right coronary artery

rCBF regional cerebral blood flow

rcp reciprocal translocation

RCT randomized controlled trial

RCU red cell utilization

RD reaction of degeneration; Registered Dietitian

rd rutherford

RDA recommended dietary allowance; right displacement of the abomasum

RDE receptor-destroying enzyme

RE radium emanation; right eye; retinol equivalent

Re rhenium

Rect. L. rectificatus (rectified)

Redig. in pulv. L. redigatur in pulverem (let it be reduced to powder)

Red. in pulv. L. reductus in pulverem (reduced to powder)

REG radioencephalography

REM rapid eye movements; reticular erythematous mucinosis

Rep. L. repetatur (let it be repeated)

RES reticuloendothelial system

RF radio frequency; rheumatoid factor

RFA right frontoanterior (position of the fetus)

RfD reference dose

RFI renal failure index

RFLP restriction fragment length polymorphism

RFP right frontoposterior (position of the fetus)

RFT right frontotransverse (position of the fetus)

RGN Registered General Nurse (Scotland)

RGO reciprocating gait orthosis

Rh rhodium

r-HuEPO recombinant human erythropoietin

RIA radioimmunoassay

RID radial immunodiffusion

RIF resistance-inducing factor; right iliac fossa; rifampin

RIND reversible ischemic neurologic deficit

RIPA radioimmunoprecipitation assay

RISC RNA-induced silencing complex

RIST radioimmunosorbent test

RLF retrolental fibroplasia

RLL right lower lobe

RMA right mentoanterior (position of the fetus)
RML right middle lobe
RMP right mentoposterior (position of the fetus)
RMT right mentotransverse (position of the fetus)
RN registered nurse
Rn radon
RNA ribonucleic acid
RNAi RNA interference
RNase ribonuclease
RNase I, RNase A pancreatic ribonuclease
RNP ribonucleoprotein
ROA right occipitoanterior (position of the fetus)
rob robertsonian translocation
ROP right occipitoposterior (position of the fetus)
ROT right occipitotransverse (position of the fetus)
RPE retinal pigment epithelium
RPF renal plasma flow
R Ph Registered Pharmacist
RPLND retroperitoneal lymph node dissection
rpm revolutions per minute
RQ respiratory quotient
RRA Registered Record Administrator
rRNA ribosomal RNA
RSA right sacroanterior (position of the fetus)
RScA right scapuloanterior (position of the fetus)
RSCN Registered Sick Children's Nurse
RScP right scapuloposterior (position of the fetus)
RSP right sacroposterior (position of the fetus)
RST right sacrotransverse (position of the fetus)
RSV respiratory syncytial virus; Rous sarcoma virus
RTA renal tubular acidosis
RTF resistance transfer factor
Ru ruthenium
RUL right upper lobe
RV residual volume; Rotavirus (or rotavirus); rotavirus vaccine
RVA rabies vaccine adsorbed
RVAD right ventricular assist device
RVH right ventricular hypertrophy
S sacral vertebrae (S1–S5); serine; siemens; smooth (colony); spherical lens; substrate; sulfur; Svedberg unit
S. L. signa (mark)
S entropy
S_1 first heart sound
S_2 second heart sound
S_3 third heart sound
S_4 fourth heart sound
S_f Svedberg flotation unit
s second
s. L. semis (half); L. sinister (left)
$\bar{s}$ L. sine (without)
s sample standard deviation
s^{-1} reciprocal second
Σ summation
σ standard deviation
σ^2 variance
SA sinoatrial
S.A. L. secundum artem (according to art)
SAAG serum-ascites albumin gradient
SACH solid ankle cushion heel
SAD seasonal affective disorder
SADS Schedule for Affective Disorders and Schizophrenia; sudden adult arrhythmia (or arrhythmic) death syndrome
S.A.L. L. secundum artis leges (according to the rules of art)
SAP sphingolipid activator protein (saposin)
SARS severe acute respiratory syndrome
SARS-CoV SARS-associated coronavirus
SB sinus bradycardia
Sb antimony (L. stibium)
SBE subacute bacterial endocarditis
SBFT small bowel follow-through
SBMA spinobulbar muscular atrophy
SC closure of semilunar valves; secretory component; subcutaneous
Sc scandium
SCAT sheep cell agglutination test
ScD L. Scientiae Doctor (Doctor of Science)
ScDA L. scapulo-dextra anterior (right scapuloanterior [position of the fetus])
scDNA single copy DNA
ScDP L. scapulo-dextra posterior (right scapuloposterior [position of the fetus])
SCFA short-chain fatty acid
SChE serum cholinesterase
SCI spinal cord injury
SCID severe combined immunodeficiency
ScLA L. scapulo-laeva anterior (left scapuloanterior [position of the fetus])
SCLC small cell lung carcinoma
ScLP L. scapulo-laeva posterior (left scapuloposterior [position of the fetus])
SCM State Certified Midwife
scr scruple
scu-PA single chain urokinase-type plasminogen antivator
SD skin dose; standard deviation
SDA L. sacro-dextra anterior (right sacroanterior [position of the fetus])
SDE specific dynamic effect
SDP L. sacro-dextra posterior (right sacroposterior [position of the fetus])
SDS sodium dodecyl sulfate
SDS-PAGE SDS–polyacrylamide gel electrophoresis
SDT L. sacro-dextra transversa (right sacrotransverse [position of the fetus])
SE standard error; sphenoethmoidal suture
Se selenium
SED skin erythema dose
semel in d. L. semel in die (once a day)
Semih. L. semihora (half an hour)
SEP somatosensory evoked potential
Sept. L. septem (seven)
seq. luce L. sequenti luce (the following day)
Ser serine
SERM selective estrogen receptor modulator
Serv. L. serva (keep; preserve)
SEWHO shoulder-elbow-wrist-hand orthosis
SF-1 steroidogenic factor 1
SFEMG single fiber electromyography
SGA small for gestational age
SGOT serum glutamic-oxaloacetic transaminase
SGPT serum glutamic-pyruvic transaminase
SHBG sex hormone–binding globulin
SHH Sonic Hedgehog (gene)
SHML sinus histiocytosis with massive lymphadenopathy (Rosai-Dorfman disease)
SI stimulation index; Système International d'Unités (International System of Units)
Si silicon
SIAD syndrome of inappropriate antidiuresis
SIADH syndrome of inappropriate antidiuretic hormone
s.i.d. L. semel in die (once a day)
SIDS sudden infant death syndrome
sig. L. signa (mark)
Sig. n. pro. L. signa nomine proprio (label with the proper name)
SIMV synchronized intermittent mandatory ventilation
sing. L. singulorum (of each)
Si non val. L. si non valeat (if it is not enough)
Si op. sit L. si opus sit (if it is necessary)
siRNA small interfering RNA
SISI short increment sensitivity index
SIV simian immunodeficiency virus
Si vir. perm. L. si vires permittant (if the strength will permit)
SK streptokinase
SKSD streptokinase-streptodornase
SKY spectral karyotype
sl slyke
SLA L. sacro-laeva anterior (left sacroanterior [position of the fetus])
SLAC scapholunate advanced collapse
SLE systemic lupus erythematosus
SLO scanning laser ophthalmoscope
SLP L. sacro-laeva posterior (left sacroposterior [position of the fetus])
SLT L. sacro-laeva transversa (left sacrotransverse [position of the fetus])
Sm samarium
Sm 153-EDTMP samarium Sm 153 lexidronam
SMC selenomethylnorcholesterol
SMO supramalleolar orthosis
SMON subacute myelo-opticoneuropathy

Appendix 2

SMR	standardized morbidity ratio; standardized mortality ratio
S.N.	L. secundum naturam (according to nature)
Sn	tin (L. stannum)
SNAP	sensory nerve action potential
SNGFR	single nephron glomerular filtration rate
snoRNA	small nucleolar RNA
snoRNP	small nucleolar ribonucleoprotein
SNP	single nucleotide polymorphism
SNRI	serotonin-norepinephrine reuptake inhibitor
snRNA	small nuclear RNA
snRNP	small nuclear ribonucleoprotein
SNS	sympathetic nervous system
SO	sphenooccipital synchondrosis
SOB	shortness of breath
SOFAS	Social and Occupational Functioning Assessment Scale
Sol.	solution
solv.	L. solve (dissolve)
SOMI	sternal-occipital-mandibular immobilizer
s. op. s., S.O.S.	L. si opus sit (if it is necessary)
sp.	L. spiritus (spirit)
SPA	sperm penetration assay
SPCA	serum prothrombin conversion accelerator (factor VII)
SPECT	single-photon emission computed tomography
SPF	specific-pathogen free; sun protection factor
sp gr	specific gravity
sph	spherical; spherical lens
spir., Spt.	L. spiritus (spirit)
SQ	subcutaneous
SR	stimulation ratio
Sr	strontium
sr	steradian
SRBC	sheep red blood cell
SRF	skin reactive factor
SRH	somatotropin-releasing hormone
SRIF	somatotropin release–inhibiting factor
SRN	State Registered Nurse (England and Wales)
SRS-A	slow-reacting substance of anaphylaxis
SRT	speech reception threshold; speech recognition threshold
SS	somatostatin
ss.	L. semis (half)
SSD	source-skin distance
ssDNA	single-stranded DNA
SSPE	subacute sclerosing panencephalitis
SSR	simple sequence repeat
SSRI	selective serotonin reuptake inhibitor
ssRNA	single-stranded RNA
SSS	sick sinus syndrome; specific soluble substance
s.s.s.	L. stratum super stratum (layer upon layer)
S.S.V.	L. sub signo veneni (under a poison label)
ST	sinus tachycardia
St	stoke
St.	L. stet (let it stand); L. stent (let them stand)
STAT	signal transducer and activator of transcription
stat.	L. statim (at once, immediately)
STD	sexually transmitted disease
STE	subperiosteal tissue expander
STEC	Shiga toxin-producing *Escherichia coli*
STEMI	ST elevation myocardial infarction
STI	sexually transmitted infection; systolic time intervals
STP	standard temperature and pressure (0°C and 760 mm Hg)
STPD	standard temperature and pressure (dry)
STR	short tandem repeat
STRP	short tandem repeat polymorphism
STS	serologic test for syphilis
su.	L. sumat (let him take)
Sub fin. coct.	L. sub finem coctionis (toward the end of boiling)
SUDS	sudden unexplained death syndrome
sum.	L. sumat (let him take); L. sumendum (to be taken)
SUNCT	short-lasting unilateral neuralgiform headache attacks with conjunctival injection and tearing
SUZI	subzonal insemination
SV	sinus venosus; simian virus; stroke volume
SV40	simian virus 40
Sv	sievert
SVC	superior vena cava
SVT	supraventricular tachycardia
Syr.	L. syrupus (syrup)
T	intraocular tension; tesla; threonine; thymine; thymidine; tetanus toxoid; thoracic vertebrae (T1–T12); triangulation number
T	absolute temperature; transmittance; twisting number
$T_{1/2}$	half-life; half-time
$\mathbf{T_1}$	tricuspid valve closure
$\mathbf{T_3}$	triiodothyronine
$\mathbf{T_4}$	thyroxine
$\mathbf{T_m}$	melting temperature; transport maximum; tubular maximum
t	translocation
t	temperature; time
$\mathbf{t_{1/2}}$	half-life; half-time
ϑ	angle
τ	mean life; torque
TA	*Terminologia Anatomica*; toxin-antitoxin
Ta	tantalum
TAA	tumor-associated antigen
TAC	tetracaine, epinephrine (adrenaline), and cocaine (solution)
TAD	6-thioguanine, ara-C (cytarabine), and daunomycin
TAT	Thematic Apperception Test; toxin-antitoxin
TB	tuberculosis
Tb	terbium
TBG	thyroxine-binding globulin
TBI	traumatic brain injury; total body irradiation
TBII	TSH-binding inhibitory immunoglobulins
TBW	total body water
TC	transcobalamin
Tc	technetium
TCDD	2,3,7,8-tetrachlorodibenzo-*p*-dioxin
$\mathbf{TCID_{50}}$	median tissue culture infective dose
TCM	traditional Chinese medicine
TCMI	T cell–mediated immunity
TCR	T cell antigen receptor; transcription-coupled repair
TCV	total cell volume
$\mathbf{TD_{50}}$	median toxic dose
Td	tetanus and diphtheria toxoids
TDA	TSH-displacing antibody
Tdap	diphtheria and reduced tetanus toxoids and acellular pertussis vaccine
TDE	tetrachlorodiphenylethane
TDI	toluene diisocyanate
T1DM	type 1 diabetes mellitus
T2DM	type 2 diabetes mellitus
t.d.s.	L. ter die sumendum (to be taken three times a day)
TdT	terminal deoxynucleotidyl transferase
Te	tellurium
TeBG	testosterone-estradiol–binding globulin
TED	threshold erythema dose
TEE	transesophageal echocardiography
TEM	transanal endoscopic microsurgery
TENS	transcutaneous electrical nerve stimulation
TEOAE	transient evoked otoacoustic emissions
TEPP	tetraethyl pyrophosphate
TESE	testicular sperm extraction
TESPA	thiotepa
TET	treadmill exercise test; tubal embryo transfer
TF	transfer factor
TFF	trefoil factor
6-TG	6-thioguanine
Tg	thyroglobulin
TGE	transmissible gastroenteritis
TGF	transforming growth factor
TGN	trans-Golgi network
TGT	thromboplastin generation test
TH	tyrosine hydroxylase
Th	thorium
THA	total hip arthroplasty
THAM	tris(hydroxymethyl)aminomethane (tromethamine)
THC	tetrahydrocannabinol
THF	tetrahydrofolate; tetrahydrofolic acid
Thr	threonine
Ti	titanium
TIA	transient ischemic attack
TIBC	total iron-binding capacity
t.i.d.	L. ter in die (three times a day)
tinct.	L. tinctura (tincture)
TIPS	transjugular intrahepatic portosystemic shunt
TIV	trivalent inactivated influenza vaccine
TJA	total joint arthroplasty
TK	thymidine kinase

TKA total knee arthroplasty
TKD tocodynamometer
TKG tocodynagraph
Tl thallium
TLC total lung capacity; thin-layer chromatography
TLI total lymphoid irradiation
TLSO thoracolumbosacral orthosis
TLV threshold limit value
Tm thulium
TMA trimellitic anhydride
TMD temporomandibular disorder
TMI transmandibular implant
TMST treadmill stress test
Tn normal intraocular tension
TND transmissible neurodegenerative disease (prion disease)
TME total mesorectal excision
TMJ temporomandibular joint
TMJD temporomandibular joint disorder
TNF tumor necrosis factor
TNM tumor-nodes-metastasis (staging)
TNS transcutaneous nerve stimulation
TNT trinitrotoluene
TORCH toxoplasmosis, other agents, rubella, cytomegalovirus, herpes simplex (syndrome)
TPA, t-PA tissue plasminogen activator
TPHA *Treponema pallidum* hemagglutination assay
TPN total parenteral nutrition; triphosphopyridine nucleotide
TPP thiamine pyrophosphate
TR tricuspid regurgitation
TRA tumor rejection antigen (tumor-specific transplantation antigen)
TRALI transfusion-related acute lung injury
TRAPS TNF-receptor–associated periodic syndrome
TRH thyrotropin-releasing hormone
Trid. L. triduum (three days)
Trit. L. tritura (triturate)
tRNA transfer RNA
troch. L. trochiscus (troche)
Trp tryptophan
TRU turbidity reducing unit
TRUS transrectal ultrasonography
TS test solution; tricuspid stenosis
TSA tumor-specific antigen
TSC tuberous sclerosis complex
TSD Tay-Sachs disease
TSE transmissible spongiform encephalopathy (prion disease)
TSF triceps skinfold
TSH thyroid-stimulating hormone
T-spine thoracic spine
TSTA tumor-specific transplantation antigen
TT therapeutic touch; thrombin time
TTV thrombotic threshold velocity
TU tuberculin unit
TUIP transurethral incision of the prostate
TULIP transurethral laser-induced prostatectomy
TUMT transurethral microwave thermotherapy
TUNA transurethral needle ablation
TUR transurethral resection
TURBT transurethral resection of bladder tumor
TURP transurethral resection of the prostate
tus. L. tussis (a cough)
TUVP transurethral vaporization of the prostate
TWZ triangular working zone
TXA_2 thromboxane A_2
TXB_2 thromboxane B_2
Tyr tyrosine
TZD thiazolidinedione
U international unit of enzyme activity; unit *(on the JCAHO "Do Not Use" List)*; uracil; uranium; uridine
u atomic mass unit
UDP uridine diphosphate
UK urokinase
ult. praes. L. ultimum praescriptus (last prescribed)
UMP uridine monophospate
ung. L. unguentum (ointment)
UPP urethral pressure profile
UPPP uvulopalatopharyngoplasty
URR urea reduction ratio
US ultrasound
USAN United States Adopted Names
USP *United States Pharmacopeia*
USRDS United States Renal Data System
Ut dict. L. ut dictum (as directed)
Utend. L. utendus (to be used)
UTI urinary tract infection
UTP uridine triphosphate
UV ultraviolet
UVA ultraviolet A
UVB ultraviolet B
UVC ultraviolet C
V valine; vanadium; vision; volt; volume
V voltage; volume
V_{max} maximum velocity of an enzyme-catalyzed reaction
V_T tidal volume
v. L. vena (vein)
v velocity; voltage
VA visual acuity
VAC vincristine, dactinomycin, and cyclophosphamide
VACTERL vertebral, anal, cardiac, tracheal, esophageal, renal, and limb (association)
VAD ventricular assist device
Val valine
VAMP vincristine, methotrexate, 6-mercaptopurine, and prednisone
var. variety
VATER vertebral defects, imperforate anus, tracheoesophageal fistula, radial and renal dysplasia (association)
VATS video-assisted thoracic (or thoracoscopic) surgery
VBG vertical banded gastroplasty
VC vital capacity
VCG vectorcardiogram
VCU voiding cystourethrography
VCUG voiding cystourethrogram; voiding cystourethrography
VD venereal disease
VDH valvular disease of the heart
VDRL Venereal Disease Research Laboratories
VEE Venezuelan equine encephalomyelitis
VEGF vascular endothelial growth factor
VEP visual evoked potential
Vesic. L. vesicula (a blister)
VF vocal fremitus
vf visual field
VFib ventricular fibrillation
VFl ventricular flutter
VHDL very-high-density lipoprotein
VIG vaccinia immune globulin
VIP vasoactive intestinal polypeptide
VISA vancomycin-intermediate *Staphylococcus aureus*
VLA very late activation (antigen)
VLBW very low birth weight (infant)
VLCD very low calorie diet
VLDL very-low-density lipoprotein
VMA vanillylmandelic acid
VMD L. Veterinariae Medicinae Doctor (Doctor of Veterinary Medicine)
VNS vagal nerve stimulation
VNTR variable number tandem repeats; variable number of tandem repeats
VP variegate porphyria
VPB ventricular premature beat
VPC ventricular premature complex
VPD ventricular premature depolarization
VPF vascular permeability factor
VPRC volume of packed red cells
VR vocal resonance
VRE vancomycin-resistant enterococci
VRSA vancomycin-resistant *Staphylococcus aureus*
VS volumetric solution
VSG variable surface glycoprotein
VT ventricular tachycardia
vv. L. venae (veins)
v/v volume (of solute) per volume (of solvent)
VVS vulvar vestibulitis syndrome
VW vessel wall
vWF von Willebrand factor
VZIG varicella-zoster immune globulin
W tryptophan; tungsten (Ger. Wolfram); watt
W work; writhing number
WAIS Wechsler Adult Intelligence Scale
Wb weber
WBC white blood cell; white blood cell count
WEE western equine encephalomyelitis
WHHL Watanabe heritable hyperlipidemic (rabbit)
WHO World Health Organization; wrist-hand orthosis

WISC	Wechsler Intelligence Scale for Children
wt	weight
w/v	weight (of solute) per volume (of solvent)
X	Kienböck unit; xanthine; xanthosine
X	reactance
$\bar{X}$	sample mean
x	abscissa
Xe	xenon
XIST	X-inactivation–specific transcript (gene)
XMP	xanthosine monophosphate
XOAN	X-linked ocular albinism (Nettleship-Falls)
XU	excretory urography
Y	tyrosine; yttrium
y	ordinate
YAC	yeast artificial chromosome
Yb	ytterbium
Z	atomic number; impedance
ZES	Zollinger-Ellison syndrome
ZIFT	zygote intrafallopian transfer
Zn	zinc
Zr	zirconium
ZSR	zeta sedimentation ratio
Zz.	L. zingiber (ginger)

APPENDIX 3

SYMBOLS

The Greek Alphabet

For more information on the Greek alphabet, including pronunciation and transliteration, see *Fundamentals of Medical Etymology*, p. xxiii.

Capital	Lower Case	Letter Name	Transcription
Α	α	alpha	a
Β	β	beta	b
Γ	γ	gamma	g
Δ	δ	delta	d
Ε	ε	epsilon	e
Ζ	ζ	zeta	z
Η	η	eta	ē
Θ	θ	theta	th
Ι	ι	iota	i
Κ	κ	kappa	k
Λ	λ	lambda	l
Μ	μ	mu	m
Ν	ν	nu	n
Ξ	ξ	xi	x
Ο	ο	omicron	o
Π	π	pi	p
Ρ	ρ	rho	r
Σ	σ, ς	sigma	s
Τ	τ	tau	t
Υ	υ	upsilon	y (sometimes u)
Φ	φ	phi	ph
Χ	χ	chi	ch (sometimes kh)
Ψ	ψ	psi	ps
Ω	ω	omega	ō

Symbols Commonly Used in Pedigrees

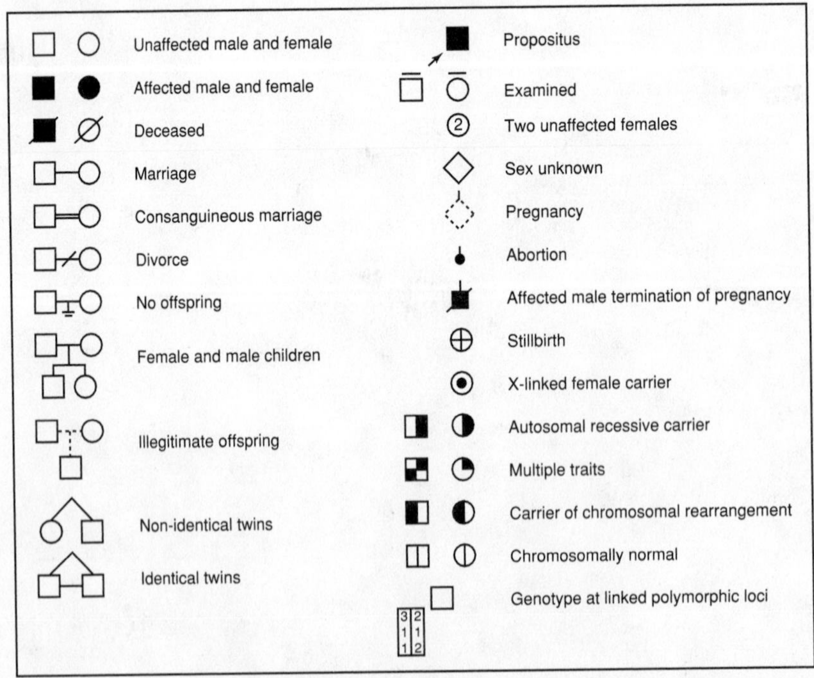

From Rimoin, DL et al., eds: Emery & Rimoin's Principles and Practice of Medical Genetics, 3rd ed. New York: Churchill Livingstone, 1995.

Appendix 3

Mathematics and Statistics

Symbol	Meaning
α	probability of Type I error
β	probability of Type II error
$1-\beta$	power (of a statistical test)
χ^2	chi-square
Cov_{AB}	covariance of A and B
CV	coefficient of variation
D	nonparametric statistic
d	parametric statistic
E	expectancy
e	base of natural logarithms
F	F statistic
f	frequency, function
H_0	null hypothesis
H_1	alternative hypothesis
H_a	alternative hypothesis
ln	natural logarithm
m	median
μ	population mean
N	population size
n	sample size
ν	degrees of freedom
P	probability
p	probability that event will occur
$P(A)$	probability that event A will occur
$P(A \mid B)$	probability that, given event A, event B will occur (conditional probability)
q	probability that an alternative event will occur (equal to $1/p$)
r	sample correlation coefficient
R	rate
ρ	population correlation coefficient
r_s	Spearman's rank correlation coefficient
Σ	summation
s	sample standard deviation
s^2	sample variance
σ	population standard deviation
σ^2	population variance
SD	standard deviation
SE	standard error
t	(Student's) *t*-test variable
x	abscissa
$\overline{X}$	sample mean
$\lvert x \rvert$	absolute value of x
y	ordinate
$+$	plus
$-$	minus
$\pm$	plus or minus
$\times$	multiplied by, times
$\div$, /	divided by
$=$	equals
$\sim$	approximately
$\cong$	congruent to, approximately equal to
$\approx$	approximately equal to
$\neq$	not equal to
$>$	greater than *(on the JCAHO "Do Not Use" List)*
$\geq$	greater than or equal to
$\ngtr$	not greater than
$<$	less than *(on the JCAHO "Do Not Use" List)*
$\leq$	less than or equal to
$\nless$	not less than
$\equiv$	identical to
$\sqrt{}$	square root
$\sqrt[3]{}$	cube root
!	factorial
%	per cent
∞	infinity
$\binom{n}{k}$, ${}_nC_k$	binomial coefficient
$*$	estimate (biased), used over a symbol
$\wedge$	estimate (unbiased), used over symbol
$\subset$	is a subset of
$\supset$	contains as a subset
$\cap$	("cap") intersection
$\cup$	("cup") union

Appendix 3

Miscellaneous Symbols

Symbol	Meaning
Ⓐ	axilla
ⓐⓧ	axilla
Ⓗ	hypodermic
ⓗ	hypodermic
ⒾⓂ	intramuscular
ⒾⓋ	intravenous
Ⓛ	left
Ⓜ	murmur
ⓜ	mouth
	by mouth
	murmur
Ⓞ	by mouth
	oral
Ⓡ	rectal
	rectum
	right
0	absent
	no response
+	acid
	and
	increased
	plus
	positive
	present
	slight trace
++	moderate
	normally active
	noticeable reaction
	trace
+++	increased
	moderately active
	moderately severe
++++	large amount
	pronounced reaction
	severe
++/+	2 plus on the right, 1 plus on the left
0/0	zero on either side
(+)	significant
−	absent
	alkaline
	decreased
	diminished
	minus
	negative
(−)	insignificant
±	plus or minus
	positive or negative
(±)	possibly significant
1×	once
×2	twice
2×	twice
/	divided by
	of
	per
°	degree
	hour
1°	first degree
	one hour
	primary
2°	secondary
	second degree
	two hours
3°	tertiary
	third degree
24°	24 hours
i̅i̅	two
′	foot
	minute
	univalent
″	bivalent
	inch
	second
:	is to
	ratio
::	as (in ratios)
∴	therefore
#	fracture
	gauge
	has been done
	has been given
	number
	pounds
@	at *(on the JCAHO "Do Not Use" List)*
∞	indefinitely more
	infinite
	infinity
Δ	change
	difference
	Gibbs free energy
	prism diopter
Δ*A*	change in absorbance
ΔpH	change in pH
Δt	time interval
↗	deviated
	displaced
	increase
	increasing
↑	elevated
	gas
	increased
	increasing
↑↑	extensor response, Babinski sign
	testes undescended
⇧	up
↘	decrease
	decreasing
↓	decreased
	decreasing
	deficiency
	deficit
	depressed
	diminished
	precipitate
↓↓	bilaterally descended
	both down
	plantar response, Babinski sign
	testes descended
⇩	down
↑V	increase due to *in vivo* effect
↓V	decrease due to *in vivo* effect
↑C	increase due to chemical interference during the assay
↓C	decrease due to chemical interference during the assay
→	causes
	distal
	no change
	reaction proceeds to the right
	results in
	transfer to
	yields
←	caused by
	derived from
	is due to
	reaction proceeds to the left
⇆	reversible reaction
?	doubtful
	equivocal
	flicker
	possible
	questionable
	unknown
‖	parallel
	parallel bars
⊖	normal
c̄	with
s̄	without
✓	check
	observe for
✓'d	checked
✓c̄	check with
φ	none

Miscellaneous Symbols *Continued*

Symbol	Meaning
∨	systolic blood pressure
∧	diastolic blood pressure
∟	right lower quadrant right angle
⌐	right upper quadrant
¬	left upper quadrant
⌟	left lower quadrant
∠	angle
∠E	angle of entry
∠X	angle of exit
○○	male
♂	male
♀	female
*	birth not verified presumed
†	dead death died
℞	recipe, take
℥	ounce
f℥	fluid ounce
℈	scruple
♏	minim
ʒ	drachm, dram
fʒ	fluidrachm, fluidram

APPENDIX 4

PHOBIAS

Fear of:	Phobia
air	aerophobia
amphibians	herpetophobia
animals	zoophobia
bacilli	bacillophobia
bad men	sclerophobia
barren space	cenophobia, kenophobia
bearing a deformed child	teratophobia
beating	mastigophobia, rhabdophobia
bees	apiphobia, melissophobia
being alone	autophobia, eremophobia, monophobia
being beaten	mastigophobia, rhabdophobia
being buried alive	taphephobia
being enclosed	claustrophobia, clithrophobia
being laughed at	catagelophobia, katagelophobia
being locked in	clithrophobia
being looked at	scopophobia, scoptophobia
being scratched	amychophobia
being touched	aphephobia, haphephobia, haptephobia
being unclean	automysophobia
being unclothed	gymnophobia, nudophobia
birds	ornithophobia
blood	hematophobia, hemophobia
blushing	ereuthophobia, erythrophobia
body defect, imaginary	dysmorphophobia
brain disease	meningitophobia
bridge, crossing	gephyrophobia
building, being inside	domatophobia
burglars	scelerophobia
burial alive	taphephobia
cancer	cancerophobia, cancerphobia, carcinomatophobia, carcinophobia
cats	ailurophobia, galeophobia, gatophobia
change	kainophobia, kainotophobia, neophobia
childbirth	maieusiophobia, tocophobia
children	pedophobia
choking	anginophobia, pnigophobia
climbing	climacophobia
coitus	coitophobia
cold	cheimaphobia, cryophobia, psychropophobia
colors	chromatophobia, chromophobia
comets	cometophobia
confinement	claustrophobia
contamination	coprophobia, molysmophobia, mysophobia, scatophobia
corpses	necrophobia
crossing a bridge or river	gephyrophobia
crossing a street	dromophobia
crowds	demophobia, ochlophobia
dampness	hygrophobia
darkness	achluphobia, noctiphobia, nyctophobia, scotophobia
dawn	esophobia
daylight	phengophobia
dead bodies	necrophobia
death	necrophobia, thanatophobia
defecation	coprophobia
deformed child, bearing	teratophobia
deformity	dysmorphophobia
demons	demonophobia
dental operations	odontophobia
depths	bathophobia
devils or the devil	demonophobia, satanophobia
dirt	coprophobia, mysophobia, rhypophobia, rupophobia
dirtiness, personal	automysophobia
disease	nosophobia, pathophobia
disease, specific	monopathophobia
disorder	ataxiophobia, ataxophobia
dogs	cynophobia
dolls	pediophobia
drafts	aerophobia, anemophobia
drugs	pharmacophobia
dust	amathophobia
eating	cibophobia, phagophobia, sitophobia
electricity	electrophobia
emptiness	cenophobia, kenophobia
enclosed spaces	claustrophobia
endlessness	apeirophobia
error	hamartophobia
everything	panophobia, panphobia, pantophobia
excrement	coprophobia, scatophobia
eyes	ommatophobia
failure	kakorrhaphiophobia
fatigue	kopophobia
fearing or fears	phobophobia
feathers	pteronophobia
feces	coprophobia
female genitals	eurotophobia
fever	febriphobia, pyrexiophobia
filth	mysophobia, rhypophobia, rupophobia
filth, personal	automysophobia
fire	pyrophobia
fish	ichthyophobia
flogging	mastigophobia, rhabdophobia
floods	antlophobia
flutes	aulophobia
flying	aviophobia
fog	homichlophobia
food	cibophobia, phagophobia, sitophobia
forests	hylophobia
fresh air	aerophobia
frogs	batrachophobia
functioning	ergasiophobia
fur	doraphobia
germs	microbiophobia, microphobia
ghosts	phasmophobia, demonophobia
girls	parthenophobia
glare	photaugiaphobia
glass	crystallophobia, hyalophobia
God	theophobia
gravity	barophobia
hair	trichopathophobia, trichophobia
heart disease	cardiophobia
heat	thermophobia
heaven	siderophobia, uranophobia
heights	acrophobia, hyposophobia
hell	hadephobia, stygiophobia
hereditary disease or heredity	patroiophobia, patriophobia
high objects	batophobia
home, returning to	nostophobia
horses	equinophobia, hippophobia
houses	domatophobia, oikophobia
human society	anthropophobia
humiliation	catagelophobia, katagelophobia
ideas	ideophobia
infinity	apeirophobia
inherited disease	patroiophobia, patriophobia

Appendix 4

Fear of:	Phobia
injury	traumatophobia
innovation	neophobia
insanity	lyssophobia, maniaphobia
insects	acarophobia, entomophobia
instrument of punishment	rhabdophobia
jealousy	zelophobia
justice	dikephobia
knives	aichmophobia
large objects	megalophobia
left or objects to the left	levophobia
light	photophobia
lightning	astraphobia, astrapophobia, keraunophobia
loneliness	eremophobia, monophobia
love	erotophobia
machinery	mechanophobia
malignancy	cancerophobia, cancerphobia, carcinomatophobia, carcinophobia
many things	polyphobia
marriage	gamophobia
medicines	pharmacophobia
men	androphobia
messiness	ataxiophobia, ataxophobia
metals	metallophobia
meteors	meteorophobia
mice	musophobia
microorganisms	microbiophobia, microphobia
mind	psychophobia
minute objects	acarophobia, microbiophobia, microphobia
mirrors	eisoptrophobia, spectrophobia
missiles	ballistophobia
mites	acarophobia
moisture	hygrophobia
money	chrematophobia
motion	kinesophobia
movement	ergasiophobia
myths	mythophobia
naked body or nakedness	gymnophobia, nudophobia
names or naming or being named	onomatophobia
needles	belonephobia
neglecting duty	paralipophobia
new things	kainophobia, kainotophobia, neophobia
night	achluphobia, noctiphobia, nyctophobia
northern lights	auroraphobia
novelty	kainophobia, kainotophobia, neophobia
nudity	gymnophobia, nudophobia
ocean	nautophobia, thalassophobia
odor, personal	automysophobia, bromidrosiphobia
odors	olfactophobia, osmophobia, osphresiophobia
one's own voice	phonophobia
oneself	autophobia, monophobia
open spaces	agoraphobia, agyiophobia
overwork	ponophobia
pain	algophobia, odynophobia
parasites	acarophobia, parasitophobia
passing high objects	batophobia
people	anthropophobia
personal odor or uncleanliness	automysophobia, bromidrosiphobia
phobia, development of	phobophobia
pins	belonephobia
places	topophobia
pleasure	hedonophobia
points or pointed objects	aichmophobia
poison	iophobia, toxiphobia, toxicophobia
poverty	peniaphobia
precipices	cremnophobia
public places	agoraphobia, agyiophobia
punishment	poinephobia
rabies	cynophobia, lyssophobia
radiation	radiophobia
railroads	siderodromophobia
rain or rainstorms	ombrophobia

Fear of:	Phobia
rectal excreta	coprophobia, scatophobia
rectum	proctophobia
red	erythrophobia
reptiles	herpetophobia
responsibility	hypengyophobia
ridicule	catagelophobia, katagelophobia
right or objects to the right	dextrophobia
rivers	potamophobia
rivers, crossing	gephyrophobia
robbers	harpaxophobia
rod	mastigophobia, rhabdophobia
ruin	atephobia
sacred objects	hierophobia
scabies	scabiophobia
scratch, receiving	amychophobia
sea	nautophobia, thalassophobia
self	autophobia
semen	spermatophobia
sex	genophobia
sexual intercourse	coitophobia, cypridophobia, cypriophobia
sexual love	erotophobia
sharp objects	aichmophobia, belonephobia
ships	nautophobia
shock	hormephobia
sickness	nosophobia, pathophobia
sin or sinning	enosiophobia, hamartophobia, peccatiphobia
sitting	thaasophobia
sitting down, the act	cathisophobia, kathisophobia
skin, animal	doraphobia
skin disease	dermatosiophobia
skin lesion	dermatophobia
sleep	hypnophobia
small objects or animals	microbiophobia, microphobia
smelling bad	automysophobia, bromidrosiphobia
smothering	pnigerophobia
snakes	ophidiophobia
snow	chionophobia
solitude	autophobia, eremophobia, monophobia
sounds	acousticophobia, phonophobia
sourness	acerophobia
speaking	glossophobia, laliophobia, lalophobia
speaking aloud	phonophobia
specific disease	monopathophobia
specific word	onomatophobia
spiders	arachnephobia, arachnophobia
spirits	demonophobia
stairs	climacophobia
standing up	stasiphobia
standing up and walking	stasibasiphobia
stars	siderophobia
stating untruths	mythophobia
stealing	kleptophobia
stories	mythophobia
strangers	xenophobia
street, crossing	dromophobia
streets	agoraphobia, agyiophobia
string	linonophobia
sunlight	heliophobia
symbolism	symbolophobia
syphilis	syphilophobia
talking	laliophobia, lalophobia
tapeworms	taemophobia
taste or tasting	geumaphobia
teeth	odontophobia
thinking	phronemophobia, psychophobia
thirteen	triskaidekaphobia
thunder	astraphobia, astrapophobia, brontophobia, keraunophobia, tonitrophobia
time	chronophobia
touching	aphephobia, haphephobia, haptephobia
trains	siderodromophobia
travel	hodophobia, dromophobia
trembling	tremophobia

Appendix 4

Fear of:	Phobia
trichinosis	trichinophobia
tuberculosis	phthisiophobia, tuberculophobia
uncleanliness, self	automysophobia
untruths	mythophobia
vaccination	vaccinophobia
vehicles	amaxophobia
venereal disease	cypridophobia, cypriphobia
voices	phonophobia
voids	cenophobia, kenophobia
vomiting	emetophobia
walking	basiphobia
water	aquaphobia, hydrophobia, nautophobia
weakness	asthenophobia
wind	anemophobia
wind instruments	aulophobia
women	gynephobia, gynophobia
word, specific	onomatophobia
work	ergasiophobia, ponophobia
writing	graphophobia
x-rays	radiophobia

APPENDIX 5

TABLE OF ELEMENTS

Name	Symbol	At. No.	At. Wt.*
Actinium	Ac	89	[227]
Aluminum	Al	13	26.982
Americium	Am	95	[243]
Antimony	Sb	51	121.760
Argon	Ar	18	39.948
Arsenic	As	33	74.922
Astatine	At	85	[210]
Barium	Ba	56	137.327
Berkelium	Bk	97	[247]
Beryllium	Be	4	9.012
Bismuth	Bi	83	208.980
Bohrium	Bh	107	[264]
Boron	B	5	10.811
Bromine	Br	35	79.904
Cadmium	Cd	48	112.411
Calcium	Ca	20	40.078
Californium	Cf	98	[251]
Carbon	C	6	12.007
Cerium	Ce	58	140.116
Cesium	Cs	55	132.906
Chlorine	Cl	17	35.453
Chromium	Cr	24	51.996
Cobalt	Co	27	58.933
Copernicium	Cn	112	[277]
Copper	Cu	29	63.546
Curium	Cm	96	[247]
Darmstadtium	Ds	110	[269]
Dubnium	Db	105	[262]
Dysprosium	Dy	66	162.50
Einsteinium	Es	99	[252]
Erbium	Er	68	167.26
Europium	Eu	63	151.964
Fermium	Fm	100	[257]
Fluorine	F	9	18.998
Francium	Fr	87	[223]
Gadolinium	Gd	64	157.25
Gallium	Ga	31	69.723
Germanium	Ge	32	72.61
Gold	Au	79	196.967
Hafnium	Hf	72	178.49
Hassium	Hs	108	[265]
Helium	He	2	4.003
Holmium	Ho	67	164.930
Hydrogen	H	1	1.008
Indium	In	49	114.818
Iodine	I	53	126.905
Iridium	Ir	77	192.217
Iron	Fe	26	55.845
Krypton	Kr	36	83.80
Lanthanum	La	57	138.906
Lawrencium	Lw	103	[262]
Lead	Pb	82	207.2
Lithium	Li	3	6.941
Lutetium	Lu	71	174.967
Magnesium	Mg	12	24.305
Manganese	Mn	25	54.938
Meitnerium	Mt	109	[268]

Name	Symbol	At. No.	At. Wt.*
Mendelevium	Md	101	[258]
Mercury	Hg	80	200.59
Molybdenum	Mo	42	95.94
Neodymium	Nd	60	144.24
Neon	Ne	10	20.180
Neptunium	Np	93	[237]
Nickel	Ni	28	58.693
Niobium	Nb	41	92.906
Nitrogen	N	7	14.007
Nobelium	No	102	[259]
Osmium	Os	76	190.23
Oxygen	O	8	15.999
Palladium	Pd	46	106.42
Phosphorus	P	15	30.974
Platinum	Pt	78	195.078
Plutonium	Pu	94	[244]
Polonium	Po	84	[209]
Potassium	K	19	39.098
Praseodymium	Pr	59	140.908
Promethium	Pm	61	[145]
Protactinium	Pa	91	231.036
Radium	Ra	88	[226]
Radon	Rn	86	[222]
Rhenium	Re	75	186.207
Rhodium	Rh	45	102.906
Roentgenium	Rg	111	[272]
Rubidium	Rb	37	85.468
Ruthenium	Ru	44	101.07
Rutherfordium	Rf	104	[261]
Samarium	Sm	62	150.36
Scandium	Sc	21	44.956
Seaborgium	Sg	106	[262]
Selenium	Se	34	78.96
Silicon	Si	14	28.086
Silver	Ag	47	107.868
Sodium	Na	11	22.990
Strontium	Sr	38	87.62
Sulfur	S	16	32.066
Tantalum	Ta	83	180.948
Technetium	Tc	43	[98]
Tellurium	Te	52	127.60
Terbium	Tb	65	158.925
Thallium	Tl	81	204.383
Thorium	Th	90	232.038
Thulium	Tm	69	168.934
Tin	Sn	50	118.710
Titanium	Ti	22	47.867
Tungsten	W	74	183.84
Uranium	U	92	238.029
Vanadium	V	23	50.942
Xenon	Xe	54	131.29
Ytterbium	Yb	70	173.04
Yttrium	Y	39	88.906
Zinc	Zn	30	65.39
Zirconium	Zr	40	91.224

*Atomic weights are corrected to conform with the 1995 values of the International Union of Pure and Applied Chemistry, expressed to the fourth decimal point, rounded off to the nearest thousandth. For elements with no stable nuclides, the mass number of the longest lived isotope of the element is shown in brackets.

APPENDIX 6

CELSIUS AND FAHRENHEIT TEMPERATURE EQUIVALENTS

Celsius—Fahrenheit

°C	°F	°C	°F	°C	°F
−40	−40.0	9	48.2	58	136.4
−39	−38.2	10	50.0	59	138.2
−38	−36.4	11	51.8	60	140.0
−37	−34.6	12	53.6	61	141.8
−36	−32.8	13	55.4	62	143.6
−35	−31.0	14	57.2	63	145.4
−34	−29.2	15	59.0	64	147.2
−33	−27.4	16	60.8	65	149.0
−32	−25.6	17	62.6	66	150.8
−31	−23.8	18	64.4	67	152.6
−30	−22.0	19	66.2	68	154.4
−29	−20.2	20	68.0	69	156.2
−28	−18.4	21	69.8	70	158.0
−27	−16.6	22	71.6	71	159.8
−26	−14.8	23	73.4	72	161.6
−25	−13.0	24	75.2	73	163.4
−24	−11.2	25	77.0	74	165.2
−23	−9.4	26	78.8	75	167.0
−22	−7.6	27	80.6	76	168.8
−21	−5.8	28	82.4	77	170.6
−20	−4.0	29	84.2	78	172.4
−19	−2.2	30	86.0	79	174.2
−18	−0.4	31	87.8	80	176.0
−17	+1.4	32	89.6	81	177.8
−16	3.2	33	91.4	82	179.6
−15	5.0	34	93.2	83	181.4
−14	6.8	35	95.0	84	183.2
−13	8.6	36	96.8	85	185.0
−12	10.4	37	98.6	86	186.8
−11	12.2	38	100.4	87	188.6
−10	14.0	39	102.2	88	190.4
−9	15.8	40	104.0	89	192.2
−8	17.6	41	105.8	90	194.0
−7	19.4	42	107.6	91	195.8
−6	21.2	43	109.4	92	197.6
−5	23.0	44	111.2	93	199.4
−4	24.8	45	113.0	94	201.2
−3	26.6	46	114.8	95	203.0
−2	28.4	47	116.6	96	204.8
−1	30.2	48	118.4	97	206.6
0	32.0	49	120.2	98	208.4
+1	33.8	50	122.0	99	210.2
2	35.6	51	123.8	100	212.0
3	37.4	52	125.6	101	213.8
4	39.2	53	127.4	102	215.6
5	41.0	54	129.2	103	217.4
6	42.8	55	131.0	104	219.2
7	44.6	56	132.8	105	221.0
8	46.4	57	134.6	106	222.8

Fahrenheit—Celsius

°F	°C	°F	°C	°F	°C
−40	−40.0	55	12.7	146	63.3
−39	−39.4	60	15.5	147	63.8
−38	−38.9	65	18.3	148	64.4
−37	−38.3	70	21.1	149	65.0
−36	−37.8	75	23.8	150	65.5
−35	−37.2	80	26.6	151	66.1
−34	−36.7	85	29.4	152	66.6
−33	−36.1	86	30.0	153	67.2
−32	−35.6	87	30.5	154	67.7
−31	−35.0	88	31.0	155	68.3
−30	−34.4	89	31.6	156	68.8
−29	−33.9	90	32.2	157	69.4
−28	−33.3	91	32.7	158	70.0
−27	−32.8	92	33.3	159	70.5
−26	−32.2	93	33.8	160	71.1
−25	−31.7	94	34.4	161	71.6
−24	−31.1	95	35.0	162	72.2
−23	−30.6	96	35.5	163	72.7
−22	−30.0	97	36.1	164	73.3
−21	−29.4	98	36.6	165	73.8
−20	−28.9	98.6	37.0	166	74.4
−19	−28.3	99	37.2	167	75.0
−18	−27.8	100	37.7	168	75.5
−17	−27.2	101	38.3	169	76.1
−16	−26.7	102	38.8	170	76.6
−15	−26.1	103	39.4	171	77.2
−14	−25.6	104	40.0	172	77.7
−13	−25.0	105	40.5	173	78.3
−12	−24.4	106	41.1	174	78.8
−11	−23.9	107	41.6	175	79.4
−10	−23.3	108	42.2	176	80.0
−9	−22.8	109	42.7	177	80.5
−8	−22.2	110	43.3	178	81.1
−7	−21.7	111	43.8	179	81.6
−6	−21.1	112	44.4	180	82.2
−5	−20.6	113	45.0	181	82.7
−4	−20.0	114	45.5	182	83.3
−3	−19.4	115	46.1	183	83.8
−2	−18.9	116	46.6	184	84.4
−1	−18.3	117	47.2	185	85.0
0	−17.8	118	47.7	186	85.5
+1	−17.2	119	48.3	187	86.1
5	−15.0	120	48.8	188	86.6
10	−12.2	121	49.4	189	87.2
15	−9.4	122	50.0	190	87.7
20	−6.6	123	50.5	191	88.3
25	−3.8	124	51.1	192	88.8
30	−1.1	125	51.6	193	89.4
31	−0.5	126	52.2	194	90.0
32	0	127	52.7	195	90.5
33	+0.5	128	53.3	196	91.1
34	1.1	129	53.8	197	91.6
35	1.6	130	54.4	198	92.2
36	2.2	131	55.0	199	92.7
37	2.7	132	55.5	200	93.3
38	3.3	133	56.1	201	93.8
39	3.8	134	56.6	202	94.4
40	4.4	135	57.2	203	95.0
41	5.0	136	57.7	204	95.5
42	5.5	137	58.3	205	96.1
43	6.1	138	58.8	206	96.6
44	6.6	139	59.4	207	97.2
45	7.2	140	60.0	208	97.7
46	7.7	141	60.5	209	98.3
47	8.3	142	61.1	210	98.8
48	8.8	143	61.6	211	99.4
49	9.4	144	62.2	212	100.0
50	10.0	145	62.7	213	100.5

APPENDIX 7

UNITS OF MEASUREMENT

Multiples and Submultiples of the Metric System

Multiples and Submultiples	Power	Prefix	Symbol
1,000,000,000,000	(10^{12})	tera-	T
1,000,000,000	(10^{9})	giga-	G
1,000,000	(10^{6})	mega-	M
1,000	(10^{3})	kilo-	k
100	(10^{2})	hecto-	h
10	(10)	deca-	da
0.1	(10^{-1})	deci-	d
0.01	(10^{-2})	centi-	c
0.001	(10^{-3})	milli-	m
0.000 001	(10^{-6})	micro-	μ
0.000 000 001	(10^{-9})	nano-	n
0.000 000 000 001	(10^{-12})	pico-	p
0.000 000 000 000 001	(10^{-15})	femto-	f
0.000 000 000 000 000 001	(10^{-18})	atto-	a

TABLES OF WEIGHTS AND MEASURES

Measures of Mass

Metric and Avoirdupois

Kilograms	Grams	Milligrams	Grains	Drams	Ounces	Pounds
1	1000	1.0×10^{6}	1.5432×10^{4}	564.3776	35.2736	2.2046
0.001	1	[illegible]000	15.4324	0.5644	0.0353	0.002205
1.0×10^{-6}	0.001	1	0.0154	5.6438×10^{-4}	3.53×10^{-5}	2.2046×10^{-6}
6.48×10^{-5}	0.0648	64.8	1	0.0366	0.0023	1.4×10^{-4}
0.0018	1.772	[illegible]771.632	27.34	1	0.0625	0.0039
0.0284	28.350	2.8350×10^{4}	437.5	16	1	0.0625
0.4536	453.5924	4.536×10^{5}	7000	256	16	1

Metric and Apothecary*

Kilograms	Grams	Milligrams	Grains	Scruples (℈)	Drams (ʒ)	Ounces (℥)	Pounds (£)
1	1000	1.0 × 1[illegible]	1.5432×10^{4}	771.6049	257.2016	32.1512	2.6792
0.001	1	1000	15.4324	0.7716	0.2572	0.03215	0.002679
1.0×10^{-6}	0.001	1	0.0154	7.7160×10^{-4}	2.5720×10^{-4}	3.2151×10^{-5}	2.6792×10^{-6}
6.48×10^{-5}	0.0648	64.8	1	0.05	0.0167	0.0021	1.7×10^{-4}
0.001296	1.296	1296	20	1	0.333	0.042	0.0035
0.003888	3.888	3888	60	3	1	0.125	0.0104
0.03110	31.103	31.103 × [illegible]4	480	24	8	1	0.0833
0.3732	373.2418	3.73 × 1[illegible]	5760	288	96	12	1

*The Joint Commission (JCAHO) prescribes the use of [illegible]etric, instead of apothecary, units.

Appendix 7

Metric and Troy

Grams	Grains	Ounces	Pounds
1	15.4324	0.03215	0.002679
1.0648	1	0.002	0.00017
31.103	480	1	0.083
373.2418	5760	12	1

Measures of Fluid Capacity

Metric and Apothecary*

Liters	Deciliters	Milliliters	Minims	Fluid Drams	Fluid Ounces	Pints	Quarts	Gallons (US)
1	10	1000	1.623×10^4	270.5	33.8	2.113	1.056	0.2641
0.1	1	100	1623	27.05	3.38	0.2113	0.1056	0.0264
0.001	0.01	1	16.23	0.2705	0.0338	0.002113	0.001056	2.6406×10^{-4}
6.161×10^{-5}	6.161×10^{-4}	0.06161	1	0.0166	0.002	1.302×10^{-4}	6.51×10^{-5}	1.628×10^{-5}
0.003697	0.03697	3.6967	60	1	0.125	0.0078	0.0039	9.7656×10^{-5}
0.02957	0.2957	29.5737	480	8	1	0.0625	0.0312	0.0078
0.4731	4.7318	473.179	7680	128	16	1	0.5	0.125
0.9464	9.4636	946.358	1.536×10^4	256	32	2	1	0.25
3.7854	37.8543	3785.434	6.1440×10^4	1024	128	8	4	1

*The Joint Commission (JCAHO) prescribes the use of metric, instead of apothecary, units.

Approximate Household Equivalents

Drops	Minims	Teaspoons	Tablespoons	Fluid Ounces	Cups (or glasses)*	Milliliters
1	1	1/60	—	—	—	0.06161
60	60	1	1/3	1/8	—	5
180	180	3	1	1/2	1/16	15
—	—	48	16	8	1	240

*A household tumbler or glass is considered equivalent to one (8 ounce) cup.

Measures of Length

Micrometers	Millimeters	Centimeters	Meters	Kilometers	Inches	Feet	Yards	Miles
1	0.001	1.0×10^{-4}	1.0×10^{-6}	1.0×10^{-9}	3.937×10^{-5}	3.281×10^{-6}	1.0936×10^{-6}	—
1.0×10^3	1	1.0×10^{-1}	1.0×10^{-3}	1.0×10^{-6}	0.03937	0.00381	0.001094	6.2137×10^{-7}
1.0×10^4	10	1	1.0×10^{-2}	1.0×10^{-5}	0.3937	0.0321	0.01094	6.2137×10^{-6}
1.0×10^6	1000	100	1	0.001	39.37	3.280	1.0936	6.2137×10^{-4}
1.0×10^9	1.0×10^6	1.0×10^5	1000	1	3.937×10^4	3280.84	1093.6121	0.6214
1.0×10^{10}	1.0×10^7	1.0×10^6	1.0×10^4	10	3.937×10^5	3.28×10^4	1.0936×10^4	6.2137
2.54×10^4	25.4	2.54	0.0254	2.54×10^{-5}	1	0.0833	0.02778	1.5783×10^{-5}
3.048×10^5	304.8	30.48	0.3048	3.048×10^{-4}	12	1	0.3333	1.8939×10^{-4}
9.144×10^5	914.4	91.44	0.9144	9.144×10^{-4}	36	3.0	1	5.6818×10^{-4}
1.6093×10^9	1.6093×10^6	1.6093×10^5	1609.34	1.6093	6.336×10^4	5280	1760	1

*The Joint Commission (JCAHO) prescribes the use of metric, instead of apothecary, units.

APPENDIX 8

REFERENCE INTERVALS FOR THE INTERPRETATION OF LABORATORY TESTS*

Reference Intervals† for Hematology

Test	Conventional Units	SI Units
Acid hemolysis (Ham test)	No hemolysis	No hemolysis
Alkaline phosphatase, leukocyte	Total score, 14–100	Total score, 14–100
Cell counts		
Erythrocytes		
Males	4.6–6.2 million/mm^3	4.6–6.2 × 10^{12}/L
Females	4.2–5.4 million/mm^3	4.2–5.4 × 10^{12}/L
Children (varies with age)	4.5–5.1 million/mm^3	4.5–5.1 × 10^{12}/L
Leukocytes, total	4500–11,000/mm^3	4.5–11.0 × 10^9/L
Leukocytes, differential counts*		
Myelocytes	0%	0/L
Band neutrophils	3–5%	150–400 × 10^6/L
Segmented neutrophils	54–62%	3000–5800 × 10^6/L
Lymphocytes	25–33%	1500–3000 × 10^6/L
Monocytes	3–7%	300–500 × 10^6/L
Eosinophils	1–3%	50–250 × 10^6/L
Basophils	0–1%	15–50 × 10^6/L
Platelets	150,000–400,000/mm^3	150–400 × 10^9/L
Reticulocytes	25,000–75,000/mm^3 (0.5–1.5% of erythrocytes)	25–75 × 10^9/L
Coagulation tests		
Bleeding time (template)	2.75–8.0 min	2.75–8.0 min
Coagulation time (glass tube)	5–15 min	5–15 min
D dimer	<0.5 μg/mL	<0.5 mg/L
Factor VIII and other coagulation factors	50–150% of normal	0.5–1.5 of normal
Fibrin split products (Thrombo-Welco test)	<10 μg/mL	<10 mg/L
Fibrinogen	200–400 mg/dL	2.0–4.0 g/L
Partial thromboplastin time, activated (aPTT)	20–25 s	20–35 s
Prothrombin time (PT)	12.0–14.0 s	12.0–14.0 s
Coombs' test		
Direct	Negative	Negative
Indirect	Negative	Negative
Corpuscular values of erythrocytes		
Mean corpuscular hemoglobin (MCH)	26–34 pg/cell	26–34 pg/cell
Mean corpuscular volume (MCV)	80–96 μm^3	80–96 fL
Mean corpuscular hemoglobin concentration (MCHC)	32–36 g/dL	320–360 g/L
Haptoglobin	20–165 mg/dL	0.20–1.65 g/L
Hematocrit		
Males	40–54 mL/dL	0.40–0.54 g/L
Females	37–47 mL/dL	0.37–0.47 g/L
Newborns	49–54 mL/dL	0.49–0.54 g/L
Children (varies with age)	35–49 mL/dL	0.35–0.49 g/L
Hemoglobin		
Males	13.0–18.0 g/dL	8.1–11.2 mmol/L
Females	12.0–16.0 g/dL	7.4–9.9 mmol/L
Newborns	16.5–19.5 g/dL	10.2–12.1 mmol/L
Children (varies with age)	11.2–16.5 g/dL	7.0–10.2 mmol/L
Hemoglobin, fetal	<1.0% of total	<0.01 of total
Hemoglobin A_{1c}	3–5% of total	0.03–0.05 of total
Hemoglobin A_2	1.5–3.0% of total	0.015–0.03 of total
Hemoglobin, plasma	0.0–5.0 mg/dL	0.0–3.2 μmol/L
Methemoglobin	30–130 mg/dL	19–80 μmol/L
Erythrocyte sedimentation rate (ESR)		
Westergren		
Males	0–15 mm/h	0–15 mm/h
Females	0–20 mm/h	0–20 mm/h
Wintrobe		
Males	0–5 mm/h	0–5 mm/h
Females	0–15 mm/h	0–15 mm/h

*From Laura J. McCloskey, PhD, Reference Intervals for the Interpretation of Laboratory Tests. In Edward T. Bope et al. (eds.), Conn's Current Therapy 2011. Philadelphia, Elsevier, 2011.
†Conventional units are percentages; SI units are absolute cell counts.
Abbreviation: SI = International System of Units.

Appendix 8

Reference Intervals* for Clinical Chemistry (Blood, Serum, and Plasma)

Analyte	Conventional Units	SI Units
Acetoacetate plus acetone		
Qualitative	Negative	Negative
Quantitative	0.3–2.0 mg/dL	30–200 mol/L
Acid phosphatase, serum (thymolphthalein monophosphate substrate)	0.1–0.6 U/L	0.1–0.6 U/L
ACTH (see Corticotropin)		
Alanine aminotransferase (ALT), serum (SGPT)	1–45 U/L	1–45 U/L
Albumin, serum	3.3–5.2 g/dL	33–52 g/L
Aldolase, serum	0.0–7.0 U/L	0.0–7.0 U/L
Aldosterone, plasma		
Standing	5–30 ng/dL	140–830 pmol/L
Recumbent	3–10 ng/dL	80–275 pmol/L
Alkaline phosphatase (ALP), serum		
Adult	35–150 U/L	35–150 U/L
Adolescent	100–500 U/L	100–500 U/L
Child	100–350 U/L	100–350 U/L
Ammonia nitrogen, plasma	10–50 μmol/L	10–50 μmol/L
Amylase, serum	25–125 U/L	25–125 U/L
Anion gap, serum calculated	8–16 mEq/L	8–16 mmol/L
Ascorbic acid, blood	0.4–1.5 mg/dL	23–85 μmol/L
Aspartate aminotransferase (AST), serum (SGOT)	1–36 U/L	1–36 U/L
Base excess, arterial blood, calculated	0 ± 2 mEq/L	0 ± 2 mmol/L
Bicarbonate		
Venous plasma	23–29 mEq/L	23–29 mmol/L
Arterial blood	21–27 mEq/L	21–27 mmol/L
Bile acids, serum	0.3–3.0 mg/dL	0.8–7.6 mmol/L
Bilirubin, serum		
Conjugated	0.1–0.4 mg/dL	1.7–6.8 μmol/L
Total	0.3–1.1 mg/dL	5.1–19.0 μmol/L
Calcium, serum	8.4–10.6 mg/dL	2.10–2.65 mmol/L
Calcium, ionized, serum	4.25–5.25 mg/dL	1.05–1.30 mmol/L
Carbon dioxide, total, serum or plasma	24–31 mEq/L	24–31 mmol/L
Carbon dioxide tension (Pco_2), blood	35–45 mm Hg	35–45 mm Hg
β-Carotene, serum	60–260 μg/dL	1.1–8.6 μmol/L
Ceruloplasmin, serum	23–44 mg/dL	230–440 mg/L
Chloride, serum or plasma	96–106 mEq/L	96–106 mmol/L
Cholesterol, serum or EDTA plasma		
Desirable range	<200 mg/dL	<5.20 mmol/L
Low-density lipoprotein (LDL) cholesterol	60–180 mg/dL	1.55–4.65 mmol/L
High-density lipoprotein (HDL) cholesterol	30–80 mg/dL	0.80–2.05 mmol/L
Copper	70–140 μg/dL	11–22 μmol/L
Corticotropin (ACTH), plasma, 8 AM	10–80 pg/mL	2–18 pmol/L
Cortisol, plasma		
8:00 AM	6–23 μg/dL	170–630 μmol/L
4:00 PM	3–15 μg/dL	80–410 μmol/L
10:00 PM	<50% of 8:00 AM value	<50% of 8:00 AM value
Creatine, serum		
Males	0.2–0.5 mg/dL	15–40 μmol/L
Females	0.3–0.9 mg/dL	25–70 μmol/L
Creatine kinase (CK), serum		
Males	55–170 U/L	55–170 U/L
Females	30–135 U/L	30–135 U/L
Creatinine kinase MB isoenzyme, serum	<5% of total CK activity <5% of ng/mL by immunoassay	<5% of total CK activity <5% of ng/mL by immunoassay
Creatinine, serum	0.6–1.2 mg/dL	50–110 μmol/L
Erythrocytes	145–540 ng/mL	330–1220 nmol/L
Estradiol-17β, adult		
Males	10–65 pg/mL	35–240 pmol/L
Females		
Follicular	30–100 pg/mL	110–370 pmol/L
Ovulatory	200–400 pg/mL	730–1470 pmol/L
Luteal	50–140 pg/mL	180–510 pmol/L
Ferritin, serum	20–200 ng/mL	20–200 μg/L
Fibrinogen, plasma	200–400 mg/dL	2.0–4.0 g/L
Folate, serum	3–18 ng/mL	6.8–4.1 nmol/L
Follicle-stimulating hormone (FSH), plasma		
Males	4–25 mU/mL	4–25 U/L
Females, premenopausal	4–30 mU/mL	4–30 U/L
Females, postmenopausal	40–250 mU/mL	40–250 U/L
Gastrin, fasting, serum	0–100 pg/mL	0–100 mg/L
Glucose, fasting, plasma or serum	70–115 mg/dL	3.9–6.4 nmol/L
γ-Glutamyltransferase (GGT), serum	5–40 U/L	5–40 U/L
Growth hormone (hGH), plasma, adult, fasting	0–6 ng/mL	0–6 μg/L
Haptoglobin, serum	20–165 mg/dL	0.20–1.65 g/L

Appendix 8

Reference Intervals* for Clinical Chemistry (Blood, Serum, and Plasma) *Continued*

Analyte	Conventional Units	SI Units
Immunoglobulins, serum (see table of Reference Intervals for Tests of Immunologic Function)		
Iron, serum	75–175 μg/dL	13–31 μmol/L
Iron-binding capacity, serum		
Total	250–410 μg/dL	45–73 μmol/L
Saturation	20–55%	0.20–0.55
Lactate		
Venous whole blood	5.0–20.0 mg/dL	0.6–2.2 mmol/L
Arterial whole blood	5.0–15.0 mg/dL	0.6–1.7 mmol/L
Lactate dehydrogenase (LD), serum	110–220 U/L	110–220 U/L
Lipase, serum	10–140 U/L	10–140 U/L
Lutropin (LH), serum		
Males	1–9 U/L	1–9 U/L
Females		
Follicular phase	2–10 U/L	2–10 U/L
Midcycle peak	15–65 U/L	15–65 U/L
Luteal phase	1–12 U/L	1–12 U/L
Postmenopausal	12–65 U/L	12–65 U/L
Magnesium, serum	1.3–2.1 mg/dL	0.65–1.05 mmol/L
Osmolality	275–295 mOsm/kg water	275–295 mOsm/kg water
Oxygen, blood, arterial, room air		
Partial pressure (PaO_2)	80–100 mm Hg	80–100 mm Hg
Saturation (SaO_2)	95–98%	95–98%
pH, arterial blood	7.35–7.45	7.35–7.45
Phosphate, inorganic, serum		
Adult	3.0–4.5 mg/dL	1.0–1.5 mmol/L
Child	4.0–7.0 mg/dL	1.3–2.3 mmol/L
Potassium		
Serum	3.5–5.0 mEq/L	3.5–5.0 mmol/L
Plasma	3.5–4.5 mEq/L	3.5–4.5 mmol/L
Progesterone, serum, adult		
Males	0.0–0.4 ng/mL	0.0–1.3 mmol/L
Females		
Follicular phase	0.1–1.5 ng/mL	0.3–4.8 mmol/L
Luteal phase	2.5–28.0 ng/mL	8.0–89.0 mmol/L
Prolactin, serum		
Males	1.0–15.0 ng/mL	1.0–15.0 μg/L
Females	1.0–20.0 ng/mL	1.0–20.0 μg/L
Protein, serum, electrophoresis		
Total	6.0–8.0 g/dL	60–80 μg/L
Albumin	3.5–5.5 g/dL	35–55 μg/L
Globulins		
α_1	0.2–0.4 g/dL	2.0–4.0 g/L
α_2	0.5–0.9 g/dL	5.0–9.0 g/L
β	0.6–1.1 g/dL	6.0–11.0 g/L
γ	0.7–1.7 g/dL	7.0–17.0 g/L
Pyruvate, blood	0.3–0.9 mg/dL	0.03–0.10 mmol/L
Rheumatoid factor	0.0–30.0 IU/mL	0.0–30.0 kIU/L
Sodium, serum or plasma	135–145 mEq/L	135–145 mmol/L
Testosterone, plasma		
Men	300–1200 ng/dL	10.4–41.6 nmol/L
Women	20–75 ng/dL	0.7–2.6 nmol/L
Pregnant	40–200 ng/dL	1.4–6.9 nmol/L
Thyroglobulin	3–42 ng/mL	3–42 μg/L
Thyrotropin (hTSH), serum	0.4–4.8 μIU/mL	0.4–4.8 mIU/L
Thyrotropin-releasing hormone (TRH)	5–60 pg/mL	5–60 ng/L
Thyroxine, free (FT_4), serum	0.9–2.1 ng/dL	12–27 pmol/L
Thyroxine (T_4), serum	4.5–12.0 μg/mL	58–154 nmol/L
Thyroxine-binding globulin (TBG)	15.0–34.0 μg/mL	15.0–34.0 mg/L
Transferrin	250–430 mg/dL	2.5–4.3 g/L
Triglycerides, serum, after 12-h fast	40–150 mg/dL	0.4–1.5 g/L
Triiodothyronine (T_3), serum	70–190 ng/dL	1.1–2.9 nmol/L
Triiodothyronine uptake, resin (T_3RU)	25–38%	0.25–0.38
Troponin I	0.05–0.50 ng/mL	0.05–0.50 ng/mL
Urate		
(FT_4) Males	2.5–8.0 mg/dL	150–480 μmol/L
(FT_4) Females	2.2–7.0 mg/dL	130–420 μmol/L
Urea, serum or plasma	24–49 mg/dL	4.0–8.2 nmol/L
Urea nitrogen, serum or plasma	11–23 mg/dL	8.0–16.4 nmol/L
Viscosity, serum	1.1–1.8 cP	1.1–1.8 mPas-s
Vitamin A, serum	20–80 μg/dL	0.70–2.80 μmol/L
Vitamin B_{12}, serum	180–900 pg/mL	133–664 pmol/L

Abbreviations: EDTA = ethylenediaminetetraacetic acid; SI = International System of Units.
*Reference values can vary depending on the method and sample source used.

Appendix 8

Reference Intervals* for Therapeutic Drug Monitoring (Serum or Plasma)

Analyte	Therapeutic Range	Toxic Concentrations	Proprietary Analyte Name(s)
Analgesics			
Acetaminophen	10–40 μg/mL	>150 μg/mL	Tylenol, Datril
Salicylate	100–250 μg/mL	>300 μg/mL	Aspirin, Bufferin
Antibiotics			
Amikacin	20–30 μg/mL	Peak >35 μg/mL Trough >10 μg/mL	Amkin
Gentamicin	5–10 μg/mL	Peak >10 μg/mL Trough >2 μg/mL	Garamycin
Tobramycin	5–10 μg/mL	Peak >10 μg/mL Trough >2 μg/mL	Nebcin
Vancomycin	5–35 μg/mL	Peak >40 μg/mL Trough >10 μg/mL	Vancocin
Anticonvulsants			
Carbamazepine	5–12 μg/mL	>15 μg/mL	Tegretol
Ethosuximide	40–100 μg/mL	>250 μg/mL	Zarontin
Phenobarbital	15–40 μg/mL	40–100 ng/mL (varies widely)	Luminal
Phenytoin	10–20 μg/mL	>20 μg/mL	Dilantin
Primidone	5–12 μg/mL	>15 μg/mL	Mysoline
Valproic acid	50–100 μg/mL	>100 μg/mL	Depakene
Antineoplastics and Immunosuppressives			
Cyclosporine A	150–350 ng/mL	>400 ng/mL	Sandimmune
Methotrexate, high dose, 48 h	Variable	>1 μmol/L, 48 h after dose	
Sirolimus (within 1 h of 2-mg dose)	4.5–14 ng/mL	Variable	Rapamune
Sirolimus (within 1 h of 5-mg dose)	10–28 ng/mL	Variable	Rapamune
Tacrolimus (FK-506), whole blood	3–20 μg/L	>15 μg/L	Prograf
Bronchodilators and Respiratory Stimulants			
Caffeine	3–15 ng/mL	>30 ng/mL	Elixophyllin
Theophylline (aminophylline)	10–20 μg/mL	>30 μg/mL	Quibron
Cardiovascular Drugs			
Amiodarone (obtain specimen more than 8 h after last dose)	1.0–2.0 μg/mL	>2.0 μg/mL	Cordarone
Digoxin (obtain specimen more than 6 h after last dose)	0.8–2.0 ng/mL	>2.4 ng/mL	Lanoxin
Disopyramide	2–5 μg/mL	>7 μg/mL	Norpace
Flecainide	0.2–1.0 μg/mL	>1 μg/mL	Tambocor
Lidocaine	1.5–5.0 μg/mL	>6 μg/mL	Xylocaine
Mexiletine	0.7–2.0 μg/mL	>2 μg/mL	Mexitil
Procainamide	4–10 μg/mL	>12 μg/mL	Pronestyl
Procainamide plus NAPA (*N*-acetyl procainamide)	8–30 μg/mL	>30 μg/mL	
Propranolol	50–100 ng/mL	Variable	Inderal
Quinidine	2–5 μg/mL	>6 μg/mL	Cardioquin, Quinaglute
Tocainide	4–10 ng/mL	>10 ng/mL	Tonocard
Psychopharmacologic Drugs			
Amitriptyline	120–150 ng/mL	>500 ng/mL	Elavil, Triavil
Bupropion	25–100 ng/mL	Not applicable	Wellbutrin
Desipramine	150–300 ngmL	>500 ng/mL	Norpramin
Imipramine	125–250 ng/mL	>400 ng/mL	Tofranil
Lithium (obtain specimen 12 h after last dose)	0.6–1.5 mEq/L	>1.5 mEq/L	Lithobid
Nortriptyline	50–150 ng/mL	>500 ng/mL	Aventyl, Pamelor

*Values can vary depending on the method and sample collection device used. Always consult the reference values provided by the laboratory performing the analysis.

Appendix 8

Reference Intervals* for Clinical Chemistry (Urine)

Analyte	Conventional Units	SI Units
Acetone and acetoacetate, qualitative	Negative	Negative
Albumin		
Qualitative	Negative	Negative
Quantitative	10–100 mg/24 h	0.15–1.5 μmol/d
Aldosterone	3–20 μg/24 h	8.3–55 nmol/d
δ-Aminolevulinic acid (δ-ALA)	1.3–7.0 mg/24 h	10–53 μmol/d
Amylase	<17 U/h	<17 U/h
Amylase-to-creatinine clearance ratio	0.01–0.04	0.01–0.04
Bilirubin, qualitative	Negative	Negative
Calcium (regular diet)	<250 mg/24 h	<6.3 nmol/d
Catecholamines		
Epinephrine	<10 μg/24 h	<55 nmol/d
Norepinephrine	<100 μg/24 h	<590 nmol/d
Total free catecholamines	4–126 μg/24 h	24–745 nmol/d
Total metanephrines	0.1–1.6 mg/24 h	0.5–8.1 μmol/d
Chloride (varies with intake)	110–250 mEq/24 h	110–250 mmol/d
Copper	0–50 μg/24 h	0.0–0.80 μmol/d
Cortisol, free	10–100 μg/24 h	27.6–276 nmol/d
Creatine		
Males	0–40 mg/24 h	0.0–0.30 mmol/d
Females	0–80 mg/24 h	0.0–0.60 mmol/d
Creatinine	15–25 mg/kg/24 h	0.13–0.22 mmol/kg/d
Creatinine clearance (endogenous)		
Males	110–150 mL/min/1.73 m^2	110–150 mL/min/1.73 m^2
Females	105–132 mL/min/1.73 m^2	105–132 mL/min/1.73 m^2
Cystine or cysteine	Negative	Negative
Dehydroepiandrosterone		
Males	0.2–2.0 mg/24 h	0.7–6.9 μmol/d
Females	0.2–1.8 mg/24 h	0.7–6.2 μmol/d
Estrogens, total		
Males	4–25 μg/24 h	14–90 nmol/d
Females	5–100 μg/24 h	18–360 nmol/d
Glucose (as reducing substance)	<250 mg/24 h	<250 mg/d
Hemoglobin and myoglobin, qualitative	Negative	Negative
Homogentisic acid, qualitative	Negative	Negative
17-Hydroxycorticosteroids		
Males	3–9 mg/24 h	8.3–25 μmol/d
Females	2–8 mg/24 h	5.5–22 μmol/d
5-Hydroxyindoleacetic acid		
Qualitative	Negative	Negative
Quantitative	2–6 mg/24 h	10–31 μmol/d
17-Ketogenic steroids		
Males	5–23 mg/24 h	17–80 μmol/d
Females	3–15 mg/24 h	10–52 μmol/d
17-Ketosteroids		
Males	8–22 mg/24 h	28–76 μmol/d
Females	6–15 mg/24 h	21–52 μmol/d
Magnesium	6–10 mEq/24 h	3–5 mmol/d
Metanephrines	0.05–1.2 ng/mg creatinine	0.03–0.70 mmol/mmol creatinine
Osmolality	38–1400 mOsm/kg water	38–1400 mOsm/kg water
pH	4.6–8.0	4.6–8.0
Phenylpyruvic acid, qualitative	Negative	Negative
Phosphate	0.4–1.3 g/24 h	13–42 mmol/d
Porphobilinogen		
Qualitative	Negative	Negative
Quantitative	<2 mg/24 h	<9 μmol/d
Porphyrins		
Coproporphyrin	50–250 μg/24 h	77–380 nmol/d
Uroporphyrin	10–30 μg/24 h	12–36 nmol/d
Potassium	25–125 mEq/24 h	25–125 mmol/d
Pregnanediol		
Males	0.0–1.9 mg/24 h	0.0–6.0 μmol/d
Females		
Proliferative phase	0.0–2.6 mg/24 h	0.0–8.0 μmol/d
Luteal phase	2.6–10.6 mg/24 h	8–33 μmol/d
Postmenopausal	0.2–1.0 mg/24 h	0.6–3.1 μmol/d
Pregnanetriol	0.0–2.5 mg/24 h	0.0–7.4 μmol/d
Protein, total		
Qualitative	Negative	Negative
Quantitative	10–150 mg/24 h	10–150 mg/d
Protein-to-creatinine ratio	<0.2	<0.2
Sodium (regular diet)	60–260 mEq/24 h	60–260 mmol/d

Reference Intervals* for Clinical Chemistry (Urine) *Continued*

Analyte	Conventional Units	SI Units
Specific gravity		
Random specimen	1.003–1.030	1.003–1.030
24-h collection	1.015–1.025	1.015–1.025
Urate (regular diet)	250–750 mg/24 h	1.5–4.4 mmol/d
Urobilinogen	0.5–4.0 mg/24 h	0.6–6.8 μmol/d
Vanillylmandelic acid (VMA)	1.0–8.0 mg/24 h	5–40 μmol/d

Abbreviation: SI = International System of Units.
*Values can vary depending on the method used.

Reference Intervals for Toxic Substances

Analyte	Conventional Units	SI Units
Arsenic, urine	<130 μg/24 h	<1.7 μmol/d
Bromides, serum, inorganic	<100 mg/dL	<10 mmol/L
Toxic symptoms	140–1000 mg/dL	14–100 mmol/L
Carboxyhemoglobin, blood	Saturation, percent	
Urban environment	<5%	<0.05
Smokers	<12%	<0.12
Symptoms		
Headache	>15%	>0.15
Nausea and vomiting	>25%	>0.25
Potentially lethal	>50%	>0.50
Ethanol, blood	<0.05 mg/dL, <0.005%	<1.0 mmol/L
Intoxication	>100 mg/dL, >0.1%	>22 mmol/L
Marked intoxication	300–400 mg/dL, 0.3%–0.4%	65–87 mmol/L
Alcoholic stupor	400–500 mg/dL, 0.4%–0.5%	87–109 mmol/L
Coma	>500 mg/dL, >0.5%	>109 mmol/L
Lead, blood		
Adults	<20 μg/dL	<1.0 μmol/L
Children	<10 μg/dL	<0.5 μmol/L
Lead, urine	<80 μg/24 h	<0.4 μmol/d
Mercury, urine	<10 μg/24 h	<150 nmol/d

Abbreviation: SI = International System of Units.

Reference Intervals for Tests Performed on Cerebrospinal Fluid

Test	Conventional Units	SI Units
Cells	<5 mm^3, all mononuclear	<5 × 10^6/L, all mononuclear
Protein electrophoresis	Albumin predominant	Albumin predominant
Glucose	50–75 mg/dL (20 mg/dL less than in serum)	2.8–4.2 mmol/L (1.1 mmol/L less than in serum)
IgG		
Children <14 y	<8% of total protein	<0.08 of total protein
Adults	<14% of total protein	<0.14 of total protein
IgG index		
$\left(\frac{\text{CSF/serum IgG ratio}}{\text{CSF/serum albumin ratio}}\right)$	0.3–0.6	0.3–0.6
Oligoclonal banding on electrophoresis	Absent	Absent
Pressure, opening	70–180 mm H_2O	70–180 mm H_2O
Protein, total	15–45 mg/dL	150–450 mg/L

Abbreviations: Ig = immunoglobulin; SI = International System of Units.

Appendix 8

Reference Intervals for Tests of Gastrointestinal Function

Test	Conventional Units
Bentiromide	6-h urinary arylamine excretion >57% excludes pancreatic insufficiency
β-Carotene, serum	60–250 ng/dL
Fecal fat estimation	
Qualitative	No fat globules seen by high-power microscope
Quantitative	<6 g/24 h (>95% coefficient of fat absorption)
Gastric acid output	
Basal	
Males	0.0–10.5 mmol/h
Females	0.0–5.6 mmol/h
Maximum (after histamine or pentagastrin)	
Males	9.0–48.0 mmol/h
Females	6.0–31.0 mmol/h
Ratio: basal/maximum	
Males	0.0–0.31
Females	0.0–0.29
Secretin test, pancreatic flud	
Volume	>1.8 mL/kg/h
Bicarbonate	>80 mEq/L
D-Xylose absorption test, urine	>20% of ingested dose excreted in 5 h

Reference Intervals for Lymphocyte Subsets, Whole Blood, Heparinized

Antigen(s) Expressed	Cell Type	Percentage	Absolute Cell Count
CD2	E rosette T cells	73–87%	1040–2160
CD3	Total T cells	56–77%	860–1880
CD3 and CD4	Helper-inducer cells	32–54%	550–1190
CD3 and CD8	Suppressor-cytotoxic cells	24–37%	430–1060
CD3 and DR	Activated T cells	5–14%	70–310
CD16 and CD56	Natural killer (NK) cells	8–22%	130–500
CD19	Total B cells	7–17%	140–370

Reference Intervals for Tests of Immunologic Function

Test	Conventional Units	SI Units
Autoantibodies, Serum, Adult		
Anti-CCP antibody	0–19 U	
Anti-dsDNA antibody	0–40 IU	0–40 IU
Antinuclear antibody	<1:40	
Rheumatoid factor (total IgG, IgA, IgM)	0–30 mg/dL	
Complement, serum		
C3	85–175 mg/dL	0.85–1.75 g/L
C4	15–45 mg/dL	150–450 mg/L
Total hemolytic (CH_{50})	150–250 U/mL	150–250 U/mL
Immunoglobulins, serum, adult		
IgA	70–310 mg/dL	0.70–3.1 g/L
IgD	0.0–6.0 mg/dL	0.0–60 mg/L
IgE	0.0–430 ng/dL	0.0–430 mg/L
IgG	640–1350 mg/dL	6.4–13.5 g/L
IgM	90–350 mg/dL	0.90–3.5 g/L

Helper-to-suppressor ratio: 0.8–1.8. *Abbreviations*: anti-CCP = anticyclic citrullinated peptide; dsDNA = double-stranded DNA; Ig = immunoglobulin; SI = International System of Units.

Appendix 8

Reference Values for Semen Analysis

Test	Conventional Units	SI Units
Volume	2–5 mL	2–5 mL
Liquefaction	Complete in 15 min	Complete in 15 min
pH	7.2–8.0	7.2–8.0
Leukocytes	Occasional or absent	Occasional or absent
Spermatozoa		
Count	60–150 × 10^6 mL	60–150 × 10^6 mL
Fructose	>150 mg/dL	>8.33 mmol/L
Morphology	80–90% normal forms	>0.80–0.90 normal
Motility	>80% motile	>0.80 motile

Abbreviation: SI = International System of Units.

CREDITS

ILLUSTRATIONS AND TABLES

Abeloff, MD et al: Abeloff's Clinical Oncology, 4th ed. Churchill Livingstone, 2008: page 755

Abrahams, P et al: McMinn's Color Atlas of Human Anatomy, 6th ed. Mosby, 2008: pages 42, top right; 111, bottom right; 286; 308; 353; 419, left; 475; 573; 632, top right; 738; 808; 813; 860, bottom right; 906; 967; 1046, bottom left; 1101, bottom right; 1106; 1107, top left; 1114; 1127; 1205; 1208; 1290; 1298; 1319; 1364, bottom right; 1395; 1401, bottom left; 1403; 1412; 1433; 1584; 1585; 1587; 1588; 1662; 1689; 1695; 1725, bottom; 1742; 1772; 1797; 1801; 1807; 1810; 1816; 1970; 2001; 2038; 2048; 2051; 2071, bottom right; 2096, middle right

Adam, A et al: Grainger and Allison's Diagnostic Radiology, 5th ed. Churchill Livingstone, 2008: pages 59, top left; 85; 174, bottom left; 580; 581; 703; 718; 980; 1372, bottom right; 1408; 1668; 1673; 2013, top right

Adkinson, NF Jr et al: Middleton's Allergy: Principles and Practices, 7th ed. Mosby, 2009: pages 231; 1128, bottom right; 1601; 1782, bottom right

Adkison, L, Brown, MD: Elsevier's Integrated Genetics. Mosby, 2007: page 698

Albert, DM et al: Albert & Jakobiec's Principles & Practice of Ophthalmology, 3rd ed. Saunders, 2008: pages 177; 556; 1185

Albert, RK et al: Clinical Respiratory Medicine, 3rd ed. Mosby, 2008: pages 253; 439; 704; 802; 1717

Aspinall, RJ, Taylor-Robinson, SD: Mosby's Color Atlas of Gastroenterology and Liver Disease. Mosby, 2002: pages 387, top right; 647

Atkinson, BF: Atlas of Diagnostic Cytopathology, 2nd ed. Saunders, 2004: pages 224; 323, top right; 689; 1638; 2019

Auerbach, PS: Wilderness Medicine, 5th ed. Mosby, 2007: pages 34; 496, left; 1439

Ballinger, PW, Frank, ED: Merrill's Atlas of Radiographic Positions and Radiologic Procedures, 10th ed. Mosby, 2003: page 879

Baren, JM et al: Pediatric Emergency Medicine. Saunders, 2008: pages 336; 461, top left; 656, top right; 869; 1034, bottom left; 2081

Barkauskas, V et al: Health & Physical Assessment, 3rd ed. Mosby, 2002: pages 655, bottom right; 717; 1148; 1430, top right; 1614; 1889; 1900; 1934; 2036

Bath-Balogh, MB, Fehrenbach, MJ: Illustrated Dental Embryology, Histology, and Anatomy, 2nd ed. Saunders, 2006: pages 450, top left; 1306

Berkovitz, BKB et al: Oral Anatomy, Histology, and Embryology, 4th ed. Mosby, 2009: pages 197, bottom right; 327; 511, top right; 871, bottom right; 1938; 1939, bottom left

Bird, DL, Robinson, DS: Torres and Ehrlich Modern Dental Assisting, 9th ed. Saunders, 2009: pages 162, top left; 199; 215; 435; 489; 1101, top left; 1630; 1738; 1957; 1969; 2082, top left

Bolognia, JL et al: Dermatology. Mosby, 2003: pages 561; 1055, top right; 1067, bottom left; 1175; 1273; 1274, bottom left; 2026, bottom right

Bolognia, JL et al: Dermatology, 2nd ed. Mosby, 2008: pages 43; 131; 195, top right; 218, bottom right; 219; 270; 344; 447, bottom right; 494, right; 495; 498; 534; 566, bottom right; 567; 714; 715, bottom left; 715, top; 747; 799; 832, top right; 838; 871, bottom left; 890; 1023; 1099, top left; 1227, bottom right; 1235; 1236; 1361; 1541; 1552; 1561; 1711; 1714; 1768; 1815, top left; 1931; 1988, top left; 2050, bottom left; 2096, top right

Bontrager, KL, Lampignano, JP: Textbook of Radiographic Positioning and Related Anatomy, 6th ed. Mosby, 2005: page 347

Bontrager, KL, Lampignano, JP: Textbook of Radiographic Positioning and Related Anatomy, 7th ed. Mosby, 2010: pages 88; 143; 159; 239; 387, bottom left; 546; 727, bottom right; 822, top right; 851, bottom left; 952; 1004, bottom left; 1260; 1565; 1788; 1793; 2007

Bope, ET et al: Conn's Current Therapy. Saunders, 2010: page 377

Boron, WF, Boulpaep, EL: Medical Physiology, 2nd ed. Saunders, 2009: pages 124; 197, top left; 401, bottom right; 796; 950; 974, top right

Boyd, LB: Dental Instruments, 3rd ed. Saunders, 2009: pages 401, top left; 656, bottom right; 822, bottom left; 865

Bradley, WG et al: Neurology in Clinical Practice, 5th ed. Butterworth-Heinemann, 2008: page 1831

Bragg, DG et al: Oncologic Imaging, 2nd ed. Saunders, 2002: page 218, top right

Brenner, BM: Brenner & Rector's The Kidney, 8th ed. Saunders, 2008: pages 240; 1165, top left; 1477; 2010

Browner, BD et al: Skeletal Trauma, 4th ed. Saunders, 2008: page 1458

Bullough, PG: Orthopaedic Pathology, 5th ed. Mosby, 2010: page 1301

Callen, JP et al: Color Atlas of Dermatology, 2nd ed. Saunders, 2000: pages 342, bottom right; 1265, bottom left

Canale, ST, Beaty, JH: Campbell's Operative Orthopaedics, 11th ed. Mosby, 2008: pages 375, bottom right; 713; 818; 820; 837; 944; 1348; 1540; 1856; 1986; 2082, bottom left

Carlson, BM: Human Embryology and Developmental Biology, 4th ed. Mosby, 2009: page 924

Carr, JH, Rodak, BF: Clinical Hematology Atlas, 3rd ed. Saunders, 2009: pages 9; 180; 204, bottom left; 233, top left; 316; 324, top right; 324, bottom left; 605, top right; 629; 833; 896; 1176; 1272; 1656; 1707

Centers for Disease Control and Prevention: pages 96; 99, bottom right; 189; 361; 456; 526; 623; 774, top left; 1159; 1229; 1375; 1401, top left; 1443; 1727; 1787; 1890; 1963; 1974

Christian, PE et al: Nuclear Medicine and PET: Technology and Techniques, 5th ed. Mosby, 2004: page 1624

Clark, DA: Atlas of Neonatology. Saunders, 2000: pages 287; 372; 511, bottom left; 574; 613; 728, bottom right; 854; 955; 1061; 1063; 1092; 1220, bottom left; 1330; 1830; 2006; 2071, top left

Cohen, BA: Pediatric Dermatology, 3rd ed. Mosby, 2005: pages 190; 592, bottom right; 1442

Cohen, J, Powderly, WD: Infectious Diseases, 2nd ed. Mosby, 2004: pages 233, bottom right (Courtesy of the Armed Forces Institute, Bethesda, Maryland); 357; 545; 684; 693 (Courtesy of Dr. M.E. Jones, Edinburgh); 761; 847; 970; 1085 (Courtesy of Dr. C.S. Ratnatunga [deceased]); 1669

Cohen, S, Hargreaves, KM: Pathways of the Pulp, 9th ed. Mosby, 2006: page 1914

Crawford, MH et al: Cardiology, 3rd ed. Mosby, 2010: page 1327

Custalow, CB: Color Atlas of Emergency Department Procedures. Saunders, 2004: page 431

Damjanov, I, Linder, J: Pathology: A Color Atlas. Mosby, 2000: pages 506; 846; 862; 902; 962, bottom right; 986; 1018, top right; 1018, bottom left; 1269; 1750; 1841 (B); 1922, bottom right; 1987

Daniel, SJ, Harfst, SA: Mosby's Dental Hygiene, 2nd ed. Mosby, 2008: pages 271; 470; 774, bottom right

DeLee, JC et al: Orthopaedic Sports Medicine, 3rd ed. Saunders, 2009: page 1757, bottom right

DiSaia, PJ, Creasman, WT: Clinical Gynecologic Oncology, 7th ed. Mosby, 2007: page 1084, bottom left

Douglas, G et al: MacLeod's Clinical Examination, 11th ed. Churchill Livingstone, 2005: page 1030, bottom left

Drake, RL et al: Gray's Anatomy for Students, 2nd ed. Churchill Livingstone, 2010: pages 42, bottom right; 111, top right; 118; 135; 139; 208; 254, top left; 278, bottom right; 355; 379; 400, bottom left; 415; 418, top right; 419; 436; 527; 632, bottom left; 678; 739; 740, bottom right; 749, top right; 829; 941; 1031; 1128, top right; 1132; 1172; 1332; 1343; 1556; 1618; 1903; 1975, top right; 2018; 2054

Eisenberg, RL, Johnson, NM: Comprehensive Radiographic Pathology, 3rd ed. Mosby, 2003: pages 1091; 1645; 1845, top right

Emond, RTD et al: Colour Atlas of Infectious Diseases, 4th ed. Mosby, 2003: pages 83 (Courtesy of Dr. E.H. Brown [deceased]); 341; 1081; 1188; 1333; 1474 (Courtesy of Dr. L.S. Carstairs [deceased]); 1593, top right; 1893, bottom left; 2017

Erlandsen, SL, Magney, JE: Color Atlas of Histology. Mosby, 1992: pages 1281; 1354

Fawcett, DW: The Cell. Saunders, 1981: page 1304

Feehally, J et al: Comprehensive Clinical Nephrology, 3rd ed. Mosby, 2007: page 302

Feldman, M et al: Sleisenger and Fordtran's Gastrointestinal and Liver Disease, 8th ed. Saunders, 2006: pages 317; 348; 384; 1163, top left (Courtesy of Dr. David N. Fredricks, Palo Alto, California); 1675, bottom right; 1965, top right (Courtesy of Director, Armed Forces Institute of Pathology, Washington, DC); 1997

Fink, MP et al: Textbook of Critical Care, 5th ed. Saunders, 2005: page 399

Credits

Firestein, GS et al: Kelley's Textbook of Rheumatology, 8th ed. Saunders, 2008: pages 503; 1025; 1065; 1291 (Courtesy of Dr. G. Hoffman)

Fitzpatrick, JE, Morelli, JG: Dermatology Secrets, 3rd ed. Mosby, 2007: page 1683

Flint, PW: Cummings Otolaryngology, 5th ed. Mosby, 2010: pages 6, top right; 459; 1006; 1029; 1836, top right

Forbes, CD, Jackson, WF: Color Atlas and Text of Clinical Medicine, 3rd ed. Mosby Ltd., 2003: pages 1168; 1426; 2080

Gabbe, SG et al: Obstetrics: Normal and Problem Pregnancies, 5th ed. Churchill Livingstone, 2007: page 332

Garden, OJ et al: Principles and Practice of Surgery, 5th ed. Churchill Livingstone, 2007: page 1227, top left

Gartner, LP, Hiatt, JL: Color Textbook of Histology, 3rd ed. Saunders, 2007: pages 74, top left; 167 (Courtesy of Dr. Alexey Khodjakov); 285; 299; 323, bottom left; 619; 631; 636; 740, top left; 998 (A); 1041; 1084, right; 1113; 1219; 1265, top right; 1288; 1415; 1519, top right; 1633, bottom left; 1697, bottom right; 1697, top right; 1925; 2026, top left

Gatzoulis, MA et al: Diagnosis and Management of Adult Congenital Heart Disease, Churchill Livingstone, 2003: page 1756, bottom left

Gerbert, J: Textbook of Bunion Surgery, 3rd ed. Saunders, 2001: page 260

Goering, R et al: Mim's Medical Microbiology, 4th ed. Mosby, 2007: pages 440; 1019, top left; 1163, bottom right; 1406, top left; 1457

Goetz, CG: Textbook of Clinical Neurology, 3rd ed. Saunders, 2007: pages 784; 1504, bottom left; 1756, top right; 2000

Goldberger, AL: Clinical Electrocardiography, 7th ed. Mosby, 2006: pages 133; 214, bottom left; 722; 835; 898; 1506; 1625; 1837; 1848; 1854; 1940; 2077, top right

Goldman, L, Ausiello, D: Cecil Medicine, 23rd ed. Saunders, 2008: pages 24; 211; 259, bottom right; 599; 660, bottom left; 861, bottom right; 1019; 1024; 1095; 1279, top left; 1554; 1558; 1640; 1944, top left

Grosfeld, JL et al: Pediatric Surgery, 6th ed. Mosby, 2006: page 14

Guyton, AC, Hall, JE: Textbook of Medical Physiology, 11th ed. Saunders, 2006: pages 10; 1449, bottom left; 2076

Habif, TP: Clinical Dermatology, 5th ed. Mosby, 2010: pages 853; 1701

Hacker, NF et al: Hacker & Moore's Essentials of Obstetrics and Gynecology, 5th ed. Saunders, 2010: page 1173, bottom right

Haines, DE: Fundamental Neuroscience for Basic and Clincal Applications, 3rd ed. Churchill Livingstone, 2006: pages 781, top right; 1071

Hemmings, HC, Hopkins, PM: Foundations of Anesthesia, 2nd ed. Mosby, 2006: page 75, top left

Henry, MC, Stapleton, ER: EMT Prehospital Care, 4th ed. Mosby, 2010: pages 185, top left; 261, bottom; 743

Herring, W: Learning Radiology: Recognizing the Basics, Mosby, 2007: page 264

Hochberg, MC et al: Rheumatology, 4th ed. Mosby, 2008: pages 874, bottom left; 1311

Hordinsky, M et al: Atlas of Hair and Nails. Churchill Livingstone, 2000: pages 1230; 1322

Iannucci, J, Jansen Howerton, L: Dental Radiography, 3rd ed. Saunders, 2006: page 1631

Ibsen, OAC, Phelan, JA: Oral Pathology for the Dental Hygienist, 4th ed. Saunders, 2004: page 460, bottom left

Ignatavicius, DD, Workman, ML: Medical-Surgical Nursing, 5th ed. Saunders, 2006: pages 181; 726, top right

Ishihara: Tests for Color Blindness, 1973: page 1892

Jacob, S: Human Anatomy. Churchill Livingstone, 2007: pages 2, top left; 11; 136; 243; 298; 370; 688, bottom left; 860, top left; 926; 1000; 1007, top; 1007; 1058; 1099, bottom right; 1105, top left; 1134; 1142, bottom right; 1145; 1165, bottom right; 1198; 1199; 1212; 1317; 1340; 1367; 1420, bottom right; 1424; 1459; 1498; 1519, bottom left; 1520; 1526; 1574; 1580; 1619; 1620; 1741; 1751, bottom right; 1872; 1973, bottom left; 1982; 1999; 2050, top right

James, WD et al: Andrews' Diseases of the Skin, 10th ed. Saunders, 2006: page 496, top right

John, DT, Petri, WA, Jr: Markell and Voge's Medical Parasitology, 9th ed. Saunders, 2006: pages 77; 524, bottom left; 1234

Johnson, WT: Color Atlas of Endodontics. Saunders, 2002: page 1150

Jorde, LB et al: Medical Genetics, 4th ed. Mosby, 2010: pages 183; 977 (Courtesy of Dr. A. Brothman); 1213

Kanski, JJ, Nischal, KK: Ophthalmology. Mosby, 1999: pages 127, top left; 499, bottom left; 628, top left

Keystone, JS et al: Travel Medicine, 2nd ed. Mosby, 2008: page 1076

Kierszenbaum, AL: Histology and Cell Biology, 2nd ed. Mosby, 2007: page 17, bottom left

Kliegman, RM et al: Nelson Textbook of Pediatrics, 18th ed. Saunders, 2007: pages 57; 74, bottom right; 296; 338; 493; 597; 857; 866; 929; 968; 1033; 1122; 1373, top left; 1420; 1451; 1495, bottom left; 1539; 1593, bottom right; 1930; 2069; 2075

Koeppen, BM, Stanton, BA: Berne and Levy Physiology, 6th ed. Mosby, 2010: pages 282; 786, top left

Kronenberg, HM et al: Williams Textbook of Endocrinology, 11th ed Saunders, 2008: page 921, bottom left

Kumar, P, Clark, ML: Clinical Medicine, 7th ed. Saunders Ltd., 2009 page 559

Kumar, V et al: Robbins and Cotran Pathologic Basis of Disease, 7th ed Saunders, 2005: page 1962, bottom right

Kumar, V et al: Robbins and Cotran Pathologic Basis of Disease, 8th ed Saunders, 2010: pages 29; 169, bottom right; 234; 374; 462; 481; 531 bottom right; 531, top right; 541; 577; 723; 763; 842, top right; 845 864, top left; 1077; 1097; 1098; 1112; 1144; 1156; 1222; 1242; 1359 1535; 1555; 1871; 1883; 1922, top left; 1980, top left; 1980 (B); 1994 2028

Kumar, V et al: Robbins Basic Pathology, 8th ed. Saunders, 2007: pages 919; 1424, top

Larsen, WJ: Human Embryology, 3rd ed. Churchill Livingstone, 2001 page 591 (Courtesy of Cincinnati Children's Hospital Medical Center)

Lawrence, CM, Cox, NH: Physical Signs in Dermatology, 2nd ed. Mosby 2001: pages 85, bottom right; 273; 494, bottom left; 540, bottom right 982; 1180; 1380

Libby, P et al: Braunwald's Heart Disease, 8th ed. Saunders, 2008: pages 82; 95; 174, top right; 206, bottom right; 228; 245; 267; 395; 437; 507 555; 601; 607, top left; 664; 701; 1064; 1228; 1603; 1604; 1770; 1861 1867; 1915; 1923

Liebgott, B: The Anatomical Basis of Dentistry, 3rd ed. Mosby, 2011 pages 56, top left; 745; 807; 1646; 2014, bottom right

Lim, EKS et al: Medicine and Surgery. Churchill Livingstone, 2007 page 18

Lissauer, T, Clayden, G: Illustrated Textbook of Paediatrics, 3rd ed Mosby, 2007: pages 15; 1715

Long, SS: Principles and Practice of Pediatric Infectious Disease, 3rd ed Churchill Livingstone, 2008: pages 1962, top right

Mahon, CR et al: Textbook of Diagnostic Microbiology, 3rd ed. Saunders 2007: pages 54; 241; 337; 406, bottom left; 484; 979; 1186; 1641; 1682 1886, top right; 1886, bottom left; 1890, top right; 1958; 2094

Male, D et al: Immunology, 7th ed. Mosby, 2006: pages 39, bottom left 104; 605, bottom left; 1431; 1622

Mandell, GL et al: Mandell, Douglas, and Bennett's Principles and Practice of Infectious Diseases, 7th ed. Churchill Livingstone, 2009 pages 280; 566, top left; 694, bottom left; 1147; 1470

Marks, JG Jr, Miller, JJ: Principles of Dermatology, 4th ed. Saunders 2006: pages 53; 116; 281; 292, top right; 292, bottom left; 391, top right; 499, top left; 805; 852; 951; 978; 1125, top left; 1166; 1217; 1405 1430, bottom left; 1542; 1547; 1654; 1896; 2012; 2085, top right

Marx, JA et al: Rosen's Emergency Medicine, 7th ed. Mosby, 2010: pages 369; 537, top right; 1476; 1791; 1857

Mason, RJ et al: Murray and Nadel's Textbook of Respiratory Medicine 4th ed. Saunders, 2005: pages 162, bottom left; 1472; 1751, top left 1762, top right; 1763; 1979; 1980 (A)

McPherson, RA, Pincus, MR: Henry's Clinical Diagnosis and Management by Laboratory Methods, 21st ed. Saunders, 2007: pages 92; 256 524, top right; 620; 885; 1220, top left; 1320, top right; 1486; 1675, top right; 1756, top left; 1762, bottom left; 1762, bottom right; 2084, top right

Mettler, FA Jr: Essentials of Radiology, 2nd ed. Saunders, 2005: pages 23 bottom left; 113; 157; 163; 171; 479; 615; 707; 914; 934, top left; 1344 1754; 1769

Mettler, FA Jr, Guiberteau, MJ: Essentials of Nuclear Medicine Imaging 5th ed. Saunders, 2006: page 1088

Miller, RD et al: Miller's Anesthesia, 7th ed. Churchill Livingstone, 2009 page 621

Moore, KL et al: Color Atlas of Clinical Embryology, 2nd ed. Saunders 2000: pages 36; 592, top left (Courtesy of Dr. A.E. Chudley)

Moore, KL, Persaud, TVN: The Developing Human, 8th ed. Saunders 2008: pages 64, bottom right; 64, top right; 125, bottom righ (Courtesy of Professor Emeritus Dr. K.V. Hinrichsen [deceased]); 60 (A), (B), (F), (G); 1164, bottom left (Courtesy of Dr. A.E. Chudley) 1666; 1734; 1735

Morse, SA et al: Atlas of Sexually Transmitted Diseases and AIDS, 3rd ed Mosby, 2003: pages 402, top right; 1276; 1328, top right; 1665

Murray, PR et al: Medical Microbiology, 6th ed. Mosby, 2009: pages 284 bottom right (Courtesy of Dr. T. Baker); 404; 444; 1109; 1471

Nadeau, SE et al: Medical Neuroscience. Saunders, 2004: pages 391 bottom; 1297; 1302; 1570

Neville, BW et al: Oral and Maxillofacial Pathology, 3rd ed. Saunders 2009: pages 93, bottom right; 400, top right; 426, top left; 450, bottom right; 461, top right; 641; 768; 775; 831; 887; 923, top left; 1125 bottom right; 1173, top left; 1274, top right; 1379; 1422; 1553; 1680 1776; 1819; 1821; 1829; 1841, top right; 1878; 1936, bottom left; 2014 top right; 2087

Newman, MG et al: Carranza's Clinical Periodontology, 10th ed Saunders, 2006: pages 261, top right; 375; 662, top left; 1516; 1672

Credits

Nishimura, H et al: Prenatal Development of the Human with Special Reference to Craniofacial Structures: An Atlas, National Institutes of Health, 1977: pages 607 (C), (D), (E), (H), (I); 1660; 2056, top right
NOAA National Centers for Coastal Ocean Science: page 522
Nolte, J: The Human Brain, 6th ed. Mosby, 2009: pages 486, top right (Courtesy of Dr. Nathaniel T. McMullen, University of Arizona College of Medicine); 1296; 1495, top right; 1794
Nolte, J, Angevine, JB Jr: The Human Brain in Photographs and Diagrams, 3rd ed. Mosby, 2007: pages 333; 418, bottom left; 609, top right; 682; 709; 735, right; 1121; 1907
Nussbaum, RL et al: Thompson & Thompson Genetics in Medicine, 6th ed. revised reprint. Saunders, 2004: page 1880 (Courtesy of Dr. S. Schwartz)
Nussbaum, RL et al: Thompson & Thompson Genetics in Medicine, 7th ed. Saunders, 2007: page 769
Orrison, WW Jr: Neuroimaging. Saunders, 2000: page 1790
Otto, CM: Textbook of Clinical Echocardiography, 4th ed. Saunders, 2009: page 295, top left
Palay, DA, Krachmer, JH: Ophthalmology for the Primary Care Physician. Mosby, 1998: pages 112, top left; 385; 2093, bottom right
Palay, DA, Krachmer, JH: Primary Care Ophthalmology, 2nd ed. Mosby, 2005: pages 5, top left; 225; 278, top left; 469; 568; 592, bottom left; 630; 649; 655, top right; 960; 1449, top left; 1468; 1508; 1546; 1615, bottom left; 1679, bottom right; 1744, bottom left; 1782, top left; 1898
Parrillo, JE, Dellinger, RP: Critical Care Medicine, 3rd ed. Mosby, 2007: page 1709
Patton, KT, Thibodeau, GA: Anatomy & Physiology, 7th ed. Mosby, 2010: pages 42, top left; 318 (Courtesy of Professor I Stotz [deceased]); 396 (Courtesy of Dr. C. Flickinger); 467; 618 (Courtesy of MM Perry); 628, bottom left (Courtesy of Dr. C. Flickinger); 726, bottom left; 779, bottom right; 839; 938, bottom right; 998 (B); 1067, top right; 1170, top left (Courtesy of Dr. B. Russell); 1267; 1633, top left; 1679, top left; 1945; 2013, bottom left
Pelley, JW: Elsevier's Integrated Biochemistry. Mosby, 2007: page 1493
Perloff, JK: Clinical Recognition of Congenital Heart Disease, 5th ed. Saunders, 2003: pages 413; 1955, bottom right; 1973, top left; 1973, top right
Perloff, JK et al: Congenital Heart Disease in Adults, 3rd ed. Saunders, 2008: page 1768, top right
Peters, W, Pasvol, G: Atlas of Tropical Medicine and Parasitology, 6th ed. Mosby, 2007: pages 41 (Courtesy of Professor M.S.R. Hutt [deceased]); 162, top right; 195, bottom left; 206, top left; 604 (Courtesy of Dr. J.F. Kassel [deceased]); 624; 1060; 1069 (Courtesy of Drs. J. Anderson and H. Fuglsang); 1215; 1336; 1868; 2089
Pollard, TD, Earnshaw, WC: Cell Biology, 2nd ed. Saunders, 2008: page 1651
Proffit, WR et al: Contemporary Orthodontics, 4th ed. Mosby, 2007: pages 120, bottom right; 125, top left; 221; 368; 434; 579; 668; 1055, bottom left; 1096; 1353; 1501, bottom left; 1523; 1693
Rakel, RE: Textbook of Family Medicine, 7th ed. Saunders, 2007: pages 1635; 1929
Regezi, JA et al: Atlas of Oral & Maxillofacial Pathology. Saunders, 2000: pages 811; 1939, top right; 2087, bottom right
Regezi, JA et al: Oral Pathology, 5th ed. Saunders, 2008: pages 59, bottom left; 293; 320; 342, top left; 520; 646; 721, bottom right; 804, top right; 804, bottom left; 836; 894; 1022; 1030, top right; 1087; 1592, top right; 1706; 1985
Roberson, TM et al: Sturdevant's Art and Science of Operative Dentistry, 5th ed. Mosby, 2006: page 1572
Rodak, BF et al: Hematology, 3rd ed. Saunders, 2007: pages 80; 358 (Courtesy of Cytogenetics Laboratory, Indiana University School of Medicine, Indianapolis, Indiana); 901; 1027, bottom left; 1027, top right
Roitt, I et al: Immunology, 6th ed. Mosby, 2001: pages 102; 106; 1600
Rosai, J: Ackerman's Surgical Pathology, 8th ed. Mosby, 1998: page 460, top right
Rosai, J: Rosai and Ackerman's Surgical Pathology, 9th ed. Mosby, 2004: pages 70; 259, top left; 486, bottom left; 533; 786, bottom right; 803; 1141; 1533; 1537; 1544; 1545; 1598; 1690; 1777; 1988, bottom right
Sapp, JP et al: Contemporary Oral and Maxillofacial Pathology, 2nd ed. Mosby, 2004: pages 488; 1139; 1158; 1313; 1628; 1941, top right
Schoenwolf, GC et al: Larsen's Human Embryology, 4th ed. Churchill Livingstone, 2009: page 505 (Courtesy of Cincinnati Children's Hospital Medical Center); 2093, top right
Seidel, HM et al: Mosby's Guide to Physical Examination, 6th ed. Mosby, 2006: pages 26; 179; 350 (Courtesy of Richard A Buckingham, MD, Clinical Professor, Otolaryngology, Abraham Lincoln School of Medicine, University of Illinois, Chicago, Illinois); 410; 429, top left; 535; 563; 662, top right; 690; 705, bottom right; 798; 889; 956; 1021, bottom left; 1059, left; 1074, bottom right; 1103; 1351; 1410; 1499; 1610; 1611; 1615, top right; 1621; 1642; 1647; 1708; 1743; 1773; 1885; 1893, top right; 1897; 1902; 1909; 1978
Shah, BR, Laude, TA: Atlas of Pediatric Clinical Diagnosis. Saunders, 2000: pages 447, top left; 1853
Spicer, WJ: Clinical Microbiology and Infectious Diseases, 2nd ed. Churchill Livingstone, 2008: pages 165; 801; 1755
Standring, S: Gray's Anatomy, 40th ed. Churchill Livingstone, 2008: pages 50; 56, bottom left; 145; 252; 300; 361, top right; 405; 417; 419, bottom right; 420; 432; 696; 861, top left; 1013; 1284
Stern, TA et al: Massachusetts General Hospital Comprehensive Clinical Psychiatry, Mosby, 2008: pages 528; 1237
Stevens, A et al: Core Pathology, 3rd ed. Mosby, 2009: page 1435, top left (Courtesy of Cincinnati Children's Hospital Medical Center)
Stoelting, RK, Miller, RD: Basics of Anesthesia, 5th ed. Churchill Livingstone, 2007: page 390
Strauss, JF, Barbieri, RL: Yen and Jaffe's Reproductive Endocrinology, 6th ed. Saunders, 2009: page 909
Swartz, MH: Textbook of Physical Diagnosis, 6th ed. Saunders, 2010: pages 20, bottom left; 275; 386, top right; 406, top left; 643, bottom left; 660, top right; 661; 945, top right; 990, bottom right; 999; 1240; 1279, bottom right; 1364, top left; 1399; 1456; 1551, bottom left; 1710; 1757, top left; 1765; 1849, top right; 1997, bottom left
Thibodeau, GA, Patton, KT: Anatomy & Physiology, 5th ed. Mosby, 2003: page 2023
Thibodeau, GA, Patton, KT: Anatomy & Physiology, 6th ed. Mosby, 2007: pages 789; 1117; 1347; 1452
Thompson, LDR: Endocrine Pathology. Churchill Livingstone, 2006: page 1294
Thompson, LDR: Head and Neck Pathology. Churchill Livingstone, 2006: page 781, bottom right
Tighe, SM: Instrumentation for the Operating Room, 7th ed. Mosby, 2007: pages 367; 520, bottom left; 732; 843; 1653; 1699; 1737; 1744, top left; 1881
Topol, EJ: Textbook of Interventional Cardiology, 5th ed. Saunders, 2008: page 1716
Townsend, CM et al: Sabiston Textbook of Surgery, 18th ed. Saunders, 2008: pages 292, bottom right; 752; 1111; 1124; 1505; 1784; 1827, bottom left
Tsokos, GC et al: Systemic Lupus Erythematosus. Mosby, 2007: page 1079
Tucker, SM: Pocket Guide to Fetal Monitoring and Assessment, 5th ed. Mosby, 2004: pages 295, bottom right; 474; 1888
Vidic, B, Suarez, FR: Photographic Atlas of the Human Body. Mosby, 1984: pages 20, top right; 203; 274; 402, bottom right; 441, bottom left; 728, top left; 730; 736; 737; 776; 795; 927; 1046, top right; 1077, bottom right; 1232; 1310; 1981
Waldman, SD: Atlas of Interventional Pain Management, 3rd ed. Saunders, 2009: page 226
Wecker, L et al: Brody's Human Pharmacology, 5th ed. Mosby, 2010: page 945, bottom right
Wein, AJ et al: Campbell-Walsh Urology, 9th ed. Saunders, 2007: pages 309; 1238; 1243; 1559; 2008
Weiss, CM, Weiss, A: Principles & Practice of Implant Dentistry. Mosby, 2001: pages 8, bottom left; 923, bottom right
Weissman, BNW: Imaging of Arthritis and Metabolic Bone Disease. Mosby, 2009: page 1543
White, SC, Pharoah, MJ: Oral Radiology, 5th ed. Mosby, 2004: page 611
Yanoff, M, Duker, JS: Ophthalmology, 3rd ed. Mosby, 2009: pages 480; 502; 721, top left; 905; 1174; 1329; 1448; 1551, top left; 1633, bottom right; 2085, bottom left
Yeo, CJ: Shackelford's Surgery of the Alimentary Tract, 6th ed. Saunders, 2007: page 962, top right
Young, NS et al: Clinical Hematology. Mosby, 2005: page 466
Zaoutis, LB, Chiang, VW: Comprehensive Pediatric Hospital Medicine. Mosby, 2007: pages 19; 642; 643, top right; 1034, top left; 1190; 1435, bottom left
Zitelli, BJ, Davis, HW: Atlas of Pediatric Physical Diagnosis, 5th ed. Mosby, 2007: pages 84; 93, top left; 304; 326; 330; 407; 428; 458; 478; 523; 537, bottom right; 540, top right; 544; 584; 589; 635; 638; 659; 662, top right; 669; 671; 694, top right; 708; 754; 757; 765; 772; 788; 832, bottom right; 850; 851, bottom right; 884; 907; 911, bottom left; 911, top right; 915; 933; 959; 992, bottom right; 1161; 1178; 1226; 1282; 1320, bottom left; 1346; 1377; 1400; 1445; 1446; 1487; 1488; 1492; 1514; 1557; 1613; 1648, top left; 1649; 1681; 1696; 1761; 1821; 1827, top right; 1828; 1833, bottom left; 1833, top right; 1836, bottom left; 1838; 1841 (A); 1845, bottom left; 1849; 1851; 1869; 1901 (Courtesy of Dr. K. Schuitt [deceased]); 1918, bottom right; 1933; 1936, top right; 1941, bottom left; 1965